Cardiovascular Drug Therapy

Editorial Board

Cardiovascular Drug Therapy

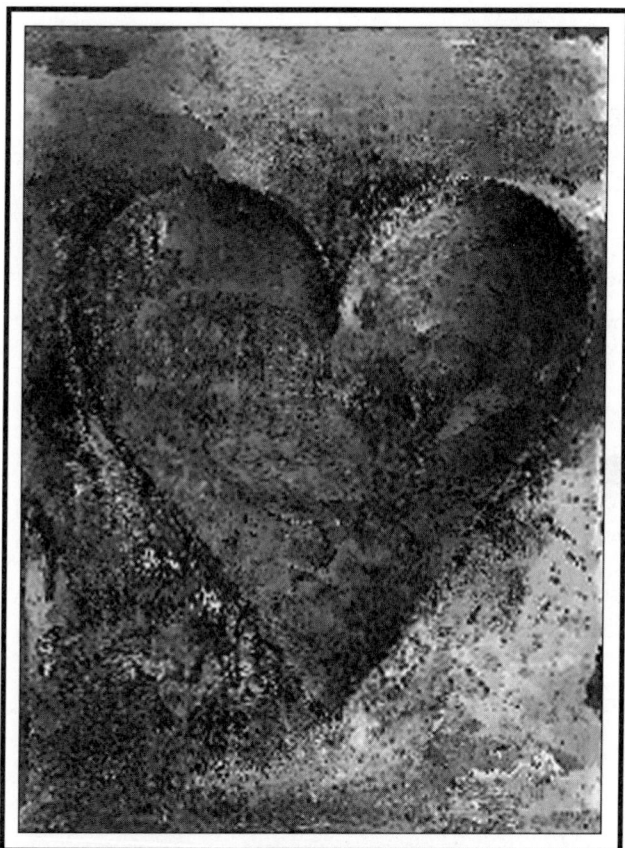

Second Edition

Franz H. Messerli, M.D.
Ochsner Clinic and Alton Ochsner Medical Foundation
New Orleans, Louisiana

*Cover illustration: Blue Heart by Jim Dine
(Collection of Walker Art Center, Minneapolis.
Gift of the artist in memory of Fred Leach,
his teacher and friend, 1988.)*

W.B. SAUNDERS COMPANY
A Division of Harcourt Brace & Company
Philadelphia London Toronto Montreal Sydney Tokyo

W.B. SAUNDERS COMPANY
A Division of Harcourt Brace & Company

The Curtis Center
Independence Square West
Philadelphia, Pennsylvania 19106

Library of Congress Cataloging-in-Publication Data

Cardiovascular drug therapy / [edited by] Franz H. Messerli.—2nd ed.

    p.   cm.

Rev. ed. of: Cardiovascular drug therapy. 1990.

Includes bibliographical references and index.

ISBN 0–7216–4814–2

1. Cardiovascular agents.   2. Heart—Diseases—Chemotherapy.   I. Messerli, Franz H.   II. Cardiovascular drug therapy.   [DNLM: 1. Cardiovascular Diseases—drug therapy. WG 166 C976 1996]

RM345.C374 1996   615′.71—dc20

DNLM/DLC   95-1013

CARDIOVASCULAR DRUG THERAPY, 2nd edition   ISBN 0–7216–4814–2

Printed in the United States of America.

Last digit is the print number: 9   8   7   6   5   4   3   2   1

To those who inspired us such as Osler, Page, Pickering, White . . .
To those who taught us such as Freis, Genest, Hurst, Laragh, Lown,
and many others.
To our patients, who continue to teach and inspire us.

Contributors

FREDDY ABI-SAMRA, M.D.
Director of Electrophysiology, Ochsner Clinic, New Orleans, LA
Moricizine

BENQT ÅBLAD, M.D., PH.D.
Professor of Pharmacology, Medical Faculty, Göteborg University, Göteborg, Sweden; Medical Director, Astra Hässle, Mölndal, Sweden
Metoprolol

FRANZ C. AEPFELBACHER, M.D.
Hypertension Laboratory, Alton Ochsner Medical Foundation, New Orleans, LA
Betaxolol; Doxazosin; Cardiac Effects of Calcium Antagonists in Hypertension; Nifedipine; Ranolazine

C. T. ALABASTER, PH.D.
Group Research Scientist, Pfizer Central Research, Sandwich, Kent, United Kingdom
Dofetilide

MICHAEL H. ALDERMAN, M.D.
Professor and Chairman, Department of Epidemiology and Social Medicine, Albert Einstein College of Medicine, Bronx, NY
Guanfacine

RICHARD P. AMES, M.D.
Clinical Professor of Medicine, Columbia University; Senior Attending Physician, St. Luke's Roosevelt Hospital Center, New York, NY
Indapamide: Does It Differ from Low-Dose Thiazides?

JEFFREY L. ANDERSON, M.D.
Professor of Internal Medicine (Cardiology), University of Utah School of Medicine; Chief, Division of Cardiology, LDS Hospital, Salt Lake City, UT
Bretylium Tosylate; Anisoylated Plasminogen-Streptokinase Activator Complex (APSAC)

FRITS W. BÄR, M.D.
Lecturer in Cardiology, University of Maastricht; Cardiologist, Academic Hospital Maastricht, Maastricht, Limburg, The Netherlands
Saruplase

JACQUES D. BARTH, M.D., PH.D.
Associate Professor of Medicine (Cardiology) and Associate Professor of Preventive Medicine, Atherosclerosis Research Institute, University of Southern California, Los Angeles, CA
Pravastatin

OLAF BEHMER, M.D.
Schwarz Pharma AG, Monheim, Germany
ACE Inhibition in Renal Impairment

CONRAD B. BLUM, M.D.
Associate Professor of Clinical Medicine, Columbia University College of Physicians and Surgeons, New York, NY
Fluvastatin

PETER BOLLI, M.D.
Health Sciences Centre, Winnipeg, Manitoba, Canada
Bisoprolol

GÖRAN BONDJERS, M.D., PH.D.
Professor of Cardiovascular Research, Dean, Faculty of Medicine, Medical Faculty, Göteborg University, Göteborg, Sweden
Metoprolol

RAY BORAZANIAN, B.S.
Technical Editor, Cleveland Clinic Journal of Medicine, The Cleveland Clinic Foundation, Cleveland, OH
Diuretics in Hypertension

HENRI BOUNAMEAUX, M.D.
Assistant Professor of Medicine, University of Geneva Medical School; Chief, Division of Angiology and Hemostasis, Department of Internal Medicine, University Hospital of Geneva, Switzerland
Fraxiparine (Nadroparin Calcium)

D. CRAIG BRATER, M.D.
Professor and Chairman, Department of Medicine, Indiana University School of Medicine, Indianapolis, IN
Torsemide

DENNIS R. BRESNAHAN, M.D., F.A.C.C., F.A.C.P.
Clinical Assistant Professor, Department of Medicine, Division of Cardiovascular Diseases, University of Missouri–Kansas City Medical School; Co-Director, Coronary Care Unit, MidAmerica Heart Institute, St. Luke's Hospital, Kansas City, MO
Nitroprusside

W. VIRGIL BROWN, M.D.
Charles Howard Candler Professor of Medicine, Director, Division of Arteriosclerosis and Lipid Metabolism, Emory University School of Medicine; Charles Howard Candler Professor of Internal Medicine, Emory University Hospital, Emory Clinic, Atlanta, GA
Bile Acid Sequestrants: Cholestyramine and Colestipol

HANS R. BRUNNER, M.D.
Professor and Chief, Division of Hypertension, University Hospital, Lausanne, Switzerland
Angiotensin-Converting Enzyme Inhibitors; Cilazapril

JAMES F. BURRIS, M.D.
Professor of Medicine, Associate Professor of Pharmacology, Georgetown University School of Medicine; Associate Dean for Research Operations, Georgetown University Medical Center, Washington, DC
Hypertensive Emergencies; Clonidine

ROBERT M. CALIFF, M.D.
Professor of Medicine, Director of Cardiac Care Unit, Duke University Medical Center, Durham, NC
Anisoylated Plasminogen-Streptokinase Activator Complex (APSAC)

A. JOHN CAMM, M.D., F.R.C.P., F.A.C.C.
Professor of Clinical Cardiology, St. George's Hospital Medical School, University of London, London, United Kingdom
Chronic Arrhythmias; Intravenous Adenosine as an Antiarrhythmic Agent

VITO M. CAMPESE, M.D.
Professor of Medicine, University of Southern California School of Medicine; Associate Chief, Division of Nephrology, Department of Medicine, Los Angeles County–University of Southern California Medical Center, Los Angeles, CA
Minoxidil

CHRISTOPHER P. CANNON, M.D.
Assistant Professor of Medicine, Harvard Medical School; Associate Physician, Cardiovascular Division, Department of Medicine, Brigham and Women's Hospital, Boston, MA
Hirulog

ROBERT M. CAREY, M.D.
Dean and James Carroll Flippin Professor of Medical Science, University of Virginia School of Medicine, Charlottesville, VA
Carmoxirole

MARK D. CARLSON, M.D.
Associate Professor of Medicine, Case Western Reserve University School of Medicine; Vice Chairman for Clinical Affairs, Department of Medicine, University Hospitals of Cleveland, Cleveland, OH
Flecainide

WILLIAM D. CARLSON, M.D., PH.D.
Assistant Professor of Medicine, Harvard Medical School; Massachusetts General Hospital, Brigham and Women's Hospital, Boston, MA
Carvedilol

STEFANO CARUGO, M.D.
Universitá Statale, Milan, Italy
Lacidipine in the Treatment of Hypertension

KANU CHATTERJEE, M.B., F.R.C.P.
Professor of Medicine, University of California, San Francisco, San Francisco, CA
Combination Therapy in Congestive Heart Failure

JACQUES E. CHELLY, M.D.
Department of Pharmacology, University of Texas, Health Sciences Center, Houston, TX
Principles and Practice of Vasodilatation

JAMES H. CHESEBRO, M.D.
Professor of Medicine, Mount Sinai School of Medicine; Director of Clinical Research; Associate Director, Cardiovascular Institute, Mount Sinai Medical Center and Mount Sinai Hospital, New York, NY
Combination Therapy in Vaso-occlusive Disease; Acute Thromboembolism; Antithrombotic Therapy for the Prevention of Cardiac and Arterial Thromboembolism; Dipyridamole

DEANNA G. CHEUNG, M.D.
Clinical Instructor of Medicine, University of California, Irvine, College of Medicine, Irvine, CA; Staff Physician, Veterans Affairs Medical Center, Long Beach, CA
Clonidine; Guanabenz

PABLO A. CHIALE, M.D.
Chief, Department of Clinical Electrocardiography and Electrophysiology, Service of Cardiology, Ramos Mejiá Hospital, Buenos Aires, Argentina
Amiodarone

ARAM V. CHOBANIAN, M.D.
Dean, Boston University School of Medicine, Boston, MA
Acebutolol; Trandolapril

JEAN-PAUL CLOZEL, M.D.
F. Hoffman-La Roche Ltd., Basel, Switzerland
Mibefradil: The First L- and T-Calcium Antagonist

JAY N. COHN, M.D.
Head, Cardiovascular Division, University of Minnesota Medical School, Minneapolis, MN

DÉSIRÉ COLLEN, M.D., PH.D.
Professor of Medicine, University of Leuven; Adjunct Head of Clinic, University Hosptials, Leuven, Belgium
Single-Chain Urokinase-Type Plasminogen Activator (Prourokinase)

TYRONE J. COLLINS, M.D.
Staff, Department of Medicine, Director, Interventional Cardiology, Ochsner Clinic, New Orleans, LA
Pharmocologic Management of the Angioplasty Patient

LUIGI COLOMBO, M.D.
Director, Day Hospital and Clinical Section of the Center E. Grossi Paoletti, S. Paolo Hospital, Milan, Italy
Ciprofibrate

WILSON S. COLUCCI, M.D.
Associate Professor of Medicine, Harvard Medical School; Director, Cardiomyopathy Center, Brigham and Women's Hospital, Boston, MA
Principles and Practice of Inotropic Therapy

LEAH COLWELL-ADAMS, PHARM.D.
Clinical Research Coordinator, Department of Medicine, Division of Arteriosclerosis and Lipid Metabolism, Emory University School of Medicine, Atlanta, GA
Bile Acid Sequestrants: Cholestyramine and Colestipol

ANTHONY J. COMEROTA, M.D.
Associate Professor of Surgery, Temple University School of Medicine; Chief, Section of Vascular Surgery, Temple University Hospital, Philadelphia, PA
Urokinase

C. RICHARD CONTI, M.D.
Eminent Scholar (Cardiology), Professor of Medicine, and Chief of Cardiology, University of Florida College of Medicine, Gainesville, FL
Angina Pectoris

MICHAEL H. CRAWFORD, M.D.
Robert S. Flinn Professor and Chief, Cardiology Division, University of New Mexico Health Sciences Center, Albuquerque, NM
Nadolol

LUIGI X. CUBEDDU, M.D., Ph.D.
Chairman, Pharmacology Department, Universidad Central de Venezuela, Caracas, Venezuela
Cardiovascular Therapy in Patients with Organ Failure

CARL DAHLÖF, M.D., Ph.D.
Associate Professor, Medical Faculty, Göteborg University, Göteborg, Sweden
Metoprolol

DWIGHT DAVIS, M.D.
University Hospital, The M.S. Hershey Medical Center, Hershey, PA
Acute Pulmonary Edema

LIVIO DEI CAS, M.D.
Professor of Cardiology, Chair of Cardiology, University of Brescia, Brescia, Italy
Ibopamine

PETER W. DE LEEUW, M.D., Ph.D.
Department of Internal Medicine, University Hospital Maastricht, Maastricht, The Netherlands
Trandolapril

JOËL DE LEIRIS, Ph.D.
Professor of Physiology, University Joseph Fourier, Grenoble, France
Trimetazidine: Experimental Aspects

VINCENT DeQUATTRO, M.D., F.A.C.C., F.A.C.P.
Professor of Medicine, University of Southern California School of Medicine; Chief, Clinical Hypertension Service, LAC–University of Southern California Medical Center, Los Angeles, CA
Fixed Combinations as Step-One Therapy in Cardiovascular Disorders; Benazepril

THOMAS G. DiSALVO, M.D.
Instructor, Harvard Medical School; Assistant in Medicine, Massachusetts General Hospital, Boston, MA
Combination Therapy in Vaso-occlusive Disease; Acute Thromboembolism; Antithrombotic Therapy for the Prevention of Cardiac and Arterial Thromboembolism; Dipyridamole

JAMES E. DOHERTY, M.D.
Professor of Medicine, College of Medicine, University of Arkansas, Little Rock, AR
Principles and Practice of Digitalis

PETER DOMINIAK, M.D.
Professor of Pharmacology, Institute of Pharmacology, Medical University of Lübeck, Lübeck, Germany
Moxonidine

A. E. DOYLE, M.D.*
Emeritus Professor of Medicine, University of Melbourne; Director, Graduate Education, Repatriation General Hospital, Heidelberg, Melbourne; Senior Physician, St. Vincent's Hospital, Fitzroy, Melbourne, Australia
Ketanserin

RAGHVENDRA K. DUBEY, Ph.D.
Assistant Professor, Department of Medicine, Center for Clinical Pharmacology, University of Pittsburgh Medical Center, Pittsburgh, PA
Endogenous and Therapeutic Nitrates

ALAN DUBROW, M.D.
Clinical Assistant Professor of Medicine, Mt. Sinai School of Medicine; Physician-in-Charge, Hemodialysis, Beth Israel Medical Center, New York, NY
Labetalol

VICTOR J. DZAU, M.D.
Chief, Division of Cardiovascular Medicine, Stanford University School of Medicine, Stanford, CA

GARABED EKNOYAN, M.D.
Professor of Medicine, Baylor College of Medicine; Chief, Renal Services, Ben Taub General Hospital, Houston, TX
Amiloride

JOHN ELLIOTT, M.B., Ch.B, Ph.D., F.R.A.C.P.
Senior Lecturer in Cardiology, Christchurch School of Medicine; Consultant Cardiologist, Christchurch Hospital, Christchurch, New Zealand
Perfluorochemicals, Specifically Fluosol

MURRAY EPSTEIN, M.D.
Professor of Medicine, Division of Nephrology, University of Miami School of Medicine; Attending Physician, Nephrology Section, Veterans Affairs Medical Center, and Jackson Memorial Medical Center, Miami, FL
Furosemide; Thiazide Diuretics, Chlorthalidone, and Metolazone

DENNIS R. FELLER, Ph.D.
Chairperson, Department of Pharmacology and Toxicology, School of Pharmacy, The University of Mississippi, University, MS
Clofibrate

ROBERTO FERRARI, M.D., Ph.D.
Associate Professor, Chair of Cardiology, University of Brescia; Divisione Di Cardiologia, Spedali Civili; Fondazione Clinica Del Lavoro, Brescia, Italy
Gallopamil

*Deceased

WALTER FLAMENBAUM, M.D.
Clinical Professor of Medicine, Mt. Sinai School of Medicine; President and CEO, Therics, Inc., New York, NY
Labetalol

RICHARD N. FOGOROS, M.D.
Associate Professor of Medicine, Medical College of Pennsylvania and Hahnemann University, Allegheny Campus; Director, Clinical Electrophysiology, Allegheny General Hospital, Pittsburgh, PA
Phenytoin

LAURA P. FOWLKES, M.D.
Fellow in Cardiovascular Disease, University of Tennessee, Memphis, TN
Cardiovascular Disease in Women and Hormonal Substitution

KIM FOX, M.D.
Senior Lecturer, National Heart and Lung Institute; Consultant Cardiologist, Royal Brompton Hospital, London, United Kingdom
Nicorandil

GARY S. FRANCIS, M.D.
Professor of Medicine, University of Minnesota Medical School, Minneapolis, MN
Use of Angiotensin-Converting Enzyme Inhibitors in the Treatment and Prevention of Congestive Heart Failure

NAHUM A. FREEDBERG, M.D.
Cardiology Fellow, St. Vincent Hospital, Indianapolis, IN
Disopyramide

EDWARD D. FREIS, M.D.
Professor of Medicine, Georgetown University School of Medicine; Chief, Hypertension Research Clinic, Department of Veterans Affairs Medical Center, Washington, DC
Hypertensive Emergencies

T. FRIEDRICH, M.D.
Director of Clinical Research, Central Research Division, Pfizer Inc., Groton, CT
Dofetilide

TED D. FRIEHLING, M.D.
Clinical Associate Professor of Medicine, Georgetown University School of Medicine, Washington, DC; Director, Electrophysiology Laboratory, Fairfax Hospital, Fairfax, VA
Ventricular Arrhythmias

WILLIAM H. FRISHMAN, M.D.
Professor and Associate Chairman, Department of Medicine, Albert Einstein College of Medicine; Montefiore Medical Center, Bronx, NY
β-Adrenergic Blocking Drugs in Cardiac Disorders; Ultrashort-Acting β-Adrenoreceptor Blocking Drug: Esmolol; Cardiovascular Uses of Calcium Antagonists; Amlodipine

EDWARD D. FROHLICH, M.D.
Professor, Department of Medicine and Department of Physiology, Louisiana State University; Clinical Professor of Medicine and Adjunct Professor of Physiology, Tulane University; Vice President for Academic Affairs, Alton Ochsner
Distinguished Scientist, Alton Ochsner Medical Foundation, New Orleans, LA
Methyldopa

VALENTIN FUSTER, M.D., Ph.D.
Arthur M. and Hilda A. Master Professor of Medicine, Mount Sinai School of Medicine, New York, NY
Combination Therapy in Vaso-occlusive Disease; Acute Thromboembolism; Antithrombotic Therapy for the Prevention of Cardiac and Arterial Thromboembolism; Dipyridamole

CLIFFORD J. GARRATT, D.M.
Senior Lecturer, University of Leicester; Consultant Cardiologist, Glenfield Hospital, Leicester, United Kingdom
Intravenous Adenosine as an Antiarrhythmic Agent

ALLAN GAW, M.B., Ph.D.
British Heart Foundation Fellow, University Department of Pathological Biochemistry, Royal Infirmary, Glasgow, United Kingdom
Fenofibrate

EDWARD E. GENTON, M.D.
Section on Cardiology, Department of Medicine, Ochsner Clinic, New Orleans, LA
Warfarin

CRISTINA GIANNATTASIO, M.D., Ph.D.
Researcher, Universitá Statale, Milan, Italy
Lacidipine in the Treatment of Hypertension

RAY W. GIFFORD, Jr., M.D.
Professor of Internal Medicine, The Ohio State University College of Medicine, Columbus, OH; Consultant, Department of Nephrology and Hypertension, The Cleveland Clinic Foundation, Cleveland, OH
Diuretics in Hypertension

EDWARD M. GILBERT, M.D.
Associate Professor of Medicine, Director of Heart Failure Treatment Program, Cardiology Section, University of Utah Medical Center, Salt Lake City, UT
Carvedilol

JASWINDER S. GILL, M.D., M.R.C.P., F.A.C.C.
Lecturer, St. George's Hospital Medical School, University of London; Senior Registrar, St. George's Hospital, London, United Kingdom
Chronic Arrhythmias

PETER GOHLKE, Ph.D.
Associate Professor, Department of Pharmacology, University of Kiel, Kiel, Germany
Ramipril

SIDNEY GOLDSTEIN, M.D.
Professor of Medicine, Case & Western Reserve University, Cleveland, OH; Head, Division of Cardiovascular Medicine, Henry Ford Hospital, Detroit, MI
Cardioprotection After Acute Myocardial Infarction

EDGAR R. GONZALEZ, Pharm.D.
Associate Professor of Medicine and Pharmacy, Virginia Commonwealth University, Medical College of Virginia;

Director, Critical Care Pharmacy, Medical College of Virginia
Hospitals, Richmond, VA
Use of Cardiovascular Drugs During Cardiopulmonary
Resuscitation

ANTONIO M. GOTTO, JR., M.D., D.PHIL.
Distinguished Professor and Chairman, Department of
Medicine, Baylor College of Medicine; Chief, Internal Medicine
Service, The Methodist Hospital, Houston, TX
Hyperlipidemias

WILLIAM F. GRAETTINGER, M.D.
Associate Professor of Medicine and Vice Chairman,
Department of Medicine, Reno Division, University of Nevada,
School of Medicine; Chief, Medical Service, Veterans Affairs
Medical Center, Reno NV
Clonidine; Guanabenz

TOMASZ GRODZICKI, M.D., PH.D.
Associate Professor, Department of Gerontology and Family
Medicine, Collegium Medicum, Jagiellonian University, Cracow,
Poland
Cardiovascular Drug Therapy in Elderly

EHUD GROSSMAN, M.D.
Associate Professor of Medicine, Sackler School of Medicine, Tel-
Aviv University, Tel-Aviv, Israel; Associate Professor of
Medicine, Hypertension Unit, The Chaim Sheba Medical Center,
Tel-Hashomer, Israel
Isradipine

SCOTT GRUNDY, M.D., PH.D.
Director, Center for Human Nutrition, University of Texas
Southwestern Medical Center at Dallas, Dallas, TX

LARRY M. HAGERMAN, B.S.
Director, Information Assets, Pharmacia, Inc., Dublin, OH
Clofibrate

DONALD HALL, M.D.
Director, Intensive and Coronary Care, Department of
Cardiology, German Heart Center, Munich, Germany
Molsidomine

W. DALLAS HALL, M.D.
Professor of Medicine, Director, Division of Hypertension,
Emory University School of Medicine, Atlanta, GA
Cardiovascular Therapy in Black Patients

LENNART HANSSON, M.D., PH.D.
Professor, University of Uppsala; Physician-in-charge,
Samariterhemmet Hospital, Uppsala, Sweden
β-Adrenoreceptor Blockers in Hypertension

JOHN W. HARBISON, M.D.
Professor of Neurology, Neurosurgery and Ophthalmology, and
Chairman, Division of Neurology, Medical College of Virginia,
Virginia Commonwealth University, Richmond, VA
Ticlopidine Hydrochloride

ANDREA HASTILLO, M.D.
Associate Professor of Medicine and Cardiology, Medical College
of Virginia, Virginia Commonwealth University; Co-Director,
Coronary Intensive Care Units, Medical College of Virginia
Hospital, Richmond, VA
Dobutamine

RICHARD W. HENTHORN, M.D.
Director, Electrophysiology Laboratory, The Christ Hospital,
Cincinnati, OH
Flecainide

DAWN HERSHMAN, M.D.
Department of Medicine, Columbia University College of
Physicians and Surgeons; Presbyterian Hospital, New York, NY
β-Adrenergic Blocking Drugs in Cardiac Disorders;
Ultrashort-Acting β-Adrenoreceptor Blocking Drug:
Esmolol; Amlodipine

MICHAEL L. HESS, M.D.
Professor of Medicine and Physiology, Chairman, Division of
Cardiopulmonary Laboratories and Research, Medical College of
Virginia, Virginia Commonwealth University; Medical College
of Virginia Hospitals, Richmond, VA
Dobutamine; Amrinone; Vesnarinone

JOHN N. HILL, M.B., F.R.A.C.P., D.D.U.
Staff Consultant Cardiologist, Princess Alexandra Hospital,
Brisbane, Queensland, Australia
Disopyramide

ÅKE HJALMARSON, M.D., PH.D.
Professor of Cardiology, Medical Faculty, Göteborg University;
Chairman, Institute for Heart and Lung Diseases, Göteborg
University, Göteborg, Sweden
Metoprolol

NORMAN K. HOLLENBERG, M.D., PH.D.
Professor, Harvard Medical School; Physician, Brigham and
Women's Hospital, Boston, MA
Diuretics in Congestive Heart Failure

RUSSELL D. HULL, M.B., B.S., M.SC.
Professor of Medicine, University of Calgary; Head, Division of
General Internal Medicine, Foothills Hospital, Calgary, Alberta,
Canada
Logiparin in the Prevention and Treatment of Deep Vein
Thrombosis

DONALD B. HUNNINGHAKE, M.D.
Professor of Medicine (Cardiology) and Pharmacology, Director,
Heart Disease Prevention Clinic, University of Minnesota,
Minneapolis, MN
Drug Treatment of Hyperlipidemia: Initial Therapy and
Combination Therapy

AKIHISA IGUCHI, M.D., PH.D.
Professor, Nagoya University School of Medicine, Nagoya,
Japan
Probucol

D. ROGER ILLINGWORTH, M.D., PH.D.
Professor of Medicine; Director, Lipid Disorders Clinic; Chief,
Section of Clinical Nutrition and Lipid Metabolism, Division of
Endocrinology, Diabetes and Clinical Nutrition, Department of
Medicine, Oregon Health Sciences University; Attending
Physician, University Hospital, Oregon Health Sciences
University, Portland, OR
Simvastatin

JONATHAN L. ISAACSOHN, M.D.
Associate Director, Metabolic Atherosclerosis Research Center,
Cincinnati, OH
Lovastatin

DOUGLAS H. ISRAEL, M.D.
Attending Physician, Yale–New Haven Hospital, Hospital of St. Raphael, New Haven, CT
Combination Therapy in Vaso-occlusive Disease;
Antithrombotic Therapy for the Prevention of Cardiac and Arterial Thromboembolism

ALLAN S. JAFFE, M.D.
Professor of Medicine, Cardiovascular Division, Washington University School of Medicine; Director, Cardiac Intensive Care, Barnes Hospital, St. Louis, MO
Acute Myocardial Infarction in Perspective; Acute Myocardial Infarction; Use of Cardiovascular Drugs During Cardiopulmonary Resuscitation

JAMES STEPHEN JENKINS, M.D.
Department of Medicine, Ochsner Clinic; Director, Diagnostic Catheterization, Ochsner Medical Institutions, New Orleans, LA
Pharmacologic Management of the Angioplasty Patient

NORMAN M. KAPLAN, M.D.
Professor of Internal Medicine, Head, Hypertension Division, University of Texas, Southwestern Medical Center, Dallas, TX
Drug Treatment of Hypertension

RALPH A. KELLY, M.D.
Assistant Professor of Medicine, Harvard Medical School; Physician, Brigham and Women's Hospital, Boston, MA
Diuretics in Renal Failure

M. J. KENDALL, M.D., F.R.C.P.
Reader in Medicine, Birmingham Medical School; Consultant Physician, Department of Medicine, Queen Elizabeth Hospital, Birmingham, United Kingdom
Imdur

ZEBULON V. KENDRICK, PH.D.
Professor of Physical Education, Director, Biokinetics Research Laboratory, Temple University, Philadelphia, PA
Cardiovascular Drug Therapy Interacting with Exercise

JULIAN P. KEOGH, PH.D.
Postdoctoral Research Scientist, Institute of Toxicology, Medical University of Lübeck, Lübeck, Germany
Moxonidine

CHARLES R. KERR, M.D.
Professor, University of British Columbia; Head, Division of Cardiology, University of British Columbia, Vancouver Hospital and Health Science Centre, Vancouver, British Columbia, Canada
Amiodarone

JOHN M. KESSLER, PHARM.D., B.C.P.S.
Clinical Associate Professor, Pharmacy Practice Division, School of Pharmacy, University of North Carolina at Chapel Hill, Chapel Hill, NC; Assistant Director of Pharmacy, Duke University Medical Center, Durham, NC
Cardiovascular Drug Therapy in Patients with Organ Failure

KWAN EUN KIM, M.D.
Professor of Medicine, Medical College of Pennsylvania and Hahnemann University; Director of Hypertension Section,

Division of Nephrology and Hypertension, Department of Medicine, Hahnemann University Hospital, Philadelphia, PA
Spironolactone

CAREY D. KIMMELSTIEL, M.D.
Assistant Professor, Tufts University School of Medicine; Assistant Physician; Assistant Director, Adult Cardiac Catheterization Laboratory, New England Medical Center; Director, Cardiac Catheterization Laboratory, Faulkner Hospital, Boston, MA
Milrinone

WOLFGANG KIOWSKI, M.D.
Professor of Medicine, University Hospital, University of Zürich, Zürich, Switzerland
Nitrendipine

IRWIN KLEIN, M.D.
Professor of Medicine, Cornell University Medical College, New York, NY; Chief, Division of Endocrinology, North Shore University Hospital, Manhasset, NY
Thyroid Hormone (T_4 and T_3)

JOHN D. KLEMPERER, M.D.
Research Fellow, Department of Cardiothoracic Surgery, New York Hospital–Cornell Medical College, New York, NY
Thyroid Hormone (T_4 and T_3)

MARVIN A. KONSTAM, M.D.
Professor of Medicine and Radiology, Tufts University School of Medicine; Director, Heart Failure and Cardiac Transplant Center; Director, Adult Cardiac Catheterization Laboratory, New England Medical Center, Boston, MA
Milrinone

MICHAEL C. KONTOS, M.D.
Assistant Professor, Medical College of Virginia, Richmond, VA
Amrinone

JOHN B. KOSTIS, M.D.
John G. Detwiler Professor of Cardiology, Professor of Medicine and Pharmacology, and Chairman, Department of Medicine, University of Medicine and Dentistry of New Jersey–Robert Wood Johnson Medical School; Chief of Medical Service, Robert Wood Johnson University Hospital, New Brunswick, NJ
Lisinopril

PETER R. KOWEY, M.D.
Professor of Medicine, Jefferson Medical College, Philadelphia, PA; Clinical Professor of Medicine and Adjunct Professor of Pharmacology, Medical College of Pennsylvania and Hahnemann University, Philadelphia, PA; Chief, Division of Cardiovascular Diseases, The Lankenau Hospital and Medical Research Center; President, Cardiology Foundation of Lankenau; President, Mainline Arrhythmia and Cardiology Consultants; President and Chairman, Board of Directors, Cardiovascular Alliance of the Delaware Valley, Wynnewood, PA
Ventricular Arrhythmias

HERBERT J. KRAMER, M.D.
Professor of Medicine and Nephrology, Faculty of Medicine, Department of Medicine, University of Bonn, Bonn, Germany
ACE Inhibition in Renal Impairment

LOUIS KURITSKY, M.D.
Clinical Assistant Professor, Department of Community Health and Family Medicine, University of Florida, Gainesville, FL
Indapamide: Does It Differ from Low-dose Thiazides?

MASAFUMI KUZUYA, M.D., Ph.D.
Assistant Professor, Nagoya University School of Medicine, Nagoya, Japan
Probucol

CHARLES R. LAMBERT, M.D., Ph.D.
Abraham Mitchell Professor of Medicine, University of South Alabama College of Medicine; Director, Cardiac Catheterization Laboratories, University of South Alabama Medical Center, Mobile, AL
Nicardipine

BERNARD LAMPORT, M.D.*
Clinical Instructor, Department of Epidemiology and Social Medicine, Albert Einstein College of Medicine, Bronx, NY
Guanfacine

JOHN H. LARAGH, M.D.
Hilda Altschul Master Professor of Medicine, Director, Cardiovascular Center and Hypertension Center, New York Hospital–Cornell Medical Center, New York, NY
Hypertension; Carmoxirole

M. LYTKEN LARSEN, M.D.
Visiting Professor, Division of Endocrinology, Diabetes and Clinical Nutrition, Department of Medicine, Oregon Health Sciences University, Portland, OR; Department of Cardiology A, Aarhus Amtssygehus Tage-Hansens Gade 2, D-8000 Aarhus C Denmark
Simvastatin

STEPHANE LAURENT, M.D., Ph.D.
Professor of Pharmacology, Paris University; Department of Pharmacology, Broussais Hospital, Paris, France
Rilmenidine

CARL J. LAVIE, M.D., F.A.C.C., F.A.C.P., F.A.C.C.P.
Clinical Assistant Professor of Medicine and Physiology, Louisiana State University School of Medicine; Medical Co-Director, Cardiac Rehabilitation and Prevention; Director, Exercise Laboratories; Associate Director, Internal Medicine Training Program, Ochsner Heart and Vascular Institute, Ochsner Clinic and Alton Ochsner Medical Foundation, New Orleans, LA
Antioxidants in the Prevention of Cardiovascular Disease; Nitroprusside; Nicotinic Acid; Gemfibrozil; Probucol; Fish Oils

DEPING LEE, M.D.
Assistant Professor of Research Medicine, University of Southern California School of Medicine; Clinical Coordination, Research Trials Division, Clinical Hypertension Service, LAC–University of Southern California Medical Center, Los Angeles, CA
Benazepril

KENNEDY R. LEES, M.D., F.R.C.P.
Senior Lecturer, Department of Medicine, and Therapeutics, University of Glasgow; Consultant Physician, Clinical Director, Acute Stroke Unit, Western Infirmary, Glasgow, United Kingdom
Perindopril

*Deceased

PAUL R. LICHTLEN, M.D.
Professor of Medicine and Cardiology, Hannover Medical School, Hannover, Germany
Combination Therapy in Angina Pectoris

H. ROGER LIJNEN, Ph.D.
Professor, Faculty of Medicine, University of Leuven, Leuven, Belgium
Single-Chain Urokinase-Type Plasminogen Activator (Prourokinase)

GÉRARD M. LONDON, M.D.
Hopital FH Manhes, Fleury–Merogis, France
Principles and Practice of Vasodilatation

CHRISTOPH J. LOSEM, M.D.
Assistant, Department of Medicine, University of Bonn, Bonn, Germany
Triamterene

DAVID T. LOWENTHAL, M.D., Ph.D.
Professor of Medicine, Pharmacology and Exercise Science, University of Florida College of Medicine; Director, Geriatric Research, Education and Clinical Center, VA Medical Center, Gainesville, FL
Cardiovascular Drug Therapy Interacting with Exercise

BENEDICT R. LUCCHESI, M.D., Ph.D.
Professor of Pharmacology, University of Michigan Medical School, Ann Arbor, MI
C7E3 Fab (abciximab)

THOMAS F. LÜSCHER, M.D.
Professor of Medicine, Division of Cardiology, University Hospitals, Bern, Switzerland
Endogenous and Therapeutic Nitrates

ANDREW I. MacISAAC, M.B.B.S., F.R.A.C.P.
Department of Cardiology, St. Vincent's Hospital, Melbourne, Victoria, Australia
Perfluorochemicals, Specifically Fluosol

GIUSEPPE MANCIA, M.D.
Professor of Medicine, University of Milan; Chair of Internal Medicine, St. Gerardo Hospital; Head of Cardiovascular Laboratory, Centro Auxologico Italiano, Milan, Italy
Lacidipine in the Treatment of Hypertension

G. B. JOHN MANCINI, M.D.
Professor and Head, Department of Medicine, University of British Columbia, Vancouver, British Columbia, Canada
Pravastatin

ARDUINO A. MANGONI, M.D.
Universitá Statale, Milan, Italy
Lacidipine in the Treatment of Hypertension

ARIE J. MAN IN'T VELD, M.D., Ph.D.
Professor of Cardiovascular Pharmacotherapy, Erasmus University, Rotterdam, The Netherlands
Pindolol

VICTOR J. MARDER, M.D.
Professor of Medicine; Chief, Hematology Unit; Associate Chair for Academic Affairs, Department of Medicine, University of

Rochester School of Medicine and Dentistry; Attending
Physician, Strong Memorial Hospital, Rochester, NY
Streptokinase

ROGER A. MARINCHAK, M.D.
Associate Professor of Medicine, Thomas Jefferson University
School of Medicine; Clinical Associate Professor of Medicine,
The Medical College of Pennsylvania/Hahnemann University,
Philadelphia, PA; Director, Clinical Cardiac Electrophysiology
Laboratory, The Lankenau Hospital and Medical Research
Center, Wynnewood, PA
Ventricular Arrhythmias

JAY W. MASON, M.D.
Professor of Internal Medicine, Chief, Division of Cardiology,
School of Medicine, University of Utah, Salt Lake City, UT
Quinidine

BARRY J. MATERSON, M.D.
Professor of Medicine, University of Miami School of Medicine;
University of Miami Medical Group, Miami, FL
Furosemide; Thiazide Diuretics, Chlorthalidone, and
Metolazone

FRANK C. McGEEHIN, III, M.D.
Clinical Assistant Professor of Medicine, Jefferson Medical
College of Thomas Jefferson University, Philadelphia, PA;
Associate, Lankenau Hospital and Medical Research Center,
Wynnewood, PA
Procainamide

MARCO METRA, M.D.
Research Associate, Chair of Cardiology, University of Brescia,
Brescia, Italy
Ibopamine

ERIC L. MICHELSON, M.D.
Professor of Medicine, Medical College of Pennsylvania and
Hahnemann University; Hahnemann University Hospital,
Philadelphia, PA
Acute Tachyarrhythmias; Procainamide

RICHARD V. MILANI, M.D., F.A.C.C.
Adjunct Assistant Professor, Department of Biostatistics and
Epidemiology, Tulane University School of Public Health and
Tropical Medicine, New Orleans, LA; Adjunct Assistant
Professor, Department of Medicine, Baylor College of Medicine,
Houston, TX; Medical Director, Cardiovascular Health Center,
Co-Director, Cardiopulmonary Rehabilitation and Prevention;
Ochsner Clinic, New Orleans, LA
Antioxidants in the Prevention of Cardiovascular Disease;
Nicotinic Acid; Gemfibrozil; Fish Oils

WILLIAM E. MITCH, M.D.
Garland Herndon Professor of Medicine, Emory University
School of Medicine, Atlanta, GA
Diuretics in Renal Failure

MURRAY A. MITTLEMAN, M.D., Dr.P.H.
Instructor in Medicine, Harvard Medical School; Staff
Physician, Cardiovascular Division, Deaconess Hospital, Boston,
MA
Circadian Rhythm, Triggering Events, and Cardiovascular
Therapy

DAVID J. MOLITERNO, M.D.
Assistant Professor of Medicine, The Ohio State University;
Director, Angiographic Core Laboratory, Cleveland Clinic
Foundation, Cleveland, OH
Thrombolytic Therapy in Acute Myocardial Infarction

JOEL MORGANROTH, M.D.
Clinical Professor of Medicine, University of Pennsylvania
School of Medicine; Adjunct Professor of Medicine, Jefferson
Medical College of Thomas Jefferson University; President,
Premier Research Worldwide, Philadelphia, PA
Moricizine

RICHARD L. MUELLER, M.D.
Clinical Instructor in Medicine, Cornell University Medical
College; Clinical Assistant Attending Physician, The New York
Hospital, New York, NY
Nitroglycerin; Long-Acting Nitrates

DAVID MULCAHY, M.D.
Senior Lecturer, Trinity College; Consultant Cardiologist,
Adelaide Hospital and Meath Hospital, Dublin, Ireland
Nicorandil

JAMES E. MULLER, M.D.
Associate Professor of Medicine, Harvard Medical School; Chief,
Cardiovascular Division, Deaconess Hospital, Boston, MA
Circadian Rhythm, Triggering Events, and Cardiovascular
Therapy

JAMES D. MURPHY, M.D.
Fellow, Division of Cardiology, University of Florida,
Gainesville, FL
Sinus Node Inhibitors: Zatebradine and Other Agents

JOSEPH MURPHY, M.B., M.R.C.P.I., F.A.C.C.
Mayo Clinic and Mayo Foundation, Rochester, MN
Nitroprusside

MICHAEL B. MURPHY, M.D.
Department of Pharmacology and Therapeutics, University
College, Cork, Ireland
Dopamine

KATHERINE T. MURRAY, M.D.
Assistant Professor of Medicine and Pharmacology, Vanderbilt
University School of Medicine, Nashville, TN
Propafenone

V. SHRINIVAS MURTHY, M.D., Ph.D.
Clinical Professor of Medicine, University of Wisconsin in
Madison, Madison, WI; Director of Outpatient Health Center,
Medical Director, Primary Care Clinic, Sinai-Samaritan Medical
Center, Milwaukee, WI
Ultrashort-Acting β-Adrenoreceptor Blocking Drug:
Esmolol

JEAN M. NAPPI, Pharm.D.
Professor of Pharmacy, College of Pharmacy, Medical University
of South Carolina, Charleston, SC
Quinidine

CONSTANCE F. NEELY, M.D.
Assistant Professor of Anaesthesiology, University of
Pennsylvania School of Medicine, Philadelphia, PA
Intravenous Nicardipine

JOEL M. NEUTEL, M.D.
Hypertension Center, Veterans Affairs Medical Center, Long Beach, CA
Doxazosin

HOWARD A. I. NEWMAN, Ph.D.
Professor of Pathology, College of Medicine, The Ohio State University, Columbus, OH
Clofibrate

D. J. NICHOLS, Ph.D.
Head, Clinical Pharmacokinetics, Early Clinical Research Group Pfizer Central Research, Sandwich, Kent, United Kingdom
Dofetilide

ALAN S. NIES, M.D.
Clinical Professor of Medicine, Robert Wood Johnson Medical School, New Brunswick, NJ; Executive Director, Clinical Pharmacology, Merck Research Laboratories, Rahway, NJ
Propranolol

MARGARETA I. L. NORDLANDER, Ph.D.
Associate Professor, Department of Physiology, University of Göteborg, Göteborg, Sweden; Associate Director, Department of Cardiovascular Pharmacology, Astra Hässle, Mölndal, Sweden
Felodipine

EDUARDO NUÑEZ, M.D.
Hypertension Research Fellow, Hypertension Laboratory, Ochsner Clinic, New Orleans, LA
Betaxolol; Terazosin

JÜRG NUSSBERGER, M.D.
Privat-Docent, Médecin-adjoint, Division of Hypertension, University Hospital, Lausanne, Switzerland
Angiotensin-Converting Enzyme Inhibitors

KAIE OJAMAA, Ph.D.
Assistant Professor of Cell Biology, Cornell University Medical College, New York, NY; Director, Molecular Endocrinology Laboratory, North Shore University Hospital, Manhasset, NY
Thyroid Hormone (T_4 and T_3)

GUNNAR OLSSON, M.D., Ph.D.
Associate Professor, Karolinska Institute, Stockholm, Sweden; Medical Director, Astra Hässle, Mölndal, Sweden
Metoprolol

LIONEL H. OPIE, M.D., D.Phil., F.R.C.P.
Professor of Medicine and Director, Heart Research Unit of the Medical Research Council, University of Capetown Medical School, Capetown, South Africa
Cardiovascular Drug Interactions; Trimetazidine: Experimental Aspects

SHMUEL OREN, M.D.
Senior Lecturer, Ben Gurion University of the Negev, Beer Sheva, Israel; Head of Internal Medicine Department, Barzilai Medical Center, Ashkelon, Israel
Isradipine

JOSEPH P. ORNATO, M.D.
Professor of Internal Medicine/Cardiology, Virginia Commonwealth University, Medical College of Virginia; Chief, Internal Medicine Section of Emergency Medical Services, Medical College of Virginia, Richmond, VA
Use of Cardiovascular Drugs During Cardiopulmonary Resuscitation

WILLIAM W. PARMLEY, M.D.
Professor of Medicine, University of California, San Francisco; Chief of Cardiology, Moffitt/Long Hospital, San Francisco, CA
Congestive Heart Failure; Calcium Antagonists in the Prevention of Atherosclerosis

DEVEN J. PATEL, M.B.B.S., M.R.C.P.
Senior Registrar, Harefield Hospital, Harefield, Middlesex, United Kingdom
Nicorandil

CARLO PATRONO, M.D.
Professor of Pharmacology University of Chieti G. D'Annunzio, School of Medicine, Chieti, Italy
Acetylsalicylic Acid

TERJE R. PEDERSEN, M.D.
Head Physician Coronary Care Unit, Medical Department, Aker Hospital, University of Oslo, Oslo, Norway
Timolol

CARL J. PEPINE, M.D.
Professor of Medicine, Co-Director, Division of Cardiovascular Medicine, University of Florida College of Medicine, Gainesville, FL
Nicardipine; Sinus Node Inhibitors: Zatebradine and Other Agents; Ranolazine

GRAHAM F. PINEO, M.D.
Professor of Medicine, University of Calgary; Director, Clinical Trials Unit, Calgary General Hospital, Calgary, Alberta, Canada
Logiparin in the Prevention and Treatment of Deep Vein Thrombosis

BERTRAM PITT, M.D.
University of Michigan Medical School; Division of Cardiology, Taubman Medical Center, Ann Arbor, MI
Mibefradil: The First L- and T-Calcium Antagonist

PHILIP J. PODRID, M.D.
Professor of Medicine, Boston University School of Medicine; Director of Arrhythmia Service, Boston University Medical Center Hospital, Boston, MA
Aggravation of Arrhythmia by Antiarrhythmic Drugs; Mexiletine

JAMES L. POOL, M.D.
Associate Professor of Medicine, Section on Hypertension and Clinical Pharmacology, Baylor College of Medicine, Houston, TX
Terazosin

PETER E. POOL, M.D.
Clinical Professor of Medicine (Cardiology), University of California, San Diego School of Medicine, La Jolla, CA; Director, Reno Cardiology Research Laboratory, Reno, NV
Diltiazem

PHILIP A. POOLE-WILSON, M.D., F.R.C.P.
Professor of Cardiology, Department of Cardiac Medicine, National Heart and Lung Institute, University of London, London, United Kingdom
Nisoldipine

ROBERT PORDY, M.D.
Associate Director, Clinical Development–Cardiovascular, Hoffmann-La Roche Inc., Nutley, NJ
Mibefradil: The First L- and T-Calcium Antagonist

B. N. C. PRICHARD, M.B., M.Sc., F.R.C.P., F.F.P.M.
Professor of Clinical Pharmacology, University College; Consultant Physician, University College Hospital, London, United Kingdom
Bisoprolol; Principles and Practice of α-Antiadrenergic Therapy; Moxonidine

ERIC N. PRYSTOWSKY, M.D.
Consulting Professor of Medicine, Duke University School of Medicine, Durham, NC; Director, Clinical Electrophysiology Laboratory, St. Vincent Hospital, Indianapolis, IN
Supraventricular Arrhythmias; Disopyramide; Propafenone

HENRY A. PUNZI, M.D., F.C.P.
Staff Physician, Trinity Medical Center; Medical Director, Trinity Hypertension Research Center, Carrollton, TX
Captopril

HENRY PURCELL, M.B.
Senior Research Fellow, Department of Cardiology, Royal Brompton Hospital, London, United Kingdom
Nicorandil

STEPHEN R. RAMEE, M.D.
Staff, Department of Medicine, Ochsner Clinic; Director, Cardiac Catheterization Laboratory, Ochsner Medical Institutions, New Orleans, LA
Pharmacologic Management of the Angioplasty Patient

JOHN L. REID, D.M., F.R.C.P.
Regius Professor, Department of Medicine and Therapeutics, University of Glasgow; Consultant Physician, Western Infirmary, Glasgow, United Kingdom
Perindopril

JAMES A. REIFFEL, M.D.
Professor of Clinical Medicine, Columbia University College of Physicians and Surgeons; Attending Physician and Director, Clinical Electrophysiology Programs, Columbia Presbyterian Medical Center, New York, NY
Propafenone

GERT-HINRICH REIL, M.D.
Associated Professor of Cardiology and Clinical Pharmacology, Städtische Kliniken Oldenburg, Oldenburg, Germany
Combination Therapy in Angina Pectoris

LEON RESNEKOV, M.D., F.R.C.P.*
Rawson Professor of Medicine (Cardiology), University of Chicago; Attending Cardiologist, University of Chicago Medical Center, Chicago, IL
Nifedipine

STUART RICH, M.D.
Professor of Medicine, University of Illinois at Chicago, College of Medicine; Chief, Section of Cardiology, University of Illinois at Chicago Medical Center, Chicago, IL
Combination Therapy in Pulmonary Hypertension

*Deceased

ROBERT ROBERTS, M.D.
Chief of Cardiology, Baylor College of Medicine, Houston, TX

JÜRGEN K. ROCKSTROH, M.D.
Academic Assistant, Department of Medicine, University of Bonn, Bonn, Germany
Triamterene

D. M. RODEN, M.D.
Professor of Medicine and Pharmacology, William Stores Professor of Experimental Therapeutics, Director, Division of Clinical Pharmacology, Vanderbilt University School of Medicine, Nashville, TN
Dofetilide

MAURICIO B. ROSENBAUM, M.D.
Chief, Service of Cardiology, Ramos Mejiá Hospital, Buenos Aires, Argentina
Amiodarone

MARTIN RUBIN, PH.D.
Emeritus Professor, Georgetown University School of Medicine, Washington, DC; President, International Chelation Research Foundation, Chevy Chase, MD
Magnesium EDTA Chelation

HEINZ RÜDDEL, M.D.
Assistant Professor, University of Bonn, Bonn, Germany
Cardiovascular Therapy and Stress

WERNER RUDOLPH, M.D.
Professor of Medicine, University of Munich School of Medicine; Chairman, Department of Cardiology, German Heart Center, Munich, Germany
Molsidomine

ROBERT B. RUTHERFORD, M.D.
Professor of Surgery, University of Colorado Health Sciences Center, Denver, CO
Urokinase

MICHEL E. SAFAR, M.D.
Professor of Therapeutics, University of Paris; Chief, Internal Medicine, Broussais Hospital, Paris, France
Rilmenidine; Principles and Practice of Vasodilatation

MARTIN ST. JOHN SUTTON, M.B.B.S., F.R.C.P.
Professor of Medicine, University of Pennsylvania School of Medicine; Director, Cardiac Imaging Program, Hospital of the University of Pennsylvania, Philadelphia, PA
ACE Inhibition in the Post–Myocardial Infarction Patient

ANDERS SANDBERG, M.Sc.
Astra Hässle, Mölndal, Sweden
Metoprolol

TIZIANA SANTAGADA, M.D.
Clinical Development of Ethical Drugs, Clinical Research Department, Byk Gulden Italia, Cormano, Milan, Italy
Urapidil

STEPHEN SCHEIDT, M.D.
Professor of Clinical Medicine, Cornell University Medical College; Director, Cardiology Training Program, The New York Hospital–Cornell Medical Center, New York, NY
Nitroglycerin; Long-Acting Nitrates

ROLAND E. SCHMIEDER, M.D.
Professor of Medicine, University of Erlangen-Nuremberg, Nuremberg, Germany
Cardiovascular Therapy and Stress; Ketanserin

JAMES SCHOENBERGER, M.D.
Emeritus Roberts Professor and Chairman, Department of Preventive Medicine, Rush–Presbyterian–St. Luke's Medical Center, Chicago, IL
Fixed Combinations as Step-One Therapy in Cardiovascular Disorders

PETER SCHULMAN, M.D., F.A.C.C.
Associate Professor of Medicine, University of Connecticut School of Medicine, Farmington, CT
Bepridil

HERMANN SCHULZ, M.D.
President, Interlab International Clinical Laboratory and Research Organization, Munich, Germany
ACE Inhibition in Renal Impairment

JAMES SHEPHERD, PH.D., F.R.C.PATH., F.R.C.P.
Professor of Pathological Biochemistry, University of Glasgow, Honorary Consultant Biochemist, Royal Infirmary, Glasgow, United Kingdom
Fenofibrate

ROBERT C. SHEPPARD, M.D.
Adjunct Assistant Professor of Medicine, Medical College of Pennsylvania and Hahnemann University, Philadelphia, PA; Director, Clinical Cardiac Electrophysiology, Bayfront Medical Center, Saint Petersburg, FL
Acute Tachyarrhythmias

SOL SHERRY, M.D.*
Emeritus Professor of Medicine and Emeritus Dean, School of Medicine, Temple University School of Medicine, Philadelphia, PA
Streptokinase

DANIEL M. SHINDLER, M.D.
Associate Professor of Clinical Medicine, Division of Cardiovascular Diseases and Hypertension, University of Medicine and Dentistry of New Jersey–Robert Wood Johnson Medical School; Director, Echocardiography, Robert Wood Johnson University Hospital, New Brunswick, NJ
Lisinopril

JOSHUA B. SHIPLEY, M.D., PH.D.
Clinical Instructor, Department of Medicine, Fellow, Division of Cardiology, Medical College of Virginia, Virginia Commonwealth University; Medical College of Virginia Hospitals, Richmond, VA
Vesnarinone

DOMENIC A. SICA, M.D.
Professor of Medicine, Chairman, Clinical Pharmacology and Hypertension, Medical College of Virginia, Virginia Commonwealth University, Richmond, VA
Fosinopril

BRAMAH N. SINGH, M.D., PH.D.
Professor of Medicine, UCLA School of Medicine; Chief of

Cardiology, VA Medical Center of West Los Angeles, Los Angeles, CA
Sotalol; d-Sotalol

CESARE R. SIRTORI, M.D., PHD.
Professor of Clinical Pharmacology, University of Milano; Director, Center E. Grossi Paoletti for Atherosclerosis Prevention and Treatment, Niguarda Hospital, Milan, Italy
Ciprofibrate

PETER SLEIGHT, M.D., F.R.C.P.
Field-Marshal Alexander Professor of Cardiovascular Medicine, University of Oxford; Cardiac Department, John Radcliffe Hospital, Oxford, United Kingdom
Treatment Strategies After Myocardial Infarction

DAVID H. G. SMITH, M.D.
Mt. Sinai Medical Center, Cleveland, OH
Doxazosin

DAVID W. SNYDER, M.D.
Staff Cardiologist, East Jefferson General Hospital, Metairie, LA
Acute Myocardial Infarction

BURTON E. SOBEL, M.D.
Amidon Professor and Chair, Department of Medicine, The University of Vermont College of Medicine; Physician-in-Chief, Fletcher Allen Health Care, Burlington, VT
Acute Myocardial Infarction in Perspective

EDMUND H. SONNENBLICK, M.D.
Olson Professor of Medicine, Director of Cardiovascular Center, Albert Einstein College of Medicine; Chief, Division of Cardiology, Weiler Hospital of The Albert Einstein College of Medicine/Bronx Municipal Hospital Center, Bronx, NY
Cardiovascular Uses of Calcium Antagonists

JOHN A. SPITTELL, JR., M.D., M.A.C.P., F.A.C.C.
Professor (Emeritus) of Medicine, Mayo Medical School; Consultant, Cardiovascular Disease, Mayo Clinic, Rochester, MN
Pentoxifylline

KELLY ANNE SPRATT, D.O.
Clinical Instructor in Medicine, Division of Cardiovascular Diseases, Medical College of Pennsylvania and Hahnemann University, Philadelphia, PA
Principles and Practice of Digitalis

BERNARDO STEIN, M.D., F.A.C.C.
Interventional Cardiologist, Morton Plant Hospital, Clearwater, FL
Combination Therapy in Vaso-occlusive Disease; Antithrombotic Therapy for the Prevention of Cardiac and Arterial Thromboembolism

EVAN A. STEIN, M.D., PH.D.
Voluntary Professor, Pathology and Laboratory Medicine, University of Cincinnati, Cincinnati, OH; President, Medical Research Laboratories, Highland Heights, KY
Lovastatin

MARIA LUISA STELLA, M.D.
Universitá Statale, Milan, Italy
Lacidipine in the Treatment of Hypertension

*Deceased

MICHAEL STIMPEL, M.D.
Assistant Professor of Internal Medicine, University of Cologne Medical School, Cologne, Germany; Head of Cardiovascular Clinical Research, Department of Cardiovascular Clinical Research, Schwarz Pharma AG, Monheim, Germany
Moexipril

JOEL A. STROM, M.D.
Professor of Medicine, Associate Professor of Radiology, Albert Einstein College of Medicine; Director, Cardiac Non-Invasive Laboratory, Jack D. Weiler Hospital, Bronx, NY
Ultrashort-Acting β-Adrenoreceptor Blocking Drug: Esmolol

DAVID C. STUMP, M.D.
Senior Director, Clinical Research, Genentech Inc., South San Francisco, CA
Single-Chain Urokinase-Type Plasminogen Activator (Prourokinase)

JAY M. SULLIVAN, M.D.
Professor of Medicine, Chief, Division of Cardiovascular Diseases, University of Tennessee, Memphis, TN
Cardiovascular Disease in Women and Hormonal Substitution; Atenolol

BORYS SURAWICZ, M.D.
Professor Emeritus and Senior Research Associate, Krannert Institute of Cardiology, Indiana University School of Medicine; Staff Member, St. Vincent Hospital Heart Institute, Indianapolis, IN
Arrhythmias

DAVID O. TAYLOR, M.D.
Assistant Professor of Medicine, Division of Cardiology, University of Utah, Salt Lake City, UT
Dobutamine

STANLEY H. TAYLOR, M.D., PH.D.
Professor of Cardiology, University of Leeds; Chairman, Department of Cardiology, The General Infirmary, Leeds, United Kingdom (Retired)
Doxazosin

UDHO THADANI, M.B.B.S., M.R.C.P., F.R.C.P.C.
Professor of Medicine, Director of Clinical Cardiology Research, Oklahoma University Health Sciences Center; Vice Chief of Cardiology and Staff Physician, University Hospital and VA Medical Center, Oklahoma City, OK
Isosorbide Mononitrate

KLAUS THURAU, M.D., PH.D.
Chairman and Professor of Physiology, University of Munich, Munich, Germany
ACE Inhibition in Renal Impairment

ALAN J. TIEFENBRUNN, M.D., F.A.C.C.
Associate Professor of Medicine, Washington University School of Medicine; Associate Physician, Barnes Hospital, St. Louis, MO
Tissue-Type Plasminogen Activator

LOUIS TOBIAN, M.D.
Professor of Medicine, University of Minnesota Medical School, Minneapolis, MN
Potassium Supplements: Dietary Potassium and Potassium Supplements

GEOFFREY H. TOFLER, M.B.B.S.
Assistant Professor of Medicine, Harvard Medical School; Co-Director, Institute for Prevention of Cardiovascular Disease, Deaconess Hospital, Boston, MA
Circadian Rhythm, Triggering Events, and Cardiovascular Therapy

CYNTHIA A. TOHER, M.D.
Research Fellow, Cardiovascular Division, University of Minnesota Medical School, Minneapolis, MN
Use of Angiotensin-Converting Enzyme Inhibitors in the Treatment and Prevention of Congestive Heart Failure

DAVID E. TOLMAN, M.D.
Assistant Professor of Medicine, Director, Cardiac Transplant/Heart Failure Program, Medical College of Virginia, Virginia Commonwealth University; Medical College of Virginia Hospitals, Richmond, VA
Vesnarinone

ERIC J. TOPOL, M.D.
Professor of Medicine, The Ohio State University; Chairman, Department of Cardiology, Cleveland Clinic Foundation, Cleveland, OH
Thrombolytic Therapy in Acute Myocardial Infarction

ALEXANDER G. G. TURPIE, M.D., F.R.C.P., F.A.C.P., F.A.C.C., F.R.C.P.C.
Professor, Department of Medicine, McMaster University; Internist, Hamilton Civic Hospitals, Hamilton, Ontario, Canada
Danaparoid; Enoxaparin (Lovenox)

THOMAS UNGER, M.D.
Professor of Pharmacology, and Director, Institute of Pharmacology, University of Kiel, Kiel, Germany
Ramipril

ANTON H. VAN DEN MEIRACKER, M.D., PH.D.
University Hospital Department of Internal Medicine I, Dyksigt, Rotterdam, The Netherlands
Pindolol

PETER A. VAN ZWIETEN, M.D., PH.D.
Professor and Chairman, Department of Pharmacotherapy, Consultant/Staff Member, Department of Cardiology, Academic Medical Centre, Amsterdam, The Netherlands
Cardiovascular Receptors and Drug Therapy

CARL J. VAUGHAN, M.B.
Research Fellow, Department of Pharmacology and Therapeutics, University College, Cork, Ireland
Dopamine

FRANK VERMEER, M.D.
Department of Cardiology, Academic Hospital Maastricht, Maastricht, The Netherlands
Saruplase

MARC VERSTRAETE, M.D., PH.D., F.R.C.P., F.A.C.P. (Honorary)
Professor of Medicine, Center for Molecular and Vascular Biology, University of Leuven, Leuven, Belgium
Heparin; Hirudin

AUGUST W. von EIFF, M.D.
Professor of Medicine, University of Bonn, Bonn, Germany
Cardiovascular Therapy and Stress

BERNARD WAEBER, M.D.
Professor, Médecin-adjoint, Division of Hypertension, University Hospital, Lausanne, Switzerland
Angiotensin-Converting Enzyme Inhibitors; Cilazapril

ALBERT L. WALDO, M.D.
The Walter H. Pritchard Professor of Cardiology and Professor of Medicine, Case Western Reserve University School of Medicine; Director, Cardiac Electrophysiology Program, University Hospitals of Cleveland, Cleveland, OH
Flecainide

J. DAVID WALLIN, M.D.
Professor of Internal Medicine, Chief, Section of Nephrology, Louisiana State University School of Medicine, New Orleans, LA
Intravenous Nicardipine

MICHAEL A. WEBER, M.D.
Professor of Medicine, University of California, Irvine, College of Medicine, Irvine, CA; Chief, Clinical Pharmacology and Hypertension, Veterans Affairs Medical Center, Long Beach, CA
Bisoprolol; Clonidine; Guanabenz; Doxazosin; Quinapril Hydrochloride; Losartan

MARK W. I. WEBSTER, M.B., Ch.B., F.R.A.C.P.
Director, Interventional Cardiology, Green Lane Hospital, Auckland, New Zealand
Acute Thromboembolism; Dipyridamole

MYRON H. WEINBERGER, M.D.
Professor of Medicine, Director, Hypertension Research Center, Indiana University School of Medicine, Indianapolis, IN
Prazosin

MATTHEW R. WEIR, M.D.
Professor of Medicine, Head, Division of Nephrology and Clinical Research Unit, Department of Medicine, University of Maryland School of Medicine, University of Maryland Hospital, Baltimore, MD
Bisoprolol; Quinapril Hydrochloride; Verapamil

J. MARCUS WHARTON, M.D.
Associate Professor of Medicine, Director of Clinical Cardiac Electrophysiology, Duke University Medical Center, Durham, NC
Disopyramide

ANDREW WHELTON, M.D.
Associate Professor of Medicine, Johns Hopkins University School of Medicine, Baltimore, MD
Bumetanide

PAUL K. WHELTON, M.D.
Associate Professor of Epidemiology, Johns Hopkins University School of Hygiene and Public Health; Associate Professor of Medicine, Johns Hopkins University School of Medicine; Johns Hopkins Hospital, Baltimore, MD
Bumetanide

WILLIAM B. WHITE, M.D.
Professor of Medicine, University of Connecticut School of Medicine; Chief, Section of Hypertension and Vascular Diseases, and Head, Division of Internal Medicine, University of Connecticut Health Center, Farmington, CT
Cardiovascular Therapy During Pregnancy and Lactation

PATRICK L. WHITLOW, M.D., F.A.C.C.
Director, Interventional Cardiology, The Cleveland Clinic Foundation, Cleveland, OH
Perfluorochemicals, Specifically Fluosol

INGELA WIKLUND, Ph.D.
Professor, Medical Faculty, University of Bergen, Bergen, Norway
Metoprolol

JOHN WIKSTRAND, M.D., Ph.D.
Professor of Clinical Physiology, Medical Faculty, Göteborg University; Director, Wallenberg Laboratory for Cardiovascular Research, Göteborg University, Göteborg, Sweden
Metoprolol

DONALD T. WITIAK, Ph.D.
Professor of Medicinal Chemistry, School of Pharmacy, University of Wisconsin–Madison, Madison, WI; Professor Emeritus, School of Pharmacy, The Ohio State University, Columbus, OH
Clofibrate

MARK A. WOOD, M.D.
Assistant Professor of Internal Medicine, Co-Director, Cardiac Electrophysiology, Medical College of Virginia, Richmond, VA
Amrinone

JAMES B. YOUNG, M.D.
Chief, Section of Heart Failure and Cardiac Transplant Medicine, Cleveland Clinic Foundation, Cleveland, Ohio
Enalapril

PRINCE K. ZACHARIAH, M.D., Ph.D.
Professor of Medicine, Mayo Medical School, Mayo Clinic, Rochester, MN; Co-Chair, Department of Medicine, Mayo Clinic, Jacksonville, FL
Verapamil

ALBERTO ZANCHETTI, M.D.
Professor of Medicine, University of Milan; Director, Centro di Fisiologia Clinica e Ipertensione, Ospedale Maggiore, Milan, Italy
Urapidil; Felodipine

ROBERT ZELIS, M.D.
Department of Medicine, University Hospital, M.S. Hershey Medical Center, Hershey, PA
Acute Pulmonary Edema

MICHAEL G. ZIEGLER, M.D.
Professor of Medicine, Division of Nephrology and Hypertension, University of California San Diego School of Medicine; Director, Clinical Research Center, University of

California San Diego Medical Center, San Diego, CA
Postural Hypotension: Initial Treatment and Combined
Therapy

DOUGLAS P. ZIPES, M.D.
*Professor of Medicine, Indiana University School of Medicine,
Indianapolis, IN*

RANDALL M. ZUSMAN, M.D.
*Associate Professor of Medicine, Department of Medicine,
Harvard Medical School; Associate Physician in Medicine,
Director, Division of Hypertension and Vascular Medicine,
Cardiac Unit, Medical Services, Massachusetts General
Hospital, Boston, MA*
Captopril

Preface

Over the past few years, we have witnessed an exceedingly rapid evolution in the treatment of cardiovascular disorders. This is true not only for invasive and surgical procedures but also for drug therapy. Dozens of new cardiovascular molecules have appeared on the market over the past decade. Only a few of these drugs are novel and unique and, therefore, offer real progress in the treatment of cardiovascular disease. The only requirements of the Food and Drug Administration for approval of a new pharmaceutical molecule are documents attesting to its efficacy and safety, but not superiority over similar agents. This often results in the marketing of many "me too" drugs and creates thereby an embarrassment of riches, which is prone to confuse the general practitioner, internist, and cardiologist. *Cardiovascular Drug Therapy* serves to create some order out of this disarray.

The basic objectives of this second edition of *Cardiovascular Drug Therapy* remain similar to those of the first edition: to provide a comprehensive but practical and authoritative guide to the drug treatment of cardiovascular disorders and related conditions. Thus, *Cardiovascular Drug Therapy* has become the standard textbook for the practicing cardiologists or internists, allowing them to critically assess the plethora of drugs currently on the market. The second edition has been completely redone and every chapter was extensively revised. It has 54 chapters more than the first edition: A total of 64 new chapters have been added, and 10 have been omitted. This change reflects not only a variety of new drugs that came to the market (and the vanishing of older ones that are no longer used), but also the addition of an entirely new section of lipid-lowering agents with which the cardiologist is to become increasingly more familiar. The section on antithrombotic therapy was considerably expanded because of the advent of several low molecular heparin derivatives. New drug classes that are currently emerging are the angiotensin receptor inhibitors (of which losartan is the first prototype), the sinus node inhibitors, and the cellular antiischemic agents. Certain drugs with less well defined mechanisms of action but that are also used to treat cardiovascular disorders were included in a special section.

I hope that this text will continue to be a useful, comprehensive, day-to-day source of information and education for many health professionals.

FRANZ H. MESSERLI, M.D.

Acknowledgments

I am deeply indebted to many talented and dedicated people for their contributions to *Cardiovascular Drug Therapy*. I would like to acknowledge the special help of Franz Aepfelbacher, M.D., the staff of the Ochsner Medical Editing Department under the direction of Marion Stafford, and my secretary, Ann Ranftle, in the completion of this project.

All the staff at W.B. Saunders have toiled endless hours in their efforts and provided us with excellent advice and support throughout this endeavor. I particularly appreciate the expertise of Richard Zorab and Arlene Friday Chappelle, who were most accommodating.

FRANZ H. MESSERLI, M.D.

Contents

PART ONE:
Therapeutic Strategies in Patients and Diseases   **1**

I. Emerging Concepts in
   Cardiovascular Drug Therapy   3

1. Acute Myocardial Infarction in
   Perspective   3
   Burton E. Sobel, M.D., and
   Allan S. Jaffe, M.D.

2. Angina Pectoris   8
   C. Richard Conti, M.D.

3. Congestive Heart Failure   10
   William W. Parmley, M.D.

4. Arrhythmias   13
   Borys Surawicz, M.D.

5. Hypertension   16
   Franz H. Messerli, M.D., and
   John H. Laragh, M.D.

6. Hyperlipidemias   19
   Antonio M. Gotto, Jr., M.D., D.Phil.

II. Drug Treatment of Chronic
    Cardiovascular Disorders:
    Initial Therapy and
    Combination Therapy   27
    Norman M. Kaplan and Bramah N. Singh

7. Combination Therapy in Angina
   Pectoris   27
   Gert-Hinrich Reil, M.D., and
   Paul R. Lichtlen, M.D.

8. Combination Therapy in
   Congestive Heart Failure   43
   Kanu Chatterjee, M.B., F.R.C.P.

9. Chronic Arrhythmias   58
   Jaswinder S. Gill, M.D., M.R.C.P., F.A.C.C.,
   and A. John Camm, M.D., F.R.C.P., F.A.C.C.

10. Drug Treatment of Hypertension   66
    Norman M. Kaplan, M.D.

11. Drug Treatment of Hyperlipidemia:
    Initial Therapy and Combination
    Therapy   75
    Donald B. Hunninghake, M.D.

12. Combination Therapy in Pulmonary
    Hypertension   82
    Stuart Rich, M.D.

13. Postural Hypotension: Initial
    Treatment and Combined Therapy   94
    Michael G. Ziegler, M.D.

14. Combination Therapy in
    Vaso-occlusive Disease   101
    Thomas G. DiSalvo, M.D.,
    Valentin Fuster, M.D., Ph.D.,
    Douglas H. Israel, M.D.,
    Bernardo Stein, M.D., F.A.C.C., and
    James H. Chesebro, M.D.

III. Drug Treatment of
     Cardiovascular
     Emergencies   119
     Robert Zelis and Eric L. Michelson

15. Acute Pulmonary Edema   119
    Dwight Davis, M.D., and
    Robert Zelis, M.D.

16. Acute Myocardial Infarction   128
    David W. Snyder, M.D., and
    Allan S. Jaffe, M.D.

17. Hypertensive Emergencies   148
    James F. Burris, M.D., and
    Edward D. Freis, M.D.

18. Acute Thromboembolism   160
Thomas G. DiSalvo, M.D.,
Mark W. I. Webster, M.B., Ch.B., F.R.A.C.P.,
James H. Chesebro, M.D., and
Valentin Fuster, M.D., Ph.D.

19. Acute Tachyarrhythmias   182
Robert C. Sheppard, M.D., and
Eric L. Michelson, M.D.

20. Use of Cardiovascular Drugs
During Cardiopulmonary
Resuscitation   206
Joseph P. Ornato, M.D.,
Edgar R. Gonzalez, Pharm.D., and
Allan S. Jaffe, M.D.

IV. Special Clinical Situations   225
Peter Sleight and Sidney Goldstein

21. Cardiovascular Drug Therapy
in the Elderly   225
Tomasz Grodzicki, M.D., Ph.D., and
Franz H. Messerli, M.D.

22. Cardiovascular Therapy in
Patients with Organ Failure   234
John M. Kessler, Pharm.D., B.C.P.S., and
Luigi X. Cubeddu, M.D., Ph.D.

23. Cardiovascular Drug Therapy
Interacting with Exercise   250
Zebulon V. Kendrick, Ph.D., and
David T. Lowenthal, M.D., Ph.D.

24. Cardiovascular Therapy and
Stress   262
Roland E. Schmieder, M.D.,
Heinz Rüddel, M.D., and
August W. von Eiff, M.D.

25. Cardiovascular Therapy During
Pregnancy and Lactation   269
William B. White, M.D.

26. Cardiovascular Therapy in Black
Patients   280
W. Dallas Hall, M.D.

27. Cardioprotection After Acute
Myocardial Infarction   291
Sidney Goldstein, M.D.

28. Treatment Strategies After
Myocardial Infarction   298
Peter Sleight, M.D., F.R.C.P.

29. Pharmacologic Management of the
Angioplasty Patient   303
James Stephen Jenkins, M.D.,
Stephen R. Ramee, M.D., and
Tyrone J. Collins, M.D.

30. Circadian Rhythm, Triggering
Events, and Cardiovascular
Therapy   311
James E. Muller, M.D.,
Geoffrey H. Tofler, M.B.B.S., and
Murray A. Mittleman, M.D., Dr.P.H.

31. Cardiovascular Disease in Women
and Hormonal Substitution   316
Laura P. Fowlkes, M.D., and
Jay M. Sullivan, M.D.

32. Antioxidants in the Prevention of
Cardiovascular Disease   324
Richard V. Milani, M.D., F.A.C.C., and
Carl J. Lavie, M.D., F.A.C.C., F.A.C.P.,
F.A.C.C.P.

33. Fixed Combinations as Step-One
Therapy in Cardiovascular
Disorders   330
Franz H. Messerli, M.D.,
Vincent DeQuattro, M.D., F.A.C.C., F.A.C.P.,
and James Schoenberger, M.D.

34. Cardiovascular Receptors and
Drug Therapy   334
Peter A. van Zwieten, M.D., Ph.D.

35. Cardiovascular Drug Interactions   347
Lionel H. Opie, M.D., D.Phil., F.R.C.P.

PART TWO:
Cardiovascular Drugs   355

V. Diuretics   357
Norman K. Hollenberg and
Ray W. Gifford, Jr.

A. Principles and Practice of Diuretic
Therapy   357

36. Diuretics in Renal Failure   357
Ralph A. Kelly, M.D., and
William E. Mitch, M.D.

37. Diuretics in Hypertension 371
Ray W. Gifford, Jr., M.D., and
Ray Borazanian, B.S.

38. Diuretics in Congestive Heart
Failure 383
Norman K. Hollenberg, M.D., Ph.D.

B. Loop Diuretics 388

39. Furosemide 388
Murray Epstein, M.D., and
Barry J. Materson, M.D.

40. Bumetanide 396
Andrew Whelton, M.D., and
Paul K. Whelton, M.D.

41. Torsemide 402
D. Craig Brater, M.D.

C. Thiazide Diuretics and
Derivatives 412

42. Thiazide Diuretics,
Chlorthalidone, and Metolazone 412
Barry J. Materson, M.D., and
Murray Epstein, M.D.

43. Indapamide: Does It Differ from
Low-dose Thiazides? 420
Richard P. Ames, M.D., and
Louis Kuritsky, M.D.

D. Potassium-Sparing Diuretics and
Potassium Substitutes 435

44. Triamterene 435
Jürgen K. Rockstroh, M.D.,
Christoph J. Losem, M.D., and
Franz H. Messerli, M.D.

45. Amiloride 443
Garabed Eknoyan, M.D.

46. Spironolactone 454
Kwan Eun Kim, M.D.

47. Potassium Supplements: Dietary
Potassium and Potassium
Supplements 461
Louis Tobian, M.D.

VI. β-Adrenoreceptor Blockers 465
John L. Reid and William H. Frishman

A. Principles and Practice of
β-Adrenoreceptor
Blockade 465

48. β-Adrenergic Blocking Drugs in
Cardiac Disorders 465
William H. Frishman, M.D., and
Dawn Hershman, M.D.

49. β-Adrenoreceptor Blockers in
Hypertension 474
Lennart Hansson, M.D., Ph.D.

B. Noncardioselective
β-Adrenoreceptor Blockers 483

50. Propranolol 483
Alan S. Nies, M.D.

51. Timolol 494
Terje R. Pedersen, M.D.

52. Acebutolol 496
Aram V. Chobanian, M.D.

53. Nadolol 500
Michael H. Crawford, M.D.

54. Ultrashort-Acting β-Adrenoreceptor
Blocking Drug: Esmolol 507
William H. Frishman, M.D.,
V. Shrinivas Murthy, M.D., Ph.D.,
Joel A. Strom, M.D., and
Dawn Hershman, M.D.

55. Pindolol 516
Arie J. Man in't Veld, M.D., Ph.D., and
Anton H. van den Meiracker, M.D., Ph.D.

C. Cardioselective β-Adrenoreceptor
Blockers 522

56. Metoprolol 522
Åke Hjalmarson, M.D., Ph.D.,
Gunnar Olsson, M.D., Ph.D.,
Göran Bondjers, M.D., Ph.D.,
Carl Dahlöf, M.D., Ph.D.,
Anders Sandberg, M.Sc.,
Bengt Åblad, M.D., Ph.D.,
Ingela Wiklund, Ph.D., and
John Wikstrand, M.D., Ph.D.

57. Atenolol 540
Jay M. Sullivan, M.D.

58. Betaxolol 550
Eduardo Nuñez, M.D.,
Franz C. Aepfelbacher, M.D., and
Franz H. Messerli, M.D.

59. Bisoprolol 557
    Matthew R. Weir, M.D., Peter Bolli, M.D.,
    B. N. C. Prichard, M.B., M.Sc., F.R.C.P.,
    F.F.P.M., and Michael A. Weber, M.D.

D. α- and β-Adrenoreceptor
   Blockers 568

60. Labetalol 568
    Walter Flamenbaum, M.D., and
    Alan Dubrow, M.D.

61. Carvedilol 583
    William D. Carlson, M.D., Ph.D., and
    Edward M. Gilbert, M.D.

VII. Antiadrenergic Drugs 601
     B. N. C. Prichard and Michael A. Weber

A. Principles and Practice of
   α-Antiadrenergic Therapy 601

62. Principles and Practice of
    α-Antiadrenergic Therapy 601
    B. N. C. Prichard, M.B., M.Sc., F.R.C.P.,
    F.F.P.M.

B. Centrally Acting Antiadrenergic
   Drugs 616

63. Methyldopa 616
    Edward D. Frohlich, M.D., and
    Franz H. Messerli, M.D.

64. Clonidine 622
    Deanna G. Cheung, M.D.,
    James F. Burris, M.D.,
    William F. Graettinger, M.D., and
    Michael A. Weber, M.D.

65. Guanabenz 628
    Deanna G. Cheung, M.D.,
    William F. Graettinger, M.D., and
    Michael A. Weber, M.D.

66. Rilmenidine 633
    Michel E. Safar, M.D., and
    Stephane Laurent, M.D., Ph.D.

67. Guanfacine 642
    Michael H. Alderman, M.D., and
    Bernard Lamport, M.D.

68. Moxonidine 651
    Peter Dominiak, M.D.,
    Julian P. Keogh, Ph.D., and
    B. N. C. Prichard, M.B., M.Sc., F.R.C.P.,
    F.F.P.M.

C. Peripherally Acting Antiadrenergic
   Drugs 661

69. Prazosin 661
    Myron H. Weinberger, M.D.

70. Terazosin 665
    James L. Pool, M.D., Eduardo Nuñez, M.D.,
    and Franz H. Messerli, M.D.

71. Urapidil 673
    Alberto Zanchetti, M.D., and
    Tiziana Santagada, M.D.

72. Doxazosin 681
    Joel M. Neutel, M.D., Stanley H. Taylor, M.D.,
    Ph.D., David H. G. Smith, M.D.,
    Michael A. Weber, M.D., and
    Franz C. Aepfelbacher, M.D.

VIII. Angiotensin-Converting
      Enzyme Inhibitors 690
      Victor Dzau and Hans R. Brunner

A. Principles and Practice of
   Angiotensin-Converting Enzyme
   Inhibitors 690

73. Angiotensin-Converting Enzyme
    Inhibitors 690
    Hans R. Brunner, M.D.,
    Bernard Waeber, M.D., and
    Jürg Nussberger, M.D.

74. Use of Angiotensin-Converting
    Enzyme Inhibitors in the
    Treatment and Prevention of
    Congestive Heart Failure 711
    Cynthia A. Toher, M.D., and
    Gary S. Francis, M.D.

75. ACE Inhibition in the
    Post–Myocardial Infarction
    Patient 717
    Martin St. John Sutton, M.B.B.S., F.R.C.P.

76. ACE Inhibition in Renal
    Impairment 722
    Herbert J. Kramer, M.D.,
    Hermann Schulz, M.D.,
    Klaus Thurau, M.D., Ph.D., and
    Olaf Behmer, M.D.

B. Specific ACE Inhibitors 726

77. Captropril   726
*Henry A. Punzi, M.D., F.C.P., and
Randall M. Zusman, M.D.*

78. Enalapril   742
James B. Young, M.D.

79. Lisinopril   750
*John B. Kostis, M.D., and
Daniel M. Shindler, M.D.*

80. Ramipril   755
Peter Gohlke, Ph.D., and Thomas Unger, M.D.

81. Perindopril   775
*Kennedy R. Lees, M.D., F.R.C.P., and
John L. Reid, D.M., F.R.C.P.*

82. Trandolapril   784
*Aram V. Chobanian, M.D., and
Peter W. de Leeuw, M.D., Ph.D.*

83. Benazepril   788
*Vincent DeQuattro, M.D., F.A.C.C., F.A.C.P.,
and Deping Lee, M.D.*

84. Quinapril Hydrochloride   794
*Matthew R. Weir, M.D., and
Michael A. Weber, M.D.*

85. Fosinopril   801
Domenic A. Sica, M.D.

86. Cilazapril   810
*Bernard Waeber, M.D., and
Hans R. Brunner, M.D.*

87. Moexipril   813
Michael Stimpel, M.D.

IX. Angiotensin Inhibitors   817

88. Losartan   817
Michael A. Weber, M.D.

X. Arteriolar and Venous
Vasodilators   826
Edward D. Frohlich and Bertram Pitt

A. Vasodilatation   826

89. Principles and Practice of
Vasodilatation   826
*Michel E. Safar, M.D.,
Gerard M. London, M.D., and
Jacques E. Chelly, M.D.*

90. Endogenous and Therapeutic
Nitrates   832
*Thomas F. Lüscher, M.D., and
Raghvendra K. Dubey, Ph.D.*

B. Arteriolar Vasodilators   853

91. Minoxidil   853
Vito M. Campese, M.D.

C. Arteriolar and Venous
Vasodilators   858

92. Nitroprusside   858
*Joseph Murphy, M.B., M.R.C.P.I., F.A.C.C.,
Carl J. Lavie, M.D., F.A.C.C., F.A.C.P.,
F.A.C.C.P., and
Dennis R. Bresnahan, M.D., F.A.C.C., F.A.C.P.*

93. Nitroglycerin   865
*Richard L. Mueller, M.D., and
Stephen Scheidt, M.D.*

94. Long-Acting Nitrates   876
*Richard L. Mueller, M.D., and
Stephen Scheidt, M.D.*

95. Isosorbide Mononitrate   881
*Udho Thadani, M.B.B.S., M.R.C.P.,
F.R.C.P.C.*

96. Imdur   885
M. J. Kendall, M.D., F.R.C.P.

XI. Calcium Antagonists   891
Robert Roberts and Alberto Zanchetti

A. Principles and Practice of
Calcium Antagonism   891

97. Cardiovascular Uses of Calcium
Antagonists   891
*William H. Frishman, M.D., and
Edmund H. Sonnenblick, M.D.*

98. Calcium Antagonists in the
Prevention of Atherosclerosis   901
William W. Parmley, M.D.

99. Cardiac Effects of Calcium
Antagonists in Hypertension   908
*Franz H. Messerli, M.D., and
Franz C. Aepfelbacher, M.D.*

B. Specific Calcium Antagonists   915

100. Verapamil 915
Matthew R. Weir, M.D., and
Prince K. Zachariah, M.D., Ph.D.

101. Gallopamil 926
Roberto Ferrari, M.D., Ph.D.

102. Diltiazem 931
Peter E. Pool, M.D.

103. Nifedipine 972
Leon Resnekov, M.D., F.R.C.P.,
Franz H. Messerli, M.D., and
Franz C. Aepfelbacher, M.D.

104. Nicardipine 979
Charles R. Lambert, M.D., Ph.D., and
Carl J. Pepine, M.D.

105. Intravenous Nicardipine 995
J. David Wallin, M.D., and
Constance F. Neely, M.D.

106. Nitrendipine 999
Wolfgang Kiowski, M.D.

107. Nisoldipine 1005
Philip A. Poole-Wilson, M.D., F.R.C.P.

108. Mibefradil: The First L- and
T-Calcium Antagonist 1009
Jean-Paul Clozel, M.D., Robert Pordy, M.D.,
and Bertram Pitt, M.D.

109. Isradipine 1016
Ehud Grossman, M.D., Shmuel Oren, M.D.,
and Franz H. Messerli, M.D.

110. Amlodipine 1024
William H. Frishman, M.D., and
Dawn Hershman, M.D.

111. Felodipine 1040
Margareta I. L. Nordlander, Ph.D.,
Franz H. Messerli, M.D., and
Alberto Zanchetti, M.D.

112. Lacidipine in the Treatment of
Hypertension 1047
Giuseppe Mancia, M.D.,
Arduino A. Mangoni, M.D.,
Stefano Carugo, M.D.,
Maria Luisa Stella, M.D., and
Cristina Giannattasio, M.D., Ph.D.

113. Bepridil 1053
Peter Schulman, M.D., F.A.C.C.

XII. Lipid-Lowering Drugs 1061
Antonio Gotto and Scott Grundy

114. Nicotinic Acid 1061
Carl J. Lavie, M.D., F.A.C.C., F.A.C.P.,
F.A.C.C.P., and Richard V. Milani, M.D.,
F.A.C.C.

115. Bile Acid Sequestrants:
Cholestyramine and Colestipol 1067
W. Virgil Brown, M.D., and
Leah Colwell-Adams, Pharm.D.

116. Clofibrate 1075
Dennis R. Feller, Ph.D.,
Howard A. I. Newman, Ph.D.,
Larry M. Hagerman, B.S., and
Donald T. Witiak, Ph.D.

117. Fenofibrate 1083
James Shepherd, Ph.D., F.R.C.Path., F.R.C.P.,
and Allan Gaw, M.B., Ph.D.

118. Ciprofibrate 1092
Cesare R. Sirtori, M.D., Ph.D., and
Luigi Colombo, M.D.

119. Gemfibrozil 1098
Richard V. Milani, M.D., F.A.C.C., and
Carl J. Lavie, M.D., F.A.C.C., F.A.C.P.,
F.A.C.C.P.

120. Probucol 1102
Masafumi Kuzuya, M.D., Ph.D.,
Akihisa Iguchi, M.D., Ph.D., and
Carl J. Lavie, M.D., F.A.C.C., F.A.C.P.,
F.A.C.C.P.

121. Lovastatin 1107
Evan A. Stein, M.D., Ph.D., and
Jonathan L. Isaacsohn, M.D.

122. Simvastatin 1114
M. Lytken Larsen, M.D., and
D. Roger Illingworth, M.D., Ph.D.

123. Pravastatin 1120
Jacques D. Barth, M.D., Ph.D., and
G. B. John Mancini, M.D.

124. Fluvastatin 1128
Conrad B. Blum, M.D.

XIII. Positive Inotropic Agents 1136
Jay N. Cohn and Wilson S. Colucci

A. Digitalization 1136

125. Principles and Practice of
Digitalis 1136
*Kelly Anne Spratt, D.O., and
James E. Doherty, M.D.*

B. Inotropic Therapy 1146

126. Principles and Practice of
Inotropic Therapy 1146
Wilson S. Colucci, M.D.

C. Specific Positive Inotropic
Agents 1151

127. Dobutamine 1151
*Andrea Hastillo, M.D.,
David O. Taylor, M.D., and
Michael L. Hess, M.D.*

128. Dopamine 1162
*Michael B. Murphy, M.D., and
Carl J. Vaughan, M.B.*

129. Amrinone 1167
*Michael C. Kontos, M.D.,
Mark A. Wood, M.D., and
Michael L. Hess, M.D.*

130. Milrinone 1177
*Marvin A. Konstam, M.D., and
Carey D. Kimmelstiel, M.D.*

131. Vesnarinone 1185
*Michael L. Hess, M.D.,
Joshua B. Shipley, M.D., Ph.D., and
David E. Tolman, M.D.*

132. Carmoxirole 1189
*Robert M. Carey, M.D., and
John H. Laragh, M.D.*

133. Ibopamine 1194
*Marco Metra, M.D., and
Livio Dei Cas, M.D.*

XIV. Antiarrhythmic Drugs 1207
Douglas Zipes and A. John Camm

A. Principles and Practice of
Antiarrhythmic Therapy 1207

134. Supraventricular Arrhythmias 1207
Eric N. Prystowsky, M.D.

135. Ventricular Arrhythmias 1215
*Peter R. Kowey, M.D.,
Ted D. Friehling, M.D., and
Roger A. Marinchak, M.D.*

136. Aggravation of Arrhythmia by
Antiarrhythmic Drugs 1229
Philip J. Podrid, M.D.

B. Specific Antiarrhythmic Drugs 1239

137. Intravenous Adenosine as an
Antiarrhythmic Agent 1239
*Clifford J. Garratt, D.M., and
A. John Camm, M.D., F.R.C.P., F.A.C.C.*

138. Amiodarone 1247
*Charles R. Kerr, M.D.,
Mauricio B. Rosenbaum, M.D., and
Pablo A. Chiale, M.D.*

139. Bretylium Tosylate 1264
Jeffrey L. Anderson, M.D.

140. Disopyramide 1273
*J. Marcus Wharton, M.D.,
John N. Hill, M.B., F.R.A.C.P., D.D.U.,
Nahum A. Freedberg, M.D.,
and Eric N. Prystowsky, M.D.*

141. Dofetilide 1296
*T. Friedrich, M.D., D. J. Nichols, Ph.D.,
C. T. Alabaster, Ph.D., and
D. M. Roden, M.D.*

142. Flecainide 1304
*Mark D. Carlson, M.D.,
Richard W. Henthorn, M.D., and
Albert L. Waldo, M.D.*

143. Mexiletine 1319
Philip J. Podrid, M.D.

144. Moricizine 1331
*Joel Morganroth, M.D., and
Freddy Abi-Samra, M.D.*

145. Phenytoin 1338
Richard N. Fogoros, M.D.

146. Procainamide 1341
*Frank C. McGeehin, III, M.D.,
and Eric L. Michelson, M.D.*

147. Propafenone 1349
*James A. Reiffel, M.D.,
Katherine T. Murray, M.D., and
Eric N. Prystowsky, M.D.*

148. Quinidine 1362
*Jean M. Nappi, Pharm.D., and
Jay W. Mason, M.D.*

149. Sotalol   1369
     Bramah N. Singh, M.D., Ph.D.

150. d-Sotalol   1380
     Bramah N. Singh, M.D., Ph.D.

  C. Sinus Node Inhibitors   1386

151. Sinus Node Inhibitors:
     Zatebradine and Other Agents   1386
     James D. Murphy, M.D., and
     Carl J. Pepine, M.D.

XV. Antithrombotic Therapy   1395

  A. Principles and Practice of
     Antithrombotic Therapy   1395

152. Antithrombotic Therapy for the
     Prevention of Cardiac and
     Arterial Thromboembolism   1395
     Thomas G. DiSalvo, M.D.,
     Douglas H. Israel, M.D.,
     Bernardo Stein, M.D., F.A.C.C.,
     James H. Chesebro, M.D., and
     Valentin Fuster, M.D., Ph.D.

153. Thrombolytic Therapy in Acute
     Myocardial Infarction   1430
     David J. Moliterno, M.D., and
     Eric J. Topol, M.D.

  B. Platelet Inhibitors   1443

154. Acetylsalicylic Acid   1443
     Carlo Patrono, M.D.

155. Dipyridamole   1451
     Thomas G. DiSalvo, M.D.,
     Mark W. I. Webster, M.B., Ch.B., F.R.A.C.P.,
     James H. Chesebro, M.D., and
     Valentin Fuster, M.D., Ph.D.

156. Ticlopidine Hydrochloride   1465
     John W. Harbison, M.D.

  C. Anticoagulants   1473

157. Heparin   1473
     Marc Verstraete, M.D., Ph.D.,
     F.R.C.P., F.A.C.P. (Honorary)

158. Logiparin in the Prevention
     and Treatment of Deep Vein
     Thrombosis   1480
     Russell D. Hull, M.B.B.S., M.Sc., and
     Graham F. Pineo, M.D.

159. Fraxiparine
     (Nadroparin Calcium)   1484
     Henri Bounameaux, M.D.

160. Hirudin   1490
     Marc Verstraete, M.D., Ph.D., F.R.C.P.,
     F.A.C.P. (Honorary)

161. Hirulog   1498
     Christopher P. Cannon, M.D.

162. Danaparoid   1505
     Alexander G. G. Turpie, M.D., F.R.C.P.,
     F.A.C.P., F.A.C.C., F.R.C.P.C.

163. Enoxaparin (Lovenox)   1511
     Alexander G. G. Turpie, M.D., F.R.C.P.,
     F.A.C.P., F.A.C.C., F.R.C.P.C.

164. Warfarin   1517
     Edward E. Genton, M.D.

  D. Thrombolytic Agents   1521

165. Streptokinase   1521
     Sol Sherry, M.D., and
     Victor J. Marder, M.D.

166. Urokinase   1542
     Robert B. Rutherford, M.D., and
     Anthony J. Comerota, M.D.

167. Anisoylated Plasminogen-
     Streptokinase Activator Complex
     (APSAC)   1553
     Jeffrey L. Anderson, M.D., and
     Robert M. Califf, M.D.

168. Tissue-Type Plasminogen
     Activator   1567
     Alan J. Tiefenbrunn, M.D., F.A.C.C.

169. Single-Chain Urokinase-Type
     Plasminogen Activator
     (Prourokinase)   1578
     H. Roger Lijnen, Ph.D.,
     David C. Stump, M.D., and
     Désiré Collen, M.D., Ph.D.

170. Saruplase   1587
     Frits W. Bär, M.D., and
     Frank Vermeer, M.D.

XVI. Cellular Antiischemic
     Agents   1594

171. Trimetazidine: Experimental
     Aspects   1594
     Joël de Leiris, Ph.D., and
     Lionel H. Opie, M.D., D.Phil., F.R.C.P.

172. Ranolazine   1600
     Franz C. Aepfelbacher, M.D.,
     Carl J. Pepine, M.D., and
     Franz H. Messerli, M.D.

XVII. Other Drugs for the
      Treatment of
      Cardiovascular Disorders   1604
      Giuseppe Mancia and Lennart Hansson

173. Pentoxifylline   1604
     John A. Spittell, Jr., M.D.,
     M.A.C.P., F.A.C.C.

174. Fish Oils   1608
     Carl J. Lavie, M.D., F.A.C.C., F.A.C.P.,
     F.A.C.C.P., and Richard V. Milani, M.D.,
     F.A.C.C.

175. Magnesium EDTA Chelation   1613
     Martin Rubin, Ph.D.

176. Perfluorochemicals, Specifically
     Fluosol   1618
     John M. Elliott, M.B., Ch.B., Ph.D.,
     F.R.A.C.P., Andrew I. MacIsaac, M.B.B.S.,
     F.R.A.C.P., and
     Patrick L. Whitlow, M.D., F.A.C.C.

177. c7E3 Fab (abciximab)   1625
     Benedict R. Lucchesi, M.D., Ph.D.

178. Nicorandil   1638
     Henry Purcell, M.B.,
     Deven J. Patel, M.B.B.S., M.R.C.P.,
     David Mulcahy, M.D., and Kim Fox, M.D.

179. Molsidomine   1645
     Werner Rudolph, M.D., and
     Donald Hall, M.D.

180. Ketanserin   1650
     Roland E. Schmieder, M.D., and
     A. E. Doyle, M.D.

181. Thyroid Hormone (T$_4$ and T$_3$)   1656
     John D. Klemperer, M.D.,
     Kaie Ojamaa, Ph.D., and
     Irwin Klein, M.D.

Index   1663

PART ONE

Therapeutic Strategies in Patients and Diseases

I.

Emerging Concepts in Cardiovascular Drug Therapy

CHAPTER 1

Acute Myocardial Infarction in Perspective

Burton E. Sobel, M.D., and Allan S. Jaffe, M.D.

HISTORICAL CONSIDERATIONS

The age-adjusted mortality rate associated with acute myocardial infarction has declined remarkably since the mid-1970s, in part because of reduction of risk factors such as hypercholesterolemia, hypertension, and smoking, and in part because of improved treatment. Nevertheless, infarction remains the leading cause of death among adults in the United States (nearly 25% of all adult deaths annually) and worldwide in developed nations. Among the 5 million Americans with suspected acute infarction each year,[1] definite infarction occurs in almost 1.5 million. Approximately 750,000 patients are hospitalized. More than 500,000 die either suddenly before hospitalization is possible or soon after reaching a hospital.[2, 3]

Better treatment has reduced the case-fatality rate of this devastating disorder. Before the advent of coronary care units in the 1960s, mortality in patients hospitalized with acute myocardial infarction was approximately 30%. Improved detection and prompt electrical defibrillation, championed by coronary care units, decreased hospital mortality by half, to approximately 15%. After the importance of infarct size as a determinant of prognosis was established in the 1970s, the incidence of cardiogenic shock and death accompanying profound heart failure declined, possibly because of the development of interventions designed to limit the extent of infarction by reducing myocardial oxygen requirements with β-adrenergic blocking agents and vasodilators. However, despite the clearly demonstrable benefit in studies in experimental animals, the overall impact of reduction of myocardial oxygen requirements in patients was modest. Thus, in the 1970s, hospital mortality remained as high as 12%.

It soon became clear that a greater positive impact would require augmentation of perfusion of ischemic myocardium as well as diminution of myocardial oxygen requirements. Despite early consideration of coronary thrombolysis as a potential therapy in the late 1950s, this approach languished. Confusion regarding the role of thrombosis as the proximate cause of infarction was one factor. Because complete occlusion of an infarct-related artery was often absent at autopsy of patients who succumbed after acute myocardial infarction, it was thought by many that thrombosis was only an epiphenomenon. In fact, however, spontaneous recanalization had occurred in many such patients and was unrecognized at autopsy. Judging from angiograms obtained during the first few hours after the onset of infarction, DeWood and coworkers[4] demonstrated that coronary thrombosis was indeed the proximate cause of acute transmural myocardial infarction in 80% or more of afflicted patients.

Another factor that caused implementation of coronary thrombolysis to languish was the lack of definitive, objective end points needed to demonstrate unequivocal benefit. Coronary angiography had been thought to be too dangerous in critically ill subjects until investigators elucidating coronary vasospasm documented its safety. Soon thereafter, allegedly ethical barriers to aggressive diagnostic angiography in critically ill patients collapsed.

ADVANCES IN KNOWLEDGE OF PATHOPHYSIOLOGY

Complete thrombotic coronary occlusion is the cause of most acute myocardial infarctions manifested by ST elevation and the evolution of Q waves on the electrocardiogram. Thrombi are generally juxtaposed to complex atherosclerotic plaques and are initiated by plaque rupture, ulceration, or fissuring with consequent activation of platelets induced by exposure of circulating blood to collagen and basement membrane on the luminal surface of vessel walls. Coronary vasospasm may be stimulated by thromboxane elaborated by activated platelets and contribute to further reduction of flow and potentiation of occlusive thrombosis because of high shear forces favoring interaction of platelets mediated by binding of the surface glycoprotein 1b-IX to von Willebrand's factor within the arterial wall.

Sequential angiography delineates clot lysis within

3

60 to 90 minutes in most patients treated with thrombolytic agents, particularly with clot-selective fibrinolytic agents. Beneficial effects of early recanalization result not only from increased delivery of oxygen to ischemic myocardium but also from washout of potentially noxious arrhythmogenic and injurious amphipathic metabolites. The benefit conferred by recanalization, regardless of the mechanism by which it is induced, depends on the rapidity and persistence of restoration of nutritive perfusion in an interval preceding extensive cell death throughout jeopardized ischemic myocardium.[5] Complete interruption of myocardial perfusion leads to cell death if sustained for 20 minutes or more.[6] Transmural necrosis is complete in the hearts of experimental animals within a few hours.

Results of numerous clinical studies are consistent with evolution of necrosis over analogous intervals in the absence of recanalization and with the temporal dependence of benefit induced by reperfusion. Thus, optimal benefit can be obtained only when recanalization is induced early after the onset of infarction, ideally within 60 to 90 minutes.[5]

Reperfusion can be induced surgically by immediate coronary artery bypass grafting, mechanically by percutaneous transluminal coronary balloon angioplasty and so-called new device angioplasty, and pharmacologically with fibrinolytic agents. Neither surgery nor immediate angioplasty is or is likely to become applicable to the large majority of afflicted patients because of inherent delays; the need for a cadre of highly skilled medical, technical, and nursing personnel virtually instantaneously; the need for immediately available facilities with specialized equipment on a 24-hour-a-day basis; and economic constraints. The potential advantages of surgical and mechanical interventions include the possibility that, under ideal circumstances, flow can be restored rapidly and at high volume.

The disadvantages of angioplasty compared with surgery and pharmacologic thrombolysis include a high incidence of restenosis (approximately 40% within 3 to 6 months, with most occurring early in this interval) that may compromise prolonged benefit. Neither initial angioplasty nor pharmacologic fibrinolysis should be viewed as the "last intervention" that will ever be offered to the patient. Regardless of the choice of initial treatment, it is, of course, necessary to follow up successfully treated patients, arrest or reverse coronary atherosclerosis medically, and consider additional procedures if deterioration occurs.

PHARMACOLOGIC THROMBOLYSIS

The results of numerous studies in the 1970s in the Soviet Union, Europe, and the United States demonstrated that intracoronary administration of activators of the fibrinolytic system could induce recanalization in many patients with acute myocardial infarction. However, regional and global left ventricular systolic function did not improve consistently. It soon became clear that functional improvement of ischemic regions depended on the brevity of ischemia sustained before reperfusion. Thus, functional improvement was obtained when reperfusion was implemented within 2 hours after the onset of infarction but often not when reperfusion was initiated later.[7] Global function did not necessarily exhibit parallel changes, because of the initial hyperfunction of nonischemic myocardium and its regression as the jeopardized ischemic zone recovered. Intracoronary fibrinolysis appeared to improve survival as well, as shown in the Western Washington Cooperative Collaborative Study, in which 30-day and 1-year survival rates were increased in treated patients with anterior infarction.[7–9]

Unfortunately, however, widespread intracoronary administration of thrombolytic agents is fraught with logistic and economic difficulties. Some delay is inevitable because of the need for cardiac catheterization and selective angiography. Even modest delay can markedly limit the extent of myocardium that can be salvaged. Accordingly, pressure intensified to induce thrombolysis by intravenous administration of fibrinolytic agents—adjudged to be more universally applicable, less expensive, and potentially more effective because of the rapidity with which coronary thrombolysis could be induced.

Intravenous administration of streptokinase within 4 hours after the onset of symptoms of acute myocardial infarction was found to recanalize approximately 50% of infarct-related arteries, as judged from results of numerous studies, including many in which preinterventional and postinterventional angiograms were available.[10] Failure to recanalize many vessels promptly is probably attributable to geometric considerations (large clot burdens, severe underlying stenosis predisposing to immediate reocclusion) and the intrinsic properties of nonclot-selective agents when given intravenously. Such intrinsic properties include universal depletion of plasminogen from blood with consequent leeching of plasminogen from thrombi[11] and consequent compromise of lysis as well as activation of the coagulation system by plasmin[12] with potentially deleterious local consequences despite vigorous anticoagulation with heparin.[13] Despite the relatively high failure rate of recanalization with intravenous administration of conventional activators of the fibrinolytic system such as streptokinase, the incidence of left ventricular failure is reduced, 21-day mortality is decreased, long-term survival is improved, and the quality of life appears to be enhanced in patients treated within 3 hours after the onset of chest pain as judged from results of many studies. In the Gruppo Italiano per lo Studio della Streptochinasi nell'Infarto Miocardico (GISSI-1) trial, early mortality was reduced by approximately 50% in patients given streptokinase during the first hour after the onset of chest pain.[14]

Enthusiasm for coronary thrombolysis was intensified by the development of activators of the fibrinolytic system exhibiting relative clot selectivity, particularly tissue-type plasminogen activator (t-PA). In contrast with intravenous streptokinase, urokinase, and acylated plasminogen streptokinase activator complexes (all of which elicit marked fibrinogenolysis in the systemic circulation, resulting in a systemic lytic state), intravenous t-PA induces coronary thrombolysis in 75% to 90% of infarct-related coronary arteries in an average of 45 minutes or less with much less degradation of circulating proteins.[15, 16] Fibrin specificity with t-PA or any other agent is, however, only a relative phenomenon. Thus, even though fibrin-associated t-PA is 10,000-fold more active than t-PA in solution, high concentrations or prolonged administration of the agent can lead to some activation of plasminogen in the circulation and to fibrinogenolysis.

Intravenous administration of t-PA generally induces coronary thrombolysis within 90 minutes without marked fibrinogenolysis or marked accumulation of fibrinogen degradation products in most patients given 100 mg IV over 1.5 to 3 hours.[17-19] It is well tolerated, without the allergic reactions and hypotension seen so often with streptokinase. The alpha phase half-life of t-PA in the circulation is only 3 to 5 minutes. Accordingly, its effects on circulating proteins can be interrupted promptly by discontinuation of intravenous infusions. In contrast, effects on thrombi are prolonged because of avid binding to fibrin in clots and protection against neutralization by circulating inhibitors. Thus, lysis continues even as concentrations in the plasma decline after termination of infusions.[20]

When similar amounts of t-PA are administered over a 90-minute interval, so-called accelerated or front-loading regimens, even higher frequencies of recanalization of infarct-related arteries are seen within 60 to 90 minutes—in some studies, exceeding 90%. Not only is overall patency increased, the magnitude of restoration of perfusion is greater as well. In the GUSTO trial,[21] grade 3 patency as defined by the Thrombolysis in Myocardial Infarction Study Group (TIMI) (restoration of apparently normal flow of angiographic dye) was induced 90 minutes after treatment in 54% of patients treated with t-PA compared with less than 30% in those treated with streptokinase.

High frequencies of recanalization are facilitated by the use of what have been called conjunctive interventions,[22] that is, administration of agents to enhance the pharmacologic effects of fibrinolytic drugs by obviating procoagulant effects invariably present locally and paradoxically increased systemically by the drugs themselves.[12] Thus, concomitant administration of aspirin and vigorous administration of heparin initiated with a bolus of 5000 to 10,000 units followed immediately by an infusion of 1000 U/hr reduces the incidence of early thrombotic reocclusion and increases the rapidity of initial recanalization. The benefits of clot-selective fibrinolytic agents and conjunctive therapy in increasing the rapidity and frequency of recanalization, established first in studies in laboratory animals and subsequently in mechanistic clinical investigations, are associated with improved outcome in patients studied prospectively as well. Thus, mortality was reduced by 14% in patients treated with t-PA compared with streptokinase, accompanied by a decrease in the incidence of congestive heart failure and arrhythmia in the GUSTO trial.[21] Benefits were evident over a wide range of age, time to treatment, and locus of infarction, and regardless of gender, previous infarction, hypertension, or risk factors such as diabetes. The ongoing development of direct-acting thrombin inhibitors such as hirudin should increase the rapidity and frequency of recanalization even more.[23] Even with conventional anticoagulants, early treatment with t-PA is remarkably effective as judged from the 99% survival in patients treated within 90 minutes in the Myocardial Infarction Triage and Intervention (MITI) trial, in which no age limitation was incorporated.[24]

Coronary artery recanalization obviously is not an end in itself. In most patients who sustain acute myocardial infarction, coronary thrombosis is a manifestation of severe underlying atherosclerosis and stenosis of the infarct-related artery. Accordingly, reocclusion can occur after initially successful coronary thrombolysis (in 5% to 12% of patients), generally early. Reocclusion is more common when residual stenosis is severe. Its incidence can be reduced by vigorous use of conjunctive agents including heparin. Further improvements can be anticipated with the use of novel, direct-acting thrombin inhibitors; inhibition of tissue factor, factor VII, and factor Xa; and use of antiplatelet agents.

Thrombolysis is remarkably safe in properly selected patients. Approximately 1% of patients with acute myocardial infarction will suffer a stroke in the peri-infusion interval, with or without fibrinolysis. The overall incidence of stroke is increased, but only minimally, with fibrinolytic drugs (by approximately 0.1% to 0.2%).[25] The risk of intracranial hemorrhage, the most severe potential complication, is increased modestly to approximately 0.4% (from approximately 0.2%) regardless of the agent (e.g., 0.3% with streptokinase and 0.4% with t-PA in the GISSI-2 trial). A slight excess of hemorrhagic strokes occurs with t-PA compared with streptokinase (0.1% to 0.2% in the GUSTO trial). Larger disparities have been seen only in studies in which higher amounts of t-PA have been used (e.g., 150 to 200 mg of duteplase, an alternative form of t-PA, in ISIS-3). Bleeding complications are more common in the elderly. Nevertheless, the reduction in mortality and net clinical benefit of thrombolysis are substantial in the elderly because of increased risk of death caused by infarction per se and despite the increased risk of complications in absolute terms associated with thrombolysis.

MODERN MANAGEMENT (THROMBOLYSIS, ADJUNCTIVE AND CONJUNCTIVE THERAPY)

Early reperfusion is the most effective, widely applicable means of interrupting evolving acute myocardial infarction, limiting infarct size, reducing the incidence and severity of sequelae, and improving survival. Accordingly, intravenous administration of clot-selective thrombolytic agents and direct angioplasty in patients with contraindications to fibrinolysis or in those who sustain infarction under unusual circumstances (e.g., in a catheterization laboratory) are the treatments of choice. Contraindications to thrombolysis include a bleeding diathesis, history of cerebrovascular accident, recent surgery or trauma, long-standing uncontrolled hypertension with hypertensive vascular disease, active peptic ulcer disease, and other conditions predisposing to hemorrhage. Patients particularly likely to benefit from early recanalization are those with anterior wall transmural myocardial infarction who can be treated within 4 hours of the onset of infarction. However, some patients may benefit from treatment later than 6 hours after the apparent onset of infarction, perhaps because of stuttering infarction, recurrent spontaneous thrombolysis and reocclusion, or unavoidable misclassification of the actual time of onset of infarction that can be delayed after the onset of chest pain.

Unfortunately, the mean time to initial treatment with thrombolytic agents (the so-called door to needle time) remains high, in the range of 1.7 hours. Optimal time to treatment is much shorter, as demonstrated conclusively in the MITI study, in which 99% survival accompanied treatment initiated within the first 90 minutes.

In addition to conjunctive treatment, such as administration of aspirin and heparin intravenously, designed to potentiate thrombolysis and accelerate and sustain recanalization induced by thrombolytic drugs, adjunctive treatment is essential to protect jeopardized ischemic myocardium. It includes adequate analgesia (to diminish deleterious sympathetic stimulation of the heart and platelet aggregation secondary to increased circulating catecholamines), provision of oxygen if arterial oxygen saturation is low, reduction of myocardial oxygen requirements with venous and arterial vasodilators as indicated by ventricular loading conditions and guided by hemodynamic monitoring when necessary, adjustment of central vascular volume to optimize cardiac performance and minimize ventricular wall stress, vigorous treatment of arrhythmias that compromise cardiac performance, and immediate defibrillation should ventricular fibrillation occur. Prophylactic lidocaine is not necessary when defibrillation can be implemented immediately and pharmacologic treatment initiated promptly as indicated.[26] However, administration of magnesium (a 1-g dose over 5 minutes followed by an 8-g infusion during the first 48 hours) appears to reduce mortality associated with infarction in patients treated with or without thrombolytic agents.[27] β-Adrenergic blocking agents decrease mortality as well and are indicated in all patients without specific contraindications and particularly in those in whom increased sympathoadrenal activity is evident (e.g., manifested by relative or absolute tachycardia, systolic hypertension).

The work of breathing should be reduced by prevention and vigorous treatment of pulmonary edema with mechanical ventilatory assistance devices when indicated. Rarely, mechanical support of the circulation may be needed when severe mitral regurgitation, ventricular septal rupture, free wall rupture, or cardiogenic shock supervenes. For these conditions, definitive diagnosis and prompt surgical intervention are essential. Prevention or prompt reversal of substantial fever, pericarditis, or loss of blood (e.g., from occult gastrointestinal tract bleeding and retroperitoneal bleeding or hemorrhage from any site) is necessary to avoid cardiac decompensation and prevent undue increases in myocardial oxygen requirements. Any patient in whom unexplained tachycardia, malignant arrhythmia, persistent or recurrent chest pain, refractory congestive heart failure, hypotension, or low cardiac output occurs may require early cardiac catheterization and angioplasty or surgery.

Recanalization after administration of thrombolytic agents can be recognized often by prompt relief of chest pain, accelerated resolution of ST-segment elevation on the electrocardiogram (ECG), early peaking of the MB creatine kinase (CK) time-activity curve in plasma, and improved regional ventricular performance. However, these phenomena are neither sufficiently sensitive nor specific enough to differentiate patients with initial recanalization and virtually immediate reocclusion or failed recanalization from those in whom recanalization is successful. Both continuous ECG monitoring of ST-segment elevation and its regression and of QRS vectors[28] and changes in the rate of appearance in plasma of macromolecular markers of myocardial injury, such as isoforms of individual isoenzymes of CK and myoglobin,[29] have been employed for rapid detection of failed recanalization or early reocclusion—both of which may justify early, "rescue" angioplasty.

Cardiac catheterization and angioplasty should be performed if hemodynamic deterioration or other manifestations of early recurrent infarction or reocclusion appear after recanalization that has been thought to be successful initially.[30] Before hospital discharge, elective coronary angioplasty is indicated if signs or symptoms of ischemia occur at rest or are induced by submaximal exercise.[31]

RESEARCH IN PROGRESS

Several agents that may possibly diminish injury to myocytes subjected to ischemia, reperfusion, or both are undergoing vigorous investigation for use as adjunctive agents. Myocytes rendered ischemic and subsequently subjected to reperfusion promptly accumulate free intracellular calcium because of the prevailing concentration gradient and the diminished barrier function of injured cell membranes. Excess intracellular calcium can impair mitochondrial oxidative phosphorylation, accelerate hydrolysis of adenosine triphosphate (ATP) by activating calcium-dependent adenosine triphosphatases (ATPases), and potentially activate lytic enzymes such as phospholipases that can elaborate amphipathic metabolites and degrade sarcolemma and other membranous cytosolic organelles. Accordingly, calcium antagonists may exert salutary effects on myocardium subjected to reperfusion. Thus, in dogs with coronary occlusion followed by reperfusion within 2 hours, salvage of myocardium is enhanced almost twofold by concomitant administration of diltiazem hydrochloride compared with salvage elicited by reperfusion alone via inhibition of lipid peroxidation.[32] β-Blockers inhibit the same processes, perhaps explaining the benefits sometimes seen with their early use (during the initial 2 to 4 hours) in reducing the extent of apparent infarction in patients treated with and without fibrinolytic agents.

In the past few decades remarkable progress has been made in the early detection and effective treatment of acute myocardial infarction. The importance of infarct size as a determinant of prognosis and of thrombosis as the proximate cause of most transmural infarctions has been established. Complex atherosclerotic plaques have been demonstrated to be the underlying culprit. Secondary prevention of the progression of coronary disease and recurrent events after acute infarction with β-adrenergic blocking agents, aspirin, and antilipidemic agents has proved to be helpful. The death rate from coronary artery disease has declined considerably, by more than 20% between 1984 and 1994 alone, as a result of improved prevention and improved treatment. Nevertheless, efforts to reduce its toll must continue.

The pivotal role of the physician cannot be overemphasized. Results of the GISSI-1, MITI, GUSTO, and numerous other studies are consistent with results of mechanistic laboratory and clinical studies showing that the benefits of thrombolysis are profoundly dependent on the rapidity of recanalization of the infarct-related artery. Patients at risk must therefore be educated to recognize promptly and interpret correctly the symptoms of acute myocardial infarction so that immediate treatment can be obtained. Provision of knowledge and preclusion of delay can transmit the proven benefit of early recanalization to many patients who will be victimized by acute myocardial infarction. Hospitals must provide prompt access and rapid transportation for the patients they serve, reduce the all-too-typical logistic delays that prevail currently, and administer appropriate treatment within minutes. Streamlined initial diagnostic evaluations must be available immediately and around the clock. Arrangements must be in place for expeditious transfer of patients requiring angioplasty or surgery to well-staffed and well-equipped tertiary-care centers that can respond promptly. The essential ingredient is prevention of delay when signs or symptoms of bona fide heart attack occur.

Anticipated Developments

Rapid progress is being made in the development of even more clot-selective fibrinolytic agents, such as molecular variants of t-PA with specifically desirable pharmacologic properties including increased fibrin specificity, resistance to inhibitors, and prolonged half-life in the circulation. Self-administration, or administration by paramedical personnel, of clot-selective fibrinolytic agents by alternative routes, such as intramuscular injection with telephonic ECG surveillance, may reduce delay time and improve outcome.[33, 34] Molecular hybrids comprising components of plasminogen activators and of antibodies targeting them to fibrin may increase therapeutic efficacy. Perhaps the most important advances in the immediate future will be improved conjunctive therapy with effective direct-acting antithrombins, antiplatelets, and novel anticoagulant agents (e.g., anti-Xa and anti–tissue factor agents). These agents will not only decrease thrombin activity, and hence platelet activation, but also diminish rebound after discontinuation of antithrombins by preventing accumulation of active procoagulants capable of generating thrombin activity.

Development of novel adjunctive agents to reduce or retard injury associated with ischemia or to enhance reperfusion, or both, such as scavengers of oxygen-derived free radicals, is another promising avenue. Mechanical repair of diseased vessels, devoid of the high incidence of restenosis now encountered, may be possible, based on the elucidation of mediation of restenosis by cytokines, growth factors, and adhesion molecules. Pharmacologic prophylaxis of sudden cardiac death in patients identified at particularly high risk may be possible as biochemical and anatomic processes underlying initiation of life-threatening arrhythmias induced by ischemia become clarified.[35]

Ultimately, improved prevention of atherosclerosis will assume a dominant role in reducing the toll from coronary artery disease. Suppression not only of hypercholesterolemia but also of elevated plasma homocysteine and plasminogen activator inhibitor type-1 and other risk factors that may be shown to be determinants of progression of vascular disease is likely to become increasingly important. Nevertheless, for the foreseeable future, the outcome for many patients with coronary artery disease will depend most on their being able to access the medical care system promptly and effectively when manifestations of acute myocardial infarction first occur. The physician has the ultimate responsibility and optimal opportunity to use powerful advances already available to increase survival and to improve the quality of life in those afflicted with acute myocardial infarction.

REFERENCES

1. Selker HP: Coronary care unit triage decision aids. How do we know they work? Am J Med 87:491, 1989.
2. Graves EJ: 1983 Summary: National Hospital Discharge Survey. Rockville, MD: National Center for Health Statistics, September 18, 1984.
3. U.S. Bureau of the Census: Statistical Abstract of the United States, 11th ed. Washington, DC: U.S. Government Printing Office, 1991, pp 82–83.
4. DeWood MA, Spores J, Notske R, et al: Prevalence of total coronary occlusion during the early hours of transmural myocardial infarction. N Engl J Med 202:897, 1980.
5. Tiefenbrunn AJ, Sobel BE: The timing of coronary recanaliza-

tion: Paradigms, paradoxes, and pertinence. Circulation 85:2311, 1992.

6. Reimer KA, Lowe JE, Rasmussen MM, et al: The wavefront phenomenon of ischemic cell death. Myocardial infarct size versus duration of coronary occlusion in dogs. Circulation 56:786, 1977.

7. Kennedy JW, Gensini GG, Timmis GC, et al: Acute myocardial infarction treated with intracoronary streptokinase: A report of the society for coronary angiography. Am J Cardiol 55:871, 1985.

8. Kennedy JW, Ritchie JL, Davis KB, et al: Western Washington randomized trial of intracoronary streptokinase in acute myocardial infarction. N Engl J Med 309:1477, 1983.

9. Kennedy JW, Ritchie JL, Davis KB, et al: The Western Washington randomized trial of intracoronary streptokinase in acute myocardial infarction. A 12-month follow up report. N Engl J Med 312:1073, 1985.

10. Winniford MD: Thrombolytic therapy for acute myocardial infarction. Cardiovasc Rev Rep 7:573, 1986.

11. Torr SR, Nachowiak DA, Fujii S, et al: "Plasminogen steal" and clot lysis. J Am Coll Cardiol 19:1085, 1992.

12. Eisenberg PR, Sherman LA, Jaffe AS: Paradoxical elevation of fibrinopeptide A after streptokinase: Evidence for continued thrombosis despite intense fibrinolysis. J Am Coll Cardiol 10:527, 1987.

13. Prager NA, Torr-Brown SR, Sobel BE, et al: Maintenance of patency after thrombolysis in stenotic coronary arteries requires combined inhibition of thrombin and platelets. J Am Coll Cardiol 22(1):296, 1993.

14. Gruppo Italiano per lo Studio della Streptochinasi nell'Infarto Miocardico (GISSI): Effectiveness of intravenous thrombolytic treatment in acute myocardial infarction. Lancet 1:397, 1986.

15. Sobel BE: Thrombolysis in the treatment of acute myocardial infarction. *In* Fuster V, Verstraete M (eds): Thrombosis in Cardiovascular Disorders. Philadelphia: WB Saunders, 1992, pp 289–326.

16. Tiefenbrunn AJ, Sobel BE: Thrombolysis and myocardial infarction. Fibrinolysis 5:1, 1991.

17. Collen D, Topol EJ, Tiefenbrunn AJ, et al: Coronary thrombolysis with recombinant human tissue-type plasminogen activator: A prospective, randomized, placebo-controlled trial. Circulation 70:1012, 1984.

18. TIMI Study Group: The thrombolysis in myocardial infarction (TIMI) trial. Phase I findings. N Engl J Med 312:932, 1985.

19. Verstraete M, Bory M, Collen D, et al: Randomized trial of intravenous recombinant tissue-type plasminogen activator versus intravenous streptokinase in acute myocardial infarction. Report from the European Cooperative Study Group for Recombinant Tissue-Type Plasminogen Activator. Lancet 1:842, 1985.

20. Eisenberg PR, Sherman LA, Tiefenbrunn AJ, et al: Sustained fibrinolysis after administration of t-PA despite its short half life in the circulation. Thromb Haemost 7:35, 1987.

21. The GUSTO Investigators: Preliminary results from the GUSTO trial. Presented at the American Federation for Clinical Research National Meeting, Washington, DC, April 30, 1993.

22. Sobel BE, Hirsh J: Principles and practice of coronary thrombolysis and conjunctive treatment [editorial]. Am J Cardiol 68:382, 1991.

23. Haskel EH, Prager NA, Adams SP, et al: Relative efficacy of antithrombin compared with antiplatelet agents in accelerating coronary thrombolysis and preventing early reocclusion. Circulation 83:1048, 1991.

24. Weaver WD, Eisenberg MS, Martin JSI, et al: Myocardial Infarction Triage and Intervention project–phase I: Patient characteristics and feasibility of prehospital initiation of thrombolytic therapy [abstract]. *In* Stump DC (ed): Coronary Thrombolysis. A Research Compendium. South San Francisco: Genentech, Inc., 1993, p 241.

25. Sobel BE, Collen D: Strokes, statistics, and sophistry in trials of thrombolysis for acute myocardial infarction. Am J Cardiol 71:424, 1993.

26. Knabb RM, Rosamond TC, Fox KAA, et al: Enhancement of salvage of reperfused ischemic myocardium by diltiazem. J Am Coll Cardiol 8:861, 1986.

27. Jaffe AS: Prophylactic lidocaine for suspected acute myocardial infarction. Heart Disease and Stroke 1:179, 1992.

28. Woods KL, Fletcher S, Roffe C, Haider Y: Intravenous magnesium sulphate in suspected acute myocardial infarction: Results of the second Leicester Intravenous Magnesium Intervention Trial (LIMIT-2). Lancet 339:1553, 1992.

29. Dellborg M, Riha M, Swedberg K, for the TEAHAT study-group: Dynamic QRS complex and ST-segment monitoring in acute myocardial infarction during recombinant tissue plasminogen activator therapy. Am J Cardiol 67:343, 1991.

30. Abendschein DR, Ellis AK, Eisenberg PR, et al: Prompt detection of coronary recanalization by analysis of rates of change of concentrations of macromolecular markers in plasma. Coron Artery Dis 2:201, 1991.

31. Topol EJ, Califf RM, Kereiakes DJ, et al: Thrombolysis and angioplasty in myocardial infarction (TAMI) trial. J Am Coll Cardiol 10:65B, 1987.

32. Topol EJ: Acute Coronary Intervention. New York: Alan R. Liss, 1987.

33. Sobel BE, Saffitz JE, Fields LE, et al: Intramuscular administration of tissue-type plasminogen activator in rabbits and dogs and its implications for coronary thrombolysis. Circulation 75:1262, 1987.

34. Sobel BE, Sarnoff SJ, Nachowiak DA: Augmented and sustained plasma concentrations after intramuscular injections of molecular variants and deglycosylated forms of tissue-type plasminogen activators. Circulation 81:1362, 1990.

35. Saffitz JE, Corr PB, Sobel BE: Arrhythmogenesis and ventricular dysfunction after myocardial infarction: Is anomalous cellular coupling the elusive link? Circulation 87:1742, 1993.

CHAPTER 2

Angina Pectoris

C. Richard Conti, M.D.

Although much is known and written about events after myocardial ischemia, key questions about pathogenesis remain unanswered. What mechanism or mechanisms trigger the individual attacks? What causes attacks of ischemia to continue recurring in some cases and to terminate spontaneously in others? The answers to these questions are not easy to discern from information currently available. Considerable speculation is made about the precise factors that initiate myocardial ischemia, but little evidence supports it. The speculation relates to the role of disordered metabolic or neurohumoral control over the coronary circulation, increased sensitivity of vascular smooth muscles at the site of an atherosclerotic plaque to substances such as thromboxane, and temporary platelet occlusion. A combination of these factors may be responsible for large-vessel coronary artery obstruction.

The sequence of endothelial (plaque) disruption, platelet activation, and thrombogenic factors, that is, the balance between the thrombolytic system and the coagulation system, determines which blood vessels thrombose and which vessels remain patent but stenotic.

In patients with significant coronary atherosclerosis and reproducible effort angina pectoris, ischemia is probably due to an increased myocardial oxygen demand (increased heart rate or blood pressure) that cannot be met because of a fixed coronary reserve. In addition, unknown factors responsible for an increase in myocardial oxygen demand that cannot be measured by routine methods must also be considered.

CLINICAL PRESENTATION

It is well known that patients with chest pain secondary to myocardial ischemia have variable histories and different clinical and laboratory features. For example, most patients with severe recurrent ischemia (unstable angina) have angina pectoris with minimal or no effort, but a few patients have normal exercise tolerance and only recurrent rest angina pectoris. Variable changes on the electrocardiogram (e.g., ST-segment depression or elevation or T-wave peaking or inversion during chest pain) may indicate different degrees of myocardial ischemia. Coronary angiographic findings are not uniform and range from normal to severely obstructed, disrupted plaques in multiple vessels. These variable clinical and laboratory expressions of the unstable state suggest that different mechanisms may be active in different patients. Thus, it is naive to think that such a complex condition as angina pectoris can be treated in the same manner in all patients.

RATIONALE FOR THERAPY

Current evidence strongly suggests that coronary atherosclerosis is a common denominator in most patients with ischemic heart disease. Accordingly, it is understandable why extracardiac factors that increase myocardial oxygen demand (e.g., tachycardia, anemia, hypertension, smoking, discontinued drugs, sympathomimetic amines) might create an acute ischemic state. In addition, the turbulence and stasis of flow caused by the atherosclerotic plaque can be responsible for intermittent platelet aggregation in diseased vessels[1] as well as intermittent coronary artery thrombosis.[2-5]

To initiate the process of thrombosis and occlusion of a blood vessel, intimal disruption occurs on the surface of an atherosclerotic plaque. Plaque susceptible to this process consists of a fibrous cap and a necrotic core. As the process of plaque disruption occurs, platelet aggregation results at the site of disruption. These aggregated platelets then release substances such as serotonin and thromboxane A_2, which are potent vasoconstrictors. In addition, injured endo-thelial cells release substances such as endothelin, another potent vasoconstrictor.

Thus, it is sensible to correct any extracardiac factors that may be aggravating the patient's angina and to consider the use of platelet-active agents for long-term management of patients[6] and intravenous heparin for short-term management.[7] The evidence is weak that isolated hemorrhages bleeding into an atheromatous plaque account for the progression of symptoms. However, because this diagnosis is obtained at autopsy, angiography is not revealing. Similarly, rapid progression of atherosclerosis can be defined only pathologically. The clinician performing serial coronary angiograms can identify only stenosis, which may have many causes, including intramural thrombosis formation.

Solid angiographic,[3, 8] pathologic,[9] and angioscopic[10] evidence now suggest that patients with acute ischemic syndromes have eccentric and irregular lesions associated with plaque rupture, with superimposed, partially occlusive thrombus, or with recanalized thrombus. Plaques tend to rupture at the weakest point of the atheroma. This is usually at the junction between the normal wall and the atheroma. Vessels most commonly involved in these events are the proximal left anterior descending coronary artery, the right coronary artery near the origin of the marginal branch, and the circumflex coronary artery proximal to and near the origin of the obtuse marginal branch. Of course, these are also the commonest sites of high-grade stenoses and thromboses. A plaque becomes vulnerable to rupture when the cap becomes thin and the soft lipid core contains low-density lipoprotein (LDL)–activated macrophages. The LDL-activated macrophages are thought to play a central role in the expansion of the necrotic core leading to erosion of the fibrous cap and ultimately to intimal disruption. Thinning of the fibrous cap can also be related to the development of superficial fissures secondary to repetitive bending of the vessel during cardiac contraction. These observations provide evidence that the use of platelet-active agents and anticoagulants is appropriate for acute and chronic management of these patients.

Proponents of the spasm hypothesis note that some patients develop transmural infarction with normal, near-normal, or patent but stenotic coronary arteries. The precise role of coronary artery spasm in the pathogenesis of acute myocardial infarction and unstable angina pectoris is still unknown. It may occur before the event, contribute to the event, or simply be an epiphenomenon. Coronary artery spasm undoubtedly is a real phenomenon.

EARLY TREATMENT

If coronary artery spasm is identified as the mechanism that produces myocardial ischemia, the use of vasodilators in the early phases of unstable angina is appropriate. However, when thrombosis is clearly defined, thrombolytic therapy in the early stages is reasonable.

Table 2–1. **Causes of the Development of Acute Myocardial Ischemia**

1. Extracardiac factors in patients with severe coronary atherosclerosis
2. Rupture of an atheromatous plaque, which may lead to
   • rapid progression of atherosclerosis
   • transient platelet aggregation
   • intermittent coronary artery thrombosis
   • abnormal constriction of an epicardial coronary artery
3. A combination of 1 and 2

If severe coronary artery disease is found (with or without thrombosis), the argument is strong for therapy with anticoagulants such as intravenous heparin during the acute phase of the illness. A similar argument could be made for the use of antiplatelet agents during the acute and convalescent phases.

If extracardiac (aggravating) factors are present, for example, hypertension or tachycardia, they must be corrected appropriately.

It may not be possible to identify the appropriate mechanism responsible for unstable angina pectoris in every case, but the clinician must attempt to do so, because the selection of appropriate therapy for an individual patient depends on the mechanism responsible for the symptoms.

SUMMARY

Unstable angina is a simple term that describes a complex group of conditions with a heterogeneous pathogenesis and prognosis. Low- and high-risk groups can be identified by simple clinical criteria such as failure to respond promptly to medical treatment and the presence or absence of electrocardiographic changes.

In patients with cardiac disease, understanding pathogenic mechanisms often influences decisions regarding prognosis and treatment. Current understanding of pathologic processes that may underlie the nature of acute myocardial ischemia and thus may influence its management is summarized here.

Potential causes of acute myocardial ischemia are listed in Table 2–1.

REFERENCES

1. Folts JD, Cromwell EB, Rowe LL: Platelet aggregation in partially obstructed vessels and its elimination with aspirin. Circulation 54:365, 1976.
2. Vetrovec CW, Leinbach RC, Gold HK, et al: Intracoronary thrombolysis in syndromes of ischemia: Angiographic and clinical results. Am Heart J 104:946, 1982.
3. Mandelkorn JB, Wolf NM, Singh S, et al: Intracoronary thrombus in nontransmural myocardial infarction and in unstable angina pectoris. Am J Cardiol 52:1, 1983.
4. Capone GJ, Meyer BB, Wolf NM, et al: Incidence of intracoronary thrombi in patients with active unstable angina pectoris. Circulation 70(Suppl 2):II-415, 1984.
5. Lawrence JR, Shepherd JT, Bone I, et al: Fibrinolytic therapy in unstable angina pectoris: A controlled clinical trial. Thromb Res 17:767, 1980.
6. Lewis HD, Davis JW, Archibald DG, et al: Protective effects of aspirin against acute myocardial infarction and death in unstable angina. N Engl J Med 309:396, 1983.
7. Telford AM, Wilson C: Trial of heparin versus atenolol in prevention of myocardial infarction in intermediate coronary syndrome. Lancet 1:1225, 1981.
8. Ambrose JA, Winters SL, Stern A, et al: Angiographic morphology and the pathogenesis of unstable angina pectoris. J Am Coll Cardiol 5:609, 1985.
9. Falk E: Unstable angina with fatal outcome: Dynamic coronary thrombosis leading to infarction and/or sudden death. Autopsy evidence of recurrent mural thrombosis with peripheral embolization culminating in total vascular occlusion. Circulation 71:699, 1985.
10. Forrester JS, Litvack F, Grundfest W, et al: A perspective of coronary disease seen through the arteries of living man. Circulation 75:505, 1987.

CHAPTER 3

Congestive Heart Failure

William W. Parmley, M.D.

Substantial progress has been made since the 1970s in the understanding of and therapy for congestive heart failure (CHF). One of the most important advances has been a growing understanding of its pathophysiology, particularly the role of hormonal factors and the peripheral circulation. As systolic function decreases, a number of important reflex mechanisms are activated, including increased levels of serum catecholamines[1] and arginine vasopressin[2] and activation of the renin-angiotensin system.[3] Hemodynamically, these changes result in an increase in heart rate, contractility, and systemic vascular resistance. Systemic vascular resistance is presumably designed to maintain blood pressure in the face of a fall in cardiac output. Although the maintenance of blood pressure is an important goal in preserving perfusion of vital organs such as the brain, heart, and kidneys, this elevation of systemic vascular resistance has deleterious effects by further increasing the resistance to ejection of blood from the left ventricle.

Thus, a vicious circle appears set in motion: Systolic dysfunction leads to reduction in stroke volume and cardiac output. In turn, reflex activation of the sympathetic nervous system (and other neurohumoral systems) increases systemic vascular resistance. This increase in resistance further reduces stroke volume as it increases afterload. A patient moves through this circle until a new steady state is achieved consisting of a lower cardiac output and a higher systemic resistance than is optimal for the patient. The best evidence to support the existence of this vicious circle is pharmacologic. When potent arteriolar vasodilators such as hydralazine are administered, a 50% increase in cardiac output occurs, with little or no reduction in arterial pressure.[4] This discrepancy suggests that arteriolar tone has been set too high and thus overshoots. Perhaps this potent reflex is better designed to meet acute emergencies such as hypotension from blood loss; it is less well tuned for chronic problems such as chronic CHF.

NEUROHUMORAL ACTIVATION

Important advances have been made in better understanding the influence of the principal neurohumoral systems activated in CHF: (1) the sympathetic nervous system, (2) the renin-angiotensin-aldosterone system, and (3) increased secretion of arginine vasopressin (antidiuretic hormone [ADH]). Each of these hormone systems contributes to peripheral vasoconstriction, but other important effects occur as well.

Increased sympathetic tone and adrenal activity contribute to a substantial increase in circulating catecholamines (principally norepinephrine). In a general way, the magnitude of increase in plasma catecholamines is related to the severity of the heart failure[5] and thus to the ultimate prognosis. When heart failure is treated appropriately and patients become better compensated, a reduction occurs in catecholamine levels, presumably because of a withdrawal of sympathetic tone. Elevated catecholamine levels appear to reflect a combination of beneficial and potentially detrimental effects. Beneficial effects of an increase in catecholamines include the following: (1) an increase in heart rate, which helps maintain cardiac output in the face of a fall in stroke volume; (2) an increase in contractility, which helps preserve stroke volume; and (3) an increase in systemic vascular resistance that may be initially beneficial in maintaining arterial pressure but that frequently enhances afterload to the degree that it reduces cardiac output, as described earlier. Other detrimental effects of elevated catecholamine levels include increases in both myocardial oxygen consumption and the frequency and severity of arrhythmias. In this context, it is interesting to speculate whether β-adrenergic blockers should be given to patients with chronic CHF. Although some evidence suggests that β-blockers might be beneficial in patients with idiopathic dilated cardiomyopathy,[6] they do not appear to aid most patients with heart failure.

Activation of the renin-angiotensin-aldosterone system has attracted considerable attention, primarily because of the advent of angiotensin-converting enzyme (ACE) inhibitors.[7] Renin release from the juxtaglomerular cells occurs with hyponatremia, decreased perfusion pressure, and increased catecholamine levels—all of which accompany CHF. Renin converts angiotensinogen to angiotensin I, an inactive decapeptide. Angiotensin I is converted to angiotensin II by converting enzyme, which is predominant in pulmonary capillary endothelial cells. Angiotensin II has potentially deleterious effects that include potent vasoconstriction, facilitation of sympathetic outflow, and increased production of aldosterone, which further retains salt and water. It is understandable why ACE inhibitors have been so beneficial in blocking these adverse effects.

The least important of the three neurohumoral systems discussed here appears to be the arginine vasopressin system. Although ADH level is increased in many patients with heart failure, a selective antagonist of its effects produced no important hemodynamic changes.[8] However, increased ADH levels may play an important role in hyponatremic patients.

VASODILATOR THERAPY

The role of vasodilators was first elucidated in acute heart failure and only later was applied to patients with chronic heart failure. A number of important principles emerged from these studies. One was the differential effects of arteriolar dilators versus venodilators. Arteriolar dilators increase cardiac output by decreasing systemic vascular resistance. Venodilators, conversely, lower right and left atrial filling pressures by redistributing blood away from the chest into the peripheral veins (capacitance reservoir of blood in the body). A combined arteriolar dilator and venodilator, such as nitroprusside, was effective both in increasing cardiac output and in reducing atrial filling pressures.[9]

The greatest percentage response to intravenous vasodilators occurred in the sickest patients with the highest filling pressures. Furthermore, the response to vasodilators was dependent on the level of pulmonary capillary wedge pressure. At high filling pressures, beneficial responses were characterized by increases in cardiac output and reductions in filling pressure. However, as filling pressure fell below 15 to 20 mmHg, a reduction in stroke volume occurred as the ventricle moved down the ascending limb of the Frank-Starling curve.[9] Thus, whenever a venodilator is given, filling pressure should be maintained above approximately 15 mmHg to avoid reduced cardiac output and hypotension. This principle is also important in the treatment of chronic heart failure.

Although intravenous vasodilators have improved hemodynamics and relieved symptoms in patients with acute heart failure due to myocardial infarction, it is less clear whether they reduce the mortality rate. Two placebo-controlled studies with nitroprusside had somewhat different results: The European study[10] showed a reduction in mortality, but the Veterans Administration Cooperative Study[11] showed no overall reduction. More specifically, when nitroprusside was given later than 12 hours after the onset of the infarction, mortality was reduced; when it was given within the first 12 hours, deleterious effects were noted. Both studies agreed that nitroprusside was effective after 12 hours.

After their demonstrated hemodynamic and clinical

benefits in acute heart failure, vasodilators were applied to chronic heart failure. Several important lessons were learned. Although arteriolar vasodilators are effective in increasing cardiac output, they have not increased exercise tolerance in placebo-controlled studies.[12, 13] In contrast, drugs with venodilating properties have increased exercise tolerance in placebo-controlled studies.[14, 15] Therefore, to achieve both goals—that is, increased cardiac output and reduced atrial filling pressure—it has become common to administer both a venodilator and an arteriolar dilator, such as isosorbide dinitrate and hydralazine.[16] This combination not only improved overall hemodynamics but also was shown in the Veterans Administration Heart Failure Trial (V-HEFT) to prolong life.[17]

ACE inhibitors have emerged in the past few years as the vasodilators most commonly used for heart failure. Although their acute hemodynamic benefits are only modest, their long-term effects have been quite salutary.[7] In double-blind, placebo-controlled trials, they have produced increases in exercise tolerance as well as improvements in symptoms. Furthermore, the work of the Consensus Trial Study Group with enalapril has shown prolongation of life in patients with severe (class IV) heart failure.[18] Results of this trial and of the V-HEFT trial established vasodilator therapy as a cornerstone in the management of chronic heart failure.

In the V-HEFT 2 trial, enalapril and isosorbide dinitrate were compared in patients with moderate heart failure already receiving digitalis and diuretics. Enalapril was slightly and statistically better in reducing mortality.[19] In the two arms of the Studies Of Left Ventricular Dysfunction (SOLVD) trial, enalapril was tested against a placebo. In asymptomatic patients with reduced ejection fractions, enalapril reduced the rate of development of CHF and tended to reduce mortality rate, although this latter effect was not statistically significant.[20] In the symptomatic arm of the SOLVD trial, enalapril reduced mortality.[21] In the Survival And Ventricular Enlargement (SAVE) trial, captopril reduced mortality compared with placebo in patients after a substantive myocardial infarction.[22] This presumably occurred by reducing the rate of left ventricular dilation, thinning, and remodeling after a large infarction. All of these data indicate why ACE inhibitors have become the premier form of vasodilator therapy.

A new combined arteriolar and venodilator, flosequinan, is effective in improving hemodynamics and exercise tolerance.[23] However, in a large multicenter mortality trial, it increased mortality at the usual dose of 100 mg, perhaps because of its concomitant inotropic effects.

NEW INOTROPIC AGENTS

Since the mid-1980s, a number of new inotropic agents for treating chronic heart failure have been investigated. Some of these agents are catecholamine derivatives. Intermittent dobutamine therapy has shown promise in some studies because hemodynamic and clinical benefits have persisted for a few weeks after a 2- to 3-day infusion.[24] Precise mechanisms of the improvement are unclear, but they may relate to a training effect from increased ventricular reserve or from a more fundamental change in mitochondrial function.[25] Because these drugs have a propensity for arrhythmias and increased oxygen consumption, however, it is unclear whether this form of therapy will be valuable for all patients. Similarly, new oral catecholamine derivatives may well have beneficial hemodynamic effects (e.g., levodopa, prenalterol), but they may also produce an unacceptably high level of arrhythmias and other side effects.[26]

More important, a whole new class of potent oral inotropic vasodilators has emerged. Amrinone is the parent compound, now available for intravenous use in critical care units.[27] Many of these new drugs appear to work primarily by inhibiting phosphodiesterase and thus increasing levels of cyclic adenosine monophosphate. They are potent drugs that produce a striking increase in cardiac output and a decrease in pulmonary capillary wedge pressure. Although short-term studies showed beneficial hemodynamic and clinical effects,[28] long-term studies were less encouraging.[29]

In a multicenter trial in patients with severe heart failure,[30] milrinone increased mortality compared with placebo. Thus, the phosphodiesterase inhibitors (milrinone and amrinone) have been restricted to short-term intravenous administration.

A new combined inotropic and vasodilator drug, vesnarinone, was associated with reduced mortality at a low dose (60 mg)[31] but with increased mortality at a high dose (120 mg). This interesting drug deserves further evaluation. Furthermore, it may be that lower doses of inotropic agents will prove to be more beneficial than higher doses.

FUTURE NEEDS

Despite the overall progress in our understanding and management of chronic heart failure, many problems remain. Most important is our need to prevent heart failure. Because coronary artery disease is the most important cause of CHF, a decline in coronary disease through preventive measures will eventually have an impact on the number of patients who develop heart failure. Because the mode of death is sudden half the time in patients with CHF, we need better antiarrhythmic drugs. Our comprehension of cardiomyopathy and its diverse causes is particularly deficient. Only when we better understand its etiology and pathophysiology can we prevent this disorder or treat it more effectively. The role of excess calcium in the pathogenesis of cardiomyopathy is especially intriguing.[32] We probably will see better pharmacologic agents for the treatment of heart failure, including β-blockers with vasodilating properties and specific neurohumoral antagonists. Immunologic therapy in cardiomyopathy with myocarditis is a promising but unproven approach. Ultimately, a more precise identification of the biochemical changes producing heart failure will be required before we can limit or reverse their effects. In short, we have just begun to understand the process of CHF. Major advances are required before a further substantial impact on this problem is possible.

REFERENCES

1. Zelis R, Davis D: The sympathetic nervous system in congestive heart failure. Heart Failure 2:21, 1986.
2. Creager MA: The role of vasopressin in congestive heart failure. Heart Failure 2:14, 1986.
3. Cody R: Issues regarding renin-angiotensin systemic activity in chronic congestive heart failure. Heart Failure 2:40, 1986.
4. Chatterjee K, Parmley WW, Massie B, et al: Oral hydralazine therapy for chronic refractory heart failure. Circulation 54:879, 1976.
5. Levine TB, Francis G, Goldsmith S, et al: Activity of the sympathetic nervous system and renin-angiotensin system assessed by plasma hormone levels and their relation to hemodynamic abnormalities in congestive heart failure. Am J Cardiol 49:1659, 1982.
6. Swedberg K, Hjalmarson A, Waagstein F, et al: Beneficial effects of long-term beta-blockade in congestive cardiomyopathy. Br Heart J 44:117, 1980.
7. Parmley WW: Captopril for heart failure. In Cohn J (ed): Drug Treatment of Heart Failure. New York: Advanced Therapeutics Communications, 1983, pp 179–198.
8. Creager MA, Faxon DP, Cutler SS, et al: Contribution of vasopressin to vasoconstriction in patients with congestive heart failure: Comparison with the renin-angiotensin system and the sympathetic nervous system. J Am Coll Cardiol 7:758, 1986.
9. Chatterjee K, Parmley WW: Vasodilator therapy for acute myocardial infarction and chronic heart failure. J Am Coll Cardiol 1:133, 1983.
10. Durrer JD, Lie KL, VanCapelle FRJ, et al: Effect of sodium nitroprusside on mortality in acute myocardial infarction. N Engl J Med 306:1126, 1982.
11. Cohn JN, Franciosa JA, Francis CS, et al: Effect of short-term infusion of sodium nitroprusside on mortality rate in acute myocardial infarction complicated by left ventricular failure. N Engl J Med 306:1129, 1982.
12. Franciosa JA, Weber KT, Levine TB, et al: Hydralazine in the long-term treatment of chronic heart failure: Lack of difference from placebo. Am Heart J 104:587, 1982.
13. Franciosa JA, Jordan RA, Wilen MM, et al: Minoxidil in patients with chronic left heart failure: Contrasting hemodynamic and clinical effects in a controlled trial. Circulation 70:63, 1984.
14. Franciosa JA, Goldsmith SR, Cohn JN: Contrasting immediate and long-term effects of isosorbide dinitrate on exercise capacity in congestive heart failure. Am J Med 69:559, 1980.
15. Cohn JN: Nitrates for congestive heart failure. Am J Cardiol 56:19A, 1985.
16. Massie B, Chatterjee K, Werner J, et al: Hemodynamic advantage of combined oral hydralazine and nonparenteral nitrates in the vasodilator therapy of chronic heart failure. Am J Cardiol 40:794, 1977.
17. Cohn JN, Archibald DG, Ziesche S, et al: Effect of vasodilator therapy on mortality in chronic congestive heart failure. N Engl J Med 314:1547, 1986.
18. Consensus Trial Study Group: Effects of enalapril on mortality in severe congestive heart failure. N Engl J Med 316:1429, 1987.
19. Cohn JN, Johnson G, Ziesche S, et al: A comparison of enalapril with hydralazine-isosorbide dinitrate in the treatment of congestive heart failure. N Engl J Med 325:303, 1991.
20. The SOLVD Investigators: Effect of enalapril on mortality and the development of heart failure in asymptomatic patients with reduced left ventricular ejection fractions. N Engl J Med 327:685, 1992.
21. The SOLVD Investigators: Effect of enalapril on survival in patients with reduced left ventricular ejection fractions and congestive heart failure. N Engl J Med 325:293, 1991.
22. SAVE Investigators: Effect of captopril on mortality and morbidity in patients with left ventricular dysfunction after myocardial infarction. N Engl J Med 327:669, 1992.
23. Cavero PG, DeMarco T, Kwasman M, et al: Flosequinan, a new vasodilator: Systemic and coronary hemodynamics and neuroendocrine effects in congestive heart failure. J Am Coll Cardiol 20:1542, 1992.
24. Liang C-S, Sherman LG, Doherty JU, et al: Sustained improvement of cardiac function in patients with congestive heart failure after short-term infusion of dobutamine. Circulation 69:113, 1984.
25. Unverferth DV, Magorien RD, Altschild R, et al: The hemodynamic and metabolic advantages gained by a three-day infusion of dobutamine in patients with congestive cardiomyopathy. Am Heart J 106:29, 1983.
26. Francis GS: The role of inotropic agents in the management of heart failure. In Cohn J (ed): Drug Treatment of Heart Failure. New York: Advanced Therapeutics Communications, 1983, pp 121–151.
27. Benotti JR, Grossman W, Braunwald E, et al: Hemodynamic assessment of amrinone: A new inotropic agent. N Engl J Med 299:1373, 1978.
28. LeJemtel TH, Keung E, Sonnenblick EH, et al: Amrinone: A new non-adrenergic cardiotonic agent effective in the treatment of intractable myocardial failure in man. Circulation 59:1098, 1979.
29. Packer M, Medina N, Yushak M: Hemodynamic and clinical limitations of long-term inotropic therapy with amrinone in patients with severe chronic heart failure. Circulation 70:1038, 1984.
30. Packer M, Carver JR, Rodemeffer RJ, et al: Effect of oral milrinone on mortality in severe chronic heart failure. N Engl J Med 325:1468, 1991.
31. Feldman AM, Bristow MR, Parmley WW, et al: Effects of vesnarinone on morbidity and mortality in patients with heart failure: Results of a multicenter trial. N Engl J Med 329:149, 1993.
32. Wikman-Coffelt J, Sievers R, Parmley WW, et al: Verapamil preserves adenine nucleotide pool in cardiomyopathic Syrian hamster. Am J Physiol 250(1 Pt 2):H22, 1986.

CHAPTER 4

Arrhythmias

Borys Surawicz, M.D.

Although credit for the most important advances in the therapy of cardiac arrhythmias made during the past 30 years must be given not to drugs but to electrical devices such as pacemakers and defibrillators, substantial progress also has been made in the pharmacologic treatment of arrhythmias. The advances in this field are related intimately to progress in the understanding of the mechanisms of cardiac arrhythmia, which are reviewed briefly before the discussion of drug therapy.

ARRHYTHMIA MECHANISMS

Conceptually, the occurrence of arrhythmia requires the presence of two factors, an appropriate substrate and a releasing trigger. In the normal heart, the substrate may be a cell capable of spontaneously firing an action potential (e.g., an automatic pacemaker fiber in the conducting tissue), and the trigger may be a neurotransmitter that brings the diastolic depolarization to the threshold of firing an ectopic impulse. This type of mechanism can produce automatic parasystolic and nonparasystolic ectopic tachycardias in the atria, atrioventricular (AV) junction, and ventricles. Although such autonomically controlled rhythms represent only a small fraction of ectopic tachycardias, they may be disabling when the activity is incessant and when the ectopic foci are protected, that is, not amenable to overdrive suppression.

In addition to automaticity resulting from depolarization beginning at the level of normal diastolic potential, repolarization can reach threshold and induce ectopic impulses by three other mechanisms: (1) slow channel–dependent automaticity in depolarized myocardium, (2) early afterdepolarizations, and (3) triggered late afterdepolarizations.

The low therapeutic efficacy of calcium antagonists on the substrate other than the AV and the sinoatrial (SA) nodes suggests that the mechanism of slow channel–dependent automaticity does not play an important role in clinical tachyarrhythmias. The significance of early afterdepolarizations is equally uncertain. *In vitro*, these afterdepolarizations can be precipitated by low levels of potassium, cesium, barium, and other substances that lower potassium conductance and inhibit full repolarization to the level of resting potential. These afterdepolarizations are believed to play a role in the genesis of torsade de pointes associated with congenital and acquired long QT syndrome, a concept that is difficult either to prove or to disprove. Late afterdepolarizations can be elicited *in vitro* in the setting of increased intracellular calcium concentration. This mechanism may operate in digitalis-induced ectopic tachycardias, but it is probably of no great importance under other circumstances.

Prevailing evidence suggests that the most common cause of tachyarrhythmias is reentry, a process requiring the presence of a reentrant pathway, unidirectional block, and slow conduction. Reentry is a proven mechanism for tachycardias using the AV bypass tracts, and it is almost certainly the mechanism of tachycardia using dual pathways within the AV node (AVN tachycardia). Reentry is also the probable mechanism of atrial flutter, atrial fibrillation, and most ventricular tachyarrhythmias. Depending on the circumstances, the site of unidirectional block may be a region of impaired conduction, prolonged refractory

period, or depressed excitability. These abnormalities frequently coexist. The possible mechanisms of slow conduction include depressed sodium channel–dependent conduction, calcium channel–dependent conduction, and electrotonus. Gardner et al.[1] have shown that reentrant tachycardia in a model of chronic myocardial infarction was associated with slow conduction caused by impulse propagation that was not parallel but perpendicular to the fiber orientation. Such anisotropic conduction probably results from the presence of structural barriers in the damaged myocardium.[2] Interestingly, slow impulse propagation in the anisotropic matrix generates normal action potentials with higher than normal velocity of depolarization. The possible role of anisotropic conduction in clinical arrhythmias is under investigation. If anisotropic conduction is proved to be of importance, it will be necessary to reassess the mechanisms of drugs acting on such substrate.

DRUG TREATMENT OF SUPRAVENTRICULAR ARRHYTHMIAS

The drug treatment of supraventricular arrhythmias is usually more satisfactory than that of ventricular arrhythmias. This difference can be explained by the availability of drugs capable of slowing impulse transmission through the AV node, a structure that controls ventricular rate in most supraventricular tachyarrhythmias. The slowing of AV nodal conduction and prolongation of the nodal refractory period can be accomplished acutely or chronically by vagal stimulation, most notably with digitalis, β-adrenergic blockade, and depression of calcium current passing through the slow channel by verapamil or diltiazem administration. An additional type of acute treatment is available in the form of adenosine or adenosine triphosphate (ATP).

The AV node is a component of the reentrant circuit of the two most common types of reentrant supraventricular tachycardias, namely, AV reentry and AVN reentry. In the case of AVN reentry, the entire circuit is probably located within the AV node and atrial approaches to AVN. In the case of AV reentry, drugs can be used to act on the AV node as well as on other components of the reentrant circuit (i.e., the atrium, the ventricular myocardium, and the His-Purkinje system). Indeed, the most effective drugs for prevention of tachycardias using accessory pathways are those that combine properties of AV nodal suppression with slowing of conduction in the atria, ventricles, and Purkinje system—that is, class IC drugs such as encainide, flecainide, and propafenone. Amiodarone also possesses these properties, and it also lengthens the refractory period of the atria and the ventricles.

Prevention of atrial fibrillation and atrial flutter requires administration of drugs that prolong the atrial refractory period or slow atrial conduction, that is, antiarrhythmic drugs with class I or class III properties. Prevention is more successful in patients without structural heart disease and with normal left atrial size. Antiarrhythmic therapy usually fails to prevent recurrences when atria become scarred or distended. However, when atrial tachyarrhythmia becomes established, ventricular rate can be controlled with drugs that act on the AV node, particularly using the combination of digitalis and a β-blocker or calcium antagonist.

DRUG TREATMENT OF VENTRICULAR ARRHYTHMIAS

In the case of ventricular arrhythmias, a discrete anatomic target such as the AV node cannot be identified without detailed intracardiac mapping. Ventricular arrhythmias may originate in the Purkinje fibers or in the ventricular myocardium, and the reentrant circuits usually involve tissues with nonhomogeneous refractory periods. Conduction within these circuits is slow and nonhomogeneous and may be isotropic or anisotropic. In most cases, the drugs probably affect the substrate, the trigger, and the cardiac tissues outside the reentrant circuit. As evidence of an altered substrate, we may consider the drug-induced slowing of the rate of ventricular tachycardia; as evidence of action on the trigger, consider the suppression of premature impulses initiating tachycardia. However, the distinction between the substrate and the trigger is blurred when the trigger originates within the abnormal substrate.

The two most important drawbacks of drug therapy for ventricular tachyarrhythmias are lack of effectiveness and the propensity to aggravate arrhythmias. Unfortunately, both phenomena tend to occur more frequently in clinical situations in which the drugs are needed most urgently, that is, in patients with depressed ventricular function and serious life-threatening arrhythmias. Some serious proarrhythmic effects are probably caused largely by increased refractory periods (torsade de pointes associated with QT_c lengthening), and some are largely due to an excessive slowing of conduction (incessant monomorphic ventricular tachycardia). Because the effectiveness of antiarrhythmic drugs is linked to their effect on the refractory period and conduction, it appears unlikely that the proarrhythmic effects caused by slow conduction or a prolonged refractory period are entirely avoidable. However, the incidence of proarrhythmic effects may be lessened by eliminating factors known to aggravate arrhythmias, such as hypokalemia and excessive bradycardia. Also, the onset of therapy requires careful supervision to detect so-called idiosyncratic reactions that usually appear during the first 5 to 7 days of drug treatment. It is possible that combining two drugs with different properties may lessen the proarrhythmic tendency, but this has not been firmly established.

The inadequacy of antiarrhythmic drugs can be attributed to the complexity of the substrate. This is suggested by the fact that in most patients with symptomatic sustained ventricular tachycardias, drugs do not protect them against arrhythmia induction by extrastimuli of low intensity delivered during programmed electrical stimulation. Arrhythmias are rendered noninducible by treatment with one of the class I drugs or amiodarone in only approximately 20% to 30% of patients.[3] Patients in whom the drugs prevent inducibility of ventricular tachycardia appear to have less complex or anatomically smaller substrates because they tend to have less impaired ventricular function and less pronounced fractionated activity detected by high-frequency, low-amplitude signals recorded in the signal-averaged electrocardiogram.

The obvious question is whether it is feasible to develop a drug that will either suppress all triggers or render the entire substrate impregnable to development of continuing reentry in the presence of a trigger. Certain clinical observations justify an attitude of cautious optimism with regard to such possibilities. One observation is past experience with quinidine in the treatment of atrial fibrillation; the other is more recent experience with amiodarone.

When quinidine was used in doses progressively increasing up to several grams per day,[4] fibrillatory activity was converted to a slow regular atrial flutter or to sinus rhythm in nearly all cases. A similar antifibrillatory effect exerted on the ventricles probably would make ventricular tachycardia sufficiently slow to be well tolerated. Unfortunately, quinidine, like other class I antiarrhythmic drugs, produces hypotension and dose-dependent depression of contractile force. These unwanted effects preclude administration of doses that would be required to drastically alter the electrophysiologic properties of the substrate.

Amiodarone meets the definition of an almost ideal universal antiarrhythmic drug by virtue of its combining nearly all known potentially antiarrhythmic properties. Amiodarone prolongs the refractory period of the atria and ventricular myocardium, presumably because of depression of time-dependent potassium current; it depresses automaticity of the SA node and the AV nodal conduction by action on the calcium channel; it is a powerful blocker of the sodium channel, with rapid-recovery kinetics from the drug-induced sodium channel block;[5] it is a noncompetitive inhibitor of α-adrenergic, β-adrenergic, and muscarinic receptors; and it inhibits thyroxine (T_4) conversion to triiodothyronine (T_3). Such a combination of several independent antiarrhythmic mechanisms appears to account for the unique effectiveness of amiodarone in treating a wide range of supraventricular and ventricular tachyarrhythmias. Unfortunately, the metabolic toxicity of amiodarone, attributed mainly to the inhibition of phospholipase, seriously limits long-term therapy in many patients who may benefit from the drug.

Clearly, substantial progress in antiarrhythmic drug therapy could be achieved by developing either a quinidine-like drug without vasodilating and negative inotropic properties or an amiodarone-like drug without its toxic metabolic effects.

NONPHARMACOLOGIC TREATMENT

While awaiting the development of new magic bullets, attention focuses on alternatives to drug therapy for patients with serious symptomatic and life-threatening arrhythmias. The most successful solution for the prevention of sudden cardiac death from ventricular fibrillation or hemodynamically intolerable ventricular tachycardia has been achieved using an automatic implantable cardioverter-defibrillator (AICD).[6] Increasing use of implantable transvenous cardioverter-defibrillators obviates the need for thoracotomy.[7] The introduction of a multiprogrammable pacemaker cardioverter-defibrillator provides, in addition to defibrillation antitachycardia pacing tiered therapy, more discriminating algorithms and backup pacing for bradycardia.[8] However, the procedure will not obviate the need for antiarrhythmic drug therapy, because the devices do not eliminate the substrate of arrhythmia.

A definitive cure of arrhythmia can be achieved only by surgical or catheter ablation of the focus of the arrhythmia, if it can be identified by mapping during an electrophysiologic study. Endocardial catheter ablation has been used to destroy arrhythmic foci in the atria, AV junction, and ventricles in patients in whom surgical therapy is not feasible. The greatest progress has been made in the ablation of the accessory pathways and portions of the AV node or perinodal atrial tissue responsible for the perpetuation of AV nodal reentrant tachycardias. The recently reported success rates for accessory pathway ablation by radiofrequency shocks are close to 99%, with complication rates below 2% and no mortality. The success rates of ablation of the slow reentrant AV nodal pathway are nearly as high.[9]

Among patients with ventricular tachycardias, surgical ablation is successful in 60% to 90% in whom tachycardia can be induced electrically and mapped during operation.[10] However, the drawbacks of a surgical mortality rate of approximately 10% to 12% and of further attrition from causes other than arrhythmias during follow-up detract from wide application of surgery unless it can be combined with other corrective procedures (e.g., aneurysmectomy or coronary artery bypass grafts). Nevertheless, surgical procedures remain attractive alternatives for patients who have monomorphic presentations of drug-resistant ventricular tachycardia.

REFERENCES

1. Gardner PI, Ursell PC, Fenoglio JJ Jr, et al: Electrophysiologic and anatomic basis for fractionated electrograms recorded from healed myocardial infarcts. Circulation 72:596, 1985.
2. Spach MS, Dolber PC: Relating extracellular potentials and their derivatives to anisotropic propagation at a microscopic level in human cardiac muscle: Evidence for electrical uncoupling of side-to-side fiber connections with increasing age. Circ Res 58:356, 1986.
3. Wellens HJJ, Brugada P, Stevenson WG: Programmed electrical stimulation: Its role in the management of ventricular arrhythmias in coronary heart disease. Prog Cardiovasc Dis 29:165, 1986.
4. Sokolow M: Some quantitative aspects of treatment with quinidine. Ann Intern Med 45:582, 1956.
5. Varro A, Nakaya Y, Elharrar V, et al: Use-dependent effects of amiodarone on V̇max in cardiac Purkinje and ventricular muscle fibers. Eur J Pharmacol 112:419, 1985.
6. Mirowski M, Mower MM: Transvenous catheter defibrillation for prevention of sudden cardiac death. J Am Coll Cardiol 11:371, 1988.
7. Bardy GH, Hofer B, Johnson G, et al: Implantable transvenous cardioverter-defibrillators. Circulation 87:1152, 1993.
8. Bardy GH, Troutman C, Poole JE, et al: Clinical experience with a tiered-therapy multiprogrammable antiarrhythmia device. Circulation 85:1689, 1992.
9. Jackman WM, Beckman KJ, McClelland JH, et al: Treatment of supraventricular tachycardia due to atrioventricular nodal reentry by radiofrequency catheter ablation of slow-pathway conduction. N Engl J Med 327:313, 1992.
10. Cox JL: The status of surgery for cardiac arrhythmias. Circulation 71:413, 1985.

CHAPTER 5

Hypertension

Franz H. Messerli, M.D., and John H. Laragh, M.D.

THE PAST

In 1935, the blood pressure of Franklin D. Roosevelt, thirty-second president of the United States, was 136/78 mmHg (Fig. 5–1). Two years later, a value of 162/98 mmHg was recorded, and his blood pressure reached 188/105 mmHg in 1941. In March 1944, left ventricular hypertrophy was noted on the electrocardiogram and cardiac enlargement on chest x-ray examination, and FDR's blood pressure was 186/108 mmHg. Throughout 1944, the President's blood pressure continued to climb, and shortly before the Yalta Conference, values of 260/150 mmHg were recorded. On April 12, 1945, while sitting for a portrait, he complained of a terrific occipital headache and became unconscious a few minutes later. Systolic pressure was well over 300 mmHg; diastolic pressure was 190 mmHg. A few hours later, the President was pronounced dead.

This famous case report illustrates all too well a disease entity that, like poliomyelitis and smallpox, is now of primarily historical interest to the practicing physician. FDR had mild hypertension for many years, developed target-organ disease, and finally progressed to an accelerated or malignant phase that ended with a massive cerebral hemorrhage. This sequence of events was a common occurrence in clinical

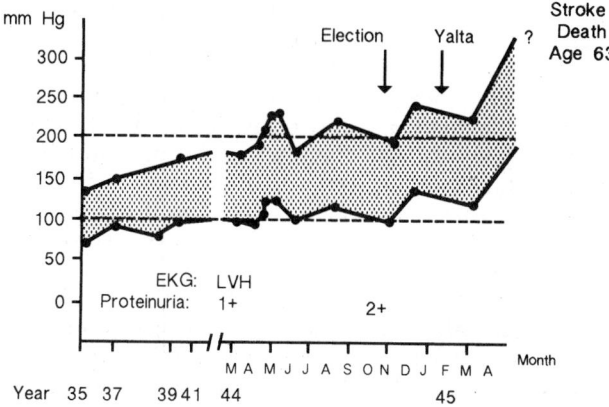

Figure 5–1. Natural history of essential hypertension (presumed) in President Franklin D. Roosevelt, 1935–1945. LVH, left ventricular hypertrophy.

practice before the availability of antihypertensive drugs, and the physician had no tool apart from severe salt restriction (which was poorly tolerated by most patients) to influence the course of hypertensive cardiovascular disease.

Thus, essential hypertension, although easily identified in clinical practice because of the ingenious invention of Riva-Rocci, remained for nearly half a century an incurable disease invariably leading to stroke, heart attack, congestive heart failure, dissecting aneurysm, and renal insufficiency.

In retrospect, it is perhaps a matter of semantics whether the dawn broke with the discovery of chlorothiazide by Karl Beyer and his colleagues at Merck Sharpe & Dohme or earlier with the development of ganglion blockers by Plonker and Zaimis, reserpine by Wilkins, hydralazine by Jonkman and guanethidine by Plummer (both at Ciba), or bretylium tosylate by Burroughs Wellcome. The thiazides were used first alone and later in combination with reserpine or methyldopa. These discoveries led to the honeymoon phase of antihypertensive therapy during which clinical evidence of benefits was convincing and clearly outweighed the cost of leaving patients untreated (Fig. 5–2). Hypertensive encephalopathy disappeared, pulmonary edema melted away, and retinopathy with papilledema, hemorrhages, and cotton-wool spots resolved in parallel with the fall in arterial pressure. Even in patients with less severe hypertension, evidence of left ventricular hypertrophy on chest x-ray film and electrocardiogram decreased, proteinuria became less pronounced, and patients subjectively improved.

Although this early period of drug treatment of hypertension was heroic and exciting, it must be remembered that most antihypertensive drugs were not developed from the outset with the goal of lowering arterial pressure. The antihypertensive properties of most of these agents were discovered accidentally by clinicians. Sulfanilamide, when used as an antimicrobial drug, was demonstrated to have beneficial effects in congestive heart failure; clinicians subsequently showed that it lowered blood pressure. The antihy-

pertensive effects of methyldopa were first observed in control subjects in a study designed to evaluate its effect as a decarboxylase inhibitor in carcinoid syndrome. The antihypertensive properties of clonidine were discovered when a patient to whom it was given for the treatment of allergic rhinitis became drowsy and fell asleep. The β-blockers and calcium antagonists entered the antihypertensive arsenal after they had been used for the treatment of angina pectoris and arrhythmias for many years. Thus, pharmacologists have had a poor record in identifying antihypertensive drugs in the laboratory. Actually, only captopril, an orally active angiotensin-converting enzyme inhibitor, was discovered through an extensive search by Squibb after the blood pressure–lowering properties of the venom of the Brazilian snake *Bothrops jararaca* were documented in humans. Therefore, captopril can possibly be considered the first "designer drug" that opened the gates to modern pharmacotherapy of essential hypertension.

THE PRESENT

When the Veterans Administration study led by Freis clearly documented the benefits of antihypertensive treatment not only in severe but also in mild essential hypertension, the modern era of antihypertensive drug treatment began. For the first time, it was shown that lowering blood pressure by stepped-care therapy in mildly hypertensive patients prolonged life and reduced the rate of strokes. The benefits of treating mild hypertension were, however, less obvious than the ones observed with more severe blood pressure elevation (see Fig. 5–2). Proponents of the stepped-care approach started to march triumphantly throughout North America and other continents. The stepped-care approach was touted as safe, efficacious, and so simple that it could be used even by nurse practitioners and physicians who did not regularly

Severity of Disease and Risk of Morbidity and Mortality

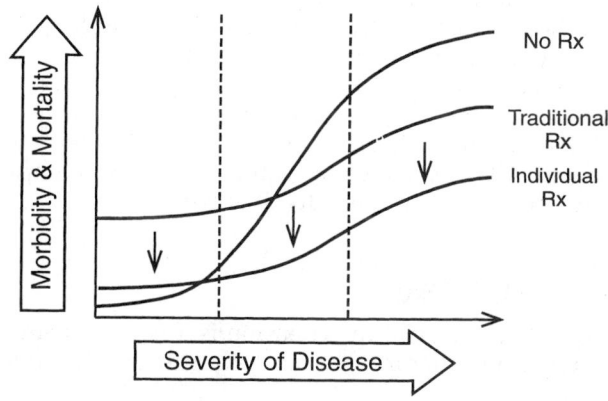

Figure 5–2. Morbidity and mortality as a function of severity of the disease: effects of therapeutic intervention. Note that even with the most specific therapy, there will be an excessive risk at very low levels of blood pressure elevation.

treat hypertensive patients, such as gynecologists or psychiatrists. Numerous studies attest to the fact that antihypertensive treatment by the stepped-care approach reduces cardiovascular morbidity and mortality.

However, it soon became apparent that stepped care was not the ultimate and only solution to essential hypertension. First, the reduction in morbidity and mortality was related mostly to a decreased incidence of strokes and perhaps renal failure, but little or no reduction in coronary artery disease was observed. Second, patients with mild essential hypertension who were asymptomatic before treatment complained about a variety of symptoms induced by antihypertensive therapy. They often were unwilling to trade a statistical increase in life expectancy by a few years for a substantial loss of quality of life for the remainder of their days. Third, it became obvious that essential hypertension was not a homogeneous disorder; therefore, a "cookbook" approach with a single recipe (i.e., stepped care) was in many instances likely to fail or be intrusive.

This latter line of thought was initiated by Laragh and colleagues in the early 1970s, when they were able to demonstrate clear-cut differences in blood pressure responsiveness that depended on the activity of the renin-angiotensin-aldosterone system. Patient profiling according to renin status was a simple, straightforward way to identify the predominant mechanism of pressure elevation—vasoconstriction in patients belonging to the high-renin category, and volume expansion in patients belonging to the low-renin category. Hyperreninemia, as induced in renovascular hypertension, and mineralocorticoid excess, as observed in patients with primary aldosteronism, are two experiments of nature that illustrate the extremes of the two pathogenetic forms of essential hypertension. These pioneering observations were subsequently extended to the adrenergic nervous system, systemic and regional hemodynamics, and cellular sodium and calcium transport. When first elucidated, each of these individual systems seemed to promise to lead us to the Holy Grail, the etiology of essential hypertension.

Sadly, further work failed to completely fulfill earlier hopes, and the ultimate cause of hypertension remains as elusive as ever. However, these pioneering observations have demonstrated that essential hypertension is a heterogeneous disorder and that mechanisms of pressure elevation vary from patient to patient. Clearly, therefore, antihypertensive therapy must be tailored to the individual patient.

THE FUTURE

Given that essential hypertension is a heterogeneous disorder and that mechanisms of pressure elevations vary from one patient to another, it follows that no single drug will be effective and safe in all patients with essential hypertension. Moreover, long-standing hypertension commonly leads to target-organ disease (i.e., left ventricular hypertrophy, coronary artery disease, renal failure, and cerebrovascular damage). Each of these target-organ diseases often follows a course of its own that is no longer related to the triggering event, i.e., the elevation of arterial pressure. For example, the occurrence of left ventricular hypertrophy, which increases by sixfold to sevenfold the risk of dying suddenly of acute myocardial infarction, may be diminished, unchanged, or increased by antihypertensive therapy, depending on the mechanism by which the drug lowers pressure. The same holds true for patients in whom hypertension has led to nephrosclerosis, renal failure, coronary artery disease, congestive heart failure, or cerebrovascular disease.

At the same time, it must be remembered that mild essential hypertension is an asymptomatic disorder and should remain so when treated. Fortunately, the newer antihypertensive agents, such as angiotensin-converting enzyme inhibitors and calcium antagonists, are remarkably free of side effects and may even give patients a feeling of increased well-being, perhaps because they maintain or improve blood flow to target organs.

Ample evidence suggests that lowering arterial pressure diminishes cardiovascular morbidity and mortality and thus prolongs life. However, we are just now learning that diminishing millimeters of mercury is not the ultimate goal in the treatment of hypertension. All antihypertensive drugs lower arterial pressure to approximately the same extent. However, the effects of these drugs on target-organ disease, metabolic derangements, and quality of life are by no means alike. The antihypertensive approach of the future should demonstrate efficacy of drug therapy in preventing or reducing target-organ damage and should preserve or improve organ function. At the same time, therapy should diminish concomitant risk factors for cardiovascular disease and improve the quality of life.

As available pharmacologic agents are now more potent and specific and have fewer side effects than ever before, we have reached a new level of therapeutic expertise. This expertise can enable us to achieve, for greater numbers of patients than ever before, the primary goal of antihypertensive therapy using the fewest number of drugs in the lowest possible dosage, thereby showing benefits of drug therapy even in patients with the mildest forms of blood pressure elevation (see Fig. 5–2). For increasing numbers of patients, monotherapy achieved by a rational process is a realizable goal. This modality will surely mean fewer side effects and a better quality of life for many patients, with reduced toxicity and optimal protection from heart attack and stroke.

CHAPTER 6

Hyperlipidemias

Antonio M. Gotto, Jr., M.D., D.Phil.

The primary indication for treatment of dyslipidemia is prevention of coronary heart disease (CHD). The other indication is treatment and prevention of pancreatitis in individuals in whom plasma triglyceride levels exceed 1000 mg/dl (11.3 mmol/L). Five classes of lipid-regulating drugs are approved for use in the United States: (1) nicotinic acid, (2) the bile acid sequestrants (colestipol and cholestyramine), (3) the 3-hydroxy-3-methylglutaryl coenzyme A (HMG-CoA) reductase inhibitors (fluvastatin, lovastatin, pravastatin, and simvastatin), (4) the fibric acid derivatives (gemfibrozil, the little-used clofibrate, and fenofibrate, which is not yet clinically available), and (5) probucol. The approved lipid-regulating agents are often referred to as lipid-lowering drugs, because their lipid indications are to lower levels of low-density lipoprotein (LDL) cholesterol and/or plasma triglyceride; however, in several of the drug classes, agents have the additional benefit of raising levels of high-density lipoprotein (HDL) cholesterol. A few generalizations can be made about lipid-regulating drug therapy.

BEFORE CONSIDERING DRUG THERAPY

As a rule, use of lipid-regulating drug therapy requires establishing a diagnosis of a primary lipid disorder, a diagnosis that involves detailed clinical and laboratory evaluation to exclude causes of secondary dyslipidemia. Treatment of underlying disorders such as hypothyroidism and diabetes mellitus needs to be carried out before proceeding with other forms of therapy (Table 6–1).

Lipid-regulating pharmacotherapy is an adjunct to nonpharmacologic measures, which include dietary

Table 6–1. General Stepwise Approach to Lipid-Regulating Therapy

1. Screening for dyslipidemia
2. Identification and characterization of dyslipidemia
3. Full clinical evaluation and laboratory workup
4. Treatment of underlying disorders (e.g., diabetes mellitus, hypothyroidism, nephrotic syndrome) and replacement or removal of any drugs (e.g., β-blockers, diuretics, estrogen, isotretinoin) that can cause secondary dyslipidemia; determination of any primary dyslipidemia
5. Lipid-regulating hygienic measures
   • Low-fat, low-cholesterol diet
   • Weight control
   • Increased physical activity
6. Addition of pharmacotherapy to hygienic measures
7. Consideration of combination drug therapy

Alternative therapy (e.g., LDL apheresis) for severe forms of dyslipidemia (e.g., homozygous familial hypercholesterolemia)

therapy, weight control, and increased physical activity. Dietary modification usually consists of restriction of total fat, saturated fat, and cholesterol, with reduction of total caloric intake when appropriate. The Step One Diet of the United States National Cholesterol Education Program[1] (NCEP) is equivalent to the dietary recommendations for the general population age 2 and older: 30% or less of calories as total fat, 8% to 10% of calories as saturated fat, and less than 300 mg/day of dietary cholesterol. The NCEP Step Two Diet is more rigorous—with saturated fat reduced to less than 7% of calories and dietary cholesterol reduced to less than 200 mg/day—but still represents moderate dietary therapy. The treatment guidelines[1, 2] of the second Adult Treatment Panel of the NCEP include a new emphasis on physical activity and weight loss as components of nonpharmacologic therapy for dyslipidemia. The panel points out that even modest weight reduction is valuable—that, for example, weight loss of 5 to 10 lb (2.3 to 4.5 kg) can double the reduction of LDL cholesterol achieved by lowering intake of saturated fat and cholesterol. In addition, weight loss lowers plasma triglyceride and raises HDL cholesterol levels.

The main problem in dietary programs is long-term adherence. It is my experience that adjunctive use of exercise is extremely important in enabling patients to achieve long-term adherence to dietary therapy, particularly to a regimen that entails weight loss. In addition, regular exercise in itself has favorable effects on lipid and carbohydrate metabolism.[3] It reduces plasma triglyceride levels and raises HDL cholesterol levels, and in some patients lowers LDL cholesterol levels. There is growing evidence that regular exercise reduces risk of death from CHD, an effect that may be mediated through benefits on body weight, blood pressure, and the coronary vasculature as well as lipids.[1]

Involvement of a registered dietitian or other nutrition professional can also be important in achieving adherence to dietary therapy, particularly with the Step Two Diet. At The Methodist Hospital in Houston, the Diet Modification Clinic is a crucial component of our antiatherosclerosis program.

CHOOSING TO INITIATE DRUG THERAPY

The decision to add a drug to a lipid-regulating therapeutic regimen is made only after 3 to 6 months of nonpharmacologic intervention, except in cases of very high risk for a CHD event or pancreatitis. Earlier drug therapy may be considered, for example, in homozygous familial hypercholesterolemia, when LDL cholesterol is high after coronary artery bypass grafting or a myocardial infarction, in a cardiac transplant recipient, or in a patient who has already experienced pancreatitis.

Assessing the risk-to-benefit ratio is very important in deciding whether to use lipid-regulating drug therapy. Among the factors to consider are the potential side effects and costs of the therapy. Commitment to lipid-regulating drug therapy usually represents a commitment to long-term or lifelong therapy.

The updated diagnosis and treatment guidelines of the NCEP[1, 2] emphasize risk stratification by whether evidence of CHD or other atherosclerotic disease has or has not been seen in a patient (secondary versus primary prevention). The guidelines recommend aggressive cholesterol-lowering intervention in hypercholesterolemic patients who have atherosclerotic disease. The NCEP's LDL cholesterol goal in these patients is 100 mg/dl (2.6 mmol/L) or lower—a low level, but one that some preclinical and clinical data have suggested must be reached to achieve the best results in terms of the regression or arrest of atherosclerotic lesions.[4] In primary prevention, the NCEP guidelines recommend that lipid-lowering drug therapy be delayed in most young men and premenopausal women with high LDL cholesterol levels who are otherwise at low risk for CHD in the near future. They call for aggressive intervention in patients without known atherosclerotic disease when LDL levels are high and there are multiple risk factors, such as smoking and hypertension; the LDL cholesterol goal in this scenario is less than 130 mg/dl (3.4 mmol/L). Target goals are, of course, only rough guidelines; therapy and its goals are individualized for patients according to clinical judgment. Current NCEP therapeutic action limits and goals are summarized in Chapter 11.

Some of the distinction between primary and secondary prevention may be artificial. The asymptomatic patient may in fact have advanced coronary disease. Reduction in CHD risk appears to be about the same whether cholesterol lowering is for primary or secondary prevention. Rossouw and colleagues in 1990 performed meta-analyses of the results of eight secondary-prevention and four primary-prevention cholesterol-lowering trials selected as the most informative in terms of size and design; they found that in primary prevention, a 10% reduction in total cholesterol led to reductions of 25%, 12%, and 22% in the number of nonfatal, fatal, and all myocardial infarctions, respectively; in secondary prevention, the corresponding reductions were 19%, 12%, and 15%.[5] Nonetheless, the high-risk patient is the one who will benefit the most from treatment, whether it is diet, exercise, pharmacotherapy, or a combination of interventions. There is a good chance that the individual who for some years has had multiple risk factors for atherosclerosis has developed atherosclerosis.

Most patients with known CHD are older than 65. Elderly patients are candidates for lipid-regulating drug therapy if they do not have a poor cardiac prognosis or coexisting medical conditions that impair quality of life or life expectancy.

Beginning drug treatment does not mean discontinuing diet and exercise therapy. Hygienic interventions should be continued to obtain the maximum benefit of pharmacotherapy. The NCEP has provided an excellent outline of tactics for enhancing adherence to lipid-lowering treatment regimens (Table 6–2).

EMPHASIS ON LDL CHOLESTEROL

The revised diagnosis and treatment guidelines issued in 1993 by the Adult Treatment Panel of the NCEP[1, 2] focus on LDL cholesterol, as did the antecedent NCEP guidelines of 1987. Extensive observational epidemiologic and interventional data show benefit for reducing elevated LDL cholesterol levels.[6–8] There is absolutely no question that aggressive reduction of LDL cholesterol level reduces CHD risk

Table 6–2. **National Cholesterol Education Program Tactics for Enhancing Adherence to Lipid-Lowering Therapeutic Regimens**

Tactic	Examples/Notes
Teach the patient to take the treatment regimen.	Instructions should be simple and concise but complete.
Help the patient identify ways to remember doses.	Tailor doses to daily rituals. Send reminders.
Develop reinforcers of adherence.	Chart of lipid responses. Continuing encouragement.
Anticipate common problems and teach patients how to manage them.	How to minimize side effects.
Involve a family member or friend in the patient's therapy program.	Develop an advocate for the patient's welfare.
Establish a supportive relationship with the patient.	Listen carefully and respond in an open, nonjudgmental manner.
Make adherence important by asking about it.	Develop an approach that is encouraging, not condemnatory.
Provide ongoing education and updates about the patient's illness and treatment.	Incorporate new data and the patient's increasing level of understanding. Be on guard for misinformation the patient has received from the media, friends, or other sources.
Provide individualized services for patients who continue to avoid adherence.	Assess barriers: Physical—e.g., poor vision, forgetfulness Access—e.g., transportation, income, time Attitude—e.g., fatalism Therapy—e.g., complexity, side effects Social—e.g., family instability Faulty health perceptions—e.g., denial, looks to symptoms to prompt treatment

Data from National Cholesterol Education Program: Second report of the Expert Panel on Detection, Evaluation, and Treatment of High Blood Cholesterol in Adults (Adult Treatment Panel II). Circulation 89:1329, 1994.

in patients at high risk for morbidity and mortality from the disease, and most likely it has benefit as well in those at lower risk. Peto has reported that cholesterol levels considered normal by treatment algorithms in the West may be elevated compared with what is biologically normal, perhaps defined by average cholesterol levels in societies, such as China, in which the diet is plant based; he suggests that reductions in CHD risk by cholesterol-lowering drugs may be worthwhile not only among hypercholesterolemics but also among "normocholesterolemics" who are otherwise at high risk for CHD.[9]

When the focus of therapy is reduction of LDL cholesterol, the drugs of choice are the HMG-CoA reductase inhibitors, the bile acid sequestrants, and nicotinic acid.

HMG-CoA Reductase Inhibitors

The HMG-CoA reductase inhibitors, or statins, are the most effective drugs for lowering LDL and are extremely valuable in reaching a target goal of 100 mg/dl. These drugs, which are easy to take, have made a remarkable difference in the treatment of elevations of total and LDL cholesterol levels. In addition, they moderately decrease plasma triglyceride levels and moderately increase HDL cholesterol levels. Their records of efficacy and safety have been outstanding, although long-term safety data are not yet available. Statins are ideal drugs for patients with established CHD who have failed to achieve adequate LDL lowering with diet and exercise. They are also particularly useful in severe forms of hypercholesterolemia.

Statins have been used as single agents or in drug combinations in several angiographically monitored cholesterol-lowering trials (i.e., "regression" trials) that have achieved stabilization or reduction of coronary stenosis, among them the Familial Atherosclerosis Treatment Study (FATS),[10] the University of California, San Francisco, Arteriosclerosis Specialized Center of Research (UCSF-SCOR) Intervention Trial,[11] and the Monitored Atherosclerosis Regression Study (MARS).[12] The mechanisms, uses, dosages, side effects, and contraindications of the HMG-CoA reductase inhibitors and other approved lipid-lowering drugs, both as single agents and in drug combinations, are fully discussed in Chapters 11 and 114 through 124.

Bile Acid Sequestrants

The bile acid sequestrants, or resins, have an excellent, well-established safety profile. In addition to substantially lowering LDL cholesterol levels, they may slightly raise HDL cholesterol levels but have no effect on or may even increase plasma triglyceride levels. They are particularly suitable for treating younger patients and patients with moderately elevated LDL cholesterol levels. The major problem with the bile acid resins is patient acceptance. Some patients object to the taste of the drugs, and the gastrointestinal side effects include bloating, nausea, and constipation. Side effects are particularly troublesome at higher doses of a bile acid resin. Large doses are often required for maximal reduction of LDL levels, because the bile acid resins are in fact not highly proficient in binding bile acids in the intestine. However, lower doses may yield adequate results.

The use of cholestyramine in the Lipid Research Clinics Coronary Primary Prevention Trial was associated with a 19% decrease in myocardial infarction or CHD death.[13] Resins as single agents or in drug combinations have been used with success in such regression trials as FATS,[10] the UCSF-SCOR Intervention Trial,[11] the Cholesterol Lowering Atherosclerosis Study (CLAS),[14] and the St Thomas' Atherosclerosis Regression Study (STARS).[15]

Nicotinic Acid

Nicotinic acid, which has favorable substantial effects on all the major lipid fractions—total, LDL, and HDL cholesterol and plasma triglyceride—is an extremely useful drug. The safety profile of its crystalline form is well established. However, use of nicotinic acid is limited by side effects and lack of acceptability to some patients (primarily because of the side effect of flushing). Nicotinic acid is not recommended as a first-line drug in diabetes mellitus because it increases insulin resistance and fasting and postprandial hyperglycemia and hyperinsulinemia. In insulin-resistant "prediabetic" patients, it may accelerate the appearance of clinical diabetes.

It is of interest that nicotinic acid reduces plasma levels of lipoprotein(a) [Lp(a)]. Elevated levels of Lp(a) have been associated with increased risk for CHD, but, unlike other lipoproteins, Lp(a) appears resistant to most conventional treatments for dyslipidemia, including diet. The only agents thus far studied that have been able to reduce Lp(a) levels are nicotinic acid, neomycin, and certain steroids, as well as perhaps, in postmenopausal women, estrogen–progestin as hormone replacement therapy.[16, 17]

Nicotinic acid was shown to reduce risk for recurrent myocardial infarction in the Coronary Drug Project[18] and, in a 15-year follow-up of that trial, was associated with reduced all-cause mortality versus placebo.[19] A significant reduction in total mortality was also seen in the Stockholm Ischaemic Heart Disease Secondary Prevention Study, which used nicotinic acid and clofibrate as an open-label intervention.[20] Among the major regression trials that have included nicotinic acid in combination drug regimens are FATS,[10] CLAS,[14] and the UCSF-SCOR Intervention Trial.[11]

Combination Drug Therapy

If the therapeutic goal has not been reached after 3 months of single-agent drug therapy, consideration may be given to adding a second agent. Combination drug therapy in many cases will increase the effectiveness of lipid-lowering therapy, decrease side effects, and improve compliance; it may also allow lower drug doses. Aggressive combination drug regimens have been successful in slowing progression or achieving regression of coronary atherosclerotic lesions.[10, 11, 14] Combination drug therapy for dyslipidemia, including potential toxicity with certain combinations, is discussed in full in Chapter 11.

Estrogen Replacement Therapy

The NCEP suggests consideration of estrogen replacement therapy in postmenopausal women with dyslipidemia, not only because orally administered estrogens moderately lower LDL cholesterol levels and moderately raise HDL cholesterol levels, but also because preliminary findings support an association of estrogen use with substantially reduced risk for CHD.[21–23] Estrogen replacement therapy, however, has not yet received a United States Food and Drug Administration indication for either lipid lowering or prevention of CHD. Estrogen use can increase levels of plasma triglyceride, particularly in women who already have elevated triglyceride levels.

Interventional trials using clinical end points and/ or angiographic monitoring will probably be necessary to establish the benefit of estrogen therapy in CHD risk. Large trials that are being developed to address this question include the multi-institutional Heart and Estrogen-Progestin Replacement Study (HERS) of the University of California, San Francisco, and a trial that is part of the Women's Health Initiative of the United States National Institutes of Health.[24]

Probucol

Probucol is generally restricted to use in patients who have not responded to or tolerated other drugs. It may also have a role in combination drug therapy, for example, combined with a resin. Its LDL-lowering effects are modest, and it lowers HDL levels as well. Its effect on triglyceride levels is variable but usually minor. Antioxidant activity has been shown in preclinical studies.[25]

The Issue of Total Mortality

Data linking very low levels of cholesterol with excess noncardiovascular mortality have been gathered from both clinical trials and observational studies.[26] It is unlikely that the two sets of data are related, because total cholesterol levels achieved in clinical trials average around 230 mg/dl (5.9 mmol/L) and the levels that have been associated with excess mortality in observational studies are well below 160 mg/dl (4.1 mmol/L).[27]

I believe the evidence thus far presented to suggest that low cholesterol causes excess mortality lacks breadth and rigor and does not outweigh the undoubtedly favorable effects of cholesterol lowering on CHD risk. The same conclusion was reached by the Adult Treatment Panel of the NCEP[1, 2] and by the European Atherosclerosis Society.[28] The associations reported may represent chance, or low cholesterol may be a consequence of disease or a confounder associated with other variables.[27, 29, 30] More research is needed to resolve this issue, but for now there is no compelling evidence to justify the change in public health policy called for by some.[31]

Strong data regarding all-cause mortality have recently become available from the 5-year, double-blind Scandinavian Simvastatin Survival Study (4S),[31a] which demonstrated that lipid lowering can reduce all-cause mortality in secondary prevention. The sole primary end point in the trial was total mortality, and use of the HMG-CoA reductase inhibitor simvastatin (20 mg/day, increased to 40 mg/day in 37% of patients) reduced total mortality 30% compared with placebo ($p = .0003$). The 4444 men and women enrolled in the trial had a history of angina pectoris or acute myocardial infarction, as well as total cholesterol of 215 to 310 mg/dl (5.5 to 8.0 mmol/L) and serum triglyceride of 220 mg/dl (2.5 mmol/L) or less after an 8-week lipid-lowering diet. The relative risk in the simvastatin group was 0.66 for a major coronary event (the secondary end point); it was 0.73 for any coronary event and 0.63 for coronary artery bypass grafting or percutaneous transluminal coronary angioplasty (tertiary end points). The simvastatin and placebo groups were comparable in numbers of noncardiovascular deaths (46 versus 49), deaths due to cancer (33 versus 35), and violent deaths (6 versus 7). Reduction of total mortality applied to both patients younger than 60 years of age and patients 60 years of age and older (study age range, 35 to 70). The 4S results emphasize the importance of treating those patients at highest risk for future cardiovascular events, particularly patients who have experienced previous cardiovascular events. A large clinical trial designed to examine the question of total mortality is still lacking for lipid lowering as primary prevention.

ELEVATED PLASMA TRIGLYCERIDE AND LOW HDL CHOLESTEROL LEVELS

Evidence has recently emerged that the occurrence of elevated plasma triglyceride levels in conjunction with low HDL cholesterol levels, even without elevation of LDL cholesterol levels, confers high risk for CHD.[32] In both the primary-prevention Helsinki Heart Study and the observational Prospective Cardiovascular Muenster (PROCAM) Study, subjects at highest risk were those with a high ratio of LDL to HDL cholesterol (>5) and elevated triglyceride levels (>200 mg/dl [2.3 mmol/L]).[33, 34]

Elevated plasma triglyceride and low HDL cholesterol levels, both exacerbated with worsening glycemic control, constitute the typical dyslipidemia of non-insulin-dependent diabetes mellitus. A 1993 American Diabetes Association consensus panel concluded that elevated triglyceride and low HDL levels are likely intrinsically related to the abnormal physiology produced by insulin resistance or inadequate insulin action and concomitant metabolic disturbances.[35] Risk for atherosclerotic disease is high in both insulin-dependent and non-insulin-dependent diabetes mellitus. The incidence of CHD is doubled in diabetic men and quadrupled in diabetic women compared with nondiabetic men and women.[36] Increased plasma triglyceride and decreased HDL cholesterol levels are also the characteristic dyslipidemia of the posited syndrome X, a constellation of metabolic risk factors for CHD defined by resistance to insulin-mediated glucose uptake and associated as well with hypertension.[37] Epidemiologic data are not available to link syndrome X directly to increased incidence of CHD, but several of its components are risk determinants.

Reanalyses of data from large angiographic studies have suggested that reduction of levels of triglyceride-rich lipoproteins and enhanced clearance of these particles are important in slowing progression or inducing regression of coronary atherosclerosis. At 2-year follow-up in CLAS, which used colestipol plus nicotinic acid as secondary prevention, benefit of therapy on global coronary stenosis score was associated with greater triglyceride lowering, an effect not due to greater reductions in LDL levels or greater increases in HDL levels.[38] At 2 years in MARS, which used lovastatin as a single agent, progression of early atherosclerotic lesions in coronary segments correlated inversely with levels of triglyceride-rich lipoproteins, whereas progression in advanced lesions correlated positively with the LDL/HDL ratio.[39]

Thus, concentrations of plasma triglyceride and HDL cholesterol are important factors to take into account when selecting lipid-regulating pharmacotherapy for a given patient. For the patient with pure hypertriglyceridemia, nicotinic acid or a fibrate appears to be the drug of choice. For purposes of simplification, patients may be divided into those in whom only total and LDL cholesterol levels are elevated, those in whom only triglyceride level is elevated, and those in whom both LDL and triglyceride levels are elevated (combined hyperlipidemia). Triglyceride elevation is often accompanied by a low HDL cholesterol level. Isolated low HDL is not considered an indication for drug therapy unless the patient has established CHD or is otherwise at very high risk[1, 2, 40]— from a strong family history of CHD, familial combined hyperlipidemia, or diabetes mellitus, for example.

Resins, as noted earlier, have fairly little effect on HDL cholesterol levels, and they have the disadvantage of raising plasma triglyceride levels in hypertriglyceridemic subjects. The available statins have modest effects in reducing triglyceride and raising HDL levels; their potency in lowering LDL levels may be diminished in patients with moderate to severe hypertriglyceridemia.

Nicotinic Acid

Nicotinic acid is an excellent drug for consideration when there is dyslipidemia in the triad of LDL, HDL,

and triglyceride. Some of the problems with patient acceptance can be overcome by beginning the drug in small doses; side effects may be reduced by the patient's taking aspirin or ibuprofen 30 minutes before the nicotinic acid and taking the nicotinic acid with meals. The limitation in the diabetic patient was stated earlier.

Fibric Acid Derivatives

Fibrates are well-tolerated drugs that are very potent in lowering triglyceride levels. They raise HDL levels by 10% to 20%, depending on the fibrate used. In the Helsinki Heart Study, a 34% reduction in CHD events was observed in the group treated with gemfibrozil,[41] and CHD events were reduced 71% with gemfibrozil therapy in the high-risk subgroup with an LDL/HDL ratio above 5 and triglyceride level of more than 200 mg/dl compared with the corresponding placebo subgroup.[33]

Two chief concerns arise with use of the fibrates. One is the increased risk for myositis with the combination of a statin and a fibrate. The second is that in hypertriglyceridemic patients, the fibrates can have little effect on LDL or can raise LDL levels.[42]

The second effect raises the very important consideration of the subfraction distribution of LDL and HDL particles. Considerable data have accumulated supporting the increased atherogenicity of small, dense LDL particles, the predominant LDL particles in LDL phenotype B (as opposed to LDL phenotype A, in which larger, more buoyant LDL particles predominate).[43, 44] Subjects with triglyceride elevation tend to have LDL phenotype B,[45] and phenotype B is twice as common in diabetic men as in nondiabetic men.[46] Available evidence suggests that the B pattern is not affected by the approved statins but can be corrected with treatment by fibrates.[47–50] Therefore, although treatment with a fibrate may result in an increase in the measured LDL cholesterol, the LDL particles may be larger and less atherogenic, a result akin in concept to the increase in large, buoyant very-low-density lipoproteins (and hence plasma triglyceride) with a vegetarian diet.[32]

LESION REGRESSION AND CLINICAL EVENTS

Angiographically monitored lipid-lowering clinical trials have indicated a potential benefit in reduction of CHD events that is greater than that predicted by the fairly modest changes in coronary diameter or stenosis. In FATS, for example, the overall percent change in coronary stenosis at 32 months was −0.9 in the patient group receiving nicotinic acid plus colestipol, and −0.7 in the group receiving lovastatin plus colestipol (versus +2.1, indicating progression, in the placebo group); CHD events were reduced 80% and 70%, respectively, in the two treatment groups.[8] In STARS at 39 months, CHD events were reduced 69% and the overall percent change in coronary stenosis was −1.1 in the diet group; corresponding values were 89% and −1.9 in the group receiving diet plus cholestyramine.[8] In the Program on the Surgical Control of the Hyperlipidemias (POSCH), which used partial ileal bypass to achieve lipid lowering, an overall coronary lesion score indicating definite progression (versus no change or regression) at 3 years was associated with approximately twofold increases in risk for all-cause mortality, CHD mortality, and clinical CHD events by 9.7-year follow-up.[51] Yet the amount of lesion change in POSCH was small.

Further data are required to confirm these findings. However, if the findings are substantiated, they will provide a strong additional rationale for the use of lipid-regulating drug therapy in patients with established CHD. Several explanations for the unexpected effectiveness of therapy have been proposed. One hypothesis is that reducing dyslipidemia stabilizes atherosclerotic plaque: for example, at a crucial stage in plaque development, a reduction in lipid content may alter its structure in such a way as to make it less susceptible to fissuring and intravascular hemorrhage. This hypothesis is compatible with the concept of reverse cholesterol transport. Moreover, reducing dyslipidemia may improve endothelial function and enable endothelial healing to occur, or it may decrease the inflammatory process that has been observed in ruptured plaques. It may also allow remodeling of the damaged coronary artery.

FUTURE DIRECTIONS

Possible future strategies for managing dyslipidemia include further refining clinical guidelines, improving current pharmacologic strategies, developing novel pharmacologic strategies, and using gene-based therapies.

Improving Current Pharmacologic Strategies

Developing agents with enhanced activity in the currently approved classes of lipid-lowering drugs should be a priority. It would be desirable to develop bile acid sequestrants that are more effective at lower dosages; these agents have the advantage of a nonsystemic mode of action, but compliance has been limited by problems with palatability. Use of nicotinic acid is also hindered by side effects. Sustained-release nicotinic acid—associated with a lower incidence of some adverse effects—is available, but its use is generally not recommended because of an association with increased hepatotoxicity.[52] Thus, another goal is the development of a nicotinic acid derivative or related compound similar in efficacy to crystalline nicotinic acid but with fewer side effects. The investigational HMG-CoA reductase inhibitor atorvastatin reportedly has more efficacy in lowering LDL cholesterol and plasma triglyceride level than currently available statins.[53] Fibrates with enhanced lipid-regulating effects might be developed as well.

Intense research interest is focused on the exact effects of exogenous estrogens on plasma lipoprotein metabolism and CHD risk. In addition, investigations need to be extended with currently available agents that have shown indications of antiatherosclerotic activity unrelated to any lipid-regulating activity, including β-adrenergic blockers, angiotensin-converting enzyme inhibitors, and calcium antagonists.

Developing Novel Pharmacologic Strategies

One potential pharmacologic strategy is to develop inhibitors of cholesterol biosynthesis other than HMG-CoA reductase inhibitors. Inhibitors of squalene synthase[54, 55] and of squalene epoxidase[56] have been described and are reported to upregulate LDL receptor activity; another potential target is squalene cyclase.

Another strategy is to alter the activity of proteins or enzymes involved in the regulation of lipoprotein metabolism. Possibilities include enhancing lipoprotein lipase activity (an action that has been attributed to fibrates) and inhibiting hepatic lipase, acyl:cholesterol acyltransferase, or possibly cholesteryl ester transfer protein.

There is a great deal of evidence that oxidation of lipoproteins plays an important role in atherogenesis. However, the clinical role of administered antioxidants has yet to be established. Two large clinical trials of antioxidants, the Alpha-Tocopherol, Beta Carotene Study[57] (not designed primarily to evaluate cardiovascular end points) and the Probucol Quantitative Regression Swedish Trial (PQRST),[58] have failed to show a clinical benefit. The approach remains under intense investigation.

Gene Therapy

Although probably some years from clinical use, the emerging technologies of gene therapy are promising in antiatherosclerosis efforts. Homozygous familial hypercholesterolemia, in which competent LDL receptors are absent, provides a model for investigating gene therapy in CHD prevention. Grossman et al. have reported sustained LDL cholesterol lowering in a subject with this disorder, after infusion of autologous hepatocytes modified *ex vivo* with a recombinant retrovirus containing the LDL receptor gene;[59] however, some workers have suggested that more rigorous criteria are required for evaluation of the success of such intervention.[60]

In Watanabe heritable hyperlipidemic rabbits (which are LDL receptor deficient), an adenoviral vector has been used to deliver human LDL receptor DNA.[61] Serum cholesterol levels were lowered substantially; however, transgene expression was stable for only 7 to 10 days, and cholesterol levels returned to baseline within 3 weeks. The development of neutralizing antibodies made subsequent treatments largely ineffective.

Inhibition of gene expression may have therapeutic application in CHD prevention. Antisense oligonucleotides can potentially be used to control gene expres-

Table 6–3. **Some Important Considerations in Lipid-Regulating Drug Therapy**

1. Control of hypercholesterolemia should be considered as important as control of hypertension. The physician and other health professionals should be strong advocates of cholesterol control and strive to achieve patient adherence to therapy.

2. Lipid-regulating drug therapy is a supplement to—not a replacement for—diet, weight control, and exercise.

3. Careful consideration must be given to a variety of factors before beginning lipid-regulating drug therapy, which is usually long-term or lifelong therapy. Assess the risk:benefit ratio.

4. Therapeutic action limits and goals are general guidelines that should be individualized according to the patient's global risk for CHD and the physician's clinical judgment.

5. A variety of safe and effective agents are available for lowering LDL cholesterol and/or plasma triglyceride levels. Many of the agents have the additional benefit of raising HDL cholesterol levels. The physician should become well versed in the heterogeneous forms of dyslipidemia and the diverse and flexible treatments and combinations of treatments available.

6. Updated guidelines for treating hypercholesterolemia in adults have been released by the United States National Cholesterol Education Program.[1,2] Focus recommendations have been presented by the American Diabetes Association[34] and the United States National Institutes of Health Consensus Development Conference on Triglyceride, High-Density Lipoprotein, and Coronary Heart Disease.[40]

sion and protein synthesis at several points; the inhibition of smooth muscle cell proliferation in the arterial wall is one possible application.

CONCLUSION

Exciting new developments such as the possibility of major clinical benefit from small amounts of atherosclerotic lesion regression point to an evolving field and to further advances in therapy for the number one cause of death and disability in our society. Despite the clear importance of lipid-lowering therapy in patients with atherosclerotic disease, however, it has been estimated that only one third of those with established CHD are undergoing treatment with diet or drugs.[62] Roberts has written that cardiologists, who should be the dominant force in secondary prevention of CHD, seem to have inadequate interest in the management of dyslipidemia.[63] LaRosa and Cleeman would also include general physicians in the group not active enough in managing dyslipidemia.[4] The NCEP's new emphasis on CHD risk in patients with established atherosclerotic disease[1,2] should be useful to these physicians in increasing their knowledge of the problem and in selecting appropriate interventions. Selected highlights regarding the use of lipid-regulating pharmacotherapy are provided in Table 6–3.

REFERENCES

1. National Cholesterol Education Program: Second report of the Expert Panel on Detection, Evaluation, and Treatment of High Blood Cholesterol in Adults (Adult Treatment Panel II). Circulation 89:1329, 1994.
2. Expert Panel on Detection, Evaluation, and Treatment of High Blood Cholesterol in Adults: Summary of the second report of the National Cholesterol Education Program (NCEP) Expert Panel on Detection, Evaluation, and Treatment of High Blood Cholesterol in Adults (Adult Treatment Panel II). JAMA 269:3015, 1993.
3. Fletcher GF, Blair SN, Blumenthal J, et al: Statement on exercise: Benefits and recommendations for physical activity programs for all Americans. A statement for health professionals by the Committee on Exercise and Cardiac Rehabilitation of the Council on Clinical Cardiology, American Heart Association. Circulation 86:340, 1992.
4. LaRosa JC, Cleeman JI: Cholesterol lowering as a treatment for established coronary heart disease. Circulation 85:1229, 1992.
5. Rossouw JE, Lewis B, Rifkind BM: The value of lowering cholesterol after myocardial infarction. N Engl J Med 323:1112, 1990.
6. Gotto AM Jr, LaRosa JC, Hunninghake D, et al: The cholesterol facts: A summary of the evidence relating dietary fats, serum cholesterol, and coronary heart disease. A joint statement by the American Heart Association and the National Heart, Lung, and Blood Institute. Circulation 81:1721, 1990.
7. Manson JE, Tosteson H, Ridker PM, et al: The primary prevention of myocardial infarction [review]. N Engl J Med 326:1406, 1992.
8. Brown BG, Zhao X-Q, Sacco DE, et al: Lipid lowering and plaque regression: New insights into prevention of plaque disruption and clinical events in coronary disease. Circulation 87:1782, 1993.
9. Peto R: The Oxford overview of cholesterol-lowering trials: Disease-specific mortality rates. In Lewis B, Paoletti R, Tikkanen MJ (eds): Low Blood Cholesterol: Health Implications. London: Current Medical Literature, 1993, pp 29–30.
10. Brown G, Albers JJ, Fisher LD, et al: Regression of coronary artery disease as a result of intensive lipid-lowering therapy in men with high levels of apolipoprotein B. N Engl J Med 323:1289, 1990.
11. Kane JP, Malloy MJ, Ports TA, et al: Regression of coronary atherosclerosis during treatment of familial hypercholesterolemia with combined drug regimens. JAMA 264:3007, 1990.
12. Blankenhorn DH, Azen SP, Kramsch DM, et al: Coronary angiographic changes with lovastatin therapy: The Monitored Atherosclerosis Regression Study (MARS). Ann Intern Med 119:969, 1993.
13. Lipid Research Clinics Program: The Lipid Research Clinics Coronary Primary Prevention Trial results. I. Reduction in incidence of coronary heart disease. JAMA 251:351, 1984.
14. Cashin-Hemphill L, Mack WJ, Pogoda JM, et al: Beneficial effects of colestipol-niacin on coronary atherosclerosis. A 4-year follow-up. JAMA 264:3013, 1990.
15. Watts GF, Lewis B, Brunt JNH, et al: Effects on coronary artery disease of lipid-lowering diet, or diet plus cholestyramine, in the St Thomas' Atherosclerosis Regression Study (STARS). Lancet 339:563, 1992.
16. Howard GC, Pizzo SV: Biology of disease: Lipoprotein(a) and its role in atherothrombotic disease. Lab Invest 69:373, 1993.
17. Soma MR, Osnago-Gadda I, Paoletti R, et al: The lowering of lipoprotein[a] induced by estrogen plus progesterone replacement therapy in postmenopausal women. Arch Intern Med 153:1462, 1993.
18. The Coronary Drug Project Research Group: Clofibrate and niacin in coronary heart disease. JAMA 231:360, 1975.
19. Canner PL, Berge KG, Wenger NK, et al: Fifteen year mortality in Coronary Drug Project patients: Long-term benefit with niacin. J Am Coll Cardiol 8:1245, 1986.
20. Carlson LA, Rosenhamer G: Reduction of mortality in the Stockholm Ischaemic Heart Disease Secondary Prevention Study by combined treatment with clofibrate and nicotinic acid. Acta Med Scand 223:405, 1988.
21. Stampfer MJ, Colditz GA, Willett WC, et al: Postmenopausal estrogen therapy and cardiovascular disease: Ten-year follow-up from the Nurses' Health Study. N Engl J Med 325:756, 1991.
22. Barrett-Connor E, Bush TL: Estrogen and coronary heart disease in women. JAMA 265:1861, 1991.

23. Martin KA, Freeman MW: Postmenopausal hormone-replacement therapy [editorial]. N Engl J Med 328:1115, 1993.
24. Kirchstein R: From the National Institutes of Health: Largest US clinical trial ever gets under way. JAMA 270:1521, 1993.
25. Walldius G: Probucol and nicotinic acid: Old drugs, new findings and new derivatives. Curr Opin Lipidol 3:34, 1992.
26. Jacobs D, Blackburn H, Higgins M, et al: Report of the Conference on Low Blood Cholesterol: Mortality associations. Circulation 86:1046, 1992.
27. Rossouw JE, Gotto AM Jr: Does low cholesterol cause death? [editorial]. Cardiovasc Drugs Ther 7:789, 1993.
28. Prevention of coronary heart disease: Scientific background and new clinical guidelines. Recommendations of the European Atherosclerosis Society prepared by the International Task Force for Prevention of Coronary Heart Disease. Nutr Metab Cardiovasc Dis 2:113, 1992.
29. Stamler J, Stamler R, Brown V, et al: Serum cholesterol: Doing the right thing [editorial]. Circulation 88:1954, 1993.
30. Castelli WP: Long-term relationship between serum cholesterol and total mortality in the Framingham Heart Study. In Lewis B, Paoletti R, Tikkanen MJ (eds): Low Blood Cholesterol: Health Implications. London: Current Medical Literature, 1993, pp 2–9.
31. Hulley SB, Walsh JMB, Newman TB: Health policy on blood cholesterol: Time to change directions [editorial]. Circulation 86:1026, 1992.
31a. Scandinavian Simvastatin Survival Study Group: Randomised trial of cholesterol lowering in 4444 patients with coronary heart disease: The Scandinavian Simvastatin Survival Study (4S). Lancet 344:1383, 1994.
32. Castelli WP: Epidemiology of triglycerides: A view from Framingham. Am J Cardiol 70(Suppl):3H, 1992.
33. Manninen V, Tenkanen L, Koskinen P, et al: Joint effects of serum triglyceride and LDL and HDL cholesterol concentrations on coronary heart disease risk in the Helsinki Heart Study: Implications for treatment. Circulation 85:37, 1992.
34. Assmann G, Schulte H: Relation of high-density lipoprotein cholesterol and triglycerides to incidence of atherosclerotic coronary artery disease (the PROCAM experience). Am J Cardiol 70:733, 1992.
35. American Diabetes Association Consensus Development Conference on the Detection and Management of Lipid Disorders in Diabetes: Detection and management of lipid disorders in diabetes. Diabetes Care 16(Suppl 2):106, 1993.
36. Kannel WB: Lipids, diabetes, and coronary heart disease: Insights from the Framingham Study. Am Heart J 110:1100, 1985.
37. Reaven GM: Role of insulin resistance in human disease (syndrome X): An expanded definition. Annu Rev Med 44:121, 1993.
38. Miller BD, Krauss RM, Cashin-Hemphill L, et al: Baseline triglyceride levels predict angiographic benefit of colestipol plus niacin therapy in the Cholesterol-Lowering Atherosclerosis Study (CLAS) [abstract 1946]. Circulation 88:I-363, 1993.
39. Hodis HN, Mack WJ, Pogoda JM, et al: Effect of triglyceride-rich lipoproteins on progression of early atherosclerotic lesions as determined by coronary angiography in the Mevinolin (Lovastatin) Atherosclerosis Regression Study (MARS) [abstract 716-3]. J Am Coll Cardiol 21(Suppl):71A, 1993.
40. NIH Consensus Development Panel on Triglyceride, High-Density Lipoprotein, and Coronary Heart Disease: Triglyceride, high-density lipoprotein, and coronary heart disease. JAMA 269:505, 1993.
41. Frick MH, Elo O, Haapa K, et al: Helsinki Heart Study: Primary-prevention trial with gemfibrozil in middle-aged men with dyslipidemia. Safety of treatment, changes in risk factors, and incidence of coronary heart disease. N Engl J Med 317:1237, 1987.
42. Grundy SM, Vega GL: Two different views of the relationship of hypertriglyceridemia to coronary heart disease: Implications for treatment [review]. Arch Intern Med 152:28, 1992.
43. Austin MA, King M-C, Vranizan KM, et al: Atherogenic lipoprotein phenotype: A proposed genetic marker for coronary heart disease risk. Circulation 82:495, 1990.
44. Austin MA, Breslow JL, Hennekens CH, et al: Low-density lipoprotein subclass patterns and risk of myocardial infarction. JAMA 260:1917, 1988.
45. McNamara JR, Jenner JL, Li Z, et al: Change in LDL particle size is associated with change in plasma triglyceride concentration. Arterioscler Thromb 12:1284, 1992.
46. Feingold KR, Grunfeld C, Pang M, et al: LDL subclass phenotypes and triglyceride metabolism in non-insulin-dependent diabetes. Arterioscler Thromb 12:1496, 1992.
47. Tikkanen MJ: Fibric acid derivatives. Curr Opin Lipidol 3:29, 1992.
48. Illingworth DR: Fibric acid derivatives. In Rifkind BM (ed): Drug Treatment of Hyperlipidemia. New York: Marcel Dekker, 1991, pp 103–138.
49. Lahdenpers S, Tilly-Kiesi M, Vuorinen-Markkola H, et al: Effects of gemfibrozil on low-density lipoprotein particle size, density distribution, and composition in patients with type II diabetes. Diabetes Care 16:584, 1993.
50. Tilly-Kiesi M, Tikkanen MJ: Low density lipoprotein density and composition in hypercholesterolaemic men treated with HMG CoA reductase inhibitors and gemfibrozil. J Intern Med 229:427, 1991.
51. Buchwald H, Matts JP, Fitch LL, et al: Changes in sequential coronary arteriograms and subsequent coronary events. JAMA 268:1429, 1992.
52. McKenney JM, Proctor JD, Harris S, et al: A comparison of the efficacy and toxic effects of sustained- vs immediate-release niacin in hypercholesterolemic patients. JAMA 271:672, 1994.
53. Black D: Atorvastatin: A step ahead for HMG-CoA reductase inhibitors [abstract]. Atherosclerosis 109:88, 1994.
54. Bergstrom JD, Kurtz MM, Rew DJ, et al: Zaragozic acids: A family of fungal metabolites that are picomolar competitive inhibitors of squalene synthase. Proc Natl Acad Sci USA 90:80, 1993.
55. Kelly MJ, Roberts SM: Combating cholesterol. Nature 373:192, 1995.
56. Hidaka Y, Hotta H, Nagata Y, et al: Effect of a novel squalene epoxidase inhibitor, NB-598, on the regulation of cholesterol metabolism in Hep G2 cells. J Biol Chem 266:13171, 1991.
57. The Alpha-Tocopherol, Beta Carotene Cancer Prevention Study Group: The effect of vitamin E and beta carotene on the incidence of lung cancer and other cancers in male smokers. N Engl J Med 330:1029, 1994.
58. Walldius G, Erikson U, Olsson AG, et al: The effect of probucol on femoral atherosclerosis: The Probucol Quantitative Regression Swedish Trial (PQRST). Am J Cardiol 74:875, 1994.
59. Grossman M, Raper SE, Kozarsky K, et al: Successful ex vivo gene therapy directed to liver in a patient with familial hypercholesterolemia. Nat Genet 6:335, 1994.
60. Brown MS, Goldstein JL, Havel R, et al: Gene therapy for cholesterol [letter]. Nat Genet 7:349, 1994.
61. Kozarsky KF, McKinley DR, Austin LL, et al: In vivo correction of low density lipoprotein receptor deficiency in the Watanabe heritable hyperlipidemic rabbit with recombinant adenoviruses. J Biol Chem 269:13695, 1994.
62. Cohen MV, Byrne M-J, Levine B, et al: Low rate of treatment of hypercholesterolemia by cardiologists in patients with suspected and proven coronary artery disease. Circulation 83:1294, 1991.
63. Roberts WC: Getting cardiologists interested in lipids. Am J Cardiol 72:743, 1993.

II.

Drug Treatment of Chronic Cardiovascular Disorders

INITIAL THERAPY AND COMBINATION THERAPY

Editors: Norman M. Kaplan and Bramah N. Singh

CHAPTER 7

Combination Therapy in Angina Pectoris

Gert-Hinrich Reil, M.D., and Paul R. Lichtlen, M.D.

HISTORICAL ASPECTS

The concept of medical treatment of angina pectoris is based, on the one hand, on the present knowledge of the pathophysiology of coronary atherosclerosis and, on the other hand, on the specific effects of the three main classes of antianginal drugs: nitrates, β-blockers, and calcium antagonists. Since the mid-1970s, a large body of information in this field has provided new and deeper insights into rational and individualized therapy. Nitrates have been known for more than a century,[1] whereas β-blockers and calcium antagonists were introduced only in the early and late 1960s, yet led to a substantial extension of antiischemic treatment.[2-9] As these three most commonly applied antianginal agents have different effects on the myocardium, the coronary circulation, and the peripheral circulation (Table 7–1), their combination in antiischemic treatment was a logical step forward. Table 7–1 demonstrates the desired and actual drug effects based on the studies mentioned in the literature. Combination therapy considerably improved the efficacy of the prophylactic treatment of ischemia[10-17]

and allowed a decrease in the individual drug dose, thus reducing unwanted side effects. An important further aspect came from more recent findings in 24-hour electrocardiography (ECG) Holter monitoring:[18] it was observed that daily ischemic episodes follow a circadian distribution and that clinically silent episodes occur approximately three times more frequently than symptomatic ones. Hence, preventive treatment had to focus not only on the suppression of symptomatic ischemic episodes but also on the more prevalent clinically silent episodes.[19, 20] This shifted the therapeutic goal toward a broader target: the prevention of all ischemic episodes[21] or a substantial reduction in the daily number of ischemic episodes and of the total ischemic burden.[22]

PATHOPHYSIOLOGIC CONSIDERATIONS OF ISCHEMIA
Basic Pathophysiology of Coronary Artery Disease

Long before coronary artery disease becomes symptomatic, early coronary atherosclerotic lesions, called

Table 7–1. **Sites and Effects of Antiischemic Drugs**

Myocardium		Coronary Circulation		Peripheral Circulation	
Desired Effect					
Decrease of regional MVO$_2$, increase of O$_2$ delivery in ischemic area		Decrease of vasomotor tone, dilation of eccentric stenoses ↓ Proximal arteries ↓ Peripheral resistance Increase in coronary flow		Afterload reduction ↓ Peripheral resistance ↓ Blood pressure Preload reduction	
Actual Drug Effect					
↓ Heart rate	BB	Dilation of epicardial arteries,	NT, CaA	↑ Capacitance arteries	NT, CaA
↓ Contractility	BB	of eccentric stenoses		↑ Arteriolar dilation	CaA
↓ Wall tension	CaA, BB, NT	Arteriolar dilation	CaA	↓ Arteriolar resistance	
↑ Cardioprotection	CaA	↑ Coronary flow	CaA	Venous dilation, pooling	NT

BB, β-blocking agents; NT, nitrates; CaA, calcium antagonists; MVO$_2$, myocardial oxygen consumption.

27

"fatty streaks," develop in the intima of the arterial wall, a process already starting at a young age.[23–26] From experimental[27, 28] and clinical studies,[24, 29–32] it became evident that fatty streaks can progress over years to typical, intraluminal atherosclerotic plaques.[33] The result of this initial "growth" of early atherosclerotic lesions is eccentric plaques (stenoses) of a low degree (percent diameter stenosis ≤50%).[24, 34] These early lesions are clinically silent; however, a few of them progressively change into a more concentric-shaped stenosis. Coronary flow reserve is still completely preserved and compensated by arteriolar dilation.[24] These plaques have a relatively high tendency to rupture their fibrous cap and to lead to thrombotic occlusion with impending acute myocardial infarction.[24, 33, 35, 36] Hence, the further increase in plaque volume leading to ischemic events is usually due to plaque complications like rupture of the fibrous cap followed by intramural bleeding and formation of an intraluminal platelet thrombus.[36, 37] These increases in total plaque volume eventually result in a percent diameter stenosis of up to 75% or more, limiting coronary flow and reserve, especially during episodes of increased oxygen demand[37, 38] (Fig. 7–1). Consequently, ischemia is the result of an increase in oxygen demand in excess of the maximal possible oxygen supply of this myocardial region with jeopardized blood flow. The most important hemodynamic events associated with a high increase in myocardial oxygen consumption and therefore likely to induce ischemia as a result of a reduced coronary reserve are increases in heart rate, in contractility, and in wall tension (blood pressure).[39] These alterations precede ST-segment depressions, the equivalent to subendocardial ischemia, which starts with a delay of several minutes.[38, 40]

The early, eccentric stenoses still possess a "normal" wall segment of various sizes with sufficiently preserved vascular smooth muscle cells[34] able to react to endogenous or exogenous vasoconstricting or vasodilating agents.[41, 42] There is convincing evidence that in coronary segments altered by atherosclerosis, both vasoconstriction of the normal wall segment as well as formation of transient platelet thrombi on complicated plaques can promptly further reduce the lumen of a stenotic area up to the provocation of ischemia.[24, 36, 37] These dynamic obstructions,[41] especially those caused by changes in vasomotor tone, usually produce a primary reduction of myocardial blood flow and oxygen supply at rest, that is, in a situation of low, stable oxygen demand. These functional and organic events at least partially explain the clinical course, especially in unstable angina (i.e., attacks of angina at rest).[43] Consequently, the clinical picture of unstable angina is characterized by a sudden increase in anginal episodes, at low levels of exercise and/or at rest.[44] In this situation, coronary reserve is variable and may alter its dynamics independently of the patient's activities.[42] This mainly oc-

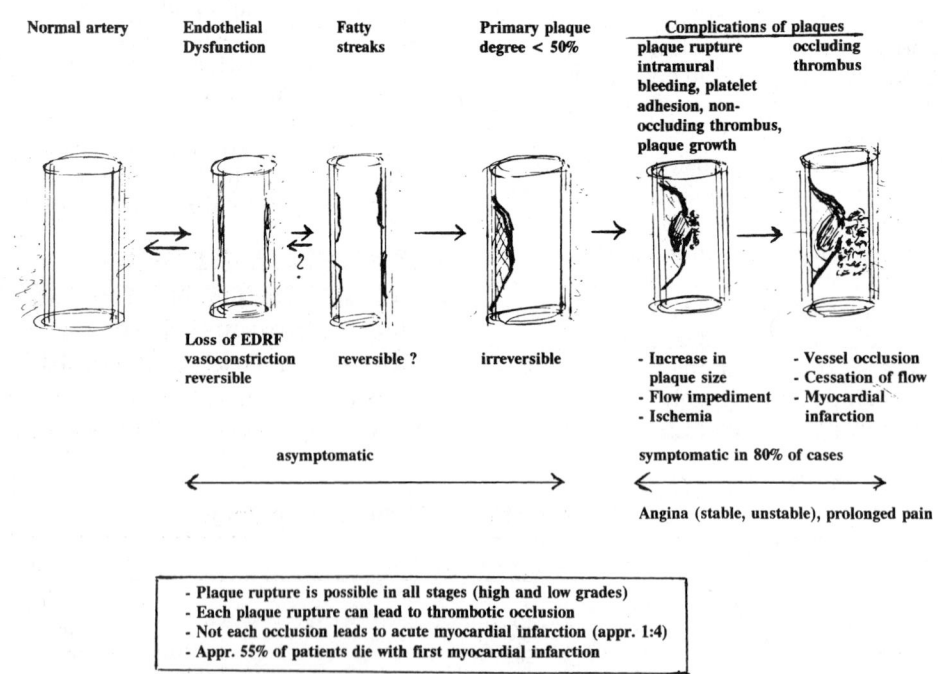

Figure 7–1. Course of coronary artery disease as demonstrated for a single plaque. The first abnormality is endothelial dysfunction in the presence of high cholesterol levels and free oxygen radicals leading to a loss of endothelium-derived relaxing factor–nitric oxide (EDRF-NO). This is followed by cholesterol deposition in the intima and the evolution of fatty streaks; these first two stages are reversible. Fatty streaks can develop into new plaques "growing" into the arterial lumen; these new plaques have a low percent diameter stenosis (<50%) and are clinically silent. The clinically symptomatic stage is induced by the complications of plaques: plaque rupture with intramural bleeding (increase in plaque volume), and platelet adhesion and nonoccluding or occluding thrombi, eventually followed by acute myocardial infarction. Note that plaque rupture is possible in all stages (in high- and low-grade lesions) and that each plaque rupture can lead to thrombotic occlusion, whereas approximately only every fourth occlusion leads to a myocardial infarction. Hence, ischemia is the result of progressing plaques with a high percent diameter stenosis (>75%), usually after plaques undergo complications.

curs in the presence of eccentric stenoses of varying degree (dynamic stenoses).[41, 43] Under clinical monitoring, it becomes evident that ST-segment changes are often the first and only indicator of ischemia.[24, 38, 45–47] Finally, at this stage of advanced coronary artery disease, further progress occurs, often ending in complete vessel occlusion due to abrupt plaque rupture with secondary thrombus formation.[36] Consequently, these events often lead to myocardial infarction or to sudden cardiac death.[48]

Symptomatic and Asymptomatic Ischemic Episodes

Ischemic episodes, both at rest as well as during exercise, can occur with or without anginal pain. Holter monitoring studies over a period of 24 to 48 hours have demonstrated that the majority of the daily ischemic episodes ($\geq 75\%$) are clinically silent.[18–20, 38, 49, 50] This is in accordance with the evidence that exercise stress tests also often produce no symptoms.[51] These findings also indicate that the generation of pain during ischemia depends not only on specific hemodynamic and metabolic changes but also on its transmission and central nervous system perception.[52, 53] In addition, the concentration of pain-producing substances may be too low, the underperfused area too small, or the flow reduction insufficient to provoke ischemia.[17, 54] In any case, these carefully designed studies failed to elucidate specific electrocardiographic and hemodynamic patterns that predict silent or painful ischemic episodes.[42] Finally, all these studies imply that the assessment and treatment of the total ischemic burden are the main goals of noninvasive antiischemic therapy.[21, 22]

INTENTIONS OF ANTIISCHEMIC TREATMENT

The main goal of therapeutic efforts is the improvement of the patient's prognosis. However, until now, no antiischemic drug therapy has been documented to influence decisively the course of coronary atherosclerosis, especially to retard serious coronary events such as nonfatal and fatal myocardial infarctions and sudden coronary death.[14, 15, 17] This, so far, is especially the case for primary prophylactic antiatherosclerotic treatment with lipid-lowering drugs, which reduce acute myocardial infarction only to a moderate extent, not sufficient for a major impact on the disease.[55–58] Furthermore, most studies failed to show a significant influence on total mortality.[59–63] The same is also true for nitrates, calcium antagonists, and, to a certain extent, angiotensin-converting enzyme (ACE) inhibitors. Accordingly, in patients with stable angina pectoris, antiischemic medical treatment proved to be inferior to bypass surgery with regard to long-term prognosis as demonstrated in randomized, prospective studies.[64–66] This is especially true for specific subgroups such as patients with high-grade stenoses of the left main coronary artery or double- and triple-vessel disease with high-grade left anterior descend-

ing artery stenoses and, above all, in the presence of severely impaired left ventricular function.[65] On the other hand, in many patients, medical treatment is highly effective in preventing ischemia without or with anginal pain. Thus, antiischemic therapy also protects against ventricular dysfunction, specifically against stunning or even hibernating myocardium, as induced by repeated ischemic episodes.[67] The decision to start medical treatment therefore depends on being able to reduce or even abolish total ischemic burden and by doing so to preserve myocyte integrity,[68, 69] to improve working capacity, and, above all, to improve the quality of life. Consequently, drug treatment can achieve important secondary goals, as has been demonstrated in numerous studies, especially when using combination therapy (for review, see references 13–17).

PHARMACOLOGY OF ANTIISCHEMIC DRUGS

Several considerations have to be taken into account when selecting drugs for special combination therapy.[15, 17] First, an attempt should be made to extrapolate from a carefully obtained history the underlying mechanisms of ischemia in an individual case. Is it induced by fixed (concentric) or dynamic (eccentric) stenoses or by an acute event like plaque rupture and platelet thrombus formation? Furthermore, one has to realize that ischemia is pathogenetically related both to the abnormal coronary system, with its anatomic and functional limitations of oxygen supply, as well as to the myocardium's major determinants for oxygen consumption: heart rate, contractility, and wall tension.[39] In addition, ischemia is also influenced by the peripheral circulation, that is, by changes in preload and afterload.[54] These three systems (myocardium, coronary circulation, and peripheral circulation) are highly susceptible to specific interactions of antiischemic compounds (see Table 7–1).

Finally, the hemodynamic changes induced by ischemia offer the basis for specific indications and contraindications of a particular drug, with regard to coronary blood flow (oxygen delivery), left ventricular function, and serious, unwanted side effects. Therefore, knowledge of the basic pharmacologic features of the most widely applied antianginal drugs is a necessary prerequisite in planning effective combination therapy.

Nitroglycerin and Organic Nitrate Esters

Nitroglycerin was introduced into the treatment of angina pectoris more than a century ago.[1] The reasons for the unique antiischemic effect of nitrates are known today. They substitute an endogenous vasodilator, the endothelium-derived relaxing factor (EDRF), today recognized as nitric oxide (NO), produced by the endothelial cells from L-arginine through NO synthase.[70–73] NO achieves its vasodilating function through stimulation of cyclic guanosine monophosphate (cGMP) in the underlying vascular smooth muscle cells. Accordingly, all nitrate compounds have to be converted to NO. However, in contrast with the endogenous NO, nitrates are not dependent on the endothelium for their action. This is of special importance because, in atherosclerosis, endothelial function (and by this, NO production) is often impaired, so that coronary vasoconstriction prevails. Hence, during exercise, coronary blood flow might be impaired, especially in areas of high-grade eccentric stenoses resulting from increased alpha tone.[73, 74] Sublingual nitroglycerin remains the "gold standard" for the relief of anginal attacks or for their prevention. Depending on the route of administration,[75] the primary effect of these agents is mediated by local or systemic venodilation and results in a decrease in venous return.[76] This reduction in preload leads to a decrease in left ventricular end-diastolic volume and pressure, owing to the decompressing effect on the endocardium (Table 7–2). Consequently, subendocardial flow is passively increased, enabling reoxygenation of the subendocardial layers. This reduces the increased wall tension in the ischemic myocardial area and finally normalizes local contractility.[77-79] Especially at higher doses, nitrates also decrease left ventricular afterload mainly by lowering cardiac output and systolic pressure, whereas arteriolar resistance remains unchanged, or even increases mildly.[80] The net effect of this class of drugs is an improvement in the ratio of oxygen demand to delivery.[79, 81] Of importance is the direct dilating effect of nitrates on normal as well as on diseased coronary artery segments,[82] especially on the still "normal" wall segment of eccentric stenoses, where dilations of percent diameter stenosis up to 60% are observed, leading to a considerable reduction in proximal coronary resistance.[34, 78, 83] By this process, nitrates shift blood to the ischemic region despite an overall decrease in coronary blood flow.[78-80, 84] Hence, there is redistribution of flow during exercise, preferably toward the subendocardial ischemic areas. Nitrates are subjected to special kinetic patterns, characterized by short half-lives (in minutes), low bioavailabilities (<5%),[85] and possible drug tolerance.[72, 86, 87] Therefore, sustained-release for-

mulations, leading to long-standing constant blood levels, as well as longer-lasting pharmacologic compounds, were introduced[88] in order to achieve more effective prophylactic antiischemic therapy. These long-lasting compounds may, however, induce tolerance,[85-87] unless a nitrate-free interval of 3 to 6 hours is established. This interval can most often be arranged during the night, especially in patients with exercise-induced angina.

β-Adrenergic Blocking Agents

β-Adrenergic blocking agents substantially decrease myocardial oxygen consumption mainly by reducing sympathetic tone. This is achieved by a decrease in heart rate at rest and during exercise,[89-91] a negative inotropic effect reducing myocardial contractility as well as wall stress,[90, 91] and a mild drop in arterial blood pressure accompanied by an increase in coronary vasomotor tone and resistance.[92, 93] Therefore, the three main determinants of myocardial oxygen consumption[39] are directly influenced by β-blocking agents, an effect resulting in the relief, especially of angina on effort (for a synoptic overview see Table 7–2). On the other hand, β-blocking agents inhibit coronary artery vasodilation and may even produce vasoconstriction,[92-94] both in epicardial coronary arteries and arterioles; they therefore might also lead to an increase in coronary vasomotor tone.[95] In addition, some β-blockers (noncardiospecific) also increase peripheral resistance, often associated with severe side effects such as cold extremities. Their antihypertensive effect is mainly due to a central action as well as a mild reduction in cardiac output.[91] Although additional properties, such as lipophilicity, intrinsic sympathomimetic activity (ISA), membrane-stabilizing properties, and cardioselectivity, have considerable therapeutic implications in selected groups of patients with concomitant diseases (e.g., diabetes mellitus, chronic airway obstructions), all β-blocking agents seem to be equally effective in the treatment of angina pectoris.[96] Hence, based on different pharmacokinetic properties,[97-99] unwanted side effects (e.g., impairment of left ventricular function, that is,

Table 7–2. **Cardiovascular Effects of Antianginal Drugs**

	Calcium Antagonists			β-Blockers	Nitrates
	D	N	V		
Myocardial O₂ supply					
Coronary flow	↑	↑	↑	↓	↓
Dynamic obstructions	↓	↓	↓	↑	↓
Myocardial O₂ demand					
Heart rate	↓	↑	↓	↓ ↓	↑
Contractility	(↓)	0	↓	↓ ↓	0
Afterload	↓	↓ ↓	↓	(↑)	0
Preload	0	0	0	(↑)	↓ ↓
Cardiac output	↑	↑ ↑	↑		↓
SA/AV conduction	↓	0	↓ ↓	↓ ↓	0
BR activity	↓	↑ ↑	↓ ↓	↓	↑

AV, atrioventricular; BR, baroreceptor response; D, diltiazem; N, nifedipine; SA, sinoatrial; V, verapamil; ↑, increase or shortening; ↓, decrease or prolongation; 0, no change; parentheses indicate somewhat of an increase or decrease.

negative inotropic effect), bradycardia (especially in elderly persons with decreased sympathetic tone), as well as coronary and peripheral vasoconstriction, β-blockers have to be used with caution.

Calcium Antagonists

These agents act both on the systemic as well as on the coronary vasculature by blocking the voltage-dependent calcium channel of vascular smooth muscle cells.[100] Based on this mechanism, these drugs relax epicardial coronary arteries, especially the normal wall segment in eccentric stenoses, and thus increase the stenotic diameter and reduce proximal coronary resistance; in addition, they dilate coronary arterioles, preferably those in the ischemic, subendocardial zone and reduce peripheral coronary resistance.[100–104] Calcium antagonists also decrease peripheral resistance and lead to a reduction of afterload and blood pressure. They vary in their efficacy on the vasculature, the myocardium, and the conduction system;[105–107] of the first-generation calcium blockers, nifedipine is the most potent and diltiazem the weakest arterial dilator.[105, 108] Calcium antagonists depress myocardial contractility in isolated, as well as *in situ*, heart muscle preparations,[5, 109] but also in human subjects when the drug is administered intracoronarily.[110] This negative inotropic effect is the result of a direct blockade of the calcium channels of myocytes,[110] resulting in reduced availability of trigger calcium-initiating contraction.[105, 110–112] After administration, the direct cardiodepressant effect is counterbalanced by a reflex increase in sympathetic tone induced by afterload reduction.[109] *In vivo*, verapamil has the most pronounced myocardial depressant effect,[111–113] because of its marked attenuation of baroreceptor reflex control.[114] In addition, verapamil and diltiazem, when administered together, can lead to a decrease in sinus node activity and depression of atrioventricular (AV) nodal conduction.[115, 116] All calcium antagonists increase coronary blood flow, however, without interfering with vascular autoregulation;[84, 100, 102–104] therefore, they do not produce a steal phenomenon, in contrast with dipyridamole, which completely blocks autoregulation.[83, 100, 103] Recent studies performed on dogs have shown that, during stress-induced subendocardial ischemia, coronary reserve is not completely exhausted,[117] yet a further arteriolar dilation and increase in flow are achieved by the administration of nifedipine and other calcium antagonists.[101] In addition, coronary flow is also improved through a marked dilation of the large epicardial arteries, especially of severe eccentric stenosis,[83] by a decrease in proximal resistance.

Hence, calcium antagonists influence both myocardial oxygen demand by reducing afterload and myocardial oxygen supply by increasing coronary blood flow (for a synoptic overview, see Table 7–2). The pharmacokinetics of these drugs differ mainly in their specific bioavailability. Because of its lipophilicity, verapamil undergoes an excessive first-pass metabolism in the liver, resulting in a bioavailability of only approximately 20% (nifedipine, 30% to 60%).[113] The biologic half-lives (range, 3 to 7 hours), as well as therapeutic plasma levels (range, 15 to 130 ng/ml), are remarkably identical for these compounds;[113] therefore, these drugs—without special galenic formulations—require a three-times-daily administration. In the last 10 years, powerful second-generation calcium antagonists, especially of the dihydropyridine type, became available,[118, 119] differing from nifedipine by higher tissue specificity (vasculature) and lipophilicity as well as longer half-lives.

Both in animals and in humans, calcium antagonists also revealed a considerable antiatherosclerotic effect.[57, 58, 120–127] Studies performed in rabbits fed a diet rich in cholesterol (blood levels up to 2000 mg/dl) showed a significant retardation of aortic atherosclerotic plaques (sudanophilic lesions) when calcium antagonists, especially nifedipine, nicardipine, or verapamil, were administered simultaneously with a diet rich in cholesterol.[123, 126, 127] In human subjects, so far only nifedipine and nicardipine have been adequately tested; when analyzed by quantitated coronary angiography, both drugs angiographically revealed a significant 30% to 65% reduction of newly formed coronary lesions in coronary segments previously "normal" (for details, see references 29, 31, 124, and 125). Calcium antagonists additionally have a significant cardioprotective effect. In animals, when given before and during ischemia, both verapamil and nifedipine were shown to reduce devastating ischemic changes such as mitochondrial damage.[127, 128] Also in animals, the two agents were shown to prevent stunned myocardium after restoration of normal flow.[67, 129, 130]

EXPERIENCE WITH COMBINATION THERAPY IN CORONARY ARTERY DISEASE

Stable Angina Pectoris

Many short-term clinical studies have been performed in patients with stable angina. The first combination, still a classic one, is the administration of β-blockers with nitrates.[12]

Figure 7–2 demonstrates the typical results of such a study performed in the early 1970s.[91, 131, 132] Left ventricular end-diastolic pressure and stroke work index were studied at rest and during bicycle ergometry in patients with severe coronary artery disease who exercised until angina and/or significant ST-segment depression ($\geq$0.1 mV) developed. When these end points were reached, end-diastolic pressure was abnormally increased to more than 30 mmHg with a rise in stroke work index to more than 80 g/m². After administration of propranolol, end-diastolic pressure remained elevated during exercise (33 mmHg); however, stroke work index decreased considerably (68 g/m²). With the addition of nitroglycerin, end-diastolic pressure significantly dropped to 22 mmHg and anginal pain and ST-segment depression were relieved

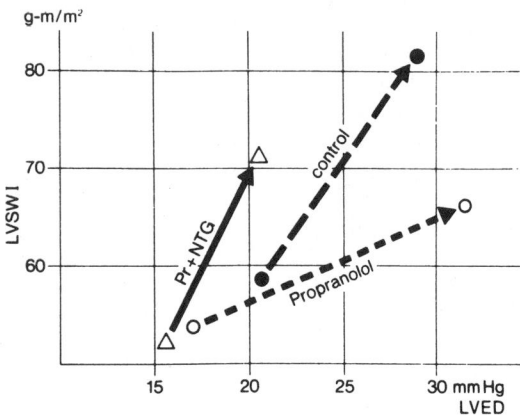

Figure 7–2. Relation between left ventricular stroke work index (g/m²) (LVSWI, ordinate) and left ventricular end-diastolic (LVED) pressure (abscissa) at rest and during exercise (mean workload, 65 watts; n = 22 patients with severe coronary artery disease). Changes in both parameters are indicated after administration of propranolol (0.007 mg/kg IV) and after additional nitroglycerin (0.8 mg sublingually). (From Lichtlen P, Albert H, Spiegel M, et al: Insuffisance coronaire: Evaluation par les tests d'effort de la fonction de ventricule gauche sous propranolol administré seul ou avec nitroglycerine. Therapie 25:252, 1970) (see text).

(see open arrows in Table 7–3). Similar results have been reported in other short-term studies.[133–135]

These trials focus on the main beneficial interaction of both drugs. β-Blockers reduce oxygen consumption by inhibiting the sympathetically mediated increase in heart rate and contractility, but, conversely, they also increase left ventricular end-diastolic volume and pressure as a result of their negative inotropic effect. Nitrates, on the other hand, counterbalance the unfavorable effect on preload by venous dilation and a reduced venous return. In addition, nitrates may increase heart rate and also myocardial contractility by reflex stimulation of sympathetic tone owing to a mild drop in blood pressure.[136] Details of the specific hemodynamic effects of both drugs either alone or in combination are demonstrated in Table 7–3. It is obvious that, both for theoretic and for practical reasons, the combination of these two compounds is not only attractive but also beneficial.[89, 137, 138] This combination is particularly useful because β-blockers administered alone can lead to heart failure in patients with impaired left ventricular function. The addition of nitrates balances the β-blocking effect (i.e., the negative inotropic effect) by reducing left ventricular end-diastolic volume and pressure; in addition, it reduces proximal coronary resistance by relaxing the normal wall segment of eccentric stenoses. In practice, adding a selective β-blocker in a low dose to a strong, long-acting nitrate is recommended.

Surprisingly, only few long-term studies of this combination are available so far, not all demonstrating a beneficial result. Jensen et al.[139] and Muller et al.[140] failed to find any improvement in clinical symptoms with the combination in comparison with either drug alone. In contrast, Schaumann[141] and Delmare[142] demonstrated a clear benefit by combining the two drugs. More controlled studies on long-term therapy with both drugs are necessary to confirm their superiority to monotherapy.[15] It should be kept in mind, however, that the therapeutic benefit depends on the right balance between the dose of the β-blocker and of the long-term nitrate.

Since the introduction of calcium antagonists into the treatment of stable angina,[8, 103] one must also consider the benefit of these drugs in combination with β-blockers. In several controlled studies, the addition of nifedipine to β-blockers was found to improve antianginal efficacy, with regard to both workload as well as exercise duration. Lynch et al.[143] found that the combination of propranolol (240 and 480 mg/day) and nifedipine (60 mg/day) was superior to either drug alone. In addition, the number of silent ischemic episodes determined by 24-hour Holter monitoring was significantly reduced. It is noteworthy that the higher dose of propranolol 480 mg/day showed no further improvement in antiischemic efficacy or hemodynamics. Interestingly, the rate-pressure product did not further decrease after adding nifedipine. Therefore, it is concluded that the benefit of nifedipine during exercise, to a great extent, is due to the increase in poststenotic, especially subendocardial, flow[84, 100, 101] (see Table 7–3). In contrast, Ekelund and Oroe[144] and Braun et al.[145] reported improvement of hemodynamic parameters with a concomitantly further decrease of the rate-pressure product when

Table 7–3. **Combination Therapy and Resulting Cardiovascular Effects**

	β-Blockers			Nitrate + β-Blocker	Nitrate +		
	D	N	V		D	N	V
Myocardial O₂ supply							
Coronary flow	(↓)	(↓)	(↓)	↓ ↓	↑	↑	↑
Dynamic obstructions	(↑)	(↑)	(↑)	0	↓ ↓	↓ ↓	↓ ↓
Myocardial O₂ demand							
Heart rate	↓ ↓	↓	↓ ↓	↓	0	↑	0
Contractility	↓ ↓	↓	↓ ↓	↓	0	↑	0
Afterload	↓	↓	↓	(↓)	↓	↓ ↓	↓
Preload	0	0	0	⇓	↓	↓	↓
Cardiac output	0	⇑	0	↓ ↓	↑	↑ ↑	↑ ↓
SA/AV conduction	↓	0	↓ ↓	↓	↑	0	↑ ↓
BR activity	↓	⇑	↓ ↓	0	⇓	↑ ↑	⇓

All symbols as indicated in Table 7–2. ⇓ or ⇑ denotes decrease or increase in primary and therapeutically favorable effect, respectively.

nifedipine was added. This effect, together with a reported increase in left ventricular ejection fraction as assessed by radionuclide ventriculography,[145] may be interpreted as left ventricular unloading (afterload reduction) caused by the additional administration of nifedipine.

Similar results have been obtained by a number of researchers.[11, 146-150] In general, it was found that the combination of β-blockers with nifedipine improved antianginal efficacy by further reducing the number and duration of ischemic events. In some cases, reduction of the dose of the adjunctive β-blocker was achieved without a loss in the drug's benefit.[11, 143, 144, 146, 151, 152]

The combination of verapamil with β-blockers has been far more controversial. A necessary prerequisite for this combination is a preserved left ventricular function and preferably a normal sinus and AV nodal function.[10, 15, 17] In patients with atrial fibrillation, the combination might, however, be beneficial owing to the negative chronotropic effect of verapamil on AV nodal conduction. Subramanian et al.[153] studied the comparative efficacy of a relatively high dose of verapamil (360 mg/day) and propranolol (240 mg/day) using treadmill exercise testing. Fourteen of 22 patients studied receiving propranolol alone remained symptomatic after monotherapy and therefore were advanced to combination therapy of verapamil (360 mg/day) and propranolol (120 mg/day). In spite of reducing the dose of propranolol to 120 mg/day, more than 50% of the patients became asymptomatic, and exercise capacity was considerably increased. The combination was superior to therapy with either drug alone. No serious adverse reactions were reported. Winniford et al.[154] and Leon et al.[155] assessed the antiischemic efficacy and left ventricular function in patients with high doses of both drugs. In both studies, the combination therapy demonstrated benefit in comparison with either drug treatment alone. However, in both studies, some cases of exertional dyspnea as well as bradycardia and second-degree atrioventricular block were documented.

Other studies with lower doses[156-158] produced favorable results. However, the salutary effects reported in all the studies were obviously not without some risks. Therefore, it is recommended that the dose of both verapamil and β-blockers be kept relatively low when they are applied in combination. Plasma levels of verapamil and propranolol in the study of Leon et al.[155] as well as in other studies exceeded the normal range by a factor of 2 to 3, when compared with the normal range given by Johnsson and Regardh.[97]

The combination of diltiazem with β-blockers was expected to be favorable by several authors, assuming that diltiazem has the least negative inotropic effect of all calcium antagonists.[159, 160] Strauss and Parisi[161] reported superiority of the combination of a high dose of diltiazem (up to 360 mg/day) with propranolol (up to 320 mg/day) with regard to both the antiischemic potency as well as exercise duration. In 12 patients, Hung et al.[162] studied exercise duration after the administration of both drugs alone and in combination; they found no difference in exercise duration after monotherapy compared with combination therapy. However, Humen et al.[163] and Boden et al.[164] reported hemodynamic improvement as well as clinical benefits after adding diltiazem to propranolol. Yet, as only few studies are available, the final evaluation of the antiischemic efficacy and safety of this combination has to wait until further controlled trials are available. Overall, the effect of this specific drug combination appears rather similar to the one obtained by applying verapamil in combination with β-blockers.

In general, the above-mentioned studies elucidate the problems of combining calcium antagonists with β-blockers. Left ventricular dynamics as well as baroreceptor reflex response to peripheral vasodilation should, however, be preserved in the interplay between these two compounds. One has to keep in mind that nifedipine, verapamil, and diltiazem differ widely in their effects on left ventricular contractility as well as on heart rate, when effective doses are applied for maintaining an equal drop in mean arterial blood pressure.[165] The greater a drug's vasodilatory effect, the more complete is the neutralization of its negative inotropic action, provided baroreceptor-mediated sympathetic reflex control is preserved.[111, 165] In relation to this specific mechanism, two excellent studies[166, 167] were performed applying combination therapy with the aim of gaining deeper insights into the interrelation between left ventricular ejection fraction (pump function) and the rate-pressure product (oxygen consumption). Both trials applied almost equivalent drug doses (propranolol 160 mg/day, verapamil 360 mg/day, nifedipine 60 mg/day, diltiazem 250 mg/day, respectively) and showed similar ejection fractions at controls (range from 58% to 63%). Interestingly, left ventricular function during exercise, either with propranolol alone or in combination with one of the three calcium antagonists, did not decrease significantly when compared with placebo. This might be explained by the stepwise reduction of the rate-pressure product, causing a parallel increase in baroreceptor-activated sympathetic tone. These trials confirm that baroreceptor reflex control can remain active, even when high doses of β-blockers and calcium antagonists are administered, suggesting a beneficial interaction of both drugs. Because the dihydropyridine-type calcium antagonists are associated with the least depression of baroreceptor function, their combination with β-blockers seems to be the combination of choice.[10, 11, 16, 17]

The importance of peripheral vasodilation in the combination with β-blockers and calcium antagonists can be derived from the studies of Kieval et al.[168] as well as of Packer et al.[169] Kieval et al.[168] studied patients with known coronary artery disease yet still normal left ventricular ejection fractions averaging 60% (determined by angiography) on long-term treatment with oral propranolol (40 to 160 mg/day leading to plasma levels of 66 to 82 ng/ml); in addition, these patients received short infusions of intravenous verapamil (14 to 30 mg reaching plasma levels of 122 to 214 ng/ml). This combination led to a 24% decrease in mean systemic vascular resistance without changes in left ventricular performance. Packer et al.[169] evaluated the same parameters, however, in the presence of high doses of oral propranolol (500 mg/day reaching plasma levels averaging 474 ng/ml) and high oral doses of verapamil (up to 120 mg three times daily). After the first dose of 120 mg of verapamil with plasma levels averaging 205 ng/ml, there was no further decrease in the rate-pressure product but a severe deterioration of left ventricular ejection fraction, resulting in pump failure. Patients were then withdrawn from oral propranolol, while the same incremental doses of verapamil were continued; this also led to a substantial recovery of patients' hemodynamics. On the other hand, when mean plasma levels of verapamil were kept high, averaging 383 ng/ml, and plasma levels of propranolol were reduced to 40 ng/ml, peripheral resistance decreased, leading to improved left ventricular function. It can therefore be concluded that peripheral vasodilation (i.e., low peripheral resistance) indirectly preserves left ventricular performance. It improves the adaptation dynamics against various unwanted hemodynamic changes induced either by negative inotropic drugs such as β-blockers or verapamil or by ischemia itself. Hence, in the search for optimal doses of this combination therapy, the preservation of vasodilatory reflex control is mandatory. Otherwise, "afterload mismatch," as described by Ross,[170] might result as the peripheral circulation fails to counterbalance the direct cardiodepressant effects of both drugs.

The combination of calcium antagonists with nitrates is used less often in stable angina,[12] and there have also been few, if any, well-conducted controlled studies to judge its clinical relevance.[15] As outlined in Table 7–2, nitrates, although leading to a redistribution of flow, reduce myocardial blood flow, whereas calcium antagonists increase flow. Nevertheless, both compounds decrease oxygen demand, the main therapeutic goal in exertional angina, nitrates more than calcium antagonists. Hence, if this combination is applied, e.g., by adding to a long-acting nitrate a long-acting calcium antagonist, verapamil or diltiazem appears more suitable than a dihydropyridine. This special combination is superior because its effect on afterload is weaker and does not lead to an overshooting baroreceptor reflex response.[15, 95, 115]

Unstable Angina Pectoris

Until recently, definition and classification of unstable angina were mainly clinical.[43, 44, 171] Deeper insights into the pathophysiologic mechanisms, describing the different types of coronary stenoses (eccentric versus concentric, and complicated, i.e., ruptured, versus uncomplicated ones) and their association with platelet aggregation and vasospasm in more detail,[33–37, 172–174] led to the present specific medical management. The changing clinical picture of angina at rest, with attacks increasing in intensity, duration, and frequency of pain as well as of exertional angina even at low

levels of exercise, can be attributed both to functional changes, such as coronary spasm (increased vasomotor tone), as well as to organic alterations such as plaque rupture and platelet thrombus formation, or to both types of events occurring simultaneously. Furthermore, extracardiac causes like anemia or hypotension are also to be considered.[44] Because of the complexity of the underlying mechanisms, the necessary therapeutic strategy cannot be extrapolated immediately and treatment might initially lack a logical and commonly accepted concept.

In view of the special pathophysiologic concept of unstable angina, agents with a strong vasodilatory effect are the first choice, especially when an abnormal increase in vasomotor tone of large epicardial arteries is clinically suspected; the increase in myocardial oxygen delivery by drugs relaxing coronary spasm is then the main goal of combination therapy. Accordingly, the combination of calcium antagonists with nitrates was shown to guarantee maximal diameter enlargement of large epicardial arteries, especially of eccentric, dynamic obstructions.[17, 83, 100, 175] As outlined in Table 7–3, this combination provides a mild increase in coronary flow as a result of the dilation of eccentric stenoses by both types of drugs and of subendocardial arterioles through calcium antagonists. In addition, nitrates reduce preload, which is not affected by calcium antagonists. Therefore, both drugs act synergistically to improve myocardial oxygen supply. Because both drugs lower blood pressure and stimulate sympathetic reflex activities, there is the risk of hypotension and an unwanted increase in heart rate. Side effects, such as headaches, palpitations, hypotension, and flush, might be avoided by starting treatment with calcium antagonists such as verapamil or diltiazem that are known to have a lesser effect on afterload reduction.

Hence, a number of studies demonstrate that calcium antagonists as well as nitrates, and also their combination, are highly effective in unstable angina.[17, 176–182] Nevertheless, in patients with low blood pressure (systolic ≤100 mmHg), caution is indicated. In the early stages of acute myocardial infarction—which often evolves from unstable angina without being recognized—a critically low driving pressure might lead to regional underperfusion and thus to an extension of the infarct zone.[17, 183, 184]

The administration of β-blockers in patients with unstable angina remains controversial, especially when applied as monotherapy. Early experience in this field, reported by Guazzi et al.,[185] was favorable and indicated a decrease in the incidence of anginal attacks as well as of ST-segment alterations in patients receiving propranolol (160 to 800 mg/day). Subsequent observations did not confirm this positive clinical experience. Robertson et al.[95] reported a severe exacerbation of angina in a controlled study of six patients with unstable angina mainly of the variant type (Prinzmetal) when receiving low doses of propranolol (160 mg/day). Interestingly, the deterioration did not progress when the dose was increased (640 mg/day), suggesting that even small doses of a β-blocker are sufficient to lead to considerable impairment of unstable angina, especially in the vasospastic group. Similar results were described by Tilmant et al.[186] in 11 patients with angiographically documented coronary spasm. These authors compared placebo, propranolol (225 mg/day), and diltiazem (360 mg/day) and their combinations. The group receiving propranolol alone had a 36% increase in silent ischemic episodes (24-hour Holter monitoring), which were completely abolished by the addition of diltiazem. Accordingly, the combination of both drugs had the same beneficial effects as diltiazem alone. Similar unfavorable results for propranolol were obtained by Parodi et al.[187] in another trial of 15 patients with unstable angina.

In summary, in unstable angina, β-blockers should be administered with caution. They might be beneficial in advanced stages of coronary artery disease, when the increase in vasomotor tone plays a minor role but fixed, mainly concentric, often complicated high-grade stenoses prevail. In this situation, especially in the presence of an increased resting heart rate, therapy should primarily aim at the decrease in myocardial oxygen demand. As both stable and unstable angina have a common pathophysiologic pathway leading to more severe, high-grade stenoses, in this advanced stage additional afterload reduction also might become a beneficial therapy. Accordingly, several studies demonstrated therapeutic efficacy with β-blockers in the management of unstable angina,[13, 188] especially when progressing to acute myocardial infarction. In general, however, with a few exceptions, β-blockers should not be the main or only drug administered in unstable angina, but should be combined with vasodilators such as calcium antagonists and/or nitrates.

Triple Therapy

Triple therapy should be applied only when carefully designed and dose-titrated monotherapy and double therapy have failed to adequately reduce symptomatic and silent episodes of ischemia. This complex treatment may be performed for the following reasons:

1. Minimization of oxygen demand. When β-blocker therapy is initiated in stable angina, afterload and preload can be further decreased by additional reduction of systemic peripheral resistance and of venous return through venodilation and venous pooling. Calcium antagonists and nitrates will achieve this goal. The potential benefit might, however, be jeopardized by an unwanted increase in heart rate through an excessive drop in arterial pressure. On the other hand, when treatment begins with vasodilators (nitrates, calcium antagonists), especially in unstable angina, additional administration of nonspecific β-blockers can be beneficial, leading to a further decrease in oxygen demand and preventing an excessive drop in blood pressure.

2. Increase in oxygen delivery. Because β-blocker therapy is associated with a decrease in oxygen consumption and myocardial blood flow,[91, 103] maintenance of or even an increase in myocardial oxygen delivery and a redistribution of flow are often desirable. Thus, the additional administration of calcium antagonists and/or nitrates might become important, with the aim of maximally dilating epicardial coronary arteries and subendocardial arterioles.

3. Reduction of adverse side effects. Overall, there is, as yet, little evidence that triple therapy reduces adverse side effects better than double therapy.[14] In contrast, in special situations it seems impossible to decide which drug is responsible for the main therapeutic action and which for the adverse reaction when applying a more complex triple therapy.

There are only a few studies reporting on experience with triple therapy. Tolins et al.[189] studied 19 patients with stable angina pectoris on long-term propranolol therapy (160 mg/day) for stable angina together with nifedipine (20 mg) and isosorbide dinitrate (ISDN, 20 mg) over a short period of time. They found that exercise duration with triple therapy was not improved when compared with double therapy applying propranolol with either nifedipine or ISDN alone. The limiting factor in this study was an excessive drop in blood pressure. Consequently, they concluded that maximal therapy is not necessarily optimal with regard to the therapeutic benefit. Two other studies obtained positive results when β-blockers and ISDN were combined with nifedipine[190] or with diltiazem.[164] It is important to note that in all these trials drug doses were carefully titrated and adjusted to the patients' tolerance; therefore, these strategies may be of particular interest in future trials with a selected group of patients.

When applying β-blockers and calcium antagonists in combination, unfavorable effects might arise by virtue of their specific synergistic and antagonistic actions. For example, nitrates might compensate for some of the adverse effects of β-blockers and calcium antagonists (e.g., the impairment of left ventricular function and the increase in preload) but precipitate others (e.g., hypotension and an unwanted increase in heart rate). Hence, triple therapy might be beneficial only if the doses of the individual drugs are reevaluated and adjusted to the patient's individual tolerance. More recently, ACE inhibitors are included in triple therapy combined either with β-blockers or with nitrates or calcium antagonists. This is done especially for remodeling of the left ventricle and prevention of (sudden) death due to heart failure (see later). In general, however, only limited clinical experience with triple therapy is available in patients with severely depressed left ventricular function or abnormalities of the cardiac conduction system. Therefore, triple therapy should be applied only in selected groups of patients in an advanced or final stage of stable and unstable coronary artery disease, except when ACE inhibitors are added.

The indications for triple therapy concern mainly the presence of additional abnormalities such as hypertension and left ventricular dysfunction. Calcium antagonists and ACE inhibitors have a marked antihypertensive effect by reducing peripheral systemic resistance without reducing cardiac output. Nitrates are effective in reducing the elevated left ventricular end-diastolic pressure in patients after extensive myocardial infarction.[191] These drugs may also be beneficial in the remodeling phase, administered alone or together with ACE inhibitors.[191, 192] All these factors have to be taken into account when patients with advanced coronary artery disease undergo medical treatment.

ACE Inhibitors

In the 1980s, a new class of compounds—angiotensin-converting enzyme (ACE) inhibitors—was introduced into cardiovascular therapy and meanwhile became a powerful tool to treat heart failure, especially ventricular dysfunction, and to reduce overall mortality.[192-197]

Based on experimental data, these drugs have a favorable hemodynamic and neurohumoral profile also favoring antiischemic therapy. ACE inhibitors decrease peripheral resistance without provoking an increase in reflex tachycardia[198, 199] and thus reduce myocardial oxygen demand. In addition, ACE inhibitors increase local concentrations of the vasodilatory peptide bradykinin, augment coronary blood flow owing to the preinstalled blood pressure level,[200] scavenge oxygen radicals especially during reperfusion injury,[198, 199, 201] and directly dilate the large epicardial coronary arteries.[199] Furthermore, collateral flow is improved by suppression of the activated renin-angiotensin-aldosterone cascade during myocardial ischemia.[198] Additionally, these drugs have special effects to prevent nitrate tolerance in humans.[202] In rats, they suppress neointimal proliferation after balloon dilatation;[203] and in dogs, they considerably decrease the extent of myocardial ischemia and reduce infarct size.[199, 204]

However, in contrast with the experimental data, most clinical studies with ACE inhibitors so far fail to show convincing evidence for a beneficial antiischemic effect in patients with stable angina pectoris. Some trials even reported an impairment of the clinical situation with regard to angina, so that ACE inhibitors had to be withdrawn.[198, 205-209] These adverse effects are mainly caused by hemodynamic disturbances resulting from a decrease in coronary perfusion pressure and flow due to drug-induced systemic hypotension. Only a few studies show positive results with ACE inhibitors in stable angina.[210-212] Therefore, the main indications to use ACE inhibitors in coronary artery disease, especially in the presence of manifest angina pectoris, concern patients with coexisting arterial hypertension or latent or overt myocardial pump failure. However, this special concept is still debated because recent studies demonstrated an inferiority of ACE inhibitors in comparison with the classic antianginal drugs when applied alone or in combination.[213, 214]

Hence, at present, there is still only limited evidence that ACE inhibitors play a significant role in prevention or relief of angina pectoris. It remains a matter of debate whether cardiovascular disease and ACE inhibitors interact unfavorably and beneficial therapeutic effects are therefore neutralized.[215, 216] It seems that ACE inhibitors as monotherapy or in combination with either group of the classic antiischemic compounds are of limited value unless there is associated left ventricular dysfunction[194, 197] or hypertension.[192]

CRITICAL VIEW OF COMBINATION THERAPY
Guidelines and Principles

Despite extensive practical experience, the clinical value of combination therapy in stable angina is still debated. In view of the complexity of the underlying pathophysiology and the large variability in dosing and in drug effects, especially in triple therapy, it is impossible to propose a commonly accepted concept applicable to all patient subsets under all clinical circumstances. Nevertheless, some guidelines for medical management can be outlined. Long-acting nitrates and β-blockers in combination are commonly accepted as a first-line treatment for stable angina, especially in patients with previous myocardial infarctions and mildly increased preload.[12, 14, 217] However, specific pharmacokinetic properties and the development of tolerance (nitrates) require additional agents to balance adverse effects.[72, 81, 86, 87, 180, 218, 219] Therefore, β-blockers have also been combined with calcium antagonists in increasing frequency during the past few years. This is especially the case in the presence of additional diseases like hypertension and/or left ventricular dysfunction, in which combination with an afterload-lowering drug, such as a calcium antagonist, might become necessary.[8, 11, 113]

In unstable angina, calcium antagonists and nitrates, either alone or in combination, should be recommended as first-line treatment; β-blocking agents, if necessary, are preferably combined with one of the two vasodilators.

During the acute phase of myocardial infarction, nitrates remain the treatment of choice, usually applied as a constant infusion of nitroglycerin (0.75 to 6 mg/hr) titrated to a systolic blood pressure not lower than 100 mmHg.[191, 220] Nitrates reduce preload and therefore support left ventricular remodeling. To what extent they decrease mortality in acute myocardial infarction is still debated.[221, 222]

Calcium antagonists should be applied with caution in acute myocardial infarction, because under special circumstances they can be detrimental.[183] This is the case especially when blood pressure is low (systolic 100 mmHg or less) and may further drop through additional afterload reduction. This can result in a cascade of events that may finally lead to expansion of the infarct size and sudden coronary death due to severe life-threatening arrhythmias.[223, 224]

In contrast, in patients with a high blood pressure (i.e., chronic hypertension), calcium antagonists may be beneficial in acute myocardial infarction because they lower blood pressure, reduce myocardial oxygen consumption, and improve myocardial blood flow (i.e., oxygen delivery) in the collateral marginal infarct zone. If calcium antagonists are applied in acute myocardial infarction, they should be administered intravenously to titrate closely the dose to an acceptable blood pressure level, a systolic value above 110 mmHg.

Because of their diverse pharmacodynamic properties, calcium antagonists should be applied selectively.[225] Verapamil and diltiazem, which slow sinus- and AV-nodal conduction and, by this, heart rate, have fewer adverse effects, especially when administered alone,[10] than dihydropyridine-type calcium antagonists. However, when combined with β-blockers, verapamil and diltiazem can induce heart failure and bradyarrhythmias.[225] In contrast, dihydropyridines, which increase heart rate as a result of their strong afterload reduction, are effective in antiischemic treatment not only when administered alone but especially in combination with β-blockers, where they show only a low incidence of side effects. In monotherapy, nifedipine, however, is accompanied by a relatively high incidence of adverse side effects, in contrast with verapamil and diltiazem;[10] this is especially the case when applied in a short-acting form with rapid changes in plasma levels. In combination with β-blockers, nifedipine is generally accepted to be safe even in patients with mildly reduced left ventricular performance.[10, 11] Unwanted changes in plasma levels can be avoided by applying the second-generation dihydropyridine calcium antagonist amlodipine; owing to its very long half-life of 35 to 50 hours, it leads to very constant blood levels and exerts a strong antiischemic effect even with once-a-day dosing of 5 or 10 mg.[226]

The interplay of β-blockers with calcium antagonists can, however, become a problem when dosing is not adjusted to the patients' needs. In this special drug combination, attempts to use higher doses can be tempered by potentially serious hemodynamic as well as electrophysiologic adverse reactions. Experience suggests that somewhat lower than normal doses of both drugs should be administered when they are applied in combination. However, this therapeutic approach remains beneficial only as long as left ventricular unloading is maintained. Therefore, at least partial preservation of baroreceptor reflex control is mandatory in this combination therapy, in order to prevent "afterload mismatch."

It should be stressed once more that triple therapy is indicated only when carefully designed double therapy has failed. This situation seems to be more common in unstable angina than in stable angina.

Evaluation of Therapy

In view of the pathophysiologic impact of ischemia and its high frequency of clinically silent episodes,[18, 19] evaluation of antiischemic treatment can no longer consist merely in counting anginal attacks or the number of nitroglycerin tablets consumed or in searching for ST-segment improvement during exercise testing.[17, 18] Therapy has to include objective and quantifiable parameters such as the assessment of the number of ischemic episodes (typical ST-segment depression ≥0.1 mV over at least 1 minute) by 24-hour Holter monitoring. As evidenced in such studies, the outcome of exercise testing is often irrelevant when compared with ischemia during daily life.[38, 49, 88, 227] Hence, control by Holter monitoring might lead to an improvement of therapeutic efficacy resulting in a further reduction of ischemic events both during daily work as well as during the night as reported by Quyyumi et al.[228] In this regard, Holter monitoring demonstrated a better reduction of symptomatic than asymptomatic, silent ischemic episodes. Of special importance is the suppression of the circadian distribution of spontaneous ischemic episodes, especially of the morning peak of ischemic events.[88, 229] Complete abolition of ischemia is, however, rarely achieved.[17] On the other hand, it is debatable whether complete suppression of ischemic episodes is necessary. So far, there is no evidence that antiischemic drug treatment per se reduces the overall morbidity or mortality of coronary heart disease, that is, prolongs life.[17] There is, however, also no evidence that ischemic episodes provoke life-threatening arrhythmias.[230] There is, however, evidence that antiischemic treatment reduces fibrosis in the poststenotic myocardial areas.[68] Hence, the major target of antiischemic drug treatment, especially in patients with stable angina, remains the well-being of the patient, freedom from pain, preservation of left ventricular function, and, by these, improvement in performance of daily activities. Nevertheless, prevention of serious coronary events such as unstable angina is only partially achieved by drug therapy; this, in part, is a result of the complex mechanisms of this type of ischemia. There is also no evidence that drug therapy prevents acute myocardial infarction, unless specific substances like acetylsalicylic acid (ASA) are added. As its antithrombotic effect is clearly demonstrated in several studies, it is recommendable today to add ASA in low doses (100 mg/day) to the antiischemic treatment unless there are severe contraindications.[19, 231]

REFERENCES

1. Murrell W: Nitroglycerin as a remedy for angina pectoris. Lancet 79:80, 1879.
2. Black JW, Stevenson JS: Pharmacology of a new adrenergic beta-receptor-blocking compound (nethalide). Lancet 2:311, 1962.
3. Epstein SE, Braunwald E: Beta-adrenergic receptor blocking drugs: Mechanisms of actions and clinical applications. N Engl J Med 275:1106, 1966.
4. Wolfson S, Gorlin R: Cardiovascular pharmacology of propranolol in man. Circulation 40:501, 1969.
5. Fleckenstein A: History of calcium antagonists. Circ Res 52:I3, 1983.
6. Krikler D: Verapamil in cardiology. Eur J Cardiol 2:3, 1974.
7. Nayler WG, Szeto J: Effect of verapamil on contractility, oxy-

gen utilization and calcium exchangeability in mammalian heart muscle. Cardiovasc Res 3:30, 1969.

8. Lichtlen P: The influence of nifedipine on left ventricular and coronary dynamics at rest and during exercise in patients with coronary artery disease. *In* Hashimoto K, Kimura E, Kobayashi T (eds): First International Nifedipine Symposium. Tokyo: University Tokyo Press, 1975, pp 114–120.

9. Lichtlen P, Ebner F: Nifedipine—historical aspects. *In* Lichtlen PR (ed): Sixth Adalat Symposium. Amsterdam: Excerpta Medica, 1986, pp 3–19.

10. Leon MB, Rosing DR, Bonow RO, et al: Combination therapy with calcium-channel blockers and beta-blockers for chronic stable angina pectoris. Am J Cardiol 55:69B, 1985.

11. Krikler DM, Harris L, Rowland E: Calcium-channel blockers and beta-blockers: Advantages and disadvantages of combination therapy in chronic stable angina pectoris. Am Heart J 104:702, 1982.

12. Hoekenga D, Abrams J: Rational medical therapy for stable angina pectoris. Am J Med 76:309, 1984.

13. Feldman RL: A review of medical therapy for coronary artery spasm. Circulation 75(Suppl V):V-96, 1987.

14. Crawford MH: The role of triple therapy in patients with chronic stable angina pectoris. Circulation 75(Suppl V):V-122, 1987.

15. Julian DG: Comparison and combinations in anti-anginal therapy. Eur Heart J 6:37, 1985.

16. Lichtlen PR: Calcium antagonists and their combination with nitrates and beta-blocking agents in the treatment of ischemic heart disease. *In* Maseri A, Sobel BE, Chierchia S (eds): Hammersmith Cardiology Workshop Series, Vol 3. New York: Raven Press, 1987, pp 243–252.

17. Lichtlen PR: The combination of antianginal drugs, effects and indications. Cardiovasc Drugs Ther 2:47, 1988.

18. Hausmann D, Lichtlen PR, Nikutta P, et al: Circadian variation of myocardial ischemia in patients with stable coronary artery disease. Chronobiol Int 8:385–398, 1991.

19. Lichtlen PR, Hausmann D: Silent ischemia, its clinical importance as seen in 1989. Z Kardiol 79(Suppl III):23–29, 1990.

20. Deanfield JE, Shea H, Ribiero P, et al: Transient ST-segment depression as a marker of myocardial ischemia during daily life. Am J Cardiol 54:1195–1200, 1984.

21. Pepine CJ, Hill JA: Medical therapy for silent myocardial ischemia. Circulation 75(Suppl II):II-43, 1987.

22. Cohn PF: Total ischemic burden: Definition, mechanism and therapeutic implications. Am J Med 81:2, 1986.

23. Stary HC: Evolution and progression of atherosclerotic lesions in the coronary arteries of children and young adults. Arteriosclerosis 9(Suppl I):I-19, 1989.

24. Lichtlen PR, Nikutta P, Jost S, et al: Anatomical progression of coronary artery disease in humans as seen by prospective, repeated, quantitated coronary angiography: Relation to clinical events and risk factors. Circulation 86:828, 1992.

25. Ross R: The pathogenesis of atherosclerosis—an update. N Engl J Med 8:488, 1986.

26. Fagiotto A, Ross R, Harker L: Studies of hypercholesterolemia in the non-human primate. Parts I and II. Arteriosclerosis 4:323, 1984.

27. Wissler RW: Morphological characteristics of the developing atherosclerotic plaque: Animal studies and studies of lesions from young people. *In* Weber PC, Leaf A (eds): Atherosclerosis Review 1991. New York: Raven Press, 1991, pp 91–103.

28. Fagiotto A, Ross R: Studies of hypercholesterolemia in the non-human primate. II: Fatty streak conversion to fibrous plaque. Arteriosclerosis 4:341, 1984.

29. Lichtlen PR, Nellessen U, Rafflenbeul W, et al: International nifedipine trial on antiatherosclerotic therapy (INTACT). Cardiovasc Drugs Ther 1:71, 1987.

30. Blankenhorn DH, Nessim SA, Johnson RL, et al: Beneficial effects of combined colestipol-niacin therapy on coronary atherosclerosis and coronary venous bypass grafts. JAMA 257:3233, 1987.

31. Waters D, Lespérance J, Francetich M, et al: A controlled clinical trial to assess the effect of a calcium channel blocker on the progression of coronary atherosclerosis. Circulation 82:1940, 1990.

32. Watts GF, Lewis B, Brunt JNH, et al: Effects on coronary artery disease of lipid-lowering diet, or diet plus cholestyramine, in the St Thomas' atherosclerosis regression study (STARS). Lancet 339:563, 1992.

33. Fuster V, Badimon L, Badimon JJ, et al: The pathogenesis of coronary artery disease and the acute coronary syndromes. N Engl J Med 326:310(B), 1992.

34. Freudenberg H, Lichtlen PR: The normal wall segment in coronary stenoses—a postmortem study. Z Kardiol 70:863, 1981.

35. Davies MJ, Thomas AC: Plaque fissuring: The cause of acute myocardial infarction, sudden ischemic death and crescendo angina. Br Heart J 53:363, 1985.

36. Davies MJ: A macro and micro view of coronary vascular insult in ischemic heart disease. Circulation 82(Suppl II):II-38, 1990.

37. Fuster V, Stein B, Ambrose JA, et al: Atherosclerotic plaque rupture and thrombosis: Evolving concepts. Circulation 82:II-47, 1990.

38. Hausmann D, Nikutta P, Hartwig CA, et al: ST-segment analysis in the 24-h Holter ECG in patients with stable angina pectoris and proven coronary artery disease. Z Kardiol 76:554, 1987.

39. Braunwald E: Control of myocardial oxygen consumption: Physiology and clinical considerations. Am J Cardiol 27:316, 1971.

40. Hausmann D, Nikutta P, Daniel WG, et al: Increase in heart rate as the predominant trigger of symptomatic and silent myocardial ischemia in patients with angina [abstract]. Circulation 76(Suppl IV):IV-390, 1987.

41. Rafflenbeul W, Lichtlen PR: Zum Konzept der "dynamischen" Koronarstenose. Z Kardiol 71:439, 1982.

42. Maseri A: Role of coronary artery spasm in symptomatic and silent myocardial ischemia. J Am Coll Cardiol 9:249, 1987.

43. Lichtlen PR: Instabile angina pectoris. *In* Verhandlungen der Deutschen Gesellschaft fur Innere Medizin. Berlin: Springer-Verlag, 1991, pp 101–102.

44. Braunwald E: Unstable angina: A classification. Circulation 80:410, 1989.

45. Cohn PF: Time for a new approach to management of patients with both symptomatic and asymptomatic episodes of myocardial ischemia. Am J Cardiol 54:1358, 1984.

46. Nellessen U, Hecker H, Danciu V, et al: Instabile angina pectoris: Krankheitsbild und Verlauf neu überprüft. Z Kardiol 75:707, 1986.

47. Hausmann D, Nikutta P, Hartwig CA, et al: Asymptomatische Myokardischämie im Belastungs-EKG: Ein Zeichen für häufige stumme Ischämie-Episoden während des täglichen Lebens? [abstract]. Z Kardiol 76(Suppl 2):74, 1987.

48. Davies MJ, Thomas A: Thrombosis and acute coronary artery lesion in sudden ischemic death. N Engl J Med 310:1137, 1984.

49. Stern S, Tzivoni D: Early detection of silent ischemic heart disease by 24 hour electrocardiographic monitoring of active subjects. Br Heart J 36:481, 1974.

50. Cohn PF: Silent myocardial ischemia: Classification, prevalance and prognosis. Am J Med 79:2, 1985.

51. Lichtlen P: The hemodynamics of clinical ischemic heart disease. Ann Clin Res 3:333, 1971.

52. Droste C, Roskamm H: Experimental pain measurements in patients with asymptomatic myocardial ischemia. J Am Coll Cardiol 1:940, 1983.

53. Maseri A, Chierchia S, Davies G: Mechanisms of ischemic pain and silent myocardial ischemia. Am J Med 79:7, 1985.

54. Lichtlen PR: Pathophysiology of coronary and myocardial function in angina pectoris: Important aspects for drug treatment. Eur Heart J 6(Suppl F):11, 1985.

55. Lichtlen PR: Können Medikamente, insbesondere Calcium-Antagonisten, eine Regression der Atherosklerose, speziell der Koronarsklerose, bewirken? Schweiz Med Wochenschr 121:1807, 1991.

56. Lichtlen PR: Medikamentose Prävention der Koronarsklerose. Schweiz Med Wochenschr 121:1922, 1991.

57. Lichtlen PR: Ca-channel blockers as primary preventive drugs in coronary atherosclerosis: Experimental and human studies, an update. *In* Born G, Schwartz CJ (eds): New Horizens in Coronary Heart Disease. London: Current Science Ltd, 1993.

58. Lichtlen PR: Calcium antagonists in human atherosclerosis. Atherosclerosis Review 25:175, 1993.
59. Oliver MF: Reducing cholesterol does not reduce mortality. J Am Coll Cardiol 12:814, 1988.
60. Oliver MF: Cholesterol and coronary disease—outstanding questions. Z Kardiol 80(Suppl 9):57, 1991.
61. Oliver MF: Might treatment of hypercholesterolemia increase non-cardiac mortality? Lancet 337:1529, 1991.
62. Ravnskov U: Cholesterol lowering trials in coronary heart disease: Frequency of citation and outcome. Br Med J 305:15, 1992.
63. Gotto AM, LaRosa JC, Hunninghake D, et al: The cholesterol facts: A summary of the evidence relating dietary fats, serum cholesterol, and coronary heart disease. Circulation 81:1721, 1990.
64. CASS Principal Investigators and their associates: Myocardial infarction and mortality in the Coronary Artery Surgery Study (CASS) randomized trial. N Engl J Med 310:750, 1984.
65. CASS Principal Investigators and their associates: Coronary Artery Surgery Study (CASS): A randomized trial of coronary artery bypass surgery: Comparability of entry characteristics and survival in randomized patients and nonrandomized patients meeting randomization criteria. J Am Coll Cardiol 3:114, 1984.
66. Varnauskas E, The European Coronary Surgery Group: Twelve-year follow-up of survival in the randomized European Coronary Surgery Study. N Engl J Med 319:332, 1988.
67. Kloner RA, Przylenk K, Rahimtoola SH, et al: Myocardial stunning and hibernation: Mechanism and clinical implications. Heart Dis Clin Update 11:241, 1990.
68. Krayenbühl HP, Hirzel H, Hess OM, et al: Hemodynamics of painless ischemia. In von Arnim T, Maseri A (eds): Silent Ischemia. Darmstadt, Germany: Steinkopff, 1987, pp 128–132.
69. Nayler WG: Dihydropyridines and the protection of the ischemic and anoxic myocardium. In Fleckenstein A, Van Breemen C, Gross R, Hoffmeister F (eds): Bayer Symposium IX, Cardiovascular Effects of Dihydropyridine Type Calcium Antagonists and Agonists. Berlin: Springer, 1985, pp 460–471.
70. Mügge A, Förstermann U, Lichtlen PR: Endothelial functions in cardiovascular disease. Z Kardiol 78:147, 1989.
71. Mügge A, Förstermann U, Lichtlen PR: Platelets, endothelium-dependent responses and atherosclerosis. Ann Med 23:145, 1991.
72. Lichtlen PR: Neuere Aspekte über Nitrate und ihre Anwendung bei stabiler und unstabiler Angina pectoris, Präinfarkt-Syndrom und Myokardinfarkt. Internist 33:684, 1992.
73. Basssenge E: Clinical relevance of endothelium-derived relaxing factor (EDRF). Br J Clin Pharmacol 34:375, 1992.
74. Feigl O: The paradox of adrenergic coronary vasoconstriction. Circulation 76:737, 1987.
75. Rowland M: Influence of route of administration on drug availability. J Pharm Sci 61:70, 1972.
76. Opie LH: Drugs and the heart. II: Nitrates. Lancet 1:750, 1980.
77. Lichtlen P: Zur Therapie der Angina pectoris in heutiger Sicht. Z Kreislaufforsch 61:193, 1972.
78. Lichtlen PR: Wirkungsmechanismus der Nitrate, Stand 1988. Z Kardiol 78(Suppl 2):3, 1989.
79. Lichtlen PR, Gattiker K, Halter I: The effects of nitrates (ISDN) on coronary and left ventricular dynamics and exercise in patients with coronary artery disease. In Kaltenbach M, Lichtlen PR (eds): Coronary Heart Disease. Stuttgart: Georg Thieme, 1973, pp 42–56.
80. Bernstein L, Friesinger GC, Lichtlen PR, et al: The effect of nitroglycerin on the systemic and coronary circulation in man and dogs: Myocardial blood flow measured with Xenon 133. Circulation 33:107, 1966.
81. Abrams J: Nitroglycerin and long-acting nitrates. N Engl J Med 302:1234, 1980.
82. Rafflenbeul W, Urthaler F, Russell RO, et al: Dilatation of coronary artery stenosis after isosorbide dinitrate in man. Br Heart J 43:546, 1980.
83. Lichtlen PR, Rafflenbeul W: Effects of calcium-antagonists on fixed and dynamic obstructions in patients with severe coronary artery disease. In Opie LH (ed): Cardiovascular Effects of Dihydropyridine-Type Calcium Antagonists and Agonists. Berlin: Springer, 1985, pp 381–407.
84. Engel HJ, Lichtlen PR: Beneficial enhancement of coronary blood flow by nifedipine: Comparison with nitroglycerin and beta-blocking agents. Am J Med 71:658, 1981.
85. Parker JO, Ferrell B, Lakey KA: Effects of intervals between doses on the development of tolerance to isosorbide dinitrate. N Engl J Med 316:1440, 1987.
86. Rudolph W, Dirschinger J, Reiniger G, et al: When does nitrate tolerance develop? What dosages and which intervals are necessary to ensure maintained effectiveness? Eur Heart J 9(Suppl A):63, 1988.
87. Rudolph W, Dirschinger J, Kraus F, et al: Nitrate therapy in patients with coronary artery disease—preparations and doses with and without development of tolerance. Z Kardiol 79(Suppl III):57, 1990.
88. Hausmann D, Nikutta P, Daniel WG, et al: Once-a-day administration of a high dose of ISDN (120 mg): Influence on circadian variation of transient, reversible ischemic episodes in patients with stable angina pectoris. Z Kardiol 78:415, 1989.
89. Opie LH: Drugs and the heart. I: Beta-blocking agents. Lancet 1:693, 1980.
90. Lichtlen P, Albert H, Moccetti T: L'influence des betablockeurs sur le debit coronaire: Investigation chez l'homme au moyen de Xenon 133. Therapie 25:403, 1970.
91. Lichtlen P, Albert H, Spiegel M: Zur Wirkung der Beta-Rezeptoren-Blockade bei Koronarinsuffizienz. II: Linksventrikuläre Dynamik bei Arbeitsbelastung unter Propranolol und der Kombination von Propranolol und Nitroglycerin. Z Kreislaufforsch 59:207, 1970.
92. Rafflenbeul W, Berger C, Jost S, et al: Constriction of coronary arteries and stenoses with propranolol. Circulation 76:276, 1987.
93. Rafflenbeul W, Berger C, Lichtlen P: Einfluss von Betarezeptorenblockern auf Koronargefässe. In Grosdanoff P, Kaindl F, Kraupp T (eds): Beta-Rezeptoren und Beta-Rezeptorenblocker. Berlin: W de Gruyter, 1987, pp 179–186.
94. Rafflenbeul W, Jost S, Berger C, et al: Wirkung von Kalziumantagonisten und Betarezeptorenblockern auf die Koronarweite. Z Kardiol 78:16–19, 1989.
95. Robertson RM, Wood AJJ, Vaughn WK, Robertson D: Exacerbation of vasotonic angina pectoris by propranolol. Circulation 65:281, 1982.
96. Thadani U: Beta-adrenergic blocking agents for exertional angina pectoris. Herz 7:179, 1982.
97. Johnsson G, Regardh CG: Clinical pharmacokinetics of beta-adrenoreceptor blocking drugs. Clin Pharmacokinet 1:233, 1976.
98. Waal-Manning HJ: Hypertension: Which beta-blocker? Drugs 12:412, 1976.
99. McDevitt DG: Comparison of pharmacokinetic properties of beta-adrenoceptor blocking drugs. Eur Heart J 8(Suppl 2):9, 1988.
100. Lichtlen PR, Engel HJ, Rafflenbeul W: Calcium entry blockers, especially nifedipine, in angina of effort: Possible mechanisms and clinical implications. In Opie LH (ed): Calcium Antagonists and Cardiovascular Disease. New York: Raven Press, 1984, pp 221–236.
101. Heusch G, Guth BD, Seitelberger R, et al: Attenuation of exercise-induced ischemia in dogs with recruitment of coronary vasodilator reserve by nifedipine. Circulation 75:482, 1987.
102. Lichtlen PR, Engel HJ: Assessment of regional myocardial blood flow using the inert gas washout technique. Cardiovasc Intervent Radiol 2:203, 1979.
103. Lichtlen P, Engel HJ, Amende I, et al: Mechanisms of various antianginal drugs: Relationship between regional flow behaviour and contractility. In Jatene AD, Lichtlen PR (eds): 3rd International Adalat Symposium. Amsterdam: Excerpta Medica, 1976, pp 14–29.
104. Lichtlen P, Engel HJ: Coronary dynamics of various antianginal drugs at rest and during exercise measured by the precordial xenon-residue-detection technique. In Lichtlen PR (ed): Coronary Angiography and Angina Pectoris. Stuttgart, Germany: Thieme Verlag, 1976, pp 365–377.
105. Nayler WG, Panagiotopoulos S, Elz JS, et al: Fundamental mechanisms of action of calcium antagonists in myocardial ischemia. Am J Cardiol 59:75B, 1987.

106. Antman E, Muller J, Goldberg S, et al: Nifedipine therapy for coronary artery spasm: Experience in 127 patients. N Engl J Med 302:1269, 1980.
107. Rowland E, Evans I, Krikler DM: Effect of nifedipine on atrioventricular conduction as compared with verapamil. Br Heart J 42:124, 1979.
108. Pepine CJ, Conti CR: Calcium blockers in coronary heart disease. Part II. Mod Concepts Cardiovasc Dis 50:67, 1981.
109. Reil GH, Ertl J, Frombach R, et al: Comparison between the effects of nifedipine and isosorbide dinitrate on changes in myocardial vascular and extravascular space and 47-calcium-exchange in vivo. Z Kardiol 75:204, 1986.
110. Amende I, Simon R, Hood WP, et al: Intracoronary nifedipine in human beings: Magnitude and time course of changes in left ventricular contraction/relaxation and coronary sinus blood flow. J Am Coll Cardiol 2:1141, 1983.
111. Ellrodt G, Christopher Y, Chew C: Therapeutic implications of slow-channel blockade in cardiocirculatory disorders. Circulation 62:669, 1980.
112. Amende I, Simon R, Seegers A: Effects of intravenous verapamil on left ventricular systolic function and diastolic filling dynamics in patients with coronary artery disease: Analysis of intramyocardial markers. Int J Card Imaging 3:169, 1988.
113. Henry PD: Comparative pharmacology of calcium antagonists: Nifedipine, verapamil, and diltiazem. Am J Cardiol 46:1047, 1980.
114. Heesch CM, Miller BM, Thames MD: Effects of calcium channel blockers on isolated carotid baroreceptors and baroreflex. Am J Physiol 245:H653, 1983.
115. Kawai C, Konishi T, Matsuyama E: Comparative effects of three calcium antagonists, diltiazem, verapamil, and nifedipine, on the sinoatrial and atrioventricular nodes. Circulation 63:1035, 1981.
116. Talajic M, Nattel S: Frequency-dependent effects of calcium antagonists on atrioventricular conduction and refractoriness: Demonstration and characterization in anesthetized dogs. Circulation 74:1156, 1986.
117. Aversano T, Becker LC: The resistance of coronary vasodilator reserve despite functionally significant flow reduction. Am J Physiol 248:H403, 1985.
118. Nayler WG: Classification of calcium antagonists. *In* Nayler WG: Calcium-Antagonists. London: Academic Press, 1988, pp 101–129.
119. Nayler WG: Second Generation of Calcium Antagonists. New York: Springer-Verlag, 1991.
120. Henry PD: Antiatherogenic effects of calcium channel blockers: Possible mechanisms of action. Cardiovasc Drugs Ther 4:1015, 1990.
121. Henry PD: Calcium channel blockers and progression of coronary artery disease. Circulation 82:2251, 1990.
122. Henry PD: Atherosclerosis, calcium, and calcium antagonists. Circulation 72:456, 1985.
123. Henry PD, Bentley K: Suppression of atherosclerosis in cholesterol-fed rabbits treated with nifedipine. J Clin Invest 68:1366, 1981.
124. Lichtlen PR, Hugenholtz PG, Rafflenbeul W, et al: Retardation of angiographic progression of coronary artery disease by the calcium channel blocker nifedipine—results of the international nifedipine trial on antiatherosclerotic therapy (INTACT). Lancet 335:1109, 1990.
125. Lichtlen PR, Rafflenbeul W, Nikutta P, et al: The influence of nifedipine on the progression of coronary artery disease in man: The INTACT study. *In* Lichtlen PR, Reale A (eds): Adalat, A Comprehensive Review. Berlin: Springer-Verlag, 1991, pp 203–212.
126. Rouleau JL, Parmley WW, Stevens J, et al: Verapamil suppresses atherosclerosis in cholesterol-fed rabbits. J Am Coll Cardiol 6:1453, 1983.
127. Nayler WG, Dillon JS, Panagiotopoulos S, Sturrock WJ: Dihydropyridines and the ischemic myocardium. *In* Lichtlen PR (ed): 6th Adalat Symposium: New Therapy of Ischemic Heart Disease and Hypertension. Amsterdam: Excerpta Medica, 1986, pp 386–397.
128. Henry PD, Shuchleib R, Davis J, et al: Myocardial contracture and accumulation of mitochondrial calcium in ischemic rabbit heart. Am J Physiol 233:H677, 1977.
129. Bolli R, Hartley CJ, Rabinovitz RS: Clinical relevance of myocardial stunning. Cardiovasc Drugs Ther 5:877, 1991.
130. Przyklenk K, Kloner RA: Calcium antagonists and stunned myocardium: Importance for clinicians? Cardiovasc Drugs Ther 5:947, 1991.
131. Lichtlen P, Halter J, Gattiker K: The effect of isosorbide dinitrate on coronary blood flow, coronary resistance and left ventricular dynamics under exercise in patients with coronary artery disease. Basic Res Cardiol 4:402, 1974.
132. Lichtlen P, Albert H, Spiegel M, et al: Insuffisance coronaire: Evaluation par les tests d'effort de la fonction de ventricule gauche sous propranolol administré—seul ou avec nitroglycerine. Therapie 25:252, 1970.
133. Schang SJ, Pepine CJ: Coronary and myocardial metabolic effects of combined glyceryl trinitrate and propranolol administration: Observations in patients with and without coronary disease. Br Heart J 40:1221, 1978.
134. Baxter RH, Lennox IM: Increased exercise tolerance with nitrates in beta-blocked patients with angina. Br Med J 2:550, 1977.
135. Legrand V, Mancini J: Comparative study of coronary flow reserve, coronary anatomy and results of radionuclide exercise tests in patients with coronary artery disease. J Am Coll Cardiol 8:1022, 1986.
136. Wiener L, Dwyer EM, Cox JW: Hemodynamic effects of nitroglycerin, propranolol, and their combination in coronary heart disease. Circulation 39:623, 1969.
137. Parmley BW: Combination of beta-adrenergic blocking agents and nitrates in the treatment of stable angina pectoris. Cardiovasc Res 3:1425, 1982.
138. Battock DJ, Alvarez H, Chidsey CA: Effects of propranolol and isosorbide dinitrate on exercise performance and adrenergic activity in patients with angina pectoris. Circulation 39:157, 1969.
139. Jensen G, Trautner F, Rasmussen S, et al: Isosorbide dinitrate in effort-induced angina pectoris despite beta-blocking treatment: Clinical and hematological effects assessed by isotope angiocardiography. Circulation 133:3247, 1982.
140. Müller G, Überbacher HJ, Glocke M: Coronary therapeutic effectiveness of low-dose IS-5-MN in comparison with the combination of IS-5-MN and metipranolol and placebo [German]. Medizinische Welt 34:321, 1983.
141. Schaumann HJ: Additional treatment of angina pectoris with ISDN-retard during basic therapy with a beta-blocker. Therapiewoche 33:2333, 1983.
142. Delmare J: Double-blind comparative study of pindolol alone and its association with a nitrate derivative. Nouv Presse Med 7:2733, 1978.
143. Lynch P, Dargie HJ, Krikler S, et al: Objective assessment of antianginal treatment: A double-blind comparison of propranolol, nifedipine, and their combination. Br Med J 2:184, 1980.
144. Ekelund LG, Oroe L: Antianginal efficiency of nifedipine with and without a betablocker, studied with exercise tests: A double-blind, randomized subacute study. Clin Cardiol 2:203, 1979.
145. Braun S, Terdiman R, Berenfeld D: Clinical and hemodynamic effects of combined propranolol and nifedipine therapy versus propranolol alone in patients with angina pectoris. Am Heart J 109:478, 1985.
146. Bassan M, Weiler-Ravell D, Sharev O: The additive antianginal action of oral nifedipine in patients receiving propranolol: Magnitude and duration of effect. Circulation 66:710, 1982.
147. Dargie HJ, Lynch PG, Krickler DM, et al: Nifedipine and propranolol: A beneficial drug interaction. Am J Med 71:676, 1981.
148. Tweddel AC, Beattie IM, Murray RG: The combination of nifedipine and propranolol in the management of patients with angina pectoris. Br J Clin Pharmacol 12:229, 1981.
149. Jenkins RM, Nagle RE: The symptomatic and objective effects of nifedipine in combination with betablocker therapy in severe angina pectoris. Postgrad Med J 58:697, 1982.
150. Uusitalo A, Arstila M, Bae EA: Metoprolol, nifedipine, and the combination in stable effort angina pectoris. Am J Cardiol 57:733, 1986.
151. Kenmure ACF, Scruton JH: A double-blind controlled trial of

the anti-anginal efficacy of nifedipine compared with propranolol. Br J Clin Pharmacol 33:49, 1979.

152. Findlay IN, Dargie JH: The effects of nifedipine, atenolol, and that combination on left ventricular function. Postgrad Med J 59:70, 1983.

153. Subramanian B, Bowles MJ, Davis AB, et al: Combined therapy with verapamil and propranolol in chronic stable angina. Am J Cardiol 49:125, 1982.

154. Winniford MD, Huxley RL, Hillis LD: Randomized, double-blind comparison of propranolol alone and propranolol-verapamil combination in patients with severe angina of effort. J Am Coll Cardiol 1:492, 1983.

155. Leon MB, Rosing DR, Bonow RO, et al: Clinical efficacy of verapamil alone and combined with propranolol in treating patients with stable angina pectoris. Am J Cardiol 48:131, 1981.

156. Nelson GI, Silke B, Akulja RC, et al: The effect on left ventricular performance of nifedipine and metoprolol singly and together on exercise-induced angina pectoris. Eur Heart J 5:67, 1984.

157. Lessem J: Combined therapy with Ca-antagonists and beta-adrenergic receptor blocking agents in chronic stable angina. Acta Med Scand 681(Suppl):83, 1984.

158. Johnston DL, Gebhardt VA, Donald A: Comparative effects of propranolol and verapamil alone and in combination on left ventricular function and volume in patients with chronic exertional angina: A double-blind, placebo-controlled, randomized, cross-over study with radionuclide ventriculography. Circulation 68:1280, 1983.

159. Stone PH, Antman EM, Muller JE, et al: Calcium channel blocking agents in the treatment of cardiovascular disorders. Part II: Hemodynamic effects and clinical applications. Ann Intern Med 93:886, 1980.

160. Walsh RA, Badke FR, O'Rourke RA: Differential effects of systemic and intracoronary calcium channel blocking agents on global and regional left ventricular function in conscious dogs. Am Heart J 102:341, 1981.

161. Strauss WE, Parisi AF: Superiority of combined diltiazem and propranolol therapy for angina pectoris. Circulation 71:951, 1985.

162. Hung I, Lamb IH, Conally SJ, et al: The effect of diltiazem and propranol, alone and in combination, on exercise performance and left ventricular function in patients with stable effort angina: A double-blind, randomized, and placebo-controlled study. Circulation 68:560, 1983.

163. Humen DP, O'Brien P, Purves P, et al: Effort angina with adequate beta-receptor blockade: Comparison with diltiazem alone and in combination. J Am Coll Cardiol 7:329, 1986.

164. Boden WE, Bouge EW, Reichmann MJ, et al: Beneficial effects of high-dose diltiazem in patients with persistent effort angina on betablockers and nitrates: A randomized, double-blind, placebo-controlled cross-over study. Circulation 71:1197, 1985.

165. Urquahrt J, Patterson RE, Bacharach SL, et al: Comparative effects of verapamil, diltiazem, and nifedipine on hemodynamics and left ventricular function during acute myocardial ischemia in dogs. Circulation 69:382, 1984.

166. Winniford MD, Fulton KL, Corbett JR, et al: Propranolol-verapamil versus propranolol-nifedipine in severe angina pectoris of effort: A randomized, double-blind, cross-over study. Am J Cardiol 55:281, 1985.

167. Johnston DL, Lesoway R, Humen DP, et al: Clinical and hemodynamic evaluation of propranolol in combination with verapamil, nifedipine, and diltiazem in exertional angina pectoris: A placebo-controlled, double-blind, randomized, cross-over study. Am J Cardiol 55:680, 1985.

168. Kieval J, Kirsten EG, Kessler KM, et al: The effects of intravenous verapamil on hemodynamic status of patients with coronary artery disease receiving propranolol. Circulation 65:653, 1982.

169. Packer M, Muller J, Medina N, et al: Hemodynamic consequences of combined beta-adrenergic and slow calcium channel blockade in man. Circulation 65:660, 1982.

170. Ross J: Afterload mismatch in aortic and mitral valve disease: Implications for surgical therapy. J Am Coll Cardiol 5:811, 1985.

171. Lichtlen PR: Unstabile Angina pectoris—Status 1985. Hämostasiologie 6:102, 1986.

172. Davies MJ, Thomas AC, Knapman PA, et al: Intramyocardial platelet aggregates in patients with unstable angina suffering sudden ischemic cardiac death. Circulation 73:418, 1986.

173. Fuster V, Badimon L, Badimon JJ, et al: The pathogenesis of coronary artery disease and the acute coronary syndromes. N Engl J Med 326:242(A), 1992.

174. Fuster V, Badimon L, Cohen M, et al: Insight into the pathogenesis of acute ischemic syndromes. Circulation 77:1213, 1988.

175. Hopf R, Pietruska M, Dowinsky S: Combined administration of various doses of nifedipine and isosorbide dinitrate in patients with angina pectoris. In Kaltenbach M, Neufeld HN (eds): Fifth International Adalat Symposium. Amsterdam: Excerpta Medica, 1983, pp 209–216.

176. Parodi O, Maseri A, Simonetti I: Management of unstable angina at rest by verapamil. A double-blind cross-over study in coronary care unit. Br Heart J 41:167, 1979.

177. Waters DD, Théroux P, Szlachcic J, et al: Provocative testing with ergonovine to assess the efficacy of treatment with nifedipine, diltiazem, and verapamil in variant angina. Am J Cardiol 48:123, 1981.

178. Johnson SM, Mauritson DR, Willerson JT, et al: Comparison of verapamil and nifedipine in the treatment of variant angina pectoris: Preliminary observations in 10 patients. Am J Cardiol 47:1295, 1981.

179. Rosenthal SJ, Ginsberg R, Lamb IH, et al: Efficacy of diltiazem for control of symptoms of coronary arterial spasm. Am J Cardiol 46:1027, 1980.

180. Kimura E, Kishida H: Treatment of variant angina with drugs: A survey of 11 cardiology institutes in Japan. Circulation 63:844, 1981.

181. Hill JA, Feldman RL, Pepine CJ, et al: Randomized double-blind comparison of nifedipine and isosorbide dinitrate in patients with coronary arterial spasm. Am J Cardiol 49:431, 1982.

182. Winniford MD, Gabliani G, Johnson SM, et al: Concomitant calcium antagonist plus isosorbide dinitrate therapy for markedly active variant angina. Am Heart J 108:1269, 1984.

183. Held PH, Yussuf S, Furberg CD: Calcium channel blockers in acute myocardial infarction and unstable angina: An overview. Br Med J 299:1187, 1989.

184. Lichtlen P: Nifedipine, a review. In Taira N, Hosoda S, Lichtlen PR (eds): Nifedipine Quarter Century Symposium, Tokyo 1993. Amsterdam: Excerpta Medica, 1994, pp 123–148.

185. Guazzi M, Fioretini C, Polese A, et al: Treatment of spontaneous angina pectoris with betablocking agents. Br Heart J 37:1235, 1975.

186. Tilmant PY, Lablanche JM, Thieuleux FA, et al: Detrimental effect of propranolol in patients with coronary arterial spasm countered by combination with diltiazem. Am J Cardiol 52:230, 1983.

187. Parodi O, Simonetti I, L'Abbate A, et al: Verapamil versus propranolol for angina at rest. Am J Cardiol 50:923, 1982.

188. Théroux P: A pathophysiologic basis for the clinical classification and management of unstable angina. Circulation 75(Suppl V):V-103, 1987.

189. Tolins M, Weir EK, Charles E, et al: Maximal drug therapy is not necessarily optimal in chronic angina patients. J Am Coll Cardiol 3:1051, 1984.

190. Nesto RW, White HD, Ganz P, et al: Addition of nifedipine to maximal betablocker-nitrate therapy: Effects on exercise capacity and global left ventricular performance at rest and during exercise. Am J Cardiol 55:3E, 1985.

191. Jugdutt BI: Nitrates in acute myocardial infarction—state of the art. Z Kardiol 78(Suppl 2):118, 1989.

192. Pfeffer MA, SAVE investigators: Effect of captopril on mortality and morbidity in patients with left ventricular dysfunction after myocardial infarction—results of the survival and ventricular enlargement trial. N Engl J Med 327:669, 1992.

193. Swedberg K, Consensus II: Effects of the early administration of enalapril on mortality in patients with acute myocardial infarction—results of the cooperative new Scandinavian Enalapril Survival Study II (Consensus II). N Engl J Med 327:678, 1992.

194. The SOLVD investigators: Effect of enalapril on mortality and the development of heart failure in asymptomatic patients with reduced left ventricular ejection fractions. N Engl J Med 327:685, 1992.

195. The Captopril Multicenter Research Group I: Cooperative multicenter study of captopril in congestive heart failure: Hemodynamic effects and long-term response. Am Heart J 110:439, 1985.

196. The Consensus Study Trial Group, Consensus II: Effects of enalapril on mortality in severe congestive heart failure: Results of the North Scandinavian enalapril survival study (CONSENSUS). N Engl J Med 316:1429, 1987.

197. The SOLVD investigators: Effects of enalapril on survival in patients with reduced left ventricular ejection fractions and congestive heart failure. N Engl J Med 293:302, 1991.

198. Daly P, Rouleau JL: Conversions-Enzym-Hemmung bei Patienten mit Angina pectoris. Münch Med Wschr 131(Suppl I):31, 1989.

199. Ertl G, Kloner RA, Alexander RW, et al: Limitations of experimental infarct size by an angiotensin-converting enzyme inhibitor. Circulation 65:40, 1982.

200. van Zwieten PA, van Meel JCA, de Jonge A, et al: Zur Pharmakologie vasodilatatorisch wirksamer Pharmaka: neue Entwicklungen. Verh Dtsch Ges Kreislaufforschung 48:78, 1982.

201. Przyklenk K, Kloner RA: Relationship between structure and effects of ACE inhibitors: Comparative effects in myocardial ischaemic reperfusion injury. Br J Clin Pharmacol 28:167S, 1989.

202. Katz RJ, Levy WS, Buff L, et al: Prevention of nitrate tolerance with angiotensin converting enzyme inhibitors. Circulation 83:1271, 1991.

203. Clozel JP, Muller RKM, Roux S, et al: Influence of the status of the renin-angiotensin system on the effect of cilazapril on neointima formation after vascular injury in rats. Circulation 88:1222, 1993.

204. Ertl G, Wichmann J, Schweisfurth H: Aktivierung des Renin-Angiotensin-Systems (RAS) nach kurzzeitigem Koronararterienverschluß (KAV): Günstige Wirkung von Converting-Enzym-Inhibiotr (CEI). Z Kardiol 71:164, 1982.

205. Daly P, Rouleau JL, Cousineau D, et al: Acute effects of captopril on the coronary circulation of patients with hypertension and angina. Am J Med 76(Suppl):111, 1984.

206. Gibbs JSR, Crean PA, Mockus L, et al: The variable effects of angiotensin converting enzyme inhibition on myocardial ischaemia in chronic stable angina. Br Heart J 62:112, 1989.

207. Gibbs JSR, Crean PA, Wright C, et al: The variable effects of angiotensin converting enzyme inhibition on myocardial ischaemia in chronic stable angina. Br Heart J 10(Suppl):82, 1989.

208. Tardieu A, Virot P, Vandroux JC, et al: Effects of captopril on myocardial perfusion in patients with coronary insufficiency: Evaluation by the exercise test and quantitative myocardial tomoscintigraphy using thallium-201. Postgrad Med J 62(Suppl I):38, 1986.

209. Vogt M, Ulbricht LJ, Motz W: Lack of evidence for antianginal effect of enalapril. Circulation 78(Suppl II):328, 1988.

210. Lai C, Onnis E, Orani E, et al: Antiischaemic activity of ACE inhibitor enalapril in normotensive patients. J Am Coll Cardiol 9:192A, 1987.

211. Rietbrock N, Thurmann P, Kirsten R, et al: Antiischamische Wirksamkeit von Enalapril bei koronarer Herzkrankheit. Dtsch Med Wochenschr 113:300, 1988.

212. Odenthal HJ, Thurmann P, Wichmann HW, et al: Behandlung der chronisch stabilen Angina pectoris durch Angiotensin-Converting-Enzym-Hemmung—Eine randomisierte, placebo-kontrollierte, Doppelblind-cross-over-Studie. Z Kardiol 80:392, 1991.

213. Klein WW, Khurmi NS, Eber B, Dusleag J: Effects of benazepril and metoprolol OROS alone and in combination on myocardial ischemia in patients with chronic stable angina. J Am Coll Cardiol 16:948, 1990.

214. Cleland JG, Henderson E, McLenachan J, et al: Effect of captopril, an angiotensin-converting enzyme inhibitor, in patients with angina pectoris and heart failure [see comments]. J Am Coll Cardiol 17:733, 1991; Comment in J Am Coll Cardiol 17:740, 1991.

215. Abrams J: Is there a role for angiotensin-converting enzyme inhibitors in the treatment of chronic myocardial ischemia? J Am Coll Cardiol 16:957, 1990.

216. Packer M, Kukin ML: Management of patients with heart failure and angina: Do coexistent diseases alter the response to cardiovascular drugs? J Am Coll Cardiol 17:740, 1991.

217. Pitt B: Comments—combinations and comparisons. Eur Heart J 6(Suppl A):47, 1985.

218. Tillmanns H, Neumann FJ, Schoeneck V: Microcirculatory disturbances in stunned myocardium. Circulation 76(Suppl IV):147, 1987.

219. Parker JO: Nitrate therapy in stable angina pectoris. N Engl J Med 316:1635, 1987.

220. Bussmann WD, Passek D, Seidel W, et al: Reduction of CK and CK-MB indices of infarct size by intravenous nitroglycerin. Circulation 63:615, 1981.

221. Yussuf S, Collins R, MacMahan S, et al: Effect of intravenous nitrates on mortality in acute myocardial infarction: An overview of the randomized trials. Lancet 1:1088, 1988.

222. ISIS 4: Randomised study of oral isosorbide mononitrate in over 50000 patients with suspected acute myocardial infarction. ISIS Collaborative Group, Oxford, UK [abstract]. Circulation 88(Suppl 4, part 2):I-394 , 1993.

223. Rafflenbeul W: Medikamentöse Prophylaxe kardiovaskulärer Erkrankungen mit Calcium Antagonisten. Z Kardiol 81(Suppl IV):211, 1992.

224. SPRINT, The Israeli Study Group: Secondary prevention reinfarction Israeli nifedipine trial. Eur Heart J 9:354, 1988.

225. Packer M, Frishman WH: Verapamil therapy for stable and unstable angina pectoris: Calcium channel antagonists in perspective. Am J Cardiol 50:881, 1982.

226. Lichtlen PR: Therapeutic options with the long-acting calcium antagonist amlodipine: Results of the CAPE study. J Cardiovasc Pharmacol 24(Suppl B):S21, 1994.

227. Resnekov L: Silent myocardial ischemia: Therapeutic implications. Am J Med 79(Suppl 3A):30, 1985.

228. Quyyumi AA, Crake T, Wright CM, et al: Medical treatment of patients with severe exertional and rest angina: Double-blind comparison of beta-blocker, calcium-antagonist, and nitrate. Br Heart J 57:505, 1987.

229. Imperi GA, Lambert CR, Loy K, et al: Effects of titrated beta blockade (metoprolol) on silent myocardial ischemia in ambulatory patients with coronary artery disease. Am J Cardiol 60:519, 1987.

230. Hausmann D, Nikutta P, Trappe H-J, et al: Incidence of ventricular arrhythmias during transient myocardial ischemia in patients with stable coronary artery disease. J Am Coll Cardiol 16:49, 1990.

231. Born GVR: Antithrombotic drugs in the treatment of coronary heart disease: The present situation with aspirin. Z Kardiol 79(Suppl III):147, 1990.

CHAPTER 8

Combination Therapy in Congestive Heart Failure

Kanu Chatterjee, M.B., F.R.C.P.

Adequate management of acute or chronic congestive heart failure frequently requires a combination of various pharmacologic agents. The more severe the heart failure is, the more likely the need for combination therapy. Until recently, diuretics and digitalis glycosides were the only pharmacologic agents at the disposal of the physician caring for patients with heart failure. Currently, however, vasodilators, newer inotropic agents, β-adrenergic blocking agents, and immunosuppressive drugs have been included in the armamentarium. In addition, the roles of nonpharmacologic therapeutic approaches, such as intraaortic balloon counterpulsation and other cardiac assistive devices and cardiac transplantation in the management of certain subsets of patients with heart failure, have been explored. The rationale and effectiveness of some of these therapeutic modalities are well established, and others are undergoing evaluation.

Combination of pharmacologic agents should be based not only on physiologic and pharmacologic principles but also on specific therapeutic goals. Familiarity with the hemodynamic effects of various vasoactive and inotropic agents optimizes hemodynamic improvement during combination therapy. It should be emphasized that the effectiveness of drugs used for the treatment of heart failure also partly depends on the cause and the pathophysiologic mechanisms of heart failure. Inotropic and vasodilator agents, for example, are rarely effective when heart failure results primarily from left ventricular diastolic dysfunction and not from impaired systolic function. To ensure appropriate combination therapy, one must consider the cause of heart failure, therapeutic goals, and the expected hemodynamic and clinical effects of the various drugs that might help patients with heart failure. This chapter reviews the rationale and practical applications of combination therapy in the management of acute and chronic heart failure.

RATIONALE FOR THE USE OF DIFFERENT THERAPEUTIC MODALITIES
Vasodilator Therapy

The major objective of vasodilator therapy is to decrease ventricular afterload, ejection impedance, and preload when these determinants of cardiac performance are disproportionately elevated and contribute to the hemodynamic derangements and symptoms of heart failure.[1, 2]

Depressed ventricular systolic function, irrespective of the primary mechanism, is the most common cause of heart failure. When impaired systolic function results from decreased contractility and is not accompanied by a decrease in left ventricular ejection impedance, end-systolic and end-diastolic volumes increase. With ventricular dilatation, ventricular wall stress (afterload) increases because hypertrophy (wall thickness) is usually inadequate to normalize the wall stress. In addition to ventricular volume and wall thickness, intraventricular pressures contribute to wall stress (Laplace relationship). Vasodilators can reduce afterload by decreasing either intraventricular pressure or ventricular volume. Some vasodilators decrease afterload primarily by lowering systolic pressure, systemic vascular resistance, or both (e.g., hydralazine). Others decrease afterload by decreasing ventricular volumes (e.g., nitrates). Some vasodilators with balanced effects on arterial and venous beds (e.g., angiotensin-converting enzyme [ACE] inhibitors, nitroprusside) reduce left ventricular afterload by decreasing both ventricular pressure and volume. As afterload decreases, systemic hemodynamics and cardiac performance improve.

Aortic or left ventricular ejection impedance is frequently elevated in patients with congestive heart failure,[3] and reduction of aortic impedance is associated with improved left ventricular performance.[4, 5] Aortic impedance is a measure of instantaneous changes of aortic pressure and flow and incorporates arterial compliance and systemic vascular resistance. Systemic vascular resistance is primarily determined by arteriolar tone, which is regulated by interacting neuroendocrine influences. Vasodilators can decrease arteriolar tone as well as increase arterial compliance, thereby reducing left ventricular ejection impedance. Vasodilators may also decrease peripheral venous tone, cause venous pooling, and reduce venous return to the heart, with consequent reduction of intracardiac volumes. Relative changes in arterial and venous tone vary and are partly related to the type of vasodilators used.

The changes in systemic hemodynamics appear to be determined largely by the peripheral vascular effects of the vasodilators. Drugs that are predominantly venodilators decrease ventricular diastolic volumes and pressures, and systemic vascular resistance may not decrease significantly. Arteriolar dilators, on the other hand, decrease systemic vascular resistance and increase stroke volume and cardiac output with little or no change in ventricular filling pressures. It is apparent that when the objectives of therapy are to decrease both afterload and preload, a combination of arteriolar and venodilator or vasodilator drugs with balanced venodilating and arteriolar dilating properties is more likely to produce optimal hemodynamic changes.

Increased peripheral vascular tone in heart failure results from activation of various interacting neuroendocrine systems.[6] Enhanced sympathetic activity is frequent and is evident from the increased levels of circulating catecholamines. Norepinephrine and dopamine levels and, occasionally, epinephrine levels are increased, particularly in patients with decompensated heart failure. Activation of the peripheral α-receptors results in increased systemic vascular tone. Cardiac and renal sympathetic activity are also increased. In approximately two thirds of patients with overt heart failure, plasma renin activity is higher than normal. The mechanism for the activation of the renin system in heart failure remains unclear and is likely to be multifactorial. Decreased renal perfusion, increased sympathetic activity, decreased tubular sodium load, and the use of diuretics all may contribute to this activation. Increased renin production is associated with increased angiotensin I and angiotensin II. The latter is the active vasoconstrictor. Angiotensin also promotes release of neuronal norepinephrine, as well as synthesis and release of aldosterone from the adrenal glands. These angiotensin-mediated neuroendocrine changes also increase systemic vascular tone. Reduction of angiotensin II is associated with peripheral vasodilation, which is the principal rationale for the use of the ACE inhibitors.

Another vasoconstrictor hormone, vasopressin, is also elevated in some patients with heart failure. Increased levels of vasopressin result despite hyponatremia and lower effective plasma osmolality, which indicates that vasopressin release in heart failure is not regulated by the osmoreceptors. Vasopressin levels tend to decrease with increased cardiac output and stroke volume. Thus, vasopressin-mediated vasoconstriction can be attenuated by improving left ventricular function. However, specific vasopressin antagonists also decrease systemic vascular resistance.

Counterbalancing vasodilating systems are activated in patients with heart failure. An increased concentration of the metabolites of the vasodilator prostaglandins has been observed in patients with increased plasma renin activity and angiotensin II levels.[7] Atrial natriuretic peptide, which also produces vasodilation in addition to diuresis and natriuresis, is released in higher concentrations, probably in response to increased atrial and ventricular wall stress.[8] Despite increased concentrations of these vasodilator substances, exogenous prostacyclin and atrial natriuretic peptides produce vasodilation in patients with heart failure.[9] Vasodilator drugs with different mechanisms of action apparently decrease peripheral vascular tone and can improve left ventricular performances (Table 8-1). However, the hemodynamic effects of these vasodilators may differ sufficiently, and the combination of some of these vasodilators provides hemodynamic advantages.

Inotropic Therapy

Depressed contractile function usually initiates pump failure in patients with dilated cardiomyopathy. A

Table 8–1. **Various Vasodilators Used in Heart Failure**

Direct-acting vasodilators
Hydralazine, minoxidil, nitroglycerin and nitrates, nitroprusside, and molsidomine
α-Adrenergic blocking agents
Prazosin, trimazosin, terazosin, phentolamine (Regitine), phenoxybenzamine, and clonidine
Angiotensin antagonists
Saralasin, teprotide, captopril, enalapril, enalaprilat, and lisinopril
β_2-Receptor agonists
Pirbuterol, terbutaline, and salbutamol
Calcium antagonists
Nifedipine, diltiazem, felodipine, and isradipine
Prostaglandins
Prostacyclin
Serotonin antagonist
Ketanserin

reduction of the myocardial functional units (myocardial infarction) or a generalized decrease in myocardial contractile function (dilated cardiomyopathy) may precipitate pump failure. The rationale for inotropic therapy is to improve pump function by increasing contractility.

Drugs with positive inotropic effects enhance contractility, either by increasing the availability of Ca^+ to the contractile myofilaments or by increasing the responsiveness of the myofilaments to Ca^{2+}.[10–12] The mechanisms by which the different inotropic agents exert positive inotropic effect are not similar. β_1-Adrenergic receptor agonists activate the adenylate cyclase system and increase cyclic adenosine monophosphate (cAMP) and intracellular calcium concentration. Phosphodiesterase inhibitors retard degradation of cAMP, increase cAMP levels, and increase the available calcium to the contractile elements. Digitalis glycosides increase the calcium transients by inhibiting the membrane-located sodium pump and activating the Na^+ and Ca^{2+} exchange mechanism. Some inotropic agents, such as sulmazole and pimobendan, appear to enhance the sensitivity of the contractile units to intracellular calcium. Forskolin, a diterpene compound, directly activates the catalytic unit of the adenylate cyclase, which produces a marked increase in cardiac cAMP production.[13] Dibutyryl cAMP is a phosphodiesterase-resistant cyclic nucleotide analogue, and its pharmacologic effects are similar to those of increased intracellular cAMP.[14] The slow calcium channel agonists exert positive inotropic effects by promoting calcium influx.[15] Inosine and adenosine have been reported to improve contractile function by facilitating myocardial adenine nucleotide repletion and improving myocardial metabolic function.[16] Coenzyme Q10, a mitochondrial respiratory chain redox component, appears to enhance cardiac performance by also improving myocardial metabolic function.[17] Some positive inotropic agents enhance contractile function by multiple mechanisms. Vesnarinone decreases inward and outward rectifying K^+ currents and increases action potential duration. It also increases intracellular Na^+ by prolonged opening of sodium channels. Vesnarinone also inhibits cardiospecific phosphodiesterase.[18, 19] The principal mechanisms for the positive inotropic effects of the various agents that either are already available for clinical use or are undergoing clinical evaluation are summarized in Table 8–2. Because the different drugs increase contractility by different mechanisms, it may be possible to combine inotropic agents of different classes for their synergistic effects.

Combination of Vasodilator and Inotropic Therapy

The rationale for combining inotropic and vasodilator drugs is to produce optimal hemodynamic effects and improve cardiac performance. The hemodynamic advantages of such combination therapy can be explained by analyzing the effects of vasodilators and inotropic agents on the left ventricular pressure-volume loops and the end-systolic pressure and volume relations[4] (Fig. 8–1). The pressure-volume loop describes left ventricular performance. During the diastolic filling phase, when both mitral and aortic valves are closed, left ventricular filling occurs along its exponential passive pressure-volume relation. After atrial contraction, it reaches end-diastolic volume or the preload point. During the isovolumic systole, ventricular pressure rises without any change in volume. After the opening of the aortic valve, left ventricular ejection starts and continues until the aortic valve closes. Left ventricular pressure then falls during the isovolumic relaxation phase. The mitral valve opens after the left ventricular pressure matches the left atrial pressure, and filling occurs again. The horizontal limbs of the loop represent the difference between end-diastolic and end-systolic volume or stroke

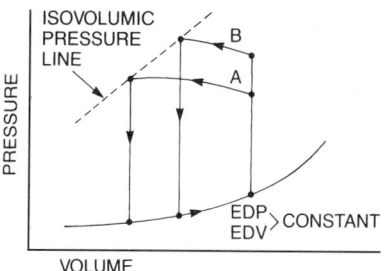

Figure 8–1. Effects of changing afterload on pressure-volume loops. The pressure-volume loop describes left ventricular performance. During the diastolic filling phase, left ventricular filling occurs along its exponential pressure-volume relation. During isovolumic systole with both mitral and aortic valves closed, ventricular pressure rises without any change in volume. The ejection phase begins with the opening of the aortic valve and continues until the aortic valve closes. The horizontal limbs of the pressure-volume loop represent the stroke volume. Left ventricular pressure then falls during the isovolumic relaxation phase, and ventricular filling recommences with mitral valve opening. The end point of ejection (i.e., end-systolic volume) and dicrotic notch pressure tend to fall on the same line, the isovolumic pressure line, irrespective of changes in afterload. A reduction in afterload is associated with a downward shift of the end ejection point on the same isovolumic pressure line. If preload (end-diastolic pressure [EDP], end-diastolic volume [EDV]) remains constant, there is an increase in stroke volume from point *B* to point *A*. (From Parmley WW, Chatterjee K: Vasodilator therapy. Curr Probl Cardiol 2:4, 1978.)

Table 8–2. Mechanisms of Action of the Positive Inotropic Drugs

Digitalis glycosides
Inhibition of "sodium pump" and activation of Na^+/Ca^{2+} exchange
β-Adrenergic
Activation of adenylate cyclase and increased cyclic adenosine monophosphate (cAMP) generation
Forskolin
Activation of the catalytic unit of adenylate cyclase and increased production of cAMP
Phosphodiesterase inhibitors
Decreased degradation of cAMP
Dibutyryl cAMP
Resistance to phosphodiesterase
Glucagon
Increased cAMP content
Calcium-channel agonists
Increased calcium influx
Sulmazole, pimobendan
Increased sensitivity of the contractile elements to calcium
Inosine, adenosine, coenzyme Q10
Improved myocardial metabolic function
Vesnarinone
Inhibition of K^+ currents and increased action potential duration
Increased NA^+ transients
Inhibition of phosphodiesterase

---

volume. Experiments in isolated hearts have demonstrated that the end point of systolic contractions (end-systolic volume and dicrotic notch pressure) tends to fall on the same line (isovolumic pressure line), regardless of changes in preload and afterload. This occurs if the contractile function remains unchanged.[20, 21] With an increase in contractile state, the isovolumic pressure line shifts up and to the left. If there is no change in end-diastolic volume, stroke volume (width of the loop) increases. Reduction of afterload is associated with a downward shift of the end-systolic pressure point on the same isovolumic pressure line. If there is no concomitant decrease in end-diastolic volume, there is a further increase in stroke volume (Fig. 8–2). If, however, end-diastolic volume also decreases during vasodilator therapy, the magnitude of increase in stroke volume during combined inotropic and vasodilator therapy is curtailed.

The rationale for vasodilator, inotropic, and combined inotropic and vasodilator therapy is further illustrated in Figure 8–3. Myocardial failure is the principal mechanism of heart failure in most patients. A reduction in overall contractile function, resulting from myocardial failure, is usually associated with decreased cardiac output. A reduction in cardiac output causes a reflex increase in systemic vascular resistance, which increases the resistance to left ventricular ejection. Because ejection impedance and stroke volume are inversely related, a further reduction in cardiac output occurs, thus establishing a vicious circle. The rationale for inotropic therapy is to break the vicious circle by increasing cardiac output by enhancing contractile function. The rationale for vasodilator therapy is to decrease resistance of left ventricular ejection and increase cardiac output. The combination

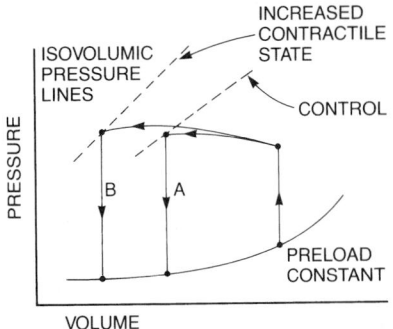

Figure 8–2. Effects of increased contractile state on pressure-volume loops and isovolumic pressure lines. With an increase in the contractile state, the isovolumic pressure line shifts to the left. *A* is the control pressure-volume loop, and *B* is the pressure-volume loop with increased contractile state. With preload constant, the horizontal limb of the pressure-volume loop increased with increased contractile state, indicating increased stroke volume. (From Parmley WW, Chatterjee K: Vasodilator therapy. Curr Probl Cardiol 2:4, 1978.)

of these two principles to increase cardiac output probably synergistically improves systemic hemodynamics and cardiac performance of patients with heart failure.

It should be emphasized that the net increase in stroke volume with vasodilator or inotropic therapy is related partly to the initial level and magnitude of the reduction in filling pressure. The ventricular function curve is curvilinear, and patients with heart failure with elevated filling pressures function on the flat portion of the ventricular function curve. In these patients, a reduction in filling pressure results in only a slight decrease in stroke volume. The net effect of the concomitant reduction in ejection impedance is usually a substantial increase in stroke volume. However, when the initial filling pressure is lower, a decrease in filling pressure of similar magnitude is associated with a greater decrease in stroke volume. The net effect is no change, a slight increase, or even a decrease in stroke volume. Venodilators decrease filling pressure more than the predominant arteriolar dilators do, which tend to decrease systemic vascular resistance by greater magnitudes. Thus, combining a vasodilator with the inotropic drugs should be based

on specific goals. If a reduction in filling pressures is desired, an agent that is predominantly a venodilator is preferable. On the other hand, if the increase in stroke volume and cardiac output is inadequate with inotropic therapy, an addition of predominantly arteriolar dilator is more likely to further increase stroke volume.

Another rationale for the combination of inotropic and vasodilator therapy is to counteract the potentially deleterious effects of vasodilator and inotropic agents on coronary hemodynamics and myocardial metabolic function. Vasodilators, in general, decrease left ventricular outflow resistance and arterial pressure and usually do not induce reflex tachycardia in patients with heart failure. They also do not exert direct positive inotropic effects. With some vasodilators, left ventricular volumes decrease. Thus, in general, myocardial oxygen consumption tends to decrease. Some vasodilators, such as nitroglycerin, sodium nitroprusside, and calcium antagonists, can cause dilation of the epicardial coronary arteries. An increase in collateral blood flow and redistribution of flow within the myocardium, with the use of some vasodilators such as nitroglycerin, may improve perfusion to the ischemic myocardium. The major disadvantage of vasodilator therapy is the reduction of coronary artery perfusion pressure, which can potentially enhance myocardial ischemia. However, the addition of vasopressor and inotropic agents to the vasodilators can maintain the perfusion pressure and prevent ischemia.

Inotropic agents in general increase myocardial oxygen consumption by increasing contractility, which is a major determinant of myocardial oxygen requirements. The addition of a vasodilator, which decreases the other determinants of oxygen requirements, may prevent an excessive increase in myocardial oxygen consumption. Thus, vasodilator and inotropic therapy can counteract the potentially deleterious effects of each other on coronary hemodynamics and myocardial metabolic function.

Diuretics

Diuretics are important in the management of heart failure and are frequently combined with vasodilator

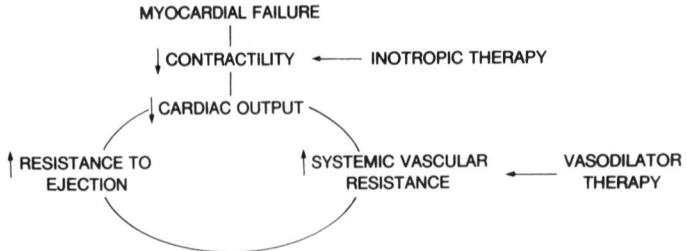

Figure 8–3. Rationale for vasodilator, inotropic, and combination of vasodilator and inotropic therapy in heart failure. Myocardial failure is associated with decreased contractile state, which decreases cardiac output. Systemic vascular resistance and resistance to left ventricular ejection increase in response to low cardiac output. Resistance to left ventricular ejection and stroke volume are inversely related. Thus, increased systemic vascular resistance causes further reduction in cardiac output. The rationale for vasodilator therapy is to increase cardiac output by decreasing systemic vascular resistance. The rationale for inotropic therapy is to increase cardiac output by increasing the contractile state. The combination of vasodilator and inotropic agents produces synergistic effects on systemic hemodynamics and cardiac performance.

and inotropic therapy. The major hemodynamic objective for diuretic therapy is to decrease intracardiac volumes, thereby decreasing systemic and pulmonary venous pressures. Reduction of filling pressure, however, is not associated with any increase in cardiac output. With an excessive decrease in filling pressure, stroke volume and cardiac output may actually decrease as the patient's cardiac function moves toward the steep portion of the ventricular function curve. In this respect, the effects of diuretics are similar to those of venodilators such as nitroglycerin. Thus, a combination of diuretics and venodilators, although effective in decreasing systemic and pulmonary venous pressures, may be inadequate to maintain cardiac output. In these circumstances, the addition of arteriolar dilators or inotropic agents may be required to increase cardiac output.

HEMODYNAMIC EFFECTS
Vasodilator Drugs

Effective combination of the various vasodilators and inotropic agents is aided by an understanding of the systemic and regional hemodynamic effects of these drugs. The systemic hemodynamic changes of the vasodilator drugs are determined primarily by their effects on the peripheral vascular beds. Drugs that are predominantly venodilators decrease systemic and pulmonary venous pressures, resulting in little or no increase in cardiac output. In patients with heart failure and elevated filling pressures, mean arterial pressure, systemic vascular resistance, and heart rate usually remain unchanged. However, in the case of arteriolar dilators, cardiac output increases along with decreased systemic vascular resistance. Systemic and pulmonary venous pressures usually do not change except in the presence of mitral regurgitation, when pulmonary capillary wedge pressure decreases along with decreased regurgitant volume. There is usually no significant change in heart rate or mean arterial pressure. The drugs with combined arteriolar and venodilating properties tend to decrease systemic and pulmonary venous pressures and increase cardiac output. The systemic hemodynamic effects of commonly used vasodilators are summarized in Table 8–3.

The regional hemodynamic effects of various vasodilator drugs may also vary. ACE inhibitors transiently decrease coronary vascular resistance and increase coronary blood flow.[22] However, subsequently, coronary blood flow and myocardial oxygen consumption tend to decrease as myocardial oxygen requirements decrease.[23] Nitroglycerin and nitrates also decrease myocardial oxygen consumption.[24] Nitroglycerin can also improve perfusion to the ischemic myocardium by causing vasodilation of the epicardial coronary arteries and increasing collateral blood flow.[25] The effects of hydralazine and prazosin on coronary hemodynamics and myocardial oxygen consumption are unpredictable. Myocardial oxygen consumption may decrease, increase, or remain unchanged.[23] In patients with chronic heart failure due to primary dilated cardiomyopathy, nifedipine, a calcium antagonist, tends to increase coronary blood flow and decrease myocardial oxygen extraction, both at rest and during exercise. There is usually no change in myocardial oxygen consumption.[26] Thus, ACE inhibitors and nitrates are particularly effective in decreasing myocardial oxygen consumption, and nifedipine is particularly effective in enhancing myocardial perfusion by decreasing coronary arterial resistance. In patients with evidence of myocardial ischemia, nitrates, ACE inhibitors, and calcium antagonists may help, because these agents can reduce myocardial ischemia.

Renal function is frequently compromised in patients with heart failure due to impaired renal perfusion. Neuroendocrine dysfunction appears to contribute to renal failure. Thus, vasodilator drugs, which can improve renal function, may be of particular benefit in the management of such patients. Hydralazine and sodium nitroprusside tend to increase renal plasma flow without causing any significant change in glomerular filtration rate.[27] ACE inhibitors also increase renal plasma flow and occasionally glomerular filtration rate if arterial pressures do not fall significantly.[28] In patients with low cardiac output and relative hypotension, ACE inhibitors may cause deterioration of renal function even when there is a modest decrease in arterial pressure.[29] This has been explained by the inhibition of the renal angiotensin II–mediated compensatory increase in the efferent

Table 8–3. **Expected Systemic Hemodynamic Effects of Commonly Used Vasodilators in Treatment of Heart Failure**

	HR	MAP	CO	PCWP	RAP
Sodium nitroprusside	↔ ↓	↓ ↔	↑ ↑	↓	↓
Nitroglycerin (IV)	↔ ↓	↓ ↔	↑ ↔	↓ ↓	↓ ↓
Nitroglycerin or nitrates	↔	↓ ↔	↔ ↑	↓ ↓	↓ ↓
Hydralazine, minoxidil	↑ ↔	↔ ↓	↑ ↑	↔ ↓	↔ ↓
Hydralazine + nitrates	↔	↔ ↓	↑ ↑	↓ ↓	↓ ↓
Prazosin, trimazosin	↔	↓	↑	↓	↓
Captopril, enalapril, and lisinopril	↔ ↓	↓	↑	↓ ↓	↓ ↓
Captopril + hydralazine	↔ ↓	↓ ↓	↑ ↑	↓ ↓	↓ ↓
Captopril + prazosin	↔	↓ ↓	↑ ↑	↓ ↓	↓ ↓

CO, cardiac output; HR, heart rate; MAP, mean arterial pressure; PCWP, pulmonary capillary wedge pressure; RAP, right atrial pressure; ↔, no change; ↓, moderate decrease; ↓ ↓, marked decrease; ↑, moderate increase; ↑ ↑, marked increase.

glomerular arteriolar tone, which tends to maintain glomerular filtration.

The calcium antagonists such as nifedipine, nisoldipine, and diltiazem can also improve renal perfusion by decreasing efferent arteriolar tone. However, a marked reduction in systemic arterial pressure may decrease renal perfusion pressure and compromise renal function.[30, 31] Limb blood flow increases in response to hydralazine, prazosin, ACE inhibitors, and calcium antagonists.[32] With nitroglycerin and nitrates, limb venous capacitance increases with little or no change in limb vascular resistance. Arteriolar dilators usually do not affect venous capacitance. Skeletal muscle blood flow usually does not increase significantly after acute administration of vasodilators; however, nitrates, a combination of hydralazine and nitrates, and ACE inhibitors improve exercise tolerance and duration of treadmill exercise during chronic maintenance therapy, indicating increased skeletal muscle blood flow.[33, 34] The potential long-term benefits of α-adrenergic blocking drugs such as prazosin and trimazosin in improving exercise tolerance of patients with chronic congestive heart failure have been evaluated in both controlled and uncontrolled studies, with conflicting results. In some studies, a substantial benefit was observed; in others, long-term clinical benefit and improvement in exercise tolerance were lacking.[35–42] When used alone, hydralazine and minoxidil, the arteriolar dilators, do not cause any significant increase in max VO_2 and exercise duration[43]; thus, these drugs should be used in combination with nitrates or ACE inhibitors when long-term clinical benefit is anticipated.

Hepatic blood flow is not significantly influenced by nitrates. Hydralazine and prazosin may increase hepatic blood flow, whereas ACE inhibitors may cause a reduction. Thus, in patients with compromised liver function, it is desirable, whenever possible, to combine ACE inhibitors with hydralazine or prazosin.

Inotropic Agents

The systemic hemodynamic effects of the inotropic agents in clinical use are qualitatively similar (Table 8–4). However, there are some differences, particularly between the hemodynamic effects of different catecholamines, which should be considered during their application in the management of acute or chronic heart failure patients. Because of potent α-receptor agonist activity and less pronounced β-agonist action, norepinephrine increases arterial pressure and systemic vascular resistance with little or no increase in cardiac output. Neo-Synephrine and methoxamine are predominantly α-receptor agonists. Their principal hemodynamic effect is an increase in systemic vascular resistance and arterial pressure. The most frequently used catecholamines in the critical care and postsurgical units are dopamine and dobutamine. Their systemic hemodynamic effects differ somewhat. Dobutamine, a synthetic catecholamine,

possesses β₁-, β₂-, and α-receptor activating properties. However, its β₁-agonist activity is far greater than its β₂- or α-receptor stimulating action. Thus, with dobutamine, there is usually a substantial increase in cardiac output with little or no change in mean arterial pressure. Systolic blood pressure, however, tends to increase with increased stroke volume, although diastolic blood pressure tends to fall as systemic vascular resistance declines.[44, 45] Tachycardia and hypotension are observed, although infrequently when large dosages of dobutamine (exceeding 10 to 15 μg/kg/min) are used. Prenalterol, a partial β-receptor agonist, and dibutyryl cAMP produce hemodynamic effects similar to those of dobutamine.[46, 47]

The systemic hemodynamic effects of dopamine vary with the dosage used.[48–50] With a very low dosage (1 to 2 μg/kg/min), renal and mesenteric vasodilation occurs along with decreased systemic vascular resistance, primarily because of activation of dopamine-2 (DA2) receptors. Decreased norepinephrine release resulting from activation of DA2 receptors may contribute to a reduction in systemic vascular tone. There is usually a modest increase in cardiac output with little or no change in mean arterial pressure or heart rate. However, renal plasma flow, renal function, and urine output tend to improve. When the dosage is increased to 5 to 10 μg/kg/min, β₁-receptors are stimulated. This is the mechanism for the positive inotropic effect of dopamine. With this dosage, cardiac output increases, pulmonary capillary wedge pressure falls, and there is usually a significant decrease in systemic vascular resistance with no change in arterial pressure. However, heart rate may increase. With further increases in the dopamine dose, α-receptors are activated, resulting in peripheral vasoconstriction, increased systemic vascular resistance, and increased arterial pressure. There is no further increase in cardiac output. Indeed, it may decrease with increasing systemic vascular resistance. With larger doses of dopamine, total pulmonary resistance and pulmonary capillary wedge pressure may also increase. In contrast, with increasing doses of dobutamine, pulmonary and systemic vascular resistance and pulmonary capillary wedge pressure tend to decrease.[44, 45] Thus, when an increase in pulmonary resistance or pulmonary capillary wedge pressure is undesirable, as in patients with predominantly right-sided heart failure, dobutamine is preferable to dopamine. However, to correct hypotension, dopamine is the drug of choice. It has been suggested that in some patients with severe pump failure, a combination of lower doses of dopamine and dobutamine may provide hemodynamic advantages without producing the potential adverse effects of each drug. However, the most frequent clinical indication of such a combination is to improve renal function with a low dose of dopamine after systemic hemodynamics have improved with dobutamine.

The hemodynamic effects of digoxin, when given intravenously in patients with chronic congestive heart failure, were similar to those following chronic

Table 8–4. **Expected Systemic Hemodynamic Effects of Inotropic or Ino-Vasodilator Agents in Treatment of Heart Failure**

	HR	MAP	CO	PCWP	RAP
Norepinephrine	↔ ↑	↑ ↑	↔ ↑	↑ ↔	↑ ↔
Isoproterenol	↑ ↑	↓	↑ ↑	↓	↓
Epinephrine	↑ ↑	↑ ↔	↑ ↑	↑ ↔	↑ ↔
Dopamine	↑	↑ ↑	↑ ↔	↑ ↔	↑ ↔
Dobutamine	↔ ↑	↔ ↓	↑ ↑	↓ ↔	↑ ↔
Salbutamol	↔ ↑	↓ ↔	↑	↔ ↓	↔ ↓
Pirbuterol	↔ ↑	↓ ↔	↑	↔ ↓	↔ ↓
Prenalterol	↔ ↓	↔ ↓	↑	↔ ↓	↔ ↓
Levodopa	↔ ↑	↔ ↑	↑	↔	↔
Ibopamine	↔ ↑	↔	↑	↑ ↔	↑ ↔
Phosphodiesterase inhibitors (amrinone, milrinone, and enoximone)	↑ ↔	↓ ↔	↑ ↑	↓ ↓	↓ ↓
Pimobendan	↑ ↔	↓ ↔	↑	↓	↓
Vesnarinone	↔ ↑	↔ ↓	↑	↓	↓

CO, cardiac output; HR, heart rate; MAP, mean arterial pressure; PCWP, pulmonary capillary wedge pressure; RAP, right atrial pressure; ↔, no change; ↓, moderate decrease; ↓ ↓, marked decrease; ↑, moderate increase; ↑ ↑, marked increase.

maintenance therapy. A substantial increase in cardiac output and a fall in pulmonary and systemic venous pressures without a significant change in mean arterial pressure and heart rate are expected.[51] In patients with acute myocardial infarction, however, intravenously administered digoxin does not produce consistent beneficial hemodynamic effects.[52] Although dobutamine causes a predictable increase in cardiac output and a decrease in pulmonary capillary wedge pressure, such changes are not usually seen with digoxin in patients with acute myocardial infarction. Furthermore, the more severe the left ventricular failure is, the less effective is digoxin. Thus, digoxin therapy is primarily indicated for the treatment of chronic heart failure rather than for heart failure accompanying acute myocardial infarction.

The systemic hemodynamic effects of the phosphodiesterase inhibitors are similar despite their structural differences.[52–60] There is usually a marked increase in cardiac output as well as decreases in systemic and pulmonary venous pressures and systemic and pulmonary vascular resistance. However, mean arterial pressure may decrease and heart rate may increase, usually only slightly. With larger doses of phosphodiesterase inhibitors (e.g., amrinone, milrinone, and enoximone), marked hypotension and tachycardia may occur. The systemic hemodynamic effects of the inotropic agents in the treatment of heart failure are summarized in Table 8–4.

Conceivably, inotropic drugs, with different mechanisms of action, could be combined to optimize the inotropic response. In clinical practice, in patients with severe refractory heart failure, newer inotropic agents are frequently added to digitalis. Addition of a phosphodiesterase inhibitor to a catecholamine is likely to produce synergistic effects on contractile function. However, dobutamine should be combined with phosphodiesterase inhibitors with caution, because hypotension can occur. The expected systemic hemodynamic effects of vasoactive and inotropic drugs in the treatment of heart failure are summarized in Table 8–5.

Diuretics

The systemic hemodynamic effects of diuretics are generally similar, regardless of the types of diuretics used and their mechanisms of action. After acute intravenous administration of furosemide in patients with acute myocardial infarction complicated by left ventricular failure, a significant reduction in systemic and pulmonary venous pressure is observed within a few minutes, even before any significant change in intravascular volume or urine output occurs.[61] This early decrease in systemic and pulmonary venous pressures has been attributed to peripheral venous pooling resulting from increased venous capacitance. There is a further decrease in right atrial and pulmonary capillary wedge pressure with increased urine output and decreased intravascular volume, usually 20 minutes or longer after intravenous administration of furosemide. Cardiac output, arterial pressure, and heart rate remain unchanged after intravenous furosemide. In some patients with chronic heart failure, there initially might even be a transient decrease in cardiac output. This results from the increased systemic vascular tone that accompanies a rise in plasma norepinephrine, vasopressin, and renin levels.

As a result of marked reduction in intravascular and intracardiac volumes with aggressive diuretic therapy, a reduction in stroke volume and cardiac output is also expected as the patient's cardiac function moves to the steep portion of the ventricular function curve. Furthermore, neuroendocrine dysfunction (elevated plasma renin activity and increased catecholamine levels) and prerenal azotemia frequently result from excessive diuretic therapy. Nevertheless, diuretics are useful drugs in relieving congestive heart failure symptoms. It is apparent that the hemodynamic effects of diuretics are similar to those

Table 8–5. **Expected Systemic Hemodynamic Effects of Combination of Commonly Used Inotropic Drugs and Vasodilators**

	HR	MAP	CO	PCWP	RAP
Dobutamine and nitroprusside	↔ ↑	↔ ↓	↑ ↑	↓ ↓	↓ ↓
Dobutamine and dopamine	↑	↔ ↑	↑ ↑	↓	↓
Norepinephrine and nitroprusside	↑ ↔	↑	↑	↓	↓
Dobutamine or dopamine and nitroglycerin	↔ ↓	↑	↑ ↑	↓ ↓	↓ ↓
Dobutamine and amrinone	↑	↓ ↓	↑ ↑	↓ ↓	↓ ↓
Dopamine and amrinone	↑	↑ ↔	↑ ↑	↓	↓
ACE inhibitors and inotropic agents (phosphodiesterase inhibitors)	↔	↓ ↓	↑ ↑	↓ ↓	↓ ↓
Levodopa or ibopamine and vasodilators	↔ ↑	↔ ↓	↑	↓	↓

ACE, angiotensin-converting enzyme; CO, cardiac output; HR, heart rate; MAP, mean arterial pressure; PCWP, pulmonary capillary wedge pressure; RAP, right atrial pressure; ↔, no change; ↓, moderate decrease; ↓ ↓, marked decrease; ↑, moderate increase; ↑ ↑, marked increase.

of nitroglycerin and nitrates. Thus, with the addition of nitrates to diuretics, a greater decrease in systemic and pulmonary venous pressures is expected. Frequently, the dose of diuretics can be reduced when nitrates are added. Thus, the potential renal and neuroendocrine adverse effects of excessive diuretic therapy can be avoided.

The hemodynamic effects of ACE inhibitors are more pronounced in patients receiving diuretics. Frequently, the dosage of diuretics should be reduced to prevent significant hypotension during therapy with ACE inhibitors. In contrast, increased dosages of diuretics are often needed to prevent secondary fluid retention during chronic therapy with hydralazine, minoxidil, or phosphodiesterase inhibitors. Long-term diuretic therapy with furosemide has been reported to increase end-systolic volume and decrease left ventricular ejection fraction in asymptomatic postinfarction patients with reduced ejection fraction.[62] These findings imply that in some patients, diuretics alone, although they may relieve congestive heart failure symptoms, cause deterioration of left ventricular function.

CLINICAL APPLICATIONS OF COMBINATION THERAPY
Acute Pulmonary Edema

The principal hemodynamic abnormality of acute cardiogenic pulmonary edema, regardless of its etiology, is acute elevation of pulmonary venous pressure exceeding oncotic pressure. For effective prompt reduction of pulmonary venous pressure and amelioration of symptoms, concurrent administration of diuretics, vasodilators, and opiates is frequently required. Very rarely, phlebotomy to decrease intravascular and intracardiac volumes is necessary. Application of a rotating tourniquet is not associated with any significant and clinically relevant reduction in pulmonary venous pressure. It should, therefore, be regarded as an obsolete treatment for pulmonary edema.

Nitroglycerin and nitrates can cause a prompt reduction of pulmonary venous pressure. Sublingual or buccal administration is preferable, because hemodynamic effects usually begin within 2 to 3 minutes.

Intravenously administered diuretics such as furosemide also decrease pulmonary venous pressure within 5 to 10 minutes in some patients and within 30 minutes in others. In addition to alleviating anxiety, the opiates, particularly morphine sulfate, also decrease pulmonary venous pressure in these patients. Administration of oxygen, if necessary, and intubation should be an integral part of the management of severe pulmonary edema.

For subsequent treatment of pulmonary edema, the etiology and pathophysiologic mechanisms of the condition should be considered. Not only do vasodilators and inotropic agents decrease regurgitant volume, left ventricular diastolic pressure, and pulmonary venous pressures in patients with mitral or aortic regurgitation, but also they increase forward stroke volume and cardiac output.[63, 64] Sodium nitroprusside is preferable to nitroglycerin in these patients. With nitroglycerin, although pulmonary venous pressure declines, forward stroke volume and cardiac output remain unchanged. As with dopamine, systemic vascular resistance may increase, which is associated with worsening regurgitation; it should be avoided until hypotension is also present. With dobutamine, systemic vascular resistance falls and regurgitant volume decreases. Therefore, dobutamine is preferable to dopamine. Thus, dobutamine should be added to nitroprusside if the response with nitroprusside alone is inadequate. If hypotension is present, dopamine infusion is started initially. Once the blood pressure increases to an acceptable level, sodium nitroprusside is added. The phosphodiesterase inhibitors amrinone, milrinone, and enoximone, when given intravenously, can cause prompt reduction in pulmonary capillary wedge pressure and an increase in cardiac output; these agents might prove useful for the treatment of pulmonary edema resulting from severe mitral or aortic regurgitation. However, their hemodynamic effects in patients with valvular regurgitation have not been adequately evaluated.

In patients with severe mitral or aortic valve stenosis, vasodilators (except nitroglycerin) should not be used, because significant hypotension associated with a reduction in cardiac output may develop. A reduction in transmitral flow, associated with a decreased transmitral pressure gradient and an increased diastolic time, reduces left atrial and pulmonary venous pressures in patients with mitral stenosis. Thus, the combination of diuretics, nitroglycerin, and drugs that can decrease heart rate (digitalis in the presence of atrial fibrillation and β-blockers) effectively reduces pulmonary venous hypertension. In patients with severe aortic valvular stenosis with fixed left ventricular outflow resistance, peripheral vasodilation with vasodilators is not accompanied by a significant increase in cardiac output; thus, hypotension develops.

In patients with hypertrophic cardiomyopathy, pulmonary venous congestion results, primarily because of abnormal diastolic function. Calcium antagonists such as verapamil, diltiazem, and nifedipine (and occasionally β-adrenergic blocking agents) may improve diastolic function and systemic hemodynamics. Therefore, these agents might aid the amelioration of congestive heart failure symptoms in these patients.

In patients with acute myocardial infarction, hemodynamics should be determined if initial therapy does not yield a prompt response. Pharmacotherapy is then guided by the hemodynamic profile. If pulmonary venous pressure remains elevated but the cardiac output and arterial pressure are normal, intravenously administered nitroglycerin and intermittent diuretic therapy are usually effective. When cardiac output remains low and arterial pressure and systemic vascular resistance are elevated, sodium nitroprusside is the vasodilator of choice. In hypotensive patients, therapy is similar to that for severe left ventricular failure and/or cardiogenic shock, described later in this chapter. Treatment of acute pulmonary edema in patients with primary myocardial disease is similar to that in patients with acute myocardial infarction.

Congestive Heart Failure in Acute Myocardial Infarction

Thrombolytic therapy, percutaneous coronary artery angioplasty, and revascularization surgery are being performed more frequently to limit "infarct size" and improve immediate and late prognoses of patients with acute myocardial infarction. Indeed, thrombolytic agents administered within a few hours of the onset of symptoms decrease short-term mortality.[65, 66] Furthermore, the incidence of congestive heart failure appears to be decreased in patients who have adequate recanalization of the infarct-related artery following thrombolytic therapy.[67] Thus, thrombolytic therapy should always be considered in appropriate subsets of patients. However, intravenous thrombolytic therapy does not appear to improve the prognosis of patients with severe left ventricular failure and cardiogenic shock. Primary angioplasty of the infarct-related artery, which can improve the prognosis, should be considered for recanalization and reperfusion therapy in these patients. Despite successful reperfusion therapy, aggressive supportive pharmacotherapy is required. In patients with persistent congestive heart failure and low-output state, hemodynamic monitoring is indicated.

Right Ventricular Infarction

Appropriate treatment of low-output state complicating predominant right ventricular infarction frequently requires combination pharmacotherapy. The principal mechanism for the decreased systemic output is reduced left ventricular preload. Reduction of left ventricular preload results from decreased right ventricular stroke volume due to right ventricular failure and the restriction of left ventricular filling due to the constraining effect of pericardium because of increased intrapericardial pressure.[68] A diastolic leftward shift of the interventricular septum also contributes to decreased left ventricular preload. The major objective in correcting a low-output state is to increase left ventricular preload by increasing right ventricular stroke volume. An increase in stroke volume can result from an increase in preload by the Frank-Starling mechanism, increased contractility, or decreased right ventricular afterload, or by a combination of these physiologic principles. Volume expansion therapy with intravenous administration of fluids is used primarily to increase right ventricular stroke volume by the Frank-Starling mechanism.[69] It is apparent that if right ventricular end-diastolic volume is already markedly increased, Frank-Starling reserve is limited. A further increase in right ventricular end-diastolic volume with volume loading is unlikely to be associated with any significant increase in right ventricular forward stroke volume. Pulmonary and systemic vasodilators (nitroprusside and nitroglycerin) can increase right ventricular stroke volume by decreasing right ventricular afterload. Drugs with positive inotropic effects can also increase right ventricular stroke volume.[70] The differences in the hemodynamic effects of the two commonly used vasoactive inotropic agents, dobutamine and dopamine, should be considered during management of a low-output state complicating right ventricular infarction. Because dopamine may increase pulmonary capillary wedge pressure and total pulmonary artery resistance, the magnitude of increase in stroke volume from increased contractility may be curtailed by the concomitant increase in right ventricular impedance. Pulmonary arterial resistance tends to decrease with dobutamine, which therefore may increase right ventricular stroke volume more effectively than dopamine. In the presence of systemic hypotension, however, dopamine should be administered initially. A vasodilator or dobutamine or an inodilator such as amrinone can then be added. Intravenous fluid administration is also necessary in these patients to maintain adequate preload. The therapeutic approach for the treatment of low-output state complicating right ventricular infarction is summarized in Table 8–6.

Acute Left Ventricular Failure

Persistent hypotension, tachycardia, pulmonary congestion, and other manifestations of low cardiac output, such as decreasing urine output and mental

Table 8–6. **Low Output Complicating Right Ventricular Infarction**

1. Right atrial and pulmonary capillary wedge pressure < 15 mmHg:
   Administer intravenous fluids.
   a. If there is an adequate increase in cardiac output, continue maintenance intravenous fluid therapy.
   b. If response is inadequate, administer dopamine in the presence of hypotension and nitroprusside or nitroglycerin in the presence of normal or elevated blood pressure; continue maintenance fluid therapy.
2. Right atrial and pulmonary capillary wedge pressure > 15 mmHg and normal or elevated arterial pressure:
   Administer nitroprusside and nitroglycerin.
   a. If there is an adequate increase in cardiac output, continue maintenance vasodilator therapy and add intravenous fluids to maintain right atrial and pulmonary capillary wedge pressure between 10 and 15 mmHg.
   b. If there is an inadequate increase in cardiac output, add dobutamine.
3. Right atrial and pulmonary capillary wedge pressure > 15 mmHg and low arterial pressure:
   Administer dopamine.
   a. If there is an adequate increase in cardiac output, continue maintenance dopamine therapy. Add intravenous fluids if right atrial and pulmonary capillary wedge pressures fall to < 15 mmHg.
   b. If there is an inadequate response, add nitroprusside or nitroglycerin when blood pressure increases to the normal range.

obtundation, are indications for hemodynamic monitoring to assess the etiology and severity of left ventricular failure. The more severe the hemodynamic abnormalities, the more frequent is the necessity for a combination of various vasoactive and inotropic agents. However, initial therapy often must be based on clinical assessment. Diuretics, nitroglycerin, and analgesics are employed in patients with manifestations of pulmonary congestion with or without persistent infarct-related chest pain. In patients with hypotension and tachycardia and clinical features of shock, intravenous vasopressor therapy with dopamine or norepinephrine is employed without delay before ventricular filling pressures and cardiac output can be determined. In the presence of severe hypotension, intraaortic balloon counterpulsation may have to be instituted concurrently with vasopressors before hemodynamic monitoring can be established. The addition or discontinuation of a given pharmacologic agent is guided by the hemodynamic response and the objective of treatment. The most useful hemodynamic parameters to guide therapy are arterial pressure, cardiac output, right atrial and pulmonary capillary wedge pressures, and systemic vascular resistance. When low cardiac index (<2.2 L/min/m^2) is associated with relatively normal or lower pulmonary capillary wedge pressure (<18 mmHg), initially, a fluid challenge is indicated to maintain left ventricular filling pressure in the optimal range (15 to 18 mmHg).[71, 72] If the increase in cardiac output is inadequate despite intravenous fluid therapy, an inotropic agent (dobutamine or dopamine) frequently must be added in relatively hypotensive patients. However, if arterial pressure is normal or elevated, with increased systemic vascular resistance (>1200 dynes/sec/cm^{-5}), vasodilator therapy, usually with intravenously administered sodium nitroprusside, is indicated along with intravenous fluid therapy. If the cardiac index is adequate but pulmonary capillary wedge pressure is elevated (>18 mmHg), a combination of diuretics and nitroglycerin or nitrates effectively lowers pulmonary capillary wedge pressure. When cardiac index is also low (<2.2 L/min/m^2), sodium nitroprusside appears to be the vasodilator of choice, provided that arterial pressure is adequate

(mean arterial pressure, >65 mmHg). Occasionally, with sodium nitroprusside, pulmonary capillary wedge pressure may remain abnormally elevated despite a substantial increase in cardiac output. The addition of intravenously administered nitroglycerin or nitrates may further reduce pulmonary capillary wedge pressure. When the increase in cardiac output with vasodilators is inadequate, addition of dobutamine may be effective. Alternatively, intravenously administered phosphodiesterase inhibitors such as amrinone, milrinone, and enoximone can be used. In hypotensive patients (systolic blood pressure, <90 mmHg), vasodilators cannot be used without maintaining arterial pressure with the concomitant administration of vasopressor or the use of intraaortic balloon counterpulsation.

Severe left ventricular failure or cardiogenic shock resulting from complications such as severe mitral regurgitation (papillary muscle infarction) or left-to-right shunt (ventricular septal rupture) is also treated with a combination of vasodilators, inotropic agents, and frequently intraaortic balloon counterpulsations to achieve hemodynamic and clinical stability before corrective surgery is performed. The severity of mitral regurgitation and its hemodynamic consequences are related not only to the extent of the anatomic derangement of the mitral valve apparatus but also to the aortic ejection impedance and resistance at the mitral valve during systole. The rationale for the use of vasodilators such as sodium nitroprusside is to increase forward stroke volume and decrease regurgitant volume by decreasing aortic impedance.[4] Effective valve orifice size also decreases, contributing to decreased regurgitant volume. A similar change in the dynamics of mitral regurgitation also occurs with inotropic agents such as dobutamine. Thus, the combination of nitroprusside and dobutamine infusion is frequently employed for the immediate pharmacologic management of severe mitral regurgitation. Inodilators such as amrinone and enoximone are also likely to be effective. In the presence of hypotension, intraaortic balloon counterpulsation therapy is instituted. Vasodilators and inotropic agents are then added as indicated and are guided by hemodynamic response.

The magnitude of left-to-right shunt resulting from rupture of the interventricular septum is related not only to the size of the defect but also to resistance in the pulmonary and systemic circulations. Because the postinfarction ventricular septal defect is usually large, resistance at the defect is usually low. Therefore, the magnitude of the left-to-right shunt is determined primarily by pulmonary and systemic vascular resistances. Increased systemic and lower pulmonary vascular resistance are associated with increased left-to-right shunt and a decline in systemic output. The major objectives of pharmacotherapy are to decrease left-to-right shunt, enhance systemic output, and decrease systemic and pulmonary venous pressures. During vasodilator therapy, left-to-right shunt may increase if the magnitude of reduction in pulmonary vascular resistance is relatively greater than that of systemic vascular resistance. Thus, vasodilator drugs with pronounced systemic arteriolar-dilating effects (hydralazine, phentolamine) have greater potential to decrease left-to-right shunt and increase systemic output. Intraaortic balloon counterpulsation selectively decreases left ventricular ejection impedance without any significant change in right ventricular outflow resistance. Thus, intraaortic balloon counterpulsation is the therapy of choice for nonsurgical reduction of left-to-right shunt. Addition of hydralazine or phentolamine may cause further reduction in left-to-right shunt. Sodium nitroprusside or nitroglycerin appears to cause significant pulmonary vasodilation and thus can increase left-to-right shunt. The systemic flow may not increase. The vasopressor and inotropic agents currently in use may also produce variable and unpredictable effects on the magnitude of left-to-right shunt and systemic output. Norepinephrine and dopamine (higher doses) increase both systemic and pulmonary vascular resistances. The net change in systemic output and left-to-right shunt is related to the magnitude of increase in systemic and pulmonary vascular resistances. In addition to exerting positive inotropic effects, dobutamine decreases both systemic and pulmonary vascular resistances. However, the magnitude of reduction of systemic vascular resistance usually is greater than that of pulmonary vascular resistance. Thus, dobutamine is preferable to other vasopressor-inotropic agents in decreasing left-to-right shunt and increasing systemic output. Combination therapy of hydralazine or phentolamine with dobutamine along with intraaortic balloon counterpulsation is necessary and is employed to establish hemodynamic stability of patients with ventricular septal rupture complicating acute myocardial infarction. Surgical repair should be considered early, as soon as patients are stabilized with pharmacotherapy.

Chronic Heart Failure

In the management of patients with chronic heart failure, combination therapy is the rule rather than the exception. Although diuretics alone can alleviate congestive heart failure symptoms in some patients with mild heart failure, neuroendocrine and renal dysfunction are more likely during diuretic therapy. Rising blood urea nitrogen and creatinine and increased plasma renin activity are frequent adverse effects of chronic diuretic therapy. Furthermore, hyperuricemia, hyperglycemia, and abnormalities of lipid profile may also occur in some patients. It has been reported that in asymptomatic postinfarction patients with depressed left ventricular dysfunction, chronic diuretic therapy may result in further left ventricular dysfunction. Furthermore, diuretics generally do not increase cardiac output in most patients with chronic heart failure. Thus, diuretics alone are not the therapy of choice even in patients with mild congestive heart failure.

The controversy regarding the role of maintenance digitalis therapy in patients with sinus rhythm has not been resolved. However, a number of studies document a beneficial effect of digitalis in appropriate subsets of patients with chronic congestive heart failure.[51, 52] Patients with depressed systolic function (reduced ejection fraction), an S_3 gallop, and evidence of pulmonary venous congestion are likely to benefit from chronic digitalis therapy.[73] Clinical trials comparing captopril and digoxin in patients with mild, chronic congestive heart failure have reported that captopril is superior to digoxin in improving exercise tolerance. However, digoxin improved left ventricular ejection fraction.[74] The relative effectiveness of digoxin and milrinone has also been assessed in a randomized, placebo-controlled clinical trial.[75] Both milrinone and digoxin improved exercise tolerance in patients with moderately severe heart failure, although maximum oxygen consumption during exercise improved only with milrinone compared with exercise tolerance in patients receiving placebo in addition to diuretics. Withdrawal of digoxin therapy from patients stabilized with digoxin, diuretics, and ACE inhibitors is associated with worsening heart failure and deterioration of clinical status and left ventricular function.[76] The Veterans Administration Cooperative Study of Heart Failure[33] reported that the prognoses of patients with mild to moderately severe chronic heart failure who were treated with a combination of hydralazine and nitrates are considerably better (38% reduction in mortality at 1 year) than those of patients receiving conventional therapy or prazosin. The benefit of combined hydralazine-nitrate therapy was also positively correlated with the improvement in ejection fraction. Captopril improved the event-free survival rate of patients with moderately severe chronic heart failure.[77] Therefore, these results favor concomitant administration of either ACE inhibitors or a combination of hydralazine and nitrates or digoxin and diuretics in all patients with mild to moderate chronic heart failure. However, digoxin should be omitted in patients who are prone to developing digitalis toxicity. In patients with significant renal failure (creatinine, >3 mg%), a combination of hydralazine, nitrates, and diuretics is preferable to ACE inhibitors, which may cause further deterioration of renal function.

In patients with more severe chronic heart failure

(New York Heart Association class IV), ACE inhibitors should be considered if there are no contraindications for their use. The CONSENSUS study[34] reported not only a significant improvement in clinical class but also prolonged survival of patients treated with enalapril (a long-acting converting enzyme inhibitor) compared with those treated conventionally or who received vasodilators (primarily nitrates). However, it should be emphasized that in the CONSENSUS trial, the average mean arterial pressure of randomized patients was 77 mmHg. Thus, these patients were not hypotensive at the initiation of treatment. In patients with hypotension (mean arterial pressure, <60 mmHg), treatment with ACE inhibitors often causes further hypotension and significant deterioration of renal function.

In relatively hypotensive patients or when ACE inhibitors or a combination of direct-acting vasodilators, hydralazine, and nitrates does not improve clinical status and cardiac performance, a combination of vasodilators and inotropic agents is frequently required. Hemodynamic monitoring to assess the severity of hemodynamic abnormalities is useful to determine the efficacy and safety of such therapy and, more important, to determine the tolerable doses of various pharmacologic agents.

The magnitude of hemodynamic improvement with the combination of captopril and hydralazine appears to be greater than that with either drug alone.[78] Similarly, the combination of captopril and prazosin may retard the development of hemodynamic tolerance to prazosin and may enhance improvement of cardiac performance. The addition of nitrates to ACE inhibitors may cause a greater reduction in pulmonary and systemic venous pressures and an increase in cardiac output. However, a combination of ACE inhibitors with other vasodilators, such as hydralazine, prazosin, and nitrates, can cause significant hypotension. Thus, this combination should be attempted only under close clinical supervision, preferably with hemodynamic monitoring.

A few nonparenteral dopaminergic and β-receptor agonists have been used to treat chronic heart failure. Levodopa, when given orally, is converted to dopamine by dopadecarboxylase, and its hemodynamic effects are similar to those of low to moderate infusions of dopamine.[79] There is usually a modest increase in cardiac output without any significant change in heart rate, mean arterial pressure, and systemic and pulmonary venous pressures. Therefore, the addition of nitrates, ACE inhibitors, or larger doses of diuretics is frequently required to decrease pulmonary and systemic venous pressures adequately. Controlled studies are not yet available to assess the long-term benefit of levodopa in patients with severe chronic heart failure. Ibopamine is a derivative of dopamine that undergoes hydrolysis to epinine (N-methyldopamine) by esterase hydrolysis. It is an orally active drug and appears to have both positive inotropic and peripheral vasodilating effects. Its systemic hemodynamic effects are similar to those of dopamine.[80] A few controlled studies have demonstrated hemodynamic and clinical improvement, including increased exercise tolerance, following treatment with ibopamine.[81, 82] However, the number of patients studied was small, and the duration of follow-up was short. Nevertheless, these studies suggest that orally administered ibopamine (100 to 200 mg three times daily) may be an effective dopaminergic agent to manage patients with chronic heart failure. However, such a regimen probably has to be combined with vasodilators to produce optimal hemodynamic effects in patients with severe heart failure. The partial β1-receptor agonist prenalterol, although producing beneficial hemodynamic effects after its acute intravenous and oral administrations, has been found to exert no sustained beneficial effects during maintenance therapy.[83] Another partial β1-receptor agonist, corwin, is also likely to be ineffective in patients with severe chronic congestive heart failure.[84] Thus, the addition of levodopa or ibopamine to vasodilators or ACE inhibitors currently is a therapeutic option in severe refractory heart failure. The effective dosage of levadopa is 1.5 to 2 g three to four times daily. Gastrointestinal intolerance occurs in almost 30% of patients receiving levodopa for chronic heart failure.

The alternative pharmacologic treatments available for severe, refractory, end-stage heart failure are limited to intermittent dobutamine infusion or the use of phosphodiesterase inhibitors. The duration of hemodynamic and clinical improvement after short-term dobutamine infusion in individual patients is quite variable and unpredictable, although some sustained clinical improvement has lasted for several days to weeks after intravenous infusion of dobutamine for 7 to 72 hours.[85, 86] Intermittent dobutamine infusion should not be practiced without monitoring because of the risk of inducing ventricular tachycardia. Intermittent amrinone infusion may also benefit patients with refractory heart failure, but it should be considered only in hospitalized patients. Furthermore, long-term intermittent dobutamine infusion therapy may be associated with increased mortality.

The systemic hemodynamic effects of the phosphodiesterase inhibitors (e.g., milrinone, enoximone) are similar despite their structural differences. One of the potential advantages of these agents is that arterial pressure either remains unchanged or falls only slightly. Therefore, they can be used in relatively hypotensive patients. However, larger doses of both milrinone and enoximone produce hypotension. Thus, dose titration is necessary to avoid undesirable side effects. Another major clinical problem is secondary fluid retention and deterioration of clinical status after initial improvement. Increasing the dose of diuretics or adding antialdosterone agents occasionally may prevent fluid retention. The mortality rate of patients with severe refractory heart failure remains very high (approximately 75% at 6 months) despite treatment with phosphodiesterase inhibitors.[87] The mortality rate may actually increase following addition of phosphodiesterase inhibitors to digitalis, diuretics, and ACE inhibitors.[88] Combination therapy with low doses of vesnarinone, ACE inhibitors, digitalis, and

Table 8–7. **Pharmacotherapeutic Approach to Chronic Heart Failure Due to Primary Myocardial Disease**

1. Determine etiology.
   a. Exclude primary valvular heart disease. Besides clinical evaluation, echo-Doppler evaluation is helpful.
   b. Exclude pericardial disease. Clinical evaluation, echocardiography, magnetic resonance imaging, computed tomography; right and left heart catheterization to establish the hemodynamic abnormalities to constrictive pericarditis.
   c. By exclusion of valvular and pericardial disease, primary myocardial disease as the cause of chronic heart failure is suspected.
2. Determine left ventricular systolic and diastolic function: Echocardiography and radionuclide ventriculography are useful noninvasive investigative techniques.
   a. Predominant diastolic dysfunction. Ejection fraction is normal or only slightly decreased; left ventricular cavity size is normal or decreased; left ventricular wall thickness is frequently markedly increased.
   b. Predominant systolic dysfunction. Ejection fraction is markedly reduced less than 40%; left ventricular cavity size is increased, with increase in diastolic and end-systolic volumes; only slight or modest increase in left ventricular wall thickness.
3. For chronic failure due to diastolic dysfunction:
   a. For mild congestive heart failure symptoms:
      Low-dose diuretics. Calcium antagonists, particularly verapamil, are added in patients with hypertrophic cardiomyopathy. β-Adrenergic blocking agents are less effective than verapamil in improving the exercise performance of patients with hypertrophic cardiomyopathy.
   b. For severe heart failure:
      Diuretics, nitrates, calcium antagonists. In obstructive hypertrophic cardiomyopathy, disopyramide may be added; digoxin is added in patients with established atrial fibrillation.
   c. In hypertrophic cardiomyopathy with significant dysrhythmias and heart failure, amiodarone is added to diuretics, nitrates, and calcium antagonists.
   d. In patients without hypertrophic cardiomyopathy, similar therapy is employed. However, the efficacy of calcium antagonists and β-blocking drugs has not been established; the role of amiodarone also remains uncertain.
4. For chronic heart failure due to systolic dysfunction:
   a. Asymptomatic left ventricular dysfunction in postinfarction patients. Although captopril improves ejection fraction and prevents left ventricular dilation, its efficacy to improve prognosis has not been established. However, its addition to conventional postinfarction drug therapy is logical.
   b. Mild to moderate heart failure—diuretics, digitalis, and combination of hydralazine and nitrates or diuretics, digitalis, and angiotensin-converting enzyme inhibitors. In patients in whom digoxin is contraindicated, diuretics and angiotensin-converting enzyme inhibitors or hydralazine nitrates are initial therapy. In hypertensive patients, dihydropyridine or calcium antagonists may be added.
   c. In patients with significant renal failure and with normal or elevated blood pressure, initial therapy is a combination of diuretics and hydralazine-nitrates. When there is an inadequate response or when there is persistent hypertension, dihydropyridine calcium antagonists may be added. In hypotensive patients, levodopa, ibopamine, milrinone, or enoximone may be of temporary benefit.
   d. Severe heart failure. Initial therapy is a combination of digitalis, diuretics, and angiotensin-converting enzyme inhibitors. When there is an inadequate increase in cardiac output or improvement in symptoms, hydralazine may be added, provided that arterial pressure is adequate. When there is an inadequate response in congestive heart failure symptoms, nitrates are added. Vesnarinone, when added, may decrease mortality.
   e. In relatively hypotensive patients, or when angiotensin-converting enzyme inhibitors cannot be used, initial therapy is a combination of diuretics, digitalis, and levodopa or of ibopamine, milrinone, and enoximone. With an adequate increase in arterial pressure, hydralazine nitrates or a low dose of angiotensin-converting enzyme inhibitors can be added.
   f. In patients with severe heart failure refractory to nonparenteral pharmacologic agents, intermittent dobutamine or amrinone infusion, with or without low-dose dopamine infusion to improve renal perfusion, is required. In some patients, a combination of nonparenteral vasodilator and inotropic agents may be reinstituted following short-term parenteral inotropic therapy.
   g. In patients with severe congestive heart failure who also have significant ventricular dysrhythmias detected by Holter monitoring, addition of a low dose of amiodarone to vasodilator and/or inotropic therapy should be considered.

diuretics, however, can decrease mortality in patients with chronic congestive heart failure.[89] Thus, for long-term combination inotropic vasodilator therapy, low-dose vesnarinone (60 mg) is preferable to other inotropic agents.

The incidence of sudden, unexpected death in chronic heart failure is high, averaging 40% to 45%.[90] In some prospective studies, the frequency of ventricular dysrhythmias has been positively correlated with total mortality.[91] Although ACE inhibitors decrease the frequency of complex ventricular arrhythmias and the rate of heart failure deaths, the incidence of sudden death remains uninfluenced.[92] A few prospective studies have indicated that low-dosage amiodarone (200 to 400 mg/day) may decrease the incidence of sudden death and overall mortality of patients who also exhibit frequent complex ventricular arrhythmias during Holter monitoring.[91, 93] Thus, the addition of amiodarone to vasodilators or ACE inhibitors should be considered at least in selected patients with severe heart failure and overt ventricular dysrhythmias. However, frequent follow-up evaluations of these patients are essential to detect serious adverse effects, including pulmonary toxicity of long-term amiodarone therapy.

When overt chronic heart failure results from left ventricular diastolic dysfunction, direct-acting vasodilators and ACE inhibitors are relatively ineffective. When systolic function is normal, positive inotropic agents such as digitalis are not indicated. Systemic and pulmonary venous hypertension associated with congestive symptoms frequently resists therapy. However, combination of a low-dose diuretic and nitrates may produce partial benefit. The calcium antagonists verapamil, diltiazem, and nifedipine have been shown to improve left ventricular diastolic function and diastolic filling characteristics in some patients with hypertrophic cardiomyopathy.[94] Thus, the addition of a calcium antagonist may cause symptomatic improvement in these patients. The presence of outflow obstruction in symptomatic patients with hypertrophic cardiomyopathy refractory to pharmacologic therapy is an indication for surgical intervention. A therapeutic approach for the treatment of chronic congestive heart failure is outlined in Table 8–7.

REFERENCES

1. Gaasch WH, Zile MR: Evaluation of myocardial function in cardiomyopathic states. Prog Cardiovasc Dis 27:115, 1984.
2. Parmley WW, Chatterjee K: Vasodilator therapy. Curr Probl Cardiol 2:4, 1978.
3. Pepine CJ, Nichols WW, Conti CR: Aortic input impedance in heart failure. Circulation 58:460, 1978.
4. Chatterjee K, Parmley WW: The role of vasodilator therapy in heart failure. Prog Cardiovasc Dis 19:301, 1977.
5. Chatterjee K: Vasodilation in heart failure. In Ledingham JGG, Warrell DA, Weatherall DJ (eds): Oxford Textbook of Medicine, Vol. II, Sec. 13. Oxford: Oxford University Press, 1983, pp 66–71.
6. Chatterjee K, Viquerat CE, Daly P: Neurohumoral abnormalities in heart failure. Heart Failure 1:69, 1985.
7. Endoh M, Yanagisawa T, Taira N, et al: Effects of new inotropic agents on cyclic nucleotide metabolism and calcium transients in canine ventricular muscle. Circulation 73(Suppl 3):111, 1986.
8. Cody RJ: The potential role of atrial natriuretic factor in the pathophysiology of congestive heart failure. Heart Failure 2:258, 1987.
9. Crozier IG, Ikram H, Gomez HJ, et al: Hemodynamic effects of atrial peptide infusion in heart failure. Lancet 2:1242, 1986.
10. Fabiato A, Fabiato F: Calcium and cardiac excitation-contraction coupling. Annu Rev Physiol 41:473, 1979.
11. Chapman RA: Control of cardiac contractility at the cellular level. Am J Physiol 245:H535, 1983.
12. Dzau VJ, Swartz SL, Creager MA: The role of prostaglandins in the pathophysiology of and therapy for congestive heart failure. Heart Failure 2:6, 1986.
13. Linderer T, Biamino G, Bruggerman T, et al: Hemodynamic effects of forskolin, a new drug with combined positive inotropic and vasodilating properties [abstract]. J Am Coll Cardiol 3:562, 1984.
14. Matsue S, Murakami E, Takekoshi N, et al: Hemodynamic effects of dibutyryl cyclic AMP in congestive heart failure. Am J Cardiol 51:1364, 1983.
15. Gross R, Schramm M, Thomas G, et al: Bay K8644, a positive inotropic dihydropyridine with Ca++ agonist properties. J Mol Cell Cardiol 15(Suppl 4):29, 1983.
16. Smiseth OA: Inosine infusion in dogs with acute ischemic left ventricular failure: Favorable effect on myocardial performance and metabolism. Cardiovasc Res 17:192, 1983.
17. Judy WV, Hall JH, Toth PD, et al: Influence of coenzyme Q10 on cardiac function in congestive heart failure [Abstract]. Fed Proc 43:358, 1984.
18. Iijima T, Taira N: Membrane current changes responsible for the positive inotropic effect of OPC-8212, a new positive inotropic agent, in single ventricular cells of guinea pig heart. J Pharmacol Exp Ther 240:657, 1987.
19. Lathrop DA, Schwartz A: Evidence for possible increase in sodium channel open time and involvement of NA/CA exchange by a new positive inotropic drug: OPC-8212. Eur J Pharmacol 117:391, 1985.
20. Suga H, Sagawa K, Shoukas A: Load independence of the instantaneous pressure-volume ratio of the canine left ventricle and effects of epinephrine and heart rate on the ratio. Circ Res 32:314, 1973.
21. Suga H, Sagawa K: Instantaneous pressure-volume relationships and their ratio in the excised, supported canine left ventricle. Circ Res 35:117, 1974.
22. DeMarco T, Daly PA, Liu M, et al: Enalaprilat, a new parenteral angiotensin-converting enzyme inhibitor: Rapid changes in systemic and coronary hemodynamics and humoral profile in chronic heart failure. J Am Coll Cardiol 9:1131, 1987.
23. Rouleau JL, Chatterjee K, Benege W, et al: Alterations in left ventricular function and coronary hemodynamics with captopril, hydralazine and prazosin in chronic ischemic heart failure—A comparative study. Circulation 65:671, 1982.
24. Chatterjee K, Rouleau JL: Hemodynamic and metabolic effects of vasodilators, nitrates, hydralazine, prazosin and captopril in chronic ischemic heart failure. Acta Med Scand Suppl 651:295, 1981.
25. Brown BG, Bolson E, Peterson RB, et al: The mechanism of nitroglycerin action: Stenosis vasodilation as a major component of the drug response. Circulation 64:1089, 1981.
26. Magorien RD, Leier CV, Kolibash AJ, et al: Beneficial effects of nifedipine on rest and exercise myocardial energetics in patients with congestive heart failure. Circulation 70:884, 1984.
27. Cogan JS, Humphreys MH, Carson CJ, et al: Afterload reduction increases renal blood flow and maintains glomerular filtration rate in patients with congestive heart failure. Clin Res 27:3A, 1979.
28. Dzau VJ, Colucci WS, Williams GH, et al: Sustained effectiveness of converting enzyme inhibition in patients with congestive heart failure. N Engl J Med 302:1373, 1980.
29. Pierpont G, Francis GS, Cohn JN: Effect of captopril on renal function in patients with congestive heart failure. Br Heart J 46:522, 1981.
30. Diamond JR, Cheung JY, Fang TL: Nifedipine-induced renal dysfunction: Alterations in renal function. Am J Med 77:905, 1984.
31. Elkayam U, Weber L, Campese VM, et al: Renal hemodynamic effects of vasodilation with nifedipine and hydralazine in patients with heart failure. J Am Coll Cardiol 4:1261, 1984.
32. Leier CV, Magorien RD, Desch CE, et al: Hydralazine and isosorbide dinitrate: Comparative central and regional hemodynamic effects when administered alone or in combination. Circulation 63:102, 1981.
33. Cohn JN, Archibald DG, Ziesche S, et al: Effect of vasodilator therapy on mortality in chronic congestive heart failure: Results of a Veterans Administration Cooperative Study. N Engl J Med 314:1547, 1986.
34. CONSENSUS Trial Study Group: Effects of enalapril on mortality in severe congestive heart failure: Results of the Cooperative North Scandinavian Enalapril Survival Study (CONSENSUS). N Engl J Med 316:1429, 1987.
35. Aronow WS, Greenfield PS, Alimadadian H, et al: Effect of vasodilator trimazosin versus placebo on exercise performance in chronic left ventricular failure. Am J Cardiol 30:789, 1977.
36. Ports TA, Chatterjee K, Wilkinson P, et al: Beneficial hemodynamic effects of a new oral vasodilator, trimazosin, in chronic heart failure [Abstract]. Clin Res 28:13A, 1980.
37. Awan NA, Hermanovich J, Whitcomb C, et al: Cardio-circulatory effects on afterload reduction with oral trimazosin in severe chronic heart failure. Am J Cardiol 44:126, 1979.
38. Elkayam U, LeJemtel T, Mathur M, et al: Marked early attenuation of hemodynamic effects of oral prazosin chronic heart failure [Abstract]. Am J Cardiol 43:403, 1980.
39. Packer M, Meller J, Gorlin R, et al: Hemodynamic and clinical tachyphylaxis to prazosin-mediated afterload in severe chronic congestive heart failure. Circulation 59:531, 1979.
40. Awan NA, Miller RR, Maxwell KS: Development of systemic vasodilator tolerance to prazosin with chronic use of the agent in ambulatory therapy of severe congestive heart failure [Abstract]. Am J Cardiol 41:367, 1978.
41. Arnold S, Williams R, Ports TA, et al: Attenuation of prazosin effect on cardiac output in chronic heart failure. Ann Intern Med 91:345, 1979.
42. Awan NA, Miller RR, DeMaria AN, et al: Efficacy of ambulatory systemic vasodilator therapy with oral prazosin in chronic refractory heart failure. Circulation 56:346, 1977.
43. Agostoni PG, DeCesare N, Doria E, et al: Afterload reduction: A comparison of captopril and nifedipine in dilated cardiomyopathy. Br Heart J 55:391, 1986.
44. Leier CV, Heban PT, Huss P, et al: Comparative systemic and regional hemodynamic effects of dopamine and dobutamine in patients with cardiomyopathic heart failure. Circulation 58:466, 1978.
45. Loeb HS, Bvedakis J, Gunnar RM: Superiority of dobutamine over dopamine in patients with low output cardiac failure. Circulation 55:375, 1977.

46. Wahr D, Swedberg K, Rabbino M, et al: Intravenous and oral prenalterol in congestive heart failure. Effects on systemic and coronary hemodynamics and myocardial catecholamine balance. Am J Med 76:999, 1984.

47. Erbel R, Meyer J, Lanberta H, et al: Hemodynamic effects of prenalterol in patients with ischemic heart disease and congestive cardiomyopathy. Circulation 66:361, 1982.

48. Goldberg LI, Rafzer SI: Dopamine receptors: Applications in clinical cardiology. Circulation 72:245, 1985.

49. Goldberg LI, Hsieh YY, Resnekow L: Newer catecholamines for treatment of heart failure and shock: An update on dopamine and a first look at dobutamine. Prog Cardiovasc Dis 4:327, 1977.

50. Goldberg LI: Cardiovascular and renal actions of dopamine: Potential applications. Pharmacol Rev 24:1, 1972.

51. Arnold SB, Byrd RC, Meister W, et al: Chronic digitalis therapy improves left ventricular function of patients with chronic heart failure. N Engl J Med 303:1443, 1980.

52. Chatterjee K: Digitalis versus newer inotropic agents: Which to use? Drug Ther 12:83, 1982.

53. Crawford MH, Richards KL, Sodums MT, et al: Positive inotropic and vasodilator effects of MDL 17043 in patients with reduced left ventricular performance. Am J Cardiol 53:1051, 1984.

54. Ludmer PL, Wright RF, Arnold MO, et al: Separation of the direct myocardial and vasodilator actions of milrinone administered by an intracoronary infusion technique. Circulation 73:130, 1986.

55. Cody RJ, Muller FB, Kubo SH, et al: Identification of the direct vasodilator effect of milrinone with an isolated limb preparation in patients with congestive heart failure. Circulation 73:124, 1986.

56. Benotti JR, Grossman W, Braunwald E, et al: Effects of amrinone on myocardial energy metabolism and hemodynamics in patients with severe congestive heart failure due to coronary artery disease. Circulation 62:28, 1980.

57. Monrad ES, Baim DS, Smith HS, et al: Effects of milrinone on coronary hemodynamics and myocardial energetics in patients with congestive heart failure. Circulation 71:972, 1985.

58. Viquerat CE, Kereiakes D, Morris DL, et al: Alterations in left ventricular function, coronary hemodynamics, and myocardial catecholamine balance with MDL 17043: A new inotropic vasodilator agent in patients with severe heart failure. J Am Coll Cardiol 5:326, 1985.

59. Kereiakes D, Chatterjee K, Parmley WW, et al: Intravenous and oral MDL 17043 (a new inotrope-vasodilator agent) in congestive heart failure: Hemodynamic and clinical evaluation in 38 patients. J Am Coll Cardiol 4:884, 1984.

60. Daly PA, Chatterjee K, Parmley WW, et al: R013-6438, a new inotrope-vasodilator: Systemic and coronary hemodynamic effects in congestive heart failure. Am J Cardiol 55:1539, 1985.

61. Dikshit K, Vyden JK, Forrester JS, et al: Renal extrarenal hemodynamic effects of furosemide in congestive heart failure after acute myocardial infarction. N Engl J Med 288:1087, 1973.

62. Sharpe N, Murphy J, Smith H, et al: Treatment of patients with symptomless left ventricular dysfunction after myocardial infarction. Lancet 1:255, 1988.

63. Chatterjee K, Ports TA, Parmley WW: Nitroprusside: Its clinical pharmacology and application in acute heart failure. In Gould L, Land B, Reddy CVR (eds): Vasodilator Therapy for Cardiac Disorders. Mt. Kisco, NY: Futura, 1979, pp 25–62.

64. Greenberg BH, Massie BM, Brundage BH, et al: Beneficial effects of hydralazine in severe mitral regurgitation. Circulation 58:273, 1978.

65. GISSI: Effectiveness of intravenous thrombolysis treatment in acute myocardial infarction. Lancet 7:387, 1986.

66. European Cooperative Study Group for Streptokinase Treatment in Acute Myocardial Infarction: Streptokinase in acute myocardial infarction. N Engl J Med 301:797, 1979.

67. Kennedy JW, Gensini GG, Timmis GC, et al: Acute myocardial infarction treated with intracoronary streptokinase: A report for the Society of Cardiac Angiography. Am J Cardiol 55:871, 1985.

68. Goldstein JA, Vlahakes GJ, Verrier EDK, et al: The role of right ventricular systolic dysfunction and elevated intrapericardial pressure in the genesis of low output in experimental right ventricular infarction. Circulation 65:513, 1982.

69. Goldstein JA, Vlahakes GJ, Verrier ED, et al: Volume loading improves low cardiac output in experimental right ventricular infarction. J Am Coll Cardiol 2:270, 1983.

70. Dell'Italia LJ, Starling MR, Blumhardt R, et al: Comparative effects of volume loading, dopamine and nitroprusside in patients with predominant right ventricular infarction. Circulation 72:1327, 1985.

71. Forrester JS, Diamond G, Chatterjee K, et al: Medical therapy of acute myocardial infarction by application of hemodynamic subsets (Part I). N Engl J Med 295:1356, 1976.

72. Forrester JS, Diamond G, Chatterjee K, et al: Medical therapy of acute myocardial infarction by application of hemodynamic subsets (Part II). N Engl J Med 295:1404, 1976.

73. Lee DC, Johnson RA, Bingham JB: Heart failure in outpatients: A randomized trial of digoxin versus placebo. N Engl J Med 306:699, 1982.

74. The Captopril-Digoxin Multicenter Research Group: Comparative effects of therapy with captopril and digoxin in patients with mild to moderate heart failure. JAMA 259:539, 1987.

75. DiBianco R, Shabetai R, Kostuk W, et al: Oral milrinone and digoxin in heart failure: Results of a placebo-controlled prospective trial of each agent and the combination. Circulation 76(Suppl 4):256, 1987.

76. Packer M, Gheorghiade M, Young JB, et al: Withdrawal of digoxin from patients with chronic heart failure treated with angiotensin-converting-enzyme inhibitors. N Engl J Med 329:1, 1993.

77. Newman TJ, Maskin CS, Denmick LG, et al: Effects of captopril on survival in patients with heart failure. Am J Med 84(Suppl 3A):140, 1988.

78. Franciosa JA, Cohn JN: Effects of minoxidil on hemodynamics of patients with congestive heart failure. Circulation 63:652, 1981.

79. Rajfer SI, Anton AH, Rossen J, et al: Beneficial hemodynamic effects of oral levodopa in heart failure: Relationship to the generation of dopamine. N Engl J Med 310:1357, 1984.

80. Rajfer SI, Rossen JD, Douglas FL, et al: Effects of long-term therapy with oral ibopamine on resting hemodynamics and exercise capacity in patients with heart failure: Relationship to the generation of N-methyldopamine and to plasma norepinephrine levels. Circulation 73:740, 1986.

81. Cantelli I, Lolli C, Bomba E, et al: Sustained oral treatment with ibopamine in patients with chronic congestive heart failure. Curr Ther Res 39:900, 1986.

82. Dei Cas L, Barilli AC, Metra M, et al: Multicenter study on the clinical efficacy of chronic ibopamine administration. Arzneimittel-Forschung 36:383, 1986.

83. Roubin GS, Choong CVP, Devenish-Meares S, et al: β-Adrenergic stimulation of the failing ventricle: A double-blind, randomized trial of sustained oral therapy with prenalterol. Circulation 66:955, 1984.

84. Bhatia SJS, Swedberg K, Chatterjee K: Acute hemodynamic and metabolic effects of ICI 118, 587 (Corwin), a selective partial beta-1 agonist in patients with dilated cardiomyopathy. Am Heart J 111:692, 1986.

85. Liang C, Sherman LG, Doherty JU, et al: Sustained improvement of cardiac function in patients with congestive heart failure after short-term infusion of dobutamine. Circulation 69:113, 1984.

86. Applefeld MM, Newman KA, Grove WR, et al: Intermittent continuous outpatient dobutamine infusion in the management of congestive heart failure. Am J Cardiol 51:455, 1983.

87. Simonton CA, Daly PA, Kereiakes D, et al: Survival in severe left ventricular failure treated with the new nonglycosidic, nonsympathomimetic oral inotropic agents. Chest 92:114, 1987.

88. Packer M, Carver JR, Rodeheffer RJ, et al: Effect of oral milrinone on mortality in severe chronic heart failure. N Engl J Med 325:1468, 1991.

89. Feldman AM, Bristow MR, Parmley WW, et al: Effects of vesnarinone on morbidity and mortality in patients with heart failure. N Engl J Med 329, 149, 1993.

90. Francis GS: Development of arrhythmias in the patient with chronic heart failure: Pathophysiology, prevalence, and prognosis. Am J Cardiol 57:3B, 1986.

91. Dargie HJ, Cleland JGF, Leckie BJ, et al: Relation of arrhythmias

and electrolyte abnormalities to survival in patients with severe chronic heart failure. Circulation 75(Suppl 4):98, 1987.
92. Cleland JGF, Dargie HJ, Hodsman GP, et al: Captopril in heart failure. Br Heart J 52:530, 1984.
93. Neri R, Mestroni L, Salvi A, et al: Ventricular arrhythmias in dilated cardiomyopathy: Efficacy of amiodarone. Am Heart J 113:707, 1987.
94. Chatterjee K, Raff G, Anderson D, et al: Hypertrophic cardiomyopathy—Therapy with slow channel inhibiting agents. Prog Cardiovasc Dis 25:193, 1982.

CHAPTER 9

Chronic Arrhythmias

Jaswinder S. Gill, M.D., M.R.C.P., F.A.C.C.,
and A. John Camm, M.D., F.R.C.P., F.A.C.C.

In the past, the use of antiarrhythmic drugs has been largely empirical. Since the 1980s, however, huge strides have been made in understanding the basis and mechanism of arrhythmias, and this has been paralleled by the recognition of the mode of action of antiarrhythmic drugs. This research has led to the appreciation that a number of necessary and critically balanced components are vital for the maintenance of an arrhythmia. Identification of the component most vulnerable to antiarrhythmic attack and selection of a suitable drug now form part of the assessment of arrhythmias in the electrophysiology laboratory. It is therefore now possible to identify and select drugs that are likely to be effective in particular situations rather than empirically searching for one to achieve suppression of the arrhythmia. The strategic basis of the selection of drugs for the treatment of arrhythmias is the concern of this chapter.

MECHANISMS OF ARRHYTHMIA

Three major mechanisms appear to exist for the generation of any form of arrhythmia: abnormal automaticity, triggered automaticity, and reentry. The cellular mechanisms of these phenomena are now more completely understood, and therefore antiarrhythmic therapy can be aimed at their vulnerable parameters.

Abnormal Automaticity

In normal myocardium, only cellular elements of the cardiac conduction system, including the sinus node, atrioventricular node, and Purkinje fibers, demonstrate automatic behavior. Atrial and ventricular cells normally have resting potentials of approximately -80 mV and do not demonstrate spontaneous activity. However, when the resting potential of such cells is reduced to reach the threshold potential, they manifest repetitive impulse initiation—depolarization-induced automaticity. The threshold potential at which automaticity is exhibited is quite variable, from -70 to -80 mV.[1] The initial reduction of membrane potential is usually due to underlying cardiac disease, most commonly cardiac ischemia.

The basis of the myocyte resting potential in most species is the delayed inward potassium rectifier current, and inactivation of this current is the most likely cause of spontaneous depolarization.[2] This can secondarily result in ion flow through either the Na^+ or Ca^{2+} channels, causing a spontaneous depolarization. At low membrane potentials, it is mainly Ca^{2+} channels that are activated, and at higher potentials, mainly Na^+. This is in keeping with the data that calcium-dependent mechanisms are important in abnormal pacemaker activity in atria at low membrane potentials.[3]

Effects of Programmed Electrical Stimulation

Typically, these forms of arrhythmia are not started or terminated by premature extrastimuli, although the rhythm may be transiently disturbed for a few cycles.[4] Abnormal automaticity is not suppressed by overdrive unless the overdrive is rapid and is maintained for a long period.[5] Indeed, short periods of overdrive may transiently accelerate the arrhythmia. This differs from normal automaticity, which is relatively easily transiently suppressed by overdrive pacing. Automatic rhythms may demonstrate a "warm up" phenomenon in which the rate gradually accelerates to a constant, and a "cool down" phenomenon as the rate gradually decelerates before termination of the arrhythmia.

Vulnerable Parameters

The potential areas of attack in an automatic rhythm include the maximum diastolic potential, the rate of phase 4 depolarization, the voltage of the threshold potential, and the action potential duration. The most easily targeted parameter appears to be the phase 4 depolarization. However, the exact processes that are involved in abnormal phase 4 depolarization in pathologic situations are not known. Therefore, there are no specifically targeted drugs that can be used in arrhythmias that are known to be of automatic origin.

Triggered Automaticity

Triggered activity is consequent upon afterdepolarizations. Afterdepolarizations are oscillations in the membrane potential that occur at the end of repolarization (early afterdepolarizations) or after repolarization has occurred (delayed afterdepolarizations).[6]

When the level of oscillation in membrane potential reaches the threshold potential, an action potential is initiated (Fig. 9–1). This may occur repeatedly, resulting in a sustained arrhythmia.

The cellular mechanism common to the occurrence of afterdepolarizations appears to be an increase in the Ca^{2+} level in myocardial cells. The classic arrhythmia dependent on triggered activity is digitalis toxicity, which causes inhibition of Na^+/K^+ pump activity.[7] This results in an increase in intracellular Na^+,[8] which subsequently causes an increase in intracellular Ca^2 through Na^+/Ca^{2+} exchange.[9] Afterdepolarizations can also be caused by catecholamines,[10] which increase calcium entry into the cell via the slow inward L-type calcium current.[11] Catecholamines also enhance uptake of Ca^{2+} by the sarcoplasmic reticulum,[12] but in the presence of increased intracellular Ca^{2+}, this may be re-released to further elevate intracellular Ca^{2+} levels (calcium-induced calcium release) and may lead to the occurrence of delayed afterdepolarizations.[13]

The current responsible for the oscillation of membrane potential after an increase in intracellular Ca^{2+} appears to be mainly dependent on entry of Na^+.[14] It is possible that calcium released from the sarcoplasmic reticulum could act on the sarcolemma to increase conductance, allowing ions to enter through concentration gradients via a nonselective cation channel.[15] Alternatively, the transient inward current could originate from the electrogenic exchange of Na^+ for Ca^{2+}.[16]

Several factors appear to influence the occurrence and magnitude of delayed afterdepolarizations, and thereby the likelihood of the development of an arrhythmia. The magnitude of afterdepolarizations is influenced by changes in cycle length, catecholamines, and parasympathetic withdrawal. The magnitude of the transient inward current, and therefore the magnitude of the delayed afterdepolarization, can be influenced by the membrane potential. The current is maximal at membrane potential levels of approximately -60 mV and diminishes at voltage levels around this.[17] The duration of the action potential also influences the occurrence of delayed afterdepolarizations[18]—the longer action potentials cause larger increases in intracellular Ca^{2+} and thereby increase the transient inward current.[19] Drugs that prolong the action potential duration, such as quinidine, therefore increase the delayed afterdepolarization amplitude,[20] whereas drugs shortening the action potential can conversely decrease the delayed afterdepolarization amplitude.[21] Any action that increases the amount of time the membrane is in the depolarized state increases the amplitude of the transient inward current and causes it to occur earlier. Thus, a decrease in the drive cycle length increases the amplitude of delayed afterdepolarizations and decreases the coupling interval to the action potential.[22] There is, therefore, a direct relationship between the drive cycle length at which triggered impulses are initiated and the coupling interval of the first triggered arrhythmic pulse and the last pulse of the drive train.

Effects of Programmed Electrical Stimulation

Triggered rhythms can be initiated by overdrive stimulation or premature extrastimuli. There should be a direct relationship between the cycle length of the stimulation and the coupling interval of the first beat of tachycardia, although lack of this relation is no absolute proof that the arrhythmia is not caused by triggered activity. Triggered rhythms may be terminated by a single extrastimulus, but it is not usually as reproducible as reentry, whereas termination with overdrive is more frequent, although this may accelerate the arrhythmia.

Vulnerable Parameters

The vulnerable parameter for delayed afterdepolarizations is cellular calcium overload. This can be prevented by drugs blocking the L-type calcium channel, decreasing action potential duration (thereby decreasing calcium entry), and decreasing sodium entry during the upstroke of the action potential.

Early Afterdepolarizations

The terminal plateau phase or the repolarization phase of the action potential may have small depolarizations that are termed early afterdepolarizations. When the magnitude of these is large enough, a net inward current is activated and an action potential ensues. Repeated activity in this manner can result in a sustained arrhythmia. Early afterdepolarizations occur more readily in Purkinje fibers than ventricular or atrial myocytes. Agents that prolong the action potential duration and increase the inward current cause early afterdepolarizations; an example of such an agent is aconitine.[6] Blockade of the outward K^+ current also delays membrane repolarization and causes early afterdepolarizations and triggered activity.[23] Drugs prolonging the action potential include sotalol,[24] *m*-acetylprocainamide,[4] and quinidine[25] and can cause early afterdepolarizations and triggered activity in isolated Purkinje fiber preparations. The occurrence of early afterdepolarizations is enhanced when the rate of stimulation is low and the K^+ concentration of the superfusate is reduced. The arrhyth-

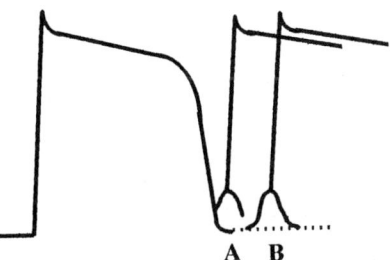

Figure 9–1. A cardiac action potential demonstrating (A) an early afterdepolarization which achieves the threshold and triggers a further action potential and (B) a delayed afterdepolarization which also triggers another action potential.

mias induced by agents that cause early afterdepolarizations resemble torsade de pointes, and this is the likely mechanism of the arrhythmia.

The mechanism of early afterdepolarizations occurring during the repolarization phase is due to either a decrease in the outward current, or an increase in the inward current, and the ionic mechanisms are likely to be similar to those discussed earlier. Afterdepolarizations occurring in the plateau phase of the action potential are likely to have a different mechanism. There is evidence that the Na^+ current through tetrodotoxin channels[26] or the L-type calcium current may be responsible.[27]

Effects of Programmed Electrical Stimulation

Arrhythmias caused by early afterdepolarizations cannot be induced by overdrive pacing or premature stimuli. They are more likely to occur at long cycle lengths and are therefore most likely to be induced by pauses. These rhythms are not generally terminated by overdrive pacing or premature stimulation.

Vulnerable Parameters

Possible ionic areas of attack for arrhythmias based on early afterdepolarizations include shortening of the action potential duration and blocking the inward current causing the triggered action potential.

Abnormal Impulse Conduction-Reentry

The occurrence of reentrant arrhythmia requires a number of particular electrophysiologic situations. There has to be a central inexcitable region, which may be anatomic, as in scar tissue, or functional, as in a region of cells that are refractory. The circuit is formed around this central obstacle by conducting paths with differential electrical properties of conduction velocity and refractoriness. Impulse conduction should have delay at some stage in the circuit to allow tissues in front to recover from refractoriness, and this is usually due to a zone of slowed conduction (Fig. 9–2). Slowed conduction can occur when the amplitude of cellular depolarization becomes reduced, and as a consequence, axial current flow is also diminished. This can occur if an impulse arises during the relative refractory period of the cells, when $Na+$ channels are still inactivated. Slowed conduction also occurs in situations in which the resting potential is low (-60 to -70 mV), when the Na^+ channels are partially inactivated and therefore unavailable to the depolarizing stimulus. At such membrane potentials, recovery from activation is markedly prolonged[28] and any consequent action potential has diminished amplitude, with reduced coaxial current flow and conduction velocity (depressed fast responses). Further inactivation of the Na^+ channel may result in a decrease in conduction velocity such that unidirectional block occurs.[29] At membrane potential levels of -50 mV, although Na^+ channels are almost totally inactivated, the L-type Ca^{2+} channel can still

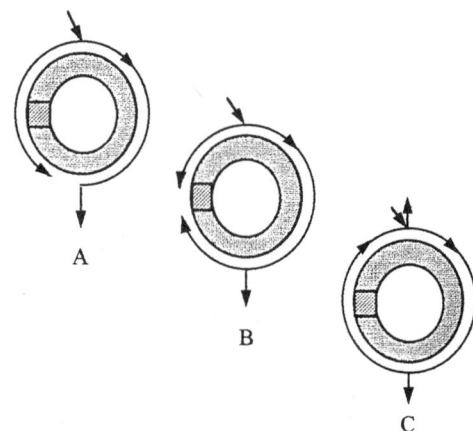

Figure 9–2. A representation of the mechanism of reentrant arrhythmias. The hatched area on the circuit around a central nonconducting obstacle represents a zone of slowed conduction. In normal circumstances, conduction proceeds through the faster pathway (A). In circumstances where there is increased delay in the slower pathway, there is retrograde penetration of this pathway by the impulse via the faster pathway (B). If the zone of conduction develops unidirectional block, then the conduction can proceed retrogradely via the slower pathway and initiate reentry (C).

be activated and result in a slowly propagated action potential (slow response).[30] Slow response action potentials can also occur in normal conduction tissue of the heart, including sinus and atrioventricular nodes, where the normal resting potential is less than -70 mV.[30] Normal myocardium exhibits anisotropic conduction, i.e., conduction in the longitudinal direction is faster than the transverse.[31] This is partially as a result of better coupling of cells in the longitudinal direction by gap junctions than transverse to the long axis of cells, leading to a lower axial resistivity than transverse.[32] Anisotropy may be uniform, where the conduction wave front is smooth, although of different velocity in all directions, or nonuniform. In nonuniform anisotropy, there are areas where transverse coupling of fibers appears to be absent, and this may be due to isolation of the bundles by fibrous septa.[31] Propagation of the impulse in the transverse direction may undergo an irregular "zigzag" sequence, which is a potent substrate for reentry.[33] Furthermore, increased resistance to axial conduction can occur when gap junction resistance becomes increased,[34] as is liable to occur when intracellular calcium levels become elevated,[35] as in myocardial ischemia.

Unidirectional Block

Unidirectional block, where conduction is blocked in one direction while remaining possible in the other, is critical to the maintenance of reentry. Unidirectional block may occur as a consequence of regional differences in recovery of excitability. In regions with the longest refractory period, a premature impulse will be blocked in this area, while conduction continues in others.[36] The premature impulse serves as a trigger, while the conditions necessary for the reentrant circuit are the substrate. In regions where conduction of impulses is depressed, a premature impulse can also result in unidirectional block.[29]

In anatomically defined circuits, conduction round the circuit is composed of a head, which is the depolarizing wave front, and the area of refractoriness that composes the tail. Between the head and the tail, there is a segment of excitable tissue on the circuit. This "excitable gap" can be small or large but allows externally delivered impulses to invade the circuit, and these may terminate the arrhythmia by making the tissue in front of the head inexcitable.

Apart from anatomically defined circuits, others may be functionally defined, as in the leading circle model of Allessie et al.[37] In this model, a central area is kept refractory because of the impulse traveling around it and constantly activating it. In this model, the head of the excitation is just able to excite the tissue ahead of it that is in the relative refractory phase; therefore, there is no gap of fully excitable tissue that can easily be accessed by premature impulses. Resetting or termination of the arrhythmia by appropriately timed impulses may therefore be difficult. Functional circuits may change in size and location. Reentry may also occur as a consequence of the anisotropic properties of cardiac muscle, where there are differences in axial resistance to impulse propagation.[38] This is most likely to be the mechanism of ventricular tachycardias in the healing and healed phases of myocardial infarction, in which the origin of these circuits is frequently in the epicardial muscle left from a transmural infarct in which the fibers are arranged in fascicles and reentrant circuits can form because of nonuniform anisotropic properties. In these regions, where activation is occurring parallel to the fiber direction, impulse transmission is rapid, whereas, in the transverse direction, the conduction is slow and may form apparent block.[39]

Effects of Programmed Electrical Stimulation

Initiation of the arrhythmia by overdrive or programmed stimulation suggests a reentrant mechanism if other characteristics eliminate the possibility of triggered activity. Demonstration of the area of slowed activity, such as fractionation of electrograms during initiation of ventricular tachycardia, is also suggestive of a reentrant mechanism. There is frequently an inverse relationship between the premature impulse coupling interval and the interval to the first impulse of tachycardia reflecting slower conduction round the circuit.[40] Reentrant arrhythmias may also be terminated by overdrive or premature stimulation. The overdrive has to be a critical rate and duration, and the premature stimulus requires a critical coupling interval. The extrastimulus has to penetrate the circuit and cause block in front of the excitation wave front. Rapid tachycardias may have a very small excitable gap that is difficult to penetrate, and functional circuits with the leading circle mechanism may have no excitable gap. Reentrant rhythms may be entrained,[41] and the demonstration of this phenomenon is strongly suggestive of such a mechanism.

Vulnerable Parameters

Drugs may prevent triggers of reentrant excitation, and these may be due to triggered activity, or may abolish the continuation of reentry. The latter is dependent on the properties of the reentrant circuit. If, for example, the excitable gap is large, it is unlikely that prolongation of refractoriness will stop reentry. The approach then would be to slow conduction to an extent that excitation is no longer maintained. If conduction is maintained by depressed fast responses, drugs blocking the sodium channel may be effective, whereas if these are due to slow responses, drugs that act as calcium antagonists may be effective. If the excitable gap is short, block within the circuit would be caused by a prolongation of the recovery from excitability of cells on the circuit.

USE OF ELECTROPHYSIOLOGIC TESTING

Electrophysiologic testing allows

1. The study of the mechanism of tachycardia, critical components, and vulnerable parameters.
2. The characterization of the electrophysiologic effects of antiarrhythmic drugs on normal and diseased tissues and on tachycardia mechanisms.
3. The specific diagnosis and description of tachycardia and evaluation of antiarrhythmic therapies in individual patients.

SUPRAVENTRICULAR TACHYCARDIA

The establishment of a clear and specific diagnosis is critical to the appropriate drug treatment of supraventricular tachycardias. Thus, documentation of the arrhythmia and electrophysiologic study form an essential part of the patient management.

Atrioventricular Nodal Reentrant Tachycardia

This is classically a reentrant tachycardia with anterograde conduction over a slow pathway and retrograde conduction over a fast pathway.[42] The existence of these is supported by electrophysiologic data, although anatomically these have not been precisely defined. The tachycardia is confined entirely to atrial tissue, and activation of the His bundle is secondary and not necessary for the maintenance of the arrhythmia. Slow channel tissue-dependent tissue (I_{Ca-L}) appears to be involved in the slow pathway, whereas the fast pathway may have fast channel–dependent (I_{Na}) cells.[43] Repolarization is dependent on I_K in both classes of cell.[44] The most vulnerable parameter is interruption of the slow pathway conduction, which can be achieved by vagal stimulation (Valsalva maneuver, carotid sinus massage) leading to M2 receptor stimulation, purinergic A2 receptor stimulation with adenosine, or calcium antagonist drugs such as verapamil or diltiazem. These approaches are useful in the acute termination of tachycardia. In some instances, β-adrenoceptor blockade or Na^+/K^+ pump inhibition with a cardiac glycoside can be used. Tachycardia recurrences can be prevented by drugs acting on the slow pathway, as well as drugs that act on the fast pathway, slowing conduction and prolonging refractoriness. These drugs include quinidine, procainamide, and disopyramide. Flecainide, propafenone, sotalol, and amiodarone are also effective. It is conventional to attempt to use calcium antagonists initially, and then move to other categories, either singly or in combination.

Wolff-Parkinson-White (WPW) Syndrome

This is characterized by the presence of accessory atrioventricular connection(s) that form a critical part of the reentrant circuit, consisting of the atrium, atrioventricular node, His-Purkinje system ventricle, and the pathway. In tachycardias with a long excitable gap, the initial approach would be to slow conduction, such that unidirectional block occurs. Data suggest that the junction between the accessory pathway and the atrium is the site at which this is likely to occur.[45] In tachycardias with a short excitable gap, prolongation of the refractory period of part of the circuit would be useful, because the depolarizing wave front would meet with refractory tissue. The atrioventricular node also forms part of the circuit and is vulnerable to attack by the agents that are relatively selective for this tissue.

In patients in tachycardia, drugs acting on the atrioventricular node are the first choice. The most ideal of these is adenosine, but calcium antagonists (verapamil and diltiazem) and β-blocking drugs are also effective. If these fail, agents acting on the accessory pathway are used, and these are sodium channel blockers, excluding mexiletine, lignocaine, and tocainide. If drug treatment fails, cardioversion should be performed. In patients with recurrent episodes of arrhythmia, suppression of the frequency of attacks is necessary. In these circumstances, agents acting on the accessory pathway (sodium channel blockers), in particular class IC drugs, are generally used. Agents acting on the atrioventricular node are avoided, because these increase the possibility that excitation proceeds preferentially through the accessory pathway rather than via the His bundle. In these circumstances, rapid atrial rhythms, in particular atrial fibrillation, can be conducted to the ventricle without the rate protective actions of the atrioventricular node and result in ventricular fibrillation. In circumstances in which class I drugs are ineffective, class III agents (amiodarone) can be extremely useful, but at increased risk of serious side effects.

Patients who continue to suffer from symptoms despite drug therapy or who are intolerant of drug treatment can be offered catheter ablation of the accessory pathway. Since the use of radiofrequency energy, this has extremely high success rates (>95% of left-sided pathways), with a low rate of complications.[46]

Mahaim Tachycardias

Right-sided connections may occur between the atrium and the distal right bundle. These pathways have properties that differ from the normal WPW type pathway. These pathways appear to only conduct anterogradely and exhibit decremental properties. Tachycardia is antidromic, with anterograde conduction over the atriofascicular connection and retrograde conduction over the right bundle branch, His bundle, atrioventricular node, and the atrium. These tachycardias can be treated with the same drug groups as for WPW syndrome, except that the pathway can respond to drugs that normally act on atrioventricular node, such as adenosine, calcium antagonists, and β-blockers. If the tachycardia is difficult to control with drugs, these pathways can be catheter ablated.[47]

Atrial Tachycardia

The mechanisms for most atrial tachycardias have not yet been adequately determined, but some appear to be reentrant, others are automatic, and yet others are due to triggered automaticity (digitalis toxicity). Drugs most likely to be effective are Na^+ channel blockers, Ca^{2+} channel blockers, and β-blocking agents. In instances in which drugs are ineffective, catheter ablation may be effective.[48]

Atypical Atrioventricular Reentry

These are reentrant tachycardias, in which the anterograde limb is through a slow pathway and the retrograde limb over the slow pathway. The retrograde P wave is therefore in the second half of the cardiac cycle. Some of these tachycardias can be over slow-slow pathways, and the retrograde P wave is central in the cardiac cycle. These arrhythmias behave as classic atrioventricular reentry in the response to drugs.

Atrial Flutter

Atrial flutter is a reentrant rhythm based on the right atrium, with the area of block based on the orifice of the inferior vena cava, and an area of functional block between this and the truncus intercavarum, although another area of slowed conduction exists between the coronary sinus and the tricuspid valve.[49] This is in keeping with the recent findings that atrial flutter can be abolished by the placement of lesions near the coronary sinus or the orifice of the inferior vena cava. Drugs that prolong refractoriness in the absence of an alteration in conduction velocity should abolish the excitable gap and hence the tachycardia. However, drugs with markedly different effects on refractoriness and conduction velocity have been shown to terminate flutter, including quinidine,[50] flecainide,[51] moricizine, and procainamide.[4] Termination of tachycardia appears to be initiated by the occurrence of block in the area of slowed conduction. These drugs and also Class III agents can suppress episodes of atrial flutter. Ablation has been attempted in patients with arrhythmia unresponsive to drug therapy, with variable reports of efficacy.

Atrial Fibrillation

The mechanism of atrial fibrillation is not understood, but early models demonstrated that placement of aconitine on the atrium led to rapid firing, and the remaining tissue is unable to follow at 1:1 activation, resulting in refractoriness and heterogeneity of conduction.[52] Recent studies of the mapping of atrial fibrillation appear to suggest that this arrhythmia may be due to one or two unstable reentrant circuits that generate very short cycle lengths and progress across the right atrial wall, temporarily disappearing and then reforming.[53] Some forms of atrial fibrillation appear to be parasympathetically mediated, and drugs with a parasympatholytic action would be indicated. Other forms of atrial fibrillation appear to be adrenergically mediated, and in these patients, β-blocking drugs are indicated.[54] Drugs that appear to be effective in patients with paroxysmal atrial fibrillation include class IC drugs (flecainide) and class III drugs (sotalol and amiodarone).

VENTRICULAR ARRHYTHMIAS
Ventricular Extrasystoles

Ventricular extrasystoles may be due to abnormal automaticity, in which phase 4 depolarization should be reduced; triggered activity, in which there should be a reduction in cellular calcium overload; or reentry, in which a decrease in conduction velocity or prolongation of refractoriness would be considered. In practice, these generally respond to β-blocking drugs, and these agents, when used after myocardial infarction, have led to a reduction in the mortality.[55] Sodium channel blocking drugs have been used, but in the presence of ischemic heart disease, these have been shown to have an adverse effect on prognosis because of the strong proarrhythmic effect.[56] Class III drugs also may be of value, and amiodarone appears from recent results to be of particular prognostic value after myocardial infarction.[57]

Ventricular Tachycardia

Ventricular tachycardia generally requires an anatomic substrate to support the tachycardia, frequently ischemic heart disease or cardiomyopathy. This substrate may be modified by a number of modulating influences, including hemodynamic changes, autonomic effects, and metabolic states. These may themselves be influenced by antiarrhythmic drugs, and because they may vary with time, they can affect the influence of drugs that are used.

Therapeutic targets for ventricular tachycardia therefore include

1. Suppression of triggering ventricular premature depolarizations
2. Alteration of the sustaining substrate
3. Blockade of transient influences

Currently, the attempts to suppress triggering ventricular ectopic beats that may serve as triggers for ventricular tachyarrhythmias have proved disappointing.[56] Drugs that alter the substrate are more effective, as long as the substrate is fixed. Drugs that affect modulating influences would, therefore, also be useful.

Idiopathic Left Ventricular Tachycardia

This is a recurrent, sustained ventricular tachycardia with a right bundle branch block configuration with a leftward axis. The arrhythmia is frequently provoked by programmed stimulation with rapid atrial pacing or by ventricular pacing. There is an inverse relationship between the coupling internal of the extrastimulus and the first beat of the tachycardia. Retrograde His activation and the relatively narrow QRS complex during tachycardia suggest that the Purkinje fiber network of the left posterior fascicle is the location of the microreentrant pathway. The arrhythmia may be terminated with programmed electrical stimulation, and entrainment may be demonstrated. Verapamil has been shown to terminate the tachycardia.

The potential vulnerable areas include the probable reentrant mechanism, and the efficacy of verapamil would suggest slow channel–dependent reentry. This agent appears to be effective in the majority of patients. Drugs prolonging repolarization can be effective in some. Na^+ channel–blocking drugs do not appear to be of great value.

Catecholamine-Dependent Tachycardias

Some forms of arrhythmia can be induced by exercise and isoprenaline infusion. Automaticity, triggered automaticity, and reentry all are enhanced by catecholamines. These arrhythmias are frequently terminated by adenosine or agents such as dipyridamole that increase tissue adenosine concentrations. Adenosine and muscarinic antagonists interfere with the electrophysiologic effects of adrenergic stimulation mediated through an increase in intracellular Ca^{2+} concentrations. Adenosine appears to be specific for arrhythmias having a response to pacing protocols that suggest triggered automaticity. Thus, as discussed previously, triggered activity and calcium overload are possible mechanisms by which catecholamines may exert their arrhythmogenic action in these arrhythmias. These arrhythmias are frequently tachycardias of a right ventricular outflow tract origin, without any evidence of underlying cardiac disease. Potential targets for antiarrhythmic drugs include the $β_1$-adrenergic receptors and actions via adenosine A1 and muscarinic M2 receptors. Prevention of calcium entry, uptake of calcium by the sarcoplasmic reticulum, and the Na^+/Ca^{2+} current are potential targets. Delayed afterdepolarizations can also be due to the Ca^{2+}-dependent nonselective inward current (I_{Na}), and this is also a potential target.

Arrhythmias in Acute Myocardial Ischemia and Infarction

In acute ischemia, rapid changes in electrophysiologic parameters can occur, creating areas of block and slowed conduction. Arrhythmias in this situation are characteristically irregular, polymorphic, and nonsustained, frequently degenerating into ventricular fibrillation. Early in ischemia, there is a decrease in the resting potential, action potential upstroke velocity (V_{max}), and action potential duration.[58] There is a rapid accumulation of K^+ in the extracellular space, which partially depolarizes the cells. In 15 to 30 minutes, the ischemic area becomes inexcitable, and there is a marked decrease in conduction velocity with eventual conduction block.[58] During later phases of ischemia, delayed afterdepolarizations and triggered activity occur and can lead to multiform ectopic rhythms, which may secondarily initiate reentrant rhythms.[59] It is likely that arrhythmias that occur in these phases relate to an endogenous release of catecholamines. Reperfusion after a period of transient ischemia is also arrhythmogenic and may result in ventricular tachycardia or ventricular fibrillation. Multiple cellular mechanisms appear to be involved in the early ischemic rhythms, but there is substantial evidence that β-blocking drugs inhibit arrhythmogenesis.[60]

Chronic Ventricular Tachycardia Related to Ischemic Heart Disease

In patients with recurrent episodes of ventricular tachycardia after myocardial infarction, these arrhythmias are generally reentrant and respond acutely to drugs that slow conduction. Data suggest that the safest and most efficacious drugs for acute termination of tachycardia include intravenous procainamide and lignocaine. Flecainide and disopyramide are more effective, although the proarrhythmic effects are greater.[61, 62] In patients in whom the arrhythmia is hemodynamically well maintained and sustained or incessant, rapid loading with intravenous amiodarone can be effective, particularly when other agents have failed.[63] Patients who do not respond to antiarrhythmic drugs, or those who are hemodynamically unstable, should have external DC cardioversion.

In patients with recurrent attacks of arrhythmia, although the occurrence of episodes can be suppressed by the use of class I drugs, these have fallen from favor because of the Cardiac Arrhythmia Suppression Trial (CAST) data, which suggest that mortality may be increased, particularly in patients with underlying cardiac structural disease and ischemia. In view of this, there has been a swing to the use of drugs that increase the action potential duration, such as sotalol, and amiodarone. Sotalol has been shown to be effective in suppressing episodes of arrhythmia,

even when these have been refractory to class I drugs.[64, 65] Amiodarone also appears to be effective in arrhythmia suppression.[66] Recent studies suggest that amiodarone has a substantial beneficial effect on mortality in patients at a high risk of life-threatening ventricular arrhythmias, although large-scale randomized trials are currently under way to test these preliminary data.[67]

Numerous combinations of antiarrhythmic drugs, both logical and illogical, have been used for the treatment of recurrent ventricular tachycardia. For example, combinations of class I agents have been attempted to achieve greater efficacy in suppression of arrhythmia,[68, 69] but the CAST study results have tempered enthusiasm for these combinations. Sotalol has been used with class I drugs, on the basis of achieving slowing of conduction in combination with a prolongation of refractoriness, and appears to be effective.[70] Amiodarone has also been used with class I drugs, and this again appears to be effective, but at an increased risk of proarrhythmic effects.[71] When amiodarone alone has failed, combination with a β-blocking agent may be useful.[72]

Patients with recurrent tachycardia even on antiarrhythmic therapy are candidates for attempted catheter ablation, provided that the arrhythmia is relatively slow and well tolerated hemodynamically. However, the results suggest that success rates are not high, even when the procedure is used in highly selected patients.[73]

The treatment of refractory ventricular arrhythmias has been made much easier by the advent of the implantable cardioverter-defibrillator. Arrhythmia that is pace terminable and infrequent episodes of arrhythmia are ideal for device therapy.[74] Preliminary data suggest that device therapy of arrhythmias offers benefits in survival in the patients at high risk of sudden cardiac death.

CONCLUSIONS

Exact mechanisms underlying many forms of arrhythmia yet remain to be precisely identified; nevertheless, some degree of understanding has resulted in the identification of drugs that are likely to be effective. Large-scale clinical trials that have been conducted and that are currently in progress will help define the role of different drugs in the treatment of these arrhythmias.

REFERENCES

1. Imanishi S, Surawicz B: Automatic activity in depolarized guinea pig ventricular myocardium. Circ Res 39:751, 1976.
2. Katzung BG, Morgenstern JA: Effects of extracellular potassium on ventricular automaticity and evidence for a pacemaker current in mammalian ventricular myocardium. Circ Res 40:105, 1977.
3. Escande D, Coulombe A, Faiure JF, et al: Two types of transient outward current in adult human atrial cells. Am J Physiol 252:H142, 1987.
4. Dangman KH, Hoffman BF: The effects of single premature stimuli on automatic and triggered rhythms in isolated canine Purkinje fibres. Circulation 71:813, 1985.

5. Hoffman BF, Dangman KH: Are arrhythmias caused by abnormal impulse generation? *In* Paes de Caravalho A, Hoffman BF, Lieberman M (eds): Normal and Abnormal Conduction in the Heart. Mount Kisco, NY: Futura Publishing, 1982, pp 429–448.

6. Cranefield PF, Aronson RS: The Conduction of the Cardiac Impulse: The Slow Response and Cardiac Arrhythmias. Mount Kisco, NY: Futura Publishing, 1988.

7. Aronson RS, Cranefield PF: The effect of resting potential on the electrical activity of canine Purkinje fibres exposed to Na-free solution or to ouabain. Pflugers Arch 347:101, 1974.

8. Dietmer JW, Ellis D: The intracellular sodium activity of cardiac Purkinje fibres during inhibition and re-activation of the Na-K pump. J Physiol (Lond) 284:241, 1978.

9. Mullins LJ: The generation of electric currents in cardiac fibers by Na/Ca exchange. Am J Physiol 236:C103, 1979.

10. Belardinelli L, Isenberg G: Actions of adenosine and isoproterenol on isolated mammalian ventricular myocytes. Circ Res 53:287, 1983.

11. Reuter H: Ion channel in cardiac cell membranes. Ann Rev Physiol 46:473,1984.

12. Mord M, Rolett EL: Relaxing effects of catecholamines on mammalian heart. J Physiol (Lond) 224:537, 1972.

13. Fabiato A: Calcium-induced release of calcium from the cardiac sarcoplasmic reticulum. Am J Physiol 245:C1, 1983.

14. Tseng G-N, Wit AL: Characteristics of a transient inward current that causes delayed afterdepolarizations in atrial cells of the canine coronary sinus. J Mol Cell Cardiol 19:1105, 1987.

15. Kass RS, Tsien RW, Weingart R: Ionic basis of transient inward current induced by strophanthidin in cardiac Purkinje fibres. J Physiol (Lond) 281:209, 1978.

16. Lipp P, Pott L: Transient inward current in guinea-pig atrial myocytes reflects a change of sodium-calcium exchange currents. J Physiol (Lond) 397:601, 1977.

17. Vassalle M, Mugelli A: An oscillatory current in sheep cardiac Purkinje fibres. Circ Res 48:618, 1981.

18. Henning B, Wit AL: The time course of action potential repolarization affects delayed afterdepolarization amplitude in atrial fibres of the canine coronary sinus. Circ Res 55:110, 1984.

19. Kass RS, Scheuer T: Slow inactivation of calcium channels in the cardiac Purkinje fibre. J Mol Cell Cardiol 14:216, 1982.

20. Wit AL, Tseng G-N, Henning B, Hanna MS: Arrhythmogenic effects of quinidine on catecholamine-induced delayed afterdepolarizations in canine atrial fibres. J Cardiovasc Electrophysiol 1:15, 1990.

21. Sheu SS, Lederer WJ: Lidocaine's negative inotropic and antiarrhythmia actions: Dependence on shortening of action potential duration and reduction of intracellular sodium activity. Circ Res 57:578, 1985.

22. Saito T, Otoguro M, Matsubara T: Electrophysiological studies on the mechanism of electrically induced sustained rhythmic activity in the rabbit right atrium. Circ Res 42:199, 1978.

23. Damiano BP, Rosen MR: Effects of pacing on triggered activity induced by early afterdepolarizations. Circulation 69:1013, 1984.

24. Carmeleit E: Electrophysiologic and voltage clamp analysis of the effects of sotalol on isolated cardiac muscle and Purkinje fibres. J Pharmacol Exp Ther 232:17, 1985.

25. Davedenko JM, Cohen L, Goodrow R, Antzelevitch C: Quinidine-induced action potential prolongation, early afterdepolarizations, and triggered activity in canine Purkinje fibres: Effects of stimulation rate, potassium, and magnesium. Circulation 79:674, 1989.

26. Coulombe A, Coraboeuf E, Deroubaix E: Computer simulation of acidosis-induced abnormal repolarization and repetitive activity in dog Purkinje fibres. J Physiol (Paris) 76:705, 1980.

27. January CT, Riddle JM: Early afterdepolarizations: Mechanism of induction and block. A role for L-type Ca^{2+} current. Circ Res 64:977, 1989.

28. Gettes LS, Reuter H: Slow recovery from inactivation of inward currents in mammalian myocardial fibres. J Physiol (Lond) 405:123, 1988.

29. Dodge FA, Cranefield PF: Nonuniform conduction of cardiac Purkinje fibres. *In* Paes de Caravalho A, Hoffman BF, Lieberman M (eds): Normal and Abnormal Conduction in the Heart. Mount Kisco, NY: Futura Publishing Co, 1982, pp 379–395.

30. Cranefield PF: The Conduction of the Cardiac Impulse: The Slow Response and Cardiac Arrhythmias. Mount Kisco, NY: Futura Publishing, 1975.

31. Spach MS, Miller WT III, Dolber PC, et al: The functional role of structural complexities in the propagation of depolarization in the atrium of the dog: Cardiac conduction disturbances due to discontinuities of effective axial resistivity. Circ Res 50:175, 1982.

32. Roberts DE, Hersch LT, Scher AM: Influence of cardial fibre orientation on wavefront conduction velocity and tissue resistivity in the dog. Circ Res 44:101, 1979.

33. Spach MS, Dolber PC: Relating extracellular potentials and their derivatives to anisotropic propagation at a microscopic level in human cardiac muscle: Evidence for electrical uncoupling of side-to-side fibre connections with increasing age. Circ Res 59:356, 1986.

34. Quan W, Rudy Y: Unidirectional block and reentry of cardiac excitation: A model study. Circ Res 66:376, 1990.

35. DeMello WC: Effects of intracellular injection of calcium and strontium on cell communication in heart. J Physiol (Lond) 250:231, 1975.

36. Sasyniuk BI, Mendez C: A mechanism for reentry in canine ventricular tissue. Circ Res 28:3, 1971.

37. Allessie MA, Bonke FIM, Schopman FJG: Circus movement in rabbit atrial muscle as a mechanism of tachycardia: III. The "leading circle" concept: A new model of circus movement in cardiac tissue without the involvement of an anatomical obstacle. Circ Res 41:9, 1977.

38. Spach MS, Dolber PC, Heidlage JF: Influence of the passive anisotropic properties on directional differences in propagation following modification of the calcium conductance in human atrial muscle: A model of reentry hased on anisotropic discontinuous propagation. Circ Res 62:811, 1988.

39. Dillon SM, Allessie MA, Ursell PC, Wit AL: Influence of anisotropic tissue structure on reentrant circuits in the subepicardial border zone of subacute canine infarcts. Circ Res 63:182, 1988.

40. Josephson ME: Tachycardia Mechanism and Management. Mount Kisco, NY: Futura Publishing, 1992.

41. Waldo AL, Plumb VJ, Arciniegas JG, et al: Transient entrainment and interruption of the atrioventricular bypass pathway type of paroxysmal atrial tachycardia: A model for understanding and identifying reentrant rhythms. Circulation 67:73, 1983.

42. Mitrani R, Klein LS, Hackett K, et al: Radiofrequency ablation for atrioventricular nodal re-entrant tachycardia: Comparison between fast (anterior) versus slow (posterior) pathway ablation. J Am Coll Cardiol 2:432, 1992.

43. Hartzell HC, Duchatelle-Gourdon I: Structure and neural modulation of cardiac calcium channels. J Cardiovasc Electrophysiol 3:567, 1993.

44. Joho RH: Toward a molecular understanding of voltage-gated potassium channels. J Cardiovasc Electrophysiol 3:589, 1993.

45. De la Fuente D, Sasyniuk B, Moe GK: Conduction through a narrow isthmus in isolated canine atrial tissue: A model of WPW syndrome. Circulation 44:803, 1971.

46. Jackman WM, Beckman KJ, McClelland JH, Lazzara R: Localization and radiofrequency catheter ablation of accessory AV pathways in Wolff-Parkinson-White syndrome. J Electrocardiol 14:24, 1992.

47. Haissaguerre M, Warin JF, Le Metayer P, et al: Catheter ablation of Mahaim fibres with preservation of atrioventricular nodal conduction. Circulation 82:418, 1990.

48. Kay GN, Epstein AE, Daily SM, Plumb VJ: Role of radiofrequency ablation in the management of supraventricular arrhythmias: Experience in 760 consecutive patients. J Cardiovasc Electrophysiol 4:371, 1993.

49. Cosio FG, Lopez-Gil M, Giocolea A, et al: Radiofrequency ablation of the inferior vena cava-tricuspid valve isthmus in common atrial flutter. Am J Cardiol 71:705, 1993.

50. Okumura K, Waldo AL: Effects of N-acetylprocainamide on experimental atrial flutter and atrial electrophysiologic properties in conscious dogs with sterile pericarditis: Comparison with the effect of quinidine. J Am Coll Cardiol 9:1332, 1987.

51. Scalabrini A, Okumura K, Olshanksky B, Waldo AL: Effects of class 1C drugs on induced atrial flutter in a dog model with sterile pericarditis. Circulation 74:ii, 1986.

52. Scherf D, Romano FJ, Terranova R: Experimental studies on auricular flutter and auricular fibrillation. Am Heart J 36:241, 1958.

53. Ortiz J, Niwano S, Abe H, et al: Mapping the conversion of atrial flutter to atrial fibrillation and atrial fibrillation to atrial flutter—insights into mechanism. Circ Res 74:882, 1994.

54. Coumel P: Neural aspects of paroxysmal atrial fibrillation. In Falk RH, Podrid PJ (eds): Atrial Fibrillation Mechanisms and Management. New York: Raven Press, 1992, pp 109–112.

55. Yusuf S, Peto R, Lewis J, et al: Beta blockade during and after myocardial infarction: An overview of the randomized trials. Prog Cardiovasc Dis 27:335, 1985.

56. The Cardic Arrhythmia Suppression Trial (CAST) Investigators: Preliminary report: Effects of encainide and flecainide on mortality in a randomized trial of arrhythmia suppression after myocardial infarction. N Engl J Med 21:406, 1989.

57. Pfisterer ME, Kiowski W, Brunner H, et al: Long-term benefit of 1 year amiodarone for treatment of persistent complex ventricular arrhythmias after myocardial infarction. Circulation 87:309, 1993.

58. Janse MJ, Kleber AG, Capucci A, et al: Electrophysiological basis for arrhythmias in acute ischemia: Role of the subendocardium. J Mol Cell Cardiol 18:339, 1986.

59. Pogwizd SM, Corr PB: Reentrant and nonreentrant mechanisms contribute to arrhythmogenesis during early myocardial ischemia: Results using 3-dimensional mapping. Circ Res 61:352, 1987.

60. Beta-blocker Heart Attack Trial Research Group: A randomized trial of propranolol in patients with acute myocardial infarction: I. Mortality results. JAMA 247:1707, 1982.

61. Kuchar DL, Rottman J, Berger E, et al: Prediction of successful suppression of sustained ventricular tachyarrhythmias by serial drug testing from data derived at the initial electrophysiologic study. J Am Coll Cardiol 12:982, 1988.

62. Griffith MJ, Linker NJ, Garratt CJ, et al: Relative efficacy and safety of intravenous drugs for termination of sustained ventricular tachycardia. Lancet 336:670, 1990.

63. Schutzenberger W, Leiuh F, Kersehner R, et al: Clinical efficacy of amiodarone in the short term treatment of recurrent sustained ventricular tachycardia and ventricular fibrillation. Br Heart J 62:367, 1989.

64. Singh SN, Cohen A, Chen YW, et al: Sotalol for refractory sustained ventricular tachycardia and nonfatal cardiac arrest. Am J Cardiol 62:399, 1988.

65. Kienzle MG, Martins JB, Wendt DJ, et al: Enhanced efficacy of sotalol for sustained ventricular tachycardia refractory to type I antiarrhythmic drugs. Am J Cardiol 61:1012, 1988.

66. Herre JM, Sauve MJ, Malone P, et al: Long-term results of amiodarone therapy in patients with recurrent ventricular tachycardia or ventricular fibrillation. J Am Coll Cardiol 13:442, 1989.

67. Schwartz PJ, Camm AJ, Frangin G, et al: Does amiodarone reduce sudden death and cardiac mortality after myocardial infarction? The European Myocardial Infarct Amiodarone Trial (EMIAT). Eur Heart J 15:620, 1994.

68. Whitford EG, McGovern B, Schoenfeld M, et al: Long-term efficacy of mexiletine alone and in combination with class 1a antiarrhythmic drugs for refractory ventricular arrhythmias. Am Heart J 115:360, 1988.

69. Yeung Lai Wah JA, Murdock CJ, Boon L, Kerr CR: Propafenone-mexiletine combination for the treatment of sustained ventricular tachycardia. J Am Coll Cardiol 20:547, 1992.

70. Dorian P, Newman D, Berman N, et al: Sotalol and type 1A drugs in combination prevent recurrence of sustained ventricular tachycardia. J Am Coll Cardiol 22:106, 1993.

71. Jung W, Mletzko R, Manz M, et al: Efficacy and safety of combination therapy with amiodarone and type 1 agents for treatment of inducible ventricular tachycardia. PACE 16:778, 1993.

72. Paul V, Griffith M, Ward DE, Camm AJ: Adjuvant xamoterol or metoprolol in patients with malignant ventricular arrhythmia resistant to amiodarone. Lancet 2:302, 1989.

73. Morady F, Harvey M, Kalbfleisch SJ, et al: Radiofrequency catheter ablation of ventricular tachycardia in patients with coronary artery disease. Circulation 87:363, 1993.

74. Bardy GH, Troutman C, Poole JE, et al: Clinical experience with a tiered-therapy, multiprogrammable antiarrhythmia device. Circulation 85:1689, 1992.

CHAPTER 10

Drug Treatment of Hypertension

Norman M. Kaplan, M.D.

In the United States in the early 1990s, the treatment of hypertension was the leading indication for visits to physicians and for the use of legal drugs.[1] Despite the tremendous growth in the numbers of hypertensives identified, treated, and well controlled since the mid-1970s, almost half of hypertensives in the United States remain untreated or inadequately controlled.[2] More of these patients will be brought under appropriate treatment, including millions of elderly hypertensives who were often left untreated because until recently there was no evidence that they benefited from therapy. Now that such evidence is available, many more of the elderly will also receive treatment, further adding to the continued growth of antihypertensive therapy.

As the use of antihypertensive drugs has increased and will continue to increase, the number of agents available has steadily expanded (Table 10–1), and newer classes have taken an increasingly larger share of the market (Fig. 10–1). This chapter addresses the choices for initial and subsequent therapy.

Before proceeding into the specifics, we need to recall the overriding purpose of the treatment of hypertension: to lower the blood pressure in order to maximally reduce cardiovascular risk without decreasing (and perhaps even improving) the enjoyment of life. Many of the drugs listed in Table 10–1 have the ability to fulfill that purpose, but none now available (or likely to become available) meets all of the criteria for perfection. Nonetheless, currently available choices come close, and when used adroitly, they can provide almost all patients protection without much bother. In our desire to provide this protection with drugs, we should not lose sight of the potential value of various nondrug therapies, used either before drug treatment is begun or after it is started.

Table 10–1. **Antihypertensive Drugs Available in the United States**

Diuretics	Adrenergic Inhibitors	
Thiazides	*Peripheral Inhibitors*	*β-Receptor Blockers*
Chlorthalidone	Guanadrel	Acebutolol
Indapamide	Guanethidine	Atenolol
Metolazone	Reserpine	Betaxolol
Thiazides	*Central α₂-Agonists*	Bisoprolol
Loop Diuretics	Clonidine	Carteolol
Bumetanide	Guanabenz	Metoprolol
Furosemide	Guanfacine	Nadolol
Torsemide	Methyldopa	Penbutolol
Potassium Sparers	*α₁-Receptor Blockers*	Pindolol
Amiloride	Doxazosin	Propranolol
Spironolactone	Prazosin	Timolol
Triamterene	Terazosin	*Combined α- and β-Blocker*
		Labetalol

Vasodilators	
Direct	*ACE Inhibitors*
Hydralazine	Benazepril
Minoxidil	Captopril
Calcium Antagonists	Enalapril
Amlodipine	Fosinopril
Diltiazem	Lisinopril
Felodipine	Quinapril
Isradipine	Ramipril
Nicardipine	
Nifedipine	
Verapamil	

THE INITIAL CHOICE

As more and more patients with milder and milder hypertension are being treated with drugs, two of their usual characteristics must be kept in mind: For the most part, they are asymptomatic; and for the majority, no overt cardiovascular harm would ensue if they were left untreated.

Therefore, the choices of therapy, particularly for the first drug, should be made with care. The first drug chosen may be taken for as long as 40 to 50 years. If it successfully lowers the blood pressure by 10 mmHg, as it will in 50% to 60% of mild hypertensives, no more drugs may be needed. Recall that the tendency of thiazide diuretics, the most commonly used antihypertensive, to raise serum cholesterol levels by 10 to 20 mg/dl was recognized only after they

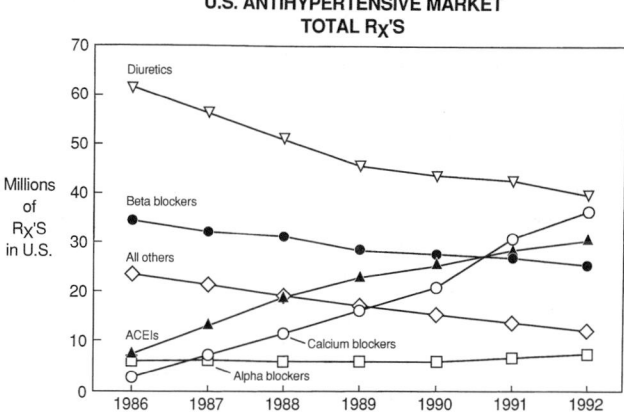

Figure 10–1. Numbers of prescriptions written for antihypertensive drugs in millions in the United States from 1986 to 1992. (From National Prescription Audit. Ambler, PA: IMS, 1993.)

were taken for up to 20 years by millions of people. The need for certainty about long-term safety, in addition to efficacy, should be obvious.

The issue has been discussed in a review of the impact of predominantly diuretic and β-blocker therapies on the blood pressure and other risk factors in 281 patients treated in a major Australian hypertension center[3] (Table 10–2). Although hypertension was well controlled, renal function, blood glucose levels, and cholesterol levels worsened. All drugs can have adverse effects, and precautions are needed in the use of any and all.

Comparative Trials

The only trials that have compared the long-term ability of different drugs to protect patients from overall and cardiovascular morbidity and mortality have essentially utilized only two classes of drugs: diuretics and β-blockers.[4] In addition, five trials have directly compared the two. Of these, three[5–7] showed no difference between them, whereas the Metoprolol Atherosclerosis Prevention in Hypertensives (MAPHY) portion of the Heart Attack Primary Prevention in Hypertensives (HAPPHY) trial[8] found that the β-blocker metoprolol provided lower coronary mortality than did a diuretic, and the Medical Research Council (MRC) trial in the elderly[9] found that a diuretic provided better coronary protection than did the β-blocker atenolol.

The issue remains unsettled and, as for now, no one class of drug has been shown to be better in protecting against morbidity or mortality than any other. Unfortunately, no data are available with any agents other than diuretics and β-blockers. A large-scale comparison between diuretics and a representative of the other three major classes—α₁-blockers, ACE inhibitors, and calcium blockers—is just under way, but the data will not be available for 6 to 8 years. Therefore, the decision to change to other drugs must be based on the possibility but not the certainty that they will be better. Some argue that, in the absence of any such data with other agents, those drugs that have been tested and found to reduce cardiovascular morbidity and mortality—namely, diuretics and β-blockers—should be chosen.[10, 11]

Table 10–2. **Effects of Therapy with Diuretics and β-Blockers in 281 Patients**

Values	Before Treatment	After 1 Year
Blood pressure (mmHg)	160/98	145/88
Weight (kg)	74	74
Potassium level (mmol/L)	4.0	4.1
Creatinine level (mmol/L)	0.08	0.11
Fasting glucose (mmol/L)	5.30	6.33
Total cholesterol (mmol/L)	5.85	6.15

From Jennings GL, Sudhir K: Initial therapy of primary hypertension. Med J Aust 152:198, 1990. © Copyright 1990, The Medical Journal of Australia. Reproduced with permission.

Joint National Committee Recommendations

The position taken in the 1993 fifth Joint National Committee Report (JNC V)[12] is illustrated in Figure 10–2. Whereas a diuretic was the sole recommendation for initial therapy in both the 1977 and 1980 reports, less than a full dose of either a thiazide-type diuretic or a β-blocker was recommended in the 1984 report. In the 1988 report, four choices were provided: diuretics, β-blocker, angiotensin-converting enzyme (ACE) inhibitor, or calcium entry blocker (CEB). In the 1993 report, six choices are provided, adding α-blockers and α-β-blockers to the list, but preference is given to diuretics and β-blockers. The report states: "Because diuretics and β-blockers have been shown to reduce cardiovascular morbidity and mortality in controlled clinical trials, these two classes of drugs are preferred for initial drug therapy. The alternative drugs—calcium antagonists, angiotensin converting enzyme (ACE) inhibitors, α_1-receptor blockers, and the α-β blocker—are equally effective in reducing blood pressure. Although these alternative drugs have potentially important benefits, they have not been used in long-term controlled trials to demonstrate their efficacy in reducing morbidity and mortality and therefore should be reserved for special indications or when diuretics and β-blockers have proved unacceptable or ineffective."[13]

The report immediately proceeds to detail a number of other factors to be considered in selection of drugs (Table 10–3). When these additional factors are taken into account, the result will be a continuation of current trends—the use of various classes with the specific drug chosen on the basis of multiple considerations, an approach best described as "individualized."

Individualized Therapy

This approach is predicated on three major principles: (1) The first choice may be one of a variety of antihy-

Table 10–3. Special Considerations for Initial Therapy As Noted in the JNC V Report

Demographic characteristics
Concomitant diseases and therapies
Quality of life
Physiologic and biochemical measurements
Cost considerations

pertensives from each class of drugs: diuretics, α-blockers, β-blockers, ACE inhibitors, or CEBs; (2) the choice can be logically based on the characteristics of the patients, in particular, certain demographic features and the presence of concomitant diseases; and (3) rather than proceeding with a second drug if the first does not work well or side effects ensue, a substitution approach is used—stop the first drug and try another from a different class.

These three principles will now be considered in detail.

Characteristics of the Drugs

Each class of drugs has different features that make its members more or less attractive (Table 10–4).

Diuretics. In the past, diuretics were almost always chosen first, because they were considered free of significant side effects, easy to take, and inexpensive. Moreover, reactive fluid retention with other drugs used without a diuretic often blunted their effect (Fig. 10–3), so the idea of using a diuretic first seemed logical. However, recognition of the "hidden" side effects and costs of diuretics, along with the lesser protection from coronary mortality in the trials in which they were used,[4] caused many to doubt the wisdom of their routine use. At the least, these factors have led to the more widespread use of lower doses of diuretics and their combinations with potassium-sparing agents.

β-Blockers. β-Blockers then became increasingly popular. However, the need for caution and the contraindications to their use, along with recognition of their potential for altering lipids adversely, put a damper on their use. The failure to find additional protection against coronary disease in trials with a β-blocker[5–7, 9] further weakened the argument for their use.

Indirect Vasodilators. Drugs that act primarily as indirect vasodilators, α-blockers, ACE inhibitors, and CEBs, are being more widely advocated for initial therapy. There seems a certain logic for the use of drugs that induce vasodilation, because an elevated peripheral resistance is the hemodynamic fault of established hypertension.[14]

Other Agents. Reserpine works as well as any of these with one dose a day. However, the concern about the subtle onset of depression and the recurrent (but unproved) claims of its carcinogenicity have caused many to stop using it.[15] The other classes of drugs are not recommended in JNC V[12] for initial therapy. The report states: "The direct-acting smooth muscle vasodilators (e.g., hydralazine, minoxidil) of-

JNC V Treatment Algorithm

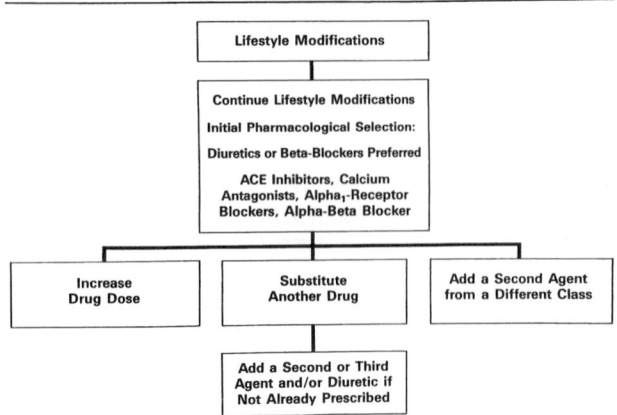

Figure 10–2. Simplified algorithm for treatment of hypertension. (From the Joint National Committee on Detection, Evaluation, and Treatment of High Blood Pressure. The fifth report of the Joint National Committee on Detection, Evaluation, and Treatment of High Blood Pressure [JNC V]. Arch Intern Med 153:154, 1993.)

Table 10–4. **Choice of Initial Therapy**

	Diuretics	Centrally Acting Agents	α-Blockers	β-Blockers	ACE Inhibitors	Calcium Antagonists
Hemodynamic Effects	Initial volume shrinkage Peripheral vasodilation	Reduce cardiac output	Peripheral vasodilation	Reduce cardiac output	Peripheral vasodilation	Peripheral vasodilation
Side Effects OVERT	Weakness Palpitations	Sedation Dry mouth	Postural dizziness	Bronchospasm Fatigue Prolong hypoglycemia	Cough Taste disturbance Rash	Flushing Local edema Constipation (verapamil)
HIDDEN	Hypokalemia Hypercholesterolemia Glucose intolerance Hyperuricemia	Withdrawal syndrome Autoimmune syndromes (methyldopa)		Glucose intolerance Hypertriglyceridemia Decrease HDL tolerance	Leukopenia Proteinuria	AV conduction (verapamil, diltiazem)
Contraindications	Preexisting volume contraction	Orthostatic hypotension Liver disease (methyldopa)	Orthostatic hypotension	Asthma Heartblock	Pregnancy	
Cautions	Diabetes mellitus Gout Digitalis toxicity			Peripheral vascular disease Insulin-requiring diabetes Allergy Coronary spasm Withdrawal angina	Renal insufficiency Renovascular disease	Heart failure
Special Advantages	Effective in blacks, elderly Enhance effectiveness of all other agents	No alteration in blood lipids No fluid retention (guanabenz)	No decrease in cardiac output No alteration in blood lipids No sedation Relieves symptoms of prostatic hypertrophy	Reduce recurrences of coronary disease Reduce manifestations of anxiety Coexisting angina, migraine, glaucoma	No CNS side effects Treat CHF Reduce recurrences of coronary disease and development of CHF Probable renal protection	Effective in blacks, elderly No CNS side effects Coronary vasodilation

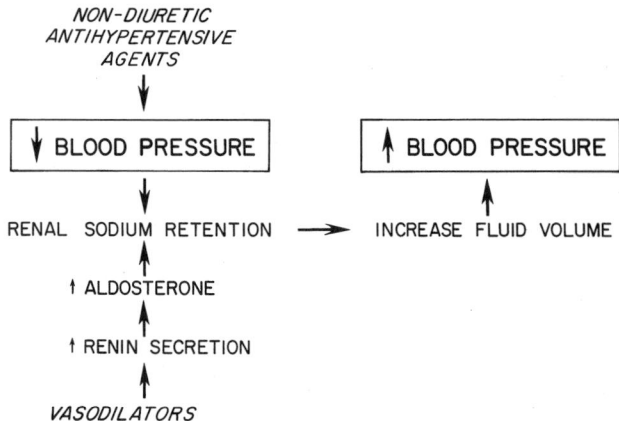

Figure 10–3. The manner by which nondiuretic antihypertensive agents may lose their effectiveness by renal sodium retention. (From Kaplan NM: Treatment of hypertension: Drug therapy. *In* Kaplan NM [ed]: Clinical Hypertension, 6th ed. Baltimore: Williams & Wilkins, 1994, p 201.)

ten induce reflex sympathetic stimulation and fluid retention. [Centrally-acting] alpha₂-agonists and peripheral acting adrenergic antagonists produce annoying side effects in a large number of patients."

Characteristics of the Patients

Demographic Features. As seen in a recent Veterans Administration cooperative study,[16] individual patients' characteristics may affect the likelihood of a good response to various classes of drugs. For example, an elderly, obese black woman will likely respond better to a diuretic than to a β-blocker or an ACE inhibitor. A younger, physically active white man would likely respond particularly well to an α-blocker or an ACE inhibitor. In general, black patients tend to do better with a diuretic, less well with a β-blocker or an ACE inhibitor, and equally well with a CEB or α-blocker than do nonblack patients. The elderly tend to respond as well as, if not better than, younger patients to most classes of antihypertensive drugs. However, for the individual patient, any drug may work well or poorly, and there is no set formula that can be used to predict certain success without side effects.

There are very few controlled crossover studies comparing two or more drugs in the same patients to explain what factors are responsible for individual variability. From the few that are available,[17–19] it is clear that some patients respond better to one type of drug than another, but no single factor explains why those who respond do so. An individual patient comparative trial[20] could be used to determine which is the best choice. Practically, if the patient's pressure is well controlled and no bothersome or potentially hazardous adverse effects are present, there is no reason to keep searching for "the best." Rather than searching for perfection, we need simply to weed out the drugs that either produce little good effect or induce significant ill effects.

Table 10–5 provides a rational approach to the choice of both initial and subsequent therapy based on demographic features and the presence of concomitant diseases.

Concomitant Conditions. Patients with hypertension, usually being middle-aged or elderly, often have other medical problems, some related to their hypertension, others coincidental.[21] As shown in Table 10–5, a hypertensive patient with angina would logically be given a β-blocker or a CEB; one with congestive heart failure (CHF), an ACE inhibitor. α-Blockers, CEBs, and ACE inhibitors are attractive choices for those in whom a diuretic or β-blocker may pose particular problems, such as diabetics or hyperlipidemic patients. In an elderly man with benign prostatic hypertrophy, an α-blocker would be a logical choice.

Plasma Renin Levels. The level of plasma renin activity (PRA) has been advocated by Laragh and coworkers, as far back as 1972[22] and persistently since,[23] as a guide to the choice of initial therapy. As attractive as the concept is, in practice it often does not work: Donnelly et al.[24] found that pretreatment PRA accounted for considerably less than 10% of the variability in response to treatment. To be sure, most studies do show that those with lower renin levels respond somewhat better to diuretics, whereas those with higher renin levels respond better to β-blockers and ACE inhibitors.[25] The elderly and blacks may respond particularly well to diuretics, perhaps because their renin levels tend to be lower, whereas younger white patients may respond well to β-blockers or ACE inhibitors, perhaps because their renin levels are higher.

Substitution Rather Than Addition

The traditional "stepped-care" approach meant that if the first drug did not work well, others would be added sequentially. This could mean that the patient is given one, two, or even three drugs, none of which works. The wisdom of substitution rather than addition seems obvious. If the first choice, even if based on all reasonable criteria, does not lower the blood pressure much or is associated with persistent, bothersome side effects, that drug should be stopped and one from another class tried. Thereby, the least number of drugs should be needed to achieve the desired fall in blood pressure with the fewest side effects.

Patients with milder hypertension often need only one drug. Therefore, substitution should work for them. For those with more severe hypertension, the first drug may do all that is expected and still not be enough. Therefore, the addition of a second or, if needed, a third drug in a stepwise manner is logical.

Cost as a Factor

For some patients, the cost of the medications used to treat hypertension may pose an obstacle to control of their disease. The cost per tablet varies from a few cents for a generic hydrochlorothiazide or reserpine to a dollar or more for a brand-name ACE inhibitor or CEB. Without clear evidence of greater efficacy or

Table 10–5. **Individualized Choices of Therapy**

Coexisting Condition	Diuretic	β-Blocker	α-Blocker	Calcium Antagonist	ACE Inhibitor
Older age	+ +	+ / −	+	+	+
Black race	+ +	+ / −	+	+	+ / −
Coronary disease	+ / −	+ +	+	+ +	+
Congestive failure	+ +	−	+	−	+ +
Cerebrovascular disease	+	+	+ / −	+ +	+
Renal insufficiency	+ +	+ / −	+	+ +	+ +
Diabetes	−	−	+ +	+	+ +
Dyslipidemia	−	−	+ +	+	+
Asthma or COPD	+	−	+	+	+

+ +, preferred; +, suitable; + / −, usually not preferred; −, usually contraindicated.

long-term benefit from the more expensive drugs, practitioners concerned about the cost might then logically choose the less expensive agent.

However, there are additional factors that need to be considered. First, the cost of the tablet may not be the major cost of the medication. If a diuretic causes hypokalemia that must be corrected, potassium supplements may cost a dollar a day or more, bringing the cost of diuretic therapy well into the range of the most expensive agents. Diuretic-induced hyperlipidemia may be an even more serious, albeit less obvious, cost.

Second, more and more agents are available in long-acting formulations, so that one tablet a day may provide full coverage. The cost may be reduced further by prescribing larger doses of tablets that can easily be broken in half. Although a dollar or more a day may pose a burden for many, the cost of medication hopefully will not interfere with the provision of what is best for most patients. Nonetheless, lacking clear proof that one type of drug is clearly more protective against cardiovascular morbidity and mortality than others, the temptation to go with the least expensive cannot be discounted.[10]

Choice of Second Drug

If a moderate dose of the first choice is well tolerated and is effective, but not enough to bring the pressure down to the desired level, a second drug can be added or the dose of the first drug increased.

As noted in JNC V,[12] "Combining antihypertensive drugs with different modes of action will often allow smaller doses of drugs to be used to achieve control, thereby minimizing the potential for dose-dependent side effects. If a diuretic is not chosen as the first drug, it will be useful as a second step agent because its addition usually enhances the effects of other agents."

The wisdom of adding a second drug rather than increasing the dose of the first has been widely accepted but inadequately tested. Nonetheless, there is no question that the addition of two drugs of dissimilar action will usually provide additional effect.[19] In patients whose diastolic blood pressure remained higher than 90 mmHg while taking the calcium blocker isradipine 2.5 mg twice daily and who were randomly assigned to receive more isradipine or to have a diuretic, a β-blocker, or an ACE inhibitor added, those given any of the second agents did better than those given more of the first drug.[26]

The choice of second drug depends largely on the nature of the first. If a diuretic is the first drug, the addition of an adrenergic inhibitor or an ACE inhibitor usually provides significant additional antihypertensive effect. The addition of an α-blocker minimizes diuretic-induced hyperlipidemia.[27] If a nondiuretic agent is the first choice, a diuretic can be used as a second drug. However, if a diuretic is to be avoided, combinations of a β-blocker and a CEB or of a CEB and an ACE inhibitor usually provide additive effects.[26]

A diuretic is particularly needed as a second drug if the use of the first agent was associated with reactive sodium retention (see Fig. 10–3). This phenomenon probably reflects a resetting of the normal pressure-natriuresis curve in the kidneys of hypertensive patients, so that any fall in pressure toward normal is interpreted as a fall to below normal, requiring a retention of fluids to bring the pressure back to what is now considered the desired pressure.

This process has been shown to occur rather often with adrenergic inhibitors that do not inhibit the renin-aldosterone mechanism, such as those acting peripherally (e.g., reserpine, guanethidine) and those acting centrally (e.g., clonidine, methyldopa). This process may also follow the use of α-blockers (e.g., doxazosin, terazosin). With direct vasodilators (e.g., hydralazine, minoxidil), the renin-aldosterone axis may be further activated by reflex sympathetic stimulation, adding further to renal sodium retention.

On the other hand, drugs that also inhibit the renin-aldosterone mechanism tend to prevent this reactive sodium retention and may actually cause some natriuresis on their own. Such drugs, including β-blockers, ACE inhibitors, and calcium entry blockers, may then be used as initial therapy with less need for the addition of a diuretic in order to preserve their effectiveness. However, for some patients, a diuretic may be needed regardless of whatever else is used. In most instances, the degree of blood pressure fall is thereby accentuated, whether the mechanism involves abolishing the reactive sodium retention or simply the antihypertensive effect of a diuretic added to that of another drug.

When an ACE inhibitor and a diuretic are combined, the two drugs may be playing off one another to mutually enhance their antihypertensive efficacy. A diuretic taken alone activates the renin-aldosterone mechanism as it shrinks fluid volume and lowers blood pressure. After an initial diuresis, this activated renin-aldosterone system works to prevent further progressive fluid loss and additional fall in blood pressure. The addition of an ACE inhibitor paralyzes the renin-angiotensin system and reduces aldosterone levels, thereby enhancing the efficacy of the diuretic. Conversely, the diuretic-induced rise in renin-angiotensin sets the patient's blood pressure up for an additional effect from the ACE inhibitor, which tends to work better in higher renin states. The same potentiation of ACE inhibitor effect occurs with dietary sodium restriction.

COUNTERACTING MULTIPLE MECHANISMS

Beyond the more pragmatic need simply to do whatever it takes to lower blood pressure adequately, there is a more theoretic reason that combination therapy often is appropriate. In approximately 95% of all patients, hypertension is of unknown cause (i.e., idiopathic, primary, or essential). Therefore, no single approach to therapy that will remove the basic cause can be formulated for the overwhelming majority of patients, unlike what can be done for the relatively few patients with secondary forms of hypertension such as those arising from renovascular disease or primary aldosteronism.

Rather than a single, specific mechanism, a multiplicity of mechanisms is likely to be involved. The various factors that influence both cardiac output and peripheral resistance, the two primary determinants of blood pressure, can be altered by various drugs. Despite our lack of knowledge as to which is primary or dominant, our therapies can nonetheless achieve a lowering of pressure. However, drugs that reduce the activity of the sympathetic nervous system may reduce pressure only a small amount, presumably because sympathetic nervous activity is playing a relatively small role in many patients' hypertension. Similarly, drugs that paralyze the renin-angiotensin mechanism may not be very efficacious because that mechanism, too, may be only partially responsible for the elevated pressure.

Our therapies are usually given without attempting to alter one or another specific pathogenetic mechanism. First, we cannot find one mechanism in most patients. Second, identification of the mechanism does not seem to matter: Approximately 50% of all patients across the board have a good response to whatever drug is chosen. As a corollary, the fact that a patient happens to respond particularly well to one form of therapy that affects one of the multiple pathogenetic mechanisms does not necessarily imply that one mechanism is the main cause of the hypertension.

Most of the mechanisms seem to be involved to some degree in most patients. Therefore, a given drug may work even if its effect is not directed against the primary mechanism.

The recognition that a high peripheral resistance, in whatever manner it is induced, is the major hemodynamic fault in almost all patients with established hypertension has led to an increasing advocacy of drugs that lower pressure by reducing peripheral resistance (e.g., vasodilators) as the more physiologically appropriate form of therapy rather than drugs that work by lowering cardiac output (e.g., β-blockers). Such vasodilators include α-blockers, direct-acting drugs such as hydralazine, ACE inhibitors, and calcium entry blockers. Because each class appears to work differently, drugs from different classes of vasodilators may be combined to achieve additional vasodilation and antihypertensive action.

Regardless of the reasons, multiple drugs may be needed, either because multiple mechanisms must be altered or because each simply adds more antihypertensive effect in a nonspecific manner. What should be obvious, however, is that the drugs should be chosen from different classes rather than from the same class. For example, it makes far better sense to choose an α-blocker and a β-blocker rather than two β-blockers if more than one drug is needed.

Two Drugs as Initial Therapy

Because one third to one half of patients end up taking two drugs, some physicians prefer to start with the combination of a diuretic and another agent. That practice is, in general, unwise for these reasons:

1. Even if the initial pressure level is fairly high, some patients respond adequately to one drug, and there is no way to know who will need more than one.

2. Except in those with dangerously high levels, a gradual, gentle lowering of pressure as can be achieved with small doses of one drug is preferable to a sudden, drastic fall resulting from two or more drugs.

3. If side effects occur, as will happen in perhaps one fourth of those given almost any antihypertensive agent, it is desirable to know which drug is responsible so it may be stopped or appropriate countermeasures taken.

4. Fixed-dose combinations, as convenient as they may be, often provide inappropriate amounts of different drugs, because most drugs have different dose-response curves. An obvious exception is the combination of a diuretic plus a potassium-sparing agent, which I consider not to be a combination of two different drugs but rather a useful way of reducing a major side effect of the diuretic. On the other hand, if the doses of the two or more drugs that many patients eventually end up with are available in a single combination tablet, this should be used to save trouble and cost.

Some patients, particularly those with fairly severe

hypertension but whose blood pressure was previously well controlled when taking two or more medications, may logically be started on more than one drug. However, such patients may also be better served by a more gradual reduction in pressure, obtainable from single-drug therapy. Only if the pressure is so high or the patient is in such immediate danger of target-organ damage as to mandate a more rapid and drastic reduction in pressure should more than one drug be given as initial therapy.

Combination Tablets

If the patient ends up on two drugs and the doses match the combinations available, such a combination tablet should be used. Of the combinations available, the addition of a potassium-sparing agent to a diuretic (Dyazide, Maxzide, Moduretic) is eminently sensible. Combinations of a diuretic plus almost every one of the other types of drugs are available, and one, with only 6.25 mg hydrochlorothiazide and the β-blocker bisoprolol (Zebeta), is approved for initial therapy as Ziac. Caution is advised not to overdose the diuretic if larger amounts of other agents are needed.

Choice of Third Drug

Various combinations usually work. In one parallel study, 93 patients uncontrolled on a diuretic and a β-blocker were randomly allocated to either nifedipine, prazosin, or hydralazine.[28] After 6 months, all three drugs lowered blood pressures significantly, and there were few differences between the three groups other than for the pattern of side effects. In a similar study, captopril, nifedipine, and hydralazine were equally effective, but the ACE inhibitor was better tolerated.[29] The key, as with two drugs, is to combine agents with different mechanisms of action.

Choice of Fourth Drug

Few patients should need more than three drugs, particularly if the various reasons for resistance to therapy are considered. For those who do, the JNC V report recommends adding a fourth drug from a different class or having the patient evaluated for the reason behind resistance.

Resistant Hypertension

The reasons for a poor response are numerous (Table 10–6), with the most likely being volume overload caused by either excessive sodium intake or inadequate diuretic.[30] In one series of 91 patients whose pressures remained above 140/90 despite use of three antihypertensive agents, the mechanisms were suboptimal drug regimen (mainly inadequate diuretic) in 43%, intolerance to medications in 22%, noncompliance in 10%, and secondary hypertension in 11%.[31] In a disadvantaged minority population, uncontrolled hypertension is most closely related to limited access

Table 10–6. **Causes for Lack of Responsiveness to Therapy**

Nonadherence to therapy
Cost of medication
Instructions not clear and/or not given to the patient in writing
Inadequate or no patient education
Lack of involvement of the patient in the treatment plan
Side effects of medication
Organic brain syndrome (e.g., memory deficit)
Inconvenient dosing

Drug-related causes
Doses too low
Inappropriate combinations (e.g., two centrally acting adrenergic inhibitors)
Rapid inactivation (e.g., hydralazine)
Drug interactions
   Nonsteroidal antiinflammatory drugs
   Oral contraceptives
   Sympathomimetics
   Antidepressants
   Adrenal steroids
   Nasal decongestants
   Licorice-containing substances (e.g., chewing tobacco)
   Cocaine
   Cyclosporine
   Erythropoietin

Associated conditions
Increasing obesity
Alcohol intake more than 1 ounce of ethanol a day

Secondary hypertension
Renal insufficiency
Renovascular hypertension
Pheochromocytoma
Primary aldosteronism

Volume overload
Inadequate diuretic therapy
Excess sodium intake
Fluid retention from reduction of blood pressure
Progressive renal damage

Pseudohypertension

From Joint National Committee: Fifth report of the Joint National Committee on Detection, Evaluation, and Treatment of High Blood Pressure (JNC V). Arch Intern Med 153:154, 1993.

to care, noncompliance with therapy, and alcohol-related problems.[32]

Before starting workup for secondary causes and altering drug therapy, blood pressures should be checked out of the office setting, because as many as half of "resistant" patients turn out to have controlled hypertension.[33]

If true resistance is present, therapy should include, in addition to adequate diuretics, an ACE inhibitor and a calcium blocker, with minoxidil reserved for those who remain resistant.[34]

One special group that may remain resistant to all available agents in any combination is elderly patients with predominantly systolic hypertension secondary to rigid atherosclerotic large arteries. Some of these patients may simply be unresponsive to whatever is given, and the only option may be to use reasonable doses of two or three medications that will, at the least, slightly lower the pressure while not causing bothersome side effects. Such poorly responsive elderly patients may, in fact, be unusual: among the initial 500 patients enrolled in the ongoing Systolic Hypertension in the Elderly Program (SHEP), all of whom had systolic pressures higher than 160 mmHg and diastolic pressures lower than 90 mmHg, 88% had a significant fall in systolic pressure after 1 year of monotherapy with just a small dose of the diuretic chlorthalidone.[35]

Stepping Down or Off Therapy

Once a good response has occurred and been maintained for a year or longer, medications may be reduced or discontinued. In most studies of patients whose medications were discontinued, the majority have their hypertension reappear in 6 to 12 months, but a significant percentage remain normotensive for 4 years or longer.[36] From their review of all published prospective studies, Schmieder et al. characterize those who remain normotensive as having mild hypertension with low pretreatment blood pressure, young age, normal body weight, low salt intake, no alcohol consumption, successful therapy with only one drug, and little or no target-organ damage. Such paragons may be hard to find, and some of them may be transient or "white coat" hypertensives whose therapy was begun before the diagnosis was established.

Whether it is worth the trouble to stop drug therapy completely is questionable. Withdrawal is certainly worthwhile in elderly patients whose blood pressures are normal on little therapy and who are free of signs of target-organ damage. The more sensible approach in well-controlled patients would be to first decrease the dose of whatever is being used. That is feasible, without loss of control, in a significant number who are well controlled on a single drug.[37] If that succeeds, withdrawal may be attempted with continued surveillance of the blood pressure.

CONCLUSION

With proper use of currently available antihypertensive medications, virtually all patients should be capable of achieving good control of their hypertension. To reach this goal, considerable time and patience may be required, but the rewards should make the effort worthwhile.

REFERENCES

1. Schappert SM: National ambulatory medical care survey: 1991 summary. From vital and health statistics of the Centers for Disease Control and Prevention/National Center for Health Statistics. Advance Data 230:1, 1993.
2. Kaplan NM: Treatment of hypertension: Drug therapy. In Kaplan NM (ed): Clinical Hypertension, 6th ed. Baltimore: Williams & Wilkins, 1994, pp 191–280.
3. Jennings GL, Sudhir K: Initial therapy of primary hypertension. Med J Aust 152:198, 1990.
4. Collins R, Peto R, MacMahon S, et al: Blood pressure, stroke, and coronary heart disease. Part 2, Short-term reductions in blood pressure: Overview of randomised drug trials in their epidemiological context. Lancet 335:827, 1990.
5. Medical Research Council Working Party: MRC trial of treatment of mild hypertension: Principal results. Br Med J 291:97, 1985.
6. IPPPSH Collaborative Group: Cardiovascular risk and risk factors in a randomized trial of treatment based on the beta-blocker oxprenolol: The International Prospective Primary Prevention Study in Hypertension (IPPPSH). J Hypertens 3:379, 1985.
7. Wilhelmsen L, Berglund G, Elmfeldt D, et al: Beta-blockers versus diuretics in hypertensive men: Main results from the HAPPHY Trial. J Hypertens 5:561, 1987.
8. Wikstrand J, Warnold I, Olsson G, et al: Primary prevention with metoprolol in patients with hypertension. Mortality results from the MAPHY study. JAMA 259:1976, 1988.
9. Medical Research Council Working Party: Medical Research Council trial of treatment of hypertension in older adults: Principal results. Br Med J 304:405, 1992.
10. Alderman MH: Which antihypertensive drugs first—and why! JAMA 267:2786, 1992.
11. Sever P, Beevers G, Bulpitt C, et al: Management guidelines in essential hypertension: Report of the second working party of the British Hypertension Society. Br Med J 306:983, 1993.
12. Joint National Committee: The fifth report of the Joint National Committee on detection, evaluation, and treatment of high blood pressure (JNC V). Arch Intern Med 153:154, 1993.
13. Neaton JD, Grimm RH Jr, Prineas RJ, et al: Treatment of mild hypertension study (TOMHS): In reply [Letter]. JAMA 270:2925, 1993.
14. Kaplan NM: Primary hypertension: Pathogenesis. In Kaplan NM (ed): Clinical Hypertension, 6th ed. Baltimore: Williams & Wilkins, 1994, pp 47–108.
15. Lederle FA, Applegate WB, Grimm RH Jr: Reserpine and the medical marketplace. Arch Intern Med 153:705, 1993.
16. Materson BJ, Reda DJ, Cushman WC, et al: Single-drug therapy for hypertension in men. A comparison of six antihypertensive agents with placebo. N Engl J Med 328:914, 1993.
17. Brunner HR, Ménard J, Waeber B, et al: Treating the individual hypertensive patient: Considerations on dose, sequential monotherapy and drug combinations. J Hypertens 8:3, 1990.
18. Edmonds D, Huss R, Jeck T, et al: Individualizing antihypertensive therapy with enalapril versus atenolol: The Zurich experience. J Hypertens 8:S49, 1990.
19. Morgan TO, Anderson A, Jones E: Comparison and interaction of low dose felodipine and enalapril in the treatment of essential hypertension in elderly subjects. Am J Hypertens 5:238, 1992.
20. Guyatt GH, Keller JL, Jaeschke R, et al: The n-of-1 randomized controlled trial: Clinical usefulness. Our three-year experience. Ann Intern Med 112:293, 1990.
21. Stewart AL, Greenfield S, Hays RD, et al: Functional status and well-being of patients with chronic conditions. Results from the medical outcomes study. JAMA 262:907, 1989.
22. Bühler FR, Laragh JH, Baer L, et al: Propranolol inhibition of renin secretion. A specific approach to diagnosis and treatment of renin-dependent hypertensive diseases. N Engl J Med 287:1209, 1972.
23. Devereux RB, Laragh JH: Angiotensin converting enzyme inhibition of renin system activity induces reversal of hypertensive target organ changes. Do these effects predict a reduction in long-term morbidity? Am J Hypertens 5:923, 1992.
24. Donnelly R, Elliott HL, Meredith PA: Antihypertensive drugs: Individualized analysis and clinical relevance of kinetic-dynamic relationships. Pharmacol Ther 53:67, 1992.
25. Niutta E, Cusi D, Colombo R, et al: Predicting interindividual variations in antihypertensive therapy: The role of sodium transport systems and renin. J Hypertens 8:S53, 1990.
26. Lüscher TF, Waeber B: Efficacy and safety of various combination therapies based on a calcium antagonist in essential hypertension: Results of a placebo-controlled randomized trial. J Cardiovasc Pharmacol 21:305, 1993.
27. Black HR: Metabolic considerations in the choice of therapy for the patient with hypertension. Am Heart J 121:707, 1991.

28. Ramsay LE, Parnell L, Waller PC: Comparison of nifedipine, prazosin and hydralazine added to treatment of hypertensive patients uncontrolled by thiazide diuretic plus beta-blocker. Postgrad Med J 63:99, 1987.
29. Bevan EG, Pringle SD, Waller PC, et al: Comparison of captopril, hydralazine and nifedipine as third drug in hypertensive patients. J Hum Hypertens 7:83, 1993.
30. Graves JW, Bloomfield RL, Buckalew VM Jr: Plasma volume in resistant hypertension: Guide to pathophysiology and therapy. Am J Med Sci 298:361, 1989.
31. Yakovlevitch M, Black HR: Resistant hypertension in a tertiary care clinic. Arch Intern Med 151:1786, 1991.
32. Shea S, Misra D, Ehrlich MH, et al: Predisposing factors for severe, uncontrolled hypertension in an inner-city minority population. N Engl J Med 327:776, 1992.
33. Mejia AD, Egan BM, Schork NJ, Zweifler AJ: Artifacts in mea-surements of blood pressure and lack of target organ involve-ment in the assessment of patients with treatment-resistant hypertension. Ann Intern Med 112:270, 1990.
34. Pontremoli R, Robaudo C, Gaiter A, et al: Long-term minoxidil treatment in refractory hypertension and renal failure. Clin Nephrol 35:39, 1991.
35. Hulley SB, Furberg CD, Gurland B, et al: Systolic Hypertension in the Elderly Program (SHEP): Antihypertensive efficacy of chlorthalidone. Am J Cardiol 56:913, 1985.
36. Schmieder RE, Rockstroh JK, Messerli FH: Antihypertensive therapy. To stop or not to stop? JAMA 265:1566, 1991.
37. Finnerty FA Jr: Stepped-down therapy versus intermittent ther-apy in systemic hypertension. Am J Cardiol 66:1373, 1990.
38. Kaplan NM: Treatment of hypertension: Drug therapy. In Kaplan NM (ed): Clinical Hypertension, 6th ed. Baltimore: Wil-liams & Wilkins, 1994, p 201.

CHAPTER 11

Drug Treatment of Hyperlipidemia
Initial Therapy and Combination Therapy

Donald B. Hunninghake, M.D.

The overwhelming purpose for the use of drugs to treat chronic dyslipidemia is to reduce the risk of coronary heart disease (CHD). The highest priority for the use of drugs is for patients who have had prior CHD or another atherosclerotic event. The bene-fits are the greatest in this high-risk group. There is also only limited disagreement about the use of drugs for primary prevention in patients who have multiple risk factors or very high blood cholesterol levels. Low-risk patients may better be treated with lifestyle modifications, and drug therapy is rarely necessary. In all patients, it is important to control other modifi-able risk factors and to ensure that the patient has been adequately instructed on diet modification, weight loss, and increased physical activity. The pa-tient should also be evaluated for secondary causes of hyperlipidemia.

After drugs such as the 3-hydroxy-3-methylglutaryl coenzyme A (HMG-CoA) reductase inhibitors have been initiated, approximately 50% of patients discon-tinue therapy within 1 year. The failure rate for other drugs, which either are more difficult to administer or have more side effects, is higher. Compliance to drug therapy may be enhanced by instructing the patient on the rationale for drug use, the expected effects and benefits, and the side effects. Patients should also be advised either that the side effects can be managed or that alternative therapies will be considered. The necessity for chronic and pro-longed therapy must be explained, and regular fol-low-up visits should be arranged. Cost presents a problem for some patients. Initiation of drug therapy without appropriate maintenance follow-up is unac-ceptable.

WHO SHOULD BE TREATED

Guidelines for the initiation of drug therapy and the target goals of therapy have been provided by the National Cholesterol Education Program (NCEP).[1,2]

Low-Density Lipoprotein Cholesterol

The primary focus for therapy is low-density lipopro-tein cholesterol (LDL-C). Other countries have pub-lished guidelines that are somewhat similar but may use total rather than LDL-C, may include triglycer-ides, or may define CHD risk in different ways.[3,4] The NCEP guidelines are provided in Table 11–1.

High-Density Lipoprotein Cholesterol

High-density lipoprotein cholesterol (HDL-C) levels below 35 mg/dl (0.9 mmol/L) are considered a major

Table 11–1. **LDL Cholesterol [mg/dl (mmol/L)]**

	Consider Drug Therapy	Suggested Target Goal
Clinical evidence of CHD or other atherosclerotic disease	≥ 130 (3.3)*	≤ 100 (2.6)
Without CHD and with two or more risk factors	≥ 160 (4.1)	< 130 (3.3)
Without CHD and with fewer than two risk factors	≥ 190 (4.9)†	< 160 (4.1)

*Clinical judgment determines whether drug therapy is initiated or drug dosage is increased when LDL-C is 100–129 mg/dl.
†Consider delaying drug therapy in men <35 years or premenopausal women without other risk factors if the LDL-C is < 220 mg/dl (5.6 mmol/L).

risk factor for CHD. Increasing HDL-C levels is the second target for therapy. If lifestyle modification is not successful, drug therapy is considered in high-risk patients such as those with CHD, multiple risk factors, diabetes mellitus, or chronic renal disease.[2, 5, 6] Clinical judgment determines the HDL-C level to be treated and the target goal. Generally, drugs that both lower LDL-C and increase HDL-C are used. The drug therapy available for effectively increasing HDL-C levels is rather limited.

Triglycerides

No trials conclusively document that lowering triglycerides is associated with a decreased risk of CHD. Epidemiologic studies indicate that patients with triglyceride levels of 200 mg/dl (2.2 mmol/L) or more are at increased risk.[5, 6] Triglyceride reduction becomes the tertiary target for drug therapy in some high-risk patients who cannot be managed with lifestyle modification only. The target goal for therapy is generally less than 200 mg/dl, with lower levels of less than 150 mg/dl (1.7 mmol/L) in diabetic patients.[6, 7]

Other

Elevated lipoprotein(a) [Lp(a)] levels have also been reported to increase the risk of CHD. Only nicotinic acid and estrogen have been reported to moderately lower Lp(a) levels. Lp(a) is not a primary target for treatment, but consideration should be given to a lower target for LDL-C levels in patients with very high Lp(a) levels. Elevated apoprotein B (Apo B) levels may also identify a high-risk group of patients, because elevated levels are frequently associated with the smaller, more dense and more atherogenic particles. Apo B is also not currently a primary target for treatment.

INITIAL SELECTION OF DRUGS

The available classes of drugs include

- HMG-CoA reductase inhibitors (statins)
- Bile acid sequestrants (resins)
- Nicotinic acid
- Fibric acid derivatives
- Estrogen in postmenopausal women
- Probucol

The suggested approach to the initial selection of a class of drugs is indicated in Table 11–2. This proposed selection of drugs generally produces the most favorable effect on the lipid/lipoprotein profile. Other factors, such as cost, the presence of diabetes mellitus, and the possibility of drug interactions, that may influence the selection of drugs are discussed later. The drugs indicated for first choice are strongly recommended for the treatment of patients with clinical evidence of CHD or other atherosclerotic vascular disease. Many of these patients also require combina-

Table 11–2. **Selection of Initial Class of Drugs Based on Lipid and Lipoprotein Levels**

LDL-C ≥ 130 mg/dl Triglycerides ≤ 400 mg/dl (4.5 mmol/L)	LDL-C < 130 mg/dl Triglycerides ≤ 400 mg/dl HDL-C ≤ 35 mg/dl (0.9 mmol/L)	Triglycerides > 400 mg/dl
	First Choice	
HMG-CoA reductase inhibitors (statins) Estrogen in postmenopausal women	Nicotinic acid (crystalline) Estrogen in postmenopausal women	Fibric acids
	Alternative Choices	
Bile acid sequestrant (if triglycerides ≤ 200 mg/dl and HDL-C > 35 mg/dl) Nicotinic acid (if triglycerides > 200 mg/dl or HDL-C < 35 mg/dl)	Statins (to lower LDL-C) Fibric acids (to lower triglycerides)	Nicotinic acid

tion therapy. The alternative choices are more likely to be used in primary prevention.

HMG-CoA Reductase Inhibitors

This class of drugs currently accounts for approximately 60% to 65% of all lipid-lowering drugs used in the United States. Their popularity is based on efficacy for lowering LDL-C, ease of administration, and very few drug-drug interactions.[2, 8, 9] With the exception of nicotinic acid, they are generally the most cost-effective drugs for lowering LDL-C. Combination therapy is less costly than using large doses of the statins as single-drug therapy. The statins can be used as the initial drug in all patients with triglyceride levels less than or equal to 400 mg/dl, but nicotinic acid, if tolerated, is preferred in patients with low HDL-C levels and when only modest reductions in LDL-C levels are required.

There are currently four marketed statins: lovastatin, pravastatin, simvastatin, and fluvastatin. At the present time, cost, desired amount of LDL-C lowering, and availability in the individual formularies primarily determine the selection of drug. There are a number of pharmacologic differences between the statins,[10, 11] but there is no conclusive evidence that any of these differences is clinically significant in terms of adverse events. Lovastatin and simvastatin are administered as prodrugs and are very lipophilic. Pravastatin and fluvastatin are administered as the parent drug and are hydrophilic. There is no definitive evidence that the lipophilic drugs cause more central nervous system symptoms or increase the risk of myopathy. Pravastatin has limited binding to plasma proteins, whereas the other three drugs are more than 90% bound. Although there are isolated reports of potentiation of the anticoagulant effect of warfarin with lovastatin and simvastatin, this does not appear to be of major clinical importance. The elimination of pravastatin involves both renal and hepatic mechanisms; the other three drugs are primarily excreted via hepatic metabolism. Again, no major clinical significance for these differences has been noted.

The usual mean reductions in LDL-C that are generally reported in clinical trials are indicated in Table 11–3.[11] Some studies suggest that daily doses of simvastatin of less than or equal to 10 mg may be somewhat more effective than indicated in Table 11–3. Individual patients may have different responses, and the dose should be titrated to achieve their target goals. The statins generally produce increases in HDL-C levels in the range of 5% to 10%. Greater increases may be seen in patients with low HDL-C levels or elevated triglyceride levels. Reductions in triglyceride levels are in the range of 5% to 15%, but greater reductions can be seen in hypertriglyceridemic patients.[12]

A single dose of a statin is always more effective if administered in the evening than in the morning. With the exception of lovastatin, these drugs are generally administered as a single bedtime dose. The bioavailability of lovastatin is better if administered with meals, and the highest daily dose (80 mg) is administered twice daily. However, lovastatin can be administered at bedtime for convenience or to avoid an interaction with the bile acid sequestrants.

A minimal decrease in LDL-C of 20% to 25% is desirable in patients with CHD. Thus, one would consider initiating therapy with the second dosage level indicated in Table 11–3. The maximal dose of the statins that should be used before switching to combination therapy is indicated by the heavy line in Table 11–3. Many would switch to combination therapy with lower doses of the statins. The dose response for LDL-C lowering with the statins is not linear. After the initial first or second dosage levels, the additional LDL-C lowering is only approximately 6% to 8% each time the dose is doubled.

Increases in transaminase levels are found with the statins in occasional patients.[12, 13] If the elevation is greater than or equal to three times the upper limits of normal (ULN) on two consecutive occasions, the dose is decreased or the drug is temporarily discontinued. If the elevation is greater than or equal to two times the ULN, the dose is decreased. Lesser elevations are simply monitored. Other causes for transaminase elevations should be explored. Other complaints may include headache, constipation, other gastrointestinal disturbances, and miscellaneous complaints. The overall frequency of side effects is low. If a patient has symptoms with one statin, another statin can be tried. Myopathy, creatine kinase level greater than 10 times ULN associated with diffuse muscle pain, is extremely rare with single-drug therapy. Myopathy has been reported more frequently when the statins are used in combination with cyclosporine, fibric acids, and occasionally with nicotinic acid and erythromycin. The frequency of myopathy is greater when higher doses of statins are used in these combinations. These combinations should be used cautiously. Patients should be instructed on the symptoms of myopathy and advised to report them immediately. The diagnosis is confirmed by greatly elevated creatine phosphokinase levels, and the statin should then be discontinued immediately.

Bile Acid Sequestrants (Resins)

The two resins that are currently available are cholestyramine and colestipol. They are both available in granular form, and colestipol is also available in tablet form. Four grams of cholestyramine (active drug) is equivalent to 5 g of colestipol (active drug). The resins have not been popular drugs because of difficulties in administration, palatability, gastrointestinal complaints, and drug-drug interactions.[9, 14] However, these drugs are effective in lowering LDL-C levels, and their long-term safety has been documented.[15] The resins are generally more costly in terms of milligrams or percent lowering of LDL-C than is nicotinic acid or the statins.

The resins are generally used as single-drug therapy in primary prevention in which reductions in LDL-C of less than 20% are desired or for initiating therapy in young adults. The reductions in LDL-C are dose dependent, but usually 60% to 65% of the maximal LDL-C lowering can be achieved with doses equivalent to 8 g of cholestyramine.[16] The percent reduction with this dose varies from 10% to 25% and is inversely related to pretreatment LDL-C levels. Patients with lower LDL-C levels may easily achieve their target LDL-C levels with low-dose resin therapy, but the resins are not used as the initial therapy in patients with very high LDL-C levels. However, they are very useful in combination with the statins. The resins are contraindicated in patients with triglyceride levels of more than 500 mg/dl (5.6 mmol/L) and type III hyperlipoproteinemia and are rarely used as single-drug therapy if triglyceride levels exceed 200 to 250 mg/dl.

The side effects of resin therapy, especially the gastrointestinal complaints, are dose dependent. The resins can also decrease the absorption of other drugs.[9]

Table 11–3. **LDL Cholesterol Reductions with the Statins (Expected Daily Dose to Produce % LDL-C Reduction)**

	% LDL-C Reduction			
	16–20	22–26	30–34	~40
Dose in mg of:				
Lovastatin	10	20	40 (PM or 20 b.i.d)	80 (40 b.i.d.)
Pravastatin	10	20	40	—
Simvastatin	5	10	20	40
Fluvastatin	20	40	—	—

The dashes indicate that this dose is generally not recommended or there are insufficient data to evaluate the required dose to achieve that effect. The heavy line dose indicates the maximal dose that should be administered before going to combination therapy. Combination therapy with lower daily doses of statins is frequently preferable.

The general recommendation is that other drugs be administered 1 hour before or 4 hours after resin. Specific drug interactions have been documented with the statins, warfarin, β-blockers, thiazide diuretics, cardiac glycosides, and exogenous thyroxine.

The most common method of administration of resin in my clinic is a dose equivalent to 8 g of cholestyramine before the evening meal. This is the most effective time for administering a single dose. It produces most of the achievable LDL-C lowering because it is frequently tolerated, and it avoids most of the drug interactions because many drugs are administered only in the morning. Larger doses are administered twice daily but are rarely used because of poor compliance.

Nicotinic Acid (Niacin)

Crystalline or Immediate-Release

Niacin decreases total and LDL-C and triglyceride levels and increases HDL-C levels.[9, 17] It is the most effective drug currently available for increasing HDL-C levels and can also modestly lower Lp(a) levels.[18, 19] The triglyceride-lowering effect is dose dependent. Daily doses in the range of 3 to 4.5 g (infrequently tolerated) are generally required to obtain a 20% to 25% reduction in LDL-C levels. A 15% to 20% reduction in LDL-C may be obtained with daily doses of 2 to 3 g.[18, 19] However, the percent increase in HDL-C levels with daily doses of 0.75 to 1 g can be 10% to 15%; 1.5 g, 20%; and 3 g or more, 30% or more.[18, 19] Thus, niacin is used primarily as single-drug therapy to increase HDL-C levels but can also modestly lower LDL-C and triglyceride levels. It is frequently used in combination with other drugs that are more effective in lowering LDL-C levels.

Niacin administration is associated with many side effects. For those patients who tolerate this drug, the availability without a prescription makes it cost-effective. Preparations that are officially approved for cholesterol lowering are more expensive. Patients should continue to take the same manufacturer's preparation and not switch preparations. Niacin therapy for dyslipidemia should be under the supervision of a physician.

The most common adverse effects of niacin are vasomotor symptoms, especially flushing. Niacin should be administered during or after meals. Inhibitors of prostaglandin synthesis may also be used to reduce vasomotor symptoms when therapy is initiated. Dose-dependent side effects include gastrointestinal complaints (primarily upper), hyperglycemia, hyperuricemia, and liver function abnormalities. There are many other less frequently reported adverse effects. Use of niacin in type I diabetes mellitus may require only a minor adjustment in insulin dosage. However, its use in type II diabetes mellitus is more problematic. It may cause major deterioration in the control of the diabetes.

Sustained-Release

Several sustained-release preparations are also available without prescription. Generally, these preparations are considered if the patient does not tolerate crystalline niacin. These preparations are easier to use, primarily because of decreased frequency of vasomotor symptoms. However, fulminant hepatotoxicity has occasionally been reported.[20] If used, daily doses of 1.5 g or less are preferred, and total daily doses exceeding 2 g are not recommended. The same manufacturer's preparation should always be used. The sustained-release preparations are more effective in lowering LDL-C levels but less effective in increasing HDL-C levels per milligram of drug administered when compared with crystalline niacin.[19, 21]

Fibric Acid Derivatives

Gemfibrozil is the most widely used drug in this class in the United States. It is generally administered in a dose of 600 mg b.i.d. Fenofibrate has been approved by the Food and Drug Administration (FDA) and should be available soon. The fibric acids are effective primarily in lowering triglyceride levels, and reductions ranging from 25% to 50% can be obtained.[22, 23] They have been used widely to increase HDL-C levels, but the increase is generally only 10% to 15%. Greater increases in HDL-C levels can be seen in patients with hypertriglyceridemia. In patients without hypertriglyceridemia, the increase in HDL-C levels with the statins is equivalent to that with the fibric acids. However, the statins are more effective in lowering LDL-C. The effect of the fibric acids on LDL-C levels is quite variable.[23] In patients without hypertriglyceridemia, reductions of 10% in LDL-C generally occur, occasionally 15%. With hypertriglyceridemia, the reduction in LDL-C levels is less, and patients with severe hypertriglyceridemia have an increase in LDL-C levels. This is due to compositional changes in LDL characterized by increased cholesterol ester content that is not thought to increase the risk of CHD.[24]

The fibric acids are easy to administer and have very few side effects. Gastrointestinal complaints are the most frequent. They also increase the lithogenicity of bile. The primary mode of excretion is renal, and the dose may have to be reduced in patients with impaired renal function. They are highly bound to serum albumin and can potentiate the effect of oral anticoagulants.

A 34% reduction in CHD events was observed with gemfibrozil in the Helsinki Heart Study, a primary prevention trial.[25] The decrease in CHD risk was partially due to the increase in HDL levels and partially due to a decrease in LDL levels. A subset of patients with LDL/HDL ratios of more than 5 and triglyceride levels of more than 200 mg/dl accounted for most of the benefit in this study.[26] When used for CHD prevention, the fibric acids are primarily used in patients with low levels of HDL-C, elevated triglyceride levels, and minimal elevations of LDL-C levels. Niacin is the preferred drug in these patients, and the fibric acids are generally used if the patient does not tolerate niacin. The enthusiasm for the fibric acids has diminished over the years. Although there has been a reduction in CHD, an increase in non-CHD deaths has been suggested in trials with clofibrate and possibly gemfibrozil.[27, 28]

Estrogen Replacement in Postmenopausal Women

Postmenopausal women have an increased risk of CHD, and this increased risk may be due to loss of estrogen.[29] Epidemiologic evidence suggests that estrogen replacement in women without evidence of CHD is associated with approximately a 50% reduction in CHD risk and that the risk may be reduced by approximately 80% in women with clinical evidence of CHD.[30–32] However, there have been no major, prospective controlled clinical trials to document this degree of risk reduction, and the potential benefits of the combination of estrogen and progestin are less well defined.

With doses equivalent to 0.625 mg of conjugated estrogen or 2 mg of micronized estradiol, approximate reductions in LDL-C by 15% and increases in HDL-C of 15% are reported.[33] Systemic estrogens have much less effect on lipoprotein levels. However, it appears that the benefits of estrogen on CHD risk are only partially related to the changes in lipoproteins and much of the benefit is due to other effects.

Estrogen administration may be used as the initial form of therapy in postmenopausal women with abnormal lipoprotein levels or can be used in combination with other lipid-altering drugs.[2, 31] Estrogen administration, especially the higher doses, can cause hypertriglyceridemia.

The choice of initial therapy requires active input from the patient. Although the benefits of estrogen appear to be dramatic, there have been no controlled trials. Also, the effect of progestin is less well defined. The required duration of estrogen replacement or whether benefit still exists if therapy is initiated many years after menopause is unknown. There are other benefits of estrogen replacement, including relief of vasomotor, genitourinary, and other menopause-associated symptoms and treatment of osteoporosis. However, fear of cancer is a major concern for many women.

The long-term effects of estrogen administration on the risk of breast cancer have not been conclusively determined. The combination of estrogen/progestin markedly attenuates the risk of endometrial hyperplasia and cancer. Appropriate monitoring for uterine and breast cancer is required for all women receiving hormonal replacement therapy.

Probucol

Probucol reduces LDL-C levels by 5% to 15% but also decreases HDL-C levels by 10% to 15%.[34] Thus, it has not been widely used as a lipid-altering drug. The greatest interest has been in its potential role as an antioxidant.[35] It is a very potent antioxidant in animal and *in vitro* studies. However, in the only clinical trial completed to date, it did not produce a beneficial effect on the progression of atherosclerosis in the femoral artery.[36] It is rarely used in patients who have not tolerated or responded to other drugs.

COMBINATION THERAPY

Combination therapy[2, 9, 37, 38] is generally used to

1. obtain a greater effect on a single lipoprotein abnormality,
2. control multiple lipid and lipoprotein abnormalities,
3. achieve target lipid and lipoprotein goals at reduced cost, or
4. reduce the likelihood of side effects owing to a smaller dose of the individual drugs that are administered.

The more commonly used drug combinations are indicated in Table 11–4.[2, 9] The proposed scheme is especially helpful in that it is applicable to almost all patients and it does not require identification of the underlying genetic abnormalities, if they should exist.

The mechanisms of action of the four classes of drugs that are commonly used are summarized in Table 11–5. The proposed drug combinations are based on their mechanisms of action.[2, 9, 37, 38] LDL-C–lowering combinations either use drugs that increase LDL receptor activity by different mechanisms or combine a drug whose major effect is to inhibit lipoprotein synthesis with one that increases LDL receptor activity. The mechanism of action of drugs that increase HDL-C levels is complex and poorly

Table 11–4. **Drug Combinations for Various Lipid and Lipoprotein Abnormalities***

LDL-C ≥ 130† TG < 200	LDL-C ≥ 130 TG 200–400	HDL-C < 35 TG ≤ 400 LDL-C < 130	TG > 400
Statin, plus 1. Resin 2. Nicotinic acid	Statin, plus 1. Nicotinic acid 2. Fibric acid	Nicotinic acid, plus 1. Fibric acid 2. Statin	Fibric acid, plus 1. Nicotinic acid 2. Statin

*All values are expressed as mg/dl.
†In primary prevention with two or more risk factors, an LDL-C of ≥ 160 mg/dl would be used.
TG, triglycerides.

Table 11–5. **Mechanisms of Action of Lipid-Lowering Drugs**

Increased LDL Receptor Activity

Statins

Inhibit the rate-limiting enzyme in cholesterol biosynthesis. The decreased hepatic and cellular concentrations of cholesterol stimulate the production of LDL receptors. The increased number of LDL receptors increases the rate of removal of LDL. There may also be a modest decrease in the intermediate-density lipoproteins, which contain more triglycerides. The net effect is a decrease in LDL-C levels with a modest reduction in triglyceride levels. (The statins may modestly decrease lipoprotein synthesis in some patients.)

Resins

Increase the fecal excretion of bile acids and decrease the enterohepatic circulation of bile acids. There is increased conversion of cholesterol to bile acids. The decreased hepatic cholesterol concentration stimulates the production of LDL receptors and increases the rate of removal of LDL.

Inhibited Lipoprotein Synthesis

Nicotinic Acid

There is decreased synthesis/secretion of VLDL, the major triglyceride-containing lipoprotein. This decreases the formation of the intermediate-density lipoproteins and LDL. The circulating levels of VLDL, intermediate-density lipoproteins, and LDL are decreased, which is manifested by decreased plasma levels of LDL-C and triglycerides.

Multiple Mechanisms

Fibric Acids

There is increased lipoprotein lipase. This enzyme enhances the removal of triglycerides from VLDL. The resultant smaller intermediate-density lipoproteins can then either be removed by the receptor or be converted to LDL, which can also be removed by the receptor. There is a decrease in circulating triglyceride levels because of the decrease in VLDL and the intermediate-density lipoproteins. LDL levels may also be decreased. (The mechanism of action of the fibric acids is not well defined, and they may also decrease lipoprotein synthesis and increase LDL receptor activity.)

---

understood and will not be discussed further. Triglyceride lowering generally involves a combination of increased lipoprotein lipase activity plus an inhibitor of lipoprotein synthesis.

Elevated LDL-C Levels and Triglycerides of 200 mg/dl or Less

The primary goal in these patients is to lower LDL-C levels, but some patients may also have low HDL-C levels. The usual combination that is used for LDL-C lowering is a statin plus a resin. Both classes of drugs increase LDL receptor activity. The LDL-C lowering of these two drugs is at least additive. The LDL lowering of the statins is not linear, and generally only a 6% additional reduction in LDL-C levels is obtained with each doubling of dose at the higher dosages.[12] Combination therapy produces a greater reduction in LDL-C levels or can produce equivalent LDL-C lowering with smaller doses of two drugs.[39–42] The total cost of the two drugs is currently less than the larger dose of statin. These principles are illustrated in Table 11–6.

The granular form of resin is not tolerated by some patients. Colestipol is currently available in tablet form. The tablets may make resin therapy more acceptable to some patients, but they may have to take

Table 11–6. **Combination of Statin and Resin for Lowering LDL-C**

	% LDL-C Lowering
Simvastatin 20 mg PM*	34
Simvastatin 40 mg PM	40
Simvastatin 10 mg PM plus 10 g colestipol†	≥40
Simvastatin 20 mg PM plus 10 g colestipol†	~50

*Or equivalent dose of other statin.
†Or 8 mg of cholestyramine.

4 to 8 tablets per day. If the target LDL-C level is not achieved with the lower doses of the two drugs, the doses of both drugs can be increased. However, the dose of statin is usually increased first because of better patient tolerance.

For patients who have low HDL-C levels, it may be preferable to combine a statin and nicotinic acid. Crystalline nicotinic acid generally produces only modest additional decreases in levels of LDL-C but significant increases in HDL-C levels. Although the risk of hepatotoxicity is greater, the sustained-release preparations produce greater decreases in LDL-C if significant increases in HDL-C are not required. Combinations of a resin and nicotinic acid can be used,[43] but the frequency of side effects is usually high.

Elevated LDL-C Levels and Triglycerides of 200 to 400 mg/dl

Patients with elevated levels of both LDL-C and triglycerides are at greater risk for CHD than patients with comparable elevations of LDL-C levels only.[5, 6] However, it is difficult to achieve the target goals for the multiple lipoprotein abnormalities, which usually also include low HDL-C levels. Nicotinic acid is the ideal drug because it favorably affects all the lipid and lipoprotein abnormalities. However, the dose of nicotinic acid that would be required is rarely tolerated. A statin, especially in patients with clinical evidence of CHD, is usually administered first. The benefits of lowering the LDL-C levels are well established, and control of LDL-C levels should be the first goal of therapy.

The combination of a statin and nicotinic acid is the first choice. The effects of nicotinic acid are additive to those of the statins. Crystalline nicotinic acid should be administered in increasing doses until target goals are achieved, or the maximal tolerated dose or a total daily dose of 3 g. The risk of myopathy appears to be very small, and there does not appear to be an increased risk of hepatotoxicity with these doses of crystalline nicotinic acid.

If nicotinic acid is not tolerated, the fibric acids are added. They generally produce little additional LDL-C lowering, but will lower triglyceride and increase HDL-C levels. The risk of myopathy is higher with increasing doses of the statins. Although there is some evidence suggesting that the risk of myopathy could be less with the combination of a fibric acid and either pravastatin or fluvastatin, there is insufficient evidence to recommend a specific statin.[44, 45]

Nicotinic acid has occasionally been used in combination with a fibric acid.[46] This combination is useful only if the dose of nicotinic acid is adequate to control LDL-C levels. The fibric acids have an additive effect on triglyceride and HDL-C levels.

HDL-C of Less Than 35 mg/dl, Triglycerides of 400 mg/dl or Less, and Lower LDL-C Levels

The ideal first drug is crystalline nicotinic acid because of its HDL-C–raising effects. Combination therapy is rarely used for increasing HDL-C levels only. If the patient is able to tolerate some nicotinic acid, a fibric acid can be used to obtain additional lowering of triglycerides or increased HDL-C levels. If the patient does not tolerate nicotinic acid, a statin is generally administered. The statins are not as effective in lowering triglycerides, but their effects on HDL-C levels are nearly equivalent to those produced by the fibric acids. Additionally, they lower LDL-C levels, and the resultant LDL-C/HDL-C ratio is more favorable than that produced with the fibric acids.

Triglycerides of 400 mg/dl or More

This patient population is only a minor contribution to the total burden of CHD. The fibric acids are used initially because many of these patients also have hyperuricemia and decreased glucose tolerance. Nicotinic acid can be used initially if these abnormalities do not exist. If the levels of triglycerides remain elevated, the fibric acids can be used in combination with nicotinic acid. If the triglyceride levels are lowered to less than 400 mg/dl with a fibric acid, elevated LDL-C levels are frequently reported. If the elevated LDL-C levels are not controlled with nicotinic acid, a small dose of a statin may be used.

TRIPLE THERAPY

Occasionally patients' hyperlipidemia cannot be controlled with two drugs, and triple therapy is required. This aggressive therapy is usually reserved for practitioners who have considerable experience with lipid-lowering drugs. Triple therapy is especially helpful in patients with very high LDL-C levels.[47, 48] However, triple therapy, with small doses of three drugs, can be used in patients with more modest lipid and lipoprotein abnormalities to correct multiple

abnormalities and at lower cost. The initial dose of any drug generally produces a much greater percentage of the maximal effect than subsequent increments in dosage.

SUMMARY

The recommended target goals for LDL-C lowering can now be achieved in most patients with the currently available drugs. Cost and side effects are the most frequent deterrents to achieving the goal. In addition, HDL-C and triglyceride levels can also be controlled in many patients. However, only modest increases in HDL-C levels can be obtained with the currently available drugs if patients do not tolerate crystalline nicotinic acid. Combination therapy is frequently required to achieve target goals in patients with CHD. In rare patients, triple therapy may be indicated. If target goals for therapy cannot be achieved in patients with CHD or other high-risk patients, consideration should be given to referral to a specialist. The benefits of treatment, especially in patients with CHD, are too great to miss this opportunity.

REFERENCES

1. Summary of the Second Report of the National Cholesterol Education Program (NCEP) Expert Panel on Detection, Evaluation, and Treatment of High Blood Cholesterol in Adults (Adult Treatment Panel II). JAMA 269:3015, 1993.
2. National Cholesterol Education Program Second Report of the National Cholesterol Education Program (NCEP) Expert Panel on Detection, Evaluation, and Treatment of High Blood Cholesterol in Adults (Adult Treatment Panel II). Circulation 89:1329, 1994.
3. Cholesterol consensus: A trans-Atlantic perspective. Proceedings of a round-table conference. Amsterdam, The Netherlands, 31 October–November 1991. Int J Cardiol 37(Suppl 1):S1, 1992.
4. Canadian Task Force on the Periodic Health Examination: Periodic Health Examination, 1993 update: 2. Lowering the blood total cholesterol level to prevent coronary heart disease. Can Med Assoc J 148:521, 1993.
5. NIH Consensus Development Panel on Triglyceride, High-density Lipoprotein, and Coronary Heart Disease: Triglyceride, high-density lipoprotein, and coronary heart disease. JAMA 269:505, 1993.
6. Assmann G, Gotto AM Jr, Paoletti R (Chairs): The hypertriglyceridemias: Risk and management. The International Committee for the Evaluation of Hypertriglyceridemia as a Vascular Risk Factor. Am J Cardiol 68(Suppl A):1A, 1991.
7. American Diabetes Association: Detection and management of lipid disorders in diabetes. Diabetes Care 16(Suppl 2):828, 1993.
8. Colosimo RJ, Nunn-Thompson C: HMG-CoA reductase inhibitors. Pharmacol Ther 18:21, 1993.
9. Hunninghake DB: Drug Treatment of dyslipoproteinemia. Endocrinol Metab Clin North Am 19:345, 1990.
10. Sirtori CR: Pharmacology and mechanism of action of the new HMG-CoA reductase inhibitors. Pharmacol Res 22:555, 1990.
11. Blum CB: Comparison of properties of four inhibitors of 3-hydroxy-3-methlyglutaryl-coenzyme A reductase. Am J Cardiol 73(Suppl):3D, 1994.
12. Bradford RH, Shear CL, Chremos AN, et al: Expanded clinical evaluation of lovastatin (EXCEL) study results. I: Efficacy in modifying plasma lipoproteins and adverse event profile in 8245 patients with moderate hypercholesterolemia. Arch Intern Med 151:43, 1991.
13. Lovastatin Study Group I through IV: Lovastatin 5 year safety and efficacy study. Arch Intern Med 153:1029, 1993.

14. LaRosa J: Review of clinical studies of bile acid sequestrants for lowering plasma lipid levels. Cardiology 76(Suppl 1):55, 1989.
15. Lipid Research Clinics Program: The Lipid Research Clinics Coronary Primary Prevention Trial results. I: Reduction in incidence of coronary heart disease. JAMA 251:351, 1984.
16. Superko HR, Greenland P, Manchester RA, et al: Effectiveness of low-dose colestipol therapy in patients with moderate hypercholesterolemia. Am J Cardiol 70:135, 1992.
17. Henkin Y, Oberman A, Hurst DC, Segrest JP: Niacin revisited: Clinical observations on an important but underutilized drug. Am J Med 91:239, 1991.
18. Illingworth DR, Stein EA, Mitchel YB, et al: Comparative effects of lovastatin and niacin in primary hypercholesterolemia: A prospective trial. Arch Intern Med 154:1586, 1994.
19. McKenney JM, Proctor JD, Harris S, et al: A comparison of the efficacy and toxic effects of sustained- vs immediate-release niacin in hypercholesterolemic patients. JAMA 271:672, 1994.
20. Etchason JA, Miller TD, Squires RW, et al: Niacin-induced hepatitis: A potential side effect with low-dose time-released niacin. Mayo Clin Proc 66:23, 1991.
21. Keenan JM, Fontaine PL, Wenz JB, et al: Niacin revisited: A randomized, controlled trial of wax-matrix sustained-release niacin in hypercholesterolemia. Arch Intern Med 151:1424, 1991.
22. Grundy SM, Vega GL: Fibric acids: Effects on lipids and lipoprotein metabolism. Am J Med 83:9, 1987.
23. Hunninghake DB, Peters JR: Effect of fibric acid derivatives on blood lipid and lipoprotein levels. Am J Med 83:44, 1987.
24. Yuan J, Tsai MY, Hunninghake DB: Changes in composition and distribution of LDL subspecies in hypertriglyceridemic patients during gemfibrozil therapy. Atherosclerosis 110:1, 1994.
25. Frick MH, Elo O, Haapa K, et al: Helsinki Heart Study: Primary-prevention trial with gemfibrozil in middle-aged men with dyslipidemia. N Engl J Med 317:1237, 1987.
26. Manninen V, Tenkanen L, Koskinen P, et al: Joint effects of serum triglyceride and LDL cholesterol and HDL cholesterol concentrations on coronary heart disease risk in the Helsinki Heart Study. Circulation 85:37, 1992.
27. Committee of Principal Investigators: WHO cooperative trial on primary prevention of ischaemic heart disease with clofibrate to lower serum cholesterol: Final mortality follow-up. Lancet 2:600, 1994.
28. Huttunen JK, Heinonen OP, Manninen V, et al: The Helsinki Heart Study: An 8.5-year safety and mortality follow-up. J Intern Med 235:31, 1994.
29. Colditz GA, Willett WC, Stampfer MJ, et al: Menopause and the risk of coronary heart disease in women. N Engl J Med 316:1105, 1987.
30. Stampfer MJ, Colditz GA: Estrogen replacement therapy and coronary heart disease: A quantitative assessment of the epidemiologic evidence. Prev Med 20:47, 1991.
31. Grady D, Rubin SM, Petitti DB, et al: Hormone therapy to prevent disease and prolong life in postmenopausal women. Ann Intern Med 117:1016, 1992.
32. Sullivan JM, Vander Zwaag R, Hughes JP: Estrogen replacement and coronary artery disease: Effect on survival in postmenopausal women. Arch Intern Med 150:2557, 1990.
33. Granfone A, Campos H, McNamara JR, et al: Effects of estrogen replacement on plasma lipoproteins and apolipoproteins in postmenopausal, dyslipidemic women. Metabolism 41:1193, 1992.
34. Hunninghake DB, Bell C, Olson L: Effect of probucol on plasma lipids and lipoproteins in type IIb hyperlipoproteinemia. Atherosclerosis 37:469, 1980.
35. Baumstark MW, Aristegui R, Zoller T, et al: Probucol incorporated into LDL particles in vivo inhibits generation of lipid peroxides more effectively than endogenous antioxidants alone. Clin Biochem 25:395, 1992.
36. Walldius G, Erikson U, Olsson AG, et al: The effect of probucol on femoral atherosclerosis: The Probucol Quantitative Regression Swedish Trial (PQRST). Am J Cardiol 74:875, 1994.
37. Larsen ML, Illingworth DR: Drug treatment of dyslipoproteinemia. Med Clin North Am 78:225, 1994.
38. Ginsberg HN: Lipoprotein metabolism and its relationship to atherosclerosis. Med Clin North Am 78:1, 1994.
39. Heudebert GR, Van Ruiswyk J, Hiatt J, et al: Combination drug therapy for hypercholesterolemia: The trade-off between cost and simplicity. Arch Intern Med 153:1828, 1993.
40. Pravastatin Multicenter Study Group II: Comparative efficacy and safety of pravastatin and cholestyramine alone and combined in patients with hypercholesterolemia. Arch Intern Med 153:1321, 1993.
41. Jacob BG, Richter WO, Scwandt P: Long-term treatment (2 years) with the HMG CoA reductase inhibitors lovastatin or pravastatin in combination with cholestyramine in patients with severe primary hypercholesterolemia. J Cardiovasc Pharmacol 22:396, 1993.
42. Weisweiler P: Simvastatin plus low-dose colestipol in the treatment of severe familial hypercholesterolemia. Curr Ther Res 44:802, 1988.
43. Blankenhorn DH, Nessim SA, Johnson RL, et al: Beneficial effects of combined colestipol-niacin therapy on coronary atherosclerosis and coronary venous bypass grafts. JAMA 257:3233, 1987.
44. Glueck CJ, Speirs J, Tracy T: Safety and efficacy of combined gemfibrozil-lovastatin therapy for primary dyslipoproteinemia. J Lab Clin Med 115:603, 1990.
45. Da Col PG, Fonda M, Fisicaro M, et al: Tolerability and efficacy of combination therapy with simvastatin plus gemfibrozil in type IIb refractory familial combined hyperlipidemia. Curr Ther Res 53:473, 1993.
46. Carlson LA, Rosenhamer G: Reduction of mortality in the Stockholm Ischaemic Heart Disease Secondary Prevention Study by combined treatment with clofibrate and nicotinic acid. Acta Med Scand 223:405, 1988.
47. Witztum JL: Intensive drug therapy of hypercholesterolemia. Am Heart J 113:603, 1987.
48. Kane JP, Malloy MJ, Tun P, et al: Normalization of low-density-lipoprotein levels in heterozygous familial hypercholesterolemia with a combined drug regimen. N Engl J Med 304:251, 1981.

CHAPTER 12

Combination Therapy in Pulmonary Hypertension

Stuart Rich, M.D.

GENERAL MEASURES

The treatment of pulmonary hypertension traditionally has been difficult. The inability to detect elevated pulmonary artery pressure (PAP) in its early stages with a simple, noninvasive test and the lack of drugs that are specific for the pulmonary vascular bed continue to hamper our efforts. However, some forms of pulmonary hypertension are treatable. Because the prognosis and response to therapy of pulmonary hypertensive states depend largely on the etiology of the disease, the management of pulmonary hypertension must be chosen in reference to the underlying cause. The use of digitalis glycosides, diuretics, and anticoagulants that have been applied to the treatment of pulmonary hypertension of several causes is addressed first.

Digoxin

As controversies have arisen regarding the effectiveness of digoxin in the chronic treatment of left ventricular failure, it is difficult, if not impossible, to prove that the use of digoxin influences the overall outcome of patients with right ventricular failure and pulmonary hypertension. Nothing is unique, however, about the sarcomeres of the right ventricle to suggest that they would be unresponsive to the inotropic properties of digoxin. In studies in animals, the prior administration of digoxin in right ventricular hypertensive states was found to lessen the reduction in contractility of the right ventricle.[1, 2] This finding would provide some rationale for administering digoxin to patients with pulmonary hypertension, even in the absence of overt right ventricular failure, unless there is a coexistent problem that would reduce the safety of taking this medication. The current value of digoxin in patients with pulmonary hypertension, however, remains uncertain.

Diuretic Therapy

Considerable controversy also exists about the usefulness of diuretics in the treatment of pulmonary hypertension. Diuretics do not possess pulmonary vasodilator properties, and thus would not be expected to lower PAP or pulmonary vascular resistance (PVR). Their role in the treatment of patients with pulmonary hypertension traditionally has been limited to patients who manifest right ventricular failure and systemic venous congestion. It has been found, however, that they are much more effective in providing symptomatic relief than one might anticipate.

Pulmonary capillary congestion and increased left ventricular filling pressures may contribute to the sensation of dyspnea and orthopnea in patients with pulmonary hypertension, because right ventricular hypertrophy tends to lead to left ventricular diastolic dysfunction.[3] Increased extravascular lung water also has been described in patients with right ventricular failure from cor pulmonale.[4] A modest reduction in the capillary wedge pressure secondary to treatment with diuretics may afford relief of orthopnea and dyspnea. More importantly, diuretics work to reduce wall stress in the right ventricle that is overloaded by volume and pressure. In the author's experience, systemic hypotension has not been a problem with diuretics in patients who have elevated right atrial pressures; thus, diuretic therapy is initiated in patients with symptoms of dyspnea and elevated jugular venous pressure, and the dose of the diuretic is titrated to the patient's symptoms. If the patient develops prerenal azotemia from judicious diuretic

therapy, it indicates a markedly reduced cardiac output and the risks of diuretic therapy may overshadow its potential benefits.

Anticoagulant Therapy

The histologic observation that diffuse microvascular thrombosis commonly exists in patients with pulmonary hypertension has led physicians to the empiric use of anticoagulants as therapy of this condition.[5] Evidence supporting the use of anticoagulants came from the work of Fuster et al.,[6] who reviewed the experience of the Mayo Clinic over a 15-year period in patients with primary pulmonary hypertension (PPH). Although retrospective in nature, their study suggested a therapeutic benefit with respect to survival in patients who were treated with anticoagulant therapy.

Subsequently, investigators have looked at assessing intravascular thrombosis in patients with PPH by measuring fibrinopeptide A (FPA) levels.[7] It was demonstrated that, in the majority of patients, FPA levels were elevated, sometimes to extraordinary heights. The administration of 5000 units of intravenous heparin brought the FPA levels down close to normal, suggesting that there is intense intravascular thrombotic activity in patients with PPH, which can be reversed with anticoagulation. More recently, the use of anticoagulants in patients with PPH was evaluated in a clinical trial assessing the influence of calcium channel blockers on survival, in which approximately half the patients received anticoagulation as well.[8] Patients with PPH who failed to respond to calcium channel blockers still had a significant improvement in survival with the use of warfarin anticoagulation compared with patients who did not receive anticoagulants. Thus, data to date strongly suggest that anticoagulation is of value in the treatment of patients with primary pulmonary hypertension, and perhaps pulmonary hypertension of other causes. The level of anticoagulation is generally recommended to establish an International Normalized Ratio (INR) of 1.5 to 2, a low-dose regimen similar to that that has been employed with success in the prophylaxis of deep vein thrombosis and recurrent pulmonary thromboembolism. Because patients with pulmonary hypertension may have right-sided heart failure and hepatic congestion, particular caution needs to be placed on the monitoring of prothrombin times. In patients whose prothrombin times are prolonged owing to hepatic congestion, the addition of anticoagulation therapy is probably not justified.

THE USE OF VASODILATORS FOR PULMONARY HYPERTENSION

Since the mid-1980s, the main focus of therapy in patients with pulmonary hypertension has been on vasodilator drugs. These drugs should not be administered without measuring pulmonary hemodynamics, of which the clinician should have a thorough understanding.

The most commonly monitored hemodynamic parameter has been pulmonary vascular resistance (PVR). Because the technology does not exist to measure resistance in the pulmonary vascular bed directly, a hydraulic equation adapted from Ohm's law has been derived to calculate PVR. In reality, the derived value is a ratio of PAP to pulmonary blood flow. Although the calculation of PVR has been helpful in characterizing the severity of many cardiovascular diseases, changes that occur in patients with PVR from interventions can be misinterpreted for several reasons. First, it is assumed that the pulmonary capillary wedge pressure used as the downstream pressure within the pulmonary arterial bed is the true closing pressure for the arterial system (Fig. 12–1). Although this appears to be the case for normal subjects, it does not necessarily hold true for patients with cardiopulmonary diseases, in which pulmonary wedge pressure often underestimates downstream pressure. This has been demonstrated in chronic obstructive lung disease and left ventricular failure.[9] In addition, when the PVR is lowered, one never knows whether it should be attributed to vasodilation or recruitment of vascular channels, because the pulmonary vasculature is not a closed system. Vasodilators usually reduce the calculated PVR by increasing cardiac output, whereas PAP is unchanged.[10] Although this effect may be interpreted to represent a reduction in right ventricular afterload, in reality, it represents an *increase* in right ventricular work and wall stress by increasing right ventricular volume in the face of a markedly elevated systolic pressure (Fig. 12–2). For example, one cannot rely solely on the numeric value

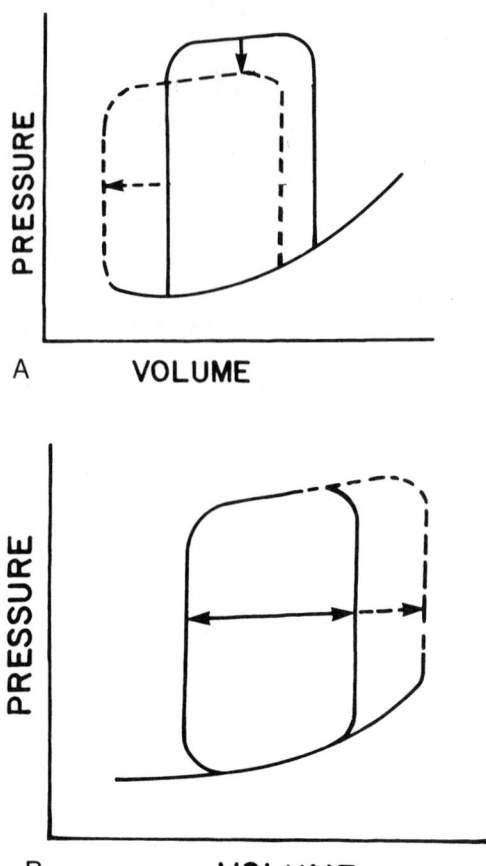

Figure 12–2. A, The effect of vasodilator drugs in a hypothetical patient with left heart failure. The stroke work of the ventricle equals the area within the pressure-volume loops. In this instance, the vasodilator increased stroke work and shifted the loop leftward so that end-systolic volume was lessened, end-diastolic volume was reduced, and stroke volume increased in response to a small reduction in systolic pressure. *B,* The effect of a vasodilator in a hypothetical patient with pulmonary hypertension. In this instance, the vasodilator also works by increasing cardiac output through a reduction in systemic blood pressure. This results in an increase in stroke work of the right ventricle that is associated with an increase in end-diastolic pressure and volume to accommodate the increased venous return. Although stroke volume goes up, right ventricular wall stress also goes up, which ultimately leads to right ventricular failure.

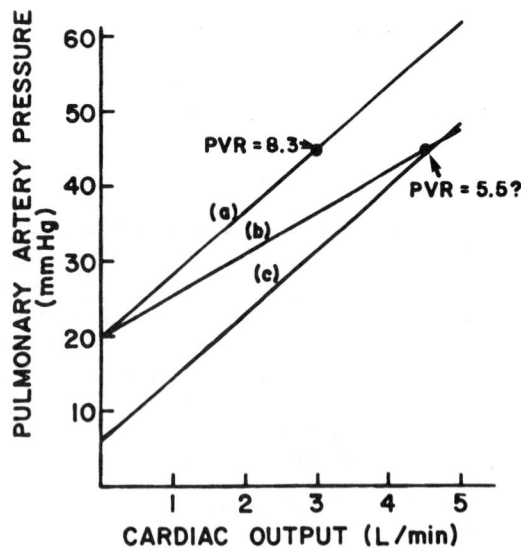

Figure 12–1. Pressure-flow plots for a hypothetic patient with pulmonary hypertension are shown. The slope of the plot can be established by measuring hemodynamics at rest and during exercise *(A).* In this instance, administration of a vasodilator caused the calculated PVR to fall from 8.3 to 5.5 units by increasing cardiac output while leaving pulmonary artery pressure unchanged. However, this is based on the assumption that the closing pressure of 20 mmHg remains unaffected *(B).* However, if the closing pressure is reduced, the slope of the pressure-flow relationship may be identical *(C),* and no actual reduction in PVR may have occurred.

for PVR, or change in resistance, as a measure of the effects of drug therapy.

Another problem in assessing the effects of vasodilators on pulmonary hypertension is that substantial hemodynamic variability exists in the pulmonary vascular bed, which can produce spontaneous changes in cardiac output and PAP.[11] This variability was evaluated specifically in patients with PPH, in whom marked swings that were not necessarily in the same direction were observed periodically in PAP and flow, suggesting constant changes in vasomotor tone within the pulmonary vascular bed. The phenomenon of variability, however, is not unique to PPH; it has been observed with many diseases and is generally proportional to the severity of the disease state. For example, variations in the frequency of ectopy in patients with heart disease, changes in arterial oxygen in patients with chronic lung disease, and changes in blood pressure in patients with systemic hypertension have been demonstrated and appear to represent a facet of the disease process in which autoregulation becomes impaired. This problem can be addressed by making evaluations based on a consistent timed effect of the drug. Thus, the time interval during which the drug appears to exert its greatest hemodynamic influence must be determined, control values must be established, and the values that occur at the specified time interval subsequently can be recorded. The use of peak drug effect is unacceptable. In a study of patients with PPH, a reduction in PAP of 22% or in PVR of 36% was required before a true drug effect was evident.

Perhaps the greatest controversy in the treatment of pulmonary hypertension concerns the definition of a beneficial drug effect. Some investigators have chosen empirically that a reduction in PVR of 20% or greater is a measure of a beneficial drug effect;[12] others have suggested that a reduction of 30%, although arbitrary, may be more reliable.[13] In either case, it is possible to produce a response in which the PAP is increased while the calculated PVR is reduced. It would be inappropriate, and actually contraindicated, to administer a drug that raised the PAP in the face of pulmonary hypertension. This is another reason why the author chooses to focus less on calculated PVR and more on directly measured variables of PAP, right atrial pressure, and cardiac output.

An important physiologic variable that is frequently overlooked is the systemic arterial oxygen content. Systemic arterial hypoxemia is common in patients with pulmonary hypertension of many causes and is attributed to the effects of low cardiac output and ventilation and perfusion inequalities in the lung. Vasodilator drugs may result in vasodilation of blood vessels supplying poorly ventilated areas of the lung and worsening of systemic hypoxemia. This complication is particularly frequent in patients with underlying chronic lung disease.[14] For that reason, systemic arterial oxygen content must be monitored before and after administration of vasodilators to screen for this potentially adverse drug effect. In patients with low cardiac output, tissue delivery of oxygen may be compromised severely and may lead to acidosis. An increase in cardiac output without a reduction in arterial oxygen saturation can result in improved oxygen tissue delivery, which theoretically may be beneficial to the patient.

Although the current experience with vasodilators suggests that some forms of pulmonary hypertension may be reversible when treated early in the course of the disease, there is a point at which drug therapy offers no hope of improvement and only exposes the patient to hazardous side effects.

VASODILATORS FOR PRIMARY PULMONARY HYPERTENSION

Primary pulmonary hypertension has served as a clinical example of a "relatively pure" pulmonary hypertensive state. The efficacy of most vasodilators has been assessed in patients with PPH only, but their effects may differ considerably in other disease states. The literature on the effects of vasodilator drugs in patients with PPH has been controversial. The major drugs that have been tested are reviewed here.

Tolazoline

Tolazoline received early attention as a possible treatment for PPH. Although classified as a histamine agonist and an α-adrenergic antagonist, it also possesses strong chronotropic properties. Tolazoline gained popularity as an agent to test the responsiveness of the pulmonary vascular bed acutely in patients with pulmonary hypertension from several causes.[15, 16] Although intravenous tolazoline may lower PAP and PVR acutely, it has not been documented to be an effective chronic oral therapy. The high incidence of side effects with oral usage, as well as its short half-life requiring dosing every 3 or 4 hours, limits its potential as an oral drug. The role of tolazoline as a pulmonary vasodilator, if it has a role, probably is limited to short-term use in patients with congenital heart disease who are undergoing surgical correction.[17]

Acetylcholine

Acetylcholine was reported in the 1950s as an agent to test the vasomotor responsiveness of the pulmonary vascular bed in patients with PPH. Acetylcholine is inactivated rapidly by the lung, which may explain why intravenous administration seems to produce selective pulmonary effects. Case reports of dramatic acute reductions of PAP have been published, but because no oral form of acetylcholine exists, chronic therapy with this drug is not feasible.[18, 19] Acetylcholine has been used as an acute intravenous test of pulmonary vasodilator reserve.[20] The response to intravenous acetylcholine appears to predict the success of the use of oral vasodilators in patients with primary pulmonary hypertension and may be useful in screening patients for testing with oral vasodilators.

Isoproterenol

Isoproterenol is a potent β-adrenergic agent that affects both systemic and pulmonary vascular beds and increases cardiac output by chronotropic and inotropic properties. Enthusiasm for using isoproterenol in patients with PPH was the result of a case report of a favorable response to chronic sublingual treatment.[21] A critical review of the literature shows that, perhaps more than any other agent, isoproterenol produces an increase in PAP in the face of a calculated reduction in PVR.[10] Thus, the increase in pulmonary blood flow seems to offset whatever vasodilation is occurring. Terbutaline has been advocated as an oral analogue of isoproterenol for chronic therapy, but there are no convincing reports that it produces any sustained beneficial effects.[22]

α-Adrenergic Blockers

The demonstration of α-adrenergic vasoconstrictive influences on the pulmonary vascular bed in laboratory animals and data suggesting similar effects in humans[23, 24] have been the basis for using α-adrenergic blockers as therapy in patients with pulmonary hypertension. Published experience on the clinical use of phentolamine and phenoxybenzamine is primarily anecdotal.[25, 26] Prazosin possesses direct, smooth muscle-relaxing properties, is an α-blocker, and is well tolerated as an oral agent. Clinical studies have failed to show a consistent beneficial response to oral prazosin, even in patients who experience reductions in pulmonary resistance from intravenous phentolamine.[27] Thus, although α-adrenergic receptors regulate pulmonary vascular tone in the normal state, it is unlikely that they play a significant role in advanced pulmonary hypertensive disease states.

Diazoxide

Diazoxide is a thiazide derivative with potent vasodilator properties that has been used widely in the treatment of hypertensive crises. Although early reports of patients with PPH showed substantial reductions in pulmonary artery pressure,[28, 29] this has not been the experience in subsequent observations.[30] Diazoxide may cause a precipitous reduction in systemic blood pressure, and the deaths that have been reported from diazoxide administration are worrisome.[30, 31] For these reasons, the author no longer tests with diazoxide and advises against challenging patients who have pulmonary hypertension.

Nitroprusside

Sodium nitroprusside is a potent vasodilator that acts on the arterial and venous beds. Like diazoxide, it gained popularity because it rapidly lowers systemic blood pressure in patients with hypertensive crises. The short half-life of the drug is an additional advantage because the effects dissipate rapidly when the infusion of the drug is stopped. Acute challenges of nitroprusside have been reported in patients with various forms of pulmonary hypertension,[32] but there are no published studies on its influence in patients with PPH. Nitroglycerin, another nitrate compound with vasodilating properties, has been tested in both intravenous and sublingual forms in patients with primary and secondary pulmonary hypertension.[33, 34] Its influence on pulmonary pressures seems to be modest at best, and its influence on cardiac output minimal. There are no long-term reports of beneficial effects using nitroglycerin preparations in patients with PPH.

Hydralazine

Rubin and Peter[35] were the first to demonstrate that hydralazine reduced PVR acutely and chronically in four patients with PPH. Lupi-Herrera et al.[36] observed that hydralazine was most effective in patients with the lowest PAPs. Others, including ourselves, have been unable to demonstrate sustained beneficial effects from hydralazine in patients with PPH.[37, 38] More recently, reports have indicated that hydralazine may increase PAP and right atrial pressure in these venous beds. Like diazoxide, it gained popularity because it rapidly lowers pressure.[39, 40] Experience with hydralazine suggests that, more than the other vasodilators, when administered chronically, it can cause deterioration of the patient's clinical condition and worsen the symptoms of dyspnea and right ventricular failure. In these cases, it appears that hydralazine increases cardiac output by reducing systemic resistance but leaves the pulmonary circulation unable to accommodate increased pulmonary blood flow. The increased venous return to the right ventricle results in increased right ventricular wall stress and, subsequently, leads to right ventricular failure. For these reasons, the author no longer uses hydralazine as a vasodilator for patients with pulmonary hypertension.

Angiotensin-Converting Enzyme Inhibitors

Because angiotensin possesses pulmonary vasoconstrictive properties, the rationale of treating patients with pulmonary hypertension with angiotensin-converting enzyme (ACE) inhibitors appears to be sound. Captopril, the most widely available ACE inhibitor, has been used in several studies in patients with PPH. As with other drugs, studies suggesting both beneficial and adverse effects have been forthcoming,[41-43] with no clear evidence that captopril is clinically useful. Captopril is indicated in improving cardiac output in patients with pulmonary hypertension secondary to left ventricular dysfunction.[44] Although captopril usually leaves the PAP unchanged, the increase in cardiac output may ameliorate some symptoms.

Calcium Antagonists

Calcium antagonists relax vascular smooth muscle by diminishing the intracellular movement of calcium during contraction, rather than by a direct effect as is seen with hydralazine and minoxidil. In laboratory animals, calcium antagonists appear to diminish the pulmonary vasoconstrictor response to hypoxia and prostaglandin $F_{2\alpha}$ ($PGF_{2\alpha}$).[45-47] The most widely tested drug in patients with PPH is nifedipine. When compared with the other classes of vasodilator drugs, nifedipine seems to result more consistently in a reduction in PAP and PVR.[37] It has been reported to exert favorable changes at rest and with exercise[48] and to improve right ventricular ejection fraction.[49] Some reports suggest that the acute effects are sustained over the long term.[50-52] However, adverse effects of nifedipine, including systemic hypotension,[53] pulmonary edema,[54] hypoxemia,[55] right ventricular failure,[56] cardiogenic shock,[56] and death,[57] also have been reported. The point has also been made that the response to nifedipine varies widely from patient to patient, which may reflect the level of underlying right ventricular function. Experience with nifedipine underscores the need for hemodynamic monitoring when initiating vasodilator therapy in patients with pulmonary hypertension. Reports on the use of diltiazem and verapamil are more limited but seem to parallel favorable[58, 59] and unfavorable[56] experiences with nifedipine. Diltiazem and verapamil can have adverse effects on heart rate and conduction as well.

Published studies regarding the effectiveness of all vasodilator drugs in patients with pulmonary hypertension generally have used conventional doses of drugs. However, because no drug has been shown to have specific effects on the pulmonary vascular bed, it should not be surprising that dose responsiveness for pulmonary vascular diseases might differ from the systemic circulation. The author evaluated a novel regimen using high doses of calcium antagonists as therapy for primary pulmonary hypertension.[60] Working from the premise that conventional doses of these agents may not be an adequate challenge to patients with PPH, a drug protocol was developed in which patients initially were challenged with conventional doses of nifedipine, 20 mg, or diltiazem, 60 mg, and then were given consecutive hourly doses until a marked fall in pulmonary vascular resistance *and* pulmonary artery pressure was achieved, or until adverse side effects became manifest. The initial drug challenges produced only marginal reductions in PAP and PVR, similar to previous published experiences. However, 17 patients (26%) responded to the treatment with a 39% fall in PAP and a 53% fall in PVR.[8] These patients were discharged on high doses of nifedipine (up to 240 mg per day) or diltiazem (up to 900 mg per day) as chronic therapy and followed up as outpatients. After 5 years, 94% of the patients responding were alive, as compared with only 55% of the patients who did not respond. The survival of the patients was also significantly better than the natural history of the disease as documented by the recent National Institutes of Health (NIH) Registry on Primary Pulmonary Hypertension. Of equal importance is that there was sustained regression in right ventricular hypertrophy and marked improvement in exercise tolerance and quality of life. In the one patient who reduced her medication back to a conventional dose, the PAP and PVR returned to pretreatment levels. Surprisingly, although adverse side effects of these drugs were anticipated with high doses, no patient taking chronic therapy had to discontinue the drug because of systemic hypotension or other intolerable side effects.

The observation that high doses of calcium antagonists can be effective in patients with PPH in which conventional doses have failed requires the reexamination of notions regarding all vasodilator drugs in this disease.

Amrinone

Amrinone is a nonglycosidic, nonadrenergic, inotropic agent that has been developed for treating congestive heart failure. Its attractiveness in the treatment of pulmonary hypertension is enhanced by its peripheral vasodilating properties. When the short-term effects of amrinone were compared with those of hydralazine and nifedipine in patients with PPH, little hemodynamic change was noted.[37] Others found a similar lack of inotropic response in patients with right ventricular failure.[61] It is possible that the inotropic response to amrinone depends on concomitant vasodilation. However, the recent observation that inotropic therapy with amrinone may accelerate ventricular dysfunction in left ventricular failure[62] should serve to temper enthusiasm for inotropic drugs as chronic therapy for pulmonary hypertension.

Oxygen

Although hypoxia can produce acute and chronic pulmonary hypertension in animals and humans, it does not appear to be an etiologic factor in patients with PPH. On the other hand, hypoxemia is common in patients with PPH, which provides an impetus to try oxygen administration as a therapy. None of the published reports on the effects of oxygen in PPH suggests that it does more than improve the patient's sense of well-being.[63] Because mild to moderate hypoxemia affects PVR only slightly, oxygen is unlikely to be of value in the typical patient with PPH. Reductions in Pa_{O_2} below 50 mmHg increase PVR dramatically,[64] and chronic oxygen administration may be an appropriate consideration in this subset of patients.

Prostaglandin Analogues in Primary Pulmonary Hypertension

Prostaglandins appear to play an important role in modulating pulmonary vascular tone in normal physiologic conditions[65] and in some forms of pulmonary hypertension.[66] Prostaglandin E_1 (PGE_1) received early attention in patients with mitral stenosis,[67] which led to its subsequent use in PPH.[68] Although modest reductions were noted in PAP and PVR, adverse reactions precluded its administration at higher doses. Prostacyclin (PGI_2) has largely replaced PGE_1 because of its greater efficacy. Like PGE_1, it requires intravenous administration and has a short half-life. It has been evaluated acutely in patients with PPH and has been shown to reduce PVR substantially.[69] Reductions in PAP also have occurred, but the maximum dose of drug that can be administered is limited by induced systemic hypotension. However, experience suggests that the acute response to a challenge with intravenous prostacyclin may be a useful way to determine the vasodilator responsiveness of the pulmonary vascular bed in patients with PPH.[70] If this is the case, it may be preferable to characterize patients based on their responses to prostacyclin before evaluating other therapeutic avenues.

Jones et al.[71] used an infusion of prostacyclin administered through an implantable intravenous infusion pump as chronic therapy for patients who responded acutely to the drug. Although substantial reductions in PAP were not achieved with this regimen, they observed symptomatic improvement in patients receiving the drug. Patients who were considered to be extremely ill were maintained on this therapy until they received heart and lung transplantation. Rubin et al. have used chronic prostacyclin as a treatment of patients who were refractory to conventional therapy.[72] The long-term results showed that patients have improved exercise tolerance, improved sense of well-being, and probable improved survival compared with patients randomized to conventional therapy or with the natural history of the disease from the NIH Registry on PPH. Because the use of the drug requires the implantation of a permanent central venous catheter and a portable infusion pump system, it currently remains a second-line therapy for patients who fail conventional vasodilators. Whether or not prostacyclin would have similar or better advantages as a first-line therapy is unknown.

The author evaluated the effects of a thromboxane synthetase inhibitor in patients with PPH.[73] On the premise that thromboxane, a vasoconstrictor, may be liberated in patients with PPH, he sought to test the acute and chronic effectiveness of the investigational agent CGS 13080, which has potent properties of thromboxane synthetase inhibition. In addition, these drugs also promote an increase in the endothelial production of PGI_2 by shunting through internal pathways. Although no acute hemodynamic effects of the thromboxane synthetase inhibitor were demonstrated, after 3 months of therapy, the drug produced a significant fall in PVR, which was further reduced by the administration of nifedipine.

The lessons learned from these studies are twofold. First, combination drug therapy for patients with PPH may be worthwhile. The use of drugs that have different pharmacologic actions that may induce a favorable environment in the pulmonary vascular bed should be pursued. Second, it may not be necessary to demonstrate acute effectiveness of an agent to show long-term benefit. By altering the physiologic environment in the pulmonary bed, perhaps with thromboxane synthetase inhibitors or prostacyclin, one might be able to promote local healing that renders the pulmonary bed more responsive to vasodilator drugs and possibly to arrest or delay the progression of the disease.

Adenosine

Adenosine is a potent naturally occurring vasodilator that produces relaxation of vascular smooth muscle and resistance in the pulmonary vascular bed. Adenosine has been evaluated as a test of pulmonary vasodilator reserve in patients with pulmonary hypertension and has marked effects by increasing cardiac output and reducing pulmonary vascular resistance.[74] Although some patients respond to adenosine and not to oral vasodilators, lack of response to intravenous adenosine appears to predict lack of response to other vasodilators. Because of its short half-life and minimal effects on systemic circulation, it appears to be a safe and ideal drug to test pulmonary vasodilator reserve. Adenosine, however, can be given only as an intravenous infusion in this regard and not a bolus injection as is used for the treatment of supraventricular tachycardias. Interestingly, when given to patients who respond to calcium antagonists, the addition of adenosine further decreases PAP and PVR.[75] This suggests that combination drug regimens for patients with severe pulmonary hypertension using vasodilators with different mechanisms may be warranted.

Nitric Oxide

Nitric oxide, whose activity appears to be similar to that of endothelium-derived relaxing factor, is another potent pulmonary vasodilator. Inhalation of nitric oxide by patients with primary and secondary forms of pulmonary hypertension has produced reductions in pulmonary vascular resistance within minutes that is dose-related and devoid of systemic effects.[76-78] It has been shown that inhalation of nitric oxide in concentrations as high as 80 ppm, for periods as long as 2 months, causes no evidence of toxicity.[78] The role of nitric oxide as a predictor of vasodilator reserve in patients with PPH, as well as its potential therapeutic role in the treatment of chronic pulmonary hypertension, is promising and needs further study.

PULMONARY HYPERTENSION SECONDARY TO LUNG DISEASE

The most common cause of pulmonary hypertension in clinical medicine is chronic lung disease, particularly chronic obstructive pulmonary disease (COPD). It has long been established that, after pulmonary hypertension develops in patients with COPD, their 3-year mortality increases to about 60%.[79] The assumption has been made that pulmonary hypertension develops because of chronic alveolar hypoxia that induces muscular hypertrophy of the pulmonary arteries. However, destruction of the pulmonary vascular bed from emphysematous changes probably also is an important contributing factor.

The only effective established treatment of pulmonary hypertension in patients with COPD has been chronic oxygen therapy.[80, 81] However, the administration of oxygen generally causes minimal reduction in mean PAP. In several trials, the chronic administration of oxygen improved survival and appeared to halt the progression of pulmonary hypertension in this setting. Some investigators have attempted to use the hemodynamic changes from acute oxygen administration as a predictor of survival in patients receiving long-term oxygen treatment.[82] These studies suggest that patients who have slight reductions in PAP from oxygen administration live longer with long-term oxygen therapy than patients who do not respond. The effectiveness of the therapy is proportional to the number of hours per day the patient uses the treatment.

Because hypoxia is a major factor in pulmonary hypertension with cystic fibrosis, kyphoscoliosis, chronic mountain sickness, and obesity-hypoventilation syndromes, there is a sound rationale for extrapolating the use of oxygen to patients who develop cor pulmonale from these conditions.

A physiologic basis exists for the administration of vasodilators, particularly calcium antagonists, to patients with pulmonary hypertension from lung disease.[45] Experimental findings indicate that hypoxia-induced pulmonary vasoconstriction requires calcium influx, which can be inhibited by certain calcium antagonists.[47] In animal studies, calcium antagonists have been shown to attenuate hypoxia-induced pulmonary hypertension and right ventricular hypertrophy.[83] Although vascular hypertrophy can be made to regress in animals that receive continuous oxygen therapy, many patients find the continuous use of oxygen difficult. Thus, it has been suggested that calcium antagonists, which inhibit hypoxic pulmonary vasoconstriction, may be effective as an alternate or adjuvant therapy to chronic oxygen.

As with PPH, many early studies have shown favorable acute hemodynamic changes from the administration of vasodilators to patients with pulmonary hypertension from chronic lung disease.[84, 85] The magnitude of these changes, however, appears less dramatic than for the changes reported in patients with PPH. More disconcerting, however, is that most recent studies not only have failed to reproduce these early favorable results but often suggest potentially harmful effects.[86, 87] Hydralazine and nifedipine are the agents that have been tested most frequently. With respect to pulmonary hemodynamics, little change in PAP and only slight reduction in PVR from an increased cardiac output are achievable from both classes of drugs. In patients with lung disease, however, particular attention must be paid to gas exchange and systemic arterial oxygenation. In patients whose arterial oxygen contents do not change with vasodilators, the argument can be made that oxygen delivery is improved by increasing the cardiac output—a potentially beneficial effect. Hydralazine appears to have a less-pronounced effect on gas exchange than nifedipine, which can cause substantial reductions in arterial oxygen saturation. This reduction is believed to result from pulmonary vasodilation in the regions of abnormal ventilation, a situation that results in increased intrapulmonary shunting. Captopril and the nitrate compounds also have been tested acutely in small numbers of patients, with few convincing effects.[34, 88]

A study in which long-term oxygen was combined with nifedipine or nitroglycerin in patients with cor pulmonale from COPD was undertaken to see whether the vasodilatory properties of the vasodilating agents, combined with improved oxygenation, could provide additive benefit to patients.[89] Despite some modest acute reductions in PVR from the vasodilators, patients who were treated with the combination therapy appeared to have the same survival rate as patients in age-controlled groups treated with long-term oxygen therapy only. Thus, convincing evidence that vasodilators have any role in the therapy for hypoxic lung disease, either as lone agents or in combination with chronic oxygen administration, is lacking.

PULMONARY HYPERTENSION SECONDARY TO COLLAGEN VASCULAR DISEASES

Pulmonary hypertension complicating collagen vascular diseases is being increasingly recognized. Pulmonary hypertension has been described in virtually every collagen vascular disease as a major clinical disorder, commonly leading to death. The mechanism for pulmonary hypertension is probably multifactorial. Most easily understood is the pathogenesis in patients who present with clinical findings of marked interstitial lung disease, confirmed by infiltrates on chest radiograph and restrictive changes on pulmonary function testing. Coexistent hypoxemia is common; therefore, pulmonary hypertension often can be explained easily on the basis of the constellation of these findings. Less common, but clearly recognized, are patients with collagen vascular disease who have moderate to severe pulmonary hypertension in the absence of any clinical parameters of restrictive lung disease. In these people, it is presumed that a vasculitis of the pulmonary vascular bed is the mechanism for the pulmonary arterial hypertension.

Unfortunately, of all the secondary forms of pulmonary hypertension, treatment of pulmonary hypertension from collagen vascular disease has been the least successful. Immunosuppressive therapy would make intuitive sense, especially for disorders in which immunosuppressive therapy is successful in treating vasculitis in other organs. A single case report of steroid-responsive pulmonary hypertension in a patient with systemic lupus erythematosus has been published.[90] Hemodynamic confirmation of a reduction in pulmonary artery pressure was used as a marker of improvement from the treatment. It was assumed that the favorable response seen in this patient was due to intervention at a relatively early stage of the disease. Other attempts to treat similar patients with steroids, however, have been unsuccessful. It would be advisable that whatever regimen is selected, it should be one that has had some measure of success for treating that collagen vascular disease and its effects on other organs. The use of exercise testing, either upright treadmill with the concomitant monitoring of pulse systemic arterial oxygen saturation or via bicycle with concomitant measurement of artery pressures from Doppler measured tricuspid regurgitation, may allow the early detection of pulmonary hypertension in patients with minimal symptoms.

The literature on the use of vasodilators in these patients is more considerable but equally disappointing. The PAP of patients with collagen vascular disease and pulmonary hypertension rarely responds to vasodilator drugs. These agents commonly induce right ventricular failure.[91–93] For this reason, one should be extraordinarily cautious before administering a vasodilator to any patient who has collagen vascular disease and pulmonary hypertension. Calcium channel blockers have been tested in patients with pulmonary hypertension from collagen vascular disease. Alpert et al. reported substantial reductions in both PAP and PVR in 9 of 10 patients with collagen vascular disease whose severity of pulmonary hypertension was mild to moderate.[94] Nootens et al. showed less effectiveness of calcium blockers on patients with more severe pulmonary hypertension, suggesting that the effectiveness of the calcium blockers in pulmonary hypertension from collagen vascular disease is affected by the duration and severity of the underlying disease process.[95]

PULMONARY HYPERTENSION SECONDARY TO MITRAL STENOSIS

Pulmonary hypertension is an expected complication of mitral stenosis. The simplest explanation is a backward transmission of increased left atrial pressure into the pulmonary vascular bed, causing secondary pulmonary hypertension. However, a subgroup of patients with mitral stenosis develops pulmonary vasoconstriction in addition to passive pulmonary hypertension from increased left atrial pressure. Depending on the severity and duration of the disease, the pulmonary vascular changes may become partially irreversible and leave the patient with residual pulmonary hypertension after mitral valve replacement.[96]

The obvious treatment of pulmonary hypertension from mitral stenosis is mitral valve surgery. Although operative morbidity and mortality increase in patients who have extreme levels of pulmonary hypertension, it has been shown that regression of even extraordinarily high levels of pulmonary hypertension occurs after mitral valve replacement or mitral valvotomy. In the series by Zener et al.,[97] patients with mitral valve disease who had pulmonary arterial systolic pressures in excess of 100 mmHg had an average reduction in pulmonary artery systolic pressure after valve surgery of approximately 50% and a reduction in PVR of approximately 70%. Thus, pulmonary hypertension complicating mitral valve disease, regardless of its severity, is no contraindication to surgical valve replacement. The treatment of mitral stenosis with balloon valvuloplasty has also been shown to cause substantial acute reductions in pulmonary artery pressure that are sustained and improved over time.[98, 99] Like mitral valve surgery, pulmonary hypertension complicating mitral stenosis is not a contraindication to balloon valvuloplasty as a therapy.

After mitral valve replacement, some patients do not experience lowered pulmonary pressure in the early postoperative period because of reactive pulmonary vasoconstriction.[100] Persisting hypertension may be due to an increase in pulmonary blood flow (after the mitral stenosis is corrected) in a pulmonary vascular bed that has been vasoconstricted previously. Perhaps as a protective measure, the pulmonary vasculature undergoes diffuse vasoconstriction that tends to keep the PAPs high even though the downstream pulmonary resistance is markedly reduced. In this setting, nitroglycerin infusions have been useful in lowering the gradient between the pulmonary wedge and left atrial pressures.[101] PGE₁ also has been infused in patients who develop refractory right ventricular failure postoperatively.[102] More recently, infusion of a thromboxane synthetase inhibitor has been shown to be effective in reducing the pulmonary hypertension that complicates the postoperative period in patients with mitral valve replacement for mitral stenosis.[103] This finding suggests that reactive vasoconstriction may be the result of thromboxane release, mediated through the platelets circulating through the lung. If the patient can be supported hemodynamically until pulmonary hypertension regresses, a marked, sustained reduction in PAP is the rule after mitral valve replacement.

PULMONARY HYPERTENSION SECONDARY TO CONGENITAL HEART DISEASE

Pulmonary vascular disease secondary to congenital heart disease is well recognized in infants and children and occasionally is seen in adults. Changes in pulmonary hemodynamics have been well described, as have the high morbidity and mortality associated with pulmonary hypertension after surgical correction of ventricular septal defects, transposition of the great arteries with ventricular septal defects, and total anomalous pulmonary venous drainage.

The increase in PVR is a function of the structural changes that decrease the cross-sectional area of the pulmonary vascular bed and occasionally have a reactive component of pulmonary vasoconstriction.[104] An increasing number of reports document pulmonary hypertension in patients with atrial septal defects, once considered to be a rare combination. Although it has been speculated that some of these patients may have PPH coexistent with their atrial septal defect, it is more likely that they are "hyperreactors" with respect to the pulmonary vascular bed and increased pulmonary blood flow.[105]

In the management of any patient with congenital heart disease and pulmonary hypertension, the fundamental principle is surgical correction. Patients with pulmonary hypertension and increased pulmonary resistance at systemic levels (Eisenmenger's reaction) are considered inoperable. The most difficult management decisions involve patients who have congenital heart defects with increased PAPs and resistance; they fall somewhere in the gray zone of operability. Operative success has been considered to be proportional to the vasodilator response of the pulmonary vascular bed to the administration of 100% oxygen or a vasodilator drug.[106] In some centers, a direct assessment of pulmonary vascular histology through open-lung biopsy may be the best predictor of operative success.[107]

The medical treatment of pulmonary hypertension in the patients with congenital heart disease occurs either after surgery or in those with Eisenmenger's physiology. It generally is presumed that PAP falls after the surgical closure of a congenital heart defect, because it is related in part to the increased pulmonary blood flow through the shunt. However, postoperative pulmonary hypertension often is seen and may lead to progressive right ventricular failure and death unless it can be counterbalanced. When managing these patients, it is important to consider the level of systemic artery pressure and cardiac output.[108] In patients with marked reduction in cardiac output, inotropic support of the right ventricle is indicated. In this setting, dopamine might be an appropriate drug, because the pulmonary vascular bed lacks dopaminergic receptors and thus should not be affected by the vasoconstrictor influences of high levels of dopamine, which affects the systemic bed. One study showed that the effect of dopamine was enhanced by combining it with nitroprusside, resulting in greater increases in cardiac output and a greater reduction in PVR than were achieved by dopamine alone.[109] In any case, it is critical to maintain systemic blood pressure when using these agents, because any reduction in right ventricular oxygen supply could lead to acute right ventricular ischemia and deterioration of right ventricular performance. Evidence of subendocardial ischemia has been demonstrated in postmortem specimens from children dying with congenital heart disease.[104]

Vasodilators have been used in the acute management of pulmonary hypertension postoperatively, but their true value is somewhat debatable. Of all the drugs, tolazoline has been used most commonly. Although promoted as having selective pulmonary effects, it also has pronounced systemic effects and sympathomimetic properties that result in an increase in cardiac output and heart rate.[17] Administration of tolazoline as a bolus (1 mg/kg), followed by an infusion of 1 to 2 mg/hr, has been reported to cause a rapid and sustained reduction in PAP in the postoperative management of some patients. Nitroprusside also has been reported useful in this setting, but the number of cases is small.[109, 110]

Some patients develop progressive pulmonary hypertension after successful operative closure of congenital heart defects with left-to-right shunts. Although it is hard to understand why these patients develop subsequent pulmonary hypertension, histologic studies show changes in the pulmonary vascular bed consistent with plexogenic arteriopathy that would otherwise be thought to result directly from the congenital heart defect. The literature on treatment of this subset of patients with vasodilators is particularly scarce. One paper reported the effects of hydralazine on two patients who had closure of a ductus arteriosus at an early age only to develop subsequent pulmonary hypertension later in life.[111] In both patients, hydralazine did not lower PVR or PAP but had systemic hypotensive effects, suggesting potential hazards for use.

Equally difficult is treatment of patients with Eisenmenger's physiology. A particular danger of using vasodilator drugs results from their lack of *selective* pulmonary vasodilating effects. Because the shunt is patent, any reduction in systemic vascular resistance is associated with a worsening of right-to-left shunting that results in systemic hypoxemia and potentially could lead to acidosis and hypotension. On the other hand, any successful reduction in PVR promotes increased left-to-right shunting. Although this short reversal might raise the systemic arterial P_{O_2} the increase in pulmonary blood flow also increases PAP and thus does not reduce the stroke work or wall stress of the right ventricle. Limited reports of the use of hydralazine and the ACE inhibitor enalapril in patients with pulmonary hypertension secondary to congenital heart disease concluded that the drugs were potentially useful,[112, 113] but the author's experience in testing vasodilators in these patients (both those who underwent successful surgery and those considered inoperable) has been uniformly disappointing. This lack of effectiveness is probably due to the chronicity of the underlying changes in the pulmonary vascular bed, which have rendered them relatively resistant to vasodilator drugs.

REFERENCES

1. Spann JF, Buccino RA, Sonnenblick EH, et al: Contractile state of cardiac muscle obtained from cats with experimentally produced ventricular hypertrophy. Circ Res 21:431, 1967.
2. Coulson RL, Rubio E, Bove AA, et al: Digoxin prophylaxis for prevention of the cardiac contractile defect produced by pressure overload [abstract]. Clin Res 23:177A, 1975.
3. Louie EK, Rich S, Brundage BH: Doppler echocardiographic assessment of impaired left ventricular filling in patients with right ventricular pressure overload due to primary pulmonary hypertension. J Am Coll Cardiol 8:1307, 1986.
4. Fishman AP: Chronic cor pulmonale. Am Rev Respir Dis 114:775, 1976.
5. Wagenvoort CA, Wagenvoort N: Primary pulmonary hypertension: A pathologic study of the lung vessels in 156 clinically diagnosed cases. Circulation 42:1163, 1970.
6. Fuster V, Steele PM, Edwards WD, et al: Primary pulmonary hypertension: Natural history and the importance of thrombosis. Circulation 70:580, 1984.
7. Eisenberg PR, Lucore C, Kaufmann E, et al: Elevations in fibrinopeptide A indicative of pulmonary vascular thrombosis in patients with primary pulmonary hypertension. Circulation 82:841, 1990.
8. Rich S, Kaufmann E, Levy PS: The effect of high doses of calcium channel blockers on survival in primary pulmonary hypertension. N Engl J Med 327:76, 1992.
9. McGregor M, Sniderman A: On pulmonary vascular resistance: The need for a more precise definition. Am J Cardiol 55:217, 1985.
10. Rich S, Martinez J, Lam W, et al: A reassessment of the effects of vasodilator drugs in primary pulmonary hypertension: Guidelines for determining a pulmonary vasodilator response. Am Heart J 105:119, 1983.
11. Rich S, D'Alonzo GE, Dantzker DR, et al: Magnitude and implications of spontaneous hemodynamic variability in primary pulmonary hypertension. Am J Cardiol 55:159, 1985.
12. Hughes JD, Rubin LJ: Primary pulmonary hypertension: An

analysis of 28 cases and a review of the literature. Medicine 65:65, 1986.

13. Reeves JT, Groves BM, Turkevich D: The case for treatment of selected patients with primary pulmonary hypertension. Am Rev Respir Dis 134:342, 1986.

14. Melot C, Hallemans R, Naeije R, et al: Deleterious effect of nifedipine on pulmonary gas exchange in chronic obstructive pulmonary disease. Am Rev Respir Dis 130:612, 1984.

15. Grover RF, Reeves JT, Blount SG Jr: Tolazoline hydrochloride (Priscoline): An effective pulmonary vasodilator. Am Heart J 61:5, 1961.

16. Rudolph AM, Paul MH, Sommer LS, et al: Effects of tolazoline hydrochloride (Priscoline) on circulatory dynamics in patients with pulmonary hypertension. Am Heart J 56:424, 1958.

17. Jones ODH, Short DF, Rigby ML, et al: The use of tolazoline hydrochloride as a pulmonary vasodilator in potentially fatal episodes of pulmonary vasoconstriction after cardiac surgery in children. Circulation 64(Suppl 2):II-134, 1981.

18. Samet P, Bernstein WH, Widrich J: Intracardiac infusion of acetylcholine in primary pulmonary hypertension. Am Heart J 60:433, 1960.

19. Charms BL: Primary pulmonary hypertension: Effect of unilateral pulmonary artery occlusion and infusion of acetylcholine. Am J Cardiol 99:94, 1961.

20. Palevsky HI, Long W, Crow J, Fishman AP: Prostacyclin and acetylcholine as screening agents for acute pulmonary vasodilator responsiveness in primary pulmonary hypertension. Circulation 82:2018, 1990.

21. Shettigar UR, Hultgren HN, Specter M, et al: Primary pulmonary hypertension: Favorable effect of isoproterenol. N Engl J Med 295:1414, 1976.

22. Person B, Proctor RG: Primary pulmonary hypertension: Responses to indomethacin, terbutaline and isoproterenol. Chest 76:601, 1979.

23. Bergofsky EH: Mechanisms underlying vasomotor regulation of regional pulmonary blood flow in normal and disease states. Am J Med 57:378, 1974.

24. Fishman AP: Autonomic vasomotor tone in the pulmonary circulation. J Anesthesiol 45:1, 1976.

25. Ruskin JN, Hutter AM Jr: Primary pulmonary hypertension treated with oral phentolamine. Ann Intern Med 90:772, 1979.

26. Pickering TG, Ritter S, Devereux RB: Beneficial effects of phentolamine and nifedipine in primary pulmonary hypertension. Cardiovasc Rev Rep 2:303, 1982.

27. Levine TB, Rose T, Kane M, et al: Treatment of primary pulmonary hypertension by alpha blockade [abstract]. Circulation 62(Suppl 3):III-26, 1980.

28. Klinke WP, Gilbert JAL: Diazoxide in primary pulmonary hypertension. N Engl J Med 302:91, 1980.

29. Hall DR, Petch MC: Remission of primary pulmonary hypertension during treatment with diazoxide. Br Med J 282:1118, 1981.

30. Hermiller JB, Bamback D, Thompson MJ, et al: Vasodilators and prostaglandin inhibitors in primary pulmonary hypertension. Ann Intern Med 97:480, 1982.

31. Buch J, Wennevold A: Hazards of diazoxide in pulmonary hypertension. Br Heart J 46:401, 1981.

32. Delaunois L, Jonard P, Kremer N, et al: Nitroglycerin and isosorbide dinitrate in pulmonary hypertension of chronic obstructive pulmonary disease. Bull Eur Physiopathol Respir 20:11, 1984.

33. Pearl RG, Rosenthal MH, Schroeder JJ, et al: Acute hemodynamic effects of nitroglycerin in pulmonary hypertension. Ann Intern Med 99:9, 1983.

34. Brent BN, Berger HJ, Matthay RA, et al: Contrasting acute effects of vasodilators on right ventricular performance in patients with chronic obstructive pulmonary disease and pulmonary hypertension: A combined radionuclide-hemodynamic study. Am J Cardiol 51:1682, 1983.

35. Rubin LJ, Peter RH: Oral hydralazine therapy for primary pulmonary hypertension. N Engl J Med 302:69, 1980.

36. Lupi-Herrera E, Sandoval J, Seaone M, et al: The role of hydralazine therapy for pulmonary arterial hypertension of unknown cause. Circulation 65:645, 1982.

37. Rich S, Ganz R, Levy PS: Comparative effects of hydralazine, nifedipine, and amrinone in primary pulmonary hypertension. Am J Cardiol 52:1104, 1983.

38. McGoon MD, Seward JB, Vliestra RE, et al: Hemodynamic response to intravenous hydralazine in patients with pulmonary hypertension. Br Heart J 50:579, 1983.

39. Kronzon I, Cohen M, Winer HE: Adverse effect of hydralazine in patients with primary pulmonary hypertension. JAMA 247:3112, 1982.

40. Packer MB, Greenberg B, Massie B, et al: Deleterious effects of hydralazine in patients with primary pulmonary hypertension. N Engl J Med 306:1326, 1982.

41. Leier CV, Bambach D, Nelson S, et al: Captopril in primary pulmonary hypertension. Circulation 67:155, 1983.

42. Ikram H, Maslowski AH, Nichols MG, et al: Hemodynamic and hormonal effects of captopril in primary pulmonary hypertension. Br Heart J 48:541, 1982.

43. Rich S, Martinez J, Lam W, et al: Captopril as treatment for patients with pulmonary hypertension: Problems of variability in assessing chronic drug treatment. Br Heart J 48:272, 1982.

44. Packer M, Medina N, Yushak M, et al: Hemodynamic patterns of response during long-term captopril therapy for severe chronic heart failure. Circulation 68:803, 1983.

45. Braunwald E: Mechanism of action of calcium channel blocking agents. N Engl J Med 307:1618, 1982.

46. Young TE, Lundquist LJ, Chesler E, et al: Comparative effects of nifedipine, verapamil, and diltiazem on experimental pulmonary hypertension. Am J Cardiol 51:195, 1983.

47. McMurty IF, Davidson AB, Reeves JT, et al: Inhibition of hypoxic pulmonary vasoconstriction by calcium antagonists in isolated rat lungs. Circ Res 31:99, 1976.

48. Olivari MT, Levine TB, Weir EK, et al: Hemodynamic effects of nifedipine at rest and during exercise in primary pulmonary hypertension. Chest 86:14, 1984.

49. Rubin LJ, Nicod P, Hillis LD, et al: Treatment of primary pulmonary hypertension with nifedipine: A hemodynamic and scintigraphic evaluation. Ann Intern Med 99:433, 1983.

50. Saito D, Haraoka S, Yoshida H, et al: Primary pulmonary hypertension improved by long-term oral administration of nifedipine. Am Heart J 105:1041, 1983.

51. Wise JR: Nifedipine in the treatment of primary pulmonary hypertension. Am Heart J 105:693, 1983.

52. Douglas JS: Hemodynamic effects of nifedipine in primary pulmonary hypertension. J Am Coll Cardiol 2:174, 1983.

53. Aromatorio GJ, Uretsky BF, Reddy PS: Hypotension and sinus arrest with nifedipine in pulmonary hypertension. Chest 87:265, 1985.

54. Batra AK, Segall PH, Ahmed T: Pulmonary edema with nifedipine in primary pulmonary hypertension. Respiration 47:161, 1985.

55. Krol RC, Evans AT, Albright DP, et al: Primary pulmonary hypertension, nifedipine, and hypoxemia. Ann Intern Med 100:163, 1983.

56. Packer M, Medina N, Yushak M: Adverse hemodynamic and clinical effects of calcium channel blockade in pulmonary hypertension secondary to obliterative pulmonary vascular disease. J Am Coll Cardiol 4:890, 1984.

57. Farber HW, Karlinsky JB, Faling LJ: Fatal outcome following nifedipine for primary pulmonary hypertension. Chest 23:708, 1983.

58. Landmark K, Refsum AM, Simonsen S, et al: Verapamil and pulmonary hypertension. Acta Med Scand 204:29, 1978.

59. Kambara H, Fujimoto K, Wakabayashi A, et al: Primary pulmonary hypertension: Beneficial therapy with diltiazem. Am Heart J 101:230, 1981.

60. Rich S, Brundage BH: High dose calcium blocking therapy for primary pulmonary hypertension: Evidence for long-term reduction in pulmonary arterial pressure and regression of right ventricular hypertrophy. Circulation 76:135, 1987.

61. Konstam MA, Cohen SR, Salem DN, et al: Effect of amrinone on right ventricular function: Predominance of afterload reduction. Circulation 74:359, 1986.

62. Packer M, Medina N, Yushak M: Hemodynamic and clinical limitations of long-term inotropic therapy with amrinone in

patients with severe chronic heart failure. Circulation 70:1038, 1984.

63. Packer M, Lee WH, Medina N, et al: Systemic vasoconstrictor effects of oxygen administration in obliterative pulmonary vascular disorders. Am J Cardiol 57:853, 1986.

64. Hyman AL, Higashida RT, Spannhake EVU, et al: Pulmonary vasoconstrictor responses to graded decreases in precapillary blood PO_2 in intact-chest cats. J Appl Physiol 51:1009, 1981.

65. Weir EK, Grover RF: The role of endogenous prostaglandins in the pulmonary circulation. Anesthesiology 48:201, 1978.

66. Said SI, Yoshida T, Kitamura S, et al: Pulmonary alveolar hypoxia: Release of prostaglandins and other humoral mediators. Science 185:1181, 1974.

67. Szczeklik J, Dubier JS, Mysik M, et al: Effects of prostaglandin E_1 on the pulmonary circulation in patients with pulmonary hypertension. Br Heart J 40:1397, 1978.

68. Halpern SM, Shah PK, Lehrman S, et al: Prostaglandin E_1 as a screening vasodilator in primary pulmonary hypertension. Chest 92:686, 1987.

69. Watkins WD, Peterson MB, Crone RK, et al: Prostacyclin and prostaglandin E_1 for severe idiopathic pulmonary artery hypertension. Lancet 1:1803, 1980.

70. Rubin LJ, Groves BM, Reeves JT, et al: Prostacyclin-induced pulmonary vasodilation in primary pulmonary hypertension. Circulation 66:334, 1982.

71. Jones DK, Higenbottam TW, Wallwork J: Treatment of primary pulmonary hypertension with intravenous epoprostenol (prostacyclin). Br Heart J 57:270, 1987.

72. Rubin LJ, Mendoza J, Hood M, et al: Treatment of primary pulmonary hypertension with continuous intravenous prostacyclin (epoprostenol). Ann Intern Med 112:485, 1990.

73. Rich S, Hart K, Kieras K, et al: Thromboxane synthetase inhibition in primary pulmonary hypertension. Chest 91:356, 1987.

74. Schrader BJ, Inbar S, Kaufmann E, et al: Comparison of the effects of adenosine and nifedipine in pulmonary hypertension. J Am Coll Cardiol 19:1060, 1992.

75. Inbar S, Schrader BJ, Kaufmann E, et al: The effects of adenosine in combination with calcium channel blockers in patients with primary pulmonary hypertension. J Am Coll Cardiol 21:413, 1993.

76. Pepke-Zaba J, Higenbottam W, Ding-Xuan T, et al: Inhaled nitric oxide as a cause of selective pulmonary vasodilation in pulmonary hypertension. Lancet 338:1173, 1991.

77. Roberts JD, Lang P, Bigatello LM, et al: Inhaled nitric oxide in congenital heart disease. Circulation 87:447, 1993.

78. Rossaint R, Falke KJ, Lopez F, et al: Inhaled nitric oxide for the adult respiratory distress syndrome. N Engl J Med 328:399, 1993.

79. Bishop JM: Hypoxia and pulmonary hypertension in chronic bronchitis. Prog Resp Res 9:10, 1975.

80. Nocturnal Oxygen Therapy Trial Group: Continuous or nocturnal oxygen therapy in hypoxemic chronic obstructive lung disease. Ann Intern Med 93:391, 1980.

81. Weitzenblum E, Sautegean A, Ehrhart M, et al: Long-term oxygen therapy can reverse the progression of pulmonary hypertension in patients with chronic obstructive pulmonary disease. Am Rev Respir Dis 131:493, 1985.

82. Ashutosh K, Dunsky M: Non-invasive tests for responsiveness of pulmonary hypertension to oxygen. Chest 92:393, 1987.

83. Kennedy T, Summer W: Inhibition of hypoxic pulmonary vasoconstriction by nifedipine. Am J Cardiol 50:864, 1982.

84. Rubin LJ, Peter RH: Hemodynamics at rest and during exercise after oral hydralazine in patients with cor pulmonale. Am J Cardiol 47:116, 1981.

85. Rubin LJ, Moser K: Long-term effects of nitrendipine on hemodynamics and oxygen transport in patients with cor pulmonale. Chest 89:141, 1986.

86. Sturani C, Bassein L, Schiavina M, et al: Oral nifedipine in chronic cor pulmonale secondary to severe chronic obstructive pulmonary disease. Chest 84:135, 1983.

87. Lupi-Herrera E, Seoane M, Verdejo J: Hemodynamic effect of hydralazine in advanced, stable chronic obstructive pulmonary disease with cor pulmonale. Chest 85:156, 1984.

88. Zielinski J, Hawrykiewicz I, Gorecka D, et al: Captopril effects on pulmonary and systemic hemodynamics in chronic cor pulmonale. Chest 90:562, 1986.

89. Morley TF, Zappasodi SJ, Belli A, et al: Pulmonary vasodilator therapy for chronic obstructive pulmonary disease and cor pulmonale. Chest 92:71, 1987.

90. Pines A, Kaplinsky N, Goldhammer E, et al: Corticosteroid responsive pulmonary hypertension in systemic lupus erythematosus. Clin Rheum 1:301, 1982.

91. Perez HD, Kramer N: Pulmonary hypertension in systemic lupus erythematosus: Report of four cases and review of the literature. Semin Arthritis Rheum 11:177, 1981.

92. Rozkovec A, Bernstein R, Asherson RA, et al: Vascular reactivity and pulmonary hypertension in systemic sclerosis. Arthritis Rheum 26:1037, 1983.

93. Niarchos AP, Whitman HH, Goldstein JE, et al: Hemodynamic effects of captopril in pulmonary hypertension of collagen vascular disease. Am Heart J 104:834, 1982.

94. Alpert MA, Pressly TA, Mukerji V, et al: Acute and long-term effects of nifedipine on pulmonary and systemic hemodynamics in patients with pulmonary hypertension associated with diffuse systemic sclerosis, the CREST syndrome and mixed connective tissue disease. Am J Cardiol 68:1687, 1991.

95. Nootens M, Kaufmann E, Rich S: The short term effectiveness of calcium channel blockers in secondary pulmonary hypertension. Am J Cardiol 71:1475, 1993.

96. Tryka AF, Godleski JJ, Schoen FJ, et al: Pulmonary vascular disease and hypertension after valve surgery for mitral stenosis. Hum Pathol 16:65, 1985.

97. Zener JC, Hancock EW, Shumway NE, et al: Regression of extreme pulmonary hypertension after mitral valve surgery. Am J Cardiol 30:820, 1972.

98. Otto CM, Davis KB, Reid CL, et al: Relation between pulmonary artery pressure and mitral stenosis severity in patients undergoing balloon mitral commissurotomy. Am J Cardiol 71:874, 1993.

99. Ribeiro PA, Al Zaibag M, Abdullah M: Pulmonary artery pressure and pulmonary vascular resistance before and after mitral balloon valvotomy in 100 patients with severe mitral valve stenosis. Am Heart J 125:1110, 1993.

100. Foltz BD, Hessel EA, Ivey TD: The early course of pulmonary artery hypertension in patients undergoing mitral valve replacement with cardioplegic arrest. J Thorac Cardiovasc Surg 88:238, 1984.

101. Halperin JL, Brooks KM, Rothlauf EB, et al: Effect of nitroglycerin on the pulmonary venous gradient in patients after mitral valve replacement. J Am Coll Cardiol 5:34, 1985.

102. D'Ambra MN, LaRaia PJ, Philbin DM, et al: Prostaglandin E_1: A new therapy for refractory right heart failure and pulmonary hypertension after mitral valve replacement. J Thorac Cardiovasc Surg 89:567, 1985.

103. Kim YD, Foegh ML, Wallace RB, et al: Effects of CGS-13080, a thromboxane inhibitor, on pulmonary vascular resistance in patients after mitral valve replacement surgery [abstract]. Circulation 76(Suppl 4):IV-389, 1987.

104. Hoffman JIE, Rudolph AM, Heymann MA: Pulmonary vascular disease with congenital heart lesions: Pathologic features and causes. Circulation 64:873, 1981.

105. Cherian G, Uthaman CB, Durairaj M, et al: Pulmonary hypertension in isolated secundum atrial septal defect: High frequency in young patients. Am Heart J 105:952, 1983.

106. Bush A, Busst CM, Shinebourne EA: The use of oxygen and prostacyclin as a pulmonary vasodilator in congenital heart disease. Int J Cardiol 9:267, 1985.

107. Braulin EA, Moller JH, Patton C, et al: Predictive value of lung biopsy in ventricular septal defect: Long-term follow-up. J Am Coll Cardiol 8:1113, 1986.

108. Burrows FA, Klinck JR, Rabinovitch M, et al: Pulmonary hypertension in children: Preoperative management. Can Anaesth Soc J 33:606, 1986.

109. Stephenson LW, Edmunds LH Jr, Raphaely R, et al: Effects of nitroprusside and dopamine on the pulmonary arterial vasculature in children after cardiac surgery. Circulation 60:104, 1979.

110. Rubin LJ, Stephenson LW, Johnston MR, et al: Comparison of

effects of prostaglandin E₁ and nitroprusside on pulmonary vascular resistance in children after open-heart surgery. Ann Thorac Surg 32:563, 1981.

111. Tripp RR, Gewitz MH, Werner JC, et al: Oral hydralazine in patients with pulmonary vascular disease secondary to congenital heart disease. Am J Cardiol 48:380, 1981.

112. Beckman RH, Rocchini AP, Rosenthal A: Hemodynamic effects of hydralazine in infants with a large ventricular septal defect. Circulation 65:523, 1982.

113. Escudero J, Navarro J, Padua A, et al: Hemodynamic changes with enalapril in pulmonary arterial hypertension secondary to congenital heart disease. Chest 91:351, 1987.

CHAPTER 13

Postural Hypotension
Initial Treatment and Combined Therapy

Michael G. Ziegler, M.D.

The maintenance of blood flow to the brain during upright posture is critical for survival. Nevertheless, a moment of lightheadedness on standing is not unusual. When one of the many mechanisms to maintain blood pressure fails, postural dizziness can become frequent and troublesome. The sympathetic nervous system integrates many of the responses that maintain blood pressure. When the sympathetic nerves fail, standing erect for any length of time may become impossible.

Postural hypotension has many causes. Successful therapy of hypotension depends on an accurate diagnosis. For example, circulatory failure from congestive heart failure is treated with salt restriction, whereas circulatory failure from hypovolemia is treated with salt. Clonidine raises blood pressure in severe autonomic insufficiency and lowers blood pressure in most other causes of postural hypotension. When the cause of a patient's hypotension is known, treatment follows logically. This chapter briefly reviews the physiology and pathology of blood pressure maintenance and discusses initial nonpharmacologic treatment and current drug therapy for postural hypotension.

BLOOD PRESSURE RESPONSE TO STANDING

When people stand up, diastolic blood pressure increases by a mean of 4 mmHg. The systolic pressure response to standing changes with age and falls in normal elderly persons. When diastolic blood pressure falls by more than 5 mmHg and postural dizziness occurs, a diagnosis of postural hypotension can be made. Maintenance of blood pressure on standing requires a complex physiologic response, because standing results in pooling of 300 to 800 ml blood in the legs. After standing for 10 minutes, there is a 10% hemoconcentration as fluid moves out of the blood vessels and into the interstitial spaces and causes swelling of the legs and feet. This "self-phlebotomy" reduces central blood volume and filling pressure to the heart. Pressure sensors in the aortic arch and

carotid bifurcation are especially sensitive to a change in arterial distention and initiate a neurogenic response in less than 0.2 second. Peripheral resistance increases and venoconstriction helps return blood to the heart. This rapid response to standing depends on several mechanisms (Fig. 13–1): (1) A neurogenic response begins at the baroreceptor. Diminished baroreceptor input to the brain stem stimulates spinal nerves that induce release of norepinephrine (NE) by the sympathetic nervous system. (2) Arterioles constrict in response to NE. (3) There is a positive cardiac inotropic and chronotropic response to NE stimulation and vagal withdrawal. (4) Constriction of capacitance vessels returns blood to the heart.

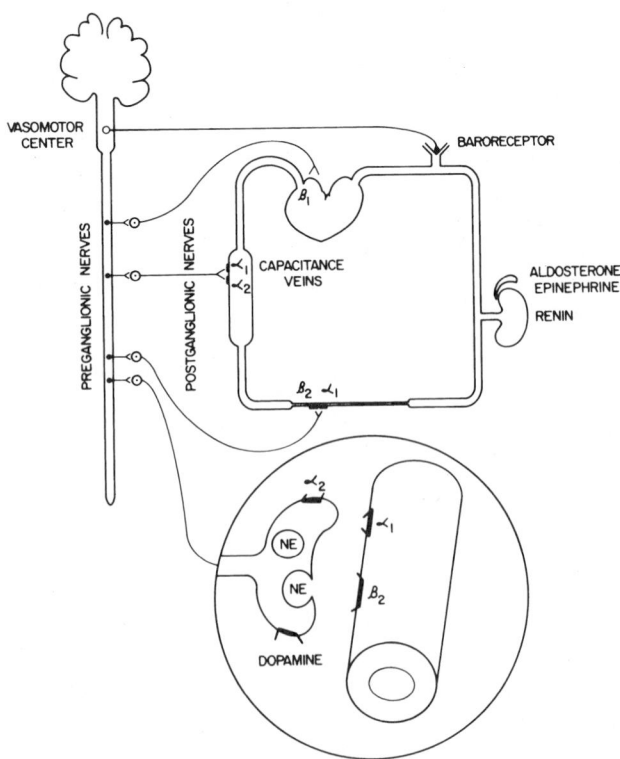

Figure 13–1. Diagrammatic representation of the neural control of blood pressure. For a detailed explanation, see the text.

In addition to this rapid response to standing, there are slower responses that maintain blood pressure. The kidney releases renin in response to low blood pressure and sympathetic nervous stimulation. Renin catalyzes angiotensin II formation, which vasoconstricts, enhances NE release from nerve endings, and releases aldosterone from the adrenal glands. Both aldosterone and sympathetic nervous stimulation of the kidney cause sodium retention.

The sympathetic nervous ending depicted in Figure 13–1 is a site of action for most drugs used to treat hypotension. The sympathetic nerves contain NE in vesicles that is released onto receptors in the blood vessels, heart, and kidneys. NE stimulates α_1- and α_2-receptors on arteries and veins to constrict these vessels. NE also stimulates β_1-receptors on the heart to increase cardiac output. Epinephrine stimulates β_2-receptors that dilate blood vessels, particularly in muscle vascular beds. The sympathetic nerve ending has presynaptic receptors that modulate the amount of NE released. The presynaptic α_2-receptors respond to NE and clonidine to diminish further NE release. Similarly, dopamine receptors inhibit NE release when stimulated by dopamine or bromocriptine. Most of the neurologic diseases that cause postural hypotension impair NE release. Both α- and β-receptors can become supersensitive when they are not stimulated by a normal amount of NE and may develop excessive responses to many adrenergic drugs in neurogenic postural hypotension.

CAUSES OF POSTURAL HYPOTENSION

Table 13–1 lists the most common causes of postural hypotension. Several diseases can cause transient hypotension with faintness or loss of consciousness. These causes must be distinguished from a seizure, which has a rapid onset and causes postictal confusion. Postural hypotension may lead to enough cerebral hypoxia to cause tonic-clonic movements, but these stop when the subject falls and blood pressure returns to normal.

The long list of diseases that cause postural hypotension may be greatly simplified by categorizing them into hypovolemic, vasodilated, and hypoadrenergic states. These physiologic categories also serve as a guide to therapy. For example, hypoadrenergic patients are unusually sensitive to pressor drugs, and hypovolemic patients respond well to mineralocorticoid drugs.

Hypovolemic States

In hypovolemic states, the heart receives inadequate blood volume. This occurs in dehydration or blood loss but also is seen commonly in patients with hypoalbuminemia from liver disease, kidney disease, or malnutrition. Vena caval thrombosis or venous blood pooling impairs blood flow to the heart. Patients with hypovolemia respond to upright posture with intense

Table 13–1. **Causes of Postural Hypotension**

Reduced Blood Supply to the Heart
Hypovolemia
  Decreased plasma volume
  Anemia
  Venous pooling
  Hemorrhage
  Adrenal insufficiency
  Vena caval obstruction
Valsalva maneuver
Cough
Atrial myxoma

Reduced Cardiac Output
Left heart
  Aortic stenosis
  Idiopathic hypertrophic subaortic stenosis
Right heart
  Pulmonary emboli
  Pulmonary stenosis
  Pulmonary tamponade
Heart failure
Arrhythmias

Vasodilation
Carcinoid
Mastocytosis
Heat
Acidosis

Neurogenic with Transient Hypotension
Vasovagal
Carotid sinus syncope
Micturition syncope
Glossopharyngeal neuralgia

Neurogenic with Persistent Hypotension
Autonomic neuropathies
  Diabetic
  Uremic
  Toxic
  Guillain-Barré syndrome
  Amyloidosis
  Idiopathic
Central nervous system defects
  Spinal (e.g., transsection, syringomyelia)
  Shy-Drager syndrome
  Degenerative disorders (e.g., parkinsonism, Huntington's chorea)
  Basilar artery disease

Drugs
Antidepressants (tricyclics, MAO inhibitors)
Diuretics
Nitrates
α-Blockers (prazosin, phenothiazines)
β-Blockers
Dopamine agonists (L-dopa, bromocriptine)
Sedatives

MAO, monoamine oxidase.

sympathetic nervous activity, tachycardia, and peripheral vasoconstriction with cool hands and feet.

Vasodilation

Vasodilation can cause postural dizziness. Pure arterial vasodilation, such as that caused by hydralazine or minoxidil, usually does not cause postural dizziness. When venodilation also is present, the combination of inadequate peripheral resistance with pooling of blood in the veins lowers blood pressure. Although the vasodilated patient has tachycardia, the extremities remain warm and pink.

Neurogenic Postural Hypotension

Neurogenic postural hypotension results from inadequate sympathetic nervous responses. These patients characteristically have recumbent hypertension and upright hypotension. Despite their low blood pressure when standing, they do not develop tachycardia or peripheral vasoconstriction. They have other abnormalities of autonomic nervous function such as incontinence, impotence, diminished sweating, and impaired pupillary constriction and dilation.

Neurogenic postural hypotension has many causes, but these can be divided into three groups, each of which has a different response to drug therapy.

Transection of the Upper Spinal Cord

Transection of the upper spinal cord leaves a quadriplegic patient with no brain input into the spinal sympathetic nerves. Pain or a full bladder may cause uncontrolled spinal reflexes and dangerous hypertension. Conversely, upright posture causes hypotension. Six weeks to 6 months after spinal injury, reflexes develop that diminish postural symptoms. A few quadriplegic patients sustain enough postural hypotension to make sitting in a wheelchair difficult, but treatment to raise the blood pressure in these patients must be tempered by the possibility that they may become severely hypertensive during episodes of autonomic dysreflexia.

Degenerative Central Nervous System Diseases

Degenerative diseases of the central nervous system (CNS) such as parkinsonism and Shy-Drager syndrome diminish central control of blood pressure and also impair spinal autonomic reflexes. These patients have CNS deficits other than those of blood pressure control. Their peripheral sympathetic nerves are intact, so they have normal basal blood levels of NE but fail to increase NE levels while standing. They have moderately increased sensitivity to NE infusions, with a pressor response to NE that is increased about fivefold.[1]

Degeneration of the Peripheral Autonomic Nerves

Many diseases, such as diabetes and uremia, cause degeneration of the peripheral autonomic nerves. Patients with fully developed peripheral autonomic neuropathy have low NE levels during rest or stress. They clear NE from their bloodstream more slowly than normal and develop a marked pressor response to NE and other α-agonists. Their lymphocytes have an increased number of β-receptors, and they develop tachycardia in response to one fifth of the dose of isoproterenol needed in normal subjects.[1] Clonidine stimulates their α_2-receptors on vascular smooth muscle and raises their blood pressure. Most patients with an autonomic neuropathy have partial degeneration of the sympathetic nerves. Basal levels of plasma NE are a bit low, and the NE response to standing is blunted. These patients have only a moderately enhanced response to β-agonists. They may develop severe postural hypotension during dehydration or fever but are asymptomatic when well. They rapidly develop symptoms of dizziness in response to α-blocking drugs or diuretics.

Drugs as a Cause of Postural Hypotension

Drugs are the most common cause of postural dizziness and fainting in the elderly.[2] Some patients have an exaggerated sensitivity to the hypotensive effects of drugs, which often indicates an underlying defect such as a mild autonomic neuropathy or volume depletion. For example, benzodiazepines, which usually do not alter blood pressure, may cause disabling postural hypotension and syncope in elderly or hypovolemic subjects.

Diuretics are one of the most common causes of postural hypotension. When combined with venodilating agents, such as nitrates or α-blockers, they can cause postural dizziness in anyone. The α-blocking drugs prazosin and labetalol cause marked venous pooling and postural hypotension after the first dose of the drug and less severe postural hypotension with subsequent doses. Many other drugs that have as their primary action blockade of dopamine, serotonin, histamine, or β-receptors also have some α-blocking activity. Chlorpromazine (Thorazine) exemplifies one drug commonly prescribed for its dopamine-blocking effects that has α-antagonist effects. When patients are first given this neuroleptic, they may stay in bed to avoid postural dizziness, and this behavior is sometimes explained as a sedative effect of the drug.

The dopamine agonist drugs L-dopa and bromocriptine relieve the motor disorders of parkinsonism and Shy-Drager syndrome, diseases that affect not only the basal ganglia but also the spinal autonomic tracts. The dopamine agonists cause hypotension by stimulating presynaptic dopamine receptors on sympathetic nerve terminals, where they inhibit NE release. The dopamine agonists usually worsen hypotension in these patients. The combination of L-dopa with carbidopa (Sinemet) causes less hypotension than bromocriptine, for two reasons. Carbidopa prevents most peripheral conversion of L-dopa to the vasodilator dopamine. Some dopamine is formed from L-dopa, however, and the body metabolizes dopamine to NE, which exerts a pressor effect.[3]

INITIAL NONPHARMACOLOGIC THERAPIES

Most pharmacologic therapies for postural hypotension raise recumbent blood pressure and increase the risk of cardiovascular disease. Nondrug therapies tend to be safer, and many are quite effective. In addition, pressor drugs are ineffective and dangerous in patients with low blood volume, because they may impair perfusion of the extremities and vital organs. Patients with autonomic insufficiency often have low blood volume.[4, 5] They develop supine hypertension and a diuresis during sleep. Hypovolemia can be minimized by elevating the head of the bed 5 to 20 degrees and by having patients rest during the day in a reclining chair rather than in bed.

The diet of most hypotensive patients should include extra salt. Many patients have their worst hypotension after meals, and this can be minimized by having small meals in the daytime and a large meal at night. Ethanol may lower blood pressure by direct vasodilation and histamine release, so it is best used at night. Caffeine has a pressor effect in these patients, and 240 mg of caffeine (two cups of fresh-brewed coffee) with breakfast can ameliorate the hypotensive effect of breakfast.[6] The patient should not consume caffeine late in the day to prevent the development of tolerance to its effects.

Support garments transfer blood from the legs and capacitance vessels to the heart. They are most useful in conjunction with a high-salt diet or fluid-retaining hormones such as fludrocortisone. Custom-fitted support garments such as Jobst stockings or antigravity suits work well if they also compress the abdomen to prevent pelvic pooling of blood. Fitted stockings alone are of small benefit, and support hose and antithromboembolism hose are of no benefit.

Heat is a potent dilator; therefore, some patients require drug therapy only in the summertime. Air conditioning should be prescribed for most patients with postural hypotension. Adequate nutrition is essential to maintain plasma albumin and blood volume. Weight loss has a diuretic effect and should be prescribed with caution.

DRUG THERAPY
Mineralocorticoids

Fludrocortisone (Florinef) is the most consistently useful drug in the treatment of postural hypotension. This mineralocorticoid increases vascular resistance and sensitizes blood vessels to NE[7] even at low doses (0.1 to 0.2 mg/day). This effect is detectable in normal subjects and is most marked in subjects with hyporeninemic hypoaldosteronism whose endogenous mineralocorticoid levels are low. It does not depend on sodium retention; its effects can be seen even in

anephric patients. Low-dose fludrocortisone therapy usually is safe and causes minimal side effects.

High doses of fludrocortisone (0.3 to 2 mg/day) do not have much more effect on vascular sensitivity to NE than do low doses, but high doses cause sodium retention, increased blood volume, and increased blood pressure in both supine and standing postures. High doses can also cause congestive heart failure, supine hypertension, and hypokalemia. The dose can be increased until it causes supine hypertension, pitting edema (1+), pulmonary congestion, or hypokalemia unresponsive to potassium supplementation. Some patients do not retain excess volume because they produce enough atrial natriuretic factor to escape the mineralocorticoid effects. After edema is present, support garments are particularly helpful in displacing fluid centrally.

Patients with the Shy-Drager syndrome have difficulty coughing up pulmonary secretions and are particularly likely to develop pulmonary congestion from fluid-retaining doses of fludrocortisone. Low doses of fludrocortisone usually are safe, whereas higher doses of the drug can be dangerous;[7] but high doses sometimes distinguish a patient confined to bed from one who is functional.

Prostaglandin Inhibition

The prostaglandins can mediate vasodilation and natriuresis. Indomethacin blocks the synthesis of prostaglandins and augments the release of NE after nerve stimulation. It can increase the excretion of NE in rats at rest or under stress and can increase vascular responses to NE.[8]

Kochar and Itskovitz[9] treated five patients with postural hypotension with indomethacin and noted an increase in blood pressure of 20 to 30 mmHg. Four of the patients had marked relief of symptoms, and one patient had a return of symptoms 48 hours after discontinuing the drug. Subsequent studies have shown clear benefit from the drug in patients with central autonomic deficits from the Shy-Drager syndrome[10-13] or with peripheral autonomic insufficiency.[10] The drug worked well in a patient with only a "patchy autonomic neuropathy"[14] and in patients with severe sympathetic nerve degeneration and low NE levels.[10] However, others have reported patients with the same diseases who failed to respond to indomethacin.[15-17] Even measurements of prostaglandin production have failed to identify which patients will respond.[10, 17]

I usually give patients with symptomatic postural hypotension a trial of a prostaglandin inhibitor to see if they will benefit. Patients are given 25 to 50 mg of indomethacin three times in 1 day, and blood pressure is measured frequently in recumbent and standing positions before and after administration of the drug. Patients who respond are given a trial of ibuprofen, because this drug often works as well as indomethacin but is less toxic. In some patients, postural hypotension is decreased; in others, bowel habits return to normal.[11] The development of recumbent hypertension is sometimes a limiting factor. A therapeutic trial of prostaglandin inhibitors is essential because a considerable fraction of patients simply fail to respond to them.

β-Blockers

Propranolol

Propranolol usually lowers blood pressure in hypertensive patients, but its effects are not uniform. It has little hypotensive effect in black patients. β-Blockers sometimes can cause a marked pressor response,[18] but this response is variable in patients with postural hypotension. Receptor sensitivity is not altered markedly in patients with parkinsonism or the Shy-Drager syndrome but is increased in patients with complete autonomic neuropathy.[1] Some patients with impaired autonomic responses develop pressor responses to propranolol; published reports suggest that this occurs in patients with supersensitive receptors. Brevetti et al.[19] and Chobanian et al.[20] reported that patients with low plasma or urinary catecholamine levels demonstrated increased blood pressure in response to propranolol. Conversely, patients with the Shy-Drager syndrome had normal NE levels while recumbent and had no blood pressure response to propranolol.[9] One group[21] suggests that hypotensive patients with low peripheral vascular resistance have a pressor response to propranolol, whereas those with low cardiac output do not.

I have not observed a satisfactory response to β-blockers in patients with postural hypotension. It has not been of symptomatic benefit nor has it increased standing blood pressure in patients with either central or peripheral autonomic failure. One patient with the Shy-Drager syndrome developed cardiorespiratory arrest after taking propranolol and required mechanical ventilation before recovering fully. The first dose of the drug should be given in the hospital to patients with postural hypotension, and the drug should not be given to patients with Shy-Drager syndrome.

β-Blockers with Intrinsic Sympathomimetic Activity

Acebutolol is a β_1-antagonist with mild intrinsic sympathomimetic activity (ISA), which means that it stimulates receptors slightly and blocks the stimulating effects of NE on β_1-receptors. It has not proved useful in patients with postural hypotension.[22] Pindolol blocks both β_1- and β_2-receptors and has more ISA than acebutolol. Xamoterol is a β_1-antagonist with even more ISA than pindolol. All these agents have been tried in the therapy of postural hypotension. The response to the ISA of these drugs depends on the sensitivity of β-receptors. Patients with parkinsonism and Shy-Drager syndrome have fairly normal β-receptor sensitivity and normal NE levels while recumbent. In contrast, patients with severe peripheral autonomic neuropathy have low resting NE levels and β-receptor sensitivity that is inversely propor-

tional to their NE levels.[4] They have brisk tachycardia in response to agents with high ISA.

Pindolol

An initial report of the successful use of pindolol for postural hypotension from diabetic autonomic neuropathy[23] was followed by other reports of successful use of the drug.[22, 24, 25] It increased both recumbent and standing blood pressure and heart rate in patients with autonomic neuropathies. However, in five patients with the Shy-Drager syndrome, pindolol was of no benefit and even precipitated congestive heart failure in two of the five.[26] Man in't Veld et al.[27] suggested that patients with CNS autonomic disease would not benefit from the drug, whereas those with peripheral neuropathies might. This suggestion was supported by the observation by Robson[28] that two of his patients with peripheral autonomic neuropathy benefited from pindolol, whereas a patient with parkinsonism had no change in postural hypotension while taking pindolol.

Xamoterol and Prenalterol

Xamoterol is a selective β_1-antagonist with a high degree of ISA. In three patients with postural hypotension, pindolol had a predominantly antagonistic effect, but xamoterol had a β-agonist effect and increased heart rate and blood pressure.[29] Prenalterol is a β-blocker with high β_1-agonist activity that increased both standing heart rate and blood pressure in a patient with Shy-Drager syndrome.[30] However, tolerance may develop eventually to prenalterol, as supersensitive β-receptors return to a normal level of sensitivity.[31]

In summary, it appears that β-blocking drugs with ISA may raise standing blood pressure in patients with supersensitive β-receptors. Patients with CNS disease of the autonomic nervous system usually respond poorly unless the agent used has high ISA, and these patients are prone to develop adverse side effects from the drugs. Drugs with high ISA can cause downregulation of the β-receptor with prolonged use[31] and may precipitate cardiac arrhythmias.[30] Drugs with low ISA may precipitate heart failure.[32] Nevertheless, these drugs may be useful, particularly in patients with severe peripheral autonomic neuropathies. They should be started in low dosage with close observation of the patient. Giving the drug once daily in the morning may delay the onset of tolerance.

Clonidine and Yohimbine

Norepinephrine stimulates both α_1- and α_2-adrenergic receptors. The α_2-receptor is the predominant α-receptor in the brain and on peripheral adrenergic nerve endings. Stimulation of the α_2-receptor in both locations inhibits neuronal release of NE. Some α_2-receptors on the vasculature cause vasoconstriction, but most vascular α-receptors are of the α_1 type. Clonidine stimulates and yohimbine blocks α_2-receptors.

In normal subjects, clonidine inhibits NE release. In patients with severe peripheral autonomic neuropathies, the sympathetic neuronal stores of NE have been destroyed. In this case, clonidine cannot inhibit NE release, and it acts to raise blood pressure through stimulation of vascular α_2-receptors. The pressor effect of clonidine is inversely proportional to plasma NE levels.[33] In these patients, clonidine still has a central sedating effect, and this limits its usefulness in treating postural hypotension.[4] Few patients with postural hypotension have sufficiently severe peripheral autonomic neuropathies to obtain a pressor response from clonidine; in most, blood pressure is lowered.

Yohimbine, in contrast, requires the presence of some sympathetic nerves to raise blood pressure. It activates the sympathetic nervous system by both central and peripheral blockade of α_2-receptors. The drug raises both blood pressure and heart rate proportionate to the increase in plasma NE it causes.[34] It has side effects of nausea, tremor, and nervousness but has proved useful in some patients.[34]

α_1-Adrenergic Agonists

The α_1-adrenergic receptor causes vasoconstriction and raises blood pressure. Many drug regimens stimulate this receptor either directly or indirectly. Patients with postural hypotension from autonomic insufficiency show varying degrees of supersensitivity to these agonists, ranging from a small increase in pressor responsiveness in parkinsonism to such enhanced sensitivity in patients with autonomic neuropathy and low NE levels that phenylephrine eye drops can cause a dramatic increase in blood pressure.[35] All these agents are capable of causing recumbent hypertension and tend to raise blood pressure more when subjects lie down than when they stand. These agents may raise blood pressure more than they relieve symptoms of postural dizziness if they constrict cerebral arteries. Patients with peripheral denervation should be warned about nasal sprays, eye drops, diet pills, and cold capsules available over the counter, which may give them dangerous hypertension even at recommended doses. Therapeutic use of these medicines to raise standing blood pressure requires caution. Medication should be taken early in the day, and patients should be warned not to lie down while the drug is effective. Blood pressure should be monitored frequently. These drugs may cause dangerous recumbent hypertension without relief of postural dizziness,[32] so it is not always safe to increase the dosage until symptoms abate.

Phenylpropanolamine and phenylephrine directly stimulate α_1-receptors. Phenylpropanolamine has a pressor effect for 1 to 3 hours.[4] Phenylephrine nasal sprays have even more short-lived action but may be useful before activities the patient finds particularly likely to cause postural dizziness.[4] Midodrine is an investigational α-agonist with a longer duration of action that has been used in patients with central and peripheral autonomic failure.[36]

Tyramine, ephedrine, amphetamine, and methylphenidate indirectly stimulate α_1-receptors by enhancing NE release. They also have some direct adrenergic agonist activity. Both tyramine and NE are metabolized by monoamine oxidase, so tyramine must be given with an inhibitor of monoamine oxidase to have much pressor effect. Although this regimen has had its advocates,[37, 38] it is difficult to control drug doses safely.[32]

Patients with parkinsonism or the Shy-Drager syndrome have a movement disorder that responds to dopamine agonists. Unfortunately, both bromocriptine and L-dopa can worsen postural hypotension. Amphetamine and methylphenidate act to release both NE and dopamine. These drugs also have a short-term beneficial effect on the depression seen in most Shy-Drager patients. The pressor effect of these drugs is mild, but the effect on a Shy-Drager patient's mobility is sometimes major because dopamine release improves the movement disorder and NE release improves blood pressure. Tolerance develops to the effects of amphetamine-like drugs, so they should be given only early in the day, in the smallest useful dose, to forestall development of drug tolerance.

Polinsky et al.[39] have developed a prototype pump to infuse NE at a rate of infusion controlled by the patient's arterial blood pressure. This technique maintained a consistent blood pressure in all postures. Attempts are under way to develop a portable device for infusion of a pressor agent.

Caffeine

A cup of fresh-brewed coffee contains 120 mg of caffeine; a cup of instant coffee or strong tea contains about half that amount. When people who ordinarily consume no caffeine are given 240 mg of the drug, plasma NE, renin, and blood pressure increase. Regular coffee drinkers, however, have no NE or blood pressure response. A pressor response is caused by 240 mg of caffeine in patients with either central or peripheral autonomic nerve failure. When administered as coffee, it is a particularly appropriate drug to prevent the postural hypotension that can follow meals in patients with autonomic insufficiency.

Normal subjects develop tolerance to the pressor effects of caffeine. Patients with autonomic failure still benefit from the drug after 240 mg each morning for 1 week.[6] It seems wise to recommend caffeine consumption only early in the day in hypotensive patients to delay the onset of tolerance to the drug.

Ergot Alkaloids

Dihydroergotamine constricts capacitance blood vessels, so it may help prevent venous pooling on standing. When given parenterally to patients with postural hypotension, dihydroergotamine increases standing blood pressure, and less than 1 mg given intravenously has a marked pressor effect, which is increased in patients receiving fludrocortisone.[40] However, the drug is poorly bioavailable, so at least

20 mg of oral dihydroergotamine is needed to obtain a pressor effect.[40, 41] Severely denervated patients may be supersensitive to the drug.[42] Its effect is enhanced by caffeine.[43]

The poor bioavailability of dihydroergotamine is a drawback to its use, but ergotamine tartrate is reported to be effective in an oral dose of 2 to 4 mg daily.[44] The ergot alkaloids may cause recumbent hypertension.[42] They may cause severe vasospasm with chronic use in patients with hypovolemia; it is not known whether they do so in patients with autonomic insufficiency.

Somatostatin and Octreotide

Intravenous somatostatin has a short half-life, but the analogue octreotide has a longer effect when given subcutaneously. The drug can raise standing blood pressure in patients with autonomic neuropathy.[45] Octreotide also inhibits insulin secretion and may cause stomach cramps; it must be given parenterally, which is not practical for most patients with postural hypotension. However, in patients with severe diabetic autonomic neuropathies, it may help normalize gastrointestinal motility and may be given with insulin. In one patient with diabetic diarrhea, the drug helped prevent fluid loss in the stool and enhanced NE release, and both of these effects diminished postural hypotension.[46]

SUMMARY

Postural hypotension may be caused by many different diseases, and optimal therapy of hypotension varies according to its cause. Peripheral autonomic neuropathy is a common cause of postural hypotension in patients with diabetes or uremia. Patients with severe neuropathy respond differently to drugs than patients with mild neuropathy.

Most drugs used to treat postural hypotension are toxic and may cause recumbent hypertension, so nondrug therapies should be tried first. When drugs are required, low-dose fludrocortisone, caffeine, and prostaglandin synthetase inhibitors have the best ratio of benefit to toxic effect for many patients, but even these agents do not work for every patient and should be given a clinical trial. Other agents such as β-blockers and α-agonists occasionally are useful but may have dangerous side effects. Some drugs, such as amphetamines and octreotide, are useful in specific diseases associated with postural hypotension. No uniformly successful therapeutic regimen exists for postural hypotension, but some therapies work in individual patients or for specific diseases that cause hypotension.

REFERENCES

1. Ziegler MG, Lake CR: Autonomic degeneration and altered blood pressure control in humans. Fed Proc 43:62, 1984.
2. Ziegler MG: Syncope and orthostatic hypotension: Syncope and faintness in the elderly. In Messerli FH (ed): Cardiovascular Disease in the Elderly. Boston: Martinus Nijhoff, 1984, pp 109–125.
3. Ziegler MG, Kennedy B, Holland OB, et al: The effects of dopamine agonists on human cardiovascular and sympathetic nervous systems. Int J Clin Pharmacol Ther 23:175, 1985.
4. Onrot J, Goldberg MR, Hollister AS, et al: Management of chronic orthostatic hypotension. Am J Med 80:454, 1986.
5. Shannon RP, Wei JY, Rosa RM, et al: The effect of age and sodium depletion on cardiovascular response to orthostasis. Hypertension 8:438, 1986.
6. Onrot J, Goldberg MR, Biaggioni I, et al: Hemodynamic and humoral effects of caffeine in autonomic failure. N Engl J Med 313:549, 1985.
7. Schatz IJ, Miller MJ, Frame B: Corticosteroids in the management of orthostatic hypotension. Cardiology 61:280, 1976.
8. Ziegler MG, Lake CR: Noradrenergic responses to postural hypotension: Implications for therapy. In Lake CR, Ziegler MG (eds): The Catecholamines in Psychiatric and Neurologic Disorders. Woburn, MA: Butterworth, 1984, pp 121–136.
9. Kochar MS, Itskovitz HD: Treatment of idiopathic orthostatic hypotension (Shy-Drager syndrome) with indomethacin. Lancet 5:1011, 1978.
10. Goldberg MR, Robertson D, FitzGerald GA: Prostacyclin biosynthesis and platelet function in autonomic dysfunction. Neurology 35:120, 1985.
11. Schlup P, Scheidegger K, Straub PW: Erfolgreiche Indomethacin-Behandlung schwere Durchfalle bei primarer orthostatischer Hypotonie. Schweiz Med Wochenschr 110:1020, 1980.
12. Tsuda Y, Kimura K, Yoneda S, et al: Hemodynamics in Shy-Drager and treatment with indomethacin. Eur Neurol 22:421, 1983.
13. Imaizumi T, Takeshita A, Ashihara T, et al: Increase in reflex vasoconstriction with indomethacin in patients with orthostatic hypotension and central nervous system involvement. Br Heart J 52:581, 1984.
14. Perkins CM, Lee MR: Flurbiprofen and fludrocortisone in severe autonomic neuropathy. Lancet 2:1058, 1978.
15. Bannister R, Davies B, Sever P: Indomethacin for Shy-Drager syndrome. Lancet 1:1312, 1978.
16. Hui KK, Conolly ME: Increased numbers of beta receptors in orthostatic hypotension due to autonomic dysfunction. N Engl J Med 304:1473, 1981.
17. Crook JE, Robertson D, Whorton AR: Prostaglandin suppression: Inability to correct severe idiopathic orthostatic hypotension. South Med J 73:318, 1981.
18. Ziegler MG, Woodsen LC: Pressor response to beta-blocking drugs. Clin Ther 7:81, 1984.
19. Brevetti G, Chiariello M, Lavecchia G, et al: Effects of propranolol in a case of orthostatic hypotension. Br Heart J 41:245, 1979.
20. Chobanian AV, Volicer L, Liang CS, et al: Use of propranolol in the treatment of idiopathic orthostatic hypotension. Trans Assoc Am Physicians 90:324, 1977.
21. Chiariello M, Brevetti G, Bonaduce D, et al: Orthostatic hypotension due to autonomic dysfunction—Different therapeutic effects of propranolol. Int J Cardiol 4:455, 1983.
22. Cleophas TJ, Kauw FH, Bijl C, et al: Effects of beta adrenergic receptor agonists and antagonists in diabetics with symptoms of postural hypotension: A double-blind, placebo-controlled study. Angiology 37:855, 1986.
23. Frewin DB, Leonello PP, Peuhall RK, et al: Pindolol in orthostatic hypotension: Possible therapy? Med J Aust 1:28, 1980.
24. Boesen F, Andersen EB, Kanstrup IL, et al: Treatment of diabetic orthostatic hypotension with pindolol. Acta Neurol Scand 66:386, 1982.
25. Man in't Veld AJ, Schalekamp MADH: Pindolol in postural hypotension. Lancet 2:1279, 1981.
26. Davies B, Bannister R, Mathias C, et al: Pindolol in postural hypotension: The case for caution. Lancet 2:982, 1981.
27. Man in't Veld AJ, Boomsma F, Moleman P, et al: Congenital dopamine-beta-hydroxylase deficiency. Lancet 1:183, 1987.
28. Robson D: Pindolol in postural hypotension. Lancet 2:1280, 1981.
29. Mahlsen J, Trap-Jensen J: Xamoterol, a new selective beta-1-

adrenoceptor partial agonist, in the treatment of postural hypotension. Acta Med Scand 219:173, 1986.

30. Goovaerts J, Verfaillie C, Fagard R, et al: Effect of prenalterol on orthostatic hypotension in the Shy-Drager syndrome. Br Med J 288:817, 1984.

31. Andersen EB, Lindskov HO, Marving J, et al: Decrease in beta-receptor density explaining the development of pindolol and prenalterol tolerance in orthostatic hypotension. Dan Med Bull 32:194, 1985.

32. Davies B, Bannister R, Sever P: Pressor amines and mono-amine-oxidase inhibitors for treatment of postural hypotension in autonomic failure: Limitations and hazards. Lancet 1:172, 1978.

33. Robertson D, Goldberg MR, Tung CS, et al: Use of alpha-2 adrenoceptor agonists and antagonists in the functional assessment of the sympathetic nervous system. J Clin Invest 78:576, 1986.

34. Onrot J, Goldberg MR, Biaggioni I, et al: Oral yohimbine in human autonomic failure. Neurology 37:215, 1987.

35. Robertson D: Contraindication to the use of ocular phenylephrine in idiopathic orthostatic hypotension. Am J Ophthalmol 87:819, 1979.

36. Schirger A, Sheps SG, Thomas JE, Fealey RD: Midodrine—A new agent in the management of idiopathic orthostatic hypotension and Shy-Drager syndrome. Mayo Clin Proc 56:429, 1981.

37. Nanda RN, Johnson RH, Keogh HJ: Treatment of neurogenic

orthostatic hypotension with a monoamine oxidase inhibitor and tyramine. Lancet 2:1164, 1976.

38. Mahar LJ, Frewin DB, Dunn DE: Idiopathic orthostatic hypotension controlled with monoamine oxidase inhibitor and 9-alpha-fluorohydrocortisone. Med J Aust 2:940, 1975.

39. Polinsky RJ, Samaras GM, Kopin IJ: Sympathetic neural prosthesis for managing orthostatic hypotension. Lancet 1:901, 1983.

40. Jennings G, Esler M, Holmes R: Treatment of orthostatic hypotension with dihydroergotamine. Br Med J 2:307, 1979.

41. Fouad FM, Tarazi RC, Bravo EL: Dihydroergotamine in idiopathic orthostatic hypotension: Short-term intramuscular and long-term oral therapy. Clin Pharmacol Ther 30:782, 1981.

42. Bellamy GR, Hunyor SN: The effect of dihydroergotamine on venous distensibility and blood pressure in idiopathic orthostatic hypotension. Aust N Z J Med 14:157, 1984.

43. Hoeldtke RD, Cavanaugh ST, Hughes JD, et al: Treatment of orthostatic hypotension with dihydroergotamine and caffeine. Ann Intern Med 105:168, 1986.

44. Chobanian AV, Tift CP, Faxon DP, et al: Treatment of chronic orthostatic hypotension with ergotamine. Circulation 63:602, 1983.

45. Hoeldtke RD, O'Dorisio TM, Boden G: Treatment of autonomic neuropathy with a somatostatin analogue SMS-201–995. Lancet 2:602, 1986.

46. Dudl RJ, Anderson DS, Ziegler MG, et al: Treatment of diabetic diarrhea and orthostatic hypotension with somatostatin analog SMS-201–995. Am J Med 83:584, 1987.

CHAPTER 14

Combination Therapy in Vaso-occlusive Disease

Thomas G. DiSalvo, M.D., Valentin Fuster, M.D., Ph.D.,
Douglas H. Israel, M.D., Bernardo Stein, M.D., F.A.C.C.,
and James H. Chesebro, M.D.

In the past 20 years, great strides in basic cardiac biochemistry and physiology have made possible unprecedented advances in cardiovascular pharmacology. At present, combination therapy with two or three drugs is common in the treatment of angina pectoris, cardiac failure, hypertension, and arrhythmias. This chapter explores the rational basis for combination antithrombotic drug therapy in vaso-occlusive disease.

COMBINATION ANTICOAGULANT AND PLATELET INHIBITOR THERAPY
Theoretical Considerations

It would appear that pathologic situations in which both platelet and coagulation cascade activation have pathogenetic importance might be optimally treated or prevented by combination therapy with anticoagulant agents and platelet inhibitors. The use of such combined therapy has been investigated in diverse cardiovascular conditions, including prosthetic valve replacement, unstable angina, myocardial infarction, coronary artery bypass grafting, and percutaneous transluminal coronary angioplasty (PTCA). After a brief review of the antithrombotic mechanisms of ac-

tion and specific platelet effects of the currently available anticoagulant agents (Table 14–1), the present role of combined anticoagulant and antiplatelet therapy and current therapeutic recommendations are presented. Mechanisms of action of currently available antiplatelet agents are briefly reviewed in the next section on therapy with combined platelet inhibitors.

Unfractionated and Fractionated (Low-Molecular-Weight) Heparin

Standard unfractionated heparin greatly accelerates the formation of antithrombin III–coagulation system

Table 14–1. **Anticoagulant Agents Under Investigation, 1994**

Standard unfractionated heparin
Fractionated (low-molecular-weight) heparin
Warfarin
Selective thrombin inhibitors
Hirudin
Hirulog
Argatroban
PPACK
MD-805
Recombinant activated protein C
Activated factor X inhibitors

serine protease complexes, thereby leading to enhanced antithrombin III–mediated inactivation of thrombin; factors XIIa, XIa, IXa, and Xa; plasmin; and kallikrein.[1] Acceleration of the inhibitory effects of antithrombin III on thrombin and factor Xa is of the greatest importance.[2] Side effects include bleeding, thrombocytopenia (on occasion associated with paradoxic thrombosis), osteoporosis, skin necrosis, alopecia, hypersensitivity reactions, and hypoaldosteronism.[1] Nomograms for dosing have been published: measurement of anticoagulant effect by protamine titration assay avoids the vagaries of different activated partial thromboplastin time reagents.[3]

Recently fractionated low-molecular-weight heparin (LMW heparin) has been widely employed in clinical studies.[4] LMW heparin is composed of heparin fractions of varying molecular weights (3000 to 9000, compared with 12,000 to 15,000 for standard unfractionated heparin). LMW heparin is prepared by partial hydrolysis of standard unfractionated heparin and subsequent isolation by gel filtration or solvent extraction. In clinical trials, LMW heparin appears as efficacious as standard heparin and possesses distinct advantages over unfractionated heparin, including (1) longer active half-life with once-a-day dosing (as a result of decreased binding to endothelial cells), (2) lower incidence of bleeding, (3) fewer platelet-associated side effects, and (4) greater bioavailability.[4] LMW heparin may be particularly useful in instances of standard heparin-induced thrombocytopenia.

Although heparin limits the effects of thrombin on fibrin synthesis and platelet activation, the direct effects of heparin on platelets are variable.[5] Heparin prevents thrombin-induced platelet aggregation *in vitro* but may potentiate aggregation induced by other agonists.[5, 6] Although the presence of prostacyclin (PGI$_2$) enhances the anticoagulant efficacy of heparin,[7] heparin has been shown to inhibit the activation of adenyl cyclase by PGI$_2$[8] and actually induces platelet aggregation in citrated platelet-rich plasma.[5] Thus, the net effect of heparin on platelets is unpredictable, with some of this variability attributable to the molecular heterogeneity of currently available heparin preparations.[9, 10] LMW heparin, unlike standard heparin, does not appear to increase platelet aggregation. In some cases, more than 60% of a standard unfractionated heparin preparation is inactive, with components of high molecular weight being less effective in activating antithrombin III and more likely to induce platelet activation.[5]

Warfarin

Warfarin inhibits vitamin K epoxide reductase and vitamin K reductase, enzymes that allow for the interconversion of vitamin KH2 to vitamin K epoxide.[11] Vitamin KH2 is an essential cofactor for vitamin K–dependent carboxylase, the enzyme responsible for the gamma-carboxylation and subsequent activation of inactive vitamin K–dependent coagulation factors II, VII, IX, and X. Warfarin has no significant direct platelet effects, but affects platelet function indirectly via its effects on thrombin.[11, 12] Side effects include bleeding and skin necrosis; this drug is contraindicated in pregnancy.[11, 12] The importance of standardization of warfarin therapy by reliance on the international normalized ratio (INR), which corrects for various thromboplastin reagents, has been emphasized.[11, 12]

Selective Antithrombins

Hirudin, a 65-amino-acid polypeptide, is the most potent selective thrombin inhibitor known.[13–18] Hirudin exhibits rapid, high-affinity binding to both thrombin's serine protease catalytic site and fibrinbinding exosite and thus blocks essentially all of thrombin's proteolytic enzymatic activity in addition to fibrin binding. Hirudin (and its recombinant analogue Hirulog) has several distinct advantages as an antithrombotic agent compared with heparin: (1) the compact molecular size of hirudin permits it to penetrate into channels within thrombi and bind and inhibit fibrin-bound thrombin that is inaccessible to the larger heparin–antithrombin III complex; (2) hirudin has no natural inhibitors, unlike heparin (which is inhibited by platelet factor-4, histidine-rich glycoprotein, or vitronectin); (3) hirudin has no direct effects on platelets or endothelial cells, unlike heparin; and (4) inactivation of thrombin by hirudin does not require a cofactor, unlike heparin (which requires antithrombin III).

In particular, inhibition of fibrin-bound thrombin is a distinct advantage of selective thrombin inhibitors compared with heparin and may confer on hirudin a distinct advantage compared with heparin in preventing arterial thrombosis.[13] Hirulog (a 20-amino-acid synthetic peptide) is more potent than hirudin in inhibiting fibrin-bound thrombin. Argatroban, another such inhibitor, has entered clinical trials.[19, 20] Bleeding complications from hirudin appear to be less common than with heparin. Intravenous and subcutaneous administration of hirudin yield predictable plasma concentrations and anticoagulant effects.[17, 18] At present, hirudin is under intense investigation in the therapy of unstable angina, as conjunctive therapy with thrombolytic agents, as preventive therapy after angioplasty or coronary artery bypass grafting, and in prevention and treatment of venous thromboembolism. Hirudin may be particularly efficacious in patients with partial or complete antithrombin III deficiency states.

COMBINATION PLATELET INHIBITOR THERAPY
Theoretical Considerations

Platelet aggregation in arterial thrombosis occurs via activation of all major platelet-activating pathways, including thrombin, collagen, adenosine diphosphate (ADP), and thromboxane A$_2$ (TXA$_2$)–dependent mechanisms.[21] Aspirin does not block all pathways of platelet activation.[22] Platelet activation and aggregation are inhibited by aspirin largely to the extent that the TXA_2-dependent mechanism is operative (although aspirin may have platelet-inhibiting effects by other than interference with TXA_2-dependent mechanisms). For example, aspirin does not inhibit platelet adhesion in single or double layers to injured endothelium or exposed subendothelium at physiologic blood flow rates, inhibit platelet secretion and activation by ADP and serotonin released from platelet alpha granules, or inhibit platelet aggregation in platelet-rich plasma to which moderate doses of thrombin or collagen have been added.[21–23] Thus, despite the unequivocal evidence of aspirin's beneficial effects in unstable angina, myocardial infarction, angioplasty, coronary artery bypass grafting, and cerebrovascular disease, in many clinical situations aspirin's antithrombotic effect may be overwhelmed by strong extrinsic stimuli to thrombosis.[22]

To increase the efficacy of antiplatelet therapy, either use of a combination of antiplatelet agents that inhibit different pathways of platelet activation by different mechanisms and sites of action or synergistic effects, or development of agents that inhibit a final common pathway of platelet activation thereby providing platelet inhibition via multiple pathways is a logical approach.[23] The mechanism of action of drugs that inhibit platelet function may be divided into four broad categories: (1) drugs that inhibit the arachidonate pathway, (2) drugs that directly increase platelet cyclic adenosine monophosphate (cAMP), (3) drugs that inhibit thrombin-induced platelet activation and aggregation, and (4) drugs that inhibit platelets through other mechanisms (Table 14–2).

Table 14–2. Antiplatelet Agents

Drugs that affect arachidonate metabolism
  Cyclooxygenase inhibitors
    Aspirin, NSAIDs
  Platelet membrane phospholipid inhibitors
    Omega-3 fatty acids
  Phospholipase A_2 inhibitors
    Quinacrine, some NSAIDs
  Thromboxane synthetase inhibitors
  TXA_2 PGH_2 receptor antagonists
    Sulotroban, ridogrel

Drugs that increase platelet cAMP
  Dipyridamole, PEG_1, PGI_2, iloprost

Drugs that inhibit thrombin
  Heparin
  Selective thrombin inhibitors
    Hirudin
    Hirulog
    Argatroban
    PPACK
Activated protein C

Drugs with other mechanisms
  Ticlopidine, clopidogrel
  Sulfinpyrazone
  Dextran
  Serotonin antagonists
    Ketanserin
  Anti–GP IIb-IIIa antibodies
    7E3
    RGD polypeptides

Drugs that Inhibit the Arachidonate Pathway

Drugs that inhibit the arachidonate pathway may be divided into the following five categories: (1) inhibitors of cyclooxygenase (aspirin and the nonsteroidal antiinflammatory drugs), (2) agents that affect platelet membrane phospholipids (omega-3 fatty acids), (3) inhibitors of phospholipase A_2 activation, (4) inhibitors of thromboxane synthetase, and (5) TXA_2 and prostaglandin H_2 (PGH_2) receptor antagonists. Agents in only the first two categories have been subjected to extensive clinical trials.

Inhibitors of Cyclooxygenase

Aspirin irreversibly acetylates the serine residue at the active site of the enzyme cyclooxygenase, thereby irreversibly inhibiting the enzymatic activity of cyclooxygenase.[22] Cyclooxygenase is found in both platelets and endothelial cells. In platelets, cyclooxygenase converts arachidonate released from platelet membrane phospholipids into TXA_2. TXA_2 stimulates platelet aggregation and vasoconstriction. In vascular endothelial cells, cyclooxygenase converts arachidonate released from endothelial membrane phospholipid into prostacyclin. Opposite in effect to TXA_2, prostacyclin inhibits platelet aggregation and promotes vasodilation. Because platelets are unable to synthesize cyclooxygenase, aspirin irreversibly inhibits cyclooxygenase and TXA_2 production for the lifetime of platelets (approximately 10 days). Endothelial cells, however, are able to resynthesize cyclooxygenase so that the effects of aspirin on endothelial cyclooxygenase activity and prostacyclin production are transitory and do not last for the entire lifetime of endothelial cells.[22]

Earlier studies suggested that low-dose aspirin preferentially inhibited platelet TXA_2 production but not endothelial cell prostacyclin production.[21, 23] This is not the case, however, because even very low doses of aspirin (35 mg/day) have been shown to inhibit both platelet TXA_2 and endothelial protacyclin synthesis.[22] Current trials of controlled-release low-dose aspirin are under way to find an aspirin preparation that will selectively inhibit platelet cyclooxygenase but not endothelial cyclooxygenase. Controlled-release low-dose preparations may be promising in this regard because (1) the continuous absorption of a controlled-release preparation may preferentially provide inhibition of platelets within the portal circulation, and (2) the low-dose preparation prevents aspirin release from the portal into the systemic circulation.[22] The use of aspirin in diverse clinical cardiovascular conditions is discussed in Chapter 152.

Omega-3 Fatty Acids

Omega-3 fatty acids (eicosapentaenoic and docosahexaenoic acids) decrease platelet aggregation responses after incorporation into platelet membranes.[23, 24] These antiaggregatory effects require several weeks to develop during long-term oral administration. In platelets, eicosapentaenoic acid competes with arachidonate for cyclooxygenase and results in the formation of endoperoxidases (TXA_3) with markedly less platelet aggregatory effects than TXA_2. In endothelial cells, eicosapentaenoic acid does not inhibit prostacyclin (PGI_2) production and also promotes production of PGI_3, which has antiplatelet and vasodilatory effects similar to prostacyclin. In animal models of restenosis after angioplasty, omega-3 fatty acids have been shown to decrease intimal hyperplasia (possibly via decreased endothelial platelet-derived growth factor production); however, several clinical trials of omega-3 fatty acids in the prevention of restenosis after angioplasty have yielded conflicting results.[25] Omega-3 fatty acids have diverse other effects, including prolongation of the bleeding time, reduction of low-density lipoprotein (LDL) cholesterol, elevation of high-density lipoprotein (HDL) cholesterol, decrease in blood viscosity, increase in erythrocyte deformability, and alteration of neutrophil and monocyte function.[24] Through these diverse mechanisms and effects, omega-3 fatty acids may promote a relative antiaggregatory and vasodilatative state. Whether or not significant antithrombotic and antiatherogenic benefits accrue will be determined in the many current trials of omega-3 fatty acids under way in diverse cardiovascular conditions.

Nonsteroidal antiinflammatory agents reversibly inhibit cyclooxygenase and have less prominent antiplatelet effects than aspirin. Although ibuprofen decreases mural thrombosis in experimental deep arterial injury, long-term indomethacin therapy has been reported to worsen myocardial ischemia in patients with known coronary disease.[23]

Phospholipase A_2 Inhibitors

Drugs that block the activation of phospholipase A_2 include the antimalarial quinacrine hydrochloride and some of the nonsteroidal antiinflammatory drugs. These agents do not have clinically important antithrombotic effects in human subjects.[26]

Thromboxane Synthetase Inhibitors

Thromboxane synthetase inhibitors with imidazole-containing structures have been developed in the hope of inhibiting TXA_2 synthesis and concomitantly preventing the suppression of PGI_2 synthesis or actually increasing its production by shunting the platelet intermediates PGG_2 and PGH_2 into prostacyclin synthesis.[27] These agents are currently being evaluated in clinical trials.[23] It appears that, on the whole, thrombin synthetase inhibitors exert a relatively weaker platelet inhibitory effect than aspirin, probably as a result of incomplete inhibition of TXA_2 synthesis as well as proaggregatory effects of PGG_2 and PGH_2 at the TXA_2 receptor level. PGH_2, which accumulates during thromboxane synthetase inhibition, interacts with platelet membrane endoperoxide receptors and activates platelets.

TXA_2 and PGH_2 Receptor Antagonists

Agents that block TXA_2 and PGH_2 receptors have been developed to circumvent the problem of proaggregatory PGG_2 and PGH_2 binding to the TXA_2 receptor.[28] These agents have been shown to inhibit the aggregation of human platelets *in vitro* while mildly prolonging the bleeding time,[29] but they do not increase PGI_2 synthesis. One such compound, sulotroban, has been reported to decrease the incidence of early occlusion of a saphenous vein coronary artery bypass graft from 11.5% to 3.1% in a small trial.[23] Another compound reduced platelet deposition on Dacron grafts in patients undergoing peripheral vascular surgery. Further clinical testing is ongoing. Combined thromboxane synthetase inhibitors and receptor blockers have also been developed. Such agents inhibit thromboxane synthesis and block the proaggregatory effects of its intermediates while shunting them into PGI_2 synthesis. These compounds result in more prolongation of the bleeding time and more inhibition of platelet aggregation than either thromboxane synthetase inhibitors or receptor blockers alone. One of these agents, ridogrel, has been reported to decrease platelet activation *in vivo*.[23] The place of these agents will require further studies.

Drugs that Increase Platelet cAMP Levels

Dipyridamole, PGE_1, and PGI_2 increase platelet cAMP level. The mechanism of action and pharmacology of dipyridamole are discussed in depth in Chapter 155. Clinical experience with dipyridamole in combination with aspirin is discussed in the next section.

PGE_1 and PGI_2 are potent vasodilators and platelet inhibitors. PGE_1 is used to maintain patency of the ductus arteriosus in neonates with congenital heart disease. PGI_2 interferes with every aspect of platelet function and is the most potent platelet inhibitor known. In addition to preventing platelet activation by all activation pathways on both biologic and artificial surfaces, PGI_2 also inhibits platelet adhesion and degranulation by increasing platelet cAMP. By limiting the release of platelet factor 4 from platelets, PGI_2 may also increase the antiplatelet effect of heparin.[23] Unfortunately, clinical use of PGI_2 is limited by its short half-life (30 minutes), requirement for intravenous administration, and strong vasodilatory side effects. Small clinical trials to date have not shown consistent benefits of PGI_2 therapy in unstable angina and myocardial infarction despite observed decreases in platelet aggregation and salutary hemodynamic effects.[23] Iloprost, a stable PGI_2 analogue, has been shown to increase the hepatic degradation of exogenous tissue-type plasminogen activator (t-PA). Thus, the role of these prostanoids as adjuncts to thrombolytic therapy is unclear despite encouraging earlier studies. Data regarding the prevention of restenosis after angioplasty have been similarly conflicting.[30] In an animal model of balloon-induced carotid artery deep arterial injury, infused PGI_2 did not prevent platelet deposition and thrombus formation.[31]

Drugs that Inhibit Thrombin

Thrombin is the most potent platelet agonist known. Thrombin perpetuates and amplifies not only thrombosis but also platelet aggregation and platelet secretion by several mechanisms. Thrombin-mediated platelet activation and aggregation is a crucial process in thrombus formation after arterial injury. Inhibition of thrombin is required to prevent platelet-rich thrombus formation after deep arterial injury in experimental models; platelet inhibition alone is insufficient.[16, 32] Collagen, although a less potent platelet agonist than thrombin, is yet a key platelet agonist. These extrinsic platelet activators thus play a crucial role in platelet function during arterial thrombosis.

Agents that have an important role in thrombin inhibition include (1) heparin, which relies for its antithrombin effect on cofactors antithrombin III and heparin cofactor I; (2) hirudin, Hirulog, argatroban, and PPACK (D-phenylalanyl-L-prolyl-L-arginyl-chloromethyl ketone), thrombin-specific inhibitors that bind and inactivate thrombin directly; and (3) activated protein C.[33-35] These agents have been previously discussed in detail. Although hirudin has no direct effects on platelets, hirudin's potent antithrombin effect has a significant effect on platelet function. In a porcine model of carotid angioplasty, hirudin reduced platelet deposition and thrombus formation to a more significant degree than high-dose heparin.[16] Hirudin in animal models also enhances thrombolysis of platelet-rich thrombi. Given these promising results, hirudin is at present under intense investigation in studies of unstable angina, myocardial infarction, and angioplasty.

Drugs with Other Mechanisms

Many other drugs exert antiplatelet effects through a variety of less clearly defined mechanisms.[26, 36, 37] Agents that have the most potential benefits are those that inhibit platelet activation by interfering with a final common biochemical pathway. Ticlopidine, approved by the Food and Drug Administration (FDA) as an antiplatelet agent, may act in this regard, although its exact mechanism of action is unknown. A thienopyridine derivative unrelated to other platelet inhibitors, ticlopidine inhibits platelet aggregation induced by high-concentration ADP and by low concentrations of other agonists including collagen, thrombin, arachidonate, epinephrine, TXA_2, and platelet activating factor.[38-40] High concentrations of agonists other than ADP, however, may overcome ticlopidine platelet inhibition. It is likely that ticlopidine interferes with the interaction of von Willebrand factor (vWF) or fibrinogen with platelets and may do so by altering platelet membrane reactivity of the glycoprotein (GP) IIb-IIIa receptor for fibrinogen.[38, 39] Several days of therapy are necessary before ticlopidine effectively inhibits platelet function; similarly, antiplatelet effects linger several days after discontinuation of the drug. As discussed in Chapter 152, ticlopidine has been shown to be effective in reducing infarction, total coronary events, and mortality compared with placebo in unstable angina, in reducing coronary artery bypass graft occlusion at 1 year compared with placebo, in reducing abrupt closure after angioplasty, and in reducing nonfatal stroke and death in cerebrovascular disease compared with placebo.[22, 41] The relatively frequent gastrointestinal side effects (diarrhea), occasional rash, rare occurrence of neutropenia, and higher cost of ticlopidine relative to aspirin have at present rendered aspirin preferable to ticlopidine except in patients with intolerance or allergy to aspirin.[22] Clopidogrel is a ticlopidine-related compound currently undergoing clinical evaluation.

Sulfinpyrazone is a competitive inhibitor of platelet cyclooxygenase and inhibits platelet adhesion to collagen, decreases thrombus formation on subendothelium, inhibits thrombus formation on artificial cannulae in experimental models, and normalizes platelet survival after prosthetic valve surgery.[23] Older studies have shown some benefit in myocardial infarction bypass surgery, although these effects are not as potent as those of aspirin.

Dextran prolongs the bleeding time by an unknown mechanism, perhaps by altering platelet membrane function and interfering with the factor VIII–vWF complex. At present, dextran is used before and after intravascular coronary stint placement to prevent thrombosis.

Serotonin is secreted from alpha granules of platelets and functions as a platelet agonist and vasoconstrictor in atherosclerotic arteries.[21] In experimental models, serotonin inhibitors decrease the cyclic flow variations caused by platelet secretion of serotonin and TXA_2 during coronary thrombolysis.[13, 42] Ketanserin, an S2 inhibitor, has been shown to be ineffective in decreasing the incidence of death, stroke, myocardial infarction, or amputation in a large randomized trial of patients with peripheral vascular disease.[23, 43]

Monoclonal antibodies directed against the GP IIb-IIIa receptor complex function as platelet receptor antagonists for fibrinogen and vWF.[44] Marked inhibition of platelet aggregation normally induced by potent agonists, such as thrombin and collagen, is thereby prevented. Prolongation of the bleeding time and hemorrhage may result with high-dose use; thus, chronic use of these antibodies may be impractical because of risk of bleeding complications. These antibodies are currently under investigation for use as adjunctive agents in the prevention of rethrombosis during coronary thrombolysis and abrupt closure during angioplasty.

Polypeptides containing the amino acid sequence RGD (Arg-Gly-Asp) are termed "disintegrins" because they inhibit the platelet GP IIb-IIIa integrin-family fibrinogen receptor.[45] One of these proteins, tigramin, is isolated from snake venom and has been shown to inhibit platelet aggregation stimulated by a large variety of platelet agonists. These compounds in animal models accelerate thrombolysis and prevent reocclusion.

CLINICAL EXPERIENCE WITH COMBINED ANTICOAGULANT AGENTS AND PLATELET INHIBITORS AND CURRENT RECOMMENDATIONS
Valvular Heart Disease and Prosthetic Heart Valves

Despite adequate anticoagulation with warfarin, patients with prosthetic heart valves still have a persistent risk of thromboembolism of up to 1% to 2% per year. Because dipyridamole exerts a potent effect on reducing platelet activation by artificial surfaces, a number of clinical studies have examined the combination of dipyridamole plus warfarin in the prevention of prosthetic valve thromboembolism. As noted in Chapter 152, six trials have demonstrated an approximate 50% reduction in the incidence of thromboembolism in patients with mechanical valvular prostheses treated with warfarin and dipyridamole combined or with warfarin alone (Table 14–3).[46–53] Dipyridamole has been approved by the FDA for use in combination with warfarin to reduce thromboembolism from mechanical prosthetic valves. In combination with warfarin, dipyridamole is given at a daily dose of 300 to 400 mg (5 to 6 mg/kg/day) because this dose in animals maximally prolongs platelet survival.[54]

The role of warfarin combined with aspirin to reduce thromboembolism in patients with prosthetic heart valves is evolving and at present is under investigation. Previous studies have shown an increased risk of bleeding complications when standard doses of aspirin (325 to 1000 mg/day) are added to standard-range anticoagulation therapy with warfarin.[46, 51, 52] In one study, 1 g of aspirin daily in addition to warfarin has resulted in a significantly increased risk of gastrointestinal bleeding.[51] Another study noted that aspirin (250 mg b.i.d.) plus warfarin increased gastrointestinal bleeding from 2% to 7% compared with warfarin alone.[52] In a randomized study of 534 patients with mechanical prostheses comparing warfarin plus aspirin (500 mg/day), warfarin plus dipyridamole (400 mg/day), and warfarin alone, an increased incidence of serious hemorrhage requiring hospitalization or transfusion in the warfarin plus aspirin group forced the investigators to discontinue this arm of the trial after 1319 patient-years of follow-up.[46]

Because the combination of warfarin and aspirin in doses of 500 to 1000 mg/day in these studies produced primarily gastrointestinal bleeding, it is likely that the cause of bleeding is direct chemical gastric irritation by aspirin.[22] The gastric irritant effects of aspirin are dose-related. Longitudinal studies have shown a small but significant increase in gastric bleeding at an aspirin dose of 75 mg/day; this risk doubles at an aspirin dose of 300 mg/day, and increases fivefold with doses of 1.8 to 2.4 g/day. Long-term therapy with the combination of aspirin and warfarin also increases the risk of gastrointestinal bleeding, especially if the aspirin dose is high (500 to 1000 mg) or the warfarin dose is high (INR, 3 to 4.5). Trials of combined aspirin and warfarin therapy have therefore employed low-dose aspirin in an attempt to decrease bleeding complications. Turpie et al.[53] randomized 370 patients in a double-blind, placebo-controlled trial to aspirin 100 mg/day plus warfarin (target INR, 3.0 to 4.5) or placebo plus warfarin (target INR, 3.0 to 4.5). After a mean follow-up of 2.5 years, the aspirin plus warfarin group compared with the placebo plus warfarin group showed significant reduction in all-cause mortality (2.8% versus 7.4%, risk reduction 63%, $p = .01$), major systemic embolism (1.6% versus 4.6%, risk reduction 65%, $p = .039$), the combined primary outcome major systemic embolism or death from vascular causes (1.9% versus 8.5%, 77% risk reduction, $p < .001$), and the combined outcome major systemic embolism, nonfatal intracranial hem-

Table 14–3. **Antithrombotic Therapy in Patients with Mechanical Prosthetic Heart Valves**

Reference	Method	Follow-up (yr)	Treatment	Dose (mg/day)	No. Patients	TE (%/yr)
Dale et al.[51]	PR, R, B	1	AC + P		38	9
			AC + ASA	1000	39	2
			ASA	1000	77	15
Sullivan et al.[50]	PR, R	1	AC + P		84	14
			AC + D	400	79	1
Kasahara[48]	PR, R	1 to 3 (mean 2.5)	AC		39	21
			AC + D	400	40	5
Groupe PACTE[47]	PR, R	1	AC		154	5
			AC + D	375	136	3
Rajah et al.[49]	PR, R	1 to 2	AC		87	13
			AC + D	300	78	4
Altman et al.[52]	PR, R	2	AC		65	20
			AC + ASA	500	57	5
Turpie et al.[53]	PR, R, B	2	AC + P		184	2.84
			AC + ASA	500	186	1.08

TE, thromboembolism: PR, prospective; R, randomized; B, blind; AC, warfarin; D, dipyridamole; ASA, aspirin; P, placebo.

orrhage, or death from hemorrhage or vascular causes (3.9% versus 9.9%, risk reduction 61%, $p = .005$). Aspirin decreased stroke (1.3% versus 4.2%, risk reduction 70%, $p = .027$) but significantly increased overall bleeding (35% versus 22%, $p = .02$). Most of the increased bleeding was minor (hematuria, epistaxis, bruising), and major hemorrhagic events were not significantly different between the two groups (8.5% versus 6.6%, $p = .43$), including intracranial bleeding (6.4% versus 5.2%, NS). Of the INRs measured, 40% were within the study target range (3 to 4.5). The authors concluded that aspirin results in a significant reduction in the combined outcome of vascular mortality and major systemic embolism when added to warfarin and that further trials are necessary to establish the efficacy of less intense anticoagulant regimens (INR, 2.0) plus low-dose aspirin. Trials of combined aspirin and warfarin therapy in prosthetic valve patients are ongoing.

There have been no trials of combined antiplatelet and anticoagulant therapy in patients with bioprosthetic heart valves.

Current Recommendations

In low-risk patients with mechanical prosthetic heart valves, warfarin should be begun 24 to 48 hours after operation (down nasogastric tube), to prolong the INR to 2.5 to 3.5, and continued indefinitely (Table 14-4). There is as yet no evidence that low-risk patients benefit from combined anticoagulant and antiplatelet therapy; the potential role of combined therapy is discussed in Chapter 152. Combination therapy is currently not recommended for routine use in low-risk patients.

In high-risk patients with mechanical prosthetic valves (prior embolism, atrial fibrillation, diminished left ventricular ejection fraction, valves implanted before 1980, anticoagulation stopped or decreased as a result of bleeding, poor patient compliance), dipyridamole has been FDA-approved for use in combination with warfarin and significantly decreases thromboembolism compared with therapy with warfarin alone. Dipyridamole dosage is 350 to 400 mg/day (5 to 6 mg/kg/day), usually given as 75 mg with meals and 150 mg at bedtime. However, because low-dose aspirin in combination with warfarin appears particu-

larly promising and may reduce vascular mortality in addition to thromboembolism, careful consideration should be given to combination therapy with low-dose aspirin and warfarin instead of combination therapy with dipyridamole and warfarin in high-risk patients. Combination therapy is discussed in detail in Chapter 152.

Patients with bioprosthetic valves have an increased risk of thromboembolism in the first 3 months after surgery; thereafter their risk of thromboembolism is low. It is recommended that warfarin be started 24 to 48 hours after surgery and maintained for 3 months (target INR, 3.0 to 4.5) in low-risk patients. For medium-risk patients (atrial fibrillation, left atrium > 50 mm), continued long-term therapy with low-dose warfarin is recommended (target INR, 2.0 to 3.0). For high-risk patients (left atrial thrombus, prior thromboembolism), high-dose long-term warfarin (target INR, 3.0 to 4.5) is recommended.

Atrial Fibrillation

There have been no trials of combined anticoagulant and antiplatelet therapy in atrial fibrillation. There is no evidence to date that combination therapy is more efficacious than therapy with anticoagulants alone. As discussed, high-risk patients with atrial fibrillation (mitral stenosis, mechanical prosthetic heart valves, previous thromboembolism, thyrotoxicosis, the elderly, depressed left ventricular function) have a risk of stroke as high as 10% per year and should be treated with anticoagulants. At the other end of the spectrum, low-risk patients younger than age 60 with atrial fibrillation but without structural heart disease or hypertension ("lone" atrial fibrillation) usually do not require anticoagulant therapy and do not appear to have an increased incidence of stroke. Medium-risk patients (nonvalvular atrial fibrillation associated with various cardiovascular conditions such as hypertension, coronary artery disease, heart failure, mitral regurgitation) have an approximately 5% risk of stroke per year. In five large trials of nonvalvular atrial fibrillation, low-dose warfarin (INR, 1.5 to 3.0) reduced the incidence of stroke by 60% from 5% to 2% per year and is thus recommended in all patients without contraindication to chronic anticoagulation.[55] The SPAF study showed that aspirin alone reduced

Table 14-4. **Recommended Antithrombotic Therapy in Patients with Prosthetic Heart Valves**

Valve	Grade-Situation	Therapy
Mechanical	Routine	MD warfarin
	Old prosthesis, TE	HD warfarin, or MD warfarin + LD ASA? or + Dip (400 mg/day)
	ACRx problems (bleeding)	LD warfarin + Dip (400 mg/day) or LD warfarin + LD ASA
	Recurrent embolism	Consider reoperation
Bioprosthetic	AVR routine—NSR	LD warfarin for 3 mo (then ASA)
	MVR routine—NSR	LD warfarin for 3 mo (then ASA?)
	AF, LA thrombus, TE	HD warfarin for 3 mo, then LD warfarin

HD warfarin, high-dose warfarin (INR, 3.0–4.5); MD warfarin, medium-dose warfarin (INR, 2.5–3.5); LD warfarin, low-dose warfarin (INR, 2.0–3.0); ACRx, anticoagulant therapy; AF, atrial fibrillation; LD ASA, low-dose aspirin (80–100 mg/day); AVR, aortic valve replacement; Dip, dipyridamole; LA, left atrium; MVR, mitral valve replacement; NSR, normal sinus rhythm; TE, previous thromboembolism.

stroke by 81% in patients younger than age 75. The AFASAK study showed no reduction in stroke with aspirin alone compared with placebo. Therapy is discussed in detail in Chapter 152.

Chronic Coronary Artery Disease

There have been no studies of combined antiplatelet and anticoagulant therapy in chronic coronary artery disease or stable angina. Platelet activation and thrombin generation are usually undetectable in the setting of chronic coronary artery disease and stable angina, although progression of coronary artery disease likely involves asymptomatic plaque disruption, asymptomatic mural thrombosis, and incorporation of mural thrombus into an enlarging atherosclerotic lesion.[56] Both aspirin and anticoagulant agents confer protection against death, myocardial infarction, and reinfarction; in this setting, aspirin is preferred and recommended (although not more efficacious) because of ease of administration, lower cost, and less need for monitoring.[22, 41] Large studies currently under way are evaluating the role of combined anticoagulant and antiplatelet agents after myocardial infarction.

Unstable Angina

Atherosclerotic plaque disruption, platelet adhesion, activation and aggregation, thrombin generation, and ultimately mural thrombus formation play key roles in the pathophysiology of unstable angina.[57] Antiplatelet therapy with aspirin or ticlopidine alone, anticoagulant therapy with heparin alone, or combined antiplatelet and anticoagulant therapy each significantly decreases the rate of death and myocardial infarction in unstable angina.[22, 41, 56] Clinical trials have focused on the additional benefit conferred by combined anticoagulant and antiplatelet therapy compared with anticoagulant therapy alone.

In the first double-blind, placebo-controlled trial by Theroux et al., heparin alone was as efficacious as heparin plus aspirin in 479 patients in the acute phase of unstable angina.[58] Thirteen percent of patients at a mean of 9.5 hours after discontinuation of heparin experienced reactivation of angina.[59] The rate of reactivation was higher in patients treated with heparin alone and was lower in patients treated with heparin plus aspirin. In the randomized, double-blind RISC trial, 796 men with unstable angina were randomized to aspirin alone 75 mg/day for 1 year, intravenous heparin alone for 4 days, aspirin for 1 year plus intravenous heparin for 4 days, or placebo.[60] The group treated with aspirin plus heparin experienced a decrease in the primary end point death and nonfatal myocardial infarction during the initial 5 days of therapy. Heparin therapy (which was discontinued at day 4) had no effect on the overall primary end point thereafter.

In their second double-blind study, Theroux et al. randomized 484 patients with unstable angina to therapy with either aspirin 325 mg b.i.d. or intravenous heparin 5000 IU bolus followed by continuous infu-sion adjusted to maintain the activated partial thromboplastin time (aPTT) at 1.5 to 2.0 times control.[61] Therapy was begun a mean 8 hours after admission and continued for at least 6 days. Patients taking aspirin at the time of hospital admission were excluded. Myocardial infarction occurred in 0.8% of the heparin-treated patients and in 3.7% of the aspirin-treated patients ($p = .035$), an odds ratio of 0.22 and risk difference of 2.9% (95% confidence interval 0.3% to 5.6%).

In a prospective open-label trial, Cohen et al. randomized 214 prior non–aspirin users within 9.5 hours of presenting with unstable angina to aspirin 162.5 mg/day or aspirin 162.5 mg/day plus intravenous heparin (aPTT two times control) followed by warfarin (INR, 2 to 3) for 12 weeks. At 2 weeks, there was significant reduction in total ischemic events in the aspirin plus anticoagulant group (10.5% versus 27%, $p = .004$), and at 12 weeks nearly significant reduction in total ischemic events (13% versus 25%, $p = .06$). Thus, a combination of aspirin and anticoagulant agents appears more efficacious than either agent alone in prior non–aspirin users.[62] An overview of the trials of Theroux, RISC, and Cohen showed that combined aspirin and heparin therapy in the acute phase of unstable angina decreased myocardial infarction by 40% compared with monotherapy with aspirin or heparin.[62]

Selective Thrombin Inhibitors Hirudin and Argatroban in Unstable Angina

Pilot trials of Hirulog, hirudin, and argatroban (discussed in detail in Chapter 152) in aspirin-treated patients have been reported.[19, 63] These agents appear efficacious, although patients may still experience refractory angina or myocardial infarction. Large studies are under way to evaluate the role of selective thrombin inhibitors and aspirin in unstable angina.

Thrombolysis in Unstable Angina

Although theoretically attractive, thrombolysis combined with aspirin or heparin therapy during unstable angina has not proved efficacious to date. Change in the angiographic appearance of the culprit lesion has been the primary end point in most studies.[57] In the TIMI IIIA trial, 306 patients with unstable angina were randomized after initial angiography to a 90-minute front-loaded infusion of t-PA (0.8 mg/kg) or placebo.[64] All patients received intravenous heparin; most patients received aspirin. Follow-up angiogram 18 to 48 hours after t-PA showed no overall advantage of t-PA in the primary end points angiographic improvement of the culprit lesion (25% versus 19%, $p = .25$) or mean change in percentage of stenosis (-6.2% versus -4.6%, $p = .16$).

Current Recommendations

Aspirin, ticlopidine, heparin, and hirudin all are effective in unstable angina. The combination of low-dose aspirin and heparin is more efficacious than either agent alone in the prevention of myocardial infarction during the acute phase of unstable angina. Although there is no conclusive evidence to date, aspirin plus heparin in the nonacute phase of unstable angina may decrease myocardial infarction compared with either therapy alone. There is no conclusive evidence to date that the combination of heparin plus aspirin decreases mortality compared with aspirin alone in either the acute or chronic phase of unstable angina. Thrombolytic agents provide no advantage in combination with antithrombotic agents. Promising selective antithrombin agents such as hirudin in combination with aspirin are presently being evaluated in large trials. Specific recommendations are provided in Table 14–5.

The duration of heparin therapy in the acute phase of unstable angina is empiric at present. As stated previously, the largest trials of heparin have continued therapy for 5 to 6 days. Reactivation of unstable angina may occur when heparin is discontinued; the incidence of reactivation can be decreased by concurrent or overlapping aspirin therapy. In the chronic phase, aspirin has been proved efficacious; the combination of aspirin and anticoagulant agents may be more effective in prior non–aspirin users than aspirin alone, and large trials are necessary.

Acute Myocardial Infarction: Absence of Concurrent Thrombolytic Therapy

Only 20% to 30% of all patients with myocardial infarction (MI) are eligible for thrombolytic therapy: the decision regarding use of antiplatelet and antithrombotic drugs in patients with MI ineligible for thrombolytic agents is one commonly faced in clinical practice. ISIS-2 conclusively established the efficacy of aspirin in acute myocardial infarction whether aspirin is administered alone or together with thrombolytic therapy.[65] When given alone without streptokinase, aspirin resulted in a highly significant 23% reduction in the primary outcome total vascular mortality (95% confidence interval -30% to -15%, $p < .00001$) and a highly significant 49% reduction in

nonfatal reinfarction. When aspirin was given with streptokinase, there was a 42% reduction in mortality, showing that aspirin had an additive beneficial mortality-lowering effect when combined with streptokinase. Mortality benefit was seen equally if aspirin was begun 0 to 4, 5 to 12, or 13 to 24 hours after symptom onset. The optimal dose, frequency of administration, and preparation of aspirin to provide maximal net benefit in acute myocardial infarction are still unsettled.

No large randomized trials of heparin alone or in combination with aspirin in myocardial infarction have been performed. Meta-analysis of older, small, largely nonrandomized trials of intravenous or subcutaneous heparin in 5700 subjects showed a 16% reduction in mortality and 22% reduction in reinfarction with heparin alone. There have been no direct comparisons of combined antiplatelet and anticoagulant therapy versus either therapy alone or placebo, but the indirect comparisons suggest a similar reduction in total mortality (approximately 20%) with either drug.

Current Recommendations

Aspirin should be given immediately to all patients with suspected evolving myocardial infarction whether or not thrombolytic therapy is planned. Non–enteric-coated aspirin 160 to 325 mg should be chewed and swallowed as soon as evolving myocardial infarction is suspected. Aspirin should be continued indefinitely. In the absence of thrombolytic therapy, all patients with suspected evolving myocardial infarction should be strongly considered for intravenous heparin in addition to aspirin. Full-dose intravenous heparin is mandatory in (1) patients at increased risk of systemic or pulmonary embolism (severe left ventricular dysfunction, history of systemic or pulmonary embolism, evidence of mural thrombus, atrial fibrillation), and (2) patients with anterior Q-wave myocardial infarction (due to risk of ventricular mural thrombosis). All patients with acute myocardial infarction should receive no less than low-dose subcutaneous

Table 14–5. **Antithrombotic Therapy in Coronary Artery Disease**

Coronary Event	Recommendations
Stable angina	Aspirin, 325 mg/day
Unstable angina	Acute phase: IV heparin plus low-dose aspirin 75–100 mg Chronic phase: aspirin 325 mg/day; consider aspirin 75–100 mg/day plus warfarin (INR, 2–3) in high-risk patients
Non-Q-wave MI	Acute phase: IV heparin plus low-dose aspirin Chronic phase: aspirin 325 mg/day
Q-wave MI: absence of thrombolytic therapy	Aspirin, 325 mg/day, in acute and chronic phases IV heparin in acute phase
Q-wave MI: presence of thrombolytic therapy	Aspirin 325 mg on admission, then 75–100 mg/day combined with adjunctive heparin* (aPTT 2–3 × control) for 2–7 days Aspirin, 325 mg/day, thereafter

aPTT, activated partial thromboplastin time; MI, myocardial infarction.
*Heparin has not yet been shown to be efficacious adjunctive therapy to streptokinase.

heparin (7500 U every 12 hours) for at least 7 days to reduce calf thrombosis.[41]

Myocardial Infarction in Presence of Concurrent Thrombolytic Therapy

The role of heparin as adjunctive therapy in streptokinase- and aspirin-treated patients is controversial. In the SCATI trial, in which none of the patients received aspirin, there was a nearly significant trend toward fewer deaths (10 deaths out of 218 patients versus 19 deaths out of 215 patients, 95% confidence interval 0.22 to 1.02) in streptokinase (SK) plus heparin (given as 2000 IU intravenous bolus followed by 12,500 IU b.i.d.) versus SK alone.[66] No differences in recurrent ischemia or nonfatal reinfarction were observed.

Thrombolytic trials since ISIS-2 have treated all patients with aspirin. In GISSI-2, the addition of subcutaneous heparin to aspirin and either SK or t-PA provided no benefit in in-hospital mortality (8.5% versus 9.0%, $p = .29$) or mortality at 35 days (9.3 versus 9.4 days, $p = .82$).[67] Minor bleeding was significantly increased by heparin, but cerebral hemorrhage was not. In ISIS-3, subcutaneous heparin did not reduce 35-day mortality (10.3% versus 10.6%, $p = .36$) or reinfarction (3.2% versus 3.5%, $p = .09$) but did significantly increase cerebral hemorrhage (0.6% versus 0.4%, $p = .03$) and noncerebral major bleeding (1.0% versus 0.8%, $p = .006$).[68] During the 7 days of heparin therapy, however, there were slightly fewer deaths in the aspirin plus heparin group than in the aspirin group alone (7.4% versus 7.9%, $p = .06$). Combining GISSI-2 and ISIS-3 and comparing the benefit of aspirin plus heparin with aspirin alone yielded no difference in death at 35 days (10.0 versus 10.2, $p = .37$), cerebral hemorrhage (0.5 versus 0.4, $p = .08$), or reinfarction (3.0 versus 3.3, $p = .06$), but a significant difference in major hemorrhage (1.0 versus 0.7, $p < .001$).[68] Thus, subcutaneous adjunctive heparin after streptokinase or t-PA confers no mortality benefit but increases the risk of bleeding. GISSI-2 and ISIS-3 have been criticized, however, for the delayed administration of heparin (4 to 12 hours after thrombolysis), the erratic absorption of subcutaneous heparin, and often suboptimal anticoagulant effect of subcutaneous heparin.

The role of intravenous adjunctive heparin with streptokinase (SK) was addressed in GUSTO.[69, 70] Comparing SK plus subcutaneous heparin (12,500 U b.i.d. begun 4 hours after SK) with SK plus intravenous heparin (5000 U bolus then 1000 U/hr with dose titrated to aPTT 60 to 85 seconds begun with SK), there were no significant differences in 24-hour mortality (2.8% versus 2.9%, NS) or 30-day mortality (7.2% versus 7.4%, $p = .731$) but nonsignificant trends toward increased nonfatal stroke, nonfatal hemorrhagic stroke, and nonfatal disabling stroke. Thus, intravenous heparin conferred no benefit in comparison with subcutaneous heparin as adjunctive therapy with streptokinase.

Studies with early infarct-related arterial angiographic patency as the primary end point have evaluated the efficacy of adjunctive heparin therapy in aspirin-treated patients after t-PA. These trials are summarized in Table 14–6.[71–75] On balance, heparin appears to improve early (18 hours) infarct-related patency after t-PA. Angiographic studies to date have not shown reduction in mortality resulting specifically from adjunctive heparin: this may reflect the small sample sizes of these trials, differences in the timing, route of administration, and dosage of heparin; use of aspirin; timing of angiography after both thrombolytic and heparin therapies; and selection and administration of thrombolytic agent. Because both early infarct-related vessel patency and patency at hospital discharge decrease mortality from myocardial infarction, the role of combination antithrombotic therapy in ensuring infarct-related patency is a crucial one.[76] Until further trials are available, it is prudent to recommend adjunctive heparin to all patients treated with t-PA and aspirin. Patients who would otherwise benefit from anticoagulation after AMI as outlined earlier should definitely receive adjunctive heparin after t-PA.

Current Recommendations

Aspirin 160 to 325 mg (chewed and swallowed) should be given immediately to all patients with suspected evolving myocardial infarction and continued indefinitely. Adjunctive intravenous heparin should be strongly considered when t-PA is administered, because improved infarct-related patency may increase survival. The risk of bleeding, including cerebral hemorrhage, is increased with t-PA plus heparin, particularly if "front-loaded" t-PA is administered. There is little evidence of any net benefit of routine adjunctive intravenous or subcutaneous heparin to streptokinase when full-dose aspirin is used. In this setting, heparin may also increase bleeding, including intracerebral hemorrhage. Patients at high risk of thromboembolic complications after myocardial infarction should receive intravenous heparin after either t-PA or SK.

Primary Prevention of Myocardial Infarction

There are no trials yet reported of combined antiplatelet and anticoagulant therapy in the primary prevention of myocardial infarction. Trials of aspirin in the primary prevention of myocardial infarction are discussed in Chapter 152. Trials of low-dose aspirin and warfarin in high-risk patients are under way.

Secondary Prevention of Myocardial Infarction

Aspirin and warfarin both are effective in the secondary prevention of MI. As discussed in Chapter 152, owing to ease of administration and monitoring and lower cost, aspirin is preferred to warfarin except in those patients intolerant of aspirin or at high risk for embolism (documented mural thrombi, severe left

Table 14–6. **Adjunctive Heparin Plus t-PA: Major Angiographic Trials**

	Trial				
	TAMI-3 [71]	*Bleich et al.* [72]	*HART* [73]	*ECSG-6* [74]	*NHSA* [75]
No. patients	134	83	205	652	241
Heparin	10,000 U IVB	5000 U IVB; 1000 U/hr	5000 IVB; 1000 U/hr	5000 U IVB; 1000 U/hr	5000 UIVB; 1000 U/hr
Heparin begun	With t-PA	With t-PA	With t-PA	With t-PA	After t-PA
Angio, timing (mean)	90 min	57 hr	18 hr	81 hr	7 days
Patency, heparin	79%	71%	82%	83%	80%
Patency, no heparin	79%	44%	51%	75%	82%
ASA given	No	Yes	Yes	Yes	Yes

*Significant at level $p < .05$.
IVB, intravenous bolus; t-PA, plasminogen activator complex; Angio, coronary angiogram; ASA, aspirin.

ventricular dysfunction, atrial fibrillation, prior thromboembolism).

There are no trials yet reported of combined antiplatelet and anticoagulant therapy in the secondary prevention of myocardial infarction. The Coumadin-Aspirin Reinfarction Study (CARS), which randomizes patients to low-dose aspirin plus low-dose coumadin after myocardial infarction, is presently under way.

Chronic Left Ventricular Aneurysm

There are no trials of combined antiplatelet and anticoagulant therapy in patients with chronic left ventricular aneurysm. Recommendations for warfarin are discussed in Chapter 152.

Percutaneous Transluminal Coronary Angioplasty (PTCA)

The plaque disruption and deep arterial injury that occur during PTCA are potent stimuli to thrombosis.[77] Therapy with antiplatelet agents has been clearly shown to reduce the risk of abrupt closure after PTCA.[22] In a randomized, double-blind placebo-controlled study from the Montreal Heart Institute, the incidence of Q-wave myocardial infarction in the group of patients treated 24 hours before PTCA with aspirin 330 mg t.i.d. plus dipyridamole 75 mg t.i.d. was 1.6% versus 6.9% ($p = .0113$) in the group treated with placebo.[78] Ticlopidine has also proved effective in the prevention of abrupt closure after PTCA.[22]

The efficacy of heparin in the prevention of abrupt closure after PTCA has not been studied in a controlled fashion, but given compelling animal studies and retrospective observational analyses of a marked reduction in abrupt closure rates, use of heparin is standard during PTCA.[79, 80] Heparin dosage, monitoring, and duration of therapy have not been established in prospective trials, and the specifics of administration during angioplasty remain largely empiric at present. To date, there is no firm evidence that heparin therapy for longer than 4 to 6 hours after routine uncomplicated PTCA prevents abrupt closure, although most patients are treated for 12 to 24 hours at present.[81] Patients undergoing complicated PTCA (unstable angina, complex lesions, multivessel angioplasty, or angiographically visible thrombus) should be treated for 16 to 24 hours before removal of vascular sheaths.[22, 80]

The specific antithrombin agents, hirudin and Hirulog, have been shown to be safe and efficacious in small studies in the prevention of abrupt closure after PTCA.[82] At present, in combination with heparin, other antiplatelet agents (GP IIa-IIB antibodies, thromboxane synthetase inhibitors, prostacyclin) are being investigated in small pilot trials to prevent abrupt closure.[25]

There have been no large studies of combined antiplatelet and anticoagulant therapy in the prevention of chronic restenosis after PTCA.[25, 80] To date, therapy with new antiplatelet agents (platelet-derived growth factor [PDGF] inhibitors, serotonin antagonists, thromboxane A_2 receptor antagonists, omega-3 fatty acids) has not proved effective in preventing chronic restenosis. Therapy of chronic restenosis is discussed in detail in Chapter 152.

Current Recommendations

Aspirin 325 mg/day should be started at least 24 hours before angioplasty and continued indefinitely. Intravenous heparin 10,000 U bolus followed by an infusion to maintain the aPTT at 1.5 to 2.0 times control should be administered during the procedure. Although there is no evidence that routine heparin therapy beyond several hours after PTCA decreases the incidence of abrupt closure, most patients should receive heparin for 12 to 18 hours; those with complex lesions, angiographic thrombus, multivessel angioplasty, or unstable angina should receive 16 to 24 hours of intravenous heparin before removal of vascular sheaths.

There is no evidence to date that aspirin, warfarin, or combined aspirin and warfarin therapy decreases chronic restenosis after PTCA. However, given the existence of residual coronary artery disease after angioplasty, patients without contraindications should be treated with aspirin 160 to 325 mg indefinitely.

Coronary Artery Bypass Surgery

The prevalence of saphenous vein bypass graft occlusion is 10% to 15% in the first month, 25% in the first year, 2% to 4% per year after the first year for the first 5 years, and then 5% per year the next 5 years.[83] At 10 years, approximately 50% of vein grafts are occluded. Graft thrombosis accounts for early closure within 1 month of surgery. Thrombotic occlusion is particularly prevalent in grafts anastomosed to small distal arteries (<1.5 mm in diameter) and grafts with low flow (<40 ml/min). After the first month and up to the first postoperative year, graft closure is typically due to the process of accelerated graft atherosclerosis, characterized by intimal hyperplasia and superimposed thrombosis. After the first postoperative year, graft occlusion mimics the process of native coronary artery atherosclerosis.

Antiplatelet therapy with aspirin, aspirin plus dipyridamole, and ticlopidine reduces graft occlusion within the first postoperative year by 30% to 50%.[84-87] Detailed discussion of the results of these combined antiplatelet trials is presented in the following section on combined antiplatelet therapy. Irrespective of dose, antiplatelet agents must be administered preoperatively or within 48 hours postoperatively to be effective.

No trials of combined antiplatelet and anticoagulant therapy in the prevention of graft occlusion have appeared. Data concerning the efficacy of warfarin compared with aspirin in the prevention of graft occlusion are conflicting. Three early, small, placebo-controlled trials were inconclusive, but randomized patients to therapy 3 to 7 days after surgery.[83] Pfisterer et al. reported no difference in the incidence of early (2 week) and late (up to 1 year) graft occlusion in 285 patients randomized to oral anticoagulants for 12 months, oral anticoagulants for 3 months followed by placebo for 9 months, dipyridamole plus aspirin, or dipyridamole plus aspirin for 3 months followed by placebo for 9 months.[88] Van der Meer et al. reported a randomized, double-blind, placebo-controlled trial of 948 patients assigned to aspirin (50 mg/day begun the night after surgery), aspirin (50 mg/day begun the night after surgery) plus dipyridamole (5 mg/kg/day for 28 hours perioperatively followed by 200 mg/b.i.d.), or oral anticoagulants begun the day before surgery (target INR, 2.4 to 4.8).[89] There were no significant differences in occlusion rates of distal anastomoses at repeat angiography (11%, 15%, 13%, respectively), myocardial infarction, death, or major bleeding at 1 year of follow-up.

No effective therapy is available for accelerated atherosclerosis of vein grafts.[90] Because patients have coexistent risk factors for coronary artery disease and residual disease after bypass surgery, long-term therapy with aspirin is recommended. Because vein grafts with low flow (40 ml/min) and anastomosis to small distal arteries (<1.5 mm) have a greater chance of thrombotic occlusion, combined long-term antiplatelet and antithrombotic therapy with low-dose aspirin and low-dose warfarin is reasonable, although this therapy has not been tested in randomized trials to date.[83]

Current Recommendations

Aspirin (160 mg) should be administered via the nasogastric tube 1 hour postoperatively and 80 to 325 mg/day continued indefinitely thereafter. After surgery, patients at high risk for thrombotic graft occlusion (flow <40 ml/min or distal artery <1.5 mm or associated endarterectomy) should be considered for combined low-dose aspirin (80 mg/day) and warfarin therapy (begun on postoperative day 1; target INR, 2 to 3) or combined aspirin (325 mg/day) plus dipyridamole (300 to 400 mg/day). In addition, until warfarin is therapeutic, low-dose heparin to maintain the aPTT just above normal may be given in the recovery room, then heparin may be increased to prolong the aPTT to 1.5 times control once chest tubes are removed.

Left Ventricular Dysfunction After Myocardial Infarction

There have been no trials of combined antiplatelet and anticoagulant therapy for left ventricular dysfunction after myocardial infarction. Anticoagulant therapy is discussed in Chapter 152.

Dilated Cardiomyopathy

To date no trials of combined antiplatelet and anticoagulant therapy in dilated cardiomyopathy have appeared.

Cerebrovascular Disease

There have been no trials of combined antiplatelet and anticoagulant therapy in cerebrovascular disease (thrombotic stroke, cardiogenic embolic stroke, transient ischemic attacks, or after carotid endarterectomy).

Peripheral Vascular Disease

There have been no long-term studies of combined antiplatelet and anticoagulant therapy in peripheral vascular disease. Although there is no evidence that antiplatelet or anticoagulant agents modify the symptoms or natural history of peripheral vascular disease, meta-analyses have shown that aspirin decreases vascular mortality by 15% ($p < .0003$) and nonfatal stroke and myocardial infarction by 30% ($p < .0001$).[91, 92] In acute thrombotic or embolic peripheral vascular occlusion, there is also no unequivocal evidence of the efficacy of antiplatelet or antithrombotic therapy, although both are often used in combination clinically in this setting. Heparin may prevent recurrent embolism after thromboembolectomy.[43]

There have been no trials of combined antiplatelet and anticoagulant therapy to prevent thrombotic occlusion after peripheral vascular reconstructive surgery. However, in an uncontrolled retrospective study using historical controls, aspirin in combination with warfarin reduced occlusions in patients undergoing a second reconstruction procedure with prosthetic grafts.[43] Trials of low-dose aspirin and low-dose warfarin to prevent thrombosis of infrainguinal bypasses are under way. Grafts anastomosed to small distal arteries (<6 mm) and grafts with low flow (<200 ml/min) are prone to thrombotic occlusion.

Current Recommendations

In patients with peripheral vascular disease, aspirin (325 mg/day) is recommended to decrease the risk of myocardial infarction and stroke but will not necessarily ameliorate the symptoms or alter the natural history of peripheral vascular disease.

Prior to peripheral vascular prosthetic reconstructive surgery, aspirin (325 mg/day) is recommended. Dipyridamole (75 mg t.i.d.) may reduce the risk of thrombotic occlusion further when added to aspirin perioperatively. Intraoperative heparin is recommended (dosage and monitoring are empiric at present). After surgery, patients should receive aspirin 325 mg/day indefinitely.

Pulmonary Embolism

There are no large randomized studies of combined antiplatelet and anticoagulant therapy in the prevention or therapy of pulmonary embolism. This entity is discussed in detail in Chapter 18.

CLINICAL USE OF COMBINED ANTIPLATELET AGENTS AND CURRENT RECOMMENDATIONS
Theoretical Considerations

Dipyridamole inhibits spontaneous platelet aggregation in stirred human blood more strongly than does aspirin.[93] In baboons, the combination of dipyridamole and aspirin limits platelet deposition in Silastic shunts more strongly than either drug alone.[94] These experimental studies, when combined with data showing normalization of platelet survival by dipyridamole in human subjects with prosthetic heart valves, led to the widespread clinical use of dipyridamole in combination with aspirin, with the hope that synergistic platelet inhibition might be achieved. Dipyridamole in combination with warfarin reduces the incidence of thromboembolism in patients with prosthetic heart valves as previously discussed and has been approved by the FDA for this use. However, there is no study that demonstrates any benefit from the use of dipyridamole alone or in combination with aspirin compared with aspirin therapy alone in situations in which the thrombogenic surface is biologic.[22] Not surprisingly, a meta-analysis of the reported antiplatelet trials to date in cardiovascular disease concluded that there is no evidence that dipyridamole is an effective antiplatelet agent either alone or in combination with aspirin.[92] There have been no large trials of combined antiplatelet therapy with agents other than aspirin, dipyridamole, and sulfinpyrazone.

Cerebral Ischemia

Two major studies have examined the role of dipyridamole and aspirin in cerebral ischemia. In the AICLA study, patients with completed stroke or transient ischemic attacks (84% and 16%, respectively) were assigned randomly to receive placebo, aspirin (330 mg t.i.d.), or aspirin (300 mg t.i.d.) plus dipyridamole (75 mg t.i.d).[95] Both active treatments significantly reduced the incidence of recurrent stroke, which occurred in 10.5% of the treated patients versus 18% of the control subjects. No difference was noted between aspirin alone and aspirin in combination with dipyridamole. The dipyridamole-aspirin trial in cerebral ischemia randomly assigned patients with carotid artery transient ischemia attacks into treatment with aspirin (325 mg q.i.d.) or aspirin (324 mg q.i.d.) plus dipyridamole (75 mg q.i.d.).[96] Owing to the significant reduction of stroke in the AICLA study, a placebo arm was omitted. No difference was seen between groups receiving aspirin and the groups receiving aspirin plus dipyridamole in the end points of stroke, retinal infarction, or total mortality. Although in the European Stroke Prevention Study aspirin combined with dipyridamole was the most effective treatment when compared with placebo, no comparison with aspirin alone was made.[97] The only study that examined the use of dipyridamole alone in the patients with transient ischemic attack failed to demonstrate any benefit of this drug in the incidence of recurrent attacks, stroke, or death despite the use of doses up to 800 mg daily.[98]

Secondary Prevention After Myocardial Infarction

PARIS I and PARIS II evaluated the efficacy of aspirin alone and aspirin in combination with dipyridamole in survivors of myocardial infarction.[99, 100] In PARIS I, aspirin alone was compared with aspirin plus dipyridamole and placebo. There was a trend toward decreased coronary events and coronary mortality in both active treatment groups, but no difference between the aspirin and aspirin-dipyridamole group. In PARIS II, more than 3000 patients who survived myocardial infarctions 4 to 16 weeks earlier were assigned randomly to receive aspirin (330 mg t.i.d.) plus dipyridamole (75 mg t.i.d.) or placebo. By the end of the study, the treatment group had a statistically significant reduction in the incidence of coronary events (24%) but only a 6% reduction in coronary mortality. Because no group received aspirin alone, no statement could be made about the efficacy of dipyridamole, but the 24% reduction in coronary events with combined aspirin-dipyridamole in PARIS II was similar to the pooled results involving second-

Table 14–7. **Antithrombotic Therapy 1994**

	Thromboembolic Risk		
Pathogenesis	*High (>6%/yr)*	*Medium (2–6%/yr)*	*Low (<2%/yr)*
Arterial system	ACS	Stable CAD	Primary prevention
	Intervention	Post-MI–Chronic	
Platelets = fibrin	PI +A/C	PI (or A/C)	PI (±)
Cardiac chambers	A-fib[1]–embolism	A-fib[1]–valv, nonvalv[2]	A-fib[1,2]–idiopathic
	A-fib[1]–mitral stenosis	Anterior MI–early	Chronic LV
	A/C (INR 2.5–3.5)	Dilated cardiomyopathy	aneurysm
Fibrin		A/C (INR 2.0–3.0)	No therapy
Prosthetic valves	Old mechanical	Recent mechanical	Bioprosthesis–NSR
	Mechanical–embolism	Bioprosthesis–A-fib	
Fibrin > platelets	A/C (INR 3.0–4.5) or	A/C (Mechanical–INR	No therapy
	(INR 2.5–3.5) + PI[3]?	2.5–3.5,[4] Bio–INR	
		2.0–3.0)	

A/C, anticoagulant; ACS, acute coronary syndrome; A-fib, atrial fibrillation; Bio, bioprosthetic; CAD, coronary artery disease; LV, left ventricular; MI, myocardial infarction; NSR, normal sinus rhythm; PI, platelet inhibitor.
[1]Cardioversion: 3 weeks before (and so on) v/s transesophageal echocardiography and decision made.
[2]ASA if associated vascular disease (AF-marker).
[3]ASA 100 mg/day; Turpie A, et al: N Engl J Med 329:524, 1993.[53]
[4]INR 2.0–3.0 + ASA 300 mg/day + Dip; Altman R, et al: J Thorac Cardiovasc Surg 101:427, 1991.[112]
Data from Stein B, Fuster V, Halperin JL, Chesebro JH: Antithrombotic therapy in cardiac disease. An emerging approach based on pathogenesis and risk. Circulation 80:1501, 1989; ACCP: Chest 102 (Suppl), 1992; and ESC: JHVD 2:398, 1993.

ary prevention of myocardial infarction using aspirin alone.[101, 102]

Unstable Angina

Two studies with high statistical power have unequivocally demonstrated the efficacy of aspirin in reducing fatal and nonfatal coronary events in unstable angina.[103, 104] Sulfinpyrazone alone was ineffective in the Canadian trial and, in combination with aspirin, did not add to the efficacy of aspirin alone.[104]

Coronary Artery Bypass

Preoperative administration of dipyridamole reduces the thrombocytopenic effects of the extracorporeal pump in pigs and preserves the platelet count during bypass in human subjects while reducing the hemostatic defect and decreasing the production of platelet microthrombi.[105, 106] Thus, preoperative dipyridamole may inhibit intraoperative platelet activation by the prosthetic materials of the cardiopulmonary bypass pump, making less likely early platelet aggregation on venous grafts. Clinical studies have failed to clearly establish a role for preoperative or postoperative dipyridamole.[83, 92] Low-dose aspirin alone (100 mg/day) was found to be effective in decreasing the risk of vein graft closure in the study by Lorenz et al.[107] In a Veterans Administration study, aspirin (325 mg/day) alone was as effective as aspirin (325 mg/day) plus dipyridamole (75 mg t.i.d.) in preventing graft occlusion.[84] In the study of Brown et al., nearly 150 patients were assigned randomly to receive aspirin (325 mg t.i.d.), aspirin (325 mg t.i.d.) plus dipyridamole (75 mg t.i.d.), or placebo.[108] Therapy was begun on the second or third postoperative day. In patients receiving treatment within 48 hours, occlusion rates were 23% in the group taking placebo, 8%

in the group taking aspirin, and 12% in the group receiving the combination.

The only study to find increased efficacy of dipyridamole in addition to aspirin was reported by Sanz et al.[109] One thousand one hundred twelve patients were enrolled in a multicenter, randomized, double-blind, placebo-controlled trial of aspirin (50 mg t.i.d.), aspirin (50 mg t.i.d.) plus dipyridamole (75 mg t.i.d.), and placebo. All patients received aspirin 100 mg q.i.d. for 48 hours before surgery and assigned treatment was begun 7 hours after surgery. Of the patients, 83% had angiography within 28 days of surgery. Aspirin plus dipyridamole significantly reduced occlusion rate compared with placebo (18% versus 12.9%, $p = .017$). Aspirin alone reduced the occlusion rate to near-significant levels (14% versus 12.9%, $p = .058$). There was increased chest tube drainage in the aspirin plus dipyridamole group, but no difference in hospital mortality or rate of early reoperation. In one trial, van der Meer et al. found no added benefit of dipyridamole 5 mg/kg per 24 hours intravenously for 28 hours preoperatively followed by 200 mg b.i.d. plus aspirin 50 mg/day compared with aspirin 50 mg/day alone in 948 patients (occlusion rate 15% versus 11% at 1 year, relative risk 0.76, 95% confidence interval 0.54 to 1.05).[89] Based on these combined data, no clear evidence supports the perioperative or long-term use of dipyridamole in the prevention of graft closure after coronary artery bypass.

Peripheral Vascular Disease

Hess et al. randomized patients with peripheral vascular disease to aspirin alone, aspirin plus dipyridamole, and placebo for 2 years.[110] Patients in the aspirin-dipyridamole group had 50% fewer occlusions than patients treated with aspirin alone. Aspirin alone was no better than placebo in preventing occlusion.

Table 14–8. **Coronary Artery Disease Antithrombotic Therapy 1994**

Syndrome	Risk	ASA	A/C	A/C + ASA <1 wk	A/C + ASA ≥1 wk
Unstable angina	High	+	+	+†	±*
MI (acute)—no lysis	High	+	±	?†	?‡
MI (acute)—lysis	High	+	±	±†	?‡
MI (acute)—LV-Ant	Medium	—	+	—	—
PTCA	High	+	+	+	—
SVBG	High	+	±	?*	?*
MI (>1 mo–3 yr)	Medium	±	+		?‡
Chronic/stable CAD	Medium	+	+		?*
Primary prevention	Low	±*	?		—

*Evolving approach in high risk: need of trials.
†GUSTO II (Hirudin)
‡Coumadin and Aspirin Reinfarction Study (CARS) (A/C + ASA low dose and fixed)

ASA, aspirin; A/C, anticoagulant; MI, myocardial infarction; LV-Ant, left ventricular anterior; PTCA, percutaneous transluminal coronary angioplasty; SVBG, saphenous vein bypass graft; CAD, coronary artery disease.

Analysis of randomization characteristics, however, revealed that patients in the aspirin group had significantly more stenoses by angiography before treatment than patients in the other groups. In a study by Schoop et al., patients were assigned randomly to receive aspirin, aspirin and dipyridamole, or placebo for 4 years.[111] In both active treatment groups, there was a significantly decreased occlusion rate compared with the rate in patients receiving placebo, but no difference between the two treatment arms was reported.

CONCLUSIONS

The selection of appropriate, effective antithrombotic therapy in cardiovascular disease is predicated on pathogenesis and risk. In high-risk situations such as unstable angina, myocardial infarction, and PTCA, use of combination antithrombotic therapy is recommended and established (Tables 14–7 and 14–8).[113] In medium-risk situations, combination therapy may be indicated in select patients if the risk of bleeding is acceptably low. In low-risk settings, the risk of combination therapy outweighs the benefits.

The role of combined antiplatelet and anticoagulant therapy is rapidly evolving. Major trials presently under way will address (1) the secondary prevention of myocardial infarction with aspirin and warfarin, (2) the prevention of mechanical prosthetic valve thromboembolism with aspirin and warfarin, (3) the prevention of thromboembolism in high-risk patients with thrombosis within cardiac chambers and atrial fibrillation with aspirin and warfarin, and (4) prevention of myocardial infarction and death in unstable angina with aspirin and selective thrombin inhibitors (Tables 14–8 and 14–9).

Major future efforts in this rapidly evolving field will include (1) establishing the increased therapeutic efficacy and cost-effectiveness of new combinations of anticoagulant agents and platelet inhibitors compared with currently available combinations of aspirin, heparin, and warfarin; (2) defining the role of low-dose aspirin and low-dose warfarin in primary prevention of myocardial infarction in high-risk patients, secondary prevention in all patients, and primary prevention of prosthetic valve thromboembolism; (3) developing

Table 14–9. **Present and Future Directions in Combination Antithrombotic Therapy**

Primary prevention (high risk)	Low-dose ASA + A/C
Chronic stable AP	Low-dose ASA + A/C LMWH + ASA
Secondary prevention S/P MI	Low-dose ASA + A/C
Unstable AP/non-Q MI: Acute	Selective thrombin inhibitors + ASA Hirudin, hirulog, argatroban Antiplatelet GP IIa/IIIb antibodies LMWH + ASA Low-dose ASA + A/C
Unstable AP/non-Q MI: Chronic	Low-dose ASA + A/C
MI: adjuncts to thrombolysis	Selective thrombin inhibitors + ASA Hirudin, hirulog, argatroban Antiplatelet GP IIa/IIIb antibodies LMWH + ASA
Coronary artery bypass surgery	Low-dose ASA + A/C
PTCA: Acute	Selective thrombin inhibitors Hirudin, hirulog, argatroban Antiplatelet GP IIa/IIIb antibodies
PTCA: Chronic	Platelet TXA_2 receptor antagonists Serotonin receptor antagonists Combined TXA_2 and GP IIa/IIIb antagonists
Prosthetic heart valve	Low-dose ASA + A/C
Atrial fibrillation	Low-dose ASA + A/C

ASA, aspirin; A/C, anticoagulants; AP, angina pectoris; S/P MI, status post–myocardial infarction; GP, glycoprotein; TXA_2, thromboxane A_2; PTCA, percutaneous transluminal coronary angioplasty; LMWH, low-molecular-weight heparin.

antiplatelet drugs that simultaneously inhibit multiple pathways of platelet activation; and (4) discovering combinations of antiplatelet and anticoagulant agents that individually inhibit separate platelet activation and coagulation system pathways and together exert a synergistic effect.

REFERENCES

1. Hirsh J: Heparin. N Engl J Med 324:1565, 1991.
2. Eisenberg P: Mechanism of action of heparin and anticoagulants therapy: Implications for the prevention of arterial thrombosis and the treatment of mural thrombosis. Coron Artery Dis 1:159, 1990.
3. Brill-Edwards P, Ginsberg J, Johnston M, et al: Establishing a therapeutic range for heparin therapy. Ann Intern Med 119:104, 1993.
4. Hirsh J: Low molecular weight heparin. Thromb Haemost 70:204, 1993.
5. Salzman E, Rosenberg R, Smith M, et al: Effects of heparin fractions on platelet aggregation. J Clin Invest 65:64, 1980.
6. Zucker M: Effects of heparin on platelet function. Thromb Diath Haemorrh 33:63, 1975.
7. Miletich J, Jackson C, Majerus P: Properties of factor Xa binding site on human platelets. J Biol Chem 253:6908, 1978.
8. Saba H, Saba S, Blackburn C, et al: Heparin neutralization of PGI2. Effects upon platelets. Science 205:499, 1979.
9. Lam L, Silbert J, Rosenberg R: The separation of active and inactive forms of heparin. Biochem Biophys Res Commun 69:570, 1976.
10. Anderson L, Barrowcliffe T, Holmer E, et al: Anticoagulant properties of heparin fractionated by affinity chromatography on matrix bound antithrombin III and by gel filtration. Thromb Res 9:575, 1976.
11. Hirsh J: Oral anticoagulant drugs. N Engl J Med 324:1865, 1991.
12. Hirsh J, Dalen J, Deykin D, et al: Oral anticoagulants: Mechanism of action, clinical effectiveness, and optimal therapeutic range. Chest 102(Suppl 4):312S, 1992.
13. Willerson J, Casscells W: Thrombin inhibitors in unstable angina: Rebound or continuation of angina after argatroban withdrawal. J Am Coll Cardiol 21:1048, 1993.
14. Deutsch E, Rao A, Colman R: Selective thrombin inhibitors: The next generation of anticoagulants. J Am Coll Cardiol 22:1089, 1993.
15. Hirudins: Return of the leech [editorial]. Lancet 340:579, 1992.
16. Heras M, Chesebro J, Webster M, et al: Hirudin, heparin, and placebo during deep arterial injury in the pig. Circulation 82:1476, 1990.
17. Verstraete M, Nurmohamed M, Kienast J, et al: Biologic effects of recombinant hirudin (CGP 39393) in human volunteers. J Am Coll Cardiol 22:1080, 1993.
18. Zoldhelyi P, Webster M, Fuster V, et al: Recombinant hirudin in patients with chronic, stable coronary artery disease. Circulation 88(part 1):2015, 1993.
19. Gold H, Torres F, Garabedian H, et al: Evidence for a rebound coagulation phenomenon after cessation of a 4-hour infusion of a specific thrombin inhibitor in patients with unstable angina pectoris. J Am Coll Cardiol 21:1039, 1993.
20. Jang I-K, Gold H, Leinbach R, et al: Persistent inhibition of arterial thrombosis by a 1-hour intravenous infusion of argatroban, a selective thrombin inhibitor. Coron Artery Dis 3:407, 1992.
21. Stein B, Fuster V, Israel D, et al: Platelet inhibitor agents in cardiovascular disease: An update. J Am Coll Cardiol 14:813, 1989.
22. Fuster V, Dyken M, Vokonas P, et al: Aspirin as a therapeutic agent in cardiovascular disease. Circulation 87:659, 1993.
23. Stein B, Fuster V: Clinical pharmacology of platelet inhibitors. In Fuster V, Verstraete M (eds): Thrombosis in Cardiovascular Disorders. Philadelphia: WB Saunders, 1992, pp 99–119.
24. Kristensen S, De Caterina R, Schmidt E, et al: Fish oil and ischaemic heart disease. Br Heart J 70:212, 1993.
25. Franklin S, Faxon D: Pharmacologic prevention of restenosis after coronary angioplasty: A review of the randomized clinical trials. Coron Artery Dis 4:232, 1993.
26. Packham M, Mustard J: Pharmacology of platelet affecting drugs. Circulation 62(Suppl V):V-26, 1980.
27. Fitzgerald G, Reilly I, Pedersen A: The biochemical pharmacology of thromboxane synthetase inhibition in man. Circulation 72:1194, 1985.
28. Vermylen J, Deckmyn H: Thromboxane synthase inhibitors and receptor antagonists. Cardiovasc Drugs Ther 6:29, 1992.
29. Saussy D, Mais D, Knapp D, et al: Thromboxane-A2 and prostaglandin endoperoxide receptors in platelets and vascular smooth muscle. Circulation 72:1202, 1985.
30. Knudtson M, Flintoft V, Roth D, et al: Effect of short-term prostacyclin administration on restenosis after percutaneous coronary angioplasty. J Am Coll Cardiol 15:691, 1990.
31. Lam J, Chesebro J, Badimon L, et al: Exogenous prostacyclin decreases vasoconstriction but no platelet thrombus deposition after arterial injury. J Am Coll Cardiol 21:488, 1993.
32. Lam J, Chesebro J, Steele P, et al: Deep arterial injury during experimental angioplasty: Relations to a positive indium-111 platelet scintigram, quantitative platelet deposition and mural thrombosis. J Am Coll Cardiol 8:1380, 1986.
33. Kiemuda K, Abiko Y: Comparative study of heparin and a synthetic thrombin inhibitor no. 805 (MD 805) in experimental antithrombin III deficient animals. Thromb Res 24:285, 1981.
34. Sturzebecher J, Markwardt F, Boight B, et al: Cyclic amides of N-alpha-arylsulfonyl-aminoacylated 4 amidinophenylalanine—tight-binding inhibitors of thrombin. Thromb Res 29:635, 1983.
35. Hanson S, Harker L: Interruption of acute platelet dependent thrombosis by the synthetic antithrombin D-phenylalanyl-L-prolyl-L-arginyl chloromethylketone (FPRMeCl). Proc Natl Acad Sci U S A 85:3184, 1988.
36. Cliveden P, Salzman E: Platelet metabolism and the effect of drugs. In Bowie EJW, Sharp AA (eds): Hemostasis and Thrombosis. London: Butterworth, 1985, pp 1–35.
37. Genton E, Gent M, Hirsh J, et al: Platelet inhibiting drugs in the prevention of clinical thrombotic disease. N Engl J Med 293:1174, 1975.
38. O'Brien J, Etherington M, Shuttleworth R: Ticlopidine—an antiplatelet drug: Effects in human volunteers. Thromb Res 18:245, 1978.
39. O'Brien J: Ticlopidine, a promise for the prevention and treatment of thrombosis and its complications. Haemostasis 13:1, 1983.
40. Wilkinson A, Hawker R, Hawker J: The influence of antiplatelet drugs on platelet survival after aortic damage or implantation of a dacron arterial prosthesis. Thromb Res 15:181, 1979.
41. Cairns J, Hirsh J, Lewis H, et al: Antithrombotic agents in coronary artery disease. Chest 102(Suppl 4):456S, 1992.
42. Willerson J, Golino P, Eidt J, et al: Specific platelet mediators and unstable coronary artery lesions: Experimental evidence and potential clinical implications. Circulation 80:198, 1989.
43. Clagett G, Graor R, Salzman E: Antithrombotic therapy in peripheral arterial occlusive disease. Chest 102(Suppl 4):516S, 1992.
44. Topol E, Plow E: Clinical trials of platelet receptor inhibitors. Thromb Haemost 70:94, 1993.
45. Verstraete M: Novel antithrombotic agents. In Fuster V, Verstraete M (eds): Thrombosis in Cardiovascular Disorders. Philadelphia: WB Saunders, 1992, pp 529–543.
46. Chesebro J, Fuster V, Elveback L, et al: Trial of combined warfarin plus dipyridamole or aspirin therapy in prosthetic heart valve replacement: Danger of aspirin compared with dipyridamole. Am J Cardiol 51:1537, 1983.
47. Groupe de Recherche PACTE: Prévention des accidents thromboemboliques systémiques chez les proteurs de prosthesis valvulaires artificielles: Essai cooperatif contrôle du dipyridamole. Coeur 9:915, 1978.
48. Kasahara T: Clinical effects of dipyridamole ingestion after prosthetic heart valve replacement—especially on the blood coagulation system. J Jpn Assoc Thorac Surg 25:1007, 1977.
49. Rajah S, Srecharan N, Joseph A, et al: A prospective trial of dipyridamole and warfarin in heart valve patients [abstract]. Acta Ther 6(Suppl 93):514, 1980.

50. Sullivan J, Harken D, Gorlin R: Pharmacologic control of thromboembolic complications of cardiac valve replacement. N Engl J Med 284:1391, 1971.

51. Dale J, Myhre E, Storstein O, et al: Prevention of arterial thromboembolism with acetylsalicylic acid: A controlled clinical study in patients with aortic ball valves. Am Heart J 94:101, 1977.

52. Altman R, Boullon F, Rouvier J, et al: Aspirin and prophylaxis of thromboembolic complications in patients with substitute heart valves. J Thorac Cardiovasc Surg 72:127, 1976.

53. Turpie A, Gent M, Laupacis A, et al: A comparison of aspirin with placebo in patients treated with warfarin after heart-valve replacement. N Engl J Med 329:524, 1993.

54. Steele P, Rainwater J, Vogel R: Platelet suppressant therapy in patients with prosthetic heart valves: Relationship of clinical effectiveness to alteration of platelet survival time. Circulation 60:910, 1979.

55. Singer D: Randomized trials of warfarin for atrial fibrillation. N Engl J Med 327:1451, 1992.

56. Fuster V, Badimon L, Badimon J, Chesebro J: The pathogenesis of coronary artery disease and the acute coronary syndromes. N Engl J Med 326:242, 1992.

57. Theroux P, Lidon R: Unstable angina: Pathogenesis, diagnosis, and treatment. Curr Prob Cardiol 17:157, 1993.

58. Theroux P, Ouimet H, McCans J, et al: Aspirin, heparin, or both to treat acute unstable angina. N Engl J Med 319:1105, 1988.

59. Theroux P, Waters D, Lam J, et al: Reactivation of unstable angina after the discontinuation of heparin. N Engl J Med 327:141, 1992.

60. The RISC Group: Risk of myocardial infarction and death during treatment with low dose aspirin and intravenous heparin in men with unstable coronary artery disease. Lancet 336:827, 1990.

61. Theroux P, Waters D, Qiu S, et al: Aspirin versus heparin to prevent myocardial infarction during the acute phase of unstable angina. Circulation 88:2045, 1993.

62. Cohen M, Adams P, Parry G, et al: Combination antithrombotic therapy in unstable rest angina and non-Q-wave infarction in nonprior aspirin users: Primary end points analysis from the ATACS Trial. Circulation 89:81, 1994.

63. Lidon R, Theroux P, Juneau M, et al: Initial experience with a direct antithrombin, hirulog, in unstable angina. Circulation 88:1495, 1993.

64. The TIMI IIIA Investigators: Early effects of tissue-type plasminogen activator added to conventional therapy on the culprit lesion in patients presenting with ischemic cardiac pain at rest: Results of the Thrombolysis in Myocardial Ischemia (TIMI IIIA) trial. Circulation 87:38, 1993.

65. ISIS-2 Collaborative Group: Randomised trial of intravenous streptokinase, oral aspirin, both, or neither among 17,187 cases of suspected acute myocardial infarction: ISIS-2. Lancet 2:349, 1988.

66. The SCATI Group: Randomised controlled trial of subcutaneous calcium-heparin in acute myocardial infarction. Lancet 2:182, 1989.

67. Gruppo Italiano per lo Studio lella Sopravvivenza nell'Infarto Miocardico: GISSI-2: A factorial randomised trial of alteplase versus streptokinase and heparin versus no heparin among 12,490 patients with acute myocardial infarction. Lancet 336:65, 1990.

68. ISIS-3 Collaborative Group: ISIS-3: A randomised comparison of streptokinase vs tissue plasminogen activator vs anistreplase and of aspirin plus heparin vs aspirin alone among 41,299 cases of suspected acute myocardial infarction. Lancet 339:753, 1992.

69. The GUSTO Investigators: An international randomized trial comparing four thrombolytic strategies for acute myocardial infarction. N Engl J Med 329:674, 1993.

70. The GUSTO Angiographic Investigators: The effects of tissue plasminogen activator, streptokinase, or both on coronary-artery patency, ventricular function, and survival after acute myocardial infarction. N Engl J Med 329:1615, 1993.

71. TAMI Study Group: A randomized controlled trial of intravenous tissue plasminogen activator and early intravenous heparin in acute myocardial infarction. Circulation 79:281, 1989.

72. Bleich S, Nichols T, Schumacher R, et al: Effect of heparin on coronary patency after thrombolysis with tissue plasminogen activator in acute myocardial infarction. Am J Cardiol 66:1412, 1990.

73. Heparin-Aspirin Reperfusion Trial (HART). A comparison between heparin and low-dose aspirin as adjunctive therapy with tissue-type plasminogen activator for acute myocardial infarction. N Engl J Med 323:1433, 1990.

74. de Bono P, Simoons M, Tijssen J, et al: Effect of early intravenous heparin on coronary patency, infarct size, and bleeding complications after alteplase thrombolysis: Results of randomised double blind European Cooperative Study Group trial. Br Heart J 67:122, 1992.

75. Thompson P, Aylward P, Federman J, et al: A randomized comparison of intravenous heparin with oral aspirin and dipyridamole 24 hours after recombinant tissue-type plasminogen activator for acute myocardial infarction. Circulation 83:1534, 1991.

76. Braunwald E: The open-artery theory alive and well again. N Engl J Med 93:329, 1993.

77. Schwartz R, Edwards W, Huber K, et al: Coronary restenosis: Prospects for solution and new perspectives from a porcine model. Mayo Clin Proc 68:54, 1993.

78. Schwartz L, Bourassa M, Lesperance J, et al: Aspirin and dipyridamole in the prevention of restenosis after percutaneous transluminal coronary angioplasty. N Engl J Med 318:1714, 1988.

79. Califf R, Fortin D, Frid D, et al: Restenosis after coronary angioplasty: An overview. J Am Coll Cardiol 17:2B, 1991.

80. Califf R, Willerson J: Percutaneous transluminal coronary angioplasty: Prevention of occlusion and restenosis. In Fuster V, Verstraete M (eds): Thrombosis in Cardiovascular Disorders. Philadelphia: WB Saunders, 1992, pp 389–408.

81. Ellis S, Roubin G, Wilentz J, et al: Effect of 18- to 24-hour heparin administration for prevention of restenosis after uncomplicated coronary angioplasty. Am Heart J 117:777, 1989.

82. Topol E, Bonan R, Jewitt D, et al: Use of a direct antithrombin, hirulog, in place of heparin during coronary angioplasty. Circulation 87:1622, 1993.

83. Chesebro J, Goldman S: Coronary artery bypass surgery: Antithrombotic therapy. In Fuster V, Verstraete M (eds): Thrombosis in Cardiovascular Disorders. Philadelphia: WB Saunders, 1992, pp 375–388.

84. Goldman S, Copeland J, Moritz T, et al: Improvement in early saphenous vein graft patency after coronary artery bypass surgery with antiplatelet therapy: Results of a Veterans Administration Cooperative Study. Circulation 77:1324, 1988.

85. Goldman S, Copeland J, Moritz T, et al: Internal mammary artery and saphenous vein graft patency: Effects of aspirin. Circulation 82(Suppl IV):IV-237, 1990.

86. Goldman S, Copeland J, Moritz T, et al: Saphenous vein graft patency 1 year after coronary artery bypass surgery and effects of antiplatelet therapy: Results of a Veterans Administration Cooperative Study. Circulation 80:1190, 1989.

87. Chesebro J, Fuster V, Elveback L, et al: Effect of dipyridamole and aspirin on late vein graft patency after coronary bypass operations. N Engl J Med 310:209, 1984.

88. Pfisterer M, Burkart F, Jockers G, et al: Trial of low-dose aspirin plus dipyridamole versus anticoagulants for prevention of aortocoronary vein graft occlusion. Lancet 1:1, 1989.

89. van der Meer J, Hillege H, Kootstra G, et al: Prevention of one-year vein-graft occlusion after aortocoronary bypass surgery: A comparison of low-dose aspirin, low-dose aspirin plus dipyridamole, and oral anticoagulants. Lancet 342:257, 1993.

90. Ip J, Fuster V, Badimon L, et al: Syndromes of accelerated atherosclerosis: Role of vascular injury and smooth muscle cell proliferation. J Am Coll Cardiol 15:1667, 1990.

91. Antiplatelet Trialists' Collaboration: Secondary prevention of vascular disease by prolonged antiplatelet treatment. Br Med J 296:320, 1988.

92. Antiplatelet Trialists' Collaboration: Collaborative overview of randomized trials of antiplatelet therapy: I, II, III. Br Med J 308:81, 1994.

93. Harrison M, Pollack S, Steiner M, et al: Inhibitors of

"spontaneous" platelet aggregation in whole blood. Athero-sclerosis 58:199, 1985.

94. Hanson K, Harker L, Bjornsson T: Effects of platelet modifying drugs on arterial thromboembolism in baboons: Aspirin potentiates the antithrombotic actions of dipyridamole and sulfinpyrazone by mechanism(s) independent of platelet cyclooxygenase inhibition. J Clin Invest 75:1591, 1985.

95. Bousser M, Eschwege E, Haguenau M, et al: "AICLA" controlled trial of aspirin and dipyridamole in the secondary prevention of atherothrombotic cerebral ischemia. Stroke 14:5, 1983.

96. American-Canadian Cooperative Study Group: Persantine aspirin trial in cerebral ischemia-Part II. Endpoint results. Stroke 16:406, 1985.

97. European Stroke Prevention Study Group: The European Stroke Prevention Study (ESPS). Principal end points. Lancet 2:1351 1987.

98. Acheson J, Danta G, Hutchinson E: Controlled trial of dipyridamole in cerebral vascular disease. Stroke 8:301, 1978.

99. Persantine-Aspirin Reinfarction Study Group: Persantine and aspirin in coronary heart disease. Circulation 62:449, 1980.

100. Klimt C, Knatterud G, Stammler J, et al: Persantine-aspirin reinfarction study—Part II. Secondary coronary prevention with persantine and aspirin. J Am Coll Cardiol 7:251, 1986.

101. Aspirin after myocardial infarction [editorial]. Lancet 1:1172, 1980.

102. Fitzgerald G: Dipyridamole. N Engl J Med 316:1247, 1987.

103. Lewis H, Davis J, Archibald D, et al: Protective effects of aspirin against acute myocardial infarction and death in men with unstable angina. N Engl J Med 309:396, 1983.

104. Cairns J, Gent M, Singer J, et al: Aspirin, sulfinpyrazone, or both in unstable angina. N Engl J Med 313:1369, 1985.

105. Becker R, Smith K, Dobell A: Effect of platelet inhibition on platelet phenomenon in cardiopulmonary bypass in pigs. Ann Surg 179:52, 1974.

106. Nuutinen L, Pihlajaniemi R, Sarrela E, et al: The effect of dipyridamole on the thrombocyte count and bleeding tendency in open heart surgery. J Thorac Cardiovasc Surg 74:25, 1977.

107. Lorenz R, Weber M, Kotzur J, et al: Improved aortocoronary bypass patency by low dose aspirin (100 mg/daily). Effects on platelet aggregation and thromboxane formation. Lancet 1:1262, 1984.

108. Brown B, Cukingnan R, DeRouen T, et al: Improved graft patency in patients with platelet inhibiting therapy after coronary artery bypass surgery. Circulation 71:138, 1985.

109. Sanz G, Pajaron A, Alegria E, et al: Prevention of early aortocoronary bypass occlusion by low-dose aspirin and dipyridamole. Circulation 82:765, 1990.

110. Hess H, Mietaschk A, Deischel G: Drug induced inhibition of platelet function delays progression of peripheral occlusive arterial disease: A prospective double blind arteriographically controlled trial. Lancet 1:415, 1985.

111. Schoop W, Levy H, Schoop B, et al: Experimentelle und klinische Studien zu der sekundaren Pravention der Peripheran Arteriosklerose. *In* Bollinger A, Rhyner K (eds): Thrombozyten Funktionschemmer. Stuttgart: Georg Thieme, 1983, pp 49–58.

112. Altman R, Rouvier J, Gurfinkel E, et al: Comparison of two levels of anticoagulant therapy in patients with substitute heart valves [see comments]. J Thorac Cardiovasc Surg 101:427, 1991.

113. Stein B, Fuster V, Halperin JL, Chesebro JH: Antithrombotic therapy in cardiac disease. An emerging approach based on pathogenesis and risk. Circulation 80:1501, 1989.

III.
Drug Treatment of Cardiovascular Emergencies

Editors: Robert Zelis and Eric L. Michelson

CHAPTER 15

Acute Pulmonary Edema

Dwight Davis, M.D., and Robert Zelis, M.D.

Acute pulmonary edema is a common medical emergency caused by the rapid accumulation of fluid in the interstitial space and alveoli of the lungs. It is caused either by severe structural or functional abnormalities of the left side of the heart or by inflammatory damage of the pulmonary microvasculature with leakage of fluid and solute into the interstitial and alveolar spaces. The gas exchange is greatly impaired, and hypoxemia develops. Pulmonary edema arising from either cardiac or noncardiac sources is a major health care and socioeconomic problem for this country. It is estimated that more than 3 million people have congestive heart failure, with approximately 400,000 new cases recognized each year. Heart failure leads to 900,000 hospital admissions each year and often is manifested by pulmonary edema.[1-3] In addition, 150,000 people are diagnosed each year with pulmonary edema from a noncardiac source.[4] Both disorders are characterized by high rates of mortality and significant morbidity. Prompt diagnosis and expeditious therapy is essential for successful patient outcome.

CARDIOGENIC PULMONARY EDEMA

The cardinal symptom of cardiogenic pulmonary edema is dyspnea. However, many other medical emergencies present similarly. The physician must first determine that the dyspneic patient is indeed suffering from pulmonary edema and, second, define the underlying pathophysiologic mechanisms. Effective therapy depends on a sound understanding of the various causes followed by a thorough and orderly approach to eliminating precipitating factors, when possible, and correction of cardiopulmonary and metabolic abnormalities.

Pathophysiology

The underlying pathophysiologic causes of pulmonary edema can be classified into two general categories: (1) hemodynamic and (2) primary alteration in the permeability of the alveolar-capillary membrane. The first involves an alteration in the Starling equation, which describes the relationship involved with the flow of liquid from pulmonary capillaries to interstitial spaces of the lung. Under normal circumstances, fluid is filtered from the pulmonary vasculature into the interstitial space and is subsequently removed by the pulmonary lymphatic system. Pulmonary edema occurs when the net flow of fluid into the interstitial space is increased and exceeds the capacity for lymphatic drainage. Normally, there is a continuous exchange of fluid, colloid, and solutes between the pulmonary vascular bed and the pulmonary interstitial space that is governed by components of hydrostatic pressure, capillary permeability, oncotic pressure, and lymphatic clearance. Hemodynamic alterations of one or several of these components or a structural abnormality of the pulmonary capillary membrane leads to the progressive development of pulmonary edema. Typically, there is an initial increase in the movement of fluid and colloid from the pulmonary capillaries into the pulmonary interstitium. At some point, this increased flow overwhelms the capacity for lymphatic drainage with net accumulation of fluid in the interstitial space. With continued accumulation of interstitial fluid and elevation of pulmonary venous pressure, fluid eventually leaks into the alveolar space.[5-7]

Hemodynamic pulmonary edema is caused by any process that elevates left atrial pressure. This process is due most commonly to left ventricular dysfunction or mitral stenosis, but other contributing factors may play secondary roles, such as arrhythmia, infection, inadvertent volume administration, or inappropriate medication with a negative inotropic agent in patients with compensated heart failure (Table 15–1). Diseases that affect the pulmonary lymphatic system, such as silicosis or bronchogenic cancer with lymphangitic spread, can also result in pulmonary edema without

Table 15–1. **Precipitating Factors for Cardiogenic Pulmonary Edema and Their Related Mechanisms**

Prolonged myocardial ischemia
 • Decreased systolic function and increased diastolic stiffness
Myocardial infarction
Excessive salt ingestion
 • Increased plasma volume
Excessive intravenous fluid administration
 • Increased plasma volume
Arrhythmia
 • Compromised cardiac output by rapid or slow heart rates, altered function by abnormal atrioventricular conduction and loss of atrial "kick"
Discontinuation of cardiac medications
 • Diuretics—increased plasma volume
 • Vasodilators—increased vascular resistance and cardiac afterload
 • Digitalis—rapid conduction, decreased inotropy
Infection, hypermetabolic states, surgery, pregnancy
 • Need for increased cardiac output or volume overload
Endocarditis
 • Valve damage with ventricular volume overload
Inappropriate drug administration, drug overdose
 • Cardiac depressant drugs (antiarrhythmic agents), β-blockers, alcohol
 • Fluid-retaining drugs (steroids, nonsteroidal anti-inflammatory agents)
Uncontrolled systemic hypertension
 • Left ventricular pressure overload
Acute physical and emotional stress
 • Increased hemodynamic burden due to tachycardia, volume overload, or systemic hypertension

significant elevation of pulmonary capillary pressures, but these causes are clinically less common.

Although left ventricular failure is the most common cause, the development of acute pulmonary edema in this setting is often the end result of many interactive processes that ultimately overwhelm protective compensatory mechanisms. Left ventricular dysfunction may progress for an extended period without overt clinical manifestations of congestive heart failure because of adaptive support from these mechanisms.

Important components of these adaptive mechanisms include myocardial hypertrophy with and without dilatation; the Frank-Starling mechanism, wherein an increase in preload helps to preserve cardiac systolic function; stimulation of the sympathetic nervous system with release of catecholamines; and activation of a number of vasoactive and nephrogenic hormones, including the renin-angiotensin-aldosterone system.[8, 9] When central adaptive processes fail, resulting in a decrease in cardiac output, peripheral mechanisms involving vasoconstriction and salt and water retention are activated to maintain organ perfusion.[10] In addition to peripheral vasoconstrictor effects, catecholamine release from sympathetic nervous system stimulation also acts centrally to increase heart rate and augment myocardial contractility. These processes eventually lead to further compromise in ventricular performance, graphically characterized by a shift downward and to the right of the ventricular function curve, which forms a new curve characterized by decreased cardiac output and ele-

vated left ventricular filling pressures (Fig. 15–1). Eventually, pulmonary edema occurs when the compensatory mechanisms are overwhelmed, usually by some precipitating event. When pulmonary edema develops, sympathetically mediated vasoconstriction is particularly prominent. Intense venoconstriction leads to plasma volume contraction with further transfer of fluid into the pulmonary interstitium, further aggravating gas exchange.

Clinical Aspects

The initial evaluation should focus on historical evidence of prior cardiovascular or pulmonary disease and, especially, recent events that might have led to decompensation (see Table 15–1). It is critical to know what medications the patient has been taking, especially any recent changes such as discontinuation of a diuretic or the addition of a negative inotropic agent. The physical examination should confirm the diagnosis of pulmonary edema and provide helpful informa-

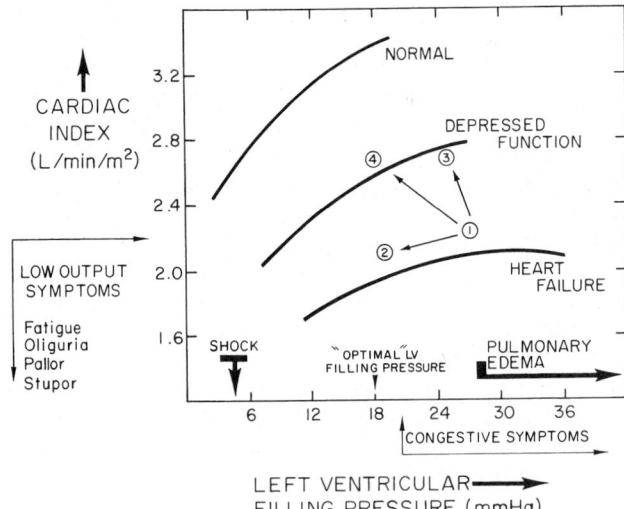

Figure 15–1. Ventricular function curves relating ventricular systolic function (cardiac index) to ventricular preload (left ventricular [LV] filling pressure, or pulmonary artery wedge pressure). The patient with decompensated heart failure has acute pulmonary edema, with markedly elevated ventricular filling pressures (*horizontal arrow*), or shock, with greatly reduced cardiac index (*vertical arrow*). Treatment of patients in pulmonary edema (position 1) consists of preload reduction (e.g., sitting posture, positive pressure breathing, and venodilating drugs such as nitroglycerin, morphine, and loop diuretics) to improve the condition of the patient to position 2. This effect predominantly reduces LV filling pressures and thereby relieves pulmonary congestive symptoms. Treatment with agents that enhance LV contractility or reduce both preload and afterload (e.g., oxygen administration, dobutamine, digoxin, nitroprusside) improves the patient's condition from position 1 to position 4. Afterload reduction (e.g., drugs with arteriolar dilating effects such as phentolamine or hydralazine) predominantly improves cardiac index and improves the patient's condition from position 1 to position 3. Afterload reduction causes the smallest decrease in LV filling pressure. In patients with pulmonary edema, knowledge of the cardiac index and LV filling pressure can help guide therapy for the best physiologic response.

tion regarding the underlying pathophysiologic condition and the patient's clinical status.

The typical patient with pulmonary edema is anxious, often struggling to stay in an upright position, with tachypneic respirations using accessory muscles; the skin is cool, clammy, and wet with perspiration; there may be coughing with production of pink, frothy sputum; and the skin is often cyanotic. The blood pressure can be either elevated because of sympathetic nervous system stimulation or depressed from severely compromised left ventricular function. The hallmark of pulmonary edema is pulmonary rales, which are normally widespread, covering most of the posterior and anterior lung fields. Common physical findings indicating compromised cardiac function include jugular venous distention, a laterally displaced apical impulse, tachycardia, and a ventricular or summation gallop. The findings of pedal edema, hepatomegaly, and ascites are helpful in generally indicating dysfunction of the right side of the heart secondary to chronic heart failure of the left side of the heart.

The preliminary history and physical examination are usually adequate to establish a diagnosis and initiate primary therapy. Patients should be questioned about factors commonly associated with ventricular dysfunction such as coronary artery disease, a prior myocardial infarction, history of a heart murmur, hypertension, diabetes, and a history of rheumatic fever. However, basic laboratory evaluation often confirms diagnosis and helps establish an underlying cause. The chest radiograph may be extremely helpful in the initial evaluation of patients with pulmonary edema. However, one guiding principle must be kept in mind—that abnormal alveolar or septal opacities may not reflect the degree of underlying pathophysiology, and the paucity of findings does not exclude severely compromised gas exchange. When abnormalities are present, they may provide clues in distinguishing pulmonary edema of cardiac origin from pulmonary edema caused by increased pulmonary capillary membrane permeability.

The chest radiograph in patients with cardiogenic pulmonary edema is characterized by a progression of findings, including redistribution of blood flow to upper segments, engorgement of pulmonary veins, early hilar distribution of fluid, prominent septal lines, pleural effusions, and cardiomegaly. In contrast, the chest radiograph in patients with noncardiogenic pulmonary edema typically demonstrates a vascular pedicle that is normal or sometimes reduced, a more peripheral pattern of fluid, no septal lines, and the absence of cardiomegaly. A number of cardiac abnormalities can produce acute pulmonary edema without cardiomegaly, including acute myocardial infarction, acute papillary muscle dysfunction, acute aortic or mitral valve dysfunction, arrhythmias in the setting of ventricular systolic and diastolic dysfunction, and acute ventricular septal defect. In addition, it is important to review the films for evidence of substantial pleural effusions, regions of collapsed or unaerated pulmonary segments, and pneumothorax. Any of these findings may complicate or alter the approach to pulmonary care.

The electrocardiogram often serves as an important screening tool in the initial evaluation of patients with pulmonary edema. Although findings can be nonspecific, many alterations indicate the underlying acute event or suggest chronic cardiac processes that may have contributed to the presentation. Myocardial infarction and ischemia are common causes of pulmonary edema and lend themselves to diagnosis by the electrocardiogram. Evolving electrocardiographic changes in addition to serial myocardial enzyme determination should be used to diagnose or exclude myocardial infarction. Ischemic-appearing repolarization abnormalities (i.e., ST-segment depression) can often represent nonspecific changes related to heart rate, conduction abnormalities, drugs, metabolic imbalances, or underlying ventricular pressure load or volume load states. Electrocardiographic evidence of right axis deviation and dilatation of the right side of the heart and/or strain should raise the possibility of acute pulmonary embolus or underlying chronic obstructive pulmonary disease.

The initial assessment and ongoing monitoring of the patient's rhythm should be a standard part of medical care. Rhythm disturbances not infrequently play a primary role in the development of pulmonary edema, particularly in the setting of underlying structural or functional cardiac abnormalities. The finding of arrhythmias producing hemodynamic instability should be addressed immediately. In certain situations, cardioversion may be required in patients with sustained atrial or atrioventricular nodal tachycardias associated with a rapid ventricular response, mitral stenosis, aortic stenosis, or impaired systolic or diastolic dysfunction. In addition, patients with ventricular tachycardia may need immediate cardioversion. In other circumstances, temporary pacing may be needed for patients with high-grade atrioventricular block or severe bradycardia.

It is important early in the evaluation to determine the degree of respiratory insufficiency. An arterial blood gas determination is invaluable in assessing the initial magnitude of hypoxemia, the presence or absence of hypercapnea, and the adequacy of pulmonary and metabolic compensatory mechanisms. If there is no significant underlying chronic lung disease, respiratory alkalosis normally develops initially, followed by respiratory acidosis; later, metabolic acidosis occurs as the patient's condition worsens. Following the preliminary blood gas evaluation and initiation of therapy, serial determinations will be needed to monitor patient response.

Metabolic abnormalities and drug toxicity may play important roles in the pathophysiology of pulmonary edema. It is helpful to evaluate blood levels of potentially toxic agents such as digitalis, antiarrhythmic drugs, bronchodilator compounds, or other medications with negative inotropic properties. Other routine laboratory blood tests may prove helpful. Abnormalities of the leukocyte count may provide early evidence of infectious processes. If significant anemia is present, the cause should be promptly identified and treated. In this regard, the need for red blood cell transfusion should be established early. Long-standing right ventricular failure can produce liver function abnormalities from high venous pressures. A diffuse nonspecific pattern of liver function abnormalities is common. The degree of hepatic dysfunction may impact significantly on clotting status and drug metabolism. Abnormalities in serum electrolytes and renal function may reflect altered perfusion from myocardial dysfunction or the state of effective intravascular volume. Alterations in calcium and magnesium can adversely affect myocardial function; therefore, serum levels should be included in the initial blood screen.

Steps in Therapy

Proper management of the typical patient with pulmonary edema requires that a number of medical issues be addressed simultaneously. The assistance of other physicians, nurses, and often ancillary support staff greatly aids in the initial stabilization period. The responsible physician needs to direct the team so that activities are prioritized and coordinated.

Effective therapy begins with expeditious but comprehensive assessment of the patient's clinical status. The first priority involves making the correct diagnosis of pulmonary edema versus other processes that may present with dyspnea and significant hypoxemia, such as respiratory failure from chronic lung disease, pulmonary embolism, severe pneumonia, or bronchial asthma. Second, it is important during the initial assessment to try to establish a diagnosis of the underlying disease process, remembering that pulmonary edema is a symptom with diverse causes that may have specific therapeutic consequences. Third, many episodes of pulmonary edema have definable precipitating causes. A management approach that addresses a specific precipitating factor will be the most effective.[11]

Although effective therapy for acute pulmonary edema must be individualized, several basic goals must be kept in mind. The initial goals are rapid relief of dyspnea and correction of hypoxemia. These goals are accomplished by a systematic approach to the basic pathophysiologic mechanisms that are present: (1) relieve pulmonary congestion (decrease preload) and thereby improve oxygenation, (2) decrease systemic vascular resistance (decrease afterload), (3) improve myocardial systolic function, (4) improve myocardial diastolic function (i.e., ventricular compliance), and (5) preserve adequate systemic arterial perfusion pressure.[12]

Initial measures should include insertion of both intravenous and arterial lines with blood sent for electrolyte, hepatic, and renal determinations in addition to blood gases. Unless there is rapid improvement in symptoms with resolution of hypoxemia, most patients will require placement of a flow-directed, balloon-tipped catheter for hemodynamic monitoring to guide cardiopulmonary therapy. The broad indications for catheterization of the right side of the heart in this setting include confirmation of a cardiac versus a noncardiac origin for pulmonary edema, evaluation of hemodynamic parameters, guidance of therapy aimed at improving cardiac function, and monitoring potential complications of therapy (such as compromised hemodynamics with positive end-expiratory pressure). If possible, sedatives are best withheld initially if the mental status is abnormal, because changes may represent hypercapnia accompanying hypoxemia.

Patients will innately assume an upright posture in which the arms support the upper chest cage. This will increase the efficiency of accessory muscles that are needed for the tremendously increased work of breathing. In addition to the pulmonary mechanical benefits of upright posture, central hemodynamics are also aided by splanchnic and lower extremity pooling of blood with a resultant decrease in venous return. When possible, therapy should be initiated with the patient in this position with the legs placed in a dependent position and a bedside table used for arm support.

Respiratory Care

When the patient with pulmonary edema is first seen, it is important to recognize the possibility of impending or progressive respiratory failure with appropriate preparation for intubation. Accordingly, the patient must be attended at all times until clinically stable. Providing supplemental oxygen is vital in the initial management, and intubation often can be avoided by thoughtful selection of concentration and method of administration. Therapy is most effective if guided by results of serial blood gas measurements.

The simple goal of supplemental oxygen therapy is to correct hypoxemia to a level of oxygen tension that meets the body's basic metabolic needs. The shape of the oxygen-hemoglobin dissociation curve is characterized by a steep and progressive decrease in arterial oxygen saturation and content when Pa_{O_2} is below 60 mmHg. Therefore supplemental oxygen is clearly warranted at this level of hypoxia or when there is a decrease in oxygen saturation to below 90%. In initiating therapy, it should also be kept in mind that providing supplemental oxygen to levels that exceed this range offers no metabolic benefit and can expose the patient to the risk of oxygen toxicity if therapy is prolonged.

In the patient without underlying chronic pulmonary disease, high-concentration humidified oxygen by face mask should be administered without delay. In contrast, patients with severe chronic pulmonary disease may have their ventilatory drive suppressed by hyperoxia. In this setting, low-flow oxygen supplementation with progressive increases until oxygen levels are at least 50 mmHg is warranted with close monitoring of clinical and laboratory parameters for alveolar hypoventilation. In this process, it is important that patients are not exposed to significant hypoxia for prolonged periods. Accordingly, a history of underlying chronic obstructive pulmonary disease or bronchial asthma is extremely helpful in planning supplemental oxygen therapy.

Nasal cannulas or Venturi masks may be appropriate for initial low-concentration oxygen therapy in selected patients. If adequate gas exchange can be obtained, nasal cannulas are usually better tolerated and can be left in place for other activities such as eating, talking, or coughing without interrupting supply. Nonrebreathing masks provide a higher concentration of oxygen but must fit tightly to function properly. This may be poorly tolerated if dyspnea is not quickly relieved, leading to the common scenario that endotracheal intubation is often necessary if an oxygen concentration above 50% is required for more than several hours.

If initial measures are not successful after a brief period, then supplemental oxygen by other noninvasive means may be effective to treat refractory hypoxemia. Continuous positive airway pressure (CPAP) delivered by a properly fitting face mask provides the next level of respiratory care. Although mortality and length of hospital stay may not be affected, oxygenation improves and the need for endotracheal intubation and mechanical ventilation is reduced.[13] A trial of CPAP for 10 to 15 minutes at 5 to 10 cm H_2O may reverse hypoxemia.[14] Effective CPAP requires a fully conscious and cooperative patient with intact airway reflexes. Individual patient responses to CPAP are unpredictable, and the risk of barotrauma and pneumothorax becomes greater with increasing levels of positive pressure. Accordingly, continuous clinical observation and serial blood gas monitoring are important.

If the respiratory response to conservative measures is inadequate, intubation should be performed as a semielective procedure before the critical situation of cardiopulmonary arrest arises. A number of general guidelines, along with close clinical assessment of the patient's status, are used to make the decision for mechanical ventilation, including (1) excessive work of breathing with progressive fatigue, (2) persistent or worsening hypoxia, (3) severe and increasing hypercapnia, (4) increasing obtundation, and (5) acidemia with worsening hemodynamic levels.

Pharmacologic Therapy

Nitroglycerin

The use of nitroglycerin has been shown to effectively and rapidly improve central hemodynamics in patients with acute pulmonary edema.[15] Typically, nitroglycerin is combined with morphine and diuretics to stabilize the patient's clinical status.[16] Nitrates provide their beneficial hemodynamic effects in pulmonary edema through potent venodilating properties when administered in low concentrations. Given sublingually, nitrates offer the advantage of convenience, rapid onset of action, and relatively short duration of effect. The onset of action is approximately 2 minutes with venodilation for 30 to 45 minutes. Serial doses

of 0.4 mg (sublingually administered tablet or lingual spray) can be administered at 10- to 15-minute intervals.[17] At higher doses, nitrates also dilate arterial resistance vessels, resulting in a decrease of both blood pressure and afterload.[18]

In patients with acute pulmonary edema and active myocardial ischemia, nitroglycerin can be administered as a continuous infusion starting at 5 μg/min with titration up by increments of 5 μg/min at 5-minute intervals. In this setting, nitrates can reduce myocardial oxygen demand by reducing left ventricular filling pressure.[19] Patient selection and clinical observation is important in the early use of nitroglycerin. Myocardial ischemia can be exacerbated if there is a profound reduction in systemic arterial pressure with resulting compromise in coronary perfusion. Hypotension is less of a problem in patients with peripheral edema and increased intravascular volume.

Three other situations warrant careful attention when considering the use of intravenous nitroglycerin. The drug should be avoided in patients with a hemodynamic profile characterized by low blood pressure, low ventricular filling pressures, and low cardiac output. Nitrates should be used with caution in patients with acute pulmonary edema associated with inferior myocardial infarction. In this setting, sudden hypotension and bradycardia can be induced, leading to significant hemodynamic instability. Lastly, nitrates are best avoided in patients with acute pulmonary edema and clinically evident right ventricular infarction.

Morphine

Morphine has a long history of use in the early management of patients with acute pulmonary edema. It has beneficial properties that oppose a number of underlying pathophysiologic abnormalities.[20] In patients with pulmonary edema, a chain of processes can create a vicious cycle of events, leading to a worsening clinical status. Increasing interstitial fluid impairs gas exchange, while decreasing pulmonary compliance produces dyspnea. With progression of the process, worsening dyspnea increases the work of breathing, which in turn increases myocardial oxygen demand. This occurs in a setting wherein myocardial function and/or oxygen supply may be extremely limited. Morphine causes central nervous system suppression of the respiratory center. There is blunting of the chemoreceptor-mediated ventilatory reflexes, leading to a decrease in the sensation of dyspnea and correspondingly a decrease in the work of breathing. In addition, morphine acts centrally to decrease sympathetic tone and thereby diminishes venous and arterial vasoconstriction.[21, 22] The net effect in most patients is a decrease in central venous return with a corresponding reduction in preload.

Morphine can be administered in intravenous doses of 2 to 5 mg over 3 to 5 minutes with close patient observation and monitoring for respiratory depression or hypotension. This regimen can be repeated at 15- to 20-minute intervals with total doses in the range of 5 to 20 mg. Subcutaneous administration should be avoided because of potentially erratic absorption. Useful end points include alleviation of anxiety and a noticeable decrease in the work of breathing. Morphine should be avoided when the potential for carbon dioxide retention is high (i.e., altered level of consciousness, chronic obstructive pulmonary disease, or bronchial asthma). An elevation of partial carbon dioxide pressure in acute pulmonary edema differs from this finding in patients with respiratory insufficiency due to chronic obstructive pulmonary disease. In pulmonary edema, respiratory acidosis is acute and caused by marked ventilation-perfusion mismatching due to fluid in the alveolar spaces. Hypoxic drive is still present, and judicious narcotic administration should not suppress respiration to the point of progressive respiratory acidosis. Responses of individual patients may vary, however, and close clinical observation is warranted.

Loop Diuretics

The use of intravenously administered loop diuretics is a standard part of initial therapy in most patients with acute pulmonary edema who have excessive intravascular volume and normal or elevated blood pressure.[23-25] Although ethacrynic acid belongs in this group, most clinical experience centers around the use of furosemide and bumetamide in this setting. The site of action is the ascending limb of the loop of Henle, where these agents inhibit sodium reabsorption from the renal filtrate. This effect increases renal salt and water excretion. Plasma volume is reduced, causing a decrease in preload and pulmonary congestion. Increases in urine flow can be noted within 5 to 10 minutes of intravenous administration, peaking at approximately 30 minutes and lasting for as long as 2 hours.

In many patients with acute pulmonary edema who are given furosemide, a decrease in pulmonary congestive symptoms can be observed within 5 minutes of administration, well before the diuretic response.[26] A part of this improvement may be the result of neurohormonal changes produced by diuretics.[27] Furosemide promotes secretion of both atrial natriuretic peptide and renal prostaglandin E_2, causing vasodilation. Data also indicate that furosemide decreases afterload and thereby contributes to relief in pulmonary edema by improving left ventricular function.[28]

The effective dose of loop diuretics varies widely. Initial doses of furosemide (30 to 60 mg) or bumetamide (1 to 3 mg) will usually generate a brisk diuresis in most patients within 15 minutes with maximal effect at 30 minutes. When determining the initial intravenous dose of a diuretic, one might find patient-supplied information regarding prior therapy extremely helpful. Patients without prior exposure to loop diuretics may be especially sensitive to them and often require small doses to effect a vigorous diuresis. In contrast, patients receiving long-term diuretic therapy, particularly with large doses, may require high intravenous doses. In patients receiving long-term diuretic therapy, an initial intravenous equivalent to the oral dose can be administered and doubled at 20- to 30-minute intervals until a brisk diuresis is induced.

The physician must guard against overzealous diuresis in patients with acute pulmonary edema. The use of diuretics becomes particularly challenging in patients with low-normal or low blood pressures and fluid overload. Here, therapy is best guided by central hemodynamic monitoring. When the patient's clinical status is tenuous and time is a factor, smaller doses of diuretics can be administered, followed by close monitoring and expeditious placement of a central catheter for direct measurement of hemodynamic parameters.

Nitroprusside

In clinical situations in which patients have not responded to initial therapeutic interventions, intravenous vasodilatory therapy may become necessary.[29] The two agents most commonly used in this setting are nitroglycerin (discussed previously) and nitroprusside. The safe and effective use of these agents in acute pulmonary edema requires monitoring of the patient's underlying hemodynamic parameters; therefore, an arterial catheter and a flow-directed balloon catheter should be placed into the pulmonary artery before initiating therapy.

Nitroprusside is a short-acting, potent venous and arteriolar dilator. It is most useful in clinical situations characterized by elevated systemic vascular resistance, increased left ventricular filling pressures, and compromised cardiac output. In patients with impaired ventricular systolic function, the decrease in systemic and pulmonary vascular resistance can greatly improve cardiac function and thereby decrease pulmonary congestion.[30]

Two other common clinical situations in which nitroprusside is useful include significant mitral valve regurgitation and severe systemic hypertension. Nitroprusside effectively reduces regurgitant volume, improves left ventricular mechanics, and augments cardiac output. In addition, the short half-life permits rapid titration for fine control of blood pressure.

Nitroprusside must be administered as a controlled continuous infusion with ongoing central hemodynamic monitoring and close patient observation. Typically, infusion is started at 0.5 to 1 µg/kg/min and titrated according to hemodynamic response. The end products of nitroprusside can cause clinical toxicity if precautions are not considered. One of these end products is thiocyanate, which is almost entirely eliminated by renal excretion. The mean elimination half-life is approximately 3 days. In patients with renal insufficiency, elimination can be markedly prolonged. In this regard, early efforts should be taken to limit the period of infusion to 24 to 48 hours. A second potentially toxic product of metabolism is cyanide, which accumulates at infusion rates greater than 2 µg/kg/min.

Dobutamine

In clinical settings in which severely depressed myocardial systolic function plays an important role in producing acute pulmonary edema, modest improvement in cardiac performance can have profound beneficial hemodynamic and clinical effects. Because of the potential for inducing life-threatening arrhythmias and increasing myocardial oxygen consumption, intervention with inotropic therapy should be considered carefully. The agent selected should match the hemodynamic needs of the patient.

Dobutamine is a parenterally administered synthetic catecholamine with primarily β_1-agonist activity and slight β_2- and α-agonist effects.[31, 32] In patients with heart failure, it consistently improves cardiac output and decreases left ventricular filling pressures without significantly increasing heart rate or blood pressure.[33] These properties make dobutamine an excellent agent for inotropic therapy in a clinical setting characterized by pulmonary edema associated with a low cardiac output, elevated left ventricular filling pressures, and elevated peripheral vascular resistance. It has had large-scale clinical use in patients with severely compromised ventricular function with or without symptoms of coronary insufficiency.

Dobutamine's half-life is 2 to 3 minutes, and it is eliminated by hepatic metabolism. Infusion is usually started at 2.5 µg/kg/min with titration guided by cardiac output, heart rate, heart rhythm, and pulmonary capillary wedge pressure. With infusion rates in the range of 15 to 20 µg/kg/min, peripheral α-adrenergic receptor stimulation may become prominent with deleterious hemodynamic and mechanical effects on myocardial performance due to increased afterload.

Dopamine

In patients with acute pulmonary edema, dopamine can often serve as a primary or adjunctive agent during the early phase of therapy.[34] The peripheral vascular and cardiac effects of dopamine are mediated by a number of distinct types of receptors with varying degrees of affinity. At low concentrations (1 to 3 µg/kg/min), the primary interaction is with dopaminergic receptors in the renal and mesenteric arterial beds causing vasodilation. There is an increase in renal blood flow, glomerular filtration rate, and sodium exertion. At slightly higher concentrations (2.5 to 10 µg/kg/min), dopamine acts as a positive inotropic agent on the myocardium through β_1-adrenergic receptors.[35] At still higher concentrations (10 to 20 µg/kg/min), dopamine activates α_1-adrenergic receptors, causing peripheral vasoconstriction.

With this distinct pharmacokinetic profile, dopamine can be titrated to a desired hemodynamic response to fit the clinical situation.[36] The enhanced renal blood flow induced by low-dose infusion of dopamine combined with diuretics has proven more effective than diuretics alone in patients with heart failure.[37] This type of use can help to generate diuresis in patients with fluid overload and low cardiac output in whom elevated sympathetic activity may significantly compromise renal function.

For inotropic support, dopamine should be started at 2.5 µg/kg/min followed by titration to an acceptable hemodynamic response. Because the drug nonselectively stimulates α_1-adrenergic receptors at high doses, patients should be closely monitored for associated changes in heart rate, blood pressure, and left ventricular filling pressures.[38] These effects can worsen cardiac and renal function as a consequence of vasoconstriction.

Dopamine, like dobutamine, can cause significant atrial and ventricular ectopy. The cardiac rhythm should be continuously monitored during infusion. In certain patients, dopamine may need to be combined with intravenous vasodilator therapy for the most beneficial hemodynamic effect.[39]

Phosphodiesterase Inhibitors

Amrinone and its congener milrinone are the latest intravenously administered inotropic agents to be approved for short-term management of severe heart failure.[40, 41] They are members of a new class of bipyridine agents with both inotropic and vasodilator properties. They act by inhibiting myocardial and vascular cyclic adenosine monophosphate (cAMP) phosphodiesterase, which increases intracellular levels of cAMP. In myocardial cells, this leads to an increase in intracellular ionized calcium, which increases contractility. The cAMP-induced protein kinase activation in vascular smooth muscle elicits another pattern of protein phosphorylation that induces vasodilation.

The hemodynamic effects include a prompt increase in cardiac output, a decrease in ventricular filling pressures, and a decrease in total peripheral resistance. These beneficial hemodynamic effects occur without a significant increase in heart rate or myocardial oxygen consumption. Milrinone is more potent than amrinone. These agents are primarily eliminated by renal excretion and should have downward dosage adjustment with renal insufficiency. Amrinone is administered with an intravenous loading dose of 0.75 mg/kg over 2 to 3 minutes followed by an infusion of 5 to 10 µg/kg/min. Based on the clinical and hemodynamic response, a second loading dose can be administered after 30 minutes. Milrinone is administered with a loading dose of 50 µg/kg over 10 minutes followed by an infusion of 0.375 to 0.75 µg/kg/min guided by patient response.

The side effects of amrinone include thrombocytopenia, nausea, vomiting, abdominal pain, anorexia, arrhythmias, hypotension, hematotoxicity, and fever. The most common side effect of milrinone is induction of non-life-threatening ventricular arrhythmias, but it does not appear to induce thrombocytopenia.

Although the mechanism of action of this class is unique, these agents do not appear to have major advantages over dobutamine in most clinical situations. In addition, the side effects of amrinone present potentially significant problems in treating typically ill patients with acute pulmonary edema.

NONCARDIAC PULMONARY EDEMA (ADULT RESPIRATORY DISTRESS SYNDROME)

Noncardiogenic pulmonary edema largely consists of adult respiratory distress syndrome (ARDS), which is a term applied to a diverse group of lung disorders characterized by widespread infiltrative pulmonary lesions and severe hypoxemia (Table 15–2).[42-44] Because of similarities in pathophysiology, adult respiratory distress syndrome is now classified as a subgroup of the multiorgan dysfunction syndrome, which is within the broad spectrum of the systemic inflammatory response syndrome. The term ARDS was selected because of similarities with the neonatal respiratory distress syndrome, even though the underlying insults are different.[45] In the adult, the clinical picture, pathophysiology, and management are similar despite the wide range of causes.[46, 47]

Pathophysiology

For all causes, the syndrome is associated with fluid accumulation in the interstitial and alveolar spaces without elevation of the pulmonary capillary pressure.[48] The grouping of ARDS with inflammatory processes recognizes that the effects of systemic mediators of inflammation are critical in the course of the disease. During the early phase, there is infiltration of neutrophils that adhere to pulmonary microvasculature. Initial damage to the vascular endothelium is mediated by products released from neutrophils and other inflammatory blood cells. With progressive disruption of the inner surface of pulmonary capillaries, permeability is increased with leakage of liquid, macromolecules, cellular components, and ultimately proteins into the interstitial and alveolar spaces. Alveoli become engorged with edematous fluid, cellular debris, and hyaline membrane.

An important consequence of ARDS in the lung is qualitative and quantitative alteration in surfactant.[49] Areas of alveolar collapse occur because of liquid accumulation and alteration in surfactant production and function. Because the lung has a limited number of ways to react to injury, the pathology is similar for the various etiologic conditions. These changes decrease lung compliance with a corresponding increase in the work of breathing while pulmonary gas exchange is severely compromised. The combination of hypoxemia and stimulation of receptors in poorly compliant lung parenchyma produces a decrease in tidal volume and a drive to increase respiratory frequency.

Clinical Aspects

From a clinical standpoint, patients are normally healthy and free of signs and symptoms for up to several hours following the precipitating insult. Typically, the first sign is an increase in respiratory frequency followed by dyspnea. The initial blood gas measurement demonstrates a decrease in P_{O_2} despite a depressed P_{CO_2}. Oxygen therapy at this stage will often significantly improve P_{O_2}. The early physical examination may be unremarkable except for perhaps soft, fine inspiratory rales. As hypoxia worsens, the patient becomes increasingly tachypneic, and cyanosis may develop. With progression, the chest radiograph demonstrates widespread alveolar and interstitial infiltrates, and the lung signs become more prominent with rales and tubular breath sounds. Hypoxemia eventually becomes refractory to simple oxygen therapy corresponding to significant right-to-left shunting of blood past collapsed and fluid filled alveoli. Mechanical ventilation is then required to stabilize and reverse hypoxemia.

When ARDS is suspected, the early placement of a flow-directed balloon pulmonary artery catheter is essential for confirmation of the diagnosis and management of the patient. Diagnosis is confirmed by evidence of pulmonary edema with a disproportionately low pulmonary capillary wedge pressure. Catheterization of the right side of the heart is then used to monitor hemodynamics and overall cardiac function during respiratory therapy. The goal is to maintain an adequate cardiac output at the lowest left ventricular filling pressure.

Respiratory Care Management

While addressing respiratory needs, it is important to identify, eliminate, or treat precipitating causes when possible. This is important because the underlying

Table 15–2. **Causes of Noncardiac Pulmonary Edema (Adult Respiratory Distress Syndrome)**

Drugs	Inhaled toxins and irritants
Thiazides	Smoke
Fluorescein	Phosgene
Propoxyphene	Ozone
Colchicine	High oxygen concentrations
Ethchlorvynol	Nitrogen dioxide
Dextran 40	Chlorine gas
Chlordiazepoxide	Cadmium
Streptokinase	Ammonia
Paraquat	
Salicylates	**Systemic reactions, nonpulmonary in origin**
Barbiturates	Fat embolism
Nitrofurantoin	Hemorrhagic pancreatitis
Morphine	Amniotic fluid embolism
Heroin	Disseminated intravascular
Methadone	coagulation
	Anaphylaxis
Infection	Thrombotic thrombocytopenic
Bacterial	purpura
Virus	
Fungus	**Miscellaneous**
Tuberculosis	Multisystem trauma
Pneumocystis carinii	Shock
Gram-negative sepsis	Ionic contrast agents
	Postcardiopulmonary bypass
Immune antigen responses	Uremia
Systemic lupus erythematosus	Diabetic ketoacidosis
Goodpasture's syndrome	Bowel infarction
	Carcinomatosis
Aspiration	Dead fetus
Near drowning	Eclampsia
Gastric acid	

disease or trauma may continue to stimulate further release of inflammatory mediators. The general therapeutic goal is to establish and maintain adequate tissue oxygenation while avoiding cardiopulmonary complications. A guiding principle for correcting hypoxemia is to use the lowest inspired fraction of oxygen to obtain adequate tissue oxygenation in an effort to avoid pulmonary complications. A P_{O_2} of 60 mmHg is generally accepted as a desirable target.

Oxygen therapy is usually initiated using a well-fitting face mask with the addition of a reservoir bag if needed with 100% oxygen at flow rates of 5 to 10 L/min. Serial blood gas measurements should be coupled with the clinical response to make adjustments. Many patients will need mechanical ventilation when noninvasive means of supplying supplemental oxygen become inadequate. This transition should be made before the patient becomes clinically unstable. The use of mechanical ventilation allows functional lung volume to be expanded, which is crucially important to open collapsed alveoli. A shift has been made to using lower tidal volumes in an effort to reduce lung damage induced by mechanical ventilation. This often requires sedation of the patient and the use of muscle relaxants.

The use of positive end-expiratory pressure (PEEP) also often plays an important role in the pulmonary management of these patients.[50] It serves two basic purposes—to improve oxygenation and to help avoid oxygen toxicity problems. A Pa_{O_2} below 60 mmHg is an indication that the FI_{O_2} should be increased to achieve this level of oxygenation. It is important to utilize the lowest level of PEEP to achieve predetermined respiratory targets in order to minimize impairment of venous return and mechanical impairment of left ventricular function.[51–53] Usually, PEEP is started at 5 mmHg and gradually increased while clinical responses, hemodynamics, and serial arterial blood gas results are followed closely. In some situations, ancillary cardiac support with vasodilators and/or inotropic agents may be needed, particularly in patients with underlying cardiac disease.

The overall goal of therapy is to establish and maintain adequate oxygenation, avoid cardiopulmonary complications, identify and remove offending precipitants, and allow time for recovery of pulmonary function. Because this process heavily depends on mediators of systemic inflammation, corticosteroids and other anti-inflammatory agents have been considered as adjunctive therapy. Unfortunately, they have not demonstrated significant beneficial effects.[54]

The mortality rate of ARDS approaches 65%, and residual restrictive impairment for pulmonary function is present in up to 30% of survivors, which emphasizes the importance of early recognition and aggressive supportive cardiopulmonary care.

Acknowledgments

The authors greatly appreciate the secretarial assistance of Mrs. Gayle E. Herrin in the preparation of this manuscript.

REFERENCES

1. Yancy CW, Firth BG: Congestive heart failure. Dis Mon 34:467, 1988.
2. Kannel WB, Belanger AJ: Epidemiology in heart failure. Am Heart J 121:951, 1991.
3. Ghali JK, Cooper R, Ford E: Trends in hospitalization rates for heart failure in the United States. Arch Intern Med 150:769, 1990.
4. Andreadis N, Petty TL: Adult respiratory distress syndrome. Problems and progress. Am Rev Respir Dis 132:1344, 1985.
5. Robin ED, Cross CE, Zelis R: Pulmonary edema. N Engl J Med 288:239, 1973.
6. Staub NC: Pulmonary edema. Physiol Rev 54:679, 1974.
7. Fishman AP: Pulmonary edema: The water-exchanging function of the lung. Circulation 46:390, 1972.
8. Davis D, Baily R, Zelis R: Abnormalities in systemic norepinephrine kinetics in human congestive heart failure. Am J Physiol 254(6 Pt 1):E760, 1988.
9. Mancini DM, Lejemtel TH, Factor F, et al: Central and peripheral components of cardiac failure. Am J Med 80:2, 1986.
10. Zelis R, Sinoway LI, Musch TI, et al: Regional blood flow in congestive heart failure: Concept of compensatory mechanisms with short and long time constants. Am J Cardiol 62:2E, 1988.
11. Ghali JK, Kadakia F, Cooper R, et al: Precipitating factors leading to decompensation of heart failure. Arch Intern Med 148:2013, 1988.
12. Forrester JS, Waters DD: Hospital treatment of congestive heart failure: Management according to hemodynamic profile. Am J Med 65:173, 1978.
13. Bersten AD, Holt AW, Vedig AE, et al: Treatment of severe cardiogenic pulmonary edema with continuous positive airway pressure delivered by face mask. N Engl J Med 325:1825, 1991.
14. Rasamen J, Heikkila J, Down J, et al: Continuous positive airway pressure by facemask in acute cardiogenic pulmonary edema. Am J Cardiol 55:296, 1985.
15. Gold HK, Leinbach RC, Sanders CA: Use of sublingual nitroglycerin in congestive heart failure following acute myocardial infarction. Circulation 46:839, 1972.
16. Bussman WD, Schupp D: Effect of sublingual nitroglycerin in emergency treatment of severe pulmonary edema. Am J Cardiol 41:931, 1978.
17. Parker JO, VanKoughnett KA, Farrell B: Nitroglycerine lingual spray: Clinical efficacy and dose-response relation. Am J Cardiol 57:1, 1986.
18. Mason DJ, Braunwald EB: The effects of nitroglycerin and amyl nitrite on anteriolar and venous tone in the human forearm. Circulation 32:755, 1965.
19. Armstrong PW, Armstrong JA, Marks GS: Pharmacokinetic-hemodynamic studies of intravenous nitroglycerin in congestive heart failure. Circulation 62:160, 1980.
20. Vismara LA, Leaman DM, Zelis R: Effects of morphine on venous tone in patients with acute pulmonary edema. Circulation 54:335, 1976.
21. Zelis R, Mansour EJ, Capone RJ, et al: The cardiovascular effects of morphine: The peripheral capacitance and resistance vessels in human subjects. J Clin Invest 54:1247, 1974.
22. Zelis R, Kinney EL, Flaim SF, et al: Morphine: Its use in pulmonary edema. Cardiovasc Rev Rep 2:257, 1981.
23. Iff HW, Flenley DC: Blood-gas exchange after furosemide in acute pulmonary edema. Lancet 1:616, 1971.
24. Berger BE, Warnock DG: Clinical uses and mechanisms of action of diuretic agents. *In* Brenner BM, Rector FC (eds): The Kidney. Philadelphia: WB Saunders, 1986, pp 433–455.
25. Gerlag PG, van Meijel JJ: High-dose furosmide in the treatment of refractory congestive heart failure. Arch Intern Med 148:286, 1988.
26. Dikshit K, Vyden JK, Forrester JS, et al: Renal and extrarenal hemodynamic effects of furosemide in congestive heart failure after acute myocardial infarction. N Engl J Med 288:1087, 1973.
27. Packer M: Neurohormonal interactions and adaptations in congestive heart failure. Circulation 77:721, 1988.
28. Wilson JR, Reichek N, Dunkman WB, et al: Effect of diuresis on the performance of the failing left ventricle in man. Am J Med 70:234, 1981.

29. Cohn JN, Burke LP: Nitroprusside. Ann Intern Med 91:752, 1979.
30. Guiha NH, Cohn JN, Mikulic E, et al: Treatment of refractory heart failure with infusion of nitroprusside. N Engl J Med 291:587, 1974.
31. Sonnenblick EH, Frishman WH, LeJemtel TH: Dobutamine: A new synthetic cardioactive sympathetic amine. N Engl J Med 300:17, 1979.
32. Leier CV, Unverferth DV: Dobutamine. Ann Intern Med 99:490, 1983.
33. Majerus TC, Dasta JF, Banman JL, et al: Dobutamine: Ten years later. Pharmacotherapy 9:245, 1989.
34. Goldberg LI, Rajfer SI: Dopamine receptors: Applications in clinical cardiology. Circulation 72:245, 1985.
35. Rajfer SI, Borow KM, Lang RM, et al: Effects of dopamine on left ventricular afterload and contractile state in heart failure: Relation to the activation of beta$_1$ adrenoceptors and dopamine receptors. J Am Coll Cardiol 12:498, 1988
36. Goldberg LI: Cardiovascular and renal action of dopamine: Potential clinical applications. Pharmacol Rev 24:1, 1972.
37. Robie NW, Goldberg LI: Comparative systemic and regional hemodynamic effects of dopamine and dobutamine. Am Heart J 90:340, 1975.
38. Stoner JD, Balen JL, Harrison DC: Comparison of dobutamine and dopamine in treatment of severe heart failure. Br Heart J 39:536, 1977.
39. Miller RR, Awan NA, Joye JA, et al: Combined dopamine and nitroprusside in congestive heart failure. Circulation 55:881, 1977.
40. Colucci WS, Wright RF, Braunwald E: New positive inotropic agents in the treatment of congestive heart failure: Mechanisms of action and recent clinical developments. N Engl J Med 314:349, 1986.
41. Braunwald E: New positive inotropic agents. Circulation 73(Suppl 3):237, 1986.
42. Rinaldo JE, Rogers RM: Adult respiratory distress syndrome: Changing concepts of lung injury and repair. N Engl J Med 306:900, 1982.
43. Bernard GR, Bringham KL: The adult respiratory distress syndrome. Annu Rev Med 36:195, 1985.
44. Hildner FJ: Pulmonary edema associated with low left ventricular filling pressures. Am J Cardiol 44:1410, 1979.
45. Ashbaugh DG, Bigelow DB, Petty TL, et al: Acute respiratory distress in adults. Lancet 2:319, 1967.
46. Raffin TA: ARDS: Mechanisms and management. Hosp Pract 22:65, 1987.
47. Bernard GR, Brigham KL: Pulmonary edema: Pathophysiologic mechanisms and new approaches to therapy. Chest 89:594, 1986.
48. Reynolds HY: Lung inflammation: Normal host defense or a complication of some disease? Annu Rev Med 38:295, 1987.
49. Petty TL, Silvers GW, Paul GW, et al: Abnormalities in lung elastic properties and surfactant function in adult respiratory distress syndrome. Chest 75:571, 1979.
50. Rizk NW, Murray JF: PEEP and pulmonary edema. Am J Med 72:381, 1982.
51. Scharf SM, Caldini P, Ingram RH Jr: Cardiovascular effects of increasing airway pressure. Am J Physiol 1:35, 1972.
52. Scharf SM, Brown R, Saunders NA, et al: Changes in left ventricular size and configuration with positive end-expiratory pressure. Circ Res 44:672, 1979.
53. Lorell BH, Palacios I, Daggitt WM, et al: Right ventricular distension and left ventricular performance. Am J Physiol 240:H87, 1981.
54. Bernard GR, Luce JM, Sprung CL, et al: High dose corticosteroids in patients with the adult respiratory distress syndrome. N Engl J Med 317:1565, 1987.

CHAPTER 16

Acute Myocardial Infarction

David W. Snyder, M.D., and Allan S. Jaffe, M.D.

Acute myocardial infarction (AMI) is caused by an imbalance between myocardial oxygen supply and demand of sufficient duration that myocardial necrosis ensues. Often it is the consequence of a dynamic process within the coronary vessel initiated by the thrombotic occlusion of a previously stenotic coronary artery.[1, 2] Regardless of the immediate cause, the resultant ischemia progresses to irreversible cell injury, beginning in the subendocardium of the central ischemic zone and spreading outward. This wave of cell death is complete by 4 hours after the onset of infarction in experimental animals[3] and in most patients, judging from the steep time dependence of benefit in therapeutic trials of coronary recanalization.[4] Thus, interventions designed to alter the course of infarction must be initiated as soon as possible. Other treatments to prevent the complications of infarction that are common during the initial hours also should be started as soon as possible. Prevention and prompt treatment of late complications such as arrhythmias, heart failure, and infarct extension are important goals throughout the remainder of the hospital course.

CONVENTIONAL MANAGEMENT

Pain and anxiety in the acute phase must be treated promptly, both to ensure patient comfort and to reverse the deleterious effects of increased sympathetic tone on the course of infarction. Morphine sulfate remains the analgesic and anxiolytic drug of choice and should be given intravenously starting with 3 to 5 mg and titrated aggressively to ensure pain relief. Hypotension and the lack of heart rate response, i.e., relative bradycardia, may occasionally follow the use of morphine and can be reversed by administration of atropine.[5] Because of this "vagotonic effect," some physicians prefer meperidine, which is vagolytic.[6] Pentazocine elevates arterial pressure and left ventricular end-diastolic pressure and therefore should be avoided in patients with AMI.[7] Because the pain of AMI reflects ongoing ischemia, definitive treatment focuses on limiting ischemia with nitrates, β-blockers, or coronary recanalization.

Mild hypoxemia is common in patients with infarction, prompting the routine use of supplemental oxygen in coronary care units (CCUs).[8, 9] Administration of oxygen results in a decrease in precordial ST segment elevation, suggesting that low-flow oxygen benefits most patients.[10] The adequacy of oxygenation should be assessed by oximetry whenever possible rather than arterial blood gas determinations, because blood gases can be associated with local bleeding if potent anticoagulants and thrombolytic agents are used.

Hypertension is common early after AMI, especially with anterior infarction, and increases the workload and oxygen demand of the heart. Initial management, including aggressive efforts to relieve pain and sedation, often lowers the blood pressure. If hypertension persists and is accompanied by other evidence of heightened sympathetic tone and if heart failure is not present, intravenous β-blockade using propranolol, metoprolol, or esmolol may lower blood pressure and limit ischemia.[11] Alternatively, if congestive heart failure and/or mitral regurgitation is present, intravenous nitroglycerin dilates venous capacitance vessels and arterial resistance vessels, favorably reducing preload and afterload while controlling blood pressure.[12] Nitroglycerin is preferred over nitroprusside when possible in patients with AMI, because nitroprusside can in some patients aggravate ischemia, probably by promoting a "coronary steal" syndrome and thereby decreasing collateral flow to the ischemic zone.[13, 14] However, in the absence of heart failure, nitroglycerin lacks arterial vasodilating properties.[15] Thus, when necessary, nitroprusside should be used rather than permitting hypertension to persist. In some studies,[16] but not all,[17] mortality has been shown to be reduced by treatment with nitroprusside, especially in hypertensive patients.

If hypertension persists after the acute phase of AMI, chronic oral antihypertensive therapy should be initiated. Unless contraindicated because of lung disease, severe peripheral vascular disease, or heart failure, β-blockers are the drugs of choice because of their ability to control hypertension and reduce the risk of reinfarction and sudden death in survivors of infarction.[18, 19] Both nonselective (e.g., propranolol, timolol) and relatively cardioselective blockers (e.g., metoprolol, practolol) prevent death and reinfarction.[20, 21] Agents with significant intrinsic sympathomimetic activity, however, do not appear to share these protective effects and should be avoided.[22] Titration of these agents to reduce heart rate into the range of 55 to 65 beats/min is advised because benefit is related to the degree of heart rate reduction.[23] β-Blockers should *not* be withheld from patients with mild heart failure, because they benefit the most from cautious administration.[24] Sublingual nifedipine should be avoided because it may precipitate an abrupt fall in arterial pressure leading to reflexive tachycardia, thereby (paradoxically) further aggravating myocardial ischemia.

Patients with heart failure and hypertension benefit long term from vasodilator therapy with control of blood pressure and improvement in cardiac function. Several large clinical trials[25, 26] have demonstrated im-proved survival in patients with heart failure who are treated with vasodilators and especially angiotensin-converting enzyme (ACE) inhibitors. Furthermore, benefit accrues to those with a reduced ejection fraction even if heart failure is not present.[27] When hypertension is not controlled with vasodilators and β-blockers alone, or if symptoms of heart failure persist, a diuretic should be added. Very low doses of diuretic often are effective for the treatment of hypertension and heart failure. Potassium-sparing preparations (thiazide plus triamterene or amiloride) avoid aggravation of arrhythmia due to potassium and magnesium depletion.

Bed rest is prescribed in the initial hours of infarction. However, prolonged bed rest promotes deconditioning and increases the risk of deep vein thrombosis. Thus, stable patients should progress to a bed-chair-bathroom regimen within 24 to 48 hours, and begin ambulation several days thereafter. Such an approach has been shown to decrease complications and allow earlier hospital discharge. Unstable patients must be mobilized cautiously, with monitoring of their hemodynamic response.

Thrombotic complications of AMI, including venous thrombosis and pulmonary embolism, occur in as many as 40% of patients with AMI who require prolonged bed rest.[28–30] These events are less common with early ambulation. However, the risk can be further reduced by the prophylactic use of small doses of heparin, which, when given subcutaneously in doses of 5000 U every 8 or 12 hours, decreases the incidence of venous thrombosis by as much as 90%.[31] Such doses of heparin do not substantially impede the formation of intracardiac thrombus (see Chapter 152).

PERICARDITIS

Asymptomatic pericardial effusions can be demonstrated echocardiographically in 30% of patients in the first week after infarction.[32–34] Effusions are more common after anterior infarction and are especially common when infarction is complicated by congestive heart failure.[32–34] Signs and symptoms of pericarditis are usually absent, and no specific treatment is indicated. Spontaneous resolution occurs slowly over a period of weeks to months.[34]

A pericardial friction rub and chest pain result in a clinical syndrome 2 to 4 days after infarction in approximately 10% of patients.[35] Typical pericardial pain (pain in the left trapezius ridge) is rarely present. Rather, the discomfort typically is pleuritic and positional in nature. At times, it may be difficult to distinguish the pain of pericarditis from that of recurrent ischemia or infarct extension. Patients with postinfarction pericarditis tend to have large Q-wave infarctions and thus also are at greater risk for the development of congestive heart failure.[36] They often do not have pericardial effusions, and the classic electrocardiographic changes of pericarditis are rarely observed.[36]

Hemopericardium is an infrequent but serious complication but is rare in the absence of Dressler's syndrome or some other pericardial process other than infarction alone.[37] Pain is not often a severe problem and can usually be treated with aspirin in full antiinflammatory doses. Nonsteroidal antiinflammatory agents should be avoided if possible because they suppress infarct healing.[38, 39]

Dressler's syndrome (postmyocardial infarction syndrome) is an immune-mediated pericarditis associated with fever and pleural and pericardial inflammation.[40, 41] It typically occurs weeks to months after myocardial infarction. The incidence of this syndrome has decreased greatly since its original description, perhaps as a result of the diminished use of anticoagulants during the acute phase of infarction.[42] Patients usually have pericardial pain, fever, elevated erythrocyte sedimentation rate, and often pleural and pericardial effusions and/or pulmonary infiltrates. Aspirin is the drug of first choice, but often treatment with nonsteroidal antiinflammatory drugs is necessary. Some patients may be refractory or have recurrent symptoms. These patients can be treated with steroids with tapering of the dosage after the sedimentation rate has normalized. However, recurrences are common as steroids are tapered.

ARRHYTHMIAS

In the 1970s, the widespread availability of CCUs for the management of AMI brought with it a decline in hospital mortality rates from 30% to less than 15%. Most of this improved survival was due to the prompt recognition and treatment of cardiac arrhythmia. Disturbances of cardiac rhythm occur in 90% of patients (Table 16–1), most commonly during the initial hours of evolution of the infarction.[43, 44] Vigorous treatment is required when arrhythmias produce hemodynamic instability, predispose to more serious arrhythmias, or aggravate ischemia through tachycardia or diminished coronary perfusion.[33] Because the

Table 16–1. **Incidence of Arrhythmias in the Coronary Care Unit**

Arrhythmia	Incidence (%)
Atrial ectopy (PACs)	80–95
Atrial fibrillation	10–20
Atrial flutter	1–5
Paroxysmal atrial tachycardia	1–5
First-degree AV block	10–15
Wenckebach second-degree AV block	5–10
Mobitz II second-degree AV block	<1
Complete heart block (AV node)	5–10
Complete heart block (infranodal)	1–3
Bundle branch block	10–20
Ventricular ectopy (PVCs)	90–100
Complex PVCs (multiform, couplets)	80–90
R wave on T wave	5–15
Ventricular tachycardia	10–20
Ventricular fibrillation	5–10

AV, atrioventricular; PACs, premature atrial contractions; PVCs, premature ventricular contractions.

extent of myocardial damage is a key factor predisposing to arrhythmias both in the CCU and late after infarction, measures to preserve myocardial viability may obviate subsequent catastrophic arrhythmias.[46, 47]

Bradycardias

Sinus bradycardia occurs in one third of patients with AMI during the first hour of symptoms[59] and is usually a reflection of increased vagal activity accompanying inferior or posterior myocardial infarction (i.e., a right coronary artery event).[48] It also can occur with coronary recanalization.[49] When asymptomatic, sinus bradycardia requires no treatment and often resolves spontaneously. If bradycardia is associated with hypotension or predisposes to ventricular arrhythmia, judicious treatment with atropine is indicated. An initial dose of at least 0.5 mg prevents paradoxic slowing of the sinus rate, generally with good therapeutic effect. Subsequently, cautious titration to achieve a heart rate of more than 60 beats/min is recommended. Only an occasional patient requires the maximal dose of 2 mg.[50] Bradycardia occurring late after infarction reflects ischemia, drug effect, or injury to the sinus or atrioventricular (AV) node. Atropine may not be effective in this setting. Insertion of a temporary pacemaker is indicated for symptomatic, marked (heart rate, <50 beats/min), or recurrent bradycardia requiring multiple doses of atropine.

Abnormalities of atrioventricular conduction also complicate the management of patients with AMI. First-degree AV block and Mobitz I second-degree AV block, like sinus bradycardia, usually accompany inferior myocardial infarction and may reflect vagotonia early during infarction or AV nodal injury.[51] Drug effects may precipitate or worsen AV block. Accordingly, digoxin, morphine, β-blockers, and calcium antagonists should be used with caution. When Mobitz I block progresses to complete heart block, it does so through progressively increasing degrees of second-degree block. Because block is at the level of the AV node, a stable junctional escape rhythm generally emerges with a rate of 45 to 60 beats/min and a narrow QRS complex. This rhythm often is well tolerated, and pacing is needed only when symptoms or hemodynamic deterioration is present.[40] In some patients, this arrhythmia is due to the buildup of adenosine and can be antagonized by administration of aminophylline.[53]

Anterior infarction less commonly results in AV conduction block and does so through a different mechanism, i.e., extensive necrosis of the interventricular septum with damage to the bundle branch system. Complete heart block can occur abruptly but is usually presaged by right or left bundle branch block, with, or more often without, Mobitz II second-degree AV block. The risk of complete heart block is highest in patients with new right bundle branch block, especially when concomitant anterior or posterior fascicular block is present.[54, 55] A temporary transvenous pacemaker should be placed prophylactically in patients with anterior infarction and Mobitz II block or bifascicular block. The availability of external pacemakers has reduced the frequency with which prophylactic temporary transvenous pacemakers are needed. When complete heart block does occur in patients with anterior infarction, the escape focus is usually below the AV node, resulting in a slow, wide complex idioventricular rhythm prone to abrupt asystole. Even with pacemaker support, the extensive myocardial necrosis underlying complete heart block results in a mortality of more than 80%.[55] Survivors of acute anterior MI complicated by transient heart block remain at high risk for a sudden death after hospital discharge. This risk can be reduced by placement of a permanent pacemaker.[56]

Abrupt asystole is a rare complication of AMI, with a mortality exceeding 90%.[43] Ventricular fibrillation, a more common cause for arrest in this setting, may be confused with asystole when fine fibrillatory waves are not evident on monitors.[57] Thus, a trial of defibrillation is justified before drug therapy with atropine and aminophylline. Persistent asystole rarely responds to external transcutaneous, transthoracic, or transvenous pacing,[73] but treatment of bradycardia before the development of asystole may be life saving.[59]

Supraventricular Tachyarrhythmias

Sinus tachycardia occurs in 30% of patients with AMI and is common in the first hours of anterior myocardial infarction, when sympathetic tone is high.[44] Causes of tachycardia, such as pain, anxiety, hypovolemia, left ventricular dysfunction, pericarditis, or the use of cardiotonic drugs, should be identified and corrected. Particular scrutiny is necessary in older patients who may have atypical signs and symptoms; this is especially the case when a diagnosis of congestive heart failure is being considered. If other causes can be eliminated, tachycardia can be treated with intravenous propranolol, metoprolol, or esmolol.[60] Anticipated benefits from β-blockade include reductions in heart rate, blood pressure, and myocardial oxygen demand with little change in left ventricular filling pressure.[12, 61]

Atrial fibrillation occurs in 10% to 20% of patients with AMI and is most common during the initial 48 hours.[62, 63] In most patients, it is a reflection of an elevated right or left atrial filling pressure.[64] Other factors predisposing to atrial fibrillation include electrolyte imbalance, drug effects, and atrial infarction.[65, 66] Correction of these factors is critical to successful treatment. Rate control can be induced with digoxin, 0.5 to 1.0 mg IV, intravenous diltiazem[82] (an infusion of 10 to 15 mg/hr after one or more boluses of 20 to 25 mg),[68] or β-blockers (propranolol up to 0.1 mg/kg IV titrated to the ventricular rate; metoprolol, up to 0.2 mg/kg; or esmolol, 50 to 300 μg/kg/min after loading with 500 μg/kg over the course of 1 minute). Esmolol is a cardioselective β-blocker that is degraded rapidly by red blood cell esterases, giving it a short half-life. Thus, it is easy to titrate and can be reversed rapidly if adverse effects occur.[69] If atrial fibrillation produces hypotension or heart failure or aggravates ischemia, immediate direct-current cardioversion is advised before drug therapy. When atrial fibrillation is recurrent or poorly tolerated, procainamide or quinidine or, in resistant or recurrent cases, propafenone, sotalol, or amiodarone can be used to maintain sinus rhythm.

Atrial flutter occurs far less commonly (in ≤5% of patients), usually in the setting of congestive heart failure or shock.[65] This arrhythmia is poorly tolerated, both because of the underlying left ventricular dysfunction usually present and because of rapid ventricular rates that are often difficult to control. Prompt cardioversion often is required. Intravenous diltiazem in doses similar to that used for atrial fibrillation is often effective.[67, 68] Verapamil also is effective and can be used in stable patients, but it can aggravate congestive heart failure or hypotension if the patient is unstable.[70] Recurrent episodes of atrial flutter can be prevented by the use of procainamide or quinidine, or can be interrupted by rapid atrial pacing.[71]

Paroxysmal atrial tachycardia in patients with AMI is rare and almost always transient, lasting only a few minutes.[65] If atrial tachycardia persists and is not terminated by vagal maneuvers or adenosine (6 or 12 mg by IV bolus),[72] intravenous diltiazem[88] or verapamil[89] terminates the arrhythmia in more than 90% of cases. However, the use of calcium antagonists is contraindicated in patients with severe left ventricular dysfunction or hypotension unrelated to the arrhythmia or in patients already treated parenterally with a β-blocker. In these patients, direct-current cardioversion with a low-energy discharge (25 J) is the best alternative. These arrhythmias also can be terminated by rapid atrial pacing.[71] Recurrent episodes may be prevented by digoxin, β-blockers, calcium antagonists, or type IA antiarrhythmic agents.

Ventricular Arrhythmias

Primary ventricular fibrillation is the major cause of death early in the course of AMI. Of patients destined to suffer primary ventricular fibrillation (occurring in the absence of heart failure or shock), 50% do so in the first hour and 80% in the first 4 hours of AMI.[75, 76] However, the incidence of primary ventricular fibrillation in the CCU, hours after the onset of pain, is less than 5%.[77, 78] Early efforts to prevent ventricular fibrillation focused on the detection and suppression of warning arrhythmias such as frequent premature ventricular contraction (PVCs), multiform PVCs, R on T PVCs, couplets, and salvos of nonsustained ventricular tachycardia.[79] However, it now has been shown clearly that such warning arrhythmias are insensitive predictors of patients who subsequently have ventricular fibrillation and are also nonspecific, occurring in an equal percentage of patients who do and those who do not go on to have primary ventricular fibrillation.[77, 78, 80, 81] Because it is not possible to predict in which patients ventricular fibrillation will develop, for many years all patients were treated prophylactically.[82, 83] However, primary ventricular fibrillation is seen in fewer and fewer patients in CCUs,[99] and lidocaine prophylaxis produces toxicity in many patients who are at low risk for arrhythmia.[85] Thus, it is not surprising that recent analyses suggest that patients who receive prophylactic lidocaine have a substantially higher mortality than those who do not.[86–88] Furthermore, primary ventricular fibrillation, when promptly managed, has little effect on the short- and long-term prognosis of patients with infarctions in most[104] but not all studies.[90] Accordingly, the prophylactic use of lidocaine is no longer deemed appropriate. β-Blockers reduce the incidence of primary ventricular fibrillation when administered during the initial 24 hours.[91, 92] Many believe that intravenous magnesium also reduces the incidence of malignant arrhythmias.[93, 94] However, a large recent randomized prospective study suggests that the reduction in mortality associated with the administration of magnesium to patients with acute infarction does not involve a reduction in arrhythmias (see later discussion).[95]

Patients who have frequent runs of ventricular tachycardia or who are symptomatic owing to arrhythmia should receive lidocaine. Lidocaine must be administered in a full dose, with a 2-mg/kg loading dose divided into two or three boluses over 10 minutes, followed by a 3-mg/min infusion. The infusion rate should be reduced to 2 mg/min after the initial 3 to 6 hours because plasma levels of lidocaine will climb because of saturation of the extravascular pool and slower lidocaine elimination after a prolonged infusion.[96] A reduced loading dose is advised in patients with heart failure or shock, and the maintenance infusion should be halved when the clearance of lidocaine is impaired by heart failure, liver disease, hypotension, or the use of drugs such as propranolol that reduce hepatic blood flow.[97] Adverse effects, most commonly central nervous system toxicity with tremor, drowsiness, or confusion, occur in as many as 50% of patients younger than age 70, even in the absence of heart failure; toxicity is more common in older and sicker populations.[98]

If frequent high-grade arrhythmias persist, procainamide can be added or substituted. Procainamide is administered as a loading dose of 10 to 15 mg/kg, given at a rate of 50 mg/min while the blood pressure and electrocardiogram are monitored. A maintenance infusion follows, at 2 to 6 mg/min, with lower doses chosen according to body size and in the presence of heart failure or renal dysfunction. Given in this manner, procainamide is remarkably well tolerated and suppresses 75% of the arrhythmias that are refractory to lidocaine.[99] For patients who do not respond to lidocaine or procainamide, a β-blocker might be considered. This therapy has been particularly useful in the subset of patients with augmented sympathetic tone, usually those with anterior infarction, who also have tachycardia and hypertension.[100]

An accelerated idioventricular rhythm (AIVR) with a rate between 60 and 120 beats/min occurs in approximately 10% of patients with AMI and may in some instances be provoked by spontaneous or induced coronary recanalization.[101, 102] In the past, AIVR was considered a benign escape rhythm seen only when the sinus rates slowed. For this reason, many were reluctant to treat it. It is now clear that in most instances, AIVR is caused by enhanced automaticity of Purkinje fibers on the endocardial surface of the infarct zone. Some patients experience rapid ventricular tachycardia with a similar morphology and a rate twice as fast as their AIVR, suggesting that rapid ventricular tachycardia with intermittent exit block is present.[103, 104] AIVR should be treated when associated with reduced cardiac output, hypotension, or rapid ventricular tachycardia.[105] Acceleration of the atrial rate with atropine or atrial pacing suppresses the AIVR, or it can be obliterated with lidocaine.

The frequency of ventricular ectopy declines rapidly with time after infarction. High-grade arrhythmias occurring after the first 24 hours of AMI generally suggest severe left ventricular injury, often with hypotension and heart failure. Such secondary arrhythmias commonly include recurrent episodes of ventricular tachycardia or ventricular fibrillation and may be refractory to treatment. Mortality in this setting is high.[101] Treatment should begin with drug therapy as outlined earlier, as well as correction of electrolyte disturbance, acid-base imbalance, or hypoxemia. Hypokalemia and hypomagnesemia predispose the patient to arrhythmias and also reduce the efficacy of antiarrhythmic drugs.[106, 107] Optimal management of congestive heart failure may also assist in arrhythmia control. When arrhythmias persist and are refractory to lidocaine and procainamide, amiodarone in a loading dose of 5 mg/kg given over 45 minutes followed by 1200 mg over 24 hours for 3 days can be effective.[108, 109] Overdrive ventricular pacing can also be useful in resistant cases.[110]

Sustained ventricular tachycardia with hypotension, or sustained ventricular fibrillation, requires immediate electrical countershock with 200 to 360 J (synchronized to the QRS complex in ventricular tachycardia, if time permits). Current recommendations include three rapid attempts at defibrillation before proceeding with cardiopulmonary resuscitation and drug therapy.[111, 112] Patients not already receiving lidocaine should be loaded with 1.5 mg/kg. An infusion can be started later.[85] Endotracheal or intravenous epinephrine (via a central line) in a dose of 1 mg (10 ml of 1:10,000 concentration) every 3 to 5 minutes may facilitate subsequent defibrillation. Attention to proper resuscitative techniques and ventilation to prevent hypoxemia and acidosis is essential, but bicarbonate is rarely needed or helpful. Because of the potential for augmenting myocardial or central nervous system injury, the administration of calcium generally is avoided unless the arrest is believed to result from hyperkalemia or to be aggravated by calcium antagonists.[113] Patients who do not respond to a dose of lidocaine may benefit from the use of bretylium (5 to 10 mg/kg). After a stable rhythm has been attained, hypotension and congestive heart failure must be aggressively treated.[114]

HEMODYNAMIC COMPLICATIONS

Hemodynamic abnormalities occur in most patients with AMI. They result from the loss of myocardial contractile elements and from impaired diastolic compliance. Signs of pulmonary congestion can be detected as rales on physical examination as well as by radiographic changes reflecting increased interstitial or alveolar fluid. Diminished cardiac output may be manifest as hypotension, cyanosis, confusion, or oliguria. The Killip classification, which separates patients into four hemodynamic classes depending on the degree of pulmonary congestion and the presence of hypoperfusion, is valuable in assessing short-term prognosis and directing therapy in patients with complicated myocardial infarction (Table 16–2).[115] However, the limitations of clinical signs are apparent, including the lack of specificity of a ventricular (S_3) gallop or pulmonary rales on physical examination and the lag phase that occurs between changes in hemodynamics and physical or radiographic findings. Direct monitoring of central venous and pulmonary capillary wedge pressures as well as cardiac output has shown that clinical estimates fail to detect significant elevations of wedge pressure (>18 mmHg) in 15% to 30% of patients.[116, 117] Hypoperfusion (cardiac index, ≤2.2 L/min/m²) is overlooked clinically in 25%.[117] This problem is particularly common in older patients.

Invasive hemodynamic monitoring is required in some patients in CCUs. Those who are clinically stable need no aggressive intervention. Those with clear evidence of pulmonary congestion usually respond well to judicious diuresis guided by the clinical response. However, if a favorable response is not demonstrated within several hours of empiric therapy, or if evidence suggests hemodynamic deterioration, placement of a pulmonary artery catheter should be considered. This approach would also be reasonable in patients in whom left ventricular failure or hypoperfusion is suspected, such as those with unexplained hypoxia or persistent tachycardia. Unstable patients who require parenteral vasodilators or agents with positive inotropic effects also benefit from hemodynamic monitoring.

HEMODYNAMIC SUBSETS

Data obtained with pulmonary artery catheterization in patients with AMI demonstrate that cardiac output is optimal with left heart filling pressures between 16 and 20 mmHg, and signs of pulmonary congestion are common with pressures of more than 18 mmHg.[116, 117, 119] Efforts to increase wedge pressure to this range can be expected to increase stroke volume, but this occurs at the expense of an increase in left ventricular radius and thus wall tension and oxygen demand. Optimizing cardiac output is only important if hypoperfusion is present; a cardiac index of less than 2.2 L/min/m² is a useful guide to physiologically inadequate perfusion.[116]

Using a wedge pressure of 18 mmHg and cardiac index of 2.2 L/min/m² as arbitrary dividing points, Forrester et al.[120] subdivided 200 patients with AMI into four hemodynamic subsets (Table 16–3). Patients with normal filling pressures (wedge pressure, ≤18 mmHg) and cardiac indexes (>2.2 L/min/m²) were clinically stable and had a mortality of only 3%.[120] Patients in subset II of the Forrester classification had elevated filling pressure and normal cardiac indexes, generally pulmonary congestion clinically, and a mortality of 9%. Subset III included all the patients with hypoperfusion (cardiac index, <2.2 L/min/m²), which was associated with a 23% in-hospital mortality. Patients with both elevated filling pressures and a depressed cardiac output (subset IV) had a 51% short-term mortality, which increased to 80% when clinical cardiogenic shock was present. The use of these hemodynamic subsets assists in prognostication and also helps direct therapeutic interventions (see Table 16–3).

Patients with normal filling pressures and normal cardiac outputs represent a low-risk group with an in-hospital mortality of less than 5%.[120] Among these are included patients with a hyperdynamic circulation typified by increased cardiac output (>3.5 L/min/m²), tachycardia, wide pulse pressure, and hypertension. These patients may have recurrent chest pain and extension of infarction. If other causes of heightened sympathetic tone such as pain, fever, or drug effect are excluded, β-blockade may be useful. Propranolol, up to 0.1 mg/kg, metoprolol, 0.2 mg/kg, or esmolol can be given intravenously to slow the heart rate, reduce blood pressure, and decrease myocardial oxygen demand. Often, beneficial changes in hemodynamics are accompanied by a decrease in chest pain. Left ventricular filling pressures that are elevated as a result of ischemia may fall after treatment with β-blockers as well.[60]

Suboptimal left ventricular filling pressures may result in hypoperfusion with hypotension and tachycardia. In the absence of an acute cause of volume loss (most commonly aggressive diuresis, but also emesis or gastrointestinal bleeding), blood volume in patients with AMI is usually normal. However, the ischemic left ventricle is relatively noncompliant and higher-than-usual filling pressures are needed to ensure adequate ventricular volume. Hypotensive patients without pulmonary congestion should be managed initially by Trendelenberg positioning and an acute volume challenge of 100 to 400 ml of crystalloid or colloid. Patients who remain hypotensive after an

Table 16–2. **Killip Classification of Patients with Acute Myocardial Infarction**

Class	Clinical Evaluation	Hospital Mortality (%)*
I	Normal	8
II	Rales <50% of lung fields or ventricular gallop	30
III	Rales >50% of lung fields, pulmonary edema	44
IV	Shock	>80

*Mortality rates reflect statistics from the 1960s.
Adapted with permission from Killip T, Kimball JT: Treatment of myocardial infarction in a coronary care unit. Am J Cardiol 20:457, 1967.

Table 16–3. **Hemodynamic Subsets in Acute Myocardial Infarction**

Subset	Pulmonary Wedge Pressure (mmHg)	Cardiac Index (L/min/m²)	Mortality (%)	Management Options
I	≤ 18	> 2.2	3	Observation (β-blockade*)
II	> 18	> 2.2	9	Diuretics, vasodilators (inotropic support)
III	≤ 18	≤ 2.2	23	Volume expansion (inotropic agents, vasodilators)
IV	> 18	≤ 2.2	51	Inotropic support, diuretic (vasopressor, vasodilator, balloon pump†)

*β-Blockade considered for limitation of infarct size, especially in patients in hyperdynamic state.

†In subset IV, the choice of vasopressor, vasodilator, or intraaortic balloon pump is dictated by the need for critical coronary perfusion pressure as well as considerations regarding myocardial oxygen demands.

Adapted from Forrester JS, Diamond G, Chatterjee K, et al: Medical therapy of acute myocardial infarction by application of hemodynamic subsets. N Engl J Med 295:1356, 1976. Copyright 1976, Massachusetts Medical Society. All rights reserved.

empiric fluid challenge should have pulmonary artery catheters and arterial catheters placed for hemodynamic monitoring. Fluid challenges with 100- to 200-ml boluses should continue until adequate cardiac output is achieved or a pulmonary capillary wedge pressure of 18 to 20 mmHg is reached.

When hypotension persists despite adequate volume expansion, usually cardiogenic shock is present. Some of these patients have marked bradycardia, which, coupled with a relatively fixed stroke volume, is responsible for low cardiac output. These patients respond to an increase in rate. Others have significant right ventricular infarction, the management of which is discussed later. Most, however, have cardiogenic shock as a result of extensive left ventricular infarction and have a short-term mortality exceeding 80%.

CONGESTIVE HEART FAILURE

Patients with mild congestive heart failure as determined by the presence of basilar rales, S_3 gallop, or radiographic signs of pulmonary congestion (Killip class II heart failure) can be managed conservatively. Treatment should include continued bed rest, oxygen, and diuresis. Only if there is no response or worsening of heart failure should the placement of a pulmonary artery catheter be considered. Patients with severe congestive heart failure (Killip class III) have diffuse rales, hypoxemia, and radiographic evidence of diffuse interstitial and alveolar edema. Emergent therapy with diuretics and vasodilators must be initiated immediately in these patients. Endotracheal intubation should be considered early to improve oxygenation and lessen the work of breathing. Hemodynamic monitoring is begun as soon as it is feasible and safe for the patient. A pulmonary wedge pressure of more than 25 mmHg is usual, as is a depressed cardiac output. Aggressive therapy with diuretics and vasodilators is continued, guided by hemodynamic responses.

In the setting of chronic congestive heart failure, diuretics improve hemodynamics through a reduction in right and left ventricular filling pressures (preload) and a decline in peripheral vascular resistance (afterload). The net result is an increase in stroke volume, preserved cardiac output, and an ameliora-

tion of pulmonary congestion.[121] Intravenous furosemide given to patients with AMI has been shown to dilate pulmonary and systemic venous capacitance beds and reduce filling pressures to the right and left sides of the heart independent of subsequent diuretic effects.[122, 123] However, there have also been reports of transient increases in peripheral vascular resistance and left ventricular filling pressures (a "pressor" effect) immediately after administration of intravenous furosemide, possibly mediated through the renin-angiotensin-aldosterone and sympathetic nervous systems.[124, 125] Which effect predominates in a given patient probably depends on the dose of furosemide given as well as the patient's state of neurohumoral activity. With acute congestive heart failure, a mild reduction in cardiac output is anticipated after a diuretic-induced reduction in preload. Excessive diuresis can result in hypotension, tachycardia, potassium depletion, and hyponatremia.

These considerations suggest caution in the use of diuretics in the treatment of patients with AMI.[126] However, one can use diuretics if judicious for the treatment of patients with mild to moderate congestive heart failure. Doses of furosemide should be limited to 0.5 mg/kg in patients with normal renal function to avoid a "pressor" response. They can be repeated every 3 or 4 hours, but a favorable response should be apparent within the first 2 hours. More severe heart failure, or a lack of response to diuresis, should prompt the use of parenteral vasodilators. Electrolytes and volume status must be watched closely to avoid aggravation of arrhythmia or an excessive decline in cardiac output.

VASODILATOR THERAPY

Myocardial infarction acutely impairs both the systolic contractile performance of the heart as well as its diastolic function. Stroke volume falls and neurohumoral mechanisms are invoked to support perfusion pressure and augment preload to the left ventricle. Release of catecholamines leads to tachycardia and an increase in contractility, while α-receptor stimulation causes peripheral vasoconstriction. This vasoconstrictor response is augmented by high levels of circulating angiotensin II as well as arginine vasopressin. These factors increase myocardial oxygen consumption and, by their effect on afterload, decrease cardiac output. Fluid retention or administration raises filling pressure in an attempt to increase cardiac output through the Frank-Starling mechanism. The initial increase in preload may improve stroke volume to a varying extent, depending on the slope of the Starling curve and preexisting filling pressures. Further increases in filling pressure beyond the plateau portion of the Starling curve serve only to increase pulmonary edema without improving cardiac output. Such increases also result in greater wall stress with the attendant propensity to infarct expansion and subsequent increased volumes during infarct remodeling.

Treatment with vasodilators ameliorate acute congestive heart failure through several mechanisms. Dilation of venous capacitance vessels reduces venous return and thereby eases pulmonary congestion. Arteriolar dilation reduces impedance, permitting increases in stroke volume and cardiac output. Reductions in left ventricular pressure and volume decrease wall stress and oxygen demand, improving subendocardial perfusion and diastolic compliance.[127] The result is that the left ventricular function curve (stroke volume versus filling pressure) is moved upward and to the left, allowing improved cardiac output at a lower filling pressure. The response to vasodilators is particularly marked in patients with mitral regurgitation, aortic insufficiency, left ventricular aneurysm, or hypertension.

Hemodynamic monitoring is essential for proper titration of parenteral vasodilators.[120, 126] Low doses of a vasodilator cause a moderate decline in peripheral vascular resistance that is offset largely by the increase in stroke volume so that little change occurs in heart rate or blood pressure. Higher doses, however, may cause excessive arterial dilation. In addition, venodilation can lower filling pressures to the steep portion of the Starling curve (below 12 to 15 mmHg), such that minor changes in preload cause an important decline in stroke volume. The result is a marked fall in blood pressure and reflex tachycardia and arterial vasoconstriction. Adverse reactions to vasodilator therapy can be avoided if hemodynamics are monitored carefully. In the failing heart, a favorable response to vasodilator therapy includes a decrease in peripheral resistance to near normal, a decline in wedge pressure to less than 20 mm Hg, and a consistent improvement in cardiac index without excessive tachycardia. Mean arterial pressure should remain at more than 70 mmHg.

Using guidelines similar to those previously outlined, patients with Killip class II or III heart failure treated with nitroprusside experience improved cardiac output and manifest a marked decline in pulmonary venous pressures without changes in heart rate and with only a minimal decline in blood pressure.[129] Reduced afterload and reduced diastolic left ventricular volume and pressure result in a decline in myocardial oxygen demand and improved subendocardial perfusion. Short-term clinical improvement[15, 129] and a reduction in hospital mortality have been reported.[130] However, these benefits were confined to patients with elevated left ventricular filling pressures. When the filling pressure is less than 15 mmHg, the addition of nitroprusside may cause a further fall in preload, a decrease in stroke volume, and resultant hypotension and tachycardia. This may be why in some studies patients with AMI treated with nitroprusside have a higher mortality.[17]

Early investigations with nitroglycerin for heart failure in patients with AMI demonstrated hemodynamic results comparable to those with nitroprusside.[131–133] Patients with elevated pulmonary venous pressures experienced decreases in filling pressures and increase in cardiac output. Those without high filling pressures often responded with excessive decreases in preload, resulting in decreased stroke volumes, hypotension, and tachycardia. As with nitroprusside, hemodynamic monitoring was essential to titrate nitroglycerin adequately for the treatment of patients with congestive heart failure.

Studies directly comparing the hemodynamic effects of nitroglycerin and nitroprusside confirm that both have venodilator and arteriolar dilating properties.[15, 134–136] Nitroglycerin, however, has relatively more potent venodilator properties and causes a greater decline in pulmonary venous pressure and a lesser increase in cardiac output than equivalent doses of nitroprusside (matched by equal effect on peripheral vascular resistance). Because of its more potent arteriolar dilating effects, nitroprusside causes a greater increase in cardiac output than nitroglycerin, especially when filling pressures fall below the optimal range. The choice between these two agents rests on the hemodynamic status of the patient and whether the primary goal is to reduce pulmonary congestion or to improve hypoperfusion. When there is no clear advantage in using one agent over the other, nitroglycerin should be selected because of its antiischemic properties, its potential to limit infarct size, and concerns[126, 136–139] that nitroprusside may exacerbate ischemia.[13]

Nitroprusside has a short plasma half-life (<3 minutes), as does nitroglycerin (approximately 5 minutes). Both are administered as continuous infusions without loading doses. Treatment with either drug is initiated at a dose of 5–10 µg/min and titrated upward every 5 to 10 minutes in 10 µg/min increments. Effective doses vary from patient to patient and cannot be predicted from baseline hemodynamics. Thus, the goal of titration is to improve cardiac index (>2.2 L/min/m²) and optimize preload (wedge pressure of approximately 16 to 18 mmHg) without a significant increase in heart rate or decline in blood pressure. If this goal cannot be met and especially if treatment is limited by hypotension, inotropic support is indicated (see later).

Hypotension complicating vasodilator therapy should be managed by a reduction in the infusion rate and moving the patient into the Trendelenburg position. Occasionally, nitroglycerin precipitates a vagal response with hypotension and bradycardia, which can be managed with atropine and a reduction in the nitroglycerin dose.[140] Both nitroglycerin and nitroprusside dilate pulmonary resistance vessels, leading to ventilation-perfusion mismatch and a fall in systemic arterial oxygen saturation.[141, 142] Methemoglobinemia with nitroglycerin and thiocyanate intoxication with nitroprusside are known complications of high-dose therapy. Prolonged infusions of nitroglycerin result in partial hemodynamic tolerance, such that the infusion rate must be titrated upward or nitroprusside must be substituted.[143, 144] Conversely, rebound deterioration of hemodynamics with abrupt termination of therapy is more common after nitroprusside administration; it can be prevented at times by gradual tapering and initiation of oral vasodilators.[15]

INOTROPIC THERAPY

Drugs with positive inotropic properties are used primarily in the treatment of cardiogenic shock but are also useful when severe congestive heart failure is refractory to treatment with vasodilators. Currently available agents include digitalis glycosides, adrenergic and dopaminergic receptor agonists, and phosphodiesterase inhibitors. Digoxin has been demonstrated to improve performance of the failing left ventricle after AMI, with little risk of aggravation of arrhythmia.[145] However, the magnitude of this effect is small, and there is little beneficial effect on preload or afterload.[146] Given the more potent effects of other agents, digoxin is now rarely used in the acute treatment of patients with AMI except to control supraventricular arrhythmias.

Catecholamines and related compounds remain the most commonly used agents for inotropic support in the CCU. Norepinephrine is a potent α-receptor agonist that causes increased peripheral resistance. This agent is used only when perfusion pressure is critically low, and then only to increase arterial systolic pressure to higher than 90 mmHg. Epinephrine and isoproterenol, because of their chronotropic and arrhythmogenic effects, should be avoided in patients with evolving myocardial infarction.

Dobutamine, a synthetic dopamine congener, is a relatively selective β1-receptor agonist with marked inotropic effects and little effect on blood pressure or heart rate at the usual doses of 10 to 15 μg/kg/min.[147, 148] At higher doses, tachycardia or an increase in blood pressure can occur. However, even low doses may accelerate the ventricular rate in atrial fibrillation. Treatment with dobutamine is normally initiated with an infusion rate of 5 μg/kg/min; the dose is then titrated according to hemodynamic response.[149] Expected benefits include an increase in cardiac output, a fall in left ventricular filling pressure, and a reflex decline in peripheral vascular resistance.[150, 151] Blood flow is increased preferentially to the coronary and skeletal muscle beds, but there is little change in renal blood flow. The reduction in left ventricular preload reduces wall stress and enhances subendocardial perfusion, offsetting increases in myocardial oxygen demand resulting from increased contractility. Clinical and experimental evidence confirm that when tachycardia is avoided, dobutamine is unlikely to aggravate ischemia or the extent of infarction.[152, 153] As with all adrenergic agents, prolonged use may result in partial tolerance as a result of downregulation of receptors. In this situation, the dobutamine infusion rate may need to be increased to elicit a stable hemodynamic response.[154]

Dopamine at a dose of 5 μg/kg/min has less effect on cardiac output than dobutamine at the same dose, but ventricular filling pressures increase even at low doses.[151] Although low doses of dopamine selectively dilate the renal arteries and improve renal blood flow, natriuresis is no better than that seen with dobutamine.[151] At higher doses, dopamine increases both arterial and pulmonary venous pressures, heart rate, and the frequency of ventricular arrhythmias.[151, 155] At higher doses, α-receptor–mediated vasoconstriction also reduces renal blood flow and increases left ventricular afterload. Dopamine should be reserved for patients with hypotension who require both inotropic and vasopressor support, or it may be used in low doses (3 μg/kg/min) for selective dilation of the renal arterial bed and promotion of the natriuretic effects of other inotropes or vasodilators. Because much of the initial response to dopamine is mediated by the release of endogenous catecholamines that are subsequently depleted, tachyphylaxis is a particular problem with this agent.[151, 156]

Amrinone, a bipyridine-derived phosphodiesterase inhibitor, has both inotropic and peripheral vasodilating properties.[157, 158] Currently approved for short-term intravenous use only, amrinone increases cardiac output while reducing cardiac filling pressure and peripheral vascular resistance. No increases in heart rate occur in patients without AMI except at high doses. Amrinone has little effect on arrhythmias. The inotropic effects of amrinone are not attenuated in patients treated with β-receptor blocking agents. Milrinone (Primacor) is a closely related phosphodiesterase inhibitor that is more potent than amrinone and avoids the high incidence of thrombocytopenia seen with that agent.[159]

Experience with amrinone and milrinone in patients with AMI is limited. The hemodynamic responses are similar to those in chronic congestive heart failure, with an increase in cardiac output, a decline in filling pressures, and modest changes in blood pressure and heart rate.[160] When compared with dobutamine in patients with elevated filling pressures but adequate cardiac output, they were more effective in lowering wedge pressures, presumably because of their vasodilator effects.[161] By lowering preload and afterload, wall tension is reduced and myocardial oxygen demands may fall. For these reasons, a beneficial effect of amrinone on myocardial oxygen consumption has been shown in a canine model of left ventricular failure.[162] In patients with congestive heart failure due to coronary artery disease, treatment with amrinone has been associated with a 20% decline in coronary blood flow as a result of a 30% reduction in myocardial oxygen demand.[163, 164] Despite these benefits, infarct size is not reduced in response to either amrinone or milrinone,[165, 166] as it is with dobutamine.[152] Furthermore, in experimental animals with coronary occlusion, exacerbation of ischemia has been reported.[167] Thus, the safety of amrinone in the setting of AMI is still unclear.

The adverse long-term effects recently reported with milrinone suggest that it may be no safer than amrinone.[168] Toxicity from amrinone includes reversible, usually mild thrombocytopenia characterized by decreased platelet survival as well as fever and liver function abnormalities. Milrinone does not cause thrombocytopenia. The plasma half-life of amrinone in normal patients is about 2.5 hours, but it may exceed 12 hours in patients with heart failure.[169] A loading dose of 0.75 to 1.5 mg/kg is given over 5 to 10 minutes followed by a maintenance infusion of 5 to 10 µg/kg/min. For milrinone, the initial dose is 50 µg/kg followed by an infusion of 0.375 to 0.75 µg/kg/min.[159]

CARDIOGENIC SHOCK

Cardiogenic shock is present when pulmonary congestion and low cardiac output are accompanied by clinical signs of hypoperfusion including hypotension, altered mental status, and oliguria. AMI may result in cardiogenic shock because of mechanical problems such as acute mitral regurgitation or ventricular septal defect (see later), significant right ventricular infarction (see later), or extensive left ventricular myocardial necrosis. The management and prognosis of cardiogenic shock vary with the underlying cause, but shock due to massive left ventricular infarction (myocardiogenic shock) proves fatal in 80% of patients, despite aggressive pharmacologic support. This dismal prognosis may be improved if early revascularization is achieved either surgically or by angioplasty.[170, 171] In some patients, temporary hemodynamic support with intraaortic balloon counterpulsation allows for an angiographic definition of anatomy, followed by revascularization, and surgical correction of mechanical lesions such as papillary muscle rupture or ventricular septal defects[172, 173] and for consideration of cardiac transplantation.

The initial goal in the treatment of cardiogenic shock is to ensure adequate coronary and central nervous system perfusion pressure. Norepinephrine (2 to 12 µg/min) is an effective vasopressor that also increases cardiac output when used in lower doses.[174] With higher doses, increasing left ventricular afterload may reduce cardiac output and aggravate ischemia. Dopamine is the preferred vasopressor when hypotension is less severe, because it has a more balanced effect on cardiac output and vascular resistance. However, both dopamine and norepinephrine increase pulmonary congestion in patients with congestive heart failure.[124] Accordingly, these agents should be used in the lowest possible doses to augment arterial pressure; dobutamine can be added for additional inotropic stimulation and to decrease filling pressures. Dopamine and dobutamine combined in the treatment of cardiogenic shock improve arterial pressure and cardiac output, promote diuresis, and reduce preload.[175]

Patients who do not improve rapidly with appropriate drug therapy should be considered for intraaortic balloon support, if there is a potentially reversible component to their pump failure. Deflation of the intraaortic balloon is timed to the cardiac cycle, at the onset of left ventricular ejection. Sudden balloon deflation reduces intraarterial volume and pressure, minimizing left ventricular afterload. At the conclusion of the ejection phase, the balloon reinflates, augmenting diastolic perfusion pressure to the coronary arteries and other arterial beds. Myocardial oxygen demands are reduced, and coronary perfusion is improved.[176, 177] Complications of balloon counterpulsation are common, including aortic rupture, arterial occlusion, and local or systemic infection. The incidence of complications has not changed with the advent of percutaneous insertion techniques.[178] In cardiogenic shock, intraaortic balloon support alone without definitive revascularization, repair of a mechanical defect, or transplantation is unlikely to influence the ultimate outcome.[179, 180] Thus, balloon support should be used as a bridging device to stabilize the shock patients to allow for diagnostic evaluation. With aggressive and expeditious implementation of pharmacologic and balloon support, progressing as indicated to emergent revascularization, mitral valve replacement, or closure of a septal defect, mortality from cardiogenic shock may be reduced to less than 50%.[171–173, 181]

RIGHT VENTRICULAR INFARCTION

Although enzymatic infarct size is similar in anterior and inferior wall infarction, left ventricular failure is far more common with anterior infarction. Occlusion of the left anterior descending coronary artery results in necrosis that is confined largely to the left ventricle, whereas a substantial portion of the damage resulting from right coronary occlusion involves the right ventricle. With right coronary occlusion proximal to the first acute marginal branch, 50% or more of the infarct may be localized to the right ventricle.[182] Patients with right ventricular hypertrophy, and perhaps patients with impaired collateral flow from the left coronary artery, may be particularly predisposed to right ventricular involvement.[183, 184]

Experimental evidence in a canine model of right ventricular (RV) infarction suggests that many hemodynamic perturbations are caused by acute enlargement of the right ventricle distending the pericardium. Intrapericardial pressures rise, the interventricular septum shifts to encroach on the left ventricular cavity, and effective transmural right and left ventricular filling pressures are limited by pericardial constraint.[185] RV function in this situation is maintained by egress of the septum into the right ventricle.[186, 187] Over time, collateral or antegrade flow results in edema and stiffening of the RV free wall, improving the efficacy of this septal egress. Eventually, RV free wall function improves.[188]

Significant right ventricular infarction should be suspected in any patient with hemodynamic compromise after inferior wall infarction. Electrocardiographic confirmation of right ventricular infarction includes the presence of ST segment elevation in the right precordial leads (V_1R through V_4R) in the acute setting or the evolution of QS complexes in the same leads when R waves are present on admission.[189, 191] Right ventricular dysfunction can also be documented by echocardiography or radionuclide angiography in 40% to 50% of patients with inferior infarction.[192]

Predominant right ventricular infarction occurs in 25% of patients with acute inferior infarction.[89, 193, 194] Classic findings include hypotension with low cardiac output, elevated central venous pressure with what appears to be (but is in reality not) a prominent Y descent in the neck veins or right atrial pressure tracing,[186, 187] and clear lungs. Classic findings may be absent, especially early in the hospital course and may be exposed only after volume loading. Hemodynamic monitoring is indicated in these patients, both to confirm the diagnosis and to assess the response to treatment.

Concomitant right atrial infarction occurs in nearly 50% of patients and exacerbates hemodynamic compromise.[187] In the absence of atrial infarction, bradycardia and particularly high-grade atrioventricular conduction block can lead to hemodynamic deterioration.[187, 195] Hemodynamics deteriorate both because of the slow rate and because the normal sequence of atrial and ventricular contraction is lost. Simple ventricular pacing does not restore proper AV sequencing, and hemodynamics do not improve. However, marked improvement occurs with AV sequential pacing owing to restoration of the atrial contribution to filling the ischemic ventricle and because properly timed atrial systole decreases atrial volume within the distended pericardium, leaving room for ventricular filling.[187, 196, 197]

Hypotension due to right ventricular infarction should be treated with volume expansion and by increasing pulmonary capillary wedge pressure to 16 to 20 mmHg. However, in response to volume expansion, intrapericardial pressures rise, and the net increase in transmural right and left ventricular filling pressures (preload) is minimized. Cardiac output and mean arterial pressure, therefore, may not improve.[198] Vasodilators and drugs that reduce preload (e.g., morphine, furosemide) may precipitate hypotension. In a controlled clinical trial, the best hemodynamic response in hypotensive patients was obtained with dobutamine infusion after appropriate, cautious volume expansion.[198] Dobutamine appears to improve stroke volume by increasing left ventricular performance and thus the egress of the septum into the RV cavity. This finding suggests that patients with disease of the left anterior descending coronary artery and/or poor left ventricular function are likely to have a worse prognosis than those without these difficulties.[203] Excessive fluid administration risks pulmonary edema, and theoretically could decrease left ventricular stroke volume if right ventricular dilatation is increased.[202]

The mortality rate with shock due to right ventricular infarction can be reduced by proper supportive care. Survivors have an excellent outlook for full functional recovery with a low incidence of chronic right or left ventricular dysfunction.

Ventricular Remodeling

A variety of processes associated with acute infarction change the geometric shape of the ventricle and can be associated with both short-term and long-term morbidity. Remodeling or its lack may be associated with myocardial rupture,[199, 200] rupture of a papillary muscle or chord of the mitral valve resulting in severe mitral regurgitation, rupture of the interventricular septum, and long-term changes in ventricular shape,[27, 201] which are associated with an adverse prognosis.

Myocardial rupture is an unusual complication of acute myocardial infarction. Although it accounts for as many as 3% of all deaths from myocardial infarction in general, given the very low mortality rate associated with acute infarction (around 10%), its overall incidence is fairly unusual.[202] Rupture occurs more frequently in older individuals and especially those with noncompliant left ventricles and those in whom myocardial infarction is the initial manifestation of ischemic heart disease.[202, 203] In some studies, rupture is associated with expansion of infarction, i.e., thinning of the infarct segment and dilation of the remaining ventricle.[199] In others, it is thought that it is the lack of expansion that leads to stress on the edges of the infarction, where normal myocardium contracts inwardly while at the same time there is paradoxical outward motion of the injured segment.[200] In this circumstance, this border zone is "bent" or "creased." As a result of the high pressure within the ventricle, blood then can seep within the interstices of the myocardium eventually reaching the pericardium. When the accumulation is sufficient, cardiac tamponade occurs. This process appears to be associated with increased wall stress and thus is more apt to occur in patients with heart failure and/or hypertension. There also is concern that rupture may occur more frequently after treatment with thrombolytic agents, especially if treatment is initiated late after the onset of infarction.[204] It should not be surprising that vasodilators such as nitroglycerin reduce the propensity to expansion and perhaps myocardial rupture as well.[138] β-Blockers also reduce the incidence of rupture.[92]

Controlled trials evaluating the treatment of rupture are lacking because of the difficulty in making the diagnosis. In general, patients with myocardial rupture have recurrent episodes of chest discomfort unassociated with electrocardiographic changes.[203] A diagnosis can be made only if the demographic characteristics of the patients are noticed and a high level of suspicion results in an echocardiogram that demonstrates an accumulating pericardial effusion. Once the diagnosis of subacute rupture is suspected, prompt therapy is required. Pericardiocentesis may be life saving, and immediate cardiac surgery is mandated; otherwise, mortality is highly likely.[205] Unfortunately, there is no absolute set of signs and symptoms that lead to this diagnosis, and thus a high degree of suspicion and expert clinical judgment are required.

A variant of myocardial rupture occurs when the rupture is sealed off locally by the pericardium. Because of the high pressures in the ventricle, the pericardium bulges and can form a large sack known as a pseudoaneurysm.[206] The pseudoaneurysm can enlarge to substantial size and act like a true aneurysm in that blood can be ejected into it reducing forward stroke volume. Rupture of the pseudoaneurysm can occur and is generally related to the size of the pseudoaneurysm, i.e., the larger the pseudoaneurysm, the greater the propensity to rupture. Accordingly, once a large pseudoaneurysm is diagnosed by echocardiogram, surgical intervention is mandated.[207] Whether pharmacologic therapy, including reduction in wall stress, would prevent rupture is speculative.

Rupture can also occur in the interventricular septum, presumably for similar reasons. In response to infarction, there is degradation of the myocardial interstitial components that have been damaged as part of the reparative process.[208] There are data also to suggest that bleeding into an infarcted area, such as might occur with late coronary recanalization, may contribute to weakness in the wall and rupture as well.[204] Conversely, the absence of collateral flow to the septum has also been reported to predispose to rupture.[209, 210] Patients with rupture of the interventricular septum generally present 2 to 7 days after acute infarction.[211] Infarction is equally frequent in the anterior and inferior locations[229] and often (40% of the time) is associated with single-vessel coronary artery disease.[213] Patients generally present with hypotension and a harsh murmur with a thrill along the left sternal border. Hemodynamic monitoring can reveal large V waves in the pulmonary artery occlusive pressure tracing, confusing the diagnosis. The diagnosis is easily made with Doppler echocardiography if the entire septum is interrogated.[214] At times, a ventricular septal defect high in the septum near the pulmonary outflow tract can be missed. In this circumstance, Swan-Ganz catheterization and blood samples for oxygen saturation usually are diagnostic. Surgical intervention can reduce the mortality associated with this abnormality by as much as 50%.[213, 215] There is considerable disagreement as to whether or not surgery should be done immediately, and the precise operation to be done, but aggressive vasodilation, including the use of intraaortic balloon counterpulsation, often is necessary to stabilize patients before definitive evaluation and surgery. However, intraaortic balloon counterpulsation alone is not effective.[195, 196]

Rupture of the mitral valve apparatus can also occur when a major head, usually of the posteromedial papillary muscle, is ruptured. In this situation (which has an incidence of about 1%), mitral regurgitation and pulmonary edema are sudden and often lead to immediate mortality.[216, 217] However, with less severe rupture, only severe mitral regurgitation may ensue. In general, patients present with hypotension and pulmonary edema. Patients have a loud murmur and often large V waves in their pulmonary artery occlusive pressure tracing. The definitive diagnosis can be made with Doppler echocardiography, which documents a flail mitral valve leaflet and severe mitral regurgitation.[214] It is important to diagnose such patients because more than 50% have single-vessel disease[233] and a modest-sized infarction[234] and therefore have the potential to be substantially improved by surgical reconstruction and/or replacement of the mitral valve. Once the diagnosis is suspected, aggressive vasodilation, including the use of intraaortic balloon counterpulsation, is mandated, with the intention to proceed to surgery when appropriate. Again, substantial controversy exists as to whether or not surgery should be done immediately or can be delayed to allow for stabilization.

A variant of these changes in ventricular geometry has recently been shown to be an important determinant of long-term prognosis. It has long been known that increases in ventricular size are associated with an adverse prognosis after acute infarction.[27] It is now apparent that such increases occur from thinning and "expansion" of the infarcted region and dilation of the remaining part of the ventricle.[27, 201, 218] This compensatory dilation that increases stroke volume to compensate for the reduced ejection fraction induced by infarction leads to increased wall stress and compensatory hypertrophy of other walls. This process has an acute phase that is mitigated by coronary recanalization but also a more chronic component that occurs insidiously over time.[219] Inhibition of this process with ACE inhibitors such as captopril has been shown to reduce mortality and morbidity.[27] Other vasodilators such as nitroglycerin have been used in experimental animals and evoke similar beneficial changes,[237] although both experimental and clinical data suggest that activation of the renin angiotensin system may play an important part in the pathogenesis of remodeling. For this reason, ACE inhibitors may be better agents and are the drugs of choice. In general, preclusion of expansion with intravenous nitroglycerin in the acute stage,[153] and in the long term, use of ACE inhibitors in traditional therapeutic doses, are recommended for all postinfarction patients who have significant reductions in ejection fraction. Obviously patients with congestive heart failure are likely to be treated with vasodilators, but even in the absence of overt heart failure, ACE inhibitors should be employed in patients with reduced ejection fractions to inhibit remodeling.[27]

Recurrent Ischemic Chest Discomfort

Recurrent ischemic chest discomfort is common in patients with acute infarction. During the early hours, it is likely a manifestation of irreversible injury, because intravenous nitroglycerin does not reduce morphine requirements.[139] Recurrent chest pain may represent a propensity to reocclusion in patients treated with thrombolytic agents, threatened reinfarction in patients with non–Q-wave infarction, pericarditis, or a propensity to myocardial rupture. Several relevant groups can be defined:

1. Patients treated with thrombolytic agents who have recurrent chest discomfort should be evaluated for the possibility of coronary reocclusion.[221] The presence of recurrent ST elevation is diagnostic, but before recurrent ECG changes, pain may occur. Patients who have received thrombolytic therapy and who are being treated with heparin should have an immediate check of the activated partial thromboplastin time (aPTT) to assess whether anticoagulation is adequate; if not, additional heparin may be necessary. If reocclusion is suspected, emergent catheterization is indicated in the absence of an immediately remediable factor (e.g., inadequate anticoagulation). If cardiac catheterization cannot be accomplished, patients are usually treated with intravenous nitroglycerin and/or β-blockers depending on their hemodynamic status.

2. Patients with non–Q-wave myocardial infarction are known to be at risk for recurrent infarction (extension of infarction), especially when they present with ST-segment changes and recurrent episodes of chest discomfort.[222] In previous trials, such patients have been shown to benefit from the adjunctive use of diltiazem in addition to nitrates and β-blockers.[223] However, in many institutions, recurrent chest pain in patients with non–Q-wave infarction mandates cardiac catheterization for the determination of coronary anatomy and the possibility of mechanical revascularization. In the absence of recurrent chest pain or ST depression, patients with non–Q-wave infarction do well.[222] However, the risk of recurrent infarction is present not only during the acute hospitalization but over time. Thus, the prognosis of patients with non–Q-wave infarction is equivalent to that of patients with Q-wave infarction by 6 months to 1 year after infarction.[224] Whether aggressive intervention would he helpful in such patients in the absence of recurrent symptoms is unclear. In some studies, β-blockers have been helpful[18] to these patients, and in others they have not.[19] Calcium antagonists may be helpful judging from clinical trials, as long as patients do not have markedly impaired hemodynamic performance.[225]

3. A subset of patients at uniquely high risk are patients with chest pain and ST-segment and/or T-wave changes in a new location distant from the site of infarction. Such patients often have multivessel coronary artery disease and are at high risk for recurrent infarction without prompt cardiac catheterization and attempts at mechanical revascularization.[226]

LIMITATION OF INFARCT SIZE

After abrupt coronary artery occlusion, irreversible cellular injury begins within the first 30 minutes in the subendocardium of the central ischemic zone and spreads outward.[3] The time to completion of the infarction varies, depending on the extent of collateral blood flow, hemodynamics, and whether transient antegrade flow (opening and closing of the infarct artery) occurs. Because the ultimate extent of myocardial necrosis is the key factor determining short- and long-term prognosis after AMI, interventions to limit infarct size and therefore decrease morbidity and mortality must be initiated as early as possible.

THROMBOLYTIC AGENTS

The most direct approach to the limitation of infarct size involves the restoration of coronary perfusion. Thrombolytic therapy with streptokinase, urokinase, tissue-type plasminogen activator, or anisoylated plasminogen streptokinase activator complex has been demonstrated to restore arterial patency in as many as 80% of patients treated within the first few hours of AMI (see Section XV, Subsection D, "Thrombolytic Agents"). Recent data support the use of these agents up to 12 hours after the onset of infarction.[227] Mortality is clearly related to both the extent and promptness of recanalization.[4, 218] Balloon angioplasty may be employed as a primary modality instead of thrombolytic agents, and some believe it is more effective than thrombolytic treatment.[229] Unfortunately, it is logistically difficult for most hospitals to offer timely angioplasty at all hours of the day and night. In patients with multivessel disease, or those with a single large-vessel occlusion that cannot be opened successfully in the catheterization suite, emergent bypass surgery may be warranted. With successful early reperfusion, mortality is diminished and left ventricular function is preserved.

Important questions regarding the use of thrombolytic agents are discussed in Chapter 152. Selection of the most appropriate agent, optimal dosage and infusion rate, benefits of combination of thrombolytic drugs, the addition of antiplatelet and antithrombin agents, the role of angioplasty in improving patency and left ventricular performance, the timing of invasive intervention, and possible benefits from drugs coadministered to diminish ischemia or limit reperfusion injury are discussed there. However, the potential benefit of revascularization is not available to all patients with evolving infarction. Clinical trials of thrombolysis generally include only a small fraction of patients screened with myocardial infarction. Some patients who are excluded might be candidates for angioplasty or surgery but only in properly equipped cardiovascular centers. Thus, other means for the limitation of ongoing infarction are needed. In addition, it is now clear that treatment often takes too long to initiate.[230] Vigorous efforts to reduce delays are essential.[231]

β-BLOCKADE

β-Adrenoceptor blockade has been tested extensively in the setting of AMI. Potential benefits of β-blockade include a reduction in myocardial oxygen demand as a result of slowing of the heart rate, a decline in arterial blood pressure, and a decrease in contractility.[11] Oxygen supply to the ischemic zone may improve because of increased collateral blood flow and a shift of flow toward the subendocardium.[61] β-Adrenergic blockade also reduces arterial concentrations of free fatty acid and limits their uptake and catabolism by the heart.[232] A shift from free fatty acid to carbohydrate catabolism allows energy production at a lower oxygen cost, favoring myocardial viability.[233, 240]

Large, well-controlled clinical trials of intravenously administered β-blockers in the early hours of AMI have demonstrated a decline in patients' mortality and a reduction in infarct size.[235-238] A large trial of metoprolol randomized patients to placebo or metoprolol, 15 mg IV followed by 50 mg PO every 6 hours. Mortality in the hospital and at 90-day follow-up was reduced, with a 47% decline in mortality after 3 months among those who continued treatment throughout the study. Overall, the mortality reduction was 36%.[235] Enzymatically estimated infarct size was 15% smaller in patients given metoprolol within 12 hours of chest pain than in patients given placebo.[236] A similar trial of intravenous timolol[254] given within 4 hours of onset of infarction resulted in a 30% reduction in infarct size based on creatine kinase release, and the electrocardiographic indexes of infarct size also were limited. No effect on infarct size was seen with propranolol in another large trial, but the timing of intervention was late. Only 2% of patients were treated within 4 hours, and 50% were treated after 8 hours.[239] As with all interventions, β-adrenergic blockade should be initiated as early as possible to affect the extent of infarction maximally. Experimental data in the dog model suggest that β-blockade can enhance myocardial salvage after coronary occlusion and reperfusion.[240, 241] Clinical trials of β-blockers in patients treated with thrombolytic agents have suggested a reduction in nonfatal infarction if β-blockers are administered early.[242]

Studies of acute β-blockade have demonstrated a decrease in the duration and severity of chest pain with the reversal of ischemia.[243-245] Ventricular ectopy, including salvos of nonsustained ventricular tachycardia, is not reliably suppressed by β-blockade, but the incidence of ventricular fibrillation is markedly reduced.[91, 245] Despite the potential negative inotropic effect, congestive heart failure is seen to a similar extent in control patients and treated patients. When β-blockade is begun early in patients with AMI, the incidence of heart failure is decreased in the treated group.[246] The frequency of myocardial rupture is similarly diminished.[238]

These promising results may not apply to all individuals with AMI. The patients included in these acute intervention studies were highly selected, and 50% to 90% of screened patients were excluded.[244, 245, 247] Many high-risk patients were excluded because of bradycardia, hypotension, heart failure, prior myocardial infarction, or current treatment with β-blockers or calcium antagonists. Despite this careful selection process, there is an excess of bradycardia, heart block, and hypotension in treated patients, especially among those with inferior infarction.[235, 237, 248] However, no increase occurs in the incidence of cardiogenic shock or the need for pacemakers, and there is a reduction in ventricular and supraventricular tachyarrhythmias.[249]

Continued β-blockade after the acute phase of infarction may reduce the incidence of infarct extension later during the hospital stay or prevent infarction in those admitted with intermediate syndrome.[249] Long-term treatment after discharge can reduce mortality in the first 2 years by approximately 25%, with a particularly marked effect on sudden cardiac death.[18-21, 250] Rates of reinfarction are reduced by 35% to 40% in most trials.[18-21, 251] β-Blockers with significant intrinsic sympathomimetic activity may not be as effective as other agents, and they should not be used routinely after myocardial infarction.[22]

Patients considered for prophylactic β-blocker therapy after myocardial infarction are those at intermediate risk for complications. Those with heart failure, inducible ischemia, or serious arrhythmias should have specific therapy directed at these complications. Those with single-vessel coronary artery disease and small, uncomplicated infarcts have excellent outlooks and little to gain from β-blockade. Thus, it has been estimated that approximately 50% of infarction survivors are eligible for chronic prophylactic therapy. Of patients treated, protection appears to apply equally regardless of age, mechanical or electrical complications of the infarct, and extent of left ventricular dysfunction. In fact, if treatment can be tolerated hemodynamically, high-risk patients, including diabetics, have the same proportionate reduction in mortality and a much greater absolute benefit from β-adrenergic blockade.[251-254]

NITROGLYCERIN

Nitroglycerin reduces myocardial oxygen demand through its effects on preload and afterload, and it may improve coronary blood flow to the ischemic zone. In animal studies, carefully controlled infusions of nitroglycerin increase collateral flow and increase the endocardial:epicardial ratio of perfusion.[255, 256] However, excessive doses, especially in the setting of low filling pressure, can cause hypotension, tachycardia, and a worsening of ischemia.[257] Early clinical studies of nitroglycerin therapy in patients with AMI confirmed the findings in animals. When given in doses that avoided hypotension, nitroglycerin could decrease ST-segment elevation and improve hemodynamics. Patients with low filling pressures were prone to hypotension, tachycardia, and worsening ischemia; these deleterious effects could be avoided when the blood pressure was supported with phenylephrine.[258, 259]

Subsequent larger, randomized clinical trials of intravenous nitroglycerin confirm a beneficial effect on enzymatically determined infarct size. In these trials, nitroglycerin infusions were titrated against the hemodynamic response, starting at 5 to 10 μg/min. End points to titration varied but basically included less than a 10% decrease in systolic or mean arterial pressure, a systolic pressure maintained at more than 90 mmHg, and an increase in heart rate of no more than 20 beats/min.[137, 139, 140, 260] Infusions were maintained for 24 to 48 hours and then tapered. Adverse reactions, which were uncommon with low-dose infusions, included hypotension, tachycardia, bradycardia, headache, nausea, and vomiting. Hypotension occurs in approximately 10% of patients, is more common in those with inferior infarction, and usually responds promptly to cessation of nitroglycerin and head-down tilt. On occasion, atropine may be necessary, and if the heart rate has not increased reflexly, it is often effective.[140] Hemodynamic monitoring to avoid a fall in filling pressure below 10 mmHg may prevent some of these hypotensive episodes.

MAGNESIUM

A variety of small clinical studies and experimental studies have suggested that intravenous administration of magnesium improves prognosis after AMI.[93, 94] Many of the clinical studies have suggested this benefit is mediated by a reduction in arrhythmias, but a recent large trial did not support this conclusion.[95] However, it did document a reduction in mortality from 10.3% to 7.8% over 30 days when all patients with AMI were treated with 1 g of magnesium over the first hour and then 8 g over the next 24 hours. Judging from a reduced frequency of congestive heart failure, benefit might have been a result of reduced infarct size.[95]

OTHER APPROACHES

Other approaches to the limitation of infarct size, including the use of calcium antagonists, hyaluronidase, oxygen–free radical scavengers, glucose-insulin-potassium infusion, antiplatelet agents, and corticosteroids, are either ineffective or unproven. However, meticulous attention to the details of "conventional" management in AMI, including pain relief, control of hypertension or hypoxemia, suppression of arrhythmia, and optimal hemodynamic support, helps limit infarct size even in patients who are not candidates for the more aggressive measures outlined earlier. The era of merely playing a supporting role for patients with evolving infarction has passed, and physicians must now consider myocardial viability as a key variable in all decisions in the CCU.

REFERENCES

1. DeWood MA, Spores J, Notske R, et al: Prevalence of total coronary occlusion during the early hours of transmural myocardial infarction. N Engl J Med 303:897, 1980.
2. Eisenberg PE, Sherman LA, Schechtman K, et al: Fibrinopeptide A: A marker of acute coronary thrombosis. Circulation 71:912, 1985.
3. Reimer KA, Lowe JE, Rasmussen MM, Jennings RB: The wavefront phenomenon of ischemic cell death. 1. Myocardial infarct size vs duration of coronary occlusion in dogs. Circulation 56:786, 1977.
4. Italian Group for the Study of Streptokinase in Myocardial Infarction (GISSI): Effectiveness of intravenous thrombolytic treatment in acute myocardial infarction. Lancet 1:397, 1986.
5. Semenkovich CF, Jaffe AS: Adverse effects due to morphine sulfate: A challenge to previous clinical doctrine. Am J Med 79:325, 1985.
6. Harvey WP, Berkman F, Leonard J: Caution against the use of meperidine hydrochloride (isonipecaine, Demerol) in patients with heart disease, particularly auricular flutter. Am Heart J 49:758, 1955.
7. Lee G, DeMaria AN, Amsterdam EA, et al: Comparative effects of morphine, meperidine, and pentazocine on cardiocirculatory dynamics in patients with acute myocardial infarction. Am J Med 60:949, 1976.
8. Gunnar RM, Loeb HS, Scanlon PJ, et al: Management of acute myocardial infarction and accelerating angina. Prog Cardiovasc Dis 22:1, 1979.
9. Sukumalchantra Y, Levy S, Danzig R, et al: Correcting arterial hypoxemia by oxygen therapy in patients with acute myocardial infarction: Effects on ventilation and hemodynamics. Am J Cardiol 24:838, 1969.
10. Madias JE, Madias NE, Hood WB: Precordial ST-segment mapping. 2. Effects of oxygen inhalation on ischemic injury in patients with acute myocardial infarction. Circulation 53:411, 1976.
11. Mueller HS, Ayers SM, Religa A, et al: Propranolol in the treatment of acute myocardial infarction: Effect on myocardial oxygenation and hemodynamics. Circulation 49:1078, 1974.
12. Flaherty JT, Magee PA, Gardner TL, et al: Comparison of intravenous nitroglycerin and sodium nitroprusside for treatment of acute hypertension developing after coronary artery bypass surgery. Circulation 65:1072, 1982.
13. Chiariello M, Gold HK, Leinbach RC, et al: Comparison between the effects of nitroprusside and nitroglycerin on ischemic injury during acute myocardial infarction. Circulation 54:766, 1976.
14. Warltier DC, Gross GT, Brooks HL: Coronary steal-induced increase in myocardial infarct size after pharmacologic vasodilation. Am J Cardiol 46:83, 1980.
15. Leier CV, Bambach D, Thompson MJ, et al: Central and regional hemodynamic effects of intravenous isosorbide dinitrate, nitroglycerin and nitroprusside in patients with congestive heart failure. Am J Cardiol 48:1115, 1981.
16. Durrer JD, Lie KI, van Cappelle FJL, et al: Effect of sodium nitroprusside on mortality in acute myocardial infarction. N Engl J Med 306:1121, 1982.
17. Cohn JN, Franciosa JA, Francis GS, et al: Effect of short-term infusion of sodium nitroprusside on mortality rate in acute myocardial infarction complicated by ventricular failure. Results of a VA Cooperative Study. N Engl J Med 306:1129, 1982.
18. Pedersen TR, Norwegian Multicenter Study Group: Six-year follow-up of the Norwegian multicenter study on timolol after acute myocardial infarction. N Engl J Med 313:1055, 1985.
19. Beta-blocker Heart Attack Trial Research Group: A randomized trial of propranolol in patients with acute myocardial infarction. I. Mortality results. JAMA 247:1707, 1982.
20. Olsson G, Rehnqvist N, Sjogren A, et al: Long-term treatment with metoprolol after myocardial infarction: Effect on 3 year mortality and morbidity. J Am Coll Cardiol 5:1428, 1985.
21. Green KG, Chamberlain DA, Fulton RM, et al: Reduction in mortality after myocardial infarction with long-term beta-adrenoceptor blockade. Br Med J 2:419, 1977.
22. Australian and Swedish Pindolol Study Group: The effect of pindolol on the two year mortality after complicated myocardial infarction. Eur Heart J 4:367, 1983.
23. Kjekshus JK: Importance of heart rate in determining beta-blocker efficacy in acute and long-term acute myocardial infarction in intervention trials. Am J Cardiol 57:43F, 1986.
24. Chadda K, Goldstein S, Byington R, Curb JD: Effect of propranolol after acute myocardial infarction in patients with congestive heart failure. Circulation 73:50310, 1986.
25. Swedberg K, CONSENSUS Trial Study Group: Effects of enalapril on mortality in severe congestive heart failure: Results of the Cooperative North Scandinavian Enalapril Survival Study (CONSENSUS). N Engl J Med 316:1429, 1987.

26. Cohn JN, Archibald DG, Ziesche S, et al: Effect of vasodilatory therapy on mortality in chronic congestive heart failure. Results of a Veterans Administration cooperative study. N Engl J Med 314:1547, 1986.
27. Pfeffer MA, Braunwald E, Moye LA, et al: Patients with left ventricular dysfunction after myocardial infarction: Results of the survival and ventricular enlargement trial. N Engl J Med 327:669, 1992.
28. Miller RR, Lies JE, Carretta RF, et al: Prevention of lower extremity venous thrombosis by early mobilization. Ann Intern Med 84:700, 1976.
29. Hayes MJ, Morris GK, Hampton JR: Comparison of mobilization after two days in uncomplicated myocardial infarction. Br Med J 3:10, 1974.
30. Maurer BJ, Wray R, Shillingford JP: Frequency of venous thrombosis after myocardial infarction. Lancet 2:1385, 1971.
31. Gallus AS, Hirsh J, Tuttle RJ, et al: Small subcutaneous doses of heparin in prevention of venous thrombosis. N Engl J Med 288:545, 1973.
32. Pierard LA, Albert A, Henrard L, et al: Incidence and significance of pericardial effusion in acute myocardial infarction as determined by two dimensional echocardiography. J Am Coll Cardiol 8:517, 1986.
33. Kaplan K, Davison R, Parker M, et al: Frequency of pericardial effusion as determined by M-mode echocardiography in acute myocardial infarction. Am J Cardiol 55:335, 1985.
34. Galve E, Garcia-DelCastillo H, Evangelista A, et al: Pericardial effusion in the course of myocardial infarction: Incidence, natural history, and clinical relevance. Circulation 73:294, 1986.
35. Lichstein E, Liu H, Gupta P: Pericarditis complicating acute myocardial infarction: Incidence of complications and significance of electrocardiogram on admission. Am Heart J 87:246, 1974.
36. Krainin FM, Flessas AP, Spodick DH: Infarction-associated pericarditis: Rarity of diagnostic electrocardiogram. N Engl J Med 311:1211, 1984.
37. Niarchos AP, McKendrick CS: Prognosis of pericarditis after acute myocardial infarction. Br Heart J 35:49, 1973.
38. Silverman HS, Pfeifer MP: Relation between the use of anti-inflammatory agents and left ventricular free wall rupture during acute myocardial infarction. Am J Cardiol 59:363, 1987.
39. Brown EJ Jr, Kloner RA, Schoen FJ, et al: Scar thinning due to ibuprofen administration following experimental myocardial infarction. Am J Cardiol 51:877, 1983.
40. Dressler W: The post-myocardial infarction syndrome: A report of 44 cases. Arch Intern Med 103:28, 1959.
41. Northcote RJ, Hutchison SJ, McGuinness JB: Evidence for the continued existence of the postmyocardial infarction (Dressler's) syndrome. Am J Cardiol 53:1201, 1984.
42. Lichstein E, Arsura E, Hollander G, et al: Current incidence of postmyocardial infarction (Dressler's) syndrome. Am J Cardiol 50:1269, 1982.
43. Pastemac RC, Braunwald E, Sobel BE: Acute myocardial infarction. In Braunwald E (ed): Heart Disease. Philadelphia: WB Saunders, 1988, pp 1222–1313.
44. O'Doherty M, Taylor DI, Quinn E: Five hundred patients with myocardial infarction—monitored within one hour of symptoms. Br Med J 286:1405, 1983.
45. Corday E, Corday SR: Advances in clinical management of acute myocardial infarction in the past 25 years. J Am Coll Cardiol 1:126, 1983.
46. Roberts R, Husain A, Ambos HD, et al: Relation between infarct size and ventricular arrhythmias. Br Heart J 37:1169, 1975.
47. Geltman EM, Ehsani AA, Campbell MK, et al: The influence of location and extent of myocardial infarction on long-term ventricular dysrhythmias and mortality. Circulation 60:805, 1979.
48. Graner LE, Gershen BJ, Orland MM, et al: Bradycardia and its complications in the prehospital phase of acute myocardial infarction. Am J Cardiol 32:607, 1973.
49. Wei JY, Markis JE, Malagold M, et al: Cardiovascular reflexes stimulated by reperfusion of ischemic myocardium in acute myocardial infarction. Circulation 67:796, 1983.
50. Das G, Talmers FN, Weissler AM: New observations on the effects of atropine on the sinoatrial and atrioventricular nodes in man. Am J Cardiol 36:281, 1975.
51. Feigl D, Ashkenazy J, Kishon Y: Early and late atrioventricular block in acute inferior myocardial infarction. J Am Coll Cardiol 4:35, 1984.
52. Biddle TL, Ehrich DA, Yu PN: Relation of heart block and left ventricular dysfunction in acute myocardial infarction. Am J Cardiol 39:961, 1977.
53. Shah PK, Nalos P, Peter T: Atropine resistant post-infarction complete AV block: Possible role of adenosine and improvement with aminophylline. Am Heart J 113:194, 1987.
54. Klein RC, Vera Z, Mason DT: Intraventricular conduction defects in acute myocardial infarction: Incidence, prognosis, and therapy. Am Heart J 108:1007, 1984.
55. Mullins CB, Atkins JM: Prognoses and management of ventricular conduction blocks in acute myocardial infarction. Mod Concepts Cardiovasc Dis 45:129, 1976.
56. Hindman MC, Wagner GS, JaRo M, et al: The clinical significance of bundle branch block complicating acute myocardial infarction. 2. Indications for temporary and permanent pacemaker insertion. Circulation 58:689, 1978.
57. Ewy GA: Ventricular fibrillation masquerading as asystole. Ann Emerg Med 13:811, 1984.
58. Cummins RO, Graves JR, Larsen MP, et al: Out-of-hospital transcutaneous pacing by emergency medical technicians in patients with asystolic cardiac arrest. N Engl J Med 328:1377, 1993.
59. Zoll PM, Zoll RH, Falk RH, et al: External noninvasive temporary cardiac pacing: Clinical trials. Circulation 71:937, 1985.
60. Forrester JA, Chatterjee K, Jobin G: A new conceptual approach to the therapy of acute myocardial infarction. Adv Cardiol 15:111, 1975.
61. Fox KM, Selwyn AP, Welman E: The effects of propranolol on myocardial perfusion and metabolism during acute regional ischemia. Clin Cardiol 3:47, 1980.
62. Jewitt DE, Baleon R, Raferty EB, et al: Incidence and management of supraventricular arrhythmias after acute myocardial infarction. Lancet 2:734, 1967.
63. Klass M, Haywood LJ: Atrial fibrillation associated with acute myocardial infarction: A study of thirty-four cases. Am Heart J 79:752, 1970.
64. Tetsuro S, Iwasaka T, Ogawa A, et al: Atrial fibrillation in acute myocardial infarction. Am J Cardiol 56:27, 1985.
65. Liberthson RR, Salisbury KW, Hutter AM Jr, et al: Atrial tachyarrhythmias in acute myocardial infarction. Am J Med 60:956, 1976.
66. Hod H, Lew AS, Keltai M, et al: Early atrial fibrillation during evolving myocardial infarction: A consequence of impaired left atrial perfusion. Circulation 75:146, 1987.
67. Salerno DM, Dias VC, Kleiger RE, et al: Efficacy and safety of intravenous diltiazem for treatment of atrial fibrillation and atrial flutter. The Diltiazem-Atrial Fibrillation/Flutter Study Group. Am J Cardiol 63:1046, 1989.
68. Ellenbogen KA, Dias VC, Plumb VJ, et al: A placebo controlled trial of continuous intravenous diltiazem infusion for 24-hour heart rate control during atrial fibrillation and atrial flutter: A multicenter study. J Am Coll Cardiol 18:891, 1991.
69. The Esmolol Multicenter Study Research Group: Efficacy and safety of esmolol vs propranolol in the treatment of supraventricular tachycardias: A multicenter doubleblind clinical trial. Am Heart J 110:913, 1985.
70. Waxman HL, Myerberg RJ, Appel R, et al: Verapamil for control of ventricular rate in paroxysmal supraventricular tachycardia and atrial flutter or fibrillation. Ann Intern Med 94:1, 1981.
71. Pittman DE, Makar JS, Kooros K, et al: Rapid atrial stimulation: Successful method of conversion of atrial flutter and atrial tachycardia. Am J Cardiol 32:700, 1973.
72. Belhasses B, Pelleg A: Acute management of paroxysmal supraventricular tachycardia: Verapamil, adenosine triphosphate, or adenosine? Am J Cardiol 54:225, 1984.
73. Huycke EC, Sung RJ, Dias VC, et al: Intravenous diltiazem for termination of reentrant supraventricular tachycardia: A placebo controlled, randomized, double-blind, multicenter study. J Am Coll Cardiol 13:538, 1989.

74. Singh BH, Ellrodt G, Peter CT: Verapamil: A review of its pharmacologic properties and therapeutic use. Drugs 15:169, 1978.

75. Pantridge JF, Webb SW, Adgey AAJ, et al: The first hour after the onset of acute myocardial infarction. In Yu PN, Goodwin JF (eds): Progress in Cardiology. Philadelphia: Lea & Febiger, 1974, pp 173–188.

76. Lawrie DM, Higgins MR, Godman MJ, et al: Ventricular fibrillation complicating acute myocardial infarction. Lancet 2:523, 1968.

77. ElSherif N, Myerburg RJ, Scherlag BJ, et al: Electrocardiographic antecedents of primary ventricular fibrillation. Br Heart J 38:415, 1976.

78. Lie KI, Wellens HJJ, Downar E, et al: Observations on patients with primary ventricular fibrillation complicating acute myocardial infarction. Circulation 52:755, 1975.

79. Lown B, Fakhro A, Hood WB, et al: The coronary care unit—new perspectives and directions. JAMA 199:188, 1981.

80. BeMett MA, Pentecost BL: Warning of cardiac arrest due to ventricular fibrillation and tachycardia. Lancet 1:1351, 1972.

81. Roberts R, Ambos HD, Loh CW, et al: Initiation of repetitive ventricular depolarizations by relatively late premature complexes in patients with acute myocardial infarction. Am J Cardiol 41:678, 1978.

82. Lie KI, Wellens HJJ, van Capelle FJ, et al: Lidocaine in the prevention of primary ventricular fibrillation: A double-blind, randomized study of 212 consecutive patients. N Engl J Med 291:1324, 1974.

83. DeSilva RA, Lown B, Hennekens CH, et al: Lidocaine prophylaxis in acute myocardial infarction: An evaluation of randomized trials. Lancet 2:855, 1981.

84. Antman EM, Berlin JA: Declining incidence of ventricular fibrillation in myocardial infarction. Implications for the prophylactic use of lidocaine. Circulation 86:764, 1992.

85. Jaffe AS: The use of antiarrhythmics in advanced cardiac life support. Ann Emerg Med 22:307, 1993.

86. MacMahon S, Collins R, Peto R, et al: Effects of prophylactic lidocaine in suspected acute myocardial infarction. An overview of results from the randomized, controlled trials. JAMA 260:1910, 1988.

87. Hine LK, Laird N, Hewitt P, Chalmers TC: Meta-analytic evidence against prophylactic use of lidocaine in acute myocardial infarction. Arch Intern Med 149:2694, 1989.

88. Volpi A, Cavalli A, Santoro E, Tognoni G: Incidence and prognosis of secondary ventricular fibrillation in acute myocardial infarction. Evidence for a protective effect of thrombolytic therapy. GISSI Investigators. Circulation 82:1279, 1990.

89. Carruth JE, Silverman ME: Ventricular fibrillation complicating acute myocardial infarction: Reasons against the routine use of lidocaine. Am Heart J 104:545, 1982.

90. Volpi A, Maggioni A, Franzosi M, et al: In-hospital prognosis of patients with acute myocardial infarction complicated by primary ventricular fibrillation. N Engl J Med 317:257, 1987.

91. Norris RM, Barnaby PF, Brown MA, et al: Prevention of ventricular fibrillation during acute myocardial infarction by intravenous propranolol. Lancet 2:883, 1984.

92. Randomised trial of intravenous atenolol among 16,027 cases of suspected acute myocardial infarction: ISIS-1. First International Study of Infarct Survival Collaborative Group. Lancet 2:57, 1986.

93. Horner SM: Efficacy of intravenous magnesium in acute myocardial infarction in reducing arrhythmias and mortality. Meta-analysis of magnesium in acute myocardial infarction. Circulation 86:774, 1992.

94. Teo KK, Yusuf S, Collins R, et al: Effects of intravenous magnesium in suspected acute myocardial infarction: Overview of randomised trials. BMJ 303:1499, 1991.

95. Woods KL, Fletcher S, Roffe C, Haider Y: Intravenous magnesium sulphate in suspected acute myocardial infarction: Results of the second Leicester Intravenous Magnesium Intervention Trial (LIMIT-2). Lancet 339:1553, 1992.

96. LeLorier J, Grenon D, Latour Y, et al: Pharmacokinetics of lidocaine after prolonged intravenous infusions in uncomplicated myocardial infarction. Ann Intern Med 87:700, 1977.

97. Collinsworth KA, Kalman SM, Harrison DC: The clinical pharmacology of lidocaine as an antiarrhythmic drug. Circulation 50:1217, 1974.

98. Rademaker AW, Kellen J, Yun KT, et al: Character of adverse effects of prophylactic lidocaine in the coronary care unit. Clin Pharmacol Ther 40:71, 1986.

99. Lima JJ, Goldfarb AL, Conti DR, et al: Safety and efficacy of procainamide infusions. Am J Cardiol 43:98, 1979.

100. Lemberg L, Castellanos A, Arcebal AG: The use of propranolol in arrhythmias complicating acute myocardial infarction. Am Heart J 80:479, 1970.

101. Norris RM, Singh BN: Arrhythmias in acute myocardial infarction. In Norris RM (ed): Myocardial Infarction. Edinburgh: Churchill Livingstone, 1982, pp 55–86.

102. Gorgels APM, Vos MA, Letsch IS, et al: Usefulness of the accelerated idioventricular rhythm as a marker for myocardial necrosis and reperfusion during thrombolytic therapy in acute myocardial infarction. Am J Cardiol 61:231, 1988.

103. Lichstein E, Ribas-Meneclier C, Gupta PK, et al: Incidence and description of accelerated ventricular rhythm complicating acute myocardial infarction. Am J Med 58:192, 1975.

104. de Soyza N, Bissett BEC, Kane JJ, et al: Association of accelerated idioventricular rhythm and paroxysmal ventricular tachycardia in acute myocardial infarction. Am J Cardiol 34:667, 1974.

105. Bigger JT, Dresdale RJ, Heissenbuttel RH, et al: Ventricular arrhythmias in ischemic heart disease: Mechanisms, prevalence, significance and management. Prog Cardiovasc Dis 19:255, 1977.

106. Nordrehaug JE, Johannessen KA, von der Lippe G: Serum potassium concentration as a risk factor of ventricular arrhythmias early in acute myocardial infarction. Circulation 71:645, 1985.

107. Dreifus LS, Azevedo IH, Watanabe Y: Electrolyte and antiarrhythmic drug action. Am Heart J 88:95, 1974.

108. Mostow ND, Vrobel TR, Noon D, et al: Rapid suppression of complex ventricular arrhythmias with high-dose oral amiodarone. Circulation 73:1231, 1986.

109. Wolfe CL, Nibley C, Bhandari A, et al: Polymorphous ventricular tachycardia associated with acute myocardial infarction. Circulation 84:1543, 1991.

110. Friedberg C, Lyon L, Donoso E: Suppression of refractory recurrent ventricular tachycardia by rapid cardiac pacing and antiarrhythmic drugs. Am Heart J 79:44, 1970.

111. Ornato J, Gonzales E, Jaffe AS: The use of cardiovascular drug during cardiopulmonary resuscitation. In Messerli FH (ed): Cardiovascular Drug Therapy, 2nd ed. Philadelphia: WB Saunders, 1996.

112. Emergency Cardiac Care Committee and Subcommittees, American Heart Association: Guidelines for cardiopulmonary resuscitation and emergency cardiac care. JAMA 268:2171, 1992.

113. Hughes WG, Ruedy JR: Should calcium be used in cardiac arrest? Am J Med 81:285, 1986.

114. Holmes HR, Babbs CF, Voorhees WD, et al: Influence of adrenergic drugs upon vital organ perfusion during CPR. Crit Care Med 8:137, 1980.

115. Killip T, Kimball JT: Treatment of myocardial infarction in a coronary care unit. Am J Cardiol 20:457, 1967.

116. Forrester JS, Diamond GA, Swan HJC: Correlative classification of clinical and hemodynamic function after acute myocardial infarction. Am J Cardiol 39:137, 1977.

117. Shell WE, DeWood MA, Peter T, et al: Comparison of clinical signs and hemodynamic state in the early hours of transmural myocardial infarction. Am Heart J 104:521, 1982.

118. Crexells C, Chatterjee K, Forrester JS, et al: Optimal level of filling pressure in the left side of the heart in acute myocardial infarction. N Engl J Med 289:1263, 1973.

119. Russell RO Jr, Rackley CE, Pombo J, et al: Effects of increasing left ventricular filling pressure in patients with acute myocardial infarction. J Clin Invest 49:1539, 1970.

120. Forrester JS, Diamond G, Chatteree K, et al: Medical therapy of acute myocardial infarction by application of hemodynamic subsets. N Engl J Med 295:1356, 1976.

121. Wilson JR, Reichek N, Dunkman WB, et al: Effect of diuresis on the performance of the failing left ventricle in man. Am J Med 70:234, 1981.

122. Dikshit K, Vyden JK, Forrester JS, et al: Renal and extrarenal hemodynamic effects of furosemide in congestive heart failure after acute myocardial infarction. N Engl J Med 288:1087, 1973.

123. Kiely J, Kelly DT, Taylor DR, et al: The role of furosemide in the treatment of left ventricular dysfunction associated with acute myocardial infarction. Circulation 48:581, 1973.

124. Francis GS, Siegel RM, Goldsmith SR, et al: Acute vasoconstrictor response to intravenous furosemide in patients with chronic congestive heart failure. Ann Intern Med 103:1, 1985.

125. Nelson GIC, Silke B, Forsyth DR, et al: Hemodynamic comparison of primary venous or arteriolar dilation and the subsequent effect of furosemide in left ventricular failure after acute myocardial infarction. Am J Cardiol 52:1036, 1983.

126. Genton R, Jaffe AS: Management of congestive heart failure in patients with acute myocardial infarction. JAMA 256:2556, 1986.

127. Chatterjee K, Parmley WW: Vasodilator therapy for acute myocardial infarction and chronic congestive heart failure. J Am Coll Cardiol 1:133, 1983.

128. Franciosa JA, Limas CJ, Guiha NH, et al: Improved left ventricular function during nitroprusside infusion in acute myocardial infarction. Lancet 1:650, 1972.

129. Chatterjee K, Parmley WW, Gans W, et al: Hemodynamic and metabolic responses to vasodilator therapy in acute myocardial infarction. Circulation 48:1183, 1973.

130. Chatterjee K, Swan HJC, Kaushik VS, et al: Effects of vasodilator therapy for severe pump failure in acute myocardial infarction on short-term and late prognosis. Circulation 53:797, 1976.

131. Flaherty JT, Come PC, Baird MG, et al: Effects of intravenous nitroglycerin on left ventricular function and ST-segment changes in acute myocardial infarction. Br Heart J 38:612, 1976.

132. Williams DO, Amsterdam EA, Mason DT: Hemodynamic effects of nitroglycerin in acute myocardial infarction: Decrease in ventricular preload at the expense of cardiac output. Circulation 51:421, 1975.

133. Bussman WD, Schofer H, Kaltenbach M, et al: Effects of intravenous nitroglycerin on hemodynamics and ischemic injury in patients with acute myocardial infarction. Eur J Cardiol 8:61, 1978.

134. Armstrong PW, Walker DC, Burton JR, et al: Vasodilator therapy in acute myocardial infarction: A comparison of sodium nitroprusside and nitroglycerin. Circulation 52:1118, 1975.

135. Kotter V, Von Leitner ER, Wunderlich J, et al: Comparison of hemodynamic effects of phentolamine, sodium nitroprusside, and glyceryl trinitrate in acute myocardial infarction. Br Heart J 39:1196 1977.

136. Bussmann WD, Passek D, Seidel W, et al: Reduction of CK and CK-MB indexes of infarct size by intravenous nitroglycerin. Circulation 63:615, 1981.

137. Jugdutt BI, Warnica JW: Intravenous nitroglycerin therapy to limit myocardial infarct size, expansion, and complications. Effect of timing, dosage, and infarct location. Circulation 78:906, 1988.

138. Jaffe AS, Geltman EM, Tiefenbrun VAJ, et al: Reduction of infarct size in patients with inferior infarction with intravenous glyceryl trinitrate. Br Heart J 49:452, 1983.

139. Flaherty JT, Becker LC, Bulkley BH, et al: A randomized prospective trial of intravenous nitroglycerin in patients with acute myocardial infarction. Circulation 68:576, 1983.

140. Come P, Pitt B: Nitroglycerin-induced severe hypotension and bradycardia in patients with acute myocardial infarction. Circulation 54:624, 1976.

141. Hales CA, Westphal D: Hypoxemia following the administration of sublingual nitroglycerin. Am J Med 65:911, 1978.

142. Mookherjee S, Keighly JFH, Wamer RA, et al: Hemodynamic, ventilatory and blood gas changes during infusion of sodium nitroprusside: Studies in patients with congestive heart failure. Chest 72:273, 1977.

143. Elkayam U, Kulick D, McIntosh N, et al: Incidence of early tolerance to hemodynamic effects of continuous infusion of nitroglycerin in patients with coronary artery disease and heart failure. Circulation 76:577, 1987.

144. Jugdutt BI, Warnica JW: Tolerance with low dose intravenous nitroglycerin therapy in acute myocardial infarction. Am J Cardiol 64:581, 1989.

145. Rahimtoola SH, Gunnar RM: Digitalis in acute myocardial infarction: Help or hazard? Ann Intern Med 82:234, 1982.

146. Goldstein RA, Passamani ER, Roberts R: A comparison of digoxin and dobutamine in patients with acute infarction and cardiac failure. N Engl J Med 303:846, 1980.

147. Gillespie TA, Ambos HD, Sobel BE, et al: Effects of dobutamine in patients with acute myocardial infarction. Am J Cardiol 39:588, 1977.

148. Leier CV, Unverferth DV: Dobutamine. Ann Intern Med 99:490, 1983.

149. Sonnenblick EH, Frishman WH, Le Jemtel TH: Dobutamine: A new synthetic cardioselective sympathetic amine. N Engl J Med 300:17, 1979.

150. Vatner SF, McRitchie RJ, Braunwald E: Effects of dobutamine on left ventricular performance, coronary dynamics, and distribution of cardiac output in conscious dogs. J Clin Invest 53:1265, 1974.

151. Leier CV, Heban PT, Huss P, et al: Comparative systemic and regional hemodynamic effects of dopamine and dobutamine in patients with cardiomyopathic heart failure. Circulation 58:466, 1978.

152. Maekawa K, Liang CS, Hood WB Jr: Comparison of dobutamine and dopamine in acute myocardial infarction. Circulation 67:750, 1983.

153. Unverferth DV, Blanford M, Kates RE, et al: Tolerance to dobutamine after a 72 hour continuous infusion. Am J Med 69:262, 1980.

154. Francis GS, Sharrna B, Hodges M, et al: Comparative hemodynamic effects of dopamine and dobutamine in patients with acute cardiogenic circulatory collapse. Am Heart J 103:995, 1982.

155. Beregovich J, Bianchi C, Rubler S, et al: Dose-related hemodynamic and renal effects of dopamine in congestive heart failure. Am Heart J 87:550, 1974.

156. Maskin CS, Ocken S, Chadwick B, et al: Comparative systemic and renal effects of dopamine and angiotensin-converting enzyme inhibition with enalaprilat in patients with heart failure. Circulation 72:846, 1985.

157. Colucci WS, Wright RF, Braunwald E: New positive inotropic agents in the treatment of congestive heart failure: Mechanism of action and recent clinical developments. N Engl J Med 314:349, 1986.

158. Benotti JR, McCue JE, Alpert JS: Comparative vasoactive therapy for heart failure. Am J Cardiol 56:19B, 1985.

159. DiBianco R: Acute positive inotropic intervention: The phosphodiesterase inhibitors. Am Heart J 121:1871, 1991.

160. Taylor SH, Verma SP, Hussain M, et al: Intravenous amrinone in left ventricular failure complicated by acute myocardial infarction. Am J Cardiol 56:29B, 1985.

161. Silke B, Verma SP, Midtbo KA, et al: Comparative hemodynamic dose-response effects of dopamine and amrinone in left ventricular failure complicating acute myocardial infarction. J Cardiovasc Pharmacol 9:19, 1987.

162. Jentzer JH, LeJemtel TH, Sonnenblick EH, et al: Beneficial effect of amrinone on myocardial oxygen consumption during acute left ventricular failure in dogs. Am J Cardiol 48:75, 1981.

163. Benotti JR, Grossman W, Braunwald E, et al: Effects of amrinone on myocardial energy metabolism and hemodynamics in patients with severe congestive heart failure due to coronary artery disease. Circulation 62:28, 1980.

164. Monrad ES, Baim DS, Smitn HS, et al: Effects of milrinone on coronary hemodynamics and myocardial energetics in patients with congestive heart failure. Circulation 71:972, 1985.

165. Campbell CA, Reddy BR, Alker KJ, et al: Effect of milrinone on acute myocardial infarct size. Am J Cardiol 60:422, 1987.

166. Campbell CA, Mehta PM, Wynne J, Kloner RA: The cardiotonic agent amrinone does not increase anatomic infarct size. J Cardiovasc Pharmacol 9:225, 1987.

167. Rude RE, Kloner RA, Maroko PR, et al: Effects of amrinone on experimental acute myocardial ischaemic injury. Cardiovasc Res 7:419, 1980.

168. Packer M, Carver JR, Rodeheffer RJ, et al: Effect of oral milrinone on mortality in severe chronic heart failure. The PROMISE Study Research Group. N Engl J Med 325:1468, 1991.

169. Edelson J, Le Jemtel TH, Alousi AA, et al: Relationship be-

tween amrinone plasma concentration and cardiac index. Clin Pharmacol Ther 29:723, 1981.

170. O'Neill W, Erbel R, Laufer N, et al: Coronary angioplasty therapy of cardiogenic shock complicating acute myocardial infarction [abstract]. Circulation 72(Suppl III):III-309, 1985.

171. Lee L, Walton JA, Bates E, et al: Cardiogenic shock complicating acute myocardial infarction: Changing therapies and prognosis [abstract]. Circulation 74(Suppl II):II-276, 1986.

172. Gunnar RM, Loeb HS: Shock in acute myocardial infarction: Evolution of physiologic therapy. J Am Coll Cardiol 1:154, 1983.

173. Hager WD, Katz AM: Management of shock in acute myocardial infarction: Changing concepts. Cardiology 74:286, 1987.

174. Abrams E, Forrester JS, Chatterjee K, et al: Variability in response to norepinephrine in acute myocardial infarction. Am J Cardiol 32:919, 1973.

175. Richard C, Ricome JL, Rirnailho A, et al: Combined hemodynamic effects of dopamine and dobutamine in cardiogenic shock. Circulation 67:620, 1983.

176. Fuchs RM, Brin KP, Brinker JA, et al: Augmentation of regional coronary blood flow by intra-aortic balloon counterpulsation in patients with unstable angina. Circulation 68:117, 1983.

177. Weiss AT, Engel S, Gotsman CJ, et al: Regional and global left ventricular function during intra-aortic balloon counterpulsation in patients with acute myocardial infarction shock. Am Heart J 108:249, 1984.

178. Alcan CE, Stertzer SH, Wallsh E, et al: Comparison of wire-guided percutaneous insertion and conventional surgical insertion of intra-aortic balloon pumps in 151 patients. Am J Med 75:24, 1983.

179. Baron DW, O'Rourke MF: Long-term results of arterial counterpulsation in acute severe cardiac failure complicating myocardial infarction. Br Heart J 38:285, 1976.

180. Cohen LS: Current status of circulatory assist devices. Am J Cardiol 33:316, 1974.

181. Keon WJ: Surgery for acute myocardial infarction and cardiogenic shock. Cardiovasc Rev Rep 2:1120, 1981.

182. Andersen HR, Falk E, Melsen D: Right ventricular infarction: Frequency, size and topography in coronary heart disease: A prospective study. J Am Coll Cardiol 10:1223, 1987.

183. Fonnan MB, Wilson BH, Sheller JR, et al: Right ventricular hypertrophy is an important determinant of right ventricular infarction complicating acute inferior left ventricular infarction. J Am Coll Cardiol 10:1180, 1987.

184. Ratliff NB, Hackel DB: Combined right and left ventricular infarction: Pathogenesis and clinicopathologic correlations. Am J Cardiol 45:217, 1980.

185. Goldstein JA, Vlahakes GJ, Verrier ED, et al: The role of right ventricular systolic dysfunction and elevated intrapericardial pressure in the genesis of low output in experimental right ventricular infarction. Circulation 65:513, 1982.

186. Goldstein JA, Tweddell JS, Barzilai B, et al: Importance of left ventricular function and systolic ventricular interaction to right ventricular performance during acute right heart ischemia. J Am Coll Cardiol 19:704, 1992.

187. Goldstein JA, Barzilai B, Rosamond TL, et al: Determinants of hemodynamic compromise with severe right ventricular infarction. Circulation 82:359, 1990.

188. Laster SB, Shelton TJ, Barzilai B, Goldstein JA: Determinants of the recovery of right ventricular performance following experimental chronic right coronary artery occlusion. Circulation 88:696, 1993.

189. Klein HO, Tordjman T, Ninio R, et al: The early recognition of right ventricular infarction: Diagnostic accuracy of the electrocardiographic V4R lead. Circulation 67:558, 1983.

190. Candell-Riera J, Figueras J, Valle V, et al: Right ventricular infarction: Relationships between ST segment elevation in V4R and hemodynamic, scintigraphic, and echocardiographic findings in patients with acute inferior myocardial infarction. Am Heart J 101:281, 1981.

191. Morgera T, Alberti E, Silvestri F, et al: Right precordial ST and QRS changes in the diagnosis of right ventricular infarction. Am Heart J 108:13, 1984.

192. Dell'Italia LJ, Starling MR, Crawford MH, et al: Right ventricular infarction: Identification by hemodynamic measurements before and after volume loading and correlation with non-invasive techniques. J Am Coll Cardiol 4:931, 1984.

193. Cohn JN, Guiha NH, Broder MI, et al: Right ventricular infarction: Clinical and hemodynamic features. Am J Cardiol 33:209, 1974.

194. Lorell B, Leinbach RC, Pohost GM, et al: Right ventricular infarction: Clinical diagnosis and differentiation from cardiac tamponade and pericardial constriction. Am J Cardiol 43:465, 1979.

195. Braat SH, de Zwaan C, Brugada P, et al: Right ventricular involvement with acute inferior wall myocardial infarction identifies high risk of developing atrioventricular nodal conduction disturbances. Am Heart J 107:1183, 1984.

196. Topol EJ, Goldschlager N, Ports TA, et al: Hemodynamic benefit of atrial pacing in right ventricular myocardial infarction. Ann Intern Med 96:594, 1982.

197. Love JC, Haffajee CI, Gore JM, et al: Reversibility of hypotension and shock by atrial or atrioventricular sequential pacing in patients with right ventricular infarction. Am Heart J 108:5, 1984.

198. Dell'Italia LJ, Starling MR, Blumhardt R, et al: Comparative effects of volume loading, dobutamine, and nitroprusside in patients with predominant right ventricular infarction. Circulation 72:1327, 1985.

199. Schuster EH, Bulkley BH: Expansion of transmural myocardial infarction: A pathophysiologic factor in cardiac rupture. Circulation 60:1532, 1979.

200. Saffitz JE, Fredrickson RC, Roberts WC: Relation of size of transmural acute myocardial infarct to mode of death, interval between infarction and death and frequency of coronary arterial thrombus. Am J Cardiol 57:1249, 1986.

201. Pfeffer MA, Lamas GA, Vaughan DE, et al: Effect of captopril on progressive ventricular dilatation after anterior myocardial infarction. N Engl J Med 319:80, 1988.

202. Dellborg M, Held P, Swedberg K, Vedin A: Rupture of the myocardium, occurrence and risk factors. Br Heart J 54:11, 1985.

203. Bates RJ, Beutler S, Resnekov L, Anagnostopoulos CE: Cardiac rupture—challenge in diagnosis and management. Am J Cardiol 40:429, 1977.

204. Mathey DG, Schofer J, Kuck K-H, et al: Transmural, haemorrhagic myocardial infarction after intracoronary streptokinase, clinical, angiographic, and necropsy findings. Br Heart J 48:546, 1982.

205. Lopez-Sendon J, Gonzalez A, Lopez E, et al: Diagnosis of subacute ventricular wall rupture after acute myocardial infarction: Sensitivity and specificity of clinical, hemodynamic and echocardiographic criteria. J Am Coll Cardiol 19: 1145, 1992.

206. Vlodaver Z, Coe JL, Edwards JE: True and false aneurysms. Circulation 51:567, 1975.

207. Shabbo FP, Dymond DS, Rees GM, Hill IM: Surgical treatment of false aneurysm of the left ventricle after myocardial infarction. Thorax 38:25, 1983.

208. Zhao M, Zhang H, Robinson TF, et al: Profound ultrastructural alterations of the extracellular collagen matrix in postischemic dysfunctional ("stunned") but viable myocardium. J Am Coll Cardiol 10:1322, 1987.

209. Mann JM, Roberts W: Acquired ventricular septal defect during myocardial infarction: Analysis of 38 unoperated necropsy patients and comparison with 50 unoperated necropsy patients without rupture. Am J Cardiol 62:8, 1988.

210. Jugdutt BI, Michorowski BL: Role of infarct in rupture of the ventricular septum after acute myocardial infarction: A two dimensional echocardiographic study. Clin Cardiol 10:641, 1987.

211. Fox AC, Glassman E, Isom OW: Surgically remediable complications of myocardial infarction. Prog Cardiovasc Dis 21:461, 1979.

212. Roberts WC, Ronan JA, Harvey WP: Rupture of the left ventricular free wall or ventricular septum secondary to myocardial infarction: An occurrence virtually limited to the first transmural myocardial infarction in a hypertensive individual [abstract]. Am J Cardiol 35:166, 1975.

213. Radford MJ, Johnson RA, Daggett WM Jr, et al: Ventricular septal rupture: A review of clinical and physiologic features and an analysis of survival. Circulation 64:545, 1981.
214. Kishon Y, Iqbal A, Oh JK, et al: Evolution of echocardiographic modalities in detection of postmyocardial infarction ventricular septal rupture and papillary muscle rupture: Study of 62 patients. Am Heart J 126:667, 1993.
215. Montoya A, McKeever L, Scanlon P, et al: Early repair of ventricular septal rupture after infarction. Am J Cardiol 45:345, 1980.
216. Nishimura RA, Schaff HV, Shub C, et al: Papillary muscle rupture complicating acute myocardial infarction: Analysis of 17 patients. Am J Cardiol 51:373, 1983.
217. Wei JY, Hutchins GM, Bulkley BH: Papillary muscle rupture in fatal acute myocardial infarction: A potentially treatable form of cardiogenic shock. Ann Intern Med 90:149, 1979.
218. Eaton LW, Weiss JL, Bulkley BH, et al: Regional cardiac dilatation after acute myocardial infarction: Recognition by two-dimensional echocardiography. N Engl J Med 300:57, 1979.
219. Jeremy RW, Allman KC, Bautovitch G, Harris PJ: Patterns of left ventricular dilation during the six months after myocardial infarction. J Am Coll Cardiol 13:304, 1989.
220. McDonald KM, Francis GS, Matthews J, et al: Long-term oral nitrate therapy prevents chronic ventricular remodeling in the dog. J Am Coll Cardiol 21:514, 1993.
221. Hsia J, Kleiman N, Aguirre F, et al: Heparin-induced prolongation of partial thromboplastin time after thrombolysis: Relation to coronary artery patency. HART Investigators. J Am Coll Cardiol 20:31, 1992.
222. Schechtman KB, Capone RJ, Kleiger RE, et al: Risk stratification of patients with non-Q wave myocardial infarction. The critical role of ST segment depression. The Diltiazem Reinfarction Study Research Group. Circulation 80:1148, 1989.
223. Gibson RS, Boden WE, Theroux P, et al: Diltiazem and reinfarction in patients with non-Q-wave myocardial infarction. Results of a double-blind, randomized, multicenter trial. N Engl J Med 315:423, 1986.
224. Nicod P, Gilpin E, Dittrich H, et al: Short- and long-term clinical outcome after Q wave and non-Q wave myocardial infarction in a large patient population. Circulation 79:528, 1989.
225. Goldstein RE, Boccuzzi SJ, Cruess D, Nattel S: Diltiazem increases late-onset congestive heart failure in postinfarction patients with early reduction in ejection fraction. The Adverse Experience Committee and the Multicenter Diltiazem Postinfarction Research Group [see comments]. Circulation 83:52, 1991.
226. Schuster EH, Bulkley BH: Ischemia at a distance after acute myocardial infarction: A cause of early postinfarction angina. Circulation 62:509, 1980.
227. Late Assessment of Thrombolytic Efficacy (LATE) study with alteplase 6–24 hours after onset of acute myocardial infarction. Lancet 342:759, 1993.
228. An international randomized trial comparing four thrombolytic strategies for acute myocardial infarction. The GUSTO investigators. N Engl J Med 329:673, 1993.
229. Grines CL, Browne KF, Marco J, et al: Original articles: A comparison of immediate angioplasty with thrombolytic therapy for acute myocardial infarction. N Engl J Med 328:673, 1993.
230. Kereiakes DJ, Weaver WD, Anderson JL, et al: Time delays in the diagnosis and treatment of acute myocardial infarction: A tale of eight cities: Report from the pre-hospital study group and the Cincinnati heart project. Am Heart J 120:773, 1990.
231. Eisenberg MS, Aghababair RV, Bossaert L, et al: Thrombolytic therapy. Ann Emerg Med 22:417, 1993.
232. Kjekshus JK, Mjos OD: Effect of inhibition of lipolysis on infarct size after experimental coronary artery occlusion. J Clin Invest 52:1770, 1973.
233. Shrago E, Shug AL, Sul H, et al: Control of energy production in myocardial ischemia Circ Res 38(Suppl 1):75, 1976.
234. Simonsen S, Kjekshus JK: The effect of free fatty acids on myocardial oxygen consumption during atrial pacing and catecholamine infusion in man. Circulation 58:484, 1978.
235. Hjalmarson A, Elmfeldt D, Herlitz J, et al: Effect on mortality of metoprolol in acute myocardial infarction. Lancet 2:823, 1981.
236. Herlitz J, Elmfeldt D, Hjalmarson A, et al: Effect of metoprolol on indirect signs of the size and severity of acute myocardial infarction. Am J Cardiol 51:1282, 1983.
237. International Collaborative Study Group: Reduction of infarct size with the early use of timolol in acute myocardial infarction. N Engl J Med 310:9, 1984.
238. ISIS-1 (First International Study of Infarct Survival) Collaborative Group: Randomized trial of intravenous atenolol among 16,027 cases of suspected acute myocardial infarction: ISIS-I. Lancet 2:57, 1986.
239. Roberts R, Croft C, Gold HEC, et al: Effect of propranolol on myocardial-infarct size in a randomized blinded multicenter trial. N Engl J Med 311:218, 1984.
240. Hammerman H, Kloner RA, Briggs LL, et al: Enhancement of salvage of reperfused myocardium by early beta-adrenergic blockade (timolol). J Am Coll Cardiol 3:1438, 1984.
241. Miyazawa K, Fukuyama H, Komatsu E, et al: Effects of propranolol on myocardial damage resulting from coronary artery occlusion followed by reperfusion. Am Heart J 111:519, 1986.
242. Roberts R, Rogers WJ, Mueller HS, et al: The TIMI investigators. Immediate versus deferred beta-blockade following thrombolytic therapy in patients with acute myocardial infarction: Results of the Thrombolysis in Myocardial Infarction (TIMI) II-B Study. Circulation 83:422, 1991.
243. Herlitz J, Hjaknarson A, Holmberg S, et al: Effect of metoprolol on chest pain in acute myocardial infarction. Br Heart J 51:439, 1984.
244. Yusuf S, Sleight P, Rossi P, et al: Reduction in infarct size, arrhythmias, and chest pain by early intravenous beta blockade in suspected acute myocardial infarction. Circulation 67(Suppl 1):32, 1983.
245. Ryden L, Ariniego R, Arnman K, et al: A double-blind trial of metoprolol in acute myocardial infarction: Effects on ventricular tachyarrhythmias. N Engl J Med 308:614, 1983.
246. Herlitz J, Hjalmarson A, Hoknberg S, et al: Development of congestive heart failure after treatment with metoprolol in acute myocardial infarction. Br Heart J 51:539, 1984.
247. MIAMI Trial Research Group: Patient population. Am J Cardiol 56:10G, 1985.
248. MIAMI Trial Research Group: Other clinical findings and tolerability. Am J Cardiol 56:39G, 1985.
249. MIAMI Trial Research Group: Development of myocardial infarction. Am J Cardiol 56:23G, 1985.
250. Singh BN, Venkatesh N: Prevention of myocardial reinfarction and of sudden death in survivors of acute myocardial infarction: Role of proplylactic beta-adrenoceptor blockade. Am Heart J 107:189, 1984.
251. Kjekshus J, Gilpin E, Cali G, et al: Diabetic patients and beta-blockers after acute myocardial infarction. Eur Heart J 11:43, 1990.
252. Gundersen T: Influence of heart size on mortality and reinfarction in patients treated with timolol after myocardial infarction. Br Heart J 50:135, 1983.
253. Gundersen T, Abrahamsen AM, Kjekshus J, et al: Timolol-related reduction in mortality and reinfarction in patients ages 65–75 years surviving acute myocardial infarction. Circulation 66:1179, 1982.
254. Furberg CD, Hawkins CM, Lichstein E, et al: Effect of propranol in postinfarction patients with mechanical or electrical complications. Circulation 69:761, 1984.
255. Swain J, Parker JP, McHale PA, et al: Effects of nitroglycerin and propranolol on the distribution of transmural myocardial blood flow during ischemia in the absence of hemodynamic changes in the unanesthetized dog. J Clin Invest 63:947, 1979.
256. Capurro NL, Kent KM, Smith HJ, et al: Acute coronary occlusion: Prolonged increase in collateral flow following brief administration of nitroglycerin and methoxamine. Am J Cardiol 39:679, 1977.
257. Jugdutt BI: Myocardial salvage by intravenous nitroglycerin in conscious dogs: Loss of beneficial effect with marked nitroglycerin-induced hypotension. Circulation 68:673, 1983.

258. Borer JS, Redwood DR, Levitt B, et al: Reduction in myocardial ischemia with nitroglycerin or nitroglycerin plus phenylephrine administered during acute myocardial infarction. N Engl J Med 293:1008, 1975.

259. Miller RR, Awan NA, De Maria AN, et al: Importance of maintaining systemic blood pressure during nitroglycerin ad-

ministration for reducing ischemic injury in patients with coronary artery disease. Am J Cardiol 40:504, 1977.

260. Jugdutt BI, Sussex BA, Warnica JW, et al: Persistent reduction in left ventricular asynergy in patients with acute myocardial infarction by intravenous infusion of nitroglycerin. Circulation 68:1264, 1983.

CHAPTER 17

Hypertensive Emergencies

James F. Burris, M.D., and Edward D. Freis, M.D.

Acute or severe blood pressure elevation may precipitate a medical emergency requiring prompt reduction of blood pressure to prevent death or progressive injury to vital organs. A hypertensive crisis is not defined by the absolute level of blood pressure elevation alone, but a diastolic pressure of more than 120 mmHg generally is associated with a greatly increased risk of imminent organ damage. Individuals with chronic hypertension may tolerate blood pressures exceeding 200/120 mmHg without immediate adverse effects as a result of an upward shift in vascular autoregulation in cerebral (Fig. 17–1), renal, and other vascular beds,[1-3] whereas previously normotensive individuals who experience rapid rises in blood pressure (as in eclampsia or acute glomerulonephritis) may sustain injury to vital organs at only moderately hypertensive blood pressures. Thus, a marked elevation of blood pressure may constitute severe hypertension alone, a hypertensive urgency, or a true hypertensive emergency, depending on the presence or absence of associated evidence of rapidly progressive target-organ damage.[4-6] Because the clinical features of hypertensive crises are often nonspecific, accurate diagnosis depends on a careful history, physical ex-

amination, and a brief laboratory screen seeking evidence of end-organ dysfunction. When evidence of progressive neurologic, cardiovascular, or renal impairment is present, immediate hospitalization and prompt reduction of the blood pressure with potent intravenous antihypertensive medications are mandatory.

The physician should not overreact to hypertension that, although severe, does not pose an immediate threat to life or target-organ function. Overzealous therapy may lower blood pressure below vascular autoregulatory limits (see Fig. 17–1), resulting in hypoperfusion of vital organs and an adverse clinical outcome.[1, 7-9] Severe hypertension and even hypertensive urgencies without evidence of ongoing target-organ damage usually can be managed with orally administered medication on an outpatient basis. The clinical status of the patient, rather than blood pressure per se, is the best guide to appropriate management.

CLASSIFICATION

Hypertensive emergencies have been defined as clinical situations in which blood pressure must be re-

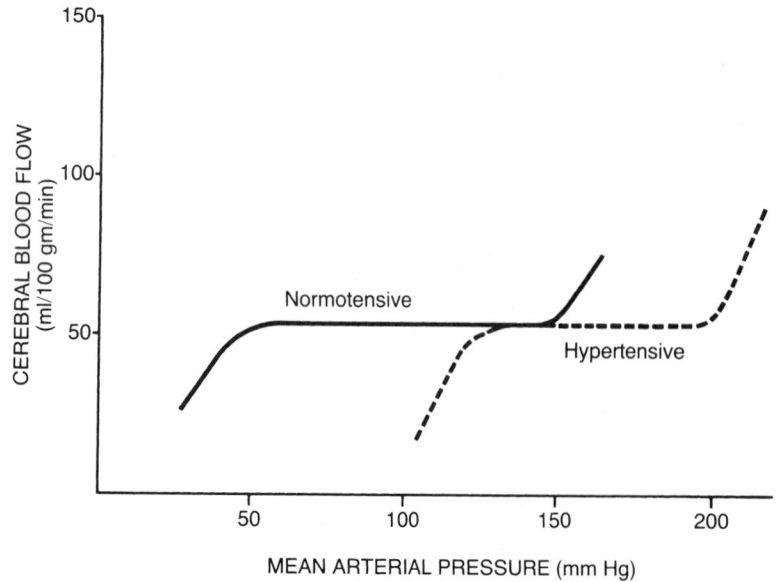

Figure 17–1. Cerebral blood flow autoregulation in normotensive and hypertensive individuals. (Adapted from Strandgaard S, Olsen J, Skinhoj E, et al: Autoregulation of brain circulation in severe arterial hypertension. Br Med J 1:507, 1973.)

duced within 1 hour to prevent hypertensive complications; hypertensive urgencies are situations in which complications are less imminent and blood pressure may be reduced within 24 hours.[4, 6, 10] The distinction is ultimately a matter of clinical judgment. True hypertensive emergencies have become relatively rare, probably as a result of more aggressive detection and treatment of hypertension in recent years. Essential hypertension is by far the most common type of hypertension; thus, untreated or uncontrolled essential hypertension is the most common underlying cause of hypertensive emergencies.[11]

In many conditions, sudden or severe elevation of blood pressure is a primary or contributing cause of a medical emergency (Table 17–1). Prompt reduction of blood pressure to safer levels is essential in all these conditions.

Accelerated and Malignant Hypertension

Severe uncontrolled hypertension of any cause may progress to the accelerated or malignant phase.[12] Most commonly, increases in circulating vasoconstrictor substances such as norepinephrine, angiotensin II, and antinatriuretic hormone are thought to precipitate a rapid increase in systemic vascular resistance, resulting in the onset of hypertensive crisis.[13] Accelerated hypertension is generally defined as severe hypertension accompanied by Keith-Wagener grade III retinopathy (hemorrhages and exudates) and azotemia, whereas malignant hypertension is characterized by grade IV retinopathy with papilledema.[2] However, the distinction is somewhat arbitrary, and both conditions indicate rapidly progressing end-organ damage. Additional clinical manifestations vary but may include headache, altered mental status, intracranial

Table 17–1. Hypertensive Emergencies: Accelerated and Malignant Hypertension

Neurologic conditions
  Hypertensive encephalopathy
  Cerebrovascular accidents
  Head injury
  Intracranial mass
  Eclampsia
Cardiovascular conditions
  Dissecting aortic aneurysm
  Angina pectoris or myocardial infarction
  Acute left ventricular failure
  Postoperative hypertension
Renal conditions
  Acute glomerulonephritis
  Chronic renal failure
  Renovascular hypertension
  Hypertension after renal transplantation
Catecholamine-associated crisis
  Pheochromocytoma
  Monoamine oxidase inhibitors
  Rebound hypertension
Miscellaneous conditions
  Severe burns
  Quadriplegia
  Disseminated vasculitis

hemorrhage, acute left ventricular failure, microangiopathic hemolytic anemia, proteinuria, and secondary hyperaldosteronism with hypokalemia.[12-16] Epistaxis and bleeding from other sites, including trachea, gastrointestinal tract, and urinary tract, may also occur.[17]

The pathologic hallmark of accelerated and malignant hypertension is generalized fibrinoid necrosing arteriolitis,[7, 18] which rapidly leads to functional deterioration of multiple target organs if blood pressure is not controlled. High blood pressure is thought to disrupt the vascular endothelium, allowing leakage of plasma into the media.[19] Along with intense vasospasm, fibrinoid change in vessel walls and platelet and fibrin deposition, loss of autoregulatory function, and narrowing of the vessel lumen impair blood flow to many organs, especially the kidneys. Untreated malignant hypertension is fatal in 80% to 90% of patients within 1 year[20, 21] and in 98% of patients within 4 years.[20] With treatment and continued blood pressure control, arteriolar necrosis will heal rapidly, permitting preservation of target-organ function and long-term patient survival.[21, 22] Aggressive treatment with potent antihypertensive agents and (when necessary) dialysis or renal transplantation has resulted more recently in 5-year survival rates of 60% to 75%.[23, 24]

Transient rises in blood urea nitrogen and creatinine due to diminished renal perfusion are commonly encountered when blood pressure is lowered, but the azotemia must not deter aggressive treatment of the hypertension.[25] Healing of renal arteriolitis and autoregulation of renal artery blood flow often permit stabilization or even improvement of renal function. Renal function usually begins to recover within 2 weeks after initiation of therapy,[23] but improvement may not be apparent for 2 to 3 months[26] and may not plateau for 6 to 12 months.[27] Renal function may deteriorate during initial treatment to the point that dialysis is necessary to maintain the patient until renal function is recovered. The more severe the impairment of renal function at the time of diagnosis, the more likely that dialysis will be necessary.[23] It may prove impossible to discontinue dialysis, but even this outcome is preferable to the neurologic and cardiac damage that uncontrolled malignant hypertension will inflict.[28]

Neurologic Conditions

Hypertensive Encephalopathy

Hypertensive encephalopathy presents as diffuse cerebral dysfunction associated with severe or sudden elevation of blood pressure, and it may complicate accelerated or malignant hypertension.[1] Alteration of cerebral vascular autoregulation with development of necrotizing vasculitis, petechial hemorrhages and small thrombi, and focal edema in the brain are the pathologic findings.[17-19] Clinical findings include marked hypertension, headache, mental confusion and apprehension, visual disturbances, nausea and vomiting, and variable transient focal neurologic deficits.[11, 14, 15] Without treatment, the syndrome may progress to convulsions, coma, and death within hours. The response to treatment is prompt and often dramatic. Failure of the patient to improve rapidly as blood pressure is lowered suggests that another condition is present; the differential diagnosis includes cerebrovascular accidents (CVAs), intracranial mass lesions, uremic or other metabolic encephalopathy, drug overdose, postictal state, encephalitis, and cerebral vasculitis associated with collagen vascular disease.[2, 29]

Lowering blood pressure too far or too rapidly may compromise cerebral blood flow,[1, 7] particularly in patients with preexisting chronic hypertension; however, this problem can be avoided by titrating intravenous therapy to lower blood pressure gradually. Cerebral hypoperfusion can be corrected quickly by placing the patient in a head-down, legs-up position by simply raising the foot end of the bed.

Hypertension Associated with Cerebrovascular Accidents

Hypertension is one of the most important risk factors for CVAs. In turn, blood pressure elevation may also be induced or exacerbated by a CVA. This latter effect is believed to be mediated by vasomotor centers in the brain as cerebral edema causes increased intracranial pressure following a stroke.[30] Severe elevation of blood pressure in a stroke patient can further impair cerebral vascular autoregulation and cause worsening of cerebral hemorrhage. Therefore, lowering of blood pressure is indicated in these patients. However, blood pressure reduction must be accomplished carefully to avoid exacerbating cerebral ischemia by reducing cerebral blood flow below the autoregulatory threshold.[7] Only medications with rapid onset but short duration of action such as nitroprusside should be used, and diastolic pressure should not be reduced below 100 mmHg initially.

A CVA may be difficult to differentiate from hypertensive encephalopathy in a patient with severe hypertension, but a stroke patient generally has fixed and often lateralizing neurologic deficits. The main differential diagnostic feature is the response to antihypertensive drug treatment:[31] patients with hypertensive encephalopathy improve promptly with blood pressure reduction, but stroke patients do not. If the neurologic deficit appears to worsen as blood pressure is lowered, presence of stroke must be presumed, and blood pressure should be allowed to rise modestly but not to severe levels. Computerized tomographic or positron-emission tomographic scanning is often helpful in diagnosing CVAs of various types.

Head Injury and Intracranial Mass

Increased intracranial pressure occurring as the result of head injury or an intracranial mass may induce severe hypertension.[32] Immediate lowering of blood pressure is often necessary to preserve function of vital organs, but definitive therapy must be directed at the underlying intracranial lesion.

Eclampsia

Eclampsia is a severe form of toxemia of pregnancy characterized by marked hypertension, convulsions, visual disturbances, oliguria, and albuminuria.[25] Definitive therapy consists of evacuation of the uterus. Sometimes delivery must be delayed because of fetal immaturity or because the mother's condition is too unstable to permit induction of labor or cesarean section; in the latter instance, parenteral antihypertensive therapy may permit stabilization of the patient and amelioration of the eclamptic state until delivery can be accomplished. Arterial vasodilators, such as hydralazine and diazoxide, are the basis of antihypertensive therapy in this condition, but convulsions are still commonly treated with intravenously administered magnesium sulfate, which also has an antihypertensive effect. Sodium nitroprusside has been used in refractory cases, but there is concern over potential fetal toxicity.[33]

Women with preexisting hypertension, chronic renal parenchymal disease, renovascular disease, hydatidiform mole, and abnormalities of pregnancy including multiple fetuses and hydramnios are at increased risk of severe hypertension during pregnancy.[32] In addition, previously normotensive women who have had toxemia of pregnancy are at increased risk of sustained hypertension later in life and, therefore, require continued observation following the pregnancy.

Cardiovascular Conditions

Dissecting Aortic Aneurysm

Severe thoracic or back pain of abrupt onset is the most characteristic symptom of aortic aneurysm dissection. Other clinical manifestations may include anxiety, headache, altered mental status, syncope, loss of vision, hemoptysis, cardiac tamponade, aortic insufficiency, various gastrointestinal symptoms, renal failure, loss of pulses, and paralysis, depending on the site and extent of the dissection.[2, 34] Prompt lowering of blood pressure is essential to arrest progression of the dissection. The immediate goal of therapy is a *systolic* blood pressure in the range of 100 to 120 mmHg or as low as tolerated without compromise of blood flow to vital organs.[28] Reduction of cardiac output and myocardial contractility to diminish shearing forces on the aortic wall is also indicated. Consequently, the preferred agents are nitroprusside combined with propranolol or, alternatively, trimethaphan camsylate. Drugs that cause reflex tachycardia, such as diazoxide, hydralazine, and sublingual nifedipine, must be avoided in this condition. Aortography should be done to determine the location and extent of the dissection after blood pressure is controlled. Patients with dissection distal to the left subclavian artery generally do best with chronic medical therapy.

Those with proximal dissections have a higher incidence of complications such as aortic insufficiency and cardiac tamponade and are best treated surgically, after progression of the dissection has been arrested with antihypertensive therapy and the patient has been stabilized. Failure to relieve thoracic pain suggests continued progression of the dissection and is an indication for more intensive hypotensive therapy and consideration of emergency surgery. Other complications that may require emergency surgery include severe aortic valvular insufficiency, leaking aneurysm, or compromise of a major vessel.[25] Emergency surgery should be avoided if possible because of its high mortality rate. Late complications of aortic dissection that may require surgery include enlarging saccular aneurysms of the aorta and progressive aortic insufficiency.[28] Continued effective antihypertensive therapy is mandatory in all cases. Antiadrenergic agents such as propranolol or clonidine are helpful in long-term medical therapy of aortic dissections to maintain reduced aortic shearing forces.

Angina Pectoris or Myocardial Infarction with Refractory Hypertension

Hypertension is a major risk factor for coronary artery disease. In turn, myocardial ischemic pain may induce transient or persistent and severe hypertension.[28] Elevation of blood pressure increases left ventricular filling pressure, diameter, and afterload, thereby increasing myocardial oxygen demand and further exacerbating myocardial ischemia.[2] Reduction of blood pressure reverses these adverse effects and may be essential to relieve pain. Some evidence suggests that lowering arterial pressure may reduce infarct size if accomplished early in the course of myocardial infarction.[35] Hypotension must be avoided, and drugs that directly or reflexively increase cardiac rate and output should not be used. Fortunately, a number of the drugs used to treat angina pectoris, such as nitrates, β-adrenergic antagonists, and calcium antagonists, also lower blood pressure and can be used both acutely and chronically for control of both conditions. Although calcium antagonists are effective antianginal agents, these drugs (especially dihydropyridines such as nifedipine) may paradoxically cause myocardial ischemia and must be used with some caution in patients with known or suspected underlying coronary artery disease. Thiazide diuretics may be added cautiously if these measures are insufficient.

Acute Left Ventricular Failure with Pulmonary Edema

Hypertension may induce or exacerbate congestive heart failure (CHF) by increasing the workload of the failing left ventricle.[28] Lowering the pressure, particularly with agents that decrease both preload and afterload, reduces cardiac work and helps restore ventricular function.[1] Furosemide should be used to reduce volume overload and potentiate antihypertensive drugs; digitalis may or may not be necessary.[17, 28]

β-Blocking drugs should be avoided in this setting. Long-term treatment of chronic hypertension is crucial to the survival of patients who have developed acute CHF.

Postoperative Hypertension

Severe postoperative hypertension is an occasional complication of operations involving the carotid artery or requiring cross-clamping of the aorta,[2, 28] including coronary artery bypass grafting and cardiac valve replacement. The condition is dangerous because even moderate hypertension may cause bleeding and disruption at vascular suture lines. Parenteral antihypertensive therapy (e.g., with nitroprusside) or sublingual therapy with nifedipine is necessary to achieve prompt reduction of blood pressure, because oral medications cannot be given in the immediate postoperative period. Hypotension must be avoided to prevent thrombosis at sites of vascular surgery.

Renal Conditions

Acute Glomerulonephritis

Acute glomerulonephritis has a number of causes, including infectious diseases, vasculitis, multisystem diseases such as systemic lupus erythematosus, and a variety of primary glomerular diseases.[36] Common clinical manifestations are hypertension, edema, hematuria, proteinuria, and azotemia. Because the hypertension often develops abruptly in previously normotensive, often younger patients, hypertensive encephalopathy may occur and requires emergency treatment as discussed previously. If the glomerulonephritis resolves, the hypertension will also abate.

Chronic Renal Failure

Chronic renal failure of any cause tends to result in hypertension owing to chronic retention of sodium and fluid. When hypertension is severe, it may precipitate any of the hypertensive crises already discussed. Measures to reduce sodium and fluid retention—including salt restriction, diuretics, and, if necessary, dialysis—are important adjuncts to antihypertensive therapy in this setting. Fear that reduction of blood pressure will compromise renal blood flow often leads to inappropriately cautious treatment of hypertensive emergencies accompanying chronic renal failure.[28] Uncontrolled hypertension can lead only to further renal damage and worsened hypertension; it also poses an imminent threat to brain and heart function. The availability of hemodialysis means that protection of irreplaceable brain and cardiac tissue must take precedence over avoidance of functional increases in blood urea nitrogen and creatinine in a life-threatening hypertensive crisis. As previously noted, initial worsening of azotemia is in fact often encountered after successful lowering of blood pressure, but renal function commonly improves with time as control of blood pressure is maintained. Adequate blood pressure control is essential for preservation or improvement of renal function.[22] One must avoid precipitous lowering of blood pressure in patients with compromised renal function whenever possible and use agents that impair renal blood flow as little as possible. Nonetheless, the primary goal of treatment is to lower blood pressure, and treatment must be vigorous enough to accomplish that goal.[37]

Renovascular Hypertension

Renovascular hypertension may progress gradually to severe hypertension, or it may occur abruptly if there is thrombosis, embolic obstruction, or dissection of the renal artery. Long-term correction of hypertension may be accomplished by transluminal angioplasty or reconstructive surgery. Antihypertensive drug therapy is used to control blood pressure prior to surgery or chronically when surgery is inappropriate. Older patients are generally managed best with medical therapy or angioplasty rather than reconstructive surgery.

Hypertension After Renal Transplantation

Successful renal transplantation often cures preexisting hypertension. However, severe hypertension may develop in these patients, and damage to the graft will result if blood pressure is not controlled promptly.[32] Stenosis at the vascular anastomotic site producing renovascular hypertension is often the cause of post-transplantation hypertension. The steroids used to prevent graft rejection also may exacerbate hypertension in transplantation patients. When feasible, reduction of steroid dosage may lessen hypertension.

Catecholamine-Associated Crises

Pheochromocytoma

Pheochromocytoma is a rare cause of hypertension, but sudden release of catecholamines from a pheochromocytoma can provoke a dramatic hypertensive crisis with extreme elevations of blood pressure and classic signs of headache, sweating, tachycardia, nausea, vomiting, and pallor.[1] Serious cardiac arrhythmias, pulmonary edema, and neurologic damage are potential complications. It must be remembered, however, that pheochromocytomas often occur with sustained rather than episodic hypertension and without the classic signs and symptoms.

The diagnosis is made by determination of plasma catecholamines, or metanephrines and catecholamines in a 24-hour collection of urine. When this diagnosis is suspected, prompt treatment with sodium nitroprusside or phenoxybenzamine followed by a β-blocker is mandatory. Correction of hypovolemia secondary to venoconstriction produced by excess circulating catecholamines is a critical adjunct to management of patients with pheochromocytoma. A β-blocker should never precede an α-blocker, because the β-blocker may aggravate peripheral vasoconstriction and result in increased hypertension. The definitive treatment for pheochromocytoma is surgical removal of the tumor. Phenoxybenzamine should be discontinued 12 hours before surgery to prevent postoperative hypotension.

Monoamine Oxidase Inhibitor–Tyramine Interaction

Monoamine oxidase inhibitors prevent degradation of tyramine, an indirectly acting sympathetic amine. When patients taking these drugs ingest foods or beverages containing large amounts of tyramine, such as Chianti wine, pickled herring, chicken livers, and unpasteurized cheeses, an acute hypertensive crisis may develop.[17, 28] Drugs such as ephedrine and amphetamines can also provoke hypertensive crisis because of release of catecholamine stores.

Rebound Hypertension After Cessation of Antihypertensive Drugs

Abrupt cessation of a number of antihypertensive medications can lead to a withdrawal syndrome characterized by anxiety, nervousness, sweating, palpitations, and rebound of blood pressure to pretreatment levels. This syndrome is associated with increased adrenergic activity and generally can be relieved by reinstituting the drug that had been discontinued. Rarely, blood pressure will "overshoot" to very high levels after abrupt cessation of therapy, requiring emergency parenteral treatment to prevent end-organ damage. Although clonidine in particular has been blamed for producing rebound hypertension, this condition has been reported after abrupt withdrawal of the other central α_2-adrenergic agonists methyldopa and guanabenz acetate, the ganglionic blockers guanethidine and bethanidine, and the β-blockers propranolol and metoprolol and oxprenolol; rebound hypertension has even been reported after withdrawal of diuretics and the angiotensin-converting enzyme (ACE) inhibitor saralasin acetate.[38, 39] Abrupt withdrawal of β-blockers may also result in exacerbation of angina pectoris and even acute myocardial infarction.[39] Exacerbations of coronary ischemia have also been reported after abrupt termination of calcium antagonists,[40–42] but the existence of a true withdrawal syndrome in this setting has been disputed.[43] The withdrawal syndrome can usually be avoided by gradually tapering medication over 1 to 2 weeks.

Miscellaneous Conditions

Severe Burns

Hypertension is an uncommon complication of severe burns.[2, 28] The mechanism of blood pressure elevation in this setting has not been established. The hypertension may be so severe as to require use of parenteral agents for initial control.

Quadriplegia

Hypertensive crises may occur in patients with high transverse lesions of the spinal cord.[1] Stimulation of muscles and skin supplied by nerves distal to the cord lesion appears to provoke increased autonomic activity, leading to hypertension that may be severe. Headache, bradycardia, CVAs, and death may result if the hypertension is not promptly controlled.

Disseminated Vasculitis

Rapidly progressive vasculitis can precipitate an acute hypertensive crisis.[17] Blood pressure must then be controlled with antihypertensive medications until therapy directed at the underlying disease becomes effective. Hypertension in this setting is often associated with renal failure caused by the underlying vascular disease.

GENERAL CONSIDERATIONS IN MANAGEMENT

The best treatment for hypertensive emergencies is prevention. Early identification and treatment of hypertension can prevent the development of most if not all hypertensive crises. When a hypertensive emergency does develop, reduction of blood pressure is the first priority. The patient should be hospitalized, preferably in an intensive care unit (ICU). A rapid evaluation, including history, physical examination, chest radiograph, electrocardiogram, complete blood count, serum electrolyte levels, blood urea nitrogen value, creatinine level, and urinalysis, should be completed. Rapidly acting antihypertensive therapy should be started immediately, without waiting for more extensive and time-consuming diagnostic testing to be carried out. In general, diastolic blood pressure should be reduced below 120 mmHg as quickly as possible to arrest rapidly progressing target-organ damage, but the therapeutic goal must be individualized. Older patients, those with long-standing hypertension, and others with underlying structural vascular changes can be harmed by excessive lowering of the blood pressure, whereas younger patients and those developing severe hypertension acutely are more likely to tolerate a more marked reduction in blood pressure. The initial goal of therapy is to abort the hypertensive crisis, not to lower blood pressure to normal. A diastolic blood pressure in the range of 100 to 110 mmHg is a reasonable initial goal of therapy in most situations.

When adequate blood pressure control has been achieved with parenteral therapy, a gradual changeover to the usual orally administered antihypertensive agents should begin as quickly as possible. Oral therapy usually can be started within the first 1 to 2 days of treatment. A common error is to switch abruptly from intravenous to oral therapy, with a consequent loss of control of blood pressure. Patients should be observed closely for postural hypotension as mobilization begins. In addition, a more extensive diagnostic evaluation can be undertaken at this time to assess possible underlying causes of the crisis. Finally, patients must be followed closely after discharge to ensure that adequate blood pressure control is maintained. Noncompliance with therapy is one of the common reasons that uncontrolled hypertension leads to hypertensive crisis and may recur following discharge. A number of well-established interventions may help to prevent, detect, and correct noncompliance in medical practice.[44] Despite advances in antihypertensive therapy, patients who have survived hypertensive emergencies are at increased risk for subsequent morbidity and mortality.

PHARMACOLOGIC TREATMENT

An ideal drug for treatment of hypertensive emergencies should have rapid onset and short duration of action, so that blood pressure can be lowered quickly and undesirable effects relieved rapidly. It should be effective in all types of hypertensive crises and able to be titrated without toxicity across a broad range of blood pressures so that smooth and precise control of the pressure can be achieved with a single agent. It should have a favorable therapeutic index and low incidence of dangerous or seriously disturbing side effects. In particular, it should not alter mental status (which confuses the assessment of patients with neurologic manifestations of hypertensive crisis) and should not decrease blood flow to vital organs or induce postural hypotension. Unfortunately, the ideal agent has not been discovered, but a number of useful drugs are available (Table 17–2). Choosing among the available agents requires careful assessment of each patient's medical condition, the urgency of lowering blood pressure, and the pharmacologic or hemodynamic effects of drugs that could be detrimental in particular situations (Table 17–3). Certain medications can be particularly recommended; some older drugs have been superseded by newer, better-tolerated agents (Table 17–4).

A common error in the treatment of hypertensive emergencies is administration of a potent diuretic, usually furosemide, as the first drug. Because most true hypertensive crises are vasoconstrictive states with normal or even reduced plasma volume, it is not surprising that this therapy often has little effect on blood pressure. Furosemide does, however, potentiate the action of the other drugs, and profound hypotension sometimes results when a second agent is added. This complication can be avoided by withholding furosemide initially and subsequently adding it in doses that take into account the reduction in blood pressure already achieved by the antihypertensive drug used first. It is often necessary to use a potent diuretic in adequate doses adjunctively in treatment of hypertensive emergencies, both to potentiate the action of other drugs and to prevent sodium and fluid retention that may be induced by other drugs.

Sedatives are contraindicated in hypertensive emergencies. They are not effective antihypertensive

Table 17–2. **Drugs Used in Treatment of Hypertensive Emergencies**

Medication			Time Course of Action			Side Effects	Special Considerations
Generic Name	*Trade Name*	**Dosage**	*Onset*	*Peak*	*Duration*		
Vasodilators							
Nitroprusside	Nipride	50–300 mg/L at rate of 0.5–8.0 µg/kg/min continuous IV infusion	Instantaneous	1–2 min	3–5 min	Nausea, vomiting, muscle twitching, sweating, flushing, hypotension	Constant monitoring required. Watch for thiocyanate toxicity. No reflex tachycardia. Solution is photosensitive.
Nifedipine	Procardia (capsule)	5–10 mg chewed and swallowed; repeated in 30 min	1–5 min	20–30 min	2–4 hr	Facial flushing, headache, postural hypotension	Puncture capsule before use. Increases cardiac output, decreases peripheral resistance.
Nitroglycerin	Nitro-Bid IV, Nitrol IV, etc.	5–100 µg/min continuous IV infusion	Within seconds	1–2 min	3–5 min	Headache, flushing, postural hypotension	Constant monitoring required. Tolerance may develop.
Diazoxide	Hyperstat I.V. Injection	5 mg/kg rapid IV bolus or 50–100 mg minibolus repeated every 5–15 min	3 min	10–15 min	4–24 hr	Nausea, vomiting, flushing, hyperglycemia, hyperuricemia, fluid retention, painful extravasation	Produces reflex tachycardia. Bolus injection may cause hypotension. May cause cessation of labor, angina.
Hydralazine	Apresoline	50–100 mg/L at rate of 10–20 mg over 20–40 min as loading dose, then 50–150 µg/min maintenance flow rate or as repeated small boluses	10–20 min	20–40 min	2–6 hr	Nausea, vomiting, tachycardia and palpitation, flushing, headache, fetal distress	Forms toxic hydrazones in sugar solutions. Increases myocardial work, may precipitate angina, ischemia, strokes, blindness.
Minoxidil	Loniten	5–40 mg PO	2 hr	4 hr	12–24 hr	Fluid retention, tachycardia	Not appropriate for acute emergencies.
Sympathetic Inhibitors							
Labetalol	Trandate Injection, Normodyne	20 mg IV bolus, then 40–80 mg bolus repeated every 10–15 min as needed, or 0.5–2 mg/min continuous IV infusion	5–10 min	10–60 min	1–8 hr	Nausea, vomiting, heart failure, bronchospasm, pain at injection site, hypotension, formication	Potential negative inotropic effect on heart. Avoid in asthmatics, CHF, heart block other than first degree.
Propranolol	Inderal Injection	1–3 mg IV at rate of 0.2 mg/min	1–2 min	5 min	3–6 hr	Bradyarrhythmias, CHF, bronchospasm	Used adjunctively with vasodilators to blunt reflex tachycardia.
Clonidine	Catapres	0.2 mg loading dose PO, then 0.1 mg PO each hr as needed	30–60 min	2–4 hr	6–12 hr	Drowsiness, dry mouth	Confuses assessment of sensorium. Not appropriate for true emergencies.
Methyldopa	Aldomet	250–500 mg IV infusion over 30 min	1–3 hr	3–5 hr	6–10 hr	Drowsiness	Confuses assessment of sensorium. Not appropriate for true emergencies.
Trimethaphan	Arfonad	0.5–1.0 g/L at rate of 1–10 mg/min continuous IV infusion	1–5 min	5–10 min	10–15 min	Urinary retention, paralytic ileus, cycloplegia, mydriasis, dry mouth, orthostatic hypotension	Constant monitoring required. No reflex tachycardia. Rapid tachyphylaxis. Diminishes renal blood flow. Respiratory paralysis at high dose.
Reserpine	Serpasil, etc.	0.25–5 mg IV	1–4 hr	3–4 hr	6–24 hr	Drowsiness, stupor, bradycardia	Confuses assessment of sensorium. Effect may be cumulative. Not appropriate for acute emergencies.
Guanethidine	Ismelin	10–25 mg PO	30–90 min	6–8 hr	12–24 hr	Postural hypotension, retrograde ejaculation	Not appropriate for acute emergencies.
Phentolamine	Regitine	5–20 mg rapid IV bolus, then infuse 100–500 mg/L at rate of 0.2–5.0 mg/min	Instantaneous	2–5 min	10 min	Tachycardia, flushing, gooseflesh, nausea, vomiting, headache, angina	Useful only for catecholamine-mediated hypertensive crises.
Phenoxybenzamine	Dibenzyline	1 mg/kg IV bolus	60–90 min	4–6 hr	12–24 hr	Similar to phentolamine	Useful only for catecholamine-mediated hypertensive crises.
Diuretics							
Furosemide	Lasix	20–40 mg IV or PO, titrate as needed	15–30 min	1–2 hr	6–8 hr	Postural hypotension, hypokalemia	Used adjunctively to potentiate other agents, prevent sodium and fluid retention.
ACE Inhibitors							
Captopril	Capoten	0.5–1.0 mg/kg IV bolus	3–5 min	20 min	4 hr	Skin rashes, proteinuria, loss of taste, acute renal insufficiency, cough	Very limited experience.
Enalaprilat	Vasotec	1.25–5 mg IV bolus every 6 hr	5–15 min	30 min	12–24 hr	Acute renal insufficiency, proteinuria, cough	Limited experience, useful in CHF.

ACE, angiotensin-converting enzyme; CHF, congestive heart failure.

Table 17–3. **Indications and Contraindications**

Medication	Indications	Comments and Contraindications
Vasodilators		
Nitroprusside	All hypertensive crises	Add β-blocker for dissecting aortic aneurysm, phenochromocytoma. Risk of thiocyanate toxicity increased in the elderly and in renal or hepatic insufficiency.
Nifedipine	Has been used in hypertensive encephalopathy, hypertensive heart disease with pulmonary edema, malignant hypertension, intracranial hemorrhage, intracranial mass lesion, severe bleeding, unstable angina pectoris, aortic dissection, and pheochromocytoma	May cause tachycardia.
Nitroglycerin	Myocardial ischemia or infarction, coronary artery bypass graft surgery	Less potent than nitroprusside, hence limited utility.
Diazoxide	Malignant hypertension, hypertensive encephalopathy, glomerulonephritis, eclampsia, severe burns, postoperative hypertension, hypertensive heart disease with pulmonary edema	Contraindicated in coronary artery or cerebral vascular disease, aortic dissections, severe diabetes. Ineffective in catecholamine-mediated crises. Often causes cessation of labor.
Hydralazine	Eclampsia, hypertensive encephalopathy, glomerulonephritis, postoperative hypertension	Contraindicated in coronary artery disease, aortic dissection. Ineffective in catecholamine-mediated crises. Add β-blocker to control reflex tachycardia.
Minoxidil	Severe hypertension associated with renal insufficiency	Contraindicated in acute emergencies requiring immediate blood pressure reduction.
Sympathetic inhibitors		
Labetalol	Malignant hypertension, hypertensive encephalopathy, postoperative hypertension, coronary insufficiency, severe burns	Contraindicated in congestive heart failure, bronchospastic disease, intracranial hemorrhage, head trauma.
Propranolol	Useful adjunctively in coronary insufficiency, aortic dissection (with sodium nitroprusside or trimethaphan), catecholamine-mediated crises (*following* nitroprusside, phentolamine, or phenoxybenzamine)	Contraindicated in congestive heart failure, asthma. May cause bradyarrhythmias.
Clonidine	Clonidine withdrawal syndrome, severe hypertension	Contraindicated as primary therapy in acute emergencies because of slow onset of action. Contraindicated when assessment of sensorium is crucial (all crises with neurologic involvement).
Methyldopa	Useful adjunctively in aortic dissection, postoperative hypertension, coronary insufficiency, severe burns	
Reserpine	Useful adjunctively in aortic dissection, postoperative hypertension, coronary insufficiency, severe burns	
Trimethaphan	Aortic dissection, hypertensive encephalopathy, hypertensive heart disease with pulmonary edema, malignant hypertension, intracerebral hemorrhage, head trauma, severe burns	Contraindicated in pregnancy, postoperative patients, lower urinary tract obstruction, glaucoma, renal insufficiency. Ineffective in catecholamine-mediated crises.
Guanethidine	Useful in resistant hypertension and adjunctively (with trimethaphan) for aortic dissection	Contraindicated as primary therapy in acute emergencies because of slow onset and prolonged duration of action.
Phentolamine / Phenoxybenzamine	Catecholamine-mediated crises	Contraindicated (ineffective) in other types of hypertensive crises.
ACE inhibitors		
Captopril, enalapril	Malignant hypertension, hypertensive encephalopathy, hypertensive heart disease with pulmonary edema, congestive heart failure	Published experience is limited. There are reports of acute renal failure in patients with renal artery stenosis.

ACE, angiotensin-converting enzyme.

agents, and they confuse the serial evaluation of neurologic symptoms.

Vasodilators

Sodium Nitroprusside

If properly used, nitroprusside is one of the most effective and safest drugs available for treatment of hypertensive emergencies. It possesses almost ideal characteristics for treatment of hypertensive crises, but rarely it induces postural hypotension. It lowers blood pressure within seconds and has almost equally rapid offset of action; if carefully monitored, it smoothly regulates blood pressure to almost any desired level. It has little or no effect on cardiac output, reduces ventricular preload and afterload, increases renal blood flow, and reduces peripheral vascular resistance.[45]

Nitroprusside must be given by constant intrave-

Table 17–4. **Recommended Treatment Regimens for Hypertensive Crises**

Preferred drugs
Parenteral: nitroprusside, labetalol, nitroglycerin
Sublingual: nifedipine
Oral: clonidine
Useful adjunctive agents
Propranolol
Furosemide
Obsolete drugs
Trimethaphan camsylate
Methyldopa and reserpine
Guanethidine
Phentolamine
Phenoxybenzamine

nous infusion with continuous blood pressure monitoring in an ICU. Because the drug is unstable in solution, it must be protected from light, and fresh solution must be prepared every 4 hours. An arterial line is not necessary, provided ICU personnel can monitor blood pressure frequently. Extravasation of the drug can cause severe local reactions. However, in such life-threatening emergencies, these inconveniences are relatively minor.

Nitroprusside can be used for prolonged periods, but when continued for more than 48 to 72 hours, the risk of thiocyanate toxicity increases.[30] Cyanide is produced by degradation of nitroprusside and is metabolized by the liver to thiocyanate, which is excreted by the kidneys. Patients with liver or kidney disease are at increased risk of thiocyanate toxicity, as are the elderly. When nitroprusside must be used for prolonged periods, blood thiocyanate levels should be measured daily, and symptoms of thiocyanate toxicity should be watched for closely.[45] Symptoms of thiocyanate poisoning include fatigue, weakness, nausea, and vomiting, progressing to confusion, hallucinations, convulsions, coma, and death.[46] Nitroprusside affects platelet function and potentiates anticoagulants. With prolonged use, it can exacerbate hypothyroidism by inhibiting iodine uptake and binding. Deaths attributed to nitroprusside toxicity usually have occurred in association with major surgical procedures.[47-52] Standard orally administered antihypertensive agents should be started as soon as the patient's condition permits so that duration of nitroprusside therapy can be minimized.

Calcium Antagonists

A substantial and proliferating literature has demonstrated that "sublingual" nifedipine is effective in acute treatment of severe hypertension and hypertensive emergencies.[53-62] Several studies have shown that absorption of nifedipine through the buccal mucosa is negligible,[63, 64] suggesting that absorption of nifedipine into the bloodstream requires delivery of the drug to the stomach by swallowing. The most rapid rise and highest peak nifedipine concentrations are achieved by chewing and swallowing the capsule.[64] When the capsule is chewed and swallowed, blood pressure begins to fall within 5 to 10 minutes. Peak effect occurs in 20 to 40 minutes, and a partial effect is sustained for up to 4 to 5 hours. Nifedipine has been used in management of hypertensive encephalopathy, hypertensive cardiac failure with acute pulmonary edema, accelerated hypertension, intracranial hemorrhage, intracranial mass lesion, severe bleeding, unstable angina pectoris, dissecting aortic aneurysm, crisis associated with renal insufficiency, pheochromocytoma, and hypertensive emergencies in children. Side effects include tachycardia and flushing, and postural hypotension has been reported.[53] Excessive hypotension appears to be a rare occurrence, but cases of myocardial ischemia and infarction attributed to nifedipine-induced hypotension have been reported.[65, 66] Nifedipine's only major disadvantage is its prolonged duration of action, which could make reversal of untoward effects difficult. Nevertheless, it is increasingly regarded as a drug of choice for hypertensive emergencies and urgencies because of its ease of administration, effectiveness, and apparently low incidence of serious adverse reactions.

Verapamil has also been used to treat hypertensive crisis but appears to be less effective than nifedipine.[58]

Nitroglycerin

Intravenously administered nitroglycerin acts rapidly to lower systemic blood pressure while maintaining or improving collateral coronary circulation.[67] Therefore, it may be useful in patients with severe hypertension associated with myocardial ischemia or infarction[67] or coronary artery bypass graft surgery.[68] However, nitroglycerin is less potent than sodium nitroprusside and is therefore of limited utility in other hypertensive emergencies.

Diazoxide

Diazoxide is an arteriolar vasodilator that has little effect on capacitance vessels;[11] at one time, it was a mainstay of treatment for hypertensive emergencies. When administered as an intravenous bolus injection, it lowers blood pressure precipitously, achieving its maximum effect within minutes and maintaining most of its hypotensive effect for several hours. The drug is effective in most hypertensive emergencies other than those due to pheochromocytoma. Its major advantages are the convenience associated with use of single intravenous boluses rather than constant infusions and its rapid lowering of blood pressure toward but rarely below normal without producing central nervous system depression. It can be used in patients with liver disease or renal insufficiency.

Diazoxide has several disadvantages. It has usually been given as a rapid 300-mg intravenous bolus injection to circumvent its high degree of protein-binding so that it can be delivered to its presumed site of action in the arteriolar wall.[69] Although frank hypotension is unusual following diazoxide injection,[70] it does occur and may be prolonged because of the drug's moderately long duration of action. Myocardial infarction and CVAs have been reported follow-ing bolus injections of diazoxide.[15, 71-74] Although early studies[75] suggested that diazoxide had to be given as a single large bolus to be effective, later studies[76-79] showed that repeated smaller boluses or constant intravenous infusions were also effective. These methods permit greater control of the magni-tude and rapidity of blood pressure reduction and thus reduce the risk of inducing serious hypotension. Diazoxide also induces reflex tachycardia and in-creased cardiac output, which can be harmful for patients with coronary or cerebrovascular insuffi-ciency, CHF, or dissecting aortic aneurysm. Diazoxide causes cessation of labor in up to 50% of eclamptic patients, but this effect can be overcome with oxyto-cin.[25] Extravasation of the drug causes a painful local reaction.

Side effects of diazoxide include sodium and fluid retention, hyperuricemia, hyperglycemia, and hyper-lipemia.[45] Serious hyperglycemia can result if the drug is used for prolonged periods, particularly in diabet-ics, and patients with gout may experience a flare of symptoms. Concomitant use of a potent diuretic will prevent sodium and fluid retention. Diazoxide should be reserved for short-term emergency treatment, and oral agents should be substituted as soon as possible.

Hydralazine Hydrochloride

Hydralazine is a direct arterial vasodilator.[12] Its ad-vantages and disadvantages are similar to those of diazoxide, but its onset of action is slower and its duration of action shorter than those of diazoxide. The drug is often used in treatment of eclampsia. Although hydralazine can be given intramuscularly, uptake may be erratic, and the intravenous route is preferred. The onset of action is usually delayed for 15 to 20 minutes after intravenous injection. Side ef-fects of short-term treatment with hydralazine include headaches, dizziness, palpitations, nausea, and diar-rhea.

Minoxidil

Minoxidil is a potent direct vasodilator that can be administered only by mouth.[80] This drug should not be used in emergencies requiring immediate blood pressure reduction, because 2 to 4 hours are required to achieve its full effect. However, it has been useful in hypertensive urgencies,[81] in patients resistant to other treatment,[82] and, after the initial emergency has been controlled, especially in patients resistant to other vasodilators.[80] Its hemodynamic effects are simi-lar to those of hydralazine, but minoxidil is more effective in reducing blood pressure, especially in pa-tients with renal insufficiency. Diuretics are required to control fluid retention, and hirsutism may be an unwelcome side effect. Contraindications are the same as those for diazoxide and hydralazine.

Sympathetic Inhibitors

Labetalol

Labetalol is a peripheral α-blocking and nonselective β-blocking drug that has shown promise in the treat-ment of hypertensive emergencies.[83-87] Labetalol is administered intravenously as a minibolus or contin-uous infusion and produces a blood pressure–lowering effect within 5 to 10 minutes; repeated bo-luses can be given until the desired reduction of blood pressure is achieved. The average effective total dose is 200 mg. Heart rate usually is modestly decreased. Labetalol may be especially useful in patients with atherosclerotic cardiovascular disease (e.g., angina pectoris, dissecting aneurysm) because it does not provoke reflex tachycardia, as do the vasodilator drugs. Orthostatic hypotension has been observed fol-lowing use of this agent. As with other β-blockers, exacerbation of bronchospasm, atrioventricular con-duction delays, bradycardia, and left ventricular fail-ure are potential hazards. Transition to oral therapy with the same drug is not difficult.

Propranolol

Propranolol is a β-adrenergic antagonist that may be used adjunctively with nitroprusside or trimethaphan in the treatment of aortic dissection or with nitroprus-side, phentolamine, or phenoxybenzamine in the treatment of catecholamine-mediated crises. Its role in these situations is to control tachycardia and ar-rhythmias. Propranolol should be avoided in patients at risk for bronchospasm or CHF.

Clonidine

This central α-adrenergic agonist has proved useful in acute treatment of severe hypertension and hyper-tensive urgencies.[88-91] Its relatively prompt onset of action permits rapid oral loading to achieve blood pressure control, and it offers the convenience of con-tinuing the same medication for chronic antihyperten-sive therapy. About half of the total loading dose required to control blood pressure acutely can be given in divided daily doses for long-term outpatient therapy.[4] Clonidine is not appropriate for use in true hypertensive emergencies because its onset of action is delayed for 30 to 60 minutes after an oral dose, its duration of action is prolonged, and sedation is a prominent side effect.[12]

Methyldopa and Reserpine

In the past, methyldopa and reserpine were used widely in the treatment of hypertensive emergencies, but these drugs have been largely superseded by newer agents.[12] In the large doses required to treat severe hypertension, both drugs produce profound somnolence that makes serial evaluation of neurologic function difficult. In addition, their slow onsets and prolonged durations of action make them inappropri-ate choices for emergencies. However, reserpine has sometimes been used adjunctively with trimethaphan camsylate in the treatment of aortic dissection.[25]

Trimethaphan Camsylate

Trimethaphan camsylate is a ganglionic-blocking drug that inhibits both sympathetic and parasympathetic autonomic activities.[2, 28] It has a rapid onset and brief duration of action and must be administered by continuous intravenous infusion with constant monitoring of blood pressure. Trimethaphan camsylate is particularly useful in aortic dissection because it can be titrated carefully to permit smooth control of blood pressure and because it decreases cardiac output and left ventricular ejection rate. Tachyphylaxis develops rapidly, making early transition to orally administered antihypertensive agents mandatory.

Adverse effects, including blurred vision, exacerbation of glaucoma due to mydriasis and cycloplegia, dry mouth, respiratory depression, nausea, constipation, fetal meconium ileus, paralytic ileus, impairment of renal blood flow with azotemia, and urinary retention, frequently complicate therapy with trimethaphan camsylate.[45] Because of the frequency and severity of the side effects associated with this drug and the availability of more effective agents, it is now rarely used.

Guanethidine

This ganglion-blocking drug is sometimes useful as adjunctive therapy with trimethaphan camsylate for aortic dissection.[28] The onset of action of guanethidine is too slow and its duration of action too prolonged for it to be useful as initial therapy. Like trimethaphan, it is seldom used today.

Phentolamine and Phenoxybenzamine

These peripheral α-receptor blockers are specifically useful in treatment of catecholamine-mediated hypertensive crises.[28] They are not consistently effective in other types of hypertensive emergencies. They do not block the β-adrenergic–mediated effects of catecholamines. Because infusions of nitroprusside are at least equally effective in catecholamine-mediated crises and are easier to manage, these drugs are now rarely used.

Angiotensin-Converting Enzyme Inhibitors

ACE inhibitors have been used with some success in treating severe hypertension and hypertensive emergencies.[62, 92–94] The delayed onset of action of available oral formulations of captopril and enalapril makes them unsuitable for use in the most acute emergencies. The hypotensive effect of ACE inhibitors has been reported to correlate with baseline plasma renin activity,[92] and a substantial proportion of patients fail to respond to these agents. This failure to respond could delay therapy with more universally effective agents such as nitroprusside.

ACE inhibitors clearly reduce morbidity and mortality in patients with CHF, making them agents of choice in patients with both hypertension and CHF. When effective and tolerated, ACE inhibitors should be employed preferentially in patients with concomitant CHF and severe hypertension or hypertensive urgencies and when making the transition from parenteral to oral therapy in those with true hypertensive emergencies in combination with CHF.[62, 95–98]

Acute renal insufficiency has been observed after administration of ACE inhibitors to patients with underlying renal disease (especially renal artery stenosis). Renal insufficiency also potentiates the risks of neutropenia, proteinuria, skin rash, and disturbances of taste sensation, which are the most important adverse effects associated with ACE inhibitors. Experience with ACE inhibitors in treatment of hypertensive emergencies is limited, and they cannot be generally recommended for this use at present.

Diuretics

Diuretics are rarely effective as sole therapy for severe hypertension, but they are useful as adjunctive therapy to potentiate the effects of other antihypertensive agents and to prevent sodium and fluid retention. Potent loop diuretics that can be given parenterally, such as furosemide, bumetanide, and ethacrynic acid, are necessary for acute treatment of hypertensive urgencies and emergencies. The longer-acting thiazide diuretics are preferred for chronic oral therapy after the crisis is controlled, but patients with renal insufficiency often require continued treatment with a loop diuretic.

REFERENCES

1. Strandgaard S, Olesen J, Skinhoj E, et al: Autoregulation of brain circulation in severe arterial hypertension. Br Med J 1:507, 1973.
2. Ram CVS: Hypertensive crises. Prim Care 10:41, 1983.
3. Mueller SM, Heistad DD: Effect of chronic hypertension on the blood-brain barrier. Hypertension 2:809, 1980.
4. Anderson RJ, Reed WG: Current concepts in treatment of hypertensive urgencies. Am Heart J 111:211, 1986.
5. Vidt DG: Current concepts in treatment of hypertensive emergencies. Am Heart J 111:220, 1986.
6. Ferguson RK, Vlasses PH: Hypertensive emergencies and urgencies. JAMA 255:1607, 1986.
7. Rajagoplan B, Ledingham JGG: Management of the hypertensive crisis. In Sleight P, Freis ED (eds): Hypertension. London: Butterworth Scientific, 1982, pp 271–292.
8. Reed WG, Anderson RJ: Effects of rapid blood pressure reduction on cerebral blood flow. Am Heart J 111:226, 1986.
9. Dangerous antihypertensive treatment [editorial]. Br Med J 2:228, 1979.
10. Joint National Committee on Detection, Evaluation, and Treatment of High Blood Pressure: The 1984 report of the Joint National Committee. Arch Intern Med 144:1045, 1984.
11. Kaplan NM: Hypertensive crisis. In Kaplan NM, Lieberman E (eds): Clinical Hypertension, 2nd ed. Baltimore: Williams & Wilkins, 1978, pp 160–177.
12. Segal JL: Hypertensive emergencies—Practical approach to treatment. Postgrad Med J 68:107, 1980.

13. Calhoun, DA, Oparil S. Treatment of hypertensive crisis. N Engl J Med 323:1177–1183, 1990.
14. Healton EB, Brust DA, Thomson GE: Hypertensive encephalopathy and the neurologic manifestations of malignant hypertension. Neurology 32:127, 1982.
15. Ledingham JGG, Rajagopalan B: Cerebral complications in the treatment of accelerated hypertension. Q J Med 47:25, 1979.
16. Gavras H, Oliver N, Aitchison J, et al: Abnormalities of coagulation and the development of malignant phase hypertension. Kidney Int 8:S252, 1975.
17. Mailloux LU: Management of hypertensive emergency. N Y State J Med 77:1290, 1977.
18. Chester EM, Agamanolis DP, Banker BQ, et al: Hypertensive encephalopathy: A clinicopathologic study of 20 cases. Neurology 28:928, 1978.
19. Tamaki K, Sadoshima S, Baumbach GL, et al: Evidence that disruption of the blood-brain barrier precedes reduction in cerebral blood flow in hypertensive encephalopathy. Hypertension 6(Suppl 1):75, 1984.
20. Keith NM, Wagener HP, Barker NW: Some different types of essential hypertension: Their course and prognosis. Am J Med Sci 197:332, 1939.
21. Harington M, Kincaid-Smith P, McMichael J: Results of treatment in malignant hypertension—A seven-year experience in 94 cases. Br Med J 2:969, 1979.
22. Herlitz H, Gudbrandsson T, Hansson L: Renal function as an indicator of prognosis in malignant essential hypertension. Scand J Urol Nephrol 16:51, 1982.
23. Lawton WJ: The short-term course of renal function in malignant hypertensives with renal insufficiency. Clin Nephrol 12:277, 1982.
24. Gudbrandsson T, Hansson L, Herlitz H, et al: Malignant hypertension—Improving prognosis in a rare disease. Acta Med Scand 206:495, 1979.
25. Finnerty FA: Treatment of hypertensive emergencies. Heart Lung 10:275, 1981.
26. Mroczek WJ: Malignant hypertension: Kidneys too good to be extirpated. Ann Intern Med 80:754, 1974.
27. Mroczek WJ, Davidov M, Gavrilovich L, et al: The value of aggressive therapy in the hypertensive patient with azotemia. Circulation 40:893, 1969.
28. Gifford RW: Management and treatment of essential hypertension, including malignant hypertension and emergencies. In Genet J, Kuchel O, Hamet P, et al (eds): Hypertension—Pathophysiology and Treatment, 2nd ed. New York: McGraw-Hill, 1983, pp 1149–1161.
29. LeSuer LM, Henry AR, Lehrner LM: Hypertensive encephalopathy—A diagnosis of exclusion. South Med J 73:379, 1980.
30. Moore MA: Hypertensive emergencies. Am Fam Phys 21:141, 1980.
31. Ram CVS: Hypertension crisis—Part 1: Causes. J Cardiovasc Med 8:645, 1983.
32. Keith TA: Hypertension crisis—Recognition and management. JAMA 237:1570, 1977.
33. Stempel JE, O'Grady JP, Morton MJ, et al: Use of sodium nitroprusside in complications of gestational hypertension. Obstet Gynecol 60:533, 1982.
34. Garrett BN, Ram CVS: Acute aortic dissection. Cardiol Clin 2:227–238, 1984.
35. Shell WE, Sobel BE: Protection of jeopardized ischemic myocardium by reduction of ventricular afterload. N Engl J Med 291:481, 1974.
36. Glassock RJ, Brenner BM: The major glomerulopathies. In Petersdorf RG, Adams RD, Braunwald E, et al (eds): Harrison's Principles of Internal Medicine, 10th ed. New York: McGraw-Hill, 1983, pp 1632–1642.
37. American Medical Association Committee on Hypertension: The treatment of malignant hypertension and hypertensive emergencies. JAMA 228:1673, 1974.
38. Garbus SB, Weber MA, Priest RT, et al: The abrupt discontinuation of antihypertensive treatment. J Clin Pharmacol 19:476, 1979.
39. Weiner N: Drugs that inhibit adrenergic nerves and block adrenergic receptors. In Gilman AG, Goodman LS, Rall TW, et al (eds): The Pharmacologic Basis of Therapeutics, 7th ed. New York: Macmillan, 1985, pp 181–214.
40. Schick EC, Liang C, Henpler FA, et al: Randomized withdrawal from nifedipine: Placebo-controlled study in patients with coronary artery spasm. Am Heart J 104:690, 1982.
41. Subramanian VB, Bowles MJ, Khurmi NS, et al: Calcium antagonist withdrawal syndrome: Objective demonstration with frequency-modulated ambulatory ST-segment monitoring. Br Med J 286:520, 1983.
42. Kozeny GA, Ragona BP, Bansal VK, et al: Myocardial infarction with normal results of coronary angiography following diltiazem withdrawal. Am J Med 80:1184, 1986.
43. Flicker MR, Quigley MA, Caldwell EG: Diltiazem withdrawal syndrome: An opposing viewpoint. Am J Med 82:1273, 1987.
44. The Working Group on Health Education and High Blood Pressure Control: The physician's guide—Improving adherence among hypertensive patients. Bethesda, MD: U.S. Department of Health and Human Services, 1987, pp 2–27.
45. Ginkus-O'Connor N: Intravenous drugs used in treating hypertensive emergencies. Heart Lung 10:848, 1981.
46. Rieves RD: Importance of symptoms in recognizing nitroprusside toxicity. South Med J 77:1035, 1984.
47. Patel CB, Laboy V, Venus B, et al: Use of sodium nitroprusside in post-coronary bypass surgery—A plea for conservatism. Chest 89:663, 1986.
48. Sarvothan SS: Nitroprusside therapy in post-open heart hypertensives—A ritual tryst with cyanide death? Chest 91:796, 1987.
49. Montoliu J, Botey A, Pons JM, et al: Fatal hypotension in normal-dose nitroprusside therapy. Am Heart J 97:541, 1979.
50. Merrifield AJ, Blundell MD: Toxicity of sodium nitroprusside. Br J Anaesthesiol 46:324, 1974.
51. Jack RD: Toxicity of sodium nitroprusside: Br J Anaesthesiol 46:952, 1974.
52. Davies DW, Kadar D, Steward DJ, et al: A sudden death associated with the use of sodium nitroprusside for induction of hypotension during anaesthesia. Can Anaesthesiol Soc J 22:547, 1975.
53. Beer N, Gallegos I, Cohen A, et al: Efficacy of sublingual nifedipine in the acute treatment of systemic hypertension. Chest 79:571, 1981.
54. Takekoshi N, Murakami E, Murakami H, et al: Treatment of severe hypertension and hypertensive emergency with nifedipine, a calcium antagonist agent. Jpn Circ J 45:852, 1981.
55. Romeo R, Sciacca AR, Finocchiaro ML, et al: Effects of nifedipine in hypertensive angina pectoris and acute pulmonary edema. Curr Ther Res 32:150, 1982.
56. Bertel O, Conen D, Radu EW, et al: Nifedipine in hypertensive emergencies. Br Med J 286:19, 1983.
57. Huysmans FTM, Sluiter HE, Thien TA, et al: Acute treatment of hypertensive crisis with nifedipine. Br J Clin Pharmacol 16:725, 1983.
58. Guazzi MD, Polese A, Fiorentini C, et al: Treatment of hypertension with calcium antagonists—Review. Hypertension 5(Suppl 2):85, 1983.
59. Erbel R, Brand G, Meyer J, et al: Emergency treatment of hypertensive crisis with sublingual nifedipine. Postgrad Med J 59(Suppl 3):134, 1983.
60. Dilmen U, Caglar MK, Senses DA, et al: Nifedipine in hypertensive emergencies of children. Am J Dis Child 137:1162, 1983.
61. Haft JI, Litterer WE: Chewing nifedipine to rapidly treat hypertension. Arch Intern Med 144:2357, 1984.
62. Angeli P, Chiesa M, Caregaro L, et al. Comparison of sublingual captopril and nifedipine in immediate treatment of hypertensive emergencies: A randomized, single-blind clinical trial. Arch Intern Med 151:678–682, 1991.
63. van Harten J, Burggraaf K, Danhof M, et al: Negligible sublingual absorption of nifedipine. Lancet 2:1363–1365, 1987.
64. McAllister RG. Kinetics and dynamics of nifedipine after oral and sublingual doses. Am J Med 81(Suppl 6A):2–5, 1986.
65. Ellrodt AG, Ault MJ, Reedinger MS, et al: Efficacy and safety of sublingual nifedipine in hypertensive emergencies. Am J Med 79:19, 1985.
66. O'Mailia JJ, Sander GE, Giles TG: Nifedipine-associated myocardial ischemia or infarction in the treatment of hypertensive urgencies. Ann Intern Med 107:185, 1987.
67. Chiariello M, Gold HK, Leinbach RC, et al: Comparison be-

tween the effects of nitroprusside and nitroglycerin on ischemic injury during acute myocardial infarction. Circulation 54:766, 1976.

68. Flaherty JT, Magee PA, Gardner TL, et al: Comparison of intravenous nitroglycerin and sodium nitroprusside for treatment of acute hypertension developing after coronary artery bypass surgery. Circulation 65:1072, 1982.

69. Seller EM, Koch-Weser J: Protein binding and vascular activity of diazoxide. N Engl J Med 281:1141, 1969.

70. Vidt DG, Gifford RW: Management of hypertensive emergencies. Cleve Clin Q 45:299, 1978.

71. O'Brien KP, Grigor RR, Taylor PM: Intravenous diazoxide in treatment of hypertension associated with recent myocardial infarction. Br Med J 4:74, 1975.

72. Graham DI: Ischaemic brain damage of cerebral perfusion type after treatment of severe hypertension. Br Med J 4:739, 1975.

73. Kanada SA, Kanada DJ, Hutchinson RA, et al: Angina-like syndrome with diazoxide therapy for hypertensive crisis. Ann Intern Med 84:696, 1976.

74. Kumar GK, Dastoor FC, Robayo JR, et al: Side effects of diazoxide. JAMA 235:275, 1976.

75. Mroczek WJ, Leibel BA, Davidov M, et al: The importance of the rapid administration of diazoxide in accelerated hypertension. N Engl J Med 285:603, 1971.

76. Johnson BF, Kapur M: The influences of rate of injection upon the effects of diazoxide. Am J Med Sci 263:481, 1972.

77. Thien TA, Huysmans FTM, Gerlag GC, et al: Diazoxide infusion in severe hypertension and hypertensive crisis. Clin Pharmacol Ther 25:795, 1979.

78. Garrett BN, Kaplan NM: Efficacy of slow infusion of diazoxide in the treatment of severe hypertension without organ hypoperfusion. Am Heart J 103:390, 1982.

79. Wilson DJ, Lewis RC, Vidt DG: Control of severe hypertension with pulse diazoxide. Cardiovasc Clin 12:79, 1982.

80. Pettinger WA: Minoxidil and the treatment of severe hypertension. N Engl J Med 303:922, 1980.

81. Alpert MA, Bauer JH: Rapid control of severe hypertension with minoxidil. Arch Intern Med 142:2099, 1982.

82. Wood BC, Sharma JN, Crouch TT: Oral minoxidil in the treatment of hypertensive crisis. JAMA 241:163, 1979.

83. Pearson RM, Havard CWH: Intravenous labetalol in hypertensive patients given by fast or slow injection. Br J Clin Pharmacol 5:401, 1978.

84. Papademetriou V, Notargiacomo AV, Khatri IM, et al: Treatment of severe hypertension with intravenous labetalol. Clin Pharmacol Ther 32:431, 1982.

85. Wilson DJ, Wallin JD, Vlachakis ND, et al: Intravenous labetalol in the treatment of severe hypertension and hypertensive emergencies. Am J Med 75:95, 1983.

86. Cressman MD, Gifford RW: Labetalol—The first combined alpha-blocker and beta-blocker. J Cardiovasc Med 9:593, 1984.

87. Lebel M, Langlois S, Belleau LJ, et al: Labetalol infusion in hypertensive emergencies. Clin Pharmacol Ther 37:615, 1985.

88. Cohen IM, Katz MA: Oral clonidine loading for rapid control of hypertension. Clin Pharmacol Ther 24:11, 1978.

89. Anderson RJ, Hart GR, Crumpler CP, et al: Oral clonidine loading in hypertensive urgencies. JAMA 246:848, 1981.

90. Houston MC: Oral clonidine loading in the treatment of hypertensive urgencies and emergencies. Cardiovasc Rev Rep 6:1249, 1985.

91. Marks AD, Adlin EV, Channick BJ: Oral clonidine for rapid control of accelerated hypertension. J Clin Pharmacol 27:193, 1987.

92. Tifft CP, Gavras H, Kershaw GR, et al: Converting enzyme inhibition in hypertensive emergencies. Ann Intern Med 90:43, 1979.

93. Ferguson RK, Vlasses PH, Koplin JR, et al: Captopril in severe treatment-resistant hypertension. Am Heart J 99:579, 1980.

94. Biollaz J, Waeber B, Brunner HR: Hypertensive crisis treated with orally administered captopril. Eur J Clin Pharmacol 25:145, 1983.

95. Chun G, Frishman WH: Rapid-acting parenteral antihypertensive agents. J Clin Pharmacol 30:195–209, 1990.

96. The CONSENSUS Trial Study Group: Effects of enalapril on mortality in severe congestive heart failure: Results of the Cooperative North Scandinavian Enalapril Survival Study (CONSENSUS). N Engl J Med 316:1429–1435, 1987.

97. The SOLVD Investigators: Effect of enalapril on survival in patients with reduced left ventricular ejection fractions and congestive heart failure. N Engl J Med 325:293–302, 1991.

98. Cohn JN, Johnson G, Zieche S, et al. A comparison of enalapril with hydralazine-isorbide dinitrate in the treatment of chronic congestive heart failure. N Engl J Med 325:303–310, 1991.

CHAPTER 18

Acute Thromboembolism

Thomas G. DiSalvo, M.D., Mark W. I. Webster, M.B., Ch.B., F.R.A.C.P., James H. Chesebro, M.D., and Valentin Fuster, M.D.

Thrombi may develop in the venous or arterial circulations. In veins, thrombi typically originate in the calf and may extend proximally. In arteries, thrombi typically originate in an area of endothelial or deeper injury. Platelet adhesion and subsequent activation of thrombin and coagulation factors result in platelet and fibrin deposition. The exuberance of this process depends on many factors, including the site and depth of initial injury and local shear forces. This process is dynamic, reflecting the balance between the body's endogenous thrombotic and fibrinolytic systems. Similar processes occur in cardiac chambers or on prosthetic vascular surfaces.

Acute embolism is frequently devastating, with a high likelihood of recurrence. Treatment focuses on prevention of both the initial event and recurrence.

Currently, three therapeutic approaches are taken: (1) inhibition of platelet function and deposition; (2) inhibition of the coagulation cascade, thereby altering the balance in favor of fibrinolysis; and (3) specific fibrinolysis of a newly formed clot.

DEEP VENOUS THROMBOSIS AND PULMONARY EMBOLISM
Primary Prevention

Rationale for the prophylaxis of deep venous thrombosis (DVT) and pulmonary embolism (PE) includes (1) the often clinically silent nature of the disease, (2) the frequent difficulty of clinical diagnosis short of invasive procedures, and (3) the narrow therapeutic

Table 18–1. Primary Prophylaxis for Deep Venous Thrombosis and Pulmonary Embolism

Low-dose subcutaneous heparin
Adjusted-dose subcutaneous heparin
Low-molecular-weight heparin
Intermittent pneumatic leg compression boots
Graduated compression stockings
Oral warfarin
Intravenous dextran
IVC interruption with filter device
Combined modalities

IVC, inferior vena cava.

window: most fatalities from PE occur 30 minutes following PE, too soon for anticoagulation to be effective.[1] A variety of prophylactic mechanical and pharmacologic measures are available for the primary prevention of DVT and PE (Table 18–1).

The specific prophylactic measure or measures employed should be determined by individual patient characteristics and risk. Table 18–2 outlines recommended prophylactic measures in medical and surgical patients.[2] The choice of prophylactic measure or measures should depend on assessment of individual risk. Low-risk patients may require only mechanical devices such as graduated compressive stockings or intermittent pneumatic compression (IPC) boots. Medium-risk patients generally require either anticoagulants or mechanical measures. High-risk medical or surgical patients should receive prophylaxis with both pharmacologic and mechanical measures.

Prophylaxis should be strongly considered in all nonambulatory hospitalized medical patients. In a trial involving 1358 consecutive patients admitted to the medical wards of an acute care hospital, the use of subcutaneous heparin (5000 U twice daily) was associated with a significant (31.1%) reduction in mortality.[3] Increasing duration of bed rest, age older than 40, congestive heart failure, myocardial infarction, cancer, chronic pulmonary disease, and significant infection all increase the risk of DVT and PE in medical patients. Primary prevention has been clearly shown to decrease the incidence of DVT and PE in selected medical patients with myocardial infarction and stroke.[1, 4, 5] In myocardial infarction, subcutaneous heparin, intravenous heparin, and oral anticoagulants all are effective in the prevention of DVT and PE (Table 18–3).[6–14]

Primary prevention also decreases the incidence of DVT and PE in surgical patients.[1, 4, 5] All surgical patients, except those younger than 40 undergoing minor surgical procedures requiring less than 30 minutes of general anesthesia, should receive some form of prophylaxis.[1] Those at highest risk include patients undergoing orthopedic hip or knee operations, gynecologic cancer or extensive intraabdominal operations, and those with multiple trauma.[1] Prophylactic therapy is cost effective in surgical patients.[15–17] Serial surveillance tests to detect DVT or PE rather than primary prophylaxis are more expensive by comparison.[1] Because risk of PE continues after hospital discharge for up to 1 month in surgical patients, prophylaxis should be continued at home for moderate- to high-risk patients.[18] All women after childbirth should receive prophylaxis.[18]

Heparin

Fixed Low-Dose Subcutaneous Unfractionated Heparin. Fixed low-dose heparin is typically administered as 5000 U of unfractionated heparin subcutaneously 2 hours preoperatively and every 8 to 12 hours thereafter (similarly in medical patients). Lower hepa-

Table 18–2. Specific Measures for the Primary Prevention of Deep Venous Thrombosis and Pulmonary Embolism in Medical and Surgical Patients

Risk	Type	Prophylaxis
Low	General medical	GCS
	Surgical, < 40 yr, no risk factors, anesthesia < 30 min	GCS
Moderate	All other general abdominal/thoracic surgery	Low-dose heparin or IPC boots or dextran
	Neurosurgery	IPC boots
	Urologic surgery	IPC boots
	Postpartum	Low-dose heparin
	Moderately debilitated medical	Low-dose heparin or IPC
High	Extensive abdominal/thoracic surgery	Oral AC ± IPC boots
	Elective hip surgery	Low-dose heparin ± IPC
		Adjusted dose heparin ± IPC
		Oral AC ± IPC
		Adjusted heparin ± IPC
		Dextran + IPC
	Emergency hip	Oral AC ± IPC
		Dextran + IPC
	Major knee	IPC
	Debilitated medical	Low-dose heparin + IPC
		Adjusted dose heparin + IPC

GCS, graduated compression stockings; IPC boots, intermittent pneumatic compression boots; AC, anticoagulants.
Adapted from Hull R, Kakkar V, Raskob G: Prevention of venous thrombosis and pulmonary embolism. *In* Fuster V, Verstraete M (eds): Thrombosis in Cardiovascular Disorders. Philadelphia: WB Saunders, 1992.

Table 18-3. **Heparin in the Prevention of Deep Vein Thrombosis and Pulmonary Embolism in Patients with Myocardial Infarction**

Trial	Emerson	Handley	VA	Drapkin	Handley	Warlow	Wary	Wright	Work Party
n	78	48	999	1136	50	146	92	800	1427
Route	SQ	IV	SQ	IVB, SQ	SQ	SQ	IV	IV	Not given
Dose	5000 q12	5000 IVB, 20,000 q12	10,000 q8–12 + AC	5000 IVB, 10,000 q8×6 + AC	5000 IVB, 7500 q12×7 days	5000 q12	40,000 SQ + AC	H ± AC	H + AC HD vs. LD
DVT, H	5%	0	—	1.5%	23%	3.2%	6.5%	2%	1.5%
DVT, C	34%	29%	—	2.6%	29%	17.2%	22%	5%	4.2%
p	<.005	.009	—	—	NS	<.025	<.05	—	—
PE, H	0	—	2%	3.8%	—	—	0	5.2%	2.2%
PE, C	12%	—	4.8%	5.3%	—	—	0	9.4%	5.6%
p	—	—	.005	—	—	—	—	—	—
Dx	I-125	I-125	V/Q	V/Q	I-125	I-125	I-125	Clinical	Clinical
Days	14	14	28	In hospital	14	10	3	30	28

DVT, deep venous thrombosis; H, heparin; C, controls; p, p value; PE, pulmonary embolism; Dx, mode of diagnosis; Days, days of duration of therapy; I-125, I-125 radiolabeled fibrinogen leg scanning; AC, anticoagulants; SQ, subcutaneous; IVB, intravenous bolus; HD, high dose; LD, low dose; V/Q, ventilation/perfusion.

rin doses are used to prevent DVT rather than to treat DVT.[2] In multiple trials, fixed low-dose heparin has been proved effective in preventing DVT in moderate- to high-risk general surgical patients without risk of increased bleeding except for minor wound hematomas.[2] In the International Multicentre Trial of 4121 patients undergoing a variety of surgical procedures, fixed low-dose heparin significantly decreased the incidence of DVT by I-125-fibrinogen scanning (24.6% to 7.7%, $p < .005$) and fatal PE (0.7% to 0.2%, $p = .005$).[19] A meta-analysis of 70 trials involving more than 16,000 patients showed that fixed low-dose subcutaneous heparin reduced the incidence of DVT by 67%, 68%, and 75% in general surgical, orthopedic, and urologic surgical patients, respectively.[4] There was a 40% reduction in the odds of nonfatal PE and a 64% reduction in the odds of fatal PE ($p < .0001$). In these trials, heparin was begun before operation and continued for several days, usually until the patient was ambulatory. Dosing subcutaneous heparin every 8 or 12 hours was equally efficacious. A second meta-analysis of 45 trials, 30 of which employed subcutaneous fixed low-dose heparin, reported the same results.[5] Thus, fixed low-dose subcutaneous heparin prevents half of perioperative PEs and two thirds of perioperative DVTs and results in a striking reduction in PE-related fatalities.

Fixed low-dose heparin has been shown effective in preventing DVT and PE in patients with myocardial infarction and stroke.[1] As mentioned earlier, fixed low-dose subcutaneous heparin may significantly decrease mortality in general medical patients admitted to acute care hospitals.[3] Fixed low-dose subcutaneous heparin also prevents DVT in medical patients with suspected myocardial infarction and heart failure.[20]

Adjusted-Dose Subcutaneous Unfractionated Heparin. Adjusted-dose subcutaneous heparin is administered to maintain the activated partial thromboplastin time (aPTT) at 1.5 to 2.0 times the upper limit of control. It has been shown to be efficacious in the highest-risk surgical patients (orthopedic hip and knee surgery) in whom fixed low-dose subcutaneous heparin is less efficacious.[2] In one trial of patients undergoing hip surgery, compared with fixed low-dose heparin, adjusted-dose heparin decreased the incidence of venographically documented DVT from 39% to 13% ($p = .003$).[21]

Fractionated Low-Molecular-Weight Heparin. The pharmacology of low-molecular-weight heparin (LMWH) is discussed in detail in Chapter 157. LMWH has several potential advantages over standard unfractionated heparin: (1) decreased bleeding complications, (2) once-daily subcutaneous dosing as a result of longer half-life, and (3) greater antithrombotic efficacy due to greater bioavailability.[22] In a meta-analysis of 52 randomized, controlled trials of LMWH in general surgical and orthopedic surgical patients, LMWH was superior to placebo ($p < .001$), dextran ($p < .001$), and unfractionated standard heparin ($p = .02$) in preventing postoperative DVT without increasing bleeding complications.[23] Another meta-analysis of 58 randomized trials of LMWH in general surgical and orthopedic patients showed that, compared with unfractionated standard heparin, LMWH significantly decreased the relative risks of DVT (0.74%, 95 percent confidence interval 0.65 to 0.86) and PE (0.43%, 95 percent confidence interval 0.26 to 0.72) without increase in major bleeding.[24] Overall in this meta-analysis, there was a 25% to 30% lower incidence of DVT with LMWH compared with standard unfractionated heparin.

In a large trial designed to test the safety of LMWH in 3809 patients undergoing major abdominal surgery, there was no difference in major bleeding with LMWH versus standard heparin, but there were fewer severe bleeding complications with LMWH (1.0% versus 1.9%, $p = .02$) and fewer wound hematomas.[25] There was no difference in this trial in the incidence of DVT or PE between groups. In a randomized, double-blind trial in 1436 patients undergoing hip or knee orthopedic surgery, LMWH was compared with adjusted low-dose warfarin (INR, 2 to 3). This use of LMWH resulted in a significant decrease in venographically documented DVT (31.4% versus 37.4%, $p = .03$), but a significant increase in bleeding complications (2.8% versus 1.2%, $p = .04$). Thus, the beneficial small reduction in DVT was offset by increased bleeding.[26] The cost-effectiveness of LMWH compared with standard heparin or warfarin is not yet established, although LMWH appears to be more efficacious than fixed low-dose unfractionated heparin in high-risk patients, and at least as efficacious as adjusted-dose subcutaneous unfractionated heparin or low-dose warfarin in high-risk patients.

Dextran

Dextran, a glucose polymer originally introduced as a volume expander, has multiple antithrombotic effects: dextran decreases platelet aggregability, blood viscosity, and platelet interaction with damaged vein walls and increases the susceptibility of fibrin-rich thrombi to undergo spontaneous lysis.[2, 27] Intravenous dextran is effective in preventing DVT and PE in moderate-risk surgical patients and in patients undergoing hip surgery.[2] Dextran may cause volume overload (especially in the elderly), bleeding, anaphylaxis, and renal toxicity.[27]

Intermittent Pneumatic Compression Boots

Intermittent pneumatic compression (IPC) boots decrease stasis by augmenting deep vein blood flow and also increase whole blood fibrinolytic activity.[1, 28–30] Sequential calf and thigh compression is effective in preventing both calf and thigh DVT in moderate-risk surgical patients.[18] IPC has a special place in preventing DVT and PE in those patients with contraindications to anticoagulation (neurosurgery, ophthalmologic surgery, active bleeding). Intermittent compression doubles the blood-flow velocity in the proximal deep veins of the legs.[18] IPC may be less effective than warfarin or heparin in high-risk surgical patients.[31]

Graduated Compression Stockings

Graduated compression stockings (GCS) apply graduated compressive pressure in the lower extremity (18 mmHg at the ankle, 14 mmHg at the calf, 8 mmHg at the knee, 10 mmHg at the lower thigh, and 8 mmHg at the midthigh) and diminish stasis.[32] GCS decrease DVT by 50% in low-risk general surgical and neurosurgical patients.[2] The role of GCS in high-risk patients is not yet established, but GCS are effective in general medical and low-risk surgical patients.[18]

Oral Anticoagulants

Oral anticoagulants are effective prophylactic agents in all risk groups.[2] In the initial study of perioperative oral anticoagulants, adjusted-dose phenindione decreased postoperative death from PE from 10% to 1%.[33] Two subsequent studies have shown that oral anticoagulants are efficacious in high-risk surgical patients.[34, 35] Oral warfarin may be started preoperatively in low dose (INR, 2 to 3) followed by postoperative moderate-dose warfarin therapy (INR, 3 to 4.5).[35]

Low-dose warfarin (INR, 2 to 2.7) postoperatively has also been shown to be effective.[36] Fixed low-dose warfarin may prevent DVT after gynecologic surgery and catheter-related thrombosis.[37, 38] Warfarin is more effective than IPC boots in high-risk surgical patients.[31] Warfarin is effective in preventing DVT and PE during myocardial infarction.[7, 11–14]

Antiplatelet Agents

Prior to the second Antiplatelet Trialists' Collaboration, there was no evidence that antiplatelet agents prevented DVT or PE.[39] In the second Antiplatelet Trialists' Collaboration meta-analysis of 53 trials completed as of March 1990, antiplatelet therapy resulted in a percent odds reduction of DVT of 39% in general surgical, traumatic and elective orthopedic surgical, and high-risk medical patients, and a percent odds reduction of 64% for PE.[40] Up to 3 weeks of therapy decreased by half the odds of DVT and decreased by two thirds the odds of PE. Mortality from PE was significantly reduced as well (0.2% versus 0.9%, $p = .0001$). It was not clear from the meta-analysis whether aspirin plus dipyridamole was more efficacious than aspirin alone. Further trials are necessary to compare antiplatelet agents and anticoagulants.

Inferior Vena Cava (IVC) Filter

Mechanical interruption of the IVC by a filter device prohibits transit of large emboli from the lower extremity veins or pelvic veins but does influence the thrombotic process.[18] IVC interruption has the following indications: (1) contraindication to anticoagulation, (2) failure of adequate anticoagulation, (3) prophylaxis in extremely high-risk patients (chronic PEs, multiple previous PEs).[1, 18] A 3% to 5% risk of recurrent PE is present as a result of enlargement of IVC collaterals despite insertion of an IVC filter.[41] In the largest series to date (469 patients), the overall rate of PE after filter insertion was 4% over 12 years.[42]

Therapy of Deep Venous Thrombosis

Anticoagulants prevent PE and recurrent DVT in the setting of established DVT.[27] Anticoagulant agents inhibit ongoing thrombosis but do not appreciably promote thrombolysis.[39] Until recently, evidence that heparin is more efficacious than oral anticoagulants in the setting of DVT is largely derived from animal studies and human studies employing historical controls.[43] A randomized, double-blind study of the safety and efficacy of intravenous heparin plus oral acenocoumarol versus oral acenocoumarol alone in the therapy of DVT was stopped early because of a significant increase in symptomatic extension and recurrence of proximal DVT in the group receiving acenocoumarol alone.[43] Thus, patients with proximal DVT require initial therapy with heparin. Subcutaneous unfractionated heparin is as efficacious as equivalent dose intravenous heparin based on meta-analysis of eight studies.[44]

Two large trials have demonstrated that the duration of intravenous heparin in the therapy of proximal DVT may be safely reduced from the traditionally recommended 10 days to 5 days without increase in recurrence or PE.[45, 46] Warfarin may be safely begun at the same time as heparin therapy and should be administered conjointly with heparin for 4 to 5 days.[45, 46] Fixed-dose subcutaneous LMWH is at least as efficacious as adjusted-dose intravenous heparin in the therapy of DVT.[47, 48] In one trial, LMWH caused significantly fewer major and minor bleeding complications.[47] The selective antithrombin agent hirudin is currently undergoing dose-ranging and pilot studies in PE.[49]

The combination of intravenous heparin followed by adequate warfarin therapy greatly reduces the recurrence of DVT (to less than 5%).[39] The duration of oral anticoagulant therapy is empiric at present and should be individualized based on risk of recurrent DVT.[39] After 2 weeks of intravenous heparin, oral warfarin is superior to fixed-dose subcutaneous heparin in the prevention of recurrent DVT and PE.[50] In low-risk patients, warfarin should be continued for 3 months; in high-risk patients, warfarin should be continued indefinitely.[18, 27, 39] The target INR for warfarin in the therapy of DVT is 2 to 3.[39]

Patients with seemingly isolated deep calf vein thrombosis have evidence of PE in 10% of cases; with serial I-125-fibrinogen–labeled leg scans, up to 23% reveal evidence of proximal DVT.[39] Such patients should either be given anticoagulant agents for 3 months or be followed up very closely with serial lower extremity noninvasive studies for 2 weeks to detect extension of thrombosis.[39]

Therapy of PE

The goal of anticoagulation after PE is to decrease the risk of recurrent PE and to inhibit propagation of existing thrombus.[41] Only one randomized trial of heparin in PE has been performed.[51] Patients with PE received either heparin, 10,000 IU every 6 hours for six doses followed by oral nicoumalone for 14 days, or no anticoagulants. The trial was stopped after enrollment of only 35 patients when interim analysis showed significantly more deaths (5 of 19 versus 0 of 16) and recurrent PE (5 of 19 versus 0 of 16) in the control group versus the treatment group ($p = .0005$ for combined end point death or recurrence). Despite heparin therapy, however, recurrent PE may occur in as many as 17% to 23% of patients.[52] With anticoagulation alone, 75% of PEs fail to resolve completely by 4 weeks, and 50% fail to resolve completely by 4 months.[52]

Patients with PE require larger doses of heparin than do patients with DVT alone.[53] The half-life of heparin is decreased and the clearance of heparin increased in the setting of PE.[27] Prospective studies have shown that recurrent PE is more likely when the aPTT is less than 1.5 times the upper limit of control.[54] Inadequate heparin dosing is common during therapy of PE: in a study from a leading academic teaching

hospital, 60% of all aPTT values were less than 1.5 times control within the first 24 hours of initiating heparin therapy.[55] Heparin tends to be underdosed during the first few days of therapy.[39] Frequent measurement of the aPTT (every 6 hours) is thus essential during heparin therapy for PE. Nomograms are available to guide dose adjustment in the setting of acute DVT and PE.[56] Failure to achieve an aPTT of more than 1.5 times control is associated with a 20% to 25% risk of recurrent venous thromboembolism.[39] The average daily intravenous heparin maintenance dose for therapy of PE is more than 31,000 U/24 hours (more than 1300 U/hr).[39]

LMWH and hirudin are currently undergoing dose-ranging studies in the therapy of PE.[57]

Thrombolytic Therapy of Pulmonary Embolism

The rationale for thrombolytic therapy of PE includes (1) possible reduction of mortality, (2) more rapid reversal of right ventricular dilation and hypokinesis than that achieved by heparin alone, (3) more rapid reversal of pulmonary vascular hemodynamic abnormalities than that achieved by heparin alone, (4) prevention of recurrent PE (due to lysis of DVT), and (5) possible prevention of chronic thromboembolic pulmonary hypertension.[52] In the early 1970s, randomized trials showed that both streptokinase and urokinase resulted in earlier angiographic improvement and relief of pulmonary hypertension than heparin alone.[58–61] More recent trials have shown that alteplase is similarly effective compared with heparin alone.[62, 63] It is estimated that approximately 10% of all PEs are currently treated with thrombolytic agents.[52]

To date, thrombolytic therapy has not been proven to reduce mortality due to acute PE: none of the individual clinical trials employing streptokinase, urokinase, or rTPA have been sufficiently large.[41] Because of the small size of these trials, thrombolytic therapy has not been clearly shown to reduce the incidence of either recurrent PE or chronic thromboembolic hypertension following PE. The primary end points of trials of thrombolytic therapy in PE to date have included the degree and time course of angiographic resolution of PE, changes in pulmonary vascular resistance or mean pulmonary arterial pressure, changes in pulmonary perfusion by serial ventilation-perfusion scanning, or echocardiographic improvement in right ventricular performance. The earliest trials of urokinase or streptokinase showed that these agents significantly decreased the severity of pulmonary artery obstruction by angiography and mean pulmonary artery pressure compared with heparin alone; such effects occurred particularly in patients with massive PE.[58–61, 64] Alteplase has been shown to reduce total pulmonary vascular resistance by 50% and angiographic severity of obstruction by 30% within 12 hours.[65] In the PIOPED study,[66] there was a trend toward improved hemodynamics after alteplase compared with therapy with heparin alone. A randomized trial of t-PA plus heparin versus heparin alone in 101 patients showed that t-PA plus heparin improved right ventricular wall motion and significantly improved pulmonary perfusion at 24 hours compared with heparin alone.[63] Despite these apparent salubrious effects, defects in pulmonary parenchymal perfusion, as shown by ventilation-perfusion scanning, do not necessarily resolve after thrombolytic therapy.[66, 67] In the Urokinase Pulmonary Embolism Trial (UPET) Phase II trial, there was no difference in results of ventilation-perfusion scans after 1 year of follow-up.[72] Like heparin, thrombolytic agents tend not to completely lyse PE; residual thrombus is frequent.[41] As shown by echocardiography, thrombolytic therapy results in more rapid resolution of right ventricular dilation and hypokinesis than heparin alone.[68] Transesophageal echocardiography may be useful in detecting emboli in the central pulmonary arteries and in monitoring response to therapy.[69] Lytic agents appear safe in carefully selected elderly patients with massive PE.[70]

At present, the thrombolytic agents, urokinase, streptokinase, and t-PA, all are approved by the United States Food and Drug Administration (FDA) for therapy of submassive or massive PE. There is likely no difference in efficacy between streptokinase (SK) and urokinase (UK).[71] In the largest trial, the UPET Phase II Study randomized 167 patients to a 12-hour urokinase infusion, 24-hour urokinase infusion, or 24-hour streptokinase infusion.[64] There was no difference between urokinase groups in severity of the primary angiographic end points of obstruction or perfusion by ventilation-perfusion scanning at 24 hours. Therapy with UK for 24 hours was associated with improvement in perfusion by ventilation-perfusion scanning but not improvement in angiographic results, compared with therapy with SK for 24 hours. There was no difference in mortality between groups. Overall, 31% of patients had "large" improvement in pulmonary angiography, perfusion lung scanning, or mean pulmonary artery pressure.[72] The UKEP study showed that a 12-hour infusion of UK at a dose of 4400 U/kg/hr followed by intravenous heparin is as effective as a 24-hour infusion of urokinase 2000 U/kg/hr plus concurrent heparin therapy.[73]

Alteplase has been compared with urokinase. In the European Multicenter Double-Blind Trial, 63 patients with massive pulmonary embolism were randomized to either urokinase 4400 U/kg/hr for 12 hours or alteplase 10 mg intravenous bolus followed by 90 mg over 2 hours.[65] During the first 2 hours of therapy, alteplase resulted in a significant decline in total pulmonary vascular resistance (PVR) compared with UK. By 12 hours, however, the magnitude of decline in PVR was equal between alteplase and UK groups. Repeat angiography at 12 to 18 hours showed a similar degree of improvement in both groups. In another trial of 45 patients, alteplase 50 mg/hr for 2 hours resulted in improvement at 2 hours in clot lysis as assessed by angiography compared with UK 2000 U/kg intravenous bolus followed by 2000 U/hr for 24 hours (82% versus 48%, $p = .008$).[67] Perfusion as assessed by perfusion lung scanning at 24 hours showed no difference between alteplase and UK. To date, then, a 2-hour infusion of alteplase appears to result in more rapid resolution of pulmonary artery thrombotic obstruction and more rapid resolution of right ventricular hypokinesis without improving results of lung perfusion scanning at 24 hours compared with a 12-hour infusion of urokinase. It may matter little which thrombolytic agent is selected as long as therapy is instituted rapidly.[71]

Thrombolytic therapy should be considered in the following circumstances: (1) hemodynamically significant PE (significant pulmonary hypertension and/or systemic hypotension), (2) hemodynamically significant PE associated with significant echocardiographic right ventricular dilation and hypokinesis, (3) hemodynamically significant PE that fails to respond to intravenous heparin. Lytic agents are beneficial up to 14 days after PE.[52] The combination of high-probability ventilation-perfusion scan results, right ventricular dilation and hypokinesis by transthoracic echocardiography, and high likelihood of previous PE by clinical assessment may obviate the need for pulmonary angiography before institution of thrombolytic therapy.[18, 41] Administration of thrombolytic agents for PE has been streamlined in recent years. Thrombolytic agents may be safely administered in step-down units; peripheral routes of administration are as efficacious as central routes; and alteplase infusion requires only 2 hours.[18, 41] Monitoring of coagulation times is not necessary when the approved dosages are used.

Surgical Therapy of PE

The role of the IVC filter has been discussed previously. Occasionally, gravely ill patients with massive PE and shock, who are not candidates for thrombolysis or in whom thrombolysis has failed, may be considered for pulmonary embolectomy. In the largest surgical series to date, operative mortality ranged from 20% to 38%: shock, prior resuscitation, prior failed thrombolysis, and advanced age all increased mortality.[74-76] In properly selected patients, results may be impressive.[76] Preliminary results of embolectomy by transvenous catheter devices appear promising in gravely ill patients who fail thrombolysis and are not surgical candidates.[77]

Current Recommendations

Recommendations for prophylaxis are displayed in Table 18–2. All medical and surgical patients (except those younger than age 40 without risk factors for DVT or PE) experiencing immobility or prolonged bed rest should receive DVT prophylaxis. Subcutaneous heparin 5000 U every 8 or 12 hours should be administered; in surgical patients, heparin should be started before the operation. Highest-risk patients (immobilized medical patients in intensive care units and surgical patients undergoing lower-extremity orthopedic, gynecologic, or extensive intraabdominal surgery) should wear compression stockings or IPC

Table 18–4. **Therapy of Deep Vein Thrombosis**

Low risk*	Intravenous heparin 5000 U bolus, then 1000 U/hr adjusted to aPTT 1.5–2.0 × control for 5 days. Begin warfarin day 1 and continue 3 months, INR 2–3.
High risk†	Intravenous heparin 10,000 U bolus then 1000–1500 U/hr adjusted to aPTT 2.0–2.5 × control for 5–10 days. Begin warfarin day 3–5 and continue indefinitely, INR 2–3.
Calf-vein‡	Intravenous heparin 5000 U bolus then 1000 U/hr adjusted to aPTT 1.5–2.0 × control for 5 days. Begin warfarin day 1 and continue 3 months, INR 2–3.

*Risk factor reversible or self-limited.
†Risk factor not reversible or self-limited, prior DVT or prior PE, present PE, massive DVT.
‡Symptomatic.

boots in addition to receiving adjusted-dose subcutaneous heparin or warfarin as outlined in Table 18–2.

Low-risk patients with DVT should receive intravenous heparin sufficient to prolong the aPTT to 1.5 to 2 times the upper limit of control for 5 days (Table 18–4). Warfarin may be begun on day 1 and continued for 3 months (INR, 2 to 3). In high-risk patients, heparin therapy should be more aggressive, aiming to prolong the aPTT to 2.0 to 2.5 times the upper limit of control. High-risk patients require higher doses of heparin, 10,000 U initial intravenous bolus and an initial infusion rate of 1000 to 1500 U/hr. The aPTT should be measured every 4 hours for the first 12 hours of therapy to ensure adequate anticoagulation. For each adjustment in dosage in heparin, the aPTT should be checked every 4 hours to document therapeutic levels. After the condition has stabilized, the aPTT should be checked daily. Warfarin may be begun on days 3 to 5 and continued indefinitely (INR, 2 to 3).

Low-risk patients with PE should receive intravenous heparin as 10,000 U initial bolus followed by 1000 to 1500 U/hr continuous infusion for 5 to 10 days (Table 18–5). It is important to remember that the heparin requirement is increased in PE. Careful

Table 18–5. **Therapy of Pulmonary Embolism**

Low risk*	Intravenous heparin 10,000 U bolus then 1000–1500 U/hr adjusted to aPTT 2.0 to 2.5 × control for 5–10 days. Begin warfarin day 3–5 and continue 3 months, INR 2–3.
High risk†	Intravenous heparin 10,000 U bolus then 1500 U/hr adjusted to aPTT 2.0 to 2.5 × control for 7–10 days. Begin warfarin day 3–5 and continue indefinitely, INR 2–3. Consider thrombolytic therapy for hypotension, right ventricular hypokinesis, pulmonary hypotension, hemodynamically significant pulmonary embolism, heparin failure.

*Risk factor self-limited or reversible.
†Risk factor not self-limited or reversible.

attention as outlined earlier should ensure that the aPTT is 2.0 to 2.5 times control soon after initiation of heparin. Warfarin may be begun on days 3 to 5 and continued for 3 months (INR, 2 to 3). In high-risk patients, heparin should be continued for 7 to 10 days. Warfarin should be begun on days 3 to 5 and continued indefinitely (INR, 2 to 3). Thrombolytic therapy should be considered in patients with acute PE and hemodynamic compromise. Standard regimens include streptokinase 250,000 U loading dose over 30 minutes followed by 100,000 U/hr constant infusion for 24 hours; urokinase 2000 U/kg bolus over 10 minutes followed by 2000 U/kg/hr for 12 to 24 hours; t-PA 100 mg over 2 hours (Table 18–6). In seriously ill patients, more rapid administration of urokinase (15,000-U/kg bolus over 10 minutes) or t-PA (10-mg bolus over 10 minutes) may be considered, although experience is limited. Heparin should be commenced at the same time as thombolytic therapy.

In general, warfarin should overlap with heparin for several days to deplete all vitamin K–dependent coagulation factors. The optimal therapeutic INR is 2 to 3; more intense regimens are no more efficacious but increase bleeding. If the underlying risk factor for thrombosis is reversible or self-limited, then treatment with warfarin should be continued for 3 months after DVT or PE (low-risk). If the underlying risk factor is not reversible or self-limited, or if there are recurrent emboli (high-risk), warfarin should be continued indefinitely.

Patients with symptomatic isolated calf vein thrombosis should receive anticoagulation for 3 months as outlined for patients with low-risk DVT.

SYSTEMIC THROMBOEMBOLISM

Autopsy studies reveal that many systemic emboli go unrecognized. Most systemic emboli originate from the heart or an atherosclerotic aorta.[78] Table 18–7 summarizes possible cardiac sources of emboli. Eighty-five percent of arterial thromboemboli of cardiac origin lodge in the brain or retina.[78] Half of these emboli cause permanent neurologic damage, and 10% may be fatal. Untreated, as many as 25% recur, often within the next month. Initial evaluation should always include an echocardiogram to search for a possible intracardiac source of systemic embolism.

Because the sequelae of cardiac thromboembolism are so serious, identification of high-risk groups who may benefit from primary prevention is critical. This

Table 18–6. **Thrombolysis for Pulmonary Embolism**

Agent	Dose*
Streptokinase	250,000 U loading dose over 30 minutes 100,000 U/hr continuous infusion for 24 hr
Urokinase	2000 U/kg loading dose over 10 minutes 2000 U/kg/hr continuous infusion for 12–24 hr
t-PA	100 mg over 2 hours continuous infusion

*With all agents, coadminister heparin 1000 U/hr without bolus at initiation of thrombolytic agent.

Table 18–7. **Sources of Systemic Embolism**

Source	Incidence
Atrial fibrillation	5%/year, not anticoagulated 2%/year, anticoagulated
Acute MI (all)	1% to 5% in weeks post MI
LV thrombus S/P MI	10% over 6–12 months
Prosthetic heart valves	2% to 4%/year, not anticoagulated 0.5%/year, anticoagulated
Dilated cardiomyopathy	Up to 3.5%/year, not anticoagulated

Other causes:
  Mitral valve prolapse
  Left atrial appendage
    thrombus
  Infective endocarditis
  Ascending aorta atheroma
  Atrial myxoma
  Marantic endocarditis
  Paradoxical via intracardiac
    shunt
	Less than 0.5%/year

MI, myocardial infarction; LV, left ventricular.

section discusses the therapy of acute thromboembolic events and prevention of recurrence with antithrombotic therapy. In an individual patient with cerebral embolism, the risk of further emboli must be weighed against the risk of worsening cerebral ischemia with anticoagulant-induced bleeding into the infected region.

Cerebral Emboli

Fifteen percent to 30% of all ischemic strokes are caused by cardiogenic emboli.[78] Classically, an embolic stroke presents as a sudden neurologic deficit maximal at onset, although 5% to 6% of embolic strokes exhibit a fluctuating course.[79] Strokes that result in hemianopia without hemiparesis, pure Wernicke aphasia, or ideomotor apraxia all are likely to be embolic in origin.[79] As many as 15% of cardiogenic emboli may cause lacunar stroke syndromes.[78] Twenty-five percent of patients with stroke and a demonstrable cardiac cause of embolism have a demonstrable noncardiac potential cause of stroke as well; 15% of patients with potential cardiac sources of embolism have severe carotid artery stenosis.[78] Thus, a definitive diagnosis of cardiogenic embolus causing stroke is often difficult to establish in individual cases.[78–81]

Approximately one third of all stroke patients have a potential cardiogenic source of emboli demonstrable by transesophageal echocardiography, 20% more than are detected by transthoracic echocardiography alone.[78] Cardiogenic emboli may be as small as 1 to 2 mm in size; such small emboli often cause transient ischemic attacks (TIAs) or transient retinal artery occlusion rather than stroke.[78] Emboli from cardiac valves tend to be small in size. In nonvalvular atrial fibrillation, emboli originate most frequently from the atrial appendage. The risk of stroke is decreased from

5% to 2% per year by chronic anticoagulant therapy. The incidence of stroke after myocardial infarction is reduced by heparin and aspirin, and possibly by thrombolytic agents: without thrombolytic or antithrombotic therapy, 10% of patients experience stroke over the 6- to 12-month interval after anterior myocardial infarction.[78]

Acute Treatment

The role of antithrombotic therapy in acute cardioembolic stroke has yet to be definitively established in large randomized, controlled clinical trials. At present, neither antiplatelet nor anticoagulant therapy has been shown to decrease mortality, infarct size, or residual neurologic deficit in acute stroke.[80, 81] Fixed low-dose subcutaneous heparin, however, has been shown to significantly reduce the incidence of DVT and PE after stroke.[80, 81] Although some trials have shown that early thrombolytic therapy in acute stroke may be efficacious, studies to date are not conclusive and proper therapy requires specialized protocols.[80, 81] Parenchymal hemorrhage of varying size may occur in as many as 4% to 9.6% of patients after thrombolytic therapy for stroke.[80] Multicenter trials of t-PA in acute ischemic stroke are under way.

Secondary Prevention

After acute cardioembolic stroke, the clinician is faced with the difficult decision of preventing recurrent embolism but risking hemorrhage by immediate anticoagulation, or preventing hemorrhage but risking recurrent embolism by withholding anticoagulation.[78, 80, 81] Pooled studies show that recurrent embolism occurs within 2 weeks in approximately 12% of cases of embolic stroke. Recurrent embolism occurs less frequently after embolic stroke due to nonvalvular atrial fibrillation (NVAF). In the absence of anticoagulation, between 20% and 40% of embolic strokes undergo some degree of spontaneous hemorrhagic transformation. Hemorrhagic transformation is more likely to occur with large strokes (involvement of more than 30% of the brain or more than one lobe of a hemisphere) and strokes associated with mass effect.[80] In the absence of anticoagulation, hemorrhagic transformation is usually clinically silent. In the absence of anticoagulation, spontaneous hemorrhagic transformation is uncommon within the first 12 hours as shown by computed tomography (CT), but by 48 hours, 75% of hemorrhagic transformations are apparent. Between 1.4% to 24% of patients treated with immediate anticoagulation after acute embolic stroke experience symptomatic neurologic deterioration as a result of hemorrhagic transformation.[80] Thus, although the risk of spontaneous hemorrhagic transformation is slightly higher than the risk of recurrent embolism, the risk of spontaneous hemorrhagic transformation declines sharply after 48 hours, whereas the risk of recurrent embolism remains constant. This temporal disparity is exploited in current recommendations of anticoagulants after embolic stroke provided in the following section.

Current Recommendations

Patients with transient ischemic attacks (TIAs) and minor ischemic strokes should be initially treated with aspirin 325 mg/day (Table 18–8).[80] Ticlopidine is more efficacious than aspirin in the treatment of TIA and minor stroke, but the greater expense and toxicity of ticlopidine render it the second-line agent. Three to 5 days of heparin anticoagulation is recommended for patients with progressing ischemic strokes, particularly when the vertebrobasilar circulation is involved.[80] In this setting, heparin should be administered to increase the aPTT to 2.0 to 2.5 times control, followed by warfarin to prolong the prothrombin time to 1.5 to 2.0 times control (target INR, 3.0 to 4.5). To date, anticoagulants have not been shown to be beneficial in completed ischemic stroke. Aspirin is recommended given its efficacy in minor stroke and TIA; prolonged anticoagulant therapy is not warranted.[80]

Given these observations, optimal anticoagulant therapy in acute embolic stroke must be individualized based on the source of embolism, the size of the stroke, and other individualized patient factors (see Table 18–8). In general, intravenous heparin should not be given for at least 48 hours after embolic stroke.[78–81] In nonhypertensive patients with less severe neurologic deficits and with small to moderate-sized strokes, if follow-up CT scanning of the head shows no hemorrhage at 48 to 72 hours, intravenous heparin without bolus may be begun. In nonhypertensive patients with severe neurologic deficits or large strokes, intravenous heparin should not be given for 5 to 14 days. A CT scan should then be performed before cautiously restarting heparin, with the aPTT 1.5 to 2.0 control value. Warfarin should be begun after 5 days of heparin therapy after small or large embolic strokes. Heparin may be discontinued when the prothrombin time is within range (target INR, 2.0 to 3.0). Exceptions to withholding heparin

for at least 48 hours in acute embolic stroke include TIA or very small strokes with high risk of recurrence.[78–81] The efficacy of antiplatelet therapy, subcutaneous adjusted dose heparin, and low-molecular-weight heparin in acute embolic stroke has not been systematically evaluated. Fixed low-dose subcutaneous heparin is indicated in all eligible patients to prevent DVT and PE.[81]

Less information is available on the optimal management of patients with hemorrhagic transformation of embolic infarcts. Starting heparin 7 to 10 days without a bolus in nonhypertensive patients appears reasonably safe if repeat CT scans show no further hemorrhage. The aPTT should be adjusted to 1.5 to 2.0 times control for 5 days before starting warfarin. Heparin is continued until the prothrombin time is therapeutic (INR, 2.0 to 3.0).

Noncerebral Emboli

Lower Extremity Emboli

The most common sites of noncerebral peripheral embolism include the lower extremities, the coronary circulation, and the viscera. Eighty-five percent of lower extremity emboli originate from the heart. Noncardiac sources include arterial aneurysm, atherosclerotic plaques in the aorta (especially when ulcerated), sites of recent vascular surgery, and paradoxical emboli.[82] Fifty percent of lower extremity emboli occlude the iliofemoral arterial segment; the rest lodge in the tibial/popliteal circulation. Fifteen percent of cardiogenic peripheral emboli travel to the upper extremities, viscera, or aortoiliac vessels. The clinical features of lower extremity embolism depend on the size of the embolus and the adequacy of extremity collateral circulation. Standard treatment is anticoagulation with heparin (aPTT, 2.0 to 2.5 times control). There is no clear benefit of antithrombotic agents in the acute setting, but recurrence may be decreased by as much as 75%.[82] Heparin may decrease thrombotic propagation from the site of occlusion if repair or extraction is delayed beyond 6 to 8 hours. Anticoagulants should be combined with surgical embolectomy or

Table 18–8. **Antithrombotic Therapy of Acute Stroke**

Type Stroke	Therapy
TIA/minor ischemic	Aspirin 325 mg/day indefinitely
	Ticlopidine 250 mg b.i.d., aspirin intolerance
Completed major ischemic	Aspirin 325 mg/day indefinitely
	Ticlopidine 250 mg b.i.d., aspirin intolerance
Progressive ischemic (especially vertebrobasilar)	Intravenous heparin 5000 U bolus, then 1000 U/hr adjusted to aPTT 2.0 to 2.5 times control if computed tomography (CT) negative
	After heparin, either warfarin INR 2 to 3 indefinitely, or aspirin 325 mg/day indefinitely
Small-moderate embolic	Intravenous heparin 1000 U/hr without bolus if CT negative at 48 hours
	Begin warfarin 3 to 5 days after heparin, INR 2 to 3 indefinitely
Large embolic	Intravenous heparin 1000 U/hr without bolus if CT negative at 5 to 14 days
	Begin warfarin 3 to 5 days after heparin, INR 2 to 3 indefinitely
Hemorrhagic transformation, embolic	Intravenous heparin 1000 U/hr without bolus if CT negative at 7 to 10 days
	Begin warfarin 3 to 5 days after heparin, INR 2 to 3 indefinitely

Adapted from Sherman DG, Dyken ML, Fisher M, et al: Antithrombotic therapy for cerebrovascular disorders. Chest 102 (Suppl 4):529S, 1992.

extraction via a Fogarty or wire loop catheter if circulation is significantly impaired. The Fogarty balloon catheter has decreased mortality by 50% and amputation by 35% and increased limb salvage by 62% to 96% in this setting.[82] Peripherally administered thrombolytic agents appear to result in partial or substantial reperfusion in 40% of cases; locally administered thrombolytic agents appear to result in successful reperfusion in 50% to 85% of cases.[82] Major bleeding complications from the local route occur in 6% to 20%. Randomized trials have not yet compared thrombolytic therapy with surgical therapy in acute lower extremity thromboembolism. Thrombolytic therapy is likely to be best used in surgically inaccessible vascular beds in patients at high-risk of surgery.

Coronary Emboli

Although their true incidence is unknown, coronary artery emboli may not be rare. In one autopsy series of more than 1000 consecutive patients dying of myocardial infarction, coronary artery emboli were found in 13%.[83] Such emboli may be clinically silent and even unrecognized.[83] The diagnosis should be especially considered when myocardial infarction occurs postpartum, or in the setting of atrial fibrillation, prosthetic heart valves, endocarditis, or underlying malignancy.[84-86] Other less common causes include atrial myxomas, nonbacterial thrombotic endocarditis, aortitis or aortic mural thrombosis, right-to-left shunts (paradoxical emboli), and intracavitary atrial or ventricular thrombi.

The left anterior descending artery is affected three to four times more commonly than the circumflex or right coronary arteries.[83] Emboli typically lodge in the distal coronary tree and result in focal transmural myocardial infarctions.[83, 85, 87] In one report, two thirds of patients with bacterial endocarditis as the cause of coronary artery embolism died suddenly; lack of collateral circulation predisposing to sudden death was likely the mechanism.[85]

Thrombolytic therapy appears efficacious. Intracoronary urokinase may result in fragmentation and downstream embolization of emboli.[88] Streptokinase was effective in patients with suspected coronary artery embolism enrolled in the GISSI-1 trial. When septic coronary artery embolism complicates native valve endocarditis, thrombolytic therapy may cause intracranial bleeding (due to the presence of mycotic aneurysms) and primary angioplasty may lead to coronary artery aneurysm formation; therapy must be carefully individualized in this instance.[89]

Mesenteric Emboli

Mesenteric emboli are less common than coronary artery emboli and underrecognized. Acute embolic splanchnic arterial occlusion typically results from emboli originating from either the heart or an atherosclerotic aorta.[90] This uncommon phenomenon occurs most often in elderly patients with multiple comorbid conditions.[90] Primary venous mesenteric thrombosis is a rare, insidious process associated with underlying prothrombotic states in 50% of cases; it does not present acutely as does embolic splanchnic arterial occlusion.[90] The signs and symptoms of acute intestinal ischemia due to embolic occlusion of splanchnic vessels are nonspecific.[91] Most commonly, pain out of proportion to physical findings (found in 80%) suggests the diagnosis; vomiting, diarrhea, and gastrointestinal bleeding occur in lesser proportion. Leukocytosis, hyperamylasemia, metabolic acidosis, and elevation of plasma creatine phosphokinase (CPK) occur.[92] The diagnosis is typically made at angiography or laparotomy; studies suggest that Duplex ultrasound of the splanchnic vessels may be efficacious.[91] When intestinal infarction occurs because of late diagnosis, mortality is 70% to 90% despite surgery.[90] Specific surgical management depends on the extent of vascular compromise and the individual patient: in young patients without frank intestinal infarction, embolectomy or revascularization procedures with "second-look" laparotomies are favored, whereas in elderly patients resection is generally preferred.[93] Postoperative anticoagulation is recommended.

Secondary Prevention of Lower Extremity, Coronary, and Mesenteric Emboli

Anticoagulation should commence immediately with heparin, 100 U/kg bolus plus an immediate infusion starting at 1000 U/hr, to prolong the aPTT to 1.5 to 2.0 times control. Subsequently, warfarin should be begun (target INR, 3.0 to 4.5) and continued indefinitely.

Paradoxical Embolism

Paradoxical embolism results from passage of an embolus from the venous circulation through a right-to-left shunt at some level to the arterial circulation. Definitive diagnosis requires that (1) a thrombus be present in the venous circulation, (2) a demonstrable right-to-left communication between the venous and arterial circulations exists, (3) clinical systemic embolism occurs, and (4) a pressure gradient promoting right-to-left shunting across the communication between the circulations is demonstrable at some point in the cardiac cycle.[94] The differential diagnosis of concurrent arterial embolism and venous thrombosis includes paradoxical embolism, right and left ventricular thrombi, biatrial myxomas, mitral and tricuspid valve disease, myocardial infarction complicated by ventricular thrombosis and congestive heart failure, and cyanotic congenital heart disease.[94]

The causes of paradoxical embolism appear in Table 18–9. Paradoxical embolism may be the presenting feature of clinically silent atrial septal defect in young adults.[95] Patent foramen ovale with right-to-left shunting is detected in as many as 40% of cases of acute cor pulmonale after myocardial infarction or hemodynamically significant PE; paradoxical embolism may result.[96, 97] Less common causes of paradoxical embolism include ventricular septal defects, pul-

Table 18–9. **Causes of Paradoxical Embolism**

Atrial septal defect
Patent foramen ovale
Ventricular septal defect
Pulmonary arteriovenous malformation
Cyanotic congenital heart disease

monary arteriovenous malformations, and congenital heart disease including Ebstein's anomaly.[98–100] Paradoxical fat emboli have been described after orthopedic surgery.[97]

The possible role of a patent foramen ovale (PFO) in paradoxical cerebral embolism has been the subject of several studies. "Pencil-patent" PFO is found in 6% and "probe-patent" PFO in 29% of all postmortem examinations, respectively.[94] PFOs range in size from 1 to 19 mm, with a mean size of 4.9 mm.[101] Emboli as small as 1 to 2 mm may cause stroke.[78] Under normal hemodynamic conditions, even in the absence of right atrial or right ventricular hypertension, right-to-left shunting across PFOs is detectable by transesophageal Doppler echocardiography.[102] Several case-control studies have shown that PFO is significantly more common in young patients with cryptogenic stroke or suspected paradoxical embolism: PFOs are found in as many as 50% of such patients by echocardiography.[101, 103–106] In one study, the presence of a PFO was independently associated with cryptogenic stroke in a multivariate logistic regression model.[104] DVT is found in as many as 57% of patients with suspected paradoxical embolism and PFO.[107]

Suspected cases of paradoxical embolism should be carefully screened for sources of both venous thrombosis and right-to-left communication.[94] Transthoracic echocardiography detects only 60% of PFOs subsequently demonstrated by cardiac catheterization or transesophageal echocardiography.[108] Contrast echocardiography during cough or Valsalva maneuvers, which elevate right atrial pressure acutely, may be helpful to demonstrate right-to-left shunting.[108] Rarely, echocardiography may show so-called impending paradoxical embolism or thrombus lodged in the PFO; such a finding necessitates prompt therapy.[109] Because emboli as small as 1 to 2 mm may cause stroke, failure to document venous or intracardiac thrombosis does not exclude the diagnosis.[101]

Therapy of paradoxical embolism depends on the cause. Significant right-to-left shunts should be closed. Closure of small PFOs after single, suspected embolic events is controversial.[110] In the presence of a PFO without DVT or elevation of right atrial pressure, it is difficult to attribute embolism to the PFO, especially in patients with other potential sources of embolism.[78] Multiple embolic events, however, warrant definitive therapy. Antiplatelet and anticoagulant therapy should be individualized depending on risk factors for thrombosis and the right-to-left communication present.[94]

Cyanotic Congenital Heart Disease

Patients with cyanotic heart disease are at risk of cerebral thrombosis, paradoxical embolism from the

venous circulation, and cerebral abscess, probably paradoxical in origin. Thrombotic episodes are most common in patients younger than 12 months but may occur at any age and relate to the degree of hypoxia.[111] Erythrocytosis by itself does not increase risk of stroke except in patients with symptoms of hyperviscosity.[112]

Current Recommendations

The underlying lesion should be corrected surgically if possible. Aggravating factors such as infection should be treated appropriately. Antithrombotic therapy should be used cautiously because of possible concomitant hemostatic defects in the patients. Patients who have no correctable lesion and have pulmonary hypertension should receive long-term anticoagulation with warfarin (prothrombin time, 1.5 to 2.0 times control; INR, 3.0 to 4.5) to reduce thromboembolic complications as well as the risk of paradoxical pulmonary emboli. In all patients with cardiac lesions, the presence of cyanosis superimposed on the underlying lesion is considered a risk factor for thrombosis and therefore increases the need for prophylactic antithrombotic therapy for the underlying lesion.

SOURCES OF THROMBOEMBOLI

A succinct summary of prophylaxis is included in this section, with treatment recommendations for each possible thromboembolic source.

Ventricular Thrombi

Myocardial Infarction

Left ventricular mural thrombosis is the major cause of acute systemic embolization after acute myocardial infarction. Ninety percent of mural thrombi occur in the setting of acute transmural anterior infarctions that involve the ventricular apex. Overall, mural thrombi occur in 40% of all anterior infarctions and 60% of large anterior myocardial infarctions involving the apex with creatine phosphokinase levels in excess of 2000 IU/L, but only 5% of inferior infarctions.[113–123] The combined effects of endocardial endothelial damage, stasis, the transient hypercoagulable state commonly observed after myocardial infarction, and presence of intensely thrombogenic ventricular residual thrombus (due largely to the activity of enzymatically active fibrin-bound thrombin) contribute to the formation of ventricular mural thrombi.[113] Embolism is twice as common with echocardiographically apparent thrombi; however, as many as 24% of cases of embolism occur in the absence of echocardiographically apparent thrombi.[124] In the absence of anticoagulant therapy, stroke occurs in 1% to 3% of all patients with myocardial infarction, 2% to 6% of patients with anterior myocardial infarction, and 10% to 20% of patients with large anteroapical infarctions.[125] Risk of stroke is highest in the first 3 months after infarction and declines sharply thereafter except in the presence of significant left ventricular dysfunction, heart failure, or atrial fibrillation. Extent of thrombus mobility (due to pedunculation) and extent of thrombus protuberance into the left ventricular cavity increase risk.[126, 127]

In a meta-analysis of 11 studies, anticoagulant therapy significantly decreased embolism (odds ratio [OR], 0.14; 95% confidence interval, 0.04 to 0.52) and decreased echocardiographically detectable mural thrombus (OR, 0.32; 95% confidence interval, 0.2 to 0.52) after myocardial infarction.[114] In this meta-analysis, thrombolytic therapy decreased mural thrombus formation (OR, 0.48; 95% confidence interval, 0.29 to 0.79), but antiplatelet therapy alone did not (OR, 1.43; 95% confidence interval, 0.04 to 56.8). It is critical not to wait for echocardiographic evidence of thrombus in patients with large transmural anterior infarctions or extensive inferior infarctions involving the apex before commencing anticoagulation therapy. Warfarin (target INR, 2.5 to 3.5) is recommended for 3 months after anterior Q-wave myocardial infarction or large inferior infarction involving the ventricular apex and indefinitely in patients with congestive heart failure, depressed left ventricular function, or atrial fibrillation (Table 18–10).

Left Ventricular Aneurysm

Mural thrombus within a left ventricular aneurysm is found in 48% to 95% of surgical patients undergoing aneurysmectomy.[128, 129] In autopsy series, mural thrombus is found within left ventricular aneurysm in 49% of cases, with up to a 40% incidence of embolism.[130] After the first 3 months after infarction, however, clinically manifest embolism in surviving patients is infrequent, occurring with an event rate of 0.35 per 100 patient-years. It is likely that intraaneurysmal thrombi form during the acute phase of myocardial infarction and persist, undergoing organization and reendothelialization. Ultimately the thrombi become laminated and adherent to the underlying aneurysmal sac.[27] Because the thrombus is contained within the noncontractile aneurysmal cul-de-sac and does not protrude into the left ventricle, it is protected from contact with the circulation. These characteristics of left ventricular aneurysm in the chronic stage probably determine the low incidence of systemic emboli.

Table 18–10. **Antithrombotic Therapy for the Prevention of Ventricular Thrombi**

Cardiac Disease	Recommendations
AMI	Intravenous heparin after large anterior AMI or inferior AMI involving the apex Warfarin for 3 months (INR 2 to 3)
LV aneurysm	Intravenous heparin followed by warfarin for 3 months after AMI (INR 2 to 3)
DCM	Warfarin (INR 2 to 3) indefinitely

AMI, acute myocardial infarction; LV, left ventricular; DCM, dilated cardiomyopathy.

At present, given the lower risk of embolism in this setting compared with thrombosis complicating acute myocardial infarction or dilated cardiomyopathy, long-term anticoagulation is not recommended (see Table 18–10). The 1% to 2% risk of hemorrhage associated with oral anticoagulants outweighs the possible benefits of anticoagulation. Therefore, routine anticoagulation is not advised beyond the first 3 months after infarction in the presence of a ventricular aneurysm. Patients with chronic left ventricular aneurysm who experience emboli should receive long-term anticoagulation therapy. Patients with left ventricular aneurysms and significantly reduced ejection fraction (less than 35%), clinical congestive heart failure, or atrial fibrillation should be given anticoagulants.

Dilated Cardiomyopathy

Intracavitary mural thrombi are common in dilated cardiomyopathy (DCM) and are found in 30% to 50% of cases at postmortem examination.[131] Echocardiography detects left ventricular thrombi in as many as 36% of cases of DCM regardless of cause.[132] Clinical embolism, found in approximately 10% to 20% of all patients with DCM, also occurs regardless of the cause of cardiomyopathy at a rate of up to 3.5% per year in nonanticoagulated patients.[133] Acute thromboembolism is thus a chronic hazard in DCM. Embolism is more frequent with coexistent atrial fibrillation. A previously detected thrombus, particularly if protuberant, may be associated with increased risk of embolism.[134] Both chronic abnormal intracavity blood flow patterns resulting in stasis and abnormalities of hemostasis contribute to the pathogenesis of intracavitary thrombosis in DCM.[135–137] Unlike in acute myocardial infarction, ventricular thrombi in DCM tend to be small, multiple, and not necessarily localized to the most dyskinetic regions. In view of the chronic risk of embolism, long-term anticoagulation with warfarin to maintain the prothrombin time at 1.5 to 2.0 times control (INR, 2.0 to 3.0) is recommended (see Table 18–10). This indication becomes stronger in the presence of atrial fibrillation, decompensated cardiac failure, or prolonged bed rest.

Atrial Thrombi

Mitral Valve Disease

Acute embolism is more frequent in rheumatic mitral valve disease than in any other type of common heart disease.[138] The incidence of embolism in nonanticoagulated patients with rheumatic mitral valve disease varies from 1% to 5% per year.[139–147] Over the entire course of rheumatic mitral disease, the incidence of systemic embolism is approximately 27%.[138] Seventy-five percent of emboli involve the cerebral circulation, and emboli may be the presenting symptom of rheumatic mitral disease in as many as 12.4% of cases.[148, 149] Isolated mitral regurgitation carries a smaller but still substantial risk. The risk of embolism is greater with increasing severity of valvular regurgitation and in patients with mixed mitral stenosis and regurgitation.[141] Thrombi occur most often in the left atrial appendage.

Atrial fibrillation increases the risk of embolism 6 to 18 times in the presence of rheumatic mitral disease.[138] Other factors that increase risk include a history of embolism, older age, and low cardiac index.[138] Left atrial size, mitral calcification, mitral valve area, and clinical functional classification do not correlate well with risk. Left atrial enlargement does not appear to be an independent risk factor for embolism, but it does increase the risk of atrial fibrillation. Because most emboli occur shortly after the onset of atrial fibrillation (a third occur within 1 month, and two thirds occur within 1 year), it is the physician's responsibility to anticipate atrial fibrillation and begin oral anticoagulation before its onset.[138] Emboli recur commonly (30% to 65%), usually within 6 months, and are associated with substantial mortality.[138, 145]

Patients with rheumatic mitral stenosis, mitral regurgitation, or mixed lesions in atrial fibrillation are at high risk for thromboembolism (Table 18–11). Anticoagulation with warfarin is advised to prolong the prothrombin time to 1.5 to 2 times control (INR, 2.5 to 3.5). Atrial fibrillation should be anticipated in patients in sinus rhythm who have marked left atrial dilation of more than 50 to 55 mm by echocardiography. These patients should receive prophylactic anticoagulation therapy. If disease is hemodynamically insignificant, no anticoagulation is required, provided no other risk factors for thromboembolism are present.

Mitral Valve Prolapse

Stroke results from embolism in the setting of mitral valve prolapse (MVP) as a result of several mecha-

nisms: (1) fibrinous nonbacterial thrombotic endocarditis of the mitral valve (seen only with significant mitral regurgitation and valvular redundancy), (2) endothelial denudation of the mitral valve with subsequent formation of leaflet fibrin thrombi, or (3) mural thrombosis of the atrium due to mitral regurgitation. Most cerebral emboli are small and result in transient ischemic attacks or small strokes.[150] Common causes of cerebral ischemia must be excluded before implicating mitral valve prolapse, especially in elderly patients.[113]

Embolic risk due to MVP is related to the severity of prolapse, leaflet redundancy, and degree of mitral regurgitation.[151] Routine prophylactic antithrombotic therapy is unwarranted in the great majority of patients with mitral valve prolapse given the low incidence of embolism in this common condition (see Table 18–11). If other risk factors for embolism (chronic or paroxysmal atrial fibrillation, left atrial size >55 mm, heart failure or severe left ventricular dysfunction, history of previous systemic embolism) are also present in patients with MVP, then appropriate prophylactic antithrombotic therapy is warranted. After a mild or transient embolic event in a patient with MVP, oral anticoagulation for 3 to 6 months is warranted while other possible causes of cerebral ischemia are investigated. If no other cause of cerebral ischemia is found, and if risk factors for future embolism as listed previously are present, patients may be treated with chronic aspirin 80 to 325 mg/day. If risk factors for embolism are present, chronic anticoagulation with warfarin (INR, 2 to 3) is indicated. If a questionable neurologic event occurs in a patient with MVP, it is appropriate to use aspirin in a dose of 80 to 325 mg/day. Investigation into other causes of cerebral ischemia should be done.

Nonvalvular Atrial Fibrillation

Nonvalvular atrial fibrillation (NVAF) is the most common cardiac disorder predisposing to cardiogenic embolism and is the cause of 45% of all cardioembolic strokes.[152] In addition, 25% to 35% of patients with NVAF have stroke; 50% to 70% of these are embolic.[153] In the absence of anticoagulation, the risk of stroke in NVAF is approximately 5% per year.[153, 154] A high risk of embolism due to NVAF occurs with coexisting rheumatic mitral valvular disease, a mechanical prosthetic valve, or thromboembolism within the previous 2 years.[113] The presence of other cardiac disease (hypertension, mitral regurgitation, congestive heart failure, ischemic heart disease), older patient age, recent onset of NVAF, and history of previous thromboembolism (beyond 2 years) all also increase risk.[153, 155] Paroxysmal NVAF may confer a slight reduction in risk compared with sustained NVAF, although this reduction is unlikely to be substantial.[153, 156] Low-risk patients with NVAF include those with "lone" atrial fibrillation: patients younger than the age of 60 who lack any signs, symptoms, or history of cardiovascular disease and who have structurally normal hearts by echocardiography. Lone atrial fibrillation in pa-

Table 18–11. **Antithrombotic Therapy in Valvular Heart Disease and Nonvalvular Atrial Fibrillation**

Cardiac Disease	Recommendations
Mitral stenosis present	Chronic warfarin (PT 1.5 to 2 times control, INR 2.5 to 3.5) if atrial fibrillation
	Consider warfarin for patients in sinus rhythm with large LA (>50 mm by M-mode echocardiogram)
Mitral regurgitation	Chronic warfarin in high-risk patients (atrial fibrillation, LV dysfunction, prior embolic events)
Mitral valve prolapse	Aspirin, 325 mg/day, if neurologic events of unclear cause occur
	Warfarin in case of obvious embolic event*
Aortic valve disease	No therapy needed in the absence of other risk factors for thromboembolism
Nonvalvular atrial fibrillation	Chronic warfarin (PT 1.2 to 1.5 times control, INR 2 to 3)
	Aspirin, 325 mg/day, in low-risk patients (lone atrial fibrillation)†

INR, international normalized ratio; LA, left atrium; LV, left ventricular; PT, prothrombin time.
*This therapy needs to be submitted to clinical trials.
†A randomized trial of low-dose warfarin, aspirin, and placebo is under way.

tients older than the age of 60 increases risk of stroke.[157] Left atrial dimension (>50 mm), spontaneous atrial contrast, and diminished left ventricular function by echocardiography define higher-risk patients with NVAF.

Results of five large trials of antithrombotic therapy in NVAF may be summarized as follows:[152-154] (1) the risk of stroke from NVAF in nonanticoagulated patients is approximately 5% per year; (2) the risk of stroke in NVAF is decreased to 2% per year (or by 60%) by warfarin; (3) high-dose and low-dose warfarin are equally efficacious; (4) aspirin, 325 mg/day, may be efficacious in preventing stroke in patients younger than the age of 75, especially if they do not have congestive heart failure; (5) neither high-dose nor low-dose warfarin increases life-threatening bleeding or intracranial hemorrhage; (6) the risk of cerebral hemorrhage due to warfarin is approximately 0.3% per year, no higher than in aspirin-treated or placebo-treated patients; (7) for every 1000 patients treated with warfarin for NVAF, warfarin prevents 20 to 30 ischemic strokes at a cost of four to six major bleeding episodes per year; and (8) two of the trials observed a decrease in vascular mortality with warfarin, including the trial with the longest follow-up.

At present, it is strongly recommended that all patients lacking contraindication to long-term warfarin therapy with sustained or paroxysmal NVAF (except patients younger than age 60 with "lone" NVAF) should be treated with long-term low-dose warfarin therapy (target INR of 2.0 to 3.0; see Table 18–11). Patients at particularly high risk of thromboembolism with NVAF include those with prior thromboembolism, significant left ventricular dysfunction, or congestive heart failure. Patients older than the age of 60 with "lone" atrial fibrillation are at risk of thromboembolism and should be considered for therapy with warfarin. Patients who have contraindications to long-term warfarin or who are poor candidates for warfarin should be treated with aspirin 325 mg once a day indefinitely.

Prosthetic Heart Valves and Thromboembolism

Mechanical Prosthetic Valves

The most important risk factor for acute thromboembolism from mechanical prosthetic heart valves is the variability and intensity of chronic anticoagulation with warfarin (Table 18–12). In patients with mitral valve prostheses, the thromboembolic event rate in those who have adequately anticoagulated blood is half that of those who have inadequately anticoagulated blood.[158-165] Fully half of all thromboembolic complications occur with inadequate anticoagulation, and half of the bleeding complications of warfarin occur with excessive anticoagulation.[159, 164, 165] The variability of the prothrombin time is probably as important as the intensity.[166]

Valves in the aortic position are at lowest risk, those in the mitral position at higher risk, and double

Table 18–12. Risk Factors for Prosthetic Valve Thromboembolism

1. Variability and intensity of anticoagulation
2. Prosthetic valve location (MV + AV > MV > AV)*
3. Atrial fibrillation
4. LA size > 50–55 mm despite sinus rhythm
5. Previous thromboembolism
6. Congestive heart failure
7. Significant left ventricular dysfunction
8. Older valve model/design†
9. Valve replacement before 1980
10. Cumulative time after operation‡

*MV, mitral valve; AV, aortic valve; LA, left atrium.
†Owing to increased turbulence of older designs and increased thrombogenicity of materials.
‡Risk of thromboembolism increases cumulatively with time after operation.

valves in the mitral and aortic positions at highest risk. Atrial fibrillation, left atrial size of more than 50 to 55 mm by M-mode echocardiography despite normal sinus rhythm, previous thromboembolism, left ventricular dysfunction, older valve design (owing to less favorable hemodynamic valve profile and construction from more thrombogenic materials), and year of valve replacement operation before 1980 (owing to referral for valve replacement later in the course of chronic valvular heart disease) all increase risk of thromboembolism.[166-170] The highest risk of thromboembolism occurs during the first postoperative year, likely because of variability in anticoagulation and the presence of nonendothelialized highly thrombogenic exposed perivalvular tissues and prosthetic surfaces.[167] However, the risk of thromboembolism persists indefinitely after operation.

Long-term therapy with anticoagulants significantly decreases the risk of thromboembolism from mechanical prosthetic heart valves.[167] With regard to warfarin dosage, the following conclusions may be drawn from the available large prospective studies: (1) a target INR of 2.5 to 3.5 appears adequate to prevent thromboembolism in most instances;[171] (2) an INR of more than 3.5 is associated with excessive bleeding but no additional protection against thromboembolism;[172] (3) an INR below 1.8 likely confers inadequate protection against thromboembolism.[173] Therapy with combined anticoagulant and antiplatelet agents is more efficacious than therapy with anticoagulants alone. Five trials have shown that the combination of the antiplatelet agent dipyridamole (375 to 400 mg/day) and warfarin is superior to warfarin alone in reducing the incidence of thromboembolism from mechanical prosthetic valves.[167, 173] Dipyridamole has been approved by the FDA for use in patients with mechanical prosthetic valves at high risk of thromboembolism. Aspirin also has additive benefit to warfarin in the prevention of thromboembolism. The combination of aspirin (500 to 1000 mg daily) and warfarin significantly increased the incidence of major hemorrhage requiring transfusion or hospitalization.[159, 174, 175] However, aspirin in lower doses appears safer.[176] Further studies are currently under way to establish the optimal doses and safety of aspirin and warfarin in combination in this setting. Antiplatelet agents alone are ineffective.[177–182]

All patients should be considered for subcutaneous heparin begun 6 hours after surgery to prolong the aPTT to the upper limit of normal (Table 18–13). Warfarin (target INR of 2.5 to 3.5) should be begun 24 to 48 hours after operation in all patients and continued indefinitely. Once the chest tubes are removed, intravenous heparin should be administered to maintain the aPTT at 1.5 to 2.0 times control until warfarin is within the therapeutic range. High-risk patients (valve implanted before 1980, previous thromboembolism, anticoagulation decreased or stopped because of bleeding, poor patient compliance, high variability in prothrombin times, patient population with an incidence of thromboembolism more than 2.0% per year on warfarin alone) should receive supplemental antiplatelet therapy. Dipyridamole 350 to 400 mg/day is FDA approved for this use. One study supports the use of low-dose aspirin 100 mg/day in high-risk patients.[176] Patients who are not at high risk and who experience bleeding problems with warfarin should be treated with low-dose warfarin (INR, 2.0 to 3.0) and either low-dose aspirin 80 to 100 mg/day or dipyridamole 375 to 400 mg/day. Patients who cannot tolerate or have absolute contraindication to warfarin should be treated with aspirin 100 to 325 mg/day plus dipyridamole 375 to 400 mg/day, although this combination has not been evaluated to date.

Bioprosthetic Valves

Thromboembolism is less frequent from bioprosthetic valves than from mechanical prosthetic valves, but it still occurs, especially in the early postoperative period.[167] The highest risk of thromboembolism occurs within the first 3 months of operation,[183] when the incidence of thromboembolism may be as high as 12% without postoperative intravenous heparin followed by warfarin.[183] Atrial fibrillation, left ventricular systolic dysfunction, and marked enlargement of the left atrium also increase the risk of bioprosthetic valve thromboembolism.[184] Platelet inhibitor therapy has not been adequately tested.

Table 18–13. **Antithrombotic Therapy for Prosthetic Valves**

Valve	Risk	Therapy
Mechanical	Low	Warfarin INR 2.5 to 3.5
	High*	Warfarin INR 3.0 to 4.5
		Warfarin INR 2.5 to 3.5 + aspirin 75–100 mg/day
		Warfarin INR 2.5 to 3.5 + dipyridamole 400 mg/day
Bioprosthetic	Low	Warfarin INR 2.0 to 3.0
	High*	Warfarin INR 3.0 to 4.5 for 3 months, then warfarin INR 2.5 to 3.5 indefinitely

*High-risk: atrial fibrillation, left atrium > 55 mm, prior thromboembolism, congestive heart failure. Consider reoperation for recurrent embolism despite adequate anticoagulation.

Warfarin should be administered to all patients within 24 to 48 hours of operation and continued for 3 months (target INR, 2.0 to 3.0; see Table 18–13). Patients at high risk of thromboembolism (previous thromboembolism, left atrial thrombus) should be treated with this dose indefinitely. Patients with moderate risk of thromboembolism (left ventricular dysfunction, atrial fibrillation, enlarged left atrium more than 50 mm by M-mode echocardiography) should receive warfarin for 3 months as stated earlier followed by warfarin at a dose to prolong the INR to 2.0 to 3.0 indefinitely after 3 months. For aortic or mitral bioprosthetic valve replacement at low risk of thromboembolism (without any of the risk factors listed earlier), patients after 3 months of warfarin (target INR, 3.0 to 4.5) may be treated with aspirin 80 mg/day indefinitely.

Arterial Thrombosis

No available antithrombotic agent at present completely prevents platelet adhesion to the subendothelium or thrombin generation after vascular injury. If the principal cause of progression of coronary artery atherosclerosis is intimal hyperplasia related to chronic and subtle endothelial damage mediated by platelet and monocyte vessel wall interactions,[185] then antithrombotic therapy in its present form may play an insignificant role in halting such progression. If, however, progression is more related to recurrent plaque rupture,[186] nonocclusive mural thrombosis, and subsequent organization and incorporation of the thrombus into the growing lesion, antiplatelet agents may play an important role.

Chronic Stable Angina Pectoris

Because plaque rupture appears to be a random event in the protracted natural history of coronary artery disease, and because platelet-rich thrombosis occurs at the site of plaque disruption, a theoretic rationale exists for the prophylactic use of platelet inhibitors in patients with stable angina pectoris. Three studies have shown that aspirin reduces the incidence of MI in patients with chronic stable angina.[187, 188] One trial showed that aspirin prevented formation of new atherosclerotic lesions but did not prevent progression of existing lesions.[187] In the first Antiplatelet Trialists' Collaboration meta-analysis of 25 trials of antiplatelet agents in patients with a history of transient ischemic attack, occlusive stroke, unstable angina, or myocardial infarction, antiplatelet therapy reduced nonfatal myocardial infarction by 32% ($p < .0001$), vascular mortality by 15% ($p = .0003$), and nonfatal stroke by 27% ($p < .0001$).[189] The second Antiplatelet Trialists' Collaboration corroborated these results.[40] Based on these results, all patients with chronic stable angina should receive aspirin 325 mg/day indefinitely (Table 18–14).

Table 18–14. **Antithrombotic Therapy in Coronary Artery Disease**

Coronary Event	Recommendations
Stable angina	Aspirin, 325 mg/day
Unstable angina	Acute phase: IV heparin plus low-dose aspirin 75–100 mg Chronic phase: aspirin 325 mg/day
Non-Q-wave MI	Acute phase: IV heparin plus low-dose aspirin Chronic phase: aspirin 325 mg/day
Q-wave MI: absence of thrombolytic therapy	Aspirin, 325 mg/day, in acute and chronic phases IV heparin in acute phase
Q-wave MI: presence of thrombolytic therapy	Aspirin 325 mg on admission, then 75–100 mg/day combined with adjunctive heparin* (aPTT 2 to 3 × control) for 2–7 days Aspirin, 325 mg/day, thereafter

aPTT, activated partial thromboplastin time; MI, myocardial infarction.
*Heparin has not yet been shown to be efficacious adjunctive therapy to streptokinase.

Unstable Angina

Convincing evidence of the benefit of aspirin in unstable angina derives from four double-blind, randomized, placebo-controlled trials.[190–193] Aspirin decreases myocardial infarction and death by approximately 50%. Ticlopidine is also efficacious.[194] Heparin alone is efficacious when administered as a continuous intravenous infusion to prolong the aPTT to 1.5 to 2.0 times control.[195–197] Comparative trials from the Montreal Heart Institute have shown that heparin alone reduces the incidence of MI in the acute phase of unstable angina compared with aspirin alone.[192, 193] Reactivation of angina may occur in as many as 13% of patients upon discontinuation of heparin but is decreased by overlapping aspirin therapy.[198] The combination of aspirin and anticoagulants is more efficacious in the acute phase and likely the chronic phase of unstable angina than either heparin or aspirin alone. In pilot studies, the selective thrombin inhibitors hirudin and argatroban appear promising in unstable angina.[199, 200] Large studies are under way to evaluate the role of selective thrombin inhibitors in unstable angina. Thrombolysis during unstable angina has not proved efficacious to date.[201] Intravenous heparin and low-dose aspirin 75 to 100 mg/day are recommended in the acute phase followed by aspirin 325 mg/day indefinitely (see Table 18–14).

Acute, Evolving Myocardial Infarction in Absence of Thrombolytic Therapy

ISIS-2 clearly established the efficacy of aspirin in evolving myocardial infarction.[202] Aspirin conferred additional survival benefit when given in combination with streptokinase. All patients with acute evolving myocardial infarction should receive aspirin whether treated with thrombolytic agents or not (see Table 18–14). Overview of the six randomized trials

of heparin in the absence of thrombolytic therapy in MI showed that anticoagulants reduced mortality by 21% in acute evolving myocardial infarction ($p < .001$).[203] Thus, anticoagulants appear similar in efficacy to aspirin in acute evolving myocardial infarction: aspirin reduces mortality by 23%, and anticoagulants reduce mortality by 16% to 22%.[204] Heparin should be considered in all patients with myocardial infarction, especially in the following subsets: (1) non-Q-wave myocardial infarction, because studies discussed earlier have established that heparin is more efficacious than aspirin in preventing infarction or reinfarction in patients with unstable angina (and non-Q-wave myocardial infarction is one end of the spectrum of unstable angina); and (2) Q-wave myocardial infarction at high risk of mural thrombosis formation (anterior infarction) or systemic embolism (atrial fibrillation, congestive heart failure, significantly depressed left ventricular function, history of prior thromboembolism) (see Table 18–14). At a minimum, all patients with myocardial infarction should receive no less than 7500 IU subcutaneous heparin for 5 days and until ambulatory to prevent venous thromboembolism.[125]

Anticoagulants in Acute, Evolving Myocardial Infarction in the Presence of Thrombolytic Therapy

After successful exogenous thrombolysis, there remains a 5% to 30% chance of reocclusion and a 4% chance of reinfarction in the absence of aspirin therapy.[125] Use of thrombolytic agents themselves results in platelet activation.[205] In animal models, maintenance of patency after thrombolysis requires combined inhibition of thrombin and platelets.[206] Thus, adjunctive antiplatelet and anticoagulant therapy plays a key role in preventing acute reocclusion after thrombolysis (see Table 18–14).

The role of routine adjunctive heparin in streptokinase and aspirin–treated patients is controversial.[207–210] Although adjunctive heparin in streptokinase and aspirin–treated patients reduces in-hospital mortality, it has not in large trials to date decreased 30- to 35-day mortality or increased early infarct-related artery patency.[211, 212] To date, no large trials with mortality as a primary end point have evaluated heparin alone or heparin as sole adjunctive therapy; in GISSI-II, ISIS-3, and GUSTO, all patients received aspirin.[207, 208] Heparin should definitely be administered in streptokinase and aspirin–treated patients who would otherwise benefit from anticoagulation after an anterior myocardial infarct, including those with atrial fibrillation, depressed left ventricular function, congestive heart failure, prior thromboembolism, or mural thrombus by echocardiography.

In t-PA and aspirin–treated patients, adjunctive heparin appears to increase early (18 hour) infarct-related patency.[213, 214] The angiographic studies to date (not including the GUSTO substudy, which was designed to evaluate the effect of accelerated t-PA on early patency and not the effect of adjunctive heparin) have been unable to show reduction in mortality due to earlier patency resulting from adjunctive heparin, but this may result from the small sample sizes of these studies. Because it is known that early infarct-related vessel patency (either early patency at 90 minutes or late patency at hospital discharge) predicts mortality, it will be crucial that future trials determine the real effects of adjunctive heparin and other antithrombin agents such as hirudin and Hirulog on infarct-related patency.[215] Until further trials are available, it is prudent to recommend adjunctive heparin to patients treated with t-PA and aspirin. Patients who would otherwise benefit from anticoagulation after an anterior MI as stated earlier should receive adjunctive heparin.

Acute Thrombotic Occlusion of a Saphenous Vein Bypass Graft

Acute thrombotic occlusion of a coronary artery saphenous vein graft (SVG) occurs in 10% to 15% of all grafts within 1 month of operation and in 25% of all grafts by 1 year.[216–219] The left internal mammary artery (LIMA) has a much lower incidence of occlusion, approximately 10% at 7 to 10 years after surgery.[220] Vein harvesting, surgical manipulation, temporal delay between vein harvesting and implantation, and vein preservation techniques result in type II vascular injury along the length of the SVG.[221, 222] Type III vascular injury may occur at sites of anastomosis between the SVG and the native coronary artery. The LIMA is protected from endothelial injury and platelet deposition owing to less extensive surgical handling, previous adaptation to arterial shearing forces, and preservation of partially intact vasa vasorum.[221] Lack of conditioning of the SVG to arterial shearing forces and further shear-induced endothelial injury on implantation increase the susceptibility of the SVG to platelet deposition.[221] Platelet deposition on the SVG is immediate and occurs as soon as blood flows through the newly implanted graft; this has been confirmed angioscopically.[223] As many as 20% of SVGs show technical faults in suturing at the distal anastomosis, which may lead to reduced graft flow and increased thrombotic risk.[223] In particular, SVGs with flow less than 40 ml/min or with a distal anastomosis to a small receiving coronary artery (less than 1.5 mm in diameter) are at increased risk for occlusion.[221]

Antiplatelet therapy with aspirin reduces the incidence of SVG occlusion after 1 month and 1 year by 30% to 50%.[221] A meta-analysis of 13 trials of antiplatelet and anticoagulants from 1966 to 1988 in humans showed that early initiation of active treatment was beneficial in preventing acute SVG occlusion (overall effect size = 0.30; confidence interval 0.21 to 0.38).[224] Low-dose aspirin (75 to 100 mg) appears as efficacious as higher-dose aspirin.[225] Ticlopidine appears effective, although its delayed onset of action (48 hours) must be considered. Dipyridamole alone is not effective, and there is no conclusive evidence to date that the combination of dipyridamole and aspi-

rin is more efficacious than aspirin alone. Antiplatelet therapy must be begun within 48 hours postoperatively to be effective. Aspirin begun as early as 1 hour postoperatively results in increased chest tube drainage and a trend toward higher rates of reoperation but not increased hospital mortality. Antiplatelet therapy is particularly efficacious in grafts at high risk of occlusion, namely those with low flow (less than 40 ml/min) or with small distal anastomoses (less than 1.5 mm). The role of aspirin combined with anticoagulants in the prevention of occlusion of high-risk grafts is theoretically attractive; either aspirin plus dipyridamole or low-dose aspirin plus warfarin should be considered in this setting (Table 18–15).

Acute Thrombotic Occlusion After Angioplasty

Angioscopy after angioplasty reveals intimal disruption, intimal dissection, and clefts in the atheroma in nearly all cases.[226, 227] Autopsy studies days after percutaneous transluminal coronary angioplasty (PTCA) reveal jagged intimal surfaces, intimal flaps, focal mural thrombosis, and fibrin deposition at the PTCA site.[228] As a result of either type II or type III vascular injury after PTCA, immediate platelet deposition occurs on the injured arterial surface.[229, 230] Such platelet deposition is not prevented by heparin or aspirin,[228–231] although aspirin has been shown to suppress transient thromboxane A_2 (TXA_2) release associated with cardiac catheterization or angioplasty.[232] Such mechanisms are responsible for a 3% incidence of acute thrombotic occlusion after PTCA.[233, 234] Acute thrombotic occlusion is more likley to occur when thrombus is present before PTCA.[228] Pre-PTCA plate-

Table 18–15. **Antithrombotic Therapy in Coronary Revascularization**

	Recommendations
SVBG surgery	Aspirin, 325 mg/day, early postoperatively and indefinitely thereafter. Also, in grafts at high risk* of occlusion, combine low-dose aspirin 75–100 mg/day with dipyridamole 400 mg/day, or low-dose warfarin (INR 2 to 3).
PTCA (acute occlusion)	Aspirin, 325 mg/day, 24 hours pre-PTCA; 325 mg/day thereafter. Intravenous heparin 10,000 U bolus at time of PTCA, then 1000 U/hr thereafter adjusted to aPTT 1.5 to 2.0 times control for 4–16 hours uncomplicated PTCA, 24 hours complicated PTCA.†
PTCA (chronic restenosis)	Current antithrombotic agents are ineffective; aspirin 75–325 mg/day should be given to all for chronic therapy of CAD.

PTCA, percutaneous transluminal coronary angioplasty; SVBG, saphenous vein bypass graft; CAD, coronary artery disease.

*Distal anastomosis < 1.5 mm or flow < 40 ml/min.

†Preceding unstable angina, visible thrombus, multivessel angioplasty, suboptimal result, dissection, intimal flap, complex lesion, acute occlusion.

let activation in the setting of unstable angina may increase the risk of acute thrombosis.[235]

Both antiplatelet agents and anticoagulants have been shown to decrease acute occlusion after angioplasty.[236] Aspirin and dipyridamole decrease by 70% transmural myocardial infarction secondary to abrupt occlusion;[237] they also decrease the need for emergency coronary artery bypass surgery.[238] Aspirin is as efficacious as aspirin plus dipyridamole.[239] Ticlopidine appears efficacious if begun 24 to 48 hours before PTCA. Trials of newer antiplatelet agents such as glycoprotein IIb/IIIa inhibitors,[240] von Willebrand antagonists, and TXA_2 inhibitors are under way in the prevention of acute occlusion.

Despite routine use in PTCA, heparin has not been studied in large randomized trials to date. In animal models, heparin decreases (but does not completely prevent) platelet deposition after deep arterial injury.[241] Observational studies in humans have shown that pretreatment with heparin before angioplasty decreases acute occlusion rates.[242] The dosage and duration of heparin therapy are empiric at present. In the one trial of uncomplicated PTCA, 18 hours of heparin was as effective as 24 hours of heparin in preventing acute occlusion.[243] Heparin can probably be safely discontinued 2 to 4 hours after an uncomplicated, low-risk PTCA. Based on current empiric standard practice, heparin should be continued for 24 hours in patients with pre-PTCA unstable angina, angiographically visible thrombus at the time of PTCA, angiographically complex lesions, the occurrence of intimal flap or dissection, multivessel angioplasty, or a suboptimal PTCA result (see Table 18–15). Preliminary trials of the selective thrombin inhibitors hirudin and Hirulog have appeared, and large trials are under way.[244, 245]

REFERENCES

1. Clagett G, Anderson F, Levine M, et al: Prevention of venous thromboembolism. Chest 102(Suppl 4):391S, 1992.
2. Hull R, Kakkar V, Raskob G: Prevention of venous thrombosis and pulmonary embolism. In Fuster V, Verstarete M (eds): Thrombosis in Cardiovascular Disorders. Philadelphia: WB Saunders, 1992.
3. Halkin H, Goldberg J, Modan M, et al: Reduction of mortality in general medical in-patients by low-dose heparin prophylaxis. Ann Intern Med 96:561, 1982.
4. Collins R, Scrimgeour A, Yusuf S, et al: Reduction in fatal pulmonary embolism and venous thrombosis by perioperative administration of subcutaneous heparin: Overview of results of randomized trials in general, orthopedic, and urologic surgery. N Engl J Med 318:1162, 1988.
5. Colditz G, Tuden R, Oster G: Rates of venous thrombosis after general surgery: Combined results of randomised clinical trials. Lancet 2:143, 1986.
6. Emerson P, Marks P: Preventing thromboembolism after myocardial infarction: Effect of low-dose heparin or smoking. Br Med J 1:18, 1977.
7. Drapkin A, Merskey C: Anticoagulant therapy after acute myocardial infarction: Relation of therapeutic benefit to patient's age, sex, and severity of infarction. JAMA 222:541, 1972.
8. Handley A: Low-dose heparin after myocardial infarction. Lancet 2:623, 1972.
9. Handley A, Emerson P, Fleming P: Heparin in the prevention of deep vein thrombosis after myocardial infarction. Br Med J 2:436, 1972.
10. Warlow C, Beattie A, Terry K, et al: A double-blind trial of low doses of subcutaneous heparin in the prevention of deep-vein thrombosis after myocardial infarction. Lancet 2:934, 1973.
11. Wray R, Maurer B, Shillingford J: Prophylactic anticoagulant therapy in the prevention of calf-vein thrombosis after myocardial infarction. N Engl J Med 288:815, 1973.
12. Wright I, Marple C, Beck D: Report of the Committee for the Evaluation of Anticoagulants in the Treatment of Coronary Thrombosis with Myocardial Infarction. Am Heart J 36:801, 1948.
13. Veterans Administration Hospitals: Anticoagulants in acute myocardial infarction: Results of a cooperative clinical trial. JAMA 225:724, 1973.
14. Assessment of short-term anticoagulant administration after cardiac infarction. Br Med J 1:335, 1969.
15. Oster G, Tuden R, Colditz G: Prevention of venous thromboembolism after general surgery: Cost-effectiveness analysis of alternative approaches to prophylaxis. Am J Med 82:889, 1987.
16. Oster G, Tuden R, Colditz G: A cost-effectiveness analysis of prophylaxis against deep-vein thrombosis in major orthopedic surgery. JAMA 257:203, 1987.
17. Salzman E, Davies G: Prophylaxis of venous thromboembolism. Ann Surgery 191:207, 1980.
18. Goldhaber S, Morpurgo M: Diagnosis, treatment, and prevention of pulmonary embolism: Report of the WHO/International Society and Federation of Cardiology Task Force. JAMA 268:1727, 1993.
19. An International Multicentre Trial. Prevention of fatal postoperative pulmonary embolism by low doses of heparin. Lancet 2:45, 1975.
20. Gallus A, Hirsh J, Tuttle R, et al: Small subcutaneous doses of heparin in the prevention of venous thrombosis. N Engl J Med 288:545, 1973.
21. Leyvraz P, Richard J, Bachmann F, et al: Adjusted versus fixed-dose subcutaneous heparin in the prevention of deep-vein thrombosis after total hip replacement. N Engl J Med 309:954, 1983.
22. Hirsh J: Rationale for development of low-molecular-weight heparins and their clinical potential in the prevention of postoperative venous thrombosis. Am J Surg 161:512, 1991.
23. Leizorovicz A, Haugh M, Chapuis F, et al: Low molecular weight heparin in prevention of perioperative thrombosis. Br Med J 305:913, 1992.
24. Nurmohamed M, Rosendaal F, Buller H, et al: Low-molecular-weight heparin versus standard heparin in general and orthopedic surgery: A meta-analysis. Lancet 340:152, 1992.
25. Kakkar V, Cohen A, Edmonson R, et al: Low molecular weight versus standard heparin for prevention of venous thromboembolism after major abdominal surgery. Lancet 341:259, 1993.
26. Hull R, Raskob G, Pineo G, et al: A comparison of subcutaneous low-molecular-weight heparin with warfarin sodium for prophylaxis against deep-vein thrombosis after hip or knee implantation. N Engl J Med 329:1370, 1993.
27. Goldhaber S, Sors H: Treatment of venous thrombosis and pulmonary embolism. In Fuster V, Verstraete M (eds): Thrombosis in Cardiovascular Disorders. Philadelphia: WB Saunders, 1992.
28. Knight M, Dawson R: Effect of intermittent compression of the arms on deep venous thrombosis in the legs. Lancet 2:1265, 1976.
29. Nicolaides A, Fernandes J, Pollock A: Intermittent sequential pneumatic compression of the legs in the prevention of venous stasis and postoperative deep venous thrombosis. Surgery 87:69, 1980.
30. Scurr J, Coleridge-Smith P, Hasty J: Regimen for improved effectiveness of intermittent pneumatic compression in deep venous thrombosis prophylaxis. Surgery 102:816, 1987.
31. Francis C, Pellegrini V, Marder V, et al: Comparison of warfarin and external pneumatic compression in prevention of venous thrombosis after total hip replacement. JAMA 267:2911, 1992.

32. Jeffery P, Nicolaides A: Graduated compression stockings in the prevention of postoperative deep vein thrombosis. Br J Surg 77:380, 1990.
33. Sevitt S, Gallagher N: Prevention of venous thrombosis and pulmonary embolism in injured patients: A trial of anticoagulant prophylaxis with phenindione in middle-aged and elderly patients with fractured necks of femur. Lancet 2:981, 1959.
34. Morris G, Mitchell J: Warfarin sodium in prevention of deep venous thrombosis and pulmonary embolism in patients with fractured neck of femur. Lancet 2:869, 1976.
35. Francis C, Marder V, Evarts M, et al: Two-step warfarin therapy: Prevention of postoperative venous thrombosis without excessive bleeding. JAMA 249:374, 1983.
36. Powers P, Gent M, Jay R, et al: A randomized trial of less intense postoperative warfarin of aspirin therapy in the prevention of venous thromboembolism after surgery for fractured hip. Arch intern Med 149:771, 1989.
37. Poller L, McKernan A, Thomson J, et al: Fixed minidose warfarin: A new approach to prophylaxis against venous thrombosis after major surgery. Br Med J 295:1309, 1987.
38. Bern M, Lokich J, Wallach S, et al: Very low doses of warfarin can prevent thrombosis in central venous catheters. Ann Intern Med 112:423, 1990.
39. Hyers T, Hull R, Weg J: Antithrombotic therapy for venous thromboembolic disease. Chest 102(Suppl 4):408S, 1992.
40. Antiplatelet Trialists' Collaboration: Collaborative overview of randomized trials of antiplatelet therapy. Parts I, II, III. Br Med J 308:81, 159, 235, 1994.
41. Wolfe M, Skibo L, Goldhaber S: Pulmonary embolic disease: Diagnosis, pathophysiologic aspects, and treatment with thrombolytic therapy. Curr Prob Cardiol 18:585, 1993.
42. Greenfield L, Michna B: Twelve-year clinical experience with the Greenfield vena caval filter. Surgery 104:706, 1988.
43. Brandjes D, Heijboer H, Buller H, et al: Acenocoumarol and heparin compared with acenocoumarol alone in the initial treatment of proximal-vein thrombosis. N Engl J Med 327:1485, 1992.
44. Holmes D, Bura A, Mazzolai L, et al: Subcutaneous heparin compared with continuous intravenous heparin administration in the initial treatment of deep vein thrombosis. Ann Intern Med 116:279, 1992.
45. Hull R, Raskob G, Rosenbloom D, et al: Heparin for 5 days as compared with 10 days in the intitial treatment of proximal venous thrombosis. N Engl J Med 322:1260, 1990.
46. Gallus A, Jackaman J, Tillett J, et al: Safety and efficacy of warfarin started early after submassive venous thrombosis of pulmonary embolism. Lancet 2:1293, 1986.
47. Hull R, Raskob G, Pineo G, et al: Subcutaneous low-molecular-weight heparin compared with continuous intravenous heparin in the treatment of proximal-vein thrombosis. N Engl J Med 326:975, 1992.
48. Prandoni P, Lensing A, Buller H, et al: Comparison of subcutaneous low-molecular-weight heparin with intravenous standard heparin in proximal deep-vein thrombosis. Lancet 339:441, 1992.
49. Parent F, Bridey F, Dreyfus M, et al: Treatment of severe venous thrombo-embolism with intravenous hirudin (HBW 023): An open pilot study. Thromb Haemost 70:386, 1993.
50. Hull R, Delmore T, Genton E, et al: Warfarin sodium versus low-dose heparin in the long-term treatment of venous thrombosis. N Engl J Med 301:855, 1979.
51. Barritt D, Jordan S: Anticoagulant drugs in the treatment of pulmonary embolism: A controlled trial. Lancet 1:1309, 1960.
52. Goldhaber S: Evolving concepts in thrombolytic therapy for pulmonary embolism. Chest 101(Suppl 4):183S, 1992.
53. Hirsh J, van Aken W, Gallus A, et al: Heparin kinetics in venous thrombosis and pulmonary embolism. Circulation 53:691, 1976.
54. Basu D, Gallus A, Hirsh J, et al: A prospective study of the value of monitoring heparin treatment with the activated partial thromboplastin time. N Engl J Med 287:324, 1972.
55. Wheeler A, Jaquiss R, Newman J: Physician practices in the treatment of pulmonary embolism and deep venous thrombosis. Arch Intern Med 148:1321, 1988.
56. Cruickshank M, Levine M, Hirsh J, et al: A standard heparin nomogram for the management of heparin therapy. Arch Intern Med 151:333, 1991.
57. Thery C, Simonneau G, Meyer G, et al: Randomized trial of subcutaneous low-molecular-weight heparin CY 216 (Fraxiparine) compared with intravenous unfractionated heparin in the curative treatment of submassive pulmonary embolism: A dose-ranging study. Circulation 85:1380, 1992.
58. Tibbutt D, Davies J, Anderson J, et al: Comparison by controlled clinical trial of streptokinase and heparin in treatment of life-threatening pulmonary embolism. Br Med J 2:343, 1974.
59. Miller G, Sutton G, Kerr I, et al: Comparison of streptokinase and heparin in treatment of isolated acute massive pulmonary embolism. Br Med J 1:681, 1971.
60. Dickie K, deGroot W, Colley R, et al: Hemodynamic effects of bolus infusion of urokinase in pulmonary thromboembolism. Am Rev Respir Dis 109:48, 1974.
61. A Cooperative Study: Urokinase Pulmonary Embolism Trial: Phase 1 results. JAMA 214:2165, 1970.
62. Dalla-Volta S, Palla A, Santolicandro A, et al: PAIMS 2: Alteplase combined with heparin versus heparin in the treatment of acute pulmonary embolism. Plasminogen Activator Italian Multicenter Study 2. Am Coll Cardiol 20:520, 1992.
63. Goldhaber S, Haire W, Feldstein M, et al: Alteplase versus heparin in acute pulmonary embolism: Randomised trial assessing right-ventricular function and pulmonary perfusion. Lancet 341:507, 1993.
64. A Cooperative Study: Urokinase-Streptokinase Embolism Trial. JAMA 229:1606, 1974.
65. Meyer G, Sors H, Charbonnier B, et al: Effects of intravenous urokinase versus alteplase on total pulmonary resistance in acute massive pulmonary embolism: A European multicenter double-blind trial. J Am Coll Cardiol 19:239, 1992.
66. A Collaborative Study by the PIOPED Investigators. Tissue plasminogen activator for the treatment of acute pulmonary embolism. Chest 97:528, 1990.
67. Goldhaber S, Heit J, Kessler C, et al: Randomised controlled trial of recombinant tissue plasminogen activator versus urokinase in the treatment of acute pulmonary embolism. Lancet 2:293, 1988.
68. Come P: Echocardiographic evaluation of pulmonary embolism and its response to therapeutic interventions. Chest 101(Suppl 4):151S, 1992.
69. Rittoo D, Sutherland G: Acute pulmonary artery thromboembolism treated with thrombolysis: Diagnostic and monitoring uses of transesophageal echocardiography. Br Heart J 69:457, 1993.
70. Meneveau N, Bassand J-P, Schieve F, et al: Safety of thrombolytic therapy in elderly patients with massive pulmonary embolism: A comparison with nonelderly patients. J Am Coll Cardiol 22:1075, 1993.
71. Thrombolysis for pulmonary embolism [editorial]. Lancet 340:21, 1992.
72. Urokinase-Pulmonary Embolism Trial: Synopsis, summary, conclusions, and recommendations. Circulation 47-48(Suppl II):II-7, 1973.
73. The UKEP Study Research Group: The UKEP Study: Multicentre clinical trial on two local regimens of urokinase in massive pulmonary embolism. Eur Heart J 8:2, 1987.
74. Meyer G, Tamisier D, Sors H, et al: Pulmonary embolectomy: A 20-year experience at one center. Ann Thorac Surg 51:232, 1991.
75. Gray H, Morgan J, Paneth M, et al: Pulmonary embolectomy for acute massive pulmonary embolism: An analysis of 71 cases. Br Heart J 60:196, 1988.
76. Clarke D, Abrams L: Pulmonary embolectomy: A 25 year experience. J Thorac Cardiovasc Surg 92:442, 1986.
77. Timsit J-F, Reynaud P, Meyer G, et al: Pulmonary embolectomy by catheter device in massive pulmonary embolism. Chest 100:655, 1991.
78. Hart R: Cardiogenic embolism to the brain. Lancet 339:589, 1992.
79. Marshall R, Mohr J: Current management of ischaemic stroke. J Neurol Neurosurg Psychiatry 56:6, 1993.
80. Sherman D, Dyken M, Fisher M, et al: Antithrombotic therapy for cerebrovascular disorders. Chest 102(Suppl 4):529S, 1992.

81. Sandercock P, van den Belt A, Lindley R, et al: Antithrombotic therapy in acute ischaemic stroke: An overview of the completed randomised trials. J Neurol Neurosurg Psychiatry 56:17, 1993.

82. Clagett G, Graor R, Salzman E: Antithrombotic therapy in peripheral arterial occlusive disease. Chest 102(Suppl 4):516S, 1992.

83. Prizel K, Hutchins G, Bulkley B: Coronary artery embolism and myocardial infarction. Ann Intern Med 88:155, 1978.

84. Wittry M, Zimmerman T, Janosik D, et al: Postpartum myocardial infarction in a patient with intermittent ventricular preexcitation. Am Heart J 117:191, 1989.

85. Wenger N, Bauer S: Coronary embolism: Review of the literature and presentation of 15 cases. Am J Med 25:549, 1958.

86. Dec W: Case 27-1986. N Engl J Med 315:111, 1986.

87. Saphir O: Coronary embolism. Am Heart J 8:312, 1932.

88. Moriuchi M, Saito S, Tamura Y, et al: Thromboembolism in an angiographically normal coronary artery. Am Heart J 118:1065, 1989.

89. Herzog C, Henry T, Simmer S: Bacterial endocarditis presenting as acute myocardial infarction: A cautionary note for the era of reperfusion. Am J Med 90:392, 1991.

90. Kitchens C: Evolution of our understanding of the pathophysiology of primary mesenteric venous thrombosis. Am J Surgery 163:346, 1992.

91. Vuyyuru L, Tikoff G, Schubert M: Towards an earlier diagnosis of intestinal infarction? Gastroenterology 103:1106, 1992.

92. Marston A: Acute intestinal ischemia: Resection rather than revascularization. Br Med J 301:1174, 1990.

93. Levy P, Krausz M, Manny J: Acute mesenteric ischemia: Improved results—a retrospective analysis of ninety-two patients. Surgery 107:372, 1990.

94. Loscalzo J: Paradoxical embolism: Clinical presentation, diagnostic strategies, and therapeutic options. Am Heart J 112:141, 1986.

95. Borow K, Karp R: Atrial septal defect: Lessons from the past, directions for the future. N Engl J Med 323:1698, 1990.

96. Kasper W, Geibel A, Tiede N, et al: Patent foramen ovale in patients with haemodynamically significant pulmonary embolism. Lancet 430:561, 1992.

97. Pell A, Hughes D, Keating J, et al: Brief report: Fulminating fat embolism syndrome caused by paradoxical embolism through a patent foramen ovale. N Engl J Med 329:926, 1993.

98. Shuiab A: Cerebral infarction and ventricular septal defect. Stroke 20:957, 1989.

99. Reguera J, Colmenero J, Guerrero M, et al: Paradoxical cerebral embolism secondary to pulmonary arteriovenous fistula. Stroke 21:504, 1990.

100. Fornace J, Rozanski L, Berger B: Right heart thromboembolism and suspected paradoxical embolism in Ebstein's anomaly. Am Heart J 114:1520, 1987.

101. Daniel W: Transcatheter closure of patent foramen ovale: Therapeutic overkill or elegant management for selected patients at risk? Circulation 86:2013, 1992.

102. Langholz D, Louie E, Konstadt S, et al: Transesophageal echocardiographic demonstration of distinct mechanisms for right to left shunting across a patent foramen ovale in the absence of pulmonary hypertension. J Am Coll Cardiol 18:1112, 1991.

103. de Belder M, Tourikis L, Leech G, et al: Risk of patent foramen ovale for thromboembolic events in all age groups. Am J Cardiol 69:1316, 1992.

104. Di Tullio M, Sacco R, Gopal A, et al: Patent foramen ovale as a risk factor for cryptogenic stroke. Ann Intern Med 117:461, 1992.

105. Harvey J, Teague S, Anderson J, et al: Clinically silent atrial septal defects with evidence for cerebral embolization. Ann Intern Med 105:695, 1986.

106. Lechat P, Mas J, Lascault G, et al: Prevalence of patent foramen ovale in patients with stroke. N Engl J Med 318:1148, 1988.

107. Stollberger C, Slany J, Schuster I, et al: The prevalence of deep venous thrombosis in patients with suspected paradoxical embolism. Ann Intern Med 119:461, 1993.

108. Gin K, Huckell V, Pollick K: Femoral vein delivery of contrast medium enhances transthoracic echocardiographic detection of patent foramen ovale. J Am Coll Cardiol 22:1994, 1993.

109. Speechly-Dick M, Middleton S, Foale R: Impending paradoxical embolism: A rare but important diagnosis. Br Heart J 65:163, 1991.

110. Bridges N, Hellenbrand W, Latson L, et al: Transcatheter closure of patent foramen ovale after presumed paradoxical embolism. Circulation 86:1902, 1992.

111. Perloff J, Child J: Congenital Heart Disease in Adults. Philadelphia: WB Saunders, 1991.

112. Perloff J, Marelli A, Miner P: Risk of stroke in adults with cyanotic congenital heart disease. Circulation 87:1954, 1993.

113. Fuster V, Verstraete M: Thrombosis in Cardiovascular Disorders. Philadephia: WB Saunders, 1992.

114. Keating E, Gross A, Schlamowitz R, et al: Mural thrombi in myocardial infarctions: Prospective evaluation by two-dimensional echocardiography. Am J Med 74:989, 1983.

115. Meltzer R, Visser C, Fuster V: Intracardiac thrombi and systemic embolization. Ann Intern Med 104:689, 1986.

116. Mikell F, Asinger R, Elsperger J, et al: Long term prospective evaluation of left ventricular thrombi in acute myocardial infarction [abstract]. Circ 64(Suppl IV):IV-93, 1981.

117. Visser C, Kan G, Lie K, et al: Left ventricular thrombus following acute myocardial infarction: A prospective serial evalution of 96 patients. Eur Heart J 4:333, 1983.

118. Tramarin R, Pozzoli M, Febo O, et al: Echocardiographic assessment of therapy efficacy in left ventricular thrombosis post myocardial infarction [abstract]. Circulation 68(Suppl III):III-331, 1983.

119. Tramarin R, Pozzoli M, Vecchio C: Trombosi ventricolare sinistra nell-infarcto miocardio recente: Studio ecocardiographico. G Ital Cardiol 12:397, 1982.

120. Friedman M, Carlson K, Marcus F, et al: Clinical correlations in patients with acute myocardial infarction and left ventricular thrombus detected by two-dimensional echocardiography. Am J Med 72:894, 1982.

121. McEntee C, Van Reet R, Winters W, et al: Incidence and natural history of mural thrombi in acute myocardial infarction by two-dimensional echocardiography [abstract]. Circulation 64(Suppl IV):IV-93, 1981.

122. Visser C, Kan G, Meltzer R, et al: Long-term follow-up of left ventricular thrombus after myocardial infarction: A two-dimensional echocardiographic study of 96 patients. Chest 86:532, 1984.

123. Fuster V, Dyken M, Vokonas P, et al: Aspirin as a therapeutic agent in cardiovascular disease. Circulation 87:659, 1993.

124. Vaitkus P, Barnathan E: Embolic potential, prevention and management of mural thrombus complicating anterior myocardial infarction: A meta-analysis. J Am Coll Cardiol 22:1004, 1993.

125. Cairns J, Hirsh J, Lewis H, et al: Antithrombotic agents in coronary artery disease. Chest 102(Suppl 4):456S, 1992.

126. Johannessen K, Nordrehaug J, von der Lippe G, et al: Risk factor for embolisation in patients with left ventricular thrombi and acute myocardial infarction. Br Heart J 60:104, 1988.

127. Jugdutt B, Sivaram C, Wortman C, et al: Prospective two-dimensional echocardiographic evaluation of left ventricular thrombus and embolism after acute myocardial infarction. J Am Coll Cardiol 13:554, 1989.

128. Reeder G, Lengyel M, Tajik A, et al: Mural thrombus in left ventricular aneurysm: Incidence, role of angiography, and relation between anticoagulation and embolization. Mayo Clin Proc 56:77, 1981.

129. Cooley D, Hallman G: Surgical treatment of left ventricular aneurysm: Experience with excision of post-infarction lesions in 80 patients. Prog Cardiovasc Dis 11:222, 1968.

130. Cabin H, Roberts W: Left ventricular aneurysm, intra-aneurysmal thrombus and systemic embolus in coronary heart disease. Chest 77:586, 1980.

131. Roberts W, Ferrans V: Pathologic aspects of certain cardiomyopathies. Circ Res 35(Suppl II):128, 1974.

132. Stratton J, Resnick A: Increased embolic risk in patients with left ventricular thrombi. Circulation 75:1004, 1987.

133. Fuster V, Gersh B, Giulani E, et al: The natural history of dilated cardiomyopathy. Am J Cardiol 47:525, 1981.

134. Falk R, Foster E, Coats M: Ventricular thrombi and thrombo-

embolism in dilated cardiomyopathy: A prospective follow-up study. Am Heart J 123:136, 1991.

135. Maze S, Kotler M, Parry W: Flow characteristics in the dilated left ventricle with thrombus: Qualitative and quantitative doppler analysis. J Am Coll Cardiol 13:873, 1989.

136. Siostrzonek P, Koppensteiner R, Kreiner G, et al: Abnormal blood rheology in idiopathic dilated cardiomyopathy. Am J Cardiol 69:1497, 1991.

137. Jafri S, Ozawa T, Mammen E, et al: Platelet function, thrombin and fibrinolytic activity in patients with heart failure. Eur Heart J 14:205, 1993.

138. Levine H, Pauker S, Salzman E, et al: Antithrombotic therapy in valvular heart disease. Chest 102(Suppl 4):434S, 1992.

139. Pumphrey C, Fuster V, Chesebro J: Systemic thromboembolism in valvular heart disease and prosthetic heart valves. Mod Concepts Cardiovasc Dis 51:131, 1982.

140. Szekely P: Systemic embolism and anticoagulant prophylaxis in rheumatic heart disease. Br Med J 1:1209, 1964.

141. Coulshed N, Epstein E, McKendrick C, et al: Systemic embolism in mitral valve disease. Br Heart J 32:26, 1970.

142. Easton J, Sherman D: Management of cerebral embolism of cardiac origin. Stroke 11:433, 1980.

143. Hart R, Miller V: Cerebral infarction in young adults: A practical approach. Stroke 14:110, 1983.

144. Deveral P, Olley P, Smith D, et al: Incidence of systemic embolism before and after mitral valvotomy. Thorax 23:530, 1968.

145. Abernathy W, Willis P: Thromboembolic complications of rheumatic heart disease. Cardiovasc Clin 5:131, 1973.

146. Askey J, Berstein S: The management of rheumatic heart disease in relation to systemic arterial embolism. Prog Cardiovasc Dis 3:220, 1960.

147. Nielson B, Galea E, Hossack K: Thromboembolic complications of mitral valve disease. Aust N Z J Med 8:372, 1978.

148. Selzer A, Cohn K: Natural history of mitral stenosis: A review. Circulation 45:878, 1972.

149. Wood P: Diseases of the Heart and Circulation. Philadephia: JB Lippincott, 1956.

150. Jackson A, Boughner D, Barnett H, et al: Mitral valve prolapse and cerebral ischemic events in young patients. Neurology 34:784, 1984.

151. Nishimura R, McGoon M, Shub C, et al: Echocardiographically documented mitral valve prolapse: Long-term follow-up in 237 patients. N Engl J Med 313:1305, 1985.

152. Laupacis A, Albers G, Dunn M, et al: Antithrombotic therapy in atrial fibrillation. Chest 102(Suppl 4):426S, 1992.

153. Nolan J, Bloomfield P: Non-rheumatic atrial fibrillation: Warfarin or aspirin for all? Br Heart J 68:544, 1992.

154. Singer D: Randomized trials of warfarin for atrial fibrillation. N Engl J Med 327:1451, 1992.

155. The Stroke Prevention in Atrial Fibrillation Investigators: Predictors of thromboembolism in artial fibrillation: I. Clinical features of patients at risk. Ann Intern Med 116:1, 1992.

156. Petersen P, Godtfredsen J: Embolic complications in paroxysmal atrial fibrillation. Stroke 17:622, 1986.

157. Brand F, Abbott R, Kannel W, et al: Characteristics and prognosis of lone atrial fibrillation: 30-year follow-up in the Framingham Study. JAMA 254:3449, 1985.

158. Barnhorst D, Oxman H, Connolly D, et al: Long-term follow up of isolated replacement of the aortic or mitral valve with the Starr-Edwards prosthesis. Am J Cardiol 35:228, 1975.

159. Chesebro J, Fuster V, Elveback L, et al: Trial of combined warfarin plus dipyridamole or aspirin therapy in prosthetic heart valve replacement: Danger of aspirin compared with dipyridamole. Am J Cardiol 51:1537, 1983.

160. Cleland J, Molloy P: Thromboembolic complications of the cloth covered Starr-Edwards prostheses No. 2300 aortic and No. 6300 mitral. Thorax 28:41, 1973.

161. Friedli B, Aerichide H, Grondin P, et al: Thromboembolic complications of heart valve replacement. Am Heart J 81:702, 1971.

162. Gadboys H, Litwak R, Niemetz J, et al: Role of anticoagulants in preventing embolization from prosthetic heart valves. JAMA 202:134, 1967.

163. Fuster V, Pumphrey C, McGoon M, et al: Systemic thrombo-

embolism in mitral and aortic Starr-Edwards prostheses: A long-term follow-up (10–19 years). Circulation 66(Suppl I):I-157, 1982.

164. Murphy D, Levine F, Buckley M, et al: A comparative analysis of the Starr-Edwards and Bjork-Shiley prostheses. J Thorac Cardiovasc Surg 86:746, 1983.

165. Perier P, Bessou J, Swanson J, et al: Comparative evaluation of aortic valve replacement with Starr, Bjork, and porcine valve prostheses. Circulation 72(Suppl II):II-140, 1985.

166. Bjork V, Henze A: Ten years' experience with the Bjork-Shiley tilting disk valve. J Thorac Cardiovasc Surg 78:331, 1979.

167. Chesebro J, Fuster V: Valvular heart disease and prosthetic heart valves. In Fuster V, Verstarete M (eds): Thrombosis in Cardiovascular Disease. Philadelphia: WB Saunders, 1992.

168. Burchfiel C, Hammermeister K, Krause-Steinrauf H, et al: Left atrial dimension and risk of systemic embolism in patients with a prosthetic heart valve. J Am Coll Cardiol 15:32, 1990.

169. Dale J, Myhre E: Can acetylsalicylic acid alone prevent arterial thromboembolism? A pilot study in patients with aortic ball valve prosthesis. Acta Med Scand 645(Suppl):73, 1981.

170. Oyer P, Stinson E, Griepp R, et al: Valve replacement with the Starr-Edwards and Hancock prostheses. Ann Surg 186:301, 1977.

171. Saour J, Sieck J, Mamo L, et al: Trial of different intensities of anticoagulation in patients with prosthetic heart valves. N Engl J Med 322:428, 1990.

172. Altman R, Rouvier J, Gurfinkel E, et al: Comparison of two levels of anticoagulant therapy in patients with substitute heart valves. J Cardiovasc Surg 101:427, 1991.

173. Stein P, Alpert J, Copeland J, et al: Antithrombotic therapy in patients with mechanical and biological prosthetic heart valves. Chest 102(Suppl 4):445S, 1992.

174. Dale J, Myhre E, Storstein O, et al: Prevention of arterial thromboembolism with acetylsalicylic acid: A controlled clinical study in patients with aortic ball valves. Am Heart J 94:101, 1977.

175. Altman R, Boullon F, Rouvier J, et al: Aspirin and prophylaxis of thromboembolic complications in patients with substitute heart valves. J Thorac Cardiovasc Surg 72:127, 1976.

176. Turpie A, Gent M, Laupacis A, et al: A comparison of aspirin with placebo in patients treated with warfarin after heart-valve replacement. N Engl J Med 329:524, 1993.

177. Ribeiro P, Al Zaibag M, Idris M, et al: Antiplatelet drugs and the incidence of thromboembolic complications of the St. Jude medical aortic prosthesis in patients with rheumatic heart disease. J Thorac Cardiovasc Surg 91:92, 1986.

178. Nair C, Mohiuddin S, Hilleman D, et al: Ten-year results with the St. Jude medical prosthesis. Am J Cardiol 65:217, 1990.

179. Myers M, Lawrie G, Crawford E, et al: The St. Jude prosthesis: Analysis of the clinical results in 815 implants and the need for systemic anticoagulation. J Am Coll Cardiol 13:57, 1989.

180. Hartz R, LoCiero JI, Kucich V, et al: Comparative study of warfarin versus antiplatelet therapy in patients with a St. Jude medical valve in the aortic position. J Thorac Cardiovasc Surg 92:684, 1986.

181. Czer L, Matloff J, Chaux A, et al: The St. Jude valve: Analysis of thromboembolism, warfarin-related hemorrhage, and survival. Am Heart J 114:389, 1987.

182. Bjork V, Henze A: Management of thromboembolism after aortic valve replacement with the Bjork-Shiley tilting disc valve. Scand J Thorac Cardiovasc Surg 9:183, 1975.

183. Turpie A, Gunstensen J, Hirsh J, et al: Randomized comparison of two intensities of oral anticoagulant therapy after tissue heart valve replacement. Lancet 1:1242, 1988.

184. Turina J, Hess O, Turina M, et al: Cardiac bioprostheses in the 1990s. Circulation 88:775, 1993.

185. Ross R: The pathogenesis of atherosclerosis: A perspective for the 1990s. Nature 362:801, 1993.

186. Fuster V, Badimon L, Badimon J, Chesebro J: The pathogenesis of coronary artery disease and the acute coronary syndromes. N Engl J Med 326:242 1992.

187. Chesebro J, Webster M, Smith H, et al: Antiplatelet therapy in coronary disease progression: Reduced infarction and new lesion formation [abstract]. Circulation 80(Suppl II):II-266, 1989.

188. Ridker P, Manson J, Gaziano M, et al: Low-dose aspirin therapy for chronic stable angina: A randomized, placebo-controlled clinical trial. Ann Intern Med 114:835, 1991.

189. Antiplatelet Trialists' Collaboration: Secondary prevention of vascular disease by prolonged antiplatelet treatment. Br Med J 296:320, 1988.

190. Lewis H, Davis J, Archibald D, et al: Protective effects of aspirin against acute myocardial infarction and death in men with unstable angina. N Engl J Med 309:396, 1983.

191. Cairns J, Gent M, Singer J, et al: Aspirin, sulfinpyrazone, or both in unstable angina. N Engl J Med 313:1369, 1985.

192. Theroux P, Ouimet H, McCans J, et al: Aspirin, heparin, or both to treat acute unstable angina. N Engl J Med 319:1105, 1988.

193. Theroux P, Waters D, Qiu S, et al: Aspirin versus heparin to prevent myocardial infarction during the acute phase of unstable angina. Circulation 88:2045, 1993.

194. Balsano F, Rizzon P, Violi F, et al: Antiplatelet treatment with ticlopidine in unstable angina: A controlled, multicenter study. Circulation 82:17, 1990.

195. Telford A, Wilson C: Trial of heparin versus atenolol in prevention of myocardial infarction in intermediate coronary syndrome. Lancet 1:1225, 1981.

196. Williams D, Kirby M, McPherson K, et al: Anticoagulant treatment in unstable angina pectoris. Br J Clin Pract 40:114, 1986.

197. Neri Serneri G, Gensini G, Poggesi L, et al: Effect of heparin, aspirin, or alteplase in reduction of myocardial ischaemia in refractory unstable angina pectoris. Lancet 335:615, 1990.

198. Theroux P, Waters D, Lam J, et al: Reactivation of unstable angina after the discontinuation of heparin. N Engl J Med 327:141, 1992.

199. Lidon R, Theroux P, Juneau M, et al: Initial experience with a direct antithrombin, hirulog, in unstable angina. Circulation 88:1495, 1993.

200. Gold H, Torres F, Garabedian H, et al: Evidence for a rebound coagulation phenomenon after cessation of a 4-hour infusion of a specific thrombin inhibitor in patients with unstable angina pectoris. J Am Coll Cardiol 21:1039, 1993.

201. The TIMI IIIA Investigators: Early effects of tissue-type plasminogen activator added to conventional therapy on the culprit lesion in patients presenting with ischemic cardiac pain at rest: Results of the Thrombolysis in Myocardial Ischemia (TIMI IIIA) trial. Circulation 87:38, 1993.

202. ISIS-2 Collaborative Group: Randomised trial of intravenous streptokinase, oral aspirin, both, or neither among 17,187 cases of suspected acute myocardial infarction: ISIS-2. Lancet 2:349, 1988.

203. Yusuf S, Wittes J, Friedman L: Overview of results of randomized clinical trials in heart disease. I. Treatments following myocardial infarction. JAMA 260:2088, 1988.

204. Hebert P, Fuster V, Hennekens C: Antiplatelet and anticoagulant therapy in evolving and myocardial infarction and primary prevention. In Fuster V, Verstarete M (eds): Thrombosis in Cardiovascular Disorders. Philadelphia: WB Saunders, 1992.

205. Rasmanis G, Vesterqvist O, Green K, et al: Evidence of increased platelet activation after thrombolysis in patients with acute myocardial infarction. Br Heart J 68:374, 1992.

206. Prager N, Torr-Brown S, Sobel B, et al: Maintenance of patency after thrombolysis in stenotic coronary arteries requires combined inhibition of thrombin and platelets. J Am Coll Cardiol 22:296, 1993.

207. Ridker P, Hepert P, Fuster V: Are both asprin and heparin justified as adjuncts to thrombolytic therapy for acute myocardial infarction? Lancet 341:1574, 1993.

208. Fuster V: Coronary thrombolysis—a perspective for the practicing physician. N Engl J Med 329:723, 1993.

209. The GUSTO Investigators: An international randomized trial comparing four thrombolytic strategies for acute myocardial infarction. N Engl J Med 329:674, 1993.

210. The GUSTO Angiographic Investigators: The effects of tissue plasminogen activator, streptokinase, or both on coronary-artery patency, ventricular function, and survival after acute myocardial infarction. N Engl J Med 329:1615, 1993.

211. Gruppo Italiano per lo Studio lella Sopravvivenza nell'Infarto Miocardico: GISSI-2: A factorial randomised trial of alteplase versus streptokinase and heparin versus no heparin among 12,490 patients with acute myocardial infarction. Lancet 336:65, 1990.

212. ISIS-3 Collaborative Group: ISIS-3: A randomised comparison of streptokinase vs tissue plasminogen activator vs anistreplase and of aspirin plus heparin vs aspirin alone among 41,299 cases of suspected acute myocardial infarction. Lancet 339:753, 1992.

213. Heparin-Aspirin Reperfusion Trial (HART): A comparison between heparin and low-dose aspirin as adjunctive therapy with tissue-type plasminogen activator for acute myocardial infarction. N Engl J Med 323:1433, 1990.

214. de Bono P, Simoons M, Tijssen J, et al: Effect of early intravenous heparin on coronary patency, infarct size, and bleeding complications after alteplase thrombolysis: Results of a randomised double blind European Cooperative Study Group trial. Br Heart J 67:122, 1992.

215. Braunwald E: The open-artery theory alive and well again. N Engl J Med 93:329, 1993.

216. Buring J, Hennekens C: Antiplatelet therapy to prevent coronary artery bypass graft occlusion. Circulation 82:1046, 1990.

217. Chesebro J, Clements I, Fuster V, et al: A platelet inhibitor drug trial in coronary artery bypass operations: Benefit of perioperative dipyridamole and aspirin therapy on early postoperative vein graft patency. N Engl J Med 307:73, 1982.

218. Goldman S, Copeland J, Moritz T, et al: Improvement in early saphenous vein graft patency after coronary artery bypass surgery with antiplatelet therapy: Results of a Veterans Administration Cooperative Study. Circulation 77:1324, 1988.

219. Verstraete M, Brown B, Chesebro J, et al: Evaluation of antiplatelet agents in the prevention of aorto-coronary bypass occlusion. Eur Heart J 7:4, 1986.

220. Spencer F: The internal mammary artery: The ideal coronary bypass graft? N Engl J Med 314:50, 1986.

221. Chesebro J, Goldman S: Coronary artery bypass surgery: Antithrombotic therapy. In Fuster V, Verstarete M (eds): Thrombosis in Cardiovascular Disease. Philadelphia: WB Saunders, 1992.

222. Luscher T: Vascular biology of coronary bypass grafts. Coron Artery Dis 3:157, 1992.

223. Grundfest W, Litvack F, Sherman T, et al: Delineation of peripheral and coronary detail by intraoperative angioscopy. Ann Surg 202:394, 1985.

224. Henderson W, Goldman S, Copeland J, et al: Antiplatelet or anticoagulant therapy after coronary artery bypass surgery: A meta-analysis of clinical trials. Ann Intern Med 111:743, 1989.

225. van der Meer J, Hillege H, Kootstra G, et al: Prevention of one-year vein-graft occlusion after aortocoronary bypass surgery: A comparison of low-dose aspirin, low-dose aspirin plus dipyridamole, and oral anticoagulants. Lancet 342:257, 1993.

226. Anderson H: Restenosis after coronary angioplasty. Disease-a-Month 29:615, 1993.

227. Califf R, Willerson J: Percutaneous transluminal coronary angioplasty: Prevention of occlusion and restenosis. In Fuster V, Verstarete M (eds): Thrombosis in Cardiovascular Disorders. Philadelphia: WB Saunders, 1992, p 389.

228. Ip J, Fuster V, Israel D, et al: The role of platelets, thrombin and hyperplasia in restenosis after coronary angioplasty. J Am Coll Cardiol 17:77B, 1991.

229. Lam J, Chesebro J, Steele P, et al: Deep arterial injury during experimental angioplasty: Relations to a positive indium-111 platelet scintigram, quantitative platelet deposition and mural thrombosis. J Am Coll Cardiol 8:1380, 1986.

230. Steele P, Chesebro J, Stanson A, et al: Balloon angioplasty: Natural history of the pathophysiologic response to injury in a pig model. Circ Res 57:105, 1985.

231. Lam J, Chesebro J, Steele P, et al: Antithrombotic therapy for deep arterial injury by angioplasty: Efficacy of common platelet inhibition compared with thrombin inhibition in pigs. Circulation 84:814, 1991.

232. Ciabattoni G, Ujang S, Sritara P, et al: Aspirin, but not heparin, suppresses the transient increase in thromboxane biosynthesis associated with cardiac catheterization or coronary angioplasty. J Am Coll Cardiol 21:1377, 1993.

233. Holmes D, Vlietstra R, Mock M, et al: Angiographic changes produced by percutaneous coronary angioplasty. Am J Cardiol 51:676, 1983.
234. Holmes D, Schwartz R: Restenosis: The clinical problem. Coron Artery Dis 4:229, 1993.
235. Tschoepe D, Schultheiz H, Kolarov P, et al: Platelet membrane activation markers are predictive for increased risk of acute ischemic events after PTCA. Circulation 88:37, 1993.
236. Franklin S, Faxon D: Pharmacologic prevention of restenosis after coronary angioplasty: A review of the randomized clinical trials. Coronary Artery Dis 4:232, 1993.
237. Schwartz L, Bourassa M, Lesperance J, et al: Aspirin and dipyridamole in the prevention of restenosis after percutaneous transluminal coronary angioplasty. N Engl J Med 318:1714, 1988.
238. White C, Knudson M, Schmidt D, et al: Neither ticlopidine nor aspirin-dipyridamole prevents restenosis post PTCA: Results from a randomized placebo-controlled multicenter trial [abstract]. Circulation 76(Suppl 4):213, 1987.
239. Lembo N, Black A, Roubin G, et al: Effect of pretreatment with aspirin versus aspirin plus dipyridamole on frequency

and type of acute complications of percutaneous transluminal coronary angioplasty. Am J Cardiol 65:422, 1990.
240. Ellis S, Tcheng J, Navetta F, et al: Safety and antiplatelet effect of murine monoclonal antibody 7E3 Fab directed against platelet glycoprotein IIb/IIIa in patients undergoing elective coronary angioplasty. Coron Artery Dis 4:167, 1993.
241. Heras M, Chesebro J, Webster M, et al: Hirudin, heparin, and placebo during deep arterial injury in the pig: The in vivo role of thrombin in platelet-mediated thrombosis. Circulation 82:1476, 1990.
242. Califf R, Fortin D, Frid D, et al: Restenosis after coronary angioplasty: An overview. J Am Coll Cardiol 17:2B, 1991.
243. Ellis S, Roubin G, Wilentz J, et al: Effect of 18- to 24-hour heparin administration for prevention of restenosis after uncomplicated coronary angioplasty. Am Heart J 117:777, 1989.
244. Topol E, Bonan R, Jewitt D, et al: Use of a direct antithrombin, hirulog, in place of heparin during coronary angioplasty. Circulation 87:1622, 1993.
245. van den Bos A, Deckers J, Heyndrickx G, et al: Safety and efficacy of recombinant hirudin versus heparin in patients with stable angina undergoing coronary angioplasty. Circulation 88:2058, 1993.

CHAPTER 19

Acute Tachyarrhythmias

Robert C. Sheppard, M.D., and Eric L. Michelson, M.D.

Any departure from sinus rhythm imparts a hemodynamic disadvantage to cardiac function. Fortunately, in most instances, the supraventricular tachyarrhythmias induce only a minor hemodynamic burden and cardiac reserve is sufficient, so patients are only minimally compromised. However, certain cardiac arrhythmias, such as ventricular tachycardia or fibrillation and occasionally supraventricular tachycardias (SVTs), may cause profound hemodynamic deterioration, particularly if they induce vasovagal reflexes or occur in the presence of valvular or severe cardiac disease, and consequently demand immediate therapy. Most importantly, life-threatening tachyarrhythmias require prompt recognition and effective management. Drug treatment of acute tachyarrhythmias is detailed in this chapter. However, several new strategies in addition to traditional pharmacologic management and external countershock are now available. The following discussion deals with the principal tachyarrhythmias that may be hemodynamically significant or have life-threatening consequences. Their description and management are emphasized. Every attempt has been made to provide timely and accurate information. However, the reader is cautioned that the drug uses and dosages described may be outside indications approved by the United States Food and Drug Administration (FDA) and may reflect relatively limited clinical or investigative experience in some cases (see Table 19–1 for the dosages of drugs discussed in this chapter). Moreover, the availability and application of antiarrhythmic drugs and other interventions in the field are evolving so rapidly that it is anticipated that specific management strategies will need frequent updating.

SUPRAVENTRICULAR TACHYARRHYTHMIAS AND THE WOLFF-PARKINSON-WHITE SYNDROME
Clinical Features

Supraventricular tachycardias may produce hemodynamic compromise and symptoms varying from minimal to marked in severity, depending on the ventricular rate, its regularity, the relative timing (or absence) of effective atrial systole with respect to ventricular systole, the hemodynamic status of the patient before the onset of the SVT, and the extent and nature of any underlying cardiac dysfunction. Several of the more common SVTs are listed in Table 19–2, and their distinguishing features are outlined in Table 19–3. Generally, the approach to acute therapy is similar for all supraventricular mechanisms, except for a few notable exceptions that are discussed specifically. The objectives of therapy are, first, to control the ventricular rate and, second, to restore and maintain sinus rhythm. In some instances, these goals are sought simultaneously; in other cases, they are sought sequentially.

Electrocardiographic Features

Initially, SVTs must be differentiated from sinus tachycardia and ventricular tachycardia. During sinus rhythm, impulses arising in the sinus node are propagated successfully to the atria via the right atrium, to the atrioventricular (AV) node, and subsequently to the ventricles via the His–bundle branch–Purkinje

Table 19–1. **Antiarrhythmic Drugs**

Drug*		Usual Dosage†	Major Adverse Effects‡
Class IA			
Disopyramide	Oral:	200–800 mg/day in 2 or 3 divided doses (depending on preparation)	CHF, anticholinergic (dry mouth, urinary retention)
Procainamide	Oral:	750–6000 mg/day in 3 or 4 divided doses (sustained release) or 4–6 divided doses (conventional)	GI (nausea), fever, lupus-like syndrome, CNS, agranulocytosis, hypotension (IV)
	IV:	5–15 mg/kg loading over 20–60 min. 2–6 mg/min maintenance	
Quinidine	Oral:	600–1600 mg/day in 2–4 divided doses (depending on preparation)	GI (diarrhea), thrombocytopenia, cinchonism, fever, hepatic, rash, proarrhythmia, drug interactions (e.g., digoxin)
Class IB			
Lidocaine	IV:	1–3 mg/kg loading in divided doses over 20 min, 1–4 mg/min maintenance	CNS (including seizures, psychosis), GI, drug interactions (e.g., propranolol, tocainide)
Mexiletine	Oral:	450–600 mg/day in 3 or 4 divided doses (with food)	GI, CNS, blurred vision, hepatic, blood dyscrasias
Phenytoin§	Oral:	14 mg/kg loading, then 200–400 mg/day in 1 or 2 divided doses	CNS, blood dyscrasias, drug interactions, hypotension (IV), fever, rash, hepatitis
	IV:	50–100 mg every 5 min to maximum 1000 mg loading, 200–400 mg/day maintenance	
Tocainide	Oral:	800–1800 mg/day in 2–4 divided doses	GI, CNS, CHF, agranulocytosis, rash, fever, interstitial pneumonitis
Class IC			
Flecainide	Oral:	100–400 mg/day in 2 divided doses	Blurred vision, CNS, GI, CHF, proarrhythmia, hypotension (IV)
Propafenone	Oral:	450–900 mg/day in 3 divided doses	GI, CS, CHF, proarrhythmia, skin rash
Moricizine	Oral:	600–900 mg/day in 3 divided doses	CNS, nausea, headache, CHF, proarrhythmia
Class II			
Acebutolol	Oral:	400–1200 mg/day in 2 divided doses	CHF, bradycardia, fatigue, hypotension, bronchospasm, lupus-like syndrome, CNS
Esmolol	IV:	10–50 mg (maximum 500 µg/kg) over 1 min loading, 1–20 mg (25–200 µg/kg)/min maintenance after titration in 1–5 mg (25–50 µg/kg)/min steps	Hypotension, CHF, bradycardia, GI, CNS, bronchospasm
Propranolol	Oral:	40–240 mg/day in 3 or 4 divided doses	CHF, bradycardia, hypotension, fatigue, bronchospasm, CNS
	IV:	0.5–1.0 mg every 5 min to maximum of 0.2 mg/kg loading	
Metoprolol§	Oral:	50–450 mg/day in divided doses	CHF, bradycardia, hypotension, CNS
	IV:	5 mg every 5 min to a maximum of 15 mg loading	
Class III			
Amiodarone	Oral:	800–1600 mg/day in divided doses for 5–14 days, then 200–800 mg/day for 5–14 days, then 100–400 mg/day thereafter	CNS, GI, thyroid, asymptomatic corneal microdeposits, skin, pulmonary fibrosis, hepatic, drug interactions (e.g., warfarin, digoxin, procainamide, quinidine, flecainide, phenytoin), hypotension, asystole (IV)
	IV:	5–10 mg/kg/20 min for 2 hr, followed by 600 mg over next 24 hr	
Bretylium	IV:	5–10 mg/kg loading, 5–10 mg/kg every 6 hr or 0.5–4.0 mg/min continuous infusion for maintenance	GI, orthostatic hypotension
Sotalol	Oral:	160–320 mg/day in 2 divided doses (must be adjusted for renal function)	CHF, proarrhythmia, bradycardia, hypotension, fatigue, bronchospasm, CNS
Class IV			
Verapamil	Oral:	160–180 mg/day in divided doses	Hypotension, CHF, bradycardia, GI (constipation)
	IV:	3–10 mg bolus over 2 or 3 min, repeated in 30 min, if necessary; 0.125 mg/min maintenance infusion	
Diltiazem	Oral:	120–300 mg in divided doses	Hypotension, CHF, bradycardia, tinnitus, GI (anorexia, constipation)
	IV:	20–25 mg bolus followed by 10–15 mg/hr maintenance infusion	
Other			
Digoxin	Oral:	0.125–0.375 mg/day in a single dose	GI, CNS, visual drug interactions, proarrhythmia
	IV:	0.25–0.5 mg initially and 0.1–0.3 mg every 4–8 hr to a total 0.5–1.0 mg loading over 24 hr	

CHF, congestive heart failure; CNS, central nervous system; GI, gastrointestinal.

*Only drugs approved by the FDA as antiarrhythmic agents are included.

†Dosages require careful, monitored individual titration and consideration of cardiac, hepatic, and renal function, possible drug interactions, and body size.

‡All antiarrhythmic drugs have the "proarrhythmic" potential to aggravate or provoke arrhythmias, and all have the potential to depress contractility and aggravate or provoke heart failure; these are listed as specific adverse effects for those drugs in which this potential has been considered exceptionally high in some patient populations. In addition, most drugs have the propensity to aggravate sinus node dysfunction and to aggravate conduction abnormalities, potentially resulting in profound bradycardia or heart block. Effects apply to both oral and intravenous forms of drug unless specifically indicated.

§Not approved as an antiarrhythmic agent but is often used in this capacity.

Table 19–2. **Supraventricular, WPW, and Atrioventricular Junctional Tachycardias**

Sinus nodal (sinoatrial) reentrant tachycardia
Intraatrial and interatrial reentrant tachycardias
Atrial fibrillation
Atrial flutter
  Typical
  Atypical
Ectopic ("automatic") atrial tachycardias
  Atrial tachycardia with or without AV nodal block
  Multifocal atrial tachycardia (chaotic atrial tachycardia)
Junctional tachycardias (nonparoxysmal junctional tachycardia)
AV nodal reentrant tachycardias
  Slow-fast form
  Fast-slow form
AV reentrant tachycardia
  WPW syndrome reciprocating tachycardia
  Concealed bypass tract reciprocating tachycardia

AV, atrioventricular; WPW, Wolff-Parkinson-White.

system. Rates of 130 to 160 beats/min create the most difficult differential diagnosis between sinus tachycardia and SVT. Rapid sinus rates are usually caused by increased activity of the cardiac sympathetic nerves and withdrawal of vagal inhibitory influences. The maximum sinus heart rate achieved during strenuous exercise varies with age and is often estimated at 220 beats/min minus the age in years. In healthy young persons, the maximum heart rate may reach more than 200 beats/min, whereas in elderly individuals, the maximum sinus heart rate rarely exceeds 150 to 160 beats/min. The sinus etiology of the tachycardia is usually recognized by a normal P-wave inscription. P waves are usually upright in leads II and aV_F, and they usually have relatively uniform, smooth contours (unless atrial hypertrophy, dilation, or an atrial conduction abnormality is also present). Furthermore, even in the presence of extreme sinus tachycardia, the rate may vary over a considerable range, whereas in paroxysmal SVTs, the rates may be rapid but are regular, usually oscillating over a range of no more than a few beats per minute.

Comparison with a previous electrocardiogram

(ECG) may be most helpful in discerning diagnostic changes in P-wave morphology in the differential diagnosis of SVT. The response to vagal maneuvers and drugs also may be diagnostic. An intravenous bolus administration of the purine nucleoside adenosine, which has a half-life of less than 10 seconds and produces transient complete AV block, can often differentiate atrial and AV nodal from ventricular tachyarrhythmias.[1] An additional important determination is whether AV dissociation is present, an indication of ventricular tachycardia, although AV nodal reentry tachycardia rarely may present with this as well (Fig. 19–1). Fusion and capture beats are virtually pathognomonic for ventricular tachycardia (Fig. 19–2). Various morphologic features have been identified that can be helpful in distinguishing ventricular tachycardia from SVT with aberrancy or bundle branch block and are described in the section on ventricular tachycardia.

PAROXYSMAL SUPRAVENTRICULAR TACHYCARDIA

Paroxysmal SVTs are a relatively common group of clinical arrhythmias that occur in otherwise normal, healthy individuals as well as in those with intrinsic cardiac disease. The attacks are usually sudden in onset and cessation. The presence or absence of a stable blood pressure does not differentiate supraventricular from ventricular tachycardia. Most cases have reentrant mechanisms initiated by fortuitously timed premature beats. In comparison, the most common types of ectopic or automatic SVTs occur more erratically, often with an initial period of gradual acceleration of the rate and a subsequent slowing of the rate at the termination of the tachycardia, with occasional dropped beats caused by variable conduction block

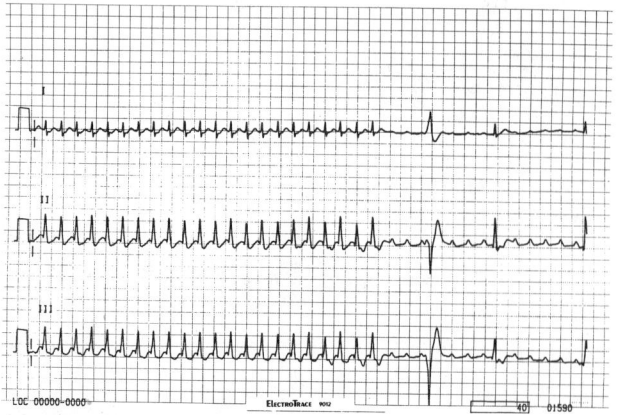

Figure 19–1. Effects of 12 mg adenosine administered by an intravenous bolus. After a few seconds, complete AV block occurs revealing an underlying atrial tachycardia as the cause of the SVT. Leads I, II, and III were recorded simultaneously.

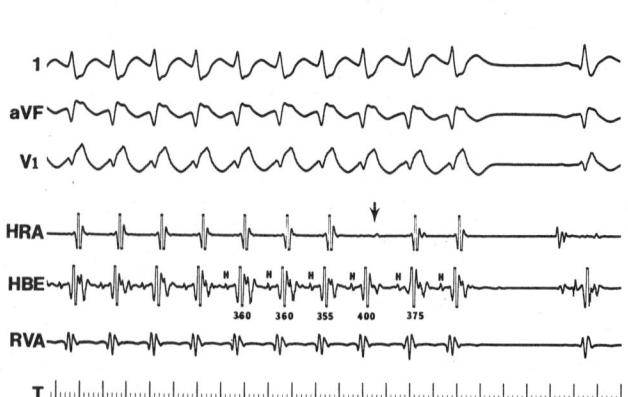

Figure 19–2. Three surface (I, aVF, and V1) and three intracardiac (high right atrium [HRA], His bundle [HBE], and right ventricular apex [RVA]) electrograms showing typical AV nodal reentry tachycardia. The arrow indicates the presence of AV dissociation with continuation of the arrhythmia (highly unusual). In addition, there are slight variations in the beat rate (numbers indicate the milliseconds of the R-R intervals).

Table 19–3. **Differential Diagnosis of Supraventricular, WPW, and Atrioventricular Junctional Tachycardias**

Sinus Nodal Reentrant Supraventricular Tachycardia
Initiation and termination by APBs independent of interatrial conduction delay or AV conduction delay
P wave identical to sinus rhythm in morphologic appearance and activation sequence
PR interval related to supraventricular tachycardia rate
AV nodal block may exist without affecting supraventricular tachycardia
Vagal maneuvers slow and then abruptly terminate supraventricular tachycardia
Atrial rate, 110–140 beats/min

Intraatrial and Interatrial Reentrant Supraventricular Tachycardia
Initiation by APBs
P wave and atrial activation sequence differ from sinus rhythm
PR interval related to supraventricular tachycardia rate
AV nodal block may exist without affecting supraventricular tachycardia
Reentry within Bachmann's bundle can be demonstrated in some instances
Vagal maneuvers may not terminate supraventricular tachycardia but may produce AV nodal block
Atrial rate, 120–240 beats/min

Ectopic Atrial Tachycardia
Cannot initiate or terminate with APBs and is independent of interatrial conduction delay or AV nodal delay
Supraventricular tachycardia "warms up"—subtle P-wave and rate alterations
P wave differs from sinus rhythm
PR interval varies with supraventricular rate
AV nodal block may exist without affecting supraventricular rate
P-wave morphologic appearance may vary with chaotic types
Vagal maneuvers do not terminate but produce AV nodal block
Atrial rate, 100–220 beats/min

AV Nodal Reentrant Supraventricular Tachycardia
Initiation and termination by APBs or VPBs, or rapid atrial pacing producing AV nodal Wenckebach cycles (in the electrophysiology laboratory)
Initiation dependent on critical increase of AH interval with shift from fast to slow pathway conduction (slow-fast type)
Retrograde P wave (negative in inferior leads) usually buried in QRS complex (slow-fast type) or immediately after QRS complex (slow-fast type), or just before QRS complex with short PR and long RP intervals (fast-slow type)
Vagal maneuvers slow or abruptly terminate supraventricular tachycardia
Rate, 140–160 beats/min

AV Junctional Tachycardia
Nonparoxysmal
Usually narrow QRS complex
P waves independent of QRS complex or retrograde with short PR or short RP intervals and negative in inferior leads
Vagal maneuvers do not terminate
Usually caused by low potassium levels, digoxin excess, or acute myocardial process
Rate, 70–130 beats/min

Atrial Flutter
Sawtoothed baseline—rates; 240–360 beats/min
Narrow QRS complex unless aberrancy or bundle branch block
AV conduction ratio usually 2:1; however, 4:1, 3:2, or other ratios are observed
Vagal maneuvers increase conduction ratio, do not terminate
Occasionally alternating cycle length of QRS complex implies concealed conduction of atrial depolarizations

Atrial Fibrillation
Varying lengths of R-R intervals
Absence of P waves; irregular; chaotic atrial activity
Vagal maneuvers slow ventricular rate, do not terminate
QRS complex usually narrow unless aberrancy or bundle branch block. Aberrancy occurs in beats terminating short cycle lengths after longer cycle lengths

Atrioventricular Reciprocating Tachycardia (Concealed Bypass Tract or WPW Syndrome)
Initiation and termination by APBs or VPBs, dependent on critical AV delay but independent of AV nodal delay
Retrograde P wave with short RP interval; P wave negative in leads reflecting atrial insertion site of bypass tract (retrograde atrial activation eccentric to the AV node)
Atrium and ventricle required to initiate and sustain reciprocating tachycardia
Ability to preexcite atrium with VPB during reciprocating tachycardia at a time when the bundle of His is refractory (in the electrophysiology laboratory)
Vagal maneuvers may slow or abruptly terminate (less sensitive than AV nodal reentrant supraventricular tachycardia)
Rate, 150–220 beats/min

AH, atrio-bundle of His; AV, atrioventricular; APBs, atrial premature beats; VPBs, ventricular premature beats; WPW, Wolff-Parkinson-White.
Note: In most cases, the initial response to intravenous adenosine parallels the response to vagal maneuvers detailed above.

or exit block out of the ectopic focus. The rate of paroxysmal reentrant SVT is usually rapid and regular at 120 to 220 beats/min. The QRS complexes are typically narrow and are usually less than 100 msec in duration, unless rate-related aberrancy develops or a bundle branch block pattern was also present during sinus rhythm. The P waves, if visible on the ECG, usually remain fixed in relationship to each QRS complex. However, the P waves may vary in their linkage to the QRS complex, depending on several important electrophysiologic mechanisms that are described briefly in a later section. The morphology of the P waves is usually clearly different from sinus rhythm, unless the mechanism is sinus nodal reentrant tachycardia, and may occur before, simultaneously with, or after the QRS complex. Vagal maneuvers may terminate the tachycardia but are not always successful.

ATRIOVENTRICULAR NODAL REENTRANT TACHYCARDIA
Slow-Fast Form

Atrioventricular nodal reentrant tachycardias are the most common form of paroxysmal SVT. Most AV nodal reentrant tachycardias are characterized by the "slow-fast" variety described here. The functional substrate for this reentrant arrhythmia is the presence of two, or dual, pathways in the AV nodal region. One pathway (dominant during sinus rhythm and thereby resulting in a normal PR interval) is able to conduct rapidly but is limited by a relatively long refractory period, which renders it more susceptible to conduction block if an atrial premature beat occurs. The other pathway is only able to conduct slowly but has a shorter refractory period. The mechanism for this arrhythmia includes sufficient delay of antegrade conduction in the slow pathway after an atrial premature beat, while unidirectional antegrade block occurs in the fast pathway. Critical delay in the slow pathway allows for recovery in the previously blocked fast pathway, resulting in reentry via retrograde engagement of the fast pathway. Initiation of the reentry mechanism can be accomplished either with rapid atrial pacing or by the extrastimulus method in the electrophysiology laboratory (Fig. 19–3). Using either method, SVT is initiated in susceptible patients by producing unidirectional block in the fast pathway

and setting up a reentrant mechanism. In this form of AV nodal reentrant tachycardia, the P waves usually are not visible in the presence of the tachycardia. Most often, the P waves are inscribed simultaneously with the QRS complex. Less commonly, the P waves may occur immediately after the QRS complex (short RP interval) and, rarely, may immediately precede the QRS complex (short PR interval); in each of these cases, the P waves are inverted in the inferior leads. The relationship of the P waves and the QRS complex is determined by the conduction time of the retrograde fast pathway versus the antegrade slow path-

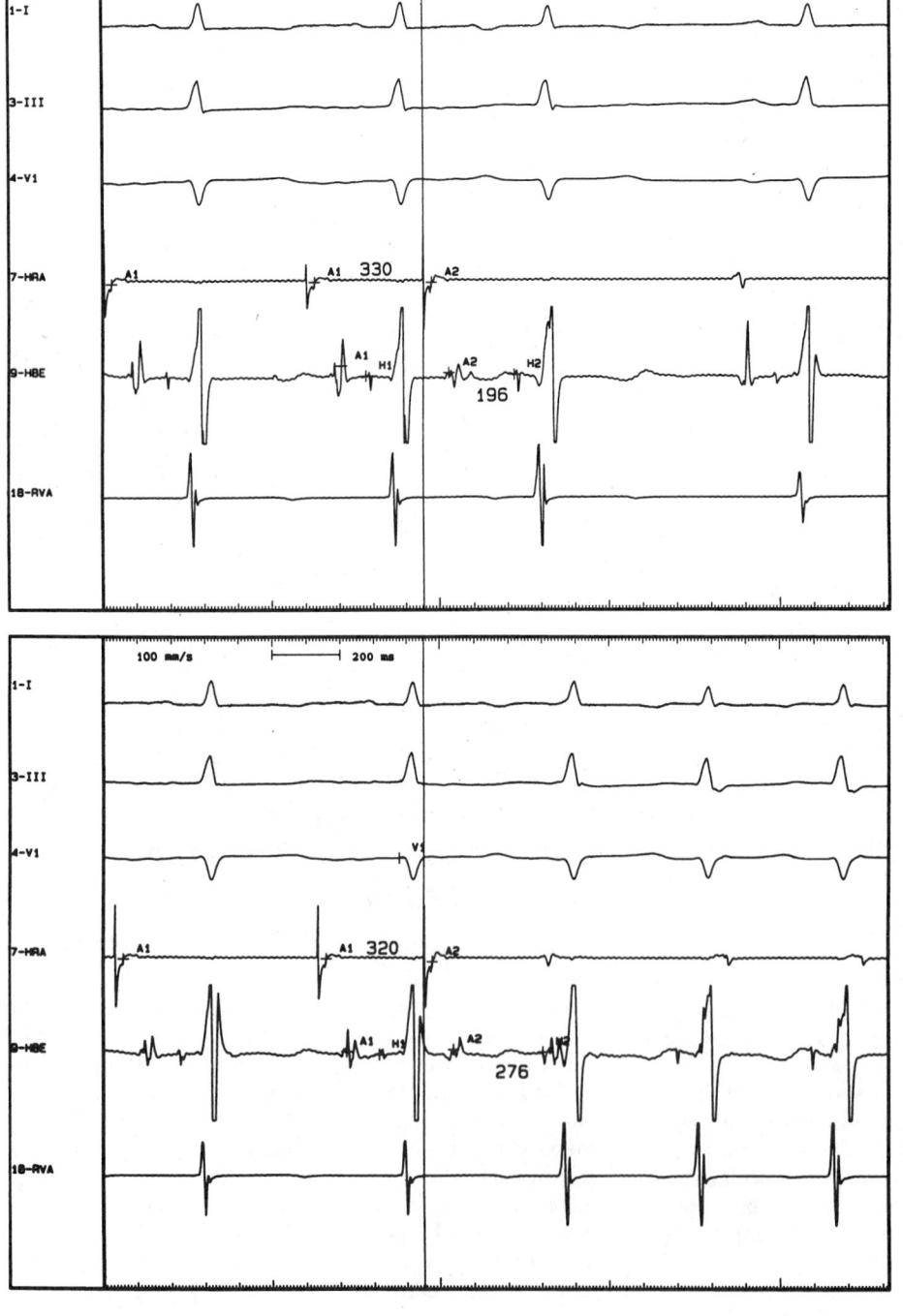

Figure 19–3. Three surface (I, III, and Vl) and three intracardiac (HRA, HBE, and RVA) electrograms showing initiation of typical AV nodal reentry tachycardia by a single atrial extrastimulus (Al–A2) producing a "jump" in AV nodal conduction onto the "slow" AV nodal pathway indicated by a marked increase in the A2-H2 interval measured on the His bundle electrogram.

way from the site of AV nodal reentry to the atria and ventricles, respectively. Retrograde dual AV nodal pathways have been demonstrated as well. Thus, in a susceptible individual, paroxysmal AV nodal reentrant SVT may be initiated by a properly timed atrial or ventricular premature beat. At times, it is difficult to distinguish this variety of SVT from those engaging a concealed retrogradely conducting bypass tract (i.e., AV reciprocating tachycardia). In AV nodal SVT, rates are typically 140 to 180 beats/min, and P waves, if discernible, are inverted in leads II, III, and aV$_F$. In AV reciprocating tachycardia, rates are often 160 to 200 beats/min, and P waves always occur after the QRS complex and are inverted in those leads closest to the atrial insertion site of the bypass tract (e.g., leads I and aV$_L$ if left-sided, aV$_R$ if right-sided). Electrophysiologic studies can identify antegrade conduction using the normal AV conduction pathway in both instances, but retrograde conduction is via the AV node in cases of AV nodal reentry and via an AV bypass tract in cases of AV reciprocating tachycardia.

In patients with refractory, recurrent SVTs, or in those patients intolerant of tachycardic episodes, electrophysiologic testing may be helpful in defining the mechanism of the arrhythmia, localizing the anatomic substrate, and suggesting therapeutic options including drugs, catheter ablative procedures, or an antitachycardia device. Recently, anatomic confirmation of dual AV nodal pathways has been described. Investigators have recorded slow and fast pathway potentials that can define appropriate sites for catheter or surgical ablation.[2, 3] Some experimental data, as well as surgical findings, indicate that these circuits involve the compact AV node as the antegrade limb and perinodal atrial tissue as the retrograde limb. Typically, the slow pathway has a more posterior and inferior position in the triangle of Koch and is closer in proximity to the os of the coronary sinus. The fast pathway often is located more anterior in the triangle in closer proximity to the attachment of the septal leaflet of the tricuspid valve.[4] The presence or absence of dual pathways or a so-called discontinuous conduction curve demonstrated at electrophysiologic testing may not always be diagnostic with regard to the apparent mechanism (AV nodal versus AV reciprocating tachycardia) or anatomic location of the arrhythmia circuit.[5, 6]

Treatment

Acutely, AV nodal reentrant SVT can often be terminated by vagal maneuvers as a first step and, if necessary, by a variety of drugs, rapid atrial pacing, or cardioversion with low energy settings (usually no more than 50 J is necessary). Even "chest thump" has been used anecdotally. Intravenous adenosine is now the single drug of choice acutely owing to its short half-life, with verapamil, β-blockers, and digoxin as second, third, and fourth choices, depending on the individual patient and circumstances. In addition, other conventional antiarrhythmic drugs such as the

class IA and IC drugs may also be used effectively, but of these, only procainamide is available for intravenous use. Pacing (using atrial bursts or the introduction of atrial and/or ventricular extrastimuli) with either temporary electrode catheters or an implanted pacemaker unit can also be used to terminate AV nodal reentrant SVT. Atrial burst pacing, however, often causes transient atrial fibrillation before restoration of sinus rhythm, so it is prudent to administer an AV nodal blocking drug first. Chronic therapy for the SVTs is discussed later. As with all tachyarrhythmias causing hemodynamic compromise, direct current cardioversion is a treatment of choice for acute management of paroxysmal SVT in a patient with hypotension.

Fast-Slow Form

In a few instances, the reentrant circuit may be reversed. Under these circumstances, antegrade conduction during a paroxysmal SVT occurs via a fast pathway and retrograde conduction via a slow pathway. The P waves (inverted in the inferior leads) are usually seen preceding QRS complex (long RP and short PR intervals). Electrophysiologic studies are often required to confirm this variety of SVT, because it can be confused with the more common cause of "long RP" tachycardia-orthodromic SVT involving an accessory AV pathway. Management is usually similar to the more common slow-fast variety. In this atypical form of paroxysmal SVT, the slow pathway has a relatively long antegrade refractory period and the fast pathway, a relatively short refractory period.

Treatment

The fast-slow form of paroxysmal AV nodal reentrant SVT tends to be sensitive to vagal maneuvers, and usually drugs are not required acutely. If necessary, the same drugs and interventions detailed earlier for the typical "slow-fast" form of SVT can be used.

WOLFF-PARKINSON-WHITE (PREEXCITATION) SYNDROME AND ATRIOVENTRICULAR RECIPROCATING TACHYCARDIAS

The Wolff-Parkinson-White (WPW) syndrome is a symptom complex that includes the ECG findings of an abnormally short PR interval in the presence of sinus rhythm and a wide QRS complex showing a characteristic initial slurring or delta wave, representing ventricular preexcitation. Afflicted individuals have a tendency to develop paroxysmal AV reciprocating tachycardias that can occur in healthy as well as diseased hearts.[7] A mechanism of sudden death associated with this syndrome has been identified as the presence of a short refractory period within the bypass fibers between the atrium and the ventricle in conjunction with paroxysms of atrial fibrillation (Fig. 19–4). Drugs such as digoxin and verapamil may

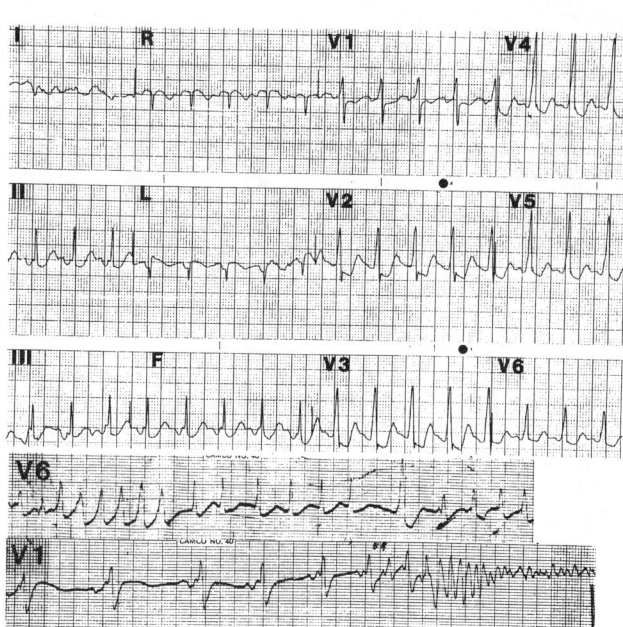

Figure 19–4. Twelve-lead ECG. *Upper portion,* WPW configuration is shown. Lead V6 shows atrial fibrillation on one occasion, and VI shows deterioration into ventricular fibrillation after several premature atrial systoles and the development of atrial fibrillation with wide QRS complexes.

enhance conduction through the bypass tract indirectly because concealed retrograde conduction via the AV node is limited by these agents; in addition, digoxin may directly shorten the refractory period of bypass tract tissue, and verapamil may elicit reflex sympathetic effects, thereby shortening refractoriness.

A typical WPW pattern is produced when an accessory pathway is located eccentric to the normal AV conduction system. If an atrial impulse is transmitted through the accessory pathway, early activation of an eccentric region of the ventricle produces a delta wave. The remaining ventricular muscle, however, is depolarized by competing excitation waves spreading through the normal His-Purkinje conduction system after incurring the usual physiologic delay within the AV node. Hence, the characteristic ventricular complex in WPW represents a fusion beat in which the relative intraatrial, interatrial, AV nodal, infranodal, and bypass tract conduction times determine in each instance the relative contribution of the normal and accessory pathways to the QRS. The ECG characteristics of WPW include (1) PR interval less than 0.12 second during sinus rhythm; (2) delta wave inscribed at the initial portion of the QRS complex, with QRS complex widening, often to more than 0.12 second; (3) secondary ST-T wave changes; (4) masking or mimicking of bundle branch or infarct patterns; and (5) susceptibility to paroxysmal arrhythmias.[7]

In the most common form of WPW tachycardia, antegrade conduction is exclusively via the normal AV nodal and infranodal pathways, and retrograde conduction from the ventricle to atrium occurs over the bypass tract completing the circuit. The AV node serves as one link in this AV reentrant tachycardia, and the QRS complex of the tachycardia is usually narrow (unless aberration or bundle branch block is present) if antegrade conduction is via the AV junction and the bundle of His. Conversely, if retrograde conduction is via the bundle of His and AV node and antegrade conduction is via the anomalous pathway, a wide QRS tachycardia is observed.

Reentrant tachycardias associated with a "concealed" bypass tract have also been described. In these cases, an accessory pathway directly connects the atrium and ventricle but conducts only in a retrograde fashion. Consequently, evidence of a delta wave (indicating ventricular preexcitation via an accessory AV connection that is bypassing the AV node), associated with the WPW syndrome, is not observed. Typically, the tachycardia rate is 150 to 220 beats/min, and the rhythm is regular, starting abruptly after a premature beat and terminating suddenly. Because these tachycardias incorporate infranodal tissue, including the ventricle, as a requisite part of the reentrant circuit, it may be more correct to refer to these rhythms as AV "reciprocating" tachycardias rather than SVTs. These arrhythmias can be initiated by either an atrial premature beat or a ventricular premature beat. For example, a properly timed ventricular premature beat may be conducted retrograde via the accessory pathway but block in a retrograde fashion in the AV node. The impulse then returns to the ventricle via the atrium through the normal antegrade AV conduction pathway (orthodromically), resulting in a narrow QRS complex. Because retrograde atrial activation proceeds from the atrial insertion site of the bypass tract to the remainder of both atria, identification of the earliest site of retrograde atrial activation can often localize the site of the bypass tract. In patients with free-wall AV bypass tracts conducting in a retrograde manner, the atria are activated eccentrically during the tachycardia and also during ventricular pacing in the electrophysiology laboratory. However, in patients with septal bypass tracts conducting retrogradely, the pattern of retrograde atrial activation may appear normal, and these rhythms may resemble those SVTs in which the reentrant circuit is confined to the AV node (Fig. 19–5).

Management of Wolff-Parkinson-White Tachycardias

Atrioventricular reciprocating tachycardias tend to have more rapid rates and are less sensitive to vagal maneuvers than AV nodal reentry SVTs. However, they often respond to intravenous adenosine or verapamil by blocking antegrade AV nodal conduction. Intravenous procainamide can be useful because of its effects on other parts of the circuit, particularly the bypass tract conduction and its atrial connection. Synchronized electrical cardioversion at low settings should be used whenever severe symptoms are present, such as chest pain or hypotension. Acutely, rapid atrial pacing can also be used but may result in a brief period of atrial fibrillation before sinus rhythm resumes. Therefore, this method should only be used for AV reciprocating tachycardias involving a concealed bypass tract (i.e., not capable of antegrade AV conduction). Importantly, the administration of either intravenous verapamil or digoxin by potentially enhancing bypass tract conduction is also contraindicated in those cases in which an AV bypass tract capable of rapid antegrade conduction is present, unless electrical countershock capability is readily available. Adenosine, although often effective in terminating AV reciprocating tachycardia, should also be used with caution in patients with the WPW syndrome because of the rebound catecholamine surge it produces after inducing complete AV nodal block, which could lead to atrial fibrillation and produce intolerably rapid, irregular ventricular rates or ventricular fibrillation resulting in sudden death (see Fig. 19–4).[8, 9]

Individuals with the WPW syndrome may respond to intravenous procainamide or to a β-blocking agent such as propranolol. The subsequent use of class IA (procainamide, quinidine, or disopyramide) or class IC (flecainide or propafenone) antiarrhythmic medications or amiodarone also may be effective. In patients with the most rapid AV conduction during atrial fibrillation or flutter (e.g., shortest RR intervals less than 240 msec), drugs often are not effective in slowing anomalous conduction, and more definitive therapy such as catheter ablation is warranted.

For subsequent management, class IA and IC drugs have been used along with drugs affecting the AV node for recurrent cases. However, the current treatment of choice for long-term management of AV reciprocating SVTs is radiofrequency catheter ablation of the accessory AV pathway. Centers have reported greater than 95% success in eliminating accessory pathway conduction with this technique with less than 1% morbidity and 0.1% mortality risk.[10] The majority of morbidity reported with early attempts at radiofrequency catheter ablation was without the use of newer steerable and deflectable tip catheters. In cases in which the bypass tract is remote from the AV node, the likelihood of needing permanent pacing after the ablation procedure is virtually nonexistent.

Electrophysiologic studies are recommended for patients with symptoms and persistent delta waves for whom the risk of rapid conduction during atrial fibrillation can be evaluated. Asymptomatic patients with ventricular preexcitation on the ECG and a benign family history should simply be watched for symptoms and/or possibly undergo an exercise stress test to assess the rapidity of antegrade AV conduction. Some individuals, by virtue of vocation or avocation may require more aggressive evaluation.

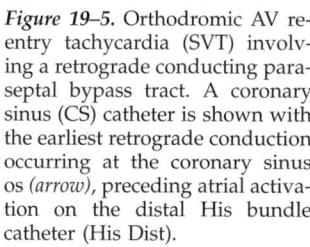

Figure 19–5. Orthodromic AV reentry tachycardia (SVT) involving a retrograde conducting paraseptal bypass tract. A coronary sinus (CS) catheter is shown with the earliest retrograde conduction occurring at the coronary sinus os *(arrow)*, preceding atrial activation on the distal His bundle catheter (His Dist).

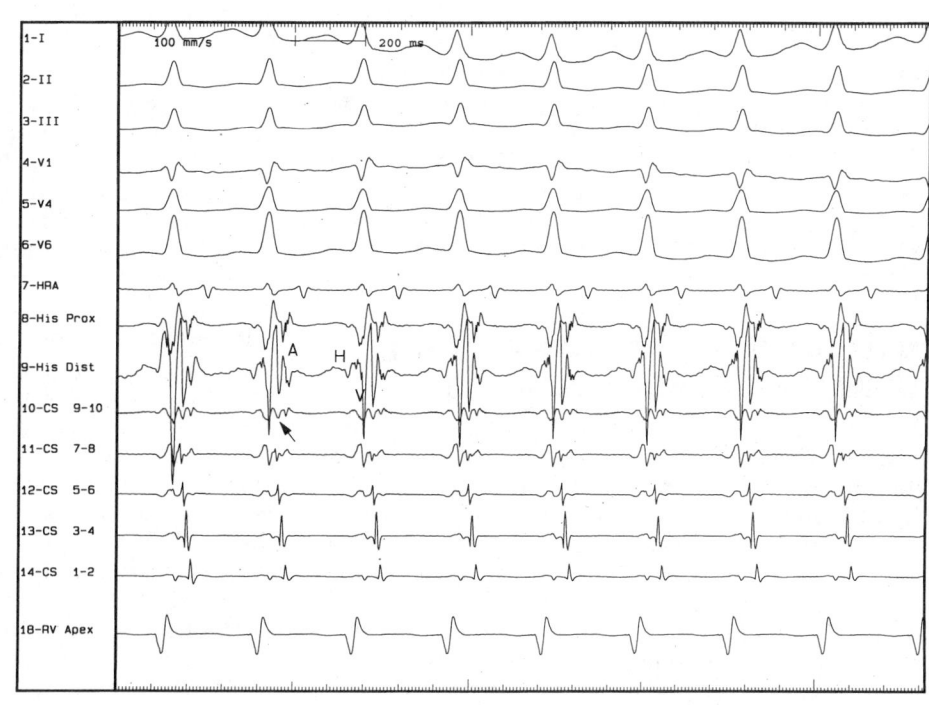

SINUS NODAL REENTRANT TACHYCARDIA

Patterns of conduction and reentry in the sinus node region have been studied extensively by many investigators, predominantly in experimental preparations,[11–13] and this mechanism may account for some of the SVTs observed in humans. The P waves are usually upright in the limb leads and indistinguishable in contour from the P waves during sinus rhythm. Clinically, the paroxysms usually show evidence of both sudden onset and sudden termination. Rates typically are in the range of 110 to 140 beats/min, but it is relatively uncommon to see sustained episodes. The rhythm may be mistaken for noncompensatory sinus tachycardia; however, it usually occurs in older patients with other manifestations of the sick sinus syndrome or, alternatively, in otherwise healthy young people. Recognition of the abrupt onset and offset, with sudden slowing of the rate, is most helpful in diagnosis. Because of its relatively slow rate, sinus nodal reentry is rarely associated with serious hemodynamic compromise.

Experimental studies by Allessie and Bonke[11] have convincingly demonstrated a point-to-point course of activation during virtually the whole interval between successive atrial beats in sinus node preparations, indicating a reentrant mechanism. Furthermore, other studies[12] suggest that conduction velocity in the anterior and posterior internodal pathways are faster than in the middle internodal pathway, providing the substrate for reentry. Experimentally, Han et al.[13] demonstrated such a reciprocal rhythm between the atria and the sinus node. Importantly, both the sinus and AV nodes have the electrophysiologic property of slow conduction that is conducive to the genesis of reentrant arrhythmias.

Treatment

Sinus nodal reentrant tachycardia seldom requires acute treatment, and it usually responds to vagal maneuvers. Acutely, intravenous adenosine, verapamil, or a β-blocker can be used either diagnostically or therapeutically, if indicated. If sick sinus syndrome is suspected, drugs depressing the sinus node are generally contraindicated without backup pacing capability.

INTRAATRIAL AND INTERATRIAL REENTRANT TACHYCARDIAS

Several forms of intraatrial and interatrial reentry also exist, in which the P-wave morphology is different from that of the sinus P wave, and the reentrant circuit is confined to atrial tissue (often at rates from 140 to 240 beats/min) and likely represents a continuum with some forms of atrial flutter. Longitudinal dissociation of Bachmann's bundle has been identified as a mechanism of SVT involving interatrial reentry.[14] Bachmann's bundle reentry may mimic sinus nodal reentry or AV nodal reentry if the P-wave con-

figuration and the right atrial activation sequence of high-to-low or low-to-high, respectively, are the only criteria considered.[15] Therefore, the exact mechanism of this arrhythmia may not be identified unless intracardiac electrograms are obtained at electrophysiologic study.

Treatment

Because the AV and sinus nodes are not integral parts of the reentrant circuit in these forms of SVT, drugs such as verapamil, adenosine, or digoxin may not be as effective in terminating or preventing the SVT, but they may increase the level of AV block, thus aiding in the differential diagnosis. An antiarrhythmic drug, such as intravenous procainamide, can be used acutely, and this or another class IA (or possibly a class IC drug if left ventricular function is normal) can be used for subsequent oral therapy, if indicated. β-Blockers may be effective if the arrhythmia is felt to be modulated by a high catecholamine state.

PAROXYSMAL ATRIAL TACHYCARDIA WITH ATRIOVENTRICULAR BLOCK

This condition was first described in 1909 by Lewis,[16] who used polygraphic records, and the first ECG studies were reported by Koplik[17] in 1917. Lown et al.[18, 19] brought this rhythm disturbance into sharp focus with pertinent observations of the association of paroxysmal atrial tachycardia (PAT) with block, digitalis intoxication, and lowered serum potassium levels. However, the name *PAT with block* is something of a misnomer, because the rhythm is uncommonly paroxysmal in onset or offset. Characteristically, PAT with block usually shows a gradual acceleration of the atrial rate that at times results in subtle deformities of the P waves. As the rhythm accelerates, various conduction delays may be observed, in part related to the effects of digitalis on the AV node, until fixed or variable block occurs.

In general, PAT with block is considered to be relatively uncommon now that digitalis toxicity is less prevalent. Nonparoxysmal AV junctional tachycardia is an associated arrhythmia that also frequently results from excess digitalis or low potassium levels. However, not all of these arrhythmias are associated with digitalis (or now more commonly, digoxin) excess. They can also be observed in the presence of coronary artery disease or acute cor pulmonale, and they have also been associated with the use of other drugs such as quinidine. PAT with block has occasionally been associated with rheumatic heart disease and may be a more serious manifestation of atrial disease than atrial fibrillation itself. Obviously, prompt diagnosis of this arrhythmia is mandatory with respect to the therapeutic implications, particularly in the presence of digoxin excess and lowered serum potassium levels. Caution must be exercised in repleting potassium, because AV nodal block may worsen acutely. An increased mortality rate associated with digitalis arrhythmias has been clearly identified.[20]

Because digitalis and low potassium levels are the most frequently cited causes of this tachycardia, it has been assumed that it has an automatic atrial mechanism. Both onset and offset of PAT with block are usually more gradual than sudden, suggesting a gradual shift of the pacemaker focus. Experimental studies have clearly shown that digitalis, especially in the presence of low potassium levels, causes enhanced phase 4 depolarization that could lead to abnormally enhanced automaticity within certain groups of atrial fibers. Alternatively, digitalis excess also facilitates socalled oscillatory afterdepolarizations reaching thres hold, leading to "triggered" tachyarrhythmias. Diseased tissue may be most susceptible to these arrhythmias, particularly in the presence of hypoxemia and catecholamine excess; consequently, patients in the period immediately after cardiothoracic surgery often are vulnerable.

Treatment

Management of PAT with block includes discontinuation of digoxin and cautious replacement of potassium. Rarely, it is necessary to use antiarrhythmic agents; phenytoin has been advocated classically because of its negligible effects on the AV node, but intravenous procainamide is an alternative to be considered for acute suppression of this arrhythmia. Lidocaine and β-blockers, with temporary pacing when necessary, are other treatment options, particularly when increased automaticity or digitalis toxicity are implicated. Digoxin-binding antibodies provide a therapeutic alternative.

MULTIFOCAL ATRIAL TACHYCARDIA

Multifocal atrial tachycardia can be diagnosed when there are frequent atrial premature systoles of at least three different contours, often in runs, marked variation in the P-P intervals, and an isoelectric baseline. The P waves differ markedly in character and frequency of discharge, apparently resulting from abnormally enhanced automaticity or possibly triggered activity (Fig. 19–6). The atrial rate is typically in the range of 100 to 200 beats/min. Varying degrees of AV block are usually present. These rhythms are closely associated with advanced pulmonary disease, hypoxemia, respiratory acidosis, cardiac decompensation, metabolic derangements, diabetes, hypokalemia, old age, and general debilitation. Notably, this form of atrial tachycardia is extremely resistant to conventional doses of digitalis preparations and conversely appears to be aggravated by excess digoxin or lowered serum potassium level. Multifocal atrial tachycardia may be difficult to distinguish from atrial fibrillation unless longer rhythm strips or several ECG leads are examined.

Treatment

Management of this arrhythmia primarily involves improvement in pulmonary hygiene and other contributing conditions. Correction of acid-base balance and pulmonary gas exchange is mandatory. Verapamil may either suppress the atrial arrhythmias or decrease AV nodal conduction in some patients. Moreover, administering 1 g of intravenous calcium gluconate just before treatment with verapamil may reduce the propensity to drug-induced hypotension without preventing the antiarrhythmic effect. Propranolol is usually contraindicated because of underlying pulmonary disease. However, newer relatively cardioselective β-blockers such as metoprolol or the ultrashort-acting esmolol have been shown to be effective, but caution must be exercised in patients with pulmonary or cardiac contraindications. Quinidine or procainamide has occasionally controlled this variety of atrial tachycardia, and, acutely, intravenous pro-

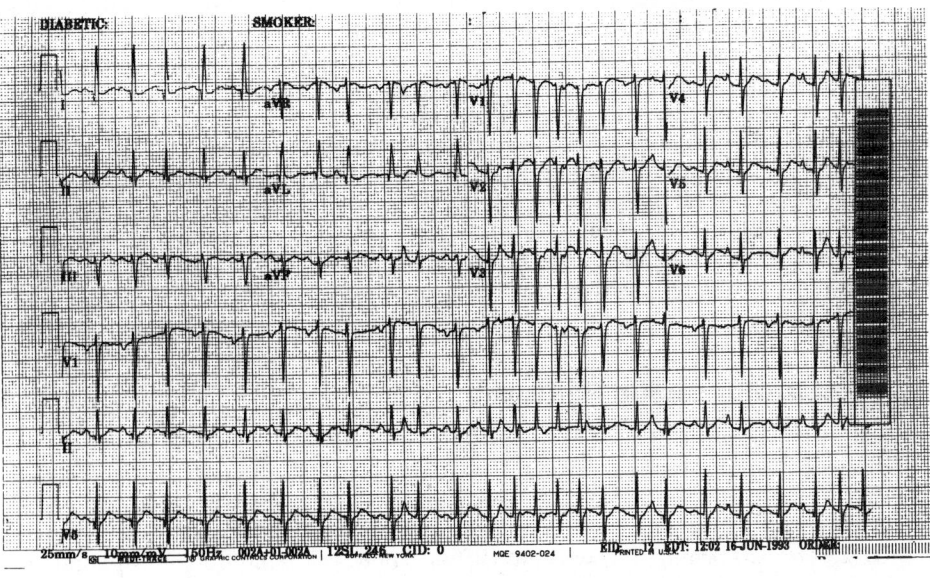

Figure 19–6. Twelve-lead ECG showing the multiple P-wave morphologies (rate is more than 100 beats/min) along the isoelectric baseline, associated with multifocal atrial tachycardia.

cainamide occasionally results in dramatic improvement.[21]

ATRIAL FLUTTER
Clinical Features

Atrial flutter is a relatively infrequent atrial arrhythmia that may be observed either as an established, incessant condition or as a paroxysmal transient rhythm. Rarely is the mechanism chronic in nature; either sinus rhythm is reestablished or atrial fibrillation ensues. Classic (type I) atrial flutter has been shown by detailed intracardiac mapping to typically involve a counterclockwise reentry loop exiting in the region between the inferior border of the coronary sinus and the inferior vena cava–right atrium border. The reentry loop extends from the region of the coronary sinus os to the free right atrial wall along the tricuspid annulus.[22]

Children have been observed to maintain atrial flutter for relatively long periods, often with spontaneous reestablishment of sinus rhythm. There is an association of atrial flutter in patients with surgically corrected congenital heart disease, and its occurrence can correlate with sudden death.[23]

Atrial flutter usually is observed in patients with moderately advanced or severe grades of myocardial involvement in the middle and older age groups. Rarely, it is observed in seemingly normal hearts. Almost any type of trauma, surgical procedure, or active pericardial-myocardial process including myocardial infarction may be associated with atrial flutter. The use of various antiarrhythmic drugs may also favor the occurrence of atrial flutter over atrial fibrillation.

The symptoms and signs depend mainly on the degree of heart damage, ventricular rate, duration of the rhythm, and, to some extent, the patient's awareness of the irregular or rapid rhythm. The most common ventricular rate in atrial flutter is 140 to 160 beats/min owing to a 2:1 AV ratio. With class IA antiarrhythmic agents, such as quinidine or procainamide, the flutter rate may slow to 200 to 240 beats/min, and 1:1 AV conduction may ensue with acceleration of the ventricular rate. This possibility is especially likely in patients who have not previously received digoxin or been given a β-blocker or calcium antagonist to slow AV nodal conduction before the initiation of a class IA antiarrhythmic agent. In addition, the available class IA drugs have vagolytic properties that may override their direct depressant effect on AV nodal conduction, further facilitating enhanced AV conduction.

Electrocardiographic Features

Typical atrial flutter is characterized by sawtooth undulations (usually inverted "flutter" waves in the inferior leads) of the baseline with rapid atrial rates in the range of 240 to 360 beats/min, but most commonly 280 to 320 beats/min, without drugs. There is usually a narrow QRS complex and a ventricular rate of 140 to 160 beats/min because of a 2:1 AV conduction ratio. Varying conduction ratios such as 3:1 and 4:1 or 2:1 alternating with 4:1 may produce grouped beating and pseudobigeminy. Typical sawtooth undulations in the baseline may not be evident, particularly with 2:1 conduction ratios, and the presence of a wide QRS tachycardia can be confused with ventricular tachycardia. Carotid sinus pressure or other vagal maneuvers or intravenous adenosine frequently reveals the presence of flutter waves and increases the AV conduction ratio transiently. In addition, slight variations in the cycle length due to various degrees of impulse penetration into the AV junction affecting the subsequent AV conduction interval are suggestive of atrial flutter. Atypical forms of flutter may be difficult to distinguish from various atrial tachycardias or atrial fibrillation, and, in some cases, these rhythms may be in flux. This situation is often evident with atrial fibrillation and flutter. In atypical atrial flutter, the flutter waves may be atypical in morphology or rate, and either slower (e.g., 210 to 280 beats/min) or more rapid (e.g., 320 to 400 beats/min) than typical flutter. The former may have several mechanisms; the latter is considered to be reentrant in nature.

Treatment

The initial goal in managing atrial flutter is to slow the ventricular rate using drugs such as digoxin, β-blocking agents such as esmolol or propranolol, or intravenous diltiazem or verapamil. To attempt chemical conversion to sinus rhythm, a β-blocker or class IA antiarrhythmic drug such as intravenous procainamide, alone or in combination, may be used. Rarely, amiodarone is a consideration, but it has been used with successful results and is preferred for patients with significantly reduced left ventricular function.[24] Recently, evidence has suggested that class IC drugs, such as flecainide and propafenone, may be useful in converting atrial flutter to sinus rhythm and in maintaining sinus rhythm, with the additional advantage of slowing AV nodal conduction. For similar purposes, the class III agent sotalol has been used effectively, although caution must be exercised in dosing and patient selection for both these class of drugs because of their risks for producing proarrhythmic ventricular tachyarrhythmias and worsening heart failure.[25, 26] Precordial shock (typically 25 to 50 J or less) may be necessary in patients demonstrating marked deterioration in cardiac hemodynamics. An alternative is to attempt rapid atrial stimulation using a transvenous electrode catheter or transesophageal atrial pacing in cases in which the tachyarrhythmia is hemodynamically relatively well tolerated. This method may result in sinus rhythm or atrial fibrillation, or it may have no effect. Factors contributing to the occurrence of atrial flutter, such as electrolyte and metabolic derangements and congestive heart failure, especially in the presence of acute myocardial infarction or open heart surgery, should be reversed.

The need for anticoagulation is not as well established for flutter as it is for atrial fibrillation.

ATRIAL FIBRILLATION
Clinical Features

Atrial fibrillation is a common cardiac arrhythmia characterized by rapid, chaotic atrial activity, variably rapid AV conduction, and irregular RR intervals. Consequently, cardiac output may be affected adversely, not only by the loss of effective atrial contractions but also by compromised ventricular filling and contraction related to variably short R-R intervals. Symptoms often parallel the resulting ventricular rate. The presence of atrial fibrillation suggests the presence of either myocardial or pericardial disease and is frequently associated with increased left atrial size and/or pressure. Although atrial fibrillation may be paroxysmal, particularly in patients with no evidence of structural heart disease (so-called lone atrial fibrillation), it is often a chronic stable rhythm and in many cases may be the final stage in the sick sinus syndrome when sinus node function becomes extremely slow or nonexistent. Patients may complain of severe palpitations or weakness in the presence of intermittent atrial fibrillation and may also be extremely symptomatic of the shifting of the cardiac rhythm from sinus to atrial fibrillation. Occasionally, intrinsic AV conduction delay may be present, and ventricular rates may be in the physiologic range in the absence of drugs that slow AV conduction. Atrial fibrillation is associated with many forms of heart disease, the most frequent being hypertensive, atherosclerotic, cardiomyopathic, and rheumatic. Paroxysmal atrial fibrillation may occur as a result of extreme vagal stimulation associated with severe diarrhea or vomiting, or it may result from ingestion of alcohol (the so-called holiday heart). In the presence of untreated atrial fibrillation, the ventricular rate may be rapid (150 to 240 beats/min) with the sudden onset of hypotension or pulmonary edema. Patients of any age with a large left atrium or valvular or cardiomyopathic heart disease may be subject to pulmonary or systemic embolization and therefore should be considered candidates for long-term anticoagulant therapy. Importantly, atrial fibrillation occurs with marked increase in frequency with advanced age and is associated with a significant propensity to cerebrovascular thromboembolic complications in the elderly, who should be considered for anticoagulant therapy. Attempts to convert atrial fibrillation to sinus rhythm with persistence of sinus rhythm are less likely to be successful in the presence of either long-standing atrial fibrillation or a large left atrium.[27, 28]

Electrocardiographic Features

Either fine or coarse undulations are seen replacing the baseline, and distinct P waves are absent. Attempts have been made using direct recordings of atrial electrograms to characterize atrial fibrillation into subtypes, based on criteria such as the regularity, polarity, amplitude, and rate of atrial depolarizations and whether the baseline is isoelectric.[29] There are also ECG correlates of specific subtypes (e.g., "coarse" versus "fine" atrial fibrillation). However, clear clinical implications with respect to either prognosis or treatment have not yet been established. Rapid irregular atrial activity with rates of 300 to 600 beats/min and normal QRS complexes duration are usually observed. The ventricular rate in the presence of untreated atrial fibrillation most often varies between 150 and 220 beats/min. It is now known that asynchronous activation of the two principal input regions to the AV node (crista terminalis and interatrial septum) may result in fragmented asynchronous conduction producing various degrees of concealment and failure of impulse propagation within the AV node, producing the irregularity of the ventricular rate.[30] The ventricular response is usually grossly irregular unless AV dissociation is present because of AV conduction block. In addition, when the ventricles are controlled by an accelerated junctional pacemaker, varying conduction ratios to the ventricles may produce grouped beating with an irregular ventricular response. Coexisting AV junctional rhythms should be suspected when the R-R intervals become regular. Digoxin excess usually is responsible, with the appearance of accelerated or escape junctional beats in association with high-grade AV conduction block. Occasionally, regularization reflects the transition from atrial fibrillation to atrial flutter. After the use of digoxin, verapamil, or a β-blocking agent, alone or in combination, the ventricular rate often slows.

An important distinction to make in atrial fibrillation is between ventricular premature depolarizations and aberrant ventricular conduction of supraventricular impulses. With the latter condition, the wide QRS beats are noted to follow a short cycle length preceded by a longer cycle length. Compensatory pauses usually are not seen because little possibility exists for concealed retrograde conduction from the ventricles into the AV junction to inhibit subsequent atrial impulses in an antegrade direction. Aberrant beats have a configuration in the right precordial leads of right bundle branch block with rSR¹ or multiphasic R¹ configurations. The initial 0.04 second of the QRS complex should be essentially identical in all leads to other narrow QRS supraventricular beats if the beat is aberrant.

Treatment

Rate control is generally the initial goal of therapy; it can be achieved within 5 to 30 minutes with either intravenous verapamil or diltiazem, a β-blocker such as esmolol or propranolol, and somewhat less rapidly with digoxin. Esmolol has the additional advantage of titratability in the acute care setting related to its half-life of only 9.2 minutes, so potential side effects such as hypotension rapidly dissipate with discontinuation of the drug. A secondary goal in atrial fibrillation of recent onset is restoration of sinus rhythm. Restoration often occurs spontaneously within hours to days if precipitating factors—including ischemia, thyrotoxicosis, hypokalemia, alcohol ingestion, catecholamine excess or substance abuse—can be reversed. A potential theoretic advantage of using drugs to hasten conversion may be to lessen the risk of thromboembolic complications associated with additional days of atrial fibrillation. Early conversion to sinus rhythm may also facilitate reduced lengths of hospital stay and decreased costs of hospitalization. In acute situations in which immediate conversion is mandatory, cardioversion with 100 J (200 J, if necessary) is the treatment of choice, but intravenous procainamide may be a useful adjunct or alternative in facilitating conversion. However, procainamide may cause more rapid AV conduction related to its vagolytic effects and via sympathetic reflexes elicited secondary to its vasodilating properties. β-Blockers such as esmolol and propranolol also offer the potential for converting the rhythm to sinus if it is of recent onset (Fig. 19–7), particularly in the setting of increased catecholamine levels, such as occurs postoperatively.[31] Oral therapy with either a class IA or IC drug may also be effective, but the response occurs over a more delayed time course of hours to days. Amiodarone and sotalol may be considered in refractory cases. A higher loading dose regimen is often used to hasten the onset of the antifibrillatory effect of amiodarone.[24]

NONCOMPENSATORY SINUS TACHYCARDIA

Although sinus tachycardia is not often thought of as a serious arrhythmia in the acute setting, it can be particularly problematic in patients with underlying ischemic, valvular, hypertrophic or other cardiomyopathic disease processes. Attention to precipitating and contributing factors such as hypovolemia, fever, pain, anxiety, and thyrotoxicosis is paramount, but additional measures may be necessary in patients who are immediately compromised by an excessive heart rate. Pathophysiologically, sinus tachycardia markedly increases myocardial oxygen requirements and reduces the time available in diastole for coronary blood flow, ventricular filling, and ventricular relax-

ation. In patients with coronary artery disease, mitral valve stenosis, or left ventricular hypertrophy or fibrosis, slowing the heart rate even modestly, from rates in excess of 110 to 120 beats/min to 70 to 80 beats/min, may be sufficient to relieve ischemia and/or improve hemodynamics, including cardiac output, blood pressure, and pulmonary capillary wedge pressure.

Treatment

Therapeutically, β-blockers are the most effective drugs available for the treatment of excessive sinus tachycardia. Clinically, management of excessive sinus tachycardia is relevant not only in the intensive care unit and emergency department, for example, to relieve myocardial ischemia, but also during preoperative anesthesia induction, intraoperatively, during invasive procedures, and in the open-heart and surgical recovery suites, as well as in the catheterization laboratory.

OVERVIEW OF THE DRUG TREATMENT OF SUPRAVENTRICULAR TACHYCARDIAS

Although SVTs can be identified and characterized by specific electrophysiologic mechanisms, the approach to management of these rhythms is similar. In general, the primary aim of therapy is to control the ventricular rate. In emergencies, particularly when evidence of deteriorating hemodynamic stability exists, rapid termination of tachycardia is mandatory. Rarely is a precordial electroshock necessary to terminate a supraventricular mechanism, but this method may be crucial in certain circumstances. Alternatively, the introduction of properly timed depolarizations either by passage of an electrode catheter or by external pacing techniques also may quickly terminate a supraventricular mechanism in certain individuals. However, because of the often significant time delays inherent in attempting to position a catheter, this treatment method should be reserved for hemodynamically stable SVTs.

Clearly, most patients with rapid SVTs require directed pharmacologic management if initial interven-

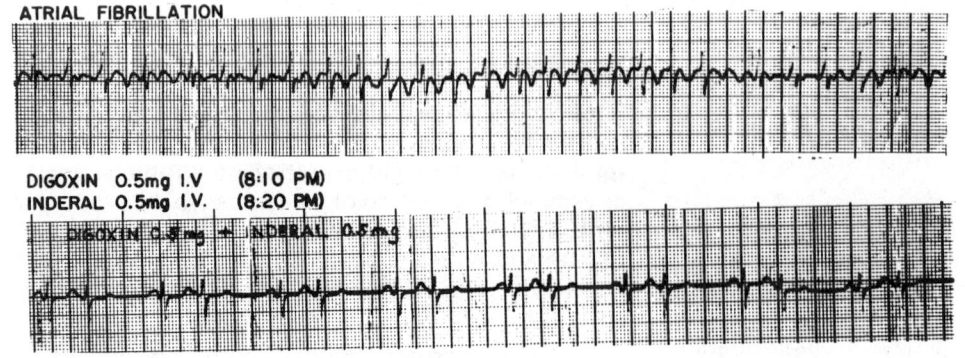

ATRIAL FIBRILLATION

DIGOXIN 0.5mg I.V   (8:10 PM)
INDERAL 0.5mg I.V   (8:20 PM)

Figure 19–7. Upper strip, Atrial fibrillation. *Lower strip,* Restoration of sinus rhythm with premature atrial systoles after administration of digoxin, 0.5 mg, and Inderal (propranolol), 0.5 mg IV.

tions such as vagal maneuvers fail. In the absence of severe hypotension, intravenous administration of at least 12 mg of adenosine terminates most reciprocating tachycardias involving the AV node as an integral part of the reentrant circuit. Because of the extremely short half-life of this agent (< 10 seconds), adenosine must be delivered via a central vein (e.g., the antecubital veins or above) to be effective. Transient hypotension, bronchospasm, sinus pauses, and precipitation of transient atrial fibrillation are among the potential adverse effects that may be enhanced by dipyridamole. Furthermore, oral theophylline preparations completely negate the antiarrhythmic effects of adenosine.[8]

Verapamil administered intravenously as a 5- to 10-mg bolus had been used as a primary drug therapy in the past. It also is effective in slowing the ventricular rate in atrial fibrillation and flutter but rarely converts either of these rhythms to sinus rhythm. Subsequent administration of oral verapamil may be necessary for continued control of the ventricular response in the presence of atrial fibrillation or flutter. Caution must be exercised to avoid inadvertently administering verapamil intravenously to patients who have ventricular tachycardias or administering either verapamil or digoxin intravenously to patients with atrial fibrillation manifesting preexcitation (WPW syndrome).[32] In both cases, hypotension and ventricular fibrillation may result. However, in rare instances, patients with specific types of ventricular tachycardias may respond well to verapamil when it is given for this purpose.[29]

Alternatively, intravenous digoxin may be administered using an initial dose of 0.25 to 0.5 mg, but in the presence of atrial flutter or fibrillation, the time required to either terminate the tachycardia or slow the ventricular rate may be considerable (20 minutes to 4 hours). Repeated administration of 0.125 to 0.25 mg of digoxin up to a total dose of 1.0 to 1.25 mg may be effective. If the tachycardia does not slow or terminate, the addition of a β-blocker such as propranolol, 0.5- to 1.0-mg doses intravenously, or esmolol has often proved to be a valuable adjunct (see Fig. 19–7).

Another agent now used as first-line therapy to control a rapid ventricular rate in atrial fibrillation is intravenous diltiazem. Most patients respond with a 20% reduction in ventricular rate to a 20- to 25-mg intravenous bolus followed by a 10 to 15 mg/hr constant infusion. Additional boluses can be delivered every 15 minutes until the desired level of AV conduction block is achieved. The AV nodal blocking effect of intravenous diltiazem is synergistic with digoxin, but unlike verapamil, another intravenous calcium antagonist, intravenous diltiazem does not increase serum digoxin levels.[33] Because the half-life of diltiazem is 2.5 hours, hypotension caused by administration of intravenous diltiazem may be considerably more difficult to manage and may not clear readily on discontinuing the infusion.

Esmolol, the ultrashort-acting cardioselective β-blocker, is also a recent addition to the therapeutic armamentarium. It is also a first-line agent for control of the ventricular rate in the presence of atrial fibrillation or flutter, and it is particularly effective in high catecholamine level states such as the period after open heart surgery or noncardiac surgery. It can also be used for noncompensatory or excessive sinus tachycardia. Its major advantages are rapid onset and offset of activity (half-life, 9.2 minutes) and ease of titration. Because it is metabolized by red blood cell esterases, its short half-life is maintained even in the presence of advanced hepatic, renal, or cardiac disease and during concomitant use of other drugs. Esmolol is usually given as an initial intravenous bolus loading infusion of 10 to 50 mg (100 to 500 µg/kg) over 1 minute, followed by a maintenance infusion of 1 to 5 mg/min (10 to 50 µg/kg/min), with further dosing increments as necessary to a maximum of about 10 to 20 mg/min (100 to 200 µg/kg/min). In those cases in which more rapid titration is desired, additional loading doses can be given at the time of each 1- to 5-mg/min dosing increment. Efficacy is usually reached at 50 to 150 µg/kg/min, and a maintenance infusion can be continued for several hours. The patient can be switched to oral maintenance therapy with an alternative agent and the esmolol infusion tapered, as indicated. Hypotension, generally mild and readily reversible with discontinuation of the infusion, occurs in 10% to 25% of patients, particularly those with systolic blood pressures below 100 mmHg initially and those receiving more aggressive dosing regimens. As with all β-blocking agents, use must be with extreme caution in patients with a history of congestive heart failure. To avoid excessive pharmacologic effect and to minimize the likelihood of hypotension, a smaller initial bolus loading infusion (10 to 20 mg, repeated as necessary) and smaller dosing increments (1 to 3 mg/min) can be used, and either subsequent loading infusions can be eliminated or the dosage reduced.

Maintenance therapy for SVTs generally is designed either to control the ventricular rate in cases in which conversion to sinus rhythm cannot be achieved or prophylactically to prevent recurrence of SVT. Chronic anticoagulation therapy is a consideration for patients in whom atrial fibrillation or flutter may recur. Among patients with atrial fibrillation or flutter of apparently recent onset, conversion to sinus rhythm can be attempted with the use of oral class IA agents (i.e., quinidine, procainamide, or disopyramide), class IC agents (flecainide or propafenone), or class III agents such as sotalol or amiodarone. Quinidine, flecainide, and amiodarone can each raise serum digoxin levels, and digoxin dosing may have to be adjusted accordingly. Patients with atrial fibrillation that persists for more than 2 days should be given adequate anticoagulation (e.g., with heparin followed by 2 to 3 weeks of warfarin) before elective chemical or electrical conversion to sinus rhythm is attempted to prevent thromboembolism. Therefore, all measures to restore sinus rhythm should be taken before this is necessary.

In patients with persistent atrial fibrillation, small

doses of digoxin in combination with a calcium antagonist or β-blocker often control the ventricular rate effectively both at rest and during exercise. Some patients with refractory and debilitating atrial fibrillation may be candidates for catheter ablation of the AV node–His bundle region. This would require subsequent implantation of a rate-responsive permanent pacemaker. Alternatively, atrial isolation surgery, such as the Maze procedure, has been done in an attempt to maintain orderly AV conduction on a limited basis.[34]

For patients with recurrent, debilitating reentrant SVTs such as AV nodal reentry tachycardia, AV reciprocating tachycardia, and typical atrial flutter, radiofrequency catheter ablation is fast becoming the treatment of choice to cure, rather than suppress, these tachycardias. In certain individuals in whom SVTs occur only rarely and are not immediately debilitating, a so-called cocktail program can be devised. For example, at the onset of SVT, the patient is advised to take an oral loading dose of digoxin, 0.5 mg, and subsequently add verapamil, 80 mg, or propranolol, 20 to 80 mg, within 1 hour if the rhythm is not controlled; or propranolol may be used as the initial agent.

Chaotic atrial tachycardias require a somewhat different method of management. These rhythms are usually associated with chronic pulmonary disease, and the use of a β-blocker is often contraindicated. These patients may respond well to verapamil, quinidine, procainamide, or the class IC agents flecainide or propafenone.

ATRIOVENTRICULAR JUNCTIONAL ARRHYTHMIAS
Clinical Features

Atrioventricular junctional rhythms, which are often benign, may occur as escape or rescue mechanisms during sinus bradycardia or as manifestations of the sick sinus syndrome. AV junctional rhythms may occur in various pathologic conditions, including myocardial infarction (particularly of the inferior wall) and myocarditis, and after open heart surgery. However, these rhythms also may occur under physiologic conditions at other times (e.g., when vagal tone is high during sleep, or at rest in young or well-conditioned persons). Independent activation of the atria and ventricles with narrow QRS complexes should suggest the presence of an AV junctional mechanism. Loss of the atrial contribution or a negative atrial kick produced by retrograde activation of the atria during ventricular systole may result in hypotension and decreased cardiac output. In contrast with escape junctional rhythms, accelerated AV junctional tachycardia can be clinically important because further administration of offending agents such as digoxin or failure to correct hypokalemia may result in more serious and potentially lethal cardiac arrhythmias. Because the rate of the normal AV junctional pacemaker is usually between 40 and 60 beats/min, junctional

rhythms demonstrating more rapid rates (typically 70 to 130 beats/min) or accelerated junctional mechanism usually reflect an additional process that may result from electrolyte imbalance, ischemia, or an excess of drugs such as digitalis.

Electrocardiographic Features

The term nonparoxysmal AV junctional rhythm has been used to describe those nonreentrant rhythms originating from the AV junctional region.[19] These rhythms apparently arise from enhanced impulse formation within the AV junctional tissues, either from enhanced automaticity or possibly from triggered activity. The AV junction is usually defined as that part of the specialized conduction system between the so-called approaches to the AV node (or the junction between the lower right atrium and AV node) and the bundle of His. Despite its small anatomic dimensions, the AV junction is composed of several different fiber types with dissimilar action potential configurations and conduction properties.[35, 36] The conduction velocity within the N region of the AV node is extremely slow, and this region is composed of specialized fibers with slow channel properties. This region is also rich in vagal innervation. The proximal portion above the N region or AN region behaves like specialized atrial myocardium, and the distal or NH region closely resembles the bundle of His. Experimental studies indicate that enhanced impulse formation can occur within the NH region, particularly in the region of the tricuspid valve.[36] Impulse formation within the AN region also has been observed, whereas enhanced impulse formation within the N region itself is still less well documented, but diastolic depolarization of these fibers has been observed experimentally in small preparations of AV nodal tissue. On ECG, AV junctional impulses most often result in a QRS configuration that is the same as the dominant supraventricular rhythm (Fig. 19–8). Occasionally, aberrant conduction of impulses formed within the AV node results in wide QRS complexes as well. Premature, narrow QRS complexes can be associated with retrograde P waves occurring either just before the QRS with a short PR interval, within the QRS complex, or after the QRS complex, depending on the relative timing of retrograde conduction to the atria versus antegrade conduction to the ventricles.

A junctional mechanism should be suspected when an apparent ectopic atrial rhythm with a short P-R interval and inverted P waves in the inferior leads is noted. Concealed junctional extrasystoles are suggested by the occurrence sometimes of nonconducted sinus or premature supraventricular beats (inverted P wave, no QRS complex) and otherwise inexplicable increases in the P-R interval at other times, including AV block, mimicking Mobitz type I or II second-degree AV block (pseudo-type II AV block). AV junctional rhythms may result in AV dissociation. Careful analysis of the ECG to ensure linkage between the QRS complex and P wave is necessary for diagnosis. Exit block can cause irregular atrial or

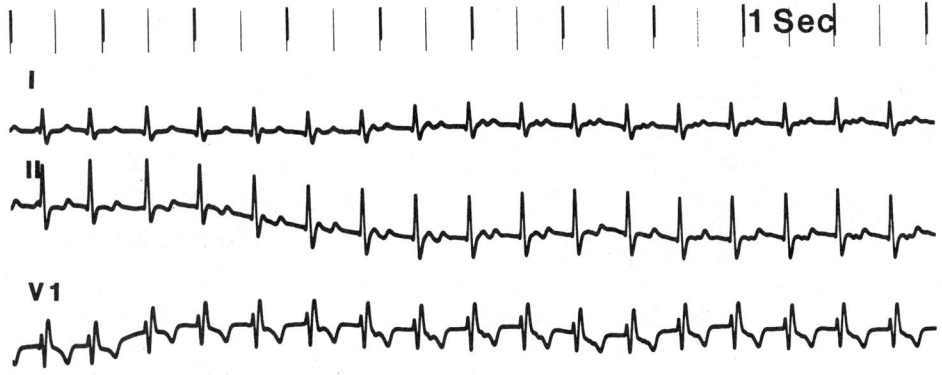

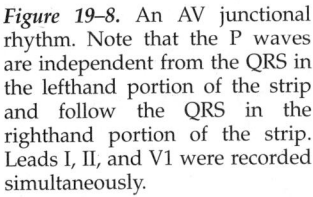

Figure 19–8. An AV junctional rhythm. Note that the P waves are independent from the QRS in the lefthand portion of the strip and follow the QRS in the righthand portion of the strip. Leads I, II, and V1 were recorded simultaneously.

ventricular rates in either a retrograde or antegrade fashion. Rarely, AV junctional parasystole can be observed.

Management

Accelerated nonparoxysmal AV junctional tachycardia is invariably a pathologic rhythm and may require therapy. Because these rhythms are usually associated with an acute process, such as recent open heart surgery, myocardial infarction, myocarditis, or active rheumatic fever, they may be difficult to terminate with any pharmacologic program. However, in cases associated with an excess of digitalis or hypokalemia, digoxin can be discontinued, potassium administered, and the use of a class I antiarrhythmic agent considered. Historically, lidocaine, phenytoin, and propranolol have been advocated, particularly in the setting of digitalis excess. Alternatively, intravenous procainamide or esmolol should be considered. In cases in which the rate is not excessive (e.g., less than 90 beats/min) and it is thought that loss of an effective atrial kick is contributing to hemodynamic compromise, overdrive atrial or AV sequential pacing can be used. Evidence suggests that class IC drugs such as flecainide may be effective in refractory cases. Rarely, an ablative procedure is necessary when such rhythms become incessant and debilitating. Such patients usually require chronic pacing after an ablative procedure. However, in many patients, these rhythms cause only modest hemodynamic compromise, in part related to loss of effective atrial transport; therefore, aggressive therapy is not indicated other than treating any reversible etiologic factors.

VENTRICULAR TACHYARRHYTHMIAS
Clinical Features

Considerable attention recently has been given to the detection and management of ventricular arrhythmias in an effort to prevent cardiovascular catastrophes and sudden death. Premature ventricular systoles are extremely common and are found in nearly all seg-

ments of the population.[37] Consequently, early descriptions of ventricular ectopic beats alternatively considered them either benign or malignant. Patients frequently complain of palpitations, thumping in the chest, or merely skipped beats. Frequently, patients become terrified by the presence of an irregular heartbeat when premature ventricular beats persist. Dizziness, syncope, or pulmonary congestion may result when these tachyarrhythmias are associated with an inadequate stroke volume. However, most patients with premature ventricular beats are totally unaware of their presence, and the physician should not emphasize them in the absence of heart disease. Often, ventricular ectopy may be seen accompanying a variety of cardiovascular problems such as coronary artery disease, hypertensive cardiovascular disease, and ischemic cardiomyopathy. Trigger mechanisms associated with ventricular arrhythmias may include metabolic derangements, particularly hypokalemia or hypomagnesemia in susceptible individuals, tobacco, caffeine, alcohol, drugs, and stress.

In the absence of underlying cardiovascular disease, the presence of ventricular premature beats usually has no significance, and the use of antiarrhythmic drugs merely for cosmetic reasons is not indicated. Furthermore, it has not been shown definitively that antiarrhythmic therapy to suppress asymptomatic premature systoles is of any clinical merit and, indeed, may be harmful.[38] In general, the frequency of premature ventricular systoles increases with age, and sporadic premature ventricular beats in persons with normal hearts do not seem to indicate an increased risk of cardiovascular events or an unfavorable prognosis.[37] Conversely, patients with ischemic heart disease or dilated or hypertrophic cardiomyopathies may represent a subset of individuals who are at high risk of sudden death.[39, 40] Following myocardial infarction, a reduced ejection fraction and the presence of ventricular arrhythmias represent individual risk factors of subsequent cardiac death.[39, 41] Patients with so-called complex or high-grade ventricular premature beats (e.g., frequent, multiform runs of premature ventricular beats, or the R wave on T wave phenomenon) associated with cardiomegaly, prior myocardial infarction, and ST-segment abnormalities are at an exceptionally high risk for cardiac death.[41]

In some patients with other specific entities, such as valvular heart disease or hypertrophic cardiomyopathy, the incidence of sudden death associated with ventricular arrhythmias is also significant. Although in the setting of acute myocardial ischemia or infarction antiarrhythmic therapy in combination with aggressive antiischemic therapy has been advocated, the treatment of isolated or even frequent premature ventricular beats rarely constitutes an acute emergency. The management of SVTs for which therapy is mandatory is discussed in an earlier section.

Electrocardiographic Features

Ventricular premature beats are characterized by QRS complexes that are premature, wide, and often bizarre in appearance. The initial QRS vector forces (0.04 second) are usually different from those of supraventricular beats. Usually the ST segment and T waves are in the opposite direction of the main QRS vector forces. The timing of a premature beat in the cycle can affect the relationship to P waves and to the subsequent QRS complex. Late-cycle premature ventricular beats may occur after the P wave and coincide with the intrinsic QRS complex, producing fusion beats, whereas early premature ventricular beats may allow retrograde conduction to the atria via the AV node, resetting the sinus node and affecting the timing of the next sinus beat. Premature ventricular beats occur most often in midcycle and leave the next P wave undisturbed (although it may be buried within the QRS complex), but they block AV conduction of this sinus beat. The next P wave occurs with normal AV conduction, generating a so-called compensatory pause. Occasionally, concealed retrograde AV conduction by the premature ventricular beat results in a slightly prolonged PR interval of the next sinus beat. Various periods of the return of the sinus cycle may be produced by sinus node reset, collision of the retrograde impulse within the atria, or collision within the AV junction.

A parasystolic ventricular rhythm should be suspected when the premature ventricular beats are not fixed in their coupling interval to the previous sinus-derived beats and when it appears that the premature beats are occurring sporadically but with relatively stable interectopic intervals that are multiples of a least common denominator. In such cases, the site of impulse formation within the ventricles or Purkinje system is presumably protected by entrance block, so that depolarization of the pacemaker site remains largely undisturbed by the dominant rhythm of the heart. These rhythms may persist for years without apparent ill effect. When a premature ventricular systole appears at the time of the sinus or dominant rhythm, the relative degree of depolarization of the ventricles by the ventricular premature beat versus the dominant rhythm may be variable. Fusion beats are a reliable indication of ventricular activation from two distinct sites. In addition to late-cycle premature ventricular beats, fusion beats are also a characteristic of ventricular preexcitation in the WPW syndrome.

The treatment of specific ventricular tachyarrhythmias is discussed in the appropriate sections later in the chapter.

SUSTAINED VENTRICULAR TACHYCARDIAS
Clinical Features

Although ventricular tachycardia is seen most frequently in patients with substantial cardiovascular disease—especially ischemic heart disease, dilated cardiomyopathies, or valvular heart disease—the symptoms associated with this arrhythmia usually depend on several factors, including the rate of the ventricular tachycardia, the relationship of P waves and atrial systole to the QRS complexes, and the degree of underlying cardiac dysfunction. At moderately rapid ventricular rates not exceeding 130 to 150 beats/min, an effective atrial kick engendered by 1:1 retrograde inscription of the P waves and atrial systole may afford adequate hemodynamic support, so that patients may not be aware of their abnormal ventricular mechanism. However, if the retrograde P waves occur within or after the QRS complex and within the ventricular systolic period, resulting in a negative atrial kick, marked hemodynamic derangements may be noted with the onset of this tachyarrhythmia. In the presence of AV dissociation with randomly occurring P waves, the symptoms engendered by compromised hemodynamics may be intermediate.

Nonsustained ventricular tachycardia, in which the number of premature ventricular beats rarely exceeds four to six in succession, may not be noticed by the patient. Frequently, nonsustained ventricular tachycardias are detected only by Holter or other ECG monitoring. More sustained (e.g., longer than 30 seconds) rapid ventricular tachycardia, with rates exceeding 150 beats/min, are most likely to be detected by the patient and are clearly symptomatic in most instances. In older individuals, lower rates of ventricular tachycardia may be hemodynamically compromising and may eventually lead to ventricular fibrillation and death. In addition, in a proportion of patients with unexplained syncope in which all neurologic causes have been excluded, particularly when cardiac disease is present, periods of ventricular tachycardia with hemodynamic derangement appear to account for neurologic symptoms.[42, 43]

Electrophysiologic Features

Traditionally, ventricular tachycardia is defined as three or more ventricular ectopic beats in succession at rates in excess of either 100 or 120 beats/min. Ventricular tachycardia is said to be sustained if it persists for more than 15 to 30 seconds and is almost invariably associated with clinical symptoms. The rate in the presence of ventricular tachycardia may vary between 100 and 280 beats/min, and the distinction between ventricular tachycardia and flutter is often difficult at rates in excess of 240 to 250 beats/min. An isoelectric baseline and effective ventricular contractions favor the diagnosis of ventricular tachycardia. However, in the presence of antiarrhythmic drugs, the morphologic distinction between ventricular tachycardia and flutter may become blurred even at relatively slow rates, and sustained ventricular tachycardia may even recur at rates less than 100 beats/min.

Many of the ECG features of ventricular tachycardia are not unique to these arrhythmias. Hence, the differential diagnosis of wide QRS tachycardias becomes a perplexing and often confounding problem for the clinician. Although the presence of AV dissociation is seen frequently in the presence of ventricular tachycardia, accelerated nonparoxysmal or paroxysmal junctional tachycardias as well as AV nodal reentry tachycardia may occasionally demonstrate this phenomenon. Occasionally, when the ventricular rate is slow, observation of ventricular capture or fusion beats may confirm the diagnosis of ventricular tachycardia. ECG features supporting the diagnosis of ventricular tachycardia include (1) a QRS complex width greater than 0.14 second if a right bundle branch block pattern is present or greater than 0.16 second if a left bundle branch block pattern is present; (2) superior axis; (3) left bundle branch block morphology with slurring of the downstroke of the S wave in lead V_1 or V_2 and a QS (peak to nadir) duration greater than 70 msec or a total QS duration exceeding 90 msec; (4) an increase in the R wave amplitude in lead V_1 compared with sinus rhythm; (5) a QR complex or a monophasic or biphasic R wave in lead V_1; (6) right bundle branch block morphology with concordance across the precordium; and (7) a deep S wave in lead V_6 in patients with tachyarrhythmias with morphologic appearance of right bundle branch block.[44-46]

Ventricular tachycardia may be classified as nonsustained or sustained, monomorphic or polymorphic. A distinctive variety of polymorphic ventricular tachycardia associated with QT (or QT_c interval) prolongation, torsade de pointes, and another distinct entity often associated with digitalis excess, so-called bidirectional ventricular tachycardia, have also been described.

Ventricular origin of the tachycardia can be documented in the electrophysiologic laboratory by a short or inverse HV interval or deflections of the bundle of His that are independent of the ventricular depolarizations. However, deflections of the bundle of His may not be readily apparent in the presence of ventricular tachycardia. In many cases, it is possible to reproduce a similar QRS contour of ventricular tachycardia by appropriate ventricular pacing, provided the ventricular tachyarrhythmia originates in proximity to the site where a ventricular pacing catheter has been advanced (Fig. 19–9). In addition, it is also possible in the electrophysiologic laboratory to distinguish ventricular tachycardia from nodofascicular reciprocating tachycardias and other rhythms that may mimic these entities.

Unfortunately, the optimum electrophysiolgic protocol to induce ventricular tachycardia is still controversial.[47] Presumably, a reentrant mechanism is the basis for most sustained ventricular tachycardias in ambulatory patients, and in the laboratory, in susceptible patients, the presence of specific anatomic and functional substrates allows for initiation of arrhythmias. In most patients, two extrastimuli are required for induction of tachycardia; however, three ventricular stimuli often are necessary. Finding an appropriate end point for the definition of significant ventricular arrhythmias and drug efficacy initially was linked to the induction of repetitive ventricular responses or nonsustained ventricular tachycardia. However, nonsustained ventricular arrhythmias do not necessarily predict subsequent sustained arrhythmias, and the induction of a sustained ventricular tachycardia or one that produces hemodynamic instability is usually the end point sought during electrophysiologic testing.[47-49] Also the definition of sustained arrhythmias remains arbitrary. Most investigators lump together tachycardias lasting longer than 15 to 30 seconds with rhythm resulting in immediate hemodynamic compromise and therefore requiring intervention with ventricular stimulation, burst pacing, or cardioversion for termination. Patients studied after resuscitation from ventricular fibrillation offer an additional level of complexity.[50, 51] Fortuitous monitoring observations, as well as data from the electrophysiologic laboratory, suggest that in most of these patients ventricular tachycardias are the initiating rhythm that subsequently degenerates into ventricular fibrillation. Furthermore, as many as 40% of these patients may not experience induced ventricular tachyarrhythmias in the laboratory even with relatively aggressive techniques.[52] The long-term outlook of these patients is still largely unknown, although there are data suggesting a poor prognosis if they are untreated.[49]

The inability to reproduce a clinically documented ventricular tachyarrhythmia poses an obvious problem in management. Every effort must be made in treatment of patients with ventricular tachyarrhythmias to identify metabolic or ischemic factors that may have precipitated the initial episode, so that the likelihood of a recurrent event or again precipitating ventricular fibrillation is minimized. The long-term fate of these patients after antiarrhythmic drug therapy cannot be predicted as easily. Furthermore, individuals showing multiple ventricular tachyarrhythmias at the time of study and follow-up present other difficult interpretive problems. This has been associated with a poor response to antiarrhythmic drug therapy, and it is still unknown whether obliteration of all of the inducible ventricular forms is necessary to prevent the recurrence of spontaneous ventricular tachycardia.[53] Ultimately, an implantable cardioverter-defibrillator is often necessary.

Although experience with electrophysiologic testing in patients with ischemic heart disease has led to some clinically useful guidelines, patients with other cardiac diagnoses associated with ventricular arrhythmias, such as idiopathic dilated cardiomyopathy or valvular heart disease, may manifest ventricular ar-

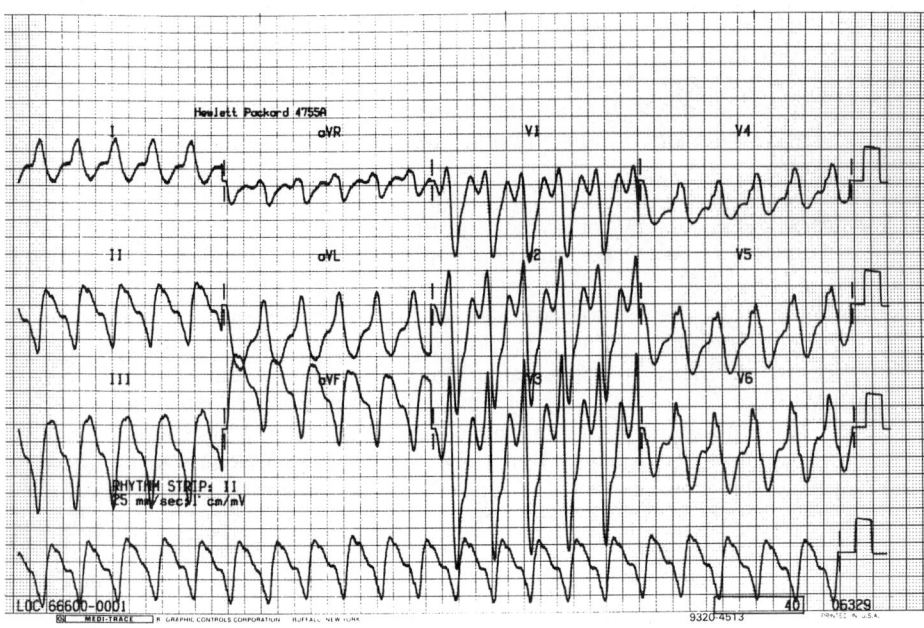

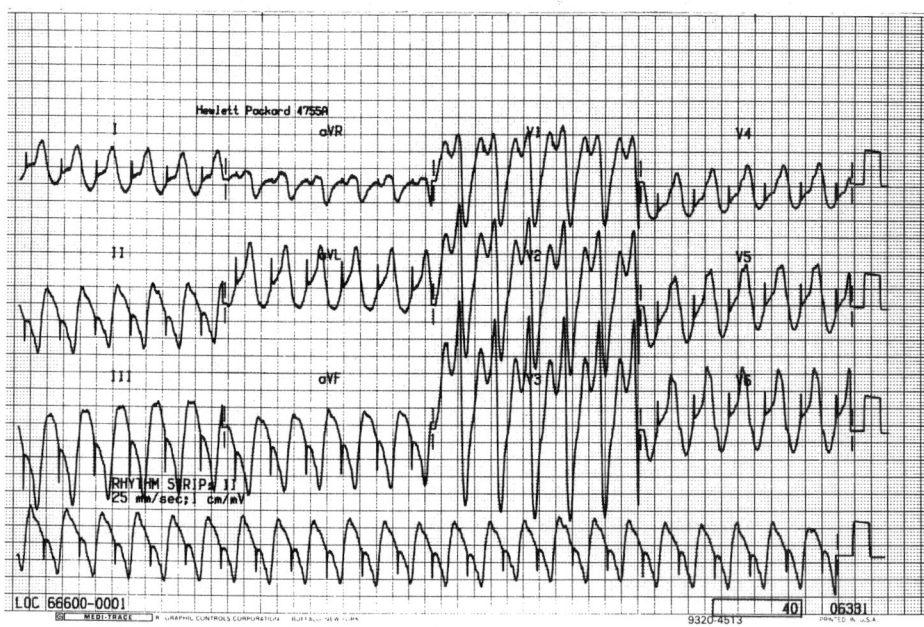

Figure 19–9. Upper portion, Twelve-lead ECG of spontaneous ventricular tachycardia. *Lower portion,* Pace-mapping. Twelve-lead ECG with pacing through a steerable catheter in the left ventricle mimicking the ventricular tachycardia morphology.

rhythmias that are more difficult to reproduce and may not have the same prognostic relevance.[52, 54] Apparent control after antiarrhythmic testing does not always ensure a favorable outcome in the long term.

Finally, it should be emphasized that patients with nonsustained ventricular tachycardia without heart disease or individuals who simply have frequent single or paired ventricular premature systoles should not be candidates for routine electrophysiologic testing. It appears that left ventricular function primarily determines whether such patients will have good or poor long-term prognoses.[49] Several ongoing clinical trials are addressing the benefits and risks of electrophysiologic guided chronic therapy in such patients.[55, 56]

TORSADE DE POINTES

The term *torsade de pointes* refers to a ventricular tachyarrhythmia characterized by QRS complexes of changing amplitude and axes that appear to twist around the isoelectric line.[57] The rates are rather rapid (often more than 200 beats/min) and the QRS complexes polymorphic (Fig. 19–10). This form of polymorphic tachycardia often occurs in the setting of a long QT (or QT_c or QTU) interval, and some consider that this feature is necessary if an arrhythmia is to be classified as torsade de pointes. Torsade de pointes may occur as part of a congenital QT prolongation syndrome but more commonly is precipitated by factors that prolong the QT interval, such as hypokalemia, class IA antiarrhythmic drugs, bradycardia, other medications, toxins, myocarditis, or ischemia, alone or in combination. This arrhythmia is frequently initiated by a premature ventricular beat occurring relatively late in diastole, particularly after a long-short sequence, associated with a prolonged TU wave. Commonly, spontaneous termination occurs. Occasionally, torsade de pointes may degenerate into ventricular fibrillation.

One of the most significant pathophysiologic features of the various forms of polymorphic ventricular tachycardia is the presence or absence of delayed repolarization, and this also has critical implications for therapy.[58, 59] When the QT interval is strictly within normal limits and polymorphic ventricular tachycardia persists or recurs despite attention to repletion of potassium, magnesium, and other remediable factors, these arrhythmias may respond favorably to conventional antiarrhythmic drugs, including the class IB agents and, if necessary, amiodarone. However, the administration of a class IA drug or agent that further prolongs the QT interval to patients with classic torsade de pointes associated with delayed repolarization may lead to disastrous consequences. In such

cases, after withdrawing any potentially offending agent and repletion of potassium and magnesium, acute management options include atrial, ventricular, or AV pacing, often at rates of 90 to 110 beats/min, and administration of isoproterenol, or paradoxically, a β-blocker if bradycardia is not present, and, in some cases, intravenous magnesium even when the serum levels are normal. Magnesium sulfate has been given intravenously for this specific purpose with success[60] and may be sufficient to suppress torsade de pointes until the effects of the offending drug have dissipated, as evidenced in part by a shortening of the QTU interval. One recommended dosing regimen is an initial 2-g bolus. In patients with an inadequate response, this bolus is followed by a second bolus 5 to 15 minutes later, and subsequently, a continuous infusion of 3 to 10 mg/min. The most common side effect is a flushed sensation, but patient monitoring for a more serious potential adverse effect, hypotension, is warranted.

In congenital QT prolongation syndromes, in which torsade de pointes is recurrent, chronic treatment with β-blockers alone, or in combination with atrial or AV pacing, may be useful. More definitive proce-

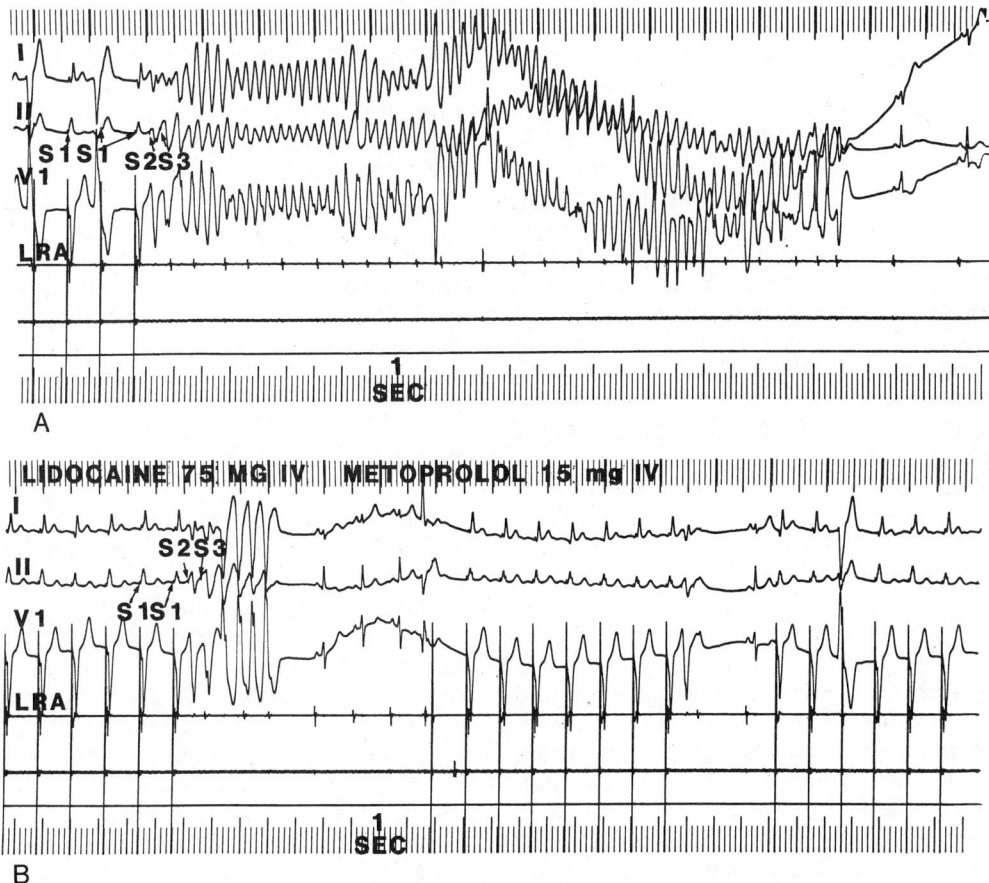

Figure 19–10. A, Programmed ventricular stimulation with two extrastimuli (S2, S3) inducing polymorphic ventricular tachycardia in a patient with long QT syndrome. B, After administration of lidocaine, 75 mg, and metoprolol, 15 mg, intravenously, there is failure of programmed pacing to produce more than a few beats of tachycardia despite the persistence of isolated premature beats occurring spontaneously.

dures including left stellectomy and left cervicothoracic sympathetic ganglionectomy have also been used with success.[61]

VENTRICULAR FIBRILLATION AND VENTRICULAR FLUTTER
Clinical Features

Ventricular flutter and fibrillation occur in a variety of cardiovascular diseases, most often associated with acute coronary insufficiency and ischemia or advanced cardiomyopathic processes. These lethal arrhythmias may also result from electrolyte imbalance, hypoxia, or antiarrhythmic drugs and perhaps from autonomic-neural and psychologic factors as well. Patients who have been resuscitated from sudden death may not show any evidence of coronary artery disease.[62-64] Furthermore, individuals who demonstrate no myocardial necrosis even in the presence of coronary artery disease remain at high risk for subsequent ventricular fibrillation. These patients require electrophysiologic studies and administration of appropriate antiarrhythmic drugs,[63] and in some cases consideration for antiarrhythmic surgery or, even more commonly, an automatic implantable cardioverter-defibrillator.

Electrocardiographic Features

Except for artifact and the rare case of WPW syndrome and rapid anomalous AV conduction during atrial fibrillation or flutter, the ECG recognition of ventricular flutter or fibrillation is usually straightforward. These rhythms usually terminate fatally within minutes unless precordial shock is delivered promptly; rarely, however, spontaneous conversion has been documented after more than 30 seconds of apparent ventricular fibrillation. Ventricular flutter resembles a sine wave with no isoelectric baseline between QRS complexes, but it can be very polymorphic as well. Rates of 150 to 350 beats/min usually are observed, but rates less than 250 beats/min tend to be associated with antiarrhythmic drug use or agonal conditions. Ventricular fibrillation manifests as rapid chaotic wavelets, often of varying amplitude, with no associated effective ventricular contractions.

Experimentally, ventricular fibrillation often occurs after abrupt proximal occlusion of a major coronary artery; even within the first 30 minutes of ischemia or infarction, arrhythmias cluster into an early and delayed phase, presumably reflecting different mechanisms.[65] In experimental models, abrupt reperfusion is also associated with a flurry of arrhythmias, including ventricular fibrillation, particularly if abrupt and complete reperfusion occurs within approximately 20 to 40 minutes of a major coronary occlusion.[66, 67] In experimental preparations, most antiarrhythmic agents are relatively ineffective in preventing ventricular fibrillation under these conditions,[68] but antiischemic interventions, including those decreasing myocardial oxygen requirements, appear to be par-

tially protective. Nevertheless, in clinical experience, ventricular fibrillation is relatively uncommon during thrombolytic therapy, even when instituted within the first hour after the onset of symptoms. Experimentally and clinically, in the subacute period of hours to days after myocardial infarction, "accelerated idioventricular rhythms" are common and apparently related to enhanced impulse formation in Purkinje fibers surviving in proximity to regions of infarction. These rhythms usually can be suppressed by most antiarrhythmic drugs, including lidocaine and procainamide, if indicated.[69] However, occasionally accelerated idioventricular rhythms are refractory to all interventions. Generally, these rhythms do not degenerate to ventricular fibrillation and only occasionally require suppression to improve hemodynamic stability. The role for prophylactic antiarrhythmic agents, either in the prehospital, acute, or subacute phase of myocardial infarction, is still controversial, but most physicians do not advocate such acute therapy other than β-blockade, based on recent meta-analyses.

In ambulatory patients, ventricular fibrillation only rarely occurs as a primary rhythm abnormality; most commonly, it follows seconds or minutes of ventricular tachycardia. In this setting, most often involving patients with chronic coronary artery disease or cardiomyopathy, the arrhythmias appear to have a reentrant mechanism and are potentially amenable to treatment and prophylaxis using drugs, devices, and various ablative procedures. Such patients can benefit from treatment only if their condition is identified before episodes of ventricular fibrillation or if they are successfully resuscitated from initial episodes. Unless a readily reversible or preventable precipitating cause (e.g., myocardial ischemia or abnormal electrolytes) can be identified in these patients, prognosis after cardiopulmonary resuscitation is guarded. For patients resuscitated from in-hospital cardiac arrest, the outlook appears even more dismal; in one typical series, only 14% of such patients lived.[70]

Treatment

Clearly, ventricular tachyarrhythmias present a most challenging and dangerous problem. Because these rhythms can rapidly deteriorate into ventricular fibrillation and are usually associated with marked hemodynamic deterioration, prompt therapy is necessary and appropriate follow-up mandatory. When the rhythm has been identified as a wide QRS tachycardia, probably ventricular in origin, the hemodynamic status of the patient must be addressed immediately. Occasionally, a sudden blow to the chest (chest thump) may terminate ventricular tachycardia (Fig. 19–11) and other reentrant tachycardias. However, some risk of precipitating ventricular fibrillation accompanies the delivery of such an impulse without benefit of synchronization with the QRS complex. In most cases, cardioversion is clearly the single most effective intervention. Prompt cardioversion may be mandatory in some instances; in others, the clinician

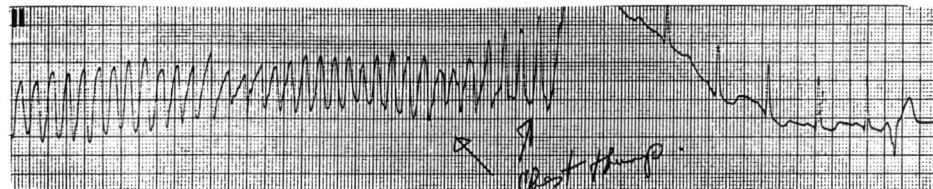

Figure 19–11. Rapid ventricular tachycardia converting to sinus rhythm with a chest thump.

may have time to attempt an intravenous bolus of lidocaine, 1 to 3 mg/kg loading dose in divided doses over 20 minutes followed by 1 to 4 mg/min maintenance infusion, as an initial approach. Alternatively, intravenous procainamide can be given using a 5 to 15 mg/kg loading dose over 20 to 60 minutes followed by a 2 to 6 mg/min maintenance infusion if lidocaine alone fails to terminate or prevent recurrence of the ventricular tachyarrhythmia or if the rhythm recurs after precordial shock. Outside the setting of an acute ischemic insult, procainamide rather than lidocaine probably should be the drug of first choice for treating ventricular tachycardia. Failure of class I antiarrhythmic agents such as lidocaine or procainamide to prevent recurrence of the ventricular tachyarrhythmia is not uncommon, and supplemental therapy may be required. Failure to recognize a wide QRS tachycardia as ventricular tachycardia and subsequently to administer a drug such as intravenous verapamil may also have deleterious consequences, including precipitation of ventricular fibrillation.[71] Adenosine, however, can be used diagnostically with considerably less risk of hemodynamic collapse, although certain uncommon forms of ventricular tachycardia may also terminate in response to adenosine, mimicking a supraventricular tachyarrhythmia.

Alternative or subsequent intravenous antiarrhythmic drug interventions include the use of β-blocking agents such as propranolol, 0.5 to 1.0 mg every 5 minutes to a maximum of 0.2 mg/kg, or the addition of bretylium, either intravenously or intramuscularly 5 to 10 mg/kg every 6 hours or a 0.5 to 4.0 mg/min (usually 1 to 2 mg/min) continuous drip of bretylium. After bretylium has been given, continued administration of lidocaine or procainamide may be unnecessary. In some instances, the combined use of lidocaine and procainamide or a class I antiarrhythmic agent and a β-blocking agent or bretylium may be required. Overdrive pacing of either the atria or ventricles may be successful in some patients, particularly in those with recurrent ventricular tachyarrhythmias associated with long QT intervals or in whom proarrhythmic effects of a class I or II antiarrhythmic agent are suspected. On an investigational basis, intravenous amiodarone has been administered as a bolus of 5 to 10 mg/kg given over 20 minutes to 2 hours and followed by a continuous drip of 300 to 600 mg over the next 24 hours for the acute treatment of refractory ventricular tachyarrhythmias. Hypotension, asystole, and conduction block are major concerns with rapid infusion of amiodarone. Digoxin antibodies should be considered in the acute management of recurrent ventricular tachyarrhythmias when digoxin toxicity is implicated.

Patients with recurrent ventricular tachyarrhythmias invariably require a precise pharmacologic program, a definitive procedure, or possibly an automatic implantable cardioverter-defibrillator after acute ventricular arrhythmias have been terminated. Electrophysiologic-directed pharmacologic therapy is successful in some 50% to 90% of selected patient populations for successful long-term (at least 1 to 3 years) management of ventricular tachyarrhythmias.[50, 72–74] However, controversies remain regarding the relative and combined validity of invasive versus noninvasive approaches to long-term management of these patients; the sensitivity, specificity, and predictive value of various electrophysiologic testing protocols; the appropriate end points of electrophysiologic testing; and the value of acute drug testing with intravenous formulations of some of the newer agents, of acute testing of oral drugs with active metabolites, of testing at all with some drugs (e.g., amiodarone), and of crossover from one drug to another within the same class.[75–78]

Although some answers are evolving, resolution and consensus are lacking on many of these and other issues. Tocainide and mexiletine (class IB) are similar to lidocaine structurally but are not identical with respect to efficacy and adverse effects.[77] The class IC agents flecainide, propafenone, and moricizine are extremely potent in suppressing premature ventricular beats; they have a relatively high propensity to proarrhythmia, particularly in patients with compromised ventricular function. In addition, they are negative inotropes. Their use in these patients without invasive electrophysiologic testing for guidance was found to increase the incidence of sudden cardiac death and recurrent ventricular tachyarrhythmias. In the Cardiac Arrhythmia Suppression Trial (CAST), these drugs were associated with a marked increase in mortality in patients after myocardial infarction.[25, 38] Amiodarone may be the single most effective agent, but it has such serious adverse effects and prolonged pharmacokinetics that its use has remained restricted to refractory cases in the United States. Furthermore, the intravenous preparation is still undergoing clinical investigation and is not readily available. Sotalol, a class III agent with β-blocker actions, appears promising as chronic therapy for selected patients with ventricular tachyarrhythmias. In one trial, sotalol was found more effective in preventing death and recurrent arrhythmias when compared with six class I antiarrhythmic drugs. However, of all the agents tested, sotalol also was associated with the most episodes of torsade de pointes.[78] Drug combinations also may have utility but, like monotherapy, require individual empirical titration and

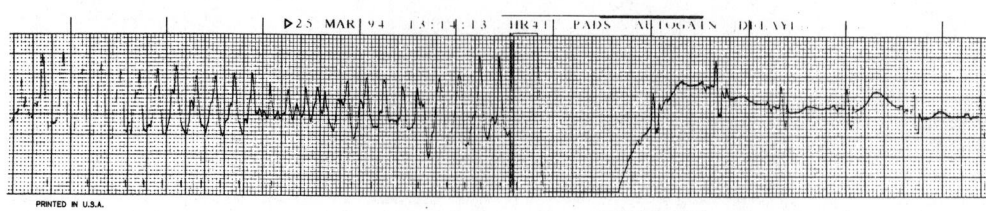

Figure 19–12. Ventricular fibrillation converting to sinus rhythm with a 20-J shock delivered by an implantable cardioverter-defibrillator.

caution to avoid additive adverse effects. Seemingly effective combinations include β-blockers plus class IA agents, or a class IA plus a class IB agent, particularly mexiletine. When amiodarone is used with other antiarrhythmic agents, an additional consideration is pharmacokinetic interaction, with increased drug levels of procainamide, quinidine, phenytoin, digoxin, and other drugs already recognized.[79, 80]

Additional options are also emerging as practical realities for patients, including catheter ablative procedures, antiarrhythmia surgery, and implantable tiered-therapy antitachycardia devices (combination of an antitachycardia pacemaker and a cardioverter-defibrillator) (Fig. 19–12). In the latter case, management of these patients requires knowledge and consideration of the device as well as of the presenting arrhythmia to avoid inadvertent patient shock or rapid pacing or failure of shocks to defibrillate effectively. For example, administration of an antiarrhythmic drug to such a patient may increase the defibrillation threshold beyond the capabilities of the defibrillator. Thus, an expert must be consulted to manage patients with implanted antiarrhythmic devices. Finally, interest is evolving in more widespread availability and application of layperson-assisted external countershock for the treatment of life-threatening arrhythmias causing cardiovascular collapse.[81] However, specific algorithms will have to be developed to ensure maximum benefit while minimizing the risk of inadvertently doing harm.

Acknowledgment

We gratefully acknowledge the contribution of Leonard S. Dreifus, M.D., to the chapter on "Acute Tachyarrhythmias" published in the first edition of this book, upon which this chapter is based.

REFERENCES

1. Sharma AD, Klein GJ, Yee R: Intravenous adenosine triphosphate during wide QRS complex tachycardia: Therapeutic efficacy, and diagnostic utility. Am J Med 88:337, 1990.
2. Jackman WM, Beckman KJ, McClelland JH, et al: Treatment of supraventricular tachycardia due to atrioventricular nodal reentry by radiofrequency catheter ablation of slow-pathway conduction. N Engl J Med 327:313, 1992.
3. Jarayeri MR, Hempe SL, Sra JS, et al: Selective transcatheter ablation of the fast and slow pathways using radiofrequency energy in patients with atrioventricular nodal reentrant tachycardia. Circulation 85:1318, 1992.
4. Iinuma H, Dreifus LS, Mazgaleo T, et al: Role of the perinodal region in atrioventricular reentry: Evidence in an isolated rabbit heart preparation. J Am Coll Cardiol 2:465, 1983.
5. Denes P, Wu D, Dhingra R, et al: Dual AV nodal pathways. A common electrophysiologic response. Br Heart J 37:1069, 1975.
6. Denes P, Wu D, Dhingra RC, et al: Demonstration of dual AV nodal pathway in patients with paroxysmal supraventricular tachycardia. Circulation 48:549, 1973.
7. Wolff L, Parkinson J, White P: Bundle branch block with short PR interval in healthy young people prone to paroxysmal tachycardia. Am Heart J 5:685, 1930.
8. McIntosh-Yellin NL, Drew BJ, Scheinman MM: Safety and efficacy of central intravenous bolus administration of adenosine for termination of supraventricular tachycardia. J Am Coll Cardiol 22:741, 1993.
9. Belhassen B, Pelleg A, Shoshani D, Laniado S: Atrial fibrillation induced by adenosine triphosphate. Am J Cardiol 53:1405, 1984.
10. Jackman WM, Wang XZ, Friday KJ, et al: Catheter ablation of accessory atrioventricular pathways (Wolff-Parkinson-White syndrome) by radiofrequency current. N Engl J Med 324:1605, 1991.
11. Allessie MA, Bonke FIM: Direct demonstration of sinus node reentry in the rabbit heart. Circ Res 44:557, 1979.
12. Satake S, Bianchi J, Dreifus LS, et al: Tachycardia and apparent sinoatrial block due to concealed sinus node reentry. PACE 6:229, 1983.
13. Han J, Malozzi AM, Moe GK: Sinoatrial reciprocation in the isolated rabbit heart. Circ Res 22:355, 1968.
14. Ogawa S, Dreifus LS, Oswick MJ: Longitudinal dissociation of Bachmann's bundle activation from the right pulmonary artery: A new technique for atrial mapping and the study of supraventricular tachycardia. Am J Cardiol 41:1089, 1978.
15. Ogawa S, Dreifus LS, Kitchen JG, et al: Catheter recording of Bachmann's bundle activation from the right pulmonary artery: A new technique for atrial mapping and the study of supraventricular tachycardia. Am J Cardiol 41:1089, 1978.
16. Lewis T: Paroxysmal tachycardia. Heart 1:42, 1909.
17. Koplik H: Paroxysmal tachycardia in children. Am J Med Sci 154:834, 1917.
18. Lown B, Marcus JF, Levin H: Digitalis and atrial tachycardias with block: A year's experience. N Engl J Med 260:301, 1959.
19. Lown B, Wyatt NF, Levin H: Paroxysmal atrial tachycardia with block. Circulation 21:129, 1960.
20. Dreifus LS, Katz M, Watanabe Y, et al: Clinical significance of disorders of impulse formation and conduction in the atrioventricular junction. Am J Cardiol 11:384, 1963.
21. Scher DL, Arsura EL: Multifocal atrial tachycardia: Mechanisms, clinical correlates, and treatment. Am Heart J 118:574, 1989.
22. Feld GK, Fleck PP, Chen P-S, et al: Radiofrequency catheter ablation for the treatment of human type I atrial flutter: Identification of a critical zone in the reentrant circuit by endocardial mapping techniques. Circulation 86:1233, 1992.
23. Vetter VL, Harowitz CN: Electrophysiologic residua and sequelae of surgery for congenital heart disease. Am J Cardiol 50:588, 1982.
24. Middlekauff HR, Wiener I, Stevenson WG: Low-dose amiodarone for atrial fibrillation. Am J Cardiol 72:75f, 1993.
25. Echt DS, Liebson PR, Mitchell LB, et al: Mortality and morbidity in patients receiving encainide, flecainide, and placebo—The Cardiac Arrhythmia Suppression Trial. N Engl J Med 324:781, 1991.
26. Alboni P, Razzolini R, Scarfo S, et al: Hemodynamic effects of oral sotalol during both sinus rhythm and atrial fibrillation. J Am Coll Cardiol 22:1373, 1993.
27. Henry WL, Marganroth J, Pearlman AS, et al: Relation between

echocardiographically determined left atrial size and atrial fibrillation. Circulation 53:273, 1976.

28. Mancini GBJ, Weinberg DM: Cardioversion of atrial fibrillation: A retrospective analysis of the safety and value of anticoagulation. Cardiovasc Rev Rep 10:18, 1990.

29. Olshansky B, Waldo AL: Atrial fibrillation: Update on mechanism, diagnosis, and management. Mod Concepts Cardiovasc Dis 56:23, 1987.

30. Mazgalev T, Dreifus LS, Bianchi J, et al: Atrioventricular nodal conduction during atrial fibrillation in rabbit heart. Am J Physiol 243:H754, 1982.

31. Michelson EL, Porterfield JK, Das G, et al: A comparison of esmolol and verapamil in the treatment of atrial fibrillation. J Am Coll Cardiol 7:157A, 1986.

32. Rankin AC, Oldroyd KG, Chong E, et al: Value and limitations of adenosine in the diagnosis and treatment of narrow and broad complex tachycardia. Br Heart J 62:195, 1989.

33. Salerno DM, Dias VC, Kleger RE, et al: Efficacy and safety of intravenous diltiazem for treatment of atrial fibrillation and atrial flutter. Am J Cardiol 63:1046, 1989.

34. Cox JL, Boineau JP, Schuessler RB, et al: Five year experience with the maze procedure for atrial fibrillation. Ann Thorac Surg 56:814, 1993.

35. Watanabe Y, Dreifus LS: Cardiac Arrhythmias. Electrophysiological Basis for Clinical Interpretation. New York: Grune & Stratton, 1977, p 78.

36. Watanabe Y, Dreifus LS: Sites of impulse formation within the atrioventricular junction of the rabbit. Circ Res 22:717, 1968.

37. Kennedy HL, Whitlock JA, Sprague MK, et al: Long-term follow-up of asymptomatic healthy subjects with frequent and complex ventricular ectopy. N Engl J Med 312:193, 1985.

38. Epstein AE, Hallstrom AP, Rogers WJ, et al, for the CAST investigators: Mortality following ventricular arrhythmia suppression by encainide, flecainide, and moricizine after myocardial infarction—the original design concept of the Cardiac Arrhythmia Suppression Trial (CAST). JAMA 270:2452, 1993.

39. Bigger JT Jr, Fleiss JL, Kleiger R, et al: The relationships among ventricular arrhythmias, left ventricular dysfunction and mortality in the 2 years after myocardial infarction. Circulation 69:250, 1984.

40. Follansbee WP, Michelson EL, Morganroth J: Nonsustained ventricular tachycardia in ambulatory patients: Characteristics and association with sudden cardiac death. Ann Intern Med 92:741, 1980.

41. Kostis JB, Byington R, Freedman LM, et al: Prognostic significance of ventricular ectopic activity in survivors of acute myocardial infarction. J Am Coll Cardiol 10:231, 1987.

42. DiMarco JP, Garan H, Hawthorne JW, et al: Role of cardiac electrophysiologic techniques in recurrent syncope of unknown cause. Ann Intern Med 95:542, 1981.

43. Teichmen SL, Felder SD, Matos JA, et al: The valve of electrophysiologic studies in syncope of undetermined origin: Report of 150 cases. Am Heart J 110:469, 1985.

44. Wellens HJJ, Bar FWHM, Lie KI: The value of the electrocardiogram in the differential diagnosis of a tachycardia with a widened QRS complex. Am J Med 64:27, 1978.

45. Kindwall KE, Brown J, Josephson ME: Electrocardiographic criteria for ventricular tachycardia in wide complex left bundle branch block morphology tachycardias. Am J Cardiol 61:1279, 1988.

46. Brugada P, Brugada J, Mont L, et al: A new approach to the differential diagnosis of a regular tachycardia with a wide QRS complex. Circulation 83:1649, 1991.

47. Fisher JD, Kim SG, Ferrick KJ, et al: Programmed electrical stimulation protocols: Variations on a theme. PACE 15:2180, 1992.

48. Sulpizi AM, Friehling TD, Kowey PR: Value of electrophysiologic testing in patients with non-sustained ventricular tachycardia. Am J Cardiol 59:841, 1987.

49. Wilber DJ, Olshansky B, Moran JF, et al: Electrophysiolgic testing and nonsustained ventricular tachycardia: Use and limitations in patients with coronary artery disease and impaired ventricular function. Circulation 82:350, 1990.

50. Morady F, Scheinman MM, Hess DS, et al: Electrophysiologic testing in the management of survivors of out-of-hospital cardiac arrest. Am J Cardiol 51:85, 1983.

51. Morady F, DiCarlo L, Winston S, et al: Clinical features and prognosis of patients with out-of-hospital cardiac arrest and a normal electrophysiologic study. J Am Coll Cardiol 4:39, 1984.

52. Josephson ME, Almendral JM, Buxton AE, Marchlinski FE: Mechanisms of ventricular tachycardia. Circulation 75(Supp III):41, 1987.

53. Mitrani RD, Biblo LA, Carlson MD, et al: Multiple monomorphic ventricular tachycardia configurations predict failure of antiarrhythmic drug therapy guided by electrophysiologic study. J Am Coll Cardiol 22:1117, 1993.

54. Naccarelli GV, Prystowsky EN, Jackman WM, et al: Role of electrophysiologic testing in managing patients who have ventricular tachycardia unrelated to coronary artery disease. Am J Cardiol 50:165, 1982.

55. Buxton AE, Fisher JD, Josephson ME, et al: Prevention of sudden death in patients with coronary artery disease: The multicenter unsustained tachycardia trial (MUSTT). Prog Cardiovasc Dis 36:215, 1993.

56. Klein H, Trappe HJ, Fieguth HG, Nisam S: Prospective studies evaluating prophylactic ICD therapy for high risk patients with coronary artery disease. PACE 16(II):564, 1993.

57. Dessertne F: La tachycardie ventriculaire a deux foyers opposes variables. Arch Mal Coeur 59:263, 1966.

58. Dontaine G, Frank R, Grosgogeat Y: Torsade de pointes: Definition and management. Mod Concepts Cardiovasc Dis 51:103, 1982.

59. Soffer J, Dreifus LS, Michelson EL: Polymorphous ventricular tachycardia associated with normal and long Q-T intervals. Am J Cardiol 49:2021, 1982.

60. Tzivoni D, Banai S, Schuger C, et al: Treatment of torsade de pointes with magnesium sulfate. Circulation 77:392, 1988.

61. Locati E, Schwartz PJ, Moss AJ, et al: Long-term survival after cervico-thoracic sympathectomy in high risk long QT syndrome patients with refractory ventricular arrhythmias. J Am Coll Cardiol 7:235a, 1986.

62. Eisenberg MS, Hallstrom AP, Copass MK, et al: Treatment of ventricular fibrillation. JAMA 251:1723, 1984.

63. Swerdlow CD, Winkle RA, Mason JW: Determinants of survival in patients with ventricular tachyarrhythmias. N Engl J Med 308:1436, 1983.

64. Lesch M, Kehoe RF: Predictability of sudden cardiac death. N Engl J Med 310:255, 1984.

65. Kaplinsky E, Ogawa S, Balke C, et al: Two periods of early ventricular arrhythmia in the canine myocardial infarction model. Circulation 60:397, 1979.

66. Kaplinsky E, Ogawa S, Michelson EL, et al: Instantaneous and delayed ventricular arrhythmias after reperfusion of acutely ischemic myocardium: Evidence for multiple mechanisms. Circulation 63:333, 1981.

67. Balke CW, Kaplinsky E, Michelson EL, et al: Reperfusion ventricular tachyarrhythmias: Correlation with antecedent coronary artery occlusion tachyarrhythmias and duration of myocardial ischemia. Am Heart J 101:449, 1981.

68. Naito M, Michelson EL, Kmetzo JJ, et al: Failure of antiarrhythmic drugs to prevent experimental reperfusion ventricular fibrillation. Circulation 63:70, 1981.

69. David D, Michelson EL, Dreifus LS: The role of animal models in electrophysiologic studies of life-threatening arrhythmias. PACE 9:896, 1986.

70. Bedell SE, Delbanco TJ, Cook EF, et al: Survival after cardiopulmonary resuscitation in the hospital. N Engl J Med 309:569, 1981.

71. Stewart RB, Bardy GH, Green HL: Wide complex tachycardia: Misdiagnosis and outcome after emergent therapy. Ann Intern Med 104:766, 1986.

72. Horowitz LN, Josephson ME, Farshidi A, et al: Recurrent sustained ventricular tachycardia. 3. Role of the electrophysiologic study in selecting antiarrhythmic drugs. Circulation 58:986, 1978.

73. Waller TJ, Kay HR, Spielman SR, et al: Reduction in sudden death and total mortality by antiarrhythmic therapy evaluated by electrophysiologic drug testing: Criteria of efficacy in patients with sustained ventricular tachycardia. J Am Coll Cardiol 10:83, 1987.

74. Steinbeck G, Andresen D, Bach P, et al: A comparison of

electrophysiologically guided antiarrhythmic drug therapy with beta-blocker therapy in patients with symptomatic, sustained ventricular tachyarrhythmias. N Engl J Med 327:987, 1992.

75. Mason JW, for the ESVEM Investigators: A comparison of electrophysiologic testing with Holter monitoring to predict antiarrhythmic drug efficacy for ventricular tachyarrhythmias. N Engl J Med 329:445, 1993.

76. Kadish AH, Buxton AE, Waxman HL, et al: Usefulness of electrophysiologic studies to determine the clinical tolerance of arrhythmia recurrences during amiodarone therapy. J Am Coll Cardiol 10:90, 1987.

77. Reiter MJ, Easley AR, Mann DE: Efficacy of class I b (lidocaine-like) antiarrhythmic agents for prevention of sustained ventricular tachycardia secondary to coronary artery disease. Am J Cardiol 59:1319, 1987.

78. Mason JW, for the ESVEM Investigators: A comparison of seven antiarrhythmic drugs in patients with ventricular tachyarrhythmias. N Engl J Med 329:452, 1993.

79. Mason JW: Amiodarone. N Engl J Med 316:455, 1987.

80. Soal AK, Werner JA, Greene HL, et al: Effect of amiodarone on serum quinidine and procainamide levels. Am J Cardiol 53:1264, 1984.

81. Weaver WD, Cobb LA, Hallstrom AP, et al: Factors influencing survival after out-of-hospital cardiac arrest. J Am Coll Cardiol 7:752, 1986.

CHAPTER 20

Use of Cardiovascular Drugs During Cardiopulmonary Resuscitation

Joseph P. Ornato, M.D., Edgar R. Gonzalez, Pharm.D., and Allan S. Jaffe, M.D.

The time from onset of cardiopulmonary arrest until restoration of an effective spontaneous circulation remains the single most important determinant of long-term, neurologically intact survival. For this reason, prompt defibrillation of ventricular fibrillation or pulseless ventricular tachycardia, when either rhythm is present, alters patient outcome more than pharmacologic maneuvers alone. However, drug treatment may be necessary during cardiopulmonary resuscitation (CPR) if initial efforts are unsuccessful.

Drugs often have to be given during resuscitation without adequate knowledge of the patient's history, preexisting conditions, or current medication. The interval before initiation of CPR is often highly variable and may not even be known. Problems with vascular access can delay initial drug administration, and the poor blood flow generated by CPR can compromise drug delivery to target end-organs. Biologic drug actions may be altered because of acidosis, hypoxemia, downregulation of receptors, target end-organ damage, impaired metabolism and excretion, and drug interactions.

PHARMACOKINETICS AND PHARMACODYNAMICS

The pharmacokinetics of most drugs are altered extensively during closed-chest CPR.[1] Severe cardiac dysfunction and circulatory collapse redistribute blood to the highly perfused organs (brain and myocardium), altering the volume of distribution of most drugs.[2] The route of administration also affects a drug's pharmacokinetic profile.[1, 3] During closed-chest compression, cardiac output falls to approximately one quarter to one third of normal,[4] and a greater percentage of blood flow is distributed to the upper part of the body (the brain and upper extremities).[2, 4] The reduced total flow and consequent prolongation of circulation time decrease venous return and slow drug delivery from the periphery into the central circulation. Thus, drug administration into the central circulation results in more rapid drug delivery to the myocardium and brain than peripheral intravenous (IV) injection.[5-12]

Central versus Peripheral Drug Administration

Little is known about the relationship between the site of drug delivery and drug bioavailability during CPR. Kuhn et al.[7] injected indocyanine green dye into the peripheral or central veins of patients who were in refractory cardiac arrest (average cardiac output, 1.3 L/min) and studied the appearance of the dye in the arterial circulation. Peak femoral artery dye concentration occurred in 90 seconds with peripheral venous injection, compared with only 30 seconds after central venous administration. Circulation time was slower with peripheral (>4 minutes) compared with central venous (3 minutes) drug administration.

Administration of equivalent drug doses of epinephrine[13] or lidocaine[5] through a central vein results in faster arterial drug appearance, higher peak arterial drug concentration, and more potent biologic effect compared with their administration into the peripheral circulation. Although there have been reports[12] suggesting that there is little biologic difference in drug effect when agents are administered by IV, intrapulmonary, and/or intracardiac central routes, a preponderance of investigators have shown that supradiaphragmatic central venous drug administration is superior to other central routes during closed-chest compression.[8, 14, 15] The use of a 20-ml saline bolus IV immediately after a drug is injected peripherally decreases its circulation time and improves its peak arterial concentration during cardiac arrest in a dog model and may improve drug delivery in patients.[16]

The American Heart Association's Guidelines do

not recommend the immediate placement of a central line but, rather, insertion of a large-bore catheter in the antecubital fossa. Because this site is above the diaphragm, it should lead to adequate drug delivery during CPR.[9, 10] It should also help avoid the following:

1. Potential problems of drug toxicity that could develop as a result of the rapid attainment of high drug concentrations[1, 15]
2. Interruption of ventilation and compression during CPR needed to place a central line
3. Inherent morbidity associated with the placement of central venous lines

However, distal wrist and hand veins are unlikely to produce efficient drug delivery when there is intense vasoconstriction. Furthermore, if a central venous line is in place at the onset of the resuscitation, it should be used for drug administration.

Whenever drugs are administered from a peripheral IV site, the extremity should be elevated and a 20-ml bolus of normal saline given to facilitate access of the agent to the central circulation.[9, 10, 16] If spontaneous circulation cannot be restored with drugs injected through peripheral veins, a central IV line should be established for further drug delivery.

Drug Diluents During CPR

Administration of IV fluids can be used to expand blood volume and to keep veins open for drug administration during CPR. Glucose-containing fluids have been the traditional vehicle for drug delivery during CPR and were thought to be beneficial because they would treat hypoglycemia if present. Recently, the administration of glucose-containing fluids during CPR has become controversial because of accumulating evidence that hyperglycemia increases production of lactic acid through anaerobic metabolism, which is detrimental to ischemic neurons.[17, 18] D'Alecy et al.[19] studied the effect of 5% dextrose administration on neurologic outcome after cardiac arrest in dogs. Dogs received 500 ml of either lactated Ringer's (LR) or 5% dextrose in LR (D5LR) prior to arrest, resulting in mean values of 129 mg/dl and 335 mg/dl, respectively. After 8 minutes of fibrillatory arrest, all six dogs who received LR and five of six dogs who had received D5LR were resuscitated. However, 2 hours after resuscitation, and thereafter, the dogs who had received the glucose load had significantly greater neurologic deficits ($p < .05$). The authors concluded that the addition of 5% dextrose significantly increased the morbidity and mortality associated with resuscitation.[19] Other studies in animals suggest that the administration of glucose during cardiac arrest increases the requirements for inotropic support and worsens neurologic outcome and mortality.[17]

Clinical data regarding the use of glucose-containing fluids are inconclusive. There is some evidence in human subjects that clinical outcome after cerebral ischemia is worsened by hyperglycemia.[17]

Patients with strokes and antecedent hyperglycemia have greater neurologic deficits when compared with other stroke patients.[20] In a retrospective study of 430 cardiac arrest victims before hospital admission, Longstreth and Inui[21] found that neurologic recovery was inversely related to the blood glucose level on admission. However, in a prospective follow-up study,[22] it was clear that blood glucose levels rose as a function of the duration of resuscitation. Thus, it is possible that hyperglycemia is a marker of a prolonged resuscitation, and the more severe neurologic deficits are a result rather than a cause of the adverse outcome.

The rise in blood glucose level during resuscitation is related in dogs to impaired glucose utilization. In one study,[23] mean blood glucose values 15 minutes after initiation of CPR ($379 + 114$ mg/dl) were significantly higher than pre-arrest values ($124 + 29$ mg/dl, $p < .01$), perhaps related to a reduction in the mean serum insulin level during CPR ($11.3 + 3.3$ μU/ml), which was significantly lower than the pre-arrest level ($16.2 + 6.0$ μU/ml, $p < .05$). The inappropriately low levels of insulin observed during CPR may adversely affect myocardial glucose utilization. It is known that hypotension reduces the release of insulin from the pancreas.[24] Further study is needed to determine whether there may be a potential role for insulin therapy in cardiac arrest victims with hyperglycemia. Until additional information is available, supplemental administration of glucose should be reserved for patients with documented hypoglycemia. Normal saline has become the preferred diluent for drugs and for intravascular fluid expansion during CPR.

Endotracheal Drug Administration

Some drugs (epinephrine, atropine, lidocaine, naloxone, bretylium, propranolol, and isoproterenol) can be given endotracheally (ET) during resuscitation when IV access cannot be secured.[25-28] In animals, ET-administered epinephrine produces effects on heart rate and blood pressure similar to those of IV epinephrine.[29] In humans, vasoconstriction after ET administration traps epinephrine in the lungs, producing a lower, slightly delayed peak plasma concentration[12, 26] but longer biologic effects[29, 30] than after IV administration. Administration of atropine endotracheally delays its onset of action but does not alter the magnitude of its effect.[27]

Drug dilution is a very important factor in ensuring a good pharmacologic response to ET drug administration.[29, 31] In the past, sterile water (SW) and normal saline (NS) have been popularly used as diluents.[32] The best diluent may depend on the drug that is being administered. For example, Greenberg et al.[32] compared the effects of ET-administered SW and NS on arterial blood gases in dogs. ET administration of SW significantly ($p < .05$) depressed arterial pH and Pa$_{O_2}$ when compared with NS. These investigators[32] concluded that ET administration of NS in dogs produces fewer detrimental effects on arterial blood gases than endotracheal administration of SW.

In contrast, a study by Hahnel et al.[33] produced opposite results. In 12 patients who received ET-administered lidocaine diluted with either SW or NS, serum lidocaine concentrations 5 and 10 minutes after the dose were significantly higher ($p < .05$) in the SW group (2.35 and 2.67 mg/L) when compared with NS (1.59 and 1.88 mg/L). The Pa_{O_2} dropped by 60 mmHg in the NS group and by 40 mmHg in the SW group ($p < .05$). Hahnel et al.[33] concluded that SW produces better absorption of lidocaine and less impairment of oxygenation than NS.

The dose of medication that should be used with ET therapy is controversial. In some studies, a dose as much as ten times greater than the IV dose is needed to duplicate the hemodynamic effects of the IV dose.[34] Because some patients may benefit from larger IV doses of epinephrine, atropine, or lidocaine during CPR,[9, 35-43] current reviews on the topic of ET drug delivery recommend an increase of 2.5 times the IV dose.[43]

Although ET drug delivery uses simple, commonly available medical equipment and is easy to perform,[25] the technique of administration markedly influences the pattern of drug absorption.[31] Most drugs should be diluted in 10 to 20 ml of NS or SW to permit distribution over the largest possible surface area. In adults or children, the mixture should be injected through a catheter or tube that extends just beyond the end of the ET tube. The drug should be injected rapidly, followed by several forceful lung inflations to distribute the material.[31]

Drug incompatibilities are particularly important during resuscitation, because multiple agents often must be administered through a single IV line. If calcium chloride and sodium bicarbonate are given together in the same IV line, calcium carbonate will precipitate. Not all chemical drug interactions are clinically relevant during the brief period of resuscitation. For example, auto-oxidation by alkaline substances (e.g., sodium bicarbonate) reduces the potency of sympathomimetic amines.[44] However, such chemical reactions occur too slowly (generally over 1 to 3 hours) to be of clinical significance if the agents are given by rapid IV injection or by continuous administration through a central line.[44] When a prolonged contact time is anticipated, alkaline solutions should not be mixed with sympathomimetic amines.

VASOPRESSORS

Epinephrine, Methoxamine, and Phenylephrine

Epinephrine, an endogenous catecholamine with both α-β-adrenergic activity, is the vasopressor of choice for use during resuscitation. Epinephrine's potent α_1- and α_2-adrenergic effects improve cerebral blood flow by preventing arterial collapse and increasing peripheral vasoconstriction.[45-48] Epinephrine also enhances coronary perfusion pressure, which is the major deter-

minant of the return of spontaneous circulation after cardiac arrest.[45, 49, 50] An aortic diastolic blood pressure of 30 to 40 mmHg markedly improves survival during resuscitation in animal models.[45, 49-51] Restoration of myocardial blood flow facilitates the resynthesis of high-energy phosphates within myocardial mitochondria and enhances cellular viability and contractile force.[52] However, the increased myocardial blood flow is at least partially antagonized by the increased myocardial oxygen consumption caused by epinephrine's β-adrenergic actions.[53]

The optimal dose of epinephrine to augment aortic diastolic blood pressure in human subjects during closed-chest compression is unknown. The American Heart Association (AHA) currently recommends a 1-mg dose based on studies in dogs weighing approximately 20 kg.[47-50] In a 70-kg man, the current recommendations provide for only 7.5 to 15 μg/kg of epinephrine every 5 minutes.

Studies concluded that dosages higher than 15 μg/kg may be required during closed-chest CPR in animal models.[35-41] Kosnik et al.[35] showed that a dose of epinephrine of 15 μg/kg (the upper range of the recommended human dose) did not maintain an aortic diastolic blood pressure above 40 mmHg during closed-chest compression in dogs. Larger doses (45, 75, and 150 μg/kg) effectively raised aortic diastolic blood pressure. High-dose (10 μg/kg) constant infusions of epinephrine have been shown to increase aortic diastolic blood pressure and coronary blood flow significantly during closed-chest compression in dogs.[36] Epinephrine (0.02, 0.2, and 2 mg/kg) also produced significant dose-dependent improvement in regional myocardial and cerebral blood flow during closed-chest compression in animal models.[37-40] Preliminary data in human subjects suggested a similar dose-dependence with respect to aortic blood pressure.[41]

From these studies, it appeared that higher doses of epinephrine might be required in human adults to improve hemodynamics and achieve successful resuscitation. Optimistic anecdotal case series and retrospective studies published in the late 1980s and early 1990s[54-57] set the stage for prospective, randomized clinical trials.[58-61]

Participants at the 1992 National Conference on CPR and Emergency Cardiac Care (ECC) reviewed preliminary results from four clinical trials.[58-61] Nine different cities provided the prehospital setting for these trials, which involved more than 2400 adult patients. One trial[60] also included in-hospital cardiac arrest. Some of these trials demonstrated increased rates of return of spontaneous circulation with higher doses of epinephrine (0.07 to 0.2 mg/kg), but none of the studies found that there was a statistically significant improvement in survival rate to hospital discharge with higher doses of epinephrine than the 1 to 1.5 mg traditional dose (Table 20–1).

Could higher doses of epinephrine be of value to some subgroups of patients and harmful to others? One of the high-dose epinephrine trials[58] showed a threefold increase in hospital discharge rates in pa-

Reference	HDE Regimen	Hosp Disch HDE	Hosp Disch SDE	p Value
Lindner et al.[58]	5 mg	14%	5%	NS
Stiell et al.[59]	7 mg	3%	5%	.38
Callaham et al.[60]	15 mg	1.7%	1.20%	.83
Brown et al.[61]	0.2 mg/kg	5%	4%	NS

HDE, high-dose epinephrine; Hosp Disch, hospital discharge rate; SDE, standard dose epinephrine.

tients with electromechanical dissociation and asystole when treated with 5 mg versus 1 mg of epinephrine as the initial dose, but this difference did not reach statistical significance. Another study[60] showed that patients older than the age of 65 and those in ventricular fibrillation did better with standard doses of epinephrine. Thus far no consistent differences in survival of any clinical subgroup have held up across the four clinical trials.

Most of the patients who survive cardiac arrest respond to early defibrillation and never receive epinephrine. What percentage of those who fail to respond are salvageable is unclear. However, because patients who are defibrillated did not qualify for these clinical trials, the survival rates of patients studied were low regardless of the dosage of epinephrine. Of some comfort is the fact that these trials did not demonstrate significant harm from higher doses of epinephrine. These studies emphasize the importance of the "standard" early interventions: airway management, chest compression, and rapid defibrillation. They suggest that epinephrine (whether at low or high dosages) as well as other late interventions represent a last desperate effort to resuscitate individuals who have a very poor chance for survival.

Based on available clinical data, there is no reason to alter the initial IV epinephrine dose of 1 mg (10 ml of a 1:10,000 solution) in adults. The use of higher doses of epinephrine after the initial 1-mg dose during resuscitation can be neither recommended nor discouraged. Regardless of which subsequent dose of epinephrine is chosen during resuscitation, epinephrine should be administered at intervals that do not exceed 3 to 5 minutes.[62] If the dose is given by peripheral injection, it should be followed by a 20-ml flush of IV fluid to ensure drug delivery into the central compartment.

The recommended pediatric epinephrine dosage for bradycardia, asystolic, or pulseless arrest is 0.01 mg/kg by the IV or intraosseous route, or 0.1 mg/kg by the ET route. Because one anecdotal case series[63] has suggested that there may be improved neurologic outcome and survival from higher doses of epinephrine in children, the AHA recommends that second and subsequent doses of epinephrine every 3 to 5 minutes should be in the range of 0.1 to 0.2 mg/kg.[9] Clinical trials need to be conducted to determine whether higher doses of epinephrine actually are beneficial.

Comparative studies between epinephrine and agents with only α-adrenergic effects in animals indicate that epinephrine's α-adrenergic effects, not its β-adrenergic effects, are important for the restoration of spontaneous circulation from ventricular fibrillation, asystole, and pulseless electrical activity (formerly known as electromechanical dissociation, or EMD).[40] Pure α-adrenergic agonists appear to be as effective as epinephrine in restoring spontaneous circulation and do not increase myocardial oxygen consumption and thereby produce or exacerbate myocardial ischemia.[36, 48, 64–69] However, studies comparing methoxamine[39] and phenylephrine[37, 70] to epinephrine at doses that raise aortic pressure comparably in experimental animals indicate that pure α-adrenergic agonists do not improve cerebral and myocardial blood flow to the same extent as does epinephrine. It may be that combined αβ-adrenergic stimulation is required to optimize myocardial and cerebral blood flow during closed-chest compression. β-Adrenergically induced dilation of cerebral microvasculature[71] and maintenance of tissue perfusion[37] may be prerequisites for achieving the increased cerebral and myocardial blood flow initiated by α-adrenergic stimulation.[45] For these reasons, although methoxamine (5 to 20 mg IV) or phenylephrine (0.1 to 0.5 mg IV) can be used during resuscitation, epinephrine is still the catecholamine of choice.[9]

Intracardiac administration should be used only during open cardiac compression or when other routes of administration are unavailable. Intracardiac injections increase the risk of coronary artery laceration, cardiac tamponade, and pneumothorax and cause interruption of external chest compression and ventilation.

During cardiac arrest, epinephrine also may be administered by continuous IV infusion. The dose should be comparable to the standard IV dose of epinephrine (1 mg every 3 to 5 minutes). This is accomplished by adding 30 mg of epinephrine hydrochloride (30 ml of a 1:1000 solution) to 250 ml of normal saline or D_5W to run at 100 ml/hr and titrating to the desired hemodynamic end point. Continuous infusions of epinephrine should be administered by central venous access to reduce the risk of extravasation and to ensure good bioavailability.

Epinephrine can also be used as a pressor and a chronotropic agent for patients who are not in cardiac arrest (e.g., septic shock, symptomatic bradycardia), although it is not a first-line agent. Epinephrine hydrochloride, 1 mg (1 ml of a 1:1000 solution), is added to 500 ml of normal saline or D_5W and administered by continuous infusion. The initial dose for adults is 1 μg/min titrated to the desired hemodynamic response (2 to 10 μg/min).

Auto-oxidation of catecholamines and related sympathomimetic compounds is pH dependent. Contact of epinephrine with other drugs that have an alkaline pH (such as sodium bicarbonate) can cause auto-oxidation, but the reaction rate is too slow to be clinically important when epinephrine is given by bolus injection or when it is infused rapidly. Epinephrine should not be added to infusion bags or bottles that contain alkaline solutions.

Even at low doses, epinephrine's positive inotropic and chronotropic effects can precipitate or exacerbate myocardial ischemia. Doses in excess of 20 mg/min or 0.3 mg/kg/min frequently produce hypertension in patients who are not in cardiac arrest. Epinephrine may induce or exacerbate ventricular ectopy, especially in patients who are receiving digitalis.

Dopamine

Dopamine hydrochloride is a chemical precursor of norepinephrine that causes dose-dependent stimulation of dopaminergic, β₁- and α-adrenergic receptors. Dopamine also triggers the release of endogenous norepinephrine. At low doses (1 to 2 µg/kg/min), dopamine produces vasodilation of renal, mesenteric, coronary, and cerebral arteries by direct dopaminergic stimulation. Urine output may increase, whereas heart rate and blood pressure are usually unchanged. Within the dosage range of 2 to 10 µg/kg/min, dopamine stimulates β₁-adrenergic receptors and increases myocardial contractility and cardiac output. Increases in cardiac output reflexly antagonize at least some of dopamine's α-adrenergic–mediated arterial vasoconstriction. This results in little change in systemic vascular resistance. The dose-response curve of the venous vasculature is more shallow, and increases in preload begin at doses as low as 2.5 µg/kg/min.[72] At doses of more than 10 µg/kg/min, dopamine predominantly stimulates α₁-receptors. This results in renal, mesenteric, peripheral arterial, and venous vasoconstriction. Doses higher than 20 µg/kg/min produce hemodynamic effects that are similar to those of norepinephrine.[72] Because of its hemodynamic effects, dopamine is an excellent pressor but is a poor agent to use for the treatment of congestive heart failure with pulmonary congestion.

Dopamine is indicated to treat hemodynamically significant hypotension in the absence of hypovolemia. One reasonable definition for the presence of significant hypotension is a systolic arterial pressure of less than 90 mmHg accompanied by evidence of poor tissue perfusion, oliguria, or changes in mental status. Dopamine should be used at the lowest dose that produces adequate perfusion of vital organs. The presence of increased vascular resistance, pulmonary congestion, or increased preload is a relative contraindication to the use of dopamine. In these settings, dopamine should be used in low doses (1 to 2 µg/ kg/min) to enhance renal blood flow.

Experimental data in animals suggest that a 40-mg dose of dopamine is comparable to a 1-mg dose of epinephrine during closed-chest compression in its ability to increase blood pressure and improve the probability of a successful resuscitation.[73] However, a more recent study,[74] using a model of prolonged cardiac arrest, demonstrates that dopamine is less effective than epinephrine at improving hemodynamics during CPR.

During resuscitation, treatment with dopamine is usually reserved for patients with hypotension and shock that occur after return of spontaneous circulation. It also can be used at low doses to treat bradycardia. When used to treat shock, norepinephrine should be added if more than 20 µg/kg/min is needed to maintain an adequate blood pressure. Gonzalez et al.[75] studied the vasopressor response to incremental doses of IV epinephrine (1, 3, and 5 mg) with and without dopamine (15 µg/kg/min) in nine cardiac arrest victims before hospital admission. Epinephrine alone produced a significant ($p < .05$) dose-dependent vasopressor effect on systolic and diastolic blood pressure. The concomitant administration of epinephrine and dopamine did not produce an additive vasopressor effect.[75]

In the immediate postresuscitation period, higher doses of dopamine may be required to induce the transient hypertension recommended to improve cerebral perfusion. It is important to remember that dopamine's α-adrenergic effects, even at low infusion rates, elevate the pulmonary artery occlusive pressure and may induce or exacerbate pulmonary congestion despite a rise in cardiac output. Vasodilators (e.g., nitroglycerin or nitroprusside) can be used to reduce preload and improve cardiac output by antagonizing increases in venous and arterial resistance produced by dopamine. The combination of dopamine and nitroprusside produces hemodynamic effects similar to those of dobutamine.[76]

Dopamine is available for IV use only. The contents of one or two ampules (400 mg per ampule) should be mixed in 250 ml of 5% dextrose. This yields a concentration of 1600 or 3200 µg/ml. The initial rate of infusion is 1 to 2 µg/kg/min. The infusion rate may be increased until blood pressure, urine output, and other parameters of organ perfusion improve. A final dosage range of 5 to 30 µg/kg/min is recommended. The lowest infusion rate that results in satisfactory hemodynamic performance should be used to minimize side effects. Dopamine should be administered via a volumetric infusion pump to ensure precise flow rates. Hemodynamic monitoring is essential for proper use of dopamine in patients who have ischemic heart disease or congestive heart failure, and it should be instituted before, or as soon as possible after, initiation of treatment. When being discontinued, dopamine should be tapered gradually to avoid hypotensive episodes thought to be related to depletion of myocardial catecholamines.

Dopamine increases heart rate and may induce or exacerbate supraventricular and ventricular arrhythmias. Furthermore, dopamine's venous and arterial vasoconstricting effects, even at low doses, can exacerbate pulmonary congestion and compromise cardiac output. Occasionally, these effects may require a dosage reduction or discontinuation of the infusion. Despite hemodynamic improvements, myocardial oxygen consumption and myocardial lactate production may increase in response to higher doses of dopamine, indicating that coronary blood supply is not sufficiently augmented to compensate for the increased cardiac work. This imbalance between supply and demand would be expected to induce or exacerbate myocardial ischemia.[37] Nausea and vomiting are frequent side effects of dopamine, especially at high doses. Like norepinephrine, dopamine also produces cutaneous tissue necrosis and sloughing if interstitial extravasation occurs. Treatment of dopamine-induced extravasation is similar to that described for norepinephrine.

Monoamine oxidase inhibitors such as isocarboxazid (Marplan), pargyline hydrochloride (Eutonyl), tranylcypromine sulfate (Parnate), and phenelzine sulfate (Nardil) may potentiate the effects of dopamine. Therefore, patients receiving these agents should be treated with one-tenth the usual dopamine dose. Agents with similar hemodynamic effects, e.g., the initial effects of bretylium tosylate, may be synergistic with dopamine. Patients receiving phenytoin may experience hypotension during concomitant administration of dopamine.[40] Like other catecholamines, dopamine may precipitate a hypertensive crisis in patients with pheochromocytoma and is contraindicated. Dopamine should not be added to solutions containing sodium bicarbonate or other alkaline IV solutions because dopamine is slowly inactivated at alkaline pH. The kinetics of this reaction are slow enough so that dopamine and alkaline solutions (aminophylline, phenytoin, sodium bicarbonate) that are administered over a short period can be infused through the same venous catheter.

Dobutamine

Dobutamine is a synthetic sympathomimetic amine with two active isomers. The D-isomer is a potent β-adrenergic agonist; the L-isomer is a potent α-adrenergic agonist. Experimental data suggest that dobutamine exerts its potent inotropic effect by stimulating β_1- and α-adrenergic receptors in myocardium with little primary effect on peripheral vasculature.[77] In contrast to norepinephrine and dopamine, dobutamine produces very little systemic arterial or venous constriction at usual clinical doses.

In general, dobutamine causes a reflex fall in peripheral vascular resistance owing to the increase in cardiac output. Pulmonary artery occlusive pressure is reduced.[72, 78] In addition, dobutamine increases heart rate only at higher doses. Although renal and mesenteric blood flow increase as cardiac output increases, dobutamine does not induce renal or mesenteric vasodilation by stimulation of dopaminergic receptors. Nonetheless, renal function seems to improve with dobutamine just as with dopamine when similar changes in cardiac output are induced, suggesting that increases in cardiac output rather than stimulation of dopaminergic receptors are the predominant determinant of renal function.[72] The net hemodynamic effects of dobutamine are similar to those of dopamine combined with a vasodilator such as nitroprusside.[76] Accordingly, dobutamine is an excellent agent for the treatment of congestive heart failure but is not nearly as potent a pressor as dopamine or norepinephrine.[77]

Dobutamine's hemodynamic actions and its lack of effect on endogenous norepinephrine release explain why dobutamine has a more favorable impact on myocardial oxygen demand than either norepinephrine or dopamine.[76, 77] Dobutamine's positive inotropic effect is balanced by increased coronary blood flow so that oxygen extraction across the heart remains unchanged.[79] However, experimental data suggest that ischemia can be induced if substantial increases in heart rate occur.[80] For that reason, and because beneficial hemodynamic responses usually are not associated with the induction of cardioacceleration, dobutamine should be titrated to avoid increases in heart rate of more than 10%.[81]

The efficacy of dobutamine as a substitute for epinephrine during resuscitation has been evaluated in dogs.[73] Resuscitation was significantly more common in dogs receiving agents with potent α-adrenergic effects such as dopamine (95%) or epinephrine (95%) than in dogs receiving dobutamine (20%) or no drug (15%). Thus, there are no data to suggest a role for dobutamine during resuscitation. It may be of benefit if inotropic support is required after return of spontaneous circulation, particularly if congestive heart failure rather than hypotension is present. At present, the AHA recommendation[9, 10] is to administer 2 to 20 µg/kg/min of dobutamine (500 mg mixed in 250 ml of D_5W or normal saline), using the smallest effective dose needed to improve hemodynamics. The maximal dose is 40 µg/kg/min.

Dobutamine can cause tachycardia, arrhythmias, and fluctuations in blood pressure, which can provoke myocardial ischemia, especially at higher doses. Other side effects include headache, nausea, tremor, and hypokalemia.

Amrinone

Amrinone is an IV inotropic and vasodilator agent whose actions are not affected by αβ-adrenergic blockade or depletion of norepinephrine. Its mechanism of action appears to be via inhibition of phosphodiesterase.[82, 83] Amrinone's positive inotropic effects occur within minutes and last 60 to 90 minutes after a single IV injection.

Amrinone has a long half-life (i.e., 4 to 6 hours). Therefore, a loading dose of amrinone of 0.75 mg/kg is recommended to achieve therapeutic levels promptly. Because the afterload-reducing effects of amrinone are directly proportional to dosage and rate of administration, the loading dose of amrinone should generally not exceed 1 mg/kg. Although the loading dose may be given over 2 to 5 minutes, it is better to give it over 15 minutes to minimize the risk of hypotension in patients who have significant left ventricular dysfunction and/or marginal blood pressure. The bolus dose is followed by a maintenance infusion begun at a rate of 2 to 5 µg/kg/min and titrated up to a rate of 10 to 15 µg/kg/min according to hemodynamic response. The initial hemodynamic response to amrinone is usually similar to that of dobutamine.[84, 85] The oral preparation of amrinone is no longer available.[86, 87]

There are no published data on the use of amrinone during cardiopulmonary resuscitation. If it has any role to play in this setting, it would likely be to treat (1) pulseless electrical activity that may be due to severe left ventricular dysfunction, or (2) congestive heart failure after return of spontaneous circulation. Because of the potential for chemical incompatibility, amrinone lactate should not be diluted with or added to dextrose-containing solutions. Amrinone may be administered directly into a venous access line flowing with dextrose-containing IV solutions. For continuous IV infusion, amrinone lactate injection should be diluted to a final concentration of 1 to 3 mg/ml in 0.45% or 0.9% sodium chloride. Amrinone infusions should be administered by means of an infusion pump that ensures a precise flow rate.

Amrinone can induce significant toxicity.[84, 86] Thrombocytopenia is common, occurring in as many as half of all patients with congestive heart failure.[86, 88, 89] The short-term IV injection and infusion can produce hypotension, arrhythmias, nausea, vomiting, liver function abnormalities, fever, and an influenza-like syndrome.[84, 86, 88] In addition, in experimental studies, amrinone exacerbates ischemia at doses that do not increase heart rate.[90] This effect may be augmented by the dose-dependent effects on heart rate that occur in patients with acute myocardial infarction.[91] Because amrinone contains metabisulfite, its use is contraindicated in patients allergic to sulfiting agents.

Isoproterenol

Isoproterenol hydrochloride is a synthetic sympathomimetic amine that is a nearly pure β-adrenergic receptor stimulator. Its potent positive inotropic and chronotropic properties generally lead to increases in cardiac output, but mean arterial pressure usually is reduced as a result of peripheral vasodilation and venous pooling. Isoproterenol markedly increases myocardial oxygen requirements and may exacerbate or induce ischemia.[92] Because pure β-adrenergic stimulation with isoproterenol causes arterial vasodilation, a fall in coronary perfusion pressure, and an increase in myocardial oxygen demand, isoproterenol is contraindicated during closed-chest compression.[9, 10, 93]

The principal indication for isoproterenol in emergency cardiac care is for the immediate and temporary control of hemodynamically significant bradycardia that is refractory to atropine in a patient with a pulse.[9, 10] Electronic (external or transvenous) pacing provides better control without the risk of inducing ischemia and should be initiated in preference to isoproterenol, or as soon as possible after initiation of therapy. When isoproterenol is used for cardioacceleration, the initial IV starting dose is 2 μg/min (1 mg of isoproterenol diluted in 250 ml of D₅W). The dose is titrated upward until the ventricular response rate is approximately 60/min. In general, this takes no more than 10 μg/min.[9, 10] Because isoproterenol increases myocardial oxygen requirements, it should be avoided whenever possible in patients with ischemic heart disease. Isoproterenol's potent chronotropic properties can induce serious arrhythmias, including ventricular tachycardia and fibrillation. Isoproterenol may also exacerbate tachyarrhythmias owing to digitalis toxicity and may precipitate hypokalemia.

VOLUME LOADING AND OTHER ADJUNCTIVE TECHNIQUES

Volume loading during closed-chest compression significantly improves forward cardiac output and arterial perfusion pressure. However, the critical determinant of coronary and cerebral flow during closed-chest compression depends on the difference between arterial and venous pressures.[4, 36-40, 48, 51, 52, 70] Volume loading (e.g., the rapid IV infusion of saline or lactated Ringer's solution) raises right atrial and cerebral venous pressure and actually diminishes critical organ blood flow during closed-chest compression.[94]

Other mechanical interventions (abdominal corset, pneumatic antishock garment, interposed abdominal compressions) can also increase central and cerebral volume and thus are unlikely to improve outcome.[9, 10, 95] Attempts to improve critical organ blood flow and survival from resuscitation have employed a vest to increase intrathoracic pressure and blood flow.[96] The proper and safe implementation of this technique will require more development; however, nearly normal myocardial and cerebral blood flows have been achieved during resuscitation in animals 20 minutes after arrest.[96] These encouraging results suggest that, with time, practical interventions may be developed to improve the efficacy of closed-chest compression.

Finally, there is substantial enthusiasm for what has been named active compression and decompression CPR (ACD-CPR), which uses a plunger to both compress and then pull the chest up. Experimental trials of this relatively simple device indicate that it can generate significantly higher blood flow than standard CPR.[97]

REFRACTORY OR RECURRENT VENTRICULAR FIBRILLATION

Electrical countershock is the treatment of choice for ventricular fibrillation (VF) and pulseless ventricular tachycardia (VT). If three initial countershocks at increasing energies (200, 200 to 300, and 360 J), intubation, epinephrine, and a fourth countershock (360 J) fail to terminate the arrhythmia (refractory VF or VT), or if, as in many cases, the arrhythmia rapidly recurs (recurrent VF or VT), antiarrhythmic drug therapy is indicated. The two most frequently used agents for this purpose are lidocaine and bretylium tosylate.

Lidocaine

Lidocaine, a potent class IB antiarrhythmic agent, is the drug of first choice for the treatment of ventricular arrhythmias in patients with acute myocardial infarction.[9-11] During resuscitation, its use results in a survival rate that is as high as that for any other FDA-approved agent,[98-100] and lidocaine does not decrease coronary perfusion pressure.

Lidocaine has antifibrillatory effects in animal models.[101] Higher plasma lidocaine concentrations (>6 mg/ml) are required to achieve an antifibrillatory effect than to control ventricular ectopy.[102, 103] Such levels are achieved routinely after a 2 mg/kg IV dose in dogs.[104] No significant elevation in ventricular fibrillation threshold is observed after a 1 mg/kg IV dose. Other studies in animals indicate that lidocaine increases the ventricular defibrillation threshold modestly, increasing the energy needed to reverse ventricular fibrillation.[105, 106] Despite these actions, lidocaine is as effective in treating ventricular fibrillation as agents that have "primary antifibrillatory effects" at lower doses (e.g., bretylium tosylate) in randomized prospective clinical trials.[98, 99] Because many episodes of apparent "refractory" VF may represent rapid recurrence rather than the persistence of the arrhythmia, the apparent benefit of lidocaine may reflect prevention of recurrence in patients who have been successfully defibrillated.[9, 10, 98, 99] Such a hypothesis suggests that positive synergism should exist between lidocaine and bretylium, as was found in one experimental study.[100]

Lidocaine reduces the incidence of primary VF in patients with acute myocardial infarction but may not necessarily alter mortality.[107, 108] A meta-analysis of 14 randomized, controlled trials of lidocaine prophylaxis during acute myocardial infarction showed that mortality was not reduced during the prehospital phase of acute myocardial infarction and suggested that mortality may be increased in patients who receive prophylactic lidocaine during the hospital phase of uncomplicated acute myocardial infarction.[108] Thus, routine prophylactic lidocaine therapy in patients with acute myocardial infarction is not advised.[108a, 108b]

The pharmacokinetics of lidocaine in patients with cardiac arrest have not been studied extensively. It is known that the volume of distribution of lidocaine is reduced owing to the low cardiac output and that clearance is delayed because of reduced hepatic blood flow.[103] Although these changes result in a higher plasma concentration, the fraction of free drug may be decreased because of increased binding to the αl-acid glycoprotein, which is released during an acute ischemic insult.[109, 110] In experimental animals, a dose of 1 mg/kg results in levels above the therapeutic range for at least 20 minutes. The very high levels, especially early after administration, are higher than those reported to be necessary to induce favorable changes in the VF threshold.[103]

Data from human studies are needed to further optimize the dosage of lidocaine during CPR. For refractory VF and pulseless VT, an initial dose of 1.5 mg/kg is suggested for all patients. Cardiac arrest victims may require only a single bolus dose of lidocaine. Plasma lidocaine concentrations should theoretically persist within the normal therapeutic range for a protracted period because of reduced drug clearance from poor blood flow during CPR.[5]

It may be advisable to give lidocaine only by bolus during cardiac arrest because of the low blood flow and prolonged circulation time.[6] After restoration of spontaneous circulation, lidocaine can then be continued by IV infusion at a rate of 30 to 50 µg/kg/min (2 to 4 mg/min). The need for additional bolus doses of lidocaine should be guided by clinical response and/or by plasma lidocaine concentrations.

In non–cardiac arrest situations, an initial bolus of 1.0 to 1.5 mg/kg followed by a maintenance infusion at a rate of 30 to 50 µg/kg/min (2 to 4 mg/min) is required to achieve therapeutic lidocaine levels rapidly. To prevent subtherapeutic plasma lidocaine levels after the initial bolus, a second bolus of 0.5 mg/kg is recommended after 10 minutes. Additional bolus injections of 0.5 to 0.75 mg/kg can be given every 5 to 10 minutes if ventricular ectopy persists, to a total dose of 3 mg/kg. The maintenance infusion should be titrated according to clinical needs and plasma lidocaine concentrations.

The maintenance dose of lidocaine should be reduced by 50% in patients with impaired hepatic blood flow (acute myocardial infarction with hemodynamic compromise, congestive heart failure, or circulatory shock), because total body clearance of lidocaine is reduced.[111, 112] Elderly patients (i.e., older than 70 years of age) have a reduced volume of distribution; in such patients, the maintenance dose should also be reduced by half.[113] Because the half-life of lidocaine increases after 24 to 48 hours of a continuous infusion, the maintenance dose should be reduced by 50% at that time. The monitoring of blood lidocaine concentrations may be helpful to avoid toxicity. Renal failure leads to the accumulation of monoethylglycylcylidine and glycinexylidide, lidocaine's metabolites, which have little antiarrhythmic activity but can produce significant neurotoxicity.[111]

Excessive doses of lidocaine can cause neurologic changes and myocardial depression. Clinical indicators of lidocaine-induced neurologic toxicity include drowsiness, disorientation, decreased hearing ability, paresthesia, and muscle twitching. Some patients may become very agitated. More serious toxic effects include focal and grand mal seizures. Severe myocardial depression can manifest itself as bradycardia, conduction disturbances, widening of the QRS, and/or hypotension.

Bretylium Tosylate

Bretylium tosylate is an adrenergic neuronal blocking drug introduced in 1950 as an antihypertensive agent. Tolerance to bretylium's antihypertensive action and its undesirable side effects limited its use as an oral agent.[114] Interest in bretylium was revived in the mid-1960s when its antifibrillatory properties were appreciated.[115]

Bretylium is a class III antiarrhythmic agent that increases myocardial electrical stability by elevating the VF threshold and by reducing the disparity in action potential duration and refractory periods between ischemic and nonischemic myocardium.[102, 103, 116-118] Some investigators have questioned the effect of bretylium on VF threshold, suggesting that its efficacy may be more dependent on the extent of sympathetic activation.[119] Bretylium does not significantly affect the ventricular defibrillation threshold,[105, 120, 121] nor does it decrease ventricular automaticity.[118] Bretylium enhances membrane responsiveness in Purkinje fibers in infarcted myocardium, improving conduction velocity.[118] This effect is probably mediated by bretylium-induced catecholamine release, which may reduce the propensity for VF to develop.[116, 122, 123]

The electrophysiologic and antifibrillatory actions of bretylium correlate better with the myocardial drug level than with its level in plasma.[124, 126] Bretylium's antiarrhythmic activity is dose-dependent; larger initial doses produce a more favorable antifibrillatory response.[104, 126, 127] High doses of bretylium (10 mg/kg) produce a more rapid and effective antiarrhythmic response compared with lower doses (5 mg/kg) in patients with ventricular arrhythmias.[126]

Some clinicians believe that bretylium is the drug of choice for the prevention and treatment of VF.[128, 129] Bretylium has been reported to induce the spontaneous conversion of VF to normal sinus rhythm,[129] although a critical review of the rhythm strips contained in these reports[129] suggests that some patients had torsade de pointes rather than VF. Chemical cardioversion with bretylium has not been reported in prospective studies.[99]

Nowak et al.[130] reported a higher rate of successful resuscitation when bretylium was used (35%) than after placebo alone (6%) in prehospital cardiac arrest victims, but their retrospective analysis leaves substantial questions concerning the comparability of the groups. Other studies also support the efficacy of bretylium for prehospital VF.[98, 131] However, no difference in clinical outcome has been observed in prospective randomized studies comparing bretylium and lidocaine for the treatment of prehospital VF,[98, 99] using IV doses of bretylium (0.5 to 1 g) and lidocaine (100 to 200 mg) in one study[99] and bretylium (10 to 30 mg/kg) and lidocaine (2 to 3 mg/kg) in another.[98] Neither study found a significant difference in the incidence of conversion from VF and tachycardia to a more organized rhythm or increased rate of survival.[98, 99] In the study by Olson et al.,[98] conversion to an organized rhythm was more common in patients who received lidocaine initially. In dogs during closed-chest compression, the antifibrillatory activity of bretylium (5 mg/kg) is more persistent than that of lidocaine (2 mg/kg) but is delayed in onset (10 minutes compared with 5 minutes).[124]

The AHA recommends the use of lidocaine as the drug of first choice for VF or pulseless VT.[9, 10] Bretylium is recommended in patients who fail to respond to at least one dose (1 mg/kg) of lidocaine. There are some data suggesting positive synergism between the two agents.[100] Bretylium is not recommended as a first-line agent because it is no more effective than lidocaine and because of its potential

for inducing hypotension, which is a common cause of morbidity in otherwise hemodynamically stable patients who are treated with doses that are lower and that are infused more gradually.[126] Bretylium-induced hypotension can be refractory to epinephrine and, in experimental models, compromises the success of resuscitative efforts for recurrent VF.[132] Bretylium induces transient hypertension early after administration (during the first 15 to 30 minutes) and hypotension thereafter.[116]

In patients with VF, a 5 mg/kg IV dose of bretylium is administered undiluted by rapid injection. The dose should be flushed with 20 ml of IV fluid if it is administered from a peripheral site. After 1 to 2 minutes to permit access to the central circulation, defibrillation is attempted again. If VF persists, the dose can be increased to 10 mg/kg and repeated at 15- to 30-minute intervals to a maximal dose of 30 to 35 mg/kg.[116]

For patients with refractory or recurrent VT, 500 mg of bretylium (10 ml) can be diluted to 50 ml, and 5 to 10 mg/kg can be injected IV over a period of 8 to 10 minutes. In the conscious patient, rapid injection can result in hypotension, nausea, or vomiting. If VT persists, a second dose of 5 to 10 mg/kg can be given in 10 to 30 minutes and, if necessary, every 6 to 8 hours thereafter.[133] Alternatively, bretylium can be administered as a continuous infusion at a rate of 2 mg/min. Although the onset of action of bretylium in VF seems to be within a few minutes, in VT it may be delayed for 20 minutes or more.

Hypertension and tachycardia are common immediately after treatment in non–cardiac arrest patients, but these effects are transient owing to the initial stimulation of norepinephrine release from adrenergic nerve terminals.[116] Nausea and vomiting can also occur after rapid injection in the awake patient. Thereafter, owing to blockage of the reuptake of catecholamines, postural hypotension is common. It is observed in as many as 60% of patients, although the mean arterial pressure infrequently falls more than 20 mmHg.[133] Treatment includes having the patient assume a supine or, if necessary, Trendelenburg position and administering IV fluids. In some cases, a vasopressor such as norepinephrine may be required. Hypotension may be refractory to epinephrine.[132] Bretylium should be used with caution in the treatment of arrhythmias accompanying digitalis toxicity because bretylium-mediated catecholamine release may exacerbate tachyarrhythmias.[116]

Procainamide

Procainamide, a class IA antiarrhythmic agent, is used in the emergency cardiac care setting most commonly to suppress symptomatic premature ventricular complexes and recurrent VT refractory to lidocaine.[134] During resuscitation, it is a second- or third-line agent (after lidocaine and/or bretylium) to treat "refractory" (or recurrent) VF or VT without a pulse. The reason for this is that a loading dose of procainamide is required, and, in general, it is not possible to achieve therapeutic levels sufficiently rapidly for procainamide to be of benefit.

Because procainamide is a presynaptic ganglionic blocker, it vasodilates and induces modest negative inotropic effects, especially in patients with left ventricular dysfunction.[135] Procainamide-induced hypotension is most pronounced after rapid IV injection or when high plasma concentrations of procainamide are present.[134, 135] It is important to monitor the electrocardiogram (ECG) and arterial blood pressure whenever procainamide is given. Adverse effects of procainamide include intraventricular conduction delays and lengthening of the PR and QT intervals. Intravenous procainamide must be administered cautiously to patients with acute myocardial infarction. Procainamide can induce or exacerbate malignant ventricular arrhythmias. This proarrhythmic propensity may be somewhat greater when hypokalemia is present.

During resuscitation,[9, 10] procainamide is usually given in a dosage of 1 g administered at a rate of 20 to 30 mg/min, followed by a maintenance infusion of 1 to 4 mg/min. An alternative regimen that achieves therapeutic levels faster (in some patients in only 15 minutes) includes a loading dose of 17 mg/kg given over 1 hour, followed by a maintenance infusion of 2.8 mg/kg/hr. In patients in whom the agent might clear slowly, the loading dose is reduced to 12 mg/kg and the infusion rate is reduced to 1.4 mg/kg/hr.[135, 136] The rate of drug administration should be reduced or stopped temporarily if hypotension or prolongation of the QT interval or QRS complex by 50% or more occurs.

ADDITIONAL CONSIDERATIONS

Occasionally, VF or VT without a pulse remains "refractory" to, or recurs incessantly, despite repeated electrical countershocks and pharmacologic treatment. In such cases, additional, less conventional treatment options should be considered. The use of β-blockers, traditionally with IV propranolol (1 mg every 5 minutes intravenously up to a total dose of 0.1 mg/kg), is worthy of consideration.[9, 10, 136a] Obviously, the potential for such treatment to compromise left ventricular function must be appreciated. For this reason, the very short-lived IV β-blocker esmolol has a theoretic advantage that remains to be proven in the setting of a cardiac arrest.

Underlying metabolic derangements should also be sought and corrected. Arterial hypoxemia should be reversed or minimized by endotracheal intubation and ventilation with 100% oxygen. Acidosis is best prevented (or treated) during closed-chest compression by optimizing CPR techniques to improve blood flow and hyperventilation. Electrolyte abnormalities are common during resuscitation, either as primary disturbances that may have triggered the arrest or as secondary phenomena due to intracellular shifts and therapeutic interventions; such electrolyte abnormalities should be corrected if present.

Resuscitation from refractory VF is less likely to be successful if hypokalemia and/or hypomagnesemia are present. Hypokalemia is common in cardiac patients and occurs in 23% to 40% of individuals treated with thiazide diuretics.[137] When loop and thiazide diuretics are used in combination, the incidence approaches 100%.[137, 138] Hypokalemia can trigger VF in experimental animal models and in patients with heart disease.[138, 139] Hypokalemia is a very potent risk factor for the development of VF in patients with acute myocardial infarction[139] as well as a common finding (as much as 50%) in survivors of out-of-hospital VF.[140, 141] Hypokalemia after resuscitation may be due to a shift in the distribution of potassium between the extracellular and intracellular space induced by metabolic events during resuscitation. Many patients (55% in one study)[141] have predisposing risk factors for the development of hypokalemia before cardiac arrest.

Hypokalemia in the patient with cardiac arrest and refractory VF must be treated aggressively. Guidelines for potassium replacement that are acceptable in the less emergent clinical circumstance may be inadequate to correct hypokalemia in a timely fashion during cardiac arrest.[142] One regimen that has been suggested includes administration of 10 mEq of potassium chloride diluted in 50 ml D_5W over 20 minutes. This dose can be repeated as necessary while rechecking serum levels.[142]

The role of magnesium homeostasis in cardiovascular disease has recently received substantial attention.[143, 144] Magnesium deficiency is associated with cardiac arrhythmias and even sudden cardiac death,[138, 143–145] and its therapeutic efficacy in patients with torsade de pointes is well established.[146] Transient hypomagnesemia is usually caused by diuretics,[147, 148] but hypomagnesemia not attributable to loss of magnesium in the urine has been observed in patients with acute myocardial infarction.[149] Hypomagnesemia is closely associated with, and is a likely determinant of, hypokalemia.[143–147] Because it may precipitate VF in experimental models in association with hypokalemia and because it can hinder the replenishment of intracellular potassium,[143] it should be corrected if present. Routine magnesium supplementation is relatively safe and has been shown to be of value prophylactically to reduce the incidence of postinfarction ventricular arrhythmias in some,[149] but not all,[150] studies.

For acute administration during VT or fibrillation, 1 or 2 g of magnesium sulfate (2 to 4 ml of a 50% solution) is diluted in 10 ml of D_5W and administered over 1 to 2 minutes. Caution should be used when magnesium is administered to safeguard against clinically significant hypotension or asystole. A 24-hour magnesium infusion (8 g $MgSO_4$ in 500 ml D_5W at 8 drops/min) should be considered in patients with documented magnesium deficiency.

Magnesium toxicity is rare, but side effects from rapid administration include flushing, sweating, mild bradycardia, and hypotension. Hypermagnesemia can produce depressed reflexes, flaccid paralysis, circulatory collapse, respiratory paralysis, or diarrhea.

Other treatment strategies can also be used in managing incessantly refractory or recurrent VF or pulseless VT. The possibility that there has been a proarrhythmic drug effect that may be exacerbating the arrhythmia must be considered.[151] Proarrhythmic drug effects, hypokalemia, and/or hypomagnesemia can induce ventricular arrhythmias such as torsade de pointes. Torsade de pointes can sometimes be prevented by phenytoin or β-blockers and can be treated with lidocaine acutely, although it is more commonly managed by pacing or other forms of overdrive suppression (including the cautious use of isoproterenol).[152, 153] A temporary pacemaker can be inserted for overdrive pacing after electrical countershock to control recurrent malignant ventricular ectopy.[153] Anecdotal treatment of ischemia with IV nitroglycerin during resuscitation has been reported.[154]

There has been a brief report concerning the use of intravenous amiodarone to treat patients with recurrent arrhythmias. Despite prolonged resuscitative efforts before the administration of IV amiodarone, 11 of 12 patients with refractory ventricular tachyarrhythmias responded, and eight left the hospital alive.[155]

BRADYASYSTOLE

Survival is poor (generally 1% to 3% or less, regardless of therapy) for patients with bradyasystole (asystole or bradycardia without a pulse). It is always important to exclude disconnection of a lead or monitor electrode before concluding that a "flat line" is the patient's rhythm. Because some patients with a "flat line" may have VF (a rhythm more amenable to treatment) masquerading as asystole,[156] the monitor lead configuration should be quickly switched to a second lead to confirm the diagnosis before treatment. If the diagnosis is still in doubt, the patient should be presumed to have VF and treated accordingly. Other general measures recommended for the treatment of bradyasystole include

1. Support of ventilation
2. Properly performed closed-chest compression
3. Frequent doses of epinephrine to maintain arterial perfusion pressure and coronary and cerebral perfusion

Atropine Sulfate

The vagolytic agent atropine sulfate is the treatment of choice for symptomatic bradycardia in patients who have a pulse.[9, 10] Atropine increases sinus node automaticity and enhances atrioventricular (AV) conduction. Atropine can restore normal AV nodal conduction and initiate electrical activity in patients with first-degree AV block or Mobitz type I AV block and in some patients with bradyasystolic cardiac arrest. However, atropine has been reported to be harmful in some patients with AV block at the His-Purkinje level (type II AV block and third-degree AV block with a new wide QRS complex).[108] Treatment with

atropine may improve outcome in patients with bradyasystolic cardiac arrest that is due to excessive vagal stimulation, but atropine is less effective when asystole or pulseless idioventricular rhythms are the result of prolonged ischemia or mechanical injury in the myocardium.[157–163]

Brown et al.[158] reported that three of eight patients survived after the administration of atropine for asystole. However, all survivors experienced cardiac arrest in the hospital (two in the catheterization laboratory and one in intensive care) and had Advanced Cardiac Life Support (ACLS) initiated within 2 minutes. Stueven et al.[159] reported a significant ($p < .04$) increase in the number of patients who survived until arrival at the emergency department after out-of-hospital cardiac arrest with asystole after receiving atropine (14% compared with 0% in those who received only epinephrine and bicarbonate), but none of the short-term survivors was discharged from the hospital. Iseri et al.[157] observed no response in 10 asystolic patients. Coon et al.[162] found that 10 of 11 patients who did not receive atropine and 8 of 10 who did receive atropine developed rhythms other than asystole, but only one patient (who did not receive atropine) was discharged alive. Unfortunately, asystolic cardiac arrest is nearly always fatal, regardless of therapy. Although there is no unequivocal proof of its value, there is little evidence that atropine is harmful in this setting. A well-designed prospective, controlled trial to determine the utility of atropine in treating asystole would be helpful.

For patients without cardiac arrest, atropine is administered intravenously in 0.5-mg aliquots. This dose may be repeated at 5-minute intervals until the desired response is achieved (i.e., an increased heart rate, usually to 60 beats/min or more, or abatement of signs and symptoms). Repeated doses of atropine should be avoided, when possible, in patients with ischemic heart disease. In patients with recurrent episodes of bradycardia, especially those with acute ischemic heart disease, the heart rate can be maintained by means of an electrical pacemaker. When the recurrent use of atropine is essential in patients with coronary artery disease, the total dose should be restricted to 2 mg, if possible, to avoid the detrimental effects of atropine-induced tachycardia on myocardial oxygen demand.[164, 165]

For patients with bradyasystolic cardiac arrest, a 1-mg dose of atropine is administered intravenously and is repeated every 3 to 5 minutes if asystole persists. In most patients, 3 mg (0.04 mg/kg) given intravenously is a fully vagolytic dose.[166] The administration of a total vagolytic dose of atropine should be reserved for patients with bradyasystolic cardiac arrest. Administration of atropine in doses of less than 0.5 mg can produce a paradoxic bradycardia owing to the central nervous system and/or peripheral parasympathomimetic effects of low doses in adults. This effect can precipitate VF.[167]

Endotracheal atropine produces a rapid onset of action similar to that observed with IV injection. The recommended adult dose of atropine for ET administration is 1.0 to 2.0 mg diluted in 10 ml of sterile water or normal saline.

Atropine always should be administered with caution in the setting of myocardial ischemia. VF and tachycardia have occurred after IV administration of atropine, especially in patients with coronary artery disease.[164, 165, 168] Excessive doses of atropine can cause delirium, tachycardia, coma, flushed and hot skin, ataxia, and blurred vision.

Calcium Chloride

Calcium plays an important role in excitation-contraction coupling of myocardial cells and in impulse formation. Although widely recommended and used in cardiac resuscitation for more than 30 years, studies[161, 169, 170] have not shown that it affects survival from bradyasystolic cardiac arrest. Furthermore, calcium administration can induce cerebral vasospasm, leading to postarrest cerebral hypoperfusion.[171-173] There is also experimental evidence that calcium efflux may markedly exacerbate reperfusion injury in the heart and the brain.[174-177] Thus, calcium chloride is not routinely indicated for the treatment of bradyasystole unless severe hypocalcemia or hyperkalemia is present or the arrest is due to calcium antagonist toxicity.[9, 10]

A 10-ml prefilled syringe or ampule of 10% solution of calcium chloride contains 13.6 mEq of calcium (100 mg = 1 ml). Calcium chloride can be given intravenously in a dose of 2 to 4 mg/kg of 10% solution (1.36 mEq of calcium per 100 mg of salt per ml) and repeated if necessary at 10-minute intervals. Two other calcium salts are available, calcium gluceptate and calcium gluconate. Calcium gluceptate can be given in a dose of 5 to 7 ml; the dose of calcium gluconate is 5 to 8 ml. Calcium chloride is preferable because it produces consistently higher and more predictable levels of ionized calcium in plasma.[178]

If the heart is beating, rapid administration of calcium can slow the heart rate. Calcium must be used cautiously in the patient receiving digitalis because it increases ventricular irritability and can precipitate digitalis toxicity. In the presence of sodium bicarbonate, calcium salts precipitate as carbonates. Thus, these drugs cannot be administered together. Calcium can produce vasospasm in coronary and cerebral arteries.

Adenosine-Blocking Drugs

Endogenous adenosine released during myocardial hypoxia and ischemia relaxes vascular smooth muscle, decreases atrial and ventricular contractility, depresses pacemaker automaticity, and impairs AV conduction.[179-186] The electrophysiologic effects that appear to be most relevant during resuscitation are caused by stimulation of the same time-independent outward potassium current that is stimulated by acetylcholine.[187, 188] Adenosine hyperpolarizes atrial muscle cells,[189] decreases the duration of the atrial action potential,[190] and decreases phase 4 diastolic depolar-

ization in sinoatrial node pacemaker cells.[191] It slows AV conduction by depressing the action potential upstroke of AV nodal "N" cells.[179] Adenosine stimulation of A1 subreceptors located on the cell surface affects both adenosine-sensitive potassium channels and cyclic adenosine monophosphate (cAMP) production by means of an inhibitory guanine nucleotide–binding (Gi) protein.[192] During normal aerobic metabolism, adenosine is formed primarily by intracellular degradation of S-adenoxyl homocysteine (SAH), catalyzed by the enzyme S-adenoxyl homocysteine hydrolase (SAH pathway).[193] During myocardial ischemia, adenosine is formed primarily by dephosphorylation of adenosine monophosphate (AMP), catalyzed by the enzyme 5'-nucleotidase (ATP pathway).[194, 195]

The cellular electrophysiologic effects of adenosine can be competitively antagonized by methylxanthines, but not by atropine. A specific adenosine antagonist (BW-A1433U) has been shown to reverse and prevent postdefibrillation bradyasystole and hemodynamic depression in a domestic pig model.[179] Aminophylline, a competitive nonspecific adenosine antagonist, has been shown to restore cardiac electrical activity within 30 seconds in 12 of 15 inhospital cardiac arrest patients whose bradyasystole was refractory to atropine and epinephrine.[196] Investigators have reported variable response to aminophylline when treating bradyarrhythmias (including AV block) due to acute myocardial infarction.[197-200] Patients with milder forms of AV block (e.g., Mobitz type I) appear to respond most consistently to aminophylline, but such individuals usually are the least compromised hemodynamically.[200]

Mechanical and Electrical Treatment

Pacing (transvenous, transthoracic, or transcutaneous) rarely influences survival in the unwitnessed cardiac arrest patient who is initially found with asystole or bradycardia without a pulse.[201-203] However, pacing is extremely useful for bradycardiac patients with a pulse and in selected patients in whom a pacemaker can be placed immediately after the development of the conduction disturbance.[202, 203] In such cases, a precordial thump can also stimulate ventricular complexes and a pulse ("fist pacing").[9, 10]

PULSELESS ELECTRICAL ACTIVITY

Pulseless electrical activity (PEA) is present when there is organized electrical activity on the ECG but no effective circulation. There are potentially many underlying causes, but the most common may involve myocardial ischemia and dysfunction due to intramyocardial increases in carbon dioxide.[204, 206] Prognosis is generally poor unless a discrete and treatable cause for PEA can be discerned and corrected. Because of the poor prognosis when a correctable cause cannot be determined, efforts should be directed toward detecting causes such as hypovolemia, tension pneumothorax, and pericardial tamponade.[9, 10] Normal saline or Ringer's lactate solution should be infused rapidly if there is evidence of hypovolemia. Suspected pneumothorax or pericardial tamponade should be confirmed by needle aspiration of the chest or pericardium, respectively. If confirmed, more definitive surgical management (chest tube or thoracotomy) is usually required.

Scrutiny of the neck veins may be helpful in attempting to define a cause for PEA. Most patients with cardiac arrest have high right-sided filling pressures and distended neck veins. When neck veins are not visible in this setting and PEA is present, hypovolemia should be suspected. In the "trauma" cardiac arrest victim (such as a patient with a gunshot wound of the chest), however, prominent neck veins should lead to the suspicion of pericardial tamponade or tension pneumothorax.[206]

General measures such as (1) support of ventilation, (2) properly performed closed-chest compression, and (3) frequent doses of epinephrine to maintain arterial perfusion pressure and coronary and cerebral perfusion are recommended for treatment of PEA.[9, 10] Bradycardia may be treated with atropine.[9, 10] Although catecholamines are frequently given, there are no data to suggest a specific benefit (other than improvement in coronary and cerebral blood flow during closed-chest compression). Calcium chloride has not been shown to affect clinical survival in controlled trials.[169, 207] In addition, the pathologically high serum calcium levels caused by its administration[172, 173] may exacerbate reperfusion injury.[174-177]

If penetrating cardiac trauma is present, open chest massage can be lifesaving.[201, 208-211] In other settings, open chest massage is rarely of value, partly because it is usually initiated late after the onset of the arrest.[212]

ACID-BASE MANAGEMENT

The marked fall in cardiac output during closed-chest massage critically reduces tissue oxygen delivery. Cells shift to anaerobic metabolism, gradually building up lactic acid as a waste product.[213-215] During anaerobic metabolism, the carbon dioxide concentration increases rapidly inside cells. Anoxic arrest of the heart causes a progressive increase in the concentration of P_{CO_2} inside heart muscle cells, which may reach very high levels (90 to 475 torr).[216] Above an intramyocardial P_{CO_2} of approximately 475 torr, pulseless electrical activity is present and the heart cannot be resuscitated.[216] Intracellular carbon dioxide eventually diffuses into capillary blood and returns to the heart and lungs in venous blood.

Central (mixed) venous blood during closed-chest compression is acidotic (pH, approximately 7.15) and hypercarbic (Pv_{CO_2}, approximately 74 torr).[217] With hyperventilation, carbon dioxide is removed as blood flows through the lungs. Accordingly, arterial blood is less acidotic. Arterial blood pH during well-performed closed-chest compression is usually normal, slightly acidotic, or mildly alkalotic.[215, 217, 219] Arterial blood can be slightly alkalotic while the venous blood

is acidotic because pulmonary blood flow is only a quarter to a third of normal amount during closed-chest compression (this phenomenon has been termed the "venous paradox").[217] It is, in fact, not a paradox but part of normal physiology that occurs when anaerobic metabolism is required (e.g., during strenuous exercise).[220] It appears that intramyocardial pH is much closer to the venous than the arterial pH.[221]

Severe arterial acidosis during closed-chest compression is usually due to inadequate ventilation.[219] The best solution is usually to improve the technique of closed-chest compression and to increase ventilation if possible. If severe acidosis is present despite hyperventilation, correct intubation, and properly performed external chest compression, an alternative method for providing assisted circulation (e.g., open-chest compressions or venoarterial bypass) may need to be considered.

In the past, administration of sodium bicarbonate ($NaHCO_3$) was recommended during closed-chest compression because of the belief that bicarbonate would buffer the H^+ ion produced during anaerobic metabolism. However, sodium bicarbonate itself contains a high concentration of carbon dioxide (260 to 280 torr).[222] In plasma, the carbon dioxide is released and diffuses into cells more rapidly than HCO_3^-, causing a paradoxic rise in intracellular P_{CO_2} and a fall in intracellular pH.[9, 10] The increases in intracellular P_{CO_2} in heart muscle cells decrease cardiac contractility, cardiac output, and blood pressure.[174, 217, 223-225] Paradoxic acidosis of cerebrospinal fluid also can occur after the use of sodium bicarbonate[226] and may be responsible for prolonged confusion after a successful resuscitation as the venous acidosis increases. Sodium bicarbonate causes other potentially harmful effects,[214, 222-225, 227] including hyperosmolality, alkalemia, and sodium overload.

At present, there are no data to suggest that treatment with sodium bicarbonate is of benefit during closed-chest compression, and it does not improve survival in experimental animals.[228-232] Therefore, sodium bicarbonate provides minimal, if any, benefit and adds significant risk. It should not be given during a routine cardiac arrest sequence.[9, 10] If used at all, bicarbonate should not be used until proven interventions such as defibrillation, cardiac compression, support of ventilation including intubation, and pharmacologic therapies such as epinephrine and antiarrhythmic agents have been employed. It has been estimated that these interventions usually require at least the first 10 minutes of the routine cardiac arrest sequence.[9, 10]

If bicarbonate therapy is considered to be necessary during CPR, the initial dose is 1 mEq/kg. No more than half of the original dose should be given every 10 minutes thereafter. Because of the markedly reduced cardiac output and the venous paradox in pH mentioned earlier, the measurement of arterial pH during closed-chest compression is rarely helpful. End-tidal CO_2 increases in keeping with the delivered load of carbon dioxide and no longer reflects pulmonary perfusion.[232a] Ready-to-use, prefilled injection syringes containing 8.4% sodium bicarbonate (50 mEq/50 ml) are recommended for use during CPR. The administration of sodium bicarbonate may help buffer hydrogen ions washed out after reestablishment of spontaneous circulation. In this situation, the use of bicarbonate should be guided by arterial blood gas measurement. However, bicarbonate in this situation may still depress cardiac function.[233, 234] In certain circumstances, such as patients with preexisting metabolic acidosis, hyperkalemia, or tricyclic antidepressant or phenobarbital overdose, bicarbonate is beneficial. Sodium bicarbonate can be administered by continuous infusion when the therapeutic goal is gradual correction of acidosis or alkalinization of blood (i.e., tricyclic antidepressant overdose) or urine (e.g., barbiturate overdose). A 5% sodium bicarbonate solution (297.5 mEq/500 ml) can be used to administer a sodium bicarbonate infusion. The infusion rate should be guided by arterial blood gas monitoring. To minimize the risk of iatrogenically induced alkalosis, complete correction of the base deficit should be avoided.

Alternative buffer agents have not yet been shown to improve survival during cardiac resuscitation. THAM (tromethamine, tris-buffer) is a potent amine buffer that actively binds H^+ ions. It combines with carbonic acid (H_2CO_3), increasing the amount of bicarbonate anion (HCO_3^-) available. THAM penetrates into cells and may neutralize acidic ions in the intracellular fluid. In dogs, THAM corrects the metabolic acidosis that occurs during cardiac arrest.[235] Anecdotal reports suggest that THAM may be of value during prolonged cardiac resuscitations in humans,[236] but more research is needed. Dichloroacetate (DCA) reduces the serum lactate concentration by stimulating pyruvate dehydrogenase, the enzyme that catalyzes the rate-limiting step in the oxidation of lactate to pyruvate.[237] It is a safe and effective adjunct for the treatment of patients with lactic acidosis[237] but does not affect intramyocardial pH during closed-chest compression in experimental animals.[221]

CEREBRAL PROTECTION DURING AND AFTER SUCCESSFUL RESUSCITATION

A primary goal of effective cardiopulmonary resuscitation is to maintain adequate cerebral circulation to sustain neuronal viability, permitting neurologically intact recovery if effective spontaneous circulation can be restored. In animal models, epinephrine appears to be the most useful pharmacologic agent because of its ability to improve cerebral and coronary blood flow during closed-chest compression.[37, 39, 46, 238, 239] Although epinephrine is widely recommended[9, 10] and used, it is unlikely that randomized trials will ever be done in humans because of reluctance to withhold epinephrine from a comparison (control) group, given its well-documented hemodynamic benefit.

After successful return of spontaneous circulation, neurologic outcome is improved if systemic blood pressure is maintained within (or, for a brief period, slightly above) the normal range.[240–242] Intracranial hypertension should be treated by hyperventilation,[9, 10] but hypocapnia induces cerebral vasoconstriction.[242a] Thus, the value of hyperventilation is unproven.[10] An adequate Pa_{O_2} should be maintained to maximize cerebral oxygen delivery using assisted ventilation if necessary. Seizure activity or fever should be treated aggressively to minimize the brain's oxygen requirement.

Several drugs have been investigated as potential cerebroprotective agents. Barbiturates improve neurologic outcome in dogs when used before global ischemia[243] and in monkeys treated immediately after global ischemia.[244] Unfortunately, a prospective multicenter study in human subjects who were comatose immediately after cardiac arrest failed to demonstrate any improvement in neurologic outcome between patients who received thiopental and those who did not.[245] The calcium antagonist lidoflazine was ineffective in altering neurologic outcome in a prospective, placebo-controlled trial involving 516 cardiac arrest survivors.[246] Other agents that are currently being studied, or are being considered for study, include prostaglandin inhibitors, phenytoin, high-dose benzodiazepines, etomidate, and deferoxamine.[9, 10] The most enthusiasm has been generated by the calcium antagonists, which are thought to improve collateral blood flow to jeopardized regions and to protect against low flow and/or reperfusion injury directly.[247–249]

REFERENCES

1. Pentel P, Benowitz N: Pharmacokinetic and pharmacodynamic considerations in drug therapy of cardiac emergencies. Drugs 9:273, 1984.
2. Voorhees WD, Babbs CF, Tacker WA: Regional blood flow during cardiopulmonary resuscitation in dogs. Crit Care Med 8:134, 1980.
3. Doan LA: Peripheral versus central venous delivery of medications during CPR. Ann Emerg Med 13:784, 1984.
4. Del Guercio LRM, Feins NR, Cohn JD, et al: Comparison of blood flow during external and internal cardiac massage in man. Circulation 31(Suppl):171, 1965.
5. Barsan WG, Levy RC, Weir H: Lidocaine levels during CPR. Ann Emerg Med 10:73, 1981.
6. Jaffe AS: The use of antiarrhythmics in advanced cardiac life support. Ann Emerg Med 22:207, 1993.
7. Kuhn GJ, White BC, Swetman RE, et al: Peripheral versus central circulation time during CPR. A pilot study. Ann Emerg Med 10:417, 1981.
8. Hedges JR, Barsan WG, Doan LA, et al: Central versus peripheral intravenous routes in cardiopulmonary resuscitation. Am J Emerg Med 2:385, 1984.
9. Standards and guidelines for cardiopulmonary resuscitation (CPR) and emergency cardiac care (ECC). JAMA 255:2905, 1986.
10. American Heart Association: Textbook of Advanced Cardiac Life Support. Dallas: American Heart Association, 1987.
11. Snyder DW, Jaffe AS: Acute myocardial infarction. In Messerli F (ed): Cardiovascular Drug Therapy, 2nd ed. Philadelphia: WB Saunders, 1995.
12. Redding JS, Asuncion JS, Pearson JW: Effective routes of drug administration during cardiac arrest. Anesth Analg 46:253, 1967.
13. Keats S, Jackson RE, Kosnik JW, et al: Effect of peripheral

versus central injection of epinephrine on changes in aortic diastolic blood pressure during closed-chest massage in dogs [abstract]. Ann Emerg Med 14:495, 1985.

14. Dalsey WC, Barsan WG, Joyce SM, et al: Comparison of superior vena caval versus inferior vena caval access using a radioisotope technique during normal perfusion and cardiopulmonary resuscitation. Ann Emerg Med 13:881, 1984.

15. Talit U, Braun S, Halkin H, et al: Pharmacokinetic differences between peripheral and central drug administration during cardiopulmonary resuscitation. J Am Coll Cardiol 6:1073, 1985.

16. Emerman CL, Pinchak AC, Hancock D, Hagen JF: The effect of bolus injection on circulation times during cardiac arrest. Am J Emerg Med 8:190, 1990.

17. Schleien CL, Berkowitz ID, Traystman R, et al: Controversial issues in cardiopulmonary resuscitation. Anesthesiology 71:133, 1989.

18. Kraig RP, Petito CK, Plum F: Hydrogen ions kill brain at concentration reached in ischemia. J Cereb Blood Flow Metab 7:379, 1987.

19. D'Alecy, Lundy EF, Barton KJ, et al: Dextrose containing intravenous fluid impairs outcome and increases death after eight minutes of cardiac arrest and resuscitation in dogs. Surgery 100:505, 1986.

20. Pulsinelli WA, Levy DE, Sigsbee B, et al: Increased damage after ischemic stroke in patients with hyperglycemia with or without established diabetes mellitus. Am J Med 74:540, 1983.

21. Longstreth WT, Inui TS: High blood glucose level on hospital admission and poor neurological recovery after cardiac arrest. Ann Neurol 15:59, 1984.

22. Longstreth WT, Diehr P, Cobb LA, et al: Neurologic outcome and blood glucose levels during out-of-hospital cardiopulmonary resuscitation. Neurology 36:1186, 1986.

23. Martin GB, O'Brien JF, Best R, et al: Insulin and glucose levels during CPR in the canine model. Ann Emerg Med 14:293, 1985.

24. Taylor SH, Saxton C, Majid PA, et al: Insulin secretion following myocardial infarction with particular respect to the pathogenesis of cardiogenic shock. Lancet 2:1373, 1969.

25. Raehl CL: Endotracheal drug therapy in cardiopulmonary resuscitation. Clin Pharmacol 5:572, 1986.

26. Hasegawa EA: The endotracheal administration of drugs. Heart Lung 15:60, 1986.

27. Scott B, Martin FG, Matchett J, et al: Canine cardiovascular responses to endotracheally and intravenously administered atropine, isoproterenol and propranolol. Ann Emerg Med 16:1, 1987.

28. Murphy KM, Caplen SM, Nowak RM, et al: Endotracheal bretylium tosylate in a canine model. Ann Emerg Med 13:87, 1984.

29. Roberts JR, Greenberg MI, Knaub M, et al: Comparison of the pharmacological effects of epinephrine administered by intravenous and endotracheal routes. J Am Coll Emerg Phys 7:260, 1978.

30. Roberts JR, Greenberg MI, Knaub MA, et al: Blood levels following intravenous and endotracheal epinephrine administration. J Am Coll Emerg Phys 8:53, 1979.

31. Mace SE: Effect of technique of administration on plasma lidocaine levels. Ann Emerg Med 15:552, 1986.

32. Greenberg MI, Baskin SI, Kaplan AM, et al: Effects of endotracheally administered distilled water or normal saline on the arterial blood gases in dogs. Ann Emerg Med 11:600, 1982.

33. Hahnel JH, Lindner KH, Schurmann C, et al: Plasma lidocaine levels and PaO2 with endotracheal administration. Dilution with normal saline or distilled water. Ann Emerg Med 19:1314, 1990.

34. Ralston SH, Tacker WA, Showen L, et al: Endotracheal versus intravenous epinephrine during electromechanical dissociation with CPR in dogs. Ann Emerg Med 14:1044, 1985.

35. Kosnik JW, Jackson RE, Keats S, et al: Dose-related response of centrally administered epinephrine on the change in aortic diastolic pressure during closed-chest massage in dogs. Ann Emerg Med 14:204, 1985.

36. Livesy JJ, Follette DM, Fey KH, et al: Optimizing myocardial supply/demand balance with alpha-adrenergic drugs during cardiopulmonary resuscitation. J Thorac Cardiovasc Surg 76:244, 1978.

37. Brown CG, Werman HA, Davis EA, et al: The effect of high-dose phenylephrine versus epinephrine on regional cerebral blood flow during CPR. Ann Emerg Med 16:743, 1987.

38. Jackson RE, Joyce K, Danosi SF, et al: Blood flow in the cerebral cortex during cardiac resuscitation in dogs. Ann Emerg Med 13:657, 1984.

39. Brown CG, Davis EA, Werman HA, et al: Methoxamine versus epinephrine on regional cerebral blood flow during cardiopulmonary resuscitation. Crit Care Med 15:682, 1987.

40. Brown CG, Werman HA, Davis EA, et al: Comparative effect of graded doses of epinephrine on regional brain blood flow during CPR in a swine model. Ann Emerg Med 15:1138, 1986.

41. Gonzalez ER, Ornato JP, Garnett AR, et al: Dose response evaluation of epinephrine during cardiopulmonary resuscitation in humans [abstract]. Drug Intell Clin Pharm 21:19, 1987.

42. Gonzalez ER: Pharmacologic controversies in CPR. Ann Emerg Med 22:317, 1993.

43. Lindemann R: Endotracheal administration of epinephrine during cardiopulmonary resuscitation [letter]. Am J Dis Child 136:753, 1982.

44. Newton DW, Fung EY, Williams DA: Stability of five catecholamines and terbutaline sulfate in 5% dextrose injection in the absence and presence of aminophylline. Am J Hosp Pharm 38:1314, 1981.

45. Pearson JW, Redding JS: Influence of peripheral vascular tone on cardiac resuscitation. Anesth Analg 44:746, 1965.

46. Michael JR, Guerci AD, Koehler RC, et al: Mechanism by which epinephrine augments cerebral and myocardial perfusion during cardiopulmonary resuscitation in dogs. Circulation 69:822, 1984.

47. Koehler RC, Michael JR, Guerci AD, et al: Beneficial effect of epinephrine infusion on cerebral and myocardial blood flow during CPR. Ann Emerg Med 14:744, 1985.

48. Otto CW, Yakaitas RW: The role of epinephrine in CPR: A reappraisal. Ann Emerg Med 13:840, 1984.

49. White RD: Defining the pressure needs of the fibrillating heart during prolonged arrest: Identification and application. Ann Emerg Med 14:587, 1985.

50. Crile G, Dolley DH: An experimental research into resuscitation of dogs killed by anesthetics and asphyxia. J Exp Med 8:713, 1906.

51. Niemann JT, Criley JM, Rosborough JP, et al: Predictive indices of successful cardiac resuscitation after prolonged arrest and experimental cardiopulmonary resuscitation. Ann Emerg Med 14:521, 1985.

52. Reimer KA, Jennings RB, Tatum AH: Pathobiology of acute myocardial ischemia. Metabolic, functional, and ultrastructural studies. Am J Cardiol 52:72a, 1983.

53. Ditchey RV: High dose epinephrine does not improve the balance between myocardial oxygen supply and demand during cardiopulmonary resuscitation in dogs [abstract]. J Am Coll Cardiol 3:596, 1984.

54. Callaham M: Epinephrine doses in cardiac arrest: Is it time to outgrow the orthodoxy of ACLS? Ann Emerg Med 18:1011, 1989.

55. Paradis NA, Koscove EM: Epinephrine in cardiac arrest: A critical review. Ann Emerg Med 19:1288, 1990.

56. Gonzalez ER, Ornato JP, Garnett AR, et al: Dose-dependent vasopressor response to epinephrine during CPR in humans. Ann Emerg Med 18:920, 1989.

57. Gonzalez ER, Ornato JP: The dose of epinephrine during cardiopulmonary resuscitation in humans: What should it be? Ann Pharmacother 25:773, 1991.

58. Lindner KH, Ahnefeld FW, Prengel AW: Comparison of standard and high-dose adrenaline in the resuscitation of asystole and electromechanical dissociation. Acta Anaesthesiol Scand 35:253, 1991.

59. Stiell IG, Hebert PC, Weitzman BN, et al: A study of high-dose epinephrine in human CPR. N Engl J Med 327:1047, 1992.

60. Callaham M, Madsen CD, Barton CW, et al: A randomized clinical trial of high-dose epinephrine and norepinephrine versus standard dose epinephrine in prehospital cardiac arrest. JAMA 268:2667, 1992.

61. Brown CG, Martin DR, Pepe PE, et al: A comparison of standard dose epinephrine and high dose epinephrine in cardiac arrest outside the hospital. N Engl J Med 327:1051, 1992.

62. Paradis NA, Martin GB, Rivers EP, et al: Coronary perfusion pressure and return of spontaneous circulation in human CPR. JAMA 263:1106, 1990.

63. Goetting MG, Paradis NA: High-dose epinephrine improves outcome from pediatric cardiac arrest. Ann Emerg Med 20:22, 1991.

64. Rothwell-Jackson RL: The adjuvant use of pressor amines during cardiac massage. Br J Surg 55:545, 1968.

65. Pearson JW, Redding JS: Epinephrine in cardiac resuscitation. Am Heart J 66:210, 1968.

66. Jude JR, Neumaster T, Kfoury E: Vasopressor-cardiotonic drugs in cardiac resuscitation. Acta Anaesthesiol Scand 29:147, 1968.

67. Ralston SH: Alpha agonist drug usage during CPR. Ann Emerg Med 13:786, 1984.

68. Yakaitis RW, Otto CW, Blitt CD: Relative importance of alpha and beta adrenergic receptors during resuscitation. Crit Care Med 7:293, 1979.

69. Brillman JA, Sanders AB, Otto CW, et al: Outcome of resuscitation from fibrillatory arrest using epinephrine and phenylephrine in dogs. Crit Care Med 13:912, 1985.

70. Brown CG, Werman HA, Davis RA, et al: Comparative effects of epinephrine and phenylephrine on regional cerebral blood flow during cardiopulmonary resuscitation [abstract]. Ann Emerg Med 15:635, 1986.

71. Edvinson L, Lacome P, Owman CH, et al: Quantitative changes in regional cerebral blood flow of rats induced by alpha- and beta-adrenergic stimulants. Acta Physiol Scand 107:289, 1979.

72. Leier CV, Heban P, Huss P, et al: Comparative systemic and regional hemodynamic effects of dopamine and dobutamine in patients with cardiomyopathic heart failure. Circulation 58:466, 1978.

73. Otto CW, Yakaitas RW, Redding JS, et al: Comparison of dopamine, dobutamine, and epinephrine in CPR. Crit Care Med 9:640, 1981.

74. Lindner KH, Ahnefeld FW, Bowdler IM: Comparison of epinephrine and dopamine during cardiopulmonary resuscitation. Intensive Care Med 15:432, 1989.

75. Gonzalez ER, Ornato JP, Levine RL: Vasopressor effect of epinephrine with and without dopamine during cardiopulmonary resuscitation. Drug Intell Clin Pharm 22:868, 1988.

76. Keung EC, Siskind SJ, Sonnenblick EH, et al: Dobutamine therapy in acute myocardial infarction. JAMA 245:144, 1981.

77. Leier CV: Acute inotropic support. In Leier CV (ed): Cardiotonic Drugs. New York: Marcel Dekker, 1986, pp 49–84.

78. Stoner JD, Bolen JL, Harrison DC: Comparison of dobutamine and dopamine in treatment of severe heart failure. Br Heart J 39:536, 1977.

76. Keung ECH, Siskind SJ, Sonneblick EH, et al: Dobutamine therapy in acute myocardial infarction. JAMA 245:144, 1981.

79. Mueller HS, Evans R, Ayers S: Effect of dopamine on hemodynamics and myocardial metabolism in man. Circulation 57:361, 1978.

80. Rude RE, Izquierdo C, Buja M, et al: Effects of inotropic and chronotropic stimuli on acute myocardial ischemic injury: Studies with dobutamine in the anesthetized dog. Circulation 65:1321, 1982.

81. Genton R, Jaffe AS: Management of congestive heart failure in patients with acute myocardial infarction. JAMA 256:2556, 1986.

82. Mancini D, Lejemtel T, Sonnenblick E: Intravenous amrinone for the treatment of the failing heart. Am J Cardiol 56:9b, 1985.

83. Scholz H: Inotropic drugs and their mechanisms of action. J Am Coll Cardiol 4:389, 1984.

84. Wynne J, Malacoff RF, Benotti JR, et al: Oral amrinone in refractory congestive heart failure. Am J Cardiol 45:1245, 1980.

85. Naccarelli GV, Gray EL, Dougherty AH, et al: Amrinone: Acute electrophysiologic and hemodynamic effects in patients with congestive heart failure. Am J Cardiol 54:600, 1984.

86. Gonzalez ER, Meyers DG: Assessment and management of cardiogenic shock. In Ornato JP (ed): Cardiovascular Emergencies. New York: Churchill Livingstone, 1986, p 128.

87. LeJemtel TJ, Keung E, Ribner JS, et al: Sustained beneficial effects of oral amrinone on cardiac and renal function in patients with severe congestive heart failure. Am J Cardiol 45:123, 1980.

88. Franciosa JA: Intravenous amrinone: An advance or wrong step? [editorial]. Ann Intern Med 102:399, 1985.

89. Klein NA, Siskind SJ, Frishman WH, et al: Hemodynamic comparison of intravenous amrinone and dobutamine in patients with chronic congestive heart failure. Am J Cardiol 48:170, 1981.

90. Chesebro JH, Harrison CE, Deets SL: Intravenous and oral amrinone therapy in refractory heart failure: Hemodynamics, exercise results, and side effects. Am J Cardiol 47:491, 1981.

91. Chesebro JH, Fuster V, Robertson JS, et al: Shortened platelet survival in cardiac failure: Predisposition to amrinone-induced platelet reduction. Circulation 66:ii, 1982.

92. Vatner SR, Baig H: Comparison of the effects of ouabain and isoproterenol on ischemic myocardium of conscious dogs. Circulation 58:654, 1978.

93. Niemann JT, Haynes KS, Garner D, et al: Postcountershock pulseless rhythms: Response to CPR, artificial cardiac pacing, and adrenergic agonists. Ann Emerg Med 15:112, 1986.

94. Ditchey RV, Lindenfeld J: Potential adverse effects of volume loading on perfusion of vital organs during closed-chest resuscitation. Circulation 69:181, 1984.

95. Niemann JT, Rosborough JP, Ung S, et al: Hemodynamic effects of continuous abdominal binding during cardiac arrest and resuscitation. Am J Cardiol 53:269, 1984.

96. Halperin HR, Guerci AD, Chandra N, et al: Vest inflation without simultaneous ventilation during cardiac arrest in dogs: Improved survival from prolonged cardiopulmonary resuscitation. Circulation 74:1407, 1986.

97. Lindner KH, Prengel AW, Pfenninger EG, et al: Vasopressin improves vital organ blood flow during closed-chest cardiopulmonary resuscitation in pigs. Circulation 91:215, 1995.

98. Olson DW, Thompson BM, Darin JC, et al: A randomized comparison study of bretylium tosylate and lidocaine in resuscitation of patients from out-of-hospital ventricular fibrillation in a paramedic system. Ann Emerg Med 13:807, 1984.

99. Haynes RE, Chinn TL, Copass MK, et al: Comparison of bretylium tosylate and lidocaine in management of out-of-hospital ventricular fibrillation: A randomized clinical trial. Am J Cardiol 48:353, 1981.

100. Hanyok JJ, Chow MS, Kluger J, Fieldman A: Antifibrillatory effects of high dose bretylium and a lidocaine-bretylium combination during cardiopulmonary resuscitation. Crit Care Med 16:691, 1988.

101. White RD: Antifibrillatory drugs: The case for lidocaine and procainamide. Ann Emerg Med 13:802, 1984.

102. Anderson JL: Antifibrillatory versus antiectopic therapy. Am J Cardiol 54:7a, 1984.

103. Chow MSS, Kluger J, DiPersio DM, et al: Antifibrillatory effects of lidocaine and bretylium immediately post cardiopulmonary resuscitation. Am Heart J 110:938, 1985.

104. Chow MMS, Ronsfeld RAA, Hamilton RA, et al: Effect of external cardiopulmonary resuscitation on lidocaine pharmacokinetics in dogs. J Pharmacol Exp Ther 224:531, 1983.

105. Kerber RE, Pandian NG, Jensen SR, et al: Effect of lidocaine and bretylium on energy requirement for transthoracic defibrillation. Experimental studies. J Am Coll Cardiol 7:397, 1986.

106. Dorian P, Fain ES, Davy JM, et al: Lidocaine causes a reversible, concentration-dependent increase in defibrillation energy requirements. J Am Coll Cardiol 8:327, 1986.

107. MacMahon S, Collins R, Peto R, et al: Effects of prophylactic lidocaine in suspected acute myocardial infarction. JAMA 260:1910, 1988.

108. Hine LK, Laird N, Hewitt P, Chalmers TC: Meta-analytic evidence against prophylactic use of lidocaine in acute myocardial infarction. Arch Intern Med 149:2694, 1989.

108a. Dunn HM, McComb JM, Kinney CD, et al: Prophylactic lidocaine in the early phase of suspected myocardial infarction. Am Heart J 110:353, 1985.

108b. Guidelines for the early management of patients with acute myocardial infarction. A report of the American College of Cardiology/American Heart Association Task Force on Assessment of Diagnostic and Therapeutic Cardiovascular Procedures (Subcommittee to Develop Guidelines for the Early Management of Patients with Acute Myocardial Infarction). J Am Coll Cardiol 16:249, 1990.

109. Routledge PA, Shand DG, Barchowsky A, et al: Relationship between alpha-1 acid glycoprotein and lidocaine disposition in myocardial infarction. Clin Pharmacol Ther 30:154, 1981.

110. Johansson BG, Kindmark CO, Trell EY, et al: Sequential changes of plasma proteins after myocardial infarction. Scand J Clin Lab Invest 29:117, 1972.

111. Thomson PD, Melmon KL, Richardson JA, et al: Lidocaine pharmacokinetics in advanced heart failure, liver disease, and renal failure in humans. Ann Intern Med 78:499, 1973.

112. Davison R, Parker M, Atkinson AJ Jr: Excessive serum lidocaine levels during maintenance infusions: Mechanisms and prevention. Am Heart J 104:203, 1982.

113. Pfeifer HJ, Greenblat DJ, Koch-Weser J: Clinical use and toxicity of intravenous lidocaine: A report from the Boston Collaborative Drug Surveillance Program. Am Heart J 92:168, 1976.

114. Dollery CT, Emslie-Smith D, McMichen E: Bretylium tosylate in the treatment of hypertension. Lancet 1:296, 1960.

115. Leveque PE: Antiarrhythmic action of bretylium. Nature 207:203, 1965.

116. Koch-Weser J: Drug therapy: Bretylium. N Engl J Med 300:473, 1979.

117. Bigger JT, Jaffe CC: The effects of bretylium tosylate on the electrophysiologic properties of ventricular muscle and Purkinje fibers. Am J Cardiol 27:82, 1971.

118. Cardinal R, Sasyniuk BI: Electrophysiological effects of bretylium tosylate on subendocardial Purkinje fibers from infarcted canine hearts. J Pharmacol Exp Ther 204:159, 1978.

119. Euler DE, Scanlon PJ: Mechanism of the effect of bretylium on the ventricular fibrillation threshold in dogs. Am J Cardiol 55:1396, 1985.

120. Tacker WA, Niebauer MJ, Babbs CR, et al: The effect of newer antiarrhythmic drugs on defibrillation threshold. Crit Care Med 8:177, 1980.

121. Koo CC, Allen JD, Pantridge JF: Lack of effect of bretylium on electrical defibrillation in a controlled study. Cardiovasc Res 18:762, 1984.

122. Sasyniuk BI: Concept of reentry versus automaticity. Am J Cardiol 54:1a, 1984.

123. Ideker RE, Klein GH, Harrison L, et al: Epicardial mapping of the initiation of ventricular fibrillation induced by reperfusion following acute ischemia. Circulation 64(Suppl 2):57, 1978.

124. Anderson JL, Patterson E, Conlon M, et al: Kinetics of antifibrillatory effects of bretylium: Correlation with myocardial concentration. Am J Cardiol 46:583, 1980.

125. Rapeport WG: Clinical pharmacokinetics of bretylium. Clin Pharmacokinet 10:248, 1985.

126. Duff HJ, Roden DM, Yacobi A, et al: Bretylium: Relations between plasma concentrations and pharmacologic actions in high-frequency ventricular arrhythmias. Am J Cardiol 55:395, 1985.

127. Lucchesi BR: Rationale of therapy in the patient with acute myocardial infarction and life-threatening arrhythmias: A focus on bretylium. Am J Cardiol 54:14a, 1984.

128. Mayer NM: Management of ventricular dysrhythmias in the prehospital and emergency department setting. Am J Cardiol 54:34a, 1984.

129. Sanna G, Arcidiacono R: Chemical ventricular defibrillation of the human heart with bretylium tosylate. Am J Cardiol 32:982, 1973.

130. Nowak RM, Bodnar TJ, Dronen S, et al: Bretylium tosylate as initial treatment for cardiopulmonary arrest: A randomized comparison with placebo. Ann Emerg Med 10:404, 1981.

131. Harrison EE, Amey BD: The use of bretylium in prehospital ventricular fibrillation. Am J Emerg Med 1:1, 1983.

132. Euler DE, Leman TW, Wallock ME, et al: Deleterious effects of bretylium on hemodynamic recovery from ventricular fibrillation. Am Heart J 112:25, 1986.

133. Anderson JL: Bretylium tosylate: Profile of the only available class III antiarrhythmic agent. Clin Ther 7:205, 1985.

134. Giardina EGV, Heissenbuttel RH, Bigger JT: Intermittent intravenous procainamide to treat ventricular arrhythmias. Ann Intern Med 78:183, 1973.

135. Koch-Weser J: Procainamide dosing schedules, plasma concentrations, and clinical effects. JAMA 215:1454, 1971.

136. Kastor JA, Josephson ME, Guss SB, et al: Human ventricular refractoriness. II: Effects of procainamide. Circulation 56:462, 1977.

136a. Anderson JL, Roder HE, Green LS: Comparative effects of beta-adrenergic blocking drugs on experimental ventricular fibrillation threshold. Am J Cardiol 51:1196, 1983.

137. Morgan DB, Davidson C: Hypokalemia and diuretics: An analysis of publications. Br Med J 280:905, 1980.

138. Hollifield JW: Potassium and magnesium abnormalities: Diuretics and arrhythmias in hypertension. Am J Med 77:28, 1984.

139. Nordrehaug JE, von der Lippe G: Hypokalemia and ventricular fibrillation in acute myocardial infarction. Br Heart J 50:525, 1983.

140. Thompson RG, Cobb LA: Hypokalemia after resuscitation from out-of-hospital ventricular fibrillation. JAMA 248:2860, 1982.

141. Ornato JP, Gonzalez ER, Starke H, et al: Incidence and causes of hypokalemia associated with cardiac resuscitation. Am J Emerg Med 3:503, 1985.

142. Ornato JP, Gonzalez ER: Refractory ventricular fibrillation. Emerg Decisions 4:35, 1986.

143. Dyckner T, Wester PO: Magnesium in cardiology. Acta Med Scand 661(Suppl):27, 1982.

144. Ebel H, Gunther T: Role of magnesium in cardiac disease. J Clin Chem Clin Biochem 21:249, 1983.

145. Rasmussen HS, Norregard P, Lindeneg O, et al: Intravenous magnesium in acute myocardial infarction. Lancet 1:234, 1986.

146. Tzivoni D, Banai S, Schuger C, et al: Treatment of torsade de pointes with magnesium sulfate. Circulation 77:392, 1988.

147. Whang R, Flink EB, Dyckner T, et al: Magnesium depletion as a cause of refractory potassium repletion. Arch Intern Med 145:1686, 1985.

148. Whang R, Oei TO, Aikawa JK, et al: Predictors of clinical hypomagnesemia. Arch Intern Med 144:1794, 1984.

149. Rasmussen HS, Aurup P, Hojberg S, et al: Magnesium and acute myocardial infarction. Arch Intern Med 146:872, 1986.

150. Woods KL, Fletcher S, Roffe C, Haider Y: Intravenous magnesium sulfate in suspected acute myocardial infarction: Results of the second Leicester Intravenous Magnesium Intervention Trial (LIMIT-2). Lancet 339:1553, 1992.

151. Bigger JT, Sahar DI: Clinical types of proarrhythmic response to antiarrhythmic drugs. Am J Cardiol 59:2e, 1987.

152. Smith WM, Gallagher JJ: "Les torsade de pointes": An unusual ventricular arrhythmia. Ann Intern Med 93:578, 1980.

153. Kowey PR, Engel TR: Overdrive pacing for ventricular tachyarrhythmias: A reassessment. Ann Intern Med 99:651, 1983.

154. Ward WG, Reid RL: High-dose intravenous nitroglycerin during cardiopulmonary resuscitation for refractory cardiac arrest. Am J Cardiol 53:1725, 1984.

155. Williams ML, Woelfel A, Cascio WE, et al: Intravenous amiodarone during prolonged resuscitation from cardiac arrest. Ann Intern Med 110:839, 1989.

156. Ewy GA, Dahl CF, Zimmerman M, et al: Ventricular fibrillation masquerading as ventricular standstill. Crit Care Med 9:841, 1981.

157. Iseri LT, Humphrey SB, Siner EJ: Prehospital brady-asystolic cardiac arrest. Ann Intern Med 88:741, 1978.

158. Brown DC, Lewis AJ, Criley MS: Asystole and its treatment: The possible role of the parasympathetic nervous system in cardiac arrest. J Am Coll Emerg Phys 8:448, 1979.

159. Stueven HA, Tonsfeldt DJ, Thompson BM, et al: Atropine in asystole: Human studies. Ann Emerg Med 13:815, 1984.

160. Myerburg RJ, Estes D, Zaman L, et al: Outcome of resuscitation from bradyarrhythmic or asystolic prehospital cardiac arrest. J Am Coll Cardiol 4:1118, 1984.

161. Ornato JP, Gonzalez ER, Morkunas AR, et al: Treatment of presumed asystole during pre-hospital cardiac arrest. Am J Emerg Med 3:395, 1985.

162. Coon GA, Clinton JE, Ruiz E: Use of atropine for brady-asystolic cardiac arrest. Ann Emerg Med 10:462, 1981.

163. Cummins RO, Graves JR, Larsen MP, et al: Out-of-hospital

transcutaneous pacing by emergency medical technicians in patients with asystolic cardiac arrest. N Engl J Med 328:1377, 1993.

164. Massumi RA, Mason DT, Amsterdam EA, et al: Ventricular fibrillation and tachycardia after intravenous atropine for treatment of bradycardias. N Engl J Med 287:336, 1972.

165. Cooper MJ, Abinader EG: Atropine-induced ventricular fibrillation: Case report and review of the literature. Am Heart J 97:225, 1979.

166. O'Rourke GW, Greene NM: Autonomic blockade and the resting heart rate in man. Am Heart J 80:469, 1970.

167. Dauchot P, Gravenstein JS: Bradycardia after myocardial ischemia and its treatment with atropine. Anesthesiology 44:501, 1976.

168. Lunde P: Ventricular fibrillation after intravenous atropine for treatment of sinus bradycardia. Acta Med Scand 199:369, 1976.

169. Stueven H, Thompson BM, Aprahamian C, et al: Use of calcium in prehospital cardiac arrest. Ann Emerg Med 12:136, 1983.

170. Stueven HA, Thompson BM, Aprahamian C, et al: Calcium chloride: Reassessment of its use in asystole. Ann Emerg Med 13:820, 1984.

171. Kirsch JR, Dean JM, Rogers MC: Current concepts in brain resuscitation. Arch Intern Med 146:1413, 1986.

172. Dembo DH: Calcium in advanced life support. Crit Care Med 9:358, 1981.

173. Carlon GC, Howland WS, Kahn RC, et al: Calcium chloride administration in normocalcemic critically ill patients. Crit Care Med 8:209, 1980.

174. Follette DM, Fey K, Buckberg GD, et al: Reducing postischemic damage by temporary modification of reperfusate calcium, potassium, pH, and osmolarity. J Thorac Cardiovasc Surg 82:221, 1981.

175. Zimmerman AN, Hulsmann WC: Paradoxical influence of calcium ions on the permeability of the cell membrane of the isolated rat heart. Nature 211:646, 1966.

176. Schanne FAX, Kane AB, Young EE, et al: Calcium dependence of toxic cell death: A final common pathway. Science 206:700, 1979.

177. Borgers E, Thone F, Xhonneux R, et al: Shifts of calcium in the ischemic myocardium. A structural analysis. In Wauquier A, Borgers M, Amery WK (eds): Protection of Tissues Against Hypoxia. Amsterdam: Elsevier, 1982, p 365.

178. White RD, Goldsmith RS, Rodriguez R, et al: Plasma ionic calcium levels following injection of chlorine, gluconate, and gluceptate salts of calcium. J Thorac Cardiovasc Surg 71:609, 1976.

179. Clemo HF, Belardinelli L: Effect of adenosine on atrioventricular conduction. I. Site and characterization of adenosine action in the guinea pig atrioventricular node. Circ Res 59:427, 1986.

180. Berne RM: Cardiac nucleotides in hypoxia: Possible role in regulation of coronary blood flow. Am J Physiol 204:317, 1963.

181. Schrader J, Baumann G, Gerlach E: Adenosine as inhibitor of myocardial effects of catecholamines. Pflugers Arch 372:29, 1977.

182. Imai S, Riley AL, Berne RM: Effect of ischemia on adenine nucleotides in cardiac and skeletal muscle. Circ Res 15:443, 1964.

183. Dobson JG: Adenosine reduces catecholamine contractile responses in oxygenated and hypoxic atria. Am J Physiol 245:H468, 1983.

184. Rubio R, Knabb MT, Tsukada T, Berne RM: Mechanisms of action of adenosine on vascular smooth muscle and cardiac cells. In Berne RM, Rall TW, Rubio R (eds): Regulatory Function of Adenosine. The Hague: Martinus Nihjoff, 1983, pp 319–332.

185. Belardinelli L, West A, Crampton R, Berne RM: Chronotropic and dromotropic effects of adenosine. In Berne RM, Rall TW, Rubio R (eds): Regulatory Function of Adenosine. The Hague: Martinus Nihjoff, 1983, pp 377–398.

186. Belardinelli L, Linder J, Berne RM: The cardiac effects of adenosine. Prog Cardiovasc Dis 32:73, 1989.

187. Belardinelli L, Giles WR, West A: Ionic mechanisms of adenosine actions in pacemaker cells from rabbit heart. J Physiol (Lond) 405:615, 1988.

188. Belardinelli L, Isenberg G: Isolated atrial myocytes: Adenosine and acetylcholine increase potassium conductance. Am J Physiol 244:h734, 1983.

189. Camm AJ, Garratt CJ: Adenosine and supraventricular tachycardia. N Engl J Med 325:1621, 1991.

190. Johnson EA, McKinnon MG: Effect of acetylcholine and adenosine on cardiac cellular potentials. Nature 178:1174, 1956.

191. West GA, Belardinelli L: Correlation of sinus slowing and hyperpolarization caused by adenosine in sinus node. Pflugers Arch 403:75, 1985.

192. Kurachi Y, Nakajima T, Sugimoto T: On the mechanism of activation of muscarinic K^+ channels by adenosine in isolated atrial cells: Involvement of GTP-binding proteins. Pflugers Arch 407:264, 1986.

193. Lerman BB, Belardinelli L: Research advances series: Cardiac electrophysiology of adenosine: Basic and clinical concepts. Circulation 83:1499, 1991.

194. Lloyd HGE, Deussen A, Wupperman H, Schrader J: The transmethylation pathway as a source for adenosine in the isolated guinea-pig hearts. Biochem J 252:489, 1988.

195. Olsson RA, Gentry MK, Townsend SR: Adenosine metabolism: Properties of dog heart microsomal 5'-nucleotidase. Adv Exp Med Biol 39:27, 1973.

196. Viskin S, Belhassen B, Roth A, et al: Aminophylline for bradyasystolic cardiac arrest refractory to atropine and epinephrine. Ann Intern Med 118:279, 1993.

197. Wesley RC Jr, Lerman BB, DiMarco JP, et al: Mechanism of atropine resistant atrioventricular block during inferior myocardial infarction: Possible role of adenosine. J Am Coll Cardiol 8:1232, 1986.

198. Shah PK, Nalos P, Peter T: Atropine resistant post infarction complete AV block: Possible role of adenosine and improvement with aminophylline. Am Heart J 113:194, 1987.

199. Gupta A, Jain A, Kala SC: Role of aminophylline in atropine resistant atrioventricular block. J Assoc Physicians India 39:214, 1991.

200. Strasberg B, Bassevich R, Mager A, et al: Effects of aminophylline on atrioventricular conduction in patients with late atrioventricular block during inferior wall acute myocardial infarction. Am J Cardiol 67:527, 1991.

201. Ornato JP, Carveth WL, Windle JR: Pacemaker insertion for prehospital bradyasystolic cardiac arrest. Ann Emerg Med 13:101, 1984.

202. Zoll PM, Zoll RH, Falk RH, et al: External noninvasive temporary cardiac pacing: Clinical trials. Circulation 71:937, 1985.

203. Falk RH, Jacobs L, Sinclair A, et al: External noninvasive cardiac pacing in out-of-hospital cardiac arrest. Crit Care Med 11:779, 1983.

204. Weisfeldt ML, Bishop RL, Greene HL: Effects of pH and PCO2 on performance of ischemic myocardium. In Roy P, Rona G (eds): International Study Group for Research in Cardiac Metabolism. The Metabolism of Contraction. Recent Advances in Studies on Cardiac Structure and Metabolism, Vol X. Baltimore: University of Maryland Press, 1975, p 355.

205. Ewy GA: Defining electromechanical dissociation. Ann Emerg Med 13:830, 1984.

206. Ornato JP: Special resuscitation situations. Circulation 74(Suppl 4):23, 1986.

207. Harrison EE, Amey BD: Use of calcium in electromechanical dissociation. Ann Emerg Med 13:844, 1984.

208. Bodai BI, Smith JP, Ward RE, et al: Emergency thoracotomy in the management of trauma. A review. JAMA 249:1891, 1983.

209. Cogbill TH, Moore EE, Millikan JS, et al: Rationale for selective application of emergency department thoracotomy in trauma. J Trauma 23:453, 1983.

210. Danne PD, Finelli F, Champion HR: Emergency thoracotomy. J Trauma 24:796, 1984.

211. Roberge RJ, Invatury RR, Stahl W, et al: Emergency department thoracotomy for penetrating injuries: Predictive value of patient classification. Am J Emerg Med 4:129, 1986.

212. Sanders AB, Kern KB, Atlas M, et al: Importance of the duration of inadequate coronary perfusion pressure in resuscitation from cardiac arrest. J Am Coll Cardiol 6:113, 1985.

213. Weil MH, Trevino RP, Rackow EC: Sodium bicarbonate during CPR—Does it help or hinder? Chest 88:487, 1985.

214. Bishop RL, Weisfeldt ML: Sodium bicarbonate administration during cardiac arrest. JAMA 235:506, 1976.

215. Grundler W, Weil MH, Yamaguchi M, et al: The paradox of venous acidosis and arterial alkalosis during CPR. Chest 86:282, 1984.

216. MacGregor DC, Wilson GJ, Holmes DE, et al: Intramyocardial carbon dioxide tension: A guide to the safe period of anoxic arrest of the heart. J Thorac Cardiovasc Surg 68:101, 1974.

217. Weil MH, Rackow EC, Trevino R, et al: Difference in acid-base state between venous and arterial blood during cardiopulmonary resuscitation. N Engl J Med 315:153, 1986.

218. McGill JW, Ruiz E: Central venous pH as a predictor of arterial pH in prolonged cardiac arrest. Ann Emerg Med 13:684, 1984.

219. Ornato JP, Gonzalez ER, Coyne MR, et al: Arterial pH in out-of-hospital cardiac arrest. Am J Emerg Med 3:498, 1985.

220. Jaffe AL: New and old paradoxes: Acidosis and cardiopulmonary resuscitation. Circulation 80:1079, 1989.

221. Kette F, Weil MH, von Planta M, et al: Buffer agents do not reverse intramyocardial acidosis during cardiac resuscitation. Circulation 81:1660, 1990.

222. Niemann JT, Rosborough JP: Effects of acidemia and sodium bicarbonate therapy in advanced cardiac life support. Ann Emerg Med 13:781, 1984.

223. Clancy RL, Cingolani HE, Taylor RR, et al: Influence of sodium bicarbonate on myocardial performance. Am J Physiol 212:917, 1967.

224. Huseby JS, Bumprecht DG: Hemodynamic effects of rapid bolus sodium bicarbonate on myocardial performance. Am J Physiol 212:917, 1967.

225. Graf H, Leach W, Arieff AI: Evidence for a detrimental effect of bicarbonate therapy in hypoxic lactic acidosis. Science 227:754, 1985.

226. Berenyi KJ, Wolk M, Killip T: Cerebrospinal fluid acidosis complicating therapy of experimental cardiopulmonary arrest. Circulation 52:319, 1975.

227. Mattar JA, Weil MH, Shubin H, et al: Cardiac arrest in the critically ill (II: Hyperosmolar states following cardiac arrest). Am J Med 56:162, 1974.

228. Redding JS, Pearson JW: Resuscitation from ventricular fibrillation. JAMA 203:255, 1968.

229. Yakaitas RW, Thomas JD, Mahaffey JE: Influence of pH and hypoxia on the success of defibrillation. Crit Care Med 3:139, 1975.

230. Redding JS, Pearson JW: Metabolic acidosis: A factor in cardiac resuscitation. South Med J 60:926, 1967.

231. Guerci AD, Chandra N, Johnson E, et al: Sodium bicarbonate does not improve resuscitation from ventricular fibrillation (VF) in dogs [abstract]. Clin Res 34:305A, 1986.

232. Guerci AD, Chandra N, Johnson E, et al: Failure of sodium bicarbonate to improve resuscitation from ventricular fibrillation in dogs. Circulation 74(Suppl IV):75, 1986.

232a. Gazmuri RJ, von Planta M, Weil MH, Rackow EC: Cardiac effects of carbon dioxide-consuming and carbon dioxide-generating buffers during cardiopulmonary resuscitation. J Am Coll Cardiol 15:482, 1990.

233. Bersin RM, Chatterjee K, Arieff AI: Metabolic and hemodynamic consequences of sodium bicarbonate administration in patients with heart disease. Am J Med 87:7, 1989.

234. Cooper DJ, Walley KR, Wiggs BR, Russell JA: Bicarbonate does not improve hemodynamics in critically ill patients who have lactic acidosis. A prospective, controlled clinical study. Ann Intern Med 112:492, 1990.

235. Minuck M, Sharma GP: Comparison of THAM and sodium bicarbonate in resuscitation of the heart after ventricular fibrillation in dogs. Anesth Analg 56:38, 1977.

236. Lee WH, Darby TD, Aldinger EE, et al: Use of THAM in the management of refractory cardiac arrest. Am J Surg 28:87, 1962.

237. Stacpoole PW, Harman EM, Curry SH, et al: Treatment of lactic acidosis with dichloroacetate. N Engl J Med 309:390, 1983.

238. Holmes HR, Babbs CF, Voorhees WD, et al: Influence of adrenergic drugs upon vital organ perfusion during CPR. Crit Care Med 8:137, 1980.

239. Ralston SH, Voorhees WD, Babbs CF: Intrapulmonary epinephrine during prolonged cardiopulmonary resuscitation: Improved regional blood flow and resuscitation in dogs. Ann Emerg Med 13:79, 1984.

240. Cantu RC, Ames A III, Dixon J, et al: Reversibility of experimental cerebrovascular obstruction induced by complete ischemia. J Neurosurg 31:429, 1969.

241. Fischer EG, Ames A: Studies on mechanisms of impairment of cerebral circulation following ischemia: Effects of hemodilution and perfusion pressure. Stroke 3:538, 1972.

242. Bleyaert AL, Sands PA, Safar P, et al: Augmentation of postischemic brain damage by severe intermittent hypertension. Crit Care Med 8:41, 1980.

242a. Todd MM, Tommasino C, Shapiro HM: Cerebrovascular effects of prolonged hypocarbia and hypercarbia after experimental global ischemia in cats. Crit Care Med 13:720, 1984.

243. Goldstein A Jr, Wells BA, Keats AS: Increased tolerance to cerebral anoxia by pentobarbital. Arch Int Pharmacodyn Ther 161:138, 1966.

244. Bleyaert AL, Neomoto EM, Safar P, et al: Thiopental amelioration of brain damage after global ischemia in monkeys. Anesthesiology 49:390, 1978.

245. Brain Resuscitation Clinical Trial I Study Group: Randomized clinical study of thiopental loading in comatose survivors of cardiac arrest. N Engl J Med 314:397, 1986.

246. Brain Resuscitation Clinical Trial II Study Group: A randomized clinical study of a calcium-entry blocker (lidoflazine) in the treatment of comatose survivors of cardiac arrest. N Engl J Med 324:1225, 1991.

247. Steen PA, Grisvold SE, Milde JH, et al: Nimodipine improves outcome when given after complete cerebral ischemia in primates. Anesthesiology 62:406, 1985.

248. Vaagenes P, Cantadore R, Safar P, et al: Amelioration of brain damage by lidoflazine after prolonged ventricular fibrillation and cardiac arrest in dogs. Crit Care Med 12:846, 1984.

249. Edmonds HL, Wauquier A, Melis W, et al: Improved short-term neurological recovery with flunarizine in a canine model of cardiac arrest. Am J Emerg Med 3:150, 1985.

IV.

Special Clinical Situations

Editors: Peter Sleight and Sidney Goldstein

CHAPTER 21

Cardiovascular Drug Therapy in the Elderly

Tomasz Grodzicki, M.D., Ph.D., and Franz H. Messerli, M.D.

The percentage of elderly subjects in the population increases continuously in all developed countries and less rapidly in developing countries as a result of decreased fertility and an increase in expected life span. In 1990, approximately 326 million persons were at least 65 years old, or approximately 6% of the world's population. In the United States, as in other highly developed countries, this figure was between 12% and 15%. Unfortunately, the aging of populations is associated with the increased number of subjects demanding long-term medical care. The practicing physician faces the question of whether age per se should influence cardiovascular drug therapy. The proper answers should be derived from the following determinants:

1. Properly documented trials
2. Age-related changes in pharmacokinetics
3. Age-related changes in cardiovascular function
4. Coexistent diseases
5. Other medications
6. Mental and socioeconomic conditions

Some of these issues are discussed here.

AGE-RELATED CHANGES IN PHARMACOKINETICS

The rapid development of various methods for the monitoring of drug levels in everyday practice helps determine the factors responsible for changes in pharmacokinetics of cardiovascular drugs in elderly patients.[1, 2]

Absorption

The absorption of most orally given agents remains unchanged in aged patients, despite reduced gastrointestinal blood flow and reduced production of gastric acid. These detrimental effects are counterbalanced by decreased motility of the gastrointestinal tract, which prolongs the time of absorption.

Distribution

The increase in fat tissue and the decrease of body water, serum albumin concentration, and lean muscle mass influence the distribution of drugs in elderly patients. The result may be an increase in concentration of a free drug that is highly protein-bound or water-soluble.

Metabolism

Decreased blood flow to the liver, as well as decreased activity of the microsomal oxidative system, leads to the decrease of liver-dependent drug metabolism in the elderly, resulting in a longer half-life. Moreover, the first-pass effect is significantly diminished. These changes lead to higher concentrations of drugs metabolized in the liver, although results of the routine tests of hepatic function remain normal.

Elimination

Glomerular filtration rate and renal blood flow decrease 1% per year from the age of 30. For the drugs eliminated by the kidneys, this means lower elimination rates and results in a longer half-life.

Age-related changes in cardiovascular and hormonal systems can be summarized as follows:

1. Increased stiffness of heart and arteries, resulting in impaired diastolic filling and increased pulse pressure
2. Disseminating atherosclerosis
3. Baroreceptor and β-receptor dysfunction
4. Lower activity of renin-angiotensin system
5. Higher levels of circulating catecholamines[3–6] because of a down-regulation of β-receptors

As stated previously, the elderly patient frequently suffers from coexisting extracardiovascular diseases that may influence the course and the outcome of cardiovascular therapy.[7] Thus, the diagnosis of pulmonary diseases, peripheral artery disease, osteoporosis, chronic osteoarthritis, renal dysfunction, malignant neoplasms, or dementia should guide our choice to proper cardiovascular therapy.

Although most of the long-term cardiovascular trials address the question of how to prolong and improve the lives of our patients, elderly patients are usually excluded. Although age is one of the most important factors influencing morbidity and mortality, it has been difficult to find aged patients that meet the strict criteria of these trials. Thus, the number of subjects over 65 years old included in the double-blind, long-term trials is very low, except in those trials focused on hypertension. A review of cardiovascular drug therapy in the elderly must, therefore, be based on short-term studies, observational papers, or subanalysis of larger trials.

DIURETICS

The entire group of diuretics should be used very cautiously in the elderly, because the total body fluid volume and intravascular volume of most elderly patients are significantly decreased.[4] Moreover, the blunted baroreceptor reaction may facilitate orthostatic hypotension and a predisposition to falls.[8] Because renal blood flow and glomerular filtration rate decrease with age, the excessive depletion in intravascular volume may lead to renal failure.

On the other hand, diuretics are the mainstay of therapy in hypertension and congestive heart failure.

Thiazide Diuretics

Thiazide diuretics in small doses (6.25 to 25 mg/day) are efficacious in elderly patients with essential hypertension. In most studies in which diuretics are the first-line therapy, a marked reduction in stroke rates is reported. Results of the British Medical Research Council study, the European Working Party on High Blood Pressure in the Elderly, the SHEP study, and the STOP trial showed significantly lower numbers of strokes in the diuretic-treated group than in the group receiving placebo.[9-11] On the other hand, diuretics are known to cause some metabolic disturbances, potentially overriding the beneficial blood-pressure–lowering effect on cardiac mortality. The most important disturbances are hypokalemia, altered metabolism of glucose and lipids, hyper-reninemia, and increased adrenergic stimulation.[12] These metabolic adverse effects of diuretics may be less important in the elderly than in the younger patient because of the shorter life expectancy. The elderly patient may simply not live long enough to experience the abolishment of the benefits of the diuretic-induced decrease in blood pressure by the hazards of the diuretic-induced metabolic changes. In patients with hypertension and diabetes, diuretics have been associated with an accelerated decline in renal function and increased mortality.[13] The undesirable effect of increase in uric acid makes diuretics unsuitable in patients suffering from gout.

In patients with left ventricular hypertrophy (LVH) and ventricular ectopy, diuretics, through hypoka-

lemia and hypomagnesemia, may aggravate electrophysiologic instability and cause more serious arrhythmias. Moreover, their influence on LVH reduction has been shown to be the smallest among antihypertensive drugs.[14]

Patients with mild to moderate congestive heart failure may respond satisfactorily to thiazide, but a loop diuretic usually is required.

Thiazide diuretics cause a long-term reduction in urinary calcium excretion, which may be desirable in elderly women. The case-control study conducted among 5137 Saskatchewan residents aged 65 years or older showed a decrease of hip fractures as thiazide use continued. Relative risks were 1.2 for less than 2 years of use, 0.8 for 2 to 5 years of use, and 0.5 for 6 or more years of use.[15] Cross-sectional studies have also shown that thiazide users have a greater bone mass than nonusers.

Loop Diuretics

In elderly patients with congestive heart failure secondary to left ventricular systolic dysfunction, as well as in patients with fluid volume overload, loop diuretics remain a cornerstone of management. However, these agents require careful supplementation of potassium and magnesium.[12] Although their influence on the prolongation of life remains disputable, loop diuretics make life easier for patients with heart failure and enhance efficacy of angiotensin-converting enzyme (ACE) inhibitors.

Loop diuretics in elderly patients with hypertension should be reserved only for those who exhibit the signs of heart or renal failure.

β-BLOCKERS

Most β-blockers lower arterial pressure by decreasing cardiac output secondary to a fall in heart rate without affecting, or even increasing, total peripheral resistance. The prevalence of heart failure, sick sinus syndrome, peripheral artery disease, glucose intolerance, and chronic obstructive pulmonary disease makes β-blockers a poor choice for treatment of elderly patients.

Conversely, it has been shown that most β-blockers (metoprolol—Goteborg study; timolol—Norwegian study; propranolol—BHAT study; and atenolol—ISIS-1) reduce the reinfarction rate and mortality after myocardial infarction, and they therefore remain a good choice in this clinical situation.[16-19] β-Blockers are also useful in combination with dihydropyridine calcium antagonists, in treating coronary artery disease, and in treating hypertension without left ventricular failure or other contraindications.[20]

Information on the newer generations of β-blockers (labetalol and carvedilol [α- and β-blockers], pindolol and bopindolol [a β-blocker with high intrinsic sympathomimetic activity (ISA)], and celiprolol [a cardioselective β-receptor antagonist with mild ISA]) in aged patients is scarce. Labetalol effectively reduced 24-hour blood pressure in 16 patients (mean age, 60 years) with isolated systolic hypertension (ISH) over 8 weeks.[21] In this single-blind, placebo-controlled trial, labetalol reduced the morning surge in systolic blood pressure as well. In another double-blind, randomized, multicenter trial, Giles et al. achieved blood pressure control in 86% of elderly patients receiving labetalol, compared with 34% of the placebo group.[22] Dropout rates were comparable in both groups (14% versus 10%, respectively).

It should be emphasized that the hemodynamic profile of newer β-blockers is different from that of the other agents. These drugs maintain cardiac output while concomitantly reducing total peripheral resistance, features that seem to be particularly attractive in the geriatric population. However, these newer agents are also not entirely free of their deleterious influence on glucose metabolism.

ANTIADRENERGIC DRUGS (METHYLDOPA, CLONIDINE, GUANABENZ)

Low doses of centrally acting antiadrenergic agents (methyldopa, clonidine, guanabenz) have been used successfully in the past to treat hypertension in the elderly. However, with the advent of more modern antihypertensive modalities with a purer side-effect profile, these drugs have been abandoned. Centrally acting antiadrenergic drugs should probably be used in combination therapy only as third- and fourth-step agents.[7]

Peripherally Acting Antiadrenergic Drugs (Doxazosin, Prazosin, Trimazosin)

These drugs, by blocking the postsynaptic α-receptors, exert their antihypertensive effect by reducing total peripheral resistance while maintaining or increasing cardiac output.[23] Because they also dilate capacitance vessels, orthostatic hypotension has been shown to occur. In elderly patients with rigid arteries and reduced baroreceptor activity, this carries a meaningful risk. Pretreatment with a diuretic (a standard practice in the past) made patients much more susceptible to this first-dose effect of prazosin. Orthostatic hypotension is uncommon with the more modern agents, such as trimazosin and doxazosin. The postsynaptic α-blockers have been shown to favorably affect dyslipoproteinemia and insulin resistance; they lower total cholesterol and increase high-density lipoprotein cholesterol and improve glucose intolerance. Although the long-term benefits of these beneficial lipid effects still remain to be determined (particularly in the elderly), postsynaptic α-blockers should be considered the first-line agents in patients with dyslipoproteinemias. Another important indication for postsynaptic α-blockers is prostatic hypertrophy. The α-blockade achieved with these agents extends to the smooth muscle in the bladder outlet and has been shown to partially diminish the symptoms of dysuria and urinary retention.

CALCIUM ANTAGONISTS

Calcium antagonists inhibit calcium entry into vascular smooth muscle and therefore lower arterial pressure by reducing total peripheral resistance. Despite this common mechanism of action, calcium antagonists vary considerably in their effects on myocardial systolic and diastolic performance, sinus and atrioventricular nodal function, and other regional circulations.[24]

Dihydropyridine Calcium Antagonists (Nifedipine, Nisoldipine, Nitrendipine, Nicardipine, Isradipine, Felodipine, and Amlodipine)

Dihydropyridine calcium antagonists are excellent antihypertensive agents in elderly patients with concomitant bradycardia. Unfortunately, when given acutely, all dihydropyridine calcium antagonists produce a reflexive increase in heart rate and cardiac output and a marked reduction in total peripheral resistance. This effect is particularly noticeable with the acute-release formulations, such as nifedipine, nitrendipine, and nicardipine.[25–27] The studies performed in patients after myocardial infarction showed an increase of mortality in patients treated with nifedipine, nisoldipine, or nicardipine when compared with placebo. These agents should, therefore, be strictly avoided after myocardial infarctions (MIs).[28, 29] Sublingual nifedipine is recommended and widely used for treatment of hypertensive emergencies; an unpredictable fall in blood pressure in elderly patients with disseminated atherosclerotic changes in arteries and decreased baroreceptor function were observed, as were fatal consequences such as stroke and MI.[30–32] We think that the sublingual administration of nifedipine can be harmful, not only in the elderly, and recommend that this practice be abandoned.

With continued administration of nifedipine, nitrendipine, and nicardipine, the cardioacceleration diminishes, and it seems to disappear completely with the newer agents (isradipine, felodipine, and amlodipine), probably as a result of baroreceptor resetting.[33–35] The sustained-released formulations make dihydropyridine calcium antagonists useful and safe in elderly patients with hypertension and angina pectoris.[36, 37] Their overall efficacy, assessed in controlled trials involving monotherapy as well as in large-scale noncontrolled studies, was slightly better in the elderly than in younger patients. Of note, these agents do not have any deleterious effects on pulmonary function and metabolism of glucose, lipids, and uric acid, which makes them desirable in most patients with coexistent diseases.[38, 39] Moreover, an increase in renal blood flow and glomerular filtration rate can be observed. Additionally, the newer calcium antagonists (isradipine, felodipine, and amlodipine) seem to have little if any negative inotropic or chronotropic effects. In contrast to other calcium antagonists, they have been shown to favorably affect systemic and regional hemodynamics in patients with congestive heart failure.

Nondihydropyridine Calcium Antagonists (Verapamil, Diltiazem, and Gallopamil)

All three of these agents have negative chronotropic and inotropic effects; that is, they slow sinus-node activity and atrioventricular (AV) node conduction and therefore should be avoided in patients with sinus and AV node disorders or congestive failure from systolic dysfunction. However, nondihydropyridine calcium antagonists, particularly verapamil, are excellent agents in patients with congestive heart failure secondary to impaired filling, because these agents improve left ventricular filling and increase coronary blood flow.[40] Impaired left ventricular filling and diastolic dysfunction are common sequelae of aging, longstanding hypertension, and LVH.[41] Verapamil, as has been demonstrated by Schulman et al., reduces left ventricular mass to a greater extent than atenolol in hypertensive elderly patients.[42]

Unlike dihydropyridine calcium antagonists, verapamil and diltiazem can be recommended in certain post-MI patients. The Danish Verapamil Infarction Trial (DAVIT-II) has documented that verapamil started 1 week after acute MI diminishes reinfarction rate and increases survival in patients without heart failure.[43] Of note, about one third of all included patients were older than 65 years, and age was not related to event rates. The decrease in reinfarction rate induced by verapamil was approximately 20%—that is, similar to that documented with β-blockers. In patients with non–Q-wave infarction without heart failure, diltiazem has also been documented to reduce reinfarction rates.[44] Although β-blockers remain the agents of choice in the management of post-MI patients, nondihydropyridine calcium antagonists should be considered when β-blockers are contraindicated or when patients cannot tolerate them.[45]

Moreover, the negative chronotropic properties of verapamil, diltiazem, and gallopamil make them (in immediate-release formulations) useful for patients with supraventricular tachyarrhythmias.[46]

Antiatheromatous Effects of Calcium Antagonists

Calcium antagonists have been shown to exert anti-atheromatous effects in certain experimental models. Some recent clinical studies with nifedipine, nicardipine, and verapamil have documented that calcium antagonists inhibit the development of new atheromatous lesions in the coronary circulation. A similar effect has been demonstrated with diltiazem in younger (mean age, 48.2 years) patients after heart transplantation.[47]

The antiatheromatous effect may be multifactorial: calcium antagonists, besides lowering blood pressure, may interfere with endothelial and platelet mecha-nisms, prevent calcium overload, inhibit smooth muscle proliferation or bind lipoproteins and esters of hydrolysis of cholesterol in liposomes, and decrease arterial wall matrix synthesis.[48] No effect on existing atheromatous plaque has been observed. These findings make calcium antagonists an attractive choice in elderly patients at risk of or suffering from atheromatosis.

In summary, the tendency to favor calcium antagonists in elderly patients with hypertension and coronary artery disease derives from the favorable actions of these agents supplementary to the reduction in blood pressure. The beneficial effects in patients with angina pectoris (both groups of calcium antagonists); the secondary prevention after MI and reduction of LVH (verapamil and diltiazem); the promising results in patients with congestive heart failure (felodipine, amlodipine); the renal protection (both groups); the lack of undesirable effects on glucose, lipid, and uric acid metabolism; the few and minor adverse effects; and the promising antiatheromatous effect make calcium antagonists the first-line cardiovascular drugs in elderly patients.

ANGIOTENSIN-CONVERTING ENZYME INHIBITORS

Despite the fact that plasma renin activity is often low and unresponsive in elderly patients, ACE inhibitors have been shown to effectively treat hypertension and congestive heart failure.[7] This suggests that the effects of ACE inhibition do not solely depend on circulating plasma renin activity. Whether this efficacy of ACE inhibitors in the elderly is mediated by a decreased breakdown of bradykinins or caused by a more marked inhibition of the tissue angiotensin system remains uncertain. ACE inhibitors lower arterial pressure by decreasing total peripheral resistance while maintaining or enhancing systemic and regional blood flow. All ACE inhibitors seem to be equally potent in the reduction of blood pressure in elderly patients, provided that the dose is adequate.[49–51] Silagy et al. published a very interesting study:[52] In this double-blind, crossover, 4-week study, the authors compared the effectiveness of the β-blocker atenolol (50 mg), the ACE inhibitor enalapril (10 mg), the diuretic hydrochlorothiazide (25 mg), and the calcium antagonist isradipine (2.5 mg) in 24 subjects (mean age, 72.3 years) with supine blood pressure of 181/79 mmHg and daytime ambulatory blood pressure of 165/82 mmHg. Although all the drugs significantly reduced supine and 24-hour blood pressure when compared with placebo, only hydrochlorothiazide and enalapril produced a consistent hypotensive effect during the entire 24-hour period. Moreover, enalapril and isradipine showed greater effect on systolic blood pressure than either of the other agents. The most common side effects were, as was expected, swollen ankles, caused by administration of isradipine; cough, caused by administration of enalapril; and breathlessness, caused by administration of atenolol. Although the study had limitations, such as its short duration, the small dose of isradipine, and the small group of patients, it remains the exclusive comparative trial in elderly patients with ISH. In another study, Espinel et al. compared the antihypertensive effects of enalapril and verapamil in 115 patients with ISH.[53] Both drugs were equally efficacious in decreasing blood pressure, and only 11 patients (9 in the verapamil group and 2 in the enalapril group) were withdrawn because of adverse effects.

Clearly, in unstable hemodynamic situations, short-acting agents (captopril) are preferable to long-acting ACE inhibitors. With prolonged administration, and in stable hemodynamic situations, the once-a-day formulations (enalapril, lisinopril, ramipril, fosinopril, and trandolapril) are more convenient than the twice-a-day or thrice-a-day ACE inhibitors. This is of particular importance in elderly, frequently demented, patients.

Major changes in the drug dosage (amount or interval) are unnecessary in elderly subjects unless their glomerular filtration rate falls below 30 ml/min.[54] Taking into account that baroreceptor function worsens with age and the frequent use of diuretics, acute hypotension may be avoided by starting therapy with lower doses and slower titration.

ACE inhibitors also seem to reduce LVH to a greater extent than any other antihypertensive drug class, which probably goes beyond pure hemodynamic effect, and they do not cause deterioration in left ventricular function.[14]

In combination therapy, ACE inhibitors are especially effective when combined with nondihydropyridine calcium antagonists or with diuretics, although the latter combination may lead to symptomatic hypotension.[7]

Because ACE inhibitors lower both the preload and the afterload to the left ventricle, they are the agents of choice in elderly patients with congestive heart failure of systolic dysfunction. ACE inhibitors are the only agents that have been shown to prolong life in patients with severe congestive heart failure (New York Heart Association [NYHA] classes III and IV). The results of the CONSENSUS study showed that enalapril therapy benefited patients who remained in NYHA class IV despite 2 weeks of prior conventional therapy.[55] The SOLVD study included patients in classes II and III with an ejection fraction below 35%.[56] The mean age of the enalapril-treated group was 60.7 years. The results of both these trials showed a significant reduction in mortality in the enalapril-treated group. Similarly, the comparison between enalapril and hydralazine-isosorbide dinitrate (mean age, 60.6 years versus 60.5 years) demonstrated a life-saving effect of ACE inhibitor therapy.[57] ACE inhibitors, when given after acute MI, have been shown to prevent progressive dilatation of the left chamber (remodeling). The multicenter Survival and Ventricular Enlargement Trial (SAVE) study, evaluating the effect of ACE inhibitors on morbidity and mortality in post-MI patients with left ventricular dysfunction (ejection fraction < 40%), showed significant reduction in both total mortality rate (19%; $p = .019$) and cardiovascular mortality rate (21%; $p = .014$), lower risk of reinfarction (25%; $p = .015$), and other cardiovascular end points in patients treated with captopril in comparison with the placebo group.[58] Conversely, it seems to be hazardous, as the CONSENSUS-2 trial has shown, to give ACE inhibitors in the very early phase of MI, especially in patients with low blood pressure.

Additionally, enalapril has been found to improve NYHA functional class, to reduce left ventricular mass, to increase blood peak flow velocity across the mitral valve, and to increase maximal treadmill exercise time in elderly post-MI patients with normal left ventricular function.[59]

The beneficial effect of ACE inhibitors on renal hemodynamics consists of increasing renal blood flow, usually without decreasing glomerular filtration rate, resulting in a reduction in microalbuminuria. Because diabetic and/or hypertensive nephropathy is common among the elderly, small doses of ACE inhibitors are recommended as renal protection.[38]

Conversely, ACE inhibitors should be used with caution, if at all, in elderly patients with significant renal impairment. In this situation, high doses of ACE inhibitors have been shown to deteriorate renal function and lead to life-threatening hyperkalemia. Milder degrees of hyperkalemia are not uncommon with ACE inhibition, because hyporeninemic hypoaldosteronism and/or renal failure often disturbs the mechanism of potassium excretion in elderly patients.

In summary, ACE inhibitors are the drugs of choice in elderly patients with congestive heart failure and hypertension. They do not harm glucose or cholesterol metabolism. Moreover, ACE inhibitors seem to be promising in the prevention of renal and heart failure. The side effects (cough, hypotension, hyperkalemia, increase in serum creatinine or blood urea nitrogen) are rare but should be carefully monitored.

DIGITALIS GLYCOSIDES

Digoxin remains the cornerstone of therapy for systolic left ventricular dysfunction and rapid atrial fibrillation. In patients with sinus rhythm, its beneficial effect is less meaningful, but recent studies suggest that the positive inotropic effect overbalances the proarrhythmic properties. However, the effects of digoxin on the morbidity and mortality of patients in congestive heart failure remain undefined.[60–62]

Digitalis glycosides should be prescribed very carefully because of their deleterious influence on the heart with diastolic dysfunction, a condition frequently observed in the elderly. The age-related decrease in renal function and the narrow therapeutic range for digitalis should be kept in mind when digoxin is being prescribed. A daily dose of 0.25 mg should be the upper limit.[63] The difficulties associated with digitalis therapy are related to the more pronounced susceptibility of the elderly to digoxin toxicity and to a relatively small predictive value of creatinine level (reflecting a reduced muscle mass) in determining the digoxin clearance. For patients with renal impairment, therapy guided by digoxin blood level is recommended.[64]

Concomitant drug therapy may influence the cardiac glycosides' pharmacokinetic parameters. The following agents significantly increase the digoxin plasma levels: amiodarone, quinidine, verapamil, diltiazem, and flecainide. In such a case, the maintenance dosage of digitalis should be reduced.[65] In contrast to calcium antagonists that lower heart rate, most dihydropyridine derivatives, as well as ACE inhibitors, seem to have no effect on digoxin plasma levels.

NONDIGOXIN INOTROPIC AGENTS

Orally administered agents that increase intracellular levels of cyclic adenosine monophosphate by inhibiting phosphodiesterase or by stimulating β-adrenergic receptors exert favorable hemodynamic effects; however, none of them has produced a consistent improvement in survival. In fact, the long-term use of selective phosphodiesterase inhibitors, such as milrinone and enoximone, in patients with severe heart failure has been associated with higher mortality when compared with patients treated with placebo.[66, 67] These drugs should be restricted to short-term therapy (for patients in shock or waiting for surgical treatment).

Vesnarinone, an orally administered inotropic agent that increases intracellular sodium and calcium and inhibits phosphodiesterase, was studied in a group of 239 patients (mean age, 58.1 years) with heart failure.[68] After 6 months of therapy, lower cardiovascular morbidity and mortality were observed in the vesnarinone-treated group as compared with the placebo-treated group ($p < .003$). Unfortunately, a higher dose of the drug (120 mg/day) was associated with an increase in mortality. Further studies are necessary to confirm these preliminary results.

β-Adrenergic agonists, such as dopamine and dobutamine, are less beneficial in elderly patients, probably because of the previously described diminished responsiveness of β-receptors in older subjects. Moreover, these drugs enhance AV conduction, which may lead to atrial fibrillation in susceptible patients.

NITRATES

Nitrate preparations exert their clinical effect through the activation of guanylyl cyclase, which catalyzes the formation of cyclic guanosine monophosphate, resulting in relaxation of venous capacity vessels and coronary arteries. Nitrates are used in patients with ischemic heart disease, heart failure, and hypertensive crises.[69] Although nitrates reduce the incidence of angina pectoris and increase exercise tolerance, the improvement of prognosis is less convincingly documented in patients with stable angina. The effects of long-acting compounds on left ventricular filling seem to be especially attractive in elderly patients, and nitrates have been used in the adjunctive therapy of congestive heart failure.[70]

The introduction of newer preparation forms, such as sustained-release granules and transdermal preparations (gel and patches), may improve compliance of the aged patient.

The problems of tolerance or nitrate-dependence do not differ when comparing elderly patients with younger ones.[71] Nitrates are generally well tolerated by elderly patients, and only postural hypotension, resulting from poor baroreceptor response and low intravascular volume, is more frequent when elderly patients are compared with younger subjects. In patients treated with diuretics and ACE inhibitors, therapy should be started with lower doses. The same applies to patients with coexistent diseases such as aortic stenosis or anemia, frequent conditions in the elderly.

ANTIARRHYTHMIC AGENTS

Regardless of the age of a patient, there are two main reasons for using the antiarrhythmic agents:

1. To reduce arrhythmia-related symptoms
2. To prevent sudden cardiac death

Taking into account the risks, such as proarrhythmic properties and negative inotropic effects, associated with all antiarrhythmic drugs, the risk-to-benefit ratio should be considered carefully.[72] In the elderly population, there is a variety of additional considerations, such as altered pharmacokinetics (reduced volume of distribution and decreased hepatic and renal elimination) and the greater risk of aggravation of arrhythmia and development of heart failure (higher prevalence of coronary artery disease, hypertension, LVH, congestive heart failure). Frequent concomitant use of proarrhythmic drugs (diuretics, digoxin) should be assessed before embarking on antiarrhythmic therapy. Further, these drugs are less effective in the elderly, and they have not been proved to prevent sudden cardiac death.

Thus, antiarrhythmic therapy is much more hazardous in the elderly, but if the benefits are well defined, therapy may continue with lower doses and slower upward titration with careful monitoring of the side effects.[73]

Class IA: Quinidine, Procainamide, Disopyramide

In the past, class IA drugs have been used intensively to achieve pharmacologic cardioversion in atrial fibrillation and for suppression of ventricular arrhythmias. Unfortunately, the proarrhythmic properties, negative inotropic effect contractility, and elevation of digoxin serum concentration make class IA drugs a poor choice in elderly patients. Aronow et al. showed that quinidine and procainamide were comparable to placebo in preventing sudden death (21% and 23%, respectively).[74] In addition, approximately 50% of patients treated with these drugs had side effects.

Class IB: Lidocaine, Tocainide, Mexiletine

Studies with these class IB agents did not show any benefits in preventing ventricular arrhythmias in elderly patients.[75, 76] This class is rarely effective when used as monotherapy, but it can be used with good results in combination therapy with sotalol.

Class IC: Encainide, Flecainide, Propafenone

The results of the CAST-1 trial showed a substantial increase in sudden death in post-MI patients treated with flecainide and encainide.[77] Flecainide can effectively restore sinus rhythm in elderly patients with atrial fibrillation. In combination therapy with amiodarone, both of these agents have been useful in suppressing episodes of ventricular tachycardia. Propafenone is a relatively new drug, but it may have certain advantages over flecainide and encainide. It can be used in pharmacologic cardioversion and in reduction of episodes of paroxysmal atrial fibrillation. However, it has weak β-adrenoreceptor antagonist properties and should probably be avoided in patients with congestive heart failure.

Class II: β-Adrenergic Blockers

β-Adrenergic blockers are highly effective in the prevention of reinfarction and sudden death in post-MI patients, but numerous side effects diminish their role in the treatment of the elderly population.

Class III: Amiodarone, Sotalol

Both of these drugs are potent and highly effective antiarrhythmic agents in supraventricular and ventricular tachyarrhythmias. Unfortunately, the use of amiodarone in the elderly is limited by some side effects. Amiodarone may aggravate thyroid disorders and can cause thickening of the pulmonary alveolar membrane and corneal microdeposits. Nevertheless, amiodarone remains the drug of choice in elderly patients with atrial fibrillation, to maintain sinus rhythm after successful cardioversion, and to suppress recurrent ventricular tachycardias.

Sotalol, in a comparison of seven antiarrhythmic drugs in patients with ventricular tachyarrhythmias (mean age, 65 years, 80% of patients with a history of MI), was found to be more effective than other agents (imipramine, mexiletine, pirmenol, procainamide, propafenone, and quinidine) in preventing death and recurrences of arrhythmia (assessed by Holter monitoring).[78] Like other β-blockers, it should be used cautiously in elderly patients.

Class IV: Diltiazem, Verapamil

Nondihydropyridine calcium antagonists (alone or in combination with digoxin) are effective in the treatment of supraventricular tachycardias and in controlling ventricular responses in patients with chronic atrial fibrillation. Of note, both drugs worsen myocardial contractility, and verapamil increases the serum digoxin level.

FIBRINOLYTIC AGENTS

Age is the most important risk factor for mortality in patients with myocardial infarction.[79] Elderly patients are prone to multivessel coronary artery disease and impaired left ventricular performance. Unfortunately, early trials of thrombolytic therapy excluded elderly patients because of hemorrhagic risk. The results of later trials clearly showed risk reduction among elderly patients treated with the thrombolytic agents (streptokinase, tissue-type plasminogen activator [t-PA], and anisoylated plasminogen streptokinase activator complex [APSAC]). Unfortunately, data from different studies show that our treatment of elderly patients with MI is biased, and advanced age remains the leading contraindication for thrombolytic therapy.[80]

A subanalysis of the ISIS-2 trial in elderly patients (70 and older) revealed a clear benefit of streptokinase over placebo.[81] The mortality rates in this age group were, respectively, 15.8% and 23.8% ($p < .001$). Similar results were obtained in the Intervention Mortality Study trial with APSAC and the Anglo-Scandinavian Study of Early Thrombolysis (ASSET) with recombinant tissue-type plasminogen activator (rt-PA).[82] The investigators of the international randomized trial comparing four thrombolytic strategies for acute myocardial infarction (GUSTO trial) presented a more open-minded approach to the problem of fibrinolysis in the elderly, including in the study more than 4000 patients older than 75 years.[83] The t-PA was slightly more effective than streptokinase in this group, a difference that was more distinct in younger subjects.

Although there is a slightly increased risk of hemorrhagic complications after thrombolytic therapy in the elderly (ISIS-2, GUSTO), it reduces mortality by 20%. This clearly demonstrates that streptokinase, t-PA, and APSAC no longer should be reserved only for young patients.[81–83]

LIPID-LOWERING THERAPY

The role of cholesterol as a cardiovascular risk diminishes with age, but it remains an important predictor of coronary heart disease.[84] However, only a few studies have looked at the influence of diet and drug therapy on lipids in the geriatric population, and no conclusive morbidity or mortality data have been generated. Thus, the role of lipid-lowering therapy in the elderly remains controversial.[85] The hydroxymethylglutaryl coenzyme A (HMG-CoA) reductase inhibitor (simvastatin) has been shown to effectively lower cholesterol levels; in higher doses, it decreases triglycerides and increases the high-density lipoprotein levels in elderly patients.[85] Also, the bile acid binding resins (cholestyramine) reduce cholesterol effectively but are poorly tolerated when compared with HMG-

CoA reductase inhibitors.[86] In the Stockholm Ischaemic Heart Disease Study, a combination of clofibrate and nicotinic acid resulted in a significant (28%) reduction in mortality in participants older than 60 years of age.[87]

Given that life expectancy is shorter in the elderly than in the middle-aged patient, the physician should carefully balance the benefit of lipid-lowering therapy (which may take years to become manifest) against the potential pitfalls—such as adverse drug reactions, impairment of quality of life, and high cost—which are present from the outset of such therapy.

REFERENCES

1. Ramsay LE, Tucker GT: Drugs and the elderly. Br Med J 282:125, 1981.
2. Montamat SC, Cusack BJ, Vestal RE: Management of drug therapy in the elderly. N Engl J Med 321:303, 1989.
3. Lakatta EG, Mitchell JH, Pomerance A, et al: Human aging: Changes in structure and function. J Am Coll Cardiol 10(Suppl A):42, 1987.
4. Messerli FH, Sundgard-Riise K, Ventura HO, et al: Essential hypertension in the elderly: Haemodynamics, intravascular volume, plasma renin activity, and circulating catecholamine levels. Lancet 2:983, 1983.
5. Kocemba J, Gryglewska B, Klich A, et al: Distribution of blood pressure and prevalence of arterial hypertension in the old population of Cracow. Mat Med Pol 23:33, 1991.
6. Swinne CJ, Shapiro EP, Lima SD, et al: Age-associated changes in left ventricular diastolic performance during isometric exercise in normal subjects. Am J Cardiol 69:826, 1992.
7. Messerli FH, Grodzicki T: Hypertension. In Messerli FH (ed): Cardiovascular Disease in the Elderly, 3rd ed. Boston: Kluwer Academic, 1993, pp 121–144.
8. Kawamoto A, Shimada K, Matsubayashi K, et al: Cardiovascular regulatory functions in elderly patients with hypertension. Hypertension 13:401, 1989.
9. Medical Research Council Working Party: MRC trial of treatment of hypertension in older adults: Principal results. Br Med J 304:405, 1992.
10. SHEP Cooperative Research Group: Prevention of stroke by antihypertensive drug treatment in older persons with isolated systolic hypertesion: Final results of the systolic hypertension in the elderly program (SHEP). JAMA 265:3255, 1991.
11. Dahlof B, Lindholm LH, Hansson L, et al: Morbidity and mortality in the Swedish Trial in Old Patients with Hypertension (STOP-Hypertension). Lancet 338:1281, 1991.
12. Gifford RW Jr: Diuretics in hypertension. In Messerli FH (ed): Cardiovascular Drug Therapy. Philadelphia: WB Saunders, 1990, pp 298–309.
13. Warram JH, Laffel LM, Valsania P, et al: Excess mortality associated with diuretic therapy in diabetes mellitus. Arch Intern Med 151:1350, 1991.
14. Dahlof B, Pennert K, Hansson L: Reversal of left ventricular hypertrophy in hypertensive patients. A metaanalysis of 109 treatment studies. Am J Hypertens 5:95, 1992.
15. Ray WA, Griffin MR, Downey W, et al: Long-term use of thiazide diuretics and risk of hip fracture. Lancet 1:687, 1989.
16. Beta-Blocker Heart Attack Trial Reasearch Group: A randomized trial of propranolol in patients with acute myocardial infarction. Mortality results. JAMA 247:107, 1982.
17. The Norwegian Multicenter Study Group: Timolol-induced reduction in mortality and reinfarction in patients surviving after myocardial infarction. N Engl J Med 304:801, 1981.
18. Hjalmarson A, Elmfeldt D, Herlitz J, et al: Effect on mortality of metoprolol in acute myocardial infarction. A double-blind randomised trial. Lancet 2:823, 1981.
19. Wikstrand J, Kendall M: The role of beta receptor blockade in preventing sudden death. Eur Heart J 13(Suppl D):111, 1992.
20. Packer M: Combined beta-adrenergic and calcium entry blockade in angina pectoris. N Engl J Med 320:709, 1989.
21. DeQuattro V, De-Ping Lee D, Allen J, et al: Labetalol blunts morning pressor surge in systolic hypertension. Hypertension 11(Suppl I):198, 1988.
22. Giles TD, Bartels DW, Silberman HM, et al: Treatment of isolated systolic hypertension with labetalol in the elderly. Arch Intern Med 150:974, 1990.
23. Leren P: The cardiovascular effects of alpha-receptor blocking agents. J Hypertens 10(Suppl 3):11, 1992.
24. Frohlich ED: Calcium antagonists. Their physiological differences. Am J Hypertens 4:430S, 1991.
25. Frampton JE, Faulds D: Nicardipine. A review of its pharmacology and therapeutic efficacy in older patients. Drugs Aging 3:165, 1993.
26. Guazzi M, Olivari MT, Polese A, et al: Nifedipine, a new antihypertensive with rapid action. Clin Pharmacol Ther 22:528, 1977.
27. Sorkin EM, Clissold SP, Brodgen RN: Nifedipine. A review of its pharmacodynamic properties and therapeutic efficacy in ischaemic heart disease, hypertension and related cardiovascular disorders. Drugs 30:182, 1985.
28. The Israeli Sprint Study Group: Secondary Prevention Reinfarction Israeli Nifedipine Trial (SPRINT). A randomized intervention trial of nifedipine in patients with acute myocardial infarction. Eur Heart J 9:354, 1988.
29. Waters D: Proischaemic complications of dihydropyridine calcium channel blockers. Circulation 84:2598, 1992.
30. Gifford RW: Management of hypertensive crises. JAMA 266:829, 1991.
31. Messerli FH, Kowey P, Grodzicki T: Sublingual nifedipine for hypertensive emergencies [letter]. Lancet 338:881, 1991.
32. Wachter RM: Symptomatic hypotension induced by nifedipine in the acute treatment of severe hypertension. Arch Intern Med 147:556, 1987.
33. Faulds D, Sorkin EM: Felodipine. A review of the pharmacology and therapeutic use of the extended release formulation in older patients. Drugs Aging 2:374, 1992.
34. Dubiel JP, Kawecka-Jaszcz K, Kocemba J, et al: Acute and long-term treatment of hypertension with nifedipine in the elderly. J Hum Hypertens 4:410, 1990.
35. Aranda P, Lopez S, Fernandez JA, et al: Nitrendipine in the therapeutic managment of elderly hypertensive patients: Results of a multicenter trial. Andalousian Hypertension Group. J Cardiovasc Pharmacol 19(Suppl 2):36, 1992.
36. Michelson EL: Calcium antagonists in cardiology: Update on sustained-release drug delivery systems. Clin Cardiol 14:947, 1991.
37. Phillips RA, Ardeljan M, Shimabukuro S, et al: Effects of nifedipine-GITS on left ventricular mass and left ventricular filling. J Cardiovasc Pharmacol 19(Suppl 2):28, 1992.
38. Bakris GL, Barnhill BW, Sadler R: Treatment of arterial hypertension in diabetic humans: Importance of the therapeutic selection. Kidney Intern 41:912, 1992.
39. Grandinetti O, Feraco E: Middle term evaluation of amlodipine vs nitrendipine: Efficacy, safety and metabolic effects in elderly hypertensive patients. Clin Exp Hypertens 15(Suppl 1):197, 1993.
40. Schmieder RE, Messerli FH, Garavaglia GE, Nunez BD: Cardiovascular effects of verapamil in patients with essential hypertension. Circulation 75:1030, 1987.
41. Dahan M, Paillole C, Ferreira B, et al: Doppler echocardiographic study of the consequences of aging and hypertension on the left ventricle and aorta. Eur Heart J 11(Suppl G):39, 1990.
42. Schulman SP, Weiss JL, Becker LC, et al: The effect of antihypertensive therapy on left ventricular mass in elderly patients. N Engl J Med 322:1350, 1990.
43. The Danish Study Group on Verapamil in Myocardial Infarction: Effect of verapamil on mortality and major events after acute myocardial infarction (The Danish Verapamil Infarction Trial II—DAVIT II). Am J Cardiol 66:779, 1990.
44. The Multicenter Diltiazem Postinfarction Trial Research Group: The effect of diltiazem on mortality and reinfarction after myocardial infarction. N Engl J Med 319:385, 1988.
45. Messerli FH: Cardioprotection—Not all calcium antagonists are created equal. Am J Cardiol 66(10):855–856, 1990.
46. Chakko S, Myerburg RJ: Antiarrhythmic drugs. Curr Opin Cardiol 5:69, 1990.

47. Schroeder JS, Gao SZ, Alderman EL, et al: A preliminary study of diltiazem in the prevention of coronary artery disease in heart-transplant recipients. N Engl J Med 328:164, 1993.
48. Parmley WW: Vascular protection from atherosclerosis: Potential of calcium antagonists. Am J Cardiol 66:161, 1990.
49. Os I, Bratland B, Dahlof B, et al: Lisinopril or nifedipine in essential hypertension? A Norwegian multicenter study on efficacy, tolerability and quality of life in 828 patients. J Hypertens 9:1097, 1991.
50. Manzato E, Capurso A, Crepaldi G: Modification of cardiovascular risk factors during antihypertensive treatment: A multicentre trial with quinapril. J Int Med Res 21:15, 1993.
51. Louis WJ, Conway EL, Krum H, et al: Comparison of the pharmacokinetics and pharmacodynamics of perindopril, cilazapril and enalapril. Clin Exp Pharmacol Physiol 19(Suppl 19):55, 1992.
52. Silagy CA, McNeil JJ, McGrath BP: Crossover comparison of atenolol, enalapril, hydrochlorothiazide and isradipine for isolated systemic hypertension. Am J Cardiol 70:1299, 1992.
53. Espinel CH, Bruner DE, Davis JR, et al: Enalapril and verapamil in the treatment of isolated systolic hypertension. Clin Ther 14:835, 1992.
54. Burnier M, Biollaz J: Pharmacokinetic optimisation of angiotensin converting enzyme (ACE) inhibitor therapy. Clin Pharmacokinet 22:375, 1992.
55. The CONSENSUS Trial Study Group: Effects of enalapril on mortality in severe congestive heart failure. N Engl J Med 316:1429, 1987.
56. The SOLVD Investigators: Effect of enalapril on survival in patients with reduced left ventricular ejection fraction and congestive heart failure. N Engl J Med 325:293, 1991.
57. Cohn JN, Johnson G, Ziesche S, et al: A comparison of enalapril with hydralazine-isosorbide dinitrate in the treatment of chronic congestive heart failure. N Engl J Med 325:303, 1991.
58. Pfeffer MA, Braunwald E, Moye LA, et al: Effect of captopril on mortality and morbidity in patients with left ventricular dysfunction after myocardial infarction. N Engl J Med 327:669, 1992.
59. Aronow WS, Kronzon I: Effect of enalapril on congestive heart failure treated with diuretics in elderly patients with prior myocardial infarction and normal left ventricular ejection fraction. Am J Cardiol 71:602, 1993.
60. Digoxin in sinus rhythm [editorial]. Br Med J 1:1103, 1979.
61. Yusuf S, Garg R, Held P, et al: Need for a large randomized trial to evaluate the effects of digitalis on morbidity and mortality in congestive heart failure. Am J Cardiol 69:64G, 1992.
62. Fleg JL, Gottlieb SH, Lakatta EG: Is digoxin really important in treatment of compensated heart failure? Am J Med 73:244, 1982.
63. Woldow A, Wang RY, Rajagopal DE, et al: The use of digoxin 0.125 mg versus 0.25 mg daily as maintenance dosage in patients older than 75 years of age. Cardiol Elderly 1:3, 1993.
64. Mooradian AD, Wynn EM: Pharmacokinetic prediction of serum digoxin concentration in the elderly. Arch Intern Med 147:650, 1987.
65. Hooymans PM, Merkus FW: Clinical relevance of pharmacokinetic interactions between cardiac glycosides and antiarrhythmic drugs. Pharm Int 252, 1986.
66. Packer M, Carver JR, Rodeheffer RJ, et al: Effect of oral milrinone on mortality in severe chronic heart failure. N Engl J Med 325:1468, 1991.
67. Uretsky BF, Jessup M, Konstam MA, et al: Multicenter trial of oral enoximone in patients with moderate to moderately severe congestive heart failure: Lack of benefit compared with placebo. Circulation 82:774, 1990.
68. Feldman AM, Bristow MR, Parmley WW, et al: Effects of vesnarinone on morbidity and mortality in patients with heart failure. N Engl J Med 329:149, 1993.
69. Davis D, Clouser KD, Zelis R: Hypertensive emergencies. In Messerli FH (ed): Cardiovascular Disease in the Elderly, 3rd ed. Boston: Kluwer Academic, 1993, p 145.
70. Rich MW: Congestive heart failure in the elderly. Cardiol Elderly 1:372, 1993.
71. Rauch B, Kubler W: Antianginal medication. Curr Opin Cardiol 6:511, 1991.
72. Podrid PJ: Safety and toxicity of antiarrhythmic drug therapy: Benefit versus risk. J Cardiovasc Pharmacol 17(Suppl 6):65, 1991.
73. Tresch DD, Litzow JT: Management of elderly patients with ventricular arrhythmias. Cardiol Elderly 1:381, 1993.
74. Aronow WS, Mercando AD, Epstein S, et al: Effect of quinidine or procainamide versus no antiarrhythmic drug on sudden cardiac death, total cardiac death in elderly patients with heart disease and complex ventricular arrhythmias. Am J Cardiol 66:423, 1990.
75. Ryden L, Arnman K, Conradson TB, et al: Prophylaxis of ventricular tachyarrhythmias with intravenous and oral tocainide in patients with and recovering from acute myocardial infarction. Am Heart J 100:1006, 1980.
76. Impact Research Group: International mexiletine and placebo antiarrhythmic coronary trial: I. Report on arrhythmia and other findings. J Am Coll Cardiol 4:1148, 1984.
77. The Cardiac Arrhythmia Suppression Trial: Preliminary report: Effect of encainide and flecainide on mortality in a randomized trial of arrhythmia suppression after myocardial infarction. N Engl J Med 321:406, 1989.
78. Mason JW: A comparison of seven antiarrhythmic drugs in patients with ventricular tachyarrhythmias. N Engl J Med 329:452, 1993.
79. Maggioni AP, Maseri A, Fresco C, et al: Age-related increase in mortality among patients with first myocardial infarctions treated with thrombolysis. N Engl J Med 329:1442, 1993.
80. Montague TJ, Ikuta RM, Wong RY, et al: Comparison of risk and patterns of practice in patients older and younger than 70 years with acute myocardial infarction in a two-year period (1987–1990). Am J Cardiol 68:843, 1991.
81. Ohman EM, O'Connor CM, Califf RM: Role of thrombolytic therapy in the treatment of acute myocardial infarction. Cardiol Elderly 1:54, 1993.
82. Maggioni AP, Franzosi MG, Santoro E, et al: The risk of stroke in patients with acute myocardial infarction after thrombolytic and antithrombotic treatment. N Engl J Med 327:1, 1992.
83. The GUSTO investigators: An international randomized trial comparing four thrombolytic strategies for acute myocardial infarction. N Engl J Med 329:673, 1993.
84. Benfante R, Reed D: Is elevated cholesterol serum level a risk factor for coronary heart disease in the elderly? JAMA 263:393, 1990.
85. Masaki KH, Petrovitch H, Rodriguez BL, et al: The value of risk factor modification in old age. Cardiol Elderly 1:391, 1993.
86. Morgan TM, Hopper J, Bertram D, et al: A study of the interaction of cholestyramine and simvastatin in the treatment of hypercholesterolemia in elderly hypertensive patients. Cardiol Elderly 1:45, 1993.
87. Carlson LA, Rosenhamer G: Reduction of mortality in the Stockholm Ischaemic Heart Disease Secondary Prevention Study by combined treatment with clofibrate and nicotinic acid. Acta Med Scand 223:405, 1988.

CHAPTER 22

Cardiovascular Therapy in Patients with Organ Failure

John M. Kessler, Pharm.D., B.C.P.S., and Luigi X. Cubeddu, M.D., Ph.D.

This chapter is intended to provide information about dosing guidelines for cardiovascular drugs in renal and liver failure. A summary of the basic principles governing drug elimination and metabolism is followed by a brief description of the relevant pharmacokinetic and pharmacodynamic characteristics of each drug. The reader is referred to the specific chapter of this book for a detailed description of the clinical pharmacology of each drug. Excellent reviews on prescribing drugs for patients in renal failure have been published.[1]

BASIC PRINCIPLES

Therapeutic drug concentration monitoring has emerged as a valuable treatment guide for drugs with therapeutic or toxic effects related to their serum concentration. Therapeutic drug concentration monitoring is most valuable for drugs with (1) a narrow margin of safety (therapeutic index), (2) large interpatient variability in response, and (3) therapeutic end points that are difficult to assess. Drug monitoring requires sensitive and specific drug assays. Most assays measure total serum drug concentrations, that is, drug bound to serum proteins plus unbound drug. The unbound drug (free drug) is often a small percentage of the total serum drug concentration. This fraction is the pharmacologically active form of the drug. In the last few years, assays that measure the pharmacologically active "unbound" concentrations of drug have become more widespread. Clinicians may prefer to assess the "unbound" concentration in special situations. These include patients with altered serum protein concentrations or altered renal and hepatic function and patients receiving combinations of drugs that may pharmacokinetically interact with each other. Disease states may change the percentage of drug bound to serum proteins. Because total drug concentration may not change, measurements of serum drug concentration may falsely represent the amount of drug available for biologic effect. Active metabolites formed from parent drugs pose additional judgmental as well as analytic problems. Laborious methods not available in most clinical laboratories are required to measure drug metabolites as well as the unbound drug. Until these methodologic problems are resolved, the clinician should interpret reported serum drug concentrations with caution or consult with a pharmacotherapy specialist to assist in interpreting these measurements.

Pharmacologic Principles

Because of the important role played by the kidneys and the liver in the elimination of drugs from the body, alterations in renal or hepatic function can produce marked decreases in drug clearance. If dose adjustments are not made, increases in drug concentration may occur, leading to toxicity. Consequently, the clinician must know which drugs require dose adjustments in patients with organ failure. Obviously, drugs that are eliminated mainly by the kidneys must be administered cautiously to patients with renal insufficiency (Table 22–1). Dose adjustment generally is not required for renally excreted drugs in subjects with hepatic insufficiency. The contrary would be true for drugs eliminated or transformed to inactive metabolites by the liver (e.g., phenytoin, heparin, reserpine, propranolol) (Table 22–2). The dose of these drugs should be reduced in patients with severe liver failure. Many drugs are eliminated or inactivated by both routes (e.g., captopril, fosinopril, methyldopa, procainamide, guanethidine). For these agents, dose adjustments often are not required unless the organ failure is severe (Table 22–3). In summary, for most drugs, decreases in dose or a reduced frequency of administration is required for patients with severe organ dysfunction. Exceptions include phenytoin and furosemide, drugs for which more frequent administration or higher doses, respectively, may be needed.

Many drugs are converted *in vivo* to active metabolites. The metabolites may contribute to the observed therapeutic or toxic effects, depending on their potency and the serum concentrations achieved. In general, metabolites are more polar than parent drugs; thus, they are eliminated to a greater extent by the kidneys. These metabolites then may accumulate in patients with renal insufficiency. For example, glycine xylide, a metabolite of lidocaine, retains part of lidocaine's pharmacologic activity and may produce toxicity in patients with severe renal failure. Conse-

Table 22–1. **Drugs Requiring Dosage Change in Renal Dysfunction**

Amiloride	Lisinopril
Aspirin?	Methyldopa
Atenolol	Mexiletine?
Benazepril	Milrinone
Bepridil?	Moricizine
Captopril	Nadolol
Clonidine	Procainamide
Diflunisal	Quinapril
Enalapril	Ramipril
Encainide	Spironolactone
Flecainide	Ticlopidine
Furosemide	Tocainide
Hydralazine	Triamterene

Table 22–2. **Drugs Requiring Dosage Change in Hepatic Dysfunction**

Bepridil	Mexiletine
Clonidine	Nifedipine
Digonin	Phenytoin
Diltiazem?	Prazosin
Disopyramide	Propafenone
Flecainide?	Propranolol
Furosemide	Quinidine?
Guanabenz	Ticlopidine
Guanfacine	Tocainide?
Isradipine	Triamterene?
Ketanserin	Verapamil
Lidocaine	

Table 22–4. **Parent Drugs and Active Metabolites with Significant Therapeutic Activity**

Parent Drug	Active Metabolite	Accumulation in Renal Failure
Captopril	Captopril disulfides*	+
Disopyramide	Monodealkyldisopyramide	+
Encainide	o-Desmethylencainide	?
Encainide	3-Methoxy-o-desmethylencainide	?
Lidocaine	Glycine xylide	+
Lidocaine	Monoethylglycinexylide	−
Methyldopa	α-Methylnorepinephrine	?
Procainamide	N-acetylprocainamide	+
Propafenone	5-Hydroxypropafenone	?
Quinidine	Dihydroquinidine	?
Spironolactone	Canrenone	−

*Metabolite inactive but converted back to parent drug; thus, metabolite accumulation enhances action produced by a dose of parent drug.

+, accumulates in renal failure; −, no accumulation in renal failure; ?, may accumulate but uncertain clinical signficance.

quently, drugs that generate active metabolites should be avoided in patients with end-stage renal disease unless assays for both drug and active metabolites are available (Table 22–4). Appearance of toxicity in the presence of nontoxic serum concentrations of the parent drug may be due to accumulation of an active metabolite.

In addition to the route of elimination, other factors determine the need for dose adjustments in patients with organ failure. A major factor is the therapeutic ratio, also known as the therapeutic index or margin of safety of the drug. The therapeutic ratio commonly is defined as toxic concentration divided by the minimal therapeutic concentration. Serum concentrations should be monitored for drugs with a small therapeutic ratio (e.g., digoxin), and close surveillance is required. For compounds with high therapeutic ratios (e.g., propranolol), moderate changes in serum concentration are less likely to result in toxicity. Dose adjustments often are not required for drugs with high therapeutic ratios.

Mechanisms of Renal Elimination

Like endogenous substances, the renal elimination of drugs may occur by either glomerular filtration or tubular secretion. Drugs present in the lumen of the kidney tubules are reabsorbed either by carrier-mediated transport mechanisms or, more frequently, by simple diffusion. The latter mechanism is favored when elevated concentrations of the drug are achieved in the tubular lumen after water reabsorp-

Table 22–3. **Drugs Not Requiring Dosage Change in Hepatic or Renal Dysfunction**

Amiodarone*	Metolazone†
Bumetanide	Metoprolol
Chlorthalidone	Minoxidil
Dipyridamole	Nitroglycerin
Doxazosin	Nitroprusside
Fosinopril	Pindolol
HMG-CoA reductase inhibitors	Propafenone
Hydrochlorothiazide†	Terazosin
Isosorbide mononitrate	Timolol
Labetalol	

*May need dose reduction based on side effects.
†With creatinine clearance greater than 25 ml/min.

tion. Parallel decreases in glomerular filtration rate and tubular functions (i.e., secretion) commonly occur in many patients with chronic renal insufficiency. Therefore, these patients would have a reduced rate of elimination for drugs excreted mainly by filtration (e.g., digoxin, aminoglycosides) as well as for drugs eliminated by secretory processes (transport of acidic compounds such as probenecid and furosemide, or of basic drugs such as disopyramide, procainamide, quinidine, amiloride, and triamterene).

Tubular secretory processes are usually carrier-mediated, active transport systems able to mobilize the drug from the blood (renal tubular cells) to the tubule lumen. Most drugs transported by these systems are polar, requiring specialized systems to cross cell membranes. When the drug is transported from the lumen to the blood, the process is known as *reabsorption*. Both processes are inhibited by agents competing with the drug for its transport protein (e.g., probenecid and penicillin interaction, uric acid and oxypurinol interaction). If the secretory processes are highly efficient, the maximal rate of elimination of a drug by renal secretion would be limited by the supply of drug to the tubular transporter sites (i.e., renal blood flow).

Mechanisms of Hepatic Elimination

As with the kidney, the hepatic clearance of a drug depends on liver blood flow (rate of delivery) and drug extraction (extraction ratio). If the drug is completely extracted from serum in a single passage through the liver (extraction ratio of 1), hepatic clearance is equal to liver blood flow (normal, 1.2 to 1.5 L/min). In this case, changes in liver blood flow would markedly affect circulating drug concentrations as well as the amount of drug that reaches the systemic circulation after oral administration (oral bioavailability). The clinician should expect a high-extraction drug when the intravenous dose is much lower than the oral dose (e.g., propranolol, verapamil). Congestive heart failure (CHF) decreases liver blood flow; therefore, its presence may be associated with decreased drug clearance and unexpected drug accumulation.

Drugs that are poorly extracted by the liver are less dependent on liver blood flow for clearance. The efficiency of extraction depends on drug supply (liver blood flow and proportion of circulating drug that is free) and the hepatic intrinsic clearance rate. The latter is an index of the liver enzyme metabolizing system. From a practical perspective, it is difficult to quantify the effects of various disease states on a drug's hepatic clearance. Alterations in serum protein binding, hepatic blood flow, and intrinsic hepatocyte function secondary to disease state affect the disposition of many drugs. The degree of change is generally unpredictable. A detailed description of how these different factors affect drug levels is beyond the scope of this chapter but is reviewed elsewhere.[2]

Pharmacodynamic Changes in Organ Failure

It may be an inappropriate assumption to make dose adjustments based solely on a drug's pharmacokinetics in patients with elimination organ dysfunction. The biologic effects of a drug (i.e., pharmacodynamics) are not always constant. For example, most antihypertensive agents with vasodilatory or sympatholytic properties produce greater blood pressure reduction in patients with renal failure. Despite the fact that the pharmacokinetic profile may dictate no need for dose adjustment, the greater hypotensive action in this patient population warrants more careful monitoring and possible reduction in dose or increase in the dosing interval. Another example of altered pharmacodynamics in patients in renal failure is that of aspirin. Aspirin produces greater prolongation of bleeding time in uremic patients than in patients with normal renal function. An increased incidence of amiodarone-induced hypothyroidism also has been reported in patients with renal insufficiency. Apparently, uremia-induced derangement of thyroid function makes the gland more sensitive to the excess iodide provided by the amiodarone. Enhanced risk of hyperkalemia has been described in patients with renal failure receiving treatment with angiotensin II–converting enzyme inhibitors. These examples indicate that changes in the pharmacodynamic effects of drugs may occur concurrently with organ dysfunction. The clinician should carefully observe the drug's effects in patients with organ failure, in addition to monitoring dose adjustments indicated by the changes in the drug's pharmacokinetics.

Dose Adjustments for Renal and Hepatic Dysfunction

Depending on the clinical urgency, drugs with long elimination half-lives may require a loading dose to ensure a more rapid therapeutic response. The loading dose varies directly with the volume of distribution and with the desired serum drug concentration. The loading dose is not determined by the elimination rate or clearance of the drug. For most drugs, the loading dose does not need to be adjusted in patients with liver or renal insufficiency (see Table 22–3). Some exceptions exist, however, in which changes in the volume of distribution of drugs have been reported in patients with impaired renal function. For example, the volume of distribution of digoxin may be reduced as much as 50% in patients in severe renal failure.[3] In addition, for drugs with a first-pass effect, a much greater amount of the drug may reach the systemic circulation after administration of loading doses in patients with severe hepatic dysfunction.

In contrast with the loading dose, maintenance doses depend greatly on the rate of drug elimination. Because renal and hepatic dysfunction may decrease drug elimination, reduced maintenance doses are required to maintain appropriate therapeutic levels.

To achieve an effective serum drug concentration in patients with organ failure, the physician could adjust the dose, the dosing interval, or both. The dosing interval may be kept constant and the dose altered, or the dose kept constant and the interval varied. In organ failure, reducing the recommended daily dose while maintaining a constant dosing interval is appropriate for drugs with long half-lives. This method avoids the large fluctuations in peak and trough levels that are otherwise produced when the total daily dose is maintained but the dosing intervals are increased. Compliance may also be enhanced with administration schedules based on a 24-hour cycle or normal daily activities, in contrast with remembering to take a drug at odd intervals (e.g., 36, 48, or 72 hours).

The next section contains recommendations for dose adjustments in patients with decreased liver or kidney function for specific drugs used to treat cardiovascular disorders. A detailed discussion of each drug's pharmacokinetics and pharmacology is found in the chapter devoted to that specific drug.

DIGOXIN

Digoxin is an effective and potent cardiotonic and antiarrhythmic agent, with a small therapeutic ratio. Digoxin is indicated for the control of supraventricular arrhythmias and for the treatment of heart failure. Therapeutic serum concentrations range from 0.8 to 2 ng/ml. Toxicity is often encountered with levels of more than 2 ng/ml. The sensitivity to digoxin's toxic effects may be seen at lower concentrations in the elderly. The usual adult maintenance dose of digoxin is between 0.125 and 0.25 mg daily when the renal function is good.

Renal Dysfunction. Nearly 70% of digoxin is eliminated by glomerular filtration; consequently, reductions in renal function prolong digoxin clearance and half-life. In anuric patients, digoxin's half-life is approximately 105 hours; its half-life in patients with normal renal function is close to 36 hours. Therefore, the maintenance dose of digoxin must be adjusted in patients with renal insufficiency.[3] Its loading dose should also be adjusted because digoxin's volume of distribution is reduced in renal dysfunction.[3] Different equations have been proposed to calculate digoxin's volume of distribution (VD, in liters) based on renal dysfunction:

$$VD = 27.0 + 3.87\ CrCl$$

where CrCl is creatinine clearance.[4] Several equations have also been described to estimate the maintenance dose (MD) in patients with renal insufficiency:

$$MD = \frac{(Css \times TBCl)}{486}$$

where maintenance dose is in mg/day. Css is average serum digoxin concentration at steady state, TBCl is total body clearance, and 486 is the constant for incomplete absorption of oral tablets. Total body clearance for patients in renal failure can be calculated as follows:[5]

$$TBCl = (1.1 \times CrCl) + 20$$

Formulas to estimate creatinine clearance based on serum creatinine levels, age, gender, and lean body weight are available.[6] These simple mathematical calculations allow the clinician to adjust digoxin dosage in patients with renal insufficiency.

Endogenous digoxin-like immunoreactive factors in serum are known to alter reported digoxin concentrations. These factors accumulate and reach higher concentrations in patients with renal failure. A recent study demonstrated that, of the commercially available assays for the measurement of serum digoxin, the SYVA and Corning assays are least affected by interference of digoxin-like immunoreactive factors.[7] A new Roche digoxin assay, "On Line," is substantially free of interference by digoxin immunoreactive factors.[7a] Because of possible interference by endogenous digoxin-like substances, a serum digoxin level should be obtained before initiating digoxin therapy in patients in severe renal failure. Blood samples to measure digoxin concentrations should be obtained at least 6 to 8 hours after dosing and ideally 12 to 24 hours after administration, regardless of the route.

Hepatic Dysfunction. Loading doses of digoxin are not significantly affected by liver failure unless concurrent renal failure exists.

The clearance of digoxin is reduced in patients with CHF. In healthy individuals, the metabolic clearance of digoxin is about 0.6 to 0.9 ml/min/kg. CHF reduces the metabolic clearance of digoxin by 50% of normal. Varying degrees of liver congestion produce a graded reduction in digoxin clearance. Sheiner et al.[8] modeled the total body clearance of digoxin in patients with CHF with the following equation:

$$MD = \frac{TBCl \times desired\ Css \times 1\ day}{F}$$

where F equals fraction of the dose absorbed. This fraction is 0.7 for oral tablets, 0.95 for soft gelatin capsules, and 1 for intravenous injections.

DISOPYRAMIDE

Disopyramide is a class IA antiarrhythmic drug, effective for the treatment of ventricular and supraventricular arrhythmias.[9] Disopyramide has a small therapeutic ratio. Serum concentrations of 2 to 6 mg/ml for the total drug and of 0.5 to 2 mg/ml for the free (unbound) drug seem to be therapeutically active.[10] The usual adult dosage is 150 mg orally every 6 hours.

Renal Dysfunction. Disopyramide requires dose adjustment in patients with renal insufficiency. The drug is eliminated partly by the kidney and partly by the liver. Nearly 50% to 70% of unbound disopyramide is cleared by the kidney. Renal tubular secretion contributes to renal elimination of the drug.

Because of the large variability and nonlinearity in the binding of disopyramide to serum proteins, measurement of free drug concentrations has been advocated.[10] Free disopyramide concentrations appear to correlate better with the drug's pharmacologic response; however, free disopyramide concentrations have been shown to vary as much as 400% over a given dose interval.[11, 12] Disopyramide is also partly metabolized in the liver to monodealkyl-disopyramide. This metabolite may contribute to the antiarrhythmic activity observed after administration of the parent compound. Furthermore, this metabolite may displace disopyramide from its binding proteins, particularly in patients with renal failure.[13]

From a practical point, patients weighing less than 50 kg should receive 100 mg every 6 hours; patients weighing more than 50 kg can receive 150 mg every 6 hours. In moderate renal insufficiency, an increase in the dosing interval to 12 to 24 hours is suggested. Dosing every 24 to 48 hours is recommended in severe renal failure. Careful evaluation of clinical response and measurement of serum concentrations are required because of disopyramide's complicated kinetics and small therapeutic ratio. Other approaches have been advocated to calculate the daily dose of disopyramide in renal insufficiency.[10] However, if the renal function is severely compromised, the doses obtained by these methods are often excessive, and a lower dose than calculated should be prescribed.

Hepatic Dysfunction. Disopyramide doses should be decreased by 25%, and serum concentrations of disopyramide should be monitored in patients with liver failure. If measurements only of total disopyramide are available, a lower therapeutic range (1 to 2.5 µg/ml) should be used and the patient should be monitored closely for signs of toxicity. These recommendations are based on the observed reductions in unbound drug clearance, decreased protein binding, and changes in albumin and α_1-acid glycoprotein levels in patients with liver dysfunction.[14–16]

LIDOCAINE

Lidocaine is a class IB antiarrhythmic drug that is effective for the prophylaxis and treatment of ventricular arrhythmias. Serum lidocaine concentrations should be routinely monitored because of the drug's small therapeutic ratio. The accepted normal therapeutic range of lidocaine is 2 to 6 µg/ml. Toxicity occurs at concentrations greater than 5 µg/ml, and poor response is often achieved between 1.5 and 2 µg/ml. A loading dose of 1 to 2 mg/kg followed by a maintenance infusion of 2 mg/min is commonly employed in otherwise healthy patients.

Renal Dysfunction. Very small amounts of lidocaine are eliminated by the kidneys.[17] Its major source of elimination is liver metabolism. Two major active metabolites are formed. Of these metabolites, glycine xylide, which has one quarter of lidocaine's potency, is more polar than lidocaine and thus may accumulate in renal insufficiency.[18] The other metabolite, monoethylglycine xylidide, retains 70% to 80% of lidocaine's activity and does not accumulate in renal failure. Although no dose adjustment is required for lidocaine in patients in renal failure, accumulation of glycine xylide may lead to lidocaine-like toxicity, despite normal serum concentrations of lidocaine.[18] For most patients, careful clinical assessment of therapeutic response and toxicity is as adequate as monitoring drug concentration, because concentration-effect relationships are poorly understood for this drug.[19]

Hepatic Dysfunction. The effects of liver disease on the pharmacokinetics of lidocaine have been studied extensively. In patients with chronic liver diseases such as cirrhosis and hepatitis, and in patients with the reduced hepatic blood flow that occurs in CHF, the dose of lidocaine should be decreased by 40% to 50% and serum concentrations should be monitored. Marked reductions in serum clearance of lidocaine have been described in these patients. Because the drug binds to α_1-acid glycoprotein, the reduction in the serum concentration of this protein in chronic liver disease affects the unbound levels of lidocaine.[17]

MEXILETINE

Mexiletine is an oral class IB antiarrhythmic agent, pharmacologically similar to lidocaine in its electrophysiologic actions. Mexiletine is effective against ventricular arrhythmias. This drug has a small therapeutic ratio because effective serum concentrations are approximately 0.5 µg/ml, and severe toxicity may occur with 2 µg/ml of mexiletine.[20] The usual adult dose is 600 to 900 mg daily in two to four divided doses.

Renal Dysfunction. Like lidocaine, mexiletine is extensively metabolized to inactive compounds in the liver. Less than 15% is excreted unchanged in the urine. Of the drug filtered, a large proportion of the unchanged drug is reabsorbed by passive diffusion. In general, in patients with chronic renal failure with creatinine clearance rates of more than 10 ml/min, no dose adjustments appear to be required. In patients with creatinine clearance rates less than 10 ml/min, increases in serum concentrations have been reported. Downward dose adjustment is recommended; however, no specific guidelines are available.

Hepatic Dysfunction. Mexiletine's elimination appears dependent primarily on the intrinsic capacity of the liver to convert the parent compound to more polar metabolites. The metabolites are believed to be inactive from a cardiac perspective. In liver insufficiency, its volume of distribution and serum protein binding are the same as those of control patients. However, mexiletine's clearance rate is lower than normal (2.31 versus 8.27 ml/kg/hr), and its elimination half-life is prolonged (28.7 versus 9.9 hours). Based on its pharmacokinetics, normal loading doses of mexiletine are administered, and the maintenance dose is adjusted to one-fourth the usual dose to achieve therapeutic concentrations in advanced alcoholic cirrhosis.[21]

TOCAINIDE

Tocainide is an oral class IB antiarrhythmic drug, pharmacologically similar to lidocaine, with clinical efficacy against ventricular arrhythmias. Tocainide has a small therapeutic ratio. Effective serum concentrations of tocainide range from 4 to 10 µg/ml. Tocainide is commonly used in dosages of 600 mg every 6 hours.

Renal Dysfunction. Nearly 30% to 50% of tocainide is eliminated unchanged by the kidneys. Thus, dose adjustments probably are required only in patients with moderate to severe renal insufficiency. The dose should be reduced by one fourth or one half, depending on the severity of renal failure. Patients with renal failure have achieved serum concentrations in the therapeutic range with maintenance doses of 600 mg daily.[22] Daily doses of 1200 mg or less are safe for most patients in renal failure.

Hepatic Dysfunction. Tocainide does not undergo significant first-pass effect after oral administration. No data are available on the effect of cirrhosis on tocainide's pharmacokinetics; however, it is reasonable to expect that this extensively (50% to 70%) metabolized drug will accumulate in patients with moderate to severe hepatocellular dysfunction. The dose may be reduced by 50% in severe hepatic disease. CHF has not been demonstrated to significantly alter the serum concentrations after normal doses. The clinician may monitor serum drug concentration to guide proper dosing with tocainide.

PHENYTOIN

Phenytoin is effective for the treatment of cardiac arrhythmias and seizure disorders. Phenytoin is a class IB antiarrhythmic agent. Its efficacy for the control of premature ventricular contractions and in digitalis-induced arrhythmias has been demonstrated. Therapeutic concentrations range from 10 to 20 µg/ml (1 to 2 µg/ml for the unbound drug). The usual adult dosage is 4 to 6 mg/kg/day; however, small changes in dosage may result in large changes in serum concentration.

Renal Dysfunction. Nearly 1% to 5% of phenytoin is eliminated unchanged in the urine. At phenytoin serum concentrations in the therapeutic range, metabolic pathways may become saturated and a greater proportion of the drug is excreted unchanged in the urine. No changes in the dose of phenytoin are required in patients with renal failure.

Hepatic Dysfunction. Phenytoin undergoes little first-pass effect; therefore, decreased hepatic blood flow is not expected to alter its pharmacokinetics significantly. Decreased hepatocyte function markedly reduces the extent of metabolism of phenytoin. Protein binding is reduced (secondary to low albumin concentrations); therefore, total clearance is increased. In general, the dose of phenytoin is expected to be decreased in the presence of cirrhosis. Total phenytoin concentrations may be falsely low relative to the free concentration, and the therapeutic range for total phenytoin may be adjusted downward. Unbound phenytoin concentrations (as opposed to total concentration) should be monitored in patients with liver disease. Clinicians should be aware of the prolonged time to reach steady-state serum concentration (1 to 2 months) so as to avoid cumulative toxicity with chronic dosing. Because phenytoin metabolism may become saturated, large changes in phenytoin serum concentrations may result from small (<10%) changes in the total daily dose. In summary, if patients with liver dysfunction require phenytoin, low daily maintenance doses are recommended. The loading dose appears to be unaffected by liver disease even in the presence of low albumin concentrations.

PROCAINAMIDE

Procainamide is a class I antiarrhythmic agent that is pharmacologically similar to quinidine in its cardiac effects. Its therapeutic ratio is small, and therapeutic serum concentrations of procainamide vary with the clinical pathology. Suppression of ventricular tachycardia requires higher concentrations (9 to 19 μg/ml) than suppression of premature ventricular depolarization in patients with chronic ischemic heart disease (8 to 10 μg/ml) or with myocardial infarction (4 to 6 μg/ml). N-Acetyl procainamide (NAPA) serum concentrations vary widely because of interpatient variation. Patients appear to be at increased risk of toxicity if the sum of procainamide and NAPA concentrations exceeds 25 to 30 μg/ml.

Renal Dysfunction. Nearly half of the administered procainamide dose is eliminated via the kidney by glomerular filtration and tubular secretion. Therefore, procainamide clearance is reduced in renal dysfunction. The dose of procainamide should be reduced in renal failure. NAPA, an equally potent and effective antiarrhythmic, is formed from the parent drug by acetylation. Nearly 85% of NAPA is eliminated by renal excretion. Compared with slow acetylators, fast acetylators excrete a higher proportion of the oral dose of procainamide than of NAPA. Excessive accumulation of NAPA may have been responsible for deaths that occurred in patients with severe renal failure receiving treatment with procainamide. Furthermore, reports of NAPA toxicity in patients in renal failure while receiving procainamide have been documented.[23] In patients with NAPA toxicity, the estimated NAPA serum half-life is 1.5 days when continuous arteriovenous hemodiafiltration is employed. This time is increased to 3.1 days with continuous arteriovenous hemofiltration and 4 to 7 days with intermittent hemodialysis. Despite these procedures, rapid return to toxic NAPA concentrations could occur in patients with large tissue deposits of procainamide. Therefore, close monitoring of NAPA serum concentrations is recommended after discontinuation of filtration or dialysis therapy in patients with toxicity due to NAPA.

In summary, in patients with normal renal function, the drug is commonly administered in divided doses at 3-hour intervals. In patients with mild, moderate, and severe renal failure, dose intervals of 4 hours, 6 to 12 hours, and 8 to 24 hours are recommended, respectively. Another approach is to reduce the maintenance dose by one third in moderate renal dysfunction and by two thirds in severe renal failure. The loading dose should also be reduced by one third in severe renal failure.[24]

Hepatic Dysfunction. No information is available about dose adjustments in liver disease. Although patients with cirrhosis have a reduced ability to metabolize procainamide, no evidence suggests that these changes in drug metabolism affect drug toxicity or efficacy.[25] Studies in which the kinetics of procainamide were related to electrophysiologic responses in patients with CHF indicated that the dose of procainamide may not have to be decreased in the presence of CHF.[26] Until more data are available, the procainamide dose may not need to be altered *a priori* in patients with liver disease. Serum concentration monitoring of both procainamide and NAPA is important, using the therapeutic ranges mentioned earlier as clinical guidelines.

QUINIDINE

Quinidine is a class I antiarrhythmic agent used for the treatment of ventricular and supraventricular arrhythmias. The drug has a small therapeutic ratio, and its effects show large interpatient variability. Therapeutic effects are commonly achieved with serum concentrations ranging from 1 to 6 μg/ml, but the levels vary with the assay employed. Wide variability among subjects in the protein binding of quinidine may be responsible for differences in response.[27] The usual adult oral dose is 400 mg every 6 hours.

Renal Dysfunction. Only 10% to 20% of quinidine is excreted renally as the parent compound. Renal clearance parallels creatinine clearance. Quinidine is not dialyzed significantly, and no dosage adjustment is necessary after peritoneal dialysis or hemodialysis.

Hepatic Dysfunction. Quinidine is metabolized extensively by the liver; however, little first-pass effect occurs. No evidence suggests that the clearance of quinidine is prolonged significantly in patients with liver failure secondary to cirrhosis or CHF.[28] Quinidine serum concentrations should be monitored to prevent toxicity due to unexpected accumulation. Dihydroquinidine, a quinidine metabolite, retains some antiarrhythmic properties of the parent drug.

FLECAINIDE

Flecainide is a class IC antiarrhythmic agent restricted for use in the treatment of life-threatening sustained ventricular tachycardia. It has a small therapeutic ratio, and its therapeutic serum concentrations range from 0.2 to 1 µg/ml. The probability of adverse reactions may increase with trough concentrations exceeding 1 µg/ml. The usual adult oral dose is 100 mg every 12 hours.

Renal Dysfunction. In healthy subjects, 10% to 40% of the dose administered appears in the urine unchanged. A positive correlation between endogenous creatinine clearance and renal flecainide clearance has been shown. The drug's half-life is prolonged from 10 hours in normal patients to 20 hours in patients in renal failure. Therefore, a reduction in the initial dose is recommended for patients in renal failure.[22] A 50% dosage reduction is recommended when the creatinine clearance is less than 35 ml/min/1.73 m^2.

Hepatic Dysfunction. Flecainide is not subject to clinically significant first-pass effects, and it is not significantly bound to serum proteins. Patients with CHF may achieve higher serum concentrations than normal because of reduced clearance.[29] Flecainide's half-life is prolonged in patients with significant hepatocellular dysfunction. Time to achieve steady-state serum concentrations may therefore be prolonged to greater than 1 week. Flecainide, unlike encainide, probably requires dosage adjustment in patients with liver dysfunction. Monitoring of the serum drug concentration is strongly recommended.

ENCAINIDE

Encainide, a class IC agent no longer routinely available in the United States, is pharmacologically related to flecainide and is indicated for the treatment of life-threatening sustained ventricular tachycardia.[30] It has a small therapeutic ratio; however, monitoring of the serum drug concentration has not been shown to predict efficacy because of the complexity of the metabolite profile and interpatient variation in response. In patients with normal renal function, the initial recommended dose is 25 mg three times daily, with increases every 3 to 5 days, up to 75 mg three or four times daily.

Renal Dysfunction. In most patients, the drug is bioactivated to o-desmethylencainide (half-life of 3 or 4 hours) and to 3-methoxy-o-desmethylencainide (half-life of 6 to 12 hours). Both metabolites are more potent than the parent drug and account for the therapeutic activity in most patients.[31] However, in poor metabolizers (10% of patients), encainide is the active drug.[32] In these individuals, encainide serum concentrations may reach levels that are 20 times greater than those attained in patients who metabolize drugs rapidly. In patients with severe renal failure, the starting dose should be decreased to 25 mg/day and titrated up to 25 mg three times daily.[33]

Hepatic Dysfunction. Individuals classified as poor metabolizers attain parent drug serum concentrations greater than 20 times those of extensive metabolizers. Dosage adjustment probably is not required in patients with hepatic cirrhosis, because their pharmacokinetic profiles are similar to those of patients with poor encainide metabolism. Electrocardiogram intervals and clinical response in cirrhotic patients are similar to those of noncirrhotic patients despite significantly reduced oral and systemic clearance of the parent compound. This similarity is explained by the lack of change in the serum concentrations of any of the pharmacologically active metabolites.[34]

MORICIZINE

Moricizine is an antiarrhythmic agent with properties similar to antiarrhythmics in Vaughan-Williams classes IA, IB, and IC. (Other class IC agents include encainide, flecainide, and propafenone.) Moricizine is indicated for the treatment of documented ventricular arrhythmias, such as sustained ventricular tachycardia, that, in the judgment of the physician, are life threatening. Effective dosages have ranged from 10 to 15 mg/kg/day in three divided doses for the suppression of ventricular premature complexes. The manufacturer advises that the usual adult dosage is between 600 and 900 mg per day (divided every 8 hours). Adjustments may be made in 150 mg/day increments at 3-day intervals. Plasma concentration monitoring cannot be used to judge the therapeutic effectiveness of moricizine. In premarketing trials, there was no correlation of peak or trough moricizine level to changes in arrhythmia. Therapeutic drug concentration monitoring may be used to document patient compliance or concentrations at which toxicity occurs. Moricizine undergoes extensive first-pass metabolism and is only 30% to 40% bioavailable. Eight moricizine metabolites have been identified in human urine; however, their possible antiarrhythmic effects are not known.[35] Approximately 56% of an administered radiolabeled moricizine dose is excreted in the feces.[36]

Renal Dysfunction. One cardiac patient with renal insufficiency had an estimated elimination half-life of 47.5 hours.[37] Well-established dosing guidelines are not published; however, it seems reasonable to expect more clinical toxicity at usual doses owing to accumulation of moricizine and its metabolites. The manufacturer recommends that starting doses of 600 mg per day or less be used in patients with renal or hepatic failure.

Hepatic Dysfunction. No specific information is available on the dosage needs of patients with liver dysfunction.

PROPAFENONE

Propafenone is a class IC antiarrhythmic drug with β-adrenoreceptor blocking actions that is indicated for documented life-threatening sustained ventricular arrhythmias. The therapeutic range has not been established, and significant overlap exists in therapeutic and toxic serum concentrations. Total daily doses of 600 mg produced mean concentrations of 490 ng/ml (range of 110 to 1780 ng/ml); 900 mg yielded 1098 ng/ml (range of 370 to 2370 ng/ml); and 1200 mg yielded 1567 ng/ml (range of 1300 to 1790 ng/ml).[38] Like encainide, propafenone's metabolic profile is highly complex and variable because it is subject to interindividual differences in genetic polymorphism.

Renal Dysfunction. Less than 1% of propafenone is excreted unchanged in the urine; therefore, no dose adjustments should be required in renal failure. However, studies in animals suggest that its 5-hydroxy metabolite is pharmacologically active. Possible accumulation of this metabolite in patients with renal insufficiency should be investigated. In one case report of two patients with end-stage renal disease (ESRD) undergoing continuous ambulatory peritoneal dialysis, the authors concluded that the pharmacokinetics were not significantly altered and the usual adult starting dose of propafenone is indicated.[39]

Hepatic Dysfunction. The initial dose of propafenone in patients with severe liver failure should be reduced by 70% to 80% because of the marked increase in bioavailability. It may also take longer to reach steady-state concentrations in such patients than in either type of metabolizer with normal hepatic function. Propafenone's pharmacokinetics are extremely complex. As with encainide, patients are classified as either poor or extensive metabolizers. Patients with hepatocellular dysfunction may act like poor metabolizers, with higher serum concentrations of the parent compound and less production of the active metabolite. Poor metabolizers may have an elimination half-life of up to 32 hours; therefore, the time to steady-state serum concentrations may be markedly prolonged.[40] However, propafenone's serum concentration does not appear to correlate with its clinical efficacy.[41, 42] Propafenone's clinical response in one study did not correlate with the presence of ascites, encephalopathy, or portal hypertension; it did correlate with measurements of albumin, total bilirubin, serum glutamic-oxaloacetic transaminase (SGOT), and prothrombin time.[43]

AMIODARONE

Amiodarone is a class III antiarrhythmic drug used to treat refractory supraventricular and ventricular tachyarrhythmia. Amiodarone has a small therapeutic ratio. Monitoring of serum drug concentrations has been proposed for patients receiving long-term amiodarone therapy.[40] The proposed therapeutic range is 1 to 2.5 mg/ml.[44]

Renal Dysfunction. Although the half-life of amiodarone is not affected in renal failure, patients seem to be more susceptible to amiodarone-induced hypothyroidism.[45] This susceptibility is due in part to the high iodide content, which becomes important when iodide excretion is reduced. It is also possible that the thyroid derangement present in uremia may make the patient more sensitive to amiodarone-induced hypothyroidism. Thus, close monitoring of thyroid function is recommended in patients with renal failure who are receiving amiodarone treatment.

Hepatic Dysfunction. No data were found describing a dosage adjustment protocol for amiodarone in patients with liver dysfunction. Empiric dosage adjustment is not anticipated, but a lower than usual maintenance dose is likely.

ANTIHYPERTENSIVE DRUGS

Because of the easy measurement of the therapeutic end point, doses are adjusted based on adequate blood pressure reduction and development of side effects. Consequently, therapeutic drug concentration monitoring of antihypertensive drugs is not used in clinical practice in patients with normal or impaired organ function. In general, greater blood pressure reduction is seen in patients with renal insufficiency treated with antihypertensive drugs. Therefore, use of smaller initial doses and more gradual escalation of doses are recommended in renal failure.

β-ADRENERGIC RECEPTOR ANTAGONISTS

The antagonists of the β-adrenergic receptors are effective antihypertensive and antianginal drugs. These agents decrease myocardial oxygen consumption and reduce blood pressure, heart rate, myocardial contractility, and serum renin activity. Selective antagonists for the β-receptors and nonselective antagonists (both β₁- and β₂-antagonists) are available for clinical use. This class of drugs has a large therapeutic ratio, and therapeutic drug concentration monitoring is not used clinically to monitor its effects.

Renal Dysfunction. No dose adjustments are required for propranolol, metoprolol, acebutolol, pindolol, labetalol, or timolol. However, clearances of atenolol and nadolol are reduced in renal insufficiency in direct proportion to the reduction in glomerular filtration rate. For either agent, reducing the dose by 50% or doubling the dosing interval appears sufficient when creatinine clearances are lower than 35 ml/min.[46, 47] Carteolol is a long-acting, nonselective β-blocker whose pharmacokinetics are affected by decreased renal function. Dosing adjustments have been recommended.[48, 49] The elimination half-life has been calculated as up to 40 hours in patients with ESRD, compared with approximately 7 hours in healthy subjects. An active metabolite of carteolol has been identified, yet it constitutes only approximately 4% of metabolized drug and therefore its clinical importance is unknown. Initial doses should start low (e.g., 2.5 mg daily) and titrate to the desired response. A 50% reduction in the usual maintenance dose may be expected in moderate to severe renal failure, and a 25% reduction may be anticipated in mild renal insufficiency.

Hepatic Dysfunction. In liver insufficiency, no dosage adjustments are required for propranolol, timolol, pindolol, metoprolol, acebutolol, and labetalol. No data were found on carteolol, yet no significant dosage adjustment is anticipated. Propranolol is metabolized extensively by the liver, and its clearance is reduced significantly in patients with cirrhosis and chronic active hepatitis. The mean clearance in one study[50] was 0.44 ml/min, compared with 0.92 ml/min in normal subjects; however, the bioavailability may vary, with unpredictable effects on serum concentrations. Propranolol's protein binding to α_1-acid glycoprotein during acute illness changes with time, affecting the pharmacologically active free concentration. Thus, doses of propranolol may be reduced during convalescence because of increased free concentrations.[51] No data were found on the effects of binding of the other β-blockers to α_1-acid glycoproteins. β-Blocker dosing should start low and be titrated to a desired clinical effect. Doses in the low-normal range should be effective for most patients.

PRAZOSIN, TERAZOSIN, AND DOXAZOSIN

These agents are selective antagonists of α_1-adrenergic receptors that reduce peripheral resistance, produce venodilation, and decrease blood pressure. Doxazosin and terazosin have longer half-lives than prazosin and may thus be used in single daily doses. Therapeutic drug concentration monitoring is not used clinically to assess therapeutic outcome for these drugs with large therapeutic ratios.

Renal Dysfunction. Prazosin is metabolized extensively by hepatic oxidative mechanisms, and the metabolites are excreted via the bile. No evidence suggests that renal failure results in accumulation of prazosin; however, some authors[52] suggest that the peak serum concentration may be elevated secondary to decreased protein binding.

Because doxazosin and terazosin are eliminated by nonrenal metabolism and no evidence exists that active metabolites are formed, there is no need for dose adjustments in patients with renal failure. As for other antihypertensive agents, greater effects may be observed with α-blockers in end-stage renal disease.

Hepatic Dysfunction. Prazosin is subject to significant first-pass metabolism; moderate to severe hepatocellular dysfunction may be expected to increase the bioavailability of prazosin and reduce its systemic clearance.[52] Final dose adjustments should be made based on hemodynamic response and patient tolerance. Both doxazosin and terazosin are eliminated by biotransformation to inactive metabolites. No information is available regarding their use in chronic liver failure. Doses should be titrated upward to the desired effect.

METHYLDOPA

Methyldopa is thought to be a centrally acting antihypertensive drug. The parent compound is inactive per se and has to be converted to active metabolites (α-methyl dopamine, norepinephrine, and epinephrine) to lower blood pressure. The active metabolites seem to stimulate centrally located α_2-adrenergic receptors to reduce sympathetic discharge. It has a large therapeutic ratio, and therapeutic drug concentration monitoring is not used clinically. The usual adult dose is 250 mg four times daily.

Renal Dysfunction. Methyldopa and its metabolites accumulate during renal failure. Furthermore, patients in renal failure are more sensitive to the hypotensive effects of methyldopa. Therefore, the following recommendations are given: increase the dosing interval to 8 to 12 hours in patients in moderate failure and to 12 to 24 hours in those in severe renal failure. Because of its small volume of distribution and its poor protein binding, methyldopa has a high dialysis clearance rate.

Hepatic Dysfunction. No information is available with regard to dosing patients in liver failure. Methyldopa is metabolized extensively in the liver and undergoes a significant first-pass effect after oral administration. Moderate to severe hepatocellular dysfunction may increase the oral bioavailability of methyldopa significantly. Final dose adjustments should be based on hemodynamic response and patient tolerance.

CLONIDINE

Clonidine is a centrally acting antihypertensive drug believed to stimulate α_2-adrenergic receptors in the medulla and perhaps in the hypothalamus and to induce a reduction in sympathetic activity. Common daily doses range from 0.1 to 1 mg divided in two or three doses. Monitoring of the therapeutic drug concentration is not used clinically to assess the effects of this drug, which has a large therapeutic ratio.

Renal Dysfunction. Dosage reduction is recommended in patients with renal failure. The dose should be reduced by 25% to 50%, maintaining the normal dosage interval.

Hepatic Dysfunction. The liver accounts for 50% of the metabolism of clonidine. Patients with moderate to severe hepatocellular dysfunction should receive the lowest possible dose of clonidine, with final dose adjustment titrated to hemodynamic effect.

GUANFACINE

Guanfacine is thought to lower blood pressure by stimulating centrally located α_2-adrenergic receptors and reducing sympathetic activity. Monitoring of the therapeutic drug concentration is not used clinically to assess the effects of this drug, which has a large therapeutic ratio. The usual initial adult dose is 1 mg daily.

Renal Dysfunction. This centrally acting α_2-adrenergic agonist has an elimination half-life of 15 to 20 hours in normal subjects. Therefore, a single daily dose is recommended for hypertension. No dosage adjustment seems necessary in patients with renal failure.[53]

Hepatic Dysfunction. No information is available on the pharmacokinetics of guanfacine in patients with liver dysfunction. No clinically significant first-pass effect occurs; however, the drug is metabolized extensively in the liver, and the metabolites are excreted in the urine. The lowest possible dose is recommended.

GUANABENZ

Guanabenz, like clonidine, is a centrally acting α_2-receptor agonist that exerts a peripheral hypotensive effect. Therapeutic drug concentration monitoring is not used clinically to assess the effects of this drug with a large therapeutic ratio. The usual dose is 4 mg twice daily.

Renal Dysfunction. This compound is metabolized extensively in the liver. For patients in renal failure, a slower rate of increase in dosage is recommended during initiation of therapy. Similar to other sympatholytic drugs, enhanced hypotensive action may be seen in patients in renal failure.

Hepatic Dysfunction. No dosing schedule has been recommended for patients in liver failure; however, the dose should be reduced in those in severe liver failure. A clinically significant first-pass effect and extensive hepatic metabolism are seen. Less than 2% of the drug is excreted intact in the urine. The lowest possible dose is recommended.

SODIUM NITROPRUSSIDE

Nitroprusside is an effective vasodilator of arterioles and venules. The drug is given intravenously and requires continuous blood pressure monitoring. The infusion rate is titrated to clinical response, and the drug has a small therapeutic ratio. Monitoring of the therapeutic drug concentration is not used clinically to assess the effects of the drug. Initial intravenous dosages are 0.25 to 2 μg/kg/min.

Renal Dysfunction. Because of the risk of possible accumulation of thiocyanate in end-stage renal disease, prolonged administration (longer than 72 hours) should be restricted. When necessary, the safety of longer infusions may be monitored by serum thiocyanate concentrations.

Hepatic Dysfunction. If the enzyme rhodanese is deficient, hepatocellular dysfunction theoretically may decrease the metabolic conversion of cyanide to thiocyanate. Because rhodanese is ubiquitous, the likelihood of clinical toxicity secondary to cyanide is remote.

MILRINONE

Milrinone is a positive inotrope and vasodilator. The vasodilating and positive inotropic effects result in reductions in preload, afterload, ventricular diastolic pressures, and coronary vascular resistance. Milrinone is indicated for short-term intravenous therapy of congestive heart failure. The majority of experience with intravenous milrinone has been in patients receiving digoxin and diuretics. In some patients, injections of milrinone and oral milrinone have been shown to increase ventricular ectopy, including nonsustained ventricular tachycardia. Both inotropic and vasodilatory effects have been observed over the therapeutic range of plasma milrinone concentration of 100 to 300 ng/ml. Therapeutic drug concentration monitoring is not used clinically to assess the effects of the drug. The primary route of excretion is via the kidney. The mean renal clearance of milrinone is approximately 0.3 L/min.

Milrinone should be administered with a loading dose followed by a continuous infusion (maintenance dose) according to the following guidelines:

Loading Dose: 50 μg/kg: Administer slowly over 10 minutes

Maintenance Dose:

Infusion Rate	Total Daily Dose (24 hr)
Minimum 0.375 μg/kg/min	0.59 mg/kg
Standard 0.50 μg/kg/min	0.77 mg/kg
Maximum 0.75 μg/kg/min	1.13 mg/kg

The infusion rate should be adjusted according to hemodynamic and clinical response. Patients should be closely monitored for hypotension and arrhythmias.

Renal Dysfunction. Dosage may be titrated to the maximal hemodynamic effect and should not exceed 1.13 mg/kg/day. Duration of therapy should depend on patient responsiveness. Reductions in infusion rate may be necessary in patients with renal impairment. For patients with clinical evidence of renal impairment, the recommended rate can be obtained using the following table:

Creatinine Clearance (ml/min/1.73 m^2)	Infusion Rate (μg/kg/min)
5	0.20
10	0.23
20	0.28
30	0.33
40	0.38
50	0.43

Hepatic Dysfunction. No specific information is available on the dosage needs of patients with liver dysfunction.

HYDRALAZINE

Hydralazine is an effective arteriolar vasodilator that is commonly used as a third-line agent for the treatment of hypertension. Therapeutic drug concentration monitoring is not used clinically to assess the effects of this drug, which has a large therapeutic ratio. The initial adult dose for hypertension is 10 mg orally three to four times daily.

Renal Dysfunction. Normal hydralazine doses vary with the acetylator characteristics of the individual. Doses from 10 to 50 mg three to four times daily are commonly prescribed for hypertensive patients with normal renal function. In mild to moderate renal failure, the dosing interval should be increased to 8 hours. However, in severe renal failure, dosing intervals of 8 to 16 hours for fast acetylators and of 12 to 24 hours for slow acetylators are recommended.

Hepatic Dysfunction. No information is available about the pharmacokinetics of hydralazine in patients with liver insufficiency. Hydralazine undergoes significant first-pass metabolism. Severe hepatocellular dysfunction theoretically may increase the bioavailability of hydralazine that is administered orally. Patients with severe chronic CHF may require a higher than normal dose of hydralazine for satisfactory clinical effect.[54] Final dose adjustments should be based on hemodynamic response and patient tolerance to the adverse effects of hydralazine.

MINOXIDIL

Minoxidil is a selective arteriolar vasodilator. It reduces peripheral resistance and blood pressure and increases renal blood flow. The drug is an effective hypotensive agent that retains its efficacy despite severe renal insufficiency. Marked fluid retention is observed during minoxidil administration; therefore, minoxidil frequently is given with a loop diuretic. Therapeutic drug concentration monitoring is not used clinically to assess the effects of this drug with a large therapeutic ratio. The usual initial adult dose is 5 mg daily.

Renal Dysfunction. Minoxidil is eliminated primarily by nonrenal routes. No dose adjustments are required in patients with renal failure. No change in minoxidil's pharmacokinetics has been reported in these patients; however, greater hypotensive effects may be produced by minoxidil in patients in renal failure.

Hepatic Dysfunction. No information is available about dosage adjustment in patients with liver failure.

CAPTOPRIL

Captopril is a sulfhydryl-containing angiotensin-converting enzyme (ACE) inhibitor. Because of the reduction in angiotensin II levels produced by captopril, a reduction in blood pressure occurs secondary to decreased arteriolar and venular constriction. The usual initial dose of captopril is 12.5 mg two or three times daily for the first 1 or 2 weeks. Therapeutic drug concentration monitoring is not used clinically to assess the effects of this drug, which has a large therapeutic ratio.

Renal Dysfunction. Captopril is eliminated mainly by the kidney. Dose adjustments should be based on glomerular filtration rate, because serum captopril concentrations are increased in proportion to the reduction in creatinine clearance. Dose reductions or longer dose intervals are adequate. A common recommendation is to reduce the dose by 50%, maintaining the dose interval constant. However, titration downward should be performed based on clinical response. As with other ACE inhibitors, the antihypertensive effects of captopril may be accentuated in patients with renal insufficiency.[55] In order to prevent exaggerated responses, titrations should be made at 1- to 2-week intervals. Captopril conjugates accumulate in renal failure. These conjugates (captopril disulfides) may be converted back to captopril in a variety of tissues, including the kidney, and they contribute to the accentuated blood pressure–lowering effect of the drug in patients in renal failure.[53]

Hepatic Dysfunction. No information was found on dosage adjustments of captopril in patients with liver dysfunction. In one reference,[56] the authors believe that captopril impairs diuretic-induced sodium excretion and suggest that this effect contraindicates the use of captopril in patients with liver cirrhosis with ascites.

ENALAPRIL

Enalapril is a nonsulfhydryl ACE inhibitor. The drug is inactive on its own and requires conversion to enalaprilat for activity. It reduces angiotensin II formation, produces arteriolar and venular vasodilation, and lowers blood pressure. Therapeutic drug concentration monitoring is not used clinically to assess the effects of this drug, which has a large therapeutic ratio. The usual daily dose of enalapril is a single dose of 10 to 40 mg.

Renal Dysfunction. Nearly 40% of enalapril is excreted in the urine as enalaprilat, the active form of enalapril. Therefore, dose reduction is required in renal failure. A reduction of the total daily maintenance dose to 5 mg is recommended for patients with creatinine clearances of less than 30 ml/min.[57] In these patients, the initial daily dose should be 2.5 mg instead of 5 mg.

Hepatic Dysfunction. No information was found on dosage adjustments of enalapril in patients with liver dysfunction. Enalapril is a prodrug that requires hepatic conversion to an active metabolite. No known population of patients is unable to convert enalapril to enalaprilat; however, patients with severe liver dysfunction have not been studied extensively.

LISINOPRIL

Lisinopril is a lysine analogue of enalaprilic acid, the active metabolite of enalapril, and is used to treat hypertension. Therapeutic drug concentration monitoring is not used clinically to assess the effects of this drug, which has a large therapeutic ratio.

Renal Dysfunction. Lisinopril has a longer half-life than enalapril and is excreted unchanged by the urine. Consequently, accumulation occurs in patients in severe renal failure. Peak lisinopril concentrations were 10 times greater in hypertensive patients with severe renal failure than in hypertensive patients with normal renal function. These higher drug levels were associated with longer antihypertensive action (72 hours), greater and longer duration of ACE inhibition, and greater degrees of hyperkalemia.[58] Although no established dosage recommendations exist, either dose reductions or increased dosing intervals are suggested for patients with renal insufficiency. Because of the long half-life of lisinopril, dosage reduction may be more appropriate.

Hepatic Dysfunction. Lisinopril is not known to be metabolized. No dosage adjustment appears to be necessary in patients with liver dysfunction.

RAMIPRIL

Ramipril, a long-acting, nonsulfhydryl ACE inhibitor, is converted in the liver to its active metabolite, ramiprilat.[59] Ramipril is used to treat hypertension and CHF. Oral doses have ranged from 5 to 20 mg daily, and the recommended starting dose in healthy adults is 2.5 mg daily.

Renal Dysfunction. Renal excretion determines ramipril's duration of action and half-life; thus, dose adjustments should be made in patients with renal failure. Ramipril's half-life increases from 5 hours in patients with creatinine clearances of more than 40 ml/min to 9 and 15 hours for creatinine clearances between 15 and 40 ml/min and less than 15 ml/min, respectively.[60] Based on the reviewed data, a 50% dosage reduction is recommended when the creatinine clearance is less than 40 ml/min, to avoid exaggerated hypotensive effects.[61]

Hepatic Dysfunction. Preliminary data suggest that, although ramipril is extensively metabolized in the liver to its active form ramiprilat, steady-state concentrations of the metabolite were not different from concentrations measured in healthy volunteers. No dosage adjustment is anticipated.

FOSINOPRIL

Fosinopril, a nonsulfhydryl, long-acting ACE inhibitor, is a prodrug that is converted by esterases to fosinoprilat. The usual starting dose for adults is 10 mg once daily, with a usual maintenance range of 20 to 40 mg daily. Divided dosing may be needed in some patients when the 24-hour blood pressure is not sufficiently controlled. A so-called dual route of elimination minimizes the need for any dosage reduction with impaired elimination organ dysfunction.

Renal Dysfunction. Fosinopril does not appear to accumulate in patients with renal dysfunction, suggesting that conversion to fosinoprilat is not impaired. Fosinoprilat's total body clearance is reportedly reduced by 50% when the creatinine clearance is less than 80 ml/min/1.73 m^2.[62] Further decreases in renal function are not associated with reduced clearance. The hepatobiliary route of elimination appears to compensate for decreased renal clearance. In summary, no dosage adjustment is anticipated.

Hepatic Dysfunction. Fosinopril is extensively metabolized by esterases in the liver, yet there are no clear data that suggest an impaired conversion to fosinoprilat. No specific guidelines were found for dosage adjustment, and no adjustments are anticipated.

QUINAPRIL

Quinapril is indicated for the treatment of hypertension; however, preliminary data suggest its effectiveness in CHF. Quinapril is a nonsulfhydryl-containing prodrug that is converted to quinaprilat, its active metabolite. The elimination half-lives of quinapril (0.8 hour) and quinaprilat (2 hours) are shorter than those of most other drugs (except captopril) in this class. Quinapril is generally administered twice daily to maintain 24-hour control of blood pressure. Doses range from 20 to 80 mg daily for hypertension and from 5 to 30 mg for CHF.

Renal Dysfunction. The kidney accounts for 50% to 60% of the elimination of quinapril (via active tubular secretion). The maximal concentration, elimination half-life, and area-under-curve (AUC) all were increased in 12 patients with ESRD.[63] Downward dose adjustments are required in renal failure, and the starting dose is reduced by 50% in patients with creatinine clearance rates of less than 60 ml/min.

Hepatic Dysfunction. No information is available on the dosage adjustment of quinapril in patients with liver dysfunction.

BENAZEPRIL

Benazepril is indicated in the treatment of hypertension, but preliminary studies have shown it to be effective for the treatment of CHF. It is a prodrug that is hydrolyzed in the liver to benazeprilat, its diacid. Like fosinopril and ramipril, the elimination half-life of benazepril is approximately 11 hours, which allows for initial once-daily dosing with subsequent adjustment to twice-daily dosing if necessary.

Renal Dysfunction. Benazepril also needs to be dose adjusted in patients with creatinine clearances of less than 30 ml/min.

Hepatic Dysfunction. No information is available on the dosage adjustment of quinapril in patients with liver dysfunction.

CALCIUM ANTAGONISTS

The calcium antagonists include a wide array of therapeutic agents with markedly different chemical and pharmacologic properties. They are used in the management of hypertension, angina pectoris, arrhythmias, and other investigational indications. Therapeutic drug concentration monitoring is not used clinically to assess the effects of these drugs, which have large therapeutic ratios.

Renal Dysfunction. Verapamil, diltiazem, nifedipine, isradipine, amlodipine, and felodipine do not require dose adjustment in patients with renal insufficiency. These drugs are extensively metabolized by the liver. The formation of renally excreted metabolites, most with minor pharmacologic activity, appears insignificant. Most information available is on verapamil. In normal subjects, norverapamil, a metabolite of verapamil, reaches serum concentrations comparable to those of verapamil. However, norverapamil is only one tenth as active as the parent compound. Only 14% of the dose of verapamil is excreted in the urine, of which 70% is as norverapamil. Therefore, it is unlikely that the metabolite would accumulate to significant concentrations in patients in renal failure. However, like other antihypertensive drugs, the blood pressure–lowering effect of calcium antagonists may be accentuated in patients with end-stage renal disease.[64] Bepridil, in contrast, has type I antiarrhythmic activity with minimal antihypertensive activity. It is extensively metabolized to metabolites that are then eliminated by the kidney and via the feces. The pharmacologic activity of the metabolites is not known. Although unstudied, dosage adjustments may be needed. Dosage titrations of bepridil should be at no less than 10-day intervals because of the long half-life for accumulation. Isradipine's bioavailability is increased by approximately 50% in patients with renal insufficiency. Despite this modest increase, the initial starting dose is not adjusted from the usual adult dose of 2.5 mg given twice daily.

Hepatic Dysfunction. Little specific information is available on dose adjustment for diltiazem, verapamil, nifedipine, isradipine, bepridil, amlodipine, or felodipine in patients in liver failure. However, each of these drugs may require dose adjustments because they are metabolized extensively by the liver. In patients with severe liver cirrhosis, one group recommends that the oral dose of verapamil be decreased by a factor of five and the intravenous dose be decreased by one half to prevent adverse effects.[65] Steady-state serum concentrations were reached after 2 days of oral administration. Nifedipine's pharmacokinetics are significantly altered in patients with severe cirrhosis. Following a single 10-mg dose, the half-life of nifedipine increased fourfold (434 ± 74 minutes in the cirrhotic group versus 102 ± 11 minutes in the control group), and the area under the curve increased twofold in the cirrhotic group. The authors conclude that there is significant risk of accumulation on multiple dosing; therefore, lower initial and maintenance doses of nifedipine are recommended.[66] The maintenance dosage of bepridil may be lower in patients with liver dysfunction, and a very slow dosage titration is recommended to avoid toxicity. The AUC for amlodipine is increased 50% in patients with liver impairment, and the initial and maintenance dosages should be decreased by 50% to 2.5 mg daily and slowly titrated upward at 14-day intervals. Isradipine's AUC is increased by approximately 50%; therefore, the final maintenance dose may be lower than the dose required in otherwise healthy nonhypertensive adults.

KETANSERIN

Ketanserin is an investigational serotonin S$_2$-antagonist with potential clinical uses in the treatment of essential hypertension, peripheral vascular disease, and portal hypertension. Therapeutic drug concentration monitoring is not used clinically to assess the effects of this drug, which has a large therapeutic ratio.

Renal Dysfunction. No information was found on the dosing of ketanserin in patients with decreased renal function.

Hepatic Dysfunction. The acute hemodynamic effects of ketanserin in patients with alcoholic cirrhosis were reported to be more pronounced and prolonged in one study.[67] The degree of effect appeared to vary with the degree of severity of cirrhosis. A formula to predict an adjusted dose of ketanserin in patients with cirrhosis is not available. Available data suggest that lower doses may be effective.

FUROSEMIDE, BUMETANIDE, AND TORSEMIDE

Furosemide, bumetanide, and torsemide are loop diuretics frequently used in patients with impaired renal and hepatic function. As antihypertensive agents, these drugs are more effective than thiazide diuretics in patients with decreased glomerular filtration rates. Furosemide's absorption from the intestines after oral administration may be erratic and incomplete in uremic patients. Renal or hepatic disease does not appear to affect the oral absorption of bumetanide. Intravenous use of furosemide may be preferred in patients with end-stage renal disease. These drugs effectively reduce fluid volume in patients in edematous states. Marked changes in electrolyte balance can occur. The usual initial adult dose of furosemide for hypertension is 40 mg twice daily. The usual initial adult dose for edema is 20 to 80 mg daily as a single dose. Patients with severe hypertension have received up to 480 mg daily, and patients with end-stage renal disease have received up to 4 g daily. The usual initial adult dose of bumetanide is 0.5 to 2 mg daily. Patients with severe hypertension or edema may require up to 10 mg daily. The usual dose of torsemide is 10 to 20 mg twice daily and is approximately equally effective to furosemide 40 mg twice daily. A small percentage of torsemide is metabolized to partially active metabolites.

Renal Dysfunction. Furosemide, bumetanide, and torsemide are rapidly eliminated by renal and nonrenal pathways in healthy subjects, and the elimination half-life is approximately 1 hour. Contrary to most drugs, the daily doses of furosemide, bumetanide, and torsemide are increased in patients with renal failure because of reduced efficacy. For patients in chronic renal failure, the usual daily doses of furosemide are 80 to 120 mg, but doses as high as 800 mg daily have been prescribed.[68] For patients in acute renal failure, oral doses up to 240 mg twice daily have been used clinically. Bumetanide doses have ranged from 1 to 10 mg daily as long-term therapy for patients in severe renal failure.[69] The usual torsemide dose is not reduced.[70]

Hepatic Dysfunction. Cirrhosis does not appear to

influence the pharmacokinetics of furosemide. However, the natriuretic response to furosemide appears to decrease with increasing liver dysfunction. An increase in dose may be expected, but furosemide should be used with caution to avoid large changes in fluid and electrolyte status. Daily doses should be titrated to effect; high daily doses of several hundred milligrams daily are not uncommon. Congestive heart failure does not appear to affect bioavailability significantly.[71-73] There is no anticipated dosage reduction for torsemide in patients with cirrhosis.[74]

HYDROCHLOROTHIAZIDE AND CHLORTHALIDONE

Thiazides and related diuretics enhance excretion of sodium, chloride, and water by interfering with sodium transport across the renal tubule in the cortical-diluting segment of the nephron. The usual dose of hydrochlorothiazide or chlorthalidone is 25 mg daily. Therapeutic drug concentration monitoring is not used clinically to assess the effects of these drugs, which have large therapeutic ratios.

Renal Dysfunction. No dose adjustments are required in patients with mild to moderate renal insufficiency. These drugs become ineffective when the glomerular filtration rates drops to lower than 25 ml/min. Thus, their use is not recommended in patients in severe renal failure.

Hepatic Dysfunction. No dosage adjustments are believed necessary for these renally eliminated drugs in patients with liver dysfunction.

TRIAMTERENE

Triamterene exerts a direct effect on distal tubule cells to inhibit sodium and potassium exchange, resulting in increased systemic potassium concentrations. Therapeutic drug concentration monitoring is not used clinically to assess the effects of this drug, which has a large therapeutic ratio. The usual adult dose is 100 mg daily given in two divided doses.

Renal Dysfunction. For patients in mild to moderate renal failure, the dose interval does not change; however, serum potassium concentrations should be monitored. The drug should be discontinued in patients in severe renal failure because of the risk of hyperkalemia.

Hepatic Dysfunction. Triamterene undergoes significant first-pass effect; therefore, its bioavailability is enhanced in patients with hepatocellular dysfunction. Systemic drug is highly metabolized in the liver, and only 15% is excreted in unchanged form. Moderate to severe liver disease is expected to decrease the clearance of triamterene; therefore, it should be used cautiously, if at all, in patients with marked organ dysfunction.

AMILORIDE

Amiloride exerts a direct effect on distal tubule cells to inhibit sodium and potassium exchange, resulting in increased systemic potassium concentrations. Therapeutic drug concentration monitoring is not used clinically to assess the effects of this drug, which has a large therapeutic ratio. The usual adult dose is 5 mg daily.

Renal Dysfunction. Like triamterene and spironolactone, amiloride should not be used in severe renal insufficiency because of the risk of hyperkalemia. Half of the dose of amiloride is excreted unchanged in the urine. Marked increases in its half-life have been observed in patients with renal failure. In patients with creatinine clearances of more than 10 ml/min, the dose should be decreased by 50% and the blood urea nitrogen, potassium, and creatinine concentrations closely monitored.

Hepatic Dysfunction. The dose of amiloride is not expected to change in patients with mild to moderate liver disease. In patients with severe liver disease, amiloride, like other diuretics, may produce hepatic encephalopathy secondary to marked shifts in electrolyte balance.

SPIRONOLACTONE

Spironolactone inhibits the physiologic effects of aldosterone on the distal tubule, causing increased sodium excretion and enhanced potassium reabsorption. Therapeutic drug concentration monitoring is not used clinically to assess the effects of this drug, which has a large therapeutic ratio. The usual adult dose is 100 mg daily given in two divided doses.

Renal Dysfunction. Like triamterene, spironolactone may increase the risk of hyperkalemia in patients with renal dysfunction. Potassium supplements should not be administered concomitantly because this further increases the risk. Spironolactone is metabolized extensively to active metabolites in the liver. No dosage adjustment is anticipated in mild to moderate renal dysfunction. Spironolactone should not be used in the presence of end-stage renal disease.

Hepatic Dysfunction. Spironolactone does not undergo significant first-pass effect; however, it is metabolized extensively to canrenone, an active metabolite that undergoes further hepatic conversion. Accumulation is expected in liver dysfunction, but high doses are tolerated by patients without unusually adverse effects. High circulating concentrations of aldosterone generally require high doses of spironolactone to produce an effect. Downward dose adjustment is not needed.

NONSTEROIDAL ANTIINFLAMMATORY DRUGS

Renal Dysfunction. Aspirin (acetylsalicylic acid) is hydrolyzed to salicylate and free acetate. Salicylic acid is excreted partly unchanged in urine and partly metabolized. Prolongation of bleeding time has been reported after aspirin administration in patients with severe renal dysfunction compared with patients with normal renal function.[75] The dose of diflunisal must be reduced in patients in renal failure, because its half-life is prolonged in this condition. Azapropazone is also eliminated 60% to 70% unchanged in the urine. The dose must be reduced by 50% in patients in renal failure. The same is true for mefenamic acid, a substance eliminated 50% unchanged in the urine. One study of 16 patients with severe renal failure did not find clinically significant changes in the elimination rate of naproxen.[76] Serum concentrations of the inactive metabolites were increased. No dose adjustment in renal failure appears necessary.[76]

Hepatic Dysfunction. The liver is the principal site of elimination of most nonsteroidal antiinflammatory agents. Indomethacin, naproxen, ketoprofen, ibuprofen, diclofenac, and piroxicam are eliminated mainly via hepatic metabolism. Very limited information is available on dosage adjustment in patients with liver dysfunction. In one study,[77] the half-life of naproxen was prolonged from 14 hours to 20 hours in a group of 11 patients with chronic hepatic impairment. The authors conclude that this is not likely to be clinically significant. Other data in patients with cirrhosis demonstrated that the clearance of unbound naproxen decreased 60% at steady state.[78] These authors recommend decreasing the maintenance dose by 50% to avoid excessive accumulation.[78] Excessive doses of some hepatically eliminated nonsteroidal antiinflammatory drugs can lead to hepatotoxicity and death.[79] Therefore, cautious use is warranted because accumulation is expected. The lowest possible doses of drugs with short half-lives should be used when necessary.

NITROGLYCERIN

Nitroglycerin is a direct-acting vasodilator used sublingually, intravenously, and transdermally in the management of angina pectoris and CHF. Nitroglycerin has a large therapeutic ratio, and therapeutic drug concentration monitoring is not used to assess its clinical effects. Nitroglycerin is metabolized extensively in the liver.

Renal Dysfunction. The dose of nitroglycerin is not expected to be altered in patients with renal disease.

Hepatic Dysfunction. The dose of nitroglycerin is not expected to be altered in patients with liver disease.

ISOSORBIDE MONONITRATE

Isosorbide mononitrate is the major active metabolite of isosorbide dinitrate. This orally active vasodilator is indicated in the management of vasospastic angina due to coronary artery disease. Isosorbide mononitrate is not subject to first-pass metabolism. The recommended initial dose is 20 mg twice daily, given 7 hours apart. A nitrate-free interval follows this schedule to minimize the onset of tolerance to the nitrate. Isosorbide mononitrate is extensively metabolized to inactive metabolites. No dosage adjustment is anticipated in patients with renal or liver dysfunction.

HYDROXYMETHYLGLUTARYL COENZYME A (HMG CoA) REDUCTASE INHIBITORS

Lovastatin and simvastatin are chemically related prodrugs that are hydrolyzed to active metabolites that interfere with cholesterol synthesis, whereas pravastatin is an active cholesterol-lowering agent in its parent form. Pharmacokinetic variables such as the AUC vary widely in patients with impaired renal and liver function; however, there is also wide variability in normal subjects. Pravastatin appears to undergo the so-called dual routes of elimination; therefore, while the total body clearance was unaffected by renal failure, the renal clearance did decline as creatinine clearance declined.[80] Serum concentration monitoring is not used to assess the therapeutic or toxic responses to HMG CoA reductase inhibitors. The starting dose of each drug is not different from the usual dose in otherwise healthy adults. No specific and accepted dosage adjustment guidelines were found in the literature.

TICLOPIDINE

Ticlopidine is a platelet aggregation inhibitor indicated for its ability to reduce the risk of thrombotic stroke (fatal or nonfatal) in patients who have experienced stroke precursors and in patients who have had a completed stroke. Ticlopidine's toxicity profile suggests that it should be reserved for patients intolerant to aspirin. For labeled indications, the adult starting dose is 250 mg twice daily, taken with food. Recommendations for dose adjustment in patients with renal and liver disease have not been published; however, pharmacokinetic data suggest that ticlopidine plasma concentrations are increased and clearance is reduced approximately 50% in patients with moderate renal failure. Bleeding times were prolonged only in patients with creatinine clearance of 20 to 50 ml/min. The effects on adenosine diphosphate–induced aggregation were not significantly increased. Ticlopidine is extensively metabolized by the liver and excreted in the feces, bile, and urine. Patients with renal or liver dysfunction should be monitored more aggressively.

REFERENCES

1. Swan SK, Bennett WM: Drug dosing guidelines in patients with renal failure. West J Med 156:633, 1992.
2. Brouwer KLR, Dukes GE, Powell JR: Influence of liver function on drug disposition. *In* Evans WE, Schentag JJ, Jusko WJ (eds): Applied Pharmacokinetics: Principles of Therapeutic Drug Monitoring. Spokane, WA: Applied Therapeutics, 1992, pp 6-1–6-69.
3. Koup JR, Jusko WJ, Elwood CM, et al: Digoxin pharmacokinetics: Role of renal failure in dosage regimen design. Clin Pharmacol Ther 18:9, 1975.
4. Keller F, Molzahn M, Ingerowski R: Digoxin dosage in renal insufficiency: Impracticality of basing it on the creatinine clearance, body weight, and volume of distribution. Eur J Clin Pharmacol 18:433, 1980.
5. Keys PW: Digoxin. *In* Evans WE, Jusko WJ, Schentag JJ (eds):

Applied Pharmacokinetics. Los Angeles: Applied Therapeutics, 1982, pp 319–349.

6. Cockroft DW, Gault MH: Prediction of creatinine clearance from serum creatinine. Nephron 16:31, 1976.

7. Graves SW, Brown B, Valdes R Jr, et al: Endogenous digoxin-like substances in renal impairment. Ann Intern Med 99:604, 1983.

7a. Jiang F, Wilhite TR, Smith CH, Landt M: A new digoxin immunoassay substantially free of interference by digoxin immunoreactive factor. Ther Drug Monit 17:184, 1995.

8. Sheiner LB, Rosenberg B, Marathe VV: Estimation of population characteristics of pharmacokinetic parameters from routine clinical data. J Pharmacokinet Biopharm 5:445, 1977.

9. Karim AZ, Nissen C, Azarnoff DL, et al: Clinical pharmacokinetics of disopyramide. J Pharmacokinet Biopharm 10:465, 1982.

10. Lima JL: Disopyramide. In Evans WE, Schentag JJ, Jusko WJ (eds): Applied Pharmacokinetics: Principles in Therapeutic Drug Monitoring. Spokane, WA: Applied Therapeutics, 1986, pp 1210–1253.

11. Lima JL, Haughley DB, Leier CV, et al: Comparison of disopyramide bioavailability and pharmacokinetics in normals and in patients with congestive heart failure. J Pharmacokinet Biopharm 12:289, 1984.

12. Svensson CK, Woodruff MN, Baxter JG, et al: Free drug concentration monitoring in clinical practice: Rationale and current status. Clin Pharmacokinet 11:450, 1980.

13. Chian W-T, von Barh C, Calissendorff B, et al: Kinetics and dynamics of disopyramide and its dealkylated metabolite in healthy subjects. Clin Pharmacol 31:73, 1986.

14. Bonde J, Graudal NA, Pedersen LE, et al: Kinetics of disopyramide in decreased hepatic function. Eur J Clin Pharmacol 31:73, 1986.

15. Echizen H, Saima S, Umeda N, et al: Protein binding of disopyramide in liver cirrhosis and in nephrotic syndrome. Clin Pharmacol Ther 40:274, 1986.

16. Pederson LE, Bonde J, Graudal NA, et al: Quantitative and qualitative binding characteristics of disopyramide in serum from patients with decreased renal and hepatic function. Br J Clin Pharmacol 23:41, 1987.

17. Thomson PD, Melmon KL, Richardson JA, et al: Lidocaine pharmacokinetics in advanced heart failure, liver disease and renal disease in humans. Ann Intern Med 78:499, 1973.

18. Collinsworth KA, Strong JM, Atkinson AJ, et al: Pharmacokinetics and metabolism of lidocaine in patients with renal failure. Clin Pharmacol Ther 18:59, 1975.

19. Stargel WW: Lidocaine. In Taylor WJ, Diers Caviness HG (eds): A Textbook for the Clinical Application of Therapeutic Drug Monitoring. Chicago: Abbott Laboratories Diagnostic Division, 1986, pp 125–131.

20. Bauman JL: Mexiletine. In Taylor WJ, Diers Caviness HG (eds): A Textbook for the Clinical Application of Therapeutic Drug Monitoring. Chicago: Abbott Laboratories Diagnostic Division, 1986, pp 125–131.

21. Pentikainen PJ, Hietakorpi S, Halinen MO, et al: Cirrhosis of the liver markedly impairs the elimination of mexiletine. Eur J Clin Pharmacol 30:83, 1986.

22. Braun J, Kolert JK, Beckeer JU, et al: Pharmacokinetics of flecainide in patients with mild and moderate renal failure compared to patients with normal renal function. Eur J Clin Pharmacol 31:711, 1987.

23. Domoto DT, Brown WW, Bruggensmith P, et al: Removal of toxic levels of N-acteylprocainamide with continuous arteriovenous hemofiltration or continuous arteriovenous hemodiafiltration. Ann Intern Med 106:550, 1987.

24. Coyle HJD, Lima JL: Procainamide. In Evans WE, Schentag JJ, Jusko WJ (eds): Applied Pharmacokinetics: Principles in Therapeutic Drug Monitoring. Spokane, WA: Applied Therapeutics, 1986, pp 137–148.

25. du Couich P, Erill S: Metabolism of procainamide and p-aminobenzoic acid in patients with acute myocardial infarction or congestive heart failure. J Am Coll Cardiol 7:1131, 1986.

26. Kessler KM, Kayden DS, Estes DM, et al: Procainamide pharmacokinetics in patients with acute myocardial infarction or congestive heart failure. J Am Coll Cardiol 7:1131, 1986.

27. Ueda CT: Quinidine. In Evans WE, Schentag JJ, Jusko WJ (eds): Applied Pharmacokinetics: Principles in Therapeutic Drug Monitoring. Spokane, WA: Applied Therapeutics, 1986, pp 712–734.

28. Kessler KM, Lowenthal DT, Warner H, et al: Quinidine elimination in patients with congestive heart failure or poor renal function. N Engl J Med 290:706, 1974.

29. Franciosa JA, Wilen M, Weeks CE, et al: Pharmacokinetics and hemodynamic effects of flecainide in patients with chronic low output heart failure. J Am Coll Cardiol 1:699, 1983.

30. Personal communications from representative of Bristol Laboratories and 3M Riker, April 1989.

31. Roden DM, Wood AJ, Wilkinson GR, et al: Disposition kinetics of encainide and metabolites. Am J Cardiol 58:4C, 1986.

32. Carey EL, Duff HJ, Roden DM, et al: Encainide and its metabolites: Comparative effects in man on ventricular arrhythmia and electrocardiographic intervals. J Clin Invest 75:539, 1984.

33. Bergstrand RH, Wang T, Roden DM, et al: Encainide disposition in patients with renal failure. Clin Pharmacol Ther 40:64, 1986.

34. Bergstrand RH, Wang T, Roden DM, et al: Encainide disposition in patients with chronic cirrhosis. Clin Pharmacol Ther 40:148, 1986.

35. Woosley RL, Morganroth J, Fogoros RN, et al: Pharmacokinetics of moricizine HCl. Am J Cardiol 60:35F, 1987.

36. Howrie DL, Pieniaszek HJ Jr, Fogoros RN, et al: Disposition of moracizine (sic) (Ethmozine) in healthy subjects after oral administration of radio labelled drug. Eur J Clin Phamacol 87:32, 607, 1987.

37. Morganroth J, Pearlman AS, Dunkman WB, et al: Ethmozin: A new antiarrhythmic agent developed in the USSR: Efficacy and tolerance. Am Heart J 98:621, 1979.

38. Hammill SC, Sorenson PB, Wood DL, et al: Propafenone for the treatment of refractory complex ventricular ectopic activity. Mayo Clin Proc 61:98, 1986.

39. Poirier JM, Joannides R, Geffroy-Josse S, et al: Propafenone pharmacokinetics in uremic patients treated by peritoneal dialysis. Clin Nephrol 38:231, 1992.

40. Siddoway LA, Roden DM, Woosley RL, et al: Clinical pharmacology of propafenone: Pharmacokinetics, metabolism and concentration-response relations. Am J Cardiol 54:9D, 1984.

41. Salerno DM, Granrud G, Sharkey P, et al: A controlled trial of propafenone for treatment of frequent and repetitive ventricular premature complexes. Am J Cardiol 53:77, 1984.

42. Connolly SJ, Kates RE, Lebsack CS, et al: Clinical pharmacology of propafenone. Circulation 68:589, 1983.

43. Lee JT, Yee YG, Dorian P, et al: Influence of hepatic dysfunction on the pharmacokinetics of propafenone. J Clin Pharmacol 27:384, 1987.

44. Rotmensch HH, Selhassen B, Swanson BN, et al: Steady-state serum amiodarone concentrations: Relationships with antiarrhythmic efficacy and toxicity. Ann Intern Med 101:462, 1984.

45. Enia G, Costante G, Catalano VC, et al: Severe hypothyroidism induced by amiodarone in a dialysis patient. Nephron 46:206, 1987.

46. Zech P, Sassard J, McAnish J, et al: Pharmacokinetics of atenolol in patients with renal impairment. Eur J Clin Pharmacol 12:175, 1977.

47. Herrera J, Vuckovich RA, Griffith DL, et al: Elimination of nadolol by patients with renal impairment. Br J Clin Pharmacol 7:S227, 1979.

48. Ameniya M, Tabei K, Furuya H, et al: Pharmacokinetics of carteolol in patients with impaired renal function. Eur J Clin Pharmacol 43:417, 1992.

49. Hasenfuss G, Schafer-Korting M, Knauf H, et al: Pharmacokinetics of carteolol in relation to renal function. Eur J Clin Pharmacol 29:461, 1985.

50. Lowenthal DJ, Affrime MB: Cardiac glycosides and antiarrhythmic drugs. In Anderson RJ, Schrier RW (eds): Clinical Use of Drugs in Patients with Kidney and Liver Disease. Philadelphia: WB Saunders, 1981.

51. Branch RA, James J, Read AE: A study of factors influencing drug disposition in chronic liver disease using the model drug (+)− propranolol. Br J Clin Pharmacol 3:243, 1976.

52. Vincent J, Meredith PA, Reid JL, et al: Clinical pharmacokinetics of prazosin-1985. Clin Pharmacokinet 10:144, 1985.

53. Kiechel JR: Pharmacokinetics of guanfacine in patients with impaired renal function and in some elderly patients. Am J Cardiol 57:18E, 1986.
54. Packer M, Meller J, Medina N, et al: Dose requirements of hydralazine in patients with severe chronic congestive heart failure. Am J Cardiol 45:655, 1980.
55. Drummer OGH, Workman BS, Miach PJ, et al: The pharmacokinetics of captopril and captopril disulfide conjugates in uremic patients on maintenance dialysis: Comparison with patients with normal renal function. Eur J Clin Pharmacol 32:267, 1987.
56. Daskalopoulos G, Pinzani M, Murray N, et al: Effects of captopril on renal function in patients with cirrhosis and ascites. J Hepatol 4:330, 1987.
57. Ulm EH, Hichens M, Gomez JH, et al: Enalapril maleate and a lysine analogue (MK-521): Disposition in man. Br J Clin Pharmacol 14:357, 1982.
58. van Schaik BAM, Geyskes GG, Boer P: Lisinopril in hypertensive patients with and without renal failure. Eur J Clin Pharmacol 32:11, 1987.
59. Ball SG, Robertson JIS: Clinical pharmacology of ramipril. Am J Cardiol 59:23D, 1987.
60. Aurell M, Delin K, Herlitz H, et al: Pharmacokinetics and pharmacodynamics of ramipril in renal failure. Am J Cardiol 59:65D, 1987.
61. Meisel S, Shamiss A, Rosenthal T: Clinical pharmacokinetics of ramipril. Clin Pharmacokinet 26:7, 1994.
62. Hui KK, Duchin KL, Kripalani KJ, et al: Pharmacokinetics of fosinopril in patients with various degrees of renal function. Clin Pharmacol Ther 49:457, 1991.
63. Wolter K, Fritschka E: Pharmacokinetics and pharmacodynamics of quinaprilat after low dose quinapril in patients with terminal renal failure. Eur J Clin Pharmacol 44(Suppl 1):S53, 1993.
64. Kleimbloesem CH, van Brummolen P, van Harten J, et al: Nifedipine: Influence of renal function on pharmacokinetics/hemodynamic relationships. Clin Pharmacol Ther 37:563, 1985.
65. Somogyi A, Albrecht M, Kleims G, et al: Pharmacokinetics, bioavailability and ECG response of verapamil in patients with liver cirrhosis. Br J Clin Pharmacol 12:51, 1981.
66. Ene MD, Roberts CHC: Pharmacokinetics of nifedipine after oral administration in chronic liver disease. J Clin Pharmacol 27:1001, 1987.
67. Hadengue A, Lee S, Moreau R, et al: Beneficial hemodynamic effects of ketanserin in patients with cirrhosis: Possible role of serotonergic mechanisms in portal hypertension. Hepatology 7:644, 1987.
68. Spilkin EX, Weller JM: Effect of frusemide in patients undergoing chronic intermittent peritoneal dialysis. Postgrad Med J 47(Suppl):36, 1971.
69. Whelton A: Long-term bumetanide treatment of renal edema: Comparison with furosemide. J Clin Pharmacol 21:591, 1981.
70. Spakn H, Knauf H, Mutschler E: Pharmacokinetics of torsemide and its metabolites in healthy controls and in chronic renal failure. Eur J Clin Pharmacol 39:345, 1990.
71. Villeneuve JP, Berbeeck RK, Wilkinson GR, et al: Furosemide kinetics and dynamics in patients with cirrhosis. Clin Pharmacol Ther 40:14, 1986.
72. Breither A, Goldman G, Edelen JS, et al: Erratic and incomplete absorption of furosemide in congestive heart failure [abstract]. Am J Cardiol 37:139, 1976.
73. Vasko MR, Brown-Cartwright D, Knochel JP, et al: Furosemide absorption altered in decompensated congestive heart failure. Ann Intern Med 102:314, 1985.
74. Schwartz S, Brater DC, Pound D, et al: Bioavailability, pharmacokinetics and pharmacodynamics of torsemide in patients with cirrhosis. Clin Pharmacol Ther 54:90, 1993.
75. Gaspari F, Vigano GL, Orisio S, et al: Aspirin prolongs bleeding time in uremia by a mechanism distinct from platelet cyclooxygenase inhibition. J Clin Invest 79:1788, 1987.
76. Anttila M, Haataja M, Kasanen A: Pharmacokinetics of naproxen in subjects with normal and impaired renal function. Eur J Clin Pharmacol 18:263, 1980.
77. Calvo MV, Domingues-Gil A, Marcias JG, et al: Naproxen disposition in hepatobiliary disorders. Int J Clin Pharmacol Ther Toxicol 18:242, 1980.
78. Williams RL, Upton RA, Cello JP, et al: Naproxen disposition in patients with alcoholic cirrhosis. Eur J Clin Pharmacol 27:291, 1984.
79. Lewis JH: Hepatic toxicity of nonsteroidal anti-inflammatory drugs. Clin Pharmacol 3:128, 1984.
80. Halstenson CE, Triscari J, DeVault A, et al: Single-dose pharmacokinetics of pravastatin and metabolites in patients with renal impairment. J Clin Pharmacol 32:124, 1992.

CHAPTER 23

Cardiovascular Drug Therapy Interacting with Exercise

Zebulon V. Kendrick, Ph.D., and David T. Lowenthal, M.D., Ph.D.

Exercise testing may be recommended for a variety of reasons, including identification of myocardial ischemia, determination of functional capacity, gathering prognostic information about patients with known coronary disease, and evaluation of therapeutic interventions such as drug therapy and revascularization surgery. Prescriptive exercise programs aid in improving functional work capacity, reducing stress, bettering the patient's general sense of well-being, lowering blood pressure, and modifying other coronary risk factors such as hyperlipidemia, glucose intolerance, and obesity. Exercise testing is recommended for the optimal planning of a rehabilitation program that maximizes a patient's residual cardiovascular potential.

For both diagnostic and prescriptive purposes, the interpretation of the graded exercise test depends on the patient's heart rate, electrocardiographic patterns, and blood pressure responses to incremental exercise stress. The interpretation of the stress test should be integrated with the patient's drug regimen. During acute exercise testing or chronic rehabilitation programs, the influence of cardiovascular drugs should be assessed carefully in terms of their effects on the determinants of myocardial oxygen demand (i.e., heart rate, myocardial wall tension, ventricular ejection time, and the contractile state of the myocardium). With the marked increase in antihypertensive and cardiac medications, these assessments become more important.

In general, the cardiovascular drugs prescribed by physicians for patients with cardiovascular disease, with the exception of β-adrenoreceptor blocking agents, permit normal exercise response. The normal response to exercise is no change or a decrease in diastolic blood pressure and an increase in systolic blood pressure, heart rate, stroke index, cardiac index, and ejection fraction. Following a rehabilitation or conditioning program, the various responses result in appropriate increases during physical activity but at an attenuated level. Furthermore, exercise intensity and duration of work performed with training can be improved significantly in patients undergoing β-blockade therapy.

Many studies have reported the effects of various drugs on subjects during acute and chronic bouts of exercise. However, a lack of uniformity in the exercise protocols used, differences in the dosage of drugs administered either acutely or chronically, and variations in the duration of chronic dosing complicate the applicability of the data. Other than heart rate and blood pressure determinations, the cardiovascular variables studied are inconsistent. Also, many studies may have limited statistical conclusions because of their small numbers of subjects. The literature also contained a few exercise studies of short duration. Because of the lack of uniformity between studies and the statistical limitations of the small number of subjects, firm conclusions could not be drawn about some of the drug-exercise interactions discussed here.

In this chapter, the pathophysiologic aspects of coronary artery disease, hypertension, and heart failure are discussed. The clinical pharmacology of nitrates, calcium antagonists, antihypertensive agents, digitalis, and antiarrhythmic agents is discussed. Each classification of drugs is related to the acute and chronic physiologic responses that occur in patients during both exercise testing and chronic exercise training programs.

CLINICAL PHARMACOLOGY OF ANTIANGINAL AGENTS

The basic principle underlying the pharmacologic treatment of angina pectoris is preservation of the balance between the oxygen supply and the demand of the heart. Antianginal drugs may improve myocardial performance, decrease the factors that increase demand, or both. These drugs reduce the afterload of the heart, lower myocardial oxygen consumption, and allow the patient to complete more work prior to the onset of angina pectoris. Vasodilators have no effect on heart rate but tend to lower blood pressure, systemic vascular resistance, and pulmonary wedge pressure. The following sections address the clinical pharmacologic considerations of the three major classes of drugs used in the management of ischemic heart disease: nitrates, β-adrenergic blocking drugs, and calcium antagonists (Tables 23–1 and 23–2).

Nitrates

The major therapeutic action of sublingual nitroglycerin (i.e., reduction of the oxygen requirement of the

heart) is achieved through alterations in peripheral circulation. Nitroglycerin reduces venous tone, thereby causing pooling of blood in the peripheral veins. Mild reductions in systemic arterial pressure and a reduction in end-diastolic and end-systolic dimensions of the intact heart occur with nitroglycerin therapy. The end-diastolic volume determines, in part, the development of myocardial wall tension and, in turn, oxygen consumption. A decrease in the tone of peripheral veins results in reduction of end-diastolic volume (preload), which decreases myocardial oxygen demand. The critical effects of nitroglycerin on the peripheral venous and arterial systems are to relieve the symptoms of angina pectoris by reducing the oxygen needs of the heart. Because stroke volume and hence cardiac output are reduced after nitroglycerin administration, it appears that venous pooling predominates over a decrease in arteriolar resistance.

The effect of nitroglycerin in lowering the triple product (systolic pressure × heart rate × ejection period) at any given level of exercise implies that it improves exercise performance by lowering myocardial oxygen consumption.[2] Therefore, the administration of nitrates increases delivery of oxygen to the ischemic myocardium.[3–5] Effort-induced angina pectoris occurs at the same triple product both before and after nitrate administration. Thus, lowering of the triple product after nitrate administration allows a patient to exercise at an increased workload before experiencing angina pectoris.

It is unclear whether nitrates exert clinically significant antianginal effects on the coronary circulation. Nitroglycerin dilates the large epicardial coronary arteries, but the clinical significance of coronary dilation on ischemic myocardium is not yet fully understood. Nitroglycerin may improve the perfusion of ischemic myocardial areas by augmenting blood supply available to collateral arterial anastomoses around the arterial obstruction. By reducing intraventricular pressures, particularly during diastole, nitrates tend to decompress subendocardial collateral vessels and potentially ischemic capillary beds.

The arteriolar vasodilating effect of acute nitrate administration during exercise can lead to a sudden decrease in peripheral vascular resistance. In a patient who is exercising and experiencing angina, administration of sublingual nitroglycerin may result in baroreceptor-mediated reflex tachycardia resulting from systemic vasodilation.

The combined effects of the increased energy demands of exercise, reflex tachycardia, and drug-induced hypotension resulting in decreased coronary blood flow could (paradoxically) result in a more severe episode of angina. Thus, a patient experiencing angina during exercise should be seated when sublingual nitroglycerin is administered.

Preferential dilation of the epicardial coronary arteries by nitrates may result in decreased perfusion of the subendocardial area. However, it has been demonstrated that, in an acutely ischemic left ventricle, nitroglycerin can increase blood supply to the subendocardial region.[6] The hypothesis that the antianginal

Table 23–1. **Primary Clinical Physiologic and Pharmacologic Rationale for the Three Classes of Drugs Used to Treat Angina Pectoris**

| | Increased Myocardial Blood Flow (Supply) | | Decreased Myocardial Oxygen Consumption (Demand) | | |
	Nitroglycerin	Calcium Antagonists	β-Blockers	Nitroglycerin	Calcium Antagonists
Dynamic coronary obstruction (spasm)	+	+	−	−	−
Fixed obstruction (atherosclerotic occlusion)	−	−	+	+	+
Combination of spasm and obstruction	+	+	+	+	+

+, active; −, not active.
From Giles TD, Lowenthal DT: Diagnosis and Management of the Patient with Angina. New York: BMI–McGraw-Hill, 1986.

effects of nitroglycerin are primarily the result of its vasodilating action on the peripheral circulation is derived from the observation that intravenously administered nitroglycerin relieves the angina syndrome despite decreased coronary blood flow.

Nitroglycerin administration reduces the elevation of left ventricular end-diastolic pressure associated with exercise-induced angina.[7] It has been demonstrated[8] that one sublingual nitroglycerin tablet may improve the patient's functional capacity by 1 metabolic equivalent during treadmill exercise. In some patients with mild to moderate angina pectoris, the administration of a long-acting nitrate reduces or eliminates the symptomatic and electrocardiographic abnormalities of myocardial ischemia during exercise stress testing.[8]

Patients with angina pectoris should *avoid sustained isometric exercise* because this type of exercise may induce left ventricular dysfunction that is reversed when the exercise is terminated.[5] During isometric exercise, left ventricular filling pressure is elevated in patients with atherosclerotic heart disease. Nitroglycerin has been shown to improve left ventricular function during isometric exercise in patients with coro-

nary artery disease by reducing left ventricular preload and afterload.[9]

β-Adrenoreceptor Blockers

The hemodynamic respiratory and metabolic changes during exercise have been intensively studied in association with β-adrenoreceptor blocking drugs.[10, 11] Response mechanisms, as they relate to isometric and dynamic activity, lead to a reduction in cardiac output with few or no peripheral vascular effects. These alterations are based on reductions in myocardial contractility and heart rate; both bring about a longer diastolic phase that allows for better coronary perfusion.[10] β-Blockade benefits patients with coronary artery disease undergoing cardiac rehabilitation: dynamic exercise performance increases by 31%[12] and patients experience fewer episodes of angina and fewer incidents of ST-segment depression.[13]

Because cardiac output is reduced to a greater extent than is blood pressure, peripheral resistance must increase with β-blockade.[14–16] This necessity, together with the fact that α-receptors are not blocked, can give rise to vasoconstriction as a result of catechola-

Table 23–2. **Pharmacologic Management of Angina Pectoris**

| Concomitant Disease or Side Effect | Nitrate | β-Adrenoceptor Blockers | Calcium Antagonists | | |
			Diltiazem	Verapamil	Nifedipine
Effort angina	+	+	+	+	+
Unstable angina—no concomitant disease	+	−	+	+	+
Rest angina	+	−	+	+	+
Asthma/COPD with bronchospasm	+	−	+	+	+
AV block	+	−	−	−	+
Symptomatic bradycardia	+	−	−	−	+
CHF	+	−	−	−	+
Depression	+	−	+	+	+
Headache	−	+	+	+	+
Hypotension	−	+	+	+	−
Insulin-dependent diabetes	+	−	+	+	+
Peripheral edema (not due to CHF)	±	+	+	+	+
Peripheral vascular disease	+	−	+	+	+
Tachycardia	−	+	+	+	−

AV, atrioventricular; CHF, congestive heart failure; COPD, chronic obstructive pulmonary disease; +, indicated; −, not indicated or should be used with caution; ±, may be used (potential side effects not extremely serious).
Modified from Giles TD, Lowenthal DT: Diagnosis and Management of the Patient with Angina. New York: BMI–McGraw-Hill, 1986.

mine release during exercise.[14] However, the effects of increased vascular resistance are thought to be obtunded by chronic β-blockade, which leads to lower blood pressure.[17, 18]

Savin et al.[19] reported that long-term β-adreno-receptor blockade during training improved exercise durations, but this improvement was smaller than that of subjects receiving placebo. It has been shown that, although the normal cardiovascular response is obtunded, a training effect can be observed in patients with ischemic heart disease who receive β-adreno-receptor blockers. This finding suggests that the duration of activity and the workload will increase. Studies by Hare et al.[20] confirmed these data and extended them into a consideration of whether elderly patients are capable of achieving a similar training effect with and without β-adrenoreceptor blocking drugs. The data show that, regardless of age (i.e., older or younger than 54 years) and β-adrenoreceptor blocker regimen, a training response is possible.

The selective β-blocker atenolol has been demonstrated to produce a better effect on the exercise response (i.e., respiratory gas exchange and less fatigue) than the nonselective β-blocker propranolol. This is as a result of less peripheral β$_2$-receptor inhibition resulting in less α-receptor–mediated vasoconstriction. The literature is replete with studies on the pharmacokinetics and pharmacodynamics of β-blockers during acute exercise that show either no change as a result of exercise or some slight modification in kinetics. We completed a 4-month exercise study of the pharmacokinetics of orally administered propranolol (80 mg) in healthy elderly subjects. No exercise training effect on the pharmacokinetics of propranolol was observed. There is also little reason to anticipate alterations in the pharmacokinetics of β-blockers as a result of exercise training in patients with coronary artery disease and/or hypertension (Table 23–3).[29, 30]

Calcium Antagonists

The administration of calcium antagonists has been reported to reduce both systolic and diastolic blood pressures during exercise in hypertensive patients,[31, 32] probably by reducing systemic vascular resistance,[31-33] although cardiac and peripheral mechanisms may explain the fall in blood pressure during exercise.[34] In normotensive, active volunteers, both nifedipine and verapamil had little effect on systolic and diastolic blood pressures during rest and during treadmill exercise. Verapamil has been reported to have a slight obtunding effect on diastolic blood pressure increases during isometric exercise.[35] Chronic treatment with newer drugs (i.e., isradipine and amlodipine) has been shown to lower blood pressure at rest and during exercise because of a reduction in systemic vascular resistance, similar to the mechanisms of all calcium antagonists.[36, 37]

In patients with chronic angina, studies have shown consistent improvement in those taking verapamil,[38, 39] nifedipine,[40] and diltiazem.[41] The reductions in exercise-induced angina and ST-segment depression seen in these patients are thought to result from a reduction in myocardial oxygen demand associated with a decrease in afterload with the calcium antagonists.[40] The enhancement of left ventricular diastolic filling observed with verapamil may also improve the angina syndrome. Diltiazem has been shown to increase exercise duration by its pharmacologic effect of decreasing the rate/pressure product during exercise.[41] The increase in coronary blood flow associated with calcium antagonists may account for some of the observed improvement in exercise tolerance.

A randomized, crossover, double-blind study using an exercise stimulus of bicycle ergometry and ambulatory 24-hour electrocardiographic monitoring for up to 8 weeks indicated that nifedipine or diltiazem, when added to β-blockers and nitrates, improved ambulatory and exercise tolerance in patients with severe yet stable angina due to multivessel coronary disease. Benefits included further prolongation of exercise duration, time to 1-mm ST-segment depression and to onset of angina, and reduction in the sum of ST-segment depressions at maximal identical load in ergometry.[42]

Table 23–3. **Effects of Exercise on Pharmacokinetics of β-Blockers**

β-Blocker	Age	Type of Exercise	Route	Effect on Plasma Concentration	Effect AUC, T½ Plasma Clearance	Reference No.
Bisoprolol	Young	Acute	PO	—	—	21
Propranolol	Young	Acute	IV	Variable	Variable	22
Penbutolol	Young	Acute	PO	—	—	23
Oxprenolol	Young	Acute	PO	—	—	24
Propranolol	Young	Acute	PO & IV	—	Vd PO	25
Pindolol	Young	Acute	PO & IV	Less inhibition of HR 50 at lower plasma concentrations	—	26
Propranolol	Young	Acute exercise of 7.5 hours	PO & IV	—	T½β with PO and with IV	27
Propranolol (present)	Old	Training	PO	—	—	28

IV, intravenous; PO, per os; AUC, area under curve; T½, elimination half-life; T½β, terminal elimination half-life; HR 50, 50% heart rate reduction; Vd PO, volume of distribution calculated from oral dosing.

No significant variance from the exercise-induced increase in serum potassium could be observed for either isometric or dynamic activity with either verapamil or nifedipine.[35] Among cardiac patients, calcium antagonist therapy during training programs seems to pose less risk of a harmful increase in blood pressure or serum potassium than does placebo.

The calcium antagonists are of particular value in patients with labile insulin-dependent diabetes in whom β-adrenoreceptor blocking therapy is relatively contraindicated or in patients with bronchospastic pulmonary disease. These drugs may also be an alternative therapy in patients who experience fatigue from β-blocking drugs.

HYPERTENSION
Hemodynamics of Hypertension During Exercise

Lund-Johansen[43] examined the hemodynamic response to bicycle ergometric exercise in both normotensive and mildly hypertensive men who trained in aerobic exercise programs. Heart rate was greater in the hypertensive group, probably because of a more pronounced adrenergic (sympathetic) response. Concurrently, small increases in stroke volume and cardiac index occurred in hypertensive subjects. Stroke volume tended to decrease progressively with age; this tendency was linked directly to a diminished increase in cardiac index in response to exercise. Total peripheral resistance was higher at all ages and at all exercise levels in hypertensive individuals, leading to greater blood pressure responses in both the systolic and diastolic components. Left ventricular stroke work was increased in both normotensive and hypertensive groups, but in the hypertensive group, it was higher after light to moderate exercise. This finding is attributed to the increased heart rate and blood pressure. However, the lack of change in stroke work at high intensities of exercise was probably due to the lower stroke volume in the hypertensive patients. Finally, the arteriovenous oxygen differential was significantly higher in patients with hypertension. This differential was also seen to increase with advancing age. The improving arteriovenous oxygen difference provides a compensatory mechanism that allows hypertensive individuals to meet the oxygen demands of the working tissue.

In other studies,[44] exercise has been shown to increase muscle blood flow in both normotensive and hypertensive patients, indicating that blood vessels in muscle share increased resistance, although probably to a lesser extent than the total circulation does. In normal subjects in the upright position, muscle blood flow measured after ischemic exercise decreases; this change is even more pronounced in hypertensive subjects.[44]

Diuretics

The hemodynamics of the diuretic effect have been studied by Lund-Johansen,[45] who found that not all diuretics have similar actions during exercise. Diuretics have several adverse biochemical and metabolic effects—such as hypokalemia, hyperglycemia, hyperuricemia, and hyperlipidemia—that must be considered prior to the initiation of exercise. These problems are less apparent with the much lower doses now being given to patients (i.e., 12.5 to 25 mg). In patients with ischemic heart disease, diuretic-induced hypokalemia and/or hypomagnesemia may result in ventricular ectopy, skeletal muscle fatigue, and possible necrosis resulting in rhabdomyolysis.

Thiazides bring about a decrease in peripheral resistance and plasma volume. Appreciable augmentation of potassium excretion, which can lead to hypokalemia, accompanies the thiazide inhibition of sodium reabsorption. Significant hypokalemia results in moderate ST-segment depression, which may mimic the changes observed with myocardial ischemia, cardiac irritability, and skeletal muscle fatigue. In one study,[46] 100 mg/day of hydrochlorothiazide resulted in an increased incidence of premature ventricular contractions that was correlated to the diuretic-induced decrease in serum potassium and magnesium. Such high doses are rarely used now for treating hypertension.

Excessive diuresis with thiazides and other diuretic drugs may accentuate exercise-induced tachycardia and postexercise hypotension. Because cardiac output is maintained during regulated diuretic therapy, the tachycardia may not occur unless the patient is hypovolemic from excessive diuretic therapy. Potassium excretion may become more pronounced when these patients prescribe for themselves low-carbohydrate, ketogenic, low-calorie diets, which increase sodium excretion. Therefore, complications in exercise responses may occur in patients undergoing diuretic therapy who are also participating in low-calorie weight-reduction programs.

During vigorous exercise, serum potassium levels increase. The increase can also occur in the setting of diuretic-induced hypokalemia, indicating that total body potassium is not depleted.[47] To ensure against potassium loss, patients taking diuretics should receive potassium supplements or potassium-sparing diuretics. With proper management, diuretic therapy results in a moderate decrease in the blood pressure response to exercise and, with adequate potassium supplementation, should not cause any drug-related risks during physical activity.

Central α-Agonists

The central α-agonist antihypertensives clonidine, α-methyldopa (methyldopa), guanabenz, and guanfacine decrease central and peripheral outflow of catecholamines and cause reductions of plasma norepinephrine in patients at rest and during exercise.[11, 48] Although these drugs can blunt the sympathetic response during exercise, they have significantly different hemodynamic effects.

In mildly hypertensive patients, methyldopa may decrease blood pressure and heart rate response during cycle ergometry.[49] Total peripheral resistance and cardiac output may[50] or may not[51] decrease. No decrease in heart rate at rest or peak exercise occurred in normal subjects taking methyldopa in multiple doses for 1 week.[52] The systolic blood pressure of these subjects was reduced at rest and during peak exercise after 1 week of treatment.[52] Clonidine has been shown to differ from methyldopa in that, in addition to reducing blood pressure and heart rate during exercise, it decreases both resting blood pressure and resting heart rate.[51, 53, 54] The decrease in heart rate through central vagal stimulation results in decreased cardiac output.[53] With chronic use of clonidine, cardiac output returns to normal.[53] Guanabenz and guanfacine are associated with similar hemodynamic changes but only minimal decreases in heart rate.[55]

To aid in patient compliance, transdermal clonidine patches can be worn on a weekly basis and allow for a smoother reduction in blood pressure and a modulation of the effects of sedation and dry mouth, which are related to the peaks of dosing with orally administered clonidine. This improvement in formulation may be better accepted by adolescents and young adult athletes with whom the daily consumption of pills may be met with noncompliance. The adherence of the patch to the skin is minimally affected by sweating and, if needed, can be reinforced with tape.

In several studies,[48, 52, 56] exercise-associated changes in serum potassium, renin, and aldosterone have been observed in normal volunteers after single and multiple doses of clonidine and methyldopa. Serum potassium and plasma aldosterone levels rose in response to dynamic exercise in both medicated and placebo conditions. Plasma renin has been reported to be suppressed in patients at rest, and the expected exercise-induced increase in plasma renin was blunted at maximal dosages of clonidine and methyldopa. No significant ST-segment changes have been shown in exercising patients using these drugs. The rise in diastolic blood pressure induced by 50% handgrip isometric activity may be decreased with methyldopa or clonidine, especially if the resting diastolic blood pressure is reduced.[55, 56] The mean change is not different from rest to peak handgrip during placebo administration and with multiple doses of these drugs. Other investigators have found a lack of blood pressure control with medication during isometric activity.[57]

β-Adrenoreceptor Blockers

Cardioselective and nonselective β-adrenergic blocking drugs decrease myocardial oxygen requirements in patients at rest and during exercise. β-Blockade therapy allows patients to perform exercise of increased intensity and duration before onset of angina. Subjects undergoing β-adrenoreceptor blocker therapy can participate in exercise programs and, despite their blunted heart rate and blood pressure response while exercising, significantly improve their exercise capacity.[29, 58-61]

Propranolol, a nonselective β-adrenoreceptor blocker, and the cardioselective β-adrenoreceptor blockers atenolol and metoprolol have been compared with placebo in normal volunteers during isotonic and isometric exercise.[48, 52, 62-64] In a study comparing propranolol, metoprolol, and placebo in a graded treadmill exercise,[70] it was shown that both heart rate and systolic blood pressure are reduced at maximum exercise. Several studies[65-70] have demonstrated a reduction in oxygen consumption or work capacity after acute and chronic administration of β-adrenoreceptor blockers. No significant changes were noted in diastolic blood pressure, oxygen consumption, or anaerobic threshold (the point at which oxygen consumption fails to increase in proportion to minute ventilation). According to Sklar et al.,[62] these results indicate that blood flow to the active muscles is unaltered.

Some small pharmacodynamic differences may exist between cardioselective and nonselective β-adrenoreceptor blocking drugs. After 9 months of administration of atenolol, metoprolol, pindolol, and sustained-release propranolol, researchers found that atenolol and metoprolol reduced exercise-induced increases in systolic blood pressure significantly, but pindolol and propranolol did not. Therefore, cardioselective β-adrenoreceptor blockers appear to be more effective than nonselective agents in blunting the increase in systolic blood pressure during dynamic physical activity. There is marked interindividual variability of β-adrenoreceptor blocking effects on heart rate and blood pressure during exercise and on oxygen consumption.[63, 64, 66, 71] Although normal volunteers given parenteral metoprolol or placebo in intraindividual crossover design using bicycle ergometry showed comparable plasm levels of metoprolol after each intravenous dose, the inhibition of exercise-induced tachycardia or increase in systolic blood pressure varied considerably among the subjects. No correlation has been found between heart rate inhibition and systolic blood pressure increase during exercise with β-adrenoreceptor blockade. The extent of a β-adrenoreceptor blocking effect on these parameters is an individual constant in both acute and chronic conditions. Trained subjects administered propranolol for 1 week had greater impairment of aerobic capacity than did the untrained subjects.[65] Atenolol administration produced no impairment of aerobic capacity in trained subjects. However, in other studies,[63, 64] atenolol administration resulted in a reduction in maximal oxygen consumption.

Studies by Lowenthal et al.[56] indicated that both resting and peak isometric exercise diastolic blood pressures of normal volunteers were reduced with high doses of atenolol and propranolol when compared with placebo. These reductions were due to a decrease in diastolic blood pressure at rest and the ensuing lower pressor response to the handgrip isometric exercise. Similar results have been observed in research with hypertensive patients taking β-blocking drugs.[68] When compared with placebo controls, both metoprolol and propranolol reduced heart rate and systolic blood pressure at rest and at peak exercise in normal patients. However, it was shown that in patients with borderline hypertensive heart failure defined by radiologic criteria (i.e., cardiac enlargement, M-mode echocardiography, and electrocardiographic findings), metoprolol, with and without prazosin vasodilatory treatment, does not safely abolish dangerous increases in blood pressure during isometric activity.[17, 57, 69, 72]

Studies on the metabolic effects of β-adrenoreceptor blockade during exercise have produced a number of provocative results. Propranolol in single and multiple doses has been reported to cause an increase in serum potassium significantly greater than that caused by placebo during dynamic exercise. This hyperkalemic effect may occur only on initial treatment during acute exercise and may be much more common with nonselective antagonists.[48] β-Adrenoreceptor blockade (propranolol, 40 mg twice a day for 1 week) also results in significantly decreased levels of renin in patients at rest and at peak exercise; when compared with placebo, this regimen has led to no changes in plasma aldosterone values. Unlike central α-agonists, propranolol and metoprolol either increase plasma norepinephrine[73] or give rise to expected normal increases in plasma values[48, 74] during physical activity. The latter observation has been attributed to the hypothesis that, during light exercise, vagal withdrawal occurs, but sympathetic activity does not increase until the heart rate rises by more than 30 beats/min.[75]

To determine the origin of exercise fatigue induced by β-adrenoreceptor antagonists in normal active individuals, Lundborg et al.[74] examined specific metabolic effects of β-blockade. After the disruption of neuromuscular transmission and decreased blood flow to working muscle were ruled out as causes of fatigue, the investigators concluded that the exercise fatigue was the result of altered substrate availability and utilization. Blood glucose, nonesterified fatty acid, and glycerol levels were found to be significantly reduced during cycling activity in patients given either propranolol or metoprolol. The reduction was followed by more rapid rises in glucagon levels in patients receiving the drugs and probably resulted from decreased muscle glycogenolysis.

It has been suggested[11, 64] that inhibition of the exercise-induced stimulation of glucose metabolism and lipolysis by β-blockers impairs exercise performance. Propranolol has been demonstrated to reduce blood glucose availability in normotensive volunteers, but atenolol has no effect on blood glucose.[69] Glycogenolysis and lipolysis depend in part on β-adrenoreceptor stimulation during exercise. The β-adrenoreceptor blocker reduction in carbohydrate and lipid substrate availability and utilization during exercise impairs normal metabolic function of the working muscle and results in an earlier perception of fatigue during the exercise task. In several studies involving β-blockade during exercise, neither propranolol nor metoprolol decreased the ventilatory response to carbon dioxide[11, 75] or the respiratory exchange ratio[4, 76] during physical activity.

In another study,[71] maximal oxygen consumption was reduced during both submaximal and maximal bicycle ergometry in normal volunteers after 80 mg of propranolol was administered in a single oral dose. Similar results have been obtained at submaximal workloads of 50% and 70%, at which ventilation, carbon dioxide, and oxygen consumption were measured. Propranolol effected an early reduction in all of these variables at 50% and 70% of maximal oxygen consumption minutes. Ventilation was greater at 5 minutes because of an increase of venous lactate. The initial reductions in oxygen consumption and carbon dioxide production were related to the reduction in cardiac output and muscle perfusion induced by propranolol.

Plasma levels of both propranolol and acebutolol increase significantly during exercise. The increased plasma concentration of these drugs may be related to pH changes during physical activity[77] or may be attributable to the exercise-induced decrease in hepatic blood flow that would affect drugs with high hepatic-extraction ratios. To date, only one study[28] has examined the effects of exercise training on the pharmacokinetics of β-blockers. All other studies have examined acute exercise and its effect on simple dose kinetics of β-blockers (see Table 23–3).

Thermoregulation During β-Adrenoreceptor Blockade

Many patients taking β-adrenoreceptor blockers may participate in regular exercise programs or have work requirements that expose them to both hot and cold environments. The β-adrenoreceptor blockers may impair thermoregulatory responses during exercise or exposure to hot and cold environments.[78-82]

During exercise, the rise in blood temperature has been shown to be accentuated by β-adrenoreceptor blockade.[79] It has been suggested that the rise in blood temperature results from a reduction in skin blood flow. The influence of β-adrenoreceptor blockade on skin blood flow during exercise may be due to an enhanced α-adrenoreceptor–induced vasoconstriction in nonactive tissue because of catecholamine-modulated peripheral vasodilation, which is mediated by the β-adrenoreceptor.[83] To dissipate heat during exercise, particularly when cutaneous blood flow is diminished, sweating must be stimulated. In normotensive volunteers receiving propranolol, sweat rate transiently increased during exercise under ambient conditions of 33°C,[84] whereas in an ambient environment of 22°C, the sweat rate was depressed and core temperature was increased.[78] Gordon et al.[80] concluded that acute administration of propranolol in coronary artery disease may accentuate the risk of hyperthermia during prolonged exercise. Sweat rate during exercise at room temperature has been shown to increase in hypertensive patients under blockade.[82]

The complaint of cool or cold and painful extremities among patients undergoing propranolol therapy lends further support to the idea of reduced skin blood flow during therapy. Propranolol may also influence the thermoregulatory response to cold exposure. Nonshivering thermogenesis is blocked by propranolol, as evidenced by rectal temperature reduction in rats.[81] Jessen[85] found that in undressed men exposed to 11°C ambient temperature, the 30% increase in oxygen consumption could be due in part to nonshivering thermogenesis. Because propranolol has been shown to inhibit nonshivering thermogenesis in rats, studies should be undertaken to determine whether propranolol adversely influences thermogenesis during cold exposure in humans.

Vasodilators

The vasodilators used in the treatment of hypertension include hydralazine, minoxidil, and peripheral α-blockers (i.e., prazosin, terazosin, and doxazosin) and calcium antagonists (discussed earlier), for which a number of exercise-related investigations have been performed. In normal volunteers, hydralazine decreased arterial pressure with resultant reflex tachycardia. This condition tends to increase cardiac output through an increase in sympathetic drive, which may lead to myocardial ischemia (e.g., an angina episode or infarction) in cardiac patients.[86] Hydralazine is also useful as an afterload reducer in patients with chronic heart failure.[87] Similarly, prazosin has been shown to decrease mean arterial pressure and total peripheral resistance in patients at rest and at dynamic workloads. Unlike hydralazine, single and multiple doses of prazosin produce neither a reflex increase in heart rate nor an exaggerated pressor response during arm-cycle ergometry.[88] During isometric activity, hydralazine neither adequately attenuates the isometric-induced increases in sympathetic activity[57, 89] nor improves skeletal muscle oxygen delivery during exercise in patients with heart failure.[90]

In normal volunteers, prazosin therapy results in reduction in both baseline and peak diastolic and systolic pressures during 50% handgrip isometric exercise at single and multiple doses.[56] During graded arm-cycle ergometric exercise, prazosin lowers systolic pressure at rest and at peak exercise and decreases diastolic pressure during dynamic exercise. The effect of prazosin on the heart rate response to dynamic exercise did not differ from that of the placebo. These data should not necessarily be extrapolated to patients with ischemic heart disease or heart failure who are participating in exercise.

In patients with chronic heart failure, hydralazine reduces arterial and pulmonary wedge pressures and increases stroke volume at rest and, to a lesser degree, during bicycle exercise.[87] The reduced effect during physical activity is thought to reflect initial impaired pump function and may explain the observation of unimproved exercise tolerance in these patients, despite improved hemodynamic parameters with orally administered hydralazine. In addition, hydralazine does not increase compromised blood flow to periph-

eral musculature during handgrip activity in patients with heart failure, indicating that its vasodilatory effect does not add to local metabolic effects.[90] Prazosin has been tested in patients with borderline hypertensive heart failure[91, 92] and has been shown to improve hemodynamics (cardiac output) and attenuate the increase in diastolic pressure associated with isometric activity. The benefit of terazosin and doxazosin over prazosin in active or inactive patients is the once-daily dosing and a lesser reflex sympathetic response.

Angiotensin-Converting Enzyme Inhibitors

The effects of captopril on dynamic exercise vary among investigators. Although Pickering et al.[93] found no changes in blood pressure or heart rate in subjects given captopril during graded treadmill activity, another study[94] indicates significant reduction in systolic and diastolic pressures during bicycle exercise that is more pronounced during physical activity than at rest.[95] Enalapril alone or with hydrochlorothiazide permits a lowering of blood pressure but an adequate cardiac response to dynamic exercise.[96] Saralasin, an angiotensin II partial antagonist, has been shown to decrease blood pressure during dynamic exercise.[97] The reduction in angiotensin II with captopril and saralasin, coupled with a varying response to blood pressure during exercise, indicates that angiotensin II is not a major determinant of blood pressure regulation during exercise in hypertensive patients. In point of fact, angiotensin-converting enzyme (ACE) inhibition does not suppress plasma angiotensin II increase during exercise in humans nor does it influence microalbuminuria with prolonged physical activity. This has significance in the management of the diabetic at rest or during exercise who has proteinuria as a manifestation of nephropathy, wherein the ACE inhibitor has been given to improve renal function.[98] Systemic vascular resistance is reduced by all (captopril, fosinopril, enalapril, quinapril, and lisinopril) ACE inhibitors.[92, 99, 100] Fosinopril has been reported to show less change in potassium at rest with increase during exercise in contrast to changes in potassium seen with other ACE inhibitors and with nonselective β-blockers. This may be due to a more lipid-soluble ACE inhibitor as a result of the phosphinic acid moiety unique to fosinopril.[101]

Manhem et al.[94] investigated the effects of captopril on catecholamines, renin activity, angiotensin II levels, and plasma aldosterone during dynamic exercise. After 4 or 5 days of high-dose captopril, both angiotensin II and plasma aldosterone levels were reduced significantly in patients at rest and during physical activity. These data conflict with the results reported recently by Aldigier et al.[98] Plasma renin activity increased over placebo at baseline and peak exercise, but the concentration of norepinephrine and epinephrine remained unchanged. Nonetheless, this class of drugs (i.e., enalapril and lisinopril) and newer-generation ACE inhibitors do not limit dynamic exercise in hypertensive patients and can blunt pressor effects during mental stress.[102]

HEART FAILURE

Patients with severe ventricular dysfunction particularly need intensive rehabilitative efforts. However, it is not unusual for these patients to be excluded from cardiac rehabilitation programs.[103] Formal cardiac rehabilitation exercise programs may produce favorable hemodynamic changes in subjects with abnormal ventricular function. An additional rationale for including such patients in physical conditioning programs has been provided by evidence from animal models and from preliminary human studies that suggest that exercise training may reduce vulnerability to ventricular fibrillation.[91] Training may enhance mechanical performance of the heart under ischemic conditions,[104] and participation in group rehabilitation programs in combination with exercise training may have psychologic benefits[105] for the patient. To interpret the therapeutic benefits of a rehabilitation program properly, frequent observation for exercise-induced arrhythmias is critical, as are determinations of antiarrhythmic drug concentrations.[106] In reviewing the previously mentioned studies, it appears that some other physiologic mechanism may account for the improvement seen in patients with ventricular dysfunction who exercise-train.

The role of exercise-induced biochemical and morphologic adaptations in skeletal muscle[107] is important in mediating cardiovascular adaptations to habitual exercise. Patients with ventricular dysfunction may be able to increase maximal oxygen consumption and residual work capacity as a result of rehabilitative exercise programs. The decreases in heart rate and mean arterial pressure associated with physical conditioning in normal subjects and coronary patients without ventricular dysfunction also occur in most patients with ventricular dysfunction.[108]

Heart failure affects both central and peripheral hemodynamic responses to exercise. Pharmacologic therapy is designed to rectify the increase in systemic vascular resistance, the decrease in skeletal muscle blood flow, an increase in oxygen uptake by skeletal muscle, and a reduction in resting heart rate and systemic blood pressure. The reductions in resting heart rate and systemic blood pressure are expectations of exercise training. The pharmacologic therapy of diuretics, digitalis, and ACE inhibitors is the mainstay for treating heart failure and can synergistically act with exercise programs to improve central and peripheral hemodynamics, decrease fatigue, and improve muscle strength. Some of the long-term effects of ACE inhibitor therapy for heart failure are similar to those of exercise training. Thus, it has been shown that ACE inhibitors can increase blood flow to the lower extremities, which may result in improved exercise capacity.

ACE inhibitors, like exercise training, have been shown to decrease sympathetic tone. Based on the exercise training–like effects of ACE inhibitors, it is reasonable that exercise training and ACE inhibitor therapy, possibly along with digoxin and/or diuretic therapy if required, may have a synergistic action over that seen with drug therapy alone.[109, 110] Furthermore, it has been demonstrated that ACE inhibitors, as a result of their primary effect on myocardium by decreasing the infarct size,[111–117] can improve survival in patients who have suffered myocardial infarction.

Digitalis

Digitalis improves work performance and may increase myocardial perfusion in patients with heart failure.[118] It may decrease the myocardial oxygen demand by lowering the left ventricular filling pressure and pulmonary capillary pressure.[119] In patients with congestive heart failure, digitalis reduces ventricular size and oxygen consumption at baseline[120] and decreases left ventricular end-diastolic pressure during exercise.[121] The decrease in myocardial oxygen demand associated with the decreases in left ventricular volume and pressure negates any concern that a digitalis-induced improvement in contractility would increase oxygen demand. In volunteers with normal coronary vessels, digitalis produces ST-segment depression during exercise.[13] Arrhythmias associated with the drug can be provoked by exercise, especially with concurrent diuretic-induced potassium and/or magnesium depletion. As a result, electrolyte values and ectopic activity of patents who take digitalis should be monitored carefully in a training program.

Digoxin plasma concentrations may vary from day to day in active persons. The most probable reason for these changes in the pharmacokinetics is a previously described increase in binding of digoxin to exercising muscles. There is reason to believe that the daily physical activity performed by digoxin-treated patients will determine to some extent the body content of digoxin. Thus, physical exercise causes a redistribution of digoxin, resulting in a fall in serum digoxin concentration with an increase in skeletal muscle digoxin concentration. The well-described quinidine-digoxin interaction could further affect the exercise-induced redistribution of digoxin by reducing skeletal muscle binding of digoxin during quinidine administration. This has been attributable to a saturation of digoxin binding sites secondary to an increase in the total body load of digoxin at steady state rather than a direct effect of quinidine on digoxin binding. Quinidine did not interfere with the effect of physical exercise in causing a redistribution of digoxin between serum and skeletal muscle.[122–124]

DRUGS USED IN THE TREATMENT OF ARRHYTHMIAS

Exercise-induced ventricular ectopy is seen in more than 25% of randomly selected patients and in almost 40% of patients with coronary disease. The prevalence of ventricular ectopy increases with age.

In patients with coronary artery disease, arrhythmias more often are ventricular in origin, are complex and sustained, occur at low heart rates, and occur during the recovery period than is the case in patients without cardiac disease. In addition, arrhythmias are seen in patients with left ventricular dysfunction, previous myocardial infarct, or multivessel disease. In this population, antiarrhythmic drug therapy is valuable for suppressing the symptoms associated with ectopy provoked by exercise.

Antiarrhythmics

Studies by Gey et al.[125, 126] showed that procainamide and quinidine produce changes in heart rate or oxygen uptake during dynamic exercise, but a slight drop in systolic blood pressure may be observed. Exercise-induced arrhythmias decreased and were less severe in most patients in the study. In another study, quinidine increased heart rate at rest and at low levels of exercise.[127] The researcher concluded that the vagolytic and the α-adrenoreceptor blocking effects of the drug, along with reflex increases in sympathetic activity, resulted in the increased heart rates. Therefore, minor cardioacceleratory effects should be anticipated during exercise testing in patients who are taking quinidine. Other investigators have pointed out that both procainamide and quinidine can mask exercise-induced ST-segment depression and produce false-negative test results.[128]

Plasma procainamide and its metabolite N-acetyl procainamide were quantified in healthy young volunteers during 4 hours of playing basketball. Although the rate of acetylation was not affected by the intense exercise, which corresponded to a submaximal workload, urinary excretions of procainamide and the N-acetylated metabolite were decreased as a result of physical activity. This is likely due to the renal clearance of procainamide being decreased commensurately with the reduction in glomerular filtration rate during physical activity. Plasma concentrations in rapid and slow acetylators of procainamide rose during exercise to a greater degree than did concentrations measured over a 4-hour period of bedrest, with the slow acetylators having a greater rise during the exercise phase than corresponding timepoints at bedrest. This effect was not correlated with electrocardiographic evidence of any added pharmacodynamic effect of procainamide in this study.[129]

Thus, in patients with demonstrable ectopy not corrected by overdrive suppression, these antiarrhythmic drugs may be used effectively during physical activity to reduce the risk of exercise-induced arrhythmias.[130] Similarly, tocainide and β-blockade are effective in suppressing ectopic activity.[131]

SUMMARY

An appreciation of the hemodynamic and biochemical changes induced by drugs during both acute and chronic exercise is important in understanding patient performance during exercise testing. Drug therapy and exercise are not mutually contraindicated in cardiovascular disease, provided that the ways in which drug therapy interacts with exercise are clearly understood.

REFERENCES

1. Giles TD, Lowenthal DT: Diagnosis and Management of the Patient with Angina. New York: Biomedical Information, 1986.
2. Georgopoulos AJ, Sones FM Jr, Page IH: Relationship between arterial pressure and exertional angina pectoris in hypertensive patients. Circulation 23:892, 1961.
3. Giles TD, Iteld BJ, Quiroz AC, et al: The prolonged effect of pentaerythritol tetranitrate on exercise capacity in stable effort angina pectoris. Chest 80:142, 1981.
4. Goldstein RE, Epstein SE: Medical management of patients with angina pectoris. Prog Cardiovasc Dis 14:360, 1972.
5. Moskowitz RM, Kinney EL, Zelis RF: Hemodynamic and metabolic responses to upright exercise in patients with congestive heart failure: Treatment with nitroglycerin ointment. Chest 76:640, 1979.
6. Harris PJ, Harrell FE Jr, Lee RL, et al: Survival in medically treated coronary artery diseases. Circulation 60:1259, 1979.
7. Roberts R: Second North American Conference on Nitroglycerin Therapy: Perspectives and mechanisms. Am J Med 76(6A):1, 1984.
8. Markis JE, Gorlin R, Mills RM, et al: Sustained effect of orally administered isosorbide dinitrate on exercise performance of patients with angina pectoris. Am J Cardiol 43:265, 1979.
9. Flessas AP, Ryan TJ: Effects of nitroglycerin on isometric exercise. Am Heart J 105:239, 1983.
10. Bruce RA, Hossack KF, Kusumi F, et al: Acute hemodynamic effect of propranolol during symptom-limited maximal exercise. Am J Cardiol 44:132, 1979.
11. Twentyman OP, Disley A, Gribbin HR, et al: Effect of beta adrenergic blockade on respiratory and metabolic responses to exercise. J Appl Physiol 51:788, 1981.
12. Pratt CM, Welton DE, Squires WG Jr, et al: Demonstration of training effect during chronic beta-adrenergic blockade in patients with coronary artery disease. Circulation 64:1125, 1981.
13. Ellestad MH: Ischemic S-T segment depression: Hemodynamic, electrophysiologic, and metabolic factors in its genesis. In Ellestad MH (ed): Stress Testing: Principles and Practice. Philadelphia: FA Davis, 1980, pp 77–96.
14. Epstein SE, Robinson BF, Kahler RL, et al: Effects of beta-adrenergic blockade on the cardiac response to maximal and submaximal exercise in man. J Clin Invest 44:1745, 1965.
15. Hamer J, Sowton E: Cardiac output after beta-adrenergic blockade in ischaemic heart disease. Br Heart J 27:892, 1965.
16. Shepherd JT: Circulatory adjustments to beta-adrenergic blockade at rest and during exercise. Am J Cardiol 55:87, 1985.
17. Hansson BG, Dymling JF, Manhem P, et al: Long-term treatment of moderate hypertension with the beta₁-receptor blocking agent metoprolol. II. Effect of submaximal work and insulin-induced hypoglycemia on plasma catecholamines and renin activity, blood pressure and pulse rate. Eur J Clin Pharmacol 11:247, 1977.
18. Talbott JH, Castleman B, Smithwick RH, et al: Renal biopsy studies correlated with renal clearance observations in hypertensive patients treated by radical sympathectomy. J Clin Invest 22:387, 1943.
19. Savin WM, Gordon EP, Kaplan SM, et al: Exercise training during long-term beta blockade treatment in healthy subjects. Am J Cardiol 55:101, 1985.
20. Hare TW, Lowenthal DT, Hakki HH, et al: The effect of exercise training in older patients in beta-adrenergic blocking drugs. Ann Sports Med 2:36, 1984.
21. LeCoz F, Sauleman P, Poirier JM, et al: Oral pharmacokinetics of bisoprolol in resting and exercising healthy volunteers. J Cardiovasc Pharmacol 18:28, 1991.
22. Frank S, Somani SM, Kohnle M: Effect of exercise on propranolol pharmacokinetics. Eur J Clin Pharmacol 39:391, 1990.
23. Brockmeier D, Hajdu P, Henke W, et al: Penbutolol: Pharmacokinetics, effect on exercise tachycardia and in vitro inhibition of radioligand binding. Eur J Clin Pharmacol 35:613, 1988.

24. Koopmans R, Oosterhuis B, Karemaker JM, et al: The effect of oxprenolol dosage time on its pharmacokinetics and hemodynamic effects during exercise in man. Eur J Clin Pharmacol 44:171, 1993.

25. Van Baak MA, Mooij JMV, Schiffers PM: Exercise and the pharmacokinetics of propranolol, verapamil and atenolol. Eur J Clin Pharmacol 43:547, 1992.

26. Jennings GL, Bobik A, Fagan ET, et al: Pindolol pharmacokinetics in relation to time course of inhibition of exercise tachycardia. Br J Clin Pharmacol 7:245, 1979.

27. Arends BG, Bohm RO, Van Kemenade JE, et al: Influence of physical exercise on the pharmacokinetics of propranolol. Eur J Clin Pharmacol 31:375, 1986.

28. Panton LB, Guillen GJ, Williams LS, et al. Effect of aerobic exercise training on propranolol pharmacokinetics in young and elderly adults [abstract]. Clin Pharmacol Ther 55:173, 1994.

29. Pollock ML, Lowenthal DT, Foster C, et al: Acute and chronic responses to exercise in patients treated with beta blockers. J Cardiopulm Rehabil 11:132, 1991.

30. Clearoux J, Leenen FH: Effects of beta blockade on muscle metabolism during prolonged exercise: A short review. Am J Hypertens 1:290S, 1988.

31. Anderson K, Vik-Mo H: Increased left ventricular emptying at maximal exercise after reduction in afterload. Circulation 69(3):492, 1984.

32. Yamakado T, Oonishi N, Kondo S, et al: Effects of diltiazem on cardiovascular responses during exercise in systemic hypertension and comparison with propranolol. Am J Cardiol 52:1023, 1983.

33. Brod J, Fencl V, Hejl Z, et al: General and regional hypertension pattern underlying essential hypertension. Clin Sci 23:399, 1962.

34. Silke B, Goldhammer E, Sharma SK, et al: An exercise hemodynamic comparison of verapamil, diltiazem, and amlodopine in coronary artery disease. Cardiovasc Drug Ther 4:457, 1990.

35. Stein DT, Lowenthal DT, Porter RS, et al: Effects of nifedipine and verapamil on isometric and dynamic exercise in normal subjects. Am J Cardiol 54:386, 1984.

36. Clearoux J, Yardley C, Marshall A, et al: Antihypertensive and hemodynamic effects of calcium channel blockers with isradipine after acute exercise. Am J Hypertens 5:84, 1992.

37. Tarazi RD, Dustan HP: Beta-adrenergic blockade in hypertension: Practical and theoretical implications of long-term hemodynamic variations. Am J Cardiol 29:633, 1972.

38. Subramanian VB, Bowles M, Lahini A, et al: Long-term antianginal action of verapamil assessed with quantitated serial treadmill stress testing. Am J Cardiol 48:529, 1981.

39. Bonow RO, Leon MB, Rosing DR, et al: Effects of verapamil and propranolol on left ventricular function and diastolic filling in patients with coronary artery disease: Radionuclide angiographic studies at rest and during exercise. Circulation 65:1337, 1982.

40. Moskowitz RM, Piccini PA, Nacarelli GV, et al: Nifedipine therapy for stable angina pectoris: Preliminary results of effects on angina frequency and treadmill exercise response. Am J Cardiol 44:811, 1979.

41. Pool PE, Seagren SC, Bonanno JA, et al: The treatment of exercise-inducible chronic stable angina with diltiazem: Effect on treadmill exercise. Chest 78:234, 1980.

42. Meluzin J, Zeman K, Stetka F, et al: Effects of nifedipine and diltiazem on myocardial ischemia in patients with severe stable angina pectoris treated with nitrates and beta blockers. J Cardiovasc Pharmacol 20:864, 1992.

43. Lund-Johansen P: Hemodynamics in early hypertension. Acta Med Scand 181(Suppl 482):1, 1967.

44. Amery A, Bossaert H, Verstraete M: Muscle blood flow in normal and hypertensive subjects: Influence on age, exercise and body position. Am Heart J 78:211, 1969.

45. Lund-Johansen P: Hemodynamic changes in long-term diuretic therapy of essential hypertension: A comparative study of chlorthalidone, polythiazide and hydrochlorothiazide. Acta Med Scand 187:509, 1970.

46. Hollifield JW: Potassium and magnesium abnormalities: Diuretics and arrhythmias in hypertension. Am J Med 77(5A):28, 1984.

47. Falkner B, Onesti G, Lowenthal DT, et al: Effectiveness of centrally acting drugs and diuretics in adolescent hypertension. Clin Pharmacol Ther 32:577, 1982.

48. Lowenthal DT, Affrime MB, Falkner B, et al: Potassium disposition and neuroendocrine effects of propranolol, methyldopa and clonidine during dynamic exercise. Clin Exp Hypertens [A] 4(9–10):1895, 1982.

49. Sannerstedt R, Varnanskes E, Werko L: Hemodynamic effects of methyldopa (Aldomet) at rest and during exercise in patients with arterial hypertension. Acta Med Scand 171:75, 1962.

50. Lund-Johansen P: Hemodynamic changes in long-term alpha methyldopa therapy of essential hypertension. Acta Med Scand 192:221, 1972.

51. Chamberlain DA, Howard J: Guanethidine and methyldopa: A haemodynamic study. Br Heart J 26:528, 1964.

52. Rosenthal L, Affrime MB, Lowenthal DT, et al: Biochemical and dynamic responses to single and repeated doses of methyldopa and propranolol during dynamic physical activity. Clin Pharmacol Ther 32:701, 1982.

53. Lund-Johansen P: Hemodynamic changes at rest and during exercise in long-term clonidine therapy of essential hypertension. Acta Med Scand 195:111, 1974.

54. Lowenthal DT, Affrime MB, Rosenthal L, et al: Dynamic and biochemical responses to single and repeated doses of clonidine during dynamic physical activity. Clin Pharmacol Ther 32:18, 1982.

55. Lowenthal DT, Kendrick ZV, Chase R, et al: Cardiovascular drugs and exercise. In Pandolf KB (ed): Exercise and Sport Sciences Reviews. New York: MacMillan, 1986, pp 67–94.

56. Lowenthal DT, Dickerman D, Saris SD, et al: The effect of pharmacological interaction on central and peripheral alpha-receptors and pressor response to static exercise. Ann Sports Med 1(3):100, 1984.

57. O'Hare JA, Murnaghan DJ: Failure of antihypertensive drugs to control blood pressure rise with isometric exercise in hypertension. Postgrad Med J 57:552, 1981.

58. Lowenthal DT, Saris SD, Packer J, et al: The mechanism of action and the clinical pharmacology of beta adrenergic blocking drugs. Am J Med 77(4A): 119, 1984.

59. Hossack KF, Bruce RA, Clark LJ: Influence of propranolol on exercise prescription of training heart rates. Cardiology 65:47, 1980.

60. Schneider MS, Kanrek DJ, Nelson KM: Positive training effects on anaerobic threshold during β-adrenergic blockade in cardiac rehabilitation. Circulation 66(Suppl 2):186, 1982.

61. Lowenthal DT, Powers SK, Pollock ML, et al: Interactions of β-blockade and exercise: Implications and applications for the elderly. Am J Geriatr Cardiol 1:42, 1992.

62. Sklar J, Johnston DG, Overlie P, et al: The effects of a cardioselective (metoprolol) and a nonselective (propranolol) beta-adrenergic blocker on the response to dynamic exercise in normal men. Circulation 65:894, 1982.

63. Hespel P, Lijnen P, Vanhees L, et al: Beta-adrenoreceptors and the regulation of blood pressure and plasma renin during exercise. J Appl Physiol 60:108, 1986.

64. Hespel P, Lijnen P, Vanhees L, et al: Differentiation of exercise-induced metabolic responses during selective beta-1 and beta-2 antagonism. Med Sci Sports Exer 18:186, 1986.

65. Hughson RL: Alterations in the oxygen deficit-oxygen debt relationships with β-adrenergic receptor blockade in man. J Physiol 349:3375, 1984.

66. Joyner MJ, Feund BJ, Jilka SM, et al: Effects of beta-blockade on exercise capacity of trained and untrained men: Hemodynamic comparison. J Appl Physiol 60: 1429, 1986.

67. Hughson RL, Russell CA, Marshall MR: Effect of metoprolol on cycle and treadmill maximal exercise performance. J Cardiac Rehab 4:27, 1984.

68. Virtanen K, Janne J, Frick MH: Response of blood pressure and plasma norepinephrine to propranolol, metoprolol and clonidine during isometric and dynamic exercise. Eur J Clin Pharmacol 21:275, 1981.

69. Lijnen PJ, Amry AK, Fagard RH, et al: The effect of beta-adrenoceptor blockade on renin, angiotensin, aldosterone and catecholamines at rest and during exercise. Br J Clin Pharmacol 7:175, 1979.

70. McLeod A, Kraus WE, Williams RS: Effects of beta-1 selective and nonselective beta-adrenoceptor blockade during exercise conditioning in healthy adults. Am J Cardiol 53:1656, 1984.

71. Tesch PA, Kaiser P: Effects of beta adrenergic blockade on O_2 uptake during submaximal and maximal exercise. J Appl Physiol 54:901, 1983.

72. Nelson GIC, Donnelly GL, Hunyor SN: Haemodynamic effects of sustained treatment with prazosin and metoprolol, alone and in combination, in borderline hypertensive heart failure. J Cardiovasc Pharmacol 4:240, 1982.

73. Christensen NJ, Brandsborg O: The relationship between plasma catecholamine concentration and pulse rate during exercise and standing. Eur J Clin Invest 3:299, 1973.

74. Lundborg P, Astrom H, Bengtsson C, et al: Effect of beta-adrenoceptor blockade on exercise performance and metabolism. Clin Sci 61:299, 1981.

75. Leitch AG, Hopkin JM, Ellis DA, et al: Failure of propranolol and metoprolol to alter ventilatory responses to carbon dioxide and exercise. Br J Clin Pharmacol 9:493, 1980.

76. Vanhees L, Fagard R, Amery A: Influence of beta adrenergic blockade on effects of physical training in patients with ischaemic heart disease. Br Heart J 48:33, 1982.

77. Henry JA, lliopoulou A, Kaye CM, et al: Changes in plasma concentrations of acebutolol, propranolol and indomethacin during physical exercise. Life Sci 28:1925, 1981.

78. Mach GW, Sharmon LM, Nahel ER: Influence of β-adrenergic blockade on the control of sweating in humans. J Appl Physiol 61:1701, 1986.

79. Brundin T: Effects of β-adrenergic receptor blockade on metabolic rate and mixed venous blood temperature during dynamic exercise. Scand J Clin Lab Invest 38:229, 1978.

80. Gordon NF, Myburgh DP, Schwellnus MP, et al: Effect of beta-blockade on exercise core temperature in coronary artery disease patients. Med Sci Sports Exer 19:591, 1987.

81. Griggio MA: The participation of shivering and nonshivering thermogenesis in warm and cold-acclimated rats. Comp Biochem Physiol [A] 73(3):481, 1982.

82. Wilcox RG, Bennett T, MacDonald IA, et al: The effects of acute or chronic ingestion of propranolol or metoprolol on the physiological responses to prolonged, submaximal exercise in hypertensive men. Br J Clin Pharmacol 17:273, 1984.

83. Rowell LB: Human cardiovascular adjustments to exercise and thermal stress. Physiol Rev 54:75, 1974.

84. Gordon NF, Kruger PE, Von Rensburg JP, et al: Effect of β-adrenoceptor blockade on thermoregulation during prolonged exercise. J Appl Physiol 58:899, 1985.

85. Jessen K: An assessment of human regulatory nonshivering thermogenesis. Acta Anaesthesiol Scand 24:138, 1980.

86. Moyer JH: Hydralazine (apresoline) hydrochloride: Pharmacological observations and clinical results in the therapy of hypertension. Arch Intern Med 91:419, 1953.

87. Ginks WR, Redwood DR: Haemodynamic effects of hydralazine at rest and during exercise in patients with chronic heart failure. Br Heart J 44:259, 1980.

88. Lund-Johansen, P, Omvik, P, White, W, et al: Long term hemodynamic effects of amlodipine at rest and during exercise in essential hypertension. Cardiology 80(Suppl 1):37, 1992.

89. Lowenthal DT, Broderman S: Hypertension and exercise. In Bove M, Lowenthal DT (eds): Exercise Medicine: Physiologic Principles and Clinical Applications. New York: Academic Press, 1984, pp 291–303.

90. Wilson JR, Untereker W, Hirshfeld J: Effects of isosorbide dinitrate and hydralazine on regional metabolic responses to arm exercise in patients with heart failure. Am J Cardiol 48:934, 1981.

91. Noakes TD, Higginson L, Opie LH: Physical training increases ventricular fibrillation thresholds of isolated rat hearts during normoxia, hypoxia, and regional ischemia. Circulation 67:24, 1983.

92. Cohn JN, Franciosa JA: Vasodilator therapy of cardiac failure. N Engl J Med 297:254, 1977.

93. Pickering TG, Base DB, Sullivan PA, et al: Comparison of antihypertensive and hormonal effects of captopril and propranolol at rest and during exercise. Am J Cardiol 49: 1566, 1982.

94. Manhem P, Bramnert M, Hulthen UL, et al: The effect of captopril on catecholamines, renin activity, angiotensin II and aldosterone in plasma during physical exercise in hypertensive patients. Eur J Clin Invest 11:389, 1981.

95. Fagard R, Lijnen P, Amery A: Hemodynamic response to captopril at rest and during exercise in hypertensive patients. Am J Cardiol 49:1569, 1982.

96. Leon AS, McNally C, Casal D, et al: Enalapril alone and combined with hydrochlorothiazide in the treatment of hypertension: Effect on treadmill exercise performance. J Cardiopulm Rehab 12:251, 1986.

97. Fagard R, Amery A. Reybrouck T, et al: Effects of angiotensin antagonism on hemodynamics, renin and catecholamines during exercise. J Appl Physiol 43:440, 1977.

98. Aldigier JC, Huang H, Dalmay F, et al: Angiotensin converting enzyme inhibition does not suppress plasma angiotensin II increase during exercise in humans. J Cardiovasc Pharm 21:289, 1993.

99. Lund-Johansen P, Omvik P: Long-term haemodynamic effects of enalapril at rest and during exercise in essential hypertension. Scand J Urol Nephrol 79(Suppl):87, 1984.

100. Omvik P, Lund-Johansen P: Combined captopril and hydrochlorothiazide therapy in severe hypertension: Long-term haemodynamic changes at rest and during exercise. J Hypertens 2:73, 1984.

101. Sullivan PA, Cervenka J, O'Conner DT, et al: Fosinopril, an angiotensin converting enzyme inhibitor and propranolol: Comparative effects at rest and exercise on blood pressure, hormonal variables and plasma potassium in essential hypertension. Cardiovasc Drug Ther 3:57, 1989.

102. Paran E, Neumann L, Cristal N, et al: Response to mental and physical stress before and during adrenoreceptor blocker and angiotensin-converting enzyme inhibitor treatment in essential hypertension. Am J Cardiol 68:1362, 1991.

103. Hetherington M, Haennel R, Teo KK, et al: Importance of considering ventricular function when prescribing exercise after acute myocardial infarction. Am J Cardiol 58:891, 1986.

104. Bersohn MM, Scheuer J: Effect of ischemia on the performance of hearts from physically trained rats. Am J Physiol 234:H215, 1970.

105. Hackett TP, Cassem NHJ: Psychological factors related to exercise. Cardiovasc Clin 9(3):223, 1978.

106. Myerburg RJ, Conde C, Sheps DS, et al: Antiarrhythmic drug therapy in survivors of prehospital cardiac arrest: Comparison of effects of chronic ventricular arrhythmias and recurrent cardiac arrest. Circulation 59:855, 1979.

107. Holloszy JO: Adaptations of muscular tissue to training. Prog Cardiovasc Dis 18:445, 1976.

108. Scheuer J, Tipton CM: Cardiovascular adaptations to physical training. Annu Rev Physiol 39:221, 1977.

109. Drexler H, Banhardt U, Meinertz T, et al: Contrasting peripheral short-term and long-term effects of converting enzyme inhibition in patients with congestive heart failure: A double-blind, placebo controlled trial. Circulation 79:491, 1989.

110. Meyer TE, Casadei B, Coates AJ, et al: Angiotensin converting enzyme inhibition and physical training in heart failure. J Intern Med 230:407, 1991.

111. The SOLVED Investigators: Effect of Enalapril on survival in patients with reduced left ventricular ejection fractions and congestive heart failure. N Engl J Med 325:293, 1991.

112. Cohn JN, Johnson G, Ziesche S, et al: A comparison of enalapril with hydralazine-isosorbide dinitrate in the treatment of chronic congestive heart failure. N Engl J Med 325:303, 1991.

113. Uretsky BF, Young JB, Shahidi FE, et al: Randomized study assessing the effect of digoxin withdrawal in patients with mild to moderate chronic congestive heart failure: Results of the PROVED trial. J Am Coll Cardiol 22: 955, 1993.

114. Cody RJ: Clinical trials of diuretic therapy in heart failure, research directions and clinical considerations. J Am Coll Cardiol 22:4(Suppl A)165, 1993.

115. Dickstein K, Aarsland T: For the Nordic enalapril exercise trial, effect of exercise performance on enalapril therapy initiated early after myocardial infarction. J Am Coll Cardiol 22:975, 1993.

116. Gheorghiade M, Hall V, Lakier JB, et al: Comparative hemody-

namic and neurohumoral effects of intravenous captopril and digoxin and their combinations in patients with severe heart failure. J Am Coll Cardiol 13:134, 1989.

117. Nordrehaug JE, Vollset SE: Reduction of exercise induced ventricular arrhythmias in mild symptomatic heart failure by benazepril. Am Heart J 125:771, 1993.

118. Vogel R, Kirch D, LeFree M, et al: Effects of digitalis on resting and isometric exercise myocardial perfusion in patients with coronary artery disease and left ventricular dysfunction. Circulation 56:355, 1977.

119. LeWinter MM, Crawford MH, O'Rourke RA, et al: The effects of oral propranolol, digoxin and combination therapy on the resting and exercise electrocardiogram. Am Heart J 93:202, 1977.

120. Gross GJ, Warltier DC, Hardman HF, et al: The effects of ouabain on nutritional circulation and regional myocardial blood flow. Am Heart J 93:487, 1977.

121. Parker JO, West RO Jr, Ledwich JR, et al: The effect of acute digitalization on the hemodynamic response to exercise in coronary artery disease. Circulation 40:453, 1969.

122. Jogestrand T, Andersson K: Effect of physical exercise on the pharmacokinetics of digoxin during maintenance treatment. J Cardiovasc Pharm 14:73, 1989.

123. Pedersen KE, Madsen J, Kjaer K, et al: Effects of physical activity and immobilization on plasma digoxin concentration and renal digoxin clearance. Clin Pharm Ther 34:303, 1983.

124. Jogestrand T, Schenck-Gustafsson K, Nordlander R, et al: Quinidine-induced changes in serum and skeletal muscle digoxin concentration: Evidence of saturable binding of digoxin to skeletal muscle. Eur J Clin Pharm 27:571, 1984.

125. Gey GP, Levy RH, Pettet G, et al: Quinidine plasma concentration and exertional arrhythmia. Am Heart J 90:19, 1975.

126. Gey GP, Levy RH, Fisher L, et al: Plasma concentration of procainamide and prevalence of exertional arrhythmias. Ann Intern Med 80:718, 1974.

127. Fenster PE, Dahl C, Marcus FI, et al: Effect of quinidine on the heart rate and blood pressure response to treadmill exercise. Am Heart J 104:1244, 1982.

128. Surawicz B, Lasseter KC: Effects of drugs on the electrocardiogram. Prog Cardiovasc Dis 13:26, 1970.

129. Ylitalo P, Hinkka H: Effect of exercise on plasma levels and urinary excretion of sulphadimidine and procainamide. Int J Clin Pharm Ther Toxicol 23:548, 1985.

130. Winkle RA, Gradman AH, Fitzgerald JW: Antiarrhythmic drug effect assessed from ventricular arrhythmia reduction in the ambulatory electrocardiogram and treadmill test: Comparison of propranolol, procainamide and quinidine. Am J Cardiol 42:473, 1978.

131. LeWinter MM, Engler RL, Karliner JS: Tocainide therapy for treatment of ventricular arrhythmias: Assessment with ambulatory electrocardiographic monitoring and treadmill exercise. Am J Cardiol 45:1045, 1980.

CHAPTER 24

Cardiovascular Therapy and Stress

Roland E. Schmieder, M.D., Heinz Rüddel, M.D., and August W. von Eiff, M.D.

"Stress is the salt of life," Selye often said; he defined stress as the nonspecific response of the body to any demand.[1, 2] Today stress is regarded as a complex physiologic syndrome of response to external and internal stimuli (stressors). The stress response includes activation of the central nervous system (CNS) and hemodynamic, neuroendocrine, and behavioral changes.[3] Two psychologic processes seem to be of particular importance in the stress response: cognitive appraisal of the stressor and coping.[4] Cognitive appraisal is the process through which a person evaluates whether a particular stressor is relevant to well-being. Coping is defined as the person's constantly changing cognitive and behavioral effort to manage external and internal demands.[5]

Cardiovascular pharmacology is concerned with the question of stress because some psychologic characteristics and certain person-environment relations seem to be important in the pathogenesis of coronary heart disease, arrhythmia, and arterial hypertension. For example, it is assumed that persons with the type A behavior pattern, hostile behavior, or inappropriate coping to everyday environmental stressors experience a pathologic degree of cardiovascular and neuroendocrine reactivity to commonly occurring stimuli (stressors) and that this pattern of reactivity mediates the development of arteriosclerosis.[6] Repeated injury of the endothelial cells in the arteries might alter permeability to lipoproteins and initiate the formation of atherosclerotic plaques.[7] Episodic increases in cardiac output elicited by stressors that require active coping and lead to β-adrenergic activation may promote elevated resistance in the peripheral vasculature.[8]

This chapter deals with the effects of stress on the heart and circulatory system and the interaction between pharmacologic agents and cardiovascular stress responses. We will discuss the impact of pharmacologic agents that influence reactivity by blocking receptors in peripheral organs. Drugs that act primarily at the level of the CNS and nonpharmacologic strategies will not be discussed in detail, although their efficacy in preventing the hazardous effects of stress on the cardiovascular system is well-established.

STRESS AS A RISK FACTOR FOR CARDIAC DISEASES
Sudden Death

Since ancient times, medical thinking and folklore have shared the view that sudden death may result from psychologic stress.[9] Because cardiac arrhythmia is considered a precursor of cardiac arrest and sudden death, numerous studies have examined the relationship of ventricular fibrillation and premature ventricular contractions to neural and psychologic mechanisms.[10] However, carefully controlled studies in humans are rare, and direct evidence of the link between stressful events and sudden death is lacking.

A retrospective analysis among 4486 widowers disclosed that, during the first 6 months after the loss of a spouse, the death rate increased by 40% above the expected rate for married men matched for age.[11] In a series of 170 reports of sudden death that had been systematically analyzed, sudden cardiac death was linked to grief or death of a close person but also to loss of self-esteem, hopeless situations, and situations of triumph and happiness.[9]

Three other well-controlled studies provide further evidence of a direct link between emotional stress and ventricular arrhythmias. In a large population of patients in a coronary care unit, social interactions at the patient's bedside and during ward rounds increased the severity and the number of ventricular arrhythmias, whereas pulse palpation by a nurse reduced ventricular ectopy.[12, 13] Taggart et al.[14, 15] systematically analyzed cardiac responses to diverse stresses induced by car racing, driving in traffic, public speaking, and emotional stress. Multiple ventricular ectopic contractions emerged in 5 of 24 patients with ischemic heart disease while they were driving their own car along a familiar route; public speaking provoked more than 6 ventricular ectopic beats/min in 6 of 23 subjects, although no cardiac disease was clinically evident. More recently, Lown et al.[16] demonstrated that psychologic stress (mental arithmetic under time pressure, reading from colored cards, and recounting an emotionally charged experience) resulted in a significant increase in ventricular premature beats in 11 of 19 patients with various types of heart disease.

However, direct evidence demonstrating a cause-and-effect relationship between emotional stress and sudden death will be difficult to establish with certainty, although individual case reports are very persuasive.[17, 18] In animal studies, for instance, exposure to an adverse environment profoundly reduced the cardiac threshold for ventricular fibrillation, and after occlusion of one coronary artery, reexposure to stressful situations resulted in diverse ventricular arrhythmias, including ventricular fibrillation.[17, 18]

Thus, there is evidence that stress significantly influences the incidence of cardiac arrhythmia and potentially triggers sudden death in patients with or without cardiac disorders.

Coronary Artery Disease

Long ignored in major epidemiologic studies, stress is gaining credibility as a risk factor in coronary artery disease. Before the turn of the century, Sir William Osler[19] described the typical patient with ischemic heart disease as a "keen and ambitious man, the indicator of whose engines is always set full speed ahead." Friedman and Rosenman[20] have emphasized the prevalence of "intense ambition, competitive drive, sense of urgency, and preoccupation with deadlines" among persons predisposed to clinical coronary artery disease. These persons were designated

as type A subjects. Their behavior, called type A behavior, is characterized by excessive rapid body movement, explosive conversational intonations, hand or teeth clenching, excessive unconscious gesturing, and a general air of impatience.

In the Western Collaborative Group Study (WCGS), type A behavior assessed by structured interview emerged as a risk factor of the same magnitude as well-known classic risk factors for the development of coronary heart disease. In addition, type A behavior was an independent risk factor for ischemic heart disease.[21] In recent years, some prospective studies corroborated the results from the WCGS study, whereas in two studies, no association between type A behavior and coronary heart disease was found.[22–24]

Subsequent analysis of the WCGS data illustrated that speed of activity, achievements, and job involvement were not related to overt manifestations of coronary heart disease. In contrast, potential for hostility, competitiveness, impatience, irritability, and vigorous voice stylistics were primarily related to coronary events.[25] Recent prospective studies emphasized the importance of hostility for the development of fatal cardiac events. Two studies[26, 27] have prospectively examined the independent contribution of hostility to coronary mortality. In both studies, an increased risk of mortality from coronary heart disease was observed among those scoring high on hostility. Thus, hostility and type A behavior seem to be important risk factors as long as other risks have not yet determined the vascular changes of arteriosclerosis.[28]

The interrelationship between stress and coronary heart disease is more complex than statistical analysis can elucidate. Clearly, emotional stress elevates blood pressure, aggravates diabetes, induces or augments hypercholesterolemia, and increases the tendency to obesity and excessive smoking.[29, 30] Consequently, emotional stress can induce or aggravate the progress of coronary heart disease by multiple pathways, and one should recognize that most accepted risk factors are strongly influenced by behavioral and psychosocial factors.

Pharmacologic Interventions for Stress-Induced Cardiac Alterations

Prevention of Sudden Death

There is substantial evidence that enhanced activity of the sympathetic nervous system and catecholamines predispose an individual to ventricular arrhythmias.[16, 17, 31, 32] Consequently, interventions increasing vagal tone and decreasing sympathetic tone of the autonomic nervous system might be beneficial in patients at risk for sudden death. A significant reduction of ventricular premature beats and a lower grade in the Lown classification were observed in ambulatory patients during sleep when compared with patients who were awake.[33] The decline in frequency and severity of ventricular arrhythmia was related to a lower level of sympathetic tone and vagotonia during sleep. Consistently, administrations of vagotonic agents or parasympathetic maneuvers in the form of carotid sinus massage lowered the incidence of premature ventricular contractions and even abolished ventricular tachycardia in certain instances.[31, 33–39]

In animal studies, behaviorally induced cardiac vulnerability was suppressed by selective β_1-adrenergic blocking drugs.[18] Consistently, a single oral dose of 40 mg of oxprenolol abolished the advanced frequency and grade of ventricular premature beats provoked by psychologic stressors, such as speaking before an audience or driving a car.[15] Decreased incidence of sudden death in patients surviving acute myocardial infarction has been documented in several prospective, double-blind studies by treatment with β-blockers initiated several days after the infarct occurred.[40–42] Interestingly, the preventive effect of β-blockers on mortality was abolished when a β-blocking agent with intrinsic sympathetic activity was used.[43]

These observations support the view that an alternation of the sympathetic drive to the heart results in diminished cardiac excitability and therefore may reduce ventricular arrhythmia. However, only in survivors of acute myocardial infarction has the wide use of β-blockers improved life expectancy. The beneficial effects of magnesium supplementation on ventricular arrhythmia has been repeatedly documented.[44–46] Magnesium supplementation increased the threshold for ventricular excitability and slowed cardiac conduction in humans. Prospective studies now recommend the use of magnesium supplementation in patients with acute myocardial infarction, because mortality was clearly reduced in this set of patients at high risk for cardiac sudden death.[47, 48]

Ventricular arrhythmias induced by long-term therapy with diuretics was not sufficiently suppressed by potassium supplementation alone; however, when magnesium was added, premature ventricular beats were abolished.[49] Vice versa, in hypertensive patients, the decrease in serum magnesium caused by diuretics correlated with the increase in premature ventricular contractions. Messerli et al.[50] have documented that hypertensive patients with left ventricular hypertrophy exhibit premature ventricular beats more frequently than normotensive patients do. Consequently, one might speculate that the high occurrence of sudden death in patients receiving large doses of thiazide diuretics was related not only to potassium but also to magnesium depletion.[51] Thus, magnesium homeostasis should be carefully maintained in cardiac patients receiving diuretics, and magnesium supplementation up to 15 mmol/day or a magnesium- or potassium-retaining agent might even be added.

Prevention of Coronary Artery Disease

The roles of nitrates, calcium antagonists, and β-blocking agents in ischemic heart disease are discussed in other chapters. However, it is interesting that of all therapeutic agents for coronary artery disease, only β-adrenoreceptor blockers inhibit or at least reduce stress-induced increases in heart rate caused by adrenergic activity. As a consequence, β-blockers diminish myocardial oxygen demand during emotional stress and might therefore be preferable in a subset of patients with coronary artery disease who exhibit exaggerated stimulation of the sympathetic nervous system.

In the management of patients with ischemic heart disease, reduction of all risk factors is a most desirable goal. When evident, diabetes and hyperlipidemia should be treated, ideal weight should be obtained and maintained, hypertension should be treated, and cigarette use should be stopped. Whether and how to treat psychosocial risk factors for coronary heart disease is controversial.[52, 53]

In therapeutic trials with hypertensive patients, a reduction of type A behavior and hostility was observed following effective antihypertensive therapy with β-blockers but not with diuretics or calcium antagonists.[54–56] Patients treated with atenolol had less pronounced type A behavior after short-term therapy compared with patients receiving diuretics or calcium antagonists. Even after long-term therapy with atenolol (1 year), hostility was less expressed than it was before therapy.[55] A similar reduction in type A behavior as a result of β-blockade was reported among coronary patients.[56] Hence, it appears to be worthwhile to administer β-blockers to patients with hypertension and marked type A behavior or hostility, thereby reducing two risk factors for coronary artery disease at the same time.

HYPERTENSION AND STRESS
Essential Hypertension

Even after thorough clinical examination, more than 90% of patients with arterial hypertension are classified as having "idiopathic," "primary," or so-called "essential hypertension." No single clinical abnormality causing sustained elevation of arterial pressure in systemic circulation can be identified in this group of patients. As early as 50 years ago, it was documented that transient or labile hypertension might progress to established hypertension.[57] Hence, one major topic of research is to elucidate pathogenetic mechanisms that convert occasionally elevated blood pressure into sustained hypertension.

The association between psychologic and environmental stress and essential hypertension has gained some support since increased cardiovascular reactivity to emotional stress has been observed in adolescents with a family history of hypertension[58–60] and in patients with borderline hypertension.[61, 62] The hemodynamic pattern resulting from exposure to mental arithmetic tasks is characterized by a rise in systolic and diastolic pressure and an increase in heart rate, stroke volume, and cardiac output, whereas total peripheral resistance decreases.[63] Increased activity of the sympathetic nervous system appears to mediate these hemodynamic changes during stress.

Prospective studies lend credence to the hypothesis

that an augmented cardiovascular reaction to stress might trigger sustained elevation of blood pressure in some persons.[64, 65] Normotensive adolescents with an augmented rise in systolic pressure in response to mental arithmetic tasks more frequently developed arterial hypertension than did those exhibiting a normal increase in blood pressure.[64] When 63 prepubertal children were categorized according to their heart rate response to mental stress, those who reacted above the median of the whole sample demonstrated a greater increase in systolic pressure after 1 year than did those whose reactions were below the median.[65] Although these findings were not entirely conclusive,[66, 67] a longitudinal follow-up study in a small sample of 35 subjects selected randomly among the residents of Bonn provided further evidence: The increment in systolic pressure in response to a standardized mental arithmetic task predicted the elevation of casual blood pressure 2½ years later.[68]

The question arises whether mental stress testing in the laboratory adequately reflects emotional stress in the natural environment. In epidemiologic studies, the impact of noise on blood pressure regulation has been noted. Subjects most heavily exposed to road or air traffic noise revealed the highest blood pressure readings and had the highest incidence of antihypertensive therapy.[69, 70] In addition, after 2½ years, average diastolic pressure increased in persons living in residential areas with high traffic noise, whereas diastolic pressure in the control group slightly decreased owing to adaptation.[68] Occupational stress also was found to influence blood pressure level: Air traffic controllers working at busy airports had an increased incidence (5.6 times) of arterial hypertension compared with persons who had low levels of occupational stress.[71]

These results suggest that stress reactions might be the starting point of the pathogenetic process leading to essential hypertension, an idea that was proposed 20 years ago in the "hypothalamus theory."[61, 72] According to this theory, internal and external stressors might affect the sympathetic hypothalamic center via the cortical limbic system, thereby eliciting an increased sympathetic nerve-fiber discharge and producing the hemodynamic alterations previously described. A progressive, repeated increase in systolic pressure might finally lead to morphologic changes in arterial walls.[73] Nevertheless, it should be emphasized that several other risk factors for the development of arterial hypertension, such as heredity, obesity, alcohol consumption, and salt intake, have been identified.[67]

Stress and the Outcome of Arterial Hypertension

In established essential hypertension, cardiovascular reactions to stress provide further specification about the risk for future cardiovascular morbid events. As in the prehypertensive stages, blood pressure response to emotional stress was found to be exaggerated in patients with sustained essential hypertension

compared with normotensive control subjects.[74, 75] Consequently, during stressful situations, pulse-pressure product, a parameter for myocardial oxygen consumption, is elevated in patients with arterial hypertension. This might be of prognostic value in patients with ischemic heart disease, because coronary reserve is already lowered in hypertensive patients with normal coronary arteries.[76, 77]

When measured during regularly recurring stressful situations, blood pressure values at the work site correlated better with the degree of left ventricular hypertrophy than did blood pressure readings made during the night or at the physician's office.[78] Furthermore, the average blood pressure at work was of greater prognostic value for hypertension-related cardiovascular damage, such as coronary artery disease, than were casual blood pressure readings.[78–80] Hence, to the degree that blood pressure readings at the work site more accurately reflect the effects of daily life stress than casual blood pressure values, the impact of antihypertensive medication on cardiovascular response to stress deserves special attention.

Antihypertensive Therapy and Stress-Induced Blood Pressure Increase

In a series of clinical trials, we investigated whether and how antihypertensive therapy diminished the increase in blood pressure resulting from mental stress. All patients examined were middle-aged, white men with mild essential hypertension World Health Organization (WHO) stage I or II. Stress testing consisted of standardized mental arithmetic tasks now in use for more than 20 years.[61] To increase stress level, each subject was distracted by affective noise (e.g., soccer game, aircraft, quarrel, jazz music) at a sound level of 90 dB(A) while performing the calculations; the challenge was further increased by announcing the elapsed time over headphones every minute during task performance.[81, 82]

The antihypertensive mechanism of diuretics does not imply *a priori* that these pharmacologic agents modify stress-induced increases in blood pressure. Indeed, in hypertensive patients, diuretics did not attenuate blood pressure or increase heart rate in response to mental stress.[83]

In contrast, β-adrenoreceptor blocking agents appeared to be more likely than diuretics to lower the cardiovascular response provoked by stress-induced stimulation of the sympathetic nervous system. However, neither cardioselective β-blockers (atenolol) nor noncardioselective β-blockers (oxprenolol, propranolol) proved capable of attenuating an increase in blood pressure during mental stress testing.[81, 83, 84] These findings were independent of the duration of antihypertensive therapy, because acute and long-term β-blockade induced similar cardiovascular stress reactions. Similar findings were reported by other research groups.[85–87]

These results provoked us to examine the cardiovascular response to stress in patients receiving antihypertensive agents that directly inhibit sympathetic outflow from hypothalamic centers to resistance vessels and to the heart. Antihypertensive therapy with clonidine leads to a decrease of peripheral catecholamine levels,[88] in particular norepinephrine concentrations,[89] and to a similar decrease of norepinephrine in the cerebrospinal fluid.[89, 90] Despite these actions attributed to centrally acting sympatholytic agents, clonidine also failed to attenuate the blood pressure response to mental challenge in hypertensive patients.[91] However, in adolescents with slightly elevated blood pressure, clonidine mitigated blood pressure increases during mental arithmetic.[92]

Antihypertensive agents acting primarily by inducing peripheral vasodilation were subsequently examined. After 6 months of effective therapy, calcium entry blockade by nitrendipine or isradipine did not diminish blood pressure increases during mental stress.[81, 93] The same held true for converting enzyme inhibitors: enalapril, lisinopril, and fosinopril administered for 3 months did not reduce stress-induced increases in systolic and diastolic pressures.[93-95]

In summary, blood pressure increases during experimental mental stress could not be attenuated by any antihypertensive regimen or by administration of sympatholytic agents.

Antihypertensive Agents and Hemodynamic Response Pattern During Emotional Stress

Although β-adrenoreceptor blockers, calcium antagonists, converting enzyme inhibitors, and diuretics all had no impact on stress-induced increases in systolic and diastolic pressures, the hemodynamic pattern producing the rise in arterial pressure was quite different. In 40 hypertensive patients randomly allocated either to β-blockers or to calcium antagonists, the pattern of hemodynamic response to mental stress was assessed before and after therapy.[81, 91] In patients receiving calcium antagonists, mental challenge provoked a physiologic response pattern: heart rate, stroke volume, and consequently cardiac output increased, whereas vascular resistance decreased. In contrast, β-adrenoreceptor blockade reversed the hemodynamic response pattern to a distinct decrease in stroke volume, heart rate, and cardiac output while total peripheral resistance increased. Because β-receptors were blocked, the increased sympathetic flow during mental challenge probably led to overriding α-receptor stimulation, thereby inducing peripheral vasoconstriction. By using a different stress test (isometric handgrip test), the same abnormal hemodynamic pattern was identified after β-blockade—that is, an increase in vascular resistance to stress.[96] Angiotensin-converting enzyme (ACE) inhibitors and diuretics also preserved the physiologic cardiovascular pattern of response to stress in the untreated patients similar to that in patients receiving calcium antagonist.[83, 93-95]

What clinical importance may be attributed to these findings? Eliot et al.[97, 98] demonstrated that patients with an exaggerated response to mental stress (evidenced by a marked increase in total peripheral resistance and no change or even a decrease in cardiac output, the so-called "hot reactors type III") were at high risk for severe cardiovascular disease. Furthermore, in a 23-year prospective study,[99] the increase in diastolic pressure in response to the cold pressor test (indicating augmented peripheral vasoconstriction) was the best single predictor for future coronary artery disease. Conceivably, peripheral vasoconstriction during stress might be harmful and can no longer be considered insignificant. Of note, the ACE inhibitors attenuated the vasoconstrictive response to the cold pressor test more effectively than calcium antagonists did.[93, 95]

Although prospective studies examining the importance of vasoconstriction during mental stress in patients receiving antihypertensive therapy are lacking, our results suggest that β-blockers for antihypertensive therapy should be prescribed with caution to patients with exaggerated, stress-induced peripheral vasoconstriction, preexisting arteriosclerotic arterial lesions, or both. In contrast, calcium antagonists and ACE inhibitors seem to preserve the "physiologic" response pattern and therefore may prove to be preferable.

Prevention of Stress-Induced Increases in Blood Pressure: Potential Role of Magnesium

The Western diet is low in magnesium and potassium[100] but high in sodium. Because magnesium is mainly an intracellular ion, measurements of serum magnesium are of little help in assessing a subclinical magnesium deficit. Magnesium deficiency is more reliably assessed by measuring the magnesium concentrations in red blood cells.[101] Experimental and preliminary clinical studies documented that low magnesium concentrations in red blood cells are related to increased blood pressure levels at rest and during stress and to vasospasms in coronary arteries.[102-105]

In a double-blind study of patients with hypertension but without target-organ damage, orally administered magnesium (15 mmol/day) was the only antihypertensive agent.[106] After 1 month of magnesium supplementation, neither systolic nor diastolic pressure changed significantly. These results were confirmed by other preliminary reports but conflicted with findings of a previous uncontrolled study.[107, 108] Whether subpopulations (e.g., high-renin hypertensive patients) profit from magnesium supplementation is the subject of ongoing investigations.

It has been suggested that oral magnesium supplementation may blunt cardiovascular hyperreactivity, which represents the typical hemodynamic pattern in the prehypertensive and hypertensive stages. In a double-blind, randomized protocol, we examined subjects with borderline hypertension characterized by a hyperreactive, exaggerated blood pressure increase during stress and by low magnesium concentrations in red blood cells. They randomly received either placebo or magnesium-L-aspartate HCl, 15 mmol/day, for 12 weeks. After 3 months, systolic pressure increases during mental challenge could be significantly attenuated with magnesium supplementation, although baseline blood pressure was not significantly different from pretreatment levels. These results suggest that magnesium supplementation indeed decelerated cardiovascular reactions to mental stress in patients with impaired magnesium homeostasis.

REFERENCES

1. Selye H: Forty years of stress research: The principal remaining problems and misconceptions. Can Med Assoc J 115:53, 1976.
2. Selye H: The stress concept. In Wheatley D (ed): Stress and the Heart. New York: Raven Press, 1977, pp 1–11.
3. Weiss SM, Matthews KA, Detre T, et al: Stress, reactivity, and cardiovascular disease. NIH Publication No. 84–2698, 1984.
4. Folkman S, Lazarus R, Dunkel-Schetter C, et al: Dynamics of a stressful encounter: Cognitive appraisal, coping and encounter outcomes. J Psychol 50:992, 1986.
5. Lazarus RS, Folkman S: Stress, Appraisal, and Coping. New York: Springer, 1984.
6. Eliot RS, Buell JC: The heart and emotional stress. In Hurst JW (ed): The Heart. New York: McGraw-Hill, 1982, pp 1637–1649.
7. Manuck SB, Kaplan JR, Clarkson TB: Atherosclerosis, social dominance and cardiovascular reactivity. In Schmidt TH, Dembroski TM, Blümchen G (eds): Biological and Psychological Factors in Cardiovascular Disease. Berlin: Springer-Verlag, 1986, pp 460–475.
8. Obrist PA, Light KC, Sherwood A, et al: Some working hypotheses on the significance of behaviorally evoked cardiovascular reactivity to pathophysiology. In Schmidt TH, Dembroski TM, Blümchen G (eds): Biological and Psychological Factors in Cardiovascular Disease. Berlin: Springer-Verlag, 1986, pp 406–417.
9. Engel GL: Sudden and rapid death during psychological stress: Folklore or folk wisdom. Ann Intern Med 74:771, 1971.
10. Lynch JJ, Paskewitz DA, Gimbel KS, et al: Psychological aspects of cardiac arrhythmia. Am Heart J 93:645, 1977.
11. Parkers CM, Benjamin B, Fitzgerald R: Broken heart: Statistical study of increased mortality among widowers. Br Med J 1:740, 1969.
12. Jarviuen KAJ: Can ward rounds be a danger to patients with myocardial infarction? Br Med J 1:318, 1955.
13. Thomas SA, Lynch JJ, Mills ME: Psychosocial influences on heart arrhythmia in a coronary case patient. Heart Lung 4:746, 1975.
14. Taggart P, Gibbons D, Sommerville W: Some effects of motor driving on the normal and abnormal heart. Br Med J 4:130, 1969.
15. Taggart P, Carruthers M, Sommerville W: Electrocardiogram, plasma catecholamines and lipids, and their modification by oxprenolol when speaking before an audience. Lancet 2:341, 1973.
16. Lown B, DeSilvia RA: Roles of psychologic stress and autonomic nervous system: Changes in provocation of ventricular premature complexes. Am J Cardiol 41:979, 1978.
17. Lown B, Verrier R, Cobalan R: Psychological stress and threshold for repetitive ventricular response. Science 182:834, 1973.
18. Lown B, Verrier R: Neural activity and ventricular fibrillation. N Engl J Med 294:1165, 1976.
19. Osler W: Lectures on angina pectoris and allied states. N Y Med J 4:224, 1896.
20. Friedman M, Rosenman RH: Association of specific overt behavior pattern with blood and cardiovascular findings: Blood cholesterol level, blood clotting time, incidence of arcus senilis, and clinical coronary artery disease. JAMA 169:1286, 1959.
21. Rosenman RH, Friedman M, Straus R, et al: Coronary heart disease in the Western Collaborative Group Study. JAMA 195:86, 1966.
22. Haynes SG, Feinleib M, Kannel WB: The relationship of psychosocial factors to coronary heart disease in the Framingham study: III. 8-year incidence of CHD. Am J Epidemiol 3:37, 1980.
23. Jenkins CD: Psychosocial and social precursors of coronary disease. N Engl J Med 284:244, 1971.
24. Rosenman RH, Brand RJ, Jenkins CD, et al: Coronary heart disease in the Western Collaborative Group Study: Final follow-up of 8½ years. JAMA 233:872, 1975.
25. Matthews KA, Glass DC, Rosenman RH, et al: Competitive drive, pattern A, and coronary heart disease: A further analysis of some data from the Western Collaborative Group Study. J Chronic Dis 30:489, 1977.
26. Shekelle RB, Gale M, Ostfeld AM, et al: Hostility, risk of coronary heart disease, and mortality. Psychosom Med 45:109, 1983.
27. Barefoot JC, Dahlstrom WC, Williams RB: Hostility, CHD incidence and total mortality: A 25-year follow-up study of 255 physicians. Psychosom Med 45:59, 1983.
28. The Review Panel on Coronary-Prone Behavior and Coronary Heart Disease: Coronary-prone behavior and coronary heart disease: A critical review. Circulation 63:1199, 1981.
29. Russek HI, Russek LG: Behavior pattern and emotional stress in the etiology of coronary heart disease: Sociological and occupational aspects. In Wheatley D (ed): Stress and the Heart. New York: Raven Press, 1977, pp 15–32.
30. Weidner G, Sexton G, McLellarn R, et al: The role of type A behaviour and hostility in an elevation of plasma lipids in adult women and men. Psychosom Med 49:136, 1987.
31. Han J, Garcia de Jalon P, Moe GK: Adrenergic effects on ventricular vulnerability. Circ Res 14:516, 1964.
32. Kliks BR, Burgess MJ, Abildskov JA: Influence of sympathetic tone on ventricular fibrillation threshold during experimental coronary occlusions. Am J Cardiol 36:45, 1975.
33. Lown B, Graboys TB, Garfein A, et al: Sleep and ventricular premature beats. Circulation 48:691, 1973.
34. Cope RL: Suppressive effect of carotid sinus on premature ventricular beats in certain instances. Am J Cardiol 4:314, 1959.
35. Lown B, Levine SA: The carotid sinus: Clinical value of its stimulation. Circulation 23:776, 1961.
36. Lorentzen D: Pacemaker-induced ventricular tachycardia: Reversion to normal sinus rhythm by carotid sinus massage. JAMA 235:282, 1976.
37. Waxman MB, Downar E, Berman D, et al: Phenylephrine (Neosynephrine) terminated ventricular tachycardia. Circulation 50:656, 1974.
38. Weiss T, Lattin GM, Engelmann K: Vagally mediated suppression of premature ventricular contractions in man. Am Heart J 89:700, 1975.
39. Nathanson MH: Action of acetyl-beta-methylcholin on ventricular rhythms induced by adrenalin. R Soc Exp Biol Med 32:1297, 1935.
40. Beta-Blocker Heart Attack Trial Research Group: A randomized trial of propranolol in patients with acute myocardial infarction: I. Mortality results. JAMA 247:1707, 1982.
41. Bigger JT, Fleiss JL, Kleiger R, et al: The multicenter postinfarction research group: The relationships among ventricular arrhythmias, left ventricular dysfunction, and mortality in the 2 years after myocardial infarction. Circulation 69:250, 1984.
42. Wilhelmsson C, Vedin JA, Wilhelmsen L, et al: Reduction of sudden deaths after myocardial infarction by treatment with alprenolol: Preliminary results. Lancet 2:1157, 1974.
43. A multicenter international study: Improvement in prognosis of myocardial infarction by long-term beta-adrenoceptor blockade using practolol. Br Med J 3:735, 1975.
44. Specter JM, Schweizer E, Goldman RH: Studies on magnesium's mechanism of action in digitalis-induced arrhythmias. Circulation 52:1001, 1975.
45. Ghani MF, Rabah M: Effect of magnesium chloride on electrical stability of the heart. Am Heart J 94:600, 1977.
46. DiCarlo LA, Moroday F, DeBuitleis M, et al: Effects of magnesium sulfate on cardiac conduction and refractoriness in humans. J Am Coll Cardiol 7:1356, 1986.

47. Woods KL, Fletcher S, Roffe C, et al: Intravenous magnesium sulphate in suspected acute myocardial infarction: Results of the second Leicester Intravenous Magnesium Intervention Trial (LIMIT-2). Lancet 339:1553, 1992.
48. Lau J, Antman EM, Jimenez-Silvia J: Cumulative meta-analysis of therapeutic trials for myocardial infarction. N Engl J Med 327:248, 1992.
49. Hollifield JW: Potassium and magnesium abnormalities: Diuretics and arrhythmias in hypertension. Am J Med 77(Suppl 5A):28, 1984.
50. Messerli FH, Ventura HO, Elizardi DJ, et al: Hypertension and sudden death: Increased ventricular ectopy activity in left ventricular hypertrophy. Am J Med 77:18, 1984.
51. Multiple Risk Factor Intervention Trial Research Group: Multiple risk factor intervention trial: Risk factor changes and mortality results. JAMA 248:1465, 1982.
52. Nunes EV, Frank KA, Kornfeld DS: Psychologic treatment for the type A behavior pattern and for coronary heart disease: A meta-analysis of the literature. Psychosom Med 48:159, 1987.
53. Friedman M, Thorensen CE, Gill JJ, et al: Alterations of type A behavior and reduction in cardiac recurrences in postmyocardial infarction patients. Am Heart J 108:237, 1984.
54. Schmieder R, Friedrich G, Neus H, et al: Effect of beta-blockers on type A coronary-prone behavior. Psychosom Med 45:417, 1983.
55. Schmieder R, Neus H, Rüddel H, et al: Alternation of type A behavior in hypertensives: A comparison between beta-blockers, diuretics and calcium antagonists. In Zanchetti A, Turner P (eds): Towards Preventive Treatment of Coronary-Prone Behavior. Toronto: Hans Huber, 1984, pp 49–55.
56. Krantz DS, Durel LA, Davia JE, et al: Propranolol medication among coronary patients: Relationship to type A behavior and cardiovascular response. J Hum Stress 8:4, 1982.
57. Levy RL, Hillman CC, Stroud WD, et al: Transient hypertension. JAMA 126:829, 1944.
58. Stern MP, Brown BW, Haskel WL, et al: Cardiovascular risk and use of estrogens or estrogen-progestagen combinations. JAMA 235:811, 1976.
59. Falkner B, Onesti G, Angelakos ET: Hemodynamic response to mental stress in normal adolescents with varying degree of genetic risk for essential hypertension. In Yamori Y, Lovenberg W, Freis E (eds): Prophylactic Approach to Hypertensive Diseases. New York: Raven Press, 1979, pp 149–156.
60. Neus H, Rüddel H, Schulte W: The long-term effect of noise on blood pressure. J Hypertens 3:31, 1985.
61. von Eiff AW: The role of the autonomic nervous system in the etiology and pathogenesis of essential hypertension. Jpn Circ J 34:147, 1970.
62. von Eiff AW, Schulte W, Hensch G: Classification of homogenous blood pressure groups and the specific hemodynamic pattern of borderline hypertension. In Yamori W, Lovenberg E, Freis D (eds): Perspectives in Cardiovascular Research: Prophylactic Approach to Hypertensive Diseases. New York: Raven Press, 1979, pp 315–319.
63. Brod J, Fencl V, Hejl Z: Circulatory changes underlying blood pressure elevation during acute emotional stress (mental arithmetic) in normotensive and hypertensive subjects. Clin Sci 18:269, 1959.
64. Falkner B, Kushner H, Onesti G: Cardiovascular characteristics in adolescents who develop essential hypertension. Hypertension 3:521, 1981.
65. von Eiff AW, Gogolin E, Jacobs U, et al: Heart rate reactivity under mental stress as a predictor of blood pressure development in children. J Hypertens 3(Suppl 4):89, 1985.
66. Radice M, Alli C, Avanzini F, et al: Role of blood pressure response to provocative tests in the prediction of hypertension in adolescents. Eur Heart J 6:490, 1985.
67. Schmieder RE, Messerli FH, Rüddel H: Risk for arterial hypertension. Cardiol Clin 4:57, 1986.
68. Neus H, Rüddel H, Schulte W, et al: The long-term effect of noise on blood pressure. J Hypertens 1(Suppl 2):251, 1983.
69. von Eiff AW, DFG-Forschungsbericht Bonn-Bad Godesberg: Fluglärmwirkungen. Eine interdisziplinäre Untersuchung über die Auswirkungen des Fluglärms auf den Menschen. Der medizinische Untersuchungsteil. Bd. I. Bolt, Boppard, 1974, pp 349–424.
70. von Eiff AW, Neus H: Verkehrslärm und Hypertonie-Risiko. Münch Med Wschr 122:894, 1980.
71. Cobb S, Rose RM: Hypertension, peptic ulcer, and diabetes in air traffic controllers. JAMA 244:489, 1973.
72. von Eiff AW: Die essentielle Hypertonie. In von Eiff AW (ed): Essentielle Hypertonie, Klinik, Psychophysiologie, und Psychopathologie. Stuttgart: Georg Thieme, 1967, pp 38–58.
73. Folkow B: Physiological aspects of primary hypertension. Physiol Rev 62:347, 1982.
74. Julius S: Borderline hypertension: Clinical and pathophysiologic significance. Adv Intern Med Pediatr 41:51, 1978.
75. Julius S, Esler M: Autonomic nervous cardiovascular regulation in borderline hypertension. Am J Cardiol 36:685, 1978.
76. Strauer BE: Ventricular function and coronary hemodynamics in hypertensive heart disease. Am J Cardiol 44:999, 1979.
77. Strauer BE: Myocardial oxygen consumption in chronic heart disease: Role of wall stress, hypertrophy and coronary reserve. Am J Cardiol 44:731, 1979.
78. Devereux RB, Pickering TG, Harshfield GA, et al: Left ventricular hypertrophy in patients with hypertension: Importance of blood pressure response to regularly recurring stress. Circulation 68:470, 1983.
79. Sokolow M, Werdegar D, Kain KH: Relationship between level of blood pressure measured casually and by portable recorders and severity of complications in essential hypertension. Circulation 34:279, 1966.
80. Perloff D, Sokolow M, Cowan R: The prognostic value of ambulatory blood pressures. JAMA 249:2792, 1983.
81. Schmieder R, Rüddel H, Neus H, et al: Disparate hemodynamic response to mental challenge after antihypertensive therapy with beta-blockers and calcium-entry blockers. Am J Med 82:11, 1987.
82. Schmieder R, Rüddel H, Schädinger H, et al: Psychophysiologic aspects in essential hypertension. How to perform mental stress tests. J Hum Hypertens 2:223, 1987.
83. Neus H, von Eiff AW, Friedrich G, et al: Der Einfluß β von Betarezeptorenblockern und Diuretika auf die Reaktivität des Blutdrucks. Z Kardiol 72:617, 1983.
84. von Eiff AW, Czernik A, Zanders H: Zur medikamentösen Beeinflussung der Sympathicushyperaktivität: Parasympathomimetikum und Betarezeptorenblocker im kurzdauernden pharmakologischen Experiment am Menschen. Klin Wochenschr 47:701, 1969.
85. Francois B, Cahen R, Gravejat MF, et al: Do beta-blockers prevent pressor responses to mental stress and physical exercise? Eur Heart J 5:348, 1984.
86. Andrén L, Hansson L: Circulatory effects of stress in essential hypertension. Acta Med Scand 646:69, 1980.
87. Nyberg G, Graham RM, Stokes GS: The effect of mental arithmetic in normotensive and hypertensive subjects and its modification by beta-adrenergic receptor blockade. Br J Clin Pharmacol 4:469, 1977.
88. Martin PR, Ebert MH, Gordon EK, et al: Effects of clonidine on central and peripheral catecholamine metabolism. Clin Pharmacol Ther 35:322, 1984.
89. Sullivan PA, de Quattro V, Foti A, et al: Effect of clonidine on central and peripheral nerve tone in primary hypertension. Hypertension 8:611, 1986.
90. Cubeddu LX, Hoffman IS, Davila J, et al: Clonidine reduces elevated cerebrospinal fluid catecholamine levels in patients with essential hypertension. Life Sci 35:1365, 1984.
91. Schmieder RE, Bater M, Langewitz W, et al: Efficacy of four antihypertensive drugs (clonidine, enalapril, nitrendipine, oxprenolol) on stress blood pressure. Am J Cardiol 63:1333, 1989.
92. Falkner B, Onesti G, Lowenthal DT, et al: The use of clonidine monotherapy in adolescent hypertension. Chest 83:425, 1983.
93. Grossman E, Schmieder R, Oren S, et al: Disparate cardiovascular responses to stress during calcium channel blockade and converting enzyme inhibition. Am J Cardiol 72:574, 1993.
94. Rüddel H, Bähr M, Langewitz W, et al: Psychophysiologische Untersuchungen bei Hypertonikern während effektiver Langzeittherapie mit Enalapril. In Brunner HR (ed): Enalapril. Stuttgart: Thieme, 1987, pp 196–208.
95. Schmieder RE, Rüddel H, Schachinger H, et al: Impact of

angiotensin converting enzyme inhibition on the hemodynamic profile during laboratory stress tests. J Hum Hypertens 6:227, 1992.

96. Garavaglia GE, Messerli FH, Schmieder RE, et al: The impact of antihypertensive therapy on cardiovascular reactivity during isometric exercise. Clin Pharmacol Ther 41:173, 1987.

97. Eliot RS, Buell JC, Dembroski TM: Biobehavioral perspectives on coronary heart disease, hypertension and sudden cardiac death. Acta Med Scand Suppl 660:203, 1982.

98. Eliot RS, Buell JL: The role of CNS in cardiovascular disorders. Hosp Pract 18:189, 1983.

99. Keys A, Simonsen E: Mortality and coronary heart disease among men studied for 23 years. Arch Intern Med 128:201, 1971.

100. Morgan KJ, Stampley GL, Zabik ME, et al: Magnesium and calcium dietary intakes of the US population. J Am Coll Nutr 4:195, 1985.

101. Ising H, Neus H, Rüddel H, et al: Intracellular magnesium and blood pressure [Abstract]. Hochdruck 6:32, 1985.

102. Rüddel H, Gogolin E, Neus H: Magnesium and kardiovasku-läre Reaktivität während Belastungsuntersuchungen. Magnesium Bull 4:98, 1982.

103. Altura BM, Altura BT: Role of magnesium ions in contractibility of blood vessels and skeletal muscles. Magnesium Bull 3:102, 1981.

104. Altura BM, Altura BT, Gebrewold A, et al: Magnesium deficiency and hypertension: Correlation between magnesium-deficient rats and microcirculatory changes in situ. Science 223:1315, 1984.

105. Schmieder R, Rüddel H, Neus H, et al: Magnesium homeostasis in hypertensives: Impact on hemodynamic pattern at rest and during challenge [Abstract]. J Am Coll Nutr 4:378, 1985.

106. Cappucio FP, Markandu ND, Beynon GW, et al: Lack of effect of oral magnesium on high blood pressure: A double-blind study. Br Med J 291:235, 1985.

107. Cohen L, Laor A, Kitzes R: Reversible retinal vasospasm in magnesium-treated hypertension despite no significant change in blood pressure. Magnesium 3:159, 1984.

108. Dyckner T, Wester PO: Effect of magnesium on blood pressure. Br Med J 286:1847, 1983.

CHAPTER 25

Cardiovascular Therapy During Pregnancy and Lactation

William B. White, M.D.

HEMODYNAMIC EFFECTS OF PREGNANCY IN HEALTHY WOMEN

Normal pregnancy induces a number of dramatic changes in systemic hemodynamics (Table 25–1), many of which enhance cardiac function to keep up with the demands of the expanding uteroplacental network of blood vessels. By the latter half of pregnancy, the uteroplacental system receives up to 40% of the cardiac output.

A 50% expansion of plasma volume occurs during the first two trimesters of pregnancy.[1, 2] The capacity of the vascular system is increased during pregnancy, apparently secondary to progesterone-induced distention of the great veins[3] and to marked growth of the venous plexus in the broad ligaments of the uterus. The increase in plasma volume is associated with an increase in glomerular filtration rate, plasma renin activity, and plasma aldosterone.[4]

The resting cardiac output increases by an average of 40% above the nonpregnant value by the twentieth week of gestation.[5] This increase in cardiac output is secondary to an augmented stroke volume that develops in the first trimester of pregnancy but is later also associated with an increased heart rate.

Systemic vascular resistance decreases during pregnancy in women without cardiac disease. Although the etiology of the reduction in systemic vascular resistance is not entirely understood, contributing factors include increased secretion of placental and ovarian steroid hormones that are vasodilatory,[6] the effects of prolactin,[7] and trophoblastic erosion of maternal endometrial vessels, causing an effect similar to an arteriovenous fistula.[6]

Systemic arterial pressure decreases near the end of the first trimester, continues to decrease modestly during the second trimester, and then begins to rise toward the prepartum values at the end of pregnancy. The fall in diastolic blood pressure generally exceeds that of the systolic blood pressure.

There are increased demands on the heart during pregnancy secondary to the hemodynamic alterations just described. Resting oxygen consumption increases proportionately less than the cardiac output, so the arteriovenous oxygen difference falls. Anemia, which is relatively common in pregnancy, causes an even greater demand on the heart to keep the peripheral tissues and the enlarged, engorged uterus properly supplied with oxygen-rich blood. Exertional activities during pregnancy demand much of the heart. Oxygen

Table 25–1. Hemodynamic Alterations During Pregnancy

Parameter	Early Pregnancy*	Late Pregnancy†
Mean arterial pressure‡	↓	↔ or ↑
Plasma volume	↑ ↑	↔
Red cell volume	↑	↑ ↑
Heart rate	↑	↑ ↑
Cardiac output	↑ ↑	↓
Stroke volume	↑ ↑	↓
Systemic vascular resistance	↓	↔

↑, Increased; ↓, decreased; ↔, maintained.
*Less than 20 weeks of gestation.
†More than 30 weeks of gestation.
‡Pulse pressure widens until the end of the second trimester.

consumption and cardiac output increase more in the pregnant than in the nonpregnant individual if the same exercise is performed. The hemodynamic compensation throughout pregnancy is an increase in the heart rate, because stroke volume decreases during the latter half of gestation.[8]

During labor, the cardiac output increases up to 40% over the third trimester values but may be modified by anesthesia and by position. The left lateral decubitus position relieves the pressure of the uterus on the inferior vena cava, improves venous return to the heart, and increases cardiac output.[9] During the second stage of labor, the cardiac output may decrease abruptly secondary to the Valsalva maneuver used to effect delivery. Subsequently, delivery results in a rapid increase in the cardiac output, because the blood volume suddenly shifts from the uteroplacental tissues to the intravascular space. Modification of an increase in central blood volume may be induced by anesthetic agents used for cesarean sections or if there is substantial blood loss immediately after delivery.[10]

CARDIAC DISEASE IN PREGNANCY

The most common cardiac disorders in pregnancy are chronic and pregnancy-induced hypertension, cardiac arrhythmias, and congestive heart failure with pulmonary vascular congestion or pulmonary edema. Ischemic heart disease is uncommon in women of child-bearing age; and the incidence of myocardial infarction in pregnant women is exceedingly low.[11] The most common cause of congestive heart failure in pregnancy has historically been rheumatic heart disease—specifically, mitral stenosis. Because mitral stenosis impairs diastolic filling, an increase in heart rate during pregnancy reduces left ventricular filling time and may induce acute pulmonary vascular congestion in a woman who was absolutely asymptomatic prior to pregnancy. Fortunately, the incidence of rheumatic valvular disease has diminished markedly over the past two decades, although it is still (apart from hypertension) the most common cardiac disorder in pregnancy, whereas congestive failure is uncommon.[7]

The most commonly used cardiac drugs during pregnancy are the antihypertensives, the antiarrhythmic agents, and the digitalis glycosides. The diuretics generally have been avoided in pregnancy, because the thiazide diuretics have been linked to possible thrombocytopenia and jaundice in the newborn, especially when used in the third trimester.[12] If absolutely essential, the loop diuretics have been used in conjunction with salt restriction, rest, and the cardiac glycosides.

This chapter focuses on the safety (to the fetus) and efficacy of the cardiac drugs in pregnancy and during lactation. The efficacy of antihypertensive drugs is assessed not only by the drugs' ability to lower blood pressure but also by their ability to improve fetal outcome. In other cardiac diseases (e.g., ventricular arrhythmias), drugs *must* be used for the welfare and safety of the mother. In these instances, sparse data

regarding safety to the developing fetus are mentioned, but controlled clinical trials with antiischemic agents, inotropic drugs, and antiarrhythmics have not been performed.

ANTIHYPERTENSIVE THERAPY DURING PREGNANCY

Growth and development of the fetus are jeopardized in the presence of maternal hypertension, and clinical trials have shown that good control of the blood pressure lowers fetal risk. What is a normal blood pressure in nonpregnant women may be considered elevated during pregnancy. The average value for seated blood pressure in the first trimester of pregnancy is about 103/56 mmHg and toward term averages 109/69 mmHg.[13] Thus, many obstetricians would consider blood pressure levels greater than 130/80 mmHg to be abnormal.

Drug therapy should be tailored to maintain the blood pressure below 135/85 mmHg throughout the pregnancy. If the patient is chronically hypertensive and already on medication, doses may have to be lowered during the first trimester as vasodilation occurs and then readjusted at the end of the second trimester or early third trimester. In pregnancy-induced hypertension, many obstetricians will observe the patient in the hospital using nonpharmacologic therapy prior to initiating antihypertensive drugs. Bedrest in the left lateral decubitus position, restriction of sodium intake to 1 or 2 g/day, and sedation are used widely. An evaluation process for fetal distress and signs of preeclampsia is performed to make decisions regarding early delivery at this time.

Diuretics

Considerable controversy exists regarding the use of diuretics in hypertensive women during pregnancy, even if the drug was effective prior to the pregnancy. A review of 25 years of randomized clinical trials of diuretic use in pregnancy in 7000 patients[14] reported that using the thiazide diuretics for hypertension and edema prevented preeclampsia, possibly secondary to the reduction of blood pressure. A diagnosis of preeclampsia requires the presence of both peripheral edema and elevated blood pressure. Thus, if these signs of preeclampsia have been removed by a diuretic, the incidence of disease reporting may have been altered even though maternal mortality and fetal outcome may have been unchanged.[14]

Hypertension during pregnancy, particularly pregnancy-induced hypertension and preeclampsia, is associated with reduced plasma volume.[15] Thus, thiazide and loop diuretics are recommended only in cases of congestive heart failure and hypertension associated with significant volume overload, such as with renal insufficiency. Potassium-sparing diuretics (e.g., spironolactone) have been reported to be effective in the management of primary hyperaldosteronism in pregnancy[16] but are relatively ineffective in pregnancy-induced hypertension.[17]

α₂-Agonists

α-Methyldopa is an effective antihypertensive agent that is used widely in treating all types of pregnancy hypertension. In addition, methyldopa has been studied rigorously in pregnant, chronically hypertensive women, both in controlled clinical trials and in comparisons with other classes of antihypertensive agents. Redman et al.[18] have performed the most extensive controlled evaluation of the effects of methyldopa on blood pressure, perinatal mortality and morbidity, and fetal loss in hypertensive women. In their report, methyldopa was found to be effective in lowering blood pressure and significantly reduced the incidence of severe or accelerated hypertension in late pregnancy or during labor. Perhaps more dramatic, however, was the reduction in perinatal fetal death: nine pregnancy losses (7.2%) occurred in the untreated group of 125 women and one fetal death (0.9%) occurred in the treated group of 117 women. Maternal side effects of methyldopa were similar to those seen in the nonobstetric population and included fatigue, dizziness, and depression.

Of the children born to the mothers in the above trial, 195 were followed-up by pediatricians for more than 7 years to evaluate the frequency of problems with physical or mental health, sight, hearing, intelligence, stature, and blood pressure.[19] Except for a small size difference between boys from the untreated group and those whose mothers were treated with methyldopa, no differences were noted in any of the above parameters in the offspring of mothers treated with methyldopa compared with the control group. This thorough long-term follow-up reinforces the efficacy and safety of methyldopa use in women with pregnancy-induced hypertension, especially if it is initiated in the middle of the second trimester or later.

In controlled studies,[20, 21] clonidine hydrochloride has also been reported to be safe in the treatment of women with hypertension during pregnancy. Horvath et al.[21] compared clonidine with methyldopa in a double-blind randomized trial in 100 women with hypertension during pregnancy. Blood pressure control was similar in each drug treatment group, and one neonatal loss (2%) occurred in each group, which was not thought to be secondary to the drugs. When 47 neonates were examined for 7 days after delivery from mothers treated with clonidine in doses of 150 to 1200 μg/day, no clinically significant hypotension or rebound hypertension was found by the same authors.[22] No long-term follow-up has been made of children born to mothers treated with clonidine during pregnancy.

α₁-Adrenergic Blocking Agents

Studies with prazosin in women with pregnancy-induced hypertension have been small and uncontrolled and generally restricted to more severe hypertension or combination therapy with β-blocking agents. Rubin et al.[23] reported that prazosin effectively controlled blood pressure in six of eight women who did not respond to β-adrenoreceptor blockade during the last trimester of pregnancy. The mean elimination half-life of prazosin is prolonged by about 30% in pregnant women in comparison with age-matched healthy men. No adverse effects of the drug were seen in the newborn.

In studies of pregnant women with severe essential hypertension that combined prazosin with the β-blocking agent oxprenolol, blood pressure control generally was improved enough to avoid parenteral drugs,[24, 25] and pregnancy was prolonged. In preeclamptic patients, however, prazosin therapy did not change the clinical outcome, and parenteral antihypertensives were required in most women. Average doses of prazosin in these studies were 1 to 2 mg three times daily.

Labetalol, which blocks α₁-, β₁-, and β₂-receptor sites, has been used for a number of years in hypertension associated with pregnancy. It appears to have its greatest value in severe essential hypertension when it is administered both in the oral form and intravenously. In a study by Michael,[26] 85 women with severe hypertension complicating pregnancy were treated with labetalol in doses of 200 to 1200 mg daily. Ninety-three percent of the patients had good control of blood pressure without significant maternal side effects. No congenital abnormalities were noted in any of the infants delivered, but intrauterine growth retardation was present in 24 of 89 neonates (27%), mainly in mothers with preeclampsia. The growth abnormality is probably secondary to the hypertensive disease process itself; radionuclide studies of uteroplacental blood flow indicate that, although labetalol significantly reduces maternal blood pressure, uteroplacental blood flow index does not change.[27] In a study of labetalol[28] in late (>32 weeks' gestation) pregnancy-induced hypertension, blood pressure and proteinuria were reduced, but the length of gestation was not prolonged and maternal outcome was unchanged.

β-Adrenergic Blocking Agents

Until recently, the β-adrenergic blocking agents were generally avoided in pregnancy because of reported maternal, fetal, and neonatal adverse side effects (Table 25–2). However, these reports were either anecdotal or based on retrospective analysis by reviewing charts, often a number of years after the

Table 25–2. **Potential Adverse Effects of β-Adrenergic Blocking Agents in Pregnancy Hypertension**

Premature or prolonged labor
Fetal or neonatal bradycardia (transient)
Delayed spontaneous breathing in the newborn (more common with intravenously administered β-blocker)
Neonatal hypoglycemia
Hyperbilirubinemia (rare)

events. In addition, β-blockers were used in women with refractory hypertension and preeclampsia, who generally have poor outcomes secondary to their underlying disease process. The large clinical trials of the marketed β-blockers that have been performed over the past few years have concluded that β-blockers are beneficial in the treatment of hypertension and cardiac disease.

A double-blind, placebo-controlled study of atenolol as a monotherapy of pregnancy-induced hypertension[29] in 120 women demonstrated that this cardioselective β-blocker in doses of 100 to 200 mg daily lowered blood pressure, whereas standard bedrest and sodium restriction had no effect. Atenolol therapy was associated with a marked reduction in the incidence of severe hypertension and the development of proteinuria (7% treated versus 100% untreated). Although transient neonatal bradycardia (none requiring intervention or therapy) was reported in the atenolol-treated group, 1-year follow-up of these children showed no difference in growth indices or development.[30] In another study with atenolol in moderate and severe hypertension during pregnancy, Fabregues et al. showed that preeclamptic patients required higher doses (100 ± 41 mg/day) than did chronic hypertensives without proteinuria (63 ± 23 mg/day) and gestational hypertensives without proteinuria (70 ± 30 mg/day) to achieve blood pressure control.[31]

The β-blocker propranolol has been used in a number of disorders other than hypertension during pregnancy. There have been reports[32] of its successful use in maternal thyrotoxicosis, obstructive cardiomyopathy, paroxysmal atrial tachycardia, dysfunctional uterine activity, and fetal tachycardia. No fetal abnormalities were reported in the various studies using propranolol for these problems. Intravenously delivered propranolol immediately prior to cesarean section appears to delay spontaneous respiration in the newborn, occasionally severely enough to require intubation.[33]

The effects of the cardioselective β-blockers atenolol and metoprolol in hypertensive, diabetic pregnant women have been studied by Olofsson et al.[34] In this report, the women were observed for a control period during which baseline blood pressure, glucose and insulin homeostasis, and fetal heart rate were established before they began therapy. Although the β-receptor blockade reduced blood pressure in 80% of the patients, no alterations of blood sugar or changes in insulin dose were noted. Fetal heart rate was reduced modestly on β-blocker therapy, but all infants had normal Apgar scores and were healthy at 1 to 4 years of age.

The long-acting, cardioselective β-blocker, betaxolol, was used to treat 22 mildly hypertensive pregnant women in a pilot study by Boutroy et al. All women carried their pregnancies to term, and mean Apgar blood pressure control was excellent in 20 of 22 women. Nine months following delivery, all 23 babies (1 twin pregnancy) were in good health.[35]

A number of studies[36, 37] have compared a β-blocker with methyldopa in the treatment of pregnancy-induced hypertension. Little difference is apparent in the blood pressure–lowering effects of oxprenolol, acebutolol, atenolol, pindolol, and propranolol compared with methyldopa. β-Blockers are better tolerated by the pregnant patient than is methyldopa; however, the thorough 7-year follow-up of the children of mothers treated with methyldopa provides an undeniable reassurance.[19]

Calcium Antagonists

Despite their widespread use in the treatment of hypertension and angina pectoris, limited data are available on the use of calcium antagonists in women with hypertension during pregnancy. Studies have been limited to evaluation of the dihydropyridines nifedipine and nitrendipine in severe or accelerated hypertension. Walters and Redman[38] reported that nifedipine was highly effective in severe hypertension of late pregnancy (blood pressure >170/110 mmHg) in oral doses of 5 to 15 mg. No effects on fetal heart rate or postpartum uterine bleeding were noted following nifedipine therapy. Limited experience with nifedipine in severe hypertension associated with preeclampsia[36] suggests that it is also effective over a 4- to 6-week period. A preliminary study[39] of a single 20-mg dose of nitrendipine demonstrated effective lowering of blood pressure (by 17/18 mmHg) in hypertensive women in the latter third of pregnancy, with no change in fetal heart rate. The apparent efficacy of these calcium antagonists in treating severe hypertension during pregnancy warrants further evaluation in controlled clinical trials.

Angiotensin-Converting Enzyme Inhibitors

Only anecdotal reports have been made of the use of angiotensin-converting enzyme (ACE) inhibitors for severe hypertension during pregnancy. A major reason for avoiding ACE inhibitors during pregnancy has been the findings of increased intrauterine death and stillbirth in pregnant animals treated with captopril.[40] Pregnancy outcome in 19 mothers following exposure to ACE inhibitors was reviewed by Piper et al.[41] Two outcomes included one preterm anemic infant requiring dialysis and a second infant that had microcephaly and an encephalocele. In a single case studied by Barr and Cohen,[42] the fetal renal abnormality following enalapril exposure was lack of proximal tubular differentiation.

Cases of successful treatment with captopril in severe hypertension were, in general, women who had not responded to more orthodox therapy or who had renovascular hypertension and repeated spontaneous abortions.[43–45] Levels of plasma renin activity and aldosterone in the baby do not appear to be greatly affected by maternal captopril administration.

Vasodilators

Hydralazine, like methyldopa, has been commonly used for the treatment of chronic, moderate hypertension during pregnancy because it has been shown to have no adverse effect on uterine blood flow.[46] Hydralazine, administered orally, is effective monotherapy for lowering blood pressure. Despite these antihypertensive effects, it does not appear to have any major impact on the fetal complications of hypertension.[47] Conversely, because hydralazine lowers blood pressure when given alone or in combination with a β-blocker,[47] it may delay the onset of preeclampsia until later in the third trimester. A recent study that compared prostacyclin (epoprostenol) with dihydralazine in severely hypertensive women showed similar efficacy in blood pressure lowering but less reflex tachycardia with epoprostenol infusion.[48]

Severe Hypertension and Preeclampsia

Severe hypertension with or without preeclampsia is usually treated with parenteral vasodilators such as hydralazine, diazoxide, labetalol, and, rarely, sodium nitroprusside (Table 25–3). In acute cases, intravenously administered hydralazine decreases systemic vascular resistance, increases heart rate, and increases cardiac index. Patients with chronic hypertension generally respond less well to parenteral hydralazine than do women with preeclampsia.[49] In addition, concern exists that hydralazine may worsen fetal risk secondary to excessive hypotension and acute uteroplacental insufficiency in preeclamptic women.

Labetalol given intravenously may be as effective or more effective than hydralazine or diazoxide for severe, accelerated hypertension during pregnancy. Labetalol is relatively predictable, causing less overshoot hypotension, not increasing maternal heart rate, and not reducing the uteroplacental blood flow index.[27, 50] Diazoxide is not generally recommended as first-line treatment for acute hypertension during pregnancy because it can induce profound and prolonged reductions in blood pressure. Small (50- to 100-mg) intravenous injections lessen the likelihood of excessive hypotension with diazoxide.[51]

The limited use of sodium nitroprusside[52] and intravenously administered nitroglycerin[53] has been reported in women with severe pregnancy-induced hypertension. Concern always exists that, although sodium nitroprusside is extremely effective in lowering blood pressure, it is a ferrocyanide that may be toxic to the fetus. One report[54] suggests that cyanide levels in the fetal liver may be below the established toxic range. Wasserman showed that there was a bimodal distribution of the effect of nitroprusside in severely hypertensive, preeclamptic women.[55] In some women, presumably with reduced effective blood volume, nitroprusside induced a fall in heart rate in association with large reductions in pressure. Cotton et al.[53] performed a hemodynamic evaluation of intravenous nitroglycerin administration in women with severe pregnancy-induced hypertension and demonstrated that volume expansion negates most of the drug's capability to lower systemic arterial pressure and pulmonary capillary wedge pressure.

Magnesium sulfate is commonly administered as a central nervous system depressant in the preeclamptic woman who is about to undergo delivery. Hemodynamic effects of magnesium sulfate given intravenously include a mild, transient decrease in mean arterial pressure coupled with a modest increase in cardiac output.[56] These parameters return to baseline and are not affected by constant infusion of the drug.

ANTIARRHYTHMIC DRUG THERAPY DURING PREGNANCY

Organic heart disease is seen more often during pregnancy both because medical and surgical management of congenital heart disease has improved and because more older women become pregnant.[57] Thus, cardiac dysfunction is increasingly common during pregnancy, and physicians must be concerned with the treatment of arrhythmias that might develop. Although the management of women with cardiac arrhythmias during pregnancy is not different from the treatment of nonobstetric patients, special consideration must be given to antiarrhythmic therapy to avoid adverse effects on the fetus. The indications for

Table 25–3. **Parenteral Antihypertensive Agents Used in Severe Essential or Pregnancy-Induced Hypertension**

Agent	Usual Dosages	Side Effects and Concerns
Diazoxide	50–100 mg IV injection, repeat once *or* 250 mg in 100 ml D₅W, infuse over 30–60 min	Precipitous maternal hypotension, fetal distress
Hydralazine	10–20 mg slow IV injection	Excessive maternal hypotension: reflex sympathetic tachycardia
Labetalol	10–20 mg slow IV injection *or* 0.25–2.0 mg/min constant infusion	Previous antiadrenergic therapy may reduce effectiveness
Nitroglycerin	0.1 μg/kg/min initially to 2.0 μg/kg/min	Effectiveness may be attenuated by increased volume
Sodium nitroprusside	0.5–3.5 μg/kg/min infusion	Thiocyanate accumulation in fetus; intensive monitoring required

the various antiarrhythmic compounds are listed in Table 25–4.

Digitalis Glycosides

Both digoxin and digitoxin cross the placenta, and serum concentrations of digoxin are similar in the newborn and mother at term.[58] No reports have been made of teratogenicity from a digitalis preparation, nor have there been untoward fetal effects from chronic maintenance digoxin therapy in the mother.[57] However, fetal deaths associated with maternal digitalis toxicity have been reported.[59]

The serum digoxin concentration in pregnant mothers is reduced by as much as 50% when compared with that of nonpregnant women[58] secondary to a rise in renal blood flow and clearance. Pharmacologic interactions of digoxin with quinidine, verapamil, or both during pregnancy are similar to those in the nonpregnant woman, and digoxin dosing may require downward adjustment if concomitant antiarrhythmic therapy is required.

Lidocaine

Most data on lidocaine in pregnancy evaluate the drug's efficacy as an anesthetic agent administered epidurally or in paracervical or pudendal blocks. A low incidence of side effects is associated with lidocaine infusions epidurally; mean neonatal plasma concentrations of lidocaine are about 50% of maternal values.[60] Lidocaine toxicity in the neonate has been associated with fetal acidosis and attributed to ion trapping.[61] The clinical signs of lidocaine toxicity in the infant include respiratory depression, apnea, bradycardia, and prolongation of the QT interval.

Disopyramide

Disopyramide crosses the placenta and is present in the newborn,[62] but data are insufficient to make generalized recommendations about this drug's utility in treating arrhythmias in pregnant women. Disopyramide may be beneficial in refractory ventricular arrhythmias,[57] but it may induce uterine contractions.[63]

Phenytoin

Phenytoin is an effective drug for both supraventricular and ventricular arrhythmias secondary to digitalis toxicity. Because phenytoin (diphenylhydantoin) is frequently used as an anticonvulsant, a substantial amount of data is available on its effects on the fetus. When phenytoin is administered to the mother during the first trimester, a syndrome of birth defects that includes mental retardation, craniofacial malformation, cleft palate, and congenital heart defects (fetal hydantoin syndrome) may develop. Thus, except for extreme cases of refractory, acute tachyarrhythmias associated with digitalis toxicity, phenytoin administration should be avoided during pregnancy.

Procainamide

Two reports[64, 65] have studied the effectiveness of procainamide in fetuses with supraventricular tachycardias. Procainamide may be effective in both maternal and fetal arrhythmias refractory to digoxin or quinidine; however, in view of the limited amount of information available in the literature, recommendations for chronic therapy with this agent are not possible.

Table 25–4. **Antiarrhythmic Drugs in Pregnancy**

Drug	Major Indications	Transplacental Passage*	Comments and Concerns
Adenosine	Supraventricular arrhythmias	—	Limited information available
Amiodarone	Refractory ventricular and supraventricular arrhythmias	0.15	Amiodarone contains large amounts of iodine; may pose fetal risk (e.g., thyroid development)
β-Blockers	Rate control or temination of atrial arrhythmias	0.5–1.5	Neonatal respiratory delay and bradycardia
Digoxin	Rate control of atrial fibrillation and treatment of PAT	1.0	Fetal distress with digitalis toxicity; adjust dose with concomitant quinidine or verapamil
Disopyramide	Atrial and ventricular ectopy	0.4	Uterine contractions may develop; little experience in newborn outcome reported
Esmolol	Supraventricular arrhythmias	—	Reduces fetal heart rate
Lidocaine	Ventricular tachyarrhythmias	0.5	Respiratory depression, apnea, bradycardia reported
Phenytoin	Ventricular ectopy secondary to digitalis toxicity	0.8	Fetal hydantoin syndrome
Procainamide	Atrial and ventricular tachyarrhythmias	0.25	Limited information available
Verapamil	PAT, rate control of atrial fibrillation	0.4	Limited experience; no adverse fetal effects reported

PAT, paroxysmal atrial tachycardia.
*Cord blood:maternal blood concentration ratio.

Quinidine

A number of reports[57, 66, 67] demonstrate the effectiveness of quinidine in treating supraventricular and ventricular tachycardia during pregnancy. No teratogenic or other adverse fetal side effects were noted in these cases. As with other antiarrhythmic drugs, clinical trials have not been performed with quinidine.

Quinidine does cross the placenta, and maternal levels of the drug may fall as much as 50% compared with nonpregnant concentrations. Fetal tachycardia readily responds to the excellent transplacental passage of quinidine and may be converted following a single maternal dose.[68] Quinidine may be added to digoxin as a second drug for cardioversion of atrial tachycardia in the fetus.

Side effects possibly attributed to quinidine include induction of premature labor, fetal eighth cranial nerve damage, and spontaneous abortion. Fortunately, these noted adverse problems are rare and are associated with toxic doses of the drug.

Verapamil

Data on the use of verapamil in pregnancy are limited to a few reports of its administration in maternal supraventricular tachycardia and fetal tachycardia. Klein and Repke[69, 70] reported success using intravenously administered verapamil (2.5 to 5.0 mg, single dose) in a 36-week pregnant, middle-aged woman with supraventricular tachycardia refractory to β-blocking agents and digoxin. The patient was not maintained on oral verapamil therapy, and no adverse fetal effects were noted.

Intrauterine supraventricular tachycardia has been successfully converted with orally administered verapamil (80 mg t.i.d.) when digoxin failed,[71, 72] and the fetal outcome has been good. An advantage of verapamil therapy for fetal supraventricular tachycardia is improved maternal tolerance over large doses of digitalis or quinidine.

Adenosine

Little is known about the endogenous purine nucleoside, adenosine, in arrhythmias during pregnancy. In a recent case report, Afridi et al. successfully treated a narrow complex supraventricular tachycardia with 12 mg of adenosine administered intravenously in a pregnant woman with Wolff-Parkinson-White syndrome. No untoward effects were reported in the infant.[73]

Amiodarone

The clinical experience with amiodarone in pregnancy is limited to a few case reports. There has been great concern that this compound, which is 39% iodine by weight, could induce thyroid disease in the fetus or have other unknown effects. Two reports[74, 75] followed women on amiodarone therapy through a large part of their pregnancies and noted no adverse effects in the neonates. Transplacental passage of amiodarone is high and may induce low birth weight, hypothyroidism, prolonged QT interval on the electrocardiogram, and brachycardias.[76, 77] Because of the limited clinical experience with amiodarone and the general toxicity of iodides in pregnancy,[78] this drug must be used during pregnancy only for life-threatening arrhythmias refractory to the other antiarrhythmic agents mentioned earlier.

Esmolol

The rapid-acting, β₁-selective adrenoreceptor blocking agent, esmolol, has been assessed in three pregnancies.[79-81] Although no fetal morbidity has been observed, esmolol is rapidly passed by the placenta, and fetal brachycardia is a possibility and may require emergency cesarean delivery.[79]

CARDIAC DRUG THERAPY DURING LACTATION

Drug transfer and concentration in breast milk depend on the physical and chemical properties of the drug. The most important factors affecting drug excretion into breast milk include degree of ionization, protein binding, molecular weight, and lipid solubility.[82, 83] Because the pH of human milk (about 7.0) is less than that of plasma (7.40), the concentration that a drug attains in milk depends largely on its pKa value. In general, the ultrafiltrate milk/plasma concentration ratio for weak acids is less than 1 and for weak bases is greater than 1.

An estimate of drug intake in an infant can be made if levels in the breast milk and maternal dose are known. Immature neonatal excretory mechanisms, maternal drug absorption, and minor variations in the breast milk may alter the estimated values.[82] Because newborn infants take in an average of 165 ml/kg/day of milk,[84] the estimated maximal dose to the infant is

$$\text{peak concentration in milk (ng/ml)} \times$$
$$165 \text{ ml/kg/day} =$$
$$\text{the daily dose (ng or ng/kg/day)}$$

Women of child-bearing age with cardiac disorders, including hypertension or cardiac arrhythmias, may wish to breastfeed their infants despite the need for antihypertensive or antiarrhythmic drug therapy. Highly sensitive assays using high-performance liquid chromatography or gas chromatographic methods with detection limits of 1 to 5 ng/ml allow us to identify most of these drugs in milk. Thus, the general recommendation would be to prescribe those agents found in minimal concentrations in the milk. After the mother discontinues breastfeeding, a change could be made to another agent that is more effective or perhaps better tolerated.

Information on excretion of cardiac drugs in breast milk is summarized in Table 25–5.

Table 25–5. **Cardiac Drug Excretion in Breast Milk**

Drug	Daily Dose (mg)	Average Concentration in Milk	Milk:Plasma Ratio	Transfer to Infant
Atenolol	100	0.6 µg/ml	3.0	10 µg/ml; may induce neonatal depression
Captopril	300	5.0 µg/ml	0.1	Not studied
Chlorthalidone	50	0.3 ng/ml	0.05	Not studied
Clonidine	0.15	1.5 ng/ml	1.5	Not studied
Digoxin	0.25	1.0 µg/ml	1.0	Not studied
Diltiazem	240	200.0 ng/ml	1.0	Not studied
Disopyramide	600	3.0 µg/ml	0.9	Not studied
Enalapril	20	1.74 ng/ml	0.01	Not studied
Flecainide	200	0.75 ng/ml	3.5	Not studied
Hydralazine	150	0.8 µg/ml	0.5	Not studied
Hydrochlorothiazide	50	100.0 ng/ml	0.4	Not detected (<1 ng/ml)
Methyldopa	1000	1.0 µg/ml	0.3	Plasma level of 0.09 µg/ml; no adverse effects noted
Metoprolol	200	1.7 µg/ml	3.0	Not studied
Mexiletine	600	—	1.5	Not known
Nadolol	80	0.35 µg/ml	5.0	Not reported
Nifedipine	90	10 ng/ml	—	Not studied
Nitrendipine	10	5.0 ng/ml	2.5	Not studied
Oxprenolol	160	130.0 ng/ml	0.3	Not elevated
Propranolol	160	50.0 ng/ml	0.6	No adverse effects noted
Quinidine sulfate	600	1.0 ng/ml	1.0	? Hepatic accumulation in premature infants
Sotalol	160	4 µg/ml	5.6	Not studied
Timolol	15	16.0 ng/ml	0.8	Not studied
Verapamil	240	20.0 µg/ml	0.4	Not detected in infants' plasma

Antihypertensive and Antiischemic Agents

Diuretics

The thiazide diuretics may suppress lactation or decrease milk production.[84] Several reports have been made of thiazide diuretics appearing in milk but in quantities highly unlikely to affect the breastfed infant.[85, 86] In the one case in which infant transfer was studied,[86] no hydrochlorothiazide was detected, and no adverse effects were noted in the baby. Despite these findings, reduction in milk volume is a relative contraindication to using diuretics for hypertension in lactating women. In the rare instance of congestive heart failure in a postpartum woman, diuretics must be used and, if administered in large doses, may necessitate supplementing breastfeeding with infant formula.

α₂-Agonists

α-Methyldopa is widely used in the treatment of hypertension in pregnancy and would be a likely drug for administration in the immediate postpartum period. In a study of three hypertensive, lactating women, the range of methyldopa concentrations in breast milk was 0.2 to 1.14 µg/ml and was related in part to the pH of the milk and the dose.[87] Infant transfer was detected, but no objective side effects were noted.

Clonidine has been reported to be detectable in breast milk when administered to the mother in doses as low as 0.15 mg daily.[82] No data are available on neonatal adverse side effects. No reports have been found on the disposition of guanabenz, prazosin, or guanadrel in human breast milk.

β-Adrenergic Blocking Agents

The β-blocking drugs are all weak bases and thus they are trapped in the milk as a result of ionization. Their milk/plasma ratio is generally greater than 1.[82] However, hydrophilic β-blockers, such as atenolol,[88] are bound weakly to plasma proteins and thus are found in higher concentration in milk than are the lipophilic β-blockers (e.g., propranolol), which are more strongly bound to the plasma proteins.[89]

Accumulation of the hydrophilic β-blockers atenolol, metoprolol, and nadolol in breast milk does not usually appear great enough to cause any notable fetal adverse side effects;[82, 88] in the case of high-dose atenolol, milk concentrations may be great enough to induce infant transfer and induce fetal symptoms.[90] Pindolol, propranolol, oxprenolol, and timolol have milk/plasma ratios less than 1 and appear in concentrations in the milk that are one third to one tenth of the levels seen with hydrophilic β-adrenergic blockers.[82, 89] Thus, it may be more appropriate to use lipophilic β-blockers during lactation as tolerated for hypertension or control of arrhythmias.

Calcium Antagonists

All data available on the excretion of calcium antagonists in human breast milk are in the form of individual case reports. Diltiazem was evaluated in a

40-year-old woman with complex ventricular arrhythmias following 4 days of administration at doses of 60 mg q.i.d. The diltiazem levels in the milk followed those in plasma and peaked 2 hours after dosing at 200 ng/ml.[91] Infant transfer was not evaluated.

A number of case studies[92–94] report the excretion of verapamil and its metabolite, norverapamil, in breast milk. The concentration of verapamil in milk ranges from 23% to 64% of the maternal plasma concentration. Verapamil was undetectable in the plasma of two infants[93, 94] when the mothers received 80 to 120 mg.

At therapeutic doses, the dihydropyridines (e.g., nifedipine) are found in concentrations ranging from 1 to 30 ng/ml in plasma,[95] making detection in milk problematic. In another single report,[96] nifedipine was detectable in milk following a maternal dosing regimen of 30 mg every 8 hours. The authors of this study estimated that the amount of nifedipine transferred into human milk was less than 5% of a therapeutic dose. The authors evaluated the excretion of the long-acting dihydropyridine calcium antagonist nitrendipine in human breast milk after a single dose of 10 mg. The milk/plasma ratio was about 2.5, with peak levels in the milk of 5 ng/ml 2 hours after dosing.[97]

ACE Inhibitors

The ACE inhibitor captopril was analyzed in the breast milk of 11 volunteers taking doses of 100 mg t.i.d.[98] Peak concentration in the milk was only 5 ng/ml, which was 0.6% of the maternal plasma concentration. Infant transfer was not studied.

Enalapril

Redman et al.[99] studied the excretion of enalapril and enalaprilat in milk in five lactating women. The milk concentrations were quite low after a 20-mg dose of enalapril. Total daily enalaprilat amounts in the milk were estimated to be under 2 mg.

Antiarrhythmic Agents

Digitalis

Digoxin is secreted into breast milk at a concentration similar to that of the steady-state serum concentration of the mother.[100] After 10 days of breastfeeding, no digoxin was detected in the nursing infant's blood following long-term administration of the drug in a mother with mitral valve disease. It was estimated that the total amount of digoxin excreted in milk would be 1 to 2 μg/day. No data are available for digitoxin or ouabain.

Disopyramide

Disopyramide was present in breast milk in a woman who was taking 200 mg t.i.d. with a calculated milk/plasma ratio of 0.9.[101] The estimated dose likely to be ingested by the infant is less than 2 mg/kg/day. Infant plasma samples after 28 days of breastfeeding while the mother was taking disopyramide showed no detectable drug. In another similar study,[102] Ellsworth et al. reported maximal transferable disopyramide doses of 3.7 mg/day (<2 mg/kg/day), assuming a milk intake of approximately 1 L.

Lidocaine

Because lidocaine is a parenteral agent used for the acute treatment of malignant ventricular arrhythmias, it is unlikely that a nursing mother receiving this drug would be in a position to breastfeed. A single report suggests that lidocaine is excreted into the breast milk at concentrations 40% of that found in maternal serum.[103]

Mexiletine

Mexiletine was excreted in the milk of a 30-year-old woman taking the drug on a dosing schedule of 200 mg every 8 hours.[104] The mean milk/plasma ratio of nine samples collected hourly was 1.45. No infant plasma samples were obtained.

Quinidine

Only one report[67] evaluates the disposition of quinidine sulfate in human breast milk. Hill and Malkasian[67] reported that quinidine is excreted in breast milk with a milk/plasma ratio of 1, and prolonged exposure may result in hepatic accumulation in the premature infant.

Sotalol

In a patient receiving sotalol, 80 mg twice daily, milk concentrations of the drug were 3 to 5 times greater than maternal serum concentrations. Infant cord serum levels were similar to internal serum levels.[105]

Flecainide

In 11 lactating women who were not nursing, the disposition of 100 mg of orally administered flecainide twice daily in milk was studied. The maximal milk concentrations of flecainide ranged from 270 to 1529 ng/μl. The infant transfer was *estimated* at 0.27 mg/kg.[106]

REFERENCES

1. Hytten FE, Paintin DB: Increase in plasma volume during normal pregnancy. J Obstet Gynaecol Br Commonw 70:402, 1963.
2. Rorinsky JJ, Jaffin H: Cardiovascular hemodynamics in pregnancy: I. Blood and plasma volumes in multiple pregnancy. Am J Obstet Gynecol 93:1, 1965.
3. Keates JS, Fitzgerald DE: Limb volume and blood flow changes during the menstrual cycle: II. Changes in blood flow and venous distensibility during the menstrual cycle. Angiology 20:624, 1969.

4. Watanabe M, Mecker CI, Gray MJ, et al: Secretion rate of aldosterone in normal pregnancy. J Clin Invest 42:1619, 1963.
5. Ueland K, Metcalfe J: Circulatory changes in pregnancy. Clin Obstet Gynecol 18:41, 1975.
6. Metcalfe J, Ueland K: Maternal cardiovascular adjustments to pregnancy. Prog Cardiovasc Dis 16:363, 1974.
7. Pearson CS: Cardiac disease in pregnancy. In Arias F (ed): High Risk Pregnancy and Delivery. St. Louis: CV Mosby, 1984, pp 181–199.
8. Ueland K, Novy MJ, Metcalfe J: Hemodynamic responses of patients with heart disease to pregnancy and exercise. Am J Obstet Gynecol 113:47, 1972.
9. Metcalfe J, McAnulty JH, Ueland K: Cardiovascular physiology. Clin Obstet Gynecol 24:693, 1981.
10. Ueland K, Hansen J: Maternal cardiovascular dynamics: III. Labor and delivery under local and caudal analgesia. Am J Obstet Gynecol 103:8, 1969.
11. Ginz B: Myocardial infarction in pregnancy. Br J Obstet Gynaecol 77:610, 1970.
12. Gray MJ: Use and abuse of thiazides in pregnancy. Clin Obstet Gynaecol 11:568, 1968.
13. MacGillivray I, Rose GA, Rowe B: Blood pressure survey in pregnancy. Clin Sci 37:395, 1965.
14. Collins R, Yusuf S, Peto R: Overview of randomised trials of diuretics in pregnancy. Br Med J 290:17, 1985.
15. Gallery EDM, Hunyor SN, Gyory AZ: Plasma volume contraction: A significant factor in both pregnancy-associated hypertension and chronic hypertension in pregnancy. Q J Med 48:593, 1979.
16. Lotgering FK, Derkz FMH, Wallenburg HCS: Primary hyperaldosteronism in pregnancy. Am J Obstet Gynecol 155:986, 1986.
17. Liedholm H, Melander A: Drug selection in the treatment of pregnancy hypertension. Acta Obstet Gynecol Scand Suppl 118:49, 1984.
18. Redman CWG, Beillin LJ, Bonnar J, et al: Fetal outcome in trial of antihypertensive treatment in pregnancy. Lancet 2:753, 1976.
19. Cockburn J, Moar VA, Ounsted N, et al: Final report of the study on hypertension during pregnancy: The effects of specific treatment on the growth and development of the children. Lancet 1:647, 1982.
20. Tuimala R, Punnomen R, Kauppila E: Clonidine in the treatment of hypertension during pregnancy. Ann Chir Gynaecol 197:47, 1985.
21. Horvath JS, Phippard A, Korda A, et al: Clonidine hydrochloride. A safe and effective antihypertensive agent in pregnancy. Obstet Gynecol 66:634, 1985.
22. Henderson-Smart DJ, Horvath JS, Phippard A, et al: Effect of antihypertensive drugs on neonatal blood pressure. Clin Exp Pharmacol Physiol 11:351, 1984.
23. Rubin PC, Butters L, Low RA, et al: Clinical pharmacology studies with prazosin during pregnancy complicated by hypertension. Br J Clin Pharmacol 16:543, 1983.
24. Lubbe WF, Hodge JV: Combined alpha- and beta-adrenoreceptor antagonism with prazosin and oxprenolol in control of severe hypertension in pregnancy. N Z Med J 94:169, 1981.
25. Domisse J, Davey DA, Roos PJ: Prazosin and oxprenolol therapy in pregnancy hypertension. S Afr Med J 64:231, 1983.
26. Michael CA: The evaluation of labetalol in the treatment of hypertension complicating pregnancy. Br J Clin Pharmacol 13(Suppl 1):127, 1982.
27. Nylund L, Lunell NO, Lewander R, et al: Labetalol for the treatment of hypertension in pregnancy: Pharmacokinetics and effects on the uteroplacental blood flow. Acta Obstet Gynecol Scand Suppl 118:71, 1984.
28. Pickles CJ, Pipkin FB, Symonds EM: A randomised placebo controlled trial of labetolol in the treatment of mild to moderate pregnancy induced hypertension. Br J Obstet Gynecol 99:964, 1992.
29. Rubin PC, Butters L, Clark DM, et al: Placebo controlled trial of atenolol in treatment of pregnancy associated hypertension. Lancet 1:431, 1983.
30. Reynolds B, Butters L, Evans J, et al: The first year of life after atenolol in pregnancy associated hypertension. Arch Dis Child 59:1061, 1984.
31. Fabregues G, Alvarez L, Jun PV, et al: Effectiveness of atenolol

in the treatment of hypertension during pregnancy. Hypertension 19(Suppl II):129, 1992.
32. Frishman WH, Rotmensch HH, Charlap S, et al: The use of beta-adrenergic blocking agents during pregnancy. In Frishman WH (ed): Clinical Pharmacology of the Beta-Adrenoreceptor Blocking Agents. Norwalk, CT: Appleton-Century-Crofts, 1985, pp 445–458.
33. Turnstall MB: The effect of propranolol on the onset of breathing at birth. Br J Anaesthesiol 41:792, 1969.
34. Olofsson P, Montan S, Sartor G, et al: Effects of beta-1 adrenergic blockade in the treatment of hypertension during pregnancy in diabetic women. Acta Med Scand 220:321, 1986.
35. Boutroy MJ, Morselli PL, Bianchetti G, et al: Betaxolol: A pilot study of its pharmacological and therapeutic properties in pregnancy. Eur J Clin Pharmacol 38:535, 1990.
36. Rubin PC: Treatment of hypertension in pregnancy. Clin Obstet Gynaecol 13:307, 1986.
37. deSwiet M: Antihypertensive drugs in pregnancy. Br Med J 291:365, 1985.
38. Walters BNJ, Redman CWG: Treatment of severe pregnancy-associated hypertension with calcium antagonist nifedipine. Br J Obstet Gynaecol 91:330, 1984.
39. Allen J, Maigaard S, Forman A, et al: Nitrendipine in hypertension of pregnancy. Br J Obstet Gynecol 94:222, 1987.
40. Broughton-Pipkin F, Symonds EM, Turner SR: The effect of captopril (SQ 14, 225) upon mother and fetus in the chronically cannulated ewe and in the pregnant rabbit. J Physiol 323:415, 1982.
41. Piper JM, Ray WA, Rosa IW: Pregnancy outcome following exposure to angiotensin-converting enzyme inhibitors. Obstet Gynecol 80:429, 1992.
42. Barr M, Cohen M: ACE inhibitor fetopathy and hypocalvaria: The kidney-skull connection. Teratology 44:485, 1991.
43. Coen G, Cugini P, Gerlin G, et al: Successful treatment of long-lasting severe hypertension with captopril during a twin pregnancy. Nephron 40:498, 1985.
44. Millar JA, Wilson PD, Morrison N: Management of severe hypertension in pregnancy by a combined drug regimen including captopril: Case report. N Z Med J 96:796, 1983.
45. Fiocchi R, Lijnen P, Fagard R, et al: Captopril during pregnancy. Lancet 2:1153, 1984.
46. Lunnell NO, Lewander R, Nylund L, et al: Acute effect of dihydralazine on uteroplacental blood flow in hypertension during pregnancy. Gynecol Obstet Invest 16:274, 1983.
47. Rosenfeld J, Bott-Kanner G, Boner G, et al: Treatment of hypertension during pregnancy with hydralazine monotherapy or with combined therapy with hydralazine and pindolol. Eur J Obstet Gynecol Reprod Biol 22:197, 1986.
48. Moodley J, Gouws E: A comparative study of the use of epoprostenol and dihydralazine in severe hypertension in pregnancy. Br J Obstet Gynecol 99:727, 1992.
49. Kuzniar J, Skret A, Piela A, et al: Hemodynamic effects of intravenous hydralazine in pregnant women with severe hypertension. Obstet Gynecol 66:453, 1985.
50. Walker JJ, Greer I, Calder AA: Treatment of acute pregnancy-related hypertension: Labetalol and hydralazine compared. Postgrad Med J 59:168, 1983.
51. Sankar D, Moodley J: Low dose diazoxide in the emergent management of severe hypertension in pregnancy. S Afr Med J 65:279, 1984.
52. Stempel JE, O'Grady PJ, Morton MJ, et al: Use of sodium nitroprusside in complications of gestation in hypertension. Obstet Gynecol 60:533, 1982.
53. Cotton DB, Longmire S, Jones MM, et al: Cardiovascular alteration in severe pregnancy-induced hypertension: Effects of intravenous nitroglycerin coupled with blood volume expansion. Am J Obstet Gynecol 154:1053, 1986.
54. Shoemaker CT, Meyers M: Sodium nitroprusside for control of severe hypertensive disease of pregnancy: A case report and discussion of potential toxicity. Am J Obstet Gynecol 149:171, 1984.
55. Wasserman N: Nitroprusside in preeclampsia: Circulatory distress and paradoxical brachycardia. Hypertension 18:79, 1991.
56. Cotton DB, Gonik B, Dorman KF: Cardiovascular alterations in severe pregnancy induced hypertension: Acute effects of

intravenous magnesium sulfate. Am J Obstet Gynecol 148:162, 1984.

57. Rotmensch HH, Elkayam U, Frishman W: Antiarrhythmic drug therapy during pregnancy. Ann Intern Med 98:487, 1983.

58. Rogers MC, Willerson JT, Goldblatt A, et al: Serum digoxin concentrations in the human fetus, neonate, and infant. N Engl J Med 287:1010, 1972.

59. Sherman JL, Locke RV: Transplacental neonatal digitalis intoxication. Am J Cardiol 6:834, 1960.

60. Abboud TK, David S, Nagappala S, et al: Maternal, fetal, and neonatal effects of lidocaine with and without epinephrine for epidural anesthesia in obstetrics. Anesth Analg 63:973, 1984.

61. Bozynski ME, Bubarth LB, Patel JA: Lidocaine toxicity after maternal pudendal anesthesia in a term infant with fetal distress. Am J Perinatol 4:164, 1987.

62. Karim A, Cook C, Campion J: Placental and milk transfer of disopyramide and its metabolites. Drug Metab Dispos 6:346, 1978.

63. Leonard RF, Braun TE, Levy AM: Initiation of uterine contractions by disopyramide during pregnancy. N Engl J Med 299:84, 1978.

64. Dumesic DA, Silverman NH, Tobias S, et al: Transplacental cardioversion of fetal supraventricular tachycardia with procainamide. N Engl J Med 307:1128, 1982.

65. Given BD, Phillipe M, Sanders SP, et al: Procainamide conversion of fetal supraventricular tachyarrhythmia. Am J Cardiol 53:1460, 1984.

66. Mendelson CL: Disorders of the heartbeat during pregnancy. Am J Obstet Gynecol 72:1268, 1956.

67. Hill LM, Malkasian GD: The use of quinidine sulfate throughout pregnancy. Obstet Gynecol 54:366, 1979.

68. Spinnato JA, Shaver DC, Flinn GS, et al: Fetal supraventricular tachycardia: In utero therapy with digoxin and quinidine. Obstet Gynecol 64:730, 1984.

69. Klein V, Repke JT: Supraventricular tachycardia in pregnancy: Cardioversion with verapamil. Obstet Gynecol 63:16S, 1984.

70. Byerly WG, Hartmann A, Foster DE, Tannenbaum AK: Verapamil in the treatment of internal paroxysmal supraventricular tachycardia. Ann Emerg Med 20:552, 1991.

71. Lilja H, Karlsson K, Lindecrantz K, et al: Treatment of intrauterine supraventricular tachycardia with digoxin and verapamil. J Perinatol Med 12:151, 1984.

72. Truccone N, Mariona F: Intrauterine conversion of fetal supraventricular tachycardia with combination of digoxin and verapamil. Pediatr Pharmacol 5:149, 1985.

73. Afridi I, Moise KJ, Rokey R: Termination of supraventricular tachycardia with intravenous adenosine in a pregnant woman with Wolff-Parkinson-White syndrome. Obstet Gynecol 80:481, 1992.

74. McKenna WJ, Harris L, Rowland E, et al: Amiodarone therapy during pregnancy. Am J Cardiol 51:1231, 1983.

75. Robson DJ, Raj MVJ, Storey GCA, et al: Use of amiodarone during pregnancy. Postgrad Med J 61:75, 1985.

76. Widerhorn J, Bhandari AK, Bugli S, et al: Fetal and neonatal adverse effects profile of amiodarone treatment during pregnancy. Am Heart J 122:1162, 1991.

77. Plomp TA, Vulsma T, de Vijlder JJM: Use of amiodarone during pregnancy. Eur J Obstet Gyneol Reprod Biol 43:201, 1992.

78. Galina MP, Avnet NL, Einhorn A: Iodides in pregnancy: An apparent cause of neonatal death. N Engl J Med 267:1124, 1962.

79. Ducey JP, Knape KG: Maternal esmolol administration resulting in fetal distress and casarean section in a term pregnancy. Anesthesiology 77:829, 1992.

80. Larson CP, Shuer LM, Cohen SE: Maternally administered esmolol decreases fetal as well as maternal heart rate. J Clin Anesth 2:427, 1990.

81. Losasso TJ, Muzzi DA, Cucchiara RF: Response of fetal heart rate to maternal administration of esmolol. Anesthesiology 74:782, 1991.

82. White WB: Management of hypertension during lactation. Hypertension 6:297, 1984.

83. Wilson J, Brown RD, Cherek DR, et al: Drug excretion in human breast milk: Principles, pharmacokinetics, and projected consequences. Clin Pharmacokinet 5:1, 1980.

84. Healy M: Suppressing lactation with oral diuretics. Lancet 1:1353, 1961.

85. Werthmann MW, Krees SV: Excretion of chlorthiazide in human breast milk. J Pediatr 81:781, 1972.

86. Miller ME, Cohn RD, Burghart PH: Hydrochlorothiazide disposition in a mother and her breast-fed infant. J Pediatr 101:789, 1982.

87. White WB, Andreoli JW, Cohn RD: Alpha-methyldopa disposition in mothers with hypertension and in their breast-fed infants. Clin Pharmacol Ther 4:387, 1985.

88. White WB, Andreoli JW, Wong SH, et al: Atenolol in human plasma and breast milk. Obstet Gynecol 63:42S, 1984.

89. Riant P, Urein S, Albergres E, et al: High plasma protein binding as a parameter in the selection of beta-blockers for lactating women. Biochem Pharmacol 24:4579, 1986.

90. Schmimmel MS, Eidelman AG, Wilsclanski MA, et al: Toxic effects of atenolol consumed during breast feeding. J Pediatr 114:476, 1989.

91. Okada M, Inoue H, Nakamura Y, et al: Excretion of diltiazem in human milk. N Engl J Med 312:992, 1985.

92. Andersen HJ: Excretion of verapamil in human milk. Eur J Clin Pharmacol 25:279, 1983.

93. Miller MR, Withers R, Bhamra R, et al: Verapamil and breast feeding. Eur J Clin Pharmacol 30:125, 1986.

94. Anderson P, Bondesson U, Mattiasson I, et al: Verapamil and norverapamil in plasma and breast milk during breast feeding. Eur J Clin Pharmacol 31:625, 1987.

95. Wong SH, Marzouk N, White WB: Measurement of calcium channel blockers by HPLC. Procedure manual on the laboratory diagnosis of cardiovascular disorders. Philadelphia: Institute for Clinical Science, 1985, pp 155–160.

96. Ehrenkranz RA, Ackerman BA, Hulse JD: Nifedipine transfer into human milk. J Pediatr 114:478, 1989.

97. White WB, Krol GJ: Nitrendipine in human plasma and breast milk. Eur J Clin Pharmacol 36:531, 1989.

98. Devlin RG, Fleiss PM: Captopril in human blood and breast milk. J Clin Pharmacol 21:21, 1981.

99. Redman CWG, Kelly JG, Cooper WD: The excretion of enalapril and enalaprilat in human breast milk. Eur J Clin Pharmacol 38:99, 1990.

100. Loughnan PM: Digoxin excretion in human breast milk. J Pediatr 92:1019, 1978.

101. Barnett DB, Hudson BA, McBurney A: Disopyramide and its N-monodesalkyl metabolite in breast milk. Br J Clin Pharmacol 14:310, 1982.

102. Ellsworth AJ, Horn JR, Raby VA, et al: Disopyramide and N-monodesalkyl disopyramide in serum and breast milk. Drug Intell Clin Pharm 23:56, 1989.

103. Zeisler JA, Gaarder TD, Demesquita SA: Lidocaine excretion in breast milk. Drug Intell Clin Pharm 20:691, 1986.

104. Lewis AM, Patel L, Johnston A, et al: Mexiletine in human blood and breast milk. Postgrad Med J 57:546, 1981.

105. Hackett LP, Wojar-Horton RE, Dusci LJ, et al: Excretion of sotalol in breast milk. Br J Clin Pharmacol 29:277, 1990.

106. McQuinn RL, Pisani A, Wata S, et al: Flecainide excretion in human breast milk. Clin Pharmacol Ther 48:262, 1990.

CHAPTER 26

Cardiovascular Therapy in Black Patients

W. Dallas Hall, M.D.

EPIDEMIOLOGY

In black persons, cardiovascular therapy centers on the management of hypertension. Hypertension is almost twice as common in blacks as in whites. Furthermore, it is more severe, begins at an earlier age, and is associated with more extensive target-organ damage,[1] particularly stroke,[2] left ventricular hypertrophy[3, 4] and end-stage renal disease.[5] Hypertensive urgencies and emergencies continue to be common in inner-city minority populations,[6] especially in the southeastern United States[7] and West Indies.[8] Use of cocaine was associated with hypertensive episodes in 7 of 20 such patients presenting with malignant hypertension in Los Angeles.[9]

Fewer data are available regarding the relative occurrence of arrhythmias and congestive heart failure in blacks than in whites. For example, the classic Framingham study on the epidemiology of congestive heart failure included only a small number of black individuals.[10] Hypertension is the most common disease associated with congestive heart failure, however, and congestive heart failure occurs with a similar incidence in hypertensive black and white individuals.[11] Isolated left ventricular diastolic dysfunction is a cause of congestive heart failure,[12] and may be especially prevalent in hypertensive blacks.[13] Overall mortality from congestive heart failure is two to three times higher in blacks than in whites.[14] In large public hospitals serving predominantly minority patients, lack of adherence to the prescribed medical regimen is common in patients requiring hospitalization for decompensated heart failure.[9, 15]

Contrary to old beliefs, angina pectoris is common in blacks. Indeed, data now document that coronary heart disease is the major cause of illness and death in the black population of the United States, accounting for 30% to 40% of all deaths in adult blacks.[16, 17]

PATHOPHYSIOLOGY[18]
Hemodynamics

The hemodynamics of hypertension do not differ significantly between blacks and whites.[19] Resting heart rates tend to be 4 to 12 beats/min slower in blacks,[19–21] which could be a reflection of higher parasympathetic tone, because the intrinsic heart rate is actually higher in blacks following autonomic blockade with atropine and propranolol.[22, 23] Elevation of total peripheral resistance is the cardinal hemodynamic feature of both racial groups. Thus, antihypertensive therapy should be directed primarily toward relief of exaggerated peripheral vasoconstriction.

Renal Anatomy and Physiology

Racial differences exist in renal hemodynamics, with blacks exhibiting lower total renal blood flow and higher renal vascular resistance.[24, 25] Blacks also have anatomic differences in the intrarenal vasculature,[24] reduced activity of the renal vasodilator kallikrein system,[26] impaired prostacyclin synthesis,[27] and decreased ability to excrete a salt load.[28, 29] Plasma catecholamine levels are generally no higher in hypertensive blacks than in whites,[20, 30–32] but some blacks have a defect in the mobilization of dopamine in response to a high salt load.[29, 33–35]

Plasma Volume

The usual inverse correlation between blood pressure and plasma or total blood volume is not always demonstrable in hypertensive blacks, who tend to demonstrate an increase rather than a decrease in plasma volume. Parrish et al.[36] reported an average plasma volume of 19.2 ml/cm height in 47 hypertensive black men and women. Chrysant et al.[37] noted expanded plasma volumes (>19 ml/cm height) in 43% of hypertensive black men versus only 21% of hypertensive white men. Thus, hypertensive blacks appear to have expanded plasma volumes compared with hypertensive whites, but not all investigators agree.[19] Several reports indicate that there is increased activity of the Na^+/H^+ antiport in blacks,[38, 39] especially hypertensive blacks with insulin resistance.[40] This could relate to the enhanced proximal tubular reabsorption of sodium.[41, 42]

Plasma Renin Activity

Plasma renin activity is typically reduced in hypertensive blacks. A low-renin profile is present in up to 65% of hypertensive blacks[43] and contrasts markedly with a low-renin state in only about 20% of hypertensive whites.[44, 45] The low-renin profile of hypertensive blacks cannot be attributed to a higher dietary intake of salt than that of whites, because multiple studies have been unable to document the notion that blacks have the higher salt intake.[46, 47] Also, the low plasma renin activity of blacks increases minimally or not at all after salt restriction or furosemide diuresis. Of interest, however, is that 10 weeks of therapy with 80 mEq/day of potassium chloride significantly increased plasma renin activity and plasma aldosterone (from 0.96 to 2.31 ng/ml/hr and from 7.6 to 15.2 ng/dl, respectively) in hypertensive blacks but not in whites.[48] Hypertensive blacks and whites have similar levels of plasma aldosterone during salt restriction, but the adrenal responsiveness of hypertensive blacks is blunted with regard to the expected increase in aldosterone following upright posture or infusion of angiotensin II.[49]

Tissue levels of renin and angiotensin II have not been studied in blacks, but it is likely that they are also suppressed because of the blunted blood pressure response to classes of drugs that act primarily on the renin-angiotensin system. Niarchos et al.[50] found no racial differences in the plasma levels of angiotensin-converting enzyme (ACE).

Intracellular Calcium

Resnick et al.[51] have demonstrated an association between low renin essential hypertension and a decreased serum level of ionized Ca^{2+}. The biologic significance of the reduced serum ionized Ca^{2+} was affirmed by higher levels of parathyroid hormone and 1,25-dihydroxyvitamin D and reduced levels of calcitonin.[52] The lower serum ionized Ca^{2+} could reflect increased intracellular Ca^{2+} in patients with low renin hypertension and in black hypertensives. However, it has not yet been demonstrated that low renin or black hypertensives have higher intracellular Ca^{2+} levels than do either normal- to high-renin black hypertensives or white hypertensives.[53]

Genetic Factors

Jeunemaitre et al.,[54] in a study of 379 nonblack sibling pairs, found evidence for a genetic linkage between the angiotensinogen gene on chromosome 1 and hypertension. Two molecular variants of the gene, M235T and T134M, were found more often in hypertensive index cases and were associated with higher plasma levels of angiotensinogen. They postulated that these mutations could be associated with a predisposition for increased blood pressure in at least 3% to 6% of nonblack patients with the onset of hypertension prior to age 60 years. Preliminary data indicate that 42% of whites but only 4% of blacks are homozygous for M235.[55] In contrast, 70% of blacks but only 12% of whites are homozygous for another mutation, T235. Barley et al.[56] had earlier reported a possible association between blood pressure and a Bg1I restriction fragment length polymorphism in the renin gene of black Afro-Caribbean subjects. No conclusions are appropriate at this time, but Kurtz and Spence[57] have published an excellent review.

Summary

In summary, the physiologic profile of most hypertensive blacks is an increase in total peripheral resistance associated with a normal cardiac output, slightly reduced heart rate, modest expansion of plasma volume, and low plasma renin activity. Hypertension is often accompanied by echocardiographic left ventricular hypertrophy and increased tortuosity of the intrarenal vasculature with a reduction in renal blood flow. All of these physiologic and anatomic features of hypertension in blacks directly affect the selection of the most appropriate cardiovascular therapy.

DRUG THERAPY
Diuretics

Diuretics are the mainstay of therapy for hypertensive blacks and are generally preferable to β-blockers, ACE inhibitors, and calcium antagonists as a choice for initial therapy.[58–60] Hypertensive blacks often exhibit an even greater blood pressure reduction with diuretic therapy than do hypertensive whites.[61] This sensitivity of blacks to the blood pressure–lowering effects of diuretic agents could relate to a more expanded plasma volume and the reduced ability of blacks to excrete a salt load naturally. In blacks studied by Holland et al.,[62] the magnitude of reduction in blood pressure following diuretic therapy was similar whether the plasma renin activity was low or normal. In contrast, the Trial of Antihypertensive Interventions and Management (TAIM) study, which reported on 397 white and 196 black hypertensives, showed that patients in the lowest renin index quartile had the greatest reduction in diastolic blood pressure with diuretic (chlorthalidone) therapy.[63] High levels of plasma renin activity occur in 6% of blacks or fewer[43] in the absence of renovascular hypertension, accelerated malignant-phase hypertension, or vasculitis.

An early Veterans Administration (VA) study documented the excellent responsiveness of black men with diastolic blood pressures between 95 and 114 mmHg to high-dose diuretic therapy.[61] As indicated in Table 26–1,[61, 64–66] hydrochlorothiazide produced an average blood pressure reduction of 20.3/13.0 mmHg in black men. This decrease was 5.0/2.1 mmHg greater than the average reduction in white men, despite a lower mean daily dosage of hydrochlorothiazide in blacks (79 mg) than in whites (114 mg). An impressive 71.3% of blacks but only 55% of whites achieved a sitting diastolic blood pressure ≤ 90 mmHg with hydrochlorothiazide monotherapy. A subsequent study conducted by the VA provided data on racial differences in response to another thiazide diuretic, bendroflumethiazide.[64] The 19.9/12.4 mmHg reduction with 5 to 10 mg daily of bendroflumethiazide was almost identical to that reported earlier with hydrochlorothiazide. Moreover, the average blood pressure reduction in 42 black men exceeded that of 26 white men by 6.6/2.2 mmHg. A more recent VA study[65] compared low-dose (25 to 50 mg daily) and high-dose (50 to 100 mg daily) hydrochlorothiazide in elderly hypertensives. Reduction in blood pressure was excellent with both dosages, 18.3/9.5 and 20.4/9.6 mmHg, respectively. In contrast to the previous three studies, the most recent VA Cooperative Study[66] found a much lower average reduction in blood pressure (-11/-11 mmHg) in diuretic-treated hypertensive blacks. This is probably explained by the shorter duration of the titration period (4 to 8 weeks vs. 8 to 12 weeks in the earlier studies) and the lower dosage of hydrochlorothiazide used (12.5 to 50 mg daily).

Table 26–1. **Blood Pressure (BP) Response to Hydrochlorothiazide (HCTZ) Therapy in Black Men with Mild to Moderate Hypertension: Four Veterans Administration Cooperative Trials**

Reference	N	Mean Age (years)	Diuretic	Dose Range (mg/day)	Duration (weeks)	Entry BP	Change BP
VA Cooperative Study Group, 1982[61]	179	50	HCTZ	50–200	10	147/101	−20.3/−13.0
VA Cooperative Study Group, 1983[64]	42	51	Bendroflumethiazide	5–10	12	149/101	−19.9/−12.4
Materson et al., 1990[65]	@ 80	64	HCTZ	25–50	8	158/99	−18.3/−9.5
	@ 88	64	HCTZ	50–100	8	157/98	−20.4/−9.6
Materson et al., 1993[66]	92	59	HCTZ	12.5–50	4–8	152/100	−11.0/−11.0*

*"Young" (mean age, 50) and "old" (mean age, 66) patients combined.

Fewer data are available regarding the response of hypertensive black women to diuretic therapy. In the study by Holland et al.,[62] the reduction of blood pressure after 4 weeks of therapy with 100 mg daily of hydrochlorothiazide in 29 hypertensive blacks (26 women) was about 28.3/14.5 mmHg. Weight loss averaged 1.7 kg (3.8 lb) from a baseline weight of 89.2 kg (199 lb). Prisant et al.[67] noted a 22/10 mmHg reduction in blood pressure in 20 black women treated for 12 weeks with 2.5 mg daily of indapamide. These decreases in blood pressure in black women are as good as or better than the excellent response of black men with similar baseline levels of blood pressure in the VA studies.

Part of the sensitivity of black women to diuretic therapy could relate to their overweight profile. In the second National Health and Nutrition Examination Survey (NHANESII), 48.1% of black women between 25 and 74 years of age were overweight, a prevalence almost twice that of white women.[68] In general, the hypertension of obesity is characterized hemodynamically by a high cardiac output and an expanded intravascular volume;[69] the latter could be associated with renal sodium retention secondary to hyperinsulinemia.[70] In obese hypertensive patients, diuretic therapy decreases blood volume, lowers cardiac preload, and reduces blood pressure.[71] The comparative efficacy of diuretic monotherapy in normal versus overweight hypertensive black women is unknown.

In the earlier VA study, an average hydrochlorothiazide dose of 114 mg daily in white men reduced serum potassium from 4.38 to 3.49 mEq/L, a decrease of 0.87 mEq/L; in black men, an average hydrochlorothiazide dose of 79 mg daily reduced serum potassium from 4.17 to 3.66 mEq/L, a decrease of 0.51 mEq/L.[61] Thus, despite the well-documented lower dietary intake of potassium in blacks,[72] no evidence was found of a greater risk of thiazide-induced hypokalemia in black men than in white men. Others,[73, 74] however, have reported an inordinate occurrence of diuretic-induced hypokalemia in black women.

The Multiple Risk Factor Intervention Trial (MRFIT) study has raised concern about the risk of sudden death and acceleration of coronary heart disease mortality with diuretic-based therapy in hypertensive patients with abnormal resting electrocardiograms (ECGs).[75] However, relatively few blacks—generally the group with the highest prevalence of abnormal ECGs—were represented in the MRFIT study. Table 26–2[75, 76] shows data from the Hypertension Detection and Follow-Up Program (HDFP) for 631 hypertensive white and 530 hypertensive black men with abnormal resting ECGs.[76] Diuretic-based therapy was associated with a 36% reduction in the risk of death from coronary heart disease in black men. Hence, there are no epidemiologic data to support the notion that diuretic therapy increases the risk of coronary heart disease mortality in hypertensive blacks.

The diuretic choice for initial therapy is a thiazide or thiazide-like drug rather than a loop diuretic. Studies comparing hydrochlorothiazide and furosemide (in predominantly black hypertensive persons) have demonstrated a greater reduction in body weight and in blood pressure with hydrochlorothiazide (Table 26–3).[77–79] Indeed, for patients with resistant hypertension but relatively normal renal function, I often switch diuretic therapy from furosemide to a thiazide-type diuretic agent before adding a new drug or increasing the dose of other antihypertensive medications. Furosemide is usually necessary for patients whose glomerular filtration rate is below 30 ml/min (roughly equivalent to a serum creatinine level above 2.0 to 2.5 mg/dl), the point at which the diuretic effectiveness of thiazides begins to wane.[80]

In hypertensive blacks, it is appropriate to begin drug therapy with 25 mg daily of hydrochlorothiazide or chlorthalidone. This dosage is about equal to 2.5 mg daily of indapamide, bendroflumethiazide, or metolazone, or to 2 mg daily of polythiazide or trichlormethiazide. In elderly patients, the initial dose

Table 26–2. **Coronary Heart Disease Mortality in White Men versus Black Men with Mild Hypertension and Abnormal Baseline ECG**

Study	Race	Group	Number of Patients	Deaths from CHD	Rate (per 1000)	Change in Mortality (%)
MRFIT[75]	White*	UC	1185	21	17.7	+65
	White*	SI	1233	36	29.2	
HDFP[76]	White	RC	318	7	22.0	+60
	White	SC	313	11	35.1	
	Black	RC	298	8	26.8	−36
	Black	SC	232	4	17.2	

*93% white.

CHD, coronary heart disease; HDFP, Hypertension Detection and Follow-up Program; MRFIT, Multiple Risk Factor Intervention Trial; RC, referred care; SC, stepped care; SI, special intervention; UC, usual care.

Table 26–3. **Hydrochlorothiazide (HCTZ)* versus Furosemide (F)† Effect on Blood Pressure (BP) in Hypertensive Blacks**

Reference	Weight Reduction (lb)		BP Reduction (mmHg)	
	HCTZ	*F*	*HCTZ*	*F*
Finnerty et al., 1977[77]	3.3	0.4	24/16	20/13
Araoye et al., 1978[78]	1.7	1.3	13/7	4/7
Holland et al., 1979[79]	4.6	2.2	40/17	27/10

*50 mg b.i.d.
†40 mg b.i.d.

of hydrochlorothiazide or chlorthalidone is reduced by 50% to 12.5 mg daily. The 25-mg daily dose is often cited as a usual ceiling dose, because the additional blood pressure–lowering effect usually accomplished with higher doses is no more than 20%. These data, however, have been compiled primarily from studies of white hypertensive persons. In a small but placebo-controlled, double-blind, crossover study of 19 hypertensive blacks, Stein et al.[81] reported a progressive reduction in both systolic and diastolic pressures with doses of 6.25, 12.5, 25, and 50 mg daily of hydrochlorothiazide (Table 26–4).

Most of the adverse effects of diuretics (including hypokalemia, hypomagnesemia, hyperuricemia, and glucose intolerance) are dose-related, and few data address whether there are ethnic differences in the occurrence of diuretic-related adverse metabolic effects.[82] Moreover, all epidemiologic studies that have failed to show a statistically significant beneficial effect of diuretic-based therapy on coronary heart disease mortality have used diuretic dosages that are considerably above the currently recommended ceiling dose for uncomplicated hypertensive patients. There is a paucity of data, especially in blacks,[83] on the adverse effects of diuretics on lipids when used in the lower daily doses such as 12.5 mg hydrochlorothiazide,[84, 85] 15 mg chlorthalidone,[86] or 2.2 mg trichlormethiazide.[87]

Serum potassium is measured at baseline and, in the absence of symptoms, again after maximal diuretic dosage is reached, usually 2 to 6 weeks later. Potassium supplementation is not prescribed routinely for normokalemic patients unless they are tak-

Table 26–4. **Progressive Reduction of Blood Pressure (BP) with Increasing Doses of Hydrochlorothiazide in 19 Hypertensive Blacks**

Dose (mg/day)	BP (mmHg)	Change in BP (mmHg)
0 (Placebo)	170.2/101.4	—
6.25	161.1/98.0	−9.1/−3.4
12.5	156.6/96.1	−13.6/−5.3
25	154.9/93.6	−15.3/−7.8
50	149.1/90.5	−21.1/−10.9

From Stein CM, Neill P, Kusemamuriwo T: Antihypertensive effects of low doses of hydrochlorothiazide in hypertensive black Zimbabweans. Int J Cardiol 37(2):231, 1992.

ing digoxin. However, potassium supplement therapy is initiated in patients whose serum potassium level falls below 3.5 mEq/L as well as in patients who have or develop ventricular ectopy or complain of new muscle weakness or paresthesias. Supplemental potassium therapy usually is prescribed in a dosage of at least 40 mEq/day. Doses of 60 mEq or more daily can sometimes be associated with further improvement in blood pressure.[74, 88, 89]

β-Blockers

The low-renin profile, lower heart rate, and expanded plasma volume of most hypertensive blacks would predict a blunted response to monotherapy with β-blockers. Table 26–5 provides data from clinical trials that have documented the blood pressure–lowering effects of monotherapy with five different β-blockers in hypertensive blacks.[61, 64, 90–93] All of these studies used relatively high dosages of β-blockers and, except for pindolol, demonstrated significant reductions in heart rate. The typical reduction in blood pressure is 6 to 10 mmHg systolic and 6 to 11 mmHg diastolic, roughly half of that documented previously with diuretic monotherapy (see Table 26–1). β-Blockers that possess additional pharmacologic properties (e.g., β-blockade with labetalol or intrinsic sympathomimetic activity with pindolol) may have a greater blood pressure–lowering effect than "regular" β-blockers in hypertensive blacks.[90, 93, 94]

Two of the VA studies allow direct comparisons of the blood pressure–lowering effects of propranolol and nadolol in hypertensive black and white men.[61, 64] With propranolol in doses up to 640 mg daily, the average blood pressure reduction in whites (13.2/12.6 mmHg) was 5.0/3.1 mmHg greater than the average blood pressure reduction in blacks. With nadolol in doses up to 240 mg daily, the blood pressure reduction in whites (17.2/15.6 mmHg) was 11.4/6.0 mmHg greater than in blacks. These data suggest that the overall blood pressure–lowering efficacy of β-blocker monotherapy in hypertensive blacks is roughly half of that in hypertensive whites with similar levels of baseline blood pressure elevation.

In hypertensive blacks, the reduction in blood pressure following β-blocker monotherapy is similar whether the patient has a low or a normal renin profile.[95] Hence, in most hypertensive blacks, renin classification is not necessary, because it will not predict the response to either diuretic or β-blocker monotherapy.[43, 95] This finding contrasts with the data of Karlberg and Tolagen[96] in hypertensive whites (and the previously mentioned TAIM trial[63] in a racially mixed population), in whom the baseline renin classification correlated directly with the response to β-blocker therapy and inversely with the response to diuretic therapy.

Little doubt exists, however, that in a subset of hypertensive black patients, perhaps 10% to 30%, the blood pressure–lowering response to β-blocker monotherapy is excellent. It is unknown whether this effect represents the relatively rare high-renin

Table 26–5. **Effects of Monotherapy with β-Blockers In Lowering Blood Pressure (BP) in Hypertensive Blacks with Mild to Moderate Hypertension**

Reference	Number of Patients	β-Blocker	Dosage (mg/day)	Initial BP (mmHg)	BP After Therapy (mmHg)	Reduction in BP (mmHg)	Reduction in Heart Rate (beats/min)
Veterans Administration, 1982[61]	172	Propranolol	80–640	@ 146.0/102.0	—	8.2/9.5	@ 16.0*
Saunders et al., 1987[90]	79	Propranolol	80–640	155.0/102.0	148.0/93.0	6.9/8.6	13.0
Veterans Administration, 1983[64]	61	Nadolol	80–240	145.1/101.2	139.3/91.6	5.8/9.6	16.1
Abson et al., 1981[91]	23	Atenolol	200	162.8/102.1	155.7/96.2	7.1/5.9	5.0
Saunders et al., 1990[92]	109	Atenolol	100	152.0/100.9	142.2/90.7	9.8/10.2	NK
Plotnick et al., 1983[93]	86†	Pindolol	15–60	152.4/102.4	138.1/91.6	14.3/10.8	3.5
Saunders et al., 1987[90]	74	Labetalol	200–1600	153.0/102.0	144.0/90.0	9.1/11.2	5.6

*Mean for both black and white study patients.
†85% of patients were black.
NK, not known.

or hyperadrenergic hypertensive black patient, or whether pharmacologic properties of β-blockers other than plasma renin inhibition are operative.

Ethnic difference in the metabolism of or sensitivity to antihypertensive drugs is not unique to the black population.[97] For example, data suggest that Chinese patients are sensitive to the β-blocking and blood pressure–lowering effects of propranolol, even though they have increased ring and side chain oxidation to 4-hydroxy-propranolol and napthoxy-lactic acid, as well as increased metabolic clearance of the drug.[98] Some observations suggest the possibility of differences between blacks and whites in the pharmacokinetic or pharmacodynamic disposition of β-blockers, at least propranolol. For example, in the Beta-Blocker Heart Attack Trial,[99] the blood level of propranolol 7 to 9 hours after drug administration was significantly lower (33 ng/ml) in black patients than in white patients (42 ng/ml). Also, Venter and Joubert[100] reported a 50% smaller reduction in exercise heart rate in blacks than in age-, weight-, and sex-matched whites after intravenous administration of about 1, 3, and 7 mg of propranolol. Johnson and Burlew[101] reported that the area under the curve was lower in normotensive blacks than in whites following an 80-mg oral dose of propranolol; they suggested possible ethnic differences in the hepatic metabolism of propranolol.

The hyporesponsiveness of most hypertensive blacks to β-blocker monotherapy becomes moot if diuretics are selected as initial therapy, because the blood pressure–lowering efficacy of β-blockers is equivalent in hypertensive blacks and whites when used in combination with diuretics.[64] Furthermore, propranolol and labetalol have equal effects on blood pressure when used in combination with diuretic therapy in hypertensive blacks.[94]

Angiotensin-Converting Enzyme Inhibitors

Weinberger and Fineberg[102] reported that race was one of the most powerful predictors of blood pressure response to ACE inhibition. Like β-blockers, a smaller reduction in blood pressure occurs in blacks on ACE inhibitor monotherapy than in whites. The reduced responsiveness of hypertensive blacks to inhibition of ACE probably is related to the low-renin profile of most hypertensive blacks, although there could be an association with the reportedly lower prostacyclin synthesis in blacks.[27]

Table 26–6 provides data on the blood pressure–lowering effects of captopril and enalapril as monotherapy in hypertensive blacks.[92, 103–107] Average reductions in blood pressure range from 5 to 13 mmHg systolic and from 4 to 10 mmHg diastolic, figures close to the earlier noted responses of hypertensive blacks to monotherapy with β-blockers. This reduction in blood pressure with monotherapy in hypertensive blacks is one half to two thirds that of hypertensive whites.[103] In blacks, however, the response to ACE inhibitor monotherapy is heterogeneous, and 20% or more of black patients can exhibit both excellent response *and* control of diastolic blood pressure to below 90 mmHg.[92]

Decreases in blood pressure are similar with either captopril or enalapril. However, in hypertensive blacks, both drugs appear to have their greatest efficacy in the higher dosage ranges.[92, 103, 104, 107–109] Little evidence exists, however, of additional benefit with the use of captopril in doses greater than 100 mg daily or of enalapril in doses of more than 20 mg daily.

In contrast to monotherapy, combination therapy with an ACE inhibitor plus a diuretic is effective in blacks. For example, in the VA study,[103] the combination of captopril plus 50 mg daily of hydrochlorothiazide reduced blood pressure by 24.8/16.4 mmHg in hypertensive blacks versus 24.0/15.7 mmHg in hypertensive whites. In the study of hypertensive blacks by Freier et al.,[107] the combination of enalapril and larger doses of hydrochlorothiazide reduced blood pressure remarkably, by 48.0/27.8 mmHg. In summary, no evidence suggests any racial difference in the blood pressure–lowering effects of ACE inhibitors used in combination with a diuretic.[108]

Because the author initiates therapy with a low-dose diuretic in most hypertensive blacks, the usual recommended starting doses of ACE inhibitors (as add-on therapy) are reduced to 12.5 mg b.i.d. for captopril, 2.5 mg q.d. for enalapril, and 5 mg q.d. for lisinopril. An alternative method is to use the usual dosages but discontinue diuretic therapy for at least 3 days.

Table 26–6. **Effects of Monotherapy with ACE Inhibitors in Lowering Blood Pressure (BP) in Hypertensive Blacks with Mild to Moderate Hypertension**

Reference	Number of Patients	ACE Inhibitor	Dosage (mg/day)	Initial BP (mmHg)	BP After Therapy (mmHg)	Reduction in BP (mmHg)
Veterans Administration, 1982[103]	151	Captopril	25–150	147.6/97.8	138.5/89.9	9.1/7.9
Moser and Lunn, 1982[104]	11	Captopril	Up to 450	166.2/106.9	152.5/101.7	13.7/5.2
Weinberger, 1985[105]	32	Captopril	75	152.7/99.2	152.0/95.1	0.7/4.1
Saunders, et al., 1990[92]	98	Captopril	50–100	150.2/100.4	142.0/90.8	8.2/9.6
Wilkins et al., 1983[106]	23*	Enalapril	10–40	150.6/97.7	145.5/88.3	5.1/9.4
Freier et al., 1984[107]	12	Enalapril	20–40	165.5/103.5	154.8/99.5	10.8/4.0

*Includes three white hypertensive patients.

Combination therapy with diuretics and ACE inhibitors has an additional advantage in that the ACE inhibitor can attenuate the adverse metabolic effects of the diuretic. Several reports have demonstrated that this combination can decrease the frequency of hypokalemia and the need for dosage of potassium supplements, reduce the incidence of hyperglycemia, and blunt the short-term rise in serum cholesterol that can sometimes accompany diuretic therapy.[105, 110–112] β-Blockers used in combination with diuretics also can reduce the frequency of diuretic-induced hypokalemia but can potentially exacerbate hyperglycemia and hyperlipidemia.

In general, ACE inhibitors have few adverse effects as evidenced by studies showing patient withdrawal rates that generally range from 4% to 11%.[113–115] This finding contrasts with withdrawal rates in the range of 13% to 20% with many of the sympatholytic agents.[116, 117] Nonetheless, there is a small but definite risk (0.1% to 0.2%) of angioedema, usually in the facial area, during the initial dosing phase. Also, the incidence of rash is about 1% to 4%, and the incidence of dry cough is 10% to 15%. The dry cough is particularly perplexing because it is typically not associated with fever, malaise, hoarseness, sputum production, or changes on the chest radiograph or laryngoscopic examination. The cough is reported mainly in middle-aged or older women, and it usually (but not always) reverses within 72 hours after discontinuation of the ACE inhibitor.[118] It recurs predictably with substitution of any alternative ACE inhibitor.

Neutropenia occurs only rarely (0.04% to 0.06%) with most ACE inhibitors used in recommended doses. However, it is well known that blacks have lower total white blood cell (WBC) counts than do whites and a higher frequency of intermittent leukopenia.[119, 120] Thus, baseline and occasional follow-up WBC counts are indicated when ACE inhibitors are prescribed in blacks.

Calcium Antagonists

In the management of hypertensive cardiovascular disease, the calcium antagonists have been elevated to one of the first-line therapies, particularly for hypertensive patients who have concomitant angina or bronchospastic pulmonary disease or who have relative contraindications to the use of diuretics or β-blockers. Compared with the other major classes of antihypertensive drugs (other than diuretics), the blood pressure–lowering efficacy of calcium antagonists in hypertensive blacks is impressive. Table 26–7 summarizes nine studies that have evaluated the blood pressure response to monotherapy with calcium antagonists in hypertensive blacks.[92, 121–128]

Average reductions in blood pressure range from 11 to 34 mmHg systolic, 10 to 18 mmHg diastolic. These changes are clearly superior to those documented previously with β-blocker or ACE inhibitor monotherapy in hypertensive blacks. Thus, calcium antagonists approach the efficacy of diuretic monotherapy. Indeed, in the small series reported by Moser et al.,[122] the blood pressure–lowering effect of monotherapy with diltiazem (34/18 mmHg) was as good as that of 50 to 100 mg daily of hydrochlorothiazide (29/21 mmHg). Similarly, in the study by Cubeddu et al.,[121] verapamil monotherapy reduced blood pressure by 16.9/12.8 mmHg in hypertensive blacks, considerably greater than the 8.1/8.6 mmHg decrease with propranolol monotherapy. Lesser differences, however, were noted in the comparison of diltiazem and propranolol monotherapy in hypertensive blacks.[123]

Two studies[129, 130] of monotherapy with calcium antagonists reported a slightly greater reduction in blood pressure in hypertensive blacks than in hypertensive whites. Most studies,[121, 123, 127] however, show equally good responses in both racial groups. Thus, in contrast to monotherapy with the β-blockers or ACE inhibitors, no convincing evidence suggests that response of blood pressure to calcium antagonists differs with race.

Nifedipine is an excellent example of effective monotherapy with a dihydropyridine-type of calcium antagonist in hypertensive blacks.[131] Its relative selectivity for the peripheral vasculature leads to impressive reductions in blood pressure, and its rapid onset of action makes it particularly useful as an orally administered agent for the treatment of hypertensive emergencies. Its onset of action begins within 10 to 30 minutes whether given by the oral, sublingual, or bite-and-swallow technique. Recent studies, however, indicate that there is minimal to no sublingual absorption of nifedipine.[132] Long-lasting preparations of nifedipine are now available. The potency of nifedipine is considerable, and one should never exceed

Table 26–7. **Effects of Monotherapy with Calcium Antagonists in Lowering Blood Pressure (BP) in Hypertensive Blacks with Mild to Moderate Hypertension**

Reference	Number of Patients	Calcium Antagonist	Dosage (mg/day)	Initial BP (mmHg)	BP After Therapy (mmHg)	Reduction in BP (mmHg)
Cubeddu et al., 1986[121]	20	Verapamil	240–480	152.8/100.1	135.9/87.4	16.9/12.8
Saunders et al., 1990[92]	100	Verapamil	240–360	151.0/100.8	137.7/87.9	13.3/12.9
Moser et al., 1985[122]	10	Diltiazem	240–360	165.0/105.0	—	34.0/18.0
Massie et al., 1987[123]	50	Diltiazem	120–360	151.0/101.0*	—	11.0/12.0
Wolfson et al., 1988[124]	16	Diltiazem	120–360	157.9/100.5	142.9/88.7	15.0/11.8
Weir et al., 1993[125]	84	Nicardipine	60–120	152.5/102.0	137.3/91.1	15.2/10.9
M'Buyamba-Kabangu et al., 1986[126]	22	Nitrendipine	20	169.0/102.0	147.0/88.0	22.0/14.0
Moser et al., 1984[127]	39	Nitrendipine	10–40	150.6/101.2	138.3/91.5	12.3/9.7
Carr and Prisant, 1990[128]	14	Isradipine	5–20	167.4/103.4	142.6/90.1	24.8/13.3

*Average baseline BP for both black (52) and white (45) participants.

the initial recommended dosage of 10 mg, because excessive hypotension can occur even with the 10-mg dosage, especially when blood pressure is unusually high.[133, 134]

Other dihydropyridine calcium antagonists are similar to nifedipine but may have a slower onset or longer duration of action. Like nifedipine, they are also useful as monotherapy in hypertensive blacks, providing effective control of blood pressure in 42% to 64% of patients.[126–128, 135]

Hypertensive hypertrophic cardiomyopathy is a condition characterized by symptoms of congestive heart failure associated with normal systolic function (ejection fraction) but impaired left ventricular diastolic function with a prolonged early diastolic filling period, often associated with left ventricular hypertrophy.[13] It is particularly common in elderly black women but can occur also in men and younger black women. Both β-blockers and calcium antagonists, used judiciously and only after documenting normal contractility, are effective treatments.[13, 136, 137]

Calcium antagonists induce no adverse effects on serum potassium, magnesium, glucose, lipids, or uric acid. In addition, they are essentially free of adverse effects such as impotence, fatigue, or impaired exercise performance. Nifedipine therapy can be associated with edema, headache, or flushing. The latter two symptoms can usually be mitigated by either switching to the long-acting formulations or taking nifedipine with meals, because the onset of action is delayed and peak serum levels are lower.[138] Therapy with verapamil is associated with constipation in 10% to 30% of patients. Both verapamil and diltiazem prolong the PR interval by an average of 0.02 to 0.03 msec and cannot be used in patients with heart block greater than the first degree or in patients with the sick sinus syndrome.

SOCIOECONOMIC CONSIDERATIONS

In 1981, the National Black Health Providers Task Force reported that some 5,000,000 American blacks, or 20% to 25% of the United States black population, had uncontrolled hypertension.[139] Although these figures have improved considerably,[140–143] hypertension remains the number one health problem in blacks residing in the United States. Data from the HDFP documented a higher 5-year mortality rate in 4846 hypertensive blacks compared with 6094 hypertensive whites[144] (Table 26–8). For example, the 5-year mortality rate in hypertensive black men was 83% to 91% greater than that of hypertensive white men.

The high rate of uncontrolled hypertension and mortality in blacks is not because cardiovascular therapy is ineffective. In fact, the data from the HDFP in Table 26–8 suggest that diuretic-based therapy of diastolic hypertension was associated with a reduction in mortality that was even more impressive in hypertensive black men (18.5%) and women (28.0%) than in hypertensive white men and women. Hence, despite the higher prevalence and risk of mortality from hypertension in blacks, the benefit of aggressive therapy was even greater in blacks than in whites. In this study, stepped-care therapy was accompanied by a strong patient support system, and therein may lie some of the explanation for the disproportionately greater benefit in hypertensive blacks. In addition, a recent study of therapy with atenolol, captopril, or verapamil SR (sustained-release) in 306 hypertensive black men and women demonstrated that blood pressure could be controlled without reducing the quality of life.[145]

Compliance and Compliance Barriers

The high percentage of patients with uncontrolled hypertension can be accounted for in part by barriers to hypertensive treatment that are prevalent in urban, black, and poor communities.[6, 146–149] Barriers related to the medical care system include inaccessibility to care, inadequate financial resources, inconveniently located health care facilities, long clinic visit waiting times, and inadequate appointment systems.

Continuity of care is a central component for the maintenance of blood pressure control. McClellan et al.[150] documented that nonattendance, defined as failure to visit a physician for hypertension care within 6 months, was reported by 29% of 907 aware hypertensive patients. The rate of uncontrolled hyperten-

Table 26–8. **Racial Differences in the 5-Year Mortality of Hypertensive Blacks and Whites: Impact of Therapy**

	Number of Subjects	5-Year Mortality (%)		Change in Mortality (%)
		Stepped Care	*Referred Care*	
Men				
Black	2148	10.53	12.92	−18.5
White	3753	5.76	6.77	−14.9
Black/white mortality (%)		183	191	
Women				
Black	2698	5.21	7.24	−28.0
White	2341	4.89	4.76	+2.7
Black/white mortality (%)		107	152	

Data from the Hypertension Detection and Follow-up Program Cooperative Group: Five-year findings of the Hypertension Detection and Follow-up Program: II. Mortality by race-sex and age. JAMA 242:2572, 1979.

sion (diastolic blood pressure above 90 mmHg) was 67% in nonattenders and 30% in attenders. The profile of nonattenders was young, male, active in the work force, and without coexisting chronic diseases. Gillum et al.[151] conducted a life-table analysis of 249 randomly selected outpatients attending a medical clinic in an urban teaching hospital. Patients who were initiating therapy or had been under care for less than 6 months had only a 50% likelihood of remaining in care 2 years later.

Patient education programs and the use of paraprofessionals have been shown to improve appointment keeping, the level of blood pressure, and the percentage of hypertensive patients with controlled blood pressure.[152–155]

Cost

McCarron et al.[156] estimate annual costs of $175 to $250 for antihypertensive medications and related laboratory charges. Stason[157] reported that, in 1986, the annual cost for the treatment of hypertension was $400 per patient; such a cost could be a burden for patients with a low income.

Shulman et al.[158] found that cost was an obstacle for blood pressure control for certain population groups. Average *per capita* income was significantly lower for black men, black women, and white men with uncontrolled hypertension than in those with controlled hypertension. Inability to afford prescription refills was reported by 36% of patients with moderate to severe hypertension but only by 16% of patients with mild or controlled blood pressure.

The Rand Health Insurance Experiment compared health outcomes in 3958 people (18% black) followed-up for 3 to 5 years after random assignment to health insurance plans that provided either free care or required enrollers to pay a share of their bills.[159] Hypertension was one of the few health measures that was influenced significantly by free care. The level of diastolic blood pressure averaged 1.9 mmHg lower in hypertensive patients receiving free care than in patients participating in cost-sharing plans.[160] The difference in the reduction of diastolic blood pressure of low-income hypertensive patients (3.5 mmHg) was significantly greater than for high-income hypertensive patients (1.1 mmHg). Free care led to an increase in the number of physician visits, an increase in the treatment rate of hypertensive patients who were not under therapy, an increase in the frequency of monitoring serum potassium levels in patients receiving diuretic therapy, an increase in the percentage of hypertensive patients with controlled blood pressure, and a higher reported compliance with dietary salt restriction.

Moser[161] has summarized the issue of cost containment in the management of hypertension, emphasizing that most major clinical trials that have demonstrated the benefit of treating hypertension have used relatively inexpensive forms of drug therapy. In addition, despite the information gains from echocardiography and 24-hour ambulatory blood pressure monitoring, neither of these procedures has been assessed completely for cost-effectiveness.

REFERENCES

1. Hall WD, Saunders E, Shulman NB: Hypertension in Blacks: Epidemiology, Pathophysiology and Treatment. Chicago: Year Book, 1985.
2. Broderick JP, Brott T, Tomsick T, et al: The risk of subarachnoid and intracerebral hemorrhages in blacks as compared with whites. N Engl J Med 326:733, 1992.
3. Dunn FG, Oigman W, Sungaard-Riise K, et al: Racial differences in cardiac adaptation to essential hypertension determined by echocardiographic indexes. J Am Coll Cardiol 1:1348, 1983.
4. Hammond IW, Alderman MH, Devereux RB, et al: Contrast in cardiac anatomy and function between black and white patients with hypertension. J Natl Med Assoc 76:247, 1984.
5. Jones CA, Agodoa L: Kidney disease and hypertension in blacks: Scope of the problem. Am J Kidney Dis 21(Suppl 1):6, 1993.
6. Shea S, Misra D, Ehrlich MH, et al: Predisposing factors for severe, uncontrolled hypertension in an inner-city minority population. N Engl J Med 327:776, 1992.
7. Felner JM, Battey LL, Jr., Hall WD: Clinical profile of 104 patients presenting to an emergency room with diastolic blood pressure ≥ 140 mmHg. Emory Univ J Med 2:102, 1988.
8. Grell GAC: The Jamaican hypertensive: Characteristics of black patients at the University Hospital of the West Indies. Pan Am Health Org Bull 19:265, 1985.
9. Patel R, Ansari A, Grim CE: Prognosis and predisposing factors for essential malignant hypertension in predominantly black patients. Am J Cardiol 66:868, 1990.
10. Kannel WB, Castelli WP, McNamara PM, et al: Role of blood

pressure in the development of congestive heart failure: The Framingham Study. N Engl J Med 297:781, 1972.

11. Aranow WS, Ahn C, Kronzon I, et al: Congestive heart failure, coronary events and atheroembolic brain infarction in elderly blacks and whites with systemic hypertension and with and without echocardiographic and electrocardiographic evidence of left ventricular hypertrophy. Am J Cardiol 67:295, 1991.

12. Bonow RO, Udelson JE: Left ventricular diastolic dysfunction as a cause of congestive heart failure: Mechanisms and management. Ann Intern Med 117:502, 1992.

13. Topol EJ, Traill TA, Fortuin NJ: Hypertensive hypertrophic cardiomyopathy of the elderly. N Engl J Med 312:277, 1985.

14. Yusef S, Thom T, Probstfield J: The public health and clinical implications of the national increase in congestive heart failure. In Morganroth J, Moore NE (eds): Congestive Heart Failure. Dordrecht: Martinus Nijhoff, 1987, pp 3–8.

15. Ghali JK, Kadakia S, Cooper R, et al: Precipitating factors leading to decompensation of heart failure: Traits among urban blacks. Arch Intern Med 148:2013, 1988.

16. Gillum RF: Coronary heart disease in black populations: I. Mortality and morbidity. Am Heart J 104:839, 1982.

17. Watkins LO: Epidemiology of coronary heart disease in black populations: Methodologic proposals. Am Heart J 108:635, 1984.

18. Hall WD: Pathophysiology of hypertension in blacks. Am J Hypertens 3(12, Pt 2):366s, 1990.

19. Messerli FH, De Carvalho JGR, Christie B, et al: Essential hypertension in black and white subjects: Hemodynamic findings and fluid volume state. Am J Med 67:27, 1979.

20. Sever PS, Peart WS, Davies IB, et al: Ethnic differences in blood pressure with observations on noradrenaline and renin: A hospital hypertensive population. Clin Exp Hypertens 1:745, 1979.

21. Liu K, Ballew C, Jacobs DR Jr, et al: Ethnic differences in blood pressure, pulse rate, and related characteristics in young adults: The CARDIA study. Hypertension 14:218, 1989.

22. Venter CP, Joubert PH, Strydom WJ: Ethnic differences in response to pharmacological denervation of the heart. IRCS Med Sci 12:903, 1984.

23. Joubert PH, Venter CP, Wellstein A: Ethnic differences in response to beta-blockade: Fact or artefact? Eur J Clin Pharmacol 34:363, 1988.

24. Levy SB, Talner LB, Coel MN, et al: Renal vasculature in essential hypertension: Racial differences. Ann Intern Med 88:12, 1978.

25. Frohlich ED, Messerli FH, Dunn FG, et al: Greater renal vascular involvement in the black patient with essential hypertension: A comparison of systemic and renal hemodynamics in black and white patients. Mineral Electrolyte Metab 10:173, 1984.

26. Margolius HS: Urinary kallikreins and prostaglandins in blacks. J Clin Hypertens 3(Suppl):51, 1987.

27. Somova LI, Mufunda JJ: Renin-angiotensin-aldosterone system and thromboxane A2/prostacyclin in normotensive and hypertensive black Zimbabweans. Ethnicity Dis 2:27, 1992.

28. Luft FC, Grim CE, Fineberg N, et al: Effects of volume expansion and contraction in normotensive whites, blacks, and subjects of different ages. Circulation 59:643, 1979.

29. Sowers JR, Zemel MB, Zemel P, et al: Salt sensitivity in blacks: Salt intake and natriuretic substances. Hypertension 12:485, 1988.

30. Rowlands DB, De Giovanni J, McLeay RAB, et al: Cardiovascular response in black and white hypertensives. Hypertension 4:817, 1982.

31. Parmer RJ, Cervenka JH, Stone RA, et al: Autonomic function in hypertension: Are there racial differences? Circulation 81:1305, 1990.

32. Bursztyn M, Bresnahan M, Gavras I, et al: Pressor hormones in elderly hypertensive persons: Racial differences. Hypertension 15(Suppl I):88, 1990.

33. Weinberger MH, Luft FC, Grim CE, et al: Sodium sensitivity and resistance of blood pressure: Racial and renal factors. J Clin Hypertens 3(Suppl):47, 1987.

34. Critchley JAJH, Sriwatanakul K, Chavuchinda C, et al: Ethnic differences in the renal dopamine response to an oral salt load. J Hum Hypertens 4:91, 1990.

35. Lee MR, Critchley JAJH, Gordon CJ, et al: Ethnic differences in the renal sodium dopamine relationship: A possible explanation for regional variations in the prevalence of hypertension? Am J Hypertens 3(6 Pt 2):100S, 1990.

36. Parrish EF, Hall WD, Wollam GL, et al: Hemodynamic and plasma volume measurement in 47 hypertensive blacks. Clin Res 31(5):844a, 1983.

37. Chrysant SG, Danisa K, Kem DC, et al: Racial differences in pressure, volume and renin interrelationships in essential hypertension. Hypertension 1:136, 1979.

38. Kuriyama S, Hopp L, Tamura H, et al: A higher cellular sodium turnover rate in cultured skin fibroblasts from blacks. Hypertension 11:301, 1988.

39. Hatori N, Gardner JP, Tomonari H, et al: Na+/H+ antiport activity in skin fibroblasts from blacks and whites. Hypertension 15:140, 1990.

40. Canessa M, Falkner B, Hulman S: Red blood cell sodium-protein exchange in hypertensive blacks with insulin-resistant glucose disposal. Hypertension 22:204, 1993.

41. Aviv A, Livnz A: The Na+/H+ antiport, cytosolic free Ca2+ and essential hypertension: A hypothesis. Am J Hypertens 1:410, 1988.

42. Aviv A: Cytosolic Ca2+, Na+/H+ antiport, protein kinase C trio in essential hypertension. Am J Hypertens 7:205, 1994.

43. Freis ED, Materson BJ, Flamenbaum W: Comparison of propranolol or hydrochlorothiazide alone for treatment of hypertension: III. Evaluation of the renin-angiotensin system. Am J Med 74:1029, 1983.

44. Brunner HR, Sealey JE, Laragh JH: Renin subgroups in essential hypertension: Further analysis of their pathophysiological and epidemiological characteristics. Circ Res 32–33(Suppl 1):99, 1973.

45. Kaplan NM, Kem DC, Holland OB, et al: The intravenous furosemide test: A simple way to evaluate renin responsiveness. Ann Intern Med 84:639, 1976.

46. Grim CE, Luft FC, Miller JZ, et al: Racial differences in blood pressure in Evans County, Georgia: Relationship to sodium and potassium intake and plasma renin activity. J Chronic Dis 33:87, 1980.

47. Frisancho AR, Leonard WR, Bollettino LA: Blood pressure in blacks and whites and its relationship to dietary sodium and potassium intake. J Chronic Dis 37:515, 1984.

48. Langford HG, Cushman WC, Hsu H: Chronic effect of KCl on black-white differences in plasma renin activity, aldosterone, and urinary electrolytes. Am J Hypertens 4:399, 1991.

49. Fisher NDL, Gleason RE, Moore TJ, et al: Regulation of aldosterone secretion in hypertensive blacks. Hypertension 23:179, 1994.

50. Niarchos AP, Resnick LM, Weinstein DL, et al: Angiotensin I converting enzyme activity in hypertension: Relationship to blood pressure, renin-sodium profiles and antihypertensive therapy. Am J Med 79:435, 1985.

51. Resnick LM, Laragh JH, Sealey JE, et al: Divalent cations in essential hypertension: Relations between serum ionized calcium, magnesium, and plasma renin activity. N Engl J Med 309:888, 1983.

52. Resnick LM, Müller FB, Laragh JH: Calcium-regulating hormones in essential hypertension: Relation to plasma renin activity and sodium metabolism. Ann Intern Med 105:649, 1986.

53. Cooper RS, Borke JL: Intracellular ions and hypertension in blacks. In Fray JCS, Douglas JG (eds): Pathophysiology of Hypertension in Blacks. New York: Oxford University Press, 1993, pp 181–213.

54. Jeunemaitre X, Soubrier F, Kotelevtsev YV, et al: Molecular basis of human hypertension: Role of angiotensinogen. Cell 71:169, 1992.

55. Lifton RP: New observations on the genetic and molecular biology of human hypertension. Am Soc Hypertens Meeting Bull, 1993, p 1.

56. Barley J, Carter ND, Cruickshank JK, et al: Renin and atrial natriuretic peptide restriction fragment length polymorphisms: Association with ethnicity and blood pressure. J Hypertens 9:933, 1991.

57. Kurtz TW, Spence MA: Genetics of essential hypertension. Am J Med 94:77, 1993.

58. Hall WD: Hypertension in blacks. *In* Wollam GL, Hall WD (eds): Management of Hypertension. Clinical Practice and Therapeutic Dilemmas. Chicago: Year Book, 1988, pp. 103–141.

59. Hall WD, Kong W: Hypertension in blacks: Nonpharmacologic and pharmacologic therapy. *In* Saunders E (ed): Cardiovascular Diseases in Blacks. Philadelphia: FA Davis, 1991, pp 157–169.

60. Wright JT Jr, Douglas JG: Drug therapy in black hypertensives. *In* Fray JCS, Douglas JG (eds): Pathophysiology of Hypertension in Blacks. New York: Oxford University Press, 1993, pp 271–291.

61. Veterans Administration Cooperative Study Group on Antihypertensive Agents: Comparison of propranolol and hydrochlorothiazide for the initial treatment of hypertension: I. Results of short-term titration with emphasis on racial differences in response. JAMA 248:1996, 1982.

62. Holland OB, Gomez-Sanchez C, Fairchild C, et al: Role of renin classification for diuretic treatment of black hypertensive patients. Arch Intern Med 139:1365, 1979.

63. Blaufox MD, Lee HB, Davis B, et al: Renin predicts diastolic blood pressure response to nonpharmacologic and pharmacologic therapy. JAMA 267:1221, 1992.

64. Veterans Administration Cooperative Study Group on Antihypertensive Agents: Efficacy of nadolol alone and combined with bendroflumethiazide and hydralazine for systemic hypertension. Am J Cardiol 52:1230, 1983.

65. Materson BJ, Cushman WC, Goldstein G, et al: Treatment of hypertension in the elderly: I. Blood pressure and clinical changes. Hypertension 15:348, 1990.

66. Materson BJ, Reda DJ, Cushman WC, et al: Single-drug therapy for hypertension in men: A comparison of six antihypertensive agents with placebo. N Engl J Med 328:914, 1993.

67. Prisant LM, Beall SP, Nichoalds GE, et al: Biochemical, endocrine, and mineral effects of indapamide in black women. J Clin Pharmacol 30:121, 1990.

68. Gillum RF: Overweight and obesity in black women: A review of published data from the National Center for Health Statistics. J Natl Med Assoc 79:865, 1987.

69. Messerli FH, Christie B, De Carvalho JGR: Obesity and essential hypertension: Hemodynamics of intravascular volume, sodium excretion and plasma renin activity. Arch Intern Med 141:81, 1981.

70. Landsberg L: Insulin and hypertension: Lessons from obesity. N Engl J Med 317:378, 1987.

71. Messerli FH, Schmeider RE: Use of diuretic agents in obese or black patients with systemic hypertension. Am J Cardiol 58(2):lla, 1986.

72. Langford HC: Dietary sodium, potassium, and calcium in black hypertensive subjects. J Clin Hypertens 3(Suppl):36, 1987.

73. Bloomfield RL, Wilson DJ, Buckalew VM Jr: The incidence of diuretic-induced hypokalemia in two distinct clinical settings. J Clin Hypertens 4:331, 1986.

74. Kaplan NM, Carnegie A, Raskin P, et al: Potassium supplementation in hypertensive patients with diuretic-induced hypokalemia. N Engl J Med 312:746, 1986.

75. Multiple Risk Factor Intervention Trial Research Group: Multiple Risk Factor Intervention Trial: Risk factor changes and mortality. JAMA 248:1465, 1982.

76. Hypertension Detection and Follow-up Program Cooperative Research Group: The effect of antihypertensive drug treatment on mortality in the presence of resting electrocardiographic abnormalities at baseline: The HDFP experience. Circulation 70:996, 1984.

77. Finnerty FA Jr, Maxwell MH, Lunn J, et al: Long-term effects of furosemide and hydrochlorothiazide in patients with essential hypertension: A two-year comparison of efficacy and safety. Angiology 28:125, 1977.

78. Araoye MA, Chang MY, Khatri IM, et al: Furosemide compared with hydrochlorothiazide: Long-term treatment of hypertension. JAMA 240:1863, 1978.

79. Holland OB, Gomez-Sanchez CE, Kuhnert L, et al: Antihypertensive comparison of furosemide with hydrochlorothiazide for black patients. Arch Intern Med 139:1015, 1979.

80. Reubi FC: Clinical use of furosemide. Ann N Y Acad Sci 139:433, 1966.

81. Stein CM, Neill P, Kusemamuriwo T: Antihypertensive effects of low doses of hydrochlorothiazide in hypertensive black Zimbabweans. Int J Cardiol 37(2):231, 1992.

82. Joffe BI, Panz VR, Seftel HC, et al: Comparative effects of diuretics in different ethnic groups. *In* Puschett JB, Greenberg A (eds): Diuretics IV: Chemistry, Pharmacology and Clinical Applications. New York: Elsevier, 1993, pp 477–482.

83. Wright JT Jr: Risk-factors in the management of the unique hypertensive patient. J Natl Med Assoc 79(Suppl):17, 1987.

84. Kohvakka A, Salo H, Gordin A, et al: Antihypertensive and biochemical effects of different doses of hydrochlorothiazide alone or in combination with triamterene. Acta Med Scand 219:381, 1986.

85. McKenney JM, Goodman RP, Wright JT: The effect of low-dose hydrochlorothiazide on blood pressure, serum potassium and lipoproteins. Pharmacotherapy 6:179, 1986.

86. Vardan S, Mehrotra KG, Mookherjee S, et al: Efficacy and reduced metabolic side effects of a 15 mg chlorthalidone formulation in the treatment of mild hypertension: A multicenter study. JAMA 258:484, 1987.

87. Sasaki J, Tominaga K, Saeki Y, et al: Effects of lisinopril and low-dose trichlormethiazide on lipoprotein metabolism in patients with mild to moderate hypertension. J Hum Hypertens 6:233, 1992.

88. Matlou SM, Isles CG, Higgs A, et al: Potassium supplementation in blacks with mild to moderate essential hypertension. J Hypertens 4:61, 1986.

89. Krishna GG, Kapoor SC: Potassium depletion exacerbates essential hypertension. Ann Intern Med 115:77, 1991.

90. Saunders E, Curry C, Hinds J, et al: Labetalol compared with propranolol in the treatment of black hypertensive patients. J Clin Hypertens 3:294, 1987.

91. Abson CP, Levy LM, Eyherabide G: Once-daily atenolol in hypertensive Zimbabwean blacks: A double-blind trial using two different doses. S Afr Med J 60:47, 1981.

92. Saunders E, Weir MR, Kong WK, et al: A comparison of the efficacy and safety of a β-blocker, a calcium channel blocker, and a converting enzyme inhibitor in hypertensive blacks. Arch Intern Med 150:1707, 1990.

93. Plotnick GD, Fisher ML, Hamilton JH, et al: Intrinsic sympathomimetic activity of pindolol. Evidence for interaction with pretreatment sympathetic tone. Am J Med 74:625, 1983.

94. Townsend RR, DiPette DJ, Goodman R, et al: Combined αβ blockade versus β₁-selective blockade in essential hypertension in black and white patients. Clin Pharmacol Ther 48:665, 1990.

95. Holland OB, Fairchild C: Renin classification for diuretic and beta-blocker treatment of black hypertensive patients. J Chronic Dis 35:179, 1982.

96. Karlberg BE, Tolagen K: The predictive value of renin profiling in the choice of treatment in primary hypertension, with special reference to patients with low renin values. *In* Laragh JH (ed): Topics in Hypertension. New York: Yorke Medical Books, 1980, pp 434–444.

97. Kalow W: Ethnic differences in drug metabolism. Clin Pharmacokinet 7:373, 1982.

98. Zhou HH, Wood AJJ: Differences in stereoselective disposition of propranolol do not explain sensitivity differences between white and Chinese subjects. Clin Pharmacol Ther 47:719, 1990.

99. Walle T, Byington RP, Furberg CD, et al: Biologic determinants of propranolol disposition: Results from 1308 patients in the Beta-blocker Heart Attack Trial. Clin Pharmacol Ther 38:509, 1985.

100. Venter CP, Joubert PH: Ethnic differences in response to β₁-adrenoceptor blockade by propranolol. J Cardiovasc Pharmacol 6:361, 1984.

101. Johnson JA, Burlew BS: Racial differences in propranolol pharmacokinetics. Clin Pharmacol Ther 51:495, 1992.

102. Weinberger MH, Fineberg NS: Variables predicting blood pressure response to enalapril. Clin Pharmacol Ther 35:281, 1984.

103. Veterans Administration Co-Operative Study Group on Antihypertensive Agents: Racial differences in response to low-dose captopril are abolished by the addition of hydrochlorothiazide. Br J Clin Pharmacol 14(Suppl 2):97, 1982.

104. Moser M, Lunn J: Responses to captopril and hydrochlorothiazide in black patients with hypertension. Clin Pharmacol Ther 32:307, 1982.

105. Weinberger MH: Blood pressure and metabolic responses to hydrochlorothiazide, captopril, and the combination in black and white mild-to-moderate hypertensive patients. J Cardiovasc Pharmacol 7(Suppl 1):52, 1985.

106. Wilkins LH, Dustan HP, Walker JF, et al: Enalapril in low-renin essential hypertension. Clin Pharmacol Ther 34:297, 1983.

107. Freier PA, Wollam GL, Hall WD, et al: Blood pressure, plasma volume, and catecholamine levels during enalapril therapy in blacks with hypertension. Clin Pharmacol Ther 36:731, 1984.

108. Parag KB, Seedat YK: Do angiotensin-converting enzyme inhibitors work in black hypertensives? A review. J Hum Hypertens 4:450, 1990.

109. Drayer JIM, Weber MA: Monotherapy of essential hypertension with a converting-enzyme inhibitor. Hypertension 5(Suppl 3):108, 1983.

110. Chrysant SG, Brown RD, Kem DC, et al: Antihypertensive and metabolic effects of a new converting enzyme inhibitor, enalapril. Clin Pharmacol Ther 33:741, 1983.

111. Weinberger MH: Influence of an angiotensin converting-enzyme inhibitor on diuretic-induced metabolic effects in hypertension. Hypertension 5(Suppl 3):132, 1983.

112. Holland OB, vonKuhnert L, Campbell WB, et al: Synergistic effect of captopril with hydrochlorothiazide for the treatment of low renin hypertensive black patients. Hypertension 5:235, 1983.

113. Veterans Administration Cooperative Study Group on Antihypertensive Agents: Low-dose captopril for the treatment of mild to moderate hypertension. Hypertension 5(Suppl 3):139, 1983.

114. Veterans Administration Cooperative Study Group on Antihypertensive Agents: Low-dose captopril for the treatment of mild to moderate hypertension: I. Results of a 14-week trial. Arch Intern Med 144:1947, 1984.

115. Groel JT, Tadros SS, Dreslinski GR, et al: Long-term antihypertensive therapy with captopril. Hypertension 5(Suppl 3):145, 1983.

116. Croog SH, Levine S, Testa MA, et al: The effects of antihypertensive therapy on the quality of life. N Engl J Med 314:1657, 1986.

117. Medical Research Council Working Party on Mild to Moderate Hypertension: Adverse reactions to bendrofluazide and propranolol for the treatment of mild hypertension. Lancet 2:539, 1981.

118. Israili ZH, Hall WD: Cough and angioneurotic edema associated with angiotensin-converting enzyme inhibitor therapy. Ann Intern Med 117:234, 1992.

119. Shaper AG, Lewis P: Genetic neutropenia in people of African origin. Lancet 2:1021, 1971.

120. McGrath CR, Hitchcock DC, van Assendelft OW: Total white blood cell counts for persons ages 1–74 years with differential leukocyte counts for adults ages 25–74 years: United States, 1971–75. Vital Health Stat [11], No. 220, DHHS Publ. No. (PHS) 82–1670, PHS. Washington, DC: U.S. Government Printing Office, January 1982, pp 1–36.

121. Cubeddu LX, Aranda J, Singh B, et al: A comparison of verapamil and propranolol for the initial treatment of hypertension: Racial differences in response. JAMA 256:2214, 1986.

122. Moser M, Lunn J, Materson BJ: Comparative effects of diltiazem and hydrochlorothiazide in blacks with systemic hypertension. Am J Cardiol 56:101h, 1985.

123. Massie B, MacCarthy EP, Ramanathan KB, et al: Diltiazem and propranolol in mild to moderate essential hypertension as monotherapy or with hydrochlorothiazide. Ann Intern Med 107:150, 1987.

124. Wolfson P, Abernethy D, DiPette J, et al: Diltiazem and captopril alone or in combination for treatment of mild to moderate systemic hypertension. Am J Cardiol 62:103g, 1988.

125. Weir MR, Wright JT Jr, Ferdinand KC, et al: Comparison of the efficacy and metabolic effects of nicardipine and hydrochlorothiazide in hypertensive black men and women. J Hum Hypertens 7:141, 1993.

126. M'Buyamba-Kabangu JR, Lepira B, Fagard R, et al: Relative potency of a beta-blocking and a calcium entry blocking agent as antihypertensive drugs in black patients. Eur J Clin Pharmacol 29:523, 1986.

127. Moser M, Lunn J, Nash DT, et al: Nitrendipine in the treatment of mild to moderate hypertension. J Cardiovasc Pharmacol 6(Suppl 7):1085, 1984.

128. Carr AA, Prisant LM: The new calcium antagonist isradipine: Effect on blood pressure and the left ventricle in black hypertensive patients. Am J Hypertens 3:8, 1990.

129. Frishman WH, Zawada ET Jr, Smith LK, et al: Comparison of hydrochlorothiazide and sustained-release diltiazem for mild-to-moderate systemic hypertension. Am J Cardiol 59:615, 1987.

130. Leary WP, Asmal AC: Treatment of hypertension with verapamil. Curr Ther Res 25:747, 1979.

131. Pacheco JP, Fan F, Wright RA, et al: Monotherapy of mild hypertension with nifedipine. Am J Med 81(Suppl 6a):20, 1986.

132. van Harten J, Burggraaf K, Danhof M, et al: Negligible sublingual absorption of nifedipine. Lancet 2:1363, 1987.

133. Wachter RM: Symptomatic hypotension induced by nifedipine in the acute treatment of severe hypertension. Arch Intern Med 147:556, 1987.

134. O'Mailia JJ, Sander GE, Giles TD: Nifedipine-associated myocardial ischemia or infarction in the treatment of hypertensive urgencies. Ann Intern Med 107:185, 1987.

135. Miller H: Isradipine: Overall clinical experience in hypertension in the United States. Am J Hypertens 4(Suppl):135, 1991.

136. Matsumoto M, Nakajima S, Fukushima M, et al: Effect of diltiazem on diastolic performance of the hypertrophied left ventricle in patients with systemic hypertension and hypertrophic cardiomyopathy. J Cardiography 13:905, 1983.

137. Dianzumba SB, DiPette D, Joyner CR, et al: Left ventricular filling in hypertensive blacks and whites following adrenergic blockade. Am J Hypertens 3:48, 1990.

138. Hirasawa K, Shen WF, Kelly DT, et al: Effect of food ingestion on nifedipine absorption and haemodynamic response. Eur J Clin Pharmacol 28:105, 1985.

139. National Black Health Providers Task Force: Final Report of the National Black Health Providers Task Force on High Blood Pressure Education and Control. DHHS Pub. No. (NIH) 81-1474, PHS. Washington, DC: U.S. Government Printing Office, 1981, p V.

140. Secretary's Task Force: Report of the Secretary's Task Force on Black and Minority Health, Vol. IV: Cardiovascular and Cerebrovascular Disease, Part 1. DHHS Publ. No. 1986-620-638: 40716, Washington, DC: U.S. Government Printing Office, 1986, pp 10–11.

141. Dannenberg AL, Drizd T, Horan MJ, et al: Progress in the battle against hypertension: Changes in blood pressure levels in the United States from 1960 to 1980. Hypertension 10:226, 1987.

142. Otten MW Jr, Teutsch SM, Williamson DF, et al: The effects of known risk factors on the excess mortality of black adults in the United States. JAMA 263:845, 1990.

143. NHLBI Data Fact Sheet: The stroke belt: Stroke mortality by race and sex. Vital Statistics, DHHS, PHS, NIH, 1989, pp 1–4.

144. Hypertension Detection and Follow-up Program Cooperative Group: Five-year findings of the Hypertension Detection and Follow-up Program: II. Mortality by race-sex and age. JAMA 242:2572, 1979.

145. Croog SH, Kong BW, Levine S, et al: Hypertensive black men and women: Quality of life and effects of antihypertensive medications. Arch Intern Med 150:1733, 1990.

146. Saunders E: Stepped care and profiled care in the treatment of hypertension: Considerations for black Americans. Am J Med 81(Suppl 6c):39, 1986.

147. James SA, Wagner EH, Strogatz DS, et al: The Edgecombe County (NC) high blood pressure control program: II. Barriers to the use of medical care among hypertensives. Am J Public Health 74:468, 1984.

148. Shulman NB: Economic issues relating to access to medications. In Saunders E (ed): Cardiovascular Diseases in Blacks. Philadelphia: FA Davis, 1991, pp 75–82.

149. Heurtin-Roberts S, Reisin E: The relation of culturally influenced lay models of hypertension to compliance with treatment. Am J Hypertens 5:787, 1992.

150. McClellan WM, Hall WD, Brogan D, et al: Continuity of care in hypertension: An important correlate of blood pressure control among aware hypertensives. Arch Intern Med 148:525, 1988.

151. Gillum RF, Neutra RR, Stason WB, et al: Determinants of dropout rate among hypertensive patients in an urban clinic. J Community Health 5:94, 1979.

152. Gillum RF, Soloman HS, Kranz P, et al: Improving hypertension detection and referral in an ambulatory setting. Arch Intern Med 138:700, 1978.

153. Zismer DK, Gillum RF, Johnson CA, et al: Improving hypertension control in a private medical practice. Arch Intern Med 142:297, 1982.

154. Gillum RF, Gillum BS: Potential for control and prevention of essential hypertension in the black community. In Matarazzo JD, Weiss SM, Herd JA, et al (eds): Behavioral Health: A Handbook of Health Enhancement and Disease Prevention. New York: John Wiley & Sons, 1984, pp 825–835.

155. Saunders E: Special management techniques for hypertension in blacks. J Clin Hypertens 3(Suppl):114, 1987.

156. McCarron DA, Hare LE, Walker BR: Therapeutic and economic controversies in antihypertensive therapy. J Cardiovasc Pharmacol 6(Suppl):837, 1984.

157. Stason WB: Opportunities for improving the cost-effectiveness of antihypertensive treatment. Am J Med 81(Suppl 6c):45, 1986.

158. Shulman NB, Martinez B, Brogan D, et al: Financial cost as an obstacle to hypertension therapy. Am J Public Health 76:1105, 1986.

159. Brook RH, Ware JE Jr, Rogers WH, et al: Does free care improve adults' health? Results from a randomized controlled trial. N Engl J Med 309:1426, 1983.

160. Keeler EB, Brook RH, Goldberg GA, et al: How free care reduced hypertension in the Health Insurance Experiment. JAMA 254:1926, 1985.

161. Moser M: "Cost containment" in the management of hypertension. Ann Intern Med 107:107, 1987.

CHAPTER 27

Cardioprotection After Acute Myocardial Infarction

Sidney Goldstein, M.D.

More than one million persons are admitted annually to the hospital in the United States as a result of an acute myocardial infarction (MI). Of those, approximately 600,000 survive the acute event and are candidates for long-term therapy to prevent or protect against a recurrent infarction. After the acute stage of MI, therapy is directed toward altering the mechanisms that contribute to ischemia, including progressive coronary atherosclerosis and coronary thrombosis, and limiting the degree of injury associated with subsequent ischemic events. Drugs that have been investigated in this regard include antiplatelet and anticoagulant agents, β-adrenergic blocking agents, antiarrhythmic drugs, and most recently, angiotensin-converting enzyme inhibitors. The results of these studies provide a rationale for the prolonged use of a number of pharmacologic agents in order to protect the myocardium from the seemingly inevitable recurrent ischemic event.

ANTIPLATELET THERAPY

The most common pathophysiologic event leading to the acute coronary event involves rupture of an atherosclerotic plaque and platelet deposition at the site of plaque rupture. The precise mechanism leading to plaque rupture remains undefined, but it is clear that the event can trigger platelet aggregation and fibrin thrombus formation. Platelet aggregation may lead to intermittent reduction in coronary flow manifesting unstable angina or progress to total occlusion as an acute MI. The intensity and duration of the thrombotic event reflect a balance between endogenous thrombotic and thrombolytic mechanisms that interact dynamically after initiation of thrombus formation. A variety of antiplatelet agents have been evaluated in order to prevent MI. These antiplatelet agents include aspirin, dipyridamole, sulfinpyrazone, and ticlopidine.

Aspirin

Aspirin is the most extensively studied antiplatelet agent both for primary prevention of coronary atherosclerotic disease and for secondary prevention after acute MI. The United States Male Physicians' Health Study reported that aspirin reduced the risk of MI but had no effect on mortality when used in primary prevention.[1] A large observational study suggested that aspirin is also beneficial in the primary prevention of cardiovascular disease in women.[2] A number of prospective trials of aspirin for secondary prevention after MI have been done. They include the Medical Research Council (MRC) in 1974[3] and 1979,[4] the Coronary Drug Project (CDP) in 1976,[5] and the Aspirin Myocardial Infarction Study (AMIS) in 1980.[6] The first MRC study failed to observe any significant benefit but reported that aspirin reduced the total mortality rate by 12% at 6 months and 25% at 12 months after infarction. A second MRC[4] trial focused on the early administration of 300 mg three times a day of aspirin and observed a decrease in mortality from 22% in the placebo group to 16% in the aspirin group. The Coronary Drug Project,[5] using a similar dose of aspirin, observed a mortality in the aspirin group of 5.8% compared with 4.3% in the placebo group. This 30% decrease in mortality did not achieve statistical significance because of the relatively small sample size. It did, however, lead to the AMIS[6] in 1980, which randomized patients with a previously documented MI to aspirin (1.0 g daily) or a placebo. Although no benefit in total mortality rate was observed (10.8% in the group taking aspirin versus 9.7% in the placebo group), there was a 22% decrease in reinfarction rate (8.1% with aspirin versus 6.3% with placebo) and a 40% decrease in definite stroke.

The effect of aspirin (325 mg three times a day) alone and in combination with dipyridamole (75 mg three times a day) was examined in the Persantine-Aspirin Reinfarction Study (PARIS-I) in 1980.[7] The mortality rate and the combined end points of death and nonfatal infarction were lower in the active treatment groups when compared with the placebo group. In the PARIS-II Trial (1986),[8] patients were randomized within 4 months after an MI. The combined end point of coronary death or nonfatal reinfarction in this study was significantly reduced by 25%. Differences in total and coronary mortality again were not statistically significant. Although not conclusive, these trends suggest that patients receive benefit from antiplatelet therapy after an MI. A meta-analysis of 31 randomized trials using a variety of antiplatelet therapies in 29,000 patients with previous heart disease revealed that there was a reduction in vascular mortality of 15% and nonfatal vascular events of 30%.[9]

In addition to its role late after an acute MI, therapy with aspirin is recommended for all patients early after the onset of myocardial ischemic syndromes including unstable angina,[10] unless contraindications for its use are present. Patients with acute MI receiving thrombolytic therapy should also receive aspirin administered in a dose of 160 mg daily, which should be continued indefinitely. None of the studies thus far have conclusively established evidence for a specific dose of aspirin. Until that time, aspirin in doses of 81 to 325 mg is recommended. Although other antiplatelet agents have been examined, conclusive beneficial results have not been achieved.

ANTICOAGULANT THERAPY

The rationale for the use of anticoagulants in patients with acute MI is to prevent expansion or propagation of the coronary artery thrombosis and, therefore, to limit the infarct size and to prevent reinfarction. In addition, anticoagulants are thought to prevent systemic emboli, a frequent complication in patients with transmural MI. They may also prevent the development of venous thrombosis and pulmonary embolism. The initial use of anticoagulants was to prevent pulmonary embolism in an era in which patients were treated with prolonged bed rest after an acute MI. Although these studies were rather primitive based on current standards for clinical trials, they tended to show some benefit. Once early ambulation after infarction became the standard, anticoagulant therapy became less relevant.

With the advent of thrombolytic therapy and the reemphasis of thrombosis as an important factor in

ischemic heart disease, the role of anticoagulants in the long-term management of patients after MI has reemerged. Much of our current knowledge is based on studies carried out almost 30 years ago, which were limited by their design, duration of follow-up, lack of placebo control, and small sample size. The Medical Research Council Trial[11] and the Sixty Plus Reinfarction Study[12] observed trends in a lower incidence of deaths, reinfarction, and embolic events. Associated with these benefits, however, there was an increased incidence of bleeding in patients receiving anticoagulant therapy, thus making anticoagulant therapy less attractive, despite the beneficial effects that were documented.

The most recent and most convincing study, the Warfarin Reinfarction Study (WARIS),[13] randomized patients to warfarin or a placebo 27 days after an acute MI (Fig. 27–1). During a mean follow-up of 37 months, decreases in mortality of 24% and recurrent MI of 34% were observed in the group treated with warfarin. In addition, the frequency of cerebrovascular accidents was lower in the warfarin-treated group. The combined incidence of major and minor bleeding episodes in the warfarin group was 0.6% per year. This carefully designed trial provides important evidence of a positive effect of warfarin on mortality and reinfarction after MI.

Anticoagulation, therefore, should be considered for its potential benefits in limiting ischemic events and preventing thromboembolic complications. Based on current information, routine use of oral anticoagulation should be considered for all survivors of an MI based on the very impressive results of the WARIS. Anticoagulant therapy should also be considered in patients at high risk of thromboembolic events, in those with anterior or apical infarct with or without a documented mural thrombus, and in patients with a dilated and hypokinetic left ventricle.[14] Therapy in that setting should be continued for about 3 months after an MI.

β-ADRENERGIC BLOCKING AGENTS

β-Adrenergic blocking agents represent the current therapeutic foundation for the treatment of patients

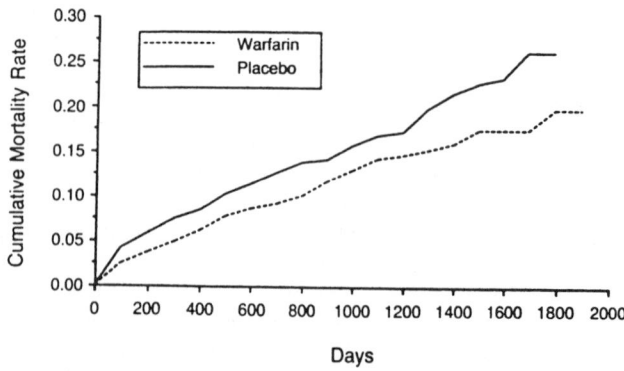

Figure 27–1. The cumulative rate of death from all causes according to original treatment assignment. (From Smith P, Arnesen II, Holme I: The effect of warfarin on mortality and reinfarction after myocardial infarction. N Engl J Med 323:147, 1990.)

with acute and chronic coronary heart disease. Although this review deals with the use of these agents in the secondary prevention after an MI, their use in the treatment of hypertension and chronic angina pectoris should also be emphasized. Investigations of β-blocker therapy in ischemic heart disease began almost three decades ago with the demonstration of the presence of β-adrenergic receptors in the cardiovascular system. The presence of β-adrenergic receptors led to the development of antianginal drugs that could block these receptors, thereby decreasing blood pressure, pulse rate, and the metabolic requirements of the heart.

The observation that β-blockers lower heart rate and blood pressure suggested that they could modify myocardial oxygen demands, resulting in a salutary effect on the jeopardized ischemic myocardial tissue. It has been proposed that the degree of bradycardia induced by β-blocker therapy is a measure of its effect on improving survival[15] (Fig. 27–2). In addition to limiting infarct size, β-blockers can decrease ventricular ectopy in both the acute and chronic phases of MI.[16, 17] Whether this is a result of a decrease in myocardial ischemia or due to an independent antiarrhythmic effect is not entirely clear. Animal studies indicate that β-blockers exhibit a dose response effect on ventricular fibrillation threshold when studied in both ischemic and nonischemic states.[18] β-Adrenergic blocking agents therefore have the potential to modify two of the major risks facing patients with ischemic heart disease: the progression of myocardial ischemia and the development of life-threatening arrhythmias.

β-Adrenergic blocking agents do differ in their physiologic and pharmacologic effects. The major difference relates to the presence of β₁ selectivity. Metoprolol, atenolol, and betaxolol, for instance, are considered drugs that have β-receptor blocking ability. These drugs tend to have a predominant, but not exclusive, effect on chronotropic and inotropic block-

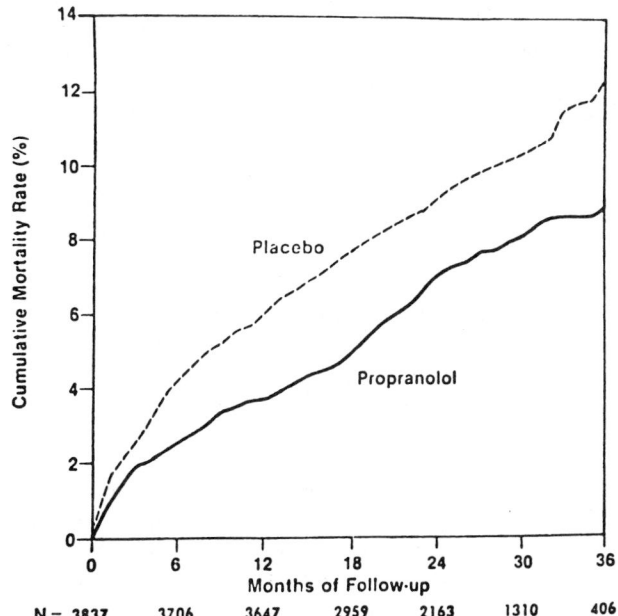

Figure 27–3. The effect of propranolol compared with placebo on cumulative mortality. (From Beta Blocker Heart Attack Trial Research Group: A randomized trial of propranolol in patients with acute myocardial infarction. I: Mortality results. JAMA 247:1707, 1982.)

ade without affecting β_2 receptors that can cause peripheral vasoconstriction and bronchial constriction. The nonselective drugs such as propranolol, timolol, and nadolol do not have this selectivity and block both β_1 and β_2 receptors.

A series of preliminary clinical studies described the benefit of β-adrenergic blocking agents in the treatment of patients who sustained an acute MI. The largest body of information has been reported by the Norwegian Multicenter Study Group[19] using timolol and the Beta Blocker Heart Attack Trial (BHAT)[20] using propranolol. Timolol was administered in doses of 10 mg twice daily and propranolol in doses of 60 to 80 mg three times a day. The results of these two studies indicate that when either drug was administered within 1 to 3 weeks after an MI, a decrease in mortality of between 25% and 36% in the first 2 years was achieved (Fig. 27–3). In addition, the Norwegian Timolol Study observed a significant reduction in reinfarction and sudden death in the active treatment group. The relative benefit of these drugs has been examined both prospectively and retrospectively in a number of different patient subsets and found to be consistently similar in almost all subgroups studied. The one exception is patients who experienced a non–Q wave MI. Here, analyses do not demonstrate significant effect of propranolol or metoprolol in patients with a non–Q wave acute MI, although the timolol-treated patients with a non–Q wave MI experienced a significant reduction in mortality.[21]

A number of different subgroups have been analyzed in order to identify those patients who can achieve the greatest benefit from β-blocker therapy. In patients between 65 and 75 years of age, timolol

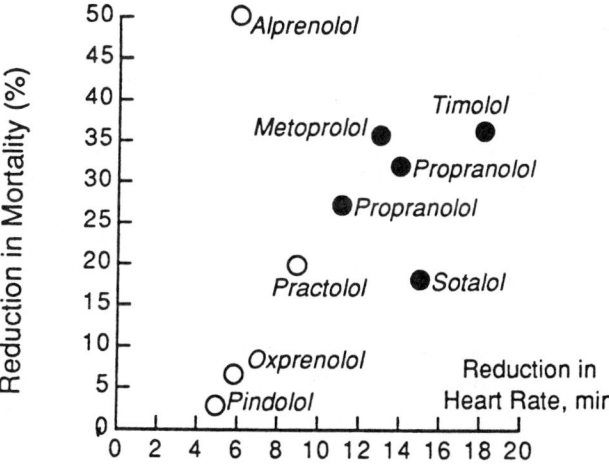

Figure 27–2. The relationship of the reduction of heart rate to reduction in mortality observed in a series of clinical trials. (From Kjekshus JK: Importance of heart rate in determining beta blocker efficacy in acute and long term myocardial infarction trials. Am J Cardiol 57:43F, 1986.)

exerted a similar decrease in reinfarction and death, indicating its efficacy regardless of age.[22] Jafri et al.[23] examined the effect of propranolol on smokers and observed that the greatest beneficial effect of propranolol on mortality was observed in individuals who were smokers before their MI and in those who continued to smoke after the event.

Ventricular ectopy has been a major predictor of both sudden death and long-term mortality in patients after MI. In the Beta Blocker Heart Attack Trial, propranolol decreased the frequency of ventricular ectopy in the first 6 weeks after the event.[16] In patients with complex ventricular ectopy, propranolol therapy resulted in a greater decrease in mortality when compared with those patients without complex ventricular premature beats.[17]

Treatment with β-blockers in postinfarction patients with left ventricular dysfunction has been of particular interest. Some concern was initially raised regarding the potential dangers of these drugs in patients with heart failure. Patients with severe left ventricular dysfunction manifested by shock and overt congestive heart failure were excluded from most β-blocker trials. In the Beta Blocker Heart Attack Trial, patients were included who had congestive heart failure but whose heart failure was stabilized with digitalis and diuretic therapy. In those patients with a history of heart failure, propranolol therapy had the greatest benefit on mortality and sudden death (Fig. 27–4).[24] There was a slight increase in heart failure in the initial phases of the treatment of these patients. In a similar study in patients with complex arrhythmias and ventricular dysfunction, propranolol was also demonstrated to decrease sudden death significantly.[25] A recent analysis of the patients who received β-blockers in the placebo arm of the Multicenter Diltiazem Postinfarction Trial further confirmed these observations.[26] In that study, patients with evidence of heart failure and a left ventricular ejection fraction of less than 30% and who received a β-blocker had a 50% decrease in mortality when compared with those who were not taking β-blockers. Although β-blockers

should be used cautiously in patients with left ventricular dysfunction, these patients have the greatest potential for benefit.

The duration of therapy in these two trials was limited to 2 to 3 years. Their beneficial effects persisted throughout that time. The Norwegian Multicenter Study[27] was extended to 6 years, during which a continued beneficial effect was observed. The effect of withdrawal of metoprolol after 2 years of therapy in patients after an MI resulted in an increase in mortality in the patients who were withdrawn from therapy compared with patients who continued therapy.[28] In patients taking a β-blocker before an MI, the risk and severity of the subsequent acute infarction was decreased.[29] Ventricular fibrillation was similar in patients regardless of prior β-blocker therapy. Patients taking a β-blocker at the time of admission had a reduced extent of infarction and risk of death during the 28-day period after an acute MI. Although there are a number of β-adrenergic blocking agents, it appears that most have a cardioprotective effect.

CALCIUM ANTAGONISTS

The term *calcium channel blocking agent* or *calcium antagonist* is used to describe a group of drugs that share a similar pharmacologic property of blocking the entrance of calcium into striated cardiac and smooth vascular muscle. These compounds are structurally and mechanistically dissimilar but share the ability to produce selective blockade of the slow inward calcium current. These compounds are potent vasodilators and have been approved for use in the treatment of hypertension, exertional angina, and vasospastic angina. At present, the compounds diltiazem, nifedipine, and verapamil have been investigated in postinfarction patients in regard to cardioprotection.

Nifedipine

Nifedipine was one of the first calcium antagonists to be tested as secondary prevention after an acute MI. The Secondary Prevention Reinfarction Israeli Nifedipine Trial (SPRINT-I)[30] randomized patients with confirmed MI to nifedipine 10 mg three times a day or placebo. No significant difference in reinfarction or mortality was observed in the two groups. Subsequently, the SPRINT-II[31] enrolled high-risk acute MI patients to nifedipine 60 mg a day or placebo. The study was terminated early because of an excess mortality noted in the nifedipine group. A number of studies have been carried out with this drug with little evidence to support its efficacy in acute or chronic ischemic heart disease, with the exception of its ability to lower blood pressure and decrease symptoms of angina pectoris.

Verapamil

In the Danish Study Group on Verapamil in Myocardial Infarction Trial (DAVIT-I),[32] verapamil was ad-

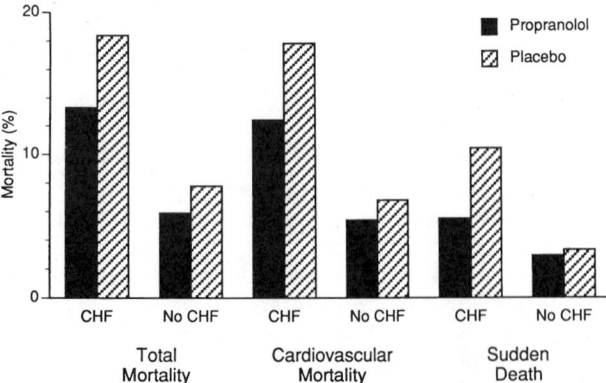

Figure 27–4. The effect of propranolol therapy on mortality in patients with and without a history of congestive heart failure at the time of randomization. (From Chadda K, Goldstein S, Byington R, et al: Effect of propranolol after acute myocardial infarction in patients with congestive heart failure. Circulation 73:503, 1986.)

ministered intravenously soon after the onset of symptoms, followed by oral verapamil. Its use resulted in increased mortality and heart failure in patients in the active treatment arm. However, patients who tolerated verapamil for the first 2 to 3 weeks after the MI had a lower morality and reinfarction rate compared with placebo. Because of these events, DAVIT-II[33] was designed to examine the role of verapamil therapy started 1 to 2 weeks after an acute MI. The study medication consisted of verapamil 120 mg three times a day or matching placebo. After 18 months, there was a statistically insignificant reduction in total mortality in the verapamil group compared with the placebo group, but there was a significant reduction in first major events in the verapamil group.

Diltiazem

Diltiazem was evaluated in the Multicenter Diltiazem Postinfarction Trial.[34] Its effect on mortality and cardiac events was examined in patients who had had a recent MI. Although the incidence of cardiac events, mortality rate, and reinfarction was 11% lower in the diltiazem group, this difference was not statistically significant. Patients receiving diltiazem had a slightly increased incidence of atrioventricular block and hypotension. Subgroup analysis showed that patients without pulmonary congestion on chest x-ray examination or a left ventricular ejection fraction of more than 40%, representing 80% of the patients enrolled, had a 30% reduction in cardiac events when compared with the placebo group. In contrast, in patients with pulmonary congestion and ejection fraction of less than 30%, diltiazem was associated with a significant 25% increase in cardiac events.

The only study to be conducted prospectively in patients with non–Q wave MI was the Multicenter Diltiazem Reinfarction Trial.[35] In this trial, patients were randomized to diltiazem, 90 mg four times a day, or placebo for 14 days. The treatment began 24 to 72 hours after onset of symptoms. In both placebo and diltiazem groups, approximately 60% of patients received β-blocker therapy and 80% were taking nitrates. During the 14-day follow-up, the rates of reinfarction and postinfarction angina were significantly lower in the diltiazem group when compared with placebo, although the 14-day mortality was not different in the two treatment groups.

A review of the trials with calcium antagonists in patients after MI suggests that nifedipine has no role in secondary prevention of reinfarction. Verapamil and diltiazem may be beneficial in reducing mortality and reinfarction when started 1 week or later after the acute event in patients with preserved left ventricular function and without signs and symptoms of heart failure. However, verapamil or diltiazem should not be used in these patients when there are signs and symptoms of heart failure, including pulmonary congestion on chest x-ray examination and/or a significant decrease in left ventricular systolic function.

ANTIARRHYTHMIC THERAPY

Although frequent and complex ventricular ectopy in patients recovering from acute MI is an important predictor of sudden death, the prognostic value of ventricular ectopy varies greatly relative to the extent of left ventricular dysfunction. As ejection fraction falls, ventricular ectopy becomes more common. In the setting of advanced ventricular dysfunction, frequent multiple multiform ventricular ectopy occurs in almost 70% of patients and is a predictor of sudden death.

A number of randomized drug trials examined the effects of phenytoin, tocainide, mexiletine, aprindine, sotalol, amiodarone, encainide, flecainide, and moricizine in the suppression of ventricular ectopy after infarction. Some of these trials were designed to investigate the use of antiarrhythmic agents regardless of ectopic beat suppression; others investigated the benefit of ectopic beat suppression alone. None of these studies observed a benefit in mortality regardless of their effect on ventricular ectopy suppression.

Sotalol

Sotalol, a β-adrenergic blocking agent with class III antiarrhythmic action, was first studied by Julian et al.[36] in survivors of acute MI. At 12 months, the mortality was 18% lower in the sotalol group than in the placebo group, but the difference was not statistically significant. More recently, the Electrophysiologic Study versus Electrocardiographic Monitoring (ESVEM)[37] Study suggested that sotalol therapy resulted in a lower risk of arrhythmia recurrence when compared with a variety of other antiarrhythmic agents. Sotalol, in its racemic form, which includes β-receptor blockade, and as D-sotalol without β-receptor-blocking effect, is now under reinvestigation as an agent to decrease death in patients at high risk after an acute MI.

Amiodarone

Amiodarone has been investigated in regard to its ability to suppress ventricular arrhythmias after acute MI.[38] Although the amiodarone significantly reduced the complex ventricular arrhythmias compared with placebo, no significant decrease in mortality occurred. The Basel Antiarrhythmic Study of Infarct Survival (BASIS)[39] was a comparison of low-dose amiodarone, conventional antiarrhythmic therapy, and placebo for 1 year after an MI in patients with high-frequency ventricular ectopy. Amiodarone was first administered at a dosage of 1000 mg for 5 days, followed by 200 mg daily for 1 year. The conventional antiarrhythmic therapy included quinidine and mexiletine plus other antiarrhythmic drugs in order to achieve ventricular beat suppression. Those patients in whom suppression was not achieved received amiodarone. A significant decrease in sudden death and arrhythmic events was achieved with amiodarone. The total mortality in the control group was 13%, 10% in the conventional therapy, and 5% in the amiodarone group. Although this study suggests that amiodarone has benefit in patients with high-frequency ventricular ectopy, it does not deal with the issue of its multisystem toxicity when used over the long term. Amiodarone has a variety of potential physiologic effects, including a β-blocking effect and an unpredictable effect on thyroid functions. A number of studies are now under way examining the benefit of amiodarone in order to provide greater insight into its potential benefit.

The CAST Study

With the development of class IC drugs with greater ability to suppress ventricular ectopy and seemingly low toxicity, the efficacy of ventricular ectopic beat suppression was investigated in the Cardiac Arrhythmia Suppression Trial (CAST).[40] The CAST enrolled asymptomatic patients who had more than six ventricular premature beats per hour and examined the effect of ventricular ectopic beat suppression on sudden death. The criteria for suppression were reduction of 80% or more in ventricular premature beats and a reduction of 90% or more in runs of ventricular tachycardia. Patients whose ventricular premature beats were suppressed by drugs were randomly assigned to receive blinded therapy: encainide, flecainide, moricizine, or placebo. The trial was prematurely discontinued because of an increased incidence in mortality in the treatment group during follow-up. Death from arrhythmias was 4.5% in the patients treated with flecainide or encainide, compared with 1.23% in patients who received placebo. The study was continued as CAST II,[41] using moricizine at three dose levels. It, too, was prematurely discontinued because of increased mortality in this treatment arm.

Electrophysiologic Guidance

There is general agreement that patients surviving cardiac arrest associated with acute MI, although associated with some increase in mortality risk, should be managed with the standard regimens outlined in this monograph. β-Adrenergic blocking agents are the foundation for that therapy. A comparison of empiric metoprolol therapy to electrophysiologically guided antiarrhythmic therapy revealed that metoprolol alone, given to previous victims of cardiac arrest, was better than guided therapy.[42]

Electrophysiologic testing for symptomatic arrhythmias, and particularly those associated with acute MI-related cardiac arrest, has also been undertaken. After an acute MI, if patients continue to have symptomatic arrhythmias in spite of maximal medical and surgical therapy for ischemia and heart failure, they should be considered for electrophysiologic study. In those symptomatic patients who are at high risk for sudden death, the use of programmed stimulation or automatic internal cardiac defibrillators is the current therapeutic standard, although these interventions have never been fully tested in clinical trials. The CAST study has challenged the wisdom of treating asymp-

tomatic patients with ventricular arrhythmias with drugs other than β-blockers, the only drug class known to decrease the incidence of sudden death.

ANGIOTENSIN-CONVERTING ENZYME INHIBITORS

Angiotensin-converting enzyme (ACE) inhibitors have been used in the treatment of congestive heart failure for some time. Recently the use of these drugs was investigated in patients after an acute MI. The initial studies demonstrated that captopril could modify the progression of left ventricular dilation after anterior MI.[43] These studies suggest that ACE inhibitors may be beneficial after an acute MI. The Survival in Ventricular Enlargement (SAVE)[44] trial examined treatment with captopril 3 to 16 days after an MI in patients with an ejection fraction of less than 40% and without evidence of heart failure or symptoms of myocardial ischemia. After an initial test dose of 6.25 mg of oral captopril, the patients were randomized to placebo or an increasing dose of captopril up to 50 mg three times daily. On this therapy, the patients receiving captopril had a 21% reduction in all-cause mortality and a 22% reduction in heart failure requiring hospitalization. Of particular interest was the observation that there was a significant decrease (by 22%) in recurrent MI in the captopril-treated patients. In the Studies of Left Ventricular Dysfunction (SOLVD),[45] treatment with captopril administered to patients with ejection fractions of less than 35% resulted in a significant reduction in the incidence of MI, unstable angina, and cardiac mortality. A subsequent investigation of ramipril in the Acute Infarction Ramipril Efficacy (AIRE)[46] study of patients with a recent MI resulted in a 27% reduction in overall mortality. From these studies, it can be concluded that in patients with clinical heart failure and/or reduced ejection fractions, a significant benefit can be obtained with ACE inhibitors when administered after an MI.

In order to examine the use of ACE inhibitors in early MI, a number of studies have been carried out. The first, The Cooperative New Scandinavian Enalapril Survival Study (CONSENSUS II),[47] examined the effect of early administration of enalapril in patients within 24 hours of acute MI. Therapy was initiated with an intravenous infusion of 1 mg of enalapril over a 2-hour period, followed by 2.5 to 5 mg orally started 6 hours after the conclusion of infusions given twice daily. This study failed to demonstrated any benefit and was prematurely stopped because of a potential increase in mortality rate. Two recent studies examined both captopril and lisinopril, also administered early after an acute MI. In both studies, a small but significant decrease in mortality was observed when these drugs were administered orally in the first 24 hours after infarctions. These studies all suggest that there are benefits to be obtained using ACE inhibitors after an acute MI, particularly when confined to patients with ejection fractions of less than 40%. It does not appear to be a major special benefit in patients with normal left ventricular function, and only a marginal benefit is associated with treatment within 24 hours after an MI.

CONCLUSION

During the last 20 years, we have made considerable advances in regard to our understanding of the mechanism and natural history of acute MI. These studies have led us up what appear to be blind alleys in our attempts to prevent recurrent infarction. Calcium antagonists and antiarrhythmic agents, at least for the present, appear to hold little promise for therapeutic benefit. In contrast, major impact has been achieved with the use of β-adrenergic blocking agents, aspirin, and, most recently, ACE inhibitors in patients with left ventricular dysfunction. More importantly, these drugs have provided biologic probes into our understanding of the pathophysiology of myocardial ischemia and infarction. As a result of these advances, clinicians have at their fingertips an expanded knowledge of the disease they are treating and a variety of effective therapeutic options from which they can choose.

REFERENCES

1. Steering Committee of the Physicians' Health Study Research Group: Final report on the aspirin component of the ongoing Physicians' Health Study. N Engl J Med 321:129, 1989.
2. Manson JE, Sampfer MJ, Colditz GA, et al: A prospective study of aspirin use and primary prevention of cardiovascular disease in women. JAMA 266:521, 1991.
3. Elwood PC, Cochrane Al, Burr MI, et al: A randomized controlled trial of acetyl salicylic acid in the secondary prevention of mortality from myocardial infarction. Br Med J 1:436, 1974.
4. Elwood PC, Sweetnam PM: Aspirin and secondary mortality after myocardial infarction. Lancet 2:1313, 1979.
5. The Coronary Drug Project Research Group: Aspirin in coronary heart disease. J Chronic Dis 29:6252, 1976.
6. Aspirin Myocardial Infarction Study Research Group: A randomized, controlled trial of aspirin in persons recovered from myocardial infarction. JAMA 243:6619, 1980.
7. The Persantine-Aspirin Reinfarction Trial Research Group: Persantine and aspirin in coronary heart disease. Circulation 62:449, 1980.
8. Klint CR, Knatterud GI, Stamler J, et al: Persantine-Aspirin Reinfarction Study. Part II: Secondary coronary prevention with persantine and aspirin. J Am Coll Cardiol 7:251, 1986.
9. Antiplatelet Trialists' Collaboration: Secondary prevention of vascular disease by prolonged antiplatelet therapy. Br Med J 296:320, 1988.
10. Lewis HD, Davis JW, Archibald DG, et al: Protective efforts of aspirin against acute myocardial infarction and death in men with unstable angina. N Engl J Med 309:396, 1983.
11. Second Report of the Working Party on Anticoagulant Therapy in Coronary Thrombosis to the Medical Research Council: An assessment on long-term anticoagulant therapy after myocardial infarction. Br Med J 2:837, 1964.
12. Sixty Plus Reinfarction Study Research Group: A double blind trial to assess long term oral anticoagulant therapy in elderly patients after myocardial infarction. Lancet 2:989, 1980.
13. Smith P, Arnesen II, Holme I: The effect of warfarin on mortality and reinfarction after myocardial infarction. N Engl J Med 323:147, 1990.
14. Weinrich DJ, Burke JF, Pauletto EJ: Left ventricular mural thrombi complicating acute myocardial infarction: Long term follow-up; with serial echocardiography. Ann Intern Med 100:789, 1984.
15. Kjekshus JK: Importance of heart rate in determining beta

blocker efficacy in acute and long term myocardial infarction trials. Am J Cardiol 57:43F, 1986.
16. Lichstein E, Morganroth J, Harrist R, et al: The BHAT Study Group: Effect of propranolol on ventricular arrhythmia: The Beta-Blocker Heart Attack Trial experience. Circulation 67(Suppl 1):5, 1983.
17. Friedman IM, Byington RP, Capone HJ, et al: Effect of propranolol in patients with myocardial infarction and ventricular arrhythmia. J Am Coll Cardiol 7:1, 1986.
18. Anderson JL, Rodier HE, Green LS: Comparative effects of beta-adrenergic blocking drugs on experimental ventricular fibrillation threshold. Am J Cardiol 51:1196, 1983.
19. The Norwegian Multicenter Study Group: Timolol-induced reduction in mortality and reinfarction in patients surviving acute myocardial infarction. N Engl J Med 304:801, 1981.
20. Beta Blocker Heart Attack Trial Research Group: A randomized trial of propranolol in patients with acute myocardial infarction. I: Mortality results. JAMA 247: 1707, 1982.
21. Gheorghiade M, Schultz I, Tilley B, et al: Effects of propranolol in non-Q-wave acute myocardial infarction in the Beta Blocker Heart Attack Trial. Am J Cardiol 60:129, 1990.
22. Gundersen T, Abrahamsen AM, Kjekshus J, et al (The Norwegian Multicentre Study Group): Timolol-related reduction in mortality and reinfarction in patients ages 65–75 years surviving acute myocardial infarction. Circulation 66:1179, 1981.
23. Jafri SM, Tilley BC, Peters R, et al: Effects of cigarette smoking and propranolol in survivors of acute myocardial infarction. Am J Cardiol 65:271, 1990.
24. Chadda K, Goldstein S, Byington R, et al: Effect of propranolol after acute myocardial infarction in patients with congestive heart failure. Circulation 73:503, 1986.
25. Furberg CD, Hawkins CM, Lichstein E, and the Beta-Blocker Heart Attack Trial Study Group: Effect of propranolol in postinfarction patients with mechanical or electrical complications. Circulation 69:761, 1984.
26. Lichstein F, Hager WD, Gregory JJ, et al: Relation between beta-adrenergic blocker use, various correlates of left ventricular function and the chance of developing congestive heart failure. J Am Coll Cardiol 16:1327, 1990.
27. Pederson TR and the Norwegian Multicenter Study Group: Six-year follow up of the Norwegian Multicenter Study of Timolol after acute myocardial infarction. N Engl J Med 313:1055, 1985.
28. Olsson G, Oden A, Johansson I, et al: Prognosis after withdrawal of chronic postinfarction metoprolol treatment: A 2–7 year follow-up. Eur Heart J 9:365, 1988.
29. Nidorf SM, Parsons RW, Thompson PI, et al: Reduced risk of death at 28 days in patients taking a beta blocker before admission to hospital with myocardial infarction. Br Med J 300:71, 1990.
30. The Israeli SPRINT Study Group: Secondary Prevention Reinfarction Israeli Nifedipine Trial (SPRINT): A randomized intervention trial of nifedipine in patients with acute myocardial infarction. Eur Heart J 9:354, 1988.
31. The SPRINT Study Group: The Secondary Prevention Reinfarction Israeli Nifedipine Trial (SPRINT II): Design, methods and results [abstract]. Eur Heart J 9(Suppl 1):350, 1988.
32. The Danish Study Group on Verapamil in Myocardial Infarction: Verapamil in acute myocardial infarction. Eur Heart J 5:516, 1984.
33. The Danish Study Group on Verapamil in Myocardial Infarction: Effect of verapamil on mortality and major events after acute myocardial infarction (The Danish Verapamil Infarction Trial II—DAVIT II). Am J Cardiol 66:779, 1990.
34. The Multicenter Diltiazem Postinfarction Trial Research Group: The effect of diltiazem on mortality and reinfarction after myocardial infarction. N Engl J Med 319:385, 1988.
35. Gibson RS, Boden WF, Therous P, et al: Diltiazem and reinfarction in patients with non-Q-wave myocardial infarction: Results of a double-blind, randomized, multicenter trial. N Engl J Med 315:423, 1986.
36. Julian DG, Prescott RJ, Jackson FS, et al: Controlled trial of sotalol for one year after myocardial infarction. Lancet 1:1142, 1982.
37. Mason JW, for the Electrophysiologic Study versus Electrocardiographic Monitoring Investigators: A comparison of electro-

physiologic testing with Holter monitoring to predict antiar-rhythmic-drug efficacy for ventricular tachyarrhythmias. N Engl J Med 329:445, 1993.

38. Hockings BEF, George T, Mahrous F, et al: Effectiveness of amiodarone on ventricular arrhythmias during and after acute myocardial infarction. Am J Cardiol 60:967, 1987.

39. Burkart F, Pfisterer M, Kiowski W, et al: Effect of antiarrhythmic therapy on mortality in survivors of myocardial infarction with asymptomatic complex ventricular arrhythmias: Basel Antiar-rhythmic Study of Infarct Survival (BASIS). J Am Coll Cardiol 16:1711, 1990.

40. Cardiac Arrhythmia Suppression Trial (CAST) Investigators: Preliminary report: Effect of encainide and flecainide on mor-tality in a randomized trial of arrhythmia suppression after myocardial infarction. N Engl J Med 321:406, 1989.

41. The Cardiac Arrhythmia Suppression Trial II Investigators: Ef-fect of the antiarrhythmic agent moricizine on survival after myocardial infarction. N Engl J Med 327:227, 1992.

42. Steinbeck G, Andresen D, Bach P, et al: A comparison of electro-physiologically guided antiarrhythmic drug therapy with beta-

blocker therapy in patients with symptomatic, sustained ven-tricular arrhythmias. N Engl J Med 327:987, 1992.

43. Sharpe N, Smith H, Murphy J, et al: Treatment of patients with symptomless left ventricular dysfunction after myocardial infarction. Lancet 1:256, 1988.

44. Pfeffer MA, Braunwald E, Moye LA, et al, on Behalf of the SAVE Investigators: Effect of captopril on mortality and mor-bidity in patients with left ventricular dysfunction after myo-cardial infarction. N Engl J Med 327:669, 1992.

45. Yusuf S, Pepine CJ, Garces C, et al: Effect of enalapril on myocardial infarction and unstable angina in patients with low ejection fractions. Lancet 340:1173, 1992.

46. The Acute Infarction Ramipril Efficacy (AIRE) Study Investiga-tors: Effect of ramipril on mortality and morbidity of survivors of acute myocardial infarction with clinical evidence of heart failure. Lancet 342:821, 1993.

47. Swedberg K, Held P, Kjekshus J, et al, on behalf of the CON-SENSUS II Study Group: Effects of the early administration of enalapril on mortality in patients with acute myocardial infarction. N Engl J Med 327:678, 1992.

CHAPTER 28

Treatment Strategies After Myocardial Infarction

Peter Sleight, M.D., F.R.C.P.

Thrombolytic treatment together with aspirin is one of the major medical successes of the 1980s. The Sec-ond International Study of Infarct Survival (ISIS-2) trial[1] (Fig. 28–1) showed that the use of these simple treatments within 4 hours of the onset of acute myo-cardial infarction (AMI) more than halved mortality; an overview of nearly all the individual patient data from the trials of any lytic agent versus control (or placebo) treatment now gives clear evidence that the finding of benefit even in patients treated later is certainly true up to 12 hours from the onset. The most recent data from ISIS-2 show that this benefit is undiminished 4 years later, even in those older than 70 at the time of randomization.

One reason for this surprisingly large benefit, in most cases without the need for any further proce-dures such as angiography and revascularization, is that the culprit lesion causing the original occlusion was likely to be a fissure in a minor nonoccluding plaque. Furthermore, the next event is more likely than not to be due to a similar event in another minor plaque. Thus, the seductive argument that early rou-tine angiography and revascularization (by angio-plasty or coronary artery bypass graft [CABG]) pre-vent future events is not as logical as first appears.

For these reasons, I believe an aggressive strategy for all patients after AMI is neither desirable nor necessary. On the other hand, we now have well-tested strategies for medical treatment to accompany or follow AMI, whether or not lytic therapy is used.

ASPIRIN

The publication of the Antiplatelet Trialists' Second Collaborative Study[2] emphasizes the importance of

this old and inexpensive therapy (Fig. 28–2). It works equally well in the presence or absence of thrombolysis (see Fig. 28–1), saving approximately 40 lives per 1000 patients treated in the first month after an AMI

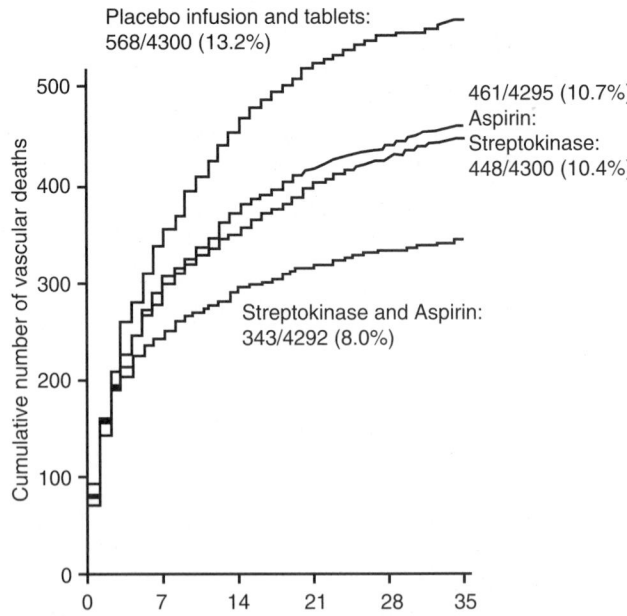

Figure 28–1. Benefits of streptokinase (up to 35 days) with and without aspirin versus placebo in patients suspected of acute MI in ISIS-2. Note that the benefit of aspirin, 160 mg chewed immedi-ately and continued daily for 1 month, is almost as great as that of SK, to which it is an additive. (From ISIS-2 [Second International Study of Infarct Survival] Collaborative Group: Randomised trial of intravenous streptokinase, oral aspirin, both, or neither, among 17,187 cases of suspected acute myocardial infarction: ISIS-2. Lancet 2:349, 1988. Copyright by The Lancet Ltd., 1988.)

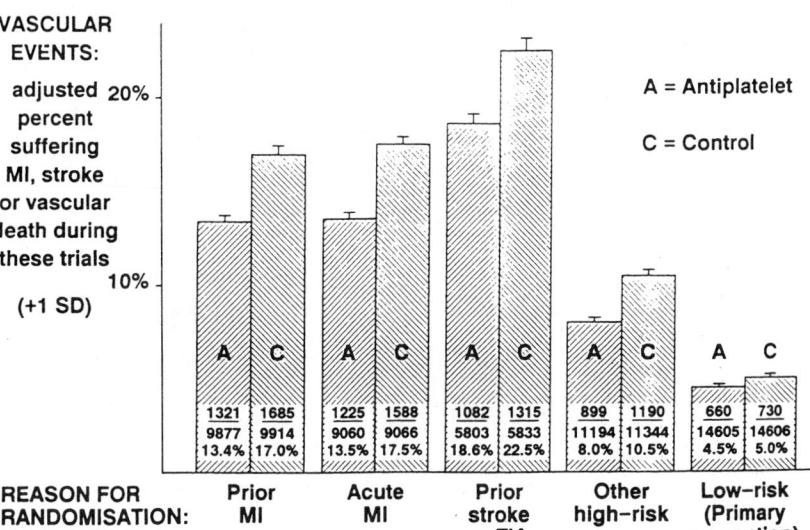

Absolute effects of ANTIPLATELET THERAPY (125 trials)
on VASCULAR EVENTS (MI, stroke or vascular death)
in four main high–risk categories and in low–risk (primary prevention)

BENEFIT (per					
1000) ± 1 sd :	36 ± 6	40 ± 5	39 ± 8	25 ± 4	5 ± 3
Months of A :	24	1	25	15	63
2P :	<0.00001	<0.00001	<0.00001	<0.00001	=0.05

VASCULAR
EVENTS:
adjusted 20%
percent
suffering
MI, stroke
or vascular
death during
these trials
10%
(+1 SD)

A = Antiplatelet

C = Control

	A	C	A	C	A	C	A	C	A	C
	1321	1685	1225	1588	1082	1315	899	1190	660	730
	9877	9914	9060	9066	5803	5833	11194	11344	14605	14606
	13.4%	17.0%	13.5%	17.5%	18.6%	22.5%	8.0%	10.5%	4.5%	5.0%

| REASON FOR RANDOMISATION: | Prior MI | Acute MI | Prior stroke or TIA | Other high–risk | Low–risk (Primary prevention) |

Figure 28–2. Benefits of short-term and longer-term aspirin in AMI. (From Antiplatelet Trialists' Collaboration: Collaborative overview of randomised trials of antiplatelet therapy. I: Prevention of death, myocardial infarction, and stroke by prolonged antiplatelet therapy in various categories of patients. BMJ 308:81,1994.)

(a reduction in mortality of about one quarter). The dose is not critical, but approximately 160 to 320 mg chewed immediately, followed by 75 to 160 mg daily, is well tested, effective, and nontoxic. Higher doses are no more effective and definitely two to three times more likely to cause bleeding or indigestion. The use of four aspirins per day—as advocated by some neurologists—is without scientific justification and appears to be based only on the fact that some earlier trials used this unnecessarily high dose.

The evidence from this latest overview strengthens the previous evidence for both the immediate use in AMI and also the longer-term use of aspirin in all patients with any form of vascular disease, in order to prevent future events. Despite this clear evidence, I still see patients admitted to a hospital with AMI after previous angina who have been treated by their physician with antianginal therapy but who have not been put on aspirin. Even if the patient gives a history of not being able to tolerate aspirin, or being "allergic" to aspirin, I rechallenge the patient with one of the newer low-dose, or slow-release, or enteric-coated aspirin formulations.

Low-dose (100 mg) slow-release preparations inhibit platelet cyclooxygenase while the platelets are in the portal circulation. When this slow "trickle" of aspirin reaches the liver, it is deacetylated on the first pass, so that no systemic aspirin is detectable, which avoids stimulation of gastric acid production by the action of aspirin in the central nervous system (CNS).

HEPARIN AND COUMADIN ANTICOAGULATION

Although there is good evidence for the use of anticoagulants in AMI in the absence of aspirin, most of the

trial evidence for heparin added to adequate aspirin comes from the GISSI-2 (Gruppo Italiano per lo Studio Della Supravivenza nell'Infarto Miocardio II) and ISIS-3 studies.[3, 4] These studies randomized subcutaneous high-dose heparin (25,000 units/day) added to 160 mg of aspirin with either tissue-type plasminogen activator (t-PA) or streptokinase (SK). Surprisingly, there was no significant long-term benefit for mortality from the addition of heparin to either agent in these trials, which included more than 60,000 patients. There was, however, a small but significant increase in hemorrhagic stroke and other bleeding, even with subcutaneous heparin (Fig. 28–3).

The results with t-PA were criticized because these trials did not use carefully titrated intravenous heparin, thought to be necessary for the short half-life t-PA. However, the Global Utilization of Streptokinase and Tissue Plasminogen Activator for Occluded Coronary Arteries (GUSTO) trial,[5] which compared the ISIS-3 subcutaneous heparin regimen with aggressive intravenous heparin, found that the subcutaneous regimen was not inferior to intravenous heparin in the prevention of reinfarction either with SK or t-PA.

My conclusions from all this new evidence are that routine use of aspirin is clearly beneficial with no evidence of serious toxicity but that the evidence for routine heparin is much less clear and is balanced by the evidence of increased risk from bleeding.

It has always been assumed that heparin was necessary with t-PA because of its short half-life, and so there are no mortality studies to throw light on the risk-to-benefit ratio. There is evidence from patency studies that heparin does add modestly to the patency achieved with t-PA and aspirin, but these studies are not big enough to address the size of the bleeding

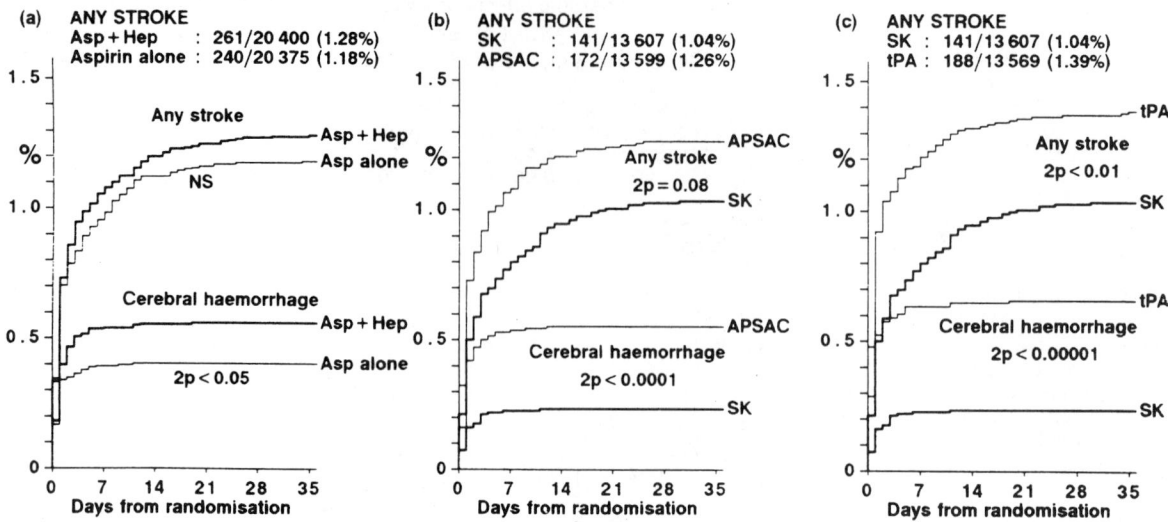

Figure 28–3. Cumulative percentage with any stroke *(upper lines)* and with (definite or probable) cerebral hemorrhage in hospital up to day 35 or prior discharge. *(a)* All patients allocated aspirin plus heparin *(thicker line)* versus all allocated aspirin alone; *(b)* all patients allocated SK *(thicker line)* versus all allocated anisoylated plasminogen-streptokinase activator complex (APSAC); *(c)* all patients allocated SK versus all allocated t-PA. (From ISIS-3 [Third International Study of Infarct Survival] Collaborative Group: ISIS-3: A randomised comparison of streptokinase vs tissue plasminogen activator vs anistreplase and of aspirin plus heparin vs aspirin alone among 41,299 cases of suspected acute myocardial infarction. Lancet 1:1, 1992. Copyright by The Lancet Ltd., 1992.)

risk involved. I continue to use intravenous heparin with t-PA, but only use heparin with SK plus aspirin in those patients at high risk of left ventricular thrombosis or systemic embolization, e.g., echo-proven mural thrombus, left ventricular (LV) failure, or arrhythmia. In such patients, I follow intravenous or high-dose subcutaneous heparin with oral anticoagulation for 3 to 6 months.

PRESERVATION OF LEFT VENTRICULAR FUNCTION

In addition to the damage caused by myocardial necrosis, LV function is also impaired by the dilation or remodeling that occurs as a result of the ischemic insult. This dilation occurs in nonischemic as well as ischemic myocardium. Dilation begins very rapidly and continues for the following weeks. Vasodilators, which facilitate left ventricular emptying, relieve symptoms of LV failure, and newer evidence suggests that, as a result, vasodilators may prevent ventricular dilation and hence improve prognosis.

ACE INHIBITION

Earlier studies in patients with heart failure (CONSENSUS-I, SOLVD)[6-8] showed the benefit of inhibiting the angiotensin-converting enzyme (ACE), which reduces vasoconstrictor angiotensin levels and also, perhaps importantly, increases plasma vasodilators such as bradykinin.

ACE Inhibition in the Postacute Phase of AMI

The SAVE study[9] randomized patients with impaired LV function at about a week or so after an MI to receive captopril or placebo. Patients receiving captopril experienced less LV dilation, and (after about 6 months) the mortality curves also diverged in favor of captopril. More recently, the Acute Infarction Ramipril Efficacy (AIRE) study,[10] coordinated in Leeds, England, by Ball, identified patients with LV dysfunction in the first 48 hours of an AMI by simple clinical criteria—pulmonary edema on chest x-ray examination or inspiratory rales (one third up the chest). Such patients gained considerable *early* benefit from the ACE inhibitor ramipril (Fig. 28–4). One month mortality in these high-risk patients was reduced by approximately 30%. These studies were carried out on pa-

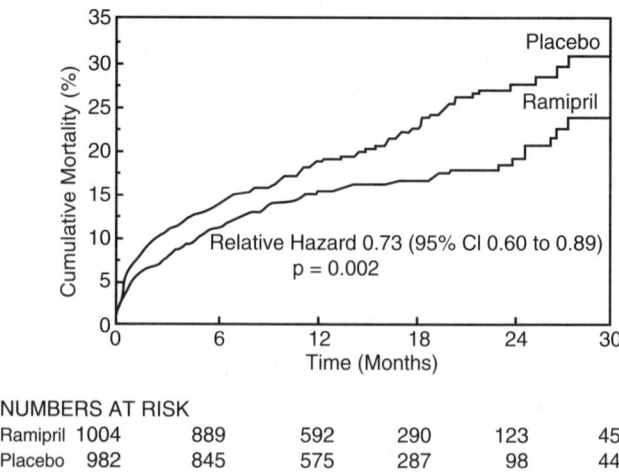

NUMBERS AT RISK

Ramipril	1004	889	592	290	123	45
Placebo	982	845	575	287	98	44

Figure 28–4. Thirty-day mortality in the AIRE study of ACE inhibition started 2 to 3 days after onset of AMI. (From The Acute Infarction Ramipril Efficacy [AIRE] Study Investigators: Effect of ramipril on mortality and morbidity of survivors of acute myocardial infarction with clinical evidence of heart failure. Lancet 342:821, 1993. Copyright by The Lancet Ltd., 1993.)

tients whose conditions had stabilized after the early stages of AMI.

ACE Inhibition in the Acute Phase of AMI

Clinicians were justifiably cautious about the possible harm (from hypotension) that might result from the use of ACE inhibition in the very early phase of AMI. This caution appeared to be justified when the CONSENSUS-II study was stopped early (at 6000 of 9000 planned patients) because no benefit was seen and there was also suspicion of some harm; the latter was not confirmed on later, more detailed analysis.[11]

After the CONSENSUS-II trial, the ISIS-4 (captopril), GISSI-3 (lisinopril), and a preliminary analysis of the Chinese captopril study reported on the use of ACE inhibitors in the early phase of MI in largely unselected patients (avoiding only those who were hypotensive: systolic blood pressure <100 mmHg) (American Heart Association [AHA] Meeting, November 1993). These trials were remarkably consistent and showed that carefully titrated oral therapy (as opposed to the intravenous enalaprilat used in CONSENSUS-II) was safe and resulted in a modest reduction in early mortality—approximately 10 to 15 fewer deaths per 1000 treated at 1 month. Judging by the earlier studies such as SAVE, this is likely to lead to further late benefit with longer follow-up. The benefit was greater in those patients who might be expected to have sustained more LV damage, i.e., those with anterior MI, a prior MI, or clinical evidence of LV failure.

We are thus left with a dilemma as to the best strategy: do we treat all nonhypotensive MI patients, withdrawing from treatment those with good LV function at the end of their hospital stay, or do we select patients who will gain the most benefit, as in the AIRE study? I suspect most clinicians, at least initially, will follow the second strategy, using ACE inhibition in the first 24 to 48 hours in high-risk patients (anterior MI, prior MI, or LV failure) after the patient's condition has stabilized.

One further benefit of ACE inhibition is that there appears to be a longer term effect that reduces reinfarction (seen in the SOLVD and SAVE trials). This effect may be a result of the reduction in angiotensin II levels in blood and tissue; angiotensin II is a known growth factor for vascular smooth muscle, so this effect is plausible, although this effect is not, at present, absolutely secure. It might simply be the result of lowered blood pressure, hence reduced risk of plaque rupture.

OTHER VASODILATORS
Nitrates

Early small trials of the use of oral or intravenous nitrates or nitroprusside suggested that there might be substantial early mortality benefit.[12] For these reasons, GISSI-3 tested intravenous nitrate infusion for 48 hours, followed by nitrate patches, and ISIS-4 examined the less expensive option of a slow-release isosorbide formulation (Imdur), which gives adequate nitrate levels for some 18 hours, followed by a nitrate-free period.

The results of these two trials (in approximately 60,000 patients) were similar and disappointing, showing only a small and statistically insignificant reduction in 5-week mortality of 2 to 3/1000 (AHA, 1993). The treatments were safe and very well tolerated apart from occasional headache. Imdur appeared to have a significant effect on early mortality (48 hours), but because this was not seen in GISSI-3 with intravenous nitrate, there is need for cautious interpretation of this early benefit.

My conclusion is that it is not necessary to use nitrates *routinely* in AMI, but that they can be used safely for the symptomatic relief of pain and/or LV failure. I would begin with oral nitrate, which should suffice for many patients, and only use intravenous preparations if the oral isosorbide fails to relieve symptoms.

Magnesium

The evidence for the use of a 24-hour infusion of magnesium sulphate was even stronger than that for nitrates,[13, 14] and it was therefore extremely perplexing when ISIS-4 was so completely negative for magnesium, with a nonsignificant excess of deaths in the magnesium arm overall. There were differences between LIMIT-2 and ISIS-4 in the patient populations, in the use of thrombolysis, and in the timing of the magnesium treatment, but examination of many subgroups in ISIS-4 (all of which were much larger than those in LIMIT-2) did not reveal any benefit. We should recall that the point estimate of a 24% reduction in mortality by intravenous magnesium in LIMIT-2 was surrounded by very wide 95% confidence intervals and that the lower estimate was only a 1% benefit. We should also remember that the original hypothesis was that a large part of the benefit of magnesium would be by an antiarrhythmic action. It was, however, shown that the benefit in LIMIT-2 was not by this mechanism but by reducing LV failure and shock. The reverse was seen in ISIS-4, namely, an increase in LV dysfunction.

We must conclude that there is now no basis for the routine use of intravenous magnesium, nor much encouragement for any use except when prior magnesium deficiency is a possibility.

β-Blockers

These agents are effective both acutely and, more commonly, long-term after AMI.[15] For the acute phase, early intravenous atenolol in ISIS-1 significantly reduced death at 5 weeks by approximately 15%. Similar results were seen with metoprolol in the MIAMI Study. Both of these results were obtained in the prethrombolytic era. Despite this evidence, their use varies markedly from country to country, perhaps because these results were overtaken by the more striking effects of thrombolysis, and perhaps also because intravenous β-blockers are contraindicated in about half the MI population, when LV function is poor. Thus, they are generally used only in the lower-risk patients.

β-Blockade lowers mortality in the acute phase mainly by a reduced risk of cardiac rupture.[16] The clinical picture of this generally fatal complication is that of electromechanical dissociation.[16] There is also a reduction of death from cerebral hemorrhage, arrhythmia, and aortic dissection. All of these are relevant to the era of thrombolysis, particularly cardiac rupture, which is an early hazard of thrombolysis.[17] Therefore, I believe β-blockers should still be used.

Long-Term β-Blockade

There is more evidence for the use of β-blockers long term, particularly to reduce sudden death and also reinfarction.[15] The reduction in risk is substantial (between ¼ and ⅓), and so they should be used more. Because of contraindications such as poor LV function and/or asthma or bronchitis, they cannot be used in more than 30% to 50% of patients; for patients with these conditions, ACE inhibitors or verapamil (see later discussion) are good alternatives. Some physicians prefer to avoid β-blockade in lower-risk patients. However, although it is possible to predict the risk of *death* post MI, it is not possible to predict that of reinfarction; therefore, this strategy seems somewhat illogical.

At the time of our review,[15] we speculated that restrospective analysis of the evidence suggested that agents without intrinsic sympathomimetic action might be more effective. This speculation is now disproved by a French study using acebutolol in high-risk patients.[18]

Calcium Antagonists

Despite variable and sometimes widespread use of calcium antagonists in AMI, there is little to support the use of any calcium antagonist in the very early phase of MI. On the other hand, there is a good deal of evidence that the dihydropyridines such as nifedipine are at best neutral and possibly harmful.[19, 20]

Although diltiazem was favorable in non–Q wave MI,[21] the larger Multicentre Diltiazem Postinfarction Trial (MDPIT)[22] of diltiazem was neutral—the benefit seen in patients who had no LV dysfunction was cancelled out by the excess mortality in those with LV failure. However, many patients in MDPIT were also taking β-blockers, which may have interacted unfavorably with the diltiazem.

The experience with verapamil in the Danish verapamil trials, DAVIT-1 and -2, was more favorable, perhaps because the verapamil was started later, at 3 days after onset, and β-blockade was not allowed. Verapamil was continued for 6 months in DAVIT-2 and significantly reduced sudden death and reinfarction to about the same extent as seen with β-blockade.[23]

In DAVIT-2, verapamil significantly reduced overall mortality in those without heart failure and was neither harmful nor beneficial in those with a history of heart failure.

Verapamil is thus a viable alternative in those patients who cannot tolerate β-blockade.

CONCLUSION

After the past decade of megatrials in acute myocardial infarction, it is now clear that we have several well-proven strategies to add to the major advance of thrombolysis. In descending order of importance and applicability are aspirin, ACE inhibitors for those with impaired LV function, and β-blockade for those with normal or mildly impaired LV function. Anticoagulation with intravenous heparin is not proved but is generally used with t-PA. After streptokinase, there is little or no role for routine use of heparin, although it may be advisable for those at high risk of LV thrombosis and embolization.

Nitrates are safe but should be used only for symptoms, beginning with oral nitrates and using intravenous nitrates only when oral treatment is insufficient. There does not seem any proven role for intravenous magnesium.

β-Blockade, verapamil, or diltiazem (the latter two started after the acute phase) are useful long-term (as is aspirin) for the prevention of reinfarction.

REFERENCES

1. ISIS-2 (Second International Study of Infarct Survival) Collaborative Group: Randomised trial of intravenous streptokinase, oral aspirin, both, or neither, among 17,187 cases of suspected acute myocardial infarction: ISIS-2. Lancet 2:349, 1988.
2. Antiplatelet Trialists' Collaboration: Collaborative overview of randomised trials of antiplatelet therapy. I: Prevention of death, myocardial infarction, and stroke by prolonged antiplatelet therapy in various categories of patients. BMJ 308:81, 1994.
3. The Gruppo Italiano per lo Studio Della Sopravivenza nell'Infarto Miocardio II (GISSI-2) and the International Study Group: A factorial randomised trial of alteplase versus streptokinase and heparin versus no heparin among 12,490 patients with acute myocardial infarction. Lancet 336:65, 1990.
4. ISIS-3 (Third International Study of Infarct Survival) Collaborative Group: ISIS-3: A randomised comparison of streptokinase vs tissue plasminogen activator vs anistreplase and of aspirin plus heparin vs aspirin alone among 41,299 cases of suspected acute myocardial infarction. Lancet 1:1, 1992.
5. The Global Utilization of Streptokinase and Tissue Plasminogen Activator for Occluded Coronary Arteries (GUSTO) Trial. N Engl J Med 329:673, 1993.
6. The CONSENSUS Trial Study Group: Effects of enalapril on mortality in severe congestive heart failure: Results of the Cooperative North Scandinavian Enalapril Survival Study (CONSENSUS). N Engl J Med 316:1429, 1987.
7. The SOLVD Investigators: Effect of enalapril on survival in patients with reduced ejection fractions and congestive heart failure. N Engl J Med 325:293, 1991.
8. The SOLVD Investigators: Effect of enalapril on mortality and the development of heart failure in asymptomatic patients with reduced left ventricular ejection fractions. N Engl J Med 327:685, 1992.
9. Pfeffer MA, Braunwald E, Moye LA, et al: Effect of captopril on mortality and morbidity in patients with left ventricular dysfunction after myocardial infarction. N Engl J Med 327:669, 1992.

10. The Acute Infarction Ramipril Efficacy (AIRE) Study Investigators: Effect of ramipril on mortality and morbidity of survivors of acute myocardial infarction with clinical evidence of heart failure. Lancet 342:821, 1993.

11. Swedburg K, Held P, Kjekshus J, et al, on behalf of the CONSENSUS II Study Group: Effects of early administration of enalapril on mortality in patients with acute myocardial infarction: Results of the Cooperative North Scandinavian Enalapril Survival Study II (CONSENSUS II). N Engl J Med 327:678, 1992.

12. Yusuf S, Collins R, MacMahon S, Peto R: Effect of intravenous nitrates on mortality in acute myocardial infarction: An overview of the randomised trials. Lancet 1:1088, 1988.

13. Teo K, Held P, Collins R, Yusuf S: Effect of intravenous magnesium on mortality in myocardial infarction. BMJ 303:1499, 1991.

14. Woods KL, Fletcher S, Roffe C, Haider Y: Intravenous magnesium sulphate in suspected acute myocardial infarction: Results of the second Leicester Intravenous Magnesium Intervention Trial (LIMIT-2). Lancet 339:1553, 1992.

15. Yusuf S, Peto R, Lewis J, et al: Beta-blockade during and after myocardial infarction: An overview of the randomised trials. Prog Cardiovasc Dis 27:335, 1985.

16. ISIS-1 (First International Study of Infarct Survival) Collaborative Group: Mechanisms for the early mortality reduction produced by beta-blockade started early in acute myocardial infarction: ISIS-1. Lancet 2:921, 1988.

17. Fibrinolytic Therapy Trialists' (FTT) Collaborative Group: Indications for fibrinolytic therapy in suspected acute myocardial infarction: Collaborative overview of mortality and major morbidity results from all randomised trials of more than 1000 patients. Lancet (In press).

18. Boissel J-P, Leizorovicz A, Picolet H, et al: APSI (Acebutolol et Prévention Secondaire de l'Infarctus): Secondary prevention after high risk acute myocardial infarction with low dose acebutolol. Am J Cardiol 66:251, 1990.

19. Holland Interuniversity Nifedipine/Metoprolol Trial (HINT) Research Group: Early treatment of unstable angina in the coronary care unit: A randomized, double blind, placebo controlled comparison of recurrent ischaemia in patients treated with nifedipine or metoprolol or both. Br Heart J 56:400, 1986.

20. Wilcox RO, Hampton JR, Banks DC, et al: Trial of early nifedipine in acute myocardial infarction: The TRENT Study. Br Med J 294:1204, 1986.

21. Gibson RS, Boden WE, Theroux P, et al: Diltiazem and reinfarction in patients with non Q-wave myocardial infarction: Results of a double blinded, randomized multicenter trial. N Engl J Med 315:423, 1986.

22. The Multicentre Diltiazem Postinfarction Trial Research Group: The effect of diltiazem on mortality and reinfarction after myocardial infarction. N Engl J Med 319:385, 1988.

23. The Danish Study Group on Verapamil in Myocardial Infarction: Verapamil in acute myocardial infarction. Eur Heart J 5:516, 1984.

CHAPTER 29

Pharmacologic Management of the Angioplasty Patient

*James Stephen Jenkins, M.D., Stephen R. Ramee, M.D.,
and Tyrone J. Collins, M.D.*

Percutaneous transluminal coronary angioplasty (PTCA) is the technique of enlarging a narrowed coronary arterial lumen by percutaneous introduction of either balloons, atherectomy devices, lasers, or stents. Since the first procedure was performed in 1977 by Andreas Gruentzig,[1] this technique has become widely accepted as an effective and safe method for treating occlusive atherosclerotic coronary artery disease, with approximately 200,000 procedures performed per year in the late 1980s and an estimated 500,000 procedures performed in 1993 alone.[2] There have been significant technologic advances in angioplasty equipment and devices aimed at providing more complete revascularization (Fig. 29–1).[3, 4] Pharmacologic therapy after angioplasty has continued to be targeted at the prevention of abrupt vessel closure, prevention of restenosis, and modification of risk factors to decrease the progression of atherosclerosis. This chapter examines the role of pharmacologic therapy in treating angioplasty patients.

PATHOPHYSIOLOGY OF ANGIOPLASTY

The morphologic effects of different interventional devices on the coronary artery lumen can be separated into two underlying processes: (1) remodeling and (2) removal.[5] Balloons and stents remodel the coronary artery lumen, displacing atherosclerotic plaque and/or thrombus by means of stretching, dissecting, splitting, or scaffolding the diseased segment. Intimal flaps, thrombus, or other obstructive material can be reattached to the adjacent vessel wall by means of thermal balloons and hot-tipped probes. Removal of obstructive atherosclerotic plaque is accomplished by atherectomy devices that excise, cut, drill, and shave or by thermal balloons and probes that heat, melt, and vaporize obstructive material. Regardless of the type of interventional device used, plaque fractures, breaks, and dissection clefts extend from the lumen into the plaque, improving blood flow by creating additional channels for coronary perfusion (Fig. 29–2).

The acute goals of medical therapy are preventing abrupt vessel closure, preventing PTCA-induced vasospasm, and enhancing thrombolysis (Figs. 29–3 and 29–4). Pharmacologic efforts are also directed at altering myocardial supply and demand to minimize the ischemic insult induced by transient coronary artery occlusion using a combination of β-blockers, calcium antagonists, and nitrates. The chronic goals of medical therapy after angioplasty are directed at preventing restenosis, preventing myocardial ischemia, and modifying risk factors.

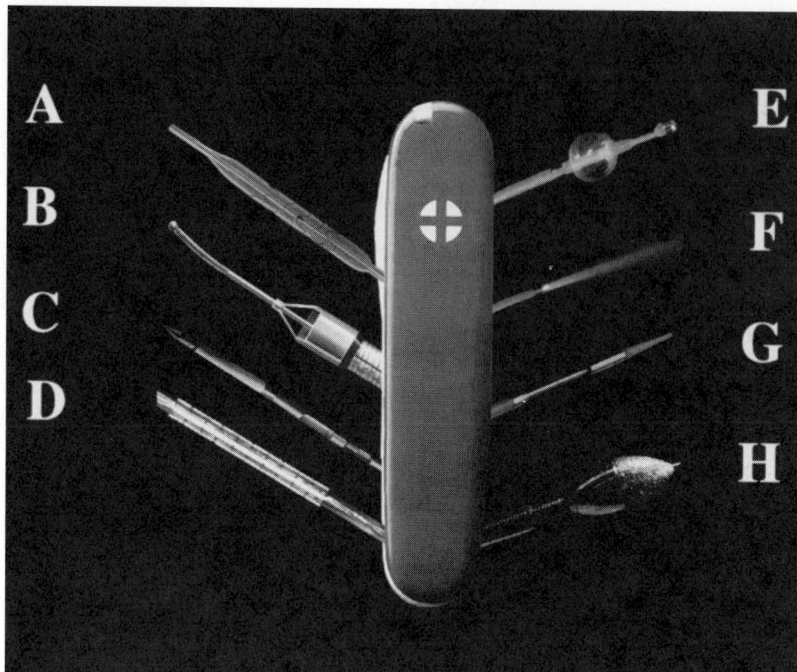

Figure 29–1. A and D, Balloon and stents. B, C, G, and H, Atherectomy catheters. E, Angioscope. F, Laser.

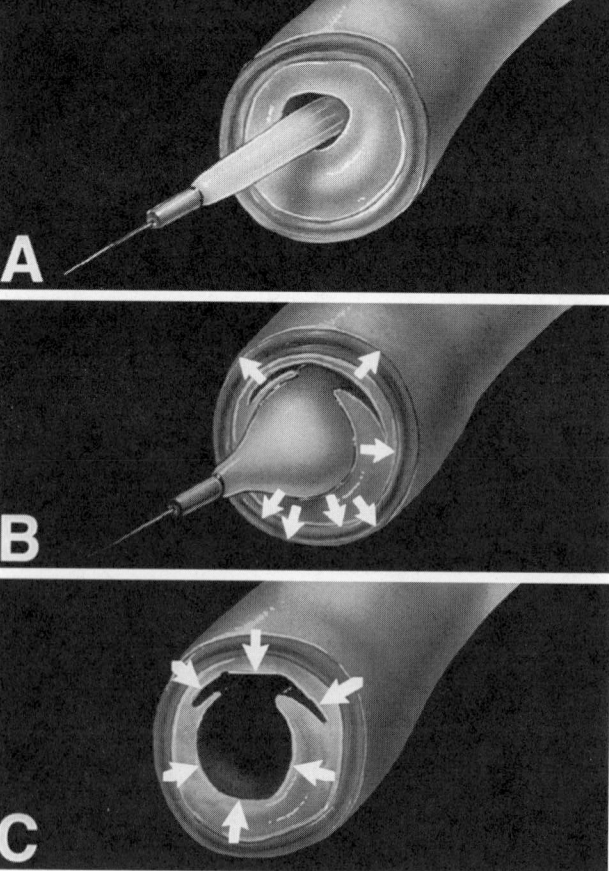

Figure 29–2. A, Coronary artery stenosis before balloon angioplasty. B, Radial forces exerted by balloon inflation. C, Elastic recoil and residual dissection after angioplasty.

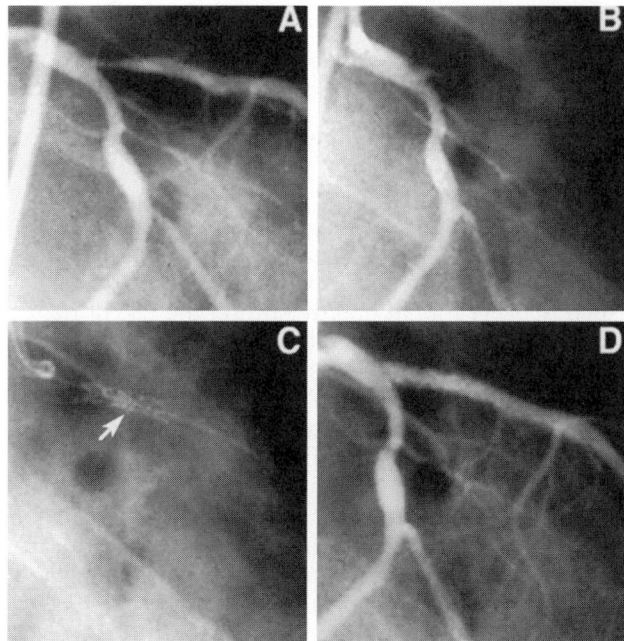

Figure 29–3. A, Coronary artery stenosis before balloon angioplasty. *B,* Abrupt vessel closure immediately after angioplasty. *C,* Intracoronary stent implantation. *D,* Successful treatment of abrupt vessel closure.

PHARMACOLOGIC AGENTS
Antiplatelet Agents
Aspirin

Percutaneous angioplasty causes severe mechanical disruption of the intima and media, making pharmacologic modification of the platelet-fibrin response to vascular trauma an important adjunct in improving success of the procedure. The efficacy of aspirin in reducing the ischemic complications and abrupt vessel closure after coronary angioplasty was established by Barnathan et al.[6] Aspirin inhibits the production of thromboxane A_2 by irreversible acetylation of platelet cyclooxygenase, thus reducing the incidence of abrupt vessel closure after PTCA by 50% to 75%.[6] Barnathan demonstrated that the incidence of occlusive intracoronary thrombi detected by angiography 30 minutes after angioplasty was significantly lower in the aspirin-treated group (1.8% versus 10.7%). In summary, the majority of data supports that aspirin is beneficial in reducing postangioplasty myocardial infarction, ischemic complications, and occlusive intracoronary thrombi.

Dipyridamole

Dipyridamole exerts its antiplatelet effect by inhibiting phosphodiesterase, the enzyme that degrades cyclic adenosine monophosphate (cAMP), blocking uptake of adenosine by the vascular endothelium and activating adenylate cyclase by prostacyclin-mediated effect on the platelet membrane. This increases the level of cAMP, which inhibits both phospholipase C and phospholipase A_2 and decreases intracellular calcium concentration, rendering platelets inactive.[7] The data to support the use of dipyridamole are not as convincing as the aspirin data. Swartz et al.[8] reported a randomized trial comparing aspirin and dipyridamole with placebo and demonstrated the incidence of Q-wave myocardial infarction to be lower in the aspirin treated group (1.6% versus 6.9%). In contrast, Mufson et al.[9] examined the influence of aspirin alone on the incidence of postprocedural myocardial infarction or emergency bypass surgery in patients with doses randomized to 80 or 1500 mg/day and found no significant differences.

Figure 29–4. Right coronary artery thrombus successfully treated with intracoronary thrombolytic infusion.

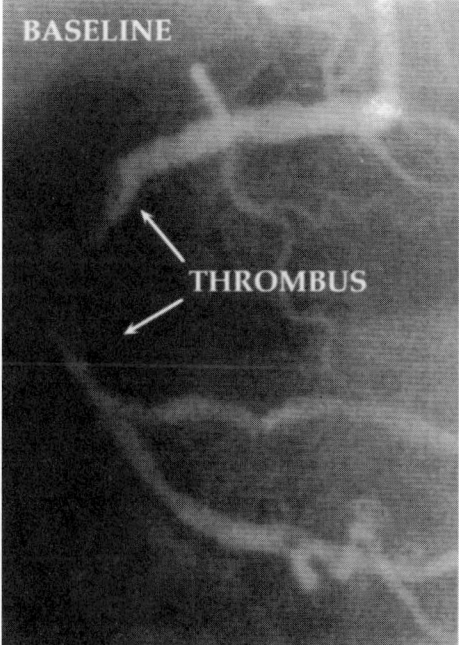

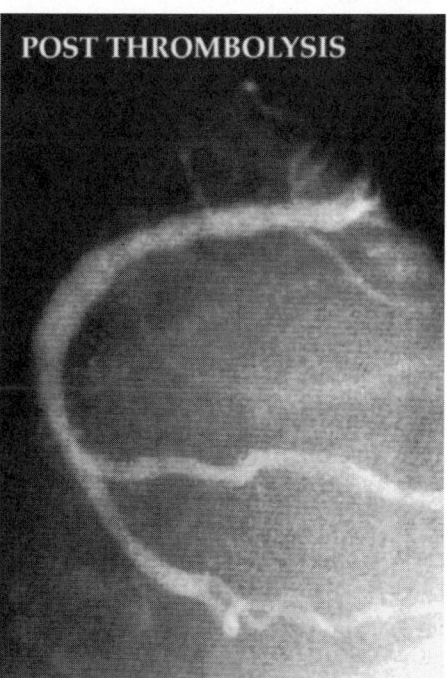

A randomized trial from Emory University by Lembo et al.[10] examined the need for administration of oral dipyridamole in combination with aspirin. They found that the addition of 75 mg of oral dipyridamole three times daily did not significantly change the incidence of ischemic complication postangioplasty when compared with aspirin alone at a dosage of 325 mg twice daily. Therefore, current data do not support the need for adjunctive treatment of the postangioplasty patient with dipyridamole.

Ticlopidine

Ticlopidine is an antiplatelet agent that interferes with platelet membrane function by inhibiting adenosine diphosphate–induced platelet-fibrinogen binding and subsequent platelet-to-platelet interactions. The Ticlopidine Study Trial demonstrated that the incidence of ischemic complications after angioplasty was reduced from 13.6% to 1.8% in the placebo-treated versus the ticlopidine-treated groups, respectively.[11] The Ticlopidine Coronary Angioplasty Trial demonstrated that the acute closure rate was significantly lower (5.1% versus 16.2%) after angioplasty in patients treated with ticlopidine than in control patients.[12] Although these data demonstrate beneficial effects of ticlopidine in the angioplasty patient, this drug is not routinely used after angioplasty at our institution because of an unfavorable side effect profile.

Dextran

Dextran is an antiplatelet agent that, when given intravenously, affects platelet adhesion after 4 to 6 hours of continuous infusion in a dose-related fashion. It works by exerting an inhibitory action on platelet membrane function[13] or by interfering with factor VIII–von Willebrand's factor (vWF) complex.[14] The antithrombotic efficacy of dextran has been shown in some studies;[15] however, clinical trials in patients undergoing coronary angioplasty have failed to demonstrate efficacy of this drug.[15] Swanson and the Mayo Clinic group[16] suggested that dextran had no effect on platelet adhesion when administered 30 minutes before balloon angioplasty. The effect of optimal administration of dextran during balloon angioplasty has not been studied. During coronary stent implantation, dextran as an adjuvant to heparin and antiplatelet therapy has been used.[17] However, side effects reported during dextran infusions, including anaphylactic reactions, acute respiratory distress syndrome, and coronary spasm, limit its present use in this selected population that has undergone stent implantation.[18]

Anticoagulant Agents

Heparin

Heparin is a family of polysaccharides with chains made of alternating residues of uronic acid and D-glucosamine of varying sulfation. Heparin functions as an anticoagulant by enhancing the rate of antithrombin III–thrombin binding by more than 1000-fold. This enhancement is also seen with all the serine proteases of the intrinsic pathway (IXa, Xa, XIa, XIIa).[19] The use of prolonged heparin infusions to decrease fibrin deposition at sites of vascular injury and to inhibit platelet aggregation[20] is somewhat controversial. Although intravenous heparin is considered essential intraprocedural pharmacotherapy, its role in the postprocedural period is less clearly established. Observational data regarding the use of heparin before PTCA in unstable patients, during PTCA, and after PTCA in vessels with suboptimal angiographic results have been obtained. Regression of angiographically visible thrombus has been reported by two groups after 6 to 7 days of continuous intravenous heparin.[21] In an uncontrolled retrospective analysis, Laskey et al.[22] reported that heparin infusion for 3 to 6 days before angioplasty in patients with unstable angina or intracoronary thrombus was associated with a significantly lower incidence of coronary occlusion than in patients not receiving heparin.

Systemic heparinization to maintain an activated clotting time (ACT) of more than 300 seconds is universally employed during coronary angioplasty. No randomized trial to determine the proper level of heparin anticoagulation during coronary angioplasty has been performed. Many factors including heparin potency, body weight, previous heparin therapy with the development of heparin antibodies, and concurrent nitroglycerin therapy may affect the adequacy of heparin anticoagulation. Lower rates of periprocedural ischemic complications have been reported in retrospective analyses by McGary et al.[23] and Dougherty et al.[24] when maintaining a partial thromboplastin time (PTT) of three or more times control or an ACT of more than 300 seconds, respectively. Receiving the standard 10,000 units heparin bolus before coronary angioplasty has not been shown to be adequate in maintaining an ACT of more than 300 seconds. Two studies[25, 26] have demonstrated that the standard bolus received by 11% and 23% of patients, respectively, was inadequate for anticoagulation. It is, therefore, recommended to routinely assess heparin anticoagulation in the cardiac catheterization laboratory.

There is also controversy regarding postangioplasty heparinization. Some operators routinely heparinize all angioplasty patients for 12 to 24 hours after the procedure, whereas others reserve prolonged heparinization for suboptimal angioplasty results. McGary et al. reported in a retrospective analysis that out-of-laboratory abrupt vessel closure rates were significantly lower in patients with PTTs more than three times control than in those with PTTs less than three times control.[23] On the contrary, three randomized trials studying a total of 959 patients failed to demonstrate a decrease in ischemic complications in patients treated with 12 to 24 hours of heparin therapy versus those receiving no heparin therapy.[27–29] These three studies, however, did not randomize patients with threatened vessel closure or suboptimal procedural results. These data suggest that heparin may prevent abrupt vessel closure after coronary angioplasty in patients with suboptimal angiographic results; however, the indications for prolonged heparin infusions and the duration of therapy have yet to be defined for patients with an uncomplicated PTCA.

Warfarin

Oral anticoagulants, the coumarins, are a group of naturally occurring lactones that are synthesized by both plants and a group of microorganisms. The most widely used of the coumarins is warfarin sodium owing to its favorable pharmacologic profile. Coumarin acts by retarding thrombin generation in both the intrinsic and extrinsic pathways of coagulation by inhibiting vitamin K–epoxide reductase in the liver. This leads to a decrease in the carboxylation of the N-terminal regions of coagulation factors II, VII, IX, and X and proteins C and S with vitamin K.[30]

The use of warfarin in the postangioplasty patient is limited mainly to stent implantation. Stent patients are anticoagulated with dextran and heparin until warfarin prolongs the prothrombin time (PT) to more than or equal to 1.5 times control or an international normalized ratio equal to 3.0 to 4.0. Continuing warfarin, in addition to aspirin and dipyridamole, for 3 months is the generally accepted regimen practiced in the United States. Subacute and acute thrombosis of stents occur in 6% to 8% of patients even with this vigorous anticoagulation practice.[31–33]

The dose-response between individuals and the many drugs that can influence the pharmacokinetics of warfarin requires close monitoring of PT levels.[34] The anticoagulant effect is potentiated by drugs inhibiting the metabolic clearance of warfarin, such as cimetidine and amiodarone, and is counteracted by drugs inducing hepatic enzyme activity, such as barbiturates and ethanol. The anticoagulant effects of warfarin are reached when the normal clotting factors are cleared from the circulation. This requires 72 to 96 hours because of the biologic half-lives of these proteins.

Thrombolytic Agents

Three thrombolytic agents have been used in conjunction with coronary angioplasty (streptokinase, recombinant tissue plasminogen activator [rtPA], and urokinase). Thrombolytic drugs as an adjunct to coronary angioplasty for preventing abrupt vessel closure is controversial. One small randomized study showed no benefit with the routine use of urokinase infusion during coronary angioplasty when compared with intracoronary heparin.[35] In patients with unstable angina or intracoronary thrombus, two groups have reported substantial resolution of large intraluminal thrombi followed by completion of successful coronary angioplasty with intracoronary streptokinase or intravenous tissue plasminogen activator[36] or with large boluses of intracoronary urokinase.[37] There were

no comparative data in patients not receiving thrombolytic agents in these two studies.

A retrospective study by Pavlidos et al.[38] compared results in 80 high-risk patients who received urokinase during angioplasty with results in 167 similar patients who did not receive intracoronary urokinase. Patients with angiographically defined intraluminal thrombus had less ischemic complications than those not receiving urokinase (3% versus 18%), whereas patients with intimal dissection were adversely affected by urokinase therapy (20.8% versus 9%). The Thrombolysis and Angioplasty in Unstable Angina Pilot study[39] randomized patients with unstable angina to low-dose urokinase versus high-dose urokinase and found no decrease in the incidence of abrupt vessel closure.

Although the apparent unfavorable effect of thrombolytic agents in the setting of dissection may be due to exaberation of subintimal hemorrhage or inhibition of intimal readherence to the vessel wall, the mechanism is unknown. In summary, thrombolytic drugs appear to have a role during PTCA in patients with large thrombus burden but do not appear to be useful during routine PTCA.

Drugs That Decrease Vessel Spasm and Prevent Ischemia

Nitrates

Nitrates have been used during coronary angioplasty to limit ischemia during balloon inflation[40] and prevent coronary spasm.[41] Doorey et al.[42] noted an increase in time to angina in patients receiving 200 μg of nitroglycerin intravenously compared with control angioplasty inflations. They also found an increase in the time to onset of 1 mm ST elevation and a blunted increase in the left ventricular end-diastolic pressure constant in patients treated with intravenous nitroglycerin before balloon inflations. The beneficial effects of nitroglycerin on these parameters could not be reproduced by Feldman et al.[43]

Although nitroglycerin provides little or no improvement in myocardial protection, intracoronary or intravenous nitroglycerin may prevent important coronary artery spasm associated with coronary angioplasty. This is especially true during directional and rotational atherectomy and intravascular ultrasound, when intense coronary artery spasm commonly occurs and can lead to hemodynamic instability. Bolus injections of 100 to 200 μg are typically given before and during the procedure, with repeat boluses given whenever spasm occurs. Intravenous nitroglycerin is used after angioplasty in patients who have demonstrated marked procedural spasm.

Calcium Antagonists

Calcium antagonists have been advocated to allow longer balloon inflations with less ischemia[44] and to prevent coronary spasm during angioplasty.[45] They decrease ischemia during balloon inflation by limiting myocardial oxygen demand and enhancing collateral flow to ischemic regions. One study in 10 patients undergoing coronary angioplasty compared parameters, including great cardiac vein flow and double product after the use of intravenous nicardipine and placebo.[46] The double product decreased by 7%, and great cardiac vein flow increased in 90% of the patients, demonstrating a decreased myocardial oxygen demand and an increase in collateral flow, respectively, when treated with nicardipine before balloon angioplasty. Serruys et al.[47] reported a marked inotropic effect and decreased anaerobic metabolism with regional nifedipine administration during PTCA. The favorable metabolic effect was thought to be due to the regional reduction in myocardial oxygen demand. Kern et al.[48] failed to demonstrate an increase in great cardiac vein flow or coronary artery occlusion pressure during balloon inflations in patients pretreated with sublingual nifedipine. It appears that some calcium antagonists given locally or intravenously may limit ischemia during balloon angioplasty.

β-Blockers

β-Blockers have been shown since as early as the 1970s to successfully limit myocardial ischemic injury in acute coronary occlusion syndromes by decreasing heart rate and myocardial contractility.[49–51] The suggestion that β-blockers may prevent myocardial ischemia has led to their use both regionally and systemically during PTCA. Two small studies addressed this issue. Feldman et al.[52] prevented or delayed myocardial ischemia in 10 of 16 patients with the use of systemic propranolol (0.1 mg/kg) administration. Zalewski et al.[53] studied the effects of regional propranolol administration during angioplasty by measuring electrocardiographic (ECG) indices of transmural injury. The time to onset of 0.1 mV ST elevation after balloon inflation and the magnitude of ST elevation after 60 seconds of coronary balloon occlusion were measured at baseline. The patients were then randomized to receive either intracoronary propranolol or saline. The time to onset of 0.1 mV ST elevation was significantly prolonged in the patients receiving intracoronary propranolol. Also, the ST segment elevation after 60 seconds of coronary occlusion was significantly decreased in the patients receiving intracoronary propranolol. No significant differences were seen in the patients who received intracoronary saline infusions. There is speculation that the beneficial effects of regional β-blockade are mediated by local protective mechanisms. Whether the relatively brief augmentation of balloon inflation duration allowed by β-blockers is important is not known.

PREVENTION OF RESTENOSIS

The pathophysiology of restenosis remains poorly understood. However, a number of mechanisms have been proposed. It is hypothesized from a substantial body of research in oncology and wound healing that restenosis is a complex expression in vascular tissue of the general biologic response to injury.[54] Clinical restenosis, defined as the return of ischemic symptoms, occurs in approximately 35% of patients. This process of wound healing, which commences shortly after the injury, progresses over several months and is complete by 3 to 6 months. The major milestones in the temporal sequence of restenosis form the current "pathophysiologic basis" for new approaches to limit restenosis and include platelet aggregation and vasospasm, inflammatory cell infiltration, release of growth factors, medial smooth muscle proliferation, proteoglycan deposition, and extracellular matrix remodeling. Research into the limitation of restenosis can be targeted at each of these steps. A host of agents, including antiplatelet agents, steroids, prostaglandins, fish oils, nitrates, calcium antagonists, ketanserin, 3-hydroxy-3-methylglutaryl coenzyme A (HMG-CoA) reductase inhibitors, angiotensin-converting enzyme inhibitors, monoclonal antibodies, and others, have been evaluated to attempt prevention of restenosis.[2] To date, no pharmacologic agent has consistently been shown to reduce restenosis.

RISK FACTOR MODIFICATION

Postangioplasty patients should be instructed about appropriate risk factor management before discharge from the hospital. Advice should include regular exercise, weight control, abstinence from tobacco, diabetic management, hypertension control, and aggressive control of serum lipids according to AHA guidelines. Clearly, patient motivation is important when attempting to modify behavior, and seldom will motivation be greater than in the period after successful angioplasty. Therefore, physicians should use this opportunity to begin programs for modifying risk factors.

Exercise testing after angioplasty can be performed

Table 29–1. **Drug Therapy for Routine PTCA**

	Preprocedure	Intraprocedure	Postprocedure	Reference
Aspirin				6
Heparin				19–29
Warfarin				30–34
Nitrates				41–43
Calcium Antagonists				44–48

▬▬▬ Mandatory   ▬▬▬ Optional

Table 29–2. **Drug Therapy for Stent Implantation**

	Preprocedure	Intraprocedure	Postprocedure	Reference
Aspirin				6
Dipyridamole				7–12
Dextran				13–18
Heparin				19–29
Warfarin				30–34
Nitrates				41–43
Calcium Antagonists				44–48

■■■ Mandatory ▒▒▒ Optional

for various reasons. It provides a baseline for functional assessment during long-term follow-up and reassures patients who are concerned about their ability to return to work. Exercise testing can also be used to confirm the relief of exercise-induced ischemia and to evaluate the importance of any residual lesions. Postangioplasty studies demonstrate improvement in exercise duration, increase in double product, improvement in ST segment depression, and resolution of angina.[55–57]

ROUTINE MEDICAL MANAGEMENT OF THE ANGIOPLASTY PATIENT
Routine Preprocedure Pharmacotherapy

At our institution, aspirin is considered essential adjunctive pharmacotherapy. Aspirin (160 to 325 mg, PO) is administered at least 1 day before elective PTCA. Calcium antagonists and/or nitrates are started the evening before angioplasty to prevent PTCA-induced vasospasm. If intravascular stenting is a consideration, dextran 40 is started at 125 cc/hr for 2 hours before the procedure and then decreased to a rate of 50 cc/hr at the time of the procedure. Sedatives and anxiolytics are given as premedication to the procedure (e.g., diazepam 2 to 10 mg, PO), and an antihistamine (diphenhydramine HCl 50 mg, PO) is administered to decrease the incidence of contrast-induced allergic reactions. Intravenous crystalloids are administered for 4 to 6 hours (50 to 150 cc/hr) to keep the patient hydrated while fasting. If a known contrast allergy exists, prednisone (50 mg), diphenhydramine HCl (50 mg), and cimetidine (300 mg) are each given orally every 8 hours for three doses before angioplasty.[58, 59] The pharmacologic management of the angioplasty patient is demonstrated chronologically in Tables 29–1 and 29–2.

Intraprocedure Pharmacotherapy

Heparin is universally employed during all interventional procedures (10,000-unit bolus), and the dosage may be repeated until an activated clotting time of more than 300 seconds is obtained. Supplemental heparin, a continuous drip or in additional hourly boluses, is given to maintain an activated clotting time of at least 300 seconds. At the time of PTCA, a continuous infusion of nitroglycerin (30 to 100 μg/min) may be used to mitigate PTCA-induced vasospasm. This is especially useful in rotational or directional atherectomy and intravascular ultrasound cases. Intracoronary nitroglycerin (200-μg boluses) may be given in addition to intravenous nitroglycerin to relieve refractory coronary spasm.

Postprocedure Pharmacotherapy

If an adequate angiographic result has been obtained, postprocedure heparin is not routinely employed. Suboptimal angiographic results suggesting persistent dissection or intraluminal thrombus warrant prolonged intravenous postprocedural heparin for 24 to 48 hours to maintain a PTT between 2.0 and 2.5 times control. In patients who develop procedural coronary spasm, intravenous nitroglycerin (30 to 100 μg/min) can be administered for 12 to 24 hours followed by oral or transdermal nitrates. Intravenous crystalloids are infused at 100 to 150 cc/hr to maintain an adequate urine output. Mannitol (12.5 to 25 g, IV) and/or lasix (20 to 40 mg, IV) are given in patients with renal insufficiency or diabetic nephropathy to prevent acute tubular necrosis. Aspirin (160 to 325 mg/day) is prescribed indefinitely, and some form of antianginal therapy (e.g., nitrates, calcium antagonist, and/or β-blocker) is prescribed for 3 to 6 months.

SUMMARY

Coronary angioplasty is a safe and effective treatment for patients with symptomatic coronary artery disease. The medical management of these patients before, during, and after the procedure is essential to a successful outcome. Future efforts need to be directed at reducing the acute complications such as bleeding and abrupt reocclusion, preventing restenosis, and modifying risk factors.

REFERENCES

1. Gruentzig A, Senning A, Siegenthaler W: Nonoperative dilation of coronary artery stenosis: Percutaneous transluminal coronary angioplasty. N Engl J Med 301:61, 1979.

2. Muller DWM, Ellis SG, Topol E: Experimental models of coronary artery stenosis. J Am Coll Cardiol 19:418, 1992.
3. Tuzcu EM, Simpfendorfer C, Dorosti K, et al: Changing patterns in percutaneous transluminal coronary angioplasty. Am Heart J 117:1374, 1989.
4. Ledley GS, Williams DO: Developments in balloon coronary angioplasty. Coronary Artery Disease 1:415, 1990.
5. Waller BF: "Crackers, breakers, stretchers, drillers, scrapers, shavers, burners, welders, melters"—the future treatment of atherosclerotic coronary artery disease? A clinical morphologic assessment. J Am Coll Cardiol 13:969, 1989.
6. Barnathan BS, Schwartz JS, Taylor L, et al: Aspirin and dipyridamole in the prevention of acute coronary thrombosis complicating coronary angioplasty. Circulation 76:125, 1987.
7. Fitzgerald GA: Dipyridamole. N Engl J Med 316:1247, 1987.
8. Swartz L, Bourassa MG, Lesperance J, et al: Aspirin and dipyridamole in the prevention of restenosis after percutaneous transluminal angioplasty. N Engl J Med 318:1714, 1988.
9. Mufson L, Black A, Roubin G, et al: A randomized trial of aspirin in PTCA: Effect of high versus low dose aspirin on major complications and restenosis [abstract]. J Am Coll Cardiol 11:236A, 1988.
10. Lembo NJ, Black AJR, Roubin GS, et al: Effect of pretreatment with aspirin versus aspirin plus dipyridamole on frequency and type of acute complications of percutaneous transluminal angioplasty. Am J Cardiol 65:422, 1990.
11. Heras M, Chesebro JH, Penny WJ, et al: Importance of adequate heparin dosage in arterial angioplasty in a porcine model. Circulation 78:654, 1988.
12. Bertrand ME, Allain H, Lablanche JM, et al: Results of a randomized trial of ticlopidine versus placebo for the prevention of acute closure and restenosis after coronary angioplasty: The TACT study [abstract]. Circulation 82:III-90, 1990.
13. Harker LA, Fuster V: Pharmacology of platelet inhibitors. J Am Coll Cardiol 8(Suppl B):21B, 1986.
14. Oberg M, Hedner U, Bergentz SE: Effect of dextran 70 on factor VIII and platelet function in von Willebrand's disease. Thromb Res 12:629, 1978.
15. Weiss HJ: The effect of clinical dextran on platelet aggregation, adhesion and ADP release in man: In vivo and in vitro studies. J Lab Clin Med 69:37, 1967.
16. Swanson KT, Vlietstra RE, Holmes DR, et al: Efficacy of adjunctive dextran during percutaneous transluminal coronary angioplasty. Am J Cardiol 54:447, 1984.
17. Schatz RA, Palmaz JC: Balloon expandable intravascular stents in human coronary arteries: Report of the initial experience [abstract]. Circulation 78(Suppl II):II-415, 1988.
18. Data LL, Nies AS: Dextran 40. Ann Intern Med 81:500, 1974.
19. Kasaki JC, Tousoulis D, Haider AW, et al: Reactivity of eccentric and concentric coronary stenosis in patients with chronic stable angina. J Am Coll Cardiol 17:627, 1991.
20. Saba HI, Saba SR, Morelli GA: Effect of heparin on platelet aggregation. Am J Hematol 17:295, 1984.
21. Douglas JS, Lutz SF, Clements SD, et al: Therapy of large intracoronary thrombi in candidates for PTCA [abstract]. J Am Coll Cardiol 11:238A, 1988.
22. Laskey MA, Deutsch E, Hirshfeld JW Jr, et al: Influence of heparin therapy on percutaneous transluminal coronary angioplasty outcome in patients with coronary arterial thrombus. Am J Cardiol 65:179, 1990.
23. McGary TF, Gottleib RS, Morganroth J, et al: The relationship of anticoagulation level and complications after successful percutaneous transluminal coronary angioplasty. Am Heart J 123:1445, 1992.
24. Dougherty KG, Marsh KC, Edelman SK, et al: Relationship between procedural activated clotting time and in-hospital post-PTCA outcome [abstract]. Circulation 82:III-189, 1990.
25. Ogilby JD, Kopelman HA, Klein LW, et al: Assessment using activated clotting times. Cathet Cardiovasc Diagn 18:206, 1989.
26. Rath B, Bennett DH: Monitoring the effect of heparin by measurement of activated clotting time during and after percutaneous transluminal coronary angioplasty. Br Heart J 63:18, 1990.
27. Ellis SG, Roubin GS, Wilentz J, et al: Effect of 18–24 hour heparin administration for prevention of restenosis after uncomplicated coronary angioplasty. Am Heart J 127:777, 1989.
28. Walford GD, Midei MM, Anversano TR, et al: Heparin after PTCA: Increased early complications and no clinical benefit [abstract]. Circulation 84:II-592, 1991.
29. Reifart N, Schmidt A, Preusler F, et al: Is it necessary to heparinize for 24 hours after percutaneous coronary angioplasty? [abstract]. J Am Coll Cardiol 19:231A, 1992.
30. Hirsh J, Genton E, Hull R: Vitamin K antagonists (oral anticoagulants). In Hirsh J, Genton E, Hull R: Venous Thromboembolism. New York: Grune & Stratton, 1981, pp 184–197.
31. Schatz RA, Baim DS, Leon M, et al: Clinical experience with the Palmaz-Schatz coronary stent: Initial results of a multicenter study. Circulation 83:148, 1991.
32. Serruys PW, Strauss BH, Beatt KJ, et al: Angiographic follow-up after placement of a self-expanding coronary artery stent. N Engl J Med 324:13, 1991.
33. Lincoff AM, Popma JJ, Ellis SC, et al: Abrupt vessel closure complicating coronary angioplasty: Clinical angiographic and therapeutic profile. J Am Coll Cardiol 19:926, 1992.
34. Hirsh J, Dalen J, Deykin D, et al: Oral anticoagulants: Mechanism of action, clinical effectiveness, and optimal therapeutic range. Chest 102:312S, 1992.
35. Zeiher AM, Kasper W, Gaissmaier C, et al: Concomitant intracoronary treatment with urokinase during PTCA does not reduce acute complications during PTCA: A double-blinded randomized study [abstract]. Circulation 82:III-189, 1990.
36. Grill HP, Brinker JA: Nonacute thrombolytic therapy: An adjunct to coronary angioplasty in patients with large intravascular thrombi. Am Heart J 118:662, 1989.
37. Kiesz RS, Hennecken JF, Bailey SR: Bolus administration of intracoronary urokinase during PTCA in the presence of intraluminal thrombus [abstract]. Circulation 84:II-346, 1991.
38. Pavlidos GS, Schreiber TL, Gangadharan V, et al: Safety and efficacy of urokinase during elective coronary angioplasty. Am Heart J 121:731, 1991.
39. Ambrose JA, Torre SR, Sharma SK, et al: Adjunctive thrombolytic therapy for angioplasty in ischemic rest angina: Results of a double-blind randomized pilot study. J Am Coll Cardiol 20:1197, 1991.
40. Horiuchi K: Improvement of ischemic tolerance during percutaneous transluminal coronary angioplasty by nicardipine and trinitroglyceride. Nippon Naika Gakkai Zasshi (Journal of Japanese Society of Internal Medicine) 78:1299, 1989.
41. Lam JYT, Chesebro JH, Fuster V: Platelets: Vasoconstriction and nitroglycerin during arterial wall injury—a new antithrombolytic role for an old drug. Circulation 78:712, 1988.
42. Doorey AJ, Mehmel HC, Schwarz FX, et al: Amelioration by nitroglycerin of left ventricular ischemia induced by percutaneous transluminal coronary angioplasty: Assessment by hemodynamic variables and left ventriculography. J Am Coll Cardiol 6:267, 1985.
43. Feldman RL, Joyal M, Conti R, et al: Effect of nitroglycerin on coronary collateral flow and pressure during acute coronary occlusion. Am J Cardiol 54:958, 1984.
44. Darius H, Schmucker B: Antianginal agents administered intracoronarily ameliorate functional impairment and extend time to ischemia during PTCA. Circulation 76(Suppl IV):IV-275, 1987.
45. Babbit DG, Perry JM, Forman MB: Intracoronary verapamil for reversal of refractory coronary vasospasm during percutaneous transluminal coronary angioplasty. J Am Coll Cardiol 12:1377, 1988.
46. Feldman RL, MacDonald RG, Hill JA, et al: Effect of nicardipine on determinants of myocardial ischemia occurring during acute coronary occlusion produced by percutaneous transluminal coronary angioplasty. Am J Cardiol 60:267, 1988.
47. Serruys PW, van den Braand W, Brower RW: Regional cardioplegia and cardioprotection during coronary angioplasty: Which role for nifedipine? Eur Heart J 4:115, 1983.
48. Kern MJ, Deligonul U, Labovitz A: Effects of nitroglycerin and nifedipine on coronary and systemic hemodynamics during transient coronary artery occlusion. Am Heart J 115:1164, 1988.
49. Maroko PR, Kjekshus JK, Sobel BE, et al: Factors influencing infarct size following experimental coronary artery occlusions. Circulation 43:67, 1971.
50. Maroko PR, Libby P, Covell JW, et al: Precordial ST segment

elevation mapping: A traumatic method for assessing alterations in the extent of myocardial ischemic injury. Am J Cardiol 29:223, 1972.

51. Gold HR, Leinbach RC, Maroko PR: Propranolol induced reduction of signs of ischemic injury during acute myocardial infarction. Am J Cardiol 38:689, 1976.

52. Feldman RL, MacDonald RG, Hill JA: Effect of propranolol on myocardial ischemia occurring during acute coronary occlusion. Circulation 73:727, 1986.

53. Zalewski A, Savage M, Goldberg S: Protection of the ischemic myocardium during percutaneous transluminal coronary angioplasty. Am J Cardiol 61:54G, 1988.

54. Forrester JS, Fishbein M, Helfant R, Fagin J: A paradigm for restenosis based on cell biology: Clues for the development of new preventative therapies. J Am Coll Cardiol 17:758, 1991.

55. Rosing DR, Cannon RO, Watson RM, et al: Three year anatomic, functional and clinical follow-up after successful percutaneous transluminal coronary angioplasty. J Am Coll Cardiol 9:1, 1987.

56. Manyari DE, Knudtson M, Klofber R, et al: Sequential thallium-201 myocardial perfusion studies after successful percutaneous transluminal coronary artery angioplasty: Delayed resolution of exercise-induced scintigraphic abnormalities. Circulation 77:86, 1988.

57. Okada RD, Lim YI, Boucher CA, et al: Clinical, angiographic, hemodynamic, perfusional and functional changes after one-vessel left anterior descending coronary angioplasty. Am J Cardiol 55:347, 1985.

58. Bielory L, Kaliner MA: Anaphylactoid reactions to radiocontrast materials. Anesthesiol Clin 23:97, 1985.

59. Zweiman B, Mishkin MM, Hildreth EA: An approach to the performance of contrast studies in contrast material-reactive persons. Ann Intern Med 83:159, 1975.

CHAPTER 30

Circadian Rhythm, Triggering Events, and Cardiovascular Therapy

James E. Muller, M.D., Geoffrey H. Tofler, M.B.B.S., and Murray A. Mittleman, M.D., Dr.P.H.

The newly recognized circadian variation and triggering of onset of acute cardiovascular disease raise three important questions for drug therapy for cardiovascular disease. First, does drug therapy alter circadian patterns of disease onset? Second, can drug therapy sever the link between a potential triggering activity, occurring at any time of day, and disease onset? Third, does the current knowledge of circadian variation of disease onset and potentially harmful physiologic processes warrant guided drug therapy?

Since the mid-1980s, many studies have documented the circadian variation and triggering of all acute cardiovascular diseases that have been studied—sudden cardiac death, nonfatal myocardial infarction, stroke, transient myocardial ischemia, and ventricular and supraventricular arrhythmias. These data documenting circadian variation of disease form the basis for addressing the important questions posed here concerning drug therapy.

EPIDEMIOLOGIC FINDINGS

The circadian pattern of myocardial infarction has been well documented to show a prominent increase in morning frequency. Both the MILIS[1] (Fig. 30–1) and the Intravenous Streptokinase in Acute Myocardial Infarction (ISAM) Study[2] (Fig. 30–2) clearly demonstrate that myocardial infarction is more likely to begin in the morning than in the late evening. The timing of myocardial infarction onset in both of these studies was determined based on the time of first appearance of creatine kinase in the plasma. Prior studies using the onset of pain as the marker for time of myocardial infarction onset were criticized because

delayed reporting of myocardial infarction onset in patients who were sleeping was thought to explain the increased morning incidence. The studies with objective timing have eliminated this possibility and firmly established the phenomenon.

In a refinement of the original reports on circadian variation, Goldberg et al.[3] have now reported that the increased incidence of myocardial infarction in the morning occurs in the first few hours after awakening.

In addition, sudden cardiac death, a condition often caused by coronary thrombosis, has a circadian pattern similar to that of nonfatal myocardial infarction,[4] reinforcing the likelihood that the two conditions share a common pathophysiologic mechanism.

TIMING AND TRIGGERS OF TRANSIENT MYOCARDIAL ISCHEMIA

Transient myocardial ischemia, a phenomenon that is more frequent than myocardial infarction, sudden cardiac death, and stroke, has been studied using Holter monitoring. This method allows precise timing of ischemic periods. Such studies have consistently demonstrated a peak incidence of ischemic episodes between 6 AM and 12 noon.[5] In addition to demonstrating this morning peak, investigations using Holter ST-segment analysis have provided insight into the possible triggers of transient ischemia. Such studies demonstrate that more than half of transient ischemic episodes are preceded by possible triggers such as mental or physical stress.[5]

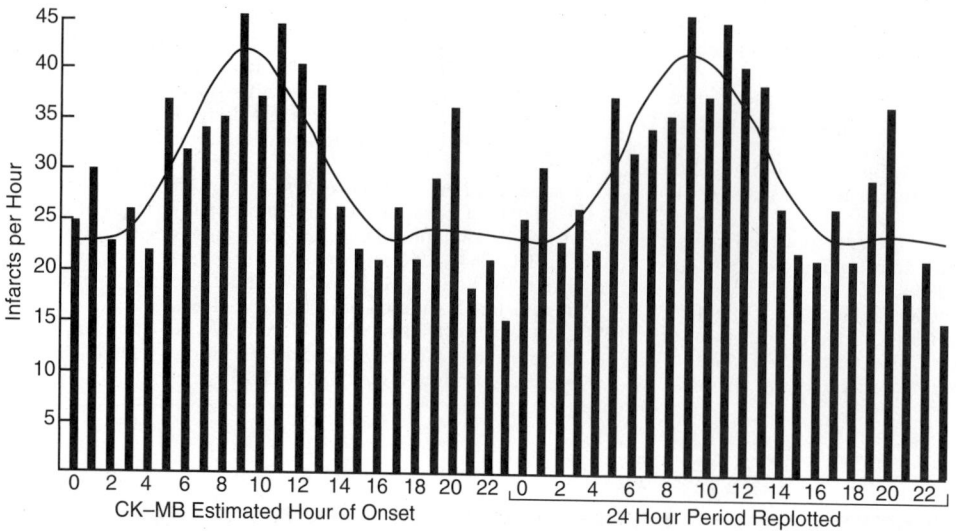

Figure 30–1. The number of infarctions beginning during each of the 24 hours of the day is plotted on the left side of the figure. On the right, the identical data are plotted again to permit appreciation of the relationship between the end and the beginning of the day. A two-harmonic regression equation for the frequency of onset of myocardial infarction has been fitted to the data *(curved line)*. A prominent circadian rhythm is present, with a primary peak incidence of infarction at 9 AM and a secondary peak at 8 PM.

EFFECT OF DRUG THERAPY ON CIRCADIAN VARIATION OF DISEASE

As the field of study of circadian variation of cardiovascular disease has progressed, investigators have attempted to determine whether various types of drug therapy alter the timing of cardiovascular events. For nonfatal myocardial infarction and sudden cardiac death, the conditions that have received the most attention, there is strong evidence that β-adrenergic blockade, a therapy well documented to prevent the occurrence of these disorders, selectively decreases the morning peak of events.

The evidence supporting this effect of β-blockade is of two types. First, studies determining the timing of infarction have shown a flattening of the morning peak in patients who happened to be receiving β-adrenergic blocking agents before their infarct[2] (Fig. 30–3). Because β-blockers were not randomly as-

signed, these studies are open to the criticism that the absence of the morning peak is a result of confounding by factors other than the therapy. The second type of evidence, which is not subject to the concerns over confounding, comes from the Beta Blocker Heart Attack Trial (BHAT), in which patients were randomly assigned to β-blockade or placebo.[6] β-Blockade demonstrated a selective beneficial effect against the occurrence of sudden cardiac death in the morning.

Evidence indicating a selective benefit of aspirin therapy in the morning has been less impressive than that for β-blockade. Observations of the timing of infarction in patients taking aspirin therapy, but not by random assignment before their infarction, have yielded mixed results. However, the single randomized study in which the effect has been studied has demonstrated a selective morning decrease in nonfatal myocardial infarction in patients receiving aspirin therapy.[7] It is possible that the randomized study is powerful enough to detect a small beneficial effect that cannot be detected by the nonrandomized, observational studies.

Studies of silent myocardial ischemia have demonstrated that β-blockade, but not a short-acting calcium antagonist, attenuates the morning increase in silent

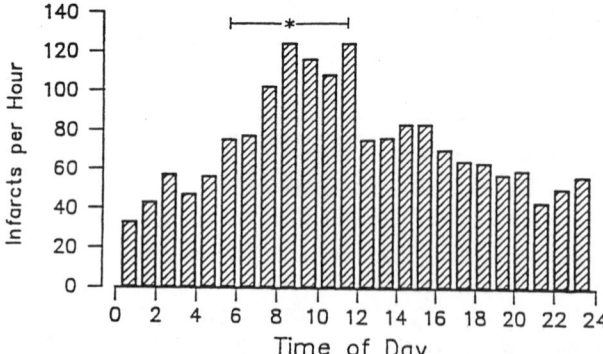

Figure 30–2. Bar graph of incidence of myocardial infarction of 1741 patients of the ISAM (Intravenous Streptokinase in Acute Myocardial Infarction) Study. There is a marked circadian variation ($p < .001$) with a peak during the morning hours. Myocardial infarction occurred 1.8 times more frequently between 6 AM and 12 noon compared with the average of other quarters of the day. The risk of myocardial infarction in the afternoon and evening was approximately equally distributed, whereas during the night a trough period occurred in the incidence of myocardial infarction.

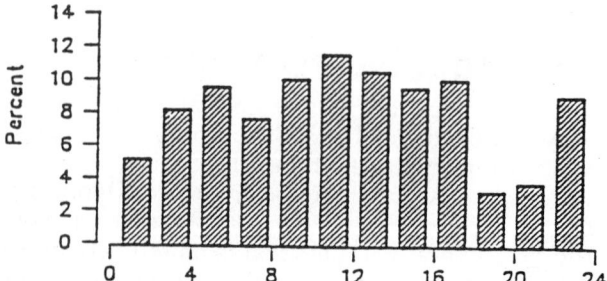

Figure 30–3. Bar graph of the incidence of myocardial infarction in the group of 206 patients in the ISAM Study receiving β-adrenergic blocker therapy before their myocardial infarction. Morning incidence of myocardial infarction did not increase. Percentage of myocardial infarctions per 2-hour interval is indicated on the y-axis, and the time of day is indicated on the x-axis (military time).

myocardial ischemia.[8] Another study has demonstrated that the morning increase in silent ischemia results from morning activities and can be prevented by nadolol therapy.[9]

These studies indicate that the answer to the first question posed in this chapter is positive—drug therapy can affect the time of day of cardiac events. However, these studies of the effects of drug therapy on time of day of events have not yet been complemented by studies of the ability of drug therapy to prevent triggering of events by heavy exertion and anger. More detailed investigation of triggering is required to answer this second question.

TRIGGERING OF CARDIOVASCULAR DISEASE

As studies of circadian variation have advanced, it has become clear that daily patterns of increases in disease onset are simply the manifestation of a more important underlying variation in the frequency of *triggering* of disease onset. Although less well characterized, the triggering of disease has even greater potential significance for drug therapy than does circadian variation.

As early as 1910, myocardial infarction onset has been attributed to external triggers. It was reported that "Direct events often precipitated the disease; the infarct began in one case on climbing a high staircase, in another during an unpleasant conversation, and in a third during emotional distress associated with a heated card game."[10] This clinical description by Obraztsov and Strazhesko was later challenged when, in the early 1960s, Master concluded that "Coronary occlusion takes place irrespective of the physical activity being performed or the type of rest taken."[11] As already mentioned, studies using modern epidemiologic methods have clearly documented increased rates of myocardial infarction onset in the morning hours.[1] This finding, combined with a new understanding of the pathogenesis of myocardial infarction, has renewed interest into the investigation of triggering. Sumiyoshi et al. reported that 53% of 416 patients admitted with infarction to the National Heart Center of Japan from 1977 to 1985 reported their infarct began during moderate-to-heavy exercise, emotional stress, or excitement.[12] This rate was similar to the MILIS group finding that 48.5% reported a possible trigger.[13]

In order to quantitate the role of potential trigger activities in the onset of infarction, various attempts have been made to obtain control data. In the Japanese National Heart Center Study,[12] the frequency of emotional or physical stress in the month prior to infarction was compared with the same month 1 year before infarction, which was designated the control period. This comparison yielded a significantly higher frequency of stress in the month before infarction than that reported during the control period (58% versus 34%, $p < .01$). However, this type of comparison is complicated by recall bias. A new study method called the case-crossover design, in which

each patient serves as his or her own control for relatively recent activities, is now being employed in a study entitled Determinants of the Onset of Myocardial Infarction, funded by the National Heart, Lung, and Blood Institute. In this study, more than 2000 patients with infarction have been interviewed to determine their activities in the hours immediately before infarction onset and in a control period 24 hours earlier. Data from this study have quantitated the risk that heavy physical exertion may trigger infarction and documented reduction of that risk by regular exertion.[14] Quantitative information on triggering of many types will eventually be available from this database.

OPPORTUNITY FOR PREVENTIVE THERAPY

Data on circadian variation and triggering, together with a better understanding of pathophysiology, suggest a new opportunity to reduce the massive number of deaths caused by cardiovascular disease. The new approach builds on the relatively recent understanding that approximately 90% of cases of nonfatal myocardial infarction (MI) and many cases of sudden cardiac death are caused by disruption of a coronary atherosclerotic plaque followed by occlusive thrombus formation. In many cases, the plaque that disrupts had not previously produced a critical stenosis.

The importance of the new approach outlined here is evident from review of the limitations of prior approaches. Identification and reduction of chronic risk factors (hypertension, hyperlipidemia, smoking, and others) have led to major gains. However, these risk factors do not fully explain the variance of disease onset in the population, and disease occurrence remains unacceptably high. Thrombolytic therapy for acute MI has received much attention, but it has been estimated that it can prevent less than 5% of the deaths from heart attack because its impact is limited by the occurrence of most deaths out-of-hospital before therapy can be initiated.[15] However, as a byproduct of thrombolytic research, much has been learned about disease onset. Recent advances in understanding of acute disease onset have created a novel possibility for prevention of onset of cardiovascular disease—an advance that would add to the gains made by chronic risk factor reduction and be effective against a far greater number of heart attack deaths than would thrombolysis.

The new information on triggering has provided the basis for a general theory of onset of coronary thrombosis.[16] It is postulated that onset occurs when a "vulnerable" atherosclerotic plaque disrupts and occlusive thrombus formation occurs. Hemodynamic stresses may cause the disruption of the plaque; hemostatic and vasoconstrictive forces may then determine whether the resultant thrombus is occlusive.

A better understanding of the mechanism by which clinical disease is produced by "vulnerable" but not necessarily "stenotic" plaques opens the possibility of major reductions in cardiovascular mortality before

MORNING INCREASE OF PHYSIOLOGIC PROCESSES THAT MIGHT TRIGGER MYOCARDIAL INFARCTION

A variety of mechanisms, alone or in combination, could account for the morning increase in myocardial infarction onset. A morning arterial pressure surge could initiate plaque disruption. An increase in coronary arterial tone could worsen the flow-reduction produced by a fixed stenosis. The combination of increases in arterial pressure and coronary tone increase could result in increased shear stress (force directed against the endothelium resulting from increased coronary blood flow velocity), thus predisposing a vulnerable plaque to disrupt. Other prothrombotic processes, including increased platelet adhesion, increased blood viscosity, and increased platelet aggregability,[17] have been implicated in the morning increase in ischemic events. Such a thrombotic tendency could increase the likelihood that an otherwise harmless mural thrombus overlying a small plaque fissure would propagate and occlude the coronary lumen.

Although a 24-hour periodicity of disease onset (see Figs. 30–1 and 30–2) and physiologic processes is well established, it remains unclear whether this periodicity results from a true endogenous circadian rhythm or from the daily rest-activity cycle. Cortisol secretion, for example, is well known to be an endogenous circadian process not dependent on daily activity,[18] whereas the morning platelet aggregability increase is abolished if the subjects remain at bedrest.[19] There may also be an interaction between circadian and rest-activity cycles, e.g., assumption of the upright posture leading to sympathetic activation may be more likely to cause intense vasoconstriction when endogenously controlled cortisol levels are high. This concept is controversial because circadian stage and sleep-wake cycles with posture change are confounded in all epidemiologic studies of infarction timing thus far reported. Investigations analyzing the relationship between an unusual wake-time on the day of myocardial infarction and standard wake-time on other days could potentially separate the wake-sleep cycle from the underlying cortisol rhythm, but such studies have not been reported.

Although the peak incidence of disease onset occurs in the morning, it is likely that similar physiologic processes trigger disease onset at other times of the day. The peak morning incidence of infarct onset probably results from the synchronization of all potential triggers in the morning, while a secondary evening peak in infarct onset observed in the MILIS data may result from synchronization of the population for an additional trigger, such as the evening meal. For other periods of the day, exposure of the population to potential triggers is random, and no other prominent peaks of incidence are observed.

OTHER POTENTIAL TRIGGERING CYCLES

The circadian (24-hour) cycle is not the only cycle that may provide clues to triggering of disease onset; seasonal variation and increases around the time of holidays and birthdays have also been reported. Mortality from ischemic heart disease shows an annual cycle with an increase in the winter.[20] In the Southern Hemisphere, seasonal variation in heart disease mortality has been confirmed, with peak mortality occurring during June, July, and August.

SIGNIFICANCE

Recognition of the circadian variation of onset of acute cardiovascular disease and potentially harmful physiologic processes has led to the third question posed here—should we now alter our drug therapy based on this knowledge? For β-blockade, the data appear sufficient to justify selection of an agent that provides adequate 24-hour protection, particularly in the morning hours. This recommendation is based on substantial evidence, but there has not been, and there is unlikely to be, a randomized trial comparing the ability of a long-acting β-blocker versus a shorter-acting agent to prevent cardiovascular events.

For aspirin, the issue of morning protection is moot, because a single dose of aspirin provides suppression of morning platelet activity for approximately 3 days. For other agents, such as coronary vasodilators and anti-hypertensive agents, the issue is unresolved. It seems reasonable that pharmacologic protection should be provided during the morning hours for patients already receiving antiischemic and antihypertensive therapy. However, studies documenting that such a regimen is more likely to prevent myocardial infarction or sudden death than a regimen providing less morning protection have not been reported and, to our knowledge, are not in progress or planned.

Because infarcts are more frequent in the morning and can be triggered by exertion, questions about the relative risk of morning exercise versus afternoon or evening exercise have been raised. It is clear that exercise is beneficial in reducing the risk of infarction, and although theoretic concerns can be raised, there is no evidence that exercise in the morning is more hazardous than exercise at other times of the day. Data from the Onset Study indicate that the relative risk of exertion in the morning is no greater than at other times of the day. The difference between the relative risk versus the absolute risk of experiencing an event during exertion is also important. Although there may exist a sixfold increase in the relative risk of an infarction during exercise in the morning hours, this translates to only a very small increase in absolute risk because baseline risk is low. Therefore, there is at present *no justification* for a recommendation that afternoon exercise is preferable to morning exercise.

The significance of the morning increase extends beyond the morning period. Complete elimination of the morning increase in onset of myocardial infarction by effective therapy would prevent only a small fraction of the total morbidity and mortality caused by this disease. This is true because, although the incidence of disease onset is greatest in the 6 AM to noon period, the majority of infarcts occur at other times of the day, and prevention of these events requires a broader therapeutic approach. For this reason, the primary significance of the recognition of circadian variation of disease onset is the support it provides for the broader concept that the onset of infarction *at any time of the day* is frequently triggered by activities of the patient. This concept provides a number of clues to the mechanisms of disease onset—clues that suggest a value of studies ranging from the epidemiologic to the molecular level.

On the epidemiologic level, studies must be conducted in which patients who experience a nonfatal myocardial infarction are interviewed to determine whether the event had an identifiable trigger. Because potentially triggering activities occur frequently without producing an event, the studies must be controlled for the frequency of potential triggers at times when an event did not occur.

The certainty with which an activity can be identified as a trigger will also vary in individual cases. In a patient whose plaque is only slightly vulnerable, the activity required to produce disease onset may be extreme, and the activity can be recognized as a trigger by its intensity. Other features that may aid in the recognition of an activity as a trigger are its occurrence immediately before the event, its ability to produce physiologic changes likely to trigger thrombosis, and its absence as part of the patient's routine activity. However, in a patient with an extremely vulnerable plaque, even nonstrenuous, routine, daily activities such as eating a heavy meal may be sufficient to trigger the cascade leading to infarction. In such instances, it may be impossible to identify the triggering activity even though it was present. Thus, the group of patients with *identifiable* triggers will be a subset of those in whom external triggering actually occurred.

On the clinical level, increased study of the relationship between daily activities and potentially triggering physiologic responses could clarify the manner in which these processes cause disease onset.

On the basic science level, there is a need for complete characterization of the control mechanisms of potentially adverse and beneficial physiologic processes. With improved understanding of these mechanisms, clinicians may eventually be able to eliminate unnecessary and potentially detrimental surges in arterial pressure, vasoconstriction, and coagulability that contribute to disease onset, and to increase the activity of potentially beneficial processes such as the fibrinolytic system. The factors determining plaque vulnerability require further characterization. The reduction in clinical events recently achieved by marked lowering of plasma cholesterol might result not only from a reduced tendency to coronary artery stenosis but also from a reduction in the formation of lipid pools within plaques that might increase the susceptibility of a plaque to rupture.

Greater understanding of triggering mechanisms should facilitate progress in the prevention of myocardial infarction. The means of prevention would not be to eliminate potential triggering activities—an undesirable and unattainable goal—but to design drug therapy and possibly nonpharmacologic measures that can be evaluated in randomized studies for their ability to sever the link between a potential triggering activity and development of myocardial infarction.

Acknowledgment

We are grateful for the assistance of Ms. Kathleen Carney in the preparation of the manuscript.

REFERENCES

1. Muller JE, Stone PH, Turi ZG, et al: Circadian variation in the frequency of onset of acute myocardial infarction. N Engl J Med 313:1315, 1985.
2. Willich SN, Linderer T, Wegscheider K, et al: Increased morning incidence of myocardial infarction in the ISAM Study: Absence with prior beta-adrenergic blockade. Circulation 80:853, 1989.
3. Goldberg R, Brady P, Muller JE, et al: Time of onset of symptoms of acute myocardial infarction. Am J Cardiol 66:140, 1990.
4. Muller JE, Ludmer PL, Willich SN, et al: Circadian variation in the frequency of sudden cardiac death. Circulation 75:131, 1987.
5. Rocco MB, Barry J, Campbell S, et al: Circadian variation of transient myocardial ischemia in patients with coronary artery disease. Circulation 75:395, 1987.
6. Beta-Blocker Heart Attack Trial Research Group: A randomized trial of propranolol in patients with acute myocardial infarction: Mortality results. JAMA 247:1707, 1982.
7. Ridker PM, Manson JE, Buring JE, et al: Circadian variation of acute myocardial infarction and the effect of low-dose aspirin in a randomized trial of physicians. Circulation 82:897, 1990.
8. Mulcahy D, Keegan J, Cunningham D, et al: Circadian variation of total ischemic burden and its alteration with anti-anginal agents. Lancet 2:755, 1988.
9. Parker JD, Testa MA, Jimenez AH, et al: Morning increase in ambulatory ischemia in patients with stable coronary artery disease: Importance of physical activity and increased cardiac demand. Circulation 89:604, 1994.
10. Obraztsov VP, Strazhesko ND: The symptomatology and diagnosis of coronary thrombosis. *In* Vorobeva VA, Konchalovski MP (eds): Works of the First Congress of Russian Therapists. Comradeship Typography of A.E. Mamontov, 1910, p 26.
11. Master AM: The role of effort and occupation (including physicians) in coronary occlusion. JAMA 174:942, 1960.
12. Sumiyoshi T, Haze K, Saito M, et al: Evaluation of clinical factors involved in onset of myocardial infarction. Jpn Circ J 50:164, 1986.
13. Tofler GH, Stone PH, Maclure M, et al: Analysis of possible triggers of acute myocardial infarction (The MILIS Study). Am J Cardiol 66:22, 1990.
14. Mittleman MA, Maclure M, Tofler GH, et al: Triggering of acute myocardial infarction by heavy physical exertion: Protection against triggering by regular exertion. N Engl J Med 329:1677, 1993.
15. Muller JE, Tofler GH: Circadian variation and cardiovascular disease onset. N Engl J Med 325:1038, 1991.

16. Muller JE, Abela GS, Nesto RW, et al: Triggers, acute risk factors, and vulnerable plaques: The lexicon of a new frontier. J Am Coll Cardiol 23:809, 1994.
17. Fuster V, Badimon L, Badimon JJ, et al: The pathogenesis of coronary artery disease and the acute coronary syndromes. N Engl J Med 326:242, 1992.
18. Weitzman ED, Fukushima D, Nogeire C, et al: Twenty-four hour pattern of the episodic secretion of cortisol in normal subjects. J Clin Endocrinol 33:14, 1971.
19. Tofler GH, Brezinski DA, Schafer AI, et al: Concurrent morning increase in platelet aggregability and the risk of myocardial infarction and sudden cardiac death. N Engl J Med 316:1514, 1987.
20. Rose G: Cold weather and ischaemic heart disease. Br J Prev Soc Med 20:97, 1966.

CHAPTER 31

Cardiovascular Disease in Women and Hormonal Substitution

Laura P. Fowlkes, M.D., and Jay M. Sullivan, M.D.

EPIDEMIOLOGIC STUDIES

Although there has been an encouraging decrease in the death rate from coronary heart disease over the past quarter century, the incidence is still very high, causing over 500,000 deaths per year in the United States alone. Much attention is given to known risk factors such as cigarette smoking, hypertension, and hypercholesterolemia, but only recently has the impact of the menopause been widely appreciated.

Data from the Framingham cohort clearly indicate that there are sex-specific differences in the manifestations of coronary heart disease. The reasons for these differences are incompletely understood. Women have a delay in onset of coronary disease by 10 years relative to men. Myocardial infarction and sudden death are delayed by 20 years and more commonly occur after age 55 in women. The first manifestation of coronary heart disease in women is much more likely to be uncomplicated angina pectoris than in men, who more often present with angina pectoris complicated by an acute myocardial infarction. Sudden death is more common among men in all age groups. Of note, the case fatality rates are higher for women than men in nearly every age stratum.[1]

Women lose their resistance to coronary disease as the menopause progresses, and this is not explained by alterations in lifestyle or risk factors (with the possible exception of lipoprotein changes that occur with the menopause). The Framingham cohort exhibited a greater than twofold age-adjusted increase in risk for coronary heart disease among postmenopausal women compared with premenopausal women. This applies to both natural and surgical menopause. Surgical menopause was classified as removal of one, both, or an unspecified number of ovaries.[2]

The apparent protective effect of estrogen replacement therapy contrasts sharply with the knowledge that early, high-dose oral contraceptive agents were associated with increased incidence of myocardial infarction in older, cigarette-smoking women. There is also evidence from the Coronary Drug Project that there is a higher incidence of subsequent coronary events in male survivors of myocardial infarction who received relatively high doses of conjugated equine estrogens compared with placebo.[3]

Hospital-Based Studies

The effect of hormone replacement therapy in coronary heart disease in postmenopausal women remains a subject of intense debate. Some of the earliest analyses have been hospital-based case-control studies. These studies have consistently failed to show a protective effect. Rosenberg et al.[4] studied 477 women aged 30 to 49 years who were hospitalized for myocardial infarction and compared them with 1832 hospitalized controls. The age-adjusted relative risk estimates for myocardial infarction for recent users of estrogen compared with nonusers was 1.0 (95% confidence interval [CI] 0.60 to 1.7) and for past users was 1.2 (CI 0.8 to 1.8) compared with nonusers. The control group included a significant number of patients with fractures. The large number of fractures in the control subjects may have been a marker of decreased exposure to estrogens, raising the question of an exposure bias that would underestimate the protective effect of estrogens.

Jick et al.[5] studied 107 women younger than age 46 who were admitted for myocardial infarction. Seventeen patients were compared with 34 hospitalized controls. Nine of 17 patients were estrogen users, compared with 4 of 34 controls, for a crude relative risk estimate of 7.5 (CI 2.4 to 24). Only one patient with myocardial infarction (MI) had never smoked. The small study size, the young age group studied, and the possible confounding effect of smoking made it difficult to determine whether any adverse cardiovascular effects recorded by the investigators were indeed related to estrogen use.

Comorbidity in the control groups in the hospital-based studies tended to make this study design less than ideal. As noted by some authors,[6] it is also possible that other sources of bias existed, such as recall bias and a bias based on prescribing practices of physicians who care for patients who have medical problems and require hospitalization. It is conceivable that physicians are reluctant to prescribe estrogens to patients who already take several medications, fearing drug interactions or diminished compliance.

Community-Based Studies

In an attempt to avoid the bias inherent in the hospital-based studies, community-based studies were devised. These studies routinely matched patients admitted to the hospital for myocardial infarction or who died from a coronary event to controls from the same community. Pfeffer et al.[7] studied 15,500 women aged 57 to 98 years in a retirement community that was known to use the same pharmacy and hospital almost exclusively. Hospital records were used to document admissions for myocardial infarction, and autopsy records confirmed a death from a coronary event. Pharmacy records documented estrogen exposure. Cases were matched three to one with controls in the community, yielding an adjusted relative risk estimate of 0.86 (CI 0.54 to 1.37) for myocardial infarction for those who had ever used estrogen, and for current users, 0.68 (CI 0.32 to 1.42), thus, failing to show a statistically significant protective effect. The short duration of estrogen use in the cases and the low mean daily dose (≤ 0.41 mg) in both groups limit the interpretation of the results.

Ross et al.[8] studied the same community and reported a misclassification of estrogen exposure if one looked at pharmacy records. They found a greater accuracy when the criteria were based on medical records compared with pharmacy records. In their study, patients were matched to both living and deceased controls, in an attempt to remove any bias that might be introduced because of extra contact that the patients may have had with the health care system before the end of their lives. The relative risk estimate of death from ischemic heart disease with estrogen use for cases compared with living control subjects was 0.43 (CI 0.24 to 0.75, $p < .01$), for deceased control subjects it was 0.57 (CI 0.33 to 0.99, $p < .05$). With the exception of the study by Ross et al.,[8] none of the community-based studies was able to show a statistically significant benefit. There was, however, a suggestion of a protective effect.

Angiographic Studies

Some investigators have used angiography to study the prevalence of significant coronary disease based on estrogen use in women. This eliminates the possibility of including patients with chest pain due to causes other than atherosclerosis. Sullivan et al.[9] studied 2188 women older than age 55 or with a history of oophorectomy who had angiography between 1972 and 1984 at the Baptist Memorial Hospital in Memphis, Tennessee. Data were obtained on admission regarding other known risk factors for coronary disease as well as current estrogen use. There were 1444

women with significant coronary disease compared with 744 who had normal coronary arteries. Only 2.7% of those with coronary disease used estrogens, in contrast with 7.7% of the control group, a difference that was statistically significant. Logistic regression analysis disclosed that the most important independent risk factors for the presence of coronary disease were age, cholesterol, smoking, diabetes mellitus, and hypertension. The only factor significantly associated with the absence of coronary disease was estrogen replacement therapy.

These observations have been confirmed by three additional angiographic studies. Gruchow et al.[10] analyzed data from the Milwaukee Cardiovascular Data Registry about 933 postmenopausal women. All underwent coronary arteriography, and coronary occlusion scores were calculated for each patient by measuring the percentage of luminal obstruction and the number of vessels involved. Estrogen use was defined at the time of angiography or within the preceding 3 months. In addition to a medical history, measurements of total, low-density lipoprotein (LDL), and high-density lipoprotein (HDL) cholesterol and triglycerides were made.

After grouping by age, estrogen users had lower occlusion scores than did nonusers in each age group, with those women older than 60 years showing the greatest difference. Occlusion scores increased significantly with age in the nonusers but not in the users. Regression analysis showed that postmenopausal estrogen use was the strongest independent predictor of occlusion scores, with a negative coefficient indicating that estrogen use was associated with lower scores. Age was the only other significant predictor of score.

The odds ratio for estrogen use was calculated for patients for low, moderate, and severe occlusion scores adjusted for age, smoking, exercise, and body mass, with those with low scores serving as the referent group. Those with moderate occlusion scores had an odds ratio for estrogen use of 0.59 (CI 0.73 to 0.48), and those with severe occlusion scores had an odds ratio of 0.37 (CI 0.46 to 0.29). Thus, women with severe disease were least likely to use estrogen.

To analyze the role of blood lipids, a statistical model was tested treating lipids as possible explanatory variables. The estrogen users had significantly higher HDL cholesterol values than did the nonusers (58.7 ± 18.1 mg/dl versus 46.4 ± 14.4 mg/dl). The inclusion of HDL cholesterol in this model reduced the negative association between estrogen use and occlusion score so that the relationship was no longer statistically significant, suggesting that the effect of estrogen on coronary disease was partially mediated by HDL cholesterol.

McFarland et al.[11] in South Carolina used a similar design to that of Sullivan et al.[9] in an analysis of 345 pre- and postmenopausal women aged 35 to 59 years. Estrogen replacement had a significant protective effect, with an odds ratio of 0.50 (CI 0.30 to 0.80).

Hong et al.[12] studied the prevalence of angiographically documented coronary artery disease in 90 postmenopausal women who came to Georgetown University Medical Center for chest pain. Coronary artery disease (CAD) was defined as stenosis of more than 25% of at least one major coronary artery. Choosing this definition of CAD was an attempt to include early disease that may predispose to future ischemic coronary syndromes, in addition to those that are presently hemodynamically significant. Mean age in the estrogen user group was 58 years (± 8) compared with 63 years (± 8) in the nonuser group. Lipid profiles were obtained on the day of the angiography. CAD was present in 4 of 18 (22%) estrogen users compared with 49 of 72 (68%) who were nonusers ($p < .001$). Estrogen use was associated with an odds ratio of 0.13 or with an 87% reduction in the prevalence of angiographic CAD. Absence of estrogen use was the most powerful independent predictor of the presence of CAD in these women.

Mean HDL cholesterol was higher in the user group (63.6 ± 6 versus 48 ± 2; $p < .01$). The ratio of total to HDL cholesterol was lower as well and was another independent predictor of the absence of CAD.

PROSPECTIVE STUDIES

Several important prospective studies have yielded statistically significant protective effects. Bush et al.[13] studied 2270 women aged 40 to 69 years for 8.5 years. Of 1677 nonusers, there were 44 deaths, compared with six deaths in 593 users, for an age-adjusted relative risk of 0.34 (CI 0.12 to 0.81), which changed little when the estimate was adjusted for risk factors. The groups were similar in the baseline prevalence of coronary disease, which was 12% in users compared with 10% in nonusers.

Lipid profiles were analyzed in both groups. Estrogen users had a higher mean HDL cholesterol level (66.7 ± 19.6 versus 57.1 ± 16.6 in nonusers). LDL cholesterol levels were also significantly lower. When HDL cholesterol was added to the regression model, the protective effect of estrogen was attenuated by more than 40%, suggesting that HDL cholesterol was partially responsible for the protective effect.

Stampfer et al.[14] reported results from the Nurses' Health Study, which monitored 32,317 female nurses aged 30 to 55 years by mailed questionnaires from 1976 to 1980. Information was obtained on cardiovascular risk factors and estrogen use, and the end points were fatal and nonfatal myocardial infarction. During the follow-up period, there were 90 women who had events. Compared with those who had never used postmenopausal hormones, the age-adjusted relative risk of CAD in those who had ever used hormones was 0.5 (CI 0.3 to 0.8; $p = .007$). The risk estimate in current users was 0.3 (CI 0.2 to 0.6; $p = .001$). Risk estimates were similar when adjusted for risk factors. There was no difference based on duration of use.

Ten-year follow-up from the Nurses' Health Study[15] involving 337,854 person-years of follow-up revealed 224 strokes, 405 cases of fatal and nonfatal major coronary events, and 1263 deaths from all causes. The age- and risk factor–adjusted relative risk estimate of

major coronary disease in current estrogen users was 0.56 (CI 0.40 to 0.80). The risk was reduced regardless of type of menopause. The risk was also conferred on women without baseline risk factors for coronary disease. The relative risk estimate for stroke among current users compared with those who never used was 0.97 (CI 0.65 to 1.45).

Henderson et al.[16] studied 8841 women aged 50 to 83 years in a retirement community by questionnaire from 1981 to 1987. The age-adjusted relative risk estimate for fatal myocardial infarction among current users was 0.47 (CI 0.20 to 1.08) and among past users was 0.62 (CI 0.43 to 0.90) compared with nonusers. There was no difference based on dose, duration of use, and type of menopause. In this study,[17] the relative risk of stroke was reduced to 0.53 ($p < .05$) in women who used estrogens for more than 15 years. In the Upsalla Health Care Region study,[18] the relative risk of stroke was 0.72 (95%; CI 0.58 to 0.88) in estrogen users and 0.61 (0.40 to 0.88) in those receiving combined estrogen-progestin therapy.

One cohort study showed an adverse effect with the use of estrogens in cardiovascular disease. Wilson et al.[19] studied the effect of estrogen use in the Framingham cohort of 1234 postmenopausal women aged 50 to 83 years who participated in the 12th biennial examinations and were followed up for 8 years. End points were grouped in certain analyses. Cardiovascular disease included coronary heart disease, cerebrovascular disease, intermittent claudication, and congestive heart failure. Coronary heart disease included angina pectoris, myocardial infarction, and coronary death or sudden death. Cerebrovascular disease included first occurrence of stroke or a transient ischemic attack.

Wilson et al. reported an age- and risk factor–adjusted relative risk estimate for total cardiovascular disease of 1.76 ($p < .01$), and for myocardial infarction, 1.87, not statistically significant. When patients were grouped according to smoking status, the increased risk for myocardial infarction was statistically significant only in the subgroup who smoked.

Interpretation of the results of the study is limited by several factors. It is known that angina pectoris is not a specific indicator of coronary artery disease, and therefore most studies of estrogen replacement therapy limit the end points to well-documented fatal and nonfatal myocardial infarction. The investigators also controlled for HDL cholesterol among the other coronary heart disease risk factors. As other studies have shown, adding HDL to the risk factor–adjusted risk estimate attenuates the protective effect of estrogens, thus demonstrating that HDL cholesterol is partially responsible for the beneficial effect. It should not be treated as a confounder in the initial risk factor–adjusted relative risk estimate.

A reanalysis of the Framingham Heart Study[20] eliminated angina pectoris as an end point and found that the relationship between estrogen replacement therapy and cardiovascular disease reported by Wilson et al.[19] was applicable only to the 12th biennial examination. Eaker and Castelli[20] analyzed the data from examinations 11 and 12. They demonstrated that among women aged 50 to 59 there was a protective effect that did not achieve statistical significance. Among women aged 60 to 69, there was an adverse effect that did not achieve statistical significance. The second analysis also controlled for HDL cholesterol, which may have resulted in an underestimate of the protective effect of estrogens.

There was one small randomized trial by Nachtigall et al.[21] that compared 84 matched pairs of patients in a hospital for patients with chronic diseases in New York. Most of the patients had a chronic disease, and there was a higher frequency of immobility than in an outpatient setting. The patients were treated with 2.5 mg conjugated equine estrogens (CEE) daily and medroxyprogesterone acetate (MPA) 10 mg per day for 7 days per month compared with a group receiving placebo. The follow-up period was 10 years.

Of the 168 patients, 10 deaths occurred. Three deaths were in the treatment group, and seven were in the control group. There were only four cases of myocardial infarction. One occurred in the treatment group and three in the control group. There was a nonsignificant reduction in the incidence of myocardial infarction in the estrogen-treated group. The short duration of estrogen use per month, the low event rate, and the high incidence of chronic disease and immobility make the results of the study difficult to extrapolate to the general population.

Wolf et al.[22] presented data from the National Health and Nutrition Examination Survey (NHANES), which monitored 1944 white women older than 55 for up to 16 years after the baseline survey in 1971 to 1975. By 1987, there were 347 deaths due to cardiovascular disease. Age- and risk factor–adjusted relative risk estimate for death from cardiovascular disease was 0.66 (CI 0.48 to 0.90). The same investigators in a separate analysis[23] reported a 31% reduction in incidence of stroke and a 63% reduction in death due to stroke. Both studies compared those who had ever taken estrogen to those who had never taken it.

Women with Coronary Artery Disease

The effects of estrogen replacement therapy on survival in women who had coronary artery disease were studied by Sullivan et al.[24] Data from the Baptist Memorial Hospital Registry were examined to determine the outcome of 2268 postmenopausal women who had had coronary angiography between the years 1972 and 1985. Subjects were divided into those who had no disease, mild to moderate disease, or severe disease. Five-year survival for the patients without coronary disease was 98% in both users and nonusers. Ten-year survival was 91% in those who had never used estrogen and 98% in the users. The difference was not statistically significant. Among patients with mild to moderate coronary lesions at baseline, survival was significantly better among 99 estrogen users than among 545 nonusers. In those who had never used estrogen, 5-year survival was 91% and 10-year survival was 85%. In those who had

used estrogen, 5-year survival was 98% and 10-year survival 96% ($p = .027$). The difference in survival was most marked in those patients with severe lesions. Here, mortality occurred at a rate of 4% per year in 1108 women who had never used estrogen replacement therapy. Five-year survival was 81% in this group and 60% at 10 years, whereas 5- and 10-year survival in those who had used estrogen was 98% ($p = .007$). However, the number of patients in this group of estrogen users was relatively small. The most important independent determinants of mortality were the number of vessels involved with more than 70% stenosis, severity of the impairment of the ejection fraction, and the age and the presence of a significant stenosis of the left main coronary artery. The only significant factor predicting survival was estrogen use. Relative risk equaled 0.16 (CI 0.04 to 0.66; $p = .11$).

Stampfer and Colditz[6] reviewed the evidence from 31 studies that had been published and noted that 25 of them showed a protective effect, which was statistically significant in 12. The cumulative relative risk including all studies based on use of estrogen at any time was 0.56 (0.50 to 0.61). Weighted summary relative risk estimates based on study design confirmed the adverse trend in the hospital- and community-based case-control studies, which, with the difficulties with bias and control selection, tended to underestimate the protective effect. The most accurate reflections of the true effect were thought to be in the two study designs using angiography and prospective studies with internal control groups. The combined relative risk estimate for the two study designs was 0.50 (CI 0.43 to 0.56).

In their discussion, Stampfer and Colditz commented that although the prospective studies with internal control groups and the angiography studies appear to come closest to measuring the degree of protection offered by estrogens, these studies are not without potential sources of bias. The question can be raised whether users of estrogens are healthier at baseline and that is why they suffer fewer cardiac events. However, several of the better designed prospective studies chose control groups that were similar in risk factor profiles to the cases, and that multivariate analysis failed to significantly change the risk estimate.

Several authors have attempted to control for frequency of clinic visits to address the issue of whether estrogen users simply are more vigilant about their health care and this is the reason why they have fewer cardiac events.[8, 15] Ross et al.[8] chose a deceased control group that had a higher likelihood of contact with the health care system than healthy living controls and was still able to demonstrate a protective effect. As reported by Stampfer and Colditz,[6] higher contact with health care providers would tend to document more coronary events in the user groups, which would result in an underestimate of the protective effect. Thus, it would seem very unlikely that the protective effect occurs simply because estrogen users are healthier or more vigilant about their health care.

There has also never been any clear evidence that socioeconomic status has a confounding effect.

Stampfer and Colditz[6] report that no study found a clear difference based on duration of use and dose of estrogen and confirmed that current users had more protection than past users. They note that, in many of the studies, estrogen use was documented at baseline and not frequently updated.

Effects of Age

The data are conflicting regarding which age group is most likely to benefit from hormone replacement therapy. Many studies reported age-adjusted relative risk estimates but did not specifically comment on the effects between age groups. It is known, however, that investigators who studied younger age groups, such as Stampfer et al.,[14] and those who studied older age groups, such as Henderson et al.,[16] were able to demonstrate a protective effect. Wilson et al.[19] reported a nonsignificant protective effect in the 50- to 59-year age group and a nonsignificant adverse trend in the 60- to 69-year age group. Sullivan et al.[9] demonstrated that estrogen therapy reduced the prevalence of coronary disease, particularly in women younger than 70. Gruchow et al.[10] reported significantly lower occlusion scores in all age groups, but the effect was most marked in the groups older than 60, a result opposite to that of Sullivan et al.[9] In the 10-year follow-up of the Nurses' Health Study, Stampfer et al.[15] reported a nonsignificant trend ($p = .19$) toward more protection among younger postmenopausal hormone users. For the oldest age group, defined as women aged 60 to 64, the relative risk was 1.35 (CI 0.65 to 2.82). At this point, it seems clear that postmenopausal women of all ages benefit to some degree from estrogen use. Further study would be needed to further assess which age groups benefit the most. The data must also be viewed with the knowledge of the natural history of coronary disease in women. The end points of most studies of estrogen replacement therapy are fatal and nonfatal myocardial infarction, events that are known to occur at an older age in women than in men.

Natural versus Surgical Menopause

The protective effect of estrogens is conveyed to women after both natural and surgical menopause. Gruchow et al.,[10] Henderson et al.,[16] and Wolf et al.[22] reported no difference based on natural or surgical menopause. However, Bain et al.[25] found a statistically significant protective effect only in the subgroup who had undergone bilateral oophorectomy. In the 10-year follow-up of the Nurses' Health Study, Stampfer et al.[15] reported a relative risk estimate among current users who had undergone natural menopause of 0.62 (CI 0.39 to 0.97) and a relative risk estimate in the group who had undergone surgical menopause of 0.40 (CI 0.22 to 0.73).

Low-Risk Patients

Evidence is conflicting whether hormone replacement therapy is cardioprotective in women who are free of coronary disease. Sullivan et al.[24] reported no survival benefits in women free of angiographically documented coronary disease. Those with moderate to severe disease benefited significantly. Stampfer et al.[15] reported that in participants of the larger Nurses' Health Study who had a low risk factor profile, there was still a protective effect, with an age-adjusted relative risk estimate of 0.53 (CI 0.31 to 0.91).

Effects of Estrogen on Lipoproteins

Previous evidence suggests that an important part of the cardioprotective effect of estrogen replacement therapy is due to an effect on serum lipids. It is known that many postmenopausal women have an HDL cholesterol level of less than 46 mg/dl, which is associated with a sixfold higher risk of coronary disease than women who have an HDL cholesterol level of more than 67 mg/dl.[26] LDL cholesterol rises with age and is higher in older women than in men. The ratio of total cholesterol to HDL cholesterol also rises with age, and higher ratios are associated with an increased risk of coronary artery disease.[2] Conjugated estrogens in menopausal replacement doses (0.625 mg) are known to decrease total cholesterol by 11%, increase HDL cholesterol by 14%, increase triglycerides by 11%, and decrease LDL cholesterol by 10%. There is a dose-response effect as well.[27] It is postulated that those women who require either cyclic or daily supplementation with progestins would experience an attenuation of the beneficial effect. Sherwin and Gelfand[28] reported that the daily administration of conjugated equine estrogens (CEE) with the cyclic coadministration of medroxyprogesterone acetate (MPA) attenuated but did not completely reverse the beneficial lipid effects of estrogens. Weinstein[29] reported the outcome of a comparison of cyclic versus low-dose daily MPA with CEE. Patients who received 2.5 mg per day of MPA with 0.625 mg per day of CEE had decreases in total and LDL cholesterol levels, no significant change in HDL cholesterol levels, and favorable endometrial pathology. Other investigators have confirmed the acceptability of this approach.[30]

The interaction of estrogens on lipoprotein pathways is complex. Estrogen increases the activity of hepatic apoprotein B and E receptors and increases the uptake of LDL cholesterol and chylomicron remnants and thus decreases LDL cholesterol levels. By increasing the synthesis of apoprotein A1 and reducing the activity of hepatic lipoprotein lipase, estrogen raises HDL cholesterol levels.[31]

Additional effects on lipoproteins are being evaluated in an effort to explain the relationship of estrogens, menopause, and protection from ischemic heart disease. One of those is lipoprotein(a) [Lp(a)], which is a complex between LDL and apolipoprotein(a) and is known to be an independent predictor of premature coronary disease.[32] There is no clear variation in Lp(a) levels with age, sex, and diet, although levels are higher in postmenopausal women compared with premenopausal women.[33]

The effects of hormonal regulation of lipoproteins, particularly lipoprotein(a), were studied in 30 elderly men with prostatic carcinoma who were randomized to receive either ethinyl estradiol and polyestradiol phosphate or orchidectomy.[34] The 15 estrogen-treated men demonstrated a mean reduction of Lp(a) of 51% ($p < .001$), compared with a mean increase of 20% in the group receiving orchidectomy ($p < .01$). There was no association noted between the percentage reduction in Lp(a) levels and the apo(a) phenotype. The investigators observed a reduction in LDL cholesterol, and an increase in HDL cholesterol and triglycerides. Multivariate analysis demonstrated that the changes in Lp(a) levels were explained in part but not completely by the changes in HDL cholesterol and triglycerides. The authors commented on the fact that elderly men with prostatic carcinoma who have been treated in the past with estrogens have been shown to experience more cardiovascular events.[35] The explanation for this apparent paradox is unknown.

There is evidence from investigators in Milan, Italy,[36] suggesting that treatment with menopausal replacement doses of conjugated equine estrogens may also improve lipid profiles by decreasing Lp(a) concentration. Thirty postmenopausal women were treated with either CEE and cyclic regimen of MPA or placebo and were followed up for 1 year. Pretreatment Lp(a) levels in the treatment group went from 21.7 (SD 9.1) to 11.1 (SD 5.2; $p < .05$) and 10.6 (SD 6.5; $p < .05$) in 6 and 12 months, respectively, and remained essentially unchanged in the placebo group, whose baseline Lp(a) level was 16.9 (SD 6.6) and was 16.3 (SD 6.9) and 16.7 (SD 6.3) at 6 and 12 months, respectively. Further study is necessary to determine the significance of these findings.

Estrogen replacement therapy increases the risk of endometrial cancer, a risk that is greatly reduced by the addition of progestin. However, progestins, particularly those that resemble androgens, attenuate the HDL cholesterol–elevating properties of estrogens, according to a number of short-term studies. Because estrogen replacement today is usually given in combination with a progestin, the available data concerning the possible cardioprotective effects of combined estrogen replacement therapy, i.e., hormone replacement therapy, should be considered. In nonhuman primates, both estrogen and estrogen with progestin were found to reduce the extent of aortic atherosclerosis in surgically menopausal monkeys fed a high-fat diet, even though HDL levels were reduced by combination therapy.[37] Combination therapy also reduced LDL cholesterol uptake by blood vessel cells to the same extent as estrogen replacement therapy.

In long-term human cohort studies, such as the Rancho Bernardo Study[38] and the Atherosclerosis Risk in Communities Study,[39] HDL levels did not differ significantly between those receiving either estrogen or hormone replacement therapy. A recent Swedish cohort study showed approximately equal reduction of cardiovascular risk in women receiving either estrogen or combination replacement.[40] The single published randomized trial of estrogen replacement, that of Nachtigall et al.,[21] showed a reduction in the rate of myocardial infarction in 84 pairs of hospitalized women who received combination therapy. However, the results of two current larger prospective, placebo-controlled trials of hormone replacement therapy for cardiovascular endpoints will not be available for years.

Other Effects of Estrogen

Observational data are limited on the effects of estrogen on metabolic parameters such as blood pressure, body mass index, fasting glucose and insulin levels, clotting factors, and so on. To date there is no evidence that the mechanism of estrogen's protective effect is mediated by any of these factors,[41] although estrogen replacement therapy reduces blood pressure on the average and improves insulin sensitivity.

Studies carried out in the 1950s have shown that estrogens can cause regression of coronary disease in cholesterol fed chicks.[42] This has been confirmed in more recent studies of ovariectomized monkeys. These effects were noted to be independent of HDL cholesterol levels.[37]

In recent years, it has been learned that the endothelium plays an important role in the modulation of blood vessel tone. Furchgott and Zawadzk[43] were the first to demonstrate that the removal of the endothelium altered the way in which a blood vessel responded to the application of acetylcholine. The response of normal healthy vessels was vasodilation, whereas, after removal of the endothelium, acetylcholine caused vasoconstriction. Subsequently it has been discovered that acetylcholine occupies receptors on the endothelial cell membrane that stimulate the release of endothelium-derived relaxing factor, a vasodilatory, platelet-repelling compound similar in effect but chemically distinct from prostacyclin. Relaxing factor is now known to be, either wholly or partially, nitric oxide, which is derived from L-arginine in the cell. Release of nitric oxide activates guanylate cyclase, which results in the synthesis of cyclic guanidine monophosphate, which in turn results in vasodilation.[44]

Ludmer et al.[45] demonstrated that acetylcholine infused into normal human coronary arteries caused vasodilation, whereas infusion of the same dose in a segment of the artery with an atherosclerotic lesion resulted in vasoconstriction of the diseased and adjacent areas, suggesting that atherosclerotic involvement of the blood vessel wall impairs endothelial function. More recently, Williams et al.[46] have demonstrated that when oophorectomized monkeys are fed a high-lipid diet, acetylcholine causes coronary vasoconstriction when infused into the coronary vessels, suggesting loss of endothelial cell function. However, when these monkeys received estrogen replacement therapy, the infusion of acetylcholine caused vasodilation as it does in normal animals.

Similar observations have been reported in women.[47] Thus, there is evidence that estrogens influence endothelial cell function, and this may play a part in their cardioprotective effect. In studies of monkeys, the estrogen-replaced animals also had much less atherosclerotic involvement despite their oophorectomies and their high-lipid diets.

The other evidence that estrogen replacement therapy alters blood vessel function is derived from studies showing that there are estrogen receptors in blood vessel walls and that estrogens stimulate the production of[48] and prolong the half-life of[49] prostacyclin.

Extracardiovascular Risk and Benefits

Thus far, during this discussion, only the cardiovascular benefits of estrogen replacement therapy have been considered. Although there are other benefits, there are risks as well.[50] The other benefits include prevention of osteoporosis and effects on vasomotor tone, genitourinary atrophy, and mood and well-being. However, the risks include an increased incidence of endometrial carcinoma in women receiving unopposed estrogens, and various idiosyncratic responses that include rare instances of elevated blood pressure or thrombotic episodes. Considerable attention has been given to the question of whether or not estrogen replacement therapy is associated with an increased incidence of breast cancer, with published studies offering conflicting answers. Two recent meta-analyses of this issue continued the controversy, one suggesting that there was no increased risk,[51] the other a 30% increased risk of breast cancer.[52]

Risk/Benefit Assessment

Goldman and Tosteson[53] compared the risks and benefits of estrogen replacement therapy based on epidemiologic data, which at this point best addresses the use of unopposed estrogens. They emphasize that relative risk estimates may not take into account that a large increase in the risk of the occurrence of a rare event may have much less impact than a small increase in the risk of occurrence of a common event. When comparing a woman's risk of dying of a disease related to estrogen deficiency, epidemiologic evidence suggests that from age 65 to 74 a woman's risk of dying of complications of hip fracture is reduced to a similar degree that her risk is increased for dying of breast cancer should she use estrogens (0.36% absolute reduction versus 0.30% absolute increase).

The same argument applies to the issue of ischemic heart disease. Goldman and Tosteson state that the absolute reduction in death from ischemic heart disease may be equal to the increase in mortality from endometrial cancer (a 2.4% absolute reduction and increase in mortality, respectively). They are careful to state that epidemiologic evidence suggests that the mortality from endometrial carcinoma is "only 10% as high for endometrial cancer associated with exogenous estrogen as for 'naturally occurring' disease, presumably because of earlier detection." They also

emphasize the need for a randomized clinical trial to compare the long-term effects in groups receiving estrogens with and without progestins.

Grady et al.[54] reported results from a meta-analysis assessing the risks and benefits of use of hormone replacement therapy in asymptomatic white postmenopausal women 50 years old in preventing disease and prolonging life. Pooled relative risk estimates from published studies comparing those who had ever used estrogen with those who had never used it yielded relative risk estimates of 2.31 (CI 2.13 to 2.51) for endometrial carcinoma, 1.01 (CI 0.97 to 1.05) for breast cancer, 0.65 (CI 0.59 to 0.71) for coronary heart disease, 0.75 (CI 0.68 to 0.84) for hip fracture, and 0.96 (CI 0.82 to 1.13) for stroke. The risk estimate for breast cancer was based on short-term use, less than 8 years. The only disease for which there were enough data to yield a pooled relative risk estimate for combined estrogen and progestin use was endometrial carcinoma, for which there was no increased risk with combination therapy.

Changes in overall life expectancy were calculated. In women without a uterus, the life expectancy for treatment with unopposed estrogen increased by 1.1 years. In women with an intact uterus, life expectancy increased by 0.9 years. To calculate the effects of adding a progestin to life expectancy, two scenarios were compared. If progestins were postulated to have no effect on overall mortality, life expectancy increased by a full 1.0 year. When a more pessimistic effect was tested—by assigning the relative risk of dying from ischemic heart disease as 0.80 instead of the predicted 0.65 with unopposed estrogens, and by using a relative estimate for breast cancer of 2.0 as opposed to 1.01—the increase in life expectancy was reduced to 0.10 years. Grady et al. concluded that estrogen replacement therapy was beneficial to women without an intact uterus who were at risk for or who had coronary disease. In contrast, there was insufficient evidence that women without coronary disease and those with an intact uterus would obtain substantial survival benefits from hormone replacement therapy.

However, there are many women for whom clear benefits have yet to be definitively established, such as those women who have no risk factors for osteoporosis or coronary artery disease, and especially for those women who have an intact uterus. For the present, the use of estrogen replacement therapy is a decision that must be made between the patient and her physician on an individual basis, weighing the risks and benefits.

REFERENCES

1. Lerner DJ, Kannel WB: Patterns of coronary heart disease morbidity and mortality in the sexes: A 26-year follow-up of the Framingham population. Am Heart J 111:383, 1986.
2. Kannel WB: Metabolic risk factors for coronary heart disease in women: Perspective from the Framingham Study. Am Heart J 114:413, 1987.
3. The Coronary Drug Project Research Group: The coronary drug

project—initial findings leading to modifications of its research protocol. JAMA 214:1303, 1970.

4. Rosenberg L, Slone D, Shapiro S, et al: Noncontraceptive estrogens and myocardial infarction in young women. JAMA 244:339, 1980.

5. Jick H, Dinan B, Rothman KJ: Noncontraceptive estrogens and nonfatal myocardial infarction. JAMA 239:1407, 1978.

6. Stampfer MJ, Colditz GA: Estrogen replacement therapy and coronary heart disease: A quantitative assessment of the epidemiologic evidence. Prev Med 20:47, 1991.

7. Pfeffer RL, Whipple GH, Kurosaki TT, et al: Coronary risk and estrogen use in postmenopausal women. Am J Epidemiol 107:479, 1978.

8. Ross, RK, Paganini-Hill A, Mack TM, et al: Menopausal oestrogen therapy and protection from death from ischemic heart disease. Lancet 1:858, 1981.

9. Sullivan JM, Vander Zwaag R, Lemp GF, et al: Postmenopausal estrogen use and coronary atherosclerosis. Ann Intern Med 108:358, 1988.

10. Gruchow HW, Anderson AJ, Barboriak JJ, et al: Postmenopausal use of estrogen and occlusion of coronary arteries. Am Heart J 115:954, 1988.

11. McFarland KF, Boniface ME, Hornung CA, et al: Risk factors and noncontraceptive estrogen use in women with and without coronary disease. Am Heart J 117:1209, 1989.

12. Hong MK, Romm PA, Reagan K, et al: Effects of estrogen replacement therapy on serum lipid values and angiographically defined coronary artery disease in postmenopausal women. Am J Cardiol 69:176, 1992.

13. Bush TL, Barrett-Conner E, Cowan LD, et al: Cardiovascular mortality and noncontraceptive use of estrogen in women: Results from the Lipid Research Clinics Program Follow-up Study. Circulation 75:1102, 1987.

14. Stampfer MJ, Willett WC, Colditz GA, et al: A prospective study of postmenopausal estrogen therapy and coronary heart disease. N Engl J Med 313:1044, 1985.

15. Stampfer MJ, Colditz GA, Willett WC, et al: Postmenopausal estrogen therapy and cardiovascular disease: Ten year follow-up from the Nurses' Health Study. N Engl J Med 325:756, 1991.

16. Henderson BE, Paganini-Hill A, Ross RK: Estrogen replacement therapy and protection from acute myocardial infarction. Am J Obstet Gynecol 159:312, 1988.

17. Henderson BE, Paganini-Hill A, Ross RK: Decreased mortality in users of estrogen replacement therapy. Arch Intern Med 151:75, 1991.

18. Falkeborn M, Persson L, Terens A, et al: Hormone replacement therapy and the risk of stroke. Arch Intern Med 153:1201, 1993.

19. Wilson PWF, Garrison RJ, Castelli WP: Postmenopausal estrogen use, cigarette smoking, and cardiovascular morbidity in women over 50: The Framingham Study. N Engl J Med 313:1038, 1985.

20. Eaker ED, Castelli WP: Coronary heart disease and its risk factors among women in the Framingham Study. In Eaker E, Packard B, Wenger NK, et al (eds): Coronary Heart Disease in Women. New York: Haymarket Doyma, 1987, pp 122–132.

21. Nachtigall LE, Nachtigall RH, Nachtigall RD, et al: Estrogen replacement therapy II: A prospective study in the relationship to carcinoma and cardiovascular and metabolic problems. Obstet Gynecol 54:74, 1979.

22. Wolf PH, Madans JH, Finucane FF, et al: Reduction of cardiovascular disease-related mortality among postmenopausal women who use hormones: Evidence from a national cohort. Am J Obstet Gynecol 164:489, 1991.

23. Finucane FF, Madans JH, Bush TL, et al: Decreased risk of stroke among postmenopausal hormone users: Results from a national cohort. Arch Intern Med 153:73, 1993.

24. Sullivan JM, Vander Zwaag R, Hughes JP, et al: Estrogen replacement and coronary artery disease—effect on survival in postmenopausal women. Arch Intern Med 150:2557, 1990.

25. Bain C, Willett WC, Henenekens CH, et al: Use of postmenopausal hormones and risk of myocardial infarction. Circulation 64:42, 1981.

26. Abbott RD, Wilson PWF, Kannel WB, et al: High density lipoprotein cholesterol, total cholesterol screening, and myocardial infarction: The Framingham Study. Arteriosclerosis 8:207, 1988.

27. Bush TL, Miller VT: Effects of pharmacologic agents used during menopause: Impact on lipids and lipoproteins. In Mishell D (ed): Menopause: Physiology and Pharmacology. Chicago: Year Book Medical Publishers, 1986, pp 187–208.

28. Sherwin BB, Gelfand MM: A prospective one-year study of estrogen and progestin in postmenopausal women: Effects on clinical symptoms and lipoprotein lipids. Obstet Gynecol 73:759, 1989.

29. Weinstein L: Efficacy of a continuous estrogen-progestin regimen in the menopausal patient. Obstet Gynecol 69:929, 1987.

30. Luciano M, Turksoy RN, Carleo J, et al: Clinical and metabolic responses of menopausal women to sequential versus continuous estrogen and progestin replacement therapy. Obstet Gynecol 71:39, 1988.

31. Ettinger B: Hormone replacement therapy and coronary heart disease. Obstet Gynecol Clin North Am 4:741, 1990.

32. Rhoads GG, Dahlen G, Berg K, et al: Lp(a) lipoprotein as a risk factor for myocardial infarction. JAMA 256:2540, 1986.

33. Guyton JR, Dahlen GH, Patsch W, et al: Relationship of plasma lipoprotein Lp(a) levels to race and to apolipoprotein B. Arteriosclerosis 5:265, 1985.

34. Henriksson P, Angelin B, Berglund L: Hormonal regulation of serum Lp(a) levels: Opposite effects after estrogen treatment and orchidectomy in males with prostatic carcinoma. J Clin Invest 89:1166, 1992.

35. Blackard CE, Doe RP, Mellinger GT, et al: Incidence of cardiovascular disease and death in patients receiving diethylstilbestrol for carcinoma of the prostate. Cancer 26:249, 1970.

36. Soma M, Fumagalli R, Paoletti R, et al: Plasma Lp(a) concentration after oestrogen and progestogen in postmenopausal women [letter]. Lancet 337:612, 1991.

37. Adams MR, Kaplan JR, Manuk SB, et al: Inhibition of coronary artery atherosclerosis by 17B estradiol in ovariectomized monkeys: Lack of an effect of added progesterone. Arteriosclerosis 10:1051, 1990.

38. Barrett-Conner E, Wingard DL, Criqui MH: Postmenopausal estrogen use and heart disease risk factors in the 1980's: Rancho Bernardo, California revisited. JAMA 267:2095, 1989.

39. Nabulsi AA, Folsom AR, White A, et al: Association of hormone-replacement therapy with various cardiovascular risk factors in postmenopausal women. N Engl J Med 328:1069, 1993.

40. Falkeborn M, Persson L, Adami H-O, et al: The risk of acute myocardial infarction after oestrogen and oestrogen-progestogen replacement. Br J Obstet Gynaecol 99:821, 1992.

41. Barrett-Conner E, Bush TL: Estrogen and coronary heart disease in women. JAMA 265:1861, 1991.

42. Pick R, Stamler J, Rodbard S, et al: Estrogen induced regression of coronary atherosclerosis in cholesterol fed chicks. Circulation 6:858, 1952.

43. Furchgott RF, Zawadzk JV: The obligatory role of endothelial cells in the relaxation of arterial smooth muscle by acetylcholine. Nature 288:373, 1980.

44. Ignarro W, Byrns RE, Buga GM, et al: Endothelium-derived relaxing factor (EDRF) released from artery and vein appears to be nitric oxide (NO) or a closely related species. Fed Proc 46:644, 1987.

45. Ludmer PL, Selwyn AP, Shook TL, et al: Paradoxical vasoconstriction induced by acetylcholine in atherosclerotic coronary arteries. N Engl J Med 315:1046, 1986.

46. Williams JK, Adams MR, Klopfenstein HS: Estrogen modulates responses of atherosclerotic coronary arteries. Circulation 81:1680, 1990.

47. Herrington M, Braden G, Downes TR, et al: Estrogen modulates coronary vasomotor responses in postmenopausal women with early atherosclerosis [abstract]. Circulation 86:I-619, 1992.

48. Fogelberg M, Vesterquist O, Diczfalusy U, Henriksson P: Experimental atherosclerosis: Effects of estrogen and atherosclerosis on thromboxane and prostacyclin formation. Eur J Clin Invest 20:105, 1990.

49. Yui Y, Aoyama T, Morishita H, et al: Serum prostacyclin stabi-

lizing factor is identical to apolipoprotein A-l(Apo A-l): A novel function of Apo A-l. J Clin Invest 82:803, 1988.
50. Ernster VL, Bush TL, Hugkins GR, et al: Benefits and risks of estrogen and/or progestin hormone use. Prev Med 17:201, 1988.
51. Dupont WD, Page DL: Menopausal estrogen replacement therapy and breast cancer. Arch Intern Med 151:67, 1991.
52. Steinberg KK, Thacker SB, Smith J, et al: A meta-analysis of the effect of estrogen replacement therapy on the risk of breast cancer. JAMA 265:1985, 1991.
53. Goldman L, Tosteson AN: Uncertainty about postmenopausal estrogen: Time for action, not debate [editorial]. N Engl J Med 325:800, 1991.
54. Grady D, Rubin SM, Petitti DB, et al: Hormone therapy to prevent disease and prolong life in postmenopausal women. Ann Intern Med 117:1016, 1992.

CHAPTER 32

Antioxidants in the Prevention of Cardiovascular Disease

Richard V. Milani, M.D., F.A.C.C.,
and Carl J. Lavie, M.D., F.A.C.C., F.A.C.P., F.A.C.C.P.

The development of atherosclerosis is a multifaceted process by which low-density lipoprotein (LDL) cholesterol infiltrates into the intima of the endothelium, resulting in foam cell and fatty streak formation. Numerous growth factors and inflammatory mediators are released that induce cell proliferation and lesion progression. Since the mid-1980s, the principal pharmacologic approach to the prevention of atherosclerosis has been based on the "lipid hypothesis," which holds that lowering serum cholesterol levels, and more specifically, LDL cholesterol levels, reduces the incidence of atherosclerotic cardiovascular disease. Further strengthening this hypothesis, several lipid intervention trials have demonstrated success in reducing the incidence of clinical coronary disease. More recent trials have demonstrated angiographic regression of coronary lesions after intense lipid-lowering therapy utilizing drugs, diet, or surgery aimed at reducing lipid levels.

Because of the multifaceted nature of atherosclerosis, pharmacologic approaches other than lipid-lowering therapy have been successful in reducing either the incidence of coronary artery disease, as with aspirin, or the demonstration of plaque formation, as with fish oils. More recent data have shown that the use of dietary antioxidants may protect against oxidative injury, which has been implicated in the pathogenesis of a long list of diseases including atherosclerosis. We review the current data regarding the "oxidative modification hypothesis" and the impact of antioxidant therapy in the prevention of coronary atherosclerosis.

FREE RADICALS

Free radicals (also called oxygen-derived free radicals or free oxygen radicals) are molecules or molecular fragments that have an unpaired electron. These molecules have a heightened reactivity that leads to abstraction of a hydrogen atom from another molecule, thereby initiating a chain reaction. The release of these reactive oxygen species results in oxidative injury to biologic systems such as lipids found in cell membranes and proteins found in blood vessels and myocardial tissues. In addition to the free radicals derived from exogenous sources (i.e., radiation, pollution, cigarette smoke), free radicals are constantly produced endogenously as a result of normal biologic and metabolic processes. For instance, under normal conditions, activated neutrophils generate superoxide anions in order to kill engulfed microorganisms. During ischemic conditions, xanthine oxidase is formed from xanthine dehydrogenase, which reacts with hypoxanthine, forming superoxide anion and other free radicals that cause lipid peroxidation (Fig. 32–1). After myocardial ischemia, neutrophils accumulate in reperfused tissues, releasing superoxide anions and other free radicals. Finally, mitochondria, endoplasmic reticulum, and nuclear membranes have been shown to produce superoxide anion after antioxidation of electron transport chain components.[1]

OXIDIZED LOW-DENSITY LIPOPROTEINS AND ATHEROSCLEROSIS

The earliest lesion of atherosclerosis is the fatty streak, which contains a large number of foam cells. Foam cells are primarily macrophages loaded with cholesterol derived from plasma lipoproteins. Although a high level of LDL cholesterol in plasma is recognized as a risk factor for atherosclerosis, a number of observations indicate that native LDL does not generally induce foam cell formation. Native LDL cholesterol is taken up by the LDL receptor originally described by the classic studies of Brown and Goldstein.[2–4] *In vivo* studies have shown that two thirds or more of the removal of LDL from plasma is mediated by the LDL receptor and that the removal occurs mostly in the liver.[5, 6] However, as Steinberg et al. suggest, two lines of evidence strongly suggest that the arterial uptake of LDL, giving rise to foam cells and fatty streaks, must be by pathways independent of the LDL receptor.[7] Lesions rich in macrophage-derived foam cells develop even in patients and animals deficient in functional LDL receptors (patients with homozygous familial hypercholesterolemia, and Watanabe heritable hyperlipidemic [WHHL] rabbits).[8, 9] Secondly, normal monocytes and monocyte-derived tissue macrophages in culture cannot be converted to foam cells by incubation with even very high concentrations of native LDL cholesterol.[10, 11] These observations suggest that cholesterol must be taken up via an alternative receptor pathway, which has since been described by Goldstein as the "scavenger receptor."[11] The scavenger receptor does not recognize native LDL but does recognize specifically modified forms of LDL such as oxidized LDL. Oxidized LDL is rapidly taken up by the scavenger receptor, leading to foam cell formation (Fig. 32–2).

One of the earliest events observed in experimental atherosclerosis is the adherence of circulating monocytes to arterial endothelial cells. Oxidatively modified LDL, but not native LDL, has been shown to be a potent chemoattractant for circulating human monocytes.[12] Oxidatively modified LDL, but not native LDL, has also been shown to be a potent inhibitor of resident macrophage motility and is cytotoxic.[13–15] This cytotoxicity may induce functional changes in endothelial cells that favor penetration of circulating monocytes or favor the movement of LDL into the

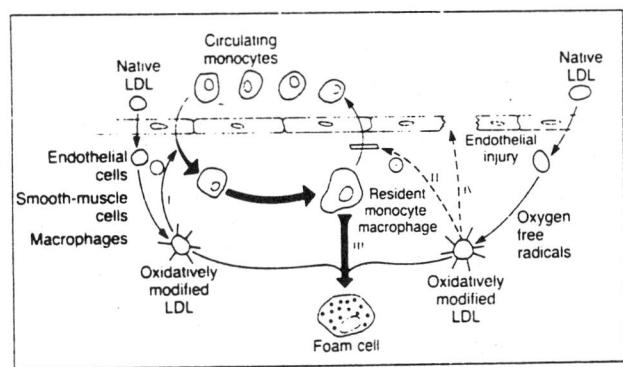

Figure 32–2. Four mechanisms by which the oxidation of LDL (catalyzed by endothelial cells, smooth muscle cells, or macrophages) may contribute to atherogenesis. Mechanisms are (I) the recruitment of circulating monocytes by means of the chemotactic factor present in oxidized LDL but absent in native LDL; (II) inhibition by oxidized LDL of the motility of resident macrophages and therefore of their ability to leave the intima; (III) enhanced rate of uptake of oxidized LDL by resident macrophages, leading to the generation of foam cells; and (IV) cytotoxicity of oxidized LDL, leading to loss of endothelial integrity. (Reprinted by permission from Steinberg D, Parthasarathy S, Carew TE, et al: Beyond cholesterol. Modifications of low-density lipoprotein that increase its atherogenicity. N Engl J Med 320:915, 1989. Copyright 1989, Massachusetts Medical Society.)

subendothelial space, thus accelerating the formation of fatty streaks.[7]

Several studies appear to document the presence of oxidatively modified LDL *in vivo.* Antibodies against "models" of oxidized LDL, or against oxidized LDL itself, show immunostaining in rabbit aortic atherosclerotic lesions but not in normal areas of the rabbit aorta.[16, 17] In addition, LDL that is eluted from aortic lesions in WHHL rabbits and subjected to polyacrylamide-gel electrophoresis and Western blotting shows cross reactivity with antibodies specific to oxidized LDL.[7] Finally, plasma from human subjects has also been shown to contain autoantibodies that react with various forms of oxidized LDL.[7]

For many years, lipid peroxides have been detected in atherosclerotic aortas at autopsy, and correlations were found between the degree of atherosclerosis and the levels of these oxidation products in arterial tissues.[18] Patients with proven coronary artery disease and peripheral vascular disease have increased serum levels of lipid peroxides, as do smokers, who are known to be at increased coronary risk. Cigarette smoking, a known risk factor for coronary artery disease, predisposes LDL to oxidation.[19]

Oxidized LDL appears to be uniquely destructive in other ways. Abnormal vasomotion has been a known vascular abnormality in patients with atherosclerosis.[20, 21] This effect appears to be related to the presence of oxidized LDL, which has been shown to directly inactivate endothelium-derived relaxing factor (EDRF) and directly promotes production of endothelin, a potent vasoconstrictor.[22–24] These events do not occur *in vitro* with exposure to native LDL and are unique to oxidized LDL. Oxidized LDL cholesterol, therefore, not only appears to induce fatty streaks

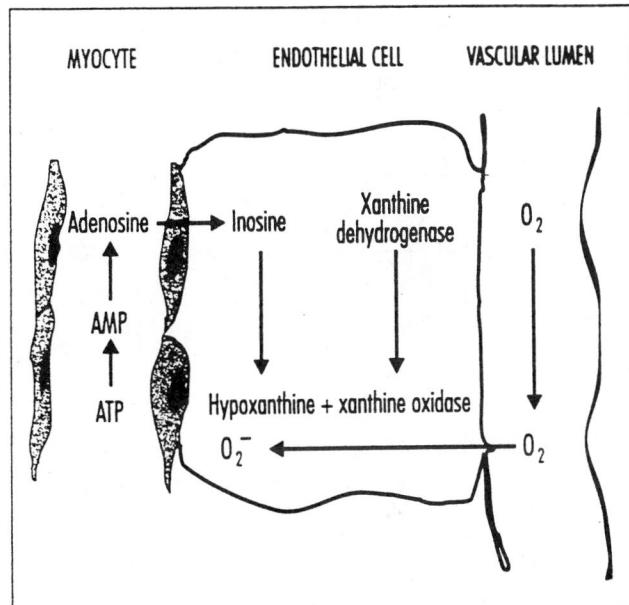

Figure 32–1. Xanthine dehydrogenase in the endothelial cells is converted to xanthine oxidase during ischemia. The reaction between xanthine oxidase and hypoxanthine, derived from the degradation of adenosine triphosphate (ATP), converts molecular oxygen (O_2) entering the vascular lumen during reperfusion into superoxide anion (O_2^-). AMP, adenosine monophosphate. (From Mehta JL, Yang BC, Nichols WW: Free radicals, antioxidants, and coronary heart disease. Journal of Myocardial Ischemia 5(8):31, 1993.)

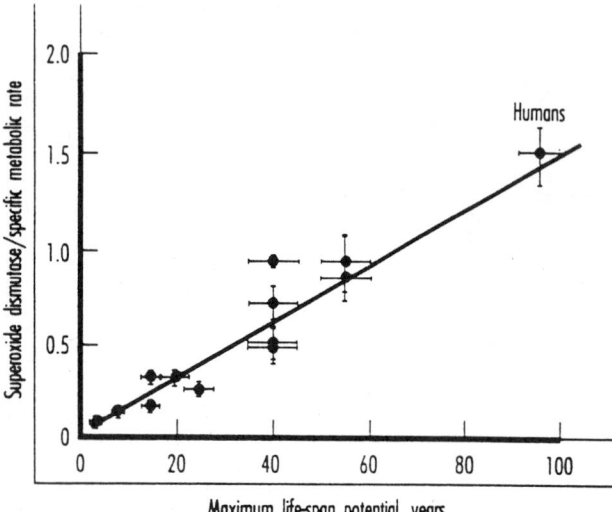

Figure 32–3. Correlation between liver superoxide dismutase content and maximum life-span potential in various species. Maximum life-span potential is an estimate of the mean (± SD) at 95% mortality. (From Mehta JL, Yang BC, Nichols WW: Free radicals, antioxidants, and coronary heart disease. Journal of Myocardial Ischemia 5(8):31, 1993.)

and plaque formation but promotes vasospasm and paradoxical vasoconstriction in patients with atherosclerotic coronary artery disease.

NATURALLY OCCURRING ANTIOXIDANTS

A number of antioxidant mechanisms are available to the body, to either scavenge free radicals or to counteract their effects. Almost all species possess antioxidant mechanisms, including the synthesis of superoxide dismutase (SOD), catalase, and glutathione peroxidase. These antioxidants have been identified in endothelial cells, platelets, hepatic cells, and neutrophils, and their purpose appears to be aimed at preventing damage caused by endogenously derived free radicals. The importance of these antioxidant mechanisms in biologic systems is underscored by the data demonstrating a direct correlation between liver superoxide dismutase (SOD) content and life-span potential in different species (Fig. 32–3).[25]

ANTIOXIDANTS AND ATHEROGENESIS

The majority of intervention studies currently available to study the effects of antioxidant therapy in atherogenesis utilize the WHHL rabbits. These animals are bred to serve as a model for the human disease, homozygous familial hypercholesterolemia, in which cells are unable to express receptors for the LDL particle. This abnormality results in markedly elevated levels of LDL cholesterol and extensive premature atherosclerosis. When this rabbit model was used to test the effects of probucol, a hypolipidemic agent with potent antioxidant properties, significant

reductions in arterial plaque occurred when compared with controls.[26] The impact of probucol therapy, therefore, was due either to its hypolipidemic effect or to its antioxidant effect.

To test which effect was predominant, WHHL rabbits were treated with either lovastatin, which lacks significant antioxidant properties, or probucol.[27] Dosages of the two drugs were adjusted to produce similar reductions in serum cholesterol levels. The results of this study indicate that although cholesterol levels in the probucol-treated animals did not fall quite as much as those of the lovastatin-treated animals, there was significantly less arterial disease and LDL degradation in the probucol group.

These results indicate that the primary mechanism behind probucol's action in reducing arterial disease was due to its antioxidant effects, which was a more potent antiatherosclerotic mechanism than its LDL-lowering effect. These data further demonstrate the importance of LDL oxidation in the development of atherosclerotic disease.

NUTRITIONAL ANTIOXIDANTS

The concentration of antioxidant micronutrients in human tissues depends primarily on dietary intake. Antioxidant nutrients for which intake has been studied in relationship to cardiovascular disease include vitamin E, vitamin C, beta-carotene, and selenium. The role of these nutrient antioxidants in protecting humans against oxidative stress can be shown in Figure 32–4.[62]

The serum levels of these dietary antioxidants reflect not only the dietary habits of the individual but in some cases the geographic location of the individual as well. For instance, the selenium content of

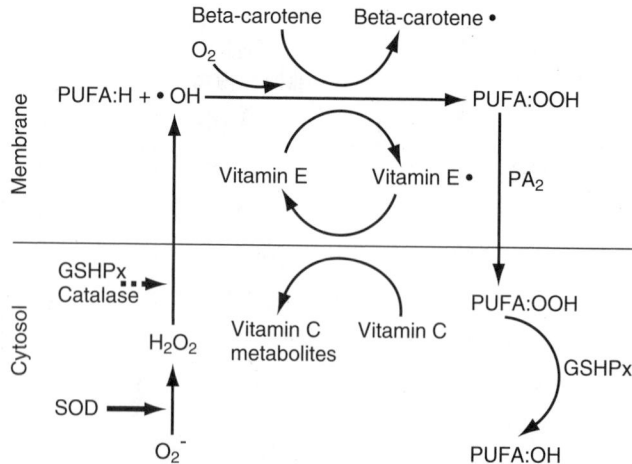

Figure 32–4. Major antioxidant defense mechanisms within the cell. Beta-carotene •, beta-carotene radical; GSHPx, glutathione peroxidase; H_2O_2, hydrogen peroxide; O_2, oxygen, O_2^- = superoxide anion; • OH, hydroxyl radical; PA_2, phospholipase A_2; PUFA:H, polyunsaturated fatty acid; PUFA:OH, fatty acid hydroxide; PUFA:OOH, fatty acid hydroperoxide; SOD, superoxide dismutase; Vitamin E •, vitamin E radical. (From Kardinaal AFM, van Poppel G, Kok FJ: The protective role of antioxidants and coronary artery disease. Journal of Myocardial Ischemia 4:64, 1992.)

various foods is often related to the selenium content of the soil where the food has been grown.

Table 32–1 lists the sources of dietary antioxidants and their recommended daily allowances.[62]

Vitamin E

Of the four major nutrient antioxidants, vitamin E has been the most extensively studied in its relation to cardiovascular disease. Vitamin E is a lipid-soluble antioxidant that is transported with other lipids inside lipoprotein particles and thus may provide antioxidant protection against LDL oxidation in close proximity to the LDL particle. Vitamin E, or more specifically α-tocopherol, the most biologically active and prevalent form of vitamin E, is the predominant lipophilic antioxidant in plasma membranes and tissue and is the most abundant antioxidant in LDL.[28]

On the average, there are six molecules of α-tocopherol per LDL particle.[29, 30] Enrichment of LDL with α-tocopherol has been shown to reduce its susceptibility to oxidation. Esterbauer et al. demonstrated that the lag phase of LDL oxidation is lengthened with increased LDL α-tocopherol content.[31] Other studies in humans have confirmed that α-tocopherol supplementation increases the oxidative resistance of LDL.[32, 33]

In the Multinational Monitoring Project of Trends and Determinants of Cardiovascular Disease, or the World Health Organization (WHO) MONICA study, plasma levels of antioxidants were compared among apparently healthy men from 16 different populations. Investigators found an inverse correlation between antioxidant levels and ischemic heart disease mortality, a relationship that was strongest for vitamin E (Fig. 32–5).[34]

Riemersma et al. have shown an inverse relationship between plasma levels of vitamin E and angina pectoris.[35] Their results indicated that individuals whose plasma vitamin E levels were in the lowest quintile had an almost threefold greater risk of angina than did those whose vitamin E levels were in the highest quintile.

Two large-scale prospective studies, one in men and one in women, showed that the use of large doses of vitamin E supplements is associated with a

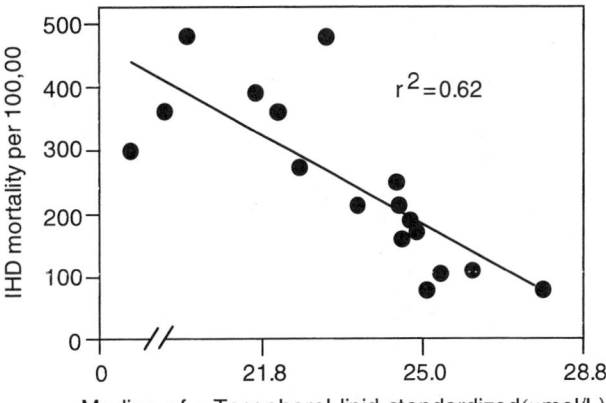

Figure 32–5. Relationship between plasma vitamin E levels and mortality due to ischemic heart disease (IHD), as determined in the Optional Vitamin Study, World Health Organization (WHO)/ MONICA project. (From Kardinaal AFM, van Poppel G, Kok FJ: The protective role of antioxidants and coronary artery disease. Journal of Myocardial Ischemia 4:64, 1992.)

significantly decreased risk of coronary heart disease. The Nurses Health Study enrolled 87,245 female nurses and assessed their consumption of a wide range of nutrients, including vitamin E, via dietary questionnaires.[36] During a follow-up period of 8 years, which was 97% complete, those in the top fifth with respect to vitamin E intake had a relative risk of major coronary disease of 0.66 after adjustment for age and smoking. Most of the variability in intake and reduction of risk was attributable to vitamin E consumed as supplements.

In the Health Professional's Follow-up Study, 39,910 United States male health professionals, aged 40 to 75 years, also completed dietary questionnaires that assessed their intake of vitamin C, beta-carotene, and vitamin E.[37] During 4 years of follow-up, those men consuming more than 60 IU of vitamin E per day had a risk reduction for coronary disease of 36% compared with those consuming less than 7.5 IU per day.

In both studies, the benefit of vitamin E was largely, if not entirely, confined to the subgroup of the population taking large amounts of supplements. In other words, within the range of vitamin E intakes afforded by natural foodstuffs, even when supplemented by multivitamins at usual doses, there was little or no protective effect.

It should be pointed out, however, that these data are observational and that confounding may partially account for the results. Clearly, studies using a double-blind, randomized, placebo-controlled method are needed to prove cause and effect relationships.

Vitamin C

Vitamin C (ascorbic acid) is a water-soluble antioxidant that reacts with superoxide, hydroxyl radicals, and singlet oxygen.[35] It can also regenerate α-tocopherol from tocopheroxyl radical form.[38]

The results of several epidemiologic studies sup-

Table 32–1. **Dietary Sources of Vitamins E and C, Beta-carotene, and Selenium and the Recommended Dietary Allowance (RDA) of Each Nutrient**

Nutrient	Dietary Sources	Recommended Daily Allowance	
		Men	*Women*
Vitamin E	Vegetable oils, soybeans, milk, eggs, fish, muscle meats, nuts, margarine	70–80 α-TE	60–65 α-TE
Vitamin C	Fresh fruits and vegetables	60 mg	60 mg
Beta-carotene	Green leafy vegetables, corn, carrots	1000 μg RE	800 μg RE
Selenium	Fish, meat, liver, grains	70 μg	55 μg

α-TE, alpha-tocopherol equivalent; RE, retinol equivalent.

port a role for low plasma vitamin C levels in atherosclerosis. The WHO/MONICA study revealed a moderately strong inverse correlation between plasma vitamin C and coronary artery disease mortality.[34] Dubick et al. reported that vitamin C concentrations are lower in the aortas of persons with atherosclerosis relative to unaffected controls.[39] In the United Kingdom, coronary artery disease mortality is high in areas where residents have relatively low vitamin C consumption.[40] In a small European study, coronary artery disease mortality was 60% higher in individuals who had low plasma vitamin C levels than in those who had high vitamin C levels; however, because of the small number of cases, this difference was not statistically significant.[41] In another epidemiologic study, those individuals who consumed 500 mg or more of vitamin C per day demonstrated an increase in life expectancy that was all due to the prevention of cardiovascular end points.[42]

Smokers and diabetics have lower vitamin C levels than do control subjects.[43-45] It is quite possible that these low levels may predispose LDL to oxidation, which could enhance atherogenesis in these higher-risk individuals.

Vitamin C is able to prevent chemical and cell-mediated oxidation of LDL, as well as protect the natural antioxidants present in LDL, such as vitamin E and beta-carotene, from oxidative stress.[46, 47] Although no double-blind, randomized, controlled trial of vitamin C has been undertaken, these data suggest the possible role for vitamin C in preventing atherosclerosis.

Beta-Carotene

Beta-carotene (provitamin A) is a member of the carotenoid family of plant pigments and is the precursor of retinol (vitamin A). When large doses are taken, a significant amount of beta-carotene escapes conversion to retinol and accumulates in the plasma lipoproteins. Beta-carotene has been shown to be able to quench singlet oxygen and free radicals.[48, 49] *In vitro* studies have demonstrated that beta-carotene prevents both LDL modification and its induction of monocyte transmigration.[50] Beta-carotene is also effective in preventing the oxidation of lipoprotein(a).[51]

Epidemiologic data have demonstrated that individuals consuming large quantities of fresh fruits and vegetables (natural sources of beta-carotene) have a reduced mortality due to coronary artery disease and a decreased risk of acute myocardial infarction.[52, 53]

Smokers have lower LDL beta-carotene levels relative to nonsmokers, and LDL levels from smokers are more prone to oxidative modification than in their nonsmoking counterparts.[54] In the Health Professionals Follow-up Study noted earlier, beta-carotene intake was not associated with a lower risk of coronary disease among those individuals who had never smoked, but it was inversely associated with coronary disease risk among current smokers (relative risk, 0.30) and former smokers (relative risk, 0.60).[37] The effect, therefore, of beta-carotene may be a threshold

phenomenon in which low levels, induced by poor intake or smoking, may enhance risk, and adequate levels may reduce it.

The best-designed study to date demonstrating the potential beneficial effects of beta-carotene occurred quite accidentally from data derived from the Physicians' Health Study. Beta-carotene was given in a double-blind, randomized placebo-controlled fashion to determine whether or not its antioxidant effect could prevent cancer formation. It was noted that those subjects randomized to consuming 50 mg of beta-carotene every other day had a 44% reduction in major coronary events compared with the control group.[55] This is the only study to date that has prospectively enrolled patients in a double-blind, placebo-controlled fashion testing the effects of an antioxidant in preventing coronary heart disease.

Selenium

Selenium is a mineral that is a cofactor of glutathione peroxidase. Several trials have examined the relationship between serum selenium concentrations and the risk of coronary artery disease. Although many of these trials demonstrated an inverse relationship between coronary events and serum selenium levels, others have shown no significant relationship.[56-59] It appears, however, that selenium concentrations must be below a threshold level before such a relationship exists. Selenium supplementation increases the activity of glutathione peroxidase in platelets of selenium-deficient humans, and this increase levels off when a plasma selenium concentration reaches approximately 100 mg/L.[60]

Part of the problem in reproducing selenium's relationship to coronary events, if any, is in measuring selenium levels in the plasma. A more effective method of measurement has been proposed using the selenium level in toenails, which reflects long-term intake. Using this technique, Kok et al. found significantly lower toenail selenium levels in patients who had suffered myocardial infarction than in healthy population control subjects.[61] This would indicate that low selenium levels were present before the infarction, thus suggesting a possible role for selenium in preventing clinical coronary artery disease.

CONCLUSIONS

Many experimental and epidemiologic data demonstrate that oxidation of LDL, or the oxidative modification hypothesis, plays a pivotal role in the development of atherosclerosis and clinical coronary artery disease. *In vitro* studies indicate that LDL oxidation can be inhibited by a variety of both endogenous and exogenous antioxidants, including nutrient antioxidants such as vitamin E, vitamin C, beta-carotene, and selenium. Epidemiologic data further suggest that either increased intake or high plasma levels of dietary antioxidants reduces risk for cardiovascular end points. Finally, a single, placebo-controlled, randomized trial of the nutrient antioxidant beta-carotene has demonstrated a significant protective effect in reducing coronary end points. These data strongly support the oxidative modification hypothesis and suggest the need for future studies to assess the effects of antioxidant nutrients on the progression of atherosclerosis in animals and on cardiovascular events in humans. If these studies confirm the oxidative modification hypothesis, dietary antioxidants will become an integral part of the regimen for primary and secondary prevention of coronary atherosclerosis.

REFERENCES

1. Mehta JL, Yang BC, Nichols WW: Free radicals, antioxidants, and coronary heart disease. Journal of Myocardial Ischemia 5(8):31, 1993.
2. Goldstein JL, Brown MS: The low-density lipoprotein pathway and its relation to atherosclerosis [review]. Annu Rev Biochem 46:897, 1977.
3. Brown MS, Goldstein JL: Receptor-mediated control of cholesterol metabolism. Study of human mutants has disclosed how cells regulate a substance that is both vital and lethal. Science 191:150, 1976.
4. Brown MS, Kovanen PT, Goldstein JL: Regulation of plasma cholesterol by lipoprotein receptors [review]. Science 212:628, 1981.
5. Kesaniemi YA, Witztum JL, Steinbrecher UP: Receptor-mediated catabolism of low density lipoprotein in man. Quantitation using glucosylated low density lipoprotein. J Clin Invest 71:950, 1983.
6. Pittman RC, Attie AD, Carew TE, et al: Tissue sites of degradation of low density lipoprotein: Application of a method for determining the fate of plasma proteins. Proc Natl Acad Sci USA 76:5345, 1979.
7. Steinberg D, Parthasarathy S, Carew TE, et al: Beyond cholesterol. Modifications of low-density lipoprotein that increase its atherogenicity [see comments]. N Engl J Med 320:915, 1989.
8. Rosenfeld ME, Tsukada T, Gown AM, Ross R: Fatty streak initiation in Watanabe Heritable Hyperlipemic and comparably hypercholesterolemic fat-fed rabbits. Arteriosclerosis 7(1):9, 1987.
9. Buja LM, Kita T, Goldstein JL, et al: Cellular pathology of progressive atherosclerosis in the WHHL rabbit: An animal model of familial hypercholesterolemia. Arteriosclerosis 3:87, 1983.
10. Brown MS, Goldstein JL: Lipoprotein metabolism in the macrophage: Implications for cholesterol deposition in atherosclerosis. Annu Rev Biochem 52:223, 1983.
11. Goldstein JL, Ho YK, Basu SK, et al: Binding site on macrophages that mediates uptake and degradation of acetylated low density lipoprotein, producing massive cholesterol deposition. Proc Natl Acad Sci USA 76:333, 1979.
12. Quinn MT, Parthasarathy S, Fong LG, et al: Oxidatively modified low density lipoproteins: A potential role in recruitment and retention of monocyte/macrophages during atherogenesis. Proc Natl Acad Sci USA 84:2995, 1987.
13. Morel DW, DiCorleto PE, Chisolm GM: Endothelial and smooth muscle cells alter low density lipoprotein in vitro by free radical oxidation. Arteriosclerosis 4:357, 1984.
14. Hessler JR, Robertson AL Jr, Chisolm GM III: LDL-induced cytotoxicity and its inhibition by HDL in human vascular smooth muscle and endothelial cells in culture. Atherosclerosis 32:213, 1979.
15. Quinn MT, Parthasarathy S, Steinberg D: Endothelial cell-derived chemotactic activity for mouse peritoneal macrophages and the effects of modified forms of low density lipoprotein. Proc Natl Acad Sci USA 82:5949, 1985.
16. Haberland ME, Fong D, Cheng L: Malondialdehyde-altered protein occurs in atheroma of Watanabe heritable hyperlipidemic rabbits. Science 241:215, 1988.
17. Palinski W, Rosenfeld ME, Yla-Herttuala S, et al: Low density lipoprotein undergoes oxidative modification in vivo. Proc Natl Acad Sci USA 86:1372, 1989.
18. Glavind J, Hartmann S, Clemmensen J, et al: Studies on role of lipoperoxides in human pathology; presence of peroxidized lipids in the atherosclerotic aorta. Acta Pathol Microbiol Scand 30:1, 1952.
19. Scheffler E, Huber L, Fruhbis J, et al: Alteration of plasma low density lipoprotein from smokers. Atherosclerosis 82:261, 1990.
20. Golino P, Piscione F, Willerson JT, et al: Divergent effects of serotonin on coronary-artery dimensions and blood flow in patients with coronary atherosclerosis and control patients [see comments]. N Engl J Med 324:641, 1991.
21. Zeiher AM, Drexler H, Wollschlager H, et al: Endothelial dysfunction of the coronary microvasculature is associated with coronary blood flow regulation in patients with early atherosclerosis. Circulation 84:1984, 1991.
22. Tanner FC, Noll G, Boulanger CM, et al: Oxidized low density lipoproteins inhibit relaxations of porcine coronary arteries. Role of scavenger receptor and endothelium-derived nitric oxide [see comments]. Circulation 83:2012, 1991.
23. Chin JH, Azhar S, Hoffman BB: Inactivation of endothelial derived relaxing factor by oxidized lipoproteins. J Clin Invest 89:10, 1992.
24. Boulanger CM, Tanner FC, Bea ML, et al: Oxidized low density lipoproteins induce mRNA expression and release endothelin from human and porcine endothelium. Circ Res 70:1191.
25. Tolmasoff JM, Ono T, Cutler RG: Superoxide dismutase: Correlation with life-span and specific metabolic rate in primate species. Proc Natl Acad Sci USA 77:2777, 1980.
26. Kita T, Nagano Y, Yokode M, et al: Probucol prevents the progression of atherosclerosis in Watanabe heritable hyperlipidemic rabbit, an animal model for familial hypercholesterolemia. Proc Natl Acad Sci USA 84:5928, 1987.
27. Carew TE, Schwenke DC, Steinberg D: Antiatherogenic effect of probucol unrelated to its hypocholesterolemic effect: Evidence that antioxidants in vivo can selectively inhibit low density lipoprotein degradation in macrophage-rich fatty streaks and slow the progression of atherosclerosis in the Watanabe heritable hyperlipidemic rabbit. Proc Natl Acad Sci USA 84:7725, 1987.
28. Jialal I, Fuller CJ: Oxidized LDL and antioxidants [review]. Clin Cardiol 16:I6, 1993.
29. Esterbauer H, Dieber-Rotheneder M, Waeg G, et al: Endogenous antioxidants and lipoprotein oxidation. Biochem Soc Trans 18:1059, 1990.
30. Esterbauer H, Dieber-Rotheneder M, Waeg G, et al: Biochemical, structural, and functional properties of oxidized low-density lipoprotein [review]. Chem Res Toxicol 3:77, 1990.
31. Esterbauer H, Dieber-Rotheneder M, Striegl G, et al: Role of vitamin E in preventing the oxidation of low-density lipoprotein. Am J Clin Nutr 53:314S, 1991.
32. Princen HM, van Poppel G, Vogelezang C, et al: Supplementation with vitamin E but not beta-carotene in vivo protects low density lipoprotein from lipid peroxidation in vitro: Effect of cigarette smoking. Arterioscler Thromb 12:544, 1992.
33. Reaven PD, Khouw A, Beltz WF, et al: Effect of dietary antioxidant combinations in humans. Protection of LDL by vitamin E but not by beta-carotene. Arterioscler Thromb 13:590, 1993.
34. Gey KF, Puska P, Jordan P, Moser UK: Inverse correlation between plasma vitamin E and mortality from ischemic heart disease in cross-cultural epidemiology. Am J Clin Nutr 53:326S, 1991.
35. Riemersma RA, Wood DA, Macintyre CC, et al: Risk of angina pectoris and plasma concentrations of vitamins A, C, and E and carotene [see comments]. Lancet 337:1, 1991.
36. Stampfer MJ, Hennekens, CH, Manson JE, et al: Vitamin E consumption and the risk of coronary disease in women [see comments]. N Engl J Med 328:1444, 1993.
37. Rimm EB, Stampfer MJ, Ascherio A, et al: Vitamin E consumption and the risk of coronary heart disease in men. N Engl J Med 328:1450, 1993.
38. Packer JE, Slater TF, Willson RL: Direct observation of a free radical interaction between vitamin E and vitamin C. Nature 278:737, 1979.
39. Dubick MA, Hunter GC, Casey SM, Keen C: Aortic ascorbic

acid, trace elements, and superoxide dismutase activity in human aneurysmal and occlusive disease. Proc Soc Exp Biol Med 184:138, 1987.

40. Armstrong BK, Mann JI, Adelstein AM, Eskin F: Commodity consumption and ischemic heart disease mortality, with special reference to dietary practices. J Chron Dis 28:455, 1975.
41. Gey KF, Brubacher GB, Stahelin HB: Plasma levels of antioxidant vitamins in relation to ischemic heart disease and cancer. Am J Clin Nutr 45:1368, 1987.
42. Enstrom JE, Kanim LE, Klein MA: Vitamin C intake and mortality among a sample of the United States population [see comments]. Epidemiology 3(3):194, 1992.
43. Stankova L, Riddle M, Larned J, et al: Plasma ascorbate concentrations and blood cell dehydroascorbate transport in patients with diabetes mellitus. Metabolism 33:347, 1984.
44. Chow CK, Thacker RR, Changchit C, et al: Lower levels of vitamin C and carotenes in plasma of cigarette smokers. J Am Coll Nutr 5(3):305, 1986.
45. Ramirez J, Flowers NC: Leukocyte ascorbic acid and its relationship to coronary artery disease in man. Am J Clin Nutr 33:2079, 1980.
46. Harats D, Ben-Naim M, Dabach Y, et al: Effect of vitamin C and E supplementation on susceptibility of plasma lipoproteins to peroxidation induced by acute smoking. Atherosclerosis 85:47, 1990.
47. Kalra J, Chaudhary AK, Prasad K: Increased production of oxygen free radicals in cigarette smokers. Int J Exp Pathol 72:1, 1991.
48. Foote CS, Denny RW: Chemistry of singlet oxygen. VII. Quenching by beta-carotene. J Am Chem Soc 90:6233, 1968.
49. Krinsky NI: Carotenoid protection against oxidation. Pure Appl Chem 51:649, 1979.
50. Navab M, Imes SS, Hama SY, et al: Monocyte transmigration induced by modification of low density lipoprotein in cocultures of human aortic wall cells is due to induction of monocyte chemotactic protein 1 synthesis and is abolished by high density lipoprotein. J Clin Invest 88:2039, 1991.
51. Naruszewicz M, Selinger E, Davignon J: Oxidative modification of lipoprotein (a) and the effect of beta-carotene. Metabolism 41:1215, 1992.
52. Palgi A: Association between dietary changes and mortality rates: Israel 1949 to 1977; a trend-free regression model. Am J Clin Nutr 34:1569, 1981.
53. Gramenzi A, Gentile A, Fasoli M, et al: Association between certain foods and risk of acute myocardial infarction in women. Br Med J 300:771, 1990.
54. Harats D, Ben-Naim M, Dabach Y, et al: Cigarette smoking renders LDL susceptible to peroxidative modification and enhanced metabolism by macrophages. Atherosclerosis 79:245, 1989.
55. Gaziano JM, Manson JE, Ridker PM, et al: Beta carotene therapy for chronic stable angina. Circulation 82:III, 1990.
56. Salonen JT, Alfthan G, Huttunen JK, et al: Association between cardiovascular death and myocardial infarction and serum selenium in a matched-pair longitudinal study. Lancet 2:175, 1982.
57. Miettinen TA, Alfthan G, Huttunen JK, et al: Serum selenium concentration related to myocardial infarction and fatty acid content of serum lipids. Br Med J 287:517, 1983.
58. Ringstad J, Jacobsen BK, Thomassen Y, Thelle DS: The Tromso Heart Study: Serum selenium and risk of myocardial infarction a nested case-control study. J Epidemiol Comm Health 41:329, 1987.
59. Kok FJ, van Poppel G, Melse J, et al: Do antioxidants and polyunsaturated fatty acids have a combined association with coronary atherosclerosis? Atherosclerosis 86:85, 1991.
60. Salonen JT: Selenium in ischaemic heart disease. Int J Epidemiol 16:323, 1987.
61. Kok FJ, Hofman A, Witteman JCM, et al: Decreased selenium levels in acute myocardial infarction [see comments]. JAMA 261:1161, 1989.
62. Kardinaal AFM, van Poppel G, Kok FJ: The protective role of antioxidants and coronary artery disease. Journal of Myocardial Ischemia 4:64, 1992.

CHAPTER 33

Fixed Combinations as Step-One Therapy in Cardiovascular Disorders

Franz H. Messerli, M.D., Vincent DeQuattro, M.D., F.A.C.C., F.A.C.P., and James Schoenberger, M.D.

Fixed combinations have been used for the treatment of hypertension for more than three decades. The first triple combination (reserpine, hydralazine, and hydrochlorothiazide) was marketed three decades ago. Ever since then, fixed combinations have had their advocates as well as their opponents. The advocates consist mainly of practicing physicians who have learned to appreciate any measure that simplifies therapy and thereby possibly enhances patient compliance. The opponents, on the other hand, consist mainly of the physicians and teachers at the academic medical centers who may not always care for patients over a prolonged period of time. Until very recently, the United States Food and Drug Administration (FDA) had allowed fixed combination therapy to be initiated only after both drug doses had been titrated to the exact amount in the fixed combination.

However, the FDA has softened its stance somewhat and now allows some fixed combinations to be used as first-line therapy.[1] Nevertheless, it is still preferred that efficacy and safety of combination therapy are documented by an elaborate factorial design analysis,[2] and therefore only a few new fixed combinations have reached the cardiovascular market over the past few years. On a theoretical basis, a variety of additional fixed combinations could be envisioned (Tables 33–1 and 33–2). In other countries with less stringent requirements, the market has been flooded with a variety of fixed combinations to the degree that the practicing physician is put at risk of no longer being able to recall the actual ingredients. Of note, however, some drugs when given together are prone to decrease tolerability and should therefore probably not be used in fixed combinations (Tables 33–1 and 33–3).

Table 33–1. **Sense and Nonsense Combination Therapy in Hypertension**

	Diuretics	α-Blockers	Arterial Dilators	β-Blockers	ACE Inhibitors
α₁-Blockers	G				
Arterial dilators	F	P			
β-Blockers	G	G	G		
ACE inhibitors	G	?	G	F	
DHP–Ca antagonist	F	?	?	G	G
HRL–Ca antagonist	F	?	?	P	G

G, good; F, fair; P, poor; DHP, dihydropyridine; HRL, heart rate lowering.

In this chapter, we discuss a few of the more common fixed combinations that are currently used in cardiovascular medicine.

PREREQUISITES FOR FIXED-DOSE COMBINATIONS

The individual drugs of fixed-dose combinations should have compatible pharmacokinetics. That is, both agents should have approximately the same duration of action and have similarly effective relatively narrow dose ranges. In drugs with incompatible pharmacokinetics but similar clearance rates, the time for each drug to reach a steady-state level will be different. Therefore, the ratio of the concentration of the two drugs in the body will vary with time. Equally important is that the absorption of each of the components is good and that one drug does not interfere with the bioavailability of the other one. Compatible pharmacokinetics are of particular concern in fixed combinations used to treat patients with renal insufficiency. Thus, the biologic half-life of both components should be affected to the same extent by a reduction in glomerular filtration rate. The same consideration is of concern in patients with hepatic dysfunction for drugs that are predominantly metabolized in the liver.

DIURETIC–DIURETIC COMBINATIONS

Fixed combinations of the thiazide diuretics with a potassium-sparing diuretic have become well established in the treatment of hypertension and to a lesser

Table 33–3. **Diminished Tolerability and Adverse Drug Reactions as the Result of Combination Therapy in Hypertension**

Drug A	Drug B	Drug B Potentially Aggravates
Diuretic	Vasodilators	Hypokalemia
Diuretic	Propranolol	Hypoglycemia, dyslipoproteinemia
HRL–Ca antagonist	β-Blocker	AV block, bradycardia
α-Blocker	Diuretic	First-dose hypotension
ACE inhibitors	Diuretic	Decrease in GFR
ACE inhibitors	Potassium-sparing diuretic	Hyperkalemia
Hydralazine	DHP–Ca antagonist	Cardioacceleration, myocardial ischemia

AV, atrioventricular; DHP, dihydropyridine; GFR, glomerular filtration rate; HRL, heart rate lowering.

extent in the treatment of congestive heart failure. The thiazide used is most commonly hydrochlorothiazide, and the potassium-sparing diuretic is spironolactone (Aldactazide, see Chapter 46), amiloride (Moduretic, see Chapter 45), or triamterene (Dyazide and Maxzide, see Chapter 44). In general, the antihypertensive effect of the potassium-sparing diuretics is minimal. Thus, little if any additional fall in arterial pressure is seen when a potassium-sparing drug is added to hydrochlorothiazide. The rationale for adding spironolactone, amiloride, or triamterene is therefore solely to prevent hypokalemia and metabolic alkalosis. However, because hypokalemia by itself triggers some counterregulatory mechanisms that increase arterial pressure,[3–5] the addition of a potassium-sparing compound may in turn facilitate the antihypertensive efficacy of hydrochlorothiazide. Of note, the risk of strokes has been shown to increase with a low dietary potassium intake, and hypokalemia may therefore be considered a risk factor for cerebrovascular disease.[6] Fixed combinations with all three potassium-sparing drugs are available and have been approved by the FDA for the initial therapy of hypertension.

DIURETIC–β-BLOCKER COMBINATIONS

Several fixed combinations of β-blockers with a diuretic are currently available. In general, an additive

Table 33–2. **Enhanced Tolerability ("Synergism") as a Result of Combination Therapy in Hypertension**

Drug A	Drug B	Drug B Potentially Improves
DHP–Ca antagonist	β-Blocker	Palpitations
β-Blocker	DHP–Ca antagonist	Bradycardia
Ca antagonist	ACE inhibitor	Edema
Diuretic	ACE inhibitor	Hypokalemia, insulin resistance
Diuretic	α-Blocker	Insulin resistance, hyperlipidemia
ACE inhibitor	Ca antagonist	Cough
Antiadrenergic	Diuretic	Edema, pseudoresistance
Vasodilator	Diuretic	Fluid retention

effect on arterial pressure is seen when the two drugs are combined. Whereas the older combinations used fairly high doses of hydrochlorothiazide (between 25 and 50 mg) and therefore often aggravated adverse metabolic effects,[7] one of the newer combinations has been shown to be remarkably effective with only 6.25 mg of hydrochlorothiazide.[8] In contrast with other β-blocker–diuretic combinations, bisoprolol/hydrochlorothiazide (Ziac) is very well tolerated and has a side effect profile similar to that of placebo.[8] Conceivably, the β-blocker antagonizes some of the compensatory mechanisms (such as an increase in the activity of the sympathetic nervous system as well as of the renin-angiotensin system) that are triggered by diuretic therapy. Thus, although the combination of a β-blocker with the diuretic has, at the most, additive effects on the fall in arterial pressure, a favorable effect (synergism) with regard to other pathophysiologic findings may be observed.

ACE INHIBITOR–DIURETIC COMBINATIONS

Most of the available angiotensin-converting enzyme (ACE) inhibitors have also been marketed as fixed combinations with hydrochlorothiazide. Similar to the situation with β-blockers, the older combinations used higher doses of hydrochlorothiazide than the newer ones. Synergism with regard to prevention of hypokalemia and other pathophysiologic findings such as insulin resistance has been documented when the two components are combined.[9] With regard to arterial pressure, factorial design analyses have shown that in general an additive effect can be expected. Of note, however, some patients whose blood pressure responds poorly to monotherapy with an ACE inhibitor (e.g., African-American patients) respond better when they are pretreated with a diuretic.[9] Conceivably, diuretic therapy, by stimulating the renin-angiotensin cascade, turns a low-renin patient into a high-renin patient and thereby elicits a better response of arterial pressure to ACE inhibition.

MacGregor et al. reported that dietary sodium restriction added to ACE inhibition therapy was as efficacious in lowering arterial pressure as adding a thiazide, but in contrast with the thiazide did not have any adverse metabolic effect.[10] This would indicate that the ACE inhibition does not completely abolish all metabolic effects of diuretic therapy. Interestingly, doses as low as 6.25 mg of hydrochlorothiazide seem to be equally effective as higher doses when added to an ACE inhibitor.[11]

ANGIOTENSIN II RECEPTOR INHIBITOR–DIURETIC COMBINATIONS

Most recently the fixed combination of low-dose hydrochlorothiazide with losartan (Hyzar) has been introduced. Given that losartan has a relatively flat dose-response curve, no up-titration of the losartan dose is advised. A patient whose blood pressure responds insufficiently to losartan monotherapy should instead be switched directly to the combination of losartan/hydrochlorothiazide. As with ACE inhibitor–diuretic combinations, the addition of an angiotensin II receptor blocker to hydrochlorothiazide seems to diminish hypokalemia and insulin resistance.[12, 13] Because hydrochlorothiazide increases uric acid and losartan has a uricosuric effect,[14] some synergistic effect of the combination with regard to uric acid metabolism can be expected. The losartan/hydrochlorothiazide combination is remarkably well tolerated and overall adverse effects are indistinguishable from those with placebo.[12, 13] It is available in the dose of 50 mg of losartan and 12.5 mg of hydrochlorothiazide.

DIHYDROPYRIDINE CALCIUM ANTAGONIST–β-BLOCKER COMBINATIONS

Fixed combinations of a dihydropyridine calcium antagonist and a β-blocker have become available outside the United States. As with most fixed combinations, the effect on arterial pressure is, at the most, additive. However, because some of the dihydropyridine calcium antagonists produce an increase in sympathetic activity leading to cardiac acceleration, the addition of a β-blocker may blunt this effect. This fixed combination is not only attractive in hypertension but should be considered in some patients with angina pectoris and coronary artery disease as well.

CALCIUM ANTAGONIST–ACE INHIBITOR COMBINATIONS

Most recently, fixed combinations containing calcium antagonists and ACE inhibitors have become available. The first such combination marketed in the United States is amlodipine/benazepril (Lotrel) in the doses of 2.5/10, 5/10, and 5/20 mg, respectively. Factorial design analyses have documented that the antihypertensive efficacy of the two drug classes is additive and occasionally supraadditive (Fig. 33–1).[15] In a single dosing study, the addition of benazepril did "unmask" the hypotensive effect of a low dose of a dihydropyridine calcium antagonist in normotensive volunteers,[16] thus demonstrating synergism of the combination with regard to blood pressure. Some synergism has also been shown with regard to side effects such as peripheral edema. Specifically, the peripheral edema that occasionally occurs with amlodipine monotherapy ("hyperfiltration" edema) has been reported to diminish in a dose-response fashion when benazepril was added.[15]

The calcium antagonist–ACE inhibitor combination is attractive not only because of its powerful blood pressure–lowering effect and excellent tolerability. Conceivably, some of the protective effects on the heart, the kidney, and the microvasculature that had been documented with either one of the two drug classes may also turn out to be additive and therefore be relatively independent of the blood pressure–low-

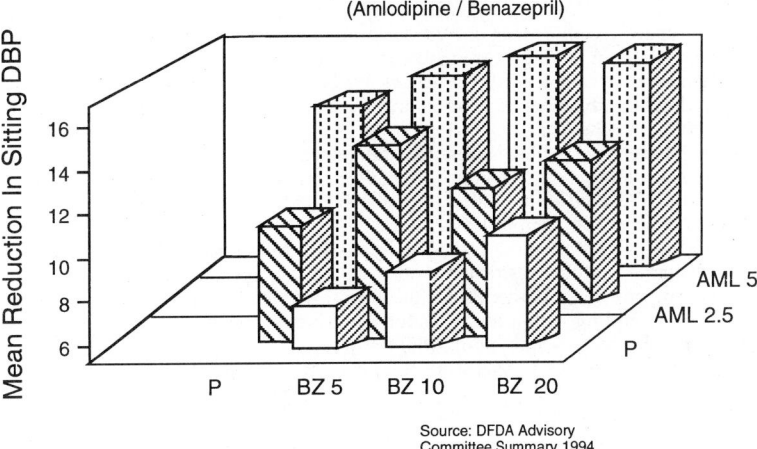

RESPONSE SURFACE ANALYSIS
(RAW DATA)
(Amlodipine / Benazepril)

Source: DFDA Advisory
Committee Summary 1994

Figure 33–1. Factorial design analysis assessing antihypertensive efficacy of amlodipine and benazepril alone and in combination. Note that the effect on blood pressure is supraadditive for some doses when placebo effects are subtracted. Blood pressure was taken at trough, 24 hours after dosing. (Data on file, Ciba.)

ering effect. Other promising fixed combinations include verapamil and trandolapril as well as diltiazem and enalapril. The combination of a heart rate–lowering calcium antagonist with an ACE-inhibitor may offer an advantage in post–myocardial infarction (MI) patients. Conversely, the combination of a calcium antagonist such as amlodipine (which has been documented to reduce morbidity and mortality in dilated cardiomyopathy) with an ACE inhibitor may be of advantage in patients with congestive heart failure.

FIXED COMBINATIONS IN DISEASES OTHER THAN HYPERTENSION

At the present time, no fixed combinations are available or indicated for the treatment of other chronic cardiovascular disorders such as congestive heart failure, coronary artery disease including angina, arrhythmias, or hyperlipidemia. However, at least on a theoretical basis, it would make sense to combine two drugs in some of these conditions, especially for hyperlipidemia.

Table 33–4. **Advantages and Disadvantages of Fixed-Dose Combinations**

Advantages
• Convenience and simplicity
• Easy titration
• Cost (occasionally less than individual drugs)
• Improved compliance
• Optimal dose of both drugs for most patients*

Disadvantages
• Incompatible pharmacokinetics (particularly in renal or hepatic failure)
• Loss of dosing flexibility
• Cost (may be more than individual drugs, particularly when one of them is generic)
• Difficulties in identifying the culprit of an adverse or idiosyncratic reaction
• Encouragement of improper or hazardous therapy

*Applies only for combinations that have been thoroughly tested by factorial design analyses.

SHOULD FIXED COMBINATION BE USED AS STEP-ONE THERAPY?

The diuretic–diuretic combinations are commonly used all over the globe as initial therapy for hypertension. The FDA recently also has given its blessing to the combinations of hydrochlorothiazide plus bisoprolol as well as of hydrochlorothiazide and captopril to be used as first-line therapy for the treatment of hypertension, whereas, surprisingly, this was denied for the newer combination of calcium antagonist and ACE inhibitors as well as of angiotensin II receptor inhibitors and hydrochlorothiazide. However, in our opinion, there is no valid reason not to consider fixed combinations such as angiotensin receptor inhibitor/hydrochlorothiazide, calcium antagonist/hydrochlorothiazide, or β-blockers/calcium antagonist as first-line therapy in certain carefully selected patients (Table 33–4). Clearly, fixed combinations will not always provide the optimal amount of both drugs serving to achieve an additive effect on blood pressure and a synergistic effect on other pathophysiologic findings. However, because most of them were extensively tested in a factorial design analysis, the practicing physician can have confidence that fixed combinations will be well tolerated in most patients even when used as initial therapy.

REFERENCES

1. Fenichel RR, Lipisky RJ: Combination products as first-line pharmacotherapy [editorial]. Arch Intern Med 154:1429, 1994.
2. Division of Cardio-Renal Drug Products (Food and Drug Administration) Proposed Guidelines for the Clinical Evaluation of Antihypertensive Drugs. Draft 6/29/1988.
3. Krishna GG, Miller E, Kapoor S: Increased blood pressure during potassium depletion in normotensive men. N Engl J Med 320:1177, 1989.
4. Krishna GG, Kapoor SC: Potassium depletion exacerbates essential hypertension. Ann Intern Med 115:77, 1991.
5. Siani A, Strazzullo P, Giacco A, et al: Increasing the dietary potassium intake reduces the need for antihypertensive medication. Ann Intern Med 115:753, 1991.
6. Khaw K-T, Barrett-Connor E: Dietary potassium and stroke-

associated mortality: A 12-year prospective population study. N Engl J Med 316:235, 1987.

7. Dornhorst A, Powell SH, Pensky J: Aggravation by propranolol of hyperglycaemic effect of hydrochlorothiazide in type II diabetes without alteration of insulin secretion. Lancet I:123, 1985.

8. Zachariah PR, Messerli FH, Mroczek W: Low-dose bisoprolol/hydrochlorothiazide: An option in first-line, antihypertensive treatment. Clin Ther 15:779, 1993.

9. Weinberger MH: Blood pressure and metabolic responses to hydrochlorothiazide, captopril, and the combination in black and white mild-to-moderate hypertensive patients. J Cardiovasc Pharmacol 7(Suppl 1):S52, 1985.

10. Singer DRJ, Markandu ND, Cappuccio FP, MacGregor GA: Moderate sodium restriction added to an angiotensin converting enzyme inhibitor is as effective in lowering blood pressure as adding a thiazide, without the adverse metabolic effects. J Hypertens 9(Suppl 6):S485, 1991.

11. Andrén L, Weiner L, Svensson A, Hansson L: Enalapril with either a "very low" or "low" dose of hydrochlorothiazide is equally effective in essential hypertension. A double-blind trial in 100 hypertensive patients. J Hypertens 1:384, 1983.

12. Weber MA, Byyny RL, Pratt JH, et al: Blood pressure effects of the angiotensin II receptor blocker, losartan. Arch Intern Med 155:405, 1995.

13. Messerli FH, Weber MA, Bruner HR: Angiotensin II receptor inhibition: A new therapeutic principle. Submitted for publication to JAMA.

14. Tsunoda K, Abe K, Hagino T, et al: Hypotensive effect of losartan, a nonpeptide angiotensin II receptor antagonist, in essential hypertension [published erratum appears in Am J Hypertens 6(5 Pt 1):451, 1993]. Am J Hypertens 6:28, 1993.

15. Data on file, Ciba.

16. Jakobsen J, Glaus L, Graf P, et al: Unmasking of the hypotensive effect of nifedipine in normotensives by addition of the angiotensin converting enzyme inhibitor benazepril. J Hypertens 10:1045, 1992.

CHAPTER 34

Cardiovascular Receptors and Drug Therapy

Peter A. van Zwieten, M.D., Ph.D.

In the recent past, pharmacology was restricted mainly to describing the effects and the basis of the systemization of drugs. This approach may be defined as "pharmacography." The aim of pharmacology today is to understand the mode of action of drugs in a physiologic and pathophysiologic sense and to interpret this mode of action on the basis of molecular, biochemical, or pathochemical processes. Insights thus obtained will contribute both to the development of new, more selective, and more effective drugs and to the proper application of these drugs as therapeutic agents.

In 1913, Ehrlich formulated the postulate *corpora non agunt nisi fixata*, which in a dynamic sense is known now as the postulate of the pharmacon-receptor interaction. For decades since then, the receptor has been mainly an operational concept, indispensable for discussing and understanding the mode of action of drugs on a molecular level. Thus, the receptor concept was of great heuristic value. Only recently has the existence of receptors been established experimentally through selective binding studies with radioactively labeled ligands; these studies have resulted in receptor localization, isolation, and identification.[1, 2]

More recently, a great deal of interest has developed in the so-called coupling of receptor signals to cellular events, which transfer the information received by stimulating the receptor with an agonist into the stimulus (nomenclature according to the Ariëns hypothesis) and hence into physiologic or pharmacologic events. A schematic view of this type of coupling process in the case of adrenoreceptors[3] is shown in Figure 34–1. The following experimental methods are available to obtain information on receptors, their function and localization, and their role in drug action:

1. *Classic molecular pharmacology with selective agonists, antagonists, and their interactions, as described by dose-response curves, shifts, and so forth.* This method has been highly rewarding despite its inability to yield any information on receptor location and density. A further limitation is its dependence on the availability of selective agonists and antagonists, which are more or less accidentally discovered. Accordingly, a hypothesis based on the selectivity of a series of agonists and antagonists for certain receptors may require revision or even rejection when new agonists or antagonists with higher selectivities are introduced.

2. *Radioligand-binding studies,[1, 2] in which drugs with high specific radioactivities are bound to specific binding sites or receptors in homogenates of certain tissues.* The method is applicable only *in vitro*. The results obtained yield information on the *affinity* of a certain drug for a particular type of receptor. However, this method does not yield any information on *functional* implications of the binding of drugs to receptors. For this reason, the results obtained in radioligand-binding studies should be considered together with functional studies that establish pharmacologic effects. Finally, radioligand-binding studies allow the calculation of the number of receptors in the tissue studied. This method is, for instance, used to establish the number of α_2-adrenoreceptors in platelets or the number of β_2-adrenoreceptors in lymphocytes.[4, 5]

3. *Investigations on the coupling processes between receptor signals and effects, as discussed earlier.* This field is only in an initial stage of development, but it is very promising. The information obtained implicates both the specificity of receptors and the translation of receptor-triggered signals into physiologic or pharmacologic effects.

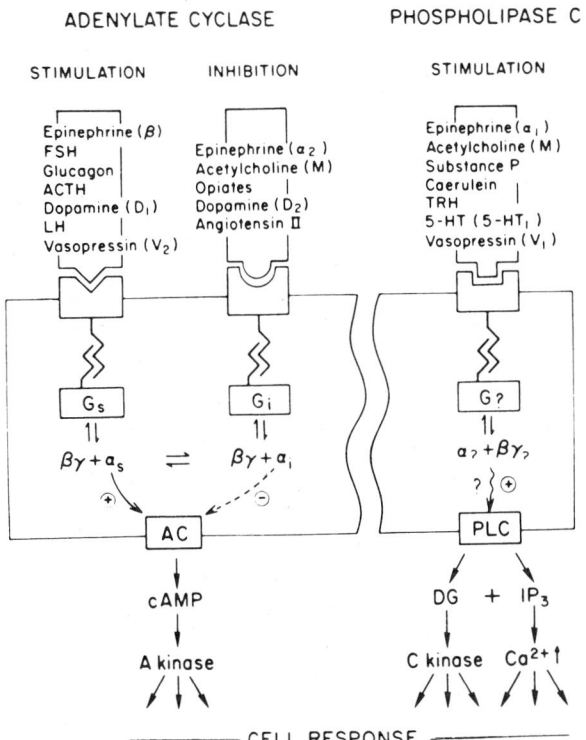

Figure 34–1. Transfer of receptor-triggered signals to physiologic and pharmacologic effects. Interaction of an agonist with a specific receptor at the cell surface induces the dissociation of a coupling protein ($G_?$, G_S, G_i). Subunits of these proteins subsequently regulate intracellular effector enzymes by inducing the formation of intracellular signal molecules: cyclic adenosine monophosphate (cAMP), inositoltriphosphate (IP_3), and diacylglycerol (DG). cAMP and DG activate their respective protein kinases, and IP_3 mobilizes intracellular calcium ions. The final cell response is triggered via the activation of specific target proteins by calcium ions and by phosphorylation of these proteins. ACTH, adrenocorticotropic hormone; 5-HT, 5-hydroxytryptamine; FSH, follicle-stimulating hormone; LH, luteinizing hormone; TRH, thyrotropin releasing hormone.

4. An important enrichment of receptor pharmacology has been the *introduction of cloning techniques as usual in molecular biology,* thus allowing us to determine the amino acid sequence of receptors.

Before discussing the various categories of cardiovascular drugs and their interactions with the corresponding receptors, most relevant receptor types in the cardiovascular system and the associated agonists and antagonists will be outlined. Moreover, some attention will be paid to changes in receptor density induced by pathologic conditions or by the prolonged use of drugs.

CARDIOVASCULAR RECEPTORS: AGONISTS AND ANTAGONISTS

This survey of the various receptor types known to occur in the cardiovascular system is limited to those receptors relevant to modern drug therapy of cardiovascular disease. As such, the α- and β-adrenoreceptors associated with the sympathetic nervous system are emphasized. Furthermore, some attention is paid to dopaminergic, serotonergic, muscarinic, and glyco-

side receptors. The discussion on the receptor types and their characteristics is extended by briefly treating the profile of the most relevant agonists and antagonists interacting with each relevant receptor type.

Peripheral Sympathetic Nervous System and Its Receptors

A schematic overview of the postganglionic sympathetic neuron and the corresponding synapse is shown in Figure 34–2. Although the preganglionic neuron is a vital part of the sympathetic system from the physiologic point of view, discussion of it will be limited because no relevant drugs owe their activity to interaction with peripheral preganglionic sympathetic structures. The sympathetic ganglia are the targets of the ganglionic blockers or ganglioplegic drugs. These structures, as well as the obsolete ganglioplegic agents, are beyond the scope of this chapter. Instead, the postganglionic α- and β-receptors are emphasized.

Presynaptic α$_2$-adrenoreceptors are located at the level of the membranes of the vesicles or varicosities—that is, the storage sites of the endogenous neurotransmitter (see Fig. 34–2). The excitation of the presynaptic α-adrenoreceptors by an agonist—either the endogenous neurotransmitter noradrenaline (or adrenaline) or a synthetic α-sympathomimetic drug—inhibits the release of endogenous noradrenaline from the vesicle. Accordingly, intrasynaptic noradrenaline inhibits its own release. This process is believed to be a negative feedback phenomenon, which may be relevant as a physiologic regulation circuit. However, firm evidence for such a role of the presynaptic adrenoceptors is lacking so far. The concept of presynaptic and postsynaptic receptors, developed mainly by Langer and Starke,[6–9] has been thoroughly investigated for α-adrenoreceptors. It has been recognized that β-adrenergic, cholinergic, dopaminergic, and angiotensin II receptors also occur at both presynaptic and postsynaptic sites.

Postsynaptic α-adrenoreceptors are located in the target organ and are particularly important as targets for neurotransmitters and drugs.

Agonists and Antagonists of α$_1$- and α$_2$-Adrenoreceptors

As with β-receptors (discussed later), it has been necessary to subdivide the α-adrenoreceptors into two subtypes, α$_1$- and α$_2$-adrenoreceptors.[10–15] This subdivision is based on the affinity of each receptor subtype for selective agonists and antagonists. In contrast to earlier views, which have led to considerable confusion, the subdivision into α$_1$ *and* α$_2$ is *not* associated with the differentiation into presynaptic and postsynaptic adrenoreceptors. That is, the terms α$_1$- *and* α$_2$-*adrenoreceptors* refer to receptor demand, whereas the terms *presynaptic* and *postsynaptic* reflect the anatomic location of the receptors.

The selectivity of agonists and antagonists is studied by means of various pharmacologic models, both *in vivo* and *in vitro.* More recently, radioligand-binding

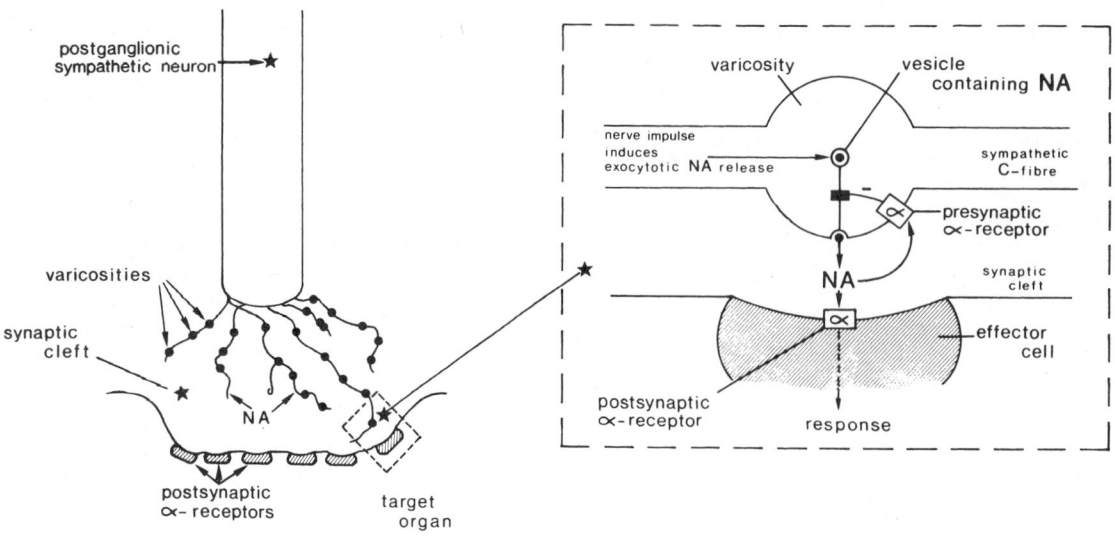

Figure 34–2. Adrenergic synapse. Nerve activity releases the endogenous neurotransmitter noradrenaline (NA) and adrenaline from the varicosities. Noradrenaline and adrenaline reach the postsynaptic α- (or β-) adrenoreceptors on the cell membrane of the target organ by diffusion. Upon receptor stimulation, a physiologic or pharmacologic effect is initiated. Presynaptic α_2-adrenoreceptors on the membrane *(insert)*, when activated by endogenous noradrenaline as well as by exogenous agonists, induce an inhibition of the amount of transmitter noradrenaline released per nerve impulse. Conversely, the stimulation of presynaptic β_2-receptors enhances noradrenaline release from the varicosities. Once noradrenaline has been released, it travels through the synaptic cleft and reaches both α- and β-adrenoreceptors at postsynaptic sites, thus causing physiologic effects such as vasoconstriction or tachycardia.

techniques have become valuable tools in such investigations, as discussed in the introduction to this chapter.

Table 34–1 presents a survey of the most important agonists and antagonists of α_1- and α_2-adrenoreceptors. Obviously, the endogenous neurotransmitters, noradrenaline and adrenaline, are nonselective ago-nists, which stimulate both α_1- and α_2-adrenoreceptors about equally well. Methoxamine, cirazoline, and, to a lesser degree, phenylephrine are prototypes of selective α_1-adrenoreceptor stimulants. The experimental agents B-HT 920, B-HT 933 (azepexole), and UK 14,304 are the best examples of highly selective α_2-adrenoreceptor agonists. With respect to the antagonistic drugs, the classic compound phentolamine is an example of a nonselective α_1- and α_2-blocker. The antihypertensive drug prazosin is a selective antagonist of α_1-adrenoreceptors at postsynaptic sites, as are its successors doxazosin, trimazosin hydrochloride, and terazosin. Selective α_2-adrenoreceptor antagonists are, for instance, the rauwolfia alkaloids rauwolscine and yohimbine (see Table 34–1) and the synthetic agent idazoxan.

Agonists and Antagonists of β_1- and β_2-Adrenoreceptors

β-Adrenoreceptors are also subdivided into presynaptic and postsynaptic subtypes. The excitation of presynaptic (prejunctional) β-adrenoreceptors facilitates the release of endogenous noradrenaline, and their blockade inhibits its mobilization (see Fig. 34–2).

β-Adrenoreceptors are located, for instance, in the heart, the bronchi, and the gut; however, various biochemical processes, such as the liberation of glucose from glycogen, also are known to be mediated by β-receptors. β-Receptors are divided into β_1- and β_2-subtypes.[16-20] The postsynaptic β_1-adrenoreceptors are involved mainly in the regulation of cardiac function. Their stimulation causes an increase in cardiac frequency and contractility. Excitation of β_2-adrenoreceptors by the appropriate agonists induces bron-

Table 34–1. α-Adrenoreceptor Agonists and Antagonists*

Agents	Receptor Stimulated or Blocked
Agonists	
Noradrenaline (neurotransmitter)	$\alpha_1 + \alpha_2 + \beta_1$
Adrenaline (neurotransmitter)	$\alpha_1 + \alpha_2 + \beta_1 + \beta_2$
Methoxamine	α_1
Clonidine (Catapres, Catapresan)	$\alpha_2 > \alpha_1$
Guanfacine	$\alpha_2 > \alpha_1$
Azepexole (B-HT 933)	α_2
B-HT 920	α_2
UK-14,304	α_2
Antagonists	
Phentolamine (Regitine)	$\alpha_1 + \alpha_2$
Tolazoline hydrochloride	$\alpha_2 > \alpha_1$
Prazosin (Minipress)	α_1
Doxazosin mesylate	α_1
Terazosin hydrochloride	α_1
Trimazosin hydrochloride	α_1
Labetalol	$\alpha_1 + \beta_1 + \beta_2$
Corynanthine ⎱ (diastereoisomer)	α_1
Rauwolscine ⎰ (diastereoisomer)	α_2
Yohimbine	α_2
Idazoxan	α_2

*Characterization with respect to their selectivity for α_1- and α_2-adrenoreceptors.

chodilatation, vasodilatation, and hyperglycemia. The classic β-adrenoreceptor agonists such as isoprenaline and orciprenaline are nonselective (i.e., they stimulate β_1- and β_2-adrenoreceptors equally well).

Presynaptic β-adrenoreceptors belong mainly to the β_2 subtype. Selective β_2-adrenoreceptor stimulants such as terbutaline, salbutamol, and fenoterol influence the bronchi without causing excessive tachycardia. Therefore, they are preferred for bronchospasmolysis over the nonselective β_1- and β_2-adrenoreceptor agonists (isoprenaline, orciprenaline), which are known to provoke tachycardia and palpitations. More recently, dobutamine has been introduced as a moderately selective β_1-adrenoreceptor agonist, but it also possesses significant α_1-agonistic potency. The neurotransmitter noradrenaline is selective as a β_1-adrenoreceptor agonist, besides its α_1- and α_2-adrenoreceptor agonistic activity. Adrenaline is nonselective with respect to both α- and β-adrenoreceptors, because it simultaneously stimulates α_1- and α_2- as well as β_1- and β_2-adrenoreceptors.

An overview of selective and nonselective β-adrenoreceptor stimulants is given in Table 34–2.

All therapeutically applied β-adrenoreceptor–blocking agents are known to block β_1-adrenoreceptors substantially. Most therapeutic effects are based on β_1-adrenoreceptor blockade as well. Certain β-blockers, the so-called nonselective β-blockers, are known to block β_2-adrenoreceptors substantially. The experimental compound ICI 118,551 has been introduced as a selective β_2-blocker without β_1 activity. In most instances the β_2-adrenoreceptor blockade is responsible for side effects. Bronchoconstriction and vasoconstriction are known to be induced by β_2-receptor blockade. Only in a few cases—that is, in the treatment of migraine and certain forms of tremor—is β_2-blockade known to be the basis of the therapeutic effect.

Apart from the blocking activity of β-sympatholytic agents, various compounds in this series possess other properties, such as membrane-stabilizing (local anesthetic) potency and intrinsic sympathomimetic activity. These properties shall be dealt with separately below, together with the so-called cardioselectivity of β-adrenoreceptor–blocking agents, which is based on the preferential antagonistic activity of certain β-blockers for β_1-adrenoreceptors. Table 34–2 also contains a survey of the most important β-adrenoreceptors, agonistic and antagonistic drugs, and their ancillary properties.

Function and Distribution of α_1-, α_2-, β_1-, and β_2-Adrenoreceptors at Presynaptic and Postsynaptic Sites

The work by various research groups has made it obvious that presynaptic α-adrenoreceptors are predominantly of the α_2 subtype. At postjunctional sites, however, both α_1- and α_2-adrenoreceptors are found in comparable proportions. Postsynaptic β-adrenoreceptors are predominantly of the β_2 subtype. At postsynaptic sites in blood vessels, β_2-adrenoreceptors are present almost exclusively. The heart contains both β_1- and β_2-adrenoreceptors, but β_1-receptors are more numerous and functionally dominant. The *functional* role of the various vascular receptor subtypes involved may be summarized as follows:

Presynaptic Receptors

Stimulation of presynaptic α_2-adrenoreceptors causes an impaired release of noradrenaline from presynaptic sites; receptor blockade by α_2- or nonselective α_1- and α_2-antagonists evokes an enhanced release of the endogenous neurotransmitter. Stimulation of presynaptic β_2-adrenoreceptors causes an accelerated release of endogenous noradrenaline, whereas the blockade of presynaptic β-adrenoreceptors by an appropriate antagonist inhibits noradrenaline release from the vesicles.

Postsynaptic Receptors

Stimulation of vascular postsynaptic α_1-adrenoreceptors in blood vessels (in particular in the arterioles) causes vasoconstriction, increased peripheral resistance, and a rise in blood pressure. The same principle holds true for the stimulation of postsynaptic α_2-adrenoreceptors. However, it should be realized that both contractile processes are probably different, as re-

Table 34–2. **β-Adrenoreceptor Agonists and Antagonists***

Agents		Receptors Stimulated or Blocked	ISA
Agonists			
Noradrenaline (neurotransmitter)		$\beta_1 + \alpha_1 + \alpha_2$	
Adrenaline (neurotransmitter)		$\beta_1 + \beta_2 + \alpha_1 + \alpha_2$	
Dobutamine (racemate)		$\beta_1 > \beta_2 + \alpha_1$	
Prenalterol		β_1 (partial agonist)	
Xamoterol		β_1 (partial agonist)	
Isoprenaline		$\beta_1 + \beta_2$	
Orciprenaline		$\beta_1 + \beta_2$	
Fenoterol		$\beta_2 \gg \beta_1$	
Pirbuterol		$\beta_2 \gg \beta_1$	
Rimiterol		$\beta_2 \gg \beta_1$	
Ritodrine		$\beta_2 \gg \beta_1$	
Salbutamol		$\beta_2 \gg \beta_1$	
Terbutaline		$\beta_2 \gg \beta_1$	
Antagonists			
Propranolol		$\beta_1 + \beta_2$	−
Alprenolol		$\beta_1 + \beta_2$	±
Pindolol	nonselective	$\beta_1 + \beta_2$	+ + +
Oxprenolol		$\beta_1 + \beta_2$	+ +
Timolol		$\beta_1 + \beta_2$	−
Sotalol		$\beta_1 + \beta_2$	−
Practolol		$\beta_1 \gg \beta_2$	+
Atenolol		$\beta_1 \gg \beta_2$	−
Metoprolol		$\beta_1 \gg \beta_2$	−
Bisoprolol		$\beta_1 \ggg \beta_2$	−
Acebutolol		$\beta_1 \gg \beta_2$	±
ICI 118, 551		$\beta_2 \gg \beta_1$	−

*Characterization with respect to their selectivity for β_1- and β_2-adrenoreceptors and to intrinsic sympathomimetic activity (ISA).

flected by the different dose-response curves, that of the α_1-vasoconstriction being much steeper than that of the α_2-adrenoreceptor–mediated vasoconstriction. Moreover, the α_1-adrenoreceptor–induced vasoconstriction occurs more rapidly than that of the α_2-adrenoreceptor–mediated process. Finally, the α_2-adrenoreceptor–mediated vasoconstriction is highly sensitive to pretreatment with calcium antagonists. This sensitivity is less obvious for the vasoconstriction mediated by α_1-adrenoreceptors. The dependency of α_2-adrenoreceptor–mediated vasoconstriction on the presence of extracellular calcium has led to the hypothesis that the formation of the α_2-adrenoreceptor agonist complex is accompanied by the inward flux of calcium ions, which can be blocked by calcium antagonists.

Evidence[21, 22] suggests that, because of its extrasynaptic position, the postsynaptic α_2-adrenoreceptor is not under direct neuronal control (Fig. 34–3). This situation contrasts with that of the postsynaptic α_1-adrenoreceptor, which is under direct neuronal control because of its position within the synapse. Accordingly, the postsynaptic α_2-adrenoreceptor is considered to be noninnervated. As such, it should be regarded as a hormone receptor that reacts predominantly to the circulating catecholamines noradrenaline and adrenaline.

In the heart, the stimulation of β_1-adrenoreceptors causes tachycardia and a rise in contractile force. However, recent studies suggest that the stimulation of postsynaptic β_2-adrenoreceptors in the heart also causes an inotropic effect, which is the basis of the activity of some newer inotropic agents. In blood vessels, in particular in the resistance vessels, the postsynaptic β-receptor is of virtually only the β_2 subtype. Its stimulation by appropriate agonists, including circulating adrenaline, causes a modest degree of vasodilatation. Conversely, its blockade leads to modest vasoconstriction. Similarly, as for the postsynaptic α_2-adrenoreceptor, the postsynaptic β_2-adrenoreceptor is not under direct neuronal control (non-

innervated) and thus should instead be considered a hormone receptor.[23]

Adrenoreceptors in the Central Nervous System

Both α- and β-adrenoreceptors have been shown to occur in various regions of the central nervous system. The role of central β-adrenoreceptors so far remains unclear and will not be discussed here. Central α-adrenoreceptors in the region of the brain stem are most likely to be involved in the central regulation of blood pressure and heart rate via the peripheral sympathetic system and possibly also the parasympathetic system. Central α-adrenoreceptors of both α_1 and α_2 subtypes are found, particularly in the pontomedullary region. Functionally important nuclei in this region are the nucleus tractus solitarii, the vasomotor center, and the nucleus of the vagus nerve. High densities of adrenergic synapses and associated receptors are found in and around these nuclei and the interconnecting neuronal pathways. Central α_2-adrenoreceptors are particularly relevant in cardiovascular drug therapy because they are the targets of centrally acting antihypertensive drugs such as clonidine, α-methyldopa, and guanfacine[24-26] (see earlier section, "Agonists and Antagonists of α_1- and α_2-Adrenoreceptors"). More recently, it has been proposed that imidazoline receptors in the central nervous system, not α_2-adrenoreceptors, are the target of clonidine (and related drugs). However, the imidazoline receptors are similar to α_2-adrenoreceptors and are also connected to the α_2-receptors. Central α_1-adrenoreceptors are less obvious as drug targets, but they probably play a role in the blunting of baroreceptor reflex activity induced by prazosin and related drugs.[27]

Dopaminergic Receptors in the Cardiovascular System and the Kidney

Dopaminergic receptors, like adrenoreceptors, also occur at both presynaptic and postsynaptic sites. In addition, a subdivision into DA1 and DA2 subtypes, based on the selectivity of agonists and antagonists, is also generally accepted, at least for peripheral dopaminergic receptors. In the central nervous system, not to be discussed in this context, the situation is much more complex. Dopamine receptors have been demonstrated to occur at postsynaptic sites in the coronary, cerebral, hepatic, and femoral vascular beds; on the juxtaglomerular cells in the kidney; on the renal tubuli; and possibly also in the adrenal cortex.[28-30] Presynaptic dopaminergic receptors are found in the sympathetically innervated arterioles and possibly also on other blood vessels. Dopaminergic receptors have been demonstrated by means of histologic studies in sympathetic ganglia. However, it remains unclear whether these receptors are located at presynaptic or postsynaptic sites. Presynaptic dopaminergic receptors differ with respect to their preference for a variety of selective agonists and antago-

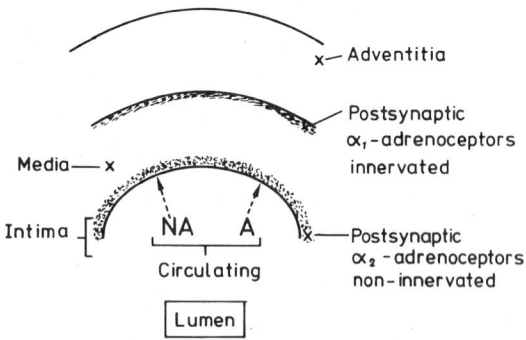

Figure 34–3. Differential positions of postsynaptic (postjunctional) α_1- and α_2-adrenoreceptors in vascular smooth muscle. The α_1-adrenoreceptor is assumed to have an intrasynaptic position and is thus under direct neuronal control. The α_2-adrenoreceptor is "noninnervated," that is, not under direct neuronal control, owing to its extrasynaptic position. It is closer to the vascular lumen and hence is influenced mainly by circulating noradrenaline (NA) and adrenaline (A). As such, it should be considered a hormone receptor, like the noninnervated β_2-adrenoreceptors.

nists. Presynaptic dopaminergic receptors at the sympathetic nerve endings are assumed to be of the DA2 subtype and hence are similar to dopaminergic receptors in several brain regions. The postsynaptic dopaminergic receptors in several vascular beds, particularly those on resistance vessels (precapillary arterioles) and those on the renal tubuli, belong to the DA1 subtype. The dopaminergic receptors at the sympathetic ganglia have not been studied in sufficient detail but are assumed to belong to the DA2 subtype.

Agonists and Antagonists of Dopaminergic Receptors

The number of selective agonists and antagonists to dopaminergic receptors is much smaller than the number of those selective for the various types of adrenoreceptors, as discussed earlier. This fact is not surprising, because the adrenergic nervous system and its receptors have been studied more thoroughly than has the dopaminergic system. However, increasing interest in dopaminergic receptors and associated drugs can be expected to lead to a rapid expansion of the compounds available, thus increasing the probability that more selective agonists and antagonists toward the dopaminergic receptor subtypes are to be anticipated in the near future. Our knowledge of dopaminergic agonists and antagonists is summarized in Table 34–3. Fenoldopam mesylate is the only selective agonist for DA1-receptors, and only two experimental compounds (Sch 23390 and SK&F 83566) are available as DA1-receptor antagonists. Domperidone is the only selective DA2-receptor antagonist used in pharmacologic analysis. Selective DA2-receptor agonists are available in larger numbers, including well-known drugs such as bromocriptine and its successors lergotrile mesylate and pergolide mesylate (ergolines) as well as a variety of N-alkylated dopamine analogues. Table 34–3 also enumerates several nonselective DA1- and DA2-receptor agonists and antagonists, including dopamine. However, besides its agonistic effect on both dopaminergic receptor subtypes (DA1 and DA2), dopamine also stimulates αβ-adrenoreceptors. This complicated receptor profile should be

taken into account when dopamine is administered as a therapeutic agent to patients in cardiogenic shock, as discussed later.[28-30]

Pharmacologic Effects Caused by the Stimulation and Blockade of Dopaminergic Receptors

Stimulation of postsynaptic DA1-receptors in blood vessels by a selective agonist causes peripheral vasodilatation, a reduction of total peripheral resistance, and a fall in blood pressure. Stimulation of postsynaptic DA1-receptors in the kidney induces enhanced natriuresis, probably resulting from an effect on the renal tubuli via DA1-receptors, and improved renal perfusion, as a result of a DA1 effect on the renal vasculature.[28-30] Stimulation of presynaptic DA2-receptors with a selective agonist induces an impaired release of noradrenaline from the sympathetic nerve endings and hence vasodilatation. This effect, however, is rather weak and hardly suitable as a basis for the development of vasodilator and antihypertensive drugs.

Blockade of either DA1- or DA2-receptors by appropriate antagonists does not greatly affect renal function or the cardiovascular system. This observation is in accordance with the extremely low, subthreshold concentration of circulating dopamine, the endogenous agonist. Obviously, the various DA1- and DA2-receptors in the vascular bed and the kidney are hardly stimulated at physiologic conditions.

Serotonin (Serotonergic) Receptors in the Cardiovascular System[31, 32]

5-Hydroxytryptamine (5HT; serotonin) is present mainly in the platelets, in the enterochromaffinic cells of the small intestine, and in the central nervous system. Peripheral 5HT probably does not play a major role in physiologic circulatory regulation processes, but this case may be different in pathologic conditions. 5HT in plasma achieves an extremely low, subthreshold concentration. However, local concentrations of 5HT, especially in the microcirculation, can become rather high following platelet aggregation, when large amounts of 5HT are released. For this reason, it is hypothesized that 5HT may play a relevant role in ischemic changes in the microcirculation (caused by atherosclerosis, diabetes mellitus, and so forth) and thus enhance preexisting vascular damage. The role of 5HT in the generation and maintenance of essential hypertension is subject to speculation only. The interest in 5HT and its receptors has been greatly stimulated by the antihypertensive and vasodilator drug ketanserin, a selective $5HT_2$-receptor antagonist (see later section, "Serotonin Receptor Antagonists"). Similar to the receptor types dealt with in preceding paragraphs, 5HT-receptors are divided into at least three distinct subtypes: $5HT_1$, $5HT_2$, and $5HT_3$. Their functional roles in circulation can be summarized briefly as follows:

Table 34–3. **Dopaminergic Receptor Agonists and Antagonists**

Agent	DA1-Receptor	DA2-Receptor
Agonists	Fenoldopam mesylate	Bromocriptine, pergolide, lergotrile, LV 141865, LV 171555, N-alkylated analogues of dopamine (A6,7 DTN, and A5,6 DTN)
Antagonists	Sch 23390 SK&F 83566	Domperidone
Nonselective agonists (DA1 and DA2)		Dopamine, dipropyldopamine, apomorphine hydrochloride
Nonselective antagonists (DA1 and DA2)		Bulbocapnine, metoclopramide hydrochloride, sulpiride, haloperidol, pimozide

1. 5HT$_1$-receptors are found in blood vessels and on the sympathetic nerve endings; their stimulation with an appropriate agonist (including 5HT) causes vasodilatation and inhibition of noradrenaline release from presynaptic sites, respectively.

2. 5HT$_2$-receptors are found on vascular smooth muscle and on platelets. When stimulated by an agonist, they induce vasoconstriction (in particular in microcirculatory vessels) and enhanced platelet aggregation.

3. 5HT$_3$-receptors occur on cardiac pacemaker cells, sympathetic nerve endings, and vagal afferents. When stimulated, they simultaneously trigger an increase in heart rate (pacemaker) and stimulation of noradrenaline release (sympathetic nerve endings).

An extremely complicated, virtually unpredictable final response will occur with the simultaneous stimulation of all 5HT-receptor subtypes, as effectuated by the nonselective endogenous agonist 5HT itself. Several more or less selective agonists and antagonists for the various 5HT-receptor subtypes have been introduced. Because almost none of them has achieved any clinical relevance in cardiovascular medicine, these experimental compounds will not be discussed here in any detail. The selective 5HT$_2$-receptor antagonist, ketanserin, is discussed in the section on serotonin receptor antagonists.

Cholinergic (Muscarinic) Receptors in the Cardiovascular System[33]

The classic subdivision of cholinergic receptors into the nicotinic (N) and muscarinic (M) subtypes has been maintained through the years. Both subtypes of cholinergic receptors are stimulated by the endogenous agonist and neurotransmitter acetylcholine. However, different antagonists are required to block either nicotinic or muscarinic receptor subtypes, such as tubocurarine and related drugs and ganglioplegic drugs for N-receptors and parasympatholytic drugs (e.g., atropine) for M-receptors. A few years ago, interest in this field was renewed by the demonstration that M-receptors are not homogeneous and should be divided into at least three subtypes (M1, M2, and M3) and possibly four (M4). A limited number of selective antagonists for these M-receptor subtypes is available, but only nonselective agonists are known. Pirenzepine is a selective M1-receptor antagonist that is used in the treatment of peptic ulcer and that may display fewer side effects on the cardiovascular system than the classic nonselective antagonist atropine.

The M-receptors in the heart are assumed to belong to the M2 subtype. The new compound AF-DX116 has been recognized as a cardioselective M2-receptor antagonist with little effect on anything other than cardiac tissues. It might be useful in the treatment of certain conditions of bradycardia. Coronary spasm, as encountered in Prinzmetal's angina and unstable angina, has been demonstrated to be triggered by cholinergic stimulation. Anticholinergic drugs with a high selectivity for the coronary system (yet to be developed) can be of potential therapeutic usefulness.

Glycoside Receptors in the Heart[34, 35]

The Na$^+$/K$^+$-activated magnesium-dependent ATPase in the membrane of cardiac cells has been considered for many years to be the specific binding partner and even the receptor for cardiac glycosides. As such, this ATPase may be regarded as a receptor, triggering the inotropic action of cardiac glycosides; therefore, a brief discussion is in order. The vast body of experimental data and attempts to interpret these may be summarized as follows: Under normal conditions of contraction frequency of the heart, there appears to be an ATPase surplus that does not participate in the maintenance of ionic homeostasis. Furthermore, in cardiac tissues, the amount of active Na$^+$/K$^+$ ATPase has been shown not to be constant but to adapt rapidly to the patient's needs, as triggered by the actual sodium load. In therapeutic doses, cardiac glycosides interact only with a specific conformation of the enzyme, which occurs only during the process of active transport. The binding of cardiac glycosides in therapeutic concentration to the Na$^+$/K$^+$ ATPase is not necessarily followed by relevant changes in ion fluxes, because the inhibition of the Na$^+$/K$^+$ pumps can be compensated for by the surplus of ATP available. However, at high concentrations of the cardiac glycosides, overall transport of Na and K is impaired, as reflected by toxic phenomena. The inotropic effect of the cardiac glycosides is assumed to be induced by improving the release of calcium ions from the lipid portion of the enzyme.

CHANGES IN RECEPTOR DENSITY: UPREGULATION AND DOWNREGULATION

The density of receptors on the cell membrane or elsewhere is not, as presumed earlier, a constant figure but is subject to variation induced by internal and external factors. Accordingly, the receptor density is determined by the rate of receptor deactivation. Exposure to agonists enhances the conversion of receptors from the responsive state (R) into the deactivated state (*R*) and thus brings about downregulation. Prevention of receptor activation (e.g., by reversible blockade through competitive antagonists, by denervation in the case of neurotransmitter receptors [autoreceptors], or by gland extirpation in the case of hormones) reduces the "receptor consumption" and thus tends to increase the density in receptors (R). This process is known as upregulation.[36]

Both downregulation and upregulation are well-known phenomena in physiology and pharmacology. Well-known examples are the increased density in β-receptors induced by prolonged exposure to the β-blocker (upregulation) and the reduction of the α$_2$-adrenoreceptor density on the platelets of patients with pheochromocytoma because of continuous exposure to high concentrations of plasma catecholamines (downregulation). With the introduction of the radioligand-binding technique, this field has been opened for quantitative investigation.[1, 2] Attempts have been made to establish the influence of age, disease, and drug treatment on receptor density. A few relevant examples of this type of investigation are discussed here.

Influence of Age on Receptor Density

The influence of age is potentially relevant in cardiovascular therapy, because most cardiovascular patients are more than 50 years of age. This problem has been studied mainly with respect to the influence of senescence on α- and β-adrenoreceptors. Despite older reports that the number of β-adrenoreceptors would decrease with age, current work indicates that the density of β-adrenoreceptor binding sites in older subjects is similar to that in young subjects.[37] It should be realized that currently available techniques allow only the determination of β_2-receptor density on *ex vivo* lymphocytes, whereas the β_2-adrenoreceptors are more closely related to cardiovascular parameters, functions, and disorders. Despite the similarity in β_2-receptor density in old and young subjects, membranes of lymphocytes from elderly patients appear to show decreases in isoprenaline-stimulated adenylate cyclase activity. This finding suggests uncoupling of the adrenoreceptor–adenylate cyclase system as the process underlying desensitization. This desensitization explains the lower adrenergic responsiveness and diminished cardiac frequency usually observed during old age. No method is available to assess the α_1-receptor density in human material with radioligand-binding techniques. For instance, using [^{3}H]-yohimbine or [^{3}H]-clonidine, it has become possible to determine the density of α_2-adrenoreceptors in *ex vivo* human thrombocytes, but the relevance of such information to hypertensive disease and its treatment is questionable. Old age does not necessarily cause changes in the density of α_2-adrenoreceptors on platelets, and most reports suggest that no change occurs at all.[38]

Influence of Disease on Receptor Density

The question of whether disease states influence receptor density has been studied predominantly in connection with essential hypertension and with congestive heart failure. Hypertensive diseases in an established phase have been reported to be associated with an increased density of α_2-adrenoreceptors on *ex vivo* thrombocytes. However, other reports indicate that in essential hypertension, the α_2-receptor density is unchanged. This issue remains unresolved.[39]

Irrespective of inconclusive changes in α-adrenoreceptor density in hypertension, it has been established that hypertensive patients show an enhanced reactivity to vasoconstrictor stimuli. Some authors claim that this hyperreactivity is limited to α_2-adrenoreceptors. Others,[40, 41] however, have established that an exaggerated vasoconstrictor response is found for both α_1- and α_2-adrenoreceptors, at least in the vascular bed of the forearm of hypertensive patients.

Congestive Heart Failure

Radioligand-binding studies with human and animal tissues in congestive heart failure, studied in tissues from obduction material, from explanted hearts, or obtained by biopsy, have focused mainly on β-adrenoreceptors.[42, 43] As congestive heart failure develops, the density of β-adrenoreceptors gradually is reduced. This finding may be interpreted as a phenomenon of downregulation caused by the usually elevated levels of plasma catecholamines in patients with congestive heart failure. More recently, it was reported that in dilated cardiomyopathy, downregulation occurs for β_1-adrenoreceptors but not for β_2-adrenoreceptors. Accordingly, the ratio of β_2-adrenoreceptors to β_1-adrenoreceptors increases steadily during the development of the disease; thus, it has been suggested that β_2-adrenoreceptor agonists would be preferable over β_1-stimulants as inotropic agents in patients with this type of congestive heart failure. Logically, the β_1-receptor downregulation causes a reduced inotropic response to β_1-adrenoreceptor agonists in patients with heart failure. It seems likely that in other types of heart failure, such as that caused by severe myocardial ischemia, β_2-receptor downregulation also occurs.

Myocardial Ischemia

A limited number of radioligand-binding studies have shown that experimental ischemia in animal models is associated with an increased density of α_1-adrenoreceptors. This finding might explain the increase of the myocardial sensitivity to the arrhythmogenic effect of catecholamines induced by ischemia (e.g., after coronary ligation). This increased sensitivity is counteracted by α-adrenoreceptor antagonists but much less by β-blockers.[44]

Changes in Receptor Density

Changes in receptor density as a result of drug treatment usually are caused by receptor upregulation or downregulation. This important issue is discussed in the forthcoming section.

RECEPTOR PROFILE OF CARDIOVASCULAR THERAPEUTIC AGENTS

This section discusses the availability of selective agonists and antagonists of the various receptor types. In addition, the receptor profiles of the most relevant and well-known cardiovascular therapeutic agents, including a few interesting experimental compounds, are characterized.

α_2-Adrenoreceptor Agonists

Noradrenaline and adrenaline, the endogenous catecholamines, are both nonselective α_1- and α_2-adrenoreceptor agonists, apart from their interaction with β-adrenoreceptors. Their stimulatory effect on both α1- and α2-adrenoreceptors at postsynaptic sites is reflected mainly by vasoconstriction. Their presynaptic effect is probably much less relevant to their overall pharmacodynamic activity. Their stimulatory activity on the heart is mediated by β-adrenoreceptors. As drugs, noradrenaline and adrenaline are hardly of therapeutic importance in cardiovascular disorders. They may be useful as vasoconstrictors, added to local anesthetic agents in anaphylactic shock, and as decongestants in conditions of rhinitis or conjunctivitis. Selective α1-adrenoreceptor agonists such as cirazoline or methoxamine are available but have not found particular therapeutic applicability. α2-Adrenoreceptor agonists like clonidine, guanfacine, and α-methylnoradrenaline (derived from α-methyldopa) are the prototypes of the centrally acting antihypertensive drugs.[10–15] Clonidine and guanfacine are nonselective α2- and α1-agonists.

α-Methylnoradrenaline is predominantly an α2-agonist. These compounds stimulate central α2-adrenoreceptors in the pontomedullary region and thus depress peripheral sympathetic activity. Their effect on peripheral presynaptic or postsynaptic α2-adrenoreceptors is weaker and not of particular importance. Sedation and a dry mouth, the most widely observed side effects of these compounds, are also mediated by α2-adrenoreceptors but in brain regions other than those triggering the fall in blood pressure. Because the same receptor types (α2) are involved, it is difficult to design new molecules with central hypotensive activity but without the aforementioned adverse reactions. Indeed, such a separation has not been achieved so far, despite considerable research effort. Newer molecules such as B-HT 933 (azepexole) are more selective for α2-adrenoreceptors than are clonidine or guanfacine, but it is unlikely that this higher degree of selectivity offers real advantages over clonidine. The peripheral α2-adrenoreceptor agonistic activity of the drugs available seems not to offer any potential therapeutic advantages.

α1-Adrenoreceptor Antagonists

The various sequelae of vasodilatation, leading to built-in adverse reactions, have always been a serious drawback to the therapeutic use of phentolamine and other classic α-adrenoreceptor blockers, and these compounds have not achieved an important position in the treatment of hypertension apart from their use in the preoperative phase of treatment for pheochromocytoma. The situation has improved with the introduction of selective α1-adrenoreceptor blocking agents, of which prazosin is the prototype. Prazosin, a vasodilator drug, causes little reflex tachycardia. This phenomenon may be explained by the fact that prazosin, because of its α1-adrenoreceptors, does not interfere with reflexes mediated via presynaptic α2-adrenoreceptors. However, it remains subject to debate whether the noninvolvement of prejunctional α2-adrenoreceptors in the case of prazosin can fully explain the unusually modest degree of reflex tachy-

cardia that is a common side effect of most other vasodilator drugs. The blockade of central α1-adrenoreceptors also may play a role in the prevention of such reflex tachycardia.

In conclusion, two mechanisms are held responsible for the phenomenon of the vasodilation caused by prazosin, doxazosin, terazosin, trimazosin, and similar α1-adrenoreceptor blockers not accompanied by significant reflex tachycardia: selective α1-receptor blockade in the periphery leaves presynaptic α2-receptor–mediated noradrenaline release unchanged (no enhancement; see Fig. 34–2); and blockade of central α1-adrenoreceptors depresses baroreceptor reflex activity (Fig. 34–4).

The pharmacologic profile of the newer selective α1-adrenoreceptor–blocking agents, such as doxazosin and terazosin, is virtually identical to that of prazosin, but pharmacokinetic differences between the various

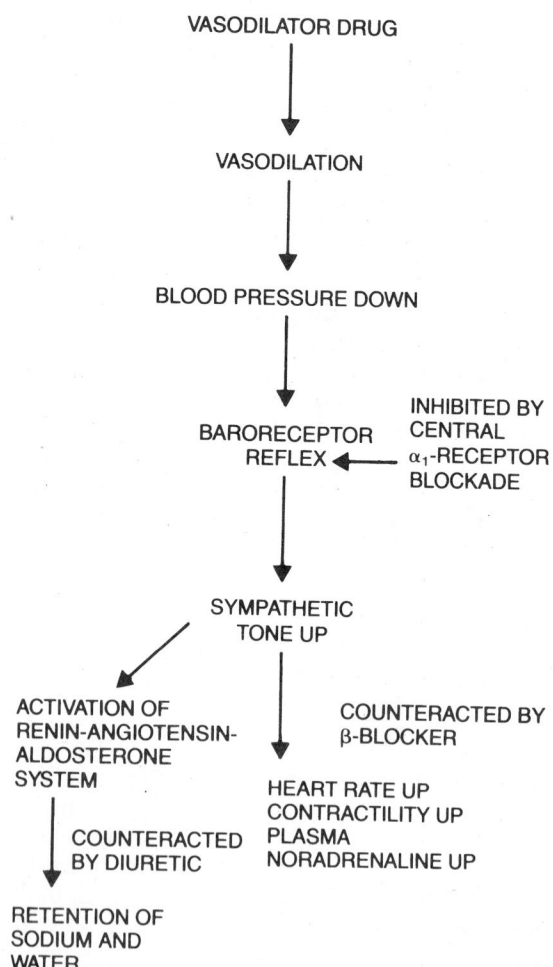

Figure 34–4. Reflex mechanisms triggered by vasodilator drugs. Reflex activation of the sympathetic system is mediated by the baroreceptors. The increased sympathetic activity causes a stimulation of the renin-angiotensin-aldosterone system. This forms the basis for retention of sodium and water. The rise in cardiac activity is counteracted by a β-blocker. Diuretics (natriuretic agents) prevent the retention of sodium and water. The blockade of central α1-adrenoreceptors by selective α1-adrenoreceptor antagonists (provided that they penetrate into the central nervous system) diminishes baroreceptor reflex activation.

α_1-blockers exist. Prazosin and related drugs are usually combined with diuretic agents or β-blockers. Their use as unloading agents in patients with congestive heart failure is still controversial.

More recently, some interest has developed in the use of α_2-adrenoreceptor blocking agents as potential antihypertensive agents. Yohimbine, the classic selective α_2-adrenoreceptor antagonist, cannot be used successfully in antihypertensive treatment because of its central effects (which may even cause a rise in blood pressure) and its interaction with dopaminergic receptors. The recently introduced selective α_2-antagonist 6-chloro-N-methyl 1-2,3,4,5-tetrahydro-1-H-3 benzazepine (SK&F 86466)[44] has been reported to lower blood pressure in various types of hypertensive rats. Its antihypertensive activity proved particularly obvious in hypertensive rats with high plasma noradrenaline levels. The hypotensive effect of SK&F 86466 was accompanied by significant reflex tachycardia that proved, however, to be transient and of shorter duration than that caused by treatment with phentolamine. It is speculated that the short duration of reflex tachycardia during treatment with SK&F 86466 is caused by an unknown mechanism in the central nervous system. The efficacy of this compound, at least in animal models of hypertension, indicates that postjunctional α_2-adrenoreceptors sufficiently contribute to vascular tone and blood pressure, whereas presynaptic mechanisms appear to be less relevant.

Finally, urapidil[45-47] should be mentioned as a newer α_1-adrenoreceptor blocking agent with a chemical structure different from that of prazosin, terazosin, and related drugs. Urapidil is a rather selective antagonist of peripheral postsynaptic α_1-adrenoreceptors. Furthermore, in animal models, the drug displays a relevant central hypotensive effect, which, unlike that of clonidine and related drugs, does not involve the excitation of central α_2-adrenoreceptors. Its central mechanism at the receptor level is explained by the stimulation of $5HT_{1A}$ receptors. Urapidil also possesses some β_1-adrenoreceptor antagonistic activity, but this component is rather weak and probably does not contribute significantly to the drug's antihypertensive potency. Although urapidil is a vasodilator because of its aforementioned pharmacologic characteristics, it does not cause reflex tachycardia, and, during antihypertensive treatment with urapidil, there is a tendency to bradycardia. The absence of reflex tachycardia despite vasodilation is probably explained by the central mechanism, involving $5HT_{1A}$-receptor stimulation.

β-Adrenoreceptor Agonists

Besides being α_1- and α_2-adrenoreceptor agonists, the endogenous neurotransmitters and catecholamines noradrenaline and adrenaline are β-adrenoreceptor stimulants. Noradrenaline activates only β_1-adrenoreceptors, but adrenaline is a nonselective β_1- and β_2-stimulant. This β-adrenoreceptor stimulating activity of noradrenaline and adrenaline has virtually no application in cardiovascular medicine, α-adrenorecep-

tor–mediated vasoconstriction being the unavoidable drawback of the catecholamines. During the past two decades, attempts have been made to introduce synthetic β-adrenoreceptor stimulants as inotropic (cardiotonic) drugs in the treatment of congestive heart failure. Because both β_1- and β_2-adrenoreceptor stimulation cause inotropic actions, agonists with β_1- and β_2- or combined β_1- and β_2-stimulatory activity have been studied. The most relevant of these compounds are listed in Table 34–2. None of the β-adrenoreceptor agonists has gained widespread clinical use in the chronic treatment of congestive heart failure. At best, a few of these compounds can be used in patients with acute heart failure. This limitation of the long-term use of β-adrenoreceptor stimulants in the treatment of heart failure is brought about by the following problems:

1. Under clinical conditions, the inotropic agents all cause a certain degree of tachycardia (but on theoretic grounds, a separation between chronotropic and inotropic activities could be possible).
2. Virtually none of the β-agonists in Table 34–2 can be administered orally; therefore, parenteral application is unavoidable.
3. Chronic administration of these compounds leads to receptor desensitization (downregulation).

A few of the compounds listed in Table 34–2 may be characterized briefly as follows:[16-20] Isoprenaline and orciprenaline are classic nonselective β_1- and β_2-agonists widely applied in bronchial asthma as broncholytics before the development of selective β_2-adrenoreceptor agonists. Because both agents cause significant tachycardia and a consequent sharp rise in oxygen consumption, they are no longer used in the treatment of congestive heart failure unless severe bradycardia occurs. Orciprenaline is longer-acting than isoprenaline. Both compounds are applied only parenterally.

Dobutamine

The inotropic agent dobutamine is reported to stimulate β_1-adrenoreceptors, to a lesser degree β_2-adrenoreceptors, and also α_1-adrenoreceptors. The (−)-isomer has greater selectivity for inotropy than has the (+)-isomer of isoprenaline. The (−)-isomer is the stronger α_1-adrenoreceptor agonist and the weaker $\beta_1 > \beta_2$-adrenoreceptor stimulant. Therefore, it is likely that α_1-adrenoreceptor stimulation is involved in the inotropic action of dobutamine apart from its β-stimulant activity. At low doses, dobutamine causes a stronger inotropic than chronotropic response, but tachycardia is observed at higher doses. Dobutamine has a short half-life and duration of action, requiring prolonged intravenous infusion as the only useful route of administration. Continuous application for more than 72 hours may lead to tolerance as a result of downregulation of β-adrenoreceptors.

The possibility of administering dobutamine by means of intermittent infusions is being studied with the aim of obtaining sufficient cardiac stimulation while avoiding β-adrenoreceptor downregulation.

Prenalterol

Prenalterol is a selective partial β$_1$-adrenoreceptor agonist with a high degree of intrinsic sympathomimetic activity. Although acute effects of prenalterol may be useful to improve cardiac performance, long-term treatment has proved disappointing, probably as a result of β-receptor downregulation. Partial agonists are more likely than full agonists to induce receptor desensitization.

Salbutamol and Terbutaline

Salbutamol and terbutaline are also β$_2$-agonistic drugs that might be expected to cause hemodynamic effects similar to those of pirbuterol. Although these agents are well-known bronchospasmolytics, scarce clinical data are available regarding their potential usefulness in the treatment of congestive heart failure. Their use may be limited by the development of tolerance as observed clinically in limited numbers of patients.

For this reason, one might also consider the use of α$_1$-adrenoreceptor stimulants in the treatment of congestive heart failure. Indeed, the inotropic activity of α$_1$-adrenoreceptor agonists seems to be maintained after desensitization of cardiac β-adrenoreceptors. However, it has not been established whether cardiac α-adrenoreceptors are downregulated after prolonged treatment with α-agonists or during congestive heart failure.

β-Adrenoreceptor Antagonists (β-Blockers) and Their Ancillary Properties[16–20, 48, 49]

Selectivity for β$_1$- or β$_2$-Adrenoreceptor Subtypes

The blockade of β$_1$-adrenoreceptors causes mainly cardiac effects, such as a decrease in cardiac frequency and contractile force as well as an impairment of atrioventricular conduction. Plasma renin is reduced as a result of β$_1$-adrenoreceptor–triggered reduction in renin release from the juxtaglomerular cells. Because all therapeutic cardiovascular effects of β-blockers are mediated by β$_1$-adrenoreceptor blockade (whereas in most cases, the blockade of β$_2$-adrenoreceptors causes unpleasant and sometimes dangerous side effects), a great effort has been invested in the development of β-adrenoreceptor–blocking drugs with a preferential affinity toward β$_1$-adrenoreceptors. Some compounds with such a preferential affinity have been developed, but the selectivity of this type of drug has remained limited. Even when the expression *β$_1$-adrenoreceptor selectivity* might be acceptable, the term *cardioselectivity* is certainly not justified for the compounds available at present.

Despite a preferential affinity for β$_1$-adrenoreceptors, the β-sympatholytic compounds classified as cardioselective still display enough affinity for β$_2$-adrenoreceptors that they are not safe in patients suffering from obstructive airway disease. Moreover, the bronchi have been demonstrated also to contain a limited density of β$_1$-adrenoreceptors. It should be recognized, however, that the severity of the impairment of ventilation is certainly less than that observed for nonselective β$_1$- and β$_2$-adrenoreceptor–blocking agents. Well-known examples of selective β$_1$-adrenoreceptor–blocking agents (at least in low doses) are atenolol, bisoprolol, metoprolol, practolol (no longer applied), and, to a lesser degree, acebutolol (see Table 34–2).

The experimental compound ICI 118,551, a selective β$_2$-adrenoreceptor–blocking agent that is being investigated as a potential therapeutic agent in certain conditions of tremor and in migraine, was mentioned earlier.

Intrinsic Sympathomimetic Activity

β-Adrenoreceptor–blocking agents cause the formation of a drug-receptor complex with β-adrenoreceptors; accordingly, all β-blockers are bound to possess affinity toward the β-receptors. Certain drugs (e.g., pindolol, oxprenolol, and alprenolol) not only display affinity toward the receptor but also are mildly agonistic. Accordingly, the receptor is blocked and inaccessible to endogenous catecholamines (noradrenaline, adrenaline), whereas the β-blocker itself mildly stimulates the β-adrenoreceptor. This phenomenon is characterized as partial agonism. β-Blockers with intrinsic sympathomimetic activity cause less bradycardia than do those devoid of this property. They have been claimed to cause less cardiac depression than β-blockers without intrinsic sympathomimetic activity, but this condition appears to hold true only under conditions of rest.

During exercise, any potential advantage of intrinsic sympathomimetic activity can be overcome by the excess noradrenaline liberated from the sympathetic nerve endings. β-Blockers with intrinsic sympathomimetic activity have been demonstrated to cause a mild degree of vasodilatation, in contrast to the nonintrinsic sympathomimetic activity blockers, which tend to induce vasoconstriction, in particular at the beginning of a treatment period. This unusual hemodynamic profile of the β-blockers with intrinsic sympathomimetic activity might be advantageous in the treatment of essential hypertension, which, in an established stage, is always associated with elevated total peripheral resistance. However, genuine clinical advantages of β-blockers with intrinsic sympathomimetic activity remain to be demonstrated.

Membrane Stabilization

Membrane stabilization, or local anesthetic activity, is an unspecific property of several β-blockers such as propranolol. This pharmacologic effect is not mediated by receptors and plays no relevant role in the usual clinical doses.

Dopaminergic Agonists

Dopamine

Dopamine, the endogenous agonist of dopaminergic DA1- and DA2-receptors, simultaneously stimulates both $\beta\alpha$-adrenoreceptors[28-30] (see earlier section, "Agonists and Antagonists of Dopaminergic Receptors"). Always given in an intravenous infusion, dopamine increases cardiac output predominantly by increasing contractile force rather than heart rate, but tachycardia also occurs at higher doses. Systemic and pulmonary vascular resistance are reduced. On theoretic grounds, renal perfusion should be expected to increase; however, in patients with chronic congestive heart failure, this is not always the case. Natriuresis is increased, possibly as a result of improved renal perfusion and a direct effect on the renal tubuli mediated by DA1-receptors. At higher doses, α_1-receptor stimulation induces vasoconstriction.

L-Dopa

L-Dopa, given by mouth, has been reported to increase cardiac performance in patients with congestive heart failure. The effect obtained is in fact caused by dopamine, formed with *in vivo* decarboxylation of the amino acid L-dopa. A potential advantage of this treatment is offered by the oral applicability of L-dopa. However, L-dopa may exhibit considerable adverse reactions, as is well known from its application in Parkinson's disease.

Ibopamine

Ibopamine is an orally active analogue of dopamine that, after absorption, is hydrolyzed to yield the active metabolite epinine (*N*-methyldopamine). Accordingly, ibopamine should be considered a prodrug. The pharmacologic and therapeutic characteristics of ibopamine are virtually the same as those of dopamine. The oral applicability of ibopamine is potentially favorable. Only short-term studies on the effect of ibopamine in congestive heart failure are available.

Dopexamine

Dopexamine, a compound derived from and pharmacologically similar to dopamine, is assumed to stimulate DA1- and DA2-receptors and β_2-adrenoreceptors. Adrenoreceptors of the β_1- and α-types are not involved. The drug can be administered only intravenously. Dopexamine causes a mild inotropic effect, reduced peripheral vascular resistance, and increased natriuresis. Heart rate is hardly influenced. As such, dopexamine is a potentially interesting drug for the treatment of acute congestive heart failure. No data are available on its usefulness when used in long-term therapy.

Fenoldopam

Fenoldopam is a selective agonist to peripheral DA1-receptors. The compound is being investigated as a potential antihypertensive agent that causes vasodilatation, improves renal perfusion, and enhances natriuresis. These various effects are mediated by the stimulation of DA1-receptors at postsynaptic sites.

Dipropyldopamine and Propylbutyldopamine

The experimental DA2-receptor agonists dipropyldopamine and propylbutyldopamine lower blood pressure in various animal models of hypertension. The antihypertensive effect is induced by the stimulation of vascular presynaptic DA2-receptors, causing a reduced release of endogenous noradrenaline from the sympathetic nerve endings.

Serotonin Receptor Antagonists

Ketanserin is a potent and highly selective blocker of serotonergic receptors of the 5HT$_2$-type. In addition, the compound is a selective α_1-adrenoreceptor–blocking agent, but this activity is much weaker than its affinity for 5HT$_2$-receptors. The well-documented antihypertensive activity of ketanserin probably is caused neither by peripheral 5HT$_2$- nor by α_1-adrenoreceptor blockade alone. A mutual enhancement of both activities is conceivable, but it is not supported by experimental evidence. More recently, a central hypotensive mechanism of ketanserin has been supported. The fall in blood pressure caused by ketanserin is caused by a reduction of total peripheral resistance. Reflex tachycardia does not occur. Ketanserin has been claimed to be particularly effective in the treatment of elderly hypertensive patients. On theoretic grounds, it is assumed to be particularly useful in hypertensive patients with systemic vascular disease due to atherosclerosis, diabetes mellitus, or old age. This issue, however, remains to be proved clinically. At present, ketanserin also is being investigated as a potentially therapeutic agent in peripheral vascular disease.

Anticholinergic Drugs

Atropine is a nonselective antagonist toward M1-, M2- and M3-cholinergic receptors. Its modest usefulness in the temporary treatment of certain forms of bradycardia has been known for many decades. More recently, attempts have been made to develop more selective antagonists toward the M-receptor subtypes (see earlier section, "Cholinergic [Muscarinic] Receptors in the Cardiovascular System"). AF-DX 116 is the first example of a cardioselective M2-receptor antagonist that might be of use in the treatment of bradyarrhythmia. No clinical data are available.

Cardiac Glycosides

Digoxin, digitoxin, ouabain, and other cardiac glycosides are classic drugs known to interfere with glycoside receptors. The clinical differences between these compounds are mainly the results of differential biotransformation and kinetic properties, but they are not explained by different types of interaction with the glycoside receptors. The cardiac glycosides (digitalis) are so well-known that no discussion is warranted here.

CONCLUSION

Receptor pharmacology is advancing rapidly, having contributed significantly to the rational design of and a better insight into the mode of action of cardiovascular drugs. The concept of receptors interacting with agonists or antagonists has facilitated a systematic classification of the drugs that stimulate or antagonize αβ-adrenoreceptors and their various subtypes. The variety of drugs involved and their action can be differentiated and classified only because of the receptor concept. A similar development is emerging for the drugs interacting with dopaminergic receptors and their subtypes, and potentially interesting therapeutic agents in this field are anticipated. Although the role serotonergic receptors and serotonin play in cardiovascular disease is drawing considerable attention, the $5HT_2$-receptor blocker ketanserin is the only cardiovascular therapeutic agent that interacts with 5HT-receptors.

The subdivision of M-cholinergic receptors into various subtypes is a recent development of some interest to cardiovascular drug designers, but no clinical data are available. Finally, although it is agreed that cardiac glycosides also act primarily by triggering glycoside receptors, many details of their mode of action at a cellular level remain to be elucidated. Information on changes in receptor density associated with age, disease, or the use of drugs has been available for only a few years as a result of the radioligand-binding technique. These investigations should be pursued actively because of their potential relevance. This recommendation holds true even more for investigations on the coupling process between receptor stimulation and drug effects, which can be studied.

REFERENCES

1. Ariëns EJ: Receptors: Perspectives in pathology and clinical medicine. J Recept Res 4:1, 1984.
2. Laduron PM: Criteria for receptor sites in binding studies. Biochem Pharmacol 33:833, 1984.
3. Lefkowitz RJ, Caron MG, Stiles GL: Mechanisms of membrane-receptor regulation. N Engl J Med 310:1570, 1984.
4. Brodde OE: Dichte und Affinität von α-adrenozeptoren bei Normotonikern und Hypertonikern. In Hayduk K, Bock KD (eds): Zentrale Blutdruckregulation durch α2-Rezeptorenstimulation. Darmstadt: Steinkopf Verlag, 1983, pp 41–56.
5. Brodde OE, Daul A, O'Hara N, et al: Increased density and responsiveness of α2- and β2-adrenoceptors in circulating blood cells of essential hypertensive patients. Hypertension 2(Suppl 3):111, 1984.
6. Langer SZ: Presynaptic regulation of the release of catecholamines. Pharmacol Rev 32:337, 1984.
7. Starke K: α-Adrenoceptor subclassification. Rev Physiol Biochem Pharmacol 88:199, 1981.
8. Langer SZ: Presynaptic receptors and their role in the regulation of transmitter release. Br J Pharmacol 60:481, 1977.
9. Starke K, Langer SZ: Presynaptic receptors. In Raspe G, et al (eds): Advances in the Biosciences. Oxford: Pergamon Press, 1981, pp 1–3.
10. Van Zwieten PA, Timmermans PBMWM: Central and peripheral α-adrenoceptors: Pharmacological aspects and clinical potential. Adv Drug Res 13:209, 1984.
11. Van Zwieten PA, Timmermans PBMWM, Van Brummelen P: Role of α-adrenoceptors in hypertension and in antihypertensive treatment. Am J Med 77:17, 1984.
12. Van Zwieten PA, Timmermans PBMWM: Cardiovascular α2-adrenoceptors. J Mol Cell Cardiol 15:717, 1983.
13. Van Zwieten PA, Van Meel JCA, Timmermans PBMWM: Calcium antagonists and α-adrenoceptor-mediated vasoconstriction. J Cardiovasc Pharmacol 4:S273, 1982.
14. Broadley KJ: Cardiac adrenoceptors. J Auton Pharmacol 2:119, 1982.
15. Van Zwieten PA, Schonbaum E: Receptors in the Cardiovascular System (Progress in Pharmacology Ser. Vol. 6). New York: VCH, 1986, pp 1–193.
16. Lands AM, Arnold A, McAuliff JP, et al: Differentiation of receptor systems activated by sympathomimetic amines. Nature 214:597, 1967.
17. Nahorski SR: Identification and significance of α-adrenoceptor subtypes. Trends Pharmacol Sci 3:95, 1981.
18. Frishman W: Clinical pharmacology of the new β-adrenoceptor blocking drugs. Part I: Pharmacodynamic and pharmacokinetic properties. Am Heart J 97:663, 1979.
19. Kenakin TP: An in vitro quantitative analysis of the α-adrenoceptor partial agonist activity of dobutamine and its relevance to inotropic selectivity. J Pharmacol Exp Ther 216:210, 1981.
20. Brodde OE, Leifert FJ, Krehl HJ: Coexistence of β1- and β2-adrenoceptors in the rabbit heart: Quantitative analysis of the regional distribution by (−)-3H-dihydroalprenolol binding. J Cardiovasc Pharmacol 4:34, 1980.
21. Langer SZ, Massingham R, Shepperson NB: Presence of postsynaptic α-2-adrenoceptors of predominantly extrasynaptic location in the vascular smooth muscle of the dog hind limb. Clin Sci 59(Suppl 6):225S, 1980.
22. Wilffert B, Timmermans PBMWM, Van Zwieten PA: Extrasynaptic location of α-2 and non-innervated β-2-adrenoceptors in the vascular system of the pithed normotensive rat. J Pharmacol Exp Ther 221:762, 1984.
23. Hawthorn MH, Broadley K: Evidence from use of neuronal update inhibition, that β1-adrenoceptors, but not β2-adrenoceptors, are innervated. J Pharm Pharmacol 34:664–666, 1982.
24. Schmitt H: Action des α-sympathomiméthiques sur les structures nerveuses. Actual Pharmacologie (Paris) 24:93, 1971.
25. Kobinger W: Central α-adrenergic systems as targets for hypotensive drugs. Rev Physiol Biochem Pharmacol 81:40, 1978.
26. Van Zwieten PA, Thoolen MJMC, Timmermans PBMWM: The hypotensive activity and side-effects of methyldopa, clonidine and guanfacine. Hypertension 6(Suppl 2):II-28, 1984.
27. Huchet AM, Velly J, Schmitt H: Role of α1- and α2-adrenoceptors in the modulation of the baroreflex vagal bradycardia. Eur J Pharmacol 71:455, 1981.
28. Goldberg LI: Dopamine receptors: Applications in clinical cardiology. Circulation 72:245, 1985.
29. Goldberg, LI, Kohli JD: Peripheral dopamine receptors: A classification based on potency series and specific antagonism. Trends Pharmacol Sci 4:64, 1983.
30. Struyker Boudier HAJ: Dopamine receptors in the cardiovascular system and in the kidney. Progr Pharmacol 6:81, 1986.
31. Saxena PR, Richardson BP, Mylecharane FJ, et al: Functional receptors for 5-hydroxytryptamine. Trends Pharmacol Sci 7:3, 1986.
32. Göthert M: Serotonin receptors in the circulatory tract. Prog Pharmacol 6:155, 1986.
33. Eglen RM, Whiting RL: Muscarinic receptor subtypes: A critique of the current classification and a proposal for a working nomenclature. J Auton Pharmacol 5:323, 1986.
34. Peters TH: Glycoside receptors in the heart. Progr Pharmacol 6:65, 1986.
35. Schwartz A: Is the cell membrane Na^+/K^+-ATPase enzyme system the pharmacological receptor for digitalis? Circ Res 39:2, 1976.

36. Hollenberg MD: Biochemical mechanisms of receptor regulation. Trends Pharmacol Sci 6:299, 1985.
37. Doyle V, O'Malley K, Kelly JG: Human lymphocyte β-adrenoceptor density in relation to age and hypertension. J Cardiovasc Pharmacol 4:738, 1982.
38. Docherty JR: Aging and the cardiovascular system. J Auton Pharmacol 6:77, 1984.
39. Motulsky HJ, O'Connor DT, Insch PA: Platelet α2-adrenergic receptors in treated and untreated essential hypertension. Clin Sci 64:265, 1983.
40. Amann FW, Bolli P, Kiowski W, et al: Enhanced α-adrenoceptor-mediated vasoconstriction in essential hypertension. Hypertension 3(Suppl 1):119, 1981.
41. Jie K, Van Brummelen P, Timmermans PBMWM, et al: Identification of vascular postsynaptic α1 and α2-adrenoceptors in man. Circ Res 54:447, 1984.
42. Bristow MR: Myocardial β-adrenergic receptor down-regulation in heart failure. Int J Cardiol 5:648, 1984.
43. Bristow MR, Ginsberg R, Minobe W, et al: Decreased catecholamine sensitivity and β-adrenergic-receptor density in failing human hearts. N Engl J Med 307:205, 1982.
44. Roester JM, McCafferty JP, DeMartinis RM, et al: Characterization of the antihypertensive activity of SK&F 86466, a selective α2-antagonist in the rat. J Pharmacol Exp Ther 236:1, 1986.
45. Schoetensack W, Bruckachen EG, Zeck K: Urapidil. In Scriabine A (ed): New Drugs Annual; Cardiovascular Drugs. New York: Raven Press, 1983, pp 19–48.
46. Van Zwieten PA, De Jonge A, Wilffert B, et al: Cardiovascular effects and interaction with adrenoceptors of urapidil. Arch Int Pharmacodyn Ther 276:180, 1985.
47. Van Zwieten PA: Pharmacological and haemodynamic profile of urapidil. In Amery A (ed): Treatment of Hypertension with Urapidil. London: Royal Society Medicine Services, 1986, pp 1–186.
48. Frishman WH: β-Adrenoceptor antagonists: New drugs and indications. N Engl J Med 305:500, 1981.
49. Fitzgerald JD: β-Adrenoceptor antagonists. In Van Zwieten PA (ed): Pharmacology of Antihypertensive Drugs. Handbook of Hypertension, Vol. 3. Amsterdam: Elsevier, 1984, pp 249–306.

CHAPTER 35

Cardiovascular Drug Interactions

Lionel H. Opie, M.D., D.Phil., F.R.C.P.

Each of the major categories of cardiovascular drugs suffers from the complexities of numerous drug interactions, which are becoming more frequent and better defined in mechanism as clinical pharmacologic studies progress. Some of the chief interactions of the various classes of cardiovascular drugs are summarized in Tables 35–1 through 35–6.[1-8]

This chapter analyzes cardiovascular drug interactions first by the major organ sites of such interactions: (1) the cardiovascular system, (2) the liver, (3) the kidney, (4) the gut, (5) the plasma proteins, and (6) the cholinergic messenger system. Second, major interactions of each drug class are highlighted.

THE HEART AS A SITE FOR DRUG INTERACTION
Sinoatrial and Atrioventricular Nodes

The pacemaker functions of the sinoatrial (SA) and atrioventricular (AV) nodes are controlled by at least three currents, two of which are susceptible to β-blockers. These currents are the slow inward calcium current and the underlying spontaneous phase 4 depolarization. Theoretically, the combination of β-blockade with calcium antagonism could arrest the heart; this event does not occur readily, either because full blocking doses of these drugs are seldom given or because calcium antagonists block the long-lasting L channels rather than the shorter transient T channels. The latter type of channel is thought to be chiefly involved in the control of the initial phase of SA depolarization. However, cardiac arrest may occur when an intravenous bolus of verapamil or diltiazem is given to patients already receiving a β-blocker,

especially when there is preexisting SA node disease. Other drugs interacting with the SA or AV node include central antiadrenergic agents (methyldopa, reserpine, clonidine), amiodarone, and the vagal stimulant, digoxin. In digitalis poisoning, intravenous verapamil must never be given for fear of precipitating complete AV block (additive effects of verapamil and digoxin on the AV node).

Intraventricular Conduction System

A number of antiarrhythmics inhibit intraventricular (His-Purkinje) conduction, including quinidine (class IA) and all class IC antiarrhythmics (e.g., flecainide, encainide, propafenone, and lorcainide). Cotherapy with these agents, sometimes required for severe ventricular arrhythmias, may precipitate serious additive intraventricular conduction defects so that the QRS width of the electrocardiogram must be monitored.

Myocardial Contraction

Numerous negative inotropic cardiovascular agents exist, the best known of which are the β-blockers. The calcium antagonists are also potentially negative inotropic; this effect usually is offset by peripheral vasodilation, especially in the case of nifedipine and other dihydropyridines. In practice, verapamil has the most negative inotropic effect of the calcium antagonists, closely followed by diltiazem and then the dihydropyridines. Of the antiarrhythmics, disopyramide and flecainide are powerful negative inotropes. Any combinations of these drugs (β-blockers with calcium antagonists, disopyramide, or flecainide) must be instituted with care and require monitoring of left ven-

Table 35–1. Drug Interactions of β-Adrenergic Blocking Agents

Cardiac Drug	Interacting Drugs	Mechanism	Consequences	Prophylaxis
Hemodynamic Interactions				
All β-blockers	Calcium antagonists (esp. nifedipine)	Added hypotension	Risk of myocardial ischemia	BP control, adjust doses
	Verapamil or diltiazem	Added negative inotropic effect	Risk of myocardial failure	Check for CHF, adjust doses
	Flecainide	Added negative inotropic effect	Hypotension	Check LV function, flecainide levels
Electrophysiologic Interactions				
All β-blockers	Verapamil	Added inhibition of SA and AV nodes	Bradycardia, asystole, complete heart block	Exclude sick sinus syndrome, AV nodal disease; adjust dose
	Diltiazem	Added negative inotropic effect	Excess hypotension	Exclude predrug LV failure
Hepatic Interactions				
Propranolol	Cimetidine	Cimetidine decreases propranolol metabolism	Excess propranolol effects	Reduce both drug doses
	Lidocaine	Low hepatic blood flow	Excess lidocaine effects	Reduce lidocaine dose
Metoprolol	Verapamil	Verapamil decreases metoprolol metabolism	Excess metoprolol effects	Reduce metoprolol dose
	Cimetidine	Cimetidine decreases metoprolol metabolism	Excess metoprolol effects	Reduce both drug doses
Labetalol	Cimetidine	Cimetidine decreases labetalol metabolism	Excess labetalol effects	Reduce both drug doses
Antihypertensive Interactions				
β-Blockers	Indomethacin NSAIDs	Indomethacin inhibits vasodilatory prostaglandins	Decreased antihypertensive effect	Omit indomethacin; use alternative drugs
Immune Interactions				
Acebutolol	Other drugs altering immune status; procainamide, hydralazine, captopril	Theoretical risk of additive immune effects	Theoretical risk of lupus erythematosus or neutropenia	Check antinuclear factors and neutrophils; low doses during cotherapy

AV, atrioventricular; BP, blood pressure; CHF, congestive heart failure; LV, left ventricular; NSAIDs, nonsteroidal antiinflammatory drugs; SA, sinoatrial.
Modified from Opie LH: Adverse cardiovascular drug interactions. *In* Hurst JW (ed): The Heart, 8th ed. New York: McGraw-Hill, 1994, with permission of The McGraw-Hill Companies.

Table 35–2. Clinical Significance of Reported Drug Interactions with Calcium Antagonists

Drug	Verapamil	Nifedipine	Diltiazem
Cardiac glycosides			
Digoxin	3 (+)	0/1 (+)	1 (+)
Digoxin	2 (+)	0	0
β-Adrenergic blockers	2 (+)	1 (+)	2 (+)
α-Adrenergic blockers	2 (+)	3 (+)	N A
Antiarrhythmic drugs			
Quinidine	2 (+)	1 (−)	1 (+)
Disopyramide	3 (+)	0	1 (+)
Nitrates	0/1 (+)	1 (+)	0/1 (+)
H₂-receptor antagonists			
Cimetidine	3 (+)	3 (+)	3 (+)
Ranitidine	0	0	0
Anticonvulsants			
Phenobarbital	3 (−)	0	N A
Phenytoin	N A	2 (+)	N A
Carbamazepine	3 (+)	N A	N A
Lithium carbonate	N A	N A	2 (+)
General anesthetics			
Halothane	3 (+)	3 (+)	N A
Isoflurane	3 (+)	N A	N A
Cytostatic agents	3 (−)	N A	N A
Theophylline	1 (+)	N A	2 (+)
Enzyme inducers			
Rifampin	3 (−)	N A	N A
Sulfinpyrazone	3 (−)	N A	N A
Social drugs			
Cigarettes	3 (−)	3 (−)	3 (−)
Ethanol	N A	1 (+)	N A

NA, no data available on specific interaction; 0, no contraindication; 1, reported interaction—questionable clinical significance; 2, significant interaction—only seen in a limited number of cases; 3, significant interaction—commonly observed; +, enhanced effect of either drug; −, decreased effect of either drug.
Modified with permission from Piepho RW, Culbertson VL, Rhodes RS: Drug interactions with the calcium-entry blockers. Circulation 75(Suppl V):V-181, 1987. Copyright 1987, American Heart Association.

Table 35–3. **Interactions of Antiarrhythmic Drugs**

Drug	Interactive Drug	Result
Class IA		
Quinidine	Digoxin	Increased digoxin level
	β-Blockers, verapamil, diltiazem	Enhanced hypotension, nodal inhibition
	Amiodarone, sotalol, disopyramide	Increased risk of torsade de pointes
	Diuretics	If hypokalemia, risk of torsade de pointes
	Verapamil	Increased quinidine level, risk of hypotension
	Nifedipine	Decreased quinidine level
	Warfarin	Enhanced anticoagulation
Procainamide	Cimetidine	Prolonged procainamide half-life (avoid possible immune effects)
	Captopril	Negative inotropism, depressed conduction
Disopyramide	Other type I antiarrhythmics	Increased hepatic disopyramide metabolism
	Phenytoin	Hypotension, negative inotropic effect
	β-Blockers, verapamil	Exaggerated anticholinergic effect
	Anticholinergics	Decreased anticholinergic effect
	Pyridostigmine	
Class IB		
Lidocaine	β-Blockers	Reduced hepatic clearance of lidocaine; toxicity
	Cimetidine	As above
	Verapamil	Combined negative inotropism
Tocainide	—	Few or no interactions
Mexiletine	Phenytoin	Increased hepatic metabolism of mexiletine
Class IC		
Flecainide	Amiodarone	Blood flecainide levels rise
	Agents inhibiting SA or AV nodes (β-blockers, verapamil, diltiazem, digoxin, amiodarone)	SA and AV nodal depression
	Agents with negative inotropic effects (β-blockers, quinidine, disopyramide)	Depressed myocardium
	Agents with depressed HV conduction (quinidine, procainamide, amiodarone)	Conduction delay
	Digoxin	Modestly increased digoxin level
Propafenone	Digoxin	Digoxin level increased
Class III		
Sotalol	Diuretics, class Ia agents, amiodarone, tricyclics, phenothiazines	Risk of torsade de pointes
Amiodarone	As for sotalol	Risk of torsade de pointes
Class IV		
Verapamil	β-Blockers, excess digoxin, myocardial depressants, quinidine	See Table 35–2

AV, atrioventricular, SA, sinoatrial.
Modified from Marcus FI, Opie LH: Antiarrhythmic agents. *In* Opie LH (ed): Drugs for the Heart, 4th ed. Philadelphia: WB Saunders, 1995, p 217.

tricular function clinically and, if necessary, by echocardiography.

QT Interval and Torsade de Pointes

The following drugs prolong the QT interval: class IA antiarrhythmics, especially quinidine and disopyramide; class III agents (amiodarone and sotalol); tricyclics; probucol; phenothiazines; and bepridil. Diuretics and agents causing diarrhea may provoke hypokalemia, which also predisposes to QT-interval prolongation; the latter in turn may set the scene for torsade de pointes. Bradycardia also predisposes to torsade. Hence, combination therapy or cotherapy of class I and III antiarrhythmics, including the β-blocker sotalol and some other agents, can be dangerous, especially in the presence of thiazide diuretic

Table 35–4. **Drug Interactions Causing High Serum Digoxin Levels**

Decreased Renal Excretion
  Excess diuretics causing hypokalemia
  Concurrent cardiac drugs (quinidine, verapamil, amiodarone)
  Potassium-retaining agents (spironolactone, triamterene, amiloride, captopril)
  Depressed renal blood flow (β-blockers)
Decreased Nonrenal Clearance May Be an Additional Factor
  Cardiac drugs (quinidine, verapamil, amiodarone)
  Potassium-retaining diuretics (spironolactone, triamterene, amiloride)
Decreased Conversion in Gut to Digoxin Reduction Products
  Antibiotics destroying bacteria-converting digoxin to inactive reduction products (erythromycin, tetracycline)

Modified from Marcus FI, Opie LH, Sonnenblick EH, et al: Digitalis and acute inotropes. *In* Opie LH (ed): Drugs for the Heart, 4th ed. Philadelphia: WB Saunders, 1995, p 148.

Table 35–5. **Antiarrhythmic Drugs That Have Little or No Pharmacokinetic Interaction with Digoxin**

Class I agents:	procainamide, disopyramide
Class IB agents:	lidocaine, phenytoin, tocainide, mexiletine, moricizine
Class IC agents:	encainide (flecainide may cause mild elevation)
Class II agents:	β-blockade, unless renal blood flow critical
Class III agents:	sotalol
Class IV agents:	diltiazem (modest elevation may occur)

Modified from Marcus FI, Opie LH, Sonnenblick EH, et al: Digitalis and acute inotropes. *In* Opie LH (ed): Drugs for the Heart, 4th ed. Philadelphia: WB Saunders, 1995, p 154.

Table 35–6. **Drug Interactions of Antithrombotic Agents**

Cardiac Drug	Interacting Drugs	Mechanism	Consequence	Prophylaxis
Aspirin	Hepatic enzyme inducers (barbiturates, phenytoin, rifampin)	Increases aspirin metabolism	Decreases aspirin effect	Avoid combination
	Sulfinpyrazone, probenecid	Aspirin decreases urate excretion	Decreases uricosuric effect of sulfinpyrazone or probenecid	Increase dose of sulfinpyrazone or probenecid
	Thiazide diuretics	Aspirin decreases urate excretion	Hyperuricemia	Check blood urate
Sulfinpyrazone	Warfarin	Aspirin is antithrombotic	Excess bleeding	Check prothrombin time
	Warfarin	Sulfinpyrazone displaces warfarin from plasma proteins	Excess bleeding	Check prothrombin time
Warfarin	Potentiating drugs			
	Allopurinol	Mechanism unknown	Excess bleeding	Check prothrombin time
	Amiodarone	Mechanism unknown	Sensitizes to warfarin for 1–2 mo	Avoid combination
	Aspirin	Added bleeding tendency	Excess bleeding	Check prothrombin time
	Cimetidine	Decreases warfarin degradation	Increases blood warfarin	Check prothrombin time
	Quinidine	Hepatic interaction	Excess bleeding	Check prothrombin time
	Sulfinpyrazone	Displaces warfarin from plasma proteins	Excess bleeding	Check prothrombin time
	Inhibitory drugs			
	Cholestyramine	Decreases absorption of warfarin	Decreases warfarin effect	Check prothrombin time

Modified from Opie LH: Calcium antagonists. Part IV. Side effects and contraindications. Drug interactions and combinations. Cardiovasc Drug Ther 2:177, 1988.

treatment.[9] For example, in the therapy of hypertension, sotalol and a thiazide diuretic should not be combined in the absence of a potassium-retaining component to the diuretic.

PERIPHERAL CIRCULATION AND DRUG INTERACTIONS

The tone of vascular smooth muscle is regulated in a complex mode, including the vasoconstrictive effects of norepinephrine released from terminal neurons; this hormone stimulates both postsynaptic α_1- and α_2-receptors to cause vasoconstriction. Monoamine oxidase inhibitors and cocaine decrease the reuptake of norepinephrine by the terminal neurons and may cause intense vasoconstriction and hypertensive crises in those predisposed to such conditions by high rates of adrenergic drive. α-Receptors are inhibited by *quinidine*, which interacts with other vasodilators. The best-documented interaction is that of quinidine and verapamil, which may be explained by peripheral vasodilation (quinidine) and the negative inotropic effect of verapamil.[10] Additionally, verapamil decreases quinidine clearance. *Prazosin* (α_1-blocker) may also interact with verapamil and nifedipine so that the added hypotensive may be excessive. *Angiotensin-converting enzyme (ACE) inhibitors* are indirect vasodilators that may have excessive hypotensive effects when overdiuresis has stimulated the formation of high circulating concentrations of renin and angiotensin II. *Nonsteroidal antiinflammatory drugs (NSAIDs)* and *indomethacin*, by their inhibition of the formation of vasodilatory prostaglandins, may detract from the antihypertensive effect of diuretics, β-blockers, ACE inhibitors, and probably all other antihypertensive agents. *Aspirin* may reduce the benefits of ACE inhibition in heart failure.[11]

HEPATIC DRUG INTERACTIONS

Many cardiovascular drugs are metabolized in the liver. These include the lipid-soluble β-blockers (especially propranolol, oxprenolol, labetalol, and metoprolol), the calcium antagonists, most antiarrhythmics, aspirin, and warfarin. In general, hepatic metabolism is via the oxidase system, which in turn can be induced by several drugs (phenytoin, barbiturates, and rifampin or rifampicin) that accelerate the breakdown of those cardiovascular drugs metabolized in the the liver. The result is that blood levels of the drugs fall, and their therapeutic efficacy decreases. Conversely, cimetidine binds to the oxidase system to inhibit the breakdown of cardiovascular drugs undergoing hepatic metabolism, including some antiarrhythmic drugs such as procainamide;[12] therefore, cimetidine increases the blood levels of the coadministered drugs and enhances their therapeutic efficacy. Other drugs interfering with the hepatic metabolism of each other are verapamil and metoprolol (risk of increased nodal inhibition and negative inotropism), verapamil and prazosin (increased hypotensive effect), and verapamil and theophylline (blood theophylline levels increase). It is simpler and possibly safer to combine verapamil with atenolol (not metabolized in the liver) than with metoprolol.[13] Nicardipine and diltiazem interact with cyclosporin, so that the hepatic metabolism of cyclosporin is inhibited and blood cyclosporin levels rise. Quinidine interacts with warfarin to allow excess warfarin levels and bleeding.

All the discussed interactions are pharmacokinetic interactions. Pharmacodynamic interactions occur when altered hepatic blood flow changes rates of first-pass liver metabolism. For example, when β-blocker and lidocaine are given together, as during acute myocardial infarction, lidocaine metabolism is reduced with risk of lidocaine toxicity.[14] Propranolol, by decreasing hepatic blood flow, decreases nifedipine metabolism so that blood nifedipine levels rise. By increasing hepatic flow, nifedipine has opposite effects so that the breakdown of propranolol is increased, resulting in lower blood levels of propranolol.

RENAL DRUG INTERACTIONS

Probably the best-known renal interactions of cardiac drugs relate to the clearance of *digoxin,* decreased by quinidine,[15] quinine, verapamil, and probably amiodarone and propafenone. All of these agents predispose to digitalis toxicity, especially in the presence of renal failure or when extrarenal clearance of digoxin is reduced by potassium-retaining diuretics (spironolactone, triamterene, amiloride). Particularly important is the concept of interactions among combined drugs and digoxin in the treatment of congestive heart failure and arrhythmias, such as quinidine, spironolactone, and digoxin, which can elevate digoxin levels significantly.[16]

Urate excretion is promoted by probenecid and sulfinpyrazone and is inhibited by aspirin and thiazide diuretics; hence, these drugs may cancel one another's effects on urate excretion.

Diuretic excretion into the renal lumen is required. For a diuretic to act, it must be excreted into the lumen of the renal nephron. This process is inhibited by probenecid, which therefore decreases diuretic efficacy. However, probenecid also decreases tubular secretion of captopril and therefore increases the blood levels of the latter agent.

Captopril, but not other ACE inhibitors, inhibits the renal excretion of furosemide with decreased diuretic potency.[17]

Cimetidine decreases renal clearance of procainamide with higher blood procainamide levels. Both agents occasionally may predispose the patient to neutropenia.

GASTROINTESTINAL INTERACTIONS

The gastrointestinal absorption of *digoxin* is decreased by interfering agents such as cholestyramine, some antacids, high-bran diets, and combinations of kaolin and pectin. The gastrointestinal breakdown of digoxin by gastrointestinal flora is inhibited by the antibiotics erythromycin and tetracycline so that blood digoxin levels rise.

The gastrointestinal absorption of *warfarin* is decreased by cholestyramine.

PLASMA PROTEIN BINDING

Probably the most important interaction is between *sulfinpyrazone and warfarin.* Sulfinpyrazone powerfully displaces warfarin so that the dose required may drop dramatically. *Prazosin* displaces digoxin from plasma proteins in dogs; a similar effect in humans has not yet been reported.

CHOLINERGIC INTERACTIONS

In the autonomic nervous system, acetylcholine stimulates cardiovascular muscarinic receptors, which, in general, have effects opposite to those of β-adrenergic stimulation, so that heart rate falls and the inotropic state decreases.

Disopyramide

Disopyramide binds directly to muscarinic receptors so that the action of acetylcholine is interfered with and heart rate and contractility rise. To a lesser extent, quinidine and (to an even lesser exent) procainamide have similar effects. In the gut, the inhibitory effect of disopyramide on muscarinic receptors causes constipation. Thus, disopyramide should be given with care to patients receiving verapamil, which also causes constipation through a different mechanism involving inhibition of calcium channels of the gut. Disopyramide also acts on the bladder to cause urinary retention, which theoretically may be lessened in patients receiving atropine. Disopyramide may predispose patients to glaucoma; β-blockers such as timolol and betaxolol may counteract this effect of disopyramide. For systemic β-blockers, there is added danger of a negative inotropic effect with disopyramide.

Pyridostigmine

Pyridostigmine has a beneficial drug interaction with disopyramide. Pyridostigmine inhibits acetylcholinesterases so that more acetylcholine becomes available, with decreased side effects of disopyramide.

Acetylcholine released as a result of the activity of muscarinic receptors promotes depolarization and initiates contraction. Quinidine binds to muscarinic receptors, presumably to decrease the amount of acetylcholine released. Such binding of quinidine with the muscarinic receptors may explain its interaction with some antibiotics to cause weakness. Furthermore, in patients with myasthenia gravis, drugs that inhibit cholinesterases act by increasing acetylcholine availability. Such drugs may have decreased therapeutic effect, again because of the binding of quinidine to muscarinic receptors. Presumably, disopyramide, which binds more tightly to muscarinic receptors than does quinidine, may have similar drug interactions.

MAJOR INTERACTIONS OF VARIOUS CLASSES OF CARDIAC DRUGS

β-Adrenergic Blocking Agents

There are two major types of interactions (see Table 35–1). First, pharmacodynamic interactions result from additive effects of various categories of drugs. β-Blockers may interact adversely with calcium antagonists to cause excess hypotension or to cause undue bradycardia or AV nodal block. In addition, the negative inotropic effect of calcium antagonists, especially of verapamil, may interact adversely with that of β-blockers. Secondly, drugs such as propranolol, metoprolol, and labetalol, which are metabolized by the liver, have many hepatic interactions. Cimetidine reduces hepatic blood flow and increases blood levels of propranolol and metoprolol. Verapamil raises blood levels of metoprolol. Conversely, by decreasing hepatic blood flow, β-blockers may increase blood levels of lidocaine.

Calcium Antagonists

The potential interactions of these drugs are reviewed in Table 35–2. The major pharmacodynamic interactions between calcium antagonists and β-blockers already have been outlined in the preceding section.

Verapamil

Verapamil has a major interaction with digoxin (see Table 35–2), increasing blood digoxin levels by more than 50%. In digitalis poisoning, intravenous bolus injections of verapamil are absolutely contraindicated, because added inhibitory effects on the AV node can be fatal. Prazosin enhances the hypotensive effect of verapamil, possibly in part through a hepatic pharmacokinetic interaction. Verapamil and quinidine may give rise to excess hypotension, possibly because both have peripheral α-adrenoreceptor blocking qualities.

Nifedipine

Nifedipine is metabolized by the liver so that its antianginal effect is decreased when liver enzymes are induced by cigarette smoking. Conversely, cimetidine decreases the hepatic breakdown and increases the pharmacologic effects of nifedipine. Nifedipine increases blood levels of propranolol, possibly by an effect on hepatic blood supply. Nifedipine has only a small effect on blood digoxin. In hypertension, nifedipine's effects are not subject to interference by NSAIDs.[19]

Other Dihydropyridines

In general, these are metabolized by the same route as nifedipine and subject to similar interactions.

Diltiazem

Metabolized by the liver, diltiazem is also subject to many of the same interactions as nifedipine, so that cimetidine increases the effect of diltiazem, and cigarette smoking decreases it. Furthermore, diltiazem interacts with cyclosporin, which is also metabolized by the liver, so that blood levels of cyclosporin increase.

Antiarrhythmic Agents

Among the numerous interactions of antiarrhythmic drugs (see Table 35–3), the most frequent are with (1) digoxin, which, when combined with verapamil, quinidine, amiodarone, or propafenone, may result in higher than expected blood levels of digoxin, (2) diuretics, which may cause QT-interval prolongation and a risk of torsade de pointes when combined with antiarrhythmics that prolong the action potential duration per se, including sotalol,[9] quinidine, disopyramide, and amiodarone,[18] and (3) hepatic enzyme inducers, which alter the metabolism of agents such as quinidine and most antiarrhythmics that are metabolized in the liver, so that cimetidine decreases hepatic metabolism, whereas phenytoin, barbiturates, and rifampicin have opposite effects.

Digoxin

Several agents—including quinidine,[15] verapamil, nitrendipine, propafenone, and amiodarone—increase blood digoxin levels (see Table 35–4). In the presence of renal failure, drugs ordinarily causing a modest or minimal rise in blood digoxin levels, such as diltiazem or nifedipine, sometimes can precipitate digoxin toxicity. Conversely, blood levels of digoxin may fall during cotherapy with cholestyramine, because gastrointestinal absorption of digoxin is decreased. Levels of digoxin not normally causing toxicity can become toxic when the blood potassium falls, as occurs during cotherapy with potassium-losing diuretics. Because of numerous interactions of digoxin with antiarrhythmic drugs, it should be noted that there are several such drugs that have little or no pharmacokinetic interactions with digoxin (see Table 35–5).

Vasodilators

Prazosin

Prazosin appears to interact with the calcium antagonists verapamil and nifedipine so that excess hypotension may result. Cotherapy should be undertaken with care; conversely, the added hypotension achieved by prazosin may be required when hypertension appears to be resistant to therapy with nifedipine.

Angiotensin-Converting Enzyme Inhibitors

In general, ACE inhibitors have few drug interactions. They are potassium-retaining and therefore should not be given together with potassium-retaining diuretics such as Moduretic, Dyazide, Maxzide, or Aldactone.

Antithrombotic Agents

Aspirin

Aspirin interacts with hepatic enzyme inducers (see Table 35–6), which increase aspirin metabolism and decrease aspirin effects. Conversely, by decreasing urate excretion, aspirin diminishes the uricosuric effects of sulfinpyrazone and probenecid. Aspirin, again by decreasing urate excretion, may promote urate retention resulting from the use of thiazide diuretics. Aspirin may limit the hemodynamic effects of ACE inhibitors in severe heart failure.[11]

Sulfinpyrazone

Sulfinpyrazone powerfully displaces warfarin from plasma proteins with risk of excess bleeding.

Warfarin

Warfarin interacts with many other drugs, so that caution is always required. Among the effect-potentiating drugs are allopurinol, amiodarone, aspirin, cimetidine, quinidine, and sulfinpyrazone. Among the effect-inhibitory drugs are cholestyramine. Whenever any drug is given to a patient receiving warfarin, one should be alert for possible effects on prothrombin time.

SUMMARY

The major pharmacodynamic interaction of cardiovascular drugs lies in the cardiovascular system itself, where added negative inotropic effects or added effects on the SA and AV nodes are risks. Hemodynamic interactions are explained by the basic cardiovascular circulatory properties of each major category of drugs, including β-blockers, calcium antagonists, and those antiarrhythmics with major circulatory effects such as quinidine, disopyramide, and flecainide.

The major pharmacokinetic interactions lie in the liver and kidney. Lipid-soluble β-blockers, all calcium antagonists, and most antiarrhythmics are metabolized chiefly by the liver. Drugs altering activity of the hepatic oxidase system, such as barbiturates or cimetidine (opposite actions), can be expected to interfere with all such cardiac drugs. Further important pharmacokinetic interactions take place in the kidney. The renal clearance of digoxin is impaired by a number of important agents, including quinidine, verapamil, and amiodarone. Gastrointestinal interactions occur largely in relation to digoxin. Plasma protein binding is the site of one well-known interaction, namely that of sulfinpyrazone with warfarin. Finally, the cholinergic system is inhibited by the antiarrhythmic drugs disopyramide and quinidine, resulting in interactions with β-blockers and with drugs used in the therapy of myasthenia gravis.

REFERENCES

1. Opie LH: Adverse cardiovascular drug interactions. In Hurst JW (ed): The Heart, 8th ed. New York: McGraw-Hill, 1994, pp 1971–1985.
2. Piepho RW, Culbertson VL, Rhodes RS: Drug interactions with the calcium-entry blockers. Circulation 75(Suppl V):V181, 1987.
3. Lessem JN: Interaction between Ca²⁺ antagonists and digitalis. Cardiovasc Drug Ther 1:441, 1988.
4. Nafziger AN, May JJ, Bertino JS: Inhibition of theophylline elimination by diltiazem therapy [abstract]. Clin Pharmacol Ther 41:203, 1987.
5. Opie LH: Calcium antagonists. Part IV: Side effects and contraindications. Drug interactions and combinations. Cardiovasc Drug Ther 2:177, 1988.
6. Marcus FI, Opie LH: Antiarrhythmic agents. In Opie LH (ed): Drugs for the Heart, 4th ed. Philadelphia: WB Saunders, 1995, p 217.
7. Marcus FI, Opie LH, Sonnenblick EH, et al: Digitalis and acute inotropes. In Opie LH (ed): Drugs for the Heart, 4th ed. Philadelphia: WB Saunders, 1995, pp 148–154.
8. Marcus FI: Pharmacokinetic interactions between digoxin and other drugs. J Am Coll Cardiol 5:82A, 1985.
9. McKibbin JK, Pocock WA, Barlow JB, et al: Sotalol, hypokalaemia, syncope, and torsade de pointes. Br Heart J 51:157, 1984.
10. Maisel AS, Motulsky HJ, Insel PA, et al: Hypotension after quinidine plus verapamil: Possible additive competition at alpha-adrenergic receptors. N Engl J Med 312:167, 1985.
11. Hall D, Zeitler H, Rudolph W: Counteraction of the vasodilator effects of enalapril by aspirin in severe heart failure. J Am Coll Cardiol 20:1549, 1992.
12. Christian CO Jr, Meredith CG, Speeg KV Jr: Cimetidine inhibits procainamide clearance. Clin Pharmacol Ther 36:221, 1984.
13. McLean AJ, Knight R, Harrison PM, et al: Clearance-based oral drug interaction between verapamil and metoprolol and comparison with atenolol. Am J Cardiol 55:1628, 1985.
14. Ochs HR, Carstens G, Greenblatt DJ: Reduction in lidocaine clearance during continuous infusion and by coadministration of propranolol. N Engl J Med 303:373, 1980.
15. Hager WD, Fenster P, Mayersohn M, et al: Digoxin-quinidine interaction: Pharmacokinetic evaluation. N Engl J Med 300:1238, 1979.
16. Fenster PE, Hager WD, Goodman MM: Digoxin-quinidine-spironolactone interaction. Clin Pharmacol Ther 36:70, 1984.
17. Toussaint C, Masselink A, Gentges A, et al: Interference of different ACE inhibitors with the diuretic action of furosemide and hydrochlorothiazide. Klin Wochenschr 67:1138, 1989.
18. Marcus FI: Drug interactions with amiodarone. Am Heart J 106:924, 1983.
19. Salvetti A, Magagna A, Abdel-Haq B, et al: Nifedipine interactions in hypertensive patients. Cardiovasc Drugs Ther 4:963, 1990.

PART TWO

Cardiovascular Drugs

V.

Diuretics

Editors: Norman K. Hollenberg and Ray W. Gifford, Jr.

A. Principles and Practice of Diuretic Therapy

CHAPTER 36

Diuretics in Renal Failure

Ralph A. Kelly, M.D., and William E. Mitch, M.D.

Diuretics are among the most commonly prescribed drugs because of their high efficacy and relative safety. Dysfunction of the kidneys necessarily results in a decline in diuretic efficacy as well as an increase in toxicity. Ironically, as renal function decreases and higher doses of diuretics become necessary, the remaining nephrons become more susceptible to damage from overdiuresis, which can accelerate the decline in renal function. Nevertheless, diuretics are valuable agents in the management of fluid and electrolyte imbalance in patients with renal disease and in the treatment of many complications of renal failure, including hypertension. As other chapters will detail the pharmacology of commonly used diuretics in cardiovascular therapy, we will focus here on the use of diuretics in the treatment and prevention of renal insufficiency and the risks these drugs pose in patients with kidney disease.

ACUTE RENAL FAILURE

Although diuretics have been used for years to enhance urine flow in patients with an acute decline in renal function, the appropriateness of this indication remains very controversial.[1] Infusions of mannitol were demonstrated to maintain urine flow and prevent a sharp decline in creatinine clearance in dogs following renal artery clamping, provided that mannitol was administered before occlusion of blood flow. Experiments in animal models of acute renal failure (ARF) have tended to support the contention that diuretics can abort or mitigate the pathophysiologic processes leading to acute renal insufficiency. The data in humans are much less conclusive. Although oliguric renal failure may be converted to a nonoliguric form, there is little evidence to suggest that the morbidity or mortality resulting from ARF is reduced

or that recovery of renal function is accelerated by diuretics.

Animal Models of Acute Renal Failure

The evidence from animal models that diuretics can preserve renal function must be evaluated with the knowledge that the renal insult may be quite different from model to model and that no one experimental model duplicates the complex physiologic and biochemical events that precipitate renal failure in humans.[2] As with human studies, the standard of success or failure of a diuretic regimen varies from report to report, making comparisons difficult.

Mannitol

Mannitol has been the diuretic most extensively evaluated for a potential role in preserving renal function. The drug is an osmotic diuretic and increases solute and water excretion by inhibiting water reabsorption in the proximal tubule, thus reducing the favorable concentration gradient for sodium reabsorption. Mannitol also increases plasma flow to the inner medulla, thereby reducing the high tonicity in the medulla that is necessary for both solute and water reabsorption in the distal nephron.[3, 4] Mannitol can increase glomerular filtration and renal blood flow in hypoperfusion models of ARF.[5] Other suggested mechanisms for a protective effect of mannitol include increasing glomerular filtration pressure to augment glomerular filtration rate (GFR), flushing out of tubular debris, reducing endothelial cell volume to allow reflow in ischemic models of ARF, protecting mitochondrial function in tubular cells, and releasing intrarenal vasoactive prostaglandins.[6–10] In ARF produced by arterial infusion of vasoconstrictor drugs such as norepinephrine, mannitol maintained renal function and solute excretion if it was administered before the catecholamine infusion.[5] In experimental ARF induced by renal artery occlusion, early studies appeared to indicate that renal function could be protected if the infusion were initiated before the artery was clamped.[1, 11] In more recent studies in which inulin clearance rather than changes in plasma creatinine and urinary flow rates were used to monitor glomerular function, no beneficial effects of mannitol could be documented.[12, 13] Other osmotic diuretics (e.g., sucrose) are also ineffective. For example, when sucrose was given alone or in combination with either an inhibitor of the generation of oxygen-derived free radicals or with a scavenger of free radicals, renal function did not improve in models of postischemia ARF.[14–16]

In nephrotoxic models of ARF, the evidence suggested that mannitol infusion may confer some benefit in rats given toxic doses of mercuric chloride[7] or cis-platinum,[17, 18] but any benefit was small compared with results in rats not receiving mannitol. In hemoglobinuric and myoglobinuric models of ARF, mannitol maintains urine flow and diminishes the severity of renal dysfunction, presumably by preventing tubular cast formation.[19, 20] Although experimental myoglobinuria generates hydroxyl radicals and mannitol can function as a scavenger of hydroxyl radicals, this action of the drug does not appear to be an important mechanism contributing to mannitol's beneficial effect on renal dysfunction.[21] Mannitol combined with an iron chelator, deferoxamine, did exert an additive benefit on reducing renal dysfuntion in experimental myoglobinuria.[21] Presumably, the added benefit was due to the action of mannitol as an osmotic diuretic.

Loop Diuretics

Loop diuretics, principally furosemide, have also been studied extensively in animal models of ARF because of their potential for inducing renal arterial vasodilation. In norepinephrine-induced ARF in dogs, furosemide was shown to increase renal blood flow and solute excretion, thereby blunting the acute decline in renal function observed in control animals.[22] Although intravenously administered thiazide diuretics induced natriuresis in these same animals, they also caused renal vasoconstriction and a decline in renal blood flow, resulting in no protective effect. The beneficial effect of furosemide in this model depended on an increase in solute excretion and not solely on vasodilation, because acetylcholine given in doses that resulted in the same degree of renal vasodilation caused by furosemide conveyed no protection.[22]

In contrast to these data, evidence for a benefit in ischemic models of ARF is less convincing. Although some preservation of renal function was demonstrated when changes in creatinine clearance were assessed,[9, 23, 24] furosemide did not prevent a decline in inulin clearance.[25] Moreover, both muzolamine and furosemide were shown to increase renal blood flow following ischemic injury, but neither drug increased the rate of recovery of the GFR.[26] In other studies,

both furosemide and piretanide increased the GFR and reduced the accumulation of Tamm-Horsfall protein in tubules of rats with ARF following renal artery clamping.[27] However, in these experiments, furosemmide or piretanide was given 24 hours before the ischemic insult and was infused throughout the following week. The authors concluded that loop diuretics can minimize renal tubular damage due to intratubular deposition of Tamm-Horsfall protein (i.e., principally in the ascending loop of Henle). The improved renal function required prolonged infusion during the days after the ischemic injury.[27, 28] It has also been suggested that loop diuretics minimize cellular damage in the ischemic nephron by inhibiting ion transport and limiting metabolic work in the loop of Henle.[29, 30] The loop of Henle is emphasized because loop diuretics exert their effects primarily on this segment, which seems especially susceptible to ischemic injury.[29]

In nephrotoxic models of ARF, the results are also conflicting. Renal function improved little in rats pretreated with a loop diuretic and then given mercuric chloride compared with control animals unless volume losses were replaced continuously by infusion of 0.9% sodium chloride,[31] emphasizing the importance of establishing a normal extracellular fluid volume in maintaining natriuresis in ARF.[32] However, rats infused with furosemide 48 hours before and again after a dose of mercuric chloride reportedly maintained renal function.[33] Furosemide was shown to minimize the nephrotoxicity of uranyl nitrate and cis-platinum *if the diuretic had been administered for several days*,[17, 34] although these findings were not confirmed by another group.[35] In contrast, experimental aminoglycoside nephrotoxicity could not be ameliorated by furosemide administration in two studies.[36, 37] Curiously, in glycerol-induced ARF in rats (in contrast with results with mannitol infusions[20, 21, 38]), furosemide accelerated the decline in inulin clearance compared with measurements in control animals. Apparently, furosemide caused a greater decline in renal blood flow.[39, 40]

Dopamine

Dopamine has a complex pharmacology owing to its actions on α_1- and β-catecholamine receptors in the heart and peripheral vasculature and on vascular dopaminergic receptors, including those in the renal artery. When infused at rates less than 2 μg/kg/min, dopamine causes natriuresis in salt-replete animals, presumably by producing renal vasodilation and inhibiting solute resorption along the nephron.[41, 42] In a renal artery occlusion model of ischemic ARF in rats, dopamine significantly increased creatinine clearance compared with that in control animals.[43] In a nephrotoxic model of ARF in dogs, the combination of dopamine and furosemide proved superior to either dopamine or furosemide alone in maintaining creatinine clearance rates and urine flow rates.[24] There may be a role for dopamine as adjunctive therapy with atrial natriuretic peptide (ANP) in the treatment of ARF.

Atrial Natriuretic Peptide

A growing body of evidence supports the beneficial effects of ANPs and related congeners in experimental models of ARF. Infusions of ANPs, either ANP (1–28) or ANP (5–28) (ANPIII), minimize the extent of renal dysfunction following ischemic[44–46] and renal cytotoxic[47–50] injury. Smaller ANP analogues, such as A68828, have effects similar to infusions of naturally occurring ANP peptides.[51–53] Even when ANP infusions were initiated up to 48 hours after acute (norepinephrine-induced) renal injury in rats, both the extent of morphologic damage to the tubule and renal function improved in treated, compared with control, animals.[54] ANP exerts complex changes in systemic and intrarenal hemodynamics and tubular function, including an increase in renal blood flow, an increase in single-nephron GFR, and probably reduced sodium and water resorption. Systemic hypotension induced by infusing ANP can be treated by concomitantly infusing dopamine at doses sufficient to maintain an adequate mean arterial pressure.[54–56] Infusions of lower doses of dopamine (e.g., <5 μg/kg/min) had no beneficial effect. Higher doses not only caused systemic hypertension, but had detrimental effects on kidney function.[53, 54] Thus, an infusion of ANP alone or in combination with dopamine (at a concentration sufficient to prevent ANP-induced hypotension) can improve renal function acutely and limit long-term renal dysfunction following ischemic and some forms of nephrotoxic injury. Urodilatin, a congener of ANP isolated from human urine, exerts similar intrarenal actions as ANP but has less effect on systemic hemodynamics. Urodilatin can also improve renal dysfunction after ischemic injury, both immediately following bilateral renal artery occlusion and after 24 hours of established ARF in rats.[57] As with ANP, the benefit from urodilatin depends in part on maintaining an adequate renal perfusion pressure by infusing dopamine.[57]

Acute Renal Failure in Humans

Despite the encouraging if inconclusive evidence for using mannitol or loop diuretics in certain animal models of ARF, the evidence in humans is much less convincing. This should not be surprising, given the more complex pathophysiology of human ARF and the fact that it is often impossible to intervene early in the evolution of the illness. Commonly, the absence of histologic or precise verification of the nature and extent of renal injury precludes any firm conclusions regarding efficacy. Nevertheless, some controlled trials, typically in patients undergoing surgical procedures that carry a high risk of ARF, demonstrate the limited efficacy and potential toxicity of diuretics in the prevention and treatment of ARF. Only data from controlled studies will be examined here; the reader is referred to reviews of the use of diuretics in ARF for a more comprehensive survey.[58–61]

Mannitol

A number of prospective controlled trials have been carried out in surgical patients receiving mannitol as prophylactic therapy.[62–66] Compared with control groups, groups given mannitol typically experienced increased urine flow rates, although mortality was not diminished. However, in a study of patients undergoing surgery for treatment of obstructive jaundice who were treated with mannitol, creatinine clearance was improved compared with the untreated control subjects.[63] In a controlled trial of mannitol infusions in patients receiving cadaveric renal transplants, hemodialysis was required significantly less often in the treatment group, although mortality and graft survival were unaffected.[65] In the only controlled trial of prophylactic mannitol infusions in cardiopulmonary bypass surgery, children receiving mannitol had significantly lower serum creatinine levels postoperatively than did control subjects given equal volumes of crystalloid. However, no patient in either group required dialysis, and mortality was unaffected.[66] In interpreting these results, it is important to emphasize that neither diuretic therapy nor fluid replacement was controlled postoperatively in mannitol-treated or untreated patients.

There have been few controlled trials of mannitol infusions in patients receiving nephrotoxins. No beneficial effect of mannitol was found in a small double-blind study of patients receiving amphotericin B in which inulin and creatinine clearance rates were measured.[67] However, in a larger trial of patients undergoing intravenous pyelography who received a 60-minute mannitol infusion following injection of the dye, there was a 50% drop in the expected decline in renal function compared with a group of historical control subjects.[68, 69]

There is little support for the use of mannitol in established ARF, and no controlled trials have been attempted. In a limited, retrospective study of children with progressive or established ARF, mannitol added to furosemide resulted in no additional diuresis and no change in the dose of loop diuretics required to maintain urine flow.[70] In a group of surgical patients with oliguric ARF given up to 60 g of mannitol over 24 hours, 54% of the patients studied responded with an increase in urine flow rates; mortality was significantly reduced in this group compared with nonresponders.[71] It is unclear from this study whether mannitol actually reversed an ongoing pathophysiologic process or merely identified a group of patients at reduced risk for advanced renal insufficiency. Volume-depleted patients with prerenal azotemia may represent some fraction of the group who appeared to respond to mannitol, as this study antedated technical advances that make routine monitoring of extracellular volume status and cardiac output possible.

Loop Diuretics

The only controlled trials of loop diuretics in humans with ARF have used furosemide. Again, there is little evidence that the drug significantly reduces morbidity or has any effect on mortality. Furosemide given to children with poststreptococcal glomerulonephritis resulted in higher urine flow rates and better control of edema, but in the same report, patients with hemolytic-uremic syndrome or acute tubular necrosis did no better following administration of the diuretic.[72] In a study of surgical patients randomized to receive either mannitol (0.5 g/kg) or furosemide (1 mg/kg) postoperatively, GFR as assessed by sequential inulin clearances actually fell in the furosemide group, although renal blood flow and urine flow rates increased.[64] No improvement in mortality or serious change in renal function was noted in either group. Most uncontrolled or retrospective studies of loop diuretics in the prophylaxis of ARF have failed to note any beneficial effect.[73, 74]

Despite this discouraging evidence for the use of furosemide in the prevention of ARF, furosemide may have a limited role in the treatment of established oliguric acute renal insufficiency. In a retrospective study of patients with ARF from a variety of causes, all of whom had been dialyzed at least twice before receiving the diuretic, the hospital courses of those receiving furosemide were compared with the hospital courses of patients receiving no diuretic. Patients receiving very high doses (up to 3200 mg/day) became nonoliguric and required fewer dialyses compared with untreated control subjects or patients receiving a 600-mg dose of furosemide daily.[75] There was no improvement in mortality, and the duration of azotemia was no shorter in the high-dose group. In a similar, large retrospective study of furosemide using lower doses (up to 500 mg/day) in ARF, there was a significant reduction in the requirement for dialysis but not in mortality or duration of azotemia and of hyperkalemia.[76] Three prospective controlled studies have reached similar conclusions.[77–79] In each case, high doses of furosemide succeeded in significantly increasing urine flow and preventing oliguria, but, again, morbidity and mortality were unaffected. Importantly, tinnitus, decreased hearing, or deafness was reported in a small number of patients treated with high-dose furosemide in each study.

Dopamine

Despite promising animal data and a number of uncontrolled trials in humans, no prospective controlled studies have investigated the use of low-dose dopamine in the treatment of ARF, either alone or in combination with diuretics. In eight patients with ARF and oliguria unresponsive to volume expansion and furosemide, dopamine resulted in a consistent increase in urine output but no decline in serum creatinine.[80] In two other uncontrolled studies, dopamine in combination with furosemide increased natriuresis and urine flow rate, but it is unclear whether this represented an improvement in the morbidity of renal insufficiency.[81, 82] The absence of any controlled trials makes it difficult to justify the common clinical practice of combining dopamine and loop diuretics, par-

ticularly if the intention is to preserve renal function or reverse or shorten the course of ARF. Although infusion rates of less than 3 μg/kg/min of dopamine should pose little risk to most patients, the drug has a high potential for producing cardiac arrhythmias; therefore, errors in judging lean body weight or dosage may result in acute cardiac toxicity and a rapid rise in peripheral vascular resistance. Whether dopamine will prove to be a useful adjunct to ANP in the treatment of ARF in humans, as has been documented in animals, remains to be demonstrated. A number of controlled trials to investigate the safety and efficacy of ANP are under way.

CHRONIC RENAL FAILURE
Pharmacology

Regardless of etiology, once a moderate degree of chronic renal failure (CRF) has occurred, renal insufficiency tends to be progressive.[83] Rates of deterioration of renal function vary widely among patients, but the rate of progression is quite constant for individual patients.[84] Because progressive renal dysfunction affects both the pharmacokinetics and the pharmacodynamics of diuretics, physicians should modify therapeutic regimens as insufficiency becomes more severe.

Osmotic Diuretics

Osmotic diuretics are filtered at the glomerulus and do not require transport into the tubular lumen by organic acid secretory mechanisms in the proximal tubule. Osmotic diuretics can maintain urine flow at low GFRs, as occurs in hypotension or dehydration, as long as the perfusion pressure in glomerular capillaries is sufficient to maintain filtration. If the tubular epithelium remains relatively impermeable, mannitol infusions will maintain the flow of salt and water to distal portions of the nephron. Nevertheless, as renal disease progresses, fewer glomeruli will be available to filter the diuretic, and the solute load in remaining nephrons will increase, thereby diminishing the pharmacologic effect of osmotically active drugs. The reduced renal clearance of mannitol or other osmotic diuretics will result in their accumulation and a potentially dangerous degree of volume expansion, leading to pulmonary edema and hyponatremia. Therefore, these drugs have little role in the treatment of patients with CRF.

Thiazide Diuretics

The thiazide diuretics include a number of agents that are chemically and pharmacologically similar, including chlorothiazide, the prototype for this class of diuretics, and chlorthalidone and metolazone, which are heterocyclic variants of the basic benzothiadiazine nucleus. The thiazides are useful in the management of mild to moderate hypertension and as single agents in the initial management of early congestive heart failure. However, their utility is limited when the depletion of the extracellular volume increases the avidity of solute resorption in proximal segments of the nephron. Thiazide diuretics are largely ineffective when the GFR is less than 30 ml/min,[85] partly because of reduced secretion into the proximal tubule due to competition for organic acid transporters by accumulating metabolic byproducts of metabolism in uremia. Decreased secretion limits delivery of the drugs to their site of action in the distal tubule. In contrast with loop diuretics, which increase renal blood flow, thiazide diuretics acutely reduce glomerular filtration, at least when administered intravenously.[86] Metolazone may cause a smaller reduction in GFR than other drugs of this class, but it is unclear whether this is a clinically important distinction.[87, 88] Indapamide, a potent sulfamoylbenzamide derivative that acts as a direct vascular smooth muscle dilator, may also pose less risk to patients with mild renal insufficiency, although the safety and efficacy of this drug in patients with renal disease have yet to be established.[89, 90]

Loop Diuretics

The loop diuretics are among the most potent diuretic agents known, potentially capable of inducing loss, at least for a short period, of up to 20% of the filtered load of sodium. This class of diuretics includes the sulfonamide derivative of anthranilic acid, furosemide, and its more potent congeners, bumetanide and piretanide, plus the structurally unrelated drugs ethacrynic acid, muzolimine, and torsemide. These diuretics maintain solute loss even in the presence of a low GFR and renal perfusion.[91] Unlike the thiazides, the loop-active agents do not acutely induce a decline in GFR, perhaps because these drugs inhibit the influx of sodium chloride into macula densa cells, thereby blocking the tubuloglomerular feedback response.[92] These drugs also are secreted into the tubular lumen by the organic acid secretory pathway, and therefore their pharmacologic effect may be delayed or diminished by drugs secreted by the same mechanism (e.g., probenecid) or endogenous inhibitors of the transporter that accumulate in uremia.

All loop diuretics have a diminished natriuretic effect in patients with extreme renal insufficiency.[93] As is the case in patients with advanced congestive heart failure, this is not the result of a reduction in bioavailability because absolute absorption is unaffected, although in CRF delivery of these drugs to their site of action is delayed and extrarenal clearance is generally enhanced.[94–105] A potential exception is the new loop diuretic muzolimine, which may not depend on secretion into the tubular lumen in order to reach its site of action in the loop of Henle.[104, 106, 107] The metabolism of torsemide also differs from that of the other loop diuretics. It undergoes extensive oxidative biotransformation in the liver, resulting in inactive, as well as active, metabolites.[108, 109] Thus, the duration of action of torsemide is largely independent of renal function. However, in CRF patients, the drug's efficacy, as in the case of most diuretics, is

directly related to GFR and the delivery of solute and the drug and its active metabolites, to the ascending limb of Henle's loop in the few, remaining functional nephrons.

Although delivery of loop diuretics may be depressed in CRF, the Na/K/2Cl cotransporters in the loop of Henle, the "molecular receptors" for these drugs, appear to be as susceptible to inhibition by these drugs as they are in normal subjects.[110] The efficacy of the loop diuretics is not normally affected by a chronic metabolic acidosis, although advanced respiratory acidosis combined with hypoxemia may substantially reduce their urinary clearance, thereby limiting their natriuretic effect.[111] In any event, larger doses of diuretic are required to attain comparable increases, in absolute terms, of solute and water excretion in patients with CRF.[112, 113] Doses of furosemide as high as 600 mg/day may be required, but the frequency of dosage usually can be reduced, owing to the prolonged half-life of these drugs in renal disease. Dosage guidelines for the use of most of these drugs in patients with renal failure have been published.[60, 114–116] One useful approach in establishing an effective dose of a loop diuretic in edematous patients with CRF is to double the intravenous dose in successive increments until a plateau in sodium and fluid excretion is reached.[93] Assuming a bioavailability of 50% for furosemide (80% for bumetanide), the oral dose can be readily calculated. The frequency of oral dosing is usually decreased because of the prolonged elimination half-life of these drugs in CRF. Continuous intravenous infusion of a loop diuretic seems to diminish the risk of ototoxicity, because the peak levels of diuretic are lower than after a bolus. Besides this potential benefit, there is no evidence that a continuous diuretic infusion increases fluid and electrolyte excretion more effectively than intermittent dosing.

An important complication of high doses of loop diuretics is ototoxicity.[117] As ethacrynic acid is more ototoxic than other loop diuretics, there is little justification for its use in patients with renal failure, except in patients with a history of drug allergy or interstitial nephritis caused by sulfonamides. Sensorineural hearing loss usually requires doses of furosemide greater than 1 g/day; transient hearing loss may be common in patients receiving large-bolus doses of furosemide.[118] Bumetanide and piretanide may be less ototoxic than furosemide. The ototoxicity of loop diuretics is synergistic with that of the aminoglycosides.

All loop diuretics cause changes in systemic hemodynamics that are initially unrelated to the degree of natriuresis they induce. The acute administration of furosemide results in a rapid increase in venous capacitance and a decline in cardiac filling pressures.[119] This effect, which is coincident with a rise in plasma renin activity, is blunted by prostaglandin synthesis inhibitors and by a high dietary salt intake.[120, 121] An apparently paradoxic rise in systemic vascular resistance and blood pressure following intravenous furosemide infusion may occur in some patients as well as in normal subjects, an effect that is blocked by inhibitors of renin release or angiotensin II formation.[122-126] Because both the rise in venous capacitance and arteriolar resistance are initiated by renin released from the kidney, the systemic hemodynamic effects of loop diuretics are reduced in severe CRF and abolished in anephric subjects. In addition to renal arterial vasodilation and increase in venous capacitance, some of the natriuretic response to loop diuretics is mediated by increased prostaglandin formation. Therefore, cyclooxygenase inhibitors such as nonsteroidal antiinflammatory drugs (NSAIDs) may reduce the potency and efficacy of these diuretics. This drug interaction may be more pronounced in patients with reduced baseline renal perfusion.[127-132] Fortunately, doses of aspirin used to selectively inhibit platelet production of thromboxane B_2 (0.5 mg/kg/day) seem to have no effect on urinary prostaglandin excretion or the natriuresis induced by furosemide.[133]

Potassium-Sparing Diuretics

This class of diuretics comprises drugs that are relatively weak natriuretic agents. Because of their pharmacologic action in the distal nephron and collecting duct, they reduce the secretion of potassium and protons into the tubular lumen. There are two classes of these agents: the aldosterone antagonists and the direct inhibitors of sodium conductance in the apical membrane of distal collecting duct epithelial cells. The classic aldosterone antagonist in common use is spironolactone, although the spironolactone congener, potassium canrenoate, and its common metabolic byproduct, canrenone, are also available commercially. Their efficacy depends on high plasma aldosterone levels. Amiloride and triamterene are structurally related agents that inhibit Na^+ entry into the collecting duct epithelia by blocking apical sodium conductance channels.[134, 135] Amiloride also blocks the sodium-hydrogen antiporter in proximal and distal nephron segments, but only at doses much higher than can be attained in humans.

A major effect of these drugs is to diminish renal potassium secretion, and this may lead to clinically important hyperkalemia, particularly in patients with renal insufficiency. These drugs may also cause mild metabolic acidosis. For these reasons, the potassium-sparing diuretics are contraindicated in patients with CRF or ARF. Indeed, Knauf et al. showed that at creatinine clearance rates below 50 ml/min, the natriuretic effect of amiloride was eliminated, but a potassium-retaining effect of the drug could still be detected.[136]

Atrial Natriuretic Peptide

As with experimental models of ARF in animals, ANPs increase solute and water excretion in nephrotoxic and subtotal nephrectomy models of CRF,[137-141] even at low-dose rates of infusion that do not affect systemic hemodynamics.[142] In a limited number of studies, short-term infusion of ANP congeners in patients with CRF showed that the hemodynamic and renal responses varied with the etiology and extent of renal dysfunction and the dose of ANP congener administered. In most patients, there were significant increases in GFR and renal excretion of sodium, chloride, phosphorus, and water during the infusion or just after a bolus injection.[142-146] The effect of a transient ANP infusion on systemic and renal vascular resistance was more pronounced and longer-lasting in CRF patients than in control subjects given similar doses of the peptide.[146] The prolonged effect was due in part to the reduced clearance and longer half-life of ANP in CRF patients.[147] ANP infusions also reduced the plasma aldosterone concentration in CRF, as well as in control patients.[147] The plasma half-life of available ANP analogues is less than 5 minutes, even in patients with CRF. This factor limits the utility of ANP for the treatment of sodium, water, or phosphorus retention in patients with chronic renal dysfunction. Newer pharmacologic approaches are becoming available, however, including inhibitors of ANP catabolism. One such agent, sinorphan, which inhibits a metalloendopeptidase called "neutral endopeptidase," decreases the clearance of endogenous ANP.[148, 149] In a single-dose, double-blind crossover trial of sinorphan in CRF patients, plasma ANP levels and cyclic guanosine monophosphate levels increased within 1 hour, whereas sodium excretion increased approximately twofold in the second and third hours following drug administration.[150] Thus, therapeutic strategies that decrease the clearance of endogenous ANP or of exogenously administered ANP analogues may prove useful in controlling fluid and solute homeostasis in CRF. Whether these agents would offer any advantage during chronic administration to existing diuretic regimens or whether they will change the progression of renal dysfunction in CRF remains to be determined.

Combined Diuretic Regimens

In patients with edema refractory to high doses of loop diuretics or when side effects such as ototoxicity occur, combinations of diuretics may result in an acceptable natriuresis at lower doses of both drugs. Indeed, the combination of a loop diuretic with a thiazide often results in a synergistic increase in solute and water excretion.[151-157] This may be due in part to an "unmasking" of the proximal tubular effect of thiazides (inhibition of carbonic anhydrase) plus inhibition of sodium chloride resorption in the loop of Henle, although additive effects in the distal tubule are probably most important.

Although the loop-thiazide combination of diuretics may be efficacious in selected patients with refractory edema, profound intravascular volume depletion and electrolyte disturbances complicate their use. First, potassium wasting is severe and potentially life-threatening, and second, advanced prerenal azotemia may occur, leading to irreversible renal insufficiency in some patients.[156] Consequently, this combination of diuretics should be initiated only in the hospital, and outpatient therapy should be carefully regulated by monitoring changes in body weight and serum electrolyte levels.

The combination of a potassium-sparing diuretic and a more proximally acting drug is among the most common drug combinations prescribed. However, this combination usually has less than an additive effect on sodium excretion for the following reasons. Triamterene, but not amiloride or spironolactone, inhibits the tubular secretion of furosemide, thus delaying and possibly limiting its pharmacologic effect. In addition, the loop diuretics tend to attenuate the inhibitory effect of amiloride or triamterene on collecting duct Na^+ conductance.[158] Nonetheless, this combination of diuretics may be useful in selected patients with mild renal insufficiency and a well-defined need to limit excessive potassium wasting (e.g., in patients with cardiac arrhythmias), provided that these patients are carefully monitored for the development of hyperkalemia and metabolic acidosis. In patients with chronic obstructive pulmonary disease, potassium-sparing diuretics, alone or in combination with other diuretics, may be preferred to diuretics that produce metabolic alkalosis and thereby diminish ventilatory drive.[159] Occasionally, patients with renal failure and metabolic alkalosis due to such factors as vomiting and prolonged nasogastric suction may respond well to acetazolamide alone or in combination with a loop diuretic.[160] Caution must be exercised here as well, because acetazolamide can induce acute metabolic acidosis in patients with early renal insufficiency.[161]

Indications for Use of Diuretics

The clinical indications for a diuretic or a diuretic combination are similar to those in patients with normal renal function and fall into two broad classes: (1) the need for a negative sodium balance and (2) a limited number of other conditions including hypercalcemia, hypercalciuria, nephrogenic diabetes insipidus, type IV renal tubular acidosis, "dialysis disequilibrium" syndrome, and prevention of altitude sickness. Because other chapters discuss specific indications in more detail, only those aspects of diuretic use particularly relevant to renal failure patients are discussed here.

Induction of a Negative Sodium Balance

Often, CRF is complicated by edema. Many patients can maintain neutral salt balance until renal insufficiency progresses to the point at which the remaining nephrons no longer increase the fractional excretion of sodium sufficiently to match dietary intake. This usually occurs at a GFR of less than 5 ml/min, although edema can occur at higher GFRs in patients with congestive heart failure, hepatic disease, or the nephrotic syndrome. In general, there is little reason to prescribe a diuretic for these patients if edema is mild, because diuretic administration carries the risk of excessive volume depletion and electrolyte abnormalities.

In the nephrotic syndrome, most patients are relatively resistant to diuretics even when the GFR is well-preserved.[162] Despite the effect of hypoalbuminemia on drug binding, this apparently is not the result of changes in pharmacokinetics, at least in the case of furosemide.[163-165] Nevertheless, a dose can usually be found that will result in natriuresis, although patients must be cautioned not to lose more than 0.5 kg/day to avoid volume depletion and a decline in GFR. Because many nephrotics have high plasma aldosterone levels, profound hypokalemia may result from diuretic therapy. Hyponatremia is also more common in these patients because of the combination of dietary salt restriction and diuretic use. Interestingly, patients with nephrotic syndrome exhibited a more pronounced diuretic and natriuretic response to short-term bolus infusions of ANP than patients with other forms of CRF.[144] Because ANP infusions also lower the plasma aldosterone,[143] ANP congeners in combination with diuretics might limit the extent of hypokalemia in nephrotic patients receiving other diuretics.

The treatment of hypertension is a common indication for diuretics in CRF. Although the mechanism for the benefits of diuretics is debated in patients with essential hypertension, hypertension in CRF clearly appears to be a volume-dependent disease process.[166-168] In dialysis patients, adequate blood pressure control is often achieved by ultrafiltration without the need for additional antihypertensive drugs.

Importantly, control of blood pressure in patients with accelerated hypertension can delay the progression of advanced renal failure.[169, 170] The addition of angiotensin-converting enzyme (ACE) inhibitors to a diuretic regimen has been found to slow the progress of deteriorating renal function and reduce glomerular albumin loss in patients with diabetic nephropathy.[171, 172] Similar data were obtained in animal models of chronic renal insufficiency.[173]

Indications for Diuretic Use Other Than Induction of a Negative Sodium Balance

Aside from increasing salt excretion, a few indications for diuretics are unique to patients with renal insufficiency. Type IV renal tubular acidosis, also called hyporeninemic, hypoaldosteronemic, metabolic acidosis, is characterized by moderate renal insufficiency, hyperkalemia, and a normal anion gap metabolic acidosis.[174] Replacement therapy with synthetic mineralocorticoids can correct the electrolyte abnormalities but may exacerbate edema and hypertension. Furosemide alone may achieve the same reduction in hyperkalemia and a reversal of metabolic acidosis in selected patients with type IV renal tubular acidosis.[175]

A relatively recent addition to the list of indications for diuretic administration is use of an osmotic diuretic during a hemodialysis procedure to minimize the rapid osmotic shifts that cause neurologic symptoms of the "dialysis disequilibrium syndrome."[176] Several agents have been employed successfully (hypertonic saline or dextrose, mannitol), but a large net shift of fluid into the extracellular space must be avoided to prevent pulmonary edema.

Complications of Diuretic Use

Many complications of diuretic use in patients with renal failure are similar to those seen in patients with normal renal function and are discussed elsewhere in this book and in several reviews.[177-184] Only the aspects of these complications that are particularly relevant to treatment of patients with renal failure are discussed here.

Excessively Rapid Reduction in Extracellular Fluid Volume

This complication can precipitate ARF and accelerate the rate of decline in renal function in CRF. Obviously, potent loop diuretics in high doses or a combination of diuretics pose a greater risk of rapidly depleting intravascular volume. However, a moderate rise in blood urea nitrogen (BUN) with diuretics does not necessarily indicate imminent prerenal azotemia, because urea clearance always declines more rapidly than the GFR in response to mild volume depletion in CRF.[185] Finally, drug interactions should be considered in patients exhibiting an abrupt rise in serum creatinine, such as the administration of loop diuretics with NSAIDs.[130, 186]

In certain patients, the combination of ACE inhibitors with a diuretic may cause a dramatic reduction in GFR.[187-193] Initially, this phenomenon was described in patients with advanced renal artery stenosis (bilateral, or unilateral stenosis with one functioning kidney) in whom a precipitous decline in GFR occurred primarily because of a fall in glomerular efferent arteriolar tone but also because of a fall in blood pressure.[187, 188] It is now recognized that many patients with advanced congestive heart failure and moderate renal insufficiency (serum creatinine, 1.5 to 2.0 mg/ dl) also can experience a rise in serum creatinine following initiation of ACE inhibitor therapy, in spite of an increase in cardiac output and a decline in left ventricular filling pressure. Although some of these patients may have renal artery stenosis, more recent evidence suggests that most are demonstrating a form of prerenal azotemia due to an excessively rapid diuresis. In one report,[190] a reduction in diuretic dose without a change in dosage of the ACE inhibitor resulted in most patients' experiencing a return to baseline renal function. Nevertheless, in certain patients with advanced congestive heart failure for whom an adequate GFR depends highly on circulating angiotensin II levels, use of long-acting ACE inhibitors may be detrimental to renal function regardless of extracellular volume status.[193, 194]

Alterations in Potassium and Magnesium Homeostasis

Although hypokalemia is a common complication of diuretic use, it is rarely life-threatening, whereas hy-

perkalemia caused by administration of potassium-sparing diuretics to patients with renal failure is life-threatening. Moreover, the natriuretic effects of these diuretics are virtually absent at a GFR below 50 ml/ min even though their potassium-retaining effects may still be present.[150] Therefore, there is little justification for the routine use of potassium-sparing diuretics in patients with renal insufficiency.

Occasionally, patients with a mild reduction in GFR show unacceptably high urinary potassium losses. For example, severe salt restriction coupled with regular diuretic use may stimulate aldosterone-induced potassium secretion.[195, 196] Renal losses of potassium also can be exacerbated with high epinephrine levels caused by stress, myocardial ischemia, pulmonary edema,[197] or the administration of insulin whether or not concomitant glucose is given.[198] In such patients, in patients with congestive heart failure receiving cardiac glycosides, or in patients with malignant arrhythmias, supplemental potassium may be necessary.[199-213] Nevertheless, the likelihood of severe hyperkalemia and worsening metabolic acidosis due to potassium-sparing diuretics is very real in patients with advanced CRF (GFR <30 ml/min), and this risk usually outweighs any other considerations. It should also be noted that administration of prostaglandin-synthesis inhibitors, β-blockers, or ACE inhibitors can result in a rise in plasma potassium levels.[214]

Loss of magnesium stores, with or without a low serum concentration of magnesium (i.e., hypomagnesemia), caused by thiazide or loop diuretics is unusual in CRF, particularly when the GFR declines to less than 30% of normal. Loss of magnesium stores can occur in patients following treatment with amphotericin B or certain aminoglycoside antibiotics. Symptomatic hypomagnesemia can be associated with concomitant diuretic use and/or a poor dietary magnesium intake. There has been increasing interest in the cardiovascular toxicity of magnesium depletion and the unreliability of an isolated serum magnesium as an index of total body magnesium content.[215-219] Magnesium deficiency can induce or exacerbate the tendency to a number of cardiac arrhythmias, including atrial fibrillation and supraventricular arrhythmias, ventricular arrhythmias (including ventricular fibrillation), and, in particular, arrhythmias elicited by so-called early afterdepolarizations (e.g., torsade de pointes).[218-223] These arrhythmias occur predominantly in CRF patients with underlying cardiac disease and/or other electrolyte and acid-base abnormalities. Hypermagnesemia is a more common complication of CRF but probably has few cardiovascular complications.

Hyponatremia

Hyponatremia is a common complication of diuretics, particularly in patients with the nephrotic syndrome, but also in patients with advanced oliguric and non-oliguric renal failure in whom free water clearance is reduced. Restriction of free water intake will usually control this complication, although more aggressive management is clearly indicated in patients who develop any neurologic symptoms.[224] Of the commonly employed diuretics, the longer-acting thiazides with or without a potassium-sparing diuretic appear to pose the highest risk for diuretic-induced hyponatremia, particularly in the elderly or in malnourished patients.

Metabolic Acidosis

The chronic metabolic acidosis of renal insufficiency can be rapidly exacerbated by administration of carbonic anhydrase inhibitors.[161] Potassium-sparing diuretics may also exacerbate a metabolic acidosis by reducing renal acid excretion.

Ototoxicity

Although loop diuretics are potent inhibitors of the Na/K/2Cl cotransporter, inhibition of this transporter on cells outside the kidney is clinically unimportant except in the cochlea. As previously discussed, all loop diuretics possess some ototoxicity, with ethacrynic acid being the most toxic. Transient hearing loss may be common in patients receiving bolus injections of furosemide because of a reversible decrease in endocochlear potential and eighth nerve action potential.[118] Most cases of diuretic-induced ototoxicity have occurred in patients with renal failure, frequently in those also receiving an aminoglycoside antibiotic.

Hyperuricemia

Hyperuricemia is a common complication of diuretic therapy. Competition by diuretics for the organic acid pathway in the proximal tubule and enhanced proximal and distal tubular resorption of uric acid caused by diuretic-induced volume contraction cause the hyperuricemia.[215] Although sustained plasma urate levels of up to 10 mg/100 ml may sometimes occur, gout or uric acid nephropathy is rarely a clinical problem.[225-227] Indacrinone, a uricosuric loop diuretic, may have some utility in patients with advanced hyperuricemia. Because of its hepatic toxicity, the uricosuric diuretic ticrynafen is no longer marketed in the United States.

Carbohydrate Intolerance and Hyperlipidemia

The effects of diuretics on carbohydrate and lipid metabolism are not qualitatively different in patients with CRF[228, 229] than in other patients, although more studies are needed in this area. Most patients with renal failure have some degree of carbohydrate intolerance and abnormal lipid metabolism even in the absence of diuretics. The impact of thiazide diuretics, particularly on serum lipid levels, remains controversial.[230-236] Elevated low-density lipoprotein (LDL) levels, including an increase in the ratio of LDL to high-density lipoprotein (HDL) cholesterol,[237] have been reported in patients receiving thiazides but not in those receiving loop diuretics.[238] Serum triglyceride levels are also significantly higher in patients receiving thiazide diuretics, even among patients receiving exercise training and strict dietary control of cholesterol and lipid intake.[228, 239-247] The risk of exacerbating hyperlipidemia, although low, should be considered before prescribing thiazide diuretics in patients with mild CRF. For example, patients with a family history of atherosclerosis or hyperlipidemia should probably avoid long-term thiazide therapy. Because these complications may be dose-related, the lowest effective dose should be administered, particularly in the case of the thiazide diuretics.

Carbohydrate intolerance has been a recognized complication of thiazide diuretics for many years. Ketoacidosis due to thiazide-induced carbohydrate intolerance is rare, but nonketotic hyperosmolar coma can occur, particularly in volume-depleted patients.[248] Peripheral insulin resistance occurs in normal subjects receiving thiazide diuretics, and this abnormality can be ameliorated by concomitant therapy with an ACE inhibitor.[249-251] Hypokalemia by itself can exacerbate glucose intolerance, but most patients with insulin resistance from thiazide therapy are not severely hypokalemic. On the other hand, insulin resistance in nonhepatic tissues is rare in normal individuals receiving loop diuretics who have normal values of serum potassium.[230]

Bullous Skin Lesions

There have been several reports of a photosensitive bullous dermatitis in CRF patients receiving high doses of furosemide.[252, 253] Porphyrin metabolism was abnormal in several affected patients, but this was not a universal finding. The mechanism for this adverse reaction is unknown; treatment involves withdrawal of the drug and application of topical steroids.

Interstitial Nephritis

All sulfamoyl-containing diuretics have been associated with interstitial nephritis in patients with normal renal function, but the incidence appears to be higher in renal failure patients.[254, 255] In patients receiving a diuretic, interstitial nephritis should always be considered a potential mechanism for unexpected deterioration of renal function.[84] A renal biopsy may be helpful in suspicious cases.

REFERENCES

1. Selkurt EE: Changes in renal clearance following complete ischemia of the kidney. Am J Physiol 144:395, 1945.
2. Honda N, Hishida A: Pathophysiology of experimental nonoliguric acute renal failure. Kidney Int 43:513, 1993.
3. Buerkert J, Martin D, Prasad J, et al: Role of deep nephrons and the terminal collecting duct in a mannitol-induced diuresis. Am J Physiol 240:F411, 1981.
4. Mathisen O, Raeder M, Kiil F: Mechanism of osmotic diuresis. Kidney Int 19:431, 1981.
5. Patak RV, Fadem SZ, Lifschitz MD, et al: Study of factors which modify the development of norepinephrine-induced acute renal failure in the dog. Kidney Int 15:227, 1979.

6. Johnston PA, Bernard DB, Perrin NS, et al: Prostaglandins mediate the vasodilatory effect of mannitol in the hypoperfused rat kidney. J Clin Invest 68:127, 1981.

7. Schrier RW, Arnold PE, Gordon JA, et al: Protection of mitochondrial function by mannitol in ischemic acute renal failure. Am J Physiol 247:F365, 1984.

8. Zager RA: Glomerular filtration rate and brush border debris excretion after mercuric chloride and ischemic acute renal failure: Mannitol versus furosemide diuresis. Nephron 33:196, 1983.

9. Hanley MJ, Davidson K: Prior mannitol infusion in a model of ischemic acute renal failure. Am J Physiol 241:F556, 1981.

10. Mason J, Joeris B, Welsch J, Kriz W: Vascular congestion in ischemic renal failure: The role of cell swelling. Miner Electrol Metab 15:114, 1989.

11. Levinsky NG, Bernard DB, Johnston PA: Mannitol and loop diuretics in acute renal failure. In Brenner BM, Lazarus JM (eds): Acute Renal Failure. Philadelphia: WB Saunders, 1983, pp 712–722.

12. Kreisberg J, Venkatachalarn M, Patel Y, et al: Failure of mannitol to protect against 40 minutes of renal artery occlusion in the rat [abstract]. Clin Res 31:516A, 1983.

13. Lewis RM, Patton MK, Osgood RW, et al: Evaluation of renal blood flow, urine flow, and the effects of mannitol, furosemide and bradykinin in acute renal failure induced by renal artery occlusion in the dog [abstract]. Clin Res 30:541A, 1982.

14. Bayati A, Kallskog O, Wolgast M: The long-term outcome of postischemic acute renal failure in the rat: I. A functional study after treatment of SOD and sucrose. Acta Physiol Scand 138:25, 1990.

15. Bayati A, Kallskog O, Nygren K, Wolgast M: The long-term outcome of postischemic acute renal failure in the rat: II. A histopathological study of the untreated kidney. Acta Physiol Scand 138:35, 1990.

16. Wolgast M, Bayati A, Hellberg O, et al: Osmotic diuretics and hemodilution in postischemic renal failure. Renal Fail 14:297, 1992.

17. Pera MD, Zook BC, Harder HC: Effects of mannitol or furosemide diuresis on the nephrotoxicity and physiological disposition of cis-dichloro-diammineplatinum-(II) in rats. Cancer Res 39:1269, 1979.

18. Cvitkovic E, Spaulding J, Bethune V, et al: Improvement of cis-dichlorodiammineplatinum: Therapeutic index in an animal model. Cancer Res 39:1357, 1977.

19. Zager RA, Gamelin LM: Pathogenetic mechanisms in experimental hemoglobinuric acute renal failure. Am J Physiol 256:F446, 1989.

20. Zager RA, Foerder CA, Bredl CR: The influence of mannitol on myoglobinuric acute renal failure: Functional, biochemical, and morphologic assessments. J Am Soc Nephrol 2:848, 1991.

21. Zager RA: Combined mannitol and deferoxamine therapy for myohemoglobinuric renal injury and oxidant tubular stress. J Clin Invest 90:711, 1992.

22. De Torrente A, Miller PD, Cronin RE, et al: Effect of furosemide and acetylcholine in norepinephrine induced acute renal failure. Am J Physiol 235:F131, 1978.

23. Kramer HJ, Neumark A, Schmidt S, et al: Renal functional and metabolic studies on the role of preventive measures in experimental acute ischemic renal failure. Clin Exp Dial Apheresis 7:77, 1983.

24. Kramer HJ Schnermann J, Wasserman C, et al: Prostaglandin-independent protection by furosemide from oliguric ischemic renal failure in conscious rats. Kidney Int 17:455, 1980.

25. Mason J, Kain H. Welsch J, et al: The early phase of experimental acute renal failure: VI. The influence of furosemide. Pfluegers Arch 392:125, 1981.

26. Satta A, Faedda R, Turrim F, et al: Prevention of acute renal failure by diuretics. Z Kardiol 74(Suppl 12):179, 1985.

27. Bayati A, Nygren K, Kallskog O, Wolgast M: The effect of loop diuretics on the long-term outcome of post-ischemic acute renal failure in the rat. Acta Physiol Scand 139:271, 1990.

28. Bayati A: A study in the maintenance phase of ischemic acute renal failure in the rat. Acta Physiol Scand 138:349, 1990.

29. Brezis M, Rosen S, Epstein FH: Acute renal failure. In Brenner BM, Rector FC Jr. (eds): The Kidney, Vol 1, 4th ed. Philadelphia: WB Saunders, 1991, p 993.

30. Brezis M, Rosen S, Silva P, Epstein FH: Renal ischemia: A new perspective. Kidney Int 26:375, 1984.

31. Ufferman RC, Jaenike JR, Freeman RB, et al: Effects of furosemide on low-dose mercuric chloride acute renal failure. Kidney Int 8:362, 1975.

32. Hishida A, Yonemura K, Ohishi K, et al: The effect of saline loading on uranium-induced acute renal failure in rats. Kidney Int 33:942, 1988.

33. De Rougemont D, Wunderlich PF, Torhorst J, et al: HgCl2-induced acute renal failure in the rat: Effects of water diuresis, saline loading, and diuretic drugs. J Lab Clin Med 95:646, 1982.

34. Ward JM, Grabin ME, Berlin E, et al: Prevention of renal failure in rats receiving cis-diamminechloroplatinum II by administration of furosemide. Cancer Res 37:1238, 1977.

35. Lindner A, Cutler RE, Goodman WG: Synergism of dopamine plus furosemide in preventing acute renal failure in the dog. Kidney Int 16:158, 1979.

36. De Rougemont A, Oeschger A, Konrad L, et al: Gentamicin-induced acute renal failure in the rat. Nephron 29:176, 1981.

37. Lawson DH, Macadam RF, Singh H, et al: Effect of furosemide on antibiotic-induced renal damage in rats. J Infect Dis 126:593, 1972.

38. Wilson DR, Thiel G, Arce ML, et al: Glycerol-induced hemoglobinuric acute renal failure in the rat: II. Micropuncture study of the effect of mannitol and isotonic saline on individual nephron function. Nephron 4:337. 1967.

39. Helgeland A, Leren P, Foss OP, et al: Serum glucose levels during long-term observation of treated and untreated men with mild hypertension. Am J Med 76:802, 1984.

40. Aranda JV, Perez J, Sitar DS, et al: Pharmacokinetic disposition and protein binding of furosemide in newborn infants. J Pediatr 93:507, 1978.

41. Robie NW, Nutter DO, Moody C, et al: In vivo analysis of adrenergic receptor activity of dopamine and dobutamine. Am Heart J 90:340, 1975.

42. Adam WR: Aldosterone and dopamine receptors in the kidney: Sites for pharmacologic manipulation of renal function. Kidney Int 18:623, 1980.

43. Goldfarb D, Iaina A, Serban L, et al: Dopamine in the early recovery phase of acute ischaemic renal failure in rats. Isr J Med Sci 17:1069, 1981.

44. Nakamoto M, Shapiro JI, Shanley PF, et al: In vitro and in vivo protective effect of atriopeptin III on ischemic acute renal failure. J Clin Invest 80:698, 1987.

45. Shaw SG, Weidmann P, Hodler J, et al: Atrial natriuretic peptide protects against acute ischemic renal failure in the rat. J Clin Invest 80:1232, 1987.

46. Schafferhans K, Heidbreder E, Grimm D, Heidland A: Human atrial natriuretic factor prevents against norepinephrine-induced acute renal failure in the rat. Klin Wochenschr 64:73, 1986.

47. Seki G, Suzuki K, Nonaka T, et al: Effects of atrial natriuretic peptide on glycerol induced acute renal failure in the rat. Jpn Heart J 33:383, 1992.

48. Capasso G, Anastasio P, Giordano D, et al: Beneficial effects of atrial natriuretic factor on cisplatin-induced acute renal failure. Am J Nephrol 7:228, 1987.

49. Gianello P, Ramboux A, Poelart D, et al: Prevention of acute cyclosporine nephrotoxicity by atrial natriuretic factor after ischemia in the rat. Transplantation 47:512, 1989.

50. Schafferhans K, Heidbreder E, Sperber S, et al: Atrial natriuretic peptide in gentamicin-induced acute renal failure. Kidney Int 34:S101, 1988.

51. Pollock DM, Opgenorth TJ: Beneficial effect of the atrial natriuretic factor analog A68828 in postischemic acute renal failure. J Pharmacol Exp Therap 255:1166, 1990.

52. Pollock DM, Holst M, Opgenorth TJ: Effect of the ANF analog A68828 in cisplatin-induced acute renal failure. J Pharmacol Exp Therap 257:1179, 1991.

53. Pollock DM, Opgenorth TJ: Beneficial effect of the ANF analog A68828 on recovery from ischemic acute renal failure. Renal Fail 14:141, 1992.

54. Conger JD, Falk SA, Hammond WS: Atrial natriuretic peptide and dopamine in established acute renal failure in the rat. Kidney Int 40:21, 1991.

55. Conger JD, Falk SA, Yuan BH, Schrier RW: Atrial natriuretic peptide and dopamine in a rat model of ischemic acute renal failure. Kidney Int 35:1126, 1989.
56. Conger JD, Robinette JB, Kelleher SP: Nephron heterogeneity in ischemic renal failure. Kidney Int 26:422, 1984.
57. Shaw S, Weidmann P, Zimmermann A: Urodilatin, not nitroprusside, combined with dopamine reverses ischemic acute renal failure. Kidney Int 42:1153, 1992.
58. Brenner BM, Lazarus JM: Acute Renal Failure. Philadelphia: WB Saunders, 1987.
59. Mann HJ, Fuks DW, Hemstrom CA: Acute renal failure. Drug Intell Clin Pharm 20:421, 1986.
60. Reineck HJ: Use in renal failure. In Eknoyan G, Martinez-Maldonado M (eds): The Physiological Basis of Diuretic Therapy in Clinical Medicine. Orlando, FL: Grune & Stratton, 1986, pp 277–291.
61. Raymond KH, Hunt JM, Stein JH: Acute and chronic renal failure. In Dirks JH, Sutton RAL (eds): Diuretics: Physiology, Pharmacology and Clinical Use. Philadelphia: WB Saunders, 1986, pp 237–258.
62. Barry KG, Cohen A, Knochel JP, et al: Mannitol infusion: II. The prevention of acute functional renal failure during resection of an aneurysm of the abdominal aorta. N Engl J Med 264:967, 1961.
63. Dawson JL: Post-operative renal function in obstructive jaundice: Effect of a mannitol diuresis. Br Med J 1:82, 1965.
64. Jarnberg PO, Eklund J, Granberg PO: Acute effects of furosemide and mannitol on renal function in the early postoperative period. Acta Anaesthesiol Scand 22:173, 1978.
65. Weimer W, Geerlings W, Bijnen AB, et al: A controlled study of the effect of mannitol on immediate renal function after cadaver donor kidney transplantation. Transplantation 35:99, 1983.
66. Ridgen SP. Dillon MJ, Kind PRN, et al: The beneficial effect of mannitol on postoperative renal function in children undergoing cardiopulmonary bypass surgery. Clin Nephrol 21:148, 1984.
67. Bullock WE, Luke RG, Nuttall CE, et al: Can mannitol reduce amphotericin B nephrotoxicity? Double-blind study and description of a new vascular lesion in kidneys. Antimicrob Agents Chemother 10:555, 1976.
68. Anto HR, Chou SY, Porush JC, et al: Infusion intravenous pyelography and renal function: Effects of hypertonic mannitol in patients with chronic renal insufficiency. Arch Intern Med 141:1652, 1981.
69. Shafi T, Chou SY, Porush JG, et al: Infusion intravenous pyelography and renal function: Effects in patients with chronic renal insufficiency. Arch Intern Med 138:1218, 1978.
70. Prandota J: High doses of furosemide in children with acute renal failure: A preliminary retrospective study. Int Urol Nephrol 23:383, 1992.
71. Luke RG, Briggs JD, Allison MEM, et al: Factors determining response to mannitol in acute renal failure. Am J Med Sci 259:168, 1970.
72. Powell HR, McCredie DA, Rotenberg E: Response to furosemide in acute renal failure: Dissociation of renin and diuretic responses. Clin Nephrol 14:55, 1980.
73. Yeboah ED, Petrie A, Pead JL: Acute renal failure and open heart surgery. Br Med J 1:415, 1972.
74. Lucas CE, Zito JH, Carter KM, et al: Questionable value of furosemide in preventing renal failure. Surgery 82:314, 1977.
75. Cantarovich F, Galli C, Benedetti L, et al: High dose furosemide in established acute renal failure. Br Med J 4:449, 1973.
76. Minuth AN, Terrell JB, Suki WN: Acute renal failure: A study of the course and prognosis of 104 patients and the role of furosemide. Am J Med Sci 271:317, 1977.
77. Kleinknecht D, Ganeval D, Gonzalez-Duque LA, et al: Furosemide in acute oliguric renal failure: A controlled trial. Nephron 17:51, 1976.
78. Brown CB, Ogg CS, Cameron JS, et al: High-dose frusemide in acute reversible intrinsic renal failure. Scott Med J 19(Suppl 1):35, 1974.
79. Brown CB, Ogg CS, Cameron JS: High-dose frusemide in acute renal failure: A controlled trial. Clin Nephrol 15:90, 1981.
80. Lindner A: Synergism of dopamine and furosemide in di-

uretic-resistant, oliguric acute renal failure. Nephron 33:121, 1983.
81. Henderson IS, Beattie TJ, Kennedy AC: Dopamine hydrochloride in oliguric states. Lancet 2:827, 1980.
82. Graziani G, Cantaluppi A, Casati S, et al: Dopamine and frusemide in oliguric acute renal failure. Nephron 37:39, 1984.
83. Mitch WE, Walser M, Buffington M, et al: A simple method of estimating progression of chronic renal failure. Lancet 1:1326, 1976.
84. Mitch WE: Measuring the progression of renal insufficiency. In Mitch WE (ed): The Progressive Nature of Renal Disease (Contemporary Issues in Nephrology Series: Vol 14). New York: Churchill-Livingstone, 1986, pp 167–188.
85. Schreiner GE, Bloomer HA: Effect of chlorothiazide on the edema of cirrhosis, nephrosis, congestive heart failure, and chronic renal insufficiency. N Engl J Med 257:1016, 1957.
86. Hook JB, Blatt AH, Brody MJ, et al: Effects of renal saliuretic-diuretic agents on renal hemodynamics. J Pharmacol Exp Ther 154:667, 1966.
87. Craswell PW, Ezzat E, Kopstein J, et al: Use of metolazone, a new diuretic, in patients with renal disease. Nephron 12:63, 1973.
88. Bennett WM, Proter GA: Efficacy and safety of metolazone in renal failure and the nephrotic syndrome. J Clin Pharmacol 13:357, 1973.
89. Slotkoff L: Clinical efficacy and safety of indapamide in the treatment of edema. Am Heart J 106:233, 1983.
90. Chaffman M, Heel RC, Brogden RN, et al: Indapamide: A review of its pharmacodynamic properties and therapeutic efficacy in hypertension. Drugs 28:189, 1984.
91. Feig PU: Cellular mechanism of action of loop diuretics: Implications for drug effectiveness and adverse effects. Am J Cardiol 57:14A, 1986.
92. Wright FS, Schnermann J: Interference with feedback control of glomerular filtration rate by furosemide, triflocin, and cyanide. J Clin Invest 53:1695, 1974.
93. Brater DC: Use of diuretics in chronic renal insufficiency and nephrotic syndrome. Semin Nephrol 8:333, 1988.
94. Grahnen A, Hammarlund M, Lundquist T. Implications of intraindividual variability in bioavailability studies of furosemide. Eur J Clin Pharmacol 27:595, 1984.
95. Beermann B, Midskov C: Reduced bioavailability and effect of furosemide given with food. Eur J Clin Pharmacol 29:725, 1986.
96. Ogata H, Kawatsu Y, Maruyama Y, et al: Bioavailability and diuretic effect of furosemide during longterm treatment of chronic respiratory failure. Eur J Clin Pharmacol 28:53, 1985.
97. Brater DC, Day B, Burdette A, et al: Bumetanide and furosemide in heart failure. Kidney Int 26:183, 1984.
98. Pentikainen PJ, Pasternack A, Lampainen E, et al: Bumetanide kinetics in renal failure. Clin Pharmacol Ther 37:582, 1985.
99. Lau HSH, Hyneck ML, Berardi RR, et al: Kinetics, dynamics, and bioavailability of bumetanide in healthy subjects and patients with chronic renal failure. Clin Pharmacol Ther 39:635, 1986.
100. Marcantonio LA, Auld WHR, Murdoch WR, et al: The pharmacokinetics and pharmacodynamics of the diuretic bumetanide in hepatic and renal disease. Br J Clin Pharmacol 15:245, 1983.
101. Walter U, Rockel A, Lahn W, et al: Pharmacokinetics of the loop diuretic piretanide in renal failure. Eur J Clin Pharmacol 29:337, 1985.
102. Marone C, Reubi FC, Perisic M, et al: Pharmacokinetics of high doses of piretanide in moderate to severe renal failure. Eur J Clin Pharmacol 27:589, 1984.
103. Berg KJ, Walstad RA, Bergh K: The pharmacokinetic and diuretic effects of piretanide in chronic renal insufficiency. Br J Clin Pharmacol 15:347, 1983.
104. Bouletreau P, Meunier J, Kerihuel JC, et al: Clinical study of muzolimine in acute renal failure, pharmacodynamics and pharmacokinetics. Z Kardiol 74:96, 1985.
105. Howlett MR, Skellern GG, Auld WHR, Murdoch WR: Metabolism of the diuretic bumetanide in healthy subjects and patients with renal impairment. Eur J Clin Pharmacol 38:583, 1990.

106. Morachiello P, Coli U, Landini S, et al: Step-dose of muzolimine at different stages of chronic renal failure: Comparison with furosemide. Z Kardiol 74:115, 1985.

107. Mastrangelo F, Rizzelli S, Corliano C, et al: Muzolimine in advanced chronic renal failure. Z Kardiol 74:109, 1985.

108. Spahn H, Knauf H, Mutschler E: Pharmacokinetics of torasemide and its metabolites in healthy controls and in chronic renal failure. Eur J Clin Pharmacol 39:345, 1990.

109. Knauf H, Mutschler E: Saluretic effect of the loop diuretic torasemide in chronic renal failure. Interdependence of electrolyte excretion. Eur J Clin Pharmacol 39:337, 1990.

110. Brater DC, Anderson SA, Brown-Cartwright D: Response to furosemide in chronic renal insufficiency: Rationale for limited doses. Clin Pharmacol Ther 40:134, 1986.

111. Babini R, DuSouich P: Furosemide pharmacodynamics: Effects of respiratory and acid-base disturbances. J Pharmacol Exp Ther 237:623, 1986.

112. Muth RG: Diuretic properties of furosemide in renal disease. Ann Intern Med 69:249, 1968.

113. Stone WJ, Bennett WM, Cutler RE: Long-term bumetanide treatment of patients with edema due to renal disease. J Clin Pharmacol 21:587, 1981.

114. Bennett WM, Muther RS, Parker RA, et al: Drug therapy in renal failure: Dosing guidelines for adults. Ann Intern Med 93:286, 1980.

115. Knauf H, Spahn H, Mutschler E: The loop diuretic torasemide in chronic renal failure. Pharmacokinetics and pharmacodynamics. Drugs 41:23, 1991.

116. Russo D, Gazzotti RM, Testa A: Torasemide, a new loop diuretic, in patients with chronic renal failure. Nephron 55:141, 1990.

117. Wigand ME, Heidland A: Ototoxic side effects of high doses of furosemide in patients with uremia. Postgrad Med J 47:554, 1971.

118. Rybak L: Furosemide ototoxicity: Clinical and experimental aspects. Laryngoscope 95(Suppl 38):1, 1985.

119. Dikshit K, Vyden JK, Forrester JS, et al: Renal and extrarenal hemodynamic effects of furosemide in congestive heart failure after acute myocardial infarction. N Engl J Med 288:1087, 1973.

120. Johnston GD, Hiatt WR, Nies AS, et al: Factors modifying the early non-diuretic vascular effects of furosemide in man: The possible role of renal prostaglandins. Circ Res 53:630, 1983.

121. Gerber JG: Role of prostaglandins in the hemodynamic and tubular effects of furosemide. Fed Proc 42:1701, 1983.

122. Kelly RA, Wilcox CS, Meyer TW, et al: Response of the kidney to furosemide: II. Effect of captopril on sodium balance. Kidney Int 24:233, 1983.

123. Nelson GIC, Aheya RC, Silke B, et al: Hemodynamic effects of furosemide and its influence on repetitive rapid volume loading in acute myocardial infarction. Eur Heart J 4:706, 1983.

124. Johnston GP, Nicholls DP, Leahey WJ, et al: The effects of captopril on the acute vascular response to furosemide in man. Clin Sci 65:359, 1983.

125. Johnston GD, O'Connor PC, Nicholls DP, et al: The effects of propranolol and digoxin on the acute vascular response to furosemide in normal man. Br J Clin Pharmacol 19:417, 1985.

126. Francis GS, Siegel RM, Goldsmith SR, et al: Acute vasoconstrictor response to intravenous furosemide in patients with chronic congestive heart failure. Ann Intern Med 103:1, 1985.

127. Blackshear JL, Davidman M, Stillman MT: Identification of risk for renal insufficiency from nonsteroidal anti-inflammatory drugs. Arch Intern Med 143:1130, 1983.

128. Nies AS, Gal S, Fadul S, et al: Indomethacin-furosemide interaction: The importance of renal blood flow. J Pharmacol Exp Ther 226:27, 1983.

129. Webster J: Interactions of NSAIDs with diuretics and beta-blockers: Mechanisms and clinical implications. Drugs 30:32, 1985.

130. Kirchner KA: Prostaglandin inhibitors after loop segment chloride uptake during furosemide diuresis. Am J Physiol 248:F698, 1985.

131. Channoavasin P, Seiwell R, Brater DC: Pharmacokinetic-dynamic analysis of the indomethacin-furosemide interaction in man. J Pharmacol Exp Ther 215:77, 1980.

132. Eriksson LO, Beermann B, Kallner M: Aspects of the effects of NSAIDs on renal function in congestive heart failure. Agents Actions 17(Suppl):99, 1985.

133. Wilson TW, McCauley FA, Wells HD: Effects of low-dose aspirin on responsee to furosemide. J Clin Pharmacol 26:100, 1986.

134. Sariban-Sohraby S, Benos DG: The amiloride-sensitive sodium channel. Am J Physiol 250:C175, 1986.

135. Sica DA, Gehr TWB: Triamterene and the kidney. Nephron 51:454, 1989.

136. Knauf H, Reuter K, Mutschler E: Limitation on the use of amiloride in early renal failure. Eur J Clin Pharmacol 28:61, 1985.

137. Luft FC, Sterzel RB, Lang RE, et al: Atrial natriuretic factor determinations and chronic sodium homeostasis. Kidney Int 29:1004, 1986.

138. Luft FC, Lang RE, Aronoff GR, et al: Atriopeptin III kinetics and pharmacodynamics in normal and anephric rats. J Pharmacol Exp Therap 236:416, 1986.

139. Hildebrant DA, Banks RO: Effect of atrial natriuretic factor on renal factor in rats with nephrotic syndrome. Am J Physiol 254:F210, 1988.

140. Sterzel RB, Luft FC, Lang RE, Ganten D: Effects of atrial natriuretic factor in rats with renal insufficiency. J Lab Clin Med 110:63, 1987.

141. Ortola FV, Ballermann B, Brenner BM: Endogenous ANP augments fractional excretion of Pi, Ca, and Na in rats with reduced renal mass. Am J Physiol 255:F1091, 1988.

142. Johns EJ, Rutkowski B: The action of atriopeptin III on renal function in two models of chronic renal failure in the rat. Br J Pharmacol 99:317, 1990.

143. Windus DW, Stokes TJ, Morgan JR, Klahr S: The effects of atrial peptide in humans with chronic renal failure. Am J Kidney Dis 13:477, 1989.

144. Burnier M, Mooser V, Wauters JP, et al: Bolus injections of synthetic atrial natriuretic peptide in patients with chronic renal failure or nephrotic syndrome. J Cardiovasc Pharmacol 13:682, 1989.

145. Woolf AS, Mansell MA, Hoffbrand BI, et al: The effects of low dose intravenous 99-126 atrial natriuretic factor infusion in patients with chronic renal failure. Postgrad Med J 65:362, 1989.

146. Meyer-Lehnert H, Bayer T, Predel HG, et al: Effects of atrial natriuretic peptide on systemic and renal hemodynamics and renal excretory function in patients with chronic renal failure. Klin Wochenschr 69:895, 1991.

147. Takagi T, Nishikawa M, Mori Y, Matsubara H, Inada M: Effects of atrial natriuretic peptide infusion and its metabolism in patients with chronic renal failure. Endocrinol Jpn 38:497, 1991.

148. Gros C, Souque A, Schwartz JC, et al: Protection of atrial natriuretic factor against degradation: Diuretic and natriuretic responses after in vivo inhibition of enkephalinase (EC 3.4.24.11) by acetorphan. Proc Natl Acad Sci U S A 86:7580, 1989.

149. Lecomte JM, Baumer P, Lim C, et al: Stereoselective protection of exogenous and endogenous atrial natriuretic factor by enkephalinase inhibitors in mice and humans. Eur J Pharmacol 179:65, 1990.

150. Dussaule JC, Michel C, Peraldi NM, et al: Inhibition of neutral endopeptidase stimulates renal sodium excretion in patients with chronic renal failure. Clin Sci 84:31, 1993.

151. Ghose RR, Gupta SK: Synergistic action of metolazone with "loop" diuretics. Br Med J 282:1432, 1981.

152. Oster JR, Epstein M, Smaller S: Combined therapy with thiazide-type and loop diuretic agents for resistant sodium retention. Ann Intern Med 99:104, 1983.

153. Brater DC, Pressley RH, Anderson SA: Mechanisms of the synergistic combination of metolazone and bumetanide. J Pharmacol Exp Ther 233:70, 1985.

154. Marone C, Muggli F, Lahn W, et al: Pharmacokinetic and pharmacodynamic interaction between furosemide and metolazone in man. Eur J Clin Invest 15:253, 1985.

155. Arnold WC: Efficacy of metolazone and furosemide in children with furosemide-resistant edema. Pediatrics 74:872, 1984.

156. Wollam GL, Tarazi RC, Bravo EL, et al: Diuretic potency

of combined hydrochlorothiazide and furosemide therapy in patients with azotemia. Am J Med 72:929, 1982.

157. Gavin EH: A comparison of combinations of diuretics in nephrotic edema. Am J Dis Child 141:769, 1987.

158. Hropot M, Fowler N, Karlmark B, et al: Tubular action of diuretics: Distal effects on electrolyte transport and acidification. Kidney Int 28:477, 1985.

159. Hill NS: Fluid and electrolyte considerations in diuretic therapy for hypertensive patients with chronic obstructive pulmonary disease. Arch Intern Med 146:129, 1986.

160. Kaye M: The effect of a single oral dose of the carbonic anhydrase inhibitor acetazolamide in renal disease. J Clin Invest 34:277, 1955.

161. Maisey DN, Brown RD: Acetazolamide and symptomatic metabolic acidosis in mild renal failure. Br Med J 283:1527, 1981.

162. Brater DC: Resistance to diuretics: Emphasis on a pharmacological perspective. Drugs 22:477, 1981.

163. Rane A, Villeneuve JP, Stone WJ, et al: Plasma binding and disposition of furosemide in the nephrotic syndrome and in uremia. Clin Pharmacol Ther 24:199, 1978.

164. Prandota J, Pruitt AW: Furosemide binding to human albumin and plasma of nephrotic children. Clin Pharmacol Ther 17:159, 1975.

165. Keller E, Hoppe-Seyler G, Schollmeyer P: Disposition and diuretic effect of furosemide in the nephrotic syndrome. Clin Pharmacol Ther 12:442, 1982.

166. Bank N, Lief PD, Piczon O: Use of diuretics in treatment of hypertension secondary to renal disease. Arch Intern Med 138:1524, 1978.

167. Kaufman AM, Levitt MF: The effect of diuretics on systemic and renal hemodynamics in patients with renal insufficiency. Am J Kidney Dis 5:A71, 1985.

168. Faubert PF, Porush JG: Managing hypertension in chronic renal disease. Geriatrics 42:49, 1987.

169. Mitchell HC, Graham RM, Pettinger WA: Renal function during long-term treatment of hypertension with minoxidil. Ann Intern Med 93:676, 1980.

170. Friedlaender MM, Rubinger D, Popovtzer MM: Improved renal function in patients with primary renal disease after control of severe hypertension. Am J Nephrol 2:12, 1982.

171. Parving HH, Andersen AR, Smidt UM, et al: Effect of antihypertensive treatment on kidney function in diabetic nephropathy. Br Med J 294:1443, 1987.

172. Marre M, LeBlanc H, Suarez L, et al: Converting enzyme inhibition and kidney function in nontensive diabetic patients with persistent microalbuminemia. Br Med J 294:1448, 1987.

173. Meyer TW, Anderson S, Rennke HG, et al: Converting enzyme inhibitor therapy limits progressive glomerular injury in rats with renal insufficiency. Am J Med 79:31, 1985.

174. Kurtzman NA: Acquired distal renal tubular acidosis. Kidney Int 24:807, 1983.

175. Sebastian A, Schambelan M: Amelioration of type 4 renal tubular acidosis in chronic renal failure with furosemide. Kidney Int 12:534A, 1977.

176. Arief AI, Lazarowitz VC, Guisado R: Experimental dialysis disequilibrium syndrome: Prevention with glycerol. Kidney Int 14:270, 1978.

177. Smith TW, Braunwald EB, Kelly RA: Management of heart failure. In Braunwald EB (ed): Heart Disease: A Textbook of Cardiovascular Medicine. Philadelphia: WB Saunders, 1987, pp 485–543.

178. Puschett JB: Clinical pharmacologic implications in diuretic selection. Am J Cardiol 57:6A, 1986.

179. Lant A: Diuretics: Clinical pharmacology and therapeutic use. Drugs Part I 29:57–87; Part II 29:162–188, 1985.

180. Kokko JP: Site and mechanism of action of diuretics. Am J Med 77:11, 1984.

181. Berger BE, Warnock DG: Clinical uses and mechanisms of action of diuretic agents. In Brenner BM, Rector FC (eds): The Kidney, Vol 1. Philadelphia: WB Saunders, 1986, pp 433–455.

182. Mudge GH, Wainer IM: Drugs affecting renal function and electrolyte metabolism. In Gilman AF, Gordman LS, Rall TW, et al (eds): The Pharmacologic Basis of Therapeutics, 7th ed. New York: Macmillan, 1985, pp 879–907.

183. Frommer JP, Wesson DE, Eknoyan G: Side effects and complications of diuretic therapy. In Eknoyan G, Martinez-Maldonado M (eds): The Physiological Basis of Diuretic Therapy in Clinical Medicine. Orlando, FL: Grune & Stratton, 1986, pp 293–309.

184. Dirks JH, Sutton RAL (eds): Section III: Complications of diuretic therapy. In Dirks JH, Sutton RAL (eds): Diuretics: Physiology, Pharmacology & Clinical Use. Philadelphia: WB Saunders, 1986, pp 287–373.

185. Dal Canton A, Fuiano G, Conte G, et al: Mechanism of increased plasma urea after diuretic therapy in uraemic patients. Clin Sci 68:255, 1985.

186. Davidman M, Olson P, Kohen J, et al: Iatrogenic renal disease. Arch Intern Med 151:1809, 1991.

187. Hricik DE, Browning PJ, Kopelman R, et al: Captopril-induced functional renal insufficiency in patients with bilateral renal-artery stenoses or renal-artery stenosis in a solitary kidney. N Engl J Med 6:308, 1983.

188. Hricik DE: Captopril-induced renal insufficiency and the role of sodium volume. Ann Intern Med 3:103, 222, 1985.

189. Funck-Bretano C, Chatellier G, Alexandre JM: Reversible renal failure after combined treatment with enalapril and frusemide in a patient with congestive heart failure. Br Heart J 55:596, 1986.

190. Packer M, Lee WH, Medina N, et al: Functional renal insufficiency during long-term therapy with captopril and enalapril in severe chronic heart failure. Ann Intern Med 106:346, 1987.

191. McMurray J, Matthews DM: Consequences of fluid loss in patients treated with ACE inhibitors. Postgrad Med J 63:385, 1987.

192. Hogg KJ, Hillis WS: Captopril/metolazone-induced renal failure. Lancet 1:501, 1986.

193. Packer M, Lee WH, Yushak M, et al: Comparison of captopril and enalapril in patients with severe chronic heart failure. N Engl J Med 315:847, 1986.

194. Giles TD, Chiaromida A, De Maric T, et al: A comparison of lisinopril and captopril in congestive heart failure [abstract]. Circulation 74(Suppl 2):11, 1986.

195. Ram CVS, Garrett BN, Kaplan NM: Moderate sodium restriction and various diuretics in the treatment of hypertension. Arch Intern Med 141:1015, 1981.

196. Wilcox CS, Mitch WE, Kelly RA, et al: Factors affecting potassium balance during furosemide administration. Clin Sci 67:195, 1984.

197. Epstein FH, Rosa RM: Adrenergic control of serum potassium. N Engl J Med 309:1450, 1983.

198. Thier SO: Potassium physiology. Am J Med 80(Suppl 4A):3, 1986.

199. Tannen RL: Diuretic-induced hypokalemia. Kidney Int 28:988, 1985.

200. Hollenberg NK: Potassium, rnagnesium and cardiovascular morbidity. Am J Med 80(Suppl 4A):1, 1986.

201. Melby JC: A symposium: Hypertension, diuretics, and diuretic-induced hypokalemia. Am J Cardiol 58:1A, 1986.

202. Papademetriou B: Diuretics, hypokalemia, and cardiac arrhythmias: A critical analysis. Am Heart J 111:1217, 1986.

203. Kassirer JP, Harrington JT: Fending off the potassium pushers. N Engl J Med 312:785, 1985.

204. Atwood JE, Gardin JM: Diuretics, hypokalemia and ventricular ectopy. Arch Intern Med 145:1185, 1985.

205. Knochel JP: Diuretic-induced hypokalemia. Am J Med 77(5A):18, 1984.

206. Packer M: Sudden unexpected death in patients with congestive heart failure: A second frontier. Circulation 72:681, 1985.

207. Dyckner T, Wester PO: Potassium/magnesium depletion in patients with cardiovascular disease. Am J Med 82(Suppl 3A):11, 1987.

208. Packer M, Gottlieb SS, Blum MA: Immediate and long-term pathophysiologic mechanisms underlying the genesis of sudden cardiac death in patients with congestive heart failure. Am J Med 82(Suppl 3A):4, 1987.

209. Packer M: Potential role of potassium as a determinant of morbidity and mortality in patients with systemic hypertension and congestive heart failure. Am J Cardiol 65:45E, 1990.

210. Podrid PJ: Potassium and ventricular arrhythmias. Am J Cardiol 65:33E, 1990.

211. Freis ED: The cardiotoxicity of thiazide diuretics: Review of the evidence. J Hypertens 8:S23, 1990.
212. Kelly RA: Cardiac glycosides and congestive heart failure. Am J Cardiol 65:10E, 1990.
213. Chakko SC, Frutchey J, Gheorghiade M: Life-threatening hyperkalemia in severe heart failure. Am Heart J 117:1083, 1989.
214. Cleland JGF, Dargie HO, East BW, et al: Total body and serum electrolyte composition in heart failure: The effect of captopril. Eur Heart J 6:681, 1985.
215. Kahn AM: Effect of diuretics on the renal handling of urate. Semin Nephrol 8:305, 1988.
216. Reinhart RA: Magnesium metabolism: A review with special reference to the relationship between intracellular content and serum levels. Arch Intern Med 148:2415, 1988.
217. Dorup I, Skajaa K, Clausen T, Kjeldsen K: Reduced concentrations of potassium, magnesium, and sodium-potassium pumps in human skeletal muscle during treatment with diuretics. Br Med J 296:455, 1988.
218. Abraham AS, Rosenman D, Meshulam Z, et al: Serum, lymphocyte, and erythrocyte potassium, magnesium, and calcium concentrations and their relation to tachyarrhythmias in patients with acute myocardial infarction. Am J Med 81:983, 1986.
219. Reinhart RA, Marx JJ, Broste SK, Hass RG: Myocardial magnesium: Relation to laboratory and clinical variables in patients undergoing cardiac surgery. J Am Coll Cardiol 17:651, 1991.
220. Gottlieb SS, Baruch L, Lukin ML, et al: Prognostic importance of the serum magnesium concentration in patients with congestive heart failure. J Am Coll Cardiol 16:827, 1990.
221. Ralston MA, Murnane MR, Unverferth DV, Leier CV: Serum and tissue magnesium concentrations in patients with heart failure and serious ventricular arrhythmias. Ann Intern Med 113:841, 1990.
222. Seelig M: Cardiovascular consequences of magnesium deficiency and loss: Pathogenesis, prevalence and manifestations—magnesium and chloride loss in refractory potassium repletion. Am J Cardiol 63:4G, 1989.
223. Iseri LT: Role of magnesium in cardiac tachyarrhythmias. Am J Cardiol 65:47K, 1990.
224. Stearns RH, Spital A: Disorders of water balance. In Kokko JP, Tannen RL (eds): Fluids and Electrolytes. Philadelphia: WB Saunders, 1990.
225. Fessel WJ: Renal outcomes of gout and hyperuricemia. Am J Med 67:74, 1979.
226. Johnson MW, Mitch WE: The risks of asymptomatic hyperuricemia and the use of uricosuric diuretics. Drugs 21:220, 1981.
227. Roubenoff R: Gout and hypertension. Rheum Dis Clin North Am 16:539, 1990.
228. Pasternack A, Leino T, Solakivi-Jaakkola J, et al: Effect of furosemide on the lipid abnormalities in chronic renal failure. Acta Med Scand 214:153, 1983.
229. Kelly RA, Mitch WE: The systemic consequence of renal failure. In Eknoyan GE, Krickel JP (eds): Nutrition. Orlando, FL: Grune & Stratton, 1984, pp 461–500.
230. Bloomgarden ZT, Ginsberg-Fellner F, Rayfield EJ, et al: Elevated hemoglobin A1C and low-density cholesterol levels in thiazide-treated diabetes. Am J Med 77:823, 1984.
231. Raftery EB: The metabolic effects of diuretics and other antihypertensive drugs: A perspective as of 1989. Int J Cardiol 28:143, 1990.
232. Thompson WG: An assault on old friends: Thiazide diuretics under siege. Am J Med Sci 300:152, 1990.
233. Ames R: Effects of diuretic drugs on the lipid profile. Drugs 36:33, 1988.
234. Johnson BF, Danylchuk MA: The relevance of plasma lipid changes with cardiovascular drug therapy. Med Clin North Am 73:449, 1989.
235. Freis ED: Critique of the clinical importance of diuretic-induced hypokalemia and elevated cholesterol level. Arch Intern Med 149:2640, 1989.
236. Luther RR, Glassman HN, Estep CB, et al: The effects of terazosin and methyclothiazide on blood pressure and serum lipids. Am Heart J 117:842, 1989.
237. Percy-Stable E, Carlis PV: Thiazide-induced disturbances in carbohydrate, lipid and potassium metabolism. Am Heart J 106:245, 1983.
238. Bloomgarden ZT, Ginsberg-Fellner F, Rayfield EJ, et al: Elevated hemoglobin A1C and low-density cholesterol levels in thiazide-treated diabetes. Am J Med 77:823, 1984.
239. Ames RP: Coronary heart disease and the treatment of hypertension: Impact of diuretics on serum lipids and glucose. J Cardiovasc Pharmacol 6:S466, 1984.
240. Hietanen E, Hamalainen H, Maki J, et al: Beta-blockers, diuretics and physical fitness as determinants of serum lipids in myocardial infarction patients. Scand J Clin Lab Invest 46:97, 1986.
241. Helgeland A: The impact in serum lipids of combinations of diuretics and alpha-blockers and of beta-blockers alone. J Cardiovasc Pharmacol 6:S474, 1984.
242. Gerber A, Weidmann P, Bianchetti MG, et al: Serum lipoproteins during treatment with the antihypertensive agent indapamide. Hypertension 7(Suppl 2):164, 1985.
243. Multiple Risk Factor Intervention Trial Research Group: Multiple Risk Factor Intervention Trial: Risk factor changes and mortality results. JAMA 248:1465, 1982.
244. Goldman AI, Steele BW, Schnaper HW, et al: Serum lipoprotein levels during chlorthalidone therapy—A Veterans Administration–National Heart, Lung, and Blood Institute cooperative study on antihypertensive therapy: Mild hypertension. JAMA 244:1691, 1980.
245. Frick MH, Elo O, Haapa K, et al: Helsinki Heart Study: Primary prevention trial with gemfibrozil in middle-aged men with dyslipidemia. N Engl J Med 317:1237, 1987.
246. Linn S, Fulwood R, Rifkind B, et al: High density lipoprotein cholesterol levels among US adults by selected demographic and socioeconomic variables. Am J Epidemiol 129:281, 1989.
247. Samuelsson O, Wilhelmsen L, Andersson OK, et al: Cardiovascular morbidity in relation to change in blood pressure and serum cholesterol levels in treated hypertension. JAMA 258:1768, 1987.
248. O'Byrne S, Feely J: Effects of drugs on glucose tolerance in non-insulin-dependent diabetics (Part I). Drugs 40:6, 1990.
249. Pollare T: Insulin sensitivity and blood lipids during antihypertensive treatment with special reference to ACE inhibition. J Diabet Compl 4:75, 1990.
250. Pollare T, Lithell H, Berne C: A comparison of the effects of hydrochlorothiazide and captopril on glucose and lipid metabolism in patients with hypertension. N Engl J Med 321:868, 1989.
251. Black HR: The coronary artery disease paradox: The role of hyperinsulinemia and insulin resistance and implications for therapy. J Cardiovasc Pharmacol 15:S26, 1990.
252. Burry JN, Lawrence JR: Phototoxic blisters from high furosemide dosage. Br J Dermatol 94:495, 1976.
253. Freydenriech G, Pindborg T, Schmidt H: Bullous dermatosis among patients with chronic renal failure on high-dose furosemide. Acta Med Scand 202:61, 1977.
254. Lyons H, Pinn VW, Cortell S, et al: Allergic interstitial nephritis causing reversible renal failure in four patients with idiopathic nephrotic syndrome. N Engl J Med 288:124, 1973.
255. Magil AB, Balloon HS, Cameron EC, et al: Acute interstitial nephritis associated with thiazide diuretics. Am J Med 69:939, 1980.

CHAPTER 37

Diuretics in Hypertension

Ray W. Gifford, Jr., M.D., and Ray Borazanian, B.S.

Nearly a decade before the introduction of effective orally administered diuretics, Megibow et al.[1] demonstrated that frequent parenteral injections of a mercurial diuretic reduced the blood pressure of patients with severe hypertension. However, until chlorothiazide was introduced in 1957, the inconvenience of frequent parenteral injections greatly limited the clinical usefulness of diuretics in the management of hypertension.

After 1958, a multitude of thiazide and related compounds became available, and diuretics assumed a leadership position among antihypertensive drugs. Clinical experience led physicians to the almost unanimous conclusion that orally administered diuretics were preferable to the alternatives available before 1975 to initiate antihypertensive therapy. The alternatives were reserpine and its derivatives, hydralazine, ganglion-blocking agents (hexamethonium, pentolinium tartrate, and mecamylamine), veratrum compounds, methyldopa, and guanethidine. All of these produced disagreeable side effects that often prevented adequate control of blood pressure; furthermore, their prolonged administration led to fluid retention and pseudoresistance.

Now that newer drugs are available—including β-adrenergic blocking agents, calcium antagonists, selective α_1-adrenergic blocking agents, an α/β-blocker, and angiotensin-converting enzyme (ACE) inhibitors, the traditional role of diuretics as initial monotherapy is being challenged. However, only the diuretics and the β-blockers have been subjected to randomized controlled clinical trials that have demonstrated reductions in morbidity and mortality.[2-4] For this reason, the report of the fifth Joint National Committee on Detection, Evaluation, and Treatment of High Blood Pressure[5] recommended that these agents be given preference in the initial monotherapy of hypertension, unless there are contraindications to their use or special indications for another class of agents.

Similar recommendations have been made by the Canadian[6] and British[7] Hypertension Societies and by a Consensus Development Conference Report to the National Advisory Committee on Core Health and Disability Support Services in New Zealand.[8] The World Health Organization–International Society of Hypertension Guidelines acknowledged that only the diuretics and β-blockers have been shown to reduce cardiovascular morbidity and mortality in randomized clinical trials but rejected this as sufficient justification for recommending that they be given preference in selecting the appropriate drug for initial therapy.[9]

MECHANISM OF ACTION

More than 35 years after the introduction of chlorothiazide, the mechanism of the antihypertensive action of diuretics has not been conclusively elucidated.[10] Several possible mechanisms are discussed in the following sections.

Depletion of Plasma Volume

Plasma volume depletion may play a role in the immediate reduction of blood pressure but probably is not the entire explanation for the chronic antihypertensive effect of orally administered diuretics.[10] During the first 4 to 6 weeks of treatment with a diuretic, it is possible to measure a reduction in extracellular fluid volume, including plasma volume, but this depletion is less obvious thereafter even though blood pressure stays down.[11-13] An intact sympathetic nervous system should be able to compensate for the chronic volume loss, just as it does acutely in blood donors after phlebotomy.

Debate still exists about whether extracellular and plasma volume eventually returns to[12-15] or remains significantly below pretreatment levels.[16-18] Vardan et al.[19] found no decrease in plasma volume at 1 month or 1 year after initiating antihypertensive therapy with 50 mg of hydrochlorothiazide (HCTZ) in 13 elderly patients with isolated systolic hypertension, even though average blood pressure decreased by 38 mmHg systolic and 13 mmHg diastolic.

Elimination of Edema in Walls of Arterioles

Tobian and Binion[20] have demonstrated that the media and intima of renal arteries obtained at autopsy have a higher sodium and water content in hypertensive than in normotensive subjects. Tobian et al.[21] also reported that the mesenteric arterioles of rats in which renovascular hypertension was created by removal of one kidney and placement of a clip on the remaining renal artery had 13% more water per 100 g of solids than did arterioles taken from rats whose renovascular hypertension had been reversed by removing the clip. It is conceivable that edema of the arteriolar wall compromises the lumen and increases peripheral vascular resistance. If diuretic therapy removes the edema from the walls of the arterioles, reduction in blood pressure might result from a reduction in total peripheral resistance. However, no direct evidence suggests that the arterioles of hypertensive human subjects are waterlogged or, if they are, that diuretic treatment will remove the fluid.

Reduction in Vascular Reactivity

Numerous studies[22-25] have shown that diuretic therapy reduces vascular reactivity to infusions of norepinephrine and that forearm blood flow paradoxically increases in normotensive subjects receiving orally administered diuretic when norepinephrine is infused. Aoki and Brody[26] demonstrated that methyclothiazide-treated rats with induced renal hypertension exhibited a significant lesser vascular responsiveness in the hind limb to lumbar sympathetic nerve stimulation than was observed in untreated hypertensive rats. Yet, spontaneous sympathetic nerve activity was not reduced by thiazide therapy in renal hypertensive rats.[26]

Therefore, it appears that diuretic treatment diminishes the responsiveness of the vascular bed to sympathetic stimulation without affecting sympathetic nerve activity per se. A decrease in venous reactivity has also been reported in hypertensive patients treated with hydrochlorothiazide.[27] This increase in venous capacitance would permit venous pooling and reduce venous return of blood to the heart, which would perhaps explain the reduction of cardiac output observed in the first few weeks of therapy with diuretics. Schohn and Jahn[28] measured blood pressure and changes in pulmonary capillary wedge pressure and pressure in the right atrium in response to infusions of norepinephrine and angiotensin II in five oliguric patients undergoing dialysis. They found that spironolactone plus altizide reduced the reactivity to these vasoconstrictors, and concluded that the antihypertensive effect of diuretics is mainly due to a direct action on the resistance and capacitance vessels. This acute experiment in oliguric patients may not be relevant to prolonged administration of diuretics to hypertensive patients with normal renal function.

The decrease in vascular responsiveness could theoretically be due to an increase in the ratio of extracellular to intracellular sodium ($Na_e : Na_i$) in the smooth muscle cells of the arterioles and veins, making them less responsive to sympathetic stimulation.[29] The shift in sodium from the intracellular to the extracellular space could occur without any net loss of total body sodium, which is consistent with studies that have failed to show a long-term decrease in total exchangeable sodium during chronic diuretic therapy.[12, 14]

Emerging evidence shows that it is the concentration of intracellular calcium ions, not sodium, that prompts vascular smooth muscle contraction.[30, 31] Prostacyclins, in particular the formation of prostanoid by the kidney, as well as the prostacyclin-stimulated formation of antihypertensive lipids have been suggested as a mechanism for the vasodilation induced by diuretics.[10]

Several observations[11, 32–34] of cardiovascular hemodynamics are consistent with the theory that the initial reduction in blood pressure during the first weeks of diuretic therapy is due to volume depletion. During this period, cardiac output falls, presumably because of decreased venous return. Total peripheral vascular resistance remains unchanged or even increases slightly, body weight usually decreases 1.0 to 1.5 kg (2 or 3 lbs), and plasma renin activity increases. Thereafter, cardiac output returns to pretreatment levels, total peripheral vascular resistance declines below

pretreatment levels, and plasma and extracellular fluid volume as well as body weight approach or return to pretreatment levels. The observations that plasma renin activity decreases and body weight and plasma volume increase abruptly when long-term treatment with a diuretic is discontinued suggest that some depletion of extracellular fluid volume continues during long-term therapy.[15, 18]

The theory that best explains these observations is that the initial reduction in blood pressure is solely the result of volume depletion, but the long-term antihypertensive effect of diuretics is the result of diminished vascular responsiveness to sympathetic nervous stimulation, which would ordinarily compensate for the small but persistent depletion of plasma volume.[18] Figure 37–1 is a schematic representation of this hypothesis.[11]

The initial decrease in blood pressure due to volume depletion may be related to dosage of the diuretic. In 18 elderly patients with isolated systolic hypertension receiving 50 mg of HCTZ daily, Vardan et al.[35] found no decrease in cardiac output at the end of 1 month even though systolic and diastolic blood pressures were significantly reduced by a decrease in total peripheral resistance.

The importance of volume control in the management of hypertension has been emphasized by Dustan et al.[36] and Finnerty et al.[37] Some nondiuretic agents, especially adrenergic-inhibiting drugs (except

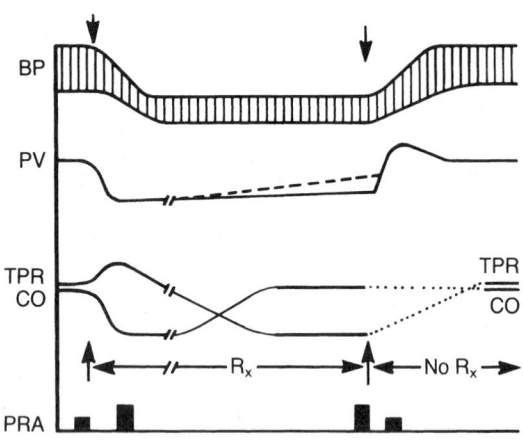

Figure 37–1. Suggested mechanism for the antihypertensive effect of chronic oral diuretic therapy. During the first 4 to 6 weeks of diuretic therapy, a measurable decrease occurs in plasma volume (PV) and extracellular fluid volume (ECFV), which presumably leads to a decrease in venous return, a fall in cardiac output (CO) and blood pressure (BP), and a rise in plasma renin activity (PRA). Thereafter, PV and ECFV tend to return toward normal, with a rise in CO to pretreatment levels and a decrease in total peripheral resistance (TPR) that presumably is mediated by impaired response of the arterioles to sympathetic stimulation. BP remains down throughout the period of treatment. The fact that PRA remains elevated as long as the diuretic is administered suggests that PV and ECFV do not return to normal. The abrupt rise in PV after discontinuation of diuretic therapy suggests that PV has not returned to normal, but overshoot may also play a part. Rx, treatment with diuretic; No Rx, no treatment. (From Tarazi RC: Diuretic drugs: Mechanisms of antihypertensive action. *In* Onesti G, Kim KE, Moyer JH [eds]: Hypertension: Mechanisms and Management. New York: Grune & Stratton, 1973, pp 251–260.)

for β-blockers) and direct vasodilators (hydralazine, minoxidil), when used as monotherapy, lead to occult fluid retention that ultimately counteracts their hypotensive effects (pseudotolerance). This is prevented by having a diuretic in the regimen from the outset, or it is corrected if a diuretic is added to the regimen when it occurs. Indeed, lack of a diuretic in the regimen is such a common cause of refractory hypertension that a widely accepted definition of resistant hypertension stipulates that blood pressure does not respond to a rational triple-drug regimen *that includes a diuretic*.[38]

PREPARATIONS AND DOSAGES

Table 37–1 is adapted from the report of the Fifth Joint National Committee,[5] listing the available diuretics and their dosages as well as some of their side effects.

The thiazide and thiazide-like compounds are all equally effective as antihypertensive agents when given in equivalent doses. Most, if not all, of these agents are effective when given once daily. They share similar metabolic side effects (see Table 37–1). The chief differences among them relate to dosage and cost. Metolazone and indapamide are presumably more effective diuretics than the others when glomerular filtration rate is impaired. The claim that indapamide has fewer and less severe metabolic side effects than the others has not been substantiated convincingly.

Careful studies[39–43] have demonstrated that effective antihypertensive dosages of diuretics are much lower than have customarily been prescribed. The range of effective antihypertensive doses is from 12.5 to 50 mg of hydrochlorothiazide or chlorthalidone and 2.5 to 5 mg of bendroflumethiazide per day. Presumably, lower doses of other thiazide and thiazide-like diuretics shown in Table 37–1 might be effective; the doses listed in that table reflect current recommendations of the Fifth Joint National Committee on Detection, Evaluation, and Treatment of High Blood Pressure.[5] The metabolic side effects shown in Table 37–1 are dose-dependent,[39–43] and a lessening of the benefit-risk ratio clearly occurs when doses above 50 mg daily are prescribed. The benefit-cost ratio also declines with doses above this level.

Except for torsemide, the loop diuretics (see Table 37–1) are short-acting and therefore must be given at least twice daily. Although they are more potent diuretics than the thiazides, they are no more effective in controlling hypertension. Their short duration of action makes them less desirable agents unless renal function is impaired, in which case they (or metolazone or indapamide) become the agents of choice. Ethacrynic acid is the only nonsulfonamide diuretic except for the potassium-sparing agents. Consequently, ethacrynic acid is useful when patients cannot tolerate sulfonamide compounds, especially when photosensitivity is a problem.

The potassium-sparing agents are not potent diuretics and are seldom used by themselves in managing hypertension. They are useful in conjunction with a thiazide-type diuretic to prevent diuretic-induced hypokalemia. The risk of hyperkalemia must be considered when prescribing these agents, because hyperkalemia is at least as lethal as hypokalemia.

Potassium-sparing diuretics should be prescribed with caution if at all for patients with renal failure; for patients who use salt substitutes, most of which contain potassium; and for patients who are receiving β-blockers, ACE inhibitors, or nonsteroidal antiinflammatory drugs, all of which tend to increase serum potassium concentration. Patients with hyporeninemic hypoaldosteronism can become severely hyperkalemic when receiving potassium-sparing diuretics. Usually, they are elderly, often with non-insulin-dependent diabetes mellitus, and their pretreatment serum potassium concentration is frequently greater than 5 mEq/L.

CHARACTERISTICS OF THE IDEAL ANTIHYPERTENSIVE DRUG

To position the diuretics in the contemporary competition for initial therapy of hypertension, it is appropriate to list the attributes of the ideal drug by which the various alternatives for initial monotherapy can be measured (Table 37–2). In an attempt to provide some objectivity by which to compare drugs, numeric values were assigned to quantitate the degree to which each class of antihypertensive drugs possesses the characteristics in Table 37–2.[44] The conclusion was that, based on these characteristics, diuretics were the agents of choice.

The fallacy in this method was that the relative importance of the different attributes shown in Table 37–2 was not considered. Obviously, if a drug is neither safe nor effective, it fails to qualify even if it has all the other attributes. The same is true if it is unsafe but effective.

The diuretics have been challenged on the basis of safety and, to some extent, symptomatic side effects. In all other categories, the diuretics score as well as or better than their alternatives. Specifically, they are less expensive than the alternatives, they are easy to titrate because of their flat dose-response curve above doses of 25 or 50 mg daily, and most have durations of action long enough to permit once-daily dosage. Diuretics are the gold standard against which other drugs are compared for effectiveness in reducing blood pressure.

Only the diuretics and β-blockers have been subjected to large randomized clinical trials and, with one exception,[45] diuretic-based therapy has been effective in reducing cardiovascular morbidity and mortality, especially strokes[2–4] (Table 37–3).[45–57] β-Blockers have been employed as monotherapy in only three long-term, placebo-controlled trials,[53, 56, 57] and the calcium antagonists, ACE inhibitors, and α₁-blocking agents have not been used in randomized trials to determine long-term effects on morbidity and mortality in primary hypertension.

Long-term observational studies led to the expecta-

Table 37–1. **Diuretics and Their Side Effects**

Agent	Usual Daily Dose (mg)*	Precautions and Special Considerations	Side Effects
Thiazides and Related Sulfonamide Diuretics			
Bendroflumethiazide (Naturetin)	2.5–5	May be ineffective in renal failure except for indapamide and metolazone; hypokalemia increases digitalis toxicity; may cause an increase in blood levels of lithium; may precipitate acute gout	Hypokalemia, hypomagnesemia, hyperuricemia, glucose intolerance, insulin resistance, hypercholesterolemia, increased LDL cholesterol, hypertriglyceridemia, hypercalcemia, sexual dysfunction, weakness, photosensitivity (except for ethacrynic acid), leukopenia, allergic skin rash, decrease in urinary calcium excretion
Benzthiazide (Exna)	12.5–50		
Chlorothiazide (Diuril)	125–500†		
Chlorthalidone (Hygroton)	12.5–50		
Hydrochlorothiazide (HydroDIURIL, Esidrix)	12.5–50		
Hydroflumethiazide (Saluron, Diucardin)	12.5–50		
Indapamide (Lozol)	1.25–5		
Methyclothiazide (Enduron)	2.5–5		
Metolazone (Zaroxolyn)	2.5–5		
Metolazone (Mykrox)	0.5–1		
Polythiazide (Renese)	1–4		
Quinethazone (Hydromox)	25–100		
Loop Diuretics‡			
Bumetanide (Bumex)	0.5–5†	Effective in chronic renal failure	As above, except for hypercalcemia and an increase in urinary calcium excretion
Ethacrynic acid (Edecrin)	25–100†		
Furosemide (Lasix)	20–320†		
Torsemide (Demadex)	2.5–20		
Potassium-Sparing Agents			
Amiloride (Midamor)	5–10	Danger of hyperkalemia in patients receiving a potassium supplement, a potassium-containing salt substitute, an ACE inhibitor, or a nonsteroidal antiinflammatory drug, as well as in patients with renal failure; can cause renal failure in patients treated with a nonsteroidal antiinflammatory drug (indomethacin + triamterene); may increase blood levels of lithium; spironolactone interferes with digoxin immunoassay; danger of renal calculi (triamterene)	Hyperkalemia Spironolactone only— gynecomastia, mastodynia, gastrointestinal irritation, drowsiness, lethargy, irregular menses or postmenopausal bleeding, hirsutism
Spironolactone (Aldactone)	25–100†		
Triamterene (Dyrenium)	50–150†		

Combination Thiazide and Potassium-Sparing Diuretic Preparations

Product	Dose (Tablets or Capsules/Day)	Product	Dose (Tablets or Capsules/Day)
Hydrochlorothiazide 25 mg + triamterene 37.5 mg (Maxzide 25)	½–2	Hydrochlorothiazide 25 mg + spironolactone 25 mg (Aldactazide 25)	1–2
Hydrochlorothiazide 50 mg + triamterene 75 mg (Maxzide 50)	½–1	Hydrochlorothiazide 50 mg + spironolactone 50 mg (Aldactazide 50)	½–1
Hydrochlorothiazide 25 mg + triamterene 37.5 mg (Dyazide)	1–2	Hydrochlorothiazide 50 mg + amiloride 5 mg (Moduretic)	½–1

ACE, angiotensin-converting enzyme; LDL, low-density lipoprotein.
*The dosage range may differ slightly from recommended dosage in *Physicians' Desk Reference* or package insert. Given once daily unless otherwise indicated.
†This drug is usually given in divided doses twice daily.
‡Larger doses of loop diuretics may be required in patients with renal failure.

tion that treating hypertension would reduce the incidence of coronary events by 20% to 25% and of strokes by approximately 40%.[58] However, although the incidence of strokes was reduced by the expected amount, coronary events were only reduced by 14% to 16%.[2, 3] Several hypotheses have been advanced to explain this discrepancy, including the possibility that the adverse metabolic effects of diuretics and β-blockers compromised their expected beneficial effects of lowering the blood pressure. However, it is possible that the treatment trials were too short to demonstrate such a reduction.[59] Most of the observational studies from which the risks of hypertension were calculated

lasted between 6 and 25 years, whereas the average duration of the treatment trials was less than 5 years.[59] Moreover, the 8.5-year follow-up data from the Hypertension Detection and Follow-Up Program (HDFP)[60] and the 10.5-year follow-up data from the Multiple Risk Factor Intervention Trial (MRFIT)[61] showed greater decreases in coronary events than did the original, shorter trials. The beneficial effect of antihypertensive treatment on preventing coronary disease may in fact require decades to achieve expected levels.[59] The Systolic Hypertension in the Elderly Program (SHEP) showed a 27% reduction in fatal and nonfatal coronary events in the diuretic-

Table 37–2. **Characteristics of the Ideal Step-One Drug**

Reduces cardiovascular morbidity and mortality in controlled
    treatment trials*
Safe
Effective as monotherapy (should normalize blood pressure as the
    sole agent for at least 50% of patients with stage 1
    hypertension)
Well tolerated by most patients (few side effects that necessitate
    cessation of therapy)
Inexpensive
Dose easy to titrate (no more than a two- or three-step titration)
Desirable hemodynamic effects (for most hypertensive patients,
    this means a reduction in total peripheral resistance with little
    or no change in cardiac output; in the few patients who have
    hyperkinetic circulation, it would mean a reduction in cardiac
    output with little or no effect on total peripheral resistance)
Minimal drug interactions
Augments the effect of other antihypertensive agents that might
    be necessary subsequently
Does not produce pseudotolerance (occult salt and water
    retention, expanding extracellular fluid volume and raising
    blood pressure)
Long-acting (one dose daily is a distinct advantage to enhance
    compliance)
Minimal contraindications

*Only diuretics and β-blockers have been shown to reduce the risk of
cardiovascular morbidity and mortality in controlled clinical trials.

treated subjects compared with those receiving placebo,[55] and the diuretic arm of the Medical Research Council (MRC) trial in the elderly showed a 44% reduction in coronary mortality compared with the placebo group.[56] Moreover, a meta-analysis of all trials in elderly patients with hypertension showed nearly a 30% reduction in coronary mortality.[4]

It is plausible that the newer agents are more effective in reducing coronary events than the diuretics. However, only large randomized clinical trials will answer this question. Until then, present evidence supports the use of diuretics in most hypertensive patients.[62]

Table 37–3. **Large Randomized Clinical Trials Using Diuretic-Based Stepped-Care Therapy**

**Trials Showing a Significant Reduction in Cardiovascular
Morbidity or Mortality**
VA Cooperative Trial, 1967* [46]
VA Cooperative Trial, 1970* [47]
US Public Health Service Trial* [48]
Hypertension Detection and Follow-up Program (HDFP)[49, 50]
Australian National Trial* [51]
European Working Party on High Blood Pressure in the Elderly
    (EWPHE)* [52]
Medical Research Council (MRC) Trial* [53]
Oslo Study[54]
Systolic Hypertension in the Elderly Program (SHEP)* [55]
MRC-Elderly* [56]
Swedish Trial in Old Patients with Hypertension
    (STOP-Hypertension)* [57]

**Trials That Did Not Show a Significant Reduction in
Cardiovascular Morbidity or Mortality**
Multiple Risk Factor Intervention Trial (MRFIT)[45]

*Placebo-controlled.

SAFETY OF DIURETICS

The issue of safety of diuretics revolves around their metabolic side effects, some of which are potentially atherogenic (dyslipidemia, hyperuricemia, hyperglycemia) or arrhythmogenic (hypokalemia, hypomagnesemia).

These metabolic derangements have been implicated in the failure of the treatment trials to reduce coronary events to anticipated levels,[63] even though the incidence of strokes, congestive heart failure, and total cardiovascular morbidity and mortality has been reduced.[2–4] In the MRFIT,[45] an excess of sudden deaths was noted among hypertensive men with abnormal resting electrocardiograms in the special intervention group who were treated with a diuretic, compared with their counterparts in the usual care group. It has been speculated that this difference was the result of diuretic-induced hypokalemia from the large dosages of diuretic used in the special intervention group. This theory is difficult to reconcile with the fact that the lowest death rate encountered in either group of hypertensive men with abnormal resting electrocardiograms was in a special intervention subgroup that received 100 mg of chlorthalidone daily.[64] It should be noted that in the SHEP trial, coronary events were reduced more in elderly patients who had resting electrocardiographic abnormalities than in those who had normal resting electrocardiograms.[55]

Effect on Lipid Metabolism

In general, trials lasting 1 year or less have shown that diuretic therapy is associated with an increase in serum cholesterol and, sometimes, triglycerides.[65–68] When measured, the high-density lipoprotein (HDL) fraction of total cholesterol was unchanged, but the low-density lipoprotein (LDL) fraction was increased.[66] Most long-term studies have failed to show any adverse effect of thiazide therapy on serum lipid concentrations[69–75] (Table 37–4), although several lacked a placebo-controlled group.[71, 73, 74] The tendency since 1975, at least in the United States, is for serum cholesterol concentration to decrease over time, so the failure of cholesterol to rise during administration of a diuretic is not necessarily synonymous with no effect. Perhaps the diuretic prevented the cholesterol from falling as much as it would have otherwise.[76, 78] On the other hand, the Trial of Mild Hypertension Study (TOMHS)[75] and the European Working Party on High Blood Pressure in the Elderly (EWPHE) trial[72] both had placebo-controlled groups, and there was no difference in the change in serum cholesterol between the placebo groups and the diuretic-treated groups.

Ames and Hill[65] showed that only 21 of 39 subjects reacted to chlorthalidone therapy with significant increases in serum cholesterol or triglyceride levels, whereas 18 experienced little if any adverse effects.

In the Veterans Administration (VA) Trial of Single Drug Therapy for Hypertension in Men, only those participants whose blood pressure did not respond to

Table 37–4. **Observations from Clinical Trials on Effect of Diuretics on Serum Cholesterol and Triglyceride Levels**

Trial and Duration	Diuretic and Daily Dose (mg)	Cholesterol			Triglycerides		
			Concentration (mg/dL)			Concentration (mg/dL)	
		N	BASELINE	Rx	N	BASELINE	Rx
VA Coop.							
10 wk[68]	HCTZ 50–100	343	224	231[a]	343	184	220
58 wk[71]	Same	167	226	223	170	189	184
Berglund and Andersson[74]							
1 yr	Bendrofluazide 10	53	267	263	53	142	142
6 yr	Same	49	267	255	49	142	151
VA-NHLBI[67]							
1 yr	Chlorthalidone 50–100	302	203	213[a]	297	152	167[a]
	Placebo	308	196	196	308	129	134
Oslo[70]							
4 yr	HCTZ	26	271	273	26	143	120
	No Rx	33	278	280	33	170	139
Ames & Hill[65]							
6 mo	HCTZ, 25–50 or chlorthalidone 50 twice a week to 100/day	39	227	238[b, c]	39	142	176[b, c]
	Diet only	35	231	220[b]	35	120	117
Grimm et al[66]							
6–12 wk[d]	HCTZ 100	39	221	236[e]	39	158	185[a]
	Chlorthalidone 100	39	221	240[f]	39	158	185[a]
	Placebo	39	221	223	39	158	151
MRC[76]							
3 yr							
Men	Bendrofluazide 10	256	246	247			
	Placebo	539	247	242[e]			
Women	Bendrofluazide 10	229	262	265			
	Placebo	417	261	258			
HDFP[73]							
5 yr	Chlorthalidone 50–100	318	231	222			
	Chlorthalidone + other agents	716	232	223			
	No Rx[g]	71	225	212			
EWPHE[72]							
1 yr	HCTZ 25 + triamterene 50	158	251	248			
	Placebo	157	253	243			
2 yr	HCTZ 25 + triamterene 50	99	261	241			
	Placebo	91	263	247			
3 yr	HCTZ 25 + triamterene 50	48	256	239			
	Placebo	42	259	238			
SHEP[55]							
4.5 yr	Chlorthalidone 12.5–25	1882	236	244[h]			
	Placebo	1821	236	236			
TOMHS[75]							
4 yr	Chlorthalidone 15–30	117		−4.5[i]	117		−14.7
	Placebo	207		−5.1	207		−14.5
STOP-Hypertension[77]							
12 mo	HCTZ 25 + amiloride 2.5	246		+6.6[j]			
	Placebo	228					

[a]$p<.001$.
[b]$p<.005$ versus pretreatment.
[c]$p<.005$ versus diet group.
[d]On each regimen.
[e]$p<.01$ (comparing change in active treatment group with change in placebo group).
[f]$p<.001$ (comparing change in active treatment group with change in placebo group).
[g]Not a prospectively designed control group.
[h]$z = 3.3$.
[i]All participants were instructed in lifestyle modifications.
[j]Compared with placebo (NS).

a diuretic had a significant increase in total serum cholesterol and triglycerides at the end of the 8- to 12-week titration period compared with men receiving placebo. There were virtually no changes in triglycerides, total cholesterol, or LDL cholesterol concentrations for patients who responded to treatment with hydrochlorothiazide.[79] Because the rise in serum cholesterol and triglyceride concentrations usually occurs in the first month,[65] the patients who are likely to respond adversely can easily and quickly be identified by measuring serum lipids before and 4 to 6 weeks after initiating diuretic therapy. In the report by Ames and Hill,[65] 100 mg of chlorthalidone daily led to an average increase in serum cholesterol level of 20 mg/dl, whereas smaller doses were accompanied by a rise of only 6 mg/dl. A low-saturated-fat diet prevented the rise in serum cholesterol level induced by diuretic therapy.[66] In the MRFIT, the average serum cholesterol concentration decreased more for men who were not receiving a diuretic (13.1 mg/dl) than for men who were receiving a diuretic (9.1 mg/dl).[78]

A study by Carlsen et al.[39] demonstrated that metabolic side effects of bendrofluazide were dose-related, including adverse lipid effects. However, blood pressure was lowered nearly the same amount regardless of dose.

A biostatistical phenomenon that must be considered when examining highly variable measurements such as serum cholesterol, blood glucose, or blood pressure in individual patients is "regression to the mean." Jeunemaitre et al.[80] reported changes in metabolic parameters following treatment with spironolactone, hydrochlorothiazide plus amiloride, or cyclothiazide plus triamterene. There were 100 subjects in each group, and they were followed up for an average of 20 months. Although average plasma cholesterol and glucose levels rose slightly from baseline in the thiazide-treated groups, the most striking finding was that when pretreatment values for cholesterol and glucose were low, they increased during treatment, but when pretreatment values were high, they decreased during treatment. The same phenomenon was noted in serum cholesterol concentrations during the HDFP trial[73] and the VA–National Heart, Lung, and Blood Institute (VA-NHLBI) trial.[67]

In summary, the evidence from controlled trials suggests that diuretic-induced increases in serum cholesterol or triglyceride levels occur only in susceptible patients, are dose-related, can be recognized within the first 4 weeks of treatment, and can be prevented or ameliorated by a low-fat diet. They are more likely to occur in patients with normal serum cholesterol concentrations than in patients with high concentrations; therefore, an elevated serum cholesterol level is not an *a priori* contraindication to the use of diuretics in the management of hypertension. Finally, long-term studies suggest that diuretic-induced hypercholesterolemia may not persist beyond the first year of therapy (see Table 37–4).

Hyperuricemia

Diuretic therapy notoriously increases serum uric acid concentrations for both men and women.[81] Despite its high frequency, diuretic-induced hyperuricemia so rarely leads to clinical gout that a hereditary trait seems likely to explain the few cases in which gout does develop *de novo* when diuretics are administered. In the HDFP trial,[81] only 15 cases of gout were re-

corded in 5 years among 3693 participants at risk. Thiazide and related diuretics, as well as loop diuretics, often aggravate preexisting gout; therefore, clinical gout (but not asymptomatic hyperuricemia) is a relative contraindication to the use of thiazide-type diuretics unless the patient is also receiving an antiuricemic agent such as allopurinol or probenecid.

Finally, in a multivariate analysis including age, systolic blood pressure, relative weight, cigarette smoking, and serum cholesterol concentration, serum uric acid did not add independently to the risk for coronary heart disease in the Framingham Study.[82]

Glucose Metabolism

By promoting insulin resistance, thiazide diuretics can increase the concentration of plasma glucose during fasting as well as after a glucose load.[83–87] However, this increase often is not apparent clinically, because the levels during treatment frequently are not abnormal—they are simply higher than they were at baseline.

Diuretic-induced glucose intolerance was first apparent at 2 and 3 years in the EWPHE trial[83] and only after 6 years in the cohort followed by the British MRC group.[85] At 14 years, glucose tolerance had deteriorated even more than at 6 years.[86] In the cohort of 34 patients followed-up for 14 years, blood glucose in fasting patients had increased from 85.5 mg/dl at baseline to 109.2 mg/dl, and the 2-hour glucose level had increased from 100.1 mg/dl at baseline to 145.6 mg/dl.[86] These changes are reversible when thiazide therapy is discontinued,[84] even after 14 years.[86]

Diuretic agents can aggravate preexisting diabetes in some susceptible patients and can precipitate clinical diabetes in predisposed patients.[88] Nevertheless, the use of thiazide diuretics did not appear to increase the incidence of clinical diabetes requiring hypoglycemic agents to a greater extent than did other antihypertensive drugs in a study of Medicaid patients.[89]

Amery et al.[83] and the VA group[84] reported a relationship between impaired glucose metabolism and potassium loss during diuretic therapy, but Lewis et al.[85] did not find this relationship.

Berglund et al.[90] found that blood glucose concentration 1 hour after a glucose load was lower in patients after 10 years of diuretic therapy than it was initially.

Fasting glucose levels tended to regress to the mean in the series reported by Jeunemaitre et al.,[80] and diuretic-induced changes in plasma glucose were dose-related in the study by Carlsen et al.[39]

Diuretic therapy has been associated with increased mortality in diabetic patients with retinopathy in nonrandomized observations in which there was no attempt to allocate treatment regimens prospectively.[91, 92] Diuretic-based therapy was used in several of the large prospective randomized trials in which diabetics were not excluded (EWPHE,[83] HDFP,[93] SHEP[55]), and no adverse effects were reported. In the HDFP[93] and SHEP[94] trials, diabetic patients received as much benefit as the nondiabetic patients did in the reduction of morbidity and mortality. Walker et al.[95] found that hydrochlorothiazide and lisinopril had the same effect on blood pressure control and the rate of decline of renal function in patients with type II diabetes mellitus and nephropathy. However, in a similar study in patients with type I diabetes and nephropathy, Lewis et al.[96] reported that patients randomized to captopril had less proteinuria and showed slower progression of renal impairment compared with a control group that received placebo and, when necessary, antihypertensive agents other than ACE inhibitors or calcium antagonists.

A consensus report of the American Diabetes Association[97] and a working group report from the National High Blood Pressure Education Program[98] have both acknowledged the usefulness of low-dose diuretic therapy in controlling hypertension in diabetic patients because insulin resistance is frequently accompanied by sodium and volume retention.[87] A consensus report from the Canadian Hypertension Society, however, warns that diuretics should not be prescribed as first-line therapy in managing hypertension in diabetic patients.[99]

Hypokalemia

The potential danger of hypokalemia to the myocardium is a nonissue, because it can be prevented by routinely prescribing a potassium-sparing diuretic in combination with the thiazide. Although more and more physicians are doing this, it is not necessary[100] and can be hazardous if the contraindications to potassium-sparing diuretics are not observed. These contraindications have already been discussed in the section "Preparations and Dosages."

The indications for initiating therapy with a combination diuretic are listed in Table 37–5. In the absence of clinical heart disease, myocardial irritability, or digitalis therapy, routine prescription of potassium-sparing agents is unnecessary, especially when low doses of thiazides are prescribed.

It is not clear whether hypokalemia induced by diuretic therapy causes ventricular arrhythmias or ectopy, especially in patients with normal hearts. Using Holter monitoring[101] or an exercise stress test,[102] ventricular ectopic activity has been shown to correlate inversely with serum potassium in patients receiving

Table 37–5. **Indications for Adding a Potassium-Sparing Diuretic to a Thiazide**

Concomitant digitalis therapy
Frequent ventricular ectopy
History of tachyarrhythmias
Abnormal resting electrocardiogram (especially left ventricular hypertrophy)
Symptomatic hypokalemia
Serum K$^+$ <3.0 mEq/L without symptoms
Before general anesthesia
During episodes of nausea, vomiting, diarrhea, anorexia

Adapted with permission from Gifford RW Jr: The role of diuretics in the treatment of hypertension. Am J Med 44(Suppl 4A):105, 1984.

diuretic therapy. The MRC study[103] has shown a correlation between thiazide therapy and ventricular ectopic activity, but it was unrelated to serum potassium concentration.

Stewart et al.[104] have reported that hypertensive patients with ischemic heart disease had more frequent ventricular ectopic activity, a higher Lown classification during ambulatory electrocardiographic monitoring, and greater myocardial electrical instability as assessed by programmed ventricular stimulation while receiving a potassium-wasting diuretic than they did while receiving a potassium-sparing agent. They concluded that in patients with ischemic heart disease, even minor decreases in serum potassium concentrations as a result of thiazide therapy can lead to potentially serious arrhythmias. Conversely, some studies[105–108] have failed to demonstrate a relationship between the frequency or severity of ventricular ectopic activity and the concentration of serum potassium in patients taking orally administered diuretics, some of whom had echocardiographic evidence of left ventricular hypertrophy.[107, 108]

Prescribing a combination tablet of a thiazide and a potassium-sparing agent is the most reliable way to prevent hypokalemia. Dietary manipulations are usually ineffective. It is practically impossible to ensure adequate potassium intake by selecting foods that are high in potassium; a more rational approach is to decrease sodium in the diet so that less sodium reaches the distal tubular site where sodium is exchanged for potassium. Potassium chloride supplements are expensive and may be poorly tolerated by patients. Between 60 and 100 mEq of potassium are required to prevent diuretic-induced hypokalemia. Seldom does the physician prescribe this much potassium chloride as a supplement—and even more seldom does the patient take it if prescribed.

Comments on Safety

No drug is absolutely safe. The physician hopes that the drug prescribed presents fewer risks than the disease being treated. Certainly, this is true for diuretics in the treatment of stages 2 to 4 (moderate to severe) hypertension, both diastolic and isolated systolic. The HDFP trial[109] suggested that it is also true for stage 1 (mild) hypertension.

Some physicians presume that the ACE inhibitors, selective α_1-adrenergic blocking agents, and calcium antagonists are inherently safer because they do not have the metabolic side effects of diuretics and β-blockers. Enthusiasm about ACE inhibitors and calcium antagonists may change when there has been 25 years' experience in millions of patients. The adverse effects of diuretics and β-blockers can be anticipated, but it took years to uncover this information. Furthermore, no long-term, randomized clinical trials have been conducted using ACE inhibitors, selective α_1-adrenergic blocking agents, or calcium antagonists to show that they reduce cardiovascular morbidity and mortality. It is unknown whether they will be more effective, less effective, or as effective as diuretics.

Such a comparative trial is presently being conducted by the National Heart, Lung, and Blood Institute of the National Institutes of Health.

Most of the data cited in this section on safety issues were collected using large doses (50 to 200 mg) of hydrochlorothiazide or chlorthalidone. Smaller doses now in use undoubtedly will minimize the adverse metabolic effects.[39]

SYMPTOMATIC SIDE EFFECTS AND QUALITY OF LIFE

Experience has shown that diuretics are usually well-tolerated by most patients. In a double-blind study, the 1-year feasibility trial of SHEP[110] found no significant difference in frequency of symptomatic side effects between 443 patients receiving chlorthalidone (25 to 50 mg daily) and 108 patients receiving placebo. Only 6 participants receiving chlorthalidone and 2 in the placebo group were withdrawn from the study because of symptomatic side effects.

In the full-scale SHEP trial, 28.1% of the subjects receiving chlorthalidone reported "any specified problem characterized as intolerable" during the 5 years of the study, compared with 20.8% of the subjects receiving placebo ($z = 5.9$).[55] Of the subjects receiving chlorthalidone, 91.8% reported "any specified problem," compared with 86.4% of those receiving placebo ($z = 6.0$). However, the investigators characterized this as a "low-order excess of adverse effects" that did not affect the course of the study.

In the Single Drug Therapy for Hypertension in Men study, a randomized double-blind trial conducted by the VA, only 3% of the men randomized to receive hydrochlorothiazide withdrew from the trial or had to have the dosage reduced because of adverse drug effects.[111] This compared with withdrawal rates of 4% for diltiazem, 5% for atenolol, 6% for placebo, 7% for captopril, 12% for prazosin, and 14% for clonidine. No drug was associated with a significant increase in the frequency of impotence or edema.

In the TOMHS trial, only 23 participants experienced serious adverse side effects requiring interruption of therapy during follow-up.[75] Fourteen of these were patients receiving one of the five drugs (2.1%), and nine were in the placebo group (3.8%). Only 1 of the 136 subjects randomized to receive chlorthalidone had to have treatment discontinued, and this was for an urticarial reaction.

An overall side-effect severity score based on 55 symptoms determined at each follow-up visit indicated that symptoms were more common among participants given placebo than among those given active drug treatment ($p = .05$). No significant differences among drug treatments were noted for this side-effect severity score.[75]

In a double-blind study comparing the effects of propranolol, methyldopa, and captopril on various parameters of quality of life in 626 men, Croog et al.[112] found that captopril interfered less with quality of life than did the other agents. Diuretics were re-

served for supplemental therapy in case blood pressure was not controlled by monotherapy. The addition of a diuretic detracted from the quality of life, but apparently not enough to prevent the authors from drawing conclusions about the other drugs. Without the diuretic, however, the study might not have been completed, because 36%, 31%, and 22% of patients receiving captopril, methyldopa, and propranolol, respectively, required the addition of a diuretic by the sixteenth week.

Subjects in the TOMHS trial[75] were graded on seven indices of quality of life. The overall test that combined the seven quality of life indices indicated that quality of life improved significantly more for participants given acebutolol ($p = .001$) and chlorthalidone ($p = .008$) than for participants given placebo; results for other active treatment groups were intermediate and did not differ significantly from those for the placebo group.

During the 1-year SHEP feasibility trial, there was no difference between subjects receiving chlorthalidone and those receiving placebo with regard to cognitive functions or level of depression.[113] At the end of the full-scale trial that lasted for an average of 4.5 years, 4.4% of persons in the active treatment group and 4.7% in the placebo group were diagnosed with depression.[55] A positive diagnosis for dementia was made for 1.6% in the diuretic-treated group, compared with 1.9% in the placebo group.

In a VA trial involving elderly men with hypertension, blood pressure reduction did not adversely affect cognitive and behavioral functions.[114] Hydrochlorothiazide in doses of 25 to 50 mg daily was prescribed as initial therapy and supplemented when necessary with hydralazine, methyldopa, metoprolol, or reserpine.

SELECTION OF THE INITIAL DRUG

Expensive and sophisticated studies of hemodynamics and hormonal measurements are not necessary to select the appropriate initial drug. The role of plasma renin activity in the selection of a diuretic for initial therapy has not been helpful.[115] Table 37–6 lists some indications that should be considered for choosing between the five classes of drugs that are appropriate for initial therapy. In general, diuretics are particularly effective in elderly patients, black patients, and patients with volume-dependent hypertension (obesity, chronic renal failure, type II diabetes mellitus, primary aldosteronism). In the VA Trial of Single Drug Therapy, hydrochlorothiazide reduced systolic blood pressure more than any other agent except for clonidine.[111] Because of the numerous advantages of diuretics, they may be prescribed whenever there is no special indication for an alternative and no contraindication to their use.

If an alternative agent is selected as initial therapy, an orally administered diuretic is an excellent choice when a second agent is required, regardless of which nondiuretic agent has been prescribed. The addition of a diuretic agent or an increase in the dose of a

Table 37–6. **Indications for Choosing Between Classes of Drugs for Initial Therapy**

Diuretics*
Chronic renal failure (loop diuretics)†
Congestive heart failure†
Black patient
Elderly patient
Obese patient
Resistant hypertension
Recurrent renal calculi (calcium) (non-loop diuretics)

β-Adrenergic Blocking Agents*
Post myocardial infarction (cardioprotective effect,
    non-ISA, non–α-blocking agents preferred)†
Young patient
Hyperkinetic circulation
Angina pectoris
Migraine headache
Senile tremor
Severe hypertrophic cardiomyopathy of the elderly
Severe asymmetric septal hypertrophy with outflow obstruction
Atrial fibrillation to control ventricular rate
Paroxysmal supraventricular tachycardia (non-ISA,
    non–α-blocking agents preferred)

Calcium Antagonists
Elderly patient
Black patient
Angina pectoris
Sexual dysfunction from other drugs
Hypertension induced by cyclosporine
Migraine, paroxysmal supraventricular tachycardia, atrial
    fibrillation to slow atrioventricular conduction (verapamil or
    diltiazem)

ACE Inhibitors
Congestive heart failure (systolic dysfunction)†
Type I diabetes mellitus with nephropathy†
Young patient
White patient
Heavy proteinuria
Chronic renal disease (especially diabetic glomerulosclerosis)
Impotence from other drugs

Selective α₁-Adrenergic Blocking Agents
Diabetes
Lipid abnormalities
Benign prostatic hypertrophy

ACE, angiotensin-converting enzyme; ISA, intrinsic sympathomimetic activity.
*Diuretics and β-blockers are preferred unless there is a contraindication to their use or a special indication for another agent.
†Primary indication.

diuretic was effective in controlling blood pressure for 17 of 34 patients who presented with resistant hypertension that was attributed to suboptimal regimens.[116]

REFERENCES

1. Megibow RS, Pollack H, Stollerman GH, et al: The treatment of hypertension by accelerated sodium depletion. J Mt Sinai Hosp 15:233, 1948.
2. Collins R, Peto R, MacMahon S, et al: Blood pressure, stroke, and coronary heart disease: Part II. Short-term reductions in blood pressure: Overview of randomised drug trials in their epidemiological context. Lancet 335:827, 1990.
3. Hebert PR, Moser M, Mayer J, Hennekens CH: Recent evidence on drug therapy of mild to moderate hypertension and decreased risk of coronary heart disease. Arch Intern Med 153:578, 1993.
4. Mulrow CD, Cornell JA, Herrera CR, et al: Hypertension in the elderly. Implications and generalizability of randomized trials. JAMA 272:1932, 1994.
5. Joint National Committee on Detection, Evaluation, and Treatment of High Blood Pressure: The fifth report of the Joint National Committee on Detection, Evaluation, and Treatment of High Blood Pressure (JNC V). Arch Intern Med 153:154, 1993.
6. Ogilvie RI, Burgess ED, Cusson JR, et al: Report of the Canadian Hypertension Society Consensus Conference 3: Pharmacologic treatment of essential hypertension. Can Med Assoc J 149:575, 1993.
7. Sever P, Beevers G, Bulpitt C, et al: Management guidelines in essential hypertension: Report of the second working party of the British Hypertension Society. Br Med J 306:983, 1993.
8. The Core Services Committee: The management of raised blood pressure in New Zealand. The National Advisory Committee on Core Health and Disability Support Services, Wellington, New Zealand, November 1992.
9. 1993 guidelines for the management of mild hypertension: Memorandum from a World Health Organization/International Society of Hypertension meeting. Hypertension 22:392, 1993.
10. van Zwieten PA: Comparative mechanisms of action of diuretic drugs in hypertension. Eur Heart J 13(Suppl G):2, 1992.
11. Tarazi RC: Diuretic drugs: Mechanisms of antihypertensive action. In Onesti G, Kim KE, Moyer JH (eds): Hypertension: Mechanisms and Management. New York: Grune & Stratton, 1973, pp 251–260.
12. Gifford RW Jr, Mattox VR, Orvis AL, et al: Effect of thiazide diuretics on plasma volume, body electrolytes, and excretion of aldosterone in hypertension. Circulation 24:1197, 1961.
13. Conway J, Lauwers P: Hemodynamic and hypotensive effects of long-term therapy with chlorothiazide. Circulation 21:21, 1960.
14. Lauwers P, Conway J: Effect of long-term treatment with chlorothiazide on body fluids, serum electrolytes, and exchangeable sodium in hypertensive patients. J Lab Clin Med 56:401, 1960.
15. Wilson IM, Freis ED: Relationship between plasma and extracellular fluid volume depletion and the antihypertensive effect of chlorothiazide. Circulation 20:1028, 1959.
16. Hansen J: Hydrochlorothiazide in the treatment of hypertension. Acta Med Scand 183:317, 1968.
17. Leth A: Changes in plasma and extracellular fluid volume in patients with essential hypertension during long-term treatment with hydrochlorothiazide. Circulation 42:479, 1970.
18. Tarazi RC, Dustan HP, Frohlich ED: Long-term thiazide therapy in essential hypertension. Evidence of persistent alteration in plasma volume and renin activity. Circulation 41:709, 1970.
19. Vardan S, Dunsky MH, Hill NE, et al: Effect of one year of thiazide therapy on plasma volume, renin, aldosterone, lipids and urinary metanephrines in systolic hypertension of elderly patients. Am J Cardiol 60:388, 1987.
20. Tobian L, Binion JT: Tissue cations and water in arterial hypertension. Circulation 5:754, 1952.
21. Tobian L, Olson R, Chesley G: Water content of arteriolar wall in renovascular hypertension. Am J Physiol 216:22, 1969.
22. Aleksandrow D, Wysznacka W, Gajewski J: Influence of chlorothiazide upon arterial responsiveness to norepinephrine in hypertensive subjects. N Engl J Med 261:1052, 1959.
23. Davidov M, Gavrilovich L, Mroczek W, et al: Relation of extracellular fluid volume to arterial pressure during drug-induced saluresis. Circulation 40:349, 1969.
24. Winer BM: The antihypertensive mechanisms of salt depletion induced by hydrochlorothiazide. Circulation 24:788, 1961.
25. Feisal K, Eckstein JW, Horsley AW, et al: Effects of chlorothiazide on forearm vascular responses to norepinephrine. J Appl Physiol 16:549, 1961.
26. Aoki VS, Brody MJ: The effect of thiazide on the sympathetic nervous system of hypertensive rats. Arch Int Pharmacodyn Ther 177:423, 1969.
27. Ogilvie RI, Schlieper E: The effect of hydrochlorothiazide on venous reactivity in hypertensive men. Clin Pharmacol Ther 11:589, 1970.

28. Schohn DC, Jahn HA: Effects of a potassium-sparing/thiazide diuretic on cardiovascular reactivity to vasopressor agents. Am J Cardiol 65:14K, 1990.

29. Friedman SM, Jamieson JD, Friedman CL: Sodium gradient, smooth muscle tone, and blood pressure regulation. Circ Res 7:44, 1959.

30. Blaustein MP: Physiological effects of endogenous ouabain: Control of intracellular Ca^{2+} stores and cell responsiveness. Am J Physiol 264:C1367, 1993.

31. Shingu T, Matsuura H, Kusaka M, et al: Significance of intracellular free calcium and magnesium and calcium-regulating hormones with sodium chloride loading in patients with essential hypertension. J Hypertens 9:1021, 1991.

32. Dustan HP, Cumming GR, Corcoran AC, et al: A mechanism of chlorothiazide-enhanced effectiveness of antihypertensive ganglioplegic drugs. Circulation 19:360, 1959.

33. Lohmoller G, Lohmoller R, Pfeffer MA, et al: Mechanism of immediate hemodynamic effects of chlorothiazide. Am Heart J 89:487, 1975.

34. Shah S, Khatri I, Freis ED: Mechanism of antihypertensive effect of thiazide diuretics. Am Heart J 95:611, 1978.

35. Vardan S, Mookherjee S, Warner R, Smulyan H: Systolic hypertension in the elderly. JAMA 250:2807, 1983.

36. Dustan HP, Tarazi RC, Bravo EL: Dependence of arterial pressure on intravascular volume in treated hypertensive patients. N Engl J Med 286:861, 1972.

37. Finnerty FA, Davidov M, Mroczek WJ, et al: Influence of extracellular fluid volume on response to antihypertensive drugs. Circ Res 26–27(Suppl l):71, 1970.

38. Gifford RW, Jr.: Resistant hypertension: Introduction and definitions. Hypertension 11(Suppl II):65, 1988.

39. Carlsen JE, Køber L, Torp-Pederesen C, Johansen P: Relation between dose of bendrofluazide, antihypertensive effect, and adverse biochemical effects. Br Med J 300:975, 1990.

40. Materson BJ, Oster JR, Michael UF, et al: Dose response to chlorthalidone in patients with mild hypertension: Efficacy of a lower dose. Clin Pharmacol Ther 24:192, 1978.

41. Tweedale MG, Ogilvie RI, Ruedy J: Antihypertensive and biochemical effects of chlorthalidone. Clin Pharmacol Ther 22:519, 1977.

42. Berglund G, Andersson O: Low doses of hydrochlorothiazide in hypertension: Antihypertensive and metabolic effects. Eur J Clin Pharmcol 10:177, 1976.

43. Vardan S, Mehrotra KG, Mookherjee S, et al: Efficacy and reduced metabolic side effects of a 15-mg chlorthalidone formulation in the treatment of mild hypertension: A multicenter study. JAMA 258:484, 1987.

44. Gifford RW, Jr.: First step therapy of essential hypertension: The advantages of initial diuretic treatment. In Whelton PK (ed): Potassium in Cardiovascular and Renal Medicine: Arrhythmias, Myocardial Infarction, and Hypertension. New York: Marcel Dekker, 1986, pp 495–505.

45. Multiple Risk Factor Intervention Trial Research Group: Multiple Risk Factor Intervention Trial: Risk factor changes and mortality results. JAMA 248:1465, 1982.

46. Veterans Administration Cooperative Study Group on Antihypertensive Agents: Effects of treatment on morbidity in hypertension: Results in patients with diastolic blood pressures averaging 115 through 129 mmHg. JAMA 202:1028, 1967.

47. Veterans Administration Cooperative Study Group on Antihypertensive Agents: Effects of treatment on morbidity in hypertension: II. Results in patients with diastolic blood pressure averaging 90 through 114 mmHg. JAMA 213:1143, 1970.

48. Smith WM: Treatment of mild hypertension: Results of a ten-year intervention trial. Circ Res 40(Suppl I):98, 1977.

49. Hypertension Detection and Follow-up Program Cooperative Group: Five-year findings of the Hypertension Detection and Follow-up Program: I. Reduction in mortality of persons with high blood pressure, including mild hypertension. JAMA 242:2562, 1979.

50. Hypertension Detection and Follow-up Program Cooperative Group: Five-year findings of the Hypertension Detection and Follow-up Program: II. Mortality by race, sex and age. JAMA 242:2572, 1979.

51. The Australian Therapeutic Trial in Mild Hypertension: Report by the Management Committee. Lancet 1:1261, 1980.

52. Amery A, Birkenhager W, Brixko P, et al: Mortality and morbidity results from the European Working Party on High Blood Pressure in the Elderly Trial. Lancet 1:1349, 1985.

53. Medical Research Council Working Party: MRC trial of treatment of mild hypertension: Principal results. Br Med J 291:97, 1985.

54. Helgeland A: Treatment of mild hypertension: A five-year controlled drug trial. The Oslo study. Am J Med 69:725, 1980.

55. SHEP Cooperative Research Group: Prevention of stroke by antihypertensive drug treatment in older persons with isolated systolic hypertension: Final results of the Systolic Hypertension in the Elderly Program. JAMA 266:3255, 1991.

56. MRC Working Party: Medical Research Council trial of treatment in older adults: Principal results. Br Med J 304:405, 1992.

57. Dahlöf B, Lindholm LH, Hansson L, et al: Morbidity and mortality in the Swedish trial in old patients with hypertension (STOP-Hypertension). Lancet 338:1281, 1991.

58. MacMahon S, Peto R, Cutler J, et al: Blood pressure, stroke, and coronary heart disease: Part I. Prolonged differences in blood pressure: Prospective observational studies corrected for the regression dilution bias. Lancet 335:765, 1990.

59. MacMahon S: Antihypertensive drug treatment: The potential, expected and observed effects on vascular disease. J Hypertens 9(Suppl VII):S239, 1990.

60. Hypertension Detection and Follow-up Program Cooperative Group: Persistence of reduction and mortality of participants in the Hypertension Detection and Follow-up Program. JAMA 259:2113, 1988.

61. The Multiple Risk Factor Intervention Trial Research Group: Mortality rates after 10.5 years for participants in the Multiple Risk Factor Intervention Trial: Findings related to a priori hypotheses of the trial. JAMA 253:1795, 1990.

62. Alderman MH: Which antihypertensive drugs first—And why! JAMA 267:2786, 1992.

63. Freis ED: The cardiovascular risks of thiazide diuretics. Clin Phamacol Ther 39:239, 1986.

64. Multiple Risk Factor Intervention Trial Research Group: Baseline rest electrocardiographic abnormalities, antihypertensive treatment, and mortality in the Multiple Risk Factor Intervention Trial. Am J Cardiol 55:1, 1985.

65. Ames RP, Hill P: Elevation of serum lipid levels during diuretic therapy of hypertension. Am J Med 61:748, 1976.

66. Grimm RH, Leon AS, Hunninghake DB, et al: Effects of thiazide diuretics on plasma lipids and lipoproteins in mildly hypertensive patients: A double-blind controlled trial. Ann Intern Med 94:7, 1981.

67. Goldman AI, Steele BW, Schnaper HW, et al: Serum lipoprotein levels during chlorthalidone therapy. A Veterans Administration—National Heart, Lung, and Blood Institute cooperative study on antihypertensive therapy: Mild hypertension. JAMA 244:1691, 1980.

68. Veterans Administration Cooperative Study Group on Antihypertensive Agents: Comparison of propranolol and hydrochlorothiazide for the initial treatment of hypertension: I. Results of short-term titration with emphasis on racial differences in response. JAMA 248: 1996, 1982.

69. Rossner S: Serum lipid changes during treatment with antihypertensive drugs. Acta Med Scand 628(Suppl):89, 1979.

70. Helgeland A, Hjermann I, Leren P, et al: High-density lipoprotein cholesterol and antihypertensive drugs: The Oslo study. Br Med J 2:403, 1978.

71. Veterans Administration Cooperative Study Group on Antihypertensive Agents: Comparison of propranolol and hydrochlorothiazide for the initial treatment of hypertension: II. Results of long-term therapy. JAMA 248:2004, 1982.

72. Amery A, Birkenhager W, Bulpitt C, et al: Influence of antihypertensive therapy on serum cholesterol in elderly hypertensive patients: Results of trial by the European Working Party on High Blood Pressure in the Elderly (EWPHE). Acta Cardiol (Brux) 37:235, 1982.

73. Williams WR, Schneider KA, Borhani NO, et al: The relationship between diuretics and serum cholesterol in Hypertension Detection and Follow-up Program participants. Am J Prev Med 2:248, 1986.

74. Berglund G, Andersson O: Beta-blockers or diuretics in hyper-

tension? A six-year follow-up of blood pressure and metabolic side effects. Lancet 1:744, 1981.

75. Neaton JD, Grimm RH, Prineas RJ, et al: Treatment of mild hypertension study: Final results. JAMA 270:713, 1993.

76. Medical Research Council Working Party on Mild to Moderate Hypertension: Adverse reactions to bendrofluazide and propranolol for the treatment of mild hypertension. Lancet 2:539. 1981.

77. Ekbom T, Dahlöf B, Hansson L, et al: Antihypertensive efficacy and side effects of three beta-blockers and diuretic in elderly hypertensives: A report from the STOP-Hypertension study. J Hypertens 10:1525, 1992.

78. Lasser NL, Grandits G, Caggiula AW, et al: Effects of antihypertensive therapy on plasma lipids and lipoproteins in the Multiple Risk Factor Intervention Trial. Am J Med 76(Suppl 2A):52, 1984.

79. Materson BJ, Lakshman MR, Nunn S, Cushman WC: Plasma lipid and lipoprotein profiles in response to six antihypertensive drugs and placebo. In Puschett JB, Greenberg A (eds): Diuretics IV: Chemistry, Pharmacology and Clinical Applications. New York: Elsevier, 1993, pp 511–513.

80. Jeunemaitre X, Charru A, Chatellier G, et al: Long-term metabolic effects of spironolactone and thiazides combined with potassium-sparing agents for treatment of essential hypertension. Am J Cardiol 62:1072, 1988.

81. Langford HG, Blaufox MD, Borhani NO, et al: Is thiazide-produced uric acid elevation harmful? Arch Intern Med 147:645, 1987.

82. Brand FN, McGee DL, Kannel WB, et al: Hyperuricemia as a risk factor of coronary heart disease: The Framingham Study. Am J Epidemiol 121:11, 1985.

83. Amery A, Berthaux P, Bulpitt C, et al: Glucose intolerance during diuretic therapy: Results of trial by the European Working Party on Hypertension in the Elderly. Lancet 1:681, 1978.

84. Veterans Administration Cooperative Study Group on Antihypertensive Agents: Propranolol or hydrochlorothiazide alone for the initial treatment of hypertension: IV. Effect on plasma glucose and glucose tolerance. Hypertension 7:1008, 1985.

85. Lewis PJ, Kohner EM, Petrie A, et al: Deterioration of glucose tolerance in hypertensive patients on prolonged diuretic treatment. Lancet 1:564, 1976.

86. Murphy MB, Lewis PJ, Kohner E, et al: Glucose intolerance in hypertensive patients treated with diuretics: A fourteen-year follow-up. Lancet 2:1293, 1982.

87. Epstein M, Sowers Jr: Diabetes mellitus and hypertension. Hypertension 19:403, 1992.

88. Goldner MG, Zarowitz H, Akgun S: Hyperglycemia and glycosuria due to thiazide derivatives administered in diabetes mellitus. N Engl J Med 262:403, 1960.

89. Gurwitz JH, Bohn RL, Glynn RJ, et al: Antihypertensive drug therapy and the initiation of treatment for diabetes mellitus. Ann Intern Med 118:273, 1992.

90. Berglund G, Andersson OK, Widgren BR: Low-dose antihypertensive treatment with a thiazide diuretic is not diabetogenic: A ten-year controlled trial with bendroflumethiazide. J Hypertens 4(Suppl V):S525, 1986.

91. Warram JH, Laffel LMB, Valsania P, et al: Excess mortality associated with diuretic therapy in diabetes mellitus. Arch Intern Med 151:1350–1356, 1991.

92. Klein R, Moss SE, Klein BE, DeMets DL: Relation of ocular and systemic factors to survival in diabetes. Arch Intern Med 149:266, 1989.

93. Langford HG, Stamler J, Wassertheil-Smoller S, Prineas RJ: All-cause mortality in the Hypertension Detection and Follow-up Program: Findings for the whole cohort and for persons with less severe hypertension, with and without other trains related to risk of mortality. Prog Cardiovasc Dis 29(Suppl 1):29, 1986.

94. The Systolic Hypertension in the Elderly Program Cooperative Group: Low dose diuretic-based antihypertensive treatment reduces risk in elderly diabetics with isolated systolic hypertension [abstract]. Circulation 88(Suppl I):386, 1993.

95. Walker WG, Hermann JA, Anderson JE: Randomized doubly blinded trial of enalapril vs hydrochlorothiazide on glomerular filtration rate in diabetic nephropathy: Early vs late results [abstract]. Hypertension 22:410, 1993.

96. Lewis EJ, Hunsicker LG, Bain RP, Rohde RD: The effect of angiotensin-converting enzyme inhibition on diabetic nephropathy. N Engl J Med 329:1456, 1993.

97. Arky RA, Caro JF, Johnson C, et al: Treatment of hypertension in diabetes. Diabetes Care 16:1397, 1993.

98. National High Blood Pressure Education Program report on hypertension in diabetes. Hypertension 23:145, 1994.

99. Dawson KG, McKenzie JK, Ross SA, et al: Report of the Canadian Hypertension Society Consensus Conference: V. Hypertension and diabetes. Can Med Assoc J 149:821, 1993.

100. Siegel D, Hulley SB, Black DM, et al: Diuretics, serum and intracellular electrolyte levels, and ventricular arrhythmias in hypertensive men. JAMA 267:1083, 1992.

101. Holland OB, Nixon JV, Kuhnert L: Diuretic-induced ventricular ectopic activity. Am J Med 70:762, 1981.

102. Hollifield JW, Slaton PE: Thiazide diuretics, hypokalemia and cardiac arrhythmias. Acta Med Scand 647(Suppl):67, 1981.

103. Greenberg G, Brennan PJ, Miall WE: Effects of diuretic and beta-blocker therapy in the Medical Research Council Trial. Am J Med 76(Suppl 2A):45, 1984.

104. Stewart DE, Ikram H, Espiner EA, et al: Arrhythmogenic potential of diuretic induced hypokalaemia in patients with mild hypertension and ischemic heart disease. Br Heart J 54:290, 1985.

105. Madias JE, Madias NE, Gavras HP: Nonarrhythmogenicity of diuretic-induced hypokalemia: Its evidence in patients with uncomplicated hypertension. Arch Intern Med 144:2171, 1984.

106. Lief PD, Belizon I, Matos J, et al: Diuretic-induced hypokalemia does not cause ventricular ectopy in uncomplicated essential hypertension [abstract]. Kidney Int 25:203, 1984.

107. Papademetriou V, Burris JF, Notargiacomo A, et al: Thiazide therapy is not a cause of arrhythmia in patients with systemic hypertension. Arch Intern Med 148:1272, 1988.

108. Narayan P, Colleran J, Kokkinos P, et al: Hydrochlorothiazide therapy and ventricular arrhythmias in hypertensive patients with advanced left ventricular hypertrophy [abstract]. J Am Coll Cardiol 19:196A, 1992.

109. Hypertension Detection and Follow-up Program Cooperative Group: The effect of treatment on mortality in "mild" hypertension: Results of the Hypertension Detection and Follow-up Program. N Engl J Med 307:976, 1982.

110. Hulley SB, Furberg CD, Gurland B, et al: Systolic Hypertension in the Elderly Program (SHEP): Antihypertensive efficacy of chlorthalidone. Am J Cardiol 56:913, 1985.

111. Materson BJ, Reda DJ, Cushman WC, et al: Single-drug therapy for hypertension in men: A comparison of six antihypertensive agents with placebo. N Engl J Med 328:914, 1993 (published correction appears in N Engl J Med 330:1689, 1994).

112. Croog SH, Levine S, Testa MA, et al: The effects of antihypertensive therapy on the quality of life. N Engl J Med 314:1657, 1986.

113. Gurland LJ, Teresi J, Smith WM, et al: Effects of treatment for isolated systolic hypertension on cognitive status and depression in the elderly. J Am Geriatr Soc 36:1015, 1988.

114. Goldstein G, Materson BJ, Cushman WC, et al: Treatment of hypertension in the elderly: II. Cognitive and behavioral function. Hypertension 15:361, 1990.

115. Wyndham RN, Gimenez L, Walker G, et al: Influence of renin levels on the treatment of essential hypertension with thiazide diuretics. Arch Intern Med 147:1021, 1987.

116. Yakovlevitch M, Black HR: Resistant hypertension in a tertiary care clinic. Arch Intern Med 151:1786, 1991.

CHAPTER 38

Diuretics in Congestive Heart Failure

Norman K. Hollenberg, M.D., Ph.D.

Diuretics were used to treat edema well before its pathogenesis was understood. Calomel (mercurous chloride) was apparently used by Paracelcus in the sixteenth century.[1] The recognition of the diuretic properties of organomercurials early in this century as a byproduct of the mercurial use to treat syphilis resulted in their introduction in the 1920s and wide use for the next three decades.[2] Indeed, the early introduction of diuretics and their wide acceptance as being fundamental in the treatment of edema may have contributed to our limited information on their therapeutic efficacy: there have been no placebo-controlled clinical trials.

We treat any disease process for one of two fundamental reasons: relief of symptoms or change in natural history. Although no placebo-controlled, double-blind trials have been made on diuretic use in the patient with congestive heart failure, no one would deny their capacity to induce diuresis, and few would deny the symptom relief that results from diuresis in the patient with pulmonary edema, orthopnea, ascites, anasarca, and profound peripheral edema. These symptoms are often limiting. In his classic analysis of the contribution of reduced sodium excretion and the resultant fluid retention to the pathogenesis of the syndrome of congestive heart failure,[3] Homer Smith pointed out that the engorgement of the cardiac chambers due to sodium retention could lead to further cardiac dilatation and exaggerate the failure of the already incompetent heart. Surely he spoke tongue in cheek when he asked, "How much, if anything, has the heart to do with chronic congestive heart failure?"

Conversely, in the absence of controlled clinical trials, no indication is available as to whether the natural history of congestive heart failure has been modified by diuretic use. In the patient near death with pulmonary edema who is rescued by diuresis, most of us would suspect strongly that life had been prolonged. Indeed, in patients with milder symptoms, diuretic use and resultant electrolyte disarray might have contributed to morbidity and mortality. This chapter emphasizes that aspect of diuretic use in heart failure, because the physician can do much to limit the important negative aspects of diuretic use.

Because substantial attention is given elsewhere to the pharmacology of the agents and their site of action, those issues will be addressed only when they are immediately relevant to specific problems in the patient with congestive heart failure. The growing use of angiotensin-converting enzyme (ACE) inhibitors in the patient with congestive heart failure has, inevitably, led to a rethinking of the strategy of diuretic use in the patient with congestive heart failure.

ACTIONS OF DIURETICS IN PATIENTS WITH HEART FAILURE
Renal Actions

The renal actions of diuretics in patients with heart failure must be viewed in the context of nephron function when enhanced sodium reabsorption occurs. Animal models have provided a confusing picture of events, perhaps because micropuncture studies are necessarily performed under anesthesia and with the kidney exposed.[4] Two lines of evidence from studies in humans have suggested that an increase in sodium resorption in heart failure occurs proximal to the ascending limb of the loop of Henle, especially in the proximal tubule. Osmotic diuretics normally reduce the kidney's capacity to generate a dilute urine. Paradoxically, in patients with advanced congestive heart failure, the administration of osmotic diuretics increased the diluting capacity.[5] The most straightforward interpretation is that the osmotic diuretics reduce sodium reabsorption at the level of the proximal tubule and thus enhance delivery of sodium to the loop of Henle, where a dilute urine is created. Bennett et al.[6] employed diuretics that act on various segments within the tubule system as an index of regional sodium reabsorption, providing further evidence for enhanced proximal and loop sodium reabsorption in the patient with advanced congestive heart failure.

Refractory Edema

The definition of refractory edema has evolved as the options for treating edema have evolved. Presumably, when the only therapy available was bed rest and digitalis, "refractory edema" might have been applied to the insertion of Southey tubes or multiple scarification of the grossly edematous leg as a nonrenal approach to relieving massive edema.[2]

With the advent of mercurial diuretics, it was quickly recognized that patients who developed alkalosis in response to these agents became refractory to further therapy, and that acidifying salts such as ammonia chloride or alternating use of a carbonic anhydrase inhibitor would restore responsiveness to mercurial diuretics because of the acidifying action. It was also recognized that acidosis limited the response to a carbonic anhydrase inhibitor.[1] Thus, a strategy evolved in which concomitant use of diuretic agents with different profiles and different limiting actions might, when combined, enhance the response.

When thiazide diuretics were introduced, it became apparent that they too demonstrated a pattern in which initial diuresis and natriuresis produced a drop in weight and total body sodium; however, with continued use, a new steady state was achieved in which sodium intake and sodium excretion were equal, but at a reduced total body sodium. In contrast with the use of mercurial diuretics and carbonic anhydrase inhibitors, however, with thiazide diuretics, no obvious mechanism such as acidosis or alkalosis limited sodium excretion. If the indication for diuretic use was edema, the patients were often free of edema when this new steady state was reached. Although long recognized, this phenomenon was given a clear conceptual context by Chonko and Grantham[7] in their lucid analysis of what they called the *braking phenomenon.* Their analysis emphasized that continued diuretic drug administration will result routinely in a state of physiologic diuretic resistance, which is of substantial therapeutic importance because it limits adverse intravascular volume depletion and its consequences. In this conceptual context, *diuretic resistance* in the edematous patient can be defined as a clinical state in which the braking phenomenon occurs before the therapeutic goal has been reached.

Drug-induced diuresis depends on a series of processes reflected in pharmacokinetics and pharmacodynamics.[8] In congestive heart failure, the pharmacokinetic limitation is best viewed in two steps. The first step involves how the administered drug reaches the kidney (extrarenal pharmacokinetics). The second step involves how the drug, having reached the kidney, is delivered to its target site of action within the nephron (intrarenal pharmacokinetics). The pharmacodynamic principle involves the interaction between a drug and the cells that results in inhibition of sodium reabsorption.

When furosemide and bumetanide were given intravenously to patients with heart failure, especially when renal function was preserved, no pharmacokinetic differences were demonstrated.[8] The usual dose of diuretic results in delivery of the usual amount of diuretic to the site of action in the kidney. To the extent that congestive heart failure results in renal failure, these patterns are altered (discussed elsewhere in this book).

In contrast to intravenous dosing, oral dosing produces clear changes in delivery. Overt malabsorption does not occur; rather, the time course of absorption is delayed so that the peak of drug appearance in urine is both considerably delayed and substantially reduced. That is, the delivery of the agent is spread over time. During a therapeutic titration, therefore, it makes good sense to administer the loop diuretics intravenously rather than to wait the many hours required to ascertain a response.

With the exception of diuretic action on the distal tubule and collecting duct, all diuretics must reach the tubular lumen to be effective. Excluding the osmotic agents, all of the available diuretic agents are organic acids that are highly bound to serum proteins and therefore do not reach the tubular lumen by glomerular filtration in significant amounts. These agents are actively secreted into the luminal compartment from the blood by way of the organic acid transport pathway of the proximal tubule. Agents that block the access of these diuretics to their site of action can diminish the response. Although probenecid is the classic blocker at this step of the process, an enormous number of widely employed drugs or organic acids are transported by this system and will compete with diuretics for access. One might anticipate, then, that a host of widely used agents, including penicillin, might blunt the delivery of loop diuretics to their site of action, but no literature is available on this contribution.

There is clear evidence of resistance to furosemide action that cannot be accounted for by drug delivery or concentration in the tubular lumen in the patient with advanced congestive heart failure. The reason for that resistance is unclear, but it presumably is related to the fundamental limitation of renal sodium handling in patients in congestive heart failure.

Azotemia is an important factor limiting the renal response to diuretics in patients with heart failure, as is hyponatremia. In a protocol designed to assess the renal and systemic response to the converting enzyme inhibitor captopril in patients with advanced heart failure, resistance to digitalis and large doses of furosemide in the patient confined to bed rest were made central entry criteria.[9] Although azotemia and hyponatremia were not entry criteria, every patient in the study[9] had progressive azotemia and hyponatremia with aggressive diuretic use. This stage seems to involve a vicious circle in which the use of large doses of diuretic will promote diuresis, but at the cost of progressive azotemia: the progressive azotemia limits the response to further doses of diuretic.

During this study, it was noted that patients who had been clinically stable often deteriorated during the initiation of therapy with a nonsteroidal antiinflammatory agent. Clinical deterioration rapidly reversed when the nonsteroidal antiinflammatory agent was discontinued. The release of ibuprofen as an over-the-counter agent has increased the frequency of this problem and made it more difficult to identify. All of these agents are organic acids and could block the delivery of the diuretics to their site of action. Although their mechanism is probably more complex, it may partly reflect the role of prostaglandins as mediators of the renal hemodynamic response to loop diuretics.[7]

Sequential Nephron Blockade

The physiologic braking phenomenon in response to continued diuretic use is well understood.[7, 8] When sodium reabsorption at one level of the nephron is impeded, the resultant sodium loss leads to a reactive response in which increased sodium reabsorption occurs elsewhere in the nephron. Thus, despite the continued action of the agent at its primary locus, increased sodium reabsorption elsewhere—proximal and distal to that locus of action—can limit the response. One would anticipate, then, that diuretic agents that work at other segments of the nephron would lead to natriuresis. By analogy with the earlier combined use of mercurial diuretics and a carbonic anhydrase inhibitor—and for the same reason—the efficacy of diuretic combinations becomes understandable.

Diuretic agents are usually grouped into four major categories according to their main site of action in the nephron. The first site is the proximal tubule, where carbonic anhydrase inhibitors decrease sodium absorption primarily by inhibiting bicarbonate transport. The second site is the thick ascending limb of Henle's loop where the loop diuretics inhibit Na^+/K^+/$2Cl$ cotransport. The third site is the distal tubule, where thiazides and quinetazone derivatives exert their main effect. The fourth locus is the cortical collecting tubule, the primary site of potassium secretion and aldosterone action. A number of factors contribute to diuretic action.[10] The natriuretic action of loop diuretics is substantially greater in patients with heart failure than in normal subjects.[11] Although loop diuretics are most potent and have the greatest natriuretic effect when measurements are made during the 6 hours of their peak action, sodium retention during the remainder of a 24-hour interval can offset the natriuretic effect unless sodium intake is restricted.[10, 12] Similarly, the natriuretic response to aldosterone antagonists or other potassium-sparing agents is substantially greater in the patient with activation of the sodium-retaining mechanisms as in heart failure than in normal subjects or patients with hypertension.[10, 11, 13]

One approach to increasing natriuresis when a severe refractory state has occurred is sequential nephron blockade. Ideally, the goal is to inhibit sodium reabsorption primarily at the nephron sites exhibiting increased sodium reabsorption, but few clinical clues are available to identify that site in the individual patient. Concomitantly, renal blood flow and glomerular filtration rate should be sustained, maintaining delivery of both sodium and drug, as discussed in the last section of this chapter, "Combination of Diuretics and Converting Enzyme Inhibitors."

A massive natriuretic response can be induced by the synergistic effect resulting from adding what appears to be a relatively small dose of a diuretic agent, acting mainly in the distal or cortical diluting segment, to a large but apparently ineffective dose of a potent loop diuretic. The introduction of metolazone, combined with furosemide and other loop diuretics, strongly confirmed earlier studies with thiazides.[14]

A 1983 editorial[14] not only provided a substantial list of references to this phenomenon, but also pointed out that this approach to the treatment of resistant edema is often far from innocuous. As described in the experience with high-dose furosemide, the advent or worsening of azotemia is common; the potential for severe electrolyte disarray, including hypokalemia and metabolic alkalosis, is substantial. When the rate of transcapillary refilling is exceeded, frank hypotension can occur, and fatalities have been reported. Certainly, when such therapy is undertaken, hospitalization is needed, and careful monitoring of urine flow, renal function, serum electrolyte, and acid base status is warranted.

ACE inhibition has provided an alternative approach to the treatment of refractory edema, especially in patients in whom diuretic therapy has resulted in azotemia or hyponatremia. The development of active endopeptidase inhibitors that act by preventing the degradation of atrial natriuretic peptide has led to preliminary evidence of sustained natriuretic and diuretic activity in patients with heart failure.[15] The development of new molecules in which ACE inhibition and neutral endopeptidase inhibition is induced by the identical chemical species is likely to be very attractive in the patient with heart failure. Precisely how to place these novel therapies in treatment today is still unclear.

Extrarenal Actions

In addition to their actions on the kidney to promote natriuresis, the extrarenal actions of diuretic agents may be important in the salutary response they induce.

One prominent action of furosemide therapy in the patient with congestive heart failure is venodilation.[16] Furosemide administered intravenously reduced left ventricular filling pressure in minutes, accompanied by a sharp increase in mean calf venous capacitance. This study confirmed the clinical impression that the relief of symptoms in the patient with acute pulmonary edema frequently preceded the diuretic effect. The vascular response occurred well before diuresis or the change in blood pressure or cardiac output. Indeed, the peak increase in urine flow and the peak natriuretic effect were seen 30 to 60 minutes later.

Biddle and Yu[17] confirmed the acute reduction in right atrial, pulmonary arterial, and pulmonary wedge pressure after administration of similar furosemide doses. Lung water, measured by a double isotope technique, was not changed up to 2 hours after administration of furosemide, but it fell significantly 4 to 24 hours after drug administration. Because dyspnea was relieved earlier, this symptom appears to be more related to chamber and intravascular pulmonary pressures than to total lung water in acute pulmonary edema. Again, venodilatation was confirmed as the major initial action of furosemide.

In long-term studies, Wilson et al.[18] documented that diuresis improved the performance of the failing ventricle primarily through a reduction in afterload without altering left ventricular diastolic dimensions. Their data suggested that the long-term diuretic action primarily reduces arteriolar resistance, which is analogous to the sequence in the patient with hypertension in whom long-term diuretic administration ultimately reduced total peripheral resistance.[1] A surprisingly poor correlation existed between the overall reduction in arterial blood pressure and improvement in myocardial performance.

An often ignored aspect of diuretic action in patients with congestive heart failure involves the functional implications of the increase in pulmonary water characteristic of that syndrome. Pulmonary congestion leads to a reduction in pulmonary compliance and an augmentation in the resistance to air flow; as a consequence, respiratory work is increased.[19, 20] Under normal conditions, the respiratory muscles use about 1% of total body oxygen uptake, but in the patient with severe congestive heart failure, the cost of breathing can be increased substantially as a consequence of the reduced pulmonary compliance and increased airway resistance. To what extent breathlessness and fatigue reflect the diversion of blood flow to the respiratory muscles remains unclear, but a diuretic-induced reduction in pulmonary water and improved pulmonary compliance and airway resistance should ultimately increase the efficiency of respiratory work.

A study by Lee et al.,[21] primarily designed to assess the role of digoxin in patients with heart failure, also clarified the interaction of digoxin with diuretics. Patients who responded to digoxin in that study had more chronic and severe heart failure, more evidence of left ventricular dilatation and a reduction in ejection fraction, and, most notably, a clear third heart sound. The third heart sound was the most powerful predictor of a salutary response to digoxin. Indeed, the presence of a third heart sound was a better correlate of digitalis response than the severity of heart failure itself. The genesis of a third heart sound of left ventricular origin probably depends on the existence of enough left ventricular dilatation to allow the heart to strike the chest wall during protodiastole. The authors suggested that digitalis would be effective primarily when diuretic therapy had caused an elevation in left atrial pressure, so that early ventricular filling was rapid and a third heart sound was thereby generated. In patients in whom diuretic treatment restored left atrial pressure to normal or near normal, the third heart sound disappeared, and no further clinical improvement could be attributed to digitalis. It is marvelous that a physical sign easily elicited at the bedside provides the clearest indication of therapeutic choice.

COMPLICATIONS OF DIURETIC USE IN CONGESTIVE HEART FAILURE

A host of complications has been well documented with diuretic use, including hyperuricemia, hyperglycemia, hyperlipidemia, ototoxicity with furosemide and ethacrynic acid, and a number of specific side effects with individual agents, such as gynecomastia with spironolactone use and osteomalacia with long-term acetazolamide use.[7, 22] Rather than provide a cursory review of a subject already well reviewed in a number of chapters and review articles,[7, 8, 22] attention will be focused on a number of problems that may have specific and important long-term implications for natural history in heart disease.

Sudden death, presumably reflecting a cardiac arrhythmia, is responsible for 50% of the mortality in congestive heart failure.[23] Unfortunately, the more severe the abnormality in left ventricular function, the less clear it is that antiarrhythmic agents are effective, and the more likely it becomes that their use will provoke further left ventricular dysfunction.[23] In the patient with heart failure who is treated with diuretics, the resultant deficits of potassium and magnesium are likely to be important. Reviews[23-26] suggest that electrolyte abnormalities are common, often unrecognized, and amenable to therapy when properly planned.

Muscle biopsy in patients with congestive heart failure indicated that measurement of serum potassium concentration often underestimated tissue potassium deficits.[24] Tissue potassium content was reduced significantly in more than half of patients so treated, often in the presence of a normal serum potassium concentration. Moreover, levels of muscle magnesium were below normal in 43% of the patients.

More than 40% of patients with hypokalemia also have hypomagnesemia.[25] Attempts to reverse the potassium deficit with potassium supplements in such patients are exceedingly unlikely to be successful. Tissue magnesium repletion is necessary before cellular potassium uptake will occur.

Potassium-sparing diuretic combinations—including triamterene, amiloride, and spironolactone—were substantially more successful in reversing both potassium deficits and magnesium deficits in patients with congestive heart failure[24] than was the application of potassium salts. Publications have paid substantial attention to the issue of potassium and magnesium sparing.[10-13, 27, 28] The possibility that amiloride is more effective than spironolactone in attenuating thiazide-induced magnesium deficits has been raised.[28] On the other hand, there is substantial evidence of a magnesium-sparing effect of spironolactone,[11] and the possibility that blocking the action of aldosterone can limit structural cardiac remodeling is receiving considerable attention.[13]

The implications of combined potassium and magnesium deficits for arrhythmogenesis have long been recognized.[29, 30] Dyckner and Wester[24] assessed the relationship between tissue content and arrhythmias in patients with congestive heart failure. The infusion of magnesium-containing solutions led to significant increases in serum and muscle concentrations of both potassium and magnesium; it also led to a reduction in the frequency of ventricular ectopic beats. Potassium infusions increased serum potassium concentration, at least transiently; however, in the presence of a magnesium deficit, they did not change tissue potassium content, nor was there an impact on prevalence of ventricular ectopic beats. All in all, it is difficult to ignore these interactions.

Because the frequency of ventricular premature beats has been the index of so many of these studies, it is reasonable to question whether they are clinically important. The area is controversial, but it should be less controversial. A host of studies[31-35] has documented a clear increase in the frequency and severity of clinically important ventricular arrhythmias and death in patients who are hypokalemic at the time of myocardial infarction. When diuretics are required in the patient with congestive heart failure, as they generally are, strategies must be employed to minimize the impact of the regimen on potassium and magnesium, both serum and cellular. One choice is the combination of a natriuretic agent with a potassium-sparing agent. Alternatively, strategies involving ACE inhibitors can be considered.

COMBINATION OF DIURETICS AND CONVERTING ENZYME INHIBITORS

The increasing use of ACE inhibitors in the patient with heart failure and the interaction of these agents with diuretics have made it necessary to develop strategies for their combined use. Early after their introduction, it became apparent that ACE inhibitors not only could relieve symptoms but also could reverse azotemia and hyponatremia in patients who had been treated with diuretics and a low-salt diet.[9] It also became evident that these agents could induce hypotension and that, when they did so, they would provoke azotemia and hyponatremia,[36] especially in patients who had been treated aggressively with diuretics.

Growing evidence that ACE inhibition not only relieves symptoms but can also change the natural history of congestive heart failure[37] makes it clear that the use of ACE inhibitors will continue to accelerate.

When using diuretics in combination with ACE inhibition, the severity of congestive heart failure; the presence or absence of concurrent hyponatremia; prior diuretic use and evidence of fluid retention; baseline blood pressure, especially when relative hypotension is present; and whether hypertension contributed to the pathogenesis of heart failure must be taken into account. More severe heart failure, especially with hyponatremia and baseline hypotension or a history of aggressive diuretic use, makes the patient prone to hypotension with ACE inhibition.

Current recommendations on the dosage of ACE inhibitors work well in the individual who is neither hypotensive nor hyponatremic and in whom blood pressure is not in the borderline low range—that is, in the healthiest of patients with heart failure.

Hypotension, progressive azotemia, and hyponatremia are the most common reasons for discontinuing use of ACE inhibitors in the patient with heart failure. No single strategy has evolved to deal with this problem. Several factors must be kept in mind. In the individual in whom increasing diuretic use has provoked volume contraction and in whom pulmonary congestion is currently rate-limiting, it is reasonable to discontinue diuretic use and liberalize sodium intake prior to instituting an ACE inhibitor. Conversely, in the patient who is still edematous and has pulmonary congestion, liberalizing sodium intake is not possible.

The alternative is to reduce the ACE inhibitor dose to low levels. Captopril doses as low as 1 or 2 mg lead to salutary hemodynamic, renal, and clinical responses without hypotension in patients with ad-

vanced heart failure.[9] Information on the equivalent dose of enalapril is not available, but, because enalapril is so much more potent than captopril, equivalent doses would have to be substantially lower than 1 mg.[38]

To achieve a 1-mg dose, pulverize a tablet and make a solution that is given by mouth. Because the preparation is probably unstable, discard the preparation at 8-hour intervals. After a day or two during which very low doses are used, the cardiovascular state of the individual stabilizes and larger doses are well tolerated.

Furosemide is required to reverse hyponatremia in the patient treated with an ACE inhibitor who begins with baseline hyponatremia.[39] Typically, furosemide therapy is stopped or doses are reduced to 20 to 40 mg daily when ACE inhibition is instituted.

The available data suggest that strategies involving multiple diuretic use to treat resistant edema will be replaced with strategies in which limited diuretic doses are combined with an ACE inhibitor. What to do in the patient in whom resistant edema develops despite the combined use of optimal doses of a diuretic and an ACE inhibitor represents the current frontier. At the moment, this condition appears to be an indication for heart transplantation. There are limits to the efficacy of medical therapy.

REFERENCES

1. Mudge GH: Diuretics and other agents employed in the mobilization of edema fluid. In Goodman LS, Gilman A (eds): The Pharmacological Basis of Therapeutics, 3rd ed. New York: MacMillan, 1965, pp 827–858.
2. Eggleston C: Treatment of cardiac failure. In Cecil LR (ed): A Textbook of Medicine. Philadelphia: WB Saunders, 1930, pp 1099–1114.
3. Smith HW: Salt and water volume receptors: An exercise in physiologic apologetics. Am J Med 23:623, 1957.
4. Hollenberg NK, Schulman G: Renal perfusion and function in the sodium-retaining states. In Seldin DW, Geibisch G (eds): Physiology and Pathology of Electrolyte Metabolism. New York: Raven Press, 1985, pp 1119–1136.
5. Bell NH, Schedl HP, Bartter FC, et al: An explanation of abnormal water retention and hypoosmolarity in congestive heart failure. Am J Med 36:351, 1964.
6. Bennett WM, Bagby GC, Antonovic JN: Influence of volume expansion on proximal tubular sodium reabsorption to saline infusion. Am Heart J 85:55, 1973.
7. Chonko A, Grantham JJ: Treatment of edema states. In Maxwell MH, Kleeman CR, Narins RG (eds): Disorders of Sodium Content and Concentration. New York: McGraw-Hill, 1987, pp 429–460.
8. Brater CD: Resistance to diuretics: Emphasis on a pharmacological perspective. Drugs 22:477, 1981.
9. Dzau VJ, Colucci WS, Williams GH, et al: Sustained effectiveness of converting-enzyme inhibition in patients with severe congestive heart failure. N Engl J Med 302:1373, 1980.
10. Reyes AJ: Effects of diuretics on renal excretory function. Eur Heart J 13(Suppl G):15–21, 1992.
11. Nicholls MG: Interaction of diuretics and electrolytes in congestive heart failure. Am J Cardiol 65:17E–21E, 1990.
12. Wilcox CS, Mitch WE, Kelly RA, et al: Response of the kidney to furosemide: I. Effects of salt intake and renal compensation. J Lab Clin Med 102:450–458, 1983.
13. Weber KT, Villarreal D: Aldosterone and antialdosterone therapy in congestive heart failure. Am J Cardiol 71:3A–11A, 1993.
14. Oster JR, Epstein M, Smoller S: Combined therapy with thia-

zide-type and loop diuretic agents for resistant sodium retention. Ann Intern Med 99:405, 1983.

15. Elsner D, Muntze A, Kromer EP, Riegger GAJ: Effectiveness of endopeptidase inhibition (Candoxatril) in congestive heart failure. Am J Cardiol 70:494–498, 1992.

16. Dikshit K, Vyden JK, Forrester JS, et al: Renal and extrarenal hemodynamic effects of furosemide in congestive heart failure after acute myocardial infarction. N Engl J Med 288:1087, 1973.

17. Biddle TL, Yu PN: Effect of furosemide on hemodynamics and lung water in acute pulmonary edema secondary to myocardial infarction. Am J Cardiol 43:86, 1979.

18. Wilson JR, Reichek N, Duniman WB, et al: Effect of diuresis on the performance of the failing left ventricle in man. Am J Med 70:235, 1981.

19. Schlant RC: Altered physiology of the cardiovascular system in heart failure. In Hurst JW, Logue RB (eds): The Heart, Arteries and Veins. New York: McGraw-Hill, 1970, pp 405–423.

20. Depeursinge FB, Depeursinge CD, Boutaleb AK, et al: Respiratory system impedance in patients with acute left ventricular failure: Pathophysiology and clinical interest. Circulation 73:386, 1986.

21. Lee DCS, Johnson RA, Bingham JB, et al: Heart failure in outpatients: A randomized trial of digoxin versus placebo. N Engl J Med 306:699, 1982.

22. Suki WN, Stinebaugh BJ, Frommer JP, et al: Physiology of diuretic action. In Seldin DW, Giebisch G (eds): The Kidney: Physiology and Pathophysiology. New York: Raven Press, 1985, pp 2127–2162.

23. Packer M, Gottlieb SS, Blum MA: Immediate and long-term pathophysiologic mechanisms underlying the genesis of sudden cardiac death in patients with congestive heart failure. Am J Med 82:4, 1987.

24. Dyckner T, Wester PO: Potassium/magnesium depletion in patients with cardiovascular disease. Am J Med 82:11, 1987.

25. Whang R: Magnesium deficiency: Pathogenesis, prevalence, and clinical implications. Am J Med 82:24, 1987.

26. Ryan MP: Diuretics and potassium/magnesium depletion: Directions for treatment. Am J Med 82:38, 1987.

27. Prichard BNC, Owens CWI, Woolf AS: Adverse reactions to diuretics. Eur Heart J 13(Suppl G):96–103, 1992.

28. Murdoch DL, Forrest G, Davies DL, et al: A comparison of the potassium and magnesium-sparing properties of amiloride and spironolactone in diuretic-treated normal subjects. Br J Clin Pharmacol 35(4):373–378, 1993.

29. Roden DM, Iansmith DHS: Effects of low potassium or magnesium concentrations on isolated cardiac tissue. Am J Med 82(3A):18, 1987.

30. Hollifield JW: Magnesium depletion, diuretics and arrhythmias. Am J Med 82(3A):30, 1987.

31. Dyckner T, Helmers C, Lundman T, et al: Initial serum potassium level in relation to early complications in prognosis in patients with acute myocardial infarction. Acta Med Scand 197:207, 1975.

32. Dyckner T, Helmers C, Wester PO: Cardiac dysrhythmias in patients with acute myocardial infarction. Acta Med Scand 216:127, 1984.

33. Solomon RJ, Cole AG: Importance of potassium in patients with acute myocardial infarction. Acta Med Scand Suppl 647:87, 1981.

34. Nordrehaug JE, von der Lippe G: Hypokalaemia and ventricular fibrillation in acute myocardial infarction. Br Heart J 50:525, 1983.

35. Johansson BW, Dziamski R: Malignant arrhythmias in acute myocardial infarction. Drugs 28(Suppl):11, 1984.

36. Hollenberg NK: Pathophysiology of congestive heart failure: The role of the kidney. In Cohn JN (ed): Drug Treatment of Heart Failure. New York: Yorke Medical Books, 1983, pp 53–71.

37. The CONCENSUS Trial Study Group: Effects of enalapril on mortality in severe congestive heart failure. N Engl J Med 316:1429, 1987.

38. Packer M, Lee WH, Yushak M, et al: Comparison of captopril and enalapril in patients with severe chronic heart failure. N Engl J Med 315:847, 1986.

39. Dzau VJ, Hollenberg NK: Renal response to captopril in severe heart failure: Role of furosemide in natriuresis and reversal of hyponatremia. Ann Intern Med 100:777, 1984.

B. Loop Diuretics

CHAPTER 39

Furosemide

Murray Epstein, M.D., and Barry J. Materson, M.D.

The loop diuretics are so named because they act principally on the thick ascending limb of the loop of Henle (TALH). This nephron segment reabsorbs 20% to 30% of the filtered load of sodium chloride. By virtue of their ability to abolish a large portion of this loop function, loop diuretics are the most potent diuretics in clinical use. Because they have a steep dose-response natriuresis curve, they have been called *high-ceiling* diuretics. The organomercurials were the first effective loop diuretics but are no longer used. The loop diuretics in wide clinical use are furosemide, ethacrynic acid, and bumetanide (Table 39–1). Other less well known and less used drugs include piretanide, muzolimine, etozolin, and indacrinone.

Furosemide is the prototype of this class of diuretics. With its introduction in 1966, furosemide represented a major breakthrough in the treatment of many patients with sodium retention. Furosemide is the standard against which all other loop diuretics are evaluated, having become an invaluable tool for physiologists and pharmacologists throughout the world.

Loop diuretics are characterized by prompt onset of action and short duration of diuresis.[1] Although the site of action of the loop diuretics is well characterized, the biochemical mechanisms of action are not

Table 39–1. **Loop Diuretics**

Generic Name	Trade Name
Azosemide	Luret
Bumetanide	Bumex
Ethacrynic acid	Edecrin
Furosemide	Lasix
Indacrinone	
Muzolimine	
Piretanide	Arlix

fully elucidated. Evidence indicates that the diuretics are secreted into the lumen of the proximal tubule and act on the luminal membrane of the TALH to inhibit NaCl reabsorption. As a result of this inhibition, reabsorption of other electrolytes that depend on NaCl transport in this segment is also inhibited. Among these electrolytes are potassium, calcium, and magnesium. As a consequence of inhibition of NaCl transport in the ascending limb, the generation and maintenance of a hypertonic interstitium is compromised. Loop diuretics thus induce not only natriuresis but also diuresis by virtue of diminishing the gradient for passive water movement from the descending limb of the loop of Henle and the medullary collecting duct. As a result, free water clearance and the ability to concentrate urine maximally are markedly decreased.

This chapter reviews the effects of furosemide, the most widely used loop diuretic, and considers the determinants of response to furosemide.

PHARMACOLOGIC CHARACTERISTICS OF LOOP DIURETICS

Although the loop diuretics exhibit similar pharmacologic spectra, the parent compounds share few chemical properties. Most are carboxylic acids. Ethacrynic acid is a derivative of aryloxyacetic acid, furosemide is a derivative of anthranilic acid, and bumetanide is derived from 3-aminobenzoic acid. Bumetanide has a higher milligram-for-milligram potency than furosemide, but the compounds are similar in other respects.[2]

The mercurial diuretics, such as mersalyl and meralluride, are also loop diuretics but are no longer commercially available. These drugs lost favor because they were not readily absorbed from the gastrointestinal tract, became ineffective following the development of metabolic alkalosis, and caused some toxic side effects at high concentrations.

Furosemide is readily absorbed from the gastrointestinal tract, binds avidly to plasma proteins, and is rapidly eliminated from the body. Furosemide is largely eliminated by renal excretion, primarily by proximal tubular secretion. About one third of the drug is excreted intact by the liver or metabolized before urinary or intestinal excretion. The onset of action occurs 30 to 60 minutes after oral administration and 2 to 5 minutes after intravenous injection. The duration of action of a single orally administered tablet is about 6 hours; a single intravenous injection lasts 3 hours.

ACUTE ACTION OF FUROSEMIDE
Diuretic Actions

Furosemide acts on the medullary and cortical segments of the TALH. Although it is clear that the site of action is the TALH, the exact mechanism of action is not fully defined. Presumably, furosemide is se-

creted into the tubular fluid by the proximal tubule and acts on the luminal side of the cells of the TALH. Furosemide is thought to act principally by inhibiting Na^+-$2Cl$-K^+ cotransport across the luminal membrane.[3, 4] It is interesting that, as a group, the loop diuretics have similar actions despite markedly different chemical structures.

Although furosemide is a potent drug, it must be emphasized that the natriuretic response varies markedly among individuals. The variability in response is due principally to differences in individual sodium balance and extracellular fluid volume (ECV). Inhibition of NaCl transport by furosemide presumably depends on the luminal concentration of the drug and thus the extracellular fluid concentration and integrity of the proximal tubule secretory system. An additional determinant of varying responsiveness is the bioavailability of furosemide, which depends on differences in absorption from the bowel.

Furosemide also affects renal water handling. Because of its principal action within the ascending limb, it usually diminishes both free water clearance and the ability to concentrate urine (free water absorption).[5, 6]

Because the loop of Henle reabsorbs about 25% of the filtered potassium, it is not surprising that furosemide affects potassium excretion. Furosemide influences renal potassium excretion by virtue of its effects on loop potassium reabsorption and distal tubular secretion. Potassium reabsorption by the loop of Henle is thought to be passive and dependent on sodium transport. Inhibition of NaCl cotransport or diminution of the transepithelial voltage leads to a decrease in potassium reabsorption by the loop. Furthermore, potassium secretion in the distal nephron highly depends on the flow rate past the secretory sites. A decrease in water absorption by the thin descending limb as a result of diminished interstitial osmolality results in enhanced fluid delivery to the distal convoluted tubule and enhanced net potassium secretion. Mineralocorticoids also markedly influence potassium secretion in the distal nephron. Accordingly, potassium may be lost continually in the urine in the course of diuretic administration because of inhibition of loop reabsorption and elevation of aldosterone-mediated distal secretion.

The loop of Henle reabsorbs some 25% of the filtered calcium and 65% of the filtered magnesium. These divalent cations are thought to be reabsorbed principally by passive mechanisms that depend on the active transport of sodium chloride.[7] Furosemide, presumably through its action on NaCl transport, inhibits calcium and magnesium reabsorption in the loop of Henle.

Other Actions

Furosemide has several physiologic actions other than natriuresis. Furosemide administration increases systemic venous capacitance; this vascular response is blocked by nonsteroidal antiinflammatory drugs, indicating involvement of prostaglandins.[8] This increase in systemic venous capacitance results in a prompt decrease in left atrial pressure and reduced cardiac preload. This attribute recommends the use of furosemide as an effective agent in the treatment of cardiogenic pulmonary edema in addition to its diuretic effect. Furosemide also increases renal blood flow and stimulates renin release.

CHRONIC RESPONSE TO LOOP DIURETICS
Braking Phenomenon

The kidney possesses compensatory mechanisms to limit the diuretic response after sustained administration of furosemide and other loop diuretics. This process is called the *braking phenomenon*. The fundamental basis for the braking or limitation of diuretic response is a decrease in the ECV. Chronic or sustained contraction of the ECV leads to an increase in salt and water reabsorption in the proximal and distal tubules. The diuretic inhibition within the loop is thus overridden. Figure 39–1[9] schematically illustrates the response of an individual given loop diuretic over a sustained period. An immediate loss of sodium and water in the urine occurs. The loss of salt and water from the ECV is reflected by a loss in body weight (a reasonable estimate of fluid volume changes). Sodium excretion gradually decreases over several days, attaining levels similar to those before diuretic administration and equal to dietary sodium intake.

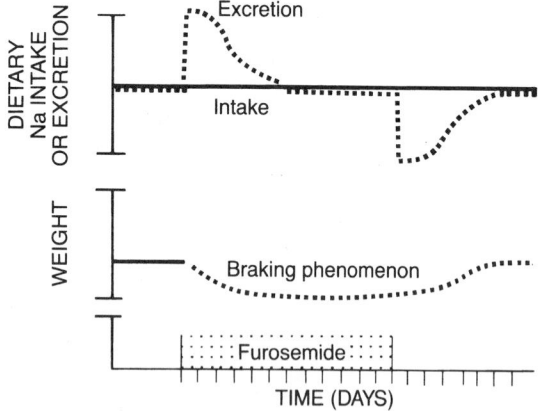

Figure 39–1. Response to continued administration of a loop diuretic in a normal subject on a constant salt intake. Initially, urinary excretion increases and extracellular fluid volume decreases concomitantly with the urinary salt and water loss. Following a lag phase, urinary salt excretion returns to normal (to equal daily intake) as proximal and distal tubular reabsorption increase to offset the diuretic action within the loop. Accordingly, a steady state is reestablished but at the expense of a contracted extracellular fluid volume. Conversely, when the loop diuretic is stopped, there is a similar lag phase during which excretion is initially decreased, resulting in a retention of salt and water and body weight gain before a normal balance is attained. (Adapted from Grantham JJ, Chonko AM: The physiologic basis and clinical use of diuretics. *In* Brenner BM, Stein JH [eds]: Sodium and Water Homeostasis. New York: Churchill Livingstone, 1978, pp 178–211.)

DETERMINANTS OF RESPONSE TO LOOP DIURETICS
Distribution, Metabolism, and Elimination

Furosemide has a number of properties that influence its effectiveness. First, it is readily absorbed by the gastrointestinal tract, which permits oral administration. Second, it is tightly bound to plasma proteins, which limits its distribution within the body fluids. Third, it is secreted efficiently by the proximal tubule into the tubular fluid. Because furosemide acts from the luminal side, it tends to be concentrated at the site of diuretic action. Finally, renal and nonrenal clearance are relatively rapid, so that drug accumulation does not normally occur. Collectively, these properties render furosemide an ideal agent for clinical use.

Furosemide is bound tightly to plasma protein and distributes with negligible tissue binding in the body in a volume smaller than the ECV.[10] Because the volume of distribution of furosemide is a function of the free unbound furosemide concentration, the distribution volume decreases in conditions associated with reduction in serum albumin concentration (e.g., aging, nephrotic syndrome, uremia, and cirrhosis), and total distribution volumes are altered in association with changes in plasma protein binding.[11] Moreover, furosemide can be displaced from the protein-binding sites by other acidic exogenous drugs or endogenous acidic anions. Displacement from serum albumin enhances diuretic action by increasing glomerular filtration of the diuretics and by increasing the amount of free diuretic available for tubular secretion. Although the predominant route of drug clearance is through the kidney, furosemide also is eliminated through the biliary tract.

Intrarenal Determinants

Furosemide can be delivered to its site of action even when renal blood flow and glomerular filtration rate are compromised. Furosemide is further concentrated in the lumen as water is lost from the tubular fluid, as it progresses down the thin descending limb of the loop of Henle.

The potency of furosemide is determined by three independent factors: (1) the pharmacokinetics of the drug, (2) its proximal secretion, and (3) the ECV and sodium balance of the patient. ECV and sodium balance are often more important factors in modifying the clinical response to diuretics than are changes in the proximal secretion or the pharmacokinetics of the diuretics.[12]

Role of Dietary Sodium Restriction as an Adjunct to Diuretic Therapy

During diuretic therapy of patients whose levels of Na intake are equivalent to those used in clinical practice, diuretic-induced Na loss is limited primarily by Na retention in the postdiuretic period. Although the administration of a loop diuretic leads to activation of the renin-angiotensin-aldosterone axis and the sympathetic nervous system, Almeshari et al.[13] have demonstrated that the period of postdiuretic Na retention does not depend solely on these two well-defined pathways for ECV homeostasis, because it is not prevented by the blockade of angiotensin II generation and aldosterone secretion with captopril or α-adrenoceptors with prazosin, even when given together.[14, 15] Rather, postdiuretic Na retention may be attributable in part to an adaptive change in tubular transport capacity mediated in part by an increase in the Na,K-ATPase activity of the distal convoluted tubule. Collectively, these findings emphasize the importance of salt restriction both during loop diuretic therapy and after its withdrawal to obviate Na retention resulting from these powerful Na-retaining mechanisms.

Extrapolating these findings to the care of patients receiving diuretic therapy, we emphasize the importance of the restriction of dietary salt, both during diuretic therapy and for some time after its withdrawal, to obviate the period of salt retention. Otherwise, the physician may reach an erroneous conclusion that the patient has a primary salt-retaining condition requiring ongoing diuretic treatment for its control.

Diuretic Insensitivity

The diuretic response to furosemide is unpredictable in a number of disease states. Although many circumstances in which patients' conditions become refractory to loop diuretics are clearly understood, some remain unexplained (Table 39–2). Insensitivity to a diuretic may occur after prolonged administration. In some instances, a diuretic response may be elicited by a change of diuretic, even to another drug acting at the same nephron site. For example, a patient whose condition is refractory to furosemide may respond to ethacrynic acid. The basis for this observation is not clear. Some clinicians use the term *insensitivity* of the nephron to the diuretics, but this term is a misnomer. It is probably not the interaction of the diuretic agent with the NaCl cotransport site that is faulty, but rather the physiologic setting that is not conducive to specific drug action. As examples, abnormalities of renal blood flow, plasma protein binding, and proximal secretion may result in ineffective concentrations of the drug within the TALH. A number of clinical observations collectively support a multifactorial resistance rather than a receptor desensitization as a basis

for unresponsiveness to diuretics. A logical step to circumvent this problem is to change loop diuretics. If a given dose is ineffective, one should increase the dose rather than merely give the same dose more frequently.

A report by Inoue et al.[16] has suggested an innovative approach to the management of furosemide resistance in patients with hypoalbuminemia. They marshalled evidence indicating that binding to albumin is essential for the delivery of furosemide to the kidney. Injection of furosemide-albumin complex (furosemide mixed with albumin solution) rapidly increased the urine volume of hypoalbuminemic patients who showed a marked resistance to furosemide alone.

Interactions Between Nonsteroidal Antiinflammatory Drugs and Loop Diuretics

Because the response to diuretics depends on an unimpaired renal prostaglandin system, administration of nonsteroidal antiinflammatory drugs, which inhibit renal cyclooxygenase activity, have been reported to reduce the diuretic and natriuretic effects of loop diuretics.[17, 18] It has been suggested that sodium balance may modulate this interaction. For example, in dogs, indomethacin impaired the natriuretic effects of furosemide in sodium-depleted but not in sodium-loaded dogs.[19]

Whereas an impairment of renal vasodilatory prostaglandins diminishes the diuretic and natriuretic effects of loop diuretics, an increased renal production of vasoconstrictor prostanoids (i.e., TXA_2) may impair the renal response to loop diuretics. Furthermore, Pinzani et al.[20] have demonstrated that the inhibition of TX-synthase activity with OKY 046 enhanced the diuretic and natriuretic effects of intravenously administered furosemide.

Effects of Aging

An additional consideration is the effect of aging on the pharmacokinetics of loop diuretics. Andreasen et al.[21] have documented significant age-related changes in the fate of unchanged furosemide in normal subjects. The serum clearance of furosemide was reduced in the elderly, and the average amount of unchanged furosemide in the urine during the initial 30 minutes after administration was decreased in elderly normal subjects. The authors concluded that the age-related changes in renal handling of furosemide may be attributable to a reduction in the tubular secretion of the drug. Because the natriuretic and diuretic ef-

Table 39–2. **Determinants of the Diuretic Response to Loop Diuretics**

Influence	Example	Diuretic Response
Fluid and sodium balance	Volume contraction	Decreased
Inhibition of proximal secretion	Organic acids (e.g., probenecid)	Decreased
Diminished proximal secretion	Renal failure	Decreased
Prostaglandin inhibition	Nonsteroidal antiinflammatory drugs	Decreased

fects of the drug are closely related to their urinary excretory pattern, these studies suggest that furosemide (and presumably other loop diuretics) may be less efficient in mobilizing sodium in the older patient.

CLINICAL USE
Indications

The indications for furosemide diuretics are listed in Table 39–3. The major use of furosemide is in patients with edematous states. Less frequent indications include the correction of symptomatic fluid and electrolyte disorders, including hyponatremia and hypercalcemia. The role of furosemide in the prophylaxis of acute renal failure remains controversial.

In planning a diuretic regimen, several general principles must be borne in mind.[22] Diuretic drugs such as furosemide should be viewed as adjuncts to other measures, including bed rest and nutritional supplementation, in the therapy of patients with edema and ascites. Diuretic treatment has two distinct goals: (1) to mobilize a large surplus of salt and water from the interstitial fluid space and peritoneal cavity and (2) to maintain a normal sodium balance in patients without edema in whom an additional reduction of sodium intake is not feasible because of cost or unpalatability of the diet. It should be remembered that the drugs initially chosen to mobilize edema fluid may be different from those diuretic agents required subsequently to maintain a normal sodium balance. Given the diversity of the underlying disease (such as in cirrhotic patients) and the degree of fluid retention, it is apparent that any diuretic regimen must be individualized for each patient. Finally, the goal of diuretic administration in the cirrhotic patient with ascites is not to render the patient free of edema and ascites but rather to remove only enough retained fluid to ensure patient comfort.[22]

Brater[23] pointed out that the usual custom of increasing the dosage of loop diuretics in a stepwise fashion to a maximum of 400 mg/day for furosemide or 10 mg/day for bumetanide appears to be without merit. Brater has shown that if administration of a loop diuretic leads to an inadequate natriuretic response, increasing the dose to 2.5 times the usual clinical dose should more than compensate for any changes that occur in the disposition of loop diuretics in patients with liver disease. Some patients are truly refractory to diuretics and do not respond to any dose. Aggressive escalation to doses greater than 2.5 times normal will not induce further natriuresis but only risk toxicity in such patients.

Table 39–3. **Indications for Furosemide**

Mobilization of edema and ascites
Treatment of severe symptomatic hyponatremia
Treatment of hypercalcemia
Possible role in prophylaxis of acute renal failure
Treatment of halide intoxication
Treatment of distal renal tubular acidosis

Precautions

Care should be exercised with respect to the rapidity with which ascites is mobilized by diuretics. Until recently, rigid constraints were placed on attempts to mobilize ascitic fluid in cirrhotic patients without concomitant edema. Such a restriction was grounded in part on the studies of Shear et al.,[24] who reported that in ascitic patients without edema, any diuresis that exceeds 900 ml/day must be mobilized at the expense of the plasma compartment, with resultant volume contraction and, eventually, electrolyte abnormalities, oliguria, and azotemia.

Several groups of investigators have reevaluated the effects of large-volume (4 to 25 L/day ascites) or total paracentesis (complete mobilization of ascites during only one paracentesis session), concluding that these modalities constitute effective and relatively safe therapy for mobilizing ascites. Extensive studies of Arroyo et al.[25, 26] have clearly established a role for large-volume paracentesis in treating refractory ascites.

Both diuresis and therapeutic paracentesis have a role in the management of patients with ascites. They are not mutually exclusive. However, the practitioner must be aware of the risks of both methods and base individualized therapy on the balance of these risks.

MANAGEMENT OF SELECTED SPECIFIC CONDITIONS

The major indications for loop diuretics are listed in Table 39–3. Most are self-explanatory, but several require further comment.

Congestive Heart Failure

Although mild congestive heart failure may be treated with thiazide diuretics, loop diuretics such as furosemide must be used to manage patients with moderate to severe failure. Chronic monotherapy with diuretics improves functional class in most patients, usually as a result of a reduction in left ventricular filling pressure but relatively unchanged cardiac output.[27]

Much of the symptomatic improvement in congestive heart failure is due to reduction in pulmonary water, improvement in pulmonary compliance, reduction in resistance to airflow, and reduction in respiratory work. In experimental animals, normal subjects, and patients with congestive failure, a single intravenous dose of a loop diuretic reduced pulmonary vascular pressure with concomitant reductions in pulmonary wedge pressure, pulmonary artery pressure, and right atrial pressure.[27]

The management of congestive heart failure is often complicated by an inability of orally administered furosemide to produce effective diuresis.[28, 29] Patients with this diuretic resistance often require intravenous furosemide administration to achieve the desired clinical response. It has been suggested that this resistance is due to malabsorption of furosemide secondary to changes induced by congestive heart failure in the gastrointestinal tract, such as edema of the gut wall, delayed gastric emptying, decreased intestinal motility, or decreased splanchnic blood flow. Vasko et al.[29] assessed whether patients with decompensated congestive heart failure had altered absorption of orally administered furosemide. They observed a qualitative alteration in furosemide absorption in patients with decompensated heart failure when compared with patients with compensated congestive heart failure. Thus, compensated patients had more rapid absorption and greater peak serum furosemide concentrations. These investigators concluded that such qualitative changes may be a contributing factor to the diuretic resistance seen in many patients with congestive heart failure.

In recent years, furosemide has been used in combination with captopril in the setting of severe congestive heart failure.[30, 31] Newer treatment strategies using the addition of captopril for afterload reduction have evolved. Although it has been shown that captopril by itself can improve survival in patients with class III or IV congestive heart failure, the addition of furosemide is required to ensure concomitant natriuresis and correction of hyponatremia, if present.[32]

Hypertension and Reduced Renal Function

Although thiazide-type medications are the diuretic agents of choice for patients with hypertension and normal renal function,[33] they may not be as effective in patients with creatinine clearances below 50 ml/min and are generally ineffective at creatinine clearances below 35 ml/min. In patients with such reduction in renal function, diuretic management of hypertension should take the form of a loop diuretic, either as a sole agent or in combination with other antihypertensive drugs.

Nephrotic Syndrome

Patients with nephrotic syndrome and symptomatic edema, especially when nephrotic syndrome is severe, may be relatively refractory to loop diuretics. Substantial amounts of furosemide bind to protein in their urine, preventing its access to the site of action in the TALH.[23] In addition, secretion of loop diuretics by the proximal tubule may diminish as a result of a major reduction in plasma albumin concentration and consequent decreased delivery of albumin-bound drug to the secretory sites in the proximal straight tubule. In such patients, the physician must use increasing doses of furosemide as stated previously. A preliminary report has advocated the administration of furosemide as a furosemide-albumin complex to overcome such diuretic resistance.[16]

Hyponatremia

An interesting application of furosemide is its adjunctive use (together with hypertonic saline) for the prompt correction, when appropriate, of severe hyponatremia.[34] Furosemide serves two purposes: (1) it tends to prevent volume overload in patients at risk, and (2) by interfering with the renal concentrating ability and thus lowering urine osmolality, it may markedly increase the loss of water. This second effect, combined administration of the concentrated solution of sodium, results in a rapid increase in serum sodium. Sodium levels that are increased too rapidly, however, have attendant risks such as central pontine myelinolysis (see Chapter 42).

Syndrome of Hyporeninemic Hypoaldosteronism

It has been suggested that the renal acidification defect frequently associated with the syndrome of hyporeninemic hypoaldosteronism (SHH; type 4 renal tubular acidosis) is the most common form of renal tubular acidosis.[35] Certainly, it is one of the most frequent causes of hyperkalemia in patients with diabetic nephropathy or chronic interstitial nephropathy and mild to moderate renal insufficiency.

The obvious therapy for SHH is chronic administration of a mineralocorticoid such as fludrocortisone. However, this method carries the risk of inducing sodium retention with subsequent worsening of congestive heart failure, hypertension, and edema, especially in elderly, chronically ill patients. Sometimes, sodium retention occurs even when potassium excretion is not enhanced. For these reasons, and because of its proven efficacy and safety when used properly, furosemide in relatively low doses (e.g., 40 to 120 mg/day) appears to be the agent of choice for the treatment of SHH.[35] Furosemide's improvement of potassium homeostasis and acidosis is based on both a renal and an extrarenal effect, because no significant correlation exists between the decrement in serum potassium concentration and the cumulative urinary excretion of potassium.[35]

Prophylaxis of Acute Renal Failure

The role of furosemide in the prophylaxis or management of acute renal failure cannot be avoided. If the patient has already undergone an acute insult, some observers advocate attempts to increase urine flow rate and renal blood flow with the use of furosemide or mannitol. Even if renal failure occurs after such therapy, some experts have advocated furosemide administration in the hope that it will induce a higher rate of urine output (e.g., nonoliguric acute renal failure), which is associated with better outcome. Conversely, the evidence that high doses of diuretic will convert low-output failure to high-output failure and improve prognosis is controversial. We believe that furosemide has only a limited role in the treatment of patients who already demonstrate evidence of *established* renal failure.[36]

ADVERSE METABOLIC EFFECTS

As a consequence of the adjustments in tubular reabsorption that follow sustained diuretic administration, a number of adverse metabolic complications may ensue (Table 39–4). In essence, most of these complications arise as consequences of contraction of the extracellular volume.

Metabolic Alkalosis

Metabolic alkalosis, usually mild, is commonly associated with the use of loop-type diuretics.[37] Its generation relates mainly to enhanced ammoniagenesis and, to a lesser extent, to the potential for a rapid loss of large amounts of bicarbonate-poor fluids (contraction alkalosis). The former is currently attributed to the combined effects of potassium depletion and secondary aldosteronism coupled with an increased delivery of sodium to the distal nephron with increased avidity for its tubular reabsorption at the same site. The factors tending to perpetuate diuretic-induced metabolic alkalosis include (1) continued use of the diuretic, (2) increased tubular secretion of hydrogen ions related to volume contraction, potassium deficiency, and perhaps chloride deficiency, and (3) reduction in glomerular filtration rate secondary to volume contraction and possibly to potassium and chloride deficiency.

Potassium Depletion

Potassium wasting and hypokalemia may complicate the sustained use of the loop diuretics.[38] Urinary potassium excretion is increased because of inhibition of potassium reabsorption in the TALH and enhanced potassium secretion in the distal nephron. Potassium reabsorption is inhibited by the loop diuretics in association with NaCl in the TALH. Distal potassium secretion is increased for the following reasons: (1) greater tubular fluid flow into the distal nephron as a result of diminished medullary osmolality, (2) elevated renin-angiotensin-aldosterone levels triggered by volume contraction, and (3) metabolic alkalosis as a result of bicarbonate conservation. Nevertheless, exaggerated kaliuresis may be curtailed, provided that the rate of fluid delivery to the distal tubule becomes sufficiently reduced by volume contraction–mediated increases in proximal tubular reabsorption. Not all patients are equally susceptible to potassium depletion.

Table 39–4. **Potential Major Complications of Furosemide**

Azotemia
Hyponatremia
Hypokalemia
Metabolic alkalosis
Ototoxicity
Cardiac dysrhythmias
Sulfonamide-type hypersensitivity

Most patients receiving loop diuretics for antihypertensive therapy do not develop significant potassium depletion. Patients receiving diuretics for edema may be more prone to potassium depletion than nonedematous subjects; thus, potassium supplementation or the concurrent use of potassium-sparing diuretics in these patients seems advisable. The risk of diuretic-induced hypokalemia is increased in subjects with relatively large salt and water intakes.

Although loop diuretics are more potent than distal diuretics, hypokalemia and potassium depletion are less marked in patients receiving loop diuretics.[38] Although the mechanism has not been established, it has been postulated that the shorter duration of action of the loop diuretic is responsible for this phenomenon.

Hyponatremia

Furosemide blocks the ability of the kidney to generate free water. This impairment of renal diluting ability is attributable to several factors. First, loop diuretics inhibit NaCl transport in the TALH. Furthermore, volume contraction, limitation of flow to the TALH, and elevated antidiuretic hormone levels diminish the ability of the kidney to excrete solute-free water. Consequently, a marked increase in water ingestion in patients receiving loop diuretics may result in hyponatremia.[39] A typical scenario may include the following sequence of events. The physician may send the patient home on a diuretic regimen with the explanation that the drug may result in dehydration. The unwary patient may drink excessive amounts of water. Patients may also respond to thirst center stimulation mediated by antidiuretic hormone and angiotensin II. Collectively, these events may lead to hyponatremia.

Furosemide, however, induces dilutional hyponatremia much less frequently than do thiazide-type diuretics. This difference has been attributed to the differing effects of the two diuretics on the loop of Henle. Thus, although both diuretics impair renal diluting capacity, furosemide also produces an impairment of concentrating ability.

Hypocalcemia and Hypomagnesemia

The loop diuretics normally increase urinary calcium and magnesium excretion in association with the increase in NaCl excretion. Thus, furosemide has a role in the treatment of hypercalcemia. Because (in analogy with NaCl excretion) the increased calcium excretion diminishes with progressive volume depletion, the acute calciuretic properties of furosemide can be sustained by maintaining volume expansion with intravenously administered saline.

Although magnesium excretion is increased by either loop or distally acting diuretics, magnesium depletion occurs primarily with the loop diuretics such as furosemide. This finding may relate to the fact that the most important site of reabsorption of magnesium in the nephron is the TALH.

DOSAGE AND ADMINISTRATION
Edema

The usual initial adult oral dose of furosemide for the management of edema is 20 to 80 mg given as a single dose, preferably in the morning. In adults who do not respond, all succeeding oral dosages may be increased in 20- to 40-mg increments every 6 to 8 hours until the desired diuretic response is obtained. We prefer not to exceed 360 mg/day, at which point we would consider adding metolazone (see Chapter 42). The effective dosage may be given once or twice daily thereafter, or, in some cases, by intermittent administration on 2 to 4 consecutive days each week.

Hypertension

The usual adult oral dosage of furosemide for the management of hypertension is 40 mg twice daily initially and for maintenance. Higher dosages may be necessary for the management of hypertension in adults with renal insufficiency. In these adults, oral furosemide dosage may be increased until the desired therapeutic response is achieved, adverse effects become intolerable, or a suggested maximal dosage of 360 mg daily, in two divided doses, is attained. The risk of adverse effects (e.g., ototoxicity) at these high dosages should be considered.

REFERENCES

1. Materson BJ: Insights into intrarenal sites and mechanisms of action of diuretic agents. Am Heart J 106:188, 1983.
2. Branch RA, Read PR, Levine D, et al: Furosemide and bumetanide: A study of responses in normal English and German subjects. Clin Pharmacol Ther 19:538, 1976.
3. Schlätter E, Greger R, Weidtke C: Effect of high-ceiling diuretics on active salt transport in the cortical thick ascending limb of Henle's loop of rabbit kidney. Pfluegers Arch 396:210, 1983.
4. Friedman PA. Biochemistry and pharmacology of diuretics. Semin Nephrol 8:198, 1988.
5. Suki W, Rector FC Jr, Seldin DW: The site of action of furosemide and other sulfonamide diuretics in the dog. J Clin Invest 44:1458, 1965.
6. Eknoyan G, Suki WN, Rector FC Jr, et al: Functional characteristics of the diluting segment of the dog nephron and the effect of extracellular volume expansion on its reabsorptive capacity. J Clin Invest 46:1178, 1967.
7. Ng RCK, Peraino RA, Suki WN: Divalent cation transport in isolated tubules. Kidney Int 22:492, 1982.
8. Gerber JG: Role of prostaglandins in the hemodynamic and tubular effects of furosemide. Fed Proc 42:1707, 1983.
9. Grantham JJ, Chonko AM: The physiologic basis and clinical use of diuretics. In Brenner BM, Stein, JH (eds): Sodium and Water Homeostasis. New York: Churchill Livingstone, 1978, pp 178–211.
10. Rane A, Villeneuve JP, Stone WJ, et al: Plasma binding and disposition of furosemide in the nephrotic syndrome in uremia. Clin Pharmacol Ther 24:199, 1978.
11. Branch RA: Role of binding in distribution of furosemide: Where is nonrenal clearance? Fed Proc 42:1699, 1983.
12. Wilcox CS, Mitch WE, Kelly RA, et al: Response of the kidney to furosemide: I. Effects of salt intake and renal compensation. J Lab Clin Med 102:450, 1983.
13. Almeshari K, Ahstrom NG, Capraro FE, Wilcox CS: A volume-independent component to postdiuretic sodium retention in humans. J Am Soc Nephrol 3:1878, 1993.
14. Kelly RA, Wilcox CS, Meyer TW et al. The response of the kidney to furosemide: II. Effect of captopril on sodium balance. Kidney Int 24:233, 1983.
15. Wilcox CS, Guzman NJ, Mitch WE: Na+, K+ and BP homeostasis in man during furosemide: Effects of prazosin and captopril. Kidney Int 31:135, 1987.
16. Inoue M, Okajima K, Itoh K, et al: Mechanism of furosemide resistance in analbuminemic rats and hypoalbuminemic patients. Kidney Int 32:198, 1987.
17. Mirouze D, Zipser RD, Reynolds TB: Effects of inhibitors of prostaglandin synthesis on induced diuresis in cirrhosis. Hepatology 3:50, 1983.
18. Planas R, Arroyo V, Rimola A, et al: Acetylsalicylic acid suppresses the renal hemodynamic effect and reduces the diuretic action of furosemide in cirrhosis with ascites. Gastroenterology 84:247, 1983.
19. Herchuelz A, Derenne F, Deger F, et al: Interaction between nonsteroidal antiinflamtory drugs and loop diuretics: Modulation by sodium balance. J Pharmacol Exp Ther 248:1175, 1988.
20. Pinzani M, Laffi G, Meacci E, et al: Intrarenal thromboxane A2 generation reduces the furosemide-induced sodium and water diuresis in cirrhosis with ascites. Gastroenterology 95:1081, 1988.
21. Andreasen F, Hansen U, Husted SE, et al: The pharmacokinetics of furosemide are influenced by age. Br J Clin Pharmacol 16:391, 1983.
22. Epstein M: Diuretic therapy in liver disease. In Eknoyan G, Martinez-Maldonado M (eds): The Physiological Basis of Diuretic Therapy in Clinical Medicine. Orlando, FL: Grune & Stratton, 1986, pp 225–246.
23. Brater DC: Pharmacodynamic and pharmacokinetic considerations in the therapy of patients with resistant edema. In Puschett JB, Greenberg A (eds): Diuretics II: Chemistry, Pharmacology and Clinical Applications. New York: Elsevier, 1987, pp 308–314.
24. Shear L, Ching S, Gabuzda GJ: Compartmentalization of ascites and edema in patients with hepatic cirrhosis. N Engl J Med 282:1391, 1970.
25. Arroyo V, Ginés P, Planas R, et al: Paracentesis in the management of cirrhotics with ascites. In Epstein M, (ed): The Kidney in Liver Disease, 3rd ed. Baltimore: Williams & Wilkins, 1988, pp 578–592.
26. Ginés P, Arroyo V, Vargas V, et al: Paracentesis with intravenous infusion of albumin as compared with peritoneovenous shunting in cirrhosis with refractory ascites. N Engl J Med 325:829, 1991.
27. Dikshit K, Vyden JK, Forrester JS, et al: Renal and extrarenal hemodynamic effects of furosemide in congestive heart failure after acute myocardial infarction. N Engl J Med 288:1087, 1973.
28. Kuchar DL, O'Rourke MF: High dose furosemide in refractory cardiac failure. Eur Heart J 6:954, 1985.
29. Vasko MR, Brown-Cartwright D, Knochel JP, et al: Furosemide absorption altered in decompensated congestive heart failure. Ann Intern Med 102:314, 1985.
30. Dzau VJ, Hollenberg NK: Renal response to captopril in severe heart failure: Role of furosemide in natriuresis and reversal of hyponatremia. Ann Intern Med 100:777, 1984.
31. Cowley AJ, Wynne RD, Stainer K, et al: Symptomatic assessment of patients with heart failure: Double-blind comparison of increasing doses of diuretics and captopril in moderate heart failure. Lancet 2:770, 1986.
32. Packer M, Lee WH, Yushak M, et al: Comparison of captopril and enalapril in patients with severe chronic heart failure. N Engl J Med 315:847, 1986.
33. Epstein M, Oster JR: Hypertension: Practical Management. Miami: Battersea, 1988.
34. Hantman D, Rossier B, Zohlman R, et al: Rapid correction of hyponatremia in the syndrome of inappropriate secretion of antidiuretic hormone: An alternative to hypertonic saline. Ann Intern Med 78:870, 1973.
35. Sebastian A, Schambelan M, Sutton JM: Amelioration of hyperchloremic acidosis with furosemide therapy in patients with chronic renal insufficiency and type 4 renal tubular acidosis. Am J Nephrol 4:287, 1984.
36. Epstein M, Schneider NS, Befeler B: Effect of intra-arterial furosemide on renal function and intrarenal hemodynamics in acute renal failure. Am J Med 58:510, 1975.
37. Bosch JP, Goldstein MH, Levitt MF, et al: Effect of chronic furosemide administration on hydrogen and sodium excretion in the dog. Am J Physiol 232:F397, 1977.

38. Tannen RL (principal discussant): Diuretic-induced hypokalemia [clinical conference]. Kidney Int 28:988, 1985.

39. Abramow M, Cogan E: Clinical aspects and pathophysiology of diuretic-induced hyponatremia. Adv Nephrol 13:1, 1984.

CHAPTER 40

Bumetanide

Andrew Whelton, M.D., and Paul K. Whelton, M.D.

HISTORY

The saluretic diuretics differ in their mechanisms of action, their sites of action, their electrolyte excretory patterns, and even their clinical utility; nonetheless, they share a structural similarity, namely, the sulfamoyl group (SO_2NH_2) that is found in the molecular configuration of many clinically important diuretics.[1, 2] This unifying feature exists because the sequential development of many diuretics was based on a serendipitous observation during trials of sulfanilamide therapy in bacterial infections (Fig. 40–1). Southworth[3] reported in 1937 that the treatment of bacterial infections with massive doses of sulfanilamide produced metabolic acidosis. Subsequently, it was identified that this effect was due to inhibition of the enzyme carbonic anhydrase. It was noted also that carbonic anhydrase was abundantly present in renal tissues and accounted for renal regeneration of filtered bicarbonate. Furthermore, the unsubstituted sulfamoyl group of sulfanilamide was found to be closely associated with its inhibitory effects on carbonic anhydrase. Attempts to find a more suitable carbonic anhydrase inhibitor led to the synthesis of acetazolamide, which remains the best diuretic of this class.[4]

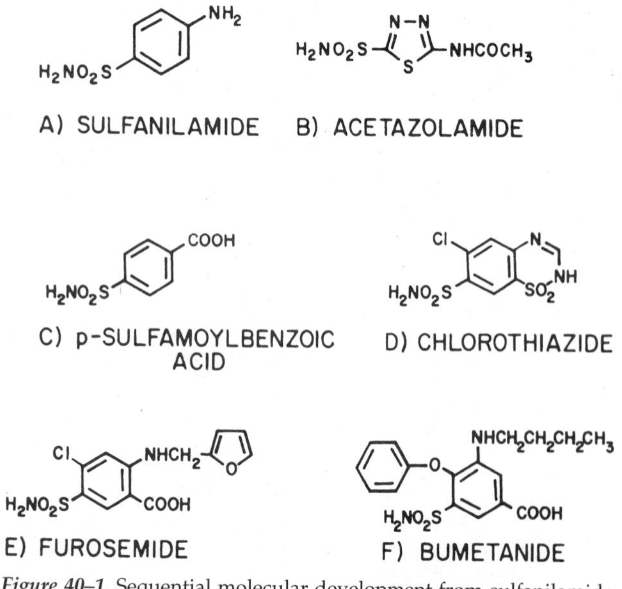

Following the use of a carbonic anhydrase inhibitor for saluretic diuretic purposes, self-limiting hyperchloremic acidosis evolves within a few days, with loss of continued diuretic effect. This characteristic of carbonic anhydrase inhibitors prompted continual modification of the sulfonamide molecule and led to the introduction of chlorothiazide, the prototype of all thiazide diuretics, in the late 1950s. The worldwide utility of this compound led to intensive interest in the development of other sulfamoyl compounds as potential diuretics. Numerous new thiazide diuretics were introduced into the clinical arena. In the early 1960s, a new variety of diuretic action was described with furosemide. Although structurally indistinct from the thiazides, furosemide has a major diuretic potency that identified it as working dominantly within the loop of Henle to produce a peak sodium excretion of as much as 25% of the filtered load. In comparison with the thiazide diuretics, which work at a more distal site within the nephron, furosemide had not only a much greater maximal saluretic response but also a substantially shorter duration of effective action. From the historical point of view, ethacrynic acid and furosemide became available for clinical use at about the same time in the early 1960s. Ethacrynic acid, a phenoxyacetic acid derivative, was identified during a screening of agents similar to the organomercurials that would react with substances containing sulfhydryl but possibly would be less toxic. Compared with the organomercurials, ethacrynic acid was not nephrotoxic, but ototoxicity was noted to be an important complication and has thereby markedly decreased ethacrynic acid's clinical popularity.

At the time of early clinical development of furosemide, Feit[5] postulated that, structurally, furosemide could be on the border between the thiazide group of diuretics and a more specific structure for high-ceiling (loop) diuretic activity. This finding led to the development of a series of 4-substituted 3-amino-5-sulfamylbenzoic acid derivatives, one of which, 3-N-butylamino-4-phenoxy-5-sulfamylbenzoic acid (bumetanide), was selected for further investigation.[6] Initial investigations in a canine model indicated that the action of bumetanide, characterized by an intense short-term diuretic effect, was similar to that of ethacrynic acid and furosemide. On a milligram-per-milligram dosing basis, oral administration of bumetanide had about 100 times the activity of furosemide, and

A) SULFANILAMIDE **B)** ACETAZOLAMIDE

C) p-SULFAMOYLBENZOIC ACID **D)** CHLOROTHIAZIDE

E) FUROSEMIDE **F)** BUMETANIDE

Figure 40–1. Sequential molecular development from sulfanilamide to bumetanide. See Feit[1] for details of the historical evolution of the molecule from sulfanilamide to bumetanide.

following parenteral administration, it was 40 to 60 times more active. These dramatic results led to its further clinical investigation and its ultimate availability for patient use. It was introduced into clinical use in the United States in 1982.

CHEMISTRY

Bumetanide is a 4-substituted derivative of sulfamylbenzoic acid. It has the chemical name 3-N-butylamino-4-phenoxy-5-sulfamylbenzoic acid.[5] As a metanilamide derivative, it differs from the sulfanilamide structure of the thiazides and furosemide. A distinct characteristic of this agent is the presence of a phenoxy group (C_6H_5O) in the position normally occupied by a trifluromethyl group (CF_3) or a chlorine atom. Feit et al.[1, 5] have demonstrated that the introduction of a phenoxy or a phenylthio moiety in place of the chlorine atom in various thiazide-type diuretics diminished diuretic activity, but a similar exchange for the chlorine atom in furosemide significantly increased diuretic potency.

Bumetanide has the chemical formula $C_{17}H_{20}N_2O_5S$ and a molecular weight of 364.41.[7] Serum protein binding is 85% to 95% at usual total serum protein concentrations.[8, 9]

PHARMACOLOGY
Animal Pharmacology and Toxicology

Early screening of bumetanide demonstrated that the dog was the most sensitive test animal and that rats showed only weak sensitivity to bumetanide and related compounds as a result of rapid metabolism of the drug.[8] In dogs, bumetanide proved to be similar to furosemide in its type of action but 30 to 50 times and 100 times more potent after intravenous and oral administration, respectively, using a clinically comparable milligram-to-milligram dosing range.[6, 9] Over a 6-hour study period, 5 to 7 mEq/kg of sodium was excreted after administration of bumetanide. Potassium excretion remained low, and the Na^+,K^+ excretory ratio was more favorable than is characteristically found with thiazides.[8] In dogs, renal clearance of bumetanide occurs at a rate exceeding glomerular filtration and approximating the clearance of para-aminohippuric acid. This finding indicates that renal elimination of the drug results from a combination of glomerular filtration and tubular secretion. Probenecid blocks tubular secretion of bumetanide and diminishes its intrarenal activity.[10] Bekersky and Popick,[11] evaluating the disposition of bumetanide in an isolated perfused rat kidney model, have further clarified the renal tubular secretory and reabsorptive kinetics of bumetanide. These investigators have suggested that the drug may undergo bidirectional active transport in the proximal renal tubule. In dogs that have undergone nephrectomy, the volume of distribution is 10% of body weight, indicating an exclusive extracellular site of drug distribution.

The direct effects of bumetanide and furosemide on the thick ascending limb of the loop of Henle (TALH) were evaluated in an *in vitro* rabbit renal tubular model by Imai.[12] Dose response analysis disclosed that bumetanide was 14 times as potent as furosemide on a weight-for-weight basis. These data and subsequent studies by Schlatter et al.[13] in the same animal model demonstrated that furosemide and bumetanide act at the Na^+-K^+-2Cl cotransport site in the TALH. Feig reviewed the historical evolution of identification of the Na^+-K^+-2Cl cotransport system within the TALH and its implications for diuretic effectiveness and adverse effects.[14]

Acute and chronic toxicity of bumetanide in several animal species has been reported to be extremely low.[8, 15-17] In view of the ototoxic potential of loop diuretics such as ethacrynic acid, extensive ototoxic evaluations have been undertaken in dogs and cats.[18-20] These data, when converted to clinically equivalent milligram-for-milligram dosing of furosemide, indicate that bumetanide in these animal species has about 10% to 20% of the ototoxic potential of furosemide.[15]

Pharmacology and Pharmacokinetics in Humans

Evaluation of normal volunteers and of patients with a variety of clinical disease states has led to a clear picture of the human pharmacology of bumetanide.[7, 8, 15, 21-28] The diuretic response to both oral and intravenous dosing with bumetanide is similar in view of almost complete (80% to 85%) absorption of the drug from the gastrointestinal tract. Furosemide, in comparison, is only 40% to 60% absorbed after oral administration. Bumetanide is rapidly absorbed following oral administration and has a prompt onset of action (20 to 40 minutes). Its peak of activity is within the first 1 or 2 hours after administration; it has a duration of action of about 6 to 8 hours and an elimination half-life of 1 hour. Bumetanide manifests a linear dose-response curve at doses of 0.25 to 2.5 mg.[15] At similar doses, it is 40 to 50 times more potent than furosemide in enhancing urine flow and electrolyte excretion after oral administration and 25 to 30 times more potent when administered intravenously.[23] Bumetanide is about 90% bound to serum protein. In addition to the differences in bioavailability between bumetanide and furosemide (already noted), the total body clearance of bumetanide (about 200 ml/min) is slightly greater than that of furosemide.

Following oral or intravenous administration of bumetanide to healthy nonedematous volunteers, the dominant electrolytes excreted in the urine are sodium, potassium, and calcium with equimolar amounts of cation and anion. The increase in sodium excretion represents about 10% to 18% of the filtered load of proton.[15] The Na^+/K^+ ratio of the urine after bumetanide administration is 3:1.[24] Quantitative excretion of potassium is slightly less with bumetanide than with furosemide given in comparable doses.[25] In addition to sodium and potassium losses, an increase in urinary calcium, magnesium, and urate is also reported, but it is typically of limited clinical significance. As a result of the influence of bumetanide on the TALH, free water clearance is significantly reduced.[26]

Bumetanide rapidly increases total renal blood flow by as much as 40% or more of baseline value, an effect that apparently is mediated by prostaglandin, because it can be inhibited by nonsteroidal antiinflammatory drugs.[27] This increase in blood flow is maintained for up to 1 hour; the predominant increase is in flow to the juxtamedullary area of the kidney.[26]

It had been speculated for some time that access to the functional site within the TALH might be different for bumetanide than for furosemide, with furosemide requiring a luminal site of action and bumetanide acting, in part at least, by blood-borne delivery to the antiluminal side of the TALH. The precise human studies of Voelker et al.[29] have made it apparent that intraluminal delivery is needed for full expression of the activity of both diuretics.

Site and Mechanism of Action Within the Nephron

In considering the influence of diuretics on sodium transport within the nephron, four dominant sites of action are of central importance: the proximal tubule, the TALH, the distal convoluted tubule, and the principal cell within the cortical-collecting duct system. Details of the cellular mechanisms of and diuretic inhibition of sodium transport have been reviewed by Jacobson[30] and by Puschett.[31] This chapter considers only the site of action of the loop diuretics, the TALH.

The major apical transport system present within the cells of the TALH is a complex electroneutral carrier system that moves Na^+, K^+, and $2Cl$ ions into the cell. The basolateral cell membrane Na^+,K^+-ATPase pump, which maintains intracellular sodium concentration at a low level and provides the energy for the apical Na^+-K^+-$2Cl$ electroneutral carrier system. $2Cl$ anions exit from the cell into the peritubular capillary via an electroneutral KCl transporter system and by a conductive pathway through a chloride channel. Because no major potassium conductance apparently occurs across the basolateral cell membrane, the potassium that enters into the cell via the apical carrier system recycles into the urine across the apical cell membrane, because the latter exhibits high potassium conductance. The recycling of potassium and the movement of chloride from the cell into the blood help to generate a transepithelial positive potential that drives sodium out of the lumen of the tubule through the paracellular space.[29] Hence, for every sodium ion transported via the apical carrier system, one is moved via the paracellular space. Bumetanide and other diuretics derived from sulfamoylbenzoic acid appear to work by binding to the apical cell-mediated carrier, in particular, the chloride-binding site.[4, 30–33] Although the Na^+-K^+-$2Cl$ cotransport

system is present in other mammalian tissues, the affinity of bumetanide for the binding site within the TALH and the metabolism, pharmacokinetics, and high intratubular concentrations of bumetanide lead to its clinical effectiveness as an inhibitor of sodium reabsorption within the nephron.

The natriuretic effect of bumetanide, like that of other loop agents, also depends on a prostaglandin-mediated increase in renal blood flow, particularly within the medulla.[26, 27] This increase in blood flow serves to decrease the interstitial concentration of solutes that participate in generating concentrated urine. Hence, there is a resultant trend to diuresis secondary to increased medullary blood flow and washout of solutes. As previously stated, the intrarenal hemodynamic effects of bumetanide can be inhibited by nonsteroidal antiinflammatory drugs. Hence, patients who have been receiving long-term bumetanide will appear to be less responsive to the diuretic if nonsteroidal antiinflammatory drug therapy is begun.

Extracellular Fluid Volume and Electrolyte Effects of Bumetanide

A responsive normal kidney will sustain a loss of 15% to 20% of glomerular filtrate under the influence of therapeutic doses of bumetanide. In response to this massive loss of fluid and electrolytes, the extracellular fluid volume (ECF) contracts significantly, initiating a series of modulating hemodynamic, hormonal, and neurologic responses. These multifactorial responses enhance sodium and water reabsorption at nephron sites other than the loop of Henle, thereby resulting in stabilization of ECF contraction and an apparent clinical decrease in activity of bumetanide. By the addition of diuretics that work at sites other than the loop of Henle, it becomes possible to reinstitute a saluretic diuresis with further ECF contraction.[31]

Characteristically, bumetanide-induced urinary sodium loss is achieved at urine sodium concentrations that are lower than those concomitantly present in the blood. This difference means that, under most clinical circumstances of bumetanide use, the loss of sodium and water within the urine is hypotonic with respect to ECF concentrations, which results in a trend toward hypernatremia. This trend is helpful in many clinical circumstances in which patients with edema have dilutional hyponatremia because, as their edema is mobilized, their serum sodium concentrations return to normal.

Water Metabolism

Water metabolism is significantly influenced by the activity of the TALH. In this portion of the nephron, reabsorption of sodium chloride and potassium chloride without reabsorption of water produces a progressively more dilute tubular fluid. If antidiuretic hormone is not produced, the maximally dilute tubular fluid is excreted, resulting in excretion of large quantities of electrolyte-free water in the urine. Bumetanide inhibits this generation of electrolyte-free water and thereby prevents maximal dilution of the urine. If an individual who is being treated with bumetanide ingests an amount of water that supersedes the reduced diluting ability of the kidney, ECF volume will expand and hyponatremia will develop. Clinically, induction of hyponatremia by reduction of urine-diluting ability is uncommon with loop diuretics but is encountered more frequently with the thiazide group of diuretics. In contrast, the TALH is also central to the generation of maximally concentrated urine. Concentrated urine is produced when there is continued tubular transport of solutes into the interstitial fluid of the renal medulla and papilla with a resultant increase in interstitial osmolality. A simultaneous release of antidiuretic hormone then provides an osmotic communication between the low osmotic activity of fluid passing through the distal nephron and the high osmotic activity of the interstitium of the medulla and papilla. Water moves out of the lumen of the tubule into the hypertonic interstitium of the medulla and papilla, and a progressively concentrated residual tubular fluid is produced, resulting in the excretion of maximally concentrated urine. Bumetanide inhibits this process by reducing solute transport into the interstitium of the medulla. Thus, bumetanide inhibits maximal concentration and maximal dilution of urine.

Potassium, Calcium, and Magnesium Excretion

Potassium wasting by the kidney is induced by all loop diuretics, and the quantitative loss profile has already been discussed. Characteristically, patients who receive once-daily chronic administration of bumetanide do not tend to become hypokalemic. This finding is in contrast with the frequent occurrence of hypokalemia in patients treated with thiazide diuretics. Bumetanide-induced potassium loss is related to a combination of events. Potassium reabsorption is directly inhibited in the TALH. In addition, as a result of the stimulus created by diuretic activation of the renin-angiotensin-aldosterone axis, distal tubular exchange of sodium for potassium is enhanced.

Bumetanide inhibits calcium reabsorption in the TALH.[34] Usually, this effect is not of clinical importance during chronic therapy. However, in emergency states of hypercalcemia, high-dose bumetanide coupled with vigorous intravenous fluid and electrolyte replacement therapy is highly effective in reducing elevated serum calcium levels as a result of significant urinary losses of calcium.[35]

Magnesium reabsorption within the TALH is also inhibited by bumetanide.[34, 36] No evidence suggests that magnesium is meaningfully depleted in routine chronic use. However, in a patient with chronic hypokalemia that is apparently difficult to replete, the possibility of a concurrent bumetanide-induced magnesium deficit should be considered.

Venous Dilatation

All loop diuretics produce an acute increase in venous capacitance by venodilatation of the large veins, particularly within the thorax. Symptomatically, this effect occurs within minutes of administration of a diuretic. A measurable reduction in cardiac preload, as reflected by a reduction of pulmonary-capillary wedge pressure, is seen within 15 minutes;[35] this effect is not well defined hemodynamically, but it is clearly independent of the renal effects of loop diuretics.

Outside the kidney, this targeted effect of bumetanide on venous capacitance vessels is the only clinically important direct effect of the drug. Although bumetanide reduces symptoms of acute pulmonary vascular overload, it does not necessarily increase cardiac output and must therefore be combined with other agents that increase contractility (e.g., cardiac glycosides, sympathomimetic compounds) or reduce myocardial workload (e.g., vasodilators).[35]

Blood Pressure

Bumetanide is not approved by the United States Food and Drug Administration for the management of high blood pressure. Few long-term studies have addressed this hemodynamic effect of the drug. Long-term clinical trials in which blood pressure has been assessed as a clinical parameter have shown a slight but significant (3% to 10%) reduction in standing systolic or mean arterial blood pressure when total body weight has been reduced concurrently.[37-39] Like other loop diuretics, it can be used as an adjunct to blood pressure control medications and may be most valuable in the therapy of hypertension in patients with chronic renal failure.

SPECIFIC DISEASE STATES
Heart Disease

Extensive trials of bumetanide in patients with congestive heart failure have studied[40-45] both oral and parenteral routes of drug delivery. Response to the drug has been uniformly excellent, with patients typically demonstrating prompt clinical improvement and relief of symptoms. The pathophysiologic mechanisms inherent to the clinical improvement in patients with congestive heart failure treated with bumetanide have already been identified. In summary, because of bumetanide's inhibition of sodium and water reabsorption in the proximal tubule and its inhibition of sodium chloride reabsorption within the loop, intravascular congestion and edema formation are impeded, and the cycle leading to chronic edema is blunted. Moreover, in the management of patients with congestive heart failure, bumetanide has been shown to be safe and well tolerated.

It had been speculated for many years that patients with extensive peripheral edema such as in congestive heart failure might demonstrate diuretic resistance on the basis of decreased absorption of the drug secondary to edema within the wall of the gut. Now it is apparent from the work of Brater et al.[28] that the degree of drug absorption is not decreased, but full absorption is delayed such that the time from drug administration to peak clinical effects may be prolonged substantially.[28]

Nephrotic Syndrome

Patients with the nephrotic syndrome respond well to bumetanide; in comparative trials of bumetanide and furosemide, the results typically have been comparable with both drugs.[7, 37, 46–50] With both drugs, the quantitative response to diuretics is significantly modified by a patient's level of renal function at the time of therapy. In many long-term trials, the reported data do not make it possible to quantify the exact number of patients with the nephrotic syndrome as the renal disease specifically contributing to edema formation. Some patients with what appears to be resistance to furosemide have responded to bumetanide.[37] However, it is impossible to document how often this response to bumetanide is seen in truly furosemide-resistant cases.

Characteristically, patients with the nephrotic syndrome may need relatively high doses of loop diuretics even at a point at which they exhibit normal renal function. The explanation for this dosing phenomenon is based on the hypoalbuminemia seen in patients with the nephrotic syndrome. Hypoalbuminemia results in a reduction in protein binding of the drug. The unbound drug diffuses into tissues, thereby increasing the volume of distribution of the compound. As a result, the levels of nonbound drug do not increase in these patients.[51, 52] An increase in drug dosing can offset these pharmacokinetic parameters. An additional consideration that might contribute to the reduced responsiveness of the kidney to diuretics in the nephrotic syndrome is that the diuretic may bind to filtered proteins, thereby reducing delivery of drug to the critical Na^+-K^+-$2Cl$ cotransport site of action within the TALH.[53] A report by Inoue et al.[54] has added considerably more information to our understanding of the reduced responsiveness of hypoalbuminemic patients to loop diuretics. These authors demonstrated that, in the case of furosemide resistance, the administration of furosemide bound to albumin (furosemide-albumin complex) produced a significant diuretic response, whereas comparable dosing with native furosemide and comparable dosing of albumin on its own were not associated with a diuretic response. This finding suggests that resistance of hypoalbuminemic patients to furosemide (and presumably to bumetanide) may result from impaired delivery of the drug to the peritubular sites of loop diuretic transport as a result of albumin deficiency. Further characterization of this albumin ligand vectorial transport to the kidney is needed.

Renal Insufficiency

Patients with significant impairment of renal function need progressively larger doses of loop diuretics to achieve diuretic response because of a combination of factors such as the renal parenchymal disease itself and its effect on diuretic pharmacokinetics. The nephron mass available to respond to the administered diuretic is reduced. In addition, the proximal tubular organic acid system of transport that actively delivers loop diuretics into the lumen of the nephron is competitively inhibited by organic acids that accumulate in chronic renal failure, thereby reducing drug delivery to its site of action within the nephron. Hence, it is necessary to increase diuretic dosing to offset this reduced tubular transport of diuretic.

It had been speculated that bumetanide might not fully depend on glomerular filtration and the proximal tubular organic acid transport system for reaching its intranephronal site of action. However, Voelker et al.[29] have demonstrated convincingly that bumetanide, like furosemide, requires intraluminal delivery (presumably by glomerular filtration and proximal tubular secretion) to produce a full expression of diuretic response.

The studies of Voelker et al.[29] have also identified clinically meaningful differences in the pharmacokinetics of furosemide and bumetanide in patients with chronic renal insufficiency. In their patients, bumetanide was cleared from the systemic circulation at a rate twice that of furosemide. This difference results from the fact that, in renal failure, nonrenal clearance of bumetanide was unchanged, whereas nonrenal clearance of furosemide was reduced by 50% with resultant greater delivery of drug into the urine of patients with chronic renal insufficiency. From the practical point of view, this disparity means that, in patients with chronic renal failure, the potency ratio between bumetanide and furosemide is 20:1, compared with the typical 40:1 ratio seen in virtually all other clinical states. The results also demonstrate an upper limit of parenteral dosing responsiveness in patients with chronic renal insufficiency. The authors recommend that bumetanide or furosemide administration be limited to 6 to 8 mg/dose and 160 mg/dose, respectively.

Rudy et al.[55] have recently evaluated the hypothesis that a continuous, low-dose infusion of a loop diuretic is more efficacious and better tolerated than conventional intermittent bolus therapy in patients with severe chronic renal insufficiency. To study this question, eight patients with severe, but stable, chronic renal impairment were randomized to receive a 12-mg intravenous dose of bumetanide, given either as two 6-mg bolus doses separated by 6 hours or as the same total dose administered as a 12-hour continuous infusion. Comparable amounts of bumetanide appeared in the urine during the study. However, the continuous infusion of the diuretic resulted in significantly greater net sodium excretion. These results suggest that continuous infusion of a loop diuretic is likely to be useful in patients with severe chronic renal impairment in whom natriuresis is inadequate or who manifest evidence of drug toxicity with standard diuretic dosing regimens.[55] The implications of these findings for patients who require loop diuretic therapy need evaluation in prospective clinical trials of individuals with severe chronic renal failure, hepatic failure, or congestive heart failure.

Liver Disease

In patients with cirrhosis and edema, the pharmacokinetics of loop diuretics are similar to those in individuals with the nephrotic syndrome. Because many of these patients are hypoalbuminemic, the issues already reviewed pertinent to this finding in the nephrotic syndrome are applicable to hypoalbuminemic cirrhotics. Typically, absorption from the gastrointestinal tract is normal.[28] Dosing regimens used in the nephrotic syndrome are appropriate. However, the drug should be administered with caution to ensure that patients do not develop excessive contraction of effective circulating intravascular volume.

ADVERSE EFFECTS

Precautions that should be considered with the use of bumetanide pertain to physiologic responses to the drug and to unforeseen idiosyncratic or hypersensitivity reactions. Physiologic side effects include hypokalemia, metabolic alkalosis, hyperuricemia, volume contraction, and, depending on the clinical circumstances, hyponatremia or hypernatremia. Typically, glucose metabolism is not influenced to an important clinical degree, and significant abnormalities in lipid metabolism have not been reported.

Bumetanide-induced hypokalemia is similar in appearance to hypokalemia caused by furosemide. It is infrequent and dose-dependent.[1] Patients in disease states that typically enhance potassium excretion or individuals with poor dietary intake of potassium are the most likely to experience bumetanide-induced hypokalemia.[56]

ADMINISTRATION AND DOSAGE

Bumetanide is available in oral (0.5-, 1.0-, and 2.0-mg tablets) and parenteral forms (0.25 mg/ml in 2-, 4-, and 10-ml vials). The usual oral dose of the drug is 0.5 to 2.0 mg/day. It may be administered one to three times per day, depending on the clinical response and the nature of the patient's disease process. The approved upper limit of daily oral dosing is 10 mg, but slightly higher dosing regimens such as 5 or 6 mg t.i.d. may prove useful in patients with edema that is difficult to mobilize. In the average adult, there appears to be no benefit in exceeding the latter dosing regimen.

Because orally administered bumetanide is almost fully absorbed, the parenteral and oral dosing schedules are similar. Parenterally administered drug may be given intramuscularly or intravenously. When the drug is given intravenously, it may be infused over a 1- or 2-minute interval. It can be administered directly or in more dilute form with physiologic saline, 5% dextrose in water, or lactated Ringer's solution.

REFERENCES

1. Feit PW: Bumetanide—The way to its chemical structure. J Clin Pharmacol 21:531, 1981.
2. Whelton A: An overview of national patterns and preferences in diuretic selection. Am J Cardiol 57:2A, 1986.
3. Southworth H: Acidosis associated with the administration of para-amino-benzene-sulfonamide (prontylin). Proc Soc Exp Biol Med 36:58, 1937.
4. Maren TH: An historical account of CO_2 chemistry and the development of carbonic anhydrase inhibitors. Pharmacologist 21:303, 1979.
5. Feit PW: Aminobenzoic acid diuretics: 2.4-substituted-3-amino-5 sulfamylbenzoic acid derivatives. J Med Chem 14:432, 1971.
6. Ostergaard EH, Magnussen MP, Nielsen CK, et al: Pharmacological properties of bumetanide, a new potent diuretic. Arzneimittelforschung 22:66, 1972.
7. Asbury MJ, Gatenby PBB, O'Sullivan S, et al: Bumetanide: Potent new loop diuretic. Br Med J 1:211, 1972.
8. Frey HH: Pharmacology of bumetanide. Postgrad Med J 51(Suppl 6):14, 1975.
9. Cohen M, Hinsch E, Vergona R, et al: A comparative and tissue distribution study of bumetanide and furosemide in the dog. J Pharmacol Exp Ther 197:697, 1976.
10. Holland SD, Williamson HE: Probenecid inhibition of bumetanide induced natriuresis in the dog. Proc Soc Exp Biol Med 161:299, 1979.
11. Bekersky I, Popick AC: Disposition of bumetanide in the isolated perfused rat kidney: Effects of probenecid and dose response. Am J Cardiol 57:33A, 1986.
12. Imai M: Effect of bumetanide and furosemide on the thick ascending limb of Henle's loop of rabbits and rats perfused in vitro. Eur J Pharmacol 41:409, 1977.
13. Schlatter E, Gregor R, Weidtke C: Effect of "high-ceiling" diuretics on active salt transport in the cortical thick ascending limb of Henle's loop of rabbit kidney. Pflugers Arch 396:210, 1983.
14. Feig PU: Cellular mechanism of action of loop diuretics: Implications for drug effectiveness and adverse effects. Am J Cardiol 57:14A, 1986.
15. Flamenbaum W, Friedman R: Pharmacology, therapeutic efficacy, and adverse effects of bumetanide, a new "loop" diuretic. Pharmacotherapy 2:213, 1982.
16. McCalin RM, Dammers KD: Toxicologic evaluation of bumetanide, a potent diuretic agent. J Clin Pharmacol 21:543, 1981.
17. Masuda H, Maita K, Kimura K, et al: The safety test of bumetanide. Ann Rep Sankyo Res Lab 25:110, 1973.
18. Brown RD: Cochlear N_1 depression induced by the new "loop" diuretic bumetanide. Neuropharmacology 14:547, 1975.
19. Brown RD: Effect of bumetanide on the positive endocochlear dc potential of the cat. Toxicol Appl Pharmacol 38:137, 1976.
20. Brown RD, Manro JE, Daigneault EA, et al: Comparative acute ototoxicity of intravenous bumetanide and furosemide in the purebred beagle. Toxicol Appl Pharmacol 48:157, 1976.
21. Henning R, Lundval O: Evaluation in man of bumetanide, a new diuretic agent. Eur J Clin Pharmacol 6:224, 1973.
22. Olsen UB: The pharmacology of bumetanide. Acta Pharmacol Toxicol 41(Suppl 3):1, 1977.
23. Cohen M: Pharmacology of bumetanide. J Clin Pharmacol 21:537, 1981.
24. Hutcheon DE, Vincent ME, Sandhu RS: Renal electrolyte excretion pattern in response to bumetanide in healthy volunteers. J Clin Pharmacol 21:604, 1981.
25. Brater DC, Fox WR, Chennavasin P: Electrolyte excretion patterns: Intravenous and oral doses of bumetanide compared to furosemide. J Clin Pharmacol 21:599, 1981.
26. Higashio T, Youichi A, Kenjiro Y: Renal effects of bumetanide. J Pharmacol Exp Ther 207:212, 1978.
27. Brater DC, Fox WR, Chennavasin P: Interaction studies with bumetanide and furosemide: Effects of probenecid and of indomethacin on response to bumetanide in man. J Clin Pharmacol 21:647, 1981.
28. Brater DC: Disposition and response to bumetanide and furosemide. Am J Cardiol 57:20A, 1986.
29. Voelker JR, Cartwright-Brown D, Anderson S, et al: Compari-

son of loop diuretics in patients with chronic renal insufficiency. Kidney Int 32:572, 1987.

30. Jacobson HR: Diuretics: Mechanisms of action and uses. Hosp Pract 22:129, 1987.

31. Puschett JB: Clinical pharmacologic implications in diuretic selection. Am J Cardiol 57:6A, 1986.

32. Greger R, Schlatter E, Lang F: Evidence for electroneutral sodium chloride cotransport in the cortical thick ascending limb of Henle's loop of rabbit kidney. Pflugers Arch 396:308, 1983.

33. Hass M, McManus TJ: Bumetanide inhibits (Na$^+$K$^+$ 2Cl) cotransport at a chloride site. Am J Physiol 245:C235, 1983.

34. White MG, van Gelder J, Eastes G: The effect of loop diuretics on the excretion of Na$^+$, Ca^{++}, Mg^{++}, and Cl$^-$. J Clin Pharmacol 21:610, 1981.

35. Narins RG, Chusid P: Diuretic use in critical care. Am J Cardiol 57:26A, 1986.

36. White MG: The effect of intravenous bumetanide in man with normal and low renal function. J Clin Pharmacol 25:581, 1981.

37. Whelton A: Long-term bumetanide treatment of renal edema: Comparison with furosemide. J Clin Pharmacol 21:591, 1981.

38. Stone WJ, Bennett WM, Cutler RE: Long-term bumetanide treatment of patients with edema due to renal disease. Cooperative studies. J Clin Pharmacol 21:587, 1981.

39. Herlong HF, Hunter FM, Koff RS, et al: A comparison of bumetanide and furosemide in the treatment of ascites. Cooperative study. J Clin Pharmacol 21:701, 1981.

40. Olsen KH, Sigurd B, Hesse B, et al: Diuretic action of bumetanide in congestive heart failure. Postgrad Med J 51(Suppl 6):54, 1975.

41. Sigurd B, Hesse B, Bollerup AC, et al: Investigations with intravenous bumetanide. Postgrad Med J 51(Suppl 6):27, 1975.

42. Kourkoukis C, Christensen O, Augoustakis D: Bumetanide in congestive heart failure. Curr Med Res Opin 4:422, 1976.

43. Abrams J: Intramuscular bumetanide and furosemide in congestive heart failure. J Clin Pharmacol 21:673, 1981.

44. Hutcheon D, Vincent ME, Sandhu RS: Clinical use of diuretics in congestive heart failure. J Clin Pharmacol 21:668, 1981.

45. Dixon DW, Barwolf-Gohlke C, Gunnar RM: Comparative efficacy and safety of bumetanide and furosemide in long-term treatment of edema due to congestive heart failure. J Clin Pharmacol 21:680, 1981.

46. Lau K, DeFronzo R, Morrison G, et al: Effectiveness of bumetanide in nephrotic syndrome: A double blind crossover study with furosemide. J Clin Pharmacol 16:489, 1976.

47. Runeberg L, Pasternack A, Borgmastars H, et al: Clinical trial of a new diuretic, bumetanide, in seriously ill patients. Ann Clin Res 6:272, 1974.

48. Berg KJ, Trosdal A, Wideroe TE: Diuretic action of bumetanide in advanced chronic renal insufficiency. Eur J Clin Pharmacol 9:265, 1976.

49. Yajnick VH, Kalawadia S, Parekh BH, et al: Bumetanide versus furosemide as a diuretic. Curr Ther Res Clin Exp 29:584, 1981.

50. Barclay JE, Lee HA: Clinical and pharmacokinetic studies on bumetanide in chronic renal failure. Postgrad Med J 51(Suppl 6):43, 1975.

51. Rane A, Villeneuve JP, Stone WJ, et al: Plasma binding and disposition of furosemide in the nephrotic syndrome and in uremia. Clin Pharmacol Ther 24:199, 1978.

52. Keller E, Hoppe-Seyler G, Schollmeyer P: Disposition and diuretic effect of furosemide in the nephrotic syndrome. Clin Pharmacol Ther 32:442, 1982.

53. Green TP, Mirkin BL: Furosemide disposition in normal and proteinuric rats: Urinary drug protein binding as a determinant of drug excretion. J Pharmacol Exp Ther 218:122, 1981.

54. Inoue M, Okajima K, Itoh K: Mechanism of furosemide resistance in analbuminemic rats and hypoalbuminemic patients. Kidney Int 32:198, 1987.

55. Rudy DW, Voelker JR, Green PK, et al: Loop diuretics for chronic renal insufficiency: A continuous infusion is more efficacious than bolus therapy. Ann Intern Med 115:360, 1991.

56. Whelton A, Watson AJ: The incidence of hypokalemia and hyperkalemia associated with diuretic use. *In* Whelton PK, Whelton A, Walker WG (eds): Potassium in Cardiovascular and Renal Medicine. New York: Marcel Dekker, 1986, pp 237–254.

CHAPTER 41

Torsemide

D. Craig Brater, M.D.

Torsemide (torasemide outside the United States) is a new loop diuretic that was approved for marketing in the United States by the Food and Drug Administration (FDA) in August of 1993. This diuretic is somewhat distinct in that, at low dosages having minimal diuretic effects, the drug is effective in and approved for the treatment of hypertension. At higher dosages, this diuretic has activity like that of other loop diuretics, though it differs somewhat in its metabolism and thereby in pharmacokinetics.

The chemical structures of torsemide and its metabolites are shown in Figure 41–1. This figure also quantifies the amounts of each of these compounds that are excreted into the urine, the quantity that is responsible for diuretic effect. Of note, only about 25% of the parent drug reaches the urine unchanged. This amount is substantially less than that which occurs with furosemide and bumetanide, wherein approximately 50% of an intravenous dose reaches the urinary site of action. It is also noteworthy that one of the torsemide metabolites has equal potency to the

parent compound, but the amount of this metabolite that reaches the urine in both healthy subjects and patients with various clinical conditions is sufficiently low that it is unlikely to contribute to efficacy. Thus, it is a reasonable assumption that diuretic effects are due to torsemide itself.

EFFICACY IN HYPERTENSION

At low doses, torsemide is an effective antihypertensive agent. If the dose is kept sufficiently low, the antihypertensive effect occurs with few of the adverse effects traditionally associated with diuretics, such as altered glucose homeostasis and increased serum lipoproteins.

Antihypertensive efficacy has been demonstrated in a double-blind randomized trial of 143 previously untreated patients who received monotherapy with torsemide.[1] Patients had entry diastolic blood pressures between 100 and 115 mmHg. They were followed up for 1 year. Unpublished studies in addi-

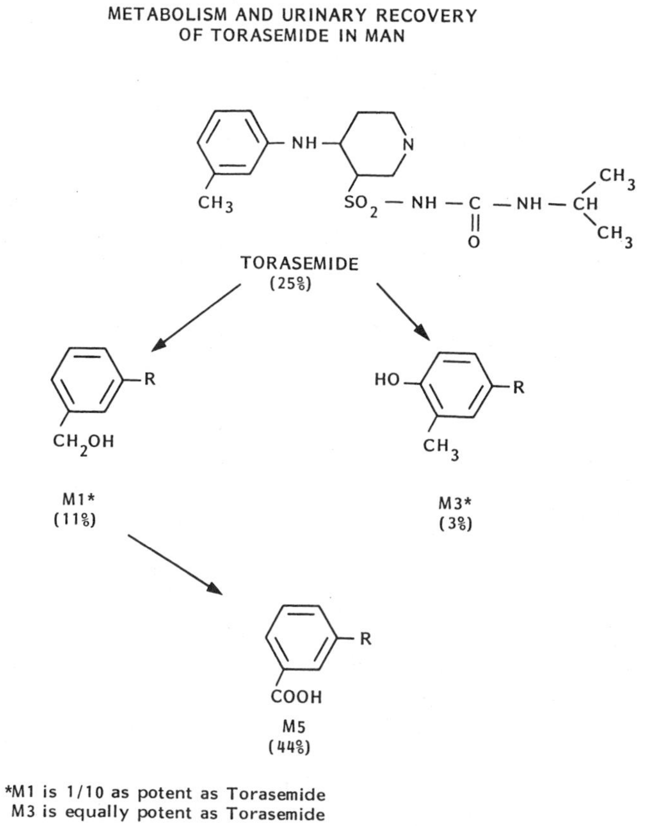

METABOLISM AND URINARY RECOVERY
OF TORASEMIDE IN MAN

*M1 is 1/10 as potent as Torasemide
M3 is equally potent as Torasemide

Figure 41–1. Chemical structure of torsemide (torasemide) and its metabolites. Values in parentheses indicate the percentage of an intravenous dose appearing in the urine.

tional patients have also been performed and submitted to the FDA as part of the approval process. In the published study, patients were divided into two groups, one of which started with a dose of 2.5 mg and the second of which started with a dose of 5 mg. After 4 weeks, the dose could be doubled if response was inadequate. Forty-five patients were dropped from the study, most for protocol violations. Only those patients completing the study were analyzed, which was one of the flaws of the study. Another flaw is that there was no placebo control.

These flaws notwithstanding, 53% of patients had an adequate response to 2.5 mg/day with a decrease in blood pressure from $177 \pm 2/105 \pm 1$ to $157 \pm 3/90 \pm 1$ at 4 weeks with blood pressures at 1 year of $153 \pm 3/86 \pm 1$. Similarly, of those patients randomized to a single dose of 5 mg/day, 66% responded to this dose at 4 weeks with a fall in blood pressure from $178 \pm 2/106 \pm 1$ to $156 \pm 2/90 \pm 1$ at 4 weeks and $154 \pm 2/86 \pm 1$ at 1 year. Moreover, in those patients who did not respond to the initial 2.5-mg dose, doubling to 5 mg/day at 4 weeks resulted in a blood pressure decrease in the previous nonresponders, so that 80% of patients reached satisfactory control. Similar results occurred in the group initially receiving 5 mg/day in whom the dose was doubled.

In all groups, there was negligible change in metabolic parameters (e.g., serum glucose and serum lipoproteins). Doses of 2.5 mg/day and 5 mg/day had

negligible effects on serum potassium concentrations, though doses of 10 mg/day not infrequently required potassium supplementation.

This study indicates a reasonable antihypertensive response to 2.5 mg or 5 mg of torsemide once a day with minimal adverse metabolic effects. However, this study did not have a placebo control, which may account for the fact that studies in the United States utilizing placebo controls were unable to demonstrate efficacy with 2.5 mg/day (FDA Cardiovascular Renal Drugs Advisory Committee Meeting, April 30, 1992). Thus, FDA-approved dosing recommendations for treatment of hypertension are to begin with 5 mg/day and increase to 10 mg/day in those patients who have not responded to the lower dose. Because the 10-mg dose is associated with the metabolic abnormalities that are considered to be traditional with higher-dose diuretics in the treatment of hypertension, it is likely that most clinicians would simply use a 5-mg dose. If the response is inadequate, rather than doubling the dose to 10 mg and risking adverse metabolic effects, most clinicians would likely either try a different agent or add another agent to the 5-mg/day dose of torsemide.

The efficacy of a single dose of torsemide has also been assessed in patients in whom it has been compared with hydrochlorothiazide[2] (Winsor, personal communication). In a study of 24 elderly patients (more than 60 years old) randomized to receive either 25 mg of hydrochlorothiazide per day or 2.5 mg of torsemide per day, patients were followed up for 19 weeks. With hydrochlorothiazide, supine blood pressures decreased from $177 \pm 17/103 \pm 5$ to $135 \pm 10/80 \pm 7$. With torsemide, blood pressures decreased from $175 + 17/105 \pm 5$ to $149 \pm 12/84 \pm 6$. This magnitude of effect on blood pressure is sufficiently striking as to question its generalizability. All of the patients treated with hydrochlorothiazide achieved a supine diastolic blood pressure of less than or equal to 90 mmHg; comparable values for torsemide were 90%. However, patients receiving hydrochlorothiazide suffered a decrease in potassium concentration on average of 0.7 mEq/L, whereas those receiving torsemide had a fall in serum potassium concentration of only 0.1 mEq/L. In addition, hydrochlorothiazide caused an increase of 0.7 mmol/L in serum glucose concentration, whereas torsemide caused a decrease of 0.1 mmol/L. In the doses used, neither of these diuretics caused a change in serum lipoproteins.

Thus, in this study in elderly subjects, a 2.5-mg/day dose of torsemide was as efficacious as 25 mg/day of hydrochlorothiazide but had fewer adverse metabolic effects.

A multicenter trial in the United States had different quantitative results but a similar qualitative outcome (Winsor, personal communication). In this study, 281 patients were randomized to five study groups of 40 to 45 patients each: placebo, 2.5 mg torsemide/day, 5 mg torsemide/day, 25 mg hydrochlorothiazide/day, and 50 mg hydrochlorothiazide/day. Trough blood pressures at 4 and 6 weeks of treatment showed that only the 50-mg dose of hydrochlorothiazide caused a significant decrease in supine diastolic blood pressure compared with placebo (-3.7 mmHg). Overall, when assessing supine and standing systolic and diastolic trough blood pressures, 2.5 mg torsemide could not be distinguished from placebo. Five milligrams of torsemide and both doses of hydrochlorothiazide significantly decreased supine systolic and both standing systolic and diastolic blood pressures. The magnitude of effect of 5 mg torsemide was similar to that of 25 mg hydrochlorothiazide. Hydrochlorothiazide appeared to cause more potassium loss than torsemide. Overall, then, this study indicated the lowest effective antihypertensive dose of torsemide to be 5 mg.

In summary, the data concerning treatment of hypertension with torsemide create a quandary, because the published studies suggest that patients will respond to 2.5 mg of torsemide per day. However, these studies were not placebo-controlled, and results were unrealistic. In contrast, from the United States data, it would appear that for most patients a starting dose of 5 mg/day is more rational. Unfortunately, these studies have not been published and have only been scrutinized through the FDA review process. In patients with an inadequate response to 5 mg, one must decide whether to double the dose to 10 mg/day with a concomitant increased risk of adverse metabolic effects as opposed to switching agents or adding another agent to the 5-mg/day dose.

EFFICACY AS A LOOP DIURETIC
Pharmacology

The chemical structures of torsemide and its metabolites are shown in Figure 41–1. As indicated in the figure, 25% of an intravenous dose of torsemide appears in the urine. As with other loop diuretics, it has been shown that torsemide must reach the lumen or urinary side of the nephron in order to inhibit solute reabsorption at the thick ascending limb of the loop of Henle.[3] As such, in vitro microperfusion of isolated thick ascending limbs of the loop of Henle has indicated that torsemide is effective when placed on the lumen side of the nephron but has negligible effects at relevant concentrations when placed on the peritubular side.[4, 5] Studies have also demonstrated in humans that using probenecid to block torsemide's secretion into the lumen of the nephron causes a shift to the right in the relationship between serum concentration and natriuretic response without affecting the relationship between amounts of diuretic in the urine and response.[3] These human data proved that in vitro studies in animal nephrons extrapolate to humans in terms of the requirement for diuretic to reach the urine to cause a response. Lastly, clearance studies in humans have demonstrated that the site of action is indeed the thick ascending limb of the loop of Henle.[6]

Because 25% of an intravenous dose reaches the urine in healthy subjects, it is apparent that renal clearance accounts for 25% of the total clearance of torsemide from the body. This also means that 75% of torsemide elimination occurs via other pathways, presumably hepatic metabolism. This pattern of metabolism is distinctly different from furosemide and bumetanide, for which renal clearance accounts for approximately 50% of elimination.[7, 8] This pattern of metabolism leads to several predictions concerning the disposition and effects of torsemide in different disease states, and as will be discussed, these predictions have proven true. For example, because renal clearance is a relatively small component of the total clearance of torsemide, one would anticipate that patients with renal insufficiency would have a negligible decrease in total clearance of the drug, because there would be sufficient hepatic metabolic activity to maintain rates of overall elimination similar to those in subjects with normal renal function. Indeed, the half-life of torsemide is not prolonged in patients with renal insufficiency, in contrast to the half-life observed with furosemide (see later discussion). One would also predict that patients with cirrhosis would have a decreased ability to eliminate torsemide by metabolism, making more of the drug available to be eliminated in the urine and to elicit a diuresis in patients with liver disease. A similar phenomenon might be expected to occur in patients with severe heart failure due to the congestive hepatopathy that occurs in such patients. Findings in these different clinical conditions are discussed later.

In summary, torsemide acts in the kidney as a typical loop diuretic. It must reach the urine to be active. It gains access to this site by active secretion via the organic acid transport pathway of the proximal tubule that can be blocked by probenecid. Torsemide has unique metabolic characteristics with a large component of metabolism in the liver (75%).

EFFICACY IN EDEMATOUS DISORDERS

Torsemide's efficacy in various clinical conditions can be demonstrated in several fashions. That torsemide is effective as a diuretic in patients with chronic renal insufficiency, in those with cirrhosis, and in those with congestive heart failure (CHF) is clear and is discussed later under "Pharmacokinetics and Pharmacodynamics." Efficacy can also be demonstrated in terms of overall sodium loss, weight loss, or decrease in symptoms associated with fluid retention. Traditionally, diuretics have not been studied in this fashion, because it has always been assumed that relief of edema and intravascular volume expansion would result in clinical improvement.

It is noteworthy that several studies have demonstrated the efficacy of torsemide in patients with CHF by assessing weight loss and improvement in signs and symptoms. I am aware of only one study of diuretics in patients with CHF that utilized a placebo group (excluding acute, single-dose studies). Patterson et al. randomized 66 patients with New York Heart Association class II (38%) or III (62%) CHF to 7 days of therapy with placebo or 5, 10, or 20 mg of torsemide.[9] Maintenance diuretics were discontinued, and the succeeding 24 hours were used to quantify baseline values of CHF signs and symptoms and urinary electrolyte excretion. Patients then were randomized as indicated and followed-up as hospital inpatients on a fixed sodium intake for 1 week. Importantly, all patients were required to have peripheral edema at the outset of the study. Patients receiving placebo had no change in weight. Those receiving 5 mg torsemide/day had an insignificant weight loss of about 0.5 kg at 1 week. Those receiving 10 and 20 mg of torsemide lost a statistically significant 0.64 kg and 0.94 kg, respectively, after 1 day of therapy. At 1 week, both of the higher doses caused approximately 1.5 kg of weight loss. This study clearly documents efficacy compared with placebo when using body weight as a primary end point.

Other studies have assessed relief of signs and/or symptoms of CHF and compared torsemide with furosemide. In a double-blind multicenter trial of 104 patients with New York Heart Association class II or III CHF, patients received either torsemide 5 mg/day (n = 34), torsemide 10 mg/day (n = 34), or furosemide 40 mg/day (n = 36).[10] After 4 weeks of therapy, 71% of those receiving 5 mg of torsemide a day lost at least 2.5 kg in body weight. Comparable values for 10 mg of torsemide a day were 76% and for furosemide were 61%. In terms of functional improvement, 62% of the group receiving 5 mg of torsemide per day experienced an improvement in New York Heart Association functional class, and none deteriorated. For the group receiving 10 mg of torsemide per day, 62% improved and, again, none deteriorated. For the group receiving 40 mg of furosemide per day, 56% improved and 1 deteriorated. Thus, this study supports the notion that loop diuretics have efficacy in patients with CHF as demonstrated by sustained weight loss and functional improvement.

Goebel reported a study of 70 patients with CHF who were stable for at least 2 weeks on 40 mg of furosemide/day.[11] Patients randomly received 10 or 20 mg of torsemide or 40 mg furosemide and were followed up for 6 weeks. Weight loss at this time averaged 2.1, 3.0, and 1.3 kg, respectively. Efficacy was also assessed in terms of severity of peripheral edema and radiographically determined heart size and degree of pulmonary congestion. The 20-mg dose of torsemide showed significant improvement in all three end points; the 10-mg dose showed efficacy in two of three variables; furosemide showed improvement in one of three variables.

Another study randomized 49 patients with New York Heart Association class III or IV CHF to single intravenous doses of 5, 10, or 20 mg of torsemide or 40 mg of furosemide.[12] Efficacy was assessed relative to a preceding 24-hour diuretic-free interval. Both 20 mg of torsemide and 40 mg of furosemide caused significant increases in 24-hour fractional excretion of sodium and significant decreases in body weight. The magnitude of effect was similar.

These latter studies are confounded by lack of placebo controls, but the collation of data strongly supports efficacy of loop diuretics in general and torsemide in particular for treatment of CHF.

Torsemide has also been assessed in terms of its hemodynamic effects. In one study of 21 patients with New York Heart Association class III to IV CHF, 20 mg of torsemide intravenously was contrasted with 20 mg of furosemide intravenously.[13] Both diuretics lowered left-ventricular filling pressure and caused prompt diuresis. In another study, 19 patients with severe CHF were administered the same doses of torsemide and furosemide as in the previous study.[14] This study entailed catherization of the left side of the heart, and it was demonstrated that both drugs decreased left-ventricular end-diastolic pressure. Although the dose of torsemide used in both of these studies is considerably greater than that of furosemide in terms of the diuresis that would ensue, it still seems likely that torsemide has the same acute hemodynamic effect as other loop diuretics.

PHARMACOKINETICS AND PHARMACODYNAMICS
Healthy Subjects

The pharmacokinetics of torsemide in healthy subjects is shown in Table 41–1.[15–19] This loop diuretic has a high bioavailability of 80% to 100%, which is similar to that of bumetanide. These values contrast with furosemide, with which bioavailability is on the order of 40% to 60%, but with great variability among patients. As indicated previously, the amount of an intravenous dose excreted unchanged in the urine is approximately 25%. The volume of distribution is small owing to a high degree of protein binding. The half-life of approximately 3½ hours is considerably longer than that of bumetanide (about 1 hour) and that of furosemide (about 1.5 hours). Though not shown in this table, torsemide is absorbed quickly, as are other loop diuretics, so that the onset of peak effect after oral dosing is usually within 30 minutes to 1 hour.

The pharmacodynamics of a loop diuretic are best assessed by relating the urinary excretion rate of the diuretic to response.[20] The urinary excretion rate represents the exposure of the active site at the thick ascending limb of the loop of Henle to the diuretic; response can be quantified as sodium excretion rate or fractional excretion of sodium. Figure 41–2 shows summary data for four different loop diuretics in order to compare their potencies. All loop diuretics have very steep response curves with an upper plateau of response that amounts to a sodium excretion rate of approximately 3.0 mEq/min. If expressed as fractional excretion of sodium, this upper asymptote occurs at a value of approximately 20%. Because the thick ascending limb of the loop of Henle normally reabsorbs only about 20% of filtered sodium, this maximal response indicates that loop diuretics are able to completely inhibit this nephron segment. From Figure 41–2, one can discern that torsemide is inter-

Table 41–1. **Pharmacokinetics of Torsemide**

	n	Reference No.	Bioavailability (%)	Half-Life (hr)	Clearance (ml/min/kg)	Volume of Distribution (L/kg)	Percentage of Dose Excreted in Urine (%)
Healthy young	12	15		3.3 ± 0.5	0.53 ± 0.20	0.14 ± 0.04	33 ± 12
	12	16	84 ± 13	3.6 ± 1.9	0.61 ± 0.20	0.17 ± 0.05	16 ± 5
	7	17		5.1 ± 4.2	0.53 ± 0.17	0.24 ± 0.07	26 ± 13
	6	18	91 ± 12	2.2 ± 0.3	0.84 ± 0.04	0.16 ± 0.03	27 ± 3
	9	19	85*	3.8	0.57	0.19	20
Elderly	11	15		3.7 ± 1.1	0.58 ± 0.15	0.18 ± 0.05	20 ± 4
Chronic renal insufficiency:							
Moderate	24	25	100	4.8 ± 1.7	0.43 ± 0.10	0.17 ± 0.04	5.4 ± 3.3
			94	5.2 ± 1.0	0.46 ± 0.08	0.20 ± 0.02	5.8 ± 2.7
			103	5.5 ± 0.9	0.46 ± 0.09	0.21 ± 0.03	5.6 ± 2.5
Severe	9	17		4.6 ± 2.2	0.54 ± 0.16	0.21 ± 0.06	11 ± 10
	90	24		4.1			1.1
	24	25	108	3.8 ± 1.8	0.86 ± 0.50	0.23 ± 0.07	2.8 ± 2.5
			104	5.2 ± 3.9	0.77 ± 0.42	0.27 ± 0.12	2.6 ± 2.2
			92	4.6 ± 3.2	1.05 ± 0.81	0.33 ± 0.24	2.8 ± 2.6
Cirrhosis	10	27		4.7	0.29		19
	12	28	96	8.1 ± 3.4	0.46 ± 0.16	0.29 ± 0.07	27 ± 11
Congestive heart failure	22	33		6.5			16
	16	34		4.2 ± 1.1			22 ± 8
				4.9 ± 2.3			21 ± 8
				5.8 ± 2.2			21 ± 9

*Single values represent median.

mediate in potency between bumetanide and furosemide and similar to piretanide.

Figure 41–3 summarizes the pharmacokinetics and pharmacodynamics of torsemide in healthy subjects. This figure will serve as a frame of reference for similar analyses in different clinical conditions that will be presented subsequently. The top panel of this figure shows plasma concentrations of torsemide versus time after both oral and intravenous dosing. It is obvious from this figure that bioavailability is virtually complete. The third graph depicts the urinary excretion rate of torsemide versus time, again indicating the similarity of delivery to the site of action after both oral and intravenous dosing. This and the previous graph also indicate the relatively long half-life of torsemide. The second graph indicates response as urinary sodium excretion rate over time. These data indicate that the response lasts about 4 hours and is similar with both oral and intravenous dosing, the only difference being a slightly delayed onset of effect after oral dosing, as one would expect. Lastly, the bottom panel indicates the relationship between urinary torsemide excretion rate and response.

Elderly Subjects

As can be seen from Table 41–1, the pharmacokinetics of torsemide in elderly patients are similar to those in healthy young subjects.[15] On average, clearance is slightly decreased, as is the percentage of dose excreted in the urine unchanged. One would predict, then, that if elderly patients are administered the same dose of torsemide as are their young counterparts, the elderly patients will experience delivery of less drug to the urine and have a diminished response, even though sensitivity of the nephron per se is likely unchanged. That this is indeed the case is shown in Figure 41–4A. This depiction indicates that the serum concentration of torsemide over time is similar in both elderly and young subjects (upper left graph), but because of decreased renal clearance of torsemide, there is diminished delivery of diuretic into the urine over time (lower left graph). As a result, there is less sodium excretion over time (upper right graph). When one assesses the pharmacodynamics of response, the relationship between amounts of torsemide in urine and response are similar in elderly and young subjects (lower right graph). Thus, the decreased overall response that occurs in elderly subjects when given the same dose of torsemide as a younger person are due to changes in pharmacokinetics, wherein renal clearance and delivery of diuretic to the site of action are diminished. Thus, elderly subjects will need a larger dose to receive the same

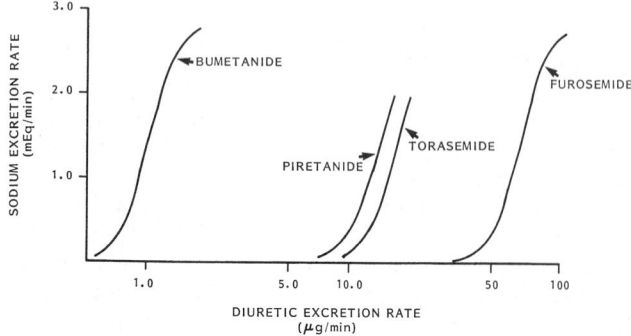

Figure 41–2. Schematized urinary diuretic excretion rate ("dose") versus response curves for loop diuretics.

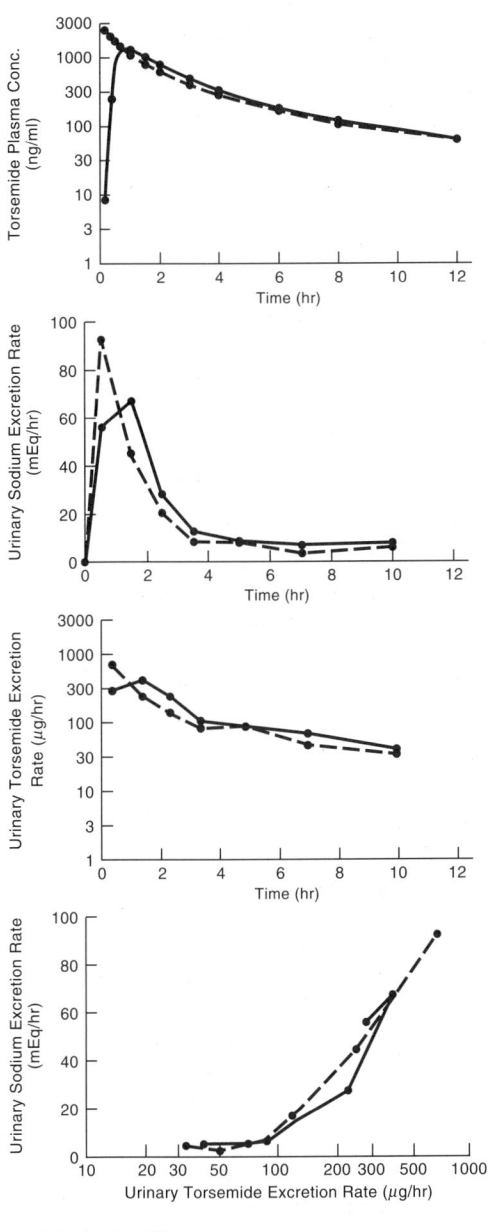

● Oral   ●--● IV

Figure 41–3. Pharmacokinetics and pharmacodynamics of torsemide after oral dosing *(solid line)* and intravenous dosing *(dashed line)* in healthy subjects. The top graph shows plasma concentration versus time, the third graph shows urinary torsemide excretion rate versus time, the second graph shows urinary sodium excretion rate versus time, and the bottom graph shows the relationship between urinary torsemide excretion rate and response.

diuretic response as a younger person. These findings are similar to those delineated with furosemide, wherein elderly subjects on average need twice as great a dose to achieve the same amount of diuretic in the urine as the young.[21, 22]

Patients with Renal Insufficiency

Because renal clearance of torsemide contributes a relatively small amount to total clearance, one would predict that in patients with renal insufficiency there

would be little change in total clearance and in half-life with declining renal function. If torsemide follows patterns similar to those of other loop diuretics, one would also predict that the decreased renal function would result in impaired delivery of torsemide to its urinary site of action.[23] One would also predict that sensitivity of remnant nephrons would be unchanged, as has been observed with furosemide and bumetanide.[23] As a consequence, the diminished response to torsemide, as with other loop diuretics, would be accounted for by the decreased amount of diuretic reaching the site of action rather than a change in sensitivity of the nephron. Table 41–1 lists pharmacokinetic parameters for torsemide in patients with moderate and with severe renal insufficiency.[17, 24, 25] With increasing severity of renal dysfunction, the percentage of dose excreted into the urine is progressively diminished; thus, larger doses must be administered to achieve "normal" amounts of diuretic in the urine.

Figure 41–4*B* shows data from patients with moderate and with severe renal insufficiency as compared with healthy subjects. As indicated in the upper left graph, there is little difference in the serum concentration versus time profile. The values for half-life in Table 41–1 substantiate the prediction that there is little change in half-life in patients with renal insufficiency compared with subjects with normal renal function. However, because of diminished renal clearance of torsemide as a function of the renal disease per se, delivery of diuretic into the urine over time is decreased considerably (lower left graph). This decreased diuretic delivery results in a greatly diminished natriuretic response (upper right graph). When one assesses the pharmacodynamics of response (lower right graph), the relationship is greatly diminished. However, if one depicts response as fractional excretion of sodium (not shown) as opposed to sodium excretion rate, the relationship for patients with renal insufficiency virtually can be superimposed on that for subjects with normal renal function. In addition, studies have been performed wherein sufficiently large doses of torsemide have been administered to define maximal response.[26] This maximal response occurs at a fractional excretion rate of 20% to 25%, indicating that the sensitivity of remnant nephrons in patients with renal insufficiency is comparable with that in subjects with normal renal function. Importantly, it is clear from such studies that a dose of 100 mg of torsemide is sufficient to reach this upper plateau of response. As such, in patients with severe renal insufficiency, 100 mg appears to be the maximum necessary dose. For patients with lesser degrees of renal dysfunction, a dose of 50 mg is likely to be a reasonable maximum, even though up to 200 or even 400 mg has been safely administered.

Figure 41–5 confirms the prediction that there is no change in the elimination half-life of torsemide in patients with renal insufficiency. This distinctly contrasts with the case of furosemide, with which elimination half-life is prolonged in patients with renal insufficiency.[7] This difference from furosemide is in

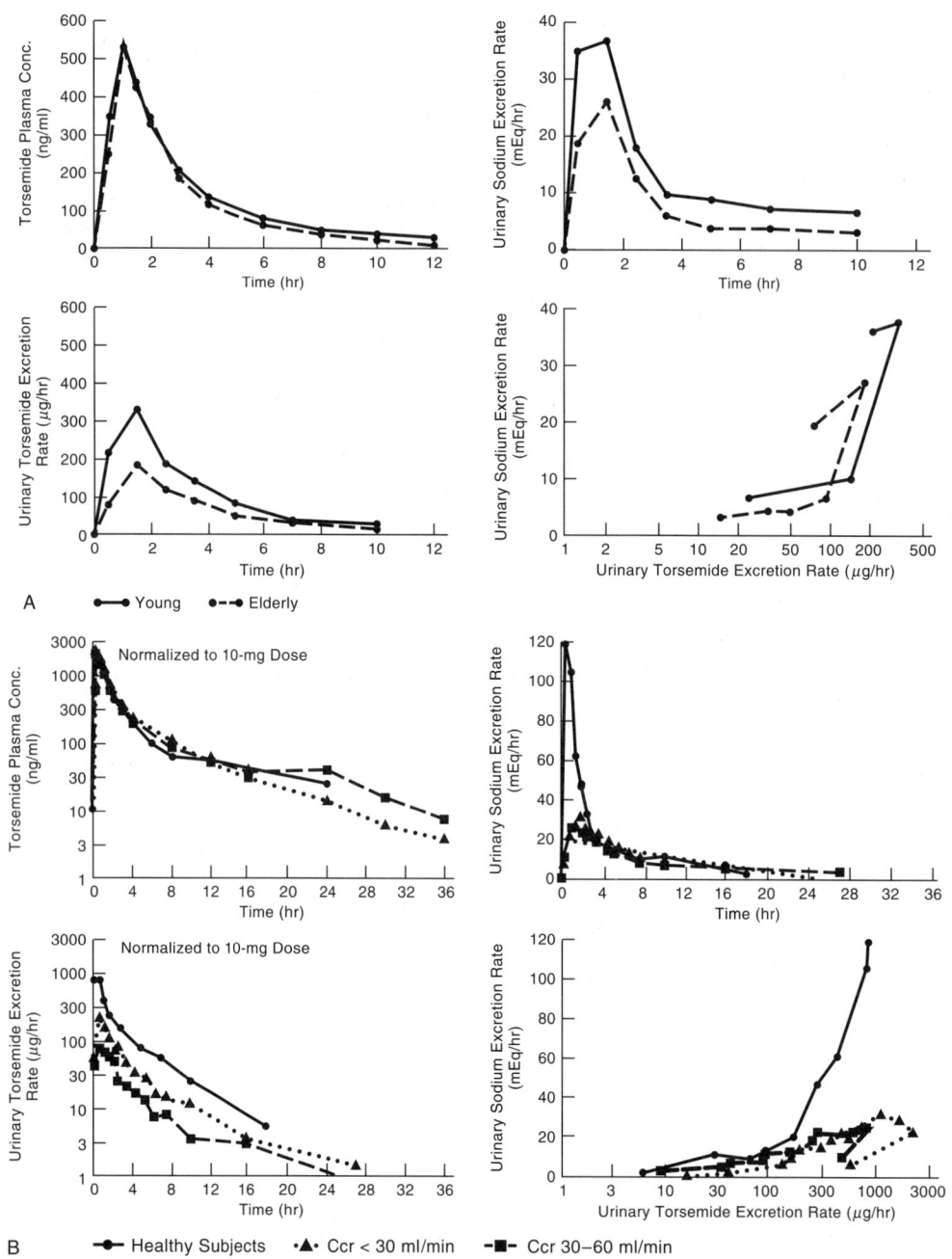

Figure 41–4. A, Pharmacokinetics and pharmacodynamics of torsemide in healthy elderly subjects *(dashed lines)* compared with young subjects *(solid lines).* Depictions are as described for Figure 41–3. *B,* Pharmacokinetics and pharmacodynamics of torsemide in patients with moderate *(dotted lines)* and severe *(dashed lines)* renal insufficiency. Depictions are as in Figure 41–3.

turn due to the fact that renal insufficiency causes a decrease in total clearance owing to both a dramatic decrease in renal clearance and a decrease in nonrenal clearance of furosemide in patients with renal insufficiency.[23] Bumetanide is similar to torsemide in patients with renal insufficiency in that hepatic metabolism of bumetanide is sufficient to minimize any half-life prolongation in patients with renal insufficiency.[23] Clinically, these observations mean that accumulation of torsemide in patients with severe renal insufficiency would be no different from that in subjects with normal renal function.

Hepatic Cirrhosis

Because hepatic metabolism constitutes approximately 75% of the elimination of torsemide, one would predict that patients with severe liver disease might have impaired elimination of this diuretic with a decrease in total clearance of the drug and a prolongation in half-life. Table 41–1 shows that this is the case.[27, 28] Figure 41–4C shows how hepatic disease affects delivery of torsemide into the urine and subsequent response. There is little difference in the serum concentration versus time profile in patients with

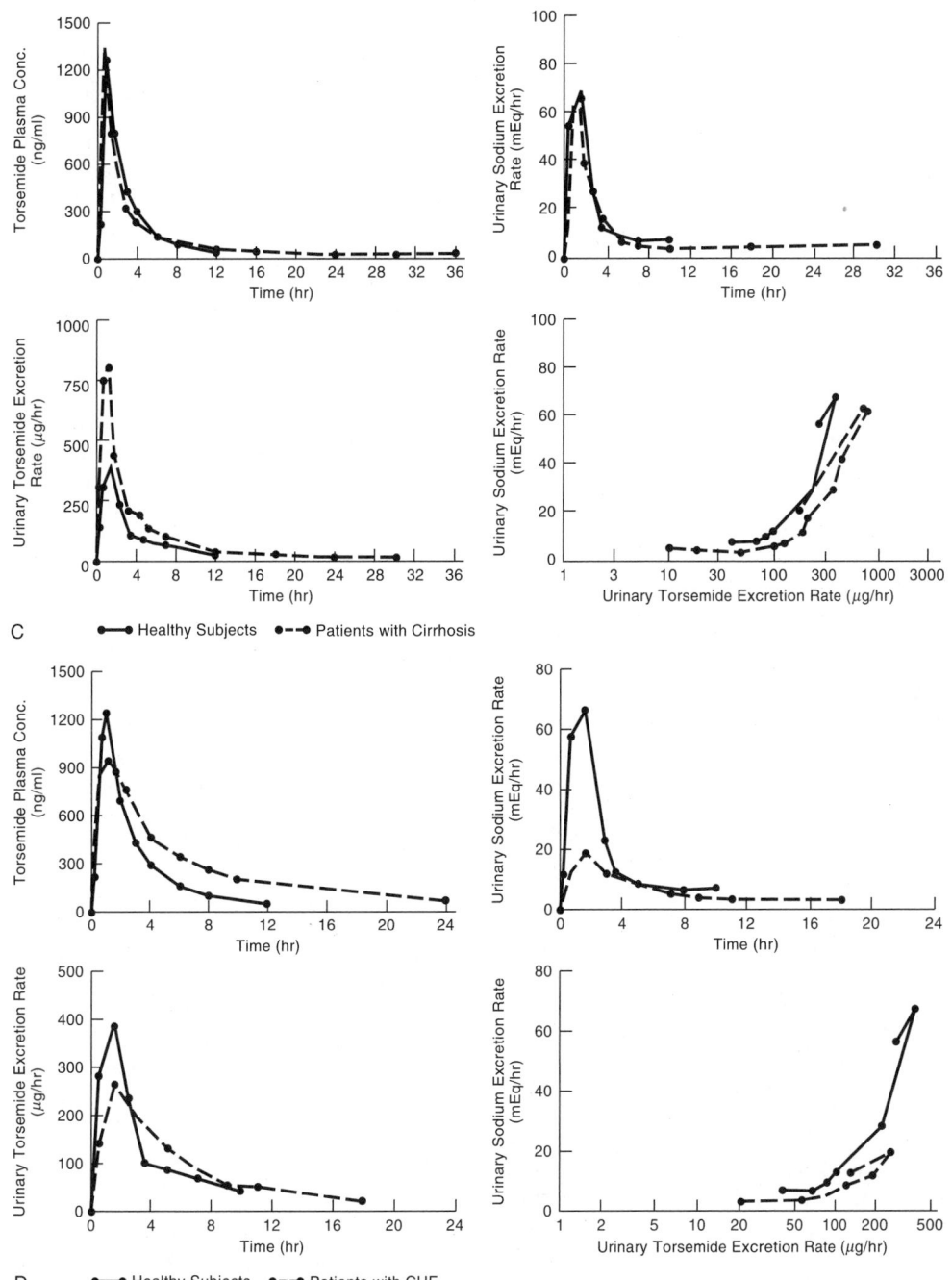

Figure 41–4 *Continued C,* Pharmacokinetics and pharmacodynamics of torsemide in patients with cirrhosis *(dashed lines).* Depictions are as in Figure 41–3. *D,* Pharmacokinetics and pharmacodynamics of torsemide in patients with congestive heart failure *(dashed lines).* Depictions are as in Figure 41–3.

liver disease, though half-life is prolonged to a small degree, as shown in Table 41–1. The decreased nonrenal clearance allows more torsemide to persist in plasma with subsequent increased delivery into the urine over time (lower left graph). Despite this increased delivery of diuretic to the urinary site of action, the sodium excretory response over time is similar in patients with cirrhosis to that in healthy subjects (upper right panel). The explanation for this disparity is that the pharmacodynamics of response is altered in patients with cirrhosis, wherein the rela-

tionship between urinary torsemide excretion rate and urinary sodium excretion rate is shifted to the right. Thus, nephrons in patients with cirrhosis have decreased sensitivity. This abnormality persists even if response if expressed as fractional excretion of sodium. The normal overall response that occurs in such patients is due to two countervailing forces, wherein the decreased responsiveness of the nephron is offset by the increased delivery of diuretic to the site of action.[28] The response demonstrated in Figure 41–4C is obtained with a 10-mg dose of torsemide.

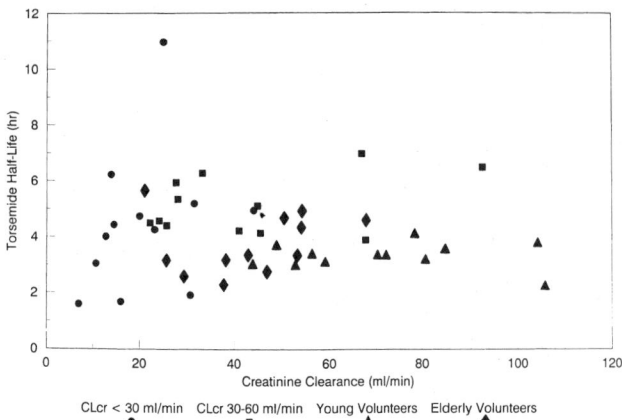

Figure 41–5. Lack of relationship between torsemide half-life and renal function.

Although this dose was not sufficient to define the maximal response that can be elicited in such patients, it is clear that the diuresis that occurred is quite brisk. It would be highly unlikely that higher doses of this potent loop diuretic would be needed in such subjects.

The decreased responsiveness of the nephron to torsemide in patients with cirrhosis is similar to that which has been observed by numerous investigators with furosemide.[29-32] The mechanism for this abnormal response is not clear but might be related to increased proximal tubular reabsorption of sodium and/or increased distal tubular reabsorption of sodium. With furosemide, however, there is no change in delivery of diuretic into the urine.[29-32] Therefore, if a patient with cirrhosis is given the same dose of furosemide as a healthy subject, delivery of furosemide into the urine is similar in the two groups, but overall response is diminished because of the decreased sensitivity of the nephron. Torsemide differs in this regard in that the decreased responsiveness is offset by the increased diuretic delivery into the urine. In turn, this change in delivery is due to the contribution of hepatic metabolism to the overall elimination of this diuretic.

Congestive Heart Failure

The pharmacokinetics of torsemide in patients with CHF appear to be a hybrid of those observed in patients with mild renal insufficiency and those observed in patients with liver disease (see Table 41–1). Though the pharmacokinetics of this diuretic in patients with heart failure is incompletely understood, preliminary information indicates that there is a decrease in the amount of drug appearing in the urine, which is most likely related to concomitant decreases in renal function in patients with severe heart failure.[33, 34] This effect in and of itself should not increase the elimination half-life of the drug. However, in the studies that have been performed in patients with CHF, it appears that the half-life is prolonged to about the same degree as has been observed in patients

with hepatic cirrhosis.[33, 34] This finding could be due to congestive hepatopathy, causing a decrease in hepatic elimination of the drug with a concomitant decrease in total clearance.

Figure 41–4D shows that the half-life is prolonged when assessing the serum concentration of torsemide versus time (upper left graph). In turn, there is a decrease in delivery of diuretic into the urine over time (lower left graph) that results in diminished sodium excretion over time (upper right graph). However, it is apparent that the decreased sodium excretory response is greater in magnitude than the decrease in delivery of diuretic into the urine. The explanation for this observation is that there is also a diminished sensitivity of the nephron to torsemide in patients with CHF (lower right graph). Thus, in patients with CHF, there is both a pharmacokinetic abnormality, wherein decreased diuretic is delivered to the site of action, and a decrease in the pharmacodynamics of response. These two abnormalities act in concert to cause a dramatic decrease in overall natriuresis after a dose of torsemide in such patients.

A study[35] has defined the pharmacodynamics of response in greater detail. Sufficiently large doses of torsemide have been administered to define maximal response in patients with heart failure, and this occurs at a fractional excretion of sodium that is about one third to one half of that which occurs in healthy subjects. This decreased pharmacodynamics of response is similar to that described for both furosemide and bumetanide in patients with CHF.[36] The mechanism for this changed pharmacodynamics is unclear but may relate to increased proximal and/or distal tubular reabsorption of sodium. Importantly, these studies have demonstrated that the maximal response to torsemide can be obtained with intravenous doses of approximately 50 mg. Larger doses are unnecessary unless concomitant renal insufficiency is present.

SUMMARY

Torsemide is a new loop diuretic that has been approved by the FDA. It has a broad pharmacologic profile in that low doses (5 to 10 mg/day) are effective in lowering arterial pressure. If 5-mg doses are used, minimal if any adverse metabolic effects occur. At these doses, the antihypertensive effect is similar to that of low-dose thiazide diuretics. On the other hand, with higher doses, a typical loop diuretic pharmacology manifests itself. As a loop diuretic, torsemide is similar to both furosemide and bumetanide, though it does have some distinctive pharmacokinetic characteristics. The maximal doses needed for different disease states have been defined sufficiently. As such, patients with severe renal insufficiency need not receive doses greater than 100 mg (or rarely 200 mg). Those with lesser degrees of renal dysfunction should receive 50 mg. In such patients, there is no prolongation of half-life, and clinicians need not worry about drug accumulation. Patients with cirrhosis show an interesting pattern wherein diminished responsiveness of the kidney is offset by increased delivery of diuretic into the urine, so that overall natriuretic response is similar to that which occurs in healthy subjects. Thus, a brisk diuresis occurs with 10-mg doses in such patients, and it is highly unlikely that higher doses would be needed. Patients with CHF show abnormalities in both kinetics and in dynamics that are additive and thereby diminish natriuretic response. Doses sufficient to achieve maximal response in such patients will only elicit a fractional excretion rate of sodium that is one third to one half what would occur in healthy subjects. Such maximal rates can be attained with doses of 50 mg of torsemide, even in patients with severe CHF; it is unlikely that higher doses would be necessary. In most clinical conditions, it appears that dosing once per day is effective. That this relatively infrequent dosing rate can be effective may be a result of the longer half-life of torsemide compared with other loop diuretics. It is highly likely, however, that many patients will not attain a sufficient natriuresis with administration of a ceiling dose once per day, and in such patients repeated dosing will be necessary in order to attain the desired cumulative response.

Where torsemide fits in the armamentarium of diuretics is unclear. If one considers the overall dosing range, this diuretic has the uniqueness of a thiazide-like effect at low doses and a loop diuretic effect at high doses. The somewhat unique pharmacokinetic characteristics may make it more readily used in some patient groups. If indeed the lower frequency of dosing that is implied from currently published clinical trials can be maintained with broader clinical use, the advantages to the patient of taking drug less often may be helpful. Further studies are needed to address these issues, which will be a critical determinant of the cost efficacy of this diuretic compared with its competitors.

REFERENCES

1. Baumgart P, Walger P, von Eiff M, Achhammer I: Long-term efficacy and tolerance of torsemide in hypertension. Prog Pharmacol Clin Pharmacol 8:169, 1988.
2. Reyes AJ, Chiesa PD, Santucci MR, et al: Hydrochlorothiazide versus a non-diuretic dose of torsemide as once daily antihypertensive monopharmacotherapy in elderly patients. A randomized and double-blind study. Prog Pharmacol Clin Pharmacol 8:183, 1988.
3. Brater DC, Leinfelder J, Anderson SA: Clinical pharmacology of torsemide, a new loop diuretic. Clin Pharmacol Ther 42:187, 1987.
4. Wittner M, Di Stefano A, Schlatter E, et al: Torasemide inhibits NaCl reabsorption in the thick ascending limb of the loop of Henle. Pflügers Arch 407:611, 1986.
5. Wittner M, Di Stefano A, Wangemann P, et al: Analogues of torasemide—Structure function relationships—Experiments in the thick ascending limb of the loop of Henle of rabbit nephron. Pflügers Arch 408:54, 1987.
6. Lupinacci L, Puschett JB: An examination of site and mechanism of action of torasemide in man. J Clin Pharmacol 28:441, 1988.
7. Brater DC: Diuretics. In Williams RL, Brater DC, Mordenti J (eds): Rational Therapeutics: A Clinical Pharmacologic Guide for the Health Professional. New York: Marcel Dekker, 1989, pp 269–315.
8. Schwartz MA: Metabolism of bumetanide. J Clin Pharmacol 21:555, 1981.
9. Patterson JH, Corder CN, Applefield MM, et al: Short-term efficacy of oral torsemide in patients with chronic congestive heart failure [abstract]. Pharmacotherapy 12:245, 1992.
10. Stauch M, Stiehl L: Controlled, double-blind clinical trial on the efficacy and tolerance of torasemide in comparison with furosemide in patients with congestive heart failure—a multicenter study. Prog Pharmacol Clin Pharmacol 8:121, 1988.
11. Goebel K-M: Six-week study of torsemide in patients with congestive heart failure. Clin Ther 15:1051, 1993.
12. Hariman RJ, Bremner S, Louie EK, et al: Dose-response study of intravenous torsemide in congestive heart failure. Am Heart J 128:352, 1994.
13. Isbary J, Achhammer I, Wetzels E: The influence of 20 mg torasemide IV and 20 mg furosemide IV on hemodynamics and diuresis in patients with high grade left heart failure. Prog Pharmacol Clin Pharmacol 8:137, 1988.
14. Langbehn AF, Achhammer I, Bolke T: Acute hemodynamic effects of 20 mg furosemide and 20 mg furosemide given intravenously to patients with congestive heart failure. Prog Pharmacol Clin Pharmacol 8:147, 1988.
15. Barr WH, Smith H, Karnes HT, et al: Comparison of bioavailability, pharmacokinetics, and pharmacodynamics of torasemide in young and elderly healthy volunteers. Prog Pharmacol Clin Pharmacol 8:15, 1988.
16. Barr WH, Smith HL, Karnes HT, et al: Torasemide dose-proportionality of pharmacokinetics and pharmacodynamics. Prog Pharmacol Clin Pharmacol 8:29, 1988.
17. Knauf H, Spahn H, Rücker HM, Mutschler E: The loop diuretic torasemide in renal failure—kinetics and dynamics. Prog Pharmacol Clin Pharmacol 8:81, 1988.
18. Lesne M: Comparison of the pharmacokinetics and pharmacodynamics of torasemide and furosemide in healthy volunteers. Drug Res 38:160, 1988.
19. Neugebauer G, Besenfelder E, von Möllendorff E: Pharmacokinetics and metabolism of torasemide in man. Drug Res 38:164, 1988.
20. Brater DC: Clinical pharmacology of loop diuretics. Drugs 41(Suppl 3):14–22, 1991.
21. Andreasen F, Hansen U, Husted SE, Jansen JA: The pharmacokinetics of furosemide are influenced by age. Br J Clin Pharmacol 16:391, 1983.
22. Kerremans ALM, Tan Y, van Baars H, et al: Furosemide kinetics and dynamics in aged patients. Clin Pharmacol Ther 34:181, 1983.
23. Voelker JR, Brown-Cartwright D, Anderson S, et al: Comparison of loop diuretics in patients with chronic renal insufficiency: Mechanism of difference in response. Kidney Int 32:572, 1987.
24. Kult J, Ziegler J, von Möllendorff E: Pharmacodynamics and kinetics of torasemide and furosemide in patients with high grade renal failure after administration of high intravenous doses. Prog Pharmacol Clin Pharmacol 8:239, 1988.
25. Gehr TWB, Rudy DW, Matzke GR, et al: The pharmacokinetics of intravenous and oral torsemide in patients with chronic renal insufficiency. Clin Pharmacol Ther 56:31, 1994.
26. Rudy DW, Gehr TWB, Matzke GR, et al: The pharmacodynamics of intravenous and oral torsemide in patients with chronic renal insufficiency. Clin Pharmacol Ther 56:39, 1994.
27. Brunner G, von Bergmann K, von Mölendorff E: Comparison of diuretic effects and pharmacokinetics of torasemide and furosemide after a single oral dose in patients with hydropically decompensated cirrhosis of the liver. Drug Res 38:176, 1988.
28. Schwartz S, Brater DC, Pound D, et al: Bioavailability, pharmacokinetics, and pharmacodynamics of torsemide in patients with cirrhosis. Clin Pharmacol Ther 54:90, 1993.
29. Traeger A, Häntzer, Penzlin M, et al: Pharmacokinetics and pharmacodynamic effects of furosemide in patients with liver cirrhosis. Int J Clin Pharmacol Ther Toxicol 23:129, 1985.
30. Villeneuve J-P, Verbeeck RK, Wilkinson GR, Branch RA: Furosemide kinetics and dynamics in patients with cirrhosis. Clin Pharmacol Ther 40:14, 1986.

31. González G, Arancibia A, Rivas Ml, et al: Pharmacokinetics of furosemide in patients with hepatic cirrhosis. Eur J Clin Pharmacol 22:315, 1982.
32. Verbeeck RK, Patwardhan RV, Villeneuve J-P, et al: Furosemide disposition in cirrhosis. Clin Pharmacol Ther 31:719, 1982.
33. von Möllendorff E, Neugebauer G: Pharmacokinetics of oral torasemide in patients with congestive heart failure. Prog Pharmacol Clin Pharmacol 8:73, 1988.
34. Vargo DL, Kramer WG, Black PK, et al: The pharmacodynamics of torsemide in patients with congestive heart failure. Clin Pharmacol Ther 56:48, 1994.
35. Vargo DL, Kramer WG, Black PK, et al: The pharmacodynamics of torsemide patients with congestive heart failure. Clin Pharmacol Ther 56:48, 1994.
36. Brater DC, Chennavasin P, Seiwell R: Furosemide in patients with heart failure. Shift of the dose-response relationship. Clin Pharmacol Ther 28:182, 1980.

C. Thiazide Diuretics and Derivatives

CHAPTER 42

Thiazide Diuretics, Chlorthalidone, and Metolazone

Barry J. Materson, M.D., and Murray Epstein, M.D.

HISTORY AND CHEMISTRY

Modern orally administered thiazide and thiazide-like diuretics owe their discovery to observations made on the mild diuretic effects of sulfanilamide in 1937 and 1938.[1-3] Schwartz[4] observed that sulfanilamide, an antimicrobial drug containing a sulfamoyl group, was useful as a diuretic in the treatment of patients with congestive heart failure. The diuretic effect was found to be caused by the weak carbonic anhydrase–inhibiting activity of sulfanilamide. Intensive investigation into carbonic anhydrase–inhibiting compounds led to the discovery of carzenid, which produced substantial diuresis in dogs[5] and saluresis in human subjects.[6] Novello and Sprague[7] pursued this work to the synthesis of chlorothiazide, the first practical orally administered thiazide diuretic, in 1957. The discovery of the more potent compound hydrochlorothiazide (HCTZ) was published the following year.[8] HCTZ became and for more than 30 years has remained the cornerstone of the thiazide diuretic group. The remainder of the discussion on thiazides in this chapter will deal exclusively with HCTZ, although there are at least six thiazides (two available in the United States) and 22 hydrothiazides (six available in the United States; Table 42–1).[9]

Chlorthalidone is not strictly a thiazide but rather an *m*-sulfamoylarylpseudocarboxamide. It was first reported in 1959.[10] Although its clinical properties are similar to those of HCTZ, chlorthalidone was developed because of its long duration of natriuretic response.

Quinethazone was developed by systematic exploration of the diuretic activity of 6-sulfamoyltetrahydroquinazolinones.[11] Metolazone is a chemical analogue of quinethazone that was developed later.[12] Metolazone differs from quinethazone by the introduction of an *o*-tolyl group in position 3 and the substitution of a methyl group for an ethyl group in position 2. It was developed as a long-acting thiazide-like diuretic and antihypertensive agent that ap-

peared to be effective even in the face of a decreasing glomerular filtration rate.[13]

Metolazone has continued to be of interest because of its unusual effects in the proximal tubule, new data on efficacy of low doses of a micronized formulation, and the effects of its combination with loop-blocking diuretics.

Metolazone increases renal phosphate excretion[14] by inhibition of phosphate reabsorption across the brush border membrane of the proximal tubule.[15] Studies by Kempson et al.[15] of isolated renal brush border membrane vesicles demonstrated that metolazone could inhibit sodium-dependent phosphate, D-glucose, and L-proline transport, whereas neither acetazolamide nor chlorothiazide caused these effects. Odlind et al.[16] dissociated the diuretic effect of metolazone from its urinary excretion rate. They suggested that its diuretic effect might be elicited primarily from the peritubular side of the nephron and that there might be a luminal, sodium-independent kaliuretic effect. These results could explain the clinical observation that it is possible to affect kaliuresis without diuresis with metolazone in severely decompensated patients with hepatic cirrhosis.[17] The proximal tubule and peritubular actions might also contribute to the effects of metolazone in patients with renal failure.

More has been learned about the mechanism of action of thiazide diuretics at the cellular, membrane, and tissue levels. Evidence points strongly to the presence of thiazide-specific receptors in the renal tubules and elsewhere.[20-22] The transport mechanism has been identified as thiazide-sensitive Na^+-Cl^- cotransport.[3-5] This results in reduction of intracellular chloride concentration and consequent hyperpolarization of the basolateral membrane voltage of distal tubule cells.[23] The acute vasorelaxant effect of HCTZ may be due to involvement of Ca^{2+}-activated K^+ channels.[24] The antihypertensive effect does not appear to depend on enhanced prostacyclin synthesis.[25]

If metolazone were similar to chlorthalidone and HCTZ in its dissociation of the dose-response curves

Table 42–1. Thiazide and Thiazide-Like Diuretics

Generic Name	Trade Name*
Thiazides	
Acetothiazide	
Benzthiazide	Naclex, Exna
Bromothiazide	
Chlorothiazide	Diuril
Flumethiazide	Ademol
Iodothiazide	
Hydrothiazides	
Althiazide	Altizid
Bemetizide	Dehydrosanol
Bendroflumethiazide	Naturetin
Benzylhydrochlorothiazide	Dehydron
Buthiazide (thiabutazide)	Salucin
Carmetizide	Myarl
Cyclopenthiazide	Navidrex
Cyclothiazide	Anhydron
Epithiazide	Thiaver
Ethiazide	Neo-Diuresal
Hydrobenzthiazide	Aquazid
Hydrochlorothiazide	HydroDIURIL, Esidrix, Oretic
Hydroflumethiazide	Saluron, Diucardin
Mebutizide	Neoniagar
Methalthiazide	
Methyclothiazide	Enduron
Parafluthiazide	
Penfluthiazide	Brizide
Polythiazide	Renese
Sumetizide	Hypotensine
Tetrachlormethiazide	Depleil
Trichlormethiazide	Naqua
Thiazide-Like Drugs	
Chlorthalidone	Hygroton, Thalitone
Clopamide	Aquex, Brinaldix
Clorexolone	Nefrolan
Fenquizone	Idrolone
Indapamide	Fludex, Natrilix, Lozol
Metolazone	Zaroxolyn, Diulo, Mykrox
Quinethazone	Hydromox
Xipamide	Aquaphor, Diurexan

*Not all trade names are included. A given generic drug may have a different trade name in each of several countries.

Data from reference 9 and other sources.

for decrements of blood pressure and serum potassium concentration, it would be useful to establish the lowest effective therapeutic dose.[26] Indeed, Curry et al.[27] published the results of two multicenter trials of a new micronized metolazone formulation. This more bioavailable form of metolazone proved to be effective in reducing blood pressure with administration of as little as 0.5 mg without inducing significant hypokalemia.

Metolazone can be combined with furosemide to treat severe congestive heart failure[28] and refractory edema.[29] The effects of the combination have been defined as additive[30] or supraadditive.[31] The combination generally worked in children with furosemide-resistant edema, but it failed in those with serum albumin levels of less than 1.5 g/L or renal insufficiency.[32] The combination of metolazone with bumetanide was also effective but not supraadditive.[33]

The structural formulas for chlorothiazide, HCTZ, chlorthalidone, and metolazone are shown in Figure 42–1.

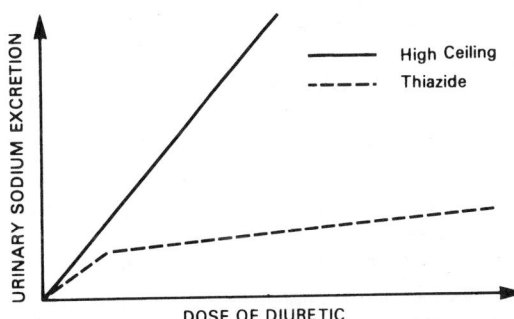

Figure 42–1. Structural formulas for selected thiazide and thiazide-like diuretics. Note that chlorthalidone and metolazone are not benzothiadiazides, but all four drugs possess identically oriented chloride and sulfamoyl groups.

PHARMACOLOGY AND PHARMACOKINETICS

The thiazide and thiazide-like diuretics are similar in overall pharmacology and mechanism of action. Some differences between them, however, have important implications for clinical practice.

Common characteristics of this group of drugs are their low ceiling, flat dose-response curve, slow onset of effect, long duration of action, and tendency to reduce urine calcium.[34] *Low ceiling* refers to the phenomenon whereby near-maximal urinary sodium excretion is achieved at relatively low doses of these diuretics and further increases in drug dose result in only small additional amounts of sodium excretion. This phenomenon, of course, also describes the shape of the dose-response curve. It is important to note that, although the shapes of the dose-response curve for urinary sodium excretion and blood pressure reduction are similar, they are not necessarily superimposable. Figure 42–2 compares the dose-response curve for the thiazide diuretics with that for the loop

Figure 42–2. Idealized dose-response curves for high-ceiling (loop) and thiazide diuretics. Urinary sodium excretion is greater after administration of higher doses of a high-ceiling diuretic. In contrast, little further increase in urinary sodium excretion can be achieved by increasing dosages of thiazide diuretics above their usually recommended levels. (From Materson BJ: Insights into intrarenal sites and mechanisms of action of diuretic agents. Am Heart J 106:188, 1983.)

(high-ceiling) diuretics.[34] An important focus of attention on the thiazide group of diuretics has been the ascending portion of the dose-response curve. In general, one should use the lowest dose possible to achieve effect while minimizing adverse effects.

Time courses of action of HCTZ, different doses of metolazone, and furosemide are depicted in Figure 42–3.[14] In contrast with the rapid onset and short duration of action of the loop diuretics, the thiazides and thiazide-like drugs tend to have a much slower onset of action and longer duration. The latter property is important in the treatment of hypertension, in which sustained reduction of extracellular fluid volume is a goal.

The chronic reduction of extracellular fluid volume is also the likely explanation for decrease in urinary calcium excretion that occurs with the thiazide diuretics. The thiazides do not interfere with distal calcium reabsorption and, by promoting increased proximal reabsorption of calcium driven by volume depletion, the amount of calcium delivered into the urine can be reduced. This quality greatly aids the treatment of renal calculus formation due to urine supersaturated with calcium.

EFFECTS ON PATHOPHYSIOLOGY
Effects on Hemodynamics

As a consequence of their natriuretic effects, all of the thiazide and thiazide-like diuretics deplete extracellular fluid volume. Patients with edematous states usually experience slow but constant weight losses as long as mobilizable extracellular fluid is present. After peripheral edema clears, it is more difficult to mobilize ascitic and pleural fluid. Depletion of intravascular volume activates counterregulatory mechanisms: increased proximal tubular reabsorption of salt and

water, aldosterone stimulation of distal sodium reabsorption and hydrogen and potassium excretion, and antidiuretic hormone-stimulated reabsorption of tubular fluid across the collecting tubule. Collectively, these events have been called the *braking phenomenon*.[35]

Nonedematous hypertensive patients will also lose 0.5 to 2.0 kg as a result of extracellular fluid volume diuresis. The counterregulatory mechanisms discussed earlier will be activated, and homeostasis will be achieved and maintained at a lower body weight. With time, total peripheral resistance will fall. Although the exact mechanism for this chain of events has not been established, possible factors include decreased sensitivity and reactivity of the resistance arterioles to vasoactive humoral agents. Additional possible factors include an effect like calcium channel blocking at the membrane level and reverse autoregulation.[36]

Effects on Ventricular Function and Structure

Thiazide diuretics improve ventricular function in patients with congestive heart failure by reducing preload, thereby allowing the ventricle to function in a more efficient range of the Frank-Starling curve. In hypertensive patients, the use of thiazide diuretics alone does decrease the mass of a hypertrophied left ventricle.[37, 38] When thiazides are used as adjuncts to other antihypertensive drugs, especially in severely hypertensive patients who have a component of congestive heart failure, the cardiac silhouette can be reduced on standard chest radiographs and the strain pattern on the electrocardiogram can be reversed.

Effects on Electrophysiology

The thiazide diuretics have no direct effect on cardiac electrophysiology. Nevertheless, the question of cardiac arrhythmias associated with metabolic changes induced by diuretics remains extremely controversial. Evidence suggests that epinephrine lowers serum potassium concentration;[39] that hypokalemia, per se, can induce and increase the frequency and severity of ventricular ectopy;[40] and that hypokalemic patients are at greater risk of serious dysrhythmias at the time of myocardial infarction.[41] Holland et al.,[42] Hollifield and Slaton,[43] and the Medical Research Council[44] have implicated diuretic-induced hypokalemia (and perhaps magnesium loss) in the induction of ventricular ectopy or sudden death. This finding fueled a controversy over the claimed need for potassium supplementation.[45]

Conversely, investigators such as Papademitriou et al.[46] and Madias et al.[47] have been unable to demonstrate diuretic-induced ventricular ectopy, even when serum potassium levels are low. Caralis et al.[48] found that ventricular ectopy could be induced only in patients with clinically apparent organic heart disease by history, physical findings, chest radiograph, or electrocardiogram. These findings led to a recommen-

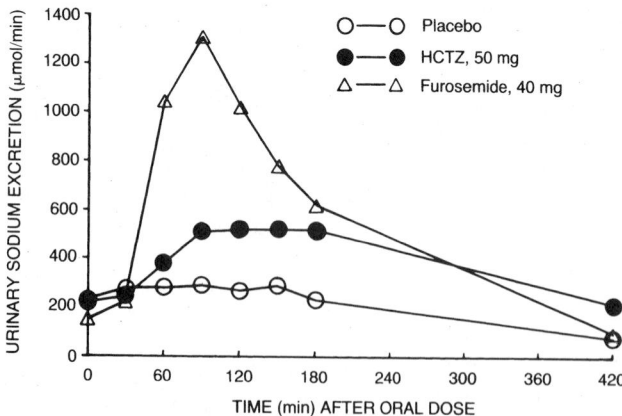

Figure 42–3. Time-course of urinary sodium excretion ($U_{Na}V$) after an oral dose of placebo, furosemide 40 mg, and hydrochlorothiazide (HCTZ) 50 mg. Each group is the mean of six subjects. Control represents the mean of the four 30-minute control periods from 8:00 to 10:00 AM. The 420-minute point represents a urine collection made by the ambulatory subjects after they were dismissed from the procedure room at 180 minutes. (Modified from Materson BJ, Hotchkiss JL, Barkin JS, et al: Oral metolazone: Effects on urine composition in water-loaded normal man. Curr Ther Res 14:545, 1972.)

dation that potassium supplementation should be reserved for patients with clinical evidence of organic heart disease.[49, 50]

Even in the absence of hypertension, hypokalemia, or treatment with thiazide diuretics, left ventricular hypertrophy per se is a risk factor for ventricular ectopy.[51]

EFFECTS ON BODY FLUIDS, VOLUME STATUS, AND ELECTROLYTES
Volume Depletion

The most fundamental effect of a diuretic drug is an increase in the output of urine. If fluid intake is restricted such that a net negative balance of water occurs, total extracellular fluid volume will be depleted. This depletion occurs first from the intravascular fluid compartment. Increased oncotic pressure due to concentration of intravascular proteins alters the Starling forces to favor reabsorption of fluid from the interstitial compartment. Therefore, edema fluid will tend to move back into the intravascular compartment, from which it can be excreted.

Low serum protein concentration, such as that found in the nephrotic syndrome and decompensated cirrhosis of the liver, will provide much less of an oncotic effect and thereby render the transit of fluid out of the interstitial space less effective. As long as the diuretic remains effective in this clinical setting, intravascular volume may become depleted, and renal blood flow and glomerular filtration rate may decrease; thus, the patient may become more susceptible to symptomatic orthostatic hypotension. As detailed in Chapter 39, the condition of patients with portal hypertension may be further complicated by sequestration of intravascular volume in the portal bed.

Hypokalemia

The effects of thiazide diuretics on serum electrolytes are well known. Hypokalemia, especially in non-edematous states, is a direct function of diuretic dose. This quality is of great clinical importance because of the need to use only the lowest effective dose of the diuretic so that the possibility of hypokalemia is minimized.[52, 53] Figures 42–4 and 42–5 illustrate two ways to examine the dose-response curves for diuretics and hypokalemia. In Figure 42–4,[26] the blood pressure–lowering effect of chlorthalidone is clearly maximal at 25 mg for a group of patients with mild hypertension, but the percentage of patients who experienced hypokalemia at any time during the study continued to increase with increasing doses. The Veterans Administration Cooperative Study on Hypertension in the Elderly[54] had a single point in the protocol at which large numbers of men 60 years of age or older had been taking 25, 50, or 100 mg of HCTZ for mild to moderate hypertension. When the percentage of patients at each concentration of serum

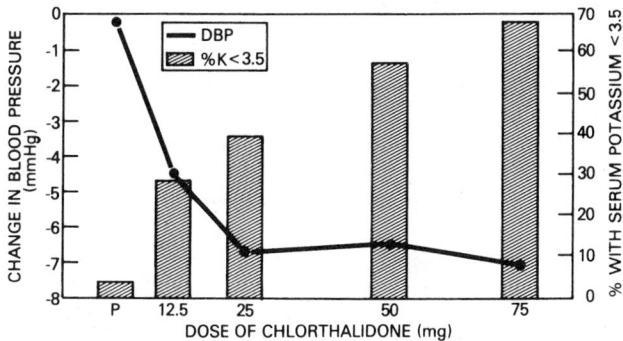

Figure 42–4. Dose-response curve for the effect of chlorthalidone on diastolic blood pressure (DBP) superimposed on its effect on serum potassium levels. The *vertical bars* depict the percentage of patients whose serum potassium was less than 3.5 mEq/L at any time during the study. The adverse effect (hypokalemia) increases with increasing drug dose, whereas there is no further therapeutic benefit beyond 25 mg. (From Materson BJ: Diuretic dose-response relationships. Mod Med 56[Suppl A]:47, 1988.)

potassium was plotted (see Fig. 42–5), a roughly Gaussian distribution for each dose of HCTZ appeared. Of interest is the shift of each curve further to the left as the dose of HCTZ is increased. Therefore, even though there is considerable overlap, the tendency toward hypokalemia with increasing diuretic dose is clear. The risk of hypokalemia can be further minimized by moderate dietary sodium restriction to about 70 to 100 mmol/day[55] and by encouraging consumption of fresh potassium-rich fruits and vegetables. Routine potassium supplementation or use of potassium-sparing diuretic drugs in patients with uncomplicated hypertension is probably not warranted.[56]

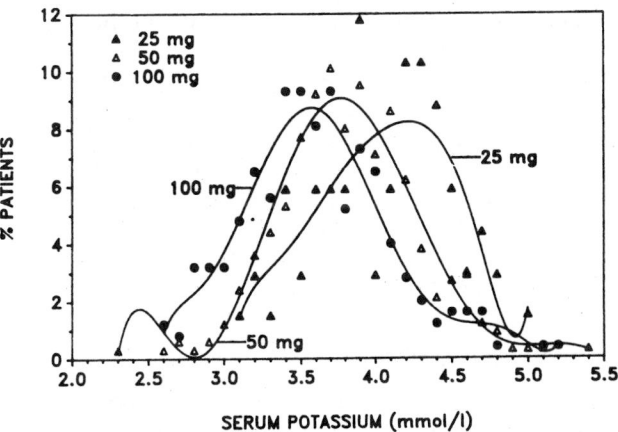

Figure 42–5. Distribution of serum potassium levels after randomization to low-dose (25 mg once or twice daily) or high-dose (50 mg once or twice daily) hydrochlorothiazide. Patients were taking either 25 mg (n = 68), 50 mg (n = 338), or 100 mg (n = 248) of hydrochlorothiazide daily. Curves were fitted to the scatter plot of the percentage of patients at each level of serum potassium for each of the three final doses. Although there is considerable overlap, the distribution curves are shifted to the left as dose increases. (Data from Materson BJ, Cushman WC, Goldstein G, et al: Treatment of hypertension in the elderly: I. Blood pressure and clinical changes. Results of a Department of Veterans Affairs cooperative study. Hypertension 15:348, 1990.)

As a consequence of diuretic-induced intravascular volume contraction and stimulation of aldosterone secretion, bicarbonate reabsorption (hydrogen ion secretion) is increased proximally, and hydrogen ion secretion is increased distally. The results are a higher serum bicarbonate concentration and lower serum hydrogen ion concentration (increased serum pH). This development represents classic hypokalemic metabolic alkalosis associated with thiazide diuretic therapy. Ordinarily, this condition is mild and of no consequence. More severe electrolyte disturbances are likely to be associated with overly vigorous diuresis.[57]

Hyponatremia

Hyponatremia due to thiazide diuretics is uncommon but of great clinical importance because it is potentially disabling or life-threatening.[58] Because all thiazides interfere with the clearance of free water, patients who take these drugs and consume large quantities of water may develop significant dilutional hyponatremia within a few days.[59] Patients taking a thiazide-type diuretic should be warned that they should contact their physician immediately if they experience headache, nausea, or vomiting. A serum sodium determination should be made at that time. Women and elderly patients appear to be particularly susceptible to hyponatremia and its consequences. Sometimes, patients who take thiazide diuretics and experience intercurrent illnesses with vomiting or diarrhea that provoke hypokalemia may be particularly susceptible to acute hyponatremia if they are able to drink and retain free water.

Deciding how rapidly to raise the serum concentration is especially difficult in severely symptomatic patients in whom the duration of hyponatremia is unclear.[60] The rate of increase must be individualized depending on the patient's clinical condition and course. The serum sodium concentration should not be increased more than 0.5 mmol/L/hr, and the concentration should not be permitted to exceed 125 mmol/L/hr in the first 24 to 36 hours.[61]

This entire topic remains highly controversial. There are arguments that hypoxemia results from prolonged hyponatremia and that the hypoxemia rather than rapid correction of hyponatremia is responsible for central pontine myelinolysis.[62, 63]

Hypercalcemia

Serum calcium levels are almost invariably increased slightly by treatment with thiazide diuretics. A purely hypothetical explanation for this phenomenon is that, by depleting the body of excess salt and water, diuretics turn off the secretion of the hypothalamic natriuretic hormone (digitalis-like substance), thereby permitting a corrective shift of intracellular to extracellular calcium. A few patients treated with thiazide diuretics develop calcium levels substantially above the normal range.[64] Some such patients are found on further investigation to have parathyroid adenomas.[65]

One of the concerns about the use of thiazide di-

uretics in the elderly was that it might increase the number of falls due to orthostatic hypotension. In fact, thiazides are not associated with any increase in falls, and there may be a tendency for fewer nonspinal fractures, such as those of the wrist and hip.[66] The latter benefit could be explained by a beneficial side effect of thiazide diuretics whereby calcium is shifted into bones, thus increasing bone density.[67]

Magnesium and Zinc Depletion

Prolonged treatment with thiazide-type diuretics also can deplete body stores of magnesium. Because serum magnesium levels reflect intracellular magnesium contents so poorly, it is difficult to perform definitive studies that determine the importance of this phenomenon. Magnesium and potassium depletion have been proposed as determinants of diuretic-associated ventricular ectopic activity, but this theory is unproved. However, the possibility of magnesium depletion should be kept in mind when thiazides are used to treat patients who have decompensated cirrhosis of the liver, because intracellular magnesium depletion is likely to be part of the basic disease process.

Zinc also may be lost in the urine during chronic thiazide diuretic treatment. This loss is more likely to take place in patients with edema than in those with hypertension. The clinical importance of zinc loss remains unknown. There is an unsubstantiated suggestion that zinc loss is associated with sexual dysfunction.[68]

ENDOCRINE AND METABOLIC EFFECTS

All thiazide diuretics activate the endocrine counter-regulatory hormonal systems. This activation includes the release of renin, angiotensin, aldosterone, antidiuretic hormone, and norepinephrine. Serum concentrations of uric acid predictably will increase by 1 to 1.5 mg/dl, and this elevation will be maintained for the duration of thiazide diuretic therapy. Carbohydrate metabolism may be impaired in some patients. When thiazide administration is terminated, plasma glucose levels tend to return quickly to baseline.[69] These mechanisms are largely related to hypokalemia but also may be partly due to decreased sensitivity of islet cells to catecholamines. It is also possible that diuretics have a direct effect on pancreatic β-cells. Hermansen et al.[70] infused furosemide and indapamide into normal dogs and studied the effects on $\beta\delta$-cell secretion. Neither drug altered somatostatin (δ-cell) secretion, but both directly inhibited insulin secretion. The clinical relevance of these observations remains uncertain. Harrower et al.[71] found no change in plasma insulin or glucose levels during glucose tolerance tests of 10 hypertensive patients whose blood pressures had been controlled successfully by indapamide for 1 year. Raggi et al.[72] found no change in fasting glycemia, postprandial glycemia, and glycosylated hemoglobin in a similar population treated with 2.5 mg of indapamide for 6 months.

The use of thiazide diuretics in patients with diabetes mellitus has become highly controversial.[73, 74] There is evidence that HCTZ is associated with a decrease in insulin sensitivity[75] in contrast with most other antihypertensive drugs.[76, 77] In a study by the Department of Veterans Affairs Cooperative Study Group on Antihypertensive Agents, mean serum glucose levels increased significantly in patients treated with HCTZ compared with those treated with other drugs or placebo.[78] The statistically significant difference remained even after 2 years of treatment.

There is strong evidence for the necessity of treating hypertension in diabetic patients.[79] Because diabetic patients are usually hypervolemic, diuretics (particularly in low-dose monotherapy or in combination with other agents)[80] have a role.[81] Others argue against the use of thiazides in diabetic patients, claiming that they are associated with increased mortality.[82, 83] On the other hand, because overall data from many more recent studies show that cardiovascular mortality was decreased on therapy with lower dosages of a thiazide diuretic, the Joint National Committee recently has recommended that thiazides and β-blockers be the first-line antihypertensive agents of choice for treating hypertension in general.[85] However, these studies generally excluded insulin-dependent or unstable diabetics.

The effect of thiazide diuretics on plasma lipids remains highly controversial. It is clear that thiazide diuretics elevate total serum cholesterol levels initially,[85, 86] perhaps by elevating the concentrations of low-density lipoprotein (LDL) cholesterol. Restriction of dietary intake of fats may prevent diuretic-associated increases in serum cholesterol.[87] Relatively few long-term studies have been made on this point. Some data[88] suggest that cholesterol levels return to baseline values after 6 months of diuretic therapy.[78] However, it is possible that a placebo-controlled baseline value may become lower with time because of regression toward the mean. Therefore, a lipid-elevating effect of thiazides might still be present. Any association of these diuretic-induced, elevated lipid levels with an increased risk of coronary heart disease is inferential and has not been proved.

Effects on Renal Hemodynamics

Because thiazide diuretics deplete intravascular volume, they predictably reduce renal blood flow and glomerular filtration rate slightly. This reduction is reflected by a small increase in the serum concentration of urea nitrogen (2 to 5 mg/dl is the usual normal range) and a trivial increase in serum creatinine concentration.

In general, thiazide and thiazide-like diuretics tend to lose their antihypertensive and diuretic efficacy as glomerular filtration rate declines.[89] Metolazone[90] and indapamide,[91] however, continue to have a beneficial effect, but it may be necessary to increase the dose. The reasons for this continued effect are not fully

understood but may have to do with the release of free metolazone from red blood cell–binding sites as the serum levels of urea nitrogen increase, the ability of free metolazone to block sodium phosphate transport in the proximal tubule, and enterohepatic recycling through the biliary system.

CLINICAL USE
Indications

The indications for thiazide and thiazide-like diuretics may be divided into those that benefit from the diuretic effect and those related to the nondiuretic effects. Use of these drugs is primarily in patients with hypertension and edematous states (discussed in Chapter 39). A Veterans Administration study[78] demonstrated that doses of HCTZ as low as 12.5 mg daily were effective in treating patients with mild to moderate hypertension. The study also showed the importance of an age-by-race interaction in predicting what types of patients would be more or less likely to respond to single-drug therapy. When compared with five other classes of antihypertensive drugs, HCTZ was most effective in older blacks and least effective in younger whites. Uses of diuretics in patients in nonedematous states are listed in Table 42–2.[92]

Yendt[93] first described the use of thiazide diuretics for treatment of nephrolithiasis. This use probably reflects a generic effect of the thiazide class of diuretics in that they increase proximal tubule calcium reabsorption as a response to extracellular fluid volume depletion and leave the distal calcium reabsorptive mechanism intact. Metolazone reduced the occurrence of nephrolithiasis in 38 men by 77% over 3

Table 42–2. **Use of Diuretics in Nonedematous States***

Neonatal Disorders
Respiratory distress syndrome
Bronchopulmonary dysplasia
Edema of prematurity
Disorders of Calcium and Phosphate Metabolism
Hypercalcemia
Hypocalcemic states—hypoparathyroidism and
  pseudohypoparathyroidism
Hypercalciuria—renal, absorptive, vitamin D–induced, renal
  tubular acidosis
Renal calcium stones—hypercalciuria, idiopathic, oxalosis
Hypophosphatemia—hypophosphatemic rickets, Fanconi
  syndrome
Disorders of Water, Electrolytes, and Acid-Base Balance
Nephrogenic diabetes insipidus
Inappropriate secretion of antidiuretic hormone
Hypokalemia—Bartter syndrome, Liddle syndrome
Renal tubular acidosis—types 1, 2, and 4
Urine alkalinization—uric acid nephropathy
Increased Intracranial and Intraocular Pressure
Hydrocephalus
Glaucoma

*Indications for all types of diuretics are included.
Modified from Alon U: Non-diuretic use of diuretics. In Pushchett JB, Greenberg A (eds): Diuretics II: Chemistry, Pharmacology and Clinical Applications. New York: Elsevier, 1987, pp 315–319. Copyright 1987 by Elsevier Science Publishing Company, Inc.

years.[94] The hypocalciuric effect of metolazone could be potentiated by dietary sodium restriction or blunted by dietary sodium excess. Volume depletion, combined with the ability of thiazides to decrease free water clearance, accounts for the reduction of urine volume in patients treated with thiazides for diabetes insipidus.[95]

Probably all other antihypertensive drugs have at least an additive beneficial effect when combined with a thiazide or thiazide-like diuretic. In addition, the tendency of thiazides to cause hypokalemia can be reduced or abolished by combination with a potassium-sparing diuretic. Some available combinations are listed in Table 42–3.

Precautions and Adverse Effects

HCTZ is associated occasionally with phototoxic skin reactions. Patients characteristically have a diffuse maculopapular rash in sun-exposed areas. The rash disappears with discontinuation of the HCTZ. We have successfully transferred patients with HCTZ-induced photodermatitis to therapy with metolazone and observed a similar beneficial therapeutic effect without recurrence of the rash. The logic for this change is that metolazone has its main ultraviolet absorption spectrum outside of the sunlight range. However, when we analyzed a large number of diuretics in the laboratory of Dr. J. Richard Taylor (unpublished data), we learned that the ultraviolet absorption spectra listed in standard reference books were peaks used primarily for analysis. All of these drugs have multiple absorption peaks, some of which are in the sunlight spectrum. Therefore, no adequate explanation exists for this successful therapeutic maneuver.

Table 42–3. **Antihypertensive Combinations with Hydrochlorothiazide or Chlorthalidone***

Antihypertensive or Diuretic	Brand Name
With Hydrochlorothiazide	
Spironolactone	Aldactazide
Methyldopa	Aldoril
Hydralazine	Apresoline-Esidrix, Apresazide
Captopril	Capozide
Triamterene	Dyazide, Maxzide
Guanethidine	Esimil
Reserpine	Hydropres, Serpasil-Esidrix
Propranolol	Inderide
Metoprolol	Lopressor HCT
Amiloride	Moduretic
Labetalol	Normozide, Transdate HCT
Deserpidine	Oreticyl
Reserpine/hydralazine	Ser-Ap-Es
Timolol	Timolide
Enalapril	Vaseretic
With Chlorthalidone	
Clonidine	Combipres
Reserpine	Regroton, Demi-Regroton
Atenolol	Tenoretic

*Not all brand names and no generic brands are listed.

Interference with Other Drugs

The drug interaction of metolazone with furosemide is of major clinical importance. Patients who have been resistant to furosemide diuresis may respond after the addition of 2.5 to 20.0 mg of metolazone. Diuresis with this combination may be brisk or even excessive and should be used with foresight and considerable caution, preferably in the hospital.[29] When properly used, this combination can be of considerable value as an adjunct to treatment of severely hypertensive patients who require minoxidil and have severe salt and water retention associated with its use. An additional indication for this combination is mobilization of excess fluid in patients with renal insufficiency.

Thiazide diuretics generally increase plasma levels of lithium and may cause lithium toxicity.[96] The combination should be used only with extreme caution, if at all.

REFERENCES

1. Southworth H: Acidosis associated with administration of para-amino-benzene-sulfonamide (prontylin). Proc Soc Exp Biol Med 36:58, 1937.
2. Marshall EK Jr, Cutting WC, Emerson K Jr: Toxicity of sulfanilamide. JAMA 110:252, 1938.
3. Strauss MB, Southworth H: Urinary changes due to sulfanilamide administration. Bull Johns Hopkins Hosp 63:41, 1938.
4. Schwartz WB: Effect of sulfanilamide on salt and water excretion in congestive heart failure. N Engl J Med 240:173, 1949.
5. Beyer KH: Factors basic to development of useful inhibitors of renal transport mechanisms. Arch Int Pharmacodyn Ther 98:97, 1954.
6. Merrill JP: Experience with dirnate, an oral diuretic agent. Am J Med 14:519, 1953.
7. Novello SC, Sprague JM: Benzothiadiazine dioxides as novel diuretics. J Am Chem Soc 79:2028, 1957.
8. de Stevens G, Werner LH, Halamandaris A, et al: Dihydrobenzothiadiazine dioxides with potent diuretic effect. Experientia 14:463, 1958.
9. Allen RC: Sulfonamide diuretics. *In* Cragoe EJ Jr (ed): Diuretics, Chemistry, Pharmacology, and Medicine. New York: John Wiley & Sons, 1983, pp 49–200.
10. Graf W, Girod E, Schmid E, et al: Zur Konstitution von Benzophenon-2-carbonsäure-Derivaten. Helv Chim Acta (Basel) 42:1085, 1959.
11. Cohen E, Klarberg B, Vaughan J Jr: Quinazolinone sulfonamides, a new class of diuretic agents. J Am Chem Soc 82:2731, 1960.
12. Belair E, Kaiser F, Van Denburg B, et al: Pharmacology of SR 720-22. Arch Int Pharmacodyn Ther 177:71, 1969.
13. Craswell PW, Ezzat E, Kopstein J, et al: Use of metolazone, a new diuretic, in patients with renal disease. Nephron 12:63, 1973.
14. Materson BJ, Hotchkiss JL, Barkin JS, et al: Oral metolazone: Effects on urine composition in water-loaded normal man. Curr Ther Res 14:545, 1972.
15. Kempson SA, Kowalski JC, Puschett JB: Direct effect of metolazone on sodium-dependent transport across the renal brush border membrane. J Lab Clin Med 101:308, 1983.
16. Odlind B, Beerman B, Lindstrom B, et al: Some effects of metolazone on electrolyte transport. Ups J Med Sci 92:19, 1987.
17. Lowenthal DT, Shear L: Use of a new diuretic agent (metolazone) in patients with edema and ascites. Arch Intern Med 132:38, 1973.
18. Ellison DH, Morrisey J, Desir GV: Solubilization and partial purification of the thiazide diuretic receptor from rabbit renal cortex. Biochim Biophys Acta 1069:241, 1991.

19. Ellison DH, Biemesderfer D, Morrisey J, et al: Immunocyto-chemical characterization of the high-affinity thiazide diuretic receptor in rabbit renal cortex. Am J Physiol 264:F141–F148, 1993.

20. Cremaschi D, Porta C, Botta G, Meyer A: Nature of the neutral Na(+)-Cl− coupled entry at the apical membrane of rabbit gallbladder epthelium: IV. Na+/H+, Cl/HCO3− double ex-change, hydrochlorothiazide-sensitive Na(+)-Cl− symport and Na(+)-K(+)-2Cl− cotransport are all involved. J Mem-brane Biol 129:221, 1992.

21. Shimizu T, Nakamura M: Ouabain-induced cell swelling in rabbit connecting tubule: Evidence for thiazide-sensitive Na(+)-Cl− cotransport. Pflugers Arch Eur J Physiol 421:314, 1992.

22. Terada Y, Knepper MA: Thiazide-sensitive NaCl absorption in rat cortical collecting duct. Am J Physiol 259:F519, 1990.

23. Stanton BA: Cellular actions of thiazide diuretics in the distal tubule. J Am Soc Nephrol 1:832, 1990.

24. Calder JA, Schachter M, Sever PS: Direct vascular actions of hydrochlorothiazide and indapamide in isolated small vessels. Eur J Pharmacol 220:19, 1992.

25. Gerber JG, LoVerde M, Byyny RL, Nies AS: The antihyperten-sive efficacy of hydrochlorothiazide is not prostacyclin depen-dent. Clin Pharmacol Ther 48:424, 1990.

26. Materson BJ: Diuretic dose-response relationships. Mod Med 56(Suppl A):47, 1988.

27. Curry CL, Janda SM, Harris R, et al: Clinical studies of a new, low-dose formulation of metolazone for the treatment of hypertension. Clin Ther 9:47, 1986.

28. Grosskopf I, Rabinovitz M, Rosenfield JB: Combination of furo-semide and metolazone in the treatment of severe congestive heart failure. Isr J Med Sci 22:787, 1986.

29. Epstein M, Lepp BA, Hoffman DS, et al: Potentiation of furose-mide by metolazone in refractory edema. Curr Ther Res 21:656, 1977.

30. Marone C, Muggli F, Lahn W, et al: Pharmacokinetic and phar-macodynamic interaction between furosemide and metolazone in man. Eur J Clin Invest 15:253, 1985.

31. Brater DC, Pressley RH, Anderson SA: Mechanisms of the synergistic combination of metolazone and bumetanide. J Phar-macol Exp Ther 233:70, 1985.

32. Arnold WC: Efficacy of metolazone and furosemide in children with furosemide-resistant edema. Pediatrics 74:872, 1984.

33. Greenberg A, Wallia R, Puschett JB: Combined effect of bumeta-nide and metolazone in normal volunteers. J Clin Pharmacol 25:369, 1985.

34. Materson BJ: Insights into intrarenal sites and mechanisms of action of diuretic agents. Am Heart J 106:188, 1983.

35. Grantham JJ, Chonko AM: The physiologic basis and clinical use of diuretics. In Brenner BM, Stein JH (eds): Sodium and Water Homeostasis. New York: Churchill Livingstone, 1978, pp 178–211.

36. Freis ED: How diuretics lower blood pressure. Am Heart J 106:185, 1983.

37. The Treatment of Mild Hypertension Research Group: The treatment of mild hypertension study: A randomized, placebo-controlled trial of a nutrional-hygienic regimen alone with vari-ous drug monotherapies. Arch Intern Med 151:1413–1423, 1991.

38. Devereux RB, Roman MJ: Hypertensive left ventricular hyper-trophy: Pathogenesis, prognostic importance, and treatment. Cardiovasc Rev Rep 13:24–33, 1992.

39. Struthers AD, Reid JL, Whitesmith R, et al: Effects of intrave-nous adrenaline on electrocardiogram, blood pressure, and se-rum potassium. Br Heart J 49:90, 1983.

40. Hulting J: In hospital ventricular fibrillation and its relation to serum potassium. Acta Med Scand 647(Suppl):109, 1981.

41. Dyckner T, Helmers CC, Lundman T, et al: Initial serum po-tassium level in relation to early complications and prognosis in patients with acute myocardial infarction. Acta Med Scand 197:207, 1975.

42. Holland OB, Nixon JV, Kuhnert L: Diuretic-induced ventricular ectopic activity. Am J Med 70:762, 1981.

43. Hollifield JW, Slaton PE: Thiazide diuretics, hypokalemia and cardiac arrhythmias. Acta Med Scand(Suppl) 647:67, 1981.

44. Medical Research Council on Mild to Moderate Hypertension: Ventricular extrasystoles during thiazide treatment: Substudy of MRC mild hypertension trial. Br Med J 287:1249, 1983.

45. Harrington JT, Isner JM, Kassirer JP: Our national obsession with potassium. Am J Med 73:155, 1982.

46. Papademetriou V, Fletcher R, Khatri IM, et al: Diuretic-induced hypokalemia in uncomplicated systemic hypertension: Effect of plasma potassium correction on cardiac arrhythmias. Am J Cardiol 52:1017, 1983.

47. Madias JE, Madias NE, Gavras HP: Nonarrhythmogenicity of diuretic-induced hypokalemia: Its evidence in patients with uncomplicated hypertension. Arch Intern Med 144:2171, 1984.

48. Caralis PV, Materson BJ, Perez-Stable E: Potassium and di-uretic-induced ventricular arrhythmias in ambulatory hyper-tensive patients. Miner Electrolyte Metabol 10:148, 1984.

49. Materson BJ, Caralis PV: Risk of cardiac arrhythmias in relation to potassium imbalance. J Cardiovasc Pharmacol 6:S493, 1984.

50. Materson BJ: Diuretic-associated hypokalemia [editorial]. Arch Intern Med 145:1966, 1985.

51. Messerli FH, Ventura HO, Elizardi DJ, et al: Hypertension and sudden death: Increased ventricular ectopic activity in left ventricular hypertrophy. Am J Med 77:18, 1984.

52. Materson BJ, Oster JR, Michael UF, et al: Dose response to chlorthalidone in patients with mild hypertension. Efficacy of a lower dose. Clin Pharmacol Ther 24:192, 1978.

53. Materson BJ: A multi-center dose-response study of chlorthali-done 25 mg in mild hypertension. In Mann RD, Guarino RA (eds): Chlorthalidone 25 mg. Lancaster, UK: MTP Press, 1979, pp 27–37.

54. Materson BJ, Cushman WC, Goldstein G, et al: Treatment of hypertension in the elderly: I. Blood pressure and clinical changes. Results of a Department of Veterans Affairs coopera-tive study. Hypertension 15:348, 1990.

55. Parijs J, Joossens JV, Van der Linden L, et al: Moderate sodium restriction and various diuretics in the treatment of hyperten-sion. Am Heart J 85:22, 1973.

56. Kassirer JP, Harrington JT: Diuretics and potassium metabo-lism: A reassessment of the need, effectiveness, and safety of potassium therapy. Kidney Int 11:505, 1977.

57. Materson BJ: Adverse effects of antihypertensive treatment. Cardiol Clin 4:105, 1986.

58. Ashraf N, Locksley R, Arieff AI: Thiazide-induced hypona-tremia associated with death or neurologic damage in outpa-tients. Am J Med 70:1163, 1981.

59. Friedman E, Shadel M, Halkin H, Farfel Z: Thiazide-induced hyponatremia: Reproducibility by single dose rechallenge and analysis of pathogenesis. Ann Intern Med 110:24–30, 1989.

60. Gross PA, Ketteler M, Hausmann C, et al: The charted and the uncharted waters of hyponatremia. Kidney Int 32(Suppl 21):S67, 1987.

61. Sterns RH: Severe symptomatic hyponatremia: Treatment and outcome. Ann Intern Med 107:656, 1987.

62. Tanneau RS, Rouhart F, BenSoussan T, et al: Brain damage following hyponatremia: What is the determinant? Am J Med 94:223, 1993.

63. Laureno R: Myelinolysis is due to rapid correction of hypona-tremia. Am J Med 94:225, 1993.

64. Parfitt AM: Chlorothiazide-induced hypercalcemia in juvenile osteoporosis and hyperparathyroidism. N Engl J Med 281:55, 1969.

65. Stote RM, Smith LH, Wilson DM, et al: Hydrochlorothiazide effects on serum calcium and immunoactive parathyroid hor-mone concentrations: Studies in normal subjects. Ann Intern Med 77:587, 1972.

66. Cauley JA, Cummings SR, Seeley DG, et al: Effects of thiazide diuretic therapy on bone mass, fractures, and falls. The Study of Osteoporotic Fractures Research Group. Ann Intern Med 118:666, 1993.

67. Giles TD, Sander GE, Roffidal LE, et al: Comparative effects of nitrendipine and hydrochlorothiazide on calciotropic hormones and bone density in hypertensive patients. Am J Hypertens 5:875, 1992.

68. Materson BJ: Sexual dysfunction during antihypertensive treat-ment. Prog Pharmacol 6:117, 1985.

69. Murphy MB, Kohner E, Lewis PJ, et al: Glucose intolerance in hypertensive patients treated with diuretics: A fourteen-year follow-up. Lancet 2:1293, 1982.

70. Hermansen K, Schmitz O, Arnfred J, et al: Effects of furosemide and indapamide upon pancreatic insulin and somatostatin secretion in vitro. Diabetes Res 3:221, 1986.
71. Harrower AD, McFarlane G, Donnelly T, et al: Effect of indapamide on blood pressure and glucose tolerance in non-insulin-dependent diabetes. Hypertension 7(Suppl II):161, 1985.
72. Raggi U, Palumbo P, Moro B, et al: Indapamide in the treatment of hypertension in non-insulin-dependent diabetes. Hypertension 7(Suppl II):157, 1985.
73. Caro JF: Diabetes and hypertension: not the final chapter. Diabetes Care 16:540, 1993.
74. Moser M, Ross H: The treatment of hypertension in diabetic patients. Diabetes Care 16:542, 1993.
75. Pollare T, Lithell H, Berne C: A comparison of the effects of hydrochlorothiazide and captopril on glucose and lipid metabolism in patients with hypertension. N Engl J Med 262:868, 1989.
76. Berne C, Pollare T, Lithell H: Effects of antihypertensive treatment on insulin sensitivity with special reference to ACE inhibitors. Diabetes Care 14(Suppl 4):39, 1991.
77. Swislocki AL, Hoffman BB, Reaven GM: Insulin resistance, glucose intolerance, and hyperinsulinemia in patients with hypertension. Am J Hypertens 2:419, 1989.
78. Materson BJ, Reda DJ, Cushman WC, et al: Single-drug therapy for hypertension in men. A comparison of six antihypertensive agents with placebo. N Engl J Med 328:914, 1993.
79. Parving H-H: Impact of blood pressure and antihypertensive treatment on incipient and overt nephropathy, retinopathy, and endothelial permeability in diabetes mellitus. Diabetes Care 14:260, 1991.
80. Epstein M, Sowers JR: Diabetes mellitus and hypertension. Hypertension 19:1, 1992.
81. Stein PP, Black HR: Drug treatment of hypertension in patients with diabetes mellitus. Diabetes Care 14:425, 1991.
82. Christlieb AR: Treatment selection considerations for the hypertensive diabetic patient. Arch Intern Med 150:1167, 1990.
83. Warram JH, Laffel LM, Valsania P, et al: Excess mortality associated with diuretic therapy in diabetes mellitus. Arch Intern Med 151:1350, 1991.
84. Joint National Committee on Detection, Evaluation, and Treatment of High Blood Pressure: The fifth report of the joint National Committee on Detection, Evaluation, and Treatment of High Blood Pressure (JNC V). Arch Intern Med 153:154, 1993.
85. Perez-Stable E, Caralis PV: Thiazide-induced disturbances in carbohydrate, lipid, and potassium metabolism. Am Heart J 106:245, 1983.
86. Ames RP, Peacock PB: Serum cholesterol during treatment of hypertension with diuretic drugs. Arch Intern Med 144:710, 1984.
87. Grimm RH Jr, Leon AS, Hunninghake DB, et al: Effects of thiazide diuretics on plasma lipids and lipoproteins in mildly hypertensive patients: A double-blind controlled trial. Ann Intern Med 94:7, 1981.
88. Freis ED, Materson BJ: Short-term versus long-term changes in serum cholesterol with thiazide diuretics alone. Lancet 1:1414, 1984.
89. Reubi FC, Cottier PT: Effects of reduced glomerular filtration rate on responsiveness of chlorothiazide and mercurial diuretics. Circulation 23:200, 1961.
90. Paton RR, Kane RE: Long-term diuretic therapy with metolazone of renal failure and the nephrotic syndrome. J Clin Pharmacol 17:243, 1977.
91. Acchiardo SR, Skautakis VA: Clinical efficacy, safety, and pharmacokinetics of indapamide in renal impairment. Am Heart J 106:237, 1983.
92. Alon U: Non-diuretic use of diuretics. In Puschett JB, Greenberg A (eds): Diuretics II: Chemistry, Pharmacology, and Clinical Applications. New York: Elsevier, 1987, pp 315–319.
93. Yendt ER: Renal calculi. Can Med Assoc J 1032:479, 1970.
94. Cunningham E, Oliveros FH, Nascimento L: Metolazone therapy of active calcium nephrolithiasis. Clin Pharmacol Ther 32:642, 1982.
95. Earley LE, Kahn M, Orloff J: The mechanism of antidiuresis associated with the administration of hydrochlorothiazide to patients with vasopressin-resistant diabetes insipidus. J Clin Invest 41:1988, 1962.
96. Crabtree BL, Mack JE, Johnson CD, Amyx BC: Comparison of the effects of hydrochlorothiazide and furosemide on lithium disposition. Am J Psychiatry 148:1060, 1991.

CHAPTER 43

Indapamide: Does It Differ from Low-dose Thiazides?

Richard P. Ames, M.D., and Louis Kuritsky, M.D.

HISTORY

Indapamide was initially investigated in the desoxycorticosterone acetate-saline hypertensive cat and dog, as well as the renally hypertensive cat, dog, and rat.[1, 2] These studies established its long-acting antihypertensive efficacy. Used in Europe since 1974,[3] indapamide received approval in the United States in 1983 as an antihypertensive and diuretic agent. Currently, it is used in more than 100 countries by more than 1.5 million patients.[4]

CHEMISTRY

Indapamide is the first of a class of antihypertensive diuretic agents known as indolines. Chemically designated 4-chloro-N-(2-methyl-indoline)3-sulfamoylbenzamide, indapamide, 1.25 and 2.5 mg per day, is a mildly natriuretic antihypertensive agent.[5–7] Its lipid solubility is greater than that of all other diuretics (5 to 80 times more than thiazides).[8] This property is believed to account for its capacity to reduce vascular reactivity to endogenous vasopressors like epinephrine,[3] norepinephrine,[8–10] and angiotensin II.[7]

Structurally, both indapamide and thiazides contain an o-chlorobenzene sulfonamide ring, but replacement of the thiazide ring with a methylindoline ring imparts higher lipid solubility (Fig. 43–1). A white to whitish-yellow crystalline powder, indapamide is a weak acid (pK$_a$ 8.8) in aqueous solution. It has a molecular weight of 365.8, and its empirical formula is $C_{16}H_{16}Cl_3O_3S$.[11]

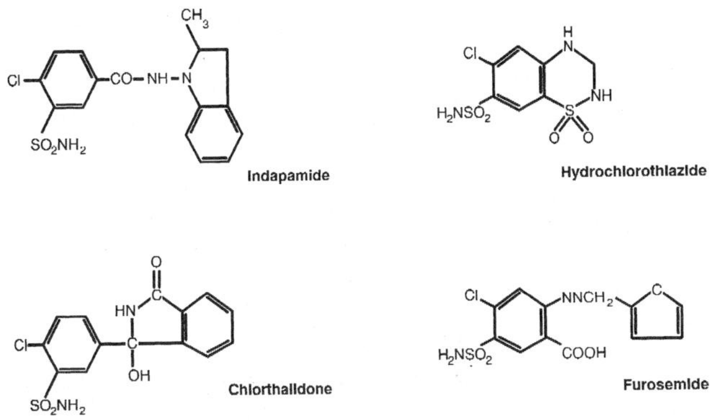

Figure 43–1. Chemical structures of indapamide and selected diuretics.

PHARMACOKINETICS

The intestinal absorption of indapamide occurs within 30 minutes to 1 hour; it is unaffected by food or antacids. Bioavailability is almost 100%.[12, 13]

Indapamide is highly bound to plasma proteins and to red blood cells. In the red cell, it binds to carbonic anhydrase without inhibiting it. High binding in the vascular compartment produces its relatively low apparent volume of distribution of 60 L. The metabolism of indapamide follows linear kinetics, with a half-life of 15 hours.[12] Steady-state plasma levels are reached within 3 to 4 days.[8] Metabolism occurs primarily in the liver, but 60% to 70% of the drug is excreted by the kidney. Only 5% to 7% of an administered dose appears in the urine as unchanged drug. The intestinal tract accounts for 20% to 30% of excretion.[2] There is little accumulation in renal insufficiency, presumably because of a shift to biliary elimination.[8]

PHARMACOLOGY

Indapamide is traditionally grouped with diuretics in classification, based on its chemical structure and its capacity to cause natriuresis and diuresis in high dosage.[13, 14] At doses most commonly used to treat hypertension (1.25 and 2.5 mg per day), indapamide exhibits substantial vasorelaxant action. Decreased peripheral resistance (mean, 10% to 18%[4, 15–20]) with indapamide is attributed to several factors: (1) blunting of responsiveness to endogenous vasopressors, including prostaglandin F_2;[21] as already stated; (2) decreased transmembrane calcium transport;[22] and (3) possibly increased levels of vasodilatory prostaglandin E_2.[23] However, the reduction in vascular reactivity to norepinephrine in patients with essential hypertension does not always correlate with the effectiveness in lowering blood pressure.[7] Hence, it is unclear that this aspect of change in vascular reactivity represents the major mode of antihypertensive action of the drug.

Indapamide reduces the passage of extracellular calcium ions across the plasma membrane; it may also affect the release of calcium from the sarcoplasmic reticulum.[22] This effect is believed to account for the inhibitory influence of indapamide on isometric contractions of smooth muscle of rat portal vein and myometrium *in vitro*. Indapamide may exert this effect by binding to calcium channels in the plasma membrane. There are actually three conformations of calcium channels: resting, open, and inactivated. Indapamide binds to resting channels, whereas verapamil and nifedipine bind to open and inactivated channels, respectively.[4] In addition, indapamide may reduce the sodium content of arterial smooth muscle cells.

PROSTAGLANDIN EFFECTS

Antagonism of thrombotic prostaglandins and enhancement of vasorelaxant prostaglandins would be positive attributes for an antihypertensive agent. Thromboxane A_2 and prostacyclin are two mediators of these prostaglandin effects, respectively. Indapamide increases prostacyclin *in vitro* in a significantly more potent fashion than furosemide or hydrochlorothiazide. Spironolactone blocks prostacyclin synthesis. In addition, indapamide inhibits thromboxane A_2 synthesis.[23] Prostaglandin homeostasis may be more important in blood pressure control than previously thought; evidence for this derives from the attenuation of antihypertensive drug effectiveness by nonsteroidal antiinflammatory drugs,[24] which block prostanoid synthesis. Renal production of prostaglandin E_2 is suppressed in essential hypertension, but indapamide can increase it.[25] In fact, after 6 weeks of treatment with indapamide, urinary prostaglandin E_2 and F_2 levels are both increased.[26] In the kidney, prostaglandin E_2 can act as a vasodilator and as an inhibitor of tubular sodium reabsorption.[27]

EFFECT ON FREE RADICALS

Indapamide can affect vascular reactivity and provide cardiac protection by another mechanism. Indapamide and its major metabolite, 5-hydroxyindapamide, possess free radical scavenging activity in a concentration-dependent manner comparable to α-tocopherol.[28] Free radicals can inactivate nitric oxide,[4] also termed endothelium-derived relaxing factor, the primary vasodilator of the coronary circulation. By quenching free radicals, indapamide preserves vasodilator activity in the coronary vascular bed.

Indapamide is not a direct stimulant of nitric oxide, but evidence suggests that it may restore the release of nitric oxide after its inhibition by impaired prostanoid production.[29]

Free radicals are also involved in lipid peroxidation.[30] This process can lead to damage of cell membranes. In experimental animals, indapamide pretreatment can lower myocardial hydroperoxide production during reperfusion after induced ischemia. Cardiac protection can be demonstrated by improved myocardial function and reduced release of lactic dehydrogenase after ischemia.[30] The reduced lactic dehydrogenase release is considered to be indicative of limited damage to cell membranes.

DIURETIC EFFECTS

The portion of indapamide's action that is diuretic occurs at the proximal segment of the distal tubule.[2, 31] At this site, it inhibits sodium reabsorption. At doses of 5 mg or more per day, this effect can be substantial.[14] At 2.5 mg per day, fractional sodium excretion is unchanged when measured after 4 weeks of treatment.[7] Twenty-four-hour urine volume does not change with indapamide 2.5 mg per day, but at 5 mg per day it increases 20%.[32–35] Urinary potassium excretion increases in the short term (1 week)[6] but returns to baseline in longer follow-up (6 weeks) when serum potassium is lower.[5] Total body sodium and potassium levels as well as plasma volume do not change, but extracellular fluid volume decreases.[2, 7, 36]

In sum, at the usual therapeutic dose of 1.25 to 2.5 mg per day, the antihypertensive effect of indapamide seems to be related as much to its various vascular effects as to its diuretic property.

EFFECTS ON BLOOD PRESSURE

Indapamide 2.5 mg per day is a highly effective antihypertensive agent. In numerous studies, systolic blood pressure has been shown to decrease by 9 to 53 mmHg and diastolic blood pressure by 3 to 43 mmHg in trials of 1 to 104 weeks in duration (Tables 43–1[5, 6, 36–66] and 43–2[67–72]). The onset of the antihypertensive effect occurs within a few days and increases gradually. Only 50% to 80% of the maximal therapeutic effect is achieved at 1 month.[40, 50] The lowering of systolic blood pressure is of greater magnitude and more rapid onset than that of diastolic blood pressure. The effect on diastolic blood pressure may be progressive for as long as 16 to 36 weeks.[50, 51, 55] The magnitude of the antihypertensive action of indapamide is related to the severity of the hypertension.[40] In a 640-patient study, blood pressure reductions of 23/14 mmHg, 35/25 mmHg, and 53/43 mmHg were observed in mild, moderate, and severe hypertension, respectively.[35] Twenty-four-hour ambulatory monitoring studies show good control of blood pressure throughout the entire day.[73, 74] There is also a suggestion of blunting of the circadian rise in blood pressure in the morning.[53, 73] Blood pressure efficacy is not affected by posture. There is no evidence of tachyphylaxis in studies of longer than 1 year in duration.[35, 46]

The new 1.25 mg dose formulation has proved more effective than placebo[65] and equally effective as the 2.5 mg dose in a parallel study of 2 months' duration (Saunders M, Rhone-Poulenc Rorer, personal communication). However, 5 and 10 mg doses have given greater reductions in diastolic blood pressure than the 1.25 mg dose.[66]

An additional antihypertensive response upon raising the dose from 2.5 to 5 mg daily has been occasionally noted. This effect has occurred in patients with moderate or severe hypertension or in those with a small response to the lower dose.[7, 44, 56] However, this finding has been disputed on the grounds that the dose was increased prematurely (4 to 8 weeks); a given dose may not exert its full effect for 16 or more weeks, as stated previously. A similar criticism of the aforementioned efficacy trials of the 1.25 mg dose formulation of indapamide could be made.[65, 66] Because the trial lasted only 8 weeks, the 1.25 mg dose may not have reached its full effect in lowering diastolic blood pressure.

Most of the reported studies of efficacy had no parallel placebo group, so the magnitude of the placebo effect, if any, could not be determined. In the absence of a placebo group, the observed blood pressure response usually overstates the actual pharmacologic effect of a drug. In Table 43–1, only 5 of the 31 studies had a parallel placebo group; in these five studies, blood pressure decreased in the placebo group. The decrease in blood pressure in the placebo groups was 20% to 50% of that in the treatment groups.[6, 48, 54, 65, 66]

EFFECTS ON CARDIAC FUNCTION AND STRUCTURE

Heart rate is usually unaffected by indapamide as reported in clinical studies (see Tables 43–1 and 43–2) and confirmed in an ambulatory intraarterial monitoring study.[73] The absence of reflex tachycardia has been attributed to a resetting of baroreceptor sensitivity or to complementary venodilation.[10] Cardiac output is usually unchanged or increased as demonstrated by M-mode echocardiography or impedance cardiography. Stroke volume is unchanged or decreased during treatment with indapamide.[7, 18, 75] These findings are consistent with a decrease in peripheral resistance, i.e., vasodilation, as the major hemodynamic consequence of indapamide therapy.[17, 18]

Most studies of thiazide diuretics show little regression of relative wall thickness in hypertensive patients who have echocardiographic left ventricular hypertrophy.[76–85] Indapamide has been demonstrated to reduce left ventricular hypertrophy within 6 months.[86–88] Left ventricular mass index, systolic and diastolic dimensions, and left ventricular wall stress all are improved; relative wall thickness is reduced, but not always significantly.[7, 57, 86–88] Weak correlation with blood pressure change indicates that mechanisms other than blood pressure lowering are probably operant.[57] Comparable reductions in left ventricular mass index to equipotent doses of nifedipine and timolol have been demonstrated in animal studies.[8]

EFFECT ON ELECTROLYTES AND FLUID VOLUME STATE

Serum potassium usually decreases modestly during treatment with indapamide 2.5 mg daily. This response varies considerably among studies. Tables 43–1 and 43–2 show the range of change in serum

Table 43–1. **Selected Clinical and Metabolic Effects of Indapamide in Hypertension**

Author (reference)	Number of Patients	Duration (weeks)	Weight (kg)	Pulse Beats (min⁻¹)	Blood Pressure (mmHg), Supine	Glucose (mg/dl)	Uric Acid (mg/dl)	Potassium (mEq/L)
					Change from Baseline			
Gerber et al. (5)	29	6	−0.7*	+2	−11*/−6*	+2	+1.2	−0.6*
Borghi et al. (6)	10	1	—	+11	−24* (mean)	—	+1.7*	−0.3*
Parallel placebo	10	1	—	+1	−5* (mean)	—	−0.6*	—
Meyer-Sabellek et al. (36)	20	26	+0.7	+4	−20*/−10*	−2	+0.1	−0.3*
Kubik and Coote (37)	27	8	—	NS	−14*/−6*	—	+1.2*	0
Horgan et al. (38)	17	24	—	—	−12*/−16*		+0.8*	−0.14
Passeron et al. (39)	644	12	NS	−3	−34*/−21*	0	—	−0.4*
Wheeley et al. (40)	1212	—	—	—	−25*/−15*	—	—	—
Beling et al. (41)	311	40	—	—	−14*/−9*	—	+0.93*	−0.45*
DeDivittiis et al. (42)	15	4	NS	−5	−30*/−16*	+5.7*	+0.4	−0.2
Ferrara et al. (43)	14	8	NS	−1	−12*/−11*	+3	0	—
Morledge (44)	8 Obese	40	—	—	−39*/−16* Standing	−5	—	—
Noble et al. (45)	5	8	—	NS	−17*/−23*	—	—	−0.4
Scalabrino (46)	15	104	—	—	−29*/−11*	−6	−0.2	+0.3
Kreeft et al. (47)	17	12	NS	+3	−9/−3	+8	+1.4*	−0.4*
Schaller et al. (48)	16	8	−0.9	+1	−15*/−8*	−4	+0.7	−0.2
Parallel placebo	15	8	+0.2	−2	−3/−2	−6	+0.1	−0.1
Cardona et al. (49)	15	16	—	—	−17*/−14*	−10	−0.4	—
Abbou (50)	905	16	—	−5*	−30*/−17*	—	—	−0.3
Chaignon et al. (51)	22	16	−0.5	+1	−12*/−11*	0	+0.1	−0.2
Von Funcke et al. (52)	2178	12	−0.6	—	−28*/−17*	−1	0	−0.1
Lacourciere (53)	30	12	—	0	−17*/−7*	—	—	−0.2
Taylor et al. (54)	15	16	−1.9	−1	−17*/−10*	—	NS	−0.2
Parallel placebo	12	16	+1.9	−5	−6/−4	—	—	+0.2
Plante and Dessurault (55)	23	48	—	—	−24*/−19*	—	+0.5*	−0.5*
Spannbrucker et al. (56)	24	12	—	NS	−25*/−23*	+7	+0.5	−0.4*
Komajda et al. (57)	18	26	—	−2	−29*/−15*	—	+0.8	−0.35*
Elliott et al. (58)	11	4	−0.9*	3	−13*/−10*	+10	+1.0*	−0.3*
Prisant et al. (59)	18	12	NS	—	−22*/−10*	+7	+0.8	+0.1
Guez et al. (60)	30	12	—	—	−26*/−16*	NS	NS	−0.3*
Athanassiadis et al. (61)	37	16	−1.2*	−3	−21*/−15*	—	+0.7*	0
Bing et al. (62)	8	16	−2.4*	—	−20*/−6*	—	—	−0.8*
Pedersen et al. (63)	11	6	—	—	−10*/−8*	—	—	—
Danielsen et al. (64)	11	6	—	0	−13*/−13*	—	—	−0.4*
Ferdinand et al. (65)								
1.25 mg	82	8	—	—	−11*/8*	—	—	—
Placebo	90	8	—	—	−3/−4	—	—	—
St. John Hammond et al. (66)								
1.25 mg	70	8	—	—	x/−9*	—	—	−0.3*
5 mg	70	8	—	—	x/−11*	—	—	−0.6*
10 mg	70	8	—	—	x/−11*	—	—	−0.8*
Placebo	70	8	—	—	x/−2	—	—	—

Indapamide dosage 2.5 mg/day except for references 65 and 66.
*p <.05 versus baseline.
NS, stated to be nonsignificant; x, no date given; —, not mentioned.

potassium to be from +0.3 to −0.8 mEq/L. This variation is attributable, in part, to oral potassium supplementation in some studies.[89, 90] In large studies, serum potassium has dropped below 3 mEq/L in fewer than 1% of patients; it decreased below 3.5 mEq/L in 6% to 14% of patients.[35, 36] In one study, adding indapamide to enalapril 5 mg daily caused potassium to drop below 3.5 mEq/L in 5 of 21 patients (24%), but it did not fall below 3 mEq/L in any patient.[91] Decreases in serum potassium in the range of 0.3 mEq/L are not associated with changes in the total body potassium.[36, 92] There is a dose-response relationship of indapamide to hypokalemia.

In comparative studies, indapamide caused decreases of serum potassium of 0.3 to 0.4 mEq/L, similar to that of hydrochlorothiazide 25 mg per day but greater than that of torasemide.[56, 58]

Indapamide caused significantly less symptomatic hyponatremia than hydrochlorothiazide 50 mg per day in one study,[55] but no differences were noted in other studies.[41, 45, 93, 94] Potassium wasters were identified in one study by measuring potassium excretion after 3 days of treatment with hydrochlorothiazide. Patients so identified were randomized between indapamide and metolazone 0.5 mg daily. Indapamide lowered serum potassium more than metolazone.[95]

Indapamide often lowers body weight slightly, apparently as a result of its diuretic effect (see Tables 43–1 and 43–2). The fluid lost appears to emanate from the interstitial compartment because extracellular fluid volume decreases but plasma volume is unchanged.[7, 9] A similar redistribution of extracellular fluid has been observed during long-term treatment with thiazides and with a furosemide-spironolactone

Table 43–2. **Selected Clinical and Metabolic Effects of Indapamide Monotherapy in Patients with Hypertension and Diabetes Mellitus**

Author (reference)	Number of Patients	Duration (weeks)	Weight (kg)	Pulse Beats (min⁻¹)	Blood Pressure (mmHg), Supine	Glucose (mg/dl)	Uric Acid (mg/dl)	Potassium (mEq/L)
			Weight (kg)	*Pulse Beats (min⁻¹)*	*Blood Pressure (mmHg), Supine*	*Glucose (mg/dl)*	*Uric Acid (mg/dl)*	*Potassium (mEq/L)*
Roux and Courtois (67)	11 type I	8	—	—	$-15^*/-7^*$	-9	—	—
	17 type II	8	—	—	$-15^*/-9^*$	$+13$	0	-0.3^*
Raggi et al. (68)	20 type II	24	-0.6	—	$-12^*/-8^*$	0	$+1.0$	$+0.3$
Harrower and McFarlane (69)	10 type II	52	-0.2	—	$-16^*/-20^*$	$+246†$	—	NS
Velussi et al. (70)	60 type II	25	—	NS	$-30^*/-17^*$	-5	0	-0.4
Gambardella et al. (71)	All type II							
	10 normal albuminurics	24	—	—	$-31^*/-14^*$	-16	—	-0.5^*
	10 micro-albuminurics	24	—	—	$-51^*/-19^*$	-8	—	-0.2
Osei et al. (72)‡	13 type II	24	-2	NS	$-18^*/-8^*$	$+77^*$	—	-0.1

Symbols are the same as those in Table 43–1.
$*p < .05$ versus baseline.
†, Area under the glucose tolerance curve in mmol/1.
‡, Mean dose of indapamide 3.5 mg per day (range, 2.5 to 7.5 mg per day).

combination regimen.[96–99] Plasma volume is reduced acutely by thiazides, but it returns nearly to normal in prolonged therapy.[100]

ENDOCRINE AND METABOLIC EFFECTS
Lipids

Indapamide is lipid neutral in studies of short, intermediate, and long duration. This fact can be ascertained from Figure 43–2, which displays the percentage change from baseline in total cholesterol, high-density lipoprotein (HDL) cholesterol, and triglycerides in 13 studies of indapamide monotherapy. Each bar in the figure represents the average change reported for an individual study. The bars are arranged in order of increasing duration of treatment with indapamide 2.5 mg per day. The five studies that report lipid values at several intervals of the study have a bar for each time point of lipid measurement.[36, 38, 41, 46, 70] There is a downtrend of total cholesterol over the 2-year time span of these studies. However, this trend is influenced heavily by the small study of Scalabrino, which comprises all the data for study of more than 10 months of follow-up.[46] Excluding the data of Scalabrino at 12 months and longer, there is no trend in levels of total cholesterol, HDL cholesterol, or triglycerides.

The average change in these lipid indices, weighted for the number of persons in each study, is displayed at the right of each row of bars. The accompanying standard deviation represents the variation of the means of the individual studies. It does not represent the average of the standard deviations reported in the studies. In determining the statistical significance of the overall mean change from baseline of each lipid index, the degree of freedom was chosen to represent the number of studies, not the sum of patients in all studies.

To be included in this analysis (see Fig. 43–2), the study had to present data for at least one of the three lipid indices and for blood pressure before and during treatment. The criterion of blood pressure measurements allows for the simultaneous assessment of efficacy of the drug in the same patients. The dual evaluation is important because, in comparing lipid effects of indapamide with those of thiazides, one needs to consider whether the reported advantage of indapamide in safety is accompanied by similar efficacy.

Regarding the lipid effects of indapamide in hypertensive patients with type IIa, IIb, and type IV hyperlipidemia, scant information is available. One small study reported no significant change in lipids during 2 years of therapy.[46] Apolipoproteins B, A_1, and A_2 may remain unchanged[5–7, 101] or may increase.[5, 102, 103]

Figure 43–2 omits data on lipid effects of indapamide 1.25 mg daily because such data are available only in preliminary form. An early report suggests that this new low-dose form of indapamide has no effect on total cholesterol, LDL cholesterol, and triglyceride levels but may lower HDL cholesterol.[66]

The adverse effects of thiazide diuretics on the lipid profile have been observed largely in studies in which high doses were used, i.e., the equivalent of 50 to 100 mg per day of hydrochlorothiazide.[104, 105] Because lower doses of thiazides are recommended today, the questions arise whether adverse effects occur at a lower thiazide dose and how this compares with indapamide. The best answer to these questions would come from a large randomized, double-blind, comparative trial. Unfortunately, no such trial has ever been reported. However, a small trial with this design found no significant difference in lipid effects when hydrochlorothiazide was used in a dose of 25 mg daily for 1 month.[58] A review of the data in this study leaves some question about the validity of the authors' conclusion. HDL cholesterol remained unchanged with indapamide 2.5 mg per day but decreased from 54 ± 4 (SEM) to 40 ± 3 mg/dl with hy-

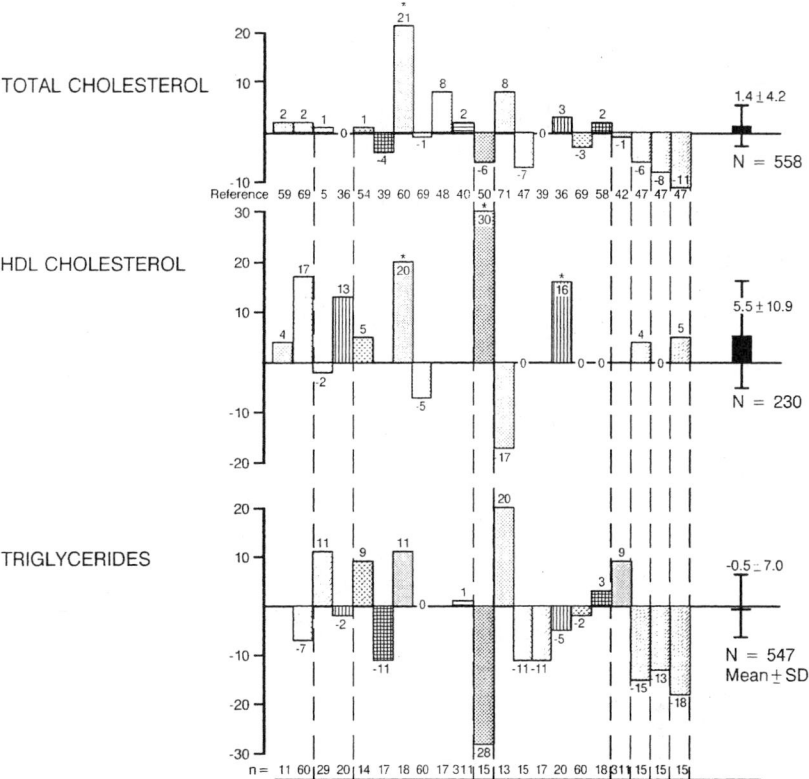

Figure 43–2. Percentage change from baseline in total cholesterol, HDL cholesterol, and triglycerides in 13 studies of indapamide 2.5 mg per day. Numbers near the top or bottom of each bar represent the actual percentage change. The reference number of each study is listed between the panels for total cholesterol and HDL cholesterol. The number of patients in each study, listed at the foot of the columns of bars, was used in obtaining the weighted mean, displayed at the right of each row. Absence of bar indicates no data. Zero indicates no change from baseline. HDL, high-density lipoprotein. *p <.05 versus baseline.

drochlorothiazide.[58] This large drop in HDL, with accompanying small value for the standard error of the mean (SEM), certainly appears statistically significant.

The only other study comparing indapamide to a low-dose thiazide had no placebo period in the study design. On directly substituting indapamide 2.5 mg per day for trichlormethiazide 2 mg daily, all lipid components increased proportionally; there was no change in the ratios of total cholesterol to HDL cholesterol or of low-density lipoprotein (LDL) cholesterol to HDL cholesterol.[102] On switching a subgroup of these patients back to trichlormethiazide, the lipid constituents decreased again; there was no change in the lipid ratios.[103] The unchanged lipid ratios suggest that there is no difference between these drugs on the risk of developing coronary heart disease.

Because of the paucity of direct clinical comparisons between indapamide and low-dose thiazides, we undertook a meta-analysis of all published reports of low-dose thiazides on the lipid profile, analogous to that for indapamide in Figure 43–2. The thiazide effects are arranged in two dosage categories: low dose and very low dose (Fig. 43–3).[58, 106–116] Low dose is the equivalent of 25 mg per day of hydrochlorothiazide. Very low dose is a dose up to 15 mg of hydrochlorothiazide per day or its equivalent in other thiazides. The same criteria for selecting studies were applied as for the indapamide meta-analysis. Figure 43–3 reveals that there is no difference in lipid effects between the low-dose and very-low-dose thiazides; consequently, the results of the two dose levels were combined to

calculate the weighted mean displayed on the far right of each row of bars. Total cholesterol and triglycerides increased modestly but significantly from baseline by 3.8% and 10.3%, respectively. Comparing the weighted means between indapamide and thiazides, there was no difference in drug effects on total cholesterol or HDL cholesterol levels. However, triglycerides increased more during treatment with thiazides than with indapamide (Fig. 43–4). Figure 43–4 also shows the summary of a similar meta-analysis of effects of high-dose thiazides on the lipid profile. High dose means a dose greater than 25 mg per day of hydrochlorothiazide or its equivalent. The mean and modal dose in these 19 studies was 50 mg per day (data from individual studies not shown).[47, 107, 109–111, 114, 115, 117–128] One-way analysis of variance (ANOVA) testing reveals that high-dose thiazides cause a greater increase in total cholesterol than indapamide but no difference from low-dose thiazides. High-dose thiazides cause a greater increase in triglycerides than both indapamide and low-dose thiazides.

To ascertain whether the more favorable effects of indapamide are accompanied by equivalent efficacy, blood pressure changes reported in each of these studies were summarized in a similar fashion (data from individual studies not shown). Figure 43–5 reveals that the effectiveness of indapamide to lower blood pressure was intermediate between that of high-dose and low-dose thiazides. Differences between indapamide and the two dose categories were not significant. The only difference in blood pressure among groups was a smaller decrease in systolic

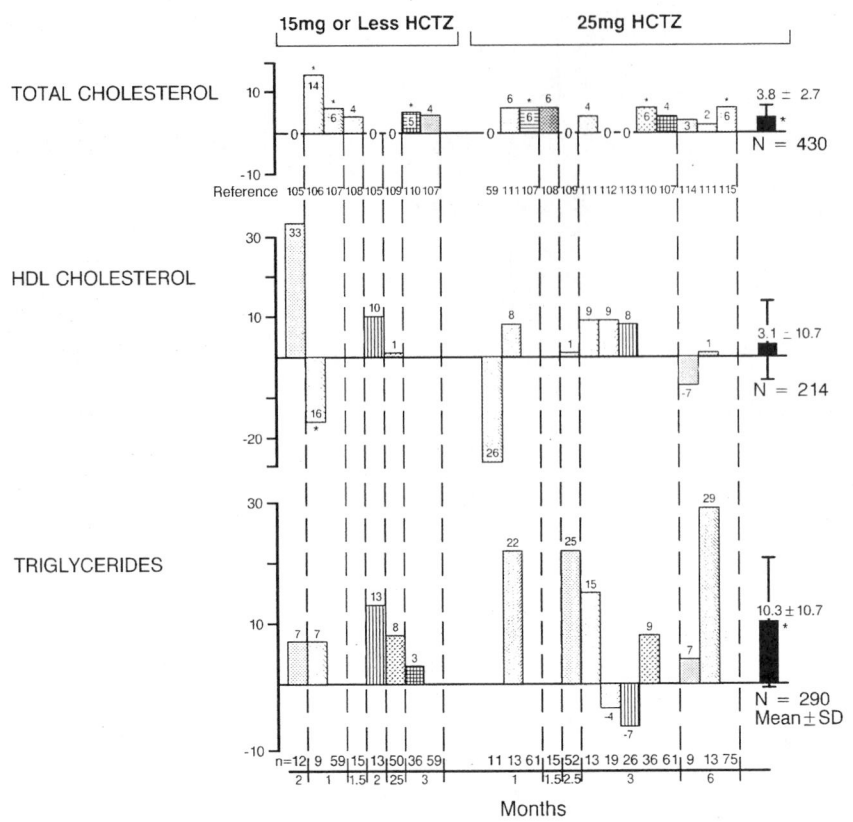

Figure 43–3. Percentage change from baseline for specific lipid indices arranged in relation to the duration of therapy with hydrochlorothiazide (7 studies), chlorthalidone (3 studies), cyclopenthiazide, and bendroflumethiazide (1 study each). Measurements of lipids at two or more time points are shown for three studies. Data for two or more dosage levels are given for four studies. Symbols and notations are the same as in Figure 43–2.

blood pressure with low-dose than with high-dose thiazides.

Our conclusion from this meta-analysis is that indapamide has a more favorable effect on the lipid profile than thiazides at any dose. That is, the advantage of indapamide is an absence of effect on triglyceride levels. It also causes less increase in total cholesterol than with high-dose thiazides. There is no trade-off in antihypertensive efficacy of indapamide in achieving this advantage in lipid effects. In addition, the data suggest that thiazide effects on triglycerides and blood pressure are dose-dependent.

This comparison is offered with the caveat that even the largest meta-analyses are inferior in scientific rigor to a randomized double-blind study of a sizable group comparing these agents head-on. The major weakness of meta-analysis is the absence of randomization. Randomization provides a degree of assurance that similar patients are being compared.

Glucose

In a dose of 2.5 mg per day, indapamide has negligible impact on fasting glucose in short-term and long-term studies (see Table 43–1). A single study reported adverse effects on glucose, C peptide, and glycohemoglobin, but large doses of indapamide (up to 7.5 mg per day) were used (mean dose, 3.5 mg per day) in patients with diabetes mellitus (see Table 43–2).[72]

In a recent multicenter study, indapamide in a dose

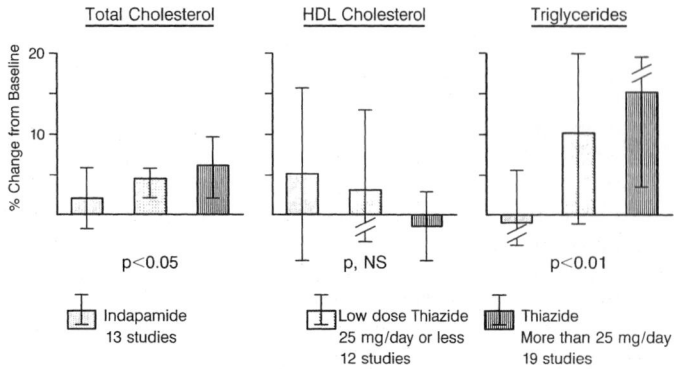

Figure 43–4. Summary of the mean change in lipids during treatment with indapamide 2.5 mg per day; two dose levels of thiazides are shown for comparison. Summary bars for indapamide are from Figure 43–2 and for low-dose thiazides from Figure 43–3. Bars represent the overall mean ± SD of the individual study means. NS, not significant.

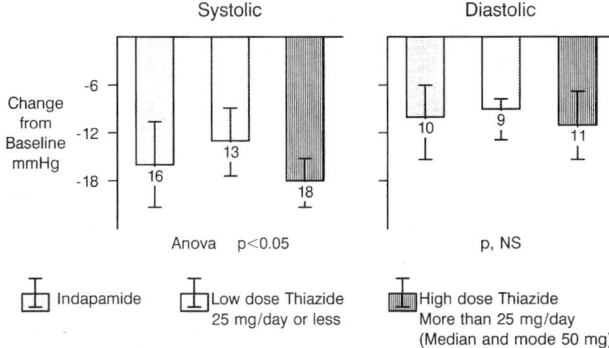

Figure 43–5. Summary of the mean changes in blood pressure during treatment with indapamide 2.5 mg per day and two dose levels of thiazides. The blood pressure data are taken from the same studies for which lipid data are given in Figures 43–2 to 43–4.

of 1.25 mg per day increased fasting glucose by only 3.5 mg/dl, whereas the 2.5 mg daily dose increased glucose by 8.6 mg/dl after 8 weeks of parallel double-blind comparison (Saunders M, Rhone-Poulenc Rorer, personal communication).

Uric Acid

Indapamide may increase serum uric acid levels, but clinical gout is rarely precipitated.[2] Inspection of Tables 43–1 and 43–2 reveals that data on serum uric acid were reported in 23 of the studies tabulated; uric acid levels increased significantly in eight of these studies. In contrast, uric acid levels decreased, albeit nonsignificantly, in only two of the studies. In one large study, only 4 of 311 patients (1.3%) discontinued indapamide because of high serum uric acid; these patients had raised uric acid levels before receiving indapamide.[41]

Preliminary findings concerning the effects of 1.25 mg per day of indapamide on serum uric acid are divergent. In one study, serum uric acid increased only 0.1 mg/dl, but in another study it increased 0.56 mg/dl from baseline after 8 weeks of therapy (Saunders M, Rhone-Poulenc Rorer, personal communication).

Calcium and Magnesium

Serum calcium level may increase in short-term study (1 to 6 weeks).[5, 6] In longer studies, serum calcium level was found to be unchanged from baseline.[5, 7, 59] Serum and red cell magnesium levels are unchanged after treatment with indapamide.[5, 54, 56]

Selenium

Serum selenium level does not change during treatment with indapamide.[59]

Phosphate

Indapamide increases urinary phosphate excretion in high dosage in humans.[129] This effect may be valuable

to explore, because studies in the United States have shown that dietary phosphate intake is inversely related to blood pressure.[130] In animals, phosphate depletion results in decreased sensitivity to vasopressor amines.[131] However, in humans, it is unclear whether the usual 2.5 mg daily dose affects phosphate excretion. No effect of indapamide was observed in one short-term study.[132] In contrast, a long-term study in elderly hypertensive patients revealed both increased urinary phosphate excretion and lowered serum phosphate levels with indapamide but not with hydrochlorothiazide. In this study, the change in blood pressure was proportional to the change in serum phosphate with indapamide but not with the thiazide.[55] This interesting finding deserves confirmation.

Circulating Pressor Substance

Thiazide diuretics in high dose and vasodilators like hydralazine have been shown to increase plasma and urinary catecholamines.[133, 134] In contrast, indapamide does not raise norepinephrine or epinephrine levels.[5, 7, 57, 135] Some investigators report a decrease in norepinephrine.[10, 136] Indapamide produces a significant reduction (23%) in plasma normetanephrine, suggesting that indapamide has a sympathoplegic effect and reduces catechol turnover.[135] Like calcium antagonists and thiazides, indapamide does activate renin and aldosterone, and this accounts, in large part, for its hypokalemic action.[5, 25, 59, 64, 135–138]

Platelets

In contrast with thiazide diuretics, indapamide inhibits phase 2 of biphasic platelet aggregation by a mechanism separate from thromboxane A_2 blockade.[139, 140] Indapamide also increases the number of α_2-receptors on platelets.[141] The clinical consequences of these effects are unclear.

RENAL EFFECTS

Indapamide does not change glomerular filtration rate (GFR) or renal blood flow as assessed by inulin and para-amino hippurate clearance in patients with hypertension.[5, 142, 143] However, using radio-labelled iothalamate and hippuran, GFR and renal blood flow decrease 9%.[63] Potassium excretion increases in the short-term and later returns to baseline, as mentioned earlier.[5, 6] Urinary calcium decreases during indapamide therapy,[6, 64] and this may, in part, account for the short-term rise in serum calcium described earlier.[5, 6] Urinary calcium decreases more than 50% in patients with idiopathic hypercalciuria.[144] It also decreases substantially in patients with essential hypertension and in those with recurrent nephrolithiasis.[6]

Urinary magnesium was unchanged in a single-dose study of indapamide.[145] In contrast, urinary magnesium increased after 1 week of treatment in both hypertensive patients and calcium stone formers.[6] Nevertheless, in longer follow-up, serum magnesium level remains unchanged, as noted previously.[5, 54, 56] This contrasts with thiazides, which can cause clinically significant hypomagnesemia.[146–148] An important manifestation of hypomagnesemia is the phenomenon of resistant hypokalemia. In this condition, serum potassium levels do not rise with potassium repletion until the concomitant magnesium deficit has been replaced.[149]

EFFECTS ON THE CENTRAL NERVOUS SYSTEM

Fatigue, dizziness, and lightheadedness can occur, but they are mild and infrequent. They are rarely a cause for discontinuation of indapamide.[39, 40, 45, 47–49, 56, 70, 138, 150]

QUALITY OF LIFE

Studies that address quality of life show a favorable impact of indapamide. Specifically, middle-aged and elderly male and female patients experience significant positive effects on depression, fatigue, and sexual function, as assessed by physicians and self-reporting in open, uncontrolled trials.[60, 151, 152] A study of middle-aged patients, in which a visual analogue scale was used in testing, demonstrated improvements in concentration, energy, and anxiety level in comparison with a preceding placebo period.[60]

The addition of indapamide in 470 patients whose blood pressure had not been adequately controlled in general practice resulted in increased sexual interest and decreased daytime fatigue, sleep disturbance, and frequency of headache.[153]

Controlled, randomized comparisons have shown captopril to be superior in quality of life issues to methyldopa, propranolol, and enalapril.[154, 155] Thus, it is particularly noteworthy that indapamide has an equally positive effect on quality of life measures as captopril. In fact, in a randomized double-blind comparison, indapamide had a superior effect on one of the well-being measures, namely, sleep latency time.[53] Nevertheless, as pointed out by others,[156] it would be premature to assume that indapamide is superior to other diuretics in regard to quality of life issues in the absence of a randomized double-blind comparative trial.

COMPARATIVE ANTIHYPERTENSIVE EFFECT

Effectiveness of indapamide monotherapy 2.5 mg per day in mild or moderate hypertension is equivalent to 25 to 50 mg of hydrochlorothiazide,[41, 44, 47, 48] 50 to 100 mg of chlorthalidone,[157, 158] 5 mg of bendroflumethiazide,[64, 159] and 0.5 mg of metolazone[95] in trials lasting from 2 months to 3 years. In elderly patients, indapamide was more effective than 50 mg of hydrochlorothiazide.[55] Figure 43–5 summarizes a meta-analysis of efficacy comparing indapamide with low- and high-dose thiazides. The figure illustrates that indapamide is intermediate in effectiveness between low

and high doses of thiazides but not significantly different from either dose category. High-dose thiazides lower systolic blood pressure more than low-dose thiazides, but the diastolic blood pressure response is similar. The antihypertensive effects of indapamide are equivalent to those of atenolol[17, 42] and pindolol.[137, 160] Indapamide proved slightly less effective than metoprolol 200 mg daily[37] and nifedipine 20 mg twice daily.[51] It lowers blood pressure as well as captopril 12.5 to 50 mg twice daily.[53]

As mentioned earlier, indapamide 1.25 mg per day is equivalent to 2.5 mg per day in antihypertensive effect (Saunders M, Rhone-Poulenc Rorer, personal communication).

COMBINATION THERAPY

Indapamide 2.5 mg per day has been combined with β-blockers and angiotensin-converting enzyme (ACE) inhibitors with additive blood pressure effects and a favorable side effect profile.[2] The specific β-blockers with which it has been successfully combined are atenolol,[42, 161] metoprolol,[37] nadolol,[162] oxprenolol, pindolol,[137] and propranolol.[61] The addition of indapamide to patients whose blood pressure was not previously controlled by propranolol or captopril alone resulted in control of 67% and 85% of patients, respectively. In the latter study, quality of life measures improved with both agents.[61] The combination of indapamide with β-blockers (n = 121), vasodilators (n = 34), or ACE inhibitors (n = 6) resulted in similar efficacy in all groups.[52] Indapamide and methyldopa in combination are well tolerated and somewhat more effective than the combination of hydrochlorothiazide and methyldopa.[45] In a large multicenter study, two thirds of patients had satisfactory blood pressure control whether taking indapamide monotherapy or a combined drug regimen.[89] In contrast with these additive effects when combining indapamide with indirect vasodilator drugs, indapamide is not additive to bendroflumethiazide and vice versa.[62]

In severe hypertension, adding indapamide 2.5 mg per day to full doses of captopril can lower blood pressure substantially.[90] In mild and moderate hypertension in which easy titration and low-dose regimens are desirable, adding indapamide can be more effective than titrating enalapril higher in patients with uncontrolled hypertension.[91] To be specific, in this latter randomized, placebo-controlled parallel study, adding indapamide 2.5 mg daily lowered blood pressure by 18/11 mmHg, whereas titrating the dose of enalapril from 5 to 10 mg decreased diastolic blood pressure only 3 mmHg and systolic pressure remained unchanged. As a result, 69% of patients receiving the combination of indapamide and enalapril reached goal blood pressure, whereas only 34% reached goal on enalapril 10 mg daily and 29% on enalapril 5 mg plus placebo. Diuretic action appeared to contribute importantly to the superior effectiveness of indapamide in this study. Evidence for this surmise includes a decrease of 4 pounds in body weight ($p <$ .05 versus baseline), a decrease in serum potassium of 0.5 mEq/L, and an increase in uric acid of 1.3 mg/dl. Surprisingly, the presence of ACE inhibition with enalapril 5 mg daily did not mitigate the hypokalemic effect of indapamide.[91]

SELECTED PATIENT GROUPS
Elderly Patients

Indapamide 2.5 mg daily has proved more effective than 50 mg of hydrochlorothiazide in elderly patients in a 48-week study. Furthermore, there was significantly less adverse impact of indapamide on sodium, potassium, and uric acid in this study.[55] The metabolic impact of indapamide can be further mitigated by reducing the dose to 1.25 mg per day without loss of antihypertensive effectiveness, as mentioned previously. In addition, 24-hour intraarterial monitoring studies show similar efficacy and safety in the elderly as in younger patients.[74] Because indapamide has a more dramatic impact on systolic than on diastolic blood pressure, elderly patients, who commonly exhibit disproportionate elevations in systolic pressure, may be favorably affected. Quality of life studies in the elderly show the therapeutic efficacy to be accompanied by improvements in physical and emotional well-being.[40, 150]

Diabetes Mellitus

Indapamide does not have the same metabolic consequences in type II diabetes mellitus as high-dose thiazide diuretics.[119, 163] Such patients studied from 1 month to 1 year with indapamide show no change in serum glucose,[67–71] insulin resistance,[68, 70] or glycohemoglobin.[68, 70] In a 6-month study of 60 previously untreated hypertensive patients with type II diabetes mellitus, indapamide decreased systolic blood pressure by 30 mmHg and diastolic blood pressure by 17 mmHg without notable change in mean daily blood glucose, glycohemoglobin, total cholesterol, HDL cholesterol, triglycerides, creatinine, sodium, potassium, or uric acid levels[70] (see Table 43–2). Fasting glucose decreased by 11% and postprandial glucose decreased by 22% in another study of diabetic patients.[52]

Microalbuminuria has been identified as a strong risk factor for the development of nephropathy and early mortality in diabetes mellitus.[164–167] In fact, microalbuminuria, i.e., albumin excretion rates of 30 to 300 mg per day, is considered the earliest stage of diabetic nephropathy. A topic of considerable interest at present is to ascertain whether drugs can cause regression of microalbuminuria and, in so doing, prevent the decline in glomerular filtration rate that characterizes diabetic nephropathy.[168, 169] Indapamide has been tested in this setting and, indeed, causes regression of microalbulminuria[170, 171] and also of immunoglobulin G4 (IgG4), another marker of diabetic nephropathy.[172] During 3 years of follow-up, glomerular filtration rate has remained stable in this group of 10 patients with type II diabetes mellitus.[172]

A similar regression of microalbulminuria and preservation of glomerular filtration (GFR) rate has been observed with the ACE inhibitor captopril in type II diabetes; in this study, a parallel control group showed a decline in GFR.[173] These data strengthen the evidence that suppressing microalbuminuria is associated with the preservation of GFR and possibly the prevention of diabetic nephropathy. Furthermore, indapamide may be as effective in this regard as ACE inhibitors.

RENAL FAILURE

Indapamide has proved effective for blood pressure control at all levels of renal function.[7, 174] In small studies, it has even been effective in functionally anephric patients who were receiving hemodialysis treatment.[175] The preserved efficacy in dialysis patients has been attributed to its vascular action.[35] The usefulness of indapamide in the setting of advanced renal failure stands in contrast with thiazides, which become ineffective at a glomerular filtration rate below 25 to 30 ml/min.

Indapamide does not accumulate appreciably in the blood in renal impairment, as mentioned previously.[8] Furthermore, the antihypertensive effect is not correlated to the concentration of indapamide in whole blood. For these reasons, no dose adjustment is necessary in renal failure. Indapamide is not removed from blood by dialysis.[8]

In a small study, creatinine clearance improved after patients with hypertension and renal insufficiency switched to indapamide from alternative therapy.[174] Thus, indapamide deserves further investigation for a potential effect of preventing or retarding the progression of renal disease.

INDICATIONS AND DOSE

Indapamide is indicated for the initial treatment of mild and moderate hypertension. It may also be used in combination with any other antihypertensive drug except diuretics to treat any level of blood pressure severity. The dose is 1.25 to 2.5 mg once daily.

Indapamide is also indicated for the treatment of sodium and water retention in congestive heart failure. The initial dose is 2.5 mg once daily. If diuresis is insufficient, the dose may be increased to 5 mg daily.

CONTRAINDICATIONS

Patients who are sensitive to indapamide or to other sulfonamide-derived drugs should not receive it.

INTERFERENCE WITH OTHER DRUGS

Special caution should be used in administering indapamide to patients who have hypokalemia or are predisposed to it. This caution applies particularly to patients who have cardiac arrhythmias or who take a digitalis preparation.

Patients taking lithium also need close monitoring.

The renal clearance of lithium may be lowered by indapamide; consequently, the dose of lithium may need to be reduced, and serum levels measured periodically. In view of the mild diuretic action of indapamide in a dose of 1.25 to 2.5 mg daily, the risk of lithium toxicity may be less marked for indapamide than for thiazides and loop diuretics.

Indapamide has been used safely in patients taking first- or second-generation sulfonylurea agents for type II diabetes mellitus, as stated earlier.[67-71] Nevertheless, glucose should be measured periodically in these patients, as in nondiabetic patients, because of the occasional occurrence of hyperglycemia (0.6% in one series).

INTERACTION OF OTHER DRUGS WITH INDAPAMIDE

Nonsteroidal antiinflammatory drugs may blunt or abolish the antihypertensive efficacy of indapamide by inhibiting prostacyclin synthesis. Indomethacin has specifically been demonstrated to cause this interaction with antihypertensive therapy,[24] but there is no direct demonstration of this interaction with indapamide.

COMPLIANCE AND COST

Indapamide is well tolerated. As stated previously, in a large general practice study of 1202 patients, only 1.3% withdrew because of side effects.[40] In a British primary care study of 470 patients with essential hypertension, 13% of patients complained of some side effects on non-indapamide therapy, but only 6 of 435 patients (1.4%) did so on indapamide.[153]

Regarding cost, indapamide represents good value among the recently introduced brand name products. Table 43-3 compares the cost of several popular antihypertensive drugs. The information in Table 43-3 was obtained in a telephone survey of seven pharmacies in the New York metropolitan and suburban area in 1993. The only associated expense difference from other nondiuretic agents would be the need for periodic electrolyte and glucose monitoring. The infrequency of hypokalemia with indapamide makes the additional expense of potassium supplementation, for the most part, avoidable.

SUMMARY AND BRIEF OVERVIEW

Indapamide possesses unique features not seen with other diuretics. It stimulates the production of prostacyclin and inhibits thromboxane A_2. It slows the passage of extracellular calcium across the plasma membrane. It scavenges free radicals and thereby facilitates the action of nitric oxide. It has been used safely in diabetes mellitus. It does not cause hypomagnesemia. There is no adverse effect on the lipid profile. Taken together, this evidence supports the concept that vascular activity is a major mechanism of indapamide's antihypertensive effect. Yet, if indapamide is primarily a vasodilator, its property of lowering serum potassium and raising uric acid distinguishes it from all other vasodilators. It should be noted that the blunting of vascular reactivity to pressor substances is not unique to indapamide; thiazides impair vasoconstrictor responses to norepinephrine in humans and animals.[176, 177] In addition, a lowering of peripheral resistance does not distinguish indapamide from other diuretics. Thiazides also produce this hemodynamic effect when studied in long-term therapy.[98]

Finally, if indapamide is indeed distinct from other diuretics, then the beneficial effect on cardiovascular morbidity and mortality demonstrated in the large-scale hypertension treatment trials, which were based mainly on thiazides as initial drug, may not be directly applicable to indapamide.[178-181] If the benefits of antihypertensive treatment are specific to the classes of drugs tested, as implied by the Joint National Committee,[182] then indapamide would need to be directly tested for its effectiveness in the prevention of cardiovascular disease.

IMPLICATIONS FOR THERAPY

Indapamide is a highly effective antihypertensive drug with excellent symptomatic and metabolic acceptability. It appears to have a better net effect on blood pressure and the lipid profile than thiazides in high or low dose. Thus, when a diuretic is indicated in the treatment of hypertension, indapamide represents a good choice.

When alternative classes of drugs are selected as initial therapy, indapamide represents an excellent add-on drug. With ACE inhibitors as the initial drug, indapamide can be added early, before upward titration of the ACE inhibitor, for best antihypertensive effect.[91] In this way, blood pressure can be lowered expeditiously, with low doses of both drugs, few titration steps, a once-daily regimen, and good tolerance. Because the Joint National Committee recommends a diuretic or β-blocker as preferred first-line therapy,[182] indapamide qualifies as initial drug for a large segment of the hypertensive population. Because of the

Table 43-3. **Cost to Patient of Selected Antihypertensive Drugs**

	Cost of 100 Brand Name Tablets	
	Average	*Minimum*
Verelan 240 mg (verapamil)	$133.14	$122.19[a]
Tenormin 50 mg (atenolol)	89.65	80.23[b]
Lotensin 10 mg (benazepril)	78.26	72.00[c, d]
Lozol 2.5 mg (indapamide)	87.74	77.29[a]
Maxzide 25/37.5 (triamterene/ hydrochorothiazide)	44.78	41.73[d]
Dyazide (triamterene/hydrochlorothiazide)	40.00	32.29[a]
Oretic/Esidrix 25 mg	11.25	6.93[a]

Seven pharmacies surveyed: four in Manhattan, three in New Jersey. Manhattan: Arrow (c), Duane Reade, Pathmark, 90th St. New Jersey: Drug Fair (d), Genovese (a), Rite Aid (b)

Note: Most pharmacies have a 10% discount for persons 62 years old or older.

favorable qualities described heretofore, indapamide can be given not only to patients with uncomplicated hypertension but also to young and elderly hypertensive patients with associated diseases such as diabetes mellitus, left ventricular hypertrophy, microalbuminuria, and renal failure. It can be used effectively in patients with hypertension associated with asthma, peripheral vascular disease, angina, and chronic obstructive pulmonary disease. When hypertension is complicated by moderate or severe heart failure, indapamide can be increased to 5 mg per day for better diuretic effect. If edema is not cleared by this dose, thiazides or loop diuretics should be substituted for indapamide.

REFERENCES

1. Hicks PE: The effects of long-term oral treatment with indapamide on the development of DOCA-salt hypertension in rats: Vascular reactivity studies. Clin Exp Hypertens 1:713, 1979.
2. Thomas JR: A review of 10 years of experience with indapamide as an antihypertensive agent. Hypertension 7(Suppl II):II-152, 1985.
3. Wilson PR, Kem DC: Indapamide. In Messerli F (ed): Cardiovascular Drug Therapy. Philadelphia: WB Saunders, 1990, pp 348–356.
4. Campbell DB, Brackman F: Cardiovascular protective properties of indapamide. Am J Cardiol 65(17):llH, 1990.
5. Gerber A, Weidmann P, Bianchetti MG, et al: Serum lipoproteins during treatment with the antihypertensive agent indapamide. Hypertension 7(Suppl II):II-164, 1985.
6. Borghi L, Elia G, Trapassi MR, et al: Acute effect of indapamide on urine calcium excretion in nephrolithiasis and human essential hypertension. Pharmacology 36:348, 1988.
7. Leenen FHH, Smith DL, Farkas RM, et al: Cardiovascular effects of indapamide in hypertensive patients with or without renal failure: A dose-response curve. Am J Med 84(Suppl lB):76, 1988.
8. Massry S: Indapamide in perspective. In Drugs in Focus. Manchester, United Kingdom: ADIS Press International, 1989.
9. Grimm W, Weidmann P, Meier A, et al: Correction of altered noradrenaline reactivity in essential hypertension by indapamide. Br Heart J 46:404, 1981.
10. Carretta R, Fabris B, Tonutti L, et al: Effect of indapamide on the baroreceptor reflex in essential hypertension. Eur J Clin Pharmacol 24:579, 1983.
11. Lozol. In: Physicians' Desk Reference, 45th ed. Montvale, NJ: Medical Economic Data Production Company, 1991, p 1782.
12. Grebow PE, Treitman JA, Barry EP, et al: Pharmacokinetics and bioavailability of indapamide: A new antihypertensive drug. Eur J Clin Pharmacol 22:295, 1982.
13. Caruso FS, Szabadi RR, Vukovich RA: Pharmacokinetics and clinical pharmacology of indapamide. Am Heart J 106:212, 1983.
14. Chaffman M, Heel RC, Brogden RN, et al: Indapamide: A review of its pharmacodynamic properties and therapeutic efficacy in hypertension. Drugs 28:189, 1984.
15. Carretta R, Fabris B, Bardelli M, et al: Resting systemic hemodynamics after chronic treatment of essential hypertension with indapamide. In Ogilvie RI, Safar M (eds): Indapamide in the Current Treatment of Hypertension. New Prospects in Hypertension. London: John Libbey Eurotext, 1986, pp 27–31.
16. Canicave JCI, Lesbrie FX: Measurement of peripheral resistance by carotid pulse wave recordings: Study of a vasopressor and an antihypertensive agent. Curr Med Res Opin 5(Suppl 1):79, 1977.
17. Velasco M, Urbina-Quintana A, Hernandes-Pieretti O: Cardiovascular haemodynamic effects of indapamide and atenolol in hypertensive patients. Curr Ther Res 31:1007, 1982.
18. Gensini G, Esente P, Giambartolomei A: A systemic hemodynamic evaluation of indapamide. Clin Ther 5:475, 1983.
19. Villareal H, Nunez-Poissot E, Anguas MC, et al: Effects of the acute and chronic administration of indapamide on systemic and renal haemodynamics in essential hypertension. Curr Med Res Opin 8(Suppl 3):135, 1983.
20. Magrini F, Buzzetti G, DeGiovanni F, et al: Systemic and pulmonary hemodynamic effects of indapamide in patients with mild arterial hypertension. J Cardiovasc Pharmacol 7:281, 1985.
21. Usui H, Kanda M, Ohsumi S, et al: Effects of indapamide, a new non-thiazide antihypertensive diuretic agent, on smooth muscles of blood vessels. Folia Pharmacol Jpn 74:389, 1978.
22. Mironneau J: Indapamide-induced inhibition of calcium movement in smooth muscles. Am J Med 84(Suppl 1B):10, 1988.
23. Grose JH, Gbeassor FM, Lebel M: Differential effects of diuretics on eicosanoid biosynthesis. Prostaglandins Leukotrienes Med 24(2–3):103, 1986.
24. Watkins J, Abbott EC, Hensby CN, et al: Attenuation of hypotensive effect of propranolol and thiazide diuretics by indomethacin. Br Med J 281:702, 1980.
25. Lebel M, Grosse JH, Belleau LJ, Langlois S: Antihypertensive effect of indapamide with special emphasis on renal prostagandin production. Curr Med Res Opin 8(Suppl 3):81, 1983.
26. Lebel M, Gbeassor FM, Grose JH: Effet antihypertenseur de l'indapamide et action sur la biosynthese des metabolites de l'acide arachidonique. JAMA (Edition Francaise) 9(Suppl 88):21, 1984.
27. FitzGerald GA: Prostaglandins and related compounds. In Wyngaarden JB, Smith LH Jr, Bennett JC (eds): Cecil Textbook of Medicine, 19th ed. Philadelphia: WB Saunders, 1992, pp 1206–1212.
28. Tamura A, Sato T, Fugii T: Quenching action of oxygen radical by indapamide and its metabolites. J Med Pharm Sci 18:1469, 1987.
29. Schini VB, Dewey J, Vanhoutte PM: Effects of indapamide on endothelium-dependent relaxations in isolated canine femoral arteries. Am J Cardiol 65(17):6H, 1990.
30. Boucher FR, Schatz CJ, Guez DM, deLeiris JG: Beneficial effect of indapamide on experimental myocardial ischemia. Am J Hypertens 5:22, 1992.
31. Materson BJ: Insights into intrarenal sites and mechanisms of action of diuretic agents. Am Heart J 106:188, 1983.
32. Goldberg B, Furman KI: Observations on the effects of a new diuretic-S1520. S Afr Med J 48:113, 1974.
33. Schlesinger P, Benchimol AB: The treatment of hypertension with indapamide: A controlled trial. In Velasco M (ed): Arterial Hypertension. Amsterdam: Excerpta Medica, 1980, pp 196–199.
34. Schlesinger P, Oignam W, Tabet FF, Benchimol AB: The treatment of hypertension with indapamide: A controlled trial. Curr Med Res Opin 5(Suppl 1):159, 1977.
35. Campbell DB: The possible mode of action of indapamide: A review. Curr Med Res Opin 8(3):9, 1983.
36. Meyer-Sabellek W, Gotzen R, Heitz J, et al: Serum lipoprotein levels during long-term treatment of hypertension with indapamide. Hypertension 7(Suppl II):II-170, 1985.
37. Kubik MM, Coote JH: Comparison of the antihypertensive effects of indapamide and metoprolol. Postgrad Med J 57(Suppl 2):44, 1981.
38. Horgan JH, O'Donovan A, Teo KK: Echocardiographic evaluation of left ventricular function in patients showing an antihypertensive and biochemical response to indapamide. Postgrad Med J 57(Suppl 2):64, 1981.
39. Passeron J, Pauly N, Desprat J: International multicenter study of indapamide in the treatment of essential arterial hypertension. Postgrad Med J 57(Suppl 2):57, 1981.
40. Wheeley M St G, Bolton JC, Campbell DB: Indapamide in hypertension: A study in general practice of new or previously poorly controlled patients. Pharmacotherapeutica 3:145, 1982.
41. Beling S, Vukovich RA, Neiss ES, et al: Long-term experience with indapamide. Am Heart J 106:258, 1983.
42. DeDivitiis O, DiSomma S, Petitto M, et al: Indapamide and atenolol in the treatment of hypertension: Double-blind com-

parative and combination study. Curr Med Res Opin 8:493, 1983.

43. Ferrara LA, Giumetti D, Fasano ML, et al: Once a day indapamide therapy in hypertension: Effects on the heart and peripheral circulation. Jpn Heart J 24:731, 1983.

44. Morledge JH: Clinical efficacy and safety of indapamide in essential hypertension. Am Heart J 106:229, 1983.

45. Noble RE, Webb EL, Godfrey JC, et al: Indapamide in the stepped-care treatment of obese hypertensive patients. Curr Med Res Opin 8(Suppl 3):93, 1983.

46. Scalabrino A: Clinical investigations on long-term effects of indapamide in patients with essential hypertension. Curr Ther Res 35(1):17, 1984.

47. Kreeft JH, Langlois S, Ogilvie RA: Comparative trial of indapamide and hydrochlorothiazide in essential hypertension, with forearm plethysmography. J Cardiovasc Pharmacol 6:622, 1984.

48. Schaller MD, Waeber B, Brunner HR: Double-blind comparison of indapamide with a placebo in hypertensive patients treated by practicing physicians. Clin Exper Hypertens 7:985, 1985.

49. Cardona R, Lopez B, Fragachan F: Effects of indapamide on the lipid profile of patients with essential hypertension. In Cardona R (ed): New Prospects in Hypertension. London: John Libbey, 1985, pp 93–97.

50. Abbou C-B: The efficacy and tolerance of indapamide in essential hypertension: A multi-centre study of 981 patients. Curr Med Res Opin 9:494, 1985.

51. Chaignon M, Lucsko M, Rapoud JP, et al: Effets compares de la nifedipine et de l'indapamide dans le traitement de l'hypertension arterielle. Arch Mal Coeur 78:67, 1985.

52. Von Funcke VH, von Bredow C, Cermakova E: Indapamide in the treatment of hypertension. Fortschr Med 104(6):133, 1986.

53. Lacourciere Y: Analysis of well-being and 24-hour blood pressure recording in a comparative study between indapamide and captopril. Am J Med 84(Suppl 1B):47, 1988.

54. Taylor DR, Constable J, Sonnekus M, Milne FJ: Effect of indapamide on serum and red cell cations, with and without magnesium supplementation, in subjects with mild hypertension. S Afr Med J 74:273, 1988.

55. Plante GE, Dessurault DL: Hypertension in elderly patients: A comparative study between indapamide and hydrochlorothiazide. Am J Med 84(Suppl 1B):98, 1988.

56. Spannbrucker N, Achhammer I, Metz P, Glocke M: Comparative study on the antihypertensive efficacy of torasemide and indapamide in patients with essential hypertension. Arzneimeittelforschung 38:190, 1988.

57. Komajda M, Klimczak K, Boutin B, et al: Effects of indapamide on left ventricular mass and function in systemic hypertension with left ventricular hypertrophy. Am J Cardiol 65:37H, 1990.

58. Elliott WJ, Weber RR, Murphy MB: A double-blind, randomized, placebo-controlled comparison of the metabolic effects of low-dose hydrochlorothiazide and indapamide. J Clin Pharmacol 31:751, 1991.

59. Prisant LM, Beall SP, Nichoalds GE, et al: Biochemical, endocrine, and mineral effects of indapamide in black women. J Clin Pharmacol 30:121, 1990.

60. Guez D, Crocq L, Safavian A, Labardens P: Effects of indapamide on the quality of life of hypertensive patients. Am J Med 84(Supp 1B):53, 1988.

61. Athanassiadis DI, Dimopoulos GC, Tsakiris AK, et al: Clinical efficacy and quality of life with indapamide alone or in combination with beta blockers or angiotensin converting enzyme inhibitors. Am J Cardiol 65(17):62H, 1990.

62. Bing RF, Russell GI, Swales JD, Thurston H: Indapamide and bendrofluazide: A comparison in the management of hypertension. Br J Clin Pharmacol 12:883, 1981.

63. Pedersen EB, Danielsen H, Spencer ES: Effect of indapamide on renal plasma flow, glomerular filtration rate and arginine vasopressin in plasma in essential hypertension. Pharmacology 26:543, 1984.

64. Danielsen H, Pedersen EB, Spencer ES: Effect of indapamide on the renin-aldosterone system, and the urinary excretion of potassium and calcium in essential hypertension. Br J Clin Pharmacol 18:229, 1984.

65. Ferdinand K, Flamenbaum W, Hall WD, et al: Lower dose indapamide therapy in the treatment of patients with mild and moderate hypertension. Am J Hypertens [abstract] 6:121A, 1993.

66. St John Hammond PG, Ratner P, Mullican W, et al: Dose-reponse study of indapamide [abstract]. J Am Soc Nephrol 4:541, 1993.

67. Roux P, Courtois H: Blood sugar regulation during treatment with indapamide in hypertensive diabetics. Postgrad Med J 57(Suppl 2):70, 1981.

68. Raggi U, Palumbo P, Moro B, et al: Indapamide in the treatment of hypertension in non-insulin-dependent diabetes. Hypertension 7(Suppl II):II-157, 1985.

69. Harrower ADB, McFarlane G: Antihypertensive therapy in diabetic patients: The use of indapamide. Am J Med 84(Suppl 1B):89, 1988.

70. Velussi M, Cernigoi AM, Miniussi PM, et al: Treatment of mild-to-moderate hypertension with indapamide in type II diabetics: Midterm (six months) evaluation. Curr Therap Res 44:1076, 1988.

71. Gambardella S, Frontoni S, Felici MG, et al: Efficacy of antihypertensive treatment with indapamide in patients with noninsulin-dependent diabetes and persistent microalbuminuria. Am J Cardiol 65(17):46H, 1990.

72. Osei K, Holland G, Falko JM, et al: Indapamide. Effects on apoprotein, lipoprotein, and glucoregulation in ambulatory diabetic patients. Arch Intern Med 146:1973, 1986.

73. Ocon J, Mora J: Twenty-four hour blood pressure monitoring and effects of indapamide. Am J Cardiol 65(17):58H, 1990.

74. Rowlands DB, Glover DR, Young MA, et al: Once daily indapamide in the treatment of the elderly and young hypertensive. Eur J Clin Pharmacol 27:397, 1984.

75. Dunn FG, Hillis WS, Tweddel A, et al: Non-invasive cardiovascular assessment of indapamide in patients with essential hypertension. Postgrad Med J 57(Suppl 2):19, 1981.

76. Ferrara LA, DeSimone G, Pasanisi F, Mancini M: Left ventricular mass reduction during salt depletion in arterial hypertension. Hypertension 6:755, 1984.

77. Giles TD, Sander GE, Roffidal LC, et al: Comparison of nitrendipine and hydrochlorothiazide for systemic hypertension. Am J Cardiol 60:103, 1987.

78. Wollam GL, Hall WD, Porter VD, et al: Time course of regression of left ventricular hypertrophy in treated hypertensive patients. Am J Med 75:100, 1983.

79. Drayer JIM, Gardin JM, Weber MA, Aronow WS: Changes in ventricular septal thickness during diuretic therapy. Clin Pharmacol Ther 32:283, 1982.

80. Khatri J, Gottdiener H, Notargiacomo A, Freis E: Effect of therapy on left ventricular function in hypertension. Clin Sci 59:435, 1980.

81. Messerli FH, Nunez BD, Nunez MM, et al: Hypertension and sudden death. Arch Intern Med 149:1263, 1989.

82. Mezzetti A, Guglielmoi MD, Mancini M, et al: Captopril improves blood pressure control and favors the regression of left ventricular hypertrophy in patients taking hydrochlorothiazide. Curr Ther Res 47:146, 1990.

83. Arora R, Nair M, Gupta GD, Gupta MP: Assessment of left ventricular changes in systemic hypertension before and after therapy. Indian Heart J 36:155, 1984.

84. Ferrara LA, deSimone G, Mancini M, et al: Changes in left ventricular mass during a double-blind study with chlorthalidone and slow-release nifedipine. Eur J Clin Pharmacol 27:525, 1984.

85. Cherchi A, Sau F, Seguro C: Regression of left ventricular hypertrophy after treatment of hypertension by chlorthalidone for one year and other diuretics for two years. J Hypertens 1(Suppl 2):278, 1983.

86. Mace PJE, Littler WA, Glover DR, et al: Regression of left ventricular hypertrophy in hypertension: Comparative effects of three different drugs. J Cardiovasc Pharmacol 7(Suppl 2):S52, 1985.

87. Rowlands DB, Glover DR, Ireland MA, et al: Assessment of left-ventricular mass and its response to antihypertensive treatment. Lancet 1:467, 1982.

88. Sami M, Haichin R: Regression of left ventricular hypertrophy in hypertension with indapamide. Am Heart J 122:1215, 1991.

89. Mimran A, Zambrowski JJ, Coppolani F: The antihypertensive action of indapamide: Results of a French multicenter study of 2,184 ambulant patients. Postgrad Med J 57(Suppl 2):60, 1981.

90. Kocijancic M, Dimkovic S: Antihypertensive effect of indapamide given in conjunction with captopril in severe hypertension. Curr Med Res Opin 10:313, 1986.

91. Ames R, Griffing G, Marbury T, et al: Effectiveness of indapamide versus enalapril as second-step therapy of systemic hypertension. Am J Cardiol 69:267, 1992.

92. Isaac R, Witchitz S, Kamoun A, Bagatini JC: A long-term study of the influence of indapamide on the exchangeable potassium and sodium pool in hypertensive patients. Curr Med Res Opin 5(Suppl 1):64, 1977.

93. Ogilvie RI: Diuretic treatment in essential hypertension. Curr Med Res Opin 8(Suppl 3):53, 1983.

94. Plante GE, Robillard C: Indapamide in the treatment of essential arterial hypertension. Curr Med Res Opin 8(Suppl 3):59, 1983.

95. McKay JH: Clinical trial of two single-entity thiazides: Microx vs Lozol. Modern Medicine 56(Suppl A):71, 1988.

96. Weidmann P, Beretta-Piccoli C, Meier A, et al: Antihypertensive mechanism of diuretic treatment with chlorthalidone. Complementary roles of sympathetic axis and sodium. Kidney Int 23:320, 1983.

97. Niarchos AP, Magrini F: Hemodynamic effects of diuretics in patients with marked peripheral oedema and mild hypertension. Clin Pharmacol Ther 31:370, 1982.

98. Shah S, Khatri I, Freis ED: Mechanism of antihypertensive effect of thiazide diuretics. Am Heart J 95:611, 1978.

99. Van Brummelen P, Schalekamp MADH: Body fluid volumes and the response of renin and aldosterone in short- and long-term thiazide therapy of essential hypertension. Acta Med Scand 207:259, 1980.

100. Conway J, Lauwers P: Hemodynamic and hypotensive effects of long-term therapy with chlorothiazide. Circulation 21:21, 1960.

101. Weidmann P, Bianchetti MG, Mordasini R: Effects of indapamide and various diuretics alone and combined with beta-blockers on serum lipoproteins. Curr Med Res Opin 8(Suppl 3):123, 1983.

102. Yoshino G, Kasama T, Iwatani I, et al: Comparison of the effects of indapamide and trichlormethiazide or lipoprotein and apolipoprotein. Curr Therap Res 39:1027, 1986.

103. Yoshino G, Iwai M, Kazum T, et al: Comparison of the long-term effects of indapamide and trichlormethiazide on lipoprotein and apolipoprotein. Curr Therap Res 42:607, 1987.

104. Ames RP: The effects of antihypertensive drugs on serum lipids and lipoproteins. I. Diuretics. Drugs 32:260, 1986.

105. Weidmann P, Ferrier C, Saxenhofer H: Serum lipoproteins during treatment with antihypertensive drugs. Drugs 35(Suppl 6):118, 1988.

106. McVeigh GE, Dulie EB, Ravenscroft A, et al: Low and conventional dose cyclopenthiazide on glucose and lipid metabolism in mild hypertension. Br J Clin Pharmacol 27:523, 1989.

107. McKenney JM, Goodman RP, Wright JT Jr, et al: The effect of low-dose hydrochlorothiazide on blood pressure, serum potassium, and lipoproteins. Pharmacotherapy 6:179, 1986.

108. Vardan S, Mehrotra KG, Mookherjee S, et al: Efficacy and reduced metabolic side effects of 15 mg chlorthalidone formulation in the treatment of mild hypertension. JAMA 258:484, 1987.

109. Burris JF, Weir MR, Oparil S, et al: An assessment of diltiazem and hydrochlorothiazide in hypertension. JAMA 263:1507, 1990.

110. Carlsen JE, Kober L, Torp-Pedersen C, Johansen P: Relation between dose of bendrofluazide, antihypertensive effect, and adverse biochemical effects. Br Med J 300:975, 1990.

111. Finnerty FA: Step-down treatment of mild systemic hypertension. Am J Cardiol 53:1304, 1984.

112. Lehtonen A, Gordin A, Salo H: Comparison of sustained release verapamil and hydrochlorothiazide in hypertension: Effect on blood pressure and metabolic variables. Int J Clin Pharmacol Ther Toxicol 25:301, 1987.

113. Lacourciere Y, Gagne C: Influence of zofenopril and low doses of hydrochlorothiazide on plasma lipoproteins in patients with mild to moderate essential hypertension. Am J Hypertens 2:861, 1989.

114. Kohvakka A, Salo H, Gordin A, Eisalo A: Antihypertensive and biochemical effect of different doses of hydrochlorothiazide alone or in combination with triamterene. Acta Med Scand 219:381, 1986.

115. Kochar MB, Landry KM, Ristow SM: Effects of reduction in dose and discontinuation of hydrochlorothiazide in patients with controlled essential hypertension. Arch Intern Med 150:1009, 1990.

116. Oberman A, Wassertheil-Smoller S, Langford HG, et al: Pharmacologic and nutritional treatment of mild hypertension: Changes in cardiovascular risk status. Ann Intern Med 112:89, 1990.

117. Pollare F, Lithell H, Berne C: A comparison of the effects of hydrochlorothiazide and captopril on glucose and lipid metabolism in patients with hypertension. N Engl J Med 321:868, 1989.

118. Johnson BF, Saunders R, Hickler R, et al: The effects of thiazide diuretics upon plasma lipoproteins. J Hypertens 4:235, 1986.

119. Ames RP: Hyperlipidemia in hypertension: Causes and prevention. Am Heart J 122:1219, 1991.

120. Middeke M, Richter WO, Schwandt P, et al: Normalization of lipid metabolism after withdrawal from antihypertensive long-term therapy with beta-blockers and diuretics. Atherosclerosis 10:145, 1990.

121. Andersen B, Snorrason SP, Ragnarsson J, Hardarson T: Hydrochlorothiazide and potassium chloride in comparison with hydrochlorothiazide and amiloride in the treatment of hypertension. Acta Med Scand 218:449, 1985.

122. Kaplan NM, Grundy S: Comparison of the effects of guanabenz and hydrochlorothiazide on plasma lipids. Clin Pharmacol Ther 44:297, 1988.

123. Farsang C, Peter M, Balas-Eltes A, Feher J: Prazosin improves atherogenic index and inhibits the deleterious effect of dihydrochlorothiazide in patients with essential hypertension. J Cardiovasc Pharmacol 10(Suppl 12):S240, 1987.

124. Distler A, Haerlin R, Hilgenstock G, Passfall J: Clinical aspects of antihypertensive therapy with urapidil. Comparison with hydrochlorothiazide. Drugs 40(Suppl 4):21, 1990.

125. Stamler R, Stamler J, Gosch FC, et al: Initial antihypertensive drug therapy. Final report of a randomized controlled trial comparing alpha-blocker and diuretic. Hypertension 12:574, 1988.

126. Trost BN, Weidmann P, Riesen W, et al: Comparative effects of doxazosin and hydrochlorothiazide on serum lipids and blood pressure in essential hypertension. Am J Cardiol 59:99G, 1987.

127. McVeigh G, Galloway D, Johnston D: The case for low dose diuretics in hypertension: Comparison of low and conventional doses of cyclopenthiazide. Br Med J 297:95, 1988.

128. Monmany J, Domingo P, Gomez JA, et al: Effects of long-term treatment with metoprolol and hydrochlorothiazide on plasma lipids and lipoproteins. J Intern Med 228:323, 1990.

129. Campbell DB, Phillips EM: Short-term effects and urinary excretion of the new diuretic, indapamide, in normal subjects. Eur J Clin Pharmacol 7:407, 1974.

130. Gruchow HW, Sobocinski KA, Baroriak JJ: Alcohol, nutrient intake and hypertension in US adults. JAMA 253:1567, 1985.

131. Plante GE, Lafreniere MC, Tam PF, Sirois P: Effect of indapamide on phosphate metabolism and vascular reactivity. Am J Med 84(Suppl 1B):26, 1988.

132. Bloch R, Steimer C, Welsch M, Schwartz J: L'effet hypocalciurique de l'hydrochlorothiazide, de la chlorthalidone, de l'indapamide et de l'acide tienilique. Therapie 36:567, 1981.

133. Lake CR, Ziegler MG, Coleman MD, Kopin J: Hydrochlorothiazide-induced sympathetic hyperactivity in hypertensive patients. Clin Pharmacol Ther 26:428, 1979.

134. Schiffl H, Weidmann P, Meier A, Ziegler WH: Relationship between plasma catecholamines and urinary catecholamine excretion rates in normal subjects and diseased states. Klin Wochenschr 3:837, 1981.

135. DeOrtiz H, DeQuattro E, Stephanian E, DeQuattro V: Long-term effectiveness of indapamide in hypertension: Neural, renin and metabolic responses. Clin Exp Hypertens 5:665, 1983.

136. Noveck RJ, McMahon FG, Quiros A, Giles T: Extrarenal contributions to indapamide's antihypertensive mechanism of action. Am Heart J 106:221, 1983.

137. Chalmers JP, Wing LMH, Grygiel JJ, et al: Effects of once daily indapamide and pindolol on blood pressure, plasma aldosterone concentration and plasma renin activity in a general practice setting. Eur J Clin Pharmacol 22:191, 1982.

138. Anavekar SN, Ludbrooke A, Louis WJ, Doyle AE: Evaluation of indapamide in the treatment of hypertension. J Cardiovasc Pharmacol 1:389, 1979.

139. Shirahase H, Suzuki Y, Kunitomo K, et al: Inhibitory effect of indapamide (Natrix) on platelet aggregation in vitro. J Med Pharm Sci 14:1614, 1985.

140. Shirahase H, Suzuki Y, Kunitomo K, et al: Platelet aggregation inhibition of indapamide (Natrix) in vitro-2. J Med Pharm Sci 18:1021, 1987.

141. Carreta R, Fabris B, Fischetti F, et al: Platelet alpha 2-adrenoceptor modifications induced by long-term treatment with indapamide in essential hypertension. Am J Med 84(Suppl lB):31, 1988.

142. Waal-Manning HJ, Doesburg RMN: Randomized cross-over trial of indapamide and conventional diuretics in hypertension: Metabolic and renal effects. N Z Med J 95:19, 1982.

143. Lemieux G, L'Homme C: The treatment of hypertension with indapamide alone or in combination with other drugs. Curr Med Res Opin 8(Suppl 3):87, 1983.

144. Lemieux G: Treatment of idiopathic hypercalciuria with indapamide. Can Med Assoc J 135:119, 1986.

145. Reyes AJ, Leary WP, van der Byl K: Urinary magnesium output after a single dose of indapamide in healthy adults. S Afr Med J 64:820, 1983.

146. Kuller L, Farrier N, Caggiulla A, et al: Relationship of diuretic therapy and serum magnesium levels among participants in the Multiple Risk Factor Intervention Trial. Am J Epidemiol 122:1045, 1985.

147. Drup I, Skajaa K, Clausen T, Kjeldsen K: Reduced concentrations of potassium, magnesium, and sodium potassium pumps in human skeletal muscle during treatment with diuretics. Br Med J 296:455, 1986.

148. Cocco G, Iselin HU, Strozzi C, et al: Magnesium depletion in patients on long-term chlorthalidone therapy for essential hypertension. Eur J Clin Pharmacol 32:335, 1987.

149. Dyckner T, Wester PO: Ventricular extra-systoles and intracellular electrolytes before and after potassium and magnesium infusions in patients on diuretic treatment. Am Heart J 97:12, 1979.

150. Hashida JG: A double-blind multicentre study of indapamide in the treatment of essential hypertension. Curr Med Res Opin 5(Suppl 1):116, 1977.

151. Werning C, Weitz T, Ludwig B: Assessment of indapamide in elderly hypertensive patients with special emphasis on well-being. Am J Med 84(Suppl 1B):104, 1988.

152. Leonetti G, Rappelli A, Salvetti A, Scapellato L: Tolerability and well-being with indapamide in the treatment of mild-moderate hypertension. Am J Med 84(Suppl 1B):59, 1988.

153. Watters K, Campbell B: Can an antihypertensive agent be both effective and improve the quality of life? Br J Clin Pract 40(6):236, 1986.

154. Croog SH, Levine S, Testa MA, et al: The effects of antihypertensive therapy on the quality of life. N Engl J Med 314:1657, 1986.

155. Testa MA, Anderson RB, Nackley JF, et al: Quality of life and antihypertensive therapy in men: A comparison of captopril and enalapril. N Engl J Med 328:907, 1993.

156. Van Hoof R, Amery A, Fagard R, Staessen J: Quality of life during treatment of hypertensive patients with diuretics. Acta Cardiol 45:393, 1990.

157. Millier P, Tcherdakott P: Antihypertensive activity of a new agent, indapamide: A double-blind study. Curr Med Res Opin 3:9, 1975.

158. Hatt PY, Leblond JB: A comparative study of the activity of a new agent, indapamide, in essential arterial hypertension. Curr Med Res Opin 3:138, 1975.

159. Zacharias FJ: A comparative study of the efficacy of indapamide and bendrofluazide given in combination with atenolol. Postgrad Med J 57(Suppl 2):51, 1981.

160. Rumboldt Z, Rumboldt M, Jurisic M: Indapamide versus betablocker therapy: A double-blind, cross-over study in essential hypertension. Curr Med Res Opin 9:10, 1984.

161. Anania V, Bartoli E, Desole MS, et al: Valutazione dell' associazione atenolol indapamide mella terapia dell'ipertensione arteriosa. Clin Ter 62:2157, 1981.

162. Houde M, Carriere S: Indapamide for out-patient treatment of hypertension: Modifications in serum catecholamine levels. Curr Med Res Opin 8(Suppl 3):68, 1983.

163. Struthers AD, Murphy MB, Dollery CT: Glucose tolerance during antihypertensive therapy in patients with diabetes mellitus. Hypertension 7(Suppl II):II-95, 1985.

164. Jarrett RJ, Viberti GC, Argyropoulus A, et al: Microalbuminuria predicts mortality in noninsulin dependent diabetes. Diabetic Med 1:17, 1984.

165. Mogensen CE: Microalbuminuria predicts clinical proteinuria and early mortality in maturity-onset diabetes. N Engl J Med 310:356, 1984.

166. Schmitz A, Vaeth M: Microalbuminuria: A major risk factor in non-insulin-dependent diabetes. A 10-year follow-up study of 503 patients. Diabet Med 5:126, 1988.

167. Nelson RG, Kunzelman CL, Pettitt DJ, et al: Albuminuria in type 2 (non-insulin dependent) diabetes mellitus and impaired glucose tolerance in Pima Indians. Diabetologia 32:870, 1989.

168. Baba T, Murabayashi S, Takebe K: Comparison of the renal effects of angiotensin converting enzyme inhibitor and calcium antagonist in hypertensive type II diabetic patients with microalbuminuria: A randomized controlled trial. Diabetologia 31:40, 1989.

169. Melbourne Diabetic Nephropathy Study Group: Comparison of perindopril and nifedipine in hypertensive and normotensive diabetic patients with microalbuminuria. Br Med J 302:210, 1991.

170. Janka HU, Weitz F, Blummer E, et al: Hypertension and microalbuminuria in diabetic patients taking indapamide. J Hypertens 78:S316, 1989.

171. Flack JR, Molyneaux L, Willey K, Yue DK: Regression of microalbuminuria: Result of a controlled study, indapamide versus captopril. J Cardiovasc Pharmacol 22(Suppl 6):S75, 1993.

172. Gambardella S, Frantoni S, Lala A, et al: Regression of microalbuminuria in type II diabetic, hypertensive patients after long-term indapamide treatment. Am Heart J 122:1232, 1991.

173. Ravid M, Savin H, Jutrin S, et al: Long-term stabilizing effect of angiotensin-converting enzyme inhibition on plasma creatinine and on proteinuria in normotensive type II diabetic patients. Ann Intern Med 118:577, 1993.

174. Brennan L, Wu MJ, Laquer UJ: A multicenter study indapamide in hypertensive patients with impaired function. Clin Therap 5:121, 1982.

175. Acchiardo SR, Skoutakis VA: Clinical efficacy, safety and pharmacokinetics of indapamide in renal impairment. Am Heart J 106:237, 1983.

176. Feisal KA, Eckstein JW, Horsley AW, Keasling HH: Effects of chlorothiazide on forearm vascular responses to norepinephrine. J Appl Physiol 16:549, 1961.

177. Eckstein JW, Wendling MG, Abboud FM: Circulatory responses to norepinephrine after prolonged treatment with chlorothiazide. Circ Res 18–19(Suppl I):I-48, 1966.

178. Collins R, Peto R, MacMahon SB, et al: Blood pressure, stroke, and coronary heart disease. Part 2. Short-term reductions in blood pressure: Overview of randomized drug trials in their epidemiological context. Lancet 335:827, 1990.

179. SHEP Cooperative Research Group: Prevention of stroke by antihypertensive drug treatment in older persons with isolated systolic hypertension. JAMA 265:3255, 1991.

180. Dahlof B, Lindholm LH, Hansson L, et al: Morbidity and mortality in the Swedish Trial in Old Patients with Hypertension (STOP-Hypertension). Lancet 338:1281, 1991.

181. MRC Working Party: Medical Research Council trial of treatment of hypertension in older adults: Principal results. Br Med J 304:405, 1992.

182. The fifth report of the Joint National Committee on Detection, Evaluation and Treatment of High Blood Pressure (JNC V). Arch Intern Med 153:154, 1993.

D. Potassium-Sparing Diuretics and Potassium Substitutes

CHAPTER 44

Triamterene

Jürgen K. Rockstroh, M.D., Christoph J. Losem, M.D., and Franz H. Messerli, M.D.

HISTORY

Triamterene, a pteridine derivative, is a weak diuretic with potassium-sparing properties. Historically, the first information about pteridines was obtained in 1891 when Frederick Gowland Hopkins succeeded in isolating the pigment xanthopterin from butterfly wings.[1] The nature of pteridine in xanthopterin was established in 1940.[2] In 1954, Haddow observed the capacity of xanthopterin to affect renal tissue.[3] This and other reports, suggesting the influence of other pteridines in diverse biologic events,[4-6] led Wiebelhaus et al.[7, 8] to test pteridines in biologic screening series in rats. Their results led to the introduction of triamterene as a diuretic agent in 1961. In the same year, Crosley et al.[9] were the first to evaluate the possible utility of triamterene in human subjects.

The most striking effect of the new agent was its potassium-sparing properties, which could not be explained by aldosterone antagonism. Because hypokalemia represents the major metabolic alteration in patients treated long term with thiazides (described in more than 40% of patients), the availability of a potassium-sparing diuretic seemed to offer obvious advantages. Although triamterene may augment the effect of other diuretics, the main reason for administering the drug is to prevent or correct hypokalemia.

CHEMISTRY

Triamterene is a triaminopteridine with a phenyl substitute at position 6. Chemically it is related to folic acid.

PHARMACOLOGY

Triamterene develops its pharmacologic diuretic activity at the luminal surface of the cortical collecting duct.[10, 11] At this specific site of the distal tubule, triamterene inhibits the reabsorption of sodium ions in exchange for potassium and hydrogen ions by abolishing the luminal negative voltage.[12] The degree of natriuresis and diuresis appears to be limited by the fact that the amount of filtered sodium reaching the collecting duct is relatively small.[13]

Because the distal nephron is not readily accessible, most studies evaluating the pharmacologic properties of triamterene have been carried out in epithelial systems. As a result of these experiments, it was shown that sodium movement in epithelial and cellular tissues *in vitro* was inhibited by triamterene or amiloride,[11, 14, 15] presumably by the same mechanism of action.[12, 13] Because of amiloride's high degree of water solubility, its diuretic properties have been studied extensively in experimental systems; however, triamterene, with its high degree of water insolubility, has only rarely been investigated. At present, interaction of amiloride and triamterene with the cell membrane remains controversial. Both drugs may serve as a plug "blocking the mouth of the sodium channels or they may act at spatially distinct modifier sites."[12, 14, 16, 17]

Triamterene has a pK_a of 6.20 and is protonated at physiologic pH. Its lower pKa than the pKa of amiloride (8.7) may explain its weaker inhibiting effects in cellular transport processes.[18]

In addition to the natriuretic, diuretic, and potassium-sparing properties of triamterene, further pharmacologic characteristics have been described. Triamterene has been shown to competitively inhibit dihydrofolate reductase.[19] Concentrations of the drug have been reported in the central nervous systems as well as in the hearts of guinea pigs.[20, 21] Furthermore, active transport of the drug out of the central nervous system has been postulated.[21] More extensive literature on the pharmacologic features of triamterene has been provided by Pruitt et al.[22]

PHARMACOKINETICS

Absorption

Since the 1960s, triamterene has been available for clinical use only as an oral agent. Orally administered triamterene is rapidly but incompletely absorbed from the gastrointestinal tract; a significant amount of the drug has been recovered in feces after oral administration.[22] As a consequence of the various forms and pharmacologic preparations in which triamterene may be administered (in combination with other diuretics, alone, orally, intravenously, or as a liquid), different absorption and bioavailability rates have been documented. When triamterene is administered as a liquid, approximately 60% appears to be

435

absorbed.[23] In a bioavailability-bioequivalence comparison of Dyazide capsules (50 mg of triamterene and 25 mg of hydrochlorothiazide) and Maxzide tablets (75 mg of triamterene and 50 mg of hydrochlorothiazide), it was demonstrated that one Dyazide capsule delivers approximately one-quarter the quantity of triamterene to the bloodstream as one Maxzide tablet.[24] The absorption rate of triamterene in Maxzide tablets was identical to the absorption rate in liquid preparations of triamterene.[24] Mutschler et al.[25] reported that triamterene had a bioavailability of 52% after intravenous administration and an 83% extent of absorption. This value was much higher than in the results of previous reports. The difference in absorption and bioavailability was assumed to be an effect of a substantial first-pass effect.

Metabolism

After its administration, triamterene is rapidly metabolized in the liver by parahydroxylation of the benzene ring.[26] Subsequently, this phase I metabolite (2,4,7-triamino-6-p-hydroxyphenylpteridine) is conjugated with active sulfate to form p-hydroxytriamterene sulfuric acid ester (phase II metabolite).[25, 27] Improvements in analytic methods revealed that the phase II metabolite is the major metabolite of triamterene in urine and possesses the same diuretic and potassium-sparing effects as native triamterene.[25, 28] The pharmacologic activity of the phase II metabolite was confirmed in various animal experiments[25, 29] and in a further study in human subjects.[30] The measured plasma concentration ratio of triamterene and its phase II metabolite was 1:10, corresponding to the ratio of excretion in urine.[24] The half-life of triamterene and its compounds in plasma was documented to be 190 minutes, and the plasma protein-binding capacity was approximately 50% to 55%.[25] Peak plasma levels of triamterene and its phase II metabolite were found 90 minutes after administration. Significant decreases in plasma and urinary triamterene and its phase II metabolite were observed after 6 to 8 hours.

Excretion

The plasma half-life of triamterene ranges from 2 to 4 hours.[12] Triamterene and its phase II metabolite are excreted in bile and urine. In the case of renal elimination, triamterene is actively secreted into the lumen of the proximal tubule[31] by the organic cation transport system.[32, 33] The sulfate conjugate is hypothesized to undergo tubular secretion[23] by means of the organic anion transport system. The renal plasma clearances of triamterene and of hydroxytriamterene sulfuric acid ester are 220 ml/min and 180 ml/min, respectively. The amount of the phase II metabolite measured by Mutschler et al.[25] that was renally excreted was 12 to 17 times greater than the measured amount of the parent compound. Urinary excretion of this metabolite has been documented up to 15 hours after oral administration.

In renal disease, an impaired pharmacologic pattern of triamterene excretion may emerge. Depending on the degree of impairment of kidney function, the phase II metabolite of triamterene accumulates. As the parenchyma of the functioning kidneys is reduced, a decrease in hydroxytriamterene sulfate excretion occurs. In renal insufficiency, biliary excretion of triamterene and its metabolites does not increase substantially.

The extent of biliary excretion of triamterene in healthy volunteers is presumed to cover one half of the administered dose.[25] (However, in patients with hepatitis, the total amount of triamterene and its related compounds is excreted renally, because patients with hepatitis are unable to excrete triamterene or its metabolites in bile.[25]) In patients with cirrhosis of the liver, the elimination of triamterene is markedly prolonged because of a decrease in the rate of hydroxylation. However, the elimination of hydroxytriamterene sulfate remains unchanged.

In the isolated perfused rat kidney, the excretion of triamterene is markedly reduced by H2-antagonists, whereas the excretion of the phase II metabolite (p-hydroxytriamterene sulfuric acid ester) is not affected. In contrast, probenecid does not influence tubular secretion of triamterene but cuts excretion of the phase II metabolite by 80%.[34]

Effects on Pathophysiology

The potassium- and magnesium-sparing and weak natriuretic properties of triamterene predominantly influence electrolyte balance and renal function. These two effects will be dealt with first, in order to provide a basis by which other systemic pathophysiologic effects may be understood.

Effects on Electrolyte Balance

In the nephron, triamterene preserves potassium by inhibiting sodium exchange in the cortical collecting duct. Triamterene was found not to act as a competitive aldosterone inhibitor because, unlike spironolactone, it increased the output of sodium in adrenalectomized dogs and rats.[35] Triamterene also possesses magnesium-sparing abilities.[36] At present, no explanation for this mechanism has been found.

The potassium- and magnesium-sparing properties are of importance in counteracting the potassium and magnesium losses associated with thiazide and loop diuretics. Forty-two percent of hypertensive patients treated with thiazide diuretics have been reported to have subnormal values of potassium, and nearly one half have been reported to have some degree of magnesium deficiency, depending on the duration and intensity of diuretic treatment.[36, 37] In some patients, magnesium depletion is only detectable by muscle micropuncture, because of the weak correlation between levels of magnesium in serum and tissue.[38] The importance of magnesium derives from its role as an activator of membrane-bound Na,K-ATPase, which controls potassium uptake at the cellular level.[39-41]

Magnesium depletion reduces enzyme activity and thereby limits cellular regulating mechanisms that are capable of preventing cellular potassium loss. This may explain why potassium supplementation, unlike the potassium- and magnesium-sparing effects of triamterene, often is ineffective in increasing levels of body potassium in magnesium-depleted patients.[36, 42] Paradoxically, the administration of potassium salts may even lead to a further loss of body potassium by increasing aldosterone activity. A 0.2 to 0.4 mEq/100 ml increase in serum potassium was documented to cause a 50% to 100% increase in aldosterone release.[43]

Muscle micropuncture studies[36] in patients with diuretic-induced hypokalemia revealed that after additional administration of triamterene, an 8% elevation in intracellular potassium and a 15% elevation of intracellular magnesium were observed. This finding was confirmed in subsequent studies.[36, 44–48]

Effects on Renal Function

In clinical studies, triamterene was documented to impair renal function. De Carvalho et al.[49] measured a mean serum creatinine elevation from 1.0 to 1.3 mg/100 ml and a blood urea nitrogen (BUN) elevation from 12 to 18 mg/100 ml. Subsequent studies confirmed these results.[50, 51] A significant decrease in creatinine clearance (30%) was also found in a combination of thiazides and triamterene.[52] However, the degree of renal impairment caused by triamterene did not lead to clinical changes in patients who had normal renal function before drug administration.[53] In patients with impaired renal function before therapy, azotemia may occur.[53]

After triamterene administration, serum uric acid level was reported to increase slightly (>0.82 mg/100 ml).[50] However, the clinical significance of this finding is uncertain. A field study of 47,000 patients receiving triamterene-thiazide combinations demonstrated that in fewer than 0.05% of patients with previous history of gout, clinical manifestation of frank gout occurred.[53] These data were questioned by a second field study recruiting 840 patients older than 60 years who were not discriminated for a previous history of gout. In the patient group treated with thiazide plus triamterene, the incidence of gout was significantly higher than in the placebo group.[54]

Because of its ability to inhibit excretion of both potassium and hydrogen, triamterene may affect the balance of blood pH. In general, this effect is insignificant, because the cortical collecting duct has low hydrogen transport capability.[13, 55] However, reduction of the regulatory capability of the kidneys may be important in patients with metabolic acidosis.

In clinical studies,[56] it has been shown that triamterene reduces renal blood flow (RBF) as much as 30%. This finding may be related to the decrease in excretion of urinary prostaglandin E (PGE) associated with combination triamterene-thiazide therapy. In contrast, urinary PGE excretion has been shown to increase during combination amiloride-thiazide therapy.[52, 57] Prostaglandin E is a vasodilator that maintains RBF

under conditions such as decreased blood pressure or increased angiotensin II activity.[58, 59] Most patients receiving diuretic therapy demonstrate increased renin activity and elevated levels of angiotensin II.[60] Therefore, increased PGE excretion should be expected during combination triamterene-thiazide therapy. Thus, the measured decrease in urinary PGE excretion with triamterene may indicate an impairment of PGE production. This hypothesis is reinforced by the fact that the simultaneous administration of a prostaglandin synthetase inhibitor, indomethacin, and triamterene has been reported to induce acute reversible renal failure.[59, 61]

Hemodynamics

As a consequence of triamterene's weak diuretic properties, no significant changes in plasma volume or body weight are observed after its administration. Subsequently, only a small increase in renin activity (<2.5 mg/ml/hr) and aldosterone release (<20 mg/24 hr) has been described.[49] In patients with essential hypertension, the decrease in mean arterial pressure after triamterene monotherapy ranged from 7 to 11 mmHg.[49, 50] In contrast, thiazide monotherapy resulted in a decrease in mean arterial pressure of 15.7 mmHg. The combination of triamterene and a thiazide revealed a total decrease in mean arterial pressure of 19.3 mmHg.[50] Apparently, the blood pressure–lowering effect of combination therapy with triamterene and a thiazide is more powerful than the effect of thiazide monotherapy. This phenomenon may be explained by the ability of triamterene to counteract some of the thiazide-induced effects of hyperaldosteronism.

Effects on Cardiac Function

More recent animal and *in vitro* studies revealed a direct antiarrhythmic effect of triamterene and its metabolites on the myocardium.[62, 63] Busch et al.[63] suggested that this effect of triamterene is independent of the drug's secondary antiarrhythmic effect on the heart by counteracting hypokalemia and hypomagnesemia. In addition, Völger summarized *in vitro* studies uncovering positive inotropic properties of triamterene.[62] This positive inotropic effect was explained by inhibition of the enzyme phosphodiesterase. However, the clinical significance of these findings has yet to be proved.

Secondary Effects on Pathophysiology

The aforementioned triamterene-induced changes in potassium and magnesium levels are especially important to electrophysiology and glucose regulation.

It is well known that intracellular and extracellular hypokalemia raise the automaticity and excitability of heart muscle cells.[64, 65] In addition, depletion of intracellular magnesium such as occurs during diuretic therapy reinforces this effect by causing further losses of intracellular potassium. Hypokalemia counteracts the antiarrhythmic effect of sodium channel–blocking drugs by increasing the action potential of heart cells.[66] During digitalis therapy, increased toxicity was found to result from a reduced effective refractory period.[67, 68]

Furthermore, digitalis induces intracellular potassium losses by impairing Na,K-ATPase activity.[69] Conversely, triamterene's magnesium-sparing effects support the activity of Na,K-ATPase and thereby increase intracellular and extracellular potassium levels. Triamterene administration in hypokalemic patients has been shown to expand the therapeutic range of digitalis[43, 67, 68, 70] and to augment the effects of antiarrhythmic agents.

Hypokalemia, which may arise during antiarrhythmic and diuretic therapy, appears to be responsible, at least to some extent, for the diabetogenic effect of several diuretics. Release of insulin from pancreatic β cells in healthy volunteers has been demonstrated to be influenced by the plasma potassium level.[71] Low plasma potassium inhibits insulin excretion, whereas high plasma potassium supports insulin release.[72, 73] Long-term investigations concluded that patients treated with a thiazide-triamterene combination obtained better glucose tolerance than patients receiving thiazide monotherapy.[71, 74] This may be explained by the potassium-sparing effect of triamterene. On the other hand, in few cases was it documented that triamterene decreased glucose tolerance in diabetic patients.[75]

INDICATIONS

In edematous states and in hypertension, triamterene is used in conjunction with more powerful diuretics to prevent or correct hypokalemia and hypomagnesemia.[38] Rare indications for triamterene monotherapy are hypokalemic periodic paralysis, Bartter's syndrome, and Liddle's syndrome.

Adjuncts to Diuretic Therapy in Essential Hypertension

Because of its weak blood pressure–lowering properties, triamterene is unsuitable as a single antihypertensive agent. This triamterene is used in combination with more powerful potassium-losing diuretics, such as thiazides, in order to balance electrolytes. By counteracting hypokalemia and hypomagnesia, triamterene or other potassium-sparing agents are expected to prevent side effects of diuretic therapy such as ventricular arrhythmias, glycoside toxicity, or impairment of glucose tolerance.[65, 71, 76, 77] The occurrence of ventricular arrhythmias is regarded as a main risk factor for sudden death in hypertensive patients.[77–82] A combination of thiazides and triamterene reduced the incidence of fatal cardiac events in hypertensive patients older than 60 years (11 events in 1000 patients within 1 year) in a large field study.[83] However, the addition of triamterene to thiazides did not reduce the incidence of ventricular arrhythmias compared with patients treated with thiazides alone in a study by Siegel et al.[84] Only a subgroup of patients (serum potassium levels, <3.0 mmol/L) treated with thiazides alone revealed an increased number of ventricular arrhythmias and thus might profit from administration of triamterene. A reduction of fatal cardiac events by additional administration of triamterene has yet to be shown. Therefore, risks and benefits of the administration of triamterene are controversial.[85, 86]

Today, indiscriminate prescribing of prophylactic potassium supplementation and potassium-sparing agents is discouraged.[87] Nonetheless, specific clinical situations exist in which diuretic-induced hypokalemia must be avoided.

The initial combination of diuretics with potassium-sparing agents therefore is acceptable in patients receiving digitalis glycosides or drugs that change the repolarization of cardiac cells (i.e., tricyclic antidepressants or phenothiazines[12]); in elderly or chronically sick patients who are likely to have anorexia or deficient dietary intake, such as alcoholics; in patients receiving concomitant therapy with corticosteroids, carbenoxolone, or laxatives;[12] in patients with myocardial ischemia or infarction; and in patients with left ventricular hypertrophy[88] or with severe hypokalemia (3.0 mEq/L).[89] Diabetic patients are prone to having hypokalemia because of their unphysiologic pattern of insulin release. However, renal failure and hyporeninemic hypoaldosteronism that may lead to hyperkalemia should be taken into consideration before potassium-sparing treatment is commenced.

Adjunctive Therapy in Edematous States

Congestive Heart Failure

In patients with congestive heart failure, profound hemodynamic and endocrine disturbances lead to major changes in electrolyte balance, with sodium and water retention and losses of total body potassium and magnesium.[90, 91] Further electrolyte imbalances are induced by the use of thiazides and loop diuretics. Potassium-sparing drugs tend to abolish metabolic alkalosis and kaliuresis induced by diuretics and secondary hyperaldosteronism. Thus, coadministration of a potassium-sparing agent such as triamterene may be particularly beneficial.[92] Again, special care should be taken in patients receiving digitalis concomitantly and in patients with renal failure.

Nephrotic Syndrome

The treatment of edema in the nephrotic syndrome consists of mild sodium restriction and, in selected patients, judicious use of diuretics. A potassium-sparing diuretic such as triamterene may be employed concomitantly with thiazide and loop diuretics.[93] Closely matched controls of potassium and creatinine are mandatory and are of particular importance in patients with progressing renal failure.

Cirrhosis

Fluid retention in hepatic cirrhosis involves hormonal and humoral disturbances.[94] The potassium deficit in patients with decompensated cirrhosis is estimated to be 10% to 30% of total body potassium. Usually, spironolactone is administered as the physiologic therapy to counteract hyperaldosteronism. As an alternative therapy, patients may receive potassium-sparing agents in combination with thiazides or loop diuretics. As previously mentioned, elimination of triamterene is markedly prolonged in cirrhosis of the liver, and accumulation of the drug may occur. An individualized diuretic regimen and careful monitoring are therefore indicated.

Rare Indications

Hypokalemic Periodic Paralysis

Because the onset of this disorder occurs before the age of 25 years, it appears to be primarily an autosomal dominant inherited condition. The pathogenesis is not fully understood, but a membrane defect is probably responsible for a shift of potassium from blood into muscle cells, while total body potassium remains constant. As a drug of second choice, triamterene may prevent paralyzing attacks.[95]

Bartter's Syndrome

A marked increase in sodium permeability of the cell membranes is believed to be the proximate cause of Bartter's syndrome. Metabolic alkalosis and hyperreninemic secondary hyperaldosteronism with hypochloremia are observed.[96–98] Blood pressure remains normal because increases in bradykinins and prostaglandins (PGE_2, PGI) seem to balance increases in angiotensin II and kallikrein. One possible therapeutic approach involves administration of indomethacin and potassium supplementation or a potassium-sparing agent.

Liddle's Syndrome

Liddle's syndrome is a hypertensive disease characterized by hypokalemic alkalosis and negligible aldosterone secretion.[99] A generalized enhanced sodium transport in cell membranes has been accepted as the primary abnormality. Triamterene, but not spironolactone, has been reported to correct the electrolyte imbalance effectively.[99, 100]

BIOCHEMICAL CHANGES AND ADVERSE EFFECTS

The side effects of triamterene are listed in Tables 44–1 and 44–2.[100–103] Triamterene and its metabolites have been identified in 181 of 50,000 renal calculi (0.4%) investigated by Ettinger et al.[104] The annual incidence of triamterene calculi was estimated to be 1 in 1500 patients treated with triamterene. In contrast,

Table 44–1. **Biochemical Changes Associated with Triamterene**

Hyperkalemia
Hyperuricemia
BUN and creatinine elevation
Urine sediment abnormalities
Impaired renal excretion of PGE_2
Hyperglycemia
Megaloblastosis, eosinophilia

BUN, blood urea nitrogen.

Jick et al.[105] could not reconfirm an increased incidence of renal stones resulting from triamterene therapy. It seems that, in the vast majority of patients, triamterene is simply embedded in the protein matrix of renal stones. Carey et al.[106] pointed out that patients receiving triamterene in whom calculi form early during treatment and with a family history of calculi are more prone to further calculi. This may explain the observation of a 35% incidence of previous renal calculi in patients in whom calculi develop while being treated with triamterene, compared with a 4% incidence of previous calculi in patients who did not. This finding suggests that the patient rather than the drug is the risk factor.[107, 108] Thus, triamterene should be used with caution in patients who form renal stones.

Gastrointestinal disturbances have occasionally been reported.[52, 109] Nausea can usually be prevented by taking the drug after meals.

Hyperkalemia

The most important and potentially lethal hazard of all potassium-sparing agents is hyperkalemia.[110] In general, the dangerous complications of hyperkalemia have been estimated to be as prevalent as 1 in 200 cases.[86] In patients with diabetes mellitus, hyperkalemia may occur in 26% of cases. Hyperkalemia was judged to be responsible for one half of preventable deaths reported in the Boston Collaborative Drug Study.[111]

Hyperuricemia

The increase in serum uric acid levels caused by triamterene has an additive effect to that produced by thiazides.[107, 109, 112] In patients treated for hypertension who received 200 mg of triamterene daily, Spiekermann et al.[113] estimated a 17% incidence of hyperuricemia. Although clinical observation of acute gout

Table 44–2. **Adverse Effects of Triamterene Administration**

Urogenital: stone formation
Renal: interstitial nephritis
Gastrointestinal: diarrhea, nausea, vomiting
Dermatologic: rash, urticaria, pruritus, photosensitivity[101]
Central nervous system and other side effects: dizziness, headache, muscle spasm, general weakness, drug fever[102, 103]

arthritis has been rare, patients who have a history of gout or pretreatment high serum levels of uric acid and an impaired renal function should not receive triamterene therapy.[83]

Blood Urea Nitrogen (BUN) Concentration and Creatinine Elevation

Some investigators[51, 56, 114, 115] have reported blood urea nitrogen and creatinine elevation as well as a decrease in renal blood flow and glomerular filtration rate during triamterene therapy, reflecting a decrease in renal function.

In as many as 50% of patients treated with triamterene, abnormalities in urinary sedimentation have been documented, suggesting tubulointerstitial damage. Occasionally, triamterene may be the primary cause of interstitial nephritis.[116–118]

Hyperglycemia

Because hypokalemia per se impairs glucose tolerance by a defect in insulin secretion, an improvement in glucose tolerance should be expected with the potassium-sparing effect of triamterene therapy. However, in several reports,[74] a hyperglycemic effect has been associated with triamterene in diabetic patients.

Megaloblastosis

Triamterene is a weak competitive inhibitor of folic acid *in vitro* but seems to exert no relevant antifolic activity *in vivo*. In patients with reduced folate stores, as in pregnancy or chronic alcoholism, the red blood cell count should be monitored.[119]

Pregnancy

No evidence of triamterene-induced fetal abnormalities has been reported. However, because our knowledge of its effect in human subjects is limited, triamterene should be prescribed cautiously in pregnancy.

CONTRAINDICATIONS AND DRUG INTERACTIONS
Contraindications

Four main contraindications to the administration of triamterene have been documented: (1) hyperkalemia, (2) concomitant therapy with other potassium-sparing agents or with potassium substitution, (3) renal dysfunction with creatinine values of more than 1.5 mg/dl or azotemia, and (4) hypersensitivity to the drug.

Drug Interactions

No interaction of triamterene with other drugs has been established. However, reversible renal failure was observed when triamterene was given in combination with indomethacin.[59, 61] This may have oc-

curred because both drugs inhibit the protective effect of prostaglandin in states of impaired renal perfusion.

Drugs that elevate sodium concentration in the distal renal tubules increase the degree of diuresis and potassium conservation of triamterene.

Ranitidine significantly reduces the renal clearance of triamterene and its phase II metabolite. Because gastrointestinal absorption of triamterene is also decreased, in healthy volunteers only mild alterations in pharmacodynamics resulted.[33, 34]

The combination of triamterene with angiotensin-converting enzyme inhibitors may cause severe hyperkalemia. Triamterene should be discontinued, and potassium levels should be monitored cautiously.

β-Blockers inhibit renin release from the juxtaglomerular cells and potassium influx into the cells, thereby possibly causing hyperkalemia.[84]

THE PLACE OF TRIAMTERENE AMONG OTHER DIURETICS

Triamterene, amiloride, and spironolactone have similar effects on potassium balance, natriuresis plasma volume, and peripheral renin activity.

In hypertension, diuretics have been a cornerstone of therapy for decades. However, the pathophysiologic understanding in this nonhomogeneous disease has grown, and the spectrum of therapeutic agents has expanded. This enables the physician to respond better to the pathophysiologic changes that differ in subgroups according to age, sex, race, obesity, and concomitant diseases.[120]

Especially in obese patients and black patients, and perhaps in women more than in men, low-dose diuretics have remained a preferred choice as step-1 therapy.[120] Coadministration of triamterene is desirable in patients with potassium waste and in patients

Table 44–3. **Situations That Require Potassium Monitoring**

1. **Reduced potassium absorption**
   a. Anorexia (alcoholism, age)
   b. Resection/inflammation of small intestine
2. **Gastrointestinal losses** due to vomiting; diarrhea (infection, vasoactive intestinal peptide, villous adenoma, fistulas)
3. **Renal losses** in primary aldosteronism (adrenocortical adenoma, hyperplasia, carcinoma); secondary aldosteronism (hypertensive states, renovascular hypertension, Bartter's syndrome, Liddle's syndrome, hepatic failure with ascites, heart failure)
   a. Excess glucocorticoids; excessive licorice ingestion; renal tubular acidosis; metabolic alkalosis
   b. Excess nonreabsorbable urinary anions (bicarbonate; lactate; acetate, carbenicillin, penicillin)
   c. Treatment with thiazides or loop diuretics
4. **Loss (shift) into cells** in alkalemia, hypokalemic periodic paralysis
5. **Chronic exercise**
6. **Increased sensitivity to hypokalemia-induced arrhythmias**
   a. Left ventricular hypertrophy
   b. Ischemia/infarction
   c. Digitalis treatment
   d. Excess catecholamines (stress, exercise, tumor)

Table 44–4. **Formulations of Triamterene for Monotherapy and Combination Therapy**

Monotherapy
Dyrenium (50- and 100-mg capsules), 100 mg twice daily after meals. Treatment should be individualized. Maximum daily dose is 300 mg.
Combination Therapy
Dyazide (50 mg of triamterene + 25 mg of HCTZ), one or two capsules twice daily after meals. Maximum daily dose is four capsules.
Maxzide (75 mg of triamterene + 50 mg of HCTZ), one tablet daily. Maximum daily dose is two tablets.

HCTZ, hydrochlorothiazide.

at risk for cardiac arrhythmias, as detailed in Table 44–3.[83]

In cirrhosis of the liver, the metabolic activation of triamterene is impaired, and hepatic clearance is reduced. As these parameters change with progression of the disease, amiloride ensures a more stable therapeutic effect.

In nephrotic syndrome with impaired renal function, amiloride seems to be advantageous in combination with a diuretic, as it does not interfere with prostaglandin synthesis. With all potassium-sparing agents, periodic monitoring of serum potassium levels is indicated.

Formulations of triamterene for monotherapy and combination therapy are provided in Table 44–4.

SOCIOECONOMIC CONSIDERATIONS AND DRUG COMPLIANCE

Diuretics such as thiazides and loop diuretics still are common agents in the treatment of essential hypertension. Triamterene has been proved effective in preventing hypokalemia and hypomagnesemia associated with diuretic therapy in specific high-risk groups. The cost of both combinations is especially attractive when compared with other potassium-sparing agents and potassium supplements.[28]

SUMMARY

Triamterene given alone has a minor effect on arterial pressure and natriuresis. In combination with more potent diuretics, it prevents hypokalemia at the expense of a decrease in renal function. Administration of triamterene as an adjunct to diuretics should be restricted to patients at risk for hypokalemia (see Table 44–3). Potassium blood levels should be monitored carefully to prevent hyperkalemia.

REFERENCES

1. Hopkins FG: Pigment in yellow butterflies. Nature 45:197, 1891.
2. Purrmann R: Die Synthese des Xanthopterins. Über die Flügelpigmente der Schmetterlinge. Liebigs Ann 546:98, 1941.
3. Haddow A: Ciba Foundation Symposium on Chemistry and Biology of Pteridines. In Wolstenholme GEW, Cameron MP (eds): Boston: Little, Brown, 1954, pp 100–102.
4. Wiebelhaus VD, Weinstock J, Maass AR, et al: The diuretic and natriuretic activity of triamterene and several related pteridines in the rat. J Pharmacol Exp Ther 149:397, 1965.
5. Doisy RJ, Roichart DA, Werterfeld WW: Comparative studies of various inhibitors of xanthine oxidase and related enzymes. J Biol Chem 217:307, 1955.
6. Albert A: Quantitative studies of the avidity of naturally occurring substances for trace metals. Biochem J 54:646, 1953.
7. Wiebelhaus VD, Weinstock J, Brennan FT, et al: Further laboratory studies on triamterene, SK&F 8524. Pharmacologist 3:59, 1961.
8. Wiebelhaus VD, Weinstock J, Brennan FT, et al: A potent, nonsteroidal orally active antagonist of aldosterone. Fed Proc 20:409, 1961.
9. Crosley AP, Ronquillo CM, Strickland WH, et al: Triamterene, a new natriuretic agent. Preliminary observations in man. Ann Intern Med 56:241, 1961.
10. Koeppeh BM, Biag BA, Biebisch GH: Intracellular microelectrode characterization in the rabbit cortical collecting duct. Am J Physiol 244:F35, 1983.
11. Baba WI, Indhope GR, Wilson GM: Site and mechanism of action of the diuretic triamterene. Clin Sci 27:181, 1964.
12. Lant A: Diuretics. Clinical pharmacology and therapeutic use (Part II). Drugs 29:162, 1985.
13. Materson BJ: Insights into intrarenal sites and mechanisms of actions of diuretic agents. Am Heart J 106:188, 1983.
14. Cuthbert AW: Aspects of the pharmacology of passive ion transfer across cell membranes. Prog Med Chem 14:1, 1977.
15. Baba WI, Lant AF, Smith AJ, et al: Pharmacological effects in animals and normal human subjects of the diuretic amiloride hydrochloride (MK-870). Clin Pharmacol Ther 9:318, 1968.
16. Cuthbert AW: Importance of guanidinium groups for blocking sodium channels in epithelia. Mol Pharmacol 12:945, 1976.
17. Sudo K, Hoshi T: Mode of action of amiloride in toad urinary bladder. J Membr Biol 32:115, 1977.
18. Cragoe EJ: Structure activity relationship in the amiloride series. In Cuthbert AW, Fanelli GM, Jr, Scriabine A (eds): Amiloride and Epithelial Sodium Transport. Baltimore: Urban & Schwarzenberg, 1979, pp 1–20.
19. Robert D, Hall TC: Drug interactions: Pteridine diuretics and antifols. I. The inhibition of dihydrofolate reductase by analogues of 2,4,7,-triaminopteridines. J Clin Pharmacol 8:217, 1968.
20. Dayton PG, Pruitt AW, McNag JLV, et al: Studies with triamterene, a substituted pteridine. Unusual brain to plasma ratio in mammals. Neuropharmacology 11:435, 1972.
21. Pruitt AW, McNag DL, Dayton PG: Transfer characteristics of triamterene and its analogs: Central nervous system, placenta and kidney. Drug Metab Dispos 3:40, 1975.
22. Pruitt AW, Winkel JS, Dayton PG: Variations in the fate of triamterene. Clin Pharmacol Ther 21:610, 1977.
23. Hasegawa J, Lin ET, Williams RL, et al: Pharmacokinetics of triamterene and its metabolite in man. J Pharmacokinet Biopharm 10:507, 1982.
24. Blume CD, Williams RL: A new antihypertensive agent: Maxzide (75 mg triamterene/50 mg hydrochlorothiazide). Am J Med 77:52, 1984.
25. Mutschler E, Gilfrich JH, Knauf H, et al: Pharmacokinetics of triamterene. Clin Exp Hypertens [A] 5:249, 1983.
26. Knauf H, Lubcke R, Wais U: Potassium-retaining diuretics. A comparative study on their mechanisms of action. In Addison GM (ed): Aldosterone Antagonists in Clinical Medicine, ICS No. 460. Amsterdam: Excerpta Medica, 1978, pp 70–76.
27. Lehmann K: Trennung, Isolierung und Identifizierung von Stoffwechselprodukten des Triamterens. Arzneimittelforschung/Drug Res 15:812, 1965.
28. Houston MC, Johnston PE: Essential hypertension: New insights and controversies in treatment with diuretics. South Med J 79:984, 1986.
29. Leilich G, Knauf H, Mutschler E, et al: Influence of triamterene and hydroxytriamterene sulfuric acid ester on diuresis and saluresis in rats after oral and intravenous application. Arzneimittelforsch 30:949, 1980.

30. Knauf H, Lubcke R, Mohrke W, et al: Saluretische und Kalium-sparende Wirkung der Phase II Metaboliten von Triamterene beim Menschen. Naunyn Schmiedebergs Arch Pharmacol (Suppl) 319:R87, 1982.

31. Kau ST: Handling of triamterene by the isolated perfused rat kidney. J Pharmacol Exp Ther 206:701, 1978.

32. Muirhead MR, Somogyi AA, Rolan PE, et al: Effect of cimetidine on renal and hepatic drug elimination: Studies with triamterene. Clin Pharmacol Ther 40:400, 1986.

33. Muirhead MR, Bochner F, Somogyi AA: Pharmacokinetic drug interactions between triamterene and ranitidine in humans: Alterations in renal and hepatic clearances and gastrointestinal absorption. J Pharmacol Exp Ther 244:734, 1988.

34. Muirhead MR, Somogyi AA: Effect of H2 antagonists on the differential secretion of triamterene and its sulfate conjugate metabolite by the isolated perfused rat kidney. Drug Metab Dispos 19:312, 1991.

35. Baba WI, Indhope GR, Wilson GM: Triamterene, a new diuretic drug. Studies in normal men and in adrenalectomized rats. Br Med J 2:756, 1962.

36. Dyckner T, Wester PO: Intracellular magnesium loss after diuretic administration. Drugs 28(Suppl 1):161, 1984.

37. Wang R, Oei TO, Airawa J, et al: Predictors of clinical hypomagnesemia-hypokalemia, hypophosphatemia, hyponatremia, hypocalcemia. Arch Intern Med 144:1794, 1984.

38. Dyckner T, Wester PO: Potassium/magnesium depletion in patients with cardiovascular disease. Am J Med 82(Suppl 3A):11, 1987.

39. Skou JC: Further investigations on a Mg + + and Na + activated adenosinetriphosphatase, possibly related to the active linked transport of Na + and K + across the nerve membrane. Biochem Biophys Acta 241:443, 1971.

40. Glynn IJ: The action of cardiac glycosides on ion movements. Pharmacol Rev 16:381, 1964.

41. Dyckner T, Wester PO: The relation between extra- and intracellular electrolytes in patients with hypokalemia and/or diuretic treatment. Acta Med Scand 204:269, 1978.

42. Dyckner T, Wester PO: Ventricular extrasystoles and intracellular electrolytes in hypokalemic patients before and after correction of the hypokalemia. Acta Med Scand 204:395, 1978.

43. Cannon PJ, Ames RP, Laragh JH: Relation between potassium balance and aldosterone secretion in normal subjects and in patients with hypertension or renal tubular disease. J Clin Invest 45:865, 1966.

44. Ryan MP: Diuretics and potassium/magnesium depletion. Am J Med 82(Suppl 3A):38, 1987.

45. Ryan MP, Philips O: Diuretic-induced calcium and magnesium excretion in the rat [abstract]. Irish J Med Sci 146:303, 1977.

46. Devane J, Ryan MP: The effects of amiloride and triamterene on urinary magnesium excretion in conscious saline-loaded rats. Br J Pharmacol 72:891, 1981.

47. Kroenke K, Wood DR, Hanley JF: The value of serum magnesium determination in hypertensive patients receiving diuretics. Arch Intern Med 147:1553, 1987.

48. Widmann L, Dyckner T, Wester PO: Effects of triamterene on serum and skeletal muscle electrolytes in diuretic-treated patients. Eur J Clin Pharmacol 33:577, 1988.

49. De Carvalho JGR, Emery AC, Frohlich ED: Spironolactone and triamterene in volume-dependent essential hypertension. Clin Pharmacol Ther 27:53, 1980.

50. Cranston WI, Semmence AM, Richardson DW, et al: Effect of triamterene on elevated arterial pressure. Am Heart J 70:455, 1965.

51. Walker BR, Hoppe RC, Alexander F: Effect of triamterene on the renal clearance of calcium, magnesium, phosphate and uric acid in man. Clin Pharmacol Ther 13:245, 1972.

52. Zawada ET: Antihypertensive therapy with triamterene-hydrochlorothiazide or amiloride-hydrochlorothiazide. Arch Intern Med 146:1312, 1986.

53. Hollenberg NK, Bannon JA: The PACT study: Post-marketing surveillance in 47,465 patients treated with Maxzide (triamterene/hydrochlorothiazide). Am J Med 80(Suppl 4A):30, 1986.

54. Fletcher AE: Adverse treatment effects in the trial of the European Working Party on High Blood Pressure in the Elderly. Am J Med 90(Suppl 3A):42S, 1991.

55. Kokko JP: Site and mechanism of action of diuretics. Am J Med 77:11, 1984.

56. Morin Y, Turmel L, Fortier J: Triamterene: Clinical studies in arterial hypertension. Am Heart J 69:195, 1965.

57. Chiba S, Abe U, Yasujima M, et al: Effect of triamterene on urinary excretion of immunoreactive prostaglandin E in essential hypertension. Tohoku J Exp Med 129:249, 1979.

58. Dunn MJ, Hood VL: Prostaglandins and the kidney. Am J Physiol 233:F169, 1977.

59. Oates JA, Fitzgerald GA, Branch RA, et al: Clinical implications of prostaglandin and thromboxane A2 formation (second of two parts). N Engl J Med 319:761, 1988.

60. Frohlich ED: Diuretics in hypertension. J Hypertens 5(Suppl 3):43, 1987.

61. Favre L, Glasson P, Vallotton MB: Reversible acute renal failure from combined triamterene and indomethacin. Ann Intern Med 96:317, 1982.

62. Völger KD: Tierexperimentelle und humanpharmakologische Untersuchungen mit dem phase II metaboliten von triamteren. Arzneimittelforschung/Drug Res 41:499, 1991.

63. Busch AE, Netzer T, Ullrich F, Mutschler E: Antiarrhythmic properties of benzyl-triamterene derivatives in the coronary artery ligated and perfused rat. Arzneimittelforschung/Drug Res 41:124, 1991.

64. Vassalle M: Cardiac pacemaker potentials at different extra and intracellular potassium concentrations. Am J Physiol 208:770, 1965.

65. Hollifield JW: Magnesium depletion, diuretics and arrhythmias. Am J Med 82(Suppl 3A):30, 1987.

66. Roden DM, Iansmith DHS: Effects of low potassium or magnesium concentrations on isolated cardiac tissue. Am J Med 82(Suppl 3A):18, 1987.

67. Lown B, Weller JM, Wyatt N, et al: Effects of alterations of body potassium on digitalis toxicity. J Clin Invest 31:648, 1952.

68. Steiness E, Olesen KH: Cardiac arrhythmias induced by hypokalemia and potassium loss during maintenance digoxin therapy. Br Heart J 38:167, 1976.

69. Cohn KE, Kleiger RE, Harrison DC: Influence of potassium depletion on myocardial concentration of titrated digoxin. Circ Res 20:473, 1967.

70. Seller RH, Greco J, Banach S, et al: Increasing the inotropic effect and toxic dose of digitalis by the administration of antikaliuric drugs—further evidence for a cardiac effect of diuretic agents. Am Heart J 90:56, 1975.

71. Amery A, Berthaux P, Bulpitt C, et al: Glucose intolerance during diuretic therapy. Results of a trial by the European Working Party on Hypertension in the Elderly. Lancet 1:681, 1978.

72. Gorden P: Glucose intolerance with hyperkalemia. Failure in short-term potassium depletion in normal subjects to reproduce the glucose and insulin abnormalities in clinical hypokalemia. Diabetes 22:544, 1972.

73. Rowe JW, Tobin JD, Rosa RM, et al: Effect of experimental potassium deficiency on glucose and insulin metabolism. Metabolism 29:498, 1980.

74. Amery A, Birkenhage W, Brixko P, et al: Glucose intolerance during diuretic therapy in elderly hypotensive patients. A second report from the European Working Party on High Blood Pressure in the Elderly. Postgrad Med J 62:919, 1986.

75. Walker BR, Capuzzi DM, Alexander F, et al: Hyperkalemia after triamterene in diuretic patients. Clin Pharmacol Ther 13:643, 1972.

76. Hollifield JW: Thiazide treatment of hypertension. Effects of thiazide diuretics on serum potassium, magnesium, and ventricular ectopy. Am J Med 80(Suppl 4A):8, 1986.

77. Lown B, Calvert AF, Armington R, et al: Monitoring for serious arrhythmias and high risk of sudden death. Circulation 52(Suppl 3):189, 1975.

78. Veterans Administration Cooperative Study Group on Antihypertensive Agents: Effects of treatment on morbidity in hypertension. JAMA 213:1143, 1970.

79. Multiple Risk Factor Intervention Trial Research Group: Baseline rest electrocardiographic abnormalities, antihypertensive treatment, and mortality in the Multiple Risk Factor Intervention Trial. Am J Cardiol 55:1, 1985.

80. Holland OB, Nixon JV, Kuhnert L: Diuretic-induced ventricular ectopic activity. Am J Med 70:762, 1981.
81. Hollifield JW, Slaton PE: Thiazide diuretics, hypokalemia and cardiac arrhythmias. Acta Med Scand [Suppl] 647:67, 1981.
82. Medical Research Council Working Party on Mild to Moderate Hypertension: Ventricular extrasystoles during thiazide treatment: Substudy of MRC mild hypertension trial. Br Med J 287:1249, 1983.
83. Fletcher A, Amery A, Birkenhäger W, et al: Risks and benefits in the trial of the European Working Party on High Blood Pressure in the Elderly. J Hypertens 9:225, 1991.
84. Siegel D, Hulley SB, Black DM, et al: Diuretics, serum and intracellular electrolyte levels, and ventricular arrhythmias in hypertensive men. JAMA 267:1083, 1992.
85. Kassirer JP, Harrington JT: Diuretics and potassium metabolism: A reassessment of the need, effectiveness and safety of potassium therapy. Kidney Int 2:505, 1977.
86. Harrington JT, Isner JM, Kassirer JP: Our national obsession with potassium. Am J Med 73:155, 1982.
87. Papademetriou V, Price M, Johnson E, et al: Early changes in plasma and urinary potassium in diuretic-treated patients with systemic hypertension. Am J Cardiol 54:1015, 1984.
88. Messerli FH, Ventura HO, Elizardi DJ, et al: Hypertension and sudden death—increased ventricular ectopic activity in left ventricular hypertrophy. Am J Med 77:18, 1984.
89. Ramsay LE, Hettiarachchi J, Fraser R, et al: Amiloride, spironolactone, and potassium chloride in thiazide-treated hypertensive patients. Clin Pharmacol Ther 27:533, 1980.
90. Dyckner T, Wester PO: Potassium-sparing diuretics. Acta Med Scand [Suppl] 707:79, 1986.
91. Porter GA: The role of diuretics in the treatment of heart failure. JAMA 240:1614, 1980.
92. Schwinger RH, Erdmann E: Heart failure and electrolyte disturbances. Methods Find Exp Clin Pharmacol 14:315, 1992.
93. Glassock RJ, Adler SG, Ward HJ, et al: Primary glomerular diseases in the kidney. In Brenner BM, Rector FC (eds): The Kidney. Philadelphia: WB Saunders, 1986, pp 929–1013.
94. Epstein M: Deranged sodium homeostasis in cirrhosis. Gastroenterology. 76:622, 1979.
95. Conn HO, Atterbury CE: Cirrhosis. In Schiff L, Schiff ER (eds): Diseases of the Liver. Philadelphia: JB Lippincott, 1987, pp 813–817.
96. Riggs JE, Griggs RC: The diagnosis and treatment of periodic paralysis. In Klawan HL (ed): Clinical Neuropharmacology, Vol 4. New York: Raven Press, 1979, pp 123–138.
97. Garrick R, Ziyadeh FN, Jorkaski D, et al: Bartter's syndrome: A unifying hypothesis. Am J Nephrol 5:379, 1985.
98. Stein JH: The pathogenetic spectrum of Bartter's syndrome. Kidney Int 28:85, 1985.
99. Mutoh S, Hirayama H, Ueda S, et al: Pseudohyperaldosteronism (Liddle's syndrome): A case report. J Urol 135:557, 1986.
100. Hoshiyama M: A 79-year-old man with hypertension, hypokalemia, hyporeninemia and hypoaldosteronemia similar to Liddle's syndrome. Nippon Naibunpi Gakkai Zasshi 68:111, 1992.
101. Fernandez de Corres F, Bernaola G, Fernandez E, et al: Photodermatitis from triamterene. Contact Dermatitis 17:114, 1987.
102. Safdi MA: Fever secondary to triamterene therapy [letter]. N Engl J Med 303:707, 1980.
103. Mackowiak PA, LeMaistre CF: Drug fever: A critical appraisal of conventional concepts. An analysis of 51 episodes in two Dallas hospitals and 97 episodes reported in the English literature. Ann Intern Med 106:728, 1987.
104. Ettinger B, Oldroyd NO, Sorgel F: Triamterene-induced nephrolithiasis. JAMA 244:2443, 1980.
105. Jick H, Dinan B, Hunter J: Triamterene and renal stones. J Urol 127:224, 1982.
106. Carey RA, Bey MMA, McNally CF, Tannenbaum P: Triamterene and renal lithiasis: A review. Clin Ther 6:302, 1989.
107. McMahon FG: Management of essential hypertension. The low-dose era. In McMahon FD (ed): Potassium-retaining Diuretics. New York: Futura Publishing, 1984, pp 183–206.
108. Woolfran RG, Mansell MA: Does triamterene cause renal calculi? BMJ 303:1217, 1991.
109. Mudge GH: Diuretics and other agents employed in the mobilization of edema fluid. In Goodman LS, Gilman A (eds): The Pharmacologic Basis of Therapeutics. New York: Macmillan, 1970, pp 839–873.
110. Hollifield JW: Potassium and magnesium abnormalities. Diuretics and arrhythmias in hypertension. Am J Med 77:28, 1984.
111. Jick H: Drugs remarkably nontoxic. N Engl J Med 84:162, 1976.
112. Chrysant SG, Chappel C, Faraham DJ, et al: Antihypertensive and metabolic effects of single and combined atenolol regimens. J Clin Pharmacol 32:61, 1992.
113. Spiekermann RE, Berge KG, Thurber DL, et al: Potassium-sparing effects of triamterene in the treatment of hypertension. Circulation 34:524, 1966.
114. Cohen AB: Hyperkalemic effects of triamterene. Ann Intern Med 65:521, 1966.
115. Shaldon S, Ryder JA: Use of a pteridine diuretic (triamterene) in the treatment of hepatic ascites. Br Med J 2:764, 1962.
116. Spence JD, Lindsay RM, Wong DG: Effects of triamterene and amiloride on urinary sediment in hypertensive patients taking hydrochlorothiazide. Lancet 2:73, 1985.
117. Fairley KF, Birch DF, Haines I: Abnormal urinary sediment in patients on triamterene. Lancet 1:421, 1983.
118. Bailey RR, Lynn KL, Drennan CJ, et al: Triamterene-induced acute interstitial nephritis. Lancet 1:226, 1982.
119. Corcino J, Waxman S, Herbert V: Mechanism of triamterene-induced megaloblastosis. Ann Intern Med 73:419, 1970.
120. Messerli FH, Schmieder RE: Use of diuretic agents in obese or black patients with systemic hypertension. Am J Cardiol 58:11A, 1986.

CHAPTER 45

Amiloride

Garabed Eknoyan, M.D.

Amiloride is an orally effective diuretic with a modest natriuretic property but a marked ability to reduce urinary potassium excretion.[1-4] Its development was prompted in the quest for potassium-sparing agents as companion drugs to overcome the undesirable side effect of potassium loss induced by the more potent natriuretic agents such as thiazides and loop diuretics.[5, 6]

In the early reports of the diuretic and antihypertensive properties of this compound, which appeared in the mid-1960s, it was referred to as amipramizide, guanamprazine, amipramidin, DCP, and MK-870.[2, 5-7] In 1967, it was given the U.S. adopted name amiloride hydrochloride. In 1969, it became available for clinical use in Europe; in 1981, it became available in the United States, where it is marketed in 5-mg tablets as

Midamor and in a fixed combination of 5 mg of amiloride with 50 mg of hydrochlorothiazide as Moduretic.

CHEMISTRY

Amiloride hydrochloride, present as the dihydrate, $C_6H_8ClN_7O \cdot HCl \cdot 2H_2O$, is a yellow to greenish yellow, odorless crystalline solid with a molecular weight of 302.12. It is an organic base with a pK of 8.7. It is soluble in water (5.2 mg/ml), methanol (19.6 mg/ml), and dimethyl sulfoxide (>200 mg/ml). It is stable in heat and light. It belongs to the group of compounds classified as pyrazinoylguanidines (Fig. 45–1).[5-9]

PHARMACOLOGY

Although amiloride and its analogues have been used experimentally as specific inhibitors of transport in various tissues,[10, 11] in the doses used clinically, it has no important pharmacologic actions except those related to the renal tubular transport of electrolytes, where it reduces the sodium permeability of cortical collecting tubules and collecting ducts.[12] Under normal conditions, the administration of amiloride increases the renal excretion of sodium chloride by as much as 2% or 3% of the filtered load of sodium.[13] At the same time, urine pH may increase moderately, which indicates reduced secretion of hydrogen.[4, 14] More importantly, however, natriuresis is associated either with only a slight increase or, depending on the dose used, with an absolute decrease in the rate of potassium excretion.[5, 6, 12] This effect of amiloride is more striking when it is given together with the other more potent natriuretic agents, such as thiazides, furosemide, and ethacrynic acid, which normally induce a severalfold increase in potassium excretion.[1, 12, 15] Under these conditions, the effect of amiloride on sodium excretion is almost additive to that of the other diuretics, but it is antagonistic with respect to potassium excretion. As a result, a positive potassium balance is maintained despite the marked natriuresis that is induced.[12, 16-18]

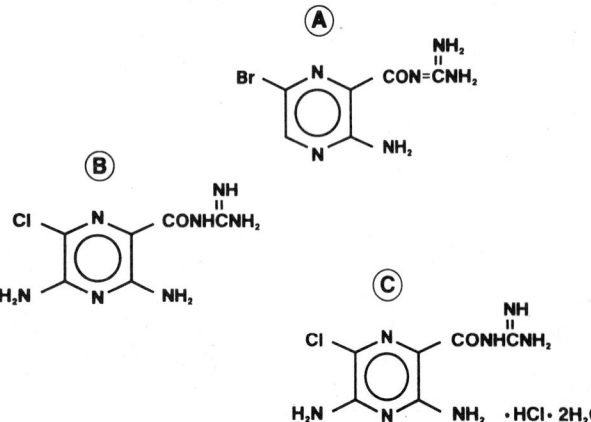

Figure 45–1. Structure of amiloride (C) and some of its analogues (A and B).

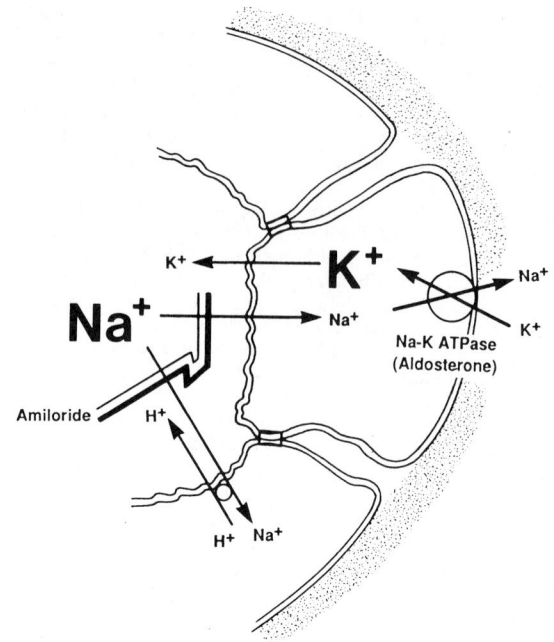

Figure 45–2. Cellular mechanism of potassium and hydrogen secretion in the late distal tubule and early collecting tubule. Amiloride inhibits sodium entry across the apical entry channels and secondarily inhibits potassium and hydrogen secretion.

This important antikaliuretic effect of amiloride that characterizes it as a potassium-sparing agent can best be appreciated in the context of normal handling of potassium by the kidney.[19, 20] Essentially, all of the filtered potassium is reabsorbed in the proximal tubule and loop of Henle. Depending on the homeostatic needs of the body, a variable amount of potassium secretion occurs in the terminal portion of the distal convoluted tubule and cortical portion of the collecting duct. As a result, the amount of potassium excreted in the urine reflects predominantly the function of the distal potassium-secreting cells (Fig. 45–2). The principal determinant of potassium secretion is the potassium concentration inside these cells, which is maintained by the uptake of potassium across the basolateral membrane by the sodium and potassium-dependent adenosine triphosphatase (Na, K-ATPase) pump located at this site. The activity of the pump is limited by the intracellular concentration of sodium and is stimulated by the levels of circulating aldosterone. To prime the pump, sodium enters the cell by passive diffusion across specific sodium channels located on the luminal membrane of the cell. The intracellular potassium is then transported across the apical membrane into the lumen down its electrochemical gradient. The amount of potassium that can be secreted depends on (1) the distal delivery of sodium, which by diffusing down its concentration gradient through the apical sodium channels into the cell provides a stimulus for potassium secretion, and (2) the rate of flow of the tubular fluid, which maintains relatively low potassium concentrations within the lumen and thus a more favorable cell-to-lumen potassium gradient.

Of the factors that regulate distal cellular potassium secretion, the most important to the effect of diuretics are the tubular fluid flow rate, the luminal fluid composition, and the level of circulating aldosterone. Diuretics that inhibit sodium reabsorption in the proximal portions of the nephron (carbonic anhydrase inhibitors, loop diuretics, thiazides) increase the tubular fluid flow rate across the distal tubule and the sodium load delivered to it and thereby stimulate increased potassium excretion. In turn, the volume depletion that ensues stimulates aldosterone secretion, which further potentiates and prolongs the potassium losses that can occur.[21] Thus, potassium losses can persist beyond the period of diuresis (Fig. 45–3). In addition, the development of systemic alkalosis during continued diuretic therapy favors the entry of potassium into the cells and, by increasing the potassium concentration in the potassium-secreting cells, provides a further stimulus for potassium loss.[14, 19] In contrast to the effect of other diuretics, amiloride, by blocking the sodium-entry channels on the luminal surface of the potassium-secreting cells, decreases the availability of intracellular sodium to the Na, K-ATPase pump and thereby limits the concentration of intracellular potassium available for secretion. In addition, by inhibiting the sodium entry pathways, it increases the luminal membrane voltage and thus decreases the electrochemical gradient for potassium exit from the cell.[12] Experiments on isolated perfused cortical collecting tubules of rabbits have clearly demonstrated that amiloride at luminal concentrations of 10^{-5} M markedly inhibits the absorption of sodium and secretion of potassium and dramatically reverts the polarity of the transepithelial voltage.[22] In all epithelia in which this effect of amiloride has been shown to be operative, the drug acts more effectively on the luminal surface than on the contraluminal surface of the epithelial cells.[10, 12] The inhibition of sodium transport is rapid and reversible, indicating that the effect is on the cellular membrane.

In addition to inhibiting the sodium entry pathway of apical cell membranes of tight epithelia, at low concentrations (<1 μM), amiloride at higher concentration inhibits yet another sodium transport pathway, namely that of Na$^+$-H$^+$ exchanger[22, 23] (see Fig. 45–2). Such an effect has been shown in a variety of cells, including the membrane vesicles of the proximal tubule microvillus,[24] the perfused proximal tubule,[25] the distal tubule,[26] and the medullary collecting duct.[27] Amiloride is not an inhibitor of carbonic anhydrase. This reversible inhibition of the sodium site of the exchanger accounts for the reduced H$^+$ excretion and increased urine pH noted in vivo.[4, 5] The peak urinary concentrations of 12 to 31 μg/ml of amiloride attained in patients after the ingestion of a 20-mg dose of amiloride[28] are within the range needed to inhibit the Na$^+$-H$^+$ exchanger.

Amiloride is not an inhibitor of membrane ATPase, except at relatively high concentrations (10^{-3} M; i.e., 1000 times the level attained in the urine), at which it has been shown to inhibit the Na, K-ATPase preparation of intact proximal tubules in suspension.[29] At these concentrations, in vitro amiloride accumulates within cells, including renal epithelial cells, and exerts its effect directly on intracellular processes rather than on the membrane.[30-32]

The effects of amiloride are independent of aldosterone and have been demonstrated in animals with their adrenal glands removed.[5, 6] However, to the extent that amiloride decreases the availability of intracellular sodium, it indirectly counters the action of aldosterone on the cortical collecting tubule cells, an effect that has been demonstrated experimentally and observed clinically.[33, 34] At higher doses, it can prevent potassium loss due to primary hyperaldosteronism, for which the daily requirement of amiloride may be as high as 40 mg.[15, 33, 34]

PHARMACOKINETICS

After oral administration, 25% to 30% of the drug is absorbed from the gastrointestinal tract. Absorption is increased to 40% to 50% if the drug is taken on an empty stomach and fasting is maintained for 4 hours.[5, 7, 28] Within 72 hours after intravenous administration, 90% of the dose is recovered in the urine, 15% to 30% of it being excreted within the first 6 hours. Amiloride is not significantly metabolized in humans, and the urinary product appears to be the intact parent compound.[5, 7, 28, 35]

The volume of distribution of amiloride in dogs is

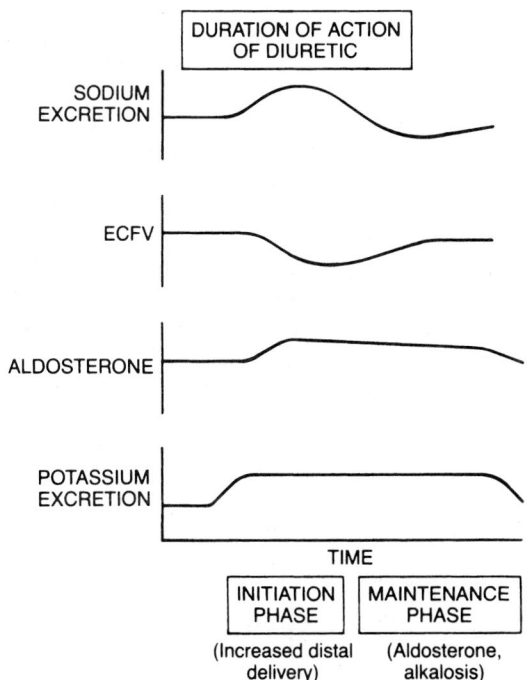

Figure 45–3. Diuretic-induced changes in the excretion of sodium and potassium and in the secretion of aldosterone. The boxes at the bottom indicate the two phases of diuretic-induced potassium loss: loss initially due to increased distal sodium delivery and flow rate during the action of the diuretic agent and subsequent loss because of the increased aldosterone secretion due to the extracellular fluid (ECFV) volume depletion after the diuretic effect on the kidney has subsided and the sodium excretion has been reduced.

15 to 18 times that of the volume of distribution of inulin, indicating extravascular sequestration of the drug. Equilibrium between the vascular and extravascular compartments is attained rapidly, within 30 minutes of ingestion, after which a stable state is reached. In rats, the drug is slowly and completely eliminated within 2 to 3 days after intraperitoneal injection and is not concentrated in any specific organ.[5, 7, 28, 35]

In human subjects, peak blood concentrations occur at 4 hours, with an elimination half-life of 7 to 12 hours.[36] Amiloride has low protein binding (less than 40%) and, given its molecular weight, should be filtered. Actually, the renal clearance of amiloride is 400 to 600 ml/min, which is about 4 or 5 times that of the glomerular filtration rate, indicating additional tubular secretion of the drug.[28] Being a basic compound, amiloride is secreted into the urine by the organic base pathway. Consequently, basic drugs such as cimetidine and procainamide interfere with its secretion.[37] Not unexpectedly, given its membrane effect, amiloride acts from the luminal side of the tubules, and its renal excretion and urinary concentrations rather than its blood levels determine its action. In humans, about 25% of a dose appears in the urine 10 hours after oral ingestion, most of which occurs at the 2- to 6-hour period after ingestion. Amiloride remains detectable in the urine for more than 24 hours after ingestion,[28] which corresponds well with the clinical response to amiloride. Its effect begins 2 hours after oral ingestion, reaches a maximum within 4 to 6 hours, and usually wanes within 12 to 24 hours, depending on the dose ingested.[5, 7, 34, 38–41] An increasing dose-response relationship is obtained in humans, with only a little increase in the effect noted at doses above 40 mg.[40]

Less than 2% of amiloride is excreted in bile; hence, unlike triamterene, neither its excretion nor its renal action is influenced by the presence of liver disease. In individuals with renal impairment, the elimination half-life of the drug is increased from 8 to 144 hours, being most prolonged in patients with the lowest renal function.[42] Because all potassium-sparing diuretics should be avoided in the presence of renal insufficiency (glomerular filtration rate <30 ml/min), the pharmacokinetics of amiloride in the presence of renal failure are of dubious value.

EFFECTS ON PATHOPHYSIOLOGY

In the usual clinical doses, the effects of amiloride on pathophysiology are secondary only to its effects on the kidney. The renal effects of this agent, therefore, are considered first to provide a basis for the explanation of its other systemic effects.

Effects on Renal Function

Amiloride results in a modest natriuresis combined with a marked reduction of potassium excretion. Clearance studies in human subjects and animals after amiloride administration demonstrate a profound decrease in the renal excretion of potassium (80% of excreted potassium) and a modest increase in sodium excretion (2% to 3% of filtered load).[28, 39, 40] Micropuncture and microperfusion experiments have localized this effect to the distal tubule and shown that amiloride in concentrations of less than 0.1 mM decreases potassium secretion and sodium reabsorption at this segment of the nephron.[12] The potassium-sparing effect is most evident when the drug is used in combination with other diuretics with a proximal site of action such as thiazides and loop diuretics.[1, 12, 13, 17, 18, 43] Thus, under experimental conditions of furosemide-induced diuresis, amiloride can reduce potassium excretion by as much as 80%, depending on the dose administered.[44] Except in occasional circumstances, the natriuretic effect of amiloride is too weak to be of use alone and requires doses large enough to increase the potential risk of hyperkalemia.[45] Amiloride's main clinical use has been that of a potassium-sparing agent when used with other diuretics, principally thiazides.

Amiloride also exerts a dose-dependent inhibitory effect on magnesium excretion, but only under experimental conditions of diuresis.[44, 46, 47] The magnesium-sparing effect of amiloride is less pronounced than the potassium-sparing effect, the reduction in the fractional excretion of magnesium being one sixth to one seventh that of its effect on the fractional potassium excretion.[44] The mechanism of its effect on magnesium excretion is not evident. It is not mediated by extrarenal factors, such as volume depletion or glomerular filtration rate, and it is immediate in onset, indicating a direct renal effect. However, no evidence exists of distal magnesium secretion, and micropuncture studies have failed to substantiate an effect of amiloride on magnesium transport in the cortical collecting tubule.[48, 49] Whatever the mechanism involved, the net effect is that the administration of amiloride with thiazide or loop diuretics also maintains a positive magnesium balance.[50–54]

Although the suggestion has been made that amiloride may be hypercalciuric in man,[55] direct micropuncture and microperfusion studies in rats indicate that amiloride increases the rate of calcium absorption in the distal tubule with a consequent decrease in calcium excretion.[56, 57] Amiloride exerts no effect on phosphate excretion.[55]

Amiloride reduces the net hydrogen secretion in the collecting tubule. Experimental studies have shown that the long-term administration of amiloride is associated with inability to lower the urine pH after an acid challenge and results in a reduction of collecting tubule P_{CO_2} (a measure of distal nephron proton secretion) during bicarbonate loading.[14, 58] Metabolic acidosis can occur during chronic amiloride administration. The metabolic acidosis is mainly the result of inhibition of distal acidification by amiloride because of its direct effect on sodium channels and Na^+-H^+ exchanger. It may be aggravated by a reduction in ammoniogenesis if hyperkalemia is present.[14]

Amiloride does not alter renal hemodynamics or cause a change in glomerular filtration.[4, 5] Amiloride facilitates receptor binding of atrial natriuretic peptide (ANP) to its receptor and potentiates the effects of ANP at a number of sites,[59] including the kidney,[60] in which it increases the natriuretic effects of ANP.[61]

Effects on Fluid Volume State and Electrolytes

By virtue of its modest diuretic effect, amiloride results in only minimal changes in extracellular fluid volume status. Although no change in body weight may be found, there may be a marked (up to 13-fold) increase in plasma aldosterone but only a small rise in plasma renin activity.[3] The adrenal stimulation appears to result from both potassium retention and renin activation consequent to natriuresis.[3, 41]

A far greater and clinically more important effect results from the capacity of amiloride to prevent or correct the hypokalemia of patients treated with thiazides.[17, 18, 20, 33, 41, 43, 44] As expected from its magnesium-sparing effect, amiloride administered with thiazides also maintains serum and tissue magnesium levels within normal range.[44, 50–53, 62]

No effect of amiloride on other electrolytes has been shown. The serum urate level remains unaltered. The drug appears to have no effect on serum lipoproteins.[63]

Effects on Ventricular Function, Electrophysiology, and Structure

Amiloride exerts no direct effect on ventricular function and structure. Neither its diuretic nor its antihypertensive effects are great enough to result in an adverse effect on ventricular function or mass. Its principal effect on cardiac function stems from its ability to prevent and correct diuretic-induced hypokalemia.

A number of carefully conducted clinical studies have linked the presence of diuretic-induced hypokalemia with the occurrence of increased ventricular arrhythmias.[64–66] The effects of potassium on the electrophysiologic properties of the heart have been studied extensively, and hypokalemia has been shown to be clearly arrhythmogenic.[67, 68] The copresence of diuretic-induced hypomagnesemia has been implicated as an added but independent variable that increases the occurrence of ventricular ectopy in these patients.[44, 69, 70] Although the detrimental effects of hypokalemia on the cardiac function of all patients in whom it develops while they are taking diuretics have been questioned by some[71, 72] and debated by others,[73] the fact remains that hypokalemia is common in diuretic-treated patients.[74] It is also clear that a subset of patients who are hypokalemic is at increased risk of ventricular ectopy, especially those with ventricular hypertrophy, those receiving concurrent digitalis therapy, and those with histories of arrhythmias and conductive defects.[66, 68, 69, 73, 75, 76] Furthermore, it is obvious that, in patients with myocardial infarction, diuretic-induced hypokalemia increases the risk of adrenaline-induced hypokalemia and ventricular fibrillation.[75–78] Hence, amiloride indirectly affects the electrophysiology of the myocardium through its capacity to prevent potassium and magnesium depletion and thereby to circumvent the principal side effect of the other diuretic agents that are the cornerstone of hypertension and edema therapy.[79, 80]

At high concentrations of amiloride, the direct effects on the myocardium can be demonstrated in vitro. Amiloride exerts a positive inotropic effect on isolated atria of guinea pigs and papillary muscle of dogs.[81–83] In canine sinoatrial nodes selectively perfused through the sinus node artery, amiloride induces a negative chronotropic and a positive inotropic effect in a concentration-dependent manner.[84] Amiloride also has been shown to prolong the action potential, or refractory period, of guinea pig atria and papillary muscles of dog Purkinje fibers.[83] The acute administration of amiloride to dogs reduces the myocardial efflux of potassium induced by acetyl strophantidin.[85] However, no change of potassium efflux occurs in the absence of cardiac glycosides.[86] In isolated rabbit papillary muscle preparation, potassium efflux is not altered by amiloride.[87] In chick heart cell cultures, amiloride partially inhibits the passive (ouabain-insensitive) potassium influx. At rather high concentrations of 10^{-3} M, amiloride inhibits myocardial microsomal Na, K-ATPase,[88] and cardiac sarcolemmal Na^+/H^+ antiporter.[89] In the isolated perfused heart, amiloride protects the myocardium from arrhythmias induced by ischemia[90] and ouabain.[91, 92]

Effect on Hemodynamics

The principal hemodynamic effect of amiloride, shown in a number of studies, is a reduction in mean arterial pressure of 7 to 14 mmHg (Table 45–1). Amiloride also has an added antihypertensive effect when given in combination with hydrochlorothiazide.[17, 18, 33, 93–97]

The mechanism of amiloride's antihypertensive effect remains undefined. The natriuresis it induces when given alone is not sufficient to provide a solid basis for its antihypertensive effect. When given with thiazides, its antihypertensive effect has been attributed to the enhanced natriuresis. However, its added antihypertensive effect in combination with thiazides is not always evident. When amiloride was combined with hydrochlorothiazide in the treatment of patients with hypertension, serum potassium levels were invariably normalized as compared with such levels when hydrochlorothiazide was given alone.[93–97] Conceivably, the correction or prevention of hypokalemia itself could account for the reduction in blood pressure, as has been found in thiazide-treated patients whose potassium deficiencies were corrected by potassium supplementation.[98]

Effects on Central Nervous System

Amiloride exerts no apparent clinical effect on central nervous system function. In experimental studies,

Table 45–1. **Effect of Amiloride Alone and in Combination with Hydrochlorothiazide (HCTZ) in Treating Mild and Moderate Hypertension**

Reference	No. of Patients	Drug and Dosage (mg)	Duration of Study (wk)	MAP (mmHg)	Δ BP (mmHg)	Mean Serum Potassium Level*
17		Placebo		111.4		4.0
	10	A 10 & HCTZ 100	8	101.1	−10.3	3.65
		Placebo		112.7		4.2
	9	HCTZ 100	8	101.4	−11.3	3.19
18		Placebo		101.9		4.0
	11	HCTZ 50 b.i.d.	8	99.5	−2.4	3.0
		Placebo		105.9		4.2
	13	A 5 & HCTZ 50 b.i.d.	8	104.5	−1.4	3.5
33		Placebo		128.1		3.96
	5	A 40	4	118.4	−9.7	4.67
93		Placebo		118.3		4.24
	44	A 5 (1 or 2)	12	108.3	−10.0	4.47
		Placebo		120.0		4.24
	45	A 5 & HCTZ 50 (1 or 2)	12	105.7	−14.3	3.86
		Placebo		118.7		4.15
	53	HCTZ 50 (1 or 2)	12	104.0	−14.7	3.56
94		Placebo		125.0		4.3
	65	HCTZ 25 (1 or 2)	12	105.3	−20.7	4.0
		Placebo		123.7		4.2
	65	A 2.5 & HCTZ 25 (1 or 2)	12	105.3	−18.4	4.2
95		Placebo		130.3		4.15
	10	HCTZ 50 b.i.d.		124.2	−6.1	3.56
	10	A 10 b.i.d.	2	126.7	−3.6	—
	10	A 10 b.i.d.	4	123.1	−7.2	4.47
	10	A 10 HCTZ 25 b.i.d.	4	114.8	−15.5	4.41
	10	HCTZ 50 b.i.d.		119.0	−11.3	3.54
96		Placebo		126.3		4.0
	19	HCTZ 25 (1 or 2)	8	111.7	−14.6	3.8
		Placebo		126.7		4.0
	18	A 2.5 & HCTZ 25 (1 or 2)	8	108.7	−18.0	4.0
97		Placebo		126.8		4.2
	10	A 5	6	111.9	−14.9	4.6
	10	HCTZ 50	6	111.9	−14.9	3.7
	10	A 5/HCTZ 50	6	110.7	−16.8	4.0

A, amiloride; Δ BP, change in mean arterial blood pressure; HCTZ, hydrochlorothiazide; MAP, mean arterial blood pressure.
*Values do not reflect the number of patients on HCTZ alone who had hypokalemia of less than 3.5 mEq/L.

amiloride has been shown to depress the rate of cerebrospinal fluid production.[99, 100]

Cellular and Membrane Effects

Because of its ability to block sodium channels, amiloride has been used extensively as a probe to study transport phenomena in a myriad of tissues and organs.[10] Most of these studies have used concentrations of the drug that are orders of magnitude higher than the micromolecular concentrations required for the inhibition of sodium transport in tight epithelia such as those in the distal nephron. At the doses used, the compound accumulates within the cell, where it has been shown to bind to nuclei, mitochondria, and purified nucleic acid.[30] Much if not all of the reported inhibitory effects of amiloride on a variety of cell functions, such as protein synthesis and Na, K-ATPase activity, are due to its intracellular effects.[101] In fact, to limit the entry of the compound into cells and prevent such undesirable side effects on cell function, polymer-bound analogues of amiloride have been developed to permit the study of its direct membrane effect.[31] Such structural modification of the compound has been shown to enhance either its electrogenic sodium-channel blocking activity or its electroneutral Na^+-H^+ antiporter.[102, 103]

CLINICAL USE

The ability of amiloride to augment modestly the natriuresis but reduce significantly the potassium loss of other more potent diuretics constitutes its principal utility in clinical medicine.

Indications

The potassium-sparing ability of amiloride has led to its use as adjunctive therapy with thiazides and loop diuretics in the treatment of hypertension and edema and alone in the management of primary aldosteronism, Bartter's syndrome, and lithium-induced nephrogenic diabetes insipidus.

Although amiloride does seem to have a mild antihypertensive effect (see Table 45–1), it is principally in combination with hydrochlorothiazide that it has proved most useful in the control of hypertension to prevent hypokalemia occurring with thiazides alone (see section on effects on renal function and fluid volume state and electrolytes). The connection between diuretics, hypokalemia, and arrhythmias continues to be the center of considerable debate, particularly in the light of overall controversy of the benefit of diuretics in the larger clinical trials of antihypertensive therapy.[104–106] However, certain facts remain well-established. First, more data support the ability of diuretics to reduce the morbidity and mortality of hypertension than support any other available antihypertensives. Second, the use of thiazides and loop diuretics increases urinary potassium losses in all patients, results in hypokalemia in a significant number of patients, and produces severe potassium depletion in some patients. The ability of potassium-sparing diuretics to circumvent this problem has been well-established and constitutes their principal attractiveness in the management of hypertension. Third, independent of the antihypertensive drug used in the initial step of antihypertensive therapy, the subsequent addition of a diuretic generally results in better control of hypertension and allows the use of smaller doses of the first-step agent, thereby reducing its side effects (which as a rule are dose-related).

While the importance of maintaining serum potassium continues to be debated, the risk for a subset of individuals who are predisposed to the arrhythmogenic effect of even modest hypokalemia is well established (see earlier section, "Effects on Ventricular Function, Electrophysiology, and Structure"). The preservation of potassium becomes absolutely essential in patients with edema due to congestive heart failure, in whom the diseased myocardium has necessitated digitalis therapy.

The edema of liver failure poses an analogous situation. The propensity of patients with liver failure to hypokalemia, whether the result of renal losses due to secondary aldosteronism or of gastrointestinal losses due to diarrhea, is well established. The induction of diuresis in these patients invariably aggravates their potassium losses. In the presence of advanced hepatic failure, the propensity of hypokalemic states to increase ammoniogenesis constitutes a real and imminent threat to hepatic encephalopathy. As such, the maintenance of normal potassium balance in patients with liver cirrhosis is essential. Amiloride has been successfully used to mobilize the edema of patients with liver cirrhosis while preventing potassium losses.[45, 107] In this regard, it has certain advantages over the other potassium-sparing agents. Unlike triamterene, it is excreted by the kidney and does not depend on hepatic clearance for its excretion, nor does it depend on hepatic metabolism for its activation.[108] Unlike spironolactone, it has a direct renal effect rather than competitively inhibiting aldosterone.[34]

The other indications of amiloride are less common but should be kept in mind. As competitive inhibitors of aldosterone, spironolactones are effective in the treatment of primary aldosteronism. However, amiloride has been shown also to be effective in controlling the hypertension and electrolyte disturbances associated with adrenal hyperplasia and adenoma.[15, 33, 34] Another use of amiloride is in the mitigation of polyuria due to lithium-induced nephrogenic diabetes insipidus.[109, 110] Amiloride, which in vitro antagonizes the inhibitory effect of lithium on vasopressin-induced water transport in a variety of epithelia,[111] also improves the defect in free water reabsorption caused by lithium in vivo.[112, 113] In this regard, it should be kept in mind that the volume depletion induced by diuretics can reduce the clearance of lithium. However, because of its small natriuretic effect, amiloride circumvents this problem in patients on lithium therapy. In combination with thiazides, amiloride can be used in the treatment of nephrogenic diabetes insipidus.[114] Amiloride is indicated in the treatment of hypokalemia in patients with Bartter's syndrome.[115, 116] Finally, bronchial inhalation of amiloride has been successfully used in the treatment of the mucoviscidosis of cystic fibrosis.[117]

Precautions and Adverse Effects

Electrolyte disorders and azotemia are the principal adverse effects associated with amiloride. Hyponatremia also may occur when amiloride is used with thiazides and loop diuretics.[118, 119] The incidence of hyponatremia induced by the combination of amiloride and hydrochlorothiazide appears to be low. It has occurred in elderly patients who have received prolonged diuretic therapy, especially when resistance to prior diuretic therapy necessitated the addition of amiloride. Azotemia has also been found in the same context, either in elderly patients or in those who previously were resistant to diuretic therapy. Both hyponatremia and azotemia are reversible after the discontinuation of diuretic therapy, restriction of water intake, restoration of volume depletion, and treatment of the underlying primary condition. Hyperkalemia is another more serious adverse effect of amiloride. Conditions that constitute a high risk for the development of hyperkalemia with amiloride use are the following:

1. Glomerular filtration rates less than 30 ml/min or serum creatinine levels higher than 2.5 to 3.0 mg/dl, particularly in patients with tubulointerstitial nephropathy who have distal tubular dysfunction

2. The presence of diabetes mellitus which, in addition to causing a reduction in glomerular filtration rate, may be associated with true hyporeninemic hypoaldosteronism or with a distal tubular defect in secreting potassium

3. Severe, relentless salt retention in patients whose avid proximal sodium reabsorption limits the distal delivery of sodium and therefore the ability to secrete potassium

4. Low-salt diets requiring salt substitutes that contain potassium or the use of other potassium supplements

5. Reduced renal function due to aging, particularly if serum creatinine concentration is not elevated because of reduced muscle mass and the renal insufficiency remains clinically undetected

6. Use of agents such as β-blockers that prevent potassium entry into cells[3, 120–123]

In the presence of normal renal function and the absence of conditions that compromise potassium metabolism, hyperkalemia is a rare complication of amiloride therapy unless doses exceed 20 mg/day.

Subacute and chronic toxicologic studies in monkeys, rats, and rabbits have revealed no organ toxicity or carcinogenicity of amiloride in dosages up to 5 mg/kg/day. No effect on the fetus was found in pregnant animals except at dosages of 8 mg/kg/day or greater. Studies in the rat have shown that amiloride is excreted in milk in concentrations higher than those found in blood.[6] Thus, the drug is not expected to adversely affect pregnancy, but its continued use in breast-feeding mothers is best avoided.

Contraindications

Amiloride is contraindicated in individuals who fall into the categories discussed in the preceding section—specifically, patients with renal insufficiency (creatinine concentration >2.5 to 3.0 mg/dl), patients with diabetic nephropathy (creatinine concentration >1.5 mg) or with tubulointerstitial nephropathy of any cause whose baseline potassium is high, patients who are taking potassium supplements or other potassium-sparing agents, and patients with known hypersensitivity to amiloride.

Interference and Interaction with Other Drugs

Amiloride per se does not interfere with other drugs. In fact, its principal use is with other drugs in its general category, diuretics, with which it can potentiate their action, particularly when secondary aldosteronism has developed such that distal sodium retention results in resistance to other diuretics. More important is its potassium- and magnesium-conserving ability, which prevents the potassium and magnesium losses associated with other diuretics. However, amiloride should not be used with other potassium-sparing diuretics, not only because its addition will be of no further therapeutic value to the patient but also because of the inherent risk of causing further potassium blocking and the potential risk of hypokalemia. The same concern has been expressed about the angiotensin-coverting enzyme inhibitors enalapril and captopril. These agents reduce hypokalemia associated with thiazide diuretics. Their administration to patients receiving amiloride not only may cause hyperkalemia but also may interfere with protection from hyperkalemia that would be provided by hyperaldosteronism from a direct effect of the elevated serum potassium levels. It is important to discontinue potassium supplements before starting amiloride ad-

ministration because of the increased risk of hyperkalemia.

By blocking the entry of potassium into cells, β-blockers may accentuate the elevated potassium level in patients taking potassium-sparing agents, particularly individuals with impaired renal function or on high potassium intake. This effect may occur even with the use of topical ophthalmic β-blockers.

The administration of corticosteroids, particularly those with mineralocorticoid activity, may increase potassium losses and decrease the natriuretic effect of amiloride, with apparent resistance to the drug. As a rule, increasing the dose of amiloride will overcome this effect of corticosteroids.[34]

Generally, nonsteroidal antiinflammatory agents, especially indomethacin, may reduce the antihypertensive effect of diuretics, probably because of the inhibition of renal prostaglandin synthesis with consequent sodium and water retention. In this regard, it might be noted that, unlike triamterene, amiloride actually enhances the renal production of prostaglandin E_2.[124]

Use in Patients with Impaired Organ Function

Potassium-sparing agents are contraindicated in patients with reduced renal function because of the risk of hyperkalemia. Amiloride is excreted unchanged by the kidney, and its half-life is prolonged in renal insufficiency. It should not be used in anyone with a serum creatinine concentration greater than 2.5 mg/dl except under special conditions, in which case the dosage should be reduced and the serum potassium closely monitored.[108, 120, 122]

Amiloride can be used in patients with liver disease. Unlike triamterene, it is neither cleared nor metabolized in the liver, nor does it depend on hepatic metabolism for activation. However, to the extent that the glomerular filtration rate may be reduced in patients with severe cirrhosis, amiloride is best administered in small doses and under careful monitoring of serum potassium concentration.[45, 108]

Place in the Antihypertensive Arsenal

The place of amiloride in the antihypertensive arsenal is its use in conjunction with hydrochlorothiazide to prevent the potassium and magnesium losses associated with thiazides used alone.

As with triamterene, the advantage of amiloride over spironolactone is its mechanism of action, which is independent of aldosterone; hence, no escape can occur. Amiloride is superior to spironolactone as a potassium-conserving agent, being as much as 15 times more potent, particularly in the first 10 hours of oral administration.[5, 6, 34] Its advantage over triamterene is its longer duration of action. A single oral dose may be sufficient to maintain potassium balance during both the initial high flow of diuresis and the subsequent period of secondary aldosteronism (see Fig. 45–3).[20] Triamterene, although effective in most instances on a once-daily basis, may have to be administered twice daily to preserve potassium.[113] In contrast to triamterene, amiloride does not interfere with folic acid metabolism or precipitate around kidney stone nuclei.[120, 126, 127]

Dosage and Administration

The usual dose of amiloride is 5 to 10 mg/day, but a lower dose of 2.5 mg may be sufficient and is preferred in the presence of reduced renal function. The maximum recommended dose of the drug is 20 mg/day. However, this dosage is rarely necessary and, should it be instituted, requires close monitoring of electrolytes. The drug is available only as an oral form in 5-mg tablets (Midamor).

The fixed-dose combination of 5 mg of amiloride hydrochloride and 50 mg of hydrochlorothiazide (Moduretic) is available in tablets. The usual dose is one or two tablets per day.

SOCIOECONOMIC CONSIDERATIONS

Diuretic agents, especially thiazides, remain the cornerstone of, if not the initial agents for, the treatment of essential hypertension, particularly when there are no special indications for other antihypertensive agents or contraindications for the use of a diuretic. Given their propensity to produce hypokalemia, the combined use of thiazides with potassium-sparing agents have proved specially effective. The combination of 50 mg of hydrochlorothiazide with 5 mg of amiloride as a once-daily agent is particularly effective in improving patient compliance.[128, 129] The cost-effectiveness of this combination is especially attractive when it is compared with alternative therapy with potassium supplements.

Some 20 to 40 mEq of potassium are required to prevent thiazide-induced hypokalemia. The cost of 1 mEq of potassium varies, but, when the amount to be used is considered, it is generally more expensive than amiloride.[130–132] In addition, potassium supplements increase the number of tablets to be ingested and the attendant problems of compliance. Finally, whereas gastrointestinal side effects of potassium supplements have been reduced with available formulations, they have in no way been eliminated and remain a real and imminent added concern.[120]

In terms of the cost of the amiloride-thiazide combination versus that of a triamterene-thiazide or spironolactone-thiazide combination, the amiloride combination saves money because of its duration of action, which is generally effective on a once-daily dosage, whereas twice-daily or more frequent dosage may be necessary with the other two potassium-sparing formulations.[125]

REFERENCES

1. Alter S, Cushman P, Hilton JG: A new guanidine diuretic, amipramizide: Reduction of the kaliuretic effect of ethacrynic acid. Clin Pharmacol Ther 8:243, 1966.
2. Wilson JD, Richmond DE, Simmonds HA, et al: MK-870: A new potassium-sparing diuretic. N Z Med J 65:505, 1966.
3. Bull MB, Laragh JH: Amiloride—A potassium-sparing natriuretic agent. Circulation 37:45, 1968.
4. Antcliff AC, Beevers DG, Hamilton M, et al: The use of amiloride hydrochloride in correction of hypokalemic alkalosis induced by diuretics. Postgrad Med J 47:644, 1971.
5. Baer JE, Jones CB, Spitzer SA, et al: The potassium-sparing and natriuretic activity of N-amidino-3,5,-diamino-6-chloropyrazine carboxamide hydrochloride dihydrate (amiloride hydrochloride). J Pharmacol Exp Ther 157:472, 1967.
6. Cragoe EJ: Pyrazine diuretics. In Cragoe EJ Jr (ed): Diuretics, Chemistry, Pharmacology, and Medicine. New York: John Wiley, 1983, pp 303–341.
7. Schmid E, Fricke G: Studies on urinary excretion of the potassium-retaining diuretic amiloride (desmethyl-pipazuroyl-guanidine, MK-870) in man. Pharmacol Clin 1:110, 1969.
8. USAN and the USP Dictionary of Drug Names. Rockville, MD: United States Pharmacopeial Conventions, 1987, p 37.
9. The Merck Index, 10th ed. Rahway, NJ: Merck, 1983, p 60.
10. Benos DL: Amiloride: A molecular probe of sodium transport in tissues and cells. Am J Physiol 242:C131, 1982.
11. Kleyman TR, Cragoe EJ: Cation transport probes: The amiloride series. Methods Enzymol 191:739, 1990.
12. Velazquez H, Wright FS: Control by drugs of renal potassium handling. Annu Rev Pharmacol Toxicol 26:293, 1986.
13. Knox FG, Hammond TG, Haramati A: Sites and mechanisms of action in the kidney and effect on monovalent ion excretion. In Eknoyan G, Martinez-Maldonado M (eds): The Physiological Basis of Diuretic Therapy. Orlando: Grune & Stratton, 1986, pp 95–108.
14. DuBose TD Jr: Effect on acid-base balance. In Eknoyan G, Martinez-Maldonado M (eds): The Physiological Basis of Diuretic Therapy. Orlando: Grune & Stratton, 1986, pp 125–137.
15. Melby JC, Griffing GT: Alterations in the renin-aldosterone system by diuretics and converting enzyme inhibitors. In Whelton PK, Whelton A, Walker WG (eds): Potassium in Cardiovascular and Renal Medicine. New York: Marcel Dekker, 1986, pp 53–65.
16. Borchgrevink PC, Holten T, Jynge P: Tissue electrolyte changes induced by high doses of diuretics in rats. Pharmacol Toxicol 60:77, 1987.
17. Ram CVS, Holland OB, Kaplan NM: Attenuation of diuretic-induced hypokalemia by amiloride, a potassium-sparing agent. J Clin Pharmacol 21:484, 1981.
18. Fernandez PG, Sharma JN, Galway AB, et al: Potassium conservation with amiloride/hydrochlorothiazide (Moduret) in thiazide-induced hypokalemia in hypertension. Curr Med Res Opin 8:120, 1982.
19. Field MJ, Berliner RW, Giebisch G: Regulation of renal potassium metabolism. In Maxwell M, Kleeman C, Narins RG (eds): Clinical Disorders of Fluid and Electrolyte Metabolism. New York: McGraw-Hill, 1987, pp 119–146.
20. Giebisch G: Some reflections on the mechanism of renal tubular potassium transport. Yale J Biol Med 48:315, 1975.
21. Melby JC: Selected mechanisms of diuretic-induced electrolyte changes. Am J Cardiol 58:1A, 1986.
22. Stoner LC, Burg MB, Orloff J: Ion transport in cortical collecting tubule: Effect of amiloride. Am J Physiol 227:453, 1974.
23. Weinman SA, Reuss L: Na$^+$-H$^+$ exchange at the apical membrane of Necturus gallbladder: Extracellular and intracellular pH studies. J Gen Physiol 80:299, 1982.
24. Kinsella JL, Aronson PS: Amiloride inhibition of the Na$^+$-H$^+$ exchanger in renal microvillus membrane vesicles. Am J Physiol 241:F374, 1981.
25. Schwartz GJ: Na$^+$-dependent H$^+$ efflux from proximal tubule: Evidence for reversible Na$^+$-H$^+$ exchange. Am J Physiol 241:F380, 1981.
26. Kunau RT Jr, Walker KA: Total CO$_2$ absorption in the distal tubule of the rat. Am J Physiol 252:F468, 1987.
27. Frommer JP, Wesson DE, Laski ME, et al: Bicarbonate reabsorption by the collecting duct of the Munich-Wistar rat. Clin Res 31:444A, 1983.
28. Weiss P, Hersey RM, Dujovne CA, et al: The metabolism of amiloride hydrochloride in man. Clin Pharmacol Ther 10:401, 1969.

29. Soltoff SP, Mandel LM: Amiloride directly inhibits the Na, K-ATPase activity of rabbit kidney proximal tubules. Science 220:957, 1983.
30. Costa CJ, Kirschner LB, Cragoe EJ Jr: Intracellular binding of spin-labeled amiloride: An alternative explanation for amiloride's effect at high concentration. J Cell Physiol 130:392, 1987.
31. Cassel D, Cragoe EJ Jr, Rotman M: A dextran-bound amiloride derivative is a selective inhibitor of Na$^+$/H$^+$ antiport: Application for studying the role of the antiporter in cellular proliferation in human fibroblasts. J Biol Chem 262:4587, 1987.
32. O'Neill RG, Dubinsky WP: Amiloride uptake into rabbit renal epithelial cells: A fluorescent study. Kidney Int 23:264, 1983.
33. Kremer D, Boddy K, Brown JJ, et al: Amiloride in the treatment of primary hyperaldosteronism and essential hypertension. Clin Exp Pharmacol Physiol 4:55, 1978.
34. McInnes GT: Relative potency of amiloride and spironolactone in healthy man. Clin Pharmacol Ther 31:472, 1982.
35. Baer JE: Role of drug metabolism in drug research and development: Basic considerations. J Pharm Sci 61:1674, 1972.
36. Smith AJ, Smith RN: Kinetics and bioavailability of two formulations of amiloride in man. Br J Pharmacol 48:646, 1973.
37. Somogyi AA, Hovens CM, Muirhead MR, Bochner F: Renal tubular secretion of amiloride and its inhibition by cimetidine in humans and in an animal model. Drug Metab Dispos Biol Fate Chem 17:190, 1989.
38. Schwartz A, Seller R, Onesti G, et al: Pharmacodynamic effects of a new potassium-sparing diuretic, amiloride. J Clin Pharmacol 9:217, 1969.
39. Lant AF, Smith AJ, Wilson GM: Clinical evaluation of amiloride, a potassium sparing diuretic. Clin Pharmacol Ther 10:50, 1969.
40. Baba WI, Lant AF, Smith AJ, et al: Pharmacological effects in animals and normal human subjects of the diuretic amiloride hydrochloride MK-870. Clin Pharm 9:318, 1968.
41. Lammintausta R, Kanto J, Mantyla R: Renin-aldosterone system and urinary electrolytes after amiloride, hydrochlorothiazide and the combination. Int J Clin Pharmacol 16:503, 1978.
42. George CF: Amiloride handling in renal failure. Br J Clin Pharmacol 9:94, 1980.
43. Davidson C, Gillebrand IM: Use of amiloride as a potassium conserving agent in severe cardiac disease. Br Heart J 35:456, 1973.
44. Ryan MP: Magnesium and potassium-sparing diuretics. Magnesium 5:282, 1986.
45. Yamada S, Reynolds TB: Amiloride (MK870) a new antikaliuretic diuretic: Comparison to other antikaliuretic diuretics in patients with liver disease and ascites. Gastroenterology 59:833, 1970.
46. Wester PO, Dyckner T: Diuretic treatment and magnesium losses. Acta Med Scand 647:145, 1981.
47. Allenberg GA, Negri AL, Rainoldi FA, et al: Acute effect of amiloride on urinary magnesium excretion in dogs. Acta Physiol Pharmacol Latinoam 36:89, 1986.
48. Shareghi GR, Agus ZS: Phosphate transport in the light segment of the rabbit cortical collecting tubule. Am J Physiol 242:F379, 1982.
49. Quamme GA, Dirks JH: Magnesium transport in the nephron. Am J Physiol 239:F393, 1980.
50. Wildman L, Dyckner T, Webster PO: Effect of moduretic and aldactone on electrolytes in skeletal muscle in patients on long-term diuretic therapy. Acta Med Scand 661:33, 1982.
51. Abraham AS, Roseman D, Meshulam Z, et al: Intracellular cations and diuretic therapy following acute myocardial infarction. Arch Intern Med 146:1301, 1986.
52. Ryan MP: Diuretics and potassium/magnesium depletion: Directions for treatment. Am J Med 82:38, 1987.
53. Dyckner T, Wester PO: Potassium-sparing diuretics. Acta Med Scand 707:79, 1986.
54. Schwinter RH, Antoni DH: Triamterene may presreve lymphocyte magnesium and potassium in patients with congestive heart failure. Magnes Res 5:29, 1992.
55. Johny KV, Lawrence JR, O'Halloran W: Amiloride hydrochloride: A hypercalciuric diuretic. Aust Ann Med 18:267, 1969.
56. Costanzo LS, Weiner IM: Relationship between clearance of Ca and Na: Effect of distal diuretics and PTH. Am J Physiol 230:67, 1976.
57. Costanzo LS: Comparison of calcium and sodium transport in early and late rat distal tubules: Effect of amiloride. Am J Physiol 246:F937, 1984.
58. Hutler HN, Ilnicki LP, Licht H, et al: On the mechanism of diminished urinary carbon dioxide tension caused by amiloride. Kidney Int 21:8, 1982.
59. Linz W, Albus U, Wiener G, et al: Amiloride potentiates the vascular effects of atrial natriuretic factor. J Hypertens 6:S300, 1988.
60. Iwata T, Hardee E, Frohlich ED, Cole FE: Amiloride enhances atrial natriuretic factor stimulation of cGMP accumulation of rat glomeruli. Peptides 10:575, 1989.
61. Seino M, Abe K, Nushiro N, et al: The effects of atrial natriuretic peptide and amiloride on renal hemodynamics and the renal kallikrein-kinin system. J Hypertens 6:321, 1988.
62. Borchgrevink PC, Jynge P: Direct effects of furosemide and amiloride on the perfused and ischaemic heart. Pharmacol Toxicol 64:100, 1989.
63. Spence JD, Wong DG: Amiloride with or without salbutamol versus placebo: Effects on lipoproteins in hypertensive patients with timolol-hydrochlorothiazide. J Hypertens 4:S515, 1986.
64. Holland OB, Nixon JV, Kuhnert L: Diuretic-induced ventricular ectopic activity. Am J Med 70:762, 1981.
65. Hollifield JW, Slaton PE: Thiazide diuretics, hypokalemia and cardiac arrhythmias. Acta Med Scand 647:67, 1981.
66. Whelton PK, Watson AJ: Diuretic-induced hypokalemia and cardiac arrhythmias. Am J Cardiol 58:5A, 1986.
67. Surawicz B, Lepeschkin E: The electrocardiographic pattern of hypopotassemia with and without hypocalcemia. Circulation 8:801, 1953.
68. Helefant RH: Hypokalemia and arrhythmias. Am J Med 80:13, 1986.
69. Solomon RJ: Ventricular arrhythmias with myocardial infarction and ischaemia: Relationship to serum potassium and magnesium. Drugs 28:66, 1984.
70. Lumme JA, Jounela AJ: Cardiac arrhythmias in hypertensive outpatients on various diuretics: Correlation between incidence and serum potassium and magnesium levels. Ann Clin Res 18:186, 1986.
71. Papademetriou V, Fletcher R, Khatri IM, et al: Diuretic-induced hypokalemia in uncomplicated systemic hypertension: Effect of plasma potassium correction on cardiac arrhythmias. Am J Cardiol 52:1017, 1983.
72. Madias JE, Madias NE, Gavras HP: Non-arrhythmogenicity of diuretic-induced hypokalemia: Its evidence in patients with uncomplicated hypertension. Arch Intern Med 144:2171, 1984.
73. Atwood JE, Gardin JM: Diuretics, hypokalemia, and ventricular ectopy: The controversy continues. Arch Intern Med 145:1185, 1985.
74. Morgan DB, Davidson C: Hypokalemia and diuretics: An analysis of publications. Br Med J 280:905, 1980.
75. Nordrehaug JE, Von Der Lippe G: Hypokalemia and ventricular fibrillation in acute myocardial infarction. Br Heart J 50:525, 1983.
76. Ikran H, Espiner EA, Nicholls MG: Diuretics, potassium and arrhythmias in hypertensive coronary disease. Drugs 4:101, 1986.
77. Struthers AD, Whitesmith R, Reid JL: Prior thiazide diuretic treatment increases adrenaline-induced hypokalemia. Lancet 1:1358, 1983.
78. Holland OB: Potassium loss, ventricular irritability, and the risk of sudden death in hypertensive patients. Drugs 4:78, 1986.
79. Maronde RF, Milgram M, Vlachakis ND, et al: Response of thiazide-induced hypokalemia to amiloride. JAMA 249:237, 1983.
80. Svendsen UG, Ibsen H, Rasmussen S, et al: Effects of combined therapy with amiloride and hydrochlorothiazide on plasma and total body potassium, blood pressure, and the renin-angiotensin-aldosterone system in hypertensive patients. Eur J Clin Pharmacol 30:151, 1986.
81. From AH, Probstfield JL, Smith TR: Ethacrynic acid induced inotropism. Proc Soc Exp Biol Med 149:1059, 1975.

82. Pousti A, Khoyi MA: Effect of amiloride on isolated guinea pig atrium. Arch Int Pharmacodyn Ther 242:222, 1979.

83. Yamashita S, Motomura S, Taira N: Cardiac effects of amiloride in the dog. J Cardiovasc Pharmacol 3:704, 1981.

84. Satoh H, Hashimoto K: An electrophysiological study of amiloride on sino-atrial node cells and ventricular muscle of rabbit and dog. Naunyn Schmiedebergs Arch Pharmacol 333:83, 1986.

85. Seller RH, Greco J, Banach S, et al: Increasing the inotropic effect of toxic dose of digitalis by the administration of antikaliuretic drugs: Further evidence for a cardiac effect of diuretic agents. Am Heart J 90:56, 1975.

86. Walter SD: Cardiac actions of kaliuretics and anti-kaliuretics without digitalis. Am Heart J 92:124, 1975.

87. Poole-Wilson PA, Cobbe SM, Fry CH: Acute effects of diuretics on potassium exchange, mechanical function, and the action potential in rabbit myocardium. Clin Sci Mol Med 55:555, 1978.

88. Gibson K, Harris P: Effect of diuretics on microsomal (Na^+K^+) ATPase in human heart and the rat heart and kidney. Cardiovasc Res 4:343, 1970.

89. Periyasamy SM: Inhibition of cardiac sarcolemmal Na^+/H^+ antiporter by opioids. Can J Physiol Pharmacol 70:1048, 1992.

90. Scholz M, Albus U, Linz W, et al: Effects of Na^+/H^+ exchange inhibitors in cardiac ischemia. J Mol Cell Cardiol 24:731, 1992.

91. Lotan CS, Miller SK, Prohost GM, Elgavish GA: Amiloride in ouabain-induced acidification, inotropy, and arrhythmia. J Mol Cell Cardiol 24:243, 1992.

92. Rabkin SW: Digitalis glycosides accentuate the depressant effect of anoxia and reoxygenation on the cardiac myocytes: Antagonism by amiloride. Arch Int Pharmacodyn Ther 313:76, 1991.

93. Multicenter Diuretic Cooperative Study Group: Multiclinic comparison of amiloride, hydrochlorothiazide, and hydrochlorothiazide plus amiloride in essential hypertension. Arch Intern Med 141:482, 1981.

94. Myers MG: Hydrochlorothiazide with or without amiloride for hypertension in the elderly. A dose-titration study. Arch Intern Med 147:1026, 1987.

95. Gombos EA, Fries ED, Moghadam A: Effects of MK-870 in normal subjects and hypertensive patients. N Engl J Med 275:1215, 1966.

96. Salmela PI, Juustila H, Kinnunen O, et al: Comparison of low doses of hydrochlorothiazide plus amiloride and hydrochlorothiazide alone in hypertension in elderly patients. Ann Clin Res 18:88, 1986.

97. Patterson JW, Dollery CT, Haslam RM: Amiloride hydrochloride in hypertensive patients. Br Med J 1:422, 1968.

98. Kaplan NM, Carnegie A, Raskin P, et al: Potassium supplementation in hypertensive patients with diuretic-induced hypokalemia. N Engl J Med 312:746, 1985.

99. Davson H, Segal MB: The effects of some inhibitors and accelerators of sodium transport on the turnover of ^{22}Na in the cerebrospinal fluid and brain. J Physiol 209:131, 1970.

100. Dormer FR: Effects of diuretics on cerebrospinal fluid formation and fluid movement. Exp Neurol 24:54, 1969.

101. Soltoff SP, Cragoe EJ Jr, Mandel LJ: Amiloride analogues inhibit proximal tubule metabolism. Am J Physiol 250:C744, 1986.

102. Friedrich T, Sablotni J, Burckhardt G: Identification of the renal Na^+/H^+ exchanger with N,N'-dicyclohexylcarbodiimide (DCCD) and amiloride analogues. J Membr Biol 94:253, 1986.

103. Li JH, Cragoe EJ Jr, Lindemann B: Structure-activity relationship of amiloride analogs as blockers of epithelial Na channels. II: Side-chain modifications. J Membr Biol 95:171, 1987.

104. Multiple Risk Factor Intervention Trial Research Group: Baseline rest electrocardiographic abnormalities, antihypertensive treatment and mortality in the Multiple Risk Factor Intervention Trial. Am J Cardiol 55:1, 1985.

105. Kaplan NM: Therapy of mild hypertension: An overview. Am J Cardiol 53:2A, 1984.

106. MRC Working Party: Medical Research Council Trial of Treatment of Hypertension in Older Adults. Br Med J 304:405, 1992.

107. Bianchi GP, Petrillo M: Prevention of diuretic induced electrolyte disturbances by amiloride in patients with ascites due to cirrhosis of the liver. Acta Cardiol 17:307, 1973.

108. Brater DC: Clinical pharmacokinetics. In Eknoyan G, Martinez-Maldonado M (eds): The Physiological Basis of Diuretic Therapy in Clinical Medicine. Orlando: Grune & Stratton, 1986, pp 27–55.

109. Battle DC, Von Riotte AB, Gaviria M, et al: Amelioration of polyuria by amiloride in patients receiving long-term lithium therapy. N Engl J Med 312:408, 1985.

110. Kosten TR, Forrest JN: Treatment of severe lithium-induced polyuria with amiloride. Am J Psychiatry 143:1563, 1986.

111. Singer I, Franko EA: Lithium-induced ADH resistance in toad urinary bladder. Kidney Int 3:151, 1973.

112. Martinez-Maldonado M, Opova-Stitzer S: Distal nephron function of the rat during lithium chloride infusion. Kidney Int 12:17, 1977.

113. Mehta PK, Sodhi B, Arruda JL, et al: Interaction of amiloride and lithium on distal urinary acidification. J Lab Clin Med 93:983, 1979.

114. Knoers N, Monnens LA: Nephrogenic diabetes insipidus: Clinical symptoms, pathogenesis, genetics, and treatment. Pediatr Nephrol 6:476, 1992.

115. Griffing GT, Komanicky P, Aurecchia SA, et al: Amiloride in Bartter's syndrome. Clin Pharmacol Ther 31:713, 1982.

116. Colussi G, Rombola G, Verde G, et al: Distal nephron function in Bartter Syndrome: Abnormal conductance to chloride in the cortical collecting tubule? Am J Nephrol 12:229, 1992.

117. Lenoir G, Willemot JM, Pradier J, et al: Amiloride hydrochloride nebulized by oxygen in the treatment of mucoviscidosis. Rev Mal Respir 9:613, 1992.

118. Strykers PH, Stern RS, Morse BM: Hyponatremia induced by a combination of amiloride and hydrochlorothiazide. JAMA 252:389, 1984.

119. Bayer AJ, Farag R, Browne S, et al: Plasma electrolytes in elderly patients taking fixed combination diuretics. Postgrad Med J 62:159, 1986.

120. Frommer JP, Wesson DE, Eknoyan G: Side effects and complications of diuretic therapy. In Eknoyan G, Martinez-Maldonado M (eds): The Physiological Basis of Diuretic Therapy in Clinical Medicine. Orlando: Grune & Stratton, 1986, pp 293–309.

121. Greenblatt DJ, Koch-Weser J: Adverse reactions to spironolactone: A report from the Boston Collaborative Surveillance Program. JAMA 225:40, 1973.

122. Kassirer JP, Harrington JT: Diuretics and potassium metabolism: A reassessment of the need, effectiveness and safety of potassium therapy. Kidney Int 11:505, 1977.

123. Yap V, Patel A, Thomsen J: Hyperkalemia with cardiac arrhythmia: Induction by salt substitutes, spironolactone and azotemia. JAMA 236:2775, 1976.

124. Zawada ET Jr: Antihypertensive therapy with triamterene-hydrochlorothiazide vs amiloride-hydrochlorothiazide. Comparison of effects on urinary prostaglandin E_2 excretion. Arch Intern Med 146:1312, 1986.

125. Ridgeway, NA, Ginn DR, Alley K: Outpatient conversion of treatment to potassium-sparing diuretics. Am J Med 80:785, 1986.

126. Werness PG, Bergert JH, Smith LH: Triamterene lithiasis: Solubility pK effect on crystal formation and matrix binding of triamterene and its metabolites. J Lab Clin Med 99:254, 1982.

127. Zimmerman J, Selhub J, Rosenberg IH: Competitive inhibition of folic acid absorption in rat jejunum by triamterene. J Lab Clin Med 108:272, 1986.

128. Myers MG: Diuretic therapy for hypertension in the elderly. Drugs 4:184, 1986.

129. Morgan TO, Nowson C, Murphy J, et al: Compliance and the elderly hypertensive. Drugs 4:174, 1986.

130. Vardan S, Rapacke J, Mookerjee S: Clinical efficacy and cost comparison of an amiloride-hydrochlorothiazide combination versus hydrochlorothiazide and wax-matrix potassium supplement in the treatment of essential hypertension. Clin Ther 8:420, 1986.

131. Stason WB: Opportunities for improving the cost-effectiveness of antihypertensive treatment. Am J Med 81(Suppl 6C):45, 1986.

132. Maronde RF, Chan LS, Vlachakis N: Hypokalemia in thiazide-treated systemic hypertension. Am J Cardiol 58:18A, 1986.

CHAPTER 46

Spironolactone

Kwan Eun Kim, M.D.

Spironolactone, a 17-spirolactone steroid, is a specific aldosterone antagonist that competitively binds to the cytoplasmic hormone receptors to prevent cellular response. Spironolactone, therefore, impairs reabsorption of sodium and secretion of potassium and hydrogen ions in the distal renal tubule, thereby producing potassium retention, natriuresis, and diuresis.

Since the introduction of spironolactone in 1959, the agent has been used successfully in the treatment of hypertension, primary aldosteronism, and edematous conditions, such as occur with congestive heart failure, cirrhosis of the liver, and nephrotic syndrome.

MECHANISM OF ACTION

The aldosterone receptors are found in the cytosol, the soluble fraction of cytoplasm of the target cells. Aldosterone receptors are present in several tissues, including the salivary glands, colon, and several segments of the nephron. In the context of the action of spironolactone, the most important target cells are those of the late distal renal tubule and renal collecting duct.

Spironolactone acts as a competitive inhibitor of the binding of aldosterone to its receptors in responsive cells of the distal nephron.[1, 2] In the presence of aldosterone, spironolactone antagonizes sodium and potassium exchange in the distal renal tubule. The end results are natriuresis, diuresis, and potassium retention.

It has also been shown that spironolactone can inhibit aldosterone synthesis *in vitro*.[3] However, such an effect may be of little significance *in vivo*, because the doses required to inhibit aldosterone biosynthesis *in vitro* are much larger than those needed to inhibit receptor binding of aldosterone.[1]

PHARMACOKINETICS

Spironolactone is extensively metabolized in human subjects.[4–6] The metabolic pathway of spironolactone is shown in Figure 46–1.[5]

Until recently, spironolactone and its metabolites were measured fluorometrically.[7–9] Canrenone had been considered the major biologically active metabolite of spironolactone.[4, 10, 11] With the introduction of high-performance liquid chromatographic methods to measure canrenone concentration in blood, it became clear that fluorometric methods were not specific for canrenone but measured other metabolites as well.[5, 12–16]

It has been shown that, following a single dose of spironolactone in humans, canrenone accounts for only 11% of the antimineralocorticoid activity at peak concentration and for 15% over 24 hours. After long-term dosing, canrenone accounts for only about 25% of activity at steady state.[12, 13, 15, 16] These findings indicate that canrenone is not a major biologically active metabolite of spironolactone.[12, 13, 15, 16] Overdiek et al.[5] and Gardiner et al.[17] showed that 7-α-thiomethylspirolactone is the major metabolite of spironolactone detectable in the plasma following a single[15, 17] or repeated doses of spironolactone.[17] This metabolite has been shown to possess a higher affinity for aldosterone receptors in rat kidney slices than canrenone does.[18] Furthermore, it has potent antimineralocorticoid activity in rats and dogs.[19] However, in a bioassay model developed to determine the renal antimineralocorticoid activity of orally administered spironolactone in humans, the activity of 7-α-thiomethylspirolactone was found to be 33% that of spironolactone.[20] Because serum concentrations of this metabolite were not determined in the study,[20] incomplete absorption or extensive first-pass metabolism could not be ruled out as a reason for this reduced *in vivo* activity.[21]

It had been reported that spironolactone is metabolized too rapidly to be detected in plasma or urine.[4, 11, 20, 22] However, unchanged spironolactone has been detected in serum.[5, 17, 21, 23, 24] In comparison to canrenone, spironolactone has a higher affinity for rat renal aldosterone receptors,[18] and it has antimineralocorticoid action in an isolated bladder system.[25] No metabolite of spironolactone has been found that is more active in human subjects than the unchanged parent drug.[5] Therefore, unmetabolized spironolactone itself might be responsible for much of its antimineralocorticoid action.[5] Further studies are necessary to clarify the pharmacokinetics of spironolactone.

Concomitant food intake has been shown to enhance its bioavailability, by increasing the absorption and decreasing the first-pass effect of spironolactone.[26]

Spironolactone has a gradual onset of diuretic action, with the maximal effect being reached the third day of therapy.[27, 28] After withdrawal of spironolactone, diuresis persists for 2 or 3 days.[28]

CLINICAL USES
Treatment of Hypertension

Spironolactone has been administered to reduce blood pressure and to prevent or correct hypokalemia induced by kaliuretic diuretics. It has been shown that spironolactone is as effective as hydrochlorothiazide or chlorthalidone in lowering blood pressure in patients with essential hypertension.[29–34] The daily doses of spironolactone, hydrochlorothiazide, and

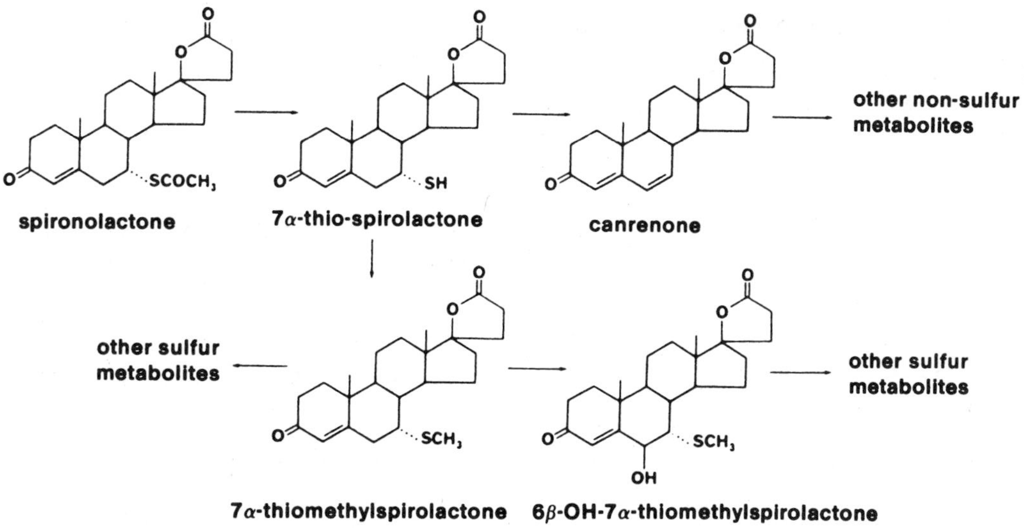

Figure 46–1. Metabolic pathway of spironolactone.

chlorthalidone administered were 50 to 400 mg, 50 to 100 mg, and 100 mg, respectively.[29–34]

Schrijver and Weinberger[30] reported that spironolactone in doses of 200 and 400 mg/day did not produce a greater antihypertensive effect than doses of 100 mg/day, and gynecomastia was encountered only in doses of 200 and 400 mg/day. Scherstén et al.[35] found that a 200-mg daily dose of spironolactone has more antihypertensive effect than a 50-mg daily dose but does not differ from the effectiveness of a 100-mg daily dose. Jeunemaitre et al.[36] also reported that blood pressure reduction was greater with 75 to 100 mg of spironolactone daily than with 25 to 50 mg of spironolactone daily, but no additional reduction was found with doses above 150 mg daily. They found that gynecomastia was reversible and dose-related; at doses of 50 mg or less, the incidence was 6.9%, but it was 52.2% for doses of 150 mg or higher.[36] Therefore, a daily dose of 50 to 100 mg spironolactone is recommended for the treatment of patients with essential hypertension.

Spironolactone may be given alone or combined with a thiazide or another kaliuretic diuretic or nondiuretic antihypertensive agent. The antihypertensive effects of spironolactone and kaliuretic diuretics are additive, and hypokalemia may be prevented or corrected when they are used in combination.[37, 38] It has also been shown that spironolactone and propranolol,[39] metoprolol,[40] methyldopa,[34] or nifedipine[41] have synergistic or additive hypotensive effects.[34, 39–41]

Spironolactone is effective for short-term preoperative control of blood pressure and serum potassium levels in patients with primary aldosteronism associated with adrenal adenoma. In patients with primary aldosteronism, long-term medical therapy with spironolactone is the treatment of choice for patients with bilateral adrenal hyperplasia or for patients with adrenal adenoma who are unable or unwilling to undergo surgery.[42] It is useful in patients who remain hypertensive after adrenal surgery.

Unlike thiazides, spironolactone alters plasma glucose, lipid, and uric acid levels little and only transiently.[43] Spironolactone can therefore be useful for patients in whom such biochemical changes may be particularly detrimental, such as those with gout.

Spironolactone is often prescribed in combination with a kaliuretic diuretic to prevent hypokalemia and obtain simultaneously an added hypotensive or natriuretic action. Many patients with diuretic-induced hypokalemia are treated with potassium chloride supplements. The ability of potassium chloride and spironolactone to raise plasma potassium cannot be accurately compared, because the dose response of potassium chloride is not parallel to that of spironolactone. Spironolactone in a daily dose of 100 mg corrected hypokalemia better than 64 mEq of potassium chloride.[44–46] Both triamterene and spironolactone have significant and parallel dose-response curves for increasing plasma potassium concentration, with a potency ratio of 4:1.[44] Thus, 100 mg of triamterene is equivalent to 25 mg of spironolactone.

The ratio of the abilities of amiloride and spironolactone to increase plasma potassium concentration is 2.8:1.0.[45] Therefore, 20 mg of amiloride is equivalent to 56 mg of spironolactone. George et al.[47] reported that the potassium-retaining effect of spironolactone was sustained, but the potassium-retaining effect of amiloride declined 1 month after administration of the drug.

Ramsay et al.[45] have shown that spironolactone is effective even when plasma aldosterone concentrations are well within the normal range. The additive antihypertensive effects of thiazide and spironolactone in a combination preparation, as well as the beneficial effects of this combination on serum potassium levels, have been reported.[29, 48, 49] However, the rise in plasma potassium concentration induced by spironolactone varies considerably among patients, so the fixed-dose thiazide-spironolactone combination tablets may not reliably prevent hypokalemia.[50]

Treatment of Congestive Heart Failure

Spironolactone, both alone and combined with a thiazide diuretic or a loop diuretic, has been effective in the treatment of patients with heart failure.[51] Spironolactone has a weak diuretic and natriuretic action, which produces a maximum fractional sodium excretion of about 2%. Spironolactone prevents or corrects diuretic-induced hypokalemia and has an additive diuretic effect when administered concomitantly with a kaliuretic diuretic that acts at different sites in the renal tubule.[52]

The most widely used diuretics in the treatment of heart failure are thiazide diuretics and loop diuretics. Both are associated with certain undesirable metabolic effects, most notably hypokalemia.[53-58]

The addition of spironolactone has been shown to produce a substantial diuresis and clinical improvement in patients with severe heart failure refractory to combination therapy with high doses of a loop diuretic, with low doses of an angiotensin-converting enzyme (ACE) inhibitor, and with or without digitalis.[59-62] The ACE inhibitor was restricted to low doses in these patients with severe congestive heart failure because of hypotension and consequent renal insufficiency.[60]

Low doses of an ACE inhibitor did not suppress aldosterone significantly.[60, 62] A low-dose ACE inhibitor and spironolactone must be combined only in the absence of hyperkalemia and significant azotemia and under careful monitoring of potassium levels and renal function.

Treatment of Cirrhotic Ascites

Hyperaldosteronism has been considered important in sodium retention in patients with cirrhosis of the liver.[63-65] However, it has been shown that plasma aldosterone concentrations of patients with cirrhosis and ascites range from normal to very high values.[63-65] Furthermore, sodium retention may persist despite lowering of the plasma aldosterone concentration to normal levels, which suggests that factors other than aldosterone play an important role in the sodium retention of cirrhosis.[65, 66] Arroyo et al.[64] found a significant inverse relationship between plasma aldosterone levels and urinary sodium excretion in patients with nonazotemic cirrhosis and ascites, suggesting that, even though aldosterone is not the only factor implicated in sodium retention, it appears to influence the degree of sodium excretion in these patients. Spironolactone has been shown to be the most effective diuretic agent in the management of cirrhotic ascites.[63] The administration of furosemide alone was followed by a satisfactory diuretic response in only 11 of 21 nonazotemic cirrhotic patients with ascites (51%), whereas spironolactone was effective in 18 of 19 patients (95%).[63] Potassium stores are frequently depleted in cirrhotic patients.[67] Therefore, the most rational and effective treatment of cirrhosis with ascites is the administration of spironolactone.

Shear et al.[68] showed that disparity between the rates of mobilization of ascitic and nonascitic fluid in cirrhotic patients was evident during spontaneous diuresis but most marked during diuretic administration. After diuretic administration, the rate of ascites absorption varied markedly but did not exceed 930 ml per 24 hours despite the excretion of up to 4.7 L of nonascitic fluid.

Pockros and Reynolds[69] showed that patients with ascites and no edema were able to mobilize more than 1 L/day of ascitic fluid during rapid diuresis, although at the expense of plasma volume contraction and renal insufficiency. Patients with ascites and edema did not develop plasma volume contraction or renal insufficiency during rapid diuresis because of preferential mobilization of edema. These patients with edema may safely undergo rapid diuresis until edema disappears.

An initial dose of 100 mg of spironolactone per day is recommended for the treatment of ascites in cirrhotic patients. If there is no satisfactory diuretic response after 3 to 5 days of treatment, the dosage of spironolactone may be increased stepwise every 3 to 5 days to a maximum of 400 mg/day. Spironolactone has a gradual onset of diuretic action, with the maximum effect being reached on the third day of therapy.[27, 28] If no satisfactory diuretic response occurs with the maximum dosage of spironolactone, a loop diuretic agent should be added. Among loop diuretics, furosemide, 40 to 80 mg/day, has been most commonly administered.[63, 70, 71] If diuretic response is unsatisfactory, the dosage of furosemide may be increased stepwise to a maximum of 240 mg/day.

Treatment of Edema Accompanying the Nephrotic Syndrome

The mechanisms of sodium retention in patients with nephrotic syndrome are complex and are not precisely known.[72-80] The plasma aldosterone concentrations in patients with nephrotic syndrome have been found to range from low to high.[72-76] Clinical and experimental studies have shown that enhanced renal tubular sodium reabsorption in patients with nephrotic syndrome occurs along the distal nephron sites[77, 78] as well as the proximal tubules.[79] It appears that the plasma aldosterone concentration and the nephron sites of enhanced sodium reabsorption in patients with nephrotic syndrome depend on the stage of sodium retention and underlying renal disease.[74, 75, 77-79]

Loop diuretics and thiazides are the most widely used diuretics in the treatment of patients with nephrotic edema. Spironolactone may prevent or correct diuretic-induced hypokalemia and may have an additive diuretic effect when administered concomitantly with a thiazide or loop diuretic. Spironolactone should not be used in patients with renal failure because of the risk of hyperkalemia.

Treatment of Hirsutism

Spironolactone has been used effectively in the treatment of hirsutism in women with polycystic ovary syndrome or idiopathic hirsutism.[81, 82] Spironolactone, an aldosterone antagonist, also has an antiandrogenic action. Spironolactone reduces testosterone biosynthesis by inhibiting 17-hydroxylase activity and microsomal cytochrome P-450 reductase in both gonads and adrenal glands.[83–85] In addition, spironolactone competitively inhibits the interaction between 5-dehydrotestosterone and its cytoplasmic receptor protein in the skin and other peripheral tissues.[83–88] Spironolactone also decreases skin 5-reductase activity.[89]

In hirsutism, spironolactone is administered in doses of 75 to 200 mg/day.[82, 91] Efficacy is not clearly improved with higher doses, but adverse reactions appear to be dose-related.[90]

Renal and Systemic Hemodynamic Effects

It has been shown that the glomerular filtration rate does not change after 3 days and after 3 months of spironolactone therapy.[91] After 4 months of spironolactone therapy, the decrease in blood pressure was associated with a significant decrease in total peripheral resistance and no change in cardiac output.[92] Spironolactone therapy increases plasma renin activity.[30, 31, 33, 34, 91, 92]

Vascular and Cardiac Effects

Studies suggest that spironolactone blocks aldosterone-mediated sodium efflux[93] and inhibits slow calcium channels in vascular smooth muscle cells.[94–96]

Elevated aldosterone levels in experimental animal models (unilateral renal ischemia or hyperaldosteronism) have been associated with excessive collagen accumulation resulting in myocardial fibrosis.[97–101] Ventricular stiffness and pathologic ventricular hypertrophy can then follow.[101] Spironolactone pretreatment in these animal models prevented myocardial fibrosis.[100]

Adverse Effects and Drug Interactions

The most serious adverse effect of spironolactone therapy is hyperkalemia. The risk of hyperkalemia is greatly increased in patients with renal insufficiency and in those who simultaneously receive potassium supplements.[102] In the Boston Collaborative Drug Surveillance Program, 8.6% of patients taking spironolactone developed hyperkalemia.[102] However, the incidence of hyperkalemia in nonazotemic patients who were not receiving potassium supplementation was only 2.8%, whereas in patients with blood urea nitrogen values of 50 mg/100 ml or greater who received potassium chloride and spironolactone, 42.1% became hyperkalemic.[102] Salt substitutes contain large amounts of potassium and may lead to hyperkalemia if taken by patients receiving spironolactone.[103]

Hyperchloremic metabolic acidosis, usually associated with hyperkalemia, may occur in patients with decompensated hepatic cirrhosis.[104] The effect of spironolactone in lowering serum bicarbonate concentra-

tion in these patients may be due to direct antagonism of aldosterone's stimulation of renal hydrogen ion secretion.[104, 105] It also has been shown that urinary ammonia excretion correlates inversely with serum potassium concentration in patients with hypoaldosteronism.[106] Therefore, spironolactone-induced hyperkalemia may suppress ammonia production, thereby contributing to the development of hyperchloremic metabolic acidosis.[104] Like other diuretic agents, spironolactone may cause hyponatremia, dehydration, and a rise in blood urea nitrogen and serum creatinine.[32–36, 102]

Long-term administration of spironolactone has been found to cause an increase,[30, 35] no change,[34, 36, 107, 108] or a transient decrease[43] in serum uric acid concentration. Schrijver and Weinberger,[30] in a comparison of spironolactone and hydrochlorothiazide, found larger increases in uric acid levels in patients treated with hydrochlorothiazide than in those treated with spironolactone. Falch and Schreiner[43] observed a decrease in the serum uric acid level after 6 months of spironolactone therapy, but the level returned to the control value after 12 months of the therapy. Roos et al.[107] reported that spironolactone therapy decreased uric acid clearance and uric acid excretion, but serum uric acid concentration did not change. These authors[107] suggested that spironolactone therapy probably inhibited endogenous uric acid production to about the same degree as it decreased clearance, so that no change in the serum uric acid level occurred.

It appears that spironolactone therapy does not produce hyperglycemia.[30, 34–36, 43] Spironolactone may induce an impaired glucose tolerance, but the impairment is small and transient.[43]

Spironolactone therapy has been found to produce no change or only small and transient changes in plasma lipid levels.[43, 108–110] Falch and Schreiner[43] reported that treatment of primary hypertension with 100 mg/day of spironolactone for 6 and 12 months produced no changes in total cholesterol and low-density lipoprotein (LDL) cholesterol concentrations but decreased high-density lipoprotein (HDL) cholesterol concentrations. Triglyceride concentrations decreased at 6 months of therapy but returned to control levels at 12 months of therapy. Ames and Hill[109] also found that spironolactone did not change total cholesterol and triglyceride concentrations; however, they did not measure HDL cholesterol concentrations. Scherstén et al.[35] and Jeunemaitre et al.[36] reported that spironolactone therapy did not change total cholesterol concentrations but increased triglyceride concentrations.

The antiandrogenic activity of spironolactone may produce some adverse endocrine effects, including gynecomastia, decreased libido, and impotence in men, and menstrual irregularities and painful breast enlargement in women.[30, 36, 84, 111, 112] These adverse effects, particularly gynecomastia and metrorrhagia, are dose-related.[30, 36, 112]

In 1975, Loube and Quirk[113] reported their concern that long-term therapy with spironolactone might cause breast cancer, but there have been no indications that spironolactone therapy causes breast cancer in human subjects.[114, 115] Like many other drugs, spironolactone can cause gastrointestinal disturbances, muscle cramps, fatigue, headache, and skin rashes.[30, 31, 34, 102, 116]

It has been shown that spironolactone inhibits the renal tubular secretion of digoxin with a consequent decrease in the renal clearance of digoxin and an increase in the serum digoxin concentration.[117–119] In addition, spironolactone and its metabolites may interfere with the radioimmunoassay of digoxin, producing spuriously elevated serum digoxin concentrations.[120, 121] Thus, careful clinical evaluation and measurement of serum digoxin concentrations are required when digoxin is combined with spironolactone.

Acetylsalicylic acid has been shown to reduce the natriuretic effect of spironolactone, possibly by reducing active renal tubular secretion of canrenone, an active metabolite of spironolactone.[122, 123] However, in one clinical trial,[124] concurrent use of acetylsalicylic acid and spironolactone did not alter the antihypertensive effect of spironolactone.

Spironolactone has been shown to reduce the half-life of antipyrine by stimulating the hepatic metabolism of that agent.[125, 126] It has been shown that spironolactone increases serum lithium levels and might augment the effect of lithium in patients with manic depressive illness.[127] Spironolactone has been shown to reduce the hypoprothrombinemic effect of warfarin.[128]

REFERENCES

1. Corvol P, Clair M, Oblin ME, et al: Mechanism of the antimineralocorticoid effects of spirolactones. Kidney Int 20:1, 1981.
2. Marver D, Kokko JP: Renal target sites and mechanism of action of aldosterone. Miner Electrolyte Metab 9:1, 1983.
3. Erbler HC: Stimulation of aldosterone production in vitro and its inhibition by spironolactone. Naunyn Schmiedebergs Arch Pharmacol 273:366, 1972.
4. Karim A: Spironolactone: Deposition, metabolism, pharmacodynamics, and bioavailability. Drug Metab Rev 8:151, 1978.
5. Overdiek JWPM, Hermens WAJJ, Merkus FWHM: New insights into the pharmacokinetics of spironolactone. Clin Pharmacol Ther 38:469, 1985.
6. Karim A: Spironolactone metabolism in man revisited. In Contemporary Trends in Diuretic Therapy. Current Clinical Practice Series No. 35. Amsterdam: Excerpta Medica, 1986, pp 22–37.
7. Gochman N, Gantt CL: A fluorometric method for the determination of a major spironolactone (Aldactone) metabolite in human plasma. J Pharmacol Exp Ther 135:312, 1962.
8. Sadée W, Dagcioglu M, Riegelman S: Fluorometric microassay for spironolactone and its metabolites in biological fluids. J Pharm Sci 61:1126, 1972.
9. Neubert P, Koch K: Simultaneous automated determination of spironolactone metabolites in serum. J Pharm Sci 66:1131, 1977.
10. Ochs HR, Greenblatt DJ, Bodem G, et al: Spironolactone. Am Heart J 96:389, 1978.
11. Weiner IM, Mudge GH: Diuretics and other agents employed in the mobilization of edema fluid. In Gilman AG, Goodman LS, Rall TW, et al (eds): Goodman and Gilman's The Pharmacological Basis of Therapeutics, 7th ed. New York: Macmillan, 1985, pp 879–907.
12. Neurath GB, Ambrosius D: High-performance liquid chromatographic determination of canrenone, a major metabolite of spironolactone, in body fluids. J Chromatogr 163:230, 1979.
13. Dahlöf CG, Lundborg P, Persson BA, et al: Re-evaluation of the antimineralocorticoid effect of the spironolactone metabolite, canrenone, from plasma concentrations determined by a new high-pressure liquid-chromatographic method. Drug Metab Dispos 7:103, 1979.
14. Overdiek JWPM, Hermens WAJJ, Merkus FWHM: Determination of the serum concentration of spironolactone and its metabolites by high-performance liquid chromatography. J Chromatogr 341:279, 1985.
15. Abshagen U, Besenfelder E, Endele R, et al: Kinetics of canrenone after single and multiple doses of spironolactone. Eur J Clin Pharmacol 16:255, 1979.
16. Merkus FWHM, Overdiek JWPM, Cilissen J, et al: Pharmacokinetics of spironolactone after a single dose: Evaluation of the true canrenone serum concentrations during 24 hours. Clin Exp Hypertens 5:239, 1983.
17. Gardiner P, Schrode K, Quinlan D, et al: Spironolactone metabolism: Steady-state serum levels of the sulfur-containing metabolites. J Clin Pharmacol 29:342, 1989.
18. Funder JW, Feldman D, Highland E, et al: Molecular modifications of anti-aldosterone compounds: Effects on affinity of spirolactones for renal aldosterone receptors. Biochem Pharmacol 23:1493, 1974.
19. Hofmann LM: Aldosterone antagonists in laboratory animals. In Wesson LG, Fanelli GM (eds): Recent Advances in Renal Physiology and Pharmacology. Baltimore: University Park Press, 1974, pp 305–316.
20. McInnes GT, Asbury MJ, Shelton JR, et al: Activity of sulfur-containing intermediate metabolites of spironolactone. Clin Pharmacol Ther 27:363, 1980.
21. Overdiek JWPM, Merkus FWHM: The metabolism and biopharmaceutics of spironolactone in man. Rev Drug Metabol Drug Interact 5:273, 1987.
22. Ramsay L, Shelton J, Harrison I: Spironolactone and potassium canrenoate in normal man. Clin Pharmacol Ther 20:167, 1976.
23. Varin F, The Minh Tu, Benoît F, et al: High-performance liquid chromatographic determination of spironolactone and its metabolites in human biological fluids after solid phase extraction. J Chromatogr 574:57, 1992.
24. Sungaila I, Bartle WR, Walker SE, et al: Spironolactone pharmacokinetics and pharmacodynamics in patients with cirrhotic ascites. Gastroenterology 102:1680, 1992.
25. Sakauye C, Felman D: Agonist and antimineralocorticoid activities of spirolactones. Am J Physiol 231:93, 1976.
26. Overdiek JWPM, Merkus FWHM: Influence of food on the bioavailability of spironolactone. Clin Pharmacol Ther 40:531, 1986.
27. Brater DC: Clinical pharmacokinetics. In Eknoyan G, Martinez-Maldonado M (eds): The Physiological Basis of Diuretic Therapy in Clinical Medicine. Orlando: Grune & Stratton, 1986, pp 27–55.
28. Shackleton CR, Wong NLM, Sutton RAL: Distal (potassium-sparing) diuretics. In Dirks JH, Sutton RAL (eds): Diuretics: Physiology, Pharmacology & Clinical Use. Philadelphia, WB Saunders, 1986, pp 117–134.
29. Berglund G, Andersson O: Hydrochlorothiazide and spironolactone alone and in a fixed combination in hypertension. Curr Ther Res 27:360, 1980.
30. Schrijver G, Weinberger MH: Hydrochlorothiazide and spironolactone in hypertension. Clin Pharmacol Ther 25:33, 1979.
31. Ferguson RK, Turek DM, Rovner DR: Spironolactone and hydrochlorothiazide in normal-renin and low-renin essential hypertension. Clin Pharmacol Ther 21:62, 1977.
32. Kreeft JH, Larochelle P, Ogilvie RI: Comparison of chlorthalidone and spironolactone in low-renin essential hypertension. Can Med Assoc J 128:31, 1983.
33. Drayer JIM, Kloppenborg PWC, Festen J: Intrapatient comparison of treatment with chlorthalidone, spironolactone and propranolol in normoreninemic essential hypertension. Am J Cardiol 36:716, 1975.
34. Walter NMA, Suthers MB, Friedman A, et al: A comparison

between spironolactone and hydrochlorothiazide with and without α-methyldopa in the treatment of hypertension. Med J Aust 1:509, 1978.

35. Scherstén B, Thulin T, Kuylenstierna J: Clinical and biochemical effects of spironolactone administered once daily in primary hypertension: Multicenter Sweden Study. Hypertension 2:672, 1980.

36. Jeunemaitre X, Chatellier G, Kreft-Jais C: Efficacy and tolerance of spironolactone in essential hypertension. Am J Cardiol 60:820, 1987.

37. Brest AN: Spironolactone in the treatment of hypertension: A review. Clin Ther 8:568, 1986.

38. Miller SA, Cobb SD, Petrulis AS, et al: Step 1½ therapy for the treatment of hypertension. Ohio State Med J 81:57, 1985.

39. Karlberg BE, Kågedal B, Tegler L, et al: Renin concentrations and effects of propranolol and spironolactone in patients with hypertension. Br Med J 1:251, 1976.

40. Lavenius B, Hansson L: A double-blind comparison of spironolactone and hydrochlorothiazide in hypertensive patients treated with metoprolol. Int J Clin Pharmacol Ther Toxicol 20:291, 1982.

41. Henry M, Wehrlen M, Pelletier B., et al: Spironolactone versus nifedipine in essential hypertension. Am J Cardiol 65(Suppl): 36K, 1990.

42. Takeda R, Yamazaki T, Ito Y, et al: Twenty-four year spironolactone therapy in an aged patient with aldosterone-producing adenoma. Acta Endocrinol (Copenh) 126:186, 1992.

43. Falch DK, Schreiner A: The effect of spironolactone on lipid, glucose and uric acid levels in blood during long-term administration to hypertensives. Acta Med Scand 213:27, 1983.

44. Jackson PR, Ramsay LE, Wakefield V: Relative potency of spironolactone, triamterene and potassium chloride in thiazide-induced hypokalemia. Br J Clin Pharmacol 14:257, 1982.

45. Ramsay LE, Hettiarachchi J, Fraser R, et al: Amiloride, spironolactone, and potassium chloride in thiazide-treated patients. Clin Pharmacol Ther 27:533, 1980.

46. Ibsen H: The effect of potassium chloride and spironolactone on thiazide-induced potassium depletion in patients with essential hypertension. Acta Med Scand 96:21, 1974.

47. George CF, Breckenridge AM, Dollery CT: Comparison of the potassium-retaining effects of amiloride and spironolactone in hypertensive patients with thiazide-induced hypokalemia. Lancet 2:1288, 1973.

48. Akbar FA, Boston PF, Chapman J, et al: Spironolactone and hydroflumethiazide in the treatment of hypertension. Br J Clin Pract 35:317, 1981.

49. Dueymes JM: Clinical update: Spironolactone and altizide as monotherapy in systemic hypertension. Am J Cardiol 65(Suppl):20K, 1990.

50. Ramsay LE, Hettiarachchi J: Spironolactone in thiazide-induced hypokalemia: Variable response between patients. Br J Clin Pharmacol 11:153, 1981.

51. Muller J: Spironolactone in the management of congestive cardiac failure: A review. Clin Ther 9:63, 1986.

52. Muller JE: Spironolactone in the management of congestive heart failure. Am J Cardiol 65(Suppl):51K, 1990.

53. Kim KE, Onesti G, Moyer JH, et al: Ethacrynic acid and furosemide: Diuretic and hemodynamic effects and clinical uses. Am J Cardiol 27:407, 1971.

54. Morgan DB, Davidson C: Hypokalemia and diuretics: An analysis of publications. Br Med J 280:905, 1980.

55. Murphy MB, Lewis PJ, Kohner E, et al: Glucose intolerance in hypertensive patients treated with diuretics: A fourteen-year followup. Lancet 2:1293, 1982.

56. Weidmann P, Gerber A: Effects of treatment with diuretics on serum lipoproteins. J Cardiovasc Pharmacol 6(Suppl 1):S260, 1984.

57. Ames RP: Coronary heart disease and the treatment of hypertension: Impact of diuretics on serum lipids and glucose. J Cardiovasc Pharmacol 6(Suppl 3):S466, 1984.

58. Weinberger MH: Diuretics and their side effects. Dilemma in the treatment of hypertension. Hypertension 11(Suppl 2):16, 1988.

59. Ikram H, Webster MWI, Nicholls MG, et al: Combined spironolactone and converting-enzyme inhibitor therapy for refractory heart failure. Aust N Z J Med 16:61, 1986.

60. Dhalström U, Karlsson E: Captopril and spironolactone therapy in patients with refractory congestive heart failure. Curr Ther Res 51:235, 1992.

61. Van Vliet AA, Donker AJM, Nauta JJP, et al: Spironolactone in congestive heart failure refractory to high-dose loop diuretic and low-dose angiotensin-converting enzyme inhibitor. Am J Cardiol 71(Suppl):21A, 1993.

62. Zannad F: Angiotensin-converting enzyme inhibitor and spironolactone combination therapy. New objectives in congestive heart failure treatment. Am J Cardiol 71(Suppl):34A, 1993.

63. Pérez-Ayuso RM, Arroyo V, Planas R, et al: Randomized comparative study of efficacy of furosemide versus spironolactone in nonazotemic cirrhosis with ascites. Relationship between the diuretic response and the activity of the renin-aldosterone system. Gastroenterology 84:961, 1983.

64. Arroyo V, Bosch J, Mauri M: Renin, aldosterone and renal haemodynamics in cirrhosis with ascites. Eur J Clin Invest 9:69, 1979.

65. Rosoff L Jr, Zia P, Reynolds T, et al: Studies of renin and aldosterone in cirrhotic patients with ascites. Gastroenterology 69:698, 1975.

66. Epstein M, Levinson R, Sancho J, et al: Characterization of the renin-aldosterone system in decompensated cirrhosis. Circ Res 41:818, 1977.

67. Podalsky S, Zimmerman HJ, Burrows BA: Potassium depletion in hepatic cirrhosis. A reversible cause of impaired growth-hormone and insulin response to stimulation. N Engl J Med 288:644, 1973.

68. Shear L, Ching S, Gabuzda GJ: Compartmentalization of ascites and edema in patients with hepatic cirrhosis. N Engl J Med 282:1391, 1970.

69. Pockros PJ, Reynolds TB: Rapid diuresis in patients with ascites from chronic liver disease: The importance of peripheral edema. Gastroenterology 90:1827, 1986.

70. Fogel MR, Sawhney VK, Neal EA: Diuresis in the ascitic patient: A randomized controlled trial of three regimens. J Clin Gastroenterol 3(Suppl 1):73, 1981.

71. Arroyo V, Ginés P, Planas R: Management of patients with cirrhosis and ascites. Semin Liver Dis 6:353, 1986.

72. Strauss J, Freundlich M, Zilleruelo: Nephrotic edema: Etiopathogenic and therapeutic considerations. Nephron 38:73, 1984.

73. Dorhout Meese EJ, Geer AB, Koomans HA: Blood volume and sodium retention in the nephrotic syndrome: A controversial pathophysiological concept. Nephron 36:201, 1984.

74. Hammond TG, Whitworth JA, Saines D, et al: Renin-angiotensin-aldosterone system in nephrotic syndrome. Am J Kidney Dis 4:18, 1984.

75. Brown EA, Markandu ND, Roulston JE, et al: Is the renin-angiotensin-aldosterone system involved in the sodium retention in the nephrotic syndrome? Nephron 32:102, 1982.

76. Brown EA, Markandu ND, Sagnella GA: Evidence that some mechanism other than the renin system causes sodium retention in nephrotic syndrome. Lancet 2:1237, 1982.

77. Ichikawa I, Rennke HG, Hoyer JR, et al: Role of intrarenal mechanisms in the impaired salt excretion in experimental nephrotic syndrome. J Clin Invest 71:91, 1983.

78. Usberti M, Federico S, Cianciaruso B, et al: Relationship between serum albumin concentration and tubular reabsorption of glucose in renal disease. Kidney Int 16:546, 1979.

79. Koomans HA, Geers AB, Meiracker AH, et al: Effects of plasma volume expansion on renal salt handling in patients with the nephrotic syndrome. Am J Nephrol 4:227, 1984.

80. Krishna GG, Danovitch GM: Effects of water immersion on renal function in the nephrotic syndrome. Kidney Int 21:395, 1982.

81. Milewics A, Silber D, Kirschner MA: Therapeutic effects of spironolactone in polycystic ovary syndrome. Obstet Gynecol 61:429, 1983.

82. Evans DJ, Burke CW: Spironolactone in the treatment of idiopathic hirsutism and the polycystic ovary syndrome. J R Soc Med 79:451, 1986.

83. Loriaux DL, Menard R, Taylor A, et al: Spironolactone and endocrine dysfunction. Ann Intern Med 85:630, 1976.

84. Stripp B, Taylor AA, Barter FC, et al: Effect of spironolactone on sex hormones in man. J Clin Endocrinol Metab 4:777, 1975.

85. Menard RH, Martin HF, Stripp B, et al: Spironolactone and cytochrome P-450: Impairment of steroid hydroxylation in the adrenal cortex. Life Sci 15:1639, 1974.

86. Corvol P, Michaud A, Menard J: Antiandrogenic effect of spironolactone: Mechanism of action. Endocrinology 97:52, 1975.

87. Boiselle A, Dione FT, Tremblay RR: Interaction of spironolactone with rat skin androgen receptor. Can J Biochem 57:1042, 1979.

88. Eil C, Ekelson SK: The use of human skin fibroblasts to obtain potency estimates of drug binding to androgen receptors. J Clin Endocrinol Metab 59:51, 1984.

89. Serafin PC, Catalino J, Lobo RA: The effect of spironolactone on genital skin 5 α-reductase activity. J Steroid Biochem 23:191, 1985.

90. Rittmaster RS, Loriaux DL: Hirsutism. Ann Intern Med 106:95, 1987.

91. Roos JC, Dorhout Mees EJ, Koomans HA, et al: Intrarenal sodium handling during chronic spironolactone treatment. Nephron 38:226, 1984.

92. Bevegård S, Castenfors J, Danielson M: The effects of four months' treatment with spironolactone on systemic blood pressure, cardiac output and plasma renin activity in hypertensive patients. Acta Med Scand 202:373, 1977.

93. Moura AM, Angeli M, Worcel M: Extrarenal effects of aldosterone and mineralocorticoid compounds. Kidney Int 34(Suppl 26):5, 1988.

94. Dacquet C, Loirand G, Mironneau G, et al: Spironolactone inhibition of contraction and calcium channel in rat portal vein. Br J Pharmacol 92:535, 1987.

95. Mironneau J, Sayet I, Rakoarisoa L, et al: Interactions of spironolactone with (+)-($_3$H)-isradipine and (−)-($_3$H) desmethoxyverapamil binding sites in vascular smooth muscle. Br J Pharmacol 101:6, 1990.

96. Mironneau J: Calcium channel antagonist effects of spironolactone, an aldosterone antagonist. Am J Cardiol 69(Suppl):7K, 1990.

97. Brilla CG, Pick R, Tan LB, et al: Remodeling of the rat right and left ventricle in experimental hypertension. Circ Res 67:1355, 1990.

98. Brilla CG, Weber KT: Reactive and reparative myocardial fibrosis in arterial hypertension in the rat. Cardiovasc Res 26:671, 1992.

99. Campbell SE, Janicki JS, Matsubara BB, et al: Myocardial fibrosis in the rat with mineralocorticoid excess: Prevention of scarring by amiloride. Am J Hypertens 6:487, 1993.

100. Brilla CG, Matsubara LS, Weber KT: Antifibrotic effects of spironolactone in preventing myocardial fibrosis in systemic arterial hypertension. Am J Cardiol 71(Suppl):12A, 1993.

101. Weber KT, Brilla CG: Pathological hypertrophy and cardiac interstitium: Fibrosis and renin-angiotensin-aldosterone system. Circulation 83:1849, 1991.

102. Greenblatt DJ, Koch-Weser J: Adverse reactions to spironolactone. A report from the Boston Collaborative Drug Surveillance Program. JAMA 225:40, 1973.

103. Yap V, Patel A, Thomsen J: Hyperkalemia with cardiac arrhythmia: Induction by salt substitutes, spironolactone, and azotemia. JAMA 236:2775, 1976.

104. Gabow PA, Moore S, Schrier RW: Spironolactone-induced hyperchloremic acidosis in cirrhosis. Ann Intern Med 90:338, 1979.

105. Knochel JP, White MG: The role of aldosterone in renal physiology. Arch Intern Med 131:876, 1973.

106. Sebastian A, Schambelan M, Lindenfeld S, et al: Amelioration of metabolic acidosis with fludrocortisone therapy in hyporeninemic hypoaldosteronism. N Engl J Med 297:576, 1977.

107. Roos JC, Boer JC, Peuker KH, et al: Changes in intrarenal uric acid handling during chronic spironolactone treatment in patients with essential hypertension. Nephron 32:209, 1982.

108. Garcia Puig J, Mirana ME, Mateos F, et al: Hydrochlorothiazide versus spironolactone: Long term metabolic modification in patients with essential hypertension. J Clin Pharmacol 31:455, 1991.

109. Ames RP, Hill P: Antihypertensive therapy and the risk of coronary heart disease. J Cardiovasc Pharmacol 4(Suppl 2):S206, 1982.

110. Weidmann P, Uehlinger DE, Gerber A: Antihypertensive treatment and serum lipoproteins. J Hypertens 3:297, 1985.

111. Rose LI, Underwood RH, Newmark SR: Pathophysiology of spironolactone-induced gynecomastia. Ann Intern Med 87:398, 1977.

112. Helfer EL, Miller JL, Rose LI: Side-effects of spironolactone therapy in the hirsute woman. J Clin Endocrinol Metab 66:208, 1988.

113. Loube SD, Quirk RA: Breast cancer associated with administration of spironolactone. Lancet 1:1428, 1975.

114. Jick H, Armstrong B: Breast cancer and spironolactone. Lancet 2:368, 1975.

115. Tremblay R: Treatment of hirsutism with spironolactone. Clin Endocrinol Metab 15:363, 1986.

116. Downham TF III: Spironolactone-induced lichen planus. JAMA 240:1138, 1978.

117. Steiness E: Renal tubular secretion of digoxin. Circulation 50:103, 1974.

118. Waldorff S, Hansen PB, Egebald H: Interactions between digoxin and potassium-sparing diuretics. Clin Pharmacol Ther 33:418, 1983.

119. Hedman A, Angelin B, Arvidsson A, Dahlqvist R: Digoxin-interactions in man: spironolactone reduces renal but not biliary digoxin clearance. Eur J Clin Pharmacol 42:481, 1992.

120. Silber B, Sheiner LB, Powers JL, et al: Spironolactone-associated digoxin radioimmunoassay interference. Clin Chem 25:48, 1979.

121. Morris RG, Lagnado PY, Lehmann DR, et al: Spironolactone as a source of interference in commercial digoxin immunoassays. Ther Drug Monit 9:208, 1987.

122. Tweeddale MG, Ogilvie RI: Antagonism of spironolactone-induced natriuresis by aspirin in man. N Engl J Med 289:198, 1973.

123. Ramsay LE, Harrison IR, Shelton JR, et al: Influence of acetylsalicylic acid on the renal handling of a spironolactone metabolite in healthy subjects. Eur J Clin Pharmacol 10:43, 1976.

124. Hollifield JW: Failure of aspirin to antagonize the antihypertensive effect of spironolactone in low-renin hypertension. South Med J 69:1034, 1976.

125. Taylor SA, Rawlins MD, Smith SE: Spironolactone—A weak enzyme inducer in man. J Pharm Pharmacol 24:578, 1972.

126. Huffman DH, Schoeman DW, Pentikälnen P, et al: The effect of spironolactone on antipyrine metabolism in man. Pharmacology 10:338, 1973.

127. Gillman MA, Lichtigfeld FJ: Synergism of spironolactone and lithium in mania. Br Med J 292:661, 1986.

128. O'Reilly RA: Spironolactone and warfarin interaction. Clin Pharmacol Ther 27:198, 1980.

CHAPTER 47

Potassium Supplements
Dietary Potassium and Potassium Supplements

Louis Tobian, M.D.

Statistically, hypertension is harmful because hypertensive people suffer three to four times more strokes, more myocardial infarctions, and more angina, congestive failure, and renal failure. However, many people have these same high levels of blood pressure and do not suffer strokes or myocardial infarctions. Their arteries are seemingly not harmed by the high blood pressure. At the opposite end of the spectrum, patients are often frightened because many of their parents or siblings have died of a stroke or have had a coronary death before the age of 50. Seemingly, the arteries of these families are exceedingly susceptible to relatively mild degrees of hypertension and other risk factors. Actually, hypertension would be much less of a problem if it did not involve extra coronary, cerebral, or renal vascular disease. Our findings strongly suggest that elevated blood pressure per se is only one of the determinants of arterial lesions. Other factors apparently are strongly involved. Considering the other factors has now almost become a necessity. Using the antihypertensive treatments of 10 years ago, various trials have indicated that lowering the blood pressure produces only a small reduction in coronary deaths. In numeric terms, coronary deaths are certainly the number one complication of hypertension, and the older methods of treatment seemingly cannot solve this problem.

We must therefore adopt a new philosophy for treating hypertension that involves twin objectives. First, we must continue to lower the blood pressure into the normal range without side effects. This eradicates the excessive stretch on the endothelial cells and smooth muscle cells and should result in several benefits. One would expect a reduction of growth factors or their receptors. One would expect an increase in the factors retarding growth along with their receptors. One would expect a recovery of a healthy capacity for the production of endothelial relaxing factor as well as a reduction in the proteins on endothelial cells that cause monocytes to stick excessively. In hypertension, one gets much vascular protection just from lowering the blood pressure. However, this objective is no longer sufficient. We must also lower the susceptibility of arteries to injury while we lower blood pressure. Several factors have now been identified as a means for making arteries more resistant to injury. The diet and lifestyle of Paleolithic man differed tremendously from ours; the biggest dietary differences were their low-fat, low-salt, and very much greater potassium (K) intakes.[1] These Paleolithic people averaged about 284 mEq of K per day,[1, 2] whereas Americans average about 64 mEq,[3] about a fourth as much as our prehistoric ancestors.

There are populations around the world that have particularly low K intakes and very poor cardiovascular health. A few years ago, the blacks in the Southeastern United States ate about 30 mEq of K per day, and they suffered more strokes and more end-stage renal disease than any group in the United States.[4, 5] The people of Scotland average about 45 mEq of K per day, and they have much more cardiovascular disease than the people of southern England, France, or Italy. In fact, the area around Glasgow is now considered the myocardial infarction leader of the world. The people in Tibet average around 20 mEq of K a day, and they have a very high stroke incidence. We can now add the people of Newfoundland, who average about 40 mEq of K per day and have a very high incidence of strokes.

Using the Dahl S rat, we found that, after they had been on a high-NaCl diet for about 5 months, they had hypertension and dilated renal tubules with casts in them. When we increased the K in the diet from 0.75% to 2.0%, the number of these tubular lesions was reduced by 50%, even though the blood pressure was not really changed at all.[6] This represents a considerable degree of renal tubular protection. In the same microscopic slides, we made another unexpected observation. Volhard showed, some 90 years ago, that hypertensive arteries have thicker walls, and they were 38% thicker in our kidney slides.[6] The Dahl S rats on the high-K diet, however, seemingly were able to avoid this thickening of the artery wall, even though their blood pressure was as high as ever.[6] The high-K diet seemed to avoid this wall lesion of hypertension, even though there was no measurable reduction of blood pressure.

It was possible that the same process was occurring in the cerebral circulation. We therefore started a colony of stroke-prone, spontaneously hypertensive (SHRsp) rats. We gave some of them a normal 0.75% K diet and some of them a high 2.1% K diet. The high K level was reminiscent of the diet of prehistoric man. After a while, there were many deaths, mainly from stroke, but it turned out that almost all of the deaths were in the group fed normal-K diets, in which the mortality rate was 83% at 4 months, whereas those on high-K diets had only a 2% mortality rate.[7] In Dahl S rats, the mortality rate was 55% for rats on regular K and 4% for rats on high K.[7] There was a big difference in survival curves with the different K intakes. In the stroke-prone rat, the high-K diet did lower the blood pressure somewhat, just as critical studies in human subjects have indicated a similar reduction in blood pressure. These studies in humans were 6-week

461

studies, not long-term studies. To investigate the implication of this, we put some stroke-prone rats on the two diets; after a few weeks, we measured the blood pressure of every rat intraarterially. Using these data, we obtained two groups with perfectly matched blood pressures but with contrasting K intakes. Ultimately, as these matched groups continued their respective diets, the mortality rate was 64% for rats on regular K and 6% for rats on high K, even though these two groups had perfectly matched blood pressures.[7] This is a 91% reduction in mortality, and it suggested that a high-K diet protects arteries from the injury of hypertension, even though blood pressure is pretty much the same in these two groups.

After 8 weeks on a regular-K diet, 72% of stroke-prone rats showed a spot of brain hemorrhage; on the high-K diet, however, only 5.5% had a brain hemorrhage.[8] We also found that 36% of the slides showed a brain infarct for the regular-K diet, whereas only 2% of the slides showed a similar infarct for the high-K diet, a 94% reduction.[8]

We studied the effect of high-K diets on arteries other than those in the kidney. In several arteries, we found that the medial layer was reduced in thickness by about 20% with a high-K diet, even though the blood pressure was much the same in these two groups.[9] That study included the aorta and the mesenteric, carotid, and basilar arteries.

Normally, the intima and endothelium of arteries have very little thickening; but in hypertension, one finds irregular thickening of the intima. We measured the thickness and damage of the intima on both high-K and normal-K diets and noticed that with the high-K diet, the thickness of the aortic intima was reduced 54%, of the mesenteric artery intima 44%, and of the carotid intima 35%.[10] There was a large reduction in the thickening of the intima in all three arteries with virtually the same blood pressure in these two groups. The thickening of the intima is so closely related to dysfunction of the endothelial cells that we decided to measure endothelial capacity for releasing relaxing factor, which is mainly nitric oxide. When we put rings of normotensive aortas contracted with norepinephrine in a muscle bath and then added acetylcholine, relaxation was 83% at 10^{-7} acetylcholine.[11] In hypertensive rats, there is the well-known damage to the arteries that seems to compromise this ability to release relaxing factor. In our SHRsp rats on a normal-K diet, relaxation was only 38%.[11] In aortic rings from other equally hypertensive SHRsp rats that were fed the high-K diet, a challenge with 10^{-7} acetylcholine brought about a normal 76% relaxation. My interpretation here is that the high-K diet preserved the health of the endothelial cells in the face of a similar degree of hypertension. This has allowed them to continue to release relaxing factor and thereby produce a normal relaxation. When non–endothelium-dependent nitroprusside is added to the bath, the relaxation was equal for both the normal-K and the high-K groups. When arteries lack relaxing factor, platelets tend to stick to the endothelium and to one another, which could be the basis of a thrombosis.[12–14] If one can preserve the

ability of these endothelial cells to continue to release nitric oxide (relaxing factor), this tendency toward thrombosis might be diminished.

Other stroke-prone SHRsp rats were fed a high-cholesterol diet.[15] They developed a degree of hypercholesterolemia of about 220 mg/dl. Some were on a regular-K diet; others were on a high-K diet. With a gas chromatograph, we measured directly the cholesterol esters depositing in the wall of the whole aorta. Rats on the high-K diet had a 64% lower deposition of cholesterol esters than those on the regular-K diet. We surmise that a high-K diet protects the endothelial cells against injury from both hypertension and hypercholesterolemia. As they are less injured, they have fewer sticking monocytes, less increased permeability, and fewer growth factors, which results in a greatly reduced deposition of cholesterol esters.

One of the ways that the arteries could be less thickened on a high-K diet is the appearance of growth-retarding humoral factors. Aortas from SHRsp rats were mounted in a chamber and perfused with tissue culture fluid containing Krebs' electrolytes. We noticed that the SHRsp rats on a high-K diet released much more of an agent that retards growth much as transforming growth factor (TGF)–β does than did the rats on a regular-K diet, a 2.5 times greater release.[16] However, administration of anti–TGF-β antibodies does not change this result. We therefore think that this difference is related to a substance that retards proliferation but is not TGF-β. If a high-K diet causes much more of it to be released, this would result in a reduced thickening of the intima.

A high-K diet also makes the SHRsp aorta less sticky to monocytes. If one infuses radioactive monocytes, about 40% fewer of them stick to the aorta in SHRsp rats on a high-K diet compared with those on a normal-K diet. Similarly, in the brain, about 52% fewer monocytes stick in the brain of the SHRsp rats on a high-K diet compared with those on a normal-K diet. If aortas are perfused for 3 hours, one finds that the aortas that come from rats on a normal-K diet and are perfused in the chamber at high pressure are the ones that have the excessive sticking of monocytes. The other groups do not.

Our setup would not permit the measurement of oxygen free radicals, so we tried to measure one of the main effects of oxygen free radicals, namely lipid peroxidation. We noted that in normotensive rats, the intima has a low degree of lipid peroxidation. One finds twice as much lipid peroxidation in the intima of the hypertensive rat. Moreover, the hypertensive rats on a high-K diet had a 23% lower level of lipid peroxidation in the intima than those on a normal-K diet; this could be one of the mechanisms by which a high-K diet protects the health of arteries in a hypertensive setting.

We also found that there is much more lipid peroxidation in the plasma of SHRsp hypertensive rats than in normotensive rats. A high-K diet reduced the high degree of lipid peroxidation in plasma of SHRsp hypertensive rats to an almost normal level (a 37% reduction), even though the blood pressure was the same in the high-K and normal-K groups. A high level of lipid peroxide in the plasma can oxidize the low-density lipoprotein molecules, making them much more atherogenic. It can also oxidize membrane lipids of endothelial cells. Thus, reducing circulating lipid peroxides could significantly improve the health of the arteries.

Khaw and Barrett-Connor[3] studied dietary K in a retirement community near San Diego in which all participants were over age 50. In women taking in less than 49 mEq of K per day, there were 5.3 stroke deaths per 100. An intermediate level of K intake cut that down by 60%. If the women had taken more than 67 mEq of K per day, there were no stroke deaths at all. Men taking less than 59 mEq a day had 3.4 stroke deaths per 100. An intermediate level of K cut that down 30%. If they took in more than 76 mEq of K per day, there were no stroke deaths at all. Seemingly, relatively small increases in K intake were associated with greatly reduced deaths from stroke, at least over the 12 years of this study. These investigators determined how much one would gain from taking 10 extra mEq of K per day. According to these investigators, this would decrease stroke deaths by about 40% and would do so without any significant change in blood pressure. This parallels the findings in our studies.

One cannot determine the protective effect of the high-K diet in stroke-prone rats by doing measurements of serum K. Striking protection can occur in rats on the high-K diet, even though the fasting serum K level does not increase at all. We found that the plasma K level does rise about 0.3 mEq/L at the finish of a large, night-time, high-K meal in these rats. However, these studies have encouraged me to insist that, for patients on thiazides, the serum K levels be kept in the 4s and not be allowed to get down into the 3s and the 2s.

A number of stroke-prone SHRsp rats were fed a 6% high-NaCl diet for 23 days. With one group of these rats, this diet contained 0.5% K, which is the same level of K per calorie that we find in the typical American diet. A second diet contained 2.1% K, which is similar to the K level in the diet of prehistoric men and women.

After 23 days, we found that the total exchangeable sodium and K and the skeletal muscle, aorta, and bone sodium and K in the stroke-prone SHRsp rats were the same in the rats on high-K diets as in the rats on regular-K diets. The plasma K level during the daylight hours was the same in the rats on high-K diets as in the rats on regular-K diets.

In contrast to its effect in skeletal muscle tissue, the high K-diet profoundly changed the concentrations of sodium and K in the renal papilla. The 15 stroke-prone SHR rats on the normal-K diet averaged 58 mEq of K/L of papilla water, whereas 15 similar stroke-prone rats on the high-K diet averaged 73 mEq K/L. Thus, the high-K diet increased the K concentration in the papilla by 24% ($p < .000001$). Some of this high K concentration could be explained by a high K concentration in the urine passing through the papillary collecting duct.

The concentration of sodium was also measured in these papillae. In the stroke-prone SHR rats on the 6% NaCl diet, the regular 0.5%-K intake was accompanied by a sodium concentration of 104 mEq/L of papilla water. When K was added to this same diet, the sodium concentration in the papilla rose to 158mEq/L of papilla water. This represents a 52% increase in the sodium concentration in the papilla in the group fed the high-K diet ($p < .000001$), and the sodium in the urine in the papillary collecting ducts cannot account for it.

In the two groups of stroke-prone SHR rats on the 6% NaCl diet, the millimoles of urea per liter of papillary water were not significantly different in the high-K diet compared with the normal K diet. In the stroke-prone SHR rats on the high-salt diets, the rats on the high-K diet led to a 25% greater osmolality in the papilla (546 mOsm/L) than in similar stroke-prone rats on a regular-K diet (436 mOsm/L; $p < .001$). Thus, the concentration of milliosmoles was also markedly elevated with the high-K diet.

The renal papilla has many interstitial cells. These cells release medullipin I and prostaglandins E_2 and F_2. These interstitial cells are quite responsive to increases in the osmolality of the papilla. Danon et al.[17] placed minced rat papillae in Krebs-Hensleit solution and added milliosmoles in the form of either sodium chloride or sucrose or urea. Their work showed that increasing the NaCl concentration to 1500 mOsm/L increased the output of prostaglandins 25-fold. An increase of osmolality also might increase the output of medullipin I from the interstitial cells.

To gain some insight into the activity of these renal papillary interstitial cells, we took advantage of the fact that these cells have two unique fatty acids in their triglycerides. These are arachidonic acid (C20:4) and adrenic acid (C22:4). With this in mind, we obtained papillae from Dahl S rats eating a diet with 2% NaCl, which is roughly similar to the American diet. Rats were on either 0.6% normal-K intake or 2.1% high-K intake. The triglyceride fraction of the lipids was extracted from the rat renal papillae, and the fatty acids in it were measured with a gas chromatograph. The amounts of arachidonic and adrenic acid in these samples were roughly equal and were added together as an index of the number of granules in the interstitial cells. The high-K diet markedly reduced these special fatty acids in the interstitial cell granules by 53% ($p < .05$). The 25-week high-K diet appeared to have a marked effect on the special fatty acids of the interstitial cells, suggesting a definite change in their rate of secretion; this likely indicates an increase in the secretory rate of medullipin I, which is a strong vasodilator. Nearly all endogenous vasoconstrictors act as growth factors for vascular smooth muscle cells, and endogenous vasodilators act as antiproliferative agents. An increased secretion of medullipin I would ultimately act as a vasodilator on vascular smooth muscle cells and would have an antiproliferative effect on these cells. Thus, the putative increased secretion of medullipin I, acting as an antiproliferative agent, could partially explain the reduced hypertrophy of the walls of arteries in hypertensive rats on high-K diets.

To summarize, many studies indicate that a high-K diet can prevent cerebral arterial and renal lesions, even though the blood pressure remains hypertensive. The high-K diet also tends to significantly lower blood pressure levels. High-K diets are a prime example of protecting arteries in a hypertensive setting. In patients at high risk, K supplements can be added to the high-K diet, with the proviso that serum K levels be monitored from time to time. This is the new dimension in hypertension therapy—protecting the arteries in addition to normalizing the blood pressure.

REFERENCES

1. Eaton SB, Konner M: Paleolithic nutrition: A consideration of its nature and current implications. N Engl J Med 312:283, 1985.
2. Denton D: Hunger For Salt, an Anthropological, Physiological and Medical Analysis. New York: Springer-Verlag, 1982, p 573.
3. Khaw KT, Barrett-Connor E: Dietary potassium and stroke associated mortality: A 12-year prospective population study. N Engl J Med 316:235, 1987.
4. Grim CE, Luft FC, Miller JZ, et al: Racial differences in blood pressure in Evans County, Georgia: Relationships to sodium and potassium intake and plasma renin activity. J Chronic Dis 33:87, 1980.
5. Langford HG: Dietary potassium and hypertension: Epidemiologic data. Ann Intern Med 98(Suppl):770, 1983.
6. Tobian L, MacNeill D, Johnson MA, et al: Potassium protection against lesions of the renal tubules, arteries and glomeruli and nephron loss in salt-loaded hypertensive Dahl S rats. Hypertension 6(Suppl 1):170, 1984.
7. Tobian L, Lange J, Ulm K, et al: Potassium reduces cerebral hemorrhage and death in hypertensive rats even when BP is not lowered. Hypertension 7(Suppl 2):110, 1985.
8. Tobian L, Lange J, Johnson MA, et al: High-K diets markedly reduce brain haemorrhage and infarcts, death rate and mesenteric arteriolar hypertrophy in stroke-prone spontaneously hypertensive rats. J Hypertens 4(Suppl 5):205, 1986.
9. Tobian L: High potassium diets reduce stroke mortality and arterial and renal tubular lesions in hypertension. American Institute of Nutrition Symposium Proceedings, Nutrition '87, 1987, p 119.
10. Tobian L, Sugimoto T, Johnson MA, et al: High K diets protect against endothelial injury in stroke-prone SHR rats. J Hypertens 5(Suppl 5):263, 1987.
11. Sugimoto T, Tobian L, Ganguli MC: High K diets protect against dysfunction of endothelial cells in stroke-prone SHR rats. Hypertension 11(6):579, 1988.
12. Radomski MW, Palmer RMJ, Moncada S: Comparative pharmacology of endothelium-derived relaxing factor, nitric oxide and prostacyclin in platelets. Br J Pharmacol 92:181, 1987.
13. Radomski MW, Palmer RMJ, Moncada S: Endogenous nitric oxide inhibits human platelet adhesion to vascular endothelium. Lancet 2:1057, 1987.
14. Radomski MW, Palmer RMJ, Moncada S: The role of nitric oxide and cGMP in platelet adhesion to vascular endothelium. Biochem Biophys Res Commun 148:1482, 1987.
15. Tobian L, Jahner T, Johnson MA: High K diets markedly reduce atherosclerotic cholesterol ester deposition in aortas of rats with hypercholesterolemia and hypertension. Am J Hypertens 3:133, 1990.
16. Sugimoto K, Tobian L, Ishimitsu T, et al: High K diets greatly increase the release of growth-inhibiting agents from aortas of stroke prone spontaneously hypertensive rats, thereby partially explaining reduced aortic wall thickening. J Hypertens 9(Suppl 6):S176, 1991.
17. Danon A, Knapp HR, Oelz O, et al: Stimulation of prostaglandin biosynthesis in the renal papilla by hypertonic mediums. Am J Physiol 234:F64, 1978.

VI.

β-Adrenoreceptor Blockers

Editors: John L. Reid and William H. Frishman

A. Principles and Practice of β-Adrenoreceptor Blockade

CHAPTER 48

β-Adrenergic Blocking Drugs in Cardiac Disorders

William H. Frishman, M.D., and Dawn Hershman, M.D.

The therapeutic efficacy and safety of β-adrenoreceptor blocking drugs has been well established in patients with angina pectoris, cardiac arrhythmias, and hypertension, and in reducing the risk of mortality and nonfatal reinfarction in survivors of acute myocardial infarction.[1-4] These drugs may be useful as primary protection against cardiovascular morbidity and mortality in hypertensive patients.[5] The drugs are also used for a multitude of other cardiac (Table 48–1)[2-4, 6-17] and noncardiac (Table 48–2)[2, 3, 18-26] conditions.

EFFECTS ON ELEVATED SYSTEMIC BLOOD PRESSURE

β-Adrenergic blockers effectively reduce the blood pressure of many patients with combined systolic and diastolic hypertension and of elderly patients with isolated systolic hypertension (Tables 48–3 and 48–4).[2, 3, 27] They were cited as first-line therapy by the Fifth Report of the Joint National Commission on Detection, Evaluation and Treatment of High Blood Pressure.[28] However, there is no consensus as to the mechanism(s) by which these drugs lower blood pressure. Some or all of the following proposed mechanisms probably play a part.

β-Blockers without vasodilatory activity appear to be more efficacious in white patients and younger patients than they are in black patients.[28, 29] A combination of very-low-dose diuretic (thiazide) and β-blocker (bisoprolol) has been approved as a new first-line antihypertensive therapy.[30, 31]

Negative Chronotropic and Inotropic Effects

Slowing of the heart rate and some decrease in myocardial contractility with β-blockers lead to a decrease in cardiac output, which in the short term and long term may lead to a reduction in blood pressure.[1] These factors might be of particular importance in the treatment of hypertension related to high cardiac output[32] and increased sympathetic tone.

Differences in Effects on Plasma Renin

The relation between the hypotensive action of β-blocking drugs and their ability to reduce plasma renin activity remains controversial. Some β-blocking drugs can antagonize sympathetically mediated renin release,[33] although adrenergic activity is not the only mechanism by which renin release is mediated. Other major determinants are sodium balance, posture, and renal perfusion pressure.

Table 48–1. **Reported Cardiovascular Indications for β-Adrenoreceptor Blocking Drugs**

Hypertension*
Angina pectoris*
"Silent" myocardial ischemia
Supraventricular arrhythmias*
Ventricular arrhythmias*
Reducing the risk of mortality and reinfarction in
 survivors of acute myocardial infarction*
Hyperacute phase of myocardial infarction*
Dissection of the aorta
Hypertrophic cardiomyopathy*
Reversing left ventricular hypertrophy
Digitalis intoxication
Mitral valve prolapse
QT-interval prolongation syndrome
Tetralogy of Fallot
Mitral stenosis
Congestive cardiomyopathy
Fetal tachycardia
Neurocirculatory asthenia

*Formally approved indications by U.S. Food and Drug Administration.

Table 48–2. Some Reported Noncardiovascular Indications for β-Adrenoreceptor Blocking Drugs

Neuropsychiatric
  Migraine prophylaxis*
  Essential tremor*
  Situational anxiety
  Alcohol withdrawal (delirium tremens)
Endocrine
  Thyrotoxicosis*
  Hyperparathyroidism
Other
  Glaucoma*
  Portal hypertension and gastrointestinal bleeding

*Formally approved indications by U.S. Food and Drug Administration.

The important question remains whether there is a clinical correlation between the β-blocker's effect on the plasma renin activity and the lowering of blood pressure. Investigators[31] have found that "high-renin" patients do not always respond or may even show a rise in blood pressure, and that "normal-renin" patients have less predictable responses. In high-renin hypertensive patients, it has been suggested that renin may not be the only factor maintaining the high blood pressure state. The exact role of renin reduction in blood pressure control remains undefined.

Central Nervous System Effect

Good clinical and experimental evidence suggests that β-blockers cross the blood-brain barrier and enter the central nervous system.[34] Although there is little doubt that β-blockers with high lipophilicity (e.g., metoprolol, propranolol) enter the central nervous system in high concentrations, a direct antihypertensive effect mediated by their presence has not been well defined. Also, β-blockers that are less lipid-soluble and less likely to concentrate in the brain than propranolol appear to be as effective in lowering blood pressure.[32, 35, 36]

Effects on Peripheral Resistance

Nonselective β-blockers have no primary action in lowering peripheral resistance and indeed may cause it to rise by leaving the peripheral α-adrenoreceptor

Table 48–3. Proposed Mechanisms to Explain the Antihypertensive Actions of β-Blockers

Reduction in cardiac output
Inhibition of renin
Central nervous system effects
Effects on prejunctional β-receptors: reductions in
  norepinephrine release
Reduction in peripheral vascular resistance
Reduction in venomotor tone
Reduction in plasma volume
Resetting of baroreceptor levels
Attenuation of the pressor response to catecholamines
  with exercise and stress

From Frishman WH: Clinical Pharmacology of the Beta-Adrenoceptor Blocking Drugs, 2nd ed. Norwalk, CT: Appleton-Century-Crofts, 1984, p 28.

stimulatory mechanisms unopposed.[37] The vasodilating effect of catecholamines on skeletal muscle blood vessels is β_2-mediated, suggesting possible therapeutic advantages in using β_1-selective blockers, agents with partial agonist activity, or β-blocking drugs with α-blocking activity. Because β_1 selectivity diminishes as the drug dosage is raised, and because hypertensive patients generally have to be given far larger doses than are required simply to block the β_1-receptors alone, β_1 selectivity[38] offers the clinician little, if any, real specific antihypertensive advantage.[38, 39]

Effects on Prejunctional β-Receptors

Apart from their effects on postjunctional tissue β-receptors, it is believed that blockade of prejunctional β-receptors may be involved in the hemodynamic actions of β-blocking drugs. The stimulation of prejunctional α_2-receptors leads to a reduction in the quantity of norepinephrine released by the postganglionic sympathetic fibers.[40, 41] Conversely, stimulation of prejunctional β-receptors is followed by an increase in the quantity of norepinephrine released by the postganglionic sympathetic fibers.[42, 43] Therefore, blockade of prejunctional β-receptors should diminish the amount of norepinephrine released, leading to weaker stimulation of postjunctional α-receptors, an effect that would produce less vasoconstriction. Opinions differ, however, on the contributions of presynaptic β-blockade to both a reduction in the peripheral vascular resistance and the antihypertensive effects of β-blocking drugs.

Other Proposed Mechanisms

Less well documented effects of β-blockers that may contribute to their antihypertensive actions include favorable effects on venous tone and plasma volume,[2] membrane stabilizing activity,[44] and resetting of baroreceptors.[45]

EFFECTS IN ANGINA PECTORIS

Ahlquist[46] demonstrated that sympathetic innervation of the heart causes the release of norepinephrine, activating β-adrenoreceptors in myocardial cells (see Table 48–4). This adrenergic stimulation causes an increment in heart rate, isometric contractile force, and maximal velocity of muscle fiber shortening, all of which lead to an increase in cardiac work and myocardial oxygen consumption.[47] On the other hand, the decrease in intraventricular volume caused by the sympathetic-mediated enhancement of cardiac contractility tends to reduce myocardial oxygen consumption by reducing myocardial wall tension (LaPlace's law).[48] Although there is a net increase in myocardial oxygen demand by adrenergic stimulation, this effect is normally balanced by a concomitant increase in coronary blood flow. Angina pectoris is believed to occur when oxygen demand exceeds supply (i.e., when coronary blood flow is restricted by coronary stenoses or spasm). Because the conditions

Table 48–4. **Pharmacodynamic Properties and Cardiac Effects of β-Adrenoreceptor Blockers**

Drug	Relative β1 Selectivity*	Partial Agonist Activity	Membrane-Stabilizing Activity	Resting Heart Rate	Exercise Heart Rate	Resting Myocardial Contractility	Resting Blood Pressure	Exercise Blood Pressure	Resting Atrioventricular Conduction	Antiarrhythmic Effect
Acebutolol	+	+	+	↓↔	↓	↓	↓	↓	↓	+
Atenolol	++	0	0	↓	↓	↓	↓	↓	↓	+
Betaxolol	++	0	0	↓	↓	↓	↓	↓	↓	+
Bisoprolol†	++	0	0	↓	↓	↓	↓	↓	↓	+
Bucindolol‡	0	+	0	↓↔	↓	↓↔	↓	↓	↓↔	+
Carteolol	0	+	0	↓↔	↓	↓↔	↓	↓	↓	+
Carvedilol§	0	0	++	↓↔	↓	↓↔	↓	↓	↓↔	+
Esmolol	++	0	0	↓	↓	↓	↓	↓	↓	+
Labetalol‖	0	+?	0	↓↔	↓	↓↔	↓	↓↓	↓↔	+
Metoprolol	++	0	0	↓	↓	↓	↓	↓	↓	+
Nadolol	0	0	0	↓	↓	↓	↓	↓	↓	+
Oxprenolol	0	+	+	↓↔	↓	↓↔	↓	↓	↓↔	+
Penbutolol	0	+	0	↓↔	↓	↓↔	↓	↓	↓↔	+
Pindolol	0	++	0	↓↔	↓	↓↔	↓	↓	↓↔	+
Propranolol	0	0	++	↓	↓	↓	↓	↓	↓	+
Sotalol	0	0	0	↓	↓	↓	↓	↓	↓	+
Timolol	0	0	0	↓	↓	↓	↓	↓	↓	+
Isomer: D-propranolol	0	0	++	↔	↔	↔↓¶	↔	↔	↔↓¶	+¶

++, strong effect; +, modest effect; 0, no effect; ↑, elevation; ↓, reduction; ↔, no change.
*β1-selectivity is only seen with low therapeutic drug combinations. With higher concentrations, β1-selectivity is not seen.
†Bisoprolol is also approved in combination with very-low-dose diuretic as a first-line antihypertensive agent.
‡Bucindolol has additional direct vascular smooth muscle relaxatory and weak α1-adrenergic blocking properties.
§Carvedilol has additional vasodilatory activity mediated by α1-adrenergic blockade and possibly calcium entry blockade.
‖Labetalol has additional α1-adrenergic blocking properties and direct β2-adrenergic vasodilatory activity.
¶Effects of D-propranolol with doses in humans well above the therapeutic level. The isomer also lacks β-blocking activity.
Data from Frishman WH: Clinical Pharmacology of the β-Adrenoceptor Blocking Drugs, 2nd ed. Norwalk, CT: Appleton-Century-Crofts, 1984, p 32; Frishman WH: The beta-adrenoceptor blocking drugs. Int J Cardiol 2:165, 1982; and Frishman WH: Beta-adrenergic blockers. Med Clin North Am 72(1):52, 1988.

that precipitate anginal attacks (e.g., exercise, emotional stress, food) cause an increase in cardiac sympathetic activity, it might be expected that blockade of cardiac β-adrenoreceptors would relieve the anginal symptoms. This was the basis for early clinical studies with β-blocking drugs in patients with angina pectoris.[49]

Four main factors—heart rate, myocardial contractility, ventricular systolic pressure, and the size of the left ventricle—contribute to the myocardial oxygen requirements of the left ventricle. Of these, heart rate and systolic pressure appear to be the most important (heart rate multiplied by the systolic blood pressure is a reliable index to predict the precipitation of angina in a given patient).[50, 51]

The reduction in heart rate effected by β-blockade has two favorable consequences: a decrease in blood pressure, thus reducing myocardial oxygen needs, and a longer diastolic filling time associated with a slower heart rate, allowing for an increased period for coronary perfusion. β-Blockade also reduces exercise-induced blood pressure increments, the velocity of cardiac contraction, and oxygen consumption at any patient workload (Fig. 48–1).[50, 51] It has been recently proposed by our group that the β-blocker effects on contractility may be more important than those on heart rate in relieving myocardial ischemia.

Studies in dogs have shown that propranolol causes a decrease in coronary blood flow.[52] However, subsequent experimental animal studies have demonstrated that shunting induced by β-blockers occurs in the coronary circulation, maintaining blood flow to ischemic areas, especially in the subendocardial region.[53] In humans, concomitant with the decrease in myocardial oxygen consumption, β-blockers can cause a reduction in coronary blood flow and a rise in coronary vascular resistance.[54] However, on the basis of coronary autoregulation, the overall reduction in myocardial oxygen needs with β-blockers may be sufficient cause for this decrease in coronary blood flow.[50, 51]

Virtually all β-blockers, whether or not they have partial agonist activity, α-blocking effects, membrane stabilizing activity, and general or selective β-blocking properties, produce some degree of increased work capacity without pain in patients with angina pectoris. Therefore, it must be concluded that this effect results from a common characteristic of β-blockers: blockade of cardiac β-receptors.[50] Both D- and L-propranolol have membrane-stabilizing activity, but only L-propranolol has significant β-blocking activity. The racemic mixture (D- and L-propranolol) causes a decrease in both heart rate and force of contraction in dogs, whereas the D-isomer has hardly any effect.[55] In human subjects, D-propranolol, which has "membrane" activity but no β-blocking properties, has been ineffective in relieving angina pectoris even at very high doses.[56]

Although exercise tolerance improves with β-blockade, the increments in heart rate and blood pressure with exercise are blunted, and the rate-pressure product (systolic blood pressure × heart rate) achieved when pain occurs is lower than that reached during a control run.[57] The depressed pressure-rate product

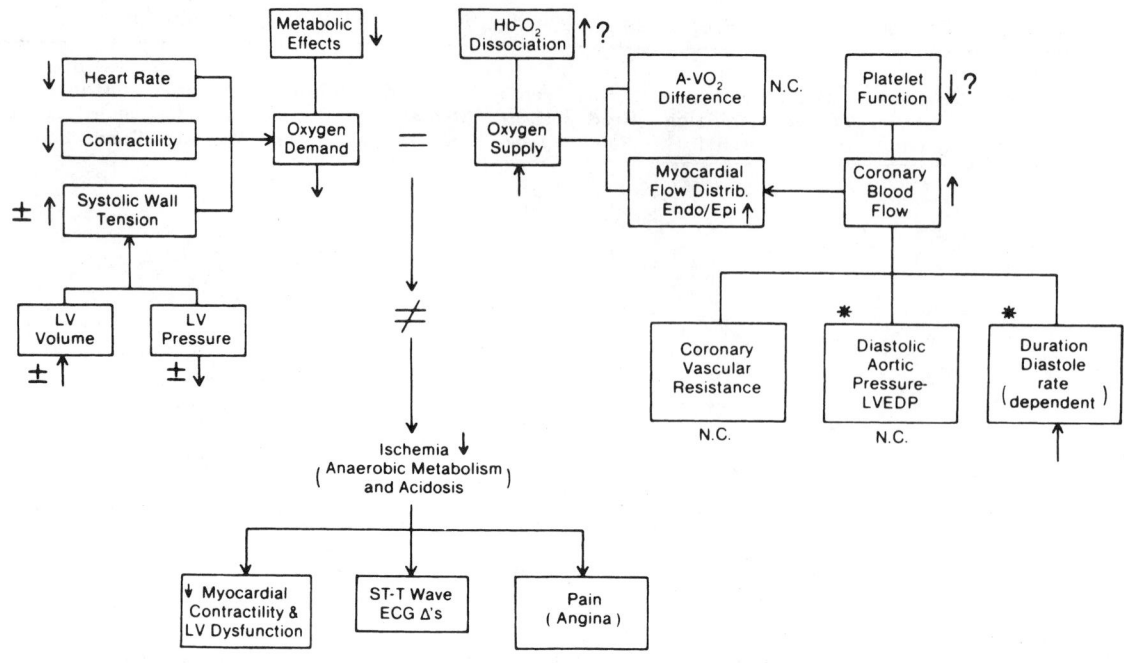

* *Limiting only in presence of coronary obstruction*

Figure 48–1. Effects of β-adrenergic blockade on myocardial oxygen supply and demand. β-Adrenergic blockers reduce overall myocardial oxygen requirements by their effects on heart rate, contractility, and blood pressure. At the same time, oxygen supply and coronary flow may be augmented by an increased diastolic perfusion time secondary to a reduction in heart rate. LVEDP, left ventricular end-diastolic pressure; NC, no change. (Adapted from Frishman WH: Beta-adrenergic blockade in the treatment of coronary artery disease. *In* Hurst JW [ed]: Clinical Essays on the Heart, Vol 2. New York: McGraw-Hill, 1983, p 25; and Frishman WH: Multifactorial actions of beta-adrenergic blocking drugs in ischemic heart disease: Current concepts. Circulation 67[Suppl 1]:11, 1983.)

at the end of exercise (about 20% reduction from control) is reported to occur with various β-blocking drugs and probably is related to both decreased cardiac output and myocardial contractility with treatment. Thus, although exercise tolerance increases with β-blockade, patients exercise less than might be expected. This may also relate to the action of β-blockers in increasing left ventricular size, causing increased left ventricular wall tension and an increase in oxygen consumption at a given blood pressure.[58]

Combined Use with Other Antianginal Therapies in Angina Pectoris

Nitrates

Combined therapy with nitrates and β-blockers may more effectively treat angina pectoris than either drug alone.[50, 59] The primary effects of β-blockers are to cause a reduction in both resting heart rate blood pressure and contractility and the changes with exercise. Because nitrates produce a reflex increase in heart rate and contractility owing to a reduction in arterial pressure, concomitant β-blocker therapy is extremely effective because it blocks this reflex increment in the heart rate. Similarly, the preservation of diastolic coronary flow with a reduced heart rate will also be beneficial.[50] In patients with a propensity for myocardial failure who may have a slight increase in heart size with the β-blockers, the peripheral venodi-

lator effects of nitrates will counteract this tendency by reducing heart size. During the administration of nitrates, the reflex increase in contractility that is mediated through the sympathetic nervous system will be checked by the presence of β-blockers. Similarly, the increase in coronary resistance associated with β-blocker administration can be ameliorated by the administration of nitrates.[50]

Calcium Antagonists

Calcium antagonists are a group of drugs that block transmembrane calcium currents in vascular smooth muscle to cause arterial vasodilatation. Some calcium antagonists (diltiazem, verapamil) also slow the heart rate and reduce atrioventricular conduction. Combined therapy with β-adrenergic and calcium antagonists can provide clinical benefits for patients with angina pectoris who remain symptomatic with either agent used alone.[60–62] Because adverse cardiovascular effects can occur, however, patients being considered for combination treatment must be selected carefully and observed closely.[60, 61]

Angina at Rest and Vasospastic Angina

Clinical studies of β-blocker therapy for angina at rest have been largely uncontrolled, with the rationale that the pathogenesis of chest pain at rest is similar to that with exertion. However, angina pectoris can be caused by multiple mechanisms, and coronary vasospasm and thrombosis appear to be responsible for ischemia in a significant proportion of patients with angina at rest.[50] Therefore, β-blockers that primarily reduce myocardial oxygen consumption but fail to exert vasodilating effects on coronary vasculature may not be totally effective in patients in whom angina is caused or increased by dynamic alterations in coronary luminal diameter.[50, 61] Despite the theoretical dangers in using the drugs in rest and vasospastic angina, β-blockers have been used successfully both as monotherapy and in combination with vasodilating agents in many patients.[50]

ANTIARRHYTHMIC EFFECTS
Electrophysiologic Effects

β-Adrenergic blocking drugs have two main effects on the electrophysiologic properties of specialized cardiac tissue (Table 48–5).[63] The first effect results from specific blockade of adrenergic stimulation of cardiac pacemaker potentials. In concentrations causing significant inhibition of adrenergic receptors, β-blockers produce little change in the transmembrane potentials of cardiac muscle. However, by competitively inhibiting adrenergic stimulation, β-blockers decrease the slope of phase 4 depolarization and the spontaneous firing rate of sinus or ectopic pacemakers and thus decrease automaticity. Arrhythmias occurring in the setting of enhanced automaticity, as seen in myocardial infarction, digitalis toxicity, hyperthyroidism, and pheochromocytoma, would therefore be expected to respond well to β-blockade.[2, 63]

The second electrophysiologic effect of some β-blockers involves membrane stabilizing action, also known as "quinidine-like" or "local anesthetic" action, which is observed only at very high dose levels. This property is unrelated to inhibition of catecholamine action and is possessed equally by both the D- and L-isomers of the drugs (D-isomers have almost no β-blocking activity).[63] Characteristic of this effect is a reduction in the rate of rise of the intracardial action potential without an effect on the spike duration of the resting potential.[63] Associated features include an elevated electric threshold of excitability, a delay in conduction velocity, and a significant increase in the

effective refractory period. This effect and its attendant changes have been explained by inhibition of the depolarizing inward sodium current.[63]

Sotalol is unique among the β-blockers in that it possesses class III antiarrhythmic properties, causing prolongation of the action potential period and thus delaying repolarization.[64] Clinical studies have verified the efficacy of sotalol in control of arrhythmias.[65] Recent studies have suggested, though, that the class III antiarrhythmic properties of sotalol may be contributing to its increased toxicity compared with other β-blockers.[64] But additional investigation will be required to determine whether its class III antiarrhythmic properties contribute significantly to its efficacy as an antiarrhythmic agent.

The most important mechanism underlying the antiarrhythmic effect of β-blockers, with the possible exclusion of sotalol, is believed to be β-blockade with resultant inhibition of pacemaker potentials. The contribution of membrane-stabilizing action does not appear to be clinically significant. *In vitro* experiments with human ventricular muscle have shown that the concentration of propranolol required for membrane stabilizing is 50 to 100 times the concentration that usually is associated with inhibition of exercise-induced tachycardia and at which only β-blocking effects occur.[63] Moreover, D-propranolol, which possesses membrane-stabilizing properties but no β-blocking action, is a weak antiarrhythmic even at high doses, whereas β-blockers devoid of membrane-stabilizing action (e.g., atenolol, esmolol, metoprolol, nadolol, pindolol) have been shown to be effective antiarrhythmic drugs.[2, 3, 66] Differences in overall clinical usefulness are related to their other associated pharmacologic properties.[2, 3]

Therapeutic Uses in Cardiac Arrhythmias

β-Adrenergic blocking drugs have become an important treatment modality for various cardiac arrhythmias (Table 48–6).[2, 3, 63] Although it has long been believed that β-blockers are more effective in treating supraventricular arrhythmias than in treating ventricular arrhythmias, it now appears that this may not be the case. These agents can be quite useful in the treatment of ventricular tachyarrhythmias in the setting of myocardial ischemia, mitral valve prolapse, and other cardiovascular conditions.[63, 67, 68]

EFFECTS IN SURVIVORS OF ACUTE MYOCARDIAL INFARCTION

β-Adrenergic blockers have beneficial effects on many determinants of myocardial ischemia (Table 48–7).[2, 51, 69] The results of placebo-controlled, long-term treatment trials with some β-adrenergic blocking drugs in survivors of acute myocardial infarction have demonstrated a favorable effect on total mortality; cardiovascular mortality, including sudden and nonsudden

---

Table 48–5. Antiarrhythmic Properties of β-Blockers

β-blockade
  Electrophysiology: depress excitability; depress conduction
  Prevention of ischemia: decrease automaticity; inhibit reentrant mechanisms
Membrane-stabilizing effects
  Local anesthetic, quinidine-like properties: depress excitability; prolong refractory period; delay conduction
  Clinically—probably not significant
Special pharmacologic properties (β₁ selectivity, intrinsic sympathomimetic activity) do not appear to contribute to antiarrhythmic effectiveness
Type III antiarrhythmic properties of sotalol may provide additional antiarrhythmic efficacy and toxicity

Table 48–6. **Effects of β-Blockers in Various Arrhythmias**

Arrhythmia	Comment
Supraventricular	
Sinus tachycardia	Treat underlying disorder; excellent response to β-blocker if there is need to control rate (e.g., ischemia).
Atrial fibrillation	β-blockers reduce rate; rarely restore sinus rhythm. May be useful in combination with digoxin.
Atrial flutter	β-blockers reduce rate; sometimes restore sinus rhythm.
Atrial tachycardia	Effective in slowing ventricular rate; may restore sinus rhythm; useful in prophylaxis.
Ventricular	
Premature ventricular contractions	Good response to β-blockers (as effective as quinidine), especially digitalis-induced and exercise (ischemia)-induced arrhythmias, mitral valve prolapse, or hypertrophic cardiomyopathy.
Ventricular tachycardia	Effective as quinidine, most effective in digitalis toxicity and exercise (ischemia)-induced arrhythmia.
Ventricular fibrillation	Electrical defibrillation is treatment of choice; β-blockers can be used to prevent recurrence in cases of excess digitalis or sympathomimetic amines; appear to be effective in reducing the incidence of ventricular fibrillation and sudden death after myocardial infarction.

From Frishman WH: Clinical Pharmacology of the Beta-Adrenoceptor Blocking Drugs, 2nd ed. Norwalk, CT: Appleton-Century-Crofts, 1984, p 100.

cardiac deaths; and the incidence of nonfatal reinfarction.[4, 70] These beneficial results with β-blocker therapy can be explained in part by both the antiarrhythmic (see Table 48–6) and the antiischemic effects of these drugs.[51, 66, 71] In addition, it has also been proposed that β-adrenergic blockers could reduce the risk of atherosclerotic plaque fissure and subsequent thrombosis.[72] Two nonselective β-blockers, propranolol and timolol, have been approved for reducing the risk of mortality in infarct survivors when started 5 to 28 days after an infarction. Metoprolol and ateno-

Table 48–7. **Possible Mechanisms by which β-Blockers Protect the Ischemic Myocardium**

Reduction in myocardial oxygen consumption, heart rate, blood pressure, and myocardial contractility
Augmentation of coronary blood flow
  Increase in diastolic perfusion time by reducing heart rate
  Augmentation of collateral blood flow
  Redistribution of blood flow to ischemic areas
Alterations in myocardial substrate use
Decrease in microvascular damage
Stabilization of cell and lysosomal membranes
Shift of oxyhemoglobin dissociation curve to the right
Inhibition of platelet aggregation

lol, two β₁-selective blockers, are approved for the same indication and can both be used intravenously in the hyperacute phase of a myocardial infarction. β-Blockers have been suggested as a treatment for reducing the extent of myocardial injury[4, 73, 74] and mortality during the hyperacute phase of myocardial infarction,[75, 76] but their exact role in this situation remains unclear.[77] Intravenously and orally administered atenolol have been shown to cause a modest reduction in early mortality when given during the hyperacute phase of acute myocardial infarction.[75] Atenolol and metoprolol reduce early infarct mortality rates by 15%,[75, 76] an effect that may be improved on when β-adrenergic blockade is combined with acute thrombolytic therapy. Metoprolol combined with acute thrombolysis has been evaluated in the Thrombolysis In Myocardial Infarction II (TIMI-II) study.[78]

SILENT MYOCARDIAL ISCHEMIA

Investigators have observed that not all myocardial ischemic episodes detected by electrocardiography are associated with detectable symptoms.[79] Positron emission imaging techniques have validated the theory that these silent ischemic episodes indicate true myocardial ischemia.[80] The prognostic importance of silent myocardial ischemia occurring at rest and/or during exercise has not been determined.[81] β-Blockers are as successful in reducing the frequency of silent ischemic episodes detected by ambulatory electrocardiogram (ECG) monitoring as in reducing the frequency of painful ischemic events.[79]

OTHER CARDIOVASCULAR APPLICATIONS

Although β-blockers have been studied extensively in patients with angina pectoris, arrhythmias, and hypertension, they have also been shown to be safe and effective for other cardiovascular conditions (see Table 48–l). The following sections describe some of these conditions.

Hypertrophic Cardiomyopathy

β-Adrenergic receptor blocking drugs have been proven effective in therapy for patients with hypertrophic cardiomyopathy and idiopathic hypertrophic subaortic stenosis.[8] These drugs are useful in controlling the symptoms: dyspnea, angina, and syncope.[2, 3] β-Blockers have also been shown to lower the intraventricular pressure gradient both at rest and with exercise.

The outflow pressure gradient is not the only abnormality in hypertrophic cardiomyopathy; more important is the loss of ventricular compliance, which impedes normal left ventricular function. It has been shown by invasive and noninvasive methods that propranolol can improve left ventricular function in this condition.[82] The drug also produces favorable changes in ventricular compliance while it relieves symptoms. Propranolol has been approved for this condition and may be combined with the calcium antagonist verapamil in patients who do not respond to the β-blocker alone.

The salutary hemodynamic and symptomatic effects produced by propranolol derive from its inhibition of sympathetic stimulation of the heart.[83] However, there is no evidence that the drug alters the primary cardiomyopathic process; many patients remain in or return to their severely symptomatic state and some die despite its administration.[8]

Dilated Cardiomyopathy

The ability of intravenously administered sympathomimetic amines to effect an acute increase in myocardial contractility through stimulation of the β-adrenoceptor has prompted hope that orally administered analogues may provide long-term benefit for patients with severe heart failure. Observations concerning the regulation of the myocardial adrenoceptor and abnormalities of β-receptor–mediated stimulation in the failing myocardium have caused a critical reappraisal of the scientific validity of sustained β_1-adrenoceptor stimulation, however.[84, 85] New evidence suggests that β_1-adrenoceptor blockade, when tolerated, has a favorable effect on the underlying cardiomyopathic process.[17, 86–88]

The excessive catecholamine stimulation of the heart that occurs in chronic congestive heart failure can cause myocardial catecholamine depletion,[89] a direct toxic effect on the heart,[90, 91] alterations in the β-adrenergic receptor/adenylate cyclase complex,[92] and downregulation of β-adrenergic receptors.[84, 85, 93] It appears that β-adrenergic blockade can correct these abnormalities and possibly improve left ventricular function.[87, 88]

Preliminary studies with chronic β-blockade have demonstrated improvement in left ventricular function in many patients with advanced cardiomyopathy.[94–97] These studies have included patients who showed dramatic improvement in their hemodynamic situations while awaiting cardiac transplantation. Recently completed and ongoing double-blind multicenter studies with the selective blockers bisoprolol and metoprolol and the vasodilating β-blockers bucindolol and carvedilol would suggest an important future role for β-blockade as a long-term adjunctive treatment to other existing therapies (digoxin, diuretics, ACE inhibitors) in patients with chronic congestive cardiomyopathy.[98]

Mitral Valve Prolapse

This auscultatory complex, characterized by a nonejection systolic click, a late systolic murmur, or a midsystolic click followed by a late systolic murmur, has been studied extensively. Atypical chest pain, malignant arrhythmias, and nonspecific ST- and T-wave abnormalities have been observed with this condition. By decreasing sympathetic tone, β-adrenergic block-

ers have been shown to be useful for relieving the chest pains and palpitations that many of these patients experience and for reducing the incidence of life-threatening arrhythmias and other ECG abnormalities.[10]

Dissecting Aneurysms

β-Adrenergic blockade plays a major role in the treatment of patients with acute aortic dissection. During the hyperacute phase, β-blocking agents reduce the force and velocity of myocardial contraction and hence the progression of the dissecting hematoma.[7] Moreover, such administration must be initiated simultaneously with the institution of other antihypertensive therapy that may cause reflex tachycardia and increases in cardiac output and myocardial force of contraction, factors that can aggravate the dissection process. Initially, propranolol is administered intravenously to reduce the heart rate to below 60 beats/min. Once a patient is stabilized and long-term medical management is contemplated, the patient should be maintained on oral β-blocker therapy to prevent recurrence.[7]

It has been demonstrated that long-term β-blocker therapy may also reduce the risk of dissection in patients prone to this complication (e.g., Marfan's syndrome).[99] Systolic time intervals are used to assess the adequacy of β-blockade in children with Marfan's syndrome.[13]

Tetralogy of Fallot

By reducing the effects of increased adrenergic tone on the right ventricular infundibulum in tetralogy of Fallot, β-blockers have been shown to be useful for the treatment of severe hypoxic spells and hypercyanotic attacks.[12, 13] With long-term use, these drugs have also been shown to prevent prolonged hypoxic spells. These drugs should be considered only palliative; definitive surgical repair of this condition is usually required.

QT-Interval Prolongation Syndrome

The syndrome of ECG QT-interval prolongation is usually a congenital condition associated with deafness, syncope, and sudden death.[11] Abnormalities in sympathetic nervous system functioning in the heart have been proposed as explanations for the electrophysiologic aberrations seen in these patients.[11] Propranolol appears to be the most effective drug for treatment of this syndrome. It reduces the frequency of syncopal episodes in most patients and may prevent sudden death.[11] This drug will reduce the ECG QT interval.

Regression of Left Ventricular Hypertrophy

Left ventricular hypertrophy induced by systemic hypertension is an independent risk factor for cardiovas-

Table 48–8. Pharmacodynamic Properties and Noncardiac Effects of β-Adrenoreceptor Blockers

Drug	Relative β₁ Selectivity*	Partial Agonist Activity	Membrane-Stabilizing Activity	Bronchial Tone	Platelet Aggregability	Plasma Renin Activity	Peripheral Vascular Resistance	RBF	GFR	HDL-C	LDL-C	VLDL-TRI
Acebutolol	+	+	+	↑↔↓								
Atenolol	+ +	0	0	↑↔↓		↓↔	↑↔	↓↔	↓↔	↔	↔	↔
Betaxolol	+	0	0	↑↔↓		↓↔	↑↔	↓↔	↓↔	↔	↔	↔
Bisoprolol	+ +	0	0	↑↔↓		↓↔	↑↔	↓↔	↔	↔	↔	↔
Bucindolol	0	+	0	↑↔↓		↓↔	↑↔	↓↔	↓↔	↔	↔	↔
Carteolol	0	+	0	↑↔↓		↓↔	↓	↑↔	↔	↔	↔	↔
Carvedilol	0	0	+ +	↑↔↓	↓	↓↔	↓↔↑	↓↔	↓↔	↔	↔	↔
Esmolol	+ +	0	0	↑↔↓		↓↔	↓	↑↔	↔	↔	↔	↔
Labetalol†	0	+?	0	↑↔↓	↔	↓↔	↑↔	?	?	?	?	?
Metoprolol	+ +	0	0	↑↔↓	↔	↓↔	↓	↔↑	↔	↔	↔	↔
Nadolol	0	0	0	↔↓		↓↔	↑	↓↔	↓↔	↔↓	↔	↑↔
Oxprenolol	0	+	+	↑↔↓		↓↔	↑	↑	↑↔	?	?	?
Penbutolol	0	+	0	↑↔↓	↓	↓↔	↑↔	↓↔	↓	?	?	?
Pindolol	0	+ +	0	↑↔↓	↓	↓↔	↔↓	?	?	?	?	?
Propranolol	0	0	+ +	↔↓	↓	↓↔↑	↔↓	↓↔	↓↔	↔	↔	↔
Sotalol	0	0	0	↔↓		↓	↑	↓	↓	↓	↔	↑
Timolol	0	0	0	↔↓	↓	↓	↑	↓	↓	?	?	?
Isomer:												
D-propranolol	0	0	+ +	↔	↓	↔	↔	↔	↔	?	?	?

GFR, glomerular filtration rate; HDL-C, high-density lipoprotein cholesterol; LDL-C, low-density lipoprotein cholesterol; RBF, renal blood flow; VLDL-TRI, very-low-density lipoprotein triglycerides; + +, strong effect; +, modest effect; 0, no effect; ↑, elevation; ↓, reduction; ↔, no change.

*β₁ Selectivity is seen only with low therapeutic drug concentrations. With higher concentrations, β₁ selectivity is not seen.

†Labetalol has additional α₁-adrenergic blocking properties and direct vasodilatory activity.

Data from Frishman WH: Clinical Pharmacology of the β-Adrenoceptor Blocking Drugs, 2nd ed. Norwalk, CT: Appleton-Century-Crofts, 1984, pp 36–37; and Frishman WH: Beta-adrenergic blockers. Med Clin North Am 72(1):61, 1988.

cular mortality and morbidity.[100] Regression of left ventricular hypertrophy with drug therapy is feasible and may improve patient outcome.[100] β-Adrenergic blockers can cause regression of left ventricular hypertrophy, as determined by echocardiography, with or without an associated reduction in blood pressure.[100]

NONCARDIOVASCULAR APPLICATIONS

β-Adrenergic receptors are ubiquitous in the human body, and their blockade affects a variety of organ and metabolic systems (Table 48–8).[2, 3, 6] Some noncardiovascular uses of β-blockers (glaucoma, migraine headache prophylaxis, essential tremor) have been approved by the Food and Drug Administration.[1]

REFERENCES

1. Frishman WH: β-Adrenoceptor antagonists: New drugs and new indications. N Engl J Med 305:500, 1981.
2. Frishman WH: Clinical Pharmacology of the β-Adrenoceptor Blocking Drugs, 2nd ed. Norwalk, CT: Appleton-Century-Crofts, 1984.
3. Frishman WH, Sonnenblick EH: β-Adrenergic blocking drugs. In Schlant RC, Alexander RW (eds): The Heart, 8th ed. New York, McGraw Hill, 1993, p 1271.
4. Frishman WH, Furberg CD, Friedewald WT: β-Adrenergic blockade for survivors of acute myocardial infarction. N Engl J Med 310:830, 1984.
5. Wikstrand J, Warnold I, Olsson G, et al: Primary prevention with metoprolol in patients with hypertension. JAMA 259:1976, 1988.
6. Cruickshank JM, Prichard BNC: Beta Blockers in Clinical Practice, 2nd ed. Edinburgh: Churchill Livingstone, 1994, p 765.
7. DeSanctis RW, Doroghazi RM, Austen WG, Buckley MJ: Aortic dissection. N Engl J Med 317:1060, 1987.
8. Cohen LS, Braunwald E: Amelioration of angina pectoris in idiopathic hypertrophic subaortic stenosis with beta-adrenergic blockade. Circulation 35:847, 1967.
9. Turner JRB: Propranolol in the treatment of digitalis-induced and digitalis-resistant tachycardia. Am J Cardiol 18:450, 1966.
10. Winkle RA, Lopes MG, Goodman DS, et al: Propranolol for patients with mitral valve prolapse. Am Heart J 93:422, 1970.
11. Schwartz PJ: Idiopathic long QT syndrome: Progress and questions. Am Heart J 109:399, 1985.
12. Kornbluth A, Frishman WH, Ackerman M: β-Adrenergic blockade in children. Cardiol Clin 5:629, 1987.
13. Garson A, Gillette PC, McNamara DG: Propranolol: The preferred palliation for tetralogy of Fallot. Am J Cardiol 47:1098, 1981.
14. Meister SG, Engel TR, Feitosa GS, et al: Propranolol in mitral stenosis during sinus rhythm. Am Heart J 94:685, 1977.
15. Bhatia ML, Shivastava S, Roy SG: Immediate hemodynamic effects of a beta-adrenergic blocking agent—propranolol—in mitral stenosis at fixed heart rates. Br Heart J 34:638, 1972.
16. Svedberg K, Hjalmarson A, Waagstein F: Beneficial effects of long-term beta-blockade in congestive cardiomyopathy. Br Heart J 44:117, 1980.
17. Sullebarger JT, Liang C-S: Beta-adrenergic receptor stimulation and inhibition in chronic congestive heart failure. Heart Failure 7:154, 1991.
18. Kraus ML, Gottlieb LD, Horwitz RI, et al: Randomized clinical trial of atenolol in patients with alcohol withdrawal. N Engl J Med 313:905, 1985.
19. Weber RB, Reinmuth OM: The treatment of migraine with propranolol. Neurology 22:366, 1972.
20. Young RR, Growdon JH, Shahani BT: Beta-adrenergic mechanism in action tremor. N Engl J Med 293:950, 1975.
21. Granville-Grossman KL, Turner P: The effect of propranolol on anxiety. Lancet 1:788, 1966.
22. Frishman WH, Razin A, Swencionis C, et al: Beta-adrenoceptor blockade in anxiety states: A new approach to therapy. Update. Cardiovasc Rev Rep "Classics of the Decade Series" 13(2):8, 1992.
23. Sellers EM, Degani NC, Silm DH, et al: Propranolol decreased noradrenaline secretion and alcohol withdrawal. Lancet 1:94, 1976.
24. Ingbar SH: The role of antiadrenergic agents in the management of thyrotoxicosis. Cardiovasc Rev Rep 2:683, 1981.
25. Caro JF, Castro JH, Glennon JA: Effect of long-term propranolol administration on parathyroid hormone and calcium con-

centration in primary hyperparathyroidism. Ann Intern Med 91:740, 1979.

26. Lebrec D, Poynard T, Hillon P, et al: Propranolol for prevention of recurrent gastrointestinal bleeding in patients with cirrhosis. N Engl J Med 305:1371, 1981.

27. The SHEP Cooperative Research Group: Prevention of stroke by antihypertensive drug treatment in older persons with isolated systolic hypertension: Final results of the Systolic Hypertension in the Elderly Program (SHEP). JAMA 265:3255, 1991.

28. The Fifth Report of the Joint National Committee on Detection: Evaluation and treatment of high blood pressure. Arch Intern Med 153:154, 1993.

29. Saunders E, Weir MR, Kong BW, et al: A comparison of the efficacy and safety of a β-blocker, a calcium channel blocker, and a converting enzyme inhibitor in hypertensive blacks. Arch Intern Med 150:1707, 1990.

30. Frishman WH, Bryzinski BS, Coulson LR, et al: A multifactorial trial design to assess combination therapy in hypertension: Treatment with bisoprolol and hydrochlorothiazide. Arch Intern Med 154:1461, 1994.

31. Frishman WH, Burris JF, Mroczek WJ, et al: First-line therapy option with low-dose bisoprolol fumarate and low-dose hydrochlorothiazide in patients with stage I and stage II systemic hypertension. J Clin Pharmacol 35:182, 1995.

32. Frohlich ED: Hyperdynamic circulation and hypertension. Postgrad Med J 52:68, 1972.

33. Laragh JH: Vasoconstriction-volume analysis for understanding and treating hypertension: The use of renin and aldosterone profiles. Am J Med 55:261, 1973.

34. Myers MG, Lewis PJ, Reid JL, et al: Brain concentration of propranolol in relation to hypotension effects in the rabbit with observations on brain propranolol levels in man. J Pharmacol Exp Ther 192:327, 1975.

35. Frishman WH: Atenolol and timolol: Two new systemic β-adrenoceptor antagonists. N Engl J Med 306:1456, 1982.

36. Frishman WH: Nadolol: A new β-adrenoceptor antagonist. N Engl J Med 305:678, 1981.

37. Prichard BNC: Propranolol as an antihypertensive agent. Am Heart J 79:128, 1970.

38. Frishman WH: β-Adrenergic blockers. In Izzo JL Jr, Black HR (eds): Hypertension Primer. Dallas: American Heart Association, 1993, p 297.

39. Koch-Weser J: Metoprolol. N Engl J Med 301:698, 1979.

40. Langer SZ: Presynaptic receptors and their role in the regulation of transmitter release. Br J Pharmacol 60:481, 1977.

41. Berthelsen S, Pettinger WA: A functional basis for classification of β-adrenergic receptors. Life Sci 21:595, 1977.

42. Yamaguchi N, de Champlain J, Nadeau RL: Regulation of norepinephrine release from cardiac sympathetic fibers in the dog by presynaptic α- and β-receptors. Circ Res 41:108, 1977.

43. Majewski HJ, McCulloch MW, Rand MJ, et al: Adrenaline activation of pre-junctional β-adrenoceptors in guinea pig atria. Br J Pharmacol 71:435, 1980.

44. Rahn KH, Hawlina A, Kersting F, et al: Studies on the antihypertensive action of the optical isomers of propranolol in man. Naunyn Schmiedebergs Arch Pharmacol 286:319, 1974.

45. Pickering TG, Gribbin B, Petersen ES, et al: Effects of autonomic blockade on the baroreflex in man at rest and during exercise. Circ Res 30:177, 1972.

46. Ahlquist RP: A study of adrenotropic receptors. Am J Physiol 153:586, 1948.

47. Sonnenblick EH, Ross J Jr, Braunwald E: Oxygen consumption of the heart: Newer concepts of its multifactorial determination. Am J Cardiol 22:328, 1968.

48. Sonnenblick EH, Skelton CL: Myocardial energetics: Basic principles and clinical implications. N Engl J Med 285:668, 1971.

49. Black JW, Stephenson JS: Pharmacology of a new adrenergic beta-receptor blocking compound (Nethalide). Lancet 2:311, 1962.

50. Frishman WH: Beta-adrenergic blockade in the treatment of coronary artery disease. In Hurst JW (ed): Clinical Essays on the Heart, Vol 2. New York: McGraw-Hill, 1983, p 25.

51. Frishman WH: Multifactorial actions of beta-adrenergic blocking drugs in ischemic heart disease: Current concepts. Circulation 67(Suppl 1):11, 1983.

52. Parratt JR, Grayson J: Myocardial vascular reactivity after β-adrenergic blockade. Lancet 1:338, 1966.

53. Becker LC, Fortuin NJ, Pitt B: Effects of ischemia and antianginal drugs on the distribution of radioactive microspheres in the canine left ventricle. Circ Res 28:263, 1971.

54. Wolfson S, Gorlin R: Cardiovascular pharmacology of propranolol in man. Circulation 40:501, 1969.

55. Barrett AM: A comparison of the effect of (±) propranolol and (+) propranolol in anesthetized dogs: β-Receptor blocking and hemodynamic action. J Pharm Pharmacol 21:241, 1969.

56. Bjorntorp P: Treatment of angina pectoris with beta-adrenergic blockade, mode of action. Acta Med Scand 184:259, 1968.

57. Frishman WH, Smithen C, Befler B, et al: Non-invasive assessment of clinical response to oral propranolol. Am J Cardiol 35:635, 1975.

58. Robinson BF: The mode of action of beta-antagonists in angina pectoris. Postgrad Med J 47(Suppl 2):41, 1971.

59. Parmley WW: The combination of beta-adrenergic blocking agents and nitrates in the treatment of stable angina pectoris. Cardiol Rev Rep 3:1425, 1982.

60. Weiner DA, Klein MD: Calcium antagonists for the treatment of angina pectoris. In Weiner DA, Frishman WH (eds): Therapy of Angina Pectoris. New York: Marcel Dekker, 1986, p 145.

61. Frishman WH, Sonnenblick EH: Calcium-channel blockers. In Schlant RC, Alexander RW (eds): The Heart, 8th ed. New York: McGraw Hill, 1993, p 1291.

62. Frishman WH: Comparative efficacy and concomitant use of bepridil and beta blockers in the management of angina pectoris. Am J Cardiol 69:50D, 1992.

63. Miura D, Frishman WH, Dangman KH: Class II drugs. In Dangman KH, Miura D (eds): Basic and Clinical Electrophysiology and Pharmacology of the Heart. New York, Marcel Dekker, 1991, p 665.

64. Cavusoglu E, Frishman WH: Sotalol: A new β-adrenergic blocker for ventricular arrhythmias. Prog Cardiovasc Dis 37(6):423, 1995.

65. ESVEM Investigators: Determinants of predicted efficacy of antiarrhythmic drugs in the Electrophysiologic Study Versus Electrocardiographic Monitoring Trial. Circulation 87:323, 1993.

66. Frishman WH, Murthy VS, Strom JA: Ultra-short acting β-adrenergic blockers. Med Clin North Am 72:359, 1988.

67. Ryden L, Ariniego R, Arnman K, et al: A double-blind trial of metoprolol in acute myocardial infarction: Effects on ventricular tachyarrhythmias. N Engl J Med 308:614, 1983.

68. Lichstein E, Morganroth J, Harrist R, et al: Effect of propranolol on ventricular arrhythmias—The beta-blockers: Preliminary data from the heart attack trial experience. Circulation 67(Suppl 1):32, 1983.

69. Braunwald E, Muller JE, Kloner RA, et al: Role of beta-adrenergic blockade in the therapy of patients with myocardial infarction. Am J Med 74:113, 1983.

70. Boissel-J-P, Leizorovicz A, Picolet H, et al: Secondary prevention after high risk myocardial infarction with low-dose acebutolol. Am J Cardiol 66:251, 1990.

71. Furberg CD, Hawkins CM, Lichstein E: Effect of propranolol in post-infarction patients with mechanical or electrical complications. Circulation 69:761, 1984.

72. Frishman WH, Lazar EJ: Reduction of mortality, sudden death and non-fatal reinfarction with beta-adrenergic blockers in survivors of acute myocardial infarction: A new hypothesis regarding the cardioprotective action of beta-adrenergic blockade. Am J Cardiol 66:66G, 1990.

73. International Collaborative Study Group: Reduction of infarct size with the early use of timolol in acute myocardial infarction. N Engl J Med 310:9, 1984.

74. Hjalmarson A, Elmfeldt D, Herlitz J, et al: Effect on mortality of metoprolol in acute myocardial infarction. Lancet 2:823, 1981.

75. ISIS-I Collaborative Group: Randomized trial of intravenous atenolol among 16,027 cases of suspected acute myocardial infarction: ISIS-II. Lancet 2:57, 1986.

76. MIAMI Trial Research Group: Metoprolol in acute myocardial infarction (MIAMI): A randomized placebo-controlled international trial. Eur Heart J 6:199, 1985.

77. Frishman WH, Skolnick AE, Miller KP: Secondary prevention post infarction: The role of β-adrenergic blockers, calcium-channel blockers and aspirin. *In* Gersh BJ, Rahimtoola SH (eds): Management of Myocardial Infarction. New York: Elsevier, 1991, p 469.

78. The TIMI Study Group: Comparison of intravenous and conservative strategies after treatment with intravenous tissue plasminogen activator in acute myocardial infarction: Results of the thrombolysis in myocardial infarction (TIMI) phase II trial. N Engl J Med 320:618, 1989.

79. Frishman WH, Teicher M: Antianginal drug therapy for silent myocardial ischemia. Am Heart J 114:140, 1987.

80. Deanfield JE, Shea MJ, Selwyn AP: Clinical evaluation of transient myocardial ischemia during daily life. Am J Med 79(Suppl 3A):18, 1985.

81. ACIP Investigators: Asymptomatic Cardiac Ischemia Pilot Study (ACIP). Am J Cardiol 70:744, 1992.

82. Hubner PJB, Ziady GM, Lane GK, et al: Double-blind trial of propranolol and practolol in hypertrophic cardiomyopathy. Br Heart J 35:1116, 1973.

83. Epstein SE, Henry WL, Clark CE, et al: Asymmetric septal hypertrophy. Ann Intern Med 81:650, 1974.

84. Bristow MR, Ginsberg R, Minobe W, et al: Decreased catecholamine sensitivity and β-adrenergic receptor density in failing human hearts. N Engl J Med 307:205, 1982.

85. Colucci WS, Alexander RW, Williams GH, et al: Decreased lymphocyte beta-adrenergic receptor density in patients with heart failure and tolerance to the beta-adrenergic agonist pirbuterol. N Engl J Med 305:185, 1981.

86. Bristow MR: The adrenergic nervous system in heart failure [editorial]. N Engl J Med 311:850, 1984.

87. Andersson E, Blomstrom-Lundquist C, Hedner T, et al: Exercise hemodynamics and myocardial metabolism during long-term betaadrenergic blockade in severe heart failure. J Am Coll Cardiol 18:1059, 1991.

88. Lichstein E, Hager WD, Gregory JJ, et al: Relation between beta-adrenergic blocker use, various correlates of left ventricular function, and the chance of developing congestive heart failure: The Multicenter Diltiazem-Post Infarction Research Group. J Am Coll Cardiol 16:1327, 1990.

89. Sole MJ, Kamble AB, Hussain MN: A possible change in the rate-limiting step for cardiac norepinephrine synthesis in the cardiomyopathic Syrian hamster. Circ Res 41:814, 1977.

90. Bloom S, Davis DL: Calcium as mediator of isoproterenol-induced myocardial necrosis. Am J Pathol 69:459, 1972.

91. Kahn DS, Rona G, Chappel CI: Isoproterenol-induced cardiac necrosis. Ann N Y Acad Sci 156:285, 1969.

92. Gilbert EM, Port JD, Hershberger RI, et al: Clinical significance of alterations in the β-adrenergic receptor-adenylate cyclase complex in heart failure. Heart Failure 5:91, 1989.

93. Heinsimer JA, Lefkowitz RJ: The beta-adrenergic receptor in heart failure. Hosp Pract 11(18):103, 1983.

94. Eichorn EJ, Bedotto JB, Malloy CR, et al: Effect of β-adrenergic blockade on myocardial function and energetics in congestive heart failure: Improvements in hemodynamic, contractile, and diastolic performance with bucindolol. Circulation 82:473, 1990.

95. Waagstein F, Caidahl K, Wallentin I, et al: Long-term β-blockade in dilated cardiomyopathy: Effects of short and long-term metoprolol treatment followed by withdrawal and readministration of metoprolol. Circulation 80:551, 1989.

96. Heilbrunn SM, Shah P, Bristow MR, et al: Increased β-receptor density and improved hemodynamic response to catecholamine stimulation during long-term metoprolol therapy in heart failure from dilated cardiomyopathy. Circulation 79:483, 1989.

97. Jessup M: Beta-adrenergic blockade in congestive heart failure: Answering the old questions. J Am Coll Cardiol 18:1067, 1991.

98. CIBIS Investigators and Committees: A randomized trial of β-blockade in heart failure: The Cardiac Insufficiency Bisoprolol Study (CIBIS). Circulation 90:1765, 1994.

99. Pyeritz RE: Protection of the aortic root by propranolol in Marfan's syndrome. J Med Genet 23:469, 1986.

100. Hachamovitch R, Sonnenblick EH, Strom VA, et al: Left ventricular hypertrophy in hypertension and the effects of antihypertensive drug therapy. Curr Prob Cardiol 13(6):375, 1988.

CHAPTER 49

β-Adrenoreceptor Blockers in Hypertension

Lennart Hansson, M.D., Ph.D.

HISTORY

In 1948, Ahlquist[1] introduced the concept of α- and β-receptors based on the response of different organ systems to various agonists. These receptors are now usually referred to as adrenoreceptors. The α-adrenoreceptors are most sensitive to stimulation with epinephrine, less to norepinephrine, and least to isoprenaline; β-adrenoreceptors are most sensitive to isoprenaline, less to epinephrine, and least to norepinephrine.[1] Later, Lands et al.[2] subdivided the β-adrenoreceptors into the β₁ and β₂ subtypes. The β₁-adrenoreceptors have equal affinity for norepinephrine and epinephrine, whereas the β₂-adrenoreceptors have greater affinity for epinephrine than for norepinephrine.[2] Expanded knowledge about the adrenoreceptors and their distribution in various organs, in combination with the hemodynamic observations by Sannerstedt[3] and Lund-Johansen[4] that increased total peripheral resistance is a hallmark of established hypertension, made it totally unexpected that β-adrenoreceptor blocking agents (β-blockers) would have a useful antihypertensive effect. In a paper published in 1968, the observed antihypertensive effect of β-blockers in patients with hypertension was considered a paradox.[5]

Observations on the first β-adrenoreceptor blocking compound had been published by 1958,[6] but not until 1964 did the first publications appear that showed that β-blockers had an antihypertensive effect. Two of these studies[7, 8] referred to pronetholol, a compound that was discontinued because of suspicions of tumorigenesis.[9] However, Prichard and Gillam[10] also published observations on the antihypertensive effect of propranolol in 1964. Because of the persistence of Prichard and Gillam, who continued publishing in this area,[11, 12] other investigators became interested and could confirm the useful antihypertensive

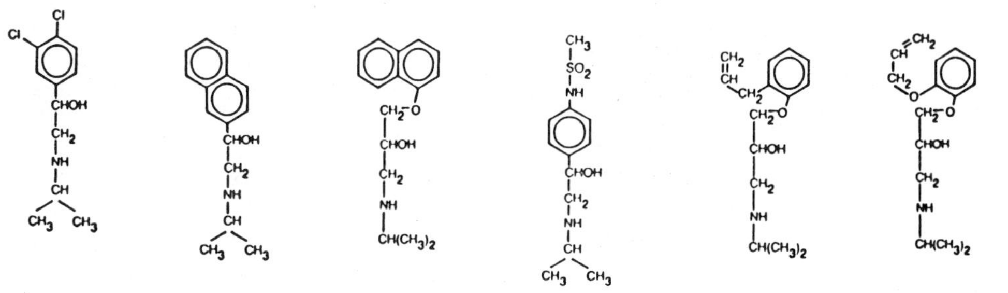

Dichloroisoprenaline (DCI) Pronethalol Propranolol Sotalol Alprenolol Oxprenolol

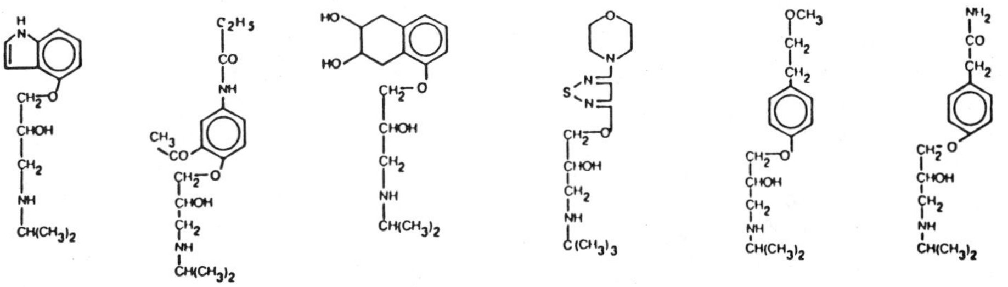

Pindolol Acebutolol Nadolol Timolol Metoprolol Atenolol

Figure 49–1. Structural formulas of 12 different β-adrenoreceptor blocking compounds.

effect of β-blockers.[13, 14] Mainly because of the favorable balance between their therapeutic and adverse effects, β-blockers became the drugs of first choice in the treatment of hypertension in some centers by the early 1970s.[15] β-Blockers have become widely accepted as first-line treatment for hypertension, as illustrated by the guidelines for the treatment of mild hypertension issued jointly by the World Health Organization and the International Society of Hypertension already in 1983 and 1986[16, 17] and by the Joint National Committee on Detection, Evaluation and Treatment of High Blood Pressure in 1984.[18]

CHEMISTRY

The chemical constitutions of the various β-blockers vary widely, but they have one general feature in common: an aminopropanol moiety linked to an aromatic system (Fig. 49–1).[19] The β-blockers can be further divided into arylethanolamines (e.g., pronethalol and sotalol) and aryloxypropranolamines (e.g., propranolol, atenolol, and pindolol).[19] It is possible to identify the structural properties that are essential for the β-blocking activity and for the relative lipophilicity of these compounds, whereas the structural requirements for partial agonisms are less clear.[19] The structural requirements for β_1 or β_2 selectivity within a chemical series of compounds can usually be predicted, but not with absolute certainty.[19]

PHARMACOLOGY

The main pharmacologic action of β-blockers is obviously to block β-adrenoreceptors. Such receptors are not uniformly distributed in the body. β_1-Adrenoreceptors predominate in cardiac and adipose tissue, whereas β_2-adrenoreceptors are of clinical relevance in numerous organs (e.g., blood vessels and bronchi) (Table 49–1). However, it should be remembered that the organ separation of β_1- and β_2-adrenoreceptors varies greatly among species as well as among individuals.[20]

In addition to their ability to block β_1- and β_2-adrenoreceptors, β-blockers have a number of ancil-

Table 49–1. **Type and Organ Distribution of β-Adrenoreceptors**

Tissue	Receptor Type	Response
Myocardium	β_1	Inotropic, chronotropic, dromotropic
Bronchial muscle	β_2	Relaxation
Vascular muscle	β_2	Relaxation
Biliary muscle	β_2	Relaxation
Skeletal muscle	β_2	Tremor
Coronary vascular muscle	β_1	Relaxation
Uterus	β_2	Relaxation
Liver	β_1	Glycogenolysis
Adipose	β_2	Release of free fatty acids

lary properties, such as an agonistic effect, often referred to as intrinsic sympathomimetic activity (ISA), membrane-stabilizing activities (MSAs), and vasodilating actions (which can be attributed to α-adrenoreceptor blockade, stimulation of vascular β$_2$-adrenoreceptors, or a direct nonadrenergic inhibition of vascular tone) (Table 49–2). The combination of tissue differentiation of the adrenoreceptors with the availability of a multitude of β-blockers with different characteristics opens up possibilities for carefully tailored therapy. However, for the treatment of patients with hypertension, it is obvious that the blockade of β$_1$-adrenoreceptors is the *sine qua non*, but properties such as selective β$_2$ ISA or other ways of obtaining vasodilatation markedly influence the hemodynamic profile of these agents.

The pharmacokinetic profile of the β-blockers is closely related to their lipophilicity.[19] Compounds such as propranolol, oxpranolol, and pindolol are rapidly and completely absorbed when given orally, whereas the absorption of nadolol varies widely depending on species, a quality that also holds true for for the β$_1$-selective agent atenolol but not for metoprolol.[19] The extent of systemic bioavailability varies considerably, depending mainly on the lipophilicity of the drug, although plasma-protein binding appears to play a role as well. The elimination half-life of most agents is 3 to 6 hours, and elimination is mainly by metabolism of the lipophilic agents, whereas the hydrophilic ones are excreted mainly by the kidneys.[19]

EFFECTS ON PATHOPHYSIOLOGY
Hemodynamics

Acute intravenous administration of propranolol to both normotensive and hypertensive individuals caused a significant reduction of cardiac output in both groups, attributable mainly to a fall in heart rate in the hypertensive group and a reduction in stroke volume in the normotensive group.[21] Similar observations have later confirmed that intravenous administration of propranolol or a similar β-blocker causes a rapid reduction in heart rate and cardiac output but no acute fall in blood pressure.[22, 23]

During prolonged oral administration of a β-blocker such as propranolol, the significant reduction in cardiac output remains, whereas the total peripheral resistance falls from an initially elevated level after the acute dose of the β-blocker to a level not significantly higher than the level initially untreated (Fig. 49–2).[22, 23] This clear dissociation between the β-blocking effect, evident from the reduced heart rate and cardiac output, and the antihypertensive effect, which appears hours or days later, has been called the delayed vasodilating effect.[24] Another illustration of the dissociation between the β-blocking and the antihypertensive effects is when treatment with β-blockers is interrupted. In this situation, heart rate rapidly returns to the initial untreated level, sometimes with a temporary overshoot, whereas blood pressure returns only gradually to the initial level.[25]

This hemodynamic pattern, illustrated in Figure 49–2, is similar to that of most β-blockers, and this pattern seems to persist during extended periods of treatment. Thus, in a 5-year hemodynamic follow-up of hypertensive patients treated with atenolol that used reliable and reproducible methods, the antihypertensive effect clearly was attributable mainly to a persisting reduction in cardiac output.[26]

However, β-blockers with marked ISA seem to differ in this respect. In an extensive review of hemodynamic studies conducted with various β-blockers in patients treated for hypertension, Man in't Veld and Schalekamp[27] showed that, after acute administration, β-blockers with ISA do not reduce cardiac output at rest. If anything, they cause an acute fall in vascular resistance and blood pressure, and this hemodynamic profile becomes clearly established during long-term treatment.

Table 49–2. **Pharmacologic Properties of β-Adrenoreceptor Blocking Compounds**

Compound	Blocks β$_1$	Blocks β$_2$	MSA	β$_1$ ISA	β$_2$ ISA	Antihypertensive Effect	Comments
Nonselective							
Propranolol	+	+	+	−	−	+	
Timolol	+	+	−	−	−	+	
Oxprenolol	+	+	+	+	+	+	
Pindolol	+	+	−	?	+	+	Marked ISA
β$_1$-Selective							
Metoprolol	+	−	−	−	−	+	
Practolol	+	−	−	+	+	+	
Epanolol	+	−	−	+	−	?	
β$_2$-Selective							
ICI 118.511	−	+	?	−	−	−	
β-Blockade + Vasodilatation							
Labetalol	+	+	+	−	−	+	α-Blocking effect
Carvedilol	+	+	−	−	−	+	Direct vasodilatation
Dilevalol	+	+	−	−	+	+	Vasodilation due to β$_2$-agonism

ISA, intrinsic sympathomimetic activity; MSA, membrane-stabilizing activity.

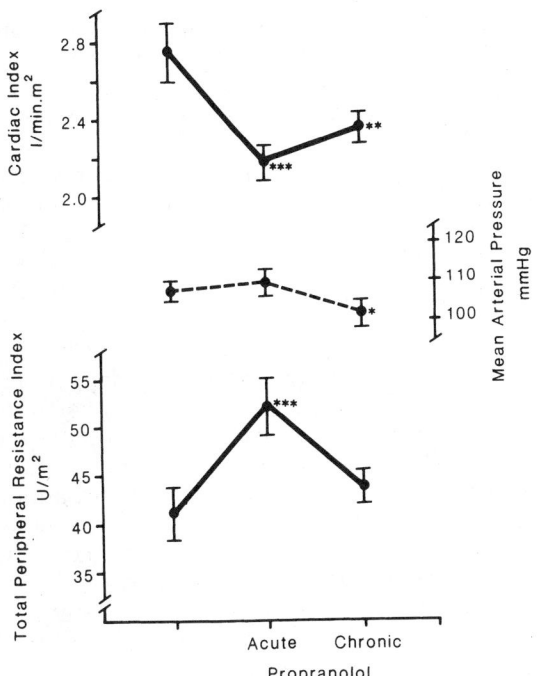

Figure 49–2. Hemodynamic changes in 15 male patients with essential hypertension. Initial values after 4 weeks of treatment with placebo. Acute values after propranolol, 0.22 mg/kg body weight IV. Chronic values after 4 weeks of propranolol, 160–320 mg/day IV. *, $p < .05$; **, $p < .01$; ***, $p < .001$. (From Hansson L: Beta-adrenergic blockade in essential hypertension: Effects of propranolol on hemodynamic parameters and plasma renin activity. Acta Med Scand 194[Suppl 550]:1, 1973.)

Mode of Action

Although the hemodynamic profile of β-blockers in the treatment of hypertension is well known, the exact mode of action remains to be elucidated.[28] In 1972, it was shown that propranolol reduced blood pressure more effectively in patients with high plasma renin activity and that the patients' untreated renin status could be used in predicting the antihypertensive response.[29] However, others could not confirm this relationship between renin status and antihypertensive responsiveness,[22] and a review of data obtained with 10 different β-blockers showed that each agent's degree of renin suppression during treatment was inversely correlated with its degree of ISA. Furthermore, the fall in blood pressure was unrelated to the change in renin.[27]

In the catecholamine theory, the antihypertensive effect of β-blockers is linked to their effect on plasma norepinephrine. However, this theory is questioned because the plasma concentration of norepinephrine may reflect differences in clearance of this amine rather than changes in sympathetic activity. Moreover, most β-blockers tend to increase the plasma concentration of norepinephrine during long-term treatment, whereas agents with marked ISA tend to lower norepinephrine.[27] Thus, analogous to the effects exerted on plasma renin activity, the effects of β-blockers on norepinephrine and on blood pressure appear to be dissociated.

In the presynaptic β-blockade theory, it is suggested that blockade of presynaptic β-adrenoreceptors would inhibit the release of norepinephrine from sympathetic nerve terminals and thereby reduce sympathetic activity to the heart, kidneys, and arterioles. Such effects could explain the reduction in vascular resistance during long-term β-blocker therapy discussed earlier. This theory is probably the most valid of any proposed thus far. It is supported by the observation that the isolated portal vein of rats, which can serve as a useful model of a precapillary arteriole, shows an attenuated response to electrical stimulation after long-term, but not short-term, administration of propranolol or metoprolol.[30]

The theory that the MSA of some β-blockers play a role in the antihypertensive effect has been discarded because of the simple observation that numerous β-blockers devoid of MSA still have potent antihypertensive effects; in addition, studies with the dextroisomer of propranolol, which is devoid of a β-blocking effect but retains the MSA, have shown that this isomer does not lower blood pressure.[31]

In view of the multitude of pharmacologic effects that can be obtained by the various β-blockers in their interplay with adrenoreceptors in different organs, it is conceivable that not one but several mechanisms are at play. Thus, it would be an oversimplification to try to find one mechanism that can explain the mode of action of these agents in all circumstances.

Effects on Blood Pressure

Following the initial observations by Prichard and others, briefly reviewed earlier,[7, 8, 10–14] the antihypertensive effect of β-blockers has been well established, and these agents have been recommended as first-line therapy by several authoritative bodies.[16–18]

In direct comparisons with placebo or other active antihypertensive agents, the efficacy of β-blockers has varied considerably. In a double-blind study originating in Jamaica, no antihypertensive effect of propranolol could be demonstrated.[32] This result contrasts with some of the early British trials, in which propranolol was considered to be at least as effective as bethanidine or guanethidine.[12, 14]

Direct comparisons between chlorthalidone and propranolol or alprenolol have shown no difference in antihypertensive potency.[33, 34] However, in a comparative study of six β-blockers and the thiazide diuretic bendroflumethiazide, the diuretic was superior to all the β-blockers (acebutolol, labetalol, pindolol, propranolol, and timolol) with the exception of atenolol.[35]

Effects on Cardiovascular Structure

The effects of antihypertensive agents on cardiovascular structure have often been disregarded. This is surprising in view of the findings that left ventricular hypertrophy is associated with an increased risk of cardiac arrhythmias and even sudden death.[36, 37] Moreover, hypertrophic structural changes of the precapillary resistance vessels tend to magnify the effect of all blood pressure–raising stimuli for simple geometric reasons.[38] Against this background, it is desirable that antihypertensive treatment reduce or normalize hypertension-induced cardiovascular structural changes.[38, 39]

The antihypertensive effect and the effect on left ventricular hypertrophy during treatment with antihypertensive agents are dissociated, but treatment with β-blockers clearly may reduce cardiac hypertrophy.[40] In a meta-analysis of all treatment studies of hypertension published before December 1990, comprising 109 studies and based on more than 2400 patients, β-blockers were found to reduce echocardiographically determined left ventricular mass by reducing left ventricular wall thickness.[41] Moreover, antihypertensive treatment with β-blockers has also been shown to reduce hypertrophic changes in the precapillary resistance vessels, but in this respect there may be differences between agents devoid of ISA and agents possessing ISA.[42]

Additional Effects

When β-blockers were given to patients who had survived acute myocardial infarctions, it was found that such therapy improved survival and reduced the risk of reinfarctions.[43-48] In particular, some of the later and well-controlled comparisons with placebos in sufficiently large numbers of patients (e.g., the Norwegian Timolol Study) proved these benefits (Fig. 49–3).[45]

Similar hopes of a preventive effect against coronary heart disease were raised in the treatment of hypertension.[15] Such hopes were reinforced by some early clinical observations. In particular, the long-term therapeutic trial in more than 1000 middle-aged hypertensive patients who were treated mainly with β-

blockers led to some expectations, because the rate of fatal and nonfatal myocardial infarctions was reduced by about 50% in the treated group.[49] However, these findings were from an open study that was not randomized or placebo-controlled.

Prospective and well-designed studies, in particular the Medical Research Council (MRC) Trial in Mild Hypertension, which compared propranolol and bendroflumethiazide;[50] the International Prospective Primary Preventive Study in Hypertension (IPPPSH), which compared treatment with oxprenolol with treatment devoid of β-blockers;[51] and the Heart Attack Primary Preventive Study in Hypertension (HAPPHY), which compared atenolol or metoprolol with a thiazide diuretic,[52] have failed to show a primary preventive effect when β-blockers are used in the treatment of hypertension. Therefore, although one would logically expect such an effect because of the experience in patients after infarction, who admittedly are at much higher risk than patients with mild to moderate hypertension, it remains to be shown beyond doubt that treatment with β-blockers will indeed confer this highly desirable effect. It could be added that the MRC, IPPPSH, and HAPPHY trials have established another important fact, namely, that β-blockers not only reduce blood pressure but also positively affect hypertension-induced morbidity (e.g., from stroke or congestive heart failure).[50-52] In elderly hypertensive patients, β-blockers, together with diuretics, have been shown to effectively reduce cardiovascular morbidity and mortality. Thus, in the Systolic Hypertension in the Elderly Program (SHEP) study, in which significant reductions in stroke and coronary heart disease morbidity were shown, 30% of all patients were treated with β-blockers.[53] Although no significant effect of the β-blocker regimen itself was demonstrated, it should be noted that the β-blocker was not given in a randomized fashion, but only to patients who did not respond to diuretic therapy.[53]

In the Swedish Trial in Old Patients with Hypertension (STOP-Hypertension), antihypertensive treatment with one of three β-blockers (atenolol, metoprolol, or pindolol) or a diuretic (hydrochlorothiazide and amiloride), usually given in combination (two thirds of all patients received combined treatment with one of the β-blockers plus the diuretic), effectively reduced stroke morbidity, all cardiovascular morbidity, and total mortality in "old elderly" (70 to 84 years) hypertensive patients.[54]

In the British Medical Research Council trial of treatment in older adults with hypertension, patients were randomized to either placebo or treatment with diuretics or β-blockade.[55] Although it was claimed that treatment with the β-blocker did not convey any benefit as compared with placebo, it should be noted that some 180 patients were excluded from the β-blocker arm because of "low heart rate" (definition not given)—that is, the potentially best responders to such therapy in terms of reduced risk of myocardial infarction or sudden death.[55] Moreover, 25% of all patients were lost to follow-up, which does not facili-

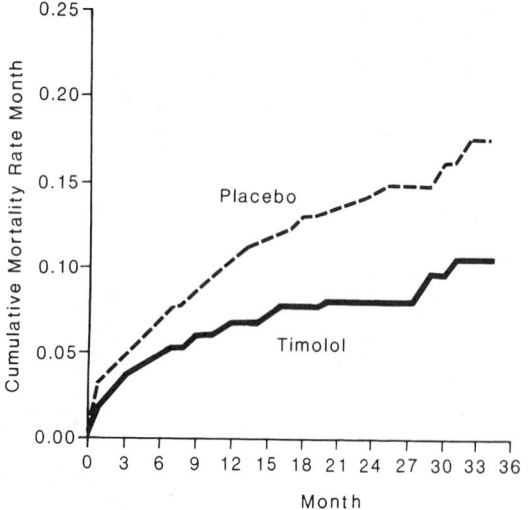

Figure 49–3. Life table cumulative rates of death from all causes in the Norwegian Post-Infarction Timolol Study. (From The Norwegian Multicenter Study Group: Timolol-induced reduction in mortality and reinfarction in patients surviving acute myocardial infarction. N Engl J Med 304:801, 1981.)

tate the demonstration of therapeutic effects. As a comparison, it can be mentioned that no patient was withdrawn from the STOP-Hypertension study because of a low pulse rate, and no patient was lost to follow-up.[54]

Other additional effects that may be of clinical relevance in some situations are the effects on serum electrolyte concentration during exposure to severe stress. When epinephrine is infused to plasma levels corresponding with those seen during severe stress, the serum potassium value has been reduced significantly. This potentially arrhythmogenic and dangerous hypokalemia can be counteracted by β-blockers possessing a β_2-adrenoreceptor blocking ability.[56, 57]

Adverse Effects

β-Blockers have been shown to be relatively well tolerated when used in the treatment of hypertension; in many of the early studies, adverse effects were considered to be few and mild.[12-14] In large-scale, placebo-controlled, double-blind studies, it has been possible to compare the rate and severity of side effects caused by β-blockers with those recorded during administration of placebo or a thiazide diuretic (e.g., in the MRC Trial in Mild Hypertension) (Table 49-3).[58] Obviously, the rate of side effects is similar during treatment with a thiazide diuretic and a β-blocker, and both of these regimens cause more adverse effects than does placebo.[58] In broad terms, side effects caused by β-blockers tend to cause subjective symptoms, as opposed to metabolic disturbances during thiazide treatment; moreover, the adverse effects induced by β-blockade are usually encountered soon after initiation of treatment, which must be regarded as advantageous.

The severe side effects caused by practolol, including severe eye and skin disorders and sclerosing peritonitis, appear to have been specific to this compound.[15] Because of these severe adverse effects, practolol was rapidly withdrawn from further long-term clinical use.

The marked differences in lipophilicity between some β-blockers (e.g., atenolol and metoprolol) result in concentrations of metoprolol in the cerebrospinal fluid several times higher after parenteral administration, but this difference is not reflected in different hemodynamic effects of the two agents.[59] It has, however, been claimed that a hydrophilic compound such as atenolol would cause fewer side effects in the central nervous system than more lipophilic agents.[60, 61] This claim is supported by the finding in two studies of sleep pattern, in which four β-blockers (atenolol, metoprolol, pindolol, and propranolol) were compared with placebo. In both studies, all β-blockers except atenolol significantly increased the number of awakenings[62] or subjective reports of dreaming and early awakening.[63] However, others have not found a difference in the incidence or degree of sedation caused by atenolol and metoprolol, with the exception that the hydrophilic compound produced a longer-lasting sedation.[64]

The potentially negative effects of various antihypertensive drugs on serum lipoproteins have attracted a certain interest, and β-blockers are no exception.[65] It has been shown that propranolol may increase serum triglyceride concentrations and reduce high-density lipoprotein (HDL) cholesterol levels, whereas prazosin in the same study reduced low-density lipoprotein (LDL) and very-low-density lipoprotein (VLDL) cholesterol levels.[66] However, the reports in the literature conflict somewhat in this area. Thus, in one series of patients given β-blockers (atenolol, pindolol, propranolol, and metoprolol), all agents caused a rise in serum triglyceride levels, which was most pronounced with atenolol.[67] In a comparison of metoprolol and atenolol, no changes were seen with atenolol, but metoprolol increased triglyceride levels and reduced HDL cholesterol concentrations.[68] In a review of 22 studies in this area, van Brummelen[69] showed that β-blockers with marked ISA caused the smallest changes in the lipid profile. It remains to be shown to what extent the minor drug-induced changes in serum lipoproteins have clinical significance.

Table 49–3. **Withdrawal of Randomized Treatment Due to Adverse Effects in Men with Mild Hypertension***

Effect	Bendroflumethiazide (2452 PY)	Propranolol (2738 PY)	Placebo (6776 PY)
Impaired glucose tolerance	9.4	3.7	2.5
Gout or serum urate > 501 μmol/L	12.2	2.6	1.0
Impotence	19.6	5.5	0.9
Raynaud phenomenon	0	5.5	0.2
Skin disorder	0.4	2.2	0.2
Dyspnea	0	8.0	0.2
Constipation	1.6	0.4	0
Lethargy	6.9	10.2	0.3
Nausea, dizziness, headaches, etc.	8.6	6.7	1.2

*In this trial, significant numbers of patients received additional therapy, mainly α-methyldopa or guanethidine. Please note that more than 1000 patients in the placebo group were on active treatment at the end of the trial. It is assumed that the reported data are in reference to patients on monotherapy. Rates are per 1000 patient years (PY).

Data from Medical Research Council Working Party on Mild to Moderate Hypertension: Adverse reactions to bendrofluazide and propranolol for the treatment of mild hypertension. Lancet 2:539, 1981.

CLINICAL USE
Indications

β-Blockers are prescribed mainly for the treatment of cardiovascular disorders, especially arterial hypertension. The general acceptance of β-blockers as first-line treatment for hypertension has made this the most widely prescribed class of compounds in many countries. Other cardiovascular indications are also of major importance, particularly the treatment of angina pectoris or as secondary prophylaxis after a myocardial infarction. Other indications are palpitations without organic heart disease, supraventricular tachyarrhythmias, hyperthyroidism, pheochromocytoma, and prophylactic treatment of migraine and tremor.

Precautions

β-Blockers may mask symptoms of hypoglycemia in patients with diabetes mellitus treated with insulin. Together with certain anesthetics, β-blockers may cause hypotension. When used together with class I antiarrhythmics, β-blockers may cause additive negative inotropic effects.

When given to pregnant women, β-blockers may cause bradycardia in the fetus. Therefore, the potential benefits for the mother should be weighed against the potential risks for the fetus. In lactating women, some β-blockers may be transferred to the child during breast-feeding, but it appears unlikely that this will have noticeable effects as long as the mother is taking doses in the therapeutic range.

Contraindications

Bronchial asthma is an absolute contraindication to all β-blockers. It could be argued that $β_1$-selective agents are safer in this respect, but it should be noted that $β_1$ selectivity is a relative phenomenon; and as has been pointed out earlier, there is not an absolute organ separation of $β_1$- and $β_2$-adrenoreceptors in various organs. Other absolute contraindications are untreated left ventricular failure and atrioventricular block II or III.

Interference

Concomitant therapy with some drugs (e.g., hydralazine) interacts with the hepatic metabolization (in particular of lipophilic β-blockers such as propranolol) so that the first-pass effect is reduced and more of the active drug reaches the general circulation.[70] Concomitant administration of cimetidine increases the plasma concentration of certain β-blockers, presumably by reducing their first-pass metabolism in the liver.

Together with class I antiarrhythmics, β-blockers may exert additional negative inotropic effects, which may lead to disturbing hemodynamic alterations, particularly in patients with reduced left ventricular function. This combination should also be avoided in patients with sick sinus syndrome and pathologic atrioventricular conduction.

In combination with verapamil, β-blockers have been known to cause severe bradycardia and hypotension.[71] The combination of β-blockers and diltiazem may have negative effects on atrioventricular conduction and sinus node function. The hypertensive reaction that sometimes follows abrupt cessation of clonidine may be augmented by β-blockers, especially nonselective agents.[72] The first-dose orthostatic effect of prazosin may be augmented by concomitant treatment with β-blockers. The hypoglycemic effects of insulin and orally administered antidiabetics of the sulphonylurea type may be augmented by β-blockers, especially nonselective agents.[15] Several nonsteroidal antiinflammatory drugs may counteract the antihypertensive effect of β-blockers. Ergotamine and β-blockers may have synergistic negative effects on peripheral perfusion, which may lead to severe peripheral ischemia. Concomitant treatment with certain inhalation anesthetics and β-blockers may lead to severe hypotension.

In addition, β-blockers are known to interact with the metabolism of theophylline, lidocaine, cimetidine, warfarin, rifampicin, chlorpromazine, disopyramide, ampicillin, and verapamil.

Use in Patients with Impaired Organ Function

In patients with severely reduced renal function, hydrophilic β-blockers such as atenolol and sotalol may reach high plasma levels, but these are not associated with clinical effects.[73] Moreover, β-blockers that are metabolized mainly in the liver (e.g., propranolol) may reach increased plasma concentrations in patients with reduced hepatic function. Although the clinical effects in these situations are not entirely clear, it may be appropriate to reduce the dosages of the respective agents in these situations.

Place of β-Blockers in the Antihypertensive Arsenal

As already described, several expert committees have recommended β-blockers as first-line treatment for hypertension,[16-18] as have many national hypertension leagues or associations. Thus, it appears likely that β-blockers will continue to play an important role in the treatment of hypertension for many years, even if a more individualized choice of antihypertensive treatment appears logical.[74, 75]

If a more ambitious therapeutic goal is to be obtained in the treatment of hypertension (i.e., strictly normotensive blood pressure levels),[76] it will undoubtedly be necessary to administer combined treatment much more frequently than in the past. In this situation, a combination of a β-blocker and a dihydropyridine calcium antagonist may be highly effective.[77, 78] Finally, if a primary preventive effect against coronary heart disease were to be shown with β-blocker treatment in patients with hypertension, the position of these agents in the antihypertensive arsenal obviously would be reinforced. Despite the negative intervention trials in this area,[50-52] it appears that the highly desirable preventive effect against coronary disease is still a realistic possibility, provided that patients at sufficiently high risk are treated.[79]

Dosage and Administration

As discussed earlier, intravenous administration of β-blockers does not reduce blood pressure. The main exception is labetalol, which, because of its combination of α- and β-adrenoreceptor blockade, can be used intravenously in the treatment of hypertensive emergencies.[15]

In the oral long-term treatment of hypertension, most β-blockers can be given once daily to most patients, which is a reflection of the dissociation between the antihypertensive and the β-blocking effects,[24] briefly discussed earlier. It could be added that some newer agents, in particular bopindolol, which is a nonselective β-blocker with a clinically relevant degree of ISA, has a duration of action measurable even 96 hours after a single oral dose.[80]

The dosage of β-blockers when used in the treatment of hypertension usually does not differ from the dosage recommended for other indications. The early proposals that propranolol had to be given in doses of 4 g daily to achieve the full therapeutic effect[12] have not been supported by further studies, and this practice has now been abandoned.

SOCIOECONOMIC CONSIDERATIONS
Compliance

Patient response to antihypertensive treatment, including compliance, is affected by a number of factors, in particular the number and severity of adverse effects in relation to the experienced or expected therapeutic effect.[81] It is also of utmost importance that treatment does not negatively affect the patient's quality of life.[82] In a large-scale comparison of several aspects of quality of life during treatment with propranolol, captopril, and α-methyldopa, it was shown that well-being was significantly lower during propranolol therapy than during captopril therapy.[83]

It can be argued that a more modern β-blocker (e.g., a β₁-selective agent) would have been more competitive in this respect, but there are reports on reduced short-term memory function after administration of atenolol as compared with enalapril.[84]

In the absence of direct comparative trials, it is difficult to discuss possible differences regarding compliance between different antihypertensive agents. The clinical impression is that compliance is relatively good with β-blockers, and the evaluation of compliance is facilitated by the lowering of resting heart rate seen with most of these agents.

Cost

The cost of antihypertensive treatment is always difficult to evaluate realistically. The costs of medication and care must be evaluated together and considered in relation to the expected benefits, such as prolongation of life expectancy and lowering of morbidity. If one limits the discussion to the direct costs of pills, β-blockers are more expensive than thiazide diuretics but less expensive than some of the newer classes of compounds such as the angiotensin-converting enzyme inhibitors. However, the total annual cost of treatment with β-blockers probably is not much higher than with thiazide diuretics, because a number of laboratory tests (e.g., of serum potassium and serum urate levels) need not be performed during β-blocker therapy. As with all antihypertensive therapies, the total costs of treatment and care are dwarfed in comparison with the expected benefits.

FUTURE POSSIBILITIES

It has already been mentioned that, if a primary preventive effect against coronary disease can be demonstrated when β-blockers are used in the treatment of hypertension, their position in the antihypertensive armamentarium would be reinforced. One other possible effect would lead to a similar result: the antiatherogenetic effect that treatment with β-blockers may confer. Results obtained in a double-blind, placebo-controlled study with metoprolol in patients after myocardial infarction indicate that not only was the rate of reinfarction and cardiac death reduced by treatment, but the number of atherosclerotic complications in the brain and the legs also was reduced.[85]

Several studies with various β-blockers[86] have reported less severe atherosclerosis in the large arteries of animals fed cholesterol. Moreover, studies in macaque monkeys subjected to severe psychosocial stress have shown that the marked coronary atherosclerosis induced by the experiment could, to a significant extent, be prevented by β-blocker treatment.[87] The mechanisms by which this positive effect was obtained are not fully known, but the effect was clearly dissociated from the antihypertensive effect. β-Adrenoreceptor–mediated inhibition of endothelial prostacyclin synthesis may have played a role.[88]

If clinical trials were to confirm that β-blockers have a significant antiatherosclerotic effect, the implications for future cardiovascular therapy would be considerable.

REFERENCES

1. Ahlquist RP: A study of the adrenotropic receptors. Am J Physiol 153:586, 1948.
2. Lands AM, Arnold A, McAuliff JP, et al: Differentiation of receptor systems activated by sympathomimetic amines. Nature 214:597, 1967.
3. Sannerstedt R: Hemodynamic response to exercise in patients with arterial hypertension. Acta Med Scand 180(Suppl 458):1, 1966.
4. Lund-Johansen P: Hemodynamics in early essential hypertension. Acta Med Scand 182(Suppl 482):1, 1967.

5. Frohlich ED, Tarazi RC, Dustan HP, et al: The paradox of beta-adrenergic blockade in hypertension. Circulation 37:417, 1968.
6. Powell CE, Slater IH: Blocking of inhibitory adrenergic receptors by a dichloro analogue of isoproterenol. J Pharmacol Exp Ther 122:480, 1958.
7. Prichard BNC: Hypotensive action of pronethalol. Br Med J 1:1227, 1964.
8. Schröder G, Werkö L: Nethalide, a beta adrenergic blocking agent. Clin Pharmacol Ther 5:159, 1964.
9. Paget GE: Carcinogenic action of pronethalol. Br Med J 2:1266, 1963.
10. Prichard BNC, Gillam PMS: The use of propranolol in the treatment of hypertension. Br Med J 2:725, 1964.
11. Prichard BNC, Gillam PMS: Propranolol in hypertension. Am J Cardiol 18:387, 1966.
12. Prichard BNC, Gillam PMS: Treatment of hypertension with propranolol. Br Med J 1:7, 1969.
13. Hansson L, Malmcrona R, Olander R, et al: Propranolol in hypertension: Report on 158 patients treated up to one year. Klin Wochenschr 50:364, 1972.
14. Zacharias FJ, Cowen KJ, Presst J, et al: Propranolol in hypertension: A study of long-term therapy 1964–1970. Am Heart J 83:755, 1972.
15. Hansson L: Drug treatment of hypertension. In Robertson JIS (ed): Handbook of Hypertension, Vol 1, Clinical Aspects of Essential Hypertension. Amsterdam: Elsevier, 1983, pp 397–436.
16. WHO/ISH Third Mild Hypertension Conference: Guidelines for the treatment of mild hypertension: Memorandum from a WHO/ISH meeting. Hypertension 5:394, 1983.
17. WHO/ISH Fourth Mild Hypertension Conference: 1986 Guidelines for the treatment of mild hypertension: Memorandum from a WHO/ISH meeting. J Hypertens 4:383, 1986.
18. The Joint National Committee on Detection, Evaluation and Treatment of High Blood Pressure: The 1984 report of the Joint National Committee on Detection, Evaluation and Treatment of High Blood Pressure. Arch Intern Med 144:1045, 1984.
19. Fitzgerald DG: Beta-adrenoreceptor antagonists. In van Zwieten PA (ed): Handbook of Hypertension, Vol 3, Pharmacology of Antihypertensive Drugs. Amsterdam: Elsevier, 1984, pp 249–306.
20. Carlsson EB, Åblad B, Brändström A, et al: Differentiated blockade of the chronotropic effects of various adrenergic stimuli in the cat heart. Life Sci 11:953, 1972.
21. Ulrych M, Frohlich ED, Dustan HP, et al: Immediate hemodynamic effects of beta-adrenergic blockade with propranolol in normotensive and hypertensive man. Circulation 37:411, 1968.
22. Hansson L: Beta-adrenergic blockade in essential hypertension: Effects of propranolol on hemodynamic parameters and plasma renin activity. Acta Med Scand 194(Suppl 550):1, 1973.
23. Tarazi RC, Dustan HP: Beta-adrenergic blockade in hypertension: Practical and theoretical implications of long-term hemodynamic variation. Am J Cardiol 29:633, 1972.
24. Hansson L: Beta-adrenoreceptor blocking drugs as antihypertensive agents. In Amery A, Fagard R, Lijnen P, et al (eds): Hypertensive Cardiovascular Disease: Pathophysiology and Treatment. The Hague: Martinus Nijhoff, 1982, pp 743–754.
25. Conway FJ, Amery A: The antihypertensive effect of propranolol and other beta-adrenoreceptor antagonists. In Davies DS, Reid JL (eds): Central Action of Drugs in the Regulation of Blood Pressure. Tunbridge, UK: Pitman, 1975, pp 277–290.
26. Lund-Johansen P: Hemodynamic consequences of long-term beta-blocker therapy: A 5-year follow-up study of atenolol. J Cardiovasc Pharmacol 1:487, 1979.
27. Man in't Veld AJ, Schalekamp MADH: Effects of 10 different beta-adrenoreceptor antagonists on hemodynamics, plasma renin activity and plasma norepinephrine in hypertension: The key role of vascular resistance changes in relation to partial agonist activity. J Cardiovasc Pharmacol 5(Suppl 1):S30, 1983.
28. Hansson L: Beta-blockers in hypertension. J Hypertens 5(Suppl 3):S61, 1987.
29. Bühler FR, Laragh JH, Baer L, et al: Propranolol inhibition of renin secretion. N Engl J Med 287:1209, 1972.
30. Ljung B, Åblad B, Dahlöf C, et al: Impaired vasoconstrictor nerve function in spontaneously hypertensive rats after long-term treatment with propranolol and metoprolol. Blood Vessels 12:311, 1975.
31. Waal-Manning HJ: Lack of effect of d-propranolol on blood pressure and pulse rate in hypertensive patients. Proc Univ Otago Med School 48:80, 1970.
32. Humphreys GS, Delvin DG: Ineffectiveness of propranolol in hypertensive Jamaicans. Br Med J 1:601, 1968.
33. Paterson JW, Dollery CT: Effect of propranolol in mild hypertension. Lancet 2:1148, 1966.
34. Bengtsson C: Comparison between alprenolol and chlorthalidone as antihypertensive agents. Acta Med Scand 191:433, 1972.
35. Wilcox RG: Randomised study of six beta-blockers and a thiazide diuretic in essential hypertension. Br Med J 2:383, 1978.
36. Kannel WB, Gordon T, Offutt D: Left ventricular hypertrophy by electrocardiography: Prevalence, incidence and mortality in the Framingham study. Ann Intern Med 71:89, 1969.
37. Messerli FH, Ventura HO, Elizardi DJ, et al: Hypertension and sudden death: Increased ventricular ectopic activity in left ventricular hypertrophy. Am J Med 77:18, 1984.
38. Folkow B, Hansson L, Sivertsson R: Structural vascular factors in the pathogenesis of hypertension. In Robertson JIS (ed): Handbook of Hypertension, Vol 1, Clinical Aspects of Essential Hypertension. Amsterdam: Elsevier, 1983, pp 133–150.
39. Hansson L: The future of pharmacological therapy for risk factor reduction. Drugs 36(Suppl 3):110, 1988.
40. Frohlich ED: The heart in hypertension. In Genest J, Kuchel O, Hamet P, et al (eds): Hypertension, 2nd ed. New York: McGraw-Hill, 1983, pp 791–810.
41. Dahlöf B, Pennert K, Hansson L: Reversal of left ventricular hypertrophy in hypertensive patients: A meta-analysis of 109 treatment studies. Am J Hypertens 5:95, 1992.
42. Hansson L, Svensson A, Gudbrandsson T, et al: Treatment of hypertension with beta-blockers with and without intrinsic sympathomimetic activity. J Cardiovasc Pharmacol 5(Suppl 1):S26, 1983.
43. Wilhelmsson C, Vedin JA, Wilhelmsen L, et al: Reduction of sudden deaths after myocardial infarction by treatment with alprenolol: Preliminary results. Lancet 2:1157, 1974.
44. Multicentre International Study: Improvement in prognosis of myocardial infarction by long-term beta-adrenoreceptor blockade using practolol: A multicentre international study. Br Med J 3:735, 1975.
45. The Norwegian Multicenter Study Group: Timolol-induced reduction in mortality and reinfarction in patients surviving acute myocardial infarction. N Engl J Med 304:801, 1981.
46. Beta-blocker Heart Attack Trial Research Group: A randomized trial of propranolol in patients with acute myocardial infarction. I: Mortality results. JAMA 247:1707, 1982.
47. Hjalmarson A, Elmfeldt D, Herlitz J, et al: Effect on mortality of metoprolol in acute myocardial infarction. Lancet 2:823, 1981.
48. ISIS-1 (First International Study of Infarct Survival) Collaborative Group: Randomized trial of intravenous atenolol among 16,027 cases of suspected acute myocardial infarction: ISIS-1. Lancet 2:57, 1986.
49. Berglund G, Wilhelmsen L, Sannerstedt R, et al: Coronary heart-disease after treatment of hypertension. Lancet 1:1, 1978.
50. Medical Research Council Working Party: MRC trial of treatment of mild hypertension: Principal results. Br Med J 291:97, 1985.
51. The IPPPSH Collaborative Group: Cardiovascular risks and risk factors in a randomized trial of treatment based on the beta-blocker oxprenolol: The International Prospective Primary Preventive Trial in Hypertension (IPPPSH). J Hypertens 3:379, 1985.
52. Wilhelmsen L, Berglund G, Elmfeldt D, et al: Beta-blockers versus diuretics in hypertensive men: Main results from the HAPPHY trial. J Hypertens 5:561, 1987.
53. SHEP Cooperative Research Group: Prevention of stroke by antihypertensive drug treatment in older persons with isolated systolic hypertension: Final results of the Systolic Hypertension in the Elderly Program (SHEP). JAMA 265:3255, 1991.
54. Dahlöf B, Lindholm LH, Hansson L, et al: Morbidity and Mortality in the Swedish Trial in Old Patients with Hypertension (STOP-Hypertension). Lancet 338:1281, 1991.
55. MRC Working Party: Medical Research Council trial of treatment of hypertension in older adults: Principal results. Br Med J 304:405, 1992.

56. Struthers AD, Reid JL, Whitesmith R, et al: The effect of cardio-selective and non-selective beta-adrenoreceptor blockade on the hypokalemic and cardiovascular responses to adrenomedullary hormones in man. Clin Sci 65:143, 1983.

57. Brown MJ, Brown DC, Murphy MB: Hypokalemia from beta$_2$-receptor stimulation by circulating epinephrine. N Engl J Med 309:1414, 1983.

58. Medical Research Council Working Party on Mild to Moderate Hypertension: Adverse reactions to bendrofluazide and propranolol for the treatment of mild hypertension. Lancet 2:539, 1981.

59. van Zwieten PA, Timmermans PBMWM: Comparison between the acute hemodynamic effects and brain penetration of atenolol and metoprolol. J Cardiovasc Pharmacol 1:85, 1979.

60. Henningsen NC, Mattiasson I: Long-term clinical experience with atenolol—A new selective beta-1-blocker with few side effects from the central nervous system. Acta Med Scand 205:61, 1979.

61. Cruickshank JM: The clinical importance of cardioselectivity and lipophilicity in beta blockers. Am Heart J 100:160, 1980.

62. Kostis JB, Rosen RC: Central nervous system effects of beta-adrenergic blocking drugs: The role of ancillary properties. Circulation 75:204, 1987.

63. Betts TA, Alford C: Beta-blocking drugs and sleep: A controlled trial. Drugs 25(Suppl 2):268, 1983.

64. Gengo FM, Huntoon L, McHugh WB: Lipid-soluble and water-soluble beta-blockers: Comparison of the central nervous system depressant effect. Arch Intern Med 147:39, 1987.

65. Tanaka N, Sagaguchi K, Oshige K, et al: Effect of chronic administration of propranolol on lipoprotein composition. Metabolism 25:1071, 1976.

66. Leren P, Foss PO, Helgeland A, et al: Effect of propranolol and prazosin on blood lipids: The Oslo study. Lancet 2:4, 1980.

67. Shaw J, England JDF, Hua ASP: Beta-blockers and plasma triglycerides. Br Med J 1:968, 1978.

68. Rössner S, Weiner L: Atenolol and metoprolol: Comparison of effects on blood pressure and serum lipoproteins, and side effects. Eur J Clin Pharmacol 24:573, 1983.

69. van Brummelen P: The relevance of intrinsic sympathomimetic activity for the beta-blocker-induced changes in plasma lipids. J Cardiovasc Pharmacol 5(Suppl 1):S51, 1983.

70. McLean AJ, Skews H, Bobik A, et al: Interaction between oral propranolol and hydralazine. Clin Pharmacol Ther 27:726, 1980.

71. Wayne VS, Harper RW, Laufer E, et al: Adverse interaction between beta-adrenergic blocking drugs and verapamil—Report of three cases. Aust N Z J Med 12:285, 1982.

72. Hansson L: Clinical aspects of blood pressure crisis due to withdrawal of centrally acting antihypertensive drugs. Br J Clin Pharmacol 15:485, 1983.

73. Sassard J, Pozet N, McAinsh J, et al: Pharmacokinetics of atenolol in patients with renal impairment. Eur J Clin Pharmacol 12:175, 1977.

74. Zanchetti A: Which drug to which patient? J Hypertens 3(Suppl 2):S57, 1985.

75. Laragh JH: When is it useful to inhibit the renin-angiotensin system for treating hypertension? J Cardiovasc Pharmacol 7(Suppl 4):S86, 1985.

76. Hansson L: What are we really achieving with long-term drug therapy? Am J Hypertens 1:414, 1988.

77. Hansson L, Dahlöf B: Antihypertensive effect of a new dihydropyridine calcium antagonist, PN 200-110 (Isradipine), combined with pindolol. Am J Cardiol 59(Suppl B):137B, 1987.

78. Hansson L, Dahlöf B, Gudbrandsson T, et al: Antihypertensive effect of felodipine or hydralazine when added to beta-blocker therapy. J Cardiovasc Pharmacol 12:94, 1988.

79. Hansson L: Primary prevention against CHD with beta-blockers ruled out by HAPPHY? J Hypertens 5:573, 1987.

80. Platzer R, Galeazzi RL, Niederberger W, et al: Simultaneous modelling of bopindolol kinetics and dynamics. Clin Pharmacol Ther 122:480, 1984.

81. Hansson L: Assessment of the patient's response. J Hypertens 3(Suppl 2):S65, 1985.

82. Robertson JIS: The treatment of hypertension and quality of life. J Hypertens 3(Suppl 2):S89, 1985.

83. Croog SH, Levine S, Testa MA, et al: The effects of antihypertensive therapy on the quality of life. N Engl J Med 314:1657, 1986.

84. Lichter I, Richardson PJ, Wyke MA: Differential effects of atenolol and enalapril on memory during treatment for essential hypertension. Br J Clin Pharmacol 21:641, 1986.

85. Olsson G, Rehnqvist N, Sjögren A, et al: Long-term treatment with metoprolol after myocardial infarction: Effect on 3-year mortality and morbidity. J Am Coll Cardiol 5:1428, 1985.

86. Östlund-Lindqvist A-M, Lindqvist P, Bräutigam J, et al: The effect of metoprolol on atherosclerosis in cholesterol-fed rabbits. In VIth International Washington Spring Symposium [abstract 147], Washington, DC, May 20–23, 1986.

87. Manuck SB, Kaplan JR, Matthews KA: Behavioral antecedents of coronary heart disease and atherosclerosis. Arteriosclerosis 6:2, 1986.

88. Adler B, Gimbrone M, Schaffer A, et al: Prostacyclin and beta-adrenergic catecholamines inhibit arachidonate release and PGI$_2$-synthesis by vascular endothelium. Blood 58:514, 1981.

B. Noncardioselective β-Adrenoreceptor Blockers

CHAPTER 50

Propranolol

Alan S. Nies, M.D.

HISTORY

The discovery of propranolol, the prototypic β-adrenergic blocker, was the result of insight, logic, and serendipity. An interesting personal account of these events has been published by Shanks.[1] In the mid-1950s, J. W. Black formulated a hypothesis that pharmacologic inhibition of the cardiac effects of the sympathetic nervous system might have therapeutic value for treatment of angina pectoris by reducing cardiac oxygen demands during periods of stress. Black pursued his hypothesis at Imperial Chemical Industries, where he embarked on a systematic search for a drug that would block the cardiac effects of epinephrine.

The first compound, pronethalol, was found to inhibit responses to isoproterenol in human subjects and, more importantly, to increase the exercise tolerance of patients with angina pectoris, thus confirming the accuracy and utility of Black's logical deduction.[2, 3] Unfortunately, pronethalol was found to cause malignant tumors in mice and was never released for general use. However, a congener of pronethalol, propranolol, was found to be more potent and less toxic.[4] Clinical studies were soon performed, and propranolol was subsequently marketed, initially in the United Kingdom and eventually worldwide.

CHEMISTRY

Propranolol has an oxypropanolamine side chain attached to the 1 position of naphthalene. All β-adrenergic blocking drugs, including propranolol, have asymmetric centers at the β-carbon to which the —OH is attached. Thus, these compounds can exist as two optical isomers (enantiomers) that are mirror images of each other. The β-adrenergic blocking properties reside predominately in one enantiomer, which in propranolol is the S—(—) isomer, commonly called l-propranolol. However, most β-adrenergic receptor blockers, including propranolol, are marketed as the racemate, which is an equimolar mixture of the two enantiomers. As far as the living organism is concerned, each enantiomer is unique and has its own metabolic fate, pharmacokinetics, and pharmacologic effects.

PHARMACOLOGY

The major effect of propranolol is to antagonize the action of norepinephrine and epinephrine at all β-adrenergic receptors. Propranolol binds reversibly with high affinity to the β-adrenergic receptor, but it can be displaced by a sufficiently high concentration of agonist. Although propranolol binds to the same site on the receptor as the agonists, the antagonist does not trigger any response, indicating that it does not have any agonist or intrinsic sympathomimetic activity.

When sympathomimetics interact with the β-adrenergic receptor, they lead to loss of receptor numbers (density) and attenuation of the effect. This phenomenon is called *downregulation* of the β-adrenergic receptor and depends on chronic stimulation with an agonist.[5] Propranolol, by blocking the chronic stimulation, can result in *upregulation* of the β-adrenergic receptor, a phenomenon that is the reversal of downregulation.[6] The greatest upregulation occurs in patients who have the highest sympathetic activity, and thus the greatest downregulation, prior to propranolol administration.[7] When propranolol therapy is discontinued, the β-adrenergic receptor density continues to be increased for a few days after propranolol has been eliminated from the body. It has been suggested that the increased density of β-adrenergic receptors results in enhanced adrenergic activity, which might account, in part, for the withdrawal syndrome described in patients with coronary artery disease or hypertrophic cardiomyopathy in whom un-

toward events develop when propranolol is discontinued abruptly.[8-11]

Of all the β-adrenergic blocking drugs, propranolol is the most lipid-soluble; therefore, it partitions into lipid-rich areas of the body such as the brain.[12] The importance of this property to the effects of propranolol is uncertain, but some of the side effects attributed to the central nervous system (CNS) may be related to this physicochemical property.

Propranolol also is a potent local anesthetic because of its ability to block sodium channels in excitable tissue and thus alter the action potential of nerves and cardiac muscle. This property is unrelated to β-adrenergic blockade, is sometimes described as *membrane-stabilizing* or *quinidine-like*, and is present equally in both enantiomers of propranolol.[13] Although this electrophysiologic effect can be easily demonstrated *in vitro* and in animal models, its clinical significance is debated.

PHARMACOKINETICS

The study of the absorption and disposition of propranolol not only has provided insight into one of the reasons for the variability in patient response, but propranolol has also become a model for drugs that are avidly cleared from the circulation by the liver.[14]

Metabolism

Propranolol is converted to a large number of metabolites resulting from oxidation or conjugation of the aromatic ring, the side chain, or both. One metabolite, 4-hydroxypropranolol, is an active β-adrenergic blocker having nearly the same activity as the parent compound and is formed in substantial quantities only after oral dosing.[15] However, the metabolite has a shorter half-life than that of propranolol, accumulates less than the parent drug, and thus does not make a substantial contribution to the β-adrenergic blockade during long-term therapy.

Intravenous Dosing

When given intravenously, approximately 90% of propranolol is extracted from the blood on a single passage through the liver, resulting in a clearance of 1.0 to 1.2 L/min, which is close to hepatic blood flow.[16] The apparent volume of distribution of propranolol is 3.6 L/kg, and the half-life after intravenous administration is 2 or 3 hours. The high hepatic extraction efficiency occurs despite the fact that propranolol is 90% bound to plasma proteins, a major one being α_1-acid glycoprotein.

Because of the high hepatic extraction of propranolol, changes in hepatic blood flow can alter the delivery of propranolol to the liver and affect the drug's clearance. Because β-adrenergic blockade with propranolol reduces cardiac output and hepatic blood flow, the drug reduces its own clearance. This effect accounts for the fact that (+)-propranolol, which does not produce β-adrenergic blockade, has a higher clearance than racemic propranolol, which reduces hepatic blood flow.[17]

Oral Dosing

When propranolol is given by mouth, it is well-absorbed into the portal circulation, where it must pass through the liver before it reaches the systemic circulation. The fraction that actually reaches the systemic blood is called the *bioavailability*. Because propranolol has a high hepatic extraction, it has a low bioavailability.[14] For small single doses, only about 10% of the dose reaches the systemic circulation. With multiple doses, the avid removal processes of the liver become saturated, so that the bioavailability increases to 20% to 50%.[18] This effect results in a lower systemic clearance of propranolol when given orally than when it is given intravenously; this kinetic change is reflected in a prolongation of half-life to 3 to 6 hours instead of 2 or 3 hours for propranolol given intravenously.

Because of the key role of the liver and the portal circulation in the disposition of propranolol, portacaval anastomosis can have important effects on the drug's bioavailability and elimination. In such cases, the bioavailability of propranolol can approach 100%, because the hepatic presystemic elimination is bypassed.[19] Thus, oral doses of a few milligrams of propranolol that would have minimal or no effect in a normal subject will have effects equivalent to those of an intravenous dose of the same amount in patients with portacaval shunting.

Duration of Action

Some investigators have indicated that the β-adrenergic blocking effects of propranolol persist longer than one would expect from the half-life of the drug. However, such claims have resulted from misinterpretation of the relationship of the pharmacokinetic half-life to the pharmacologic effect. The most commonly used index of β-adrenergic blockade in man is a reduction of exercise-induced tachycardia. A maximal reduction of exercise tachycardia is achieved at a plasma concentration of about 100 ng/ml.[20] Furthermore, the relationship of the reduction of exercise tachycardia to the log of the plasma propranolol concentration is such that half of the maximal effect of propranolol remains at a plasma level of 8 to 12 ng/ml.[21] Thus, if a patient is taking a dose of propranolol that results in a plasma concentration of 200 ng/ml, several half-lives will be required before half of the effect is lost. At one half-life, the concentration will be 100 ng/ml, and there will be no loss of β-adrenergic blocking effect as judged by reduction in exercise tachycardia. After the second half-life, the concentration will be 50 ng/ml; after the third, 25 ng/ml; and after the fourth, 12 ng/ml. At 12 ng/ml, propranolol still produces 50% of its maximal effect on exercise tachycardia. If the half-life is 4 hours, a loss of one half of the effect will take 16 hours. No evidence suggests that β-adrenergic receptor blockade persists after propranolol has been eliminated from the body.

Because propranolol may be well-tolerated at high concentrations, large doses can be used as a strategy for increasing the interval between doses to 12 to 24 hours, even though the drug has a relatively short half-life.

EFFECTS ON PATHOPHYSIOLOGY
Effects on Hemodynamics

After the first dose of propranolol, cardiac output and heart rate are reduced with a reflex rise in peripheral vascular resistance, such that arterial pressure is little changed. In experimental animals, blood flow to most organs is reduced, with the exception of the brain.[22] By reducing blood flow to the splanchnic vasculature, propranolol can reduce portal venous pressure in patients with hepatic cirrhosis. Clinical trials of propranolol for the prevention of variceal bleeding have produced mixed results, but a 1992 meta-analysis suggests a benefit from the prophylactic use of propranolol in patients with cirrhosis and high-risk varices who have no history of hemorrhage.[23]

In some patients, peripheral vascular resistance returns to pretreatment values with continued propranolol administration even though cardiac output remains reduced. This decrease in resistance in the face of a reduced cardiac output accounts for the fall in arterial pressure and the effectiveness of propranolol as an antihypertensive drug.

The magnitude of propranolol's effect on heart rate depends on the sympathetic activity. At rest, there is little sympathetic tone, and the heart rate is primarily under the influence of the parasympathetic nervous system. Thus, changes in resting heart rate cannot be used as an accurate index of β-adrenergic receptor blockade. When the sympathetic nervous system is activated, as with exercise, the effect of propranolol will be most apparent, and a reduction in exercise heart rate is a good way to gauge the degree of β-adrenergic receptor blockade.[24]

Effects on Ventricular Function and Structure

At clinically used doses, propranolol has little direct effect on ventricular function. Rather, it reduces cardiac rate, force of contraction, and speed of conduction in the sinoatrial (SA) and atrioventricular (AV) nodes by blocking the effects of catecholamines at β-adrenergic receptors. Similarly, propranolol has no direct effect on ventricular structure but can inhibit the development of focal myocardial necrotic lesions and electrocardiographic abnormalities associated with excessive sympathetic stimulation, such as may occur following subarachnoid hemorrhage.[25] Propranolol can also reduce ventricular wall thickness in hypertensive patients with ventricular hypertrophy.[26]

Effects on Electrophysiology

Propranolol has effects at usual doses that result from β-adrenergic receptor blockade at the SA and AV nodes. As a consequence, propranolol can slow the sinus rate, reduce conduction through the AV node, increase the functional refractory period of the AV node, and produce varying degrees of SA and AV block.

At clinically attained plasma concentrations in excess of those required to produce high degrees of β-adrenergic receptor blockade, propranolol can produce a reduction in the action potential duration, a shortening of the QT_c interval, and an increase in the ratio of the ventricular effective refractory period to the action potential duration.[27] Massive overdoses of propranolol can lead to intraventricular conduction delay.[28] These latter effects are not related to β-adrenergic receptor blockade but may be clinical reflections of the membrane-stabilizing effects of propranolol.[29]

Effects on Coronary Blood Flow

Propranolol reduces coronary blood flow as a physiologic adjustment to the drug-induced reduction in cardiac work and oxygen demands, but blood flow to ischemic regions is maintained.[30, 31] However, concern exists that, during intense sympathetic stimulation, propranolol may potentiate the rise in coronary resistance as a result of unopposed α-adrenergic vasoconstriction.[32] The possibility of excessive vasoconstriction is supported by the observation that, in some individuals with vasospastic angina, propranolol seems to increase coronary vasoconstriction.[33] Also, although patients who are receiving propranolol for classic angina pectoris can increase their exercise performance, pain usually occurs at a lower pressure-rate product than prior to therapy. However, this effect does not necessarily reflect a reduction in oxygen delivery to the myocardium, because propranolol can increase ventricular size, which will increase myocardial wall tension and increase cardiac oxygen demands for any given pressure-rate product. Intracoronary infusion of propranolol does not worsen the local stenosis of a coronary artery but, in fact, increases the luminal area of the diseased artery at rest and during exercise.[34]

Effects on Arteries and Veins

Although propranolol does not have direct effects on blood vessels, it can produce vasoconstriction by two mechanisms. First, by reducing cardiac output, propranolol results in reflex vasoconstriction that acutely increases peripheral vascular resistance. Second, if epinephrine is circulating when propranolol is given, the vascular resistance will increase markedly, because the vasodilator effect of epinephrine mediated via β2-adrenergic receptors will be blocked, unmasking the potent α-adrenergic receptor–mediated vasoconstriction. In this situation, arterial pressure will rise, and reflex bradycardia will result.[35] Clinical situations in which propranolol can produce hypertension include pheochromocytoma, hypoglycemia, clonidine withdrawal, and administration of epineph-

rine for therapy of asthma or urticaria. However, it is important to realize that, although epinephrine concentrations are increased during exercise, propranolol does not inhibit the vasodilation that occurs in working muscles.[36]

Effects on Fluid Volume and Electrolytes

Propranolol produces minor changes in fluid volume in most patients, although it lowers arterial pressure and cardiac output.[37] Perhaps there is little fluid retention because propranolol reduces renin secretion (discussed later) and thereby reduces the formation of angiotensin II and aldosterone, the latter being the major regulatory hormone influencing sodium retention. In patients with marginal cardiac function, propranolol can cause sodium retention as part of the syndrome of heart failure precipitated by the drug.

Serum electrolytes are changed little by propranolol, but serum potassium concentration may increase slightly.[38] There are two potential explanations for the increase in serum potassium. First, propranolol reduces plasma renin activity and thereby reduces aldosterone secretion that will reduce renal potassium loss. Second, and probably more important, propranolol can alter transcellular movement of potassium. Stimulation of β2-adrenergic receptors increases the movement of potassium into skeletal muscle cells, thus decreasing serum potassium. By blocking this effect, propranolol can prevent the fall in serum potassium associated with adrenergic stimulation.[39]

Endocrine and Metabolic Effects

β-Adrenergic receptors are involved in a number of metabolic functions. Renin secretion is stimulated by activation of the β-adrenergic receptors in response to epinephrine released from the adrenal glands or norepinephrine released from adrenergic neurons. Both β1- and β2-adrenergic receptors are responsible for renin release,[40] and both are blocked by propranolol. This action on renin may account for some of the antihypertensive effects of propranolol.[41]

β2-Adrenergic receptor activation can affect glucose homeostasis by stimulating insulin release and glycogenolysis. The clinical importance of β-adrenoreceptor–mediated release of insulin is questionable. In normal individuals, no deficit in insulin secretion can be attributed to propranolol.[42] Anecdotal reports of hyperosmolar coma associated with propranolol in patients with type II diabetes have not been related unequivocally to the effect of propranolol on insulin secretion or its inhibition of hormone-stimulated lipolysis.[43] More important to glucose homeostasis is the ability of propranolol to block β2-adrenoreceptor–stimulated glycogenolysis. Normal individuals have multiple mechanisms to mobilize glucose, and propranolol produces little or no change in the recovery from hypoglycemia.[44] However, in patients with diabetes, the role of β-adrenoreceptor–mediated glycogenolysis becomes important, because the secretion of glucagon that normally protects against hypoglycemia is often impaired;[45] in such patients, propranolol can prolong an episode of hypoglycemia.[46] In addition, propranolol can blunt the feeling of anxiety and the tremor that accompanies sympathetic activation.

Propranolol and other β-adrenergic receptor blocking drugs have been found to produce small changes in blood lipids; triglyceride is increased, high-density lipoprotein (HDL) cholesterol is decreased, and total and low-density lipoprotein (LDL) cholesterol are unchanged.[47] The finding that propranolol reduces HDL cholesterol has produced some concern that long-term effects of the drug may result in an increased risk of coronary artery disease. However, in patients who have suffered myocardial infarction, the established benefit of propranolol far outweighs the theoretic risk.[48]

Propranolol also can inhibit catecholamine-stimulated lipolysis, resulting in a reduction of free fatty acid concentration that is particularly evident during exercise. This metabolic change leads to increased reliance of exercising muscles on carbohydrate fuels.[49]

Propranolol can alter the metabolism of thyroxine by reducing its conversion to triiodothyronine (T_3) such that more thyroxine is converted to inactive reverse T_3.[50] Whether this effect is related to β-adrenergic receptor blockade is questionable because (+)-propranolol has a similar effect, and nadolol, another nonselective β-adrenergic receptor blocking drug, does not.[51] This effect does not reduce the metabolic rate.[52]

Effects on Renal Function

When given acutely, propranolol reduces renal blood flow because of the reduction in cardiac output and the reflex rise in vascular resistance.[53] When given chronically, propranolol may continue to produce small reductions in renal blood flow and glomerular filtration rate. These effects are usually of no clinical consequence, but there are occasional reports of patients who have had clinically significant reductions in glomerular filtration rates during propranolol therapy.[54]

Effects on the Central Nervous System

Propranolol gains ready access to the brain because of its lipophilicity, and it can produce side effects attributable to CNS function. The genesis of these side effects is unclear. Do they occur because of propranolol interacting with β-adrenergic receptors in the brain, or are they related to nonspecific effects of the drug? Water-soluble β-blockers are said to have fewer side effects attributable to CNS dysfunction, but this is not a constant finding.[55] It has been suggested that the magnitudes of the CNS effects of the lipophilic and hydrophilic drugs are similar, but the time course of these effects varies. Gengo et al.[56] found that the CNS effects of the water-soluble drug atenolol had a more protracted time course than did the effects of the lipid-soluble drug, metoprolol. This finding suggests that, although entry into the cerebrospinal fluid is slower with the hydrophilic drugs, the exit of these drugs from the brain may also be slower and may account for the prolonged effect.

CLINICAL USE
Indications

Propranolol is approved for more indications than any other β-adrenergic receptor blocking drug. The three major areas of use in cardiovascular medicine are the management of coronary artery disease, the treatment of hypertension, and the treatment and prophylaxis of supraventricular and ventricular arrhythmias. In addition, propranolol has many other uses and has had a major impact on areas of medicine remote from cardiology and hypertension.

Angina Pectoris

By reducing the response of the heart to sympathetic stimulation, propranolol reduces the heart rate, contractility, and systolic arterial pressure during exercise; these effects decrease cardiac oxygen demands at any grade of exercise.[57] The effects of propranolol on ventricular wall tension are not always predictable. Wall tension may decrease because of a fall in arterial pressure, but because left ventricular size may increase, wall tension may also increase, because wall tension is a direct function of both ventricular size and cavitary pressure. It has been suggested that if cardiac enlargement develops in a patient on propranolol, digitalis may offset this effect and increase the antianginal effect by reducing wall tension.[58]

Other potentially beneficial effects in patients with angina pectoris are an increase in diastolic filling time during which coronary blood flow occurs,[57] a redistribution of the coronary blood flow toward the ischemic area,[30] a shift in the oxyhemoglobin dissociation curve so that more oxygen can be released to the tissues,[59] and a reduction in platelet aggregation.[60] The last effect is not reproducible with platelets *in vitro* except with excessively high concentrations of propranolol, suggesting that the effect seen *in vivo* is not a direct effect of the drug.

For therapy of angina pectoris, the initial propranolol doses should be small (40 mg/day), and the dose should be increased until there is adequate β-adrenergic receptor blockade or pain relief as judged by exercise tolerance and patient diaries. If the dose is too small, β-adrenergic receptor blockade will not be adequate and less than maximal benefit will accrue. A reduction in exercise heart rate rather than resting heart rate must be used as the index of β-adrenergic receptor blockade so that the drug will not be discarded prematurely.[61] If too large a dose is used, exercise tolerance may paradoxically decrease, perhaps because exercise is limited by fatigue, a side effect of propranolol. β-Adrenergic receptor blockade must be adequate throughout the dosing interval, which requires twice-daily administration of the standard formulation or a single daily dose of the sustained-release preparation.[62] Propranolol is useful alone or when added to other therapies for angina pectoris.

In patients with *variant angina pectoris,* in which coronary vasospasm causes the ischemia, propranolol is frequently not helpful, and the condition of some patients clearly deteriorates on propranolol, which can increase the intensity and length of vasospastic episodes.[33]

In patients with crescendo or *unstable angina pectoris,* propranolol is usually used in addition to nitrates, calcium antagonists, and aspirin, and it frequently is helpful in relieving pain.[63] In this setting, the effect of propranolol on the resting sympathetic tone is apparently of benefit.

Myocardial Infarction

No doubt exists that propranolol, 60 to 80 mg three times daily, will improve survival and reduce the reinfarction rate when it is begun 1 or more weeks after a myocardial infarction and is continued for 3 years or longer.[64, 65] The exact mechanism whereby propranolol reduces mortality is unknown. The benefit is probably multifactorial, with the antiischemic, antihypertensive, and antiarrhythmic effects of propranolol all playing a role.[66, 67] In patients with low mortality risk after an infarction, the incremental benefit provided by propranolol is small. This fact has persuaded some to suggest that the drug should be reserved for the subset of patients at higher risk who have histories of congestive heart failure, persistent signs of ischemia, or myocardial dysfunction or electrical instability during hospitalization for myocardial infarction.[68, 69]

Antiarrhythmic Effects

Propranolol is useful for the management of both ventricular and supraventricular arrhythmias. Propranolol slows the ventricular response to atrial fibrillation and atrial flutter by prolonging the functional refractory period of the AV node, an effect that is additive to digitalis and calcium antagonists.[70] Propranolol does not have a primary action to convert atrial fibrillation and flutter to sinus rhythm. Propranolol, 1 to 5 mg IV, often converts paroxysmal supraventricular tachycardia to sinus rhythm. This arrhythmia is usually a reentry rhythm in which the AV node is involved in at least one limb of the reentry. By blocking the AV node, the reentry can be aborted and the abnormal rhythm terminated. Chronic propranolol therapy can be used to prevent recurrence of paroxysmal supraventricular tachycardia. In patients with Wolff-Parkinson-White syndrome and recurrent atrial fibrillation or flutter with antegrade conduction over the aberrant bundle, propranolol will not slow the ventricular response. However, propranolol will not make the arrhythmia worse, which can happen with digitalis or verapamil.

Propranolol can also slow a sinus tachycardia, but it should rarely be used for this purpose, because sinus tachycardia is usually a physiologic response to an underlying abnormality, such as cardiac failure, bronchospasm, or circulatory shock, all of which may be made worse by the addition of propranolol. Sinus tachycardia that accompanies thyrotoxicosis can be safely managed with propranolol, unless there is associated cardiomyopathy or heart failure.

Propranolol also has a role in the management of ventricular arrhythmias. Propranolol is particularly effective in arrhythmias that arise from excessive sympathetic stimulation or increased cardiac sensitivity to catecholamines, such as may be produced by some inhalation anesthetics. If used in patients with pheochromocytoma, propranolol must be preceded by adequate α-adrenergic receptor blockade to avoid a hypertensive crisis that can result from unopposed α-adrenergic stimulation produced by excessive amounts of circulating epinephrine.

Although ventricular arrhythmias usually do not have obvious sympathetic components, propranolol may still be useful in their treatment. In patients with coronary artery disease and stable, nonsustained ventricular arrhythmias, propranolol at the usual doses for producing β-adrenergic blockade effectively suppresses arrhythmias in about 40% of patients. At doses higher than those required to produce maximal suppression of exercise-induced tachycardia, propranolol controls another 40% of stable ventricular arrhythmias.[71] These doses produce concentrations of propranolol that have been shown to have effects on the cardiac action potential unrelated to β-adrenergic blockade.[27] It is likely that the antiarrhythmic effect requiring high doses of propranolol is due to effects other than β-adrenergic receptor blockade.[72]

Hypertension

When β-adrenergic receptor blocking drugs were being developed, no one predicted that they would be useful for managing hypertension. Prichard[73] noticed an antihypertensive effect of pronethalol in patients with angina pectoris, and this effect was confirmed in hypertensive patients. Subsequently, propranolol was found to be effective as monotherapy for hypertension and to offer many advantages over drugs that were currently available.[74]

The precise mechanism whereby propranolol lowers arterial pressure has not been determined. Among the theories that have been proposed to explain the antihypertensive effects of propranolol[75, 76] are effects on renin secretion, catecholamine release from adrenergic neurons, baroreceptor sensitivity, CNS control of arterial pressure, autoregulation of the circulation, and prostaglandin and nitric oxide synthesis. Probably, there are multiple modes of action, and one or another predominates in any given patient. Because all β-adrenergic receptor blockers are effective antihypertensive drugs and (+)-propranolol does not reduce blood pressure, the property responsible for this therapeutic effect is undoubtedly due to β-adrenergic receptor blockade. Black patients and smokers are least responsive to the antihypertensive effects of propranolol.[77, 78]

When added to other antihypertensive drugs, propranolol can produce a further reduction in arterial pressure. Part of the mechanism of the additional antihypertensive effect of propranolol is due to its ability to block the normal reflexes that limit the response to the other antihypertensive agents.[79, 80]

Propranolol is effective as an antihypertensive agent when given once daily, despite its half-life of 3 to 6 hours.[81] Part of the reason for this apparent discrepancy between blood levels and effect may be explained by the concepts discussed earlier in this chapter, but the observation that propranolol can be taken up into adrenergic neurons to be subsequently released on sympathetic stimulation may also be important in this regard.[82]

Hypertension in pregnant women is a special situation in which one must consider not only the patient but also the fetus. Propranolol is well-tolerated in pregnancy, and the initial fears about premature labor, neonatal hypoglycemia, or infants who are small for gestational age have not turned out to be significant problems in controlled trials.[83]

Aortic Dissection

Propranolol is frequently used for acute and chronic medical management of aortic dissection because it can reduce arterial pressure and the rate of rise of pressure in the aorta, both of which are important in the propagation of the tear. If a vasodilator, such as sodium nitroprusside, is used in hypertensive patients with aortic dissection, the concurrent use of a β-adrenergic receptor blocker such as propranolol is mandatory to counteract the potentially damaging effects of reflex sympathetic stimulation.[84]

Cardiomyopathy

Propranolol has been the pharmacologic treatment of choice for patients with hypertrophic cardiomyopathy.[85] In addition to its antiarrhythmic and antiischemic effects, propranolol can reduce the dynamic obstruction that may occur in these patients by reducing contractility and increasing ventricular diameter. Propranolol does not appear to improve abnormal diastolic function. Abrupt withdrawal of propranolol can cause marked deterioration of the clinical course of these patients.[11]

There is also interest in the use of β-adrenergic receptor blockers for the treatment of dilated cardiomyopathies and heart failure.[86] The use of β-adrenergic receptor blockade for this purpose is experimental, because β-adrenergic receptor stimulation may be deleterious in these patients because of increased oxygen demands, arrhythmias, and catecholamine-induced myocardial necrosis.

Mitral Valve Prolapse

Patients with mitral valve prolapse may have a number of symptoms suggesting β-adrenergic hypersensitivity that can be ameliorated by propranolol.[87] These patients are typically anxious, and reassurance along with the antiarrhythmic and antianxiety effects of propranolol can often greatly improve the ability of such patients to function effectively.

Thyrotoxicosis

Propranolol is useful in reducing the adrenergic manifestations of thyrotoxicosis until more definitive antithyroid therapy or surgery can be undertaken. Propranolol quickly controls tachycardia and improves the tremor, anxiety, and myopathy of thyrotoxicosis. However, it has no effect on the underlying disease and should not be considered sole or primary therapy. Moreover, propranolol may be dangerous in patients with cardiomyopathy or heart failure.[88, 89]

Migraine

An important indication for propranolol is the prophylaxis of migraine headaches. The mechanism of this effect is unknown, but several other β-adrenergic receptor blocking drugs are also effective.[90] Propranolol does not interact with the antimigraine drug, sumatriptan.[91]

Tremor

Propranolol is effective in controlling familial essential tremor, probably by blocking β$_2$-adrenergic receptors on skeletal muscle.[92]

Psychiatric Uses

Propranolol is being used more often for anxiety, particularly performance anxiety (stage fright). The theory of detrimental performance anxiety is that the syndrome represents a positive feedback system in which the β-adrenoreceptor–mediated manifestations of anxiety, including tachycardia (palpitations), tremor, and hyperventilation, beget more anxiety and more symptoms until, at some level, performance abruptly deteriorates.[93] Propranolol is thought to achieve its beneficial effect in performance anxiety by antagonizing the peripheral adrenergic manifestations of anxiety rather than affecting the brain. In this way, propranolol interrupts the positive feedback loop. Double-blind, controlled trials have shown that certain types of performance, particularly those in which tremor is detrimental, can be improved objectively by propranolol or several other β-adrenergic receptor blockers.[93, 94] The appropriate oral dose of propranolol in this syndrome is 40 mg, 30 to 60 minutes prior to the performance.

Propranolol has also been used in neurotic anxiety, wherein its main effect is probably on the adrenergically mediated symptoms. In this setting, the benzodiazepines are probably more effective for long-term use.[95]

Adverse Effects

Most of the serious adverse effects of propranolol are manifestations of β-adrenergic receptor blockade in patients who are critically dependent on sympathetic function; thus, many of the life-threatening side effects are not dose-related.[96] These effects occur when the drug is first given. If a small amount of the drug can be tolerated, much larger amounts usually will also be safe. Patients who are at increased risk for the adverse effects of β-adrenergic receptor blockade can often be determined in advance, and the drug can be avoided.

Cardiac

Patients with compensated heart failure often have increased sympathetic nervous activity. Propranolol can precipitate acute exacerbation of congestive heart failure in such patients. Nonetheless, with caution, propranolol can often be used safely in patients with histories of heart failure controlled with medical management, and some investigators believe that β-adrenergic blockers can actually improve cardiac function over the long term.[86] In some patients, cardiac failure gradually develops after propranolol is started; these patients can usually be managed with digitalis, diuretics, and afterload-reducing agents with continuation of the propranolol if necessary.

Propranolol may also produce adverse effects related to reduced automaticity of the SA pacemakers or reduced conduction in the SA or AV node. Although sinus bradycardia is a frequent effect of propranolol, it is usually asymptomatic and worries the physician more than the patient. However, these effects can reduce cardiac output and produce syncope in patients with SA or AV nodal disease or those who take other drugs that affect these structures. In patients with sick sinus syndrome, the AV nodal pacemakers that would normally take over the cardiac rhythm when the SA node is suppressed are also suppressed by propranolol, resulting in a hemodynamically inadequate, slow idioventricular rhythm that may require a pacemaker.[97] Similarly, in patients with AV nodal disease, propranolol can produce second- or third-degree heart block.

A feeling of fatigue is common in patients receiving propranolol. It may be related to reduced peripheral blood flow, an effect on the CNS, an effect on fuel delivery to working skeletal muscle because of inhibition of lipolysis and glycogenolysis,[98] or an effect that inhibits exercise-induced increase in respiratory gas exchange.[99] The decreased ability to perform endurance exercise while receiving propranolol may have a similar cause and may not be related solely to a reduced cardiac output.

Pulmonary

Propranolol effectively blocks the β₂-adrenergic receptors that mediate bronchodilation. Bronchospastic pulmonary disease may be exacerbated by propranolol, and such attacks are resistant to therapy with β-adrenergic receptor agonists. Thus, propranolol should *never* be given to an asthmatic patient.

Central Nervous System

Side effects attributable to CNS dysfunction are relatively common with propranolol.[100] These effects commonly are sleep disturbances; bizarre, vivid dreams; and fatigue, but more serious side effects, such as visual hallucinations and depression, may occur.[101, 102] Drug-induced depression may account for the association of increased antidepressant use in patients who are receiving β-adrenergic receptor blocking drugs for hypertension,[103] but not all investigators have found evidence of an increased prevalence of depression in patients receiving these drugs.[104] Nonetheless, if depression occurs in a patient receiving propranolol, the drug should be promptly discontinued. When taken in massive overdose, propranolol can produce seizures.[28]

Peripheral Vasculature

Anecdotal reports suggest that the condition of patients with intermittent claudication or Raynaud's syndrome may deteriorate on administration of propranolol. Controlled studies have not shown this to be the case.[105, 106] However, cold hands and feet are relatively common in patients who receive propranolol in cold weather, and this effect is likely to result from reduced skin blood flow produced by β-adrenergic receptor blockade.

Metabolic

The metabolic effects of propranolol were discussed earlier in this chapter. Of greatest potential concern in diabetic patients who are taking hypoglycemic drugs is the ability of propranolol to prolong episodes of hypoglycemia, mask adrenergic symptoms accompanying hypoglycemia, and increase arterial pressure during hypoglycemia.

Propranolol can produce a slight rise in serum potassium that is usually of no clinical consequence but occasionally is significant when propranolol is given concurrently with other drugs that can increase serum potassium concentration.

Other

Impotence occurs with propranolol, but to a lesser degree than with many other drugs that affect the sympathetic nervous system. In the Medical Research Council (MRC) trial, propranolol was associated with impotence, necessitating withdrawal from the study of 6.3 per 1000 men, a lower incidence than in men who received a diuretic (12.6/1000) but higher than in patients receiving placebo (1.3/1000).[77]

Contraindications

Propranolol is contraindicated clinically when continued β-adrenergic receptor stimulation is required for maintenance of life. Thus, patients who have decompensated heart failure or active bronchospasm should not receive propranolol or any β-adrenergic receptor blocker. All other contraindications are relative, but, in general, propranolol should not be used in patients with diabetes who are receiving hypoglycemia drugs, patients with chronic pulmonary disease involving bronchospasm as a part of the syndrome, or patients with depression.

Drug Interactions

Propranolol can decrease the clearance of lidocaine by reducing hepatic blood flow.[107] The reduction in clearance results in lidocaine concentrations that are higher for any given infusion rate. It has been suggested that propranolol can also interfere with oxidative metabolism independent of its effects on hepatic blood flow, but clinical examples of such an interaction are unknown. Cigarette smoking and drugs that induce hepatic drug-metabolizing enzymes—such as phenytoin, phenobarbital, rifampin, and halofenate—can increase the presystemic elimination of propranolol given orally and thereby reduce its bioavailability.[108] Cimetidine, by inhibiting the drug-metabolizing enzyme activity, can increase the bioavailability of propranolol.[109]

The major interactions involving propranolol are pharmacodynamic rather than pharmacokinetic. Nonsteroidal antiinflammatory drugs can reduce the antihypertensive effects of propranolol without influencing the β-adrenergic receptor blocking effects of the drug.[110] Propranolol can add to the effect of other drugs—such as verapamil, diltiazem, and digoxin—that reduce conduction velocity and increase the functional refractory period of the AV node, and the combination sometimes results in AV block. Drugs that have direct negative inotropic effects, such as disopyramide and calcium antagonists, can produce more severe cardiac depression in the presence of propranolol because the normal sympathetic compensation is blocked, but this is unlikely to be a problem in patients with good cardiac function.

Use in Patients with Renal or Hepatic Dysfunction

Hepatic dysfunction can decrease the clearance of propranolol because of reduced metabolic enzyme activity and reduced hepatic blood flow.[19] As discussed earlier, shunts connecting the portal vein directly to the vena cava will increase the bioavailability of propranolol as the liver is bypassed during the absorption process.

Renal dysfunction produces little change in propranolol kinetics. Clearance of the drug is unchanged and, if anything, the half-life tends to be slightly shorter because the apparent volume of distribution is somewhat reduced.[111] The inactive metabolites of propranolol accumulate in patients with renal failure and can interfere with some of the laboratory methods for detection of bilirubin.[112]

Place in Antihypertensive Arsenal

Propranolol remains an excellent drug for the treatment of hypertension and, with the exception of thiazide diuretics and hydralazine, has accumulated more years of experience than any other antihypertensive drug in common use. Additionally, β-blockers and thiazide diuretics are the only classes of drugs that have been shown in controlled clinical trials to reduce the morbidity and mortality attributable to hypertension. Direct comparisons of antihypertensive drugs are few, but monotherapy with propranolol has been compared with a thiazide diuretic in large studies performed by the Veterans Administration (VA) and the MRC of the United Kingdom.[77, 78] In the VA study, hydrochlorothiazide was more effective than propranolol as an antihypertensive drug, particularly in black patients. Propranolol was more effective in white than in black patients. Study termination for lack of efficacy or side effects was greater with propranolol than with hydrochlorothiazide. In the MRC trial, the thiazide diuretic also was more effective as an antihypertensive in the entire population and reduced the incidence of strokes more than propranolol did. Propranolol was effective only in reducing the incidence of strokes in nonsmoking patients. Overall, coronary events were not reduced; however, in nonsmoking male patients, the incidence of coronary vascular events was lowest in patients receiving propranolol. The incidences of side effects were similar for the two active treatment groups.

The VA has also compared propranolol with verapamil.[113] Verapamil was more effective as an antihypertensive in the entire population. Propranolol was much less effective in black than in white patients, whereas verapamil was equally effective in patients of both races. The incidences of side effects were similar in the two groups.

Finally, in a comparative study designed to evaluate the effect of antihypertensive therapy on the quality of life, propranolol was compared with methyldopa and captopril.[114] Captopril was the best tolerated of these drugs, followed by propranolol and methyldopa. This study was not designed to compare the beneficial effects of the drugs on morbidity resulting from hypertension.

The Joint National Committee for the treatment of hypertension now recommends β-adrenergic receptor blockers or diuretics as drugs that should be considered for initial management of hypertension.[115] When these agents are inappropriate, ineffective, or poorly tolerated, alternative initial drugs include the angiotensin-converting enzyme inhibitors, calcium antagonists, and α/β-adrenergic inhibitors. Patients likely to respond well to monotherapy with propranolol are younger, nonsmoking whites. Patients who have one of the other indications for propranolol are also logical candidates for the drug. The choice of propranolol over other β-adrenergic receptor blockers is based on individual patient tolerance, because the antihypertensive effects of all β-adrenergic receptor blocking drugs are the same. If propranolol is not chosen as monotherapy, it can be added to other antihypertensive drugs. It is particularly effective when combined with a diuretic, with or without a vasodilator.

Dosage and Administration

The usual dose range for propranolol given orally for most indications is 80 to 480 mg daily. Although often given twice daily, the drug may be effective when administered once a day for hypertension in the standard formulation, and it is certainly effective once daily in the sustained-release preparation (Inderal-LA) for most indications. Propranolol has been suggested as the most cost-effective treatment for hypertension.[116] When used intravenously to produce acute β-adrenergic receptor blockade, such as in adults with dissecting aortic aneurysm, propranolol is given in an initial 1-mg test dose that is followed by a loading dose of 5 to 10 mg and a sustaining infusion of 3 mg/hr. This administration regimen will achieve a high degree of β-adrenergic receptor blockade in most patients.[117]

REFERENCES

1. Shanks RG: The discovery of beta-adrenoceptor blocking drugs. Trends Pharmacol Sci 62:405, 1984.
2. Black JW, Stephenson JS: Pharmacology of a new adrenergic β-receptor blocking compound (nethalide). Lancet 2:311, 1962.
3. Alleyne GAO, Dickinson CJ, Dornhorst AC, et al: Effect of pronethalol in angina pectoris. Br Med J 2:1226, 1963.
4. Black JW, Crowther AF, Shanks RG, et al: A new adrenergic beta-receptor antagonist. Lancet 1:1080, 1964.
5. Stiles GL, Caron MG, Lefkowitz RJ: β-Adrenergic receptors: Biochemical mechanisms of physiological regulation. Physiol Rev 64:661, 1984.
6. Aarons RD, Nies AS, Gal J, et al: Elevation of β-adrenergic receptor density in human lymphocytes after propranolol administration. J Clin Invest 65:949, 1980.
7. Fraser J, Nadeau J, Robertson D, et al: Regulation of human leukocyte beta receptors by endogenous catecholamines: I. Relationship of leukocyte beta receptor density to the cardiac sensitivity to isoproterenol. J Clin Invest 67:1777, 1981.
8. Miller RR, Olson HG, Amsterdam EA, et al: Propranolol withdrawal rebound phenomenon. N Engl J Med 293:416, 1975.
9. Nattel S, Rangno RE, VanLoon G: Mechanism of propranolol withdrawal phenomena. Circulation 59:1158, 1979.
10. Krukemyer JJ, Boudoulas H, Binkley PF, et al: Comparison of hypersensitivity to adrenergic stimulation after abrupt withdrawal of propranol and nadolol: Influence of half-life differences. Am Heart J 120:572, 1990.
11. Gilligan DM, Chan WL, Stewart R, et al: Adrenergic hypersensitivity after beta-blocker withdrawal in hypertrophic cardiomyopathy. Am J Cardiol 68:766, 1991.
12. Woods PB, Robinson ML: An investigation of the comparative liposolubilities of β-adrenoceptor blocking agents. J Pharm Pharmacol 33:172, 1981.
13. Vaughan Williams EM: A classification of antiarrhythmic actions reassessed after a decade of new drugs. J Clin Pharmacol 24:129, 1984.
14. Nies AS, Shand DG: Clinical pharmacology of propranolol. Circulation 52:6, 1975.
15. Paterson JW, Conolly ME, Dollery CT, et al: The pharmacodynamics and metabolism of propranolol in man. Pharmacol Clin 2:127, 1970.
16. Shand DG, Evans GH, Nies AS: The almost complete hepatic extraction of propranolol during intravenous administration in the dog. Life Sci 10:1417, 1971.
17. Nies AS, Evans GH, Shand DG: The hemodynamic effects of beta-adrenergic blockade on the flow-dependent hepatic clearance of propranolol. J Pharmacol Exp Ther 184:716, 1973.
18. Routledge PA, Shand DG: Clinical pharmacokinetics of propranolol. Clin Pharmacokinet 4:73, 1979.
19. Branch RA, Shand DG: Propranolol disposition in chronic liver disease: A physiological approach. Clin Pharmacokinet 1:264, 1976.
20. Coltart DJ, Shand DG: Plasma propranolol levels in the quantitative assessment of β-adrenergic blockade in man. Br Med J 3:731, 1970.
21. Chidsey C, Pine M, Favrot L, et al: The use of drug concentration measurements in studies of the therapeutic response to propranolol. Postgrad Med J 52(Suppl 4):26, 1976.
22. Nies AS, Evans GH, Shand DG: Regional hemodynamic effects of beta-adrenergic blockade with propranolol in the unanesthetized primate. Am Heart J 85:97, 1973b.
23. Pagliaro L, D'Amico G, Sorensen TIA, et al: Prevention of first bleeding in cirrhosis. A meta-analysis of randomized trials of nonsurgical treatment. Ann Intern Med 117:59, 1992.
24. McDevitt DG: The assessment of β-adrenoceptor blocking drugs in man. Br J Clin Pharmacol 4:413, 1977.
25. Cruickshank JM, Neil-Dwyer G, Lane J: The effect of oral propranolol upon the ECG changes occurring in subarachnoid hemorrhage. Cardiovasc Res 9:236, 1975.
26. Lavie CJ, Ventura HO, Messerli FH: Regression of increased left ventricular mass by antihypertensives. Drugs 42:945, 1991.
27. Duff HJ, Roden DM, Brorson L, et al: Electrophysiologic actions of high plasma concentrations of propranolol in human subjects. J Am Coll Cardiol 2:1134, 1983.
28. Buiumsohn A, Eisenberg ES, Jacob H, et al: Seizures and intraventricular conduction defect in propranolol poisoning. Ann Intern Med 91:860, 1979.
29. Henry JA, Cassidy SL: Membrane stabilizing activity: A major cause of fatal poisoning. Lancet 1:1414, 1986.
30. Becker L, Pitt B: Regional myocardial blood flow, ischemia and antianginal drugs. Ann Clin Res 3:353, 1971.
31. Prida XE, Feldman RL, Hill JA, et al: Comparison of selective (beta₁) and nonselective (beta₁ and beta₂) beta-adrenergic blockade on systemic and coronary hemodynamic findings in angina pectoris. Am J Cardiol 60:244, 1987.
32. Kern MJ, Ganz P, Horowitz JD, et al: Potentiation of coronary vasoconstriction by beta-adrenergic blockade in patients with coronary artery disease. Circulation 67:1178, 1983.
33. Robertson RM, Wood AJJ, Vaughn WK, et al: Exacerbation of vasotonic angina pectoris by propranolol. Circulation 65:281, 1981.
34. Gaglione A, Hess OM, Corin WJ, et al: Is there coronary vasoconstriction after intracoronary beta-adrenergic blockade in patients with coronary artery disease? J Am Coll Cardiol 10:299, 1987.
35. Houben H, Thien T, van't Laar A: Effect of low-dose epinephrine infusion on hemodynamics after selective and nonselective β-blockade in hypertension. Clin Pharmacol Ther 31:685, 1982.
36. Hiatt WR, Fradl DC, Zerbe GO, et al: Selective and nonselective β-blockade of the peripheral circulation. Clin Pharmacol Ther 35:12, 1984.
37. Tarazi RC, Frohlich ED, Dustan HP: Plasma volume changes with long-term beta-adrenergic blockade. Am Heart J 82:770, 1971.
38. Traub YM, Rabinov M, Rosenfeld JB, et al: Elevation of serum potassium during beta blockade: Absence of relationship to the renin-aldosterone system. Clin Pharmacol Ther 28:765, 1980.
39. Struthers AD, Reid JL: The role of adrenal medullary catecholamines in potassium homeostasis. Clin Sci 66:377, 1984.
40. Olson RD, Nies AS, Gerber JG: Beta-adrenergically mediated release of renin in the dog is not confined to either beta-1 or beta-2 adrenoceptors. J Pharmacol Exp Ther 222:606, 1982.
41. Hollifield JW, Sherman K, Vander Zwagg R, et al: Proposed mechanisms of propranolol's antihypertensive effect in essential hypertension. N Engl J Med 295:68, 1976.
42. Totterman K, Groop L, Groop P-H, et al: Effect of beta-blocking drugs on beta-cell function and insulin sensitivity in hypertensive non-diabetic patients. Eur J Clin Pharmacol 26:13, 1984.

43. Podolsky S, Pattavina CG: Hyperosmolar nonketotic diabetic coma: A complication of propranolol therapy. Metabolism 22:685, 1973.
44. Clarke WL, Santiago JV, Thomas L, et al: Adrenergic mechanisms in recovery from hypoglycemia in man: Adrenergic blockade. Am J Physiol 236:E147, 1979.
45. Popp DA, Shah SD, Cryer PE: Role of epinephrine-mediated β-adrenergic mechanisms in hypoglycemia glucose counter-regulation and posthypoglycemic hyperglycemia in insulin-dependent diabetes mellitus. J Clin Invest 69:315, 1982.
46. Lager I, Blohme G, Smith U: Effect of cardioselective and non-selective β-blockade on the hypoglycemic response in insulin-dependent diabetics. Lancet 1:458, 1979.
47. Ames RP: The effects of antihypertensive drugs on serum lipids and lipoproteins. II. Non-diuretic drugs. Drugs 32:335, 1986.
48. Byington RP, Worthy J, Craven T, et al: Propranolol-induced lipid changes and their prognostic significance after a myocardial infarction: The Beta Blocker Heart Attack Trial experience. Am J Cardiol 65:1287, 1990.
49. Juhlin-Dannfelt A: Metabolic effects of β-adrenoceptor blockade on skeletal muscle at rest and during exercise. Acta Med Scand (Suppl) 665:113, 1982.
50. Verhoeven RP, Visser TJ, Docter R, et al: Plasma thyroxine, 3,3′,5′-triiodothyronine and 3,3′,5′-triiodothyronine during β-adrenergic blockade in hyperthyroidism. J Clin Endocrinol Metab 44:1002, 1977.
51. Reeves RA, From GLA, Paul W, et al: Nadolol, propranolol, and thyroid hormones: Evidence for a membrane-stabilizing action of propranolol. Clin Pharmacol Ther 37:157, 1985.
52. Zwillich CW, Matthay M, Potts DE, et al: Thyrotoxicosis: Comparison of effects of thyroid ablation and beta-adrenergic blockade on metabolic rate and ventilatory control. J Clin Endocrinol Metab 46:491, 1978.
53. Sullivan JM, Adams DF, Hollenberg NK: Beta-adrenergic blockade in essential hypertension. Reduced renin release despite renal vasoconstriction. Circ Res 39:532, 1976.
54. Wilkinson R: β-Blockers and renal function. Drugs 23:195, 1982.
55. Dahlöf C, Dimenäs E: Side effects of β-blocker treatments as related to the central nervous system. Am J Med Sci 299:236, 1990.
56. Gengo FM, Huntoon L, McHugh WB: Lipid-soluble and water-soluble β-blockers. Arch Intern Med 147:39, 1987.
57. Prichard BNC: β-Adrenergic receptor blocking drugs in angina pectoris. Drugs 7:55, 1974.
58. Crawford MH, LeWinter MM, O'Rourke RA, et al: Combined propranolol and digoxin therapy in angina pectoris. Ann Intern Med 83:449, 1975.
59. Schrumpf JD, Sheps DS, Wolfson S, et al: Altered hemoglobin-oxygen affinity with long-term propranolol therapy in patients with coronary artery disease. Am J Cardiol 40:76, 1977.
60. Frishman WH, Weksler B, Christodoulou JP, et al: Reversal of abnormal platelet aggregability and change in exercise tolerance in patients with angina pectoris following propranolol. Circulation 50:887, 1974.
61. Jackson G, Atkinson L, Oram S: Reassessment of failed beta-blocker treatment in angina pectoris by peak exercise heart rate measurements. Br Med J 3:616, 1975.
62. Jones GR, Mir MA: Comparison of antianginal efficacy of one conventional and three long acting beta-adrenoceptor blocking agents in stable angina pectoris. Br Heart J 46:503, 1981.
63. Gottlieb SO, Weisfeldt ML, Ouyang P, et al: Effect of the addition of propranolol to therapy with nifedipine for unstable angina pectoris: A randomized, double-blind, placebo-controlled trial. Circulation 73:331, 1986.
64. Beta-Blocker Heart Attack Trial Research Group: A randomized trial of propranolol in patients with acute myocardial infarction. I. Mortality results. JAMA 247:1707, 1982.
65. Beta-Blocker Heart Attack Trial Research Group: A randomized trial of propranolol in patients with acute myocardial infarction. II. Morbidity results. JAMA 250:2814, 1983.
66. Frishman WH, Lazar EJ: Reduction of mortality, sudden death and non-fatal reinfarction with beta-adrenergic blockers in survivors of acute myocardial infarction—a new hypothesis regarding the cardioprotective action of beta-adrenergic blockade. Am J Cardiol 66:G66, 1990.
67. Olsson G, Ryden L: Prevention of sudden death using beta-blockers—review of possible contributory actions. Circulation 84(Suppl 6):33, 1991.
68. Furberg CF, Hawkins CM, Lichstein E (for the Beta-Blocker Heart Attack Trial Study Group): Effect of propranolol in postinfarction patients with mechanical or electrical complications. Circulation 69:761, 1984.
69. Viscoli CM, Horwitz RI, Singer BH: Beta-blockers after myocardial infarction: Influence of first-year clinical course on long-term effectiveness. Ann Intern Med 118:99, 1993.
70. Harrison DC, Griffin JR, Fiene TJ: Effects of beta-adrenergic blockade with propranolol in patients with atrial arrhythmias. N Engl J Med 273:410, 1965.
71. Woosley RL, Kornhauser D, Smith R, et al: Suppression of chronic ventricular arrhythmias with propranolol. Circulation 60:819, 1979.
72. Murray KT, Reilly C, Koshakji RP, et al: Suppression of ventricular arrhythmias in man by D-propranolol independent of beta-adrenergic receptor blockade. J Clin Invest 85:836, 1990.
73. Prichard BNC: Hypotensive action of pronethalol. Br Med J 1:1227, 1964.
74. Prichard BNC, Gillam PMS: Use of propranolol (Inderal) in treatment of hypertension. Br Med J 2:725, 1964.
75. Prichard BNC, Owens CWI: Mode of action of beta-adrenergic blocking drugs in hypertension. Clin Physiol Biochem 8:1, 1990.
76. Man in't Veld AJ: Vasodilation, not cardiodepression, underlies the antihypertensive effect of beta-adrenoceptor antagonists. Am J Cardiol 67:13B, 1991.
77. Medical Research Council Working Party: MRC trial of treatment of mild hypertension: Principal results. Br Med J 291:97, 1985.
78. Veterans Administration Cooperative Study Group on Antihypertensive Agents: Comparison of propranolol and hydrochlorothiazide for the initial treatment of hypertension. I. Results of short-term titration with emphasis on racial differences in response. JAMA 248:1996, 1982.
79. Gilmore E, Weil J, Chidsey C: Treatment of essential hypertension with a new vasodilator in combination with beta-adrenergic blockade. N Engl J Med 282:521, 1970.
80. Pettinger WA, Mitchell HC: Renin release, saralasin and the vasodilator-beta-blocker drug interaction in man. N Engl J Med 292:1214, 1975.
81. van den Brink G, Boer P, van Asten P, et al: One and three doses of propranolol a day in hypertension. Clin Pharmacol Ther 27:9, 1980.
82. Russell MP, Webb JG, Walle T, et al: Adrenergic nerve stimulation-induced release of propranolol from the perfused hindlimb and spleen of the dog and associated changes in postjunctional response. J Pharmacol Exp Ther 226:324, 1983.
83. Rubin PC: Beta-blockers in pregnancy. N Engl J Med 305:1323, 1981.
84. DeSanctis RW, Doroghazi RM, Austen WG, et al: Aortic dissection. N Engl J Med 317:1060, 1987.
85. Maron BJ, Bonow RO, Cannon RO, et al: Hypertrophic cardiomyopathy. Interrelations of clinical manifestations, pathophysiology, and therapy. N Engl J Med 316:844, 1987.
86. Bristow MR: Pathophysiologic and pharmacologic rationales for clinical management of chronic heart failure with beta-blocking agents. Am J Cardiol 71:12C, 1993.
87. Davies AO, Mares A, Pool JC, et al: Mitral valve prolapse with symptoms of beta-adrenergic hypersensitivity. Am J Med 82:193, 1987.
88. Woeber KA: Thyrotoxicosis and the heart. N Engl J Med 327:94, 1992.
89. Geffner DL, Hershman JM: β-Adrenergic blockade for the treatment of hyperthyroidism. Am J Med 93:61, 1992.
90. Holroyd KA, Penzien DB, Cordingley GE: Propranolol in the management of recurrent migraine: A meta-analytical review. Headache 31:333, 1991.
91. Scott AK, Walley T, Breckenridge AM, et al: Lack of an interaction between propranolol and sumatriptan. Br J Clin Pharmacol 32:581, 1991.

92. Winker GF, Young RR: Efficacy of chronic propranolol therapy in action tremors of the familial, senile or essential varieties. N Engl J Med 290:984, 1974.
93. James IM: Practical aspects of the use of beta-blockers in anxiety states: Situational anxiety. Postgrad Med J 60(Suppl 2):19, 1984.
94. Brantigan CO, Brantigan TA, Joseph N: Effect of beta blockade and beta stimulation on stage fright. Am J Med 72:88, 1982.
95. Peet M: Beta-blockade in anxiety. Postgrad Med J 60(Suppl 2):16, 1984.
96. Greenblatt DJ, Koch-Weser J: Adverse reactions to β-adrenergic receptor blocking drugs: A report from the Boston Collaborative Drug Surveillance Program. Drugs 7:118, 1974.
97. Strauss HC, Gilbert M, Svenson RH, et al: Electrophysiologic effects of propranolol on sinus node function in patients with sinus node dysfunction. Circulation 54:452, 1976.
98. McLeod AA, Brown JE, Kuhn C, et al: Differentiation of hemodynamic, humoral and metabolic responses to β_1- and β_2-adrenergic stimulation in man using atenolol and propranolol. Circulation 67:1076, 1983.
99. McLeod AA, Knopes KD, Shand DG, et al: β_1-selective and non-selective β-adrenoceptor blockade, anaerobic threshold and respiratory gas exchange during exercise. Br J Clin Pharmacol 19:13, 1985.
100. Kostis JB, Rosen RC: Central nervous system effects of β-adrenergic-blocking drugs: The role of ancillary properties. Circulation 75:204, 1987.
101. Fleminger R: Visual hallucinations and illusions with propranolol. Br Med J 1:1182, 1978.
102. Petrie WM, Maffucci RJ, Woosley RL: Propranolol and depression. Am J Psychiatry 139:92, 1982.
103. Avorn J, Everitt DE, Weiss S: Increased antidepressant use in patients prescribed β-blockers. JAMA 255:357, 1986.
104. Bright RA, Everitt DE: β-blockers and depression. Evidence against an association. JAMA 267:1783, 1992.
105. Coffman JD, Rasmussen HM: Effects of β-adrenoceptor-blocking drugs in patients with Raynaud's phenomenon. Circulation 72:466, 1985.
106. Radack K, Deck C: β-Adrenergic blocker therapy does not worsen intermittent claudication in subjects with peripheral arterial disease. A meta-analysis of randomized controlled trials. Arch Intern Med 151:1769, 1991.
107. Ochs HR, Carstens G, Greenblatt DJ: Reduction in lidocaine clearance during continuous infusion and by coadministration of propranolol. N Engl J Med 303:373, 1980.
108. Branch RA, Herman RJ: Enzyme induction and β-adrenergic receptor blocking drugs. Br J Clin Pharmacol 17:77S, 1984.
109. Wood AJJ, Feely J: Pharmacokinetic drug interactions with propranolol. Clin Pharmacokinet 8:253, 1983.
110. Houston MC: Nonsteroidal anti-inflammatory drugs and antihypertensives. Am J Med 90:42S, 1991.
111. Wood AJJ, Vestal RE, Spannuth CL, et al: Propranolol disposition in renal failure. Br J Clin Pharmacol 10:561, 1980.
112. Stone WJ, Walle T: Massive propranolol metabolite retention during maintenance hemodialysis. Clin Pharmacol Ther 28:449, 1980.
113. Cubeddu LX, Aranda J, Singh B, et al: A comparison of verapamil and propranolol for the initial treatment of hypertension. Racial differences in response. JAMA 256:2214, 1986.
114. Croog SH, Levine S, Testa MA, et al: The effects of antihypertensive therapy on the quality of life. N Engl J Med 314:1657, 1986.
115. The Joint National Committee: The fifth report of the Joint National Committee on Detection, Evaluation and Treatment of High Blood Pressure (JNCV). Arch Intern Med 153:154, 1993.
116. Edelson JT, Weinstein MC, Tostoson ANA, et al: Long term cost effectiveness of various initial monotherapies for mild to moderate hypertension. JAMA 263:407, 1990.
117. McAllister RJ Jr: Intravenous propranolol administration: A method for rapidly achieving and sustaining desired plasma levels. Clin Pharmacol Ther 20:517, 1976.

CHAPTER 51

Timolol

Terje R. Pedersen, M.D.

Timolol was first described in 1970 in its racemic form[1] and is now available as a maleate in the pure L-isomeric form. In the United States, timolol is available in oral form under the trade name Blocadren and as an ophthalmic solution (Timoptic) for the treatment of glaucoma. In some countries, timolol is also marketed for intravenous use. Orally administered timolol is not a commonly used β-blocker in the United States.

PHARMACOLOGY

Timolol is a nonselective β-adrenergic blocking agent; the affinity to β_1- and to β_2-receptors is almost equal.[2] It has no membrane-stabilizing and only negligible partial agonist activity.[3] In humans, it is 8 to 10 times more potent than propranolol in reducing resting heart rate, and it is 14 times more potent in suppressing tachycardia induced by isoproterenol infusion.[4, 5]

PHARMACOKINETICS

When timolol tablets are administered orally, 90% to 100% of the drug is rapidly absorbed, uninfluenced by food ingestion.[6] Peak plasma levels occur 1 to 2 hours after intake. Plasma half-life is approximately 2 to 4 hours. Between 5% and 10% is excreted unchanged in the urine; the rest is broken down into several inactive metabolites that are subsequently excreted through the kidneys. Plasma half-life is not influenced by moderate renal failure. Bioavailability studies show that 50% to 75% of the drug reaches the central circulation after first pass through the hepatorenal system. Plasma levels may vary sixfold or sevenfold after a given oral dose. In plasma, only 10% is bound to proteins. Timolol has moderate lipid solubility.

EFFECTS ON PATHOPHYSIOLOGY

Timolol's hemodynamic and electrophysiologic effects are similar to those of other β-adrenergic blocking agents.[7-10] It improves exercise tolerance in patients with angina pectoris.[11] It substantially reduces the long-term risk of sudden death and reinfarction in patients surviving acute myocardial infarction.[12] It has been shown to reduce the size of an acute myocardial infarction when given intravenously within 4 hours after onset of symptoms.[13] It is effective in the treatment of supraventricular arrhythmias[14] and in certain cases of recurrent ventricular tachycardia.[15] The number of cases with primary heart arrest in the Norwegian Multicenter Study on Timolol after Myocardial Infarction was only 26 in the group treated with timolol against 74 among those receiving placebo, indicating a strong antifibrillatory effect.[16] In animal experiments, timolol in doses as low as 0.003 mg/kg has increased the ventricular fibrillation threshold substantially.[17] This might be analogous to some of the cardioprotective effect of timolol in patients who have survived an acute myocardial infarction. In these experiments, protection against ventricular fibrillation has been obtained, even though the heart rate was maintained at a constant level through pacing. The hypokalemia induced by increased plasma levels of epinephrine is prevented by timolol.[18, 19] Plasma uric acid usually increases by approximately 10% during long-term therapy. On average, plasma triglycerides are increased by 20% to 30% and plasma high density lipoproteins are reduced by approximately 10%, whereas total cholesterol levels remain unchanged.[20]

CLINICAL USE

In hypertension, timolol may be used either alone or in combination with most other antihypertensive agents. Combination with verapamil should be avoided because of the effect on atrioventricular node conduction. The usual dose is 10 to 30 mg/day, administered in two doses. In some cases, 60 mg/day may be necessary. In angina pectoris, doses of 5 mg b.i.d. may prove sufficient for optimal increase of exercise tolerance, especially in elderly patients.

As a secondary measure for prevention of cardiac death and reinfarction after acute myocardial infarction, treatment may be started as soon as the patient is hemodynamically stable. A starting dosage of 5 mg b.i.d. is recommended, increasing to 10 mg b.i.d. after 2 days. Treatment is usually well tolerated, even in patients with large infarctions complicated with severe heart failure in the acute stage. Such patients should be stabilized with diuretics, digitalis, and vasodilating drugs before receiving timolol. If the systolic blood pressure is less than 100 mmHg, timolol is usually not tolerated. In a 6-year follow-up of patients using timolol after infarction, there was no indication of a diminishing protective effect on mortality.[21]

Timolol seems particularly indicated in patients with hypertension and/or angina after an acute myocardial infarction because of the combined effect on those conditions. It also has a protective effect in diabetic patients after myocardial infarction.[22] In cardiac arrhythmias and in acute myocardial infarction,

a dose of 1 mg is administered intravenously. This dose may be repeated within 10- to 20-minute intervals. To achieve sustained levels of β-adrenergic blockade, a constant infusion rate of 0.6 mg/hr is usually sufficient.

Timolol has the same contraindications and side effects as other noncardioselective β-adrenergic blocking agents. It can be used without dosage restriction in patients with moderate renal failure.

The cost of timolol treatment is comparable with that of other β-adrenergic blocking agents.[23]

REFERENCES

1. Hall RA, Robson RD, Share NN: A new potent beta-adrenergic blocking agent, (3-morpholino-4-83-t-butylamino-2-hydroxy-propoxy)-1,2,5-thiadiazole hydrogen maleate. Proc Can Fed Biol Soc 13:33, 1970.
2. Sweet CS, Britt PM, Solar JJ, et al: Peripheral vascular interactions of timolol and other beta-adrenergic receptor antagonists in anesthetized dogs. In Hanson L, Julius S, Richardson PJ (eds): Proceedings of the Timolol Intercontinental Symposium, Stockholm. Stockholm: MSDI, 1979, pp 111–129.
3. Frishman W: Clinical pharmacology of the new beta-adrenergic blocking drugs: Part 1. Pharmacodynamic and pharmacokinetic properties. Am Heart J 97:663, 1979.
4. Ulrych M, Franciosa J, Conway J: Comparison of a new beta-adrenergic blocker (MK950) and propranolol in man. Clin Pharmacol Ther 13:232, 1972.
5. Achong MR, Piafky KM, Ogilvie RI: Comparison of cardiac effects of timolol and propranolol. Clin Pharmacol Ther 19:148, 1976.
6. Mäntylä R, Männistö P, Nykänen S, et al: Pharmakokinetic interactions of timolol with vasodilating drugs, food and phenobarbitone in healthy human volunteers. Eur J Clin Pharmacol 24:227, 1983.
7. Lund-Johansen P: Hemodynamic long-term effects of timolol at rest and during exercise in essential hypertension. Acta Med Scand 199:263, 1976.
8. Pawlowski GJ: Treatment of essential hypertension with a new beta-blocking drug, timolol: Experience with a b.i.d. dosage regimen. Curr Ther Res 22:846, 1977.
9. Rofman B, Kulaga S, Gabriel M, et al: Multiclinic evaluation of timolol in the treatment of mild-to-moderate essential hypertension. Hypertension 2:643, 1980.
10. Ezri MD, Marchlinski FE, Buxton AE, et al: Electrophysiologic effects of intravenous timolol. Int J Cardiol 3:329, 1983.
11. Aronow WS, Turbow M, Van Camp S, et al: The effect of timolol vs placebo on angina pectoris. Circulation 61:66, 1980.
12. The Norwegian Multicenter Study Group: Timolol-induced reduction in mortality and reinfarction in patients surviving acute myocardial infarction. N Engl J Med 304:801, 1981.
13. The International Collaborative Study Group: Reduction of infarct size with the early use of timolol in acute myocardial infarction. N Engl J Med 310:9, 1984.
14. Sweany AE, Moncloa F, Vickers FF, et al: Antiarrhythmic effect of intravenous timolol in supraventricular arrhythmias. Clin Pharmacol Ther 37:124, 1985.
15. Ribeiro LGT, Price BA, Pool PE, et al: Efficacy of timolol in the treatment of malignant ventricular arrhythmias. Clin Res 32:681A, 1984.
16. Pedersen TR: A multicenter study on timolol in secondary prevention after myocardial infarction. Acta Med Scand Suppl 674:1, 1983.
17. Anderson JL, Rodier HE, Green LS: Comparative effects of beta-adrenergic blocking drugs on experimental ventricular fibrillation threshold. Am J Cardiol 51:1196, 1983.
18. Reid JL, Whyte KF, Struthers AD: Epinephrine-induced hypokalemia: The role of beta adrenoceptors. Am J Cardiol 57:23f, 1986.
19. Nordrehaug JE, Johannnessen K-A, von der Lippe G, et al:

Effect of timolol on changes in serum potassium concentration during acute myocardial infarction. Br Heart J 53:388, 1985.

20. Gundersen T, Kjekshus J, Stokke O, et al: Timolol maleate and HDL cholesterol after myocardial infarction. Eur Heart J 6:840, 1985.

21. Pedersen TR: Six-year follow-up of the Norwegian Multicenter Study on Timolol after Myocardial Infarction. N Engl J Med 313:1055, 1985.

22. Gundersen T, Kjekshus J: Timolol treatment after myocardial infarction in diabetic patients. Diabetes Care 6:285, 1983.

23. Frishman WH: Atenolol and timolol, two new systemic β-adrenoceptor antagonists. N Engl J Med 306:1456, 1982.

CHAPTER 52

Acebutolol

Aram V. Chobanian, M.D.

Acebutolol is a β-adrenergic receptor antagonist that is approved in the United States for the treatment of hypertension and of ventricular arrhythmias. It is cardioselective and causes only partial inhibition of the β2-receptor. Furthermore, it has intrinsic sympathomimetic activity (ISA), with both partial agonist and antagonist effects.

CHEMICAL STRUCTURE AND METABOLISM

Acebutolol is a derivative of isopropylaminopropane and, as such, is structurally similar to many other β-blockers. In humans, it is converted primarily to acetolol, which is then converted to diacetolol. Diacetolol is the major product of acebutolol metabolism and is probably responsible for many of the effects associated with acebutolol administration.[1]

Acebutolol undergoes a "first-pass effect," as has been observed with propranolol and certain other β-blockers.[2] Most of the drug is absorbed after oral administration,[3] and the major portion of absorbed drug probably reaches the systemic circulation. Both acebutolol and diacetolol are removed primarily by excretion in urine and feces.[4] Little conjugation to sulfate and glucuronide derivatives occurs, and excretion occurs primarily as free acebutolol or diacetolol.[5] Acebutolol is secreted into bile and has an enterohepatic circulation.

PHARMACOKINETICS

Following an oral dose of acebutolol, peak plasma levels of acebutolol are achieved within 3 hours, and peak plasma levels of its diacetolol metabolite are achieved within 4 hours. Absorption from the gastrointestinal tract does not appear to be influenced by food.[6] The plasma disappearance of acebutolol is more rapid than that of diacetolol[7] (Fig. 52–1). This difference appears to be related at least in part to continued conversion of the parent drug to its metabolite. The plasma half-life of acebutolol is relatively similar to that of propranolol or metoprolol[7–9] and shorter than that of nadolol or atenolol.[10, 11] However, the β-blockade lasts longer than the half-life of acebu-

tolol would suggest because of the more prolonged half-life of diacetolol.

With chronic administration of acebutolol in clinically relevant doses, the plasma levels of diacetolol are usually more than double those of unchanged acebutolol.[2] The presence of hepatic disease does not appreciably alter the pharmacokinetics of either acebutolol or diacetolol.[7] In patients with renal failure, diacetolol clearance may be decreased and its blood levels increased.[12] However, the disposition of acebutolol usually is only minimally affected. Reduction of drug dosage is generally unnecessary in patients with either severe renal or hepatic failure. Both acebutolol and diacetolol are removed during hemodialysis.

One study on the effects of age on acebutolol pharmacokinetics suggested that acebutolol achieves higher blood levels and slower rates of clearance in elderly than in younger subjects.[13] However, a subsequent investigation failed to demonstrate significant differences between young and old subjects.[14]

Only 10% to 20% of acebutolol is bound to plasma proteins,[15] and few drug interactions have been observed with it. It appears that acebutolol does not affect the pharmacokinetics of warfarin, digoxin, orally administered contraceptive drugs, hydrochlorothiazide, and hydralazine.[6, 16, 17]

PHARMACOLOGIC PROPERTIES
β1-Receptor Selectivity

Experimental studies involving blockade of vasodilator or bronchodilator responses to isoproterenol have

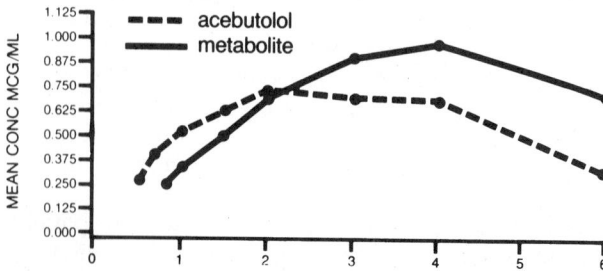

Figure 52–1. Plasma concentration-time curves of acebutolol and its metabolite, diacetolol, after a single 400-mg dose of acebutolol. MCG, micrograms. (From Ryan JR: Clinical pharmacology of acebutolol. Am Heart J 109:1131, 1985.)

demonstrated relative β1-selectivity or cardiac selectivity with both acebutolol and diacetolol.[18, 19] In patients with reversible obstructive pulmonary disease, acebutolol has less potential for inducing bronchoconstriction and less inhibitory effect on β2-stimulated bronchodilation than nonselective β-blockers.[20, 21] The degree of β1-selectivity at clinically effective doses of acebutolol appears to be similar to that observed with both atenolol and metoprolol. However, with all three drugs, such selectivity is usually decreased when large doses are used.

β-Blockers may inhibit the rate of recovery of insulin-induced hypoglycemia in insulin-treated diabetes, an effect mediated through inhibition of the β2-receptor. This problem is lessened with β1-selective agents such as acebutolol compared with their nonselective counterparts.[22]

Intrinsic Sympathomimetic Activity (ISA)

Acebutolol not only combines with and inhibits β-adrenoreceptors, but it also stimulates the activation site of the receptor. All currently available β-antagonists have chemical structures similar to that of isoproterenol, and those with associated agonistic properties share with isoproterenol the hydroxyl groups in positions 3 and 4 of the aromatic ring. Acebutolol is somewhat weaker than pindolol in ISA properties.

Several pharmacologic effects have been attributed to the effects of acebutolol as a partial agonist. Despite β-blockade, resting heart rate is reduced much less than with β-blockers lacking ISA.[23] Stroke volume and cardiac output are similarly less affected by acebutolol than by drugs such as propranolol.[24] This feature is clearly related to the ISA effects of acebutolol and not to its cardioselective action. In patients with impaired cardiac function, acebutolol and other β-blockers with ISA have been shown acutely to produce less depression of left ventricular performance when compared with propranolol and other nonselective agents.[25, 26] The clinical importance of these observations is still unclear.

When given acutely, acebutolol may increase total peripheral resistance somewhat, but on a chronic basis no reduction is apparent.[27] Some published data have suggested that β-antagonists with ISA or β1-selectivity produce fewer problems than nonselective β-antagonists in patients with Raynaud's phenomenon or peripheral vascular insufficiency secondary to arteriosclerosis obliterans. However, not all studies have supported these conclusions, and the clinical significance of these findings remains uncertain.

Membrane-Stabilizing Effects and Electrophysiologic Properties

As with some other β-blockers, acebutolol's membrane-stabilizing effect resembles that of quinidine or of local anesthetics. However, membrane stabilization generally does not occur with β-blockers unless very high blood levels are achieved. Such an effect is prob-

ably of little clinical importance. Acebutolol does have a relatively potent quinidine-like action on cardiac conduction.[28] Multicenter controlled trials have compared the effects of acebutolol, propranolol, quinidine, and placebo in patients with multiple premature ventricular contractions.[29] Acebutolol was found to be effective as an antiarrhythmic agent (Fig. 52–2) with potential comparable to that of propranolol or quinidine.[29] Therefore, it can be a useful antiarrhythmic drug.

ANTIHYPERTENSIVE ACTIONS

A wide variety of clinical studies have demonstrated the effectiveness of acebutolol as an antihypertensive agent. In a large, double-blind, multicenter study involving patients with mild and moderate hypertension, acebutolol induced a significant reduction in blood pressure, averaging 15.9/14.9 mmHg. This reduction was comparable with that achieved with hydrochlorothiazide.[30] The mean dose used in this study was 757 mg daily of acebutolol and 68 mg daily of hydrochlorothiazide. The drug appears to be effective in various hypertensive subgroups, including the elderly;[31] in one large study, it was found to be as potent as hydrochlorothiazide in elderly patients.[32] However, like other β-antagonists lacking α-blocking properties,[33] acebutolol appears to be less effective in black patients than in white patients.

The antihypertensive effect of acebutolol appears to be comparable with that of other β-blockers.[34, 35] The reasons that β-blockers lower blood pressure are not well-understood. Explanations have included suppression of renal renin release and reduction of angiotensin levels, cardiodepression or other inhibitory action on postsynaptic β-receptors, central nervous system effects, and inhibition of presynaptic β-receptors. Acebutolol and other β-blockers with ISA properties differ from other β-blockers with respect to cardiodepressant action, ability to suppress plasma renin, and effects on β-receptor density.[36, 37] Further-

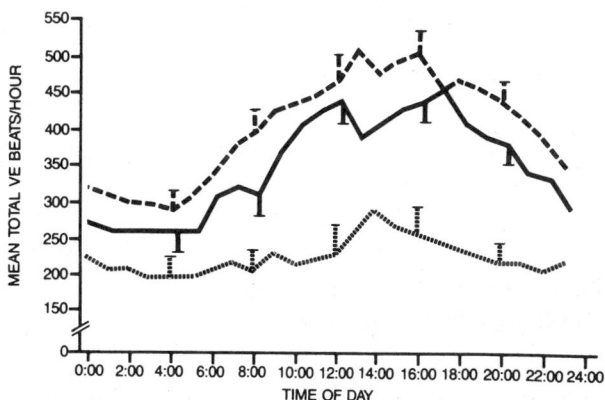

Figure 52–2. Diurnal variation of mean total ventricular contractions per hour (mean ± SEM) at baseline (---), during placebo administration (—), and with acebutolol (···). VE, ventricular ectopic. (From Chandraratna PAN: Comparison of acebutolol with propranolol, quinidine, and placebo: Results of three multicenter arrhythmia trials. Am Heart J 109:1198, 1985.)

more, wide differences in solubility and ability to penetrate into the brain have raised questions as to whether β-blockers have any primary effect on central nervous system function. Thus, the action of β-blockers remains unknown.

Many studies have compared the effects of acebutolol with the effects of other types of antihypertensive drugs. The best study in this regard, the Treatment of Mild Hypertension Study (TOMHS), involved a comparison of acebutolol, enalapril, chlorthalidone, amilodipine, and doxazosin, as well as placebo.[38] Nutritional-hygienic lifestyle intervention was instituted in all patient groups as well. The blood pressure effects of acebutolol were clearly comparable with those of the other drugs.

Acebutolol adds to the antihypertensive effects of other drugs with different mechanisms of action. Studies have shown excellent blood pressure responses to acebutolol combined with nifedipine,[39] captopril,[40] clonidine,[41] or diuretics.[42]

DOSAGES OF ACEBUTOLOL IN HYPERTENSION

The smallest effective dose of acebutolol in adults is approximately 200 mg daily, and the average dose when used alone is 200 to 400 mg daily. In hypertension, once-daily administration is generally adequate for blood pressure control.[43] The half-life of acebutolol is relatively brief, but the half-life of the active metabolite diacetolol is prolonged.

EFFECTS IN SPECIAL HYPERTENSIVE POPULATIONS
Diabetic Patients

Acebutolol is effective in diabetic patients with hypertension and does not appear to influence diabetic control significantly.[44] However, in nondiabetic patients, acebutolol has been shown to inhibit glucose tolerance following an acute glucose load but does not affect the changes in plasma insulin.[45] Acebutolol should be used cautiously in insulin-treated diabetic patients because of its potential effect of delaying the rate of recovery of blood glucose during hypoglycemic episodes. However, because this action is mediated primarily via β2-receptor inhibition, acebutolol and other cardioselective β-blockers are less of a problem than nonselective β-antagonists.

Patients with Peripheral Vascular Insufficiency

All β-blockers may induce adverse effects in patients with peripheral arterial insufficiency and should be used with caution in them. A study in hypertensive patients with intermittent claudication showed no significant reductions in ankle blood pressure or in maximum walking and claudication distances with acebutolol therapy.[46] The benefits of partial agonistic ac-

tivity or of cardioselectivity in the treatment of such patients have not been established conclusively.

Patients with Left Ventricular Hypertrophy

In hypertensive patients, acebutolol may have a beneficial action on the regression of cardiac hypertrophy. Hypertensive patients treated with acebutolol for 6 to 12 months experienced significant decreases in left ventricular mass and posterior wall and ventricular septal thickness as determined by echocardiography.[47]

Patients with Left Ventricular Dysfunction

Although β-blockers may induce congestive heart failure, reports suggest that a subgroup of patients with left ventricular failure are candidates for β-blocker therapy. Much of the work supporting the latter approach has utilized metoprolol, which, like acebutolol, has β1-receptor selectivity. This field continues to evolve rapidly, and the value of either acebutolol or other β-blockers in such patients requires further delineation.

Patients with Angina Pectoris

Acebutolol is an effective antianginal drug,[48] even when administered once daily.[49] Acebutolol induces reductions in blood pressure and heart rate both at rest and following exercise, although the decreases in resting heart rate are not as great as with propranolol and other β-blockers lacking ISA. Left ventricular function is maintained in patients with coronary disease treated with acebutolol.[26] A major concern regarding β-blockers with ISA properties has been their effects in the secondary prevention of myocardial infarction. Prior studies with oxyprenolol and pendolol failed to demonstrate reduced mortality following myocardial infarction.[50, 51] However, a more recent controlled trial of acebutolol in patients with a history of myocardial infarction showed a 48% reduction in total mortality.[52] Thus, acebutolol may provide secondary protection of myocardial infarction despite its ISA properties.

Patients with Hypertension in Pregnancy

Limited information is available regarding the use of acebutolol in pregnant patients. One study comparing acebutolol with methyldopa in 20 hypertensive pregnant patients revealed no major problems with acebutolol therapy.[53] Both acebutolol and diacetolol are present in much higher concentrations in milk than in plasma in lactating mothers and therefore represent potential risks to breastfed infants.[54]

ADVERSE EFFECTS

As with all β-adrenoreceptor antagonists, acebutolol may cause such problems as bronchoconstriction, bradyarrhythmias, left ventricular dysfunction, central nervous system side effects, coolness of the extremities, sexual dysfunction, and excessive fatigue. Some potential advantages attributed to β_1-selectivity and ISA have already been discussed. Acebutolol is less lipophilic than propranolol and metoprolol, but the lipophilicity of β-blockers has not been clearly associated with clinically significant central nervous system side effects.

Acebutolol and other cardioselective β-blockers have potential advantages over nonselective agents with respect to metabolic effects during exercise. The nonselective agents appear to cause more severe exercise-induced hypoglycemia, which might be of clinical importance in selected patients.[55]

Antinuclear antibody tests might yield positive results in a small percentage of patients treated with acebutolol. However, no clinical consequence of this serologic abnormality has been reported.

EFFECTS ON PLASMA LIPIDS AND LIPOPROTEINS

Some β-blockers have been shown to affect adversely plasma lipids and lipoproteins. Drugs such as propranolol, metoprolol, nadolol, and atenolol increase plasma triglycerides and very-low-density lipoproteins and reduce high-density lipoproteins. On the other hand, acebutolol is relatively free of such adverse effects, presumably because of its ISA property. In the TOMHS study, acebutolol produced no adverse effects on serum lipids and lipoproteins as compared with placebo.[38] In fact, low-density lipoprotein cholesterol levels were significantly lower in the acebutolol group than in the placebo group.

SUMMARY AND CONCLUSIONS

Acebutolol is a β-adrenergic antagonist with β-cardioselective and partial agonistic activities. It is converted primarily to diacetolol, an active metabolite, and undergoes a prominent "first-pass" effect in the liver. Both acebutolol and diacetolol are eliminated primarily by urinary excretion.

Acebutolol is an effective antihypertensive drug when used either alone or in combination with other blood pressure–lowering medications. It also has potent antianginal effects and may provide secondary prevention against myocardial infarction. Furthermore, acebutolol has quinidine-like antiarrhythmic action and may be useful in some patients with ventricular arrhythmias. The duration of the effect of acebutolol is such that once-daily administration is usually adequate for the treatment of most hypertensive and anginal patients. However, twice-daily dosing is required for antiarrhythmic therapy.

The cardioselective properties of acebutolol exist primarily at relatively low doses. The clinical benefits of cardioselectivity are limited to somewhat less bronchoconstriction and less prolongation of insulin-induced hypoglycemia than are caused by nonselective β-blockers.

Because of its partial agonistic effects, acebutolol induces less slowing of resting heart rate and somewhat less depression of left ventricular function compared with β-blockers lacking ISA. Acebutolol does not adversely affect plasma lipids and lipoproteins.

REFERENCES

1. Thibonnier M, Flabeau C, Thouvenin M, et al: Antihypertensive effect of diacetolol in essential hypertension. Br J Clin Pharmacol 13:533, 1982.
2. Winkle RA, Meffin PJ, Ricks WB, Harrison DC: Acebutolol metabolite plasma concentration during chronic oral therapy. Br J Clin Pharmacol 4:519, 1977.
3. Kaye CM, Kumana CR, Leighton M, et al: Observations on the pharmacokinetics of acebutolol. Clin Pharmacol Ther 19:416, 1976.
4. Gabriel R, Kaye CM, Sankey MG: Preliminary observations on the excretion of acebutolol and its acetyl metabolite in the urine and feces of man. J Pharm Pharmacol 33:386, 1981.
5. Gulaid AA, James IM, Kaye CM, et al: The pharmacokinetics of acebutolol in man, following the oral administration of acebutolol HCl as a single dose (400 mg), and during and after repeated oral dosing (400 mg, b.i.d.). Biopharm Drug Dispos 2:103, 1981.
6. Ryan JR: Clinical pharmacology of acebutolol. Am Heart J 109:1131, 1985.
7. DeBono G, Kaye CM, Roland E, Summers AJ: Acebutolol: Ten years of experience. Am Heart J 109:1211, 1985.
8. Gomeri R, et al: Pharmacokinetics of propranolol in normal healthy volunteers. J Pharmacokinet Biopharm 5:183, 1977.
9. Regardh CG, Borg KO, Johansson R, et al: Pharmacokinetic studies on the selective beta1-receptor antagonist metoprolol in man. J Pharmacokinet Biopharm 2:347, 1974.
10. Dreyfuss J, Griffith DL, Singhvi SM: Pharmacokinetics of nadolol, a β-receptor antagonist: Administration of therapeutic single- and multiple-dosage regimens to hypertensive patients. J Clin Pharmacol 19:712, 1979.
11. Mason WD, Winer N, Kochak G, et al: Kinetics and absolute bioavailability of atenolol. Clin Pharmacol Ther 25:408, 1979.
12. Smith RS, Warren DJ, Renwick AG, George CF: Acebutolol pharmacokinetics in renal disease. Br J Clin Pharmacol 16:253, 1983.
13. Roux A, Henry JF, Fouache Y, et al: A pharmacokinetic study of acebutolol in aged subjects as compared to young subjects. Gerontology 29:202, 1983.
14. Vincon G, Albin H, Demotes MF, et al: Influence of age on the pharmacokinetics of acebutolol. J Pharmacol (Paris) 15:123, 1984.
15. Coombs TJ, Coulson CJ, Smith VJ: Blood plasma binding of acebutolol and diacetolol in man. Br J Pharmacol 9:395, 1980.
16. Roux A, Le Liboux A, Delhotal B, et al: Pharmacokinetics in man of acebutolol and hydrochlorothiazide as simple agents and in combination. Eur J Clin Pharmacol 24:801, 1983.
17. Jack DB, Kendall MJ, Dean S, et al: The effect of hydralazine on the pharmacokinetics of three different beta adrenoceptor antagonists: Metoprolol, nadolol, and acebutolol. Biopharm Drug Dispos 3:47, 1982.
18. Basil B, Jordan R, Loveless AH, et al: β-Adrenoceptor blocking properties and cardioselectivity of M & B 17,803A. Br J Pharmacol 48:198, 1973.
19. Daly MJ, Flook JJ, Levy GP: The selectivity of β-adrenoceptor antagonists on cardiovascular and bronchodilator responses to isoprenaline in the anesthetized dog. Br J Pharmacol 53:173, 1975.
20. Decalmer PB, Chatterjee SS, Cruickshank JM, et al: Beta-blockers and asthma. Br Heart J 40:184, 1978.
21. Greefhorst APM, van Heerwaarden CLA: Comparative study of the ventilatory effects of three beta-1-selective blocking agents in asthmatic patients. Eur J Clin Pharmacol 20:417, 1981.
22. Deacon SP, Karunanayake A, Burnett D: Acebutolol, atenolol and propranolol and metabolic responses to acute hypoglycemia in diabetics. Br Med J 2:1255, 1977.

23. Wahl J, Turlapaty P, Singh BN: Comparison of acebutolol and propranolol in essential hypertension. Am Heart J 109:313, 1985.

24. Svendsen TL, Trap-Jensen J, Carlsen JE, McNair A: Immediate central hemodynamic effects of five different beta-adrenoceptor-blocking agents, acebutolol, atenolol, pindolol, practolol, and propranolol in patients with ischemic heart disease. Am Heart J 109:1145, 1985.

25. Katz RJ, DiBianco R, Singh S, et al: Acebutolol and left ventricular function: Assessment by radionuclide angiography. Clin Pharmacol Ther 29:149, 1981.

26. Singh SN, DiBianco R, Katz RJ, et al: Effect of acebutolol on left ventricular performance. Am Heart J 109:1151, 1985.

27. Tsukiyama H, Otsuka K, Higuma K: Effects of β-adrenoceptor antagonists on central hemodynamics in essential hypertension. Br J Clin Pharmacol 13(Suppl):269, 1982.

28. Mason JW, Winkle RA, Meffin PJ, Harrison DC: Electrophysiological effects of acebutolol. Br Heart J 40:35, 1978.

29. Chandraratna PAN: Comparison of acebutolol with propranolol, quinidine, and placebo: Results of three multicenter arrhythmia trials. Am Heart J 109:1198, 1985.

30. Wahl J, Singh BN, Thoden WR: Comparative hypotensive effects of acebutolol and hydrochlorothiazide in patients with mild to moderate hypertension: A double-blind multicenter evaluation. Am Heart J 111:353, 1986.

31. Boyles PW: Effects of age and race on clinical response to acebutolol in essential hypertension. Am Heart J 109:1184, 1985.

32. Salvetti A, Lucchini M, Airoldi G, et al: Multicentre comparison of the antihypertensive effect of acebutolol and hydrochlorothiazide in uncomplicated mild-moderate hypertension in the elderly. Eur J Clin Pharmacol 29:275, 1985.

33. Veterans Administration Cooperative Study Group on Antihypertensive Agents: Comparison of propranolol and hydrochlorothiazide for the initial treatment of hypertension. JAMA 248:2004, 1982.

34. Turner AS, Brocklehurst JC: Once-daily acebutolol and atenolol in essential hypertension: Double-blind crossover comparison. Am Heart J 109:1178, 1985.

35. Abengowe CU: A double-blind comparison of acebutolol (Sectral) and propranolol (Inderal) in the treatment of hypertension in black Nigerian patients. J Int Med Res 13:116, 1985.

36. Man in't Veld AJ, Schalekamp MA: Hemodynamic consequences of intrinsic sympathomimetic activity in relation to changes in plasma renin activity and noradrenaline during beta-blocker therapy for hypertension. Postgrad Med J 59(Suppl 3):140, 1983.

37. Basso A, Piantelli L, Cognini G, et al: Acebutolol-induced decrease of mononuclear leukocyte beta-adrenoceptors in hypertension. Pharmacology 31:278, 1985.

38. The Treatment of Mild Hypertension Research Group. The treatment of mild hypertension study. Arch Intern Med 151:1413, 1991.

39. Lejeune P, Gunselmann W, Hoppe I, et al: Effects of a fixed combination of low-dose nifedipine and acebutolol on essential hypertension: Comparison with standard dose of acebutolol. Clin Exp Hypertens 7:1541, 1985.

40. DeDivitiis O, Petitto M, Di Somma S, et al: Therapeutic approach to arterial hypertension: Comparison and combination of acebutolol with nifedipine and captopril. Cardiologia 30:469, 1985.

41. Plouin PF, Degoulet P, Fermé I, et al: Clonidine, acebutolol and their interaction in essential hypertension: Effects on blood pressure and the control of water and electrolyte balance. Eur Heart J 4(Suppl G):7, 1983.

42. Gorkin JU, Elijovich F, Dziedzic SW, Krakoff LR: Addition of acebutolol to diuretics in hypertension. Clin Pharmacol Ther 30:739, 1981.

43. Weber MA, Drayer JI: Once-daily administration of acebutolol in treatment of hypertension. Am Heart J 109:1175, 1985.

44. Fraser DM, Nimmo GR, Poloniecki JD: Acebutolol in the treatment of diabetic patients with hypertension. Curr Med Res Opin 10:122, 1986.

45. Lehtonen A: The effect of acebutolol on plasma lipids, blood glucose and serum insulin levels. Acta Med Scand 216:57, 1984.

46. Svendsen TL, Jelnes R, Tønnesen KH: The effects of acebutolol and metoprolol on walking distances and distal blood pressure in hypertensive patients with intermittent claudication. Acta Med Scand 219:161, 1986.

47. Trimarco B, Ricciardelli B, De Luca N, et al: Effect of acebutolol on left ventricular hemodynamics and anatomy in systemic hypertension. Am J Cardiol 53:791, 1984.

48. DiBianco R, Singh S, Singh JB, et al: Effects of acebutolol on chronic stable angina pectoris: A placebo-controlled, double-blind, randomized crossover study. Circulation 62:1179, 1980.

49. Pina IL, Smith EV, Weidler DJ: Low-dose acebutolol given once daily in the treatment of chronic angina pectoris. J Clin Pharmacol 28:427, 1988.

50. The European Infarction Study Group (EIS): A secondary prevention study with slow release oxyprenolol after myocardial infarction: Morbidity and mortality. Eur Heart J 5:189, 1984.

51. Australian and Swedish Pindolol Study Group: The effects of pindolol on the two years mortality after complicated myocardial infarction. Eur Heart J 4:367, 1983.

52. Boissel J-P, Leizorovicz A, Picolet H, Peyrieux J-P: Secondary prevention after high-risk acute myocardial infarction with low-dose acebutolol. Am J Cardiol 66:251, 1990.

53. Williams ER, Morrissey JR: A comparison of acebutolol with methyldopa in hypertensive pregnancy. Pharmatherapeutica 3:487, 1983.

54. Boutroy MJ, Bianchetti G, Dubruc C, et al: To nurse when receiving acebutolol: Is it dangerous for the neonate? Eur J Clin Pharmacol 30:737, 1989.

55. Koch G, Franz IW, Gubba A, Lohmann FW: Beta-adrenoceptor blockade and physical activity: Cardiovascular and metabolic aspects. Acta Med Scand Suppl 672:55, 1983.

CHAPTER 53

Nadolol

Michael H. Crawford, M.D.

HISTORY

Nadolol (SQ 11725) was developed in 1973 in the United States at the Squibb Institute for Medical Research. It was discovered as part of a search for β-adrenergic blocking agents with more selectivity or greater safety than propranolol.[1] It was initially considered a potential antiarrhythmic agent; however, it received United States Food and Drug Administration approval for the treatment of angina and hypertension under the trade name of Corgard in 1979.[2] It was the third orally administered β-blocker approved for use in hypertension (after propranolol and metoprolol) and the second to be approved for angina pectoris.

CHEMISTRY

Although all currently established β-blocking drugs share some structural features, they can roughly be divided into two basic structural types: A secondary amino group adjacent to an alcohol group on a two-carbon chain attached to either an aryl group or an aryloxymethylene group. Nadolol—2,3,-cis-1,2,3,4-tetrahydro-5-[om17.2][2-hydroxy-3-(tert-butylamino)propoxy]-2,3-naphthalenediol—falls into the latter group and is related structurally to propranolol.

PHARMACOLOGY

Nadolol is a nonselective β-blocker that possesses no intrinsic sympathomimetic activity and no membrane-stabilizing activity.[3] Its lipid solubility is low, second only to atenolol.[4] Its dose-ratio potency relative to propranolol (1.0) is 0.2 intravenously and 0.8 orally.[5, 6]

PHARMACOKINETICS

After oral administration, approximately 30% of the dose of nadolol is absorbed, and maximum concentrations in the plasma are achieved after 1 to 4 hours. Approximately 20% of the absorbed dose is bound to plasma proteins. Nadolol is excreted 70% unchanged in the feces because of the relatively low absorption, although there is probably some enterohepatic circulation. Twenty percent of the total dose, or two thirds of what has been absorbed, is excreted unchanged in the urine. The terminal elimination half-life of nadolol is 14 to 17 hours, with a total body clearance of 157 ml/min.[7] The half-life is shorter in children: 4 hours in those younger than 22 months, 7 to 16 hours in older children.[8]

Nadolol follows linear kinetics after a single dose of up to 80 mg, which corresponds most closely to an open two-compartment model. After multiple doses, plasma concentrations increase by a factor of 2.5, which suggests nonlinearity at steady state.[9] Nadolol is widely distributed to body tissues with an apparent volume of distribution of 2 L.[10] There is little liver metabolism, but renal failure does impair excretion of the drug and must be considered in dosing. Despite this dependence on renal clearance, no adjustment for the age of the patient seems to be necessary.

EFFECTS ON PATHOPHYSIOLOGY
Hemodynamics

After either intravenous or oral administration, the major hemodynamic effect of nadolol is a decrease in sinus node frequency, which results in a reduced heart rate. Heart rate reductions are greater during maximum exercise (between 15% and 20%) than at rest (between 6% and 8%).[5, 11] The reduced heart rate results in a concomitant decrease in cardiac output.[12]

Ventricular Function

Animal studies have suggested that nadolol has less myocardial contractility depressant activity than propranolol and other β-blockers.[1] However, in normal persons after an acute intravenous bolus of nadolol, reductions in stroke-work index, ejection fraction, rate of rise in left ventricular pressure (dP/dt), and V_{max} have been observed.[13] Usually, there is no net change in left ventricular end-diastolic pressure in normal individuals. On the other hand, patients with depressed left ventricular function at baseline may show an increase in pulmonary capillary wedge pressure after the intravenous administration of nadolol. LeWinter et al.[5] compared intravenous nadolol with propranolol in equipotent blocking doses in 10 subjects with ischemic heart disease. Both drugs produced similar decreases in heart rate and left ventricular ejection fraction and increases in mean pulmonary artery wedge pressure. There were no statistically significant differences between the two drugs with respect to their effect on any of the variables measured.

Electrophysiology

Nadolol decreases sinoatrial impulse formation but does not impair atrial conduction or that of accessory pathways.[14] Atrioventricular nodal effective and functional refractory periods are increased.[15] Nadolol also decreases the diastolic depolarization rate of ectopic pacemakers and can decrease ventricular arrhythmias by this mechanism. In addition, nadolol effectively suppresses rate-dependent ventricular tachycardias caused by catecholamine-sensitive automaticity or other trigger mechanisms.[16] Finally, it decreases the electrical instability associated with prolongation of the QT interval. These antiarrhythmic effects of nadolol are common to all β-blockers except for sotalol, which has class III antiarrhythmic activity.[17]

Coronary Blood Flow

The effect of nadolol on coronary blood flow is similar to that of other β-blocking agents. It produces a decrease in resting coronary blood flow that is proportional to the decrease in myocardial oxygen demand produced mainly by a decrease in heart rate.[18]

Arteries and Veins

Because nadolol is a nonselective β-blocker, the β_2 vasodilator stimulation of the peripheral arteries is blocked, resulting in a slight increase in systemic vascular resistance.[1] This effect is rarely associated with a change in mean arterial pressure in normal individuals. Furthermore, pulmonary vascular resistance is increased slightly, and significant increases in pulmonary artery pressure have been observed following intravenous nadolol administration.[5]

Fluid Volume State and Electrolytes

Acute nadolol administration can produce a mild increase in plasma volume similar to that noted with propranolol. However, long-term monotherapy with β-blockers is not associated with increased plasma volume.[19] Unlike the β_1-selective blockers, nadolol prevents the epinephrine-induced decrease in serum potassium level.[20] The potassium-lowering effect of epinephrine is caused by β_2-stimulation, which is blocked by all nonselective β-blockers. Whether this is of any clinical benefit during periods of stress, when epinephrine levels increase, has not been proved. However, β_2-blockade is a theoretic advantage of nonselective blockers such as nadolol in patients with ischemic heart disease.

Endocrine System and Metabolism

Nadolol, like all β-blockers, antagonizes the effect of thyroxin, which is in part mediated by β-adrenergic stimulation.[21] Nadolol has no effect on hepatic function despite the fact that the reduction in cardiac output leads to a reduction in hepatic blood flow. During nadolol treatment of hyperthyroidism, increases in plasma cholesterol and triglycerides have been reported.[22]

Nadolol affects plasma lipoprotein levels like other β-blockers do. In one study, there was a mild increase in total serum cholesterol and a 29% increase in very-low-density lipoprotein cholesterol. Also, decreases were noted in triglyceride levels, low-density lipoprotein cholesterol levels, and high-density lipoprotein cholesterol levels. The increase in very-low-density lipoprotein cholesterol was statistically significant, but none of the other effects were.[22] In one report on nadolol, increased triglyceride levels resulted in pancreatitis.[24] Whether these changes in lipoprotein levels are important clinically remains to be proved.

Renal Function

One of the unique properties of nadolol is that, unlike other β-blockers, it preserves renal blood flow.[12] Textor et al.[25] studied 15 hypertensive subjects with normal glomerular filtration rates by oral administration of nadolol. Blood pressure and cardiac index decreased significantly, and total peripheral resistance increased. However, renal blood flow and glomerular filtration rate were maintained rather than decreased, as is seen with other β-blockers. Also, the fraction of renal blood flow over cardiac output increased, indicating a redistribution of a lower cardiac output to the kidneys. These data suggest that nadolol has a direct renal vasodilator effect. Results of studies in patients with mild renal impairment have been similar.[26, 27] Thus, mild renal failure in patients with hypertension is not a contraindication to nadolol therapy.

Central Nervous System

Nadolol does not cross the blood-brain barrier well because of its low lipid solubility.[22] Hence, central nervous system β-blocker effects are seen less often with nadolol. Nadolol is useful for blocking peripheral sympathetic effects, because it is somewhat more potent per milligram than propranolol as a nonselective β-adrenergic blocker.

CLINICAL USE
Indications

Hypertension

Nadolol is an effective antihypertensive agent for patients with mild to moderate essential hypertension. Like other β-blockers, the exact mechanism of action is unknown but is unlikely to be related to changes in vascular tone, because β-blockers produce mild increases in systemic vascular resistance. Some of the antihypertensive effect is undoubtedly related to a decrease in cardiac output, and, in some patients, there may be effects on renal renin release.

Oral nadolol administration can be expected to decrease the diastolic blood pressure approximately 10%, systolic blood pressure approximately 15%, and mean arterial pressure approximately 18% in patients with hypertension.[29] It is equally effective on supine or upright measurements. Postural hypotension is unusual. The long half-life of nadolol results in little difference between peak and trough serum levels and provides uniform blood pressure control for 24 hours.[30] Like all β-blockers, nadolol is more efficient when it is combined with a thiazide diuretic. In a Veterans Administration Cooperative Study,[31] nadolol monotherapy reduced diastolic blood pressure below 90 mmHg in 49% of patients, compared with 46% who responded to thiazide diuretic alone. Combination therapy was successful in 85%. Like other β-blockers, nadolol was less effective in black patients than in white patients in this study. However, a study of 21 Nigerian patients with hypertension showed a better than 90% success rate for treatment with nadolol.[32] Nadolol is equally effective in young and old patients,[33] and no tolerance to the effects of nadolol has been observed in studies in which it remained effective for up to 2 years.[19]

Angina Pectoris

Studies have demonstrated that nadolol is highly efficacious versus placebo in the treatment of chronic stable angina pectoris.[3] Like other β-blockers, the mechanism of action is mainly related to a decrease in myocardial oxygen demand, especially with exertion or other stresses. Because of its long half-life, nadolol was administered once daily (compared with propranolol, which was given four times a day) and was efficacious in several studies.[18, 34–36] In addition, studies comparing once-daily nadolol to once-daily conventional and long-acting preparations of propranolol, oxprenolol, pindolol, and atenolol found nadolol superior for controlling angina and exercise heart rate.[37, 38] In comparative studies with calcium antagonists, nadolol has shown efficacy equal to that of monotherapy.[39, 40] In addition, it is useful in combination with nitrates or calcium antagonists.[41, 42] Nadolol has been efficacious for long-term therapy in angina pectoris; no tolerance has been observed in studies lasting for 3 years or more. It is also quite effective in patients with angina and hypertension.[43]

Nadolol has not been used extensively in hospitalized patients with unstable angina pectoris, because it is generally believed that a short-acting β-blocker is better in this situation. If the patient develops myocardial infarction or heart failure or needs emergency surgery, the effects of the shorter-acting agents dissipate more quickly. However, in the long-term management of a patient whose condition has been stabilized with medical therapy, nadolol could be substituted for shorter-acting β-blockers to provide a more convenient method of β-blocker administration for the long-term control of angina pectoris.

Arrhythmias

Although nadolol was first developed as a potentially unique β-blocker antiarrhythmic drug, its clinical efficacy with arrhythmias is not different from that of other β-blockers.[44] It has been shown to be useful for the prevention of supraventricular tachycardia in adults and children and to control the heart rate of patients with chronic atrial tachyarrhythmias.[45–47] Nadolol has also been shown to be useful for treating certain ventricular arrhythmias, especially those associated with acute ischemia.[48, 49] It has been demonstrated in a dog model to prevent ventricular tachycardia induced by coronary artery ligation.[2, 16] In addition, it appears that nadolol is effective in decreasing the frequency of premature ventricular contractions in doses as low as 20 mg/day or less.[50] However, in patients with ejection fractions of less than 40%, it is less effective for controlling ventricular tachycardia.[51, 52]

Other Indications

Nadolol, like other nonselective β-blockers, is quite effective in controlling anxiety-related and essential tremor.[53–56] Nadolol also has been shown to be useful for control of certain migraine headaches and has been used successfully to control sympathetic overactivity associated with hyperthyroidism.[21, 57, 58] In addition, nadolol has been used successfully to reduce aggressive and violent behavior in patients with chronic psychiatric disorders and in combination with psychostimulants for attention deficit hyperactivity disorder.[59–61]

Nadolol has been used to control portal pressure in patients with hepatic cirrhosis and esophageal varices because of its ability to lower hepatic blood flow.[62] In a randomized, placebo-controlled trial of 589 patients with cirrhosis and esophageal varices, nadolol effectively prevented the first episode of bleeding and reduced mortality associated with gastrointestinal bleeding.[63] Whether nadolol would be useful prophylactically following myocardial infarction has not

been tested. However, other nonselective β-blockers have been found useful in this regard, and in animal models,[64, 65] nadolol's myocardial preservation properties have been comparable with those of other β-blockers. By reducing the heart rate and blood pressure response to exercise and mental stress in the morning hours, once-daily nadolol administration may favorably alter potential triggers of myocardial infarction.[66]

Precautions and Adverse Effects

Cardiovascular System

The cardiovascular adverse effects of nadolol all are related to the pharmacologic effects of β-blockers.[67] In this regard, nadolol can produce a decrease in heart rate, cardiac index, stroke work, and ejection fraction and can lead to hypotension in selected patients. By far the most common adverse cardiovascular effect is excessive bradycardia (3% incidence); rarely, susceptible individuals experience second- and third-degree heart block. Hypotension is unusual as an adverse effect (<1%) but has been reported, especially in association with severe bradycardia. Left ventricular dysfunction can occur in susceptible individuals, and congestive heart failure may result. However, heart failure rarely occurs when the usual clinical doses are used in patients with normal baseline left ventricular function. Also, there are no withdrawal β-adrenergic hypersensitivity reactions with nadolol because of its long half-life.[68] Thus, nadolol can be discontinued abruptly, unlike shorter-acting β-blockers.

Central Nervous System

The adverse central nervous system effects of other β-blockers are less common with nadolol but have been observed. These include fatigue, dizziness, lassitude, vivid dreams, insomnia, impotence, paresthesias, and irritability. Fatigue is the most common side effect, occurring in approximately 2% of patients.[3]

Gastrointestinal Side Effects

There are no unique gastrointestinal side effects of nadolol, but as with all β-blockers, there have been reported cases of gastrointestinal disturbance, such as diarrhea, nausea, vomiting, and constipation. These occur in fewer than 1% of patients.[3]

Other Adverse Effects

Other reported adverse effects have included dry mouth, dry eyes, increased sweating, and skin rash in a few patients. Also, bronchospasm and a sensation of cold extremities have occurred in a few instances.[67]

Contraindications

There are only two absolute contraindications to the use of nadolol or any β-blocker: severe bradyarrhythmias and bronchospasm. Bradyarrhythmias are a contraindication because the most prevalent adverse effect of nadolol administration is reduced heart rate. Thus, in patients who already have bradyarrhythmias, the drug is contraindicated. Also, because nadolol is a nonselective β-blocker, it does block the bronchodilatory $β_2$-receptors and can aggravate bronchospasm in susceptible individuals.

There are several relative contraindications to nadolol. The first is overt congestive heart failure. Although some might consider this an absolute contraindication, it is noteworthy that patients with heart failure have been shown in some studies to actually benefit from β-blocker administration. Whether this is due to its antiarrhythmic effects or to effects on the number of β-receptors in the myocardium is currently unclear but is undergoing further clinical investigation. Another relative contraindication is severe peripheral vascular disease and claudication. Blockade of vasodilatory $β_2$-receptor stimulation may aggravate this condition and lead to increased claudication or a feeling of cold extremities. Another relative contraindication is severe diabetes mellitus, especially if patients experience hypoglycemic episodes. Nadolol, like other nonselective β-blockers, can decrease the gluconeogenic stimulus of the sympathetic nervous system, but more important, it will impair the patient's ability to recognize hypoglycemia by blocking piloerection, tachycardia, and other sympathetic symptoms that signify that the blood sugar is falling to dangerously low levels. Nadolol is not contraindicated in most diabetics, even those who are insulin-dependent, but is contraindicated in patients with severe brittle diabetes who are subject to hypoglycemic episodes.

Interference with Other Drugs

There are no unique pharmacologic interactions with other drugs. All drug interactions involving nadolol are predictable because its pharmacologic action is that of a β-blocker. Because the major adverse effect of nadolol is slowing of the heart rate, it is predictable that in combination with drugs such as digoxin and verapamil, there would be an increased tendency toward excessive bradycardia or even heart block. Also, because nadolol is a mild cardiac depressant, it can accentuate the cardiac depressant effects of other drugs, such as disopyramide and verapamil. Although nadolol alone rarely produces hypotension unless severe bradycardia is caused, it can potentiate the hypotensive effects of other drugs such as vasodilators. Because nadolol is not metabolized in the liver, blood levels of nadolol are not affected by cimetidine or other agents that induce hepatic enzymes, such as phenobarbital.[69] Finally, nadolol does not affect theophylline metabolism in smokers.[70]

Use in Patients with Impaired Organ Function

Because nadolol is largely excreted by the kidneys, decreased renal function affects the clearance of the drug. Studies in patients with chronic renal failure who are receiving dialysis have shown that the half-life of the drug can be prolonged to 20 to 36 hours. Thus, it is feasible to give nadolol once after each dialysis and achieve a prolonged effect.[71]

Because nadolol is not metabolized by the liver, it can be given to patients with impaired liver function. Interestingly, despite the fact that nadolol reduces hepatic blood flow because of a decrease in cardiac output, there is no evidence that nadolol impairs liver function. Also, because nadolol increases blood flow to the kidney, the portohepatic gradient actually decreases, which may be important in the treatment of patients with esophageal varices.[62, 63]

Nadolol concentrates fivefold in human breast milk, which should be kept in mind when prescribing the drug to lactating women.[72]

Nadolol in the Antihypertensive Arsenal

Nadolol has the same relative place in the antihypertensive arsenal as other β-blockers. It is useful in treating mild to moderate hypertension, and its effect is potentiated by the coadministration of diuretics. Nadolol is useful when there are contraindications to other antihypertensive agents or when the patient cannot tolerate alternative agents. It is also useful in treating patients with concomitant diseases such as angina pectoris and arrhythmias, because it reduces exercise blood pressure and heart rate more effectively than angiotensin-converting enzyme inhibitors.[73] In addition, nadolol is extremely useful for patients with labile hypertension and associated anxiety states.

Nadolol has several unique advantages among the β-blockers. First, it is the only β-blocker that has a pharmacologic half-life long enough so that once-daily therapy is accomplished without major peaks and valleys in the plasma concentration. This makes for consistent blood pressure control, even in patients with labile hypertension. Second, it is unique among the β-blockers in preserving renal blood flow. Because renal function is an important determinant of prognosis in hypertensive patients, this may be an important consideration. However, there is currently little clinical evidence that this potential benefit of nadolol is of any clinical significance. Third, as a nonselective β-blocker, it does not potentiate the epinephrine-induced hypokalemia that can be seen with the selective β-blockers. Again, there is no strong evidence that this is important clinically. Finally, because of nadolol's low lipid solubility, it has fewer side effects than other β-blockers. This is important in treating hypertensive patients, because most patients with hypertension do not feel ill. Thus, motivating them to take their medication is often difficult, and compliance can be a problem. Studies have shown that side effects are the major reason that patients discontinue their antihypertensive medication. In regard to compliance, nadolol seems to be unique among the β-blockers in that it can be administered once a day and has a low incidence of side effects relative to many other β-blockers.

Dosage and Administration

Nadolol is available only as an oral preparation, but it is supplied in a variety of tablet sizes for convenient dosing. The dose of nadolol that produces an equivalent β-blocking effect is approximately equal to or slightly lower than that of propranolol: the average ratio of nadolol to propranolol is 0.8 for daily doses.[6] For treating anxiety states, essential tremor, and tachyarrhythmias, doses as low as 20 mg/day may be effective. For the treatment of hypertension, 80 mg/day or more usually is required. Maximum doses of nadolol for the treatment of hypertension have ranged up to 640 mg/day. For the treatment of angina pectoris, the dose is usually 120 mg/day or more. However, the usefulness of doses higher than 240 mg/day in the treatment of angina has not been established.

SOCIOECONOMIC CONSIDERATIONS
Compliance with Regimen

Nadolol has two unique features that enhance compliance. First is its long pharmacologic half-life, which truly permits once-daily administration with adequate blood levels for the entire day. Second is the lower incidence of side effects relative to many β-blockers because of the drug's low lipid solubility. These advantages are also important to patients with angina pectoris. Effective once-daily dosing can alleviate anxiety concerning the possibility of missing a dose. Also, because side effects are common with many antianginal agents, nadolol helps ensure compliance.

Cost

Nadolol is intermediate in cost among the β-blockers available in the United States. β-Blockers in general are less costly than some of the newer antihypertensive agents, such as the angiotensin-converting enzyme inhibitors. β-Blockers are also less expensive than some of the newer antianginal medications, such as calcium antagonists and the topical nitrate patches. In addition, β-blockers are less expensive than many of the newer antiarrhythmic agents. Therefore, in terms of cost, β-blockers are often the low-cost alternative for treating patients.

Acknowledgment

The help of Karen Porrini, Pharm. D., of E. R. Squibb and Sons, in compiling the list of studies on nadolol is appreciated.

REFERENCES

1. Lee RJ, Evans DB, Baky SH, et al: Pharmacology of nadolol (SQ 11725), a beta-adrenergic antagonist lacking direct myocardial depression. Eur J Pharmacol 33:371, 1975.
2. Evans DB, Peschika MT, Lee RJ, et al: Anti-arrhythmic action of nadolol, a beta-adrenergic receptor blocking agent. Eur J Pharmacol 35:17, 1976.
3. Heel RC, Brogden RN, Pakes GE, et al: Nadolol: A review of its pharmacological properties and therapeutic efficacy in hypertension and angina pectoris. Drugs 20:1, 1980.
4. Wood AJJ: Pharmacologic differences between beta blockers. Am Heart J 108:1070, 1984.
5. LeWinter MM, Curtis GP, Engler RL, et al: Effects of equiblocking doses of nadolol and propranolol on left ventricular performance. Clin Pharmacol Ther 26:162, 1979.
6. Miller LA, Crawford MH, O'Rourke RA: Nadolol compared to propranolol for treating chronic stable angina pectoris. Chest 86:189, 1984.
7. Dreyfuss J, Griffith DL, Singhvi S, et al: Pharmacokinetics of nadolol, a beta-receptor antagonist: Administration of therapeutic single- and multiple-dose regimens to hypertensive patients. J Clin Pharmacol 19:712, 1979.
8. Mehta AV, Chidambaram B, Rice PJ: Pharmacokinetics of nadolol in children with supraventricular tachycardia. J Clin Pharmacol 32:1023, 1992.
9. Krukemyer JJ, Boudoulas H, Binkley PF, Lima JJ: Comparison of single-dose and steady-state nadolol plasma concentrations. Pharm Res 7:953, 1990.
10. Dreyfuss J, Brannick LJ, Vukovich RA, et al: Metabolic studies in patients with nadolol: Oral and intravenous administration. J Clin Pharmacol 17:300, 1977.
11. Vukovich RA, Foley JE, Brown B, et al: Effect of beta-blockers on exercise double product (systolic blood pressure × heart rate). Br J Clin Pharmacol 7:167S, 1979.
12. DuPont AG, Vanderniepen P, Bossuyt AM, et al: Nadolol in essential hypertension: Effect on ambulatory blood pressure, renal haemodynamics and cardiac function. Br J Clin Pharmacol 20:93, 1985.
13. Frishman WH: Nadolol: A long-acting beta-adrenoceptor blocking drug. In Frishman WM (ed): Clinical Pharmacology of the Beta-Adrenergic Blocking Drugs. New York: Appleton-Century-Crofts, 1980, pp 163–170.
14. Chang MS, Sung RJ, Tai TY, et al: Nadolol and supraventricular tachycardia: An electrophysiologic study. J Am Coll Cardiol 2:894, 1983.
15. Cohen IS, Widrich W, Duchin KL, et al: Acute electrophysiologic effects of nadolol. J Clin Pharmacol 23:93, 1983.
16. Patterson E, Scherlag BJ, Lazzara R: Mechanism of prevention of sudden death by nadolol: Differential actions on arrhythmia triggers and substrate after myocardial infarction on the dog. J Am Coll Cardiol 8:1365, 1986.
17. Manley BS, Alexopoulos D, Robinson GJ, Cobbe SM: Subsidiary class III effects of beta-blockers? A comparison of atenolol, metoprolol, nadolol, oxprenolol, and sotalol. Cardiovasc Res 20:705, 1986.
18. Burke SE, Murthy VS: Effects of nadolol on myocardial oxygen consumption and ischemic ST-T changes during coronary occlusion in anesthetized dogs. Fed Proc 37:235, 1978.
19. Frohlich ED, Messerli FH, Deslinski GR, et al: Long-term renal hemodynamic effects of nadolol in patients with essential hypertension. Am Heart J 108:1141, 1984.
20. Brown MJ, Brown DC, Murphy MB: Hypokalemia from beta$_2$-receptor stimulation by circulating epinephrine. N Engl J Med 309:1414, 1983.
21. Wilkinson R, Burr WA: A comparison of propranolol and nadolol pharmacokinetics and clinical effects in thyrotoxicosis. Am Heart J 108:1160, 1984.
22. Littley MD, Kingswood JC, John R, Lazarus JH: Effect of nadolol on plasma lipids in hyperthyroidism. Horm Metab Res 21:331, 1989.
23. Johnson BF: The emerging problem of plasma lipid changes during antihypertensive therapy. J Cardiovasc Pharmacol 4:S213, 1982.
24. O'Donoghue DJ: Acute pancreatitis due to nadolol-induced hypertriglyceridaemia. Br J Clin Pract 43:74, 1989.
25. Textor SC, Fouad FM, Bravo EL, et al: Redistribution of cardiac output to the kidneys during oral nadolol administration. N Engl J Med 307:601, 1982.
26. Fallo F, Gregianin M, Bui F, et al: Comparison of the antihyper-

tensive and renal effects of tertatolol and nadolol in hypertensive patients with mild renal impairment. Eur J Clin Pharmacol 40:309, 1991.

27. van Zyl A, Jennings AA, Byrne MJ, Opie LH: Effects of therapy on renal impairment in essential hypertension. S Afr Med J 82:407, 1992.

28. Cruickshank JM: The clinical importance of cardioselectivity and lipophilicity in beta-blockers. Am Heart J 100:160, 1980.

29. Duchin KL, Vukovich RA, Dennick LG, et al: Effects of nadolol beta-blockade on blood pressure in hypertension. Clin Pharmacol Ther 27:57, 1980.

30. Mancia G, Ferrari A, Pomidossi G, et al: Twenty-four-hour blood pressure profile and blood pressure variability in untreated hypertension and during antihypertensive treatment by once-a-day nadolol. Am Heart J 108:1078, 1984.

31. Veterans Administration Cooperative Study Group on Antihypertensive Agents: Efficacy of nadolol alone and combined with bendroflumethiazide and hydralazine for systemic hypertension. Am J Cardiol 52:1230, 1983.

32. Iyun AO: Clinical experience with nadolol in Nigerian patients with essential hypertension. West Afr J Med 8:18, 1989.

33. Mitenko PA, McKenzie JK, Sitar DS, et al: Nadolol antihypertensive effect and disposition in young and elderly adults with mild to moderate essential hypertension. Clin Pharmacol Ther 46:56, 1989.

34. Furberg B, Dahlqvist A, Raak A, et al: Comparison of the new beta-adrenoceptor antagonist, nadolol, and propranolol in the treatment of angina pectoris. Curr Med Res Opin 5:388, 1978.

35. Ling ASC, Groel JT: Improved physical performance as a therapeutic objective in patients with angina. Br J Clin Pharmacol 7:161s, 1979.

36. Prager G: Angina pectoris: Effective therapy once daily. J Int Med Res 7:39, 1979.

37. Jones GR, Mir MA: Comparison of antianginal efficacy of one conventional and three long-acting beta-adrenoreceptor blocking agents in stable angina pectoris. Br Heart J 46:503, 1981.

38. Kostis JB, Lacy CR, Krieger SD, et al: Atenolol, nadolol, and pindolol in angina pectoris on effort: Effect of pharmacokinetics. Am Heart J 108:1131, 1984.

39. Singh S, Doherty J, Udhoji V, et al: Amlodipine versus nadolol in patients with stable angina pectoris. Am Heart J 118:1137, 1989.

40. Singh S: Long-term double-blind evaluation of amlodipine and nadolol in patients with stable exertional angina pectoris. The Investigators of Study 152. Clin Cardiol 16:54, 1993.

41. Miller WE, Vittitoe JA, O'Rourke RA, et al: Nadolol versus diltiazem and combination for preventing exercise-induced ischemia in severe angina pectoris. Am J Cardiol 62:372, 1988.

42. Tirlapur VG, Afzal M: Cardiorespiratory effects of isosorbide dinitrate and nifedipine in combination with nadolol: A double-blind comparative study of beneficial and adverse antianginal drug interactions. Am J Cardiol 53:487, 1984.

43. Alexander JC, Christie MH, Vernam KA, et al: Long-term experience with nadolol in treatment of hypertension and angina pectoris. Am Heart J 108:1136, 1984.

44. Sung RJ, Tai DY, Svinarich JT: Beta-adrenoceptor blockade: Electrophysiology and antiarrhythmic mechanisms. Am Heart J 108:1115, 1984.

45. Saksena S, Klein GJ, Kowey PR, et al: Electrophysiologic effects, clinical efficacy and safety of intravenous and oral nadolol in refractory supraventricular tachyarrhythmias. Am J Cardiol 59:307, 1987.

46. DiBianco R, Morganroth J, Freitag JA, et al: Effects of nadolol on the spontaneous and exercise-provoked heart rate of patients with chronic atrial fibrillation receiving stable dosages of digoxin. Am Heart J 108:1121, 1984.

47. Mehta AV, Chidambaram B: Efficacy and safety of intravenous and oral nadolol for supraventricular tachycardia in children. J Am Coll Cardiol 19:630, 1992.

48. Nademanee K, Schleman MM, Singh BN, et al: Beta-adrenergic blockade by nadolol in control of ventricular tachyarrhythmias. Am Heart J 108:1109, 1984.

49. Coumel P, Escoubet B, Attuel P: Beta-blocking therapy in atrial and ventricular tachyarrhythmias: Experience with nadolol. Am Heart J 108:1098, 1984.

50. Morganroth J, Duchin KL: Effectiveness of low-dose nadolol for ventricular arrhythmias. Am J Cardiol 58:273, 1986.

51. Leclercq JF, Leenhardt A, Lemarec H, et al: Predictive value of electrophysiologic studies during treatment of ventricular tachycardia with the beta blocking agent nadolol. The Working Group on Arrhythmias of the French Society of Cardiology. J Am Coll Cardiol 16:413, 1990.

52. Munsif AN, Saksena S: Efficacy of nadolol alone or in combination with a type IA antiarrhythmic drug in sustained ventricular tachycardia: A prospective study. PACE 12:1816, 1989.

53. James I, Savage I: Beneficial effect of nadolol on anxiety-induced disturbances of performance in musicians: A comparison with diazepam and placebo. Am Heart J 108:1150, 1984.

54. Koller WC: Nadolol in essential tremor. Neurology 33:1076, 1983.

55. Foster NL, Newman RP, LeWitt PA, et al: Treatment of resting tremor by beta-adrenergic blockade. Am Heart J 108:1173, 1984.

56. Blom MW, Sommers DK: The effects of baclofen, nadolol and propranolol on tremor amplitudes in geriatric patients with essential tremor. Med Sci Res 20:835, 1992.

57. Ryan RE: Comparative study of nadolol and propranolol in prophylactic treatment of migraine. Am Heart J 108:1156, 1984.

58. Herman VS, Joffe BI, Kalk WJ, et al: Clinical and biochemical responses to nadolol and clonidine in hyperthyroidism. J Clin Pharmacol 29:1117, 1989.

59. Ratey JJ, Sorgi P, O'Driscoll GA, et al: Nadolol to treat aggression and psychiatric symptomatology in chronic psychiatric inpatients: A double-blind, placebo-controlled study. J Clin Psychiatry 53:41, 1992.

60. Ratey JJ, Greenberg MS, Lindem KJ: Combination of treatments for attention deficit hyperactivity disorder in adults. J Nerv Ment Dis 179:699, 1991.

61. Alpert M, Allan ER, Citrom L, et al: A double-blind, placebo-controlled study of adjunctive nadolol in the management of violent psychiatric patients. Psychopharmacol Bull 26:367, 1990.

62. Merkel C, Sacerdoti D, Finucci GF, et al: Effect of nadolol on liver haemodynamics and function in patients with cirrhosis. Br J Clin Pharmacol 21:713, 1984.

63. Poynard T, Calcs P, Pasta L, et al: Beta-adrenergic-antagonist drugs in the prevention of gastrointestinal bleeding in patients with cirrhosis and esophageal varices [abstract]. N Engl J Med 324:1532, 1991.

64. Frishman WH, Furberg CD, Friedewald WT: Beta-adrenergic blockade for survivors of acute myocardial infarction. N Engl J Med 310:830, 1984.

65. Burmeister WE, Reynolds RD, Lee RJ: Limitation of myocardial infarct size by atenolol, nadolol, and propranolol in dogs. Eur J Pharmacol 75:7, 1981.

66. Jimenez AH, Tofler GH, Chen X, et al: Effects of nadolol on hemodynamic and hemostatic responses to potential mental and physical triggers of myocardial infarction in subjects with mild systemic hypertension. Am J Cardiol 72:47, 1993.

67. Frishman WH: Nadolol: A new beta-adrenoceptor antagonist. N Engl J Med 305:678, 1981.

68. Krukemyer JJ, Boudoulas H, Binkley PF, Lima JJ: Comparison of hypersensitivity to adrenergic stimulation after abrupt withdrawal of propranolol and nadolol: Influence of half-life differences. Am Heart J 120:572, 1990.

69. Duchin KL, Stern MA, Willard BA, et al: Comparison of kinetic interactions of nadolol and propranolol with cimetidine. Am Heart J 108:1084, 1984.

70. Corsi CM, Nafziger AN, Pieper JA, et al: Lack of effect of atenolol and nadolol on the metabolism of theophylline. Br J Clin Pharmacol 29:265, 1990.

71. Michaels RS, Duchin KL, Akbar S, et al: Nadolol in hypertensive patients maintained on long-term hemodialysis. Am Heart J 108:1091, 1984.

72. Devlin RG, Duchin KL, Fleiss PM: Nadolol in human serum and breast milk. Br J Clin Pharmacol 12:393, 1981.

73. Kostis JB, Shindler DM, Moreyra AE, et al: Differential exercise effects of captopril and nadolol in patients with essential hypertension. Angiology 43:647, 1992.

CHAPTER 54

Ultrashort-Acting β-Adrenoreceptor Blocking Drug: Esmolol*

William H. Frishman, M.D., V. Shrinivas Murthy, M.D., Ph.D., Joel A. Strom, M.D., and Dawn Hershman, M.D.

β-Adrenergic blockers are important therapeutic drugs in cardiovascular and noncardiovascular diseases.[1] However, some physicians have been reluctant to use these drugs in seriously ill patients because of potentially adverse effects (i.e., bradycardia, hypotension, aggravation of heart failure, and bronchospasm). These adverse effects, which are more common after intravenous (IV) than after oral administration of β-blocking drugs,[2, 3] stem from β-adrenergic blockade in patients who depend on their sympathetic tone to compensate for cardiopulmonary inadequacies. Unfortunately, it is often difficult to assess the magnitude of this catecholamine dependency. Once an IV β-blocking agent such as atenolol, metoprolol, or propranolol is administered, its pharmacologic effects persists for several hours after the drug is discontinued.[4] Deterioration of a patient's condition with IV β-blockade or the development of adverse reactions may be difficult to reverse.

To circumvent the prolonged activity of conventional β-blockers, two new β-blockers were developed for continuous IV infusion: esmolol, which is relatively β1-selective, and flestolol, which is nonselective, each having ultrashort durations of pharmacologic action.[5-8] In December 1986, esmolol (Brevibloc) was approved in the United States for emergent parenteral treatment of rapid ventricular rates in patients with atrial fibrillation or atrial flutter and for treatment of sinus tachycardia when control of rate is desirable. Esmolol is the fourth β-blocker to be approved for IV clinical use. Esmolol differs from these agents because it can be rapidly titrated, and its pharmacologic effects dissipate within 30 minutes after the drug is discontinued.[9]

ESMOLOL
Chemistry and Pharmacokinetics

The chemical structure of esmolol is similar to that of metoprolol and propranolol (Fig. 54–1). However, it differs from these agents in that it has an ethylene-extended methyl ester group in the paraposition of the phenyl ring. The addition of the ester group makes the molecule susceptible to rapid hydrolysis by esterases, resulting in a β-blocker with a short duration of action (terminal half-life, 9.2 minutes).[9]

Esmolol is rapidly metabolized by erythrocyte es-

terases via hydrolysis of the methyl ester.[10, 11] An unidentified plasma factor is required for the full expression of this esterase activity, and there may be some drug metabolism by tissue esterases.[12] Unlike most ester-containing drugs (e.g., succinylcholine), esmolol is not metabolized by plasma cholinesterase. The hydrolysis of esmolol results in the formation of a weakly active acid metabolite (1/1500 the potency of esmolol) and methanol.[9] The amount of methanol formed is within the normal range seen in humans and, therefore, is clinically insignificant.[13]

Other pharmacokinetic properties of esmolol have been investigated in healthy volunteers after 2-hour drug infusions of 50, 150, and 400 μg/kg/min.[10] The steady-state blood concentration of esmolol correlated significantly with dose.[10] Using an open, two-compartment model, the drug was found to have a rapid distribution half-life of 2.03 minutes and an elimination half-life of 9.19 minutes. The total body clearance of esmolol was 285 ml/kg/min and was independent

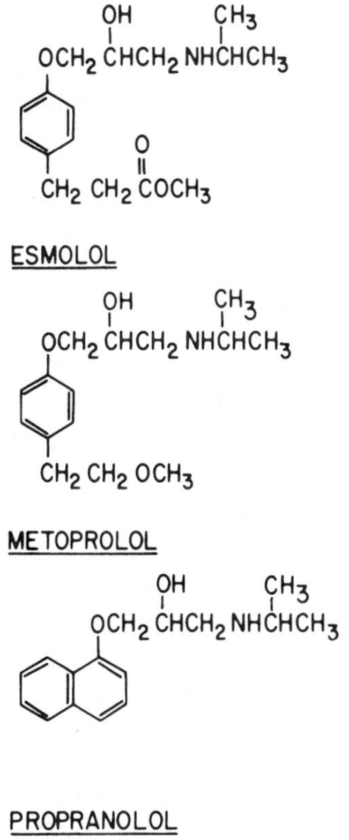

ESMOLOL

METOPROLOL

PROPRANOLOL

Figure 54–1. Chemical structures of propranolol, metoprolol, and the ultrashort-acting β-blocker, esmolol.

This chapter was adapted from Frishman WH, Murthy VS, Strom JA: Ultrashort-acting β adrenergic blocking drugs: Esmolol and flestolol. Med Clin North Am 72:359, 1988.

of dose and plasma drug levels (dose-dependent kinetics).[10] Within 24 hours, 73% to 88% of an infused dose of esmolol was eliminated in the urine as its acid metabolite, whereas less than 1% of the parent compound was excreted unchanged.[10, 14]

After a 1-minute infusion of the loading dose (500 µg/kg/min), steady-state blood levels of esmolol for doses of 50 to 300 µg/kg/min are reached within 5 minutes; steady-state is reached in 30 minutes without the loading dose. Elimination kinetics are dose-independent over this range.[10] Esmolol is 55% protein bound,[13] has a volume distribution of 3.43 L/kg,[13] and is weakly lipid soluble.[13] The comparative pharmacology of intravenously administered esmolol and propranolol is presented in Table 54–1.

The pharmacokinetic properties of esmolol have also been investigated in patients with end-stage renal[14] and hepatic diseases, and they did not differ significantly from those observed in normal subjects. However, the elimination half-life of the inactive acid metabolite was significantly prolonged in end-stage renal disease.[15]

The clearance of ASL 8123, the metabolite of esmolol, by hemodialysis, is significant, whereas continuous ambulatory peritoneal dialysis (CAPD) has a minimal effect on elimination of the metabolite from the body. Blood pressure and pulse determinations are not affected in the CAPD patient despite increased levels of the metabolite, demonstrating again that the metabolite has minimal β-blocking effects.[16]

Pharmacodynamics

The β-blocking effects of esmolol have been confirmed in both animal[9, 12] and human studies.[10, 17] The drug reduces heart rate at rest and during exercise and attenuates isoproterenol-induced changes in heart rate and blood pressure. In humans, the magnitude of these effects correlates strongly with steady-state levels of esmolol.[10, 17]

In animal studies, esmolol has been found to be 50 times less potent than propranolol and 6 times less potent than metoprolol.[5, 13] However, in humans, esmolol appears to be 1/15 as potent as propranolol.[17] Esmolol is relatively β1-selective,[18] is devoid of intrinsic sympathomimetic activity,[19] and has 1/100 the local anesthetic effect of propranolol.[17]

In human studies,[20] an esmolol infusion of 500 µg/kg/min for 4 minutes followed by a maintenance infusion of 300 µg/kg/min for 10 minutes caused significant decreases in heart rate and systolic blood pressure. Esmolol reduced the index of contractility by 18%, cardiac index by 17%, left ventricular (LV) stroke work index by 20%, and LV ejection fraction by 18%. There were small but statistically significant increases in mean right atrial pressure, mean right ventricular pressure, mean pulmonary artery pressure, pulmonary capillary wedge pressure, and LV end-diastolic pressure. At steady state, arterial blood concentration of esmolol was 3.91 ± 0.43 µg/ml. The hemodynamic changes and blood esmolol concentration returned to baseline within 30 minutes after discontinuation of esmolol.[20]

In other clinical studies, the magnitude of β-blockade produced by IV infusions of 50 to 300 µg/kg/min of esmolol was comparable to that produced by IV injections of 3 to 6 mg of propranolol.[21, 22] An esmolol infusion of 300 µg/kg/min and an oral propranolol dose of 40 mg every 8 hours were equally effective in inhibiting exercise-induced tachycardia.[17]

In resting patients with coronary artery disease, a loading dose infusion of 500 µg/kg/min of esmolol for 5 minutes followed by a maintenance dose of 300 µg/kg/min for up to 24 minutes produced decreases in arterial pressure, heart rate, LV contractility, and cardiac index and increases in LV systolic volume and pulmonary vascular resistance, findings similar to those of other β-blockers. However, in contrast with other β-blockers, discontinuation of the esmolol infusion produced a rapid reversal of these hemodynamic effects within 30 minutes, consistent with its short elimination half-life.[23]

The comparative hemodynamic effects of propranolol and esmolol during rest and exercise have been compared in patients with coronary artery disease and preserved LV function.[22] Esmolol was infused at a loading dose of 500 µg/kg/min for 2 minutes followed by a maintenance infusion of 200 µg/kg/min; 4 mg of propranolol was infused over 4 minutes. After 12 minutes of treatment, both drugs had pro-

Table 54–1. **Comparative Pharmacologic Properties of Esmolol and Propranolol**

Property	Esmolol	Propranolol
β-Blockade potency	0.07	1.0
Therapeutic plasma levels	400–1200 ng/ml	30–380 ng/ml
Relative β1-selectivity	+	0
Intrinsic sympathomimetic activity	0	0
Membrane-stabilizing activity	0	+
Lipid solubility	+	+ +
Distribution half-life (min)	~2	~5
Elimination half-life	~9 min	~4.5 hr
Metabolism	Blood esterases	Hepatic
Active metabolites	No	Yes
Onset of intravenous β-blockade (min)	~0.07	~0.12
Time to maximal intravenous β-blockade (min)	~1.0	~6.0
Time to 50% recovery after treatment (min)	~10	~40
Time to 100% recovery after treatment (min)	~30	>60

duced comparable decreases in resting heart rate, systolic blood pressure, cardiac index, and ventricular ejection fractions. Both drugs attenuated exercise-induced increments in heart rate, systolic blood pressure, and cardiac index; esmolol had a greater effect on systolic blood pressure.[22]

Esmolol has also been studied in patients with severe LV dysfunction.[24] Using doses of 200 μg/kg/min in these patients, ventricular ejection fraction and cardiac output decreased, and pulmonary capillary wedge pressure increased without evidence of overt congestion. The hemodynamic effects of the drug were rapidly reversed within 10 to 30 minutes after the infusion was discontinued.

The electrophysiologic effects of esmolol have been evaluated in patients,[25] and findings are characteristic of those observed with other β-blockers.[26, 27] The drug has significant effects on the sinoatrial and atrioventricular nodes, with little pharmacologic activity on His-Purkinje and ventricular tissues. After a 1-minute loading dose of 500 μg/kg/min and a maintenance dose of 300 μg/kg/min, the electrophysiologic effects of therapy were evident within 5 minutes.[25] A similar time course of action has been documented after IV doses of metoprolol[28] and acebutolol.[29] However, recovery from esmolol-induced effects occurred significantly earlier after treatment cessation.[25]

Clinical Applications

Esmolol has been evaluated in the treatment of supraventricular tachyarrhythmias,[30, 31] for rapid control of heart rate and reduction in myocardial oxygen consumption in patients with acute myocardial ischemia,[32] in the management of perioperative tachycardia and hypertension,[33] and for treatment of postoperative hypertension.[34]

Supraventricular and Ventricular Tachyarrhythmias

The efficacy of β-blockers in the management of supraventricular tachyarrhythmias has been well documented.[26–29, 35] Therapeutic benefits result from their effects in reducing automaticity of normal and ectopic pacemaker cells and in slowing conduction of impulses through the atrioventricular node.[26, 27]

The safety and efficacy of esmolol were evaluated in the treatment of supraventricular tachycardias in two multicenter, double-blind control studies[21, 36] and in one multicenter, open-label, baseline control study.[37] Patients studied had atrial fibrillation (approximately 60%), atrial flutter (approximately 20%), sinus tachycardia (approximately 13%), and supraventricular tachycardia due to other causes (7%).[21, 36, 37] In each of these studies, the dose of esmolol was titrated using an initial 1-minute loading dose of 500 μg/kg/min, which preceded six consecutive titration steps of 50, 100, 150, 200, 250, and 300 μg/kg/min.[21, 36, 37] Each titration step lasted 5 minutes in the double-blind studies[21, 36] and 5 to 15 minutes in the open-label study.[37] The loading dose preceding each titration step

was used to rapidly achieve a steady-state blood level of esmolol.

In the first double-blind trial,[36] the effects of esmolol were compared with those of placebo; in the second double-blind study,[21] the effects of the drug were compared with those of propranolol. Propranolol was administered at a rate of 1 mg/min for 3 minutes during the first 5 minutes and for an additional 3 minutes during the next 5 minutes, providing a total dose of 6 mg. In the double-blind trials, a therapeutic response was defined as a decrease in the ventricular rate by 20%,[21, 36] a decrease in ventricular response to less than 100 beats/min, or conversion to sinus rhythm. In the open-label trial,[37] a therapeutic response was defined as a 15% decrease in ventricular rate or conversion to sinus rhythm.

In these trials, 247 patients received esmolol, 55 received propranolol, and 31 received placebo.[21, 36, 37] With esmolol, a dose-dependent increase in therapeutic response rate was seen between 50 and 200 mg/kg/min, with little additional benefit observed with higher doses.[21, 36, 37] In a large proportion of patients responding to esmolol during the titration period, the therapeutic response was sustained during maintenance periods ranging from 4 to 24 hours.[21, 36] The average doses of esmolol producing therapeutic responses in these three trials were 97.5,[36] 115,[21] and 95[37] μg/kg/min. In the placebo-controlled study,[36] 66% of patients treated with esmolol responded favorably versus 8% treated with placebo. Esmolol and propranolol were equally effective (72% and 69% response rates, respectively).[21] Fourteen percent of esmolol-treated patients converted to normal sinus rhythm during dose titration; 16% reverted to normal rhythm on propranolol.[21] During maintenance, an additional 10% converted to normal rhythm on esmolol; this occurred in 8% treated with propranolol.[21] Thus, in these studies, 50 to 200 μg/kg/min of esmolol was found to be comparable to an IV dose of 3 to 6 mg of propranolol in the treatment of supraventricular tachycardia.[21] However, the fluid volumes infused to achieve comparable β-blockade were considerably larger with esmolol. After the termination of esmolol treatment, its effects on heart rate tended to dissipate within 20 minutes, whereas the effects of propranolol on heart rate persisted for at least 4 to 5 hours.[36]

The therapeutic response rate of esmolol in patients with supraventricular tachyarrhythmias was comparable to those seen with other β-blockers used intravenously.[29, 38] In an open-label comparison study, esmolol appeared to be as effective as intravenously administered verapamil (5 to 10 mg) for treatment of supraventricular arrhythmias,[39] but verapamil had a continued pharmacologic effect lasting 4 hours after termination of treatment.

In the first prospective trial in which esmolol was compared with verapamil in the treatment of patients with atrial fibrillation/flutter having a rapid ventricular rate, esmolol compared favorably in terms of both efficacy and safety.[40] There was a 28% decrease in the ventricular response in the esmolol group, similar to a 30% decrease in the verapamil group. However, 14 of the 28 patients (50%) treated with esmolol converted to sinus rhythm, whereas only 2 of the 17 verapamil-treated patients (12%) converted. Both the esmolol and verapamil treatment groups experienced a gradual drop in systolic blood pressure (12% and 14%, respectively). Between the two groups, there was no difference in the percentage of patients whose systolic blood pressure dropped below 90 mmHg and no difference in adverse events. However, asymptomatic hypotension was noted in 50% of the patients in each study group.

Shettigar et al.[41] examined the combined use of esmolol and digoxin in the treatment of patients with atrial fibrillation/flutter. The conversion rate was 33% with satisfactory control of heart rate achieved at a mean interval of 21 minutes. When the results were compared with those of Platia et al.,[40] heart rate control with combination therapy was found to be superior to either esmolol or verapamil alone. In addition, the incidence of asymptomatic hypotension (systolic blood pressure, <90 mmHg) occurred in 10% of the patients on dual therapy as compared with 48% and 46% for esmolol and verapamil monotherapy, respectively.

Esmolol has been used successfully for the rapid control of heart rate in patients with postoperative supraventricular tachyarrhythmias[42] when infused for up to 24 hours, and in some patients with congestive heart failure and asthma, in whom β-blockade would usually be contraindicated.[37]

Esmolol has been shown to raise the ventricular fibrillation threshold in dogs with acute myocardial ischemia.[13] Some β-blockers have been shown to reduce the frequency of ventricular fibrillation episodes observed in the coronary care unit in patients surviving an acute myocardial infarction.[43] However, there have been no studies in humans examining the effects of esmolol on ventricular arrhythmias.

Myocardial Ischemia

By blocking catecholamine-induced increments in heart rate, in velocity and extent of myocardial contraction, and in blood pressure, esmolol,[12, 17, 44-46] like other β-blockers,[47-49] reduces determinants of myocardial oxygen consumption, making it a potentially useful drug for treating acute myocardial ischemia and for reducing the extent of damage caused by myocardial infarction. Results of placebo-controlled trials using intravenously administered atenolol,[50] metoprolol,[43, 51] and timolol[52] have demonstrated beneficial effects of β-blockade in patients with suspected or diagnosed myocardial infarcts by reducing the duration of chest pain, the incidence of ventricular arrhythmias, and possibly the extent of myocardial damage.

The effects of esmolol were evaluated in 19 patients with acute myocardial ischemia who were in sinus rhythm.[32] Esmolol was infused in stepwise incremental doses of 50 to 300 μg/kg/min. Each titration dose was infused for 30 minutes and was preceded by a 1-minute loading dose of 500 μg/kg/min. After the titration period, the patients were maintained on esmolol for up to 7 hours. Esmolol reduced the heart rate by approximately 15 beats/min (maximal effect on heart rate occurred with 150 μg/kg/min). Systolic blood pressure decreased by 15%, cardiac index by 21%, and the rate-pressure product by 33%. No significant effects on systemic and pulmonary vascular resistances, pulmonary capillary wedge pressure, and electrocardiographic PR interval were observed. Hypotension developed in 10 patients but was quickly reversed within 30 minutes of reducing the dose of esmolol or terminating treatment. At the end of the study, all hemodynamic parameters returned to preinfusion values within 30 minutes of discontinuing esmolol treatment.[32] Most patients were subsequently started on oral β-blocker therapy, without loss of therapeutic benefit. This study demonstrated the possibility that IV treatment with esmolol might predict tolerance to oral β-blocker use in patients with acute myocardial ischemia.[32] If adverse effects develop with esmolol, they can be reversed quickly.

The beneficial effects of β-adrenergic blocking agents in the treatment of unstable angina pectoris result from their effects on reducing heart rate, blood pressure, and myocardial contractility.[1] Short-acting β-blockers have potential utility secondary to the rapid reversal of these hemodynamic alterations when the drug is discontinued. Despite the previously mentioned study demonstrating the utility of esmolol for the treatment of myocardial infarction,[32] only a few studies have investigated esmolol's effect in patients with unstable angina.[53, 54]

The safety and efficacy of esmolol was determined by comparing β-blockade achieved with either continuous infusion of esmolol or increasing oral doses of propranolol in 23 patients with unstable angina.[53] Both treatment groups experienced a similar decrease in heart rate, mean arterial pressure, diastolic blood pressure, and rate-pressure product. Chest pain was significantly reduced in both study groups. In the esmolol group, chest pain episodes decreased from 4.6 ± 3.3 over 24 hours to 1.4 ± 1.8 in the first 48-hour study period, and in the propranolol group chest pain episodes decreased from 2.6 ± 1.4 over 24 hours to 1.0 ± 1.5 in a 48-hour study period. Five of 9 esmolol patients and 6 of 10 propranolol patients who were maintained on the drug for more than 24 hours had no further episodes of chest pain. There were no differences in frequency of adverse reactions between the two groups.

The use of esmolol as a complement to conventional therapy of unstable angina with nitrates and calcium antagonists was evaluated in a multicenter, prospective, randomized, placebo-controlled study.[54] Hemodynamic and antiischemic variables were evaluated in 113 patients—59 randomized to esmolol, and 54 to placebo treatment. Esmolol significantly decreased heart rate and systolic and diastolic blood pressures. There was no difference between the groups in reports of recurrent angina during the infusion period, but there was a trend toward a lower number of episodes of silent ischemia in the esmolol-treated patients. Thirty-nine percent of the esmolol patients, as compared with 22% of the placebo patients, experienced an adverse effect. Most frequently these effects consisted of hypotension, bradycardia, and gastrointestinal upset and resolved quickly with withdrawal of medication.[54]

The hemodynamic response to esmolol was also examined in 16 patients with myocardial ischemia and compromised LV function.[55] The rate-pressure product decreased by 33%, similar to decreases found in other studies. There was no change in pulmonary capillary wedge pressure or AV conduction, but the cardiac index fell by 14%. There were no new episodes or exacerbations of congestive heart failure or clinically symptomatic hypotension or bradycardia.[55]

Esmolol is not yet approved for clinical use in acute myocardial ischemia, but it can be used for the treatment of sinus tachycardia in the patient with myocardial ischemia if heart rate reduction is desired.

Perioperative Tachycardia and Hypertension

In patients with cardiovascular disease, surgical procedures performed under anesthesia can produce perioperative cardiovascular instability resulting from changes in sympathoadrenal activity.[56] Various stressors, such as laryngoscopy, endotracheal intubation, skin incision, and manipulation of internal organs, can lead to increased catecholamine release.[56-58] Patients with coronary artery disease may be unable to tolerate an increase in heart rate or blood pressure.[59, 60] β-Blockers such as propranolol[61, 62] effectively manage these hemodynamic changes, but these drugs may be undesirable because of their relatively long durations of action after IV infusion is terminated. Esmolol has been shown to blunt increments in intubation-induced tachycardia and blood pressure when compared with placebo in patients undergoing noncardiac[63-66] and cardiac surgical procedures.[67-70]

In a placebo-controlled study in patients undergoing coronary bypass surgery,[70] esmolol infusion began with a loading dose of 500 μg/kg/min for 2 minutes before induction of anesthesia, followed by a maintenance infusion of 200 μg/kg/min until the patient was on cardiac bypass. Esmolol significantly attenuated the cardioaccelerator effects of induction of anesthesia, intubation, sternotomy, and aortic dissection when compared with placebo.[70]

Aside from studies showing a beneficial effect of prophylactic treatment with esmolol in preventing intraoperative tachycardia and hypertension, several studies have investigated esmolol for the treatment of intraoperative tachycardia and hypertension.[71] Thirty patients were randomized in a placebo-controlled, double-blind study design.[71] With a loading dose of 80 mg and infusion of 12 mg/min, the esmolol-treated patients showed a 20% to 24% decrease in heart rate compared with a 3% to 13% decrease in the placebo group. The treatment groups showed no significant differences in blood pressure change. No adverse events were reported. The effects on intraoperative tachycardia were confirmed in a study that compared

placebo with esmolol therapy in IV boluses of 50 and 100 mg.[72] The results suggest that a dose of 50 mg adequately controls tachycardia during surgery.

The increase in heart rate that occurs during extubation can be successfully treated by bolus injections of esmolol. In a double-blind study comparing hemodynamic effects after 1-, 1.5-, and 2-mg/kg bolus doses of esmolol given 2 minutes after reversal of neuromuscular blockade,[73] a 1.5-mg/kg dose of esmolol blocked the maximal increase in heart rate and controlled systolic blood pressure, whereas a 1-mg/kg dose was insufficient to block increases in systolic blood pressure and a 2-mg/kg dose produced a significant decrease in blood pressure (>20%).[83]

Esmolol is not yet approved for prevention of perioperative tachycardia, but it can be used for management of perioperative supraventricular tachyarrhythmias.[42]

Postoperative Hypertension

After coronary bypass surgery, systolic hypertension is common,[74] and increased sympathetic activity has been implicated as the cause for this rise in blood pressure.[75] In patients with this condition, intravenously administered sodium nitroprusside, nitroglycerin, and labetalol can be used to reduce elevated blood pressure.[76, 77] Esmolol has been compared with nitroprusside in patients after coronary bypass surgery.[34] After the measurements of baseline hemodynamics, patients were randomized to receive either 0.5 to 10 μg/kg/min of nitroprusside or esmolol titrated from 25 to 300 μg/kg/min, with each esmolol titration step preceded by a 1-minute loading dose of 500 μg/kg/min. The titration end point was a 15% reduction in systolic blood pressure or a systolic blood pressure value of less than 120 mmHg. After a 20-minute washout phase, the patients were crossed over to the other drug used in the study, and the titration sequence and hemodynamic measurements were repeated. Both drugs reduced blood pressure and LV stroke index. Nitroprusside reduced diastolic pressure to a greater extent. Esmolol decreased the heart rate and cardiac index, whereas nitroprusside caused a slight increment in these parameters. Systemic vascular resistances and arterial oxygen tension were reduced by nitroprusside, and no changes were seen with esmolol.

Esmolol has been compared with labetalol in the treatment of postoperative hypertension after intracranial surgery.[78] No difference was found in terms of effectiveness in controlling hypertension, frequency of future hypertensive episodes in the recovery room, or frequency or severity of hypotension. However, bradycardia in the recovery period occurred in 60% of the labetalol group compared with 10% of the esmolol group.[78]

Esmolol is not approved for clinical use in the treatment of postoperative hypertension but can be used to treat postoperative supraventricular tachyarrhythmias.[42]

Esmolol has been found to be a suitable agent for

the purposeful induction of hypotension in a small group of patients undergoing spinal fusion and neurosurgery for cerebral arteriovenous malformations.[79] Esmolol has also been found to be successful in attenuating the tachycardia and hypertension associated with electroconvulsive therapy.[80]

Cocaine Cardiotoxicity

β-Blocker therapy has been suggested as a first-line treatment for cocaine cardiotoxicity, but unopposed β-activity may contribute to an adverse response. The first discussion of the use of esmolol in the treatment of cocaine-induced cardiotoxicity appeared in a case report describing a patient in whom cocaine was applied topically to the nasal mucosa during nasal polypectomy.[81] The cocaine induced a rapid increase in the patient's heart rate and blood pressure, and ST-segment depression appeared on the precordial electrocardiographic leads. Infusion of esmolol produced a rapid reversal of these effects. In a study of seven patients who received esmolol therapy for cocaine-induced cardiovascular toxicity,[82] three patients had a favorable response, whereas treatment failed in three patients. The authors concluded that there was no consistent hemodynamic benefit of esmolol therapy for cocaine-induced cardiotoxicity.[82]

Thyrotoxic Crisis

The cardiovascular complications of thyrotoxic crisis include tachyarrhythmias, chest pain, dyspnea, and congestive heart failure.[83] Propranolol has been the drug of choice for managing these cardiac effects. The advantages of using esmolol over propranolol stem from the rapid reversal of hemodynamic collapse with esmolol in patients experiencing congestive heart failure. In a case report, the maximal dose of esmolol was found to decrease heart rate, tremulousness, and agitation while having no effect on blood pressure.[83] Additional studies are needed to evaluate the use of esmolol in the treatment of thyrotoxicosis.

Neurogenic Syncope

β-Blockers have been used in the treatment of neurocardiogenic syncope determined by positive results on a head-up tilt test. Because the presenting symptoms can worsen, an effective therapeutic strategy must be identified quickly. A study was done in 21 patients with neurogenic syncope to determine whether response to esmolol was a predictor of response to metoprolol.[84] All of the patients with negative tilt test results during the esmolol infusion continued to have negative results with oral metoprolol administration. Of the patients that had a positive response during esmolol administration, 90% continued to have a positive response with oral metoprolol therapy. It was concluded that when patients have positive head tilt test results with esmolol challenge,

alternative treatment strategies from β-blockade should be considered.[84]

Adverse Effects

Hypotension, defined as systolic blood pressure below 90 mmHg and diastolic blood pressure below 50 mmHg, has been the most frequent adverse effect observed with esmolol, with a reported incidence ranging from 12% to 44%.[21, 36, 37] Similar doses of esmolol were used in each trial; however, the duration of infusion varied. Systolic hypotension was more common and was dose-related.[21, 36] Thirty percent of the hypotensive patients were symptomatic, with complaints of nausea, dizziness, headache, and dyspnea. Hypotension did resolve in most patients spontaneously with dose adjustment or with termination of therapy. With discontinuation of esmolol, 95% of patients became normotensive within 30 minutes.[21, 36, 37] Hypotension caused by esmolol may be avoided by careful titration to the minimum effective dose.

Hypotension has been reported as an adverse effect in studies in which intravenously administered metoprolol, timolol, and acebutolol were used to treat supraventricular tachyarrhythmias.[28, 29, 38] In a comparative trial, the incidence of hypotension was higher with esmolol treatment (36%) than with propranolol treatment (6%), despite similar therapeutic efficacies.[21] The mechanism for this relative difference in incidence is unknown. However, the duration of hypotension is much shorter after termination of esmolol treatment.

Esmolol, like the β_1-selective blockers metoprolol[85] and atenolol, should be used with caution in patients with bronchospastic disease. In a double-blind study of patients with bronchial asthma, the effects of esmolol on airway resistance were compared with those of the nonselective β-blocker propranolol and placebo.[86] No significant change in airway resistance occurred with either esmolol (300 µg/kg/min) or placebo. In contrast, 50% of propranolol-treated patients developed clinically significant bronchoconstriction.[86]

In another study of 50 patients with active cardiac disease and chronic obstructive pulmonary disease (COPD), esmolol was administered to determine if β-blockade could be achieved in this high-risk population.[87] The dosage was titrated in three increments of 8, 16, and 24 mg/min at 10-minute intervals. Hemodynamic and pulmonary end points were specified as heart rate less than 60 beats/min, systolic blood pressure less than 95 mmHg (or decline to 80% of baseline value), FEV_1 80%, wheezing, or dyspnea, resulting in discontinuation of the esmolol infusion. Heart rate decreased from 84 to 60 beats/min, systolic blood pressure decreased from 124 to 106 mmHg, and diastolic blood pressure decreased from 70 to 62 mmHg. Despite the expected hemodynamic effect, ventilatory function was not significantly affected. Pulmonary end points were reached in three patients (6%) who were all asymptomatic with a decrease in FEV_1 of more than 20%. No other adverse effects were observed. This study suggests that patients with

COPD and for whom β-blockade is indicated can be treated with esmolol with little risk of bronchospasm.[87] Sheppard et al.[86] found a small but significant risk of increased airway resistance and increased bronchomotor sensitivity to dry air in 10 asthmatic patients given esmolol and placebo in a double-blind crossover study. Specific airway resistance values did not differ between the two groups. However, the doses used in this study were not sufficient to affect blood pressure and heart rate.

If esmolol is used in patients at risk for bronchospasm, the infusion should be terminated immediately. A β$_2$-agonist may be administered concurrently but should be used with caution in patients with rapid ventricular rates.

As with all other β-blockers, esmolol is contraindicated in patients whose myocardium and cardiac conduction system depend on β-adrenergic stimulation.[1] If esmolol leads to clinical evidence of LV dysfunction or conduction abnormalities, these adverse effects can be reversed by reducing or discontinuing the infusion, and, if necessary, by administering atropine, dopamine, glucagon, dobutamine, amrinone, or milrinone.

Other side effects of esmolol that are unrelated to hypotension and are generally mild and infrequent include nausea, vomiting, headache, fatigue, and somnolence.[37] The development of phlebitis at the site of esmolol infusion has been reported in 8% of patients and may be related to duration of infusion.[21, 36, 37] Whenever irritation at the infusion site is observed, a change of site should be considered.

Drug Interactions

Medications commonly used in acute care situations have been evaluated for possible interactions with esmolol. Esmolol inhibits the hydrolysis of benzylcholine by human plasma cholinesterase in vitro.[88, 89] Plasma cholinesterase is responsible for the hydrolysis of succinylcholine, a muscle relaxant used during anesthesia, and concomitant esmolol use has led to clinically insignificant prolongation of the succinylcholine's duration of action.[88, 90]

Digoxin plasma levels increased slightly when the drug was concomitantly administered with esmolol.[91] However, digoxin has no effect on the pharmacokinetics of esmolol.[91] When esmolol and morphine were concomitantly administered intravenously in normal subjects, no effect on morphine blood levels was observed, but esmolol blood levels were increased slightly, without any effect on other pharmacokinetic parameters.[91] In a similar study, no significant interaction between esmolol and warfarin was observed.[91]

Clinical Use

Esmolol hydrochloride (Brevibloc) is available as a parenteral preparation containing 2.5 g of drug in a 10-ml solution per ampule. For the treatment of supraventricular tachycardia, two ampules of esmolol are diluted in 500 ml of IV fluid to provide a solution of 10 mg/ml. The manufacturer warns that esmolol should never be infused in concentrations greater than 10 mg/ml because of potential venous irritation. The amount of fluid necessary to infuse 100 μg/kg/min of esmolol into a 70-kg man would be approximately 40 ml/hr, in contrast with the 3-ml volume used to administered 3 mg of propranolol. Over 24 hours, the esmolol infusion would require administering 1 L of fluid. Diluted esmolol is stable for up to 24 hours at room temperature, and the drug is compatible with all commercially available IV solutions except for sodium bicarbonate (5%). The drug should not be infused through a butterfly IV needle to avoid irritation at the infusion site.

Infusion of esmolol solution should be initiated with a loading dose of 500 μg/kg/min for 1 minute, followed by a maintenance dose of 50 μg/kg/min for 4 minutes. If the therapeutic response is not adequate with this dose, the loading dose should be repeated and the maintenance dose increased to 100 μg/kg/min and infused for another 4 minutes. If a therapeutic response is not seen within 5 minutes, the titration process should be continued as needed, using the loading dose followed by increments in the maintenance dose of 50 μg/kg/min until the maximal infusion rate of 200 μg/kg/min is achieved. Although the maintenance dose can be increased to 300 μg/kg/min, such a dose yields little additional benefit.[21, 36, 37] As the desired therapeutic response is approached, or if there is concern about the development of hypotension, the loading infusion should be omitted, and the incremental dose in maintenance should be reduced to 25 μg/kg/min at intervals longer than 4 minutes. Once a therapeutic response is achieved, infusion can be maintained for up to 24 to 48 hours; no data support the safety of infusions beyond this point.

Esmolol is not approved for bolus administration, although there is preliminary evidence that this treatment mode may be useful.[92] Some studies have indicated that dosing with an IV esmolol bolus may be a simple alternative to loading and maintenance infusion of the drug. When esmolol was administered as an IV bolus injection at doses of 100 and 150 mg, it was found that the drug slowed atrioventricular conduction without altering sinus rate or blood pressure. This implies that IV bolus therapy with esmolol may be useful in the treatment of acute supraventricular tachycardias.[92]

Most patients with supraventricular tachycardia in whom control of the heart rate with esmolol is adequate and clinical status is stable can then be placed on alternative oral antiarrhythmic regimens, which can include propranolol, digoxin, or verapamil. The esmolol infusion should be reduced by 50% within 30 minutes of oral antiarrhythmic drug administration; if the patient status remains stable after the second oral dose, the infusion should be discontinued 1 hour later.

If an adverse effect occurs with an esmolol infusion, the dose should be reduced or the infusion should be terminated; the adverse effects usually dissipate within 30 minutes.[37] Abrupt withdrawal of esmolol has not been reported to produce the adverse effects reported with chronic β-blocker therapy in patients with coronary artery disease;[93] however, caution should still be maintained.

Esmolol, like other β-blockers, reduces the rate of discharge of the sinoatrial node and delays conduction through the atrioventricular node in children. Esmolol has been shown to prevent recurrences of supraventricular tachycardia in children but has not been shown to terminate supraventricular tachycardia.[94] Similar to its effects in adults, it also decreases blood pressure and heart rate significantly. Two studies have demonstrated that the dosage required to produce β-blockade is higher in children,[94, 95] ranging from 300 to 1000 μg/kg/min, as compared with adults, in whom the dosage is 100 to 300 μg/kg/min.

It is well known from animal studies that esmolol can produce a dose-dependent decrease in maternal and fetal heart rates.[96] The effects of esmolol on the human fetus have been reported in two case studies with conflicting results. Losasso et al.[97] described the use of esmolol in a pregnant woman at 22 weeks' gestation with no resultant morbidity or mortality. In response to the administration of four bolus doses of esmolol, 500 μg/kg each, and a stepwise increase in esmolol infusion from 50 to 200 μg/kg/min over the course of 10 minutes, fetal heart rate decreased less than 7%. Ducey reports a case of esmolol use in a 29-year-old woman at term who developed supraventricular tachycardia.[98] Esmolol, 0.5 mg/kg, was administered intravenously over 5 minutes, followed by an infusion of 50 μg/kg/min. Twenty minutes after the esmolol bolus was begun, fetal heart rate increased from 160 to 175 beats/min, then dropped 4 minutes later to 70 to 80 beats/min. Fetal bradycardia persisted despite termination of the infusion. Emergency caesarean section was performed. The safety of esmolol in pregnancy still needs to be established.

Dose adjustments of esmolol are not necessary in patients with hepatic or renal dysfunction.

CONCLUSION

Ultrashort-acting β-blockade is a potentially useful pharmacologic modality. A drug such as esmolol allows careful titration of β-blockade and the ability to terminate therapy with rapid dissipation of its clinical effects. Esmolol may provide a relative safety advantage over other parenteral β-blockers in patients who depend on β-adrenergic stimulation.

REFERENCES

1. Frishman WH: β-Adrenoceptor antagonists: New drugs and new indications. N Engl J Med 305:500, 1981.
2. Luria MH, Adelson EI, Miller AJ: Acute and chronic effects of an adrenergic beta-receptor blocking agent (propranolol) in the treatment of cardiac arrhythmias. Circulation 34:767, 1966.
3. Greenblatt DJ, Koch-Weser J: Adverse reactions to beta-adrenergic receptor blocking drugs: A report from the Boston Collaborative Drug Surveillance Program. Drugs 7:118, 1974.
4. McDevitt DG: Adrenoceptor blocking drugs: Clinical pharmacology and therapeutic use. Drugs 17:267, 1979.
5. Zaroslinski J, Borgman RJ, O'Donnell JP, et al: Ultra-short acting beta-blockers: A proposal for the treatment of the critically ill patient. Life Sci 31:899, 1982.
6. Erhardt PW, Woo CM, Gorczynski RJ, et al: Ultrashort-acting beta-adrenergic receptor blocking agents. 1. (Aryloxy)propanolamines containing esters in the nitrogen substituent. J Med Chem 25:1402, 1982.
7. Erhardt PW, Woo CM, Anderson WG, et al: Ultra-short acting beta-adrenergic receptor blocking agents. 2. (Aryloxy)propanolamines containing esters on the aryl function. J Med Chem 25:1408, 1982.
8. Gorczynski RJ, Voung A: Cardiovascular pharmacology of ACC 9089—a novel, ultrashort-acting beta-adrenoceptor antagonist. J Cardiovasc Pharmacol 6:555, 1984.
9. Gorczynski RJ: Basic pharmacology of esmolol. Am J Cardiol 56:3F, 1985.
10. Sum CY, Yacobi A, Kartzinel R, et al: Kinetics of esmolol, an ultrashort-acting beta blocker and of its major metabolite. Clin Pharmacol Ther 34:427, 1983.
11. Quon CY, Stampfli HF: Biochemical properties of blood esmolol esterase. Drug Metab Dispos 13:420, 1985.
12. Murthy VS, Hwang TF, Zagar ME, et al: Cardiovascular pharmacology of ASL 8052, an ultrashort-acting β blocker. Eur J Pharmacol 94:43, 1983.
13. Reynolds RD, Gorczynski RJ, Quon CY: Pharmacology and pharmacokinetics of esmolol. J Clin Pharmacol 26:A3, 1986.
14. Achari R, Drissel D, Matier WL, et al: Metabolism and urinary excretion of esmolol in humans. J Clin Pharmacol 26:44, 1986.
15. Flaherty J, Wong B, LaFollette G, et al: Kinetics of esmolol and ASL 8123 in normals and in renal failure [abstract]. Clin Pharmacol Ther 39:192A, 1986.
16. Flaherty JF, Wong B, LaFollette G, et al: Pharmacokinetics of esmolol and ASL-8123 in renal failure. Clin Pharmacol Ther 45:321, 1989.
17. Reilly CS, Wood M, Koshakji RP, et al: Ultrashort-acting beta blockade: A comparison with conventional beta blockade. Clin Pharmacol Ther 38:579, 1985.
18. Gorczynski RJ, Shaffer JE, Lee RJ: Pharmacology of ASL 8052—a novel beta-adrenergic receptor antagonist with an ultrashort duration of action. J Cardiovasc Pharmacol 5:668, 1983.
19. Gorczynski RJ, Murthy VS, Hwang TF: Beta-blocking and hemo-dynamic effects of ASL 8052. J Cardiovasc Pharmacol 6:1048, 1984.
20. Askenazi J, MacCosbe PE, Hoff J, et al: Hemodynamic effects of esmolol, an ultrashort-acting beta blocker. J Clin Pharmacol 27:567, 1987.
21. Abrams J, Allen J, Allin D, et al: Efficacy and safety of esmolol versus propranolol in the treatment of supraventricular tachyarrhythmias: A multicenter double-blind clinical trial. Am Heart J 110:913, 1985.
22. Iskandrian AS, Hakki AH, Laddu A: Effects of esmolol on cardiac function: Evaluation by non-invasive techniques. Am J Cardiol 56:27F, 1985.
23. Askenazi J, Hoff JV, Turlapaty P, et al: The effects of esmolol on cardiac hemodynamic function [abstract]. Clin Res 33:167A, 1985.
24. Iskandrian AS, Bemis CE, Hakki AH, et al: Effects of esmolol on patients with left ventricular dysfunction. J Am Coll Cardiol 8:225, 1986.
25. Greenspan AM, Spielman SR, Horowitz LN, et al: Electrophysiology of esmolol. Am J Cardiol 56:19F, 1985.
26. Singh BN, Jewitt DE: Beta-adrenergic blocking drugs in cardiac arrhythmias. Drugs 7:426, 1974.
27. Frishman WH, Silverman R: Physiologic and metabolic effects. In Frishman WH (ed): Clinical Pharmacology of the β-Adrenergic Blocking Drugs, 2nd ed. Norwalk, CT: Appleton-Century-Crofts, 1984, pp 27–49.
28. Moller B, Ringquist C: Metoprolol in the treatment of supraventricular tachyarrhythmias. Ann Clin Res 11:34, 1979.
29. Williams DO, Tatebaum R, Most AS: Effective treatment of supra-ventricular arrhythmias with acebutolol. Am J Cardiol 44:521, 1979.
30. Klein G, Wirtzfield A, Alt E, et al: Antiarrhythmic activity of esmolol (ASL 8052)—a novel ultrashort-acting beta-adrenoceptor blocking agent. Int J Clin Pharmacol Ther Toxicol 22:112, 1984.

31. Byrd R, Sung RJ, Marks J, et al: Safety and efficacy of esmolol (ASL 8052: An ultrashort-acting beta-adrenergic blocking agent) for control of ventricular rate in supraventricular tachycardias. J Am Coll Cardiol 3:394, 1984.

32. Kirshenbaum JM, Kloner RA, Antman EM, et al: Use of an ultrashort-acting β blocker in patients with acute myocardial infarction. Circulation 72:873, 1985.

33. Reves JG, Flezzani F: Perioperative use of esmolol. Am J Cardiol 56:57F, 1985.

34. Gray RJ, Bateman TM, Czer LSC, et al: Comparison of esmolol and nitroprusside for acute post-cardiac surgical hypertension. Am J Cardiol 59:887, 1987.

35. White HD, Antman EM, Glynn MA, et al: Efficacy and safety of timolol for prevention of supraventricular tachyarrhythmias after coronary artery bypass surgery. Circulation 70:479, 1984.

36. Anderson S, Blanski L, Byrd R, et al: Comparison of the efficacy and safety of esmolol, a short-acting beta blocker with placebo in the treatment of supraventricular tachyarrhythmias. Am Heart J 111:42, 1986.

37. The Esmolol Research Group: Intravenous esmolol for the treatment of supraventricular tachyarrhythmias: Results of a multicenter, baseline controlled safety and efficacy study of 160 patients. Am Heart J 112:498, 1986.

38. Sweany AE, Moncola F, Vickers FF, et al: Antiarrhythmic effects of intravenous timolol in supraventricular tachyarrhythmias. Clin Pharmacol Ther 37:124, 1985.

39. Michelson EL, Porterfield JK, Das G, et al: A comparison of esmolol and verapamil in the treatment of atrial fibrillation/flutter [abstract]. J Am Coll Cardiol 7:157A, 1986.

40. Platia EV, Michelson EL, Porterfield JK, et al: Esmolol versus verapamil in the acute treatment of atrial fibrillation or atrial flutter. Am J Cardiol 63:925, 1989.

41. Shettigar UR, Toole JG, O'Came Appunn D: Combined use of esmolol and digoxin in the acute treatment of atrial fibrillation or flutter. Am Heart J 126:368, 1993.

42. Gray RJ, Bateman TM, Czer LSC, et al: Esmolol: A new ultrashort-acting beta-adrenergic blocking agent for rapid control of heart rate in postoperative supraventricular tachyarrhythmias. J Am Coll Cardiol 5:1451, 1985.

43. Ryden L, Arniego R, Arnman K, et al: A double-blind trial of metoprolol in acute myocardial infarction. N Engl J Med 308:614, 1983.

44. Lange R, Kloner RA, Braunwald E: First ultrashort-acting beta-adrenergic blocking agent: Its effect on size and segmental wall dynamics of reperfused myocardial infarcts in dogs. Am J Cardiol 51:1759, 1983.

45. Lange R, Kloner RA, Braunwald E: Enhancement of functional recovery of "stunned," reperfused myocardium by a new ultrashort-acting beta blocker. J Am Coll Cardiol 3:545, 1984.

46. Kloner RA, Kirshenbaum J, Lange R, et al: Experimental and clinical observations on the efficacy of esmolol in myocardial ischemia. Am J Cardiol 56:40F, 1985.

47. Mueller HS, Ayres SM: The role of propranolol in the treatment of acute myocardial infarction. Prog Cardiovasc Dis 19:405, 1977.

48. Braunwald E, Muller JE, Kloner RA, et al: Role of beta-adrenergic blockade in the therapy of patients with acute myocardial infarction. Am J Med 74:113, 1983.

49. Frishman WH, Furberg CD, Friedewald WT: β-Adrenergic blockade for survivors of acute myocardial infarction. N Engl J Med 310:830, 1984.

50. Yusuf S, Sleight P, Rossi P, et al: Reduction in infarct size, arrhythmias and chest pain by early intravenous beta-blockade in suspected acute myocardial infarction. Circulation 67(Part 2):I32, 1983.

51. Hjalmarson A, Elmfeldt D, Herlitz J, et al: Effect on mortality of metoprolol in acute myocardial infarction: A double-blind randomized trial. Lancet 2:823, 1981.

52. International Cooperative Study Group: Reduction in infarct size with the early use of timolol in acute myocardial infarction. N Engl J Med 310:9, 1984.

53. Wallis DE, Pope C, Littman WJ, et al: Safety and efficacy of esmolol for unstable angina pectoris. Am J Cardiol 62:1033, 1988.

54. Hohnloser SH, Meinertz T, Klingenheben T, et al: Usefulness of esmolol in unstable angina pectoris. Am J Cardiol 67:1319, 1991.

55. Kirshenbaum JM, Kloner RJ, McGowan N, et al: Use of an ultrashort-acting beta-receptor blocker (esmolol) in patients with acute myocardial ischemia and relative contraindications to beta-blockade therapy. J Am Coll Cardiol 12:773, 1988.

56. Reves J: Adrenergic response to cardiopulmonary bypass. Mt Sinai J 52:511, 1985.

57. Stoelting RK, Peterson C: Circulatory changes in patients with coronary artery disease following thiamylal-succinylcholine and tracheal intubation. Anesth Analg 55:232, 1976.

58. Stoelting RK: Circulatory changes during direct laryngoscopy and tracheal intubation: Influence of duration of laryngoscopy with or without prior lidocaine. Anesthesiology 47:381, 1977.

59. Roy WL, Edelist G, Gilbert B: Myocardial ischemia during noncardiac surgical procedures in patients with coronary artery disease. Anesthesiology 51:393, 1979.

60. Slogoff S, Keats A: Does perioperative myocardial ischemia lead to postoperative myocardial infarction? Anesthesiology 62:107, 1985.

61. Slogoff S: Beta-adrenergic blockers. In Kaplan JA (ed): Cardiac Anesthesia, Vol 2, Cardiovascular Pharmacology. New York: Grune & Stratton, 1983, pp 181–208.

62. Oka Y, Frishman W, Becker R, et al: Clinical pharmacology of the new β-adrenoceptor blocking drugs. Part 10. Beta-adrenoceptor blockade and coronary artery surgery. Am Heart J 99:255, 1980.

63. Gold MI, Brown M, Coverman S, et al: Heart rate and blood pressure effects of esmolol after ketamine induction and intubation. Anesthesology 64:718, 1986.

64. Cucchiara RF, Benefiel DJ, Matteo RS, et al: Evaluation of esmolol in controlling increases in heart rate and blood pressure during endotracheal intubation in patients undergoing carotid endarterectomy. Anesthesiology 65:528, 1986.

65. Liu PL, Gatt S, Gugino LD, et al: Esmolol for control of increases in heart rate and blood pressure during tracheal intubation after thiopentone and succinylcholine. Can Anaesth Soc J 33:556, 1986.

66. Murthy VS, Hwang TF, Sandage BW, et al: Esmolol and the adrenergic response to perioperative stimuli. J Clin Pharmacol 26:A27, 1986.

67. Menkhaus PG, Rever JG, Kissin I, et al: Cardiovascular effects of esmolol in anesthetized humans. Anesth Analg 64:327, 1985.

68. Newsome LR, Roth JV, Hug CC, et al: Esmolol attenuates hemodynamic responses during fentanyl-pancuronium anesthesia for aortocoronary bypass surgery. Anesth Analg 65:451, 1986.

69. Shulman B, Tys DM, Girard D, et al: Hemodynamic effects of esmolol during anesthesia for myocardial revascularization [abstract]. Anesthesiology 63(3A):A64, 1985.

70. Newsome LR, Roth JV, Hug CC, et al: Esmolol attenuates hemodynamic responses to intubation and surgical stimulation during open heart surgery [abstract]. Anesthesiology 63(3A):A62, 1985.

71. Gold MI, Sacks DJ, Grosnoff DB, et al: Use of esmolol during anesthesia to treat tachycardia and hypertension. Anesth Analg 68:101, 1989.

72. Whirley-Diaz J, Gold MI, Helfman SM, et al: Can esmolol manage surgically-induced tachycardia? Bolus esmolol treatment of intra-operative tachycardia due to surgical stimulation. Anaesthesia 220:46, 1991.

73. Dyson A, Isaac PA, Pennant JH, et al: Esmolol attenuates cardiovascular responses to extubation. Anesth Analg 71:675, 1990.

74. Estafanous F, Tarazi R: Systemic arterial hypertension associated with cardiac surgery. Am J Cardiol 46:685, 1980.

75. Reves JG, Karp RB, Buttner EE, et al: Neuronal and adrenomedullary catecholamine release in response to cardiopulmonary bypass in man. Circulation 66:49, 1982.

76. Flaherty JT, Magee PA, Gardner TL, et al: Comparison of intravenous nitroglycerin and sodium nitroprusside for treatment of acute hypertension developing after coronary bypass surgery. Circulation 65:1072, 1982.

77. Morel DR, Forster A, Suter PM: Labetalol in the treatment of hypertension following coronary artery surgery. Br J Anaesth 54:1191, 1982.

78. Muzzi DA, Black S, Losasso TJ, et al: Labetalol and esmolol in the control of hypertension after intracranial surgery. Anesth Analg 70:68, 1990.

79. Ornstein E, Matteo RS, Schwartz AE: The use of esmolol for deliberate hypotension [abstract]. Anesthesiology 65(3A):A575, 1986.
80. O'Flaherty D, Husain MM, Moore M, et al: Circulatory responses during electroconvulsive therapy. The comparative effects of placebo, esmolol and nitroglycerin. Anaesthesia 47:563, 1992.
81. Pollan S, Tadjziechy M: Esmolol in the management of epinephrine- and cocaine-induced cardiovascular toxicity. Anesth Analg 69:663, 1989.
82. Sand IC, Brody SL, Wrenn KD, et al: Experience with esmolol for the treatment of cocaine-associated cardiovascular complications. Am J Emerg Med 9:161, 1991.
83. Brunette DD, Rothong C: Emergency department management of thyrotoxic crisis with esmolol. Am J Emerg Med 9:232, 1991.
84. Sra JS, Murthy VS, Jazayeri MR, et al: Use of intravenous esmolol to predict efficacy of oral beta-adrenergic blocker therapy in patients with neurocardiogenic syncope. J Am Coll Cardiol 19:402, 1992.
85. Koch-Weser J: Metoprolol. N Engl J Med 301:698, 1979.
86. Sheppard D, DiStefano S, Byrd RC, et al: Effects of esmolol on airway function in patients with asthma. J Clin Pharmacol 26:169, 1986.
87. Gold MR, Dec GW, Cocca-Spofford D, et al: Esmolol and ventilatory function in cardiac patients with COPD. Chest 100:1215, 1991.
88. Murthy VS, Patel KD, Elangovan RG, et al: Cardiovascular and neuromuscular effects of esmolol during induction of anesthesia. J Clin Pharmacol 26:351, 1986.
89. Barabas E, Kirkpatrick T, Zsigmond EK: Inhibitory effects of esmolol on human plasma cholinesterase in vitro [abstract]. Anesthesiology 6l(3A):A308, 1984.
90. McCammon RL, Hilgenberg JC, Sandage BW, et al: The effects of esmolol on the onset and duration of succinylcholine-induced neuromuscular blockade [abstract]. Anesthesiology 63(3A):A31, 1985.
91. Lowenthal DT, Porter RS, Saris SD, et al: Clinical pharmacology, pharmacodynamics and interactions with esmolol. Am J Cardiol 56:14F, 1985.
92. Sintetos AL, Hulse J, Pritchett ELC: Pharmacokinetics and pharmacodynamics of esmolol administered as an intravenous bolus. Clin Pharmacol Ther 41:112, 1987.
93. Frishman WH: Beta-adrenergic blocker withdrawal. Am J Cardiol 59(13):26F, 1987.
94. Trippel DL, Wiest DB, Gillette PC: Cardiovascular and antiarrhythmic effects of esmolol in children. J Pediatr 119:142, 1991.
95. Wiest DB, Trippel DL, Gillette PC, et al: Pharmacokinetics of esmolol in children. Clin Pharmacol Ther 49:618, 1991.
96. Ostman PL, Chestnut DH, Robillerd JE, et al: Transplacental passage and hemodynamic effects of esmolol in the gravid ewe. Anesthesiology 69:738, 1988.
97. Losasso TJ, Muzzi DA, Cucchiara RF: Response of fetal heart rate to maternal administration of esmolol. Anesthesiology 74:782, 1991.
98. Ducey JP, Gordon Knape K: Maternal esmolol administration resulting in fetal distress and cesarean section in a term pregnancy. Anesthesiology 77:829, 1992.

CHAPTER 55

Pindolol

Arie J. Man in't Veld, M.D., Ph.D., and Anton H. van den Meiracker, M.D.

HISTORY

The development of β-adrenoceptor antagonists began in 1948 with Ahlquist's discovery that sympathetic nervous activity is controlled by a single transmitter with two receptors, called α (alpha) and β (beta).[1] The α-receptors are generally associated with peripheral vasoconstriction, stimulation of the uterus, and pupillary dilation. β-Receptors control bronchodilation, vasodilation, uterine relaxation, and myocardial stimulation. The first therapeutic β-blocker (pronethalol) became available in 1962.[2] This was rapidly superseded by propranolol in 1964.[3] Pindolol, launched in Britain about 1969, was developed because of its relatively marked intrinsic sympathomimetic activity (ISA).[4]

CHEMISTRY

Structurally similar to isoproterenol and propranolol, pindolol (Fig. 55–1) is known chemically as 1-(1H-indol-4-yloxy)-3-[(1-methylethyl)amino]-2-propanol.

PHARMACOLOGY

Pindolol is a nonselective β-adrenoceptor antagonist. In addition to blocking β-adrenergic receptors, pindo-lol exerts some partial agonist activity, also referred to as ISA.[5] Evidence suggests that this ISA is selective for the β_2-adrenoceptor.[6] Pindolol has no membrane-stabilizing activity.[5]

PHARMACOKINETICS

After oral administration, pindolol is rapidly and almost completely absorbed. Food does not affect significantly the extent of absorption, but the rate may be increased.[7] The bioavailability after oral administration ranges from 50% to 100%, and the reported volume of distribution ranges between 1.2 and 2.0 L/kg.[8] Peak plasma concentrations are obtained within 2 hours after an oral dose.[9–13]

Approximately 50% to 70% of pindolol is bound to plasma proteins. Pindolol crosses the blood-brain barrier as reflected by changes in mood, sleep pattern, and the electroencephalogram.[5] It also crosses the placenta, and measurable concentrations are found in human milk.[14]

Elimination of pindolol is a first-order process with a half-life of 2.5 to 4.0 hours.[15] Approximately 35% to 50% of each dose of pindolol is excreted unchanged in the urine. In uremic patients (creatinine clearance, 1.2 L/hr), this value may be less than 15%. The part

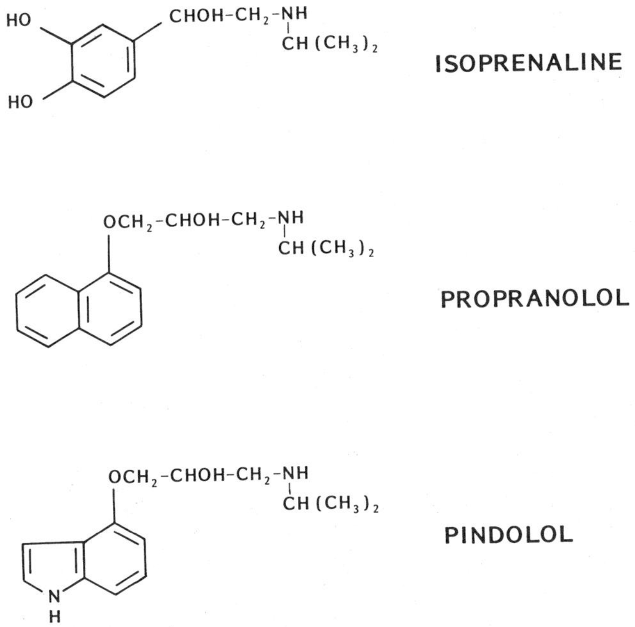

Figure 55–1. Chemical structures of isoprenaline, propranolol, and pindolol.

of pindolol not excreted in the urine is metabolized in the liver, principally to inactive conjugated glucuronides and sulfates; no active metabolites have been identified.[5]

In patients with severe hepatic impairment, clearance of pindolol may be reduced,[16] and dose reduction sometimes is required.[5] In patients with mild to moderate renal impairment, dosage adjustment is usually not necessary, because altered drug absorption and volume of distribution and increased nonrenal elimination may compensate for the reduction in renal excretion.

EFFECTS ON PATHOPHYSIOLOGY
Effects on Hemodynamics

Related to its relatively marked degree of ISA, the hemodynamic effects of pindolol differ from β-blockers lacking this property.[17–22] Thus, in contrast to β-blockers lacking ISA, acute administration of pindolol in a resting subject does not suppress heart rate unless cardiac sympathetic tone is relatively high. The threshold is between about 70 and 90 beats/min: below 70 beats/min, the heart rate increases; above 90, the heart rate decreases.[23] Also, unlike β-blockers without ISA, acute administration of pindolol to resting normotensive or hypertensive subjects has no suppressive effect on stroke volume or cardiac output.[19, 21, 24] Because of this absent cardiodepression, baroreflex-mediated vasoconstriction, which typically occurs after acute administration of β-blockers devoid of ISA, is not seen after acute administration of pindolol.[18, 20, 21]

During long-term administration of pindolol to hypertensive patients, cardiac output remains unchanged or increases slightly despite a reduction in blood pressure. This means that the hemodynamic mechanism underlying the blood pressure fall is a reduction in total systemic vascular resistance.[20, 22]

It should be noted that under circumstances of an increased cardiac sympathetic drive, as during exercise, pindolol acts much like other β-blockers, reducing exercise-induced increases in heart rate, cardiac output, and blood pressure.[25]

Effects on Ventricular Function and Structure

Under resting conditions, pindolol does not cause the depression of ventricular function associated with β-blockers devoid of ISA.[23] Thus, cardiac output, ejection fraction, and maximal rate of change of intraventricular pressure during isovolumetric contraction (dp/dt_{max}) are not reduced,[26] whereas left ventricular end-diastolic pressure, pulmonary artery pressure, and pulmonary capillary wedge pressure are not increased.[21, 24]

In hypertensive patients with impaired left ventricular fractional shortening as assessed by echocardiography, administration of pindolol for 15 weeks was associated with an improvement of ventricular function, whereas hypertensive patients with a normal pretreatment fractional shortening showed a small deterioration.[27] In a small study in patients with ischemic heart disease and a reduced resting ventricular ejection fraction, pindolol was associated with a higher ejection fraction, both at rest and during maximal exercise, compared with propranolol.[28] These beneficial effects of pindolol are most likely related to its ISA.

Studies on the effects of pindolol on left ventricular hypertrophy are scarce. Sau et al. showed a significant reduction in ventricular mass within 6 months of the initiation of therapy.[29] Vyssoulis et al. also demonstrated regression of left ventricular hypertrophy in 35 hypertensive patients treated with pindolol for an average of 31 weeks.[30]

Effects on Electrophysiology

At rest, pindolol has no effect on atrial conduction velocity, sinus node and corrected sinus node recovery times, or atrioventricular (AV) nodal or His-Purkinje conduction velocity, whereas acebutolol and atenolol prolong sinus node function and AV nodal conduction velocity.[31] However, during submaximal exercise, the effect of pindolol on sinus node and AV node function is similar to that of atenolol and acebutolol.

Although pindolol, like other β-blockers, has antiarrhythmic properties,[32] a single case report has described an increase in ventricular ectopic beats during pindolol treatment.[33]

Effects on Arteries and Veins

Plethysmographic studies in hypertensive patients have shown that long-term administration of pindolol, in contrast with metoprolol, is associated with a decrease in the resistance of the calf vascular bed.[34] Maarek et al.[35] reported an increase in brachial artery diameter, brachial artery blood flow, and forearm blood flow and a decrease in forearm vascular resistance and venous tone in hypertensive individuals treated with pindolol for 12 weeks.

Most likely, the vasodilatory effect of pindolol on peripheral arteries is partly mediated through stimulation of vascular β$_2$-adrenoceptors.[36]

In patients with intermittent claudication, resting calf blood flow does not change, and postexercise calf blood flow availability is decreased by pindolol.[37]

Metabolic and Endocrine Effects

Although blood glucose levels are usually not altered by pindolol, a decrease in insulin sensitivity during treatment with pindolol is detectable by the euglycemic clamp technique.[38] Catecholamine-induced glycogenolysis is impaired by pindolol, and blood glucose levels during and after ergometric exercise are lower with pindolol than with placebo or the β$_1$-selective blockers atenolol and acebutolol.[39]

Pindolol, unlike β-blockers devoid of ISA, has neutral or minimal effects on plasma triglyceride or total cholesterol levels.[40-42] In some studies, a favorable slight increase in high-density lipoprotein (HDL) cholesterol was detected.[42, 43] However, Vyssoulis et al. did not show any effect of pindolol on HDL cholesterol in either normolipidemic or dyslipidemic hypertensive patients.[44]

Pindolol appears to have less suppressing effect on plasma renin activity than β-blockers devoid of ISA,[18, 45] but stimulated plasma renin activity is suppressed equally by pindolol and propranolol.[46]

Resting plasma catecholamine concentrations are usually unaffected or moderately decreased during administration of pindolol.[18, 47-49] As with other β-blockers, the already elevated plasma catecholamine concentrations in response to exercise increase further during administration of pindolol.[49]

Effects on Renal Function

Rosenfeld et al. showed that acute administration of pindolol reduces the glomerular filtration rate and renal blood flow in patients with essential hypertension.[50] Because heart rate was also decreased in these patients, the authors attributed these negative effects to decreased cardiac output or increased renal vascular resistance. These data contrast with several long-term studies showing that pindolol has no adverse effects on glomerular filtration rate or renal blood flow.[24, 51, 52]

Effects on the Central Nervous System

Pindolol crosses the blood-brain barrier and causes central nervous system side effects.[5] It is hypothesized that part of the antihypertensive effect of pindolol is mediated via central vasomotor centers. Several stud-ies have shown that pindolol reduces plasma norepinephrine concentrations.[18] However, whether this reduction reflects a decrease in sympathetic nerve activity or an increase of the overall clearance of norepinephrine is not known.

CLINICAL USE
Indications

The principal indications for pindolol are hypertension, exercise-induced angina pectoris, and cardiac arrhythmias.

Hypertension

The antihypertensive effect of pindolol is similar to that of other β-blockers.[18] Pindolol monotherapy lowers daytime blood pressure by about 15%. Compared with this figure, the antihypertensive effect of pindolol is somewhat attenuated during the night, when sympathetic tone is low.[53] Like other β-blockers, pindolol does not cause orthostatic hypotension. Marks et al. have shown the efficacy of pindolol in controlling blood pressure in general practice.[54] In the Swedish Trial in Old Patients with Hypertension (STOP-Hypertension), the antihypertensive efficacy of pindolol has been compared with that of metoprolol, atenolol, and the combination of hydrochlorothiazide plus amiloride.[55] In these elderly hypertensive patients, pindolol was as effective as the other two β-blockers in terms of both blood pressure–lowering effect and responder rate.

In contrast with β-blockers devoid of ISA, the onset of the antihypertensive effect of pindolol after initiation of therapy is immediate.[56] Possibly, this is related to the absence of the initial reflex vasoconstriction in response to the fall in cardiac output, which occurs with β-blockers devoid of ISA.

Exercise-Induced Angina Pectoris

Because of the lack of heart rate reduction, or even increases in heart rate in patients with low sympathetic tone, pindolol should probably be avoided in patients with angina pectoris at rest or at low levels of exertion.[14]

However, in most cases of angina, pindolol protects the myocardium from the adverse effects of adrenergic hyperactivity, as in exercise or stress, and reduces cardiac oxygen consumption. Several placebo studies have shown that pindolol, 10 to 40 mg daily, reduces the frequency of angina attacks and nitroglycerin consumption.[5]

Cardiac Arrhythmias

The antiarrhythmic properties of pindolol result from antagonism of the effects of catecholamines on automaticity.[14] Fears that the ISA of pindolol would reduce its efficacy appear to be groundless. The drug is effective against both supraventricular and ventricular tachyarrhythmias as well as against thyrotoxicosis-induced arrhythmias.[14]

In patients with sick sinus syndrome who require β-blocker therapy for tachycardia or angina pectoris, pindolol, rather than propranolol, may be the drug of choice, because pindolol causes less sinus-node depression, which may obviate the need for prophylactic permanent pacemakers.[57]

Other Indications

In myocardial infarction, intravenous administration of pindolol, as opposed to a β-blocker devoid of ISA, does not reduce infarct size.[58] In the Australian and Swedish Pindolol Study Group,[59] early treatment (fewer than 5 days after infarct) with pindolol increased mortality compared with placebo, but later treatment (more than 12 days) was clearly beneficial in reducing the risk of death (12.9% versus 27.6% mortality rates).

Patients with hyperthyroidism experienced less nervousness and fewer palpitations with pindolol.[60] However, pindolol is less effective than propranolol in reducing thyrotoxic tachycardia.[61]

Like other β-blockers, pindolol reduces intraocular pressure in open-angle glaucoma when applied locally.[62, 63]

Precautions and Adverse Reactions

Congestive Heart Failure

Initiation of β-blockade in patients with a high sympathetic tone is associated with myocardial depression, even with pindolol. Sympathetic tone may be high to maintain cardiac output in patients with incipient heart failure. If pindolol is given to such patients, decompensation may occur. Severe pulmonary edema and circulatory collapse have been reported with pindolol.[5] Extreme caution should therefore be exercised in the institution of pindolol treatment in patients who show any sign of incipient heart failure.

Bronchospastic Disorders

In asthmatic patients in remission, pindolol, like other β-blockers, has little or no effect on forced expiratory volume in 1 second (FEV_1).[64] In asthmatics not in remission, administration of pindolol can cause a marked fall in FEV_1.[64] Furthermore, pindolol impairs the bronchodilatory effect of therapeutic doses of sympathomimetic agents.[45, 65, 66] Accordingly, pindolol should not be given to patients with bronchospastic disease.

Diabetes Mellitus

Pindolol should be used with caution in diabetes mellitus, because the hypoglycemic effects of insulin may be enhanced and prolonged. Furthermore, the symptoms of hypoglycemia, such as tachycardia, may be masked. Severe hypoglycemic incidents have occurred in diabetic patients taking pindolol.[5]

Atrioventricular Block

Experimentally, pindolol increases AV nodal conduction time; clinically, it may cause AV dissociation or cardiac arrest in patients with digitalis-induced AV node conduction disturbances.[5]

Withdrawal of Treatment

Pindolol should be withdrawn cautiously, particularly in patients with angina pectoris, because it may increase the frequency of angina attacks.[5] Treatment should therefore be tapered off over at least 2 weeks. Compared with β-blockers devoid of ISA, pindolol may be safer in this respect, because the drug does not upregulate β-adrenoreceptors and does not cause supersensitivity to catecholamines.[67–69]

Pregnancy

Because relevant data are inadequate, the use of pindolol in early pregnancy cannot be recommended. Montan et al. showed that pindolol, in contrast with atenolol, had no adverse effects on fetal hemodynamics in women with pregnancy-induced hypertension who were in the third trimester of pregnancy, despite a similar reduction in blood pressure.[70] Placental weight was significantly lower in the atenolol than in the pindolol group, but there was no difference in birthweight.

Adverse Reactions

The adverse effects commonly observed with pindolol are summarized in Table 55–1. These effects are generally mild, are not dose-related, and occur relatively early in treatment.[5] In a general practice study in more than 7000 patients, the incidence of side effects tended to decrease over the course of the 6-week study.[54]

Weight gain in patients on pindolol is believed to be unrelated to treatment, but edema has been reported more frequently with pindolol than with placebo.[14] Persistent but minor increases in serum transaminases occur in approximately 7% of patients.[14] No adverse hematologic or renal effects of pindolol have been reported.[5]

Contraindications

Pindolol should not be used in patients with bronchial asthma, second- or third-degree AV block, severe bradycardia, or heart failure. Because pindolol is excreted in breast milk, its use should be avoided in nursing mothers.

Interference with Other Drugs

Cimetidine stereoselectively inhibits the renal clearance of pindolol, and coadministration of pindolol and cimetidine is associated with a 36% increase in pindolol blood levels.[71]

Table 55–1. **Reported Adverse Effects of Oral Pindolol Therapy**

	Frequency of Reporting (%)		
Adverse Effect	Golightly	Rosenthal	Crowder & Cameron
Cardiovascular			
Palpitations	0.4	—	0.6
Central Nervous System			
Fatigue, lassitude	4.8	3.00	4.7
Unusual dreams or nightmares	6.2 ⎫		—
Insomnia or sleep disturbances	3.2 ⎬	3.50	1.7
Dizziness	3.1	8.10	9.0
Depression	1.5	—	0.8
Headache	1.7	4.90	3.5
Nervousness or irritability	0.8	—	—
Hallucinations	0.3	—	—
Lightheadedness	—	—	2.4
Gastrointestinal			
Nausea, indigestion, or abdominal discomforts	2.0	7.50	7.5
Dry mouth or nose	1.4	0.20	0.5
Diarrhea or loose stools	0.4	—	0.7
Genitourinary			
Impotence or decreased libido	0.8	0.03	—
Musculoskeletal			
Muscle or leg cramps	2.7	—	2.0
Cold extremities	0.8	—	0.8
Tremor	0.5	1.00	0.7
Pulmonary			
Dyspnea or wheezing	0.9	0.80	—

Data from Golightly LK: Pindolol: A review of its pharmacology, pharmacokinetics, clinical uses, and adverse effects. Pharmacotherapy 2:134, 1982.

Although pindolol has been reported to cause a decrease in plasma digoxin levels,[72] the suppressive effect of digitalis on AV conduction and pindolol's effects are additive; close electrocardiographic monitoring is advised if the two drugs are used together.[5]

Care should be exercised when using insulin or oral hypoglycemic drugs in combination with pindolol because of the potential for masking and augmenting the hypoglycemic effects of these agents.[5]

Use in Patients with Impaired Organ Function

Dosage reduction of pindolol is not necessary in patients with mild or moderate renal insufficiency. In patients with *severe* renal failure, the elimination half-life of pindolol is increased two to five times;[73] in this situation, a twofold dosage reduction is recommended.

In patients with liver cirrhosis and low antipyrine clearance, pindolol is accumulated.[16] Accordingly, a reduction of the dosage of pindolol in this condition is necessary.

Dosage and Administration

The recommended starting oral dosage for pindolol in hypertension is 5 mg daily with increases of 5 mg daily at 1- or 2-week intervals. Because of the flat dose-response curve,[74] little additive blood pressure–lowering effect might be expected from dosages above 20 mg daily. When antihypertensive response is inadequate, one should consider combination with one of the other classes of antihypertensive agents rather than increasing the dosage of pindolol above 20 mg daily.

In angina pectoris, the recommended oral dosage of pindolol is 5 mg three times daily, and in arrhythmias, the recommended oral dosage is 5 to 10 mg three times daily.

REFERENCES

1. Ahlquist RP: A study of adrenotropic receptors. Am J Physiol 153:586, 1948.
2. Black JW, Stephenson JS: Pharmacology of a new adrenergic beta-receptor blocking compound. Lancet 2:311, 1962.
3. Kendall MJ, Smith SR: Adrenergic blocking agents. J Clin Hosp Pharm 8:155, 1983.
4. Northcote RJ: The clinical significance of intrinsic sympathomimetic activity. Int J Cardiol 15:133, 1987.
5. Golightly LK: Pindolol: A review of its pharmacology, pharmacokinetics, clinical uses, and adverse effects. Pharmacotherapy 2:134, 1982.
6. Clark B: Pharmacological analysis of the intrinsic sympathomimetic activity of pindolol: Evidence for selective beta-2-adrenoceptor stimulation. Triangle 23:33, 1984.
7. Kiger JL, Lavene D, Guillaume MF, et al: The effect of food and clopamide on the absorption of pindolol in man. Int J Clin Pharmacol Biopharm 13:228, 1976.
8. Riddell JG, Harron DWG, Shanks RG: Clinical pharmacokinetics of beta-adrenoceptor antagonists: An update. Clin Pharmacokinet 12:305, 1987.
9. Gugler R, Bodem G: Single and multiple dose pharmacokinetics of pindolol. Eur J Clin Pharmacol 13:13, 1978.
10. Gugler R, Herold W, Dengler HJ: Pharmacokinetics of pindolol in man. Eur J Clin Pharmacol 7:17, 1974.
11. Jennings GL, Bobik A, Faga ET, et al: Pindolol pharmacokinetics in relation to time course of inhibition of exercise tachycardia. Br J Clin Pharmacol 7:245, 1979.

12. Salako LA, Falase AO, Aderoumu AF: Comparative beta-adrenoceptor-blocking effects and pharmacokinetics of propranolol and pindolol in hypertensive Africans. Clin Sci 57(Suppl 5):393S, 1979.

13. Salako LA, Falase AO, Ragon A, et al: Beta-adrenoceptor blocking effects and pharmacokinetics of pindolol: A study in hypertensive Africans. Eur J Clin Pharmacol 15:299, 1979.

14. Frishman WH: Pindolol: A new beta-adrenoceptor antagonist with partial agonist activity. N Engl J Med 308:940, 1983.

15. American Hospital Pharmacists Society: Pindolol. In McEvoy GK, McQuarrie GM (eds): Drug Information. Bethesda, MD: American Society of Hospital Pharmacists, 1987, pp 852–854.

16. Ohnhaus EE, Munch U, Meier J: Elimination of pindolol in liver disease. Eur J Clin Pharmacol 22:247, 1982.

17. Clark BJ: The pharmacology of pindolol: Analysis of its intrinsic sympathomimetic acitivity. Vasc Med 3:17, 1985.

18. Man in't Veld AJ, Schalekamp MADH: How intrinsic sympathomimetic activity modulates the haemodynamic responses to beta-adrenoceptor antagonists: A clue to the nature of their antihypertensive mechanism. Br J Clin Pharmacol 13(Suppl 2):245S, 1982.

19. Svendsen T, Hartling O, Trap Jensen J: Immediate haemodynamic effects of propranolol, practolol, pindolol, atenolol and ICI 89,406 in healthy volunteers. Eur J Clin Pharmacol 15:223, 1979.

20. Man in't Veld AJ, van den Meiracker AH, Schalekamp MADH: The effect of beta-blockers on total peripheral resistance. J Cardiovasc Pharmacol 8(Suppl 4):S49, 1986.

21. van den Meiracker AH, Man in't Veld AJ, Ritsema van Eck HJ, et al: Hemodynamic and hormonal adpatations to beta-adrenoceptor blockade: A 24-hour study of acebutolol, atenolol, pindolol and propranolol in hypertensive patients. Circulation 78:957, 1988.

22. van den Meiracker AH, Man in't Veld AJ, Boomsma F, et al: Hemodynamic and β-adrenergic receptor adaptations during long-term β-adrenoceptor blockade. Studies with acebutolol, atenolol, pindolol, and propranolol in hypertensive patients. Circulation 80:903, 1989.

23. Kostis JB, DeFelice EA: The hemodynamic effect of pindolol. Curr Ther Res Clin Exp 33:494, 1983.

24. van den Meiracker AH, Man in't Veld AJ, Ritsema van Eck HJ, et al: Systemic and renal vasodilation after beta-adrenoceptor blockade with pindolol: A hemodynamic study on the onset and maintenance of its antihypertensive effect. Am Heart J 112:368, 1986.

25. Lund Johansen P: Central haemodynamic effects of beta-blockers in hypertension. A comparison between atenolol, metoprolol, timolol, penbutolol, alprenolol, pindolol and bunitrolol. Eur Heart J 4(Suppl D):1, 1983.

26. Rousseau MF, Pouleur H, Debaisieux JC, et al: Contrasting effects of two beta-adrenoceptor partial agonists, pindolol and Corwin, on left ventricular diastolic function. Eur Heart J 5(Suppl 1):273, 1984.

27. Plotnick GD, Fisher ML, Wohl B, et al: Improvement in depressed cardiac function in hypertensive patients during pindolol treatment. Am J Med 76:25, 1984.

28. Gebhardt VA, Wisenberg G: The role of beta blockade, with and without intrinsic sympathomimetic activity, in preserving compromised left ventricular function in patients with ischemic heart diasease. Am Heart J 109:1013, 1985

29. Sau F, Seguro C, Cherchi A: Regression of left ventricular hypertrophy after antihypertensive therapy by pindolol [abstract]. 11th Scientific Meeting of the International Society of Hypertension, Heidelberg, 1986, p 413.

30. Vyssoulis GP, Karpanou EA, Pitsavos CE, et al: Regression of left ventricular hypertrophy in systemic hypertension with beta blockers (propranolol, atenolol, metoprolol, pindolol and celiprolol). Am J Cardiol 70:1209, 1992.

31. Hombach V, Braun V, Höpp HW, et al: Electrophysiological effects of cardioselective and non-cardioselective beta-adrenoceptor blockers with and without ISA at rest and during exercise. Br J Clin Pharmacol 13:285S, 1982.

32. Podrid PJ, Lown B: Pindolol for ventricular arrhythmia. Am Heart J 104:491, 1982.

33. Binkley PF, Lewe R, Lima J, et al: Enhanced ventricular ectopy following pindolol: An adverse effect of a beta-blocker with intrinsic sympathomimetic activity. Am Heart J 112:424, 1986.

34. Svensson A, Gudbrandsson T, Sivertsson R, Hansson L: Haemodynamic effects of metoprolol and pindolol: A comparison in hypertensive patients. Br J Clin Pharmacol 13:259S, 1982.

35. Maarek B, Simon A Ch, Levenson J, et al: Chronic effects of pindolol on the arterioles, large arteries, and veins of the forearm in mild to moderate essential hypertension. Clin Pharmacol Ther 39:403, 1986.

36. Chang P, Van Brummelen P: Acute vasodilator action of pindolol in humans. Hypertension 1:146, 1988.

37. Roberts DH, Tsao Y, McLoughlin GA, Beckenbridge A: Placebo-controlled comparison of captopril, atenolol, labetolol, and pindolol in hypertension complicated by intermittent claudication. Lancet 2:650, 1987.

38. Litthell HOL: Effect of antihypertensive drugs on insuline, glucose and lipid metabolism. Diabetes Care 14:203, 1991.

39. Koch G, Franz IW, Lohmann FW: Effects of short-term and long-term treatment with cardio-selective and non-selective beta-receptor blockade on carbohydrate and lipid metabolism and on plasma catecholamines at rest and during exercise. Clin Sci 61(Suppl 7):433S, 1981.

40. Ames RP: The effects of antihypertensive drugs on serum lipids and lipoproteins II: Non-diuretic drugs. Drugs 32:335, 1986.

41. Chanu B, Rouffy J, Noseda G, et al: Comparative study of the effects of pindolol and atenolol on blood lipids. Cur Ther Res 49:588, 1991

42. Pasotti C, Capra A, Fiorelli G, et al: Effects of pindolol and metoprolol on plasma lipids and lipoproteins. Br J Clin Pharmacol 13:435S, 1982.

43. Sasaki J, Saku K, Ideishi M, et al: Effects of pindolol on serum lipids, apolipoproteins, and lipoprotiens in patients with mild to moderate essential hypertension. Clin Ther 11:219, 1989

44. Vyssoulis GP, Karpanou EA, Pitsavos CE, et al: Differentiation of β-blocker effects on serum lipids and apolipoproteins in hypertensive patients with normolipidaemic or dyslipidaemic profiles. Eur Heart J 13:1506, 1992.

45. Morgan TO, Roberts R, Carney SL, et al: Beta-adrenergic blocking drugs, hypertension and plasma renin. Br J Clin Pharmacol 2:159, 1975

46. Harms HH, Gooren L, Spoelstra AJG, et al: Blockade of isoprenaline-induced changes in plasma free fatty acids, immunoreactive insulin levels and plasma renin activity in healthy human subjects, by propranolol, pindolol, practolol, atenolol, metoprolol and acebutolol. Br J Clin Pharmacol 5:19, 1976.

47. Anavekar SN, Louis WJ, Morgan TO, et al: The relationship of plasma levels of pindolol in hypertensive patients to effects on blood pressure, plasma renin and plasma noradrenaline levels. Clin Exp Pharmacol Physiol 2:203, 1975.

48. Kirsten R, Heintz B, Bohmer D, et al: Relationship of plasma catecholamines to blood pressure in hypertensive patients during beta-adrenoceptor blockade with and without intrinsic sympathomimetic activity. Br J Clin Pharmacol 13:397S, 1982.

49. Dominiak P, Grobecker H: Elevated plasma catecholamines in young hypertensive and hyperkinetic patients: Effect of pindolol. Br J Clin Pharmacol 13:318S, 1982.

50. Rosenfeld J, Boner G, Wianer E: Renal function during acute and long-term pindolol treatment in hypertensive patients with normal and decreased glomerular filtration. Br J Clin Pharmacol 13:238S, 1982.

51. Pasternach A, Pörsti P, Pöyhönen L: Effect of pindolol and propranolol on renal function of patients with hypertension. Br J Clin Pharmacol 13:241S, 1982.

52. Wilcox CS, Lewis PS, Peart WS, et al: Renal function, body fluid volumes, renin, aldosterone and noradrenaline during treatment of hypertension with pindolol. J Cardiovasc Pharmacol 3:598, 1981.

53. Mann S, Millar Graig MW, Balasubramanian V, Raftery EB: Once daily beta-adrenoceptor blockade in hypertension: An ambulatory assessment. Br J Clin Pharmacol 12:223, 1981.

54. Marks AD, Finestone A, Sobel E, et al: An office based primary care trial of pindolol ("Visken") in essential hypertension. Curr Med Res Opin 10:296, 1986.

55. Ekbom T, Dahlöf B, Hansson L, et al: Antihypertensive efficacy and side effects of three beta-blockers and a diuretic in eldery hypertensives: A report from the STOP-Hypertension study. J Hypertens 10:1525, 1992.
56. van den Meiracker AH, Man in't Veld AJ, Ritsema van Eck HJ, et al: Direct 24-hour haemodynamic monitoring after starting beta-blocker therapy: Studies with pindolol in hypertension. J Hypertens 2(Suppl 3):581, 1984.
57. Strickeberger SA, Fish RD, Lamas GA: Comparison of effects of propanolol versus pindolol on sinus rate and pacing frequency in sick sinus syndrome. Am J Cardiol 71:531, 1993.
58. Owensby DA, O'Rourke MF: Failure of intravenous pindolol to reduce the hemodynamic determinants of myocardial oxygen demand or enzymatically determined infarct size in acute myocardial infarction. Aust N Z J Med 15:704, 1985.
59. Australian and Swedish Pindolol Study Group: The effect of pindolol on the two years mortality after complicated myocardial infaction. Eur Heart J 4:367, 1983.
60. Schelling JL, Scazziga B, Dufour RJ, et al: Effect of pindolol, a beta-adrenoceptor antagonist, in hyperthyroidism. Clin Pharmacol Ther 14:158, 1973.
61. Turner P: Beta-adrenergic blocking drugs in hyperthyroidism. Drugs 7:48, 1974.
62. Smith RJH, Blamires T, Nagasubramanian S, et al: Addition of pindolol to routine medical therapy: A clinical trial. Br J Ophthalmol 66:102, 1982.
63. Andreasson S, Jensen KM: Effect of pindolol on intraocular pressure in glaucoma: Pilot study and a randomised comparison with timolol. Br J Ophthalmol 67:228, 1983.
64. Benson MK, Berrill WT, Cruickshank JM, Sterling GS: A comparison of four beta-adrenoceptor antagonists in patients with asthma. Br J Clin Pharmacol 5:415, 1978.
65. Christensen CC, Boye NP, Erikson H, Hansen G: Influence of pindolol (Visken) on respiratory function in 20 asthmatic patients. Eur J Clin Pharmacol 13:9, 1978.
66. Ruffin RE, McIntyre ELM, Latimer KM, et al: Assessment of beta-adrenoceptor antagonists in asthmatic patients. Br J Clin Pharmacol 13:325S, 1982.
67. van den Meiracker AH, Man in't Veld AJ, Molinoff PB, et al: Effects of pindolol and propranolol on haemodynamics and lymphocyte beta-receptors in essential hypertension. J Cardiovasc Pharmacol 10(Suppl 4):S55, 1987.
68. Rangno RE, Langois S: Comparison of withdrawal phenomena after propranolol, metoprolol and pindolol. Am Heart J 104:473, 1982.
69. Walden RJ, Hernandez J, Yu Y, et al: Withdrawal of beta-blocking drugs. Am Heart J 104:515, 1982.
70. Montan S, Ingemarsson I, Marsál K, Sjöberg NS: Randomised controlled trial of atenolol and pindolol in human pregnancy: Effects on fetal haemodynamics. Br Med J 304:946, 1992.
71. Mutschler E, Spahn H, Kirch W: The interaction between H₂-receptor antagonists and beta-adrenoceptor blockers. Br J Clin Pharmacol 17(Suppl 1):51S, 1984.
72. Schwarz HJ: Pharmacokinetics of pindolol in humans and several animal species. Am Heart J 104:357, 1982.
73. Ohnhaus EE, Heidemann H, Meier J, Maurer G: Metabolism of pindolol in patients with renal failure. Eur J Clin Pharmacol 22:423, 1982.
74. Frishman WH, Costis J: The significance of intrinsic sympathomimetic activity in beta-adrenoceptor blocking drugs. Cardiovasc Rev Rep 3:503, 1982.

C. Cardioselective β-Adrenoreceptor Blockers

CHAPTER 56

Metoprolol

Åke Hjalmarson, M.D., Ph.D., Gunnar Olsson, M.D., Ph.D., Göran Bondjers, M.D., Ph.D., Carl Dahlöf, M.D., Ph.D., Anders Sandberg, M.Sc., Bengt Åblad, M.D., Ph.D., Ingela Wiklund, Ph.D., and John Wikstrand, M.D., Ph.D.

Several comprehensive review articles describe in detail the pharmacokinetic and pharmacodynamic properties of metoprolol.[1-3] This chapter, therefore, focuses mainly on the important long-term therapeutic effects of metoprolol. Important reported data that have not been previously reviewed also are included.

Since metoprolol was introduced in 1975, the drug has been shown to be of value in hypertension,[4-8] angina pectoris,[9-15] certain arrhythmias,[16-27] primary[5] and secondary prevention of cardiovascular diseases,[16, 17, 28-33] and migraine.[34, 35] Furthermore, long-term administration for hypertension reduces left ventricular hypertrophy[7, 8] and decreases total peripheral resistance.[7, 8] Long-term data on safety are good. The therapeutic range and tolerance have been improved by controlled-release preparations.

PHARMACOKINETIC AND PHARMACODYNAMIC PROPERTIES

Metoprolol is the first described β₁-selective blocker devoid of intrinsic sympathomimetic activity.[2] The drug has little or no membrane-stabilizing activity. The octanol-water partition coefficient at pH 7.4, +37°C is 0.98. Metoprolol is a basic drug with a pKₐ of 9.6. The volume of distribution is approximately 5.6 L/kg. Protein binding is less than 10%. Metoprolol is extensively metabolized by the hepatic monooxygenase system and is excreted, only to a minor degree, via urine (approximately 3%). Its biologic half-life is approximately 3 to 4 hours; no active metabolites exist.[36]

Absorption from the gastrointestinal tract is almost

complete, although extensive first-pass hepatic metabolism reduces systemic availability by approximately 50%. The duodenum, jejunum, ileum, and colon have similar capacities for absorption, apparently by first-order kinetics. After long-term treatment, systemic availability increases. Partial saturation of the first-pass effect, reduced hepatic blood flow, or both may explain this change.

In an extensive study with the radioligand binding technique,[37] using tissue from rats, guinea pigs, and humans, the affinity of metoprolol for β_1-adrenoreceptors was shown to be about 30 times higher than its affinity for β_2-adrenoreceptors. The results of *in vivo* studies in humans and animals show that metoprolol is a potent inhibitor of β-receptor–mediated effects mainly involving β_1-adrenoreceptors. Such effects include not only reduction of exercise-induced tachycardia but also antihypertensive and cardiac antianginal and antiarrhythmic effects.[1–3] On the other hand, compared with nonselective β-blockers, metoprolol has been shown to cause only minor inhibition of mainly β_2-receptor–mediated effects, such as the vasodilator response to epinephrine and the bronchodilator response to terbutaline.[1–3]

So far, there is no basis for assuming that the clinical effects described for metoprolol involve actions other than those due to β-blockade. It is important to note, however, that the integrated pattern of metoprolol's effects may be influenced by the pharmacokinetic properties of the drug. As a moderately lipophilic drug, metoprolol has been shown to be rapidly and effectively distributed into underperfused tissues such as ischemic myocardium after acute coronary artery occlusion in dogs, pigs, and cats.[37] Comparative studies were done with the hydrophilic blocker atenolol, which has the same degree of β_1-selectivity as metoprolol.[37] Atenolol was distributed much less effectively to the ischemic myocardium than was metoprolol. This distribution difference was associated with a marked divergence in antiischemic effects in the ischemic regions of the left ventricle as studied in cats with constant heart rate. Metoprolol exerted an antiischemic effect, as shown by biochemical, electrocardiographic, and hemodynamic data. Atenolol, however, did not cause any corresponding effect.

PRIMARY PREVENTION OF CORONARY ARTERY DISEASE
Hypertension

The goal of treating patients with hypertension is to prevent morbidity and mortality associated with high blood pressure and to control blood pressure by the least intrusive means possible.[38] Pooled analyses of all studies performed with thiazide diuretics in patients with hypertension have shown a 40% reduction in stroke but only a modest 8% to 10% beneficial effect on coronary events.[39] The lack of a risk reduction in coronary events is a great problem because the risk for coronary events is even greater than the risk for

stroke in most patients with hypertension.[40] The high mortality rate from coronary artery disease in hypertensive patients can be substantially reduced only if the treatment can reduce the risk of sudden death.[41] Clinical trials have not yet produced long-term prognostic data on the effects of angiotensin-converting enzyme (ACE) inhibitors, calcium antagonists, or α-blockers on cardiovascular complications and sudden death in hypertensive patients.[38] There are many possible mechanisms, apart from the antihypertensive effect, by which a β-blocker may lower the risk for coronary events in hypertensive patients. These include antiatherosclerotic effects, antithrombotic effects, cardiac antiischemic effects, and antifibrillatory effects.[42]

In the Metoprolol Atherosclerosis Prevention in Hypertensives (MAPHY) study,[5, 40, 43, 44] a primary preventive study in 3234 hypertensive men aged 40 to 64 years with untreated diastolic blood pressure above 100 mmHg, the main aim was to investigate whether metoprolol given as initial treatment would prevent coronary events better than thiazide diuretics. The results showed that total mortality was lower in patients randomized to metoprolol than in those randomized to thiazide diuretics ($p = .028$).[5] The reduction in relative risk was independent of absolute risk and demographic differences (Fig. 56–1).[40] The explanation for the reduced risk for total mortality was a reduced risk for sudden cardiovascular deaths ($p = .017$) (Fig. 56–2).[44]

The morbidity results support the conclusions from the mortality data.[40] Altogether, 255 patients suffered a definite coronary event—sudden death or a fatal or definite nonfatal acute or silent myocardial infarction—during the course of the trial. The incidence of coronary events was significantly lower during follow-up in patients randomized to metoprolol than in patients randomized to diuretics: 111 versus 144 cases, respectively ($p = .001$), and a risk ratio of 0.76 for metoprolol-treated patients at the end of the trial (95% confidence interval for end of trial data, 0.58 to 0.98) (Fig. 56–3). There was no difference in stroke rates between the two treatment groups (see Fig. 56–3).

Post hoc subgroup analyses also showed that the incidence of all first definite coronary events (fatal plus nonfatal) was significantly lower in nonsmoking patients receiving metoprolol than in nonsmoking patients receiving diuretics ($p = .0008$).[40] Furthermore, total mortality and coronary artery disease mortality were significantly lower in smokers receiving metoprolol than in smokers receiving diuretics ($p = .012$ and $p = .021$, respectively).[5, 43] In addition, the risk for combined fatal and definite nonfatal coronary events tended to be lower in smokers receiving metoprolol, although the difference in risk did not reach the level of formal statistical significance ($p = .09$).[40] In the whole study population, as well as in subgroups of nonsmokers and smokers, the incidence of all first definite and possible coronary events was significantly lower in patients receiving metoprolol compared with patients receiving diuretics.[40]

An analysis of cost-effectiveness of hypertensive

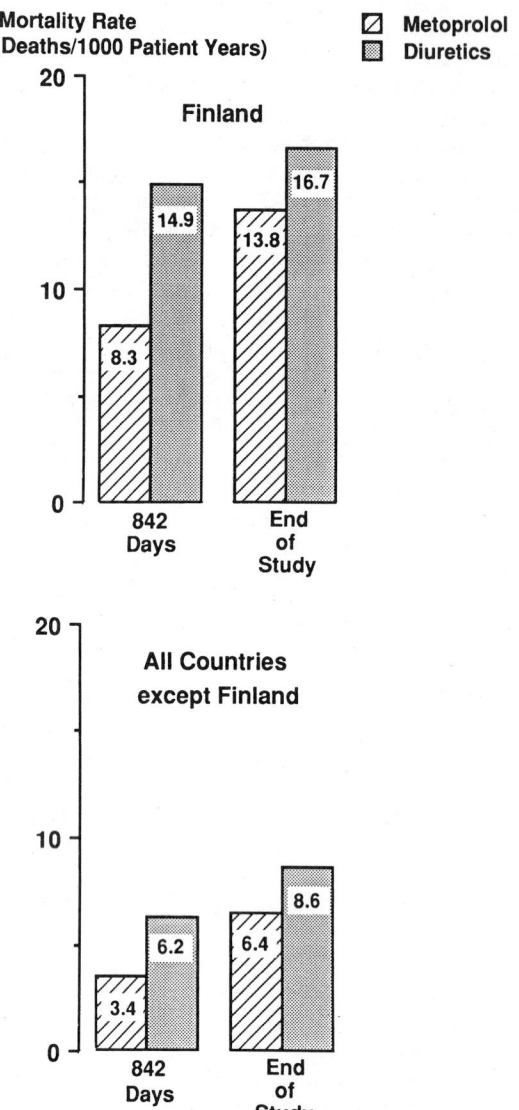

Figure 56–1. Cumulative mortality rates in patients from Finland and in patients from other countries except Finland at shortest common follow-up period for all patients (842 days) and at the end of the Metoprolol Atherosclerosis Prevention in Hypertensives (MAPHY) study. The reduction in relative risk by metoprolol was similar in different risk groups and thus seemed to be independent of risk level. (Reproduced with permission from Wikstrand J, Warnold I, Tuomilehto J, et al: Metoprolol versus thiazide diuretics in hypertension. Morbidity results from the MAPHY study. Hypertension 17:579, 1991. Copyright 1991 American Heart Association.)

treatment based on the results from the MAPHY study showed that metoprolol was more cost-effective than thiazide diuretics because of the more favorable effect on coronary events.[45]

Comment

Results from primary and secondary preventive studies with β-blockers have not been uniform, and the publication of the results from the MAPHY study aroused great interest as well as a number of comments in the literature.[40, 42, 46] Investigators have sought to understand the role of β-blockers, particu-

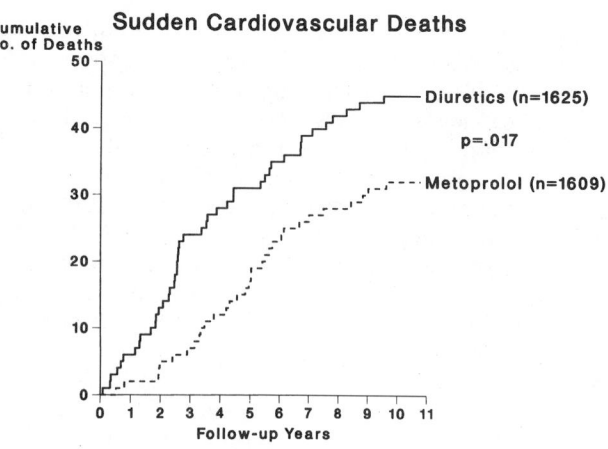

Figure 56–2. Cumulative numbers of sudden cardiovascular deaths in the MAPHY study. The p value refers to the difference in the survival experience between the two randomization groups during the entire study period. (From Olsson G, Tuomilehto J, Berglund G, et al: Primary prevention of sudden cardiovascular death in hypertensive patients: Mortality results from the MAPHY study. Am J Hypertens 4:151, 1991.)

larly in relation to sudden death; clinical and experimental data indicate that not only sympathetic tone but also vagal tone is important in the control of cardiac electrical stability and the risk of sudden death.[46] A preliminary report on studies in animals found that metoprolol counteracted a stress-induced reduction in vagal tone and that such an effect might contribute to the prevention of spontaneous ventricular fibrillation and sudden death.[47] Skinner[48] and Parker et al.[49] have presented a theoretical model for brain regulation of cardiac vulnerability. Their experimental data indicate that β_1-blockade within the brain

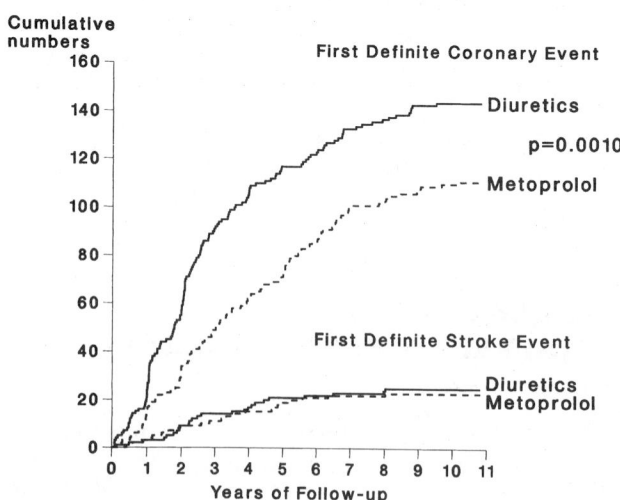

Figure 56–3. Cumulative numbers for all first definite coronary events and stroke events in the two randomization groups. The p value refers to difference in risk between the two randomization groups during the entire study period. (Reproduced with permission from Wikstrand J, Warnold I, Tuomilehto J, et al: Metoprolol versus thiazide diuretics in hypertension. Morbidity results from the MAPHY study. Hypertension 17:579, 1991. Copyright 1991 American Heart Association.)

may decrease the risk of ventricular fibrillation and sudden death by favorably affecting central nervous system control of cardiac electrical stability. Sudden death is the leading cause of death in patients with hypertension, and a reduced risk of sudden death is the major reason for the reduction in total mortality seen with β-blockers.[50] To date, the best documented data cover the lipophilic β-blockers, and it is speculated that counteracting a stress-induced reduction in cardiac vagal tone in combination with cardiac β₁-blockade and antiischemic action results in a reduction in sudden death risk as seen with these β-blockers.[46]

Hypertension in the Elderly

In a randomized, double-blind study of 562 elderly hypertensive patients (60 to 75 years of age), a traditional antihypertensive treatment schedule, starting with hydrochlorothiazide, 25 mg once daily, which was doubled if there was an unsatisfactory response, was compared with antihypertensive treatment with metoprolol, 100 mg once daily, adding hydrochlorothiazide, 12.5 mg daily, if the response was not satisfactory with metoprolol alone.[6]

Both regimens reduced systolic and diastolic blood pressures equally well. Approximately 70% of previously untreated patients responded to the metoprolol regimen after 4 weeks of treatment. A positive response was defined as diastolic blood pressure less than or equal to 95 mmHg or mean arterial pressure reduction greater than or equal to 10%. The response rate was similar in different age groups. In nonresponders to metoprolol monotherapy, the addition of a low-dose diuretic controlled blood pressure.

There were no differences between the two groups in total change in the pattern of symptoms. Sleep disturbances that have been associated with β-blockers were not a problem for patients on the metoprolol regimen; on the contrary, reports of insomnia were significantly fewer in the group treated with metoprolol in single or combination therapy compared with baseline. Dyspnea and other symptoms related to physical activity were no more common after metoprolol therapy than after hydrochlorothiazide therapy. This may be explained by the β-blocker–induced decrease in heart rate, resulting in increases in both diastolic filling time and coronary perfusion time. This effect may be particularly important in an aging, stiff, hypertensive heart. No serious metabolic side effects were observed with metoprolol, whereas more patients taking diuretics showed hypokalemia and hyperuricemia.

An efficacy-tolerance index that accounted for blood pressure response, subjective symptoms, and metabolic side effects favored the metoprolol regimen, both in the total study population and in previously untreated patients.[6] The results from this large-scale, double-blind study show that metoprolol in single or combination therapy is efficient, safe, and well-tolerated in elderly hypertensive patients. Furthermore, results from the MAPHY study[5, 40, 43, 44]

and from the Swedish Trial in Old Patients with Hypertension (STOP-Hypertension) study[51] indicate a favorable effect on the prognosis for both myocardial infarction and sudden cardiovascular death, as well as for stroke. This is clinically important because of the high risk for cardiovascular complications in elderly hypertensive patients.

Cardiovascular Effects of Very-long-term Treatment

Ultimately, therapy in patients with hypertension should not only lower blood pressure but also cause regression of structural adaptive changes, restore normotensive homeostasis, and improve long-term prognosis. Two studies of long-term metoprolol therapy with repeat echocardiographic examinations have shown reversal of left ventricular hypertrophy and restoration of normal hemodynamics. In the first study, the examinations were performed every 6 months over a 2-year period.[7] In the other study, examinations were performed before and after 7 years of treatment.[8] In the first study, an initial decrease in cardiac output was recorded 6 months after initiation of treatment and was caused by reduced heart rate and stroke volume. The reduction in stroke volume was due to a decrease in left ventricular end-diastolic diameter and not to an increase in end-systolic volume or a decrease in contractility. Thus, the positive effect of a decrease in afterload induced by metoprolol overrides any negative effect of β-blockade on left ventricular contractility.

As shown in Figure 56–4, the hemodynamic conditions of patients during the initial year of treatment differed in several respects from those after 2 years, when cardiac output had returned to pretreatment levels. This late increase in cardiac output reported by Wikstrand et al.[7] in this study was explained by an increase in left ventricular end-diastolic volume, probably reflecting improvement in left ventricular compliance. In agreement with this observation, Hartford et al.,[8] in another study, reported normalization of disturbances in left ventricular relaxation, left ventricular filling pattern, and distensibility after 7 years of metoprolol treatment.

Both studies showed that long-term metoprolol treatment reduces left ventricular thickness and peak and end-systolic wall stress, the latter resulting in an increase in coronary reserve. Thus, the long-term effect on oxygen supply and demand in the left ventricle clearly is beneficial.

The blood pressure reduction after long-term antihypertensive treatment with metoprolol is explained by a decrease in total peripheral resistance.[7, 8] This has been observed both in patients receiving metoprolol as monotherapy in the study published by Wikstrand et al.[7] and in those receiving combination therapy, as in the study by Hartford et al.[8] In the latter study, minimal vascular resistance in the calf at maximal dilation was reduced, indicating reversal of hypertrophy in arterial resistance vessels.

A strong case can be made for the importance of

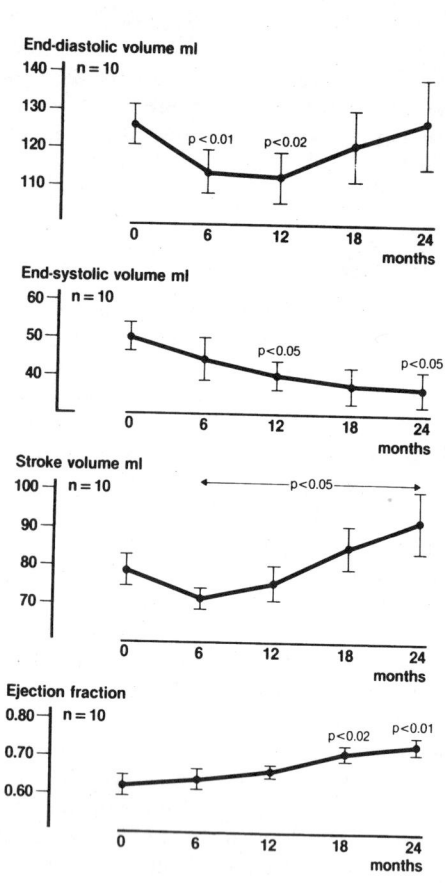

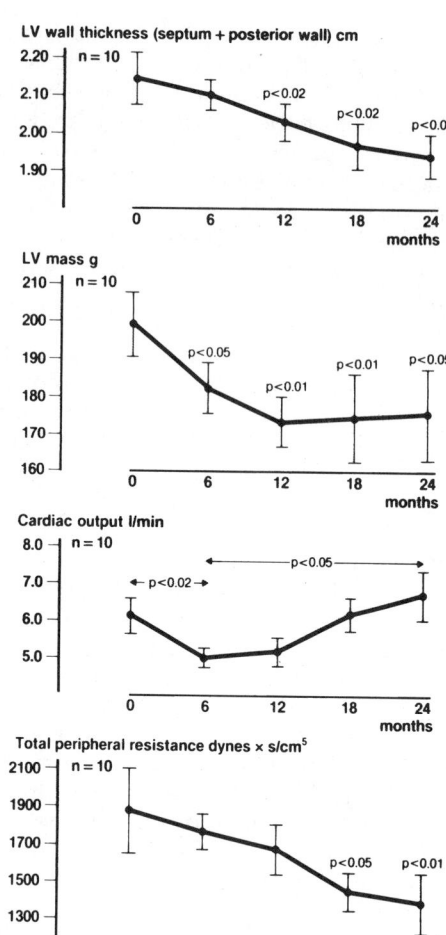

Figure 56–4. Changes in hemodynamics registered by repeat echocardiographic examinations during metoprolol antihypertensive treatment. LV, left ventricular. (Data from Wikstrand J, Trimarco B, Buzzetti G, et al: Increased cardiac output and lowered peripheral resistance during metoprolol treatment. Acta Med Scand Suppl 672:105, 1983.)

long-term adrenergic influences, both in the development of hypertrophy and in its reversal by medical treatment. This obviously applies to both cardiac hypertrophy and hypertrophy in resistance vessels. Antihypertensive drugs that lower heart rate and inhibit neurohormone-mediated trophic effects might well offer special benefits in terms of regression of cardiovascular changes, independent of their blood pressure–lowering effect. In the long run, this remodeling of the cardiovascular system leads to a reduction in total peripheral resistance, to normalized cardiac output (because of improved diastolic filling), and to an increase in coronary reserve.

Renal Effects of Very-long-term Treatment

Glomerular filtration rate is usually maintained at or close to normal levels in mild and moderate primary hypertension, whereas renal blood flow is usually reduced, and the renal vascular resistance is characteristically elevated.[52] Renal involvement in hypertension may also lead to increased urinary albumin excretion. Clinical proteinuria in patients with primary hypertension is associated with a poorer prognosis.[52]

In the 7-year follow-up study already mentioned,[8, 52] renal function was also studied. Renal function and urinary albumin excretion were examined in a random sample of men with newly diagnosed primary hypertension and in normotensive men of the same age. The hypertensive subjects were treated with metoprolol, either as monotherapy or combined with hydrochlorothiazide or hydralazine. Glomerular filtration rate, renal blood flow, renal vascular resistance, and the 24-hour albumin excretion were determined.

The reduction in glomerular filtration rate during 7 years of follow-up was not significantly greater in the hypertensive subjects treated with metoprolol in monotherapy or combination therapy than in the normotensive group. As judged from the study of a subgroup of the hypertensive subjects, a decrease in glomerular filtration rate occurred early as an immediate, drug-induced, functionally explained effect. Renal vascular resistance was significantly reduced in the hypertension group, and the changes in renal blood flow and renal vascular resistance after 7 years of treatment did not differ significantly from those due to normal aging. The urinary albumin excretion in the hypertensive group was significantly reduced after 7 years but remained higher than in the normotensive group. In conclusion, the effects of antihypertensive treatment with metoprolol on renal vascular resistance and microalbuminuria were favorable; furthermore, the changes in renal function and hemodynamics seen after long-term treatment with metoprolol in primary hypertension were not significantly different from the changes caused by normal aging in normotensive subjects.[52]

SECONDARY PREVENTION IN CORONARY HEART DISEASE
Acute Myocardial Infarction

Acute myocardial infarction is a critical condition with a high risk of mortality and a high incidence of complications such as pain, arrhythmias, and heart failure. Mortality and morbidity are closely related to the severity of myocardial damage. Cardioprotective interventions are essential and should be instituted as early as possible. Many animal experimental studies have suggested interventions suitable for the prevention and limitation of infarct development. Several of these interventions have been studied in clinical settings, but in few have results been conclusive.

One of the best documented cardioprotective therapies is the use of β-blocking agents in patients with threatened or definite acute myocardial infarction. The first study to demonstrate a significant reduction in mortality and morbidity after the onset of symptoms of acute myocardial infarction was the Goteborg Metoprolol Trial.[28] After that report, two very large multicenter international trials were performed, including many thousands of patients: the Metoprolol in Acute Myocardial Infarction (MIAMI) Trial on metoprolol[29] and the First International Study of Infarct Survival (ISIS-I) Trial on atenolol.[53] Today, a total of 28 controlled trials of β-blockers in acute myocardial infarction involve more than <27,000 patients, and, considering all the studies together, the hospital mortality rate is significantly reduced (approximately 13%). The following sections review the effects of metoprolol in acute myocardial infarction.

Chest Pain, Electrocardiographic Changes, and Infarct Size

During the early 1970s, studies performed in patients with acute myocardial infarction showed a favorable effect of β-blockers on the severity of myocardial ischemia.[54] In view of this study and other observations, the large placebo-controlled Goteborg Metoprolol Trial[28] was planned. In this trial, 1395 patients with suspected acute myocardial infarctions were included and randomized to metoprolol or placebo; treatment started immediately after arrival at the hospital. Metoprolol was given intravenously in a total dose of 15 mg (5 mg intravenously at 2-minute intervals) and was followed by 200 mg orally daily for 3 months. Similarly, placebo was given to half of the patients. Intravenous injections of metoprolol caused a prompt reduction in the severity of chest pain and in ST-

segment elevation.[16] Among patients treated within 12 hours after onset of symptoms, metoprolol therapy limited infarct development as judged from serum enzyme curves as well as from Q- and R-wave changes from precordial mapping. The effects on infarct limitation were most marked among patients with initially elevated heart rate and systolic blood pressure. The observations in the Goteborg Metoprolol Trial[16, 28] were later confirmed in the even larger multicenter international MIAMI Trial[17, 29] including 5778 patients with suspected acute myocardial infarctions. Similar results were obtained in the Belfast Metoprolol Trial.[30]

Infarct Development

In the Goteborg Metoprolol Trial,[16, 28] a subgroup of patients to whom metoprolol was given within 12 hours and in whom heart rate was greater than 70 beats/min at entry, had significant protection against the development of an early definite infarction. This finding was confirmed in the larger MIAMI Trial.[17, 29] The distribution of "definite," "possible," or "no" acute myocardial infarction within 3 days differed significantly between the two treatment groups. Patients given placebo had more "definite" and less "possible" or "no" infarctions than the metoprolol group did. A larger proportion of patients in the placebo group also developed Q-wave infarction. In addition to the early effect of treatment, there was significant prevention of late infarct development (after day 3) in both studies,[16–19, 28, 29] supporting the idea that metoprolol may prevent infarct development when instituted sufficiently early.

Arrhythmias

Several studies have reported that β-blockers reduce supraventricular and ventricular arrhythmias in patients with acute myocardial infarctions. This was clearly demonstrated in the Goteborg Metoprolol Trial,[16] in which supraventricular and ventricular tachycardias, electrically converted or treated overall, were reduced by more than 50%. In the MIAMI trial, the incidence of supraventricular tachyarrhythmias and the need for antiarrhythmic agents such as lidocaine for ventricular arrhythmias was reduced significantly. In patients specially monitored for ventricular arrhythmias, metoprolol was shown to reduce the frequency of ventricular ectopic beats.[18, 19] In the Goteborg trial, metoprolol significantly reduced the incidence of ventricular fibrillation during hospital stay.[16, 20] In the MIAMI trial, there was a reduced incidence of ventricular fibrillation during days 5 through 15 in patients treated with metoprolol,[17, 29] although this trend was not statistically significant.

Mortality

The Goteborg Metoprolol Trial[28] was the first large, placebo-controlled trial to report a significant reduction in early mortality after administration of a β-blocker shortly after onset of a heart attack. The main objective of this trial was to assess the 90-day mortality rate, which was reduced by 36% with metoprolol ($p = .024$) (Fig. 56–5). An analysis of data from the first 2 weeks of treatment indicates a similar but insignificant reduction in mortality even at that time. In order to study the earliest phase of acute myocardial infarction, the multicenter international MIAMI trial was planned.[29] The study was designed to target that subset of patients in the Goteborg Metoprolol Trial who seemed to benefit more than others. These were patients with initial heart rates greater than 65 beats/min without certain contraindications. Using data from the Goteborg Metoprolol Trial, the MIAMI investigators predicted a 7% placebo mortality rate after 15 days; a 35% reduction was expected with active treatment. However, the MIAMI trial included far more low-risk patients than anticipated, and the mortality rate among patients taking the placebo was only 4.9%, compared with the calculated 7%. The mortality rate in the metoprolol group was 4.3%; thus, a difference of 13% (95% confidence interval −8 to 33) was found to be statistically insignificant. In the very large international ISIS trial on atenolol,[53] which included 16,105 patients, the reduction in mortality after 7 days was similar to that of the MIAMI trial.

Eight important risk factors among entry variables in the MIAMI trial were used to create a subgroup with the highest mortality risk that consisted of one third of all patients. In this group of older and/or sicker patients, the placebo mortality rate of 8.5% was reduced to about 6% with active treatment, a difference of 30%. This difference was similar to the one observed in all patients in the Goteborg trial. Among patients with a low mortality risk, there was no clear-cut advantage of metoprolol over placebo during this period. Thus, the two studies taken together clearly demonstrate that among older and/or sicker patients, metoprolol reduced the mortality rate by 30% to 45% during the initial 15 days following onset of infarction (Fig. 56–6).[16, 17]

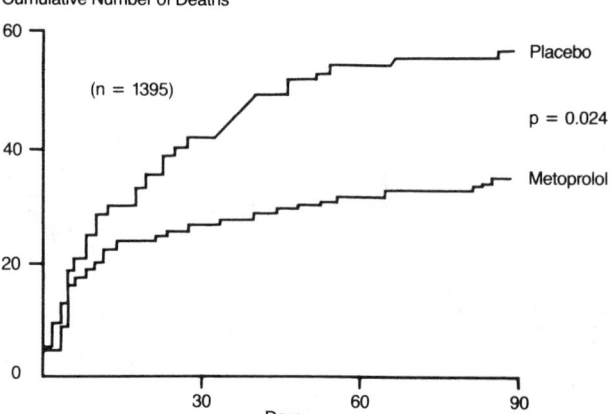

Figure 56–5. Cumulative number of deaths in the Göteborg Metoprolol Trial. (Adapted from Hjalmarson Å, Elmfeldt D, Herlitz J, et al: Effect on mortality of metoprolol in acute myocardial infarction. Lancet 2:823, 1981.)

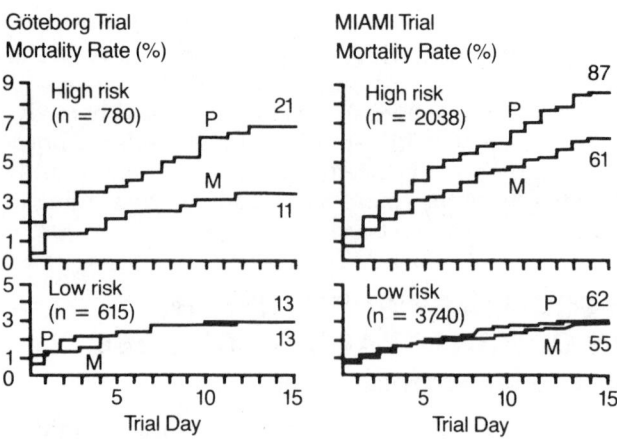

Figure 56–6. Mortality according to risk stratification in the Göteborg and Metoprolol in Acute Myocardial Infarction (MIAMI) trials. P, placebo; M, metoprolol. (Data from Hjalmarson Å [ed]: MIAMI: Metoprolol in acute myocardial infarction. Am J Cardiol 56:1G, 1985; and Hjalmarson Å, Elmfeldt D, Herlitz J, et al: Effect on mortality of metoprolol in acute myocardial infarction. Lancet 2:823, 1981.)

Tolerance and Adverse Reactions

It is well known that β-blockers cannot be given to all patients with suspected acute myocardial infarction. Definite contraindications are well demonstrated in studies in which all consecutive eligible patients have been considered for entry.[16, 17, 28, 29] Approximately 15% of patients with suspected acute myocardial infarction have definitive contraindications to β-blockade. In the Goteborg trial, 6.4% of patients treated with metoprolol were not given a full intravenous or full initial oral dose, and 9.7% were withdrawn because of cardiovascular adverse experiences, compared with 5.2% in the placebo group. Similar observations were made in the MIAMI trial. The two studies showed no significant differences regarding incidence of atrioventricular blocks II and III, congestive heart failure, or cardiogenic shock between metoprolol-treated and control groups. The major causes of dose reduction or withdrawal of metoprolol treatment were hypotension and bradycardia. In most patients, no treatment other than dose reduction or withdrawal of metoprolol was needed. Treatment was reinstituted later in several patients. Treatment of hypotension or bradycardia with atropine or inotropic agents was slightly more common (2%) in metoprolol groups than in the placebo groups. An invasive hemodynamic substudy in about 200 patients during the first 24 hours of the MIAMI trial indicated good cardiovascular tolerance of metoprolol in acute myocardial infarction, based on objective variables.[55]

β-Blockers Combined with Thrombolytic Therapy

Studies have been published on the use of intravenous administration of metoprolol in combination with the thrombolytic agents streptokinase and recombinant tissue-type plasminogen activator (rt-

PA).[56-58] In these studies, metoprolol was well tolerated. Hypotension and other potentially adverse events did not occur more often in the β-blocker–treated patients regardless of simultaneous placebo or rt-PA treatment. In the Thrombolysis in Myocardial Infarction Phase II (TIMI-2) trial,[58] metoprolol significantly reduced the number of recurrent ischemic episodes and nonfatal reinfarctions, both within 6 days and 6 weeks of follow-up, a reduction of about 60%. In the Thrombolysis Early in Acute Heart Attack Trial (TEAHAT),[57] intravenous metoprolol was given acutely to 66% of all patients suitable for treatment with rt-PA. The administration of rt-PA compared with placebo showed significant limitation of infarct size and improved 30-day measures of left ventricular function, as judged from ejection fraction. The best effects of rt-PA were obtained among patients given combined treatment with metoprolol shortly after arrival in hospital. Thus, it can be concluded that metoprolol is well suited to be given together with thrombolytic agents to improve early myocardial protection without adverse reactions.

Conclusions

Early intravenous administration of metoprolol followed by oral maintenance treatment reduces mortality, morbidity, and infarct complications in patients with suspected acute myocardial infarctions. The treatment is generally well tolerated and can be safely administered to about 80% of all eligible patients. Metoprolol has been found to be one important means of salvaging the ischemic myocardium, instituted alone or combined with other treatment modalities such as thrombolytics, in order to improve prognosis in patients with acute myocardial infarction.

After Myocardial Infarction

Following an acute myocardial infarction, the mortality rate after discharge from the hospital is approximately 10% during the first year, increasing an additional 5% to 6% in the next 3 years.[59] Chronic metoprolol treatment (100 to 200 mg daily) for secondary prevention has been shown to reduce mortality by approximately 25%.[28, 30-33] The reduction in mortality was similar in men and women (Fig. 56–7) and was due primarily to a reduction in sudden cardiac deaths,[50] which was most evident in elderly patients and patients with large infarcts or cardiac enlargement (i.e., high-risk patients).[31, 60] Nonfatal reinfarctions have also been shown to be reduced by approximately 25% (Fig. 56–8).[28, 30-33] The reduction in reinfarction rate was most obvious in patients with a history of hypertension prior to infarction.[61] Additional benefits included a lower incidence of cerebrovascular events, a reduced need for coronary artery bypass surgery because of disabling angina pectoris,[31] a reduction in readmissions to the hospital for cardiovascular reasons (heart failure, angina pectoris, or

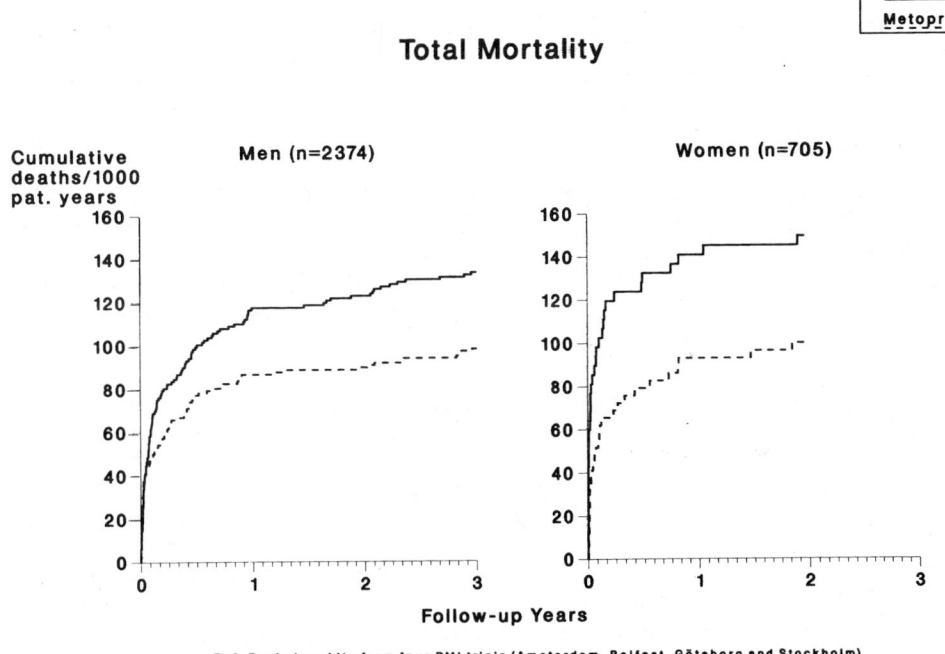

Total Mortality

Ref: Pooled results from four PMI trials (Amsterdam, Belfast, Göteborg and Stockholm)

Figure 56–7. Mortality in men and women participating in double-blind, randomized, placebo-controlled postinfarction trials with treatment for secondary prevention. (Data from Hjalmarson Å, Elmfeldt D, Herlitz J, et al: Effect on mortality of metoprolol in acute myocardial infarction. Lancet 2:823, 1981; Salathia KS, Barber JM, McIlmoyle EL, et al: Very early intervention with metoprolol in suspected acute myocardial infarction. Eur Heart J 6:190, 1985; Olsson G, Rehnqvist N, Sjögren A, et al: Long-term treatment with metoprolol after myocardial infarction: Effect on 3-year mortality and morbidity. J Am Coll Cardiol 5:1428, 1985; and Manger Cats V, van Capelle FLJ, Lie KL, et al: The Amsterdam Metoprolol Trial. Effect of treatment with metoprolol on first-year mortality in a single center study with low placebo mortality rate after myocardial infarction [abstract]. Drugs 29[Suppl 1]:8, 1985.)

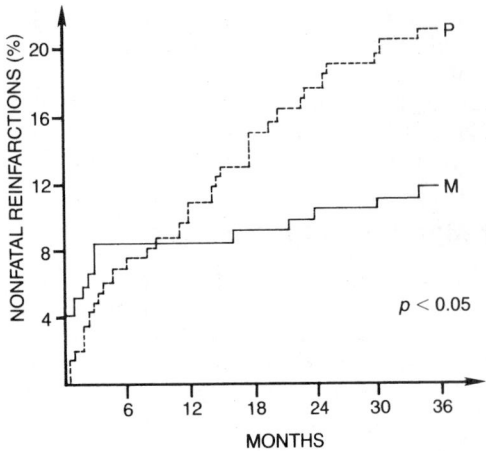

Figure 56–8. Reduction in the incidence of nonfatal reinfarction reported in the Stockholm Metoprolol Trial. P, placebo; M, metoprolol. (Adapted from Olsson G, Rehnqvist N, Sjögren A, et al: Long-term treatment with metoprolol after myocardial infarction: Effect on three-year mortality and morbidity. J Am Coll Cardiol 5:1428, 1985.)

symptomatic arrhythmias), and an increased proportion of patients who remained free of cardiac symptoms during the postinfarction period.[62, 63]

Postinfarction Arrhythmias

After institution of metoprolol to patients after infarction, the frequency of ventricular arrhythmias was reduced.[21] Patients showing an initial positive antiarrhythmic response to treatment ($\geq 75\%$ reduction in ventricular arrhythmias) seemed to have a more favorable prognosis if treatment was continued than untreated patients did.[21] In addition, long-term treatment counteracted the spontaneous increase in the frequency and complexity of chronic ventricular arrhythmias seen after an infarction with increasing time of follow-up.[21] This may be a reflection of a beneficial effect of metoprolol on the progression rate of the underlying disease (see the section on atherosclerosis).

Postinfarction Angina

In patients with exercise-induced signs of myocardial ischemia in the early postinfarction period (ST-segment depressions or angina pectoris), chronic metoprolol treatment improved prognosis so that the risk of dying or having a reinfarction was reduced.[14] Diastolic function in postinfarction patients was improved by metoprolol, probably because of its antiischemic action. This effect might have counteracted the negative inotropic effect of the β-blockade per se.[64]

Overall Effect of Postinfarction Therapy

In an effort to evaluate what prophylactic postinfarction metoprolol treatment really means to the average patient, a quality-adjusted life expectancy analysis was performed in the Stockholm Metoprolol

Postinfarction Trial.[62] In that analysis, in addition to prolonging survival, long-term metoprolol treatment significantly improved the quality of life in terms of prolongation of time spent in an optimal functional state and reduction of time spent in a disabled state after a new thromboatherosclerotic complication.

Economic Consequences of Prophylactic Postinfarction Therapy

To evaluate the economic consequences of widespread prophylactic postinfarction treatment with β-blockade, a cost-effect analysis was performed in the Stockholm Metoprolol Postinfarction Trial.[63] In that analysis, the costs of the β-blocker, of drug therapy for heart failure, and of rehospitalization due to cardiac disease, as well as indirect costs, calculated as the value of loss of productivity resulting from sick leave or early retirement due to cardiac disease, were analyzed. This analysis concluded that instead of adding costs, prophylactic treatment with metoprolol for three years following an acute myocardial infarction in fact reduced total cost by 13% per patient because of reduced morbidity.

Duration of Postinfarction Therapy

Whether long-term postinfarction therapy with β-blockade should be terminated after a certain treatment period or should be continued indefinitely has been debated. Data now indicate that long-term mortality is increased following withdrawal of chronic postinfarction metoprolol therapy,[65] suggesting that treatment should be continued for as long as no side effects develop. Actually, withdrawal of prophylactic postinfarction metoprolol treatment three years after the acute event resulted in a doubling of the risk for subsequent death.[65] Furthermore, morbidity (expressed as the need for readmission to the hospital because of cardiac reasons) increased following withdrawal of treatment. These findings are of great importance because continuation of postinfarction β-blocker therapy has been shown to result in the maintenance of initially achieved benefits from treatment.[66, 67]

Angina Pectoris

β-Blockers have been a mainstay of treatment in angina pectoris for many years. The acute beneficial effect is exerted by decreasing systemic arterial pressure and heart rate and a mild reduction in contractility, resulting in reduced myocardial oxygen demand. In addition, acute administration of metoprolol intravenously reduces uptake of free fatty acids by the normal and ischemic myocardium, the latter becoming less ischemic perhaps because of reduced myocardial oxygen consumption due to altered substrate utilization.[68]

The prolongation of diastole due to heart rate reduction may possibly facilitate blood flow through poorly perfused regions of the myocardium. Furthermore, in animal models, a redistribution of myocardial blood flow in the ischemic heart has been shown to result from reduced blood flow in normal epicardial myocardium and increased blood flow in the ischemic subendocardium.[69, 70] Thus, the antiischemic effect of metoprolol could be ascribed both to an increased blood flow supply and to a reduced metabolic demand of the myocardium.

Stable Exertional Angina

Metoprolol, 100 to 200 mg daily, effectively improved exercise tolerance and reduced the frequency of anginal attacks and the need for nitrates in stable exertional angina.[9, 10] In patients with obstructive coronary artery disease and documented episodes of silent ischemia, the number, as well as the length, of these episodes was reduced.[11] In postinfarction patients with signs of exercise-induced myocardial ischemia (ST-segment depression and angina pectoris), chronic metoprolol treatment improved prognosis.[14] In one long-term study of stable angina (18 months), chronic metoprolol treatment seemed to reduce the magnitude of exercise-induced myocardial ischemia with time,[12] supporting the idea of additional beneficial long-term effects apart from the acute β-blocking effects (see later section, Effects on Atherosclerosis).

Unstable Angina

In a large study on unstable angina, acute treatment with metoprolol, 200 mg daily, was shown to have a beneficial short-term effect in the prevention of recurrent myocardial ischemia, progression to myocardial infarction, or both.[13] These findings agree with the reported lower incidence of development to definite myocardial infarction in patients receiving metoprolol in whom suspected acute myocardial infarction was observed in the Goteborg Metoprolol Trial and the MIAMI trial[16, 17] (discussed earlier).

Spontaneous Rest Angina

In a randomized study by Polese et al.,[15] the conditions of patients with spontaneous rest angina improved after metoprolol treatment, as compared with those receiving placebo treatment.

Patients Undergoing Surgery

Patients with coronary artery disease who have been taking β-blockers for long periods and who are about to undergo surgery should be given a preoperative dose appropriate to the duration and stressful nature of the procedure in order to prevent so-called rebound phenomena.[71, 72] Furthermore, metoprolol treatment in patients with ischemic heart disease undergoing major surgery has been reported to reduce the risk of preoperative myocardial infarction or arrhythmia.[73]

Effects of Withdrawal of Therapy

Sudden termination of β-blocker therapy may precipitate so-called rebound phenomena, manifested as exacerbation of symptoms and increased sensitivity to β-adrenergic stimuli. These phenomena occur approximately 2 to 8 days after abrupt withdrawal,[74] and after even longer periods after gradual withdrawal.[75] Gradual withdrawal may prevent or attenuate rebound effects. The clinical significance of these phenomena is probably greatest in patients with ischemic heart disease. The mechanism for the rebound phenomena is a transient period of hypersensitivity of β-adrenoreceptors following long-term treatment.[74, 75] If withdrawal of chronic metoprolol treatment is intended, it may be preferable to withdraw the drug over a period of at least 2 weeks. If increased cardiac symptoms occur, they can be readily reversed by reinstitution of the drug. Furthermore, it must be emphasized that withdrawal of postinfarction metoprolol treatment resulted in worsened long-term prognosis (see "After Myocardial Infarction") even if patients experienced no acute withdrawal phenomena.[65]

Comment

Prophylactic long-term metoprolol treatment after acute myocardial infarction improves prognosis. Mortality and reinfarction risk are reduced by approximately 25%. This mortality reduction is most obvious in so-called high-risk patients. The reduction in reinfarction is most evident in patients with a history of hypertension. At present, no data identify patients who will benefit from treatment in terms of increased well-being. The beneficial prophylactic effects are demonstrated for up to 3 years but seem to be continuous, because in subsequent years, withdrawal of treatment results in increased mortality and morbidity. Postinfarction treatment with metoprolol is cost effective. The antianginal efficacy of metoprolol is well documented. Furthermore, silent ischemia is reduced by metoprolol treatment. Metoprolol treatment has been shown to improve prognosis in patients with unstable angina and in patients with postinfarction angina.

ANTIARRHYTHMIC EFFECTS
Electrophysiologic Effects in Man

In healthy volunteers, a single intravenous dose (15 mg) of metoprolol did not affect right ventricular repolarization time.[76] However, the same dose given after 5 weeks of oral medication (400 mg daily) prolonged repolarization time.[77] In patients with paroxysmal tachycardia, a bolus injection of 0.2 mg/kg significantly increased the sinus node recovery time (conduction time from the lower right atrium to the bundle of His). Sinus cycle length and refractoriness of the atrioventricular node also increased, whereas conduction time and atrial and ventricular effective refractory periods were unaffected.[78] Metoprolol significantly reduced the prolongation of the QT interval caused by thiopentone and suxamethonium when given prior to laryngoscopy.[79]

Clinical Effects

β-Blockers are useful in the management of arrhythmias resulting from excessive catecholamine release, acute and chronic supraventricular tachycardias, and ventricular arrhythmias unresponsive to first-choice agents.

Metoprolol treatment has been effective in acute supraventricular tachycardias (atrial tachycardia, atrial flutter, atrial fibrillation).[22-24] This effect was the result of conversion to sinus rhythm or reduction in ventricular rate. In chronic atrial fibrillation, the combination of metoprolol and digitalis treatment effectively reduces ventricular rate.[25-27]

Ventricular arrhythmias induced by physical exercise are most often successfully treated with metoprolol. Metoprolol often acts as an adjunct to other antiarrhythmic agents[24] in patients with symptomatic ventricular arrhythmias of uncertain origin. The antiarrhythmic effects of metoprolol in acute myocardial infarction and in the postinfarction phase have been discussed.

EFFECTS ON DILATED CARDIOMYOPATHY

Patients with severe heart failure due to idiopathic dilated cardiomyopathy have been reported to improve after institution of metoprolol treatment.[80-82] Similar findings have also been reported in patients with unspecified severe heart failure.[83-85] In the first reported study,[80] heart failure deteriorated following withdrawal of the β-blocker therapy.[86] A double-blind, randomized study with metoprolol studying the effect on mortality and the need for heart transplantation (due to aggravated heart failure) as primary end points, and cardiac function, exercise tolerance, and quality of life as secondary end points, has been completed. In a 1993 report,[87] it was concluded that metoprolol had a beneficial effect on progressive heart failure, observed as a significant reduction in patients deteriorating to the point that a heart transplant was required, together with better overall cardiac function in the metoprolol group, as well as a better quality of life.

In the initial studies, there was a selection of patients with resting sinus tachycardia. In later series, improvement was also observed in patients without resting tachycardia. A remarkable response has also been seen in patients with pacemaker treatment due to atrioventricular block. With these patient categories, it is important to start with very low doses (e.g., 12.5 to 25 mg daily) and then gradually titrate the dose over weeks to the maximal tolerated dose. Most often, improvement is not seen until weeks to months after institution of treatment. As a rule, β-blockade should not be instituted in untreated heart failure. Initially, the condition should be treated by conventional means, and β-blockade might be added after stabilization under careful supervision in the hospital.

EFFECTS ON SERUM LIPIDS

In view of the significance of lipoprotein disorders in atherogenesis, it is not surprising that the effects of antihypertensive drugs on lipoprotein levels have been subject to considerable interest. For β-receptor antagonists, this interest has focused on treatment-induced changes in triglycerides and high-density lipoproteins (HDLs) (see Day et al.[88] for review). Thus, both nonselective and β1-selective antagonists induce an increase in triglycerides and a decrease in HDLs. Both high triglyceride and low HDL levels are related to an increased incidence of clinical complications of atherosclerosis, in cross-sectional as well as prospective epidemiologic studies.[89] Because there is evidence that several β1-selective, as well as nonselective, antagonists have an antiatherogenic effect (see Effects on Atherosclerosis), the potentially undesirable effects of these drugs on lipoproteins may appear confusing. However, the actual mechanisms by which high triglyceride levels increase atherogenesis are unknown. Likewise, even though it has been suggested that HDL may be significant in eliminating cholesterol from arterial tissue (for review, see Bondjers et al.[90]), the actual data supporting this suggestion are weak. In addition, no prospective intervention data suggest that a favorable change in triglycerides or HDLs actually affects morbidity in clinical complications of atherosclerosis. Therefore, when evaluating the potential effects of β-blockers on clinical complications of atherosclerosis, more attention should be paid to the demonstrated effects of these drugs on atherosclerosis-related vascular diseases than on any potentially undesirable effects on lipoprotein levels.

Deposition of cholesterol in arterial tissue is one of the hallmarks of atherosclerosis. The mechanisms involved in this process are now being unraveled to the molecular level. It appears that low-density lipoproteins (LDLs) are of particular significance. LDL binds with high affinity to the arterial proteoglycan, a major component of the extracellular matrix of the vascular wall (for review, see Camejo[91]). A specific peptide sequence in the apolipoprotein of LDL binds with high affinity to the glycosaminoglycan component of the proteoglycan. The binding sequence is located in the putative ligand for the LDL receptor.[92] Binding of LDLs to arterial proteoglycans not only leads to extracellular deposition of the lipoprotein but also enhances lipoprotein uptake in arterial macrophages[93] and smooth muscle cells.[94] This uptake is partly mediated by mechanisms that are not subject to feedback control mechanisms.[94] Therefore, foam cell transformation may be induced when cells are exposed to proteoglycan-treated LDLs, both in macrophages[93] and in smooth muscle cells.[94] Thus, the interaction of LDLs with arterial proteoglycans may be a key process in various aspects of lipid accumulation in atherogenesis.

The affinity of LDLs for proteoglycans varies among individuals[91, 92] and is particularly high in persons who have sustained a myocardial infarction at an early age.[95] In fact, in one cross-sectional study of persons who suffered a myocardial infarction before the age of 50 years, the LDL affinity for arterial proteoglycans was an independent discriminator of myocardial infarction patients, with a higher discriminating power than any of the established risk factors. However, the significance of LDL affinity for proteoglycans in prospective studies remains to be demonstrated.

When healthy volunteers were subjected to short-term treatment with metoprolol, triglycerides increased and HDL cholesterol decreased in accord with a number of previous studies. However, in parallel with these effects, LDL affinity for proteoglycans was decreased.[96] This effect, central in the progress of atherogenesis as it might be, would be easier to reconcile with the demonstrated antiatherogenic effects of β-blockers.[97] Therefore, perhaps it might be appropriate to discuss the desirable effects that may be induced with β-blockers, or at least metoprolol, on lipoproteins.

EFFECTS ON ATHEROSCLEROSIS

In long-term prevention trials, metoprolol has been found to reduce the incidence of coronary and cerebrovascular complications in hypertensive patients,[6] as well as in patients surviving myocardial infarction.[50] The mechanisms involved in these preventive effects of metoprolol are not clear. The results obtained could be ascribed only in part to the well-established antihypertensive, cardiac antiischemic, and antiarrhythmic effects of metoprolol.[3] The reductions observed in the incidence of stroke and myocardial infarction suggest that additional contributing factors may prevent arterial thromboembolic events. This may involve prevention of the final thromboembolic process, retarded progression of atherosclerotic lesions, or both. The possible role of an antiatherogenic effect of metoprolol is supported by the results of several animal studies.[98]

Effects on Experimental Atherosclerosis

Metoprolol treatment of rabbits fed cholesterol resulted in a significant decrease in developed coronary and aortic atherosclerosis.[99, 100] This antiatherogenic effect was not associated with any significant changes in serum levels of cholesterol or other major lipids. Apart from metoprolol, it has been reported that propranolol, oxprenolol, and sotalol also reduce development of atherosclerosis in cholesterol-fed animals.[97] Because these four β-blockers have in common β1-adrenoreceptor blockade, the reported antiatherosclerotic effects may be ascribed mainly to inhibition of β1-adrenoreceptors. This hypothesis is supported by some observations by Manuck et al.[101] in studies on atherosclerotic development in monkeys exposed to psychosocial stress. The authors described an increased atherogenic effect in monkeys with augmented β1-mediated responsiveness as reflected by an exaggerated heart rate response to brief stress. In addition to these findings, metoprolol was shown to prevent platelet deposition at the intima of aortic ramifications in studies with rabbits.[102] This result suggests a role for β1-mediated factors in atherogenic processes involving platelet-endothelium interactions.

Thus, some evidence suggests that sympathetic activation, mainly by stimulation of β1-mediated mechanisms, is a separate risk factor for atherosclerosis operating apart from established factors such as hypercholesterolemia and hypertension.

Mechanisms of Antiatherogenic Effect

The specific β1-mediated mechanisms causing accelerated atherogenesis have not been identified, but both hemodynamic factors and various biochemical processes appear to be involved. As a working hypothesis,[98] we ascribe the observed antiatherogenic effects of metoprolol to a combination of β1-blockade (1) in the central nervous system, leading to a reduction in peripheral sympathetic nerve discharge, (2) in the heart, leading to hemodynamic changes, and (3) in biochemical systems, leading to reduced atherogenic activity.

HEMODYNAMIC EFFECTS

The hemodynamic effects of metoprolol may contribute to retarded atherogenesis, especially at arterial bends and branching points (i.e., the well-known predilection sites for atherosclerosis). Blood flow patterns are heterogeneous at these locations, and recent reports suggest that atherosclerotic lesions predominate at sites with low shear stress (i.e., regions with nonlaminar low flow).[103] A decrease in heart rate—for instance, by β-blockade—has been suggested to reduce local atherogenesis by counteracting flow aberrations at these sites.[104] Pressure-related factors may also contribute to the prevalence of atherosclerotic lesions at arterial branching sites, where wall stress has been shown to be at least four times higher than at unbranched aortic segments.[105] Thubrikar et al.[105] showed that chronic mechanical reduction of arterial intramural stress and cyclic stretching prevented development of atherosclerosis. Treatment with a β-blocker such as metoprolol can be expected to reduce arterial intramural stress and cyclic stretching as a result of reduced heart rate, decreased pulse pressure, and a lower arterial pressure. Therefore, these hemodynamic effects might contribute to the antiatherogenic effect of metoprolol.

BIOCHEMICAL FACTORS

Reports suggest that some biochemical factors may contribute to the antiatherogenic effect of metoprolol. Results reported by Lindén et al.[96] (see earlier section, Effects on Serum Lipids) indicate that metoprolol treatment in human subjects caused structural changes in plasma LDL, resulting in a reduction of its potential for deposition in the arterial wall. This finding may help explain the observation in animal studies that metoprolol decreased cholesterol accumulation in arterial intima without associated reductions in plasma lipid levels.[99, 100]

Furthermore, metoprolol caused an increased biosynthesis of prostacyclin in stressed rabbits.[106] Besides being a potent vasodilator and antithrombotic agent, prostacyclin has antiatherogenic actions that cause reduced fibrosis and cholesterol accumulation in arterial intima.[104] The results obtained in rabbits suggest that increased prostacyclin biosynthesis may contribute to the antiatherosclerotic, antihypertensive, and cardiac antiischemic effects of metoprolol. The clinical significance of this mechanism has not been clarified, but preliminary results in patients suggest that metoprolol treatment is associated with increased prostacyclin production.[107]

These results suggest that both hemodynamic and biochemical factors may contribute to the antiatherogenic effect of metoprolol. Some described effects (increased prostacyclin biosynthesis, prevention of platelet adhesion, reduced blood flow dynamics, decreased arterial cyclic stretching) may also suggest a contributory role of metoprolol in the prevention of acute formation of arterial thrombus.

It is obviously important to establish the contribution of potential antiatherogenic and antithrombolitic actions of metoprolol to its well-documented preventive effects in cardiovascular diseases.

SOCIOECONOMIC CONSIDERATIONS
Safety and Tolerability

Considering long-term drug treatment in patients with hypertension and ischemic heart disease, the aspects of safety and tolerability are extremely important. The experience of metoprolol treatment is impressive in this respect. Approximately 60 million patient-years of treatment have been accumulated to date. The safety of treatment is exemplified by long-term studies that indicated primary and secondary prevention of cardiovascular diseases and no tendency to increase noncardiovascular deaths.[5, 50]

Tolerance of metoprolol is good. Most subjective symptoms caused by metoprolol can be ascribed to β-adrenoreceptor blockade. Thus, side effects are attenuated most often by dose reduction or occasionally by administration of a β-agonist or atropine. Likewise, overdosing or intoxication for suicidal reasons is handled by careful supervision and, when indicated, administration of a β-agonist or atropine.

Subtle subjective symptoms, usually thought to be related to the central nervous system, have been reported during treatment with metoprolol as well as with other β-blockers.[108, 109] The mechanism behind these symptoms is poorly understood, and the question of whether there are differences in the symptom profile among β-blockers with different pharmacokinetic properties is still controversial. Results of published studies conflict, which might be explained by factors such as study design and comparison of differ-

ent dose regimens. However, as studies report, effects related to the central nervous system seemed to be correlated with the degree of peripheral β-blockade.[110, 111] Thus, some subjective symptoms may be due to the central nervous system perception of peripheral β-blockade rather than to blockade of β-receptors in the central nervous system per se. This view is supported by findings that the moderately lipophilic blocker metoprolol and the more hydrophilic agent atenolol exert similar effects on the central nervous system.[111] However, the effect of atenolol lasted longer than that of metoprolol because of the longer half-life of atenolol.[112]

Patients with obstructive pulmonary disease that is not well controlled with β_2-stimulants should avoid β-blockers. Glucose tolerance is not changed by metoprolol (100 to 200 mg/day for at least 1 week) in hypertensive and postinfarction patients with or without non-insulin-dependent diabetes mellitus.[113-115] In insulin-dependent diabetic patients, acute administration of metoprolol does not aggravate prolonged hypoglycemia.[116] Metoprolol also may be given in ordinary doses to patients with severe renal and hepatic failure.[117, 118] However, the dose should be reduced in patients with portacaval shunts.

For further details regarding contraindications, interactions, and use in pregnancy, information can be obtained from previous review articles[1-3] and ordinary package leaflets.

Quality of Life

The main reason to assess the quality of life of patients receiving antihypertensive drug therapy is to ensure the acceptability of the treatment. It is generally agreed that relevant aspects of quality of life in hypertension include the impact on well-being and symptomatic complaints.[119] Drug effects on vitality, sexual life, sleep, and cognitive function are other equally important areas.

Results from several studies in hypertension indicate a lower frequency of central nervous system symptoms when β_1-selective adrenoceptor agonists are used. Relatively β_1-selective blockers, such as metoprolol and atenolol, reduce the incidence and severity of unwanted side effects. In contrast, the nonselective agent propranolol has been reported to cause central nervous system symptoms.[111, 120-122] Similarly, adverse effects on quality of life, such as general well-being, vitality, and depression, have only been confirmed with propranolol treatment.[123] Well-being and tolerability of treatment with selective β-blockers are equal to those reported with treatment with ACE inhibitors or calcium antagonists[124, 125] and should not be confounded with results derived from propranolol treatment.[126]

Studies comparing metoprolol and atenolol suggest that irrespective of hydrophilicity or lipophilicity, both drugs may similarly cause mild subjective symptoms, which seems to be consistent with the half-life of the drugs. In fact, it has been suggested that the degree of lipophilicity seems to be of minor importance for the occurrence of central nervous system subjective symptoms.[127-131]

Metoprolol in a Once-Daily Controlled-Release System

Advances in pharmaceutical technology and biopharmaceutical research during the last few decades have enabled the development of novel and improved delivery systems for many drugs. The aim of such development is to realize the full potential of the drug by controlling the rate of input into the body.

Important potential benefits include achievement of steady drug concentrations within the therapeutic range, decreased frequency of administration, reduced adverse effects, and thereby improved patient compliance. This is relevant to β-adrenoreceptor blockers, because they may produce too great an effect on β_1-receptors or may cause unwanted effects mediated by blockade of the β-receptors when administered in conventional tablet form. Controlled delivery of a β_1-selective blocker so as to avoid high plasma concentrations therefore should facilitate the full benefits of β_1-blockade with a low number of adverse effects.

Several factors make metoprolol suitable for administration in a controlled-release (CR) delivery system: (1) The drug is rapidly and completely absorbed throughout the gastrointestinal tract;[132, 133] (2) it has a relatively short plasma elimination half-life of about 3 to 4 hours, which prevents the drug from being accumulated; and (3) there is a well-defined relationship between plasma concentrations and the β_1-blocking effect.[134, 135] Preferably, a formulation should deliver metoprolol in order to achieve even plasma concentrations and β_1-blocking effect over a 24-hour period after once-daily administration. Two different approaches to achieve this goal, an osmotic pump system and a formulation containing multiple units of the drug, have been described.[136, 137] The biopharmaceutical and clinical properties of the latter are described as follows.

Biopharmaceutical Properties

In the multiple-unit system, each pellet (i.e., drug unit) represents a discrete system that delivers the drug at a predetermined rate. One important feature of the multiple-unit system is that the dose is spread over a large area of the gastrointestinal tract, thus avoiding exposure of the mucosa to high concentrations of the drug. The pellets were designed to deliver metoprolol at a near-constant rate for about 20 hours, independent of physiologic factors such as pH and peristalsis. Therefore, continuous absorption of the drug over the main part of the dosage interval can be obtained regardless of the given dose (50 to 200 mg) or concomitant food intake.[138] Figure 56–9 illustrates the resultant steady-state plasma concentrations and percentage of reduction in exercise heart rate relative to placebo after once-daily administration with the multiple-unit metoprolol CR formulation.[139] CR ad-

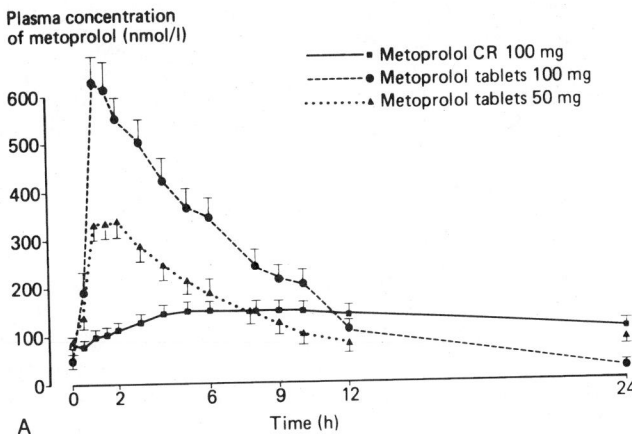

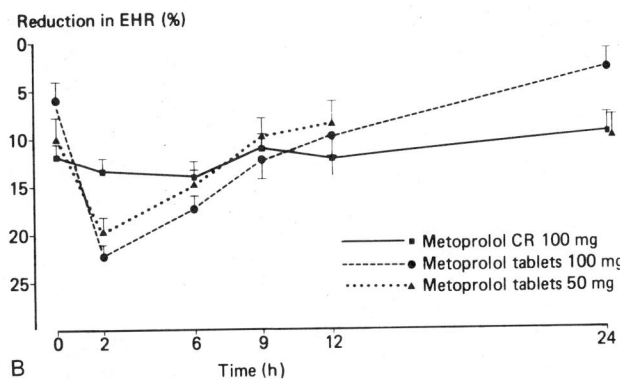

Figure 56–9. Mean (SEM) plasma concentrations of metoprolol (*A*) and mean (SEM) percentage reduction in exercise heart rate (EHR) (*B*) in 12 healthy subjects after 5 days' treatment with metoprolol CR, 100 mg once daily, and conventional metoprolol tablets, 100 mg once daily and 50 mg twice daily. (Adapted from Sandberg A, Blomqvist I, Jonsson UE, et al: Pharmacokinetic and pharmacodynamic properties of a new controlled-release formulation of metoprolol: A comparison with conventional tablets. Eur J Clin Pharmacol 33[Suppl]:S9, 1988.)

ministration maintains an appreciable plasma concentration and β_1-blocking effect for 24 hours after administration with considerably less fluctuation than is seen with conventional metoprolol tablets given in a once- or twice-daily regimen.

Clinical Implications

In outpatients with mild to moderate essential hypertension, the metoprolol CR formulation of 100 mg produces significantly greater β_1-blockade and considerably higher plasma concentrations 24 hours after administration than a conventional metoprolol tablet of 100 mg after 4 weeks of once-daily treatment.[140] Blood pressure control with 100 mg of the CR formulation has been shown to be equal to or slightly better than that obtained with 100 mg of conventional metoprolol tablets.[140, 141] In addition, 50 mg of metoprolol CR has been shown to be effective as monotherapy in reducing blood pressure;[142, 143] 50 mg of metoprolol CR has been shown to be as effective as 100 mg of the conventional metoprolol tablet.[144] Thus, the development of the CR formulation with its effect on the 24-hour plasma profile has made it possible to halve the daily dose of metoprolol in the treatment of essential hypertension and yet achieve the same blood pressure control. In the treatment of angina pectoris, a once-daily regimen of the CR formulation has been shown to be at least as effective as conventional metoprolol tablets given twice daily.[145]

Because undesirable effects with β-blockers mainly derive from blockade of $β_2$-receptors, the potential advantages of the CR formulation are its ability to maintain $β_1$-selectivity over 24 hours but with relative lack of peak plasma concentrations, thus avoiding decreased clinical $β_1$-selectivity as seen at high plasma concentrations. Accordingly, Kendall et al. demonstrated that terbutaline-induced hypokalemia ($β_2$-mediated) was significantly less affected by the CR formulation than by atenolol and conventional metoprolol, each at 100 mg. Löfdahl et al.[146] performed a study in asthmatic patients, evaluating the relative involvement of $β_2$-receptors at maximal plasma concentrations after single-dose administration of metoprolol in the CR formulation of 100 and 200 mg and conventional 100-mg tablets of atenolol. The effect on ventilator capacity forced expiratory volume in 1 second (forced expiratory volume in 1 second [FEV_1] and functional vital capacity [FVC]) after infusion and inhalation of terbutaline, a $β_2$-adrenoreceptor agonist, was significantly less with either dose of the CR formulation than with atenolol. The lower number of $β_2$-receptor–mediated adverse effects obtained in the study with the CR formulation can probably be attributed to the considerably reduced peak plasma concentration, because there were no reported differences in effect on the ventilatory function in asthmatic patients between metoprolol and atenolol when the drug was given as conventional tablets of 100 mg.[147]

Yet another effect of $β_2$-blockade is a decreased exercise capacity due to metabolic effects resulting in leg fatigue. Perceived exertion and leg fatigue assessed during exercise tests were shown to be greater with atenolol and conventional metoprolol tablets than with metoprolol CR.[144, 148, 149] Interestingly, there was no difference between metoprolol CR (50 mg) and placebo.[149] These effects on exercise capacity were parallel to inhibited muscle lipolysis and enhanced ammonium production as a measure of catabolism.[149] In a placebo-controlled, double-blind study in hypertensive men, using the glucose clamp technique, metoprolol CR did not affect glucose uptake.[150]

These examples illustrate how several years of clinical experience with a drug can be successfully interlinked with modern pharmaceutical technology to improve and simplify therapeutic use.

SUMMARY

Metoprolol is a safe and well-tolerated $β_1$-adrenoreceptor blocker proven to be beneficial as an antihypertensive, antianginal, and antiarrhythmic drug. Its therapeutic range and tolerance have been further improved by pharmaceutical development of a once-daily, slow-release preparation. Metoprolol treatment has been shown to improve prognosis when used as primary prevention in hypertension and as secondary prevention in the acute phase of a myocardial infarction, as well as during the postinfarction period. The beneficial effects on prognosis are probably due to a combination of early hemodynamic actions as well as to late effects (after long-term treatment) on cardiovascular function and structure. The initial responses to treatment include reduction in heart rate and blood pressure together with changes in certain metabolic processes, resulting in improved balance of myocardial oxygen demand and supply. In addition, important antiarrhythmic/antifibrillatory actions are achieved, probably due to a combination of counteracting stress-induced reduction in cardiac vagal tone, a reduction in sympathetic stimulation of the heart, and myocardial antiischemic effects. The beneficial effects observed after long-term treatment (in hypertension and in postinfarction prophylaxis) are most probably due to beneficial effects on the underlying disease. In hypertensive patients, long-term treatment with metoprolol has been shown to reduce left ventricular systolic wall stress, to reverse left ventricular hypertrophy, to improve left ventricular compliance, to decrease the stiffness of large arteries, and to reduce total peripheral resistance and albuminuria. Animal experiments and certain studies in humans support the hypothesis that part of the beneficial effect is due to antiatherosclerotic actions that retard atherosclerosis. This action may be related to effects of metoprolol on lipid metabolism, resulting in reduced cholesterol accumulation in arterial intima wall, and effects on prostacyclin biosynthesis and platelet interaction with arterial intima. Further research in this field is required.

REFERENCES

1. Åblad B, Carlsson E, Johnsson G, et al: Metoprolol. *In* Scriabine A (ed): Pharmacology of Antihypertensive Drugs. New York: Raven Press, 1980, pp 247–262.
2. Åblad B, Borg KO, Carlsson E, et al: Animal and human pharmacological studies on metoprolol—a new selective adrenergic beta-1-receptor antagonist. Acta Pharmacol Toxicol 36(Suppl 5):5, 1975.
3. Benfield P, Clissold SP, Brogden RN: Metoprolol: An updated review of its pharmacodynamic and pharmacokinetic properties, and therapeutic efficacy, in hypertension, ischemic heart disease and related cardiovascular disorders. Drugs 31:376, 1986.
4. Brogden RN, Heel RC, Speight TM, et al: Metoprolol: A review of its pharmacological properties and therapeutic efficacy in hypertension and angina pectoris. Drugs 14:321, 1977.
5. Wikstrand J, Warnold I, Olsson G, et al: Primary prevention with metoprolol in patients with hypertension. Mortality results from the MAPHY study. JAMA 259:1976, 1988.
6. Wikstrand J, Westergren G, Berglund G, et al: Antihypertensive treatment with metoprolol or hydrochlorothiazide in patients aged 60 to 75 years: Report from a double-blind international multicenter study. JAMA 255:1304, 1986.
7. Wikstrand J, Trimarco B, Buzzetti G, et al: Increased cardiac output and lowered peripheral resistance during metoprolol treatment. Acta Med Scand Suppl 672:105, 1983.
8. Hartford M, Wendelhag J, Berglund G, et al: Cardiovascular

and renal effects of long-term antihypertensive treatment. JAMA 259:2553, 1988.

9. Uusitalo A, Kyryläinen O, Johnsson G: A dose response study on metoprolol in angina pectoris. Ann Clin Res 13(Suppl 30):54, 1981.

10. Uusitalo A, Arstila M, Bae E, et al: Metoprolol, nifedipine and the combination in stable effort angina pectoris. Am J Cardiol 57:733, 1986.

11. Imperi GA, Lambert CR, Coy K, et al: Effects of titrated beta-blockade (metoprolol) on silent myocardial ischemia in ambulatory patients with coronary artery disease. Am J Cardiol 60:519, 1987.

12. Comerford MB, Besterman EMM: An eighteen month study of the clinical response to metoprolol, a selective beta-1-receptor blocking agent, in patients with angina pectoris. Postgrad Med J 52:481, 1976.

13. HINT, the Holland Interuniversity Nifedipine/Metoprolol Trial Research Group: Early treatment of unstable angina at the coronary care unit: A randomized, double-blind, placebo-controlled comparison of recurrent ischaemia in patients treated with nifedipine and/or metoprolol. Br Heart J 56:400, 1986.

14. Olsson G, Rehnqvist N, Freysehuss U, et al: Influence of long-term metoprolol treatment on early and late exercise test performance after acute myocardial infarction. Am J Cardiol 61:519, 1988.

15. Polese A, de Cesare N, Bartoletti A, et al: Cardioselective beta-blockade with metoprolol in spontaneous rest angina [abstract 2721]. In X World Congress of Cardiology [abstract book]. Washington, DC: American Heart Association, 1986, p 470.

16. The Goteborg Metoprolol Trial in Acute Myocardial Infarction: Am J Cardiol 53:1D, 1984.

17. Hjalmarson Å (ed): MIAMI: Metoprolol in acute myocardial infarction. Am J Cardiol 56:1G, 1985.

18. Murray DP, Murray RG, Littler WA: The effects of metoprolol given early in acute myocardial infarction on ventricular arrhythmias. Eur Heart J 7:217, 1986.

19. Rehnqvist N, Olsson G, Erhardt L, et al: Metoprolol during acute myocardial infarction reduces ventricular arrhythmias both in the early stage and after the acute event. Int J Cardiol 15:301, 1987.

20. Rydén L, Ariniego R, Armnan K, et al: A double-blind trial of metoprolol in acute myocardial infarction. N Engl J Med 308:614, 1983.

21. Olsson G, Rehnqvist N: Evaluation of anti-arrhythmic effect of metoprolol treatment after acute myocardial infarction. Relationships between treatment response and survival during a 3-year follow-up. Eur Heart J 7:312, 1986.

22. Rehnqvist N: Clinical experience with intravenous metoprolol in supraventricular tachyarrhythmias. Ann Clin Res 13(Suppl 30):68, 1981.

23. Stroobandt R, Kesteloot H: Intravenous metoprolol for the treatment of acute supraventricular tachyarrhythmias. Acta Cardiol 3:155, 1981.

24. Wasir HS, Mahapatra RK, Bathia ML, et al: Metoprolol—a new cardioselective beta-adrenoreceptor blocking agent for treatment of tachyarrhythmias. Br Heart J 39:834, 1977.

25. Mitrovic V, Neuss H, Buss J, et al: Senkung der Herzfrequenz bei chronischem Vorhofflimmern, durch Beta-rezeptoren-blockade. Herz Kreisl 13:493, 1981.

26. Khalsa A, Edvardsson N, Olsson SB: Effects of metoprolol on heart rate in patients with digitalisis-treated chronic atrial fibrillation. Clin Cardiol 1:91, 1978.

27. Burgersdijk C, van der Meer FJM, van der Vijer JCM: Effects of metoprolol on digitalis-resistant atrial tachyarrhythmias in chronic obstructive pulmonary disease. Neth J Med 27:283, 1984.

28. Hjalmarson Å, Elmfeldt D, Herlitz J, et al: Effect on mortality of metoprolol in acute myocardial infarction. Lancet 2:823, 1981.

29. Metoprolol in Acute Myocardial Infarction Trial Research Group: Metoprolol in acute myocardial infarction (MIAMI). A randomized placebo-controlled international trial. Eur Heart J 6:199, 1985.

30. Salathia KS, Barber JM, McIlmoyle EL, et al: Very early intervention with metoprolol in suspected acute myocardial infarction. Eur Heart J 6:190, 1985.

31. Olsson G, Rehnqvist N, Sjögren A, et al: Long-term treatment with metoprolol after myocardial infarction: Effect on 3-year mortality and morbidity. J Am Coll Cardiol 5:1428, 1985.

32. Manger Cats V, van Capelle FLJ, Lie KL, et al: The Amsterdam Metoprolol Trial. Effect of treatment with metoprolol on first-year mortality in a single center study with low placebo mortality rate after myocardial infarction [abstract]. Drugs 29(Suppl 1):8, 1985.

33. Lopressor Intervention Trial Research Group: The Lopressor Intervention Trial: Multicentre study of metoprolol in series of acute myocardial infarction. Eur Heart J 8:1056, 1987.

34. Kangasniemi P, Hedman C: Metoprolol and propranolol in the prophylactic treatment of classical and common migraine. A double-blind study. Cephalalgia 4:91, 1984.

35. Andersson PG, Dahl S, Hansen JH, et al: Prophylactic treatment of classical and non-classical migraine with metoprolol—a comparison with placebo. Cephalalgia 3:207, 1988.

36. Åblad B, Borg KO, Carlsson E, et al: Metoprolol. In Goldberg ME (ed): Pharmacological and Biochemical Properties of Drug Substances, Vol 2. Washington, DC: American Pharmaceutical Association, 1979, pp 186–227.

37. Abrahamsson T, Ek B, Nerme V: The $beta_1$- and $beta_2$-adrenoreceptor affinity of atenolol and metoprolol: A receptor-binding study performed with different radioligands in tissues from the rat, the guinea pig, and man. Biochem Pharmacol 37:203, 1988.

38. The Fifth Report of the Joint National Committee on Detection, Evaluation, and Treatment of High Blood Pressure (JNC V). Arch Intern Med 153:154, 1993.

39. MacMahon SW, Cutler JA, Furberg CD, Payne GH: The effects of drug treatment for hypertension on morbidity and mortality from cardiovascular disease: A review of randomized controlled trials. Prog Cardiovasc Dis 29(Suppl 1):99, 1986.

40. Wikstrand J, Warnold I, Tuomilehto J, et al: Metoprolol versus thiazide diuretics in hypertension. Morbidity results from the MAPHY study. Hypertension 17:579, 1991.

41. Kannel WB, Thomas HE Jr: Sudden coronary death: The Framingham study. In Greenberg HM, Dwyer EM Jr (eds): Sudden Coronary Death. New York: New York Academy of Sciences, 1982, pp 3–20.

42. Wikstrand J, Berglund G, Tuomilehto J: Beta-blockade in the primary prevention of coronary heart disease in hypertensive patients. Review of present evidence. Circulation 84(Suppl 6):93, 1991.

43. Tuomilehto J, Wikstrand J, Olsson G, et al: Decreased coronary heart disease in hypertensive smokers. Mortality results from the MAPHY Study. Hypertension 13:773, 1989.

44. Olsson G, Tuomilehto J, Berglund G, et al: Primary prevention of sudden cardiovascular death in hypertensive patients: Mortality results from the MAPHY study. Am J Hypertens 4:151, 1991.

45. Johanulesson M, Wikstrand J, Jönsson B, et al: Cost-effectiveness of antihypertensive treatment. Metoprolol versus thiazide diuretics. Pharmacoeconomics 3:36, 1993.

46. Wikstrand J, Kendall M: The role of beta receptor blockade in preventing sudden death. Eur Heart J 13(Suppl D):111, 1992.

47. Åblad B, Bjurö T, Björkman J-A, et al: Role of central nervous beta-adrenoceptors in the prevention of ventricular fibrillation through augmentation of cardiac vagal tone. Am Coll Cardiol 117:165A, 1991.

48. Skinner JE: Regulation of cardiac vulnerability by the cerebral defense system. J Am Coll Cardiol 5:88B, 1985.

49. Parker GW, Michael LH, Hartley CJ, et al: Central $beta$-adrenergic mechanisms may modulate ischemic ventricular fibrillation in pigs. Circ Res 66:259, 1990.

50. Olsson G, Wikstrand J, Warnold I, et al: Metoprolol induced reduction in postinfarction mortality: Pooled results from five double-blind randomized trials. Eur Heart J 13:28, 1992.

51. Dahlöf B, Lindholm LH, Hansson L, et al: Morbidity and mortality in the Swedish Trial in Old Patients with Hypertension (STOP-Hypertension). Lancet 338:1281, 1991.

52. Ljungman S, Wikstrand J, Hartford M, et al: Effects of long-

term antihypertensive treatment and aging on renal function and albumin excretion in primary hypertension. Am J Hypertens 6:554, 1993.

53. ISIS-1 (First International Study of Infarct Survival) Collaborative Group: Randomized trial of intravenous atenolol among 16,027 cases of suspected acute myocardial infarction. Lancet 2:57, 1986.

54. Waagstein F, Hjalmarson Å: Double-blind study of the effect of cardioselective beta-blockade on chest pain in acute myocardial infarction. Acta Med Scand 587:201, 1976.

55. Held P, Corbeij HMA, Dunselman P, et al: Hemodynamic effects of metoprolol in acute myocardial infarction. A randomized, placebo-controlled multicenter study. Am J Cardiol 56:47G, 1985.

56. Vlay SC, Lawson WE: The safety of combined thrombolysis and betaadrenergic blockade in patients with acute myocardial infarction: A randomized study. Chest 93:716, 1988.

57. TEAHAT Study Group: Very early thrombolytic therapy in suspected acute myocardial infarction: A randomized placebo controlled trial. Am J Cardiol 65:401, 1990.

58. The TIMI Study Group: Comparison of invasive and conservative strategies after treatment with intravenous tissue plasminogen activator in acute myocardial infarction: Results of the thrombolysis in myocardial infarction (TIMI) Phase II Trial. N Engl J Med 320:618, 1989.

59. Rotmensch HH, Vlasses PH, Ferguson RK: Prophylactic use of beta-adrenergic blockade in survivors of myocardial infarction. Heart Lung 13:366, 1984.

60. Olsson G, Rehnqvist N: Effect of metoprolol in post infarction patients with increased heart size. Eur Heart J 7:468, 1986.

61. Olsson G, Rehnqvist N: Reduction of nonfatal reinfarctions in patients with a history of hypertension by chronic postinfarction treatment with metoprolol. Acta Med Scand 220:33, 1986.

62. Olsson G, Lubsen J, van Es GA, et al: Quality of life after myocardial infarction: Effects of chronic metoprolol treatment on mortality and morbidity. Br Med J 292:1491, 1986.

63. Olsson G, Levin LÅA, Rehnqvist N: Economic consequences of postinfarction prophylaxis with betablockers. A cost-effect study of metoprolol. Br Med J 294:339, 1987.

64. Lindvall K, Olsson G, Rehnqvist N: Left ventricular function following withdrawal of chronic metoprolol treatment in patients with ischemic heart disease. A double-blind study. Eur Heart J 7:1045, 1986.

65. Olsson G, Odén A, Johansson L, et al: Prognosis after withdrawal of chronic post infarction metoprolol treatment: A 2 to 7 year follow-up. Eur Heart J 9:365, 1988.

66. Herlitz J, Hjalmarson Å, Swedberg K, et al: The influence of early intervention in acute myocardial infarction on long-term mortality and morbidity as assessed in the Göteborg Metoprolol Trial. Int J Cardiol 10:291, 1986.

67. Pedersen T (for the Norwegian Study Group): Six year follow-up of the Norwegian Multicenter Study on timolol after acute myocardial infarction. N Engl J Med 313:1055, 1985.

68. Van Der Wall DD, Westera G, Visser FC, et al: Influence of metoprolol on myocardial uptake of free fatty acids in experimental myocardial ischemia. Curr Ther Res 32:653, 1982.

69. Buck JD, Hardman HF, Warltier DC, et al: Changes in ischemic blood flow distribution and dynamic severity of a coronary stenosis induced by beta blockade in the canine heart. Circulation 64:708, 1981.

70. Åblad B, Abrahamsson T, Björkman JA, et al: Effects of metoprolol on ischemic myocardial regional function and oxygen supply/demand ratio in the dog. In Hugenholtz PG, Goldman BS (eds): Unstable Angina, Current Concepts and Management. New York: Schattauer, 1985, pp 159–170.

71. Pontén J, Biber B, Bjurö T, et al: Beta-receptor blockade and spinal anaesthesia. Withdrawal versus continuation of long-term therapy. Acta Anaesthesiol Scand Suppl 76:62, 1982.

72. Pontén J, Biber B, Henriksson BA, et al: Beta-receptor blockade and neuroleptanaesthesia. Withdrawal versus continuation of long-term therapy in gallbladder and carotid artery surgery. Acta Anaesthesiol Scand 26:576, 1982.

73. Pasternack PF, Imparato AM, Bauman FG, et al: The hemodynamics of beta-blockade in patients undergoing abdominal aortic aneurysm repair. Circulation 76(Suppl 3):1, 1987.

74. Rangno RE, Langlois S, Lutterodt A: Metoprolol withdrawal phenomena: Mechanism and prevention. Clin Pharmacol Ther 31:8, 1982.

75. Olsson G, Hjemdahl P, Rehnqvist N: Rebound phenomena following gradual withdrawal of chronic metoprolol treatment in patients with ischemic heart disease. Am Heart J 108:454, 1984.

76. Edvardsson N, Hirsch I, Olsson SB: Acute effects of lignocaine, procainamide, metoprolol, digoxin and atropine on human myocardial refractoriness. Cardiovasc Res 18:463, 1984.

77. Edvardsson N, Olsson SB: Effects of acute and chronic beta-receptor blockade on ventricular repolarisation in man. Br Heart J 45:628, 1981.

78. Camm AJ, Ward DE, Withmarsh VB: The acute electrophysiological effects of intravenous metoprolol. Clin Cardiol 5:327, 1982.

79. Saarnivaara L, Lindgren L, Hynynen M: Effects of practolol and metoprolol on QT interval, heart rate and arterial pressure during induction of anaesthesia. Acta Anaesthesiol Scand 28:644, 1984.

80. Waagstein F, Hjalmarsson A, Swedberg K, et al: Beta-blockade in dilated cardiomyopathies: They work. Eur Heart J 4(Suppl A):173, 1983.

81. Engelmeier RS, O'Connell JB, Walsh R, et al: Improvement in symptoms and exercise tolerance by metoprolol in patients with dilated cardiomyopathy: A double-blind, randomized placebo-controlled trial. Circulation 72:536, 1985.

82. Anderson JL, Lutz JR, Gilbert EM, et al: A randomised trial of low-dose beta-blockade therapy for idiopathic dilated cardiomyopathy. Am J Cardiol 55:471, 1985.

83. Weber KT, Likoff MJ, McCarthy D: Low-dose beta-blockade in the treatment of chronic cardiac failure. Am Heart J 104:877, 1982.

84. Fowler MB, Bristow MR, Laser JA, et al: Betablocker therapy in severe heart failure: Improvement related to beta₁-adrenergic receptor up regulation [abstract]. Circulation 70(Suppl 2):112, 1984.

85. Waagstein F, Blomström-Lundquist C, Andersson B, et al: Long-term effects of metoprolol in severe heart failure due to ischemic cardiomyopathy, primary valve disease and diabetes [abstract]. Circulation 76(Suppl 4):358, 1987.

86. Swedberg K, Hjalmarson ÅA, Waagstein F, et al: Adverse effects of beta-blockade withdrawal in patients with congestive cardiomyopathy. Br Heart J 44:134, 1980.

87. Waagstein F, Bristow MR, Swedberg K, et al for the Metoprolol in Dilated Cardiomyopathy (MDC) Trial Study Group: Beneficial effects of metoprolol in idiopathic dilated cardiomyopathy. Lancet 342:1441, 1993.

88. Day JL, Metcalf J, Simpson N, et al: Adrenergic mechanisms in the control of plasma lipids in man. Am J Med 76:94, 1984.

89. Gordon T, Kavvel WB, Castelli WP, et al: Lipoproteins, cardiovascular disease and death. Arch Intern Med 141:1128, 1981.

90. Bondjers G, Wiklund O, Olofsson SO, et al: Relationship between high-density lipoproteins and atherosclerosis. In Day CE (ed): High-Density Lipoprotein. New York: Marcel Dekker, 1981, pp 463–504.

91. Camejo G: The interaction of lipids and lipoproteins with the intercellular matrix of arterial tissue: Its possible role in atherogenesis. Adv Lipid Res 19:1, 1982.

92. Camejo G, Olofsson SO, Lopez F, et al: Identification of apoB-100 segments mediating the interaction of low-density lipoproteins with arterial proteoglycans. Arteriosclerosis 8:368, 1988.

93. Hurt E, Camejo G: Effects of arterial proteoglycans on the interaction of LDL with human monocyte-derived macrophages. Atherosclerosis 67:115, 1987.

94. Bondjers G, Wiklund O, Olofsson SO, et al: Low-density lipoprotein interaction with arterial proteoglycans: Effect on lipoprotein interactions with arterial cells. In Suckling KE, Groth PHE (eds): Hyperlipidemia and Atherosclerosis. London: Academic Press, 1988, pp 135–48.

95. Lindén T, Bondjers G, Camejo G, et al: Affinity of LDL to human arterial proteoglycan among male survivors of myocardial infarction. Eur J Clin Invest 19:38, 1989.

96. Lindén T, Camejo G, Wiklund O, et al: Effect of short-term

beta-blockade on serum lipid levels and on the interaction of LDL with human arterial proteoglycan: A comparison between metoprolol-CR and atenolol. *In* Lindén T: Retention and accumulation of apo-lipoprotein B and lipids in human arterial tissue [Ph.D. thesis]. Goteborg: Vasastadens, 1988 (ISBN 91-7900-480-6).

97. Kaplan JR, Manuck SB, Adams MR, et al: The effect of beta-adrenergic blocking agents on atherosclerosis and its complications. Eur Heart J 8:928, 1987.

98. Åblad B, Björkman JA, Gustafsson D, et al: The role of sympathetic activity in atherogenesis—effects of beta-blockade. Am Heart J 116:322, 1988.

99. Östlund-Lindqvist AM, Lindqvist P, Bräutigam J, et al: The effect of metoprolol on diet-induced atherosclerosis in rabbits. Arteriosclerosis 8:40, 1988.

100. Lindqvist P, Olsson G, Nordborg C, et al: Atherosclerosis in rabbits identified as high and low responders to an atherogenic diet and the effect of treatment with a beta-1-blocker. Atherosclerosis 72:163, 1988.

101. Manuck SB, Kaplan JR, Matthews RA: Behavioural antecedents of coronary heart disease and atherosclerosis. Arteriosclerosis 6:2, 1986.

102. Pettersson K, Åblad B: Metoprolol inhibits platelet deposition at arterial bifurcations in rabbits with sympathetic activation. FASEB J 2:A1580, 1988.

103. Zarins CK, Giddens DP, Bharadray BK, et al: Carotid bifurcation atherosclerosis. Quantitative correlation of plaque localisation with flow velocity profiles and wall shear stress. Circ Res 53:502, 1983.

104. Willis AL, Smith DL, Vigo C: Suppression of principal atherosclerotic mechanisms by prostacyclins and other eicosanoids. Prog Lipid Res 25:645, 1986.

105. Thubrikar MJ, Baker JW, Nolans SP: Inhibition of atherosclerosis associated with reduction of arterial intramural stress in rabbits. Arteriosclerosis 8:410, 1988.

106. Åblad B, Björkman JA, Edvardsson N, et al: A beta-adrenergic mechanism in the arterial wall possibly involved in genesis of cardiovascular disease. Fed Proc 46:974, 1987.

107. Winther K, Hedman C: Beta-adrenoceptor blockade, platelets, and rheologic factors. Cephalalgia 6(Suppl 15):33, 1986.

108. Lewis RV, Jakson, Ramsay LE: Side-effects of beta-adrenoceptor blocking drugs assessed by visual analogue scale. Br J Clin Pharmacol 19:255, 1985.

109. Currie D, Lewis A, McDevitt DG: Central effects of the beta-adrenoceptor antagonists propranolol and metoprolol. Br J Clin Pharmacol 25:124, 1988.

110. Dahlöf C, Dimenäs E: CNS-related subjective symptoms of beta-blockers evaluated by visual analogue scales (VAS). *In* III World Conference on Clinical Pharmacology and Therapeutics [abstract book]. Copenhagen: Munksgaard, 1986.

111. Gengo FM, Ermer JC, Carey C, et al: The relationship between serum concentrations and central nervous system effects of metoprolol. J Neurol Neurosurg Psychiatry 48:101, 1985.

112. Gengo FM, Huntoon P, McHugh WB: A comparison of the CNS depressant effect of a lipid-soluble and water-soluble beta-blocker. Arch Intern Med 147:39, 1987.

113. Groop L, Tötterman KJ, Harno K, et al: Influence of beta-blocking drugs on glucose metabolism in patients with non-insulin dependent diabetes mellitus. Acta Med Scand 211:7, 1982.

114. Micossi P, Pollavini G, Raggi U, et al: Effects of metoprolol and propranolol on glucose tolerance and insulin secretion in diabetes mellitus. Horm Metab Res 16:59, 1984.

115. Olsson G, Rehnqvist N: Effects of metoprolol treatment on glucose tolerance after myocardial infarction. Eur J Clin Pharmacol 33:311, 1987.

116. Clausen-Sjöblom N, Lins PE, Adamson U, et al: Effects of metoprolol on the counter-regulation and recognition of prolonged hypoglycaemia in insulin-dependent diabetics. Acta Med Scand 222:57, 1987.

117. Jordö L, Attman PO, Aurell M, et al: Pharmacokinetic and pharmacodynamic properties of metoprolol in patients with impaired renal function. Clin Pharmacokinet 5:169, 1980.

118. Regåardh CG, Jordo L, Ervik M, et al: Pharmacokinetics of metoprolol in patients with hepatic cirrhosis. Clin Pharmacokinet 6:375, 1981.

119. Bulpitt CJ, Fletcher AE: Quality of life evaluation of antihypertensive drugs. Pharmacoeconomics 1:95, 1992.

120. Kostis JB, Rosen RC: Central nervous system effects of beta-adrenergic blocking drugs: The role of ancillary properties. Circulation 75:204, 1987.

121. Beta Blocker Heart Attack Trial Research Group: A randomized trial of propranolol in patients with acute myocardial infarction. JAMA 247:1707, 1982.

122. Contant J, Engler R, Janowsky D, et al: Central nervous system side effect of β-adrenergic blocking agents with high and low lipid solubility. J Cardiovasc Pharmacol 13:656, 1989.

123. Hjemdahl P, Wiklund I: Quality of life on antihypertensive drug therapy: Scientific end-point or marketing exercise? J Hypertens 10:1437, 1992.

124. Nugent L, Miola S, Walker F: Comparison of enalapril and metoprolol as initial therapy for mild to moderate hypertension. J Clin Pharmacol 27:461, 1987.

125. Zachariah PK, Bolulet G, Chrysant SG, et al: Evaluation of antihypertensive efficacy of lisinopril compared to metoprolol in moderate to severe hypertension. J Cardiovasc Pharmacol 9(Suppl 3):S53, 1987.

126. McAreavey D, Vermeulen R, Robertson JI: Newer beta blockers and the treatment of hypertension. Cardiovasc Drug Ther 5:577, 1991.

127. Kendall M: Metoprolol CR/ZOK—its role and efficacy: A review article. J Clin Pharmacol 30:S57, 1990.

128. Dahlof C, Dimenäs E, Kendall M, Wiklund I: Quality of life in cardiovascular disease. Emphasis on β-blocker treatment. Circulation 84(Suppl 6):108, 1991.

129. Dimsdale JE: Reflections on the impact of antihypertensive medications on mood, sedation, and neuropsychologic functioning. Arch Intern Med 152:35, 1992.

130. Gengo FM, Huntoon L, McHugh WB: Lipid-soluble and water-soluble beta-blockers. Comparison of the central nervous system depressant effect. Arch Intern Med 147:39, 1987.

131. Dahlöf C, Dimenäs E: Side effects of β-blocker treatment as related to the central nervous system. Am J Med Sci 299:236, 1990.

132. Godbillon J, Edvard D, Vidon N, et al: Investigation of drug absorption from the gastrointestinal tract of man. III. Metoprolol in the colon. Br J Clin Pharmacol 19(Suppl 2):113S, 1985.

133. Jonsson UE, Sandberg A: Absorption study of metoprolol with positioned release capsule. *In* Prescott LF, Nimmo WS (eds): Abstract Book from Second International Conference on Drug Absorption 1983: Rate Control in Drug Therapy. Edinburgh: Churchill Livingstone, 1985, p 68.

134. Johnsson G, Regåardh CG, Sölvell L: Combined pharmacokinetic and pharmacodynamic studies in man of the adrenergic beta-1-receptor antagonist metoprolol. Acta Pharmacol Toxicol 36(Suppl 5):31, 1975.

135. Harron DWG, Balnave K, Kinney CD: Effects on exercise tachycardia during forty-eight hours of a series of doses of atenolol, sotalol, and metoprolol. Clin Pharmacol Ther 29:295, 1981.

136. Theeuwes F, Swanson D, Guittard G, et al: Osmotic delivery systems for the beta-adrenoceptor antagonists metoprolol and oxprenolol: Design and evaluation of systems for once-daily administration. Br J Clin Pharmacol 19:69S, 985.

137. Ragnarsson G, Sandberg A, Jonsson UE, et al: Development of a new controlled-release metoprolol product. Drug Devel Indust Pharmacy 13:1495, 1987.

138. Sandberg A, Ragnarsson G, Jonsson UE, et al: Design of a new multiple-unit controlled-release formulation of metoprolol. Eur J Clin Pharmacol 33(Suppl):S3, 1988.

139. Sandberg A, Blomqvist I, Jonsson UE, et al: Pharmacokinetic and pharmacodynamic properties of a new controlled-release formulation of metoprolol: A comparison with conventional tablets. Eur J Clin Pharmacol 33(Suppl):S9, 1988.

140. Rydén L, Kristensson BE, Westergren G: Effect of metoprolol CR on blood pressure and exercise heart rate in hypertension: A comparison with conventional tablets. Eur J Clin Pharmacol 33(Suppl):S33, 1988.

141. Houtzagers J Jr, Smilde JG, Creytens G, et al: Efficacy and tolerability of a new controlled-release formulation of metoprolol: A comparison with conventional metoprolol

tablets in mild to moderate hypertension. Eur J Clin Pharmacol 33(Suppl):S39, 1988.

142. Jäättelä A, Baandrup S, Houtzagers J, Westergren G: The efficacy of low dose metoprolol CR/ZOK in mild hypertension and in elderly patients with mild to moderate hypertension. J Clin Pharmacol 30(Suppl):S66, 1990.

143. Wahlqvist I, Olofsson B, Olsson G, Westergren G: Low dose metoprolol CR/ZOK—Effective and well tolerated treatment in hypertension [abstract]. Am J Hypertens 4:23A, 1991.

144. Omvik P, Leer J, Istad H, Westergren G: Equal efficacy and improved tolerability with 50 mg controlled release metoprolol compared with 100 mg conventional metoprolol in hypertensive patients. Am J Therapeut 1:65, 1994.

145. Egstrup K, Gundersen T, Härkönen R, et al: The antianginal efficacy and tolerability of controlled release metoprolol once daily: A comparison with conventional metoprolol tablets twice daily. Eur J Clin Pharmacol 33(Suppl):S45, 1988.

146. Löfdahl CG, Dahlöf C, Westergren G, et al: Controlled-release metoprolol compared with atenolol in asthmatic patients: Interaction with terbutaline. Eur J Clin Pharmacol 33(Suppl): S25, 1988.

147. Löfdahl CG, Svedmyr N: Cardioselectivity of atenolol and metoprolol. A study in asthmatic patients. Eur J Respir Dis 62:396, 1981.

148. Blomqvist I, Westergren G, Sandberg A, et al: Pharmacokinetics and pharmacodynamics of controlled-release metoprolol: A comparison with atenolol. Eur J Clin Pharmacol 33(Suppl): S19, 1988.

149. Akhlaghi S, Maxwell SRJ, Kendall MJ, et al: A comparison of the β1-selectivity of conventional metoprolol and metoprolol CR during exercise in healthy volunteers. J Clin Pharm Ther 18:259, 1993.

150. Landin K, Tengborn L, Smith U: Metformin and metoprolol CR treatment in non-obese men. J Intern Med 235:335, 1994.

CHAPTER 57

Atenolol

Jay M. Sullivan, M.D.

HISTORY

The development of the first selective β-receptor blocker, dichloroisoproterenol, was reported by Powell and Slater[1] in 1958, eventually leading to wide acceptance of Ahlquist's 1948 classification of adrenergic receptors.[2] Although this agent could effectively block the β-stimulatory effects of sympathomimetic amines, it also possessed relatively powerful β-agonist effects, leading to stimulation of receptors before inducing blockade, a property called *intrinsic sympathomimetic activity* (ISA).

Knowing that the inotropic and chronotropic effects of catecholamines on the heart were mediated by β-adrenergic receptors, Black and Stephenson[3] proposed that β-adrenoreceptor blocking drugs would effectively treat patients with atherosclerotic heart disease and angina pectoris by blunting the normal increase in sympathetic activity during exertion or emotion, which ordinarily causes an increase in heart rate and myocardial contractility, thereby preventing the increase of myocardial oxygen demand to a level exceeding the capacity of a diseased coronary artery to increase blood flow.

Black et al.[3, 4] developed the β-blockers pronethalol and propranolol in 1962 and 1965, respectively. Clinical trials proved the latter to be an effective antianginal agent.[5] However, propranolol was also found to aggravate asthma because of blockade of β2-receptors in the bronchioles, thus preventing sympathetically mediated bronchodilation. This observation, plus the knowledge that β-receptors in various tissues could be stimulated differentially,[6] led to a search for agents that could block β1-receptors selectively. The first such agent was practolol, which was withdrawn from use because of adverse effects. Of the agents developed subsequently, atenolol, introduced in 1976, appears to be among the most cardioselective.[7]

CHEMISTRY

Most β-adrenoreceptor blocking agents resemble the agonist isoproterenol in that they possess an aromatic ring linked by an OCH$_2$ group to a substituted ethanolamine side chain. The synthetic β-adrenergic receptor blocker atenolol has a molecular weight of 266 daltons and is designated chemically as benzeneacetamide, 4-{2'-hydroxy-3'-[(1 methylethyl)amino]propoxyl}. The compound is polar and hydrophilic and has a water solubility of 26.5 mg/ml at 37°C. Its logarithmic partition coefficient is 0.23 (octanol/water). Atenolol is freely soluble in acid solution.

PHARMACOLOGY
Adrenergic Receptors

Adjacent to various effector cells, such as those of vascular smooth or cardiac muscle, lies a sympathetic neuron that can synthesize, store, release, and resequester norepinephrine. Together, these structures constitute the adrenergic neuroeffector junction. Sir Henry Dale[8] first proposed that catecholamines act at unique receptor sites on the effector cells after observing that ergot alkaloids inhibited the pressor effect of epinephrine, suggesting that the two compounds competed for occupancy at the same effector sites. Subsequently, after studying the effect of several sympathomimetics on different organ systems, Ahlquist[2] proposed that not all adrenergic receptors were the same and labeled those mediating different responses as αβ-adrenoreceptors. Later, Lands et al.[6] advanced the concept that β-adrenoreceptors consisted of two subtypes, β1 and β2, the former predominating in heart and kidney and the latter occurring largely in vascular smooth muscle, bronchioles, and the uterus. Further investigation suggested that the β1-receptors were innervated, responding to the release of norepinephrine at a neuroeffector junction, whereas the β_2-receptors were not innervated and responded to circulating epinephrine released by the adrenal medulla.

Still, further research has shown that there are two types of α-receptors as well: α_1-receptors at the postsynaptic site, which mediate smooth muscle contraction and respond to stimulation by norepinephrine, and α_2-receptors on the presynaptic neuron, which inhibit norepinephrine release from the nerve terminal.[9] More recently, α_2-receptors have also been found in postsynaptic sites. In addition, β-receptors have also been identified on the presynaptic sympathetic nerve terminal that, when stimulated, enhance the release of norepinephrine from the nerve terminal.

When norepinephrine is released from the nerve terminal, it combines with the receptor to form a complex, resulting in an activation of adenyl cyclase, an enzyme on the internal surface of the cell membrane. When activated, adenyl cyclase increases the intercellular formation of cyclic adenosine monophosphate, which in turn acts to stimulate or inhibit several pathways[9] (Table 57–1).

Properties Common to All β-Adrenoreceptor Blocking Agents

All β-receptor blocking agents are competitive antagonists—that is, they can be displaced from binding sites on the β-receptor by increasing the concentration of agonist. For example, the degree of blockade imposed by a β-blocking agent is usually estimated by determining how much the dose of isoproterenol must be increased to raise the heart rate by a certain amount before and after β-blockade. One explanation for the wide variation in doses of different β-blockers required to obtain a desired clinical result is differences in their efficacy of blockade. There appears to be a maximum blood concentration of β-blockers, or plateau, beyond which further increases in dosages do not result in more β-blockade, possibly because sympathetic activation cannot be increased beyond certain limits.[5] At equivalent β-blocking concentrations (i.e., doses reducing maximum exercise heart rate equally), all β-blockers appear to have the same clinical efficacy.

Table 57–1. **Effect of Stimulation of Adrenergic Receptors**

Receptor	Tissue	Response
α_1	Uterus	Contraction
	Vascular smooth muscle	Vasoconstriction
α_2	Blood platelets	Aggregation
β_1	Adipose cells	Lipolysis
	Cardiac tissue	Increased heart rate, force of contraction, and atrioventricular conduction
β_2	Bronchial smooth muscle	Bronchodilation
	Vascular smooth muscle	Vasodilation

Table 57–2. **Selectivity of β-Blockers**

Nonselective	Cardioselective
Carteolol	Acebutolol
Labetalol	Atenolol
Nadolol	Betaxolol
Oxprenolol	Metoprolol
Penbutolol	
Pindolol	
Propranolol	
Sotalol	
Timolol	

Properties by Which β-Blocking Agents Differ

Selectivity

Certain of the β-blocking agents have greater affinity for the innervated β_1-receptors than for the β_2-receptors, whereas other drugs block both β_1- and β_2-receptors equally (Table 57–2). Examples of β_1-selective agents are atenolol and metoprolol. Propranolol, nadolol, timolol, and others block both β_1- and β_2-receptors and are called *nonselective* β-blockers. Drugs that primarily block β_1-receptors are called *cardioselective*. With regard to this property, two important qualifications must be kept in mind. First, cardioselectivity is only relative. Thus, when the concentration of any β_1-selective agent is sufficiently high, the compound will block the β_2-receptors as well. Second, most tissues contain both β_1- and β_2-receptors, but the relative amounts vary in different tissues. For example, the heart contains β_1-receptors but also some β_2-receptors, and the bronchioles contain mainly β_2-receptors but also some β_1-receptors. The latter probably explains why even low doses of cardioselective agents decrease forced expiratory volume at 1 second (FEV_1) at rest, because the β_1-receptors of the bronchi are blocked. Higher doses block the bronchial β_2-receptors, causing a still greater decrease in resting FEV_1. Although the decrease in resting FEV_1 is relatively small in most patients receiving cardioselective agents, there have been reported cases of severe asthmatics developing bronchospasm when treated with β-blocking drugs. Thus, many clinicians avoid using β-blocking drugs in the treatment of patients with asthma, largely because alternative agents are available to treat associated conditions (e.g., calcium antagonists for the treatment of angina pectoris, hypertension, or supraventricular arrhythmias).

In the peripheral vasculature, blockade of both β_1- and β_2-receptors leaves α_1-receptors unopposed when they are stimulated by circulating epinephrine. Thus, tissue perfusion sometimes diminishes in patients with peripheral vascular disease when nonselective agents are used. However, decreased perfusion can occur even with low doses of selective agents because of the fall in cardiac output.

Differences in selectivity have clinical implications in the treatment of diabetic patients in two respects. First, during hypoglycemia, epinephrine is released, which, by stimulating unopposed α-receptors during nonselective β-blockade, can cause hypertension and subsequent reflex bradycardia, which is potentially hazardous in diabetics with coronary artery disease. Second, epinephrine increases glycogenolysis and gluconeogenesis in the liver and skeletal muscle by stimulating β2-receptors. Thus, the use of nonselective β-blocking agents can prolong recovery from hypoglycemia in insulin-dependent diabetic patients. Further, because the tachycardia induced by sympathetic discharge is blocked, the patient loses one of the warning signs of hypoglycemia. However, sweating in response to epinephrine release is maintained or even enhanced.

One further important aspect of relative β1-selectivity is the fact that such agents, even when given in doses high enough to effect β2-receptors, do not bind to these receptors with the same avidity as do nonselective β-blockers. Therefore, they can be displaced by lower levels of β2-agonists. Thus, patients with bronchospastic disease who encounter difficulties while receiving β1-selective agents can be more easily treated with β2-agonists such as terbutaline.[10]

Intrinsic Sympathomimetic Activity

All β-receptors contain both binding sites and activation sites. A pure agonist, such as isoproterenol, is bound avidly to both the attachment and the activation sites. In contrast, a pure antagonist, such as atenolol and most other β-receptor blockers, interacts avidly with attachment sites but not with activation sites. Certain β-blocking drugs attach avidly to binding sites but have relatively low affinity for the activation site. Therefore, they stimulate the receptor mildly while blocking the effect of released catecholamines. Because of this property, when sympathetic activation is low, such as when a patient is at rest, partial stimulation of the activation site is evident clinically because of less slowing of heart rate than is seen with a β-blocker without ISA. In contrast, during exercise, when sympathetic activation is high, blocking effects predominate, and the heart rate does not increase to the extent that it would without β-blockade. In contrast with β-blockers without ISA, such as atenolol, β-blockers with this property cause a reduction in peripheral vascular resistance with little change in cardiac output. This difference may be due to activation of peripheral β2-receptors by agents with ISA. This effect on peripheral vasculature offers theoretical advantages in the treatment of patients with peripheral vascular disease or obstructive airway disease.[11] However, the long-term impact of such treatment with agents with ISA has not been established.

Membrane-Stabilizing Activity

Some β-adrenoreceptor blocking drugs, notably propranolol, have quinidine-like effects in that they impair the capacity of excitable tissues to undergo depolarization. This effect is due to the capacity of these compounds to interact with sodium channels in cell membranes. With clinically available compounds, this property becomes apparent only at doses much higher than those required for maximal β-adrenergic blockade. At high doses, propranolol has been found to cause a shortening of both the ventricular effective refractory period and the duration of the monophasic action potential and to have ventricular antiarrhythmic effects that were not apparent when lower β-blocking doses were given.

Certain of the β-blockers, such as metoprolol and pindolol, have only weak membrane-stabilizing activity. Others, atenolol included, have no membrane-stabilizing activity. Membrane-stabilizing activity is not necessary for most therapeutic effects of β-blockers.

PHARMACOKINETICS

Most β-receptor blocking drugs are soluble in lipids (Table 57–3). A few, such as atenolol and nadolol, are more soluble in water. Lipid-soluble agents penetrate cell membranes easily and cross the blood-brain barrier rapidly. Thus, their volumes of distribution within the body tend to be larger. Lipid-soluble drugs are highly bound to plasma proteins and are metabolized by the liver at a relatively rapid rate. For example, about 95% of an orally administered dose of propranolol is metabolized on its first passage through the liver from the gut. In contrast, water-soluble agents are excreted by the kidney without metabolic change. Although lipid- and water-soluble β-blockers do not appear to differ in clinical efficacy, the difference in their solubilities has clinical implications.[12] Lipophilic β-blockers have been found to have higher ratios of brain/plasma concentration, reflecting the ease with which they penetrate the blood-brain barrier. The side effects of fatigue, insomnia, and nightmares have been attributed to high central nervous system concentrations of lipophilic β-receptor blocking drugs. Kostis and Rosen[13] have shown that higher nocturnal wakefulness, restlessness, and depression scores were created in volunteers taking propranolol and pindolol than in those receiving atenolol, metoprolol, or placebo. In that study, other measures of psychomotor and sexual function failed to show a consistent difference.

Closely related to the differing solubility properties of the β-blockers are their pharmacokinetics. In general, water-soluble agents are absorbed from the gastrointestinal tract at variable rates and are excreted by

Table 57–3. **Solubility of β-Blockers**

Lipid	Water
Metoprolol	Acebutolol
Oxprenolol	Atenolol
Penbutolol	Betaxolol
Pindolol	Carteolol
Propranolol	Labetalol
Timolol	Nadolol
	Sotalol

the kidney without undergoing hepatic metabolism. Their rate of excretion depends on renal function and is diminished as glomerular filtration falls. Water-soluble β-blockers tend to have relatively longer half-lives.

Lipid-soluble β-blockers are rapidly absorbed from the gastrointestinal tract and metabolized by the liver at varying rates during their first pass. Drugs such as propranolol and metoprolol are rapidly cleared from the liver, whereas agents such as timolol and pindolol are cleared less quickly. Individuals vary considerably in the amount of a β-blocker that is metabolized during the first pass through the liver; thus, a greater dose titration is required. Because of the rapid hepatic clearance of these drugs, their half-lives tend to be relatively short.

The clinical implications of the differing pharmacokinetics of the β-blockers are reflected in the required dose intervals. Because the water-soluble compounds are excreted slowly, they need be given only once daily, whereas the lipid-soluble compounds are metabolized more rapidly and must be given two or three times daily to maintain clinically efficacious β-blockade. It is believed that patients comply better with once-daily dosing than with programs requiring multiple doses.

EFFECTS ON PATHOPHYSIOLOGY
Effects on Hemodynamics

Many investigators have found that atenolol reduces heart rate, cardiac index, and blood pressure. The results of studies of total peripheral resistance have been less uniform. Acute intravenous administration is usually followed by an increase in total peripheral resistance of 20% to 30%.[14] Studies during chronic oral administration of atenolol have found either no change in vascular resistance[15, 16] or an increase of about 5%.[17] In long-term studies, Lund-Johansen[18] has demonstrated that the hemodynamic effects of atenolol are unchanged after 1 and 5 years of therapy.

Predictably, atenolol blunts the reflex-mediated increase in heart rate that usually follows the Valsalva maneuver or abrupt tilting to the upright position.[17]

Effects on Ventricular Function and Structure

Most studies of intravenously administered atenolol have shown that this agent reduces indices of isovolumic contraction and systolic function in both normal subjects and patients with coronary artery disease.[19–21] However, a negative inotropic effect was not seen when atenolol was given to experimental animals.[22] Echocardiographic studies of hypertensive patients with normal ventricular function during long-term oral administration of atenolol did not reveal a reduction of fractional shortening or ejection fraction, whereas ejection fraction was reduced in patients with coronary artery disease.[23]

Dunn et al.[24] used echocardiography and electrocardiography to study the effect of atenolol on left ventricular hypertrophy in hypertensive patients. Wall thickness decreased significantly within 4 weeks, but left ventricular mass and QRS voltage did not decrease significantly until after 6 months of therapy. The improvement was still present after 1 year of therapy.

In a study of the effect of combination atenolol-enalapril therapy on left ventricular mass and function in 21 hypertensives, Ketelhut et al.[25] found that left ventricular mass decreased gradually over 3 years, even though blood pressure fell much earlier. Left ventricular pump function remained well preserved.

Effects on Electrophysiology

Atenolol prolongs sinus node recovery time and lengthens the RR interval. An increase in atrial refractory period follows administration of atenolol. β-Blockade also prolongs atrioventricular conduction. Atenolol does not possess membrane-stabilizing activity.

Effects on Coronary Blood Flow

Atenolol causes a reduction in coronary blood flow in both normal and atherosclerotic coronary arteries, the decrease being greatest in the diseased vessels.[20, 26] Although atenolol reduces myocardial oxygen demand, this effect is due to a reduction of heart rate. When heart rate is held constant by atrial pacing, oxygen demand does not decrease.[19] It has been proposed that atenolol redistributes blood flow to ischemic areas of the myocardium, but this has not yet been proved.

Effects on Arteries and Veins

Nonselective β-blockers affect vascular β_2-receptors. Thus, when plasma catecholamine levels rise (e.g., during stress or cigarette smoking), vascular α_1-receptors are stimulated without the countering influence of β_2-receptors, resulting in vasoconstriction without modulating vasodilation. This condition in turn causes elevation of blood pressure and reflex bradycardia. Atenolol, in small doses, does not block β_2-receptors; therefore, this potential problem is circumvented.

Effects on Fluid Volume and Electrolytes

Atenolol has no effect on plasma volume, exchangeable sodium or potassium, or total body potassium.[17, 26] However, because it does not block peripheral β_2-receptors, which mediate the transport of potassium from extracellular to intracellular compartments, it does not prevent the fall in serum potassium levels that can occur when plasma catecholamine levels rise.[27]

Endocrine and Metabolic Effects

Like other β-blocking agents, atenolol inhibits the release of renin, resulting in a decrease in angiotensin II production and aldosterone secretion. Atenolol causes plasma norepinephrine levels to rise by about 30% but does not affect epinephrine levels.[17]

Blockade of β_1-receptors inhibits lipolysis, which in turn results in decreased release of free fatty acids and glycerol when epinephrine levels rise during stress.[28] Lowered release of free fatty acids during exercise could worsen fatigue. Atenolol, like other β-blockers, causes an increase in plasma triglyceride levels and a fall in high-density lipoprotein concentration.[29] The effect appears to be dose-dependent.

When given in doses large enough to block β_2-receptors, the resulting reduction of glucose production in response to catecholamine release can prolong hypoglycemia induced by insulin.[30]

Effects on Renal Function

Atenolol has been found to reduce renal vascular resistance in hypertensive patients.[17] No effect on creatinine clearance, glomerular filtration rate, or renal blood flow has been observed. In contrast, nonselective β-blockers have been found to reduce renal function in hypertensive patients.

Microalbuminuria is thought to be an early indicator of hypertension-induced renal damage and vascular permeability. Bianchi et al.[31] compared the effects of enalapril, nitrendipine, atenolol, or diuretic on 48 hypertensive patients with urinary albumin extraction and found that only enalapril decreased urinary albumin. In a similar study, Samuelsson et al.[32] compared the effects of lisinopril and atenolol on urinary albumin excretion and found no differences.

Effects on the Central Nervous System

Although atenolol does not pass the blood-brain barrier freely, some of the compound reaches the central nervous system.[12] The following symptoms, possibly related to a central nervous system effect, have been reported by patients receiving atenolol: dizziness, vertigo, light-headedness, tiredness, fatigue, lethargy, drowsiness, depression, and vivid dreams. A study[33] compared the effects of atenolol and enalapril on memory in a group of hypertensive patients. Enalapril was found to have no effect on memory, whereas a slight impairment of memory was measured in atenolol-treated patients. However, Madden et al.[34] found no effect on memory caused by atenolol or propranolol.

CLINICAL USE
Indications

Arteriosclerotic Heart Disease with Angina Pectoris

Angina pectoris results when myocardial oxygen demands exceed the capacity of the coronary circulation to supply oxygen. During exercise or emotional stress, angina occurs in patients with significant obstructive coronary artery disease because sympathetic activation increases myocardial contractility, heart rate, and systolic blood pressure, all of which increase myocardial oxygen demands. All β-blocking compounds studied to date appear to be effective in the treatment of angina pectoris when given in appropriate doses.[35] Relief of angina can occur even at lower than full β-blocking doses. The choice of agent usually depends on other considerations, such as concomitant illnesses requiring a particular type of β-blocker (e.g., migraine headache requiring a nonselective agent or the presence of another condition that a nonselective β-blocker might aggravate, such as insulin-dependent diabetes mellitus, with which a cardioselective agent might be better tolerated). Angina pectoris can result also from coronary vasospasm, and limited evidence suggests that nonselective β-blockade or large doses of selective β-blockers can aggravate angina in patients with coronary vasospasm due to unopposed stimulation of α-receptor.[36]

Wikstrand et al.[37] have examined the published evidence that β-blockers are effective in the primary prevention of coronary heart disease in hypertensive patients. Atenolol, metoprolol, oxprenolol, and propranolol have been studied. Metoprolol, oxprenolol, and propranolol were shown to reduce the risk of coronary events significantly, but only in men who do not smoke. In the Metoprolol Atherosclerosis Prevention in Hypertensives (MAPHY) trial, the reduction of coronary events was 24%[38] compared with diuretics, which lowered blood pressure equally, suggesting that the mechanism of protection involved antiatherosclerotic, antithrombolic, antiischemic, or antifibrillatory effects. However, in the similar Heart Attack Primary Prevention in Hypertension (HAPPHY) study, no favorable effect was found for atenolol.[39] The reasons for these discrepant results are not clear.

Approximately one patient in five with coronary artery disease has episodes of silent ischemia during daily life. Atenolol, 100 mg daily, has been used in a placebo-controlled trial to determine if treatment of silent ischemia effects outcome.[40] In a study of 306 patients, it was found that treatment with atenolol increased event-free survival. Compared with placebo, the relative risk of a first event was 0.44 (95% confidence interval is 0.26 to 0.75; $p = .001$). Four other trials are underway to provide a definitive answer to this important question.

Hypertension

After the demonstration of antihypertensive efficacy, β-blocking agents grew in popularity because of a relative lack of side effects when compared with previously available orally active antisympathetic drugs, such as reserpine and methyldopa. The mechanisms of antihypertensive action of the β-blockers remain under investigation.[15–18] These agents are known to lower cardiac output, to inhibit renin release, and to alter baroreceptor sensitivity. It has also been postulated that they might act to lower blood pressures through an effect on the central nervous system or by altering catecholamine release. The weight of evidence points to the reduction of cardiac output as the major antihypertensive mechanism. Shortly after institution of therapy, cardiac output falls, but peripheral vascular resistance rises. With time, peripheral resistance decreases but remains higher than pretreatment levels. The decrease in cardiac output can result in reduced exercise performance, particularly in endurance athletes. As monotherapy, the β-blocking agents lower systolic and diastolic blood pressure by as much as 15 mmHg and are more effective when given with a diuretic or a vasodilator. Part of the efficacy of these combinations is explained by the ability of β-blockers to prevent the compensatory responses to diuretics and vasodilators by inhibiting both renin release and the baroreceptor reflex, which are ordinarily activated as blood pressure is lowered. Evidence suggests that the response to β-blockers is related to plasma renin activity: patients with higher renin activity show the greatest drop in blood pressure with β-blockers as monotherapy. Thus, patients such as blacks and the elderly, who ordinarily have low plasma renin activity, tend to have smaller responses. However, it has been suggested that the reduced antihypertensive effect in these groups can be overcome by increased dosage.

The Systolic Hypertension in the Elderly Program[41] compared active treatment with chlorthalidone (with atenolol added if necessary) and placebo in 473 patients with systolic pressure over 160 mmHg and diastolic pressure less than 90 mmHg. During 4.5 years of follow-up, average treated systolic pressure was 143 mmHg, and diastolic pressure was 69 mmHg. The relative risk of stroke was reduced to 0.64 ($p = .0003$), and the relative risk of fatal and nonfatal myocardial infarction was 0.73. Thus, lowering blood pressure in elderly patients improved outcome instead of precipitating strokes or heart attacks.

Silagy et al.[42] compared the antihypertensive effects of atenolol, enalapril, hydrochlorothiazide, and isradipine in patients with isolated systolic hypertension and found that isradipine and enalapril had the greatest effect on systolic blood pressure, whereas only hydrochlorothiazide and enalapril were effective over an entire 24-hour period.

The Medical Research Council trial of hypertension in older adults[43] compared atenolol, hydrochlorothiazide plus amiloride, and placebo in the treatment of 4396 hypertensives, aged 65 to 74 years. During a follow-up of 5.8 years, the diuretic group had a 31% reduction of strokes ($p = .04$) and a 44% reduction of coronary events ($p = .0009$), whereas the same end points were not significantly reduced in the atenolol group. This controversial study suggests that it may be advantageous to use diuretics as first-line treatment of the older hypertensive.

Atenolol has been found to be an effective agent for the management of hypertension during pregnancy. In a placebo-controlled, double-blind study, Rubin et al.[44] observed the development of proteinuria significantly less often in hypertensive pregnant women treated with atenolol without an increase in neonatal adverse outcomes.

Montan et al.[45] compared the effects of atenolol and pindolol, a compound with ISA, on the uteroplacental circulation of 29 women with pregnancy-induced hypertension. They found that although the two agents had comparable antihypertensive effects, atenolol decreased umbilical vein blood flow and increased fetal aortic and umbilical artery pulsatility index, a measure of vascular resistance. Pindolol did not share this effect and was associated with higher placental weights but similar birthweights. Thus, the clinical implications of these observations remain speculative.

Cardiac Arrhythmias and Myocardial Infarction

Withdrawal of sympathetic tone at the atrioventricular junction results in decreased conduction and automaticity and in lengthening of the refractory period. These effects are useful in terminating and preventing supraventricular atrial tachycardia as well as in converting or controlling the ventricular response rate in cases of atrial flutter or atrial fibrillation. Although sinus tachycardia slows in response to β-blockers, this effect is useful primarily in the treatment of conditions such as thyrotoxicosis and anxiety states. Other situations ordinarily require correction of the underlying cause of the tachycardia (e.g., volume depletion). However, in patients with acute myocardial infarction, treatment of sinus tachycardia secondary to anxiety and pain can result in reduced myocardial oxygen demand and thus prevent recurrence of angina or extension of the area of infarction.

The β-receptor blocking drugs have also been found useful in the treatment of ventricular premature complexes, particularly when caused by catecholamine excess, and some have been shown to raise the threshold for induction of ventricular fibrillation.[46] An effect on ventricular extrasystoles and fibrillation has been proposed as one explanation of the reduction in sudden death seen in survivors of acute myocardial infarction treated chronically with β-blockers. This important long-term therapeutic effect has been demonstrated clearly for propranolol and timolol.[47, 48] A short-term reduction in death rate from acute myocardial infarction has been demonstrated also when therapy with atenolol or metoprolol was started soon after the onset of symptoms of infarction.[49, 50]

Hypertrophic Obstructive Cardiomyopathy

Interventions that decrease cardiac size or increase cardiac contractility increase the left ventricular outflow tract gradient and worsen the symptoms of patients with hypertrophic obstructive cardiomyopathy. In contrast, agents that decrease contractility and heart rate, such as β-blocking agents[51] and certain calcium antagonists, relieve symptoms in this disorder. Agents that decrease peripheral vascular resistance, such as nitroglycerin, β-blockers with ISA, and β-blockers with α-receptor blocking properties, may not be effective in the treatment of this disorder.

Dissecting Aneurysm of the Aorta

Pharmacologic therapy of this disorder calls for lowering blood pressure and reducing the rate of ventricular ejection, thus lowering the shearing force of blood that tends to enlarge the aneurysm. The negative inotropic effect of β-blockers and their blood pressure–lowering effects tend to make them useful in the treatment of this disorder.[52] In contrast, agents that lower vascular resistance in addition to inducing β-blockade might not be as desirable therapeutically.

Pheochromocytoma

Blockade of β_2-receptors mediating vasodilation in the presence of high circulating catecholamine levels leads to unbalanced stimulation of α-receptors and can worsen blood pressure elevation in patients with pheochromocytoma. However, in patients with pheochromocytoma who receive adequate doses of α-blocking agents, the addition of β-blockade is sometimes needed for the treatment of tachycardia and cardiac arrhythmias.[53]

Miscellaneous Conditions

β-Blockade, particularly with nonselective agents, has proved to be effective in the prevention of migraine headaches[54] and familial tremor.[55] The tremor and palpitations associated with anxiety are also relieved by β-blockade, as are those of alcohol and drug withdrawal.[56–58] β-Blockers are also useful in controlling the symptoms of hyperthyroidism.[59]

Precautions, Adverse Effects, and Contraindications

A number of cardiovascular disorders present absolute or relative contraindications to the use of atenolol and other β-adrenoreceptor blocking agents. Patients with congestive heart failure due to impaired myocardial contractility ordinarily experience a worsening of symptoms when compensatory sympathetic drive to the heart is blocked. Thus, the use of β-blockers in such patients is contraindicated.[60] However, manifestations of failure, such as an S_4 cardiac gallop and minimal pulmonary rales, can be caused by increased stiffness of the heart in the setting of acute myocardial infarction or chronic hypertension. β-Blockade in patients with acute myocardial infarction whose rales clear with diuretics is not invariably associated with a worsening of symptoms of failure.[61] Similarly, reduction of blood pressure in patients with chronic hypertension usually leads to a reduction of afterload and improvement in cardiac function. During 4 years of treatment with atenolol, only 2 of 547 hypertensive patients experienced heart failure.[62]

A number of clinical trials have examined the effect of β-blockers in patients with idiopathic or ischemic dilated cardiomyopathy and have found that certain patients experience increased exercise time, cardiac output, and ejection fraction, whereas others have no response or even deteriorate.[63] No clinical characteristics have been identified that predict response. A number of agents have been studied, including acebutolol, alprenolol, atenolol, bucindolol, carteolol, labetolol, metoprolol, practolol, and propranolol. A newer compound, xamoterol, has been associated with worsening of congestive heart failure. In a multicenter trial of 381 patients with idiopathic dilated cardiomyopathy, metoprolol reduced mortality and clinical deterioration by 34% compared with placebo. Ejection fraction increased by 0.12 in the treated group and 0.06 in the placebo group ($p < .0001$).[63]

Because β-adrenoreceptor blockers slow atrioventricular conduction, they should not be used in patients with advanced grades of heart block, such as second- or third-degree atrioventricular block, because of the risk of producing complete heart block and a ventricular response rate inadequate to maintain the integrity of the circulation.[64] Similarly, a patient with symptomatic sinus bradycardia will experience a worsening of symptoms when the heart rate is further slowed by therapy with β-blockers.

In patients with peripheral vascular disease, β-adrenergic blockade can lower blood pressure and cardiac output, thus decreasing perfusion of the extremities, an effect that may be worsened by the unbalanced α-tone that results with the use of nonselective β-blockers.[65] Cardioselective agents, when used in low doses, or agents with ISA or associated α-blocking properties, may not lower limb blood flow to the same degree as nonselective agents.

Nonselective β-blocking agents and high doses of selective agents also decrease skin temperature and can cause cold extremities, acrocyanosis, or aggravation of Raynaud's phenomenon. These symptoms appear to be less noticeable when small doses of selective agents or agents with ISA or α-blocking properties are used.

Bronchospastic Disease

As noted earlier, all β-blocking agents cause increased airway resistance, even in normal subjects. The effect is more marked when nonselective β-blockers are used. This effect can cause severe problems in patients with active bronchospastic disease, particularly those who depend on theophylline or β-agonists. β-Blockers should not be used in the management of such patients unless the reasons are compelling.

Diabetes Mellitus

In patients with insulin-dependent (type I) diabetes, β-blockers can obscure the tachycardia ordinarily associated with hypoglycemia and prolong the duration of hypoglycemia.[30] These effects are particularly noticeable when nonselective agents are used.[66] However, larger doses of cardioselective agents cause similar results, which does not invariably result in a major clinical problem. β-Blockers have also been reported to inhibit insulin release in type II diabetics, but this does not necessarily lead to deterioration of the patient's clinical status.[67]

Many hypertensive patients have hyperinsulinemia and obesity. Santucci and Ferris[68] have reviewed the literature relevant to the effect of antihypertensive drugs on insulin sensitivity. They concluded that only angiotensin-converting enzyme inhibitors improve sensitivity, whereas thiazides, atenolol, and metoprolol diminish insulin sensitivity, and calcium antagonists have no effects.

Hyperlipidemia

β-Blocking agents can elevate plasma triglyceride levels and lower high-density lipoprotein levels, thus adversely affecting a patient's cardiovascular risk profile.[29] This effect is most prominent with large doses of nonselective agents. The effect tends to diminish with time, but it does not disappear entirely and is relatively minor when small doses of atenolol are used. Agents with ISA have no effect on triglyceride concentrations and can increase high-density lipoprotein levels. The implications of these observations on the outcomes of patients with cardiovascular disease remain to be determined.

Carruthers et al.[69] compared the effects of atenolol and doxazosin on overall cardiovascular risk in 191 hypertensive patients with normal serum lipids. They observed the risk profile to be reduced to 92.4% of baseline by atenolol and to 74.6% by doxazosin ($p = .0074$). However, more patients had to withdraw from the α-blocker because of side effects or poor response.

In the Trial of Antihypertensive Interventions and Management,[70] which involved overweight hypertensives, atenolol plus diet-induced weight loss lowered cardiovascular risk to 0.85, whereas the risk was 1.04 after 6 months in those following a chlorthalidone-diet regimen.

Miscellaneous Metabolic Effects

Because blockade of peripheral β_2-receptors leads to unbalanced α-adrenergic stimulation when plasma catecholamine levels rise, nonselective β-blockade sometimes can be associated with elevation of blood pressure. This may occur when plasma catecholamine concentrations rise during insulin-induced hypoglycemia or when catecholamine levels rise in response to cigarette smoking or stress.[71]

In contrast, nonselective β-blockade frequently is associated with a minor rise in serum potassium level. β-Blockade diminishes the increase in sodium-potassium transport across cell membranes that usually occurs when β-adrenergic receptors are stimulated. In patients receiving small doses of cardioselective agents, increases in catecholamines (e.g., in response to stress) can result in a decrease in serum potassium levels due to activation of the membrane pump's moving potassium into cells.[27] This effect could be a

problem, especially for patients who are potassium-depleted as a result of chronic diuretic therapy.

Chronic Fatigue

Many patients complain of fatigue, insomnia, nightmares, depression, or loss of energy and concentration when receiving selective or nonselective β-blockers. These effects are thought to be due to accumulation of these compounds in the central nervous system, because most β-blockers are lipid-soluble and readily pass the blood-brain barrier. Anecdotal experience suggests that the water-soluble compounds, atenolol and nadolol, are associated with fewer side effects related to the central nervous system. The occurrence of sleep disturbances has been supported by a controlled study.[13]

Contraindications

Because of the considerations discussed in the previous section, certain conditions are believed to be contraindications to the use of atenolol, including sinus bradycardia and atrioventricular block greater than first degree, because, in both conditions, β-blockade could slow the ventricular rate to the extent that cardiac output is inadequate to sustain blood pressure. Because patients with overt cardiac failure or cardiogenic shock depend on sympathetic stimulation of the heart to maintain circulatory integrity, β-blockade with atenolol or other agents is contraindicated, although a growing body of evidence indicates that certain patients with dilated cardiomyopathy benefit from β-blockade.

Interactions with Other Drugs

When used concomitantly with drugs causing catecholamine depletion such as reserpine, atenolol and other β-blockers can have an additive effect, resulting in hypotension and severe bradycardia.

If atenolol is given when a short-acting central α_2-agonist such as clonidine is withdrawn, the resulting increase in sympathetic outflow in the presence of peripheral β_2-receptor blockade can result in severe hypertension. Caution is advised when atenolol and other β-blockers are combined with agents potentially exerting negative inotropic or chronotropic effects, such as the calcium antagonists.

Use in Patients with Impaired Renal Function

Because atenolol is excreted unchanged by the kidney, serum levels are increased in patients with impaired renal function. Atenolol does not accumulate significantly until creatinine clearance falls to levels less than 35 ml/min/1.73 m², at which point the maximum daily dose of atenolol should be limited to 50 mg. When creatinine clearance is less than 15 ml/min/1.73 m², the elimination half-life rises to more than 27 hours. Therefore, dosage should be limited to

25 mg daily. Patients who require hemodialysis should receive 25 or 50 mg after each period of dialysis.

Atenolol's Place in the Antihypertensive Arsenal

Atenolol has several advantages as an antihypertensive agent. Because it is water-soluble, it is excreted relatively slowly by the kidney; therefore, it need be given no more than once daily in most cases. Furthermore, its hydrophilicity results in limited passage through the blood-brain barrier, thus resulting in fewer central nervous system–related side effects compared with lipophilic β-blockers.

Evidence suggests that atenolol is among the most β_2-receptor–selective of the β-blocking agents; therefore, as long as the daily dose is sufficiently low, side effects related to blockade of β_2-receptors—such as increased airway resistance, bronchospasm, prolongation of insulin-induced hypoglycemia, and cold extremities—are seen less frequently.

Dosage and Administration

For patients with hypertension or angina pectoris, therapy is usually started with an oral dose of 50 mg administered once a day. If the desired therapeutic response does not occur within 1 week, the dose should be increased to 100 mg once daily. Further dose increments do not benefit the resistant hypertensive patient, who should receive a second agent such as a diuretic, vasodilator, α_1-receptor blocker, or central α_2-agonist. Patients with angina can benefit from doses up to 200 mg/day because there is less attenuation of beneficial effect at 24 hours at the higher dose.

SOCIOECONOMIC CONSIDERATIONS
Compliance

During chronic β-blockade, the density of β-adrenoreceptors in various tissues increases. If β-blocking agents are discontinued abruptly, the increased number of receptors makes patients more sensitive to the effect of catecholamines.[72] This effect has resulted in aggravation of angina pectoris and ventricular arrhythmias, myocardial infarction, and death in patients whose β-blocking agents are stopped without prior downward tapering of the dose. These agents should be tapered over 2 or more weeks. If patients have histories of poor compliance with medical programs, the use of β-blockers should be considered carefully, because patients may discontinue therapy on their own. When patients frequently forget to take doses of β-blockers, an agent with a long duration of action allowing once-daily administration, such as atenolol, may be used.

Cost

When the daily costs of the starting doses for hypertension recommended by the manufacturers of several β-blocking agents were compared—rating generic propranolol as 1.0—the following relative costs were found: β-blockers such as proprietary propranolol, metoprolol, nadolol, pindolol, and atenolol cost about twice as much as generic propranolol, whereas timolol was almost three times more expensive. In contrast, the relative cost of treating patients with hypertension with generic hydrochlorothiazide would be only 15% of the cost of generic propranolol (Table 57–4).

Table 57–4. Relative Cost of β-Blocking Agents (per Medium-Strength Tablet)

Generic	
Hydrochlorothiazide	0.15
Propranolol	1.00
Timolol	3.35
Pindalol	7.90
Proprietary	
Labetalol	3.90
Betaxolol	4.74
Metoprolol	4.85
Propranolol	5.00
Timolol	5.00
Penbutolol	7.80
Acebutolol	8.00
Atenolol	8.50
Carteolol	8.50
Pindolol	8.80
Nadolol	9.25
Sotolol	30.00

REFERENCES

1. Powell CE, Slater IH: Blocking of inhibitory adrenergic receptors by a dichloro analogue of isoproterenol. J Pharmacol Exp Ther 122:480, 1958.
2. Ahlquist RP: A study of the adrenotrophic receptors. Am J Physiol 153:586, 1948.
3. Black JW, Stephenson JS: Pharmacology of a new adrenergic beta-receptor blocking compound (Nethalide). Lancet 2:314, 1962.
4. Black JW, Duncan WA, Shanks R: Comparison of some properties of pronethalol and propranolol. Br J Pharmacol 25:577, 1965.
5. Chidsey C, Pine M, Farot L, et al: The use of drug concentration measurements in studies of the therapeutic response to propranolol. Postgrad Med J 52:26, 1976.
6. Lands AM, Luduena FP, Buzzo HJ: Differentiation of receptors responsive to isoproterenol. Life Sci 6:2241, 1967.
7. Harms HH: Isoproterenol antagonism of cardioselective beta adrenergic blocking agents: A comparative study of human and guinea pig cardiac and bronchial beta adrenergic receptors. J Pharmacol Exp Ther 199:329, 1976.
8. Dale HH: On some physiologic actions of Ergot. J Physiol (Lond) 34:163, 1906.
9. Frishman WH: Clinical Pharmacology of the β-Adrenoceptor Blocking Drugs, 2nd ed. Norwalk, CT: Appleton-Century-Crofts, 1984.
10. Ellis ME, Sahay JN, Chatterjee SS, et al: Cardioselectivity of atenolol in asthmatic patients. Eur J Clin Pharmacol 21:173, 1981.
11. Svensson A, Gudrandsson R, Sivertsson R, et al: Metoprolol and pindolol in hypertension: Different effects on peripheral haemodynamics. Clin Sci 61:425S, 1981.
12. Taylor EA, Jefferson D, Carrol JD, et al: Cerebrospinal fluid concentrations of propranolol, pindolol and atenolol in man: Evidence for central action of beta-adrenoceptor antagonists. Br J Clin Pharmacol 12:549, 1981.

13. Kostis JB, Rosen RC: Central nervous system effects of beta-adrenergic-blocking drugs: The role of ancillary properties. Circulation 75:204, 1987.

14. Astrom H, Vallin H: Effect of a new beta-adrenergic blocking agent, ICI 66082, on exercise haemodynamics and airway resistance in angina pectoris. Br Heart J 36:1194, 1974.

15. Astrom H, Vallin H: Effect of atenolol on exercise haemodynamics in angina pectoris and hypertension. Postgrad Med J 53(Suppl 3):84, 1977.

16. Brown HC, Carruthers SG, Johnson GD, et al: Clinical pharmacologic observations on atenolol, a beta-adrenoceptor blocker. Clin Pharmacol Ther 20:524, 1976.

17. Dreslinski GR, Messerli FH, Dunn FG, et al: Hemodynamics, biochemical and reflexive changes produced by atenolol in hypertension. Circulation 65:1365, 1982.

18. Lund-Johansen P: Hemodynamic long-term effects of a new β-adrenoceptor blocking drug, atenolol (ICI 66082), in essential hypertension. Br J Clin Pharmacol 3:445, 1976.

19. Lichtlen P, Simon R, Amende I, et al: Left ventricular function and regional myocardial blood flow after atenolol in normals and patients with coronary artery disease. Postgrad Med J 53(Suppl 3):85, 1977.

20. Thompson DS, Naqui N, Juul SM, et al: Haemodynamic and metabolic effects of atenolol in patients with angina pectoris. Br Heart J 43:668, 1980.

21. Amende I, Simon R, Hood WP, et al: The effects of beta-blocker atenolol and nitroglycerin on left ventricular function and geometry in man. Circulation 60:836, 1979.

22. Harry JD, Knapp MF, Linden RJ: The actions of a new beta-adrenergic blocking drug, ICI 66082, on the rabbit papillary muscle and on the dog heart. Br J Pharmacol 51:169, 1974.

23. Ibrahim MM, Madkour A, Mossallam R: Effect of atenolol on left ventricular function in hypertensive patients. Circulation 62:1036, 1980.

24. Dunn FG, Ventura HO, Messerli FH, et al: Time course of regression of left ventricular hypertrophy in hypertensive patients treated with atenolol. Circulation 76:254, 1987.

25. Ketelhut R, Franz IW, Behre U, et al: Preserved ventricular pump function after a marked reduction of ventricular mass. J Am Coll Cardiol 20:864, 1992.

26. Wilkinson R, Stevens IM, Pickering M, et al: A study of the effect of atenolol and propranolol on renal function in patients with essential hypertension. Br J Clin Pharmacol 10:51, 1980.

27. Vincent HH, Boomsa F, Man in't Veld AJ, et al: Effect of selective and non-selective β-agonists on plasma potassium and norepinephrine. J Cardiovasc Pharmacol 6:107, 1984.

28. Smith U: Adrenergic control of human adipose tissue lipolysis. Eur J Clin Invest 10:343, 1980.

29. Weidmann P, Vehlinger DE, Gerber A: Antihypertensive treatment and serum lipoproteins. J Hypertens 3:297, 1985.

30. Smith V: Effect of beta-adrenergic blocking drugs on the reaction to hypoglycemia and the physical working capacity. Cardiovasc Rev 2:563, 1981.

31. Bianchi S, Bigazzi R, Baldar G, et al: Microalbuminuria in patients with essential hypertension: Effects of several antihypertensive drugs. Am J Med 93:525, 1993.

32. Samuelsson O, Hedner T, Ljungman S: A comparative study of lisinopril and atenolol on low degree urinary albumin excretion, renal function and haemodynamics in uncomplicated, primary hypertension. Eur J Clin Pharmacol 43:469, 1992.

33. Lichter I, Richardson PJ, Wyke MA: Differential effects of atenolol and enalapril on memory during treatment for hypertension. Br J Clin Pharmacol 21:641, 1986.

34. Madden DJ, Blumenthal JA, Ekelund LG: Effects of beta-blockade and exercise on cardiovascular and cognitive functioning. Hypertension 11:470, 1988.

35. Gerber JG, Nies AS: Beta-adrenergic blocking drugs. Annu Rev Med 36:145, 1985.

36. Robertson RM, Wood AJJ, Vaughn WK, et al: Exacerbation of vasotonic angina pectoris by propranolol. Circulation 65:281, 1982.

37. Wikstrand J, Berglund G, Tuomilehto J: Beta-blockade in the primary prevention of coronary heart disease in hypertensive patients. Review of present evidence. Circulation 84(Suppl):193, 1991.

38. Wikstrand J, Warnold I, Tuomilehto J, et al: Metoprolol versus thiazide diuretics in hypertension. Morbidity results from the MAPHY Study. Hypertension 17:579, 1991.

39. Wilhelmsen L, Berglund G, Elmfeldt D, et al: Beta-blockers versus diuretics in hypertensive men: Main results from the HAPPHY trial. J Hypertens 5:561, 1987.

40. Pepine CJ, Cohn PF, Deedwania PC, et al: Effects of treatment on outcome in mildly symptomatic patients with ischemia during daily life. The Atenolol Silent Ischemia Study. Circulation 90(2):762, 1994.

41. SHEP Cooperative Research Group: Prevention of stroke by antihypertensive drug treatment in older persons with isolated systolic hypertension. Final results of the Systolic Hypertension in the Elderly Program (SHEP). JAMA 265:3255, 1991.

42. Silagy CA, McNeil JJ, McGrath BP: Crossover comparison of atenolol, enalapril, hydrochlorothiazide and isradipine for isolate systolic systemic hypertension. Am J Cardiol 70:1299, 1992.

43. MRC Working Party: Medical Research Council trial of treatment of hypertension in older adults: Principal results. Br Med J 304:405, 1992.

44. Rubin PC, Clark DM, Sumner DJ, et al: Placebo-controlled trial of atenolol in treatment of pregnancy-associated hypertension. Lancet 1:431, 1983.

45. Montan S, Ingemarsson I, Marsál K, Sjöberg NO: Randomised controlled trial of atenolol and pindolol in human pregnancy: Effects on fetal haemodynamics. Br Med J 304:946, 1992.

46. Woosley RL, Komhauser D, Smith R, et al: Suppression of chronic ventricular arrhythmias with propranolol. Circulation 60:819, 1979.

47. Norwegian Multicenter Study Group: Timolol-induced reduction in mortality and reinfarction in patients surviving acute myocardial infarction. N Engl J Med 304:801, 1981.

48. Beta-blocker Heart Attack Trial Research Group: A randomized trial of propranolol in patients with acute myocardial infarction: I. Mortality results. JAMA 247:1707, 1982.

49. Hjalmarson A, Herlitz J, Holmberg S, et al: The Goteborg metoprolol trial: Effects on mortality and morbidity in acute myocardial infarction. Circulation 67(Suppl 1):26, 1983.

50. ISIS-1 (First International Study of Infarct Survival) Collaborative Group: Randomised trial of intravenous atenolol among 16,027 cases of suspected acute myocardial infarction: ISIS-1. Lancet 2:57, 1986.

51. Cohen LS, Braunwald E: Amelioration of angina pectoris in idiopathic hypertrophic subaortic stenosis with beta-adrenergic blockade. Circulation 35:847, 1967.

52. Wheat MW Jr: Treatment of dissecting aneurysms of aorta: Current status. Prog Cardiovasc Dis 16:87, 1977.

53. Manger WM, Gifford RW: Current concepts of pheochromocytoma. Cardiovasc Med 3:289, 1978.

54. Weber RB, Reinmuthom JL: The treatment of migraine with propranolol. Neurology 22:366, 1972.

55. Young RR, Growdon JH, Shanhani BT: Beta adrenergic mechanisms in action tremor. N Engl J Med 293:950, 1975.

56. Editorial: Beta-blockers in anxiety and stress. Br Med J 1:415, 1976.

57. Sellers EM, Degan NC, Zilm DH, Macleod SM: Propranolol-decreased noradrenaline excretion and alcohol withdrawal. Lancet 1:94, 1976.

58. Grosz HJ: Narcotic withdrawal symptoms in heroin users treated with propranolol. Lancet 2:564, 1972.

59. Ingbar SH: The role of antiadrenergic agents in the management of thyrotoxicosis. Cardiol Rev Respir 2:683, 1981.

60. Prichard BNC, McDevitt DG, Shanks RG: Uses of beta-adrenoceptor blocking drugs. J R Coll Physicians Lond 11:35, 1976.

61. Yusuf S, Peto R, Bennett D, et al: Early intravenous atenolol treatment in suspected acute myocardial infarction. Lancet 2:273, 1980.

62. Zacharias FJ, Cowan KJ, Cuthbertson PJR, et al: Atenolol in hypertension, a study of long term therapy. Postgrad Med J 53(Suppl 3):102, 1977.

63. Waagstein F, Bristow MR, Swedberg K, et al: Beneficial effects of metoprolol in idiopathic dilated cardiomyopathy. Lancet 342:1441, 1993.

64. Conolly ME, Kersting F, Dollery CT: The clinical pharmacology of beta-adrenoceptor blocking drugs. Prog Cardiovasc Dis 19:203, 1976.

65. Rodger JC, Sheldon CD, Lerski RA, et al: Intermittent claudication complicating beta-blockade. Br Med J 1:1125, 1976.
66. Lager I, Blohme G, Smith U: Effect of cardioselective and nonselective β-blockade on the hypoglycemic response in insulin-dependent diabetes mellitus. Lancet 1:458, 1979.
67. Myers MG, Hope-Gill HF: Effect of *d*- and *dl*-propranolol on glucose-stimulated insulin release. Clin Pharmacol Ther 25:303, 1979.
68. Santucci A, Ferri C: Insulin resistance and essential hypertension: Pathophysiologic and therapeutic implications. J Hypertens 10(Suppl):S9, 1992.
69. Carruthers G, Dessain P, Fodor G, et al: Comparative trial of doxazosin and atenolol on cardiovascular risk reduction in systemic hypertension. The Alpha Beta Canada Trial Group. Am J Cardiol 71:575, 1993.
70. Wassertheil-Smoller S, Oberman A, Blaufox MD, et al: The Trial of Antihypertensive Interventions and Management (TAIM) Study. Final results with regard to blood pressure, cardiovascular risk, and quality of life. Am J Hypertens 5:37, 1992.
71. Deacon SP, Barnet D: Comparison of atenolol and propranolol during insulin-induced hypoglycaemia. Br Med J 2:272, 1976.
72. Lindenfeld J, Crawford MH, O'Rourke RA, et al: Adrenergic responsiveness after abrupt propranolol withdrawal in normal subjects and in patients with angina pectoris. Circulation 62:704, 1980.

CHAPTER 58

Betaxolol

Eduardo Nunez, M.D., Franz C. Aepfelbacher, M.D., and Franz H. Messerli, M.D.

HISTORY

In 1975, Synthelabo, a French pharmaceutical firm, embarked on a project aimed at developing a highly cardioselective β-adrenoreceptor blocker with low membrane-stabilizing activity, prolonged duration of action, and high bioavailability after oral administration. An agent possessing all of these properties would be unique within this class of drugs. A formulation enabling once-daily dosing with minimal side effects would be beneficial for treating patients with chronic disorders in whom noncompliance is a frequent problem. This β-blocker would be potentially useful in the long-term treatment of patients with hypertension, angina pectoris, arrhythmias mediated by excessive stimulation of cardiac β1-adrenoreceptors, and glaucoma.

CHEMISTRY

Betaxolol (2-propanol,1-[4-[2-(cyclopropyl/methoxy)-ethyl]phenoxy]3[(1-methylethyl)amino]) is chemically related to other β1-specific adrenergic blocking compounds such as atenolol, metoprolol, and acebutolol. Its synthesis from *p*-hydroxyphenylacetic acid requires eight steps. A nonhygroscopic powder with a molecular weight of 343.9, betaxolol is 35% soluble in water and 100% soluble in ethanol and has a pH of 6 (in 2% solution) and a pK_a of 9.4.[1]

PHARMACOLOGY

The pharmacologic properties of betaxolol have been investigated extensively in animal models. The relative potency of its β-adrenoreceptor blockade, cardioselectivity, partial agonist activity, and antihypertensive and hemodynamic effects have been summarized by Cavero et al.[2] From these investigations, it is apparent that betaxolol is a relatively potent β1-adrenoreceptor blocking agent with weak membrane-stabilizing activity and no partial agonist effect.

PHARMACODYNAMICS
β-Adrenoreceptor Activity

The inhibitory effect of betaxolol on isoproterenol-induced tachycardia has been demonstrated *in vitro* in studies of guinea pig atria.[2] Betaxolol was found to be twice as potent as metoprolol, seven times as potent as acebutolol, and similar in potency to propranolol. Similar comparative studies supported these findings. In isolated spontaneously beating rat atria, betaxolol was equipotent to propranolol, and it was 8, 9, and 63 times as potent as metoprolol, atenolol, and practolol, respectively, in suppressing tachycardia.

In a comparative study performed on rats anesthetized with pentobarbital, intravenously administered betaxolol, metoprolol, and propranolol had similar effects on heart rate.[2] However, when these agents were administered orally (5 mg/kg), betaxolol produced a superior and more sustained effect on heart rate in comparison with the other two agents. More recently, a similar reduction on exercise heart rate in humans was found for betaxolol, atenolol, and nadolol when given orally.[3]

Cardioselectivity

Betaxolol has greater affinity for β1-adrenoreceptors than does propranolol, which blocks both β1- and β2-adrenoreceptors nonselectively. It appears to have relatively greater affinity for cardiac β1-adrenoreceptors than does metoprolol or atenolol. This greater selectivity for β1-adrenoreceptors has been confirmed using radioligand-binding techniques in guinea pig, bovine, and human lung tissue.[4, 5]

This characteristic was also demonstrated in studies of dogs treated with isoprenaline. The effects of intravenously administered betaxolol on the resultant tachycardia and hypotension, which are mediated by both subtypes of β-adrenoreceptors, were evaluated.[2]

Intravenous administration of betaxolol, 35 µg/kg, resulted in a 50% reduction in heart rate (β_1-mediated response), but there was no discernible effect on blood pressure (β_2-mediated response), even when doses as high as 1.0 mg/kg IV were used.

The specificity of betaxolol's β_1-blocking action is evidenced by its failure to inhibit either the vasodilatory effects of acetylcholine or histamine or the vasoconstrictive effects of 5-hydroxytryptamine or norepinephrine.[2]

The β_1 selectivity of betaxolol in man has been shown in three ways:[6] (1) In normal subjects, 10- to 40-mg oral doses reduced resting heart rate at least as much as 40 mg of propranolol and produced less inhibition of isoproterenol-induced increases in forearm blood flow and finger tremor than propranolol. In this study, 10 mg of betaxolol was at least comparable to 50 mg of atenolol. (2) In normal subjects, single intravenous doses of betaxolol and propranolol that produced equal effects on exercise-induced tachycardia had differing effects on insulin-induced hypoglycemia: propranolol, but not betaxolol, prolonged the hypoglycemia compared with placebo. Neither drug affected the maximal extent of the hypoglycemic response. (3) In a single-blind crossover study in 10 asthmatics, 30-minute intravenous infusion of low doses of betaxolol (1.5 mg) and propranolol (2 mg) had similar effects on resting heart rate but had differing effects on forced expiratory volume at 1 second (FEV_1) and forced vital capacity (VC): propranolol caused significant reduction (10% to 20%) from baseline in mean values for both parameters, whereas betaxolol had no effect on mean values.

As with propranolol and metoprolol, intrinsic β-sympathomimetic stimulation does not occur with betaxolol. This is in contrast with pindolol and acebutolol, which exhibit partial agonist activity.[2]

Hemodynamic Effects

In the spontaneously hypertensive rat, orally administered betaxolol decreased both heart rate and blood pressure, effects that persisted for several hours.[2] After pithing, arterial pressure was raised by electrically stimulating the spinal cord. Betaxolol effectively inhibited these pressor effects, but hypertensive responses to norepinephrine and α-adrenoreceptor agonists were unaffected, indicating a possible peripheral mechanism. One study suggests that betaxolol possesses a direct vasodilating action, probably due to the inhibition of Ca^{2+} influx across the cell membrane.[7]

Betaxolol produces the hemodynamic effects characteristic of β_1-adrenoreceptor blockers that lack intrinsic β-sympathomimetic activity. In anesthetized dogs treated with morphine, betaxolol diminished cardiac output and left ventricular work load. Compared with the same dose of propranolol, betaxolol had a lesser effect on cardiac output. Both propranolol and betaxolol increased total peripheral resistance and depressed left ventricular contractility.[2]

In a study of 10 hypertensive patients, intrave-

nously administered betaxolol (600 µg/kg) reduced resting heart rate, cardiac output, arterial pressure, and myocardial contractility. Pulmonary arterial and wedge pressures were unchanged. Total peripheral resistance was mildly increased.[8] In another experimental study,[9] intravenously administered betaxolol did not differ from atenolol and propranolol in decreasing (dose-dependent) heart rate, maximum left ventricular dP/dt, cardiac output, mean arterial pressure, and myocardial oxygen consumption; however, betaxolol decreased the total peripheral resistance, whereas atenolol and propranolol increased it. This hemodynamic profile makes betaxolol more beneficial than atenolol and propranolol in the treatment of hypertension and ischemic heart disease. The hemodynamic findings in other studies involving patients with coronary artery disease were similar.[10, 11]

Electrophysiologic Effects

Consistent with its negative chronotropic effect, due to β-blockade of the sinoatrial (SA) node and lack of intrinsic sympathomimetic activity, betaxolol increases sinus cycle length and sinus node recovery time. Conduction in the atrioventricular (AV) node is also prolonged.[12] In a study of 21 patients, the electrophysiologic effects of intravenously administered betaxolol (150 µg/kg) were compared with those of intravenously administered propranolol (200 µg/kg). Both drugs produced a moderate suppression of sinus node activity and prolongation of A-H interval; however, the change in A-H interval was more marked with propranolol, but not significantly so. Betaxolol had minimal effect on retrograde AV conduction and no effect on the His-Purkinje system.[13]

Renal Effects

The renal effects of intravenously administered betaxolol (150 µg/kg) and intravenously administered propranolol (200 µg/kg) were compared in a study of 12 patients. Renal blood flow and glomerular filtration rate were unaffected. The renal excretion of sodium and chloride was not reduced significantly; phosphorus and potassium excretion was increased. With propranolol, urinary excretion of sodium and chloride fell while other electrolytes remained unaffected. Hypertensive patients demonstrated decreased plasma renin levels with long-term administration of betaxolol; in patients with renal insufficiency and in the elderly, the elimination half-life was prolonged.[14–16]

Another study showed decreased renal vascular resistance with betaxolol, a desired effect of antihypertensive agents. This effect could be mediated by an increase in atrial natriuretic peptide during treatment.[17]

Respiratory Effects

The potential for impaired ventilation in patients with reversible, obstructive airways disease is well recognized. The effects of intravenously administered betaxolol (22.5 µg/kg) and intravenously administered propranolol (30 µg/kg) on ventilatory parameters were studied in 10 patients with asthma and 10 patients with chronic bronchitis.[18] In asthmatics, mean FEV_1 and VC were unaffected by betaxolol; in contrast, propranolol significantly decreased FEV_1 and VC. However, analysis of individual responses showed that a minority of betaxolol-treated subjects experienced a noteworthy fall in FEV_1 and VC (three and two subjects, respectively).

Similarly, betaxolol reduced FEV_1 in only one subject with chronic bronchitis, whereas propranolol caused a significant fall in FEV_1. Betaxolol caused no variation in VC, whereas 2 of the 10 chronic bronchitis patients given propranolol experienced a decrease in VC exceeding 15%.

A separate study comparing the effects of betaxolol versus propranolol during exercise revealed that pulmonary function and peak expiratory flow rate were unaffected by betaxolol but diminished by propranolol.[8]

Effects on Carbohydrate Metabolism

β-Adrenergic blockade may blunt premonitory signs and symptoms (e.g., tachycardia, blood pressure changes) of acute hypoglycemia. Nonselective β-blockers may potentiate insulin-induced hypoglycemia. This is less likely with cardioselective agents. Betaxolol does not potentiate insulin-induced hypoglycemia and, unlike nonselective β-blockers (propranolol), does not delay recovery of blood glucose to normal levels.[19, 20] Betaxolol has been compared with propranolol, a noncardioselective β-blocker, and acebutolol, a $β_1$-cardioselective agent indicated for use in diabetic patients. In a study of 30 hypertensive nondiabetic patients, oral glucose tolerance tests were unaffected by betaxolol, acebutolol, and propranolol.[21] In another study, betaxolol did not change fasting or postprandial glucose-insulin relationships during simultaneous treatment with either the sulphonylurea glibenclamide or the biguanide metformin.[22]

Effects on Lipid Metabolism

Studies of the lipid effects of two selective β-adrenoreceptor blockers, metoprolol and atenolol, were inconclusive, but a significant reduction in high-density lipoprotein (HDL) cholesterol was common to both agents. Selective β-adrenoreceptor blockers appear to have a less pronounced effect on triglyceride levels. In 10 hypertensive patients treated with betaxolol, total cholesterol and low-density lipoprotein (LDL) were only moderately elevated (<8%) after 1 year of therapy. Interestingly, HDL cholesterol, the protective moiety, was unaffected. In addition, levels of apoprotein B, the essential protein component of the atherogenic lipoproteins, were not adversely affected.[23] In another study, none of 71 patients treated with betaxolol experienced significant changes in total choles-

terol, HDL, LDL, or serum triglycerides after 6 months of therapy.[24] Similar results were found in obese hypertensive patients under therapy with betaxolol.[25]

Hematologic Effects

Platelet aggregation and clotting time were not affected *in vitro*.[26]

PHARMACOKINETICS

A thorough understanding of the pharmacokinetic profile of a new agent is crucial to the design of appropriate clinical trials to assess full therapeutic potential. The pharmacokinetics of betaxolol have been studied extensively in animals and humans.[26-28] Betaxolol is the only $β_1$-blocker to have both a long half-life and a high degree of bioavailability.[26, 29] Table 58–1 compares selected pharmacokinetic properties of the various β-adrenoreceptor blocking agents.

After low-dose (10 to 40 mg) oral administration, betaxolol is rapidly and completely absorbed from the gastrointestinal tract, is about 50% protein-bound, and has a plasma half-life of some 16 hours. Betaxolol has no active metabolites. Tissue distribution is wider than for other β-adrenergic blockers (4.0 to 7.3 L/kg). Peak drug plasma concentrations are achieved 3 or 4 hours after administration, are highly consistent, and are proportional to the administered dose. The relationship between dose and drug concentration is linear, and dose-drug concentration correlates well with reductions in heart rate and arterial pressure. Steady-state blood levels are reached 5 days after therapy is initiated.

Betaxolol has excellent bioavailability (89%), which is evidenced by studies comparing the effects of different routes of administration.[30] After oral administration, the degree of β-blockade is only slightly less than it is after intravenous administration. Bioavailability is unaffected by alterations in hepatic blood flow, and, unlike propranolol and atenolol, it is unaffected by the simultaneous ingestion of food or ethanol. First-pass effect is minimal, and elimination of the drug is governed by hepatic biotransformation. The combination of these factors results in highly consistent plasma drug concentrations.[8, 26, 27]

With its pharmacokinetic profile, it is anticipated that the cardioselective β-blocker betaxolol may offer the following distinct clinical advantages.

Lipid Solubility

Betaxolol is more lipophilic than atenolol, but less so than propranolol. Whether lipid solubility increases adverse central nervous system effects of β-blockers is unclear.[31-33]

Low Dosage

With excellent absorption and bioavailability, good potential exists for effective low-dose therapy. Oral

Table 58–1. **Comparison of Pharmacokinetic Parameters of β-Adrenoreceptor Blocking Agents**

Drugs	T_{max} (hr)	$T_{1/2}$ (hr)	F (%)	Protein Binding (%)	Urinary Elimination of Unchanged Product (%)	Active Metabolite
Betaxolol*	2.0–6.0	16–22	80–90	50	15	None
Acebutolol*	1.0–3.0	3–5	20–60	10	15	N-Ac-A
Alprenolol	0.5–1.5	2–4	1–10	35	<1	4-OH-A
Atenolol*	2.0–4.0	3–6	40–60	10	40	None
Labetalol	1.0–2.0	4	40	50	5	None
Metoprolol*	0.5–1.5	3–6	40–50	88	9	None
Nadolol	2.0–4.0	14–24	30–50	30	10–70	None
Oxprenolol	0.5–1.0	1–3	25–60	90	5	None
Pindolol	1.5–2.0	2–4	85–95	45	50	None
Propranolol	1.0–3.0	3–5	20–30	90–95	<1	4-OH-P
Sotalol	2.0–4.0	5–13	90–100	10	75	None
Timolol	2.0–3.0	3–5	75	10	5–20	None

*Cardioselective; T_{max}, time to maximum effect; $T_{1/2}$, half-life; F, bioavailability (%).

From Ferrandes B, Durand A, Andre-Fraisse J, et al. Pharmacokinetics and metabolism of betaxolol in various animal species and man. *In* Morselli PL, Kilborn JR, Carero I, et al (eds): Betaxolol and Other β₁-Adrenoceptor Antagonists. New York: Raven Press, 1983, pp 51–64.

administration of betaxolol, 10 to 40 mg once daily, has been shown to produce an effect on heart rate and blood pressure comparable to that of propranolol, 40 to 160 mg twice daily,[34] and atenolol, 25 to 100 mg once daily.[24]

Bioavailability

Betaxolol has a higher bioavailability than propranolol, acebutolol, metoprolol, atenolol, and nadolol.[30] It is equivalent in bioavailability to pindolol and sotalol, both of which are nonselective β-blockers.[27]

Duration of Action

Advertisements for betaxolol emphasize its relatively long half-life compared with other β-blockers, but the correlation between half-lives of β-blockers and their duration of action in treating hypertension is poor. The mechanism of action of these drugs in lowering elevated blood pressure is unknown; antihypertensive effects may last longer than β-blockade. The long elimination half-life of betaxolol (mean 16 hours) and prolonged duration of action allow once-daily dosing with reliable, consistent, full 24-hour control of blood pressure.[24, 30, 34, 35] These features are desirable in the treatment of chronic cardiovascular disorders, especially when noncompliance is a potential problem. In a comparative study, betaxolol demonstrated less plasma level fluctuation, intersubject variability, and intrasubject variability than atenolol.[35]

When used in the treatment of angina pectoris, betaxolol significantly reduced exercise-induced ST-segment depression in the trough phase of the plasma level when compared with propranolol[36] or atenolol.[37]

Dose-Plasma Concentration

The stable relationship between dose and plasma concentration should result in predictable, reliable drug concentrations that can be titrated easily for optimal therapeutic effect.

CLINICAL USE

Extensive study of the pharmacodynamics and physiologic effects of betaxolol has confirmed that it shares the general characteristics of β-adrenoreceptor blockers. The short- and long-term effects of betaxolol have been studied in controlled and comparative trials involving more than 7300 patients in Europe and the United States. In addition, clinical efficacy and patient tolerance have been assessed in thousands of patients in open trials. Betaxolol was generally well tolerated, with an adverse events profile comparable with those of similar agents.

ESSENTIAL HYPERTENSION

β-Blockers have been used in the treatment of hypertension since the late 1960s, and in many centers they have been used as first-line therapy. Their role in this position appears stronger than earlier in view of the results of the three large intervention trials in elderly hypertensive patients (SHEP, STOP-Hypertension, and MRC), which all used β-blockers as one of their therapeutic alternatives.[38]

Comparative Clinical Studies

In placebo-controlled studies, betaxolol was found to lower arterial pressure significantly in hypertensive patients during short- and long-term administration. In comparative trials, betaxolol was found to be as effective as propranolol and atenolol in reducing heart rate and arterial pressure within the dose ranges used. Data from the United States trials demonstrate the efficacy of an initial dose of 10 mg once daily for the treatment of mild and moderate hypertension.[16, 24, 34] In some patients, increases in dosage to 20 mg/day may be required to attain better control of arterial pressure.

Betaxolol, 20 mg, was found to be superior to propranolol LA, 160 mg, in terms of duration of action[39] and hypotensive effect.[40] A 1-year, double-blind Finnish study of 100 patients showed that betaxolol, 20 mg once daily, was comparable with atenolol, 100 mg once daily, for the treatment of hypertension.[41] In a 24-week, randomized, double-blind study of 146 hypertensive patients, a single daily dose of betaxolol, 10 to 40 mg, was found to have a hypotensive effect comparable with a once-daily dose of atenolol, 25 to 100 mg. Also, the cumulative response rates in supine diastolic pressure (90 mmHg or less, or a minimum reduction of 10 mmHg) at the highest doses used in the study were markedly higher in the betaxolol-treated group—83% versus 65% of the atenolol-treated group. Similarly, at the highest doses used in the study, analysis of the cumulative response rates found that 72% of the betaxolol group achieved normotension, versus 52% of the atenolol group.[24]

In a multicenter, randomized, double-blind trial in 117 patients, betaxolol (10 to 40 mg/day) was equal or superior to atenolol (25 to 100 mg/day) in its effect on blood pressure; 41 (72%) of 57 betaxolol-treated patients achieved normotension, compared with 31 (52%) of 60 patients treated with atenolol.[30] In another controlled trial in 93 patients, betaxolol (10 to 40 mg once daily) was equal in effectiveness to propranolol (40 to 160 mg b.i.d.) for treatment of mild to moderate hypertension.[34] Other randomized clinical comparisons of betaxolol found the drug at least as effective as atenolol, propranolol, or acebutolol.[42, 43]

ISCHEMIC HEART DISEASE
Experimental Evidence

In one study, betaxolol attenuated the ischemia-induced myocardial acidosis in dog hearts and was more effective in improving myocardial acidosis with a relatively weak effect on myocardial contractile function than were atenolol and propranolol.[44] In another study, using dog hearts subjected to an occlusion of the left anterior descending coronary artery and pretreated with betaxolol IV, betaxolol delayed the onset of myocardial metabolic change from aerobic to anaerobic during ischemia, hence reducing the severity of myocardial ischemic injury.[45]

Comparative Clinical Studies: Angina Pectoris

Betaxolol was compared with placebo in a study of 18 men with exertional angina pectoris. At doses capable of relieving angina and enhancing exercise tolerance, no significant effect on left ventricular systolic function was found.[46] The hemodynamics of intravenously administered betaxolol at rest and during exercise were studied in 14 patients with coronary artery disease. With doses of 0.15 and 0.30 mg/kg, left ventricular filling pressure increased slightly at rest without impairment of left ventricular function. No evidence was found of a clinically significant negative inotropic effect during exercise.[10]

In a double-blind, randomized study of patients with stable angina pectoris, betaxolol, 20 mg, had the same antianginal effect and a comparable antiischemic effect as atenolol, 100 mg, at 3 hours. Twenty-four hours after drug ingestion, the β-blocking, antianginal, and antiischemic effects of atenolol significantly decreased. Betaxolol maintained its β-blocking and antianginal activities at 24 hours and compared favorably with atenolol in antiischemic activity ($p < .05$), suggesting prolonged effects compared with atenolol.[47]

Other studies have confirmed that betaxolol appears to be as useful as atenolol and propranolol for the therapy of angina pectoris.[36, 48, 49]

ARRHYTHMIAS
Clinical Studies

In several studies in humans, and with electrophysiologic testing, betaxolol has been proven to be effective in the treatment of supraventricular tachycardia by prolonging the antegrade functional refractory period of the A-V node.[12] Its potential usefulness in antiarrhythmic therapy needs to be proved with additional clinical studies.

NONCARDIOVASCULAR INDICATIONS

Betaxolol has been proven effective for the treatment of glaucoma[50] and neuroleptic-induced akathisia.[51, 52]

CLINICAL PROFILE

Although betaxolol's pharmacokinetic profile differs from that of other β-blockers, it shares the clinical characteristics of other β-adrenoreceptor antagonists. As such, it can be anticipated that the standard contraindications and precautions recommended for drugs in this class will be applicable.

Contraindications

Contraindications include known hypersensitivity to β-blockers, sinus bradycardia, greater than first-degree AV block, cardiogenic shock, and overt congestive heart failure.

Warnings and General Precautions

Patients should be advised that reductions in intraocular pressure may interfere with glaucoma screening tests. In certain patients, acute withdrawal may precipitate acute angina pectoris or myocardial infarction.

Hepatic and Renal Systems

Betaxolol is primarily metabolized in the liver to metabolites that are inactive, and then it is excreted by the kidneys; dosage reductions have not routinely been necessary with hepatic and/or renal insufficiency, but patients with such conditions should be observed. Patients on dialysis require a reduced dose.

Respiratory System

Because of the risk of bronchospasm, all use of β-adrenoreceptor antagonists in patients with chronic respiratory disease is discouraged. However, because betaxolol has demonstrated increased cardioselectivity, it may prove to be a safer alternative to other β-blocking agents when these agents must be used.

Endocrine System

β-Blockade may also mask some symptoms of hypoglycemia and thyrotoxicosis.

Pediatric Use

Indications for pediatric use have not yet been established.

Adverse Effects

Serious adverse effects have been uncommon but, as with all β-blockers, the major serious adverse effects associated with therapy with betaxolol are bradycardia (more frequent in elderly patients), high-degree AV block, bronchospasm, acute pulmonary edema, and hypotension. The profile of adverse effects of betaxolol, including central nervous system effects (fatigue and depression),[24] is similar to that of atenolol.[24, 34] Betaxolol, like other β-blockers, has been associated with the appearance of antinuclear antibodies. In general, the side effects associated with the clinical use of betaxolol have generally been minimal or mild and are common to other selective β-blockers (Table 58–2).

Although animal studies have shown a lack of teratogenic potential, adequate studies have not been conducted in pregnant women. Only if the potential benefit exceeds the potential risk should the use of β-blockers be considered in pregnant women.

Drug Interactions

The combination of any β-blocker with a catecholamine-depleting drug such as reserpine may seriously depress sympathetic activity, which may be manifested clinically as hypotensive episodes and bradycardia. In patients receiving digitalis, β-blockade can increase the risk of bradycardia and AV block.

Specific studies of betaxolol have examined the effect of concomitant use of some commonly prescribed drugs.[8] No pharmacokinetic interactions were identified with either hydrochlorothiazide or chlorthalidone. In contrast with propranolol and metoprolol, betaxolol is not susceptible to enzyme inhibition by cimetidine. Coadministration of nifedipine, which elevates propranolol concentration, had no effect on the pharmacokinetics of betaxolol, an observation that is consistent with a low first-pass effect. Prothrombin time in patients on chronic warfarin therapy was not affected by betaxolol. Literature reports suggest that orally administered calcium antagonists may be used in combination with β-adrenergic blocking agents when heart function is normal but should be avoided in patients with impaired cardiac function. Hypotension, AV conduction disturbances, and left ventricular failure have been reported in some patients receiving β-adrenergic blocking agents when an orally administered calcium antagonist was added to the treatment regimen.

Potential Therapeutic Advantages of Betaxolol Therapy

Because of betaxolol's enhanced β₁-specificity, side effects due to β₂-blockade should be minimized. When a decision is made to use β-blocker therapy, with appropriate caution, in patients at risk for complications (e.g., patients with chronic respiratory disease, diabetes mellitus, or peripheral vascular insufficiency), β₁-cardioselective agents such as betaxolol may offer advantages over less-selective agents. Compliance should be better with once-daily dosing than with multidose β-blocker regimens. Because betaxolol has low protein binding and minimal hepatic metabolism, its potential for drug interactions is likely lower than that of other agents.

Finally, the pharmacokinetics of betaxolol appear to result in a more complete 24-hour effect, resulting in a more consistent response; this quality may provide more efficient control of blood pressure. If this evidence is substantiated, betaxolol will prove to be a significant addition to the β-blocker armamentarium (Table 58–3).

Table 58–2. **Side Effects of Betaxolol**

Dermatologic: Rash
Respiratory: Dyspnea, pharyngitis, rhinitis, upper respiratory infection
Neuropsychiatric: Headache, dizziness, fatigue, paresthesias, lethargy, nervousness, insomnia, vivid dreams, depression
Gastrointestinal: Dyspepsia, nausea, diarrhea
Musculoskeletal: Joint and muscle pain

Table 58–3. **Potential Clinical Applications of Betaxolol**

- As initial monotherapy in patients with mild and moderate hypertension
- In the poorly compliant or partially compliant patient on multidose β-blocker therapy
- In the stable hypertensive diabetic patient for whom a highly β₁-specific blocker is preferred
- In low doses and with caution in the patient with coexistent mild bronchospastic disease when β-blockers must be used
- In combination with a thiazide diuretic in the patient with moderate to severe hypertension (diastolic pressure 105 to 129 mmHg)
- In the patient with mild to moderate renal dysfunction (creatinine clearance >20 ml/min)
- As a component of triple therapy for hypertension (i.e., with diuretic, vasodilator, and β-blocker) in the refractory patient

CONCLUSION

Betaxolol is an effective once-a-day β_1-blocker for treatment of hypertension and offers clinical advantages over other β-blockers marketed for this indication in relation to its particularly long duration of action and marked cardioselectivity. For other indications, however, there are not enough data.

REFERENCES

1. Manoury P: Betaxolol: Chemistry and biological profile in relation to its physicochemical properties. In Morselli PL, Kilborn JR, Cavero I, et al (eds): LERS Monograph Series, Vol 1. Betaxolol and Other β1-Adrenoceptor Antagonists. New York: Raven Press, 1983, pp 13–19.
2. Cavero I, Lefevre-Borg F, Manoury P, et al: In vitro and in vivo pharmacological evaluation of betaxolol, a new, potent, and selective β1-adrenoceptor antagonist. In Morselli PL, Kilborn JR, Cavero I, et al (eds): LERS Monograph Series, Vol 1. Betaxolol and Other β1-Adrenoceptor Antagonists. New York: Raven Press, 1983, pp 31–42.
3. Lipworth BJ, Irvine NA, Mc Devitt DC: The effects of chronic dosing on the beta 1 and beta 2-adrenoceptor antagonism of betaxolol and atenolol. Br J Clin Pharmacol 31(2):154, 1991.
4. Engel G: Subclasses of beta-adrenoceptors—a quantitative estimation of beta 1 and beta 2-adrenoceptors in guinea pig and human lung. Postgrad Med J 57(Suppl 1):77, 1981.
5. Satoh E, Narimatsu A, Hosohata Y, et al: The affinity of betaxolol, a beta 1-adrenoceptor-selective blocking agent, for beta-adrenoceptors in the bovine trachea and heart. Br J Pharmacol 108:484, 1993.
6. Physicians' Desk Reference. Montvale, NJ: Medical Economics Data, 1994.
7. Besho H, Suzuki I, Tobe A: Vascular effects of betaxolol, a cardioselective beta-adrenoceptor antagonist, in isolated rat arteries. Jpn J Pharmacol 55(3):351, 1991.
8. Data on file, Lorex Pharmaceuticals, Skokie, Illinois.
9. Satoh N, Suzuki J, Bessho H, et al: Effects of Betaxolol on cardiohemodynamics and coronary circulation in anesthetized dogs: Comparison with atenolol and propranolol. Jpn J Pharmacol 54(2):113, 1990.
10. Biamino G: Hemodynamics of betaxolol at rest and during exercise in patients with ischemic heart disease. In Morselli PL, Kilborn JR, Cavero I, et al (eds): LERS Monograph Series, Vol 1. Betaxolol and Other β1-Adrenoceptor Antagonists. New York: Raven Press, 1983, pp 251–256.
11. Harrison DC: Clinical testing of β-adrenergic blockade in angina pectoris. In Morselli PL, Kilborn JR, Cavero I, et al (eds): LERS Monograph Series, Vol 1. Betaxolol and Other β1-Adrenoceptor Antagonists. New York: Raven Press, 1983, pp 243–250.
12. Kuhlkamp V, Ickrath O, Haasis R, et al: Comparison of the effects of intravenous and oral betaxolol on antegrade and retrograde conduction in patients with atrioventricular nodal reentrant and atrioventricular reentrant tachycardia. Eur Heart J 10(6):493, 1989.
13. Lekieffre J, Libersa C, Caron J, et al: A study of the electrophysiologic effects of parenteral betaxolol. In Morselli PL, Kilborn JR, Cavero I, et al (eds): ERS Monograph Series, Vol 1. Betaxolol and Other β1-Adrenoceptor Antagonists. New York: Raven Press, 1983, pp 167–170.
14. Fillastre JP, Godin M, Cazor JL, et al: Renal effects of betaxolol. In Morselli PL, Kilborn JR, Cavero I, et al (eds): LERS Monograph Series, Vol 1. Betaxolol and Other β1-Adrenoceptor Antagonists. New York: Raven Press, 1983, pp 183–194.
15. Bauer JH, Reams GP, Lau A: A comparison of betaxolol and nadolol on renal function in essential hypertension. Am J Kidney Dis 10:109, 1987.
16. Reams GP, Bauer JH, Lau A: The acute and chronic effects of betaxolol on blood pressure, renin—aldosterone and renal function in essential hypertension. J Clin Pharmacol 27:118, 1987.
17. Hollenbeck M, Plum J, Heerg P, et al: Influence of betaxolol on renal function and atrial natriuretic peptide in essential hypertension. J Hypertens 19:819, 1991.
18. Hugues FC, Julien D, Marche J: Influence of betaxolol and atenolol on airways in chronic obstructive lung disease: Comparison with propranolol. In Morselli PL, Kilborn JR, Cavero I, et al (eds): LERS Monograph Series, Vol 1. Betaxolol and Other β1-Adrenoceptor Antagonists. New York: Raven Press, 1983, pp 195–205.
19. Benn JJ, Brown PM, Beckwith LJ, et al: Glucose turnover in type I diabetic subjects during exercise. Effect of selective and nonselective beta-blockade and insulin withdrawal. Diabetes Care 15(11):1721, 1992.
20. Janka HU, Ziegler AG, Larrat V, et al: The effect of the beta 1 selective beta blocker, betaxolol, on metabolism in type II diabetics. Arzneimittelforschung 39(5):615, 1989.
21. Frances Y, Luccioni R, Vague P, et al: Effects of betaxolol, propranolol, and acebutolol on the glycoregulation after oral glucose tolerance test in hypertensive patients. In Morselli PL, Kilborn JR, Cavero I, et al (eds): LERS Monograph Series, Vol 1. Betaxolol and Other β1-Adrenoceptor Antagonists. New York: Raven Press, 1983, pp 213–220.
22. Sinclair AJ, Davies IB, Warrington SJ: Betaxolol and glucose-insulin relationships: Studies in normal subjects taking glibenclamide or metformin. Br J Clin Pharmacol 330(5):699, 1990.
23. Jaillard J, Rouffy J, Sauvanet JP: Long-term influence of betaxolol on plasma lipids and lipoproteins. In Morselli PL, Kilborn JR, Cavero I, et al (eds): LERS Monograph Series, Vol 1. Betaxolol and Other β1-Adrenoceptor Antagonists. New York: Raven Press, 1983, pp 221–231.
24. Mroczek WJ, Burris JF, Hogan LB, et al: Comparison of the antihypertensive effects of betaxolol to atenolol. Am J Cardiol 61:807, 1988.
25. van Os JS, van Brummelen P, Woittez AJ: Betaxolol in obese hypertensive patients. Long-term effects on blood pressure and serum lipids. Neth J Med 40:227, 1992.
26. Warrington SJ, Turner P, Kilborn JR, et al: Blood concentrations and pharmacodynamic effects of betaxolol, a new β-adrenoceptor antagonist, after oral and intravenous administration. Br J Clin Pharmacol 10:60, 1980.
27. Fernandes B, Durand A, Andre-Fraisse J, et al: Pharmacokinetics and metabolism of betaxolol in various animal species and man. In Morselli PL, Kilborn JR, Cavero I, et al (eds): LERS Monograph Series, Vol 1. Betaxolol and Other β1-Adrenoceptor Antagonists. New York: Raven Press, 1983, pp 51–64.
28. Stagni G, Davis PJ, Ludden PM: Human pharmacokinetics of betaxolol enantiomers. J Pharm Sci 80(4):321, 1991.
29. Balnave JD, Neil JD, Russell CJ, et al: Observations on the efficacy and pharmacokinetics of betaxolol, a cardioselective β-adrenoceptor-blocking drug. Br J Clin Pharmacol 11:171, 1981.
30. Ludden TM, Boyle DA, Gieseker D, et al: Absolute bioavailability and dose proportionality of betaxolol in normal healthy subjects. J Pharmacol Sci 77:779, 1988.
31. Dimsdale JE, Newton RP, Joist T, et al: Neuropsychological side effects of beta-blockers. Arch Intern Med, 149:514, 1989.
32. Conant J, Engler R, Janowsky D, et al: Central nervous system side effects of β-adrenergic blocking agents with high and low lipid solubility. J Cardiovasc Pharmacol 13:656, 1989.
33. Dahlof C, Dimenas E: Side effects of β-blocker treatment as related to the central nervous system. Am J Med Sci 299:236, 1990.
34. Davidov ME, Glazer N, Wollam G, et al: Comparison of betaxolol, a new beta-1-adrenergic antagonist, to propranolol in the treatment of mild to moderate hypertension. Am J Hypertens 1:206S, 1988.
35. Kunka, RL, Wong Y, Anderson RL, et al: Steady-state fluctuation and variability of betaxolol and atenolol plasma levels. Ther Drug Monit (In press).
36. Narahara KA, and Betaxolol Investigators Group: Double-blind comparison of once daily betaxolol versus propranolol four times daily in stable angina pectoris. Am J Cardiol 65:577, 1990.
37. Mc Lenachan JM, Findlay IN, Wilson JT, et al: Twenty-four-hour beta-blockade in stable angina pectoris: A study of atenolol and betaxolol. J Cardiovasc Pharmacol 20(2):311, 1992.
38. Hansson L: Treatment of hypertension in the elderly. J Hypertens Suppl 11(4):S25, 1993.

39. Kesteloot H, Missotten A, Coupez-Lopinot R, et al: Effect of betaxolol on heart rate at rest and during exercise. Acta Cardiol (Brux) 37:117, 1982.

40. Coupez JM, Bachy C, Coupez-Lopinot R: Comparison of the effects of betaxolol and long-acting propranolol in the hypertensive patient at rest and during a dynamic exercise test. In Morselli PL, Kilborn JR, Cavero I, et al (eds): LERS Monograph Series, Vol 1. Betaxolol and Other β1-Adrenoceptor Antagonists. New York: Raven Press, 1983, pp 315–324.

41. Salonen JT, Palminteri R, Salonen R: Long-term treatment of hypertension with fixed doses of betaxolol and atenolol. In Rosenfeld JB, Silverberg DS, Viskoper R (eds): Hypertension Control in the Community. London: John Libbey, 1985, pp 267–269.

42. Beresford R, Heel RC: Betaxolol. A review of its pharmacodynamic and pharmacokinetic properties, and therapeutic efficacy in hypertension. Drugs 31(1):6, 1986.

43. Burris JF, Davidod ME, Jenkins P, et al: Comparison of the antihypertensive effects of betaxolol and chlorthalidone as monotherapy and in combination. Arch Intern Med 149(11):2437, 1989.

44. Abe Y, Narimatsu A, Tobe A: Betaxolol, a cardioselective beta-adrenoceptor antagonist, attenuates ischemic myocardial acidosis in dogs. Jpn J Pharmacol 53(2):185, 1990.

45. Abe Y, Narimatsu A, Tobe A: Effects of betaxolol, a cardioselective beta-adrenoreceptor antagonist, on ischemic myocardial

46. Alpert MA, Singh A, Homes RA, et al: Effect of beta blockade with betaxolol on left ventricular systolic function in chronic stable angina pectoris and left ventricular dysfunction. Am J Cardiol 57:721, 1986.

47. de Backer G, Derese A: Double-blind study of betaxolol in patients with stable angina pectoris. In Morselli PL, Kilborn JR, Cavero I, et al (eds): LERS Monograph Series, Vol 1. Betaxolol and Other β1-Adrenoceptor Antagonists. New York: Raven Press, 1983, pp 261–266.

48. MacLenachan JM, Findlay IN, Wilson JT, et al: Twenty-four-hour β-blockade in stable angina pectoris: A study of atenolol and betaxolol. J Cardiovasc Pharmacol 20:311, 1992.

49. Alpert MA, Mukerji V, Villarreal D, et al: Efficacy of betaxolol in the treatment of stable exertional angina pectoris: A dose-ranging study. Angiology 41(5):365, 1990.

50. Berropsi A, Leibowitz H: Betaxolol. A new beta-adrenergic blocking agent for treatment of glaucoma. Arch Ophthalmol 100:943, 1982.

51. Dumon JP, Catteau J, Lanvin F, et al: Randomized, double-blind, crossover, placebo-controlled comparison of propranolol and betaxolol in the treatment of neuroleptic-induced akathisia. Am J Psychiatry 149(5):647, 1992.

52. Adler LA, Angrist B, Rotrosen J: Efficacy of betaxolol in neuroleptic-indiced akathisia. Psychiatry Res 39(2):193, 1991.

CHAPTER 59

Bisoprolol

Matthew R. Weir, M.D., Peter Bolli, M.D., B. N. C. Prichard, M.B., M.Sc., F.R.C.P., F.F.P.M., and Michael A. Weber, M.D.

β-Adrenoreceptor blocking drugs were first introduced into therapeutics in 1963. Since then, there has been continuous development of nonselective and cardioselective β-blockers as well as nonselective β-blockers that also possess α-blocking capabilities (Table 59–1). All these drugs are competitive inhibitors of the effect of catecholamines on the β-receptor. Important differentiating characteristics among these drugs include selectivity between β1- and β2-receptors, whether or not they possess intrinsic sympathomimetic activity, as well as whether or not the drugs possess α-adrenoreceptor blocking capability. Bisoprolol is a highly β1-selective (cardioselective) β-adrenoreceptor blocker that does not possess any intrinsic sympathomimetic activity.[1] It was first synthesized and developed by the pharmaceutical research department of E. Merck, Darmstadt, Federal Republic of Germany. It is approved in nearly all European markets as well as in parts of Asia and Japan. It is also available in the United States.

PHARMACOLOGIC CHARACTERISTICS

Bisoprolol, like other β-blockers, has a propanolamine side chain that determines its affinity for β-adrenoreceptors. The L-form is the active compound, and its β-blocking potency is 30 to 40 times higher than that of the D-form.[2] Bisoprolol antagonizes the β-adrenoreceptor toward β-adrenoreceptor agonists competitively. Bisoprolol is devoid of intrinsic sympathomimetic activity,[3] local anesthetic activity, or calcium antagonistic effects.[4, 5]

The β1-selectivity of bisoprolol indicates the high degree of affinity that the drug has for the β1 adrenoreceptor and explains why there is less of a rise of blood pressure in response to pressor stimuli involving high levels of catecholamines, nearly no increase in airways resistance in asthmatic subjects, nearly no interference of various metabolic functions, nearly no alteration of lipoprotein metabolism, and less of a block on cardiac effects of isoprenaline as compared with nonselective and less β1-selective agents.

β1-Adrenoreceptor Selectivity

One of the outstanding pharmacologic properties of bisoprolol is its high degree of β1-adrenoreceptor selectivity. This effect has been demonstrated in several tissues of various animal species. *In vitro* studies using (-)-[^{125}I]iodocyano-pindolol in rat and in rabbit lung membranes showed that bisoprolol had about 100 times greater affinity to β1-adrenoreceptors than to β2-adrenoreceptors.[3] Inhibition of ^{3}H-dihydroalprenolol binding by bisoprolol and other β-blockers on plasma membranes from rat heart and lung showed that bisoprolol had a greater β1:β2 selectivity

Table 59–1. **Classification of β-Adrenoreceptor Blocking Drugs**

	Partial Agonist Effect (Intrinsic Sympathomimetic Effect)	Membrane Stabilizing Effect (Quinidine-like Effect)
Division I: Nonselective ($\beta_1 + \beta_2$) block		
Group I		
Oxprenolol	+	+
Alprenolol		
Penbutolol		
Group II		
Propranolol	−	+
Group III		
Pindolol	+	−
Carteolol		
Group IV		
Sotalol	−	−
Timolol		
Nadolol		
Division II: Cardioselective block (β_1)		
Group I		
Acebutolol	−	+
Group III		
Practolol	−	−
Group IV		
Atenolol	−	−
Bisoprolol		
Metoprolol		
Division III: Nonselective block + α block/vasodilator		
Group III		
Labetalol	−	−
Division IV: Cardioselective block + α block		
No example yet available		

From Prichard BNC: Bisoprolol: A new beta-adrenoreceptor blocking drug. Eur Heart J 8(Suppl M):121, 1987.

ratio than atenolol, betaxolol, or propranolol.[2, 6] Selectively and with high affinity, ^{3}H-bisoprolol binds to β_1-adrenoreceptors in dog heart and in rabbit lung membrane preparations.[7–9] The radioligand binding model uses rat reticulocytes and membrane preparations of the rat parotid gland (β_1-receptors). Using a radiolabeled ligand that binds nonspecifically to β-receptors, the β_1-receptor of the parotid gland suspension and the β_2-receptor of the reticulocyte suspension were fully occupied. This cell suspension was then mixed with the serum of patients or healthy volunteers being treated with different β-blockers: atenolol, betaxolol, propranolol, and bisoprolol. The nonspecific radioligand was then displaced by the different β-blockers. Inhibition constants (c_i values) of a characteristic magnitude for each β-blocker and receptor type could be determined from these tests. The ratio of $c_i/\beta_1:c_i/\beta_2$ was 1:75 for bisoprolol, 1:35 for atenolol and betaxolol, and 1.4:1 for propranolol. Therefore, bisoprolol proved to be the β-blocker with the highest affinity to β_1-receptors in this model as well.[9a, 10]

The dose of bisoprolol that inhibits the β_2-adrenoreceptor–mediated vasodilator effects of isoprenaline in dogs is 147 times higher than the dose that affects the β_1-adrenoreceptor–mediated tachycardic effect of isoprenaline. In guinea pigs, the dose of bisoprolol

that reduces heart rate is 124 times lower than the dose that affects bronchial tone.[2] In these experimental models, the β_1-adrenoreceptor–mediated effects were greater than those found with other β-blockers.[2] In cats, which are considered to be critical predictors for pharmacologic effects in humans, the $\beta_1:\beta_2$ selectivity ratio was between 12 and 21 and of the order found in binding studies in rats and dogs,[2] but the ratio was four times higher than that of atenolol in the same preparation.[11, 12]

In humans, evidence for β_1-selectivity has been obtained in a number of clinical pharmacologic studies. β_1-Selectivity was assessed by ability of bisoprolol to reduce exercise-induced tachycardia. This quality was compared with its inhibitory effect on isoprenaline-induced β_2-adrenoreceptor–mediated vasodilation, as demonstrated by the fall in diastolic blood pressure. Compared with propranolol, bisoprolol showed a 12 times greater reduction in exercise-induced tachycardia than in an isoprenaline-induced fall in diastolic pressure. Thus, a higher $\beta_1:\beta_2$ ratio was obtained for bisoprolol than with the cardioselective β-blockers acebutolol and metoprolol (Fig. 59–1).[13] In the human forearm arterial bed, isoprenaline-induced vasodilation was countered less by bisoprolol than by atenolol,[14, 15] but the reduction in heart rate was similar with both drugs.[15] This lesser blocking effect of vascular β_2-adrenoreceptors may reduce the possibility of unopposed vasoconstriction mediated by α-adrenoreceptors. In humans, bisoprolol has a twofold higher β_1-selectivity than atenolol[10] and is 9 to 15 times more potent.[16]

High β_1-receptor selectivity of bisoprolol is also reflected by its relatively minor effects on pulmonary function parameters in patients with chronic obstructive lung disease and asthma even beyond therapeutic dosage (5 to 10 mg) and by the reversibility of

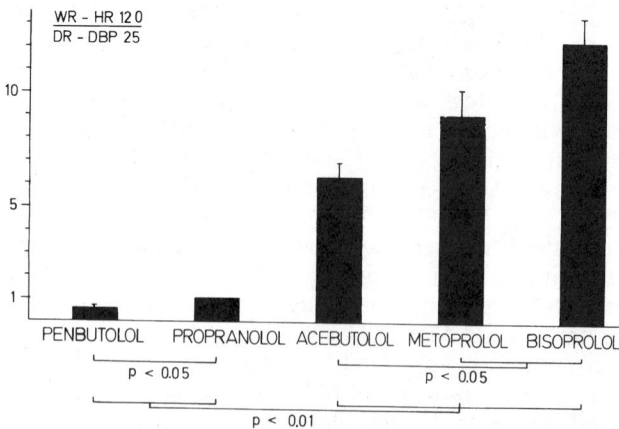

Figure 59–1. Comparison of the relative β_1-selectivity of penbutolol, propranolol, acebutolol, metoprolol, and bisoprolol. WR–HR 120, workload ratio for exercise tachycardia of 120 beats/min on β-blockade as compared with that before β-blockade. DR–DBP 25, isoprenaline dose ratio for a decrease in diastolic blood pressure by 25 mmHg on β-blockade as compared with that before β-blockade for a decrease in diastolic blood pressure by 25 mmHg. (From Krämer B, Balser J, Stubbig K, et al: Comparison of bisoprolol with other beta-adrenoceptor blocking drugs. J Cardiovasc Pharmacol 8[Suppl 11]:S46, 1986.)

these β_2-receptor–mediated effects by β_2-agonists.[17–19] Another proof for high β_1-selectivity and its clinical benefits is that bisoprolol generally induces no change in the cholesterol fractions in long-term therapy and that bisoprolol generally has no influence on the carbohydrate metabolism.[20–22] Because bisoprolol does not bind to human lymphocyte β_2-adrenoreceptors, their density did not change during bisoprolol treatment.[3, 23] In contrast, propranolol and pindolol bind to lymphocyte β_2-adrenoreceptors, resulting in an increase[3, 24] or decrease,[3, 25] respectively, in their density.

Hemodynamic Effects

Intravenous injections of bisoprolol in anesthetized dogs demonstrated the typical effects of acute β-blockade (i.e., a dose-dependent decrease in heart rate); with higher doses, a decrease in cardiac contractility and blood pressure was followed by an increase in peripheral resistance and a rise in left ventricular end-diastolic pressure.[2, 5]

Bisoprolol lowered blood pressure and heart rate in renal hypertensive rats and dogs.[2, 5] Blood pressure fell after the first day of administration, and the maximal antihypertensive effect was obtained after two or three once-daily medications.[2] In young spontaneously hypertensive rats, chronic treatment with bisoprolol for 14 weeks attenuated the development of hypertension and decreased heart rate in a dose-related manner.[2, 5] Bisoprolol also blunted the increase in blood pressure induced by salt intake.[2]

In volunteers, bisoprolol caused a dose-dependent decrease in heart rate, blood pressure, and pressure-rate product.[26] Bisoprolol, 10 and 20 mg, lowered exercise heart rate by 24% and 25%, respectively, which was similar to the effects of 200 mg metoprolol (-26%) but greater than the effects of 80 mg propranolol (-20%). There was much less of an effect on bronchial β_2-adrenoreceptors with bisoprolol than with 80 mg propranolol, and 20 mg of bisoprolol appeared to have about the same effect on bronchial β_2-adrenoreceptors as 200 mg of metoprolol.[27]

In patients with ischemic heart disease, single doses of 5 and 20 mg oral bisoprolol reduced heart rate and cardiac index while total peripheral resistance increased.[28, 29] There was no significant change in systolic blood pressure, but there was a marked decline in the rate-pressure product, although there was a slight increase in pulmonary capillary wedge pressure and a decrease in ejection fraction. These changes were not significant.

Bisoprolol, when dosed chronically to hypertensive patients, has been demonstrated to be associated with a decrease in left ventricular mass index and an improvement in left ventricular diastolic filling as assessed by echocardiography.[30]

Noninvasive studies of single doses of 10, 20, and 40 mg of bisoprolol in hypertensive subjects demonstrated a dose-dependent fall in systolic and diastolic blood pressure both at rest and during exercise. There was some increase in left ventricular echocardiographic dimension, and left ventricular systolic time intervals were increased at the higher doses, but the pre-ejection period–to–left ventricular ejection time ratio as an index of left ventricular performance was not changed.[31] Chronic therapy with bisoprolol versus placebo in hypertensive subjects has demonstrated no significant change in mean ejection fraction either at peak or trough measurement.[32]

Other investigators have shown that bisoprolol inhibits the tachycardia of exercise in normal volunteers as well as in hypertensive subjects.[33] In comparative studies with propranolol, using Doppler techniques, propranolol increased arm and vascular resistance, whereas bisoprolol therapy resulted in only a small increase in femoral resistance.[34]

In animal experiments, bisoprolol decreased renal vascular resistance and increased renal blood flow and glomerular filtration rate (GFR), whereas filtration fraction remained unchanged; these effects were more marked than with other β-blockers given at doses that lowered heart rate to a similar extent.[3]

Acute intravenous administration of 10 mg of bisoprolol to hypertensive patients reduced effective renal plasma flow by 23% and GFR by 14%, with a decrease in heart rate of 23% and of plasma renin activity of 25%, without affecting blood pressure greatly.[35] These results are similar to those obtained with acute administration of other β-blockers.[36] Reduction in renal function is considered to be the result of a fall in cardiac output after acute administration of β-blockers. Although data on renal function during chronic bisoprolol treatment are not yet available, it might be inferred from the results of other cardioselective β-blockers that, during long-term treatment, no significant reduction occurs in GFR and effective renal plasma flow.[37]

Effect on Presynaptic β-Adrenoreceptors

Bisoprolol does not block presynaptic β-adrenoreceptors in blood vessels and hence does not interfere with facilitation of presynaptic β-adrenoreceptor–mediated noradrenaline release,[1] which is in agreement with numerous findings that presynaptic β-adrenoreceptors are of the β_2-subtype.[38]

PHARMACOKINETICS AND METABOLISM

The prominent pharmacokinetic features of bisoprolol are its high bioavailability, long plasma half-life, and metabolic and renal clearance characteristics that involve hepatic and renal pathways nearly equally. The pharmacokinetics of bisoprolol are linear over a wide range of doses (2.5 to 100 mg), independent of age.[39] Given orally, it develops a dose-dependent β-blocking effect in the dose range between 2.5 and 20 mg, with only minor increases in potency above 20 mg.[26] Studies in healthy volunteers showed that after oral intake of 10 mg, bisoprolol peak plasma levels of about 40 ng/ml were reached in 2 to 4 hours; thereaf-

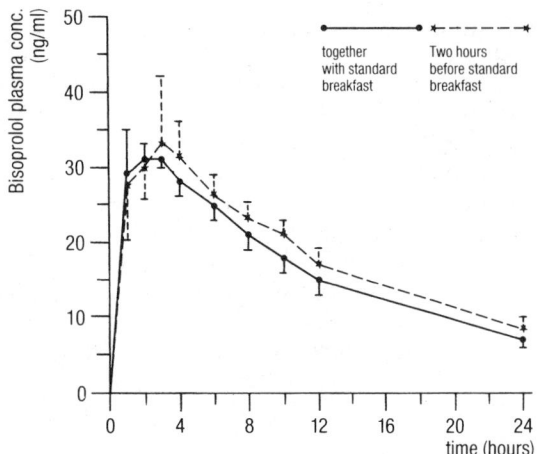

Figure 59–2. Plasma concentration time course of bisoprolol after single oral administration of 10 mg to six healthy male subjects 2 hours before *(solid line)* and together with standard breakfast *(dashed line)*. Crossover design; mean values ± SD. (From Leopold G: Balanced pharmacokinetics and metabolism of bisoprolol. J Cardiovasc Pharmacol 8[Suppl 11]:S16, 1986.)

ter, plasma levels fell gradually to 10 ng/ml after 24 hours with a half-life of 10 or 12 hours (Fig. 59–2). Because there is a residual plasma concentration after 24 hours, bisoprolol administered once daily has a calculated accumulation factor of 1.2, which compensates for its small first-pass effect.[39] Bisoprolol is almost completely absorbed by the intestines and, because of its small first-pass effect (<10%), results in a 90% absolute bioavailability. Therefore, plasma concentrations of bisoprolol show only small variations within and among individuals and are not altered by concomitant food intake (see Fig. 59–2).[39, 40] Furthermore, because of low protein binding (30%), bisoprolol kinetics are insensitive to protein-binding interactions.[41]

After oral administration, bisoprolol is 50% metabolized by the liver and 50% excreted unaltered by the kidney. Therefore, in case of failure of one of the two clearance pathways, the half-life of bisoprolol will at the most double, as was the case during chronic treatment with bisoprolol in patients with renal insufficiency or in patients with cirrhosis of the liver.[42] The metabolism of bisoprolol is not affected by liver enzyme inhibition with cimetidine or by liver enzyme induction with rifampicin and is independent of genetic oxidation polymorphism.[39, 43] In accordance with its metabolic and renal clearance characteristics, the lipophilicity:hydrophilicity ratio of bisoprolol lies in the middle between the lipophilic β-blocker propranolol and the hydrophilic β-blocker atenolol.[39] The metabolism of bisoprolol in humans consists of dealkylation followed by oxidation to three inactive carboxylic acid metabolites that do not accumulate relative to the parent drug and that are predominantly excreted by the kidneys.[40, 41] A stereoselective metabolism of bisoprolol was excluded.[10]

Studies in rats demonstrated that bisoprolol penetrates the blood-brain barrier. The concentration of unchanged drug in the brain is about the same as in

plasma. The concentration of unchanged bisoprolol in rat brain is higher than after administration of atenolol but is lower than the concentration after administration of metoprolol or propranolol.[41] However, no evidence proves that bisoprolol has major behavioral effects or other side effects influencing the central nervous system.[5, 44]

Bisoprolol has limited penetration through the placental barrier in rats; ^{14}C-labeled bisoprolol studies showed that concentrations in the fetus were about half of those in maternal plasma.[41] Using the same methodology, less than 1% of radioactivity contained in plasma is found in the milk of lactating Wistar rats after oral administration of ^{14}C-bisoprolol.[41]

TREATMENT OF ANGINA PECTORIS

Like other β-blockers, bisoprolol exerts its antianginal effect by lowering myocardial oxygen consumption through negative chronotropic and inotropic effects.[45] These parameters were determined in two studies[28, 29]

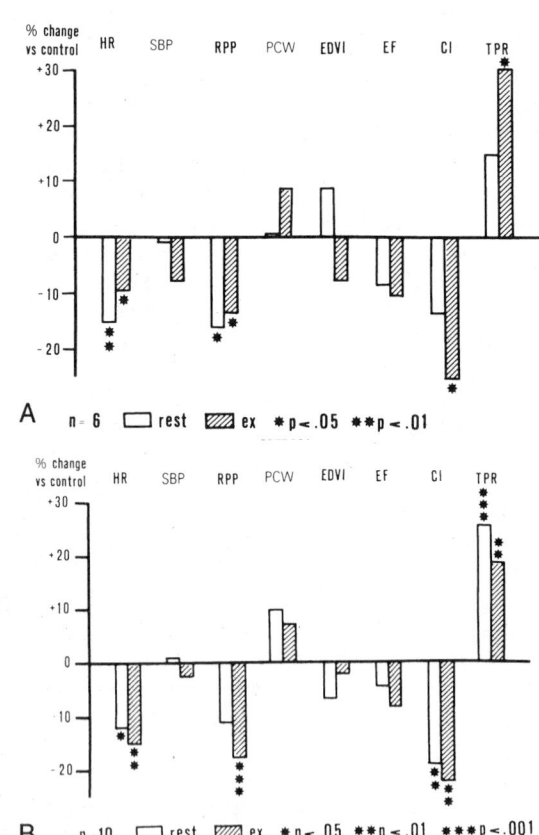

Figure 59–3. Percentage changes (from baseline values) of hemodynamic parameters at rest *(open bars)* and during the last 2 minutes of 5 minutes of steady-state supine bicycle exercise *(hatched bars)* in patients with chronic ischemic heart disease, 2 hours after a single oral dose of 5 mg of bisoprolol *(A)* (n = 6) and after 20 mg of bisoprolol *(B)* (n = 10). HR, heart rate; SBP, systolic blood pressure; RPP, rate-pressure product; PCW, pulmonary capillary wedge pressure; EDVI, end-diastolic volume index; EF, ejection fraction; CI, cardiac index; TPR, total peripheral resistance. (From Burkart F, Pfisterer M, Steinmann E: Effects of bisoprolol in relation to metoprolol and bufuralol on left ventricular hemodynamics at rest and during exercise in chronic ischemic heart disease. J Cardiovasc Pharmacol 8[Suppl 11]:S78, 1986.)

on left ventricular hemodynamics in patients with stable angina pectoris. Burkart et al.[28] found that 2 hours after administration of 5 mg of bisoprolol heart rate and pressure-rate product fell significantly, but the negative inotropic effect was minimal, as judged from minor changes in pulmonary capillary wedge pressure, end-diastolic volume index, and ejection fraction (Fig. 59–3). After administration of 20 mg of bisoprolol, the changes of all hemodynamic parameters were of similar magnitude, except for heart rate and cardiac index, which decreased further to a significant degree, demonstrating the dose dependency of the negative chronotropic effect. Similar observations were made by Bonelli and Staribacher[29] using 10 and 40 mg bisoprolol, although the 40-mg dose was found not to be of additional therapeutic benefit, particularly in view of its greater negative inotropic effect. The antianginal effect of bisoprolol at doses between 5 and 20 mg has been well documented in numerous studies.[46–51] In a placebo-controlled, double-blind, crossover study in patients with stable angina pectoris, exercise heart rate, systolic blood pressure, and pressure-rate product were decreased and anginal symptoms as well as the degree of ST-segment depression reduced 2.5 hours after single oral doses of 5, 10, or 20 mg of bisoprolol.[46] With administration of bisoprolol, 10 and 20 mg (Fig. 59–4), the subjects' maximal workloads were significantly greater than with placebo therapy. In a series of studies on increased exercise tolerance, a reduction in ST-segment depression could still be demonstrated 24 hours after administration of bisoprolol, 5 and 10 mg, during chronic treatment.[49, 51] Administration of bisoprolol, 10 mg o.d., and atenolol, 100 mg o.d., for 12 weeks in 157 patients with stable angina pectoris had comparable effects. Both therapeutic regimens significantly increased exercise tolerance and decreased the pressure rate product.[52] Bisoprolol, 10 to 20 mg once daily, had an antianginal effect comparable with that of verapamil, 80 to 120 mg three times daily, but the pressure-rate product was lower with bisoprolol because of its greater reduction of heart rate.[50]

In a randomized, double-blind study with two parallel groups, the effects of bisoprolol (10 mg, 20 mg o.d.) on transient myocardial ischemia were compared with those of nifedipine s.r. (20 mg, 40 mg b.i.d.) in 330 patients with history of chronic stable angina, positive exercise tolerance test, and at baseline more than two transient ischemic episodes/48 hr of Holter monitoring (central evaluation).

There were two treatment phases of 4 weeks each, with 48-hour Holter monitoring after each phase. During phase 1, patients received either 10 mg of bisoprolol daily or 20 mg of nifedipine s.r. twice daily. During phase 2, they received either 20 mg of bisoprolol daily or 40 mg of nifedipine s.r. twice daily.

In phase 1 of the trial, 4 weeks of bisoprolol therapy (10 mg daily) reduced the mean ($\pm$SD) number of transient ischemic episodes from 8.1 ± 0.6 to 3.2 ± 0.4/48 hr. Nifedipine reduced transient ischemic episodes from 8.3 ± 0.5 to 5.9 ± 0.4/48 hr. Reductions were statistically significant for both drugs; the difference between bisoprolol and nifedipine was highly significant ($p < .0001$). Doubling of the dose in phase 2 of the trial had small additive effects.

The percentage of patients who responded to treatment with a reduction in number of episodes was significantly higher in the bisoprolol group than in the nifedipine group. At the end of phase 1, 40.6% of bisoprolol-treated patients and 14.8% of nifedipine-treated patients had no ischemic episodes in the 48-hr Holter monitoring (100% responder). At the end of phase 2 (4 weeks: bisoprolol 20 mg o.d.; nifedipine s.r. 40 mg b.i.d.), the percentage of the 100% responder was 52.5% in the bisoprolol group and 15.6% in the nifedipine group. The difference between bisoprolol and nifedipine was highly significant ($p < .0001$). Compared with the nifedipine effect, the bisoprolol effect on the circadian variation of ischemic episodes is markedly pronounced.[53]

Therefore, with administration of bisoprolol, 10 mg once daily, most patients remain free of angina.[49] In many patients, as little as 5 mg of bisoprolol was effective; with 10 mg, maximal effects were achieved.[48, 49] By increasing the daily dose to 20 mg or higher, additional beneficial effects may be small.[49]

TREATMENT OF HYPERTENSION
Antihypertensive Effects

Bisoprolol has been demonstrated to be a highly effective antihypertensive drug in numerous trials.[31, 33, 53–59] In double-blind studies in patients with mild to moderate essential hypertension who were randomized to 5, 10, and 20 mg of bisoprolol daily, Weiner and Frithz,[33] Kirsten et al.,[23] and Ikeda et al.[58] found a dose-dependent fall in blood pressure and heart rate. Blood pressure continued to decrease over the first 2

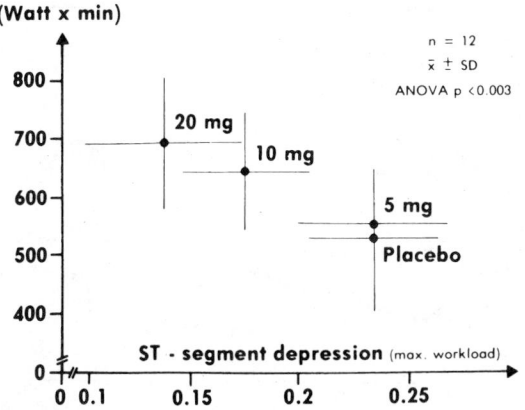

Figure 59–4. Correlation between maximum exercise performance (Watt $\times$ min) and ST-segment depression 2.5 hours after single oral administration of placebo or 5, 10, or 20 mg of bisoprolol to 12 patients with coronary heart disease. Mean values $\pm$ SD; $p < .003$ for dose-response relationship (ANOVA). (From Schnellbacher K, Marsovszky E, Roskamm H: Effect of bisoprolol on exercise tolerance in patients with coronary heart disease: Placebo-controlled double-blind crossover study. J Cardiovasc Pharmacol 8[Suppl 11]:S143, 1986.)

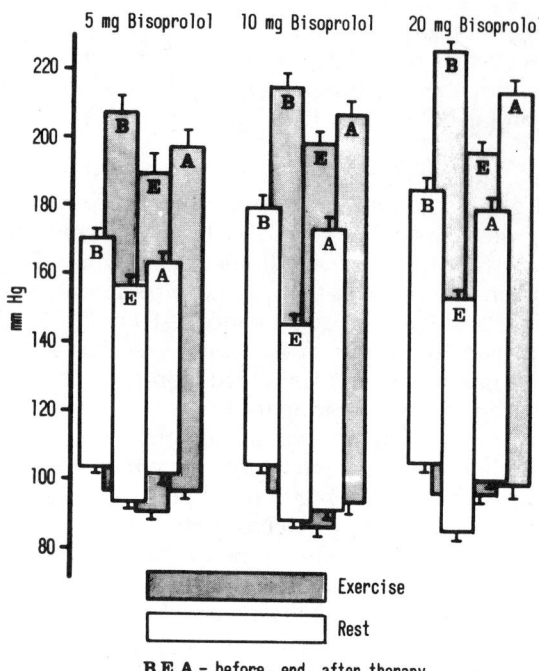

Figure 59–5. Systolic and diastolic blood pressure *(top and bottom of the bars)* at rest *(open bars)* and at peak exercise *(shaded bars)* at the end of the initial placebo phase (B), after 12 weeks' active treatment with 5, 10, or 20 mg of bisoprolol (E), and following 1 week on placebo (A) (mean, SEM; n = 15). (From Kirsten R, Neff J, Heintz B, et al: Influence of different bisoprolol doses on hemodynamics, plasma catecholamines, platelet aggregation, and alpha-2 and beta-receptors in hypertensive patients. J Cardiovasc Pharmacol 8[Suppl 11]:S113, 1986.)

weeks, which coincides largely with the buildup of the plateau phase of plasma bisoprolol concentrations.[23] Some patients' pressure can be controlled with daily doses as low as 2.5 mg.[57] Orthostatic regulation is not impaired, and the diurnal variation of blood pressure is not influenced.[58] Bisoprolol has also demonstrated efficacy in diverse population groups, including young, old, black, and nonblack hypertensive patients. Neutel et al.[60] demonstrated that bisoprolol was equally effective in old (average age, 66 years) and young (average age, 47 years) hypertensive patients. In this same study, investigators demonstrated that bisoprolol was effective in reducing blood pressure in black hypertensives (n = 35, −10 ± 5/ −9 ± 3 mmHg). However, this antihypertensive effect was not as great as that seen in the whole cohort of younger patients (n = 84, −15 ± 1/ −11 ± 1 mmHg) and older hypertensives (n = 23, −16 ± 2/ −10 ± 1 mmHg). In a follow-up for up to 1 year, blood pressure and heart rate remained stable on bisoprolol therapy.[33, 57] Response rates for a target diastolic pressure no higher than 90 mmHg were about 60% to 70%; for no higher than 95 mmHg, they were about 80%.[23, 33, 57, 58] Once-daily administration of 5 to 20 mg of bisoprolol provides sustained (24 hours) lowering of blood pressure, during rest and during exercise (Fig. 59–5).[23, 59]

Three years of experience with bisoprolol in the treatment of mild to moderate hypertension by Gie-

secke and Buchner-Moll[61] demonstrated a sustained therapeutic effect. At the end of this 3-year period, 22.6% of the patients required 5 mg or less, 63.7% needed 10 mg or less, and 13.7% of the patients required 20 mg. Only 34 of the 164 patients in the study experienced adverse events, and only two of those patients required early study withdrawal.

Comparison with Other Antihypertensive Drugs

Several studies compared the antihypertensive effects of bisoprolol with those of atenolol,[54, 55] metoprolol,[62] nifedipine,[63, 64] and a diuretic.[65] The Bisoprolol International Multicenter Study (BIMS)[54] included 104 patients, and a study by Lithell et al.[55] included 309 patients with essential hypertension. Patients were treated in a double-blind fashion for 8 weeks with bisoprolol, 10 to 20 mg, or atenolol, 50 to 100 mg daily,[54] and for 6 months with bisoprolol, 5 or 10 mg, or atenolol, 50 mg daily.[55] Response rates were consistent with those found in other β-blocker studies,[66] although they were somewhat greater for bisoprolol than for atenolol (Fig. 59–6). Most hypertensive patients can be treated with 5 mg[55] or 10 mg[54] daily, and bisoprolol, 5 mg, seems equipotent to atenolol, 50 mg.[55] In the BIMS,[54] patients younger than age 60 responded more often to both β-blockers than pa-

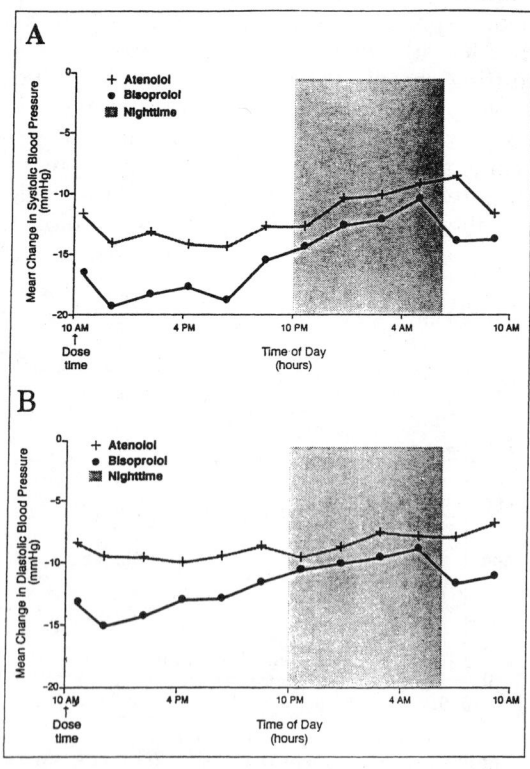

Figure 59–6. Mean changes from baseline to end of treatment in ambulatory systolic *(A)* and diastolic *(B)* blood pressures over the 24-hour monitoring period in patients receiving bisoprolol (n = 107) or atenolol (n = 96). (Reprinted with permission from Neutel JM, Smith DHG, Rom CVS, et al: Application of ambulatory blood pressure monitoring in differentiating between antihypertensive agents. Am J Med 94:181, 1993.)

tients older than age 60. Once-daily doses of bisoprolol, 10 mg, controlled exercise blood pressure, heart rate, and pressure-rate product within 3 hours, in a manner similar to that of metoprolol, 100 mg. However, after 24 hours, the response to bisoprolol was better than the response to metoprolol,[62] thus demonstrating that bisoprolol administered once daily provides 24-hour efficacy with regard to blood pressure reduction. Bisoprolol has also been compared with atenolol using 24-hour ambulatory blood pressure monitoring. Neutel et al.[67] noted that whereas conventional blood pressure measurements obtained in the physician's office did not detect significant differences in the antihypertensive effects of bisoprolol and atenolol, ambulatory blood pressure monitoring revealed significant treatment differences in both the efficacy and duration of action of these two agents (see Fig. 59–6). What was most interesting was the fact that bisoprolol therapy reduced ambulatory systolic and diastolic blood pressure by 43% and 49%, respectively, more than atenolol during the early morning hours. This particular observation by these investigators may have potential clinical importance, because the early morning rise in blood pressure may be associated with an increased risk for myocardial ischemia. Bisoprolol has also been compared with nifedipine in the treatment of essential hypertension in the elderly in two different trials.[63, 64] Both trials demonstrated similar antihypertensive efficacy of the two agents, with fewer side effects in the bisoprolol treated group. Efficacy results in one trial[64] demonstrated changes in blood pressure with bisoprolol of $-22 \pm 16/-15 \pm 9$ mmHg and with nifedipine of $-24 \pm 17/-17 \pm 7$ mmHg. Diastolic blood pressure was normalized in 79% of the patients on bisoprolol and 86% of the patients on nifedipine ($p = NS$).

In another trial, bisoprolol was compared with enalapril in terms of antihypertensive efficacy and influence on perception of quality of life.[68] In this particular study, patients were crossed over to receive each antihypertensive therapy. At the end of each therapy period, the patients completed a quality of life questionnaire. The antihypertensive effects of each drug were similar. The quality of life perception as measured with the Inventory of Subjective Health was comparable for the two drugs. Adverse events were more commonly reported in the enalapril-treated group.

In a double-blind, placebo-controlled study in 36 patients, the effects of 10 mg bisoprolol o.d. or 20 mg nitrendipine o.d. on 24-hour blood pressure were compared. Both substances lowered the daytime blood pressure effectively, whereas during the night only treatment with bisoprolol produced a significant antihypertensive effect. This study shows that, in contrast with nitrendipine, a single dose of bisoprolol guarantees effective lowering of the blood pressure over 24 hours.[69]

With chronic treatment, Honore[65] found a distinctly better blood pressure response to bisoprolol 10 mg than to hydrochlorothiazide 50 mg plus amiloride 5 mg daily.

Thus, the overwhelming clinical evidence suggests that bisoprolol possesses comparable antihypertensive efficacy to other commonly used agents.

More recent clinical trials with bisoprolol have studied its antihypertensive effect in combination with low doses of hydrochlorothiazide.[70] The combination of 2.5, 5, or 10 mg of bisoprolol with 6.25 mg of hydrochlorothiazide was very effective in reducing both systolic and diastolic blood pressure in patients with mild to moderate hypertension. The response rates were 61%, 73%, and 80%, respectively. The side-effect profile was comparable to that with placebo, and there was no adverse influence on the patients' perception of quality of life.[71]

ANTIARRHYTHMIC AND ELECTROPHYSIOLOGIC PROPERTIES

Like other β-blockers, bisoprolol acts on parts of the conduction system that are influenced by the sympathetic nervous system. Therefore, bisoprolol prolongs sinus rhythm cycle length, increases sinus node recovery time, depresses atrioventricular conduction, and prolongs the refractory period of the atrioventricular (AV) node. However, no effects on atrial or ventricular conduction intervals or refractory periods were noted.[72] As expected in a small number of patients with Wolff-Parkinson-White syndrome, bisoprolol did not change the refractory periods of the accessory AV pathways.[72] However, bisoprolol may effectively reduce heart rate in patients with chronic atrial fibrillation and unsatisfactory responses to digitalis alone.[72] Like propranolol,[73] bisoprolol reduced premature atrial and ventricular contractions in about half of patients with doses between 2.5 and 10 mg (rarely 20 mg) given once daily.[74]

BISOPROLOL IN CARDIAC INSUFFICIENCY

In the past, β-blockers were considered as clearly contraindicated in the treatment of cardiac insufficiency, owing to their negative inotropic properties. Now there is a reversal of this attitude because of the results of recently performed large-scale studies investigating the therapeutic potential of β-blockers in the management of cardiac insufficiency.[75–78]

Numerous β-blocker studies in postinfarction patients have already shown a decrease in mortality with β-blockade, especially in patients with ventricular dysfunction. With progress of understanding the underlying pathophysiologic mechanisms of cardiac insufficiency, it became clear that the excessive sympathetic activation plays a major role in the progression of chronic heart failure. The antagonization of deleterious catecholamine effects obtained by β-blocker is therefore considered as having a favorable influence on the symptoms and on the progression of cardiac insufficiency.

The therapeutic potential of bisoprolol in patients

with heart failure was investigated in a large-scale mortality study.[79, 80] CIBIS (Cardiac Insufficiency Bisoprolol Study) was a double-blind, placebo-controlled, randomized multicenter European study in which two parallel groups of patients with chronic heart failure were compared. The primary end point was mortality, and the secondary end point was tolerability.

A total of 641 patients with cardiac insufficiency of New York Heart Association (NYHA) stage III or IV were enrolled. In one half of the patients, the cardiac insufficiency condition was due to dilated cardiomyopathy, and in the other half to an ischemia-related heart disease. In addition to their standard therapy with a diuretic or a vasodilator, the patients also received either bisoprolol or placebo. The initial dose of 1.25 mg of bisoprolol, administered once daily, was increased step by step to a terminal dose of 5 mg, also administered once daily. The follow-up observation phase lasted on average 2 years.

There were fewer deaths in the bisoprolol group than with placebo (16.6% as compared with 20.9%), which, however, was not significant. Certain groups of patients profited in particular from treatment with bisoprolol, showing a statistically significant drop in mortality as compared with those patients treated with placebo, namely patients without a history of myocardial infarction, patients with dilated cardiomyopathy, and patients with a ventricular rate of more than 80 beats/min.

The regression by at least one NYHA category at the end of the study in comparison with the study start was achieved in 21% of the patients receiving bisoprolol as compared with 15% of those treated with placebo. In addition, admissions to hospitals due to cardiac decompensation were significantly less frequently necessary for patients in the bisoprolol group than for those receiving placebo. Nevertheless, another trial was mandatory to prove the beneficial effect on mortality. Therefore, a further mortality study with bisoprolol, CIBIS II, is planned to start soon with a total of 2500 patients.

ADVERSE EFFECTS

The pattern and frequency of adverse effects of bisoprolol were found to be similar to those of other cardioselective β-blockers.[22, 49, 54, 56, 62, 67] Overall, tolerability was described as good, and discontinuation of the drug as a result of side effects occurred in about 1%[54] to 3%[49] of patients with hypertension and angina pectoris, respectively.

Cardiovascular adverse effects reported most frequently were dizziness and fatigue.[22, 33, 55-58] Bradycardia rarely led to discontinuation of bisoprolol.[81]

Adverse effects relating most likely to the central nervous system included headaches[23, 33, 58] and disturbance of sleep;[23, 33, 57] depression was rare[33] and questionably drug related.[54] Tiredness, fatigue, and weakness[22, 23, 33, 56, 58] were the most frequently reported central nervous system side effects, although these symptoms could be cardiovascular as well.

Gastrointestinal side effects, mainly indigestion and rarely nausea or vomiting,[56, 58] were reported about as frequently as were cold extremities; however, in other studies, such side effects were not noted.[54] Overall, no difference was seen in the side effect profiles of patients treated for hypertension and of those treated for angina pectoris.[47-49]

However, because most adverse effects were reported spontaneously or were elicited by doctors, their frequency and relationship to bisoprolol are difficult to assess. In this respect, the evaluation of patients' well-being by self-assessment questionnaire in the BIMS[54] is informative. Accordingly, many reported side effects occurred more frequently during the placebo phase and seemed to improve on treatment with β-blockers, with the exception of tiredness, which was more frequent on bisoprolol therapy. Additionally, bisoprolol appears to have an adverse event profile that is as good or better than other commonly used hypertensive agents, such as nifedipine or enalapril.[63, 64, 68]

In a study by Kirsten et al.,[23] no evidence for hypertension rebound symptoms was found up to 1 or 2 weeks after abrupt discontinuation of antihypertensive bisoprolol treatment. Resting blood pressure and heart rate returned gradually to nearly pretreatment values, whereas peak exercise heart rate was still reduced after 2 weeks. Resting and exercise-induced plasma noradrenaline and adrenaline concentrations did not differ from pretreatment values. Platelet α_2-adrenoreceptor density, which had decreased nonsignificantly during treatment, returned to near pretreatment values, and there were no changes in lymphocyte β_2-receptors. Adrenaline-induced platelet aggregation, which was decreased in a dose-dependent manner during bisoprolol treatment, was not enhanced after its discontinuation. Similarly, Asmar et al.[82] found a significant reduction of blood pressure and heart rate consistently up to 40 hours after discontinuation of bisoprolol. Therefore, the long plasma half-life of bisoprolol may seem to represent some safeguard against a rebound phenomenon.

BISOPROLOL IN PATIENTS WITH CHRONIC OBSTRUCTIVE LUNG DISEASE

In patients with angina pectoris and chronic obstructive lung disease, bisoprolol, 5 to 20 mg daily, may provide the desired antianginal effect without impairment of pulmonary function, whereas doses of 30 and 40 mg increased airway resistance and reduced FEV_1 (forced expiratory volume in 1 second).[17] In asthmatic and hypertensive patients, single oral doses of bisoprolol, 10 to 20 mg, lowered blood pressure and heart rate to an extent similar to atenolol, 100 mg. Whereas airway resistance remained practically unchanged on bisoprolol therapy, it increased on administration of atenolol; peak expiratory flow rate and FEV_1 were slightly but not differently reduced by the two drugs.[19] Findings were similar when bisoprolol was compared with atenolol in the treatment of patients with chronic obstructive lung disease.[83] In smokers with chronic airway obstruction receiving bisoprolol, 10 mg, or acebutolol, 400 mg, specific airway conductance did not change with either drug. Whereas the bronchodilator response to salbutamol was not affected by bisoprolol, it was reduced by acebutolol.[84] The effects on pulmonary function parameters in asthmatic patients of administration of bisoprolol, 10 and 20 mg, were comparable to those observed on administration of metoprolol, 100 mg.[18] Because of high β_1-selectivity, bronchoconstriction could easily be reversed with inhalation of β_2-agonistic compounds.[18, 19] Therefore, as with other cardioselective β-blockers,[85] adverse effects related to β_2-adrenoreceptor blockade are dose-dependent,[86] but the high ratio for β_1:β_2 blockade of bisoprolol seems to provide a therapeutic window for high antianginal and antihypertensive doses (5 to 20 mg) without producing bronchoconstriction. Patients with obstructive lung disease who, despite a wide choice of antianginal and antihypertensive drugs, require β-blockade may be given bisoprolol cautiously with the concomitant prescription of β_2-agonists if necessary. In an individual patient, the risks and benefits of such treatment must be weighed carefully to justify the need for β-blockade.

BISOPROLOL IN PATIENTS WITH ENDOCRINE DISORDERS

The use of β-blockers in patients with diabetes mellitus is debated because the agents may lead to reduced awareness of and delayed recovery from hypoglycemia.[87] Because counterregulatory mechanisms to hypoglycemia are mediated predominantly by β_2-adrenoreceptors, β_1-selective blockers should interfere less with these recovery mechanisms.[88] This effect has been demonstrated with bisoprolol in healthy subjects for insulin-induced hypoglycemia.[26] Furthermore, whereas propranolol greatly suppressed hypoglycemia-induced tachycardia, this effect was less marked with bisoprolol.[26] Bisoprolol, 10 mg daily, given for 2 weeks to hypertensive patients with type II diabetes did not alter blood glucose, hemoglobin A_1 concentration, or glucosuria.[22]

In hyperthyroid patients, bisoprolol, 10 mg daily, given for 1 week did not influence plasma concentrations of free thyroxin and free triiodothyronine.[89] The pharmacokinetic characteristics of bisoprolol were not affected by the hyperthyroid state, presumably because of bisoprolol's low metabolic clearance; hyperthyroid patients improved subjectively.[89] Therefore, bisoprolol, like other β-blockers, is indicated (1) for initial treatment of symptoms of hyperthyroidism in addition to antithyroid therapy, (2) for temporary treatment until the onset of euthyroidism after radioiodine treatment, (3) for short-term presurgical treatment for toxic goiter, and (4) in thyrotoxic crisis.[89]

METABOLIC AND HORMONAL EFFECTS

Presumably as a result of β_1-selectivity,[90] no significant changes were observed in total plasma cholesterol concentrations or high-density lipoprotein (HDL) and low-density lipoprotein (LDL) cholesterol fractions, but there was an increase in plasma triglyceride concentrations.[33, 54, 57] In a randomized comparative study, 70 hypertensive patients received propranolol, 160 mg/day, atenolol 100 mg/day, mepindolol 10 mg/day, or bisoprolol 10 mg/day. They were followed up for 3 years. The HDL decrease and the increase in triglyceride levels were statistically significant for atenolol and propranolol, whereas the changes induced by bisoprolol and mepindolol did not reach statistical significance.[91] In the BIMS,[54] plasma triglyceride concentrations increased approximately 25% in patients taking bisoprolol, 10 to 20 mg daily, and 40% in patients taking atenolol, 50 to 100 mg daily, while cholesterol concentrations remained unchanged. Lithell et al.,[56] in a detailed study comparing bisoprolol, 10 and 20 mg, and atenolol, 50 and 100 mg, daily over 3 months, found small increases in plasma very-low-density lipoprotein (VLDL) cholesterol levels and a slight fall of 5% to 10% in HDL cholesterol concentrations that were similar with both drugs. Plasma triglyceride concentrations increased significantly during treatment with both drugs. There were also some minor changes in apolipoprotein fractions. The behavior of plasma lipids did not depend on pretreatment concentrations. An increase in plasma triglyceride concentration does not seem to be uncommon with β-blocker treatment and could be due to unopposed α-adrenoreceptor activity counteracting lipoprotein-lipase activity.[89, 90, 92] Prolonged therapy with bisoprolol of 3 years' duration has demonstrated no significant effect on total cholesterol or LDL cholesterol levels. However, bisoprolol did increase triglycerides from 20% to 28% but did not significantly affect HDL cholesterol.[93] As shown in Figure 59–7, 3 years of therapy had little effect on various metabolic parameters.

Resting and exercise-induced plasma epinephrine concentrations remained unchanged during antihypertensive treatment with daily doses of 5, 10, and 20 mg of bisoprolol. Although remaining unchanged under resting conditions, plasma norepinephrine concentrations increased during physical exercise in patients taking 10 or 20 mg daily.[23]

Consistent with other β-blockers,[94] bisoprolol was found to lower basal plasma renin activity[16] and to reverse isoprenaline-induced increases in humans completely.[3]

SUMMARY

Bisoprolol is a new β-adrenoreceptor blocking compound with high β_1-adrenoreceptor selectivity, a high bioavailability, and a plasma half-life of 10 or 12 hours allowing for once-daily dosage. It has a small liver first-pass effect and is equally hydrophilic and

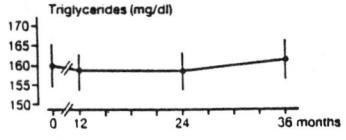
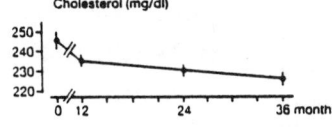
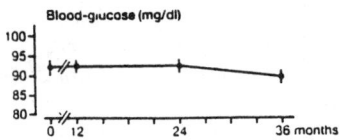
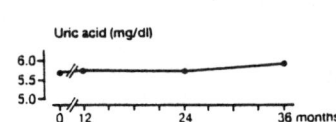

Figure 59–7. Course of changes in laboratory parameters in 164 hypertensive patients after 12, 24, and 36 months of bisoprolol therapy (data graphed as mean ± SEM). (From Giesecke HG, Buchner-Möll D: Three years of experience with bisoprolol in the treatment of mild to moderate hypertension. J Cardiovasc Pharmacol 16[Suppl 5]:S175, 1990.)

lipophilic; therefore, it is metabolized to about 50% by the liver and excreted to about 50% unchanged by the kidney. Protein binding is low, and drug absorption is not influenced by food intake.

Bisoprolol (5 or 10 mg, administered once daily) is used for the treatment of angina pectoris and hypertension. The therapeutic range lies between 5 and 20 mg given once daily. Doses of 5 to 10 mg seem to suffice for β_1-blockade without exerting a relevant β_2-receptor blocking effect, whereas doses higher than 20 mg seem to add little therapeutic effect. Bisoprolol has a favorable profile of adverse effects and does not change glucose levels in diabetics or thyroid hormone levels in hyperthyroid patients. Except for a slight rise in triglyceride concentrations, plasma lipids are unaffected. So far, no evidence exists of rebound hypertensive symptoms after abrupt discontinuation of antihypertensive bisoprolol treatment.

Bisoprolol appears to be well tolerated and safe. It represents an alternative to other β-blockers, particularly when a high degree of β_1-adrenoreceptor selectivity is required. Additionally, bisoprolol and hydrochlorothiazide used in very low doses may prove to be a very useful fixed combination that may have utility in terms of its potent antihypertensive effect, yet also be largely devoid of side effects.

REFERENCES

1. Prichard BNC: Bisoprolol: A new beta-adrenoreceptor drug. Eur Heart J 8(Suppl M):121, 1987.
2. Haeusler G, Schliep H-J, Schelling P, et al: High beta-1 selectivity and favourable pharmacokinetics as the outstanding properties of bisoprolol. J Cardiovasc Pharmacol 8(Suppl 11):S2, 1986.
3. Brodde O-E: Bisoprolol (EMD 33512), a highly selective beta-1 adrenoreceptor antagonist: In vitro and in vivo studies. J Cardiovasc Pharmacol 8(Suppl 11):S29, 1986.
4. Schliep H-J, Harting J: Beta-1 selectivity of bisoprolol, a new beta-adrenoceptor antagonist, in anesthetized dogs and guinea pigs. J Cardiovasc Pharmacol 6:1156, 1984.
5. Harting J, Becker KH, Bergmann R, et al: Pharmacodynamic profile of the selective beta-1-adrenoceptor antagonist bisoprolol. Arzneimittelforschung 36(1):200, 1986.
6. Klockow M, Greiner HE, Haase A, et al: Studies on the receptor profile of bisoprolol. Arzneimittelforschung 36:197, 1986.
7. Manalan AS, Besch HR, Watanabe AM: Characterization of [³H](+/−)carazolol binding to beta-adrenergic receptors. Application to study of beta-adrenergic receptor subtypes in canine ventricular myocardium and lung. Circ Res 49:326, 1981.
8. Kaumann AJ, Lemoine H: Direct labelling of myocardial beta-1-adrenoceptors. Comparison of binding affinity of ³H-(-)-bisoprolol with its blocking potency. Naunyn Schmiedebergs Arch Pharmacol 331:27, 1985.
9. Wang XL, Brinkmann M, Brodde OE: Selective labelling of beta-1-adrenoceptors in rabbit lung membranes by (-)[³H]bisoprolol. Eur J Pharmacol 114:157, 1985.
9a. Wellstein A, Palm D, Belz GG: Affinity and selectivity of β-adrenoceptor antagonists in vitro. J Cardiovasc Pharmacol 8(Suppl 11):36, 1986.
10. Wellstein A, Palm D, Belz GG, et al: Concentration kinetics of propranolol, bisoprolol and atenolol in humans assessed with chemical detection and a subtype-selective beta-adrenoceptor assay. Cardiovasc Pharmacol 8(Suppl 11):S41, 1986.
11. Schliep HJ, Schulze E, Harting J, et al: Antagonistic effects of bisoprolol on several beta-adrenoceptor-mediated actions in anaesthetized cats. Eur J Pharmacol 123:253, 1986.
12. Letts LG, Richardson DP, Temple DM, et al: The selectivity of beta-adrenoceptor antagonists on isoprenaline-induced changes in heart rate, blood pressure, soleus muscle contractility and airways function in anaesthetized cats. Br J Pharmacol 80:323, 1983.
13. Krämer B, Balser J, Stubbig K, et al: Comparison of bisoprolol with other beta-adrenoceptor blocking drugs. J Cardiovasc Pharmacol 8(Suppl 11):S46, 1986.
14. Chang PC, van Veen S, Vermeij P, et al: Double-blind comparison of the beta-1 selectivity of single doses of bisoprolol and atenolol. J Cardiovasc Pharmacol 8(Suppl 11):S58, 1986.
15. Wellstein A, Palm D, Belz GG, et al: Reduction of exercise tachycardia in man after propranolol, atenolol and bisoprolol in comparison to beta-adrenoceptor occupancy. Eur Heart J 8(Suppl M):3, 1987.
16. Bolli P, Müller FB, Linder L, et al: Cardiac and vascular beta-adrenoceptor-mediated responses before and during treatment with bisoprolol or atenolol. J Cardiovasc Pharmacol 8(Suppl 11):S61, 1986.
17. Dorow P: Beta-1/beta-2 splitting of bisoprolol. J Cardiovasc Pharmacol 8(Suppl 11):S65, 1986.
18. Lammers JW, Folgering HT, van Herwaarden CL: Respiratory tolerance of bisoprolol and metoprolol in asthmatic patients. J Cardiovasc Pharmacol 8(Suppl 11):S69, 1986.
19. Chatterjee SS: The cardioselective and hypotensive effects of bisoprolol in hypertensive asthmatics. J Cardiovasc Pharmacol 8(Suppl 11):S74, 1986.
20. Frithz G, Weiner L: Effects of bisoprolol, dosed once daily, on blood pressure and serum lipids and HDL-cholesterol in patients with mild to moderate hypertension. Eur J Clin Pharmacol 32:77, 1987.
21. Frithz G, Weiner L: Long term effects of bisoprolol on blood pressure, serum lipids and HDL-cholesterol in patients with essential hypertension. J Cardiovasc Pharmacol 8(Suppl 11):134, 1986.
22. Janka HU, Ziegler AG, Disselhoff G, Mehnert H: Influence of bisoprolol on blood glucose, glucosuria and haemoglobin A_1 in noninsulin-dependent diabetics. J Cardiovasc Pharmacol 8(Suppl 11):96, 1986.
23. Kirsten R, Neff J, Heintz B, et al: Influence of different bisoprolol doses on hemodynamics, plasma catecholamines, platelet aggregation, and alpha-2 and beta-receptors in hypertensive patients. J Cardiovasc Pharmacol 8(Suppl 11):S113, 1986.
24. Aarons RD, Nies AS, Gal J, et al: Elevation of beta-adrenergic receptor density in human lymphocytes after propranolol administration. J Clin Invest 65:949, 1980.
25. Molinoff PB, Aarons RD: Effects of drugs on beta-adrenergic

receptors on human lymphocytes. J Cardiovasc Pharmacol 5(Suppl 1):S63, 1983.

26. Leopold G, Ungethüm W, Pabst J, et al: Pharmacodynamic profile of bisoprolol, a new beta-1 selective adrenoceptor antagonist. Br J Clin Pharmacol 22:293, 1986.

27. Tattersfield AE, Cragg DJ, Bacon RJ: Assessment of beta-adrenoceptor selectivity of a new beta-adrenoceptor antagonist, bisoprolol, in man. Br J Clin Pharmacol 18:343, 1984.

28. Burkart F, Pfisterer M, Steinmann E: Effects of bisoprolol in relation to metoprolol and bufuralol on left ventricular hemodynamics at rest and during exercise in chronic ischemic heart disease. J Cardiovasc Pharmacol 8(Suppl 11):S78, 1986.

29. Bonelli J, Staribacher H: Haemodynamic effects of bisoprolol in patients with coronary heart disease: Influence of various bisoprolol plasma concentrations. J Cardiovasc Pharmacol 8(Suppl 11):S83, 1986.

30. Guller B, Jacques P, Reeves RL: Cardiovascular effects of bisoprolol and atenolol hypertension. Am J Hypertens 4:22A, 1991.

31. Esper RJ, Esper RC, Burrieza OH, et al: Noninvasive assessment of left ventricular performance after administration of bisoprolol. J Cardiovasc Pharmacol 8(Suppl 11):S87, 1986.

32. Prisant I M, Carr AA, Desnoyers M, et al: Multicenter evaluation of the hemodynamic effects of bisoprolol in patients with mild to moderate hypertension. J Clin Pharm 30:1096, 1990.

33. Weiner L, Frithz G: Dose-effect relationship and long-term effects of bisoprolol in mild to moderate hypertension. J Cardiovasc Pharmacol 8(Suppl 11):S106, 1986.

34. Bailliart O, Kedra AW, Bonin P, et al: Effects of bisoprolol on some local vascular resistances. Eur Heart J 8(Suppl M):87, 1987.

35. Glück Z, Reubi FC: Acute changes in renal function induced by bisoprolol, a new cardioselective beta-blocking agent. Eur J Pharmacol 31:107, 1986.

36. Sullivan JM, Adams DF, Hollenberg NK: Beta-adrenoceptor blockade in essential hypertension: Reduced renin release despite renal vasoconstriction. Circ Res 39:532, 1976.

37. Wool-Manning HJ, Bolli P: Atenolol v. placebo in mild hypertension: Renal, metabolic and stress antipressor effects. Br J Pharmacol 9:553, 1980.

38. Majewski H: Modulation of noradrenaline release through activation of presynaptic beta-adrenoceptors. J Auton Pharmacol 3:47, 1983.

39. Leopold G: Balanced pharmacokinetics and metabolism of bisoprolol. J Cardiovasc Pharmacol 8(Suppl 11):S16, 1986.

40. Leopold G, Pabst J, Ungethüm W, et al: Basic pharmacokinetics of bisoprolol, a new highly beta1-selective adrenoceptor antagonist. J Clin Pharmacol 26:616, 1986.

41. Bühring KU, Sailer H, Faro HP, et al: Pharmacokinetics and metabolism of bisoprolol-^{14}C in three animal species and in humans. J Cardiovasc Pharmacol 8(Suppl 11):S21, 1986.

42. Kirch W, Rose I, Demers HG, et al: Pharmacokinetics of bisoprolol during repeated administration to normal subjects and patients with kidney or liver disease. Clin Pharmacokinet 13:110, 1987.

43. Kirch W, Rose I, Klingmann I, et al: Interaction of bisoprolol with cimetidine and rifampicin. Eur J Clin Pharmacol 31:59, 1986.

44. Görtelmeyer R, Klingmann I: Vergleichende Untersuchung zur zentralnervosen Wirkung der beta-Rezeptorenblocker Pindolol und Bisoprolol. Arzneimittelforschung 35:1707, 1985.

45. Opie LH: Drugs and the heart. Lancet 1:1011, 1980.

46. Schnellbacher K, Marsovszky E, Roskamm H: Effect of bisoprolol on exercise tolerance in patients with coronary heart disease: Placebo-controlled double-blind crossover study. J Cardiovasc Pharmacol 8(Suppl 11):S143, 1986.

47. Kohli RS, Lahiri A, Raftery EB: Management of chronic stable angina with once-daily bisoprolol or atenolol and long-term efficacy of bisoprolol. J Cardiovasc Pharmacol 8(Suppl 11):S148, 1986.

48. Kato K, Niitani H, Kanazawa T, et al: Clinical evaluation of bisoprolol in patients with stable angina pectoris: A preliminary report. J Cardiovasc Pharmacol 8(Suppl 11):S154, 1986.

49. Wagner G: Summary of short- and long-term studies with bisoprolol in coronary heart disease (CHD). J Cardiovasc Pharmacol 8(Suppl 11):S160, 1986.

50. de Divitiis O, Liguori V, Di Somma S, et al: Bisoprolol in the treatment of angina pectoris: A double-blind comparison with verapamil. Eur Heart J 8:41, 1987.

51. de Muinck E, Wagner G, v.d. Ven LL, Lie KI: Comparison of the effects of two doses of bisoprolol on exercise tolerance in exercise-induced stable angina pectoris. Eur Heart J 8(Suppl M):31, 1987.

52. de Muinck ED, Buchner-Moell D: Comparison of the safety and efficacy of bisoprolol versus atenolol in stable exercise-induced angina pectoris: A multicenter international randomized study of angina pectoris (MIRSA). J Cardiovasc Pharmacol 19:870, 1992.

53. von Arnim Th, for the TIBBS Investigators: Medical treatment to reduce total ischemic burden: Total Ischemic Burden Bisoprolol Study (TIBBS), a multicenter trial comparing bisoprolol and nifedipine. J Am Coll Cardiol 25:231, 1995.

54. Bühler FR, Berglund G, Anderson OK, et al: Double-blind comparison of the cardioselective beta-blockers bisoprolol and atenolol in hypertension: The Bisoprolol International Multicenter Study (BIMS). J Cardiovasc Pharmacol 8(Suppl 11):S122, 1986.

55. Lithell H, Selinus I, Hosie J, et al: Efficacy and safety of bisoprolol and atenolol in patients with mild to moderate hypertension. Eur Heart J 8:53, 1987.

56. Lithell H, Weiner L, Selinus I, et al: A comparison of the effects of bisoprolol and atenolol on lipoprotein concentrations and blood pressure. J Cardiovasc Pharmacol 8(Suppl 11):S128, 1986.

57. Frithz G, Weiner L: Long-term effects of bisoprolol on blood pressure, serum lipids, and HDL-cholesterol in patients with essential hypertension. J Cardiovasc Pharmacol 8(Suppl 11):S134, 1986.

58. Ikeda M, Inagaki Y, Iimura O, et al: Clinical evaluation of bisoprolol in patients with hypertension: Interim report. J Cardiovasc Pharmacol 8(Suppl 11):S139, 1986.

59. Weiner L, Frithz G: Antihypertensive effects of bisoprolol during once daily administration in patients with essential hypertension. A dose-ranging study with parallel groups. Eur J Clin Pharmacol 29:517, 1986.

60. Neutel JM, Smith DHG, Ram CVS, et al: Comparison of bisoprolol with atenolol for systemic hypertension in four population groups (young, old, black and nonblack) using ambulatory blood pressure monitoring. Am J Cardiol 72:41, 1993.

61. Giesecke HG, Buchner-Möll D: Three years of experience with bisoprolol in the treatment of mild to moderate hypertensives. J Cardiovasc Pharmacol 16(Suppl 5):S175, 1990.

62. Haasis R, Bethge H: Exercise blood pressure and heart rate reduction 24 and 3 hours after administration in hypertensive patients following 4 weeks of treatment with bisoprolol and metoprolol: A randomized multicenter double-blind study (BISOMET). Eur Heart J 8:97, 1987.

63. Martinez JO, Garcia MJM, Botaro AR, et al: Bisoprolol and nifedipine SR in the treatment of hypertension in the elderly. J Cardiovasc Pharmacol 16(Suppl 5):S95, 1990.

64. Amabile G, Serradimigni A: Comparison of bisoprolol with nifedipine for treatment of essential hypertension in the elderly: Comparative double-blind trial. Eur Heart J 8:63, 1987.

65. Honore P: Bisoprolol versus hydrochlorothiazide + amiloride in essential hypertension, a randomized double-blind study. Eur Heart J 8:89, 1987.

66. Bühler FR: Antihypertensive actions of betablockers. In Laragh JH, Bühler FR, Seldin DW (eds): Frontiers in Hypertension Research. New York: Springer, 1981, pp 423–435.

67. Neutel JM, Smith DHG, Ram CVS, et al: Application of ambulatory blood pressure monitoring in differentiating between antihypertensive agents. Am J Med 94:181, 1993.

68. Breed JGS, Ciampricotti R, Tromp GP, et al: Quality of life perception during antihypertensive treatment: A comparative study of bisoprolol and enalapril. J Cardiovasc Pharmacol 20:750, 1992.

69. Mengden T, Schubert M, Jeck T, et al: Casual versus ambulatory 24-hour blood pressure measurements in a comparative study with bisoprolol or nitrendipine. J Hypertens 8(Suppl 4):91, 1990.

70. Lewin AJI, Lueg MC, Targum S, Cardenas P: A clinical trial evaluating the 24 hour effects of bisoprolol/hydrochlorothia-

zide 5 mg/6.25 mg combination in patients with mild to moderate hypertension. Clin Cardiol 16:732, 1993.

71. De Quattro V, Weir MR: Bisoprolol fumarate/hydrochlorothiazide 6.25 mg: A new low-dose option for first-time antihypertensive therapy. Adv Therapy 10:179, 1993.

72. Neuss H, Conrad A, Mitrovic V, et al: Electrophysiologic effects of an acute beta-blockade induced by bisoprolol in patients with supraventricular tachycardia as assessed by his-bundle electrograms. J Cardiovasc Pharmacol 8(Suppl 11):S167, 1986.

73. Woosley RL, Kornhauser D, Smith R, et al: Suppression of chronic ventricular arrhythmias with propranolol. Circulation 60:819, 1979.

74. Sugimoto T, Hayakawa H, Osada H, et al: Clinical evaluation of bisoprolol in the treatment of extrasystoles and sinus tachycardia: An interim report. J Cardiovasc Pharmacol 8(Suppl 11):S171, 1986.

75. Waagstein F, Hjalmarson A, Varnauskas E, Wallentin I: Effects of chronic beta-adrenergic receptor blockade in congestive cardiomyopathy. Br Heart J 37:1022, 1975.

76. Currie PJ, Kelly MJ, McKenzie A, et al: Oral beta-adrenergic blockade with metoprolol in chronic severe dilated cardiomyopathy. J Am Coll Cardiol 3:203, 1984.

77. Waagstein K, Caidahl K, Wallentin I, et al: Long-term beta-blockade in dilated cardiomyopathy: Effects of short- and long-term metoprolol treatment followed by withdrawal and readministration of metoprolol. Circulation 80:551, 1989.

78. Waagstein F, Bristow MR, Swedberg K, et al, for the Metoprolol in Dilated Cardiomyopathy (MDC) Trial Study Group: Beneficial effects of metoprolol in idiopathic dilated cardiomyopathy. Lancet 342:1441, 1993.

79. Lechat P: Beta-blockade treatment in heart failure: The Cardiac Insufficiency Bisoprolol Study (CIBIS) project. J Cardiovasc Pharmacol 16:158, 1990.

80. Lechat P: A randomized trial of beta-blockade in heart failure: The Cardiac Insufficiency Bisoprolol Study (CIBIS). Circulation 90:1765, 1994.

81. Höffler D, Meyer W, Heusinger H: Monotherapy of hypertension with long-acting beta-blockade. Therapiewoche 38:3891, 1988.

82. Asmar R, Hugues CH, Pannier J, et al: Duration of action of bisoprolol after cessation of a 4 week treatment and its influence on pulse wave velocity and aortic diameter: A pilot study in hypertensive patients. Eur Heart J 8(Suppl M):115, 1987.

83. Dorow P, Bethge H, Tönnesmann U: Effects of single oral doses of bisoprolol and atenolol on airway function in nonasthmatic, chronic obstructive lung disease and angina pectoris. Eur J Clin Pharmacol 31:143, 1986.

84. Macquin-Mavier I, Roudot-Thoraval F, Clerici C, et al: Comparative effects of bisoprolol and acebutolol in smokers with airway obstruction. Br J Clin Pharmacol 26:279, 1988.

85. McDevitt DG: Beta-adrenoceptor antagonists and respiratory function. Br J Clin Pharmacol 5:97, 1978.

86. Fleming GM, Chester EH, Schwartz HJ, et al: Beta-adrenergic blockade of the lung. Dose-dependent cardioselectivity of tolamolol in asthma. Chest 73:807, 1978.

87. Lager I: Adrenergic blockade and hypoglycaemia. Acta Med Scan (Suppl) 672:63, 1983.

88. Lager I, Blohme G, Smith U: Effect of cardioselective and nonselective beta-blockade on the hypoglycaemic response in insulin-dependent diabetes. Lancet 1:458, 1979.

89. Pfannenstiel P, Rummeny E, Baew-Christow T, et al: Pharmacokinetics of bisoprolol and influence on serum thyroid hormones in hyperthyroid patients. J Cardiovasc Pharmacol 8(Suppl 11):S100, 1986.

90. Day JL, Metcalfe J, Simpson CN: Adrenergic mechanisms in control of plasma lipid concentrations. Br Med J 284:1145, 1982.

91. Fogari R, Zoppi A, Tettamanti F, et al: β-Blocker effects on plasma lipids in antihypertensive therapy: Importance of the duration of treatment and the lipid status before treatment. J Cardiovasc Pharmacol 16(Suppl 5):76, 1990.

92. Waal-Manning HJ: Metabolic effects of beta-adrenoceptor blockers. Drugs 2(Suppl 1):121, 1976.

93. Fogari R, Zoppi A, Pasotti C, et al: Plasma lipids during chronic antihypertensive therapy with different β-blockers. J Cardiovasc Pharmacol 14(Suppl 7):S28, 1989.

94. Bühler FR, Burkart F, Lutold BE, et al: Antihypertensive beta-blocking action as related to renin and age: A pharmacological tool to identify pathogenic mechanisms in essential hypertension. Am J Cardiol 36:53, 1975.

D. α- and β-Adrenoreceptor Blockers

CHAPTER 60

Labetalol

Walter Flamenbaum, M.D., and Alan Dubrow, M.D.

Labetalol hydrochloride is the first of a new group of β-adrenergic blocking agents that act as competitive antagonists at both αβ-adrenoreceptors.[1] Before the development of labetalol, pharmacologic agents were available that acted at either αβ-adrenoreceptors but not at both. In addition, labetalol is the prototype of a β-blocker possessing vasodilatory properties, either direct or mediated via β-agonist activity. Labetalol appears to combine the advantages of αβ-blockers while minimizing the unwanted effects of both types of agents.

Since the initial description of the drug's pharmacology in 1972, worldwide experience regarding the clinical applications of labetalol has become extensive.[2] Developed as both an oral and an intravenous agent, labetalol has been used successfully for the treatment of essential hypertension,[3] with particular efficacy in black patients,[4] hypertension associated with pregnancy, pheochromocytoma, and angina pectoris.[3, 5, 6] The drug has also been extensively used to lower blood pressure during general anesthesia.[3]

The combination of two separate drugs with αβ-blocking properties to treat hypertension proved initially to be impractical because of the high incidence of associated major side effects, the most frequent of which were postural hypotension and tachyphylaxis from α-blockers. Phenoxybenzamine, a noncompetitive, nonspecific α-blocker, in combination with propranolol, resulted in orthostatic hypotension.[7] The combination of a β-blocker with either the postsynaptic α-blocking agent prazosin or the direct vasodilator hydralazine has been more efficacious but equally cumbersome. Labetalol is a single drug possessing a selective, postsynaptic α-blocking effect plus nonselective β-blocking activity that has been associated with a low incidence of postural hypotension and tachyphylaxis. The drug also is simple to administer. This chapter reviews the pharmacology of labetalol and its clinical utility.

CHEMICAL STRUCTURE

Labetalol hydrochloride is a 2-hydroxy-5-[1-hydroxy-2-(1-methyl-3-phenylpropyl)aminoethyl]-benzamide hydrochloride. The drug is an equal mixture of four diastereoisomers.[8] Stereoisomer RR is a nonselective, competitive β-adrenoreceptor antagonist possessing direct vasodilatory activity but virtually no α-blocking activity. The SR stereoisomer is an α-blocker with minimal β-blocking activity. Stereoisomers SS and RS possess weak αβ-blocking activity, respectively. N-alkylation of the ethanolamine moiety appears to be necessary for labetalol's combined αβ-blocking actions.[9]

CLINICAL PHARMACOLOGY

Several comprehensive reviews of the pharmacology of labetalol in animal experimental models are available.[10-12] The known pharmacologic effects are summarized in Table 60–1.[12] Labetalol possesses competitive pharmacologic blocking activity at both αβ-adrenergic receptors.[12] Differences in degree of efficacy are influenced by experimental conditions, the method of administration, and the animal species studied or tissue preparations used. Labetalol, over a wide range of tests in vitro and in vivo, seems to be 6 to 10 times less potent than phentolamine at α-adrenoreceptors; 1 to 4 times less potent than propranolol at β-adrenoreceptors; and 4 to 16 times less potent itself at α-adrenoreceptors than at β-adrenoreceptors.[10] Labetalol has been shown to possess partial β2-agonist properties,[12-14] as well as the ability to produce direct vasodilation.[15] To fully appreciate the effects of labetalol, however, one should consider its hemodynamic and antihypertensive actions.

Studies of Adrenoreceptor Blockade in Humans

In human studies, as in animal experiments, labetalol has been shown to be an effective competitive antagonist at both αβ-adrenoreceptors. Richards[16] demonstrated that labetalol causes a parallel shift to the right of the dose-response curve of isoproterenol-induced increases in heart rate and decreases in diastolic blood

pressure. These effects occurred after both oral and intravenous administration. The nonselective nature of labetalol's β-blocking properties was implied by the similarities in magnitude of the heart rate-response and diastolic blood pressure curves. On a milligram-for-milligram basis, propranolol was a four to six times more potent β-antagonist than labetalol. After either oral or intravenous administration, labetalol causes a parallel shift to the right of the cumulative log dose-response curves of phenylephrine- and norepinephrine-induced blood pressure increases, demonstrating competitive α-adrenoreceptor antagonism. Labetalol was three times less potent at α-adrenoreceptors than at β-adrenoreceptors after oral administration; it was 6.9 times less potent at α-receptors after intravenous administration. It has not been demonstrated clearly whether the ratio between the αβ-blocking properties of labetalol is affected by the dosage of the drug.[16-20]

Results of a study by Mehta and Cohn[21] agree with those of Richards et al.[20] indicating that at an oral dose of labetalol, 800 to 1600 mg/day, appeared to be four to six times more potent in blocking isoproterenol-induced tachycardia in hypertensive patients than in blocking phenylephrine-induced diastolic hypertension.

Immersion of the hand in ice water for 60 seconds (the cold-pressor test) causes blood pressure elevations through α-adrenergic stimulation. Labetalol, but not phentolamine, blocks the cold-pressor response in normotensive humans,[22] suggesting that prejunctional α-blockade does not occur with labetalol. After either oral or intravenous administration, labetalol causes a dose-related reduction of blood pressure and heart rate in response to treadmill and bicycle exercises,[18] tachycardia induced by the Valsalva maneuver,[19] and tachycardia induced by 80-degree tilt.[16]

Hemodynamic Effects in Humans

β-Blockers such as propranolol cause a decrease in heart rate and cardiac output, a widened arteriovenous oxygen difference, and, at least initially, an increase in total systemic vascular resistance. This increased peripheral vascular resistance prevents a decrease in blood pressure after acute intravenous or oral administration. Stroke volume and left ventricular filling pressures either remain unchanged or become slightly elevated. With chronic administration, blood pressure falls while elevated total peripheral vascular resistance tends to return toward pretreatment levels.[23]

Table 60–2[24] summarizes the results of several studies of the acute hemodynamic effects of intravenously administered labetalol.[25-33] In contrast with responses seen with traditional β-blockers, both blood pressure and systemic vascular resistance fall immediately after acute intravenous administration of labetalol. Cardiac output and stroke volume tend to remain unaffected, and heart rate either remains unchanged or decreases slightly. When cardiac output falls, the

Table 60–1. **Labetalol: Pharmacologic Properties**

Nonspecific β-blockade, both β1- and β2-receptors
α1-Adrenoceptor blockade
β2-Adrenoceptor agonism
Inhibition of neuronal uptake mechanism

The Diastereoisomers:
RR: Nonselective β-adrenoceptor antagonist direct vasodilatory activity
SR: α-Adrenoceptor antagonism
SS, RS: Weak adrenoceptor-blocking activity

Table 60–2. **Intravenous Labetalol in Hypertensives: Hemodynamics**

Author	Dose		Blood Pressure	Heart Rate	Cardiac Output	Vascular Resistance
Pritchard et al.[30]	0.5 mg/kg	(S)	(−)	(0)	(0)	(−)
Jockers and Thompson[27]	0.5–1.0 mg/kg	(S)	(−)	(0)	(0)	(−)
Koch[28]	50 mg	(S)	(−)	(0)	(0)	(0)
		(U)	(−)	(−)	(−)	(−)
		(E)	(−)	(−)	(−)	(−)
Bahlmann et al.[31]	0.6–1.6 mg/kg	(S)	(−)	(0)	(0)	(−)
Svendsen et al.[29]	50 mg	(S)	(−)	(0)	(0)	(−)
		(U)	(−)	(−)	(0)	(−)
		(E)	(−)	(−)	(0)	(0)
Trap-Jensen et al.[32]	0.75 mg/kg	(S)	(−)	(0)	(0)	(−)
		Psychic stress	(−)	(−)	(+)	(0)
Agabiti-Rosei et al.[26]	100 mg	(S)	(−)	(−)	(0)	(−)
Omvik and Lund-Johansen[33]	0.2–0.8 mg/kg	(S)	(−)	(−)	(−)	(−)

(S), supine; (U), upright; (E), exercise; (+), significant increase; (−), significant reduction; and (0), no significant change.
Adapted from Frishman WH: Clinical Pharmacology of the β-Adrenoreceptor Blocking Drugs. Norwalk, CT: Appleton-Century-Crofts, 1984.

decline is due entirely to decreases in heart rate. Heart rate generally falls when the patient stands, and heart rate increases during exercise are blunted. A similar hemodynamic profile may be obtained with intravenous administration of propranolol combined with hydralazine or prazosin.[34] The cardiodynamic changes after oral labetalol administration parallel those observed with parenteral administration.

Antihypertensive Effects in Humans

Table 60–3[24] summarizes the effects of oral labetalol administration in hypertensive patients in studies ranging in duration from 1 week to 6 years.[21, 28, 29, 34–37] Following long-term dosing, 300 to 2400 mg daily, supine and standing heart rate were slightly lowered, and blood pressure remained reduced. Koch,[28] in a

study of 21 months' duration, showed that stroke volume in the supine and standing positions rose to compensate for heart rate, thereby preserving cardiac output. Peripheral vascular resistance decreased further with long-term dosing. Lund-Johansen[37] demonstrated that exercise-induced blood pressure increases were blunted and heart rate was reduced. This reduction in the double product (heart rate × systolic blood pressure) tends to provide a favorable hemodynamic profile for hypertensive patients who have angina.[5]

After intravenous administration of labetalol, pulmonary artery pressures measured at rest decreased in both the supine and standing positions, but pulmonary artery pressures during exercise were unaffected.[28] In patients with coronary artery disease and stable angina pectoris, heart rate, "double-product,"

Table 60–3. **Oral Labetalol Therapy in Hypertensives: Hemodynamics**

Author	Max. Daily Dose (g/day)		Blood Pressure	Heart Rate	Cardiac Output	Vascular Resistance
Edwards and Raftery[35]	0.8	(S)	(−)	(−)	(0)	(0)
		(E)	(−)	(−)	(−)	(0)
Mehta and Cohn[21]	1.6	(S)	(−)	(−)	(0)	(−)
		(U)	(−)	(−)	(0)	(−)
		(E)	(−)	(−)	ND	ND
Fagard et al.[36]	0.3–2.4	(S)	(−)	(−)	(−)	(0)
		(U)	(−)	(−)	(−)	(−)
		(E)	(−)	(−)	(−)	(−)
Lund-Johansen[34]	0.2–0.8	(S)	(−)	(−)	(0)	(−)
		(U)	(−)	(−)	(−)	(0)
		(E)	(−)	(−)	(−)	(−)
Koch[25]	0.6–2.4	(S)	(−)	(−)	(0)	(−)
		(U)	(−)	(−)	(0)	(−)
		(E)	(−)	(−)	(0)	(−)
Svendsen et al.[29]	0.6–0.9	(S)	(−)	(−)	(0)	(−)
		(U)	(−)	(−)	(0)	(−)
		(E)	(−)	(−)	(−)	(0)
Lund-Johansen[37]	0.2–0.8	(S)	(−)	(−)	(0)	(−)
		(U)	(−)	(−)	(0)	(−)
		(E)	(−)	(−)	(0)	(−)

Abbreviations as in Table 60–2. ND, not measured.
Adapted from Frishman WH: Clinical Pharmacology of the β-Adrenoreceptor Blocking Drugs. Norwalk, CT: Appleton-Century-Crofts, 1984.

and pulmonary vascular resistance all decreased during labetalol administration. Pulmonary wedge pressures and cardiac output were unchanged. Coronary sinus blood flow increased significantly.[38] Propranolol produced significantly greater depression of cardiac function, both at rest and during exercise, than did labetalol in patients with angiographically demonstrated coronary artery disease.[39]

During chronic administration, labetalol and other β-blocking drugs did not reduce cerebral blood flow despite significant blood pressure reduction.[40] This may be ascribed to autoregulation of the cerebral vasculature.

PHARMACODYNAMICS AND PHARMACOKINETICS

In normal subjects and hypertensive patients, a hypotensive response to orally administered labetalol was seen within 2 hours and was maximal within 3 hours.[41-43] The drop in blood pressure was dose-related, and the effect was still apparent 8 hours after a single 400-mg dose. Continuous intraarterial blood pressure recording in patients receiving chronic labetalol treatments three times daily demonstrated smooth control of blood pressure over the full 24-hour period.[44, 45] Twice-daily administration appears equally effective in achieving 24-hour control,[46-48] whereas a single dose of labetalol was markedly less effective.[49]

Drops in supine systolic and diastolic blood pressures were seen in normotensive men within 3 minutes of receiving an intravenous labetalol dose of 1.5 mg/kg.[16] Hypertensive patients have responded within 5 minutes of intravenous administration of a bolus dose of 1 to 2 mg/kg of labetalol.[50, 51] Blood pressure was reduced for as long as 6 hours; 3 hours was the average duration of the antihypertensive effect.

The dose of labetalol and the plasma concentration achieved appear to be related.[16] Although wide interpatient variation limits the predictive value of plasma labetalol levels with respect to hypotensive effect,[48] patients with lower steady-state levels receiving a fixed dose of labetalol tended to require higher maintenance doses to control blood pressure.[52]

Studies using radiolabeled labetalol have shown that after a large oral dose, uptake by the tissue occurs rapidly, and the drug is quickly cleared by both renal and biliary excretion. Labetalol is rapidly and almost completely absorbed after oral administration.[53] Sixty percent of the radioactivity is excreted in the urine, and 40% is excreted in the feces.

Labetalol undergoes extensive first-pass metabolism, with a great proportion of drug inactivated by the liver and intestinal wall. An intravenous dose, therefore, is less extensively metabolized than an oral dose.[53] The major labetalol metabolite in humans is an alcoholic glucuronide, a product formed by the action of uridine diphosphate–glucuronide transferase. There are no active metabolites of the drug, and only 3% is excreted unchanged in the urine.

The bioavailability of labetalol is increased by food ingestion.[54, 55] Concomitant administration of cimetidine also increases labetalol bioavailability.[56] Because a major portion of plasma clearance results from hepatic detoxification of the drug, dosages should be decreased in patients with significant hepatic dysfunction.[57] Extensive tissue uptake is reflected in the drug's large volume of distribution. In humans, only 50% of labetalol is plasma-bound, and no drug adjustment is required in patients with renal insufficiency.[57, 58] However, some authors recommend that labetalol be slowly uptitrated when administered to patients with end-stage renal disease and that blood pressure be followed closely.[59] A study also indicates that hemodialysis does not influence drug disposition.[60] In elderly patients, both bioavailability and elimination half-life are increased,[61] although clearance may be comparable and no change in dosage may be necessary.

Labetalol is much less lipid-soluble than propranolol, and negligible amounts cross the blood-brain barrier.[53] Likewise, there is little passage of radiolabeled drug across the placenta. At delivery, fetal cord blood contains much lower concentrations of the drug than maternal plasma. Of note, fetal bradycardia has not been observed with maternal treatment. Levels of labetalol found in breast milk, although highly variable, are consistently much lower than those in maternal plasma.

High-performance liquid chromatographic assays have demonstrated results consistent with a two-compartment model, with first-order drug absorption. The terminal elimination half-life of labetalol appears to be close to 6 hours.[48] As a result of hepatic metabolism, the absolute bioavailability of labetalol is 25%. A comparison of elderly and young hypertensives revealed no changes in pharmacokinetic values as a function of age.[62]

PHYSIOLOGIC EFFECTS OF LABETALOL
Antiarrhythmic Properties

Experimental Settings

Labetalol possesses weak membrane-stabilizing activity, a property shared with other β-blockers. Propranolol, however, has much greater membrane stabilization effects.[63] In an animal model, Vaughan Williams et al.[64] described the electrophysiologic effects of labetalol on atrial, ventricular, and Purkinje cells under normal and hypoxic conditions. Labetalol displayed considerable class I antiarrhythmic activity on atrial and ventricular tissues. A class III effect, slowing of all phases of repolarization in normal ventricular tissue, was also noted. No atrioventricular conduction slowing or negative inotropy was associated with labetalol. However, another investigation[65] showed a labetalol-induced increase in the functional refractory period of the atrioventricular node in anesthetized dogs. Finally, studies in the anesthetized cat[66] and isolated rat heart[67] have shown that labetalol reduces the number of premature ventricular contractions and the incidence of ventricular fibrillation during coronary artery occlusion and reperfusion.

Electrophysiology and Antiarrhythmic Effects in Humans

Labetalol appears to have less effect on the sinoatrial or atrioventricular node than propranolol, atenolol, or acebutolol.[68–71] The atrioventricular nodal conduction time and atrial effective refractory period are slightly prolonged, with only small changes in heart rate. No effects on the His-Purkinje system have been described. In the clinical setting, labetalol seems less likely than traditional β-blockers to produce pathologic bradycardia or heart block. More studies are needed in high-risk patients, such as those with acute cardiac ischemia, before the electrophysiologic effects of labetalol can be understood.

Several studies have documented that labetalol has an antiarrhythmic effect in hypertensive patients with premature ventricular contractions (PVCs). In a daily dose of 800 mg, labetalol lowered blood pressure and significantly reduced PVCs within 2 weeks after oral therapy was begun.[71] In a crossover trial,[72] labetalol appeared superior to propranolol in reducing ventricular arrhythmias in patients with mitral valve prolapse and stress-induced arrhythmias. Intravenously administered labetalol has also successfully restored sinus rhythm in hypertensive patients with a variety of dysrhythmias.[73]

Effects of the Renin-Angiotensin-Aldosterone System

A number of clinical studies have reported that long-term, oral labetalol administration in doses of 150 to 2400 mg daily produces decrements in supine and standing plasma renin activities.[74–76] The net renin suppressive effects were apparent at low doses of labetalol and appeared to be proportional to baseline renin levels. Exercise-induced increases in plasma renin activity were also suppressed by oral labetalol therapy.[74] Significant reductions in plasma angiotensin II concentrations and plasma and urinary aldosterone levels have been reported with intravenous or oral labetalol therapy.[76]

Other investigators, in contrast, have not been able to demonstrate an influence of orally administered labetalol on the renin-angiotensin-aldosterone axis.[77–79] Louis et al.[77] administered labetalol intravenously and still observed no effect on supine plasma renin activity. Plasma aldosterone concentrations have been unchanged in other studies as well.[75]

Plasma and Urinary Catecholamines

Caution must be exercised in interpreting apparently elevated levels of plasma catecholamines during labetalol therapy.[80] A metabolite of labetalol has been shown to interfere with the fluorometric assay for catecholamines and the photometric assay for metanephrines, leading to falsely elevated values of these compounds in certain patients.[81] Unless a specific assay is available based on high-performance liquid chromatography (HPLC) (discussed later), it seems advisable to defer measurement of plasma epinephrine for at least 4 days after labetalol is discontinued in patients being evaluated for pheochromocytomas.

Other Clinical Effects of Labetalol

Plasma Glucose and Lipids

Plasma glucose levels rose significantly following labetalol administration, but no changes were noted in growth hormone, free fatty acids, or C-peptide levels. Intravenous labetalol administration may cause a rise in plasma glucose by virtue of its β₂-adrenoreceptor agonist activity.[82] Hypertensive men who underwent 4 weeks of labetalol therapy in daily doses ranging from 300 to 1200 mg experienced a small increase in mean fasting glucose, with no alteration in insulin activity or response to oral glucose tolerance tests.[83]

No adverse effects on plasma lipid levels have been reported with labetalol. Frishman et al.[84] observed no significant alterations in plasma cholesterol, triglycerides, high-density lipoprotein (HDL) cholesterol, low-density lipoprotein (LDL) cholesterol, or HDL/total cholesterol ratios after 4 months of labetalol therapy. Rouffy,[85] in a double-blind, placebo-controlled crossover study, found no changes in plasma lipids, lipoproteins, or apolipoproteins after 90 days of therapy.

Effects on Body Fluid Volumes and Renal Function

Findings have varied with regard to the effects of labetalol on body fluid volumes. Over a 6-week period during which increasing doses of labetalol were administered, Weidmann et al.[75] observed increases in body weight, plasma volume, and blood volume of 1.7%, 2.1%, and 1.7%, respectively. Another study[86] of 13 hypertensive patients reported an increase in plasma volume (294 ml) after 8 weeks of labetalol monotherapy (585 mg/day), whereas propranolol monotherapy did not increase plasma volume. In contrast with these findings, however, are the results of a long-term, multicenter study by Michaelson et al.[87] that failed to demonstrate any major changes in body weight or fluid accumulation with chronic labetalol therapy (up to 48 weeks). Thus, fluid retention might occur with labetalol monotherapy, but it is unlikely to be of clinical significance. As with any vasodilator, any fluid retention that occurs will respond to therapy with a diuretic.

Many investigators have demonstrated that short-term or long-term administration of labetalol to hypertensive patients does not result in decrements of glomerular filtration rate or renal plasma flow.[88–93] Four groups reported no significant alterations in glomerular filtration rate, renal plasma flow, filtration fraction, or free-water clearance in patients receiving up to 2400 mg of labetalol daily.[88, 90, 91, 94] Labetalol has been associated with an increase in renal plasma flow when given to hypertensives with chronic renal failure.[95] Pure β-blockers, on the other hand, have been reported to decrease renal plasma flow and glomerular filtration rate.[90, 96] Labetalol's α-blocking property may prevent deleterious alterations in renal function. Labetalol has not been shown to decrease renal function in hypertensive patients with chronic renal insufficiency and has been used successfully to treat patients with varying degrees of renal dysfunction.[89, 92, 97, 98]

Respiratory Function

Because labetalol has nonspecific β-blocking activity, one might expect it to significantly impair pulmonary function in patients with chronic obstructive lung disease. Since α-adrenoreceptor inhibitors may have a bronchodilating action of their own and they have been shown to enhance the bronchodilating effects of isoproterenol,[99] it is conceivable that labetalol's mild α-blocking action, with or without β₂-agonistic effects, might mitigate some of the bronchoconstrictor effects on β-blockade.

In healthy human volunteers, propranolol caused a reduction in timed forced expiratory volume in 1 second (FEV₁), as well as a reduction in postexercise peak expiratory flow rate. These adverse effects on pulmonary function were not observed with labetalol.[100, 101] In asthmatic patients receiving equipotent blood pressure β-blocking doses, resting FEV₁ dropped significantly after the intravenous administration of 5 mg of propranolol but not after labetalol, 20 mg, or placebo.[102, 103] It has also been reported[103] that FEV₁ fell significantly in asthmatic patients known to be sensitive to propranolol following a single dose of metoprolol but not after an equipotent dose of labetalol. Another group of asthmatic hypertensive patients sensitive to propranolol showed no change in FEV₁ after periods of labetalol therapy up to 4 weeks, with doses up to 1200 mg/day.[104]

Labetalol administration has, however, been reported to result in bronchospasm.[105] Although most studies demonstrate no clinically significant deterioration in respiratory status after labetalol administration, it may still be prudent to use caution, as with β-selective blocking drugs, in patients with clinically overt bronchospasm.

CLINICAL USE
Treatment of Essential Hypertension

Labetalol has been in clinical use in Europe since 1975 for the control of mild, moderate, and severe hypertension. Several excellent reviews have summarized the clinical experience.[6, 106, 107] Labetalol appears to be at least as effective an antihypertensive agent as a wide range of other drugs. When used either alone or in combination with a diuretic, labetalol has successfully lowered blood pressure after other regimens, including β-blockers, have failed.[108, 109]

Studies comparing labetalol with placebo have shown that labetalol has a significant antihypertensive effect.[110, 111] In comparative studies, it has been shown that labetalol is equivalent or superior to a thiazide diuretic.[112] Adding labetalol to a standard diuretic regimen has resulted in a further dose-related fall in blood pressure.[113, 114]

A number of studies have compared labetalol with other β-adrenoreceptor blockers in the treatment of hypertension.[115–121] In 18 previously untreated patients with severe hypertension, labetalol resulted in a greater fall in standing blood pressure and less bradycardia than was observed in patients receiving propranolol.[120] A randomized crossover study of 24 hypertensive patients receiving thiazide diuretic therapy[86] showed comparable antihypertensive effects of labetalol (maximum dose 2400 mg/day) and propranolol (maximum dose 960 mg/day), but labetalol was associated with a greater incidence of side effects. When smaller doses of the same antihypertensive agents were used, the antihypertensive effect of labetalol was found to be greater than that of propranolol.

A variable-dose, comparative trial of atenolol, metoprolol, pindolol, and labetalol[122] demonstrated similar control of blood pressure for all four agents. Side effects were similar but numerically less frequent with labetalol than with atenolol or pindolol. Although labetalol and metoprolol were equally effective in reducing supine and standing blood pressures, metoprolol produced a greater reduction in resting heart rate than labetalol in a study by Frishman et al.[118] of patients with mild to moderate hypertension. Labetalol appears to be at least as effective an antihypertensive agent as pure or traditional β-blockers.

Labetalol monotherapy has been compared with the combination of a β-blocker and a direct-acting vasodilator. In a fixed-dose, randomized study, labetalol, 600 mg daily, was as effective as propranolol, 60 mg daily, plus hydralazine, 100 mg daily, in lowering standing blood pressure. The drug combination, however, reduced supine blood pressure more effectively.[123] A randomized crossover trial found that labetalol plus hydrochlorothiazide was as effective as the combination of propranolol, hydralazine, and hydrochlorothiazide.[124] A dose of labetalol, 600 mg twice daily, was equivalent to the combination of pindolol, 15 mg daily, and hydralazine, 150 mg daily, in mild to moderately severe hypertensive patients.[125]

As an antihypertensive medication, labetalol has been shown to be at least as effective as methyldopa, a diuretic-methyldopa combination, clonidine, various adrenergic neuronal blockers, or the calcium antagonist verapamil. More recently, labetalol has been found to achieve more rapid control of blood pressure than the angiotensin-converting enzyme (ACE) inhibitor captopril in mild to moderate hypertensive patients.[126] In a study of 31 hypertensive patients,[127] labetalol alone appeared to be as effective as a previously used combination of different β-blocking drugs and the α-blocker prazosin.[127] Dargie et al.[108] satisfactorily substituted labetalol for methyldopa, clonidine, and adrenergic neuronal blockers in patients with severe, resistant hypertension. Wallin et al.,[128] in a large, parallel, dose-titration study, found that labetalol, 200 to 2400 mg/day with or without furosemide, was as effective as methyldopa, 500 to 2000 mg/day, combined with furosemide. In a randomized, crossover study comparing labetalol with clonidine in 17 patients treated with a thiazide diuretic,[129] doses of each medication were titrated until the patients became normotensive or until intolerable side effects developed. At average daily doses of 476 mg of labetalol and 0.355 mg of clonidine, 12 patients complained of fatigue and dry mouth from clonidine. One patient complained of limb weakness, and two experienced unsteadiness during labetalol therapy. Labetalol, 200 mg twice daily, was found to be similar to verapamil, 160 mg twice daily, in a double-blind comparative study.

Elderly hypertensives are another subgroup of patients in whom labetalol appears to be particularly useful. The hemodynamic changes effected by labetalol, in which blood pressure is decreased primarily by reducing total peripheral resistance (TPR) with little effect on cardiac output, appear to be well-suited to the needs of elderly hypertensive patients in whom TPR is high and cardiac output is low. In a trial comparing the use of labetalol monotherapy (100 to 400 mg b.i.d.) in young and older hypertensive patients,[130] blood pressure was controlled in 18 of 20 elderly patients with isolated systolic hypertension (standing systolic blood pressure >160 mmHg with standing diastolic blood pressure ≤95 mmHg) or diastolic hypertension (standing diastolic blood pressure of 95 to 104 mmHg). A larger (n = 133) multicenter study revealed similar findings.[131] In 14 of 20 elderly patients (70%), blood pressure was controlled with labetalol, 100 mg b.i.d., during titration, a significant increase ($p < .05$) over the number of younger patients whose hypertension was controlled at this dose level. In another study,[132] all 25 elderly patients (aged 60 to 80 years) in whom standing diastolic blood pressure was between 90 and 110 mmHg, standing systolic blood pressure was greater than 160 mmHg, or both achieved control of blood pressure during titration with labetalol, and 20 of these patients required doses up to 200 mg b.i.d. Furthermore, 24-hour ambulatory monitoring showed that labetalol was more effective than enalapril in maintaining reduced blood pressure throughout the day.[133, 134] Evidence from these studies indicates that elderly hypertensive patients may require less medication than younger patients to achieve blood pressure control, and that control may be achieved without producing significant orthostatic changes.[135]

A growing body of evidence points to the usefulness of labetalol in black hypertensive patients. El-Ackad[136] showed that labetalol had a greater antihypertensive effect than propranolol after 8 weeks of maintenance therapy. In a parallel study,[137, 138] we reported that blacks obtained more marked blood pressure reduction with labetalol than with propranolol and that more propranolol-treated patients required the addition of a diuretic agent to obtain control of blood pressure. We and others[139] have speculated that in black patients, labetalol's α-adrenergic properties contribute to its antihypertensive effect. Labetalol has also been demonstrated to reduce left ventricular mass in previously untreated black hypertensives.[140]

In a study designed to parallel clinical practice, Cubberly et al.[138] demonstrated the effectiveness of labetalol as monotherapy in a group of black hypertensive patients requiring *both* a β-blocker and a diuretic to achieve blood pressure control. After "off-titrating" of both the diuretic and the β-blocker in patients with persistent hypertension, blood pressure was controlled with labetalol alone. The ability of a single drug—labetalol—to replace two drugs—a β-blocker and a diuretic—is consistent with the lesser efficacy of β-blockers alone.

The sum of clinical studies reveals that labetalol, whether administered alone or in combination with diuretics, is as effective an antihypertensive agent as are most currently available medications. Prolonged administration of the drug for up to 6 years appears not to be associated with drug tolerance.[141]

Hypertensive Emergencies

Owing in large measure to its α-blocking activity, labetalol rapidly lowers blood pressure when given either orally or intravenously, and it has been used effectively in the management of hypertensive emergencies. Blood pressure declines within 2 hours of oral treatment with 300 to 400 mg of labetalol and may respond to lower doses. Oral treatment has proved efficacious in treating accelerated hypertension and hypertensive encephalopathy.[142, 143] In a study of 36 patients with severly elevated blood pressure (199/132 mmHg),[144] labetalol was at least as effective as clonidine.

When very prompt blood pressure reduction is desired or when the patient cannot take medication orally, intravenous administration is feasible. In contrast with other parenteral antihypertensive agents that may be more effective, such as diazoxide, labetalol permits steady, controlled lowering of blood pressure without changes in heart rate or cardiac output. The drug may be given safely to patients with coronary artery disease, even after recent coronary artery bypass grafting.[145] Intravenously administered labetalol does not significantly reduce cerebral blood flow and may be the drug of choice for certain patients with cardiovascular disease.[146] Labetalol has also been administered intravenously to children and effectively reduced blood pressure regardless of renal function.[147]

One large multicenter study[148] evaluated 59 patients with supine blood pressures averaging 211/134 mmHg. Patients received intravenous pulsed doses of labetalol, starting with a 20-mg test dose and gradually increasing doses to a total of up to 300 mg. Table 60–4 summarizes the effects of intravenous labetalol administration in this study. Fifty-three of 59 patients reached the therapeutic goal of a diastolic blood pressure less than 95 mmHg or a decrease of at least 30

Table 60–4. **Intravenous Labetalol in Severe Hypertension**

Variable	Mean Results
Age (years)	49.4 (range = 21–78)
Males	31
Females	28
Symptomatic	23
Asymptomatic	36
Baseline blood pressure (mmHg)	211/134
BP after labetalol, 20 mg IV	188/120 mmHg
BP after last injection (mmHg)	143/93
Mean decrement in BP (mmHg)	68/41
Total dose of labetalol (mean)	197 mg (range = 20–300 mg)

BP, blood pressure.
Adapted by permission of the publisher from Wilson DJ, Wallin JD, Wlachkis ND, et al: Intravenous labetalol in the treatment of severe hypertension and hypertensive emergencies. Am J Med 75:95, 1983. Copyright 1983 by Excerpta Medica Inc.

mmHg. No serious adverse effects were reported, even in patients with left ventricular failure, angina pectoris, acute myocardial infarction, or encephalopathy.[148] Nausea, with or without vomiting, occurred most frequently (in eight patients); six patients experienced paresthesias; four reported sweating; and two complained of a variety of side effects. Following parenteral administration, labetalol may be given orally for long-term blood pressure control.

Many additional reports support the use of labetalol in severe hypertension and hypertensive emergencies; intravenous bolus doses and continuous-flow infusion (2 mg/min) have proved safe and effective.[149, 150] The hypertensive response to intravenously administered labetalol may be reduced in patients who are already receiving treatment with $\beta\alpha$-blocking drugs.[151–154]

Intravenous bolus administration of labetalol is generally followed by a hypotensive response within 5 minutes and a maximum response 10 minutes after administration.[155] The antihypertensive effect may persist for 6 hours or more after a single bolus injection.[156] The degree of blood pressure reduction is independent of the rate of injection, but the rate of reduction appears to vary directly with the rate of injection. Blood pressure reduction is also magnified by standing.

Pheochromocytoma and the Clonidine Withdrawal Syndrome

Labetalol has been used in the management of pheochromocytoma and in the treatment of clonidine withdrawal hypertension, two clinical situations characterized by catecholamine excess in which blockade of both $\alpha\beta$-adrenergic receptors may be desirable. Several reports, in fact, document labetalol's success in the treatment of pheochromocytoma.[157–160] Labetalol appeared to be more effective in patients whose tumors secreted epinephrine predominantly and in patients with sustained rather than paroxysmal hypertension. However, there are at least two reports[161, 162] that labetalol provoked a hypertensive crisis in such patients, requiring treatment with phentolamine and phenoxybenzamine. In these patients, the pressor response to labetalol may have resulted from the predominance of β-blockade after oral therapy, leaving α-adrenoreceptor stimulation relatively unopposed.

Similar caution must be exercised before recommending labetalol for the management of hypertensive crisis following clonidine withdrawal, although labetalol has been used successfully in both its treatment and its prophylaxis.[157, 163] Rebound hypertension has occured despite labetalol therapy.[164] Orally administered labetalol should probably not be given unless α-blockade has already been achieved with intravenous phentolamine.

Ischemic Heart Disease

Labetalol has favorable hemodynamic effects in normotensive patients with documented coronary artery disease and seems less likely than conventional β-blockers to cause myocardial depression.[38, 39, 165] The α-blocking properties of labetalol may act to minimize coronary artery spasm, whereas β-blockade may suppress any arrhythmias that might develop secondary to α-adrenoreceptor-stimulator vasodilatation. Condorelli et al.[166] studied the effect of labetalol, 100 mg twice daily, on exercise tolerance in 19 normotensive subjects with angiographically proven coronary artery disease. Compared with placebo, labetalol produced significant reductions in systolic and diastolic blood pressures, heart rate, and double-product. In addition, exercise tolerance was increased, and ST-segment depression was reduced by labetalol. Oral labetalol administration has been used effectively in hypertensive patients with coexisting angina.[167–169] In contrast with conventional β-blockers, abrupt withdrawal of labetalol does not appear to result in an increase in blood pressure or anginal symptoms.[170]

Overall, initial reports on the use of labetalol in patients with myocardial infarction are encouraging.[171] Incremental infusion of labetalol lowered blood pressure safely and effectively in 15 hypertensive patients with acute myocardial infarction. However, occasional drug-associated hypotension limits the utility of the drug.

Hypertension in Pregnancy

Labetalol has been found to satisfactorily control blood pressure and reduce proteinuria in pregnant women.[172] Although labetalol crosses the placental barrier, it does not appear to adversely affect the fetus antenatally, during labor, or in the postpartum period,[173, 174] although some degree of fetal β-blockade does occur after maternal treatment.[175] Clinically significant fetal hypoglycemia, bradycardia, or respiratory depression has not been reported with maternal labetalol therapy. Hypertension during pregnancy may be controlled effectively by oral doses of labetalol ranging from 300 to 1800 mg daily.[176, 177] Labetalol compared favorably with methyldopa in three randomized studies. In one study, Lamming et al.[177]

achieved better blood pressure control with labetalol, 400 to 800 mg/day, than with methyldopa, 750 to 1500 mg daily. The perinatal mortality rate was less than 5%, and no congenital malformations were noted in any of the infants born to labetalol-treated mothers. Redman[178] described similar blood pressure control in two groups of patients treated with either labetalol, 300 to 1200 mg daily, or methyldopa, 1 to 4 g daily. Sibai et al.[179] observed no differences in serial tests of renal function or fetal status.

In situations requiring rapid blood pressure reduction, such as severe preeclampsia or eclampsia, intravenously administered labetalol appears to offer advantages over intravenously administered hydralazine or diazoxide.[180, 181] Despite favorable reports on the use of labetalol to treat hypertension in pregnancy, its use must still be considered investigational until more data confirm its safety and superiority over more established medications.[182]

Use in General Anesthesia

Labetalol has been shown to be useful for correcting uncontrolled hypertension before anesthesia, during surgery, and in the immediate postoperative period, when it can be administered either intravenously or orally.[183, 184] This has also been demonstrated in elderly persons undergoing ambulatory surgery.[185] Induced hypotension is frequently desirable to minimize blood loss during surgical procedures, and labetalol achieves this goal[186] without increasing heart rate, cardiac output, or intrapulmonary shunting.[187]

Typically used agents, such as nitroprusside and ganglionic blockers, may be accompanied by undesirable tachycardia and tachyphylaxis. Labetalol has been effective when used with halothane (less than 3%) and other anesthetic agents for controlled hypotensive anesthesia during a variety of surgical procedures, including coronary bypass surgery, coarctation repair, and otologic operations. Stable control of blood pressure and heart rate was maintained throughout anesthesia.[188–191]

SIDE EFFECTS

Side effects of labetalol, usually mild and self-limited, fall into three categories: (1) nonspecific, (2) related to α-blockade, and (3) related to β-blockade. As is true with most antihypertensive agents, more side effects were observed in the initial, pivotal studies using forced titration to control blood pressure.

Nonspecific Side Effects

Gastrointestinal side effects, including nausea, abdominal pain, dyspepsia, flatulence, vomiting, and diarrhea, have been reported in up to 15% of patients. Fatigue and headache occur less frequently. Although rare, a variety of skin rashes have been attributed to labetalol therapy.[192–194]

Side Effects Related to α-Adrenoreceptor Blockade

Dizziness, occurring in perhaps 5% of patients receiving labetalol, develops most frequently in the early stages of treatment, especially with higher initial drug dosages, or in susceptible individuals such as patients receiving diuretics concomitantly.[106] Less frequent side effects related to α-blockade include scalp tingling and nasal stuffiness. Genitourinary disorders including impotence and retrograde ejaculation are side effects related to α-blockade that rarely occur with labetalol,[195] as does hyperkalemia.[196]

Side Effects from β-Adrenergic Blockade

The side effects of β-blockade tend to be less severe and occur less frequently during treatment with labetalol than during therapy with pure β-blocking drugs. Dream disturbances, asthma, and muscle cramps are infrequent. Heart failure, intermittent claudication, and Raynaud's phenomenon occur rarely.[195]

Alterations and Contraindications During Labetalol Therapy

Antinuclear antibodies may rarely become positive in low titers during labetalol therapy, but they are not associated with clinical diseases. Approximately 8% of patients developed transaminase elevations to twice normal levels in one long-term study.[87] In half of these patients, the abormalities resolved while labetalol therapy was continued, but 2% of patients discontinued treatment because of persistently elevated transaminase levels. Hepatotoxicity[197] is a very rare event.

Labetalol should be relatively contraindicated in situations in which β-blockade is undesirable, although labetalol appears less likely than propranolol to exacerbate existing conditions when therapeutic doses are given. Heart failure and asthma are best treated with antihypertensive agents other than β-blockers. Patients with suspected or proven pheochromocytoma should receive an α-blocking agent before oral therapy is considered.

DOSAGE

The recommended starting dose of oral labetalol therapy, either alone or with a diuretic, is 100 mg twice daily. The dose may be doubled after 2 days, with upward titration continuing every 2 to 3 days, until an optimal response is obtained. A more conservative approach with weekly or biweekly increments in dose may also be utilized. The usual maintenance dose is 200 to 400 mg twice daily, although some patients may require up to 2400 mg/day, possibly in combination with a thiazide diuretic, to achieve satisfactory control of blood pressure.

Labetalol may be given intravenously, either by repeated bolus injection or by slow continuous infusion. A solution for slow infusion should be prepared by diluting 200 mg of labetalol in 200 ml of a 5% dextrose solution. The recommended rate of infusion is 2 mg of labetalol (2-ml solution) per minute. The infusion should be stopped once a satisfactory response is obtained. The infusion may be repeated every 6 to 8 hours to maintain blood pressure control. If labetalol is administered by bolus injection, an initial dose of 20 mg should be given over 2 minutes.

Additional bolus injections of 40 to 80 mg may be given at 10-minute intervals. The maximum recommended total dose of labetalol by either method of parenteral administration is 300 mg. To minimize postural hypotension, patients should remain supine for 3 hours after intravenous administration.[106] Maintenance oral dosing may begin after adequate blood pressure control by parenteral administration.

GENERAL CONSIDERATIONS

An antihypertensive agent matures by a process of evaluation and reevaluation. This not-so-gentle evolution takes place over many years, allowing development of a perspective regarding the drug's use in the general hypertensive population and identification of its place in the therapeutic arsenal. In addition to better definition of the specific therapeutic benefits, side effects become better understood. This understanding relates to the frequency and severity of side effects observed during initial drug development, when protocols may force the use of larger doses than those commonly used in clinical practice, as well as to the emergence of additional side effects as a function of time and experience.

Since the approval of labetalol for the treatment of hypertension within the United States market, the place of this agent in the antihypertensive arsenal has become clearer. This is, after all, the age of the "vasodilatory" antihypertensive; agents correcting the pathophysiology of hypertension, an increase in TPR, have come to the therapeutic forefront. As such, labetalol joins the ranks of ACE inhibitors, calcium antagonists, and other direct vasodilators. However, it does not leave behind its characteristics as a β-blocker. Thus, there remain relative or absolute contraindications to treatment in patients with bronchospasm and heart failure, despite recent work suggesting a possible role for labetalol in those patients.[198-201]

It should also be noted that labetalol may be efficacious in some clinical applications for which there is no official approval. As noted, labetalol has been used effectively to treat hypertension associated with pregnancy. This utility continues to be reaffirmed with an expanding body of data,[202-206] yet no change is anticipated in labeling. A similar observation can be made regarding the use of labetalol in patients with angina pectoris.[207-210] Although there seems to be a very limited place for labetalol therapy in catecholamine-related hypertension,[211, 212] its effect on catecholamine assays resulting in false-positive results has become better appreciated,[213-215] a problem that can be avoided using cation exchange HPLC.[216]

Labetalol has also matured as a treatment for the broad spectrum of hypertensive conditions: from monotherapy in mildly hypertensive patients, through its use as a first or second agent in patients with moderate hypertension requiring two drugs, to its use in patients with urgent or emergent hypertension. Much of this additional experience has allowed fine tuning of the use of labetalol in severe hypertension and, more particularly, in specific subgroups of hypertensive patients. The ongoing experience in patients with severe hypertension requiring rapid but controlled reduction in blood pressure has supported the initial experience with this drug.[217-219] However, of equal importance has been experience with parenteral labetalol for perioperative use, available because of the drug's efficacy in hypertensive emergencies. This use has been expanding, both in the treatment of perioperative hypertension and in the induction of hypotension for surgical reasons.[220-225]

Labetalol seems particularly useful for the treatment of hypertension occurring in black patients,[226-229] the elderly,[130, 227, 229-234] and patients undergoing cardiodynamic stress from exercise or other stimuli.[235] The latter topic is important from another point of view: the cardiodynamic stress that results in left ventricular hypertrophy, associated with enhanced morbidity or mortality, and the "surge" changes in the cardiovascular system occurring in the early morning hours. Ambulatory blood pressure monitoring has demonstrated an around-the-clock therapeutic response to labetalol[236] and, more importantly, blunting of the pressor surge in blood pressure.[237] The reduction of left ventricular mass observed with labetalol treatment may be related to this cardiodynamic protection.[238, 239]

However, regardless of these results, an antihypertensive agent is effective only if it is used. Efficacy alone is not an issue, because all "approved" antihypertensive agents have been demonstrated to lower blood pressure. Certainly, the broader the range of hypertension (from mild to emergent) and the wider the application among subgroups of patients (race and age considerations), the wider the applicability of any drug. However, all these attributes can be voided by side-effect profiles, compliance issues, and cost. The last element includes not only the direct cost of the therapeutic agent but also the indirect costs associated with laboratory tests, physician visits, side effects, and other issues. In this regard, the "true" cost of antihypertensive agents may vary less than the direct cost of the drug. As an extreme example, one need only consider the use of diuretics as monotherapy. Although the cost of the drug is low, especially if a generic equivalent is prescribed, the indirect costs from laboratory fees (measurement of potassium and other biochemical parameters) and additional therapeutic agents (potassium supplements or antikaliuretics) rapidly wipe out the apparent savings. In addition, if there is an adverse long-term effect from either altered lipids or the cardiovascular risk of alterations in electrolytes, cost-effectiveness disappears.

This was amply demonstrated by Oster et al.[240] in an analysis of the cost-effectiveness of labetalol. Utilizing data from previously published clinical trials comparing the blood pressure reductions achieved using labetalol with those achieved using propranolol, these investigators examined the cost of reducing morbidity and mortality by preventing strokes through the treatment of hypertension in black patients. The authors observed two to seven times fewer strokes with labetalol monotherapy, and a lower direct dollar cost of therapy (either as monotherapy or in combination with a diuretic) at equivalent therapeutic dosages. Prospective, rather than theoretical, expansion of such analyses will assist all clinicians in developing an optimal therapeutic perspective for antihypertensive agents.

REFERENCES

1. Frishman W, Halprin S: Clinical pharmacology of the new beta-adrenergic blocking drugs. Part 7. New horizons in beta-adrenoreceptor blockade therapy: Labetalol. Am Heart J 98:660, 1979.
2. Farner JB, Kennedy I, Levy GP, et al: Pharmacology of AH5158: A drug which blocks both alpha- and beta-adrenoreceptor blocking drugs. Br J Clin Pharmacol 45:660, 1972.
3. Wallin JD, O'Neill WM: Labetalol. Arch Intern Med 143:485, 1983.
4. Flamenbaum W: Propranolol versus labetalol: Interesting differences in efficacy. J Natl Med Assoc 77:14, 1985.
5. Frishman WH, Strom JA, Kirschner M, et al: Labetalol therapy in patients with systemic hypertension and angina pectoris: Effects of combined alpha- and beta-adrenoreceptor blockade. Am J Cardiol 48:917, 1981.
6. McCarthy EP, Bloomfield SS: Labetalol: A review of its pharmacology, pharmacokinetic clinical uses and side effects. Pharmacotherapy 3:193, 1983.
7. Berlin LJ, Joel-Jensen BE: Alpha- and beta-adrenoreceptor blockade in hypertension. Lancet 1:979, 1972.
8. Brittain RT, Drew GM, Levy GP: The alpha- and beta-adrenoreceptor blocking potency of labetalol and its individual stereoisomers in anesthetized dogs and in isolated tissues. Br J Pharmacol 77:105, 1982.
9. Aggerbick M, Guellaen G, Hanoune J: N-alkyl substitution increases the affinity of adrenergic drugs for the alpha-adrenoreceptor in rat liver. Br J Pharmacol 65:15, 1979.
10. Brittain RT, Levy GP: A review of the animal pharmacology of labetalol, a combined alpha- and beta-adrenoreceptor blocking drug. Br J Clin Pharmacol 3(Suppl 3):681, 1976.
11. Blakeley AG, Summers RJ: The pharmacology of labetalol, an alpha- and beta-adrenoreceptor blocking agent. Gen Pharmacol 9:399, 1978.
12. Baum T, Sybertz EJ: Pharmacology of labetalol on experimental animals. Am J Med 75(Suppl 4A):15, 1983.
13. Cary B, Whalley ET: Labetalol possesses beta-adrenoreceptor agonist action on the isolated rat uterus. J Pharm Pharmacol 31:791, 1979.
14. Cary B, Whalley ET: Beta-adrenoreceptor agonist activity of labetalol on the isolated rat uterus. Br J Pharmacol 67:13, 1979.
15. Dage RC, Hsich CP: Direct vasodilatation by labetalol in anesthetized dogs. Br J Pharmacol 70:287, 1980.
16. Richards DA: Pharmacologic effects of labetalol in man. Br J Clin Pharmacol 3(Suppl 3):721, 1976.
17. Richards DA, Prichard BNC, Dobbs RJ: Adrenoreceptor blockade of the circulatory responses to intravenous isoproterenol. Br Heart J 39:99, 1977.
18. Richards DA, Prichard BNC, Boakes AJ, et al: Pharmacological

19. Richards DA, Prichard BNC, Hernandez R: Circulatory effects of noradrenalin and adrenaline before and after labetalol. Br J Pharmcol 7:37, 1977.
20. Richards DA, Tuckman J, Prichard BNC: Assessment of alpha- and beta-adrenoreceptor blocking actions of labetalol. Br J Clin Pharmacol 3:849, 1976.
21. Mehta J, Cohn JN: Hemodynamic effects of labetalol, an alpha- and beta-adrenergic blocking agent, in hypertensive subjects. Circulation 55:370, 1977.
22. Maconochie JG, Richards DA, Woodings EP: Modification of pressor responses induced by "cold" [abstract]. Br J Clin Pharmacol 4:389, 1977.
23. Frishman WH, MacCarthy EP, Kimmel B, et al: A new beta-adrenergic blocker-vasodilator. Drugs (Suppl) 205:121, 1984.
24. Frishman WH: Clinical Pharmacology of the β-Adenoreceptor Blocking Drugs. Norwalk, CT: Appleton-Century-Crofts, 1984.
25. Koch G: Hemodynamic changes after acute and long-term combined alpha- and beta-adrenoreceptor blockade with labetalol as compared with beta-receptor blockade. Cardiovasc Pharmacol 3(Suppl 1):530, 1981.
26. Agabiti-Rosei E, Alicaudri CL, Beschi M, et al: The acute and chronic hypotensive effect of labetalol and the relationship with pretreatment plasma noradrenalin levels. Br J Clin Pharmacol 13(Suppl 2):87s, 1982.
27. Jockers AM, Thompson FD: Acute hemodynamic effects of labetalol and its subsequent use as an oral hypotensive agent. Br J Clin Pharmacol 3(Suppl 3):789, 1976.
28. Koch G: Cardiovascular dynamics after acute and long-term alpha- and beta-adrenoreceptor blockade at rest, supine and standing, and during exercise. Br J Clin Pharmacol 8(Suppl 2):101s, 1979.
29. Svendsen TL, Rasmussen S, Hartling OJ: Sequential haemodynamic effects of labetalol at rest and during exercise in essential hypertension. Postgrad Med J 56(Suppl 2):21, 1980.
30. Prichard BNC, Thompson FD, Boakes AJ, et al: Some haemodynamic effects of compound AH 5158 compared with propranolol, propranolol plus hydralazine, and diazoxide: The use of AH 5158 in the treatment of hypertension. Clin Sci Mol Med 48:97s, 1975.
31. Bahlmann J, Brod J, Hubrich W, et al: Effect of an alpha- and beta-adrenoreceptor blocking agent (labetalol) on haemodynamics in hypertension. Br J Clin Pharmacol 8(Suppl 2):113s, 1979.
32. Trap-Jensen J, Clausen JP, Hartling OJ, et al: Immediate effects of labetalol on central, splanchnic-hepatic, and forearm haemodynamics during pleasant emotional stress in hypertensive patients. Postgrad Med J 56(Suppl 2):37, 1980.
33. Omvik P, Lund-Johansen P: Acute hemodynamic effects of labetalol in severe hypertension. J Cardiovasc Pharmacol 4:915, 1982.
34. Lund-Johansen P: Comparative haemodynamic effects of labetalol, timolol, prazosin, and the combination of tolamolol and prazosin. Br J Clin Pharmacol 8(Suppl 2):107s, 1979.
35. Edwards RC, Raftery EB: Haemodynamic effects of long-term oral labetalol. Br J Clin Pharmacol 3(Suppl 3):733, 1976.
36. Fagard R, Amery A, Reybrouck T, et al: Response of the systemic and pulmonary circulation to alpha- and beta-receptor blockade (labetalol) at rest and during exercise in hypertensive patients. Circulation 60:1214, 1979.
37. Lund-Johansen P: Acute and chronic (six-years) hemodynamic effects of labetalol in essential hypertension. Am J Med 75(Suppl 4A):24, 1983.
38. Gagnon RM, Morisette M, Presant S, et al: Hemodynamic and coronary effects of intravenous labetalol in coronary artery disease. Am J Cardiol 49:1267, 1982.
39. Taylor SH, Silke B, Nelson GIC, et al: Haemodynamic advantages of combined alpha-blockade and beta-blockade alone in patients with coronary heart disease. Br Med J 285:325, 1982.
40. Griffith DNW, James IM, Newbury PA, et al: The effect of beta-adrenergic receptor blocking drug on cerebral blood flow. Br J Clin Pharmacol 7:491, 1979.
41. Richards DA, Maconochie JG, Bland RE, et al: Relationship between plasma concentrations and pharmacological effects of labetalol. Eur J Clin Pharmacol 11:85, 1977.

42. Serlin MJ, Orme MC, Maciver M, et al: Rate of onset of hypotensive effect of oral labetalol. Br J Clin Pharmacol 7:165, 1979.
43. Rossi A, Ziacchi V, Lomanto B: The hypotensive effect of a single daily dose of labetalol: A preliminary study. Int J Clin Pharmacol Ther Toxicol 20:438, 1982.
44. Bala-Subramanian V, Mann S, Raftery EB: The effect of labetalol on continuous ambulatory blood pressure. Br J Clin Pharmacol 8(Suppl 2):119s, 1979.
45. Sanders GL, Murray A, Rawlins MD: Interdose control of beta-blockade and arterial blood pressure during chronic oral labetalol treatment. Br J Clin Pharmacol 8(Suppl 2):27s, 1982.
46. Mancia G, Pomidossi G, Parati G, et al: Blood pressure responses to labetalol in twice and three times daily administration during a 24-hour period. Br J Clin Pharmacol 13(Suppl 1):27s, 1982.
47. Ferrari A, Buccino N, DiRienzo M, et al: Labetalol and 24-hour monitoring of arterial blood pressure in hypertensive patients. J Cardiovasc Pharmacol 3(Suppl 1):42s, 1981.
48. Maronde RF, Robinson D, Vlachakis N, et al: A study of single and multiple dose pharmacokinetic/pharmacodynamic modeling of the antihypertensive effects of labetalol. Am J Med 75(Suppl 4A):40, 1983.
49. Wilcox R: Randomized study of six beta-blockers and a thiazide diuretic in essential hypertension. Br Med J 2:383, 1978.
50. Ronne-Rasmussen JO, Andersen GS, Bowel Jensen N, et al: Acute effect of intravenous labetalol in the treatment of systemic arterial hypertension. Br J Clin Pharmacol 3(Suppl 3):805, 1976.
51. Cumming AMM, Brown JJ, Lever AF, et al: Treatment of severe hypertension by repeated bolus injections of labetalol. Br J Clin Pharmacol 8(Suppl 2):199s, 1979.
52. McNeil JJ, Andersen AE, Louis WJ, et al: Labetalol steady-state pharmacokinetics in hypertensive patients. Br J Clin Pharmacol 13(Suppl 1):75s, 1982.
53. Martin LE, Hopkins R, Bland R: Metabolism of labetalol by animal and man. Br J Clin Pharmacol 3(Suppl 3):695, 1976.
54. Mantyla R, Allonen H, Kanto J, et al: Effect of food on the bioavailability of labetalol [letter]. Br J Clin Pharmacol 9:435, 1980.
55. Daneshmend TK, Roberts CJC: The influence of food on the oral and intravenous pharmacokinetics of a high clearance drug: A study with labetalol. Br J Clin Pharmacol 14:73, 1982.
56. Daneshmend TK, Roberts CJC: Cimetidine and bioavailability of labetalol [letter]. Lancet 1:565, 1981.
57. Homeida M, Jackson L, Roberts CJC: Decreased first-pass metabolism of labetalol in chronic liver disease. Br Med J 2:1048, 1978.
58. Wood AJ, Ferry DG, Bailey RR: Elimination kinetics of labetalol in severe renal failure. Br J Clin Pharmacol 13(Suppl):81s, 1982.
59. Luke DR, Awni WM, Halstenson CE, et al: Bioavailability of labetalol in patients with end stage renal disease. Ther Drug Monit 14:203, 1992.
60. Matzke GR: Effects of hemodialysis (HD) on labetalol (L) disposition [abstract]. Clin Pharmacol Ther 39:209, 1986.
61. Abernathy DR, Schwartz JB, Plachetka JR, et al: Pharmacodynamics and disposition of labetalol in elderly hypertensive patients. Am J Cardiol 60:697, 1987.
62. Rocci ML Jr, Vlasses PH, Cressman MD, et al: Pharmacokinetics and pharmacodynamics of labetalol in elderly and young hypertensive patients following single and multiple doses. Pharmacotherapy 10:92, 1990.
63. Frishman WH: Beta-adrenoreceptor antagonists: New drugs and new indications. N Engl J Med 305:500, 1981.
64. Vaughan Williams EM, Millar JS, Campbell TJ: Electrophysiological effects of labetalol on rabbit atrial, ventricle, and Purkinje cells, in normoxia and hypoxia. Cardiovasc Res 16:233, 1982.
65. Ambio JP: A study of the labetalol-induced changes in conductivity and refractoriness of the dog heart in situ. Cardiovasc Res 12:646, 1978.
66. Pogurize SM, Sharma AD, Corr PB: Influence of labetalol, a combined alpha- and beta-adrenergic blocking agent on the dysrhythmias induced by coronary occlusion and re-perfusion. Cardiovasc Res 16:398, 1982.
67. Lubbs WF, Nguyea T, Edwards MF: Antiarrhythmic action of labetalol and its effect on adenosine metabolism in the isolated rat heart. J Am Coll Cardiol 1:296, 1983.
68. Seides SF, Josephson ME, Batsford WP, et al: The electrophysiology of propranolol in man. Am Heart J 88:733, 1974.
69. Robinson C, Birkhead J, Crook B, et al: Clinical electrophysiological effects of atenolol, a new cardio-selective beta-blocking agent. Br Heart J 40:14, 1978.
70. Mason JW, Winkle RA, Meffin PJ, et al: Electrophysiological effects of acebutolol. Br Heart J 40:35, 1978.
71. Romano S, Orfei S, Pozzoni L, et al: Pulmonary clinical trial on hypotensive and antiarrhythmic effect of labetalol. Drugs Exp Clin Res 7:65, 1981.
72. Butrous GS: Management of ventricular arrhythmias associated with mitral valve prolapse by combined alpha- and beta-blockade. Postgrad Med J 62:259, 1986.
73. Mazzola C, Ferrario N, Calzavara MP, et al: Acute antihypertensive and antiarrhythmic effects of labetalol. Curr Ther Res 29:613, 1981.
74. Lijnen PJ, Amery AK, Fagard RH, et al: Effects of labetalol on plasma renin, aldosterone, and catecholamine in hypertensive patients. J Cardiovasc Pharmacol 1:625, 1979.
75. Weidmann P, DeChatel R, Zeigler WH, et al: Alpha- and beta-adrenergic blockade with orally administered labetalol in hypertension. Am J Cardiol 41:570, 1978.
76. Salvetti A, Pedrinelli R, Sassano P, et al: Effect of increasing dose of labetalol on blood pressure, plasma renin activity and aldosterone in hypertensive patients. Clin Sci 57:401s, 1979.
77. Louis WJ, Christophidis N, Brignell M, et al: Labetalol: Bioavailability, drug plasma levels, plasma renin, and catecholamine in acute and chronic treatment of resistant hypertension. Aust N Z J Med 8:602, 1978.
78. Larochelle P, Hamet P, Hoffman B, et al: Labetalol in essential hypertension. J Cardiovasc Pharmacol 2:751, 1980.
79. Kornerup HJ, Pedersen EB, Christensen NJ, et al: Effect of oral labetalol on plasma catecholamine, renin, and aldosterone in patients with severe arterial hypertension. Eur J Clin Pharmacol 16:305, 1979.
80. Mihano L, Kolloch R, De Quattro V: Increased catecholamine excretion after labetalol therapy: A spurious effect of drug metabolites. Clin Chim Acta 95:211, 1979.
81. Bouloux PM: Interference of labetalol metabolites in the determination of plasma catecholamine by HPLC with electrochemical detection. Clin Chim Acta 150:111, 1985.
82. Riley AJ: Some further evidence for partial agonist activity of labetalol [letter]. Br J Clin Pharmacol 9:517, 1980.
83. Anderson O, Berglaud G, Hansson L: Antihypertensive action, time of onset and effects on carbohydrate metabolism of labetalol. Br J Clin Pharmacol 3(Suppl 3):757, 1976.
84. Frishman W, Michaelson E, Johnson B, et al: Effects of beta-adrenergic blockade on plasma lipids: A double-blind randomized placebo-controlled multicenter comparison of labetalol and metoprolol in patients with hypertension [abstract]. Am J Cardiol 49:984, 1982.
85. Rouffy J: Effects of labetalol (400 mg/day) on plasma lipids, lipoproteins in hypertensive patients: A double-blind drug versus placebo study. J Hypertens 3:545, 1985.
86. Humyor SN, Bauer GE, Ross M, et al: Labetalol and propranolol in mild hypertensives: Comparison of blood pressure and plasma volume effects. Aust N Z J Med 10:162, 1980.
87. Michaelson EL, Frishman WH, Lewis JE, et al: Multicenter clinical evaluation of the long-term efficacy and safety of labetalol in the treatment of hypertension. Am J Med 75(Suppl 4A):68, 1983.
88. Rasmussen S, Nielsen PE: Blood pressure body fluid volume, and glomerular filtration rate during treatment with labetalol in essential hypertension. Br J Clin Pharmacol 12:349, 1981.
89. Thompson FD, Jockes AM, Hussein MM: Monotherapy with labetalol for hypertensive patients with normal and impaired renal function. Br J Clin Pharmacol 8(Suppl 2):129s, 1979.
90. Pedersen EB, Larsen JS: Effect of propranolol and labetalol on renal haemodynamics at rest and during exercise in essential hypertensive. Postgrad Med J 2(Suppl):27, 1980.
91. Cruz F, O'Neill WM, Clifton G, et al: Effects of labetalol and methyldopa on renal function. Clin Pharmacol Ther 30:57, 1981.

92. Valvo E, Previato G, Tessitore N, et al: Effects of the long-term administration of labetalol on blood plasma, hemodynamics, and renal function in essential and renal hypertension. Curr Ther Res 29:634, 1981.

93. Malini PL, Strocchi E, Negroni S, et al: Renal haemodynamics after chronic treatment with labetalol and propranolol. Br J Clin Pharmacol 13(Suppl 1):123s, 1982.

94. Wallin JD: Adrenoreceptors and renal function. J Clin Hypertens 1:217, 1985.

95. Innes A, Gemmell HG, Smith FW, et al: The short term effects of oral labetalol in patients with chronic renal disease and hypertension. J Hum Hypertens 6:211, 1992.

96. Epstein M, Oster JR: Beta-blockers and the kidney. Mineral Electrolyte Metab 8:237, 1982.

97. Bailey RR: Labetalol in the treatment of patients with hypertension and renal function impairment. Br J Clin Pharmacol 8(Suppl 2):135s, 1979.

98. Wallin JD: Antihypertensives and their impact on renal function. Am J Med 46:4A, 1983.

99. Patel KR, Kerr JW: Alpha-receptor blocking drugs in bronchial asthma. Lancet 1:348, 1975.

100. Richards DA, Woodings EP, Maconochie JG: Comparison of the effects of labetalol and propranolol in healthy men at rest and during exercise. Br J Clin Pharmacol 4:15, 1977.

101. Maconochie JG, Woodings EP, Richards DA: Effects of labetalol and propranolol on histamine-induced bronchoconstriction in normal subjects. Br J Clin Pharmacol 4:157, 1977.

102. Skinner C, Gaddie J, Palmer KNV: Comparison of intravenous AH5158 (labetalol) and propranolol in asthma. Br J Med 2:59, 1975.

103. El-Ackad TM: The effects of labetalol and metoprolol on ventilatory function in patients with bronchial asthma sensitive to propranolol. Clin Res 32:330A, 1984.

104. George RB: Effects of labetalol in asthmatics with demonstrated propranolol sensitivity. Chest 86:318, 1984.

105. Larsen K: Influence of labetalol, propranolol, and practolol in patients with asthma. Eur J Respir Dis 63:221, 1982.

106. Brogden RN, Heel RC, Speight TM, et al: Labetalol: A review of its pharmacology and therapeutic uses in hypertension. Drugs 15:251, 1978.

107. Prichard BNC, Richards DA: Comparison of labetalol with other antihypertensive drugs. Br J Clin Pharmacol 13(Suppl 1):41s, 1982.

108. Dargie HJ, Dollery CT, Daniel J: Labetalol in resistant hypertension. Br J Clin Pharmacol 3(Suppl 3):751, 1976.

109. Milne BJ, Logan AG: Labetalol: Potent antihypertensive agent totally blocks both alpha- and beta-adrenergic receptors. Can Med Assoc J 123:1013, 1980.

110. Davidov ME, Moir GD, Poland MP, et al: Monotherapy with labetalol in the treatment of hypertension: A double-blind study. Am J Med 75:62, 1983.

111. Kane J, Gregg I, Richards DA: A double-blind trial of labetalol. Br J Clin Pharmacol 3(Suppl 3):737, 1976.

112. Horvath JC, Caterson RJ, Collett P, et al: Labetalol and bendrofluazide: Comparison of their antihypertensive effects. Med J Aust 1:626, 1976.

113. Bloomfield SS, Lucas CS, Gantt P, et al: Step II treatment with labetalol for essential hypertension. Am J Med 75:81, 1983.

114. Lifshitz AA, McMahon FG, Jain AK, et al: Combined trichlormethiazide and labetalol therapy in moderate to severe hypertension. Clin Pharmacol Ther 23:118, 1978.

115. Romo M, Haltunnen P, Saarinen P, et al: Labetalol and pindolol in the treatment of hypertension: A comparative study. Ann Clin Res 11:249, 1979.

116. Pugsley DJ, Nassim M, Armstrong BK, et al: A controlled trial of labetalol (Trandate), propranolol and placebo in the management of mild to moderate hypertension. Br J Pharmacol 7:63, 1979.

117. Kofod P, Kjaer K, Vejo S, et al: Labetalol and alprenolol: A comparative investigation of antihypertensive effect. Postgrad Med J 56(Suppl 2):69, 1980.

118. Frishman WH, Michaelson EL, Johnson BF, et al: A multiclinic comparison of labetalol to metoprolol in the treatment of mild to moderate systemic hypertension. Am J Med 75:54, 1983.

119. Bjerle P, Fransson L, Koch G, et al: Pindolol and labetalol in hypertension: Comparison of the antihypertensive effects with particular respect to conditions in the upright posture and during exercise. Curr Ther Res 27:516, 1980.

120. Pugsley DJ, Armstrong BK, Nassim MA, et al: Controlled comparison of labetalol and propranalol in the management of severe hypertension. Br J Clin Pharmacol 3:777, 1976.

121. Nicholl DP, Husaini MH, Bulpitt CJ, et al: Comparison of labetalol and propranolol in hypertension. Br J Pharmacol 9:233, 1980.

122. McNeil JJ, Louis WJ: A double-blind cross-over comparison of pindolol, metoprolol, atenolol, and labetalol in mild to moderate hypertension. Br J Clin Pharmacol 8(Suppl 2):1673s, 1979.

123. West MJ, Wing LMH, Mulligan R, et al: Comparison of labetalol, hydralazine, and propranolol in the therapy of moderate hypertension. Med J Aust 1:224, 1982.

124. Van der Veur E, ten Berge BS, Donker AJ, et al: Comparison of labetalol, hydralazine and propranolol in hypertensive outpatients. Eur J Clin Pharmacol 21:457, 1982.

125. Barnett AJ, Kalowski S, Guest C: Labetalol compared with pindolol plus hydralazine in the treatment of hypertension: A double-blind cross-over study. Med J Aust 2:105, 1978.

126. Dessl-Fulgheri P: Labetalol and captopril combined with chlorthalidone in the treatment of mild to moderate hypertension. Curr Ther Res 37:873, 1985.

127. MacDonald I, Hua ASP, Thomas GW, et al: Use of labetalol in moderate to severe hypertension. Med J Aust 1:325, 1980.

128. Wallin JD, Wilson D, Winer N, et al: Treatment of severe hypertension with labetalol compared to methyldopa and furosemide: Results of a long-term, double-blind, multicentric trial. Am J Med 75(Suppl 4A):87, 1983.

129. Anavekar SN, Barter C, Adam WR, et al: A double-blind comparison of verapamil and labetalol in hypertensive patients with coexisting chronic obstructive airways disease. J Cardiovasc Pharmacol 4:s374, 1982.

130. Forette F, Amar M, D'Allens H, et al: A double-blind comparison between labetalol and clonidine in the treatment of hypertension in the elderly: A multicentre study. Therapie 42:277, 1987.

131. Giles TD, Weber M, Bartels DW, et al: Treatment of isolated systolic hypertension with labetalol in the elderly. Arch Intern Med 150:974, 1990.

132. Nugent CA, Bleicher JM, Plachetka JR: Labetalol in the treatment of elderly patients with mild essential hypertension. J Am Osteopath Assoc 88:359, 1988.

133. Applegate WB, Borhani N, DeQuattro V, et al: Comparison of labetalol versus enalapril as monotherapy in elderly patients with hypertension: Results of 24-hour ambulatory blood pressure monitoring. Am J Med 90:198, 1991.

134. Weidler DJ, Vidt DG, Toth PD, et al: Comparison of labetalol and hydrochlorothiazide in elderly patients with hypertension using 24-hour ambulatory blood pressure monitoring. J Clin Pharmacol 30:524, 1990.

135. Giles TD, Weber M, Bartels DW, et al: Evaluation of labetalol in elderly patients with essential hypertension. J Clin Pharmacol 31:556, 1991.

136. El-Ackad TM: Comparison of the antihypertensive efficacy of labetalol with that of propranolol in black hypertensive patients. Clin Res 32:330A, 1984.

137. Flamenbaum W, Weber MA, McMahon FG, et al: Monotherapy with labetalol compared with propranolol: Differential effects by race. J Clin Hypertens 1:56, 1985.

138. Cubberly RB: Labetalol as monotherapy in hypertensive black patients. J Clin Hypertens 1:304, 1987.

139. Wong CK, Lau CP, Leung WH, et al: Usefulness of labetalol in chronic atrial fibrillation. Am J Cardiol 66:1212, 1990.

140. Foster E, Plehn JF, Bernard SA, et al: Regression of left ventricular hypertrophy in "previously untreated" hypertensive blacks after 6 months of blood pressure reduction with alpha- and beta-adrenergic blockade and thiazide therapy. Cardiovasc Drug Ther 6:147, 1992.

141. Prichard BNC, Boakes AJ, Hernandez R: Long-term treatment of hypertension with labetalol. Br J Clin Pharmacol 8(Suppl 2):171s, 1979.

142. Ghose RR, Sampson A: Rapid onset of action of oral labetalol in severe hypertension. Curr Med Res Opin 5:147, 1977.

143. Davies AB, Bal Subramanian V, Gould B, et al: Rapid reduction of blood pressure with acute oral labetalol. Br J Clin Pharmacol 13:705, 1982.

144. Atkin SH, Jaker MA, Beaty P, et al: Oral labetalol versus oral clonidine in the emergency treatment of severe hypertension. Am J Med Sci 303:9, 1992.

145. Sladen RN, Klamerus KJ, Swalfford MW, et al: Labetalol for the control of elevated blood pressure following coronary artery bypass grafting. J Cardiothorac Anesth 4:210, 1990.

146. Pearson RM, Griffith DNW, Woollard M, et al: Comparison of effects on cerebral blood flow of rapid reduction in systemic arterial pressure by diazoxide and labetalol in hypertensive patients: Preliminary findings. Br J Clin Pharmacol 8(Suppl):195s, 1979.

147. Bunchman TE, Lynch RE, Wood EG: Intravenously administered labetalol for treatment of hypertension in children. J Pediatr 120:140, 1992.

148. Wilson DJ, Wallin JD, Wlachkis ND, et al: Intravenous labetalol in the treatment of severe hypertension and hypertensive emergencies. Am J Med 75:95, 1983.

149. Lebel M: Antihypertensive effectiveness of labetalol infusion in hypertensive emergencies. Clin Invest Med 80:60A, 1985.

150. Wright JT: Labetalol by continuous infusion in severe hypertension. J Clin Hypertens 1:39, 1986.

151. MacCarthy EP, Frost GW, Stokes GS: Labetalol in hypertensive emergencies. Med J Aust 1:399, 1978.

152. McGrath, Matthews PG, Walter NM, et al: Emergency treatment of severe hypertension with intravenous labetalol. Med J Aust 2:410, 1978.

153. Anderson CC, Gabriel R: Poor hypotensive response and tachyphylaxis following intravenous labetalol. Curr Med Res Opin 5:424, 1978.

154. Yeung CK, Thomas GW, Whitworth JA, et al: Comparison of labetalol, clonidine and diazoxide intravenously administered in severe hypertension. Med J Aust 2:499, 1979.

155. Trust PM, Agabeti-Rosei E, Brown JJ, et al: Effect on blood pressure, angiotensin II and aldosterone concentrations during treatment of severe hypertension with intravenous labetalol: Comparison with propranolol. Br J Pharmacol 3(Suppl 3):799, 1976.

156. Pearson RM, Harvard CWH: Intravenous labetalol in hypertensive patients treated with beta-adrenoceptor blocking drugs. Br J Clin Pharmacol 3(Suppl 3):795, 1976.

157. Agabiti-Rosei E, Brown JJ, Trust PM, et al: Treatment of pheochromocytoma and of clonidine withdrawal hypertension with labetalol. Br J Clin Pharmacol 3(Suppl 3):809, 1976.

158. Kaufman L: Use of labetalol during hypotensive anesthesia and in the management of pheochromocytoma. Br J Clin Pharmacol 8(Suppl 2):229s, 1979.

159. Reach G, Thibonnier M, Chevillard C, et al: Effect of labetalol on blood pressure and plasma catecholamine concentrations in patients with pheochromocytoma. Br Med J 1:1300, 1980.

160. Takeda T, Kaneko Y, Omae T, et al: The use of labetalol in Japan: Result of multicentre clinical trials. Br J Clin Pharmacol 13(Suppl 1):49s, 1982.

161. Briggs RST, Birtwell AJ, Pohl JEF: Hypertensive response to labetalol in phaeochromocytoma [letter]. Lancet 1:1045, 1978.

162. Feek CM, Earnshaw PM: Hypertensive response to labetalol in phaeochromocytoma [letter]. Br Med J 2:387, 1980.

163. Rosenthal T, Rabinowitz B, Boichis H, et al: Use of labetalol in hypertensive patients after discontinuation of clonidine therapy. Eur J Pharmacol 20:237, 1981.

164. Hurley DM, Vandongen R, Beilin LJ: Failure of labetalol to prevent hypertension due to clonidine withdrawal. Br Med J 1:1122, 1979.

165. Silke B, Nelson GI, Ahwja RC, et al: Comparative hemodynamic dose response effects of propranolol and labetalol in coronary heart disease. Br Heart J 48:364, 1982.

166. Condorelli M, Brevitti G, Chiarello M, et al: Effects of combined alpha- and beta-blockade in patients with coronary artery disease. Br J Clin Pharmacol 13(Suppl 1):101s, 1982.

167. Lubbe WF, White DA: Labetalol in hypertensive patients with angina pectoris: Beneficial effect of combined alpha- and beta-adrenoceptor blockade. Clin Sci Mol Med 55:283s, 1978.

168. Besterman EMM, Spencer M: Open evaluation of labetalol in the treatment of angina pectoris occurring in hypertensive patients. Br J Clin Pharmacol 8(Suppl 2):205s, 1979.

169. Nyberg G, Bjuor I, Hagman M, et al: Relation between ST-segment depression and chest pain in patients with coronary artery disease receiving no treatment and after beta-blockade and combined alpha- and beta-blockade. Acta Med Scand 644(Suppl):30, 1981.

170. Prichard BNC, Walden RJ: The syndrome associated with the withdrawal of beta-adrenergic blocking drugs. Br J Clin Pharmacol 13(Suppl 2):337s, 1982.

171. Marx PG, Reid DS: Labetalol infusion in acute myocardial infarction with systemic hypertension. Br J Clin Pharmacol 8(Suppl 2):233s, 1979.

172. Pickles CJ, Broughton Pipkin F, Symonds EM: A randomised placebo controlled trial of labetalol in the treatment of mild to moderate pregnancy induced hypertension. Br J Obstet Gynaecol 99:964, 1992.

173. Michael CA: Use of labetalol in the treatment of severe hypertension during pregnancy. Br J Clin Pharmacol 8(Suppl 2):217s, 1979.

174. Lamming GD, Symonds EM: Use of labetalol and methyldopa in pregnancy-induced hypertension. Br J Clin Pharmacol 8(Suppl 2):217, 1979.

175. Harper A, Murnaghan GA: Maternal and fetal haemodynamics in hypertensive pregnancies during maternal treatment with intravenous hydralazine or labetalol. Br J Obstet Gynaecol 98:453, 1991.

176. Coevoet B, Leuliet P, Comoy E: Labetalol for hypertension in pregnancy. Second Congress of the International Society for the Study of Hypertension in Pregnancy, Cairo, 1980.

177. Lamming GD, Broughton Pipkin F, Symonds EM: Comparison of the alpha- and beta-blocking drug, labetalol, and methyldopa in the treatment of moderate and severe pregnancy-induced hypertension. Clin Exp Hypertens 2:865, 1980.

178. Redman CWG: A randomized comparison of methyldopa (Aldomet) and labetalol (Trandate) for the treatment of severe hypertension in pregnancy [abstract]. Clin Exp Hypertens B1:345, 1982.

179. Sibai BM, Mabie WC, Shamsa F, et al: A comparison of no medication versus methyldopa or labetalol in chronic hypertension during pregnancy. Am J Obstet Gynecol 162:960, 1990.

180. Garden A, Davey DA, Dommisse J: Intravenous labetalol and dihydralazine in severe hypertension in pregnancy. Clin Exp Hypertens B1:371, 1982.

181. Michael CA: Intravenous labetalol and intravenous diazoxide in severe hypertension complicating pregnancy. Aust N Z Obstet Gynaecol 26:18, 1986.

182. Olsen KS, Beier-Holgersen R: Fetal death following labetalol administration in pre-eclampsia. Acta Obstet Gynecol Scand 71:145, 1992.

183. Scott DB: The use of labetalol in anesthesia. Br J Clin Pharmacol 13(Suppl 1):133s, 1982.

184. Morel DR, Forster A, Suter PM: Labetalol in the treatment of hypertension following coronary artery surgery. Br J Anaesthesiol 54:1191, 1982.

185. Singh PP, Dimich I, Sampson I, et al: A comparison of esmolol and labetalol for the treatment of perioperative hypertension in geriatric ambulatory surgical patients. Can J Anaesth 39:559, 1992.

186. Toivonen J, Virtanen H, Kaukinen S: Labetalol attenuates the negative effects of deliberate hypotension induced by isoflurane. Acta Anaesthesiol Scand 36:84, 1992.

187. Goldberg ME, McNulty SE, Azad SS, et al: A comparison of labetalol and nitroprusside for inducing hypotension during major surgery. Anesth Analg 70:537, 1990.

188. Cope DHP, Crawford MC: Labetalol in controlled hypotension. Administration of labetalol when adequate hypotension is difficult to achieve. Br J Anaesthesiol 51:359, 1979.

189. Jones SEF: Coarctation in children. Controlled hypotension using labetalol and halothane. Anaesthesia 34:1052, 1979.

190. Kanto J, Pakkanen A, Allen H, et al: The use of labetalol as a moderate hypotensive agent in otological operations—plasma concentrations after intravenous administration. Int J Pharmacol Ther Toxicol 18:191, 1980.

191. Dubois C: Use of labetalol for intra- and post-operative pre-

vention of arterial hypertension during coronary artery bypass surgery. J Hypertens 2:432, 1984.

192. Gange RW, Wilson Jones E: Bullous lichen planus caused by labetalol. Br Med J 1:816, 1978.

193. Finlay AY, Waddington E: Cutaneous reactions to labetalol [letter]. Br Med J 1:987, 1978.

194. Branford WA, Hunter JAA, Muir AL: Cutaneous reactions to labetalol. Practitioner 221:765, 1978.

195. Waal-Manning HJ, Simpson FO: Review of long-term treatment with labetalol. Br J Clin Pharmacol 13(Suppl 1):65s, 1982.

196. Arthur S, Greenberg A: Hyperkalemia associated with intravenous labetalol therapy for acute hypertension in renal transplant recipients. Clin Nephrol 33(6):269, 1990.

197. Clark JA, Zimmerman HJ, Tanner LA: Labetalol hepatotoxicity. Ann Intern Med 113:210, 1990.

198. Chahine RA, Pinar Johnson T: Effect of labetalol on abnormal left ventricular function in patients with hypertension and compensated heart failure. Clin Res 35:2A, 1987.

199. Dianzumba SB, Dipette DJ, Weber M, et al: The role of alpha-adrenergic blockade on left ventricular diastolic filling in mild hypertension. Hypertension 9:547, 1987.

200. Kreutner W, Rizzo C: Labetalol protects against the potentiation by propranolol of the bronchospasm to norepinephrine in guinea pigs. Arch Int Pharmacodyn 285:117, 1987.

201. Clerici C, Harf A, Macquin-Mavier I: Failure of enhancement by labetalol of bronchopulmonary effects of histamine in guinea pigs: Independence of alpha-adrenoceptor antagonism. Br J Pharmacol 91:487, 1987.

202. Lees KR, Rubin PC: Treatment of cardiovascular diseases. Br Med J 294:258, 1987.

203. Ashe RG, Moodley J, Richardo AM: Comparison of labetalol and dihydralazine in hypertension emergencies of pregnancy. S Afr Med J 71:354, 1987.

204. Sibai BM, Gonzalez AR, Malone WC, et al: A comparison of labetalol plus hospitalization versus hospitalization alone in the management of preeclampsia remote from term. Obstet Gynecol 70:323, 1987.

205. Marie WC: A comparative trial of labetalol and hydralazine in the acute management of severe hypertension complicating pregnancy. Obstet Gynecol 70:328, 1987.

206. Rasmussen K: Fetal hemodynamics before and after treatment of maternal hypertension in pregnancy. Dan Med Bull 34:80, 1987.

207. Prida XE, Himja Feldman RL: Systemic and coronary hemodynamic effects of combined alpha- and beta-adrenergic blockade (labetalol) in normotensive patients with stable angina pectoris and positive exercise stress test responses. Am J Cardiol 59:1084, 1987.

208. Messner P, Peuch P, D'Allens P, et al: Comparative evaluation of labetalol and acebutolol in exertional angina. Semaine Hôpital Paris 63:701, 1987.

209. Kanto JH: Labetalol in the treatment of angina pectoris. Int J Clin Pharmacol Ther Toxicol 25:166, 1987.

210. Koch G, Fransson L: Hemodynamic effects at rest and during exercise of combined alpha/beta blockade alone in patients with ischemic heart disease. J Cardiovasc Pharmacol 10:474, 1987.

211. Mehta JL, Lopez LM: Rebound hypertension following abrupt cessation of clonidine and metoprolol. Treatment with labetalol. Arch Intern Med 147:389, 1987.

212. Ishikawa Y, Shimo Cori A, Yasuda G, et al: A case of malignant pheochromocytoma: A trial of blood pressure control with labetalol and alpha-methyl-tyrosine. Curr Ther Res 44:542, 1987.

213. Feldman JM: Falsely elevated level of urinary excretion of catecholamine and metanephrines in patients receiving labetalol therapy. J Clin Pharmacol 27:288, 1987.

214. Hollister AS, Mitchel ER, Baja A: False-positive urinary catecholamine assays caused by labetalol. Clin Res 35:17A, 1987.

215. Manon M, Hauger WD: Erroneous diagnosis of pheochromocytomas in a hypertensive patient on labetalol. Clin Res 35:751A, 1987.

216. Binder SR, Biaggine E: Analysis of urinary catecholamine by high-performance liquid chromotography in the presence of labetalol metabolites. J Chromotogr 385:241, 1987.

217. Ngole PM: Intravenous labetalol in the management of resistant hypertension emergency. Drug Intell Clin Pharmacol 21:512, 1987.

218. Frithz G: Treatment of severe hypertension with peroral labetalol. Ups Med J 92:75, 1987.

219. Garcia JY, Vidt DG: Current management of hypertensive emergencies. Drugs 34:263, 1987.

220. Grubb BP, Sirio C, Zelis R: Intravenous labetalol in acute aortic dissection. JAMA 258:78, 1987.

221. Roth S, Run S: Safe use of induced hypotension in a patient with chronic liver disease. Can J Anesthesiol 34:186, 1987.

222. McNulty S, Sharifi-Hzad S, Farole A: Induced hypotension with labetalol for orthognathic surgery. J Oral Maxillofac Surg 45:309, 1987.

223. Saarnivaara L, Klemola Lindgron L: Labetalol as a hypotensive agent for middle ear surgery. Acta Anesthesiol Scand 31:196, 1987.

224. Leslie JB, Kalayjian RW, Surgo MA, et al: Intravenous labetalol for the treatment of postoperative hypertension. Anesthesiology 67:413, 1987.

225. Roelofse JA, Shipton EA, Toubert JJ, et al: A comparison of labetalol, acebutolol, and lidocaine for controlling the cardiovascular responses to endotracheal intubation for oral surgical procedures. J Oral Maxillofac Surg 45:835, 1987.

226. Saunders E, Curry C, Hinds T, et al: Labetalol compared with propranolol in the treatment of black hypertensive patients. J Clin Hypertens 3:294, 1987.

227. Flamenbaum W: Management of unique hypertensive situations: A focus on difficult, problematic, elderly black patients. J Natl Med Assoc 79:31, 1987.

228. Wright JT, McKenney TM, Lambert RM, et al: Comparison of response to labetalol and atenolol by race. Clin Res 35:442A, 1987.

229. Wallin JD, Shah SV: Beta-adrenergic blocking agents in the treatment of hypertension. Choice based on pharmacologic properties and patient characteristics. Arch Intern Med 147:654, 1987.

230. Abernathy DR, Schwartz JB, Plachetka JR, et al: Comparison for young and elderly patients of pharmacodynamics and disposition of labetalol in systemic hypertension. Am J Cardiol 69:697, 1987.

231. Abernathy DR, Bartos P, Plachetka JR: Labetalol in the treatment of hypertension in the elderly and younger patients. J Clin Pharmacol 27:902, 1987.

232. Buell JC, Eliot RS, Plachetka JR, et al: Hemodynamic effects of labetalol in older adult hypertensives. J Clin Pharmacol 28:327, 1988.

233. Forette F, Henry D'Allens A, et al: Treatment of arterial hypertension in the elderly by labetalol, an alpha- and beta-blocker. Ann Cardiol Angiol (Paris) 36:103, 1987.

234. Rocci ML, Masses PH, Cressmen M, et al: Pharmacodynamics and disposition of labetalol in elderly vs young. Clin Pharmacol Ther 42:171, 1987.

235. Plachetka JR, Elliot RS, Buell JC: Blood pressure control with labetalol at rest and under three stressful stimuli. Clin Pharmacol Ther 41:190, 1987.

236. Garrett B, DeQuattro V, Plachetka J: Usefulness of 24-hour ambulatory BP monitoring in the evaluation of antihypertensive compounds. Clin Pharmacol Ther 41:228, 1987.

237. DeQuattro V, Lee DD, Allen J, et al: Labetalol blunts morning pressor surge in systolic hypertension. Hypertension 11:I198, 1988.

238. Plehn JF, Bernard SA, Batenelli V: Regression of left ventricular mass in black hypertensive patients after alpha- and beta-blockade: Analysis of diastolic function. Clin Res 35:447A, 1987.

239. DeQuattro V, Lee D, Allen J, et al: The effects of labetalol on ambulatory blood pressure and left ventricular mass and function in patients with isolated systolic hypertension. Hypertension 9:549, 1987.

240. Oster G, Huse DM, Delea TE, et al: Cost effectiveness of labetalol and propranolol in the treatment of hypertension among blacks. J Natl Med Assoc 79:1049, 1987.

CHAPTER 61

Carvedilol

William D. Carlson, M.D., Ph.D., and Edward M. Gilbert, M.D.

Carvedilol was discovered when scientists working at Boehringer Mannheim Pharmaceuticals in West Germany found that several novel β-blockers they had synthesized exhibited vasodilatory effects in addition to β-blockade.[1] These compounds belong to a class of β-blockers called phenoxyethylamines. It has been shown that peripheral resistance is elevated in essential hypertension.[2] However, in patients with hypertension, treatment using β-blockers decreases cardiac output rather than reducing peripheral resistance.[3] The addition of a vasodilator to the β-blocker increases the success rate in the treatment of hypertension over monotherapy.[4, 5] Investigators at Boehringer reasoned that these phenoxyethylamines could be potentially useful as antihypertensive agents because they had both β-blocking and vasodilating properties. They also reasoned that these compounds might be effective in the treatment of angina pectoris if vasodilation reduced the workload on the heart by reducing peripheral resistance or improved coronary blood flow. They investigated the relative efficacy of β-blockade and vasodilation to find a compound that had both properties in the same concentration range. The compound that the researchers found to have the most advantageous properties was carvedilol. Since its discovery, carvedilol has been the subject of a large number of studies to characterize its effects and develop it for therapeutic use in treating hypertension and exertional angina. The majority of studies have been carried out in Europe with the support of Boehringer Mannheim Pharmaceuticals. However, SmithKline Beecham has entered into an agreement for the development of carvedilol in the United States and has begun studies to support an application to the United States Food and Drug Administration for use of carvedilol as an antihypertensive agent.

CHEMICAL STRUCTURE

Carvedilol is a chemical compound that was synthesized as a congener of propranolol and belongs to a class of compounds called phenoxyethylamines. This class of compounds exhibits both β-blocking activity and vasodilatory activity. Carvedilol has the chemical formula $C_{24}H_{26}N_2O_4$ and a molecular weight of 406.5. The chemical name is (+)-1-(carbazol-4-yloxy)-3-[[2-(O-methoxyphenoxy) ethyl]amino]-2-propanol.

PHARMACODYNAMICS

Carvedilol has been shown to have nonselective competetive β-blocking activity in both *in vitro* and *in vivo* models. *In vitro* experiments[6] were carried out using isolated rabbit atria to determine β₁-blocking activity

and guinea pig tracheal chains to determine β₂-blocking activity. The inhibitory activity of carvedilol on the isoprenaline-induced increase in the contraction rate of rabbit atria and the relaxation of the tracheal chain preparation indicate that it has both β₁- and β₂-blocking activity. *In vivo* experiments in rabbits, dogs, and the spontaneously hypertensive strain of rats (SHR) confirmed the nonselective β-blocking activity of carvedilol.[6] In these experiments, carvedilol produced a parallel shift to the right of the dose-response curve for isoprenaline-induced tachycardia. A 50% reduction in isoprenaline-induced tachycardia was observed at intravenous doses of 0.1 to 1 mg/kg carvedilol, as shown in Figure 61–1. In a conscious rabbit model, carvedilol was approximately three times more potent than propranolol and 20 times more potent than labetalol on a milligram-to-milligram basis.[6]

The intrinsic sympathomimetic activity of carvedilol was investigated using rats pretreated with reserpine. The increase in heart rate induced by carvedilol was determined. In these studies, pindolol increased the rate by 100 beats/min at a concentration of 0.3 mg/kg, whereas propranolol and carvedilol failed to increase the rate at 1 mg/kg. Thus, it appears that carvedilol has no intrinsic sympathomimetic activity in the dose range within which it produces its β-blocking activity.

In contrast with the data derived from animal studies, studies of human heart suggest that carvedilol's β-antagonist effects are mildly selective for β₁-adrenergic receptors (approximately 10- to 40-fold selective, depending on the method of determining selectivity).[7, 8] The differences between human and animal studies are likely a result of the marked interspecies differences in cardiac receptor pharmacology.[9]

The membrane-stabilizing activity of carvedilol was investigated in rabbits by determining the intravenous dose required to raise the electrical threshold for the induction of ventricular tachycardia by 100 μA.[6] The doses found to be equally effective were (1) 1.9 mg/kg for carvedilol, (2) 0.91 mg/kg for propranolol, and (3) 2.12 mg/kg for quinidine. Table 61–1 summarizes the characterization of carvedilol as a β-blocker.

Activity of the enantiomers was investigated in conscious rabbits for β₁-blocking activity, in rat aortic strips for vasodilation, and in spontaneously hypertensive rats for its hypotensive action.[10] β-Blockade was found to be limited to the levorotatory enantiomer. Equipotent vasodilation was observed with both enantiomers in the norepinephrine-induced contraction of rat aortic strips. In the SHR, the levorotatory enantiomer reduced blood pressure at doses similar to the doses that produced β-blockade (0.02 mg/

583

Basal Heart Rate (HR) and
Isoprenaline-Induced Tachycardia
(HR Iso) after Incremental Doses

Mean Arterial Pressure (Pa_m)

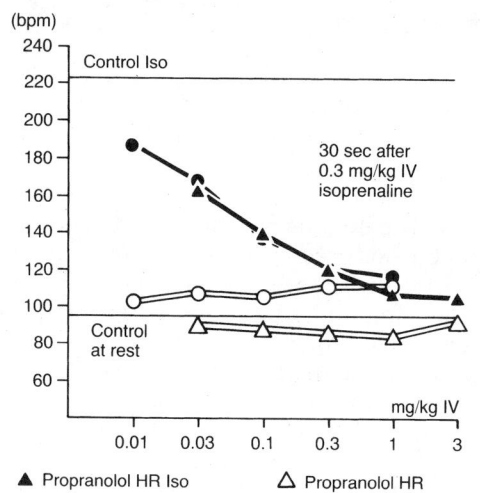

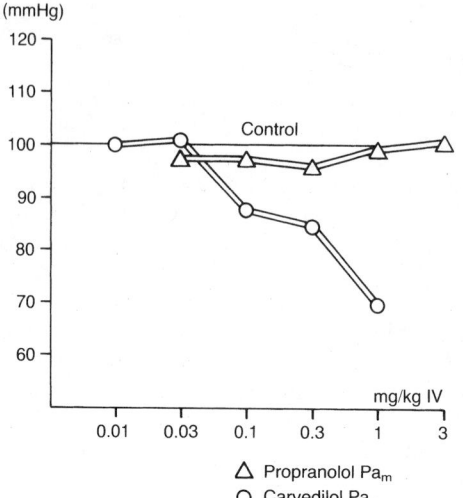

▲ Propranolol HR Iso   △ Propranolol HR
● Carvedilol HR Iso   ○ Carvedilol HR

△ Propranolol Pa_m
○ Carvedilol Pa_m

Figure 61–1. Hemodynamic effects of carvedilol (*circles*) and propranolol (*triangles*) in conscious dogs. Left panel shows resting heart rate and blockade. Right panel shows effects on mean arterial blood pressure. n = 10. (From Abshagen U: A new molecule with vasodilating and β-adrenoceptor blocking properties. J Cardiovasc Pharmacol 10[Suppl 11]:S23, 1987.)

kg), but no activity was seen with the dextrorotatory form at doses up to 0.2 mg/kg. These results suggest that the hypotensive effect of the racemic mixture is the result of the combined effects of β-blockade and vasodilation.

EFFECT ON BLOOD PRESSURE IN ANIMAL MODELS

In spontaneously hypertensive rats, carvedilol lowered blood pressure at doses of 0.1 mg/kg given intravenously and 1 mg/kg given orally. The doses required to lower blood pressure by 30 mmHg were found to be 0.37 mg/kg when given intravenously and 3.6 mg/kg when given orally. In this study, carvedilol was found to be equipotent to dihydralazine but did not produce the reflex tachycardia that was observed with dihydralazine.[4] In experiments with conscious rabbits, doses of 0.1 mg/kg were found to lower blood pressure when administered intravenously. In experiments using carotid artery occlusion in anesthetized rabbits, a dose of 0.11 mg/kg was required to lower blood pressure by 30 mmHg. Comparable effects on blood pressure were observed with doses of 0.18 mg/kg of dihydralazine and 0.98

mg/kg of labetalol administered intravenously. The hypotensive effect of intravenously administered carvedilol occurs at lower doses than with dihydralazine or labetalol and at ten times lower than the oral dose required for blood pressure reduction in these single-dose animal studies.

Mechanism of Acute Hypotensive Effect

The mechanism responsible for the acute hypotensive effect of carvedilol given either intravenously or by an oral route has been the subject of considerable study. In conscious normotensive dogs, intravenously administered carvedilol, 0.25 mg/kg, has been shown to lower blood pressure significantly.[6] Hemodynamic studies, summarized in Figure 61–2, have shown that cardiac output was maintained while total peripheral resistance decreased. Because propranolol has been shown to increase peripheral vascular resistance while decreasing blood pressure, the mechanism of the carvedilol-induced drop in blood pressure must involve an additional effect besides simple β-blockade. This additional effect is consistent with the observed effects of vasodilation in animal models. The

Table 61–1. **Characterization of β-Blocking Activity of Carvedilol and Propranolol**

Criterion		Model	Carvedilol	Propranolol
Potency	IC$_{50}$ (nM)	β$_1$-Receptor binding Guinea pig atria	2.6	21
	In vitro pA$_{10}$	Atrium	7.44 ⎱ Ratio	6.77 ⎱ Ratio
		Trachea	6.54 ⎰ 7.94	6.56 ⎰ 1.62
	In vivo ED$_{50}$ (μg/kg)	Rabbits IV	138	335
		Dogs IV	62	79
Duration of action	(hr)	Dogs PO	16	12
Intrinsic sympathomimetic activity		Tachycardia in reserpinized rats	No	No
Membrane-stabilizing activity		Antiarrhythmic potency in rabbits	+	+

From Abshagen U: A new molecule with vasodilating and β-adrenoceptor blocking properties. J Cardiovasc Pharmacol 10(Suppl 11):S23, 1987.

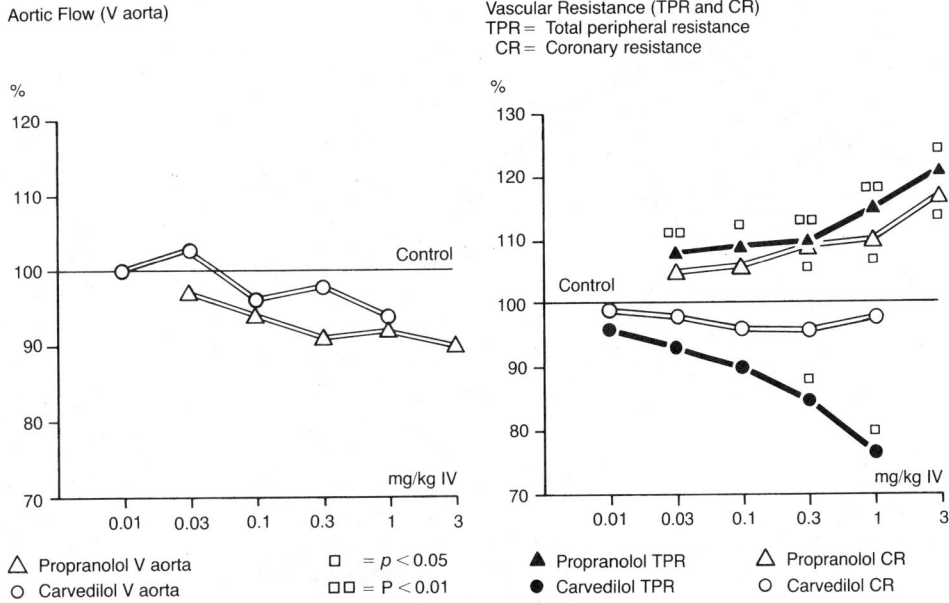

Figure 61–2. Hemodynamic effects of carvedilol *(circles)* and propranolol *(triangles)* in conscious dogs. Left panel shows aortic blood flow. Right panel shows vascular resistance. n = 10. (From Abshagen U: A new molecule with vasodilating and β-adrenoceptor blocking properties. J Cardiovasc Pharmacol 10[Suppl 11]:S23, 1987.)

exact mechanism of vasodilation, however, has not yet been clearly delineated.

To investigate the possibility that vasodilation was caused by β2-agonist activity,[6] experiments with isolated guinea pig tracheal chains were conducted. However, these experiments failed to show significant β2-agonist activity for carvedilol, whereas control experiments with pindolol showed β2-agonist activity. These results convincingly exclude β2-agonist activity as carvedilol's mechanism of vasodilation. Similarly, experiments in nictitating rat membrane preparations[10] have ruled out ganglionic-blocking activity as the mechanism responsible for the vasodilatory effect of carvedilol.

In contrast, in experiments in both isolated tissue and intact animal models, carvedilol appears to exhibit α-adrenergic–blocking activity. The norepinephrine dose-response curves in pithed rats were shifted to a similar extent by carvedilol and phentolamine. In isolated rabbit aortic strips, carvedilol blocked the response to norepinephrine to a greater extent than did labetalol but to an extent similar to that of prazosin, suggesting the presence of α1-antagonist properties. In these experiments, the ratio of the pA2 values for βα-blockade was 1:23 for carvedilol and 1:13 for labetalol, as seen in Figure 61–3. In *pithed* rats, carvedilol inhibited the actions of methoxamine and, to a lesser degree, phentolamine. Experiments in conscious rats showed that the response to phenylephrine could be antagonized by carvedilol in doses of 0.1 mg/kg IV and 0.3 mg/kg PO. Labetalol was effective intravenously in these experiments at doses comparable to those of carvedilol. This work demonstrates that carvedilol has α-adrenergic–blocking activity at concentrations close to those at which it demonstrates β-blocking activity. However, it does not prove that the vasodilatory effects in animals are due entirely to this effect.

Interestingly, carvedilol was effective in causing re-

laxation in rat aortic strips that had been contracted by (1) a thromboxane antagonist, (2) potassium chloride, and (3) norepinephrine. In these experiments, carvedilol thus acted more like the direct vasodilator glyceryl trinitrate than the α1-blocker prazosin.

The current data do not unequivocally define the mechanism of action for carvedilol. The data support significant effects of (1) nonselective β-blockade, (2) α1-blockade, and (3) an undefined effect that may be calcium channel blockade, a direct effect on smooth muscle through mechanisms similar to nitrates or through the prostaglandins. Further work is necessary to define clearly the vasodilatory mechanisms in animal models.

GENERAL PHARMACOLOGY
Cardiovascular Function

The effect of carvedilol on hemodynamics in conscious and anesthetized dogs has been investigated, using propranolol as a control. In conscious dogs, carvedilol and propranolol produced a similar inhibition of isoprenaline-induced tachycardia, but only carvedilol produced a decrease in blood pressure at comparable doses.[6] Cardiac output was decreased by less than 5% by carvedilol at doses of up to 1 mg/kg IV, whereas at equivalent doses, it was decreased by propranolol by 10% to 12%. Of more significance, total peripheral vascular resistance (PVR) was decreased by carvedilol and was increased by propranolol in a dose-dependent fashion. A maximum decrease of 12% in PVR for carvedilol was seen at the highest dose of 1 mg/kg. Likewise, a maximum increase of 20% in PVR for propranolol was observed at the highest dose of 3 mg/kg. Hindlimb perfusion was reduced by both carvedilol and propranolol, but renal perfusion was not affected by carvedilol despite the decrease in blood pressure.

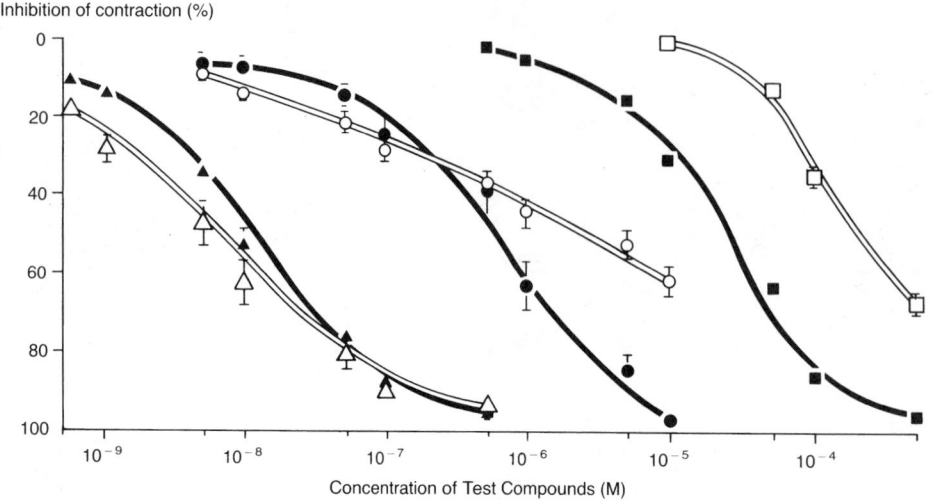

Inhibition of contraction (%)

Concentration of Test Compounds (M)

△ Sodium nitroprusside
○ Carvedilol
□ Labetalol

n = 6; means ± SEM

▲ ● ■ Precontracted with norepinephrine 10^{-5} M
△ ○ □ Precontracted with K$^+$ 4×10^{-2} M

Figure 61–3. Relaxation of rat aortic strips by test compounds. Triangles represent sodium nitroprusside. Circles represent carvedilol. Squares represent labetalol. Open symbols are precontracted with K$^+$ 40 nM. Closed symbols are precontracted with norepinephrine 10^{-5} M. (From Abshagen U: A new molecule with vasodilating and β-adrenoceptor blocking properties. J Cardiovasc Pharmacol 10[Suppl 11]:S23, 1987.)

The electrophysiologic behavior of carvedilol has been tested on sinus node preparations, Purkinje fibers, and ventricular muscle cells.[11] In the concentration range of 10^{-6} mol/L, small negative inotropic and chronotropic effects were observed. Action potential waveform, excitation, and conduction parameters were altered only slightly at these concentrations. Concentrations of 10^{-5} mol/L were found to damage cell function. These concentrations are well above the levels necessary for β-blocking activity, which occurs at 3×10^{-8} mol/L. Whether these effects might be seen with chronic oral dosing because of compartmentalization or differential penetration of carvedilol into various tissues has not yet been investigated.

Carvedilol did not demonstrate local anesthetic effects in the concentrations investigated; thus, it differs from class I antiarrhythmics. It does not significantly prolong the action potential and can thus be distinguished from class III antiarrhythmics. Calcium channel–blocking activity is not observed except at concentrations higher than those tested here and was not considered relevant at these concentrations. Thus, carvedilol cannot be classified as a class IV antiarrhythmic. β-Blockers have been observed to reduce automaticity, conduction velocity, and excitability and to increase refractory time. The electrophysiologic effects of carvedilol at relevant concentrations thus appear to be attributable to its β-blocking properties.

In vivo experiments looking at the drug's effects on the conduction system in the heart have been performed in rabbits and dogs.[12] Intravenous infusions of carvedilol at a dose of 1 mg/kg over 2 minutes produced no changes in heart rate, electrocardiographic intervals, or morphology of electrocardiographic complexes. Infusions at doses of 3 mg/kg over 30 minutes slowed the heart rate but did not affect the electrocardiogram except to reduce heart rate. When infusions of 3 mg/kg were administered over 10 minutes, the PR interval lengthened to the point of first-degree or second-degree atrioventricular

block. During the infusion of 3 mg/kg of carvedilol over 2 minutes, complete suppression of atrial activity was observed for a period of time, and a slow ventricular rhythm replaced the sinus rhythm. It is not clear whether this is a direct effect of carvedilol on the conduction tissue of the heart or enhanced vagal tone produced by profound adrenergic blockade. Similar effects have been observed for other β-blockers at high doses, but the mechanism is still unknown.[13]

Central Nervous System Function

Because carvedilol is lipid soluble, it would be expected to cross the blood-brain barrier and to exhibit some of the central nervous system effects common to some other β-blockers. In conscious rats, rabbits, and dogs, no indication of excitant or sedative effects were observed.[12] However, during the IRWIN test in rats, oral doses of 30 mg/kg produced ptosis and disorders of coordination. Some rat studies showed ptosis after oral doses of 3 mg/kg and 10 mg/kg. These effects are not unexpected for a β-blocker with high lipid solubility.

Renal Function

In experiments on rats,[12] 3 mg/kg of carvedilol administered orally was associated with a small decrease in urinary sodium excretion. Oral doses of 10 mg/kg also produced decreases in urinary potassium and chloride excretion. These effects were not increased at oral doses of 30 mg/kg. In experiments on dogs, carvedilol produced increases in urine volume after oral administration of 3, 10, and 30 mg/kg. The effect was not dose-dependent, and electrolyte excretion was not significantly affected. At a dose of 1 mg/kg, no effect on urine volume or electrolyte excretion was observed. These effects are consistent with increases in renal perfusion but may also be due to direct effects on various transport mechanisms.

PHARMACOKINETICS AND METABOLISM

The pharmacokinetics and disposition of carvedilol given orally and intravenously has been studied in 20 normal volunteers.[6] After intravenous administration of 12.5 mg over 1 hour, peak serum levels averaged 173 ng/ml at 1 hour. Figure 61–4 shows that the serum concentration is a function of time after oral and intravenous administration. The serum concentration fell rapidly after termination of the infusion but then showed an elimination half-life of 2.4 hours and a range of 1.9 to 4.2 hours. The total clearance reached 589 ml/min, and the volume of distribution of carvedilol was 132 L.

After oral administration of 25-mg and 50-mg doses, the elimination half-life was found to substantially increase to 6.4 and 7 hours, respectively. Carvedilol was rapidly absorbed, and peak concentrations were reached after 1.5 to 1.2 hours for the 25-mg and 50-mg doses. Average maximum concentrations for the 25-mg and 50-mg doses were 21 and 66 ng/ml, respectively, with large variability. The area under the concentration curves showed similar differences between the two doses and similarly large variability, with averages of 157 and 348 ng/ml/hr. Absolute bioavailability was found to be 22% to 24% for the two doses, with expectedly high variation. The data are shown in Table 61–2.[14]

The metabolism of carvedilol was studied in the 50-mg oral dose by administering ^{14}C carvedilol and measuring excretion and serum concentration of the parent compound, certain metabolites, and the [14]C.[14] The major metabolites are shown in Figure 61–5. The total reactivity of ^{14}C in plasma far exceeded the concentration of carvedilol or its major metabolite BM 14,242, and the area under the curve was 20 times greater. The elimination half-life of the radioactivity was substantially longer than that of carvedilol, averaging 39 hours in its unaltered form.

Carvedilol is subject to substantial first-pass effect in the liver, and evidence suggests that a substantial amount of enterohepatic circulation occurs. After either oral or intravenous administration, only a small percentage of carvedilol is recovered unchanged in the urine, and biliary excretion was found to be the major route of elimination. In one experiment in rats, less than 2% of ^{14}C carvedilol was recovered in the urine. The metabolites of carvedilol were studied in plasma and urine after the oral administration of ^{14}C carvedilol to 20 healthy volunteers.[12] The major components found in this study were carvedilol and its glucuronide. Together these two components accounted for 31% of the radioactivity in plasma 1.5 hours after dosing and 34% of the radioactivity in the urine 12 hours after dosing. Four other metabolites are formed by stepwise oxidative cleavage of the β-blocker side chain. A metabolite with a hydroxylated phenyl ring was present in urine in two isomeric forms with their respective sulfated conjugates. In addition, o-demethylation produces a metabolite that retains pharmacologic activity, denoted by BM 14,242 in Figure 61–5, but this appears to be less than 1% of the carvedilol dose. Approximately 16% of the metabolites were cleared by the kidney, but 60% were cleared by a fecal route.

The plasma protein binding of ^{14}C carvedilol was determined *in vitro* by equilibrium dialysis.[12] At initial concentrations of carvedilol over a range of 50 to 1000 ng/ml, the binding ratio was independent of drug concentration. In human plasma, 95% was bound to protein. Comparable values were found in animal studies. These values are generally higher than those observed for other β-blockers and are consistent with the lipophilic nature of carvedilol.

The effects of eating on absorption and metabolism were investigated after oral administration of carvedilol (Table 61–3).[15] A 25-mg capsule was given orally 30 minutes before a standard breakfast and after an overnight fast. When given with food, a delay of

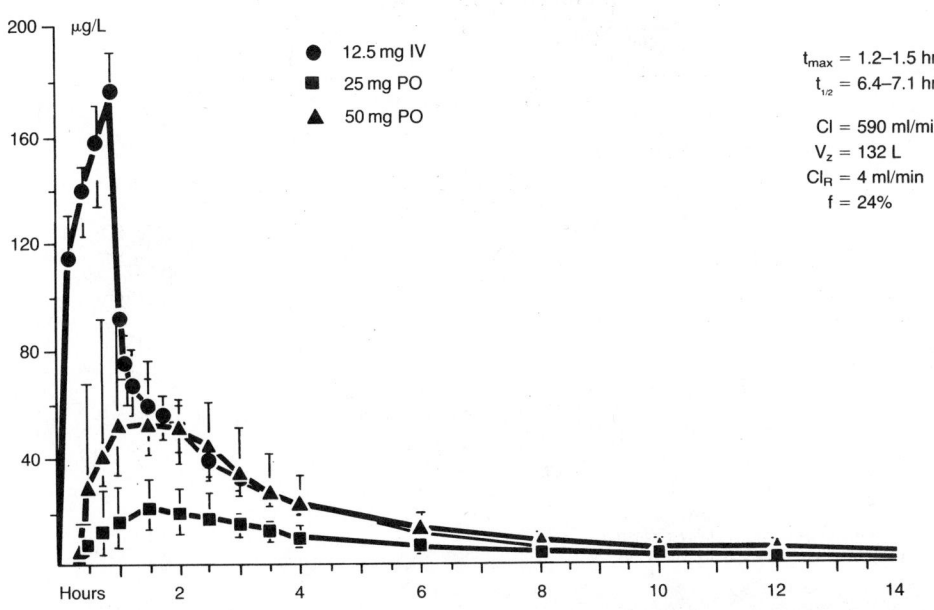

Figure 61–4. Concentration-time curves after intravenous and oral administration of carvedilol to normal human volunteers. (From Abshagen U: A new molecule with vasodilating and β-adrenoceptor blocking properties. J Cardiovasc Pharmacol 10[Suppl 11]:S23, 1987.)

Table 61–2. **Pharmacokinetic Parameters After Intravenous Infusion and Oral Administration of Carvedilol in Healthy Subjects (Median and Range)**

	AUC (ng/ml/hr)	MIRC[a] (µg/L/hr)	C_{max} (ng/ml)	T_{max} (hr)	$T_{1/2}$ (hr)	MRT[b] (ml/min)
12.5 mg IV (n = 20)	354 (246–556)	272 (104–430)	173 (109–234)	1.00 (0.67–1.00)	2.38 (1.95–4.17)	2.79 (2.16–4.76)
50 mg PO (n = 19)	348 (170–611)	194 (29–630)	66 (34–130)	1.20 (0.65–2.25)	6.35 (4.05–14.58)	7.23 (3.41–13.16)
25 mg PO (n = 18)	157 (64–374)	63 (7–873)	21 (5–99)	1.47 (0.68–3.10)	7.06 (1.97–20.93)	7.18 (2.93–26.21)

	MAT[c] (hr)	Cl[d] (ml/min)	V_z[e] (L)	F[f] (%)	Ae_{0-24hr}[g] (%)	Cl_R[h] (ml/min)
12.5 mg IV (n = 20)	—	589 (375–848)	132 (92–255)	—	—	—
50 mg PO (n = 19)	4.98 (1.62–11.50)	—	—	24 (12–46)	1[i]	4[i]
25 mg PO (n = 18)	4.76 (0.10–23.99)	—	—	22 (10–49)	—	—

[a]Mean initial rise in concentration.
[b]Mean residence time.
[c]Mean absorption time.
[d]Total clearance.
[e]Distribution volume.
[f]Absolute bioavailability.
[g]Amount excreted in urine.
[h]Renal clearance.
[i]Different study.
Adapted from Neugebauer G, Akpan W, Mollendorf EV, et al: Pharmacokinetics and disposition of carvedilol in humans. J Cardiovasc Pharmacol 10(Suppl 11):S85, 1987.

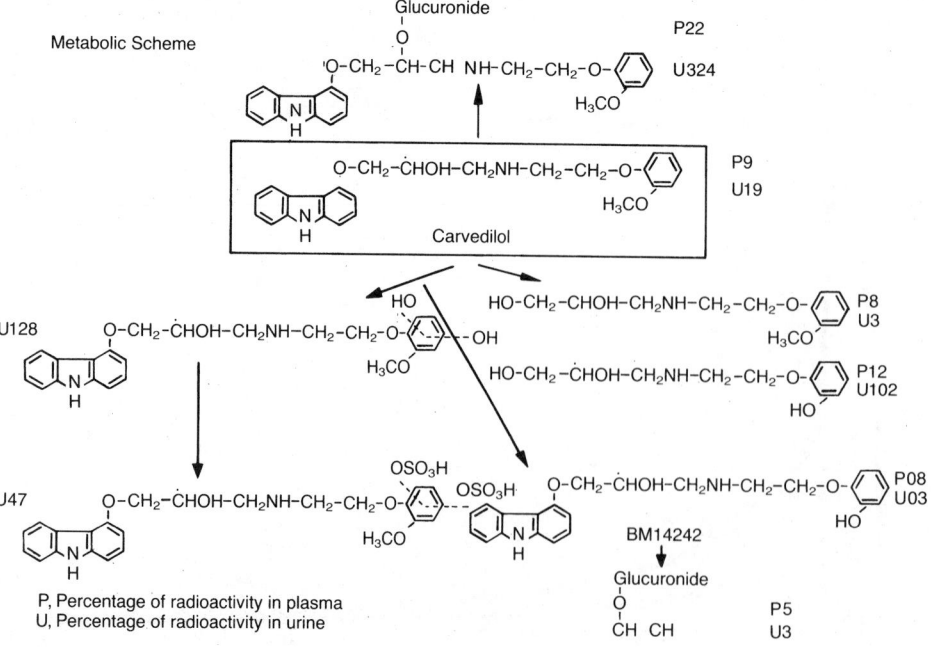

Figure 61–5. Metabolic scheme of carvedilol biotransformation in humans and the relative concentrations found in urine (U) and plasma (P). (From Neugebauer G, Akpan W, Mollendorf EV, et al: Pharmacokinetics and disposition of carvedilol in humans. J Cardiovasc Pharmacol 10[Suppl 11]:S85, 1987.)

Table 61–3. **Pharmacokinetic Parameters Derived from Plasma Carvedilol Data**

Dosage	C_{max} (ng/ml)	T_{max} (min)	AUC (ng/ml/hr)
25 mg	67 ± 13	58 ± 16	337 ± 140
50 mg	122 ± 22	58 + 12	717 ± 270
50 mg + food	128 ± 22	77 ± 16	741 ± 370
5 mg IV			184 ± 36

C_{max}, maximal concentration; T_{max}, maximal time; AUC, area under the curve.

From Louis WJ, McNeil JJ, Workman BS, et al: A pharmacokinetic study of carvedilol (BM 14,190) in elderly subjects: Preliminary report. J Cardiovasc Pharmacol 10(Suppl 11):S89, 1987.

absorption from 0.45 to 0.75 hour was observed. In addition, the peak serum concentrations obtained in fasting subjects was approximately twice that obtained in subjects who had ingested food. However, the area under the curve for the serum concentration was unaffected by the ingestion of food. The delay in absorption of carvedilol when it is administered with food and the lower serum concentrations attained may help control side effects and provide a more consistent therapeutic profile.

CLINICAL STUDIES
Hemodynamic Effects in Normal Volunteers

From the results of studies in animals, it appeared that carvedilol combined properties of β-blockade and vasodilation. Before large-scale studies could be undertaken, the hemodynamic effects produced in animal models had to be confirmed in humans. To this end, a number of small-scale trials were undertaken to investigate the hemodynamic effects of carvedilol in normal volunteers.[16] The first of these studies compared the effects of carvedilol with labetalol administered intravenously. In a single-blind, parallel design study of 24 volunteers, subjects were randomly assigned to one of three groups: saline, 15 mg of carvedilol, or 40 to 80 mg of labetalol. The effect of these treatments on the responses of blood pressure and heart rate to angiotensin II, isoproterenol, and phenylephrine were studied. Carvedilol reduced blood pressure from 138/64 to 105/50 mmHg at the end of the infusion. Heart rate did not change significantly, going from 54 to 59 beats/min. Labetalol reduced blood pressure from 135/68 to 120/58 mmHg and increased heart rate from 59 to 67 beats/min. Angiotensin II and phenylephrine produced mean increases of 20 to 25 mmHg in both systolic and diastolic pressures and a slowing of the heart rate by 10 beats/min for angiotensin II and 18 beats/min for phenylephrine. Isoproterenol had no effect on systolic pressure but reduced the diastolic pressure by 18 mmHg and increased the heart rate by 30 beats/min. Carvedilol antagonized the positive chronotropic effects and hypotensive effects of isoproterenol in addition to the pressor effects of phenylephrine. It failed to alter the effects of angiotensin II. These effects

suggest that carvedilol has properties of nonselective β-blockade and α₁-blockade. The effects also suggest that carvedilol does not have significant effects as a calcium antagonist in this dose range, at least during acute intravenous administration.

The vasodilatory and hemodynamic effects of carvedilol given orally have been investigated by several groups.[17–19] In one study, carvedilol was compared with propranolol, pindolol, and labetalol in a double-blind, placebo-controlled trial: Six healthy volunteers were given single doses of carvedilol from 12.5 to 200 mg, propranolol from 40 to 320 mg, pindolol from 2.5 to 20 mg, labetalol from 50 to 400 mg, and placebo. Heart rate and blood pressure were measured with subjects supine and standing and during exercise on a bicycle ergometer at 1 and 2 hours after drug administration. There was a dose-dependent reduction in heart rate during exercise that was greater for propranolol and pindolol than for carvedilol and labetalol. The exercise-induced rise in systolic pressure was also reduced, but the differences between the drugs in dose-response curves were less significant. Supine and standing heart rates were reduced by propranolol only, but supine systolic pressure was reduced by all four drugs. Standing blood pressure was reduced by carvedilol and pindolol (Figs. 61–6 to 61–8). The effects observed for these four drugs suggest that carvedilol has an effect on heart rate and blood pressure similar to that of labetalol and different from that of propranolol or pindolol. They support the conclusion that carvedilol acts as a combined vasodilator and β-blocker that is potentially useful in the treatment of hypertension and exercise-induced angina.

To further delineate the hemodynamic effects of carvedilol, a double-blind, crossover trial of carvedilol (50 mg), pindolol (10 mg), and propranolol (80 mg) given orally was conducted.[20] Thirteen healthy volunteers were given drug or placebo twice daily for 1 week and then received placebo for 1 week before

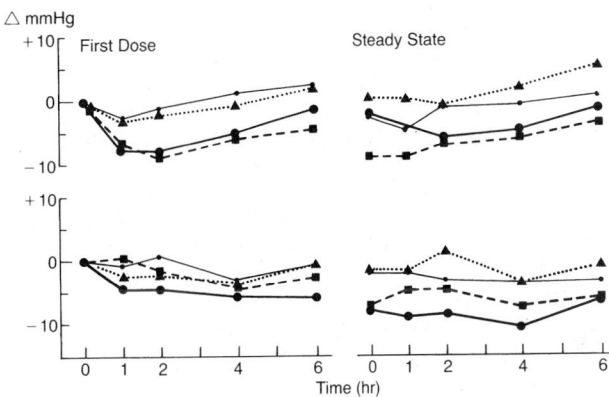

Figure 61–6. Changes in systolic and diastolic blood pressure after the first dose and at steady state. The changes are depicted as deviations from the mean basal value in mmHg. Placebo is shown in dots. Carvedilol is shown in solid circles. Pindolol is shown in triangles. Propranolol is shown in squares. (From Sundberg S, Tiihonen K, Gordin A: Vasodilatory effects of carvedilol and pindolol. J Cardiovasc Pharmacol 10[Suppl 11]:S81, 1987.)

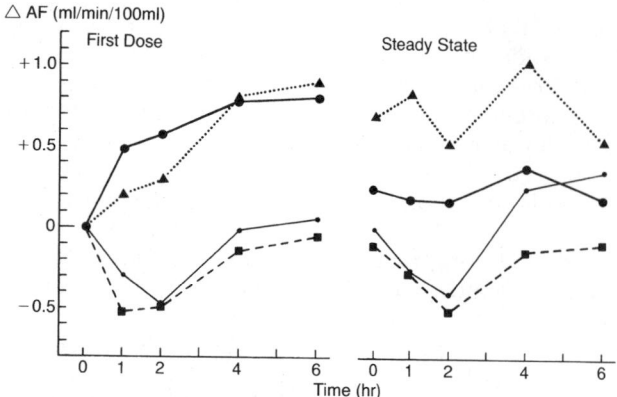

Figure 61–7. Changes in arterial calf blood flow (AF) after the first dose and at steady state. The changes are depicted as deviations from the mean basal value. Placebo is shown in dots. Carvedilol is shown in solid circles. Pindolol is shown in triangles. Propranolol is shown in squares. (From Sundberg S, Tiihonen K, Gordin A: Vasodilatory effects of carvedilol and pindolol. J Cardiovasc Pharmacol 10[Suppl 11]:S81, 1987.)

going on to the next drug in the study. Each subject received all four study drugs in this fashion. Heart rate, blood pressure, arterial calf blood flow, and pulmonary functions were measured on the first and last days of each drug treatment and placebo. Heart rate and blood pressure were lower when patients received carvedilol and propranolol than when they received pindolol or placebo. Both carvedilol and pindolol increased arterial blood flow by approximately 40% and reduced peripheral vascular resistance by approximately 35%. Both effects persisted after 1 week of treatment. None of the medications had a significant effect on pulmonary function. Carvedilol had a more significant hypotensive effect than pindolol or propranolol. These results support the conclusion that carvedilol has vasodilatory action that is not caused by intrinsic sympathomimetic activity, as with pindolol, and that it has nonselective β-blocking properties. By reducing peripheral resistance and preserving renal blood flow, these vasodilatory properties of carvedilol may provide additional beneficial effects compared with simple β-blockers for the treatment of hypertension.

Hemodynamic Effects in Hypertension

A number of studies have been undertaken to evaluate the effects of carvedilol on the hemodynamics of patients with essential hypertension, in which patients received various doses for periods of 1 week to several months. Some have studied the effects on peripheral vascular resistance, renal blood flow, and cardiac output; some have followed only blood pressure and heart rate.

In a 1-week study of carvedilol, 12 patients received carvedilol, 25 mg PO twice daily, in an open-label study.[21] Heart rate, blood pressure, plasma norepinephrine levels, and plasma renin levels were measured in patients at rest and during exercise after acute and repeated administration for 1 week after a

1-week placebo phase. During the placebo phase, the average supine blood pressure was 178/107 mmHg. One hour after the first dose, blood pressure was 162/99 mmHg. On the seventh day of treatment, again 1 hour after drug administration, blood pressure showed a further decline to 158/96 mmHg. Blood pressure measured during exercise on a bicycle ergometer rose significantly 1 hour after the first dose but showed little effect 12 hours after the dose. On the seventh day of treatment, the systolic pressure rise during exercise was significantly reduced at both 1 and 12 hours. The rise in heart rate during exercise was not significantly altered either 1 or 12 hours after the first dose, but the rise was significantly blunted at both 1 and 12 hours after 1 week of treatment. The rise in plasma norepinephrine during exercise was enhanced by treatment with carvedilol after 1 and 12 hours equally on the first and seventh days of treatment. Plasma renin level was lowered by treatment with carvedilol, and the rise during exercise was blunted as well. This effect appeared to be more pronounced after 1 week of therapy. The effects of carvedilol on hypertensive patients in this study suggest vasodilation and β-blockade. They also suggest that the β-blockade effectively blunts any reflex tachycardia that would be induced by the vasodilation. The effects on heart rate during exercise should make carvedilol effective in the treatment of exercise-induced angina, but these effects may be induced only after chronic treatment.

In another open study of oral carvedilol,[22] 24-hour blood pressure was measured intraarterially, along with left ventricular ejection fraction and the response of blood pressure and heart rate to exercise. Twelve patients with essential hypertension received 25 mg of carvedilol twice a day for 2 weeks and, if the target blood pressure was not achieved, 50 mg of carvedilol for another 2 weeks. At the conclusion of the study, blood pressure was reduced by 25/19 mmHg. Heart rate was reduced by 22 beats/min. Left ventricular

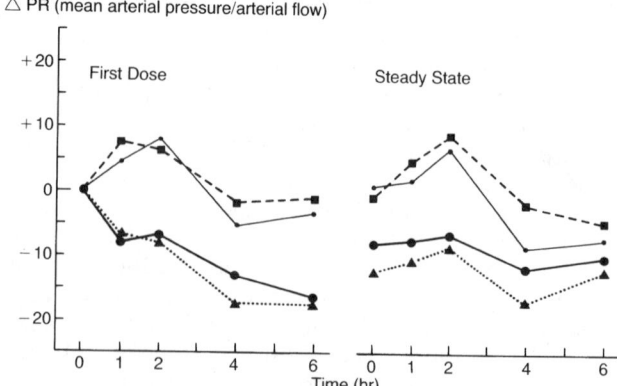

Figure 61–8. Changes in calculated peripheral resistance (PR) after the first dose and at steady state. The changes are depicted as deviations from the mean basal value in mmHg. Placebo is shown in dots. Carvedilol is shown in solid circles. Pindolol is shown in triangles. Propranolol is shown in squares. (From Sundberg S, Tiihonen K, Gordin A: Vasodilatory effects of carvedilol and pindolol. Cardiovasc Pharmacol 10[Suppl 11]:S81, 1987.)

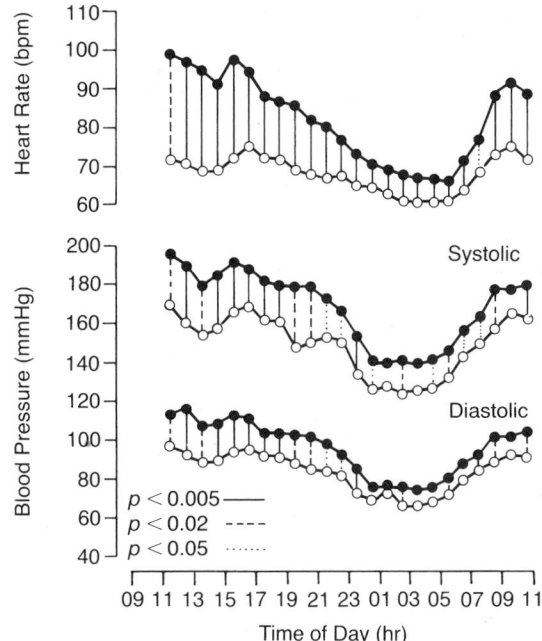

Figure 61–9. Circadian variation of blood pressure and heart rate. Dots are pretreatment values, and circles are values after 4 weeks of treatment with carvedilol. (From Heber ME, Brigden GS, Caruana MP, et al: Carvedilol for systemic hypertension. J Cardiovasc Pharmacol 10[Suppl 11]:S113, 1987.)

In a randomized, double-blind, placebo-controlled study,[24] the effects of carvedilol were assessed over a period of 4 weeks of treatment of 20 patients with essential hypertension (Tables 61–4 and 61–5). Carvedilol was given orally in a single daily dose of 50 mg. Effective renal plasma flow, glomerular filtration rate, plasma renin levels, plasma aldosterone levels, and left ventricular ejection fraction were measured, as well as blood pressure and heart rate. As observed by others, blood pressure and heart rate decreased after treatment. Renal vascular resistance decreased modestly, but renal blood flow, glomerular filtration rate, plasma renin levels, plasma aldosterone levels, and ventricular ejection fraction remained unchanged by treatment. A variety of studies have established that treatment of hypertension with β-blockers results in a decrease in renal blood flow and glomerular filtration rate.[25, 26] In contrast, as this study demonstrates, carvedilol preserves renal blood flow and glomerular filtration rate, just as the combined αβ-blocker labetalol does.[27, 28] The results suggest that carvedilol would have some advantages over standard β-blockers in the treatment of hypertension, especially in patients with compromised renal function.

The effects of chronic treatment on patients with essential hypertension have been investigated in a double-blind study of 33 patients.[29] In this study, 33 patients were given placebo for 4 weeks and then were randomized to carvedilol, 50 mg/day, or metoprolol, 100 mg twice daily. Blood pressure and heart rate, both supine and standing, and forearm blood flow by venous plethysmography were measured throughout the study just prior to the next dose. After the first dose, carvedilol produced a fall in blood pressure from 168/98 to 155/93 mmHg, and metoprolol produced a fall from 171/98 to 155/90 mmHg. Heart rate changed from 68 to 76 in patients receiving carvedilol, and from 73 to 82 in patients receiving metoprolol. After 4 weeks of treatment, carvedilol produced a further fall in blood pressure to 147/85 mmHg, with a heart rate of 57, and metropolol produced a fall to 153/85 mmHg, with a heart rate of 60. Chronic treatment with either carvedilol or metoprolol produced no significant effects on forearm resis-

ejection fraction was unchanged by treatment at rest and during exercise, but radionuclide scintigraphy did show a reduction in systolic and diastolic volumes after treatment. The early morning increase in blood pressure that has been shown to be present despite treatment with β-blockers and has been abolished with combined αβ-blockers was blunted by carvedilol (Fig. 61–9). This study suggests that carvedilol may work in part as a combined αβ-blocker that may be beneficial, without precipitating heart failure, in the treatment of hypertensive patients with decreased ejection fractions. It might also find a place in the treatment of angina by blocking the morning surge in catecholamines that has been hypothesized to account for the increased incidence of myocardial infarction in the morning hours.[23]

Table 61–4. **Acute Effect of Carvedilol (n = 10) or Placebo (n = 10) on Renal Hemodynamics, PRA, and Plasma Aldosterone**

Parameters	Carvedilol Group		Placebo Group	
	Before	*After 2 hr*	*Before*	*After 2 hr*
Mean BP (mmHg)	126.0 ± 2.7	105.4 ± 5.0*	126.6 ± 2.4	127.1 ± 2.0
RBF (ml/min/1.73 m²)	670.6 ± 30.8	681.4 ± 42.0	586.2 ± 51.1	585.9 ± 55.2
PVR (mmHg/ml/min/1.73 m²)	0.202 ± 0.015	0.162 ± 0.014*	0.235 ± 0.026	0.238 ± 0.026
GFR (ml/min/1.73 m²)	114.7 ± 4.8	105.8 ± 4.7*	107.0 ± 4.0	104.0 ± 5.5
FF (%)	31.1 ± 1.4	28.1 ± 1.9*	35.0 ± 2.5	33.7 ± 2.0
PRA (ng/ml/hr)	2.67 ± 0.70	2.07 ± 0.60	1.40 ± 0.30	1.40 ± 0.30
Plasma aldosterone (ng/l)	128.4 ± 8.2	115.6 ± 12.2	141.1 ± 23.3	130.4 ± 12.6

RBF, renal blood flow; RVR, renal vascular resistance; GFR, glomerular filtration rate; FF, filtration fraction; PRA, plasma renin activity.
Mean ± SEM.
*$p < .01$ from baseline.
From Dupont AG, Van der Niepen P, Taeymans Y, et al: Effect of carvedilol on ambulatory blood pressure, renal hemodynamics, and cardiac function in essential hypertension. J Cardiovasc Pharmacol 10(Suppl 11):S130, 1987.

Table 61–5. **Response of Renal Hemodynamics and the Other Measured Parameters to Chronic Treatment with Carvedilol (n = 10) or Placebo (n = 10)**

Parameters	Carvedilol Group		Placebo Group	
	Week 0	Week 4	Week 0	Week 4
Mean BP (mmHg)	126.0 ± 2.7	111.5 ± 4.2*	126.6 ± 2.4	126.7 ± 2.4
RBF (ml/min/1.73 m²)	670.6 ± 30.8	660.7 ± 37.9	586.2 ± 51.1	627.1 ± 54.7
RVR (mmHg/ml/min/1.73 m²)	0.202 ± 0.015	0.176 ± 0.015†	0.235 ± 0.026	0.218 ± 0.022
GFR (ml/min/1.73 m²)	114.7 ± 4.8	120.8 ± 4.2	107.0 ± 4.0	109.1 ± 4.2
FF (%)	31.1 ± 1.4	33.1 ± 0.9	35.0 ± 2.5	33.3 ± 2.2
Body weight (kg)	82.1 ± 2.9	82.2 ± 2.7	81.0 ± 3.6	81.4 ± 3.6
Urinary sodium excretion (mEq/24 hr)	127 ± 16	141 ± 23	134 ± 24	129 ± 23
PRA (ng/ml/hr)	2.67 ± 0.70	1.65 ± 0.28†	1.40 ± 0.30	1.70 ± 0.40
Plasma aldosterone (ng/L)	128.4 ± 82	104.2 ± 7.2†	141.1 ± 23.3	152.4 ± 62.1
LVEF (%)	54.7 ± 2.8	51.8 ± 2.0	60.2 ± 3.3	53.0 ± 4.6
CO (counts/ml/1.73 m²)	3696 ± 266	2952 ± 197*	3444 ± 235	3453 ± 237

RBF, renal blood flow; RVR, renal vascular resistance; GFR, glomerular filtration rate; FF, filtration fraction; PRA, plasma renin activity; LVEF, left ventricular ejection fraction; CO, cardiac output.
Mean ± SEM.
*$p < .01$.
†$p < .05$ from baseline.
From Dupont AG, Van der Niepen P, Taeymans Y, et al: Effect of carvedilol on ambulatory blood pressure, renal hemodynamics, and cardiac function in essential hypertension. J Cardiovasc Pharmacol 10(Suppl 11):S130, 1987.

tance or peripheral resistance. Peak effects of the drugs were measured with 25 mg of carvedilol and 100 mg of metoprolol. Carvedilol caused a more marked effect on blood pressure than metoprolol in this part of the study and also showed more marked orthostatic effects; two patients became symptomatic, and one withdrew from the study. The authors concluded that carvedilol was effective as an antihypertensive agent that preserved peripheral blood flow without an increase in peripheral resistance. They cautioned that the drug would probably be better tolerated if given twice daily, perhaps in a sustained release formulation to avoid orthostatic effects.

A more invasive study of the acute and chronic effects of carvedilol was carried out in 30 patients with essential hypertension during a 4-week treatment phase.[30] In this study, patients received 25 mg of carvedilol twice daily, 50 mg of carvedilol twice daily, or 80 mg of propranolol twice daily. Blood pressure, heart rate, and forearm plethysmography were followed during the study with invasive measurements of cardiac output and peripheral resistance after the 4-week placebo phase and the first dose of 25 mg of carvedilol. After the first dose of carvedilol, a significant drop in blood pressure from 156/84 to 148/81 mmHg and no significant change in heart rate were recorded. Forearm resistance fell after administration of carvedilol, from 39 to 33 units, with insignificant changes in peripheral resistance, peripheral blood flow, and cardiac output. After 4 weeks of treatment, all regimens yielded decreased blood pressure and heart rate without significant changes in peripheral resistance. However, peripheral blood flow was unchanged with carvedilol but fell with propranolol. Ninety minutes after administration of a 50-mg dose of carvedilol, a further decrease in blood pressure and peripheral resistance was seen. Unfortunately, the effects of propranolol were not similarly measured. This study suggests that the vasodilatory

effect of carvedilol prevents the rise in peripheral resistance that occurs with pure β-blockers.[31] Both acute and chronic hypotensive effects were demonstrated with carvedilol and propranolol, and it may be that the hemodynamic effects of carvedilol will be advantageous in the treatment of hypertension when peripheral resistance is found to be elevated.[32]

The effects of carvedilol on the circadian blood pressure have been studied by several groups in patients with essential hypertension. In both open trials[33] and double-blind trials,[34] the blood pressure of patients with essential hypertension was reduced throughout a 24-hour period with either once- or twice-daily dosing. The physiologic circadian rhythm of blood pressure that has been observed in normal volunteers and hypertensive patients was preserved. These studies suggest that carvedilol may be effective as a once-daily treatment for hypertension if side effects of higher doses are not prohibitive.

Long-term Trials in Hypertension

At present, only one long-term trial of carvedilol has been published.[35] This trial was an open trial of carvedilol, 25 mg twice daily over a period of 1 year. Patients underwent a 2-week washout phase followed by a 2-week placebo phase before entering the treatment phase. Blood pressure was measured every 4 weeks while the patients were sitting and standing 2 hours after the dose was given. Of the 154 patients who were screened, 86 completed the entire study. The median blood pressure (standing) before the drug was administered in the morning was decreased from 165/105 to 145/88 mmHg. When patients were seated, median blood pressure decreased from 170/105 to 145/90 mmHg. There was a significant change in these blood pressure recordings from the first week of active treatment to the completion of the study, but its magnitude was small. No changes were found in body weight or serum levels of total, high-density lipoprotein, or low-density lipoprotein cholesterol during the study. Eight patients were withdrawn from the study because of side effects. Three patients had to be withdrawn because of unacceptable decreases in blood pressure. Most side effects observed were characteristic of β-blockers (e.g., lethargy, headache, and slow heart rate). Two patients had myocardial infarction, one patient had a subdural hematoma, and one patient had a perforated ulcer. None of the serious events were attributed to the treatment with carvedilol. From this study, carvedilol appears to be both safe and effective for the long-term treatment of hypertension.

Effect on Exercise-Induced Angina

In a single-blind, randomized, placebo-controlled, crossover study,[36] 15 patients were given a single dose of carvedilol, 25 mg. The effects of the drug treatment on treadmill exercise were compared with those of the placebo control. Patients with stable exercise-induced angina were selected from a population of patients who had undergone coronary angiography and coronary angioplasty. Two control exercise tests were done at the beginning and at the end of the second week with patients receiving no therapy. Patients were then randomized to receive either carvedilol or placebo. After receiving the coded drug, patients remained semisupine while blood pressure and heart rate were monitored every 10 minutes. After 90 minutes, the patients underwent treadmill exercise testing on a standard Bruce protocol. All patients had ST-segment depression of more than 1 mm and chest pain during control and placebo testing. Heart rate and blood pressure before exercise were significantly more reduced by carvedilol than by the placebo. Heart rate and blood pressure were also decreased at peak exercise more by carvedilol than by the placebo. Exercise duration and time to 1-mm ST-segment depression were prolonged more by carvedilol than by the placebo. However, heart rate at 1-mm ST-segment depression was not changed by treatment with carvedilol compared with placebo. The results are shown in Table 61–6. The authors concluded that these results suggest that carvedilol is effective in preventing exercise-induced angina and improving both exercise-related ischemia and exercise tolerance in patients with stable exertional angina. The authors also suggest that the mechanism includes both systemic and coronary vasodilation, although this is not substantiated by their results. The mechanism of carvedilol's effect appears to be primarily β-blockade, and the arguments for coronary vasodilation are weak. This study supports the conclusion that carvedilol is an effective treatment for stable exertional angina and exerts its effect primarily through β-blockade.

There is only one published study of carvedilol in exercise-induced angina in which patients received more than a single dose.[37] In this single-blind, placebo-controlled study, 20 patients were treated for 2-week periods with placebo, carvedilol (25 mg twice daily), carvedilol (50 mg twice daily), and then placebo. Treadmill exercise testing was carried out at the end of each 2-week phase. The authors found that the time to 1-mm ST-segment depression during exercise testing for both carvedilol doses was significantly longer than for the first placebo phase, but this was true only for the 50-mg dose of carvedilol when compared with the second placebo phase. These results are consistent with the single-dose studies of carvedilol's effect on exercise-induced angina and suggest that it is an effective treatment at the 50-mg dose level. The extension of this study to include radionuclide left ventriculography showed an increase in the resting ejection fraction, peak filling rate, and ejection rate with the 50-mg dose (Fig. 61–10).[38] Significant decreases in diastolic and systolic volumes were found for both the 25-mg and 50-mg doses (Fig. 61–11). The ejection fraction at peak exercise was not significantly different for either dose of carvedilol compared with placebo. The authors suggest that the beneficial effects of carvedilol on the ejection fraction at rest might confer advantages in the long-term treatment of patients with angina. Indeed, it might have advantages for patients with exercise-induced angina

Table 61–6. **Exercise Testing**

	1-mm ST Depression				Peak Exercise				
	Time (min)	HR (beats/min)	BP (mmHg)	HR-BP Product (10^{-3})	Time (min)	HR (beats/min)	BP (mmHg)	HR-BP Product (10^{-3})	ST ↓ (mm)
Control 1	7.8	112	167	18	10.5	127	176	22	−1.9
(SD)	(± 4)	(± 16)	(± 26)	(± 4)	(± 4)	(± 24)	(± 32)	(± 6)	(± 0.7)
Control 2	9.5	110	166	18	12.0	131	176	23	−1.8
(SD)	(± 4)	(± 15)	(± 17)	(± 3)	(± 4)	(± 21)	(± 28)	(± 5)	(± 0.6)
Placebo	9.5	114	162	18	11.7	129	167	22	−1.7
(SD)	(± 3)	(± 14)	(± 23)	(± 3)	(± 4)	(± 22)	(± 25)	(± 5)	(± 0.6)
Carvedilol	11.7	116	150	17	12.8	122	155	19	−1.2
(SD)	(± 4)	(± 15)	(± 16)	(± 4)	(± 4)	(± 19)	(± 15)	(± 4)	(± 0.7)
p (carvedilol vs. placebo)	< .01	= .9	< .05	= .05	< .05	= .1	< .05	< .05	< .01

BP, systolic blood pressure; HR, heart rate; SD, standard deviation.
From Kaski JC, Rodrigues-Plaza L, Brown J, et al: Efficacy of carvedilol in exercise-induced myocardial ischemia. J Cardiovasc Pharmacol 10(Suppl 11):S137, 1987.

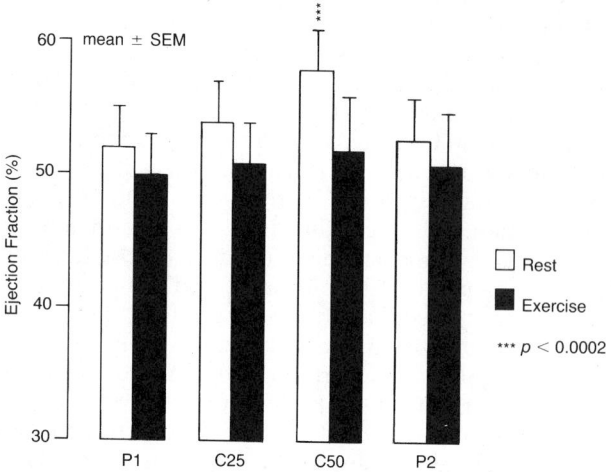

Figure 61–10. Rest and exercise ejection fraction values in patients receiving placebo or carvedilol. C25 and C50 are carvedilol, 25 mg and 50 mg twice daily. P1 and P2 are placebo 1 and 2. SEM is standard error of the mean. (From Lahiri A, Rodriguez EA, Al-Khawaja I, et al: Effects of a new vasodilating beta-blocking drug, carvedilol, on left ventricular function in stable angina pectoris. Am J Cardiol 59:769, 1987.)

and depressed ventricular function. Further studies must be done to substantiate the hemodynamic effects and to evaluate carvedilol's effect in patients with decreased ventricular function.

In another randomized, double-blind, placebo-controlled, crossover trial[39] of exercise-induced angina, 12 patients were given two single doses of 25 mg and 50 mg of carvedilol to determine the dose response of carvedilol in effort-related angina. Patients were selected from a population with documented angina and ST-segment depression on exercise testing. The patients were withdrawn from antianginal medications for at least 5 days before entering the random-

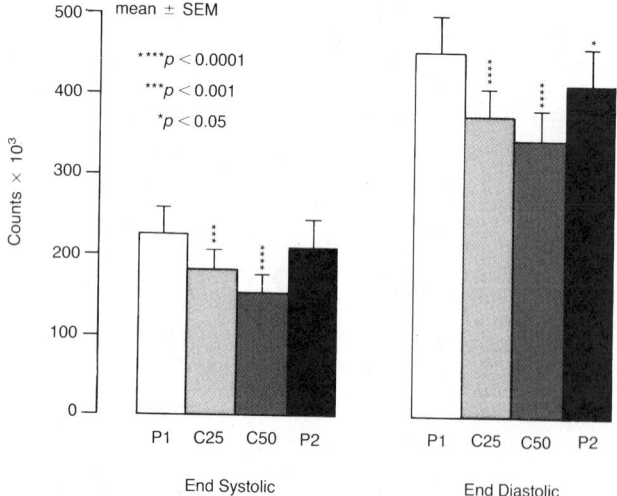

Figure 61–11. Relative left ventricular volumes are represented by end-systolic and end-diastolic counts. C25 and C50 are carvedilol, 25 mg and 50 mg twice daily. P1 and P2 are placebo 1 and 2. SEM is standard error of the mean. (From Lahiri A, Rodriguez EA, Al-Khawaja I, et al: Effects of a new vasodilating beta-blocking drug, carvedilol, on left ventricular function in stable angina pectoris. Am J Cardiol 59:769, 1987.)

ized phase. Baseline exercise testing and treatment testing were done according to a modified Naughton protocol 2 hours after receiving either drug or placebo. Carvedilol increased the time to 1-mm ST-segment depression and the exercise time in a dose-dependent fashion. The heart rate at 1-mm ST-segment depression was unchanged, whereas the blood pressure at 1-mm ST-segment depression was reduced by carvedilol. Using analysis of variance, the authors pointed out that in most instances the improvements in exercise performance and ischemia after the 25-mg dose of carvedilol did not reach statistical significance, and this may represent a type II error. They speculated on the mechanism of carvedilol's role in the treatment of angina and whether the vasodilatory properties would be beneficial. The study supports the role of carvedilol as effective treatment for exercise-induced angina at the 50-mg dose but does not shed any light on the possible benefits of its vasodilatory effects.

In the extension of this study, atenolol[40] was included to provide a comparison with a pure β-blocker. Such a comparison may allow inferences about the vasodilatory action of carvedilol. In this study, 12 patients were given single doses of placebo, 25 mg of carvedilol, 50 mg of carvedilol, and 50 mg of atenolol after a placebo control period. Maximal exercise time and time to 1-mm ST-segment depression were increased more by atenolol than by carvedilol. Heart rates at 1-mm ST-segment depression and at maximal exercise were not significantly changed by either carvedilol or atenolol. The double product of heart rate and blood pressure at 1-mm ST-segment depression was decreased for 50 mg of carvedilol but not for atenolol. These results suggest that the major effect of carvedilol on exercise-induced angina is produced by its β-blocking properties and that at a dose of 50 mg carvedilol is not as effective a β-blocker as 50 mg of atenolol. In addition, the results suggest that the vasodilatory effect of carvedilol occurs predominantly in the peripheral vasculature rather than in the coronary vasculature. Conceivably, however, some patients in whom exercise-induced angina is related to an increased oxygen demand because of an exaggerated rise in blood pressure during exercise probably would benefit more from carvedilol than from a pure β-blocker. In patients in whom exercise-induced angina is related to the increase in myocardial oxygen demand and decreased coronary perfusion, carvedilol appears to be less beneficial than a pure β-blocker.

Side Effect Profile

The side effect profile has been established from studies conducted in Europe and supervised by Boehringer Mannheim Pharmaceutical Corporation.[6] The data include all patients who have received the drug in acute and chronic studies, totaling more than 900 subjects. The side effect profile that is emerging is very similar to that of other β-blockers. Most of them are not serious side effects (e.g., headache, dizziness, tiredness, and weakness) (Fig. 61–12). Of the adverse events listed, only orthostatic hypotension should be

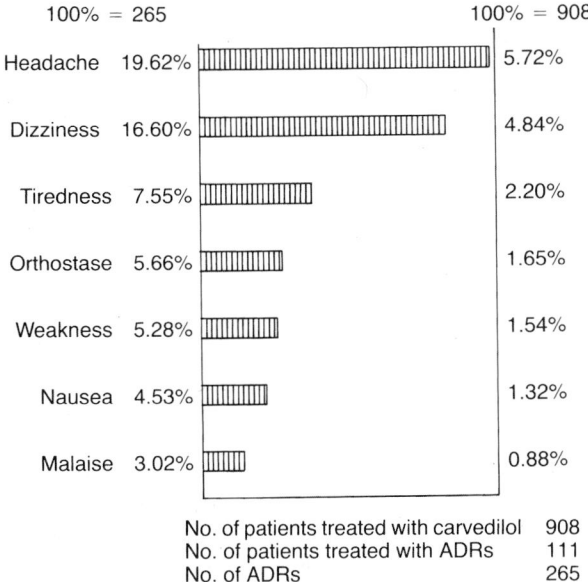

	100% = 265	100% = 908
Headache	19.62%	5.72%
Dizziness	16.60%	4.84%
Tiredness	7.55%	2.20%
Orthostase	5.66%	1.65%
Weakness	5.28%	1.54%
Nausea	4.53%	1.32%
Malaise	3.02%	0.88%

No. of patients treated with carvedilol 908
No. of patients treated with ADRs 111
No. of ADRs 265

Figure 61–12. Adverse drug reactions (ADRs) during treatment with carvedilol. (From Abshagen U: A new molecule with vasodilating and β-adrenoceptor blocking properties. J Cardiovasc Pharmacol 10[Suppl 11]:S23, 1987.)

considered serious. The incidence of 1.65% is higher than that reported for other β-blockers but is comparable with that reported for prazosin.

Other serious adverse events that have been reported to the FDA that occurred during clinical trials in Europe and the United States include

1. Three episodes of thrombocytopenia that all were reversible and were not clearly caused by the drug.
2. Two episodes of urticaria without hypotension or vascular collapse, one of which required treatment with antihistamines and steroids.
3. One episode of complete heart block and asystole that occurred during intravenous administration and resolved spontaneously.
4. One cerebrovascular accident not thought to be related to the drug.
5. One myocardial infarction possibly related to drug treatment.
6. One subdural hematoma not thought to be related to the drug.

All these events have been reported with other β-blockers as well and have acceptably low incidence. They may simply represent the natural incidence of these events in the population receiving the drug, because no control group was used for comparison.

The only real concern with carvedilol appears to be orthostatic hypotension, which may have been potentiated by several factors:

1. Taking the drug on an empty stomach, which produces more rapid absorption and a higher serum level than taking it with food.
2. Giving it to patients who have been volume depleted by the concomitant use of diuretics.

3. High intrasubject variability in bioavailability, which produces high serum levels in patients started on high doses of the drug without having received lower doses first.

These factors can be controlled to prevent orthostatic hypotension and further reduce its already low incidence. Current experience with carvedilol promises that it will have an acceptable safety profile and will be well tolerated.

Treatment of Congestive Heart Failure

Chronic β-blockade may improve hemodynamic and clinical function in patients with heart failure.[41–47] Several factors may contribute to the observed improvement with β-blocker therapy, including protection from the cardiotoxic effects of increased catecholamines,[48] upregulation of myocardial β$_1$-adrenergic receptors (which would improve myocardial responsiveness to β-agonist stimulation during times of stress[49]), improved myocardial energetics, favorable alterations of coronary blood flow, improved ventricular diastolic function, and perhaps peripheral effects, such as reduced renin release.[50]

The initiation of β-blocker therapy in patients with heart failure is difficult because of the hemodynamic deterioration that may accompany acute administration of these agents. This problem can be reduced by beginning therapy with very low doses. Some investigators have advocated the use of β$_1$-selective antagonists.[41] They argue that β$_1$-selective β-blockers should be better tolerated than nonselective β-blockers because peripheral β$_2$-adrenergic receptor blockade increases vasoconstriction. A theoretical limitation of the use of β$_1$-selective antagonists in heart failure is the fact that β$_2$-adrenergic receptors constitute up to 40% of the total myocardial β-receptor population in the failing human heart.[51] It follows that nonselective or mildly selective β-blocking agents might provide greater clinical benefits because of greater protection from the cardiotoxic effects of catecholamines. The tolerability of nonselective β-blocking agents in heart failure could be improved by the addition of vasodilatory properties. Based on this reasoning, carvedilol might be an ideal β-blocker for the therapy of heart failure, because it should give maximum cardioprotection yet still possess a favorable tolerability as a result of its α-blocking (vasodilatory) properties.

The acute hemodynamic effects of carvedilol and the β$_1$-selective antagonist metoprolol were compared in a single-blind randomized trial.[52] Fifty-five subjects with symptomatic heart failure and a left ventricular ejection fraction of less than 0.35 entered the study. Both drugs were given orally at a dose of 6.25 mg every 12 hours (only one fourth to one half of normal starting doses for hypertension). The results are summarized in Table 61–7. There was a similar decrease in heart rate in both treatment groups, suggesting a similar degree of β-blockade from carvedilol and placebo. Compared with metoprolol, carvedilol ad-

Table 61–7. **Acute Hemodynamic Effects of Carvedilol and Metoprolol in Subjects with Heart Failure (Mean ± SEM)**

	Carvedilol (n = 30)		Metoprolol (n = 25)	
	Baseline	*Therapy**	*Baseline*	*Therapy**
Heart rate (beats/min)	85 ± 3	83 ± 3	84 ± 2	81 ± 3†
Mean right atrial pressure (mmHg)	6 ± 1	6 ± 1	6 ± 1	6 ± 1
Mean systemic artery pressure (mmHg)	87 ± 2	83 ± 2†	86 ± 2	86 ± 2
Mean pulmonary artery pressure (mmHg)	28 ± 2	26 ± 2†‡	29 ± 2	29 ± 2
Mean pulmonary wedge pressure (mmHg)	17 ± 2	15 ± 1‡	17 ± 2	17 ± 2
Cardiac index (L/min/m²)	2.2 ± 0.1	2.2 ± 0.1	2.5 ± 0.1	2.5 ± 0.1
Systemic vascular resistance (Wood units)	20 ± 1	19 ± 1	17 ± 1	17 ± 1

*Average hemodynamic measurements 2 and 4 hours after oral intake of 6.25 mg of study medication.
†$p < .05$ versus baseline.
‡$p < .05$ for Δ carvedilol versus Δ metoprolol.

ministration was associated with statistically significant decreases in pulmonary artery pressure and pulmonary wedge pressure as well as trends to decrease systemic artery pressure (significant by within group analysis) and systemic vascular resistance. Thus, even at very low doses, carvedilol exhibits vasodilatory properties not observed with metoprolol. These effects would be expected to be beneficial in patients with heart failure, but it must be remembered that acute hemodynamic responses do not predict long-term efficacy of drugs used to treat heart failure.

The results of three placebo-controlled, randomized studies of carvedilol therapy in patients with heart failure were recently presented.[53–55] Subjects were required to have symptomatic heart failure secondary to either idiopathic dilated cardiomyopathy or postinfarction cardiomyopathy and a left ventricular ejection fraction of 35% or less for entry into any of these studies. Target carvedilol dose was 25 to 50 mg b.i.d. Compared with the placebo group, subjects receiving carvedilol experienced improvement in symptoms assessed by the physician (New York Heart Association functional class) or by the patient (assessed with a self-administered symptom questionnaire). In addition, significant improvements were observed in cardiac function in all three studies. The results reported by Olsen et al.[53] are summarized in Table 61–8. Similar findings were also reported by Krum et al.[54] and Metra et al.[55] Compared with pla-

cebo, carvedilol therapy was associated with significant reductions in heart rate and pulmonary wedge pressure and marked increases in stroke volume, left ventricular stroke work, and left ventricular ejection fraction. Cardiac output did not change significantly, probably because of the reduction in resting heart rate. These dramatic improvements in symptoms and left ventricular function appear to be sustained.[56] In addition, subjects treated with carvedilol appear to have an excellent prognosis. For example, the 3-year actuarial survival of 57 subjects completing the randomized study at Utah and treated with open-label carvedilol was 92% (Fig. 61–13).[56]

These clinical studies provided an opportunity to assess the effects of chronic carvedilol administration on adrenergic nervous system activation in heart failure. The Utah group compared the effects of carvedilol and metoprolol on myocardial β-receptor density during the course of placebo-controlled trials of these drugs.[57] Left ventricular ejection fraction significantly increased with both metoprolol and carvedilol ther-

Table 61–8. **Effects of Chronic Carvedilol Therapy in Subjects with Heart Failure—The Utah Experience (Percentage Change from Baseline Given as Mean ± SEM)**

	Carvedilol (n = 34)	Placebo (n = 23)
Heart rate (beats/min)	−22.4 ± 2.0*	1.4 ± 2.4
Mean pulmonary wedge pressure (mmHg)	−10.2 ± 9.2†	26.4 ± 17.6
Cardiac index (L/min/m²)	14.2 ± 4.1	4.1 ± 4.9
Stroke volume index (ml/beat/m²)	53.3 ± 9.2*	4.9 ± 7.8
LV stroke work index (g–m/m²)	63.5 ± 11.6*	−2.1 ± 9.4
LV ejection fraction (%)	52.8 ± 7.5*	0.7 ± 5.5

*$p < .001$ for Δ carvedilol versus Δ placebo.
†$p < .05$ for Δ carvedilol versus Δ placebo.
LV, left ventricular.

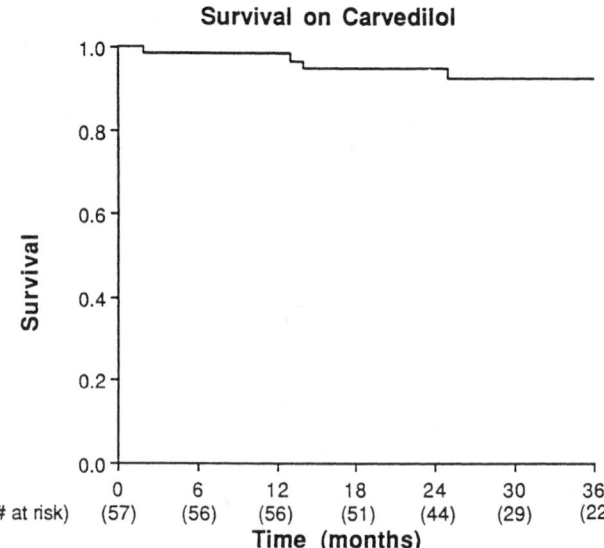

Figure 61–13. Actuarial survival of 57 subjects treated with open-label carvedilol. All subjects had symptomatic heart failure and left ventricular ejection fraction of 35% or less. The number of subjects at risk with respect to time on carvedilol therapy is given in parenthesis.

apy, but not with either drug's placebo control. Myocardial β-receptor density increased 46% with metoprolol therapy but not with carvedilol therapy or therapy with either placebo group (Fig. 61–14). Why was β-receptor upregulation not observed with carvedilol therapy? Carvedilol possesses the property of guanine nucleotide modulated binding, and, unlike metoprolol, incubation with carvedilol results in downregulation of β-receptors in cultured chick cells (personal communication, M. R. Bristow). This property would be expected to cause downregulation of myocardial β-receptors in patients treated with carvedilol. However, carvedilol therapy is also associated with a decrease in coronary sinus norepinephrine concentration,[58] a marker of cardiac sympathetic activation. Presumably, the withdrawal of an endogenous signal for downregulation (decreased myocardial norepinephrine exposure) balanced the addition of an exogenous signal for downregulation (carvedilol exposure). These data suggest that improvement in resting left ventricular function with β-blockade can occur in the absence of β-receptor upregulation.

Parasympathetic activity is decreased in patients with heart failure, resulting in a reduction in baroreceptor responsiveness. The effects of carvedilol on parasympathetic activity have been studied by the technique of heart rate variability analysis. Carvedilol therapy compared with placebo increases heart rate variability in patients with heart failure and thus shifts parasympathetic activity toward normal levels.[59, 60]

The efficacy of carvedilol is being further evaluated in three major multicenter trials: The Australia/New Zealand trial of carvedilol in ischemic cardiomyopathy[61] has randomized 415 patients with stable heart failure of ischemic etiology to receive carvedilol or placebo. After 6 months, left ventricular ejection fraction did increase by 5.2% (2 $p <.0001$), and left ventricular dimensions were reduced in the carvedilol group compared with the placebo group. Exercise performance was maintained at a lower rate pressure product, but symptoms assessed by functional classes were slightly worsened.

In the PRECISE trial,[62] carvedilol therapy was associated with improvements in left ventricular ejection fraction (Δ LVEF = 0.07 for carvedilol, Δ LVEF = 0.02 for placebo; $p = .0001$), NYHA functional class, and in both the patient's and the physician's global assessment of the patient's well-being. Fifteen percent of placebo patients, but only 3% of carvedilol patients, experienced worsening symptoms of heart failure. In addition, there were significantly fewer hospitalizations for cardiovascular causes in the group randomized to receive carvedilol (15% versus 26%, $p = .02$). There was a trend to improvement in submaximal exercise as assessed by 6-minute walk test with carvedilol therapy, but this did not achieve statistical significance.

In the MOCHA trial,[63] there was a dose-related increase in left ventricular ejection fraction as well as dose-related reductions in mortality and hospitalizations for worsening heart failure. This study found the most favorable effects occurred in subjects receiving the highest dose of carvedilol (25 mg b.i.d.). There were no differences between groups for submaximal exercise duration or quality-of-life scores.

Subjects with only mild limitations of submaximal exercise were randomized into a protocol that was separate from the MOCHA and PRECISE trials.[64] The primary end point of this 1-year study was clinical progression of heart failure as defined in hierarchical order as (1) heart failure mortality, (2) hospitalization for heart failure, or (3) an increase in heart failure medications. Significantly fewer patients randomized to receive carvedilol experienced progression of heart failure (12.4% for carvedilol versus 24.5% for placebo, $p = .011$). The individual end points of mortality and increases in heart failure medications were also significantly reduced with carvedilol therapy. As observed with the other trials, left ventricular ejection fraction significantly improved with carvedilol therapy (Δ LVEF = 0.09 for carvedilol, Δ LVEF = 0.03 for placebo; $p = .00001$).

All subjects in the four United States carvedilol heart failure trials (including the three described here) were followed prospectively by a Data and Safety Monitoring Board with the intention to demonstrate the safety of carvedilol therapy.[65] A total of 1052 patients were enrolled into these trials. After 25 months of enrollment, the Data and Safety Monitoring Board recommended termination of the randomized trials because of a favorable effect of carvedilol on survival. By intention-to-treat, mortality was 8.2% in the placebo group but only 2.9% in the carvedilol group ($p = .0001$), a 67% reduction in mortality. The treatment effect was similar in patients with class II and class III-IV symptoms and similar in ischemic heart disease and nonischemic heart disease.

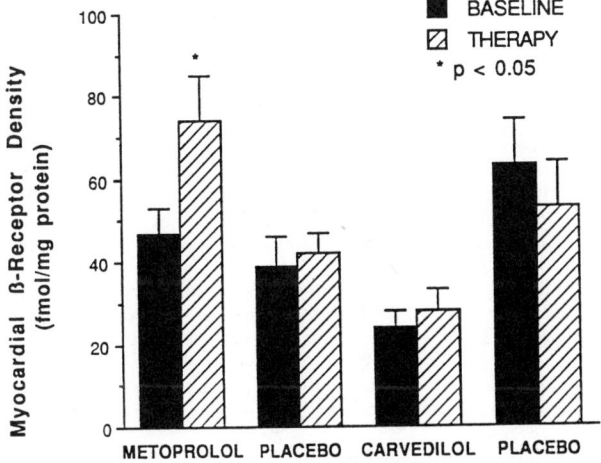

Figure 61–14. Myocardial β-receptor density at baseline *(solid bars)* and after chronic therapy *(crosshatched bars)* with metoprolol, carvedilol, and their matching placebos. Metoprolol significantly increased β-receptor density by within-group analysis and by between-group analysis compared with the metoprolol placebo group and the carvedilol group. (From Gilbert EM, Olsen SL, Renlund DB, Bristow MR: Beta-adrenergic receptor regulation and left ventricular function in idiopathic dilated cardiomyopathy. Am J Cardiol 71:23C, 1993.)

Thus, the preliminary data from the United States carvedilol heart failure trials suggest that carvedilol may play an important role in the treatment of heart failure. Carvedilol therapy results in improvements in left ventricular function and symptoms of heart failure as well as dramatic reductions in hospitalization and death from heart failure.

THE PLACE OF CARVEDILOL IN THERAPY

To date, long-term, placebo-controlled trials meeting FDA guidelines have not yet been completed for carvedilol, but preliminary data suggest that carvedilol will be effective in the treatment of hypertension, exercise-induced angina, and perhaps congestive heart failure. Carvedilol has some unique properties that should make it particularly attractive for selected populations with these disorders.

In the treatment of hypertension, current studies support its efficacy at doses of 25 to 50 mg taken twice daily. It may also be effective at lower doses and possibly in a once-daily dosing regimen. The incidence of orthostatic hypotension is higher than that for other β-blockers, as would be expected for a combined β-blocker–vasodilator. This problem may be minimized by taking medication with food and titrating doses when initiating therapy. Because evidence supports the conclusion that carvedilol reduces peripheral vascular resistance, it may have an advantage over pure β-blockers in the treatment of hypertension by preventing end-organ damage. The fact that it preserves renal blood flow may also provide an advantage in the treatment of patients with hypertension and compromised renal function.

For the treatment of exercise-induced angina, current studies suggest that carvedilol will be effective at a dosage of 50 mg given twice daily. The currently available results suggest that its effectiveness may increase with prolonged therapy. If this is true, it may be effective at lower doses. Unfortunately, the unique properties of vasodilation that carvedilol possesses appear to be a disadvantage in the treatment of exercise-induced angina, when the drug is compared with other β-blockers. The vasodilation appears to be primarily peripheral and probably shunts blood flow away from the coronaries. In a subset of patients with exercise-induced angina and decreased left ventricular function, an exaggerated hypertensive response to exercise, or perhaps both angina and hypertension, carvedilol may theoretically have some advantage over standard β-blockers, but this has yet to be substantiated.

The treatment of heart failure is perhaps one of the most interesting applications of carvedilol. Moderate-sized pilot studies have demonstrated the safety and tolerability of carvedilol in patients with heart failure. Carvedilol appears to dramatically improve left ventricular function in these subjects. In addition, carvedilol appears to have favorable effects on neurohormonal activation in heart failure, including a reduction in cardiac sympathetic drive and an increase in cardiac parasympathetic drive. Several important multicenter trials are currently assessing carvedilol's effects on exercise tolerance, and results should be available by January 1995. These trials have the power to establish the efficacy of carvedilol for the treatment of heart failure. Carvedilol promises to be an interesting and important addition to our armamentarium of treatments for a variety of cardiovascular disorders and should help sharpen our focus of treatment for the underlying causes of these major disease entities.

REFERENCES

1. Strein K, Sponer G, Muller-Beckmann B, et al: Pharmacological profile of carvedilol, a compound with β-blocking and vasodilating properties. J Cardiovasc Pharmacol 10(Suppl 11):S33, 1987.
2. Lund-Johansen P: Hemodynamic trends in untreated essential hypertension. Acta Med Scand (Suppl) 602:68, 1977.
3. Hansson L: Effects of beta-adrenoceptor blocking agents on haemodynamic parameters. Acta Med Scand (Suppl) 606:49, 1977.
4. Sannerstedt R, Stenberg J, Vedin A, et al: Chronic beta-adrenergic blockade in arterial hypertension: Hemodynamic influences of dihydralazine and dynamic exercise and clinical effects of combined treatment. Am J Cardiol 29:718, 1972.
5. Zacest R, Gilmore E, Koch-Weser J: Treatment of essential hypertension with combined vasodilation and beta-blockade. N Engl J Med 286:617, 1972.
6. Abshagen U: A new molecule with vasodilating and β-adrenoceptor blocking properties. J Cardiovasc Pharmacol 10(Suppl 11):S23, 1987.
7. Bristow MR, Larrabee P, Minobe W, et al: Effects of carvedilol on adrenergic receptor pharmacology in human ventricular myocardium and lymphocytes. Clin Investig 70:S105, 1992.
8. Bristow MR, Larrabee P, Minobe W, et al: Receptor pharmacology of carvedilol in the human heart. J Cardiovasc Pharmacol 19(Suppl 1):S68, 1992.
9. Hershberger RE, Bristow MR: Receptor alterations in failing human heart. Heart Failure 3:230, 1988.
10. Sponer G, Strein K, Muller-Beckmann B, et al: Studies on the mode of vasodilating action of carvedilol. J Cardiovasc Pharmacol 10(Suppl 11):S42, 1987.
11. Achenbach C, Nuckel B, Weimer J: Effects of the vasodilating beta-blocker carvedilol on isolated cardiac tissues. Eur Heart J 5(Suppl 1):1175, 1984.
12. Smith, Kline and French Pharmaceuticals Investigator Brochure for Carvedilol. Philadelphia: Smith, Kline and French, 1987, pp 1–60.
13. Prichard BNC, Battersby LA, Cruickshank JM: Overdosage with beta-adrenergic blocking agents. Adverse Drug React Acute Poisoning Rev 3:91, 1984.
14. Neugebauer G, Akpan W, Mollendorf EV, et al: Pharmacokinetics and disposition of carvedilol in humans. J Cardiovasc Pharmacol 10(Suppl 11):S85, 1987.
15. Louis WJ, McNeil JJ, Workman BS, et al: A pharmacokinetic study of carvedilol (BM 14,190) in elderly subjects: Preliminary report. J Cardiovasc Pharmacol 10(Suppl 11):S89, 1987.
16. Cubeddu LX, Fuenmayor N, Varin F, et al: Mechanism of the vasodilatory effect of carvedilol in normal volunteers: A comparison with labetalol. J Cardiovasc Pharmacol 10(Suppl 11):S81, 1987.
17. Tomlinson B, Cronin CJ, Graham BR, et al: Haemodynamics of carvedilol in normal subjects compared with labetalol. J Cardiovasc Pharmacol 10(Suppl 11):S69, 1987.
18. Tomlinson B, Cronin CJ, Graham BR, et al: Haemodynamics and pharmacokinetics of carvedilol (BM 14,190). Br J Clin Pharmacol 19:566, 1985.
19. Tomlinson B, Cronin CJ, Graham BR, et al: Acute haemodynamics of carvedilol compared to propranolol, labetalol, and pindolol. Br J Clin Pharmacol 21:581, 1986.
20. Sundberg S, Tiihonen K, Gordin A: Vasodilatory effects of

carvedilol and pindolol. J Cardiovasc Pharmacol 10(Suppl 11):S76, 1987.

21. Leonetti G, Sampieri L, Cuspidi C, et al: Resting and postexercise hemodynamic effects of carvedilol, a β-adrenergic blocker and precapillary vasodilator in hypertensive patients. J Cardiovasc Pharmacol 10(Suppl 11):S94, 1987.

22. Heber ME, Brigden GS, Caruana MP, et al: Carvedilol for systemic hypertension. J Cardiovasc Pharmacol 10(Suppl 11):S113, 1987.

23. Muller JE, Ludmer PL, Willich SN, et al: Circadian variation in the frequency of sudden cardiac death. Circulation 75:131, 1987.

24. Dupont AG, Van der Niepen P, Taeymans Y, et al: Effect of carvedilol on ambulatory blood pressure, renal hemodynamics, and cardiac function in essential hypertension. J Cardiovasc Pharmacol 10(Suppl 11):S130, 1987.

25. Epstein M, Oster JR: Beta-blockers and the kidney. Mineral Electolyte Metab 8:237, 1982.

26. Epstein M, Oster JR: Beta-blockers and renal function: A reappraisal. J Clin Hypertens 1:65, 1985.

27. Rasmussen S, Nulsen PE: Blood pressure, body fluid volume and glomerular filtration rate during treatment with labetalol in essential hypertension. Br J Clin Pharmacol 12:349, 1981.

28. Cruz F, O'Neill WM, Clifton G, et al: Effects of labetalol and methyldopa on renal function. Clin Pharmacol Ther 30:57, 1981.

29. Morgan T, Snowden R, Butcher L: Effect of carvedilol and metoprolol on blood pressure, blood flow, and vascular resistance. J Cardiovasc Pharmacol 10(Suppl 11):S124, 1987.

30. Eggertsen R, Sivertsson R, Andren L, et al: Acute and long-term hemodynamic effects of carvedilol, a combined β-adrenoceptor blocking and precapillary vasodilating agent, in hypertensive patients. J Cardiovasc Pharmacol 10(Suppl 11):S97, 1987.

31. Hansson L, Zweifler AJ, Julius S, et al: Hemodynamic effects of acute and prolonged beta-blockade in essential hypertension. Acta Med Scand 196:27, 1974.

32. Freis ED: Hemodynamics in hypertension. Physiol Rev 40:27, 1960.

33. Ogihara T, Ikeda M, Goto Y, et al: The effect of low-dose carvedilol on circadian variation of blood pressure in patients with essential hypertension. J Cardiovasc Pharmacol 10(Suppl 11):S108, 1987.

34. Meyer-Sabellek W, Schulte KL, Distler A, et al: Circadian antihypertensive profile of carvedilol (BM 14190). J Cardiovasc Pharmacol 10(Suppl 11):S119, 1987.

35. Schnurr E, Widmann L, Glocke M: Efficacy and safety of carvedilol in the treatment of hypertension. J Cardiovasc Pharmacol 10(Suppl 11):S101, 1987.

36. Kaski JC, Rodriguez-Plaza L, Brown J, et al: Efficacy of carvedilol in exercise-induced myocardial ischemia. J Cardiovasc Pharmacol 10(Suppl 11):S137, 1987.

37. Rodriguez EA, Lahiri A, Hughes LO, et al: Antianginal efficacy of carvedilol, a beta-blocking drug with vasodilating activity. Am J Cardiol 58:916, 1986.

38. Lahiri A, Rodriguez EA, Al-Khawaja I, et al: Effects of a new vasodilating beta-blocking drug, carvedilol, on left ventricular function in stable angina pectoris. Am J Cardiol 59:769, 1987.

39. Jamal SM, Freedman SB, Thompson A, et al: Antianginal efficacy of carvedilol, a new β-blocker with vasodilating action. J Cardiovasc Pharmacol 10(Suppl 11):S141, 1987.

40. Freedman SB, Jamal S, Harris PJ, et al: Comparison of carvedilol and atenolol for angina pectoris. Am J Cardiol 60:499, 1987.

41. Waagstein F, Hjalmarson A, Swedberg K, Wallentin L: Betablockers in dilated cardiomyopathy: They work. Eur Heart J 4:173, 1983.

42. Engelmeier RS, O'Connell JB, Walsh R, et al: Improvement in symptoms and exercise tolerance by metoprolol in patients with dilated cardiomyopathy: A double-blind, randomized, placebo controlled trial. Circulation 72:536, 1985.

43. Anderson JL, Lutz JR, Gilbert EM, et al: A randomized trial of low-dose beta-blockade therapy for idiopathic dilated cardiomyopathy. Am J Cardiol 55:471, 1985.

44. Gilbert EM, Anderson JL, Deitchman D, et al: Long-term β-blocker vasodilator therapy improves cardiac function in idiopathic dilated cardiomyopathy: A double-blind, randomized study of bucindolol versus placebo. Am J Med 88:223, 1990.

45. Woodley SL, Gilbert EM, Anderson JL, et al: β-Blockade with bucindolol in heart failure caused by ischemic versus idiopathic dilated cardiomyopathy. Circulation 84:2426, 1991.

46. Waagstein F, Bristow MR, Swedberg K, et al: Beneficial effects of metoprolol in idiopathic dilated cardiomyopathy. Lancet 342:1441, 1993.

47. Bristow MR, O'Connell JB, Gilbert EM, et al: Dose-response of chronic β-blocker treatment in heart failure from either idiopathic dilated or ischemic cardiomyopathy. Circulation 89:1632, 1994.

48. Reichenbach DD, Benditt EP: Catecholamines and cardiomyopathy: The pathogenesis and potential importance of myofibrillar degeneration. Hum Pathol 1:125, 1970.

49. Heilbrunn SM, Shah P, Bristow MR, et al: Increased β-receptor density and improved hemodynamic response to catecholamine stimulation during chronic metoprolol therapy. Circulation 79:483, 1989.

50. Gilbert EM, O'Connell JB, Bristow MR: Therapy of idiopathic dilated cardiomyopathy with chronic β-adrenergic blockade. Heart Vessels 6(Suppl):33, 1991.

51. Bristow MR, Ginsburg R, Fowler M, et al: β1 and β2 adrenergic receptor subpopulations in normal and failing human ventricular myocardium: Coupling of both receptors subtypes to muscle contraction and selective receptor down-regulation in heart failure. Circ Res 59:297, 1869.

52. Di Lenarda A, Gilbert EM, Olsen SL, et al: Acute hemodynamic effects of carvedilol versus metoprolol in idiopathic dilated cardiomyopathy [abstract]. J Am Coll Cardiol 17:142A, 1991.

53. Olsen SL, Gilbert EM, Renlund DG, et al: Carvedilol improves symptoms and left ventricular function in patients with congestive heart failure due to ischemic or idiopathic dilated cardiomyopathy [abstract]. J Am Coll Cardiol 21:114A, 1993.

54. Krum H, Schwartz B, Sackner-Bernstein J, et al: Double-blind, placebo-controlled study of the long-term efficacy of carvedilol in patients with severe heart failure treated with converting-enzyme inhibitors [abstract]. J Am Coll Cardiol 21:114A, 1993.

55. Metra M, D'Aloia A, Panina G, et al: Effects of acute and chronic carvedilol on resting and exercise hemodynamics of patients with idiopathic cardiomyopathy [abstract]. J Am Coll Cardiol 21:114A, 1993.

56. Gilbert EM, Olsen SL, Renlund DR, et al: Chronic β-blockade with carvedilol results in sustained improvements in left ventricular function in patients with heart failure [abstract]. Circulation 88:1, 1993.

57. Gilbert EM, Olsen SL, Renlund DB, Bristow MR: Beta-adrenergic receptor regulation and left ventricular function in idiopathic dilated cardiomyopathy. Am J Cardiol 71:23C, 1993.

58. Bristow MR, Olsen SL, Larrabee P, Gilbert EM: The β-blocking agents metoprolol and carvedilol affect cardiac adrenergic drive differently in subjects with heart failure from idiopathic dilated cardiomyopathy [abstract]. J Am Coll Cardiol 21:314A, 1993.

59. Schramm MS, Marks ML, Olsen SL, Gilbert EM: Chronic β-blocker therapy with carvedilol increases parasympathetic drive in heart failure [abstract]. Circulation 88:1, 1993.

60. Goldsmith RL, Krum H, Bigger JT, et al: Beta-blockade increases parasympathetic activity in chronic heart failure [abstract]. Circulation 88:1, 1993.

61. Australia-New Zealand Heart Failure Research Collaborative Group: Effects of carvedilol, a vasodilator-beta-blocker, in patients with congestive heart failure due to ischemic heart disease. Circulation 92(2):212, 1995.

62. Packer M, Colucci WS, Sackner-Bernstein J, et al: Prospective randomized evaluation of carvedilol on symptoms and exercise tolerance in chronic heart failure: Results of the PRECISE trial [abstract]. Circulation (In press).

63. Bristow MR, Gilbert EM, Abraham WT, et al: Multicenter oral carvedilol heart failure assessment (MOCHA): A six-month dose-response evaluation in class II-IV patients [abstract]. Circulation (In press).

64. Colucci WS, Packer M, Bristow MR, et al: Carvedilol inhibits clinical progression in patients with mild heart failure [abstract]. Circulation (In press).

65. Packer M, Bristow MR, Cohn JN, et al: Effect of carvedilol on the survival of patients with chronic heart failure [abstract]. Circulation (In press).

VII.

Antiadrenergic Drugs

Editors: B. N. C. Prichard and Michael A. Weber

A. Principles and Practice of α-Antiadrenergic Therapy

CHAPTER 62

Principles and Practice of α-Antiadrenergic Therapy

B. N. C. Prichard, M.B., M.Sc., F.R.C.P., F.F.P.M.

Reduction in vascular tone by α-adrenergic inhibition can be achieved at many sites.[1,2] The inhibition may be central at ganglia, sympathetic nerve endings, or the receptor site. Those drugs acting centrally and at the α-receptor are the groups in current widespread use. The use of those agents acting at sympathetic nerve endings (e.g., guanethidine) has declined greatly, and the use of ganglion-blocking drugs is obsolete as a result of associated unwanted effects from parasympathetic blockade. It is also suggested that other drugs such as calcium antagonists and angiotensin-converting enzyme (ACE) inhibitors may at least partly achieve their antihypertensive effect by influencing the sympathetic nervous system.

CARDIOVASCULAR CONTROL

Hypertension probably results from a complexity of genetic and environmental influences. It is a multifactorial disease process, and there are advantages to be gained by attending to other aspects, notably lipid profile and glucose metabolism[3-5] (also see Chapters 70 and 72).

Various candidates, however, have been suggested as being principally responsible for raised blood pressure. One is the postulate of the central role of the sympathetic nervous system. This may not be mediated only via influence on α_1 vascular receptors but also via influences on insulin metabolism and insulin release (see Chapter 72).

Sympathetic tone and reflexes mediated via peripheral α_1-receptors are crucial to control of the blood pressure. Regardless of the site of action, any drug that inhibits the innervation of the α-receptor may be expected to produce a greater effect under physiologic conditions that require increased α-mediated sympathetic activity to maintain blood pressure. There is, thus, the potential for a fall in blood pressure

on standing, after exercise, in a hot environment, after eating, or with reduced blood volume. Clearly, it is important that the degree of interference with the innervation of the α-receptor should not be such as to prevent the function of cardiovascular reflexes. It is desirable that α-mediated tone is reduced at low rates of sympathetic stimulation, e.g., resting supine, so that blood pressure is lowered. However, the inhibition should not be so great as to excessively inhibit the increased sympathetic stimulation required to avoid an excessive fall of blood pressure under certain physiologic conditions. The degree of inhibition of increases in sympathetic traffic varies widely. For instance, phenoxybenzamine, because of its noncompetitive α-receptor block, prevents compensatory reflexes and therefore results in a considerable orthostatic effect,[6] whereas centrally acting methyldopa has a relatively small postural effect, considerably less than the adrenergic neurone inhibitory drugs.[7] Even within the class of adrenergic neurone inhibitory drugs, cat nictitating membrane experiments demonstrated that bethanidine resulted in a greater block of higher frequencies of sympathetic traffic than guanethidine.[8] This has been paralleled in clinical investigations that have revealed a greater postural effect from bethanidine than from guanethidine.[7]

HEMODYNAMICS

Established hypertension is associated with an increase in peripheral resistance[9-11] that is widely distributed throughout various vascular beds (see Chapter 63). The increased vascular tone may initially increase venous return and thus cardiac output, but usually in established hypertension, cardiac output and regional blood flow are normal (see Chapter 63). It might be argued that drugs that inhibit the α-receptor innervation and thus reduce peripheral resistance represent a group that acts to reverse the most prominent hemodynamic change of hypertension. There is a reduction in vascular tone of both arteries and veins. Arteriolar dilation tends to increase cardiac output, whereas venous dilation results in venous pooling and a reduction in venous return and tends to reduce cardiac output. Overall cardiac output is usually unchanged with α-blockade.[12]

CONTROL OF BLOOD PRESSURE

The control of blood pressure in both the normotensive and hypertensive is most complex. The autonomic nervous system plays a major part in the moment-to-moment regulation of blood pressure.[13] Hormonal and renal factors become more important in long-term regulation of blood pressure, as Guyton has stressed that the pressor effect from sympathetic vasoconstriction would be overcome by volume adjustment through the kidney.[14] There are, however, many ways in which the nervous system can influence renal function.[15]

The origin of sympathetic neurones that supply the heart and blood vessels, the "vasomotor center," is situated in the lateral part of the reticular formation and the bulbar area of the brain stem. It should be considered "as the most caudal link in a series of longitudinal systems in the brain ending as high as the cortex."[16] It is now clear that there are numerous central transmitter substances. They can be divided up into simple amino acids, such as glutamate and gamma-aminobutyric acid (GABA); amines, such as noradrenaline, adrenaline, dopamine, and 5-hydroxytyramine (serotonin, 5HT);[17] and peptides, such as angiotensin, the opioid peptides, oxytonin, vasopressin, and substance P. A neurone that liberates one transmitter type may alternate with a neurone that releases a different transmitter.[17–19] More recently a clonidine-displacing substance that is thought to be the natural agonist at the imidazoline I_1 receptor has been described (see Chapter 68). It is also apparent that whereas it used to be thought that a neurone released only one transmitter, in fact, several transmitters may be released, one transmitter being exceptional.[20]

The axons from the neurones of the vasomotor center make up the bulbospinal tract, which descends in the interomedial lateral columns to the preganglionic cells in the arteriolateral columns. The balance of stimulation and inhibition provides the control of vasomotor tone by modulating the number of impulses traveling by the final common pathway, the preganglionic neurone. This neurone synapses in paravertebral ganglionic liberating acetylcholine, to activate the postganglionic neurone. Stimulation of these nerves causes vasoconstriction of resistance vessels and veins, vasodilation being largely achieved by fewer vasoconstrictor impulses.[11] In contrast with the importance of sympathetic tone to blood vessels, at rest parasympathetic tone to the heart predominates. However, even in the supine position, there is significant sympathetic tone, as demonstrated by the

dose-dependent reduction in heart rate achieved by the administration of a β-adrenoceptor blocking drug.[21]

ADRENERGIC RECEPTORS

The α-receptors have been subdivided into α_1- and α_2-receptors according to their responses to various agonists and antagonists.[22, 23] Methoxamine, the most selective, and phenylephrine are selective α_1-stimulants; clonidine, guanfacine, and guanabenz are α_2-stimulants; and adrenaline and noradrenaline stimulate both receptor subtypes. Prazosin, doxazosin, and trimazosin are selective α_1-blocking drugs; yohimbine, rauwolscine, and the more selective idazoxan block α_2-receptors; phentolamine blocks both α_1- and α_2-receptors. The α_1-receptors predominate postsynaptically in most vascular smooth muscle; α_2-receptors are also important. In some vascular beds, e.g., cerebral arteries of the dog, α_2-receptors are more numerous, and there is considerable species variation.[24] Both α_1- and α_2-receptors are present in the human forearm.[23] Postsynaptic α_1-receptors in vascular smooth muscle are involved in the mediation of nerve impulse; α_2-receptors, although also mediating contraction in response to hormonal stimulation, are extrasynaptic. Presynaptic α_2-receptors inhibit neuronal release of noradrenaline and constitute a negative feedback mechanism.[22] The α_1-receptors in vascular smooth muscle appear to be found in the adventitial layer, whereas the α_2-receptors are found closer to the interior, where they are acted upon by circulatory catecholamines.[25]

CENTRAL RECEPTORS

Central α_2-adrenergic postsynaptic receptors are the predominant α-receptors in the central nervous system (CNS). Stimulation results in a fall in blood pressure and bradycardia. Central α_1-receptors have also been demonstrated by receptor-binding techniques.[23] It is possible that central α_1-receptors are involved in mediating baroreceptor reflex function, and blockade of these receptors may be responsible for the relative lack of reflex tachycardia from prazosin.[26] More recently, however, it has been found that imidazolines, like clonidine, in contrast with the absence of effect from noradrenaline or other α-stimulants, were hypotensive in effect in the medullary nucleus reticularis lateralis. A membrane imidazoline receptor population has been defined at this site.[27] Clonidine, guanabenz, guanfacine, moxonidine, and rilmenidine bind on to the imidazoline I_2 receptors as well as α_2-receptors[28–30] (also see Chapter 68). It is likely that the imidazoline I_2 receptors are important in the antihypertensive effect of these drugs, this being more so with those agents that have a high specificity for the imidazoline I_1 receptor compared with their effect on the α_2-receptor.

There are also central presynaptic α_2-receptors that mediate a reduction in transmitter release.[22] The central α_2-receptors are found in various parts of the brain, but it appears that the medulla oblongata is important where there is a high concentration of α_2-receptors. Most work has been performed with clonidine, and a number of sites of action, mainly in the medulla, have been proposed; the most likely is the lateral reticular nucleus.[31] Other sites possess α_2-receptors, including the forebrain, where stimulation increases blood pressure, and also the spinal cord, which has been suggested as a site of action, as clonidine has been shown to exert a hypotensive effect from stimulation of these receptors in animal investigations.[32] However, a spinal site does not seem important in humans, because clonidine was without hypotensive effect in tetraplegic patients.[33] Investigations in animals with ligand-binding studies and destruction of CNS noradrenergic neurones with 6-hydroxydopamine indicate that presynaptic sites do not play a part in the hypotensive action of clonidine.[31]

METHYLDOPA

α-Methyldopa was for several years the most widely prescribed antihypertensive drug.

Mode of Action

Methyldopa inhibits dopa-decarboxylase and consequently reduces catecholamine synthesis. However, because other inhibitors of the enzyme are not antihypertensive, this was not thought to be the explanation of the antihypertensive effect of methyldopa.[34] It was noted, however, that only the *l*-isomer was decarboxylated and only the *l*-isomer lowered the blood pressure,[35] and thus further studies were conducted with this isomer. It was found that α-methyldopa is metabolized to α-methyldopamine and then to α-methylnoradrenaline. Day and Rand[36] thus suggested that α-methyldopa exerted its hypotensive action by being converted to α-methylnoradrenaline, which then acts as a false transmitter when liberated at sympathetic nerve endings. However, α-methylnoradrenaline is approximately equipotent to noradrenaline in the cat and dog[37] and in human smooth muscle is only slightly less potent than noradrenaline.[38] Moreover, although the acute administration of α-methyldopa depresses the function of sympathetic nerves depressing the response of the cat nictitating membrane to nerve stimulation,[39] no effect was seen on the responses after long-term treatment. This also suggests that a peripheral effect on nerve function is not the explanation for the antihypertensive effect of methyldopa.[40] The formation of a false transmitter is, however, relevant to the central mode of action of methyldopa (see later discussion).

Henning and van Zwieten[41] observed that a small dose of α-methyldopa injected into the vertebral artery of the cat produced a fall of blood pressure at doses that had no effect intravenously. Ingenito et al.[42] found that the administration of α-methyldopa to the vascularly isolated perfused cat brain reduced blood pressure in the rest of the animal. Thirdly, Baum et al.[43] demonstrated a reduced sympathetic

nerve traffic from methyldopa in renal hypertensive rats. It has been shown that the fall in blood pressure after a single dose of methyldopa correlates with the fall in plasma noradrenaline in humans.[44] The 24-hour urinary excretion of noradrenaline is also reduced by methyldopa in patients with essential hypertension. Further evidence for a central site of action is obtained from the observation that the antihypertensive action is inhibited by large doses of isoleucine, which competitively inhibits the transport of methyldopa across the blood-brain barrier.[45]

α-Methylnoradrenaline is formed from the metabolism of α-methyldopa in the brain,[46, 47] which then stimulates the central α_2-adrenergic receptors, most likely in the nucleus tractus solitarii of the medulla.[48] The resultant hypotensive effect is blocked by α-adrenoceptor blockade.[49, 50] Inhibition of the metabolism by a centrally active dopa-decarboxylase inhibitor abolishes the antihypertensive effect, but not by a dopa-decarboxylase inhibitor that fails to penetrate the brain.[47] Observations in humans are in agreement, as peripheral decarboxylase inhibition with α-methylhydrazine does not alter the hypotensive response to methyldopa.[51] Likewise, inhibition of α-methylnoradrenaline synthesis by the destruction of central adrenergic neurones by intraventricular 6-hydroxydopamine prevents the hypotensive effect of α-methyldopa,[52] whereas intravenous 6-hydroxydopamine reduced, but did not prevent, the hypotensive effect.[50, 53] Finally, absence of peripheral effect of methyldopa is illustrated by the observation that after doses of α-methyldopa that produce hypotension, the pressor response that is seen when the entire sympathetic outflow is stimulated is not reduced.[50]

Renin release is suppressed by methyldopa (see Chapter 63). However, the antihypertensive action of methyldopa does not appear to be due to its renin-suppressing action.[48, 54]

Hemodynamics

There are several factors, such as severity of the hypertension treated and dosage used, to account for the variability of hemodynamic effects reported from the administration of methyldopa. It appears, however, that the dominant effect is a fall in peripheral resistance with little change in cardiac output (see Chapter 63). Some investigators, however, have observed a venodepressor effect, and thus venous pooling may play a part with higher doses (2.0 to 5.0 g daily) of methyldopa.[55] Somewhat in contrast with other work, when Lund-Johansen[56] studied a series of 13 patients with mild hypertension before and after treatment with α-methyldopa for 1 year (500 to 1500 mg/day, average 896 mg/day), he found that the fall in blood pressure at rest, standing, and on exercise was associated with a fall in cardiac output, no change in peripheral resistance being observed. There was no postural drop in blood pressure; the blood pressures after α-methyldopa were supine 139/84 mmHg and standing 150/93 mmHg. Prolonged methyldopa administration reduces left ventricular mass (see Chapter 63).

Renal and splanchnic blood flow is maintained after methyldopa, and a fall in cerebral vascular resistance has been described. An increase in coronary blood flow has been reported (see Chapter 63).

There is little effect on heart rate after intravenous administration,[57] whereas after oral administration there is a modest reduction, supine, standing, and after exercise.[56, 58] The heart rate while taking α-methyldopa, however, is higher than while taking the adrenergic neurone inhibitory drugs bethanidine or guanethidine for a similar antihypertensive effect.[7]

A reversal of left ventricular hypertrophy has been demonstrated in the rat model (see Chapter 63).

Cardiovascular Reflexes

As might be predicted from drugs that interfere with α-adrenergic tone, higher doses of α-methyldopa used in the treatment of hypertension are associated with postural and exercise hypotension, although less than that seen with sympathetic inhibiting drugs bethanidine or guanethidine.[7, 59] There is also an alteration of the cardiovascular response to Valsalva's maneuver in a way characteristic of inhibition of vasoconstriction, overshoot is abolished,[60, 61] and the rise in blood pressure during the effort phase is inhibited.[62] However, other investigators have reported interference with cardiovascular reflexes, and indeed postural hypotension is seldom a problem with the clinical use of methyldopa (see Chapter 63).

Clinical Use

The antihypertensive effect of methyldopa was first observed by Oates et al.[59] It is similar in efficacy to adrenergic neurone inhibitory drugs. Johnson et al.[63] observed a fall in blood pressure in 37 patients receiving α-methyldopa that was similar to that found in 66 patients having hypertension of similar severity receiving guanethidine. This confirmed a previous within-patient study in 19 patients of Oates et al.,[59] who found that α-methyldopa, guanethidine, and pargyline had a similar antihypertensive action. Likewise, Prichard at al.[7] in a within-patient study of 30 patients found that α-methyldopa produced similar control to bethanidine and guanethidine, although six of these patients could not tolerate α-methyldopa. In a further study, it has been confirmed that α-methyldopa produced similar control of the standing blood pressure to bethanidine and also to propranolol.[64]

The usual starting dose of methyldopa is 250 mg two to three times daily, although others begin with smaller doses (e.g., 125 mg b.i.d.) to minimize initial side effects, unless blood pressure is unduly high, and particularly if the patient is already receiving other antihypertensive drugs. Side effects tend to become less as a lower blood pressure is maintained.[7] Increments of 250 mg per dose may be made. Some

physicians use only up to 2 g/day; others have in the past used higher doses, e.g., 6 g/day.[65] A diuretic should be used in addition if any side effects such as sedation occur, and most usually would be added in any case if a daily dosage of 2 g is reached. Methyldopa combines well with β-blocking drugs.[66] The development of tolerance is not uncommon, but it can usually be overcome by increasing the dose.[67]

In a 15-year survival study of patients treated with methyldopa, the mortality of those older than 60 years of age was similar to that of the general population; however, in patients younger than 50 years, the mortality was higher than in the general population.[68]

Methyldopa has been widely used and is effective in the lowering of blood pressure in pregnancy, reducing maternal morbidity and improving perinatal mortality. No detrimental fetal effects have been observed.[69] Many regard methyldopa as the drug of choice for the management of chronic hypertension in pregnancy.[70]

Side Effects

Cardiovascular side effects from methyldopa are uncommon, postural or essential hypotension being unusual,[71] although it has been reported to be more frequent in younger patients with elevated blood urea levels.[72] There have been isolated reports of severe rebound hypertension after the cessation of methyldopa treatment (see Chapter 63). In the first year after methyldopa treatment was stopped (n = 131), there was a significant increase of mortality in women (4.91 risk; CI 1.83 to 13.20) compared with those remaining on treatment (n = 167); a trend in men (1.51 risk) was not significant.[73] Diarrhea occurs in approximately 4% to 8% of patients[71] and has been reported in association with dilation of the small bowel and malabsorption.[74]

The most common side effects from methyldopa are those affecting the central nervous system; tiredness is the most common dose-limiting factor.[71] Reduced mental activity and depression are not uncommon[71] (also see Chapter 63).

Methyldopa has been associated with several immunologic abnormalities (see Chapter 63). The direct Coombs' test may be positive in as many as 20% of cases.[14] There is a suggestion of a dose-dependent relationship, the incidence being 9% at a dose of 1 g a day of methyldopa, but rising to 36% at more than 3 g daily.[75] Hemolytic anemia is rare, possibly occurring in approximately 0.02% of patients.[76] Other abnormalities reported include positive lupus and rheumatoid factors, leukopenia, thrombocytopenia, and a wide variety of hepatic disorders (see Chapter 63).

Unusual reactions to methyldopa that have been reported include myocarditis, retroperitoneal fibrosis, various skin rashes, and extrapyramidal signs. Depression of dopamine removes its inhibition of prolactin, and thus galactorrhea may occur[71] (also see Chapter 63).

Place of Methyldopa in Antihypertensive Treatment

Methyldopa has a relatively high incidence of side effects, and the general quality of life of those receiving this drug is less than that of those receiving more recently introduced alternatives such as captopril.[77] Methyldopa is no longer regarded as a first-choice drug for new patients, but it still has a place, in combination, in some resistant patients.

CLONIDINE AND NEWER CENTRALLY ACTING DRUGS

These drugs were first thought to act by stimulating central α_2-receptors; more recent evidence has suggested the hypotensive action may be dependent to a varying degree on imidazoline I_1 receptors[27, 30] (also see Chapters 66 and 68). Clonidine (see Chapter 64) was the first drug of this type described, and subsequently the search for similar compounds with fewer, particularly central nervous system, side effects has continued. Several compounds have been widely evaluated, e.g., guanabenz (see Chapter 65), guanfacine (see Chapter 67), moxonidine (see Chapter 68), and rilmenidine (see Chapter 66).

Mode of Action

Clonidine lowers the blood pressure by a direct stimulant effect on postsynaptic α-receptors in the brain stem; its action is blocked by pretreatment with α-blocking drugs[71, 78] (also see Chapter 64). The receptors are of the α_2 subtype.[78, 79] Various sites of action in the medulla have been suggested, the most likely site being the lateral reticular nucleus.[31] Clonidine thus results in an inhibition of efferent sympathetic activity and an increase in vagal tone.[71] There is a reciprocal relationship between stimulation of the inhibitory sympathetic part of the vasomotor center and activation of the dorsal motor nucleus of the vagus, leading to the increase in vagal tone (see Chapter 64). Clonidine appears to facilitate reflex baroreceptor slowing in response to angiotensin injection in the anesthetized dog.[80] Baroreceptor denervation reduces the cardiac slowing seen after clonidine.[81] Reversal of impaired baroceptor function has been reported both in hypertensive animals and in patients after receiving clonidine (see Chapter 64). Evidence of reduced central sympathetic activity is provided by measurement of plasma catecholamine levels. Clonidine,[82] guanfacine[83] (also see Chapter 67), guanabenz (see Chapter 65), and moxonidine (see Chapter 68) all have been shown to reduce plasma catecholamine levels. There is reduced noradrenaline release in response to a cold pressor stimulus.[84]

Notwithstanding some *in vitro* investigations to the contrary, it appears that neither central nor peripheral presynaptic α_2-receptors play an important part in the hypotensive effect of clonidine.[71] Clonidine still reduces inhibition of sympathetic nervous activity in animals whose hind brain noradrenaline is depleted by reserpine or 6-hydroxydopamine or when noradrenaline synthesis is inhibited by α-methyl-p-tyrosine.[85, 86] It has also been shown that stimulation of peripheral sympathetic nerves causes normal release of noradrenaline in animals treated with clonidine.[87, 88]

The absence of any effect from 6-hydroxydopamine or α-methyl-p-tyrosine is also evidence that the action of clonidine, unlike methyldopa, is not dependent on an intact noradrenaline synthesis pathway; it is a direct α-stimulant.[71]

Stimulation of peripheral postsynaptic α_2-receptors results in vasoconstriction.[23, 89] Thus, clonidine intravenously results in an initial pressor response in animals[88, 89] and humans.[90] It has also been observed that although oral administration of increasing doses of clonidine results in a progressive dose-dependent fall in blood pressure, this dose-response relationship is lost when plasma concentrations exceed 1.5 to 2 µg/L. At levels higher than 3 µg/L, it appears that peripheral α-stimulation is even more prominent because clonidine may then increase blood pressure.[91]

Animal experiments have shown that guanfacine is also a central α_2-stimulant drug, its action being blocked by phentolamine. It is approximately 12 times more selective for α-adrenoceptors than the α_1-receptor compared with clonidine, a ratio of 1:3400 compared with 1:280[83, 92] (also see Chapter 67). Similar to clonidine, postsynaptic α_2-stimulation is suggested by the initial rise in blood pressure after intravenous administration[83] (also see Chapter 67).

Guanabenz is chemically clearly related to clonidine, and its main antihypertensive effect is by stimulation of central α_2-adrenoceptors[93] (also see Chapter 65). However, it also reduces the response to peripheral sympathetic nerve stimulation, and there is some evidence for an adrenergic neurone-blocking action[93] (also see Chapter 65).

Imidazoline Binding Sites

Initially it was thought that imidazolines lowered the blood pressure by activation of central α_2-receptors. Besides in the medulla oblongata, α_2-receptors are distributed widely; they occur in the frontal cortex and locus coeruleus, where the sedative action of clonidine analogue is probably mediated (see Chapter 66). Subsequently, the ventrolateral medulla (VLM) was found to be an important connecting component of the baroreceptor reflex. Microinjection of clonidine into the VLM reduced blood pressure, whereas the α_2-stimulant α-methylnoradrenaline was ineffective.[27, 94]

The postulated imidazoline binding sites were demonstrated by Ernsberger et al.[95] Moxonidine binds with the imidazoline I_1 sites with 33 times greater selectivity for I_1 sites than for α_2 sites, whereas clonidine is only 3.8 times as selective. This selectivity is important because α_2-stimulation is thought to be responsible for important side effects (see Chapter 68).

Efaroxan is a selective antagonist for the I_1 receptors that blunts the hypotensive effect of moxonidine, whereas α_2-blockade has little effect.[30] A clonidine displacing substance (CDS) has been described that appears to be the endogenous ligand for the imidazoline receptor. In the VLM, CDS has been shown to increase blood pressure and inhibit the hypotensive action of clonidine.

Rilmenidine is another more recently developed centrally acting drug (see Chapter 66). It also appears that occupation of imidazoline I_1 receptors is more relevant to its hypotensive action, as it has a 30-fold selectivity for binding to these receptors compared with α_2-receptors. Additionally, its hypotensive effect when applied to the VLM of the rat was not blocked by α_2-blockade but was inhibited by idazoxan, a ligand for imidazoline as well as α_2-receptors.[96, 97] Rilmenidine is more selective for the imidazoline I_1 receptors in relation to its α_2-blocking activity compared with clonidine.[98] The selectivity of rilmenidine for the imidazoline I_1 receptor compared with its α_2-stimulation is the likely basis for the dissociation between antihypertensive action and central nervous system side effects due to α_2-blockade. Animal work indicates far less sedative effect than is seen with clonidine (see Chapter 66).

In summary, therefore, while an action at α_2-receptors and imidazoline I_1 receptors lowers the blood pressure, an antihypertensive effect mediated via imidazoline I_1 receptors in the VLM, with agents selective for that receptor in distinction to an action at α_2-receptors, results in a hypotensive effect with less centrally mediated side effects.

The imidazoline I_1 receptors have also been described in the kidney, platelets, and adrenal chromaffin cells (see Chapter 66). Experiments in rats indicated that stimulation of renal I_1 receptors leads to an increase in salt and water excretion.[99]

As discussed earlier, these drugs all reduce plasma catecholamine levels. Clonidine also decreases renin activity as part of the reduction in sympathetic tone; additionally, it reduces aldosterone secretion. The lack of salt and water retention usually seen with clonidine may be a consequence of the suppression of the renin-aldosterone axis (see Chapter 64), although fluid retention has been reported.[71] Guanfacine also suppresses renin activity, but this does not correlate with its antihypertensive effect[83] (also see Chapter 67). Similarly, rilmenidine results in a fall in renin activity with acute and chronic administration (see Chapter 66). Moxonidine also reduces renin levels (see Chapter 68). Renin levels, however, are not reduced by guanabenz, although some inhibition of release can be deduced, as the fall in blood pressure from guanabenz is not associated with an increase in renin that would otherwise be expected from inhibition of vascular tone (see Chapter 65).

Hemodynamics

The acute oral administration of clonidine in the supine position leads to a reduction in blood pressure, heart rate, and cardiac output owing to reduced venous return consequent on venodilation. There is no change in peripheral resistance[100, 101] (also see Chapter 64). A greater fall in blood pressure has been reported in the 45-degree tilt position, associated with a fall in vascular resistance compared with values in the same position before the drug.[100] The hemodynamic changes on exercise, the rise in heart rate and cardiac output, are not reduced by clonidine (see Chapter 64); the same is true after transdermal administration.[82]

The chronic administration of clonidine decreases blood pressure and heart rate similar to that occurring after acute administration, but there is in addition a reduction in peripheral resistance (see Chapter 64). There is some evidence that clonidine causes some regression of left ventricular hypertrophy (see Chapter 64), but evidence from the spontaneously hypertensive rat suggests this effect is not so marked as with methyldopa, only being seen with large doses.[102]

The use of clonidine is associated with a preservation of renal blood flow and glomerular filtration. There is not an important effect on creatinine levels even in patients with advanced renal impairment.[71] There is little evidence for an effect of clonidine on coronary arteries, although an antianginal action has been reported, but this may be due to a reduction of the rate pressure product (see Chapter 64).

The reduction in blood pressure from the chronic administration of guanfacine is also associated with a fall in peripheral resistance with little effect on cardiac output. The hemodynamic effect of acute administration is probably not dissimilar from that of clonidine[83] (also see Chapter 67). It is probable that the hemodynamic changes from guanabenz are similar to those of clonidine, the antihypertensive effect of chronic administration being associated with a fall in peripheral resistance with little effect on cardiac function[93] (also see Chapter 65). Acute administration of guanabenz is, however, associated with a fall in renal function, but this is not observed with long-term treatment[93] (also see Chapter 65). Similarly, the fall in blood pressure from moxonidine is associated with a reduction in peripheral resistance, while cardiac hemodynamics are unchanged (see Chapter 68). The use of moxonidine for 6 months has been associated with a reversal of left ventricular hypertrophy (see Chapter 68). Likewise, the initial antihypertensive effect of rilmenidine is associated with a reduction in cardiac output, with a tendency for peripheral resistance to even increase; subsequently peripheral resistance falls. Again, similar to clonidine, there is no effect on water and electrolyte balance. Renal blood flow and glomerular filtration rates are reduced in normal subjects; renal function is well preserved in long-term studies in hypertensive patients (see Chapter 66). Long-term administration of rilmenidine is associated with a reversal of left ventricular hypertrophy (see Chapter 66).

Cardiovascular Reflexes

The central α_2-adrenoceptor–stimulating drugs, at least with long-term administration, seldom interfere with the increase in adrenergic tone required to avoid a postural fall in blood pressure. Some postural effect has been reported after acute administration of clonidine,[71] but with long-term administration postural hypotension is rare.[71, 103] Similarly, there is no fall in blood pressure on exercise; after clonidine, the usual increment of blood pressure is observed[71] (also see Chapter 64). Likewise, the use of rilmenidine is rarely associated with a postural fall of blood pressure (see Chapter 66). The same applies to guanabenz (see Chapter 65).

Clinical Use

Clonidine alone controls the blood pressure in approximately half of the patients with mild hypertension (see Chapter 64). There have been some studies that have reported a larger proportion of patients controlled with transdermal clonidine; however, other studies reveal a similar efficacy to oral clonidine.[82] Clonidine has been found similar in efficacy to propranolol, alone and in combination with a diuretic and hydralazine. Other investigations suggest it is more effective than acebutolol, similar to labetalol, but with more side effects.[66] Transdermal clonidine has also been found to be similar in efficacy to propranolol.[82] Intravenous clonidine has the disadvantage of producing an initial rise of blood pressure, although this can be prevented by prior administration of 5 mg of phentolamine. There are, however, more appropriate drugs for hypertensive emergencies.[71] The initial dose of clonidine is usually 0.1 mg twice daily. Satisfactory control is often obtained in patients with mild hypertension with a total dose of 0.4 mg daily, the usual range is 0.2 to 0.6 mg b.i.d. (see Chapter 64), although doses up to 6 mg/day have been given.[71]

Clonidine is frequently given in combination with a diuretic, by which as many as 80% of patients may be controlled.[104] Clonidine, by reducing heart rate, is useful in combination with a direct-acting vasodilator, such as minoxidil or hydralazine (see Chapter 64). Although clonidine has been used in combination with various β-blocking agents with additive effects, because β-blocking agents enhance any pressor withdrawal reaction (see later), the combination is not advised.[66]

Guanfacine controls hypertension in approximately 60% of patients. It is probably similar in efficacy to clonidine, but some trials have shown guanfacine to be more effective. It may also be similar in efficacy to methyldopa, but again some studies suggest it is more effective (see Chapter 67). It is similar in efficacy to prazosin.[105] Guanfacine has a long half-life and can be given once daily; 1 mg is often effective, and at this dose the withdrawal syndrome is not seen (see Chapter 67). Guanfacine may be used in combination with a diuretic. In combination with a diuretic, there is a useful additional fall in blood pressure and it appears similar in efficacy to clonidine or methyldopa[83] (also see Chapter 67). Guanfacine may be useful in combination with direct-acting vasodilators to inhibit the tachycardia that otherwise occurs.[83] Tolerance does not occur with guanfacine.[83]

Guanabenz is similar in efficacy to clonidine, possibly slightly more effective than methyldopa, and similar in efficacy to propranolol. A useful additive effect has been reported in combination with hydrochlorothiazide or captopril[93] (also see Chapter 65).

Moxonidine, used once or twice daily, has been shown to be effective in hypertension. It is similar in efficacy to drugs in current use: diuretics, α_1-blocking drugs, calcium antagonists, ACE inhibitors, and β-blockade. It is also of similar efficacy to clonidine, but with fewer side effects. Studies showing an additional fall in blood pressure with a diuretic have been reported. It is well tolerated in patients with heart failure or asthma. It is effective in renal insufficiency, in which the prolonged half-life means that a lower dosage may be sufficient[106] (also see Chapter 68).

Rilmenidine probably controls mild and moderate hypertension in about 60% of patients[98] (also see Chapter 66).

Effect on Lipids

Clonidine appears to have little effect on the lipid profile, with both increases and decreases of approximately 5% in cholesterol being reported. There have been reports of a reduced low-density lipoprotein (LDL) level and improved LDL/HDL (high-density lipoprotein) ratio, but others find no change. Glucose tolerance is not affected (see Chapter 64). Guanfacine also does not appear to have adverse effects on lipids or glucose (see Chapter 67). Cholesterol and triglycerides are reduced by guanabenz; glucose is not affected (see Chapter 65).

Rilmenidine does not affect lipid or glucose metabolism (see Chapter 66). Insulin dependent diabetics with hypertension did not show any effect on lipid or glucose metabolism. Diabetic control was not affected.[107]

Side Effects

Clonidine rarely causes significant postural or exercise hypotension. Dry mouth is common in nearly half of patients initially, but in most it subsides after 4 to 6 weeks. Constipation may occur but is usually minor[71, 82] (also see Chapter 64). Sedation is the most troublesome side effect. The reported incidence varies widely.[71] Between 11% and 18% has been reported in studies of transdermal clonidine.[82] There are considerably fewer side effects with the transdermal patch, but this advantage is reduced by the incidence of skin allergy in as many as 20% of patients[82] (also see Chapter 64). A number of relatively rare side effects have been described: parotid pain, Raynaud's phenomenon, blurring of vision, rashes, sleep reversal, among others.[71]

Side effects from guanfacine are similar to those from clonidine—dry mouth, sedation, fatigue—generally at doses of more than 1 to 2 mg/day. The incidence of sedation may be less than with guanabenz[83] (also see Chapter 67) or with clonidine.[83] In a large multicenter trial (n = 580) using an average dose of 4.7 mg/day for the first year, there was a 60% incidence of dry mouth, 33% of sedation from guanfacine. In the second year of treatment, with an average dose of 3.6 mg, the incidences were 2.6% and 7.6%, respectively.[108] In the first year, guanfacine was discontinued in 52 patients, including the following reasons: dry mouth (n = 20), tiredness or weakness (n = 12), and constipation (n = 7).[108] In one comparative study, no cases of somnolence were reported in patients receiving guanfacine (n = 51), but in three cases of those receiving prazosin (n = 51).[105]

Side effects from guanabenz are similar to those of other α_2-adrenoceptor agonists, sedation and dry mouth being most common (see Chapter 65).

Laboratory tests reveal very little sedative effect from moxonidine. It does not affect driving skills (see Chapter 68). In accord with the greater selectivity for imidazoline I_1 receptors, considered responsible for the antihypertensive effect, compared with the central α_2-receptors, thought to be responsible for the sedative effect, trials indicated that moxonidine has a less sedative effect than clonidine (see Chapter 68).

Rilmenidine, unlike earlier centrally acting drugs, can lower the blood pressure at the 1-mg dose with a low level of central nervous system side effects. Sedation is less than with equally effective doses of methyldopa or clonidine and similar to that with placebo, atenolol, or hydrochlorothiazide. Dry mouth is also less than that occurring with clonidine or methyldopa[98, 109] (also see Chapter 66). However, in one study, more sleepiness was reported with rilmenidine than with methyldopa. Dry mouth increased on both drugs; psychological well-being tended to improve on rilmenidine and worsen on methyldopa. Ten patients (of 79) stopped methyldopa because of adverse effects; three (of 79) stopped rilmenidine. Of those completing the study, psychological well-being was similar.[110] Animal studies indicated that rilmenidine was of greater potency (approximately 2.5 times) for the imidazoline I_1 receptors but had much less effect (some 50-fold) on areas of the brain where the sedative effects of clonidine are thought to reside.[98]

Withdrawal Syndrome

Discontinuation of antihypertensive drugs results in blood pressure remaining at treated levels for a time and then slowly returning to pretreated levels, or a rapid return to pretreated levels, or finally an overshoot to higher levels than those previously observed. Signs and symptoms of sympathetic overactivity may occur without an overshoot of blood pressure.

The incidence of overshoot after abrupt withdrawal of clonidine is hard to assess. It does not occur after low doses are stopped; the incidence may be more important at levels of 0.9 mg/day.[71] The syndrome can be avoided by gradually reducing drug dosage over a few weeks (see Chapter 64). The withdrawal syndrome has also been reported after guanfacine, in 4 of 17 patients in one study receiving more than 3 mg daily (see Chapter 67). Animal experiments suggest that the withdrawal phenomenon is less likely to occur with guanfacine than clonidine.[83] There have also been reports of withdrawal symptoms after guanabenz; the incidence may be less than seen with clonidine[93] (also see Chapter 65).

There is no evidence of the withdrawal syndrome after the cessation of treatment with moxonidine (see Chapter 68) or rilmenidine (see Chapter 66).

Place of Centrally Acting Drugs in Antihypertensive Treatment

These drugs have a relatively high incidence of sedation and other CNS symptoms and dry mouth. There has been a continuing search for agents in which there is a dissociation between the antihypertensive effect and CNS side effects. Although it is too early to be sure, it seems this may have possibly been achieved with rilmenidine. The relatively high incidence of side effects has meant that α_2-agonists have not generally been regarded as first-line agents but more as second-line drugs often useful in combination. They are, however, effective drugs and have the advantage of not interfering unfavorably with cardiovascular reflexes. Additionally, there are few contraindications other than previous allergic reactions to these drugs. They have a broad spectrum of activity. Because the possible hazards of abrupt cessation of treatment, at least with larger doses, remains, compliance is especially important. However, the incidence of the withdrawal overshoot of blood pressure may have sometimes been overestimated.

α_1-RECEPTOR BLOCKING DRUGS

The α-receptor inhibitory drugs that have been evaluated in hypertension can be divided into those that are noncompetitive (e.g., phenoxybenzamine) and those that are competitive. The competitive agents may be further divided into nonselective (i.e., α_1 and α_2 block) and α_1-selective drugs. The noncompetitive α-receptor–blocking drugs, whether used alone or in combination, are associated with a fall in blood pressure on standing and other physiologic conditions requiring increased α_1-mediated vasoconstriction to maintain the blood pressure. The noncompetitive nature of the blockade prevents any compensatory vasoconstrictor impulses (to the erect posture, for instance) leading to any vasoconstriction because the receptor is blocked with no reversal in response to increased stimulus possible.[6] If the block is competitive, the increased sympathetic traffic associated with standing and other factors may result in some reversal of the α-receptor inhibition so that a postural fall of blood pressure may not so readily be seen. However, at a high drug dosage, even the competitive block may be great enough to prevent sufficient compensatory vasoconstriction, and therefore a fall in blood pressure may then occur on standing.[111]

Several α_1-blocking drugs have been described and evaluated in hypertension: prazosin[112] (also see Chapter 69), terazosin[113] (also see Chapter 70), doxazosin[114, 115] (also see Chapter 72), and urapidil (see Chapter 71). The last-named drug possibly also lowers the blood pressure by mechanisms other than α-blockade.[116]

Mode of Action

α₁-Blockade lowers the blood pressure by inhibiting the action of neuronally liberated noradrenaline on the postsynaptic α₁-receptor[112-114] (also see Chapters 69, 70, and 72). The α₁-receptors mediate the influence of centrally generated sympathetic tone responsible for the control of blood pressure (see earlier). Hand vein experiments have shown some inhibitory action of the constriction activity of prostaglandin $F_{2\alpha}$ by prazosin.[117]

The useful α-blocking drugs are α₁-selective,[118] not blocking the α₂-receptor. There is thus no prejunctional α₂-receptor block cutting off the negative feedback mechanism that results in an increased noradrenaline output that would antagonize the postjunctional α₁-blockade, resulting in a tachycardia from increased β-receptor stimulation, and likewise increased renin release[112-114] (also see Chapter 69). Some acute studies, however, have shown an increase in heart rate (see first-dose effect in later discussion).[112]

Renin and aldosterone levels do not appear to be affected by prazosin[112] (also see Chapter 69). Acute single-dose studies with α₁-blockade may, however, show an increase in renin and noradrenaline, in contrast with the absence of effects with prolonged administration as shown by studies with terazosin.[113] Doxazosin also has little effect on renin levels.[114] Plasma noradrenaline has been shown to be elevated with urapidil, but possibly larger doses reduce catecholamine excretion.[116]

Urapidil also is an α₁-receptor–blocking drug[116] (also see Chapter 71). There is evidence that it also has some central effect, possibly mediated by central 5-HTIA receptors (see Chapter 71). In support of a possible central action, it has been reported that single doses of urapidil lower blood pressure with some increase in heart rate, whereas higher doses reduce blood pressure but without any fall in heart rate (see Chapter 71), with no peripheral β-blocking effect occurring.[116]

Hemodynamic Effects

α₁-Receptor inhibition reduces peripheral resistance, and thus blood pressure falls. There is a reduction in vascular tone of both arteries and veins. Arteriolar dilation speeds circulation and tends to increase cardiac output, whereas venous dilation results in venous pooling and a reduction in venous return and tends to reduce cardiac output. Overall cardiac output is usually unchanged with α-blockade whether from prazosin,[12] terazosin,[113] doxazosin,[114] or urapidil[116] (also see Chapter 71).

Consequent on the absence, or relative absence, of tachycardia, presumably due to there being no presynaptic α₂-blockade, and also the reduction in afterload from α₁-blockade, prazosin has been shown to reduce myocardial oxygen consumption on exercise with no change in heart rate (see Chapter 69). Prazosin did not reduce exercise performance in hypertensive joggers. At lower levels of exercise, diastolic pressure was reduced, whereas systolic blood pressure was not reduced in contrast with atenolol, which also reduced exercise performance.[119]

Left ventricular hypertrophy is an important consequence of hypertension, and its development is associated with a worsened prognosis (see Chapter 72). There is evidence that prazosin (see Chapter 69), doxazosin,[120-122] and terazosin (see Chapter 70) cause a regression of left ventricular hypertrophy.

Fluid retention rarely occurs with prazosin (see Chapter 69). Renal blood flow and glomerular filtration rate are maintained as renal vascular resistance is reduced to balance the fall in blood pressure from prazosin (see Chapter 69). Similar findings have been reported after urapidil[116] (also see Chapter 71). An increase in blood volume and extracellular volume and a reduction in blood viscosity have been reported with prazosin. Although some investigators have not found an increase in body weight (see Chapter 69), others have observed an increase that was associated with a lesser fall of blood pressure from prazosin.[123]

Cardiovascular Reflexes

With agents such as the α₁-receptor–blocking drugs that act by interfering with vasoconstrictor tone, there is the possibility that even with competitive agents there is sufficient α₁-blockade to significantly inhibit reflex responses. Larger doses so obstruct the increased sympathetic stimulation generated by various physiologic stimuli that it is not able to overcome the inhibition sufficiently to avoid an increased fall in blood pressure. The reflexes associated with erect posture are most readily inhibited, enough to give a postural fall in blood pressure. This is seen with the first-dose phenomenon, in which the circulation is especially sensitive to α₁-blockade (see later). Although a postural drop of blood pressure is not often a clinical problem, a tendency for a lower pressure standing than supine is often seen with prazosin[124, 125] or other α₁-blocking drugs such as doxazosin[114] or urapidil.[116] Symptoms of postural hypotension such as dizziness may result in discontinuation of treatment with prazosin,[112] terazosin,[113] doxazosin,[114] and, possibly with a lower incidence, urapidil (see Chapter 71).

Clinical Use

Many trials have assessed the effect of prazosin in hypertension, although generally fewer than half of the patients in the series have been treated with prazosin alone.[112] The number of patients controlled with prazosin alone varies considerably. Turner et al.[126] achieved satisfactory control with prazosin alone in 24 of 50 hypertensive patients, whereas prazosin was used alone in only 9 of 100 patients treated for 3 years by Stokes et al.[127] Other quinazoline α-blocking drugs have been found to be effective antihypertensive agents: doxazosin[12, 114, 121, 122] and terazosin[113] (also see Chapter 70). Terazosin can be used intravenously to control the blood pressure.[128] Urapidil is also an effective antihypertensive agent (see Chapter 71), as is indoramin, another α$_1$-receptor–blocking drug that also has antihistaminergic effects that may be responsible for its not uncommon side effect of sedation.[129]

In a double-blind placebo-controlled study, terazosin titrated up to 20 mg once daily was compared with prazosin, also titrated up to the same total daily dose but given twice daily.[130] The blood pressures were assessed in 155 patients, 24 hours after terazosin and 12 hours after prazosin. The fall of diastolic blood pressure while taking terazosin (7.6 mmHg supine, 8.3 mmHg standing) was greater than after placebo (4.1 mmHg and 2.2 mmHg, respectively [$p < .05$]). The fall of supine diastolic pressure while taking prazosin (4.9 mmHg) was not significantly different from placebo, but the fall in the standing position (6.1 mmHg) was significantly greater while taking prazosin. Side effects were similar with prazosin and terazosin. Ruoff[131] showed that prazosin and terazosin gave similar falls in blood pressure when added to hydrochlorothiazide. Doxazosin, studied in a large double-blind, placebo-controlled multicenter study with dose titration between 1 and 16 mg once daily, gave similar control of the blood pressure as prazosin titrated between 0.5 and 10 mg twice daily. Falls in diastolic blood pressure 24 hours after dosage with doxazosin (average, 11.3 mg daily) were 9.1 mmHg supine and 10 mmHg standing; 12 hours after prazosin (average, 13.8 mg daily), falls were 8.6 and 10.4 mmHg, respectively, both significantly greater than the falls after placebo of 4.6 and 4.0 mmHg.[132] In another multicenter double-blind investigation, doxazosin and terazosin were found to have similar efficacy.[133] Prazosin and indoramin gave similar further falls in blood pressure when added to hydrochlorothiazide.[134] A single-blind study suggests that urapidil and prazosin are similar in efficacy.[135]

Some studies have suggested that a thiazide diuretic has a greater antihypertensive effect than prazosin,[136] but others have found a tendency for a greater fall in blood pressure after prazosin than after bendrofluazide when they were added to the treatment of patients whose hypertension was not adequately controlled with β-blockade alone.[137] Terazosin has been found similar to hydrochlorothiazide (see Chapter 70). Some, but not all, studies have indicated that doxazosin also is as efficacious as hydrochlorothiazide.[114] Urapidil appears similar in efficacy to thiazides, although some studies suggest that the latter has a slightly greater effect (see Chapter 71). Prazosin has given similar results to hydralazine in studies in which each agent was added to a diuretic, or, in other investigations, to a β-blocking drug.[112] Urapidil is similar in efficacy to dihydropyridine calcium antagonists (see Chapter 71).

Prazosin appears to give similar control of blood pressure to propranolol, atenolol, or metoprolol. Pos-sibly it has less effect than labetalol.[66] Doxazosin, overall, also gives similar control to that of various β-adrenoreceptor–blocking drugs,[114] such as atenolol.[138] Urapidil has been found to give similar blood pressure responses to various β-blockers (see Chapter 71).

Prazosin has been found to be of similar efficacy to methyldopa, clonidine,[112] and guanfacine.[105] Urapidil has been found to control hypertension in a similar number of patients as compared with methyldopa and clonidine (see Chapter 71). Studies of urapidil have shown a similar effect to captopril (see Chapter 71).

The α$_1$-blocking drugs have been evaluated in combination with a variety of drugs with useful additive effects: with diuretics[113, 139] (also see Chapter 70), calcium antagonists,[140] β-blocking drugs[141] (also see Chapter 70), and methyldopa,[139] and as part of a triple regimen with a diuretic and a β-adrenoceptor–blocking drug.[112, 142, 143]

As with many, if not all, antihypertensive drugs, it is important to employ a dose-response approach to obtain optimal results in the treatment of hypertension with α$_1$-receptor–blocking drugs. A small starting dose is particularly desirable with α$_1$-receptor–blocking drugs to avoid any first-dose effect (see later).

Blood pressure increases rapidly during the early morning to midmorning hours, a phenomenon characterized by an increase in α-adrenergic drive. There is evidence of an increase in myocardial infarction and stroke at this time in the day (see Chapter 72). Doxazosin seems to have its greatest effects during these early morning hours, although it is not known whether this is translated into special protection against cardiovascular events (see Chapter 72).

Urapidil has been found to be comparable to sodium nitroprusside or diazoxide when used intravenously to control the blood pressure in severe hypertension. Its value in preeclampsia and eclampsia has also been shown, as has its use in the control of hypertensive episodes associated with surgery (see Chapter 71).

The pharmacokinetic profile of prazosin, with a half-life of approximately 4 hours, requires multiple dosing to control the blood pressure satisfactorily throughout the day (see Chapter 69). However, the longer duration of action, with a half-life of approximately 12 hours, of the more recently introduced agents, doxazosin[114] and terazosin (see Chapter 70), allows once-daily administration.

The first-dose effect may be minimized with prazosin by taking a small dose, 0.5 to 1 mg, at bedtime. It is prudent to avoid the drug if the patient is volume depleted. A maximum of 40 mg/day may be given (see Chapter 69), but not many patients benefit from dosages higher than a total of 20 mg daily.[112] Dosage with terazosin should commence at 1 mg, also at bedtime, and increase as required up to 20 mg/day; although 40 mg has sometimes been used, the usual range is 1 to 5 mg daily[113] (also see Chapter 70). Similarly, the starting dose of doxazosin is 1 mg, with 2 to 4 mg the most usual maintenance dose; doses up to 16 mg have been used.[114] Studies with urapidil have generally used between 30 and 90 mg twice daily (see Chapter 71).

Heart Failure

A number of vasodilators have been evaluated in the treatment of congestive heart failure, including various α₁-blocking drugs. Prazosin has been found to produce hemodynamic, symptomatic improvement and to increase exercise tolerance[112] (also see Chapter 69). Tolerance may develop to the benefit from prazosin, but it can be overcome by an increase in dose or by the addition of spironolactone to the treatment.[112] Preliminary studies with terazosin (see Chapter 70) and urapidil[144] show similar results.

Benign Prostatic Hypertrophy

Approximately 40% of the prostate in benign prostatic hypertrophy is smooth muscle where α-receptors are abundant. Terazosin has been found to improve symptoms in more than 90% of patients, and 40% to 50% show improvement in peak and mean urine flow rates. This effect from α₁-blockade is most useful in acute retention and in poor surgical candidates (see Chapter 70).

Effect on Lipids and Other Metabolic Parameters

Certain changes in the lipid profile indicate an increased risk of cardiovascular disease[114] (also see Chapters 69 and 72), which is favorably affected by α₁-blocking drugs. The mechanisms involved have been discussed in detail[145] (also see Chapter 72).

Prazosin has been reported to reduce triglyceride[146–148] or to have no effect[146–151] and to reduce LDL and VLDL, increasing the cholesterol ratio.[146–150, 152] Serum cholesterol is lowered.[150] Lithell et al.,[153] however, did not observe any change in the lipids in a 1-year study of prazosin in postmenopausal women. Prazosin has been found to decrease lipid deposition in the aorta of cholesterol-fed rabbits, as does propranolol.[154] Cholesterol, the LDL, and the VLDL lipoprotein fraction all are decreased significantly, HDL is raised, and the cholesterol ratio is increased by terazosin[152, 155] (also see Chapter 70). Doxazosin also increases HDL and the HDL/total cholesterol ratio and decreases total cholesterol and triglyceride levels[114, 122, 145, 156] (also see Chapter 72). There is overall reduction in coronary risk factors with doxazosin as compared with atenolol[156] or enalapril.[157] Doxazosin also improves activity of the fibrinolytic system in contrast to atenolol.[158] It also appears that urapidil has a favorable effect on the lipid profile, reducing total cholesterol, triglycerides, and LDL cholesterol, with a small increase in HDL levels (see Chapter 71).

In contrast with some other antihypertensive drugs, α₁-blocking drugs do not adversely affect glucose or urate metabolism[112] (also see Chapters 69, 70, and 72); indeed, an improved metabolic clearance of glucose has been found in hypertensive non-insulin-dependent diabetic patients.[159] Glucose and insulin levels were reduced in nondiabetic hypertensive patients with doxazosin.[160]

Side Effects

Potentially the most important side effects induced by α₁-receptor blockers are those associated with too much inhibition of the α-receptor, principally postural hypotension. Too rapid a commencement of α-receptor inhibition produces the first-dose phenomenon[112] (also see Chapter 69) that was of considerable trouble in the early stages of the use of prazosin. The first-dose phenomenon is the occurrence, after the first dose, of symptoms of severe postural hypotension.[124, 161, 162] Loss of consciousness occurred in several instances, so that a specific effect on cerebral blood flow was suggested; however, prazosin does not appear to alter cerebral blood flow.[163] This first-dose phenomenon shows some dose dependence.[124, 162] The use of a low commencing dose of 0.5 mg, particularly if given just before bedtime, is likely to result in only minimal dizziness, if any, and to eliminate any first-dose phenomenon.[112] When prazosin is chronically administered, there is probably an increase in systemic blood volume,[164] and excessive sensitivity to the α-blockade declines. Certain maneuvers, besides a low commencing dose, influence the first-dose phenomenon. A low-sodium diet provokes, and a high-sodium diet abolishes, the phenomenon.[124] The previous administration of a diuretic or a β-adrenoceptor–blocking drug may increase the fall of blood pressure associated with the initial dose of prazosin.[112, 165] The first-dose phenomenon appears uncommon with terazosin[142] or urapidil (see Chapter 71).

Symptoms of orthostatic hypotension from prazosin[112] vary and greatly depend on how carefully increments of dose are made. The reported incidence from prazosin is approximately 10% to 20%.[112] There is an excess incidence of dizziness with terazosin over placebo of approximately 10%, and when results from double-blind trials were pooled, it was reported that 3.2% of patients withdrew because of dizziness.[113] The incidence of dizziness with doxazosin is probably similar.[114] Dizziness is possibly seen in approximately 5% of patients treated with urapidil (see Chapter 71). Peripheral edema may occur, as with other vasodilators; an incidence of 4% greater than placebo has been reported with terazosin.[166] The α₁-receptor–blocking drugs have, otherwise, a relatively low incidence of side effects (see Chapter 69). In a large study, 9.2% of the terazosin patients withdrew from therapy because of side effects, compared with 3.9% receiving placebo.[166]

Nausea has been reported to occur in approximately 5% of patients receiving prazosin[112] or terazosin,[176] possibly slightly less in patients receiving doxazosin[114] or urapidil (see Chapter 71).

Lack of energy, drowsiness, and weakness have an incidence of approximately 7% in patients receiving prazosin according to Stanaszek et al.,[112] and a similar incidence has been found with terazosin.[166] However, exercise tolerance does not appear to be limited by α_1-blockade.[3] Sexual dysfunction is relatively rare (3.2%) and has been reported with doxazosin.[114] Impotence occurs less with prazosin than with hydrochlorothiazide.[167] Fatigue has been reported in 1.4% of patients receiving urapidil (see Chapter 71).

Overall, side effects are probably less with prazosin than with methyldopa or clonidine. Some studies support a similar overall incidence to hydralazine, but with orthostatic symptoms, sexual dysfunction, and nightmares reported more often with prazosin.[112] The overall incidence of side effects with prazosin and terazosin[113] or doxazosin[114] appears similar. Side effect incidences with atenolol and doxazosin were found to be similar, but more patients were withdrawn from doxazosin.[114]

Other side effects are relatively minor and compare favorably with other antihypertensive drugs.[112] No withdrawal reaction after stopping α_1-receptor–inhibitory drugs would be expected, and this has indeed been shown to be the case after stopping terazosin.[131]

Place of α_1-Receptor–Blocking Drugs in Antihypertensive Treatment

The α-blocking drugs have three possible important advantages in the treatment of hypertension: their hemodynamic profile, the relative ease of patient selection, and the apparent absence of long-term adverse metabolic side effects, in fact a favorable effect on lipid profiles.

The α-receptor–inhibitory drugs reverse the pathologic hemodynamic changes of hypertensive patients toward those seen in normotensive subjects, the main change being a reduction in peripheral resistance. Unlike some other first-line antihypertensive drugs, they increase HDL, improve the HDL/LDL cholesterol ratio, and have other favorable effects on lipid profile.

Provided care is taken to minimize the first-dose phenomenon, particularly in susceptible patients, such as the elderly, there are no problems in patient selection. Important contraindications to β-adrenoceptor–blocking drugs are not present. α-Blocking drugs do not cause heart failure in susceptible patients; on the contrary, they are useful in its treatment. Similarly, they do not worsen asthma; in fact, they may have a modest antiasthmatic effect.[112] α-Blocking drugs increase peripheral blood flow[168] and have been used in treatment of Raynaud's phenomenon.[169]

CONCLUSIONS

Reduction of vascular tone by inhibition of the innervation of the α-adrenergic receptor became an important mode of action to lower the blood pressure in the treatment of hypertension with the advent of methyldopa and adrenergic neurone inhibitory drugs.[71] These latter drugs are now seldom used. Methyldopa is employed much less than previously, because it appears to have more side effects than

many alternative treatments. Because most patients can have their blood pressure lowered by several distinctive pharmacologic approaches, side effects and difference in quality of life between drugs become more important. It appears that methyldopa does not score well in this respect.[170]

Clonidine, a central α_2-stimulant drug, has a high incidence of sedation, and it has not been generally regarded as a first-line drug. It may be that some recently described analogues have succeeded in dissociating central sedative and antihypertensive effects.

Provided that care is taken with initial dosage and that the dosage is not sufficiently high to prevent increases in α-adrenergic tone required to compensate for the erect posture, the α_1-receptor–blocking drugs are well tolerated. They have a favorable effect on lipid profile, patient selection is relatively simple, they are often suitable as first-line agents, and they have become more widely used in recent years.[10]

REFERENCES

1. Prichard BNC, Owens CWI: Drug treatment of hypertension. *In* Genest J, Kuchel O, Hamet P, Cantin M (eds): Hypertension: Physiology and Treatment, 2nd ed. New York: McGraw-Hill, 1983, pp 1171–1210.
2. Weber MA, Drayer JI: Single-agent and combination therapy of essential hypertension. Am Heart J 108:311, 1984.
3. Swales JD: Overview of essential hypertension. *In* Swales JD (ed): Textbook of Hypertension. London: Blackwell, 1994, pp 655–660.
4. Ward R: Familial aggregation and genetic epidemiology of blood pressure. *In* Laragh JH, Brenner BM (eds): Hypertension: Pathophysiology, Diagnosis and Management, 2nd ed. New York: Raven, 1995, pp 67–88.
5. Wilson PWF, Kannel WB: Hypertension, other risk factors, and the risk of cardiovascular disease. *In* Laragh JH, Brenner BM (eds): Hypertension: Pathophysiology, Diagnosis and Management, 2nd ed. New York: Raven, 1995, pp 99–114.
6. Beilin LJ, Juel-Jensen BE: Alpha and beta adrenergic blockade in hypertension. Lancet 1:979, 1972.
7. Prichard BNC, Johnston AW, Hill ID, Rosenheim ML: Bethanidine, guanethidine, and methyldopa in treatment of hypertension: A within-patient comparison. Br Med J 1:135, 1968.
8. Boura ALA, Green AF: Adrenergic neurone blockade and other acute effects caused by N-benzyl-N'N''-dimethyl guanidine and its ortho-chloro derivative. Br J Pharmacol 20:36, 1963.
9. Tarazi RC, Conway J: The haemodynamics of hypertension. *In* Genest J, Kuchel O, Hamet P, Cantin M (eds): Hypertension: Physiopathology and Treatment, 2nd ed. New York: McGraw-Hill, 1983, pp 15–42.
10. Kaplan NM: Clinical Hypertension, 6th ed. Baltimore: Williams & Wilkins, 1994.
11. Julius S: The changing relationship between autonomic control and haemodynamics of hypertension. *In* Swales JD (ed): Textbook of Hypertension. London: Blackwell, 1994, pp 77–84.
12. Lund-Johansen P, Omvik P, Haugland H: Acute and chronic haemodynamic effects of doxazosin in hypertension at rest and during exercise. Br J Clin Pharmacol 21(Suppl 1):45S, 1986.
13. Baum T: Fundamental principles governing regulation of circulatory function. *In* Antonaccio MJ (ed): Cardiovascular Pharmacology, 2nd ed. New York: Raven Press, 1984, pp 1–34.
14. Guyton AC, Coleman TG, Cowley AW Jr, et al: A systems analysis approach to understanding long-range arterial blood pressure control and hypertension. Circ Res 35:159, 1974.
15. DiBona GF, Kopp UC: Neural control of renal function: Role in human hypertension. *In* Laragh JH, Brenner BM (eds):

Hypertension: Pathophysiology, Diagnosis and Treatment, 2nd ed. New York, Raven Press, 1995.

16. Antonaccio MJ: Central transmitters: Physiology, pharmacology and effects on the circulation. *In* Antonaccio MJ (ed): Cardiovascular Pharmacology. New York: Raven Press, 1984, pp 155–195.

17. Korner PI, Badoer E, Head GA: Neural transmitters and central mechanisms in primary hypertension. *In* Kaufmann W, Bönner G, Lang R, Meurer KA (eds): Primary Hypertension. Berlin: Springer-Verlag, 1986, pp 38–52.

18. Ganten D, Luft FC, Lang RE, et al: Brain peptides in cardiovascular regulation. *In* Kaufmann W, Bönner G, Lang R, Meurer KA (eds): Primary Hypertension. Berlin: Springer-Verlag, 1986, pp 53–61.

19. Pickel VM, Joh TH, Reis DJ: A serotonergic innervation of noradrenergic neurons in nucleus locus coeruleus: Demonstration by immunocytochemical localization of the transmitter specific enzymes tyrosine and tryptophan hydroxylase. Brain Res 131:197, 1977.

20. Chalmers JP, West MJ: The nervous system in the pathogenesis of essential hypertension. *In* Robertson JIS (ed): Handbook of Hypertension, Vol 1: Clinical Aspects of Essential Hypertension. Amsterdam: Elsevier, 1983, pp 64–96.

21. Prichard BNC, Gillam PMS: Assessment of propranolol in angina pectoris: Clinical dose response curve and effect on electrocardiogram at rest and on exercise. Br Heart J 33:473, 1971.

22. Langer SZ, Duval N, Massingham R: Pharmacologic and therapeutic significance of alpha-adrenoceptor subtypes. J Cardiovasc Pharmacol 7(Suppl 8):S1, 1985.

23. van Zwieten PA, Jie K, Van Brummelen P: Post synaptic α_1- and α_2-adrenoceptor changes in hypertension. J Cardiovasc Pharmacol 10(Suppl 4):S68, 1987.

24. Langer SZ, Hicks PE: Alpha-adrenoreceptor subtypes in blood vessels: Physiology and pharmacology. J Cardiovasc Pharmacol 6(Suppl 4):S547, 1984.

25. Langer SZ, Shepperson NB: Recent developments in vascular and smooth muscle pharmacology: The postsynaptic alpha2-adrenoceptor. Trends Pharmacol Sci 3:440, 1982.

26. Huchet AM, Doursout MF, Chelly J, Schmitt H: Possible role of central α_1-adrenoceptors in the control of the autonomic nervous system in normotensive and spontaneously hypertensive rats. Eur J Pharmacol 85:239, 1982.

27. Bousquet P, Feldman J, Tibirica E, et al: New concepts on the central regulation of blood pressure: Alpha$_2$-adrenoceptors and "imidazoline receptors." Am J Med 87:10S, 1989.

28. Reis DJ, Regunathan S, Meeley MP: Imidazole receptors and clonidine-displacing substance in relationship to control of blood pressure, neuroprotection and adrenomedullary secretion. Am J Hypertens 5:51S, 1992.

29. Hamilton CA: Adrenergic and nonadrenergic effects of imidazoline and related antihypertensive drugs in the brain and periphery. Am J Hypertens 5:58S, 1992.

30. Haxhiu MA, Dreshaj I, Schafer SG, Ernsberger P: Selective antihypertensive action of moxonidine is mediated mainly by I$_1$-imidazoline receptors in the rostral ventrolateral medulla. J Cardiovasc Pharmacol 24(Suppl 1):S1, 1994.

31. Gillis RA, Gatti PJ, Quest JA: Mechanism of the antihypertensive effect of alpha$_2$-agonists. J Cardiovasc Pharmacol 7(Suppl 8):S38, 1985.

32. Guyenet PG, Cabot JB: Inhibition of sympathetic preganglionic neurones by catecholamines and clonidine: Mediation by an alpha-adrenergic receptor. J Neurosci 1:908, 1981.

33. Reid JL, Wing LMH, Mathias CJ, et al: The central hypotensive effect of clonidine: Studies in tetraplegic subjects. Clin Pharmacol Ther 21:375, 1977.

34. Levine RJ, Sjoerdsma A: Dissociation of the decarboxylase-inhibiting and norepinephrine-depleting effects of α-methyldopa, α-ethyldopa, 4-bromo-3-hydroxy-benzyloxyamine and related substance. J Pharmacol Exp Ther 146:42, 1964.

35. Gillespie L Jr, Oates JA, Crout JR, Sjoerdsma A: Clinical and chemical studies with α-methyl-dopa in patients with hypertension. Circulation 25:281, 1962.

36. Day MD, Rand MJ: A hypothesis for the mode of action of α-methyldopa in relieving hypertension. J Pharm Pharmacol 15:221, 1963.

37. Trinker FR: The significance of the relative potencies of nor-adrenaline and α-methyl-noradrenaline for the mode of action of α-methyldopa. J Pharm Pharmacol 23:306, 1971.

38. Coupar IM, Turner P: Relative potencies of some false transmitters on isolated human smooth muscle. Br J Pharmacol 38:463P, 1970.

39. Day MD, Rand MJ: Some observations on the pharmacology of α-methyldopa. Br J Pharmacol 22:72, 1964.

40. Haefely W, Hurlimann A, Thoenen H: Adrenergic transmitter changes and response to sympathetic nerve stimulation after differing pretreatment with α-methyldopa. Br J Pharmacol 31:105, 1967.

41. Henning M, van Zwieten PA: Central hypotensive effect of α-methyldopa. J Pharm Pharmacol 20:409, 1968.

42. Ingenito AJ, Barrett JP, Procita L: A centrally mediated peripheral hypotensive effect of α-methyldopa. J Pharmacol Exp Ther 175:593, 1970.

43. Baum T, Shropshire AT, Varner LL: Contribution of the central nervous system to the action of several antihypertensive agents (methyldopa, hydralazine and guanethidine). J Pharmacol Exp Ther 182:135, 1972.

44. Struthers AD, Brown MJ, Adams EF, Dollery CT: The plasma noradrenaline and growth hormone response to alpha-methyldopa and clonidine in hypertensive subjects. Br J Clin Pharmacol 19:311, 1985.

45. Bobik A, Jennings G, Jackman G, et al: Evidence for a predominantly central hypotensive effect of alpha-methyldopa in humans. Hypertension 8:16, 1986.

46. Carlsson A, Lindqvist M: In-vivo decarboxylation of α-methyldopa and α-methyl metatyrosine. Acta Physiol Scand 54:87, 1962.

47. Henning M, Rubenson A: Evidence that the hypotensive action of methyldopa is mediated by central actions of methyl-noradrenaline. J Pharm Pharmcol 23:407, 1971.

48. Frohlich ED: Methyldopa—mechanisms and treatment 25 years later. Arch Intern Med 140:954, 1980.

49. Heise A, Kroneberg G: α-Sympathetic receptor stimulation in the brain and hypotensive activity of α-methyldopa. Eur J Pharmacol 17:315, 1972.

50. Finch L, Haeusler G: Further evidence for a central hypotensive action of α-methyldopa in both the rat and cat. Br J Pharmacol 47:217, 1973.

51. Sjoerdsma A, Vendsalu A, Engelman K: Studies on the metabolism and mechanism of action of methyldopa. Circulation 28:492, 1963.

52. Uretsky NJ, Iversen LL: Effects of 6-hydroxydopamine on catecholamine containing neurones in the rat brain. J Neurochem 17:269, 1970.

53. Korner PI, Head GA, Bobik A, et al: Central and peripheral autonomic mechanisms involved in the circulatory actions of methyldopa. Hypertension 6(5):II63, 1984.

54. Leonetti G, Terzoli L, Morganti A, et al: Relation between the hypotensive and renin-suppressing activities of alpha-methyldopa in hypertensive patients. Am J Cardiol 40:762, 1977.

55. Mason DT, Braunwald L: Effects of guanethidine, reserpine, and methyldopa on reflex venous and arterial constriction in man. J Clin Invest 43:1449, 1964.

56. Lund-Johansen P: Hemodynamic changes in long term α-methyldopa therapy of essential hypertension. Acta Med Scand 192:221, 1972.

57. Onesti G, Brest AN, Novack P, et al: Pharmacodynamic effects of α-methyldopa in hypertensive subjects. Am Heart J 67:32, 1964.

58. Chamberlain DA, Howard J: Guanethidine and methyldopa: A haemodynamic study. Br Heart J 26:528, 1964.

59. Oates JA, Seligmann AW, Clark MA, et al: The relative efficacy of guanethidine, methyldopa, and pargyline as antihypertensive agents. N Engl J Med 273:729, 1965.

60. Wilson WR, Fisher FD, Kirkendall WM: The acute hemodynamic effects of α-methyldopa in man. J Chronic Dis 15:907, 1961.

61. Dollery CT, Harington M, Hodge JV: Haemodynamic studies with methyldopa: Effect on cardiac output and response to pressor amines. Br Heart J 25:670, 1963.

62. Prichard BNC, Gillam PMS, Graham BR: Beta receptor antagonism in hypertension: Comparison with the effect of adrenergic neurone inhibition on cardiovascular responses. Int J Clin Pharmacol 4:131, 1970.

63. Johnson P, Kitchin AH, Lowther CP, Turner RWD: Treatment of hypertension with methyldopa. Br Med J 1:133, 1966.

64. Prichard BNC, Boakes AJ, Graham BR: A within patient comparison of bethanidine, methyldopa and propranolol in the treatment of hypertension. Clin Sci Mol Med 51(Suppl 3):567S, 1976.

65. Hamilton M, Kopelman H: Treatment of severe hypertension with methyldopa. Br Med J 1:151, 1963.

66. Cruickshank JM, Prichard BNC: Beta-Blockers in Clinical Practice, 2nd ed. New York: Churchill Livingstone, 1994.

67. Smirk H: Hypotensive action of methyldopa. Br Med J 1:146, 1963.

68. Dollery CT, Hartley K, Bulpitt PF, et al: Fifteen year survival of patients beginning treatment with methyldopa between 1962 and 1966. Hypertension 6(5):II82, 1984.

69. Lowe SA, Rubin PC: The pharmacological management of hypertension in pregnancy. J Hypertens 10:201, 1992.

70. Lindheimer MD: Hypertension in pregnancy. Hypertension 22:127, 1993.

71. Prichard BNC, Owens CWI, Tuckman J: Clinical features of adrenergic agonists and antagonists. In Szekeres L (ed): Handbook of Experimental Pharmacology, Vol 54, part 2. Berlin: Springer-Verlag, 1981, pp 559–697.

72. Lawson DH, Gloss D, Jick H: Adverse reactions to methyldopa with particular reference to hypotension. Am Heart J 96:572, 1978.

73. Franks PJ, Hartley K, Bulpitt PF, et al: Mortality in patients who have their antihypertensive therapy changed. J Hypertens 7:577, 1989.

74. Shneerson JM, Gazzard BG: Reversible malabsorption caused by methyldopa. Br Med J 2:1456, 1977.

75. Carstairs KC, Breckenridge A, Dollery CT, Worlledge SM: Incidence of a positive direct Coombs Test in patients on α-methyldopa. Lancet 2:133, 1966.

76. Worlledge SM, Carstairs KC, Dacie JV: Autoimmune haemolytic anaemia associated with α-methyldopa therapy. Lancet 2:135, 1966.

77. Croog SH, Levine S, Testa MA, et al: The effects of antihypertensive therapy on the quality of life. N Engl J Med 314:1657, 1986.

78. van Zwieten PA, Thoolen JMC, Timmermans PBMWM: The hypotensive activity and side-effects of α-methyldopa, clonidine and guanfacine. Hypertension 6(Suppl 2):28, 1984.

79. Weiner N: Drugs that inhibit adrenergic nerves and block adrenergic receptors. In Gilman AG, Goodman LS, Rall TW, Murad F (eds): The Pharmacological Basis of Therapeutics, 7th ed. New York: Macmillan, 1985, pp 181–214.

80. Kobinger W, Pichler L: Localization in the CNS of adrenoceptors which facilitate a cardioinhibitory reflex. Naunyn Schmiedebergs Arch Pharmacol 286:371, 1975.

81. Shaw J, Hunyor SN, Korner PI: The peripheral circulatory effects of clonidine and their role in the production of arterial hypotension. Eur J Pharmacol 14:101, 1971.

82. Langley MS, Heel RC: Transdermal clonidine: A preliminary review of its pharmacodynamic properties and therapeutic efficacy. Drugs 35:123, 1988.

83. Sorkin EM, Heel RC: Guanfacine: A review of its pharmacodynamic and pharmacokinetic properties, and therapeutic efficacy in the treatment of hypertension. Drugs 31:301, 1986.

84. Koshiji M, Ito H, Minatoguchi S, et al: A comparison of guanfacine, bunazosin, atenolol and nadolol on blood pressure and plasma noradrenaline responses to cold pressor testing. Clin Exp Pharm Physiol 19:481, 1992.

85. Haeusler G: Clonidine-induced inhibition of sympathetic nerve activity: No indication for a central presynaptic or an indirect sympathomimetic mode of action. Naunyn Schmiedebergs Arch Pharmacol 286:97, 1974.

86. Finch L: The central hypotensive action of clonidine and BAY 1470 in cats and rats. Clin Sci Mol Med 48:273S, 1975.

87. Von Hoefke W, Kobinger W: Pharmakologische Wirkungen des 2-(2,6-Dichloro-phenyl-amino)-2-Imidazolin-Hydrochlorids einer neuen, antihypertensiven substanz. Arzneimittelforschung 16:1038, 1966.

88. Rand MJ, Wilson J: Mechanisms of the pressor and depressor actions of ST 155 (2(2,6-Dichlorophenylamine-)-2-imidazoline hydrochloride, catapres). Eur J Pharmacol 3:27, 1968.

89. Houston MC: Clonidine hydrochloride: Review of pharmacologic and clinical aspects. Prog Cardiovasc Dis 23:337, 1981.

90. Rudd P, Blaschke TF: Antihypertensive drugs and the drug therapy of hypertension. In Gilman AG, Goodman LS, Rall TW, Murad F (eds): The Pharmacological Basis of Therapeutics, 7th ed. New York: Macmillan, 1985, pp 784–805.

91. Frisk-Holmberg M, Paalzow L, Wibell L: Relationship between the cardiovascular effects and steady-state kinetics of clonidine in hypertension. Eur J Clin Pharmacol 26:309, 1984.

92. Mosqueda-Garcia R: Guanfacine: A second generation alpha₂ adrenergic blocker. Am J Med Sci 299:73, 1990.

93. Holmes B, Brogden RN, Heel RC, et al: Guanabenz: A review of its pharmacodynamic properties and therapeutic efficacy in hypertension. Drugs 26:212, 1983.

94. Bousquet P, Feldman J, Schwartz J: Central cardiovascular effects of alpha adrenergic drugs: Differences between catecholamines and imidazolines. J Pharmacol Exp Ther 253:232, 1984.

95. Ernsberger P, Meeley MP, Mann JJ, Reis DJ: Clonidine binds to imidazole binding sites as well as alpha₂ adrenoceptors in the ventrolateral medulla. Eur J Pharmacol 134:1, 1987.

96. Gomez RE, Ernsberger P, Feinland G, Reis DJ: Rilmenidine lowers arterial pressure via imidazole receptors in brainstem C1 area. Eur J Pharmacol 195:181, 1991.

97. Bousquet P, Feldman J, Tibirica E, et al: Imidazoline receptors—a new concept in central regulation of the arterial blood pressure. Am J Hypertens 5:47S, 1992.

98. Walter D, Harron G: Distinctive features of rilmenidine possibly related to its selectivity for imidazoline receptors. Am J Hypertens 5:91S, 1992.

99. Allan DR, Penner SB, Smyth DD: Renal imidazoline preferring sites and solute excretion in the rat. Br J Pharmacol 108:870, 1993.

100. Onesti G, Schwartz AB, Kim KE, et al: Pharmacodynamic effects of a new antihypertensive drug, catapres (ST 155). Circulation 39:219, 1969.

101. Brod J, Horbach L, Just H, et al: Acute effects of clonidine on central and peripheral haemodynamics and plasma renin activity. Eur J Clin Pharmacol 4:107, 1972.

102. Messerli FH, Oren S, Grossman E: Left ventricular hypertrophy and antihypertensive therapy. Drugs 35(Suppl 5):27, 1988.

103. Graettinger WF, Cheung DG, Weber MA: Clonidine. In Messerli FH (ed): Cardiovascular Drug Therapy. Philadelphia: WB Saunders, 1990, pp 652–659.

104. Onesti G, Schwartz AB, Kim KE, et al: Antihypertensive effect of clonidine. Circ Res 28(Suppl 2):53, 1971.

105. Lewin A, Alderman MH, Mathur P: Antihypertensive efficacy of guanfacine and prazosin in patients with mild to moderate essential hypertension. J Clin Pharmacol 30:1081, 1990.

106. Ollivier J-P, Christen MO: I₁-imidazoline receptor agonists in the treatment of hypertension: An appraisal of clinical experience. J Cardiovasc Pharmacol 24(Suppl 1):S39, 1994.

107. Lambert AE, Mpoy M, Vandeleene B, Ketelslegers J-M: Treatment of hypertension in diabetic patients. Am J Med 87:30S, 1989.

108. Jerrie P: Clinical experience with guanfacine in long-term treatment of hypertension. Part II: Adverse reactions to guanfacine. Br J Clin Pharmacol 10(Suppl 1):157, 1980.

109. Mahieux F: Rilmenidine and vigilance: Review of clinical studies. Am J Med 87:67S, 1989.

110. Fletcher AE, Beevers DG, Dollery CT, et al: The effects of two centrally-acting anti-hypertensive drugs on the quality of life. Eur J Clin Pharmacol 41:397, 1991.

111. Prichard BNC, Boakes AJ: Labetalol in long-term treatment of hypertension. Br J Clin Pharmacol 3(Suppl 3):743, 1976.

112. Stanaszek WF, Kellerman D, Brogden RN, Romankiewicz JA: Prazosin update: A review of its pharmacological properties and therapeutic use in hypertension and congestive heart failure. Drugs 25:339, 1983.

113. Titmarsh S, Monk JP: Terazosin: A review of its pharmacodynamic and pharmacokinetic properties, and therapeutic efficacy in essential hypertension. Drugs 33:461, 1987.

114. Young RA, Brogden RN: Doxazosin: A review of its pharmaco-dynamic and pharmacokinetic properties, and therapeutic efficacy in mild or moderate hypertension. Drugs 35:525, 1988.

115. Babamoto KS, Hirokawa WT: Doxazosin: A new alpha₁ adrenergic antagonist. Clin Pharm 11:415, 1992.

116. Prichard BNC, Tomlinson B, Renondin JC: Urapidil, a multiple-action alpha blocking drug. Am J Cardiol 64:11D, 1989.

117. Beermann C, Schloos J, Belz GG: Oral administration of carvedilol and prazosin inhibits the prostaglandin F2a and noradrenaline-induced contraction of human hand veins in vivo. Clin Investig 70:S13, 1992.

118. Graham RM: Selective alpha₁-adrenergic antagonists: Therapeutically relevant antihypertenslve agents. Am J Cardiol 53:16A, 1984.

119. Thompson PD, Cullinane EM, Nugent AM, et al: Effect of atenolol or prazosin on maximal exercise performance in hypertensive joggers. Am J Med 86(Suppl lB):104, 1989.

120. Agabiti-Rosei E, Muiesan ML, Rizzoni D, et al: Reduction of left ventricular hypertrophy after longterm antihypertensive treatment with doxazosin. J Hum Hypertens 6:9, 1992.

121. Taylor SH: Efficacy of doxazosin in specific hypertensive patient groups. Am Heart J 121:286, 1991.

122. TOMHS—Treatment of Mild Hypertension Study: Final results. JAMA 270:713, 1993.

123. Izzo JL, Horwitz D, Keiser HR: Physiologic mechanisms opposing the hemodynamic effects of prazosin. Clin Pharmacol Ther 29(1):7, 1981.

124. Stokes GS, Graham RM, Gain JM, Davis PR: Influence of dosage and dietary sodium on the first-dose effects of prazosin. Br Med J 1:1507, 1977.

125. MacCarthy EP, Thornell IR, Stokes GS: Prazosin: Long-term therapy of hypertension. J Cardiovasc Med 6(Suppl):70, 1981.

126. Turner AS, Watson OF, Brocklehurst JE: Prazosin in hypertension. Part I: Clinical experience in 100 patients. N Z Med J 86:282, 1977.

127. Stokes GS, Gain JM, Mahony JF, et al: Long-term use of prazosin in combination or alone for treating hypertension. Med J Aust Special Supplement 2:13, 1977.

128. Cohen A: Efficacy and safety of intravenous terazosin in hypertensive patients: A preliminary report. Am J Med 80(Suppl 5B):86, 1986.

129. Holmes B, Sorkin EM: Indoramin: A review of its pharmacodynamic and pharmacokinetic properties, and therapeutic efficacy in hypertension and related vascular, cardiovascular and airway diseases. Drugs 31:467, 1986.

130. Deger G: Comparison of the safety and efficacy of once-daily terazosin versus twice-daily prazosin for the treatment of mild to moderate hypertension. Am J Med 80(Suppl 5B):62, 1986.

131. Ruoff G: Comparative trials of terazosin with other antihypertensive agents. Am J Med 80(Suppl 5B):42, 1986.

132. Torvik D, Madsbu H-P: Multicentre 12-week double-blind comparison of doxazosin, prazosin and placebo in patients with mild to moderate essential hypertension. Br J Clin Pharmacol 21(Suppl 1):69S, 1986.

133. Hayduk K, Schneider HT: Antihypertensive effects of doxazosin in systemic hypertension and comparison with terazosin. Am J Cardiol 59:95G, 1987.

134. Overlack A, Stumpe KO: Comparison of the effect of indoramin and prazosin in blood pressure and lipid profiles in essential hypertension. J Cardiovasc Pharmacol 8(Suppl 2):S53, 1986.

135. Kaneko Y, and The Urapidil Study Group in Japan: Double blind comparison of urapidil and prazosin in the treatment of patients with essential hypertension. Drugs 35(Suppl 6):156, 1988.

136. Schirger A, Sheps SG: Prazosin—new hypertensive agent: A double-blind crossover study in the treatment of hypertension. JAMA 237:989, 1977.

137. Marshall AJ, Pocock J, Barritt DW, Heaton ST: Evaluation of beta blockade, bendrofluazide, and prazosin in severe hypertension. Lancet 1:271, 1977.

138. Talseth T, Westlie L, Daae L: Doxazosin and atenolol as monotherapy in mild and moderate hypertension: A randomized, parallel study with a three-year follow-up. Am Heart J 121:280, 1991.

139. Stokes GS: Prazosin. *In* Doyle AE (ed): Handbook of Hypertension, Vol 5: Clinical Pharmacology of Antihypertensive Drugs. Amsterdam: Elsevier Science Publishers, 1984, pp 350–375.

140. Donnelly R, Elliott HL, Meredith PA, et al: Combination of nifedipine and doxazosin in essential hypertension. J Cardiovasc Pharmacol 19:479, 1992.

141. Lund-Johansen P: Haemodynamic long-term effects of prazosin plus tolamolol in essential hypertension. Br J Clin Pharmacol 4:141, 1977.

142. Pool JL: Terazosin. *In* Messerli FH (ed): Cardiovascular Drug Therapy. Philadelphia: WB Saunders, 1990, pp 698–707.

143. de Planque BA: A double-blind comparative study of doxazosin and prazosin when administered with β-blockers or diuretics. Am Heart J 121:304, 1991.

144. Messerli FH: Haemodynamic effects of urapidil in arterial hypertension and congestive heart failure. Drugs 35(Suppl 6):70, 1988.

145. Pool JL: Effects of doxazosin on serum lipids: A review of the clinical data and molecular basis for altered lipid metabolism. Am Heart J 121:251, 1991.

146. Leren P, Eide I, Foss OP, et al: Antihypertensive drugs and blood lipids: The Oslo Study. J Cardiovasc Pharmacol 4(Suppl 2):S222, 1982.

147. Velasco M, Silva H, Morillo J, et al: Effect of prazosin on blood lipids and on thyroid function in hypertensive patients. J Cardiovasc Pharmacol 4(Suppl 2):S225, 1982.

148. Goto Y, Tanabe T, Ogasawara Y, et al: The effects of prazosin and propranolol in combination with thiazide diuretics on blood pressure and serum lipids: A multicentre study. Eur J Clin Pharmacol 33:339, 1987.

149. Kokubu T, Itoh I, Kurita H, et al: Effect of prazosin on serum lipids. J Cardiovasc Pharmacol 14(Suppl 2):S228, 1982.

150. Velasco M, Silva H, Feldstein E, et al: Effects of prazosin and alpha-methyldopa on blood lipids and lipoproteins in hypertensive patients. Eur J Clin Pharmacol 28:513, 1985.

151. Havard CWH, Khokhar AM, Flax JS: Open assessment of the effect of prazosin on plasma lipids. J Cardiovasc Pharmacol 4(Suppl 2):S238, 1982.

152. Deger G: Effect of terazosin on serum lipids. Am J Med 80(Suppl 5B):82, 1986.

153. Lithell H, Waern U, Vessby B: Effect of prazosin on lipoprotein metabolism in premenopausal, hypertensive women. J Cardiovasc Pharmacol 4(Suppl 2):S242, 1982.

154. Blau A, Neusy AJ, Lowenstein J: The effects of propranolol and prazosin on plasma lipids and aortic atherosclerosis in cholesterol-fed rabbits. J Hypertens (Suppl 5):S485, 1986.

155. Holtzmann JL, Kaihlanen PM, Rider JA, et al: Concomitant administration of terazosin and atenolol for the treatment of essential hypertension. Arch Intern Med 148:539, 1988.

156. Carruthers G, Dessain P, Fodor G, et al: Comparative trial of doxazosin and atenolol on cardiovascular risk reduction in systemic hypertension. The Alpha Beta Canada Trial Group. Am J Cardiol 71:575, 1993.

157. Wessels F: Double-blind comparison of doxazosin and enalapril in patients with mild or moderate essential hypertension. Am Heart J 121:299, 1991.

158. Jansson J-H, Johansson B, Boman K, Nilsson TK: Effects of doxazosin and atenolol on the fibrinolytic system in patients with hypertension and elevated serum cholesterol. Eur J Clin Pharmacol 40:321, 1991.

159. Huupponen R, Lehtonen A, Väkäyalo M: Effect of doxazosin on insulin sensitivity in hypertensive non-insulin dependent diabetic patients. Eur J Clin Pharmacol 43:365, 1992.

160. Lehtonen A: Doxazosin effects on insulin and glucose in hypertensive patients. The Finnish Multicenter Study. Am Heart J 121:1307, 1991.

161. Bendall MJ, Baloch KH, Wilson PR: Side effects due to treatment of hypertension with prazosin. Br Med J 2:727, 1975.

162. Rosendorff C: Prazosin: Severe side effects are dose-dependent. Br Med J 2:508, 1976.

163. Rutland MD, Nimmon CC, Lee TY, et al: Measurement of the effects of a single dose of prazosin on the cerebral blood flow in hypertensive patients. Postgrad Med J 56:818, 1980.

164. Falch DK, Paulsen AQ, Odegaard AE, Norman N: Central

and renal circulation, renin and aldosterone in plasma during prazosin treatment in essential hypertension. Acta Med Scand 206:489, 1979.

165. Seideman P, Grahnen A, Haglund K, et al: Prazosin first dose phenomenon during combined treatment with a beta-adrenoceptor blocker in hypertensive patients. Br J Clin Pharmacol 13:865, 1982.

166. Sperzel WD, Luther RR, Glassman HN: Clinical trials with terazosin: General methods. Am J Med 80(5B):25, 1986.

167. Scharf MB, Mayleben DW: Comparative effects of prazosin and hydrochlorothiazide on sexual function in hypertensive men. Am J Med 86:110, 1989.

168. Coleman AJ: Evidence for increase in peripheral blood flow by indoramin in man. Br J Clin Pharmacol 12:79S, 1981.

169. Clement DL: Effect of indoramin on finger blood flow in vasospastic patients. Eur J Clin Pharmacol 14:331, 1978.

170. Schoenberger JA: Quality of life under antihypertensive treatment. Drugs 35(Suppl 5):74, 1988.

B. Centrally Acting Antiadrenergic Drugs

CHAPTER 63

Methyldopa

Edward D. Frohlich, M.D., and Franz H. Messerli, M.D.

Almost coincidental with the development of the thiazide congeners in the late 1950s was the synthesis of the first derivatives of DL-phenylalanine, the α-methyl-α-amino acids.[1] Within 5 years, the antihypertensive efficacy of methyldopa was reported in humans.[2] Many of the early antihypertensive compounds have been discarded in favor of newer agents, but the thiazides and methyldopa remain among the more utilized agents. For methyldopa, this long clinical experience has led to greater understanding of its mechanisms of action and the role of the adrenergic nervous system in essential hypertension. Through methyldopa, we have learned about false adrenergic neurotransmission, the interaction of the adrenergic and renopressor angiotensin systems, presynaptic and postsynaptic adrenergic receptors, central α-adrenoreceptors, and adrenergic control of arterial pressure.[3] Although methyldopa is used less frequently in the United States, it still remains very important clinically elsewhere around the world.

ADRENERGIC CONTROL OF ARTERIAL PRESSURE

Cardiovascular function is under continuous autonomic control through a balance of sympathetic and parasympathetic mechanisms. Regulation of neural control of arterial pressure is influenced by many factors, including sensory neural receptors, their afferent pathways and central internuncial connections, efferent pathways, altered catecholamine biosynthesis through effects on enzyme systems and metabolites, and different effector adrenergic receptors at vascular smooth muscle and myocardial cell membranes.[4] Afferent impulses from heart and vessels are directed to brainstem centers and then integrated in central internuncial circuits, eventually resulting in efferent responses[5] through epinephrinergic, norepinephrinergic, dopaminergic, serotoninergic, and other chemospecific[6] preganglionic neurons that synapse with postganglionic neurons.

Eventually, the norepinephrine released from a nerve ending stimulates postsynaptic $\alpha\beta$-adrenergic receptor sites on myocardial or vascular smooth muscle cells or, alternatively, presynaptic receptor sites on the nerve ending itself. Released norepinephrine may be metabolized at the synaptic cleft or systemically, or it may reenter the nerve ending for metabolism or storage.[7] Postsynaptic vascular α_1-receptor stimulation by norepinephrine results in vasoconstriction; however, stimulation of presynaptic α_2-receptors on the nerve ending inhibits further neural release of norepinephrine, providing a negative feedback system that regulates tonic adrenergic control of vessel caliber and, therefore, of vascular resistance and arterial pressure.[8]

This concept has been complicated still further with demonstration of postsynaptic α_2-receptors in specific brain centers.[9] Stimulation of these central α-receptors, particularly in the region of the nucleus tractus solitarii, results in central inhibition of adrenergically mediated efferent impulses.[10] Other brain centers are sensitive to angiotensin II stimulation and may increase adrenergic cardiovascular outflow.[11]

Thus, it is apparent that a compound such as methyldopa is capable of altering cardiovascular function through a myriad of possible mechanisms.

MECHANISMS OF ACTION

Over the years, various modes of action have been proposed for methyldopa. Although these modes may participate in methyldopa's overall antihypertensive action, its central action in the brain is presently favored.

Methyldopa Decarboxylation

Methyldopa was first synthesized in 1955 from amino acid derivatives of phenylalanine for treating certain endocrinologically active neoplastic diseases.[1] One of these derivatives was thought to inhibit serotonin and thereby arrest carcinoid tumor growth.[12, 13] Fortunately, the study of patients with carcinoid syndrome was conducted in the laboratory of Sjoerdsma, who was also interested in the treatment of hypertension.[2] These investigators reasoned that methyldopa, acting as a decarboxylase inhibitor, lowered arterial pressure by interfering with dopamine formation, the catecholamine precursor of norepinephrine.

Prolonged reduction of arterial pressure was demonstrated with the racemic compound (α-D, L-methyldopa) without associated postural hypotension.[14] The decarboxylating effect of methyldopa resided only with the L-isomer,[15] as did its antihypertensive effect;[14] therefore, subsequent work in hypertension was pursued with the L-isomer.

Initial antihypertensive studies showed that its hypotensive action was associated with increased urinary excretion of 5-hydroxytryptophan and decreased excretion of 5-hydroxyindoleacetic acid. *In vivo* studies demonstrated depletion of 5-hydroxytryptamine, dopamine, and norepinephrine stores in brain, myocardium, and most other tissues except for adrenal medulla.[16, 17] Further experimental and clinical work either indicated that other compounds that inhibited decarboxylase did not lower pressure or demonstrated a discrepancy between the duration of enzyme inhibition and the antihypertensive action.[14, 17] An alternative hypothesis was therefore necessary.

False Neurotransmission

The initial metabolic product of the decarboxylation of α-methyldopa was α-methyldopamine, a compound also capable of reducing tissue norepinephrine content.[18] This focused attention on the metabolites of methyldopa, specifically α-methyl-norepinephrine, which was demonstrated in brain tissue.[19] Both α-methyl-norepinephrine and norepinephrine enter postganglionic adrenergic nerve endings, both are later released with nerve stimulation, and both compete for the same α-adrenergic receptor site at the effector cell membrane.[20, 21] A new antihypertensive action of methyldopa was hypothesized, that of a weaker (i.e., "false") α-adrenergic neurotransmitter than the natural catecholamine.[20, 21]

Renin Release Inhibition

All antihypertensive adrenergic inhibitors suppress renin release from the kidney.[22] Because decreased adrenergic input to the kidney inhibits renin release, one might reasonably expect that methyldopa would inhibit renin release and plasma renin activity, and it does experimentally[23-27] and clinically.[27-30] Whether the pressure reduction with therapy results from suppressed release of renin or by its broader systemic adrenergic inhibition remains unresolved.

Central α-Receptor Stimulation

The mechanism of central α-receptor stimulation is now considered the most probable for methyldopa's antihypertensive action. Through its metabolite, α-methyl-norepinephrine, it stimulates postsynaptic α-adrenotropic receptors in the brain, a mechanism that more directly affects the other centrally acting antihypertensive agents.[31, 32] One specific medullary center, the nucleus tractus solitarii, contains postsynaptic α-receptors that, when stimulated, reduce adrenergic outflow to the cardiovascular system and kidneys to reduce arterial pressure and circulating plasma renin activity.[33-38] Moreover, inhibition of these α-receptors with phentolamine prevents this action as well as the antihypertensive effect of methyldopa.[39]

Only the L-isomer of methyldopa reduces pressure when administered centrally;[40] however, it must first enter the brain cells of the nucleus tractus solitarii, where it is transformed into its active metabolite, α-methyl-norepinephrine.[41] Moreover, because α-methyl-norepinephrine does not cross the blood-brain barrier, it must be formed within the central nervous system.[42] Thus, it seems reasonable to assume that following its administration, methyldopa enters the neurons of the nucleus tractus solitarii, where it is metabolized into an active neurotransmitter, α-methyl-norepinephrine, which serves as an agonist to postsynaptic α-adrenotropic receptors.

PHARMACOKINETICS

Methyldopa is rapidly, but variably, absorbed following its oral administration, and its plasma levels are substantially lower than when methyldopa is given intravenously.[43] A number of reports have indicated great variability in methyldopa absorption[44-46] that is roughly proportional to the dose administered.[45]

When ^{14}C-methyldopa was administered intravenously, nearly all radioactivity was recovered in the urine, of which half is free methyldopa and the remaining half is unidentified metabolites.[43, 44, 47] There appears to be little association between plasma levels and methyldopa's antihypertensive activity in patients.[46] In patients with renal failure, urinary excretion of free methyldopa is decreased, and plasma levels of methyldopa, particularly the sulfate conjugate, are increased.[48-50] Hence, smaller doses may be indicated in renal failure patients, and it can be removed by dialysis.[51]

HEMODYNAMIC EFFECTS
Concept

Most hypertensive diseases are characterized hemodynamically as being produced by a generalized increase in the vascular smooth muscle tone that increases arteriolar resistance and reduces venular capacitance.[4, 52] The increased total peripheral resistance is, for the most part, uniformly distributed throughout the component regional circulations.[53] Increased venular smooth muscle tone redistributes intravascular volume from the periphery to the central circulation, thereby augmenting venous return and cardiac output.[4, 50, 54-56] As hypertension progresses in severity, vascular resistance progressively increases, raising arterial pressure and promoting two primary adaptations: (1) the heart and vessels structurally adapt to the increasing workload by increasing cardiac mass and vascular wall thickness, and (2) intravascular volume contracts.[4, 53, 57-59] When the heart and vessels no longer can adapt structurally and functionally, secondary hormonal adaptations occur, and eventually cardiac and circulatory failure ensue, with associated impaired renal excretory function.[4, 53, 55, 56, 58]

As a result, the ideal antihypertensive agent should (1) reduce vascular smooth muscle tone to decrease total peripheral and organ vascular resistances, (2) maintain normal cardiac output and organ blood flows, (3) not stimulate reflexively the heart (to increase heart rate, cardiac contractility, or metabolic requirements) in response to the reduced pressure, and (4) not expand intravascular volume in response to the reduced pressure.

Systemic Hemodynamics

The reduced arterial pressure associated with methyldopa is due to a reduced total peripheral resistance without a significant change in cardiac output and heart rate.[60-66] Myocardial function is preserved, and because of adrenergic inhibition, there is little reflex cardiac stimulation or altered myocardial metabolism.[61, 62, 66-68]

Arterial pressures fall within 6 hours of oral administration, and associated with this effect is a fall in total peripheral resistance and no change or a slight reduction in cardiac output.[60-63] Resting heart rate is not slowed as with other adrenergic-inhibiting agents, and stroke volume, cardiac output, and myocardial contractility are maintained.[68, 69] However, if ventricular function is borderline or slightly impaired, cardiac output may be reduced.[68, 70]

With prolonged methyldopa treatment, arterial pressure remains reduced, and this is associated with a fall in total peripheral resistance and possibly a slight decrease in cardiac output,[64, 66, 67] but intravascular volume tends to expand, diminishing its antihypertensive effectiveness.[71-73] This can be minimized by adding small doses of a diuretic.

Differences in hemodynamic effects with prolonged methyldopa therapy have been reported between younger and older patients with essential hypertension.[66, 67] Although arterial pressure was reduced in both groups, its fall was mediated through a reduced total peripheral resistance in younger patients, whereas cardiac output and heart rate were reduced in the older patients. However, regardless of whether cardiac output was reduced or remained unchanged, renal blood flow, circulating intravascular volume, and cardiovascular reflexes remained unchanged.

Regional Blood Flows

Even if cardiac output is slightly reduced with prolonged treatment, renal blood flow does not decline.[61, 63, 74] Indeed, renal blood flow and renal parenchymal excretory function remain unchanged,[63, 74, 75] and glomerular filtration rate may even increase with prolonged therapy in some patients with chronic renal

insufficiency,[74] although other studies have demonstrated reduced glomerular filtration rate and unchanged renal blood flow of therapy.[76]

Other reports have demonstrated reduced cerebral vascular resistance in all patients studied after 2 weeks of methyldopa therapy;[77, 78] myocardial blood flow increased with methyldopa[79] because of coronary vasodilation, improved myocardial function, and changes in myocardial dimensions; splanchnic blood flow remained unchanged in patients with prolonged methyldopa.[80]

Circulatory Reflexive Changes

Normal cardiovascular responses to posture, Valsalva's maneuver, and handgrip exercise with unchanged responses of baroreceptor mechanisms have been reported with methyldopa.[67, 69, 80, 81] These responses are unlike those observed with other adrenergic-inhibiting agents.[69, 82-85] Indeed, both methyldopa and clonidine produce a greater fall of arterial pressure in the supine position than these other agents, and postural hypotension is not a major clinical finding with these centrally acting agents.[67, 69, 80, 82] However, methyldopa produces less hypotension during and after exercise than those agents.[61, 62, 68]

REVERSAL OF VENTRICULAR HYPERTROPHY

Many studies have shown that there is a definite decrease in cardiac mass with methyldopa.[57, 86-91] It is noteworthy that unlike many other antihypertensive agents, methyldopa reduces the mass of nonhypertrophied chambers as well as the hypertrophied chambers.[92] The early experimental work with methyldopa has opened a fascinating new area of investigation. Some studies have shown that control of arterial pressure with one agent was associated with a significant reduction in cardiac mass, whereas even better pressure control with other agents was not associated with changed cardiac mass.[87, 90, 93] The effect of decreasing cardiac mass is not solely dependent on physiologic unloading of the myocardium, because potent vasodilating agents (e.g., hydralazine, minoxidil) that effectively reduce left ventricular overload have no effect on cardiac mass.[87, 90, 93]

This regression of cardiac mass following methyldopa therapy was associated with the reduced muscle mass and increased collagen[93] that occur in treated normotensive rats without any hemodynamic changes.[87, 91] In contrast to these studies with the L-isomer, the D-isomer of methyldopa was without effect on hemodynamics or cardiac mass.[87] This effect of methyldopa on left ventricular mass may be age-dependent and influenced by intracellular biochemical factors that are related to the development of hypertrophy.[94] That these disparate findings were not explained only by the central antihypertensive action of methyldopa was shown by the absence of diminished cardiac mass with clonidine in similarly effective antihypertensive doses having the same hemodynamic alterations.[87] Cardiac mass decreased only when the clonidine dose was increased, so that clonidine acted as a peripheral α-adrenergic receptor agonist, thereby increasing total peripheral resistance.[87] One might conclude that there was something unique about the levoisomer of methyldopa that produced regression in cardiac mass; however, other types of antihypertensive agents have also reduced cardiac mass in hypertensive as well as normotensive animals.[95–99]

Ventricular hypertrophy increases the independent cardiovascular risk in patients with hypertension.[100] This may be related to an enhanced predisposition to cardiac arrhythmias and sudden death.[100–102] Whether this is related to the increased muscle mass, increased collagen deposition, or related ischemia, and whether pharmacologic regression of the hypertrophy improves that risk, remain purely speculative.[103]

OTHER EFFECTS

All the hemodynamic effects described may be explained by inhibition of adrenergic input to the cardiovascular system. Reduced plasma renin activity associated with methyldopa therapy may also reflect reduced adrenergic input to the juxtaglomerular apparatus of the kidney.[104] Reduced adrenergic control of the kidney can also affect sodium and water balance. Other central nervous system effects of the drug may explain the side effects of somnolence, fever, and dry mouth. Because the agent inhibits adrenergic function in other organs (in some instances, leaving unopposed parasympathetic function), patients receiving prolonged methyldopa therapy may experience a variety of other effects, including abdominal cramps, diarrhea, sexual dysfunction, and nasal stuffiness.[70, 105, 106] Methyldopa does not produce obstructive airway symptoms associated with its adrenergic-inhibitory effects, unlike other agents that inhibit β-adrenergic receptors. Methyldopa may suppress the prolactin-inhibiting hormone, dopamine; in doing so, it may permit an enhanced release of prolactin in certain patients, thereby inducing pseudolactation.[107, 108]

Several forms of immunologic alterations have been observed with methyldopa therapy. In general, they have been considered to be hypersensitivity changes that have ranged in frequency from the common development of a direct positive Coombs' test,[109] to the rare occurrence of Coombs'-positive hemolytic anemia,[110, 111] to the still less common occurrences of positive lupus and rheumatoid factors,[112] impaired hepatic function with frank hepatocellular disease with necrosis,[113–117] myocarditis,[118] retroperitoneal fibrosis,[119] leukopenia,[120] and thrombocytopenia.[121]

The most frequent immunologic alteration is development of the direct positive Coombs' test associated more with prolonged therapy (usually after longer than 6 to 12 months) in 10% to 20% of patients receiving at least 1 g of methyldopa daily.[122] This is not a contraindication to methyldopa, and it does not mean that hemolytic anemia will ensue or that the therapy

needs be discontinued. However, it is wise to periodically administer a Coombs' test and hemograms during the course of prolonged therapy (perhaps twice annually) to ensure prompt recognition of hemolytic anemia if it develops.

The antibody associated with the hemolytic anemia and Coombs' test positivity is attached to the patient's red blood cells and is of the immunoglobulin G (IgG) class with specificity for the Rh locus.[110] This abnormality may persist for months after methyldopa therapy is discontinued, even if anemia never develops. A positive Coombs' test should alert the clinician to potential problems in typing and cross-matching the patient's blood; if this occurs, expert hematologic and transfusion consultation must be available for these patients.

Development of hepatic abnormalities has also been ascribed to hypersensitivity reactions. These may be manifested as abnormal hepatic function as a result of hepatocellular disease appearing clinically as a viral[117] or granulomatous hepatitis,[116] submassive hepatic necrosis,[114] or cirrhosis.[123] Other hypersensitivity reactions may include myocarditis[120] or fever.[124] If such reactions develop, methyldopa should be discontinued and not readministered, because fatal hepatic necrosis has been reported.[114, 117]

Although rare, additional reactions to methyldopa have been reported, including bilateral renal calculi in two patients receiving prolonged methyldopa therapy,[125] in which the urine contained a brown pigment that precipitated with time and was identified as methyldopa. Other problems include reduced mental acuity,[126] muscle weakness, extrapyramidal signs, and parkinsonism.[127] Severe rebound hypertension has been reported following abrupt cessation of methyldopa therapy,[126–131] which may be similar (although apparently less common) in mechanism to the rebound hypertension observed with clonidine. Treatment of this problem includes reinstitution of the drug and/or infusion of α-adrenergic receptor blocking drugs for the severe hypertension and β-adrenergic blocking therapy for associated cardiac dysrhythmias.[132]

REFERENCES

1. Stein GA, Bronner HA, Pfister K: α-Methyl α-amino acids: II. Derivatives of DL-phenylalanine. J Am Chem Soc 77:700, 1955.
2. Oates JA, Gillespie L, Udenfriend S, et al: Decarboxylase inhibition and blood pressure reduction by α-methyl-3, 4-dihydroxy-DL-phenylalanine. Science 131:1890, 1960.
3. Frohlich ED: Methyldopa: Mechanisms and treatment 25 years later. Arch Intern Med 140:954, 1980.
4. Frohlich ED, Messerli FH, Re RN, et al: Mechanisms controlling arterial pressure. In Frohlich ED (ed): Pathophysiology: Altered Regulatory Mechanisms in Disease, 3rd ed. Philadelphia: JB Lippincott, 1984, pp 45–81.
5. Jarecki M, Thoren PN, Donald DE: Release of renin by the carotid baroreflex in anesthetized dogs. Role of cardiopulmonary vagal afferents and renal arterial pressure. Circ Res 42:614, 1978.
6. Chalmers JP: Brain amines and models of experimental hypertension. Circ Res 36:469, 1975.
7. Langer SZ, Cavero I, Massingham R: Recent developments in noradrenergic neurotransmission and its relevance to the

mechanisms of action of certain antihypertensive agents. Hypertension 2:372, 1980.

8. Langer SZ, Shepperson NB, Massingham R: Preferential noradrenergic innervation of alpha-adrenergic receptors in vascular smooth muscle. Hypertension 3(Suppl 1):112, 1981.

9. Glossman H, Hornung R: Alpha₂-adrenoceptors in rat brain. Naunyn-Schmiedebergs Arch Pharmacol 314:101, 1980.

10. Reis DJ: The nucleus tractus solitarii (NTS) and experimental neurogenic hypertension. In Hughes MJ, Barnes CD (eds): Neural Control of Circulation. New York: Academic Press, 1980, pp 81–102.

11. Lowe RD, Scroop GC: The cardiovascular response to vertebral artery infusion of angiotensin in the dog. Clin Sci 37:593, 1969.

12. Sourkes TL: Inhibition of dihydroxyphenylalanine decarboxylase by derivatives of phenylalanine. Arch Biochem Biophys 51:444, 1954.

13. Westerman E, Balzer H, Knell J: Hemmung der Serotoninbildung durch α-methyl-dopa. Arch Exp Pathol (Berlin) 234:194, 1958.

14. Gillespie L Jr, Oates JA, Crout JR, et al: Clinical and chemical studies with α-methyl-dopa in patients with hypertension. Circulation 25:281, 1962.

15. Porter CC, Totaro JA, Leiby CM: Some biochemical effects of α-methyl-3, 4-dihydroxyphenylalanine and related compounds in mice. J Pharmacol Exp Ther 134:139, 1961.

16. Hess SM, Connamacher RH, Ozaki M, et al: The effects of alpha-methyldopa and alpha-methyl-meta-tyrosine on the metabolism of norepinephrine and serotonin in vivo. J Pharmacol Exp Ther 134:129, 1961.

17. Van Zwieten PA: Centrally mediated action of alpha-methyldopa. In Onesti G, Fernandes M, Kim KE (eds): Regulation of Blood Pressure by the Central Nervous System. New York: Grune & Stratton, 1976, pp 293–301.

18. Weissbach H, Lovenberg W, Udenfriend S: Enzymatic decarboxylation of alpha-methyl amino acids. Biochem Biophys Res Commun 3:225, 1960.

19. Carlsson A, Lindquist M: In vivo decarboxylation of alpha-methyldopa and alpha-methyl metatyrosine. Acta Physiol Scand 54:87, 1962.

20. Day MD, Rand MJ: A hypothesis for the mode of action of alpha-methyldopa in relieving hypertension. J Pharm Pharmacol 15:221, 1963.

21. Day MD, Rand MJ: Some observations on the pharmacology of alpha-methyldopa. Br J Pharmacol 22:72, 1964.

22. Mancia G, Romero JC, Shepherd JT: Continuous inhibition of renin release in dogs by vagally innervated receptors in the cardiopulmonary region. Circ Res 36:529, 1975.

23. Mohammed S, Fasola AP, Privitera PJ, et al: Effect of methyldopa on plasma renin activity in man. Circ Res 25:543, 1969.

24. Privitera PJ, Mohammed S: Studies on the mechanisms of renin suppression by alpha-methyldopa. In Aosaykeen TA (ed): Control of Renin Secretion. New York: Plenum, 1972, pp 93–101.

25. Halusha PV, Keiser HR: Acute effects of alpha-methyldopa on mean blood pressure and plasma renin activity. Circ Res 35:458, 1974.

26. Sweet CS, Wenger HC, O'Malley TA: Antagonism of hydrochlorothiazide-induced elevations in plasma renin activity by methyldopa in conscious renal-hypertensive dogs. Can J Physiol Pharmacol 52:1036, 1974.

27. Weidmann P, Maxwell MH, Lupu AN, et al: Plasma renin activity and blood pressure in terminal renal failure. N Engl J Med 285:757, 1971.

28. Catt KJ, Cran E, Zimmet PZ, et al: Angiotensin II blood levels in human hypertension. Lancet 1:459, 1971.

29. Imbs JL, Spach MO, Schwartz J: Baisse de l'activite renine plasmatique apres traitment par l'alpha-methyldopa. Nouv Presse Med 1:1995, 1972.

30. Weidmann P, Hirsch D, Maxwell MH, et al: Plasma renin and blood pressure during treatment with methyldopa. Am J Cardiol 34:671, 1974.

31. Van Zwieten PA: Pharmacology of centrally acting hypotensive drugs. Br J Clin Pharmacol 10:13s, 1980.

32. Hüsler G: Central α-adrenoceptors involved in cardiovascular regulation. J Cardiovasc Pharmacol 4(Suppl 1):S72, 1982.

33. Jaju PB, Tangri KK, Bhargava KP: Central vasomotor effects of alpha methyl-dopa. Can J Physiol Pharmacol 44:687, 1966.

34. Haefely W, Hurlimann A, Thoeneu H: Adrenergic transmitter changes and response to sympathetic nerve stimulation after differing pretreatment with alpha-methyldopa. Br J Pharmacol 31:105, 1967.

35. Henning M, Van Zwieten PA: Central hypotensive effect of alpha-methyldopa. J Pharm Pharmacol 19:403, 1967.

36. Henning M, Svensson L: Adrenergic nerve function in the anesthetized rat after treatment with alpha-methyldopa. Acta Pharmacol 26:425, 1968.

37. Van Zwieten PA: The central action of antihypertensive drugs mediated via central alpha receptors. J Pharm Pharmacol 23:89, 1973.

38. Van Zwieten PA: Antihypertensive drugs with a central action. Prog Pharmacol 1:1, 1975.

39. Finch L, Haeusler G: Further evidence for a central hypotensive action of alpha-methyldopa in both the rat and cat. Br J Pharmacol 47:217, 1973.

40. Henning M: Studies on the mode of action of alpha-methyldopa. Acta Physiol Scand Suppl 322:1, 1969.

41. Day MD, Roach AG, Whiting RL: The mechanisms of the antihypertensive action of alpha-methyldopa in hypertensive rats. Eur J Pharmacol 21:271, 1973.

42. Heise A, Kroneberg G: Alpha-sympathetic receptor stimulation in the brain and hypotensive activity of alpha-methyldopa. Eur J Pharmacol 17:315, 1972.

43. Kwan KC, Foltz EL, Breault GO, et al: Pharmacokinetics of methyldopa in man. J Pharmacol Exper Ther 198:264, 1976.

44. Saavedra JA, Reid JL, Jordan W, et al: Plasma concentration of alpha-methyldopa and sulphate conjugate after oral administration of methyldopa and intravenous administration of methyldopa and methyldopa hydrochlorothiazide ethyl ester. Eur J Clin Pharmacol 8:381, 1975.

45. Barnett AJ, Bobik A, Carson V, et al: Pharmacokinetics of methyldopa: Plasma levels following single intravenous, oral, and multiple oral dosage in normotensive and hypertensive subjects. Clin Exp Pharmacol Physiol 4:331, 1977.

46. Au WYW, Dring LG, Grahame-Smith DG, et al: The metabolism of ¹⁴C-labeled alpha-methyldopa in normal and hypertensive human subjects. Biochem J 129:1, 1972.

47. Stenbaek O, Myhre E, Rugstad HE, et al: Pharmacokinetics of methyldopa in healthy man. Eur J Clin Pharmacol 12:117, 1977.

48. Buhs RP, Beck JL, Speth OC, et al: The metabolism of methyldopa in hypertensive human subjects. J Pharmacol Exp Ther 143:205, 1964.

49. Myhre E, Brodwall EK, Stenbaek O, et al: The renal excretion of methyldopa. Scand J Clin Lab Invest 29:201, 1972.

50. Myhre E, Brodwall EK, Stenbaek O, et al: Plasma turnover of methyldopa in advanced renal failure. Acta Med Scand 191:343, 1972.

51. Myhre E, Stenbaek O, Brodwall EK, et al: Conjugation of methyldopa in renal failure. Scand J Clin Lab Invest 29:195, 1972.

52. Frohlich ED: Haemodynamics of hypertension. In Genest J, Koiw E, Kuchel O (eds): Hypertension: Physiopathology and Treatment. New York: McGraw-Hill, 1977, pp 15–49.

53. Messerli FH, de Carvalho JGR, Christie B, et al: Systemic and regional hemodynamics in low, normal, and high cardiac output in borderline hypertension. Circulation 58:441, 1978.

54. Ulrych M, Frohlich ED, Dustan HP, et al: Cardiac output and distribution of blood volume in central and peripheral circulations in hypertensive and normotensive man. Br Heart J 31:570, 1969.

55. Frohlich ED: Hemodynamic factors in the pathogenesis and maintenance of hypertension. Fed Proc 41:2400, 1982.

56. Frohlich ED, Tarazi RC, Dustan HP: Clinical-physiological correlations in the development of hypertensive heart disease. Circulation 44:446, 1971.

57. Frohlich ED: The heart in hypertension. In Genest J, Kuchel O, Hamet P, et al (eds): Hypertension: Physiopathology and Treatment, 2nd ed. New York: McGraw-Hill, 1983, pp 791–810.

58. Tarazi RC, Frohlich ED, Dustan HP: Plasma volume in men with essential hypertension. N Engl J Med 278:762, 1968.

59. Tarazi RC, Dustan HP, Frohlich ED, et al: Plasma volume and chronic hypertension: Relationship to arterial pressure levels in different hypertensive diseases. Arch Intern Med 125:835, 1970.

60. Wilson WR, Fisher FD, Kirkendall WM: The acute hemodynamic effects of alpha-methyldopa. J Chronic Dis 15:907, 1962.

61. Sannerstedt R, Varnauskas F, Werko L: Hemodynamic effects of methyldopa (Aldomet) at rest and during exercise in patients with arterial hypertension. Acta Med Scand 171:75, 1962.

62. Dollery CT, Harington M, Hodge JV: Haemodynamic studies with methyldopa: Effect on cardiac output and response to pressor amines. Br Heart J 25:670, 1963.

63. Onesti G, Brest AN, Novack P, et al: Pharmacodynamic effects of alpha-methyldopa in hypertensive subjects. Am Heart J 67:32, 1964.

64. Lund-Johansen P: Hemodynamic changes in long-term alpha-methyldopa therapy in essential hypertension. Acta Med Scand 192:221, 1972.

65. Safar ME, London GM, Levenson JA, et al: Effect of alpha-methyldopa on cardiac output in hypertension. Clin Pharmacol Ther 25:266, 1979.

66. Messerli FH, Dreslinski GR, Husserl FE, et al: Anti-adrenergic therapy: Special aspects in hypertension in the elderly. Hypertension 3(Suppl 2):226, 1981.

67. Frohlich ED, Messerli FH, Pegram BL, et al: Hemodynamic and cardiac effects of centrally acting antihypertensive drugs. Hypertension 6(Suppl 2):76, 1984.

68. Chamberlain DA, Howard J: Guanethidine and methyldopa: A haemodynamic study. Br Heart J 26:528, 1964.

69. Frohlich ED: Inhibition of adrenergic function in the treatment of hypertension. Arch Intern Med 133:1033, 1974.

70. Krantz PD, Haft JJ, Venkatachalapathy D, et al: Orally administered methyldopa: Hemodynamic effects in the presence and absence of congestive heart failure. Arch Intern Med 134:478, 1974.

71. Weil JV, Chidsey CA: Plasma volume expansion resulting from interference with adrenergic function in normal man. Circulation 37:54, 1968.

72. Dustan HP, Tarazi RC, Bravo EL: Dependence of arterial pressure on intravascular volume in treated hypertensive patients. N Engl J Med 286:861, 1972.

73. Chrysant SG, Frohlich ED, Adamopoulos PN, et al: Pathophysiologic significance of relative polycythemia in essential hypertension. Am J Cardiol 37:1069, 1976.

74. Mohammed S, Hanenson IB, Magenheim HG, et al: The effects of alpha-methyldopa on renal function in hypertensive patients. Am Heart J 76:21, 1968.

75. Weil MN, Barbour BH, Chesne RB: Alpha-methyldopa for the treatment of hypertension: Clinical and pharmacodynamic studies. Circulation 28:165, 1963.

76. Grable M, Nussbaum P, Goldfarb S, et al: Effects of methyldopa on renal hemodynamics and tubular function. Clin Pharmacol Ther 27:522, 1980.

77. Meyer JS, Sawada T, Kitamura A, et al: Cerebral blood flow after control of hypertension in stroke. Neurology 18:772, 1968.

78. Lavy S, Stern S, Tzivoni D, et al: Effect of methyldopa on regional cerebral blood flow in hypertensive patients. Isr J Med Sci 16:456, 1980.

79. Colien A, Maxmen JS, Ragheb M, et al: Effects of alpha-methyldopa on the myocardial blood flow, utilizing coincidence counting method. J Clin Pharmacol 7:77, 1967.

80. Messerli FH, Aristimuno G, de Carvalho JGR, et al: Physiologic studies of methyldopa in essential hypertension. In Villareal H (ed): Proceedings of the International Symposium on Methyldopa, Mexico City, Mexico. New York: Biomedical Information Corporation Publications, 1980, pp 79–90.

81. Mancia G, Ferrari A, Gregorini L, et al: Methyldopa and neural control of the circulation in essential hypertension. Am J Cardiol 45:1237, 1980.

82. Freis ED, Rose JC, Partenope EA, et al: The hemodynamic effects of hypotensive drugs in man: III. Hexamethonium. J Clin Invest 32:1285, 1953.

83. Richardson DW, Wyso EM, Magee JH, et al: Circulatory effects of guanethidine: Clinical, renal and cardiac responses to treatment with a novel antihypertensive drug. Circulation 22:184, 1960.

84. Chrysant SG, Nishiyama K, Adamopoulos PN, et al: Systemic hemodynamic effects of bethanidine in essential hypertension. Circulation 52:137, 1975.

85. Sannerstedt R, Conway J: Hemodynamic and vascular responses to antihypertensive treatment with adrenergic blocking agents: A review. Am Heart J 79:122, 1970.

86. Ishise S, Pegram BL, Frohlich ED: Disparate effects of methyldopa and clonidine on cardiac mass and haemodynamics in rats. Clin Sci 59(Suppl 6):449s, 1980.

87. Pegram BL, Ishise S, Frohlich ED: Effect of methyldopa, clonidine, and hydralazine on cardiac mass and hemodynamics in Wistar-Kyoto and spontaneously hypertensive rats. Cardiovasc Res 16:40, 1982.

88. Tarazi RC, Ferrario CM, Dustan HP: The heart in hypertension. In Genest J, Koiw E, Kuchel O (eds): Hypertension: Physiopathology and Treatment. New York: McGraw-Hill, 1977, pp 738–755.

89. Frohlich ED: Hemodynamics and other determinants in development of left ventricular hypertrophy: Conflicting factors in its regression. Fed Proc 42:2709, 1983.

90. Sen S, Tarazi RC, Khairallah PA, et al: Cardiac hypertrophy in spontaneously hypertensive rats. Circ Res 35:775, 1974.

91. Kuwajima I, Kardon MB, Pegram BL, et al: Regression of left ventricular hypertrophy in two-kidney, one-clip Goldblatt hypertension. Hypertension 4(Suppl 2):113, 1982.

92. Sasaki O, Kardon MB, Pegram BL, Frohlich ED: Aortic distensibility and left ventricular pumping ability after methyldopa in Wistar-Kyoto and spontaneously hypertensive rats. J Vasc Med Biol 1(2):59–66, 1989.

93. Sen S, Tarazi RC, Bumpus FM: Biochemical changes associated with development and reversal of cardiac hypertrophy in spontaneously hypertensive rats. Cardiovasc Res 10:254, 1976.

94. Tomanek RJ: Selective effects of α-methyldopa on myocardial cell components independent of cell size in normotensive and genetically hypertensive rats. Hypertension 4:499, 1982.

95. Sen S, Tarazi RC, Bumpus FM: The effect of converting enzyme inhibitor (captopril) on cardiac hypertrophy in spontaneously hypertensive rats. Hypertension 2:169, 1980.

96. Ibrahim MM, Madkour MA, Mossallum R: Factors influencing cardiac hypertrophy in hypertensive patients. Clin Sci 61:1055, 1981.

97. Kazda S, Garthoff B, Thomas G: Antihypertensive effect of a calcium antagonist drug: Regression of hypertensive cardiac hypertrophy by nifedipine. Drug Dev Res 2:313, 1982.

98. Dunn FG, Bastian B, Lawrie L: Effect of blood pressure control on left ventricular hypertrophy in patients with essential hypertension. Clin Sci 59:441s, 1980.

99. Fouad FM, Nakashima Y, Tarazi RC, et al: Reversal of left ventricular hypertrophy in hypertensive patients treated with methyldopa: Lack of association with blood pressure control. Am J Cardiol 49:795, 1982.

100. Frohlich ED: Left ventricular hypertrophy as a risk factor. In Messerli FH, Amodeo C (eds): Cardiology Clinics, Vol. 4. Philadelphia: WB Saunders, 1986, pp 137–144.

101. Messerli FH, Ventura HO, Elizardi DJ, et al: Hypertension and sudden death: Increased ventricular ectopic activity in left ventricular hypertrophy. Am J Med 77:18, 1984.

102. McLenachan JM, Henderson E, Morris KI, et al: Ventricular arrhythmias in hypertensive left ventricular hypertrophy. N Engl J Med 317:787, 1987.

103. Frohlich ED: Cardiac hypertrophy in hypertension. N Engl J Med 317:831, 1987.

104. Leonetti G, Terzoli L, Morganti A, et al: Relation between the hypotensive and renin-suppressing activities of alpha methyldopa in hypertensive patients. Am J Cardiol 40:762, 1977.

105. Furkoff AK: Adverse reactions with methyldopa: A decade's reports. Acta Med Scand 203:425, 1978.

106. Itskowitz HD: Long-term treatment of hypertension with methyldopa: A retrospective multiclinic study. J Cardiovasc Pharmacol 3(Suppl 2):s75, 1981.

107. Vaidya RA, Vaidya AB, VanWoert MH, et al: Galactorrhea and Parkinson-like syndrome: An adverse effect of alpha-methyldopa. Metabolism 19:1068, 1970.

108. Pettinger WA, Horwitz D, Sjoerdsma A: Lactation due to methyldopa. Br Med J 1:1460, 1963.
109. Carstairs KC, Breckenridge A, Dollery CT, et al: Incidence of a positive direct Coombs test in patients on alpha-methyldopa. Lancet 2:133, 1966.
110. LoBuglio AF, Jandl JH: The nature of the alpha-methyldopa red-cell antibody. N Engl J Med 276:658, 1967.
111. Worlledge SM, Carstairs KC, Dacie JV: Autoimmune haemolytic anaemia associated with alpha-methyldopa therapy. Lancet 2:135, 1966.
112. Sherman JD, Love DE, Harrington JF: Anemia, positive lupus and rheumatoid factors with methyldopa. Arch Intern Med 120:321, 1967.
113. Elkington SG, Schreiber WM, Conn HO: Hepatic injury caused by L-alpha-methyldopa. Circulation 40:589, 1969.
114. Rehman OU, Keith TA, Gall EA: Methyldopa-induced submassive hepatic necrosis. JAMA 224:1390, 1973.
115. Hoyumpa AM Jr, Connell AM: Methyldopa hepatitis. Am J Dig Dis 18:213, 1973.
116. Miller AC Jr, Reid WM: Methyldopa-induced granulomatous hepatitis. JAMA 235:2001, 1976.
117. Rodman JS, Deutsch DJ, Gutman SE: Methyldopa hepatitis: A report of six cases and review of the literature. Am J Med 60:941, 1976.
118. Mullick FG, McAllister HA: Myocarditis associated with methyldopa therapy. JAMA 237:1699, 1977.
119. Iversen BM, Johannesen JW, Nordahl E, et al: Retroperitoneal fibrosis during treatment with methyldopa. Lancet 2:302, 1975.
120. Hallwright GP: Agranulocytosis caused by methyldopa (Aldomet). N Z Med J 60:567, 1961.
121. Manohitharajah SM, Jenkins WJ, Roberts PD, et al: Methyldopa and associated thrombocytopenia. Br Med J 1:494, 1971.
122. Brest AN: The management of uncomplicated hypertension and the role of Aldomet. In Maxwell MH (ed): Aldomet (Methyldopa, MSD) in the Management of Hypertension. West Point, PA: Merck Sharp & Dohme, 1978, pp 85–103.
123. Hyer SL, Knell AJ: Side effects of drugs: Cirrhosis and haemolysis complicating methyldopa treatment. Br Med J 1:879, 1977.
124. Valnes K, Hillestad L, Hansen T, et al: Alpha-methyldopa and drug fever: A study of the metabolism of alpha-methyldopa in patients and normal subjects. Acta Med Scand 204:21, 1978.
125. Murphy KJ: Bilateral renal calculi in patients receiving methyldopa. Med J Aust 2:20, 1976.
126. Alder S: Methyldopa-induced decrease in mental activity. JAMA 230:1428, 1974.
127. Lawson DH, Gloss D, Jick H: Adverse reactions to methyldopa with particular reference to hypotension. Am Heart J 96:572, 1978.
128. Feldman W, Hillman D, Baliah T, et al: Hypertension and seizures following methyldopa infusion. Pediatrics 37:781, 1967.
129. Levine RJ, Strauch BS: Hypertensive responses to methyldopa. N Engl J Med 275:946, 1966.
130. Westervelt FB Jr, Atuk NO: Methyldopa-induced hypertension [letter]. JAMA 227:557, 1974.
131. Frewin DB, Penhall PK: Rebound hypertension after sudden discontinuation of methyldopa therapy. Med J Aust 1:659, 1977.
132. Husserl FE, de Carvalho JGR, Batson HM, et al: Hypertension after clonidine withdrawal. South Med J 71:496, 1978.

CHAPTER 64

Clonidine

Deanna G. Cheung, M.D., James F. Burris, M.D.,
William F. Graettinger, M.D., and Michael A. Weber, M.D.

HISTORY AND CHEMISTRY

Clonidine hydrochloride, an imidazoline derivative, was originally developed as a nasal decongestant and vasoconstrictor.[1] Its hypotensive and bradycardic effects were first serendipitously appreciated in 1962. It is a centrally acting adrenergic agonist that lowers blood pressure by decreasing basal sympathetic nervous system activity. It was introduced first in Europe in 1966 and subsequently in the United States for use as an antihypertensive agent.

PHARMACOKINETICS

Clonidine is rapidly absorbed from the gastrointestinal tract. The onset of action occurs within 30 to 60 minutes, with the peak antihypertensive effect occurring 2 to 4 hours after oral administration. Peak plasma levels occur at 90 minutes, and the plasma half-life is 6 to 15 hours.[1, 2] Clonidine is metabolized mainly by the liver. Approximately 40% to 60% of an oral dose is excreted unchanged in the urine within 24 hours. In the presence of renal insufficiency, renal clearance is markedly reduced, with 95% of excretion in the urine and feces in 72 hours and total clearance in 5 days. Clonidine is also well absorbed through the skin as a result of its low molecular weight and high lipid solubility. It is released from a transdermal preparation at a constant rate for a 7-day period. After initial application of a transdermal clonidine patch, stable plasma concentrations are reached after 2 to 3 days. Clonidine accumulates in a skin reservoir that continues to release the drug after removal of the patch, resulting in a slow decline in the plasma level. When a new patch is applied at another site, the combined absorption from both sites maintains a constant plasma level. Plasma clonidine concentrations vary less after transdermal administration than after oral administration.[3] Skin permeability to clonidine varies slightly with the site used. The skin on the chest and upper outer arms is most permeable to clonidine and is associated with the most constant absorption rates. Skin pretreatment with 0.5% hydrocortisone may result in a slight reduction in absorption.[4] The metabolism and renal clearance of clonidine can be expected to be unaffected by the mode of administration.

MECHANISM OF ACTION

The mechanism of the antihypertensive action of clonidine is thought to be stimulation of postsynaptic α-adrenergic receptors in the nucleus tractus solitarii of the medulla oblongata. This inhibits basal efferent sympathetic vasoconstrictor effects on the peripheral and renal vasculature.[3] The same α-adrenergic-stimulating properties that cause the centrally mediated reduction of blood pressure have the opposite effect on the peripheral vasculature. A biphasic blood pressure response has been demonstrated in anesthetized dogs after intravenous infusion of clonidine. A brief initial increase in blood pressure is followed quickly by a prolonged period of lowered blood pressure and bradycardia.[1] A similar response to orally administered clonidine may be observed in hypertensive patients. Within minutes of an oral dose of clonidine, there may be a small increase in blood pressure universally followed by prolonged reduction in blood pressure as the central antihypertensive effects quickly overwhelm the peripheral pressor effect.[5] It has been suggested that this peripheral pressor effect may persist over a wider range of clonidine blood levels than the central antihypertensive effect; that is, the centrally mediated antihypertensive action of clonidine may reach a plateau stage, whereas the peripheral pressor effect may continue to increase with increasing dosages. If this is correct, it is possible that with very high doses of clonidine, the peripheral pressor effect may lessen the overall antihypertensive efficacy and, in fact, be counterproductive.[1]

The role of the sympathetic nervous system as one of a number of important blood pressure regulating factors is well established.[6] A direct relationship between blood pressure and plasma catecholamine level has been demonstrated in hypertensive patients. Hypertensive patients have been shown to have an exaggerated sympathetic nervous system response to stress. Additionally, it has been suggested that sympathetic mechanisms may contribute to elevations in blood pressure by blunting the sensitivity of the carotid baroreceptors. Clonidine may restore baroreceptor sensitivity by its central action. Reversal of impaired baroreceptor function has been demonstrated both in hypertensive animals and in patients with essential hypertension.[7, 8] The frequently observed moderate decrease in heart rate during clonidine therapy reflects vagal stimulation or sinoatrial nodal inhibition.[9, 10] This comes about as a result of a reciprocal relationship between the sympathetic vasomotor center and the dorsal motor nucleus of the vagus nerve; stimulation of the inhibitory sympathetic neurons results in increased vagal tone.

In addition to its postsynaptic action, clonidine has presynaptic α-agonist activity. This presynaptic stimulating activity may inhibit neurotransmitter release and contribute to the decrease in plasma norepinephrine concentrations found during clonidine therapy.[11]

HEMODYNAMIC EFFECTS

Oral administration of clonidine acutely reduces blood pressure, heart rate, cardiac output, and stroke volume, without any consistent change in calculated total peripheral resistance. The decrease in cardiac output is due primarily to the reduction of heart rate and venous return (due to venodilation), with no change in myocardial contractility.[1] Incremental increases in cardiac output and heart rate in response to exercise are preserved, probably because the central sympathetic inhibitory action of clonidine is more prominent than the peripheral constrictor action, allowing peripheral effector mechanisms to remain intact.[1, 12] Renal blood flow and glomerular filtration rate are preserved during treatment with clonidine, as a result of compensation for reduced renal perfusion pressure by renal autoregulation.[13] Clonidine is effective in controlling hypertension associated with renal insufficiency and does not appear to further worsen renal function.[14] However, because of the importance of the renal clearance of clonidine, the dosage may need to be adjusted in the presence of severe renal insufficiency.

Chronic administration of clonidine results in decreases in blood pressure and resting heart rate similar to those observed with acute administration. The reduction in resting heart rate is seen in both the supine and the upright positions.[15] Supine and standing blood pressures are similar, and symptoms of orthostatic hypotension are unusual and decidedly less frequent than with ganglionic blockers and peripherally acting vasodilators. Total peripheral resistance is reduced during chronic administration, but despite this persistent reduction, cardiac output returns to normal within 4 to 6 weeks.[1]

CARDIAC EFFECTS

Left ventricular hypertrophy is a common manifestation of end-organ damage from hypertension and constitutes an independent cardiovascular risk factor.[16, 17] Left ventricular mass is correlated with plasma norepinephrine concentrations in spontaneously hypertensive rats. Therapy with sympathetic blocking agents can produce a reduction in left ventricular mass in these rats that is independent of the agents' effects on blood pressure.[18] Although vasodilating agents lower blood pressure in rats[18] and in humans,[19] these agents do not cause regression of left ventricular mass. In humans, regression of left ventricular hypertrophy has been observed with clonidine therapy with and without a low-dose diuretic.[20, 21] Therapy with other centrally acting agents used as monotherapy may be more effective in reducing left ventricular mass.[22] Diastolic left ventricular filling, which reflects diastolic ventricular function, has been found to be abnormal in hypertensive patients[23] and may improve during short-term (12 weeks) clonidine therapy.[24]

The effects of clonidine on coronary arterial blood flow have not been well studied. In one study of 29 patients with exertional angina, 48% of patients demonstrated a decrease in anginal symptoms during clonidine therapy.[25] Possible mechanisms include reduction of heart rate and blood pressure (both prime determinants of myocardial oxygen consumption), reduction of left ventricular mass, and possible coronary vasodilation. Further evidence for beneficial effects of clonidine therapy in patients with obstructive coronary artery disease was found in another study in which 12 patients with chronic stable effort angina were treated with clonidine for 3 weeks. Clonidine administration lowered the rate-pressure product at rest and during exercise and increased exercise duration.[26]

There are no known direct electrophysiologic effects of clonidine. Any demonstrable electrophysiologic effects may be attributed to decreased resting sympathetic and increased resting parasympathetic tone.

EFFECTS ON RENIN AND ALDOSTERONE

Clonidine decreases plasma renin activity, presumably as a result of the decrease in sympathetic activity. However, it may directly inhibit the renal release of renin.[27] The inhibition of renin release contributes to the antihypertensive effect of clonidine. A renin-independent antihypertensive effect has also been demonstrated in patients with low renin levels in whom clonidine did not cause changes in plasma renin activity.[28] Clonidine causes suppression of aldosterone production, which may also contribute to its blood pressure–lowering effects.[1] The notable lack of salt and water retention seen with clonidine therapy is probably a result of the inhibition of the renin-aldosterone axis.

METABOLIC EFFECTS

With the growing suspicion that the metabolic effects of antihypertensive agents may be related to the pathogenesis of atherosclerosis and/or its complications, the metabolic effects of clonidine and other antihypertensive agents have been increasingly evaluated.[29–32] The effects of clonidine administration are controversial, with total serum cholesterol levels decreasing by 5% to 6% in two studies[28, 31] and increasing by 6% in another study.[30] Clonidine therapy has been noted to reduce the atherogenic low-density lipoprotein (LDL) concentrations without changing the cardioprotective high-density lipoprotein (HDL) concentrations, with a decrease in the LDL/HDL ratio and a resultant decrease in predicted cardiovascular risk.[31] However, both LDL and HDL cholesterol levels were decreased in another study, with a neutral effect on cardiovascular risk.[32] Clonidine does not adversely affect glucose tolerance.[1] This lack of consistent adverse metabolic effects on lipid metabolism, glucose tolerance, and potassium balance makes clonidine monotherapy preferable to diuretics in selected patients.

TRANSDERMAL CLONIDINE

The transdermal formulation of clonidine consists of a self-adhesive water-resistant patch that is usually applied to the chest or upper outer arms. The evenness of clonidine concentrations during transdermal therapy is a major advantage of this method of administration. The use of conventional oral medications is associated with fluctuations in plasma concentrations characterized by a peak after dose ingestion and a trough immediately before the next dose. Because plasma levels of clonidine correlate directly with the magnitude of side effects,[2, 33] especially sedation and dry mouth, it is not surprising that when transdermal clonidine has been substituted for the oral form of the agent, there has been a marked reduction in the incidence of side effects.[34–37]

Because the frequency and severity of side effects diminish adherence to treatment,[36] the transdermal formulation of clonidine may allow the use of this drug in patients who might otherwise be noncompliant. Furthermore, the once-weekly dosing schedule for this formulation has been associated with a high degree of medication compliance, with only minimal effects on quality of life.[38] In a study comparing transdermal clonidine with twice-daily verapamil,[38] the transdermal clonidine was worn as directed by 96% to 100% of patients, compared with correct dosing in only 70% of patients receiving verapamil. Similar results were observed in studies comparing transdermal clonidine with oral captopril[37] and with oral enalapril.[39] Transdermal clonidine has been successfully used with high compliance rates in patient populations at risk for poor compliance[40] and has been associated with improved compliance and reduced health care expenditures when compared with twice-daily oral agents.[41]

Multiple clinical trials with transdermal clonidine have shown its efficacy across the full demographic spectrum of hypertensive patients.[24] It has been found to work well in elderly patients as well as in the young and to be equally effective in black and in white patients. Moreover, it works well in patients with renal insufficiency,[14] patients on chronic hemodialysis,[42] and those with diabetes mellitus. As with other forms of antihypertensive therapy, it is effective as monotherapy in approximately 60% of patients with mild to moderate essential hypertension. Transdermal clonidine may be used as part of a multiple drug regimen to reduce clonidine-associated side effects and to simplify the dosing schedule.

The greatest benefit of the transdermal delivery system is its convenience and low incidence of side effects. The attractiveness of taking this medication on a once-weekly basis appears to be strong; it allows patients to go for a week without being reminded of their requirements for medical support. It is of practical value in some older or infirm patients who, for physical or emotional reasons, cannot be responsible for taking their own medications. The administration of this treatment can easily be undertaken in such individuals by a relative or other person. The advantages of transdermal administration should make it attractive in a substantial portion of hypertensive patients. In studies comparing transdermal clonidine with oral agents, a majority of patients indicated a preference for transdermal medication.[36, 38] In a survey of more than 3000 patients, a majority of those who switched from oral regimens to transdermal clonidine were satisfied or highly satisfied.[44] Whereas unwanted side effects, poor compliance, or inadequate results have occurred with conventional forms of treatment, the transdermal clonidine preparation might offer a good alternative for achieving satisfactory and well-tolerated control of blood pressure.

CLINICAL USE
Indications

Clonidine may be used in treating all forms of hypertension; its clinical efficacy has been well documented.[1, 24, 29, 30] When used as monotherapy, clonidine reduces blood pressure to normal levels in approximately one half of patients with mild hypertension.[1] Satisfactory control of blood pressure can be attained with low doses of clonidine (0.4 mg or less) in many instances. The combination of clonidine and a diuretic is even more effective than monotherapy, and the combination controls blood pressure in more than 70% of patients with mild to moderate hypertension.[44]

The use of transdermal clonidine in combination with enalapril[12, 39] and diltiazem[20, 45] has been effective and well accepted by patients. A combination of transdermal clonidine with similar agents can be expected to have comparable results. Transdermal clonidine should be effective in most situations in which oral clonidine is indicated, with the exception of the acute treatment of high blood pressure requiring urgent treatment.

Clonidine is not indicated in hypertensive emergencies when more rapidly acting and predictable agents are available. However, rapid clonidine loading is useful in treating urgent hypertensive situations or severe hypertension unaccompanied with alterations in mental status or other signs of severe end-organ dysfunction.[46] The initial dose is 0.1 to 0.2 mg PO, followed by 0.1 mg hourly until blood pressure is reduced to safe levels, or to a total dose of 0.5 mg. This approach is effective in 70% to 80% of patients within 2 to 3 hours.

Combination Therapy

Clonidine therapy can be effectively combined with many other available antihypertensive agents. In addition to the effective diuretic-clonidine combination, clonidine can be used together with directly acting vasodilators such as hydralazine or minoxidil. The centrally mediated heart rate–lowering effect of clonidine blocks the reflex tachycardia induced by other vasodilators, often obviating the need for a β-blocker. In addition, clonidine blocks the renin-stimulating effects of vasodilators, which may make such combinations more effective.

In its transdermal form, clonidine has been used successfully with both angiotensin-converting enzyme inhibitors[39] and calcium antagonists.[43]

The combination of clonidine and a β-blocker may produce variable results. Improved efficacy,[24] increased side effects, and even antagonism[1] have been reported. Propranolol appears to have additive antihypertensive and heart rate–lowering effects when combined with clonidine.[24] These additive effects suggest different mechanisms of action on the vasculature and heart for each drug. Withdrawal of both clonidine and β-blockers may lead to sympathetic overactivity, and abrupt discontinuation of combined therapy may be particularly hazardous.

The combination of clonidine with α-adrenergic blocking agents is unlikely to result in any improvement over therapy with either agent alone. α-Adrenergic blocking agents exert their antihypertensive effects by blocking peripheral postsynaptic α-receptors that reduce sympathetic vasoconstrictor tone. Although the site of action of prazosin and other α-adrenergic blocking agents differs from that of clonidine, ultimately both agents have the effect of blocking vasoconstriction produced by sympathetic nervous system stimulation of postsynaptic α-receptors. In this light, the failure of prazosin to augment the antihypertensive effects of clonidine is not unexpected.[47]

Precautions and Adverse Effects

There are no known contraindications to clonidine therapy other than known prior sensitivity. The most frequent side effects encountered with clonidine therapy are dry mouth (as many as 48% of patients), drowsiness (approximately one third of patients), and sedation (approximately 8% of patients). These side effects are manifestations of its central nervous system actions and can be minimized by giving the greater part or total daily dose at bedtime. The drowsiness and dry mouth abate in a majority of patients after 4 to 6 weeks of continued therapy. Approximately 7% of patients discontinue therapy because of intolerable side effects.[48] The transdermal patch appears to significantly reduce all the significant systemic side effects. However, a cutaneous reaction directly under the patch occurs in 10% to 20% of patients.[24, 38] This occurs 3 weeks to 9 months after starting therapy and can range from a superficial irritation to a localized contact dermatitis. The skin eruption may be associated with small vesicles or superficial ulcerations. Cessation of therapy results in disappearance of the skin lesions. Subsequent oral therapy in patients with mild skin eruptions has not been followed by systemic allergic manifestations. In addition, rechallenging patients who have had prior skin reactions with large oral dosages of clonidine has provoked new or reactivated previous skin eruptions in only one or two patients. Fair-skinned patients and women appear to be slightly more prone to allergic skin reactions. Dermal pretreatment with 0.5% hydrocortisone cream may reduce the incidence of this reaction.[4] A slight reduction in drug absorption associated with this dermal pretreatment is probably of negligible clinical significance. Pretreatment with magnesium-aluminum hydroxide suspension did not significantly reduce patch-associated dermatitis in this study. Rare gastrointestinal, dermatologic, and central nervous system adverse reactions have been reported. Sexual dysfunction, frequently seen with antihypertensive therapy, is an infrequent complication of clonidine therapy. Further delineation of the less frequent adverse reactions can be found in the prescribing information.

Discontinuation Syndrome

Much has been written about the deleterious effects of sudden discontinuation of clonidine, and a detailed review is beyond the scope of this article. An excellent review can be found elsewhere.[44] Early reports of increases in blood pressure occurring 24 to 72 hours after discontinuation of therapy to levels that were higher than pretreatment levels were of great concern. The incidence of this type of response to abrupt discontinuation of clonidine is very low and perhaps even lower than that seen after β-blocker withdrawal.

It is possible to describe three patterns of responses to abrupt discontinuation of clonidine. These probably apply to many other antihypertensive agents as well.[49] The first response to discontinuation of therapy is a gradual asymptomatic increase in blood pressure to pretreatment levels after a variable period of stable blood pressure. The second and perhaps most frequently observed response to discontinuation of clonidine therapy is for the blood pressure to remain at treated levels or to rise slowly, with signs and symptoms of sympathetic overactivity (e.g., anxiety, tachycardia, headache, and sleeplessness) predominating. The third type of response is a rapid rise in blood pressure to near-pretreatment levels within hours of discontinuation of therapy. An overshoot above pretreatment levels is unusual. The signs and symptoms of sympathetic overactivity may or may not be present with this pattern. The picture is frequently clouded by the presence of other antihypertensive agents.[49]

Because discontinuation syndromes are rare when low dosages of medication are discontinued, clonidine and other adrenergic inhibitors should be tapered, and all patients should be cautioned to the possible dangers of unsupervised discontinuation of antihypertensive medication. Particular caution should be exercised when stopping combined therapy of clonidine and other antihypertensive agents, especially centrally acting adrenergic inhibitors and β-blockers, as they may interact to cause a more severe reaction. Particular care should be used in patients with both angina and hypertension who are taking a combination of clonidine and β-blockers, because discontinuation of both agents may increase cardiac sympathetic stimulation. When discontinuation is indicated, the β-blocker should be gradually withdrawn before tapering clonidine, if possible. In case of a hypertensive crisis after acute discontinuation of clonidine in the presence of a β-blocker (unopposed α-adrenoreceptor-mediated vasoconstriction), treatment with labetalol (combined α-β-blockade) is appropriate.

The most specific therapy for signs and symptoms of withdrawal is the reinstitution of the agent that was discontinued. If severe hypertension occurs, intravenous administration of sodium nitroprusside may be necessary.

Place in Armamentarium

While the Joint National Committee on the Detection, Evaluation, and Treatment of High Blood Pressure has recommended the use of β-blockers and thiazide diuretics as first-line therapy for hypertension,[50] in fact, a significant portion of patients requiring antihypertensive treatment may have contraindications to or be unable to tolerate these agents.[51] In these patients, individualization of therapy requires consideration of underlying conditions and demographic characteristics that may influence their ability to tolerate certain medications and the likelihood of an adequate response to therapy. A comparison of clonidine to some classes of antihypertensive drugs is given in Table 64–1. Sufficient clinical experience has been accumulated to allow creation of generalized clinical profiles that may increase the likelihood of initially selecting a successful antihypertensive agent for patients in specific groups. It is reasonable to select an initial agent based on clinical experience and to increase it until blood pressure is controlled or side effects become unacceptable. If blood pressure is not lowered to acceptable levels, then another class of antihyper-

Table 64–1. **Clinical Effects of Five Types of Antihypertensive Agents**

	Clonidine	β-Blockers	Diuretic	Angiotensin-Converting Enzyme Inhibitors	Calcium Antagonists
Young	Effective	Effective	Less effective	Effective	Less effective
Elderly	Effective	Less effective	Effective	Effective	Effective
Black	Effective	Less effective	Effective	Effective	Effective
White	Effective	Less effective	Less effective	Effective	Effective
Patients with diabetes	Safe and effective	Caution with insulin RX	May affect glucose control	Recommended	Safe and effective
Serum cholesterol	Decrease	Increase	Increase	No change	No change
Serum	No effect	No effect	Usually	No effect	No effect
Exercise tolerance	No change	Decrease	Decrease	No change	No change

tensive agents may be substituted and titrated as previously discussed. Combination of agents should be reserved for the remaining patients whose blood pressure is not controlled by monotherapy.

Clonidine works well at any stage of antihypertensive therapy, is generally safe, and is limited only by its side effects. As has already been stated, clonidine also works well with the addition of a low-dose diuretic, an angiotensin-converting enzyme inhibitor, a calcium antagonist, a β-blocker, or a directly acting vasodilator such as hydralazine and minoxidil. The major limitations on its use are the side effects of dry mouth and sedation.

Dosage and Administration

The usual starting dose of oral clonidine is 0.1 mg b.i.d., which may be gradually increased by 0.1 mg per dose per week. The usual dose range is 0.2 to 0.6 mg b.i.d., although doses above 0.6 mg b.i.d. are usually unnecessary. The side effects of dry mouth and sedation can be minimized by giving the major portion of the dose at bedtime. In the elderly, once-daily administration at bedtime is a very effective and convenient way of lowering blood pressure and avoiding unpleasant side effects.

Transdermal clonidine can be substituted for the oral formulation, provides exceptional convenience, and greatly reduces the incidence of the major side effects of sedation and dry mouth.[13] Different sizes of the patch are programmed to yield 0.1 mg, 0.2 mg, or 0.3 mg of clonidine per day for 7 days. When switching a patient from oral clonidine to the transdermal patch, one selects the patch that represents the total daily dose and applies it to the upper outer arms or torso. As there is considerable intrapatient variability regarding the oral and transdermal absorption of clonidine, this is merely a safe starting point, and adjustment of the transdermal dosage is frequently required. Because it takes 2 to 3 days for blood levels of the drug to become stable, oral clonidine should be continued at the same dose for the first day that the first patch is in place. The oral clonidine should be reduced to one-half the dose on the second day and then discontinued on the third day. The patch should be replaced weekly at different sites.

Compliance

The adverse effects of clonidine can be minimized by starting with a low dose (0.1 mg) at bedtime and very slowly increasing the dosage. In most patients, side effects tend to disappear after the first few weeks of therapy. If the patient who is having troublesome side effects can be convinced to continue the medication for the 2 to 6 weeks that the side effects may take to resolve, from then on compliance will be markedly improved. The transdermal formulation significantly improves compliance by virtue of only having to be applied once a week.

REFERENCES

1. Houston J: Clonidine hydrochloride: Review of pharmacologic and clinical aspects. Prog Cardiovasc Dis 23:337, 1981.
2. Dollery CT, Davies DS, Draffan GH, et al: Clinical pharmacology and pharmacokinetics of clonidine. Clin Pharmacol Ther 19:11, 1976.
3. Lilja M, Juustila H, Sarna S, et al: Transdermal and oral clonidine. Ann Med 23:265, 1991.
4. Ito MK, O'Connor DT: Skin pretreatment and the use of transdermal clonidine. Am J Med 91(1A):42S, 1991.
5. Van Zuiten PA: Pharmacology of centrally acting drugs. Br J Clin Pharmacol 10:13s, 1980.
6. Tuck ML: The sympathetic nervous system in essential hypertension. Am Heart J 112:877, 1986.
7. Guthrie GP Jr, Kotchen TA: Effects of oral clonidine on baroreflex function in patients with essential hypertension. Chest 83(Suppl):327, 1983.
8. Lubbe WF: Clonidine in the management of uncontrolled hypertension. S Afr Med J 48:391, 1974.
9. Kobinger W, Walland A: Facilitation of vagal reflex bradycardia by an action of clonidine on cerebral alpha receptors. Eur J Pharmacol 19:210, 1972.
10. Kroner PI, Oliver JR, Sleight P, et al: Assessment of cardiac automatic excitability in renal hypertensive rats using clonidine-induced resetting of the baroreceptor-heart rate reflex. Eur J Pharmacol 33:353, 1975.
11. Sullivan PA, DeQuattro V, Foti A, et al: Effects of clonidine on central and peripheral nerve tone in primary hypertension. Hypertension 8:611, 1986.
12. Brest AN: Hemodynamic and cardiac effects of clonidine. J Cardiovasc Pharmacol 2(Suppl 1):39, 1980.
13. Schwartz AB, Kim KE, Swartz C, et al: Cardiac and renal effects of clonidine. In Onesti G (ed): Hypertension. New York: Grune & Stratton, 1973, p 381.
14. Lowenthal DT, Saris SD, Paran E, et al: The use of transdermal clonidine in the hypertensive patient with chronic renal failure. Clin Nephrol 39(1):37, 1993.
15. Brod J, Horbach L, Just H: Acute effects of clonidine on central and peripheral hemodynamics and plasma renin activity. Eur J Pharmacol 4:107, 1972.
16. Kannel WB: The Framingham study. Am J Med 75:4, 1983.
17. Casale GA, Pickering TG, Laragh JH: Value of echocardiographic measurement of left ventricular mass in predicting cardiovascular morbid events in hypertensive men. Ann Intern Med 105:173, 1986.
18. Tarazi RC, Sen S, Saracoga M, et al: The multifactorial role of catecholamines in hypertensive cardiac hypertrophy. Eur Heart J 3(Suppl A):103, 1982.
19. Reichek N, Franklin BB, Chandler T, et al: Reversal of ventricular hypertrophy by antihypertensive therapy. Eur Heart J 3(Suppl A):165, 1982.
20. Arevalo JV: Clonidine and left ventricular function in patients with arterial hypertension. Tribuna Med 68:29, 1983.
21. McMahon FC, Ryan MR Jr, LaCorte WSTJ, et al: Regression of left ventricular hypertrophy in 19 hypertensive patients treated with clonidine for 18 months: A prospective study. In Weber MA, Drayer JIM, Kolloch R (eds): Low Dose Oral and Transdermal Therapy of Hypertension. Darmstadt, Germany: Steinkopff-Verlag, 1985, p 81.
22. Drayer JIM, Weber MA, Gardin JM: Mediators of changes in left ventricular mass during antihypertensive therapy. In Keurs HEDJ, Schipperheyn JJ (eds): Cardiac LVH. Boston: Martinus-Nijhoff, 1984, p 224.
23. Gardin JM, Drayer JIM, Weber MA, et al: Pulsed Doppler echocardiographic assessment of left ventricular systolic and diastolic function in mild hypertension. Hypertension 9(Suppl 2):1190, 1987.
24. Weber MA, Graettinger WF, Drayer JIM: The adrenergic inhibitors. Med Clin North Am 71:1, 1987.
25. Raftos J, Bauer GE, Lewis RG: Clonidine in the treatment of severe hypertension. Med J Aust 1:786, 1973.
26. Thomas MG, Quiroz AC, Rice JC, et al: Antianginal effects of clonidine. J Cardiovasc Pharmacol 8(Suppl 3):S69, 1986.
27. Pettinger WA, Keeton TK, Campbell WB, et al: Evidence for

a renal adrenergic receptor inhibiting renin release. Circ Res 38:338, 1976.

28. Bolme P, Fuxe K: Pharmacologic studies on the hypotensive effects of clonidine. Eur J Pharmacol 13:168, 1971.
29. Kirkendall WM, Hammond JJ, Thomas JC, et al: Prazosin and clonidine for moderately severe hypertension. JAMA 240:2553, 1978.
30. Karlberg BE, Lins LE, Rossner S: Clonidine in mild hypertension: Effects on blood pressure and on serum lipids. J Hypertens 3(Suppl):S69, 1985.
31. Moerl H, Diehm C: Lipid metabolism and antihypertensive treatment with particular reference to clonidine. In Hayduk K, Bock KD (eds): Central Blood Pressure Regulation Clonidine Workshop. Miami: Symposia Specialists, 1983, pp 255–260.
32. Grimm RH, Collins G, Neaton JD: Clonidine and blood lipids: A double-blind placebo-controlled cross-over study. Circulation 76(Suppl 4):434, 1987.
33. Karanen A, Nykanen S, Tashinen J: Pharmacokinetics and side-effects of clonidine. Eur J Clin Pharmacol 13:97, 1978.
34. Weber MA, Drayer JIM: Clinical experience with rate-controlled delivery of antihypertensive therapy by a transdermal system. Am Heart J 108:231, 1984.
35. Burris JF, Mroczek WJ: Transdermal administration of clonidine: A new approach to antihypertensive therapy. Pharmacology 6:30, 1986.
36. McMahon FG, Jain AK, Vargas R, et al: A double-blind comparison of transdermal clonidine and oral captopril in essential hypertension. Clin Ther 12:88, 1990.
37. Weber MA, Drayer J, Brewer DD, et al: Transdermal continuous antihypertensive therapy. Lancet 1:9, 1984.
38. Burris JF, Papademetriou V, Wallin JD, et al: Therapeutic adherence in the elderly: Transdermal clonidine compared to oral verapamil for hypertension. Am J Med 91(Suppl IA):1S, 1991.
39. Weidler D, Wallin JD, Cook E, et al: Transdermal clonidine as an adjunct to enalapril: An evaluation of efficacy and patient compliance. J Clin Pharmacol 32(5):444, 1992.
40. Branche GC Jr, Batts JM, Dowdy VM, et al: Improving compliance in an inner-city hypertensive patient population. Am J Med 91(1A):37S, 1991.
41. Sclar DA, Skaer TL, Chin A, et al: Utility of a transdermal delivery system for antihypertensive therapy: Part I. Am J Med 91(1A):50S, 1991.
42. Rosansky SJ, Johnson KL, McConnel J: Use of transdermal clonidine in chronic hemodialysis patients. Clin Nephrol 39(1):32, 1993.
43. Hollifield J: Clinical acceptability of transdermal clonidine: A large scale evaluation by practitioners. Am Heart J 112:900, 1986.
44. Toubes DB, McIntosh TJ, Kirkendall WM, et al: Hypotensive effects of clonidine and chlorthalidone. Am Heart J 82:312, 1971.
45. Lueg MC, Herron J, Zellner S: Transdermal clonidine as an adjunct to sustained-release diltiazem in the treatment of mild-to-moderate hypertension. Clin Ther 13(4):471, 1991.
46. Cohen IM, Katz MA: Oral clonidine loading for rapid control of hypertension. Clin Pharmacol Ther 24:11, 1978.
47. Hubbell FA, Weber MA, Drayer JIM: Neutralization of prazosin's antihypertensive effect in the presence of clonidine [abstract]. Clin Res 29:272A, 1981.
48. McMahon FG: Management of Essential Hypertension. Mt. Kisco, NY: Futura, 1978.
49. Weber MA: Discontinuation syndrome following cessation of treatment with clonidine and other antihypertensive agents. J Cardiovasc Pharmacol 2(Suppl 1):S73, 1980.
50. The Fifth Report of the Joint National Committee on Detection, Evaluation, and Treatment of High Blood Pressure (JNC V). Arch Intern Med 153:154, 1993.
51. Weber MA, Laragh JH: Hypertension: Steps forward and steps backward. Arch Intern Med 153:149, 1993.

CHAPTER 65

Guanabenz

Deanna G. Cheung, M.D., William F. Graettinger, M.D., and Michael A. Weber, M.D.

Guanabenz (2,6-dichlorobenzylidene aminoguanidine acetate) is an orally active central α_2-adrenoreceptor agonist. It is an aminoguanidine structurally similar to clonidine (Fig. 65–1). Suppression of sympathetic discharge and lowering of blood pressure by the drug were demonstrated in animal studies in the early 1970s.[1, 2] Subsequent clinical trials demonstrated the antihypertensive efficacy of guanabenz as a single agent and in combination with hydrochlorothiazide.[3–5] Guanabenz has been available for therapeutic purposes in the United States since 1982.

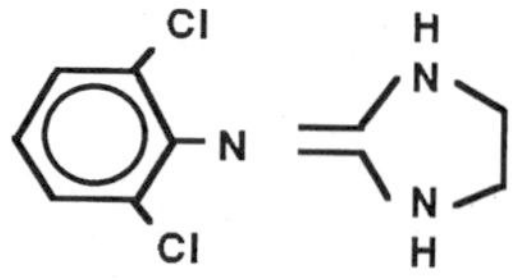

PHARMACOLOGY AND PHARMACOKINETICS

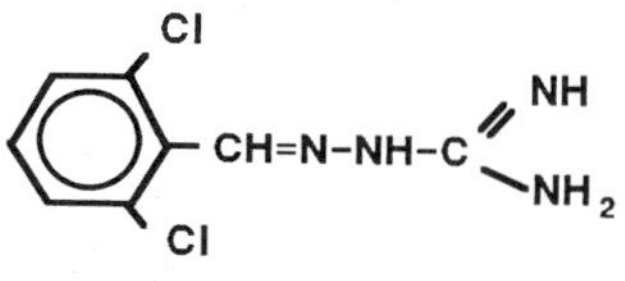

Guanabenz stimulates central postsynaptic α-adrenoreceptors, causing a reduction in sympathetic outflow from the brain stem.[1, 2, 6] This effect has been shown to be a direct, central effect rather than a reflex action.[7, 8] While guanabenz has been found to reduce the response to peripheral sympathetic nerve stimulation,[9, 10] indicating that it does have some peripheral adrenergic neuron-blocking activity, the central effect is of overriding importance to its antihypertensive effect in humans.[8, 11] Direct central α-adrenoreceptor stimulation causes reduction of norepinephrine synthesis and release from central noradrenergic neu-

Figure 65–1. Chemical structures of clonidine and guanabenz.

CLONIDINE

GUANABENZ

rons, resulting in subsequent reductions in plasma epinephrine and norepinephrine levels. Guanabenz appears to interact with the same adrenoreceptor that mediates the action of clonidine.[12] Guanabenz has also been reported to exert some β-blocking activity in red blood cell preparations;[13] however, β-blockade probably does not contribute significantly to its antihypertensive efficacy. Some evidence indicates that stimulation of nonadrenergic sites may contribute to the antihypertensive properties of this agent.[14–16] Guanabenz may also have some inhibitory effects on aldosterone synthesis.[17]

Guanabenz is readily and completely absorbed from the gastrointestinal tract and rapidly metabolized,[18] possibly by an extensive first-pass mechanism.[14, 19] The onset of action occurs within approximately 2 hours, with a duration of action of approximately 10 hours, after oral administration.[20] Peak plasma levels of 2.5 to 2.9 ng/ml are reached 2 to 5 hours after oral administration.[18, 21] A half-life of 6 hours can be expected. No data concerning the correlation between plasma concentrations and clinical activity are available. The volume of distribution has been estimated to be as large as 7400 L with a 16-mg dose and 13,400 L with a 32-mg dose in patients with mild to moderate hypertension. It is 90% bound to plasma proteins.[18]

Guanabenz is metabolized in the liver, primarily by hydroxylation followed by glucuronidation. The major metabolite (E)-p-hydroxyguanabenz is inactive, and the majority of the metabolites are excreted in the urine. The renal clearance of guanabenz is between 0.09 and 0.13 L/min.[21] Clearance may be slightly reduced in patients with moderate renal insufficiency.[22] As much as 32% of the dose may be excreted in feces. Small amounts of unchanged drug (1.4%) are excreted in urine.

PATHOPHYSIOLOGIC EFFECTS OF GUANABENZ
Hemodynamics and Cardiac Function

The antihypertensive action of guanabenz has been well documented in many clinical studies.[18, 23] A smooth dose-response relationship for blood pressure lowering has been demonstrated for doses between 2 and 16 mg.[23] Guanabenz reduces blood pressure to clinically acceptable levels in 60% to 80% of patients with mild to moderate hypertension.[24] Diastolic blood pressure reductions of 10 to 20 mmHg during chronic therapy have been observed in clinical trials.[18] These blood pressure reductions appear to be sustained during chronic therapy for periods of 6 months to 12 years.[24, 25]

Guanabenz has been shown to reduce heart rate and myocardial contractility in animals.[26, 27] However, in hypertensive patients, blood pressure appears to be lowered via a reduction in peripheral resistance with minimal effects on heart rate and contractility.[18] Single oral doses of as much as 16 mg caused no significant depression of echocardiographically measured cardiac function in hypertensive patients.[20] Likewise, after 1 month and 6 months of chronic therapy with 16 to 64 mg of guanabenz daily, no echocardiographically detectable changes in left ventricular function were found in patients. In fact, guanabenz may actually reverse hypertensive left ventricular hypertrophy.[28]

Pulse rate has been observed to decrease slightly in patients treated with guanabenz for periods longer than 1 month.[29] This may be partly related to the actions of guanabenz on peripheral adrenergic neurons.[30]

The electrophysiologic effects of guanabenz have been studied in dogs.[1] Intravenous guanabenz was found to have little effect on intraatrial or intraventricular conduction rates at doses of 0.1 to 1 mg/kg, but prolongation of atrioventricular conduction with PR interval prolongation was noted at doses of 0.01 mg/kg and higher. Decreased ventricular irritability and prolonged refractory periods were also observed. Alterations in T waves and slight ST depression were also noted in these animals. Direct effects of guanabenz on coronary blood flow have not been described in the available literature.

Fluid and Electrolyte Balance

Clinically, fluid and electrolyte homeostasis appears to be minimally affected by guanabenz therapy.[31] Weight gain and edema formation have not been reported. In fact, a slight decrease in body weight during the first several months of treatment with guanabenz has been described.[25] The mechanism of this weight loss has not been established but is thought to be related to natriuresis mediated by the effect of guanabenz on chloride resorption in the papillary collection duct.[32]

Although single oral doses of guanabenz have been reported to decrease glomerular filtration, renal plasma flow, free water clearance, and sodium excretion,[33] chronic oral administration does not significantly reduce glomerular filtration rate, sodium balance, serum sodium concentration, or body fluid volume.[22, 28, 33–35] In fact, increases in fractional excretion of sodium and free water clearance 24 hours after acute administration of guanabenz to salt-loaded hypertensive patients have been described, associated with a return to baseline within 1 week of chronic therapy.[36] Such an increase in free water clearance may be related to inhibition of vasopressin secretion by central α-adrenoreceptor stimulation[31, 37] or by antagonizing vasopressin receptors on end organs.[38]

Renal Function

Significant renal toxicity during guanabenz therapy is improbable. Long-term administration of guanabenz for periods of 6 months to 2 years resulted in no significant change in blood urea nitrogen or creatinine in a multicenter study involving 329 patients.[25] During a 12-week period, no changes in body weight or creatinine clearance were observed in patients with moderate renal insufficiency.[39] Renal vasoconstriction has been associated with α-adrenoreceptor agonist therapy[40] and does occur with guanabenz.[41] This renal vasoconstrictive response appears to be calcium dependent and is attenuated by verapamil in animal preparations.

Plasma renin activity does not appear to be suppressed by guanabenz therapy.[25, 42] However, inhibition of renin secretion has been observed during therapy with α2-agonists,[43–45] which may be related to baseline renin levels in patients with essential hypertension.[43] Even though measured plasma renin activity is not decreased, an inhibitory effect of α2-agonists on renin secretion may be inferred from the absence of an increase in renin activity in the face of reduced blood pressures.

Metabolism and Endocrinologic Function

The most noteworthy metabolic action of guanabenz is a reduction in total cholesterol levels.[35, 46, 47] Total cholesterol is usually lowered by 10% to 20%. In patients treated with guanabenz for 2 to 6 months, serum cholesterol and triglyceride levels were reduced by 19 mg/dl and 33 mg/dl, respectively.[24] Low-density lipoprotein levels can be expected to decrease.[48] The mechanism of cholesterol reduction may be related to inhibition of hepatic cholesterol production and triglyceride synthesis as well as stimulation of fatty acid oxidation.[49]

In contrast with the other two available α-adrenergic agonists, clonidine and methyldopa, glucose intolerance has not been associated with chronic treatment with guanabenz.[25, 47, 50, 51] In fact, no effect on insulin, glucagon, growth hormone, or prolactin levels was found in a group of 45 nondiabetic patients taking guanabenz for 2 years.[51] No changes in diabetic control were attributed to guanabenz therapy in diabetic patients taking the drug for periods of up to 2 years.[52]

Central Nervous System

The effect of guanabenz on the central nervous system is characterized by the mechanism of its therapeutic antihypertensive action. Guanabenz penetrates the central nervous system and has been shown to reduce cerebral norepinephrine, dopamine, and serotonin tissue contents in animal preparations.[1, 2] The therapeutic mechanism of action probably underlies the prominence of the centrally mediated side effects of sedation and dry mouth. Impairment of cerebral blood flow has not been described.

CLINICAL USE
Indications

Guanabenz is indicated in the treatment of chronic hypertension. Used as a single agent to lower blood pressure, it compares well with other agents in its class.[18] Because of its somewhat delayed onset of action relative to clonidine, guanabenz is less useful than that drug as a diagnostic tool in evaluating the presence of pheochromocytoma by catecholamine suppression. Guanabenz is not indicated for the emergent treatment of malignant or accelerated hypertension.

Side Effects and Adverse Reactions

Guanabenz shares with other centrally acting α-agonists the common side effects of sedation and dry mouth. These occur in approximately 20% to 30% of patients,[25] although in one study these side effects were reported to occur in 36% to 48%.[24] These effects usually occur within the first 2 weeks of therapy and tend to dissipate with long-term administration. Weakness, dizziness, and headache have also been reported,[24, 25] but postural hypotension, insomnia, impotence, and gastrointestinal complaints are rare (<2%). Adverse effects appear to be dose related and are less common at dosages of 8 mg/day or less. However, as many as 14% of patients may discontinue the drug because of side effects.[25]

Abrupt cessation of guanabenz therapy may be associated with a discontinuation syndrome similar to that seen with clonidine.[53–55] Blood pressure may acutely rise 5 to 20 mmHg above pretreatment values, with an associated increase in heart rate and plasma catecholamine levels after discontinuation of therapy. Sympathetic overactivity in this situation may cause symptoms of palpitations, tremulousness, dizziness, diaphoresis, anxiety, and nausea.[55] These effects usually occur within 72 hours after discontinuation of the drug. The incidence and severity of withdrawal signs and symptoms appear to be slightly less for guanabenz than for clonidine.[54] In fact, in one series of 10 patients, no evidence of a withdrawal syndrome was observed 48 hours after discontinuation of guanabenz, 16 to 48 mg daily.[56] Patients receiving high doses of antihypertensive agents and those who require concomitant β-blocker therapy may be at increased risk for a discontinuation syndrome.[57] This syndrome is of particular concern in patients who forget to take their medication and in patients undergoing anesthesia and surgery. It may be avoided by gradually withdrawing treatment whenever possible and by withdrawing β-blockers before discontinuing central α-adrenergic agents such as guanabenz.

No significant abnormalities of renal or liver function tests have been associated with acute or chronic therapy in a number of clinical trials.[18]

Contraindications

Guanabenz is contraindicated in patients with known hypersensitivity to the drug. The use of guanabenz during pregnancy has not been studied clinically and should be avoided whenever possible; an increased incidence of skeletal abnormalities, fetal loss, and low birth weights have been observed in animal studies.[18] Although guanabenz has been safely administered to children aged 12 years and older,[58] clinical studies in younger children are lacking.

Interactions with Other Pharmacologic Agents

The therapeutic action of guanabenz can be expected to enhance the blood pressure–lowering effects of other antihypertensive agents. The central nervous system depressant effects of this drug may also potentiate the action of sedative drugs such as alcohol, barbiturates, and benzodiazepines. In addition, guanabenz may increase the absorption of hydrochlorothiazide when given concomitantly; however, plasma levels of guanabenz are not significantly affected by hydrochlorothiazide. Ethanol may specifically interfere with the blood pressure–lowering effects of guanabenz and other centrally acting antihypertensive agents.[59]

During abrupt withdrawal of guanabenz from patients taking β-blocking agents, increases in plasma catecholamine levels may induce marked vasoconstriction because peripheral α-receptors are unopposed by peripheral vasodilatory β-receptors. Consequently, the use of guanabenz in combination with β-blockers should probably be restricted to patients who are well informed and reliable.

Use of Guanabenz in Patients with Impaired Organ Function

Guanabenz may be used safely in patients with chronic renal insufficiency,[39] chronic liver disease,[60] diabetes mellitus,[50–52] and asthma and other forms of obstructive pulmonary disease.[61] Although renal excretion of guanabenz and pharmacologically active metabolites is minimal,[19, 21] dosage reduction is recommended in patients with renal insufficiency. In contrast, in a series of 10 patients with alcoholic liver disease, both oral dose clearance and the volume of distribution of guanabenz were lower than in healthy volunteers,[60] resulting in increased bioavailability of the drug. Lower doses of guanabenz may be required in patients with hepatic disease; in these patients, the dose should be individually titrated and the antihypertensive response carefully monitored.

Role of Guanabenz in the Treatment of Hypertension

Although it has been justly pointed out that β-blockers and thiazide diuretics are the only antihypertensive agents that have been demonstrated to reduce morbidity and mortality in large trials,[62] in fact, a significant number of hypertensive patients may be unable to tolerate these classes of drugs as a result of side effects or concomitant conditions that preclude their use.[63] In treating individual patients, consideration of their unique clinical picture often warrants the use of different classes of antihypertensive drugs. In this context, the use of guanabenz may be indicated. Guanabenz does not cause the fluid retention

seen with other adrenergic blocking drugs. The antihypertensive efficacy of guanabenz is well established, and it can be used alone or in combination with other drugs. An additive blood pressure–lowering effect has been reported for the use of guanabenz in combination with diuretics[64] and with captopril[65] and can be expected with other agents that lower blood pressure by different mechanisms than guanabenz.

Therapy with guanabenz is safe and efficacious in a wide variety of patients, including the elderly,[65] adolescents,[58] diabetic patients,[50–52] asthmatic patients,[61] and patients with chronic renal insufficiency.[39] Neither cardiovascular disorders nor chronic liver disease (alcoholic) preclude the use of guanabenz. The advantages of this broad spectrum of efficacy and safety must be weighed against a high incidence of unpleasant side effects, particularly sedation and dry mouth, that may occur more frequently with guanabenz therapy than with clonidine and that may affect as many as 50% of patients. On the other hand, guanabenz is not associated with the fluid retention seen with clonidine or with the hepatic or hematologic abnormalities associated with methyldopa. At doses of 8 mg twice daily and lower, the incidence of side effects may be less than 28%.

Although β-blockers and thiazide diuretics probably have fewer side effects,[23] adverse effects on glucose metabolism and cholesterol levels associated with their use are not problems with guanabenz therapy. In fact, the cholesterol-lowering effect of guanabenz may confer on it a special role in treating hypertensive patients with hypercholesterolemia.

Because of the absence of orthostatic effects in elderly patients with predominantly systolic hypertension,[66] guanabenz should be considered for use in this patient population.

Dosage and Administration

The total daily dose of guanabenz is 8 to 64 mg given in divided doses. An increase in therapeutic response is seen in doses up to 16 mg/day; higher doses may be necessary in patients with severe hypertension. The drug is administered orally.

SOCIOECONOMIC CONSIDERATIONS

When costs of office visits, medications, supplemental medications (i.e., potassium for patients taking diuretics), and laboratory tests are considered, guanabenz is slightly more expensive than clonidine or methyldopa.[67] Therapy with α-adrenergic agonists costs about the same as therapy with angiotensin-converting enzyme (ACE) inhibitors, calcium antagonists, β-blocking agents, peripheral α-blocking agents, or diuretics plus potassium supplementation. Only patients who require no potassium supplementation when taking diuretics enjoy a cost advantage with diuretic monotherapy. On the other hand, concerns about the risks of metabolic derangement and lack of efficacy in certain patient populations may limit this advantage to a relatively small group of patients.

SUMMARY

Guanabenz effectively lowers blood pressure by a centrally mediated reduction in sympathetic tone in a broad patient population. The efficacy and cost of therapy are comparable to those of most other antihypertensive agents. Side effects, which are similar to those seen with clonidine, constitute the primary limitation on its use. The major advantages of guanabenz are lack of fluid retention and a beneficial effect on serum lipids.

REFERENCES

1. Baum T, Shropshire AT: Inhibition of spontaneous sympathetic nerve activity by the antihypertensive agent Wy 8678. Neuropharmacology 9:503, 1970.
2. Baum T, Shropshire AT: Studies on the centrally mediated hypotensive activity of guanabenz. Eur J Pharmacol 37:31, 1976.
3. Nash D: Clinical trial with guanabenz, a new antihypertensive agent. J Clin Pharmacol 13:416, 1973.
4. McMahon FG, Cole PA, Boyles PW, et al: Study of a new antihypertensive (guanabenz). Curr Ther Res 16:389, 1974.
5. Annanian Figueira da Silva J, Privato de Oliveira Capaceia J, Cohen I: Assessment of a new antihypertensive agent, 2,6-dichlorobenzylidene amino guanidine acetate (guanabenz): A double-blind, cross-over trial against placebo. Pharmatherapeutica 1:1, 1976.
6. Bonham AC, Trapani AG, Portis LR, et al: Studies on the mechanism of the central antihypertensive effect of guanabenz and clonidine. J Hypertens 2(Suppl 2):543, 1984.
7. Koss MC: Analysis of CNS sympathoinhibition produced by guanabenz. Eur J Pharmacol 90:19, 1983.
8. Baum T, Shropshire AT: Aspects of the antihypertensive action of indoramin and guanabenz. In Scriabine A, Sweet CS (eds): New Antihypertensive Drugs. New York: Spectrum Publications, 1976, pp 369–386.
9. Baum T, Shropshire AT, Rowles G, et al: General pharmacologic actions of the antihypertensive agent 2,6-dichlorobenzylidene amino-guanidine acetate (Wy-8678). J Pharmacol Exp Ther 171:276, 1970.
10. Farnebo LO, Hamberger B: Influence of alpha- and beta-adrenoceptors on the release of noradrenaline from field stimulated atria and cerebral cortex slices. J Pharm Pharmacol 26:644, 1974.
11. Buhler FR, Bolli P, Amann WF, et al: Sympathetic nervous system in essential hypertension and antihypertensive response to alpha-2 adrenoceptor stimulation. J Cardiovasc Pharmacol 6:S753, 1984.
12. Fluck ER, Homon CA, Knowles JA, et al: Differential binding of guanabenz and its metabolites to cerebral alpha2-receptors: The basis for a radiological assay specific for the drug. Drug Dev Res 3:91, 1983.
13. Diamant S, Agranat I, Goldblum A, et al: Beta-adrenergic activity and conformation of the antihypertensive specific alpha-2 agonist drug, guanabenz. Biochem Pharmacol 34:491, 1985.
14. Hamilton CA: Adrenergic and nonadrenergic effects of imidazoline and related antihypertensive drugs in the brain and periphery. Am J Hypertens 5:58S, 1992.
15. Hamilton CA, Yakubu MA, Howie CA, Reid JL: Do centrally-acting antihypertensive drugs act at non-adrenergic as well as alpha-2 adrenoceptor sites? Clin Exper Hypertens 14:815, 1992.
16. Hamilton CA, Yakubu MA, Howie CA, et al: Desensitization and down-regulation of brain alpha 2-adrenoceptors by centrally acting antihypertensive drugs. Br J Clin Pharmacol 30(Suppl 1):131S, 1990.
17. Brochu M, Ong H, De Lean A: Sites of action of angiotensin II, atrial natriuretic factor and guanabenz, on aldosterone biosynthesis. J Steroid Biochem Mol Biol 38:575, 1991.
18. Holmes B, Brogden RN, Heel RC, et al: Guanabenz: A review of its pharmacodynamic properties and therapeutic efficacy in hypertension. Drugs 26:212, 1983.
19. Meacham RH, Chiang ST, Kick CJ, et al: Pharmacokinetic disposition of guanabenz in the rhesus monkey. Drug Metab Dispos 9:509, 1981.
20. Shah RS, Walker BR, Vanov SK, et al: Guanabenz effects on blood pressure and non-invasive parameters of cardiac performance in patients with hypertension. Clin Pharmacol Ther 19:732, 1976.
21. Meacham RH, Emmett M, Kyriakopoulos AA, et al: Disposition of ^{14}C-guanabenz in patients with essential hypertension. Clin Pharmacol Ther 27:44, 1980.
22. Cox M, Walker BR, Braden G: Effects of guanabenz on Na$^+$, K$^+$ and water homeostasis. Kidney Int 21:186, 1982.
23. Weidler DJ, Garg DC, Jallad NS: Dose-response relationship of single oral doses of guanabenz in hypertensive patients. J Cardiovasc Pharmacol 6:S762, 1984.
24. Morgan TO: Comparison of a centrally acting antihypertensive agent and beta-adrenergic blocking agent for the treatment of hypertension. J Cardiovasc Pharmacol 6:S808, 1984.
25. Walker BR, Deitch MW, Schneider BE, et al: Long-term therapy of hypertension with guanabenz. Clin Ther 4:217, 1981.
26. Marmo E, Saini RK, Caputi AP, et al: Cardiovascular profile of BR-750 (2,6,dichlorobenzylidene-aminoguanidine acetate). Res Commun Chem Pathol Pharmacol 6:391, 1973.
27. Saini RK, Caputi AP, Marmo E: Cardiovascular profile of BR 750 (2,6-dichlorobenzylidene aminoguanidine acetate). Farmaco Edizione Pratica 28:359, 1973.
28. Mosley C, O'Connor DT, Taylor A, et al: Comparative effects of antihypertensive therapy with guanabenz and propranolol on renal vascular resistance and left ventricular mass. J Cardiovasc Pharmacol 6:S757, 1984.
29. Walker BR, Shah RS, Ramanathan KB, et al: Effect of guanabenz and methyldopa on hypertension and cardiac performance. Clin Pharmacol Ther 22:868, 1977.
30. Misu Y, Kubo T: Central and peripheral cardiovascular responses of rats to guanabenz and clonidine. Jpn J Pharmacol 32:925, 1982.
31. Bauer JH: Effects of guanabenz therapy on renal function and body fluid composition. Arch Intern Med 143:1163, 1983.
32. Stein J, Osgood R: Delineation of the site of action of guanabenz in the renal tubule. J Cardiovasc Pharmacol 6:S787, 1984.
33. Bosanac P, Dubb J, Walker BR, et al: Renal effects of guanabenz: A new antihypertensive. J Clin Pharmacol 16:631, 1976.
34. Golub MS, Eggena P, Barrett JD, et al: Fluid volumes during antihypertensive therapy with guanabenz in mild hypertension. Clin Pharmacol Ther 31:320, 1982.
35. Kaplan NM: Alpha2-adrenoceptor agonists in the treatment of hypertension. J Cardiovasc Pharmacol 7(Suppl 8):S64, 1985.
36. Gehr M, MacCarthy EP, Goldberg M: Natriuretic and water diuretic effects of central alpha2-adrenoceptor agonists. J Cardiovasc Pharmacol 6:S781, 1984.
37. Reid IA, Nolan PL, Wolf JA, et al: Suppression of vasopressin secretion by clonidine: Effects of alpha-adrenoceptor antagonists. Endocrinology 104:1403, 1979.
38. Strandhoy JW, Steg BD, Buckalew VM Jr: Antagonism of the hydroosmotic effect of vasopressin by the antihypertensive guanabenz. Life Sci 27:2513, 1980.
39. Dubrow A, Mittman N, DeCola P, et al: Safety and efficacy of guanabenz in hypertensive patients with moderate renal insufficiency. J Clin Hypertens 1:322, 1985.
40. Marchand GR, Willis LR, Williamson HE: Relationship of sodium retention produced by Catapres to changes in renal hemodynamics. Proc Soc Exp Biol Med 138:943, 1971.
41. Wolff DW, Buckalew VM Jr, Strandhoy JW: Renal alpha-1 and alpha-2 adrenoceptor mediated vasoconstriction in dogs: Comparison of phenylephrine, clonidine, and guanabenz. J Cardiovasc Pharmacol 6:S793, 1984.
42. Holland OB, Fairchild C, Gomez-Sanchez CE: Effect of guanabenz and hydrochlorothiazide on blood pressure and plasma renin activity. J Clin Pharmacol 21:133, 1981.
43. Weber MA, Drayer JIM, Hubbell FA: Effects on the renin-angiotensin system of agents acting at central and peripheral adrenergic receptors. Chest [Suppl] 83:374, 1983.

44. Golub MS, Thananopavarn C, Eggena P, et al: Hormonal and hemodynamic effects of short- and long-term clonidine therapy in patients with mild-to-moderate hypertension. Chest [Suppl] 83:380, 1983.
45. Pedrinelli R, Ugenti P, Abdel Haz B, et al: Humoral and haemodynamic effects of low, increasing doses of guanabenz in patients with essential hypertension. Int J Clin Pharmacol Res 2(Suppl 1):57, 1982.
46. Walker BR, Deitch MW, Gold JA, et al: Evaluation of guanabenz added to hydrochlorothiazide therapy in hypertension. J Int Med Res 10:131, 1982.
47. Walker BR, Schneider BE, Gold JA: A two-year evaluation of guanabenz in the treatment of hypertension. Curr Ther Res 27:784, 1980.
48. Kaplan NM: Effects of guanabenz on plasma lipid levels in hypertensive patients. J Cardiovasc Pharmacol 6:S841, 1984.
49. Capuzzi DM, Cevallos WH: Inhibition of hepatic cholesterol and triglyceride synthesis by guanabenz acetate. J Cardiovasc Pharmacol 6:S847, 1984.
50. Weber MA, Drayer JIM, McMahon FG, et al: Transdermal administration of clonidine for the treatment of high blood pressure. Arch Intern Med 144:1211, 1984.
51. Eldridge JC, Strandhoy J, Buckalew VM Jr: Endocrinologic effects of antihypertensive therapy with guanabenz or hydrochlorothiazide. J Cardiovasc Pharmacol 6:S776, 1984.
52. Weber MA, Drayer JIM, Deitch MW: Hypertension in patients with diabetes mellitus: Treatment with a centrally acting agent. J Cardiovasc Pharmacol 6:S823, 1984.
53. Ram VCS, Holland B, Fairchild C, et al: Withdrawal syndrome following cessation of guanabenz therapy. J Clin Pharmacol 19:148, 1979.
54. Winer N, Carter CH: Effects of abrupt discontinuation of guanabenz and clonidine in hypertensive patients. Clin Pharmacol Ther 31:282, 1982.
55. Bauer JH, Burch RN: Comparative studies: Guanabenz versus propranolol as first-step therapy for the treatment of primary hypertension. Cardiovasc Rev Rep 4:9, 1983.
56. Buckalew VM Jr, Burgess R, Strandhoy JW: Effect of guanabenz withdrawal on blood pressure and plasma catecholamines. J Cardiovasc Pharmacol 6:S830, 1984.
57. Lilja M, Jounela AJ, Juustila HJ, et al: Withdrawal syndromes and the cessation of antihypertensive therapy [letter]. Arch Intern Med 207:173, 1980.
58. Walson PD, Graves P, Rath A, et al: Effects of guanabenz in adolescent hypertension. J Cardiovasc Pharmacol 6:S814, 1984.
59. Abdel-Rahman AA, Carroll RG, el-Mas MM: Role of the sympathetic nervous system in the alcohol-guanabenz hemodynamic interaction. Can J Physiol Pharmacol 70:1217, 1992.
60. Lasseter KC, Shapse D, Pascucci VL, et al: Pharmacokinetics of guanabenz in patients with impaired liver function. J Cardiovasc Pharmacol 6:S766, 1984.
61. Deitch MW, Littman GS, Pascucci VL: Antihypertensive therapy with guanabenz in patients with chronic obstructive pulmonary disease. J Cardiovasc Pharmacol 6:S818, 1984.
62. Joint National Committee on Detection, Evaluation, and Treatment of High Blood Pressure: The Fifth Report of the Joint National Committee on Detection, Evaluation, and Treatment of High Blood Pressure (JNC V). Arch Intern Med 153:154, 1993.
63. Weber MA, Laragh JH: Hypertension: Steps forward and steps backward. The Joint National Committee Fifth Report. Arch Intern Med 153:149, 1993.
64. Walker BR, Hare LE, Deitch MW, et al: Comparative effects of guanabenz alone and in combination with hydrochlorothiazide as initial antihypertensive therapy. Curr Ther Res 31:764, 1982.
65. Baez MA, Woo-Ming RB, Garg DC, et al: Dose-ranging study to delineate the additive antihypertensive effect of guanabenz and captopril. J Clin Pharmacol 31:312, 1991.
66. Weber MA, Drayer JIM: Treatment of hypertension in the elderly. South Med J 79:323, 1986.
67. McCarron DA, Hare LE, Walker BR: Therapeutic and economic controversies in antihypertensive therapy. J Cardiovasc Pharmacol 6:S837, 1984.

CHAPTER 66

Rilmenidine

Michel E. Safar, M.D., and Stephane Laurent, M.D., Ph.D.

HISTORY

Rilmenidine (S 3341) is a new antihypertensive agent developed by Servier International Research Institute. It was registered in France in 1987, and to date in more than 20 other countries, for the first-line therapy of hypertension.

CHEMISTRY

Rilmenidine, or 2-(dicyclopropylmethyl) amino-2-oxazoline, is a new antihypertensive agent, the first oxazoline derivative. The chemical structure of rilmenidine is characterized by the oxazoline structure and differs in comparison with known centrally acting antihypertensive agents such as imidazoline and guanidine derivatives. Rilmenidine is a weak base with a molecular weight of 180.25, with a pK_a of approximately 9; at physiologic pH of 7.4, only 1% exists as the un-ionized form. However, rilmenidine is mildly lipid soluble and has a true partition coefficient between octanol and water of approximately 2.

For clinical administration, rilmenidine is used as the phosphate salt, which is freely soluble in water.

RECEPTOR SELECTIVITY

Because of its original structure, a wide range of receptors have been tested in binding studies, showing first that rilmenidine is able to displace only specific ligands from α_2-adrenoceptors in rat brain with a 10 times lower affinity than clonidine, but binds to α_1-adrenoceptors with an affinity 100 to 1000 times lower[1] than to α_2 subtype. In a variety of isolated blood vessels or organs, the selectivity and potency of the drug were then assessed, and although rilmenidine appears to be a partial agonist to α_2-adrenoceptors, its selectivity for both pre- or postjunctional α_2-adrenoceptors as opposed to postjunctional α_1 subtype was five times higher than that of clonidine.[2, 3]

More recent data have, however, indicated that rilmenidine could demonstrate a higher affinity for the newly described nonadrenergic imidazoline I_1 receptor.[4-7] Several studies in various species, including humans,[8-11] have established that rilmenidine has a relative affinity for I_1 compared with α_2-adrenergic sites varying from 1:1 to 200:1 depending on the preparation and experimental conditions and has a selectivity ratio for I_1 versus α_2-adrenergic receptors approximately 2.5 to 10 times higher than that of clonidine.

A distinctive imidazoline site, I_2, has also been extensively investigated,[6, 7] the function of which is, as yet, unknown. Rilmenidine demonstrated only a poor affinity for the I_2 subtype.

HEMODYNAMIC EFFECTS IN ANIMALS

After acute intravenous administration, rilmenidine[2] induced a transient hypertensive phase followed by a marked, durable, and dose-dependent reduction in blood pressure and heart rate in genetically spontaneous hypertensive rats (SHR) (Fig. 66–1)[2, 12, 13] and in various other preclinical animal models.[14-17] After oral administration in the rat, rilmenidine (0.15 to 0.60 mg/kg) significantly induced a long-lasting hypotensive action without any significant early rise in blood pressure or modification in heart rate.[2]

Chronic administration of rilmenidine in deoxycorticosterone acetate (DOCA)/salt hypertensive rats caused a dose-proportional reduction of blood pressure[15] and was shown to reduce the left ventricular cardiac hypertrophy and collagen content after 7 weeks of 10 mg/kg/day dose of rilmenidine.[18] Acute cessation of administration of rilmenidine was less frequently associated with the occurrence of rebound hypertension or behavioral disturbances than was clonidine.[12, 19, 20]

After chronic administration in the anesthetized SHR, rilmenidine did not modify renal function, including glomerular filtration rate (inulin clearance), renal blood flow (para-aminohippuric acid [PAH]

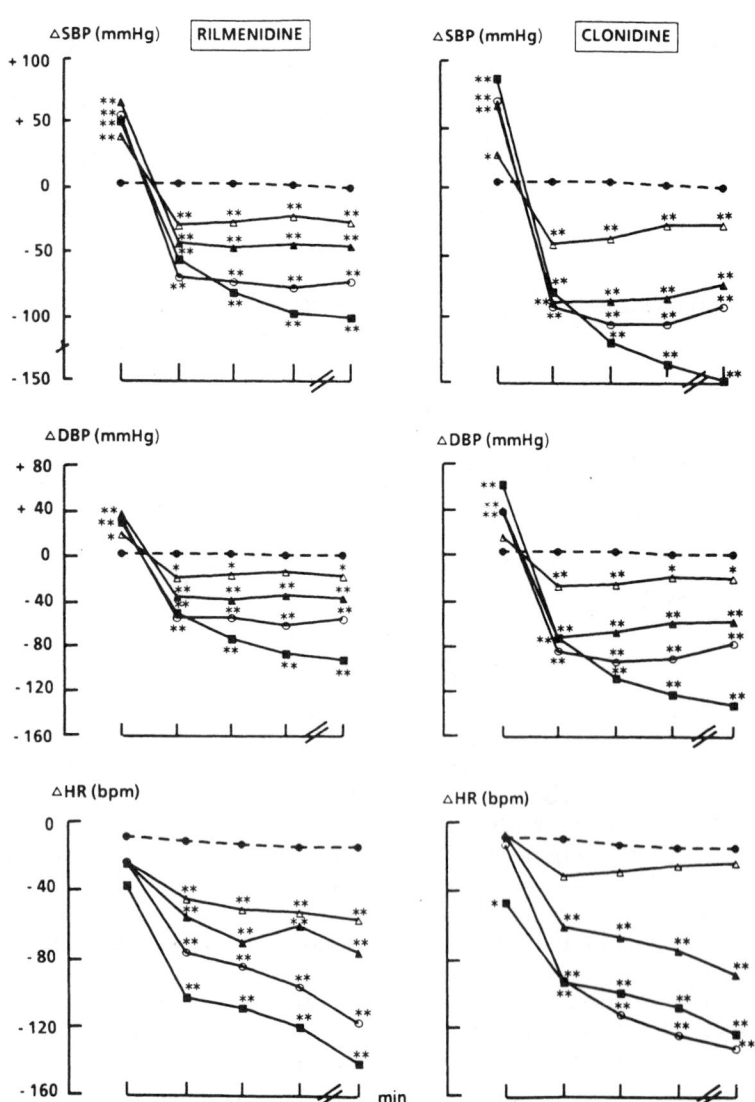

Figure 66–1. Hemodynamic effects of intravenous injections of rilmenidine ($\triangle$, 0.1 mg/kg; $\blacktriangle$, 0.2 mg/kg; $\circ$, 0.3 mg/kg; $\bullet$, 1 mg/kg), clonidine ($\triangle$, 0.003 mg/kg; $\blacktriangle$, 0.005 mg/kg; $\circ$, 0.01 mg/kg; $\bullet$, 0.03 mg/kg), and saline ($\square$) in the anesthetized, spontaneously hypertensive rat. Results are mean differences versus baseline values (n = 6 to 8). *p < .05; **p < .01 versus saline (two-way analysis of variance followed by Newman-Keuls test). SBP, systolic blood pressure; DBP, diastolic blood pressure; HR, heart rate. (From Koenig-Bérard E, Tierney C, Beau B, et al: Cardiovascular and central nervous system effects of rilmenidine [S 3341] in rats. Am J Cardiol 61:22D, 1988.)

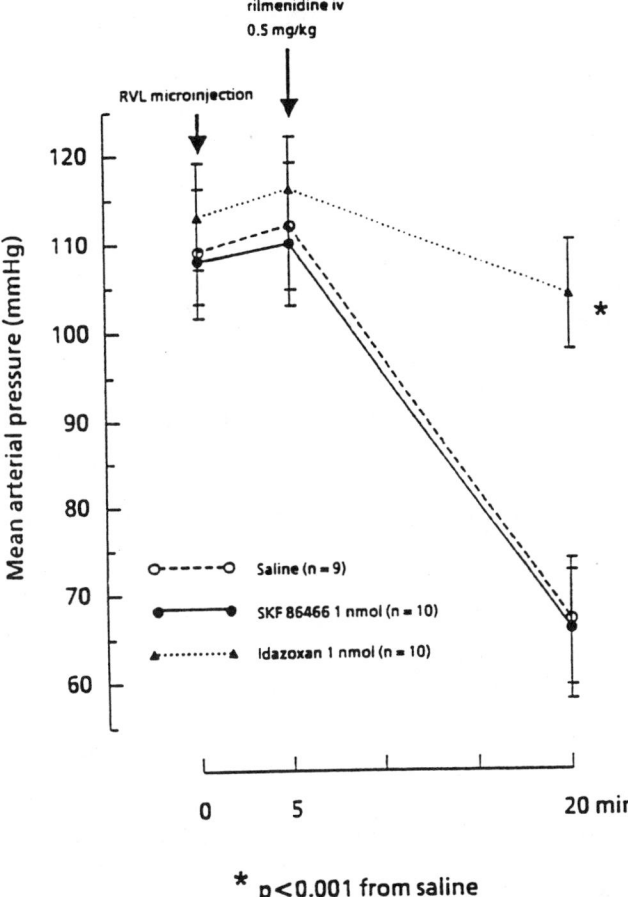

rilmenidine iv
0.5 mg/kg

RVL microinjection

o—----o Saline (n = 9)

•———• SKF 86466 1 nmol (n = 10)

▲·········▲ Idazoxan 1 nmol (n = 10)

Mean arterial pressure (mmHg)

0   5   20 min

* p < 0.001 from saline

Figure 66–2. Effect of antagonists microinjected into the rostral ventrolateral medulla (RVL) on the vasodepressor response elicited by rilmenidine injected IV. The rats received a bilateral microinjection of an isotonic solute of SKF 86466 (α_2-antagonist) or idazoxan (imidazoline antagonist) in the RVL, then 5 minutes later, an injection of rilmenidine (0.5 mg/kg). Idazoxan blocked the hypotensive effect of rilmenidine. (Adapted from Gomez RE, Ernsberger P, Feinland G, et al: Rilmenidine lowers arterial pressure via imidazole receptors in brainstem C1 area. Eur J Pharmacol 195:181, 1991.)

clearance), and urinary output.[21] However, renal function was studied in rat with innervated/denervated kidney to assess the influence of renal sympathetic nerve activity. At a moderate hypotensive dose (20 μg/kg/min, IV), rilmenidine induced a natriuresis and diuresis associated with a marked inhibition in renal nerve activity.[22] Rilmenidine reduced plasma renin activity from 35% in conscious normotensive dogs[14] to 50% in SHR.[21]

Evidence of the central component of rilmenidine's hypotensive effect was noted after injection of low doses into the left thoracic vertebral artery of chloralose-anesthetized cats. Low doses (10 to 30 μg/kg) of rilmenidine thus applied caused a pronounced and long-lasting hypotensive action. However, similar and even tenfold higher doses, when administered systemically, remained virtually ineffective. These experiments provide convincing evidence of the central hypotensive activity of rilmenidine.[15, 23]

Studies conducted in either normotensive[9] and barodenervated anesthetized[17] rat or in anesthetized[24]

and conscious[25] rabbit have indicated the involvement of central I_1 receptors in the hypotensive activity of rilmenidine. Indeed idazoxan, which develops a high affinity for I_1 receptors when injected centrally or locally into the rostral part of ventrolateral medulla (RVLM) (Fig. 66–2), preferentially antagonized the vasodepressor response to systemically or centrally administered rilmenidine. Conversely, various selective α_2-adrenoceptor antagonists were less active when administered in comparable conditions.

CENTRAL EFFECTS OF RILMENIDINE

A very obvious difference between rilmenidine and clonidine was rilmenidine's lack of or minimal sedative activity in animal experiments. In its preclinical evaluation, rilmenidine was studied using classic experiments for sedation. In mice,[15, 23] in which the degree of sedation produced by drugs to be tested is reflected by the prolongation of the hexobarbitone sleeping time (loss of righting reflex), Van Zwieten showed that, in contrast with clonidine (0.3 mg/kg IP), rilmenidine (10 mg/kg IP) did not significantly prolong the hexobarbitone-induced sleeping time. These results were confirmed in rats:[2] Rilmenidine (10 mg/kg IP) did not induce any significant alteration of the sleeping time induced by pentobarbitone, whereas clonidine (0.125 mg/kg IP) produced a significant potentiation of the sleeping time (Fig. 66–3). In 2-day-old chicks,[2] sedative effects of drugs administered intramuscularly (IM) or intraperitoneally (IP) are

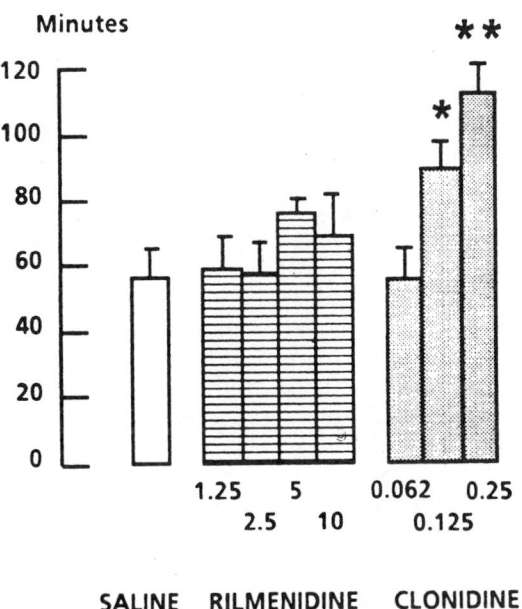

Minutes

120
100
80
60
40
20
0

1.25   5   0.062   0.25
    2.5   10   0.125

SALINE   RILMENIDINE   CLONIDINE
mg/kg, ip   mg/kg, ip

Figure 66–3. Effects of rilmenidine and clonidine on the pentobarbitone-induced (30 mg/kg) sleeping time in the rat. Mean values ± standard error of the mean (n = 8). *$p < .05$; **$p < .01$ versus saline (Dunnett test). ip, intraperitoneally. (Adapted with permission from Koenig-Bérard E, Tierney C, Beau B, et al: Cardiovascular and central nervous system effects of rilmenidine [S 3341] in rats. Am J Cardiol 61:22D, 1988.)

studied with efficacy because the blood-brain barrier is poorly developed; administration of rilmenidine up to doses of 1 mg/kg IM had no sedative effects. Rilmenidine at higher doses failed to produce the expected bell-shaped curve observed with other α_2-agonists such as clonidine, which is thought to be as a result of partial agonist activity. In rats,[2] rilmenidine reduced motor activity (open field) at doses approximately 80 times greater than clonidine, while showing identical antihypertensive properties at doses approximately 30 times greater. This ratio was confirmed in the holeboard test.[26]

Rilmenidine was free of any addictive effect. Particularly, it reduced the morphine withdrawal syndrome with an activity 100 times less than clonidine.[27]

PHARMACOLOGIC PROFILE OF RILMENIDINE

Agents that act to limit the sympathetic outflow at the target organ level undoubtedly represent an interesting approach to treat hypertension and probably cardiovascular diseases;[28] β-α_1-adrenergic blockers can illustrate this current view.

Another attractive possibility consists of reducing sympathetic activity directly at its point of genesis, i.e., the medulla oblongata located within the brain stem. α_2-Agonists have been used for decades in therapeutics to this end, but despite being clinically effective antihypertensive agents, their adverse effects (sedation, rebound effect) are too frequently observed in treated patients. Classically, the related adverse effects are also attributed to the activation of α_2-adrenoceptors and are consequently undissociable from the mode of therapeutic action. Indeed, α_2-adrenoceptors are widely distributed within the brain and particularly in the frontal cortex and the locus caeruleus that probably mediates the sedative action of clonidine analogues.[23, 29]

A recent concept has emerged since the 1980s from original studies[4, 6] that emphasized the unique vasodepressive effects of centrally acting imidazolines or related agents when injected into the RVLM in animals. Conversely, catecholamines were without influence on blood pressure in the same conditions. Furthermore, imidazoline receptors have been characterized in a restricted area in the brain[5, 8, 30] and lately subclassified as I_1 subtype.[6, 7] When occupied by rilmenidine or related agents, they selectively induce hypotension independently of α_2-adrenoceptors by sympathoinhibition as assessed by direct measurement of renal sympathetic nerve activity.[17, 25]

PERIPHERAL EFFECTS OF RILMENIDINE

In the periphery, I_1 receptors can also be detected in the kidney,[11, 31] in platelets,[32] and in adrenal chromaffin cells.[33] An *in vivo* study confirms the importance of renal I_1 receptors.[34] When injected intrarenally, drugs with a high affinity to I_1 sites were shown to increase urine flow rate secondary to an increase in sodium excretion.

As a consequence of such a unique receptorial selectivity, rilmenidine demonstrated a neat dissociation between antihypertensive activity and central nervous system side effects.[2, 15, 23, 26, 27] This pharmacologic profile is best exemplified in clinical studies (see later discussion).

Finally, preclinical studies have shown that sympathoinhibition and possibly a natriuretic effect are at the basis of the antihypertensive activity of rilmenidine.

HUMAN PHARMACOKINETICS

Because of the low dosage administered (1 to 2 mg per day), rilmenidine plasma levels were assayed by combined gas chromatography and mass spectrometry (GC-MS).[35, 36]

Studies using labeled and unlabeled compounds showed that rilmenidine was rapidly and extensively absorbed, with a bioavailability factor close to 1.[37] The relative bioavailability factors of various pharmaceutical forms (solution, tablet, capsule) were comparable and were not significantly changed by food intake. The main pharmacokinetic parameters of rilmenidine are shown in Table 66–1.[37]

Distribution was characterized by a large volume of distribution of approximately 5 L/kg (315 L), reflecting the good tissue affinity of rilmenidine. Rilmenidine was weakly bound to plasma proteins (< 10%). The weak involvement of protein binding minimizes the risk of pharmacokinetic interactions with any drug coadministered with antihypertensive agents.

Rilmenidine was mainly excreted through the kidneys. The unchanged compound (urinary fraction of rilmenidine) was approximately 65%, and no metabolite plasma levels were detected. Metabolism was poorly involved in the elimination process. This allows the assumption that no hepatic first-pass effect occurs after oral administration, as confirmed by the absolute bioavailability.

After acute administration, the linearity of the pharmacokinetics was demonstrated within the 0.5- to 2-mg range. After repeated administration, the linear disposition of rilmenidine with dose was confirmed.[37]

As antihypertensive drugs are widely used not only in the elderly but also in various physiopathologic hypertensive populations, it was of interest to verify the effects of hypertension itself and various conditions (i.e., age, renal failure, and hepatic insufficiency) on the basic pharmacokinetic parameters of rilmenidine found in healthy subjects.

Hypertension was not found to influence the absorption, distribution, or elimination processes of rilmenidine when compared with healthy subjects.[38]

In the elderly, the elimination rate was reduced, as demonstrated by a prolongation of the elimination half-life (13 ± 1 hours), an increase in the mean residence time, and a decreased total apparent clearance. When considering the extent of renal elimina-

Table 66–1. **Pharmacokinetic Parameters of Rilmenidine in Hypertensive Patients After Oral Administration, Comparison with Healthy Subjects (Mean ± SEM)**

	Healthy Subjects* (n = 8)	Hypertensive Patients (n = 11)	
	1 mg	1 mg	2 mg
t_{lag} (hr)	0.34 ± 0.11	0.39 ± 0.03	0.32 ± 0.06
C_{max} (ng/ml^{-1})	3.25 ± 0.26	3.28 ± 0.21	7.85 ± 0.70
T_{max} (hr)	1.94 ± 0.64	1.77 ± 0.17	1.33 ± 0.22
V/F (L)	332.92 ± 32.49	286.08 ± 12.78	246.55 ± 12.47
T½, z (hr)	7.00 ± 0.86	7.29 ± 0.54	6.85 ± 0.50
MRT (hr)	10.46 ± 1.22	11.18 ± 0.79	10.15 ± 0.56
CL/F (ml/min^{-1})	570.80 ± 34.92	468.05 ± 27.76	451.20 ± 36.87
CL_R (ml/min^{-1})	—	311.00 ± 40.65	313.97 ± 42.49
fe (%)	—	65.78 ± 7.89	68.10 ± 4.60

*From linearity study after single dose.

CL/F, apparent total clearance; CL_R, renal clearance; C_{max}, maximum plasma concentration; fe, fraction of the unchanged drug excreted in urine; MRT, mean residence time; SEM, standard error of the mean; t_{lag}, lag time of absorption; T_{max}, time to reach the maximum plasma concentration; T½, z, terminal half-life; V/F, apparent volume of distribution.

tion in the clearance of rilmenidine, which involves both glomerular filtration and tubular secretion, the physiologic decrease in glomerular filtration rate in the elderly is likely to be involved in the reduction of the observed clearance. This fall in total clearance is responsible for the rise in terminal elimination half-life. These modifications in the biodisposition of rilmenidine in the elderly do not require an adaptation of the dosage regimen.[38]

In patients with renal failure, the absorption of rilmenidine was not modified except in patients with severe renal failure (clearance, 5 to 15 ml/min^{-1}). The modifications of T_{max} (2.17 ± 0.31 hours), C_{max} (5.33 ± 0.56 hours), and elimination half-life (34 ± 3 hours) in severe renal failure are likely to be due to the decrease in elimination rate.[38] Indeed, elimination parameters were directly correlated to the degree of renal failure. A recent pharmacokinetic study involving patients with severe renal failure (creatinine clearance, <15 ml/min) showed that rilmenidine could be given at the dose of 1 mg every other day, because at that dose, the accumulation ratio was similar after repeated and single administration (accumulation ratio of 1.74).[39]

In patients with hepatic failure, the modifications of rilmenidine disposition after acute administration were weak. Variations in absorption and distribution confirm that rilmenidine has a minimal first-pass effect. The decrease in apparent total clearance could be caused by an alteration in metabolic function due to renal changes induced by liver disease; it seems reasonable that the decrease in the elimination rate is related to impairment of both hepatic and renal function. No adaptation of the dosage regimen is required in hepatic insufficiency.[38] Monitoring of rilmenidine plasma levels in long-term clinical studies has never shown any accumulation.[40]

EFFECTS ON PATHOPHYSIOLOGY
Effects on Hemodynamics

Rilmenidine decreased blood pressure in a dose-dependent manner[41, 42] in normotensive subjects as well as in hypertensive patients. The antihypertensive effects of acute oral administration of rilmenidine were directly related to the dose and log of the plasma concentration.[42] In hypertensive patients, acute[43] (25 and 50 µg/kg) and chronic[44] (1 mg once or twice daily) oral administration of rilmenidine led to biphasic effects on cardiac output and peripheral resistance: cardiac output decreased shortly after administration then returned to baseline values. Peripheral resistance tended to increase initially, then significantly decreased and remained below the basal levels[43] (Fig. 66–4). Chronic administration showed the same effects with lesser amplitude in cardiac index variation. The reduction in total peripheral resistance started 3 hours after administration of the drug and remained significantly lower than in baseline conditions 24 hours after administration.[44] Rilmenidine had no negative inotropic effect, as shown by the absence of any significant reduction in stroke index. Rilmenidine also preserved the physiologic increase in blood pressure and cardiac output during exercise.[45] Response to erect posture was unaltered. Fewer than 1% of patients reported an orthostatic hypotension in long-term surveillance.[40] The low rate of orthostatic hypotension may be related to an enhancement in baroreflex sensitivity after rilmenidine administration.[46]

Effects on Ventricular Function and Structure

After acute administration of rilmenidine 1 mg, the systolic time intervals did not change in normotensive subjects, thus demonstrating that no change occurred in cardiac performance with rilmenidine.[41] After repeated oral administration of 1 mg, once or twice daily, left ventricular function, assessed 3 hours after administration on systolic time intervals and M-mode shortening fraction, was in the normal range in the hypertensive patients.[44]

Although no change in left ventricular end-diastolic diameter and wall thickness was observed after a short duration (28 days) of treatment,[44] one study

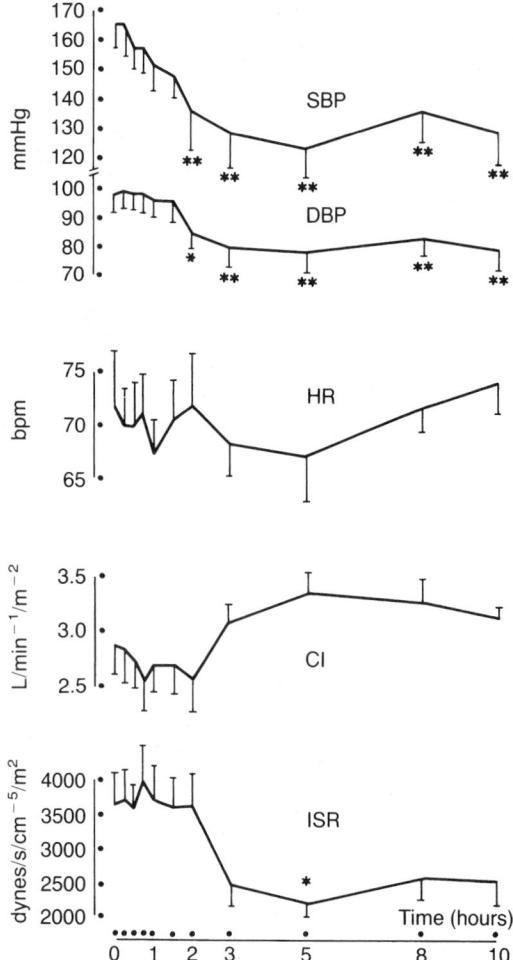

Figure 66–4. Hemodynamic effects of rilmenidine over 10 hours after oral administration of 25 µg/kg (n = 8). Values are mean ± standard error of the mean. CI, cardiac index; DBP, diastolic blood pressure; HR, heart rate; ISR, indexed systemic resistance; SBP, systolic blood pressure; *p < .05; **p < .01 versus before administration (variance analysis and Newman-Keuls test). No significant variation in heart rate and cardiac index. (Reprinted with permission from Zannad F, Aliot E, Florentin J, et al: Hemodynamic and electrophysiologic effects of a new alpha-2 adrenoceptor agonist, rilmenidine, on systemic hypertension. Am J Cardiol 61:67D, 1988.)

showed that a 1-year treatment with rilmenidine significantly decreased the left ventricular mass (LV mass) in patients with left ventricular hypertrophy and improved both the hemodynamic and hormonal profiles.[47] Indeed, the ratio between the reduction in LV mass (in grams) and the fall in mean arterial pressure (in mmHg) was 2 g/mmHg, a value quite similar to that found with angiotensin-converting enzyme inhibitors in the meta-analysis carried out by Dahlöf et al.[48] Similarly, the ratio of the early and late mitral blood flow peak velocities (E/A ratio), an index of diastolic function, significantly improved. In the same study, plasma atrial natriuretic factor (ANF) levels decreased, in parallel with the reversal of LV mass.[47]

Effects on Electrophysiology

In hypertensive patients, the electrophysiologic parameters were not modified 2 hours after oral

administration of 25 and 50 µg/kg doses of rilmenidine.[43]

Effects on Large Artery Function

After acute[49] or chronic oral administration of rilmenidine 1 mg[47] in hypertensive patients, the hypotensive effect was accompanied by a reduction in the pulse wave velocity, without any change in artery diameter. Rilmenidine treatment was therefore associated with an increase in artery compliance, significant only after chronic administration.[47]

Treatment Withdrawal Surveillance

The effects of treatment withdrawal were specifically investigated in three separate studies: during the first days after rilmenidine withdrawal, an asymptomatic rise in diastolic blood pressure (DBP) was observed in only 1 of 129 patients, including 24 elderly patients, treated for 6 to 12 weeks.[50–52] No symptom suggesting a withdrawal syndrome was reported in any other clinical trial.[40, 53–57]

Endocrine and Metabolic Effects

Endocrine effects of rilmenidine were studied in healthy subjects and hypertensive patients. In healthy subjects,[58, 59] growth hormone levels increased briefly after acute oral administration of rilmenidine (2 mg) and then returned to normal values; prolactin levels initially decreased and then returned to normal values.[59] In hypertensive patients, plasma prolactin levels remained unchanged after a 12-week period of administration of rilmenidine (1 mg once a day and 1 mg b.i.d.).[52]

Rilmenidine had no influence on carbohydrate or lipid metabolism, even in insulin-dependent diabetic hypertensive patients. Laboratory surveillance of diabetic patients did not reveal any variations in carbohydrate (fasting or postprandial blood glucose, glycosylated hemoglobin, blood sugar cycle) and lipid metabolisms.[60]

A further postregistration study involving more than 2600 patients followed up for 1 year showed no adverse metabolic effects of rilmenidine, even in cases of previous alteration of carbohydrate or lipid metabolism.[57]

Effects on Fluid Volume State and Electrolytes

Acute and repeated administration of rilmenidine (1 mg) in healthy subjects significantly reduced blood pressure but did not modify water and electrolyte balance.[61, 62] After chronic administration in hypertensive patients at the dose of 1 mg per day or 1 mg b.i.d., rilmenidine caused no variation in blood mass or weight and induced no variation in urine output, urinary osmolarity, Na^+/K^+ ratio, or electrolyte excretion rates.[63]

In short-term (1 to 4 months)[50–56] and long-term (1

to 2 years)[40, 57] studies, no changes were seen in plasma electrolytes. No significant change or a slight but significant decrease in body weight was observed in patients treated with rilmenidine. In particular, in the comparative study with hydrochlorothiazide, the mean body weight significantly decreased with rilmenidine and hydrochlorothiazide ($p < .02$) by 0.38 and 0.46 kg, respectively.[56] These results are in keeping with the absence of acquired tolerance after long-term treatment.[40, 57]

Effects on Renal Function

Acute and repeated administration of rilmenidine (1 mg) in healthy subjects[62] significantly reduced blood pressure but did not modify glomerular filtration rate (inulin clearance) and renal blood flow (PAH clearance). After repeated administration in hypertensive patients at a daily dose of 1 mg per day or 1 mg b.i.d., rilmenidine caused no change in urea, creatinine, or uric acid clearances.[63] In short-term (1 to 4 months) clinical trials,[50–56] no significant variation was seen in creatinine, urea, uric acid, or electrolyte plasma levels. In long-term (1 to 2 years)[40, 57] treatment surveillance, no changes were seen in creatinine plasma levels in patients treated with rilmenidine as a single therapy. In patients with higher plasma creatinine levels (> 100 mmol/L), plasma creatinine significantly decreased throughout 1 year of therapy with rilmenidine.[57]

Rilmenidine induced a significant fall in plasma renin activity by 58% and 44% after acute[62] and repeated administration,[63] respectively. No significant changes were shown in plasma aldosterone levels.[63]

Effects on Central Nervous System

At therapeutic doses, rilmenidine effects are characterized by a dissociation between the antihypertensive activity and central side effects.[41, 42]

The dose-effect and concentration-effect relationships of rilmenidine were evaluated in healthy subjects and hypertensive patients. Sedative effects were related directly to the dose and the log of the plasma concentration of rilmenidine. There was no significant linear dose-effect relationship for salivary flow or dry mouth. With the 1-mg dose, satisfactory antihypertensive activity was associated with a low level of central nervous system side effects.[42]

The incidence of daytime drowsiness observed with rilmenidine (1 mg per day or 1 mg b.i.d) did not differ from that observed with placebo,[53] hydrochlorothiazide,[56] or atenolol[55] and was two to three times less than that observed at equihypotensive doses of clonidine, 0.15 mg or 0.30 mg per day[54] (Fig. 66–5), and methyldopa, 0.5 g or 1 g per day[52] (Fig. 66–6).

The incidence of dry mouth with rilmenidine 1 mg per day was not significantly different from that observed with placebo.[53] With rilmenidine 1 mg b.i.d., dry mouth tended to occur at the start of treatment but was transient and disappeared as treatment continued.[53] The rate of dry mouth was consistently less

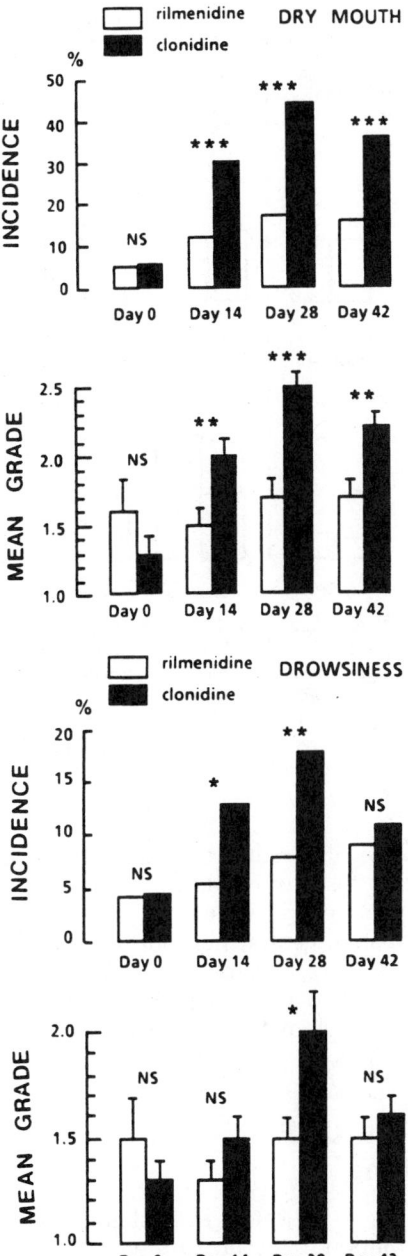

Figure 66–5. Incidence (percentage) and intensity (mean grade) of dry mouth with rilmenidine and clonidine. Incidence is the percentage of the patients presenting a dry mouth in the rilmenidine group (n = 162) and in the clonidine group (n = 171); ***$p < .001$ between groups (chi-squared test). On day 42, these data do not include 12 patients withdrawn from the study because of dry mouth. Mean grades are calculated from the patients complaining of dry mouth; **$p < .01$; ***$p < .001$ between groups (Mann-Whitney test). NS, not significant.
Incidence (percentage) and intensity (mean grade) of drowsiness with rilmenidine and clonidine. Incidence is the percentage of the patients presenting with drowsiness in the rilmenidine group (n = 162) and in the clonidine group (n = 171); *$p < .05$; **$p < .01$ between groups (chi-squared test). On day 42, these data do not include seven patients withdrawn from the study because of drowsiness. Mean grades are calculated from the patients complaining of drowsiness; *$p < .05$ between groups (Mann-Whitney test). NS, not significant. (From Fillastre JP, Letac B, Galinier F, et al: A multicenter double-blind comparative study of rilmenidine and clonidine in 333 hypertensive patients. Am J Cardiol 61:81D, 1988.)

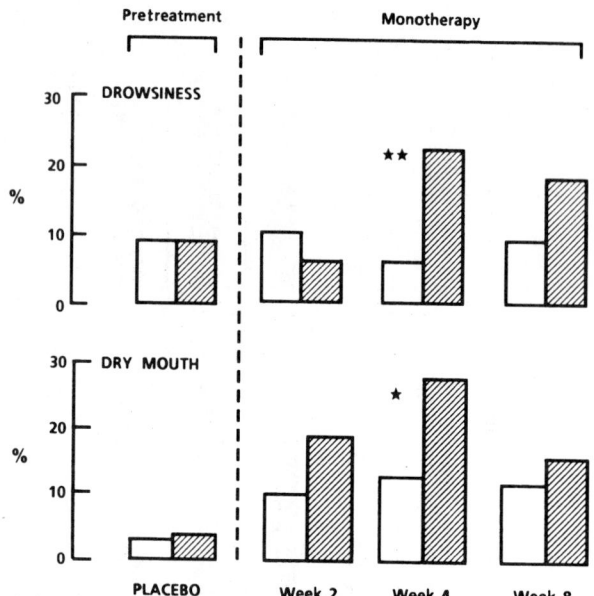

Figure 66–6. Percentage of patients reporting an aggravation or onset of symptoms; $*p < .05$; $**p < .01$ chi-squared test between treatment groups. (*Open box,* rilmenidine; *hatched box,* methyldopa.) (From UK Working Party on Rilmenidine: Rilmenidine in mild to moderate essential hypertension: A double-blind randomized, parallel-group, multicenter comparison with methyldopa in 157 patients. Curr Ther Res 47:194, 1990.)

frequent with rilmenidine than that observed at equihypotensive doses of clonidine[50, 53] (see Fig. 66–5) or methyldopa[52] (see Fig. 66–6).

In conclusion, central nervous system side effects were significantly less frequent (two to three times less frequent) and of weaker intensity with rilmenidine than with clonidine and methyldopa at equihypotensive doses.

CLINICAL USE
Indications

Rilmenidine is indicated in systemic hypertension. The dissociation between antihypertensive activity and side effects, not found with reference drugs at equihypotensive doses, supports rilmenidine as a single therapy in treatment of hypertension. By virtue of its good clinical and laboratory acceptability, rilmenidine may be recommended in elderly subjects and diabetic patients.

Precautions

During pregnancy, as with any new drug, administration of rilmenidine should be avoided, although no teratogenic or embryotoxic effects have been observed in animal experiments. Because rilmenidine is excreted in milk, its administration is not recommended for breastfeeding mothers.

In children, the use of rilmenidine should be avoided in the absence of documented experiments.

As with all antihypertensive agents, in patients presenting with recent vascular diseases (stroke, myocardial infarction), the administration of rilmenidine requires periodic medical monitoring.

Ingestion of alcohol is not recommended during treatment.

Adverse Effects

Adverse effects observed at therapeutic doses with rilmenidine are rare, benign, and transient. At the dose of 1 mg per day, in controlled studies, the incidence of adverse effects was comparable to that observed with placebo.[53] At the dose of 1 mg or 1 mg b.i.d., controlled comparative studies versus clonidine (0.15 to 0.30 mg per day)[51, 54] or methyldopa (500 to 1000 mg per day)[52] showed that the incidence of side effects was significantly lower with rilmenidine than that observed with clonidine or methyldopa.

Side effects are rare (4% to 8%), benign, and transient at therapeutic doses: fatigue, insomnia, dizziness, drowsiness, dry mouth, palpitations, epigastric pain, diarrhea, skin rashes, and, in exceptional cases (< 2%), cold extremities, orthostatic hypotension, sexual disturbances, anxiety, depression, pruritus, edema, cramps, nausea, constipation, and hot flushes.

Contraindications

Rilmenidine is currently contraindicated in case of severe depression or severe renal failure (creatinine clearance, < 15 ml/min).

Interference with Other Drugs

Concurrent treatment with monoamine oxidase inhibitors has not been investigated and thus is not recommended. Combined therapy with tricyclic antidepressants should be carried out with caution, because in that case the antihypertensive activity of rilmenidine may be partly antagonized.[64]

Association with diuretics has been investigated in pharmacoclinical and therapeutic studies. Rilmenidine did not modify the urinary effects of hydrochlorothiazide (25 mg), except for a counteraction of urinary excretion of magnesium induced by the diuretic.[61] Addition of a diuretic to rilmenidine had synergistic effects: while both rilmenidine and hydrochlorothiazide alone controlled blood pressure in 57% of patients, their combination allowed blood pressure to normalize in 35.5% of extra patients.[61]

Use in Patients with Impaired Organ Function

In case of renal failure, if creatinine clearance is greater than 15 ml/min, rilmenidine has been shown to be efficient and well tolerated in a 6-month trial.[65] The pharmacokinetic parameters of rilmenidine in patients with more severe renal failure (creatinine clearance, < 15 ml/min) may authorize its careful use at the dose of 1 mg every other day.[39] However, until now, its use should be restricted to patients with creatinine clearance greater than 15 ml/min.

The Place of Rilmenidine in the Antihypertensive Armamentarium

Rilmenidine as monotherapy leads to the normalization of approximately 60% of mild and moderate hypertension, with no acquired tolerance in long-term surveillance.[40] The acceptability of rilmenidine has been well demonstrated: low incidence of side effects, rarity of drop-outs because of side effects, and maintenance of well-being of hypertensive patients. This dissociation between the antihypertensive activity and the few central nervous system side effects is a distinctive original feature of rilmenidine.

Rilmenidine appears to cause minimal physiologic disturbances of cardiac and renal function and to maintain the physiologic response to exercise and erect posture. But the aim of an antihypertensive treatment should also include reduction of cardiovascular mortality and morbidity. Rilmenidine does not appear to aggravate risk factors involved in cardiovascular morbidity, such as glucose tolerance, hypertriglyceridemia, or hyperuricemia.[50, 52-54] Given the few contraindications of rilmenidine coupled with its efficacy in hypertension, its actions on the structure and function of the heart and large vessels, and the general well-being of patients while on treatment, rilmenidine can be advocated for first-line treatment of a wide spectrum of the hypertensive population, including patients at high risk.

Dosage and Administration

Recommended dosage is 1 tablet (1 mg) per day in a single dose in the morning. In case of insufficient results after a treatment period of 1 month, dosage may be increased to 2 tablets per day in two doses (1 tablet b.i.d.).

REFERENCES

1. Guicheney P, Dausse JP, Meyer P: Affinités respectives du S 3341 et de la clonidine pour les récepteurs adrénergiques alpha 1 et alpha 2 du cerveau du rat. J Pharmacol (Paris) 3:255, 1981.
2. Koenig-Bérard E, Tierney C, Beau B, et al: Cardiovascular and central nervous system effects of rilmenidine (S 3341) in rats. Am J Cardiol 61:22D, 1988.
3. Verbeuren TJ, Koenig-Bérard E, Jordaens FH, et al: Interaction of rilmenidine and clonidine with pre- and postjunctional alpha 2-adrenoceptors in rat and rabbit blood vessels and in rat kidneys. Arch Int Pharmacodyn 300:114, 1989.
4. Bousquet P, Feldman J, Schwartz J: Central cardiovascular effects of alpha adrenergic drugs: Differences between catecholamines and imidazolines. J Pharmacol Exp Ther 230:232, 1984.
5. Ernsberger P, Meeley MP, Mann JJ, et al: Clonidine binds to imidazoline binding sites as well as α_2-adrenoceptors in the ventrolateral medulla. Eur J Pharmacol 134:1, 1987.
6. Hieble JP, Ruffolo RR: Imidazoline receptors: Historical perspective. Fundam Clin Pharmacol 6 (Suppl I):7s, 1992.
7. Reis DJ, Regunathan S, Wang H, et al: Imidazoline receptors in the nervous system. Fundam Clin Pharmacol 6 (Suppl I):23s, 1992.
8. Bricca G, Dontenwill M, Molines A, et al: Rilmenidine selectivity for imidazoline receptors in human brain. Eur J Pharmacol 163:373, 1989.
9. Gomez RE, Ernsberger P, Feinland G, et al: Rilmenidine lowers arterial pressure via imidazole receptors in brainstem C1 area. Eur J Pharmacol 195:181, 1991.
10. Ernsberger P, Damon TH, Graff LM, et al: Moxonidine, a centrally acting antihypertensive agent, is a selective ligand for I_1-imidazoline sites. J Pharmacol Exp Ther 264(1):172, 1993.
11. Hamilton CA, Yakubu MA, Jardine E, et al: Imidazole binding sites in rabbit kidney and forebrain membranes. J Auton Pharmacol 11:277, 1991.
12. Sannajust F, Julien C, Barrès C, et al: Cardiovascular effects of rilmenidine, a new alpha-adrenoceptor agonist, and clonidine in conscious spontaneously hypertensive rats. Clin Exp Pharmacol Physiol 16:837, 1989.
13. Smits JFM, Struyker-Boudier HAJ: Regional hemodynamic effects of rilmenidine and clonidine in the conscious spontaneously hypertensive rat. Fundam Clin Pharmacol 5:651, 1991.
14. Laubie M, Poignant JC, Scuvée-Moreau J, et al: Pharmacological properties of (N-dicyclopropylmethyl) amino-2-oxazoline (S 3341) an alpha-2 adrenoceptor agonist. J Pharmacol (Paris) 16(3):259, 1985.
15. Van Zwieten PA, Thoolen MJMC, Jonkman FAM, et al: Central and peripheral effects of S 3341 (N-dicyclopropylmethyl)-amino-2-oxazoline in animal models. Arch Int Pharmacodyn Ther 279(1):130, 1986.
16. Valet P, Tran MA, Damase-Michel C, et al: Rilmenidine (S 3341) and the sympatho-adrenal system: Adrenoceptors, plasma and adrenal catecholamines in dogs. J Auton Pharmacol 8:319, 1988.
17. Mayorov D, Chernobelski M, Medvedev O: Sympathoinhibitory action of rilmenidine in conscious sinoaortically denervated rats. J Cardiovasc Pharmacol 22:314, 1993.
18. Callens-El Amrani F, Paolaggi F, Swynghedauw B: Remodelling of the heart in DOCA-salt hypertensive rats by propranolol and by an alpha-2 agonist, rilmenidine. J Hypertens 7:947, 1989.
19. Jarrott B, Lewis SJ: Discontinuation syndrome in rats chronically treated with centrally acting alpha-adrenoceptor agonists. Trends Pharmacol Sci 8:244, 1987.
20. Jarrott B, Lewis SJ, Doyle AE, et al: Effects of continuous infusions (10 days) and cessation of infusions of clonidine and rilmenidine (S 3341) on cardiovascular and behavioral parameters of spontaneously hypertensive rats. Am J Cardiol 61:39D, 1988.
21. Garattini S, Remuzzi G, Perico N, et al: Effects of chronic administration of oxaminozoline (S 3341) on renal function and on renal prostaglandins in spontaneously hypertensive rats (SHR). First International Symposium on Oxaminozoline, Heidelberg, 1986, p 48.
22. Kline RL, Cechetto DF: Renal effects of rilmenidine in anesthetized rats: Importance of renal nerves. J Pharmacol Exp Ther 266(3):1556, 1993.
23. Van Zwieten PA: Pharmacology of the alpha 2-adrenoceptor agonist rilmenidine. Am J Cardiol 61:6D, 1988.
24. Feldman J, Tibirica E, Bricca G, et al: Evidence for the involvement of imidazoline receptors in the central hypotensive effect of rilmenidine in the rabbit. Br J Pharmacol 100:600, 1990.
25. Sannajust F, Head GA: Rilmenidine-induced hypotension involves imidazoline-preferring receptors in conscious rabbits. J Cardiovasc Pharmacol 23:42, 1994.
26. Johnston AL, Koenig-Bérard E, Cooper TA, et al: A comparison of the effects of clonidine, rilmenidine and guanfacine in the holeboard and elevated plus-maze. Drug Dev Res 15:405, 1988.
27. Tierney C, Nadaud D, Koenig-Bérard E, et al: Effects of two alpha 2 agonists, rilmenidine and clonidine, on the morphine withdrawal syndrome and their potential addictive properties in rats. Am J Cardiol 61:35D, 1988.
28. Van Zwieten PA: Development and trends in the drug treatment of essential hypertension. J Hypertens 10(7):S1, 1992.
29. Reid JL: Central alpha-2 receptors and the regulation of blood pressure in humans. J Cardiovasc Pharmacol 7:S45, 1985.
30. Tibir ica E, Feldman J, Mermet C, et al: Selectivity of rilmenidine for the nucleus reticularis lateralis, a ventrolateral medullary structure containing imidazoline-preferring receptors. Eur J Pharmacol 209:213, 1991.
31. Ernsberger P, Feinland G, Meeley MP, et al: Characterization and visualization of clonidine-sensitive imidazole sites in rat kidney which recognize clonidine-displacing substance. Am J Hypertens 3:90, 1990.
32. Piletz JE, Andorn AC, Unnerstall JR, et al: Binding of [^{3}H]-p-

aminoclonidine to α_2-adrenoceptor states plus a non-adrenergic site on human platelet plasma membranes. Biochem Pharmacol 42(3):569, 1991.

33. Molderings GJ, Moura D, Fink K, et al: Binding of [³H]clonidine to I₁-imidazoline sites in bovine adrenal medullary membranes. Naunyn Schmiedebergs Arch Pharmacol 348:70, 1993.

34. Allan DR, Penner SB, Smyth DD: Renal imidazoline preferring sites and solute excretion in the rat. Br J Pharmacol 108:870, 1993.

35. Murray S, Watson D, Davies DS: Bistrifluoromethylaryl derivatives for drug analysis by gas chromatography electron capture negative ion chemical ionization mass spectrometry: Application to the measurement of (N-dicyclopropylmethyl) amino-2-oxazoline in plasma. Biomed Mass Spectrom 5:230, 1985.

36. Ehrhardt JD: Gas chromatographic negative ion mass spectrometric assay of 2-dicyclopropylmethylamino-2-oxazoline (S 3341), a new antihypertensive drug. Biomed Mass Spectrom 10:593, 1985.

37. Genissel P, Bromet N, Fourtillan JB, et al: Pharmacokinetics of rilmenidine in healthy subjects. Am J Cardiol 61:47D, 1988.

38. Singlas E, Ehrhardt JD, Zech P, et al: Pharmacokinetics of rilmenidine. Am J Cardiol 61:54D, 1988.

39. Aparicio M, Dratwa M, Fillastre JP, et al: Pharmacokinetics of rilmenidine in patients with chronic renal insufficiency and in hemodialysis patients. Am J Cardiol 74(13):44A, 1994.

40. Beau B, Mahieux F, Paraire M, et al: Efficacy and safety of rilmenidine for arterial hypertension. Am J Cardiol 61: 95D, 1988.

41. Weerasuriya K, Shaw E, Turner P: Preliminary clinical pharmacological studies of S 3341, a new hypotensive agent, and comparison with clonidine in normal males. Eur J Clin Pharmacol 27:281, 1984.

42. Dollery CT, Davies DS, Duchier J, et al: Dose and concentration-effect relations for rilmenidine. Am J Cardiol 61:60D, 1988.

43. Zannad F, Aliot E, Florentin J, et al: Hemodynamic and electrophysiologic effects of a new alpha 2-adrenoceptor agonist, rilmenidine, for systemic hypertension. Am J Cardiol 61:67D, 1988.

44. N'Guyen Van Cao A, Levy B, Slama R: Noninvasive study of cardiac structure and function after rilmenidine for essential hypertension. Am J Cardiol 61:72D, 1988.

45. De Devitiis O, Di Somma S, Liguori V, et al: Effort blood pressure control in the course of antihypertensive treatments. Am J Med 87(3C):46S, 1989.

46. Harron DWG: Antihypertensive drugs and baroreflex sensitivity: Effect of rilmenidine. Am J Med 87(3C):57S, 1989.

47. Trimarco B, Rosiello G, Sarno D, et al: Effects of one-year treatment with rilmenidine on systemic hypertension-induced left ventricular hypertrophy in hypertensive patients. Am J Cardiol 74(13):36A, 1994.

48. Dahlöf B, Pennert K, Hansson L: Reversal of left ventricular hypertrophy in hypertensive patients: A metaanalysis of 109 treatment studies. Am J Hypertens 50:95, 1992.

49. Pannier B, Safar ME: Effects of rilmenidine on arterial function in essential hypertension. Arch Mal Coeur 82(V):47, 1989.

50. Galley P, Manciet G, Hessel JL, et al: Antihypertensive efficacy and acceptability of rilmenidine in elderly hypertensive patients. Am J Cardiol 61:86D, 1988.

51. Velasco M, Soltero I, Sukerman M, et al: Double-blind, randomized study of the efficacy, tolerance, and rebound effects of the antihypertensive drug rilmenidine: Comparative evaluation with clonidine. Curr Ther Res 54(2):202, 1993.

52. UK Working Party on Rilmenidine: Rilmenidine in mild to moderate essential hypertension: A double-blind, randomized, parallel-group, multicenter comparison with methyldopa in 157 patients. Curr Ther Res 47:194, 1990.

53. Ostermann G, Brisgand B, Schmitt J, et al: Dose and concentration-effect relations for rilmenidine. Am J Cardiol 61:60D, 1988.

54. Fillastre JP, Letac B, Galinier F, et al: A multicenter double-blind comparative study of rilmenidine and clonidine in 333 hypertensive patients. Am J Cardiol 61:81D, 1988.

55. Dallochio M, Gosse P, Fillastre JP, et al: La rilmenidine, un nouvel antihypertenseur dans le traitement de prem ière intention de l'hypertension artérielle essentielle. Presse Med 20:1265, 1991.

56. Fiorentini C, Guillet C, Guazzi M: A multicentre double-blind trial comparing rilmenidine 1 mg and hydrochlorothiazide 25 mg in 244 patients. Arch Mal Coeur 82(V):39, 1989.

57. Pillion G, Février B, Codis P, et al: Long-term control of blood pressure by rilmenidine in high-risk populations. Am J Cardiol 74(13):58A, 1994.

58. Grossman A, Weerasuriya K, Damluji S, et al: Alpha 2 adrenoceptor agonists stimulate growth hormone secretion but have no acute effects on plasma cortisol under basal conditions. Horm Res 25:65, 1987.

59. Kuhn JM, Wolf LM: The effects of oxaminozoline (S 3341) on the hypothalamo-pituitary axis in the healthy subject. First International Symposium on Oxaminozoline, Heidelberg, 1986, p 81.

60. Mpoy M, Vandeleene B, Ketelslegers JM, et al: Treatment of systemic hypertension insulin-treated diabetes mellitus with rilmenidine. Am J Cardiol 61:91D, 1988.

61. Leary WP: Renal excretory actions of antihypertensive agents: Effects of rilmenidine. Am J Med 87(3C):63C, 1989.

62. De Broe ME, Verpooten G, Thomas JR, et al: Renal effects of oxaminozoline (S 3341), a new alpha-2 agonist, after single administration in the healthy subject. First International Symposium on Oxaminozoline, Heidelberg, 1986.

63. Zech P, Pozet N: Effects of a new alpha-2 agonist, oxaminozoline (S 3341), on renal function. First International Symposium on Oxaminozoline, Heidelberg, 1986.

64. Mahieu F, Paraire M, Brisgand B, et al: Effets sur la pression artérielle et la vigilance d'un nouvel alpha-2 agoniste, la rilmenidine: Influence d'un prétraitement par l'imipramine. Arch Mal Coeur 81:325, 1988.

65. Lins R, Daelemans R, Dratwa M, et al: Acceptability of rilmenidine and long-term surveillance of plasma concentrations in hypertensive patients with renal insufficiency. Am J Med 87(3C):41S, 1989.

CHAPTER 67

Guanfacine

Michael H. Alderman, M.D., and Bernard Lamport, M.D.

HISTORY

The control of blood pressure is complex, and the mechanisms by which antihypertensive drugs lower blood pressure involve various physiologic sites and organ systems. It is not surprising, therefore, that no single agent provides universally effective treatment.[1]

It was first recognized in the late 1960s that centrally acting α-adrenoreceptor agonists such as clonidine and methyldopa could reduce blood pressure. In the early 1970s, a new centrally acting α-adrenoreceptor agonist, guanfacine, was synthesized.[2] The drug was shown to lower blood pressure in both normotensive and hypertensive animals.

In hypertensive rats, guanfacine was found to have a significant antihypertensive effect after oral doses of 1 mg/kg, and the response was dose dependent up to 5 mg/kg. In anesthetized animals, doses that were too small to have a systemic effect after intravenous administration effectively lowered blood pressure when injected directly into the vertebral artery or cerebral ventricles. Moreover, the drug was well tolerated in animal studies. At doses up to 3 mg/kg, guanfacine produced moderate sedation, whereas clonidine has a marked sedative effect at doses of 0.3 mg/kg.[3]

CHEMISTRY

Guanfacine hydrochloride, *N*-amidino-2-(2,6-dichlorophenyl)-acetamide hydrochloride, has a molecular weight of 282.56. It is a colorless and tasteless, water-soluble, crystalline powder that is stable at room temperature.[4] Guanfacine is a relatively weak base with a pK$_a$ of 7.1 and, at physiologic pH, exists predominantly (67%) in the lipid-soluble base form.

PHARMACOLOGY

Guanfacine's blood pressure–lowering effects are mediated by α$_2$-adrenoreceptor activation in the central nervous system. Central stimulation of α-receptors decreases the sympathetic outflow, subsequently resulting in reduced vascular tone and a slight reduction in heart rate. In addition, stimulation of peripheral presynaptic α$_2$-adrenoreceptors, which inhibits sympathetic neurotransmission, may to some extent contribute to the overall antihypertensive effect.[5, 6] Guanfacine has a preferential affinity for α$_2$-adrenoreceptors. Binding studies indicate that guanfacine binds preferentially to α$_2$-adrenoreceptor sites in the cerebral cortex, with little or no binding at dopamine-, serotonin-, histamine H1-, and β$_1$- or β$_2$-adrenoreceptor sites.[7] The relative distribution of guanfacine between α$_1$- and α$_2$-adrenoreceptors is 1:3400, whereas the same ratio for clonidine is 1:280, indicating that guanfacine is about 12 times more selective for α$_2$-adrenoreceptors than is clonidine.

In anesthetized dogs, administration of guanfacine into the vertebral artery at a rate of 1 μg/kg/min resulted in a fall of blood pressure within 40 minutes. An intravenous infusion of guanfacine in such a small dosage did not produce a fall in blood pressure within the same time frame.[3] The hypotensive effect of an intracerebroventricular injection of guanfacine is largely abolished by the α-adrenoreceptor–blocking drug phentolamine when given in the same manner. A central site of action was further confirmed by the decreased electrical activity demonstrated in preganglionic sympathetic nerves after intraventricular guanfacine administration.[8] Guanfacine has also been shown to decrease the turnover of cerebral norepi-

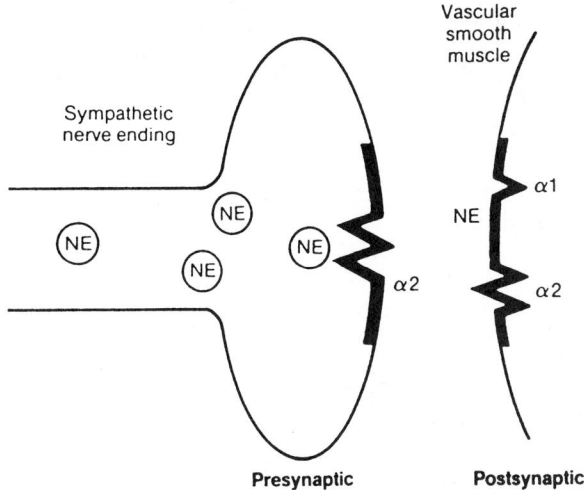

Figure 67–1. The α-adrenoreceptors. NE, norepinephrine. (Reprinted with permission from Reid JL: Alpha-adrenergic receptors and blood pressure control. Am J Cardiol 57:6E, 1986.)

nephrine, which is characteristic of central α-adrenoreceptor stimulation.[9]

Although guanfacine produces its pharmacologic effects mainly through central α$_2$-adrenoreceptors, it also appears to have a peripheral action. Intravenous administration of guanfacine in doses of 3 to 100 μg/kg in anesthetized normotensive cats produced an initial small transient pressor effect that was promptly followed by a prolonged fall in blood pressure.[3] After intravenous administration of 0.02 mg/kg of guanfacine in patients with hypertensive crisis, blood pressure rose from 239/124 to 252/130 mmHg ($p < .05$) after 2 minutes, but then decreased in 15 minutes.[10] At present, α$_2$-adrenoreceptors in peripheral sympathetic nerve endings, as in the brain, are believed to have a presynaptic and postsynaptic location (Fig. 67–1).[5] The initial transient rise of blood pressure can be explained by the increased peripheral sympathetic flow caused by the stimulation of *postsynaptic* α$_2$-adrenoreceptors in blood vessels (see Fig. 67–1). Intravenous administration of 2 mg of guanfacine to healthy individuals reduced blood pressure and plasma norepinephrine concentration before increases in plasma growth hormone concentration (an indicator of central α-adrenoreceptor stimulation)[11] were noted.[12] The decrease is likely caused by stimulation of peripheral *presynaptic* α$_2$-adrenoreceptors (see Fig. 67–1), which inhibits sympathetic nerve function.[13, 14]

PHARMACOKINETICS

At physiologic pH (7.4), guanfacine is present predominantly (67%) as the lipid-soluble base (versus 24% with clonidine), which promotes its rapid absorption after oral administration and permits penetration of the blood-brain barrier.[15] The absolute bioavailability of guanfacine is approximately 80%.[16] Maximum plasma concentrations after oral administration are reached in 1 to 4 hours.[17] Oral doses of 1, 2, 3, and 4 mg of guanfacine produce peak plasma concentrations of 3.1, 3.5, 9.1, and 12.0 μg/L, respectively.[18] Steady-state plasma concentrations are reached in most patients approximately 4 days after beginning therapy.[19, 20]

Guanfacine is approximately 64% to 72% bound to plasma proteins.[15, 16] The drug is extensively distributed, with highest concentrations found in the kidneys and liver.

Guanfacine is mainly excreted by the kidneys after extensive hepatic biotransformation into inactive metabolites; approximately half of a single oral dose is excreted unchanged in urine. The elimination half-life of guanfacine ranges from 12.1 to 22.8 hours.[18] In comparison, the half-life of clonidine ranges from 8.6 to 25.0 hours and that of methyldopa is less than 2 hours. Renal excretion of unchanged guanfacine is decreased in elderly patients and patients with impaired renal function, but plasma concentrations of the drug are only slightly increased in such patients.[21]

PHYSIOLOGIC EFFECTS
Hemodynamic and Cardiac Effects

Oral administration of guanfacine reduces systemic vascular resistance by dilating small arteries and arterioles, and this is its principal mode of action.[22, 23] The reduced vascular resistance decreases cardiac afterload and improves left ventricular performance.[22]

In one uncontrolled study, guanfacine therapy appeared to reverse left ventricular hypertrophy (LVH).[24, 25] Ibrahim et al.[25] used echocardiography to evaluate the effect of guanfacine on LVH in seven hypertensive patients. Guanfacine administered for 10 weeks induced regression of LVH and decreased left ventricular mass without influencing contractile performance of the left ventricle. These favorable observations have not been confirmed in any controlled study.

Endocrine Effects

Plasma Renin and Aldosterone

In an 8-week study, no effect on plasma volume or aldosterone levels was noted at a guanfacine dosage of 1 mg daily.[26] In contrast, plasma renin activity (PRA) was reduced by the third day of treatment at a dosage of 3 mg daily;[27] the reduction may be sustained over months of regular therapy.[28] No correlation has been noted, however, between pretreatment PRA or changes in PRA and the extent of blood pressure reduction during guanfacine therapy.[22, 29, 30]

Norepinephrine

Plasma norepinephrine concentrations were significantly decreased after intravenous and oral guanfacine administration and remained at lower concentrations than pretreatment values for the duration of treatment.[29] Because decreases in norepinephrine concentrations preceded any central effects, the antihypertensive effect of guanfacine appears to be partially mediated by inhibition of peripheral sympathetic nervous activity.

Prolactin and Growth Hormone

Hypertensive patients with elevated prolactin levels may experience reductions in serum prolactin levels during guanfacine therapy.[31] Single doses of guanfacine acutely stimulate growth hormone secretion, but no sustained effect on growth hormone secretion occurs with long-term therapy.[32]

Lipid and Glucose Metabolism

Guanfacine has not been found to increase serum lipids in short- or long-term studies.[26] In fact, in uncontrolled studies, guanfacine therapy has been shown to decrease lipid levels in hyperlipidemic patients.[31, 33] Guanfacine may reduce glucose tolerance after acute administration, but long-term therapy does not appear to affect glucose metabolism adversely.[34]

Other Pharmacologic Effects

Guanfacine therapy had no adverse effect on the hematologic and biochemical indices.[35, 36] Decreases in gastric acid levels[37] and increases in the liberation of histamine from cultured human mast cells[38] have been associated with guanfacine. When given intrathecally to rats, guanfacine also produced a moderate general analgesic effect.[39] This effect has also been observed after epidural administration in humans.[40] Acute intravenous injection of guanfacine to hypertensive patients may produce a marked decrease in glomerular filtration rate, renal blood flow, diuresis, and electrolyte clearance;[41] however, prolonged oral therapy does not adversely affect renal function in patients with normal renal function or preexisting renal impairment.[35, 42]

Effects on Central Nervous System

As a centrally acting α-adrenoreceptor agonist, guanfacine has sedative effects that are reported to be less pronounced than those produced by clonidine.[3, 17, 43] Guanfacine does not appear to impair reaction time, optomotor coordination, or concentration performance to visual or acoustic stimuli[44] or the ability to drive a motor vehicle.[45] However, the rise in blood pressure induced in hypertensive patients by central sympathetic nervous stimuli such as loud noise is not prevented by guanfacine.[46]

CLINICAL USE
Open Studies

In a variety of observational studies, the safety, tolerance, and hypertensive effects of guanfacine were demonstrated.[24, 31, 36, 46–49]

Controlled Trials

Comparisons with Placebo

A few well-designed studies have compared guanfacine with placebo as monotherapy or a second agent in the treatment of hypertension (Table 67–1). Results of these studies have indicated a significant antihypertensive effect after 1 week of treatment with 0.5 to 3 mg of guanfacine daily. Decreases in systolic and diastolic blood pressures from 17 to 57 mmHg and from 14 to 28 mmHg, respectively, were reported.[26, 50–52]

Materson et al.[51] reported a double-blind parallel study testing the effectiveness of guanfacine as a second agent in 362 patients receiving diuretic therapy (seated diastolic blood pressures between 95 and 114 mmHg). Patients were randomly assigned to treatment with 25 mg of chlorthalidone daily plus either placebo or 0.5, 1, 2, or 3 mg of guanfacine daily for 12 weeks. Combination therapy containing guanfacine dosages of 1, 2, and 3 mg/day was effective in further reducing diastolic blood pressure and was significantly different from the hypotensive effect of the combined diuretic and placebo regimen. Blood pressure reductions with 0.5 mg/day of guanfacine were not significantly different from the diuretic and placebo combination. The responses were maximized at 4 weeks of treatment.

Comparison with Other Drugs

Diuretics

Few studies have been done to compare the antihypertensive effectiveness of guanfacine and diuretics as monotherapy or in combination. Seedat[53] studied 18 patients with moderate to severe essential hypertension receiving either cyclopenthiazide 0.5 mg or hydrochlorothiazide 50 mg daily. The addition of guanfacine 2 to 15 mg daily further decreased sitting blood pressure by 39/33 mmHg over a 12-month period.

The effectiveness of using guanfacine as a step-2 antihypertensive drug in combination with a diuretic was demonstrated in a 12-week double-blind, placebo-controlled multicenter study of 249 patients with diastolic blood pressures between 95 and 114 mmHg.[52] All patients received daily doses of clorthalidone 25 mg before the study. Guanfacine (1 to 3 mg) or placebo was added to the chlorthalidone regimen. Guanfacine significantly decreased sitting diastolic and systolic blood pressure and mean arterial pressure compared with placebo. The study also demonstrated that the antihypertensive effect of guanfacine was well maintained for up to 24 hours with once-daily dosing.

Centrally Acting Drugs

Guanfacine has been compared as monotherapy or a second agent with the other centrally acting drugs methyldopa and clonidine (see Table 67–1).[54–59]

Methyldopa. Guanfacine monotherapy has been shown to be at least as effective as methyldopa monotherapy in the treatment of mild to moderate hypertension in a number of comparative studies;[58–60] however, in some studies, guanfacine produced a greater antihypertensive effect than methyldopa.[58, 59]

The addition of either methyldopa or guanfacine to the regimen of patients whose blood pressures were uncontrolled with bendrofluazide, 5 mg daily for 4 weeks,[43] resulted in similar pressure reductions. This extraordinary decline was probably due to the fact that the final but not the pretreatment pressures were recorded after 36 hours in the hospital.

Clonidine. Guanfacine monotherapy has been shown to be at least as effective as clonidine monotherapy in the treatment of mild to moderate hypertension in a number of comparative studies.[56, 57, 60] In addition, guanfacine appeared to be better tolerated.

Clonidine and guanfacine were compared as second agents in 509 patients with an average age of 53 years.[54, 55] The mean blood pressure after 4 to 5 weeks of treatment with 25 mg/day of chlorthalidone was 150/100 mmHg. Either guanfacine 1 mg/day or clonidine 0.1 mg twice daily was then added to the regimens for 6 months. The dosage of guanfacine could be increased as required to 3 mg/day and clonidine to 0.6 mg/day (administered in divided doses). Among the guanfacine- and clonidine-treated patients, the mean blood pressure fell to comparable levels (Table 67–2). Thus, the addition of guanfacine or clonidine appears to have an equivalent additive effect when given to patients already receiving diuretics.

Guanabenz

A double-blind randomized parallel trial comparing the antihypertensive effects of guanfacine, 1 mg daily, and guanabenz, 4 mg twice daily for the first week and 8 mg twice daily for the remaining 7 weeks, yielded no differences in sitting and standing diastolic and systolic blood pressures between treatment groups. Thus, when used alone, the drugs were equally effective; however, guanfacine was less sedating.[26]

Other Drugs

Few studies have evaluated the comparative or additive effects of guanfacine with other antihypertensives such as vasodilators or β-blockers. A recent comparison of five monotherapeutic agents involving clonidine as the centrally acting α-agonist revealed it to be less tolerable but equally effective at lowering blood pressure.[61] Velasco et al.[62] reported that the combination of guanfacine, 2 to 6 mg daily, and hydralazine hydrochloride, 50 to 300 mg daily, had a greater antihypertensive effect than guanfacine alone. After 4 weeks of monotherapy with guanfacine, blood pressure was reduced from 179/112 to 151/90 mmHg

Table 67–1. **Clinical Trials with Guanfacine as Monotherapy**

Reference	Control Agent	Duration (mo)	Patients*	Compared Group			Guanfacine Group			
				Dose†	BP (mmHg) Initial	Final	Dose	BP (mmHg) Initial	Final	ΔBP
Placebo-Controlled Studies										
Lochaya et al., 1980[50]	Placebo	2	17/19	—	159/110	159/108	4–12/2–3	161/111	128/90	33‡/19‡
Fillingim et al., 1986[26]	Placebo	2	9/17	—	—	Unchanged	1/1	149/97	140/84	9§/13‡
			21/21	—	—	DBP ↓ 1.6	1/1	—	DBP ↓ 12.6	BP ↓ 11.0¶
Comparative Studies										
Lauro et al., 1980[56]	Clonidine	1	13/15	0.45/3	187/107	154/93	2–4/1	184/110	146/88	7§/18‖
Distler et al., 1980[57]	Clonidine	1	7/9	0.35–0.45/2–3	179/126	150/109	1–2/3	187/127	160/111	–2§/–1§
					166/118	137/99		167/121	133/99	5§/3§
Roeckel & Heidland, 1980[58]	Methyldopa	1.5	10/10	500–2250/3	203/124	180/114	2–6/2–3	201/122	143/95	35‡/17‡
					187/117	152/104		193/118	145/94	13‡/11‡
Rengo et al., 1980[59]	Methyldopa	3	15/15	750–2000/3	187/111	177/103	1–5/2	189/110	163/95	16**/7**

BP, blood pressure; ΔBP, change in blood pressure; DBP, diastolic blood pressure.
*Control/guanfacine.
†mg daily/times a day.
‡$p <.001$.
§Not significant.
‖$p <.02$.
¶$p <.0001$.
**$p <.01$.
↓, decrease.

Table 67–2. **Clinical Trials with Guanfacine as a Second Drug in a Stepped-Care Program***

| | | | | Compared Group | | | Guanfacine Group | | | |
| | | | | | BP (mmHg) | | | BP (mmHg) | | |
Reference	Control Agent	Duration (mo)	Patients*	Dose‡	Initial	Final	Dose‡	Initial	Final	ΔBP
Placebo-Controlled Studies										
Materson et al., 1980[51]	Placebo	3	63/63	—	141/100	135/93	0.5/1	137/94	133/94	−2§/−2§
			—/64	—	141/100	135/93	1/1	141/100	127/87	8‖/6‖
			—/58	—	141/100	135/93	2/1	139/100	128/86	5‖/7‖
			—/59	—	141/100	135/93	3/1	140/101	124/88	10‖/6‖
Kennan et al., 1986[52]	Placebo	3	63/65	—	147/100	141/94	1–3/1	142/99	128/88	7‖/5‖
Comparative Studies										
Bune et al., 1981[43]	Methyldopa¶	1.5	9/9	250/3	180/114	126/86	2/3	172/109	126/84	−11§/−3§
Wilson et al., 1986[54]	Clonidine	6	236/231	0.35–0.45/2–3	147/104	133/87	1/1	150/102	134/91	2§/−6§
Jain et al., 1985[55]	Clonidine	6	20/22	1/2	150/100	136/92	1/1	151/101	133/92	4§/1§

BP, blood pressure; ΔBP, change in blood pressure.
*The first drug was chlorthalidone, 25 mg/day, for 5 weeks before administration of guanfacine and thereafter.
†Control/guanfacine.
‡mg daily/times a day.
§Not significant.
‖$p <.01$.
¶For the first drug, patients received bendrofluazide, 5 mg/day, for 1 month before administration of guanfacine and thereafter received bendrofluazide and guanfacine in combination.

($p < .05$) with the addition of oral hydralazine. Guanfacine was also able to counteract sympathetic nervous tone increases induced by arteriole vasodilators such as hydralazine and thus may be an alternative to β-blocking agents for this purpose.

Special Populations

Guanfacine has been used safely for the treatment of hypertension in the elderly. Among 2805 patients, most between the ages of 60 and 70, treatment with guanfacine, 2 mg/day, was associated with effective blood pressure control with an acceptable incidence of adverse effects. Dry mouth and drowsiness were the most common; 9.3% of the patients discontinued the drug because of adverse effects.[63]

Although some α-adrenergic agonist drugs have been shown to affect insulin secretion or glucose metabolism, thereby complicating the management of diabetic hypertensive patients, guanfacine has been found to have little effect on pancreatic β-cell function, glycosylated hemoglobin levels, or glucose tolerance.[34, 64]

Adverse Effects

The adverse reactions that occur with guanfacine are generally dose or dose-frequency dependent. Most reactions are reported during the initiation of therapy, especially when large doses are given or other drugs are added to treatment. Because guanfacine is predominantly a centrally acting drug, the most common adverse reactions are central in origin and include dry mouth and sedation. Fatigue, dizziness, and insomnia are also reported.[47, 65]

The adverse effect profile of guanfacine has been compared with that of placebo, clonidine, methyldopa, and guanabenz.[26, 54–59] In general, the adverse effect profile of guanfacine, 1 mg/day, is indistinguishable from that of placebo. Combining the results of two studies,[56, 57] the comparison of clonidine, 0.45 mg, with guanfacine, 1 to 4 mg, in 44 patients for 1 month yielded more dry mouth (18 versus 10) and sedation (9 versus 4) in the clonidine group, but more fatigue (7 versus 4) in the guanfacine group. The number of patients who discontinued treatment because of side effects was similar in both groups (two patients in each group). When guanfacine, 1 to 6 mg daily, was compared with methyldopa, 0.5 to 2.25 g daily, for 1.5 to 3 months in 50 patients,[58, 59] dry mouth was common to both treatment groups, whereas dizziness was rarely observed. When guanfacine, 1 mg daily, was compared with guanabenz, considerably more somnolence occurred in patients receiving guanabenz. Morning drowsiness was reported by 4 (15%) of the 27 guanfacine-treated patients, compared with 15 (54%) of the 28 guanabenz-treated patients.[26]

When guanfacine was given to healthy individuals or to patients with glucose intolerance for as long as 2 years, no hyperglycemic episodes were reported.[66] Although guanfacine is capable of producing brady-cardia in animals and humans,[3] no clinically significant bradycardia has been observed.[26, 53]

Withdrawal Syndrome

A withdrawal syndrome characterized by rapidly increasing blood pressure, headache, tremor, restlessness, and nausea is associated with the sudden cessation of therapy after long-term administration of centrally acting antihypertensive drugs such as clonidine.[55, 67, 68] As many as 80% of patients treated with clonidine doses higher than 1.2 mg/day have experienced the withdrawal syndrome within 18 to 20 hours after stopping therapy.[55, 65, 68, 69]

The withdrawal syndrome observed after rapid cessation of guanfacine therapy occurs in a smaller number of patients. In a study of 580 patients with essential hypertension who received guanfacine (mean dose, 4.7 mg daily) for up to 2 years, a withdrawal syndrome was reported in 3% of the patients.[65] Maximal increases in blood pressures were 17%. Factors favoring the development of the withdrawal syndrome included uncontrolled high blood pressure during therapy, a tendency to exhibit tachycardia, and doses higher than 4 mg/day. Catecholamine concentrations after discontinuation of guanfacine were greater than pretreatment values, but they were not accompanied by the severe symptoms often observed with clonidine therapy.[68–70] Supine and standing systolic and diastolic pressures increased by 13/14 and 33/16 mmHg, respectively, over treatment levels before returning to baseline values. These pressure changes were not accompanied by symptoms generally associated with clonidine withdrawal.[56, 68] Although biochemical indices suggest that increased sympathetic activity occurs after withdrawal of guanfacine, mild subjective symptoms of sympathetic stimulation are observed only in some patients after withdrawal.[55, 68, 69]

Wilson et al.[54] showed that, in the first 3 days after the abrupt cessation of guanfacine and clonidine therapy in patients with essential hypertension, significantly higher increases in systolic and diastolic blood pressures were measured in those patients who had previously received clonidine. Clonidine withdrawal also induced abrupt, significantly higher increases in pulse rate than did guanfacine during the first 4 days after withdrawal. Furthermore, more patients withdrawn from clonidine therapy reported headache, fatigue, and nausea. Five patients in the guanfacine group and eight patients in the clonidine group were removed from the study because of withdrawal complications before completing the planned 7-day withdrawal evaluation period. The longer half-life of guanfacine versus that of clonidine may be responsible for the lower incidence and lesser severity of withdrawal symptoms of guanfacine.

Indications

Clinical trials have demonstrated that guanfacine is an effective antihypertensive agent both alone or in combination with a diuretic. Guanfacine has been shown to provide an antihypertensive effect comparable with, if not greater than, that of clonidine or methyldopa. Furthermore, because of its long half-life, guanfacine can be given once daily.

Currently, it is recommended that guanfacine be used in patients with essential hypertension who are already receiving a thiazide-type diuretic. Confirmation that guanfacine can in fact lower cholesterol and triglyceride levels in hypertensive patients and glucose levels in hypertensive patients with diabetes might significantly enhance its value. A recent Swedish trial suggests that when both cholesterol and blood pressure are reduced, a significant decline in myocardial infarction occurs.[71]

Contraindications

The available literature suggests no specific contraindications to the use of guanfacine.

Drug Interactions

There is little indication that guanfacine interferes with the pharmacologic effects or metabolism of other drugs. Specifically, no adverse effects were observed during the use of guanfacine with cardiac glycosides, hypoglycemic agents, sedatives and hypnotics, coronary vasodilators, analgesics, anticoagulants, antilipemics, or bronchodilators.[4] However, the potential for increased sedation when guanfacine is administered with central nervous system depressants should be considered. Moreover, it has been reported that the antihypertensive effect of guanfacine is antagonized by tricyclic antidepressants, presumably because they reduce guanfacine uptake.[72]

Other Precautions

In elderly patients and those with impaired renal function, the total clearance, serum levels, elimination rate constant, and half-life of guanfacine were not significantly changed;[21] moreover, guanfacine did not further impair renal function. Thus, changes in guanfacine dosage do not appear to be necessary in the elderly or in patients with reduced renal function.

Dosage and Administration

The recommended dosage of guanfacine in patients already receiving a thiazide-type diuretic is 1 mg given once daily at bedtime to minimize somnolence. If it is necessary to increase the dosage, increments of 0.5 to 1 mg/day are recommended no sooner than 2 weeks after the initial dose, and at intervals of not less than 1 or 2 weeks. If the patient develops a rise in blood pressure near the end of the once-daily dosing interval, a divided dosing regimen may be used.[35] If guanfacine is used as monotherapy and the desired reduction in blood pressure is not achieved with a single daily dose of 2 or 3 mg, a diuretic should be added in the smallest recommended dose. Guanfacine

dosages higher than 3 mg daily are not recommended because of substantial increases in adverse reactions and a lack of evidence for enhanced efficacy at these dosages.[35] A dosage of 0.5 mg daily may be effective in some patients such as the elderly or those with renal insufficiency.

SOCIOECONOMIC CONSIDERATIONS
Compliance

A dose that may be taken once daily at bedtime, together with mild and reversible side effects, makes guanfacine an attractive centrally acting agent in the antihypertensive armamentarium.

Cost

The cost of treatment with the usual dosage of guanfacine is similar to that of other centrally acting α_2-adrenoreceptor agonists, but it is lower when used in the recommended initial daily dose of 1 mg.[26, 51] Treatment with guanfacine (Tenex), 1 mg/day for 30 days, costs $9.30; with clonidine, 0.1 mg twice daily, the average generic cost is $10.76; Catapres, 0.1 mg twice daily, costs $14.28; guanabenz (Wytensin), 4 mg twice daily, costs $15.93; for methyldopa, 250 mg twice daily, the average generic cost is $9.66; and Aldomet, 250 mg twice daily, costs $14.13.[73]

SUMMARY

A review[73] suggests that guanfacine is effective and safe in the treatment of patients with mild to moderate hypertension. It is at least as effective as other centrally acting α-adrenoreceptor agonists. Evidence has suggested that the use of a low guanfacine dose of 1 mg daily is associated with a low incidence and severity of side effects, which improves patient compliance. Dosages higher than 3 mg daily may not increase efficacy and are associated with increased adverse effects. Guanfacine does not affect total cholesterol and triglyceride concentrations, nor does it raise glucose levels. Guanfacine may produce less somnolence than clonidine and methyldopa. The withdrawal symptoms and morning drowsiness that often complicate the cessation of clonidine therapy are less common and less severe with guanfacine. There are no specific contraindications to its use. By the same token, there is no particular patient profile that can be used as an indication for selection of guanfacine. No evidence is available about the comparative efficacy or acceptability of guanfacine as either a first or second drug in relation to diuretics, calcium antagonists, β-blockers, peripheral antiadrenergic drugs, or angiotensin-converting enzyme inhibitors. Nevertheless, its efficacy as sole therapy has been adequately demonstrated.

In conclusion, guanfacine has been shown to extend the spectrum of effective agents and thus widens the range of therapeutic choices for the treatment of essential hypertension.

REFERENCES

1. Laragh JH: Two forms of vasoconstriction in systemic hypertension. Am J Cardiol 60:82G, 1987.
2. Bream JB, Lauener H, Picard CW, et al: Substituted phenylacetylguanidines: A new class of antihypertensive agents. Arzneimittelforschung 25:1477, 1975.
3. Scholtysik G, Lauener H, Eichenberger E, et al: Pharmacological actions of the antihypertensive agent N-amidino-2-(2,6-dichlorophenyl) acetamide hydrochloride (BS 100-141). Arzneimittelforschung 25:1482, 1975.
4. Scholtysik G, Jerie P, Picard CW: Guanfacine. In Scriabine A (ed): Pharmacology of Antihypertensive Drugs. New York: Raven Press, 1980, pp 79–98.
5. Reid JL: Alpha-adrenergic receptors and blood pressure control. Am J Cardiol 57:6E, 1986.
6. Van Zwieten PA: Overview of alpha2-adrenoceptor agonists with a central action. Am J Cardiol 57:3E, 1986.
7. Dausse JP, Cardot A, Meyer P: Specific binding of ³H-guanfacine to alpha2-adrenoceptors in rat brain: Comparison with clonidine. J Pharmacol 14:35, 1983.
8. Waite R: Inhibition of sympathetic nerve activity, resulting from central alpha-adrenoceptor stimulation. In Milliez P, Sofar M (eds): Recent Advances in Hypertension, Vol 2. Reims: Boehringer Ingelheim, 1975, pp 27–31.
9. Anden NE, Grabowska M, Strombom U: Different alpha-adrenoceptors in the central nervous system mediating biochemical and functional effects of clonidine and receptor blocking agent. Naunyn Schmiedebergs Arch Pharmacol 292:43, 1976.
10. Rosenthal J, Schafer N, Rauh J, et al: Hamodynamische Untersuchungen mit dem neuen Antihypertensivum Guanfacin. Dtsch Med Wochenschr 105:1680, 1980.
11. Lovinger R, Holland J, Kaplan S, et al: Pharmacological evidence for stimulation of growth hormone secretion by a central noradrenergic system in dogs. Neuroscience 1:443, 1976.
12. Brown MJ, Harland D, Murphy MB, et al: Effect of centrally acting alpha-adrenergic agonists on sympathetic nervous system function in humans. Hypertension 6(Suppl II):57, 1984.
13. Scholtysik G: Animal pharmacology of guanfacine. Am J Cardiol 57:13E, 1986.
14. Takeuchi K, Kogure M, Hashimoto T: Comparison of agonistic and antagonistic action of guanabenz and guanfacine on alpha 1- and alpha 2-adrenoceptors in isolated smooth muscle. Jpn J Pharmacol 43:267, 1987.
15. Kiechel JR: Pharmacokinetics and metabolism of guanfacine in man: A review. Br J Clin Pharmacol 10(Suppl 1):25S, 1980.
16. Carchman SH, Crowe JT Jr, Wright GJ: The bioavailability and pharmacokinetics of guanfacine after oral and intravenous administration to healthy volunteers. J Clin Pharmacol 27:762, 1987.
17. Dollery CT, Davies DS: Centrally acting drugs in antihypertensive therapy. Br J Clin Pharmacol 10(Suppl 1):5S, 1980.
18. Carchman SH, Crowe JT, Wright GJ: Steady-state plasma levels and pharmacokinetics of guanfacine in hypertensive patients with normal renal function [abstract]. Clin Pharmacol Ther 37:186, 1985.
19. Weiss YA, Levine DL, Safar ME, et al: Guanfacine kinetics in patients with hypertension. Clin Pharmacol Ther 25:283, 1979.
20. Hedner T, Nyberg G, Mellstrand T: Guanfacine in essential hypertension: Effects during rest and isometric exercise. Clin Pharmacol Ther 35:604, 1984.
21. Kiechel JR: Pharmacokinetics of guanfacine in patients with impaired renal function and in some elderly patients. Am J Cardiol 57:18E, 1986.
22. Rosenthal JH: Hemodynamic and endocrine responses to guanfacine in normotensive volunteers and hypertensive patients. Am J Cardiol 57:22E, 1986.
23. Kravchenko IG, Liashenko MM, Tarnakin AG, Chirkov SN: Use of the hypotensive drug guanfacine in the treatment of patients with hypertension [in Russian; English abstract]. Kardiologiia 26:41, 1986.
24. Jerie P: Clinical experience with guanfacine in long-term treatment of hypertension. Part I: Efficacy and dosage. Br J Clin Pharmacol 10(Suppl 1):37S, 1980.
25. Ibrahim MM, Emile H, Madkour MA, et al: Contractile performance following regression of left ventricular hypertrophy in hypertensive patients [abstract]. Ric Scient Educ Perm Suppl 49:243, 1985.
26. Fillingim JM, Blackshear JL, Strauss A, et al: Guanfacine as monotherapy for systemic hypertension. Am J Cardiol 57:50E, 1986.
27. Pagani G, Fiorella G, Benko R, et al: Comparison of the effects of short-term treatment with guanfacine and clonidine on glucose metabolism, plasma renin activity and some anterior pituitary hormones. Curr Ther Res 36:155, 1984.
28. Farsang C, Varga K, Vajda L, et al: Effects of clonidine and guanfacine in essential hypertension. Clin Pharmacol Ther 36:588, 1984.
29. Collart F, Staroukine M, Verniory A: Relationships between blood pressure, heart rate and plasma epinephrine, norepinephrine, angiotensin II concentrations, plasma renin activity during chronic guanfacine therapy in patients with essential arterial hypertension. Acta Cardiol 40:269, 1985.
30. Rosenthal J: Effect of guanfacine on blood pressure and renin activity in hypertensive patients. Br J Clin Pharmacol 10(Suppl 1):91S, 1980.
31. Hauger-Klevene JH, Balossi EC, Scornavacchi JC: Effect of guanfacine on growth hormone, prolactin, renin, lipoproteins and glucose in essential hypertension. Am J Cardiol 57:27E, 1986.
32. Lancranjan I, Marbach P: New evidence for growth hormone modulation by the alpha-adrenergic system in man. Metabolism 26:1225, 1977.
33. Hauger-Klevene JH: Hypolipaemic effect of guanfacine: 2 years' follow-up. Drugs Exp Clin Res 10:133, 1984.
34. Hauger-Kleven JH, Scornavacchi JC: Improvement of glucose tolerance in hypertensive diabetic patients treated with guanfacine one year. Eur J Clin Pharmacol 29:391, 1985.
35. Jerie P: Long-term evaluation of therapeutic efficacy and safety of guanfacine. Am J Cardiol 57:55E, 1986.
36. Jerie P: Low, single daily doses of guanfacine in the ambulatory treatment of hypertension. Br J Clin Pharmacol 15(Suppl 4):479S, 1983.
37. Kukes VG, Spasskii AV, Tsoi AN, et al: Extracardiac systemic pharmacodynamic effects of estulic (guanfacine) [in Russian]. Klin Med (Mosk) 65:46, 1987.
38. Lindgren BR, Grundstrom N, Andersson RG: Comparison of the effects of clonidine and guanfacine on the histamine liberation from human mast cells and basophils and on the human bronchial smooth muscle activity. Arzneimittelforschung 37:551, 1987.
39. Post C, Gordh T Jr, Minor BG, et al: Antinociceptive effects and spinal cord tissue concentrations after intrathecal injection of guanfacine or clonidine into rats. Anesth Analg 66:317, 1987.
40. Nalda-Felipe MA, Gonzalez-Machado JL: Analgesic effect of epidural guanfacine [abstract]. International Congress of Anesthesiology, Washington DC, 1988.
41. Roeckel A, Heidland A: Acute and chronic renal effects of guanfacine in essential and renal hypertension. Br J Clin Pharmacol 10(Suppl 1):141S, 1980.
42. Kirch W, Kohler H, Braun W: Elimination of guanfacine in patients with normal and impaired renal function. Br J Clin Pharmacol 10(Suppl 1):33S, 1980.
43. Bune AJ, Chalmers JP, Graham JR, et al: Double-blind trial comparing guanfacine and methyldopa in patients with essential hypertension. Eur J Clin Pharmacol 19:309, 1981.
44. Heidbreder E, Pagel G, Roeckel A, et al: Effect of guanfacine on vigilance. Br J Clin Pharmacol 10(Suppl 1):169S, 1980.
45. Klebel E: Effect of guanfacine on skills related to driving. Br J Clin Pharmacol 10(Suppl 1):173S, 1980.
46. Eggertsen R, Svensson A, Magnusson M, et al: Hemodynamic effects of loud noise before and after central sympathetic nervous stimulation. Acta Med Scand 221:159, 1987.
47. Jerie P, Lasance A: Long-term efficacy and tolerance of the antihypertensive agent guanfacine. Int J Clin Pharmacol Ther Toxicol 22:170, 1984.

48. Frisk-Holmberg M, Wibell L: Concentration-dependent blood pressure effects of guanfacine. Clin Pharmacol Ther 39:169, 1986.
49. Philipp E: Guanfacine in the treatment of hypertension due to pre-eclamptic toxaemia in thirty women. Br J Clin Pharmacol 10(Suppl 1):137S, 1980.
50. Lochaya S, Thongmitr V, Suvachittanont O: Antihypertensive effect of BS 100-141, a new central acting antihypertensive agent. Am Heart J 99:58, 1980.
51. Materson BJ, Kessler WB, Alderman MH, et al: A multicenter, randomized, double-blind dose-response evaluation of step-2 guanfacine versus placebo in mild to moderate hypertension. Am J Cardiol 57:32E, 1986.
52. Keenan RE, Black PL, Freudenburg JC, et al: Usefulness of low dose guanfacine, once a day, for 24-hour control of hypertension. Am J Cardiol 57:38E, 1986.
53. Seedat YK: Long-term treatment of hypertension with guanfacine (BS 100-141) alone and in combination therapy. Curr Ther Res 24:288, 1978.
54. Wilson MF, Haring O, Lewin A, et al: Comparison of guanfacine versus clonidine for efficacy, safety and occurrence of withdrawal syndrome in step-2 treatment of mild to moderate essential hypertension. Am J Cardiol 57:43E, 1986.
55. Jain AK, Hiremath A, Michael R, et al: Clonidine and guanfacine in hypertension. Clin Pharmacol Ther 37:271, 1985.
56. Lauro R, Reda G, Spallone L, et al: Hypotensive effect of guanfacine in essential hypertension: A comparison with clonidine. Br J Clin Pharmacol 10(Suppl 1):81S, 1980.
57. Distler A, Kirch W, Luth B: Antihypertensive effect of guanfacine: A double-blind cross-over trial compared with clonidine. Br J Clin Pharmacol 10(Suppl 1):49S, 1980.
58. Roeckel A, Heidland A: Comparative studies of guanfacine and methyldopa. Br J Clin Pharmacol 10(Suppl 1):55S, 1980.
59. Rengo F, Ricciardelli B, Volpe M, et al: Long-term comparative study of guanfacine and alpha-methyldopa in essential hypertension. Arch Int Pharmacodynam Ther 244:281, 1980.
60. Sorkin EM, Heel RC: Guanfacine: A review of its pharmacodynamic and pharmacokinetic properties, and therapeutic efficacy in the treatment of hypertension. Drugs 31:301, 1986.
61. Materson BJ, Reda DJ, Cushman WC, et al: Single drug therapy for hypertension in men: A comparison of 6 (six) antihypertensive agents with placebo. The Department of Veterans Affairs Cooperative Study Group on Antihypertensive Agents. N Engl J Med 328:914, 1993.
62. Velasco M, Urbina-Quintana A, Morillo J, et al: Systemic and cardiac hemodynamic interaction between guanfacine and hydralazine in hypertensive patients. Eur J Clin Pharmacol 27:393, 1984.
63. Gence B: The use of guanfacine in elderly hypertensive patients in everyday practice. Acta Gerontol 8:29, 1982.
64. Coves MJ, Gomis R, Goday A, et al: Antihypertensive treatment with guanfacine in patients suffering from type II diabetes mellitus. Med Clin 88:315, 1987.
65. Jerie P: Clinical experience with guanfacine in long-term treatment of hypertension. Part II: Adverse reactions to guanfacine. Br J Clin Pharmacol 10(Suppl 1):157S, 1980.
66. Sailer S, Lisch HJ, Patsch W: Guanfacine and glucose metabolism. Br J Clin Pharmacol 10(Suppl 1):123S, 1980.
67. Spiegel R, Devos JE: Central effects of guanfacine and clonidine during wakefulness and sleep in healthy subjects. Br J Clin Pharmacol 10(Suppl 1):165S, 1980.
68. Reid JL, Zamboulis C, Hamilton CA: Guanfacine: Effects of long-term treatment and withdrawal. Br J Clin Pharmacol 10(Suppl 1):183S, 1980.
69. Zamboulis C, Reid JL: Withdrawal of guanfacine after long-term treatment in essential hypertension: Observations on blood pressure and plasma and urinary noradrenaline. Eur J Clin Pharmacol 19:19, 1981.
70. Reid JL, Wing LMH, Dargie HJ, et al: Clonidine withdrawal in hypertension: Changes in blood-pressure and plasma and urinary noradrenaline. Lancet 1:1171, 1977.
71. Samuelsson O, Wilhelmsen K, Andersson OK, et al: Cardiovascular morbidity in relation to change in blood pressure and serum cholesterol levels in treated hypertension: Results from the primary prevention trial in Goteborg, Sweden. JAMA 258:1768, 1982.
72. Buckley M, Felly J: Antagonism of antihypertensive effects of guanfacine by tricyclic antidepressants [letter]. Lancet 337:1173, 1991.
73. Guanfacine for hypertension. Med Lett Drugs Ther 29:49, 1987.

CHAPTER 68

Moxonidine

Peter Dominiak, M.D., Julian P. Keogh, Ph.D., and B. N. C. Prichard, M.B., M.Sc., F.R.C.P., F.F.P.M.

Imidazoline derivatives such as oxymetazoline and clonidine have long been considered as potent α_2-adrenoceptor agonists.[1] Their peripheral effects include an increase in smooth muscular tone, resulting in raised peripheral vascular resistance, and thereafter increased blood pressure. Because of these effects, imidazolines have been employed primarily as nasal decongestants.

Although clonidine, via this mechanism, induces a transient increase in blood pressure after injection, this is followed by a longer-term blood pressure reduction. The observation of this effect stimulated intensive research into the role of α_2-adrenoceptors in central regulation of blood pressure. As a result, a concept was developed describing how centrally acting hypertensive agents excite central α_2-adrenoceptor inhibitory neurones in the nucleus tractus solitarii (NTS), the activation of which results in a reduction of peripheral sympathetic activity.[2] The actions of α-methylnorepinephrine have also been suggested to be mediated through this mechanism. The success of clonidine as an antihypertensive agent led to the synthesis of a number of other, similar compounds, such as the guanidine compounds guanfacine and guanabenz, which could also provoke activation of central α_2-adrenoceptors in the NTS.[1]

In the late 1970s and early 1980s, differences in the pharmacologic effects of phenylethylamine and imidazolines on α_2-adrenoceptors were first reported.[3] These studies at least suggested the existence of α_2-adrenoceptor subtypes. Later it was discovered that the ventrolateral medulla (VLM) in the C_1 region was an important connecting component of the baroreceptor reflex.[4] The VLM possesses imidazoline-binding sites and α_2-adrenoceptors.[4, 5] Because imidazolines such as clonidine, but not phenylethylamine-type α_2-

adrenoceptor agonists, decrease blood pressure after injection into the VLM, it was therefore concluded that specific imidazoline receptors must have been present in that region and that these were responsible for mediating the blood pressure reduction.[6] At the same time, other compounds were synthesized that led to the production of rilmenidine, a moxazoline derivative, and moxonidine, an imidazoline derivative. Preliminary pharmacologic studies characterized moxonidine as an α_2-adrenoceptor agonist with possible activity toward specific α_2-adrenoceptor subtypes.[7]

PHARMACOLOGY
Mechanisms of Action

Moxonidine is a 4-chloro-N(4,5-dihydro-1H-imidazol-2-yl)-6-methoxy-2-methyl-5-pyrimidinamine and therefore belongs to the imidazoline family of compounds. Imidazolines have long been considered to act as potent agonists or antagonists at α_2-adrenoceptors. Because clonidine has been very successfully used as a centrally acting antihypertensive agent, attempts have been made to synthesize chemical analogues, such as other imidazolines or guanidines, as efficient as clonidine, but if possible with fewer side effects.[1] With moxonidine, this goal has apparently been achieved, and as Armah et al.[7] had originally believed, its main target of action appears to be α_2-adrenoceptors in the central nervous system (CNS) and peripheral vasculature.[11]

Imidazoline Receptors

The first evidence for different sites of action for phenylethylamines and imidazolines was presented by Ruffolo et al.[8-10] and Bousquet et al.,[4] who reported a number of differences in the responses induced by these substances, although they were still discussed as having arisen from effects on α_2-adrenoceptors. Moxonidine was also described originally as having selectivity for α_2-adrenoceptors.[7, 11] Irrefutable evidence for a new receptor subtype came from Bous-

quet et al.,[4] who reported on the hypotensive effects of clonidine after microinjection into the VLM. In the same experimental model, the catecholamine α-methylnoradrenaline showed no blood pressure–reducing properties. The authors had therefore concluded that there must have been binding sites in the VLM that preferentially bind imidazolines[4] (Fig. 68–1). From binding studies in the VLM, Ernsberger et al.[5] showed selective binding sites for imidazolines and thus confirmed the presumptions of Bousquet et al.[4] (see also Kamisaki et al.[12]). The combination of functional studies with receptor binding studies clearly showed later that almost exclusively I_1-receptors, and not α_2-adrenoceptors, were responsible for mediating blood pressure reduction (Fig. 68–2).[13] Curiously, application of idazoxan, an I_2-receptor antagonist, can blunt the effects of clonidine induced in the VLM. However, α_2-adrenoceptor antagonists that do not possess imidazoline moieties are devoid of this property.[13]

It can be shown that moxonidine possesses high selectivity toward I_1-receptors.[14, 15] In the VLM, moxonidine binds I_1-binding sites with a 33-fold higher selectivity than for α_2-adrenoceptors. Clonidine has only a 3.8-fold higher selectivity in this respect. This selectivity is important, because it is the I_1-receptors that mediate blood pressure reduction in the VLM and the α_2-adrenoceptors that mediate expression of drowsiness and dry mouth, typical side effects of clonidine therapy.[15] The selectivity of moxonidine at I_1-receptors in binding at different organs is therefore variably pronounced and amounts to a factor 600- to 700-fold higher in the kidney.[15, 16] Chromaffin cells of the adrenal medulla possess almost exclusively I-receptors.[14, 15, 17, 18] Furthermore, the clinical effectiveness of imidazolines correlates closely with their binding affinities at I_1-receptors in the VLM.[15]

The comparative ability of imidazolines to displace either tritiated clonidine or tritiated idazoxan binding can be used to distinguish I_1- from I_2-type binding sites.[3] Moxonidine possesses selectivity almost exclusively for the I_1 and, after efaroxan, is the most selective substance that has been shown for this receptor (Fig. 68–3).[14]

Moxonidine has been considered to be a selective agonist and efaroxan a selective antagonist for the I_1-receptor. Haxhiu et al.[19] demonstrated the effects of moxonidine on I_1 binding sites in the VLM and its specific displacement by efaroxan in functional blood pressure studies. Efaroxan can totally blunt the hypotensive effects of moxonidine after bilateral injection of these substances in the VLM.

Until now, we have extensively discussed binding sites only, and not the actual imidazoline receptors. To study the existence of receptors, it is of interest to demonstrate specific effects, binding sites, and the abilities of these to be antagonized. Of growing interest and importance are the cloning of receptors, deduction of their amino acid sequences, and the search for their normal endogenous ligands. A protein with a molecular size of 70 kDa has been isolated from chromaffin cells of the adrenal medulla that shows specific binding sites for imidazolines but not α_2-

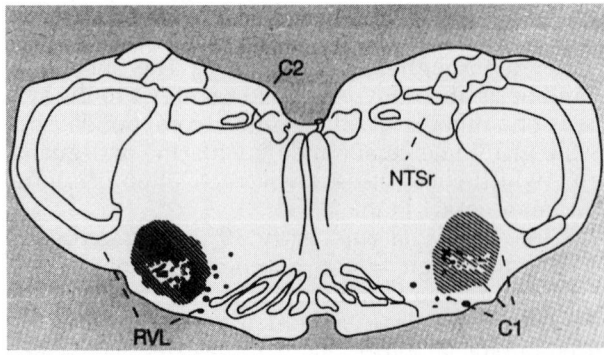

Figure 68–1. Location and site of actions of imidazoline-binding sites in the rostral ventrolateral medulla (RVL) of the C1 region. NTSr, nucleus tractus solitarii. (Modified from Bousquet P, Feldman J, Schwartz J: Central cardiovascular effects of alpha adrenergic drugs: Differences between catecholamines and imidazolines. J Pharmacol Exp Ther 253:232, 1984.)

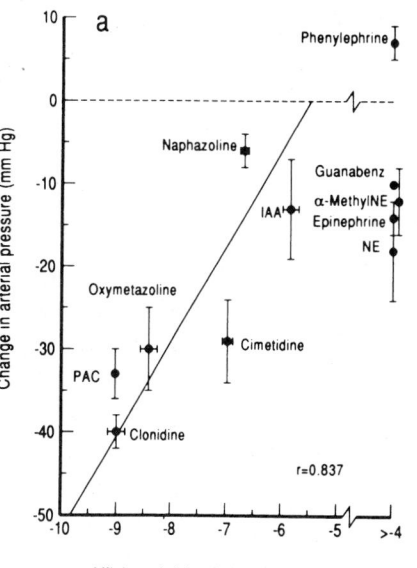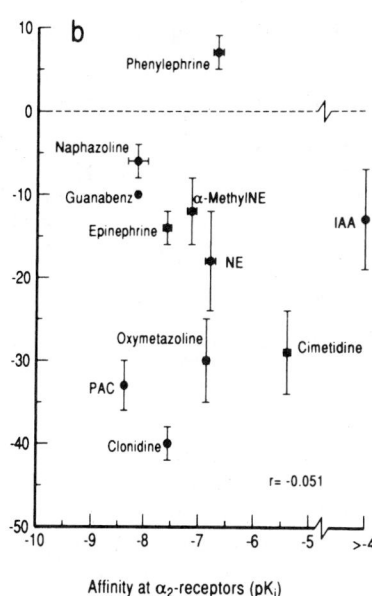

Figure 68–2. Relationship between changes in arterial blood pressure and binding affinity at imidazoline-binding sites (a) or α_2-adrenoceptors (b) for a series of clonidine-like compounds. (From Ernsberger P, Giuliano R, Willette RN, et al: Role of imidazole receptors in the vasodepressor response to clonidine analogs in the rostral ventrolateral medulla. J Pharmacol Exp Ther 253:408, 1990.)

adrenoceptor ligands.[20, 21] The endogenous ligand for this receptor was discovered only recently.

Endogenous Ligands

In 1984, a substance was isolated from calf brain that was described as "clonidine-displacing substance"

$$\text{Log } (K_i \text{ at } I_2/K_i \text{ at } I_1)$$

Efaroxan
Moxonidine
p-NH$_2$-Clonidine
Cimetidine
Clonidine
Oxymetazoline
Piperoxan
Phentolamine
CDS
Rilmenidine
Imidazole acetate
Yohimbine
Phenoxybenzamine
Guanfacine
SK&F 104078
Phenylephrine
Cirazoline
Norepinephrine
UK 14,304
Epinephrine
SK&F 86466
Idazoxan
Naphazoline
Guanabenz

Figure 68–3. Ranking of selectivity ratios for I_1- versus I_2-binding sites. Data represent the ratio of affinity constants (K_i) at I_2-binding sites in various tissues versus I_1-binding sites in the bovine VLM and are plotted on a log scale. (From Ernsberger PR, Westbrooks KL, Christen MO, Schafer SG: A second generation of centrally acting antihypertensive agents act on putative I1-imidazoline receptors. J Cardiovasc Pharmacol 20[Suppl 4]:S1, 1992.)

(CDS). This substance had a molecular weight of 500 and could displace clonidine, yohimbine, and rauwolscine from α_2-adrenoceptors.[22, 23] CDS had no effect on adenylate cyclase. Further studies conducted in the VLM showed that CDS could increase blood pressure and was able to shift the dose-response curve for clonidine's blood pressure–reducing activity to the right.[24] The investigators described the effect of CDS as antagonistic toward the blood pressure–reducing properties of clonidine. Furthermore, CDS may also be effective on smooth muscle, as could be observed on rat gastric fundi strips, on which CDS led to a dose-dependent increase in contraction.[25] It could also be reported that an extract of CDS prepared from human serum contracted rat aorta in a manner similar to clonidine.[26] On the contrary, a dose-dependent decrease in blood pressure was seen after administration of CDS into the VLM.[27] The notion of an imidazoline receptor with an endogenous ligand, namely CDS, was developed in the following way: A similarity exists between α_2-adrenoceptors and I-receptors, because guanidines possess a high affinity for both types of receptor. Because phenylethylamines do not bind to imidazoline receptors, the I-receptor is therefore by definition not an α_2-adrenoceptor subtype. The interaction of CDS with α_2-adrenoceptors and I-receptors speaks for a structural similarity between both receptor types. Because CDS is an endogenous substance, it is therefore the natural agonist for the imidazoline receptor.[25]

The structure of at least one CDS was elucidated and found to be identical with that of agmatine, a diamine that has long been known in the fields of bacterial and botanical research.[26] Agmatine binds to both α_2-adrenoceptors and imidazoline receptors and stimulates catecholamine release from the adrenal medulla. It is generated from arginine by the activity of an arginine decarboxylase and may therefore function as a putative neurotransmitter. Its affinity for I_1-

Table 68–1. **Summary of the Pharmacokinetics of Moxonidine**

1. Rapidly, almost completely absorbed
2. Absolute bioavailability 88%
3. Mostly excreted unchanged—biotransformation unimportant
4. T½, 2 hours—? retained in CNS
5. Chronic treatment—no accumulation
6. Not affected by food; age has little effect
7. Renal impairment, C_{max} T½ increased
8. No interactions with digoxin, hydrochlorothiazide, glibenclamide

Data from Weimann HJ, Rudolph ML: Clinical pharmacokinetics of moxonidine. J Cardiovasc Pharmacol 20(Suppl 4):S37, 1992.

receptors is approximately six times higher than its affinity for α_2-adrenoceptors, and 1.4 times higher than that for I_2-receptors.[26]

When one takes this finding fully into account, it is clear that both moxonidine and clonidine can no longer be designated as agonists, but rather as modulators, at I_1-receptors.

Thus, one can postulate as a mechanism of action for moxonidine a selective modulation at I_1-receptors both in organs such as the VLM where such receptors have been confirmed and in the adrenal medulla, which may also possess these receptors. Consequently, moxonidine may act by modulating the effects of the CDS agmatine in the VLM and thereby reduce blood pressure.

Moxonidine is well absorbed, bioavailability approaches 90%, and T_{max} is in approximately 1 hour. The pharmacokinetics has been reviewed by Weimann and Rudolph[28] (Table 68–1). Mitrovic et al.,[29] in a study in hypertensive patients of single doses of 0.4 mg, observed a maximum concentration of 2319 pg/ml at 1 hour, after which concentration declined. Kirch et al.[30] investigated three groups of patients (n = 8) with varying renal function. Those with normal function (glomerular filtration rate [GFR] > 90 ml/min) had a T½ of 2.6 hours; with patients having a GFR of 30 to 60 ml/min, the T½ was 3.5 hours, whereas with a GFR of less than 30 ml/min, the T½ of moxonidine had increased to 6.9 hours. Studies in five subjects indicated that the concentration of moxonidine in breast milk is between 50% and 100% of the plasma concentration.[31]

The maximum effect of moxonidine on the blood pressure is seen approximately 2 to 4 hours after the maximum blood concentration.[32]

Interaction studies have failed to reveal any effect of moxonidine on blood levels of digoxin, hydrochlorothiazide, or glibenclamide.[28]

Effects on Pathophysiology

Effects on Hemodynamics

Anesthetized and Spinalized Animal Models

In anesthetized cats, after intravenous injection, moxonidine induces a clear-cut dose-dependent reduction in arterial blood pressure. The heart rate is also re-

duced in a similar fashion.[7] As was already known for clonidine, a transient small increase in blood pressure is noticed immediately after an injected dose, which can be explained by a stimulation of peripheral postsynaptic α_2-adrenoceptors.[1, 7] Armah et al.[7] reported that after intraarterial injection of moxonidine to the arteria vertebralis, a comparable hypotensive effect was produced at doses 3.3 times lower than those effective after intravenous injection. This was clear evidence of a centrally targeted action for this substance. Experiments using spinalized cats in which only an increase in blood pressure was recorded after moxonidine injection left no doubt that this substance's normal major target of action was in the CNS.[7]

Several experiments using pithed rats, a model similar to that of the spinalized cat, revealed that moxonidine's hypertensive effect was approximately 10 times weaker than that of clonidine on a dose-to-dose basis (Fig. 68–4). Hence, all these studies confirmed that the site of action for moxonidine in bringing about blood pressure reduction was the CNS.

Similar responses to those described here have also been observed in rabbits.[7] From a comparison between moxonidine and clonidine, the investigators observed that after intravenous injection of these agents into anesthetized rabbits, clonidine is threefold more potent than moxonidine at reducing blood pressure. Conversely, after intracisternal injection, moxonidine was 4.5-fold more potent than clonidine in this respect. These contrasting data led the authors to speculate that moxonidine probably affected an α_2-adrenoceptor subtype that must have been in the CNS.

In recognition that the VLM possibly contains I_1-receptors, Haxhiu et al.[33] investigated the dose-dependent effects of moxonidine on heart rate and blood pressure in anesthetized, spontaneously hypertensive rats and compared them with those of clonidine. Each substance was applied to the VLM by bilateral injection. The ED_{50} for the blood pressure reduction induced by moxonidine was approximately twice that

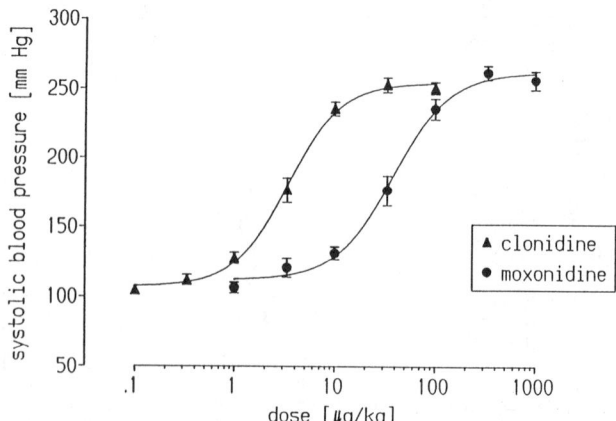

Figure 68–4. Dose-response curves of clonidine and moxonidine on systolic blood pressure of pithed spontaneously hypertensive rats. (Data from Häuser W, Gütting G, Nguyen T, Dominiak P: Influence of imidazolines on catecholamine release in pithed spontaneously hypertensive rats. Ann NY Acad Sci 763:573, 1995.)

of clonidine administered under the same conditions. Concentrations of 10 nM for each substance produced similar reductions in blood pressure.[11]

Conscious Experimental Animal Models

The effects of moxonidine on blood pressure have also been investigated in conscious, spontaneously hypertensive rats, renal-hypertensive rats, and renal-hypertensive dogs. Subcutaneous injection and oral administration of moxonidine led to a clear-cut long-term reduction in blood pressure in spontaneously hypertensive rats, which, as is the case in anesthetized models, was characterized initially by a transient small increase in blood pressure immediately after injection. Although blood pressure remained constantly reduced for a minimum of 6 hours, after 3 hours the heart rate began to increase and return to levels observed before treatment. Clonidine caused a more pronounced bradycardia in comparison with moxonidine, an effect that was maintained as long as the blood pressure reduction.[7] In renal-hypertensive dogs and rats, similar effects were also observed.[7] In spontaneously hypertensive rats receiving reserpine, moxonidine causes a dose-dependent increase in arterial blood pressure, which is clear evidence for the peripheral targets of action on α_2-adrenoceptors in the vascular smooth musculature.

In overview, moxonidine in a dose-dependent fashion reduces arterial blood pressure in a number of conscious and anesthetized animal models. The blood pressure–reducing effects of moxonidine have therefore been comprehensively confirmed in a variety of experimental animal models of hypertension. In comparison with clonidine, moxonidine is between 2 and 10 times weaker when one considers their relative ED_{50} values. Moxonidine, in comparison with clonidine, induces a weaker and shorter-lasting bradycardia. The target site for moxonidine's action is localized within the CNS, and its character of action is therefore, for the present, comparable with that of clonidine.

Single oral dose studies both in normotensives[34]

Table 68–2. **Hemodynamics of Moxonidine (0.4 mg Oral) (n = 10)**

	HR (min^{-1})	BP (mmHg)	CO (L/min)	SV (ml)	SVR (dyne·sec·cm^{-3})
Control	69	176/105	6.1	93	1695
3 hr	72	156/96	6.6	92	1446*

*$p < .01$

HR, heart rate; BP, blood pressure; CO, cardiac output; SV, stroke volume; SVR, systemic vascular resistance.

Adapted from Mitrovic V, Patyna W, Hüting J, Schlepper M: Hemodynamic and neurohormonal effects of moxonidine in patients with essential hypertension. Cardiovasc Drugs Ther 5:967, 1991.

and in hypertensive subjects[29, 32] indicate that moxonidine administration results in a fall in blood pressure due to a reduction in peripheral resistance, consequent to an inhibition of peripheral adrenergic tone, whereas the cardiac hemodynamics are essentially unchanged (Table 68–2).

Hüting et al.[35] performed a double-blind parallel group 4-week study in hypertensive patients comparing moxonidine and nifedipine; the hemodynamic findings were very similar (Fig. 68–5). Hüting et al.[35] additionally observed a decline in left ventricular and systolic volume (from 75 to 64 ml) and end-diastolic volume (from 164 to 151 ml), while LV ejection fraction was unchanged. Whereas single doses of moxonidine had no effect,[29] after 4 weeks' administration of moxonidine, pulmonary artery resistance, like systemic resistance, was reduced, although pulmonary artery pressure was unchanged.[35] The administration of moxonidine for 6 months is associated with a reversal of left ventricular hypertrophy.[36, 37]

Effects on the Sympathetic System

Animal Models

It is well known that clonidine exerts a strong effect on presynaptic α_2-adrenoceptors (autoreceptors), which is characterized by a significantly reduced norepinephrine release from the sympathetic varicosi-

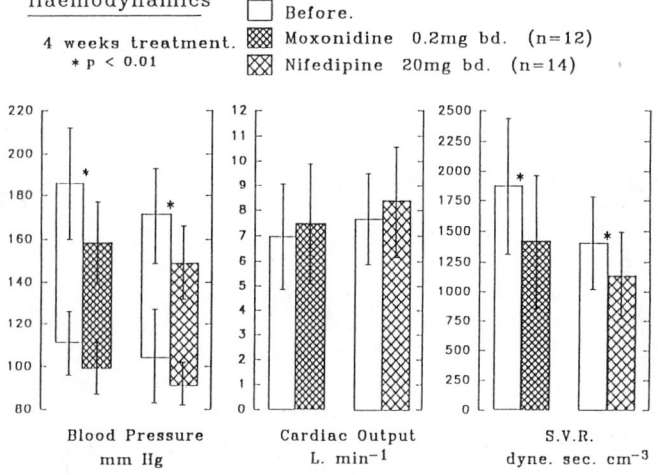

Figure 68–5. Hemodynamic double-blind comparative study of 4 weeks oral moxonidine or nifedipine treatment in patients with hypertension. Pulmonary artery pressure was unchanged, but pulmonary resistance was reduced by moxonidine (from 76 ± 24 mmHg to 61 ± 36 mmHg; $p < .01$) and by nifedipine (from 81 ± 70 mmHg to 68 ± 30 mmHg; $p < .01$). (Data from Hüting J, Mitrovic V, Bahavar H, Schlepper M: Vergleich der Wirkungen von Moxonidin und Nifedipin auf die linksventrikuläre Funktion bei Monotherapie der essentiellen Hypertonie. Herz Kreislauf 24:132, 1992.)

ties.[38-40] The reduction of plasma noradrenaline concentration that occurs during clonidine therapy is partly a result of this effect.[41] Several studies have been published investigating the effects of moxonidine on norepinephrine release.[42-46] Moxonidine in a dose-dependent fashion reduces release of [^{3}H]norepinephrine in isolated organ preparations such as the rabbit pulmonary artery and the isolated rat kidney.[42-46] The half maximal effect was seen at a 10-fold higher concentration than was observed with clonidine. After both inhibition of norepinephrine reuptake and, for example, rauwolscine-induced autoreceptor (presynaptic α_2-adrenoceptor) blockade, moxonidine shows a further inhibitory effect on release of tritiated norepinephrine, although this effect is clearly less pronounced.[42-46] The investigators could therefore not completely exclude moxonidine's effects on presynaptic imidazoline receptors in this study.

Some experiments on pithed rats, in which norepinephrine release was electrically stimulated and in which the native norepinephrine in the plasma was thus measured as "overflow," completely confirmed that moxonidine causes a clear inhibition of norepinephrine release. Once again, moxonidine was approximately 10-fold less potent than clonidine in elaborating this effect. Inhibition of reuptake and autoreceptor blockade, despite higher rauwolscine concentrations, led to a dose-dependent inhibition of plasma norepinephrine "overflow."

Summarizing, it therefore appears that moxonidine, independent of its ability to act on α_2-adrenoceptors, inhibits specific binding sites at the sympathetic varicosities. The receptor subtype responsible for mediating this effect remains to be identified.

Humans

Supporting a central reduction in adrenergic tone, studies in humans have demonstrated a reduction in renin and catecholamine levels.

Single oral dose studies in hypertensive patients have demonstrated a fall in noradrenaline levels.[29, 32] Resting adrenaline levels fall,[32] although not in all studies significantly.[29] A fall in exercising noradrenaline levels after single doses of 0.4 mg moxonidine from 541 to 407 pg/ml ($p < .01$) was reported by Mitrovic et al.,[29] but again the decline in adrenaline (110 to 81 pg/ml) was not significant.

Effect on Other Hormones

Single doses of moxonidine reduce resting renin levels[29, 32] and also with exercise.[29] Falls of resting angiotensin II and aldosterone levels were not significant.[29] Resting atrial natriuretic factor (ANF) level was unchanged, but it fell by 23% on exercise.[29]

Transient increases in growth hormone have been reported from 0.3 mg moxonidine,[47] but no change in thyroid-stimulating hormone, prolactin, gonadotropins, or adrenocorticotropic hormones.[47]

Myocardial Protection

The pharmacotherapy of arterial hypertension does not necessarily lead to prevention of hypertensive heart disease.[48, 49] For this reason, the effects of moxonidine on myocardial structure in spontaneously hypertensive rats have also been investigated using qualitative morphologic procedures. Spontaneously hypertensive rats were treated with either 8 mg/kg moxonidine per day for 3 months, or as control studies with vehicle solutions. In addition, two groups of Wistar-Kyoto rats served as normotensive controls.[48, 49] Microarteriopathy and myocardial fibrosis were significantly reduced, and the capillary supply to the hypertensive hearts was further normalized by moxonidine. The degree of hypertrophy was also reduced approximately 30% by moxonidine. The study further revealed that the reduction in left ventricular weight observed after therapy was due to a regression of hypertrophy and not to prevention of edema.[48, 49] The effects observed were thus comparable with those induced by the calcium antagonist nifedipine. Moxonidine was therefore able, like calcium antagonists and angiotensin-converting enzyme (ACE) inhibitors, to prevent the development of myocardial fibrosis. This effect could not be evoked by dihydralazine. Mall et al.[49] explained these results by saying that reduction of blood pressure alone is not sufficient to prevent the development of myocardial fibrosis. Rather, the inhibition of sympathetic activity and of the renin-angiotensin systems may have diminished growth factor production, which could have led to those effects. Many proliferative effects have been described for norepinephrine and angiotensin II.[50, 51]

In summary, the cited findings confirm that moxonidine possesses cardioprotective activity.

Effects on the Kidney (Diuretic Effects)

α-Adrenoceptors participate in regulation of tubular sodium reabsorption in the kidney.[3, 52] As an example, α_2-adrenoceptor agonists improve sodium retention.[53] It was, therefore, of interest to study the effects of moxonidine on diuresis and natriuresis. Moxonidine increases natriuresis and water excretion in hydrated and one-sided nephrectomized rats.[7, 16] The increase in urinary volume could be explained by an increased osmotic clearance.[16] The moxonidine effect on the kidneys, however, could be attributed to the high affinity for I_1-receptors, which in the kidney is about 600 times higher than that of α_2-adrenoceptors.[16]

Effects on Gastric Secretion

Whereas clonidine induced a clear reduction in gastric acid secretion, resulting in pH levels raised to alkaline levels in the gastric contents of pylorus-ligated rats, moxonidine had no such effect.[7]

Insulinotropic Effects

It has been reported that α_2-adrenoceptors located on pancreatic B cells can inhibit insulin release.[53a, 53b] On the other hand, the α-adrenoceptor antagonist phentolamine increases basal insulin release. It was discussed by Schulz and Hasselblatt[53c] that this effect of phentolamine is not related to α_2-adrenoceptor-antagonistic action but to its imidazoline structure. Up to now, neither preclinical nor clinical data exist about the action of moxonidine on insulin release.

It is, therefore, of interest that agmatine, which was recently reported to be one of the clonidine-displacing substances (CDS), caused a dose-dependent stimulation of insulin secretion from rat pancreatic islets.[53d]

Effects on Animals Fed Hypercaloric Diets

Administration of hypercaloric diets to normotensive rats resulted in definite increases in both blood pressure and heart rate.[54] Simultaneous addition of moxonidine to the hypercaloric diet prevented the onset of these effects.[54] The investigators discussed this in the light of the special ability of moxonidine to inhibit the central sympathetic tone, arguing that this effect should be more important than a pure mechanical reduction in blood pressure.

CLINICAL USE
Open Studies in Hypertension

There were several preliminary open studies performed with moxonidine in hypertension,[55, 56] the largest being a multicenter study reported by Schwarz and Kandziora.[57] There were 161 patients entered in the study; 141 patients completed a 12-month follow-up. After a placebo washout, if diastolic blood pressure was 95 mmHg or higher, 0.2 mg moxonidine was commenced and dosage was increased to control blood pressure to lower than 90 mmHg, with most patients being controlled by 0.2 or 0.4 mg daily. There was a reduction in standing blood pressure from $170 \pm 13.6/103.2 \pm 6.3$ mmHg on placebo to $147.5 \pm 12.1/88.4 \pm 5.9$ mmHg on moxonidine. There were similar results reported in another study, with 185 patients out of an original 223 patients completing an open 1-year follow-up. Here, sitting blood pressure fell from 176.1/103.5 to 148.0/87.0 at 52 weeks on moxonidine. There was an 84.2% response rate (fall 10 mmHg or < 90 mmHg) in the protocol completers. Laboratory measurements were not adversely affected.[58]

Combination Studies

Frei et al[59] reported a double-blind parallel group study of moxonidine and hydrochlorothiazide in combination in a double-blind trial in 177 hypertensive patients, where the fall in blood pressure was more than with either regimen alone (see later).

Comparative Studies

The efficacy of moxonidine in the treatment of hypertension has been defined by studies comparing it with representatives from each class of antihypertensive drugs in current use. There have been studies comparing moxonidine with the pharmacologically most comparable drug, the centrally acting clonidine, diuretics, the various classes of vasodilators, α_1-receptor blocking drugs, calcium antagonists, and angiotensin-converting enzyme inhibitors, and finally a study has been reported of moxonidine against β-blockade.

Centrally Acting Drugs

Plänitz[60] described a large double-blind parallel group study in which moxonidine (n = 122) was compared with clonidine (n = 30). A 6-week drug administration followed an initial washout period. The dosage in each case was titrated during the first week to give a diastolic blood pressure of less than 90 mmHg. The dose profile was very similar to that used in the large open study of Schwarz and Kandziora.[57] Moxonidine resulted in a fall in blood pressure from 177/100 to 151/87 in the 115 patients who completed moxonidine treatment. There were two patients who were withdrawn because of dry mouth, and five were excluded for reasons unrelated to the drug. The administration of clonidine resulted in a fall in blood pressure from 176/99 to 147/87 in the 27 patients who completed treatment; three of these clonidine-treated patients were withdrawn because of side effects.

Diuretics

In a double-blind parallel group study,[61] 35 patients were treated with moxonidine and 38 patients with hydrochlorothiazide. There were 28 patients who completed 8 weeks on moxonidine; 11 had 0.2 mg a day, and 17 received 0.4 mg a day. Thirty-four patients completed treatment with hydrochlorothiazide; 16 patients took 25 mg a day, and 18 patients took 50 mg a day. The blood pressure control was very similar in the two groups. Supine blood pressure fell from 160.1/103.0 on placebo to 147.6/91.9 on moxonidine and from 167.3/103.3 to 151.4/92.1 with hydrochlorothiazide.

Frei et al.[59] reported a double-blind parallel group trial that compared a group of patients on placebo (n = 37), moxonidine (n = 35), hydrochlorothiazide (n = 37), and treated with the combination (n = 38). The reduction in blood pressure after 8 weeks on moxonidine 0.4 mg compared with a 4-week placebo baseline was 20/12 mmHg. This was significantly greater than the fall on placebo of 13/9 mmHg. It was similar to the fall with hydrochlorothiazide (25 mg) of 22/13 mmHg, and the side effect profile was comparable. The use of the combination of both moxonidine and hydrochlorothiazide for 8 weeks led to a fall in blood pressure of 27/16 mmHg. When the response rate was defined as a 10 mmHg fall in diastolic blood pressure and/or a fall to less than 90 mmHg, moxonidine and hydrochlorothiazide each gave a response rate of 70%, and the combined treatment response rate was 88%.

α_1-Blockers

In an open study, Plänitz[62] reported a crossover study of moxonidine and prazosin in 30 patients. After a placebo washout, patients were given moxonidine for 4 weeks, and then after a further washout, prazosin was administered for 4 weeks.

The supine blood pressure fell from 184/100 on placebo to 149/89 on moxonidine, and on prazosin from 180/100 to 150/87, although three patients did not tolerate prazosin. Patients felt better on moxonidine (15 of the 30 patients); only one felt better on prazosin ($p < .001$). Conclusions must be very tentative from this study as it was not randomized or double blind.

Calcium Antagonists

A large multicenter parallel group double-blind study was reported by Wolf[63] in which moxonidine (n = 116, 0.2 mg daily in 57%, 0.2 mg b.i.d. in 43%) was compared with nifedipine sustained release (n = 113, 20 mg daily in 53%, 20 mg b.i.d. in 47%). The fall in blood pressure was similar: in the moxonidine group, blood pressure fell from 168/102 mmHg in the placebo period to 145/86 mmHg after 26 weeks of moxonidine; and in the nifedipine group, blood pressure fell from 168/102 mmHg to 140/83 mmHg after 26 weeks of treatment.

Broadly similar results were obtained in a single-blind study comparing moxonidine and nifedipine[64] and in a smaller double-blind study.[35]

Angiotensin-Converting Enzyme Inhibitors

Chrisp and Faulds[65] described a hitherto unpublished double-blind study of Lotti and Gianrossi[66] of moxonidine 0.2 mg daily or b.i.d. compared with captopril 25 mg daily or b.i.d. Responder rates, i.e., diastolic blood pressure less than 90 mmHg, were similar for moxonidine (72%) and captopril (68%). In a larger study in 100 patients, moxonidine again resulted in similar blood pressure control as with captopril. Average pressure fell from 176/101 to 155/91 with moxonidine and from 170/99 to 150/89 with captopril administration.[67]

In an ambulatory blood pressure double-blind study, Kraft and Vetter[68] compared moxonidine 0.2 mg b.i.d. and captopril 25 mg b.i.d. The 24-hour blood pressures after 4 weeks single-blind placebo were 144.6/91.4 mmHg; they then fell to 139.7/86.8 mmHg after 28 days of moxonidine treatment (n = 13, completed patients). In the captopril group (n = 10, completed patients), the pressures were 146.7/91.5 mmHg after 4 weeks of placebo and, after captopril, 141.0/87.1 mmHg. Thus, the fall in pressure was similar, as measured by both day and night blood pressures. The incidence of side effects was similar in the two groups; but while 23 patients completed the study, three others were withdrawn, two because of adverse events, one from each group, one for a nonmedical reason.

β-Blockers

In a parallel group double-blind trial of moxonidine versus atenolol, patients received a titrated dose of either moxonidine (0.2 mg daily or 0.2 mg b.i.d.) or atenolol (50 or 100 mg daily) for 8 weeks after a single-blind washout. In the moxonidine group, 25 patients were treated according to the protocol, using a dose of 0.2 mg b.i.d. in 28%, while the remaining patients had 0.2 mg daily. The dose in the atenolol group was 100 mg in 21% of the 28 patients who were treated according to the protocol; the remainder received 50 mg daily. The blood pressures at the end of the single-blind placebo in the moxonidine group were $167 \pm 8/101 \pm 3$ mmHg; they fell after 8 weeks treatment with moxonidine to $148 \pm 22/89 \pm 10$ mmHg. In the atenolol group, blood pressures fell from $169 \pm 12/102 \pm 4$ on placebo to $145 \pm 17/87 \pm 8$ mmHg after atenolol. In the atenolol group, five patients were withdrawn, one because of leg pain, possibly a drug effect, and one because of cold extremities, most probably drug related.[69]

Moxonidine in Special Patient Populations

Moxonidine appears well tolerated in patients with heart failure[70] and asthma.[71] As discussed earlier, the T½ of moxonidine is increased in renal insufficiency.[30] In a study of the antihypertensive effect of moxonidine in renal impairment, the blood pressure fall after 7 days treatment, 24 hours post dose, was 9.5/9.4 mmHg in patients with normal renal function (n = 8), 8.1/16.9 mmHg for those with a glomerular filtration rate (GFR) between 30 and 60 ml/min (n = 8), and 14.3/10.6 mmHg for those with a GFR of less than 30 ml/min (n = 8).[72]

Adverse Effects

In order to gauge the tolerance of a drug, a placebo group is needed to obtain evidence of the absolute

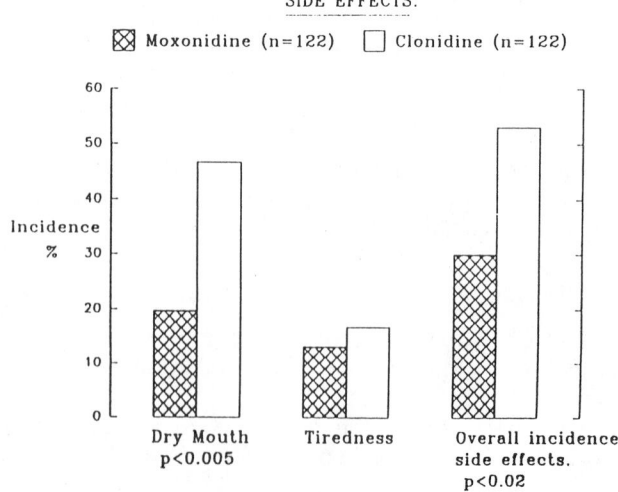

Figure 68–6. Incidence of side effects in a 6-week double-blind study comparing moxonidine and clonidine. (Modified from Plänitz V: Comparison of moxonidine and clonidine HCl in treating patients with hypertension. J Clin Pharmacol 27:46, 1987.)

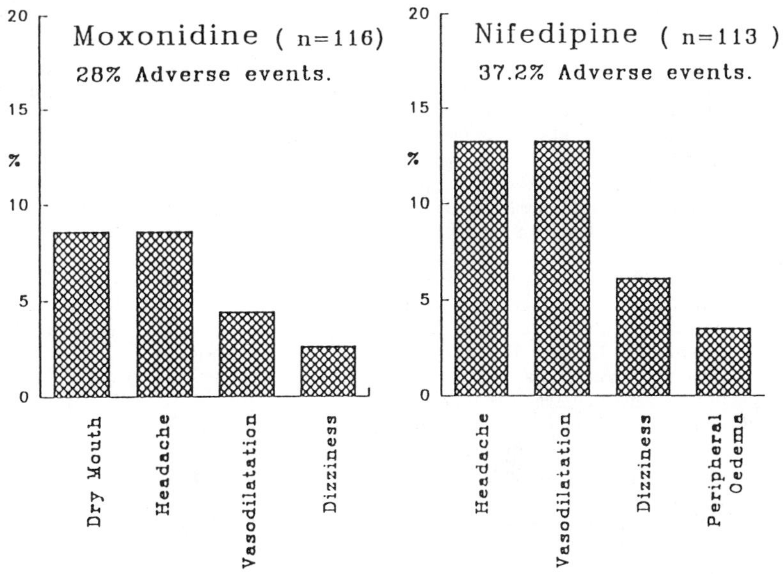

Figure 68–7. Adverse event profile in a double-blind study comparing moxonidine (n = 116) and nifedipine (n = 113). A total of 28% of patients experienced an adverse event on moxonidine and 37.2% on nifedipine. (Modified from Wolf R: The treatment of hypertensive patients with a calcium antagonist or moxonidine: A comparison. J Cardiovasc Pharmacol 20 [Suppl 4]:S42, 1992.)

incidence of side effects; as in any population, there is an incidence of spontaneous symptoms. Another useful approach is the double-blind comparative study to assess the incidence of side effects compared with existing treatment. None of the various studies have found a greater incidence of adverse events on moxonidine compared with the comparator agent. Single drug studies have supported the view that moxonidine does not have a high level of side effects,[57] as has postmarketing surveillance.[73]

There are two large double-blind parallel group studies that provide important evidence on the incidence of side effects. Plänitz[60] noted that the incidences of dry mouth, 20% and 47%, and overall incidences of side effects, 30% and 53%, respectively, were significantly less with moxonidine compared with clonidine (Fig. 68–6). In a study that compared moxonidine with nifedipine, the overall incidence of adverse events was 28% with moxonidine, whereas it was 37.2% with nifedipine (Fig. 68–7). Dry mouth and headache were the most frequent side effects seen with moxonidine, headache and vasodilation with nifedipine.

Plänitz[74] described a crossover double-blind study of moxonidine and clonidine in 20 patients. Tiredness was reported in 15% versus 60% and dry mouth in 20% versus 75% of the patients receiving moxonidine and clonidine, respectively. The total incidence of side effects (30%) on moxonidine was significantly less than on clonidine (85%) (p = .003). When well-being was assessed, 12 patients reported that they felt better on moxonidine, two on clonidine, and six expressed no preference (p = .01).

The effects of moxonidine (0.2 to 0.4 mg daily) on driving skills were evaluated by Schmidt et al.[75] in an open controlled study in hypertensive patients compared with a group of normotensive patients. There was no adverse effect of moxonidine on any of the parameters tested.

The withdrawal of clonidine has been reported to be associated with an overshoot of blood pressure if treatment was stopped abruptly. Plänitz[74] studied the rate of rise of blood pressure in the 3 days after moxonidine and clonidine were stopped. The blood pressures with clonidine rose over the first day and over 2 days after moxonidine was stopped.

SUMMARY

Moxonidine is an effective antihypertensive agent. It appears to be well tolerated compared with other antihypertensive drugs; it is similar and in several instances possibly superior, with a more favorable side effect profile.

There have been comparative studies representing all the major classes of drugs that have indicated that moxonidine is of similar efficacy to atenolol, captopril, nifedipine, clonidine, hydrochlorothiazide, and prazosin, i.e., representatives of all major groups of antihypertensive drugs.

It appears, therefore, that the I_1 imidazoline receptor selectivity in contrast with its weak agonist action at the α_2-receptor of moxonidine[14] appears indeed to fulfil what might be expected, a lower incidence of sedation.[60, 74] This is in contrast with clonidine, which has a relatively low efficacy at the I_1 imidazoline receptor in contrast with its α_2-receptor agonism[14] and its higher incidence of sedation.[59, 60]

REFERENCES

1. Kobinger W, Pichler L: Centrally acting drugs (clonidine, methyldopa, guanfacine). *In* Ganten D, Mulrow PJ (eds): Pharmacology of Antihypertensive Therapeutics. Heidelberg: Springer-Verlag Berlin, 1990, pp 227–262.
2. Reis DJ, Granata AR, Joh TH, et al: Brain stem catecholamine mechanisms in tonic and reflex control of blood pressure. Hypertension 6(Suppl II):II7, 1984.
3. Hamilton CA: The role of imidazoline receptors in blood pressure regulation. Pharmacol Ther 54:231, 1992.
4. Bousquet P, Feldman J, Schwartz J: Central cardiovascular ef-

fects of alpha adrenergic drugs: Differences between catecholamines and imidazolines. J Pharmacol Exp Ther 253:232, 1984.

5. Ernsberger P, Meeley MP, Mann JJ, et al: Clonidine binds to imidazole binding sites as well as α_2-adrenoceptors in the ventrolateral medulla. Eur J Pharmacol 134:1, 1987.

6. Dominiak P: Historic aspects in the identification of the I_1-receptor and the pharmacology of imidazolines. Cardiovasc Drugs Ther 8:21, 1994.

7. Armah BI, Hofferber E, Stenzel W: General pharmacology of the novel centrally acting antihypertensive agent moxonidine. Arzneimittelforschung/Drug Res 38:1426, 1988.

8. Ruffolo RR, Fowble JW, Miller DD, et al: Binding of [^{3}H]dihydroazapetine to alpha adrenoceptor-related proteins from rat vas deferens. Proc Natl Acad Sci USA 73:2730, 1976.

9. Ruffolo RR, Turowski BS, Patil PN: Lack of cross desensitisation between structurally dissimilar α-adrenoceptor agonists. J Pharm Pharmacol 29:378, 1977.

10. Ruffolo RR, Rice PJ, Patil PN, et al: Differences in the applicability of the Easson-Stedman hypothesis to the α_1- and α_2-adrenergic effects of phenylethylamines and imidazoles. Eur J Pharmacol 86:471, 1983.

11. Ferry D, Armah BI, Goll A, et al: Characteristics of the binding of the antihypertensive agent moxonidine to α_2-adrenoceptors in rat brain membranes. Arzneimittelforschung/Drug Res 38:1442, 1988.

12. Kamisaki Y, Ishikawa T, Takao Y, et al: Binding of [^{3}H]p-aminoclonidine to two sites, α_2-adrenoceptors and imidazoline binding sites: Distribution of imidazoline binding sites in rat brain. Brain Res 514:15, 1990.

13. Ernsberger P, Giuliano R, Willette RN, et al: Role of imidazole receptors in the vasodepressor response to clonidine analogs in the rostral ventrolateral medulla. J Pharmacol Exp Ther 253:408, 1990.

14. Ernsberger PR, Westbrooks KL, Christen MO, Schäfer SG: A second generation of centrally acting antihypertensive agents act on putative I_1-imidazoline receptors. J Cardiovasc Pharmacol 20(Suppl 4):S1, 1992.

15. Ernsberger P, Damon TH, Graff LM, et al: Moxonidine, a centrally acting antihypertensive agent, is a selective ligand for I1-imidazoline sites. J Pharmacol Exp Ther 264:172, 1993.

16. Allan DR, Penner SB, Smyth DD: Renal imidazoline preferring sites and solute excretion in the rat. Br J Pharmacol 108:870, 1993.

17. Molderings GJ, Moura D, Fink K, et al: Binding of [^{3}H]clonidine to I_1-imidazoline sites in bovine adrenal medullary membranes. Naunyn Schmiedebergs Arch Pharmacol 348:70, 1993.

18. Regunathan S, Meeley MP, Reis DJ: Expression of non-adrenergic imidazoline sites in chromaffin cells and mitochondrial membranes of bovine adrenal medulla. Biochem Pharmacol 45:1667, 1993.

19. Haxhiu MA, Dreshaj I, Schäfer SG, Ernsberger P: Selective antihypertensive action of moxonidine is mediated by I1-imidazoline receptors in the rostral ventrolateral medulla. J Cardiovasc Pharmacol 24(Suppl 1):S1, 1994.

20. Wang H, Regunathan S, Meeley MP, et al: Isolation and characterization of imidazoline receptor protein from bovine adrenal chromaffin cells. Mol Pharmacol 42:792, 1992.

21. Wang H, Regunathan S, Ruggiero DA, et al: Production and characterization of antibodies specific for the imidazoline receptor protein. Mol Pharmacol 43:509, 1993.

22. Atlas D, Burstein Y: Isolation of an endogenous clonidine-displacing substance from rat brain. FEBS Lett 170:387, 1984.

23. Atlas D, Burstein Y: Isolation and partial purification of a clonidine-displacing endogenous brain substance. Eur J Biochem 144:287, 1984.

24. Bousquet P, Feldman J, Atlas D: An endogenous non-catecholamine clonidine antagonist increases mean arterial blood pressure. Eur J Pharmacol 124:167, 1986.

25. Atlas D: Clonidine-displacing substance (CDS) and its putative imidazoline receptor: New leads for further divergence of α_2-adrenergic receptor activity. Biochem Pharmacol 41:1541, 1991.

26. Li G, Regunathan S, Barrow CJ, et al: Agmatine: An endogenous clonidine-displacing substance in the brain. Science 263:966, 1994.

27. Meeley MP, Ernsberger PR, Granata AR, Reis DJ: An endoge-

nous clonidine displacing substance from bovine brain: Receptor binding and hypotensive actions in the ventrolateral medulla. Life Sci 38:1119, 1986.

28. Weimann H-J, Rudolph M: Clinical pharmacokinetics of moxonidine. J Cardiovasc Pharmacol 20(Suppl 4):S37, 1992.

29. Mitrovic V, Patyna W, Hüting J, Schlepper M: Hemodynamic and neurohumoral effects of moxonidine in patients with essential hypertension. Cardiovasc Drugs Ther 5:967, 1991.

30. Kirch W, Hutt H-J, Plänitz V: The influence of renal function on clinical pharmacokinetics of moxonidine. Clin Pharmacokinet 15:245, 1988.

31. Klink F: Clinical investigation of the passage of Moxonidine from the maternal bloodstream to the breast milk in patients with hypertension. Beiersdorf AG Study No. 200.029-5895-2228-52, 1988.

32. Kirch W, Hutt H-J, Plänitz V: Pharmacodynamic action and pharmacokinetics of moxonidine after single oral administration in hypertensive patients. J Clin Pharmacol 30:1088, 1990.

33. Haxhiu MA, Dreshaj I, Erokwu B, et al: Vasodepression elicited in hypertensive rats by the selective I_1-imidazoline agonist moxonidine administered into the rostral ventrolateral medulla. J Cardiovasc Pharmacol 20(Suppl 4):S11, 1992.

34. MacPhee GJA, Howie CA, Elliot HL, Reid JL: A comparison of the haemodynamic and behavioural effects of moxonidine and clonidine in normotensive subjects. Br J Clin Pharmacol 33:261, 1992.

35. Hüting J, Mitrovic V, Bahavar H, Schlepper M: Vergleich der Wirkungen von Moxonidin und Nifedipin auf die linksventrikuläre Funktion bei Monotherapie der essentiellen Hypertonie. Herz Kreislauf 24:132, 1992.

36. Eichstädt H, Richter W, Bäder W, et al: Demonstration of hypertrophy regression with magnetic resonance tomography under the new adrenergic inhibitor moxonidine. Cardiovasc Drugs Ther 3:583, 1989.

37. Eichstädt H, Gatz G, Schröder R, Kreuz D: Linksventrikulare Hypertrophieregression unter einer Therapie mit Moxonidine. J Pharmacol Therapy 1:12, 1991.

38. Starke K: Regulation of noradrenaline release by presynaptic receptor systems. Rev Physiol Biochem Pharmacol 77:1, 1977.

39. Starke K: α-Adrenoceptor subclassification. Rev Physiol Biochem Pharmacol 88:199, 1981.

40. Starke K: Presynaptic α-autoreceptors. Rev Physiol Biochem Pharmacol 107:73, 1987.

41. Bravo EL, Cressman MD, Pohl MA: Cardiovascular and neurohumoral effects of long-term oral clonidine monotherapy in essential hypertensive patients. In Weber MA, Drayer JIM, Kolloch R (eds): Low Dose Oral and Transdermal Therapy of Hypertension. Darmstadt, Germany: Steinkopff, 1985, p 3.

42. Göthert M, Molderings GJ: Involvement of presynaptic imidazoline receptors in the α_2-adrenoceptor-independent inhibition of noradrenaline release by imidazoline derivatives. Naunyn Schmiedebergs Arch Pharmacol 343:271, 1991.

43. Göthert M, Molderings GJ: Modulation of norepinephrine release in blood vessels: Mediation by presynaptic imidazoline receptors and α_2-adrenoceptors. J Cardiovasc Pharmacol 20(Suppl 4):S16, 1992.

44. Göthert M, Molderings GJ: Neue Aspekte zum Wirkungsmechanismus von Antihypertensiva mit Imidazolin- oder Oxazolinstruktur. In Hayduk K, Stumpe KO (eds): Ein neues Therapieprinzip zur Behandlung der Hypertonie. Stuttgart, Germany: Schattauer, 1992, pp 11–22.

45. Molderings GJ, Hentrich F, Göthert M: Pharmacological characterization of the imidazoline receptor which mediates inhibition of noradrenaline release in the rabbit pulmonary artery. Naunyn Schmiedebergs Arch Pharmacol 344:630, 1991.

46. Bohmann C, Schollmeyer P, Rump LC: Effects of imidazolines on noradrenaline release in rat isolated kidney. Naunyn Schmiedebergs Arch Pharmacol 349:118, 1994.

47. Mill G, Gödde-Salz E, Heidemann HT, Schulte HM: Effects of a new alpha$_2$-adrenergic agonist moxonidine on anterior pituitary hormone secretion in comparison to clonidine and GHRH. Acta Endocrinol 120(Suppl 1):80, 1989.

48. Amann K, Greber D, Gharehbaghi H, et al: Effects of nifedipine and moxonidine on cardiac structure in spontaneously hypertensive rats: Stereological studies on myocytes, capillaries, arteries, and cardiac interstitium. Am J Hypertens 5:76, 1992.

49. Mall G, Greber D, Gharehbaghi H, et al: Effects of nifedipine and moxonidine on cardiac structure in spontaneously hypertensive rats (SHR)—stereological studies on myocytes, capillaries, arteries, and cardiac interstitium. Basic Res Cardiol 86(Suppl 3):33, 1991.

50. Kohlbeck-Rühmkorff C, Zimmer H-G: Molecular mechanisms of the cardiac effects of norepinephrine. Pharm Pharmacol Lett 3:123, 1993.

51. Holtz J: Angiotensin actions within the heart. Pharm Pharmacol Lett 3(Suppl):46, 1993.

52. Limon I, Coupry I, Tesson F, et al: Renal imidazoline-guanidinium receptive site: A potential target for antihypertensive drugs. J Cardiovasc Pharmacol 20(Suppl 4):S21, 1992.

53. Nord EP, Howard MJ, Hafezi A, et al: Alpha₂ adrenergic agonists stimulate Na⁺/H⁺ antiport activity in the rabbit renal proximal tubule. J Clin Invest 80:1755, 1987.

53a. Nakaki T, Kakadate T, Kato R: α₂-Adrenoceptors modulating insulin release from isolated pancreatic islets. Naunyn Schmiedebergs Arch Pharmacol 313:151–153, 1980.

53b. Langer J, Panten U, Zielmann S: Effect of adrenoceptor antagonists on clonidine-induced inhibition of insulin secretion by isolated pancreatic islets. Br J Pharmacol 79:415, 1983.

53c. Schulz A, Hasselblatt A: An insulin-releasing property of imidazoline derivatives is not limited to compounds that block α-adrenoceptors. Naunyn Schmiedebergs Arch Pharmacol 340:321, 1989.

53d. Sener A, Lebrun P, Blachier F, Malaisse WJ: Stimulus-secretion coupling of arginine-induced insulin release. Insulinotropic action of agmatine. Biochem Pharmacol 38:327, 1989.

54. Rupp H, Turcani M, Jacob R: Caloric intake and radio telemetrically assessed high blood pressure: I. Effect of the centrally acting antihypertensive drug moxonidine. Pharm Pharmacol Lett 3:103, 1993.

55. Frisk-Holmberg M, Plänitz V: A selective alpha₂-adrenoreceptor agonist in arterial essential hypertension. Clinical experience with moxonidine. Curr Ther Res 42:138, 1987.

56. Plänitz V, Kandziora J: Wirksamkeit und Vertraglichkeit des neuen Antihypertensivums Moxonidin bei vorwiegend alteren Patienten. Therapiewoche 34:6426, 1984.

57. Schwarz VW, Kandziora J: Langzeiterfahrungen mit Moxonidin, einem neuen Antihypertensivum. Fortschritte der Medizin 108:616, 1990.

58. Trieb G: Open-labelled, Uncontrolled Multicenter Study of the Anithypertensive Effects of Moxonidine in Hypertensive Patients. Study No. 220-5011. Hannover, Germany: Kali-Chemie Pharmaceuticals, 1991.

59. Frei M, Küster L, Gardosch von Krosigk PP, et al: Moxonidine

and hydrochlorothiazide in combination: A synergistic antihypertensive effect. J Cardiovasc Pharmacol 24:S25, 1994.

60. Plänitz V: Comparison of moxonidine and clonidine HCl in treating patients with hypertension. J Clin Pharmacol 27:46, 1987.

61. Larrat V: Efficacy and tolerance of moxonidine in comparison with a standard therapy with hydrochlorothiazide. Beiersdorf AG Report No. 200.029-28-54, 1990.

62. Plänitz V: Intra-individual comparison of moxonidine and prazosin in hypertensive patients. Eur J Clin Pharmacol 29:645, 1986.

63. Wolf R: The treatment of hypertensive patients with a calcium antagonist or moxonidine: A comparison. J Cardiovasc Pharmacol 20(Suppl 4):S42, 1992.

64. Mangiameli S, Privitera A, Jonte G, Löw-Kröger A: Behandlung der leichen bis mittelschweren Hypertonie: Moxonidin versus nifedipin retard. Zeit Allgemeinmed 68:862, 1991.

65. Chrisp P, Faulds D: Moxonidine: A review of its pharmacology and therapeutic use in essential hypertension. Drugs 44:993, 1992.

66. Lotti G, Gianrossi R: Moxonidin versus Captopril bie Leichter bis mittelschwerer Hypertonie. Fortschritte der Medizin 111:429, 1993.

67. Ollivier JP, Christen MO, Schäfer SG: Moxonidine: A second generation of centrally acting drugs—an appraisal of clinical experience. J Cardiovasc Pharmacol 20(Suppl 4):S31, 1992.

68. Kraft K, Vetter H: Twenty-four-hour blood pressure profiles in patients with mild-to-moderate hypertension: Moxonidine versus captopril. J Cardiovasc Pharmacol 24:S29, 1994.

69. Prichard BNC, Simmons R, Rooks MJ, et al: A double-blind comparison of moxonidine and atenolol in the management of patients with mild to moderate hypertension. J Cardiovasc Pharmacol 20(Suppl 4):S45, 1992.

70. Mitrovic V: Haemodynamic effects of moxonidine in patients with congestive heart failure during the first three hours after administration of a single 0.4 mg dose. Kali-Chemi AG Study No. 220.5003, 1989.

71. Wilkens H, Wilkens JH, Fabel H: Die Wirkung von Moxonidin—einem zentral wirksamen Antihypertensivum—auf Atemregulation und Histaminreaktivität. Kardio 10(11):1, 1992.

72. Kirch W, Plänitz V: Klinisch aspect Aspectke der Therapie mit einem zentral wirksamen Alpha₂-adrenozeptor-agonisten bie Patienten mit arterieller Hypertonie. Cor et Vasa 5(3):1, 1991.

73. Ongyert D, Dotzer F: Wirksamkeit und Verträglichkeit von Moxonidin. Zeit Allgemeinmed 69:S56, 1993.

74. Plänitz V: Crossover comparison of moxonidine and clonidine in mild to moderate hypertension. Eur J Clin Pharmacol 27:147, 1984.

75. Schmidt U, Frerick H, Kraft K, et al: Hypertension: A possible risk in road traffic. J Cardiovasc Pharmacol 20(Suppl 4):S50, 1992.

C. Peripherally Acting Antiadrenergic Drugs

CHAPTER 69

Prazosin

Myron H. Weinberger, M.D.

HISTORY, CHEMISTRY, AND PHARMACOLOGY

Prazosin is a quinazoline derivative (1-[4-amino-6,7-dimethyoxy-2-quinazoline]-4-[2-furoyl]-piperazine) agent that was approved for use in the treatment of hypertension in the United States in 1976. Preliminary studies with this agent in experimental animals in the early 1970s indicated that it lowered blood pressure and reduced peripheral resistance by a vasodilatory effect. Initially, these effects were thought to be due to a direct action of the agent on vascular smooth muscle, perhaps mediated by inhibition of phosphodiesterase. Subsequent studies revealed that the effect of this newly identified vasodilating agent was mediated by α-adrenergic blockade.[1] A variety of α-adrenergic blocking agents have been identified. Careful differentiation of the precise actions of these α-adrenergic blockers has enabled greater understanding of their differential effectiveness in various disease states.

We now recognize two types of α-adrenergic receptors, identified as α_1 and α_2.[2] In general, α_2-receptors represent the presynaptic receptors of the sympathetic nerve ending that inhibit norepinephrine release, providing feedback control of neuronal release of catecholamines. α_1-Receptors are most frequently postsynaptic in location and are present on vascular smooth muscle cells. Stimulation of the postsynaptic α_1-receptor causes contraction of vascular smooth muscle and an increase in vascular resistance and blood pressure. α_2-Receptors can also be found at the postsynaptic level. These postsynaptic α_2-receptors appear to be remote from sympathetic nerve endings, whereas the postsynaptic α_1-receptors are generally found on vascular smooth muscle in close proximity to nerve endings.

α-Adrenergic receptors are classified on the basis of their affinity for various drugs. As an example, α_1-receptors have a very high affinity for prazosin and a low affinity for drugs such as clonidine and yohimbine. On the other hand, α_2-receptors have the reverse affinity, favoring clonidine or yohimbine and having a low affinity for prazosin. Because the presynaptic α_2-receptor governs the feedback inhibition of catecholamine release from nerve endings, blockade of this receptor would be expected to lead to increased circulating catecholamine levels, which might counteract any effects on α_1-receptor blockade. The effectiveness of prazosin in reducing blood pressure apparently is related to its high specificity for postsynaptic α_1-receptors and its low blocking affinity for α_2-receptors. The α-receptors have other actions that include the blockade of serotonin or dopamine receptors as well as sympathomimetic, histamine-like, or antihistaminic effects. However, prazosin has little or none of these nonspecific actions. The advantage of selective α_1-receptor blockade is emphasized by the systemic effects of increased catecholamine release, which would result from concomitant presynaptic α_2-blockade. This might be undesirable in patients with cardiovascular disease in whom increased norepinephrine release could increase adrenergic stimulation of the heart and offset the vasodilatory effects of the postsynaptic vascular α_1-receptor blockade.

PHARMACOKINETICS

Prazosin is rapidly absorbed from the gastrointestinal tract, and peak plasma levels of the drug can be demonstrated 2 to 3 hours after oral administration. The plasma half-life of prazosin is approximately 4 hours, and the biologic effect lasts much longer. The drug is primarily metabolized by the liver. Ninety percent is excreted in feces, the rest by the kidney. There is significant first-pass metabolism by the liver.[3] The absorption and attainment of peak plasma concentrations of prazosin appear not to be influenced by food in the gastrointestinal tract. Prazosin has been shown to be over 90% bound to plasma protein. Renal insufficiency may prolong the activity of prazosin

and reduce the amount of protein-bound chemical.[3, 4] Levels of prazosin appear not to be influenced by hemodialysis.[4] No relationship has been demonstrated between the plasma concentration and the blood pressure response to prazosin. Thus, the concentration of drug at the α_1-receptor site of vascular smooth muscle is the major determinant of blood pressure response. This observation further emphasizes the variability of mechanisms involved in blood pressure elevation among hypertensive patients.

PATHOPHYSIOLOGY

Prazosin lowers blood pressure by reducing systemic vascular resistance as a result of postsynaptic α_1-receptor blockade and subsequent vasodilation. In contrast with other α-antagonists, prazosin has no effect on presynaptic (neuronal) α_2-receptors, and thus catecholamine release is not increased. In studies of hypertensive men, prazosin was shown to decrease myocardial oxygen consumption and increase stroke volume with exercise without a significant change in heart rate.[5] These observations markedly conflict with the effects of the direct-acting vasodilators, hydralazine and minoxidil, which increase myocardial oxygen consumption while inducing vasodilation by a direct action on the vasculature. This increase in myocardial work appears to be mediated by baroreceptor-induced increases in catecholamine release. Because prazosin has no blocking effects on the α_2-receptor, such an increase in catecholamine release is not observed with this agent.

Left Ventricular Hypertrophy and Function

Antihypertensive agents that increase the levels of vasoactive substances, such as angiotensin II and catecholamines, have been shown to cause progression of left ventricular hypertrophy in hypertensive animals. Treatment with prazosin has been shown to decrease left ventricular hypertrophy and to increase exercise tolerance, particularly in patients with congestive heart failure.[6] In hypertensive men with echocardiographic evidence of left ventricular hypertrophy,[7] the effects of vasodilators were examined by comparing the direct-acting agent hydralazine with the indirect-acting α-antagonist prazosin. Prazosin treatment was associated with a regression in left ventricular hypertrophy after 3 months of treatment and continuing over the 12-month course of study. No significant change in left ventricular hypertrophy was observed with hydralazine despite a comparable reduction in afterload.[7] Comparative studies using β-antagonists, methyldopa, clonidine, and prazosin show that only prazosin could normalize central hemodynamics and induce a persistent decrease in peripheral resistance with long-term treatment.[5] In contrast with β-blockers, which reduce cardiac output, prazosin was shown to increase the cardiac ejection fraction with exercise in hypertensive men.[8] Prazosin causes a generalized decrease in systemic vascular resistance, and as a consequence, blood viscosity has been shown to decrease with this agent.[9] Unlike other antihypertensive agents, prazosin is not associated with adverse effects on cardiac electrophysiology. The agent appears to dilate both capacitance and resistance vessels, thus providing a balanced dilator effect that accounts for the marked decrease in peripheral resistance observed with prazosin.

Effects on Extracellular Fluid Volume

Accompanying the vasodilation of most comparable agents, particularly the direct-acting vasodilators hydralazine and minoxidil, marked sodium and water retention and volume expansion result from marked activation of the renin-aldosterone system. This phenomenon is referred to as pseudotolerance and often develops with direct-acting vasodilators unless effective diuretic therapy is given concomitantly.[10] Unlike direct-acting vasodilators, prazosin has minimal effects on fluid retention; thus, pseudotolerance is rarely a problem with this agent, except during the treatment of congestive heart failure. When pseudotolerance is observed in the latter situation, it can be overcome by administration of diuretics. Over a 5-year period, patients receiving prazosin demonstrated consistent and equivalent blood pressure reduction, further indicating that tolerance to prazosin's antihypertensive effect does not develop.[11] These observations were confirmed in a 4- to 7-year follow-up of 172 patients taking prazosin reported by the New Zealand Hypertension Study Group in 1980.[12] Further, in marked contrast to experience with diuretics, prazosin has no known adverse effect on electrolytes.

Renal Effects

The effects of antihypertensive agents on renal hemodynamics and function are matters of increasing concern. The kidney may participate in the pathogenesis of hypertension and may be damaged by elevated blood pressure or adversely affected by drugs used to reduce blood pressure. Thus, the impact of antihypertensive agents on renal function and renal hemodynamics is appropriately a matter of scrutiny. A variety of studies have demonstrated that prazosin has no adverse effect on glomerular filtration rate or renal blood flow following short-term or long-term treatment.[13] In marked contrast to the increase in renal vascular resistance typically associated with β-blockade or diuretic therapy, those findings showed that acute administration of prazosin significantly decreased renal vascular resistance. In this study, the investigators observed expansion of plasma volume and extracellular fluid volume but no evidence of tolerance in patients in whom an antihypertensive effect was noted.[13] Other investigators have reported increases in body fluid volumes during long-term prazosin therapy.[14] Interestingly, despite the observed increase in plasma and extracellular fluid volume, an increase in weight was not observed, and, indeed, one study reported an actual decrease in body weight.[13] In

several studies, prazosin has been shown to improve blood pressure in patients with impaired renal function.[15] A careful review of these studies demonstrated no consistent effect of prazosin on plasma renin activity, plasma aldosterone, or sodium homeostasis.

Effects on Metabolic Factors

Metabolic aberrations, such as increases in blood sugar, uric acid, and lipid levels, have long been known to place hypertensive individuals at increased risk for coronary artery disease.[16] Diuretic-induced electrolyte changes have also been known to increase the risk of sudden death in hypertensive patients, particularly those with left ventricular hypertrophy or other electrocardiographic abnormalities, presumably because of induction of potassium and magnesium loss.[17] Thus, the impact of antihypertensive agents on these metabolic factors has become an issue of increasing concern.

Lipoproteins

National efforts have been mounted to increase public awareness and concern for lipid levels, much like the public education campaign initiated in the early 1970s regarding the problem of elevated blood pressure. Not only are hypertensive patients more likely to fall victim to increased vascular disease in association with elevated lipid levels, but antihypertensive agents themselves frequently may have an adverse effect on some of these lipid components. Our understanding of the nature and mechanisms by which alterations in lipids may increase the risk of cardiovascular disease has been improved by epidemiologic and cellular biology studies. We now know that increases in total cholesterol, triglyceride, low-density lipoprotein (LDL), and its carrier apoprotein B or decreases in the scavenger lipid, high-density lipoprotein (HDL), and its carrier apoprotein A1 are associated with an increased risk of cardiovascular disease. Multiple mechanisms can enhance or reduce atherogenesis. It is important to recognize the blood pressure–independent actions of major antihypertensive agents on these components. Genetic alterations in lipid levels as well as changes in the number or affinity of lipid receptors, the metabolic fate, and cellular incorporation of circulating lipids all are matters of intense current scientific inquiry. For example, diuretics raise cholesterol, triglyceride, and LDL levels, and β-antagonists generally reduce high-density lipids. β-Antagonists with intrinsic sympathomimetic activity or with α-adrenergic blocking properties may not reduce HDL.[18] Prazosin's impact on lipid levels and the various components constituting cardiovascular disease risk has been carefully studied. Prazosin has been shown to decrease total cholesterol, triglycerides, and LDL and to significantly increase HDL. The impact of these effects is most dramatically demonstrated by a study in which total cholesterol and a variety of lipid fractions were measured in hypertensive men randomly assigned to receive prazosin or the cardioselective β-adrenergic drug atenolol.[19] Even when prazosin was combined with a diuretic, beneficial effects on lipids were still discernible.[20]

Blood Sugar

Another major concern regarding antihypertensive therapy is the impact of these agents on blood glucose concentrations, because increases in blood sugar are known to be associated with an increased risk of atherosclerosis and cardiovascular disease. Moreover, insulin resistance and glucose intolerance are common in hypertensive patients. α-Antagonists have no direct adverse effect on insulin release, glucose utilization, or blood sugar levels. Furthermore, the use of an α-antagonist, which will reduce renal vascular resistance and increase renal blood flow, can be predicted to prevent the usual decline in renal function in hypertensive diabetic patients. This decline in renal function is particularly likely to be induced by agents that, despite their blood pressure–lowering effect, increase renal vascular constriction as a consequence of their pharmacologic effects or compensatory action. Agents of this type include β-blockers and diuretics. Prazosin has been shown to improve insulin sensitivity in hypertensive patients.

Benign Prostatic Hypertrophy

Urinary function at the level of the bladder sphincter is influenced by α-adrenergic tone. Prazosin has been shown to improve the symptoms of prostatic hypertrophy and to decrease the polyuria and nocturia often associated with this common problem in mature men.[21]

Adverse Effects

Prazosin has been reported to have minimal central nervous system effects or side effects.[22] It does share with most all other antihypertensive agents an identifiable frequency of headaches, drowsiness, nausea, dry mouth, fluid retention, rash, urinary incontinence, and polyarthralgia.[22] However, these side effects are generally mild and relatively infrequent compared with most other first-line antihypertensive agents. More specifically, prazosin has been reported to result in a very low incidence of impotence in hypertensive men, again in marked contrast to the majority of other antihypertensive agents. Recently, it has been recognized that diuretics produce sexual dysfunction in more than 25% of hypertensive men,[23] and experience has been similar with sympatholytic agents and β-blockers.

CLINICAL USE

Prazosin received unrestricted approval and indication for use in the treatment of hypertension. It is a reasonable first-choice agent for the vast majority of hypertensive patients. There are no absolute contraindications to its use, and, unlike other popular first-step antihypertensive drugs such as diuretics and β-blockers, it is not contraindicated for patients with gout, asthma, pulmonary disease, congestive heart failure, or peripheral vascular disease. Because it improves insulin sensitivity, glucose tolerance, and lipid levels, prazosin is a good initial choice for hypertensives with diabetes or lipid abnormalities. A major adverse effect of prazosin has been the so-called first-dose phenomenon. In approximately 0.15% of patients, shortly after the first dose of prazosin is administered, a phenomenon of weakness, dizziness, and near syncope has been reported. This first-dose effect appears to be enhanced by volume depletion and concomitant diuretic therapy and is dose-dependent.[24] The first-dose effect is more frequently encountered among older hypertensive patients in whom the positional reflexes and baroreceptor responses may be blunted. The first-dose effect may be minimized by initiating therapy with no more than 1 mg of prazosin per day given initially at bedtime and by increasing the dose at an appropriate rate after a few doses have been given. It is also prudent to avoid administration of the drug to patients who are excessively volume-depleted. It may be convenient to withdraw diuretic therapy in patients receiving such agents for 2 to 3 days before initiating treatment with prazosin to further reduce the likelihood of the first-dose phenomenon. After prazosin has been given for 2 to 3 days, diuretic therapy can be resumed if needed for blood pressure control. Patients should be reminded that the first-dose effect occurs in roughly 1 of 600 patients, and that it may occur if they discontinue prazosin therapy for a time and then resume it at a higher dose level or with concomitant diuretic therapy.

As indicated previously, the usual starting dose is 1 mg given twice a day with incremental increases to a maximum of 40 mg/day. In actual practice, a total daily dose of 10 mg/day is generally not exceeded, because at that level, second-step agents such as diuretics or calcium antagonists are added. There is some evidence that once-daily administration may be sufficient to control blood pressure for a 24-hour period in approximately 50% of patients with uncomplicated hypertension, and that twice-daily administration provides effective 24-hour blood pressure control in the overwhelming majority.[25]

COMBINING PRAZOSIN WITH OTHER ANTIHYPERTENSIVE AGENTS

When monotherapy with prazosin is not sufficient to reduce blood pressure to the desired levels, addition of second agents is often effective. Diuretics are usually selected for this purpose, because they treat the component of extracellular fluid volume expansion frequently encountered in hypertension. The prazosin-diuretic combination is the most effective one and has been used most frequently in combination studies. Less information is available regarding addition of calcium antagonists, angiotensin-converting enzyme inhibitors, β-blockers, or centrally acting sympatholytic drugs with prazosin. It appears that safety is not an issue with these combinations, but their efficacy is less well established than that of prazosin and diuretics.

SUMMARY

In summary, prazosin is a postsynaptic α_1-antagonist that has been shown to be effective in all forms of hypertension. Prazosin reduces blood pressure primarily by reducing systemic vascular resistance as a result of α_1-receptor blockade of catecholamine-induced contraction of vascular smooth muscle. It has a minimal effect on α_2-receptors and thus may be used to avoid many of the limitations of increased catecholamine levels seen with α_2-blockade. Prazosin reduces vascular resistance and increases blood flow to the regional vascular beds, including those of the heart and kidney. By reducing afterload, it reduces left ventricular work and left ventricular hypertrophy. This indirect-acting vasodilator has no adverse metabolic effects that would worsen the risk of cardiovascular disease, and it actually has been found to favorably influence glucose tolerance and the lipid profile, making it an ideal agent for hypertensive individuals at increased risk of coronary artery disease. Twice-daily administration, a low degree of impotence, and an acceptable side effect profile with minimal central nervous system effects account for its broad patient acceptance and compliance.

REFERENCES

1. Graham RM, Oates HF, Stokes IM, et al: Alpha blocking action of the antihypertensive agent, prazosin. J Pharmacol Exp Ther 201:747, 1977.
2. Hoffman BB, Lefkowitz RJ: Alpha adrenergic receptor subtypes. N Engl J Med 302:1390, 1981.
3. Wood AJ, Bolli P, Simpson FO: Prazosin in normal subjects: Plasma levels, blood pressure and heart rate. Br J Clin Pharmacol 3:199, 1976.
4. Baer L, Laragh JH: Hypertension and chronic renal disease. Cardiovasc Rev Rep 3:149, 1982.
5. Lund-Johansen P: Hemodynamic changes at rest and during exercise in long-term prazosin therapy for essential hypertension. Postgrad Med 58:45, 1975.
6. Awan NA, Miller RR, Miller MP, et al: Clinical pharmacology and therapeutic application of prazosin in acute and chronic refractory congestive heart failure: Balanced systemic venous and arterial dilation improving pulmonary congestion and cardiac output. Am J Med 65:146, 1978.
7. Leenen FHH, Smith DL, Farkas RM, et al: Vasodilators and regression of left ventricular hypertrophy: Hydralazine versus prazosin in hypertensive humans. Am J Med 82:969, 1987.
8. Scharf SC, Lee HB, Wexler JP, et al: Cardiovascular consequences of primary antihypertensive therapy with prazosin hydrochloride. Am J Cardiol 53:32A, 1984.
9. Letcher RL, Chien S, Laragh JH: Changes in blood viscosity accompanying the response to prazosin in patients with essential hypertension. J Cardiovasc Pharmacol 1:S8, 1979.
10. Okun R: Effectiveness of prazosin as initial antihypertensive therapy. Am J Cardiol 51:644, 1983.
11. Walker RG, Whitworth JA, Saines D, et al: Prazosin: Long-term treatment of moderate and severe hypertension and lack of tolerance. Med J Aust 2:146, 1981.
12. New Zealand Hypertension Study Group: Four to seven year follow-up of patients on prazosin. N Z Med J 92:341, 1980.
13. Bauer JH, Jones LB, Gaddy P: Effects of prazosin therapy on blood pressure, renal function and body fluid composition. Arch Intern Med 144:1196, 1984.
14. Koshy MC, Mickley D, Bourgoignie J, et al: Physiological evaluation of a new antihypertensive agent: Prazosin HCL. Circulation 55:533, 1977.
15. Brogden RN, Heel RC, Speight TM, et al: Prazosin: A review of the pharmacological properties and therapeutic efficacy in hypertension. Drugs 14:163, 1977.
16. Weinberger MH: Antihypertensive therapy and lipids: Paradoxical influences on cardiovascular disease risk. Am J Med 80:64, 1986.
17. Weinberger MH: Diuretics and their side effects: Dilemma in the treatment of hypertension. Hypertension 11(Suppl 2):16, 1988.
18. Weinberger MH: Antihypertensive therapy and lipids: Evidence, mechanisms and implications. Arch Intern Med 145:1102, 1985.
19. Rouffy J, Jaillard J: Comparative effects of prazosin and atenolol on plasma lipids in hypertensive patients. Am J Med 76:1105, 1984.
20. Johnson BF, Romero L, Johnson J, et al: Comparative effects of propranolol and prazosin upon serum lipids in thiazide-treated hypertensive patients. Am J Med 76:109, 1984.
21. Kirby RS: Alpha-adrenoceptor inhibitors in the treatment of benign prostatic hyperplasia. Am J Med 87(2A):265, 1989.
22. Graham RM, Pettinger WA: Prazosin. N Engl J Med 300:232, 1979.
23. Medical Research Council Working Party: Adverse reactions to bendroflumethiazide and propranolol for the treatment of mild hypertension. Lancet 2:539, 1981.
24. Rosendorff C: Prazosin: Severe side effects are dose-dependent. Br Med J 2:508, 1976.
25. Weber MA, Toukon MJ, Klein RC: Effect of antihypertensive therapy on the circadian blood pressure pattern. Am J Med 82:50, 1987.

CHAPTER 70

Terazosin

James L. Pool, M.D., Eduardo Nuñez, M.D., and Franz H. Messerli, M.D.

Terazosin hydrochloride (Abbott-45975), 2[4-{(tetrahydro-2-furanyl) carbonyl}-1-piperazinyl]-6,7-dimethoxy-4-quinazolinamine hydrochloride, a congener of prazosin, is one of several quinazoline derivatives that are selective postsynaptic α_1-antagonists.[1-8]

In 1976, prazosin was the first of this group of compounds to be approved in the United States for the treatment of hypertension. As shown in Figure 70–1, the structural difference between these two compounds is the saturated furan ring in terazosin.[7]

Saturation of the terazosin furan ring enhances dramatically the water solubility of the molecule. Tera-

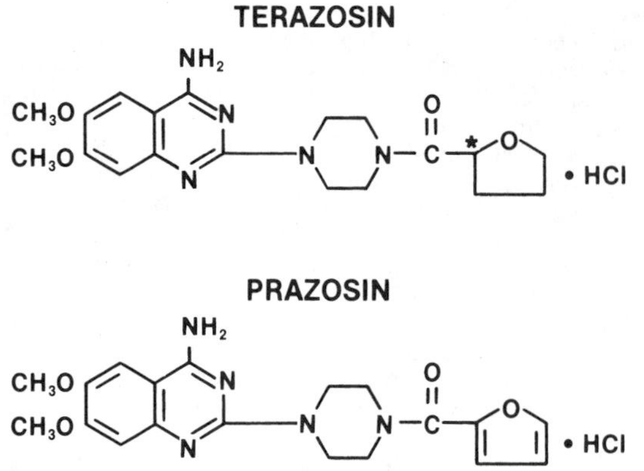

TERAZOSIN

PRAZOSIN

Figure 70–1. Chemical structures of terazosin and prazosin. The asterisk indicates the position of the optically active center of terazosin on the tetrahydrofuran ring. (Adapted with permission from Kyncl JJ: Pharmacology of terazosin. Am J Med 80[Suppl 5B]:12, 1986.)

zosin is 25 times more water soluble than prazosin. The high water solubility of terazosin is the most remarkable physicochemical difference between terazosin and prazosin. In addition, the saturated furan configuration provides the molecule with one optically active chemical center so that, unlike prazosin, terazosin can exist in two enantiomeric forms. Although both enantiomers of terazosin are pharmacologically active, unique characteristics of each enantiomer are largely unknown because animal and human studies have been performed with the terazosin racemate. The water solubility of terazosin permits parenteral administration and promotes a longer duration of action. Prazosin is not suitable for parenteral formulation.

As an α_1-antagonist, terazosin inhibits catecholamine-mediated vasoconstriction and lowers arterial blood pressure by reducing peripheral vascular resistance.[7, 8] Because increased peripheral vascular resistance plays an important role in hypertension, terazosin alone or in combination with other antihypertensive agents has been shown to be effective in the reduction of high blood pressure.[9]

PHARMACOLOGY

Several types of α-antagonists have been introduced, including nonselective α_1- and α_2-antagonists, presynaptic α_2-antagonists, and postsynaptic α_1-antagonists. Like prazosin, terazosin lowers blood pressure primarily by blocking postsynaptic α_1-adrenoreceptors.[7, 8] Terazosin has been shown to lower blood pressure in spontaneously hypertensive rats without increasing heart rate, which is characteristic of most postsynaptic α_1-antagonists.[1] In this respect, selective α_1-antagonists differ from nonselective α-antagonists like phenoxybenzamine and phentolamine. Presynaptic α_2-adrenoreceptors inhibit norepinephrine release. Nonspecific α-blockade causes these receptors to increase norepinephrine release with β-receptor–mediated tachycardia, enhanced renin secretion, and attenuation of postsynaptic α_1-inhibition. α_1-Antago-

nists may reduce vascular tone in capacitance vessels as well as resistance vessels to provide a balance of preload and afterload reduction, thus avoiding vasodilation (afterload reduction) without venodilation (preload reduction) that would promote an increase in cardiac output and heart rate.

After oral administration, the hypotensive efficacy was equal for terazosin and prazosin, but terazosin exhibited a more gradual reduction of blood pressure than did prazosin.[7] Terazosin also showed a more uniform and linear dose-response curve and less variable duration of action than prazosin. Tolerance to terazosin was not observed during 5 days of repeated oral administration in spontaneously hypertensive rats. In anesthetized male beagles, hemodynamic studies with intravenous terazosin demonstrated blood pressure reductions primarily by reduction of peripheral vascular resistance.[3, 7, 8, 10] In these experiments, terazosin decreased arterial blood pressure, left ventricular systolic pressure, and total peripheral resistance. Transient increases in heart rate, cardiac output, and left ventricular contractile force (dP/dt_{max}) were observed immediately after drug administration but returned to baseline within several minutes.

Early experiments in terazosin-treated dogs showed modifications of autonomic challenges that suggested α-blockade. Like prazosin and nonselective α-antagonists, terazosin reverses pressor responses to epinephrine administration. Pretreatment of dogs with a nonselective α-antagonist (phenoxybenzamine, 10 mg/kg IV) markedly reduced the hypotensive effect of terazosin; pretreatment with a β-antagonist (propranolol, 0.5 mg/kg IV) or an anticholinergic agent (atropine, 1 mg/kg IV) did not significantly alter the action of terazosin. Norepinephrine overflow techniques and radioligand-binding studies confirmed that terazosin was a competitive, selective α_1-antagonist with a low affinity for α_2-adrenoreceptors.[3, 7, 8, 10] Terazosin racemate affinity for the α_1-receptor was one third that of prazosin. In vitro α_1-receptor binding affinity constants (mean ± standard error of the mean) were 2.86 ± 0.36 nM for terazosin and 1.05 ± 0.27 nM for prazosin. For both agents, α_2-receptor affinities were equal and extremely low, with a more than 100-fold greater affinity for α_1-receptors than α_2-receptors. Also, in vitro studies demonstrate minimal if any antagonism by terazosin on the hemodynamic effects of acetylcholine, angiotensin II, barium chloride, calcium chloride, isoproterenol, and serotonin.

PHARMACOKINETICS AND METABOLISM

As shown in Figure 70–2, the disposition of terazosin after intravenous administration is characteristic of a two-compartment, open pharmacokinetic model that is linear and independent of dose in both normotensive volunteers and hypertensive subjects.[11] However, hypertensive patients have a significantly lower ($p < .05$) mean plasma clearance than normotensive subjects. Mean plasma elimination half-lives were in-

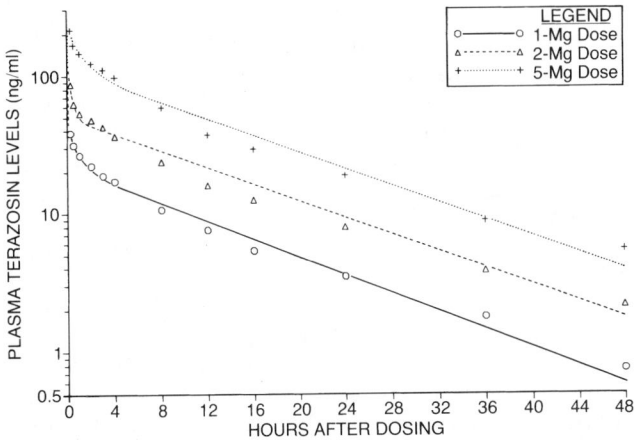

Figure 70–2. Plasma terazosin levels in hypertensive patients (n = 12) after 1-, 2-, and 5-mg doses of intravenous terazosin. (Adapted with permission from Sonders RC: Pharmacokinetics of terazosin. Am J Med 80[Suppl 5B]:20, 1986.)

dependent of intravenous dose. In normotensive subjects, mean plasma half-lives ranged from 8.9 to 12.4 hours after intravenous terazosin of 0.5-, 1.0-, and 2.0-mg doses, whereas mean half-lives in hypertensive patients varied from 11.8 to 13.3 hours after intravenous doses. Less than 15% of terazosin was recovered in the urine from both groups 24 to 48 hours after intravenous administration. The fraction of the intravenous drug excreted in the urine was independent of dose. After oral administration, terazosin absorption (90%) from the gastrointestinal tract was rapid, consistent, and nearly complete. In contrast, prazosin has a lower mean absorption (57%), with individual variability ranging from 44% to 69%. Additionally, prazosin may be affected by first-pass hepatic metabolism.[12] Oral terazosin absorption is not affected significantly by food. Peak terazosin plasma concentrations appear 1 to 2 hours after oral administration; plasma drug concentrations increase proportionally with doses up to 5 mg. Approximately 90% to 94% of the drug is bound to plasma proteins. Volume of drug distribution is 25 to 30 L. Hepatic drug metabolism is extensive, with the major route of excretion through the biliary tract. Small amounts of terazosin are excreted by the kidneys. Plasma clearance is 80 ml/min, but renal clearance is only 10 ml/min. The mean plasma elimination half-life of oral terazosin is 12 hours, which is consistent with its elimination half-life after intravenous administration. The elimination half-life of terazosin is three to four times longer than the half-life of prazosin. With a longer drug half-life, terazosin can be given orally once daily.

Because it is excreted primarily through the biliary tract, the clearance and plasma half-life of terazosin are not altered significantly in patients with moderate to severe renal insufficiency.[13] The plasma half-life of terazosin is increased and plasma clearance is decreased slightly in elderly subjects, but drug dosage adjustments have not been necessary.[14] Absorption, plasma half-life, and clearance of terazosin remain unchanged in patients with congestive heart failure.[15] Metabolism and clearance of terazosin in patients with significant liver disease have not been published.

Biotransformation of terazosin in human subjects has been studied with C^{14} isotope labeling of the 2-position of the quinazolone ring.[11] Terazosin undergoes hepatic metabolism that yields four identified metabolites: 6-O-demethyl terazosin, 7-O-demethyl terazosin, a piperazine compound, and a diamine metabolite of the piperazine compound. Metabolism predominantly involves hydrolysis of the amide linkage to produce the free piperazine derivative with some O-demethylation and, minimally, opening of the piperazine ring and N-dealkylation.

INDICATIONS
Treatment of Hypertension

Contrary to its previous reports, in 1993 the Joint National Committee (JNC V) included the postsynaptic α_1-antagonists together with the diuretics, β-antagonists, ACE-inhibitors, and calcium antagonists as initial therapeutic agents in patients with essential hypertension.[16]

Mechanism of Action

Terazosin lowers arterial pressure by blocking α_1-adrenergic receptors, thereby causing vasodilation in both resistance and capacitance vessels. Like prazosin, terazosin has little effect on α_2-receptors and therefore is unlikely to cause reflex tachycardia.[17] The fact that both resistance as well as capacitance vessels are dilated can manifest itself in one of the adverse effects of the α_1-antagonists, i.e., orthostatic hypotension.

There is now overwhelming evidence to suggest that essential hypertension is not really a hemodynamic disorder only, i.e., confined to an elevation of arterial pressure, but associated with a whole host of metabolic disease processes.[18] Thus, a variety of other cardiovascular risk factors are commonly present in the hypertensive patient. The importance of identification and management of these risk factors has now been recognized.[19, 20] The Lipid Research Clinics Program[21] documented that even a modest reduction in serum cholesterol level was associated with an impressive reduction in the prevalence of coronary heart disease. Consistent but small decreases in the serum cholesterol and triglyceride levels and an increase in high-density lipoprotein (HDL) cholesterol levels have been observed with all three α_1-antagonists, i.e., prazosin, terazosin, and doxazosin. Indeed, a decrease in total and low-density lipoprotein (LDL) cholesterol and triglyceride levels, as well as an increase in HDL cholesterol by approximately 2% to 5% resulting in a 5% to 10% decrease in the ratio of total cholesterol to HDL cholesterol, has been documented with α-antagonist therapy.[22, 23] The exact mechanism underlying these favorable lipid changes remains to be documented. Some possibilities include (1) an increase in lipid protein lipase activity, (2) an increase in the activity of the low-density lipid protein receptor (as was reported in cultured skin fibroblasts), and (3) a decrease in the catabolic rate of HDL cholesterol. Clearly, therefore, terazosin is particularly useful in patients who have only modest abnormalities in their lipid profile, because terazosin may control arterial pressure and dyslipoproteinemia simultaneously. Although this is a very attractive therapeutic concept, the beneficial effects of the α_1-antagonists on cardiovascular morbidity and mortality will have to be documented. Specifically, there is no study available showing that these lipid-lowering effects exert a benefit that exceeds the one conferred by the lowering of blood pressure alone.

Selective α_1-antagonists also have a favorable effect on glucose metabolism by reducing insulin resistance.[24] In most instances, the increase in insulin sensitivity was measured by the euglycemic insulin clamp technique. Of note, no effects of α_1-antagonist on insulin resistance have been documented to surpass the ones with angiotensin-converting enzyme (ACE) inhibitors and calcium antagonists. The exact pathogenetic mechanism accounting for the improvement in insulin resistance remains speculative. Julius and others hypothesized that these drugs could improve insulin resistance through vasodilation in skeletal muscle.[25] However, α_1-antagonists have been documented to surpass the beneficial effects of ACE inhibitors and calcium antagonists in patients with this disorder or patients who are asymptomatic.

Clinical Trials

In numerous clinical trials, terazosin has been shown to be effective alone or in combination for the treatment of patients with hypertension.[4, 9, 13, 14, 26–52] During the initial 40 clinical studies of essential hypertension, 1885 patients received terazosin once or twice daily. Women with no childbearing capability and men between 18 and 72 years of age and with supine diastolic blood pressures between 95 and 119 mmHg (inclusive) were included in these studies.[9, 44] Of these patients, there were 1151 men (61%) and 734 women (39%), with white (71%), black (23%), and Asian (6%) subjects. Comprehensive reviews of these studies have been published.[29, 51, 52] Double-blind, controlled, short-term studies (up to 16 weeks) included dose-titration, fixed-dose, and randomized withdrawal experimental designs. In addition, eligible patients from short-term studies entered an unblinded, long-term study for up to 4.7 years.[37]

Blood pressure was measured approximately 24 hours after once-daily terazosin administration or 12 hours after twice-daily oral administration. In all these studies, the initial dose of terazosin was limited to 0.5 to 1.0 mg at bedtime to minimize the possibility of syncope with the first dose. The maximal daily dose of terazosin was 40 mg. In short-term, dose-titration studies, the dose of terazosin or control (placebo or active reference drug) was increased gradually until supine diastolic blood pressure was reduced

to less than 90 mmHg or the maximal dose of terazosin (20 or 40 mg/day) was reached. The duration of some studies was variable, whereas other studies had a fixed length. Terazosin, either as monotherapy or as concurrent treatment with a thiazide diuretic (i.e., hydrochlorothiazide and methyclothiazide), was administered once or twice daily and compared with placebo. Terazosin was also compared with prazosin. In five placebo-controlled, fixed-dose studies, terazosin monotherapy was gradually increased to a fixed level for a fixed length of time regardless of blood pressure response. Terazosin was added to ongoing methyclothiazide in one of these studies. During two randomized withdrawal studies, patients were assigned randomly to either terazosin or placebo after either short-term (4 to 8 weeks) monotherapy or several months of terazosin monotherapy.[42] Finally, all patients who entered the unblinded long-term study were required to have had at least a 7 mmHg decrease in supine diastolic blood pressure from baseline to final visit during short-term studies.[37]

Terazosin Monotherapy versus Placebo

Terazosin monotherapy was significantly more effective than placebo administration. During five randomized, double-blind placebo-controlled studies with terazosin monotherapy, 351 patients with mild to moderate essential hypertension received terazosin, 1 to 40 mg/day, for 5 to 12 weeks.[9, 51] In all five studies, terazosin caused a significant decrease in supine or standing blood pressures from baseline to the final visit. No significant increase was noted in pulse rate between the group receiving terazosin and that receiving placebo. Seventy-one percent of subjects who received terazosin had supine diastolic blood pressures less than 90 mmHg or a decrease in diastolic blood pressure of more than 10 mmHg compared with baseline values. Among the patients with this response to terazosin monotherapy, two thirds achieved blood pressure control after 5 mg or less per day of terazosin; three fourths of these patients maintained this control with 10 mg or less per day. On the basis of these studies, once-daily terazosin monotherapy was shown to be effective in the treatment of mild to moderate hypertension. The circadian pattern of blood pressure in 13 patients with essential hypertension has been investigated before and after terazosin or placebo.[49] Terazosin reduced blood pressure for 24 hours and produced a downward shift in the pretreatment circadian pattern of blood pressures. Placebo did not change either the blood pressures or the circadian pattern.

Terazosin versus Prazosin

During a comparison of terazosin and prazosin, 155 patients received either once-daily terazosin (1 to 20 mg/day) or twice-daily prazosin (2 to 10 mg/day).[38] Once-daily terazosin therapy resulted in significant ($p < .05$) reductions in supine and standing diastolic blood pressures when compared with placebo. Prazosin twice daily did not cause a significant decrease in supine diastolic blood pressure but did significantly decrease standing diastolic blood pressure compared with placebo. Terazosin once daily was as effective as prazosin twice daily. Adverse experiences in terazosin, prazosin, and placebo treatment groups were similar.

Terazosin versus Hydrochlorothiazide

Terazosin, 1 to 10 mg twice daily, was compared with hydrochlorothiazide, 25 to 50 mg twice daily, in a double-blind parallel study (up to 12 weeks) in 37 patients with mild to moderate essential hypertension.[41] Both terazosin and hydrochlorothiazide produced similar, significant reductions in mean supine and standing systolic and diastolic blood pressures compared with baseline values ($p \leq .05$). The mean reductions in supine blood pressures were 16.7/10.6 mmHg for the terazosin-treated patients and 24.5/17.8 mmHg for the hydrochlorothiazide-treated patients. In this small patient group, a significantly greater reduction occurred in supine diastolic blood pressure in the group treated with hydrochlorothiazide. The mean reductions in standing blood pressure were 17.8/10.9 mmHg for the terazosin-treated group and 22.0/12.3 mmHg for the hydrochlorothiazide-treated patients, with no significant difference between groups for the standing blood pressures.

Terazosin in Combination Therapy

In three short-term studies, terazosin was added to an established diuretic regimen of hydrochlorothiazide, methyclothiazide, chlorthalidone, furosemide, amiloride, triamterene, metolazone, or spironolactone.[40] For all terazosin-treated patients in these three studies, mean supine diastolic blood pressure decreases (4.5 to 8.9 mmHg) were greater than the reductions in placebo-treated patients (0.4 to 5.8 mmHg). Terazosin and prazosin were compared in patients with supine diastolic blood pressure of 95 mmHg or less who received hydrochlorothiazide, 25 mg twice daily for 4 weeks.[41] Both α_1-antagonists combined with hydrochlorothiazide produced significant blood pressure reductions, and there was no significant difference between the two regimens. The addition of terazosin 2, 5, or 10 mg once daily to methyclothiazide produced a relatively flat dose-response curve of blood pressure reduction, indicating that all three doses of terazosin had similar antihypertensive efficacy.[40]

In a comparison study of 138 patients, terazosin, 20 mg/day, or placebo was combined with other antihypertensive drugs.[39] Background antihypertensive therapy included β-antagonists with or without diuretics and several other agents, including methyldopa, clonidine, captopril, guanethidine, hydralazine, and nifedipine. Terazosin-treated patients achieved a significantly greater reduction in supine diastolic blood pressure (7.3 mmHg; $p \leq .05$) than placebo-treated subjects (0.6 mmHg). After atenolol, 50 mg once daily for 8 weeks, the addition of terazosin reduced supine and standing systolic and diastolic blood pressures by an additional 8 to 11 mmHg. In another multicenter, placebo-controlled, double-blind study, Holtzman et al.[28] treated patients with essential hypertension with atenolol, 50 mg daily for 8 weeks. Terazosin (titration 1, 2, 5, and 10 mg once daily) or placebo was added at 2-week intervals until a maximal dose was reached or until supine diastolic blood pressure was reduced to less than 90 mmHg. Compared with placebo, terazosin produced a significant decrease (8 to 11 mmHg) in supine and standing blood pressures from mean baseline values.

Terazosin Withdrawal Studies

A novel evaluation of antihypertensive efficacy is the randomized withdrawal of some patients from drug therapy to placebo followed by assessment of blood pressure changes during several weeks. In two randomized, double-blind, placebo-controlled drug withdrawal studies, terazosin was not associated with an accelerated blood pressure withdrawal syndrome (i.e., diastolic blood pressure increase of more than 20 mmHg compared to pretreatment blood pressure).[42] After discontinuation of terazosin in these patients with mild to moderate essential hypertension, a progressive increase in blood pressure was observed in many cases to hypertensive levels. After 7 to 12 months of terazosin (< 40 mg once daily), 27 patients were monitored for 8 weeks on either placebo therapy or continuation of terazosin therapy. The terazosin group had no significant change in blood pressure; the placebo group developed a 7 mmHg increase in both supine systolic and diastolic blood pressures. During a second withdrawal study, 69 patients who received terazosin (20 mg once daily) for 4 to 8 weeks were assigned randomly to continue terazosin or begin placebo therapy for 6 weeks. Once-daily terazosin efficacy was confirmed, and rebound hypertension was not observed.

Long-term Therapy with Terazosin

Long-term, open-label terazosin therapy included 364 patients who received total daily doses of 1 to 40 mg for up to 4.7 years.[37] In this study, 244 patients received terazosin monotherapy. Sustained mean systolic and diastolic blood pressure reductions in both supine and standing positions were observed with both terazosin monotherapy and combination with other antihypertensive agents. Fifty-two percent of patients received terazosin monotherapy without the addition of other antihypertensive agents. When additional medication was required, it was introduced usually within the first 6 months of therapy. Throughout this study with terazosin monotherapy, blood pressures were reduced consistently from baseline, with mean decreases of supine systolic 9 to 12 mmHg, supine diastolic 10 to 13 mmHg, standing systolic 12 to 18 mmHg, and standing diastolic 11 to 14 mmHg. By comparison, terazosin combined with other drugs produced slightly greater reductions of identical parameters with 12 to 16 mmHg, 12 to 15 mmHg, 16 to 22 mmHg, and 13 to 19 mmHg, respectively.

Congestive Heart Failure

Limited, short-term studies with oral terazosin in small numbers of patients with congestive heart failure (CHF) have been conducted.[15, 53–55] In one study, oral terazosin, 2, 5, or 10 mg, was administered to six patients with CHF and functional class III disease (New York Heart Association classification) who received a digitalis preparation and diuretic.[15] Acute resting, supine, hemodynamic effects of terazosin in CHF included (1) significant reductions of systemic vascular resistance (10% to 25%) and total pulmonary vascular resistance, (2) a modest fall in systemic blood pressure (5% to 12%) and pulmonary artery pressure, (3) an increase in stroke volume and cardiac index with little or no increase in heart rate, and (4) a significant decline in mean right atrial pressure (a measurement of right ventricular filling pressure) and pulmonary capillary wedge pressure (a reflection of left ventricular filling pressure). Although terazosin did not significantly increase exercise capacity in these patients, exercise hemodynamics were improved after the initial dose. However, no differences were noted between the three doses in terms of pressure, resistance, stroke volume, cardiac output, and heart rate responses.

These short-term results were similar to those observed with prazosin. Like other α_1-antagonists, such as prazosin and trimazosin, terazosin has been shown to promote venodilation and vasodilation, which improve cardiac performance. The changes in exercise hemodynamics after long-term terazosin treatment in four patients (> 2 months) were comparable or improved when compared with acute drug therapy. During another acute study with eight patients with severe chronic heart failure, oral terazosin produced hemodynamic changes with improvements in left ventricular function that were similar to intravenous nitroprusside.[55] Sustained efficacy of terazosin in patients with chronic CHF has not been established. With prazosin, therapeutic tolerance develops in patients with CHF after repeated doses and hemodynamic benefits decline.

Effects on Plasma Lipids

α_1-Antagonists, including prazosin, terazosin, trimazosin, and doxazosin, have been shown to produce beneficial effects on plasma lipid levels in hypertensive patients.[56–61] Clinical trials with terazosin have demonstrated variable reductions in total cholesterol, LDL cholesterol, and very-low-density lipoprotein (VLDL) cholesterol plus beneficial increases in the HDL cholesterol–to–total cholesterol ratio.[62–65] The mechanisms for these favorable effects on lipids remain undefined, but possibilities that have been postulated include (1) an increase in low-density lipoprotein receptor activity, as seen in cultured skin fibroblasts;[66] (2) an increase in lipoprotein lipase activity;[67] and (3) a decrease in the fractional catabolic rate of HDL cholesterol.[68] LDL cholesterol is considered the most atherogenic lipid in human subjects, contributing the greatest lipid risk of coronary artery disease. HDL cholesterol is believed to be the most antiatherogenic lipid, promoting a decrease in mortality from coronary artery disease.

The role of various antihypertensive drugs in the alteration of endogenous lipid metabolism has been studied by numerous investigators.[69] The major antihypertensive drug categories, thiazide diuretics and β-antagonists, have been shown to influence adversely plasma lipid levels, possibly causing a long-term adverse effect on coronary artery disease risk. Thiazide diuretics have been shown to elevate levels of total cholesterol, total triglycerides, LDL cholesterol, and VLDL cholesterol, with a variable effect on HDL cholesterol levels. β-Antagonists can increase total triglyceride and VLDL levels, decrease HDL cholesterol levels, and have a variable effect on total cholesterol concentration.

Effects on Left Ventricular Hypertrophy

Left ventricular hypertrophy frequently occurs in untreated hypertensive patients and has been associated with a higher incidence of various cardiovascular complications. Reduction of left ventricular hypertrophy has been documented with most antihypertensive agents, including terazosin.[70] Similar findings have been reported with other α_1-antagonists.

Benign Prostatic Hypertrophy

The average component of smooth muscle tissue in benign prostatic hypertrophy (BPH) amounts to 40%. This finding, in conjunction with the demonstration by several authors[71] that human prostate contains a relative abundance of α-receptors, has led to the treatment of BPH symptoms with α-antagonists. This treatment with α-antagonists has been shown to decrease resistance along the prostatic urethra by relaxing the smooth muscle component of the prostate. α-Antagonists that have been evaluated for the therapy of BHP may be subgrouped according to receptor subtype selectivity and duration of serum elimination half-life. Phenoxybenzamine, prazosin, and terazosin are commercially available in the United States, but none of these agents is currently approved for the indication of treatment of BPH. The overall proportion of patients who demonstrate improvement in urinary symptoms on treatment ranges from 75% to 82% to 93%, respectively, for nonselective, selective α_1, and long-acting selective α_1-antagonists (terazosin).[72] A 49% improvement in Boyarsky symptom scores and a mean improvement in maximal urinary flow rate of approximately 44% have been reported for patients treated with terazosin.[72] Lepor et al.[73] recently summarized the clinical experience with terazosin for symptomatic BPH in 163 patients enrolled in open-label and single-blind studies.

Peak and mean urinary flow rates improved by 41% and 43%, respectively. Irritative, obstructive, and total symptom scores improved 63%, 33%, and 50%, respectively. In another randomized, placebo-controlled multicenter study, Lepor et al.[74] determined the efficacy and safety of terazosin in 285 men with symptomatic BPH. All terazosin groups exhibited significantly greater decreases in the total Boyarsky symptom score than placebo group. The percentage changes in total Boyarsky symptom score for the placebo and 2-, 5-, and 10-mg treatment groups using an intention-to-treat analysis were 23%, 32%, 32%, and 44%, respectively. This study unequivocally supports the short-term efficacy and safety of terazosin for the treatment of symptomatic BPH. The clinical response to selective α-blockade with terazosin is dose-related, and the clinical response did not reach a plateau within the dose range evaluated (2 to 10 mg). In recognition of these studies, the FDA considers symptomatic BPH to be an indication for treatment with terazosin even when blood pressure is normal.

In patients who are poor surgical candidates or unwilling to have surgery, treatment with the $α_1$-antagonist terazosin is currently the preferred therapy for the symptoms of BPH, including acute urinary retention. Because an α-antagonist may also have an effect directly on the bladder, relief of symptoms is possible even if no direct effect occurs on the prostate.

ADVERSE DRUG EFFECTS

Generally, terazosin was well tolerated during short- and long-term clinical trials.[35] Most adverse effects tended to be mild and transient. The most common adverse effects during terazosin treatment have been dizziness, headache, asthenia, and nasal congestion. In placebo-controlled clinical trials, 567 patients received terazosin, and 309 subjects received placebo. Sixty (10.6%) patients receiving terazosin compared with 18 (5.8%) placebo subjects withdrew because of adverse effects. Additional patient complaints included blurred vision, nausea, somnolence, palpitations, and peripheral edema. During the long-term study, a 1-kg increase in mean body weight was reported, but there was no attenuation of antihypotensive efficacy. When compared with placebo, terazosin did not produce significant changes in supine or standing heart rates.

The first-dose phenomenon, i.e., hypotension and syncope after the first dose of an $α_1$-antagonist, is well known. However, syncope with terazosin monotherapy was uncommon, occurring in less than 1% of patients when the initial dose (1 mg or less) was taken at bedtime. In the analysis of unblinded, long-term treatment, 364 patients received terazosin monotherapy or combination therapy with diuretics or β-antagonists for up to 4.7 years. In this study, 262 patients were treated for at least 1 year, and 139 were treated for 2 years or more. Only one patient discontinued the study because of syncope. The symptoms that most commonly caused discontinua-

tion of terazosin therapy were asthenia (2%), nasal congestion (2%), and dizziness (1%).[37]

In controlled trials with terazosin, there were no indications of clinically important adverse effects on laboratory tests. Terazosin does not alter levels of serum electrolytes, blood urea nitrogen, creatinine, glucose, or uric acid. There was no significant effect on renal function in hypertensive patients with normal, moderate, or severe renal impairment.[13] In comparison with placebo subjects, a greater percentage of terazosin patients had small decreases in hematocrit, hemoglobin, white blood cell count, total protein, and albumin levels from baseline values. Except for the white blood cell count, these changes have been attributed to hemodilution secondary to hemodynamic changes and mild fluid retention. The reduction of white blood cells with terazosin remains unexplained, but individual reductions have been small, and prolonged drug treatment has not been associated with progressive reductions in the white blood cell count. For both laboratory and clinical adverse effects, there is no drug-dose relationship.

SUMMARY

Terazosin is a new, long-acting, selective $α_1$-antagonist. As effective as prazosin in the treatment of mild to moderate essential hypertension, terazosin has pharmacokinetic and pharmacodynamic characteristics that are similar to those of prazosin, except that terazosin has a longer plasma elimination half-life, which allows once-daily administration. Because terazosin has better and more predictable absorption from the gastrointestinal tract, it may permit easier and more reliable dosage adjustments. No clinically significant laboratory abnormalities have been noted with long-term administration. Terazosin is approved for the treatment of patients with hypertension as initial monotherapy or in combination with diuretics and other antihypertensive drugs. Terazosin is also approved for the treatment of symptomatic prostatic hypertrophy. Of note, terazosin has a particularly favorable effect on insulin resistance and hypolipidemia.

To minimize the first-dose phenomenon, all patients should receive 1 mg at bedtime as their initial dose. The single daily dose of terazosin can be increased gradually for optimal blood pressure response. If long-term terazosin therapy is interrupted for several days, the initial 1-mg bedtime dose should be given and followed by dose titration. The normal dosage range is 1 to 5 mg once daily. However, some patients may benefit from up to 20 mg/day or twice-daily doses. The dose-response curve for terazosin is relatively flat; therefore, excessive dosage increases may not achieve greater blood pressure reduction. When terazosin is added to other antihypertensive drugs, caution and dose reduction may be necessary to avoid symptomatic hypotension.

REFERENCES

1. Kyncl JJ, Hollinger RE, Oheim WK, et al: (Abbott-45975), 2-[4-[(tetrahydro-2-furanyl) carbonyl]-1-piperazinyl]-6,7-dimethoxy-

4-quinazolinamine HCl, new antihypertensive agent of the quinazoline type [abstract]. Pharmacologist 22:272, 1980.

2. Oates HF: A new prazosin analogue, Abbott-45975 (A-45975) [letter]. N Z Med J 94:67, 1981.

3. Kyncl JJ, Bush EN, Buckner SA: Alpha-adrenergic blocking properties of terazosin [abstract]. Fed Proc 41:1648, 1982.

4. Mizogami S, Hanazuka M: Antihypertensive effect of 2-[4-(tetrahydro-2-furanyl) carbonyl-1-piperazinyl]-6,7-dimethoxy-4-quinazolinamine hydrochloride dihydrate (terazosin) [abstract]. Jpn J Pharmacol 32(Suppl 1):174P, 1982.

5. Kondo K, Ohashi K, Ebihara A: Pharmacokinetics and pharmacological effects of terazosin, a new alpha-blocker. Jpn J Clin Pharmacol Ther 13:137, 1982.

6. Kondo K, Ohashi K, Ebihara A: The pharmacokinetics and pharmacological effects of terazosin, a new alpha-blocking agent, in normotensive volunteers [abstract]. Jpn J Clin Pharmacol Ther 14:147, 1983.

7. Kyncl JJ: Pharmacology of terazosin. Am J Med 80(Suppl 5B):12, 1986.

8. Kyncl JJ, Sonders RC, Sperzel WD, et al: In Scriabine A (ed): New Cardiovascular Drugs. New York: Raven Press, 1986, pp 1–17.

9. Moser M (ed): Advances in the management of hypertension: Focus on terazosin, a new alpha-1-adrenergic antagonist. May 3–5, 1985, Boca Raton, Florida. Am J Med 80(Suppl 5B):1, 1986.

10. Kyncl JJ, Bush EN, Buckner SA: Terazosin, a new quinazoline antihypertensive agent. II. Alpha-adrenergic blocker properties. In Rosenthal J (ed): Focus on Alpha Blockade and Terazosin. Munich: Zuckschwerdt Verlag, 1986, pp 16–32.

11. Sonders RC: Pharmacokinetics of terazosin. Am J Med 80(Suppl 5B):20, 1986.

12. Reid JL, Vincent J: Clinical pharmacology and therapeutic role of prazosin and related alpha-adrenoreceptor antagonists. Cardiology 73:164, 1986.

13. Jungers P, Ganeval D, Pertuiset N, Chauveau P: Influence of renal insufficiency on the pharmacokinetics and pharmacodynamics of terazosin. Am J Med 80(Suppl 5B):94, 1986.

14. McNeil JJ, Drummer OH, Conway EL, et al: Effect of age on pharmacokinetics and blood pressure responses to prazosin and terazosin. J Cardiovasc Pharmacol 10:168, 1987.

15. Leier CV, Patterson SE, Huss P, et al: The hemodynamic and clinical responses to terazosin, a new alpha blocking agent, in congestive heart failure. Am J Med Sci 292:128, 1986.

16. Anonymous: The fifth report of the Joint National Committee on Detection, Evaluation, and Treatment of High Blood Pressure (JNCV) [see comments]. Arch Intern Med 153:154, 1993.

17. Khoury AF, Kaplan NM: α-Blocker therapy of hypertension. An unfulfilled promise. JAMA 266:394, 1991.

18. Laurenzi M, Mancini M, Menotti A, et al: Multiple risk factors in hypertension: Results from the Gubbio Study. J Hypertens 8(Suppl 1):S7, 1990.

19. Lasser NL, Grandits G, Gaggiula AW, et al: Effects of antihypertensive therapy on plasma lipids and lipoproteins in the multiple risk factor intervention trial. Am J Med 76(2A):52, 1984.

20. Weinberger MH: Antihypertensive therapy and lipids: Paradoxical influences on cardiovascular disease risk. Am J Med 80(Suppl 2A):64, 1986.

21. Lipid Research Clinics Program: The Lipid Research Clinics Coronary Primary Prevention Trial results. II. The relationship of reduction in incidence of coronary heart disease in cholesterol lowering. JAMA 251:365, 1984.

22. Lytle T, Coles S, Waite MA: A multicentre, hospital study of the efficacy and safety of terazosin and its effects on the plasma cholesterol levels of patients with untreated essential hypertension. J Hum Hypertens 5:35, 1991.

23. Working Group on Management of Patients with Hypertension and High Blood Cholesterol: National Education Programs Working Group Report on the Management of Patients with Hypertension and High Blood Pressure. Ann Intern Med 114:224, 1991.

24. Waite MA: Alpha1 blockers: Antihypertensives whose positive metabolic profile with regard to hyperinsulinemia and lipid metabolism cannot be ignored. J Intern Med 229(Suppl 2):113, 1991.

25. Julius S, Gudbrandsson P, Jamerson K, et al: The hemodynamic link between insulin resistance and hypertension. J Hypertens 9:983, 1991.

26. Tomoda F, Takata M, Hirai A, et al: Hemodynamic and endocrinologic effects of a new selective alpha-1 blocking agent, terazosin, in patients with essential hypertension: Results of long-term treatment. J Am Coll Cardiol 7(2):26A, 1986.

27. Nelson EB, Pool JL, Taylor AA, et al: Evaluation of terazosin in the treatment of essential hypertension. Clin Pharmacol Ther 31(2):255, 1982.

28. Holtzman JL, Kaihlanen PM, Rider JA, et al: Concomitant administration of terazosin and atenolol for the treatment of essential hypertension. [Published erratum appears in Arch Intern Med 148:1960, 1988.] Arch Intern Med 148:539, 1988.

29. Titmarsh S, Monk JP: Terazosin: A review of its pharmacodynamic and pharmacokinetic properties, and therapeutic efficacy in essential hypertension [review]. Drugs 33:461, 1987.

30. Hayduk K, Schneider HT: Antihypertensive effects of doxazosin in systemic hypertension and comparison with terazosin. Am J Cardiol 59:95G, 1987.

31. Hayduk K: Efficacy and safety of doxazosin in hypertension therapy. Am J Cardiol 59:35G, 1987.

32. Luther RR, Glassman HN, Sperzel WD, et al: Terazosin: A new alpha 1-blocker for the treatment of hypertension: A review of randomized, controlled clinical trials of once-daily administration as monotherapy [review]. J Hypertens 4(Suppl):S494, 1986.

33. Ferrier C, Beretta-Piccoli C, Weidmann P, et al: Alpha-1-adrenergic blockade and lipoprotein metabolism in essential hypertension. Clin Pharmacol Ther 40:525, 1986.

34. Cohen A: Efficacy and safety of intravenous terazosin in hypertensive patients. A preliminary report. Am J Med 80(Suppl 5B):86, 1986.

35. Sperzel WD, Glassman HN, Jordan DC, et al: Overall safety of terazosin as an antihypertensive agent. Am J Med 80(Suppl 5B):77, 1986.

36. Luther RR, Glassman HN, Jordan DC, et al: Efficacy of terazosin as an antihypertensive agent. Am J Med 80(Suppl 5B):73, 1986.

37. Luther RR, Glassman HN, Estep CB, et al: Terazosin, a new selective alpha 1-adrenergic blocking agent. Results of long-term treatment in patients with essential hypertension. Am J Hypertens 1(3 Pt 3):237S, 1988.

38. Deger G, Cutler RE, Dietz AJ Jr, et al: Comparison of the safety and efficacy of once-daily terazosin versus twice-daily prazosin for the treatment of mild to moderate hypertension. Am J Med 80(Suppl 5B):62, 1986.

39. Chrysant SG: Experience with terazosin administered in combination with other antihypertensive agents. Am J Med 80(Suppl 5B):55, 1986.

40. Rudd P: Cumulative experience with terazosin administered in combination with diuretics. Am J Med 80(Suppl 5B):49, 1986.

41. Ruoff G: Comparative trials of terazosin with other antihypertensive agents. Am J Med 80(Suppl 5B):42, 1986.

42. Ruoff G: Effect of withdrawal of terazosin therapy in patients with hypertension. Am J Med 80(Suppl 5B):35, 1986.

43. Dauer AD: Terazosin: An effective once-daily monotherapy for the treatment of hypertension. Am J Med 80(Suppl 5B):29, 1986.

44. Sperzel WD, Luther RR, Glassman HN: Clinical trials with terazosin. General methods. Am J Med 80(Suppl 5B):25, 1986.

45. Beretta-Piccoli C, Ferrier C, Weidmann P: Alpha 1-adrenergic blockade and cardiovascular pressure responses in essential hypertension. Hypertension 8:407, 1986.

46. Abraham PA, Halstenson CE, Matzke GR, et al: Antihypertensive therapy with once-daily administration of terazosin, a new alpha 1-adrenergic-receptor blocker. Pharmacotherapy 5:285, 1985.

47. Patterson SE: Terazosin kinetics after oral and intravenous doses. Clin Pharmacol Ther 38:423, 1985.

48. Chrysant SG, Bal IS, Johnson B, et al: Antihypertensive effectiveness of terazosin: A new long-acting alpha-adrenergic inhibitor. Clin Cardiol 8:486, 1985.

49. Drayer JI, Weber MA, DeYoung JL, et al: Long-term BP monitoring in the evaluation of antihypertensive therapy. Arch Intern Med 143:898, 1983.

50. Rosenthal J: Terazosin in mild hypertension: Experience in open

trials. Br J Clin Pract [Symposium Supplement] 41(Suppl 54):32, 1987.

51. Pool JL, Nelson EB, Taylor AA, et al: Terazosin (Hytrin): Cumulative experience of clinical trials in the USA for the treatment of mild to moderate hypertension. Br J Clin Pract [Symposium Supplement] 41 (Suppl 54):9, 1987.

52. Frishman WH, Eisen G, Lapsker J: Terazosin: A new long-acting alpha 1-adrenergic antagonist for hypertension [review]. Med Clin North Am 72:441, 1988.

53. Grant PK, Reuben SR, Jones R, et al: Pharmacodynamics of terazosin in heart failure. Eur Heart J 4(Suppl E):111, 1983.

54. O'Rourke M, Avolio A, Nichols W, et al: Terazosin hemodynamics in patients with cardiac failure [abstract]. J Am Coll Cardiol 5(2):543, 1985.

55. Lui HK, Awan NA, Needham K, et al: Comparative evaluation of the new oral systemic vasodilator terazosin and nitroprusside in severe chronic heart failure [abstract]. Clin Res 33:207A, 1985.

56. Kirkendall WM, Hammond JJ, Thomas JC: Prazosin and clonidine for moderately severe hypertension. JAMA 240:2553, 1978.

57. Leren P, Foss PO, Helgeland A, et al: Effect of propranolol and prazosin on blood lipids: The Oslo study. Lancet 2:4, 1980.

58. Havard CW, Khokhar AM, Flax JS: Open assessment of the effect of prazosin on plasma lipids. J Cardiovasc Pharmacol 4(Suppl 2):S238, 1982.

59. Singleton W, Taylor CR: Effect of trimazosin on serum lipid profiles in hypertensive patients. Am Heart J 106(5 Pt 2):1265, 1983.

60. Rouffy J, Jaillard J: Comparative effects of prazosin and atenolol on plasma lipids in hypertensive patients. Am J Med 76(Suppl 2A):105, 1984.

61. Pool JL: Plasma lipid lowering effects of doxazosin, a new selective alpha-1 adrenergic inhibitor for systemic hypertension. Am J Cardiol 59:46G, 1987.

62. Pool JL, Nelson EB, Taylor AA, et al: Alpha-1 adrenergic blockade changes plasma lipids in man [abstract]. Clin Res 30(Suppl 2):213A, 1982.

63. Deger G: Effect of terazosin on serum lipids. Am J Med 80(Suppl 5B):82, 1986.

64. Dauer AD, Deger G, Fleming L: Terazosin: An effective once-a-day antihypertensive agent with an apparent beneficial effect on cholesterol. Today's Therapeutic Trends 4(1):1, 1986.

65. Silke B: Effect of antihypertensive therapy on plasma lipoproteins in essential hypertension. Br J Clin Pract [Symposium Supplement] 41(Suppl 54):56, 1987.

66. Leren TP. Doxazosin increase low density lipoprotein receptor activity. Acta Pharmacol Toxicol (Copenh) 56:269, 1985.

67. Rubba P, De Simone B, Marotta T, et al: Adrenergic blocking agents and lipoprotein lipase activity. J Endocrinol Invest 12:119, 1989.

68. Sheu WH, Swislocki AL, Hoffman BB, et al: Effect of prazosin treatment on HDL kinetics in patients with hypertension. Am J Hypertens 3:761, 1990.

69. Weidmann P, Uehlinger DE, Gerger A: Antihypertensive treatment and serum lipoproteins [review]. J Hypertens 3:297, 1985.

70. Yasumoto K, Takada M, Toshida K, et al: Reversal of left ventricular hypertrophy by terazosin in hypertensive patients. J Hum Hypertens 4:13, 1990.

71. Caine M, Raz S, Zeigler M: Adrenergic and cholinergic receptors in the human prostate, prostatic capsule and bladder neck. Br J Urol 47:193, 1975.

72. Schlegel PN: Medical management of prostatic diseases [review]. Adv Intern Med 39:569, 1994.

73. Lepor H, Henry D, Laddu AR: The efficacy and safety of terazosin for the treatment of symptomatic BPH. Prostate 18:345, 1991.

74. Lepor H, Auerbach S, Puras-Baez A, et al: A randomized, placebo-controlled multicenter study of the efficacy and safety of terazosin in the treatment of benign prostatic hyperplasia. J Urol 148:1467, 1992.

CHAPTER 71

Urapidil

Alberto Zanchetti, M.D., and Tiziana Santagada, M.D.

Urapidil, chemically derived from uracil, has been recognized as an antihypertensive drug since the 1970s, and its clinical efficacy as monotherapy, or in combination with other antihypertensive drugs, is now well documented.

The pharmacologic effect of urapidil is mainly attributed to blockade of peripheral postsynaptic α-adrenoceptors with an additional central activity.

The therapeutic use of urapidil results in a significant reduction of blood pressure without altering heart rate and renal function. The most common adverse effects associated with urapidil therapy are dizziness, nausea, and fatigue, as expected for a vasodilator drug.

MECHANISM OF ACTION

Urapidil is an antihypertensive drug, characterized by multifactorial mechanisms of action, including peripheral α₁-adrenoceptor blockade and central serotoninergic receptor activation. The primary mode of action of urapidil is based on a selective, vascular, postsynaptic α_1-antagonism, causing a reduction in peripheral resistance.[1] Furthermore, urapidil acts on central cardiovascular regulation by stimulating $5HT_{1A}$-receptors located on somatodendritic sites of serotoninergic neurons in the B1/B3 region of the ventral medulla.[2] The latter effect leads to a decrease in sympathetic nerve activity and is additive to the blood pressure reduction resulting from peripheral α_1-adrenergic blockade; this effect may be responsible for the absence of reflex tachycardia despite pronounced vasodilation.

Interactions of urapidil with either presynaptic or postsynaptic α_2-adrenoreceptors and β-adrenoreceptors appear to be of minor importance and clinically irrelevant.[3]

PHARMACOKINETICS

The pharmacokinetics of urapidil are linear. Peak serum concentrations occur approximately 4 hours after oral administration of sustained-release capsules of urapidil. Plasma protein binding amounts to 80%.

About 20% undergoes first-pass metabolism by the liver. The mean apparent terminal plasma half-life after oral administration is about 5 hours. Bioavailability is not influenced by food intake. Urapidil is extensively metabolized in the liver, especially by parahydroxylation. Animal studies have demonstrated that the major metabolite in humans, M1, has a negligible antihypertensive activity. In contrast, the pharmacologic action of the minor metabolites M2 and M3 is similar to that of urapidil, which might contribute to its antihypertensive effect. Within 24 hours, 50% to 70% of an orally administered dose is excreted in the urine; only 10% to 15% of urapidil is found unaltered in the urine.[4, 5]

The effect of age on urapidil pharmacokinetics was investigated in 24 elderly patients (72 to 96 years old) with mild to moderate hypertension. The absorption rate was not affected, whereas the elimination half-life increased approximately twofold after intravenous or oral administration of urapidil.[6] The only available data concerning the effect of liver function impairment on urapidil pharmacokinetics result from a study evaluating the pharmacokinetics of a 30-mg single oral dose in four patients with alcoholic cirrhosis.[7] An increase in the mean half-life compared with healthy subjects (8.1 to 20.5 versus 2.5 to 3.7 hours) was the only pharmacokinetic parameter constantly altered in these patients.

No significant differences in the pharmacokinetics of a 25-mg urapidil bolus injection were found between hypertensive patients with moderately impaired renal function (creatinine clearance, 41 ± 12 ml/min)[8] and patients with hypertension and normal glomerular filtration rate. Zitta et al.[9] demonstrated that there are no relevant differences between patients with moderate renal insufficiency (creatinine clearance, 25 to 50 ml/min) and patients with severe renal impairment (creatinine clearance, <20 ml/min) in terms of volumes of distribution, total body clearance, and elimination half-life of urapidil.

However, the mean total body clearance of urapidil was reduced in these patients if compared with the values reported in healthy young subjects and patients with hypertension and normal kidney function.[4, 8] Slingeneyer et al.[10] assessed the pharmacokinetics of a single oral dose of urapidil (30 mg) in 14 patients with hypertension and end-stage renal disease requiring hemodialysis (creatinine clearance, <4 ml/min). There were increases in maximum concentration (C_{max}) (40%), half life ($T_{1/2}$) (30%), and area under the curve (AUC) (90%) when compared with healthy subjects.[4] It is possible, however, that the reduced clearance of urapidil observed in the studies of Zitta et al.[9] and Slingeneyer et al.[10] may be also due to the fact that patients involved in these studies were older than the control subjects.

HEMODYNAMICS
Arterial Pressure

Both acute and long-term administration of urapidil produce a decrease in total peripheral resistance, resulting in a reduction of arterial pressure.

After intravenous administration, urapidil significantly reduces blood pressure in hypertensive subjects, both when administered as an intravenous bolus injection (doses ranging from 10 to 50 mg) and when administered by continuous infusion (doses ranging from 40 to 160 µg/min). The antihypertensive action reaches its peak within the first 60 minutes. The pharmacologic effect starts 5 to 15 minutes after the administration, lasting up to 6 hours.[11-16]

In a randomized, double-blind, placebo-controlled trial, Culbertson et al.[17] observed an increasing reduction in systolic and diastolic blood pressure with single oral doses of 60, 90, and 120 mg in hypertensive patients. The pharmacologic effect lasted from 4.5 to 8 hours. The maximal reduction in diastolic blood pressure occurred at 3 to 5 hours after dosing.

Heart Rate

At therapeutic doses, the blood pressure–lowering effect of urapidil is not generally associated with significant changes in heart rate. Only a few cases showed a slight and transient increase after acute administration.[11, 18-22] Moreover, for similar antihypertensive effects, acute administration of urapidil always induced a smaller heart rate increase in comparison with prazosin.[21, 22]

The fall in blood pressure is then largely unopposed by baroreceptor reflexes. In fact, intravenous administration of 25 mg of urapidil has been shown not to affect cardiopulmonary reflexes and to reset arterial baroreflexes at lower blood pressure levels.[23]

Central Hemodynamics

After acute and chronic administration of urapidil, the cardiac output remains unchanged or is only slightly elevated.[24] The effects of urapidil on right and left ventricular functions are documented in 20 patients with chronic coronary artery disease and mild hypertension who were randomly assigned to receive a single intravenous administration of either urapidil (0.4 mg/kg) or clonidine (2.5 µg/kg). Both urapidil and clonidine induced a 15% decrease in mean arterial pressure with no simultaneous changes in left and right ejection fractions.[20]

The effects on cardiac morphology and function, as well as the hemodynamic changes, in hypertensive patients under long-term treatment with urapidil have been investigated in a series of echocardiographic studies.[25-29] Table 71–1 summarizes the results of the four major studies. All four studies are consistent with a reduction in left ventricular hypertrophy: in particular, a reduction in left ventricular posterior wall thickness was observed in all four studies; two studies also showed a reduction in interventricular septum thickness; and two studies showed a reduction in left ventricular mass index. The only study that explored the right ventricular wall thickness reported a significant decrease. Systolic and diastolic function indices remained unchanged.

Table 71–1. Effects of Urapidil on Cardiac Morphology: Results of Four Major Echocardiographic Studies

Time Point	1 Month	3 Months		6 Months			12 Months
Reference	28	29	27	25	28	27	25
LVM	—	—	—	—	—	↓	—
LVMI	↓		—		↓↓	↓	
IVST	—	]— ↓		—	↓↓		
PWT	↓			↓	↓↓		↓↓
RVWT		↓				↓	
LVIDd	↑	—		↑↑			—
LVIDs		—					—
LVVd	↑			↑↑			—
LVVs		—					—

LVM, left ventricular mass; LVMI, left ventricular mass index; IVST, interventricular septum thickness; PWT, posterior wall thickness; RVWT, right ventricular wall thickness; LVIDd, left ventricular internal diameter (end of diastole); LVIDs, left ventricular internal diameter (end of systole); LVVd, left ventricular volume (end of diastole); LVVs, left ventricular volume (end of systole).

↑ / ↓, significant ($p < .05$) increase or decrease versus baseline; ↑↑ / ↓↓, significant ($p < .01$) increase or decrease versus baseline; —, no significant change.

Peripheral Hemodynamics

The reduction in blood pressure induced by acute urapidil administration is accompanied by an increase in forearm[23] and splanchnic blood flow.[19] Because forearm blood flow is largely distributed to skeletal muscles, its increase is likely to help prevent symptoms such as fatigue or reduced tolerance to exercise, which often occur in patients undergoing antihypertensive therapy.

Unlike direct vasodilators such as hydralazine, urapidil also lowers "preload" by its dilating action on the venous side of the circulation, as reported by Messerli et al.[19] and Downer et al.[30] This action on preload is consistent with the observations by Lepage et al.[20] and Hirata et al.[31] of a reduction in the plasma levels of atrial natriuretic factor following urapidil administration.

METABOLIC EFFECTS

Some data suggest a favorable effect of urapidil on serum lipids and glucose metabolism. In a review of six clinical trials involving 1482 hypertensive patients, Pattenier and von Heusinger[32] concluded that treatment with urapidil, 60 mg b.i.d. for 3 months, significantly reduced total cholesterol (−10%), total triglycerides (−13%), and low-density lipoprotein (LDL) cholesterol (−10%) and increased high-density lipoprotein (HDL) cholesterol (+7%).

Similarly, in a 12-week parallel group comparison including more than 300 patients, Fariello et al.[33] showed that urapidil can correct the atherogenic plasma lipid profile characteristic of non-insulin-dependent diabetes mellitus and improve blood glucose control. The addition of a thiazide diuretic abolished these favorable effects.

Goto[34] assessed the effects of urapidil on lipid metabolism in a group of 28 patients with essential hypertension and hyperlipidemia. Urapidil (30 to 90 mg/day) was administered for 12 weeks. Total serum cholesterol, LDL cholesterol, and apolipoprotein B significantly decreased, whereas the levels of triglycerides, HDL cholesterol, apolipoprotein AI, apolipoprotein AII, and lecithin-cholesterol acyltransferase activity did not change significantly during the treatment.

Although the results of studies investigating the effects of antihypertensive agents on lipid metabolism are open to some criticism because of the failure to standardize confounding factors (dietary intake, body weight, smoking habits, exercise) or the failure to standardize the conditions of storage and measurement of samples, there is an impressive consistency concerning the possibility that urapidil, like other α-adrenergic blockers, can improve the plasma lipid profile.

EFFECTS ON RENAL FUNCTION

Intravenous injection of urapidil significantly reduces renal vascular resistance[11, 14, 16, 31] and augments[11, 31, 35] or does not change renal plasma flow.[14, 16] Exchangeable sodium, body weight, and circulating blood volume remained within the normal range after a 4-week treatment with urapidil (30 mg b.i.d.).[36]

Data from Exaire et al.[37] showing a fall in fractional excretion of sodium after a 6-month oral administration of urapidil are not supported by the results of long-term studies wherein body weight remained unchanged and no signs of sodium and water retention could be observed.[38, 39]

In contrast with the results of studies of acute administration[11, 14–16] documenting a trend toward a rise in plasma renin activity and in plasma aldosterone, a 12-day oral treatment with urapidil[31] (60 to 90 mg/day) and a 6-week oral treatment (30 mg once or twice daily)[40] were reported to leave plasma renin and aldosterone unchanged.

CLINICAL USE

The primary indication for oral urapidil administration is the therapy of hypertension, whereas the intravenous formulation is mainly suitable for use in treatment of hypertensive crises, congestive heart failure, and perioperative hypertension.

Oral Administration

The efficacy of urapidil is well established in all grades of hypertension, either as monotherapy or combined with other antihypertensive drugs.

Double-Blind, Randomized, Controlled Studies

Comparisons with Placebo

Volpe et al.[41] assessed the efficacy and the tolerability of urapidil (60 mg b.i.d.) in 40 patients with essential hypertension (supine diastolic blood pressure ranging from 100 to 120 mmHg) in a double-blind, randomized, placebo-controlled, parallel group study. After a 2-week placebo run-in phase, the patients were treated with urapidil, 60 mg b.i.d, or placebo for a further 3 weeks. Blood pressure was measured at 4 and 12 hours after drug administration. The difference between urapidil and placebo was statistically significant after 1, 2, and 3 weeks of treatment. Responder rate (supine diastolic blood pressure, <90 mmHg) was 60% in the urapidil group and 25% in the placebo group ($p < .05$).

Genovesi-Ebert et al.[27] demonstrated the efficacy of urapidil (60 to 90 mg b.i.d) in a randomized, double-blind, placebo-controlled, parallel-group trial. After 2 weeks of a placebo run-in period, 20 patients were treated with placebo or urapidil for 12 weeks. The treatment was then continued for 12 additional weeks with urapidil in both groups. Systolic and diastolic blood pressures were significantly reduced in the urapidil group after 6 and 12 weeks, and these reductions were maintained in the subsequent period of open urapidil administration. In the placebo group, blood pressure did not change during the 12 weeks of placebo and was significantly reduced after the first 6 weeks of open treatment with urapidil, but the reduction fell short of statistical significance after the following 6 weeks.

In a double-blind, parallel-group study, Rosendorff[42] compared the effects of a 6-week treatment with three different doses of urapidil (30, 60, and 90 mg b.i.d.) and placebo. Unfortunately, the results of this study are inconclusive because of the unusually large placebo effect and the great blood pressure variability in all treatment groups.

Comparisons with β-Blockers

Table 71–2 summarizes the results of four double-blind trials comparing urapidil and β-blockers.

In these short-term studies (6 to 10 weeks), urapidil produced falls in blood pressure similar to those of acebutolol,[43] metoprolol,[44] metipranolol,[45] and atenolol[46] in patients affected by all grades of hypertension (diastolic blood pressure values ranging from 95 to 130 mmHg). Although the responder rate varied

among studies, no significant differences were observed among the treatments being compared.

Consistent with other evaluations, urapidil lowered blood pressure without producing significant changes in heart rate. In contrast, β-blockers caused reduction in heart rate (mean change of −10 to −15 beats/min).

Comparisons with Thiazide Diuretics

Urapidil has been compared with hydrochlorothiazide in two randomized, double-blind studies[47–48] (see Table 71–2).

In particular, the aims of the study conducted by Fariello et al.[47] were to assess the antihypertensive effects of urapidil and hydrochlorothiazide as well as to investigate the efficacy of the combined therapy in nonresponders to monotherapy with either agent. In this multicenter study, after a 2-week, single-blind, placebo run-in phase, 113 patients were randomly allocated to receive an 8-week treatment with urapidil (60 mg b.i.d.) or hydrochlorothiazide (25 mg b.i.d.) according to a double-blind, parallel-group design. After 8 weeks, supine blood pressure was similar in both treatment groups and significantly lower than placebo run-in pressure.

At the end of the double-blind period, 24 of 47 patients had not responded to urapidil and 17 of 49 had not responded to hydrochlorothiazide. In patients whose blood pressure remained unsatisfactorily controlled, a combination therapy consisting of urapidil (60 mg b.i.d.) and hydrochlorothiazide (12.5 mg b.i.d.) was undertaken. The proportion of patients uncontrolled by monotherapy and achieving supine blood pressure of 90 mmHg or lower after the combination treatment was 39%, which shows that the two drugs act synergistically.

Distler et al.[48] showed that an 8-week treatment with urapidil (30 to 90 mg b.i.d.) significantly lowered systolic and diastolic blood pressure, although the effect of hydrochlorothiazide was slightly more pronounced. Urapidil produced a reduction of diastolic blood pressure to 90 mmHg or lower or a decrease of at least 10 mmHg in 36% of patients.

Both in the study by Fariello et al.[47] and in the study by Distler et al.,[48] urapidil, as well as hydrochlorothiazide, did not cause any clinically significant changes in heart rate.

Comparisons with Calcium Antagonists

Two double-blind studies,[49, 50] including a total of 255 patients, compared urapidil with the calcium antagonists nifedipine and nitrendipine. The efficacy of the treatments was comparable. The three drugs significantly reduced blood pressure, and responder rate ranged from 43% to 67% (see Table 71–2).

Comparisons with Centrally Acting Drugs

Eisel and Härlin[51] compared urapidil with clonidine in a double-blind study involving 20 patients; Feldstein et al.,[29] in a similar study, compared urapidil

Table 71–2. **Response Rates of Urapidil versus Other Antihypertensive Drugs (Double-Blind Studies)**

Comparative Treatment (Reference)	Number of Patients	Duration of Treatment (weeks)	Dosage (mg/day)		Responders (%)	
Acebutolol (43)	40	10	U	30–90	U	80
			A	200–400	A	60
Metoprolol (44)	40	4	U	60	U	35
			M	200	M	42
Atenolol (46)	43	8	U	60–120	U	23
			ATEN	50–100	ATEN	48
Metipranolol + butizide (45)	30	6	U	30–60	U	60
			MET	20–40	MET +	87
			B	2.5–5	B	
Slow-release nifedipine (49)	168	12	U	120	U	43
			NIF	40	NIF	57
Nitrendipine (50)	87	6	U	120	U	67
			N	20	N	49
Prazosin (52)	222	12	U	30–120	U	64
			P	1.5–6	P	64
Prazosin + thiazide diuretics (52)			U	30–120	U	67
			P	1.5–6	P	65
Clonidine (51)	20	5	U	30–60	U	50
			C	0.15–0.30	C	50
α-Methyldopa (29)	35	12	U	120–180	U	54
			METH	100–1500	METH	62
Captopril (53)	295	12	U	120	U	62
			C	50	C	58
Hydrochlorothiazide (47)	113	8	U	60	U	49
			HCT	25	HCT	65
Hydrochlorothiazide (48)	165	8	U	60–180	U	36
			HCT	25–50	HCT	56

and α-methyldopa in a group of 35 patients. Both studies showed no significant differences in reduction of blood pressure or in responder rates, defined as supine diastolic blood pressure of 95 mmHg or lower (see Table 71–2).

Comparisons with Prazosin

Kaneko et al.[52] compared the effects of urapidil and prazosin in a multicenter, randomized, double-blind study. Following a single-blind, 4-week placebo period, 412 patients with mild to moderate hypertension were treated for 12 weeks by monotherapy or in combination with thiazide diuretics. The results indicate that urapidil in monotherapy or in combination with diuretics is as effective as prazosin, because both drugs produced a significant reduction in blood pressure, and response rates in the subgroups were similar (see Table 71–2).

Comparisons with Captopril

Rosenthal and Härlin,[53] in a multicenter, double-blind, randomized parallel-group study, compared the efficacy and tolerability of 60 to 90 mg of urapidil and 25 to 50 of mg captopril twice daily. Both drugs significantly reduced blood pressure, and responder rates were similar in the two treatment groups (see Table 71–2).

Open Studies

Postmarketing surveillance studies involving more than 17,500 patients[32, 38, 39, 54–57] also can be used to document the performance of urapidil in routine practice. The daily dose range of urapidil in these trials was 30 to 180 mg for periods ranging from 4 weeks to 3 years. These studies demonstrate that the magnitude of the therapeutic effect of urapidil, both as monotherapy and in combined therapy, is of the order expected from controlled studies. In the largest of these studies,[54] involving 6825 patients, urapidil was shown to be effective regardless of the age of the patients and concomitant illnesses or medications.

Intravenous Administration

The therapeutic efficacy of urapidil administered intravenously was mainly investigated in the following conditions:

- Hypertensive crises, including cases of preeclampsia and eclampsia
- Perioperative prevention of acute pressure increases in perioperative and postoperative phases
- Congestive heart failure

Hypertensive Crises

Four controlled studies considered 75 patients affected by hypertensive crises or by severe hypertension.

Two studies,[58, 59] conducted in a single-blind manner so that the initial administration of placebo was followed by the administration of 25 mg of urapidil, documented that urapidil is more effective than placebo.

A crossover randomized study involving 10 patients showed that the antihypertensive effect of urapidil (0.5 to 1.5 mg/min) is comparable with that of sodium nitroprusside (40 to 120 mg/min).[60] No significant differences were found between the efficacy of urapidil boluses and diazoxide boluses.[61]

The results of six noncontrolled studies[62–67] confirm that either bolus injection or continuous infusion of urapidil significantly reduces blood pressure.

Dame et al.[68] proved that intravenously administered urapidil significantly lowers arterial pressure in patients affected by preeclampsia and eclampsia, even when there is no response to dihydralazine treatment. No negative effect was observed on the fetus or the mother.

Congestive Heart Failure

In four open clinical trials, urapidil was administered intravenously to a total of 41 patients with severe congestive heart failure (classes II through IV of the New York Heart Association).[69–72] These studies document a reduction in both mean pulmonary arterial pressure and pulmonary vascular resistance. Furthermore, urapidil did not affect either myocardial oxygen consumption or myocardial lactate extraction.[70, 71]

Preoperative and Postoperative Control and Prevention of Acute Pressure Increases

Sixteen studies, nine controlled and seven uncontrolled, involving more than 600 patients have assessed the efficacy of urapidil in the prevention or control of perioperative and postoperative hypertension during various surgical interventions.[30, 73–87]

Urapidil has been shown to be more effective than placebo[73] or no treatment[74] in prevention of pressure increases during general and regional anesthetic procedures.

Furthermore, comparative studies with sodium nitroprusside,[32, 75, 76] phentolamine,[77] clonidine,[78] nifedipine and nitroglycerin,[79] and isradipine[80] proved that urapidil has the same efficacy in the control of pressure increases but, unlike several of the reference drugs, did not cause tachycardia.

ADVERSE DRUG REACTIONS

At dosages usually given for the control of hypertension, urapidil appears to be well tolerated.

In short-term (2 to 12 weeks), double-blind, comparative studies[42–53] involving more than 700 patients, the frequency of reported adverse reactions ranged between 0% and 38% in patients receiving urapidil. The incidence of side effects in patients treated with reference drugs was similar, ranging from 0% (acebutolol, metoprolol + butizide) to 44% (α-methyldopa). The most frequent symptoms were dizziness, nausea, headache, fatigue, and palpitations.

In an open, uncontrolled, multicenter trial conducted in Germany,[40] more than 900 patients were treated for 1 year with urapidil (30 to 90 mg b.i.d).

Side effects were mild, transient, and similar to those reported in the other studies, including mainly dizziness (5.5%), nausea (3.4%), headache (2.5%), and fatigue (1.4%).

Safety assessment during both uncontrolled and comparative studies has also included regular monitoring of the main laboratory values. No clinically relevant urapidil-induced abnormalities have been identified.

There is no evidence that urapidil causes a first-dose hypotension, as currently experienced with prazosin.

CONTRAINDICATIONS

Urapidil should not be administered orally to pregnant or nursing women, because clinical experience in human subjects is still inadequate in this respect; animal experiments revealed no teratogenicity.

Urapidil should not be used intravenously in patients with aortic isthmus stenosis or arteriovenous shunt.

DRUG INTERACTIONS

No clinically relevant interactions with other drugs have been observed for urapidil. Concomitant administration of other antihypertensive drugs or alcohol may cause hypotension.

CONCLUSION

The clinical efficacy of urapidil is well established. In the management of hypertension, the efficacy of urapidil is comparable with that of other antihypertensive agents. However, unlike other drugs, urapidil produces its pharmacologic effect without altering heart rate, cardiac output, and renal function. Additionally, urapidil appears to have favorable interactive effects with known cardiovascular risk factors, such as left ventricular hypertrophy, carbohydrate intolerance, and dislipidemia. These characteristics, combined with an acceptable safety profile, show that urapidil offers important clinical benefits in the treatment of hypertension.

REFERENCES

1. Gillis RA, Dretchen KL, Namath I, et al: Hypotensive effect of urapidil: CNS site and relative contribution. J Cardiovasc Pharmacol 9:103, 1987.
2. Kolassa N, Beller KD, Sanders KH: Involvement of brain 5-HT$_{1A}$ receptors in the hypotensive response to urapidil. Am J Cardiol 64:7D, 1989.
3. van Zwieten PA: Pharmacodynamic backgrounds to the antihypertensive activity of and adverse reactions to urapidil. London: Royal Society of Medicine Services, 1992, pp 13–20.
4. Zech K, Steinijans VW, Radtke HW: Pharmacokinetics of urapidil in normal subjects. In Amery A (ed): Treatment of Hypertension with Urapidil. London: Royal Society of Medicine Services, 1986, pp 29–38.
5. Kirsten R, Nelson K, Volker V, et al: Clinical pharmacokinetics of urapidil. Clin Pharmacokinet 14:129, 1988.
6. Michel JP, Hessel L, Zech K, et al: Pharmacokinetics and phar-

macodynamics of urapidil in the elderly. *In* Amery A (ed): Treatment of Hypertension with Urapidil. London: Royal Society of Medicine Services, 1986, pp 39–46.

7. Bories P, Ampelas M, Bauret P, et al: The pharmacokinetics of Urapidil in liver impairment. *In* Amery A (ed): Treatment of Hypertension with Urapidil. London: Royal Society of Medicine Services, 1986, pp 53–56.

8. Godehardt E, Wambach G, Heitz W, et al: Pharmacokinetics of urapidil in patients with normal and impaired renal function. *In* Amery A (ed): Treatment of Hypertension with Urapidil. London: Royal Society of Medicine Services, 1986, pp 71–86.

9. Zitta S, Holzer H, Zech K, et al: Pharmacokinetics of urapidil in patients with impaired renal function. Drugs 40(Suppl 4):67, 1990.

10. Slingeneyer A, Mourad G, Zech K, et al: Pharmacokinetics of urapidil in end stage renal failure. *In* Amery A (ed): Treatment of Hypertension with Urapidil. London: Royal Society of Medicine Services, 1986, pp 57–62.

11. de Leeuw PW, van Es PN, de Bruyn HAM, et al: Renal haemodynamic and neurohumoral responses to urapidil in hypertensive man. Drugs 35(Suppl 6):74, 1988.

12. Magometschnigg D, Bacher S: Acute haemodynamic responses to single intravenous doses of urapidil in essential hypertensive patients. *In* Amery A (ed): Treatment of Hypertension with Urapidil. London: Royal Society of Medicine Services, 1986, pp 47–52.

13. Kirsten R, Nelson K, Neff J, et al: Pharmacodynamics and pharmacokinetics of three different doses of urapidil infused in hypertensive patients. Eur J Clin Pharmacol 30:549, 1986.

14. Wambach G, Godehardt E, Lang R, et al: Pharmacodynamics of urapidil in essential hypertension and in chronic renal failure. *In* Amery A (ed): Treatment of Hypertension with Urapidil. London: Royal Society of Medicine Services, 1986, pp 63–70.

15. Levenson J, Simon AC, Bouthier JD, et al: Postsynaptic alpha-blockade and brachial artery compliance in essential hypertension. J Hypertens 2:37, 1984.

16. Leonetti G, Terzoli L, Rupoli L, et al: Effects of intravenous urapidil on blood pressure, renal plasma flow and responsiveness to vasoconstrictor agents in hypertensive patients. *In* Amery A (ed): Treatment of Hypertension with Urapidil. London: Royal Society of Medicine Services, 1986, pp 11–18.

17. Culbertson VL, Bryant PJ, Cady WJ, et al: Acute effects of increasing doses of urapidil in patients with hypertension. Clin Pharmacol Ther 39:690, 1986.

18. Belz GG, Matthews JH, Graf D, et al: Dynamic responses to intravenous urapidil and dihydralazine in normal subjects. Clin Pharmacol Ther 37:48, 1985.

19. Messerli FH, Kobrin I, Amodeo C, et al: Immediate cardiovascular effects of urapidil in essential hypertension. *In* Amery A (ed): Treatment of Hypertension with Urapidil. London: Royal Society of Medicine Services, 1986, pp 87–91.

20. Lepage JY, Pinaud M, Hélias J, et al: Effects of urapidil on right and left ventricular functions. *In* van Zwieten PA (ed): Central and Peripheral Sympathetic Mechanisms in Hypertension: Pathophysiological and Therapeutic Aspects: Focus on Urapidil. London: Royal Society of Medicine Services, 1992, pp 29–34.

21. Moore N, Fresel J, Joannides R, et al: Compared hemodynamic effects of urapidil, prazosin and clonidine in healthy volunteers. Blood Pressure 3(Suppl 4):31, 1994.

22. Grassi G, Mancia G, Zanchetti A: Comparison of the hemodynamic and neurohumoral effects of urapidil and prazosin in patients with mild to moderate essential hypertension. Blood Pressure 3(Suppl 4):13, 1994.

23. Grassi G, Parati G, Pomidossi G, et al: Neural control of circulation before and after intravenous urapidil in essential hypertension. Drugs 35(Suppl 6):104, 1988.

24. Leonetti G, Terzoli L, Zanchetti A: Systemic haemodynamic and humoral changes during urapidil treatment in hypertensive patients. J Hypertens 6(Suppl 2):S25, 1988.

25. Trimarco B, Ricciardelli B, Cuocolo A, et al: Effects of one year of antihypertensive treatment with urapidil on left ventricular haemodynamics and anatomy. *In* Amery A (ed): Treatment of Hypertension with Urapidil. London: Royal Society of Medicine Services, 1986, pp 101–110.

26. Guffanti E, Vaccarella A, Mazzola C, et al: M-Mode echocardiographic evaluation of haemodynamic effects of urapidil. *In* Amery A (ed): Treatment of Hypertension with Urapidil. London: Royal Society of Medicine Services, 1986, pp 93–100.

27. Genovesi-Ebert A, Marabotti C, Palombo C, et al: Effect of a new multifactorial antihypertensive on heart morphology and function in mild to moderate essential arterial hypertension. Eur Heart J 13(Suppl A):45, 1992.

28. Sheiban I, Arosio E, Tonni S, et al: Favourable haemodynamic effects of a new multifactorial antihypertensive on left ventricular dimension, wall thickness and function in hypertensive patients. Eur Heart J 13(Suppl A):37, 1992.

29. Feldstein CA, Olivieri AO, Porto-Sabarls R: Comparison between the effects of urapidil and methyldopa on left ventricular hypertrophy and haemodynamics in humans. Drugs 35(Suppl 6):90, 1988.

30. Downer J, Williams DJM, Major E, et al: Urapidil in the treatment of hypertension: A comparison with sodium nitroprusside following coronary artery bypass surgery. *In* Amery A (ed): Treatment of Hypertension with Urapidil. London: Royal Society of Medicine Services, 1986, pp 115–119.

31. Hirata Y, Hayakawa H, Suzuki E, et al: Renal and endocrine effects of urapidil in patients with essential hypertension. Curr Ther Res 49:961, 1991.

32. Pattenier JW, von Heusinger FC: Effects of urapidil treatment on lipid metabolism in patients with hypertension. *In* van Zwieten PA (ed): Central and Peripheral Sympathetic Mechanisms in Hypertension: Pathophysiological and Therapeutic Aspects: Focus on Urapidil. London: Royal Society of Medicine Services, 1992, pp 61–66.

33. Fariello R, Boni E, Corda L, et al: Influence of a new multifactorial antihypertensive on blood pressure and metabolic profile in essential hypertension associated with non-insulin-dependent diabetes mellitus. Eur Heart J 13(Suppl A):65, 1992.

34. Goto Y: Effects of sustained-release urapidil on essential hypertension and hyperlipidemia: A multicenter clinical trial. Curr Ther Res 51:870, 1992.

35. Kobrin I, Amodeo C, Ventura HO, et al: Immediate hemodynamic effects of urapidil in patients with essential hypertension. Am J Cardiol 55:722, 1985.

36. Gerber A, Weidmann P, Marone C, et al: Cardiovascular and metabolic profile during intervention with urapidil in humans. Hypertension 7:963, 1985.

37. Exaire E, Chàvez HM, Pérez A, et al: Effects of chronic urapidil treatment on renal function. International Symposium on Urapidil, Recife, Brazil, 1987.

38. Liebau H, Solleder P, Harden I, et al: Drei Jahre Therapie mit Urapidil. Offene multizentrische prospektive Prufung zur Verträglichkeit, Sicherheit und Wirksamkeit von Urapidil. Byk Gulden Pharmaceuticals, Research Report 323, 1988.

39. Härlin R, Engelstätter R, Henze F, et al: Treatment of primary and secondary hypertension. Long-term use of urapidil (Ebrantil). Clin Trials J 22:215, 1985.

40. von Jendralski AH, Planz G, Kindler J, et al: Effect of urapidil (Ebrantil) on plasma catecholamines in essential hypertension. Nieren- und Hochdruckkrankheiten 15:313, 1986.

41. Volpe M, Trimarco B, Rosiello G, et al: Antihypertensive effect of urapidil: A randomized, double-blind study in mild or moderate hypertensive patients. *In* Amery A (ed): Treatment of Hypertension with Urapidil. London: Royal Society of Medicine Services, 1986, pp 135–142.

42. Rosendorff C: Urapidil in the treatment of hypertension. Drugs 35(Suppl 6):188, 1988.

43. Tzincoca C, Levenson J, Petitet A, et al: Therapeutic assessment of acebutolol and urapidil in essential hypertension under double-blind conditions. Curr Ther Res 38:579, 1985.

44. Leonetti G, Mazzola C, Boni S, et al: Comparison of the antihypertensive effect of urapidil and metoprolol in hypertension. Eur J Clin Pharmacol 30:637, 1986.

45. Schäfer N: Doppelblindstudie einen vergleichenden antihypertensiven Behandlung mit Urapidil gegen eine Kombination von Metilpranolol und Butizid. *In* Kaufman W, Bruckschen EG (eds): Urapidil: Darstellung einer neuen antihypertensiven Substanz. Amsterdam: Excerpta Medica, 1982, pp 243–250.

46. Török E, Wagner M, Podmaniczky M: Comparison of urapidil and atenolol in hypertension. Drugs 35(Suppl 6):164, 1988.

47. Fariello R, Dal Palù C, Pessina A, et al: Antihypertensive efficacy of urapidil versus hydrochlorothiazide alone in patients with mild to moderate essential hypertension and of their combination in nonresponders to monotherapy. Drugs 40(Suppl 4):60, 1990.

48. Distler A, Härlin R, Hilgenstock G, et al: Clinical aspects of antihypertensive therapy with urapidil: Comparison with hydrochlorothiazide. Drugs 40(Suppl 4):21, 1990.

49. Stumpe E, Feldhaus P, Harlin R: Antihypertensive Wirksamkeit und Verträglichkeit von Urapidil. Fortschr Med 107:54, 1989.

50. Winn K: Klinische Erfahrungen mit Urapidil und Nitrendipin. In Ganten D, Hayduk K, Hitzenberger G (eds): Beitrage zur Hypertonie: Klinische Aspekte der modernen Hochdruckbehandlung. Frankfurt am Main: Universimed, 1988, pp 50–53.

51. Eisel K, Härlin R: Double-blind, parallel group study with urapidil and clonidine in 20 patients with essential hypertension (grade III–IV). Byk Gulden Pharmaceuticals, Research Report 489, 1979.

52. Kaneko Y and the Urapidil Study Group in Japan: Double-blind comparison of urapidil and prazosin in the treatment of patients with essential hypertension. Drugs 35(Suppl 6):156, 1988.

53. Rosenthal J, Härlin R: Therapeutic assessment of urapidil or angiotensin-converting enzyme inhibition in systemic hypertension. Am J Cardiol 64:25D, 1989.

54. Meurer KA: Efficacy, tolerability and therapeutic spectrum of the antihypertensive agent urapidil (Ebrantil) in daily practice. Therapiewoche 36:4005, 1986.

55. Kaneko Y, Yasuda H, Yoshinaga K, et al: Experience with urapidil in Japan: Results of a multicentre open study in hypertensive patients. In Amery A (ed): Treatment of Hypertension with Urapidil. London: Royal Society of Medicine Services, 1986, pp 155–164.

56. Bauknecht C, Pattenier J: Urapidil in Kombination mit ACE-Hemmern. Der Allgemeinarzt 3:180, 1993.

57. Bauknecht C, Grass U: Hypertoniebehandlung und Glucosestoffwechsel. Der Karsewarzt 49:43, 1994.

58. Di Perri D: Efficacy of urapidil i.v. in patients with severe hypertension. Byk Gulden Pharmaceuticals, External Report 347E, 1987.

59. Serra P: Efficacy of urapidil i.v. in patients with severe hypertension. Byk Gulden Pharmaceuticals, External Report 384E, 1987.

60. Rosenthal J: Urapidil versus sodium nitroprusside in 10 patients with primary and secondary hypertension. Byk Gulden Pharmaceuticals, Internal Research Report RR 370, 1979.

61. Vrhovac B, Rumboldt Z, Gasparovic V: Single-blind comparative study of urapidil and diazoxide in the treatment of malignant hypertension of hypertensive crises. In Proceedings of the 10th Scientific Meeting of the International Society of Hypertension, Interlaken, 1984, pp 899–900.

62. Gless KH, Cram M, Helmstädter V: The effect on intravenously administered urapidil on blood pressure in patients with seriously increased blood pressure. Therapiewoche 28:6266, 1978.

63. Schuster P, Sturm A: Use of antihypertensive Ebrantil in hypertensive crises. Klinikarzt 10:202, 1981.

64. Zähringer J, Klepzig M, Greif J, et al: Treatment of hypertensive emergencies with urapidil: Varying responses in patients with and without coronary heart disease. Fortschr Med 22:624, 1984.

65. Thuma G: Urapidil as basic therapeutic agent in the treatment of severe hypertension. Fortschr Med 22:457, 1986.

66. Giuntoli F, Gabbani S, Natali A, et al: Treatment of hypertensive emergencies with urapidil. Curr Ther Res 49:296, 1991.

67. Späh F, Grosser KD, Thieme G: Acute haemodynamic effects of urapidil and nifedipine in hypertensive urgencies and emergencies. Drugs 40(Suppl 4):58, 1990.

68. Dame WR, Burkart W, van Aken H, et al: Treatment of pregnancy-induced hypertension by a new antihypertensive agent: urapidil. In Amery A (ed): Treatment of Hypertension with Urapidil. London: Royal Society of Medicine Services, 1986, pp 121–126.

69. Tebbe U, Sciagra R, Scholz KH, et al: Acute effects of urapidil in patients with severe heart failure. Z Kardiol 74(Suppl 5):29, 1985.

70. Metcalfe JM, Smyth P, Monaghan MM, et al: Urapidil in the treatment of congestive cardiac failure. In Amery A (ed): Treatment of Hypertension with Urapidil. London: Royal Society of Medicine Services, 1986, pp 111–114.

71. Wang RYC, Chow JSF, Chan KH, et al: Acute haemodynamic and myocardial metabolic effects of intravenous urapidil in severe heart failure. Eur Heart J 5:745, 1984.

72. Reiterer W: Longterm effects of urapidil on exercise haemodynamics in patients with hypertension and left heart failure. 11th Scientific Meeting of the International Society of Hypertension, Heidelberg, August 31–September 7, 1986.

73. Quéré JF, Ozier Y, Bringier J, et al: Does urapidil attenuate the blood pressure response to tracheal intubation for general anaesthesia? Drugs 40(Suppl 4):80, 1990.

74. Lehmann KA, Heimig Th: Circulatory response to urapidil (Ebrantil) during general and regional anesthesia: A study with normo- or hypertensive patients. Anaesthesist 34:435, 1985.

75. Junger H, van Deyk K, Kopp M: Hemodynamics during antihypertensive therapy with urapidil and sodium nitroprusside. In Kaufmann W, Bruckschen EG (eds): Urapidil: Darstellung einer neuen antihypertensiven Substanz. Amsterdam: Excerpta Medica, 1982, pp 199–146.

76. van der Stroom JG, van Wezel HB, Vroom MB, et al: Comparison of the effect of urapidil and sodium nitroprusside on hemodynamics and myocardial function in hypertensive patients recovering from coronary artery surgery. Anesthesiology 77:A126, 1992.

77. Hess W, Schulte-Sasse U, Tarnow J, et al: Comparison of phentolamine and urapidil in controlling acute intraoperative hypertension in patients subjected to coronary artery bypass surgery. Eur J Anaesth 2:21, 1985.

78. Hess W: Urapidil versus clonidine: Acute haemodynamic effects during control of intraoperative hypertensive episodes. Drugs 40(Suppl 4):77, 1990.

79. Möllhof T, van Aken H, Mulier JP, et al: Effects of urapidil, ketanserin and sodium nitroprusside on venous admixture and arterial oxygenation following coronary artery bypass grafting. Br J Anaesth 64:493, 1990.

80. Samain E, Philip I, Marti J, et al: Comparison of the hemodynamic effects of isradipine and urapidil used for the treatment of sternotomy induced hypertension. Anesthesiology 77:A113, 1992.

81. Francke N, Schmucker P, van Ackern K, et al: Antihypertensive treatment with urapidil during anaesthesia. Therapiewoche 30:880, 1980.

82. Francke N, Schmucker P, Vogel H, et al: Changes in haemodynamics and myocardial oxygen consumption during intraoperative blood pressure reduction with urapidil. In Kaufmann W, Bruckschen EG (eds): Urapidil: Darstellung einer neuen antihypertensiven Substanz. Amsterdam: Excerpta Medica, 1982, pp 113–118.

83. Barankay A, Goeb E, Richter JA: Treatment of hypertension in coronary bypass surgery clinical experience with urapidil. Arzneimittelforschung 31:849, 1981.

84. Alvarez CB: Urapidil i.v. in reactive hypertension during aorto-coronary bypass surgery. Byk Gulden Pharmaceuticals, External Research Report 465E, 1984.

85. Marty J, Pansard Y, Lancon JP: Urapidil for the treatment of sternotomy induced hypertension. Anaesthesiology 73:A88, 1990.

86. Fontana F, Allaria B, Brunetti B, et al: Cardiac and circulatory response to the intravenous administration of urapidil during general anaesthesia. Drugs Exp Clin Res 16:315, 1990.

87. Le Bret F, Vrints Y, Daas G, et al: Treatment of postoperative hypertensive attacks with urapidil in coronary patients: Effects on cardiac function evaluated by transesophageal echocardiography. Ann Fr Anaesth Reanim Suppl 9:R103, 1990.

CHAPTER 72

Doxazosin

Joel M. Neutel, M.D., Stanley H. Taylor, M.D., David H. G. Smith, M.D., Michael A. Weber, M.D., and Franz C. Aepfelbacher, M.D.

HISTORY

Drugs that inhibit sympathoadrenal stimulation of α-adrenoreceptors can be credited with opening two new therapeutic eras in the treatment of cardiovascular disorders. In the late 1940s, they were among the first compounds to receive serious consideration as antihypertensive agents.[1] In 1971, they ushered in a new and lasting era in the treatment of heart failure.[2] In both instances, phentolamine was the drug used initially, but a number of other chemically unrelated compounds with similar pharmacologic activity were later developed. However, all these early compounds were nonselective, blocking both presynaptic and postsynaptic α-adrenoreceptors, which resulted in many undesirable hemodynamic and symptomatic side effects and precluded their further development. Clinical interest in the therapeutic potential of this class of drugs has been reawakened during the past decade by major advances in knowledge of the mechanisms underlying adrenergic transmission and, in particular, by the recognition of pharmacologically distinct adrenoreceptor subtypes.[3] A natural pharmaceutical progression has been the development of more selective antagonists such as doxazosin that concentrate their activity at postsynaptic α₁-adrenoreceptor sites. A number of reviews of doxazosin with extensive bibliography have been published.[4, 5]

CHEMISTRY AND METABOLISM

Doxazosin [1-(4-amino-6,7-dimethoxy-2-quinazolinyl)-4-(1, 4-benzodioxan-2-ylcarbonyl)-piperazine monomethanesulphonate] is a water-soluble quinazoline derivative of prazosin (Fig. 72–1).

After oral ingestion in humans, absorbed doxazosin

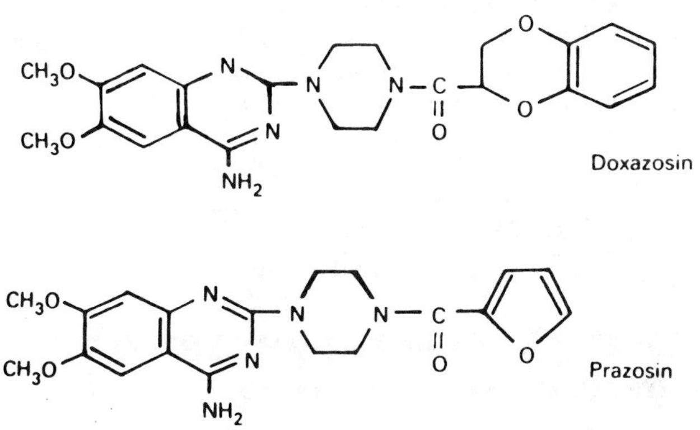

Figure 72–1. Comparison of the chemical structures of doxazosin and prazosin.

is subject to extensive biotransformation in the liver. The major routes of metabolism involve O-demethylation of the quinazoline side chain (23%) or C-hydroxylation of the benzdioxane moiety (12%; Fig. 72–2).[6–8] Both metabolites are pharmacologically inert.

PHARMACOLOGY

The selective α₁-antagonists prazosin and terazosin are well established for use in clinical practice. Doxazosin, which has a long plasma half-life that facilitates its once-daily administration,[7] is the most recently available drug in this class. Studies of its site of action indicate its selectivity for postjunctional α₁-receptors. These receptors, situated at intrajunctional locations,[9] are primary mediators of the pressor effects of norepinephrine. Doxazosin may also have antihypertensive effects beyond its blockade of sympathetically mediated vasoconstriction. In rabbit aorta preparations, it enhances the anticontractile efficacy of the endothelium-derived relaxing factor (EDRF) released by other mechanisms. It also has the ability to inhibit tissue growth in arterial structures,[10] which may reduce vascular tone.

PHARMACOKINETICS

The pharmacokinetic characteristics of doxazosin have been described for both the intravenous and oral routes of administration in numerous studies involving both young and elderly normotensive volunteers.[6, 7, 11–14] Extensive pharmacokinetic studies have also been carried out in hypertensive patients after both single and incremental doses[15] and after sustained administration.[16, 17] The pharmacokinetics of the drug have been studied in normotensive patients with renal failure[11] and in hypertensive patients with renal insufficiency.[18] From these studies, a comprehensive picture of the pharmacokinetic profile of doxazosin has been established. Details of the many pharmacokinetic studies carried out with doxazosin have been detailed by Young and Brogden.[4]

Doxazosin is well absorbed after oral administration. In normotensive young volunteers, bioavailability of the drug ranged from 62% to 69%.[6, 12, 13] A similar level of bioavailability has also been found in elderly patients.[6, 14]

In normotensive healthy volunteers, a single oral dose of 1 mg of doxazosin resulted in a mean peak plasma concentration of 8 μg/L within 3.6 hours of ingestion.[19] In hypertensive patients treated with doxazosin for 4 or more weeks, mean peak plasma con-

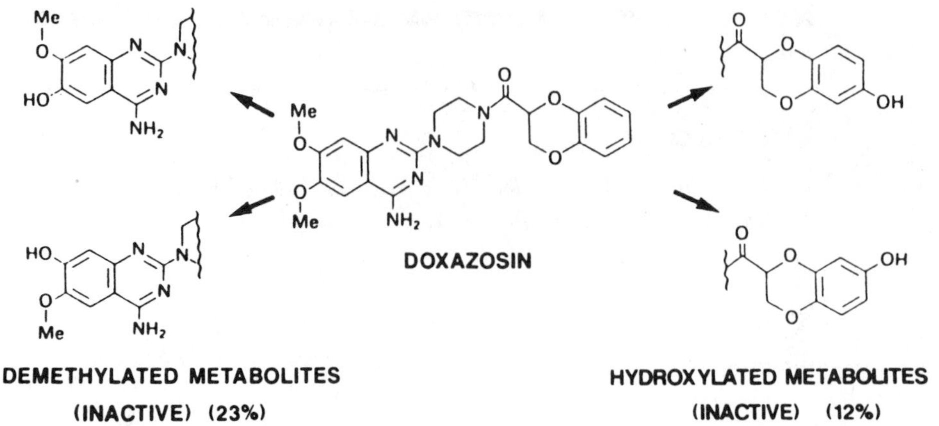

Figure 72–2. Major metabolic pathways of metabolism for doxazosin in humans. (From Elliott HL, Meredith PA, Vincent J, et al: Clinical pharmacological studies with doxazosin. Br J Clin Pharmacol 21:275, 1986.)

centrations of 150 µg/L were observed within 3 hours of administration of a single 16 mg oral dose.[16]

Doxazosin has a relatively long plasma concentration half-life. Early studies with the drug in normal volunteers appeared to show a plasma concentration half-life of between 9 and 13 hours after a single oral or intravenous dose.[6, 11, 12, 14] However, the calculated half-life in these early studies was based on a relatively short sampling period, and more recent studies indicate that the plasma concentration half-life of the drug measured during steady-state administration in hypertensive patients is between 19[15] and 22 hours.[20] The elimination half-life of doxazosin does not appear to be influenced by age[6, 14] or renal dysfunction.[11, 18]

After oral ingestion, the peak plasma concentration of doxazosin was achieved within 2 or 3 hours, irrespective of the size of dose administered.[16, 19] The peak plasma concentration increased proportionally with doubling doses of the drug between 1 and 16 mg in hypertensive patients.[15, 16] After sustained administration of the drug, the plasma concentrations and area under the plasma concentration time curve were significantly greater than after single oral doses. The degree of doxazosin accumulation was consistent with its extended plasma concentration half-life.[15] The drug is rapidly and nearly completely bound to plasma protein, regardless of the dose administered.[7] This quality accounts for its retention in the plasma during hemodialysis in patients with renal insufficiency.[11]

The apparent volume of distribution of the drug was found to be somewhat greater in elderly than in younger normotensive volunteers; this effect is probably related to the reduced lean body mass of the former.[6] The tissue distribution of doxazosin has not been studied in humans.

In humans, some 5% of the oral doxazosin dose administered is eliminated unchanged in the feces, and 5% of unchanged drug is excreted in the urine. Approximately 65% of the drug is eliminated as metabolites in the feces.[7] The plasma clearance of doxazosin by the liver is significantly less than that by hepatic blood flow.[21] This quality is a major factor

contributing to the relatively long plasma half-life of doxazosin. The total clearance of doxazosin is slightly greater in elderly patients than in young subjects. However, because the volume of distribution is also greater in the elderly, plasma drug concentrations after similar doses are of a comparable order in the young and old.[6]

The relationship between the plasma concentration of the drug and its pharmacodynamic activity is complex. In single-dose studies, the decrease in blood pressure after either intravenous or oral administration of doxazosin occurred some hours later than the achievement of the peak plasma drug concentration.[11, 13] However, during sustained administration, a relatively simple linear relationship develops between the plasma concentration of doxazosin and its antihypertensive effects.[16]

PHARMACODYNAMICS

On a weight-for-weight basis, doxazosin is about half as potent as prazosin in blocking postsynaptic α_1-adrenoreceptors in animals[22, 23] and in humans.[24, 25] Although the major pharmacodynamic and circulatory effects of doxazosin are direct consequences of its blockade of postsynaptic α_1-adrenoreceptors in the peripheral vasculature, some part of its activity may be due to inhibition of α_1-adrenoreceptors located in the central nervous system.[26]

Studies on isolated animal tissues such as the rabbit pulmonary artery and guinea pig ileum have demonstrated the very high degree of selectivity of doxazosin for α_1- as opposed to α_2-adrenoreceptors.[27] Confirmation of the postsynaptic α_1-adrenoreceptor blocking activity of doxazosin is provided by the attenuation of the vasoconstrictive effect of catecholamines on the forearm blood vessels in humans.[28]

EFFECTS ON PATHOPHYSIOLOGY
Effects on Hemodynamics

The antihypertensive efficacy of selective α-adrenergic blockers has been well established. Much early experience has been gained with terazosin[29] as well as prazosin. Large-scale clinical trials with prazosin indicated that its effects were maintained during long-term therapy[30, 31] and its efficacy was equivalent to that of the β-blocker atenolol.[31] It also had an efficacy comparable to that of the angiotensin-converting enzyme (ACE) inhibitor enalapril, although a crossover study found that patients tended to respond preferentially to either one drug or the other.[32] This suggests that the α-antagonist and the ACE inhibitor acted through different mechanisms and that each may be appropriate for different types of individual patterns.

Hemodynamic studies have confirmed the expected effects of α_1-blockade. The antihypertensive action of doxazosin is associated with a clear reduction in the total peripheral resistance index, whereas cardiac output remains essentially unaffected.[8] Doxazosin significantly reduces blood pressure in both the supine and seated positions, and also during 100-watt exercise. Yet, the drug does do not diminish the appropriate increases in systolic blood pressure and heart rate during exercise, thereby preserving exercise tolerance. In view of the frequency of renal insufficiency in patients with hypertension, it is also noteworthy that α-blockers such as doxazosin do not have adverse effects on renal function and are effective in patients with chronic renal failure.[33]

Effects on Ventricular Function and Structure

Changes in the function and structure of the left ventricle have become a topic of interest in hypertension. There is evidence that inherited differences in diastolic function[34] and left ventricular muscle mass[35] can actually precede the appearance of clinically increased blood pressure. Echocardiographic evidence of left ventricular hypertrophy occurs in as many as 50% of hypertensive patients[36] and markedly worsens the cardiovascular prognosis.[37] Factors such as increased activity of the sympathetic nervous system[38, 39] or renin-angiotensin system may produce these left ventricular changes through direct myocardial effects independent of changes in blood pressure. The sympathetic nervous system may therefore be a primary underlying mediator of these changes in left ventricular mass.

Treatment with drugs that block either the sympathetic nervous system or the renin-angiotensin system can produce regression of left ventricular hypertrophy.[40] It should be recognized, however, that the desirability of regression of left ventricular hypertrophy has yet to be fully established in clinical hypertension.

Several clinical studies have demonstrated that doxazosin can induce regression of left ventricular hypertrophy in patients with mild to moderate essential hypertension.[41–43] After 12 to 24 weeks of treatment, left ventricular mass was significantly decreased by 7% to 17%, and these changes were usually accompanied by preserved systolic and significantly improved diastolic function. Thus, doxazosin exhibits favorable effects on left ventricular structure and function similar to those seen with ACE inhibitors and calcium antagonists.

Effect on the Vascular System

Arteries are affected early in the course of hypertension. Arterial compliance, a measure of elasticity of distensibility of these vessels is significantly lower in patients with borderline or established hypertension than in normal volunteers.[44] This effect applies to small distal arteries as well as to the major vessels. The decrease in compliance is independent of the aging process and tends to be more marked in some individuals, including those with normal blood pressures, than in those with a family history of hypertension.[45]

Treatment with differing antihypertensive agents can improve arterial compliance. Clinical studies of the effects of doxazosin on compliance will be of great interest, especially because long-term treatment with this drug in the spontaneously hypertensive rat significantly inhibits collagen synthesis in vascular tissue, independent of the effects of the drug on blood pressure.[10]

Additional animal studies have revealed other mechanisms by which doxazosin may modify atherosclerosis. Thus, for example, the drug not only decreases plasma lipid concentrations but markedly inhibits the number and size of foam cells in the vascular walls of hyperlipidemic hamsters and reduces the area of stainable fatty streaks in the aorta of these animals.[46] It is not entirely clear whether the marked inhibition of foam cells in these studies was due to the suppressive effects of doxazosin on lipids or whether the drug had a direct effect in the vascular wall. However, other studies have shown that lower doses of doxazosin decrease the size of fatty streaks without changing lipid levels, whereas high doses continue to limit the streak area even when the drug effect on the plasma lipid concentration has reached a plateau.[47] One possible explanation of this effect could be linked to oxidized low-density lipoprotein (LDL), which promotes monocyte chemotaxis and the formation of foam cells from macrophages and stimulates local vascular growth factors. The potential antioxidant effects of drugs and their potential clinical effects are yet to be defined.

A further action of doxazosin is its inhibition of platelet interaction with the vascular endothelium. This effect appears to be related to the drug inhibition of adenosine diphosphate (ADP) or epinephrine-mediated platelet aggregation produced in human platelet-rich plasma.[48] Indeed platelet disaggregation can occur in the presence of higher doses of doxazosin.[49] Moreover, doxazosin has been shown to have a stimulatory action on tissue-type plasminogen activator (t-PA) in human subjects,[50] thus providing an added mechanism by which this drug could inhibit coagulation mechanisms. Of interest in this regard is recent work demonstrating that changes in coagulation factors may be an intrinsic characteristic of hypertension.[51] These preliminary studies, done largely in experimental animal models, indicate that doxazosin can directly affect the structure and function of arterial tissue and may also inhibit atherosclerotic and coagulation processes. These basic findings, together with the observations in human subjects, may reflect a direct tissue effect of doxazosin or may alternatively result from the actions on such vascular risk factors as high blood pressure and lipid abnormalities. Although these early data are interesting, they must be regarded as speculative. Clearly, there is no specific primary indication for doxazosin or other drugs of this class in preventing the vascular changes associated with hypertension.

Effect on Lipid Metabolism

There is now wide clinical experience showing the beneficial effects of α-antagonists on the plasma lipid profile. These drug-induced changes are generally of modest amplitude, and it would be inappropriate to prescribe these agents primarily for the treatment of lipid disorders. However, when compared with other commonly used classes of antihypertensive agents, specifically the diuretics and β-blockers, the α-antagonists are associated with significantly better lipid values. It has been argued that the adverse effects of such agents as diuretics on lipids may only be transitory, but careful comparative studies that have gone beyond a year of observation have indicated that these differential drug effects appear to last indefinitely. One long-term comparative study of prazosin and hydrochlorothiazide, for example, showed that the two agents had similar antihypertensive effects, but that after more than a year of treatment, the plasma concentrations of total cholesterol and traditional triglycerides were significantly lower with the α-antagonists than with the diuretic.[52] The 1-year report of data from the large-scale Treatment of Mild Hypertension Study (TOMHS) has shown similar significant advantages for doxazosin as compared with a diuretic, especially in the high-density lipoprotein (HDL) cholesterol/total cholesterol ratio.[53]

Studies have demonstrated that doxazosin decreases total cholesterol levels, decreases triglyceride concentrations, and increases the HDL/total cholesterol ratio.[54] These changes, although not large, are consistent from one study to another. The mechanisms by which doxazosin produces effects on lipids have been examined primarily in animal models. In the cholesterol-fed golden hamster treated with doxazosin for 8 weeks, there was a significant reduction in hepatic content of cholesterol and triglycerides.[55] This constituted a reduction of approximately 40% in the synthesis of cholesterol and in 3-hydroxy-3-methylglutaryl-coenzyme A (HMG-CoA) reductase activity. Studies of cultured human skin fibroblasts, in which doxazosin was found to increase the activity of low-density lipoprotein (LDL) receptors,[56] suggests a possible explanation for these findings. Moreover, further studies of the effect of doxazosin on cholesterol synthesis have indicated that this agent pro-

duces a dose-dependent increase in the binding of radiolabeled LDL cholesterol to hepatic LDL receptors, a finding that is associated with the dose-dependent decrease in cholesterol synthesis.[57]

However, doxazosin appears to reduce cholesterol synthesis independently of its effects on the binding of LDL cholesterol to hepatic receptors. Thus, it clearly reduces the production of cholesterol in fibroblasts that lack LDL receptors.[57] This finding has led to the hypothesis that doxazosin directly inhibits hepatic cholesterol synthesis, which in turn leads to an upregulation of hepatic LDL receptors. Subsequently, there is an increase in cholesterol clearance from the blood, with a resulting decrease in plasma cholesterol concentrations.[57] Additionally, doxazosin increases lipoprotein lipase activity in adipose tissue and also increases the activity of hepatic lipase.[58, 59]

Abnormalities in insulin metabolism, resulting in hyperinsulinemia, are commonly associated with lipid abnormalities observed in hypertension. It is not clear whether the state of insulin resistance directly provokes lipid abnormalities or whether the changes in both insulin and lipid levels result from an increase in sympathetic drive. This latter supposition is consistent with the observation that α-antagonists appear to reduce plasma concentrations of both LDL cholesterol and insulin.

Increased cholesterol concentrations can amplify the vascular reactivity to pressor substances.[60–62] Through this mechanism, the effects of doxazosin on cholesterol could actually contribute to its antihypertensive properties and also have antiatherogenic effects.[63] It has been reported that chronic stress in animals can accelerate the formation of atherosclerotic lesions.[64] Because these changes are presumably mediated by enhanced sympathetic activity, they could theoretically be inhibited by α-adrenergic blockade. It should be emphasized, however, that the effects of α-antagonists on either sympathetic mechanisms or lipids have not been shown to directly influence vascular pathology in human subjects.

Effects on Insulin and Glucose Metabolism

Both type I and type II diabetes mellitus often coexist with hypertension. This is especially true of type II diabetes in middle-aged and elderly patients. Given this, it is clearly desirable that antihypertensive agents not adversely affect glucose metabolism. α-Antagonists have been shown not to significantly alter glucose tolerance or plasma insulin concentrations during long-term therapy in patients with non-insulin-dependent diabetes mellitus.[65]

In a study comparing doxazosin with atenolol in patients with non-insulin-dependent diabetes mellitus, it is evident that doxazosin does not significantly alter either glucose or hemoglobin A1 concentrations. Both of these parameters are slightly but significantly increased by the β-blockers.[66]

Other studies have not only confirmed these findings[67] but have also suggested that long-term therapy with doxazosin can slightly decrease plasma concentrations of glucose and insulin.[68]

Treatment with doxazosin significantly ameliorates the lipid abnormalities characteristically observed with type II diabetes.[68, 69] These findings are consistent with the relationship between hyperinsulinemia and lipid abnormalities. If human subjects are divided into those with higher and lower plasma concentrations of insulin, those with the higher values are characterized by increased plasma concentrations of triglycerides and LDL cholesterol, whereas HDL cholesterol is decreased in this group.[70] Studies in the OB/OB mouse, which like human hypertensive patients is characterized by insulin resistance, have shown that doxazosin inhibits the stimulatory effects of insulin on plasma triglyceride concentrations.[71] Sympathetic mechanisms may therefore mediate the effect of insulin on triglycerides via α_1-receptors. The beneficial effects of doxazosin on the lipid profile may also be partly mediated by the effects of the drug on insulin.

A key study in human hypertensive subjects has examined the effect of prazosin on daily plasma insulin concentrations. In this study, it is evident that α-blocker therapy significantly reduces plasma insulin concentrations in a manner that is sustained throughout the day.[72] This is accompanied by decreased fasting concentrations of triglycerides and total cholesterol. In contrast, β-blockers appear to worsen the insulin resistance of hypertension,[73] perhaps explaining the tendency of these agents to have unwanted effects on glucose and lipid metabolism.

CLINICAL USE
Treatment of Hypertension

In patients with uncomplicated essential hypertension, the blood pressure–lowering activity of doxazosin is due solely to the relaxation of the concentrically constricted arteriolar resistance vessels throughout the systemic circulation. This antihypertensive effect of the drug is not offset by reflex cardiac stimulation. Thus, the only detectable change induced by the drug in the hemodynamic profile of a hypertensive patient is a reduction in systemic blood pressure and vascular resistance; heart rate and cardiac output remain unchanged.[8] These changes, measured in 14 patients, persisted during dynamic exercise and were not attenuated during extended treatment with oral doxazosin (2 to 16 mg OD) for 1 year.

A variety of studies indicate that the efficacy of doxazosin is closely similar to that of diuretics,[74] β-blockers,[16] other α-antagonists,[75] and ACE inhibitors.[76] Moreover, doxazosin was found to be as effective in black as in white patients and to work as well in older patients as in younger patients. It is also effective as monotherapy or in combination with other agents.[77]

Another important issue in the efficacy of antihypertensive drugs is their ability to maintain antihypertensive effects during the rapid increase in blood pressure that occurs during the early to mid-morning hours, indicating 24-hour efficacy. This increase seems to depend primarily on activity of the sympathetic nervous system (SNS) and is characterized by an increase in α-adrenergic drive. It also may contribute to the increased incidence of adverse cardiovascular events including myocardial ischemia or infarction[78, 79] and stroke[80, 81] that have been documented during this early morning period. Drugs that antagonize the rapid increase in sympathetic activity during these morning hours may therefore be potentially helpful in reducing the frequency of cardiovascular events. Studies indicate that doxazosin maintains its efficacy throughout the full 24-hour period of the day, with the greatest effect occurring during the important early morning hours.[82] However, there are no data to indicate whether this antihypertensive effect of the drug actually provides protection against cardiac or cerebrovascular events.

Consequences of the antihypertensive activity of a drug on the quality of life and everyday functioning of patients are clearly important. It has been shown that in elderly patients, prazosin, despite its clear antihypertensive effects, does not affect cerebral blood flow.[83] In careful studies of cognitive function and psychomotor performance in a large group of young to middle-aged men, prazosin also tended to be associated with better outcomes than those observed with either propranolol or hydrochlorothiazide.[84] Additionally, early studies with prazosin indicated its safety in patients with chronic lung disease or asthma.[85] More recently, doxazosin was found to be useful in patients with airways disease; in fact, measurements of forced expiratory volume during the first second (FEV_1) were, if anything, slightly improved.[86] The α-blockers also do not seem to adversely affect male sexual function; in comparison with hydrochlorothiazide, patients taking prazosin were less likely to complain of a reduction in libido and also less likely to experience problems in maintaining penile rigidity.[87]

Another key issue for many hypertensive patients is exercise tolerance. As indicated, the α-antagonists should not have any adverse effects on exercise capacity. In a study of hypertensive male joggers, prazosin was found not to limit performance. This was in clear contrast to a β-blocker, which decreased both the duration of exercise and maximal oxygen uptake.[88] Not surprisingly, the majority of patients preferred treatment with prazosin over that with the β-blockers. More recent studies with doxazosin have confirmed its lack of adverse effect on exercise tolerance.[89] α-Antagonists such as prazosin, although effective, lost favor among physicians because of its relatively common adverse side effect profile. However, newer-generation α-antagonists such as doxazosin that are taken once a day and maintain constant blood levels of drug are extremely well tolerated and have many fewer side effects than those seen with prazosin.

Treatment of Heart Failure

α-Antagonists ushered in a new approach to the treatment of heart failure nearly two decades ago.[2] Their hemodynamic benefits in this situation are now beyond doubt. Prazosin, the forerunner of the modern generation of selective α_1-adrenoreceptor blocking drugs, has been demonstrated to induce marked hemodynamic benefits in both acute and chronic heart failure. Doxazosin has not been extensively explored in this respect. An initial study in patients with congestive heart failure suggests that oral doxazosin may increase exercise tolerance and may extend survival.[90] Intravenous doxazosin has also been demonstrated to reverse rapidly the abnormal hemodynamic profiles of patients with acute left ventricular failure complicating myocardial infarction.[91] The slow absorption of the drug and the absence of first-dose postural effects enhance its clinical applicability in patients in heart failure, but its specific role in such patients should be established by further studies.

Treatment of Benign Prostatic Hyperplasia

The function and distribution of adrenergic receptors in the lower urinary tract form the rationale for the use of α-antagonists in the treatment of benign prostatic hyperplasia (BPH). The smooth muscle tone in the male bladder neck area, proximal urethra, prostatic capsule, and edematous tissue is mediated primarily by α_1-adrenoceptors, and by blocking these receptors a reduction of obstructive symptoms can be achieved.

Recently, a number of studies have confirmed the beneficial effects of doxazosin in patients with BPH.[92, 93] In a double-blind, placebo-controlled study,[94] patients treated with 4 mg doxazosin once daily for 9 weeks reported a significant improvement of voiding difficulties and frequency, as compared with the control group, and there was a trend toward an improved maximum urinary flow rate. When this study was extended to 29 weeks,[95] the improvement, both in obstructive and irritative symptoms, was even more marked as compared with week 9. Another double-blind study demonstrated significantly increased mean urinary flow rate and decreased voiding pressure after 12 weeks of therapy with doxazosin, resulting in marked improvements in hesitancy, frequency, nocturia, and urgency.[96] Adverse effects, most frequently dizziness, headache, and fatigue, were usually mild and transient, and there were no discernible adverse effects of doxazosin on sexual function. In addition, a recent study suggests that evening dosing does not diminish efficacy, yet may enhance toleration of doxazosin.[97] Treatment of normotensive patients with doxazosin resulted in minor, clinically nonsignificant reduction of blood pressure.[98] Although more complete data on long-term treatment have to be awaited, these data indicate that doxazosin could become a valuable new treatment option for the many patients with mild to moderate BPH, particularly for those who require pharmacologic therapy for hypertension.

SAFETY AND SIDE EFFECT PROFILE

Many studies have reported on the safety and side effect profile of doxazosin during chronic treatment of hypertensive patients.[99-103] The incidence of reported side effects in doxazosin-treated patients has depended on the number of patients studied and the method of reporting. The total incidence of adverse reactions in doxazosin-treated hypertensive patients has ranged from 0% to 75%, but, generally, side effects have been mild and rarely have necessitated stopping treatment.

Monitoring of side effects in 1548 hypertensive patients during long-term treatment with oral doxazosin demonstrated no predilection for any organ system.[5]

Most adverse reactions that have been reported during long-term treatment with doxazosin could be attributed to the direct pharmacologic activity of the drug. These effects include occasional postural dizziness, lethargy and fatigue, fluid retention, blurred vision, and dry mouth. Other symptoms reported during monitoring studies are common to most antihypertensive drugs and include such symptoms as headache, sedation, abdominal discomfort, and constipation.

When compared with the incidence of side effects reported from double-blind comparison trials with other antihypertensive drugs, no substantial differences were observed among placebo, prazosin, hydrochlorothiazide, or the β-blocking drugs atenolol, nadolol, and metoprolol (NDA data; Fig. 72–3).[5]

SUMMARY

Doxazosin is a highly selective α_1-antagonist that is well absorbed and that has a long duration of pharmacodynamic action after oral ingestion. Its major pharmacodynamic sites of direct circulatory activity are the systemic arteriolar resistance vessels and those of the venous capacitance system, particularly in regional circulations with extensive α-adrenoreceptor populations. The indirect effects of such a vascular relaxation reduce cardiac preload and afterload, ventricular wall stress, and myocardial oxygen consumption, particularly in the absence of reflex cardiac stimulation. Changes in the blood lipid profile associated with the long-term administration of doxazosin enhance its primary prevention potential in the hypertensive patient by augmenting the reduction in coronary heart disease risk profile. The therapeutic efficacy of doxazosin in the treatment of patients with high blood pressure has been confirmed in many studies irrespective of the severity of the hypertension, age and race of the patient, or the presence of renal impairment or diabetes mellitus. Several studies attest to efficacy and safety of doxazosin for the treatment of benign prostatic hypertrophy. Doxazosin's side effect profile shows no predilection for any particular organ system and is not substantially different from that experienced with other commonly used antihypertensive drugs. Therefore, doxazosin and other selective α_1-antagonists represent an important

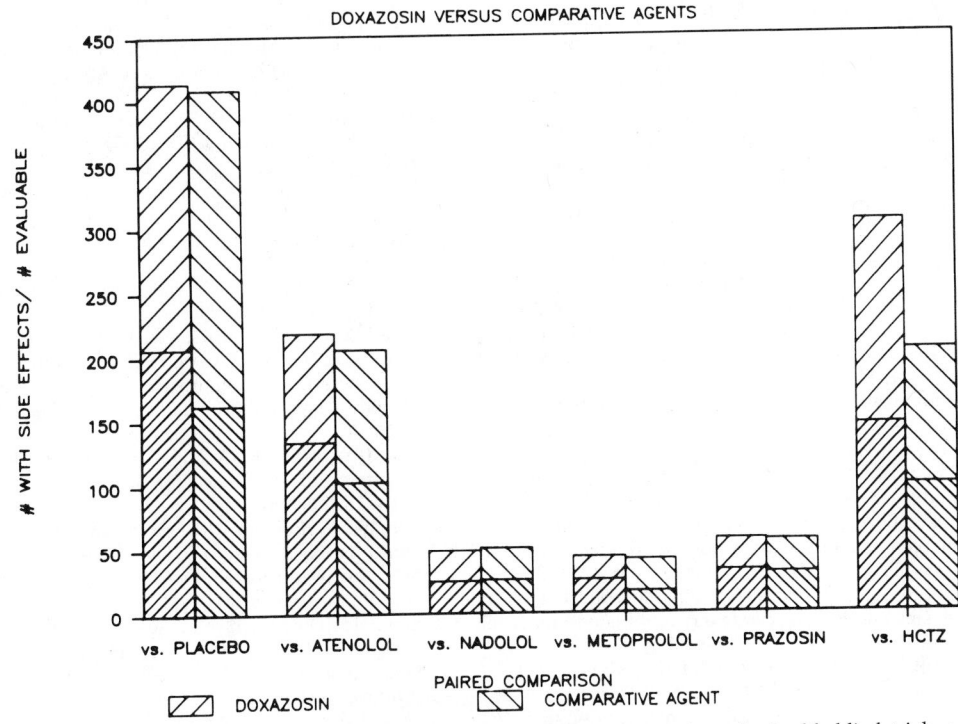

Figure 72–3. The comparative incidence of side effects experienced by hypertensive patients in double-blind trials of doxazosin versus placebo, atenolol, nadolol, metoprolol, prazosin, and hydrochlorothiazide (HCTZ). (Data from Taylor SH: Pharmacotherapeutic stature of doxazosin and its role in coronary risk reduction. Am Heart J 116[Suppl]:173S, 1988.)

first-line treatment for the management of essential hypertension.

REFERENCES

1. Taylor SH, Gould LA (eds): Phentolamine in Heart Failure and Other Cardiac Disorders. Bern: Hans Huber, 1976.
2. Majid PA, Sharma B, Taylor SH: Phentolamine for vasodilator treatment of severe heart failure. Lancet 2:719, 1971.
3. Davey M: Mechanism of alpha blockade for blood pressure control. Am J Cardiol 59:18G, 1987.
4. Young RA, Brogden RN: Doxazosin: A review of its pharmacological properties and therapeutic efficacy in mild or moderate hypertension. Drugs 35:525, 1988.
5. Taylor SH: Pharmacotherapeutic stature of doxazosin and its role in coronary risk reduction. Am Heart J 116(Suppl):173S, 1988.
6. Elliott HL, Meredith PA, Vincent J, et al: Clinical pharmacological studies with doxazosin. Br J Clin Pharmacol 21:27S, 1986.
7. Kaye B, Cussans NJ, Faulkner JK, et al: The metabolism and kinetics of doxazosin in man, mouse, rat and dog. Br J Clin Pharmacol 21:19S, 1986.
8. Lund-Johansen P, Omvik P, Haugland H: Acute and chronic haemodynamic effects of doxazosin in hypertension at rest and during exercise. Br J Clin Pharmacol 21:45S, 1986.
9. Van Brummelen P, Jie K, Van Zwieten PA: α-Adrenergic receptors in human blood vessels. Br J Clin Pharmacol 21:33S, 1986.
10. Chichester CO, Rodgers RL: Effects of doxazosin on vascular collagen synthesis, arterial pressure and serum lipids in the spontaneously hypertensive rat. J Cardiovasc Pharmacol 190(Suppl 9):S21, 1987.
11. Carlsson RV, Bailey RR, Begg EJ, et al: Pharmacokinetics and effect on blood pressure of doxazosin in normal subjects and patients with renal failure. Clin Pharmacol Ther 40:561, 1986.
12. Meredith PA, Elliott HL, Kelman AW, et al: Application of quinazoline alpha-adrenoceptor antagonists in normotensive volunteers. J Cardiovasc Pharmacol 7:532, 1985.
13. Vincent J, Elliott HL, Meredith PA, et al: Doxazosin, an alpha-1-adrenoceptor antagonist: Pharmacokinetics and concentration-effect relationships in man. Br J Clin Pharmacol 15:719, 1983.
14. Vincent J, Elliott HL, Meredith PA, et al: The pharmacokinetics of doxazosin in elderly normotensives. Br J Clin Pharmacol 21:521, 1986.
15. Cubeddu LX, Fuenmayor N, Caplan N, et al: Clinical pharmacology of doxazosin in patients with essential hypertension. Clin Pharmacol Therap 41:439, 1987.
16. Frick MH, Halttunen P, Himanen P, et al: A long-term double-blind comparison of doxazosin and atenolol in patients with mild to moderate essential hypertension. Br J Clin Pharmmacol 21:55S, 1986.
17. Shionoiri H, Yasua G, Uneda S, et al: Antihypertensive effects and pharmacokinetics after both single and consecutive administration of doxazosin [abstract 47A]. Presented at the 1st Annual Meeting of the American Society of Hypertension. May 29–30, 1986.
18. Bailey RR, Begg E, Carlson R, et al: Single-dose pharmacokinetics of doxazosin in healthy volunteers and patients with renal insufficiency. N Z Med J 98:248, 1985.
19. Rubin PC, Brunton J, Meredith PA: Determination of the vasodilator UK 33274 by HPLC using fluorescence detection. J Chromatogr 221:193, 1980.
20. Elliot HL, Meredith PA, Reid JL: Pharmacokinetic overview of doxazosin. Am J Cardiol 59:78G, 1987.
21. Greenway CV, Stark RD: Hepatic vascular bed. Physiol Rev 51:23, 1971.
22. Timmermans PBMWM, Kwa HY, Karmat AF, et al: Prazosin and its analogues UK-18,596 and UK-33,274: A comparative study on cardiovascular effects and alpha-adrenoceptor blocking activities. Arch Int Pharmacol Ther 245:218, 1980.
23. Timmermans PB, van Kemenade JE, Batink HD, van Zwieten PA: Selectivity of benzodioxane alpha-adrenoceptor antagonists for alpha-1 and alpha-2-adrenoceptors determined by binding affinity. Pharmacology 26:258, 1983.

24. Singleton W, Caxton CAPD, Hernandex J, et al: Postjunctional selectivity of alpha-blockade with prazosin, trimazosin and UK-33,274 in man. J Cardiovasc Pharmacol 4:S145, 1982.

25. De Leeuw PW, Ligthart JJ, Smout AJPM, et al: Within patient comparison of prazosin and UK-33,274. A new alpha-adrenoceptor-antagonist. Eur J Clin Pharmacol 23:397, 1982.

26. Ramage AG: A comparison of the effects of doxazosin and alfuzosin with those of urapidil on preganglionic sympathetic nerve activity in anaesthetised cats. Eur J Pharmacol 129:307, 1986.

27. Alabaster VA, Davey MJ: The α1-adrenoceptor antagonist profile of doxazosin: Preclinical pharmacology. Br J Clin Pharmacol 21:9S, 1986.

28. Jie K, Van Brummelen PP, Vermey P, et al: Identification of vascular postsynaptic alpha-1 and alpha-2 adrenoceptors in man. Circ Res 54:447, 1984.

29. Weber MA: Sympathetic nervous system and hypertension. Am J Hypertens 2:147S, 1989.

30. Komajda M: Prazosin and lipids. A multicenter study of the effects of prazosin on blood lipids in hypertensive patients. Am J Med 86(Suppl 1B):70, 1989.

31. Rouffy J, Jaillard J: Effects of two antihypertensive agents on lipids, lipoproteins and apoproteins A and B. Comparison of prazosin and atenolol. Am J Med 80(Suppl 2A):100, 1986.

32. Cheung DG, Gasster JL, Weber MA: Assessing the duration of the antihypertensive effects with whole-day automated blood pressure monitoring. Arch Intern Med 149:2021, 1989.

33. Anderton JL, Motghi A: An evaluation of the efficacy and safety of doxazosin in the treatment of hypertension associated with renal insufficiency. J Hum Hypertens 4(Suppl 3):52, 1990.

34. Graettinger WF, Weber MA, Gardin JM, Knoll ML: Diastolic blood pressure as a determinant of Doppler left ventricular filling indices in normotensive adolescents. J Am Coll Cardiol 10:1280, 1987.

35. Celentano A, Galderisis M, Garafalo M, et al: Blood pressure and cardiac morphology in young children of hypertensive subjects. J Hypertens 6(Suppl 4):S107, 1988.

36. Savage DD, Drayer JM, Henry WL, et al: Echocardiographic assessment of cardiac anatomy and function in hypertensive subjects. Circulation 59:623, 1979.

37. Levy D, Garrison RJ, Savage DD, et al: Prognostic implications of echocardiographically determined left ventricular mass in the Framingham Heart Study. N Engl J Med 322:1561, 1990.

38. Julius S, Li Y, Brant D, et al: Neurogenic pressor episodes fail to cause hypertension, but do induce cardiac hypertrophy. Hypertension 13:422, 1989.

39. Corea L, Ventivoglio M, Verdechia P, Motolese M: Plasma norepinephrine and left ventricular hypertrophy in systemic hypertension. Am J Cardiol 53:1299, 1984.

40. Weber MA, Drayer JIM, Baird WM: Echocardiographic evaluation of left ventricular hypertrophy. J Cardiovasc Pharmacol 8:S61, 1986.

41. Monsalve P, Vera O, Acuna FP, et al: Echocardiographic assessment of doxazosin on left ventricular mass in patients with essential hypertension. Am Heart J 121:356, 1991.

42. Corral JL, Lopez NC, Pecorelli A, et al: Doxazosin in the treatment of mild or moderate essential hypertension: An echocardiographic study. Am Heart J 121:352, 1991.

43. Agabiti-Rosei E, Muiesan ML, Rizzoni D, et al: Reduction of left ventricular hypertrophy after longterm antihypertensive treatment with doxazosin. J Hum Hypertens 6:9, 1992.

44. Weber MA, Smith DHG, Neutel JM, Graettinger WF: Arterial properties of early hypertension. J Human Hypertens 5:417, 1991.

45. Simon AC, Pithois-Merli I, Levenson J: Physiopharmacological approach to mechanical factors of hypertension in the atherosclerotic process. J Hum Hypertens 5(Suppl 1):15, 1991.

46. Kowala MC, Nicolosi RJ: Effect of doxazosin on plasma lipids and atherogenesis. A preliminary report. J Cardiovasc Pharmacol 13(Suppl 2):S45, 1989.

47. Foxal T, Shwaery GT, Stucchi AF, et al: Dose-related effects of doxazosin on plasma lipids and aortic fatty streak formation in the hypercholesterolemic hamster model. Am J Pathol 140:1357, 1992.

48. Hernandez R, Carvajal AR, Pajuelo JG, et al: The effect of doxazosin on platelet aggregation in normotensive subjects and patients with hypertension. An in vitro study. Am Heart J 121:389, 1991.

49. Nicolosi RJ, Weiner EJ: The effect of doxazosin on hemostasis in nonhuman primates. Third Cardura MoA Workshop Proceedings, Colorado Springs, CO, 1991.

50. Jansson JH, Johansson B, Boman K, Nilsson TK: Effects of doxazosin and atenolol on the fibrinolytic system in patients with hypertension and elevated serum cholesterol. Clin Pharmacol 40:321, 1991.

51. Smith DHG, Vaziri ND, Winer RL, et al: Interrelationship of blood pressure, arterial compliance and the hemostatic system. J Am Soc Nephrol 2:498, 1991.

52. Stamler R, Stamler J, Gosch FC, et al: Initial antihypertensive drug therapy: A comparison of alpha-blocker (prazosin) and diuretic (hydrochlorothiazide). Am J Med 86(Suppl 1B):24, 1989.

53. The Treatment of Mild Hypertension Research Group: The treatment of mild hypertension study. Arch Intern Med 151:1413, 1991.

54. Young RA, Brogden RN: Doxazosin. Drugs 35:525, 1988.

55. Jansen H, Birkenhager JC: The effects of doxazosin on hepatic lipid levels and metabolism in the golden hamster. J Cardiovasc Pharmacol 18:354, 1991.

56. Leren TP: Doxazosin increases low density lipoprotein receptor activity. Acta Pharmacol Toxicol (Copenh) 56:269, 1985.

57. D'Eletto RD, Javitt NB: Effect of doxazosin on cholesterol synthesis in cell culture. J Cardiovasc Pharmacol 13(Suppl 2):S1, 1989.

58. Jansen H, Lammers R, Baggen MG, Birkenhager JC: Effects of doxazosin on lipids, lipoprotein lipases, and cholesterol synthesis in the golden hamster. J Cardiovasc Pharmacol 13(Suppl 2):5, 1989.

59. Jansen H, Lammers R, Baggen MG, et al: Inhibition of hepatic cholesterol synthesis by the α1-adrenoceptor blocker doxazosin in the hypercholesterolemic golden hamster. Life Sci 44:103, 1989.

60. Rosendorff C, Hoffmann JIE, Verrier ED, et al: Cholesterol potentiates the coronary artery response to norepinephrine in anesthetized and conscious dogs. Circ Res 48:320, 1981.

61. Kawachi Y, Tomoike H, Maruoka Y, et al: Selective hypercontraction caused by ergonovine in the canine coronary artery under conditions of induced atherosclerosis. Circulation 69:441, 1984.

62. Bloom DS, Bomzon L, Rosendorff C, Kew MC: Renal blood flow in obstructive jaundice—an experimental study in baboons. Clin Exp Pharmacol Physiol 3:461, 1976.

63. Ohanian J, Nicolosi RJ, Vatner SF, et al: Altered adrenergic control in hypercholesterolemia. J Cardiovasc Pharmacol 19(Suppl 9):S11, 1987.

64. Ferrara LA, Marotta T, Rubba P, et al: Effects of α-adrenergic and β-adrenergic receptor blockade on lipid metabolism. Am J Med 80(Suppl 2A):104, 1986.

65. Maruyama H, Saruta T, Itoh H, et al: Effect of α-adrenergic blockade on blood pressure, glucose and lipid metabolism in hypertensive patients with non-insulin dependent diabetes mellitus. Am Heart J 121:1302, 1991.

66. Feher MD, Henderson AD, Wadsworth J, et al: Alpha-blocker therapy: A possible advance in the treatment of diabetic hypertension. Results of a crossover study of doxazosin and atenolol monotherapy in hypertensive non-insulin dependent diabetic subjects. J Hum Hypertens 4:571, 1990.

67. Levy P: Effects of prazosin on blood pressure and diabetic control in patients with type II diabetes mellitus and mild essential hypertension. Am J Med 86(Suppl 1B):59, 1989.

68. Lehtonen A, and the Finnish Multicenter Study Group: Lowered levels of serum insulin, glucose and cholesterol in hypertensive patients during treatment with doxazosin. Curr Ther Res 47:278, 1990.

69. Castrignano R, D'Angelo A, Pati T, et al: A single-blind study of doxazosin in the treatment of mild-to-moderate essential hypertensive patients with concomitant non-insulin-dependent diabetes mellitus. Am Heart J 116:1778, 1988.

70. Zavaroni I, Bonora E, Pagliara M, et al: Risk factors for coro-

nary artery disease in healthy persons with hyperinsulinemia and normal glucose tolerance. N Engl J Med 320:702, 1989.

71. Swindell AC, Valentine JJ: Interactions of doxazosin with insulin or glucagon in the ob/ob mouse. J Cardiovasc Pharmacol 13(Suppl 2):S20, 1989.

72. Swislocki ALM, Hoffman BB, Sheu WHH, et al: Effect of prazosin treatment on carbohydrate and lipoprotein metabolism in patients with hypertension. Am J Med 86(Suppl 1B):14, 1989.

73. Pollare T, Lithell H, Selinus I, Berne C: Sensitivity to insulin during treatment with atenolol and metoprolol: A randomised, double-blind study of effects on carbohydrate and lipoprotein metabolism in hypertensive patients. Br Med J 298:1152, 1989.

74. Cox DA, Leader JP, Milson JA, Singleton W: The antihypertensive effects of doxazosin. A clinical overview. Br J Clin Pharmacol 21:83S, 1986.

75. Torvik D, Madsbu HP: Multicentre 12-week double-blind comparison of doxazosin, prazosin and placebo in patients with mild to moderate essential hypertension. Br J Clin Pharmacol 21:69S, 1986.

76. Wessels F: Double-blind comparison of doxazosin and enalapril in patients with mild or moderate essential hypertension. Am Heart J 121:299, 1991.

77. Englert RG, Barlage U: The addition of doxazosin to the treatment regimen of patients with hypertension not adequately controlled by β-blockers. Am Heart J 121:311, 1991.

78. Mulcahy D, Keegan J, Cunningham D, et al: Circadian variation of total ischemic burden and its alteration with antianginal agents. Lancet 2:755, 1988.

79. Thompson DR, Blandford RL, Sutton TW, Marchant PR: Time of onset of chest pain in acute myocardial infarction. Int J Cardiol 7:139, 1985.

80. Tsementzis SA, Gill JS, Hitchcock ER, et al: Diurnal variation of and activity during the onset of stroke. Neurosurgery 17:901, 1985.

81. Marler JR, Prince TR, Clark FL, et al: Morning increase in onset of ischemic stroke. Stroke 20:473, 1989.

82. Pickering TP, et al: Personal communication.

83. Ram CVS, Meese R, Kaplan NM, et al: Antihypertensive therapy in the elderly. Effects on blood pressure and cerebral blood flow. Am J Med 82(Suppl 1A):53, 1987.

84. Lasser NL, Nash J, Lasser VI, et al: Effects of antihypertensive therapy on blood pressure control, cognition, and reactivity. A placebo-controlled comparison of prazosin, propranolol, and hydrochlorothiazide. Am J Med 86(Suppl 1B):98, 1989.

85. Chodosh S, Tuck J, Pizzuto D: Prazosin in hypertensive patients with chronic bronchitis and asthma. Am J Med 86(Suppl 1B):91, 1989.

86. Biernacki W: Doxazosin therapy in patients with chronic obstructive airways disease. J Human Hypertens 3:419, 1989.

87. Scharf MB, Mayleben DW: Comparative effects of prazosin and hydrochlorothiazide on sexual function in hypertensive men. Am J Med 86(Suppl 1B):110, 1989.

88. Thompson PD, Cullinane EM, Nugent AM, et al: Effects of atenolol or prazosin on maximal exercise performance in hypertensive joggers. Am J Med 86(Suppl 1B):104, 1989.

89. Gillin AG, Fletcher PJ, Horvath JS, et al: Comparison of doxazosin and atenolol in mild hypertension, and effects on exercise capacity, hemodynamics and left ventricular function. Am J Cardiol 63:950, 1989.

90. DiBianco R, Parker JO, Chakko S: Doxazosin for the treatment of chronic congestive heart failure: Results of a randomized double-blind and placebo-controlled study. Am Heart J 121(1 Pt 2):372, 1991.

91. Verma SP, Silke B, Taylor SH: Usefulness of doxazosin in acute myocardial infarction. (Unpublished observations.)

92. Kirby RS: Profile of doxazosin in the hypertensive man with benign prostatic hyperplasia. Br J Clin Prac [Symposium Supplement] 74:23, 1994.

93. Fawzy A, Sullivan J, Cook M, Gonzalez F: A multicenter sixteen-week double-blind placebo-controlled dose-response study using doxazosin tablets for the treatment of benign prostatic hyperplasia in patients with mild to moderate essential hypertension [abstract]. J Urol 149(Suppl A):323A, 1993.

94. Christensen MM, Bendix Holme J, Rasmussen PC, et al: Doxazosin treatment in patients with prostatic obstruction. A double-blind placebo-controlled study. Scand J Urol Nephrol 27:39, 1993.

95. Bendix Holme J, Christensen MM, Rasmussen PC, et al: 29-week doxazosin treatment in patients with symptomatic benign prostatic hyperplasia. A double-blind placebo-controlled study. Scand J Urol Nephrol 28:77, 1994.

96. Chapple CR, Carter P, Christmas TJ, et al: A three month double-blind study of doxazosin as treatment for benign prostatic bladder outlet obstruction. Br J Urol 74:50, 1994.

97. Kaplan SA, Soldo KA, Olsson CA: Effect of dosing regimen on efficacy and safety of doxazosin in normotensive men with symptomatic prostatism: A pilot study. Urology 44:348, 1994.

98. Kirby RS, Chapple CR, Christmas T: Doxazosin: Minimal blood pressure effects in normotensive BPH patients. J Urol 149(Suppl A):434A, 1993.

99. Hayduk K, Schneider HT: Antihypertensive effects of doxazosin in systemic hypertension and comparison with terazosin. Am J Cardiol 59:95G, 1987.

100. Ott P, Storm TL, Krussel LR, et al: Multicenter, double-blind comparison of doxazosin and atenolol in patients with mild to moderate hypertension. Am J Cardiol 59:73G, 1987.

101. Nash DT, Schonfeld G, Reeves RL, et al: A double-blind parallel trial to assess the efficacy of doxazosin, atenolol and placebo in patients with mild to moderate systemic hypertension. Am J Cardiol 59:87G, 1987.

102. van den Hogen ALCJ: Doxazosin in the treatment of mild and moderate essential hypertension in general medical practice. Am Heart J 116(Suppl):1757, 1988.

103. Rosenthal J: Clinical experience with doxazosin in general medical practice. Am Heart J 116(Suppl):1748, 1988.

VIII.

Angiotensin-Converting Enzyme Inhibitors

Editors: Victor Dzau and Hans R. Brunner

A. Principles and Practice of Angiotensin-Converting Enzyme Inhibitors

CHAPTER 73

Angiotensin-Converting Enzyme Inhibitors

Hans R. Brunner, M.D., Bernard Waeber, M.D., and Jürg Nussberger, M.D.

Angiotensin I, a decapeptide and main product of the interaction of the enzyme renin with its substrate, has no vasoconstrictive action per se. Renin secretion exerts a pressor effect only if angiotensin I is metabolized by the converting enzyme to the octapeptide pressor hormone angiotensin II. Accordingly, inhibition of this key intermediate enzyme provides a unique opportunity to block the complete renin-angiotensin cascade. This concept was appreciated when investigators found some components that specifically inhibited converting enzyme in the venom extract of the snake *Bothrops jararaca*.[1] Some of the polypeptides extracted from this snake venom were later synthesized[2] and used in early clinical investigation.[3, 4] Original work at the Squibb Institute in Princeton, New Jersey, led to the development of orally active potent inhibitors of angiotensin-converting enzyme (ACE).[5]

The availability of relatively specific antagonists of the renin-angiotensin system has had many important effects on modern cardiovascular medicine. First, the antagonists have provided a tool for exploring and later establishing the importance of the renin-angiotensin system in cardiovascular homeostasis. It is commonly known that the renin-angiotensin system is one of the key mechanisms involved in blood pressure regulation. It is already often forgotten that our understanding of the role of renin was acquired mainly from research based on the use of ACE inhibitors. Second, the long-term use of ACE inhibitors to treat hypertension (and congestive heart failure), which became possible only with these new orally active compounds, has provided results far exceeding the expectations of even the firmest believers in an important cardiovascular role of the renin-angiotensin

system. Although most ACE inhibitors are still only in the developmental state, the few that are generally available have already firmly established themselves as key parts of the armamentarium used to treat clinical hypertension.

APPROACHES TO INHIBITION OF THE RENIN-ANGIOTENSIN SYSTEM

The converting enzyme is not the only crossroad at which the renin-angiotensin system can be blocked. At least theoretically, other possibilities include inhibition of various steps leading to renin synthesis (including its activation from the prohormone), inhibition of renin release into the circulation, and the use of competitive antagonists masquerading as false substrates. This latter approach is under development, but orally active compounds are not yet available for clinical use.

Another approach to inhibit the renin-angiotensin effects is to prevent angiotensin II from reaching its receptor at different target organs. Indeed, the first clinically available inhibitors of the renin-angiotensin system were synthetic octapeptide analogues of angiotensin II, which operated on this principle.[6] By infusing these analogues, it has been possible specifically to inhibit the renin-angiotensin system in normotensive volunteers[7] and patients.[8-10] Because these compounds were polypeptides with relatively short half-lives, they had to be administered by continuous intravenous infusion. Furthermore, in addition to their antagonistic actions, they all had more or less evident agonistic, angiotensin II–like effects. For this reason, these analogues were rather limited as therapeutic agents. Nevertheless, these compounds allowed us to demonstrate for the first time that, at least in some hypertensive patients, the renin-angiotensin system may play an important role in sustaining elevated blood pressure and that blockade of this system may normalize blood pressure. In addition, the exquisite antihypertensive efficacy of a combination of inhibition of the renin-angiotensin system and sodium depletion by a diuretic has been demonstrated[9] (Fig. 73–1). Thus, these studies have provided the groundwork for subsequent broad clinical use of ACE inhibitors. They have also prompted the development of a nonpeptide, orally active angiotensin II antagonist, losartan, a compound lacking intrinsic agonistic property.[11] Long-term antagonism of the renin-angiotensin system with this agent seems to be effective and well tolerated in the management of hypertension and congestive heart failure.[12]

EFFECT ON THE RENIN-ANGIOTENSIN SYSTEM

The first ACE inhibitor to be used in humans was teprotide.[2, 3] This compound is a nonapeptide that is

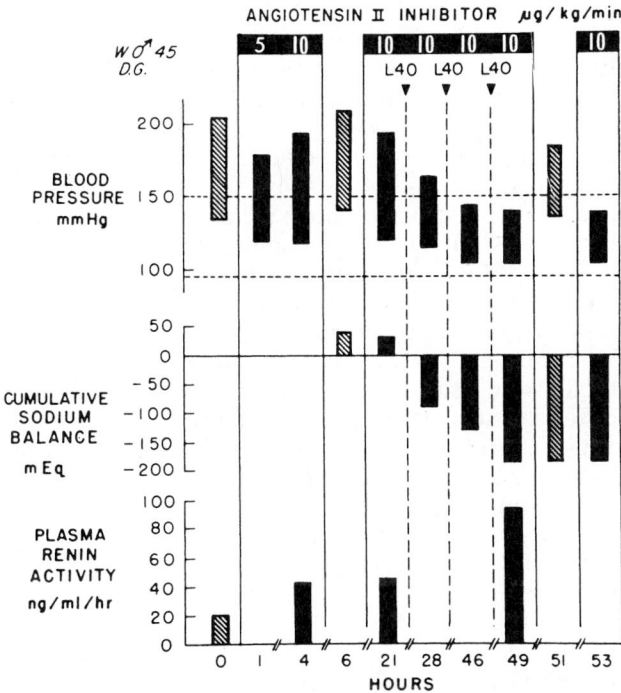

ANGIOTENSIN II BLOCKADE IN A PATIENT WITH BILATERAL RENAL ARTERY STENOSIS

Additive effect of sodium depletion on blood pressure reduction

Figure 73–1. Blood pressure reductions induced by angiotensin II blockade and concomitant salt depletion in a patient with hypertension. L40 indicates the administration of furosemide, 40 mg IV. The angiotensin II inhibitor (saralasin) alone reduced blood pressure insufficiently, and concomitant sodium depletion was necessary to control blood pressure. Even after salt depletion, discontinuation of angiotensin II blockade induces a rapid rise in blood pressure, presumably due to the very high plasma renin activity. (Reproduced with permission from Brunner HR, Gavras H, Laragh JH, et al: Hypertension in man: Exposure of the renin and sodium components using angiotensin II blockade. Circ Res 34, 35[Suppl I]:35, 1974. Copyright 1974, American Heart Association.)

effective only when administered parenterally. Numerous orally active inhibitors were subsequently developed.[5, 13] Captopril and enalapril have been studied most extensively. Captopril has a fast onset of action and can block ACE activity maximally within 15 to 30 minutes after oral administration, but it has a short plasma half-life (2 hours).[14] Unlike captopril, enalapril has a delayed onset of action. With this agent, maximal inhibition of ACE activity is achieved within 2 to 4 hours.[15, 16] Enalapril maleate, the form used for oral administration, must be hydrolyzed to its active diacid form, enalaprilat, after intestinal absorption. The plasma half-life of enalaprilat (11 hours) is much longer than that of captopril.

There are several ways to evaluate the potential for a drug to inhibit ACE activity. One way is to demonstrate blockade of the pressor response to exogenous angiotensin I. This method provides direct evidence of the efficacy of any ACE inhibitor but has the disadvantage that pharmacologic doses of angiotensin I must be injected. A more convenient way is to measure plasma ACE activity.[17] In the case of captopril, enzyme activity must be determined immediately after drawing blood because, *in vitro*, the captopril-ACE complex tends to dissociate, which may lead to underestimation of the extent to which ACE is inhibited.[18] ACE in the endothelium, not circulating ACE, is responsible for the bulk of the conversion of angiotensin I to angiotensin II;[19] thus, its activity should be corroborated by simultaneous determinations of plasma angiotensin II. Plasma angiotensin II can be determined reliably, but the assay remains laborious, because potentially interfering cross-reacting precursors and metabolites and *in vitro* production of angiotensin II have to be taken into account[20–22] (Fig. 73–2).

Role of Angiotensin II

In an individual hypertensive patient, it is difficult to assess the precise role of angiotensin II in maintaining high blood pressure by stimulating receptors of vascular smooth muscle cells. A given level of circulating angiotensin II may indeed cause different degrees of blood vessel contraction. For example, increasing total body sodium is known to enhance blood pressure responsiveness to this peptide.[23] Vascular hyperreactivity to angiotensin II is also present in hypertensive patients in whom blood vessels have undergone structural changes.[24] On the other hand, it is possible that a vasodilating prostaglandin, such as prostacyclin synthesized in the vascular wall,[25, 26] blunts the pressor effect of angiotensin II.[27] A similar modulating action might be exerted by circulating bradykinin.[28, 29]

One would expect that ACE inhibition would cause a fall in blood pressure proportional to the activity of the renin-angiotensin system. Indeed, the magnitude of the initial blood pressure reduction induced by ACE inhibitors is related to pretreatment plasma renin activity and levels of plasma angiotensin II.[30–34] However, with long-term therapy, the relationship between the fall in blood pressure and the pretreatment

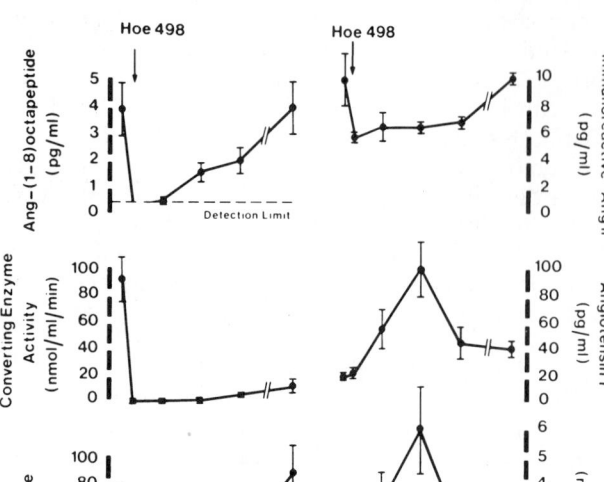

Acute ACE-Inhibition by Hoechst 498 in Normal Volunteers

Mean ± SEM n = 4

Figure 73–2. Response of the renin-angiotensin-aldosterone system to short-term ACE inhibition with a single oral dose of ramipril (HOE 498, 10 or 20 mg) in four normal volunteers. Ang-(1–8) octapeptide (true angiotensin II) virtually disappeared from plasma, whereas immunoreactive angiotensin II decreased by only 44%. PRA, plasma renin activity. (Reproduced with permission from Nussberger J, Brunner DB, Waeber B, et al: True versus immunoreactive angiotensin II in human plasma. Hypertension 7[Suppl I]:1, 1985. Copyright 1985, American Heart Association.)

levels of renin and angiotensin II becomes weak.[34–36] In many patients, sustained ACE inhibition for several weeks lowers blood pressure gradually to levels beyond those achieved at the beginning of treatment. Therefore, renin profiling appears to be of relatively little practical value in predicting whether an ACE inhibitor is likely to normalize blood pressure in a particular patient.[37] Nevertheless, good responders to acute ACE inhibition tend to continue to respond well to long-term therapy.

Angiotensin II is a well-established stimulus of aldosterone secretion.[38, 39] Therefore, it is not surprising that the rate of aldosterone production is decreased during ACE inhibition.[31, 32, 40] This effect may be of great benefit to hypertensive patients. It favors natriuresis and consequently helps to prevent sodium retention when blood pressure is lowered. Indeed, in hypertensive patients, total body sodium content was found to be reduced after prolonged ACE inhibition.[41, 42] There has been some question as to whether aldosterone secretion depends on angiotensin II and therefore is reduced during long-term treatment.[43, 44] Closely studying plasma aldosterone and angiotensin II levels after long-term (2 years) ACE inhibition, investigators found that both parameters were still markedly reduced and that changes in these parameters were closely correlated.[45]

Long-term treatment of animals with captopril or enalapril has been reported to increase the concentration of ACE in serum and in the lungs.[46–48] Induction of ACE biosynthesis by captopril has been demonstrated in cultures of human endothelial cells.[49] ACE production also appears to be induced during long-term administration of captopril or enalapril in hypertensive patients.[50, 51] This adaptive increment in plasma ACE concentration passes completely unnoticed when ACE activity is measured unless the ACE inhibitor is removed in the test tube by dialysis or dilution. ACE activity remains inhibited during long-term treatment with captopril and enalapril.[45, 50, 51] Because ACE induction occurs mainly with repeated administration of an ACE inhibitor, evidence of increased ACE concentration proves that the drug has been taken consistently and not only on the day of the office visit. After withdrawal of therapy with an ACE inhibitor, ACE concentration in plasma returns to normal over a period of days or weeks.[50] No evidence suggests that the induction of ACE activity by its inhibitors has any harmful effect.

The concentration of enzymatically active renin rises during short- and long-term ACE inhibition.[30–32] This effect is thought to be due to interruption of feedback inhibition of renin release by angiotensin II.[52] The active form of renin represents only one part of the total amount of renin found in the circulation. Indeed, an inactive form of renin (prorenin) is considered the precursor of active renin.[53] Plasma concentration of total renin used to be assessed by measuring plasma renin activity after *in vitro* activation of prorenin. Inactive renin was calculated as the difference between total and active renin levels. Using this approach, it is possible to show that both active and inactive renin concentrations increase during ACE inhibition.[54–56] It became apparent, however, that the pattern of the changes in the two types of renin differed with time: active renin tends to increase more rapidly than inactive renin. These observations could be confirmed by direct quantitation of active and total renin, using monoclonal antibodies specific for different sites of the renin molecule.[57] The rise in angiotensin I resulting from ACE inhibition appears to be due to an enhanced release of active renin rather than to an accumulation of angiotensin I.[58] The renin response to ACE inhibition is blunted by β-adrenoreceptor blockade[59] as well as by cyclooxygenase inhibition.[60, 61]

EFFECT ON OTHER PRESSOR AND DEPRESSOR SYSTEMS

Elevated plasma vasopressin levels have been reported in patients with malignant and severe hypertension.[62, 63] In these patients, vasopressin secretion may be reduced during treatment with an ACE inhibitor.[64, 65] Whether this effect contributes to the antihypertensive action of ACE inhibition in these patients remains unclear. Furthermore, for most hypertensive patients who have apparently normal vasopressin levels, there is no evidence that ACE inhibition affects vasopressin release.

The plasma concentration of atrial natriuretic peptides is increased in some hypertensive patients.[66, 67] Synthetic atrial natriuretic peptides have recently been infused during ACE inhibition in hypertensive patients.[68] ACE inhibition seemed to enhance the natriuretic and diuretic effects, but not the blood pressure–lowering effect of the investigational peptide. In contrast, in normotensive volunteers, ACE inhibition attenuated the natriuresis induced by the atrial natriuretic peptide.[69]

Acute ACE inhibition with teprotide has been reported to increase prostaglandin levels in arterial blood of hypertensive patients.[70] Subsequent studies have provided similar findings, such as significant increases in plasma levels of prostaglandin E_2 (PGE$_2$) metabolites after treatment with a single oral dose of captopril. However, plasma levels of 6-keto-prostaglandin F_1-α (PGF$_1$-α), a stable metabolite of prostaglandin I_2, were not influenced by captopril 6-keto-prostaglandin F-α (PGF-α).[71, 72] In normotensive subjects, the peak blood pressure–lowering effect of captopril correlated well with the changes in plasma PGE$_2$ metabolites but not with the changes in plasma angiotensin II, which were not found to be reduced by the ACE inhibitor.[71] In one study of hypertensive patients, only those with elevated plasma concentrations of PGE$_2$ metabolites during long-term captopril treatment had lowered blood pressure.[73] However, in another investigation of hypertensive patients, no change in plasma prostaglandin levels could be detected during long-term treatment with captopril.[74]

Administration of the cyclooxygenase inhibitor indomethacin was shown to reduce the antihypertensive effect of captopril.[60, 72, 74, 75] When captopril and indomethacin are given together, the order of administration appears to be critical to the antihypertensive effect of the ACE inhibitor.[60] The blood pressure–lowering effect of captopril was attenuated in hypertensive patients pretreated with the cyclooxygenase inhibitor, whereas it was unaffected when captopril treatment preceded the administration of indomethacin. The results obtained with enalapril are less conclusive. Administration of a cyclooxygenase inhibitor was found by some[61] but not by others[76] to blunt the antihypertensive effect of this agent. In normal subjects, acute ACE inhibition with enalapril does not modify plasma levels of PGE$_2$ metabolites.[73] These observations raise the question of whether all ACE inhibitors are equal in terms of their action on prostaglandin metabolism. For instance, captopril but not enalapril has been shown to stimulate PGE$_2$ biosynthesis in a culture of renomedullary interstitial cells.[77] In this in vitro experiment, the tissues were exposed to drug concentrations comparable with those achieved in the plasma of humans. Captopril, unlike enalapril, contains a sulfhydryl group in its chemical structure. Whether this sulfhydryl group is responsible for activation of phospholipase A_2 must be clarified. It should be stressed, however, that even enala-

pril may affect prostaglandin production in vivo, because increased urinary excretion of 6-keto-PGF$_1$-α has been detected in hypertensive patients treated for several weeks with this compound.[76] Recently, a thromboxane A_2 synthetase inhibitor was administered with captopril.[78] This agent enhanced the fall in blood pressure, but the final blood pressure reached was not different whether captopril was administered with the thromboxane A_2 synthetase inhibitor or with placebo.

Prostaglandins are presumably involved in the regulation of extracellular fluid volume. Indeed, compelling evidence suggests that renal prostaglandins promote water and sodium excretion.[79] Prostaglandin-related mechanisms seem to participate in the regulation of renal perfusion and the distribution of intrarenal blood flow.[80] Renal prostaglandins are also known to antagonize the glomerular actions of angiotensin II[81] and the tubular effects of antidiuretic hormone.[82] Therefore, prostaglandins might theoretically be involved in the renal response to ACE inhibition. In hypertensive patients, cyclooxygenase inhibition by indomethacin administration for several days decreased urinary sodium and prostaglandin excretion.[75] Some investigators demonstrated that several weeks of treatment with captopril or enalapril had no effect on urinary excretion of 6-keto-PGF$_2$-α.[83] On the other hand, a selective increase in urinary PGE$_2$ was observed in hypertensive patients treated for a few days with captopril.[84] In these patients, the increases in urinary PGE$_2$ and sodium excretion were correlated significantly and positively. This finding is interesting, given that PGE$_2$ is believed to be the main prostaglandin synthesized in the kidney.[85]

The contribution of prostaglandins to the antihypertensive effect of ACE inhibitors still must be clarified. It should be remembered in this context that prostaglandins may be involved in the blood pressure–lowering effect of various drugs other than ACE inhibitors.[73]

The renin-angiotensin-aldosterone and the kallikrein-kinin systems are significantly interrelated. Most evident is the common pathway of angiotensin II generation and bradykinin inactivation. Mineralocorticoids constitute another link between the two hormonal systems. These salt-retaining steroids are known to increase release of renal kallikrein.[86, 87] Furthermore, the vasoconstrictive effect of angiotensin II seems to be opposed by bradykinin,[29] and both angiotensin II and bradykinin stimulate prostaglandin synthesis.[88–90] Finally, it is possible that kallikrein is involved in the activation of prorenin.[91, 92]

Whether ACE inhibition results in accumulation of bradykinin and whether such an accumulation might substantially contribute to the antihypertensive effect of ACE inhibitors is still debated. Some investigators have reported increases in circulating bradykinin during acute ACE inhibition with teprotide and captopril.[71, 93] In most studies, however, no consistent changes in circulating bradykinin could be detected during short- or long-term inhibition of the bradykinin-processing enzyme kininase II.[74, 94–96] Interestingly, a decrease in the number of bradykinin tissue receptors was observed after prolonged captopril administration.[95] The same investigators also demonstrated downregulation of these receptors by exogenous bradykinin. These results led to speculation that bradykinin may accumulate in tissues. Acute and long-term ACE inhibition enhances the vascular responses to exogenous bradykinin.[97, 98] The finding of an increased thickness of weals caused by intradermal injection of bradykinin during ACE inhibition is interesting in this respect, because it suggests reduced bradykinin inactivation.[99, 100]

Approaches other than measurement of circulating kinins have been used to explore the cardiovascular role of the kallikrein-kinin system during ACE inhibition. In hypertensive animals, specific antikinin antibodies acutely attenuated the antihypertensive effect of captopril,[101] whereas the use of competitive antagonists of bradykinin gave conflicting results.[102, 103] Other experiments do not substantiate a contribution of kinins to the blood pressure–lowering effect of ACE inhibition. For instance, ACE inhibition did not lower blood pressure in rats rendered hypertensive by an infusion of angiotensin II for more than 1 week.[104] Conversely, the concept that an accumulation of bradykinin may modulate the antihypertensive effect of ACE inhibitors was suggested by a study in which aprotinin, an inhibitor of serine proteases, was administered to patients treated with captopril and found to reverse part of the antihypertensive effect of the ACE inhibitor.[105]

The renal kallikrein-kinin system presumably participates in renal sodium handling.[106–108] In sodium-loaded animals, treatment with aprotinin reduced sodium excretion.[109] Urinary kallikrein is reduced by ACE inhibition,[60, 110] probably as a result of decreased levels of aldosterone. During acute ACE inhibition, urinary kinin excretion was increased without a concomitant change in circulating bradykinin.[70] Indeed, these authors observed a correlation between the blood pressure response to acute ACE inhibition and the simultaneous rise in urinary kinin excretion, whereas no significant relationship emerged between changes in blood pressure and in plasma bradykinin levels. However, captopril administered by other investigators for several days did not change urinary kinin levels.[60] Thus, whether the renal kallikrein-kinin system facilitates the natriuresis while ACE is inhibited remains speculative.

The sympathetic nervous system participates in the regulation of human cardiovascular function under resting conditions.[111] It is thought to be hyperactive in patients with high blood pressure.[112–114] Much has been learned over the past few years on interactions between the sympathetic nervous and angiotensin-renin systems.[115] The two systems influence one another: the activation of one amplifies the activity of the other.

One possible interplay between the sympathetic nervous and the renin-angiotensin systems occurs in the brain. Angiotensin II increases sympathetic efferent nerve activity when administered centrally.[116, 117] It is uncertain whether circulating angiotensin II gains access to the brain, for instance, through some areas such as the circumventricular organs, the area postrema, and the subfornical organ, which lack tight blood-brain barriers.[118, 119] Moreover, the possible effects of ACE inhibitors on the brain-renin-angiotensin system are ill-defined.[120] Some evidence suggests that captopril penetrates the blood-brain barrier in humans in sufficient amounts to inhibit ACE in cerebrospinal fluid.[121] Hence, at least theoretically, captopril might block ACE activity in areas of the brain involved in blood pressure regulation.

At the periphery, angiotensin II seems to interact with the sympathetic nervous system, both at prejunctional and at postjunctional receptors. It has been suggested that angiotensin II inhibits the reuptake of catecholamines.[122] One possibly significant action of angiotensin II is enhancement of norepinephrine release by terminal nerve endings.[123] Angiotensin II also potentiates the effect of norepinephrine postjunctionally.[124] In humans, a postsynaptic interaction between norepinephrine and angiotensin II has been demonstrated with regard to systolic but not diastolic blood pressure.[125] Finally, angiotensin II is a well-established mediator of epinephrine release from the adrenal medulla.[126]

The influence of ACE inhibitors on cardiovascular responses to sympathetic activation has been studied in animals and humans. Captopril has been shown experimentally to blunt the pressor effect of both sympathetic nerve stimulation[127–129] and α-adrenoreceptor stimulation with exogenous norepinephrine.[130–132] Captopril has been demonstrated to attenuate the blood pressure effect of norepinephrine in normal subjects,[133] but this observation has not been confirmed by others.[134] A reduced pressor effect of norepinephrine during captopril treatment was also demonstrated in hypertensive patients.[135, 136] This observation is of particular interest because hypertensive patients are expected to have enhanced cardiovascular pressor reactivity when compared with normotensive subjects.[137]

ACE inhibitors interfere minimally with circulatory reflexes in normotensive and hypertensive subjects.[138–144] However, no change in, a resetting of, a potentiation of, and an increased sensitivity of the baroreflex activity have been described with ACE inhibition.[141–144] In most hypertensive patients, the blood pressure and heart rate response to changes in posture is not impaired.[140, 145–148] Nevertheless, there is a risk of postural hypotension in excessively sodium-depleted patients and normotensive subjects.[7, 147] In hypertensive patients, a normal adaptive response of blood pressure to changes in body position seems to be better maintained during long-term[145, 146] than during acute ACE inhibition.[149] One possible explanation for this effect is an enhanced reflex sympathetic response to standing that develops during long-term ACE inhibition. The postural increase in plasma norepinephrine appears to be greater during long-term than during acute treatment with captopril.[145, 146, 149] This corresponds with clinical experience, demonstrating that patients chronically treated with an ACE inhibitor given either alone or in combination with a diuretic rarely complain of orthostatic symptoms.[150-153]

An important characteristic of ACE inhibitors is that they lower blood pressure without inducing an increase in heart rate.[140, 141, 145, 154] They usually induce no consistent change in circulating catecholamines.[140, 155, 156] The fact that blockade of the renin-angiotensin system does not functionally enhance the cardiovascular role of the sympathetic nervous system certainly contributes to the antihypertensive efficacy of ACE inhibitors.

It has been suggested that the acceleration of heart rate that accompanies arteriolar dilatation is partly a consequence of a reflex withdrawal of vagal tone.[157] Parasympathetic system activity clearly increased in normotensive subjects during acute and long-term ACE inhibition.[144, 158-160] This action of ACE inhibitors cannot be explained by an inhibition of acetylcholinesterase. *In vitro*, neither captopril nor enalapril inhibits bovine erythrocyte acetylcholinesterase activity.[160] The parasympathomimetic effect of ACE inhibitors is probably a direct consequence of the disappearance of angiotensin II. It can indeed be reversed by infusion of subpressor doses of angiotensin II.[160] Angiotensin II has been shown experimentally to inhibit vagal responses both centrally and peripherally.[161, 162] The stimulation of vagal activity by captopril has been observed not only in normotensive subjects but in hypertensive patients as well.[138] The hemodynamic response to ACE inhibitors could therefore be related partly to an increase in vagal tone.

HEMODYNAMIC EFFECTS

Like heart rate, cardiac output remains essentially unchanged when blood pressure is lowered by an ACE inhibitor[145, 154, 163-165] (Fig. 73-3). During prolonged treatment, cardiac output may actually increase in some patients.[163] This effect is most likely to occur in patients with malignant hypertension in whom cardiac output is already reduced.[167] The fall in systemic vascular resistance resulting from ACE inhibition may be associated with a decrease in cardiac filling pressures.[163, 166] This observation reflects either a relaxant effect of ACE inhibitors on capacitance blood vessels or improved cardiac performance. Pulmonary vascular resistance is not affected by ACE inhibitors.[163, 164] Adding a diuretic to an ACE inhibitor usually does not alter the hemodynamic profile of ACE inhibition.[168] In hypertensive patients subjected to moderate or strenuous physical exercise, both captopril and enalapril reduce the peak blood pressure increase, whereas they have no effect on the heart rate response.[169, 170] ACE inhibition does not alter the increase in cardiac output in response to dynamic exercise.[170] However, when an ACE inhibitor is administered with a diuretic, the increase in cardiac output may be blunted during exercise.[168]

In the kidney, angiotensin II exerts multiple regulatory functions, including modulation of renal blood

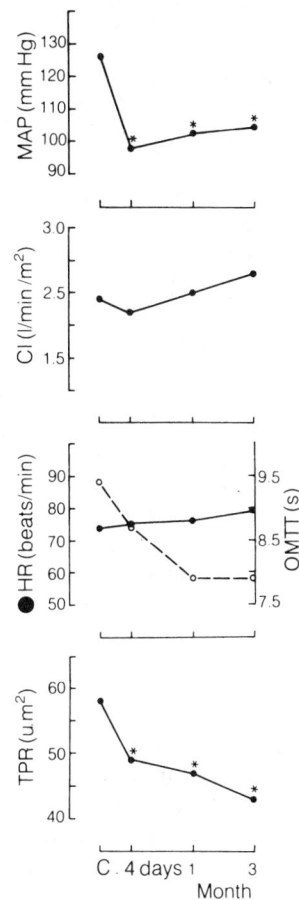

Figure 73–3. Hemodynamic pattern observed in six patients who responded to enalapril treatment and in whom blood pressure was controlled for up to 3 months. Mean arterial pressure (MAP) reduction was related to a significant change in total peripheral resistance (TPR) with no significant change in either cardiac index or heart rate (HR). (Adapted from Fouad FM, Tarazi RC, Bravo EL: Cardiac and haemodynamic effects of enalapril. J Hypertens 1[Suppl I]:135, 1983.)

flow, glomerular filtration rate (GFR), tubular reabsorption of sodium, and inhibition of renin release.[171-176] Angiotensin II acts on both the afferent and the efferent arterioles.[177] Angiotensin II is not required to maintain normal renal excretory function in subjects with normal perfusion pressure.[178] However, increased renal blood flow can be demonstrated in normotensive patients receiving ACE inhibitors.[179]

Renal vascular tone is elevated abnormally in a substantial number of hypertensive patients.[180, 181] In these patients, renal plasma flow is increased by blockade of angiotensin II generation. This effect has been shown during acute as well as during long-term ACE inhibition.[179, 182-186] The increases in renal blood flow resulting from ACE inhibition are accentuated in patients with activated renin-angiotensin systems.[179, 183] Also, when combined with a diuretic, long-term ACE inhibition enhances renal blood flow.[187] The hyperreninemia induced by a diuretic given alone would be expected to have no or even an opposite renal hemodynamic effect. The rise in renal plasma flow evoked by ACE inhibitors is characterized by preferential vasodilatation of the efferent arterioles of the glomeruli.[183, 186]

The coronary vasoconstrictive action of angiotensin II is well established.[188] In hypertensive patients, as in normotensive subjects, coronary blood flow largely depends on autoregulatory mechanisms that adjust oxygen supply to the needs of the myocardium. Under certain circumstances, angiotensin II may modulate the tone of the coronary tree of hypertensive patients and consequently impair coronary perfusion. Such an influence of angiotensin II has been confirmed.[189] In this study, diuretic therapy reduced coronary blood flow. This effect could be reversed by acute ACE inhibition despite a concurrent fall in blood pressure (Fig. 73–4), confirming similar earlier observations made in dogs given teprotide.[190] This fact suggests that angiotensin II actively participates in control of coronary vascular tone if the renin-angiotensin axis is activated.

A major concern when lowering blood pressure is maintenance of adequate cerebral perfusion. Over a wide range of blood pressures, cerebral blood flow is kept constant by autoregulation.[191] When blood pressure falls acutely below the lower limit of autoregulation, there is a risk of a harmful drop in cerebral blood flow. This condition is most likely in hypertensive patients, because they exhibit an autoregulation curve with higher blood pressure levels than those of normotensive subjects. These patients appear to be particularly prone to impaired cerebral perfusion when a very high blood pressure is reduced rapidly. ACE inhibitors lower blood pressure without diminishing cerebral blood flow.[192, 193] In one study,[193] cerebral blood flow increased after a few days; this increase appeared to be most pronounced in patients who responded to ACE inhibition with the biggest reductions in blood pressure. In another study of hypertensive patients with unilateral cerebrovascular disease, captopril actually enhanced cerebral blood flow to the affected hemisphere despite a 10% fall in blood pressure.[194] In an experimental model of hypertension, ACE inhibition acutely reduced the lower limit of cerebral autoregulation by 20 to 30 mmHg.[195]

METABOLIC EFFECTS

Concern is growing about the potentially adverse impact of antihypertensive drugs on lipid and glucose metabolism and circulating levels of potassium and uric acid.[196] Increases in plasma lipids, glucose, and uric acid levels are linked to an increased risk of ischemic heart disease.[197] Potassium depletion may trigger cardiac arrhythmias.[198]

ACE inhibitors have no effect on serum levels of total cholesterol,[199–201] very-low-density lipoprotein cholesterol, low-density lipoprotein cholesterol,[201] triglycerides,[200, 201] and glucose,[199, 200] whereas some evidence suggests that serum apolipoproteins A-I and A-II, major apolipoproteins of the high-density lipoprotein fraction, are increased by ACE inhibition.[201] In contrast, thiazide diuretics have untoward effects on lipid and glucose metabolism.[199, 202] They cause increases in total serum cholesterol concentrations while reducing the concentration of high-density lipoproteins. Interestingly, ACE inhibitors may actually prevent diuretic-induced hyperlipidemia and hyperglycemia.[199, 200]

ACE inhibitors also seem to exert a uricosuric action.[203] They reduce serum uric acid concentrations in patients with hyperuricemia. Diuretic-induced hyperuricemia is attenuated by ACE inhibition.[199, 200]

In patients with normal renal function, the reduction of aldosterone synthesis induced by ACE inhibition generally does not lead to a clinically relevant increase in serum potassium[199, 204, 205] (Fig. 73–5). The risk of developing severe hyperkalemia during ACE inhibition seems to exist mainly in patients with terminal renal failure.[204, 205] ACE inhibitors have a clear potassium-sparing effect when combined with a diuretic.[199, 200] Intracellular potassium increases when an ACE inhibitor is coadministered with a diuretic,[206] whereas it falls when a diuretic is given alone.[207] This tendency seems to indicate that the pool of intracellular potassium is preserved during ACE inhibition despite concomitant diuretic therapy. In a few patients, addition of a potassium-sparing diuretic to an ACE inhibitor may be desirable to correct hypokalemia induced by a diuretic (most often by a loop diuretic). This addition often can be made safely in patients with normal renal function.[208] However, the combination should be stopped as soon as there is any evidence of renal failure. Caution should also be exer-

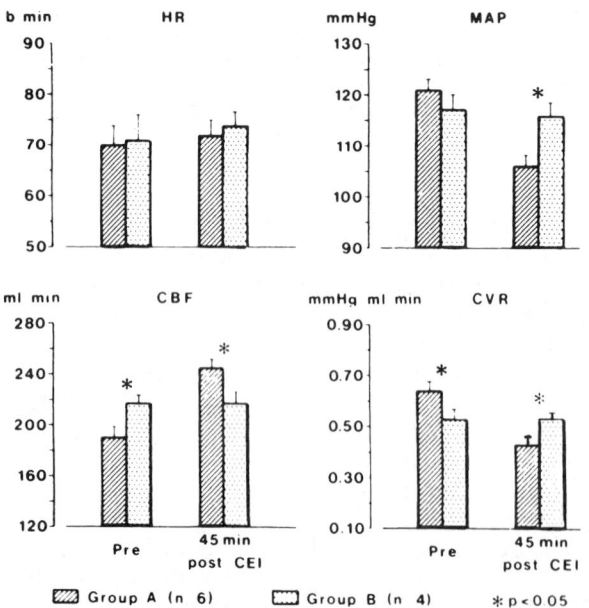

Figure 73–4. Patients who were taking furosemide (group A) had a significantly lower coronary blood flow (CBF) and higher vascular resistance (CVR) than patients on placebo (group B). After one oral dose of captopril, group A had a significant increase in CBF and decrease in CVR despite the modest fall in mean arterial pressure (MAP). HR, heart rate. (Reproduced with permission from Magrini F, Shimizu M, Roberts N, et al: Angiotensin converting enzyme inhibition and coronary blood flow. Circulation 75[Suppl I]:168, 1987. Copyright 1987, American Heart Association.)

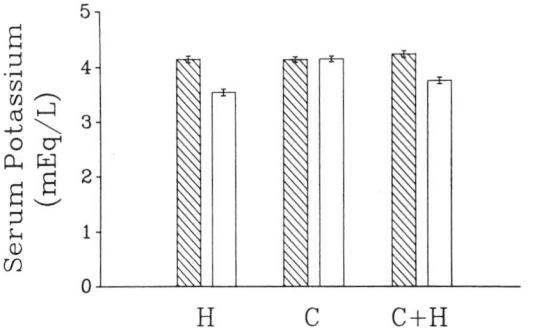

Figure 73–5. Effect of 6 weeks of treatment on serum potassium levels. Results at the end of placebo are indicated by *hatched bars.* Results after 6 weeks of active therapy are represented by *open bars.* Therapy consisted of hydrochlorothiazide (H), 15 mg t.i.d.; captopril (C), 25 mg t.i.d.; or captopril and hydrochlorothiazide (C + H). (From Weinberger MH: Blood pressure and metabolic responses to hydrochlorothiazide, captopril, and the combination in black and white mild-to-moderate hypertensive patients. J Cardiovasc Pharmacol 7[Suppl I]:52, 1985.)

cised when supplementing potassium in a patient treated with an ACE inhibitor.[209] Physiologically, it is interesting that the stimulation of aldosterone secretion by potassium is not abolished in hypertensive patients treated with ACE inhibitors;[210] perhaps because these homeostatic mechanisms of potassium metabolism are still functional in the face of ACE inhibition, serious hyperkalemia is rarely observed in hypertensive patients.

TREATMENT OF HYPERTENSION
Essential Hypertension

Essential hypertension is by far the most common form of clinical hypertension. During the last decade, a considerable number of reports have been published on the effect of ACE inhibitors in patients with essential hypertension.[211–215] These agents given alone effectively lower blood pressure in more than half of patients with mild to moderate hypertension.[199, 216–218] White hypertensive patients tend generally to respond better to treatment than do black patients.[199] Some attenuation of the clinical efficacy of ACE inhibition has been reported during long-term treatment with captopril or enalapril.[218–220] Adding a diuretic to the ACE inhibitor restored the maximal response.[220] However, a major advantage of ACE inhibitors is their ability to maintain satisfactory blood control for years when used in monotherapy.

With aging, renin secretion tends to fall.[221] This finding has led to the implication that therapy with an ACE inhibitor is less likely to be efficacious in elderly than in young hypertensive patients.[222] In fact, this hypothesis has not been confirmed by large-scale clinical studies.[223–225] The blood pressure reductions obtained with captopril or enalapril turned out to be equal in the different classes of age. However, in elderly and in young hypertensive patients, the blood pressure–lowering effect of ACE inhibition is influenced by race: white patients respond better than nonwhite patients.[226]

Renovascular Hypertension

In patients with renovascular hypertension due to unilateral renal artery stenosis, plasma renin levels are frequently increased.[227] Renovascular hypertension is usually a condition difficult to treat with conventional antihypertensive agents. In these patients, acute and long-term ACE inhibition often effectively reduce blood pressure.[228–231] ACE inhibitors generally control blood pressure without requiring additional drugs.

The fact that circulating angiotensin II is markedly diminished after ACE inhibition may adversely affect function of the kidney behind the stenosis. When perfusion pressure to the glomeruli is considerably reduced, angiotensin II may be vital to maintain adequate filtration pressure, because angiotensin II exerts its vasoconstrictor action predominantly on the efferent arterioles. That renal problems may occur during ACE inhibition was first demonstrated in patients with bilateral renal artery stenosis and patients with renal artery stenosis of a single kidney. In patients with these disorders, azotemia developed when blood pressure was lowered by captopril.[232–235] Experience to date suggests that impairment of renal function caused by such a mechanism is reversible after withdrawal of the ACE inhibitor. Ironically, hypertension in patients with bilateral renal artery stenosis or renal artery stenosis of a single kidney often responds poorly to ACE inhibition alone. Frequently, other antihypertensive drugs must be combined with an ACE inhibitor to normalize blood pressure. When blood pressure is reduced successfully, the risk of azotemia becomes most imminent.

Glomerular filtration also may cease because of unilateral renal artery stenosis, but renal failure does not develop because the intact contralateral kidney compensates[236] (Fig. 73–6). The function of the kidneys can be assessed with radionuclide techniques. However, using this approach, the GFR of the stenotic kidney is not always severely compromised by ACE inhibitors.[236, 237] Among the main determinants of the response of a stenotic kidney to ACE inhibition are the level of systemic pressure, the severity of the renal artery stenosis, the functional state of the contralateral kidney, and the degree of activation of the renin-angiotensin system. The risk of persistent damage to the stenotic kidney—for instance, by facilitating renal artery thrombosis—seems to exist only when renal blood flow is markedly diminished as a result of ACE inhibition.[238] Nevertheless, the presence of unilateral renal artery stenosis does not preclude the use of ACE inhibitors. These agents may be helpful in patients who cannot undergo reconstructive surgery or angioplasty. It is recommended that renal function be checked a few days after initiation of ACE inhibition in patients with hypertension that is difficult to control by conventional therapy. The probability that

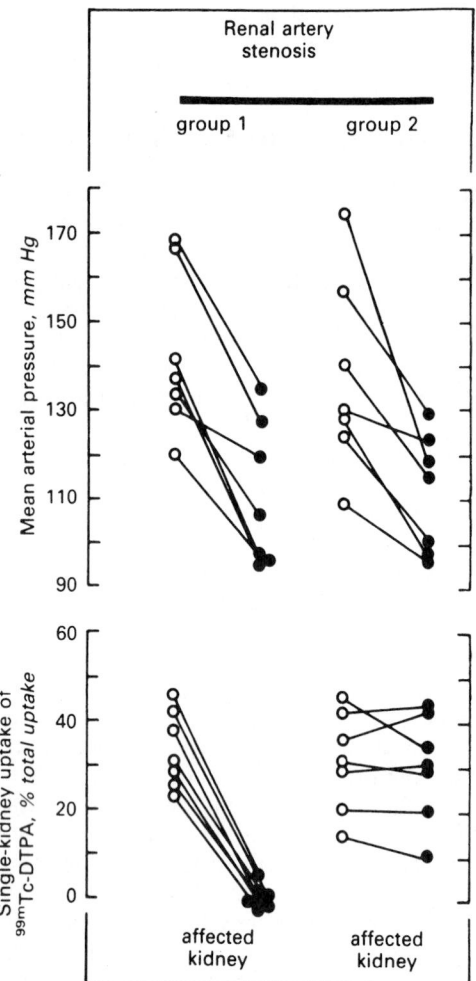

Figure 73–6. Effect of long-term captopril, 150 mg daily, on blood pressure and single kidney uptake of ^{99m}Tc-DTPA in 14 patients with unilateral renal artery stenosis. Patients with renal artery stenosis were divided into two groups according to change in diethylenetriamine pentaacetic acid uptake. Mean arterial pressure was calculated as diastolic pressure + 0.3 × pulse pressure. (From Wenting GJ, Derkx FHM, Tan-Tjiong LH, et al: Risks of angiotensin converting enzyme inhibition in renal artery stenosis. Kidney Int 31[Suppl 20]:S180, 1987.)

these patients have renovascular hypertension is not negligible.[239]

In patients with renal artery stenosis, it would seem appropriate to evaluate the renin secretory response to ACE inhibition rather than the basic renin profile. Increments in plasma renin activity induced acutely by ACE inhibitors are more pronounced in patients with renovascular hypertension than in those with essential hypertension.[240] However, the degree of hyperreninemia observed during long-term inhibition of ACE does not appear to predict the blood pressure achieved by surgical cure of renal artery stenosis.[229] ACE inhibitors, because of their stimulating effects on renin secretion, raise the sensitivity of the renal vein renin sampling test, making it more likely to uncover an asymmetry of renal renin secretion.[241]

The extent to which blood pressure is reduced by acute ACE inhibition is not always a reliable indicator

of the outcome of renal artery repair or nephrectomy in an individual patient.[228, 229] In contrast, the blood pressure response to long-term ACE inhibition has some prognostic value. Thus, blood pressure is likely to be controlled with surgery or angioplasty in a patient with proven renal artery stenosis in whom blood pressure could be normalized with an ACE inhibitor given as sole therapy for several weeks.[229] However, do not treat a patient with ACE inhibitor for long before correcting the stenosis.

Primary Aldosteronism

Renin secretion is typically suppressed in hypertensive patients with primary aldosteronism. Therefore, it is not surprising that acute ACE inhibition fails to lower blood pressure in most patients.[242–244] Nevertheless, blood pressure may be slightly lowered in some patients during either acute or prolonged ACE inhibition. Because, in many patients, essential hypertension may not respond to ACE inhibition, the lack of a drop in blood pressure cannot be used to identify patients with primary aldosteronism. However, acute ACE inhibition with captopril may be useful to differentiate patients with aldosterone-producing adenomas from those exhibiting bilateral micronodular hyperplasia. In the former, aldosterone production is supposed to be completely autonomous; for this reason, blockade of angiotensin II generation does not reduce abnormally elevated plasma aldosterone levels. In the latter, it is known that aldosterone secretion can be stimulated by angiotensin II. Thus, these patients tend to respond to captopril with some decrease in circulating aldosterone concentration.[243, 244] Whether this simple test ought to be performed systematically in patients with primary aldosteronism remains to be further explored.

Other Conditions

Renin-producing tumors are a rare cause of hypertension. In this prototype of angiotensin II–dependent hypertension, ACE inhibitors usually reduce blood pressure to normal levels.[245] However, the failure to normalize blood pressure in response to ACE inhibition does not necessarily rule out the presence of a renin-secreting tumor.

Plasma renin activity tends to be elevated in patients with pheochromocytoma.[246] ACE inhibition has occasionally lowered blood pressure substantially in these patients.[247, 248]

The use of ACE inhibitors in hypertensive pregnant women should be avoided. In pregnant rabbits and ewes, captopril has increased the rate of stillbirths.[249] In pregnant rabbits, placental perfusion is reduced by ACE inhibition.[250] Captopril administered during human pregnancy seems to affect both the maternal and fetal renin-angiotensin systems.[251] Neonatal anuria has been described after treatment with captopril[252] or enalapril[253] during pregnancy. In the latter case, peritoneal dialysis has proved life-saving. ACE inhibition during pregnancy may impair closing of a ductus arteriosus.[254] However, a number of pregnancies had favorable outcomes despite administration of ACE inhibitors.[254]

A number of studies have demonstrated the usefulness of ACE inhibitors in the management of hypertensive patients unresponsive to multiple drug combinations.[255-259] In these patients, addition of a thiazide or even a loop diuretic is often necessary to control blood pressure. ACE inhibitors can also be administered successfully to patients with malignant hypertension.[167, 257]

ACE inhibition is a rational approach to the treatment of patients who require blood pressure reduction within a few hours. For this indication, rapidly acting captopril is preferable to enalapril. Captopril may be given either by the usual oral route[260] or sublingually.[261] Substantial blood pressure reductions can be obtained within 15 minutes of oral captopril administration. In patients who are unresponsive to acute ACE inhibition alone, addition of a loop diuretic with quick onset of action usually controls blood pressure in a fast but progressive manner.[260] Parenterally administered ACE inhibitors have also been used with good results to manage hypertensive emergencies.[262-264] Caution is necessary in patients suspected of having a markedly activated renin-angiotensin system (e.g., by previous excessive diuretic administration), because sudden hypotension may develop.[260]

TREATMENT OF HYPERTENSION ASSOCIATED WITH OTHER DISORDERS
Renal Disease

Although renal disease is a major cause of hypertension, abnormally high blood pressure levels also have a deleterious effect on renal function. In some patients with chronic renal failure, the renin-angiotensin system may contribute to the development of hypertension.[265] However, in most patients, the impaired sodium-handling capacity of the kidney plays the predominant role in the pathogenesis of hypertension.[266] Plasma renin activity is often normal or even low in these patients.[255, 267, 268] There is some suggestion, however, that renin secretion, although seemingly not elevated, is inappropriately high in relation to associated sodium retention.[255, 267] Moreover, it is possible that peripheral plasma renin activity does not accurately reflect the amount of angiotensin II formed locally within the kidney.[269] In the presence of underlying renal disease, ACE inhibitors given as monotherapy normalize blood pressure less frequently than when renal function is intact.[151, 186]

Theoretically, ACE inhibitors might improve the natural history of renal disease, not only because of their antihypertensive effects, but also because of their actions on intrarenal hemodynamics and the glomerular cells.[173, 175-177] Thus, these agents are expected to prevent the development of glomerular hyperperfusion and hyperfiltration—that is, of alterations that occur with the loss of functional nephrons

and presumably contribute to further injury of the remnant glomeruli.[270] In hypertensive patients with normal renal function, the GFR has risen in response to ACE inhibition.[42, 271] In a long-term survey, however, no such effect could be demonstrated.[186] As assessed by plasma creatinine levels, GFR may also deteriorate slightly.[151] The potential of ACE inhibitors to stabilize or improve renal function in hypertensive patients with chronic renal failure is difficult to investigate, because the progression of renal disease may be largely unrelated either to the quality of blood pressure control or to the drugs used to achieve blood pressure normalization. In patients with impaired renal function, long-term ACE inhibition does not appear to alter GFR.[272] Conversely, a favorable effect on renal function cannot be ruled out, because the follow-up of a large number of hypertensive patients with impaired renal function has provided evidence for a decrease in the plasma concentration of creatinine.[151] In patients with essential hypertension who exhibit modest degrees of renal failure, strict blood pressure control with an ACE inhibitor is followed by either stabilization of or improvement in renal function.[273] In hypertensive patients with no signs of renal failure, long-term blood pressure reduction resulting from ACE inhibition is accompanied by decreases in urinary protein excretion.[186, 274] Similar results have been obtained in patients with hypertension complicated by renal parenchymal disease.[186]

When arterial hypertension is associated with terminal renal failure, it usually can be corrected by hemodialysis and ultrafiltration of extracellular fluid. Patients who do not respond to sodium depletion tend to have inappropriately high plasma renin activity.[275] In such patients, long-term ACE inhibition is an effective alternative to bilateral nephrectomy.[276, 277] ACE inhibitors are potentially useful in some patients who develop hypertension after renal transplantation.[278, 279] However, in such cases, hypertension may be due to a stenotic artery of the graft; thus, blood pressure reduction induced by an ACE inhibitor can lead to the development of renal failure.

Left Ventricular Hypertrophy

Left ventricular hypertrophy may be regarded as a compensatory process, which maintains cardiac function for some time despite increased ventricular afterload caused by sustained high blood pressure levels. Factors other than arterial pressure per se probably influence the development of ventricular hypertrophy.[280] For instance, renin and angiotensin II binding sites have been found in the cardiac myocytes.[281, 282] Angiotensin II has a positive inotropic effect on the myocardium[283] and possibly exerts a mitogenic action.[284] Whether circulating or locally generated angiotensin II is involved in the development of cardiac hypertrophy remains uncertain. Thus, there are no obvious differences in left ventricular muscle mass between hypertensive patients with high and those with low renin levels.[285] Like most antihypertensive agents, ACE inhibitors induce a regression of left ventricular hypertrophy in the face of prolonged blood pressure reduction.[154, 185, 280, 286]

Congestive Heart Failure

ACE inhibitors have markedly improved the treatment of patients with severe congestive heart failure.[287–289] These patients most often have rather low blood pressure before initiation of treatment, and they respond to ACE inhibition with an additional drop in blood pressure. Typically, hemodynamic changes induced by blockade of the renin-angiotensin system consist of reductions in total peripheral resistance, left ventricular filling pressure, and right atrial pressure; an increase in cardiac output; and no change in heart rate.[290, 291] In hypertensive patients with congestive heart failure, any reduction of blood pressure would be expected to greatly benefit cardiac function.

Coronary Artery Disease

ACE inhibitors have been administered to hypertensive patients with coronary artery disease.[292–295] Coronary blood flow and myocardial oxygen consumption decreased during acute ACE inhibition, but these changes occurred in parallel with a reduction in the double product (i.e., systolic blood pressure × heart rate), which means that the metabolic balance of the heart was not altered.[292, 294] In one study, long-term ACE inhibition even appeared to attenuate ST-segment depression observed at the maximal double product during ergometry.[293] In normotensive patients with coronary artery disease treated for a few days with captopril, myocardial perfusion was improved overall during exercise, but there may have been coronary steal in some cardiac areas.[294] A main advantage of ACE inhibition in patients with angina may be the lack of a reflex increase in myocardial sympathetic tone.[296] ACE inhibitors attenuate the progressive ventricular dilation and prevent the development of heart failure after anterior myocardial infarction.[297–299] These effects are associated with improved survival in patients with symptomatic heart failure.

Peripheral Vascular Disease

ACE inhibitors dilate both small and large arteries when lowering blood pressure.[300] Systemic arterial compliance seems to be increased by these agents.[300] Long-term ACE inhibition leads to a regression of arteriolar hypertrophy, as reflected by a reduction of the media/lumen ratio determined in subcutaneous resistance arteries obtained by gluteal biopsies.[301] Interestingly, long-term therapy with captopril in patients with hypertension associated with claudication may increase blood flow to the limbs, as reflected by an improvement in both the pain-free interval and the maximum walking distance.[302, 303]

Diabetes Mellitus

Blood pressure of hypertensive patients with diabetes mellitus should be normalized to preserve renal function as long as possible.[304]

Hypertensive patients with uncomplicated diabetes seem to respond to ACE inhibition as well as do patients with essential hypertension.[305] Lowering blood pressure of hypertensive diabetics reduces urine protein excretion without modifying renal function.[306, 307] Such a favorable effect on proteinuria has been demonstrated even in normotensive diabetics with azotemia.[308] ACE inhibition for 2 years slowed the rate of renal deterioration in patients with diabetic nephropathy.[309] These beneficial effects have been attributed to a decrease in glomerular capillary pressure that presumably is abnormally increased in diabetics, as suggested by micropuncture studies in diabetic rats.[270] The protecting effect of ACE inhibitors against deterioration in renal function in patients with diabetic nephropathy was confirmed in a prospective trial.[310] The beneficial effect is greater than expected with the blood pressure control alone. Captopril may also enhance insulin responsiveness in muscle tissue of patients with non-insulin-dependent diabetes mellitus.[311] This phenomenon could be explained by a captopril-induced accumulation of local bradykinin.[312]

Chronic Obstructive Lung Disease

Hypertensive patients suffering from chronic obstructive lung disease have been treated successfully with ACE inhibitors.[313] In this study, respiratory function tests showed no deleterious effect of ACE inhibition. Most important, antihypertensive therapy with ACE inhibitors was also revealed to be safe in asthmatic patients.[314–316] Bronchial provocation testing was performed in asthmatics treated with an ACE inhibitor. Bronchial reactivity to metacholine[315] and bradykinin[316] was not enhanced by kininase II inhibition.

DOSAGE, QUALITY OF LIFE, AND SIDE EFFECTS

During the early developmental phase of captopril, investigators used daily doses ranging from 600 to 1000 mg, even though the first study of captopril in humans showed clearly that maximal ACE blockade could be obtained with 20 mg by mouth.[14] It was realized that it is not necessary to suppress ACE activity throughout the day to achieve satisfactory blood pressure control;[50, 317] subsequently, much lower doses of captopril were tested.[216, 318–323] In one study, 25 mg of captopril twice a day lowered blood pressure to the same extent as 50 mg three times a day.[318] In another trial, 50 mg of captopril twice a day appeared more efficacious than 25 mg twice a day, but it provided results equivalent to 100 mg twice a day.[216] Hypertensive patients receiving either 50 mg of captopril once a day or 50 mg of captopril twice a day had equal blood pressure reduction.[322] As a single morning dose, 50 mg of captopril produced blood pressure reduction comparable with 10 mg of enalapril.[321, 323]

With enalapril, there is a dose-response relationship with regard to arterial pressure in hypertensive patients for daily doses ranging from 2.5 to 20 and maybe 40 mg.[324] However, doses lower than 10 mg/day may be unsatisfactory for blood pressure control. Administration of a given amount of this compound once daily appears to be as effective as giving one half of that dose twice daily.[217, 325] Captopril and enalapril are excreted by the kidney.[326, 327] Accordingly, the doses of these agents should be reduced in patients with impaired renal function.

The goal of modern antihypertensive therapy should be to lower blood pressure without impairing the patient's enjoyment of life.[328] Early in the evaluation of ACE inhibitors, it became apparent that these drugs are highly acceptable because of minimal interference with the well-being of patients. It was even suspected that ACE inhibitors produce euphoria. However, this assertion turned out to be untrue in hypertensive patients treated with captopril.[329] In normal subjects, evidence for a modest increase in alertness was found after 2 weeks of treatment with enalapril.[330] In hypertensive patients, ACE inhibition by enalapril did not alter memory function, whereas this aspect was slightly but consistently impaired by atenolol.[331] Using elaborate standardized questionnaires, it was demonstrated in hypertensive patients that captopril induces a sense of well-being and improves work performance and cognitive function but has no influence on other indices of quality of life, such as physical symptoms, sexual function, sleep, life satisfaction, and social participation.[332] This finding agreed with earlier results obtained in captopril-treated patients by less sophisticated methods.[333]

Hypotension, hyperkalemia, and renal impairment typically are side effects of angiotensin II blockade (Fig. 73–7). They all are discussed in detail elsewhere in this chapter. These adverse effects usually are seen when ACE inhibitors are misused. On one occasion, a hypotensive episode caused by ACE inhibition led to ischemic cardiovascular complications.[334] As expected, dehydration favors the occurrence of hypotension in patients treated with an ACE inhibitor.[335, 336] Infusion of either saline or angiotensin II can restore normal blood pressure, but giving a saline infusion is much simpler and therefore is preferable. In the absence of renal artery stenosis, renal insufficiency is unlikely unless vascular lesions in the kidneys are severe and widespread.[337]

Dry, nonproductive cough has been recognized as a side effect of ACE inhibitors. Postmarketing surveillance of enalapril in a large number of patients has suggested a 1% prevalence of cough.[338] For captopril, postmarketing surveillance showed that 0.2% of patients had to interrupt therapy because of irritable throat or cough.[339] This figure may be somewhat too optimistic. Experience with lisinopril indicates that cough is a problem in 3.4% of hypertensive patients, compared with 1.2% in placebo-treated patients.[340] The mechanisms responsible for this adverse effect are under investigation. In one report, normal subjects acutely treated with an ACE inhibitor became hypersensitive to inhalation of a cough-inducing substance.[341] One possibility for this is that the cough inducer releases kinins or substance P (peptides known to be degraded by ACE).[342, 343] These peptides might accumulate and trigger the cough reflex. This is compatible with the observation that inhalation of bradykinin produces cough in humans.[344] Bradykinin is a well-established activator of prostaglandin synthesis.[88–90] This highlights the finding that cyclooxygenase inhibition reduces cough in hypertensive patients receiving an ACE inhibitor.[345]

During captopril's development, excessively high doses were used. This therapy was associated with a rather high incidence of unwanted effects.[151, 204] The risk of suffering a serious adverse effect turned out to be particularly important in patients with some degree of renal failure and in those with associated connective tissue disease. The most troublesome was leukopenia, which was fatal in a few patients.[346, 347] There was also some worry about the renal effects of captopril. Some patients developed proteinuria while on captopril treatment,[348, 349] and there was fear of immune complex glomerulopathy.[350] Taste disturbance and a variety of skin eruptions were observed not infrequently in patients taking excessive doses of captopril. The incidence of all these adverse effects has declined drastically with the reduction of the total daily dose of captopril administered.[151, 224, 339] In particular, leukopenias are not a problem anymore.[224, 339] Based on a broad survey, the occurrence of a cutaneous rash or dysgeusia necessitates withdrawal of captopril in some 0.80% and 0.35% of patients, respectively.[339] Captopril may rarely cause cholestatic jaundice[351] or angioneurotic edema.[352] At the doses recommended today, captopril is believed not to have any direct nephrotoxic effect.[353]

The safety profile of enalapril is in many aspects

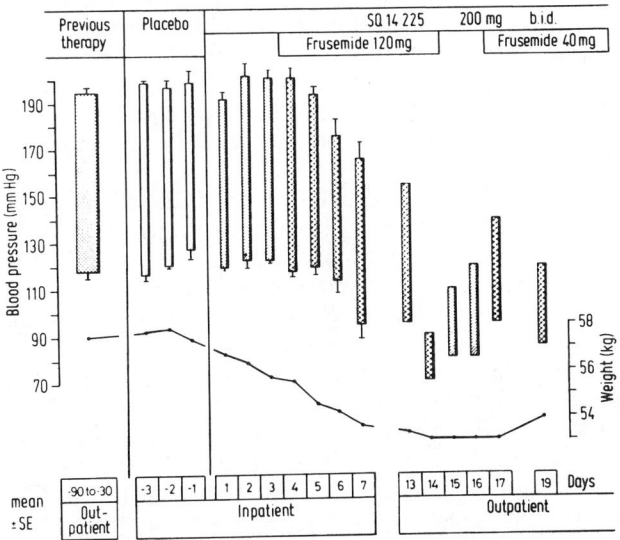

Figure 73–7. Effect of captopril (SQ 14,225) alone and in combination with frusemide (furosemide) on blood pressure and weight in a 29-year-old hypertensive patient with diabetes mellitus and chronic renal failure. Because of excessive diuretic therapy, hypotension occurred and was easily corrected by reducing the dose of frusemide without interrupting ACE blockade. (From Brunner HR, Waeber B, Wauters JP, et al: Inappropriate renin secretion unmasked by captopril [SQ 14225] in hypertension of chronic renal failure. Lancet 2:704, 1978. © by The Lancet Ltd., 1978.)

similar to that of captopril.[152, 217] However, the incidence of rash and taste disturbance tends to be lower with enalapril than with captopril.[354, 355] Interestingly, a number of patients who experienced skin rash while on captopril could be maintained on long-term enalapril therapy with no recurrence of the adverse effect.[356, 357] However, whether this condition is due to the fact that enalapril, unlike captopril, is free of a sulfhydryl group remains speculative. Enalapril may also cause angioneurotic edema,[338, 358] but even extremely high doses of this agent are well tolerated.[359]

Elderly hypertensive patients are particularly likely to experience side effects during antihypertensive therapy, but not with ACE inhibitors.[223, 224]

ACE INHIBITORS AS MONOTHERAPY OR COMBINED WITH OTHER ANTIHYPERTENSIVE AGENTS

Because a number of highly effective antihypertensive agents are now available, and because each carries an inherent albeit small risk of side effects, pharmacologic antihypertensive therapy should, whenever possible, be started by assessing the efficacy of one or several drugs given as monotherapy. Diuretics and β-blockers are well established as first-line drugs in the treatment of hypertension. ACE inhibitors and calcium antagonists also may be used as alternatives for initiating antihypertensive therapy.[360] A key point when considering the use of ACE inhibitors as a first-step treatment is their clinical efficacy compared with other classes of antihypertensive agents.

A number of studies have shown that captopril or enalapril given as monotherapy has an antihypertensive effect similar to that of the thiazide diuretics.[153, 361, 362] Both agents are also equally potent in the elderly.[363, 364] The blood pressure–lowering effect of ACE inhibitors also appears to be similar to that of β-blockers, but ACE inhibitors clearly decrease systolic pressure at rest more than do β-adrenoreceptor blocking agents.[365–370] However, during exercise, systolic blood pressure seems to be lower with β-adrenoreceptor blockade than with ACE inhibition.[371] The average blood pressure reduction in hypertensive patients taking ACE inhibitors is close to that achieved during calcium antagonism.[372–376] The results of these trials show that ACE inhibitors administered alone are effective antihypertensive drugs that can be proposed as first-line antihypertensive agents.

Initiating treatment with an ACE inhibitor may have the advantage of simplifying the therapeutic approach to the hypertensive patient. This conclusion is based on the findings of a double-blind controlled study in which ACE inhibition was the first-step treatment of mild to moderate uncomplicated essential hypertension.[51] Patients were randomly allocated to either enalapril or a placebo as the first step of therapy, followed when necessary by the successive addition of a thiazide diuretic, a β-blocker, and the vasodilator hydralazine. During the 6-month follow-up,

enalapril given as the first drug in the stepped-care approach to treatment of hypertension provided a better degree of blood pressure control than the comparative treatment. This result was achieved with a smaller number of tablets compared with conventional therapy.

The antihypertensive efficacy of ACE inhibitors is greatly enhanced by coadministration of a diuretic.[3, 153, 199, 255, 361–363, 377] When ACE inhibition alone fails to normalize blood pressure, reduction of total body sodium (for instance, by a diuretic) triggers the release of renin and consequently makes maintenance of high blood pressure depend on angiotensin II. Very low doses of diuretics may suffice to reduce blood pressure when they are combined with an ACE inhibitor.[378] In fact, the hypertensive patient whose generation of angiotensin II is blocked by ACE inhibition will become hypotensive if a critical level of sodium depletion is exceeded.[34, 255, 260] To minimize the risk of hypotension when introducing an ACE inhibitor in a patient already on diuretic therapy, it is strongly recommended that the diuretic be withdrawn or at least decreased in dosage for a few days prior to administration of the first dose. In hypertensive patients with ongoing diuretic therapy, it also seems possible to avoid hypotension by starting with small oral doses of ACE inhibitors (6.25 or 12.5 mg of captopril or 5 mg of enalapril).[379, 380] As expected, a sodium-restricted diet also potentiates the blood pressure response to ACE inhibition.[381] In this study, enalapril treatment caused a net natriuresis in salt-depleted as well as in salt-repleted hypertensive patients.

The addition of a β-blocker to an ACE inhibitor is often thought to be irrational. However, some hypertensive patients may benefit from such an association.[59, 382] Blockade of renal β-adrenoreceptors blunts hyperreninemia in response to ACE inhibition.[57] Perhaps partly by this mechanism, β-blockers sometimes induce a supplementary reduction in blood pressure. Addition of a β-blocker seems to prolong the blood pressure–lowering effect of the short-lasting inhibitor captopril.[382]

The antihypertensive effect of ACE inhibitors is consistently enhanced by calcium antagonists.[374, 375, 382–387] It has been proposed that calcium antagonists may replace diuretics in combination with an ACE inhibitor,[374] but clear evidence of equal antihypertensive efficacy with this combination has not been provided so far. Interestingly, ACE inhibition buffers the counter-regulation induced by acute calcium antagonism.[387] ACE inhibition might also attenuate the reflex increase in the tone of the sympathetic nervous system during long-term treatment with a calcium antagonist. This possibility is suggested by the observation that the incidence of adverse effects of the calcium antagonist nifedipine tends to be diminished by the concomitant administration of captopril.[373]

CONCLUSIONS

The goal of any antihypertensive therapy is to normalize blood pressure and thereby reduce the enhanced risk of major cardiovascular complications. This effect should be obtained without causing any potentially dangerous side effect. Equally important, because the patient will probably have to take antihypertensive medication for life, his or her feeling of well-being should be maintained despite drug intake. The development of ACE inhibitors has provided investigators with a magnificent tool by which to investigate the role of the renin-angiotensin system in the pathogenesis of hypertension. Furthermore, in a short time, this class of drugs has combined a high degree of efficacy with a low prevalence of side effects, interfering with the patient's quality of life only minimally.

REFERENCES

1. Ferreira SH: A bradykinin-potentiating factor (BPF) present in the venom of Bothrops jararaca. Br J Pharmacol Chemother 24:163, 1965.
2. Ondetti MA, Williams NJ, Sabo EF, et al: Angiotensin converting enzyme inhibitors from the venom of Bothrops jararaca: Isolation, elucidation of structure and synthesis. Biochemistry 10:4033, 1971.
3. Gavras H, Brunner HR, Laragh JH, et al: An angiotensin converting enzyme inhibitor to identify and treat vasoconstrictor and volume factors in hypertensive patients. N Engl J Med 291:817, 1974.
4. Sancho J, Re RN, Burton J, et al: Role of the renin angiotensin system in cardiovascular homeostasis in normal human subjects. Circulation 53:400, 1976.
5. Ondetti MA, Rubin B, Cushman DW: Design of specific inhibitors of angiotensin converting enzyme: New class of orally active antihypertensive agents. Science 196:441, 1977.
6. Pals DT, Masucci FD, Sipos F, et al: A specific competitive antagonist of the vascular action of angiotensin II. Circ Res 29:664, 1971.
7. Posternak L, Brunner HR, Gavras H, et al: Angiotensin II blockade in normal man: Interaction of renin and sodium in maintaining blood pressure. Kidney Int 11:197, 1977.
8. Brunner HR, Gavras H, Laragh JH, et al: Angiotensin II blockade in man by Sar¹-ala⁸-angiotensin II for understanding and treatment of high blood pressure. Lancet 2:1045, 1973.
9. Brunner HR, Gavras H, Laragh JH, et al: Hypertension in man: Exposure of the renin and sodium components using angiotensin II blockade. Circ Res 34, 35(Suppl I):35, 1974.
10. Streeten DHP, Anderson GH, Freiberg JM, et al: Use of an angiotensin II antagonist (saralasin) in the recognition of angiotensinogenic hypertension. N Engl J Med 292:657, 1975.
11. Timmermans PB, Carini DJ, Chiu AT, et al: The discovery of a new class of highly specific nonpeptide angiotensin II receptor antagonists. Am J Hypertens 4(4 Part 2):275S, 1991.
12. Brunner HR, Numberger J, Waeber B: Angiotensin II antagonists. In Robertson JIS and Nicholls MG (eds): The Renin-Angiotensin System. London: Gower Medical, 1993, pp 86.1–86.14.
13. Brunner HR, Nussberger J, Waeber B: The present molecules of converting enzyme inhibitors. J Cardiovasc Pharmacol 7(Suppl I):2, 1985.
14. Ferguson RK, Brunner HR, Turini GA, et al: A specific orally active inhibitor of angiotensin converting enzyme in man. Lancet 1:775, 1977.
15. Biollaz J, Burnier M, Turini GA, et al: Three new long-acting converting enzyme inhibitors: Relationship between plasma converting enzyme activity and response to angiotensin I. Clin Pharmacol Ther 29:665, 1981.
16. Brunner DB, Desponds G, Biollaz J, et al: Effect of a new angiotensin converting enzyme inhibitor MK421 and its lysine analogue on the components of the renin system in healthy subjects. Br J Clin Pharmacol 11:461, 1984.
17. Cushman DW, Cheung HS: Spectrophotometric assay and

properties of the angiotensin converting enzyme in the rabbit lung. Biochem Pharmacol 20:1637, 1971.
18. Roulston JE, McGregor GA, Bind R: The measurement of angiotensin-converting enzyme in subjects receiving captopril. N Engl J Med 303:397, 1980.
19. Ng KKF, Vane JR: Conversion of angiotensin I to angiotensin II. Nature 216:762, 1967.
20. Nussberger J, Brunner DB, Waeber B, et al: True versus immunoreactive angiotensin II in human plasma. Hypertension 7(Suppl I):1, 1985.
21. Nussberger J, Brunner DB, Waeber B, et al: Specific measurement of angiotensin metabolites and in vitro generated angiotensin II in plasma. Hypertension 8:476, 1986.
22. Nussberger J, Brunner DB, Waeber B, et al: In-vitro renin inhibition to prevent generation of angiotensins during determination of angiotensin I and II. Life Sci 42:1683, 1988.
23. Brunner HR, Chang P, Wallach R, et al: Angiotensin II vascular receptors: Their activity in relationship to sodium balance, the autonomic nervous system and hypertension. J Clin Invest 51:58, 1972.
24. Folkow B: The haemodynamic consequence of adaptive structural changes of the resistance vessels in hypertension. Clin Sci 41:1, 1971.
25. Terragno DA, Crowshaw K, Terragno NA, et al: Prostaglandin synthesis by bovine mesenteric arteries and veins. Circ Res 36, 37(Suppl I):76, 1975.
26. Dusting GJ, Moncada S, Vane JR: Prostacyclin (PGX) is the endogenous metabolite responsible for relaxation of coronary arteries induced by arachidonic acid. Prostaglandins 13:3, 1977.
27. Lonigro AJ, Itskovitz HD, Crowshaw K, et al: Dependency of renal blood flow on prostaglandin synthesis in the dog. Circ Res 32:712, 1973.
28. Vinci JM, Zusman RM, Izzo JL, et al: Human urinary and plasma kinins: Relationship to sodium-retaining steroids and plasma renin activity. Circ Res 44:1228, 1979.
29. Aubert JF, Waeber B, Nussberger J, et al: Influence of endogenous bradykinin on blood pressure response to vasopressors in normotensive rats assessed with a bradykinin-antagonist. J Cardiovasc Pharmacol 11:51, 1988.
30. Gavras H, Brunner HR, Turini GA, et al: Antihypertensive effect of oral angiotensin converting enzyme inhibitor SQ 14225 in man. N Engl J Med 298:991, 1978.
31. Case DB, Atlas SA, Laragh JH, et al: Clinical experience with blockade of the renin-angiotensin-aldosterone system by an oral converting-enzyme inhibitor (SQ 14,225 or captopril) in hypertensive patients. Prog Cardiovasc Dis 21:195, 1978.
32. Brunner HR, Gavras H, Waeber B, et al: Oral angiotensin-converting enzyme inhibitor in long term treatment of hypertensive patients. Ann Intern Med 90:19, 1979.
33. Hodsman GP, Isles CG, Murray GD, et al: Factors related to first dose hypotensive effect of captopril: Prediction and treatment. Br Med J 286:832, 1983.
34. Atkinson AB, Brown JJ, Cumming AMM, et al: Captopril in renovascular hypertension: Long-term use in predicting surgical outcome. Br Med J 284:689, 1982.
35. Case DB, Atlas SA, Laragh JH, et al: Use of first dose response or plasma renin activity to predict the long-term effect of captopril: Identification of triphasic pattern of blood pressure response. J Cardiovasc Pharmacol 2:339, 1980.
36. Waeber B, Gavras I, Brunner HR, et al: Prediction of sustained antihypertensive efficacy of chronic captopril therapy: Relationships to immediate blood pressure response and control plasma renin activity. Am Heart J 103:384, 1982.
37. Brunner HR, Waeber B, Nussberger J: Does pharmacological profiling of a new drug in normotensive volunteers provide a useful guideline to antihypertensive therapy? Hypertension 5(Suppl III):101, 1983.
38. Laragh JH, Angers M, Kelly WG, et al: Hypotensive agents and pressor substances: The effect of epinephrine, norepinephrine, angiotensin II and others on the secretory rate of aldosterone in man. JAMA 174:234, 1960.
39. Biron P, Koiw E, Nowaczynski W, et al: The effects of intravenous infusion of saline-5-angiotensin II and other pressor agents on urinary electrolytes and corticosteroids, including aldosterone. J Clin Invest 40:338, 1961.

40. Atlas SA, Case DB, Sealey JE, et al: Interruption of the renin-angiotensin system in hypertensive patients by captopril induces sustained reduction in aldosterone secretion, potassium retention and natriuresis. Hypertension 1:274, 1979.

41. Sanchez RA, Marco E, Gilbert HB, et al: Natriuretic effect and changes in renal hemodynamics induced by enalapril in essential hypertension. Drugs 30(Suppl I):49, 1985.

42. De Zeeuw D, Navis GJ, Donker AJM, et al: The angiotensin converting enzyme inhibitor enalapril and its effects on renal function. J Hypertens 1(Suppl I):93, 1983.

43. Biollaz J, Brunner HR, Gavras I, et al: Antihypertensive therapy with MK 421: Angiotensin II-renin relationships to evaluate efficacy of converting enzyme blockade. J Cardiovasc Pharmacol 4:966, 1982.

44. Griffing GT, Sindler BH, Aurecchia SA, et al: Temporal enhancement of renin-aldosterone blockade by enalapril, an angiotensin-converting enzyme inhibitor. J Clin Pharmacol Ther 32:592, 1982.

45. Brunner HR, Waeber B, Nussberger J, et al: Long-term clinical experience with enalapril in essential hypertension. J Hypertens 1(Suppl I):103, 1983.

46. Fyhrquist F, Forslund T, Tikkanen I, et al: Induction of angiotensin I-converting enzyme in rat lung with captopril (SQ 14225). Eur J Pharmacol 67:473, 1980.

47. Forslund T, Fyhrquist F, Grönhagen-Riska C, et al: Induction of angiotensin-converting enzyme with the ACE inhibitory compound MK-421 in rat lung. Eur J Pharmacol 80:121, 1982.

48. Ulm EH, Vassil TC: Total serum angiotensin converting enzyme activity in rats and dogs after enalapril maleate (MK-421). Life Sci 30:1225, 1982.

49. Fyhrquist F, Grönhagen-Riska C, Hortling L, et al: The induction of angiotensin converting enzyme by its inhibitors. Clin Exp Hypertens A5:1319, 1983.

50. Boomsma F, De Bruyn JHB, Derkx FHM, et al: Opposite effects of captopril on angiotensin I-converting enzyme "activity" and "concentration": Relation between enzyme inhibition and long-term blood pressure response. Clin Sci 60:4911, 1981.

51. Sassano P, Chatellier G, Billaud E, et al: Treatment of mild to moderate hypertension with or without the converting enzyme inhibitor enalapril: Results of a six-month double-blind trial. Am J Med 83:227, 1987.

52. Vander AJ, Geelhoed GW: Inhibition of renin secretion by angiotensin II. Proc Soc Exp Biol Med 120:399, 1965.

53. Leckie BJ: Inactive renin: An attempt at a perspective. Clin Sci 60:119, 1981.

54. Sealey JE, Overlack A, Laragh JH, et al: Effect of captopril and aprotinin on inactive renin. J Clin Endocrinol Metab 53:626, 1981.

55. Goldstone R, Horton R, Carlson EJ, et al: Reciprocal changes in active and inactive renin after converting enzyme inhibition in normal man. J Clin Endocrinol Metab 56:264, 1983.

56. Malatino LS, Manhem P, Ball SG, et al: Twenty-four hour changes in active and inactive renin after various oral doses of the converting enzyme inhibitor ramipril (HOE 498) in normal man. J Clin Hypertens 3:231, 1986.

57. Nussberger J, de Gasparo M, Juillerat L, et al: Rapid measurement of total and active renin: Plasma concentrations during acute and sustained converting enzyme inhibition with CGS 14824A. Clin Exp Hypertens A9:1353, 1987.

58. Nussberger J, Brunner DB, Waeber B, et al: Lack of angiotensin I accumulation after converting enzyme blockade by enalapril or lisinopril in man. Clin Sci 72:387, 1987.

59. Staessen J, Fagard R, Lijnen P, et al: The hypotensive effect of propranolol in captopril-treated patients does not involve the plasma renin-angiotensin-aldosterone system. Clin Sci 61:441S, 1981.

60. Quilley J, Duchin KL, Hudes EM, et al: The antihypertensive effect of captopril in essential hypertension: Relationship to prostaglandins and the kallikrein-kinin system. J Hypertens 5:121, 1987.

61. Salvetti A, Abdel-Hag B, Magagna A, et al: Indomethacin reduces the antihypertensive action of enalapril. Clin Exp Hypertens A9:559, 1987.

62. Padfield PL, Brown JJ, Lever AF, et al: Blood pressure in acute and chronic vasopressin excess. Studies of malignant hypertension and the syndrome of inappropriate antidiuretic hormone secretion. N Engl J Med 304:1067, 1981.

63. Thibonnier M, Aldigier JC, Soto ME, et al: Abnormalities and drug-induced alterations of vasopressin in human hypertension. Clin Sci 61:149, 1981.

64. Thibonnier M, Soto ME, Ménard J, et al: Reduction of plasma and urinary vasopressin during treatment of severe hypertension by captopril. Eur J Clin Invest 11:449, 1981.

65. Santucci A, Luparini RL, Ferri C, et al: Relationship between vasopressin and the renin-angiotensin-aldosterone system in essential hypertension: Effect of converting enzyme inhibitor on plasma vasopressin. J Hypertens 3(Suppl II):133, 1985.

66. Arendt RM, Gerbes AL, Ritter D, et al: Atrial natriuretic factor in plasma of patients with arterial hypertension, heart failure or cirrhosis of the liver. J Hypertens 4(Suppl II):131, 1986.

67. Sugawara A, Nakao K, Sakamoto M, et al: Plasma concentration of atrial natriuretic polypeptide in essential hypertension. Lancet 2:1426, 1985.

68. Agabiti-Rosei E, Castellano M, Beschi M, et al: Effects of infusing alpha-atrial natriuretic peptide in primary hypertension during converting enzyme inhibition. J Cardiovasc Pharmacol 10(Suppl 7):151, 1987.

69. Gaillard CA, Koomans HA, Dorhout-Mees EJ: Enalapril attenuates natriuresis of atrial natriuretic factor in humans. Hypertension 11:160, 1988.

70. Vinci JM, Horowitz D, Zusman RM, et al: The effect of converting enzyme inhibition with SQ 20, 881 on plasma and urinary kinins, prostaglandin E and angiotensin II in hypertensive man. Hypertension 1:416, 1979.

71. Swartz SL, Williams GH, Hollenberg NK, et al: Captopril-induced changes in prostaglandin production. Relationship to vascular responses in normal man. J Clin Invest 65:1257, 1980.

72. Moore TJ, Crantz FR, Hollenberg NK, et al: Contribution of prostaglandins to the antihypertensive action of captopril in essential hypertension. Hypertension 3:168, 1981.

73. Swartz SL: The role of prostaglandins in mediating the effects of angiotensin converting enzyme inhibitors and other antihypertensive drugs. Cardiovasc Drugs Ther 1:39, 1987.

74. Ogihara T, Maruyama A, Hata T, et al: Hormonal responses to long-term converting enzyme inhibition in hypertensive patients. Clin Pharmacol Ther 30:328, 1981.

75. Omata K, Abe K, Tsunoda K, et al: Role of endogenous angiotensin II and prostaglandins in the antihypertensive mechanism of angiotensin converting enzyme inhibitor in hypertension. Clin Exp Hypertens A9:569, 1987.

76. Oparil S, Horton R, Wilkins LH, et al: Antihypertensive effect of enalapril (MK 421) in low renin essential hypertension: Role of vasodilator prostaglandins [abstract]. Clin Res 31:538A, 1983.

77. Zusman RM: Regulation of prostaglandin biosynthesis in cultured renal medullary interstitial cells. In Dunn MJ, Patrono C, Cinotti GA (eds): Prostaglandins and the Kidney. New York: Plenum, 1983, pp 17–25.

78. Kudo K, Chiba S, Sato M, et al: Role of thromboxane A2 in the hypotensive effect of captopril in essential hypertension. Hypertension 11:147, 1988.

79. Dunn MJ, Hood VL: Prostaglandins and the kidney. Am J Physiol 233:F169, 1977.

80. Itskovitz HD, Terragno NA, McGiff JC: Effect of renal prostaglandin on distribution of blood flow in the isolated canine kidney. Circ Res 34:770, 1974.

81. Dunn MJ, Scharschmidt LA: Prostaglandins modulate the glomerular actions of angiotensin II. Kidney Int 31(Suppl 20):95, 1987.

82. Grantham JJ, Orloff J: Effect of prostaglandin E1 on the permeability response of the isolated collecting tubule to vasopressin, adenosine 3′,5′-monophosphate, and theophylline. J Clin Invest 47:1154, 1968.

83. Vlasses PH, Ferguson RK, Smith JB, et al: Urinary excretion of prostacyclin and thromboxane A2 metabolites after angiotensin converting enzyme inhibition in hypertensive patients. Prostaglandins Leukot Med 11:143, 1983.

84. Hornych A, Safar ME, Simon A, et al: Effects of captopril on prostaglandin and natriuresis in patients with essential hypertension. Am J Cardiol 49:1524, 1982.

85. Lee JB, Crowshaw K, Takman BH, et al: Identification of prostaglandins E2, F2α and A2 from rabbit kidney medulla. Biochem J 105:1251, 1967.

86. Margolius HS, Horwitz D, Geller RG, et al: Urinary kallikrein excretion in normal man. Relationship to sodium intake and sodium-retaining steroids. Circ Res 35:812, 1974.

87. Margolius HS, Chao J, Kaizu T: The effects of aldosterone and spironolactone on renal kallikrein. Clin Sci Mol Med 51:279S, 1976.

88. Zusman RM, Keiser HR: Prostaglandin biosynthesis by rabbit renomedullary interstitial cells in culture: Stimulation by angiotensin II, bradykinin, and arginine vasopressin. J Clin Invest 60:215, 1977.

89. McGiff JC, Terragno NA, Malik KU, et al: Release of prostaglandin E-like substance from canine kidney by bradykinin. Circ Res 31:36, 1972.

90. Blumberg AL, Denny SE, Marshall GR, et al: Blood vessel hormone interactions: Angiotensin, bradykinin, and prostaglandins. Am J Physiol 232:305, 1977.

91. Sealey JE, Atlas SA, Laragh JH, et al: Human urinary kallikrein converts inactive to active renin and is a possible physiological activator of renin. Nature 275:144, 1978.

92. Derkx FHM, Tan-Tjiong HL, Man in't Veld AJ, et al: Activation of inactive plasma renin by tissue kallikreins. J Clin Endocrinol Metab 49:765, 1979.

93. Crantz FR, Swartz SL, Hollenberg NK, et al: Differences in response to the peptidyldipeptidase hydrolase inhibitors SQ 20,881 and SQ 14,225 in normal-renin essential hypertension. Hypertension 2:604, 1980.

94. Hulthén UL, Hökfelt B: The effect of the converting enzyme inhibitor SQ 20,881 on kinins, renin-angiotensin-aldosterone and catecholamines in relation to blood pressure in hypertensive patients. Acta Med Scand 204:497, 1978.

95. Johnston CI, Clappison BH, Anderson WP, et al: Effect of angiotensin-converting enzyme inhibition on circulating and local kinin levels. Am J Cardiol 49:1401, 1982.

96. Johnston CI, McGrath BP, Millar JA, et al: Long-term effects of captopril (SQ 14225) on blood pressure and hormone levels in essential hypertension. Lancet 2:493, 1979.

97. Green LJ, Camargo ACM, Kreiger EM, et al: Inhibition of the conversion of angiotensin I to angiotensin II and potentiation of bradykinin by small peptides present in Bothrops jararaca venom. Circ Res 31(Suppl II):62, 1972.

98. Kiowski W, van Brummelen P, Hulthén UL, et al: Antihypertensive and renal effects of captopril in relation to renin activity and bradykinin-induced vasodilation. Clin Pharmacol Ther 31:677, 1982.

99. Ferner RE, Simpson JM, Rawlins MD: Effects of intradermal bradykinin after inhibition of angiotensin converting enzyme. Br Med J 294:1119, 1987.

100. Fuller RW, Warren JB, McCusker M, et al: Effect of enalapril on the skin response to bradykinin in man. Br J Clin Pharmacol 23:88, 1987.

101. Carretero OA, Miyazaki S, Scicli AG: Role of kinin in the acute antihypertensive effect of the converting enzyme inhibitor, captopril. Hypertension 2:18, 1981.

102. Waeber B, Aubert JF, Vavrek RJ, et al: Role of bradykinin in blood pressure regulation of conscious spontaneously hypertensive rats. J Hypertens 4(Suppl 6):597, 1986.

103. Benetos A, Gavras H, Stewart JM, et al: Vasodepressor role of endogenous bradykinin assessed by a bradykinin antagonist. Hypertension 8:971, 1986.

104. Textor SC, Brunner HR, Gavras H: Converting enzyme inhibition during chronic angiotensin II infusion in rats: Evidence against a non-angiotensin mechanism. Hypertension 3:269, 1981.

105. Mimran A, Targhetta R, Laroche B: The antihypertensive effect of captopril: Evidence for an influence of kinins. Hypertension 2:732, 1980.

106. Levinsky NG: The renal kallikrein-kinin system. Circ Res 44:441, 1979.

107. Carretero OA, Scicli AG: The renal kallikrein-kinin system. Am J Physiol 238:F247, 1980.

108. Fuller PJ, Funder JW: The cellular physiology of glandular kallikrein. Kidney Int 29:953, 1986.

109. Seto S, Kher V, Scicli AG, et al: The effect of aprotinin (a serine protease inhibitor) on renal function and renin release. Hypertension 5:893, 1983.

110. Ohman KP, Karlberg BE, Nilsson OR, et al: Captopril, aldosterone and urinary kallikrein in primary hypertension. Clin Exp Hypertens 5:523, 1983.

111. Reynolds TB, Paton A, Freeman M, et al: The effect of hexamethonium bromide on splanchnic blood flow, oxygen consumption and glucose output in man. J Clin Invest 32:793, 1953.

112. Ammann FW, Bolli P, Kiowski W, et al: Enhanced α-adrenoreceptor mediated vasoconstriction in essential hypertension. Hypertension 3(Suppl I):119, 1981.

113. Goldstein DS: Plasma catecholamines and essential hypertension. An analytical review. Hypertension 5:86, 1983.

114. Esler MD, Hasking GJ, Willett IR, et al: Noradrenaline release and sympathetic nervous system activity. J Hypertens 3:117, 1985.

115. Zimmerman BG, Sybertz EJ, Wong PC: Interaction between sympathetic and renin-angiotensin system. J Hypertens 2:581, 1984.

116. Bickerton RK, Buckley JP: Evidence for a central mechanism in angiotensin induced hypertension. Proc Soc Exp Biol Med 106:834, 1961.

117. Falcon JP, Philips MI, Hoffman WE, et al: Effects of intraventricular angiotensin II mediated by sympathetic nervous system. Am J Physiol 235:H392, 1978.

118. Broadwell RD, Brightman MW: Entry of peroxydase into nervous systems from extracerebral and cerebral blood. J Comp Neurol 166:257, 1976.

119. Simpson JB: The circumventricular organs and the central action of angiotensin. Neuroendocrinology 32:248, 1981.

120. Paul M, Hermann K, Printz M, et al: The brain angiotensin system: Subcellular localization and interferences with converting enzyme inhibitors. J Hypertens 1(Suppl I):9, 1983.

121. Geppetti P, Spillantini MG, Frilli S, et al: Acute oral captopril inhibits angiotensin converting enzyme activity in human cerebrospinal fluid. J Hypertens 5:151, 1987.

122. Khairallah DA: Action of angiotensin in adrenergic nerve endings: Inhibition of norepinephrine uptake. Fed Proc 31:1351, 1972.

123. Zimmerman BG: Actions of angiotensin on adrenergic nerve endings. Fed Proc 37:199, 1978.

124. Zimmerman BG: Blockade of adrenergic potentiating effects of angiotensin by 1-sar, 8-ala angiotensin. J Pharmacol Exp Ther 183:486, 1973.

125. Struthers AD, Pai S, Seidelin PH, et al: Evidence in humans for a postsynaptic interaction between noradrenaline and angiotensin II with regard to systolic but not diastolic blood pressure. J Hypertens 5:671, 1987.

126. Feldberg W, Lewis GP: The action of peptides on the adrenal medulla. Release of adrenaline by bradykinin and angiotensin. J Physiol 171:98, 1964.

127. Antonaccio MJ, Kerwin L: Pre- and post-junctional inhibition of vascular sympathetic function by captopril in SHR. Hypertension 3(Suppl I):154, 1981.

128. Hatton R, Clough DP: Captopril interferes with neurogenic vasoconstriction in the pithed rat by angiotensin-dependent mechanisms. J Cardiovasc Pharmacol 4:116, 1982.

129. De Jonge A, Knape JTA, Van Meel JCA, et al: Effect of captopril on sympathetic neurotransmission in pithed normotensive rats. Eur J Pharmacol 88:231, 1983.

130. Spertini F, Brunner HR, Waeber B, et al: The opposing effects of chronic angiotensin-converting enzyme blockade by captopril on the response to exogenous angiotensin II and vasopressin versus norepinephrine in rats. Circ Res 48:612, 1981.

131. Mimran A, Casellas D, Chevillard C, et al: Evidence for a postsynaptic effect of captopril in isolated perfused rabbit kidney. Am J Cardiol 49:1540, 1982.

132. Okuno T, Kondo K, Konishi K, et al: SQ 14,225 attenuates the vascular response to norepinephrine in the rat mesenteric arteries. Life Sci 25:1343, 1979.

133. Imai Y, Abe K, Seino M, et al: Captopril attenuates pressor responses to norepinephrine and vasopressin through depletion of endogenous angiotensin II. Am J Cardiol 49:1537, 1982.

134. Vierhapper H, Witte PU, Waldhaeusl W: Unchanged pressor effect of norepinephrine in normal man following the oral administration of two angiotensin converting enzyme inhibitors, captopril and HOE 498. J Hypertens 4:9, 1986.

135. Imai Y, Abe K, Seino M, et al: Attenuation of pressor responses to norepinephrine and pitressin and potentiation of pressor response to angiotensin II by captopril in human subjects. Hypertension 4:444, 1982.

136. Fruncillo RJ, Rotmensch HH, Vlasses PH, et al: Effect of captopril and hydrochlorothiazide on the response to pressor agents in hypertensives. Eur J Clin Pharmacol 28:5, 1985.

137. Grimm M, Weidmann P, Meier A, et al: Correction of altered noradrenaline reactivity in essential hypertension by indapamide. Br Heart J 46:404, 1981.

138. Sturani A, Chiarini C, Degli-Esposito E, et al: Heart rate control in hypertensive patients treated by captopril. Br J Clin Pharmacol 14:849, 1982.

139. Millar JA, Derk FTM, McLean K, et al: Pharmacodynamics of converting enzyme inhibition: The cardiovascular, endocrine and autonomic effects of MK-421 (enalapril) and MK-521. Br J Clin Pharmacol 14:347, 1982.

140. Niarchos AP, Pickering TG, Morganti A, et al: Plasma catecholamines and cardiovascular responses during converting enzyme inhibition in normotensive and hypertensive man. Clin Exp Hypertens A4:761, 1982.

141. Mancia G, Parati G, Pomidossi G, et al: Modification of arterial baroreflexes by captopril in essential hypertension. Am J Cardiol 49:1415, 1982.

142. Ibsen H, Egan B, Osterziel K, et al: Reflex-hemodynamic adjustments and baroreflex sensitivity during converting enzyme inhibition with MK-421 in normal humans. Hypertension 5:184, 1983.

143. Giudicelli JF, Berdeaux A, Edouard A, et al: The effect of enalapril on baroreceptor mediated reflex function in normotensive subjects. Br J Clin Pharmacol 20:211, 1985.

144. Ajayi AA, Campbell BC, Howie CA, et al: Acute and chronic effects of the converting enzyme inhibitors enalapril and lisinopril on reflex control of heart rate in normotensive man. J Hypertens 3:47, 1985.

145. Cody RJ, Tarazi RC, Bravo E, et al: Haemodynamics of orally-active converting enzyme inhibitor (SQ14225) in hypertensive patients. Clin Sci Mol Med 55:453, 1978.

146. Cody RJ, Bravo E, Fouad F, et al: Cardiovascular reflexes during long-term converting enzyme inhibition and sodium depletion. Am J Med 71:422, 1981.

147. Morganti A, Pickering TG, Lopez-Ovejero JA, et al: Endocrine and cardiovascular influences of converting enzyme inhibition with SQ14225 in hypertensive patients in the supine position and during head-up tilt before and after sodium depletion. J Clin Endocrinol Metab 50:748, 1980.

148. Zanella MT, Bravo E, Fouad F, et al: Long-term converting enzyme inhibition and sympathetic nerve function in hypertensive humans. Hypertension 3(Suppl II):216, 1981.

149. Morganti A, Sala C, Turolo L, et al: Participation of the renin-angiotensin system in the maintenance of blood pressure during changes in posture in patients with essential hypertension. J Hypertens 3:55, 1985.

150. Lederle RM: Captopril and hydrochlorothiazide in the fixed combination multicenter trial. J Cardiovasc Pharmacol 7(Suppl I):63, 1985.

151. Jenkins AC, Dreslinski GR, Tadros SS, et al: Captopril in hypertension: Seven years later. J Cardiovasc Pharmacol 7(Suppl I):96, 1985.

152. McFate Smith W, Kulaga SF, Moncloa F, et al: Overall tolerance and safety of enalapril. J Hypertens 2(Suppl II):113, 1984.

153. Vidt DG: A controlled multiclinic study to compare the antihypertensive effects of MK-421, hydrochlorothiazide, and MK-421 combined with hydrochlorothiazide in patients with mild to moderate essential hypertension. J Hypertens 2(Suppl II):81, 1984.

154. Fouad FM, Tarazi RC, Bravo EL: Cardiac and haemodynamic effects of enalapril. J Hypertens 1(Suppl I):135, 1983.

155. Bravo EL, Tarazi RC: Converting enzyme inhibition with an orally active compound in hypertensive man. Hypertension 1:39, 1979.

156. Nicholls MG, Espiner EA, Miles KD, et al: Evidence against an interaction of angiotensin II with the sympathetic nervous system in man. Clin Endocrinol 15:423, 1981.

157. Man in't Veld AJ, Wenting GJ, Boosma F, et al: Sympathetic and parasympathetic components of reflex cardiostimulation during vasodilator treatment of hypertension. Br J Clin Pharmacol 9:547, 1980.

158. Campbell BC, Sturani A, Reid JL: Parasympathomimetic activity of captopril in normotensive man. J Hypertens 1(Suppl II):246, 1983.

159. Reid JL, Millar JA, Campbell BC: Enalapril and autonomic reflexes and exercise performance. J Hypertens 1(Suppl II):129, 1983.

160. Ajayi AA, Campbell BC, Meredith PA, et al: The effect of captopril on the reflex control heart rate: Possible mechanisms. Br J Clin Pharmacol 20:17, 1985.

161. Lee WB, Ismay MJ, Lumbers ER: Mechanisms by which angiotensin II affects the heart rate of conscious sheep. Circ Res 40:286, 1980.

162. Potter EK: Angiotensin inhibits action of the vagus nerve at the heart. Br J Pharmacol 75:9, 1982.

163. Fagard R, Amery A, Reybrouck T, et al: Acute and chronic systemic and hemodynamic effects of angiotensin converting enzyme inhibition with captopril in hypertensive patients. Am J Cardiol 46:295, 1980.

164. Tarazi RC, Bravo EL, Fouad FM, et al: Hemodynamic and volume changes associated with captopril. Hypertension 2:576, 1980.

165. Muiesan G, Alicandri CL, Agabiti-Rosei E, et al: Angiotensin-converting enzyme inhibition, catecholamines and hemodynamics in essential hypertension. Am J Cardiol 49:1420, 1982.

166. Wenting GJ, De Bruyn JHB, Man in't Veld AJ, et al: Hemodynamic effects of captopril in essential hypertension, renovascular hypertension and cardiac failure: Correlations with short- and long-term effects on plasma renin. Am J Cardiol 49:1453, 1982.

167. Saragoca MA, Homsi E, Ribeiro AB, et al: Hemodynamic mechanism of blood pressure response to captopril in human malignant hypertension. Hypertension 5(Suppl I):53, 1983.

168. Omvik P, Lund-Johanson P: Combined captopril and hydrochlorothiazide therapy in severe hypertension: Long-term haemodynamic changes at rest and during exercise. J Hypertens 2:73, 1984.

169. Manhem P, Bramnert M, Hulthén UL, et al: The effect of captopril on catecholamines, renin activity, angiotensin II and aldosterone in plasma during physical exercise in hypertensive patients. Eur J Clin Invest 11:389, 1981.

170. Morioka S, Simon G, Cohn JN: Cardiac and hormonal effects of enalapril in hypertension. Clin Pharmacol Ther 34:583, 1988.

171. Navar LG, Rosivall L: Contribution of the renin-angiotensin system to the control of intrarenal hemodynamics. Kidney Int 25:857, 1984.

172. Levens NR, Peach MJ, Carey RM: Role of the intra-renal renin-angiotensin system in control of renal function. Circ Res 48:157, 1981.

173. Ichikawa I, Brenner BM: Glomerular actions of angiotensin II. Am J Med 76:43, 1984.

174. Ardaillou M, Staer J, Chansel D, et al: The effects of angiotensin II on isolated glomeruli and cultered glomerular cells. Kidney Int 31(Suppl 20):74, 1987.

175. Navar LG, Carmines PK, Huang WC, et al: The tubular effects of angiotensin II. Kidney Int 31(Suppl 20):81, 1987.

176. Mendelsohn FAO: Localization and properties of angiotensin receptors. J Hypertens 3:307, 1985.

177. Blantz RC, Gabbai FB: Effect of angiotensin II on glomerular hemodynamics and ultrafiltration coefficient. Kidney Int 31(Suppl 20):108, 1987.

178. Brunner HR, Waeber B, Nussberger J: Angiotensin converting enzyme inhibition and the normal kidney. Kidney Int 31(Suppl 20):104, 1987.

179. Hollenberg NK, Meggs LG, Williams GH, et al: Sodium intake and renal responses to captopril in normal man and in essential hypertension. Kidney Int 20:240, 1981.

180. Hollenberg NK, Adams DF, Solomon H, et al: Renal vascular tone in essential and secondary hypertension: Hemodynamic

and angiographic response to vasodilators. Medicine 54:29, 1975.

181. Hollenberg NK, Bourcki LJ, Adams DF: The renal vasculature in early essential hypertension: Evidence for a pathogenetic role. Medicine 57:167, 1978.

182. Williams GH, Hollenberg NK: Accentuated vascular and endocrine response to SQ 20881 in hypertension. N Engl J Med 297:184, 1977.

183. Mimran A, Brunner HR, Turini GA, et al: Effect of captopril on renal vascular tone in patients with essential hypertension. Clin Sci 57:421S, 1979.

184. Simon G, Morioka S, Snyder DK, et al: Increased renal plasma flow in long-term enalapril treatment of hypertension. Clin Pharmacol Ther 34:459, 1983.

185. Dunn FG, Oigman W, Ventura HO, et al: Enalapril improves systemic and renal hemodynamics and allows regression of left ventricular mass in essential hypertension. Am J Cardiol 53:105, 1984.

186. Bauer JH, Reams GP: Renal effects of angiotensin converting enzyme inhibitors in hypertension. Am J Med 81(Suppl 4C):19, 1986.

187. Bauer JH, Reams GP: Hemodynamic and renal function in essential hypertension during treatment with enalapril. Am J Med 79(Suppl 3C):10, 1985.

188. Britton S, Di Salvo J: Effects of angiotensin I and angiotensin II on hindlimb and coronary vascular resistance. Am J Physiol 225:1226, 1973.

189. Magrini F, Shimizu M, Roberts N, et al: Angiotensin converting enzyme inhibition and coronary blood flow. Circulation 75(Suppl I):168, 1987.

190. Gavras H, Liang C, Brunner HR: Redistribution of regional blood flow after inhibition of the angiotensin-converting enzyme. Circ Res 43(Suppl I):59, 1978.

191. Strandgaard S: Autoregulation of cerebral blood flow in hypertensive patients. Circulation 58:720, 1975.

192. Frei A, Müller-Brand J: Cerebral blood flow and antihypertensive treatment with enalapril. J Hypertens 4:365, 1986.

193. Minematsu K, Yamaguchi T, Tsuchiya M, et al: Effect of angiotensin converting enzyme inhibitor (captopril) on cerebral blood flow in hypertensive patients without a history of stroke. Clin Exp Hypertens A9:551, 1987.

194. Britton KE, Granowska M, Nimmon CC, et al: Cerebral blood flow in hypertensive patients with cerebrovascular disease: Technique for measurement and effect of captopril. Nucl Med Commun 6:251, 1985.

195. Barry DI, Jarden JO, Paulson OB, et al: Cerebro-vascular aspects of converting enzyme inhibition: I. Effects of intravenous captopril in spontaneously hypertensive and normotensive rats. J Hypertens 2:589, 1984.

196. Ames RP, Hill P: Antihypertensive therapy and the risk of coronary heart disease. J Cardiovasc Pharmacol 4(Suppl II):206, 1982.

197. Castelli WP, Anderson K: A population at risk: Prevalence of high cholesterol levels in hypertensive patients in the Framingham study. Am J Med 80(2A):23, 1986.

198. Hollifield JW: Thiazide treatment of hypertension. Effects of thiazide diuretics on serum potassium, magnesium, and ventricular ectopy. Am J Med 80(Suppl 4A):8, 1986.

199. Weinberger MH: Blood pressure and metabolic responses to hydrochlorothiazide, captopril, and the combination in black and white mild-to-moderate hypertensive patients. J Cardiovasc Pharmacol 7(Suppl I):52, 1987.

200. Malini PL, Strochi E, Ambrosioni E, et al: Long-term antihypertensive, metabolic and cellular effects of enalapril. J Hypertens 2(Suppl II):101, 1984.

201. Sasaki J, Arakawa K: Effect of captopril on serum lipids, lipoproteins, and apolipoproteins in patients with mild essential hypertension. Curr Ther Res 40:898, 1986.

202. Weinberger MH: Antihypertensive therapy and lipids: Evidence, mechanisms and implications. Arch Intern Med 145:1102, 1985.

203. Leary WP, Reyes AJ: Angiotensin I converting enzyme inhibitors and the renal excretion of urate. Cardiovasc Drugs Ther 1:29, 1987.

204. Waeber B, Gavras I, Brunner HR, et al: Safety and efficacy of chronic therapy with captopril in hypertensive patients: An update. J Clin Pharmacol 21:508, 1981.

205. Textor SC, Bravo EL, Fouad FM, et al: Hyperkalemia in azotemic patients during angiotensin converting enzyme inhibition and aldosterone reduction with captopril. Am J Med 73:719, 1982.

206. Costa FV, Borghi C, Boshi S, et al: Differing dosages of captopril and hydrochlorothiazide in the treatment of hypertension: Long-term effects of metabolic values and intracellular electrolytes. J Cardiovasc Pharmacol 7(Suppl I):70, 1985.

207. Ryan MP, Ryan MF, Counihan TB: The effect of diuretics on lymphocyte magnesium and potassium. Acta Med Scand 209:153, 1981.

208. Mooser V, Waeber G, Bidiville J, et al: Kalemia during combined therapy with an angiotensin converting enzyme inhibitor and a potassium-sparing diuretic. J Clin Hypertens 3:510, 1987.

209. Burnakis TG, Mioduch HJ: Combined therapy with captopril and potassium supplementation. A potential for hyperkalemia. Arch Intern Med 144:2371, 1984.

210. Barnes JN, Drew PJT, Furniss SS, et al: Effect of angiotensin converting enzyme inhibition on potassium-mediated aldosterone secretion in essential hypertension. Clin Sci 68:625, 1985.

211. Atkinson AB, Robertson JIS: Captopril in the treatment of clinical hypertension and cardiac failure. Lancet 2:836, 1979.

212. Heel RC, Brogden RN, Speight TM, et al: Captopril: A preliminary review of its pharmacological properties and therapeutic efficacy. Drugs 20:409, 1980.

213. Ferguson RK, Vlasses PH, Rotmensch HN: Clinical applications of angiotensin converting enzyme inhibitors. Am J Med 77:690, 1984.

214. Edwards CRW, Padfield PL: Angiotensin converting enzyme inhibitors: Past, present, and bright future. Lancet 1:30, 1985.

215. Tood PA, Heel RC: Enalapril: A review of its pharmacodynamic and pharmacokinetic properties, and therapeutic use in hypertension and congestive heart failure. Drugs 31:198, 1986.

216. Drayer JIM, Weber MA: Monotherapy of essential hypertension with a converting enzyme inhibitor. Hypertension 5(Suppl III):108, 1983.

217. Davies RO, Irvin JD, Kramsch DK, et al: Enalapril worldwide experience. Am J Med 77(2A):23, 1984.

218. Johns DW, Baker KM, Ayers CR, et al: Acute and chronic effect of captopril in hypertensive patients. Hypertension 2:567, 1980.

219. Veterans Administration Cooperative Study Group on Antihypertensive Agents: Low-dose captopril for the treatment of mild to moderate hypertension. Hypertension 5(Suppl III):139, 1983.

220. Ferguson RK, Vlasses PH, Swanson BN, et al: Effects of enalapril, a new converting enzyme inhibitor, in hypertension. Clin Pharmacol Ther 32:48, 1982.

221. Weidmann P, De Muyttenaere-Bursztein S, Maxwell MH, et al: Effect of aging on plasma renin and aldosterone in normal man. Kidney Int 8:325, 1975.

222. Bühler FR, Bolli P, Kiowski W, et al: Renin profiling to select antihypertensive baseline drugs. Renin inhibitors for high-renin and calcium-entry blockers for low-renin patients. Am J Med 77(2A):36, 1984.

223. Ball SG: Age-related effects of converting enzyme inhibitors: A commentary. J Cardiovasc Pharmacol 14(Suppl 4):53, 1989.

224. Saner H, Brunner HR: Antihypertensive Wirksamkeit und Verträglichkeit von Captopril. Ergebnisse einer Schweizer Feldstudie. Therapiewoche Schweiz 2:157, 1988.

225. Cooper WD, Glover DR, Kimber GR: Influence of age on blood pressure response to enalapril. Gerontology 33(Suppl I):48, 1987.

226. Schnaper HW, Stein G, Schoenberger JA, et al: Comparison of enalapril with thiazide diuretics in the elderly hypertensive patient. Gerontology 33(Suppl I):24, 1987.

227. Vaughan ED Jr, Bühler FR, Laragh JH, et al: Renovascular hypertension: Renin measurements to indicate hypersecretion and contralateral suppression, estimate renal plasma flow, and score for surgical curability. Am J Med 55:402, 1973.

228. McGrath BP, Matthews PG, Johnston CI: Use of captopril in the diagnosis of renal hypertension. Aust N Z J Med 11:359, 1981.

229. Staessen J, Bulpitt C, Fagard R, et al: Long-term converting enzyme inhibition as a guide to surgical curability of hypertension associated with renovascular disease. Am J Cardiol 51:1317, 1983.

230. Hollenberg NK: Medical therapy of renovascular hypertension: Efficacy and safety of captopril in 269 patients. Cardiovasc Rev Rep 4:854, 1983.

231. Smith RD, Franklin SS: Comparison of effects of enalapril plus hydrochlorothiazide versus standard triple therapy on renal function in renovascular hypertension. Am J Med 79(Suppl 3C):14, 1985.

232. Hricik DE, Browning PJ, Kopelman RI, et al: Captopril-induced functional renal insufficiency in patients with bilateral renal artery stenoses or renal artery stenosis in a solitary kidney. N Engl J Med 308:373, 1983.

233. Chrysant SG, Dunn M, Marples D, et al: Severe reversible azotemia from captopril therapy. Arch Intern Med 143:437, 1983.

234. Jackson B, Matthews PG, McGrath BP, et al: Angiotensin converting enzyme inhibition in renovascular hypertension: Frequency of reversible renal failure. Lancet 1:225, 1984.

235. Bussien JP, Schaller MD, Nussberger J, et al: Insuffisance rénale aiguë après inhibition de l'enzyme de conversion de l'angiotensine par différents agents. Schweiz Med Wochenschr 114:236, 1984.

236. Wenting GJ, Derkx FHM, Tan-Tjiong LH, et al: Risks of angiotensin converting enzyme inhibition in renal artery stenosis. Kidney Int 31(Suppl 20):S180, 1987.

237. Reams GP, Singh A, Logan KW, et al: Total and split renal function in patients with renovascular hypertension: Effects of angiotensin converting enzyme inhibition. J Clin Hypertens 3:153, 1987.

238. Williams PS, Hendy MS, Krill A: Captopril-induced renal artery thrombosis and persistent anuria in a patient with documented pre-existing renal artery stenosis and renal failure. Postgrad Med J 60:561, 1984.

239. Davis BA, Crook JE, Vestal RE, et al: Prevalence of renovascular hypertension in patients with grade III or IV hypertensive retinopathy. N Engl J Med 301:1273, 1979.

240. Case DB, Laragh JH: Reactive hyperreninemia following angiotensin blockade with either saralasin or converting enzyme inhibitor: A new approach to screen for renovascular hypertension. Ann Intern Med 91:153, 1979.

241. Re RN, Novelline R, Escourron MT, et al: Inhibition of angiotensin converting enzyme for diagnosis of renal artery stenosis. N Engl J Med 298:582, 1978.

242. Brunner HR, Gavras H, Waeber B, et al: Clinical use of an orally acting converting enzyme inhibitor: Captopril. Hypertension 2:558, 1980.

243. Thibonnier M, Sassano P, Joseph A, et al: Diagnostic value of a single dose of captopril in renin- and aldosterone-dependent surgically curable hypertension. Cardiovasc Rev Rep 3:1659, 1982.

244. Lyons DF, Kern DC, Brown RD, et al: Single dose captopril as a diagnostic test for primary aldosteronism. J Clin Endocrinol Metab 57:892, 1983.

245. Baruch D, Corvol P, Alhenc-Gelas F, et al: Diagnosis and treatment of renin-secreting tumors: Report of three cases. Hypertension 6:760, 1984.

246. Harrison TS, Birbari A, Seaton JR: Malignant hypertension in pheochromocytoma: Correlation with plasma renin activity. Johns Hopkins Med J 130:329, 1972.

247. Lonte G, Guffens P, Waucquez JL, et al: Effect of captopril on hypertension due to pheochromocytoma. Lancet 2:175, 1984.

248. Plouin PF, Rougeot MA, Chatellier G, et al: Système rénine-angiotensine-aldostérone au cours du phéochromocytome: Un rôle dans l'élévation tensionelle? Arch Mal Coeur 78:1734, 1985.

249. Broughton-Pipkin F, Symonds EM, Turner SR: The effect of SQ 14,225 (captopril) upon mother and fetus in the chronically cannulated ewe and in the pregnant rabbit. J Physiol 87:533, 1986.

250. Ferris TF, Wein EK: Effect of captopril on uterine blood flow and prostaglandin E synthesis in the pregnant rabbit. J Clin Invest 71:809, 1983.

251. Bontroy MJ, Vert P, Hurault De Ligny B, et al: Captopril administration in pregnancy impairs fetal angiotensin converting enzyme activity and neonatal adaptation. Lancet 2:935, 1984.

252. Rothberg AD, Lorenz R: Can captopril cause fetal and neonatal renal failure? Pediatr Pharmacol 4:189, 1984.

253. Schubiger G, Flury G, Nussberger J: Enalapril for pregnancy-induced hypertension: Acute renal failure in a neonate. Ann Intern Med 108:215, 1988.

254. Kreft-Joris C, Plouin PF, Tchobroutsky C: Angiotensin converting enzyme inhibitors during pregnancy. J Hypertens 5(Suppl 5):553, 1987.

255. Brunner HR, Waeber B, Wauters JP, et al: Inappropriate renin secretion unmasked by captopril (SQ 14,225) in hypertension of chronic renal failure. Lancet 2:704, 1978.

256. Atkinson AB, Lever AF, Brown JJ, et al: Combined treatment of severe intractable hypertension with captopril and diuretic. Lancet 2:105, 1980.

257. Case DB, Atlas SA, Sullivan PA, et al: Acute and chronic treatment of severe and malignant hypertension with the angiotensin converting enzyme inhibitor captopril. Circulation 64:765, 1981.

258. Raine AEG, Ledingham JGG: Clinical experience with captopril in the treatment of severe drug-resistant hypertension. Am J Cardiol 49:1475, 1982.

259. Havelka J, Vetter H, Studer A, et al: Acute and chronic effects of the angiotensin converting enzyme inhibitor captopril in severe hypertension. Am J Cardiol 49:1467, 1982.

260. Biollaz J, Waeber B, Brunner HR: Hypertensive crisis treated with orally administered captopril. Eur J Clin Pharmacol 25:145, 1983.

261. Tschollar W, Belz GG: Sublingual captopril in hypertensive crisis. Lancet 2:34, 1985.

262. Tifft CP, Gavras H, Kershaw GR, et al: Converting enzyme inhibition in hypertensive emergencies. Ann Intern Med 90:43, 1979.

263. Di Pette DJ, Ferraro JC, Evans RR, et al: Enalaprilat, an intravenous angiotensin-converting enzyme inhibitor, in hypertensive crises. Clin Pharmacol Ther 38:199, 1985.

264. Strauss R, Gavras I, Vlahakos D, et al: Enalaprilat in hypertensive emergencies. J Clin Pharmacol 26:39, 1986.

265. Ledingham JGG: Effects of angiotensin II and angiotensin converting enzyme inhibition in chronic renal failure. Kidney Int 31(Suppl 20):112, 1987.

266. Weidmann P: Pathogenesis of hypertension associated with chronic renal failure. Contrib Nephrol 41:47, 1984.

267. Wilkinson R, Scott DF, Udall PR, et al: Plasma renin and exchangeable sodium in the hypertension of chronic renal failure. Q J Med 39:377, 1970.

268. Davies DL, Beevers DG, Briggs JD, et al: Abnormal relationship between exchangeable sodium and the renin-angiotensin system in malignant hypertension and in hypertension with chronic renal failure. Lancet 1:683, 1973.

269. Mendelsohn FAO: Angiotensin II: Evidence for its role as an intrarenal hormone. Kidney Int 22(Suppl 12):78, 1982.

270. Hostetter TH, Rennke HG, Brenner BM: The case for intrarenal hypertension in the initiation and progression of diabetic and other glomerulopathies. Am J Med 72:375, 1982.

271. Hollenberg NK, Swartz SL, Passan DR, et al: Increased glomerular filtration rate after converting enzyme inhibition in essential hypertension. N Engl J Med 301:9, 1979.

272. Cooper WD, Doyle GD, Donohoe J, et al: Enalapril in the treatment of hypertension associated with impaired renal function. J Hypertens 3(Suppl 3):471, 1985.

273. Bauer JH, Reams GP, Lal SM: Renal protective effect of strict blood pressure control with enalapril therapy. Arch Intern Med 147:1397, 1987.

274. De Venuto G, Andreotti C, Mattarei M, et al: Long-term captopril therapy at low-doses reduces albumin excretion in patients with essential hypertension and no sign of renal impairment. J Hypertens 3(Suppl II):143, 1985.

275. Lifschitz MD, Kirschenbaum MA, Rosenblatt SG, et al: Effect of saralasin in hypertensive patients on chronic dialysis. Ann Intern Med 88:23, 1977.

276. Vaughan ED Jr, Carey RM, Ayers CR, et al: Hemodialysis-

resistant hypertension: Control with an orally active inhibitor of angiotensin converting enzyme. J Clin Endocrinol 48:869, 1979.

277. Wauters JP, Waeber B, Brunner HR, et al: Uncontrollable hypertension in patients on hemodialysis: Long-term treatment with captopril and salt subtraction. Clin Nephrol 16:86, 1981.

278. Hamilton DV, Evans DB, Maidment G, et al: Captopril in refractory hypertension in patients with chronic renal failure and renal transplantation. J R Soc Med 74:357, 1981.

279. Curtiss JJ, Luke RG, Whelchel JD, et al: Inhibition of angiotensin-converting enzyme in renal transplant recipients with hypertension. N Engl J Med 308:377, 1983.

280. Frohlich ED: Pathophysiological considerations in left ventricular hypertrophy. J Clin Hypertens 3:54, 1987.

281. Wright GB, Alexander RW, Eckstein LS, et al: Characterization of rabbit ventricular myocardial receptors for angiotensin II: Evidence for two sites with different affinities and specificities. Mol Pharmacol 24:213, 1984.

282. Dzau VJ, Re RN: Evidence for the existence of renin in the heart. Circulation 75(Suppl I):134, 1987.

283. Koch-Weser J: Nature of the inotropic action of angiotensin on ventricular myocardium. Circ Res 16:230, 1965.

284. Re RN, La Biche RA, Bryan SE: Nuclear-hormone mediated changes in chromatin solubility. Biochem Biophys Res Commun 110:61, 1983.

285. Devereux RB, Pickering TG, Cody RJ, et al: Relation of renin-angiotensin system activity to left ventricular hypertrophy and function in experimental and human hypertension. J Clin Hypertens 3:87, 1987.

286. Dahlöf B, Pennert K, Hansson L: Reversal of left ventricular hypertrophy in hypertensive patients: A meta-analysis of 109 treatment studies. Am J Hypertens 5:95, 1992.

287. Captopril Multicenter Research Group: A placebo-controlled trial of captopril in refractory chronic congestive heart failure. J Am Coll Cardiol 2:755, 1983.

288. The Consensus Trial Study Group: Effects of enalapril on mortality in severe congestive heart failure. N Engl J Med 23:1429, 1987.

289. Deedwania PC: Angiotensin-converting enzyme inhibitors in congestive heart failure. Arch Intern Med 150:1798, 1992.

290. Turini GA, Brunner HR, Ferguson RK, et al: Congestive heart failure in normotensive man: Haemodynamics, renin, and angiotensin II blockade. Br Heart J 40:1134, 1978.

291. Turini GA, Brunner HR, Gribic M, et al: Improvement of chronic congestive heart failure by oral captopril. Lancet 1:1213, 1979.

292. Daly P, Rouleau JL, Cousineau D, et al: Acute effects of captopril on the coronary circulation of patients with hypertension and angina. Am J Med 76(5B):111, 1984.

293. Strozzi C, Cocco G, Portaluppi F, et al: Ergometric evaluation of the effects of captopril in hypertensive patients with stable angina. J Hypertens 3(Suppl 2):147, 1985.

294. Mettauer B, Rouleau JL, Daly P: The effect of captopril on the coronary circulation and myocardial metabolism of patients with coronary artery disease. Postgrad Med J 62(Suppl 1):54, 1986.

295. Tardieu A, Virot P, Vandroux JC, et al: Effects of captopril on myocardial perfusion in patients with coronary insufficiency: Evaluation by the exercise test and quantitative myocardial tomoscintigraphy using thallium-201. Postgrad Med J 62(Suppl 1):38, 1986.

296. Daly P, Mettauer B, Rouleau JL, et al: Lack of reflex increase in myocardial sympathetic tone after captopril: Potential antianginal effect. Circulation 71:317, 1985.

297. Pfeffer MA, Lamas GA, Vaughan DE et al: Effect of captopril on progressive ventricular dilatation after anterior myocardial infarction. N Engl J Med 319:80, 1988.

298. Cohn JN: The prevention of heart failure—a new agenda. N Engl J Med 327:725, 1992.

299. Sutton MSJ: Should angiotensin converting enzyme (ACE) inhibitors be used routinely after infarction? Perspectives from the Survival and Ventricular Enlargement (SAVE) Trial. Br Heart J 71:115, 1994.

300. Safar ME, Bouthier JA, Levenson JA, et al: Peripheral large arteries and the response to antihypertensive treatment. Hypertension 5(Suppl III):63, 1983.

301. Schiffrin EL, Deng LY, Larochelle P: Effects of a beta-blocker or a converting enzyme inhibitor on resistance arteries in essential hypertension. Hypertension 23:83, 1994.

302. Libretti A, Catalano M: Captopril in the treatment of hypertension associated with claudication. Postgrad Med J 62(Suppl I):34, 1986.

303. Roberts DH, Tsao Y, McLoughlin GA, et al: Placebo-controlled comparison of captopril, atenolol, labetolol, and pindolol in hypertension complicated by intermittent claudication. Lancet 2:650, 1987.

304. Christlieb AR, Warram JH, Krowleski AS, et al: Hypertension: The major risk factor in juvenile onset insulin-dependent diabetics. Diabetes 30(Suppl II):90, 1981.

305. Sullivan PA, Kelleher M, Twomey M, et al: Effects of converting enzyme inhibition on blood pressure, plasma renin activity (PRA) and plasma aldosterone in hypertensive diabetics compared to patients with essential hypertension. J Hypertens 3:359, 1985.

306. Gambaro G, Morbiato F, Cicerello E, et al: Captopril in the treatment of hypertension in type I and type II diabetic patients. J Hypertens 3(Suppl II):153, 1985.

307. Matthews DM, Wathen CG, Bell D, et al: The effect of captopril on blood pressure and glucose tolerance in hypertensive non-insulin dependent diabetics. Postgrad Med J 62(Suppl I):73, 1986.

308. Taguma Y, Kitamoto Y, Futaki G, et al: Effect of captopril on heavy proteinuria in azotemic diabetics. N Engl J Med 313:1617, 1985.

309. Björck S, Nyberg G, Mulec H, et al: Beneficial effects of angiotensin converting enzyme inhibition on renal function in patients with diabetic nephropathy. Br Med J 293:471, 1986.

310. Lewis EY, Hunsicker LG, Bain RP: The effect of angiotensin-converting-enzyme inhibition on diastolic nephropathy. N Engl J Med 329:1456, 1993.

311. Jauch KW, Hartl W, Guenther B, et al: Captopril enhances insulin responsiveness of forearm muscle tissue in non-insulin-dependent diabetes mellitus. Eur J Clin Invest 17:448, 1987.

312. Dietze GJ, Rett K, Jauch KW, et al: Captopril bei Hypertonikern mit Diabetes mellitus Typ II. Herz 12(Suppl I):16, 1987.

313. Bertoli L, Fusco M, Micallef RE, et al: Treatment of essential hypertension with captopril in patients with chronic obstructive pulmonary disease. J Hypertens 3(Suppl II):153, 1985.

314. Riska H, Stenius-Aarniala B, Sovijärvi ARA: Comparison of the efficacy of an ACE inhibitor and a calcium channel blocker in hypertensive asthmatics. A preliminary report. Postgrad Med J 62(Suppl I):52, 1986.

315. Sala H, Abad J, Juanmiguel L, et al: Captopril and bronchial reactivity. Postgrad Med J 62(Suppl I):76, 1986.

316. Dixon CMS, Fuller RW, Barnes PJ: The effect of an angiotensin converting enzyme inhibitor, ramipril, on bronchial responses in asthmatic subjects. Br J Clin Pharmacol 23:91, 1986.

317. Waeber B, Brunner HR, Brunner DB, et al: Discrepancy between antihypertensive effect and angiotensin converting enzyme inhibition by captopril. Hypertension 2:236, 1980.

318. Veterans Administration Cooperative Study Group on Antihypertensive Agents: Low-dose captopril for the treatment of mild to moderate hypertension. Arch Intern Med 144:1947, 1984.

319. De Gaudemaris R, Battistella P, Siche JP, et al: Comparative study of the efficacy of captopril at a single daily dose of 100 mg and at a twice daily dose of 50 mg by measuring ambulatory pressure over 24 hours. Postgrad Med J 62(Suppl I):97, 1986.

320. Fogari R, Zoppi A, Corradi L, et al: Hypotensive effect of once-daily administration of captopril. Curr Ther Res 40:500, 1986.

321. Garanin G: A comparison of once-daily antihypertensive therapy with captopril and enalapril. Curr Ther Res 40:567, 1986.

322. Schoenberger JA, Wilson DJ: Once-daily treatment of essential hypertension with captopril. J Clin Hypertens 4:379, 1986.

323. De Cesaris R, Ranieri G, Salzano EV, et al: Once daily therapy with angiotensin converting enzyme inhibitors in mild hypertension: A comparison of captopril and enalapril. J Hypertens 5(Suppl 5):595, 1987.

324. Bergstrand R, Herlitz H, Johansson S, et al: Effective dose range of enalapril in mild to moderate essential hypertension. Br J Clin Pharmacol 19:605, 1985.

325. Bergstrand R, Johansson S, Vedin A, et al: Comparison of once-a-day and twice-a-day dosage regimens of enalapril (MK-421) in patients with mild hypertension. Br J Clin Pharmacol 14:136P, 1982.
326. Kripalani KJ, McKinstry DN, Singhvi SM, et al: Disposition of captopril in normal subjects. Clin Pharmacol Ther 27:636, 1980.
327. Fruncillo RJ, Rocci ML, Vlasses PH, et al: Disposition of enalapril and enalaprilat in renal insufficiency. Kidney Int 31(Suppl 20):117, 1987.
328. Hollenberg NK: Initial therapy in hypertension: Quality-of-life considerations. J Hypertens 5(Suppl I):3, 1987.
329. Callender JS, Hodsman GP, Hutcheson MJ, et al: Mood changes during captopril therapy for hypertension: A double-blind pilot study. Hypertension 5(Suppl III):90, 1983.
330. Olajide D, Lader M: Psychotropic effects of enalapril maleate in normal volunteers. Psychopharmacology 86:374, 1985.
331. Lichter I, Richardson PJ, Wyke MA: Differential effects of atenolol and enalapril on memory during treatment for essential hypertension. Br J Clin Pharmacol 21:641, 1986.
332. Croog SH, Levine S, Testa MA, et al: The effects of antihypertensive therapy on the quality of life. N Engl J Med 314:1657, 1986.
333. Hill JF, Bulpitt CJ, Fletcher AE: Angiotensin converting enzyme inhibitors and quality of life: The European trial. J Hypertens 3(Suppl II):91, 1985.
334. Baker KM, Johns DW, Ayers CR, et al: Ischemic cardiovascular complications concurrent with administration of captopril. Hypertension 2:73, 1980.
335. Benett PR, Cairns SA: Captopril, diarrhoea, and hypotension. Lancet 1:1105, 1985.
336. Coulshed DJ, Davies SJ, Turney JH: Prolonged hypotension after fever during enalapril treatment. Lancet 2:222, 1985.
337. Thind GS: Renal insufficiency during angiotensin-converting enzyme inhibitor therapy in hypertensive patients with no renal artery stenosis. J Clin Hypertens 4:337, 1985.
338. Cooper WD, Sheldon D, Brown D, et al: Post-marketing surveillance of enalapril: Experience in 11,710 hypertensive patients in general practice. J R Coll Gen Pract 37:346, 1987.
339. Chalmers D, Dombey SL, Lawson DH: Post-marketing surveillance of captopril (for hypertension): A preliminary report. Br J Clin Pharmacol 24:343, 1987.
340. Rush JE, Merrill DD: The safety and tolerability of lisinopril in clinical trials. J Cardiovasc Pharmacol 9(Suppl III):99, 1987.
341. Morice AH, Lowry R, Brown MJ, et al: Angiotensin-converting enzyme and the cough reflex. Lancet 2:1116, 1987.
342. Erdös EG: Angiotensin I converting enzyme. Circ Res 36:247, 1975.
343. Thiele EA, Strittmatter SM, Snyder SH: Substance K and substance P as possible endogenous substrates of angiotensin converting enzyme in the brain. Biochem Biophys Res Commun 128:317, 1985.
344. Fuller RW, Dixon CMS, Cuss FMC, et al: Bradykinin-induced bronchoconstriction in humans. Annu Rev Respir Dis 135:176, 1987.
345. Nicholls MG, Gilchrist NL: Sulindac and cough induced by converting enzyme inhibitors. Lancet 1:872, 1987.
346. Cooper RA: Captopril-associated neutropenia. Who is at risk? Arch Intern Med 143:659, 1983.
347. Ersley AJ, Alexander JC, Caro J, et al: Hematologic side effects of captopril and associated risk factors. Cardiovasc Rev Rep 3:660, 1982.
348. Prins EJL, Hoorntje SJ, Weening JJ, et al: Nephrotic syndrome in a patient on captopril. Lancet 2:306, 1979.
349. Case DB, Atlas SA, Mouradian JA, et al: Proteinuria during long-term captopril therapy. JAMA 244:346, 1980.
350. Hoorntje SJ, Kallenberg CGM, Weening JJ, et al: Immune-complex glomerulopathy in patients treated with captopril. Lancet 2:1212, 1980.
351. Rahmat J, Gelfand RL, Gelfand MC, et al: Captopril-associated cholestatic jaundice. Ann Intern Med 102:56, 1985.
352. Jett GK: Captopril-induced angioedema. Ann Emerg Med 13:489, 1984.
353. Donker AJM: Nephrotoxicity of angiotensin converting enzyme inhibitors. Kidney Int 31(Suppl 20):132, 1987.
354. Irvin JD, Viau JM: Safety profiles of the angiotensin converting enzyme inhibitors captopril and enalapril. Am J Med 8(Suppl 4C):46, 1986.
355. Case DB: Angiotensin-converting enzyme inhibitors: Are they all alike? J Clin Hypertens 3:243, 1987.
356. Gavras I, Gavras H: Captopril and enalapril. Ann Intern Med 88:556, 1983.
357. Rotmensch HH, Vlasses PH, Ferguson RK: Resolution of captopril-induced rash after substitution of enalapril. Pharmacotherapy 3:131, 1983.
358. Singer DRJ, McGregor GA: Angioneurotic oedema associated with two angiotensin converting enzyme inhibitors. Br Med J 293:1243, 1986.
359. Waeber B, Nussberger J, Brunner HR: Self poisoning with enalapril. Br Med J 288:287, 1984.
360. Zanchetti A: A re-examination of stepped-care: A retrospective and a prospective. J Cardiovasc Pharmacol 7(Suppl I):126, 1985.
361. Wing LMH, Chalmers JP, West MJ, et al: Treatment of hypertension with enalapril and hydrochlorothiazide or enalapril and atenolol: Contrasts in hypotensive interactions. J Hypertens 5(Suppl 5):603, 1987.
362. Pool JL, Gennari J, Goldstein R, et al: Controlled multicenter study of the antihypertensive effects of lisinopril, hydrochlorothiazide, and lisinopril plus hydrochlorothiazide in the treatment of 394 patients with mild to moderate essential hypertension. J Cardiovasc Pharmacol 9(Suppl 1):36, 1987.
363. Muiesan G, Agabiti-Rosei E, Buoninconti R, et al: Antihypertensive efficacy and tolerability of captopril in the elderly: Comparison with hydrochlorothiazide and placebo in a multicenter, double-blind study. J Hypertens 5(Suppl 5):599, 1987.
364. Shapiro DA, Liss CL, Walker JF, et al: Enalapril and hydrochlorothiazide as antihypertensive agents in the elderly. J Cardiovasc Pharmacol 10(Suppl 7):S160, 1987.
365. O'Connor DT, Mosley CA, Cervenka J, et al: Contrasting renal haemodynamic responses to the angiotensin converting enzyme inhibitor enalapril and the β-adrenergic antagonist metoprolol in essential hypertension. J Hypertens 2(Suppl II):89, 1984.
366. Andren L, Karlberg BE, Svensson A, et al: Long-term effects of captopril and atenolol in essential hypertension. Acta Med Scand 217:155, 1985.
367. Edmonds D, Knorr M, Greminger P, et al: ACE inhibitor versus β-blocker in the treatment of essential hypertension. Nephron 47(Suppl I):90, 1987.
368. Bolzano K, Arriaga J, Bernal R, et al: The antihypertensive effect of lisinopril compared to atenolol in patients with mild to moderate hypertension. J Cardiovasc Pharmacol 9(Suppl III):43, 1987.
369. Zachariah PK, Bonnet G, Chrysant SG, et al: Evaluation of antihypertensive efficacy of lisinopril compared to metoprolol in moderate to severe hypertension. J Cardiovasc Pharmacol 9(Suppl III):53, 1987.
370. Wing LMH, Chalmers JP, West MJ, et al: Enalapril and atenolol in essential hypertension: Attenuation of hypotensive effects in combination. Clin Exp Hypertens 10:119, 1988.
371. Franz IW, Behr U, Ketelhut R: Resting and exercise blood pressure with atenolol, enalapril and a low-dose combination. J Hypertens 5(Suppl III):37, 1987.
372. Stornello M, Di Rao G, Iachello M, et al: Hemodynamic and humoral interactions between captopril and nifedipine. Hypertension 5(Suppl III):154, 1983.
373. Salvetti A, Innocenti PF, Iardella M, et al: Captopril and nifedipine interactions in the treatment of essential hypertensives: A crossover study. J Hypertens 5(Suppl IV):139, 1987.
374. Mörlin C, Baglivo H, Boeijinga JK, et al: Comparative trial of lisinopril and nifedipine in mild to severe essential hypertension. J Cardiovasc Pharmacol 9(Suppl III):48, 1987.
375. Gennari C, Nami R, Bianchini C, et al: Nitrendipine and the angiotensin converting enzyme inhibitors in the treatment of hypertension. J Cardiovasc Pharmacol 9(Suppl IV):245, 1987.
376. Bidiville J, Nussberger J, Waeber G, et al: Are good antihypertensive responses to converting enzyme inhibitors or calcium antagonists mutually exclusive? Hypertension 11:166, 1988.
377. Brunner HR, Gavras H, Waeber B: Enhancement by diuretics

of the antihypertensive action of long-term angiotensin converting enzyme blockade. Clin Exp Hypertens 2:639, 1980.

378. Andren L, Weiner L, Svensson A, et al: Enalapril with either a "very low" or "low" dose of hydrochlorothiazide is equally effective in essential hypertension: A double-blind trial in 100 hypertensive patients. J Hypertens 1(Suppl II):384, 1983.

379. Thind GS, Mahapatra RK, Johnson A, et al: Low-dose captopril administration in patients with moderate-to-severe hypertension treated with diuretics. Circulation 67:1340, 1983.

380. Webster J, Robb OJ, Witte K, et al: Single doses of enalapril and atenolol in hypertensive patients treated with bendroflu-azide. J Hypertens 5:457, 1987.

381. Navis GJ, De Jong PE, Donker AJM, et al: Diuretic effects of angiotensin-converting enzyme inhibition: comparison of low and liberal sodium diet in hypertensive patients. J Cardiovasc Pharmacol 9:743, 1987.

382. McGregor GA, Markandu ND, Smith SJ, et al: Captopril: Contrasting effects of adding hydrochlorothiazide, propranolol, or nifedipine. J Cardiovasc Pharmacol 7(Suppl I):82, 1985.

383. Brouwer RML, Bolli P, Erne P, et al: Antihypertensive treatment using calcium antagonists in combination with captopril rather than diuretics. J Cardiovasc Pharmacol 7(Suppl I):88, 1985.

384. Donnelly R, Elliott HL, Reid JL: Nicardipine combined with enalapril in patients with essential hypertension. Br J Clin Pharmacol 22:283S, 1986.

385. Lang R, Degenhardt S, Ollenschläger G, et al: Effect of a low-dose combination nitrendipine/enalapril in less-severe degrees of hypertension. J Cardiovasc Pharmacol 9(Suppl IV):254, 1987.

386. Singer DRJ, Markandu ND, Shore AC, et al: Captopril and nifedipine in combination for moderate to severe essential hypertension. Hypertension 9:629, 1987.

387. Bellet M, Sassano P, Guyenne TT, et al: Sympatho-inhibitory effect of angiotensin converting enzyme inhibition during counter-regulation induced by dihydropyridine. J Hypertens 5(Suppl 5):583, 1987.

CHAPTER 74

Use of Angiotensin-Converting Enzyme Inhibitors in the Treatment and Prevention of Congestive Heart Failure*

Cynthia A. Toher, M.D., and Gary S. Francis, M.D.

Congestive heart failure is a common syndrome arising from a variety of pathologic processes and characterized by a wide range of clinical manifestations. It is diagnosed in approximately 400,000 patients annually, and the prevalence approaches 10% in patients older than the age of 75.[1] Despite its widespread occurrence, this syndrome defies facile definition. Heart failure has been defined as the heart's inability to meet the body's circulatory demands. By focusing on the circulatory consequences of the failing heart, this definition belies the complex pathophysiology of heart failure: circulatory compromise alone cannot explain the pathogenesis and the progression of congestive heart failure. Congestive heart failure is, rather, a multifaceted syndrome characterized not only by hemodynamic compromise, but also by complex cellular, molecular, metabolic, and neuroendocrine abnormalities.[2]

Neuroendocrine abnormalities, such as the activation of the renin-angiotensin system, play a central role in the pathogenesis of congestive heart failure.[3] Characterization of the role of the renin-angiotensin system, although as yet incomplete, has provided a conceptual framework to explain the striking efficacy of angiotensin-converting enzyme (ACE) inhibitors in the treatment of congestive heart failure. It will be useful to begin with a brief overview of that framework, because ACE inhibitors are now the cornerstone of therapy in congestive heart failure.[4] The remainder of this review focuses on the clinical efficacy of ACE inhibitors in treating and preventing congestive heart failure.

A CONCEPTUAL FRAMEWORK: THE RENIN-ANGIOTENSIN SYSTEM IN HEART FAILURE

The renin-angiotensin system is acknowledged to be important in the pathogenesis of congestive heart failure.[5, 6] A growing body of evidence[7] suggests that the renin-angiotensin system is both a classic circulating hormone system and an autocrine and paracrine system localized to a wide variety of tissues, including cardiac tissue. The circulating renin-angiotensin system has well-characterized hemodynamic effects in congestive heart failure that, although initially beneficial,[8] are ultimately deleterious.[3, 9] The tissue renin-angiotensin system has autocrine and paracrine effects that have not been characterized fully; however, there is a growing awareness that angiotensin II, the biologically active product of the renin-angiotensin system, may have important properties related to cellular growth and development, in addition to its pressor and sodium retentive properties.

The circulating renin-angiotensin system is one of several tightly integrated neuroendocrine systems that are activated in response to a decrease in cardiac output.[10] Reduced cardiac output is associated with the activation of an enzymatic cascade leading to the formation of angiotensin II. Among the effects of angiotensin II in congestive heart failure is the

Reprinted from Toher CA, Francis GS: The use of angiotensin-converting enzyme inhibitors in the treatment and prevention of congestive heart failure. Coron Artery Dis 14:37, 1993.

mediation of an increase in preload via sodium retention and an increase in afterload via systemic vasoconstriction.[11] In heart failure, increases in preload cannot augment systolic function, because the failing heart has reduced preload reserve.[12] In response to an increase in afterload, the normal heart can increase contractility to maintain cardiac output.[13] The failing heart is less able to do so, and enhancement of afterload may lead to compromise of cardiac output.[14, 15] Therefore, the circulating renin-angiotensin system, which is activated in congestive heart failure in an attempt to maintain cardiac output, ultimately may precipitate worsening myocardial function.

Activation of the circulating renin-angiotensin system in patients with congestive heart failure varies with the degree of clinical compensation: in compensated heart failure, plasma renin activity and angiotensin II levels are normal.[16] Nonetheless, ACE inhibitors are effective in compensated heart failure as well as in states characterized by low or normal plasma renin levels.[17, 18] Additionally, other investigators have found no temporal correlation between the inhibition of plasma ACE and the hemodynamic effects of ACE inhibitors.[19] These observations suggest that ACE inhibitors do not exert their effects solely by inhibiting the circulating renin-angiotensin system.

Speculation has arisen regarding the existence of a local renin-angiotensin system with autocrine and paracrine effects. In vitro molecular studies have subsequently confirmed the presence of the components of the renin-angiotensin cascade in cardiac tissue.[7] Thus, angiotensin II can be produced by cardiac tissue, in which it is likely to exert an array of local effects. These effects have not been completely elucidated in vivo; however, in vitro studies suggest that, among its other effects, angiotensin II may promote hypertrophy of cardiac myocytes.[20] Extrapolation from work done in vascular smooth muscle cells has helped to clarify the putative mechanism by which angiotensin II promotes growth: angiotensin II, via increased intracellular calcium levels and activation of protein kinase C, stimulates increased transcription of proto-oncogenes (such as c-fos and c-myc), which, in turn, may code for a variety of proteins integral to the growth and hypertrophy of cells.[21-24] If substantiated, this mechanism may be critical to understanding the role of the local renin-angiotensin system in promoting ventricular remodeling and progression of heart failure.

In summary, the role of the renin-angiotensin system in heart failure is more complex than had been supposed. The renin-angiotensin system is a dual system: a circulating classic hormonal system and a local autocrine and paracrine system localized to a variety of tissues, including cardiac tissue. The former mediates the restoration of hemodynamic homeostasis in acute and recently decompensated heart failure; however, its effects are not sufficient to explain the progression of congestive heart failure, which occurs even in the absence of activation of the circulating renin-angiotensin system. When completely characterized, the tissue renin-angiotensin system may explain this apparent paradox: its ongoing activation may contribute to the pathogenesis of congestive heart failure by locally promoting growth and hypertrophy of cardiac tissue.

ACE INHIBITORS AS TREATMENT: THE SURVIVAL TRIALS

The role of the renin-angiotensin system in congestive heart failure is not without clinical relevance. An understanding of the renin-angiotensin system provides a framework within which to place the results of recent clinical trials in congestive heart failure. If hemodynamic compromise alone is the defining feature of heart failure (the hemodynamic hypothesis), then it follows that the amelioration of hemodynamic abnormalities with direct vasodilators should be effective in the treatment of congestive heart failure; however, if congestive heart failure is a syndrome defined by hemodynamic compromise and neuroendocrine abnormalities (such as the activation of the renin-angiotensin system), then ACE inhibitors should be more effective than vasodilators. Over the last decade, several large prospective clinical trials have assessed the efficacy of direct-acting vasodilators and ACE inhibitors in prolonging the lives of patients with congestive heart failure.

Vasodilator Heart Failure Trial I

The Vasodilator Heart Failure Trial I (V-HEFT I) was the first prospective randomized clinical trial to test the hemodynamic hypothesis by assessing the effect of vasodilator drugs on mortality in congestive heart failure.[25] This study randomized 642 men with moderately severe congestive heart failure to one of three treatment arms: placebo, prazosin, or hydralazine and isosorbide dinitrate. Among patients receiving hydralazine and isosorbide, there was a 34% reduction in mortality when compared with placebo (Fig. 74–1). Notably, prazosin was the only agent to produce a significant and sustained reduction in blood pressure, but its use failed to improve survival when compared with either placebo or hydralazine-isosorbide. It is unclear why no survival benefit was conferred to patients treated with prazosin despite a greater and more prolonged reduction in blood pressure. Nonetheless, the V-HEFT I study tested the hemodynamic hypothesis and found support for the role of vasodilators in prolonging survival in patients with congestive heart failure.

Cooperative North Scandinavian Enalapril Survival Study

Although V-HEFT I first tested the efficacy of direct vasodilator therapy in congestive heart failure, it did not assess the effects of inhibition of the renin-angiotensin system. The Cooperative North Scandinavian

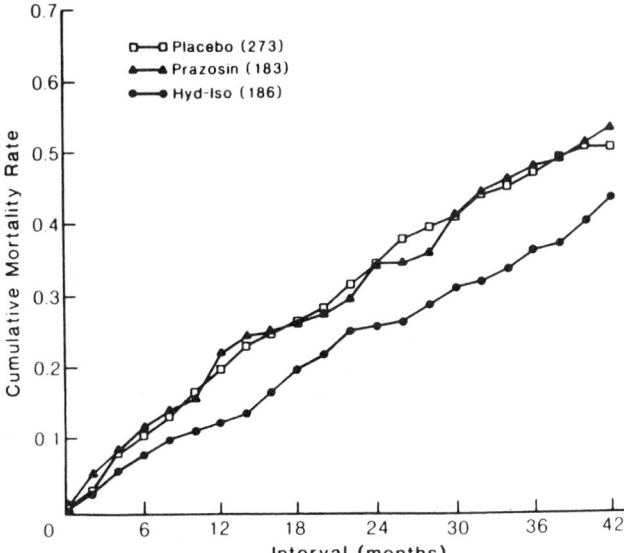

Figure 74–1. Of historical interest, V-HEFT I demonstrated for the first time that vasodilator therapy, in form of hydralazine and isosorbide dinitrate (Hyd-Iso), disrupted the natural history of congestive heart failure and prolonged survival. (Reprinted by permission from Cohn JN, Achibald DG, Ziesche S, et al: Effect of vasodilator therapy on mortality in chronic congestive heart failure: Results of a Veterans Administration Cooperative Study. N Engl J Med 314:1547, 1986. Copyright 1986, Massachusetts Medical Society.)

Enalapril Survival Study (CONSENSUS) was the first large survival study to examine the effects of ACE inhibition in congestive heart failure.[26] The trial was designed to evaluate the effects of enalapril versus placebo on survival in patients with severe congestive heart failure (New York Heart Association class IV). Two-hundred fifty-three patients receiving digitalis and diuretics were randomized to receive either enalapril or placebo. The mean age of these patients was 70 years (compared with V-HEFT I, wherein the mean age was 58 years), and approximately 50% of these patients were receiving other vasodilator therapy. This study was terminated prematurely after 18 months because of the marked reduction in mortality seen in patients treated with enalapril. Enalapril reduced mortality by 40% at 6 months and by 31% at 12 months (Fig. 74–2). Additionally, there was a dramatic reduction (50%) in the number of deaths due to pump failure in the group treated with enalapril.

Subsequent analysis of neuroendocrine activation in patients participating in CONSENSUS demonstrates a positive association between baseline levels of a variety of neuroendocrine substances (including angiotensin II) and subsequent mortality.[27] Mortality was reduced more markedly in patients with evidence of greater neuroendocrine activation.[28] These results support the use of ACE inhibitors in patients with the most pronounced abnormalities of the neuroendocrine system (as characterized by elevated baseline levels of plasma renin activity, norepinephrine, epinephrine, atrial natriuretic factor, and aldosterone). Such patients are most likely to derive a survival benefit from ACE inhibitors.

Studies of Left Ventricular Dysfunction

Prior to the publication of the Studies of Left Ventricular Dysfunction (SOLVD), data were not available to assess the survival benefits of ACE inhibitors in patients with mild heart failure or asymptomatic left ventricular dysfunction. SOLVD was thus designed to assess the effects of enalapril on mortality and morbidity in patients with NYHA class II and III heart failure.[29] SOLVD was a prospective, randomized, double-blind study that compared the effects of enalapril (in doses targeted to reach 10 mg twice per day) with those of placebo in patients with ejection fractions of less than 35%. Patients with evidence of overt congestive heart failure were assigned to the treatment arm, and those without overt congestive heart failure were assigned to the prevention arm.

In the treatment arm,[30] 2569 patients with NYHA class II and III heart failure were randomized to either placebo or enalapril. These patients were otherwise conventionally treated with vasodilators, diuretics, and digitalis. Among the treated patients, the risk of death was reduced by 16%; differences between the two groups were most marked in the first 24 months (Fig. 74–3). At 1 year, there was a 22% reduction in deaths due to the progression of heart failure and a 40% reduction in the number of hospitalizations in the enalapril-treated group. These benefits were most pronounced in the patients with the lowest ejection fractions.

The prevention arm of SOLVD demonstrated that patients with left ventricular dysfunction in the absence of overt heart failure derived no survival benefit from treatment with enalapril, although enalapril appeared to forestall the development of overt heart failure and the need for subsequent hospitalization. Thus, the results of SOLVD are consistent with those of CONSENSUS: interference with neuroendocrine systems such as the renin-angiotensin system confers survival benefit to patients with heart failure.

Subgroup analysis of baseline neuroendocrine activation in the SOLVD patients revealed normal plasma renin activity in patients entering both arms of the study.[31] This lack of activation of circulating renin-angiotensin system in the baseline state suggests that the beneficial effects of ACE inhibition may be related to interference with the tissue renin-angiotensin system.

Vasodilator Heart Failure Trial II

V-HEFT II[32] was designed to assess the life-saving effects of enalapril versus the hydralazine-nitrate combination that had been demonstrated to improve survival in V-HEFT I. To that end, 804 patients with heart failure (primarily NYHA class II or III) were assigned randomly in a double-blind fashion to receive either enalapril (20 mg/day) or hydralazine and isosorbide dinitrate (300 mg/day and 160 mg/day, respectively). Nearly all of the patients in V-HEFT II were also treated with diuretics and digitalis. At 2 years, there was a significant reduction in mortality

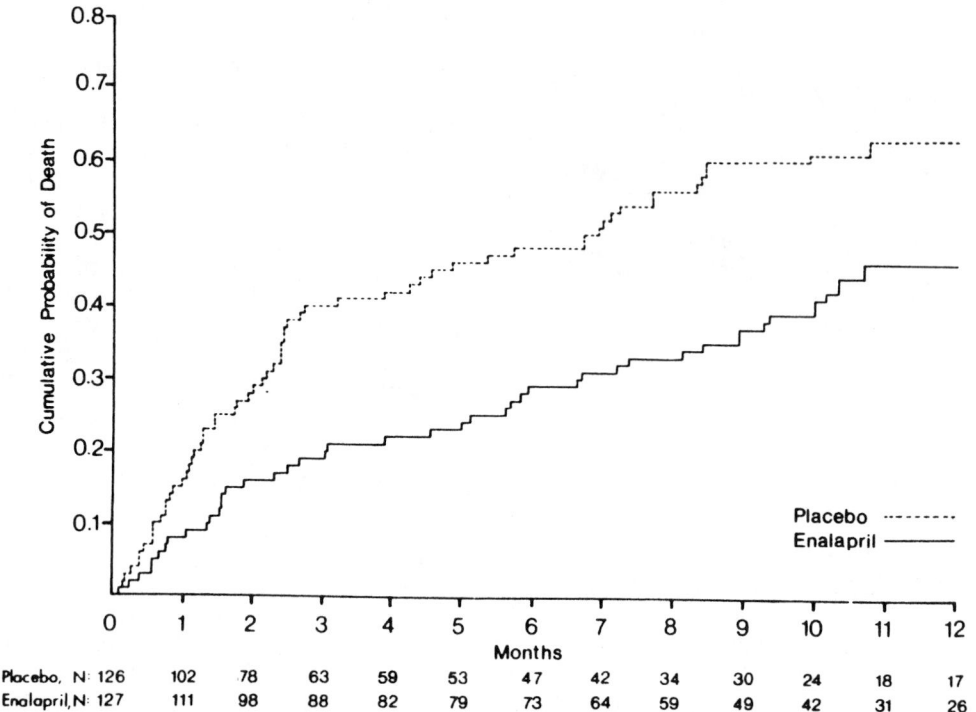

| | Placebo, N: | 126 | 102 | 78 | 63 | 59 | 53 | 47 | 42 | 34 | 30 | 24 | 18 | 17 |
| | Enalapril,N: | 127 | 111 | 98 | 88 | 82 | 79 | 73 | 64 | 59 | 49 | 42 | 31 | 26 |

Figure 74–2. Data from CONSENSUS demonstrating a marked reduction in mortality in patients with NYHA class IV heart failure who were randomized to enalapril. (Reprinted by permission from The CONSENSUS Trial Study Group: Effects of enalapril on mortality in severe congestive heart failure: Results of the Cooperative North Scandinavian Enalapril Survival Study (CONSENSUS). N Engl J Med 316:1429, 1987. Copyright 1987, Massachusetts Medical Society.)

among the patients treated with enalapril when compared with those treated with hydralazine and isosorbide dinitrate (Fig. 74–4). The decreased mortality in patients treated with enalapril was attributed to a reduction in the incidence of sudden death. This is in contrast to CONSENSUS and SOLVD, in which enalapril reduced incidences of death from progressively worsening heart failure. The reasons for these differences are not clear, but may relate to differences in study design (i.e., there was no placebo group in

V-HEFT II) and to the difficulties in classifying the mechanism of death.

Vasodilator Heart Failure Trial III

In light of these recent trials, it is clear that both direct-acting vasodilators and ACE inhibitors improve survival. The combination of a direct-acting vasodilator and ACE inhibitors may have synergistic effects in prolonging survival. This hypothesis is be-

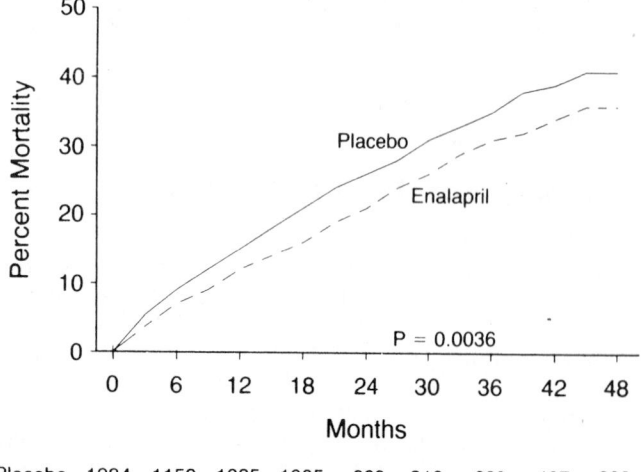

| Placebo | 1284 | 1159 | 1085 | 1005 | 939 | 819 | 669 | 487 | 299 |
| Enalapril | 1285 | 1195 | 1127 | 1069 | 1010 | 891 | 697 | 526 | 333 |

Figure 74–3. Data from the treatment arm of SOLVD indicating that enalapril confers a significant survival benefit to patients with NYHA class II and III congestive heart failure. (Reprinted by permission from The SOLVD Investigators: Effect of enalapril on survival in patients with reduced left ventricular ejection fractions and congestive heart failure. N Engl J Med 325:293, 1991. Copyright 1991, Massachusetts Medical Society.)

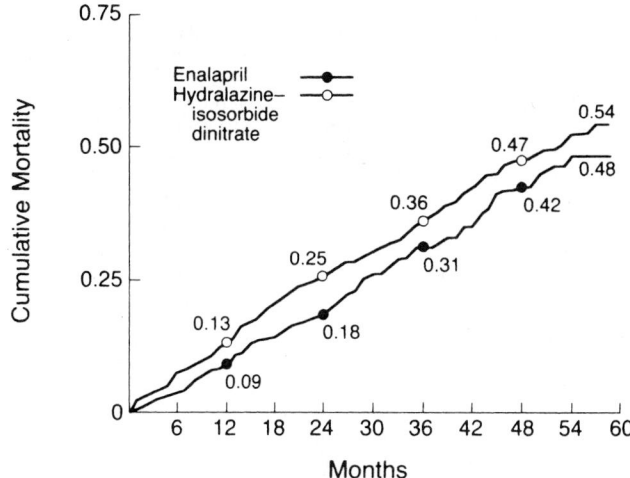

	Number Alive				
Enalapril	403	344	262	165	85
Hydralazine– isosorbide dinitrate	401	329	239	152	84

Figure 74–4. Cumulative mortality rates in patients treated with enalapril or with hydralazine–isosorbide dinitrate (V-HEFT II). At 2 years, enalapril treatment was associated with a significant (p = .016) reduction in mortality. (Reprinted by permission from Cohn JN, Johnson G, Ziesche S, et al: A comparison of enalapril with hydralazine-isosorbide dinitrate in the treatment of chronic congestive heart failure. N Engl J Med 325:303, 1991. Copyright 1991, Massachusetts Medical Society.)

ing tested in V-HEFT III with the combination of a second-generation vasculoselective calcium antagonist, felodipine, with enalapril.

Summary

In summary, a review of recent survival trials underscores the progress that has been made in the past decade in the treatment of patients with congestive heart failure. Direct vasodilators were the first therapy demonstrated to prolong life in patients with congestive heart failure. Subsequent trials have demonstrated the superiority of ACE inhibitors in prolonging life when compared with direct vasodilators. This superiority reflects the dual mechanism of action of ACE inhibitors: vasodilation and inhibition of neuroendocrine activation. Many aspects of the use of ACE inhibitors, including the mechanism of action, remain unexplored. Nonetheless, these agents have emerged as the preeminent therapy for congestive heart failure.

ACE INHIBITORS IN PREVENTION

Although ACE inhibitors have become the mainstay of treatment in congestive heart failure, there is growing interest in using these agents to prevent congestive heart failure after myocardial infarction. Left ventricular dysfunction and dilatation after myocardial infarction portend a poor prognosis[33] and may antedate the development of congestive heart failure. The mechanism of this dilatation is complex and, in its

early stages, is a consequence of infarct expansion. As the infarcted tissue elongates and stretches secondary to myocyte slippage,[34] myocyte drop-out,[35] and loss of intermyocyte collagen struts,[36] the infarct expands and may continue well after healing of the infarcted tissue.[37] Additional changes occur in the noninfarcted myocardium, including early myocyte hypertrophy,[38] myocyte slippage without dilatation,[39] and abnormal collagen deposition with subsequent myocardial fibrosis and disruption of the extracellular matrix.[40] Collectively, this process is known as ventricular remodeling.[41–43] The early increase in left ventricular volume after a large myocardial infarction may be adaptive in allowing for an increase in stroke volume in the face of diminishing myocardial contractility. Moreover, hypertrophy normalizes increased wall stress. The means by which this compensatory hypertrophy is accomplished is unclear, although mechanical stress and the cardiac renin-angiotensin system with its potential growth-promoting properties may be implicated.[44, 45] Ventricular remodeling may have long-term detrimental effects, however, and may be associated with chronic congestive heart failure.[2]

The favorable influence of ACE inhibitors in experimental[46] and clinical[47–50] myocardial injury suggests that the cardiac renin-angiotensin system may be involved in ventricular remodeling. Less remodeling occurs after treatment with captopril in patients who sustain anterior myocardial infarction.[51] When such patients were followed up, treatment with captopril was associated with lower left ventricular end-diastolic volumes, lower left ventricular filling pressures, and increased exercise capacity. In a prospective double-blind study of 100 patients with a recent Q-wave myocardial infarction and no overt congestive heart failure, Sharpe et al. demonstrated that those treated with placebo showed significant increases in left ventricular volumes when compared with patients randomized to captopril (50 mg three times daily).[52] Although the Survival and Ventricular Enlargement (SAVE) trial corroborates the benefit of captopril in preventing the development of congestive heart failure following acute myocardial infarction, CONSENSUS II indicates that intravenously administered enalaprilat followed by orally administered enalapril provides no additional survival benefit when compared with placebo.

Collectively, these studies suggest that ACE inhibitors may prove useful in preventing the development of congestive heart failure by attenuating the processes of infarct expansion and ventricular remodeling; however, further experience with ACE inhibitors after myocardial infarction (especially as regards the timing of the initiation of therapy) will be necessary to define their role in this context. The Acute Infarction Ramipril Efficacy (AIRE) study investigators reported that ramipril (1.25 to 5 mg twice daily) resulted in a substantial reduction in instances of premature death when initiated in the hospital between days 3 and 10 after acute myocardial infarction in patients with clinical evidence of heart failure.[53]

CONCLUSIONS

ACE inhibitors have emerged as increasingly important agents in the treatment and prevention of congestive heart failure. Critical questions remain unanswered: What is the mechanism of action of these agents? Do these agents have a class effect, or do some agents have specific attributes that are responsible for their action? To what extent does inhibition of the tissue renin-angiotensin system contribute to the action of these agents? Are doses other than those used in these trials effective? What is the optimal time to institute treatment with ACE inhibitors after a recent myocardial infarction? Ongoing trials may provide additional information regarding these issues.

REFERENCES

1. McFate Smith W: Epidemiology of congestive heart failure. Am J Cardiol 55:3A, 1985.
2. Katz AM: Cardiomyopathy of overload: A major determinant of prognosis in congestive heart failure. N Engl J Med 322:100, 1990.
3. Francis GS, Goldsmith SR, Levine TB, et al: The neurohormonal axis in congestive heart failure. Ann Intern Med 101:370, 1984.
4. Braunwald E: ACE inhibitors—a cornerstone of the treatment of heart failure. N Engl J Med 325:S51, 1991.
5. Davis JO: Adrenocortical and renal hormonal function in experimental cardiac failure. Circulation 25:1002, 1962.
6. Curtiss C, Cohn JN, Vrobel T, et al: Role of the renin-angiotensin system in the systemic vasoconstriction of chronic congestive heart failure. Circulation 58:763, 1978.
7. Lindpaintner K, Ganten, D: The cardiac renin-angiotensin system: An appraisal of present experimental and clinical evidence. Circ Res 68:905, 1991.
8. Harris, P: Congestive cardiac failure: Central role of the arterial blood pressure. Br Heart J 58:190, 1987.
9. Tan LB, Jalil JE, Pick R, et al: Cardiac myocyte necrosis induced by angiotensin II. Circ Res 69:1185, 1991.
10. Harris P: Evolution and the cardiac patient. Cardiovasc Res 17:313, 373, 437, 1983.
11. Cody RJ, Laragh JH: The role of the renin-angiotensin-aldosterone system in the pathophysiology of chronic heart failure. *In* Cohn JN (ed): Drug Treatment of Heart Failure. New York: Advanced Therapeutics Communications, Inc., 1983, p 35.
12. Ross J: Afterload mismatch and preload reserve: A conceptual framework for the analysis of ventricular function. Prog Cardiovasc Dis 18:255, 1976.
13. Fenn WO: The relation between the work performed and the energy liberated in muscular contraction. J Physiol 58:373, 1923.
14. Cohn JN: Vasodilator therapy for heart failure: The influence of impedance on left ventricular performance. Circulation 48:5, 1973.
15. Cohn JN: Vasodilator therapy of cardiac failure. N Engl J Med 297:27, 254, 1977.
16. Dzau VJ, Colucci W, Hollenberg NK, et al: Relationship of the renin-angiotensin-aldosterone system to clinical state in congestive heart failure. Circulation 61:645, 1981.
17. Creager MA, Faxon DP, Halperin JL, et al: Determinants of clinical response and survival in patients with congestive heart failure treated with captopril. Am Heart J 104:1147, 1982.
18. Wenting GJ, Blankestijn PJ, Poldermans D, et al: Blood pressure response of nephrectomized subjects and patients with essential hypertension to ramipril: Indirect evidence that inhibition of tissue angiotensin converting enzyme is important. Am J Cardiol 59:92D, 1987.
19. Unger T, Ganten D, Lang R, et al: Is tissue converting enzyme inhibition a determinant of the antihypertensive efficacy of converting enzyme inhibitors? Studies with the two different
20. Khairallah P, Kanabus J: Angiotensin and myocardial protein synthesis. *In* Tarazi RC, Dunbar JB (eds): Perspectives in Cardiovascular Research. New York: Raven Press, 1983, 8:337.
21. Griendling K, Tsuda T, Berk BC, et al: Angiotensin II stimulation of vascular smooth muscle. J Cardiovasc Pharmacol 14(Suppl 6):S27, 1986.
22. Taubman MB, Berk BC, Izumo S, et al: Angiotensin II induces c-fos mRNA in aortic smooth muscle: Role of calcium mobilization and protein kinase C activation. J Biol Chem 264:526, 1989.
23. Naftilan AJ, Pratt RE, Eldridge CS, et al: Angiotensin II induces c-fos expression in smooth muscle via transcriptional control. Hypertension 13:706, 1989.
24. Hoh E, Komuro I, Kurabayashi M, et al: The molecular mechanisms of angiotensin II induced c-fos gene expression on rat cardiomyocytes. Circulation 82(Suppl III):351, 1990.
25. Cohn JN, Archibald DG, Ziesche S, et al: Effect of vasodilator therapy on mortality in chronic congestive heart failure: Results of a Veterans Administration Cooperative Study. N Engl J Med 314:1547, 1986.
26. The CONSENSUS Trial Study Group: Effects of enalapril on mortality in severe congestive heart failure: Results of the Cooperative North Scandinavian Enalapril Survival Study (CONSENSUS). N Engl J Med 316:1429, 1987.
27. Swedberg K, Eneroth P, Kjekshus J, et al, for the CONSENSUS Trial Study Group: Effects of enalapril and neuroendocrine activation on prognosis in severe congestive heart failure (Follow-up of the CONSENSUS trial). Am J Cardiol 66:40D, 1990.
28. Swedberg K, Eneroth P, Kjekshus J, et al, for the CONSENSUS Trial Study Group: Hormones regulating cardiovascular function in patients with severe congestive heart failure and their relation to mortality. Circulation 82:1730, 1990.
29. The SOLVD Investigators: Studies of left ventricular dysfunction (SOLVD)—Rationale, design and methods: Two trials that evaluate the effect of enalapril in patients with reduced ejection fraction. Am J Cardiol 66:315, 1990.
30. The SOLVD Investigators: Effect of enalapril on survival in patients with reduced left ventricular ejection fractions and congestive heart failure. N Engl J Med 325:293, 1991.
31. Francis GS, Benedict C, Johnstone DE, et al: Comparison of neuro-endocrine activation in patients with left ventricular dysfunction with and without congestive heart failure: A substudy of the Studies of Left Ventricular Dysfunction (SOLVD). Circulation 82:1724, 1990.
32. Cohn JN, Johnson G, Ziesche S, et al: A comparison of enalapril with hydralazine-isosorbide dinitrate in the treatment of chronic congestive heart failure. N Engl J Med 325:303, 1991.
33. White HD, Norris RM, Brown MA, et al: Left ventricular end-systolic volume as the major determinant of survival after recovery from myocardial infarction. Circulation 76:44, 1987.
34. Weisman HF, Bush DE, Mannisi JA, et al: Cellular mechanisms of myocardial infarction expansion. Circulation 78:186, 1988.
35. Olivetti G, Capasso JM, Meggs LG, et al: Cellular basis of chronic ventricular remodeling after myocardial infarction in rats. Circ Res 68:856, 1991.
36. Whittaker P, Boughner DR, Kloner RA: Role of collagen in acute myocardial infarct expansion. Circulation 84:2123, 1991.
37. Connelly CM, McLaughlin RJ, Vogel WM, et al: Reversible and irreversible elongation of ischemic, infarcted, and healed myocardium in response to increases in pre-load and afterload. Circulation 84:387, 1991.
38. Anversa P, Loud AV, Levicky V, et al: Left ventricular failure induced by myocardial infarction: I. Myocyte hypertrophy. Am J Physiol 248:H876, 1985.
39. Olivetti G, Capasso JM, Sonneblick EH, et al: Side-to-side slippage of myocytes participates in ventricular wall remodeling acutely after myocardial infarction in rats. Circ Res 67:23, 1990.
40. Weber KT: Cardiac interstitium in health and disease: The fibrillar collagen network. J Am Coll Cardiol 13:1637, 1989.
41. Weber KT, Anversa P, Armstrong PW, et al: Remodeling and reparation of the cardiovascular system. J Am Coll Cardiol 20:3, 1992.
42. Pfeffer MA, Braunwald E: Ventricular remodeling after myocardial infarction: Experimental observations and clinical implications. Circulation 81:1161, 1990.

43. McKay RG, Pfeffer MA, Pastemak RC, et al: Left ventricular remodeling after myocardial infarction: A corollary to infarct expansion. Circulation 74:693, 1986.
44. Weber KT, Janicki JS: Angiotensin and the remodelling of the myocardium. Br J Clin Pharmacol 28:41S, 1989.
45. Drexler H, Lindpaintner K, Lu W, et al: Transient increase in the expression of cardiac angiotensinogen in a rat model of myocardial infarction and failure. Circulation 80(Suppl II):1824, 1989.
46. Pfeffer JM, Pfeffer MA, Braunwald E: Influence of chronic captopril therapy on the infarcted left ventricle of the rat. Circ Res 57:84, 1985.
47. Sigurdsson A, Held P, Andersson G, et al: Enalaprilat in acute myocardial infarction: Tolerability and effects on the renin-angiotensin system. Int J Cardiol 33:115, 1991.
48. Bonaduce D, Petretta M, Anichiello P, et al: Effect of captopril treatment on left ventricular remodeling and function after anterior myocardial infarction: Comparison with digitalis. J Am Coll Cardiol 19:858, 1992.

49. Nabel EG, Topol EJ, Galeana A, et al: A randomized placebo-controlled trial of combined early intravenous captopril and recombinant tissue-type plasminogen activator therapy in acute myocardial infarction. J Am Coll Cardiol 17:467, 1991.
50. Oldroyd KG, Pye MP, Ray SG, et al: Effects of early captopril administration on infarct expansion, left ventricular remodeling and exercise capacity after acute myocardial infarction. Am J Cardiol 68:713, 1991.
51. Pfeffer MA, Lamas GA, Vaughan DE, et al: Effect of captopril on progressive ventricular dilatation after anterior myocardial infarction. N Engl J Med 319:80, 1988.
52. Sharpe N: Early preventive treatment of left ventricular dysfunction following myocardial infarction: Optimal timing and patient selection. Am J Cardiol 68:64, 1991.
53. The Acute Infarction Ramipril Efficacy (AIRE) Study Investigators: Effect of ramipril on mortality and morbidity of survivors of acute myocardial infarction with clinical evidence of heart failure. Lancet 342:821, 1993.

CHAPTER 75

ACE Inhibition in the Post–Myocardial Infarction Patient

Martin St. John Sutton, M.B.B.S., F.R.C.P.

Since the 1980s, intense interest has centered on the limitation of myocardial infarction size, because the number of myocytes that undergo necrosis relates directly to left ventricular function,[1] which in turn is the strongest independent predictor of prognosis.[2-6] Most patients recover from acute myocardial infarction uneventfully, but some develop complications during the acute phase that can be categorized as either electrical or mechanical instability. The impact of electrical disturbances of cardiac rhythm has been partly ameliorated by the propitious use of antiarrhythmic agents; only comparatively recently have the mechanisms of early and late heart failure been understood, allowing attempts to prevent or reverse these conditions.

PATHOGENESIS OF HEART FAILURE IN THE POST–MYOCARDIAL INFARCTION

The cascade of myocellular processes that lead to heart failure begins early after the acute coronary artery occlusion. Within the first 72 hours, the infarction zone undergoes expansion[7] due to slippage of necrotic myofilaments[8,9] before the tensile strength of the infarct is augmented by the deposition of a collagen matrix as the necrotic zone undergoes repair.[9] Infarct expansion results in early left ventricular dilatation, which by Laplace's law is associated with an acute increase in wall stress. Increased wall stress is a powerful stimulus for hypertrophy of the noninfarcted left ventricular myocardium, which, if sufficient to counteract the increased wall stress, prevents further dilatation.[10] However, if the hypertrophy is insufficient to normalize the acute increase in wall stress, there is further dilatation,[10] so that dilatation begets dilatation. Concomitant left ventricular dilatation and increased wall stress result directly in depressed contractile function[11] and initiate a progressively downhill course to congestive heart failure, which has a poor prognosis.[4-6]

These alterations in left ventricular size, shape, degree of hypertrophy, and contractile function after myocardial infarction are integral components of a dynamic process that has been called left ventricular remodeling,[12, 13] which may continue for weeks or months. Left ventricular enlargement after infarction is determined by the size of the initial infarction, and the risk of death increases in direct proportion to the increase in left ventricular size.[14] After myocardial infarction, end-systolic left ventricular size and ejection fraction are the strongest predictors of adverse cardiovascular events at long-term follow-up,[2-6, 15] even more so than the extent of coronary artery disease.[15] In addition to the acute changes in the material properties of the necrotic myocardium within the infarct zone and of the adjacent, mechanically dysfunctional but viable myocardium, neurohormonal activation—especially of the adrenergic and renin-angiotensin systems—which follows acute infarction in most patients is believed to play a key role in the left ventricular remodeling of the myocardium geographically remote from the infarct zone.[16]

LIMITATION OF INFARCT SIZE

Because myocardial infarction is the most prevalent cause of death in the Western world, intense interest has focused on developing therapeutic strategies to limit the initial size of the infarction and to minimize infarction expansion and left ventricular remodeling, thus reducing mortality and long-term adverse cardiovascular events. These strategies have invoked two basic physiologic mechanisms. The first involves restoration of blood flow in the infarct-related coronary artery, either pharmacologically with thrombolysis or mechanically by percutaneous angioplasty or coronary bypass surgery.[17–26] Patency of the infarct-related coronary arteries has been demonstrated to increase survival acutely and in the long term,[22, 23] although by an unexplained mechanism. The second therapeutic strategy involves reduction of left ventricular loading conditions early after myocardial infarction to prevent left ventricular dilatation;[24, 25] this has also been associated with improved survival.[26, 27] Reduction of mean arterial pressure to 80 mmHg immediately after myocardial infarction by the intravenous administration of nitrates was first demonstrated to decrease infarction size assessed biochemically in the canine infarction model.[25] Further depression of mean arterial pressure (<80 mmHg) was associated with extension of the initial infarction.[25] In humans, the controlled decrease in mean arterial pressure with intravenously administered nitrates after infarction not only reduced the extent of left ventricular enlargement post infarction[26, 27] but translated into improved long-term survival.[26, 28] Subsequently, a number of pharmacologic agents have been used early after infarction to alter left ventricular loading conditions to improve survival, including β-adrenergic receptor blocking agents, calcium antagonists, and vasodilators. Calcium antagonists, although effective in reducing left ventricular loading conditions, have not been shown to reduce the mortality or reinfarction rate in the long term,[29] and in some hemodynamic postinfarction circumstances, they have been associated with an increased incidence of adverse cardiovascular events.[24, 30, 31] By contrast, β-adrenergic receptor blocking agents have prolonged long-term survival in several multinational postinfarction trials[32–34] and have thus become a part of conventional cardiologic practice.

RENIN-ANGIOTENSIN SYSTEM IN THE POST–MYOCARDIAL INFARCTION PATIENT

The efficacy of renin-angiotensin converting enzyme inhibition post myocardial infarction was first explored in animals as one of a number of different pharmacologic agents, including β-adrenergic blockers, antiinflammatory agents, and vasodilators, that were investigated with the specific purpose of limiting infarction size.[35–39] The combination of reduction in left ventricular loading conditions and partial inhibition of neurohormonal activation afforded by angiotensin-converting enzyme (ACE) inhibitors was theoretically advantageous in limiting infarction size compared with conventional vasodilators. Pfeffer et al.[40] first demonstrated in the rat model of myocardial infarction that ACE inhibition with captopril not only limited left ventricular dilatation post infarction, but that this reduction in remodeling was associated with prolonged survival in rats with moderate-sized infarcts (involving $<40\%$ of the left ventricle).[41] The findings in this study provided the substrate on which the first trials of renin-angiotensin converting enzyme inhibitors in survivors of acute myocardial infarction were initiated.

EFFECTS OF ACE INHIBITION IN THE POST–MYOCARDIAL INFARCTION PATIENT

A pilot study to investigate the effects of captopril in patients who had survived acute infarction demonstrated reduction in left ventricular diastolic pressure and in pulmonary artery systolic and pulmonary capillary wedge pressures with concurrent attenuation of left ventricular chamber enlargement at 1 year after infarction.[42] After this pilot trial, the combination of ACE inhibition and thrombolysis was assessed and was shown to reduce left ventricular enlargement as early as 1 week post infarction.[43] Subsequently, longitudinal echocardiographic studies of small numbers of patients with acute anterior myocardial infarction randomized either to ACE inhibition with captopril or to placebo in addition to conventional therapy[44, 45] showed significant attenuation in the progressive enlargement in left ventricular volumes and improvement in ejection fraction at 3 months of follow-up in the patients treated with captopril compared with those treated with placebo.[44, 45]

Several large, double-blind trials involving many thousands of survivors of acute myocardial infarction have randomized them to renin-angiotensin converting enzyme inhibitors with varying pharmacologic properties, to intravenously or transdermally administered nitrates, to placebo, or, most recently, to magnesium. The Survival and Ventricular Enlargement (SAVE) trial was the first large trial to test the hypothesis that long-term ACE inhibition with captopril (mean period of 3.5 years) would improve survival and decrease adverse cardiovascular events.[46] The adverse cardiovascular events were defined prospectively as death, heart failure requiring hospitalization, heart failure requiring open-label ACE inhibitor therapy, and reinfarction.[46] The SAVE trial demonstrated that oral administration of captopril begun between 3 and 16 days (mean 11 days), titrated to a maximum dose of 50 mg three times each day and continued for a minimum of 2 years (mean 3.5 years), not only reduced mortality but also significantly decreased the incidence of all the predefined adverse cardiovascular events (Fig. 75–1).[46] These beneficial effects of continued ACE inhibition in the SAVE patients occurred irrespective of ejection fraction at baseline and whether or not they received thrombolysis, β-adrenergic blocking agents, or aspirin therapy.[46] The second Cooperative Scandinavian Enalapril Survival Study (CONSENSUS II) assessed whether intravenous administration of the ACE inhibitor enalapril within 24 hours of myocardial infarction and titrated to a maximum dose of 20 mg/day by the fifth day would combine the theoretical benefits of reducing early infarction expansion with prevention of later left ventricular remodeling.[47] CONSENSUS II showed no clinical benefit (Fig. 75–2) and was terminated prematurely, because the actuarial projections showed no likelihood of a different clinical outcome in terms of survival between the enalapril and placebo treatment groups at 6 months and because of a greater incidence of early hypotensive episodes in the enalapril-treated group.[47] Thus, these first two multicenter clinical trials produced diametrically different results, which could not be easily ascribed to any major difference between the modes of pharmacologic action of captopril and enalapril.

There are several potential reasons for the discrepant findings between these first two large multicenter trials, which involve differences in patient selection, dosage, and duration, route, and timing of administration of the two ACE inhibitors. First, the SAVE trial

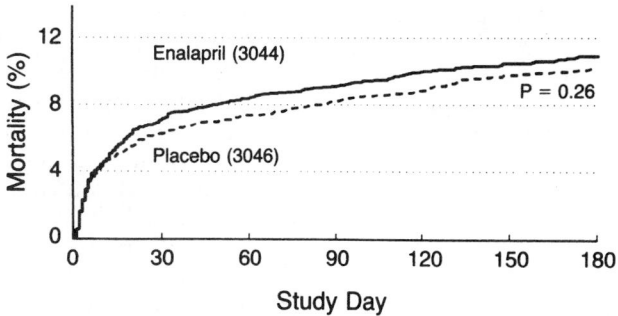

Figure 75–2. Life-table mortality curves showing no difference between the placebo and enalapril treatment groups in the Cooperative New Scandinavian Enalapril Survival Study II (CONSENSUS II). (From Swedberg K, Held P, Kjekshus J, et al, on behalf of the Consensus II Study Group: Effects of the early administration of enalapril on mortality in patients with acute myocardial infarction. Results of the Cooperative Scandinavian Enalapril Survival Study II (Consensus II). N Engl J Med 327:678, 1992. Reprinted by permission of the New England Journal of Medicine.)

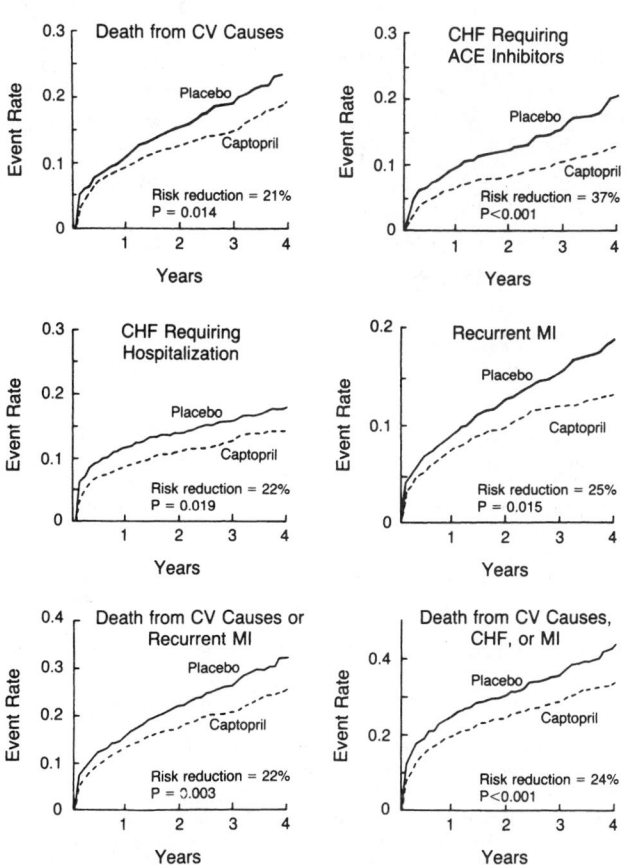

Figure 75–1. Life tables for cumulative fatal and nonfatal cardiovascular events in the Survival and Ventricular Enlargement (SAVE) trial. CV, cardiovascular; CHF, congestive heart failure; MI, myocardial infarction. (From Pfeffer MA, Braunwald E, Moye LA, et al: Effect of captopril on mortality and morbidity in patients with left ventricular dysfunction after myocardial infarction. Results of the Survival and Ventricular Enlargement Trial. The SAVE Investigators [see comments]. N Engl J Med 327:669, 1992. Reprinted by permission of the New England Journal of Medicine.)

only enrolled patients with left ventricular dysfunction at baseline (ejection faction <40%),[47] because the evidence from preliminary animal studies[41] indicated that this group of patients was at high risk and therefore most likely to benefit. By contrast, CONSENSUS II had no prerequisite regarding left ventricular function[47] but enrolled all patients with proven myocardial infarction. Second, in CONSENSUS II, the ACE inhibitor enalapril was administered intravenously within 24 hours of acute infarction;[47] in SAVE, captopril was administered orally at a mean time of 11 days after infarction.[46] Administration of the ACE inhibitor captopril was delayed in SAVE because, when the trial began, there was concern regarding the provocation of hypotension and thus possible extension of the initial infarction. The SAVE trial selected survivors of acute myocardial infarction with left ventricular dysfunction but who did not have heart failure at baseline,[46] because ACE inhibitors had been shown to be efficacious in the treatment of heart failure.[48–52] Third, patients with ongoing ischemia in SAVE were excluded because ACE inhibition with captopril was not believed to confer any therapeutic benefit for myocardial ischemia, which was best treated either by percutaneous coronary angioplasty or by coronary artery bypass surgery. Additionally, these salutary effects in SAVE were not found in CONSENSUS II because the hypotensive episodes with their associated increased early mortality offset the potential longer-term clinical benefits over the considerably shorter follow-up period.

COMBINATION OF ACE INHIBITION AND OTHER THERAPEUTIC STRATEGIES

The benefit of combining thrombolysis and ACE inhibitors in the immediate postinfarction period, which was initially suggested to increase benefit over the use of either agent alone,[43] has not been confirmed in more recently reported trials in which streptokinase or tissue plasminogen activator was used with captopril—the Captopril and Thrombolysis Study (CATS) and the Captopril plus tPA following Acute Myocardial Infarction (CAPTIN) trials, respectively, the results of which await publication. This appears to be due to the fact that the early use of thrombolysis in the entire population largely obviated left ventricular dilatation. In addition, the patient cohorts were diminutive, and the follow-up periods in both of these trials were relatively short—thus, the event rate was low, and the trials were not powerful enough to detect any possible effect. By contrast, the Acute Infarction Ramipril Efficacy (AIRE)[53] trial—in which patients who developed clinical congestive heart failure at any time post infarction were treated with up to 5 mg of orally administered ramipril, twice daily, begun at 3 to 5 days and continued for a minimum of 6 months—demonstrated a 17% reduction in mortality that first became apparent at 30 days.[53] Similar efficacy was demonstrated in the Survival of Myocardial Infarction Long-term Evaluation (SMILE) with zophinopril when the combined clinical end points of death and heart failure were assessed. In the AIRE trial, thrombolysis was administered in 65% of patients; in the SMILE trial, no patient received thrombolytic therapy.

Two megatrials—Gruppo Italiano per lo Studio della Streptochinasi nell' Infarto Miocardico III (GISSI III) and the Fourth International Study of Infarct Survival (ISIS IV), in which the early use of orally administered ACE inhibitors lisinopril (10 mg once daily) and captopril (50 mg twice daily), respectively, were compared with nitrates (and, in ISIS IV, with magnesium) in unselected patients after acute myocardial infarction—have reported their preliminary results. These two trials together enrolled over 70,000 patients and demonstrated that ACE inhibitors unequivocally improved survival at 5 to 6 weeks after infarction regardless of the use of thrombolytic therapy, which was employed in approximately 70% of patients overall and independently of left ventricular ejection fraction.

A number of clinical trials have considered the mechanism by which ACE inhibitors improve survival after acute myocardial infarction and reduce the incidence of adverse cardiovascular events; this mechanism appears to be a complex interaction of several factors. The survival of patients with left ventricular dysfunction was significantly prolonged by treatment with ACE inhibitors compared with equipotent vasodilators, suggesting a mode of action in addition to that of simply reducing left ventricular loading conditions.[49] The reduction in left ventricular loading in patients surviving acute myocardial infarction has been shown to reduce remodeling and ventricular dilatation.[44, 45] In the SAVE trial, the initial left ventricular size was highly predictive of clinical outcome, and the patients in whom adverse cardiovascular events predominated were those who developed progressive left ventricular dilatation over the course of the year after myocardial infarction.[54] ACE inhibition with captopril decreased both the incidence of postinfarction left ventricular dilatation and the

incidence of adverse cardiovascular events,[54] indicating for the first time the link between left ventricular remodeling and clinical outcome. Preliminary investigation of the possible relationship between left ventricular dilatation measured noninvasively by cross-sectional echocardiography and neurohormonal activation in the SAVE trial has shown no interaction. Neurohormonal activation in the postinfarction period was not only important but strongly predictive of long-term clinical outcome.[55] However, the combination of major initial left ventricular dilatation and neurohormonal activation heralded a poor prognosis.[55] The role of tissue-specific versus plasma ACE inhibition in the postinfarction period in explaining the efficacy is unclear but is being explored.[56, 57]

CONCLUSIONS

Although the precise mechanisms by which ACE inhibition renders its efficacy remain controversial, one indisputable conclusion has emerged from the many completed clinical trials: ACE inhibitors should be used in all patients who sustain myocardial infarction regardless of infarction size, location or transmurality, left ventricular size, ejection fraction, or use of thrombolytic therapy unless these drugs are specifically contraindicated. They should be administered orally within the first 48 hours of myocardial infarction, although one unresolved issue is how long ACE inhibitor therapy should be continued. There is now a consensus that ACE inhibitors have secured a place on the list of medications prescribed for all survivors of myocardial infarction along with aspirin and β-adrenergic receptor blocking agents.

REFERENCES

1. Pfeffer MA, Pfeffer JM, Fishbein MC, et al: Myocardial infarct size and ventricular function in rats. Circ Res 44:503, 1979.
2. Hammermeister KE, DeRouen TA, Dodge HT: Variables predictive of survival in patients with coronary disease: Selection of univariate and multivariate analysis from the clinical, electrocardiographic, exercise, arteriographic, and quantitative angiographic evaluations. Circulation 59:421, 1979.
3. Multicenter Post-Infarction Research Group: Risk stratification and survival after myocardial infarction. N Engl J Med 309:331, 1983.
4. Gottlieb S, Moss AJ, McDermott M, et al: Interrelation of left ventricular ejection fraction, pulmonary congestion and outcome in acute myocardial infarction. Am J Cardiol 69:977, 1992.
5. Kostuk WJ, Kazamias TM, Gander MP, et al: Left ventricular size after acute myocardial infarction: Serial changes and their prognostic significance. Circulation 47:1174, 1973.
6. Ahnve S, Gilpin E, Henning H, et al: Limitations and advantages of the ejection fraction for defining high risk after acute myocardial infarction. Am J Cardiol 58:872, 1986.
7. Erlebacher JA, Weiss JL, Weisfeldt ML, et al: Early dilation of the infarcted segment in acute transmural myocardial infarction: Role of infarct expansion in acute left ventricular enlargement. J Am Coll Cardiol 4:201, 1984.
8. Olivetti G, Capasso JM, Sonnenblick EH, et al: Side-to-side slippage of myocytes: Participates in ventricular wall remodeling acutely after myocardial infarction in rats. Circ Res 67:23, 1990.
9. Anversa P, Olivetti G, Capasso JM: Cellular basis of ventricular

remodeling after myocardial infarction. Am J Cardiol 68:7d, 1991.

10. Grossman W, Jones D, McLauren LP: Wall stress and patterns of hypertrophy in the human left ventricle. J Clin Invest 56:56, 1975.

11. Borow KM, Green LH, Grossman W, et al: Left ventricular end-systolic stress shortening and stress-length relations in humans: Normal values and sensitivity to ionotropic state. Am J Cardiol 50:1301, 1982.

12. McKay RJ, Pfeffer MA, Pasternak RC, et al: Left ventricular remodeling following myocardial infarction: A corollary to infarct expansion. Circulation 74:693, 1986.

13. Pfeffer MA, Braunwald E: Ventricular remodeling after myocardial infarction. Experimental observations and clinical implications. Circulation 81:1161, 1990.

14. Pfeffer MA, Pfeffer JM: Ventricular enlargement and reduced survival after myocardial infarction. Circulation 75(Suppl IV):93, 1987.

15. White HD, Norris RM, Brown MA, et al: Left ventricular end-systolic volume as the major determinant of survival after recovery from myocardial infarction. Circulation 76:44, 1987.

16. Rouleau JL, Moye LA, de Champlain J, et al: Activation of neurohumoral systems following acute myocardial infarction. Am J Cardiol 68:80d, 1991.

17. Gruppo Italiano per lo Studio della Streptochinasi nell' Infarto Miocardico (GISSI): Effectiveness of intravenous thrombolytic treatment in acute myocardial infarction. Lancet 1:397, 1986.

18. ISIS-2 (Second International Study of Infarct Survival) Collaborative Group: Randomized trial of intravenous streptokinase, oral aspirin, both, or neither among 17,187 cases of suspected acute myocardial infarction: ISIS-2. Lancet 2:349, 1988.

19. AIMS Trial Study Group: Effect of intravenous APSAC on mortality after acute myocardial infarction: Preliminary report of a placebo-controlled clinical trial. Lancet 1:545, 1988.

20. Wilcox RG, von der Lippe G, Olsson CG, et al, for the ASSET Study Group: Trial of tissue plasminogen activator for mortality reduction in acute myocardial infarction: Anglo-Scandinavian Study of Early Thrombolysis (ASSET). Lancet 2:525, 1988.

21. Sheehan FH, Braunwald E, Canner P, et al: The effect of intravenous thrombolytic therapy on left ventricular function: A report on tissue-type plasminogen activator and streptokinase from the Thrombolysis in Myocardial Infarction (TIMI) phase I trial. Circulation 75:817, 1987.

22. Jeremy RW, Hackworthy RA, Bautovich G, et al: Infarct artery perfusion and changes on left ventricular volumes in the month after acute myocardial infarction. J Am Coll Cardiol 9:989, 1987.

23. Warren SE, Royal HD, Martins JE, et al: Time course of left ventricular dilation after myocardial infarction: Influence of infarct related artery and success of coronary thrombolysis. J Am Coll Cardiol 11:12, 1988.

24. Jugdutt BI, Becker LC, Hutchins GM: Effect of intravenous nitroglycerin on collateral blood flow and infarct size in the conscious dog. Circulation 63:17, 1981.

25. Jugdutt BI: Myocardial salvage by intravenous nitroglycerin in conscious dogs: loss of beneficial effect with marked nitroglycerin-induced hypotension. Circulation 68:673, 1983.

26. Jugdutt BI, Warnica JW: Intravenous nitroglycerin therapy limited to myocardial infarction size, expansion, and complications: Effect of timing, dosage, and infarct location. Circulation 78:906, 1988.

27. Jaffe AS, Gettman EM, Tiefenbrun AJ, et al: Reduction of infarct size in patients with inferior infarction and intravenous GTN: A randomized trial. Am Heart J 106:452, 1983.

28. Jugdutt BI: Intravenous nitroglycerin in acute myocardial infarction. Am J Cardiol 68:52d, 1991.

29. Held PH, Yusuf S, Furberg CD: Calcium channel blockers in acute myocardial infarction and unstable angina: An overview. Br Med J 293:1187, 1986.

30. The Danish Study Group on Verapamil in Myocardial Infarction: Effect of verapamil on mortality and major events after acute myocardial infarction (the Danish Verapamil Infarction Trial II DAVITII). Am J Cardiol 66:779, 1990.

31. Goldstein RE, Boccuzzi SJ, Cruess D, et al: Diltiazem increases late-onset congestive heart failure in postinfarction patients

with early reduction in ejection fraction. Circulation 83:52, 1991.

32. The Norwegian Multicenter Study Group: Timolol-induced reduction in mortality and re-infarction in patients surviving acute myocardial infarction. N Engl J Med 304:801, 1981.

33. Beta-Blocker Heart Attack Trial Research Group: A randomized trial of propranolol in patients with acute myocardial infarction: Mortality results. JAMA 247:1707, 1982.

34. Herlitz J, Elmfeldt D, Holmberg S, et al: Goteborg Metoprolol Trial: Mortality and causes of death. Am J Cardiol 53:9d, 1984.

35. Ertl G, Kloner RA, Alexander RW, et al: Limitations of experimental infarct size by an angiotension converting enzyme inhibitor. Circulation 65:40, 1982.

36. Rasmussen MM, Reimer KA, Kloner RA, et al: Infarct size reduction by propanolol before and after coronary ligation in dogs. Circulation 56:794, 1977.

37. Warltier DC, Gross GJ, Brooks HL: Coronary steal-induced increase in myocardial infarction size after pharmacological coronary artery dilatation. Am J Cardiol 46:83, 1980.

38. Hammerman H, Kloner RA, Schoen FJ, et al: Indomethacin-induced scar thinning after experimental myocardial infarction. Circulation 67:1290, 1983.

39. Hammerman H, Kloner RA, Hale S, et al: Dose-dependent effects of short-term methyl prednisolone on myocardial infarct extent, scar formation and ventricular function. Circulation 68:446, 1983.

40. Pfeffer JM, Pfeffer MA, Braunwald E, et al: Influence of chronic captopril on the infarcted left ventricle of the rat. Circ Res 57:84, 1985.

41. Pfeffer MA, Pfeffer JM, Steinberg C, et al: Survival after an experimental myocardial infarction: Beneficial effects of long-term therapy with captopril. Circulation 72:406, 1985.

42. Pfeffer MA, Lamas GA, Vaughan DE, et al: Effect of captopril on progressive left ventricular dilatation after anterior myocardial infarction. N Engl J Med 319:80, 1988.

43. Nabel EG, Topol EJ, Galaena A, et al: A randomized placebo-control trial of combined intravenous captopril and recombinant tissue-type plasminogen activator therapy in acute myocardial infarction. J Am Coll Cardiol 17:467, 1991.

44. Sharpe M, Smith H, Murphy J, et al: Early prevention of left ventricular dysfunction after myocardial infarction with angiotensin-converting enzyme inhibition. Lancet 337:872, 1991.

45. Oldroyd KG, Pye MP, Ray SG, et al: Effects of early captopril administration on infarct expansion, left ventricular remodeling and exercise capacity after acute myocardial infarction. Am J Cardiol 68:713, 1991.

46. Pfeffer MA, Braunwald E, Moye LA, et al: Effect of captopril on mortality and morbidity in patients with left ventricular dysfunction after myocardial infarction. Results of the Survival and Ventricular Enlargement Trial. The SAVE Investigators [see comments]. N Engl J Med 327:669, 1992.

47. Swedberg K, Held P, Kjekshul J, et al, on behalf of the Consensus II Study Group: Effects of the early administration of enalapril on mortality in patients with acute myocardial infarction: Results of the Cooperative Scandinavian Enalapril Survival Study II (Consensus II). N Engl J Med 327:678, 1992.

48. The Consensus Trial Study Group: Effects of Enalapril on mortality in severe congestive heart failure: Results of the Cooperative North Scandinavian Enalapril Survival Study (Consensus). N Engl J Med 316:1429, 1987.

49. Cohn JN, Archibald DG, Ziesche S, et al: A Comparison of Enalapril with hydralazine-isosorbide dinitrate in the treatment of congestive heart failure. N Engl J Med 325:303, 1991.

50. Cohn JN, Archibald DG, Ziesche S, et al: Effect of vasodilator therapy on mortality in congestive heart failure: Results of Veterans Administration Cooperative Study. N Engl J Med 314:1547, 1986.

51. The SOLVD investigators: Effect of enalapril on the survival in patients with reduced left ventricular ejection fraction and congestive heart failure. N Engl J Med 325:293, 1991.

52. Yusuf S, Pepine CJ, Garces C, et al: Effect of enalapril on myocardial infarction on unstable angina in patients with low ejection fractions. Lancet 340:1173, 1992.

53. Effect of Ramipril on mortality and morbidity of acute myocardial infarction with clinical evidence of heart failure. Acute

Infarction Ramipril Efficacy (AIRE Study Investigators). Lancet 342:821, 1993.

54. St. John Sutton M, Pfeffer MA, Plappert T, et al: Quantitative two dimensional echocardiographic measurements are major predictors of adverse events following acute myocardial infarction: The protective effects of captopril. Circulation 89:68, 1994.

55. Sussex BA, Arnold JM, Parker JO, et al: Independent and interactive prognostic information of neuro-hormones and

echocardiogram in high risk post-MI patients [abstract]. J Am Coll Cardiol 19:205, 1992.

56. Sweet CS: Issues surrounding a local cardiac renin system and the beneficial actions of angiotensin-converting enzyme inhibitors in ischemic myocardium. Am J Cardiol 65:111, 1990.

57. Weber MA, Neutel JM, Smith DHG: Circulatory and extracirculatory effects of angiotensin-converting enzyme inhibition. Am Heart J 123:1414, 1992.

CHAPTER 76

ACE Inhibition in Renal Impairment

Herbert J. Kramer, M.D., Hermann Schulz, M.D., Klaus Thurau, M.D., Ph.D., and Olaf Behmer, M.D.

In recent years, the number of angiotensin-converting enzyme (ACE) inhibitors approved for the treatment of high blood pressure has increased rapidly. Comparison of the various agents shows that they may differ in their pharmacokinetics, but these differences appear to be of minor clinical relevance. Exceptions are (1) captopril, because its shorter plasma half-life facilitates dose titration especially in patients at risk, and (2) fosinopril, because of its dual and compensatory renal and biliary elimination.[1]

The active metabolites of most ACE inhibitors are excreted predominantly by the kidney. Thus, when given to patients with impaired renal function, their dose must be carefully adjusted to avoid accumulation in plasma. The fact that substantial accumulation of the active moiety already occurs with moderate impairment of renal function (i.e., creatinine clearance of 60 to 30 ml/min) aggravates this problem for the attending physician.

The difficulty of quantifying renal function in outpatient practice by measuring the endogenous creatinine clearance—a clinically useful index of the glomerular filtration rate (GFR)—has led to the use of readily measurable serum creatinine concentration as an estimate of GFR and renal function. However, in the so-called creatinine-blind range, serum creatinine concentration is a poor measure of renal function. In the absence of individual control values, serum creatinine may still fall into the normal range, while renal function may have declined to 50% of normal. Moreover, loss of muscle mass—commonly occurring in elderly individuals—leads to lower creatinine production and thus lower serum creatinine concentration, falsely suggesting normal renal function. Therefore, in the elderly and in others suffering from overt chronic renal failure, treatment of hypertension with those ACE inhibitors that are predominantly excreted via the kidney requires individual adjustment of dosage and continuous monitoring (Table 76–1). These problems may be circumvented by the use of an ACE inhibitor that, in addition to the renal excretory pathway, is also eliminated from the body by other routes.

ELIMINATION KINETICS OF ANGIOTENSIN-CONVERTING ENZYME (ACE) INHIBITORS

Comparison of the elimination kinetics of the various ACE inhibitors requires quantitative assessment of the excretion of the parent drug and the active and/or inactive metabolite(s) by the different pathways. After oral administration, a certain proportion of the substance may not be absorbed. Therefore, simply measuring the amount of drug recovered in feces cannot distinguish between nonabsorbed substance and that fraction that has been added to feces by hepatobiliary excretion. In contrast, intravenous administration of the ACE inhibitor excludes the presence of nonabsorbed ACE inhibitor in feces and ensures that all drug found in feces is excreted via the hepatobiliary route.

This technique thus allows quantification of the fraction excreted by the liver and that excreted by the kidney. The sum of both hepatic and renal clearance can be regarded as total body clearance, because elimination via lung and skin is negligible. To address these questions, we reviewed the data from the literature and compared the fractions of various ACE inhibitors eliminated in urine and feces as percentage of the total dose administered intravenously (Table 76–2).[1-15]

Experimental data from animal studies, which can-

Table 76–1. **Daily Oral Dose of Some Representative ACE Inhibitors in Patients with Renal Functional Impairment**

	Creatinine Clearance (m/min)	
	30–60	*10–30*
Captopril (mg)	12.5 b.i.d.	6.25–12.5 b.i.d.
Enalapril (mg)	5 o.d.	2.5 o.d.
Lisinopril (mg)	10 o.d.	5 o.d.
Ramipril (mg)	1.25–2.5 o.d.	1.25 o.d.
Fosinopril (mg)	10 o.d.	10 o.d.

Adapted from Carter BL: Dosing of antihypertensive medications in patients with renal insufficiency. J Clin Pharmacol 35:81, 1995.

Table 76–2. **Renal and Extrarenal Excretion of ACE Inhibitors as a Percentage of the Administered Dose Measured by Cumulative Recovery in Urine and Feces After Intravenous Application of the Main Active Metabolite to Healthy Subjects**

| ACE Inhibitor | Cumulative Recovery (% of administered dose) After IV Administration | | References |
	Urine (Period of Recovery) (hr)	Feces (Period of Recovery) (hr)	
Fosinoprilat	44 (96 hr)	46 (96 hr)	3
Fosinoprilat	40. 7 ± 5.1 (120 hr)	42.9 ± 9.6 (120 hr)	1
Benazeprilat	84.1 ± 5.9 (72 hr)		4
Captopril	86.8 ± 3.4 (96 hr)	0.4 ± 0.1 (96 hr)	5
Captopril	86.9 (72 hr)	0.8 (72 hr)	6
Captopril	92–95 (48 hr)		7
Enalaprilat	Mainly renal excretion		8
Lisinopril	88 ± 7 (72 hr)		9
Lisinopril	100% renal excretion		10
Cilazaprilat	66–84 (24 hr)		11
Cilazaprilat	91 (72 hr)		12
Perindoprilat	Mainly renal excretion		13
Libenzapril	Mainly renal excretion		14
Zofenoprilat	76.0 ± 2.5 (96 hr)	16.0 ± 1.1 (96 hr)	15

not directly be extrapolated to human conditions, have not been included in this review. Also, data obtained in humans but available only in abstract form or as "data on file" have not been included because of lack of detailed information regarding the methods employed.

ELIMINATION PATTERNS OF ACE INHIBITORS IN HEALTHY SUBJECTS

The available data obtained after intravenous administration suggest that most ACE inhibitors are excreted primarily by the kidney (see Table 76–2). Renal elimination of ACE inhibitors, which are weak acids that are protein-bound to a significant degree, such as captopril, enalapril, and ramipril (Table 76–3),[16] occurs primarily by proximal tubular secretion via the organic anion pump mechanism. In contrast, ACE inhibitors that reveal little protein binding, such as lisinopril (see Table 76–3), are eliminated to a large degree via glomerular filtration.

It can be easily recognized from Table 76–2 that,

Table 76–3. **Approximate Values for Intestinal Absorption, Bioavailability, and Protein Binding of Some Representative ACE Inhibitors After Their Oral Administration**

	Intestinal Absorption (%)	Bioavailability (%)	Protein Binding (%)
Captopril	60	70	30
Enalapril (at)	60	40	60
Lisinopril	25	25	<10
Ramipril (at)	60	40	60
Fosinopril (at)	36	30	>95

Modified from Kramer HJ: Angiotensin-Konversionsenzym-Hemmer in der Hockdrucktherapie. Med Welt 42:981, 1991.

after intravenous administration of radiolabeled ACE inhibitors or their active metabolites, fosinoprilat shows the highest fractional extrarenal excretion. It is present in nearly equal proportions in both urine and feces in subjects with normal renal function, i.e., fosinoprilat is excreted in healthy subjects in approximately equal amounts by the kidney and the liver.

ELIMINATION PATTERNS OF ACE INHIBITORS IN SUBJECTS WITH IMPAIRED KIDNEY FUNCTION

There is no close relationship between renal and extrarenal elimination of fosinoprilat. In patients suffering from renal disease, the extrarenal excretion of fosinoprilat increases roughly in proportion to the reduction in kidney function. As a result, a distinctly larger fraction of fosinoprilat administered intravenously appears in the feces of subjects with impaired renal function than in that of patients with normal renal function[1] (Fig. 76–1).

Further evidence for this enhanced biliary excretion compensating for the reduced renal elimination is provided by the time course of plasma levels and total body clearance at various degrees of deterioration of renal function. Although there was a reduction in total body clearance after intravenous administration of fosinoprilat in patients with renal impairment as compared with subjects with normal renal function, the plasma kinetics of the active metabolite of fosinopril were similar for the various degrees of renal impairment despite its decreased renal excretion.[1] These results suggest that a slight increase in plasma fosinoprilat levels—although within the therapeutic range—is required to stimulate the hepatocellular and biliary excretory mechanisms resulting in the hepatic compensation for reduced renal excretion. The conclusion is underlined by the fact that total body clearance

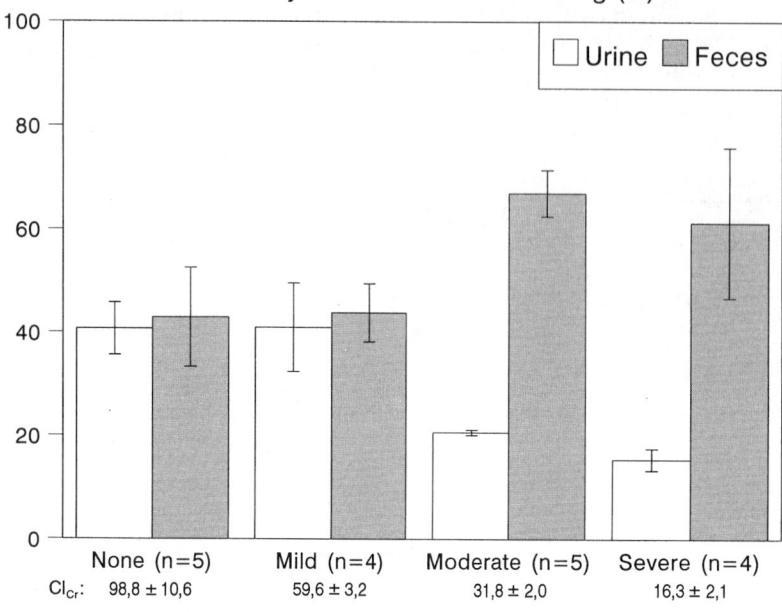

Figure 76–1. Cumulative recovery of radioactivity in urine and feces during 120 hours after application of the total dose of fosinoprilat (7.5 mg ^{14}C-fosinoprilat) administered intravenously to patients with various degrees of renal impairment.[1] Cl_{Cr}, endogenous creatinine clearance (ml/min/1.73 m²). (From Hui KK, Duchin KL, Kripalani KJ, et al: Pharmacokinetics of fosinopril in patients with various degrees of renal function. Clin Pharmacol Ther 49:457, 1991.)

remains unchanged despite the degree of renal insufficiency.[1]

As shown in Table 76–4, neither area under the curve (AUC) nor total body clearance of fosinoprilat depends on the degree of renal impairment in patients with endogenous creatinine clearance values of 11 to 72 ml/min/1.73 m². This indicates that the amount of active drug eliminated from the body per unit of time is essentially unchanged in patients in whom the renal clearance is reduced and extrarenal excretion has increased compensatorily. Even in patients with severe renal dysfunction, the AUC of fosinoprilat was only 1.6-fold greater than in subjects with normal renal function.[1] In contrast, plasma concentration of ACE inhibitors that are not eliminated extrarenally increases in patients with renal impairment,[17] as shown in Figure 76–2. Some ACE inhibitors, e.g., enalapril or benazepril, may be eliminated to a limited extent also by the liver. Nevertheless, their rather limited dual elimination pattern does not prevent significant drug accumulation in patients with severe renal impairment.[18] Although it is obvious that drug accumulation is undesirable, its consequences with respect to ACE inhibitors have not been thoroughly studied. It became evident that reduction of the originally high doses of captopril that had been given to hypertensive subjects led to a dramatic decrease in the occurrence of unwanted effects. Some of these side effects have no longer been observed since the lower doses of the drug have been applied. Futhermore, in a more anecdotal fashion, personal experiences show that side effects, e.g., cough,[19] may occur more often with conventional ACE inhibitors in patients with both hypertension and chronic renal insufficiency. Although such observations must be regarded cautiously, they suggest that these side effects may be due to drug accumulation and to clinically relevant kinin- and non-kinin-dependent interactions of ACE inhibitors with other hormonal systems.[20, 21] It is for this reason that ACE inhibitors may be hazardous in patients with severe renal impairment.

The difficulties in adjusting the dosage of an ACE inhibitor to prevent accumulation in patients at risk have been shown by Sica et al.[22] In patients with

Table 76–4. **Area Under the Plasma Concentration–Time Curve (AUC) and Total Body Clearance (CL) of Fosinoprilat After Intravenous Application of 7.5 mg ^{14}C-Fosinoprilat**

	Degree of Renal Impairment			
Fosinoprilat	None*	Mild†	Moderate‡	Severe§
AUC (ng · hr/ml)	5133 ± 590	9747 ± 1580	9380 ± 971	8401 ± 1575
CL (ml/min)	25.8 ± 3.1	13.7 ± 2.1	13.3 ± 1.7	14.3 ± 2.3

*Cl_{Cr} = 98.8 ± 10.6 ml/mm/1.73 m² (SEM; n = 5)
†Cl_{Cr} = 59.6 ± 3.2 ml/min/1.73 m² (SEM; n = 4)
‡Cl_{Cr} = 31.8 ± 2.0 ml/min/1.73 m² (SEM; n = 5)
§Cl_{Cr} = 16.3 ± 2.1 ml/min/1.73 m² (SEM; n = 4)
Cl_{Cr}, endogenous creatinine clearance.
From Hui KK, Duchin KL, Kripalani KJ, et al: Pharmacokinetics of fosinopril in patients with various degress of renal function. Clin Pharmacol Ther 49:457, 1991.

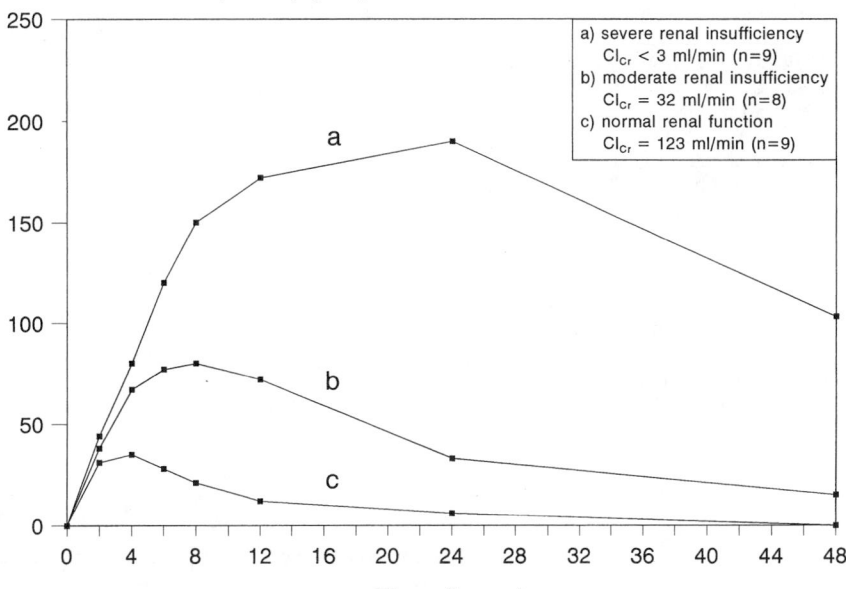

Figure 76–2. Dependency of plasma concentrations of enalapril after oral administration of 10 mg on renal function as estimated from endogenous creatinine clearance (Cl_{cr}). (Data from Lowenthal DT, Irvin JD, Merrill D, et al: The effect of renal function on enalapril kinetics. Clin Pharmacol Ther 38:661, 1985.)

moderate-to-severe renal impairment (endogenous creatinine clearance, <30 ml/min), significant accumulation of the active substance occurred as early as 10 days after starting treatment with lisinopril and enalapril, although the dosage of both substances had been reduced by 50% to 75% according to the recommendations of the United States Food and Drug Administration (FDA). In contrast, the administration of 10 mg/day of fosinopril, the dose recommended for hypertensive patients with intact renal function, did not lead to relevant drug accumulation.[3] The accumulation index (ratio of area under the plasma concentration–time curve [AUC] on day 10 and day 1) of fosinoprilat, enalaprilat, and lisinopril after oral administration of fosinopril (10 mg), enalapril (2.5 mg), or lisinopril (5 mg) once daily for 10 days approximated 1.3, 1.8, and 2.7, respectively.[22]

THERAPEUTIC IMPLICATIONS OF THE PHARMACOKINETIC DIFFERENCES BETWEEN ACE INHIBITORS

As can be seen from the study of Sica et al.,[22] dose adjustment often does not prevent the active metabolites from accumulating in patients with renal dysfunction. The particular pharmacokinetic pattern of fosinopril with its dual and compensatory elimination, however, increases the long-term therapeutic safety and simplifies the treatment of a particular group of hypertensive patients with an ACE inhibitor. In addition, the frequency of clinical and biochemical examinations during long-term treatment can be significantly reduced.

Beyond the excellent safety profile of ACE inhibitors, enhancing the compensatory biliary excretory pathway, as is the case with fosinoprilat, in patients

with reduced renal excretion function reduces the risk of increasing the plasma level above the therapeutic range. This, however, does not suspend the attending physician from carefully monitoring the patient during initial ACE inhibitor treatment with its potential side effects that are intrinsic to inhibition of the angiotensin-converting enzyme (and kininase II), e.g., the risk of acute renal failure in patients with bilateral renal artery stenosis.[23] These side effects may occur with any ACE inhibitor, irrespective of its route(s) of elimination or the plasma concentrations.

REFERENCES

1. Hui KK, Duchin KL, Kripalani KJ, et al: Pharmacokinetics of fosinopril in patients with various degrees of renal function. Clin Pharmacol Ther 49:457, 1991.
2. Carter BL: Dosing of antihypertensive medications in patients with renal insufficiency. J Clin Pharmacol 35:81, 1995.
3. Singhvi SM, Duchin KL, Morrison RA, et al: Disposition of fosinopril sodium in healthy subjects. Br J Clin Pharmacol 25:9, 1988.
4. Dieterle W, Ackermann R, Kaiser G: Pharmacokinetics of benazeprilat after intravenous administration in healthy volunteers. Eur J Clin Pharmacol 36:A303, 1989.
5. Duchin KL, Singhvi SM, Willard DA, et al: Captopril kinetics. Clin Pharmacol Ther 31:452, 1982.
6. Singhvi SM, Duchin KL, Willard DA, et al: Renal handling of captopril: Effect of probenecid. Clin Pharmacol Ther 32:182, 1982.
7. Creasey WA, Morrison RA, Singhvi SM, et al: Pharmacokinetics of intravenous captopril in healthy men. Eur J Clin Pharmacol 35:367, 1988.
8. Hockings N, Ajayi AA, Reid JL: Age and the pharmacokinetics of angiotensin converting enzyme inhibitors enalapril and enalaprilat. Br J Clin Pharmacol 21:341, 1986.
9. Till AE, Dickstein K, Aarsland T, et al: The pharmacokinetics of lisinopril in hospitalized patients with congestive heart failure. Br J Clin Pharmacol 27:199, 1989.
10. Beermann B, Till AE, Gomez HJ, et al: Pharmacokinetics of lisinopril (IV/PO) in healthy volunteers. Biopharm Drug Dispos 10:397, 1989.

11. Whitehead EM, Walters GE, Williams PEO, et al: Pharmacokinetics of intravenous cilazaprilat in normal volunteers. Br J Clin Pharmacol 27:873, 1989.
12. Williams PEO, Brown AN, Rajaguru S, et al: The pharmacokinetics and bioavailability of cilazapril in normal man. Br J Clin Pharmacol 27:181S, 1989.
13. Devissaguet JP, Ammoury N, Devissaguet M, et al: Pharmacokinetics of perindopril and its metabolites in healthy volunteers. Fundam Clin Pharmacol 4;175, 1990.
14. Kochak GM, Choi RL, deSilva JK, et al: Pharmacodynamic dependent disposition of the angiotensin converting enzyme inhibitor, libenzapril. J Clin Pharmacol 30:138, 1990.
15. Singhvi SM, Foley JE, Willard DA, et al: Disposition of zofenopril calcium in healthy subjects. J Pharm Sci 79:970, 1990.
16. Kramer HJ: Angiotensin-Konversionsenzym-Hemmer in der Hockdrucktherapie. Med Welt 42:981, 1991.
17. Lowenthal DT, Irvin JD, Merrill D, et al: The effect of renal function on enalapril kinetics. Clin Pharmacol Ther 38:661, 1985.
18. Sica DA: Kinetics of angiotensin-converting enzyme inhibitors in renal failure. J Cardiovasc Pharmacol 20(Suppl 10):S13, 1992.
19. Sorooshian M, Eynon CA, Webb DJ, Eastwood JB: Cough associated with ACE inhibitors: Increased frequency in renal failure. Eur J Int Med 2:15, 1991.
20. Heller J, Kramer HJ, Horacek V: Bradykinin and prostaglandins in the renal hemodynamic responses to ACE inhibition. Micropuncture studies in anesthetized dogs. Pflugers Arch (Eur J Physiol) 427:219, 1994.
21. Kramer HJ, Glänzer T, Meyer-Lehnert H, et al: Kinin- and non-kinin-mediated interactions of converting enzyme inhibitors with vasoactive hormones. J Cardiovasc Pharmacol 15(Suppl 6):S91, 1990.
22. Sica DA, Cutler E, Parmer RJ, et al: Comparison of the steady-state pharmacokinetics of fosinopril, lisinopril and enalapril in patients with chronic renal insufficiency. Clin Pharmacokinet 20:420, 1991.
23. Kramer HJ: Hemmung des Angiotensin-Konversionsenzyms—Einfluß auf Nierenfunktion und Elektrolythaushalt. Z Kardiol 77(Suppl 3):39, 1988.

B. Specific ACE Inhibitors

CHAPTER 77

Captopril

Henry A. Punzi, M.D., F.C.P., and Randall M. Zusman, M.D.

HISTORICAL PERSPECTIVE

In 1898, the German physicians Tigerstadt and Bergman[1] demonstrated that an extract derived from rabbit kidneys elicited a very potent pressor response. This active substance extracted from kidneys was subsequently called renin. In 1934, Goldblatt et al.[2] showed that sustained hypertension could be produced by clamping the renal artery of a dog. They noted atherosclerotic changes in the renal circulation of patients with hypertension at autopsy and proposed that hypertension might be secondary to renal ischemia. In their quest for the duplication of this mechanism of essential hypertension, the renal artery clamp technique was developed.

In 1940 in the United States, Page and Hemler[3] observed that the substance called renin required another factor that was present in the plasma to promote vessel constriction. They named this active substance renotensin. At the same time in Buenos Aires, Argentina, Braun-Menendez et al.[4] purified a pressor substance obtained from ischemic rabbit kidney that they called angiotonin. In tribute to both groups of investigators, this substance was called angiotensinogen. In 1954, Skeggs et al.[5] illustrated that the reaction of crudely purified porcine renin with angiotensinogen resulted in a mixture of two peptide hormones, inactive decapeptide (angiotensin I) and the active octapeptide, angiotensin II. The mechanism of this conversion was found to be due to an enzyme that cleaved a dipeptide from the carboxyl terminal of angiotensin I.

In 1965, Ferreira[6] described bradykinin-potentiating factor, which was present in the venom of the Brazilian pit viper, *Bothrops jararaca*. Subsequently, Ng and Vane[7] demonstrated that angiotensin I was transformed to angiotensin II during passage through the pulmonary circulation. Further work revealed that the converting enzyme was a component of the vascular endothelium, and that its intimate contact with blood passing through the pulmonary circulation accounted for the rapid metabolism of angiotensin I to angiotensin II.[8] Although Ferreira and Vane[9] attributed the effects of bradykinin-potentiating factor to its inhibition of kininase activity, the same substance was also found to inhibit angiotensin-converting activity. Subsequently known as the angiotensin-converting enzyme (ACE), this dipeptidyl carboxypeptidase cleaves a dipeptide from the carboxyl terminal of polypeptides, such as bradykinin, and it is inhibited by peptides present in snake venom. Teprotide,[10, 11] the first of the ACE inhibitors studied in humans, was shown to have antihypertensive properties. Teprotide is a synthetic nonapeptide that is effective only intravenously. Although teprotide blocked the physiologic response to angiotensin I and significantly reduced blood pressure in patients with elevated plasma renin activity, its clinical utility was limited by its intravenous administration. Systematic research to find an orally active ACE inhibitor led to the discovery of captopril by Cushman and Ondetti and their colleagues in 1975.[12]

CHEMISTRY

From this research, it was discovered that ACE was a peptidase similar to carboxypeptidase A and that both enzymes are zinc-containing metalloproteins that function by similar mechanisms.[13] Based on these findings, Cushman and Ondetti[12] attempted to design a compound that would optimize the binding between the inhibitor and the active site of ACE (Fig. 77–1). For example, captopril's sulfhydryl group enhances inhibitory potency, because the sulfur moiety binds tightly to the zinc ion of ACE. Consequently, captopril is a very potent competitive inhibitor of converting enzyme activity; it binds to ACE with an affinity that is 30,000 times greater than that of angiotensin I, the compound that competes for the active site.

PHARMACOLOGY

The renin-angiotensin system plays an important role in regulating cardiovascular homeostasis. The generation of angiotensin II results in a very powerful vasoconstrictive effect by acting primarily on the arterial bed; it also stimulates the secretion of aldosterone.[14] The primary mechanism of action of captopril is to inhibit ACE, which is responsible for the conversion of angiotensin I to angiotensin II, thus acting in the cascade of the renin-angiotensin-aldosterone system[14–17] (Fig. 77–2). Renin is stored and secreted from the renal juxtaglomerular cells located in the wall of the afferent arteriole and is contiguous to the macula densa. Renin is an acid protease that acts on the substrate angiotensinogen to release angiotensin I.[18–20]

Angiotensinogen is a glycoprotein that is synthesized in the liver. The decapeptide angiotensin I is biologically inactive and must be converted into angiotensin II by ACE in order for its activity to be expressed. ACE cleaves a dipeptide from the carboxyl terminal of the peptide angiotensin I, transforming it into the active compound angiotensin II. In the cascade of the renin-angiotensin-aldosterone system, captopril causes a predictable inhibition of plasma and tissue ACE activity, resulting in increased angiotensin I concentration, decreased concentration of angiotensin II, and increased plasma renin activity.[21] There is also a predictable decrease in plasma aldosterone concentration and urinary aldosterone excretion,

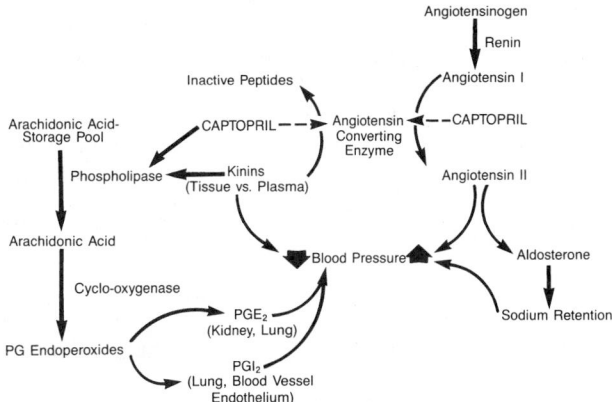

EFFECT OF CAPTOPRIL ON THE RELATIONSHIP OF RENIN-ANGIOTENSIN-ALDOSTERONE, KININS, AND PROSTAGLANDINS

Figure 77–2. Renin-angiotensin-aldosterone cascade. Interaction with captopril, kinins, prostaglandins, and the effect on the renin-angiotensin-aldosterone system. (From Zusman RM: Angiotensin converting enzyme inhibitors: Evidence for renin-dependent and renin-independent mechanisms of action. *In* Kaplan NM, Brenner BM, Laragh JH [eds]: Perspectives in Hypertension, Vol 1. The Kidney in Hypertension. New York: Raven Press, 1987, pp 161–177.)

although with prolonged captopril administration plasma aldosterone levels may return to baseline.[22–24] The converting enzyme is also responsible for the degradation of the potent vasodilator bradykinin, whose accumulation results in decreased vascular resistance, thereby lowering systemic pressure.[25, 26] The administration of converting enzyme inhibitors has not consistently affected circulating kinin concentrations.[27] However, because kinins are predominantly present in tissues, changes in their synthesis or degradation may not be reflected by changes in their plasma concentration.

Initially, pretreatment plasma renin activity was thought to be a major factor determining the efficacy of the converting enzyme inhibitors.[28] Although the effects of ACE inhibition on blood pressure are most pronounced in patients with high pretreatment plasma renin activity,[29] patients with low pretreatment renin levels also respond well to these agents. The mechanisms underlying the antihypertensive properties of captopril in low-renin hypertension are most probably not mediated by renin.[17] The elevation of bradykinin levels with captopril reported in several studies may contribute to these effects.[25, 26] In addition, the work of Vinci et al. in 1979[30] suggested that prostaglandin release may account for these non–renin-mediated actions of converting enzyme inhibition. Increased bradykinin activity indirectly stimulates prostaglandin biosynthesis and thus raises the concentration of the vasodilator prostaglandin PGE$_2$ and prostacyclin.[31] Consequently, the production of vasodilatory prostaglandins may contribute to the hypotensive actions of captopril. Captopril has been shown to possess antiplatelet aggregability properties that may result from its effects on prostacyclin.[32] In hypertensive patients, platelet aggregation is increased, and this may have an important role in the pathogenesis of atherosclerosis and vascular dis-

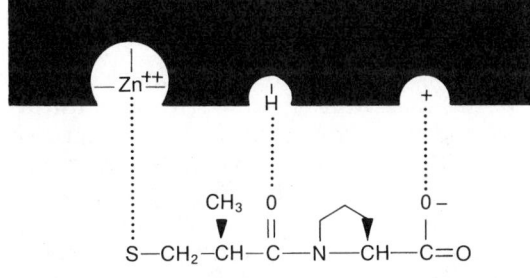

ACTIVE SITE OF ANGIOTENSIN CONVERTING ENZYME

CAPTOPRIL

Figure 77–1. The structure of captopril and its interaction with the active site on the angiotensin-converting enzyme molecule. The sulfhydryl group of captopril binds to the zinc ion of the angiotensin-converting enzyme, leading to the inhibition of the converting enzyme activity. (From Cushman DW, Ondetti MA: Inhibitors of angiotensin-converting enzyme. Prog Med Chem 174:411, 1980.)

eases.[29] Long-term administration of captopril has been associated with a reduction in plasma and urinary vasopressin levels in hypertensive subjects.[33] However, further study is required to determine the clinical significance of this finding.

The ability of captopril to stimulate vasodilatory prostaglandin production seems to be associated with its sulfhydryl component. Zusman[34] reported that the stimulation of prostaglandin biosynthesis is not an effect of the class of ACE inhibitors but instead is related to the sulfhydryl component of captopril. When captopril was incubated with renomedullary interstitial cells in tissue culture, prostaglandin biosynthesis was increased 30-fold. In contrast, the addition of enalapril (non–sulfhydryl-containing ACE inhibitor) to the interstitial cells had no effect on prostaglandin biosynthesis (Fig. 77–3).[34]

Until recently, the renin-angiotensin system was known as a circulating endocrine system.[35] It is now known that components of the renin-angiotensin system are also present in many local tissues (kidney, blood vessel, heart, adrenal gland, brain, pituitary gland, ovary, testes, uterus, placenta, gut, and salivary glands).[35] Angiotensin receptors exist throughout the vasculature, in smooth muscle, and possibly in endothelial cells. Angiotensin is synthesized not only in the circulation but also locally in many tissues. Vascular angiotensin II may contribute to vascular tone and could be a factor in the maintenance of hypertension and vascular growth, such as that occurring in the atherosclerotic process.[36]

Conversely, pharmacologic intervention in local angiotensin production may partially explain the antihypertensive activity of captopril in patients with low-renin hypertension. The magnitude and duration of blood pressure reduction appear to correlate better with the inhibition of ACE activity at the tissue level rather than in the plasma.[37, 38] This mechanism helps explain why the duration of the antihypertensive effect often exceeds the duration of ACE inhibition in the blood.

PHARMACOKINETICS

Because sulfhydryl-containing compounds are unstable in biologic fluids, quantitation of captopril levels has been difficult and several assays have been developed.[39] The pharmacokinetics of captopril have been determined by using radiochromatography and gas-liquid chromatography–selected ion monitoring mass spectrometry.[40] Even though high-performance liquid chromatography (HPLC) and radioimmunoassay techniques have been developed to measure total and free serum levels of captopril (total captopril is composed of unchanged captopril, captopril disulfide dimer, disulfide conjugates of captopril with low molecular weight thiol-containing compounds, and captopril bound to protein), the main drawback of HPLC is the utilization of sulfhydryl groups for detection purposes. Because the sulfhydryl group must be stabilized prior to HPLC, wide chromatographic peaks are frequently observed.[39]

The intravenous administration of radiolabeled captopril, using doses of 2.5, 5, and 10 mg, demonstrated that the kinetics of both unchanged and total captopril were linear and that the areas under the plasma concentration–time curves (AUC) for these dosages were similar.[41] The urinary elimination of radioactivity was dose independent over the range of 2.5 to 10 mg, with 80% of the dose excreted within 6 hours. There was an almost complete recovery of the dose 96 hours after dosing; 86.3% was recovered in the urine, and 0.3% in the feces. The mean body clearance values of doses of 2.5, 5, and 10 mg of captopril given intravenously range from 0.71 to 0.74 L/kg/hr in healthy subjects.[41] Mean renal clearance values range from 313 to 371 ml/min, clearly exceeding the glomerular filtration rate. Because the primary route of elimination of captopril is the kidneys, captopril is actively secreted into urine. Steady-state volume of distribution ranged from 0.7 to 0.84 L/kg.[39]

After oral administration of radiolabeled captopril, 71% of the dose was absorbed by healthy fasting subjects, and the bioavailability of unchanged captopril was 62%.[41] Maximum blood concentrations of unchanged captopril were approximately 0.8 to 0.9 mg/L and 1.6 to 1.9 mg/L for total captopril after a single 100-mg dose, which occurred between 0.7 and 0.9 hour after administration.[41, 42] Plasma protein binding averaged 23% and 31% at 0.5 and 2 hours, respectively.[43] Total recovery of the radiolabeled drug over a 72-hour period averaged 91% of the 100-mg dose. Captopril was found in both urine and feces, and the primary route of excretion was the kidneys. Elimination of the drug was relatively rapid, with 50% of the

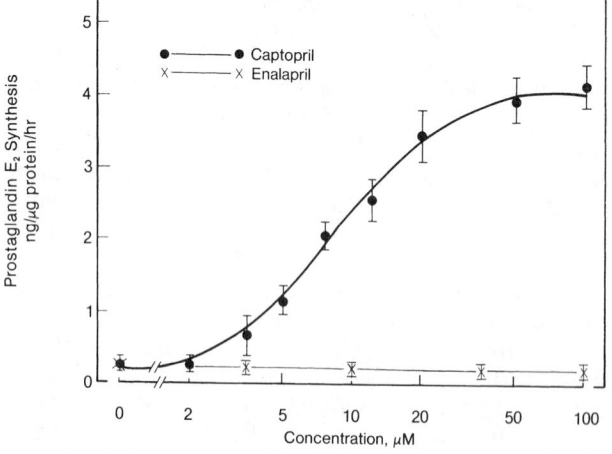

Effect of Captopril and Enalapril on Prostaglandin E$_2$ Biosynthesis

Figure 77–3. Effect of captopril on prostaglandin biosynthesis compared with that of enalapril, demonstrating a 30-fold increase in prostaglandin biosynthesis of renomedullary interstitial cells in tissue culture. (From Zusman RM: Effects of converting enzyme inhibitors on the renin-angiotensin-aldosterone, bradykinin, and arachidonic acid prostaglandin systems: Correlation of chemical structure and biologic activity. Am J Kidney Dis 10[Suppl 1]:13, 1987.)

active dose excreted in the urine in the first 4 hours. The majority (75.7%) of the drug was eliminated in the urine, and a minor amount (15.6%) was excreted in the feces.

Food appears to reduce the bioavailability of captopril, resulting in lower circulating concentrations of both unchanged and total drug.[42, 44] However, blood pressure control is not altered. It has been suggested that captopril may be ionized by the elevated gastric pH or that constituents of food may form disulfides with captopril that may not be absorbed. Captopril given with or without food has similar effects on plasma renin, aldosterone, and serum ACE activity, as well as blood pressure control.[45] Concomitant administration of antacids may interfere with the absorption and bioavailability of captopril but does not block its antihypertensive effect.[45, 46]

The pharmacokinetic parameters for captopril are not altered in the elderly. Creasey et al.[47] reported parameters for healthy elderly male subjects with normal renal function that were comparable with those found in young healthy male subjects in a fasting state. Thus, the patient's age per se is not a reason for dosage adjustment.

In humans, captopril is partially metabolized in the form of mixed disulfides with endogenous thiol-containing compounds, such as L-cysteine, glutathione, and other serum proteins. This effect may account for the differences between the pharmacokinetic and pharmacodynamic half-lives of the drug.[39] Unchanged captopril and its metabolites (e.g., captopril-cysteine disulfide) are excreted in the urine. Probenecid, by decreasing captopril's renal clearance, may increase its plasma concentrations; however, no clinical significance of this interaction has been reported.[42]

Renal Failure

In patients with impaired renal function, the pharmacokinetics of captopril are modified. The elimination half-life of captopril is increased in proportion to the patient's degree of diminished renal function, and the clearance is reduced.[47] Total captopril concentration accumulates to a greater extent than the unchanged drug in renal failure. As renal insufficiency worsens, there is significant accumulation of both unchanged and total captopril. In the study by Duchin et al.,[48] there was a correlation between creatinine clearance and total clearance of unchanged captopril. Mean AUC values of unchanged captopril increased three-fold or more in patients with severe renal dysfunction compared with those with mild renal dysfunction. Drummer et al.[49, 50] found that the peak plasma concentrations of unchanged and total captopril were three and seven times higher, respectively, in uremic patients than in those with normal renal function. The renal elimination of the unchanged captopril fell progressively as renal function worsened. Duchin et al.[48] demonstrated that captopril absorption was not influenced by uremia; over a 96- to 120-hour period, urinary excretion of total captopril was similar in patients with normal renal function and in those with mild to severe dysfunction, although it was delayed in the latter group. Approximately 30% to 40% of a dose of captopril is removed during a 4-hour hemodialysis procedure;[48] peritoneal dialysis also removes the drug.[51] As a result of the decrease in captopril's elimination, patients with impaired renal function reach higher steady-state levels for a given daily dose than patients with normal renal function. Therefore, reduced dosages or increased dosing intervals, according to the degree of renal impairment, should be used in these patients, with the end point being satisfactory blood pressure control.

Congestive Heart Failure

The pharmacokinetics of captopril would be expected to change in patients with congestive heart failure as a result of the many pathophysiologic abnormalities of the disease. When captopril, 25 mg, was administered intravenously to 14 patients with heart failure, Rademaker et al.[52] found that plasma levels of unchanged captopril over a 90-minute period were related to the percentage reduction of systemic vascular resistance. The average values for half-life, volume of distribution, and body clearance were 3.4 hours, 4 L/kg, and 0.8 L/kg/hr, respectively. In a study by Cody et al.[53] of patients with congestive heart failure, blood concentrations of captopril were similar after the first 25-mg dose, and after 3 consecutive days of therapy. Shaw et al.[54] found that the absorption of a dose of captopril, 25 mg, was rapid in 20 patients with severe heart failure, with mean peak plasma concentrations of unchanged captopril occurring 45 minutes after the dose. Some patients had a slower absorption, ranging from 90 to 140 minutes. The minimal elimination half-life was 7 hours. In this study, there was an initial correlation between the rise in plasma concentrations of unchanged captopril and the fall in systemic vascular resistance. However, with long-term therapy, hemodynamic improvement was sustained, although steady-state levels of unchanged drug did not correspond to the reduction in vascular resistance.[54]

The correlation between the pharmacokinetic and pharmacodynamic half-lives of captopril is weak. This may be secondary to reversible covalent binding of captopril, causing a reservoir-type effect, or it may be due to the inhibition of tissue ACE activity, accounting for more prolonged effects. Monitoring of the free or bound plasma concentrations of ACE inhibitors is rarely clinically indicated. Dosage should be titrated individually according to the hemodynamic response.[39]

PATHOPHYSIOLOGY AND HEMODYNAMICS

The cardiac hemodynamics of the renin-angiotensin-aldosterone system are an intricate part of fluid homeostasis and blood pressure regulation. Captopril specifically inhibits the generation of angiotensin II by blocking ACE. A single oral dose of captopril is absorbed rapidly, and hemodynamic changes are seen within 30 minutes, with maximal effects within 1 hour. These changes may persist for 8 to 12 hours. The magnitude of these hemodynamic changes is dependent on the degree of activation of the renin-angiotensin system and the patient's sodium and fluid status. In patients with elevated pretreatment plasma renin levels, a more pronounced reduction of the total peripheral resistance and subsequent lowering of blood pressure are evident. After captopril administration, systolic and diastolic blood pressures are reduced by 10% to 20% in both supine and standing positions without significant changes in cardiac output. A progressive further decrease in blood pressure has been reported with continued therapy. Sodium depletion, either by restricting dietary intake or by concomitant diuretic administration, enhances the blood pressure reduction produced by ACE inhibitors in patients with normal and low-renin hypertension.[55-58]

Unlike nonspecific arterial vasodilators, captopril produces no reflex tachycardia. Multiple explanations have been offered to account for this effect. ACE inhibitors may enhance parasympathetic activity[59] as a result of the withdrawal of angiotensin II, which may reset baroreceptor sensitivity[60] in both normotensive and hypertensive individuals. In addition, an ACE inhibitor–induced venodilatory effect may account for the minimal changes in heart rate.[61] Norepinephrine concentrations have been noted to be either unchanged[60, 62, 63] or significantly decreased during captopril therapy.[64] However, changes in the level of circulating catecholamines appear not to account for the lack of cardioacceleration. Similarly, cardiovascular response to autonomic reflexes does not appear to be modified when challenged by the cold pressor test, Valsalva maneuver, or isometric exercise.[62] The mean pulmonary artery and pulmonary capillary wedge pressures may decrease with the administration of captopril, whereas pulmonary vascular resistance appears to be unchanged.[26, 61, 65] In patients with left ventricular hypertrophy, captopril reduces left ventricular mass.[66] This may be secondary to the decreased afterload or, more important, to local structural changes caused by the drug's effects on the intracellular cardiac renin-angiotensin system. No rebound hypertension is seen after abrupt cessation of long-term ACE inhibition.[55, 56]

In patients with severe heart failure, the renin-angiotensin-aldosterone system is markedly activated secondary to a reduced cardiac output, often resulting in increased plasma angiotensin II and aldosterone levels. This results in peripheral vasoconstriction and volume expansion. Vasoconstriction further augments the afterload of the left ventricle, thereby adding to its hemodynamic burden. The vicious circle of heart failure ensues.[67] Administration of captopril in this setting causes a decrease in peripheral vascular resistance of 10% to 30%, with an increase in cardiac output and stroke volume of 40% to 50%. There is also a significant reduction in mean pulmonary artery pressure, capillary wedge pressure, and right atrial pressure.[68] Thus, both preload and afterload to the left ventricle are reduced as a result of ACE inhibitor therapy.

REGIONAL CIRCULATION

Captopril reduces systemic vascular resistance in patients with hypertension and congestive heart failure. Although the vasodilatory actions of captopril were originally attributed to arteriolar dilation, large arteries dilate as well, resulting in increased compliance. Venodilation may also play a contributory role in unburdening the left ventricle. Major changes in redistribution of regional blood flow have not been found during captopril administration. In general, blood flow to the liver decreases, while that to other areas, such as the brain, muscle, and extremities, is unchanged or increased.

Mean hepatic blood flow has been shown to be either unchanged or reduced with ACE inhibitors. In healthy subjects and in those with hepatic cirrhosis, single oral doses of captopril produced no effect on mean hepatic blood flow.[69, 70] In patients with hypertension and in those with congestive heart failure, blood flow was diminished by 25% and up to 30%, respectively, after single oral doses of captopril.[71, 72] Long-term effects, which might be different from the acute results, were not determined in these studies. After single and repeated doses of captopril, cerebral blood flow was either unchanged or increased in patients with hypertension or heart failure.[73-76] Captopril's effect on cerebral blood flow may prove to be especially beneficial in the management of elderly patients with cardiovascular diseases.[75]

RENAL EFFECTS

The renal hemodynamic effects of captopril are complex and dependent on many factors, such as sodium and water homeostasis and the presence of renal artery stenosis. Angiotensin II has a greater vasoconstrictive effect on the efferent arteriole than on the afferent arteriole. In patients with essential hypertension, glomerular filtration rate is increased during short-term captopril administration but remains unchanged with long-term therapy.[76] On administration of ACE inhibitors to patients with renal artery stenosis, renal blood flow is usually maintained on the stenotic side and may even increase on the nonstenotic side of patients with unilateral lesions.[77] When captopril is administered, the glomerular filtration rate decreases on the stenotic side. Consequently, in patients with bilateral renal artery stenosis or stenosis of the renal artery in a solitary kidney, the glomerular filtration rate may rapidly diminish, resulting in azotemia.[77] In hypertensive patients after renal transplantation, the effective renal plasma flow increased after captopril therapy, with no change in glomerular filtration rate.[78] Sodium and potassium excretion are usually unaltered after long-term administration of ACE inhibitors, resulting in no change in body weight or plasma volume in hypertensive patients.[33, 77]

HYPERTENSION— INDICATIONS FOR USE

Captopril was initially approved for use in patients with severe or refractory hypertension. Because of its efficacy, captopril was prescribed either when there was a minimal response to standard triple-drug therapy or when the adverse side effects from these drugs impaired compliance.[79] Since that time, the results of numerous clinical trials have documented the efficacy of captopril in the treatment of all degrees of hypertension.[80-83] In its Fifth Report, the Joint National Committee on the Detection, Evaluation, and Treatment of High Blood Pressure recommends monotherapy for stage I and stage II hypertension.[84] Even though diuretics and β-blockers are preferred by the committee for initial drug therapy, ACE inhibitors, calcium antagonists, α_1-receptor blockers, and β-blockers are equally efficacious in decreasing blood pressure. The lack of metabolic abnormalities as well as the safety profile associated with captopril has led to its suitability as initial drug therapy. In patients in whom nondrug therapies have failed to produce a response, captopril can be used interchangeably with the other five groups of drugs to treat hypertension.

Although pretreatment plasma renin activity is important in predicting the magnitude of the blood pressure response to ACE inhibitors, it is not related to their efficacy.[85] Multiple factors, such as fluid volume, renal blood flow, and catecholamine excess, affect pretreatment plasma renin activity. Consequently, captopril is also effective in patients with normal or low pretreatment plasma renin values, such as in black or elderly patients.[86] Mild to moderately hypertensive patients respond very well to captopril monotherapy. Numerous studies have demonstrated that blood pressure is normalized in approximately 50% of these patients.[87-89] When selecting the initial antihypertensive therapy, one must consider that in the majority of patients, hypertension can be controlled with one drug. Because the patient will most probably remain on this drug for his or her lifetime, factors such as efficacy, safety, and the effect on the patient's quality of life become important considerations in the selection of the initial antihypertensive agent.

Many trials have compared captopril with other antihypertensive agents. In double-blind, randomized trials, captopril was as effective as or more effective than thiazide diuretics.[90-92]

In other comparisons with β-blockers such as propranolol[93] and atenolol,[94] the αβ-blocker labetalol,[95] calcium antagonists,[96, 97] and other ACE inhibitors,[98, 99] captopril has demonstrated equivalent efficacy. In one study, when captopril was compared with enalapril in a double-blind, randomized fashion, patients with mild to moderate hypertension received either 100 mg of captopril or 10 mg of enalapril once daily. Captopril and enalapril administered once daily produced similar blood pressure responses and were equally well tolerated.[100] Tolerance does not develop to the antihypertensive effect of captopril, and blood pressure control is maintained during long-term ad-

ministration.[101, 102] Ambulatory blood pressure monitoring has demonstrated that captopril, either in a once- or twice-daily regimen, controls blood pressure throughout a 24-hour period.[103, 104]

Short- and long-term studies of captopril have demonstrated that it is lipid neutral or has modestly beneficial effects.[105] Captopril has also been shown to neutralize hydrochlorothiazide-induced hypercholesterolemia; therefore, captopril is a good choice in hypertensive patients with hyperlipidemia.

Left Ventricular Hypertrophy

A significant increase in morbidity and mortality from coronary events is associated with the presence of left ventricular hypertrophy (LVH).[106] Clinically, LVH can be identified by chest x-ray film and electrocardiography. However, these methods have underestimated the incidence of LVH in the hypertensive population. With the use of echocardiography, LVH has been detected in as many as 50% of hypertensive patients.[107] A higher incidence of LVH is found in the elderly. Although the stimulus for the increase in ventricular mass in the elderly is not known, there is a significant increase in cardiac risk in this population.[106, 108]

In hypertensive patients, LVH is an important independent risk factor for untoward cardiac events, including congestive heart failure, myocardial infarction, and sudden death.[108] An elevation in blood pressure is the most important condition linked to LVH. The Framingham data demonstrate that left ventricular mass increases for each age group commensurate with the elevation of systolic blood pressure.[106, 108]

Although blood pressure control may be achieved, regression of left ventricular enlargement does not occur with all antihypertensive agents.[109] LVH was thought to be a compensatory adaptation of the heart to the increased afterload. Clinical trials have demonstrated that adequate control of both systolic and diastolic blood pressures with diuretics failed to produce a regression of LVH as demonstrated by echocardiography.[110] Direct vasodilators, such as hydralazine and minoxidil, have not been shown to decrease LVH and may even increase left ventricular mass.[111] ACE inhibitors,[66, 112, 113] β-blockers without intrinsic sympathomimetic activity,[112] some of the calcium antagonists,[107] and some of the antiadrenergic agents[107] have been associated with regression of LVH.

Captopril has been extensively evaluated with respect to its effect on the left ventricular anatomy and function in hypertensive patients. Muiesan et al.[114] evaluated the effects of captopril administration for 1 year in 15 hypertensive patients with LVH. The patients were evaluated by echocardiography at 3, 6, and 12 months of treatment. The investigators demonstrated that left ventricular mass was progressively reduced to the normal range when captopril treatment was administered for 6 months. This was accompanied by normal left ventricular systolic function at rest and when the load on the heart was increased during isometric exercises and cold pressor testing. An improvement in left ventricular relaxation and filling pattern was associated with the regression of LVH, resulting in improved diastolic function.

The reversal of cardiac hypertrophy may be related to factors such as stability of blood pressure, duration of treatment, and hemodynamic changes.[66] The degree of cardioadrenergic stimulation and activation of the renin-angiotensin-aldosterone system are also very important, because angiotensin II and norepinephrine have been demonstrated to initiate LVH. Suppression of angiotensin II by ACE inhibition is associated with a decrease in the tone of the sympathetic nervous system. The interaction of these two systems may play a role in the regression of LVH and the decrease in cardiac mass reported with captopril.[66, 114-116] In addition, the reduction of myocardial muscle mass by ACE inhibition may be beneficial in decreasing arrhythmias that are commonly associated with LVH.[117]

In a recent meta-analysis of 109 treatment studies,[118] ACE inhibitors, β-blockers, and calcium antagonists reduced LV mass by reversing wall hypertrophy, but the effect was most pronounced with ACE inhibitors. Multiple mechanisms may contribute to the superior effect of the ACE inhibitors.

Combination Therapy

The combination of an ACE inhibitor and a diuretic produces additive and probably synergistic effects. With diuretics, captopril controls blood pressure consistently in more than 80% of patients treated, producing a greater reduction than that achieved by either drug alone.[119] In addition, captopril neutralizes diuretic-induced hyperglycemia and hypercholesterolemia.[120]

Low Plasma Renin Hypertension

African Americans do not respond as well as whites to equivalent doses of captopril because of diminished activity of the renin-aldosterone-angiotensin system. However, by increasing the dose of captopril[121] or adding hydrochlorothiazide to captopril, this racial difference is abolished.[122] A synergistic blood pressure–lowering effect is seen in African American patients receiving captopril plus a diuretic.[123] The synergistic effects of captopril and hydrochlorothiazide therapy can be explained by the fact that diuretics stimulate the secretion of renin and the formation of angiotensin II, which is subsequently blunted by the ACE inhibitor.[119] Metabolic side effects secondary to diuretics, such as hyperglycemia, hypercholesterolemia, hyperkalemia, hyperuricemia, and hypomagnesemia, are blunted by the concomitant administration of captopril.[120]

Refractory Hypertension

In patients with refractory hypertension, captopril was given in combination with either a diuretic, a centrally acting agent, or a β-blocker, and compared with the combination of a diuretic, a β-blocker, and hydralazine. The treatment with an ACE inhibitor was by far superior in the percentage blood pressure reduction and in the number of patients who responded to therapy.[124-127] In patients with severe hypertension, the concomitant administration of minoxidil, 5 to 40 mg daily, and captopril, 50 to 300 mg daily, successfully reduced blood pressure.[128-130]

In hypertensive patients with renal impairment, a loop diuretic, such as furosemide, should be used concomitantly with captopril.[129] Potassium-sparing diuretics have been a very popular first-line therapy for the treatment of patients with hypertension, but caution should be taken when using these diuretics with ACE inhibitors, because hyperkalemia may occur in predisposed patients.[92] For the same reason, potassium supplementation should be administered cautiously, if at all, to patients receiving ACE inhibitors, especially patients with renal impairment.[131]

The combination of β-blockers and ACE inhibitors produces less of a synergistic effect than that of the diuretic-captopril combination.[132] ACE inhibitors plus calcium antagonists also seem to have a synergistic effect on the lowering of blood pressure, and their concomitant use may have a significant role in the treatment of hypertension.[133] Because both enhance the elasticity of the arterial wall with reductions in blood pressure, these effects may prove to be very beneficial in the treatment of hypertension, especially in the elderly.

Hypertensive Therapy in Selected Subgroups

Geriatric Hypertension

The hemodynamic profile of captopril in the elderly is very desirable, because it is not associated with reflex tachycardia, fluid retention, or reduction in coronary, renal, or cerebral blood flow. Elderly hypertensive patients have numerous associated illnesses and consume a large number of medications for these conditions.[134] ACE inhibitors are a logical first choice of antihypertensive therapy because of their compatibility in the presence of chronic obstructive pulmonary disease, peripheral vascular disease, heart failure, or diabetes mellitus.

Because elderly hypertensive patients exhibit low plasma renin levels, they would not be expected to respond to ACE inhibitors as well as young patients. However, multiple studies have demonstrated that there is a marked similarity in blood pressure response in these age groups.[135, 136] In a study by Corea et al.,[137] elderly hypertensive patients responded as well to captopril as they did to chlorthalidone, but without diuretic-induced metabolic derangements.

In a multicenter study,[138] blood pressure was normalized in more than 50% of 99 elderly hypertensive subjects who received low doses of captopril (25 to 50 mg twice daily). With the addition of small doses of hydrochlorothiazide, 75% of the patients achieved blood pressure control. In this trial, efficacy was similar in black patients and white patients, and there was a relatively low withdrawal rate (5%). Similarly, Creisson et al.[139] found that the combination of captopril and hydrochlorothiazide normalized blood pressure in 96% of elderly hypertensive patients. Two other studies have further substantiated the efficacy and safety of captopril in the elderly.[92, 136] Captopril was found to be better tolerated than hydrochlorothiazide in these studies and was often effective in a single daily dose, thereby enhancing patient compliance. Results obtained from the Quality of Life Assessment Study undertaken in more than 30,000 hypertensive patients demonstrated a significant reduction in systolic blood pressure with captopril monotherapy in patients with isolated systolic hypertension.[140]

Diabetes and Hypertension

In 1982, Hostetter et al.[141] suggested that increased intraglomerular pressure was responsible for the deterioration of renal function in diabetic patients, experimentally demonstrating that glomerular capillary hyperperfusion and hypertension caused glomerular structural injury.[142] ACE inhibitors produced favorable effects by reducing not only systemic pressures but also intraglomerular pressure as a result of dilating the postglomerular arteriole.[143, 144] In 1983, Parving et al.[145] demonstrated that strict control of blood pressure was more important in the preservation of renal function than strict metabolic control in diabetic hypertensive patients with renal impairment. Subsequent studies by Zatz et al.[146] demonstrated that not all antihypertensive agents are equally effective in retarding renal damage in hypertensive diabetic rats. In this rat model, triple-drug antihypertensive therapy failed to halt the progression of renal disease even though systemic blood pressure was reduced, whereas captopril-treated rats had a marked reduction in proteinuria.

In patients with diabetic nephropathy, captopril reduced severe proteinuria that did not correlate with a fall in systemic pressure.[147] Similarly, long-term studies (>2 years) with captopril in hypertensive diabetic patients demonstrated that there was a slowdown in the progression of renal dysfunction (Fig. 77–4).[148] In 409 patients with renal disease and diabetes, captopril not only demonstrated decline in the progression of renal impairment but also reduced mortality and renal morbidity by 50% in these patients when compared with placebos.[149] ACE inhibitors may improve renal function even in normotensive diabetic patients with nephropathy.[149a] In a 4-year study of insulin-dependent diabetics, captopril reduced the urinary excretion of albumin, which increased in the control group ($p < .05$). None of the patients treated with captopril progressed to diabetic nephropathy, whereas approximatley one third of the control group did develop the disease ($p < .05$).[150] Beneficial effects on carbohydrate metabolism support the first-line use of ACE inhibitors in hypertensive diabetic patients. In studies using the glucose

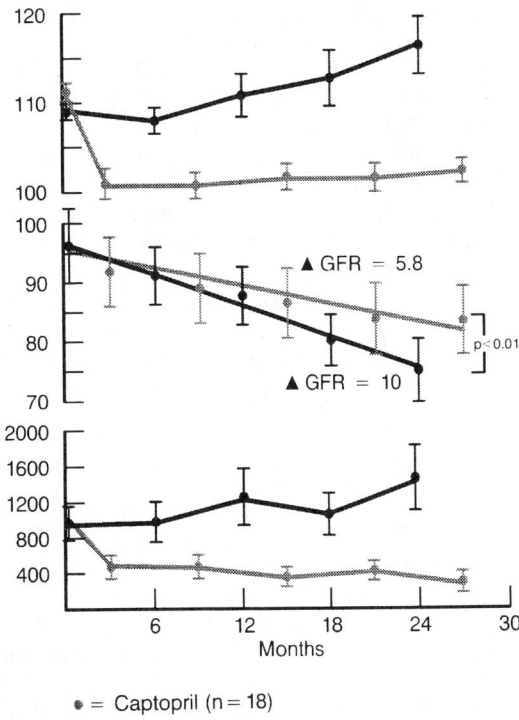

Figure 77–4. Long-term reduction in blood pressure, glomerular filtration rate, and albuminuria in hypertensive diabetic patients treated with captopril when compared with control subjects. (From Parving HH, Hommel E, Smidt UM: Protection of kidney function and decrease in albuminuria by captopril in insulin-dependent diabetics with nephropathy. Br Med J 297:1086, 1988.)

clamp technique, captopril enhanced insulin sensitivity and muscle glucose uptake, thereby improving glucose control.[151] Lower doses of insulin may be needed to maintain metabolic control in diabetic patients treated with captopril.[152]

Renal Parenchymal Disease

Increases in blood pressure are frequently seen in patients with chronic renal failure, and this may be the initial manifestation of their illness. Blood pressure elevations may be secondary to increased intrarenal levels of angiotensin II, causing an increase in glomerular capillary as well as systemic pressure, with subsequent destruction of nephrons.[142] Stabilization and improvement of renal parameters in these patients seem not to be merely functions of lowering systemic blood pressure;[153] reductions in angiotensin II levels with decreased intraglomerular pressures, or locally mediated effects of ACE inhibitors, may play a role. Captopril has been used with success in patients with advanced renal disease and in dialysis-resistant hypertension.[154] Hypertension in these patients should be closely monitored. Some studies have demonstrated that captopril reduces or halts the progression of renal disease in patients with chronic renal impairment.[155]

Renovascular Hypertension

A large body of evidence demonstrates that the estimated incidence of renovascular hypertension may be misleading at this time.[156] Medical therapy for these patients is sometimes warranted, and the use of captopril has been shown to be very efficacious.[157, 158] In patients with bilateral renal artery stenosis, or stenosis of a solitary kidney, blood pressure control with ACE inhibitors may be achieved, but there is a greater risk of drug-induced renal impairment.[159] This is due to a blunting of the angiotensin II concentration and the loss of the stimuli to keep the pressure gradient across the stenosis.[160]

Renal Transplantation

With the increased frequency of renal transplantation, a greater number of patients subsequently develop elevated blood pressures. Numerous antihypertensive regimens have been efficacious, but a small percentage of patients may be resistant to triple-drug therapy. Captopril, a diuretic, and in some cases an additional agent, have provided satisfactory antihypertensive effects in refractory hypertension associated with renal transplantation.[161] If captopril is started within 1 year of surgery, blood pressure is better controlled and renal function is improved when compared with captopril therapy that is started more than 1 year after surgery.[162] In patients who have stenosis of the renal artery to the transplanted kidney, there is a higher instance of azotemia if captopril is administered with diuretics or if patients are hypovolemic.[163]

Pediatric Hypertension

Treatment of hypertension in the pediatric population is usually refractory to conventional antihypertensive therapy. Captopril in daily doses of 0.5 to 5 mg/kg, combined with either a diuretic, a β-blocker, or both, seems to be efficacious in controlling blood pressures in children aged 2 months to 18 years. The majority of these patients had refractory hypertension associated with renal disease or vascular abnormalities.[154, 164–168]

Scleroderma Renal Crisis

This condition, characterized by an abrupt onset and rapid progression of hypertension in the presence of renal failure, is thought to be renin mediated. It occurs in 7% of patients with scleroderma. Captopril is the drug of choice for this condition. Its blood pressure–lowering effects are well tolerated, renal function is stabilized, and progression of renal failure and subsequent death are prevented.[169–171]

Quality-of-Life Studies

In 1986, Croog et al.[172] evaluated quality of life in a 24-week multicenter study of more than 400 patients randomized to receive captopril, propranolol, or methyldopa. The parameters studied were well-being,

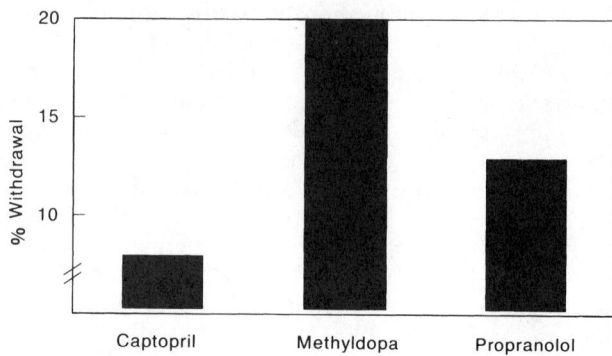

WITHDRAWAL FROM ANTIHYPERTENSIVE THERAPY DUE TO ADVERSE REACTIONS (QOL STUDY)

Figure 77–5. Percentage of withdrawal due to adverse effects during antihypertensive therapy with captopril, methyldopa, and propranolol. Captopril demonstrated a statistically lower withdrawal rate. (Reprinted by permission of The New England Journal of Medicine from Croog SH, Levine S, Testa MA, et al: The effects of anti-hypertensive therapy on the quality of life. N Engl J Med 314:1657, 1986. Copyright 1986, Massachusetts Medical Society.)

sexual function, physical symptoms, sleep patterns, cognitive skills, life satisfaction, and social participation. Patients treated with captopril but not the other agents had an improvement in their general well-being and indexes of work performance. Of interest is that all three treatment modalities provided similar blood pressure control, but differences were noted in the discontinuation rate secondary to adverse side effects (Fig. 77–5). Eight percent withdrew from the captopril group because of side effects; 13% from the propranolol group; and 20% from the methyldopa group. The difference in withdrawal rate between captopril and methyldopa was statistically significant ($p < .001$). In all three groups, the addition of hydrochlorothiazide resulted in poorer scores on the quality-of-life measures.

Studies suggest that baseline quality of life has a profound effect on a patient's response to antihypertensive therapy. In addition, the type of response depends on the agent used, even with individual agents from the same drug class. When the two ACE inhibitors captopril and enalapril were evaluated for their effects on quality of life in hypertensive men, there were considerable differences between the two agents. Overall, patients on captopril had an improvement in their quality of life, whereas patients treated with enalapril exhibited a worsening. The results of the study were analyzed by the patients' baseline quality of life. Those with low quality of life remained stable or improved with either therapy. However, those with high baseline quality of life remained stable on captopril but worsened with enalapril.[173]

HEART FAILURE— INDICATIONS FOR USE

The efficacy of long-term captopril therapy in patients with congestive heart failure has been well documented.[174] The initial studies with captopril were undertaken in patients who had severe heart failure (New York Heart Association [NYHA] classes III–IV) who were not adequately responding to digitalis glycoside and diuretics.[175, 176] However, its efficacy in milder forms of the disease has been clearly established.

The results of a major multicenter trial[177] in 92 patients with moderate to severe heart failure demonstrated that, compared with placebo, captopril significantly improved exercise tolerance time and ejection fraction. NYHA class and clinical symptoms were significantly improved in the captopril-treated patients. Overall, 80% of patients receiving captopril but only 27% of patients receiving placebo exhibited clinical improvement ($p < .001$). During this 90-day study, 21% (11 of 52 patients) of the placebo-treated patients died, compared with 4% (2 of 53 patients) of the patients receiving captopril ($p < .001$).[178]

During a long-term multicenter trial (up to 55 months), captopril was evaluated in 124 patients with NYHA class III–IV heart failure.[179] There was an improvement in exercise tolerance and ejection fraction as well as a significant reduction in heart size and the symptoms of the disease. The hemodynamic benefits of captopril included increases in cardiac index (35%), stroke index (44%), and stroke work index (34%). During this long-term study, sustained clinical improvements and increased exercise tolerance were reported in patients treated with captopril. Therefore, in contrast with nonspecific vasodilators, tolerance to the clinical and hemodynamic benefits of captopril does not appear to limit its long-term efficacy.

In patients with mild heart failure (NYHA classes II–III), captopril is clinically effective, as demonstrated by improvements in exercise performance and NYHA class rating and a significant reduction in ventricular arrhythmias.[180] Captopril administered early in the course of congestive heart failure slowed the progress of heart failure and favorably altered the natural history of the disease.[181]

Asymptomatic left ventricular dysfunction that occurs after myocardial infarction may progress to frank heart failure.[182] In order to determine whether ACE inhibition would prevent the development of heart failure, captopril was initiated during the acute phases to patients with anterior or inferior wall myocardial infarction.[183] In these patients, studied for 12 months, captopril attenuated progressive ventricular enlargement compared with the group receiving a placebo. In a similar postinfarction study, Sharpe et al.[184] found that captopril increased ejection fraction and stroke volume in patients whose ejection fractions were below 45%, compared with those treated with furosemide or placebo. Results of an ongoing multicenter SAVE trial have demonstrated that captopril initiated in the acute phases after myocardial infarction not only reduces mortality but also reduces sudden death, recurrent myocardial infarction, and ventricular arrhythmias. In addition, the captopril-treated patients had a reduction in hospitalizations for heart failure, fewer recurrent myocardial infarctions, and fewer patients with congestive heart failure requiring open-label captopril therapy.[185, 186]

The most common side effect reported with ACE inhibitors in heart failure is hypotension, which is seen on initiating therapy, especially in volume-depleted patients. The magnitude and duration of the hypotensive response are greater with the long-acting ACE inhibitors[186] than with captopril. Therefore, patients treated with other ACE inhibitors require a longer period of blood pressure monitoring than captopril-treated patients during initiation of therapy.[187] To avoid hypotension, captopril should be started in a low dose (6.25 to 12.5 mg twice daily), and the diuretic should be withheld on the day before initiation.

The improvements reported with captopril in patients with severe and milder forms of heart failure[177–180] support its use for early intervention to halt or delay the progression of this disease.

SIDE EFFECTS

Table 77–1 lists the side effects reported with captopril. Although early clinical trials used high dosages of captopril in severely ill hypertensive patients,[188] subsequent experience has been with lower doses in uncomplicated cases. Although the types of adverse effects have not changed, the incidence is markedly reduced compared with early clinical studies.[189]

Skin Rash

This is the most commonly reported side effect.[190] Manifestations include a mild pruritic, maculopapular rash localized to the arms and trunk. Urticarial or erythematous eruptions have also been reported. The rash may appear within the first few days to months of therapy and is the most frequent cause for discontinuation of therapy. The occurrence of rash is related to the dosage prescribed and the degree of renal impairment present. In patients receiving less than 150 mg of captopril per day with a serum creatinine level less than 1.6 mg/dl, the withdrawal rate from captopril due to rash was only 1.4%. When the dose was

Table 77–1. **Incidence of Most Frequent Adverse Events as Compared with Placebo in Controlled Clinical Studies with a Captopril Total Daily Dose of 100 Mg or Less**

	Captopril n = 1174	Placebo n = 448
Headache	61 (5.2)	31 (6.9)
Rash	43 (3.7)	11 (2.5)
Dizziness	41 (3.5)	9 (2.0)
Nausea	38 (3.2)	9 (2.0)
Fatigue/malaise	36 (3.1)	9 (2.0)
Taste alteration	18 (1.5)	5 (1.1)
Gastric upset	16 (1.4)	3 (0.7)
Diarrhea	13 (1.1)	5 (1.1)

Data include adverse effects for captopril with an incidence of more than 1% in patients with normal renal function.

greater than 150 mg and the creatinine level was greater than 1.6 mg/dl, the incidence increased to 5.1%. Although captopril-induced rash may disappear when enalapril is substituted, and vice versa, experience in Japanese patients has demonstrated a similar incidence of rash with both drugs.[191] There have been four cases of onycholysis with captopril therapy.[192]

Taste Disturbance

Dysgeusia, or impaired taste, has been reported with ACE inhibitor therapy. The incidence with captopril (κ 150 mg daily) ranges from 1.4% to 2.1%.[190] A variant of dysgeusia includes a metallic or sour taste in the mouth. Taste disturbances occur within the first few weeks of therapy, and spontaneous remission frequently occurs despite continued therapy. Rarely is discontinuation of therapy necessary. It is thought that taste abnormalities associated with captopril may be secondary to interference of the drug with zinc metabolism.[193-195] The incidence of taste disturbance varies with the method of side effect reporting. For example, Edwards et al.,[196] by using a specific questionnaire to identify taste abnormalities, reported a high incidence of this reaction: loss of taste occurred in 15.1% of nifedipine-treated patients and 9.1% of captopril-treated patients. Other gastrointestinal disturbances with ACE inhibitors include mouth ulcers, nausea, diarrhea, cholestatic jaundice, and, very rarely, hepatocellular injury.[190]

Cough

The most recently recognized adverse side effect from ACE inhibitors has been cough.[197-199] This cough is nonproductive and is associated with a tickling sensation in the throat and occasionally with nasal stuffiness. Cough has been observed with captopril, enalapril, and lisinopril. The frequency of its occurrence and the time to resolution increase with the duration of action of the ACE inhibitor. Thus, cough is more frequent with both enalapril and lisinopril than with captopril.[200-202] It has been difficult to assess the absolute frequency of cough, because it has been reported with similar frequency in ACE inhibitor and control groups.[203] Cough is not related to the development of airway obstruction or bronchial hyperresponsiveness.[204, 205] The effects of ACE inhibition on bradykinin or prostaglandin production may be responsible for the cough. Suppression of cough with antiinflammatory agents has been reported.[206]

Angioedema

The rare appearance of angioedema is of importance because it may lead to respiratory failure. Symptoms usually occur within the first month of therapy and sometimes after the first dose.[207] Angioedema occurs two to three times more frequently with the longer-acting ACE inhibitors (enalapril, lisinopril) than with captopril.[203] Potentiation of the effects of bradykinin may cause angioedema. Recognition of the early warning signs, such as localized edema, may minimize the consequences of this adverse reaction.

Neutropenia

In a review of 6000 patients receiving captopril therapy, Cooper[208] demonstrated that reduction in white blood cell count in these earlier reports was similar to neutropenia induced by other types of drugs. Neutropenia rarely occurs in captopril-treated patients with normal renal function. When it occurs, it is generally reversible, occurring within 60 to 90 days after the initiation of ACE inhibitor therapy and reversing within 3 weeks of discontinuation of therapy.[209] Bone marrow biopsies have demonstrated myeloid hypoplasia with a tendency toward immaturity. Evidence of red blood cell reduction was present in 25% of these patients, and a small percentage of them had a decrease in platelet number. Neutropenia did not recur in a small group of patients who were rechallenged with captopril after their initial event.[209] The risk of neutropenia is related to the dose of captopril and the presence of renal or collagen vascular diseases. The incidence of neutropenia in patients with uncomplicated hypertension is 0.01% but increases to 0.3% in patients with renal dysfunction (creatinine, > 1.6 mg/dl).[190] In renally impaired patients with collagen vascular disease, such as lupus erythematosus and scleroderma, the incidence of neutropenia was 3.7%.[191]

Renal Effects

Functional renal insufficiency may occur in patients treated with ACE inhibitors who have bilateral renal artery stenosis or stenosis in a solitary kidney.[190] This reversible side effect is secondary to dilation of the glomerular efferent arteriole and an inability to maintain glomerular filtration rate. It is uncertain whether captopril is associated with structural kidney disease. In early clinical studies, proteinuria was reported more frequently in severely hypertensive patients with preexisting renal impairment receiving captopril than in those with normal renal function. However, a comparison of biopsy specimens from hypertensive patients receiving captopril with those from untreated hypertensive patients found that subclinical glomerulonephritis was frequently present, and it is difficult to attribute this finding to drug therapy.[210, 211] On the basis of available data, it appears that long-term captopril in doses not exceeding 150 mg/day does not aggravate and may even improve mild renal impairment in most hypertensive patients.[209, 212]

DOSAGE

The effective oral dose of captopril is 50 mg daily, administered as a single dose or as two divided doses.[104, 105, 213] Lower doses, such as 6.25 to 12.5 mg twice daily, may be effective in patients with congestive heart failure or renovascular hypertension and/

or those who are volume depleted.[163, 212] Although it is recommended that captopril be taken 1 hour before meals, because food can interfere with its bioavailability, blood pressure reduction is not affected by food ingestion.[44, 45] The dose should be increased gradually at 2- to 4-week intervals to a maximum dose of 150 mg daily. Long-term effects on blood pressure may occur over several weeks even though there is a rapid onset of action. Consequently, dosage adjustments should not be any more frequent than every 2 weeks.[212] Concomitant administration of a diuretic should be attempted before increasing the dosage of captopril above 150 mg daily. If the blood pressure response is still not adequate with maximal diuretic dosage, a third agent should be added. Captopril dosage may be increased further under special circumstances, although it should not exceed 450 mg/day.[212] The risk of an acute hypotensive response can be minimized by avoiding a low-salt diet or diuretics immediately before initiation of the ACE inhibitor, because both activate the renin-angiotensin system. These should be withheld 3 days before beginning administration of an ACE inhibitor. If diuretic therapy cannot be withheld, captopril should be initiated with one quarter or one half of the original dose.[212] If patients are receiving multiple antihypertensive therapy in these situations, diuretics should be continued, but the other antihypertensives should be tapered gradually, then stopped and replaced by captopril.[212] In patients with accelerated hypertension, incremental increases of captopril dosage can be made every 24 hours or even more frequently under medical supervision until satisfactory blood pressure response is achieved.[212] In patients whose creatinine clearance is below 30 ml/min, the initial captopril dose should be reduced by 50% to 70%.[212] If concomitant diuretic therapy is instituted, a loop diuretic such as furosemide would be the drug of choice. Potassium supplementation and potassium-sparing diuretics are to be avoided in renal failure because hyperkalemia may occur as a result of captopril's effect on reducing aldosterone production.[212]

ADVANTAGES OVER OTHER AGENTS

Captopril has many advantages over other antihypertensive agents. This drug has been shown to improve quality-of-life measures and is free of many of the subjective side effects associated with other agents, such as mental depression, inability to concentrate, fatigue, sexual dysfunction, and loss of libido.[214] ACE inhibitors can be used in hypertensive patients with concomitant illnesses, such as congestive heart failure, peripheral vascular disease, and chronic obstructive pulmonary disease. Captopril may be the drug of choice in hypertensive patients with impaired insulin sensitivity or with diabetes.[215] Adverse metabolic effects such as hyperlipidemia, which are characteristic of diuretics and β-blockers, are not seen with ACE inhibitor therapy.[216]

FUTURE DIRECTIONS FOR ACE INHIBITORS

Experimental and clinical research supports the concept that ACE inhibitors may emerge as the cardioprotective agents of the 1990s.[217] In hypertension, captopril may reduce the risk of developing coronary heart disease by preventing, or causing the regression of, cardiac and vascular hypertrophy. Unlike other antihypertensive agents, ACE inhibitors have a neutral metabolic profile and therefore have no negative effects on cardiovascular risk factors.[217] In addition, captopril has been shown to inhibit atherogenesis and prevent atherosclerosis and myointimal proliferation in experimental animal models.[217a] In heart failure, captopril's beneficial effects include improvements in exercise tolerance and functional capacity and reductions in ventricular ectopy. Improved survival of heart failure patients taking ACE inhibitors has been well documented.

Because ACE inhibitors unload the heart and reduce ventricular wall stress, they have been evaluated in patients after myocardial infarction for the prevention of ventricular dysfunction and heart failure. An attenuation of left ventricular enlargement and an improvement in exercise capacity were reported in these patients after 1 year of captopril therapy. In the long-term SAVE study, captopril reduced mortality and moridity when administered to patients after an acute myocardial infarction.[185]

Captopril has been shown to produce coronary vasodilation and to increase angina threshold in patients with coronary artery disease. Van Gilst et al.[218] reported that captopril (sulfhydryl-containing ACE inhibitor), but not ramipril (non–sulfhydryl-containing ACE inhibitor), potentiated the vasodilatory effects of isosorbide dinitrate. They postulated that the sulfhydryl group of captopril serves as a tissue sulfhydryl donor, increasing the formation of cyclic guanosine monophosphate. Westlin and Mullane,[219] in a canine model of myocardial ischemia, found that captopril but not enalapril (non–sulfhydryl-containing) prevented left ventricular dysfunction after ischemia. Captopril, as a scavenger of free oxygen radicals, may prevent cellular injury due to the radical generation that occurs during reperfusion of the ischemic myocardium. In experimental animal models, ACE inhibition limited the size of myocardial infarcts.[220]

Linz et al.[221] reported a reduction in ventricular arrhythmias with ACE inhibitors during coronary ischemia in an isolated heart preparation as a result of inhibiting the cardiac renin-angiotensin system. Similarly, Westlin and Mullane[219] demonstrated that ACE inhibitors prevented ventricular arrhythmias during coronary ischemia in a canine model. In concert, these studies substantiate the importance of the renin-angiotensin system in cardiovascular diseases and the contention that its inhibition, through ACE inhibitors, is cardioprotective.

Ferranini et al.[222] demonstrated elevated circulating insulin levels secondary to peripheral tissue insulin resistance in a group of 13 patients with untreated essential hypertension who had normal body weight and normal glucose tolerance. This peripheral insulin resistance was directly correlated with the severity of hypertension.

The cause of the hyperinsulinemia secondary to insulin resistance that occurs in hypertension is not known. Conceivably, hyperinsulinemia could cause sodium reabsorption, increased sympathetic nervous system activity, vascular hypertrophy, and a cellular cation transport defect, all of which may increase arterial pressure.

Pollare et al.[223] showed that captopril increased the insulin-mediated disposal of glucose by enhancing insulin sensitivity by 11%, whereas hydrochlorothiazide administration resulted in a decrease in insulin sensitivity of similar magnitude. Therefore, captopril therapy with its improved insulin sensitivity may enhance the patient's metabolic risk-factor profile and thus provide a distinct advantage over other antihypertensive agents.

CONCLUSION

The ACE inhibitor captopril has been clinically demonstrated to be a superior antihypertensive agent. Its efficacy, favorable metabolic profile, relative freedom from side effects, and improvement in quality of life, which are important factors to be taken into consideration in selecting an antihypertensive drug, support its usefulness as first-line therapy in the treatment of hypertension.

Acknowledgments

We would like to thank our staff for all their secretarial assistance, Janith Mills, PA-C, for her support, and Karen Porrini, Pharm.D., for invaluable editorial assistance.

REFERENCES

1. Tigerstadt R, Bergman PG: Niere and Kreilauf. Scand Arch Physiol 8:223, 1898.
2. Goldblatt H, Lynsh J, Hanzal R, et al: Studies on experimental hypertension. I. The production of persistent elevation of systolic blood pressure by means of renal ischemia. J Exp Med 59:347, 1934.
3. Page F, Hemler O: A crystalline pressor substance resulting from the reaction between renin and renin activator. J Exp Med 71:29, 1940.
4. Braun-Menendez E, Fasciolo J, Leloir C, et al: La substancia hypertensora de la sangre del rinon isquemiado. Rev Soc Argent Biol 15:420, 1939.
5. Skeggs LT, Jr, Marsh W, Kahn J, et al: The existence of two forms of hypertension. J Exp Med 99:275, 1954.
6. Ferreira SA: A bradykinin-potentiating factor (BPF) present in the venom of *Bothrops jararaca*. Br J Pharmacol 24:163, 1965.
7. Ng KK, Vane JR: Conversion of angiotensin I to angiotensin II. Nature 215:762, 1967.
8. Ng KK, Vane JR: Fate of angiotensin I in the circulation. Nature 218:144, 1968.
9. Ferreira SA, Vane JR: The disappearance of bradykinin and eledoisin from the circulation and vascular beds of the cat. Br J Pharmacol Chemother 30:417, 1967.
10. Antonaccio MJ: Angiotensin converting enzyme (ACE) inhibitors. Am Rev Pharmacol Toxicol 22:57, 1982.
11. Cushman DW, Cheung HS, Sabo EF, et al: Design of potent competitive inhibitors of angiotensin-converting enzyme. Biochemistry 16:548, 1977.
12. Cushman DW, Ondetti MA: Inhibitors of angiotensin-converting enzyme. Prog Med Chem 174:411, 1980.
13. Cushman DW, Cheung HS, Sabo EF, et al: Design of new antihypertensive drugs: Potent and specific inhibitors of angiotensin-converting enzyme. Prog Cardiovasc Dis 21:176, 1978.
14. Sotter RL: Angiotensin-converting enzyme and the regulation of vasoactive peptides. Annu Rev Biochem 45:73, 1976.
15. Peach MJ: Renin angiotensin system: Biochemistry and mechanisms of action. Physiol Rev 57:313, 1977.
16. Suddy RR, Lapworth R, Bird R: Angiotensin-converting enzyme and its clinical significance: A review. J Clin Pathol 36:938, 1983.
17. Zusman RM: Angiotensin converting enzyme inhibitors: Evidence for renin-dependent and renin-independent mechanisms of action. *In* Kaplan NM, Brenner BM, Laragh JH (eds): Perspectives in Hypertension, Vol 1. The Kidney in Hypertension. New York: Raven Press, 1987, pp 161–177.
18. Davis JO, Freeman RH: Mechanisms regulating renin release. Physiol Rev 56:1, 1976.
19. Keeton TK, Campbell WB: The pharmacologic alteration of release. Pharmacol Rev 32:81, 1980.
20. Kaplan NM: Primary (essential) hypertension: Pathogenesis. *In* Kaplan NM (ed): Clinical Hypertension. Baltimore: Williams & Wilkins, 1986, pp 56–122.
21. Brunner HR, Gavras H, Waeber B, et al: Oral angiotensin converting enzyme inhibitor in long-term treatment of hypertensive patients. Ann Intern Med 90:19, 1979.
22. Atkinson AB, Cumming AMM, Brown JJ, et al: Captopril treatment: Inter-dose variations in renin, angiotensins I and II, aldosterone, and blood pressure. Br J Clin Pharmacol 13:855, 1982.
23. Faure L, Frazer MG, Hollifield JW: An orally active angiotensin I converting enzyme inhibitor for therapy of hypertension. Clin Res 26:23A, 1978.
24. Lijen P, Staessen J, Fagards R, et al: Increase in plasma aldosterone during prolonged captopril treatment. Am J Cardiol 49:1561, 1982.
25. Anderson GH, Springer J, Tiunan E: Hypotensive mechanisms of captopril. Clin Res 28:328A, 1980.
26. Mookherjee S, Anderson GH, Eich R, et al: Acute effects of captopril on cardiopulmonary hemodynamics and renin angiotensin-aldosterone and bradykinin profile in hypertension. Am Heart J 105:106, 1983.
27. Johnston CI, McGarth BP, Millar JA, et al: Long-term effects of captopril (SQ 14225) on blood pressure and hormone levels in essential hypertension. Lancet 2:492, 1979.
28. Atlas SA, Case DB, Scaley JE, et al: Interruption of the renin-angiotensin system in hypertensive patients by captopril induces sustained reduction in aldosterone secretion, potassium retention and natriuresis. Hypertension 1:274, 1979.
29. Nyrop M, Zweifler AJ: Platelet aggregation in hypertension and the effects of antihypertensive treatment. J Hypertens 6:263, 1988.
30. Vinci JM, Horowitz D, Zusman RM: The effects of converting enzyme inhibition with SQ 20881 on plasma and urinary kinins, prostaglandin E and angiotensin II in hypertensive man. Hypertension 1:416, 1979.
31. Omata K, Abe K, Tsuneda K, et al: Role of endogenous angiotensin II and prostaglandins in the antihypertensive mechanism of angiotensin converting enzyme inhibitor in hypertension. Clin Exp Hypertens [A] 9:569, 1987.
32. Someya N, Morotomi Y, Kodema K: Suppressive effect of captopril on platelet aggregation in essential hypertension. J Cardiovasc Pharmacol 6:840, 1984.
33. Aldigier JC, Plouin PF, Guyere TT, et al: Comparison of the hormonal and renal effects of captopril in severe essential and renovascular hypertension. Am J Cardiol 49:14, 1982.
34. Zusman RM: Effects of converting enzyme inhibitors on the renin-angiotensin-aldosterone, bradykinin, and arachidonic acid-prostaglandin systems: Correlation of chemical structure and biologic activity. Am J Kidney Dis 10(Suppl 1):13, 1987.
35. Dzau VJ: Cardiac renin angiotensin system: Molecular and functional aspects. Am J Med 84(Suppl 3A):22, 1988.
36. Dzau VJ: Implications of local angiotensin production in car-

diovascular physiology and pharmacology. Am J Cardiol 59:59A, 1987.

37. Unger T, Scholkens BA, Ganten D, et al: Tissue converting enzyme inhibition and cardiovascular effects of converting inhibitors. Clin Exp Hypertens [A] 9(2 and 3):417, 1987.

38. Kostis JB: Angiotensin-converting enzyme inhibitors: Emerging differences and new compounds. Am J Hypertens 2:57, 1989.

39. Duchin KL, McKinstry DN, Cohen AI, et al: Pharmacokinetics of captopril in healthy subjects and in patients with cardiovascular diseases. Clin Pharmacokinet 14:241, 1988.

40. Cohen AI, Devlin RG, Ivashkiv E, et al: Determination of captopril in human blood and urine by GLC—selected ion monitoring mass spectrometry after oral coadministration with its isotopomer. J Pharmacol Sci 71:1251, 1982.

41. Duchin KL, Singhvi SM, Willard DA, et al: Captopril kinetics. Clin Pharmacol Ther 31:452, 1982.

42. Singhvi SM, Duchin KL, Willard DA, et al: Renal handling of captopril: Effect of probenecid. Clin Pharmacol Ther 32:182, 1982.

43. McKinstry DN, Singhvi SM, Kripalani KJ, et al: Disposition and cardiovascular endocrine effects of an orally active angiotensin-converting enzyme inhibitor, SQ 14,225, in normal subjects. Clin Pharmacol Ther 23:121, 1978.

44. Mantyla R, Mannista PT, Vuorela A, et al: Impairment of captopril bioavailability by concomitant food and antacid intake. Int J Clin Pharm Ther Toxicol 22:626, 1984.

45. Muller HH, Overback A, Heck I, et al: The influence of food intake on pharmacodynamics and plasma concentrations of captopril. J Hypertens 3(Suppl 2):S135, 1985.

46. Salvetti A, Redrinelli R, Magagna A, et al: The influence of food on acute and chronic effects of captopril in essential hypertensive patients. J Cardiovasc Pharmacol 7:S25, 1985.

47. Creasey WA, Funke PT, McKinstry DN, et al: Pharmacokinetics of captopril in elderly healthy male volunteers. J Clin Pharmacol 26:264, 1986.

48. Duchin KL, Pierides AM, Heald A, et al: Intravenous captopril in patients with renal failure. Kidney Int 25:942, 1984.

49. Drummer OH, Miach PJ, Workman B, et al: The pharmacokinetics of single-dose captopril in uremic patients on maintenance dialysis. J Hypertens 1:381, 1983.

50. Drummer OH, Workman BS, Miach PJ, et al: The pharmacokinetics of captopril and captopril disulfide conjugates in uremic patients on maintenance dialysis: Comparison in patients with normal renal function. Eur J Clin Pharmacol 32:267, 1987.

51. Fujimara A, Kajiyama H, Ebihara A, et al: Pharmacokinetics and pharmacodynamics of captopril in patients undergoing continuous ambulatory peritoneal dialysis. Nephron 44:324, 1986.

52. Rademaker M, Shaw TRD, Williams BC, et al: Intravenous captopril treatment in patients with severe cardiac failure. Br Heart J 55:187, 1986.

53. Cody RJ, Schaer GL, Covitt AB, et al: Captopril kinetics in chronic congestive heart failure. Clin Pharmacol Ther 32:721, 1982.

54. Shaw TRD, Duncan FM, Williams BC, et al: Plasma-free captopril concentrations during short- and long-term treatment with oral captopril for heart failure. Br Heart J 54:160, 1985.

55. Bravo EL, Tarazi RC: Converting enzyme inhibition with an orally active compound in hypertensive man. Hypertension 1:39, 1979.

56. Vlasses PH, Koffer H, Ferguson RK, et al: Captopril withdrawal after chronic therapy. Clin Exp Hypertens 3:929, 1981.

57. DiBianco R: Angiotensin converting enzyme inhibition. Postgrad Med 78:229, 1985.

58. Edwards CRW, Padfield PL: Angiotensin-converting enzyme inhibitors: Past, present and bright future. Lancet 1:30, 1985.

59. Sturani A, Chiarini C, Degli Eposti E, et al: Captopril. N Engl J Med 307:59, 1982.

60. Warren SE, O'Connor DT, Cohen IM: Autonomic and baroreflex function after captopril in hypertension. Am Heart J 105:1002, 1983.

61. Fagard R, Bulpitt C, Lijnen P, et al: Response of the systemic and pulmonary circulation to converting enzyme inhibition (captopril) at rest and during exercise in hypertensive patients. Circulation 65:33, 1982.

62. Muiesan G, Alicandri CL, Agabiti Rosei E, et al: Angiotensin-converting enzyme inhibition, catecholamines, and hemodynamics in essential hypertension. Am J Cardiol 49:1420, 1984.

63. Fujita T, Ando K, Noda H, et al: Hemodynamics and endocrine changes associated with captopril in diuretic-resistant hypertensive patients. Am J Med 73:341, 1982.

64. Mitchell HC, Pettinger WA, Gianotti L, et al: Further studies of the hyperadrenergic state of treated hypertensives: Effect of captopril. Clin Exp Hypertens [A] 5:1611, 1983.

65. Schalekamp MADH: Clinical experience with captopril in hypertension. Prog Pharmacol 5:69, 1984.

66. Ventura HO, Frohlich ED, Messerli FH, et al: Cardiovascular effects and regional blood flow distribution associated with angiotensin converting enzyme inhibition (captopril) in essential hypertension. Am J Cardiol 55:1023, 1985.

67. Braunwald E: Clinical manifestation of heart failure. In Braunwald E (ed): Heart Disease: A Textbook of Cardiovascular Medicine. Philadelphia: WB Saunders, 1984, pp 488–502.

68. Romankiewicz JA, Brogden RN, Heel RC, et al: Captopril: An update review of its pharmacological properties and therapeutic efficacy in congestive heart failure. Drugs 25:6, 1983.

69. Shepard AN, Hayes PC, Jacyna M, et al: The influence of captopril, the nitrates and propranolol on apparent liver blood flow. Br J Clin Pharmacol 19:393, 1985.

70. Eriksson LS, Kagedal B, Wahrer J: Effects of captopril on hepatic venous pressure and blood flow in patients with liver cirrhosis. Am J Med 76:66, 1984.

71. Crossley IR, Bihari D, Gimson AES, et al: Effects of converting enzyme inhibitor on hepatic blood flow in man. Am J Med 76:62, 1984.

72. Levine TB, Olivari MT, Cohn JN: Hemodynamic and regional blood flow response to captopril in congestive heart failure. Am J Med 76:38, 1984.

73. Britton KE, Granowska M, Nimmon CC, et al: Cerebral blood flow in hypertensive patients with cerebrovascular disease: Technique for measurement and effect of captopril. Nucl Med Commun 6:251, 1985.

74. Minematsu K, Yamaguchi T, Tsuchiya M, et al: Effect of angiotensin converting enzyme inhibitor (captopril) on cerebral blood flow in hypertensive patients without a history of stroke. Clin Exp Hypertens A9:551, 1987.

75. Paulson OB, Jarden JO, Vorstrup S, et al: Effect of captopril on the cerebral circulation in chronic heart failure. Eur J Clin Invest 16:124, 1986.

76. Hollenberg NK: Renal hemodynamics in essential and renovascular hypertension: Influence of captopril. Am J Med 76:22, 1984.

77. Miyamori I, Yasuhara S, Takeda Y, et al: Effects of converting enzyme inhibitor on split renal function in renovascular hypertension. Hypertension 8:415, 1986.

78. Ribstein J, Mourad G, Mion C, et al: Chronic angiotensin converting enzyme inhibition as an alternative to native kidney removal in posttransplant hypertension. J Hypertens 4:S255, 1986.

79. Kaplan NM: Treatment of hypertension: Drug therapy. In Kaplan NM (ed): Clinical Hypertension. Baltimore: Williams & Wilkins, 1986, pp 180–272.

80. Atkinson AB, Brown JJ, Lever AF, et al: Combined treatment of severe intractable hypertension with captopril and diuretic. Lancet 2:105, 1980.

81. Ferguson RK, Vlasses PH, Koplin JR, et al: Captopril in severe treatment-resistant hypertension. Am Heart J 99:579, 1980.

82. Koffer H, Vlasses PH, Ferguson RK, et al: Captopril in diuretic-treated hypertensive patients. JAMA 244:25, 1980.

83. Veterans Administration Cooperative Study Group on Antihypertensive Agents: Low-dose captopril in the treatment of mild to moderate hypertension. Hypertension 5(Suppl III):319, 1983.

84. The Fifth Report of the Joint National Committee on Detection, Evaluation, and Treatment of High Blood Pressure (JVNC). Arch Intern Med 153:154, 1993.

85. Packer M, Medina N, Yushak M: Relation between serum sodium concentration and the hemodynamic and clinical responses to converting enzyme inhibition with captopril in severe heart failure. J Am Coll Cardiol 3:10, 1984.

86. Weber MA: The renin-angiotensin-aldosterone system and hypertension. *In* Kostis JB, DeFelice EA (eds): Angiotensin Converting Enzyme Inhibitors. New York: Alan R Liss, 1987, pp 55–92.

87. Gavras H, Brunner HR, Turini GA, et al: Antihypertensive effect of oral angiotensin-converting enzyme inhibitor SQ 14225 in man. N Engl J Med 298:991, 1978.

88. Gavras I, Gavras H: The use of ACE inhibitors in hypertension. *In* Kostis JB, DeFelice EA (eds): Angiotensin Converting Enzyme Inhibitors. New York: Alan R Liss, 1987, pp 93–122.

89. Vidt DG, Bravo EL, Fouad FM: Captopril. N Engl J Med 306:214, 1982.

90. Aberg H, Frithz G, Morlin C: Comparison of captopril (SQ 14225) with hydrochlorothiazide in the treatment of essential hypertension. Int J Clin Pharmacol Ther Toxicol 19:368, 1981.

91. Weinberger MH: Comparison of captopril and hydrochlorothiazide alone and in combination in mild to moderate essential hypertension. Br J Clin Pharmacol 14:12, 1982.

92. Woo J, Wod KS, Kin T, et al: A single-blind randomized crossover study of angiotensin-converting enzyme inhibitor and triamterene hydrochlorothiazide in the treatment of mild to moderate hypertension in the elderly. Arch Int Med 147:1386, 1987.

93. Captopril Research Group of Japan: Clinical effects of low-dose captopril plus a thiazide diuretic on mild to moderate essential hypertension. A multicenter double-blind comparison with propranolol. J Cardiovasc Pharmacol 7(Suppl 1):S77, 1985.

94. Andren L, Karlberg BE, Svensson A, et al: Long-term effects of captopril and atenolol in essential hypertension. Acta Med Scand 217:155, 1985.

95. Dessi-Fulgheri P, Bandiera F, Glorioso N, et al: Labetalol and captopril combined with chlorthalidone in the treatment of mild to moderate essential hypertension. Curr Ther Res 37:873, 1985.

96. Potter JF, Beevers DG: Comparison of nifedipine and captopril as third-line agents in hypertensive patients uncontrolled with a beta-blocker and diuretic therapy. J Clin Pharmacol 27:410, 1987.

97. Salvetti A, Innocenti PF, Iardella M, et al: Captopril and nifedipine interactions in the treatment of essential hypertension: A crossover study. J Hypertens 5(Suppl 4):S139, 1987.

98. Witte PU, Walter U: Comparative double-blind study of ramipril and captopril in mild to moderate essential hypertension. Am J Cardiol 59:115D, 1987.

99. Vlasses PH, Conner DP, Rotmensch HH, et al: Double-blind comparison of captopril and enalapril in mild to moderate hypertension. J Am Coll Cardiol 7:651, 1986.

100. Garanin G: A comparison of once-daily antihypertensive therapy with captopril and enalapril. Curr Ther Res 40:567, 1986.

101. Groel JT, Tadros SS, Dreslinski GR, et al: Long-term antihypertensive therapy with captopril. Hypertension 5(Suppl III):145, 1983.

102. Ohman P, Aurell M, Aspund J, et al: A long-term follow up of patients with essential hypertension treated with captopril. Acta Med Scand 216:53, 1984.

103. Sirgo MA, Mills RJ, Dequattro V: Effects of antihypertensive agents on circadian blood pressure and heart rate patterns. Arch Intern Med 148:25, 1988.

104. Schoenberger JA, Wilson DJ: Once-daily treatment of essential hypertension with captopril. J Clin Hypertens 4:379, 1986.

105. Weber MA: Clinical experience with converting enzyme inhibitors in hypertension. Am J Kidney Dis 10(Suppl 1):45, 1987.

106. Levy D, Garrison RJ, Savage DD, et al: Left ventricular mass and incidence of coronary heart disease in the elderly cohort. The Framingham heart study. Ann Intern Med 110:101, 1989.

107. Weber JR: Left ventricular hypertrophy: Its prime importance as a controllable risk factor. Am Heart J 116:272, 1988.

108. Levy D, Anderson KM, Savage DD, et al: Echocardiographically detected left ventricular hypertrophy: Prevalence and risk factors. Ann Intern Med 108:7, 1988.

109. Lomband M, Faini G, Pastori F, et al: Left ventricular mass and function before and after antihypertensive treatment. J Hypertens 1:215, 1983.

110. Drayer JI, Gardin, JM, Weber MA, et al: Changes in ventricular septal thickness during diuretic therapy. Clin Pharmacol Ther 32:283, 1982.

111. Fouad Tarazi F, Liebson P: Echocardiographic studies of regression of left vertricular hypertrophy in hypertension. Hypertension 7:1165, 1987.

112. Nakashima Y, Fouad FM, Tarazi RE: Regression of left ventricular hypertrophy from systemic hypertension by enalapril. Am J Cardiol 53:1044, 1984.

113. Wikstrand J, Trimarco B, Buffetti A, et al: Increased cardiac output and lowered peripheral resistance during metoprolol treatment. Acta Med Scand 672(Suppl):105, 1983.

114. Muiesan ML, Agabiti-Rosei E, Romanelli G, et al: Beneficial effects of one year's treatment with captopril on left ventricular anatomy and function in hypertensive patients with left ventricular hypertrophy. Am J Med 84(Suppl 3A):129, 1988.

115. Sheiban I, Arcaro G, Coui R, et al: Regression of cardiac hypertrophy after antihypertensive therapy with nifedipine and captopril. J Cardiovasc Pharmacol 10(Suppl 10):S187, 1987.

116. Michel JB, Dussaule JC, Alherc-Gelas E, et al: Can inhibition of the renin-angiotensin system have a cardioprotective effect? J Cardiovasc Pharmacol 7(Suppl 2):S75, 1985.

117. McLenachan JM, Henderson E, Morris KI, et al: Ventricular arrhythmias in patients with hypertensive left ventricular hypertrophy. N Engl J Med 317:787, 1987.

118. Dahlöf B, Pennert K, Hansson L: Reversal of left ventricular hypertrophy in hypertensive patients: A metaanalysis of 109 treatment studies.Am J Hypertens 5:95, 1992.

119. Ambrosini E, Borghi C, Costa FU: Captopril and hydrochlorothiazide: Rationale for their combination. Br J Clin Pharmacol 23:435, 1987.

120. Weinberger MH: Influence of an angiotensin converting enzyme inhibitor on diuretic-induced metabolic effects in hypertension. Hypertension 5(Suppl III):132, 1983.

121. Drayer J, Weber MA: Monotherapy of essential hypertension with a converting enzyme inhibitor. Hypertension 5(Suppl III):108, 1983.

122. Veterans Administration Cooperative Study Group on Antihypertensive Agents: Racial differences in response to low-dose captopril are abolished by the addition of hydrochlorothiazide. Br J Clin Pharmacol 14:975, 1982.

123. Holland OB, Von Kuhnert L, Campbell WB, et al: Synergistic effect of captopril with hydrochlorothiazide for the treatment of low renin hypertensive black patients. Hypertension 5:235, 1983.

124. Case DB, Atlas SA, Marion RM, et al: Clinical experience with captopril in moderate to severe hypertension. Cardiovasc Rev Rep 3:435, 1982.

125. Havelka J, Vetter H, Studer A, et al: Acute and chronic effects of the angiotensin-converting enzyme inhibitor captopril in severe hypertension. Am J Cardiol 49:1467, 1982.

126. Lahor MS, Regan PO, O'Donohoe JE, et al: Captopril for refractory hypertension in patients with impaired renal function. J R Soc Med 78:367, 1985.

127. Schrader J, Schoel G, Scheler F: Results of a 5-year study of captopril in patients with severe therapy-resistant hypertension. Klin Wochenschr 64:695, 1986.

128. Pessina AC, Palatini P, Sperti G, et al: Synergistic effect of minoxidil and captopril in patients with refractory hypertension. Curr Ther Res 35:269, 1984.

129. Seedat YK, Rawat R: Captopril combined with minoxidil, beta-blockers and furosemide in the treatment of refractory hypertension. Eur J Clin Pharmacol 25:9, 1983.

130. Traub YM, Levey BA: Combined treatment with minoxidil and captopril in refractory hypertension. Arch Intern Med 143:1142, 1983.

131. Burnakis TG, Mioduch J: Combined therapy with captopril and potassium supplementation. A potential for hyperkalemia. Arch Intern Med 144:2371, 1984.

132. Costa FU, Borghi C, Ambrosioni E: Captopril and oxprenolol in a fixed combination with thiazide diuretics: Comparison of their antihypertensive efficacy and metabolic effects. Clin Ther 6:708, 1984.

133. Brouwer RML, Bolli P, Erne P, et al: Antihypertensive treatment using calcium antagonist in combination with captopril rather than diuretics. J Cardiovasc Pharmacol 7:S88, 1985.

134. Anderson RJ, Kirk LM, Reed WG: Therapeutic options in the control of hypertension in the elderly: An update. Cardiovasc Rev Rep 4:63, 1987.
135. Baker SL: A study of the use of captopril in elderly hypertensive patients. Age Aging 17:17, 1988.
136. Muiesan G, Agabiti-Rosei E, Buoninconti R, et al: Anti-hypertensive efficacy and tolerability of captopril in the elderly: Comparison with hydrochlorothiazide and placebo in a multicenter, double-blind study. J Hypertens 5(Suppl 5):S598, 1987.
137. Corea L, Bentivoglio M, Verdecchia P, et al: Converting enzyme inhibition vs diuretic therapy as first therapeutic approach to the elderly hypertensive patient. Curr Ther Res 36:347, 1984.
138. Tuck ML, Katz LA, Kirkendall WM, et al: Low-dose captopril in mild to moderate geriatric hypertension. J Am Geriatr Soc 34:693, 1986.
139. Creisson C, Baulac L, Lenfant B: Captopril/hydrochlorothiazide combination in elderly patients with mild-to-moderate hypertension: A double-blind, randomized, placebo-controlled study. Postgrad Med J 62:139, 1986.
140. Schoenberger JA, Testa M, Ross AD, et al: Efficacy, safety, and quality-of-life assessment of captopril antihypertensive therapy in clinical practice. Arch Intern Med 150:301, 1990.
141. Hostetter TH, Rennke HG, Brenner BM: The case of intrarenal hypertension in the initiation and progression of diabetic and other glomerulopathies. Am J Med 72:375, 1982.
142. Brenner BM: Nephron adaptation to renal injury or ablation. Am J Physiol 249:F324, 1985.
143. Hommel E, Parving HH, Mathiesen E, et al: Effect of captopril on kidney function in insulin-dependent diabetic patients with nephropathy. Br Med J 293:467, 1986.
144. Bjorck S, Nyberg G, Mulec H, et al: Beneficial effects of angiotensin converting enzyme inhibition on renal function in patients with diabetic nephropathy. Br Med J 293:471, 1986.
145. Parving HH, Andersen AR, Smidt UM, et al: Early aggressive antihypertensive treatment reduces rate of decline in kidney function in diabetic nephropathy. Lancet 2:1175, 1983.
146. Zatz R, Dunn BR, Meyer TW, et al: Prevention of diabetic glomerulopathy by pharmacological amelioration of glomerular capillary hypertension. J Clin Invest 77:1925, 1986.
147. Taguma Y, Kitamoto Y, Futaki G, et al: Effect of captopril on heavy proteinuria in azotemic diabetics. N Engl J Med 313:1617, 1985.
148. Parving HH, Hommel E, Smidt UM: Protection of kidney function and decrease in albuminuria by captopril in insulin-dependent diabetics with nephropathy. Br Med J 297:1086, 1988.
149. Lewis EJ, Hunsicker LG, Bain RP, et al: The effect of angiotensin-converting-enzyme inhibition on diabetic nephropathy. N Engl J Med 329:20, 1993.
149a. Marre M, LeBlanc H, Suarez L, et al: Converting enzyme inhibition and kidney function in normotensive diabetic patients with persistent microalbuminuria. Br Med J 294:1448, 1987.
150. Mathiesen ER, Hommel E, Giese J, Parving HH: Efficacy of captopril in postponing nephropathy in normotensive insulin dependent diabetic patients with microalbuminuria. BMJ 303:81, 1991.
151. Jauch KW, Hartl W, Guenther B, et al: Captopril enhances insulin responsiveness of forearm muscle tissue in non–insulin-dependent diabetes mellitus. Eur J Clin Invest 17:448, 1987.
152. Shionoiri H, Miyakawa T, Takasaki I, et al: Glucose tolerance during chronic captopril therapy in patients with essential hypertension. J Cardiovasc Pharmacol 9:160, 1987.
153. Anderson S, Meyer TW, Rennke HG, et al: Control of glomerular hypertension limits glomerular injury in rats with reduced renal mass. J Clin Invest 76:612, 1985.
154. Callis L, Villa A, Catala J, et al: Long-term treatment with captopril in pediatric patients with severe hypertension and chronic renal failure. Clin Exp Hypertens [A] 8:847, 1986.
155. Ruilope LM, Miranda B, Morales JM, et al: Converting enzyme inhibition in renal failure. Am J Kidney Dis 13:120, 1989.
156. Gifford RW: Epidemiology and clinical manifestations of reno-
vascular hypertension. In Stanley JC, Ernst CB, Fry WJ (eds): Renovascular Hypertension. Philadelphia: WB Saunders, 1984, pp 77–99.
157. Hollifield JW, Moore LC, Winn SD, et al: Angiotensin converting enzyme inhibition in renovascular hypertension. Cardiovasc Rev Rep 3:673, 1982.
158. Hollenberg NK: Medical therapy of renovascular hypertension: Efficacy and safety of captopril in 269 patients. Cardiovasc Rev Rep 4:852, 1983.
159. Hricik DE, Browning PJ, Kopelman R, et al: Captopril induced functional renal insufficiency in patients with bilateral renal artery stenosis or renal artery stenosis in a solitary kidney. N Engl J Med 308:373, 1986.
160. Blythe WB: Captopril and renal autoregulation. N Engl J Med 308:390, 1983.
161. Chan MK, Sweny P, Nahas AM, et al: Captopril in hypertension after renal transplantation. Postgrad Med J 60:132, 1984.
162. Herlitz H, Ahlomen J, Aurell M, et al: Captopril in hypertension after renal transplantation. Scand J Urol Nephrol 79(Suppl):111, 1984.
163. Gagnadoux MF, Niaudet P, Bacri JL, et al: Captopril and transplant renal artery stenosis in children. Transplant Proc 17:187, 1985.
164. Bouissou F, Meguira B, Rostin M, et al: Long-term therapy by captopril in children with renal hypertension. Clin Exp Hypertens 8:841, 1986.
165. Mirkin BL, Newman TJ: Efficacy and safety of captopril in the treatment of severe childhood hypertension: Report of the International Collaborative Study Group. Pediatrics 75:1091, 1985.
166. Sagat T, Sasinka M, Furkova K, et al: Treatment of renal hypertension in children by captopril. Clin Exp Hypertens 8:853, 1986.
167. Sinaiko AR, Kashtan CE, Mirkin BL: Antihypertensive drug therapy with captopril in children and adolescents. Clin Exp Hypertens A8:829, 1986.
168. Sigstrom L, Aurell M, Jodal U: Angiotensin converting enzyme inhibitor treatment of hypertension in infancy and childhood. Scand J Urol Nephrol 79(Suppl):107, 1984.
169. Zawada ET, Clements PJ, Furst DA, et al: Clinical course of patients with scleroderma renal crisis treated with captopril. Nephron 27:74, 1981.
170. Thurm RH, Alexander JC: Captopril in the treatment of scleroderma renal crisis. Arch Intern Med 144:733, 1984.
171. Beckett VL, Donadio JV, Brennan LA, et al: Use of captopril as early therapy for renal scleroderma: A prospective study. Mayo Clin Proc 60:763, 1985.
172. Croog SH, Levine S, Testa MA, et al: The effects of antihypertensive therapy on the quality of life. N Engl J Med 314:1657, 1986.
173. Testa MA, et al: Quality of life and antihypertensive therapy in men: A comparison of captopril with enalapril. N Engl J Med 328:907, 1993.
174. Packer M: Converting-enzyme inhibitor for severe chronic heart failure: Views from a skeptic. Int J Cardiol 7:111, 1985.
175. Dzau VJ, Colucci WS, Williams GH, et al: Sustained effectiveness of converting enzyme inhibition in patients with severe congestive heart failure. N Engl J Med 302:1373, 1980.
176. Ricci S, Zaniol P, Teglio V, et al: Sustained hemodynamic and clinical effects of captopril in long-term treatment of severe chronic congestive heart failure. Br J Clin Pharmacol 14:209S, 1982.
177. Captopril Multicenter Research Group: A placebo-controlled trial of captopril in refractory chronic congestive heart failure. J Am Coll Cardiol 2:755, 1983.
178. Newman JJ, Maskin CS, Dennick LG, et al: Effects of captopril on survival in patients with heart failure. Am J Med 84(Suppl 3A):140, 1988.
179. Captopril Multicenter Research Group I: A cooperative multicenter study of captopril in congestive heart failure: Hemodynamic effects and long-term response. Am Heart J 110:439, 1985.
180. Captopril Multicenter Research Group: Comparative effects of therapy with captopril and digoxin in patients with mild to moderate heart failure. JAMA 259:539, 1988.

181. Kleber FX: Influence of captopril on life expectancy in chronic congestive heart failure. Herz 12:38, 1987.

182. Pfeffer J, Pfeffer MA, Braunwald E: Hemodymanic benefits and prolonged survival with long-term captopril therapy in rats with myocardial infarction and heart failure. Circulation 75(Suppl 1):149, 1987.

183. Pfeffer MA, Lamas GA, Vaughan DE, et al: Effect of captopril on progressive ventricular dilatation after anterior myocardial infarction. N Engl J Med 319:80, 1988.

184. Sharpe N, Murphy J, Smith H, et al: Treatment of patients with symptomless left ventricular dysfunction after myocardial infarction. Lancet 1:255, 1988.

185. Pfeffer MA, Braunwald E, Moyé LA, et al: Effect of captopril on mortality and morbidity in patients with left ventricular dysfunction after myocardial infarction. N Engl J Med 327:669, 1992.

186. Packer M, Davis B, Haumm P, et al: Effect of captopril on cause-specific mortality in patients with left-ventricular dysfunction after acute myocardial infarctions: Results of the SAVE trial. Circulation 86:4, 1992.

187. Rotmensch HH, Vlasses PH, Ferguson RK: Angiotensin-converting enzyme inhibitors. Med Clin North Am 72:399, 1988.

188. Frohlich ED, Cooper RA, Lewis EJ: Review of the overall experience of captopril in hypertension. Arch Intern Med 144:1441, 1984.

189. Irvin JD, Vian JM: Safety profiles of the angiotensin-converting enzyme inhibitors captopril and enalapril. Am J Med 81(Suppl 4C):46, 1986.

190. DiBianco R: Adverse reactions with angiotensin converting enzyme (ACE) inhibitors. Med Toxicol 1:122, 1986.

191. Omae T, Kawano Y, Yoshias K: Side effects and metabolic effects of converting enzyme inhibitors. Clin Exp Hypertens A9:635, 1987.

192. Brueggemeyer CD, Ramirez G: Onycholysis associated with captopril. Lancet 1:1352, 1984.

193. Abu-Handan D, Desai H, Sandheimer J, et al: Taste acuity and zinc metabolism in captopril-treated male hypertensive patients. Clin Res 35:437A, 1987.

194. Smit AJ, Hoorntje SJ, Donker AJM: Zinc deficiency during captopril treatment. Nephron 34:196, 1983.

195. Zumkley H, Bertram HP, Vetter H, et al: Zinc metabolism during captopril treatment. Horm Metab Res 17:256, 1985.

196. Edwards JR, Coulter DM, Beasly DMG, et al: Captopril: Four years of postmarketing surveillance of all patients in New Zealand. Br J Clin Pharmacol 23:529, 1987.

197. McNally EM: Cough due to captopril. West J Med 146:226, 1987.

198. Rossetto BJ: Side effects of captopril and enalapril. West J Med 146:102, 1987.

199. Sesoko S, Kaneko Y: Cough associated with the use of captopril. Arch Intern Med 145:1524, 1985.

200. Hood S, Nicholls MG, Gilchrist NL: Cough with angiotensin-converting enzyme inhibitors. N Z Med J 100:67, 1987.

201. Rush JE, Merrill DD: The safety and tolerability of lisinopril in clinical trials. J Cardiovasc Pharmacol 9(Suppl 3):99, 1987.

202. Coulter DM, Edwards JR: Cough associated with captopril and enalapril. Br Med J 294:1521, 1987.

203. Williams GH: Converting enzyme inhibitors in the treatment of hypertension. N Engl J Med 319:15, 1988.

204. Boulet LP, Milot J, Lampron N, et al: Pulmonary function and airway responsiveness during long-term therapy with captopril. JAMA 261:413, 1989.

205. Semple PF, Herd GW: Cough and wheeze caused by inhibitors of angiotensin-converting enzyme. N Engl J Med 314:61, 1986.

206. Nicholls MG, Gilchrist NL: Sulindac and cough induced by converting enzyme inhibitors. Lancet 1:872, 1987.

207. Jett GK: Captopril-induced angioedema. Ann Emerg Med 13:489, 1984.

208. Cooper RA: Captopril-associated neutropenia. Who is at risk? Arch Intern Med 143:659, 1983.

209. Jenkins AC, Dreslinski GR, Tadros SS, et al: Captopril in hypertension: Seven years later. J Cardiovasc Pharmacol 7:S96, 1985.

210. Case DB, Atlas SA, Mouradian JA, et al: Proteinuria during long-term therapy. JAMA 244:346, 1980.

211. The Captopril Collaborative Study Group: Does captopril cause renal damage in hypertensive patients? Lancet 1:988, 1982.

212. Brogden RN, Todd PA, Sorkin EM: Captopril: An update of its pharmacodynamic and pharmacokinetic properties, and therapeutic use in hypertension and congestive heart failure. Drugs 36:540, 1988.

213. Deyoung JP, Ruedy N, Wright JM: Antihypertensive efficacy of captopril given once, twice, and three times daily. Curr Ther Res 41:464, 1987.

214. Williams GH: Beyond blood pressure control. Effect of antihypertensive therapy on quality of life. Am J Hypertens 1:3635, 1988.

215. Tuck M: Management of hypertension in the patient with diabetes mellitus. Focus on the use of angiotensin converting enzyme inhibitors. Am J Hypertens 1:3845, 1988.

216. Ames RP: Antihypertensive drugs and lipid profiles. Am J Hypertens 1:421, 1988.

217. Kostis JB: Angiotensin converting enzyme inhibitors. II. Clinical use. Am Heart J 6:1591, 1988.

217a. Omoigui N, Dzau VJ: Differential effects of antihypertensive agents and human atherosclerosis. Am J Hypertens 6:30S, 1993.

218. van Gilst WH, deGraeff PA, Scholters E, et al: Potentiation of isosorbide dinitrate-induced coronary dilatation by captopril. J Cardiovasc Pharmacol 9:254, 1986.

219. Westlin W, Mullane K: Does captopril attenuate reperfusion-induced myocardial dysfunction by scavenging free radicals. Circulation 77(Suppl I):I30, 1988.

220. Ertl G, Kloner RA, Alexander W, et al: Limitation of experimental infarct size by an angiotensin converting enzyme inhibitor. Circulation 65:40, 1982.

221. Linz W, Scholkers BA, Han YF: Beneficial effects of the converting inhibitor ramipril in ischemic rat hearts. J Cardiovasc Pharmacol 8(Suppl 10):591, 1986.

222. Ferranini E, Buzzigoli G, Bonadonna R, et al: Insulin resistance in essential hypertension. N Engl J Med 317:350, 1989.

223. Pollare T, Lithell H, Berne C: A comparison of the effects of hydrochlorothiazide and captopril on glucose and lipid metabolism in patients with hypertension. N Engl J Med 321:868, 1989.

CHAPTER 78

Enalapril

James B. Young, M.D.

Enalapril was one of the first orally active angiotensin-converting enzyme (ACE) inhibitors to become commercially available. It has U.S. regulatory agency approval for treating hypertension and congestive heart failure, as well as for reducing mortality in patients with symptomatic left ventricular dysfunction and delaying development of overt heart failure in asymptomatic individuals with depressed ejection fraction. Enalapril is a prodrug requiring hydrolysis after absorption to form the active ACE inhibitor enalaprilat.[1] Enalapril is a prototype of the ACE inhibitor class and has been the source of much of our experimental and clinical experience with this drug class. Thus, it is an important compound in the study of ACE inhibitors.

PHARMACOLOGY

Enalapril, after hydrolysis to enalaprilat, inhibits ACE in animals and human subjects. Enalaprilat is an extremely potent inhibitor of ACE but is not absorbed from the gastrointestinal tract and is therefore suitable only for parenteral administration. The ester form (enalapril) is readily absorbed after oral administration and is then deesterified by hydrolysis in the liver into the active compound. Most data support the hypothesis that the beneficial hemodynamic effects of enalapril are caused by ACE inhibition and the consequent reduction in angiotensin II, which either directly or indirectly results in vessel dilatation and reduced peripheral vascular resistance.[2] Also, reduction of angiotensin II leads to diminished aldosterone secretion. Although the latter decrease is small, it results in minimal increases of serum potassium that sometimes are clinically significant and that can be beneficial or detrimental. Accumulating evidence suggests that tissue ACE, particularly in the vasculature, rather than circulating ACE, is the primary determinant of hemodynamic effects. Some studies suggest that the sympathetic system and changes in vasoactive kinins or prostanoids also have a role.[3]

Decreased total peripheral vascular resistance following administration of enalapril is not accompanied by any change in heart rate or cardiac output. The lack of reflex tachycardia is related to a resetting of the baroreflex rather than a reduction in its sensitivity.[4] Although enalapril is thought to lower blood pressure primarily through suppression of the renin-angiotensin-aldosterone system, enalapril is still antihypertensive in patients with low-renin hypertension. Age does not affect the bioavailability of this agent, nor does the presence of food in the alimentary tract.[5] After oral administration, enalapril reaches peak serum concentrations in approximately 1 hour. Based on urinary metabolic recovery, the extent of absorption of enalapril is approximately 60%.[6] Although this drug was antihypertensive in all races studied, the average response to enalapril monotherapy was smaller in black hypertensive patients (usually a low-renin, high-salt-modulator, hypertensive population) than in nonblack patients. A given dose shows a greater hypotensive effect and prolonged action in elderly subjects, apparently resulting from a decreased clearance rate and a reduced volume of distribution. Delayed bioactivation of enalapril to enalaprilat and altered protein or tissue binding of the latter may also, in part, account for these findings and for the fact that elderly hypertensive patients require smaller doses than middle-aged patients.[7]

In individuals with congestive heart failure, the onset of action is sometimes delayed, and its duration may be prolonged as a result of impaired liver function and decreased renal perfusion.[8] Therefore, in patients with concomitant liver and renal dysfunction, as well as in patients with severe congestive heart failure, initial doses of enalapril are often lowered to avoid the potential adverse effects (hypotension, azotemia, and hyperkalemia).[9]

PHARMACOKINETICS

Administered as the maleate salt, enalapril was designed to improve systemic bioavailability of the active ACE inhibitor enalaprilat. After oral dosing, enalapril reaches peak serum concentrations in approximately 1 hour, with approximately 60% of the dose absorbed. The peak serum concentration of enalaprilat occurs 3 to 4 hours after the oral dose of enalapril maleate. Excretion of enalapril is primarily renal, with approximately 94% of the dose recovered in the urine and feces as enalaprilat or enalapril. The principal component in urine is enalaprilat, which accounts for approximately 40% of the dose. No metabolites of enalapril, except enalaprilat, have been identified.[10] Enalaprilat undergoes polyphasic elimination with an initial elimination phase half-life of approximately 5 hours but a prolonged terminal phase of 30 to 35 hours, reflecting the strong binding of enalaprilat to plasma ACE.[11] Enalaprilat appears to penetrate most tissues (kidneys and vascular tissue in particular), although it is unclear whether the central nervous system is penetrated with therapeutic dosages.[12] Enalapril has been shown, however, to decrease circulating plasma catecholamine levels and the turnover of brain tissue catecholamines.[10, 13] Breast milk is minimally penetrated, but fetal transfer can be significant after administration to pregnant females.

Systemic clearance of enalaprilat is reduced by renal insufficiency. This metabolite may accumulate excessively in patients with moderate to severe renal dysfunction (creatinine clearance, <30 ml/min), and the dosage must be reduced in such patients. Both enalapril and enalaprilat are removed during hemodialysis. No clinically significant change in enalaprilat disposition occurs in patients with hepatic impairment, which would require routine dosage reduction.

EFFECTS ON PATHOPHYSIOLOGY

Most evidence suggests that enalapril reduces blood pressure by inhibiting the vasoconstrictor effects of angiotensin II in arterioles and arteries. However, enalapril also has a mild natriuretic effect, leading to a reduction in cardiac preload. Despite this reduction in preload and afterload, reflex tachycardia does not ensue. This is likely due to a resetting of the baroreceptor and baroreflex.[14] This resetting leads to a decrease in total peripheral vascular resistance and blood pressure, because there is little or no change in heart rate or cardiac output in patients with normal cardiac function.[15] However, in patients with decompensated heart failure, cardiac output increases substantially but with a decrease in heart rate.[16] Long-term treatment with enalapril improves arterial compliance and causes regression of left ventricular hypertrophy.[17] Many studies have confirmed the regression of left ventricular hypertrophy in hypertensive patients without deterioration in pump function.[18-20] Improved left ventricular function is manifested by increased stroke volume but decreased central venous pressure, right atrial pressure, pulmonary capillary wedge pressure, and left ventricular end-diastolic pressure. There is a sustained reduction in the rate-pressure product, usually without change in coronary sinus blood flow or myocardial oxygen consumption. There is evidence of reduced myocardial oxygen extraction and augmented coronary sinus oxygen saturation. Long-term enalapril treatment in patients with mild to moderate essential hypertension also has reduced the prevalence of ventricular and supraventricular ectopic beats, with multiform ectopic beats and couplets abolished in some studies.[21]

The effects of enalapril on renal function are complex and variable; they depend on numerous factors, such as sodium balance, intrinsic renal dysfunction, ancillary diseases (such as diabetes), and concomitant medications. Enalapril decreases renal vascular resistance and increases renal blood flow with no change in glomerular filtration rate.[15, 22, 23] It increases fractional sodium excretion and leads to a natriuretic and uricosuric effect with a tendency toward potassium retention.

Renal function is stabilized or improved in most patients with preexisting renal impairment, with only occasional cases of deterioration. This can be partly explained by the reduction of intrarenal vascular resistance and the loss of the constrictive effect of angiotensin on efferent arterioles. Dilatation of the efferent arteriole may help retard progression of damage to remaining nephrons. Diabetic patients show a marked decrease in urinary protein or albumin excretion during enalapril treatment regardless of blood pressure status. This antiproteinuric effect appears to be independent of any lowering of systemic blood pressure and may be related to changes in intrarenal hemodynamics that result in decreased glomerular filtration pressure.[24, 25] However, in the presence of bilateral renal artery stenoses or stenosis of the renal artery of a solitary kidney, wherein pressure barely can maintain glomerular filtration, relaxation of the efferent arterioles will further diminish the rate of filtration and can lead to acute renal insufficiency or dramatic hypotension, which is reversible only by discontinuation of drug treatment.

Enalapril and enalaprilat have been shown to cause dose-proportional inhibition of *in vitro* adenosine diphosphate–induced platelet aggregation. *Ex vivo* spontaneous platelet aggregation was decreased by approximately 15% (a statistically significant observation) after 4 weeks' treatment with enalapril in patients with hypertension (20 mg once daily).[26] Long-term treatment with enalapril has not demonstrated a potentially detrimental influence on the blood lipid profile, and some studies have shown an actual improvement in cholesterol level.[27-29]

THERAPEUTIC USE IN HYPERTENSION

Enalapril provides effective 24-hour blood pressure control whether administered once or twice daily. The drug does not alter the normal diurnal variation in blood pressure.[30] Titrated doses of enalapril, 5 to 40 mg/day as monotherapy, reduce mean systolic and diastolic blood pressure by 15% to 25% with adequate control (diastolic pressure <90 mmHg) in approximately 50% to 75% of patients, depending on the initial severity of hypertension.[3, 7, 31, 32] In approximately 30% of elderly white patients, a single 5-mg daily dose is sufficient, whereas black patients tend to be more resistant and require higher doses.[33, 34] Addition of a diuretic potentiates the effect of ACE inhibition and increases the rate of success to as much as 95%.[35] This combination of enalapril and a diuretic also abolishes the differences in the responsiveness of black and white patients. Furthermore, this combination attenuates some of the adverse metabolic alterations, such as hypokalemia, seen with thiazide monotherapy. There is no indication of attenuation of the antihypertensive response to enalapril during long-term therapy, and many patients have been treated for several years with this drug.[36, 37] The general lack of drug interactions with most other agents (with the exception of potassium-sparing diuretics and lithium) makes enalapril particularly suitable for patients with concomitant illnesses requiring long-term medication.[38]

USE IN SPECIAL POPULATIONS WITH HYPERTENSION
Diabetes

Because of the favorable effects of ACE inhibitors on metabolism in hypertensive diabetics, these drugs are now recommended by some as first-line therapeutic options over diuretics and β-blockers.[39] Global metabolic control of diabetes (blood pressure, insulin and glycosylated hemoglobin levels, and diabetic medication requirement) has generally remained stable or has actually improved during treatment with enalapril.[40, 41] These effects may be particularly important in patients with diabetic nephropathy and proteinuria.

Children and Pregnancy

All ACE inhibitors carry a warning for pregnancy categories C (first trimester) and D (second and third trimesters).[42] Published experience with enalapril is extremely limited in children and pediatric patients, and the drug is not presently indicated for use in children. In pediatric populations, ACE inhibition with captopril has been used successfully to treat severe hypertension secondary to such conditions as renal failure and collagen diseases, and one could expect enalapril to be as safe with the benefit of a parenterally administered dosage form in the form of enalaprilat.[43, 44] Miller et al.[45] reported their experience in 15 pediatric patients with secondary hypertension who received enalapril, 2.5 to 30 mg/day, for 5 to 12 months or longer. Blood pressure was adequately controlled in all patients, and renal function improved in seven. No clinically significant adverse effects were seen, although two patients developed mild proteinuria.

Concomitant Disorders

Hypertensive patients with gout, chronic obstructive airways disease, coronary insufficiency, renal failure, or collagen diseases seem to tolerate treatment with ACE inhibitors well. The hypertensive effect of enalapril was not blunted with the use of indomethacin and sulindac in arthritic patients.[46] Bronchial asthma and chronic bronchitis are not generally affected by ACE inhibition.[47] As a group, these compounds have been reported to cause cough.[42, 48–52]

Hall et al.[53] suggested that the vasodilator effects of enalapril observed in patients with severe heart failure could be counteracted by aspirin therapy. This is an important point, because aspirin is a frequent component of treatment protocols in which patients might concomitantly receive ACE inhibitors. Indeed, in the Survival and Ventricular Enlargement Trial,[54] 73% of patients received antiplatelet drugs, and 59% received aspirin. The Cooperative New Scandinavian Enalapril Survival Study II (CONSENSUS-II)[55] reported that 86% of patients received antiplatelet therapy; in the Prevention Trial of SOLVD,[56] 53% received aspirin therapy; and in the Treatment Trial of SOLVD,[57] 34% received such therapy. The study by Hall et al.[53] suggested that when enalapril was given before aspirin, significant decreases occurred in systemic vascular resistance, left ventricular filling pressure, and total pulmonary resistance with an increase in cardiac output. When given concomitantly with aspirin or the day after aspirin therapy, enalapril did not elicit statistically significant changes in these variables. It was speculated that in severe heart failure, aspirin-mediated inhibition of prostaglandin synthesis counteracted the systemic arterial vasodilation induced by ACE inhibition. The study, however, was small (18 patients) and limited by many factors, including the short period of observation following drug administration, absence of washout periods between study days, and data analysis after only acute administration of enalapril. It is important to point out that in the SOLVD Treatment[57] and Prevention[56] Trials, an equal distribution of antiplatelet (and presumably aspirin) therapy was reported in placebo and treatment cohorts, with beneficial effects apparent despite the fact that the patients were receiving these drugs. Definitive conclusions on concomitant aspirin or antiplatelet drug therapy in patient populations expected to receive enalapril or other ACE inhibitors await further insight. Some patients might benefit more if they were not receiving concomitant aspirin and ACE inhibitor therapy.

ENALAPRIL IN CONGESTIVE HEART FAILURE

Several large clinical trials in which mortality was the end point have used enalapril as the study drug (Table 78–1). These studies clearly demonstrate that enalapril is important for the treatment of symptomatic heart failure, usually in combination with diuretics and digitalis.[16, 57, 58] In fact, the combination of an ACE inhibitor, digoxin, and a diuretic seems most effective in preventing deterioration with increased congestive heart failure. In these patients, enalapril improves symptoms, increases survival, and decreases the frequency of hospitalization. The recommended starting dose is 2.5 mg administered once or twice daily, titrating up to a target dose of 10 mg twice daily in several weeks. The usual therapeutic dosing range is 5 to 20 mg daily, given as a single dose or two divided doses; most clinical studies have used twice-daily dosing.

It is important to distinguish between using this drug to treat hypertension and using it to treat heart failure. In hypertensive patients, the dose is generally titrated to an easily measured efficacy end point: blood pressure. On the other hand, dosing in patients with heart failure should resemble the protocols used in clinical trials to determine efficacy. Titration of the enalapril dose should be to a target level rather than to symptomatic improvement. Side effects or drug-related metabolic difficulties should prompt a decrease in dose. The most common target dose for enalapril has been 10 mg given twice daily.[16, 56–58] It can be argued that lower doses are likely to be efficacious; however, this is only a hypothesis, because higher doses have generally been used in the clinical trials. In symptomatic patients participating in the SOLVD Treatment Trial,[57] the mean daily prescribed dose of enalapril was 16.6 mg. Almost one half of the

Table 78–1. **Enalapril as Treatment for a Spectrum of Heart Failure**

Trial	No.	Risk Reduction %	
		NYHA Class	Mortality Rate
SOLVD Prevention[56]	4227	I–II	18%
SOLVD Treatment[57]	2569	II–III	6%
VHEFT-II[58]	804	III	28%
CONSENSUS-I[16]	253	IV	40%

Trial	Risk Reduction %		
	MI	CHF/HOSP	Developed CHF
SOLVD Prevention[56]	24%	36%	37%
SOLVD Treatment[57]	23%	36%	N/A
VHEFT-II[58]	N/A	N/A	N/A
CONSENSUS-I[16]	N/A	N/A	N/A

CHF, congestive heart failure; HOSP, hospitalizations; MI, myocardial infarction; NYHA, New York Heart Association.

randomized population received 10 mg twice daily, with only 1.8% of the patients in the enalapril group getting 2.5 mg once daily. After 1 year of follow-up, using 10 mg twice daily as the target dose, 80% of the enalapril group were receiving at least 75% of the prescribed dose. After 3 years, almost 70% were receiving at least three quarters of the prescribed enalapril dose. In patients with asymptomatic left ventricular dysfunction studied in the SOLVD Prevention Trial,[56] the mean daily dose of enalapril was 16.7 mg; in CONSENSUS,[16] it was 18.4 mg.

In CONSENSUS,[16] enalapril was shown to reduce mortality in New York Heart Association (NYHA) functional class IV patients by 40% at the end of 6 months. The NYHA classification also improved in the enalapril group, together with a reduction in heart size and requirement for additional medications to treat heart failure.

In a comparison study of hydralazine-isosorbide dinitrate with enalapril in the treatment of chronic congestive heart failure (VHEFT-II),[58] the mortality rate after 2 years was significantly lower in the enalapril arm (18%) than in the hydralazine-isosorbide dinitrate arm (25%) ($p = .016$, reduction in mortality = 28%). In this clinical trial, the lower mortality rate in the enalapril arm was due to a reduction in the incidence of sudden death, and this beneficial effect was more prominent in patients with less severe symptoms (NYHA class I or II).[58] This observation is different from that made in CONSENSUS[16] and SOLVD,[56, 57] which demonstrated reduction in heart failure–related deaths but no major impact on presumed arrhythmic deaths.

In the SOLVD Treatment Trial[57] (symptomatic patients), addition of enalapril to conventional therapy also significantly reduced mortality and hospitalization for heart failure in patients with chronic congestive failure and ejection fractions less than 35%. Approximately 90% of the patients were in NYHA functional classes II and III. As mentioned, the largest reduction occurred in deaths attributed to progressive heart failure, with little apparent effect of treatment on deaths classified as due to arrhythmia without pump failure. Also, fewer patients were hospitalized for worsening heart failure.

In the SOLVD Prevention Trial,[56] enalapril was shown to delay significant symptomatic heart failure in patients with left ventricular dysfunction who did not yet have symptoms or were minimally symptomatic. These patients also had substantial left ventricular dysfunction with ejection fractions of less than 35%. The majority of patients, however, were in NYHA functional class I. The SOLVD investigators described a trend toward fewer cardiovascular deaths in patients taking enalapril, but this was not statistically significant. The most important observation in this study was that the risk of symptomatic congestive heart failure was reduced by 37% in patients taking enalapril compared with patients receiving placebo. In addition, there was a 36% reduction in risk of hospitalization in patients taking enalapril.

The SOLVD Trials also demonstrated substantial antiischemic myocardial protective effects of enalapril when used in patients with left ventricular dysfunction.[59] Indeed, some of the principal effects of enalapril therapy were reported to be on the incidence of major ischemic events. In SOLVD, the 1-year mortality rate among the 650 patients experiencing acute myocardial infarction during the study was nearly eight times that seen in the 6147 patients not having this difficulty (mortality rate, 55.4% versus 7.3%; $p < .001$). After excluding deaths occurring within 7 days of a myocardial infarction, myocardial infarction still was associated with a 3.5-fold increase in mortality rate. Furthermore, myocardial infarction was accompanied by more than a doubling of the rate of hospital admissions for heart failure (20.5% versus 8.6%). Enalapril reduced the incidence of myocardial infarction in the combined SOLVD studies by 23%, hospitalization for unstable angina pectoris by 20%, and the combined end point of cardiac death, nonfatal myocardial infarction, or hospital admission for unstable angina pectoris by 22%. All observations were highly statistically significant.

A second clinical trial, CONSENSUS-II,[55] was also designed to evaluate effects of enalapril after myocardial infarction. In this trial, intravenous enalaprilat administration was begun within 24 hours of an acute myocardial infarction and segued rapidly to orally administered enalapril. Left ventricular dysfunction was not, however, an entry criterion in CONSENSUS-II,[55] as it was in SOLVD,[56, 57] and follow-up lasted only 6 months. No statistically significant effect on mortality or reinfarction rate was observed. However, fewer patients required change of therapy because of heart failure in the enalapril group (27% versus 30%; $p < .006$). Comparing the findings of CONSENSUS-II with those of SOLVD, it becomes important to recall that ACE inhibitor therapy affected mortality and morbidity in asymptomatic patients with left ventricular dysfunction only after long-term (>6 months) enalapril therapy. Longer follow-up of the CONSENSUS-II population, which had less ventricular dysfunction than the SOLVD population, may have demonstrated reduced mortality and/or ischemic events. Observations made in these clinical trials suggest that long-term treatment is required to realize the benefits of enalapril with regard to antiischemic events in patients with heart failure. This point should be contrasted with trials of β-blockers administered after infarction, which demonstrated earlier beneficial impact. β-Blockers, in contrast with ACE inhibitors, probably have a major impact on arrhythmias and sudden death after infarction and, therefore, demonstrate efficacy earlier.

Laboratory and experimental evidence point to many mechanisms that may be important to understanding the ability of ACE inhibitors in general and enalapril in particular to reduce the risk of the adverse events of coronary heart disease. These mechanisms include the antiproliferative action of ACE inhibitors on myocardium and the vascular wall, hemodynamic effects (lowering of blood pressure in particular), antiatherogenic actions, neurohormonal

Table 78–2. **Side Effects Reported in Controlled Clinical Trials of Enalapril for Hypertension**[42]

Side Effects	% Enalapril (n = 2314)	% Placebo (n = 230)
Orthostatic effects	1.2 (<0.1)*	0.0
Headache	5.2 (0.3)	9.1
Dizziness	4.3 (0.4)	4.3
Cough	1.3 (0.1)	0.9
Skin rash	1.4 (0.4)	0.4

*Number in parentheses is percentage of patients discontinuing drug because of side effects.

attenuation, and certain genetic issues. Experimental data and clinical trial information will likely shed greater insight on this observation.

Collective data from the CONSENSUS, VHEFT-II, and two SOLVD clinical trials show, then, that enalapril can help a broad range of patients with left ventricular dysfunction regardless of cause, use of other drugs, gender, age, and presence or severity of symptoms.

ADVERSE REACTIONS

Enalapril is well tolerated. In clinical trials, discontinuation of therapy was required in 3.3% of the patients with hypertension (Table 78–2) and in 5.7% of the patients with heart failure (Table 78–3). The frequency of adverse experiences was not related to total daily dosage within usual ranges. In patients with hypertension, the overall percentage of patients treated with enalapril reporting adverse experiences was often comparable with the percentages of those receiving placebo. Hypotension, dizziness, and headache are the most frequently reported side effects. One peculiar and relatively rare reaction is angioedema.[42, 56, 57]

ACE inhibitors have been associated with chronic cough and wheezing.[48–51] In theory, these agents potentiate bradykinin, which is known to have a bronchoconstrictor effect, and they increase prostaglandin production, leading to an increased pulmonary inflammatory response in susceptible individuals.[48, 49] In addition, evidence suggests that sulindac can abolish ACE inhibitor–induced cough.[50, 51]

A question has been raised about the association of solid tumors, particularly gastrointestinal tract malignancy, to enalapril therapy.[56, 57] In the SOLVD trials,[56, 57] there were gastrointestinal tract malignancies

in 3410 patients receiving placebo (0.0185 incidence) and 80 malignancies occurring in 3396 patients receiving enalapril (0.0236 incidence). In the Prevention Trial,[56] there were 40 malignancies in the placebo group and 42 in the enalapril group; the Treatment Trial[57] showed 23 gastrointestinal cancers in the placebo group and 38 in the enalapril-treated group. It is believed that the small and insignificant difference in the sum of nonfatal cancers of the gastrointestinal tract was due to chance because of the multiplicity of sites involved and the large number of comparisons made. The frequency of cancer of the gastrointestinal system did not increase proportionately with time of enalapril exposure. If there was a causal relationship between enalapril therapy and neoplasia, one would expect a higher incidence of malignancy with higher drug doses and longer drug exposure.

When hypertension is due to renal artery stenosis and patients receive enalapril, renal function may deteriorate secondary to decreased renal perfusion.[23] Because some patients with heart failure have renal perfusion dependent on high renin and angiotensin levels, these patients may also be at risk for an increase in blood urea nitrogen and creatinine levels, reflecting deterioration of renal function.[60] Indeed, in a very early heart failure trial that compared 150 mg daily of captopril to very high doses (40 mg daily) of enalapril (for heart failure),[61, 62] adverse effects such as hypotension, reduced creatinine clearance, and hyperkalemia were observed more frequently with enalapril.[61–65] This observation concerned early investigators using ACE inhibitor therapy in heart failure; however, experience indicates that lower doses of enalapril (5 to 20 mg daily) are safe, well-tolerated, and effect the desired beneficial end points.[56, 57] Indeed, in the combined SOLVD trials, there was a 0.1% incidence of renal dysfunction in patients receiving placebo and a 0.2% incidence in those receiving enalapril. This was an insignificant difference. Of particular concern would be adverse effects in relatively asymptomatic patients with left ventricular dysfunction. Focusing on the subset of patients in the SOLVD Prevention Trial, the incidence of renal dysfunction was 0.2% in enalapril-treated patients versus 0.0% in those individuals receiving placebo (p <.031). Though this difference was statistically significant, the low incidence of renal dysfunction in this study emphasizes the fact that lower doses of enalapril are safe and generally well tolerated. It is, furthermore, important to reem-

Table 78–3. **SOLVD Combined Trial (n = 6797): Side Effects Reported at Any Postrandomization Visit**

Side Effects	% Placebo	% Enalapril	Difference	Two-sided p Value
Dizziness/fainting	43.4	50.2	+6.8	<.001
Renal dysfunction	0.1	0.2	+0.1	NS
Taste disturbance	13.6	11.7	−1.8	<.028
Cough	28.8	35.0	+6.2	<.001
Angioneurotic edema	2.3	2.3	0.0	NS

NS, not significant.
Data from references 58 and 59.

phasize the fact that we can often characterize individuals who are at risk of hypotension or renal insufficiency during ACE inhibitor therapy. Patients with severe left ventricular dysfunction and congestive heart failure who have low serum sodium, who have been aggressively diuresed, or who are receiving multiple diuretics, may be at higher risk. Care should be used whenever ACE inhibitors are begun in these individuals, and low doses should be considered. One technique is to start enalapril at 2.5 mg daily, with the first dose given at bedtime. Patients can then be asked to report any symptoms that occur in the morning after rising. If excessive dizziness or orthostatic complaints are absent, 2.5 mg twice daily is usually well tolerated. Repeat clinic visits can be scheduled for 1 or 2 weeks, and biochemical safety parameters (electrolytes, blood urea nitrogen, serum creatinine) can be reevaluated and the dose accelerated to the target of 10 mg twice daily.

Medications taken to prevent difficulties from hypertension or left ventricular dysfunction must not compromise quality of life. A controversial study compared captopril with enalapril in a hypertensive population.[64, 65] Conclusions from this trial suggested that though the two ACE inhibitors were indistinguishable in terms of clinical efficacy and safety parameters, enalapril had a different impact on quality of life measurements that had been calibrated with life events. It was suggested that captopril is associated with more favorable change in overall quality of life than enalapril. It has been subsequently pointed out,[66-69] however, that this trial was probably flawed in terms of methodologic design, using assessment instruments that had been considerably amended and analyzed in a controversial fashion. Studies of enalapril mostly have shown no detriment to measures of quality of life, and significant improvements from baseline values occasionally have been observed.[70-73] Still, this subject is important, because attenuation of angiotensin II (as would occur with ACE inhibitors) may improve cognitive function and may be anxiolytic.[65]

SOCIOECONOMIC CONSIDERATIONS

As our population continues to age, more individuals are surviving life-threatening myocardial infarctions through early and more effective intervention. Furthermore, long-standing hypertensive heart disease is more common in older patients. Ventricular dysfunction and then symptomatic heart failure follow in many of these patients. Indeed, congestive heart failure is on the increase; it is now the number one cause of hospital admissions for patients older than 65 years. Because of the decrement in hospitalizations effected by enalapril and other ACE inhibitors, as well as the likely concomitant reduction in medications taken, reduced number of fatal and nonfatal ischemic events, and reduced risk of heart failure, it is important to consider the possible socioeconomic impact of the strategies outlined in the clinical trials

reviewed.[16, 56-58] Although one might expect all ACE inhibitors to share these effects, clinical trials establishing dosages necessary for reduction in mortality, major ischemic events, progression to clinically manifested heart failure, and hospitalizations must be undertaken with all new agents. Only carefully designed, well-executed clinical trials will accurately depict efficacy and side effect profiles. When this is accomplished, comparisons can be made within the ACE inhibitor group.

Acknowledgment

The author would like to thank Clyde James, R.Ph., and Marlane Kayfes for their editorial and secretarial expertise and assistance.

REFERENCES

1. Patchett AA, Harris E, Tristam EW, et al: A new class of angiotensin converting enzyme inhibitors. Nature 288:280, 1980.
2. Todd PA, Goa KL: Enalapril: A reappraisal of its pharmacology and therapeutic use in hypertension. Drugs 43(3):346, 1992.
3. Todd PA, Heel RC: Enalapril: A review of its pharmacodynamic and pharmacokinetic properties and therapeutic use in hypertension and congestive heart failure. Drugs 31:198, 1986.
4. Ajayi AA, Campbell BC, Howie CA: Acute and chronic effects of enalapril and MK521 on reflex control and heart rate in normotensive subjects. Br J Clin Pharmacol 17:602, 1984.
5. Brunner DB, Desponds G, Biollaz J, et al: Effect of a new angiotensin converting enzyme inhibitor MK-421 and its lysine analogue on the components of the renin system in healthy subjects. Br J Clin Pharmacol 11:461, 1981.
6. Ulm EH, Hichens M, Gomez HJ, et al: Enalapril maleate and a lysine analogue (MK-521): Disposition in man. Br J Clin Pharmacol 14:357, 1987.
7. Gavras H: A multicenter trial of enalapril in the treatment of essential hypertension. Am J Med 81:28, 1986.
8. Schwartz JB, Taylor A, Abernethy D, et al: Pharmacokinetics and pharmacodynamics of enalapril in patients with congestive heart failure and patients with hypertension. J Cardiovasc Pharmacol 7:767, 1985.
9. Kjekshus J, Swedberg K: Tolerability of enalapril in congestive heart failure. Am J Cardiol 62:67A, 1988.
10. de Leeuw PW, Birkenhäger WH: Changes in the pathophysiologic profile of blood pressure determinants during short-term enalapril administration. J Cardiovasc Pharmacol 8(Suppl 1):S26, 1986.
11. Donnelly R, Meredith PA, Elliott HL, et al: Kinetic-dynamic relations and individual responses to enalapril. Hypertension 15:301, 1990.
12. Unger T, Ganten D, Lang RE: Pharmacology of converting enzyme inhibitors: New aspects. Clin Exp Hypertens A5:1333, 1983.
13. Kohlmann O Jr, Bresnahn M, Gavras H: Central and peripheral indices of sympathetic activity after blood pressure lowering with enalapril (MK-421) or hydrazine in normotensive rats. Hypertension 6(Suppl 1):1, 1984.
14. Rotmensch HH, Vlasses PH, Ferguson RK: Angiotensin-converting enzyme inhibitors. Med Clin North Am 72:399, 1988.
15. Dupont AG, Vanderniepen P, Bossuyt AM, et al: Effect of enalapril on ambulatory blood pressure renal hemodynamics and cardiac function in essential hypertension. Acta Cardiologica 41:353, 1986.
16. The Consensus Trial Study Group: Effects of enalapril on mortality in severe congestive heart failure. Results of the Cooperative North Scandinavian Enalapril Survival Study (consensus). N Engl J Med 316(23):1429, 1987.
17. Safar M, Cournot P, Duchier J: Evaluation de l'efficacite d'une association cicletanine-enalapril chez des patients hypertendus.

Archives des Maladies du Coeur et de Vaisseaux 1989;82:119–124.

18. Fouad FM, Tarazi RC: Restoration of cardiac function and structure by converting enzyme inhibition possibilities and limitations of long-term treatment in hypertension and heart failure. J Cardiovasc Pharmacol 8(Suppl 1):S53, 1986.

19. Gosse P, Roudaut R, Herrero G, et al: Beta-blockers vs angiotensin converting enzyme inhibitors in hypertension: Effects on left ventricular hypertrophy. J Cardiovasc Pharmacol 16(Suppl 5):145, 1990.

20. Sampson MJ, Chambers JB, Sprigings DC, et al: Regression of left ventricular hypertrophy with 1 year of antihypertensive treatment in type 1 diabetic patients with early nephropathy. Diabet Med 8:106, 1991.

21. Melina D, Guerrera G, Colivicchi F, et al: Enalapril monotherapy in mild hypertensive heart disease: A 12-month clinical experience. Curr Ther Res 49:616, 1991.

22. Valvo E, Gammaro L, Bedogna V, et al: Systemic and renal hemodynamic changes after two-month treatment with enalapril in patients with essential hypertension. Int J Clin Pharmacol Ther Toxicol 25:656, 1987.

23. Hollenberg NK: Angiotensin-converting enzyme inhibition and renal protection. Arch Intern Med 153:2526, 1993.

24. Moore MP, Elliott TW, Nicholls MG: Hormonal and metabolic effects of enalapril treatment in hypertensive subjects with NIDDM. Diabetes Care 11:397, 1988.

25. Morelli E, Loon N, Meyer T, et al: Effects of converting-enzyme inhibition on barrier function in diabetic glomerulopathy. Diabetes 39:76, 1990.

26. Lindstrom E, Ajlner J, Axelsson KL, et al: Enalapril inhibits platelet aggregation in vitro and during long-term treatment in patients with primary hypertension. Curr Ther Res 47:665, 1990.

27. Leren P, Foss PO, Nordvik B, et al: The effect of enalapril and timolol on blood lipids: A randomized multicenter hypertension study in general practice in Norway. Acta Med Scand 223:321, 1988.

28. Perani G, Muggia C, Martignoni A, et al: Increase in plasma HDL-cholesterol in hypertensive patients treated with enalapril. Clin Ther 9:5, 1987.

29. Sasaki J, Arakawa K: Effects of enalapril on serum lipoproteins in mild essential hypertension. Clin Ther 11:38, 1989.

30. Gadsboll N, Damkjaer-Nielsen MD, Giese J, et al: Diurnal monitoring of blood pressure and the renin-angiotensin system in hypertensive patients on long-term angiotensin converting enzyme inhibition. J Hypertens 8:733, 1990.

31. Davies RO, Irvin JD, Kramsch DK, et al: Enalapril worldwide experience. Am J Med 77:23, 1984.

32. Thind GS, Johnson A, Bhatnagar D, et al: A parallel study of enalapril and captopril and 1 year of experience with enalapril treatment in moderate-to-severe essential hypertension. Am Heart J 109:852, 1985.

33. Mulinari R, Gavaras I, Gavras H: Efficacy and tolerability of enalapril monotherapy in mild-to-moderate essential hypertension in older patients compared to younger patients. Clin Ther 9:678, 1987.

34. Weinberger MH: Blood pressure and metabolic responses to hydrochlorothiazide, captopril, and the combination in black and white mild-to-moderate hypertensive patients. J Cardiovasc Pharmacol 7:S52, 1985.

35. Vidt DG (for the Multiclinic Study Group): A controlled multiclinic study to compare the antihypertensive effects of MK-421, hydrochlorothiazide, and MK-421 combined with hydrochlorothiazide in patients with mild-to-moderate essential hypertensive patients. J Cardiovasc Pharmacol 7:S52, 1985.

36. Higaki J, Mikami H, Otsuka A, et al: Effect of two years of enalapril treatment on the quality of life of elderly patients with essential hypertension complicated by other diseases. Curr Ther Res 47:620, 1990.

37. Reams GP, Bauer JH: Long term effects of enalapril monotherapy and enalapril/hydrochlorothiazide combination therapy on blood pressure, renal function, and body fluid composition. J Clin Hypertens 1:55, 1986.

38. Shionoiri H: Pharmacokinetic drug interactions with ACE inhibitors [review]. Clin Pharmacokinet 25:20, 1993.

39. Joseph JC, Schuna AA: Management of hypertension in the diabetic patient [review]. Clin Pharmacy 9:864–873, 1990.

40. Cheng IKP, Ma JTC, Yeh GR, et al: Comparison of captopril and enalapril in the treatment of hypertension in patients with non-insulin dependent diabetes mellitus and nephropathy. Int Urol Nephrol 22:295, 1990.

41. Panzalis MMC, Daccordi HA, Martello MA, et al: Effect of an angiotensin converting enzyme inhibitor (enalapril) on the glycemia of diabetic patients. Diabetes 40(Suppl 1):506A, 1991.

42. Physicians' Desk Reference, 46th ed. Montvale, NY: Medical Economics Company, 1992, pp 1565–1567.

43. Sigstrom L, Aurell M, Jodal U: Angiotensin converting enzyme inhibitor treatment of hypertension in infancy and childhood. Scand J Urol Nephrol 79(Suppl 1):107, 1984.

44. Mirkin BL, Newman TJ: Efficacy and safety of captopril in the treatment of severe childhood hypertension. Report of the International Collaborative Study Group. Pediatrics 75:1091, 1985.

45. Miller K, Atkin B, Rodel Jr PV, et al: Enalapril: A well tolerated and efficacious agent for the pediatric hypertensive patient. J Cardiovasc Pharmacol 10(Suppl 7):S154, 1987.

46. Gomez HJ, Cicero S, Busnardo I: Enalapril: A review of human pharmacology. Drugs 30(Suppl 1):13, 1985.

47. Bertoli L, Lo Cicero S, Busnardo I: Treatment of essential hypertension with captopril in patients with chronic obstructive pulmonary diseases. J Hypertens 3:S153, 1985.

48. Bucknall CE, Neilly JB, Carter R, et al: Bronchial hyperreactivity in patients who cough after receiving angiotensin converting enzyme inhibitors. Br Med J 296:86, 1988.

49. Mue S, Tamura G, Yamauchi K, et al: Bronchial responses to enalapril in asthmatic, hypertensive patients. Clin Ther 12:335, 1990.

50. McEwan JR, Choudry N, Street R, et al: The effect of sulindac on the abnormal cough reflex. J Pharmacol Exp Ther 255:161, 1990.

51. Nicholls MG, Gilchrist NL: Sulindac and cough induced by converting enzyme inhibitors. Lancet 1:872, 1987.

52. Hallwright GP, Maling TB, Town GI: Enalapril and cough: A case report. N Z Med J 99:66, 1986.

53. Hall D, Zeitler H, Rudolph W: Counteraction of the vasodilator effects of enalapril by aspirin in severe heart failure. J Am Coll Cardiol 20:1549, 1992.

54. Pfeffer MA, Braunwald E, Moye LA, et al: Effect of captopril on mortality and morbidity in patients with left ventricular dysfunction after myocardial infarction—results of the Survival and Ventricular Enlargement (SAVE) Trial. N Engl J Med 327:669, 1992.

55. Swedberg K, Held P, Kjekshus J, et al: Effects of the early administration of enalapril on mortality in patients with acute myocardial infarction—results of the Cooperative New Scandinavian Enalapril Survival Study II (CONSENSUS-II). N Engl J Med 327:678, 1992.

56. The SOLVD Investigators: Effect of enalapril on mortality and the development of heart failure in asymptomatic patients with reduced left ventricular ejection fractions. N Engl J Med 327:685, 1992.

57. The SOLVD Investigators: Effect of enalapril on survival in patients with reduced left ventricular ejection fractions and congestive heart failure. N Engl J Med 325:293, 1991.

58. Cohn JN, Johnson G, Ziesche S, et al: A comparison of enalapril with hydralazine-isosorbide dinitrate in the treatment of chronic congestive heart failure. N Engl J Med 325:303, 1991.

59. Yusuf S, Pepine CJ, Garces C, et al: Effect of enalapril on myocardial infarction and unstable angina in patients with low ejection fractions. Lancet 340:1173, 1992.

60. Suki WN: Renal hemodynamic consequences of angiotensin-converting enzyme inhibition in congestive heart failure. Arch Intern Med 149:669, 1989.

61. Feld H, Greenberg MA: Inhibition of angiotensin-converting enzyme in congestive heart failure [letter]. N Engl J Med 316:879, 1987.

62. Jaffe ME: Inhibition of angiotensin-converting enzyme in congestive heart failure [letter]. N Engl J Med 316:879, 1987.

63. Packer M, Lee WH, Yushak M, et al: Comparison of captopril and enalapril in patients with severe chronic heart failure. N Engl J Med 315:847, 1986.

64. Testa MA, Anderson RB, Nackley JF, et al: And the quality-of-life hypertension study group: Quality of life and antihypertensive therapy in men. A comparison of captopril with enalapril. N Engl J Med 328:907, 1993.
65. Oparil S: Antihypertensive therapy—efficacy and quality of life [editorial]. N Engl J Med 328:959, 1993.
66. Santanello NC, Guess H, Heyse JF: Captopril, enalapril, and quality of life [letter]. N Engl J Med 329:505, 1993.
67. Kaplan NM: Captopril, enalapril, and quality of life [letter]. N Engl J Med 329:505, 1993.
68. Waud DR: Captopril, enalapril, and quality of life [letter]. N Engl J Med 329:505, 1993.
69. Fletcher A, Ware JE, Testa MA, et al: Captopril, enalapril, and quality of life [letter]. N Engl J Med 329:505, 1993.
70. Steiner SS, Friedhoff AJ, Wilson BL, et al: Antihypertensive therapy and quality of life: A comparison of atenolol, captopril, enalapril and propranolol. J Hum Hypertens 4:217, 1990.
71. Omvik P, Thaulow E, Herland OB, et al: Double-blind, parallel, comparative study on quality of life during treatment with amlodipine or enalapril in mild or moderate hypertensive patients: A multi-centre study. J Hypertens 11:103, 1993.
72. The Treatment of Mild Hypertension Research Group: The treatment of mild hypertension study: A randomized, placebo-controlled trial of a nutritional-hygienic regimen along with various drug monotherapies. Arch Intern Med 151:1413, 1991.
73. Dahlof C, Dimenas E: General well-being during treatment with different ACE-inhibitors: Two double-blind, placebo-controlled, cross-over studies in healthy volunteers. Eur J Clin Pharmacol 43:375, 1992.

CHAPTER 79

Lisinopril*

John B. Kostis, M.D., and Daniel M. Shindler, M.D.

Lisinopril is the third angiotensin-converting enzyme (ACE) inhibitor to be used in clinical practice. Among the three ACE inhibitors available, lisinopril is the only one that is not a prodrug and does not have a sulfhydryl in its chemical structure.[1-5] The impetus for the development of ACE inhibitors was the discovery of natural peptides in the venom of the Brazilian snake *Bothrops jararaca* that inhibited kininase II and the realization that kininase II and the enzyme that converts angiotensin I to angiotensin II were the same.[6, 7] Cushman et al.[8] synthesized captopril, the first orally active ACE inhibitor with a sulfhydryl moiety acting as a zinc ligand. Because the sulfhydryl moiety (SH) seems to be responsible for some of the side effects of captopril, especially skin and taste disturbances, and contributes to its short half-life owing to easy oxidation and disulfide reactions, ACE inhibitors without SH were synthesized.[1] Enalapril, the second orally active ACE inhibitor to be marketed, has a carboxyl group as a zinc ligand. It is more potent than captopril because of additional binding sites to the enzyme (ACE), and it has a longer duration of action (Fig. 79–1). However, enalaprilat, the active compound of enalapril, is not absorbed from the gastrointestinal tract. For this reason, it is administered as its ethyl ester (enalapril) and must be bioactivated (hydrolyzed) primarily in the liver before it becomes active; it is therefore a prodrug. This need for bioactivation may result in increased interpatient variability and delayed bioactivation when disease (e.g., cirrhosis) or decreased hepatic blood flow (e.g., severe congestive heart failure [CHF]) is present.[9-11] The lysine analogue of enalapril, lisinopril, is easily absorbed and can be administered as the unesterified (diacid) form and therefore does not require bioactivation after absorption.

BIOCHEMISTRY

Lisinopril (1-[N²-[(s)-1-carboxy-3-phenylpropyl]-L-lysyl]-L) proline dihydrate was a product of an effort to synthesize ACE inhibitors not containing sulfhydryl.[1] It is a competitive inhibitor of purified ACE derived from rabbit lung.[12] The carboxyl (carbonyl) group serves as the zinc ligand to ACE, while an additional six binding sites attach lisinopril to the enzyme (see Fig. 79–1).

PHARMACOKINETICS

After oral administration, lisinopril is absorbed unchanged. Its bioavailability is about 25% and its oral absorption is 30% or greater. Maximum concentrations occur at 4 to 6 hours.[13-16] It is not bound to plasma proteins other than ACE and is not metabolized.[4] It is excreted unchanged in the urine.

The effective accumulation half-life is 12.6 hours, longer than that of captopril and slightly longer than that of enalapril. A steady-state concentration is achieved in 2 to 3 days. The elimination half-life is long, exceeding 30 hours, and shows a polyphasic relationship between plasma concentration and time, with a prolonged terminal phase that may result from binding of lisinopril to ACE (Fig. 79–2).[17, 18] The absorption of lisinopril, a rather hydrophilic compound,[19] is slower than that of enalapril. Its absorption is not influenced by the presence of food.[15]

A relationship between creatinine clearance and lisinopril clearance has been observed.[20] As expected, the clearance of lisinopril is diminished when renal function is impaired; the same is true in renal insufficiency, advanced age, and severe CHF.[20-24] In these situations, lower doses should be used.

PHARMACODYNAMICS

ACE inhibitors may exert their effects by several mechanisms, including the inhibition of the formation

*Supported in part by the John G. Detwiler Fund.

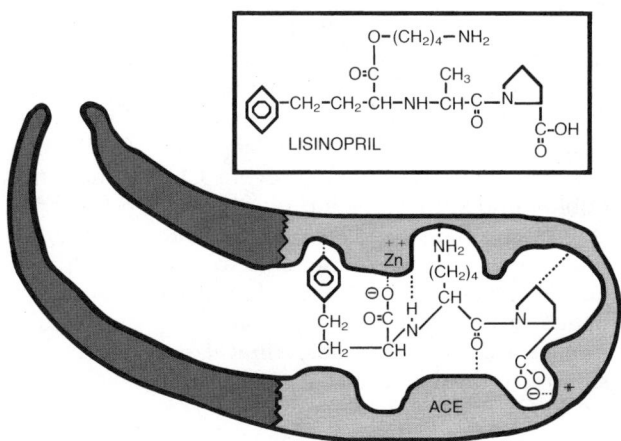

Figure 79–1. Lisinopril: chemical structure and interaction with ACE.

of angiotensin II in plasma and a variety of tissues including the heart, kidneys, and blood vessels; the prevention of the degradation of bradykinin; and the formation of prostaglandins.[25–39] Thus, the majority of the pharmacodynamic effects of lisinopril may be predicted from the known effects of angiotensin II and bradykinin. A positive relationship exists between lisinopril concentration, or the log of lisinopril concentration, and inhibition of circulating ACE, or the ratio of angiotensin I to angiotensin II.[13, 40] Lisinopril is more potent than captopril (and slightly more than enalapril) when potency is studied in vitro by measuring the dissociation half-lives of the enzyme-inhibitor complex.[17, 41] Single oral doses of lisinopril (5 to 10 mg) result in maximum ACE inhibition, decreased levels of angiotensin II, increased renin activity, increased levels of angiotensin I, decreased plasma aldosterone levels, and antagonism of the pressor response to angiotensin I but not to angiotensin II.[40, 42–48] These effects become apparent 2 to 3 hours after oral administration, reach a maximum at approximately 6 hours, and persist for as long as 24 hours, depending on the dose administered.[49]

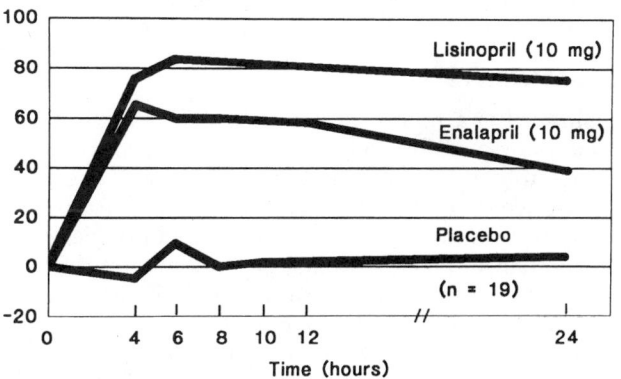

Figure 79–2. Duration of inhibition of ACE activity by lisinopril and enalapril. (From Ajayi AA, Campbell BC, Keiman AW, et al: Pharmacodynamics and population pharmacokinetics of enalapril and lisinopril. Int J Clin Pharmacol Res 5:419, 1985, with permission of Bioscience Ediprint Inc.)

The clinical effects of lisinopril depend on the state of activation of the renin-angiotensin system and the underlying hemodynamics in normal subjects. Lisinopril causes arteriolar, venous, and arterial dilatation resulting in systolic and diastolic blood pressure decrements of about 15%.[47–50] Reflex tachycardia does not occur, probably because of vagal stimulation and carotid arterial dilation resulting from improved compliance and resetting of the baroreceptors without loss of sensitivity.[47, 48, 51, 52] Cardiac output, stroke volume, and indices of left ventricular function are not altered significantly.[53] Renal plasma flow may increase while the glomerular filtration rate remains unchanged because of decreases in filtration fraction and filtration pressure.[54–57] In patients with essential hypertension, the effects are similar to those previously described, with a decrease in systemic resistance and blood pressure, a decrease in renal vascular resistance, and an increase in renal plasma flow.[44, 47, 53, 58, 59]

In patients with congestive heart failure, more pronounced changes in blood pressure may be observed.[60–63] This is accompanied by increased cardiac output and lower filling pressures, indicating improved left ventricular function. Systemic resistance is decreased but there are no marked changes in heart rate.

CLINICAL USE

Although many new indications for ACE inhibitors are evolving, the approved indications and the major clinical use are in the treatment of hypertension and CHF.[5, 64]

Use in Hypertension

Lisinopril is useful in the treatment of hypertension either as monotherapy or in combination with diuretics. As monotherapy, lisinopril, 5 to 20 mg daily, has been found to lower blood pressure effectively in both open-label studies and double-blind, placebo-controlled trials. Blood pressure is lowered for up to 24 hours after the dose when 10 or 20 mg is given. Doses higher than 20 mg daily usually do not result in added benefit.[65–67] The antihypertensive effects have been documented to persist for up to 6 months without evidence of tachyphylaxis. Although most studies have been performed in patients with essential hypertension, lisinopril has also been found useful in renal impairment as well as in renovascular hypertension.[22, 40, 68, 69]

The addition of thiazide diuretics to fixed-dose lisinopril resulted in further lowering of blood pressure in several well-conducted studies. In addition, the percentage of patients who responded with appropriate blood pressure reduction (diastolic blood pressure of less than 85 or 10 mmHg change) was higher with the combination than with either drug alone. In one study, nonblack patients responded better to lisinopril monotherapy than black patients, while in another, no difference was observed.[70] Both patient groups responded well to combination therapy.[71] Hypokalemia from hydrochlorothiazide was mitigated by the addition of lisinopril. In these studies, lisinopril was more efficacious than hydrochlorothiazide, and their combination was superior to either therapy alone.[65, 66, 71–73]

Lisinopril has also been compared with the β_1-selective blockers, atenolol and metoprolol. Although similar reductions in diastolic blood pressure were observed with lisinopril and the β-blockers, more pronounced lowering of systolic blood pressure was seen with lisinopril (Fig. 79–3).[74] This has been attributed to improved vascular compliance caused by lisinopril and to the bradycardic effect of the β-blockers.[75] Lisinopril does not significantly affect LV systolic performance, while β-blockers depress it[76] and may be superior in terms of a patient's quality of life.[77] The combination of ACE inhibitors and β-blockers is not as favorable as that of ACE inhibitors and diuretics or calcium antagonists,[74, 78, 79] but an added benefit is observed.[80] Lisinopril was found to be similar to nifedipine in terms of its efficacy in controlling essential hypertension, but was accompanied with fewer side effects.[49, 81–83] It was also found to be as effective as verapamil.[84] Both drugs were well tolerated. Lisinopril was found effective in reducing left ventricular mass and improving diastolic function in patients with hypertension.[85, 86]

Use in Congestive Heart Failure

In patients with CHF, lisinopril in an initial dose of 2.5 mg daily has been found to improve symptoms, favorably affect hemodynamics (as previously discussed), and increase exercise tolerance.[55–57, 60, 87–89] Although long duration of action allowing once-daily dosing is a beneficial feature of lisinopril in the treatment of patients with hypertension, the desirability of a long duration of action in patients with CHF is controversial. Long-acting enalapril, when given in high fixed doses to patients with severe CHF, caused

prolonged lowering of blood pressure and more central nervous system and renal side effects than short-acting captopril.[90] On the other hand, enalapril was found to decrease mortality in the Cooperative New Scandinavian Enalapril Survival Study (CONSENSUS) trial of patients with severe CHF,[91] and, in a double-blind study,[89] lisinopril improved ejection fraction and exercise tolerance more than captopril, although with slightly worse renal function. Compared with doxazosin, lisinopril was found to be more efficacious in improving exercise tolerance[92] and similar to enalapril.[93] The available clinical experience with lisinopril indicates that it is effective and well tolerated in CHF.

SIDE EFFECTS

Lisinopril is usually well tolerated and in clinical practice is not associated with unacceptable side effects. The classic side effects of ACE inhibitors may be observed with lisinopril. They include hypotension, especially in patients with severe CHF and borderline blood pressure who are receiving diuretics; azotemia, especially in dehydrated hypertensive patients or those with bilateral renal artery stenosis; hyperkalemia, especially in patients with renal insufficiency or diabetes or those taking both potassium supplements and potassium-sparing diuretics; cough; and, in susceptible individuals, nonfatal or even fatal angioneurotic edema.[24, 94] With the exception of cough, these side effects occur infrequently and can be avoided with proper selection of patients. The most frequent side effects reported in patients with hypertension were headache, dizziness, cough, and diarrhea. They occurred in 3.1% to 6.2% of patients and were more frequent than during administration of placebo (1.2% to 3.7%), although the exposure to placebo was shorter.[95] Lisinopril does not affect adversely lipoprotein metabolism.[96]

More frequent side effects were reported in patients with congestive heart failure, resulting in discontinuation of treatment in 7.4% of patients. In addition to the subjective side effects previously mentioned, the expected biochemical alterations (hyperkalemia, azotemia) were observed in a small number of patients.

SUMMARY

Lisinopril is a relatively new oral ACE inhibitor, not containing a sulfhydryl group and not a prodrug, that is effective in the treatment of hypertension and CHF on a once-daily regimen. In hypertension, it may be used as monotherapy (more effective in nonblack patients than in black patients) or combination therapy, especially with diuretics or calcium antagonists. It may also be used in CHF in conjunction with digitalis and diuretics. In addition, physicians use ACE inhibitors in patients with less severe heart failure and those with left ventricular dysfunction without CHF, although definite evidence of a benefit regarding mortality in these patient subsets is not available yet. The side-effect profile is favorable, provided that caution

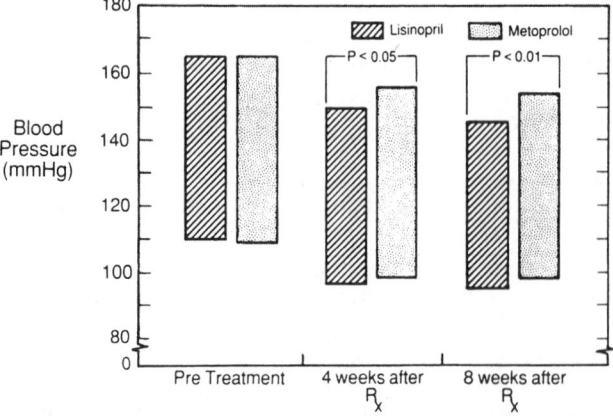

Figure 79–3. Effect of lisinopril and metoprolol on blood pressure response in moderate to severe hypertension. (From Zachariah PK, Bounet G, Chrysant SG, et al: Evaluation of antihypertensive efficacy of lisinopril compared to metoprolol in moderate to severe hypertension. J Cardiovasc Pharmacol 9(Suppl 3):S53, 1987.)

is exercised when prescribing the drug, especially to patients with CHF or renal insufficiency, or in conjunction with diuretics or potassium supplements.

REFERENCES

1. Patchett AA, Harris E, Tristram EW, et al: A new class of angiotensin converting enzyme inhibitors. Nature 228:280, 1980.
2. Biollaz J, Burnier M, Turini GA, et al: Three new long-acting converting-enzyme inhibitors: Relationship between plasma converting-enzyme activity and response to angiotensin I. Clin Pharmacol Ther 29:665, 1981.
3. DeFelice EA, Kostis JB: New ACE inhibitors. In Kostis JB, DeFelice EA (eds): Angiotensin Converting Enzyme Inhibitors. New York: Alan R Liss, 1987, pp 213–261.
4. Gomez HJ, Cirillo VJ, Moncloa F: The clinical pharmacology of lisinopril. J Cardiovasc Pharmacol 9:S27, 1987.
5. Armayor GM, Lopez LM: Lisinopril: A new angiotensin-converting enzyme inhibitor. Drug Intell Clin Pharm 22:365, 1988.
6. Ferreira S: A bradykinin-potentiating factor (BPF) present in the venom of Bothrops jararaca. Br J Pharmacol 24:163, 1965.
7. Yang HY, Erdos EG, Levin Y: A dipeptidyl carboxypeptidase that converts angiotensin I and inactivates bradykinin. Biochim Biophys Acta 214:374, 1970.
8. Cushman D, Cheung H, Sabo E, et al: Design of potent competitive inhibitors of angiotensin-converting enzyme carboxyalkanoyl and mercaptoalkanoyl amino acids. Biochemistry 16:5484, 1987.
9. Patchett AA: The chemistry of enalapril. Br J Clin Pharmacol 18:201S, 1984.
10. Todd PA, Heel RC: Enalapril: A review of its pharmacodynamic and pharmacokinetic properties, and therapeutic use in hypertension and congestive heart failure. Drugs 31:198, 1986.
11. Dzau VJ, Colucci WS, Williams GH, et al: Sustained effectiveness of converting-enzyme inhibition in patients with severe congestive heart failure. N Engl J Med 302:1373, 1980.
12. Bull HG, Thornberry NA, Cordes MHJ, et al: Inhibition of rabbit lung angiotensin-converting enzyme by N2-[(S)-1-carboxy-3-phenylpropyl]L-alanyl-L-proline and N2-[(S)-1-carboxy-3-phenylpropyl] L-lysyl-L-proline. J Biol Chem 260:2952, 1985.
13. Biollaz J, Schelling JL, Jacot Des Combers B, et al: Enalapril maleate and a lysine analogue (MK521) in normal volunteers: Relationship between plasma drug levels and the renin-angiotensin system. Br J Clin Pharmacol 14:363, 1982.
14. Ulm EH, Hichens M, Gomez HJ, et al: Enalapril maleate and lysine analogue (MK521) disposition in man. Br J Clin Pharmacol 14:357, 1982.
15. Mojavernan P, Rocci ML, Vlassers PH, et al: Effect of food on the bioavailability of lisinopril, a nonsulfhydryl angiotensin-converting enzyme inhibitor. J Pharmacol Sci 75:395, 1986.
16. Tocco DJ, Leary WP, Gomez HJ, et al: Physiological disposition and metabolism of ACE inhibitors in human subjects [abstract 487]. Second World Conference on Clinical Pharmacology & Therapeutics, Washington, D.C., July 31–Aug 5, 1983, p 83.
17. Ajayi AA, Campbell BC, Keiman AW, et al: Pharmacodynamics and population pharmacokinetics of enalapril and lisinopril. Int J Clin Pharmacol Res 5:419, 1985.
18. Beerman B, Junggren I, Cocchetto D, et al: Lisinopril steady-state kinetics in healthy subjects [abstract]. J Clin Pharmacol 25:471, 1985.
19. Ranadive SA, Chen AX, Serajuddin AT: Relative lipophilicities and structural-pharmacological considerations of various angiotensin-converting enzyme (ACE) inhibitors. Pharm Res 11:1480, 1992.
20. Gautam PC, Vargas E, Lye M: Pharmacokinetics of lisinopril (MK521) in healthy young and elderly subjects, and in elderly patients with cardiac failure. J Pharm Pharmacol 39:929, 1987.
21. Cirillo VJ, Till AE, Gomez HJ, et al: Effect of age on lisinopril pharmacokinetics [abstract B5]. Clin Pharmacol Ther 39:187, 1986.
22. Cirillo VJ, Gomez HJ, Cummings SW, et al: Lisinopril in hypertensive patients with renal dysfunction [abstract 8]. J Clin Pharmacol 27:706, 1987.
23. Kelly JG, Doyle G, Donohoe J, et al: Acute and chronic dose pharmacokinetics of lisinopril, effects of renal impairment. Br J Clin Pharmacol 23:629P, 1987.
24. Donohoe JF, Laher M, Doyle GD, et al: Lisinopril treatment of hypertension in patients with impaired renal function. Gerontology 33:36, 1987.
25. Zussman RM: Renin and nonrenin mediated antihypertensive action of converting enzyme inhibitors. Kidney Int 25:969, 1984.
26. Ganten D, Balz W, Hense HW, et al: Characterization and regulation of angiotensin (ANG) peptides in tissue of rabbits and primates. J Hypertens 3:5552, 1985.
27. Scholkens BA, Tilly H: Inhibition of converting enzyme in isolated arterial preparations with intact or disrupted endothelium. Naunyn Schmiedebergs Arch Pharmacol 332(Suppl R60):46, 1986.
28. Linz P, Petry P, Albus U, et al: The angiotensin converting enzyme inhibitor ramipril reduces reperfusion arrhythmias in the isolated working rat heart. Z Kardiol 75(Suppl 36):112, 1986.
29. Unger T, Ganten D, Lang R: Effect of converting enzyme inhibitors on tissue converting enzyme and angiotensin II: Therapeutic implication. Am J Cardiol 59:18D, 1987.
30. Campbell DJ: The site of angiotensin production. J Hypertens 3:199, 1985.
31. Velletri P, Bean B: The effects of captopril on rat aortic angiotensin-converting enzyme. J Cardiovasc Pharmacol 4:315, 1982.
32. Johnston CI, Cubela R, Sakaguchi K, et al: Angiotensin converting enzyme inhibition in plasma and tissues. Clin Exp Hypertens [A] 9:307, 1987.
33. Nakamura Y, Nakamura K, Nakamura K: Difference in response of vascular angiotensin converting enzyme activity to cilazapril in SHR. Clin Exp Hypertens [A] 9:351, 1987.
34. Dzau VJ: Implications of local angiotensin production in cardiovascular physiology and pharmacology. Am J Cardiol 59:59A, 1987.
35. van Gilst WH, deGraeff PA, Wesseling H, et al: Reduction of reperfusion arrhythmias in the ischemic isolated rat heart by angiotensin converting enzyme inhibitors: A comparison of captopril, enalapril, and HOE 498. J Cardiovasc Pharmacol 8:722, 1986.
36. Sinz W, Scholkens BA, Han YF: Beneficial effects of the converting enzyme inhibitor, ramipril, in ischemic rat hearts. J Cardiovasc Pharmacol 8(Suppl 10):S91, 1986.
37. Rochette L, Ribuot C, Belichard P, et al: Protective effect of angiotensin converting enzyme inhibitors (CEI) captopril and perindopril on vulnerability to ventricular fibrillation during myocardial ischemia and reperfusion in rats. Clin Exp Hypertens [A] 9:365, 1987.
38. Unger T, Scholkens BA, Ganten D, et al: Tissue converting enzyme inhibition and cardiovascular effects of converting enzyme inhibitors. Clin Exp Hypertens [A] 9:417, 1987.
39. Norman JA, Lehmann M, Goodman FR, et al: Central and peripheral inhibition of angiotensin converting enzyme (ACE) in the SHR: Correlation with the antihypertensive activity of ACE inhibitors. Clin Exp Hypertens [A] 9:461, 1987.
40. van Schaik Geyskes GG, Boer P: Lisinopril in hypertensive patients with and without renal failure. Eur J Clin Pharmacol 32:11, 1987.
41. Bull HG, Thornberry NA, Cordes EH: Purification of angiotensin-converting enzyme from rabbit lung and human plasma by affinity chromatography. J Biol Chem 260:2963, 1985.
42. Brunner B, Desponds G, Biollaz J, et al: Effect of a new angiotensin-converting enzyme inhibitor MK421 and its lysine analogue on the components of the renin system in healthy subjects. Br J Clin Pharmacol 11:461, 1981.
43. Nussberger J, Brunner DB, Waeber B, et al: Lack of angiotensin I accumulation after converting enzyme blockade by enalapril or lisinopril in man. Clin Sci 72:387, 1987.
44. Millar JA, Derkx FHM, McLean K, et al: Pharmacodynamics of converting enzyme inhibition: The cardiovascular endocrine and autonomic effects of MK421 (enalapril) and MK521. Br J Clin Pharmacol 14:347, 1982.
45. Hodsman GP, Zabludowski JR, Zoccali C, et al: Enalapril (MK421) and its lysine analogue (MK521): A comparison of acute and chronic effects on blood pressure, renin-angiotensin

system and sodium excretion in normal man. Br J Clin Pharmacol 17:233, 1984.

46. Semple PF, Cumming AMM, Meredith PA, et al: Onset of action of captopril, enalapril, enalaprilic acid and lisinopril in normal man. Cardiovasc Drugs Ther 1:45, 1987.

47. Ajayi AA, Campbell BC, Howie CA, et al: Acute and chronic effects of the converting enzyme inhibitors enalapril and lisinopril on reflex control of heart rate in normotensive man. J Hypertens 3:47, 1985.

48. Ajayi AA, Reid JL: The effect of enalapril on baroreceptor-mediated reflex function in normotensive subjects. Br J Clin Pharmacol 21:338, 1986.

49. Lees KR, Meredith PA, Reid JL: A clinical pharmacological study of nifedipine and lisinopril alone and in combination. J Cardiovasc Pharmacol 10:S105, 1987.

50. Amodeo C, Messerli FH, Ventura HO, et al: Disparate cardiac effects of afterload reduction in hypertension. J Hypertens 3:S371, 1985.

51. Dupont AG, Van der Niepen P, Volckaert A, et al: Improved renal function during chronic lisinopril treatment in moderate to severe essential hypertension [abstract No. 0399]. Eleventh Scientific Meeting of the International Society of Hypertension, Heidelberg, Aug. 31–Sept. 6, 1986.

52. Donohoe JF, Laher M, Doyle GD, et al: Lisinopril in hypertension associated with renal impairment. J Cardiovasc Pharmacol 9:S66, 1987.

53. Giorgi DMA, Giorgi MCP, de Almeida Burdmann E, et al: Effects of MK521 (lisinopril) on the renal plasma flow and renin-angiotensin-aldosterone system in patients with essential hypertension. J Hypertens 4:S420, 1986.

54. Laher MS, Donohoe JF, Kelly JG, et al: Antihypertensive and renal effects of lisinopril in older patients with hypertension. Am J Med 85(Suppl 3B):38, 1988.

55. Dickstein K, Aarsland T, Tjeita K, et al: A comparison of hypotensive responses after oral and intravenous administration of enalapril and lisinopril in chronic heart failure. J Cardiovasc Pharmacol 9:705, 1987.

56. Dickstein K, Aarsland T, Woie L, et al: Acute haemodynamic and hormonal effects of lisinopril (MK521) in congestive heart failure. Am Heart J 112:121, 1986.

57. Uretsky BF, Lawless CE, Rahko PS, et al: Treatment of severe heart failure with lisinopril: Acute and chronic hemodynamic echocardiographic and clinical responses [abstract 1624]. Circulation 72:406, 1985.

58. Reams GP, Bauer JH: Effect of lisinopril monotherapy on renal hemodynamics. Am J Kidney Dis 11:499, 1988.

59. Degaute JP, Leeman M, Reuse C, et al: Acute and chronic effects of lisinopril on renal and systemic hemodynamics in hypertension. Cardiovasc Drug Ther 6:489, 1992.

60. Stone CK, Uretsky BF, Linnemeier TJ, et al: Persistent hemodynamic effects of lisinopril after chronic therapy in congestive heart failure [abstract]. J Am Coll Cardiol 9:104A, 1987.

61. Materson BJ: New indications for ACE inhibitors. In Kostis JB, DeFelice EA (eds): Angiotensin Converting Enzyme Inhibitors. New York: Alan R Liss, 1987, pp 187–211.

62. Cirillo VJ, Gomez HJ, Salonen J, et al: Lisinopril: Dose-peak effect relationship in essential hypertension. Br J Clin Pharmacol 25:533, 1988.

63. Nelson EB, Chrysant SG, Gradman AH, et al: Dose-response study of lisinopril efficacy in hypertension [abstract]. J Clin Pharmacol 25:470, 1985.

64. Kostis JB: Angiotensin converting enzyme inhibitors. I: Pharmacology. II: Clinical use. Am Heart J 116(6 Pt 1):1580, 1988.

65. Pool JL, Gennari J, Goldstein R, et al: Controlled multicentre study of the antihypertensive effects of lisinopril, hydrochlorothiazide and lisinopril plus hydrochlorothiazide in the treatment of 394 patients with mild to moderate essential hypertension. J Cardiovasc Pharmacol 9:536, 1987.

66. Kochar MS, Bolek G, Kalbfleish JH, et al: A 52-week comparison of lisinopril, hydrochlorothiazide and their combination in hypertension. J Clin Pharmacol 27:373, 1987.

67. Whelton A, Dunne B Jr, Glazer N, et al: Twenty-four hour blood pressure effect of once-daily lisinopril, enalapril, and placebo in patients with mild to moderate hypertension. J Hum Hypertens 6:325, 1992.

68. Kuntziger HE, Pouthier D, Bellucci A: Treatment of hypertension with lisinopril in end-stage renal failure. J Cardiovasc Pharmacol 10:S157, 1987.

69. Fyhrquist F, Gronhagen-Riska C, Tikkanen I, et al: Long-term monotherapy with lisinopril in renovascular hypertension. J Cardiovasc Pharmacol 9:S61, 1987.

70. Weir MR, Lavin PT: Comparison of the efficacy and tolerability of Prinivil and Procardia XL in black and white hypertensive patients. Clin Ther 5:730, 1992.

71. Seedat YK, Venava Y, Cohen JD, et al: Evaluation of the antihypertensive effect of lisinopril compared to atenolol in black, mixed and Indian patients with mild-to-moderate essential hypertension. Curr Ther Res 41:852, 1987.

72. Merrill DD, Byymy RL, Carr A, et al: Lisinopril/HCTZ in essential hypertension [abstract P111]. Clin Pharmacol Ther 41:227, 1987.

73. Mehta J, Lopez LM, Thorman AD: Lisinopril versus lisinopril plus hydrochlorothiazide in essential hypertension. Am J Cardiol 61:803, 1988.

74. Zachariah PK, Bounet G, Chrysant SG, et al: Evaluation of antihypertensive efficacy of lisinopril compared to metoprolol in moderate to severe hypertension. J Cardiovasc Pharmacol 9(Suppl 3):S53, 1987.

75. Pannier BE, Garabedian VG, Madonna O, et al: Lisinopril versus atenolol: Decrease in stystolic versus diastolic blood pressure with converting enzme inhibition. Cardiovasc Drug Ther 5:775, 1991.

76. Zusman RM, Christensen DM, Higgins J, et al: Comparison of the effects of isradipine and lisinopril on left ventricular structure and function in essential hypertension: Therapeutic implications. J Cardiovasc Pharmacol 20:216, 1992.

77. Frimodt-Moeller J, Poulsen DL, Kornerup HJ, et al: Quality of life, side effects and efficacy of lisinopril compared with metoprolol in patients with mild to moderate essential hypertension. J Hum Hypertens 5:215, 1991.

78. Thind GS: Lisinopril versus atenolol alone and with hydrochlorothiazide in the treatment of mild to moderate essential hypertension. J Hypertens 4:S423, 1986.

79. Bolzano K, Arriaga J, Bernal R, et al: The antihypertensive effect of lisinopril compared to atenolol in patients with mild to moderate hypertension. J Cardiovasc Pharmacol 9:S43, 1987.

80. Soininen K, Gerlin-Piira L, Suihkonen J, et al: A study of the effects of lisinopril when used in addition to atenolol. J Hum Hypertens 6:321, 1992.

81. Mortin C, Baglivo H, Boerjinga JK, et al: Comparative trial of lisinopril and nifedipine in mild to severe essential hypertension. J Cardiovasc Pharmacol 9:S48, 1987.

82. Richardson PJ, Meany B, Breckenridge AM, et al: Lisinopril in essential hypertension: A six-month comparative study with nifedipine. J Hum Hypertens 1:175, 1987.

83. Hart W, Clarke RJ: ACE inhibition versus calcium antagonism in the treatment of mild to moderate hypertension: A multicentre study: Ireland-Netherlands Lisinopril-Nifedipine Study Group. Postgrad Med J 69:450, 1993.

84. Weir MR, Lavin PT: Comparison of the efficacy and tolerability of lisinopril and sustained-release verapamil in older patients with hypertension. Clin Ther 13:401, 1991.

85. Modena MG, Mattioli AV, Parato VM, et al: Effectiveness of the action of lisinopril on left ventricular mass and diastolic filling. Eur Heart J 13:1540, 1992.

86. Bielen EC, Fagard RH, Lijnen PJ, et al: Comparison of the effects of isradipine and lisinopril on left ventricular structure and function in essential hypertension. Am J Cardiol 69:1200, 1992.

87. Likoff MJ, Spielman SR, Hare TW, et al: Lisinopril in the treatment of chronic cardiac failure: A controlled trial [abstract 2035]. Circulation 74:510, 1986.

88. Chalmers JP, West MJ, Cyran J, et al: Placebo-controlled study of lisinopril in congestive heart failure: A multicentre study. J Cardiovasc Pharmacol 9:S89, 1987.

89. Powers ER, Chiaramida A, DeMaria AN, et al: A double-blind comparison of lisinopril with captopril in patients with symptomatic congestive heart failure. J Cardiovasc Pharmacol 9:S82, 1987.

90. Packer M, Lee WH, Yashak M, et al: Comparison of captopril

and enalapril in patients with severe chronic heart failure. N Engl J Med 315:847, 1986.

91. CONSENSUS Trial Study Group: Effects of enalapril on mortality in severe congestive heart failure: Results of the Cooperative North Scandinavian Enalapril Survival Study (CONSENSUS). N Engl J Med 316:1429, 1987.

92. Herlitz J: Comparison of lisinopril versus digoxin for congestive heart failure during maintance diurectic therapy: The Lisinopril-Digoxin Study Group. Am J Cardiol 70:84C, 1992.

93. Zannad F, van den Broek SA, Bory M: Comparison of treatment

with lisinopril versus enalapril for congestive heart failure. Am J Cardiol 70:78C, 1992.

94. Ulmer JL, Garvey, Garvey MJ: Fatal angioedema associated with lisinopril. Ann Pharmacother 26:1245, 1992.

95. Rush JE, Merrill DD: The safety and tolerability of lisinopril in clinical trials. J Cardiovasc Pharmacol 9:S99, 1987.

96. Sasaki J, Tominaga K, Saeki Y, et al: Effects of lisinopril and low-dose trichlormethiazide on lipoprotein metabolism in patients with mild to moderate hypertension. J Hum Hypertens 6:233, 1992.

CHAPTER 80

Ramipril

Peter Gohlke, Ph.D., and Thomas Unger, M.D.

HISTORY

Angiotensin-converting enzyme (ACE) inhibitors have been divided into three general chemical classes according to their zinc ligands, which coordinate to the Zn^{2+} ions in the active centers of ACE. Ramipril belongs to the class of carboxyl-containing ACE inhibitors, first represented by the compound enalapril. In an attempt to improve the inhibitory potency of this type of ACE inhibitor, the proline residue in the enalapril molecule was replaced by more lipophilic surrogates, e.g., by bicyclic iminocarboxylic acids, in order to provide stronger hydrophobic interactions with the corresponding sites in the ACE molecule. The most promising compound in this respect proved to be Hoe 498 (ramipril).

CHEMISTRY

Ramipril is characterized chemically as 2-[N-[(S)-1-ethoxycarbonyl-3-phenylpropyl]-L-alanyl](1S,3S,5S)-2-azabicyclo[3.3.0]octane-3-carboxylic acid and contains five asymmetric centers in S-configuration (Fig. 80–1). The correct stereochemistry is crucial for the pharmacologic properties of the compound.[1] Ramipril crystallizes in colorless, felty needles. The compound is easily soluble in methanol and ethanol but less soluble in water, with a partition coefficient in 1-octanol–phosphate buffer of 0.6 at pH 7.00. The molecular weight of ramipril is 416.5. Ramipril was designed as a monoethyl ester prodrug that has to be converted to the active diacid derivative, ramiprilat (molecular weight, 388.5), to develop full inhibitory potency (see Fig. 80–1). Ramiprilat is a hydrophylic compound with a partition coefficient in 1-octanol–phosphate buffer of 0.006 at pH 7.00.[2, 3]

PHARMACOLOGY

Ramiprilat, the active moiety of ramipril, is a slow- and tight-binding competitive inhibitor of ACE active at concentrations similar to those of the target enzyme, ACE, itself. The binding of ramiprilat to ACE purified from rabbit lung tissue has been described

by a two-step mechanism. In a first step, the inhibitor rapidly binds to ACE to form an initial enzyme-inhibitor complex with an inhibition constant K_i of 10.8 nmol/L. Thereafter, the enzyme-inhibitor complex undergoes a slow isomerization reaction to yield a stable enzyme-inhibitor complex with a slow dissociation velocity. The K_i value for the overall inhibition has been reported to be 7 ± 3 pmol/L, and the rate constant k_4 for the dissociation of the enzyme-inhibitor complex has been calculated to be 1.8×10^{-5} s^{-1}.[4, 5] From the value of k_4, the half-life of the enzyme-inhibitor complex was estimated to be 640 minutes for ramiprilat as compared with 29 minutes for captopril and 105 minutes for enalaprilat. Thus, the potency and long duration of action of ramiprilat are largely determined by the low dissociation rate of the final isomerized enzyme-inhibitor complex.

The *in vitro* potencies of ramipril and ramiprilat have been determined by incubation studies using purified ACE from rabbit lung as well as rat and human plasma and were expressed by the concentrations needed to inhibit 50% of the enzymatic activity (IC_{50}). Ramiprilat was shown to be a potent inhibitor of purified ACE from rabbit lung, with calculated IC_{50} values of 1.5 nmol/L[3] and 4.2 nmol/L.[6] Comparable inhibitory potencies were also obtained using rat

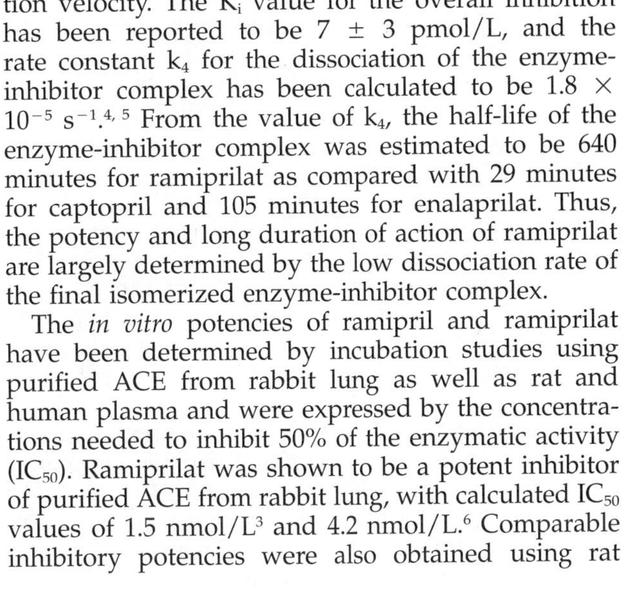

Figure 80–1. Structure and metabolism of ramipril. The most important metabolic step is the hydrolysis of the ethyl ester ramipril to the active diacid ramiprilat. Both ramipril and ramiprilat can be further metabolized to the corresponding diketopiperazines or glucuronide conjugates.

plasma (IC_{50} value, 2 nmol/L)[3] and rat serum (IC_{50} value, 0.5 nmol/L).[7] The prodrug, ramipril, is 1600 times less potent against purified ACE from rabbit lung than ramiprilat (IC_{50} value, 2500 nmol/L),[3] although an earlier study revealed a relatively high *in vitro* potency of ramipril (IC_{50} value, 26 nmol/L), probably due to a partial hydrolysis to the active diacid compound within the incubation mixture.[6] Thus, ramipril has to be activated *in vivo* in order to develop its full inhibitory activity. In rat plasma, ramipril can be partially hydrolyzed to ramiprilat, yielding a high *in vitro* potency with an IC_{50} value of 8 nmol/L.[3]

Studies in Animals

The *in vivo* potencies of ramipril and ramiprilat have been studied in different animal models after oral or intravenous drug application. Inhibition of the pressor responses to intravenously (IV) injected angiotensin I and potentiation of the depressor responses to IV bradykinin were used as a bioassay to determine the *in vivo* ACE inhibition. In anesthetized dogs and conscious stroke-prone spontaneously hypertensive rats (SHRSP), ramipril administration abolished or markedly inhibited the pressor responses to IV angiotensin I without affecting the pressor responses to IV angiotensin II and induced or potentiated the depressor responses to IV bradykinin.[8, 9]

Acute and chronic oral treatment with ramipril reduced ACE activity in plasma and in several tissue homogenates (e.g., lung, kidney, heart, aorta, mesenteric arteries, adrenal gland, and brain).[7, 9–14] As an expected consequence of ACE inhibition, plasma angiotensin II was lowered and angiotensin I was increased. Because of the withdrawal of the negative feedback of angiotensin II, plasma renin activity was increased, leading to decreased plasma angiotensinogen concentrations as a result of enhanced substrate consumption.

The recovery of ACE activity in tissue homogenates after drug withdrawal was delayed when compared with plasma. After 4 weeks of oral treatment of SHRSP with ramipril (3 mg/kg/day) and 1 week after drug withdrawal, plasma ACE activities in ramipril-treated animals were increased to levels above those of control animals, while ACE activity was still reduced in homogenates of kidney and mesenteric arteries.[10] In a further study, SHRSP were treated for 2 weeks with ramipril at a dose of 1 mg/kg/day. One week after drug withdrawal, ACE activity was still significantly inhibited in the kidney, lung, and aorta in the ramipril-treated group, but had returned to higher control values in plasma.[11] Similarly, 2 days after acute ramipril application (1 mg/kg/day) to SHRSP, there was still a significant inhibition of ACE activity in lung and kidney homogenates, whereas plasma ACE had fully recovered.[10] In general, the hemodynamic effects of ramipril correlated more closely with the inhibition of ACE activitiy within tissue homogenates than with plasma ACE activity. These observations suggest that inhibition of ACE in the vascular endothelium of the lung and in the vascular endothelium of other target organs such as the vascular wall or the kidney, which represent the paracrine/autocrine part of the renin-angiotensin system (RAS), may predominantly determine extent and duration of the cardiovascular actions of ramipril.

Ramipril has been shown to penetrate the blood-brain barrier in rats after acute oral administration of rather high doses (10 to 30 mg/kg/day), with a subsequent activation to ramiprilat.[3, 14]

Because ACE is identical with the bradykinin-degrading enzyme kininase II, ACE inhibition can theoretically potentiate the vasodepressor effects of endogenous bradykinin mediated by nitric oxide or prostacyclin. The contribution of bradykinin to the acute and chronic antihypertensive actions of ramipril has been investigated in different animal models of hypertension using specific bradykinin B_2-receptor antagonists.[15–19] Acute blockade of bradykinin B_2-receptors attenuated the responses to ramipril in two kidney–one clip (2K1C) renovascular hypertensive rats as well as in SHR.[15, 18] However, although chronic blockade of bradykinin B_2-receptors with icatibant (Hoe 140) markedly attenuated the antihypertensive actions of ramipril in 2K1C hypertensive rats, it was ineffective in spontanously hypertensive rats (SHR) and SHRSP.[16, 17, 19]

Thus, under chronic treatment conditions, bradykinin potentiation seems to gain more importance in the antihypertensive action of ramipril in renovascular hypertension associated with a stimulated renin-angiotenin system than in genetic hypertension. On the other hand, bradykinin potentiation has been shown to be implicated in a number of ramipril-induced cardiac and vascular actions in SHR and SHRSP as well as in rats with renovascular hypertension due to aortic banding, as will be outlined later.

Studies in Human Subjects

The inhibitory actions of ramipril on ACE activity in plasma, with the resulting alterations of the parameters of the renin-angiotensin system, have also been studied in normotensive and hypertensive patients as well as in patients with congestive heart failure. These studies widely confirmed the results derived from animal studies. Ramipril maximally inhibited plasma ACE activity at doses of 5 to 10 mg once daily within 1 to 4 hours after acute dosage. The duration of action lasted for more than 24 hours. The inhibition of ACE activity was frequently paralleled by decreased plasma angiotensin II and increased plasma angiotensin I concentrations and by increased plasma renin activities.[20–29] However, changes in plasma angiotensin II did not always parallel the time course of ACE inhibition. For example, in studies by Manhem et al.[22] and Nussberger et al.,[23] in which normotensive patients were treated with ramipril at doses of 5 to 50 mg and 10 to 20 mg, respectively, plasma angiotensin II levels recovered to control levels 24 hours after drug administration, although plasma ACE activity remained suppressed. Methodologic problems in measuring angiotensin peptides may account for some of these discrepancies, because angiotensin peptides were often not properly separated by high performance liquid chromatography (HPLC) for the measurement of angiotensin (1–8) octapeptide ("true" angiotensin II) (for details, see references 23 and 30). On the other hand, it has been suggested that inhibition of ACE at the level of the target organs and thus inhibition of the paracrine/autocrine RAS or local potentiation of endogenous kinins may be an important factor for the overall effects of ramipril that is not always reflected in decreased plasma angiotensin II concentrations.

In normotensive and hypertensive patients, ACE inhibitors including ramipril potentiated the blood pressure–lowering effect of bradykinin by approximately 20- to 50-fold.[31]

Measurements of ACE activity in human tissue samples of renal cortex, heart, and blood vessels were performed in patients undergoing surgical procedures.[32] The results revealed high levels af ACE activity in the renal cortex (125 nmol/mg protein per min) compared with heart, veins, and arteries (0.2, 0.23, and 0.8 nmol/mg protein per min, respectively). Oral administration of ramipril (2.5 mg twice daily) resulted in a marked inhibition of ACE activity in renal cortex (99.7%) and arteries (97.5%) 2 hours after last dosing, whereas ACE activity in homogenates of heart and veins was inhibited to a lesser extend (35% and 60.9%, respectively).

PHARMACOKINETICS

The pharmacokinetics of ramipril have been extensively reviewed[33–36] and are only summarized here. The principal pharmacokinetic characteristics of ramipril and ramiprilat in humans are listed in Table 80–1.

Ramipril can be administered to humans in solution, capsule, or tablet form, with little difference in its rate of absorption.[33] After oral application of 10 mg of ramipril, peak plasma concentrations were reached in about 0.3 to 1 hour.[22, 37, 38] The mean peak concentrations were slightly higher in the elderly than in young volunteers (62 µg/L and 52.2 µg/L, respectively).[38] After absorption, ramipril is mainly hydrolyzed to its active diacid form, ramiprilat. The primary site of conversion in humans is the liver, although hydrolysis also occurs in plasma and within other organs, depending on the presence of esterases. Mean peak plasma concentrations of ramiprilat were reached within 1.5 to 3 hours after a single oral dose of 10 mg ramipril and ranged between 24 µg/L and 33.6 µg/L in young volunteers[38, 39] and 40.6 µg/L in the elderly.[38] Comparable, but delayed, peak concentrations of the active drug were reached in patients with cardiac insufficiency (New York Heart Association class II–IV). Peak plasma levels of ramiprilat of 27.9 µg/L were detected 4.6 hours after a single oral dose of 5 mg ramipril.[40]

The rate of absorption of ramipril has been determined by Eckert et al.[37] after administration of a single dose of 10 mg/kg ^{14}C radioactively labeled ramipril to three healthy volunteers by measuring recovery of radioactivity in urine and feces. The rate of absorption calculated as the sum of radioactivity excreted renally (minimal absorption) and recovered after more than 72 hours after dosing ranged from 54% to 65%. Absorption could be even higher, because part of the drug or its metabolites may also be excreted in bile, as observed in the rat (36.1% of an oral dose) and dog.[37] Ramipril is mainly excreted by the kidney, although a significant contribution of biliary excretion has been suggested.[37] Ramipril is extensively metabolized, and only negligible amounts of unchanged drug were excreted in urine. The major metabolites of ramipril have been identified in urine as ramiprilat and the inactive glucuronide and diketopiperazine derivatives of ramiprilat. Further metabolites, which could be detected in small amounts in urine, include the diketopiperazine derivative and the glucuronide conjugate of ramipril.[38, 41]

Ramipril and ramiprilat were found to be 73% and 56% bound to human serum proteins in the concentration range of 0.01 to 10 mg/L as measured by the method of equilibrium dialysis.[37] The tissue distribution pattern of orally and intravenously administered radioactively labeled ramipril has been investigated in a quantitative study in rats. At the time of maximal blood levels, high concentrations of radioactivity could be detected in all tissues studied, with particularly high values in liver, kidneys, and lungs. The elimination of radioactivity occurred more rapidly in blood than in most tissues and was found to be particularly slow in lungs, where ACE is predominantly localized, and in subcutaneous fat, with half-lives of 63 hours and 47 hours, respectively.

Table 80–1. **Pharmacokinetics of Ramipril and Ramiprilat**

Bioavailability	54%–65%
Time to peak blood level	
Ramipril	0.3–1 hr
Ramiprilat	1.5–3 hr
Maximum blood level	
Ramipril	52–62 µg/L
Ramiprilat	22–41 µg/L
Half-life (ramiprilat)	
Initial	1.1–4.4 hr
Effective	13–17 hr
Terminal	85–190 hr
Time to onset of action	1–2 hr
Elimination	renal + (hepatic)
Protein binding	
Ramipril	73%
Ramiprilat	56%
Major metabolites	
Ramipril	Ramiprilat
	Ramipril-diketopiperazine
Ramiprilat	Ramiprilat-glucuronide
	Ramiprilat-diketopiperazine

The ability of ramipril and other ACE inhibitors to pass the blood-brain barrier was indirectly investigated in rats by measuring ACE activity in the cerebrospinal fluid after oral administration of the drugs as well as by measuring the inhibitory effect of heat-inactivated cerebrospinal fluid (CSF) of ramipril-treated rats on an enzyme reaction mixture.[3, 14, 42] The results revealed that the access of ACE inhibitors to brain structures inside the blood-brain barrier is related to the lipid solubility of the drugs. Ramipril was shown to penetrate the blood-brain barrier in rats after acute oral administration with threshold doses of 3 to 10 mg/kg/day, with a subsequent activation to ramiprilat. However, in view of its low lipophilicity, the access of ramiprilat itself to brain areas inside the blood-brain barrier appears to be limited.[3] Thus, central effects of ramipril probably depend on the actual degree of peripheral deesterification after oral application.

The placental transfer and the excretion in milk of ramipril were studied in pregnant and lactating rats after administration of radioactively labeled drug. At the time of maximal maternal blood levels, approximately 0.05% of the administered dose was detected in amniotic fluid, fetal liver, and remaining fetal carcass, suggesting a slight, transient placental transfer in rats. Approximately 0.25% of an oral dose of ramipril was calculated to be excreted with the milk.[37]

The mean half-life of ramiprilat in healthy subjects was calculated by Witte et al.[39] Serum levels of ramiprilat were measured up to 14 days after administration of a single oral dose of 10 mg ramipril to 10 normal healthy volunteers. The plasma concentration-time curve of ramiprilat declined polyphasically with an initial rapid decline after the peak level and a subsequent long terminal phase at low concentrations of ramiprilat. Calculated half-lives ranged between 1.1 and 4.5 hours for the initial distribution and elimination phase and 85 and 190 hours (mean, 113 hours) for the terminal phase. The initial rapid elimination phase probably reflects the clearance of excess non-ACE-bound ramiprilat, whereas the prolonged terminal half-life has been attributed to the saturable binding to ACE, reflecting the high affinity of ramiprilat to ACE and corresponding to the clearance of the ACE-bound drug. In spite of the long terminal half-life, no drug accumulation has been found after repeated once-daily administration of ramipril, even at the high dose of 20 mg.[33, 43, 44] The effective half-life of ramiprilat was calculated after administration of ramipril at a dose of 5 or 10 mg (once daily) for 15 days to a small group of patients and ranged between 13 and 17 hours.[34]

Several investigators studied the effects of renal impairment on the pharmacokinetics of ramipril and ramiprilat in single-dose studies[41, 45, 46] and after multiple dosing.[44] Although renal impairment did not markedly change the pharmacokinetic properties of the parent compound, ramipril, these studies demonstrated a marked influence of renal function on the kinetics of the active metabolite, ramiprilat. In general, impaired renal function was associated with higher peak plasma ramiprilat concentrations, longer time to reach peak levels, and prolonged initial half-lives, leading to an enhanced duration of action. The renal clearance of ramiprilat was significantly correlated with the creatinine clearance. Thus, dosage adjustment is necessary in patients with advanced renal failure because of the decreased rate of elimination of the active metabolite, ramiprilat.

Hepatic impairment resulted in elevated plasma concentrations of the parent drug, ramipril, owing to a diminished hepatic metabolization. However, plasma concentrations of the active metabolite, ramiprilat, appeared to be unaltered when compared with those of healthy volunteers, although maximal plasma levels were reached later.[34]

EFFECTS ON PATHOPHYSIOLOGY
Effects on Hemodynamics

The hemodynamic effects of ramipril have been investigated in anesthetized normotensive and hypertensive animals. In anesthetized normal and sodium-depleted (diuretic-pretreated) dogs, blood pressure decreased by 10 ± 1 mmHg and 30 ± 6 mmHg, respectively, after intravenous injection of 1 mg/kg of ramipril, and remained low during the 3-hour experiment. Blood pressure reduction was associated with decreases of total peripheral resistance of 12% and 16% in normal and sodium-depleted animals, respectively. Besides a marginal fall in dP/dt_{max} in sodium-depleted dogs, all other cardiovascular parameters (cardiac output, heart rate, coronary blood flow, pulmonary artery pressure) were not significantly altered under these treatment conditions.[8] Similar findings have been obtained by Richer et al.[47] in anesthetized SHR pretreated with ramipril for 8 days. Ramipril treatment at doses of 1 and 5 mg/kg/day decreased arterial blood pressure by 12% and 30%, respectively. The effect of the higher dose was related to a decrease in total peripheral resistance, while heart rate and cardiac index remained unchanged. Ramipril at a dose of 1 mg/kg/day significantly increased kidney and spleen blood flow despite an almost unchanged cardiac index and decreased vascular resistance in kidney, spleen, and liver without a significant effect on total peripheral resistance (Fig. 80–2). The higher dose of 5 mg/kg/day did not further potentiate these effects but, in addition, decreased vascular resistances in skin and muscles (see Fig. 80–2).

In anesthetized normotensive rats, ramipril (0.1 mg/kg) injected close to the origin of the renal artery increased renal blood flow by 18% for 30 minutes and decreased renal vascular resistance without changing systemic blood pressure.[8] Thus, the hemodynamic effects of ramipril are characterized by a decrease in total peripheral resistance, with renal blood flow and renal vascular resistance being particularly sensitive to ACE inhibition.

In animal studies, the effects of ramipril and ramiprilat on cardiac function and metabolism, as well as

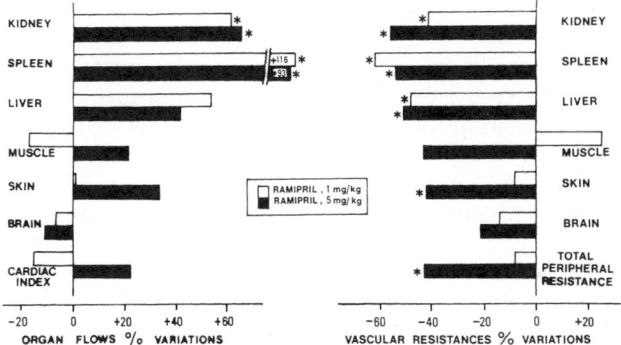

Figure 80–2. Percentage of variations from corresponding control group of the regional blood flows and of the regional vascular resistances after oral treatment of spontaneously hypertensive rats with two different doses of ramipril. *, significant difference from corresponding control value ($p < .05$). (Reprinted with permission from Richer C, Doussau M-P, Giudicelli J-F: Systemic and regional hemodynamic profile of five angiotensin I converting enzyme inhibitors in the spontaneously hypertensive rat. Am J Cardiol 59:12D, 1987.)

on reperfusion arrhythmias, have been investigated in isolated normal and ischemic heart preparations. The results of these experiments are discussed in a later section.

In human subjects, the acute and chronic effects of ramipril on the peripheral arterial hemodynamics have been studied in healthy volunteers and in patients with mild to moderate hypertension. Administration of a single dose of 10 mg ramipril to normotensive healthy volunteers significantly increased brachial artery blood flow, brachial artery diameter, and carotid artery blood flow and decreased forearm vascular resistance between 3 and 8 hours after drug intake. The arterial vasodilating effects were more pronounced in the muscular resistance vessels. Heart rate and blood pressure were not significantly affected by ramipril treatment except for diastolic blood pressure (-10 mmHg) 6 hours after drug intake.[48]

In patients with mild to moderate primary hypertension, acute treatment with ramipril (5 mg daily) did not affect brachial artery hemodynamics. However, chronic treatment (4 weeks) with ramipril was followed by a long-lasting increase in brachial artery diameter and a decrease in forearm vascular resistance.[49] Arterial distensibility was evaluated noninvasively in three different arterial segments after 4 weeks of treatment with ramipril (5 mg daily) by measuring the pulse wave velocity. Arterial distensibility was improved in carotid-femoral segments, indicating an increase in aortic compliance, whereas arterial distensibility in other arterial segments (femorotibial and brachioradial) remained unchanged.[49]

In patients with congestive heart failure, acute administration of single doses of 5 or 10 mg ramipril caused a moderate decrease in blood pressure and total peripheral resistance. Most importantly, the decrease in blood pressure was not accompanied by reflex tachycardia.[26, 50] The lack of reflex tachycardia was attributed to a ramipril-induced sensitization of the parasympathetic baroreceptor heart rate reflex

without influence on sympathetically mediated peripheral vasodilation.[50] In a small group of patients with moderate to severe congestive heart failure (NYHA classes II–IV), pulmonary capillary wedge pressure was markedly reduced up to 8 hours and remained below baseline 24 hours after administration of ramipril at doses of 5 or 10 mg. In the same study, a short-lasting increase in cardiac output with a maximum at 2 hours after ramipril administration was observed.[26] In view of the severe hypotension that may occur in some patients, an initial dose of 2.5 mg or less has been recommended with a subsequent individualized dosage scheme. After long-term treatment (3 months) with 5 mg ramipril, the 24-hour hemodynamic profile was comparable with that after the first dose, but the hypotensive response was less marked.[51]

Long-term administration of ramipril (5 to 10 mg daily for 6 weeks) to patients with stabilized congestive heart failure receiving diuretic treatment resulted in a decline in overall sympathetic tone as assessed by whole body (^{3}H)-noradrenaline kinetics. This effect was less pronounced after short-term treatment (48 hours).[52]

Regional hemodynamics in congestive heart failure have been studied 2 hours after administration of 10 mg ramipril. Despite a slight, nonsignificant reduction of mean arterial blood pressure by 7 mmHg, renal blood flow rose markedly by 93%, accompanied by a decrease in renal vascular resistance of 52%. Coronary blood flow and cerebral blood flow increased slightly but nonsignificantly by 10% and 5%, respectively, whereas forearm blood flow was unchanged.[28]

The effects of ramipril on blood pressure have been investigated in normotensive animals as well as in different animal models of hypertension. As expected, ACE inhibition by ramipril proved to be particularly effective in cases in which the RAS was stimulated, for example, in experimental models of renin-dependent hypertension or after diuretic pretreatment leading to sodium depletion. Single oral pretreatment with ramipril at a dose of 0.1 mg/kg completely prevented the blood pressure increase that occurred after release of the occlusion of a renal pedicle. Similarly, prolonged oral treatment with ramipril at a dose of 1 mg/kg/day effectively prevented the development of hypertension in rats with aortic banding when treatment was started immediately after experimental induction of hypertension.[53, 54] Furthermore, blood pressure was normalized in 2K1C hypertensive rats and in rats with aortic banding when treatment was started after hypertension had fully developed.[16, 54] These effects could be partly attributed to the bradykinin-potentiating effect of the ACE inhibitor.[16, 54]

In normotensive rats, intravenous injection of ramipril (0.1 and 1 mg/kg) caused a pronounced decrease in blood pressure that lasted for maximally 18 minutes. The duration of action of ramipril was markedly enhanced when the RAS was activated by sodium depletion (pretreatment with a diuretic).[8] Similar results were shown in anesthetized dogs as reported earlier.[8]

Several studies have demonstrated the antihypertensive efficiency of ramipril in animal models of hypertension not associated with elevated plasma renin levels (SHR, SHRSP, two-kidney, two wrapped hypertension). Repeated oral administration of ramipril (1 mg/kg/day) for 5 days as well as a single dose of 10 mg/kg/day of ramipril reduced blood pressure in conscious renal hypertensive dogs with both kidneys wrapped in cellophane (two-kidney, two wrapped hypertension).[8]

In SHRSP, ramipril produced a dose-dependent fall in blood pressure at doses of 0.1 to 10 mg/kg/day during 4 weeks of overnight drug treatment in the drinking water. Blood pressure was normalized after the highest dose of 10 mg/kg/day.[10] Similar results were obtained in SHR after 4 weeks gavage treatment at doses of 0.01 to 10 mg/kg/day. The threshold antihypertensive dose under these conditions was 0.01 mg/kg/day.[8]

Several studies in SHR and SHRSP demonstrated a persistent antihypertensive effect of ramipril after drug withdrawal.[8, 10, 11] In these studies, blood pressure was markedly lowered or normalized during 4 weeks of oral treatment with ramipril at doses of 1 and 10 mg/kg/day, respectively. Maximal blood pressure reduction was reached within 1 week. After drug withdrawal, blood pressure recovered slowly but was still significantly decreased 1 to 2 weeks after cessation of treatment when compared with vehicle-treated controls.[8, 10, 11]

Long-term early-onset treatment with 1 mg/kg/day of ramipril completely prevented or markedly attenuated hypertension development in SHR and SHRSP, respectively, whereas a dose of 0.01 mg/kg/day was without effect on blood pressure.[19, 55]

These studies demonstrate that ramipril is an effective antihypertensive drug even in cases of hypertension associated with normal or low plasma renin levels. Thus, a stimulated plasma RAS is not a prerequisite for the antihypertensive action of this drug.

Studies in normotensive sodium-replete human subjects have shown that oral administration of a single dose of ramipril had no effect on blood pressure and heart rate or caused only marginal reductions in blood pressure even at high doses of 20 to 50 mg.[20-22] However, in patients with primary hypertension, acute administration of ramipril caused significant reductions in systolic and diastolic blood pressure at doses of 2.5 to 20 mg. The maximal reduction of blood pressure after a dose of 5 mg occurred after 4 to 6 hours.[24, 56-58]

Studies using invasive and noninvasive methods of 24-hour blood pressure monitoring have revealed an effective blood pressure–lowering action of ramipril throughout the 24-hour period. Significant 24-hour blood pressure reduction was observed after a dose of 2.5 mg, with quantitatively higher effects at higher doses. The antihypertensive action of ramipril occurred after acute administration and was maintained during long-term treatment. In addition, these studies demonstrated that ramipril did not interfere with the normal circadian blood pressure pattern in patients with essential hypertension.[59-64]

The results of several clinical trials investigating the antihypertensive efficacy of ramipril during short-term and long-term treatment are summarized in Table 80–2. These studies show that ramipril monotherapy at oral doses of 1.25 to 10 mg once daily reduced blood pressure to normotensive levels in approximately 50% to 80% of the patients.[25, 57, 59, 65-72]

In a 2-year multicenter, open-label study, 555 hypertensive patients were treated with ramipril at a starting dose of 5 mg. The dosage of ramipril was then adjusted in accordance to the response of treatment and ranged from 1.25 to 20 mg. Of the patients, 23% additionally received hydrochlorothiazide. In the 415 patients whose blood pressure was controlled (diastolic blood pressure, $\leq$ 90 mmHg) by ramipril monotherapy at the end of the 2-year treatment period, 44% were taking 2.5 mg of ramipril and 41% were taking 5 mg of ramipril. A subgroup of 202 patients who had been classified as responders (diastolic blood pressure, $\leq$ 90 mmHg after ramipril monotherapy) in previous short-term double-blind studies, were analyzed for efficacy maintenance. The results indicated that ramipril maintained its antihypertensive efficacy during long-term therapy in 95% to 98% of the patients without development of tolerance. Heart rate was not significantly changed after acute and long-term administration of ramipril in these studies.

Effects on Ventricular Function and Structure

Since the mid-1980s, several studies have shown that acute ACE inhibitor treatment can prevent postischemic reperfusion arrhythmias and reperfusion injuries.[73-78] These studies were performed in isolated working rat hearts with acute regional myocardial ischemia induced by occlusion of the left coronary artery followed by reperfusion. Perfusion of the isolated rat hearts with ramiprilat (2.6×10^{-8} mol/L to 2.6×10^{-7} mol/L) as well as acute pretreatment with a single dose of 1 mg/kg ramipril reduced the incidence and duration of reperfusion arrhythmias. These effects were paralleled by an ACE inhibitor–induced increase in cardiodynamic parameters such as coronary flow, left ventricular pressure, and dP/dt_{max}. The activities of the cytosolic enzymes, lactate dehydrogenase and creatine kinase, as well as lactate output were decreased in the coronary effluent of the perfused hearts. In addition, ramipril treatment preserved the energy-rich phosphates adenosine triphosphate (ATP) and creatine phosphate and increased glycogen concentrations in the myocardium. Almost identical results were obtained in isolated ischemic hearts after 2-week pretreatment of rats with a nonantihypertensive dose of 0.01 mg/kg/day ramipril.[79]

Furthermore, in guinea pigs, ramipril protected the hearts against cardiac arrhythmias induced by digoxin infusion.[80] However, *in vitro* studies did not

Table 80–2. **Clinical Trials Investigating the Effect of Short-term and Long-term Administration of Ramipril in Patients with Mild to Moderate Hypertension**

Study Design	Treatment Duration (weeks)	Dosage (mg)	No. of Patients	Mean Reduction in Supine/Sitting BP		Patients Responding (%)[a]	Reference
				Systolic (mmHg)	Diastolic (mmHg)		
Single-blind	2	5	10	16	12	80	Stumpe et al., 1986[57]
Double-blind Randomized	6	1.25 2.5 5	52 53 53	23 23 23	16 17 20	64 63 77	Walter et al., 1987[65]
Open	8	1.25→10	46	23	14	28→78	Fukiyama et al., 1987[66]
Open	3	1→1→1[b] 1→2→2 1→2→4	20	31 31 42	19 18 11	80	Felder and Witte, 1987[67]
Open	0.5–2	2.5→10 1.25→5[c]	18 21	16 20	7 12		Kaneko et al., 1987[59]
Double-blind Randomized	4	0 2.5 5	27 28 29	8 9 13	3 7 9	41 50 48	Villamil et al., 1987[68]
Single-blind	52	10[d]	10	44	30	60	De Leeuw and Birkenhager, 1987[69]
Randomized	4	5 10	11 12	14[e] 22[e]	3[e] 9[e]		Karlberg et al., 1987[25]
Open	2 104	5 1.25←5→10[f]	201 181[f]	29 28	21 22		Schreiner et al., 1991[71]
Double-blind	12	0 1.25 2.5 5 10	41 44 43 42 43	0.5 2.2 5 5.1 8.2	2.7 4.3 6.2 6.6 7.4		Kostis, 1991[70]
Single-blind	3	2.5	569	16.3	11.2	57	Carré et al., 1992[72]
	6 (3→3) 12 (3→3→3)	2.5→2.5 2.5→2.5→2.5	306 225	 4.7 vs 3w	 1.4 vs 3w	91 94	
	6 (3→3) 12 (3→3→3)	2.5→5 2.5→5→5	225 117	9.9 vs 3w 2.6 vs 6w	7.2 vs 3w 0.6 vs 6w	56 87	
Double-blind	12 (3→3→3) 12 (3→3→3)	2.5→5→10 2.5→5→5 + Di	38 38	8.9 vs 6w 11.5 vs 6w	8.1 vs 6w 8.2 vs 6w	45 47	

[a]Usual criteria for definition of response: diastolic blood pressure ≤ 90 mm Hg (Stumpe et al., 1986: ≤ 95 mmHg) and/or blood pressure reduction > 5 mmHg (Stumpe et al., 1987); ≥ 20/10 (Fukiyama et al., 1987); ≥ 10 mmHg (Villamil et al., 1987).
[b]Ramipril was administered twice daily. The dose of ramipril were doubled if reduction of diastolic blood pressure to ≤ 90 mmHg had not been achieved after 1 week treatment.
[c]Ramipril was administered twice daily.
[d]In four subjects, hydrochlorothiazide had to be added after 1 month.
[e]Blood pressure was measured 24 hours after drug intake.
[f]Treatment started with 5 mg of ramipril per day. Dosage was then adjusted in accordance with response to treatment. 1.25 mg: n = 6; 2.5 mg: n = 85; 5 mg: n = 79; 7.5 mg: n = 2; 10 mg: n = 9.
Di, diuretic; w, week.

provide evidence for a direct antiarrhythmic activity of ramipril, because the drug was without effect on action potentials of isolated guinea pig papillary muscle or rabbit sinus node.[80]

In another model of cardiac ischemia, hearts from guinea pigs and SHR were subjected to in vivo hypoxia followed by a 5-minute period of global in situ ischemia. Myocardial function was then determined ex vivo in isolated hearts.[81] Under these conditions, ramipril pretreatment improved external heart work by approximately 40% and increased cardiac output and maximal pressure development. The effects of the ACE inhibitor were attributed to an induction of prostacyclin synthesis because they were abolished by simultaneous administration of indomethacin.[81]

Free radicals generated during ischemia and reperfusion may cause myocardial injury. In isolated working rat hearts, ramipril protected against free radical–induced injury. However, this effect was only achieved at very high concentrations of 1.25×10^{-5} mol/L. The effects of ramipril were abolished by administration of indomethacin.[82]

Evidence has been accumulated that most of the effects of ramipril in ischemic hearts are mediated by potentiation of endogenous bradykinin actions as the result of ACE inhibition. Bradykinin is continuously formed in the isolated heart and can be measured in the coronary effluent.[83] The bradykinin outflow was found to be increased under ischemic conditions as well as after perfusion with ramiprilat.[83] Bradykinin in concentrations as low as 1×10^{-9} mol/L produced almost the same pattern of beneficial effects in the isolated ischemic rat heart as observed with ramipril.[84] In addition, combined perfusion with low concentrations of bradykinin (1×10^{-12} mol/L) and ramiprilat (2.6×10^{-9} mol/L), which were ineffective when applied alone, resulted in a marked reduction in the duration of ventricular fibrillation. The specificity of the bradykinin-mediated effects by ACE inhibition with ramiprilat is underlined by the fact that the octyl-ester of ramiprilat, which lacks any ACE inhibitory activity, did not produce cardioprotective effects in isolated ischemic rat hearts.[76] Furthermore, the cardiac effects of bradykinin, as well as of ramipril and ramiprilat, were obliterated by bradykinin receptor blockade.[75–77]

Inhibition of sympathetic transmission in the heart has to be considered as an additional factor involved in the cardiac actions of ramipril. In isolated hearts, ramipril reduced noradrenaline overflow upon ischemia[78, 85, 86] and antagonized the effects of sympathetic nerve stimulation on coronary flow and contractility.[87]

Long-term chronic ACE inhibition by ramipril does not induce a supernormal cardiac performance in a normal heart but improves cardiac function and metabolism under pathophysiologic conditions such as myocardial ischemia or cardiac hypertrophy induced by chronic hypertension. In a recent study, we demonstrated that ramipril did not affect myocardial function and metabolism in normoxic hearts isolated from normotensive Wistar rats even after 8 weeks of treatment at a high dose of 1 mg/kg/day.[19] On the other hand, long-term treatment of SHRSP with ramipril improved cardiac function and metabolism even at a low dose that did not affect the development of hypertension and left ventricular hypertrophy. In this study, SHRSP were treated prenatally and, subsequently, up to 20 weeks of age with ramipril at doses of 0.01 mg/kg/day and 1 mg/kg/day. After the end of the treatment period, the hearts were isolated and cardiac parameters were measured under normoxic conditions. The results demonstrated that ramipril produced almost identical changes in cardiodynamics and cardiac enzymatic and metabolic parameters as

observed in ischemic hearts after acute treatment with ramipril[19] (Fig. 80–3). These effects of the ACE inhibitor were due to bradykinin potentiation, because they were abolished by concomitant bradykinin receptor blockade (see Fig. 80–3). In a further study, under identical treatment conditions, ramipril was shown to induce myocardial capillary growth in SHR even at doses too low to affect the development of hypertension and left ventricular hypertrophy[55] (Fig. 80–4).

Experimental and clinical studies have demonstrated a protective role of ACE inhibitors, including ramipril, after acute myocardial infarction. Hartman et al.[88, 89] showed that treatment with ramiprilat reduced myocardial infarct size by approximately 50% when compared with vehicle-treated animals in an anesthetized rabbit model of acute coronary occlusion. This effect was shown to be independent of inhibition of angiotensin II synthesis, because direct stimulation of angiotensin II receptors by angiotensin II infusion, as well as angiotensin II receptor blockade with losartan, did not alter the degree of myocardial necrosis when compared with vehicle treatment. On the other hand, the effect of ramiprilat to reduce infarct size was abolished by concomitant blockade of bradykinin receptors, suggesting that bradykinin is

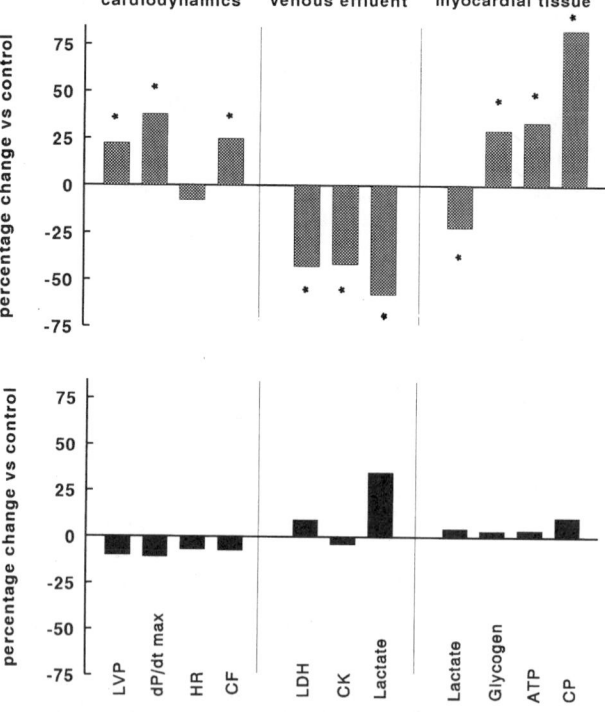

Figure 80–3. Effect of early-onset long-term oral treatment of stroke-prone spontaneously hypertensive rats with a subantihypertensive dose of 0.01 mg/kg per day ramipril alone *(dotted bars)* and after cotreatment with the bradykinin B_2-receptor antagonist Hoe 140 (500 μg/kg/day, SC) *(black bars)* on myocardial function and myocardial metabolism. LVP, left ventricular pressure; dP/dt max, differentiated left ventricular pressure; HR, heart rate; CF, coronary flow; LDH, lactate dehydrogenase; CK, creatine kinase; ATP, adenosine triphosphate; CP, creatine phosphate. * $p < .05$ compared with the vehicle-treated control group. (Adapted from Gohlke P, Linz W, Schölkens BA, et al: Angiotensin converting enzyme inhibition improves cardiac function: Role of bradykinin. Hypertension 23:411, 1994.)

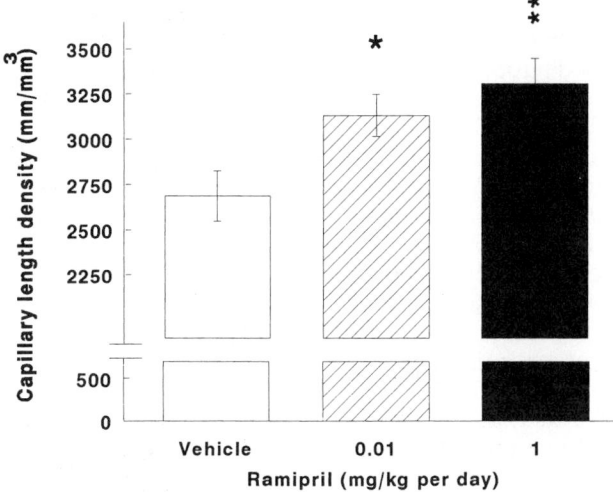

Figure 80–4. Effect of early-onset long-term treatment with two oral doses of ramipril in spontaneously hypertensive rats on myocardial capillary length density (LV cap/tiss) as determined with the orientator method. Data are mean ± SEM, n = 12 per group. * $p <$ .05, ** $p <$ .01. (Adapted from Unger T, Mattfeldt T, Lamberty V, et al: Effect of early onset ACE inhibition on myocardial capillaries in SHR. Hypertension 20:478, 1992.)

important for the myocardial protective actions of ramiprilat. Similar data were obtained in a study in anesthetized dogs, showing that ramiprilat reduced the myocardial infarct size induced by ligation of the left coronary artery for 6 hours. As in the studies by Hartman et al., the effects were reversed by bradykinin receptor blockade and, in addition, were mimicked by bradykinin infusion.[90]

Beneficial cardiac effects of ramipril were also observed in a dog model of acute left ventricular failure induced by repeated embolization. Administration of ramipril during acute ischemic left ventricular failure improved hemodynamics by a reduction in both preload and afterload parameters such as pulmonary capillary pressure, left ventricular end-diastolic pressure, and total peripheral resistance.[91]

The clinical importance of these cardiac effects of ramipril has been documented in a recent multicenter study (Acute Infarction Ramipril Efficacy [AIRE] Study).[92] In this study, ramipril was given to patients with clinical evidence of heart failure on the second to ninth day after myocardial infarction. Patients were followed up for an average of 15 months. The results showed a 27% reduction in all-cause mortality in patients who received ramipril as compared with placebo-treated patients. The effects on mortality became apparent within weeks after initiating treatment and continued to diverge from control (Fig. 80–5).

Hypertension-induced left ventricular hypertrophy (LVH) is an independent risk factor for cardiovascular diseases[93, 94] and is frequently associated with a diminished capillary density, leading to relative ischemia. These pathologic changes can predispose patients to myocardial ischemia and left ventricular failure. Thus, prevention or regression of LVH should be a primary goal in the long-term treatment of hypertensive hearts.

The effect of treatment with ramipril on the prevention and regression of LVH has been investigated in renally hypertensive rats with aortic banding. This form of hypertension-induced hypertrophy is characterized by a markedly activated RAS during the development of hypertension and cardiac hypertrophy (up to 6 weeks after aortic constriction) and normal plasma renin levels once LVH is established. Daily treatment of rats for 6 weeks with ramipril at an antihypertensive dose of 1 mg/kg/day and a subantihypertensive dose of 0.01 mg/kg/day was started either immediately after aortic constriction (prevention study) or 6 weeks after aortic constriction when cardiac hypertrophy had developed (regression study). Antihypertensive treatment with ramipril effectively reduced LVH in both the prevention and regression studies, whereas equipotent antihypertensive doses of the calcium antagonist nifedipine and the arterial vasodilator dihydralazine did not affect LVH when compared with control subjects.[53] Notably, the low dose of 0.01 mg/kg/day ramipril, although not affecting blood pressure, significantly reduced LVH.[53, 54] The effect of low- and high-dose ramipril on LVH could be abolished by chronic bradykinin receptor blockade in the prevention study but not in the regression study.[54, 95]

In a longer-term study (more than 1 year), ramipril at doses of 1 mg/kg/day and 0.01 mg/kg/day prevented the development of LVH as well as the development of myocardial fibrosis. Interestingly, LVH and myocardial fibrosis did not recur in animals during 6 months withdrawal of treatment.[96]

The antihypertrophic effects of ramipril were also tested in SHR and SHRSP, two models of genetic hypertension associated with normal to low plasma renin levels. In prevention studies, the animals were treated prenatally and subsequently up to 20 weeks of age with 1 mg/kg/day and 0.01 mg/kg/day of

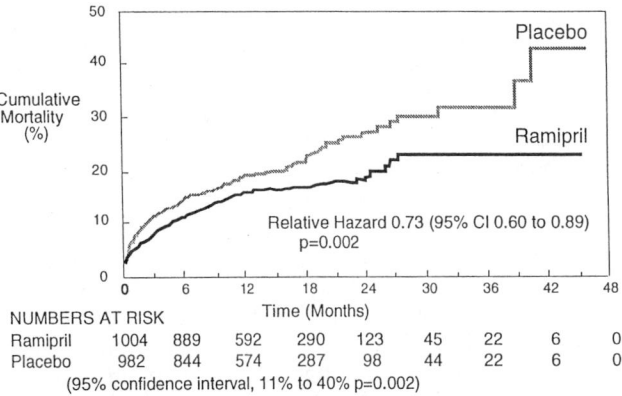

Figure 80–5. Effect of ramipril on mortality of survivors of acute myocardial infaction with clinical evidence of heart failure (AIRE study). Patients were randomly allocated to double-blind treatment with either placebo or ramipril on day 3 to 10 after acute myocardial infaction. Mortality curves illustrate the primary end point of all-cause mortality analyzed by intention to treat. (Adapted from The Acute Infarction Ramipril Efficacy (AIRE) Study Investigators: Effect of ramipril on mortality and morbidity of survivors of acute myocardial infarction with clinical evidence of heart failure. Lancet 342:821, 1993. © by The Lancet Ltd, 1993.)

ramipril.[19, 55] In a regression study, the same drug regimen was applied to 16-week-old SHR with established LVH and treatment was continued for a further 16 weeks.[97] In all studies, antihypertensive treatment with the high dose of ramipril prevented or reduced LVH. However, in contrast with rats with aortic banding, low-dose ramipril treatment did not affect LVH in the prevention study[19, 55] but reduced LVH in the regression study.[97] In addition, the degree of blood pressure reduction as well as the effects of ramipril on LVH were not influenced by chronic bradykinin receptor blockade, suggesting that bradykinin potentiation is less important for the antihypertrophic effects of ramipril in this type of genetic hypertension.[19]

Eichstaedt et al.[98] studied the regression of LVH in 32 hypertensive patients (diastolic blood pressure, > 95 mmHg) treated with ramipril (5 mg daily) for 3 months. The ACE inhibitor achieved a reduction in diastolic blood pressure to levels of 90 mmHg or lower in all patients and caused a significant reduction (approximately 22%) of LVH as demonstrated by nuclear magnetic resonance imaging as well as by echocardiography.

In a double-blind, placebo-controlled clinical study in hypertensive patients with echocardiographically detected LVH, ramipril at doses of 1.25 or 5 mg once daily caused a regression of LVH after 6 months of treatment. Because systolic and diastolic ambulatory blood pressures were not significantly decreased after the low dose, the effect on LVH appeared to be independent of the antihypertensive action of the ACE inhibitor. However, it is possible that these patients responded more sensitively to the ACE inhibitor because they had been pretreated with furosemide, leading to an activation of the RAS.[99]

Effects on Coronary Blood Flow

Numerous animal studies in isolated ischemic heart preparations have demonstrated that ramipril pretreatment or perfusion of isolated hearts with ramiprilat increased coronary blood flow.[73, 75–78] The results of some of these studies have already been described in the previous section. In these studies, the perfusion pressure was kept constant, and the effects of ramipril can best be explained by the decrease in coronary resistance caused by reversal of angiotensin II–mediated vasoconstriction or by enhanced bradykinin-induced vasodilation.

In contrast, in one study, ACE inhibitors, including ramipril, did not modify the distribution of regional myocardial blood flow in ischemic and nonischemic zones measured by radioactive microspheres during intermittent coronary artery occlusion in anesthetized dogs.[100]

Pretreatment of rats with ramipril at a dose of 1 mg/kg/day for 1 week was shown to reduce infarct size and total heart weight–to–body weight ratio and to increase myocardial blood flow after left coronary artery ligation when compared with vehicle-treated rats. These effects were mediated by potentiation of bradykinin, because they were prevented by bradyki-

nin B2-receptor blockade but remained unaltered after angiotensin AT1-receptor blockade. An improved blood supply to the marginal zone of the infarct most likely contributed to the reduction of infarct size.[101]

In isolated normoxic rabbit hearts perfused under constant flow conditions, bradykinin induced a coronary vasodilation with a maximal reduction in coronary perfusion pressure of 27%, which was associated with an enhanced release of 6-keto-PGF$_{1\alpha}$, the stable metabolite of prostacyclin, from the coronary bed. Both effects were enhanced after a 30-minute infusion of ramiprilat $(3 \times 10^{-7}$ M$)$.[102] Furthermore, pretreatment of guinea pigs with 10 mg/kg ramipril enhanced the bradykinin-induced increase in coronary flow in normoxic hearts isolated 1 hour after drug administration.[103] This effect was attenuated by the addition of the proteinase inhibitor aprotinin.

Comparable effects were also observed in normoxic isolated hearts of SHRSP excised after long-term treatment with ramipril. In this study, ramipril caused an increase in coronary blood flow even at a dose of 0.01 mg/kg/day, which was too low to affect the development of hypertension and LVH[19] (see Fig. 80–3). In this study and in some of the previously mentioned studies, the action of ramipril on coronary blood flow could be attributed to bradykinin potentiation, because the effects were abolished by bradykinin receptor blockade (see Fig. 80–3). The effect of the ACE inhibitor on coronary blood flow may also explain our observations of an increased capillary length density in hearts of SHR after long-term treatment with ramipril at doses of 1 mg/kg/day and 0.01 mg/kg/day (see Fig. 80–4).

Together, these animal studies almost unequivocally demonstrate that ramipril induces an increase in coronary blood flow under *in vitro* and *ex vivo* conditions in ischemic and nonischemic isolated hearts, and that this effect is most likely due to bradykinin potentiation.

Human studies on the effect of ramipril on coronary blood flow are scarce as yet. In 11 patients with congestive heart failure, ramipril produced a slight but nonsignificant increase in coronary blood flow from 116 ± 25 to 128 ± 29 ml/min.[28]

Effects on Arteries and Veins

The vascular wall is one of the most important target sites for ACE inhibitors, because ACE has been shown to be predominantly localized at the luminal side of the vascular endothelium.[104–106] Ramipril inhibited ACE activity in different vessel homogenates after acute or chronic oral administration[7, 9–12] and inhibited the contractile responses to angiotensin I in isolated artery strips.[107, 108] Furthermore, ramipril completely blocked the conversion of intraluminally instilled angiotensin I to angiotensin II in the isolated rabbit thoracic aorta.[106] In the same *in vitro* model, ramipril was shown to attenuate vascular bradykinin breakdown, not only by inhibition of endothelial ACE but also by inhibition of other bradykinin-degrading enzymes in deeper layers of the vascular wall.[109] Intraluminal administration of radioactively labeled ramiprilat into the isloated rabbit thoracic aorta revealed a quick diffusion of the ACE inhibitor through the vascular wall with an accumulation in the endothelium[105] (Fig. 80–6).

Ramipril was shown to exert beneficial effects on the vasculature during pathophysiologic situations such as hypertension, hyperlipidemia, and atherosclerosis.

The development of hypertension is associated with structural and functional changes of the vascular wall. Structural alterations include the development of medial hypertrophy and/or hyperplasia of small and large arteries and the loss of microvessels. Func-

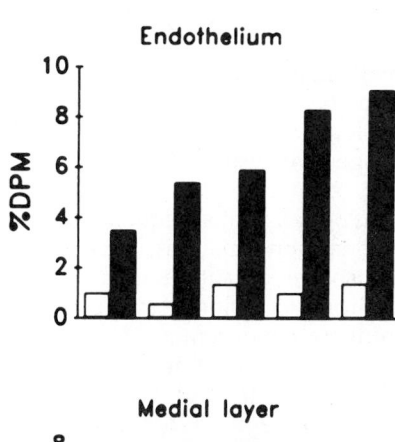
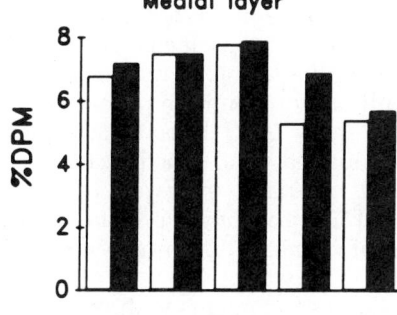
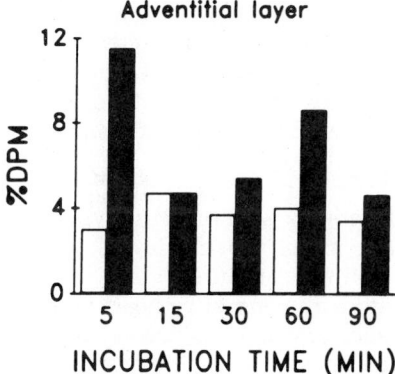

Figure 80–6. Time-dependent distribution of radioactivity in the vascular wall after administration of 3H-ramiprilat into the lumen of the rabbit thoracic aorta at two concentrations of 10^{-7} mol/L *(white columns)* and 10^{-9} mol/L *(black columns)*. The radioactivity at the start of each incubation period was taken as 100%, and the results were expressed as the percentage amount of radioactivity. (From Gohlke P, Unger T, Bünning P: Distribution of the angiotensin converting enzyme inhibitor ramiprilat in the blood vessel wall. Pharm Pharmacol Lett 2:66, 1992.)

tional changes of the vasculature are characterized by endothelial dysfunction, including an impaired endothelium-dependent relaxation to different agonists such as acetylcholine and bradykinin.

Long-term early-onset treatment of SHR with ramipril prevented the development of medial hyperplasia in mesenteric arteries as demonstrated by the decreased media-to-lumen ratio and the decreased number of smooth muscle layers in the medial layer.[110] The effect appeared to be dependent on the blood pressure–lowering action of the ACE inhibitor, because low-dose, subantihypertensive treatment with ramipril had no effect on vascular structure. On the other hand, in adult SHR with established vascular structural alterations, ramipril did not affect mesenteric vascular hyperplasia even after treatment for 16 weeks at antihypertensive doses.[97] However, despite the lack of effect on vascular structure of resistance vessels, ramipril treatment altered vascular function of compliance vessels as demonstrated by a decreased vasoconstrictor response of aortic strips to norepinephrine and a decreased vasodilator response to acetylcholine.[97] The beneficial effect of ramipril on vascular function was apparent even after low-dose treatment with 0.01 mg/kg/day, which had no effect on blood pressure. Similar results were obtained after long-term early-onset treatment of SHR and SHRSP with ramipril at doses of 0.01 mg/kg/day and 1 mg/kg/day.[108] In addition, ramipril increased aortic cyclic guanosine monophosphate (cGMP) content as a marker for nitric oxide production after long-term treatment of SHRSP independently of its antihypertensive action.[108] Furthermore, acute administration of ramipril to normotensive rats stimulated prostacyclin synthesis in the isolated rat aorta.[111] The effects on vascular cGMP and prostacyclin were found to be secondary to changes in the kinin system.

In further studies in cultured human and bovine endothelial cells, ramiprilat dose- and time-dependently increased the formation of both nitric oxide and prostacyclin[112, 113] and caused a long-lasting increase in resting intracellular calcium.[113] Again, the effects were due to the bradykinin-potentiating action of ramipril, because they were abolished by bradykinin receptor blockade. Thus, results from *in vivo* and *in vitro* studies suggest that ramipril can improve vasodilator capacity by potentiation of bradykinin-induced formation of nitric oxide and prostacyclin.

Animal experiments also revealed an attenuation of the atherosclerotic process by ACE inhibitor treatment. The development of atherosclerosis is associated with endothelial dysfunction characterized by an attenuated relaxation of atherosclerotic vessels to endothelium-dependent agents. For example, in rabbits fed an atherogenic diet, relaxation to acetylcholine in aortic rings was shown to be markedly attenuated, whereas endothelium-independent relaxation to nitroglycerin was not altered.[114, 115] Treatment with ramipril (3 mg/kg/day) preserved the endothelium-dependent relaxation to acetylcholine and prevented the reduction of basal aortic cGMP content.[114, 115] Moreover, ramipril treatment led to an increase in the plasma high-density lipoprotein (HDL) cholesterol fraction without affecting low-density lipoprotein (LDL) and very-low-density lipoprotein (VLDL) cholesterol fractions or total cholesterol.[114, 116] The improvement of aortic function by ramipril appeared to be independent of morphologic changes induced by atherogenic diet, because ramipril did not affect the percentage of aortic surface covered with lipid streaks.[114]

Ramipril has been shown to inhibit neointima formation in response to endothelial injury in rat arteries.[117, 118] The ACE inhibitor was significantly more effective compared with the angiotensin AT_1-receptor antagonist losartan, and the effect was markedly attenuated after blockade of bradykinin receptors.[117, 118] Thus, the effect of ramipril on neointima formation can be attributed to both inhibition of angiotensin II formation and kinin degradation.

Endocrine and Metabolic Effects

As a consequence of inhibition of ACE activity at different target sites, ramipril markedly influences the RAS as well as the kallikrein-kinin system. As outlined previously, ramipril reduces the formation of angiotensin II from angiotensin I, with subsequent activation of renin release from the kidney and an enhanced consumption of angiotensinogen. As angiotensin II is a potent stimulus for aldosterone secretion from the adrenals, inhibition of ACE by ramipril treatment causes a decrease in plasma aldosterone. The second major consequence of ACE inhibition by ramipril is the reduction of bradykinin degradation, because ACE is one of the most important bradykinin-degrading enzymes. Some effects of ACE inhibitor–induced bradykinin potentiation are reported in previous sections.

Ramipril was shown to exert no adverse effects on glucose and lipid metabolism. In diabetic and insulin-resistant hypertensive patients, administration of ramipril did not alter plasma lipid levels of LDL and VLDL cholesterol and triglycerides, and total cholesterol was unaltered or slightly decreased. HDL cholesterol was either unaltered or even increased after ramipril.[119–121] In a clinical study in 86 insulin-resistant hypertensive patients, 2 weeks of treatment with different ACE inhibitors, including ramipril (5 mg daily), improved insulin sensitivity as demonstrated by a fasting sample intravenous glucose tolerance test. Plasma insulin and plasma glucose levels were within the normal range in all groups of patients.[121] In another study, short-term treatment with ramipril did not influence glucose tolerance, insulin secretion, and insulin sensitivity in nondiabetic patients.[122]

In experimental studies in rabbits fed an atherogenic diet, ramipril treatment resulted in an increase in plasma HDL cholesterol levels, whereas plasma LDL, VLDL, and total cholesterol remained unchanged.[114, 115]

Effects on Renal Function

Animal studies have shown that ramipril can increase renal blood flow and decrease renal vascular resistance even at doses that had no effect on blood pressure or total peripheral resistance, as discussed in the section on hemodynamics.[8, 47]

In anesthetized dogs, acute IV administration of ramiprilat decreased blood pressure, followed by renal vasodilation and an increase in glomerular ultrafiltration coefficient. The effect on renal vasodilation was demonstrated by increased single nephron glomerular as well as total renal blood flow and decreased afferent and efferent arteriolar resistance. Bradykinin receptor antagonism did not affect the ACE inhibitor actions in dogs fed a normal sodium diet. However, in sodium-depleted dogs, the effects of ramipril on renal blood flow and glomerular ultrafiltration coefficient were found to be more pronounced and were attenuated by bradykinin B_2-receptor blockade.[123]

In human subjects, renal function with ramipril treatment has been studied under normal as well as pathophysiologic conditions such as primary hypertension, congestive heart failure, renal insufficiency, or diabetes.

Primary hypertension is frequently associated with renal functional abnormalities. This has been attributed to a disorder of autoregulatory control of the cortical nephron blood flow.[124] In a placebo-controlled study, administration of ramipril (10 mg daily) for 2 to 4 weeks to seven patients with primary hypertension lowered blood pressure and caused a significant increase in cortical nephron flow. The percentage of flow to cortical nephrons increased by 6%.[125] These data suggested that ramipril can correct the reduced cortical nephron flow found in primary hypertension. In a further study in 21 hypertensive patients with normal or impaired renal function, ramipril at doses of 2.5 to 10 mg daily increased renal blood flow despite a fall in mean blood pressure and markedly reduced renal vascular resistance by 43% after a treatment period of 12 weeks.[126]

Several studies in patients with primary hypertension have demonstrated that acute administration of ramipril at doses of 2.5 to 20 mg had no effect on urinary excretion of sodium, creatinine, or potassium.[20, 56, 58] Similar results were obtained after long-term treatment with ramipril at doses of 1.25 to 20 mg daily. The ACE inhibitor, at therapeutic doses, did not cause any clinically relevant changes in laboratory variables.[65, 127–129] For example, during a 1-year clinical trial in 331 patients with primary hypertension, ramipril did not affect plasma levels of sodium, potassium, creatinine, and urea.[128]

In patients with congestive heart failure, a deterioration of renal function has been observed with ACE inhibitor treatment.[130, 131] The effect can be explained by the importance of the RAS for the renal adaptation to cardiac failure and can be controlled by careful individual dosing and avoidance of volume depletion.

In a study by Crozier et al.,[28] 10 patients with severe congestive heart failure stabilized on digitalis and furosemide were treated with 10 and 20 mg ramipril on two consecutive days. The ACE inhibitor caused a marked increase in renal blood flow (93%) and a decrease in renal vascular resistance (52%) accompanied by a decrease in glomerular filtration rate (29%) 2 hours after the first dose. The effects were attributed to a reversal of angiotensin II–mediated vasoconstriction of the efferent arteriole. Furthermore, urinary sodium and potassium excretion tended to decrease and plasma urea and plasma creatinine levels tended to increase after acute ramipril treatment, although the changes were not significant. After 7 weeks of therapy, the NYHA functional class improved from 3.4 to 1.8, and plasma creatinine levels returned to control values. In one of the patients, renal impairment developed that was reversible after reduction of both the furosemide and the ramipril doses. In further long-term studies in patients with congestive heart failure, no renal impairment was observed after administration of ramipril at a dose of 5 mg for 10 to 12 weeks.[51, 132] Furthermore, plasma creatinine and potassium levels remained stable during ramipril treatment.

Several clinical studies have investigated the effect of acute and chronic adminstration of ramipril to hypertensive patients with various degrees of renal failure.[44, 45, 126, 133] Ramipril decreased blood pressure in all groups, unrelated to renal function, although plasma ramipril levels were higher in patients with severe renal failure.[44, 45] Serum creatinine levels remained unchanged after ramipril treatment, and a slight increase in serum potassium was found in one study. After 12 weeks of treatment with ramipril at doses of 2.5 to 10 mg daily, the glomerular filtration rate increased in patients with impaired renal function from a mean of 62 to 89 ml/min per 1.73 m^2.[126] In 23 patients with glomerulonephritis and nephrotic syndrome, proteinuria was significantly reduced from 10.4 to 8.4 g/day after 24 weeks of ramipril therapy at low doses of 1.25 mg every alternate day up to 2.5 mg daily.[134] Apart from a slight but reversible deterioration in renal function after 2 weeks, there were no negative effects on renal functions over the 24-week treatment period.

ACE inhibition in patients with bilateral renal artery stenosis or stenosis of the renal artery of a solitary kidney may cause renal dysfunction because the RAS plays a crucial role in the regulation of glomerular filtration rate when perfusion pressure is low. In patients with unilateral renal artery stenosis, it has been suggested that ACE inhibition may cause a deterioration of the stenosed kidney function, which will remain unnoticed in the presence of a normal contralateral kidney. Tillman et al.[29] studied the effect of ramipril treatment on three hypertensive patients with unilateral renal artery stenosis. The ACE inhibitor was administered for 4 weeks at a high dose of 20 mg daily. There was little change in renal plasma flow on the stenotic side, but filtration fraction was reduced in two patients. Serum potassium and urea were slightly increased, with no change in serum potassium and creatinine. The glomerular filtration rate was not consistently changed by ramipril treatment.

The long-term prognosis of diabetic patients is associated with the development of diabetic nephropathy. Effective blood pressure reduction with β-blockers and diuretics has been shown to improve survival in diabetic nephropathy.[135] ACE inhibitors like ramipril may have advantages in the treatment of hypertension in insulin-dependent and non-insulin-dependent diabetic patients because of the lack of adverse effects on glucose and lipid metabolism.[119, 120] Moreover, ACE inhibitors may exert additional beneficial actions in diabetic nephropathy as a result of reduction of efferent arteriolar resistance accompanied by a reduction in hydraulic pressure within the glomerular capillaries. In a double-blind crossover study in 10 insulin-dependent diabetic patients with early diabetic nephropathy, ramipril (5 mg) or placebo was added to ongoing antihypertensive treatment with β-blockers and diuretics for a period of 4 months.[136] The addition of ramipril resulted in a significant reduction of the rate of urinary albumin excretion and fractional albumin excretion. Renal resistance was reduced, whereas renal plasma flow tended to increase and glomerular filtration rate remained unchanged. Ambulatory blood pressure measurements revealed no further blood pressure reduction after ramipril. In a further 6-week study in insulin-dependent diabetic patients with early diabetic nephropathy, ramipril was administered at doses of 1.25 and 5 mg daily.[137] Both doses reduced the urinary albumin excretion rate, which correlated with changes in filtration rate. Blood pressure was reduced only after 5 mg ramipril. Thus, the reducing effect of ramipril on urinary albumin excretion rate appeared to be unrelated to blood pressure changes.

Effects on the Central Nervous System

The presence of a complete intrinsic brain RAS is now firmly established.[138] Brain angiotensin has been implicated in central cardiovascular and osmotic control by influencing hormone release from the pituitary gland, sympathetic activity, autonomic reflexes, and renal salt excretion. A stimulated RAS has been suggested to contribute to the maintenance of hypertension in SHR.[138] Inhibition of angiotensin II generation in the central nervous system by intracerebroventricular application of different ACE inhibitors including ramiprilat lowered blood pressure in SHR and SHRSP as well as in renal hypertensive rats.[139–142] In addition, centrally administered ramiprilat was shown to sensitize the baroreceptor reflex in SHR.[143]

However, the effects of ACE inhibition in the brain comprise more than a reduction in angiotensin II, because ACE acts on several peptide substrates that all are present in the brain, including kinins, substance P, and enkephalins.[144] Thus, ACE inhibitors may exert a number of angiotensin-related or unrelated actions in the central nervous system, even an improvement of cognitive function, as suggested by animal studies. Furthermore, cognitive enhancing effects in mice and rats were observed after peripheral application of ramiprilat-octil, a substance closely related to ramiprilat but without inhibitory effect on plasma ACE.[145, 146] These studies suggest that ramipril may exert central effects independently of its ACE inhibitory action.

However, it is still controversial whether or not ACE inhibitors gain access to the central nervous system on systemic administration. Several animal studies have demonstrated a significant inhibition of ACE activity in tissue homogenates of different brain regions after oral administration of ramipril.[9, 10, 13, 14] A better approach for measuring access of orally applied ACE inhibitors to the central nervous system is the determination of ACE inhibition in the cerebrospinal fluid (CSF), because interferences with blood plasma and brain vasculature can be ruled out. Using this approach, we have demonstrated that ramipril penetrates the blood-brain barrier in sufficient amounts to inhibit ACE activity in CSF 1 hour after acute oral administration to rats within a dose range of 3 to 10 mg/kg.[3, 14] The presence of ramipril in the CSF was also demonstrated by the inhibitory effect on an enzyme reaction mixture of heat-inactivated CSF from ramipril-treated rats.[3, 42] Moreover, ramipril can be partly hydrolyzed to ramiprilat within the CSF. This was demonstrated by comparison of the IC_{50} values of ramipril in CSF (100 nmol/L) and purified ACE from rabbit lung (2500 nmol/L).[3] Ramiprilat was shown to be a highly potent inhibitor of ACE in CSF, with an IC_{50} value of 0.5 nmol/L.[3]

Human studies on the central nervous system effects of ramipril are still lacking.

CLINICAL USE
Indications

Ramipril has become an established agent in the treatment of mild, moderate, and severe hypertension. As outlined in "Effects on Hemodynamics," ramipril decreases elevated systemic vascular resistance without induction of reflex sympathetic activation and without development of tolerance. Several clinical trials have demonstrated the short- and long-term antihypertensive efficacy of ramipril monotherapy at oral doses of 2.5 to 10 mg once daily (see Table 80–2). Significant 24-hour blood pressure reduction was achieved by once-daily ramipril without interference with normal circadian blood pressure pattern as shown by 24-hour blood pressure monitoring (see "Effects on Hemodynamics").

When compared with other antihypertensive agents, ACE inhibitors like ramipril offer additional advantages in hypertensive patients with concomitant diseases like renal impairment, diabetes mellitus, or LVH, as is outlined in "Use in Patients with Impaired Organ Function."

Like other ACE inhibitors, ramipril has proved to be useful in the treatment of congestive heart failure. The acute hemodynamic effects of ramipril in patients with congestive heart failure are given in "Effects on Hemodynamics." Besides a reduction in peripheral vascular resistance and mean arterial blood pressure,

ramipril reduced pulmonary artery pressure and pulmonary capillary wedge pressure and increased cardiac output. During long-term treatment of patients with congestive heart failure (NYHA functional class III–IV) pretreated with digitalis and diuretics, ramipril exerted similar hemodynamic action as observed after short-term treatment, i.e., ramipril increased ejection fraction and cardiac index and improved NYHA functional class and exercise duration.[28, 51]

The results of the AIRE study (see "Effects on Ventricular Function and Structure") revealed that patients with acute myocardial infarction and clinical evidence of heart failure will benefit, *quoad vitam*, from treatment with ramipril. In this study, a substantial reduction in premature deaths from all causes was obtained in patients with clinical evidence of heart failure after myocardial infarction when treatment with ramipril was initiated between the second and ninth days after myocardial infarction. The effects on mortality became apparent within weeks after initiating therapy.[92]

Precautions and Adverse Effects

Several clinical trials have shown that ramipril is a well-tolerated and safe drug in the long-term treatment of hypertension. The incidence of adverse effects was generally low, and the nature and severity of adverse effects were comparable with those of other ACE inhibitors.[34, 71, 72, 128, 147] Table 80–3 summarizes the typical side-effect profile of ramipril observed in four clinical trials.

Headache, dizziness, and nausea have been reported to be common adverse effects associated with ramipril. However, in a double-blind placebo-controlled study, their incidence rates were equal or even below those observed with placebo.[34]

Cough is the most frequently occurring, class-specific adverse effect of ramipril. The variation in the incidence of cough after ramipril treatment (see Table 80–3) may be due to differences in assessment: Cough, although present, is frequently not recognized as a side effect associated with ACE inhibitor treatment. On the other hand, cough due to intercurrent respiratory infections may be falsely ascribed to ACE inhibitor treatment. The highest incidence of cough (4.3%) was reported in the study by Carré et al.,[72] in which cough was investigated by direct questioning. In this study, the incidence of cough was not influenced by age, smoking, or respiratory tract disease and was higher in women than in men.

Angioneurotic edema is a very rare class-specific side effect of ramipril (see Table 80–3) but is particularly important because of the potential dangerous consequences.

Taste disturbance is also a very rare event in patients treated with ramipril. In a case report, replacement of captopril by ramipril abolished the captopril-induced taste disturbance and weight loss.[148]

Analysis of laboratory parameters during clinical trials did not reveal significant variations.[71, 72, 128]

Table 80–3. **Clinical Trials Investigating the Most Frequent Adverse Effects of Ramipril in Patients with Mild to Moderate Hypertension**

Adverse Effect	Carré et al.[72] (1992) n = 770, %	Schreiner et al.[71] (1991) n = 426, %	Todd and Benfield[34] (1990) n = 2211, %	Bauer et al.[128] (1989) n = 331, %	Kaplan et al.[147] (1993) n = 593, %
Cough	4.3	0.2	0.9	1.8	2.4
Headache	1.7	0.5	3.2	2.7	1.2
Dizziness	1.7	4.7	3.4	5.1	1.7
Fatigue/weakness	—	—	1.9	—	0.5
Asthenia	2.5	1.4	—	3.6	—
Nausea	1.0	2.6	1.7	—	—
Rash	—	0.2	0.6	—	—
Skin disorders	—	—	—	1.5	—
Gastrointestinal pain/disorder	—	0.7	0.6	2.7	0.3
Diarrhea	0.5	—	0.4	0.3	—
Hypotension	—	—	0.4	—	—
Pruritus	0.1	—	0.3	—	—
Taste disturbance	—	—	0.1	—	—
Heart problems	—	—	—	1.5	0.3
Insomnia	—	—	—	—	0.8
Cramps	0.5	—	—	—	—
Angioneurotic edema	—	—	0.05	—	—

Moreover, no cases of neutropenia attributable to ramipril treatment were observed.[72]

Hypotension has been rarely observed in hypertensive patients, especially shortly after initiation of therapy. The risk of symptomatic hypotension is higher in patients with volume and salt depletion (e.g., prolonged diuretic pretreatment, dietary salt restriction) and in patients with congestive heart failure. Therefore, diuretic treatment should be discontinued before starting ramipril therapy, and treatment of patients with severe congestive heart failure should be initiated under clinical supervision. Generally, the initial dose of ramipril should be reduced in these cases. Dosage adjustment also is required in patients with preexisting renal insufficiency, together with a close monitoring of renal function. The risk of renal impairment is also increased in patients with congestive heart failure and, in particular, in patients with bilateral renal artery stenosis or renal artery stenosis in a solitary kidney as well as after kidney transplantation. In cases of hepatic impairment plasma levels of the parent drug, ramipril, may increase as a result of a diminished hepatic metabolization to ramiprilat.

The risk of hyperkalemia is increased in patients with renal insufficiency and during concomitant treatment with potassium-sparing diuretics.

Contraindications

Contraindications to ramipril include cases of hypersensitivity to ramipril as well as a history of angioneurotic edema. Prescription of ramipril to patients with bilateral renal artery stenosis or renal artery stenosis in a solitary kidney as well as after kidney transplantation may be hazardous. Furthermore, ramipril should not be used in patients with primary hyperaldosteronism. In view of the absence of adequate clinical studies, ramipril should not be given to pregnant and breastfeeding women or to children.

Interference with Other Drugs

In an open-label study in 12 normotensive healthy volunteers receiving steady-state digoxin medication, ramipril (5 mg once daily) was coadministered for 14 days. There were no significant differences in serum digoxin levels throughout the treatment period as well as after withdrawal of ramipril.[43] Thus, ramipril does not affect digoxin serum levels in healthy volunteers.

Ramipril also did not affect the anticoagulant activity of acenocoumarol or phenprocoumon when coadministered at a dose of 5 mg once daily. This has been demonstrated in a placebo-controlled study[149] in 25 patients pretreated with acenocoumarol or phenprocoumon for at least 3 months before concomitant ramipril treatment as well as in a study by Verho et al.[150] after coadiministration of ramipril and phenprocoumon.

Other human studies have shown no effect of concomitant antacid administration on the pharmacokinetics of ramipril as well as no pharmacodynamic and pharmacokinetic interactions between indomethacin and ramipril (data on file, Hoechst). Concomitant treatment of ramipril with potassium-sparing diuretics may increase the risk of hyperkalemia, particularly in patients with renal insufficiency.

Combination of ramipril with other antihypertensive agents enhances their antihypertensive responses. The effects of diuretics are based on increased sodium and water loss resulting in a diminished blood volume with subsequent activation of the RAS and the sympathetic nervous system, both of which can compromise the antihypertensive action of these drugs. Coadministration of an ACE inhibitor like ramipril inhibits the RAS and, to a lesser extent, the sympathetic nervous system and thus enhances the antihypertensive actions of diuretics. In a double-blind, comparative multicenter study in patients with mild to moderate hypertension, the combination of ramipril 5 mg plus hydrochlorothiazide 25 mg was compared with ramipril monotherapy (5 or 10 mg).[151] Patients were pretreated with ramipril (2.5 to 5 mg) for 4 weeks, and those patients whose diastolic blood pressures were still higher than 90 mmHg were included in the study. During the 4 weeks of treatment, the mean reductions in supine systolic and diastolic blood pressures were more pronounced in the combination group (11.6/10.6 mmHg at end point) as compared with ramipril 5 mg (6.2/5.9 mmHg at end point) and ramipril 10 mg (7.4/7.1 mmHg at end point). No relevant changes in serum triglyceride, cholesterol, and blood glucose levels as well as in hematologic, biochemical, or electrolyte values were detected in this study.

Use in Patients with Impaired Organ Function

In patients with impaired renal function, ramipril increased renal blood flow and glomerular filtration rate after 12 weeks of treatment.[126] Furthermore, proteinuria was reduced in patients with glomerulonephritis and nephrotic syndrom[134] (see "Effects on Renal Function").

In patients with early diabetic nephropathy, ramipril reduced urinary albumin excretion rate and fractional albumin excretion without affecting glomerular filtration rate.[136, 137] Furthermore, no adverse effects on glucose and lipid metabolism have been observed after ramipril administration[119, 120] (see "Effects on Re-

nal Function"). In addition, ramipril was shown to cause effective regression of LVH in hypertensive patients, even at doses that do not affect blood pressure[99, 152] (see "Effects on Ventricular Structure and Function").

Place in Antihypertensive Arsenal

In double-blind, randomized clinical trials in patients with mild to moderate hypertension, the antihypertensive action of ramipril was compared with other ACE inhibitors (captopril, enalapril, and lisinopril) as well as with the β-blocker atenolol and the calcium antagonist nitrendipine (Table 80–4). The results revealed similar antihypertensive efficacy of ramipril when compared with the other antihypertensive agents at the dosage regimen used (see Table 80–4).[127, 151, 153–156] Most studies showed comparable response rates to either antihypertensive drug therapy. In the study by Koenig et al.,[154] ramipril 2.5 mg once daily was as effective as lisinopril 10 mg once daily in reducing systolic and diastolic blood pressures (27/15 mmHg and 23/11 mmHg, respectively). However, the responder rate on ramipril 2.5 mg was higher than on lisinopril 10 mg (66% versus 47%). Moreover, ramipril appeared to be better tolerated than lisinopril. The incidence of adverse effects after exclusion of patients who had already reported adverse effects during placebo treatment was 24% on ramipril and 44% on lisinopril.[154] Similarly, comparison of once-daily administration of ramipril 5 mg and nitrendipine 20 mg showed higher response rates on ramipril

Table 80–4. **Double-blind Clinical Trials Comparing and Combining the Effects of Ramipril with Other Antihypertensive Drugs in Patients with Mild to Moderate Hypertension**

Drug	Treatment Duration (weeks)	Dosage (mg)	No. of Patients	Mean Reduction in Supine BP (mm Hg)		Patients Responding (%)[b]	Reference
				Systolic[a]	Diastolic[a]		
Comparative studies							
Ramipril	6	1 × 10	129	20	15	65	Witte and Walter, 1987[127]
Captopril		2 × 50	119	17	14	65	
Ramipril	8	1 × 5–10	90	15–17	11	55	Zabludowski et al., 1988[153]
Enalapril		1 × 10–20	88	15–17	11	59	
Ramipril	4	1 × 2.5	58	27	15	67	Koenig et al., 1992[154]
Lisinopril		1 × 5	34	3	2	—	
		1 × 10	55	23	11	49	
Ramipril	6	1 × 10	69	21	15	71	Data on file, Hoechst
Atenolol		1 × 100	70	19	14	71	
Ramipril	12		28	16	9	43	Lenox-Smith et al., 1991[155]
Atenolol			29	13	9	41	
Ramipril[c]	6	1 × 5	26	13	11	58	Weidmann et al., 1992[156]
Nitrendipine		1 × 20	26	8	8	35	
Combination studies							
Ramipril	6	1 × 5	87	20	12	59	Data on file, Hoechst
R + Piretanide		1 × R5 + P3	84	22	15	69	
Ramipril[d]		1 × 5	54	6	6	48	Heidbreder et al., 1992[151]
		1 × 10	53	7	7	62	
R + Hydrochlorothiazide		1 × R5 + H25	57	12	11	72	

[a]Pressure reduction compared with baseline after a 4-week run-in period on placebo.
[b]Usual criteria for definition of response: diastolic blood pressure, ≤ 90 mmHg.
[c]This study was carried out by practicing physicians.
[d]Patients were intially treated single-blind for 1 week with ramipril 2.5 mg and 3 weeks with ramipril 5 mg.
Nonresponders (diastolic BP > 90 mmHg) were randomized to one of the three double-blind treatments.

than on nitrendipine (58% versus 35%) with fewer adverse effects.[156]

In a double-blind, randomized crossover study in 20 patients with mild hypertension (diastolic blood pressure, 90 to 104), the antihypertensive efficacy of ramipril 5 mg and enalapril 10 mg were compared by noninvasive, 24-hour ambulatory blood pressure monitoring.[157] The results demonstrated comparable reductions in 24-hour systolic and diastolic blood pressures after ramipril and enalapril (10/5 versus 4/4 mmHg).[157]

In further clinical trials, the addition of the diuretics piretanide (3 mg) or hydrochlorothiazide (25 mg) to ramipril (5 mg) therapy has been demonstrated to be more effective than ramipril alone (see Table 80–4). Moreover, combination therapy with ramipril (5 mg) plus hydrochlorothiazide (25 mg) appeared to be more effective than doubling the ramipril dosage to 10 mg[151] (see Table 80–4). Furthermore, addition of ramipril was shown to prevent or attenuate the adverse effects that occurred during diuretic (hydrochlorothiazide 25 or 50 mg once daily) monotherapy.[158]

Thus, ramipril has been established as an effective, safe, and well-tolerated modern antihypertensive drug, which may have some advantages over its competitors of the same and other drug classes with respect to unwarranted effects. As with other ACE inhibitors, the combination of ramipril with diuretics improves its antihypertensive action.

Dosage and Administration

The usual therapeutic doses of ramipril range from 2.5 to 10 mg once daily. In hypertensive patients not receiving diuretics, the recommended initial dosage is 2.5 mg once daily. Depending on the patient's response, dosage can be increased at intervals of 1 to 2 weeks to 5 mg and up to a maximum of 10 mg once daily. Diuretic treatment should be discontinued 2 to 3 days before starting ramipril therapy. If discontinuation of diuretic therapy is not possible, the starting dose of ramipril should be decreased to 1.25 mg once daily to avoid symptomatic hypotension.

In patients with renal impairment, dosage adjustment is necessary because of the decreased rate of elimination of the active metabolite, ramiprilat. In patients with mild to moderate renal impairment (creatinine clearance, $\leq$ 30 ml/min; serum creatinine, $\geq$ 165 μmol/L), the initial dose of ramipril should be 1.25 mg once daily and can be increased up to a maximum of 5 mg once daily. In patients with severe renal impairment (creatinine clearance, $\leq$ 10 ml/min; serum creatinine, 400 to 650 μmol/L), the recommended initial dose is also 1.25 mg once daily; the maximal dose should not exceed 2.5 mg once daily.

SOCIOECONOMIC CONSIDERATIONS
Compliance with Regimen

Ramipril can be administered to patients in relatively low doses of 2.5 to 10 mg once daily to achieve therapeutic efficacy. The possibility of once-daily dosage and the fact that ramipril is well tolerated, effective, and safe facilitate the compliance with the drug.

Cost

In general, the costs of drug therapy using ACE inhibitors are higher when compared with diuretics, β-blockers, or digitalis. However, the higher treatment costs may be offset by greater effectiveness of ACE inhibitors with respect to reducing end-organ damage, e.g., in reversing left ventricular hypertrophy. This has been suggested by a study that evaluated the long-term cost effectiveness of treatment of patients with hypertension and associated left ventricular hypertrophy from pooled data of 25 studies.[159] In this study, the overall costs of antihypertensive treatment were estimated, including average costs of drug therapy and follow-up care as well as direct costs of lost productivity owing to untoward outcomes. The authors calculated that the long-term costs of treatment with ACE inhibitors were similar to those with β-blockers. They concluded that the higher treatment costs of ACE inhibitors were offset by the greater effectiveness in reducing left ventricular hypertrophy.

In a further study, the socioeconomics of the therapy of congestive heart failure were evaluated by comparison of ACE inhibitor and digitalis therapy[160] in a retrospective evaluation of statistical material from 1986, including the drug costs as well as the costs of all medical services. The isolated study of drug treatment showed markedly higher costs for ACE inhibitors than for digitalis. However, the results revealed considerably lower costs for stationary treatment with ACE inhibitor therapy than with digitalis therapy. Overall therapy of congestive heart failure with ACE inhibitors caused considerably lower costs for medical treatment than digitalis therapy. Other factors like improvement of prognosis and subjective improvement in health were not considered in this study.

REFERENCES

1. Teetz V, Geiger R, Henning R, et al: Synthesis of a highly active angiotensin converting enzyme inhibitor: 2-[N-[(S)-1-ethoxycarbonyl-3-phenylpropyl]-L-alanyl]-(1 S,3S,5S)-2-azabicyclo[3.3.0]octane-3-carboxylic acid (Hoe 498). Arzneimittelforschung/Drug Res 34(II):1399, 1984.
2. Vasmant D, Bender N: The renin-angiotensin system and ramipril, a new converting enzyme inhibitor. J Cardiovasc Pharmacol 14(Suppl 4):S46, 1989.
3. Gohlke P, Urbach H, Schölkens BA, et al: Inhibition of converting enzyme in the cerebrospinal fluid of rats after oral treatment with converting enzyme inhibitors. J Pharmacol Exp Ther 249:609, 1989.
4. Bünning P: Inhibition of angiotensin converting enzyme by 2-[N-[(S)-l-carboxy-3-phenylpropyl]-L-alanyl]-(lS,3S,5S)-2-azabicyclo[3.3.0]octane-3-carboxylic acid (Hoe 498 diacid): Comparison with captopril and enalaprilat. Arzneimittelforschung/Drug Res 34(II):1406, 1984.
5. Bünning P: Kinetic properties of the angiotensin converting enzyme inhibitor ramiprilat. J Cardiovasc Pharmacol 10(Suppl 7):S31, 1987.

6. Becker RHA, Schölkens BA, Metzger M, et al: Pharmacological properties of the new orally active angiotensin converting enzyme inhibitor 2-[N-[(S)-1-ethoxycarbonyl-3-phenylpropyl]-L-alanyl]-(lS,3S,5S)-2-azabicyclo[3.3.0]octane-3-carboxylic acid (HOE 498). Arzneimittelforschung/Drug Res 34(II):1411, 1984.

7. Cushman DW, Wang FL, Fung WC, et al: Comparison in vitro, ex vivo, and in vivo of the actions of seven structurally diverse inhibitors of angiotensin converting enzyme (ACE). Br J Clin Pharmacol 28:115S, 1989.

8. Schölkens BA, Becker RHA, Kaiser J: Cardiovascular and antihypertensive activities of the novel non-sulfhydryl converting enzyme inhibitor 2-(N-((S)-l-ethoxycarbonyl-3-phenylpropyl)-L-alanyl)-(lS,3S,5S)-2-azabicyclo(3.3.0)octane-3-carboxylic acid (HOE498). Arzneimittelforschung/Drug Res 34(II):1417, 1984.

9. Unger T, Ganten D, Lang RE, et al: Is tissue converting enzyme inhibition a determinant of the antihypertensive efficacy of converting enzyme inhibitors? Studies with the two different compounds, HOE498 and MK421, in spontaneously hypertensive rats. J Cardiovasc Pharmacol 6:872, 1984.

10. Unger T, Fleck T, Ganten D, et al: 2-[N-[(S)-ethoxycarbonyl-3-phenylpropyl-L-alanyl]-(lS,3S,5S)-2-azabicyclo[3.3.0]octane-3-carboxylic acid (Hoe 498): Antihypertensive action and persistent inhibition of tissue converting enzyme activity in spontaneously hypertensive rats. Arzneimittelforschung/Drug Res 34(II):1426, 1984.

11. Unger T, Ganten D, Lang RE, et al: Persistent tissue converting enzyme inhibition following chronic treatment with HOE 498 and MK 421 in spontaneously hypertensive rats. J Cardiovasc Pharmacol 7:36, 1985.

12. Unger T, Ganten D, Lang RE: Tissue converting enzyme and cardiovascular actions of converting enzyme inhibitors. J Cardiovasc Pharmacol 8(Suppl 10):S75, 1986.

13. Moursi MG, Ganten D, Lang RE, et al: Antihypertensive action and inhibition of tissue converting enzyme (CE) by three prodrug CE inhibitors, enalapril, ramipril and perindopril in stroke-prone spontaneously hypertensive rats. J Hypertens 4(Suppl 3):S495, 1986.

14. Gohlke P, Schölkens BA, Henning R, et al: Inhibition of converting enzyme in brain tissue and cerebrospinal fluid of rats following chronic oral treatment with the converting enzyme inhibitors ramipril and Hoe 288. J Cardiovasc Pharmacol 14:S32, 1989.

15. Danckwardt L, Shimizu I, Bönner G, et al: Converting enzyme inhibition in kinin-deficient Brown Norway rats. Hypertension 16:429, 1990.

16. Bao G, Gohlke P, Qadri F, et al: Chronic kinin receptor blockade attenuates the antihypertensive effect of ramipril. Hypertension 20:74, 1992.

17. Bao G, Gohlke P, Unger T: Role of bradykinin in chronic antihypertensive actions of ramipril in different hypertension models. J Cardiovasc Pharmacol 20(Suppl 9):S96, 1992.

18. Cachofeiro V, Sakakibara T, Nasjletti A: Kinins, nitric oxide, and the hypotensive effect of captopril and ramiprilat in hypertension. Hypertension 19:138, 1992.

19. Gohlke P, Linz W, Schölkens BA, et al: Angiotensin converting enzyme inhibition improves cardiac function: Role of bradykinin. Hypertension 23:411, 1994.

20. Witte PU, Metzger H, Eckert HG, et al: Tolerance and pharmacokinetics of the angiotensin converting enzyme inhibitor 2-(N-((S)-1-ethoxycarbonyl-3-phenylpropyl)-L-alanyl)-(lS,3S,5S)-2-azabicyclo(3.3.0)octane-3-carboxylic acid (Hoe 498) in healthy volunteers. Arzneimittelforschung/Drug Res 34(II):1448, 1984.

21. Bussien JP, Nussberger J, Porchet M, et al: The effect of the converting enzyme inhibitor HOE 498 on the renin angiotensin system of normal volunteers. Naunyn Schmiedebergs Arch Pharmacol 329:63, 1985.

22. Manhem PJO, Ball SG, Morton J, et al: A dose-response study of Hoe 498, a new nonsulphhydryl converting enzyme inhibitor, on blood pressure, pulse rate and the renin-angiotensin-aldosterone system in normal man. Br J Clin Pharmacol 20:27, 1985.

23. Nussberger J, Brunner DB, Waeber B, et al: True versus immunoreactive angiotensin II in human plasma. Hypertension 7(Suppl I):I-1, 1985.

24. Lenz T, Distler A, Haller H, et al: Humoral and blood pressure effects of the angiotensin converting enzyme inhibitor ramipril in essential hypertension. Arzneimittelforschung/Drug Res 36(II):1693, 1986.

25. Karlberg BE, Lindström T, Rosenqvist U, et al: Efficacy, tolerance and hormonal effects of a new oral angiotensin converting enzyme inhibitor, ramipril (Hoe 498), in mild to moderate primary hypertension. Am J Cardiol 59:104D, 1987.

26. De Graeff PA, Kingma JH, Dunselman PHJM, et al: Acute hemodynamic and hormonal effects of ramipril in chronic congestive heart failure and comparison with captopril. Am J Cardiol 59:164D, 1987.

27. Crozier IG, Ikram H, Nicholls MG, et al: Acute hemodynamic, hormonal and electrolyte effects of ramipril in severe congestive heart failure. Am J Cardiol 59:155D, 1987.

28. Crozier IG, Ikram H, Nicholls G, et al: Global and regional hemodynamic effects of ramipril in congestive heart failure. J Cardiovasc Pharmacol 14:688, 1989.

29. Tillman DM, Adams FG, Gillen G, et al: Ramipril for hypertension secondary to renal artery stenosis: Changes in blood pressure, the renin-angiotensin system and total and divided renal function. Am J Cardiol 59:133D, 1987.

30. Waeber B, Nussberger J, Juillerat L, et al: Angiotensin converting enzyme inhibition: Discrepancy between antihypertensive effect and suppression of enzyme activity. J Cardiovasc Pharmacol 14(Suppl 4):S53, 1989.

31. Bönner G, Preis S, Schunk U, et al: Hemodynamic effects of bradykinin on systemic and pulmonary circulation in healthy and hypertensive humans. J Cardiovasc Pharmacol 15(Suppl 6):S46, 1990.

32. Erman A, Winkler J, Chen-Gal B, et al: Inhibition of angiotensin converting enzyme by ramipril in serum and tissue of man. J Hypertens 9:1057, 1991.

33. Ball SG, Robertson JIS: Clinical pharmacology of ramipril. Am J Cardiol 59:23D, 1987.

34. Todd PA, Benfield P: Ramipril: A review of its pharmacological properties and therapeutic efficacy in cardiovascular disorders. Drugs 39:110, 1990.

35. Kelly JG, O'Malley K: Clinical pharmacokinetics of the newer ACE inhibitors: A review. Clin Pharmacokinet 19:177, 1990.

36. Salvetti A: Newer ACE inhibitors: A look at the future. Drugs 40:800, 1990.

37. Eckert HG, Badian MJ, Gantz D, et al: Pharmacokinetics and biotransformation of 2-(N-((S)-1-ethoxycarbonyl-3-phenylpropyl)-L-alanyl)-(lS,3S,5S)-2-azabicyclo(3.3.0)octane-3 carboxylic acid (Hoe 498) in rat, dog and man. Arzneimittelforschung Drug Res 34(II):1435, 1984.

38. Meyer BH, Muller FO, Badian M, et al: Pharmacokinetics of ramipril in the elderly. Am J Cardiol 59:33D, 1987.

39. Witte PU, Irmisch R, Hajdu P, et al: Pharmacokinetics and pharmacodynamics of a novel orally active angiotensin converting enzyme inhibitor (Hoe 498) in healthy subjects. Eur J Clin Pharmacol 27:577, 1984.

40. Gerckens U, Grube E, Mengden T, et al: Pharmacokinetic and pharmacodynamic properties of ramipril in patients with congestive heart failure. J Cardiovasc Pharmacol 13(Suppl 3):S49, 1989.

41. Debusmann ER, Pujadas JO, Lahn W, et al: Influence of renal function on the pharmacokinetics of ramipril (Hoe 498). Am J Cardiol 59:70D, 1987.

42. Mellstrom B, Iadarola MJ, Yang H-YT, et al: Inhibition of Met5-enkephalin-Arg6-Phe7 degradation by inhibitors of dipeptidyl carboxypeptidase. J Pharmacol Exp Ther 239:174, 1986.

43. Doering W, Maass L, Irmisch R, et al: Pharmacokinetic interaction study with ramipril and digoxin in healthy volunteers. Am J Cardiol 59:60D, 1987.

44. Schunkert H, Kindler J, Gassmann M, et al: Steady-state kinetics of ramipril in renal failure. J Cardiovasc Pharmacol 13(Suppl 3):S52, 1989.

45. Shionoiri H, Ikeda Y, Kimura K, et al: Pharmacodynamics and pharmacokinetics of single dose ramipril in hypertensive patients with various degrees of renal function. Curr Ther Res 40:74, 1986.

46. Aurell M, Delin K, Herlitz H, et al: Pharmacokinetics and pharmacodynamics of ramipril in renal failure. Am J Cardiol 59:65D, 1987.

47. Richer C, Doussau M-P, Giudicelli J-F: Systemic and regional hemodynamic profile of five angiotensin I converting enzyme inhibitors in the spontaneously hypertensive rat. Am J Cardiol 59:12D, 1987.

48. Thuillez C, Richer C, Guidicelli J-F: Pharmacokinetics, converting enzyme inhibition and peripheral arterial hemodynamics of ramipril in healthy volunteers. Am J Cardiol 59:38D, 1987.

49. Benetos A, Asmar R, Vasmant D, et al: Long lasting arterial effects of the ACE inhibitor ramipril. J Hum Hypertens 5:363, 1991.

50. Vogt A, Unterberg C, Kreuzer H: Acute effects of the new angiotensin converting enzyme inhibitor ramipril on hemodynamics and carotid sinus baroreflex activity in congestive heart failure. Am J Cardiol 59:149D, 1987.

51. De Graeff PA, Kingma JH, Viersma JW, et al: Acute and chronic effects of ramipril and captopril in congestive heart failure. Int J Cardiol 23:59, 1989.

52. McCance AJ, Forfar JC: Decreased sympathetic tone in patients with chronic heart failure treated with ramipril. In McGregor GA, Sever PS (eds): Current Advances in ACE Inhibition 2. Edinburgh: Churchill Livingstone, 1991, pp 278–281.

53. Linz W, Schölkens BA, Ganten D: Converting enzyme inhibition specifically prevents the development and induces regression of cardiac hypertrophy in rats. Clin Exp Hypertens [A] 11:1325, 1989.

54. Linz W, Schölkens BA: A specific B2-bradykinin receptor antagonist HOE 140 abolishes the antihypertrophic effect of ramipril. Br J Pharmacol 105:771, 1992.

55. Unger T, Mattfeldt T, Lamberty V, et al: Effect of early onset ACE inhibition on myocardial capillaries in SHR. Hypertension 20:478, 1992.

56. Böhm ROB, Van Baak MA, Rahn KH: Studies on the antihypertensive effect of single doses of the angiotensin converting enzyme inhibitor ramipril (HOE 498) in man. Eur J Clin Pharmacol 30:541, 1986.

57. Stumpe KO, Overlack A, Kolloch R, et al: Effects of the new angiotensin-converting enzyme inhibitor, ramipril, in patients with essential hypertension. Klin Wochenschr 64:558, 1986.

58. De Leeuw PW, Lugtenburg PL, Van Houten H, et al: Preliminary experiences with HOE 498, a novel long-acting converting enzyme inhibitor, in hypertensive patients. J Cardiovasc Pharmacol 7:1161, 1985.

59. Kaneko Y, Omae T, Yoshinaga K, et al: Effect of ramipril, a new angiotensin converting enzyme inhibitor, on diurnal variations of blood pressure in essential hypertension. Am J Cardiol 59:86D, 1987.

60. Tochikubo O, Asahina S, Kaneko Y: Effect of ramipril on 24-hour variability of blood pressure and heart rate in essential hypertension. Am J Cardiol 59:83D, 1987.

61. Heber ME, Brigden GS, Caruana MP, et al: First dose response and 24-hour antihypertensive efficacy of the new once-daily angiotensin converting enzyme inhibitor, ramipril. Am J Cardiol 62:239, 1988.

62. Burris JF: Lessons learned with ambulatory blood pressure monitoring: A focus on ramipril. Clin Ther 15:476, 1993.

63. Spieker C, Zidek W, Vetter H, Rahn KH: Ambulatory 24-h blood pressure monitoring in essential hypertensives treated with the angiotensin-converting enzyme inhibitor ramipril. J Int Med Res 19:39, 1991.

64. McCarron D, The Ramipril Multicenter Study Group: 24-Hour blood pressure profiles in hypertensive patients administered ramipril or placebo once daily: Magnitude and duration of antihypertensive effects. Clin Cardiol 14:737, 1991.

65. Walter U, Forthofer R, Witte PU: Dose-response relation of the angiotensin converting enzyme inhibitor ramipril in mild to moderate essential hypertension. Am J Cardiol 59:125D, 1987.

66. Fukiyama K, Omae T, Kaneko Y, et al: Efficacy and safety of ramipril (HOE 498) in the treatment of hypertension: Dose finding study. Am J Cardiol 59:121D, 1987.

67. Felder K, Witte PU: Effects of the new oral angiotensin converting enzyme inhibitor 2-[N-[(S)l-ethoxycarbonyl-3-phenyl-propyl]-L-alanyl]-(1S,3S,5S)-2-azabicyclo[3.3.0]octane-3-carboxylic acid (HOE 498) in essential hypertension. Arzneimittelforschung/Drug Res 34(II):1452, 1984.

68. Villamil AS, Cairns V, Witte PU, et al: A double-blind study to compare the efficacy, tolerance and safety of two doses of the angiotensin converting enzyme inhibitor ramipril with placebo. Am J Cardiol 59:110D, 1987.

69. De Leeuw PW, Birkenhäger WH: Short- and long-term effects of ramipril in hypertension. Am J Cardiol 59:79D, 1987.

70. Kostis JB: Double-blind study of ascending doses of ramipril in patients with mild to moderate hypertension. Adv Ther 8:52, 1991.

71. Schreiner M, Berendes B, Verho M, et al: Antihypertensive efficacy, tolerance, and safety of long-term treatment with ramipril in patients with mild-to-moderate essential hypertension. J Cardiovasc Pharmacol 18(Suppl 2):S137, 1991.

72. Carré A, Zannad F, Vasmant D: The French multicentre study of ramipril in ambulatory patients with mild-to-moderate hypertension. Clin Physiol Biochem 9:105, 1992.

73. Linz W, Schölkens BA, Han YF: Beneficial effects of the converting enzyme inhibitor, ramipril, in ischemic rat hearts. J Cardiovasc Pharmacol 8(Suppl 10):S91, 1986.

74. Linz W, Schölkens BA: Influence of local converting enzyme inhibition on angiotensin and bradykinin effects in ischemic rat hearts. J Cardiovasc Pharmacol 10(Suppl 7):S75, 1987.

75. Linz W, Martorana PA, Grötsch H, et al: Antagonizing bradykinin (BK) obliterates the cardioprotective effects of bradykinin and angiotensin-converting enzyme (ACE) inhibitors in ischemic hearts. Drug Dev Res 19:393, 1990.

76. Linz W, Wiemer G, Schölkens BA: ACE-inhibition induces NO-formation in cultured bovine endothelial cells and protects isolated ischemic rat hearts. J Mol Cell Cardiol 24:909, 1992.

77. Schölkens BA, Linz W, König W: Effects of the angiotensin converting enzyme inhibitor ramipril in isolated ischaemic rat heart are abolished by a bradykinin antagonist. J Hypertens Suppl 6(4):S25, 1988.

78. Van Gilst WH, De Graeff PA, Wesseling H, et al: Reduction of reperfusion arrhythmias in the ischemic isolated rat heart by angiotensin converting enzyme inhibitors: A comparison of captopril, enalapril and Hoe 498. J Cardiovasc Pharmacol 8:722, 1986.

79. Schölkens BA, Linz W, Martorana PA: Experimental cardiovascular benefits of angiotensin converting enzyme inhibitors: Beyond blood pressure reduction. J Cardiovasc Pharmacol 18(Suppl 2):S26, 1991.

80. Linz W, Schölkens BA, Kaiser J, et al: Cardiac arrhythmias are ameliorated by local inhibition of angiotensin formation and bradykinin degradation with the converting enzyme inhibitor ramipril. Cardiovasc Drugs Ther 3:873, 1989.

81. Becker BF, Heier M, Gerlach E: Experimental evidence for cardioprotection afforded by ramipril, an inhibitor of angiotensin converting enzyme. In Schultheiss H-P (ed): New Concepts in Viral Heart Disease. Berlin: Springer-Verlag, 1988, pp 465–474.

82. Pi X, Chen X: Captopril and ramiprilat protect against free radical injury in isolated working rat hearts. J Mol Cell Cardiol 21:1261, 1989.

83. Baumgarten CR, Linz W, Kunkel G, et al: Ramiprilat increases bradykinin outflow from isolated hearts of rat. Br J Pharmacol 108:293, 1993.

84. Linz W, Martorana PA, Schölkens BA: Local inhibition of bradykinin degradation in ischemic hearts. J Cardiovasc Pharmacol 15(Suppl 6):S99, 1990.

85. Carlsson L, Abrahamsson T: Ramiprilat attenuates the local release of noradrenaline in the ischemic myocardium. Eur J Pharmacol 166:157, 1989.

86. Albus U, Kujath W: Effect of angiotensin-converting enzyme inhibitor ramipril on noradrenaline-overflow from isolated working rat hearts subjected to myocardial ischemia and reperfusion [abstract]. Naunyn Schmiedebergs Arch Pharmacol 335(Suppl):R82, 1987.

87. Xiang JZ, Linz W, Becker H, et al: Effects of converting enzyme inhibitors: Ramipril and enalapril on peptide action and sympathetic neurotransmission in the isolated heart. Eur J Pharmacol 113:215, 1985.

88. Hartman JC, Hullinger TG, Wall TM, et al: Reduction of myocardial infarct size by ramiprilat is independent of angiotensin II synthesis inhibition. Eur J Pharmacol 234:229, 1993.

89. Hartman JC, Wall TM, Hullinger TG, et al: Reduction of myocardial infarct size in rabbits by ramiprilat: Reversal by the bradykinin antagonist HOE 140. J Cardiovasc Pharmacol 21:996, 1993.

90. Martorana PA, Kettenbach B, Breipohl G, et al: Reduction of infarct size by local angiotensin-converting enzyme inhibition is abolished by a bradykinin antagonist. Eur J Pharmacol 182:395, 1990.

91. Schölkens BA, Martorana PA, Gobel H, et al: Cardiovascular effects of the converting enzyme inhibitor ramipril (Hoe 498) in anesthetized dogs with acute ischemic left ventricular failure. Clin Exp Hypertens [A] 8:1033, 1986.

92. The Acute Infarction Ramipril Efficacy (AIRE) Study Investigators: Effect of ramipril on mortality and morbidity of survivors of acute myocardial infarction with clinical evidence of heart failure. Lancet 342:821, 1993.

93. Messerli FH, Ketelhut R: Left ventricular hypertrophy: An independent risk factor. J Cardiovasc Pharmacol 17(Suppl 4):S59, 1991.

94. Levy D, Garrison RJ, Savage D, et al: Echocardiographically determined left ventricular mass and incidence of coronary heart disease in an elderly cohort: The Framingham Heart Study. Ann Intern Med 110:101, 1989.

95. Linz W, Gohlke P, Unger T, et al.: Experimental evidence for effects of ramipril on cardiac and vascular hypertrophy beyond blood pressure reduction. Arch Mal Coeur 88(II):31, 1995.

96. Linz W, Schaper J, Wiemer G, et al: Ramipril prevents left ventricular hypertrophy with myocardial fibrosis without blood pressure reduction: A one year study in rats. Br J Pharmacol 107:970, 1992.

97. Gohlke P, Linz W, Schölkens BA, et al: Effect of chronic high- and low-dose ACE inhibitor treatment on cardiac and vascular hypertrophy and vascular function in spontaneously hypertensive rats. Exp Nephrol 2:93, 1994.

98. Eichstaedt H, Danne O, Langer M, et al: Regression of left ventricular hypertrophy under ramipril treatment investigated by nuclear magnetic resonance imaging. J Cardiovasc Pharmacol 13(Suppl 3):S75, 1989.

99. Lievre M, Gueret P, Delair S, et al: ACE-inhibitor-induced reduction in left ventricular mass independent of changes in blood pressure in hypertensive patients with left ventricular hypertrophy [abstract]. Hypertension 22:419, 1993.

100. Berdeaux A, Bonhenry C, Guidicelli JF: Effects of four angiotensin I converting enzyme inhibitors on regional myocardial blood flow and ischemic injury during coronary artery occlusion in dogs. Fundam Clin Pharmacol 1:201, 1987.

101. Stauss HM, Zhu YC, Redlich Th, et al: Angiotensin-converting enzyme inhibition in infarct-induced heart failure in rats: Bradykinin versus angiotensin II. J Cardiovasc Risk 1:255, 1994.

102. Lamontagne D, König A, Bassenge E, et al: Prostacyclin and nitric oxide contribute to the vasodilator action of acetylcholine and bradykinin in the intact rabbit coronary bed. J Cardiovasc Pharmacol 20:652, 1992.

103. Schölkens BA, Linz W: Local inhibition of angiotensin II formation and bradykinin degradation in isolated hearts. Clin Exp Hypertens [A] 10:1259, 1988.

104. Ryan US, Ryan JW, Whitaker C, et al: Localization of angiotensin converting enzyme (kininase II). II: Immunocytochemistry and immunofluorescence. Tissue Cell 8(1):125, 1976.

105. Gohlke P, Unger T, Bünning P: Distribution of the angiotensin converting enzyme inhibitor ramiprilat in the blood vessel wall. Pharm Pharmacol Lett 2:66, 1992.

106. Gohlke P, Bünning P, Unger T: Distribution and metabolism of angiotensin I and II in the blood vessel wall. Hypertension 20:151, 1992.

107. Schölkens BA, Xiang J-Z, Tilly H: Influence of the converting enzyme inhibitors Hoe 498, enalapril and captopril on vascular reactivity of isolated arterial preparations. Clin Exp Hypertens [A] 6:1807, 1984.

108. Gohlke P, Lamberty V, Kuwer I, et al: Long-term low-dose angiotensin converting enzyme inhibitor treatment increases vascular cyclic guanosine 3′,5′-monophosphate. Hypertension 22:682, 1993.

109. Gohlke P, Bünning P, Bönner G, et al: ACE inhibitor effect on bradykinin metabolism in the vascular wall. In Bönner G, Fritz H, Schölkens BA, et al (eds): Agents and Actions (Suppl) Vol 38/III, Recent Progress on Kinins. Basel: Birkhäuser Verlag, 1992, pp 178–185.

110. Gohlke P, Lamberty V, Kuwer I, et al: Vascular remodeling in systemic hypertension. Am J Cardiol 71:2E, 1993.

111. Scherf H, Pietsch R, Landsberg G, et al: Converting enzyme inhibitor ramipril stimulates prostacyclin synthesis by isolated rat aorta: Evidence for a kinin-dependent mechanism. Klin Wochenschr 64:742, 1986.

112. Wiemer G, Schölkens BA, Becker RHA, et al: Ramiprilat enhances endothelial autacoid formation by inhibiting breakdown of endothelium-derived bradykinin. Hypertension 18:558, 1991.

113. Hecker M, Dambacher T, Busse R: Role of endothelium-derived bradykinin in the control of vascular tone. J Cardiovasc Pharmacol 20(Suppl 9):S55, 1992.

114. Finta KM, Fischer MJ, Lee L, et al: Ramipril prevents impaired endothelium-dependent relaxation in arteries from rabbits fed an atherogenic diet. Atherosclerosis 100:149, 1993.

115. Becker RHA, Wiemer G, Linz W: Preservation of endothelial function by ramipril in rabbits on a long-term atherogenic diet. J Cardiovasc Pharmacol 18(Suppl 2):S110, 1991.

116. Becker RHA: ACE inhibitors and atherosclerosis in animal experiments. In Schölkens BA, Unger T (eds): ACE Inhibitors, Endothelial Function and Atherosclerosis. Chichester, Sussex, UK: Media Medica Publications, 1993, pp 83–92.

117. Farhy RD, Ho K-L, Carretero OA, et al: Kinins mediate the antiproliferative effect of ramipril in rat carotid artery. Biochem Biophys Res Commun 182:283, 1992.

118. Farhy RD, Carretero OA, Ho K-L, et al: Role of kinins and nitric oxide in the effects of angiotensin converting enzyme inhibitors on neointima formation. Circ Res 72:1202, 1993.

119. Schwartz SL, Hanson C, Lucas C, et al: Double-blind, placebo-controlled study of ramipril in diabetics with mild to moderate hypertension. Clin Ther 15:79, 1993.

120. Janka HU, Nuber A, Mehnert H: Metabolic effects of ramipril treatment in hypertensive subjects with non-insulin-dependent diabetes mellitus. Arzneimittelforschung/Drug Res 40(I):432, 1990.

121. Paolisso G, Gambardella A, Verza M, et al: ACE inhibition improves insulin-sensitivity in aged insulin-resistant hypertensive patients. J Hum Hypertens 6: 175, 1992.

122. Ludvik B, Kueenburg E, Brunnbauer M, et al: The effects of ramipril on glucose tolerance, insulin secretion, and insulin sensitivity in patients with hypertension. J Cardiovasc Pharmacol 18(Suppl 2):S157, 1991.

123. Heller J, Kramer HJ, Horacek V: Roles of bradykinin and prostaglandins in the canine renal haemodynamic responses to ACE inhibition. In McGregor GA, Sever PS (eds): Current Advances in ACE Inhibition 2. Edinburgh: Churchill Livingstone, 1991, pp 195–197.

124. Britton KE: Essential hypertension: A disorder of cortical nephron control? Lancet 2:900, 1981.

125. Al-Nahhas AM, Nimmon CC, Britton KE, et al: The effect of ramipril: A new angiotensin-converting enzyme inhibitor on cortical nephron flow and effective renal plasma flow in patients with essential hypertension. Nephron 54:47, 1990.

126. Moiseyev VS, Ivleva AJ, Antija ID, et al: Cardiovascular and renal effects of ramipril. Lancet 1:846, 1989.

127. Witte PU, Walter U: Comparative double-blind study of ramipril and captopril in mild to moderate essential hypertension. Am J Cardiol 59:115D, 1987.

128. Bauer B, Lorenz H, Zahlten R: An open multicenter study to assess the long-term efficacy, tolerance, and safety of the oral angiotensin converting enzyme inhibitor ramipril in patients with mild to moderate essential hypertension. J Cardiovasc Pharmacol 13(Suppl 3):S70, 1989.

129. Predel H-G, Dusing R, Bäcker A, et al: Combined treatment of severe essential hypertension with the new angiotensin converting enzyme inhibitor ramipril. Am J Cardiol 59:143D, 1987.

130. Funck-Brentano C, Chatellier G, Alexandre JM: Reversible renal failure after combined treatment with enalapril and furosemide in a patient with congestive heart failure. Br Heart J 55:596, 1986.

131. Cody RJ: Clinical and hemodynamic experience with enalapril in congestive heart failure. Am J Cardiol 55:36, 1985.
132. Kholeif MA, Pringle S, Kesson E, et al: A comparison of the efficacy and safety of ramipril and digoxin added to maintenance diuretic treatment in patients with chronic heart failure. J Cardiovasc Pharmacol 18(Suppl 2):S180, 1991.
133. Ocon Pujadas J, Debusmann ER, Jane F, et al: Pharmacodynamic effects of a single 10 mg dose of the angiotensin converting enzyme inhibitor ramipril in patients with impaired renal function. J Cardiovasc Pharmacol 13(Suppl 3):S45, 1989.
134. Goetz R, Drechsler U, Heidbreder E, et al: Influence of the angiotensin converting enzyme inhibitor ramipril on proteinuria, blood pressure and renal function in histologically proven glomerulonephritis with nephrotic syndrome. Z Kardiol 77(Suppl 3):65, 1988.
135. Mathiesen ER, Borch-Johnsen K, Jonsen DV, et al: Improved survival in patients with diabetic nephropathy. Diabetologia 32:884, 1989.
136. Mau Pedersen M, Hansen KW, Schmitz A, et al: Effects of ACE inhibition supplementary to beta blockers and diuretics in early diabetic nephropathy. Kidney Int 41:883, 1992.
137. Marre M, Hallab M, Billiard A, et al: Small doses of ramipril to reduce microalbuminuria in diabetic patients with incipient nephropathy independently of blood pressure changes. J Cardiovasc Pharmacol 18(Suppl 2):S 165, 1991.
138. Unger T, Badoer E, Ganten D, et al: Brain angiotensin: Pathways and pharmacology. Circulation 77(Suppl I):I-40, 1988.
139. Stamler JF, Brody MJ, Phillips MI: The central and peripheral effects of Captopril (SQ 14225) on the arterial pressure of the spontaneously hypertensive rat. Brain Res 186:499, 1980.
140. Unger T, Kaufmann-Bühler I, Schölkens BA, et al: Brain converting enzyme inhibition: A possible mechanism for the antihypertensive action of captopril in spontaneously hypertensive rats. Eur J Pharmacol 70:467, 1981.
141. Suzuki H, Kondo K, Handa M, et al: Role of the brain isorenin-angiotensin system in experimental hypertension in rats. Clin Sci 61:175, 1981.
142. Phillips MI, Kimura B: Converting enzyme inhibitors and brain angiotensin. J Cardiovasc Pharmacol 8(Suppl 10):S82, 1986.
143. Moursi M, El-Dakhakhny M, Schölkens BA, et al: Interference with the autonomic nervous system by the converting enzyme inhibitor ramipril in conscious spontaneously hypertensive rats. J Cardiovasc Pharmacol 10(Suppl 7):S125, 1987.
144. Skidgel RA, Defendi R, Erdös EG: Angiotensin I converting enzyme and its role in neuropeptide metabolism. *In* Turner AJ (ed): Neuropeptides and Their Peptidases. Chichester, England: Ellis Horwood, 1988, pp 165–182.
145. Gerhardt P, Hasenohrl RU, Hock FJ, et al: Mnemogenic effects of injecting RA-octil, a CE-inhibitor derivate, systemically or into the basal forebrain. Psychopharmacology (Berl) 111:442, 1993.
146. Hock FJ, Gerhards HJ, Wiemer G, et al: Effects of the novel compound Hoe 065 upon impaired learning and memory in rodents. Eur J Pharmacol 171:79, 1989.
147. Kaplan NM, Sproul E, Mulcahy WS, et al: Large prospective study of ramipril in patients with hypertension. Clin Ther 15:810, 1993.
148. Mauersberger H, Witte PU: Disappearance of captopril-induced taste disturbance substitution with angiotensin-converting-enzyme inhibitor HOE 498. Lancet 1:517, 1985.
149. Boeijinga JK, Matroos AW, Van Maarschallerweerd MW, et al: No interaction shown between ramipril and coumarin derivative. Curr Ther Res 44:902, 1988.
150. Verho M, Malerczyk V, Grötsch H, et al: Absence of interaction between ramipril, a new ACE-inhibitor, and phenprocoumon, an anticoagulant agent. Pharmatherapeutica 5:392, 1989.
151. Heidbreder D, Froer K-L, Breitstadt A, et al: Combination of ramipril and hydrochlorothiazide in the treatment of mild to moderate hypertension. Part 1: A double-blind, comparative, multicenter study in nonresponders to ramipril monotherapy. Clin Cardiol 15:904, 1992.
152. Eichstädt HW, Felix R, Langer M, et al: Use of nuclear magnetic resonance imaging to show regression of hypertrophy with ramipril treatment. Am J Cardiol 59:98D, 1987.
153. Zabludowski U, Rosenfeld J, Akbary MA, et al: A multi-centre comparative study between ramipril and enalapril in patients with mild to moderate essential hypertension. Curr Med Res Opin 11:93, 1988.
154. Koenig W, Multicentre Study Group: Ramipril vs lisinopril in the treatment of mild to moderate primary hypertension: A randomized double-blind muticentre trial. Drug Invest 4:450, 1992.
155. Lenox-Smith AJ, Street RB, Kendall FD: Comparison of ramipril against atenolol in controlling mild-to-moderate hypertension. J Cardiovasc Pharmacol 18(Suppl 2):S150, 1991.
156. Weidmann P, Frank J, Graf W, et al: Monotherapie mit dem ACE-Hemmer Ramipril oder dem Calcium-Antagonisten Nitrendipin bei essentieller Hypertonie. Schweiz Med Wochenschr 122:1497, 1992.
157. Modesti PA, Said AM, Cecioni I, et al: Twenty-four-hour antihypertensive efficacy of ramipril and enalapril. Curr Ther Res 53:137, 1993.
158. Weinberger MH: Angiotensin converting enzyme inhibitors enhance the antihypertensive efficacy of diuretics and blunt or prevent adverse metabolic effects. J Cardiovasc Pharmacol 13(Suppl 3):Sl, 1989.
159. Eagle KA, Blank DJ, Aguiar E, et al: Economic impact of regression of left venricular hypertrophy by antihypertensive drugs. J Hum Hypertens 7:341, 1993.
160. Rohrbacher R, Schrey A: Sozioökonomie der chronischen Herzinsuffizienz—eine Krankheitskosten-Studie. Herz Kreislauf 22:426, 1990.

CHAPTER 81

Perindopril

Kennedy R. Lees, M.D., F.R.C.P., and John L. Reid, D.M., F.R.C.P.

HISTORY

Perindopril was first synthesized by Servier Laboratories in the early 1980s[1] and was identified to have inhibitory effects on angiotensin-converting enzyme (ACE). The *tert*-butylamine salt of perindopril was marketed in France in 1988 and subsequently worldwide. It has been studied extensively in human volunteers and in patients with hypertension or heart failure.

CHEMISTRY

The structure of perindopril *tert*-butylamine is given in Figure 81–1.[2] The empirical formula is $C_{19}H_{32}N_2O_5$, $C_4H_{11}N$, and thus the molecular weight of perindopril *tert*-butylamine is 442. It forms a white microcrystalline powder that is soluble in water up to 60% (weight by volume [w/v]) and in chloroform up to 15% (w/v). It is soluble in methanol and ethanol. If stored

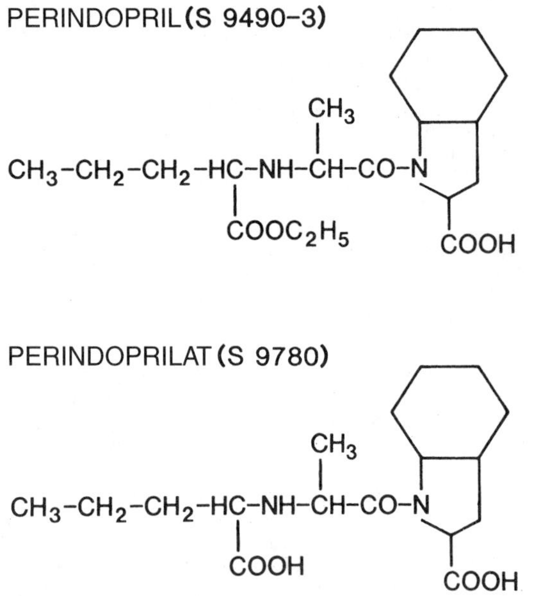

PERINDOPRIL (S 9490-3)

CH₃–CH₂–CH₂–HC–NH–CH–CO–N with CH₃, COOC₂H₅, COOH

PERINDOPRILAT (S 9780)

CH₃–CH₂–CH₂–HC–NH–CH–CO–N with CH₃, COOH, COOH

Figure 81–1. The chemical structures of perindopril and its active diacid metabolite perindoprilat.

in dry conditions at room temperature, the compound is stable for longer than 1 year.

Perindopril has been identified in several reports by the numbers S-9490 (for the free acid) or S-9490-3 (for the *tert*-butylamine salt). The active metabolite of perindopril is its deesterified form, known as perindoprilat or S-9780 (see Fig. 81–1), having a molecular weight of 339. Assays have been developed for measurement of perindopril and perindoprilat in biologic fluids.[3, 4]

PRECLINICAL PHARMACOLOGY

Perindoprilat is a potent competitive inhibitor of ACE *in vitro*, but the parent compound, perindopril, is only weakly active. Guinea pig ACE is 50% inhibited by 3000 ± 200 nmol/L perindopril (compared with 4900 ± 400 nmol/L enalapril and 24 ± 3 nmol/L captopril) but by only 2.4 ± 1 nmol/L perindoprilat (compared with 3.8 ± 0.1 nmol/L enalaprilat).[5] As is the case with several other agents including enalapril, deesterification *in vivo* thus produces a thousand-fold increase in potency.

After intravenous administration of perindopril or perindoprilat, the doses required to produce 50% inhibition of the pressor response to angiotensin I in a variety of species ranged from 2.7 ± 0.4 µg/kg (rabbit) to 148 ± 15 µg/kg (dog) for perindopril and from 1.2 ± 0.2 µg/kg (rabbit) to 13.1 ± 1.7 µg/kg (guinea pig) for perindoprilat. These figures are lower than were required with enalapril and enalaprilat, respectively,[5] and are consistent with the view that perindoprilat is more potent than enalaprilat. The conversion from perindopril to perindoprilat appears to be efficient in rabbits but less so in other species.

Angiotensin-converting enzyme is also termed kininase II because of its inactivating action on bradyki-

nin. Perindopril also potentiates the vasodilatation produced by exogenous bradykinin in anesthetized dogs.[5]

Anesthetized dogs showed a fall in blood pressure after intravenous perindopril administration, and this was enhanced if sodium restriction had previously been imposed. Conscious dogs responded to perindopril with a fall in blood pressure only when sodium was depleted. Heart rate was unchanged, plasma renin activity rose significantly, and plasma aldosterone levels fell.[5]

The duration of action, measured by inhibition of the pressor response to angiotensin I (AI), was prolonged: 1 mg/kg produced 90% inhibition in dogs, and nearly 40% inhibition persisted after 24 hours. The absorption of perindopril appeared to be rapid, with a peak effect after 1 hour in dogs. Data on the oral absorption of perindoprilat were not presented, but the absorption rate is assumed to be low.

DiNicolantonio and Doyle[6] compared the effects of perindopril with those of enalapril in spontaneously hypertensive rats (SHRs). Perindopril caused a significantly greater hypotensive response than enalapril and showed more potent inhibition of plasma ACE and AI pressor responses at each of the doses studied. Whereas ACE inhibition was maximal 1 hour after oral administration, both drugs caused a slow, progressive fall in blood pressure until 4 hours that remained maximal up to 12 hours. The fall in blood pressure was not predicted by either plasma renin activity (PRA) or ACE inhibition, even in a salt-depleted group. Inhibition of the pressor response to AI correlated with plasma ACE inhibition rather than with a fall in blood pressure. Their results in SHRs suggested that perindopril was more potent as an ACE inhibitor and more potent in lowering blood pressure than enalapril, although these two effects were dissociated in onset and duration.

A similar study has been reported by Unger et al.,[7] who compared captopril with the active diacid metabolites of perindopril, ramipril and enalapril, in rat plasma. They confirmed the order of potency to be ramipril diacid ≥ perindoprilat > enalaprilat > captopril. They also examined the effects of 1 month of treatment with the parent compounds in SHRs and confirmed that 1 mg/kg/day of perindopril or ramipril was as effective as 30 mg/kg/day of enalapril in lowering blood pressure. The blood pressure lowering effect could not be directly related to inhibition of the renin-angiotensin system in the plasma. ACE activity was measured in tissues after 4 weeks of treatment with perindopril. Not all tissues were equally affected: kidney showed the greatest inhibition (96%), followed by aortic wall (64%), heart (52%), lung (36%), hypophysis (30%), and brain cortex (26%). ACE activity was unchanged in the adrenal gland, medulla oblongata, and hypothalamus. Thus, there is evidence from two observations that plasma ACE levels may not be a reliable measure of the pharmacologic effect of these drugs: (1) the time course for lowering blood pressure is different from the time course for plasma ACE inhibition, and (2) ACE from different sites displays different degrees of inhibition following long-term oral therapy.

In terms of the effects on hemodynamics, perindopril has been shown to lower total peripheral resistance without affecting cardiac index in SHRs[8] and thus to lower blood pressure. Once again, heart rate did not increase.[9]

When the relative changes in resistance were compared in different vascular beds, they were found to be decreased by perindopril in the following order: renal > splenic = liver > skin > total peripheral > muscle = brain. Renal vasodilator effects were seen with doses that produced no measurable systemic effect.[10]

Richer et al.[8] also examined the pressor response to α_1- and α_2-agonists (cirazoline and UK 14304, respectively) in the presence and absence of perindopril in SHRs. Perindopril reduced the pressor effects to both drugs, but especially to the α_2-agonist. In addition, the pressor response to neural stimulation was also decreased by perindopril. This effect on the neural response was maintained if nephrectomized, pithed SHRs were studied, but in these animals, the α-pressor effects were not inhibited by perindopril. This was cited as evidence that perindopril exerts a prejunctional inhibitory effect on sympathetic transmission, which is not kidney-dependent, and that perindopril also exerts a kidney-dependent sympathoinhibitory effect on the postjunctional α-adrenoceptors.

As well as confirming the effects of perindopril in lowering blood pressure, Barres et al.[11] reported enhancement of baroreflex sensitivity in chronically treated animals after exposure to phenylephrine but not after exposure to nitroglycerin. They confirmed that perindopril reduced the pressor effect of phenylephrine and further noted that left ventricular (LV) weight was reduced.

A reduction in LV weight has been seen in other studies and associated with a decrease of vascular hypertrophy.[12-14] Levy et al.[12] reported that perindopril treatment reversed aortic media hypertrophy and the decrease of arterial compliance in renovascular hypertensive rats. Cadilhac and Giudicelli[15] reported a reduction of cardiac and aortic hypertrophy in SHRs with perindopril. Finally, Christensen et al.[14] and Harrap et al.[13] confirmed similar benefits in resistance vessels of SHRs and showed that perindopril treatment was more potent than other antihypertensive therapies. A further cardiac effect is that treatment with perindopril before coronary artery occlusion in rat hearts reduces the incidence of ventricular arrhythmias and mortality resulting from ventricular fibrillation.[16-18] The same effect is seen with other ACE inhibitors, but the dose required with all these drugs is higher than that used in clinical practice.

The effect of hypertension on accelerated arteriosclerosis has been studied in a rat model of arterial graft rejection.[19] Perindopril lowered blood pressure and reduced intimal damage associated with hypertension; it had no effect on the immune injury. In an atherosclerosis model produced by dietary manipulation in pigs, long-term perindopril treatment showed a significant preventive action on the deleterious effects to vascular wall function and structure induced by atherosclerosis.[20]

In summary, perindopril lowers blood pressure with little or no reflex tachycardia; it inhibits plasma and tissue ACE (especially renal ACE); it inhibits the pressor response to AI and to spinal cord stimulation; and in the presence of normal kidneys, it inhibits the pressor response to α-agonists, particularly the α_2 subtype. The response to bradykinin is enhanced by perindopril. Perindopril is 1000 times less potent in vitro than the diacid metabolite, perindoprilat, which is, in turn, slightly more potent in vivo and in vitro than enalaprilat.

There is evidence that perindopril may prevent the cardiac and vascular hypertrophy caused by hypertension and that in high doses it may reduce arrhythmias caused by acute coronary artery occlusion. In view of the varying inhibition achieved in different tissues and in plasma, it is not clear which is the major site of action responsible for the hypotensive effect of perindopril.

PHARMACOKINETICS

In normal subjects given 8 mg, the oral bioavailability of perindopril is 95%. Approximately 20% of the available parent drug is slowly metabolized to the active metabolite, perindoprilat.[21] In another study,[22] apparent clearance was estimated at 43.4 ± 9.7 L/hr, and the apparent volume of distribution was 313 ± 129 L. The time to peak perindoprilat concentration after oral perindopril was dose-dependent: 0.4 ± 0.6 hour after 4 mg, 2.1 ± 0.9 hours after 8 mg, and 2.9 ± 0.6 hours after 16 mg. No change in pharmacokinetics was detected after repeated administration for one week.

Following intravenous bolus administration of perindoprilat, the plasma profile of perindoprilat concentrations was fitted best by a three-compartment model that had half-lives for the alpha, beta, and gamma phases as follows: 0.2 ± 0.04 hours, 1.24 ± 0.2 hours, and 31 ± 17 hours, respectively. The areas under the plasma concentration-time curve for perindoprilat were 206 ± 31 hr/ng/ml after 1 mg, 411 ± 3 hr/ng/ml after 2 mg, and 822 ± 125 hr/ng/ml after 4 mg. Clearance may therefore be estimated to be approximately 4.9 L/hr.

As with enalapril, the terminal elimination half-life derived from intravenous studies may not predict the accumulation profile during repeated dosing.[23, 24] After tracer doses in animals, extensive tissue binding of the drug occurs,[25] which is less marked after larger doses. Saturable protein binding is thus probable and will influence the pharmacokinetics accordingly. In particular, it appears that both tissue and plasma ACE binding exert an influence on the pharmacokinetics and that modeling of these influences may be used to derive sensible inferences about the distribution of enzyme in humans.[26] Bree et al.[27] have shown that in the therapeutic range, perindopril was 74% bound to serum involving a nonsaturable process but that perindoprilat is only weakly bound to serum albumin, about 18%, with specific and high binding to ACE.

Further pharmacokinetic studies with perindopril have been undertaken in elderly subjects,[28] in patients with compensated hepatic cirrhosis,[29, 30] and in patients with heart failure[31] (Table 81–1). Aging appears to be associated with increased conversion of perindopril to perindoprilat and thus higher levels of active drug. Active drug clearance is correlated with renal function.[28] Indeed, studies performed in patients with renal failure after single oral administration of perindopril,[32] repeated oral administration of perindopril,[33] and in chronic hemodialyzed patients[34] have shown that renal failure had little influence on perindopril pharmacokinetics, in accordance with its essentially metabolic elimination, but that the apparent half-life of perindoprilat was inversely correlated to renal function.

EFFECTS ON PATHOPHYSIOLOGY
Hemodynamics

There are a number of reports showing that perindopril lowers blood pressure with little or no effect on heart rate[3, 35–37] at doses of 4 or 8 mg. Only studies using very small numbers of normal subjects have failed to demonstrate a significant effect of perindopril on blood pressure.[38, 39] The report by Richer et al.[39] showing a nonsignificant fall in blood pressure after administration of perindopril was conducted in only six subjects; similarly, Bussien et al.[38] gave 4 mg of perindopril to six subjects and 8 mg to six subjects and recorded a nonsignificant fall in blood pressure.

Ajayi et al.[35] compared the acute response of perindopril, 8 mg PO, with placebo in a double-blind trial in salt-replete normotensive subjects. Supine systolic and diastolic blood pressures were lowered significantly, but heart rate was not altered. In another study,[36] during repeated oral dosing with perindopril, 1 to 16 mg daily, or placebo in 36 salt-replete normotensive subjects, a significant fall in diastolic blood pressure was detected, most marked after 16 mg daily. Heart rate rose only slightly with this dose. In normal subjects, acute intravenous administration of perindo-

prilat was associated with a reduction in blood pressure and no change in heart rate.[3] A small phase-II study in patients with essential hypertension demonstrated a fall in blood pressure after 4 mg of perindopril from 164/93 mmHg to 145/84 acutely; and after 1 month receiving perindopril (4 mg or 8 mg daily), the blood pressure remained at 142/82 mmHg.[40] No postural hypotension or tachycardia was found. Because these were salt-replete patients, a greater hypotensive effect would be anticipated if salt restriction or a diuretic were added.[5, 6, 41, 42]

Richer et al.[39] studied peripheral hemodynamics in healthy subjects. Brachial artery blood flow, as measured by a pulsed Doppler technique, was increased by perindopril (4 to 16 mg) in a dose-related manner. The maximal increase was 61% 2 to 3 hours after dosing. Forearm vascular resistance was reduced by 41% at this time. Similarly, carotid artery blood flow was increased by 22% with 8 mg and by 24% with 16 mg of perindopril, although carotid artery diameter was not altered.

Ventricular Function and Structure

Animal studies on the effects of perindopril on LV function and structure have been discussed above.[11, 15–18] Asmar et al. studied the effects of perindopril on cardiac mass in 14 hypertensive patients, using M-mode echocardiography.[43] The study was single-blind, with a 12-week dose titration period (2, 4, or 8 mg once daily) followed by a 4-week placebo period; data from an additional 9-month open treatment period have also been presented for seven patients who had a good blood pressure response.[44] End-diastolic volume, septal and posterior wall thickness, and both LV mass index and mass/volume were significantly reduced after 3 months' treatment with perindopril. During the subsequent placebo period, blood pressure rose significantly toward baseline values, whereas cardiac mass measurements remained unaltered (Table 81–2). In the selected subgroup of seven patients who continued on active treatment, these measurements had improved further after 12 months.[44] Although the single-blind, sequential design and the unreported patient withdrawals leave basis for criticism, this study suggests that perindo-

Table 81–1. **Summary of Pharmacokinetic Data from Observations by the Authors**

	Healthy Young	Healthy Elderly	Compensated Hepatic Cirrhosis
Age (years)	29 ± 3	71 ± 3	59 ± 9
Bioavailability of perindopril (%)	66 ± 27	60 ± 27	64 ± 10
Perindopril to S-9780 conversion (%)	32 ± 15	61 ± 20	47 ± 4
Bioavailability of S-9780 after oral perindopril (%)	19 ± 7	35 ± 17	30 ± 6
Renal recovery of S-9780 after intravenous S-9780 (%)	70 ± 16	57 ± 25	61 ± 14

n = 8 in each group.
Mean ± SD.
Data from Lees KR, Green ST, Reid JL: Influence of age on the pharmacokinetics and pharmacodynamics of perindopril. Clin Pharmacol Ther 44:418, 1988; Tsai HH, Lees KR, Howden CW, et al: The pharmacokinetics and pharmacodynamics of perindopril in patients with hepatic cirrhosis. Br J Clin Pharmacol 28:53, 1989.

Table 81–2. **Changes in Echocardiographic Results in the 14 Patients Who Achieved the Second Placebo Period (M4)**

	M0 (Placebo)	M3 (Active Treatment)	M4 (Placebo)
End diastolic diameter (cm)	5.27 ± 0.12	5.15 ± 0.14	5.17 ± 0.14
End systolic diameter (cm)	3.30 ± 0.15	3.13 ± 0.16	3.14 ± 0.15
End diastolic volume (ml)	135.0 ± 6.9	128.0 ± 8.1*	129.6 ± 8.1
End systolic volume (ml)	39.0 ± 5.1	33.8 ± 5.2	34.0 ± 4.8
Ejection fraction (%)	0.723 ± 0.003	0.75 ± 0.02	0.75 ± 0.02
Velocity of circumferential fiber shortening (circ/sec)	1.32 ± 0.07	1.39 ± 0.07	1.40 ± 0.06
Left ventricular fractional shortening (%)	0.37 ± 0.02	0.39 ± 0.02	0.39 ± 0.02
Septal thickness (cm)	1.13 ± 0.02	1.03 ± 0.02†	1.07 ± 0.02‡
Posterior wall thickness (cm)	1.08 ± 0.03	0.99 ± 0.02†	1.04 ± 0.02§
Mass index (g/m²)	147.2 ± 6.4	124.5 ± 7.2†	134.5 ± 6.4†
Mass/volume (g/ml)	2.04 ± 0.08	1.81 ± 0.07†	1.95 ± 0.05§

Values are mean ± SD.
*$p < .05$ and †$p < .01$, M3 versus M0 and M4.
‡$p < .01$ and §$p < .05$, M3 versus M0.
From Asmar RG, Pannier B, Laurent S, et al: Haemodynamic effects of perindopril in essential hypertension. J Hum Hypertens 4(Suppl 4):35, 1990.

pril has beneficial effects on LV structure during long-term treatment. Other studies in hypertensive patients have confirmed reductions in LV mass with perindopril.[45–47]

The acute systemic and regional hemodynamic responses to perindopril (4 mg orally) have been investigated in ten patients with congestive heart failure using right-sided heart catheterization.[48] An open design was used, with only a pretreatment control measurement. Systemic vascular resistance, right atrial pressure, and mean pulmonary capillary wedge pressure were reduced for more than 24 hours; cardiac index and brachial and renal blood flow each increased (Fig. 81–2). Flammang et al.[31] presented data on 15 patients treated for 3 months, confirming that the hemodynamic benefits persist during long-term treatment.

One double-blind, placebo-controlled, parallel group study[49] in 125 patients with New York Heart Association grade II–III heart failure demonstrated symptomatic improvement after 3 months (exercise tolerance and symptom score) in perindopril-treated patients and a reduction in radiologic cardiothoracic ratio. A later report refers to a subgroup of the same patients.[50]

Effects on Arteries and Veins

As discussed, Richer et al.[39] demonstrated a peripheral vasodilating effect of perindopril. Ajayi et al.[35] reported an increase in pulse pressure during exercise after perindopril compared with placebo, presumably a consequence of peripheral arteriolar dilatation. Arterial or venous selectivity has not been reported.

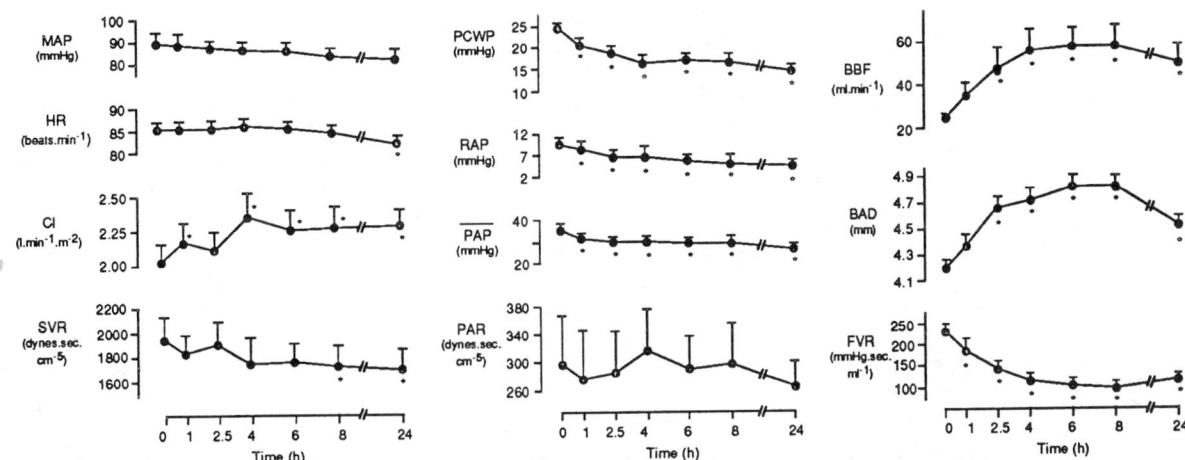

Figure 81–2. Effects of a single oral dose (4 mg) of perindopril on mean arterial pressure (MAP), heart rate (HR), cardiac index (CI), systemic vascular resistance (SVR), mean pulmonary capillary wedge pressure (PCWP), mean right atrial pressure (RAP), mean pulmonary arterial pressure (PAP), pulmonary arteriolar resistance (PAR), brachial blood flow (BBF), brachial artery diameter (BAD), and forearm vascular resistance (FVR) over the 24-hour period following its administration to patients with congestive heart failure. Results are mean ± SEM. (*Significantly different from basal value; $p < .05$). (From Thuillez C, Richard C, Loueslati H, et al: Systemic and regional hemodynamic effects of perindopril in congestive heart failure. J Cardiovasc Pharmacol 15:527, 1990.)

The effects of perindopril on left ventricular mass have been discussed above. In the same study, Asmar et al.[43] examined arterial compliance. Using pulsed Doppler techniques on the brachial artery, they found that arterial compliance was increased by 3 months' treatment with 2, 4, or 8 mg perindopril daily. The effect regressed during subsequent placebo treatment but reappeared during long-term active treatment (Fig. 81–3).[44]

Sihm et al.[51] presented data on the media-lumen ratio of human resistance vessels from hypertensive patients treated for nine months with perindopril.[51] Isradipine, hydralazine, or both could be added to achieve satisfactory blood pressure control. The media-lumen ratio fell from 9.8% ± 2.6% (mean ± SD) to 7.8% ± 1.9% (P); normotensive controls had a ratio of 7.9% ± 2.9%. This is the first indication from invasive studies of human hypertensive patients that arterial remodeling occurs.

Endocrine and Metabolic Effects

Perindopril consistently inhibits plasma ACE, causes a rise in PRA and AI, causes lower plasma AII levels, and less consistently reduces plasma aldosterone concentrations.

The inhibition of ACE is dose-related in the range of 1 to 16 mg perindopril: peak inhibition of 90% was achieved after 4 hours after administration of 16 mg,[36, 39] and 70% inhibition persisted at 24 hours (Fig. 81–4). The maximal rise in renin activity also occurred 4 to 6 hours after dosing; again, the effect on renin was dose-related between 1 and 16 mg of perindopril. Both studies showed a small decrease in aldosterone levels.

Using a different assay for plasma ACE, Bussien et al.[38] found greater inhibition at the same doses. They also demonstrated increases in PRA after 4 hours,

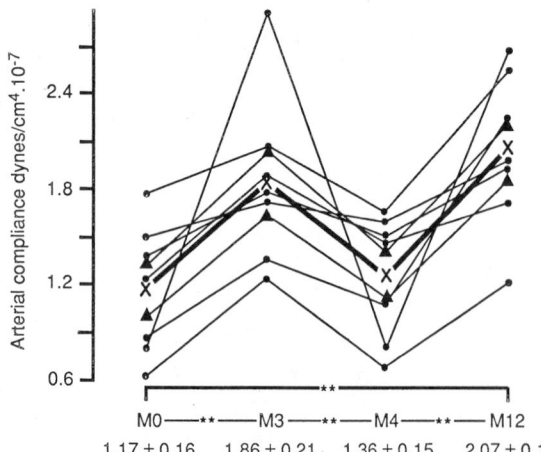

Figure 81–3. Changes in arterial compliance. ● — ●, individual values, ▲ — ▲, SEM; and × — ×, mean values. **$p < .01$; M0, end of placebo period; M3, end of 3 months' active treatment; M4, end of second placebo period; M12, end of 12 months' active treatment period. (From Asmar RG, Pannier B, Laurent S, et al: Haemodynamic effects of perindopril in essential hypertension. J Hum Hypertens 4[Suppl 4]:35, 1990.)

associated with a rise in AI, a fall in AII, and a fall in aldosterone levels.

After repeated oral dosing, there is some evidence of diminished sensitivity of plasma ACE to inhibition by perindopril.[40, 52] This is a small and clinically insignificant change. It probably represents induction of plasma ACE and also has been reported with enalapril.[53]

A double-blind, crossover study of 6 weeks' treatment with perindopril versus placebo in random order has demonstrated that perindopril has no adverse effect on plasma lipids, glucose tolerance or insulin sensitivity in hypertensive patients with non-insulin-dependent diabetes mellitus;[54] neutral effects on plasma lipids have been confirmed over longer periods.[55, 56]

Effects on Renal Function

Anderson and Morgan[57] have presented work on 32 patients with essential hypertension in whom renal function was measured during treatment with perindopril or placebo. No change was detected in 24-hour urine protein levels, glomerular filtration rate, plasma urea concentrations, or plasma creatinine levels.

Reyes et al.[58] found that perindopril, 4 or 8 mg, significantly increased urinary sodium flow and instantaneous renal clearance of sodium and chloride up to 24 hours after dosing. There was no significant change in magnesium or urate excretion, although the latter tended to increase. Chaignon et al.[59] reported an increase in renal blood flow with no change in glomerular filtration rate in hypertensive patients after receiving perindopril (8 mg) for 5 days. Quaglia et al.[60] also found no effect on renal function.

During 3 to 12 months' treatment with perindopril (2 to 8 mg once daily), 36 patients with renal impairment showed no significant change in renal function, although proteinuria decreased from 1.9 ± 0.6 to 0.9 ± 0.2 g/24 hr ($p < .01$).[61] Treatment was withdrawn for six patients; in two because of adverse events and in four because of intercurrent diseases. Long-term treatment of diabetic patients with ACE inhibitors has been linked to improvement in urinary microalbuminuria, a marker of glomerular damage. In a study of 39 hypertensive insulin-treated patients, perindopril reduced proteinuria in subjects with normal urinary albumin excretion rate or microalbuminuria, but not in those with macroalbuminuria.[62] A 12-month randomized study suggested that this effect was not specific to the ACE inhibitor.[63] The same group,[64] however, has recently presented preliminary data from normotensive diabetic microalbuminuric patients which showed a reduction in microalbuminuria with perindopril but not nifedipine.

Effects on the Central Nervous System

No effects on the brain have been reported. Ajayi et al.[35] reported the effects of perindopril on autonomic function. In a group of normal subjects, there was no evidence of any alteration in sympathetic activity

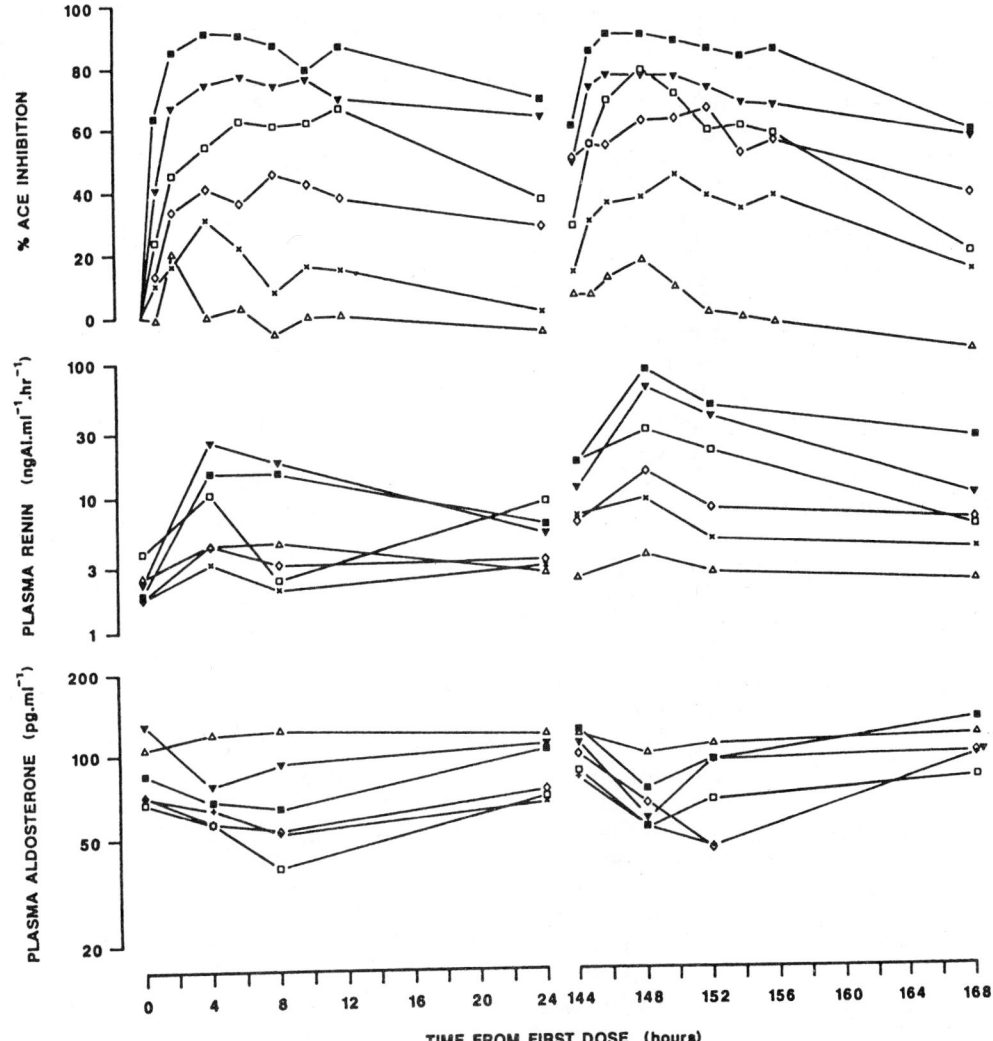

Figure 81–4. Plasma angiotensin-converting enzyme inhibition, renin activity, and aldosterone concentrations following the first and seventh daily administrations of placebo (△) and of 1 mg (×), 2 mg (◇), 4 mg (□), 8 mg (▼), and 16 mg (■) of perindopril orally. The effects were significant by analysis of variance: ACE inhibition ($p < .001$); renin activity ($p < .001$); and aldosterone ($p < .05$). Each point represents the mean for six subjects. (From Lees KR, Reid JL: Haemodynamic and humoral effects of oral perindopril, an angiotensin converting enzyme inhibitor, in man. Br J Clin Pharmacol 23:159, 1987.)

after perindopril, but a vagomimetic action was noted. This is not unique to perindopril; it has also been found with captopril and enalapril.[65–67]

CLINICAL USE

Aspects of the clinical use of perindopril have been discussed under several of the earlier headings. This section will concentrate on tolerability, antihypertensive action, and dose selection.

Initial reports showed perindopril to be well tolerated and without adverse biochemical or severe side effects.[3, 28, 29, 38–40] Additional reports on small groups of patients[68] have since been supplemented by reviews on several hundred hypertensive subjects.[69, 70] However, the largest survey of tolerability comes from postmarketing surveillance of 23,460 patients with mild to moderate hypertension.[71] There were no changes in mean serum sodium, potassium, or

creatinine levels. Side effects were infrequent, with withdrawal rates ranging from 6.1% in elderly patients to 4.2% in those aged 69 years or less. There were slightly more withdrawals among patients taking nonsteroidal antiinflammatory drugs or psychotropic medication than in other groups (6.1% and 5.3%, respectively, versus 4.1%). Cough was the reason for withdrawal in 2.6% of patients, and was more common in elderly patients and in nonsmokers.

The usual dose used in the patients reported above was 2 or 4 mg/day. A small dose-ranging study suggested that 4 or 8 mg once daily should be adequate for the majority of hypertensive patients. A larger dose-ranging study examined doses ranging from 2 to 16 mg once daily and compared once-daily with twice-daily regimens.[72] No advantage of twice-daily dosing was apparent, and the additional benefit from 12 or 16 mg/day was limited, compared with 8 mg once daily. Although higher doses may occasionally be necessary, 4 or 8 mg of perindopril once daily appears to be the optimal dose in mild to moderate hypertension.

Several studies compared the antihypertensive efficacy and tolerability of perindopril with other agents, such as captopril,[46, 47, 73] enalapril,[74] and atenolol.[74, 75] Perindopril 4 to 8 mg once daily was tolerated as well as atenolol 50 to 100 mg once daily and had an equal[74] or greater effect[75] at the doses used. Perindopril 4 to 8 mg once daily was tolerated as well as captopril 25 to 50 mg twice daily and had an equal[46] or greater effect[47, 73] on blood pressure at the doses used. In particular, 24-hour control of blood pressure appears better with once-daily perindopril than with twice-daily captopril.[76] Compared with enalapril 10 to 20 mg once daily, perindopril 4 to 8 mg once daily had the same effect on blood pressure at the time of peak effect (usually 3 to 4 hours after dosing) but a greater effect on trough (24 hour) blood pressure. The trough-peak ratio for blood pressure effect was 0.55 for enalapril and 0.78 for perindopril.[74] There is thus good evidence for the use of perindopril once daily as a first line antihypertensive treatment.

The long-term tolerability of perindopril in patients with heart failure has been summarized by Desche et al.[77] In view of the uncontrolled nature of the report, limited conclusions may be drawn regarding the incidence of adverse events and symptomatic improvements. Of the 320 patients, 3.1% died during the follow-up period and 2.8% deteriorated; the most common reason for treatment withdrawal was cough (2.8%). Symptomatic hypotension or dizziness led to treatment withdrawal in 6 patients (1.9%). Cough was reported in 6.3% of patients and dizziness in 4.1%.

In patients with congestive heart failure who have been treated with loop diuretics, particularly if they are elderly, first dose hypotension may be a problem with some ACE inhibitors. The recommended starting dose of perindopril in such patients, as in all elderly patients or those with renal impairment, is 2 mg. A double-blind, placebo-controlled study confirmed that a 2-mg dose does not normally cause a blood pressure reduction acutely, whereas captopril 6.25 mg or enalapril 2.5 mg orally is associated with significant blood pressure falls.[78]

SUMMARY

There is now extensive experience with perindopril in the treatment of mild to moderate hypertension. It is well tolerated and once-daily treatment with 4 or 8 mg gives adequate 24-hour control of blood pressure in most cases. There is evidence that long-term treatment with perindopril is associated with improvements in arterial compliance and structure, with regression of LV hypertrophy and with reductions in microalbuminuria. Perindopril appears to be lipid-neutral and to cause little effect on serum electrolytes or renal function. Experience in patients with heart failure is more limited, but first-dose hypotension appears less likely with perindopril than with captopril or enalapril.

REFERENCES

1. Vincent M, Redmond G, Portevin B, et al: Stereoselective synthesis of a new perhydroindole derivative of chiral iminodiacid, a potent inhibitor of angiotensin converting enzyme. Tetrahedron Lett 23:1677, 1982.
2. Mannhold R: Perindopril. Drugs of the Future 10:636, 1985.
3. Lees KR, Reid JL: Effects of intravenous S-9780, an angiotensin-converting enzyme inhibitor, in normotensive subjects. J Cardiovasc Pharmacol 10:129, 1987.
4. van den Berg H, Resplandy G, de Bie AThHJ, et al: A new radioimmunoassay for the determination of the angiotensin-converting enzyme inhibitor Perindopril and its active metabolite in plasma and urine: Advantages of a lysine derivative as immunogen to improve the assay specificity. J Pharm Biomed Anal 7:517, 1991.
5. Laubie M, Schiavi P, Vincent M, et al: Inhibition of angiotensin I converting enzyme with S-9490: Biochemical effects, interspecies differences and role of sodium diet in the haemodynamic effects. J Cardiovasc Pharmacol 6:1076, 1984.
6. DiNicolantonio R, Doyle AE: Comparison of the actions of the angiotensin-converting enzyme inhibitors enalapril and S-94903 in sodium-deplete and sodium-replete spontaneously hypertensive rats. J Cardiovasc Pharmacol 7:937, 1985.
7. Unger T, Moursi M, Ganten D, et al: Antihypertensive action of the converting enzyme inhibitor perindopril (S-9490-3) in spontaneously hypertensive rats: Comparison with enalapril (MK421) and ramipril (HOE 498). J Cardiovasc Pharmacol 8:276, 1986.
8. Richer C, Doussau MP, Giudicelli F: Perindopril, a new converting enzyme inhibitor: Systemic and regional hemodynamics and sympathoinhibitory effects in spontaneously hypertensive rats. J Cardiovasc Pharmacol 8:346, 1986.
9. Barres C, Curutti C, Devissaguet M, et al: Cardiovascular effects of S-9490-3, a new converting enzyme inhibitor: A computerized study in conscious spontaneously hypertensive rats. J Hypertens 3(Suppl 3):S207, 1985.
10. Richer C, Doussau MP, Giudicelli JF: Systemic and regional hemodynamic profile of five angiotensin I converting enzyme inhibitors in the spontaneously hypertensive rat. Am J Cardiol 59:12D, 1987.
11. Barres C, Cerutti C, Paultre CZ, et al: Antihypertensive effects of S-9490-3, a new converting enzyme inhibitor, in the conscious spontaneously hypertensive rat. Clin Sci 70:167, 1986.
12. Levy BI, Michel J-B, Salzmann J-L, et al: Effects of chronic inhibition on converting enzyme on mechanical and structural properties of arteries in rat renovascular hypertension. Circ Res 63:227, 1988.
13. Harrap SB, van der Merwe WM, Griffin SA, et al: Brief angiotensin converting enzyme inhibitor treatment in young spontaneously hypertensive rats reduces blood pressure long-term. Hypertension 16:603, 1990.
14. Christensen KL, Jespersen LT, Mulvany MJ: Development of blood pressure in spontaneously hypertensive rats after withdrawal of long-term treatment related to vascular structure. J Hypertens 7:83, 1989.
15. Cadilhac M, Giudicelli JF: Myocardial and vascular effects of perindopril, a new converting enzyme inhibitor, during hypertension development in spontaneously hypertensive rats. Arch Int Pharmacodyn Ther 1:114, 1986.
16. Ribuot C, Rochette L: Converting enzyme inhibitors (captopril, enalapril, perindopril) prevent early postinfarction ventricular fibrillation in the anaesthetized rat. Cardiovasc Drug Ther 1:51, 1987.
17. van Wijngaarden J, Tobe TJM, Weersink EGL, et al: Effects of early angiotensin-converting enzyme inhibition in a pig model of myocardial ischemia and reperfusion. J Cardiovasc Pharmacol 19:408, 1992.
18. Muller CA, Opie LH, Peisach M, et al: Antiarrhythmic effects of the angiotensin converting enzyme inhibitor perindoprilat in a pig model of acute regional myocardial ischemia. J Cardiovasc Pharmacol 19:748, 1992.
19. Plissonier D, Amichot G, Duriez M, et al: Effect of converting enzyme inhibition on allograft-induced arterial wall injury and response. Hypertension 18(Suppl II):II-47, 1991.

20. Charpiot P, Rolland PH, Friggi A, et al: ACE inhibition with perindopril and atherogenesis-induced structural and functional changes in minipig arteries. Arterioscler Thromb 13:1125, 1993.

21. Devissaguet JP, Ammoury N, Devissaguet M, et al: Pharmacokinetics of perindopril and its metabolites in healthy volunteers. Fundam Clin Pharmacol 4:175, 1990.

22. Lees KR, Kelman AW, Meredith P, et al: Pharmacokinetics of the angiotensin converting enzyme inhibitor, perindopril, after repeated oral dosing. Br J Clin Pharmacol 2:233, 1986.

23. Till AE, Gomez HJ, Hichens M, et al: Pharmacokinetics of repeated single oral doses of enalapril maleate (MK-421) in normal volunteers. Biopharm Drug Dispos 5:273, 1984.

24. Louis WJ, Workman BS, Conway EL, et al: Single-dose and steady-state pharmacokinetics and pharmacodynamics of perindopril in hypertensive subjects. J Cardiovasc Pharmacol 20:505, 1992.

25. Borghi H, Fillastre JP, Morin JP: Rat and rabbit renal and tissular distributions of perindopril (S-9490-3) a new angiotensin-converting enzyme inhibitor. Clin Exp Hypertens A9:1952, 1987.

26. Lees KR, Kelman AW, Whiting B, et al: Pharmacokinetics of S-9780 in man: Evidence of tissue binding. J Pharmacokinet Biopharm 17:529, 1989.

27. Bree E, Nguyen P, Urien S, et al: Specific and high affinity binding of perindoprilat, but not of perindopril to blood ACE. Int J Clin Pharmacol Ther Toxicol 30:325, 1992.

28. Lees KR, Green ST, Reid JL: Influence of age on the pharmacokinetics and pharmacodynamics of perindopril. Clin Pharmacol Ther 44:418, 1988.

29. Tsai HH, Lees KR, Howden CW, et al: The pharmacokinetics and pharmacodynamics of perindopril in patients with hepatic cirrhosis. Br J Clin Pharmacol 28:53, 1989.

30. Thiollet M, Funck-Brentano C, Grange J-D, et al: The pharmacokinetics of perindopril in patients with liver cirrhosis. Br J Clin Pharmacol 33:326, 1992.

31. Flammang D, Waynberger M, Chassing A: Acute and long-term efficacy of perindopril in severe chronic congestive heart failure. Am J Cardiol 71:48E, 1993.

32. Verpooten GA, Genissel PM, Thomas JR, et al: Single dose pharmacokinetics of perindopril and its metabolites in hypertensive patients with various degrees of renal insufficiency. Br J Clin Pharmacol 32:187, 1991.

33. Sennesael J, Ali A, Sweny P, et al: The pharmacokinetics of perindopril and its effects on serum angiotensin converting enzyme activity in hypertensive patients with chronic renal failure. Br J Clin Pharmacol 33:93, 1992.

34. Guerin A, Resplandy G, Marchais S, et al: The effect of haemodialysis on the pharmacokinetics of perindoprilat after long-term perindopril. Eur J Clin Pharmacol 44:183, 1993.

35. Ajayi AA, Lees KR, Reid JL: Effects of angiotensin converting enzyme inhibitor, perindopril, on autonomic reflexes. Eur J Clin Pharmacol 30:177, 1986.

36. Lees KR, Reid JL: Haemodynamic and humoral effects of oral perindopril, an angiotensin converting enzyme inhibitor, in man. Br J Clin Pharmacol 23:159, 1987.

37. Frances Y, Schwab C, Luccioni R: Dose antihypertensive effect relationship for the angiotensin converting enzyme inhibitor: Perindopril. Clin Exp Hypertens A8:147, 1986.

38. Bussien JP, Fasanella D'Amore T, Perret L, et al: Single and repeated dosing of the converting enzyme inhibitor perindopril to normal subjects. Clin Pharmacol Ther 39:554, 1986.

39. Richer C, Thuillez C, Giudicelli JF: Perindopril, converting enzyme blockade, and peripheral arterial hemodynamics in the healthy volunteer. J Cardiovasc Pharmacol 9:94, 1987.

40. Lees KR, Reid JL: The haemodynamic and humoral effects of treatment for one month with the angiotensin converting enzyme inhibitor perindopril in salt-replete hypertensive patients. Eur J Clin Pharmacol 31:519, 1987.

41. Case DV, Wallace JM, Keim HJ, et al: Possible role of renin in hypertension as suggested by renin-sodium profiling and inhibition of converting enzyme. N Engl J Med 296:641, 1977.

42. Man in't Veld AJ, Schicht IM, Derkx FHM, et al: Effect of an angiotensin-converting enzyme inhibitor (captopril) on blood pressure in anephric subjects. Br Med J 1:280, 1980.

43. Asmar RG, Pannier B, Santoni JP, et al: Reversion of cardiac hypertrophy and reduced arterial compliance after converting enzyme inhibition in essential hypertension. Circulation 78:941, 1988.

44. Asmar RG, Pannier B, Laurent S, et al: Haemodynamic effects of perindopril in essential hypertension. J Hum Hypertens 4(Suppl 4):35, 1990.

45. Sihm I, Schroeder P, Morn B, et al: Greater regression of left ventricular mass in essential hypertension with a perindopril based than with a thiazide based antihypertensive regimen [abstract]. Sixth European Meeting on Hypertension, Milan, Italy, June 4–7, 1993.

46. Grandi AM, Venco A, Barzizza F, et al: Double-blind comparison of perindopril and captopril in hypertension. Am J Hypertens 4:516, 1991.

47. Agabiti-Rosei E, Ambrosioni E, Finardi G, et al: Perindopril versus captopril: Efficacy and acceptability in an Italian multicenter trial. Am J Med 92(Suppl 4B):79S, 1992.

48. Thuillez C, Richard C, Loueslati H, et al: Systemic and regional hemodynamic effects of perindopril in congestive heart failure. J Cardiovasc Pharmacol 15:527, 1990.

49. Bounhoure JP, Bottineau G, Lechat P, et al: Value of perindopril in the treatment of chronic congestive heart failure: Multicenter double-blind placebo-controlled study. Clin Exp Hypertens [A] 11(Suppl 2):575, 1989.

50. Lechat P, Garnham SP, Desche P, et al: Perindopril for mild to moderate chronic congestive heart failure. Am Heart J 126(Suppl):798, 1993.

51. Sihm I, Schroeder AP, Aalkjoor C, et al: Normalisation of media to lumen ration of human subcutaneous arteries during antihypertensive treatment with a perindopril based regimen. [abstract 63]. Eur Heart J 14:520, 1993.

52. Lees KR, Kelman AW, Reid JL: Effect of repeated dosing on concentration-effect relationships with the angiotensin converting enzyme inhibitor, perindopril. Br J Clin Pharmacol 2:234, 1986.

53. Lees KR, Reid JL: Age and the pharmacokinetics and pharmacodynamics of chronic enalapril treatment. Clin Pharmacol Ther 41:597, 1987.

54. Bak JF, Gerdes LU, Sorensen NS, et al: Effects of perindopril on insulin sensitivity and plasma lipid profile in hypertensive non-insulin-dependent diabetic patients. Am J Med 92(Suppl 4B):69S, 1992.

55. Giuntoli F, Gabbani S, Natali A, et al: Effects of perindopril on carbohydrate and lipoprotein metabolism in essential hypertension. Am J Med 92(Suppl 4B):95S, 1992.

56. Jandrain B, Herbaut C, Depoorter JC, et al: Long-term (1 year) acceptability of perindopril in type II diabetic patients with hypertension. Am J Med 92(Suppl 4B):91S, 1992.

57. Anderson A, Morgan T: Response to perindopril in people on different sodium intake [abstract 0289]. Eleventh Scientific Meeting of the International Society of Hypertension, Heidelberg, Germany, August 31–September 6, 1986.

58. Reyes AJ, Leary WP, van der Byl K: Renal excretory actions of perindopril in healthy subjects. Hypertension 9:528, 1987.

59. Chaignon M, Barrou Z, Ayad M, et al: Effects of perindopril on renal haemodynamics and natriuresis in essential hypertension. J Hypertens 6(Suppl 3):S61, 1988.

60. Quaglia G, Periti M, Salvalaggio A, et al: Evaluation of a new angiotensin converting enzyme inhibitor (S-9490) [abstract]. Third National Congress of the Italian Society of Arterial Hypertension, Brescia, October 3–4, 1986.

61. Dratwa M, Sennesael J, Taillard F, et al: Long-term tolerance of perindopril in hypertensive patients with impaired renal function. J Cardiovasc Pharmacol 18(Suppl 7):S40, 1991.

62. Hermans MP, Brichard SM, Colin I, et al: Long-term reduction of microalbuminuria after 3 years of angiotensin-converting enzyme inhibition by perindopril in hypertensive insulin-treated diabetic patients. Am J Med 92(Suppl 4B):102S, 1992.

63. Melbourne Diabetic Nephropathy Study Group: Comparison between perindopril and nifedipine in hypertensive and normotensive diabetic patients with microalbuminuria. Br Med J 302:210, 1991.

64. Melbourne Diabetic Nephropathy Group: Effects of different antihypertensive agents in normotensive microalbuminuric

type I and type II diabetic patients. Presented at XIIth International Congress of Nephrology, Jerusalem, Israel, June 13–18, 1993.

65. Sturani A, Chiairini C, Degli Esposti E, et al: Heart rate control in hypertensive patients treated by captopril. Br J Clin Pharmacol 14:849, 1982.

66. Campbell BC, Sturani A, Reid JL: Evidence of parasympathetic activity of the angiotensin converting enzyme inhibitor, captopril, in normotensive man. Clin Sci 68:49, 1985.

67. Ajayi AA, Campbell BC, Howie CA, et al: Acute and chronic effects of converting enzyme inhibitors on reflex control of heart rate in normotensive man. J Hypertens 3:47, 1985.

68. Forette F, McClaran J, Delesalle MC, et al: Value of angiotensin converting enzyme inhibitors in the elderly: The example of perindopril. Clin Exp Hypertens AII(Suppl 2):587, 1989.

69. Brown CI: The safety and acceptability of perindopril. J Hum Hypertens 4(Suppl 4):51, 1990.

70. Degaute JP, Leeman M, Desche P: Long-term acceptability of perindopril: European multicenter trial on 856 patients. Am J Med 92(Suppl 4B):84S, 1992.

71. Fressinaud P, Berrut G, Gallois H: Antihypertensive activity and acceptability based upon clinical and laboratory parameters of perindopril: Chief results in 23,460 mild to moderate

hypertension patients treated for 6 months in general practice. Ann Cardiol Angeiol (Paris) 42(1):1, 1993.

72. Chrysant ZG, McDonald RH, Wright JT, et al: Perindopril as monotherapy in hypertension: A multicenter comparison of two dosing regimens. Clin Pharmacol Ther 53:479, 1993.

73. Lees KR, Reid JL, Scott MGB, et al: Captopril versus perindopril: A double blind study in essential hypertension. J Hum Hypertens 3:17, 1989.

74. Morgan T, Anderson A: Clinical efficacy of perindopril in hypertension. Clin Exper Pharmacol Physiol 19(Suppl 19):61, 1992.

75. Thurston H, Mimran A, Zanchetti A, et al: A double blind comparison of perindopril and atenolol in essential hypertension. J Hum Hypertens 4:547, 1990.

76. Herpin D, Santoni JPh, Pouyollon F, et al: Efficacy of perindopril and captopril in the treatment of mild to moderate hypertension. Curr Ther Res 45(4):576, 1989.

77. Desche P, Antony I, Lerebours G, et al: Acceptability of perindopril in mild-to-moderate chronic heart failure; results of a long-term open study in 320 patients. Am J Cardiol 71(Suppl):IE, 1993.

78. MacFadyen RJ, Lees KR, Reid JL: Differences in first dose response to angiotensin converting enzyme inhibition in congestive heart failure: A placebo controlled study. Br Heart J 66:206, 1991.

CHAPTER 82

Trandolapril

Aram V. Chobanian, M.D., and Peter W. de Leeuw, M.D., Ph.D.

Trandolapril is a relatively new angiotensin-converting enzyme (ACE) inhibitor that has been under clinical investigation since 1985 and is available in several European countries but not yet for clinical use in the United States. Available clinical trial data suggest that the drug will become useful for the management of hypertension, congestive heart failure, and postmyocardial infarction.

CHEMICAL PROPERTIES

Trandolapril is [(2S-(1(R*(R*)), 2ααβ))-1-(2-((1-(ethoxycarbonyl)-3-phenylpropyl) amino)1-oxopropyl)octahydro-lH indole-2-carboxylic acid]. It has a molecular weight of 430.

Trandolapril is a nonsulphydryl prodrug that is converted by deesterification to its active metabolite, trandolaprilat,[1] and to inactive diketopiperazine derivatives. Such conversion can occur rapidly in the mucosa of the gastrointestinal tract as well as in the blood and liver.

Trandolapril is weakly soluble in H_2O. Both trandolapril and trandolaprilat are relatively lipophilic compared with several other ACE inhibitors.[2] Such lipophilicity has been proposed to explain the drug's long duration of action.

PHARMACOKINETICS

Trandolapril is rapidly absorbed from the gastrointestinal tract after oral administration. The drug is detectable in plasma within 30 minutes of administra-

tion, and inhibition of serum ACE activity reaches peak levels in 2 to 4 hours.[1] No interaction with food is apparent with respect to either absorption of the drug or its conversion to trandolaprilat.[3]

The pharmacokinetics of trandolapril are broadly similar to those of other ACE-inhibiting prodrugs such as enalapril, ramipril, and cilazapril. However, the duration of action of orally administered trandolapril appears to be the longest of the currently available ACE inhibitors. In normal subjects, the effective half-life of accumulation is approximately 24 hours.[3] Following long-term administration, inhibition of ACE activity may persist for as long as 8 days after the last dose.[1]

Approximately 80% of circulating trandolapril is bound to plasma proteins in humans, dogs, and rats.[4] Both trandolapril and trandolaprilat are conjugated to glucuronide derivatives excreted in both urine and feces. Following oral administration of radiolabeled trandolapril in normal subjects, approximately one third of the radioactivity is excreted in urine, and two thirds is excreted in feces.[5] The excretion is in the form of free and conjugated trandolapril and trandolaprilat in both urine and feces. Despite the fecal excretion of trandolapril and trandolaprilat, renal clearance can be important in trandolapril removal from the body. Impaired renal function can reduce its plasma clearance and lead to its accumulation in humans.[6] In patients with creatinine clearances of less than 30 ml/min, initial doses of trandolapril should be lower than those used in patients with normal renal function.

Age does not appear to significantly affect the pharmacokinetics of either trandolapril or trandolaprilat.[7] Dose adjustment in the elderly with normal renal function is therefore not required.

DRUG INTERACTIONS

Interactions between trandolapril and a variety of other drugs have been studied in normal subjects. To date, no significant pharmacokinetic interactions have been observed between trandolapril and nifedipine, warfarin, digoxin, or furosemide.[2]

TISSUE BINDING

Trandolapril binds to ACE itself in a variety of tissues, including brain, kidney, heart, lung, adrenal gland, and arterial wall.[8, 9] The binding is specific, of high affinity, and saturable. The specific binding is increased by chloride ions and inhibited by chelators of zinc.[10] Similar binding characteristics have been observed with other ACE inhibitors, and it is uncertain whether clinically significant differences are present between them with respect to tissue penetration, binding, or dissociation from ACE. Displacement studies with slices of caudate putamen incubated with triated trandolapril have shown marked differences among tested compounds in their affinity to converting enzyme. Probably as a result of its high lipophilicity and its high affinity to be enzyme, tissue binding of trandolapril is far greater than that of enalapril.[11]

HEMODYNAMIC ACTIONS

As has been demonstrated with other ACE inhibitors, trandolapril is a potent vasodilator that reduces total peripheral vascular resistance and blood pressure without causing an increase in heart rate.[12] In normal subjects and in patients with uncomplicated hypertension, cardiac output is minimally affected by trandolapril. Vascular resistance is reduced in most organs, including the kidney.[13] Studies in normal dogs have demonstrated that trandolapril induces dose-dependent reductions in cardiac work. Some of the vasodilator effects of trandolapril may be related to its bradykinin-enhancing as well as its angiotensin II–inhibiting properties. The depressor response of infused bradykinin in the rat is potentiated by concurrent administration of trandolapril.[14]

ANTIHYPERTENSIVE EFFECTS
Preclinical Studies

Acute oral administration of trandolapril in doses of 0.3, 3, and 30 mg/kg caused dose-dependent reductions in mean arterial pressure in the spontaneously hypertensive rat.[14] On a dosage basis, trandolapril was more potent than enalapril.

Clinical Studies

Trandolapril is an effective antihypertensive drug in humans.[15] A large, double-blind, placebo-controlled study involving 216 subjects with mild and moderate hypertension examined the effects of 2, 4, and 8 mg of trandolapril administered once daily for 8 days.[16] The responses in all three treatment groups were significantly greater than that of the placebo group, with average decreases in blood pressure of 4.5/3.7, 12.8/8.1, 13.0/8.9, and 13.4/8.3 mmHg in the placebo, 2-mg, 4-mg, and 8-mg groups, respectively.

A second double-blind, placebo-controlled trial of 191 patients examined the effects of 0.5, 1.0, and 2.0 mg of trandolapril given once daily for 28 days.[17] The 1- and 2-mg dose groups experienced significant reductions in supine diastolic blood pressure compared with the placebo group, but adminstration of 0.5 mg/day of trandalopril did not cause a significant decrease.

The available data therefore suggest that the maintenance dose range for trandolapril in the treatment of hypertension is generally 1 to 4 mg daily, with 2 mg being the most common. The drug has a long duration of action and can be administered once daily.

Trandolapril appears to be as effective in lowering blood pressure as other ACE inhibitors, including captopril, enalapril, and lisinopril,[15] although the doses required for trandolapril are lower than those used for these other agents. The efficacy of trandolapril also appears to be similar to that of hydrochlorothiazide, nifedipine, and atenolol.[15] No long-term tolerance to the antihypertensive effects of trandolapril has been observed.

Combining trandolapril with hydrochlorothiazide increases its antihypertensive effects.[17] Data from other ACE inhibitors suggest that combining trandolapril with antihypertensive drugs of other classes will add to its blood pressure–lowering effect.

In studies with 24-hour ambulatory blood pressure monitoring, 2 mg of trandolapril administered once daily for 6 weeks caused significant reductions in systolic and diastolic blood pressure compared with a placebo administered over 24 hours of monitoring and maintained the natural circadian rhythm.[18] The blood pressure control has been shown to extend beyond 24 hours and to be significant for up to 36 hours after dosing.[18] The findings confirm the once-daily use of the drug in hypertensive subjects.

EFFECTS IN SPECIAL HYPERTENSIVE POPULATIONS
Elderly Persons

Trandolapril is effective in elderly hypertensives, although controlled studies are as yet unavailable for comparing its effects with those of other antihypertensive drugs in elderly patients and in those with isolated systolic hypertension.

Overweight Hypertensives

The efficacy of trandolapril in overweight hypertensives—a subgroup with a considerably increased risk—is well documented. Trandolapril reduces blood pressure in overweight hypertensives, defined as weight above 130% of ideal weight at baseline (Lorentz formula). Blood pressure was normalized in 70% and controlled in 46% of patients with 2 mg trandolapril alone in a long-term study.[19]

Left Ventricular Hypertrophy

Trandolapril has been reported to induce significant reductions in left ventricular mass and function in hypertensive persons treated with 1 to 4 mg of the drug daily.[12] Left ventricular mass was reduced by 23% after 3 months of therapy, and wall thickness was reduced by 12% after 6 months. Left ventricular diastolic function improved significantly, and systolic function remained intact. The findings are broadly similar to those reported for other ACE inhibitors.[20]

Renal Disease

Renal clearance of trandolapril is proportional to creatinine clearance, and plasma levels of trandolapril or trandolaprilat may be increased in patients with impaired renal function. In patients with renal failure and creatinine clearance levels less than 30 ml/min, the usual starting dose probably should not exceed 0.5 mg/day.

Experimental studies in spontaneously hypertensive rats and their Wistar-Kyoto controls made diabetic by streptozotocin administration showed that trandolapril reduces proteinuria to an extent similar to that induced by captopril in both normotensive and hypertensive diabetic rats.[21] Studies involving the potential renal protective effects of trandolapril in humans have not been reported.

EFFECTS ON CONGESTIVE HEART FAILURE

In rats with congestive heart failure induced by ligation of the left coronary artery, trandolapril therapy caused reductions in systemic blood pressure and left ventricular end-diastolic pressure and an increase in cardiac output.[22] After 6 months of therapy, cardiac fibrosis and myocardial remodeling were also reduced by trandolapril, as was total mortality.

Studies are in progress regarding the use of trandolapril in patients with congestive heart failure and post myocardial infarction.

POST MYOCARDIAL INFARCTION

As a class, ACE inhibitors have been shown to have a beneficial effect in the post myocardial infarction (MI) patient. The short- and long-term prognoses after acute myocardial infarction have been correlated with the residual left ventricular function; patients with the poorest left ventricular function had the highest mortality. The Trandolapril Cardiac Evaluation (TRACE) Study[22a] was designed to assess the effects of trandolapril in post-MI patients with left ventricular dysfunction. Patients were screened echocardiographically and included only if they had a wall motion index corresponding to an ejection fraction of 35% to 40%. A total of 1749 patients were randomized to either placebo or trandolapril in the dose of 1 to 4 mg/day. In these high-risk patients, the overall 1 year mortality was 24%. All-cause mortality on an intention-to-treat analysis was significantly lower ($p > .001$) in patients with trandolapril as compared with placebo. Trandolapril reduced the risk of mortality by 22%. Most interestingly, trandolapril significantly reduced the incidence of sudden death (133 on placebo, 105 on trandolapril, $p > .03$; risk reduction .76, with a confidence interval of .59 to .98).

VASCULAR ACTIONS

Experimental studies in the Watanabe heritable hyperlipidemic (WHHL) rabbit with hypercholesterolemia secondary to a genetic defect in the low-density lipoprotein receptor have indicated that trandolapril can reduce the development of atherosclerosis without affecting serum lipids or lipoproteins.[23] The findings were very similar to those previously observed with captopril.[24] The antiatherosclerotic action was associated with a significant reduction in cellularity of the atherosclerotic lesions and reduced thickness of both intima and media. Captopril has also been reported to inhibit atherosclerosis in cholesterol-fed monkeys.[25] The potential vasculoprotective action of ACE inhibitors is currently under investigation in humans, and data on such effects should be forthcoming in the next few years.

In the spontaneously hypertensive rat, trandolapril caused a reversal of certain changes in the arterial media induced by hypertension.[26, 27] Medial thickness was reduced significantly, and both compliance and internal diameter of resistance vessels were increased by trandolapril. Compliance of the large arteries also has been reported to increase, and pulse wave velocity has been reported to decrease, in hypertensive patients treated with trandolapril.[28, 29]

METABOLIC EFFECTS

Trandolapril does not appear to adversely affect plasma lipids and lipoproteins, blood glucose, and plasma insulin.[30] In the absence of exercise, trandolapril significantly reduced free fatty acid and glycerol levels; however, the exercise-induced increments in free fatty acid were not affected significantly by trandolapril.[30]

As with other ACE inhibitors, serum potassium levels may be increased by trandolapril, particularly in patients with significant renal disease or those receiving potassium supplements or potassium-retaining diuretics. The effect appears to be related predominantly to inhibition of aldosterone secretion, which is induced by ACE inhibitors.

ADVERSE EFFECTS

Trandolapril is well tolerated, and few adverse effects have been reported. Like other ACE inhibitors, it can cause angioneurotic edema, a potentially serious but rare complication. It is contraindicated in persons who have developed this problem while taking other ACE inhibitors.

Preclinical studies have demonstrated increased maternal and fetal mortality in rabbits treated with trandolapril.[31] Although similar data have not been reported in humans, ACE inhibitors should be contraindicated during pregnancy.

Cough is a significant side effect of trandolapril administration, as with all ACE inhibitors, with a reported incidence in one large study of 3.9%.[15]

Hypotension is a potential consequence of ACE inhibition, particularly with diuretic therapy or in volume-depleted states. ACE inhibitors may also cause deterioration of renal function in patients with bilateral renovascular disease or with severe unilateral disease in a solitary kidney.

SUMMARY

Trandolapril is a new nonsulphydryl ACE inhibitor and is a prodrug that is converted readily to its active metabolite, trandolaprilat. Trandolaprilat binds with high affinity to ACE and has a very prolonged duration of action in humans. It is an effective antihypertensive drug that requires only once-daily administration. It has been shown to decrease left ventricular mass and improve cardiac function in patients with left ventricular hypertrophy. In experimental studies, it also appears to reverse vascular hypertrophy and improve arterial compliance in hypertensive rats and to reduce albuminuria in hypertensive diabetic rats. In addition, trandolapril has been shown to inhibit atherosclerosis in the WHHL rabbit. Thus, trandolapril appears to be a promising new agent for the treatment of hypertension.

REFERENCES

1. Patat A, Sarjus A, LeGo A, et al: Safety and tolerance of single oral doses of trandolapril (RU 45,570), a new angiotensin converting enzyme inhibitor. Eur J Clin Pharmacol 36:17, 1989.
2. Nguyen CL, Brunner HR: Trandolapril in hypertension: Overview of a new angiotensin-converting enzyme inhibitor. Am J Cardiol 70:27D, 1992.
3. Danielson B, Querin S, LaRochell P, et al: Pharmacokinetics and pharmacodynamics of trandolapril after repeated administration of 2 mg to patients with chronic renal failure and healthy control subjects. J Cardiovasc Pharmacol 23(Suppl 4):S50, 1994.
4. Bree F, N'Guyen P, Tillemant JB: Study of blood binding of trandolaprilat in man. Data on file. Roussel Uclaf, report 89/1278/CN, 1989.
5. Mannhold R: Trandolapril. Drugs of Today 28:479, 1992.
6. Bevan EG, McInnes GT, Aldigier JC, et al: Effect of renal function on pharmacokinetics and pharmacodynamics of trandolapril. Br J Clin Pharmacol 35:128, 1993.
7. Arner P, Wade A, Engfeld P, et al: Pharmacokinetics and pharmacodynamics of trandolapril after repeated administration of 2 mg to young and older patients with mild to moderate hypertension. J Cardiovasc Pharmacol 23(Suppl 4):S44, 1994.
8. Bardelay C, Mack E, Worcel M, et al: Angiotensin-converting enzyme in rat brain and extraneural tissues visualized by quantitative autoradiography using 3H-trandolaprilate. J Cardiovasc Pharmacol 14:511, 1989.
9. Bree F, Hamon G, Tillement JP: Evidence for two binding sites on membrane-bound angiotensin-converting enzymes (ACE) for exogenous inhibitors except in testis. Life Sci 51:787, 1992.
10. Cumin F, Vellaud V, Corvol P, et al: Evidence for a single active site in the human angiotensin I-converting enzyme from inhibitor binding studies with 3H-trandolaprilat: Role of chloride. Biochem Biophys Res Commun 163:718, 1989.
11. Chevillard C, Brown NL, Mathieu MN, et al: Differential effects of oral trandolapril and enalapril on rat tissue angiotensin-converting enzyme. Eur J Pharmacol 147:23, 1988.
12. Guller B, Hall J, Reeves RL: Cardiac effects of trandolapril in hypertension. Am Heart J 125:1536, 1993.
13. Richer CH, Doussau MP, Guidicelli JF: Systemic and regional hemodynamic profile of five angiotensin-converting inhibitors in spontaneously hypertensive rats. Am J Cardiol 59:12D, 1987.
14. Brown NL, Badel M, Benzoni F, et al: Angiotensin-converting enzyme inhibition, anti-hypertensive activity and hemodynamic profile of trandolapril (RU 44570). Eur J Pharmacol 148:79, 1988.
15. Gaillard CA, deLeeuw PW: Clinical experiences with trandolapril. Am Heart J 125:1542, 1993.
16. A double-blind, placebo-controlled multicenter study evaluating 2 mg, 4 mg, and 8 mg doses of trandolapril administered for 8 days. Data on file. Knoll Pharmaceuticals, 1993.
17. A double-blind, placebo-controlled multicenter study evaluating doses of 0.5 mg, 1 and 2 mg of trandolapril administered for 28 days. Data on file. Knoll Pharmaceuticals, 1993.
18. Mancia G, De Cesaris R, Fogari R, et al: Evaluation of the antihypertensive effect of once-a-day trandolapril by 24-hour ambulatory blood pressure monitoring. Am J Cardiol 70:60D, 1992.
19. Backhouse CI, Orofiamma B, Pauly NC, for the Investigator Study Group: Long-term therapy with trandolapril, a new nonsulfhydryl ACE inhibitor in hypertension: A multicenter international trial. J Cardiovasc Pharmacol 23(Suppl 4):S86, 1994.
20. Dahlof B, Pennert K, Hansson L: Reversal of left ventricular hypertrophy in hypertensive patients: A meta analysis of 109 treatment studies. Hypertension 5:95, 1992.
21. Kohzuki M, Yasujima M, Yoshida K, et al: The kidney protecting effect of trandolapril in normotensive and hypertensive diabetic rats. Oyo Yakuri/Pharmacometrics 44:309, 1992.
22. Fornes P, Richer C, Pussard E, et al: Beneficial effects of trandolapril on experimentally induced congestive heart failure in rats. Am J Cardiol 70:43D, 1992.
22a. Trandolapril Cardiac Evaluation (TRACE) Study. N Engl J Med (In press).
23. Chobanian AV, Haudenschild CC, Nickerson C, et al: Trandolapril inhibits atherosclerosis in the Watanabe Heritable Hyperlipidemic rabbit. Hypertension 20:473, 1992.
24. Chobanian AV, Haudenschild CC, Nickerson C, et al: Anti-atherogenic effect of captopril in the Watanabe Heritable Hyperlipidemic rabbit. Hypertension 15:327, 1990.
25. Aberg G, Ferrer P: Effects of captopril on atherosclerosis in cynomolgous monkeys. J Cardiovasc Pharmacol 15(Suppl 5):S65, 1990.
26. Freslon J, Pourageaud F, Lecaque D, et al: Effects of trandolapril on vascular morphology and function during the established phase of systemic hypertension in the spontaneously hypertensive rat. Am J Cardiol 70:35D, 1992.
27. Belmin J, Michel J, Curmi PA, et al: Reduction of transmural 125I-albumin concentration in rat aortic media by chronic hypertension. Arterioscler Thromb 11:334, 1991.
28. Armar RG, Benetos A, Darne BM, et al: Converting enzyme inhibition: Dissociation between antihypertensive and arterial effects. J Hum Hypertens 6:381, 1992.
29. De Luca N, Rosiello G, Lamneza F, et al: Reversal of cardiac and large artery structural abnormalities induced by long-term antihypertensive treatment with trandolapril. Am J Cardiol 70:52D, 1992.
30. Predel H, Rohden C, Heine O, et al: Influence of the nonsulfhydryl angiotensin-converting enzyme inhibitor trandolapril on lipid and carbohydrate metabolism related to exercise capacity in healthy subjects. Am Heart J 125:1532, 1993.
31. McIntyre T: Oral (gavage) teratology study in rabbit. Data on file. Roussel Uclaf, report 5379–5527, 1987.

CHAPTER 83

Benazepril

Vincent DeQuattro, M.D., F.A.C.C., F.A.C.P., and Deping Lee, M.D.

Benazepril hydrochloride (known as CGS-14824A,[1] trade name Lotensin), an angiotensin-converting enzyme (ACE) inhibitor,[2, 3] via deesterification to benazeprilat, is an effective antihypertensive agent with once-daily dosing.[4] Structurally (Fig. 83–1A, B), it somewhat resembles lisinopril (Fig. 83–1C). Benazepril maintains a lofty position in the hierarchy of binding affinities to ACE in the plasma, lung, and atrium of the rat. Benazeprilat inhibits ACE in these tissues in a manner related to its avidity to the enzyme: benazeprilat > ramilprilat, > perindolprilat, > lisinopril, > enalaprilat.[5] Benazeprilat was the first ACE inhibitor introduced in the United States with significant nonrenal metabolism. This pathway, probably via the liver, may be a safeguard in patients with impaired renal function.[6]

The Joint National Committee on Detection, Evaluation, and Treatment of High Blood Pressure (JNC-IV) accorded ACE inhibitors first-line therapy status for patients with hypertension in 1988.[7] In 1993, the JNC-V recommended ACE inhibitors more specifically for patients with complicated hypertension.[8] These agents reduce morbidity and mortality in patients with left ventricular dysfunction[9, 10] and after myocardial infarction (MI).[11] Thus far, in the United States, the Food and Drug Administration (FDA) has approved eight or nine ACE inhibitors, including benazepril, for therapy of hypertension. Four inhibitors are approved for the treatment of congestive heart failure: captopril, enalapril, lisinopril, and quinapril. One inhibitor—captopril—has been approved for therapy after MI, both to preserve myocardium and to reduce mortality. Although all approved ACE inhibitors lower arterial pressure effectively in patients with systemic hypertension and are likely to be equally cardioprotective, earnest efforts are under way to uncover possible differences. For example, preliminary data suggest that cilazepril is more effective than captopril in reducing intimal hyperplasia in the aorta of an animal model with atherosclerosis.[12] Lisinopril appears to be more effective than captopril in improving brachial artery compliance in older patients with systolic hypertension.[13]

CHEMISTRY

Benazepril hydrochloride, produced as the SS diasterioisomer, is a prodrug designed for oral administration (see Fig. 83–1A). Once absorbed, the prodrug is hydrolyzed *in vivo* to its active carboxylic acid metabolite benazeprilat (see Fig. 83–1B), a strong nonsulfhydryl inhibitor of ACE.[14] Benazeprilat is poorly absorbed after oral administration.

PHARMACOLOGY
In Vitro

Both benazepril and benazeprilat inhibit rabbit lung ACE (IC_{50} [concentration at which 50% inhibition of ACE occurs] = 425 and 2 nm, respectively). Benazeprilat antagonizes angiotensin I competitively, preventing contraction of the rabbit thoracic aorta, but benazeprilat has no effect on vessels contracted with angiotensin II, potassium chloride, norepinephrine, or serotonin.

In Vivo

Benazepril inhibits angiotensin I–induced pressor effects in normotensive dogs and rats after either intravenous (0.01 to 0.3 mg/kg) or oral administration (0.3 to 3.0 mg/kg) in a dose-dependent fashion. The pressor responses of angiotensin II are not affected. Further, benazepril potentiates the vasodepressor responses to bradykinin, evidence of its action as an inhibitor of kininase II.

Antihypertensive Action

Benazepril, administered orally in doses of 0.1 to 10 mg/kg, reduced systolic blood pressure in spontaneously hypertensive rats (SHRs) with peak activity occurring at 1 hour.[14a] Acute bradycardia occurred in a non–dose-response pattern. Blood pressure was lowered for up to 10 hours after dosing. When the drug was given daily to conscious SHRs, blood pressure was lowered effectively for several days. Benazepril was studied in several other animal models of hypertension, and its effects are summarized in Table 83–1.

Thus, although no tolerance was seen, the lack of benazepril's effect on pressor response to angiotensin I suggests that inhibition of plasma ACE has little to do with its long-term effects. Benazepril reduced the development of proteinuria and glomerulosclerosis in rats of reduced renal mass. Tissue ACE was affected differentially by benazepril. Dose-related reductions in ACE activity occurred in rat aorta, lung, and kidney, but not in brain and testes, after benazepril administration.[5] The lack of effect on ACE in these two organs suggests that benazeprilat may not readily cross the blood-brain or the blood-testes barriers. Tissue ACE seems to be inhibited longer than plasma ACE, suggesting that benazeprilat is tightly bound to the active enzyme site in the tissue and is slow to dissociate.[5]

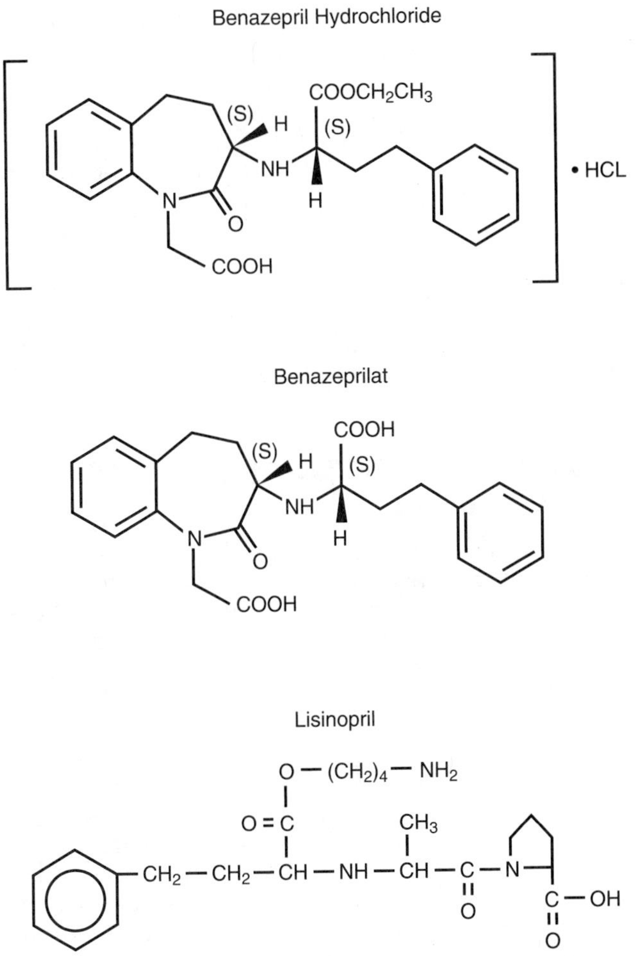

Benazepril Hydrochloride

Benazeprilat

Lisinopril

Figure 83–1. Chemical structures of benazepril hydrochloride (*A*), its active metabolite benazeprilat (*B*), and lisinopril (*C*). (From Kaiser G: Benazepril: Profile of a new ACE inhibitor. *In* Brunner JR, Salvetti A, Sever PS [eds]: Royal Society of Medicine Services International Congress and Symposium Series No. 166, 1990, pp 29–39.)

PHARMACOKINETICS
In Normal Subjects

Benazepril is rapidly absorbed (minimum of 37%) with peak absorption at 30 minutes.[14] Benazepril is converted to benazeprilat rapidly, probably by enzymatic hydrolysis in the liver,[15] and benazeprilat reached its peak at 1.5 hours.[15] Benazepril was eliminated from the plasma at four hours, and benazeprilat was eliminated biphasically (initial half-life of 3 hours, terminal half-life of 24 hours), the latter event probably reflecting avid binding of benazeprilat to ACE (Fig. 83–2).[15] Less than 1% of benazepril is excreted unchanged in urine, compared with 20% of the benazeprilat dose.[15]

In the Elderly

Findings in two studies indicate that, in elderly patients, the pharmacokinetics of benazepril are not significantly altered, but that benazeprilat is eliminated

Table 83–1. **Blood Pressure Reduction After Benazepril in Various Animals**

Animal Models	Effect	Comment
Spontaneously hypertensive rat	Present	Angiotensin I pressor
2 kidney 1 clip rat	Present	High salt, absent
Normotensive rats	Absent	Decreased peripheral vascular resistance but increased cardiac output
Normotensive rats, salt-depleted	Present	Reduced afferent and efferent arteriole resistance
Reduced renal mass rats	Present	Reduced afferent and efferent arteriole resistance
Normotensive dogs	Present	Anesthetized; increased renal blood flow, increased glomeruler filtration rate, natriuresis

less rapidly.[16, 17] Clearance of enalaprilat was similarly delayed.[17]

In Renal Impairment

The kinetics of unchanged benazepril were not influenced by renal function. On the other hand, in severe renal failure (creatinine clearance less than 30 ml/min), the area under the curve (AUC) was substantially increased, and intersubject variation was great (Fig. 83–3). When the apparent total plasma clearance of benazeprilat is correlated with creatinine clearance of patients with varying renal function, it can be seen that, even with zero creatinine clearance, there is a residual nonrenal elimination (Fig. 83–4). This is thought to be hepatic.[14] Thus, there is usually no need to adjust benazepril dosing until the creatinine clearance is 30 ml/min or less (or creatinine of 3.0 mg %).

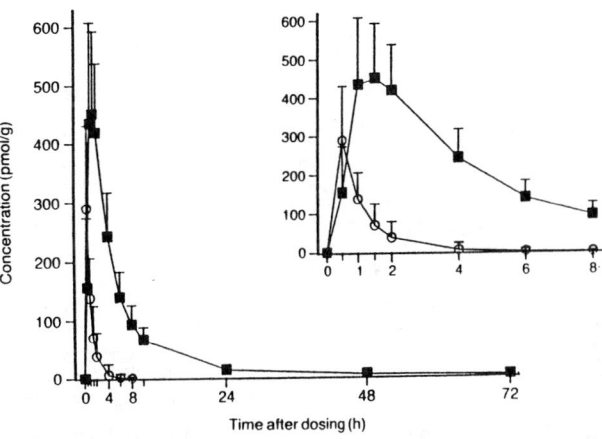

Figure 83–2. Plasma concentration-time profiles of unchanged benazepril (*open circles*) and its active metabolite benazeprilat (*filled squares*) in healthy male volunteers after a single oral 10-mg dose of benazepril HCl. Mean ± S.D., n = 36–61. (From Kaiser G, Ackermann R, Brechbuhler S, et al: Pharmacokinetics of the angiotensin-converting enzyme inhibitor benazepril HCl [CGS 14 824 A] in healthy volunteers after single and repeated administration. Biopharm Drug Dispos 10:365, 1989.)

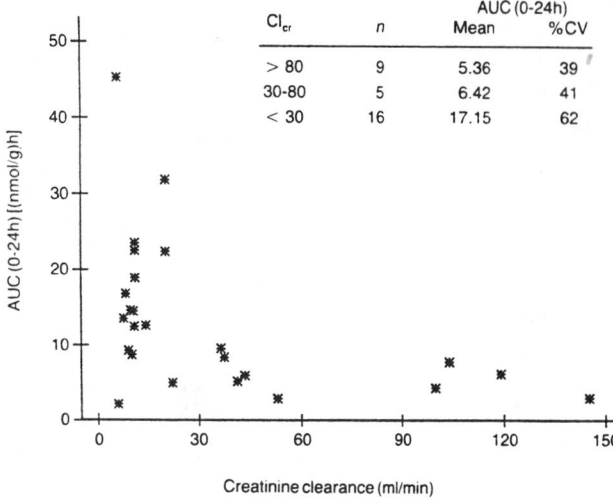

Cl$_{cr}$	n	AUC (0-24h) Mean	%CV
> 80	9	5.36	39
30-80	5	6.42	41
< 30	16	17.15	62

Figure 83–3. Correlation between the area under the curve (AUC) of benazeprilat and the creatinine clearance (Cl$_{cr}$) in patients with different levels of renal function. The 24-hour AUC (AUC[0-24h]) is after seven repeated once-daily 10-mg doses of benazepril HCl. %CV, coefficient of variation, in percentage. (From Kaiser G: Benazepril: Profile of a new ACE inhibitor. *In* Brunner JR, Salvetti A, Sever PS [eds]: Royal Society of Medicine Services International Congress and Symposium Series No. 166, 1990, pp 29–39.)

In Hepatic Cirrhosis

Benazepril concentrations in plasma were doubled in patients with cirrhosis, but the apparent conversion to benazeprilat was not affected.[18]

During Lactation

After the last of three consecutive daily doses of 20 mg of benazepril, extremely low concentrations of

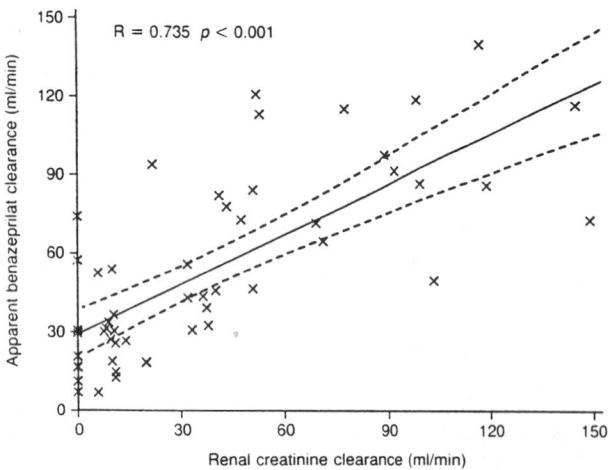

Figure 83–4. Correlation between the apparent total plasma clearance of benazeprilat (benazepril HCl dose over area under the curve of benazeprilat) and the creatinine clearance in patients with different levels of renal function. All patients received a single oral 10-mg dose of benazepril HCl. Note the linear regression line and 95% confidence limits. (From Kaiser G: Benazepril: Profile of a new ACE inhibitor. *In* Brunner JR, Salvetti A, Sever PS [eds]: Royal Society of Medicine Services International Congress and Symposium Series No. 166, 1990, pp 29–39.)

benazeprilat were found in the breast milk of normotensive lactating women.[19] The mean peak concentrations in milk were 2 and 5 picomoles/g of benazepril and benazeprilat, respectively, compared with plasma concentrations of 862 and 1614 picomoles/g, respectively. The AUC for breast milk was 1% of that in plasma for both benazepril and benazeprilat. Assuming a milk intake of 150 ml/kg/day by the infant, the maximal dose is 0.4% of the weight-adjusted maternal dose. Although 0.1% of the maternal benazepril dose may be ingested by the infant in the form of benazeprilat, the latter is not absorbed. Thus, it appears that benazepril may be administered safely to lactating mothers with nursing infants.[19]

EFFECTS ON PATHOPHYSIOLOGY
Blood Pressure

Benazepril in doses of 2 to 20 mg did not lower blood pressure in normotensive volunteers.[2] On the other hand, benazepril improved aortic compliance in these volunteers synergistically[20] when administered with a vasodilator. Benazepril controlled blood pressure in several diverse hypertensive populations.[21] Ten and 20 mg were the most effective minimal doses. Using ambulatory monitoring, Agabiti-Rosei et al.[22] found that the effects diminished at 16 hours. Most studies show a reduction of 4 to 7 mmHg at 24 hours (trough) compared with placebo. Combination therapy with hydrochlorothiazide extended the magnitude and duration of benazepril's efficacy.[21] In one study, Pessina et al.[23] found that the efficacy of once-daily benazepril improved when it was given in the morning instead of the evening. Benazepril, in 10-mg doses given in the morning, lowered mean intraarterial blood pressure over 24 hours from 155/93 to 131/83 mmHg, compared with 137/87 mmHg following evening administration.[23]

Heart Rate

Although benazepril did not affect heart rate in patients with primary hypertension[22] or in normotensive volunteers,[24] it did attenuate the heart rate increase produced by intravenous administration of the calcium antagonist nicardipine[25] and both increased[26] and decreased[27] heart rate in patients with congestive heart failure.

Cardiac Output: Pulmonary Wedge Pressure

Benazepril in doses of 2, 5, and 10 mg increased cardiac output, reduced pulmonary wedge pressure, and decreased right atrial pressure for 2 to 24 hours. The peak effects were seen at 5 to 7 hours for patients with congestive heart failure after 1 week[28] and maintained at 1 month of therapy.[26]

Left Ventricular Mass and Function

Benazepril reduced left ventricular mass in animals[29] and human subjects with hypertension.[30–32] Left ventricular diastolic function[30] and systolic and diastolic wall stress[27] were improved in patients with hypertension and those with left ventricular dysfunction, respectively. Although benazepril and concomitant digitalis and diuretic therapy[33] improved exercise tolerance in patients with congestive heart failure, it has not been approved by the FDA for the indication of congestive heart failure.

Coronary Flow

Benazeprilat was infused intravenously into mice 1 minute before and 4 and 24 hours after ligation of the left main coronary artery. Creatine kinase elevation was blunted 26% after occlusion, suggesting preservation of left ventricular muscle.[34] Studies with captopril have revealed that it potentiates the coronary vasodilator properties of nitroglycerin.[35] Benazepril reduced silent ischemic episodes approximately 50% in patients with stable angina.[36] It was ineffective as monotherapy in other patients with silent ischemia[37, 38] and in patients with angina.[36]

Left Ventricular Failure

Several studies indicate that benazepril is effective in congestive heart failure.[39–41] Benazepril improved exercise tolerance by 95 seconds, compared with 37 seconds in placebo-treated patients, in over 100 patients who were treated with digoxin and diuretic. Overall clinical status improved, as did the signs and symptoms of congestive failure in benazepril-treated patients compared with the control subjects. There were three deaths in the placebo-treated patients and none in benazepril-treated patients ($p < .05$); the overall incidence of adverse effects was identical in the two groups.[39] In a study of patients with mild heart failure 6 to 24 months after MI, benazepril was compared with placebo in patients who were not on concomitant therapy. Treatment was for a 3-month period with a double-blind, crossover design. Benazepril improved the New York Heart Association functional class in 59% of patients, whereas hydrochlorothiazide therapy produced no improvement.[40]

In another trial of patients with systolic dysfunction and ejection fractions of less than 0.40, benazepril improved treadmill exercise duration at 12 weeks ($p < .001$). There was improvement in global symptomatic status in 67% of patients.[41]

Endocrine and Metabolic Effects

Captopril reduced plasma insulin levels in patients studied with the glucose clamp technique.[42] Benazepril lowered fasting blood sugar and postprandial glucose in non-insulin-dependent diabetics,[43] and both insulin and glucose were lowered during oral glucose tolerance tests, compared with placebo. Benazepril, like other ACE inhibitors, also lowered cholesterol by 4.3%, compared with increases seen after hydrochlorothiazide therapy of 3.7%.[44] Although benazepril increased bradykinin and prostacyclin levels,

their role in the antihypertensive effects of benazepril are unknown.[45]

Effects on Renal Function

In several studies, captopril, enalapril, and other ACE inhibitors have reduced proteinuria in both patients with hypertension and patients with diabetes and have preserved renal function in these disorders.[46–48] Benazepril improved renal plasma flow[49] and urinary sodium excretion[50] and reduced urinary protein excretion[51] without adverse effects on renal function in patients with hypertension. The ultimate role of benazepril and other ACE inhibitors in patients with hypertension and diabetes awaits studies to evaluate long-term effects on both protein excretion reduction and preservation of renal function. However, a 2.5-year trial with captopril in diabetic patients with nephropathy and proteinuria in excess of 500 mg/day revealed a 50% reduction in the rate of renal failure.[52]

CLINICAL USE
Indications

Benazepril is approved for use in hypertension. Its use may be expanded to include a separate indication for congestive heart failure. Benazepril, effective in once-daily doses, is started at 10 mg and gradually increased to 40 mg/day. Benazepril is a more effective antihypertensive agent when combined with hydrochlorothiazide, and doses as small as 5 mg of benazepril plus 6.25 mg of hydrochlorothiazide control blood pressure.[21] Combination therapy with benazepril and nifedipine in doses of 10 mg of benazepril and 20 to 60 mg of nifedipine have resulted in improved blood pressure control and reduced side effects such as edema and headache[22] (Fig. 83–5).

Blood pressure control may be improved after combination therapy of β-receptor blockers and ACE inhibitors in at least two clinical situations: congestive heart failure, wherein low-dose β-blocker therapy has shown promise, and after MI, wherein larger-dose β-blocker therapy effectively reduced reinfarction, morbidity, and mortality. ACE inhibitor therapy reduces left ventricular hypertrophy in patients with hypertension, but the FDA has not approved any drug for this indication. Finally, one of the future roles of ACE inhibitor therapy is to improve coronary flow by enhancing endothelial-mediated vasodilation. Evidence from the Survival and Ventricular Enlargement (SAVE) trial,[11] in which patients were treated with captopril after MI, and from the SOLVD trials,[9] in which patients with either symptomatic or asymptomatic congestive heart failure were treated with enalapril, strongly suggests that ACE inhibitor therapy reduces coronary ischemic events and MI by improved flow and reduces morbidity and mortality in relation to ischemic heart disease. Another possible indication for ACE inhibitor therapy as described by Asmar et al.[13] is improved arterial compliance, although evidence is preliminary. Apparently, ACE in-

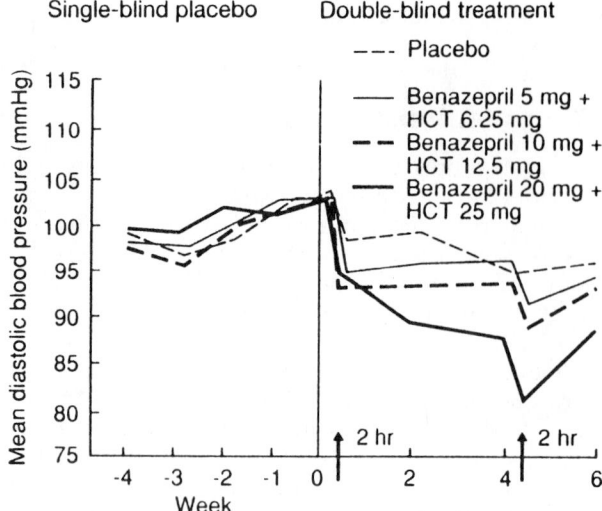

Figure 83–5. Comparison of treatment with placebo and benazepril in combination with hydrochlorothiazide (HCT) in a 4:5 ratio: mean sitting diastolic blood pressure. (Sitting diastolic blood pressures were measured just before the next daily dose and 2 hours after the daily dose at weeks 0 and 4). (From DeQuattro V: Benazepril: Profile of a New ACE Inhibitor. London/New York: Royal Society of Medicine Service, 1990.)

hibitors, calcium antagonists, and α-blocking therapy can improve arterial compliance in older patients with systolic hypertension. There is evidence of a hierarchy of affinity to vascular ACE by the various ACE inhibitors, suggesting that those most avidly bound improve arterial compliance more. In that regard, benazepril appears to have a strong affinity for the rat enzyme compared with other ACE inhibitors. If this property holds for the human enzyme, benazepril should be useful in patients after MI, those with angina, and those with reduced compliance, especially elderly patients.

Precautions

The major precautions with benazepril therapy are those of the ACE inhibitor class—cough occurs with an incidence of 6% to 12%. Certainly, the percentage of cough in patients with hypertension seems greater

Table 83–2. Eight Most Frequently Reported Adverse Experiences Considered to be Drug-Related

	Benazepril Alone		Placebo	
	n	%	n	%
Patients, total	1693	100	458	100
Headache	90	5	21	17
Dizziness	53	3	13	3
Fatigue	48	2	12	1
Cough increased	33	1	5	1
Nausea	25	1	5	<1
Postural dizziness	18	1	1	<1
Somnolence	17	1	2	<1
Vertigo	16	1	2	<1

From MacNab M, Mallows S: Safety profile of benazepril in essential hypertension. Clin Cardiol 14(Suppl IV):33, 1991.

Table 83–3. Drug-Drug Interactions with Benazepril

No Clinically Significant Deleterious Interactions With:	
Class	*Drugs*
Diuretic	Hydrochlorothiazide, chlorthalidone, furosemide
β-Blocker	Propranolol, atenolol
Calcium antagonist	Nifedipine, nicardipine
Nonsteroidal antiinflammatory drugs	Aspirin, naproxen
Anticoagulant	Warfarin, acenocoumarol
Antiulcer	Cimetidine
Digitalis	Digoxin

From MacNab M, Mallows S: Safety profile of benazepril in essential hypertension. Clin Cardiol 14(Suppl IV):36, 1991.

than that given in the package insert of only a few percent. Other common side effects of ACE inhibitor therapy are angioedema (0.2%) and headache and dizziness (approximately 2% to 6%)[52] (Table 83–2).

Drug Interactions

No clinically significant interactions were found in the course of several trials in which many various medications were coadministered with benazepril. Pharmacokinetic studies were performed with specific agents, but no drug interactions were observed (Table 83–3).

SUMMARY

Benazepril is an effective antihypertensive agent administered in once-daily doses of 10 to 40 mg/day. Dosages should be reduced in elderly patients, those of small stature, patients receiving diuretics, and those with a creatinine clearance of less than 30 ml/min. Combination therapy of doses as small as 5 mg of benazepril and 6.25 mg of hydrochlorothiazide has effectively reduced blood pressure compared with placebo. Benazepril, like other ACE inhibitors, is effective with few side effects; thus, dosing should be increased until blood pressure is controlled.

REFERENCES

1. Miller DM, Hopkins MF, Tonnesen MJ, et al: Antihypertensive assessment of CGS 14824A, an orally effective angiotensin-converting enzyme (ACE) inhibitor [abstract 9]. Pharmacologist 25:102, 1983.
2. Schaller MD, Nussberger J, Waeber B, et al: Haemodynamic and pharmacological effects of the converting enzyme inhibitor CGS 14 824A in normal volunteers. Eur J Clin Pharmacol 28:267, 1985.
3. Waeber G, Fasanella S'moew R, Nussberger J, et al: Effect on blood pressure and the renin-angiotensin system of repeated doses of the converting enzyme inhibitor CGS 14 824 A. Eur J Clin Pharmacol 31:643, 1987.
4. Brunner HR, Salvetti A, Sever PS (eds): Benazepril: Profile of a New ACE Inhibitor. London/New York: Royal Society of Medicine Services, 1990.
5. Chen B, Perich R, Jackson B, et al: Inhibition of tissue ACE by benazepril. *In* Brunner HR, Salvetti A, Sever PS (eds): Benazepril: Profile of a New ACE Inhibitor. London/New York: Royal Society of Medicine Services, 1990, pp 17–27.

6. Gengo FM, Brady E: The pharmacokinetics of benazepril relative to other ACE inhibitors. Clin Cardiol 14(Suppl IV):44, 1991.

7. The 1988 Joint National Committee on Detection, Evaluation, and Treatment of High Blood Pressure: The 1988 report of the Joint National Committee on Detection, Evaluation and Treatment of High Blood Pressure. Arch Intern Med 148:1023, 1988.

8. The Fifth Report of the Joint National Committe on Detection, Evaluation and Treatment of High Blood Pressure (JNC V). Arch Intern Med 153:154, 1993.

9. SOLVD Investigators: Effect of enalapril on survival in patients with reduced left ventricular ejection fractions and congestive heart failure. N Engl J Med 325:293, 1991.

10. CONSENSUS Trial Study Group: Effects of enalapril on mortality in severe congestive failure: Results of the Cooperative North Scandinavian Enalapril Survival Study (CONSENSUS). N Engl J Med 316:1429, 1987.

11. Pfeffer MA, Braunwald E, Moye LA, et al: Effect of captopril on mortality and morbidity in patients with left ventricular dysfunction after myocardial infarction. Results of the survival and ventricular enlargement trial. N Engl J Med 327(10):669, 1992.

12. Powell JS, Clozel JP, Muller RKM, et al: Inhibitors of angiotensin converting enzyme prevent myointimal proliferation after vascular injury. Science 245:186, 1989.

13. Asmar RG, Iannascoli F, Benetos A, Safar ME: Dose optimization study of arterial changes associated with ACE-I in hypertension. J Hypertens 10(Suppl):l3, 1992.

14. Waldmeier F, Schmidt K: Disposition of [^{14}C]-benazepril hydrochloride in rat, dog and baboon: Absorption, distribution, kinetics, biotransformation and excretion. Arzneimittelforschung/Drug Res 39(I):62, 1989.

14a. Lehmann M, Norman J, Zimmerman MB, et al: Comparative effects of angiotensin converting enzyme (ACE) inhibitors on tissue ACE activity and blood pressure in the conscious spontaneously hypertensive rat (SHR) [abstract]. Pharmacologist 27:192, 1985.

15. Kaiser G, Ackermann R, Brechbuhler S, et al: Pharmacokinetics of the angiotensin-converting enzyme inhibitor benazepril HCl (CGS 14 824 A) in healthy volunteers after single and repeated administration. Biopharm Drug Dispos 10:365, 1989.

16. Kaiser G, Ackermann R, Dieterle W, et al: Pharmacokinetics and pharmacodynamics of the ACE inhibitor benazepril hydrochloride in the elderly. Eur J Clin Pharmacol 38:379, 1990.

17. Macdonald NJ, Elliott HL, Howie CA, et al: Age and the pharmacodynamics and pharmacokinetics of benazepril. Br J Clin Pharmacol 27:707P, 1989.

18. Kaiser G, Ackermann R, Sioufi A: Pharmacokinetics of a new angiotensin-converting enzyme inhibitor, benazepril hydrochloride, in special populations. Am Heart J 117:746, 1989.

19. Kaiser G, Ackermann R, Dieterle W, et al: Benazepril and benazeprilat in human plasma and breast milk. Eur J Clin Pharmacol 36(Suppl):A303, 1989.

20. Brunel P, Guyene TT, Howald H, et al: Arterial and endocrine effects of a combination of an angiotensin converting enzyme inhibitor and a vasodilator in normotensive healthy volunteers. J Cardiovasc Pharmacol 18:175, 1991.

21. DeQuattro V: Benazepril compared with other antihypertensive agents, singly and in combination—a review. In Brunner HR, Salvetti A, Sever PS (eds): Benazepril: Profile of a New ACE Inhibitor. London/New York: Royal Society of Medicine Services, 1990, pp 91–98.

22. Agabiti-Rosei E, Rizzoni D, Zulli R, et al: Sustained antihypertensive effects of benazepril demonstrated by ambulatory monitoring: Placebo-controlled trial at two dosage levels. In Brunner HR, Salvetti A, Sever PS (eds): Benazepril: Profile of a New ACE Inhibitor. Royal Society of Medicine Services International Congress and Symposium Series No. 166, Royal Society of Medicine Services, 1990, pp 59–65.

23. Pessina AC, Mormino P, Palatini P, et al: Morning or evening benazepril administration in hypertension? A randomized study using intra-arterial blood pressure monitoring. In Brunner HR, Salvetti A, Sever PS (eds): Benazepril: Profile of a New ACE Inhibitor. Royal Society of Medicine Services International Congress and Symposium Series No. 166, Royal Society of Medicine Services, 1990, pp 51–57.

24. Nussberger J, de Gasparo M, Juillerat L, et al: Rapid measurement of total and active renin: Plasma concentrations during acute and sustained converting enzyme inhibition with CGS 14824A. Clin Exp Hypertens Part [A] 9:1353, 1987.

25. Bellet M, Sassano P, Guyenne T, et al: Converting-enzyme inhibition buffers the counter-regulatory response to acute administration of nicardipine. Br J Clin Pharmacol 24:465, 1987.

26. Milvis DM, Insel J, Boland MJ, et al: Chronic therapy for congestive heart failure with benazepril HCl, a new angiotensin converting enzyme inhibitor. Am J Med Sci 300:354, 1990.

27. Rousseau MF, Gurne O, van Eyll C, et al: Effects of benazeprilat on left ventricular systolic and diastolic function and neurohumoral status in patients with ischemic heart disease. Circulation 81(Suppl III):111, 1990.

28. Insel J, Mirvis DM, Boland MJ, et al: A multicentre study of the safety and efficacy of benazepril hydrochloride, a long-acting angiotensin-converting enzyme inhibitor, in patients with chronic congestive heart failure. Clin Pharmacol Ther 45:312, 1989.

29. Takemori E, Hasegawa Y, Katahira J, et al: Effect of benazepril hydrochloride on cardiac hypertrophy in spontaneously hypertensive rats. Arzeimittelforschung/Drug Res 41:612, 1991.

30. Porcellati C, Verdecchia P, Schillaci G, et al: Long-term effects of benazepril on ambulatory blood pressure, left ventricular mass, diastolic filling and aortic flow in essential hypertension. Int J Clin Pharmacol Ther Toxicol 29:187, 1991.

31. Guller B, Reeves RL, deSilva J: Hemodynamics during long-term use of benazepril alone or with concomitant hydrochlorothiazide [abstract 62]. J Clin Pharmacol 29:847, 1989.

32. Lee D, DeQuattro V, Brosnihan B, et al: Benazepril therapy in hypertension: LVH regression related to neural tone, blood pressure non responders have reflex increase in angiotensin 1–7 peptide. Am J Hypertens 5(5 Part 2):113A, 1992.

33. Taylor S, Kusiak V, Milmer K, et al: Double-blind comparison of once daily benazepril and thrice daily captopril in congestive heart failure [abstract P2015]. Philippines J Cardiol 19(Suppl I):1, 1990.

34. Smith III EF, Egan JW, Goodman FR, et al: Effect of two nonsulfhydryl angiotensin-converting enzyme inhibitors CGS 14831 and GGS 11617, on myocardial damage and left-ventricular hypertrophy following coronary occlusion in the rat. Pharmacology 37:254, 1988.

35. Meredith IT, Alison JF, Zhang FM, et al: Captopril potentiates the effects of nitroglycerin in the coronary vascular bed. J Am Coll Cardiol 22(2):581, 1993.

36. Klein WW, Khurmi NS, Eber B, et al: Effects of benazepril and metoprolol OROS alone and in combination on myocardial ischemia in patients with chronic stable angina. J Am Coll Cardiol 16:948, 1990.

37. Ikram H, Low CJS, Shirlaw TM, et al: Antianginal efficacy of angiotensin converting enzyme inhibition and calcium channel blockade and their combination in chronic stable angina [abstract]. J Am Coll Cardiol 17:188A, 1991.

38. Muiesan ML, Boni E, Cefis M, et al: Efficacy of transdermal nitroglycerin in combination with an ACE-inhibitor in patients with chronic stable angina pectoris [abstract]. J Am Coll Cardiol 17:377A, 1991.

39. Colfer HT, Ribner HS, Gradman A, et al: Effects of once-daily benazepril therapy on exercise tolerance and manifestations of chronic congestive heart failure. The Benazepril Heart Failure Study Group. Am J Cardiol 70(3):354, 1992.

40. Nordrehaug JE, Omsj IH, Vollset SE: A 3-month double-blind crossover study of the effect of benazepril and hydrochlorothiazide on functional class in symptomatic mild heart failure. J Intern Med 231(6):589, 1992.

41. Ribner HS, Sagar KB, Glasser SP, et al: Long-term therapy with benazepril in patients with congestive heart failure: Effects on clinical status and exercise tolerance. J Clin Pharmacol 30(12):1106, 1990.

42. Pollare T, Lithell H, Berne C: A comparison of the effects of hydrochlorothiazide and captopril on glucose and lipid metabolism in patients with hypertension. N Engl J Med 321:868, 1989.

43. Bolli GB, Torlone E, DeFeo P, et al: Rationale for ACE inhibition in hypertension associated with diabetes mellitus. In Brunner

HR, Salvetti A, Sever PS (eds): Benazepril: Profile of a New ACE Inhibitor. Royal Society of Medicine Services International Congress and Symposium Series No. 166, Royal Society of Medicine Services, 1990, pp 123–128.

44. Gomez HJ, Glazer R, Mallows S, et al: Benazepril in the treatment of older and elderly hypertensive patients. *In* Brunner HR, Salvetti A, Sever PS (eds): Benazepril: Profile of a new ACE inhibitor. Royal Society of Medicine Services International Congress and Symposium Series No. 166, Royal Society of Medicine Services, 1990, pp 111–120.

45. Salvetti A: Newer ACE inhibitors: A look at the future. Drugs 40:800, 1990.

46. Mimran A, Insua A, Ribstein J, et al: Comparative effect of captopril and nifedipine in normotensive patients with incipient diabetic nephropathy. Diabetic Care 11(10):850, 1988.

47. Bjorck S, Mulec H, Johnsen SA, et el: Renal protective effects

of enalapril in diabetic nephropathy. Br Med J 304(6823):339, 1992.

48. Bakris GM: Effects of diltiazem or lisinopril on massive proteinuria associated with diabetes mellitus. Ann Intern Med 112:707, 1990.

49. Noormohamed FH, Fuller GN, Lant AF: Effect of salt balance on the renal and hemodynamic actions of benazepril in normal men. J Clin Pharmacol 29(10):928, 1989.

50. Reams GP, Lau A, Bauer JH: Effect of benazepril monotherapy in subjects with hypertension associated with renal dysfunction. J Clin Pharmacol 29(7):609, 1989.

51. Bedogna V, Valvo E, Casagrande P, et al: Effects of ACE inhibition in normotensive patients with chronic glomerular disease and normal renal function. Kidney Int 38:101, 1990.

52. Lewis EJ, Hunsicker LG, Bain RP, et al: The effect of angiotensin coverting enzyme inhibition on diabetic nephropathy. N Engl J Med 329(20):1456, 1993.

CHAPTER 84

Quinapril Hydrochloride

Matthew R. Weir, M.D., and Michael A. Weber, M.D.

Quinapril hydrochloride is a nonsulfhydryl angiotensin-converting enzyme (ACE) inhibitor that is hydrolyzed after absorption to form its major active diacid metabolite, quinaprilat, and two minor inactive metabolites. Unlike other ACE inhibitor prodrugs, both quinapril and quinaprilat decrease plasma levels of angiotensin II and aldosterone and potentiate bradykinin activity. Quinaprilat is three times as potent an ACE inhibitor as quinapril, on a weight basis.[1, 2]

In a landmark study[3] designed to address "quality of life" issues in hypertensive patients, captopril, the first ACE inhibitor introduced into clinical practice, was found to significantly improve patients' overall sense of well-being, including physical/emotional state, sexual and social functioning, and work performance, as compared with other commonly used antihypertensive agents such as the β-blockers (e.g., propranolol) and sympatholytics (e.g., methyldopa). Although captopril was found to be effective in treating hypertension, its few drawbacks have prompted the search for newer agents. These drawbacks include decreased absorption when administered with food; short duration of action requiring administration two to three times daily; rapid onset of action, leading to first-dose hypotension in some patients; and a sulfhydryl moiety responsible for side effects, including rash and taste disturbances. Subsequently, new ACE inhibitors (e.g., enalapril, lisinopril, and ramipril) lacking the sulfhydryl moiety have been introduced. These agents may provide advantages over captopril in that they possess a longer half-life and a longer duration of action and therefore allow for once-daily dosing in many patients with hypertension.

However, because the duration of action of these newer ACE inhibitors extends for up to 60 hours, as in the case of ramipril, issues regarding safety and drug accumulation have arisen. Specifically, investigators[4, 5] have reported that very-long-acting ACE inhibitors may more adversely affect renal function than short-acting ACE inhibitors and may increase the incidence of certain side effects, such as prolonged hypotension, that may be associated with prolonged suppression of ACE activity.

Quinapril, unlike other ACE inhibitors given once daily, has a short accumulation half-life (3 hours) and a 24-hour duration of action attributed to its potent binding affinity for tissue ACE. Specifically, quinaprilat binds to ACE with greater affinity than captopril, enalapril (enalaprilat), or lisinopril[6, 7] (see Comparative Tissue and Plasma ACE Binding Potency).

PHARMACOKINETICS/ PHARMACODYNAMICS

All ACE inhibitors are pharmacodynamically similar; however, they differ in such aspects as the chemical group serving as the binding ligand, pharmacokinetics, duration of action, prodrug activity, and tissue bioavailability.

Three distinct chemical classes of ACE inhibitors are in clinical use: the sulfhydryl-containing inhibitors (e.g., captopril), the carboxyalkyldipeptides (e.g., quinapril, enalapril, benazepril, lisinopril, and ramipril), and the phosphinic acid compounds (e.g., fosinopril). The clinical significance of the differences between the chemical classes has not been established.

Absorption of quinapril following oral administration in healthy volunteers is approximately 60%; hydrolysis to quinaprilat is rapid, with peak quinapril and quinaprilat concentrations occurring 1 and 2 hours after the dose, respectively.[2] In dogs, monkeys, and humans, hydrolysis of quinapril to quinaprilat appears to occur in the gastrointestinal tract, the liver, and other extravascular sites. Metabolism to compounds other than quinaprilat is not extensive. Two diketopiperazine metabolites of quinapril have been identified in plasma and urine, with approximately 6% of an administered dose excreted in urine as each of these metabolites. Neither metabolite inhibits ACE activity.[1]

[14]C-labeled quinapril has been utilized to determine the metabolism and disposition of quinapril. Recovery of total radiolabel was virtually complete (98%); 61% was recovered in urine, and 37% was recovered in feces. Approximately 97% of either quinapril or quinaprilat circulating in plasma is bound to proteins.[2]

Absorption of quinapril and conversion to quinaprila is not affected by food in the gastrointestinal tract;[2] however, coadministration of food may increase the time to maximum plasma concentrations of quinapril and quinaprilat by approximately 30 minutes.[8] In patients with renal insufficiency, clearance of quinaprilat is reduced in direct proportion to declining renal function as assessed by creatinine clearance. Quinapril doses should therefore be decreased in direct proportion to the severity of impaired renal function.[9] Pharmacokinetic studies in patients with end-stage renal disease on chronic hemodialysis or chronic ambulatory peritoneal dialysis indicate that quinapril and quinaprilat are not eliminated by dialysis (unpublished data, Medical Affairs Department, Parke-Davis).

In patients with hepatic dysfunction (e.g., alcoholic cirrhosis), the rate and extent of quinapril deesterification to quinaprilat are decreased, resulting in lower plasma quinaprilat concentrations and up to a twofold increase in quinaprilat half-life. The rate of quinaprilat elimination is not altered. Increased dosage of quinapril should be considered in hypertensive patients with hepatic impairment.[10, 11]

TISSUE VERSUS THE CIRCULATING RENIN–ANGIOTENSIN SYSTEM

The principal effect of ACE inhibitors is to block the conversion of angiotensin I to angiotensin II. Traditionally, the renin-angiotensin system (RAS) has been considered an endocrine or circulating system. However, there is now substantial evidence that the RAS is also tissue-based, with activation occurring not only in the circulation but also locally. In fact, research employing molecular biologic techniques has produced data documenting that 90% to 99% of ACE in the body is found in tissue (heart, lung, kidney, and blood vessels) and that only 1% to 10% is found in the circulation.[12]

The implication of the discovery of tissue components of the RAS is that angiotensin II can be formed locally in or around blood vessels and may have vasoconstrictive effects. These tissue systems result in the autocrine-paracrine effects of local angiotensin II formation.[13, 14]

It has been hypothesized that the circulating RAS acts acutely during cardiovascular decompensation activity, such as dehydration, hemorrhage, and heart failure, to maintain blood pressure (via vasoconstriction and aldosterone secretion) and salt and water homeostasis. These are short-term effects. The circulating RAS is subject to feedback inhibition and is turned off as soon as the cardiovascular system reaches a compensated state. In contrast, the tissue RAS exerts long-term actions that affect cardiovascular function and structure in addition to its vasoconstriction and sodium and water effects.[12, 15] Thus, reversal of the structural changes secondary to cardiovascular disease may be important long-term antihypertensive actions that are possibly mediated by inhibition of the tissue RAS.

Considerable evidence indicates that the brain RAS is regulated differentially and independently of the circulating RAS.[16] Brain RAS is one of several tissue RASs described in a number of organs, including the vascular wall, the kidney, the adrenal gland, and the heart. The discovery of brain RAS has pioneered new concepts regarding the actions of angiotensin II. Besides being a circulating hormone, angiotensin II is now also considered a neuropeptide in the central nervous system acting as a neurohormone or neurotransmitter. Angiotensin II generated in the brain is involved in the central control of volume homeostasis, including water intake and salt appetite, as well as the release of vasopressin, oxytocin, adrenocorticotropin (ACTH), and other pituitary hormones.[17] Overactive brain RAS has been identified as one of the factors contributing to the pathogenesis and maintenance of animal models of essential hypertension. In a review article on the effects of ACE inhibitors on tissue RASs, Lee et al.[18] reported that, in spontaneously hypertensive rats, ACE inhibitors have been shown to inhibit brain RAS independently from plasma RAS.

INHIBITION OF TISSUE RAS: EFFECTS ON HYPERTENSION AND CONGESTIVE HEART FAILURE

A number of investigators have demonstrated the importance of tissue ACE inhibition in regard to the clinical efficacy of ACE inhibitors. Studies[1, 19] have revealed a better correlation between the magnitude and duration of blood pressure reduction and inhibition of ACE activity in certain tissues than with the inhibition of plasma ACE activity. Kaplan et al.[1] have shown that the blood pressure response to quinapril much more closely parallels aortic ACE inhibition than plasma ACE inhibition in renal hypertensive rats (Fig. 84–1). Moreover, ACE inhibitors have exhibited significant blood pressure–lowering effects among patients with little or no circulating renin.[13, 20]

Further studies have revealed that many of the therapeutic effects of ACE inhibitors may be related to inhibition of ACE within body tissues, especially with chronic treatment. This action, more specifically that occurring in cardiovascular tissue, may also contribute to the ability of ACE inhibitors to reduce hypertension-induced cardiac and vascular hypertrophy.[14, 21]

Evidence of the existence of RAS in the heart and

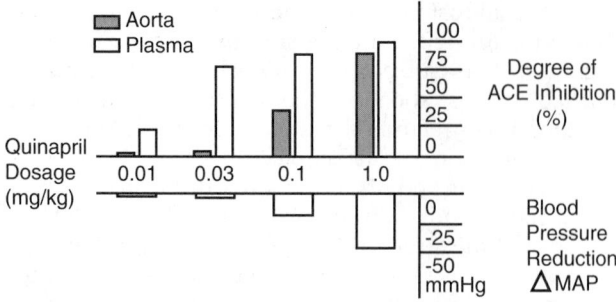

Figure 84–1. Relationship between mean arterial blood pressure (MAP) reduction and ACE inhibition with quinapril in renal hypertensive rats (n = 4). (From Kaplan HR, Taylor DG, Olson SC, et al: Quinapril—A preclinical review of the pharmacology, pharmacokinetics, and toxicology. Angiology 40:335, 1989.)

vasculature suggests a possible role for ACE inhibitors in the prevention/regression of hypertension-induced cardiac and vascular hypertrophy.[21] It has been suggested that ACE inhibition in cardiovascular tissues is responsible for the reduced mortality associated with ACE inhibitor treatment of advanced stages of congestive heart failure (CHF) and the prevention of cardiac remodeling that follows myocardial infarction.[20] Studies have supported the hypothesis that an inhibition of cardiac ACE may be involved in the beneficial hemodynamic and metabolic actions of ACE inhibitors in CHF independent of the circulating angiotensin II.[13]

Schunkert et al.[22] evaluated the functional significance of cardiac ACE in hypertrophied rat hearts. Results indicate that conversion of angiotensin I to angiotensin II is amplified in hearts with left ventricular hypertrophy, and that ACE inhibition reduces the *intracardiac* angiotensin I conversion and functional related changes in coronary resistance and diastolic function. The authors hypothesize that cardiac ACE-dependent angiotensin II production occurs in humans and may contribute to abnormal diastolic function and the development of CHF.

Dzau and Pratt[23] examined the role of tissue RAS in experimental restenosis after vascular injury. Their results indicate that tissue ACE is significantly correlated with formation of the neointima following vascular injury. The authors speculate that ACE inhibitors capable of penetrating vascular tissues and exhibiting a high affinity for and slow dissociation from tissue ACE may have unique efficacy in inhibiting vascular smooth muscle cell proliferation. Thus, ACE inhibitors that effectively inhibit tissue ACE may play a critical role in the prevention of restenosis after balloon angioplasty. The authors note that results of the Multicenter European Research trial with Cilazipril after Angioplasty to prevent Transluminal coronary Obstruction and Restenosis (MERCATOR) trial failed to show that *low* doses of cilazipril inhibit restenosis. However, they indicated that the protocol design of the MERCATOR trial was significantly different from that of the positive animal studies, which demonstrated that the inhibition of tissue ACE activi-

ties requires a higher dose or long-term pretreatment with ACE inhibitors.

The ongoing Quinapril Ischemic Event Trial (QUIET) study[24] is currently evaluating the ability of quinapril to reduce the incidence of cardiac ischemic events in patients with coronary artery disease, *independently* of effects on blood pressure (i.e., perhaps through *local* antiatherogenic effects).

Inhibition of tissue ACE may explain why the effect of some ACE inhibitors lasts longer than would be expected from the blood levels; quinapril produces significant inhibition of ACE in lung, heart, and kidney tissue when blood levels are undetectable.

COMPARATIVE TISSUE AND PLASMA ACE BINDING POTENCY

Evidence[25, 26] suggests that increased potency of binding to tissue ACE may provide a protective effect in local tissues, because structural changes occurring during the chronic state of hypertension, such as cardiovascular hypertrophy, are possibly mediated by activation of tissue RAS.

Nash[27] reviewed the comparative properties of ACE inhibitors and noted that different ACE inhibitors vary significantly in their abilities to penetrate tissue and bind to converting enzyme. In addition, he stated that current research strongly supports the concept that tissue renin-angiotensin systems are likely to be very important in the control of blood pressure.

Using a radioligand binding technique, Johnston et al.[6] studied the potency of various ACE inhibitors against both plasma and tissue ACE. The relative potency of the various ACE inhibitors was assessed by radioinhibitor binding displacement, and the potency of each agent was expressed by the ID_{50} (inhibitory concentration found to produce 50% displacement of ^{125}I-351A from ACE). Specific binding of ^{125}I to plasma, heart, kidney, lung, aorta, and testes was then determined.

In binding to rat plasma ACE, quinaprilat was more potent than benazeprilat, perindoprilat, lisinopril, or fosinoprilat.[6] The binding potency of quinaprilat to human plasma ACE was 214 times greater than that for captopril and 14 times greater than that for enalaprilat (Fig. 84–2).[7] Kaplan et al.[28] evaluated the ability of quinapril, enalapril, and captopril to inhibit ACE from guinea pig serum and found that the molar concentration of quinapril required to achieve 100% inhibition of ACE was less than 10% of that required to achieve the same inhibition level with either enalapril or captopril.

Quinaprilat was also found to be highly potent in binding to tissue ACE (Fig. 84–3). Comparative *in vitro* studies of the binding potency of various ACE inhibitors have identified the following rank order of ACE inhibitor potency: quinaprilat = benazeprilat > perindoprilat > lisinopril > enalaprilat > fosinoprilat.[6, 7] An *ex vivo* study in human atrial membranes showed that quinaprilat was a more potent inhibitor of cardiac ACE than lisinopril or enalaprilat.[29]

Nakajima et al.[30] compared the ability of quinapril

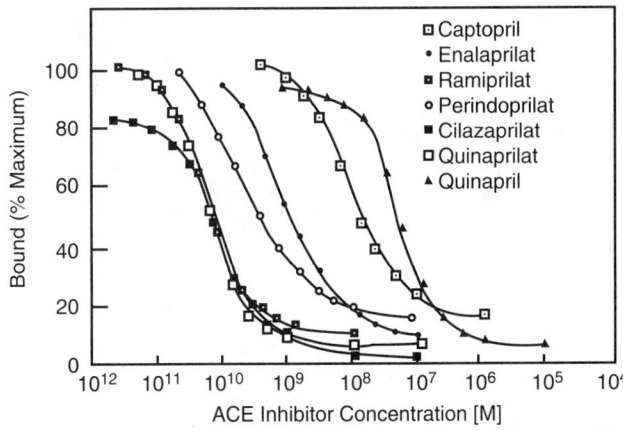

Figure 84-2. Binding displacement curves of ^{125}I-351A from human plasma ACE. (From Fabris B, Chen B, Pupic V, et al: Inhibition of angiotensin-converting enzyme [ACE] in plasma and tissue. J Cardiovasc Pharmacol 15[Suppl 2]:S6, 1990.)

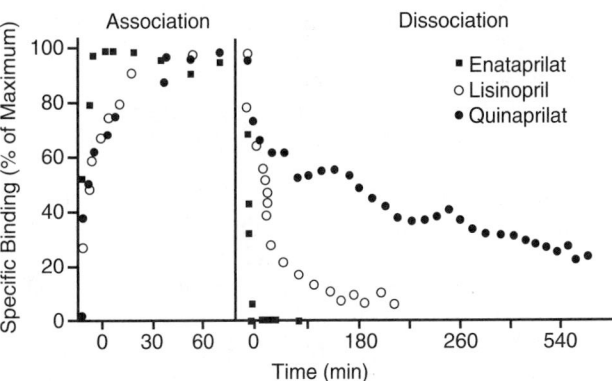

Figure 84-4. ACE inhibitor dissociation ("off") rates in human atrial membranes. (Reproduced with permission from Kinoshita A, Urata H, Bumpus FM, et al: Measurement of angiotensin I converting enzyme inhibition in the heart. Circ Res 73:51, 1993. Copyright 1993, American Heart Association.)

and enalapril to inhibit plasma and tissue ACE in spontaneously hypertensive rats. Quinapril inhibited cardiac ACE more than enalapril did.

Kinoshita et al.[29] at the Cleveland Clinic compared the rates at which enalapril, lisinopril, and quinapril bound (or associated) with tissue ACE and the rates at which the drugs dissociated from the ACE binding sites (the "off" rates). These studies were conducted in both animal (hamster ventricle) and human (atrial) tissue. The investigators found that the drugs were approximately equal in their ACE association, or "on" rates, but there were major differences in how long the drugs remained bound to tissue ACE. Enalaprilat dissociated from tissue ACE very quickly, whereas quinaprilat had a substantially longer dissociation rate than enalaprilat or lisinopril in both animal and human tissue (Fig. 84-4).

The investigators also showed that the differences in off rates paralleled differences in the duration of ACE inhibition. Specifically, quinapril was the slowest to dissociate from cardiac ACE and had the longest duration of action in terms of inhibiting ACE.

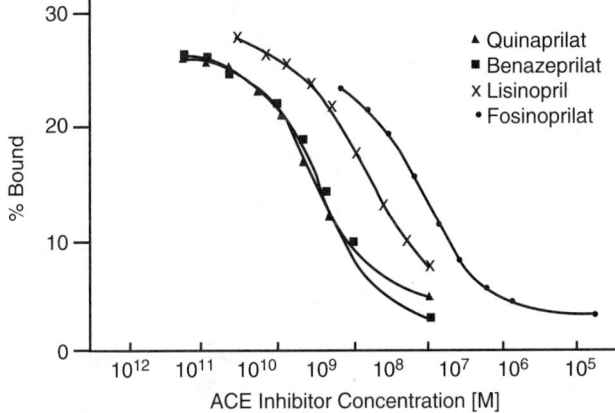

Figure 84-3. Binding displacement curves of ^{125}I-351A from cardiac ACE. (From Johnston CI, Fabris B, Yamada H, et al: Comparative studies of tissue inhibition by angiotensin converting enzyme inhibitors. J Hypertens 7[Suppl S]:S11, 1990.)

FACTORS AFFECTING TISSUE ACE BINDING POTENCY

Several factors may influence the tissue availability of ACE inhibitors. These include (1) plasma concentration, (2) the rate of conversion of ester to diacid and the potential for local conversion in tissue sites, (3) the relative number of plasma and tissue-binding sites for the ACE inhibitor, and (4) the lipophilicity of the drug.[26]

In a review article, Nash[27] concluded that reported differences in the ability of ACE inhibitors to penetrate tissues and to bind to converting enzyme may be closely related to the relative lipophilicity of these agents. Ondetti[31] compared the lipid solubility of quinapril with that of various other ACE inhibitors (ramipril, captopril, enalapril, and lisinopril) and found quinapril to be the most lipophilic; enalapril and lisinopril were considerably less lipophilic.

CLINICAL EFFICACY IN HYPERTENSION

The efficacy and safety of quinapril have been studied extensively in patients with hypertension or CHF.[32] Most studies have compared the effects of quinapril with placebo or other ACE inhibitors (such as captopril or enalapril). The comparison trials were usually randomized, double-blind, and included a washout period of up to 4 weeks. The targeted response was a decrease of diastolic blood pressure to 90 mmHg or less, or a reduction of at least 10 mmHg. Several trials added a diuretic during the washout period and in the treatment regimen if the targeted response was not reached.

Results of these studies indicate that quinapril monotherapy is safe and effective as initial therapy for the treatment of mild to moderate hypertension. Studies have shown that quinapril administered once or twice daily is equally safe and effective.[33-36]

Comparative studies[37, 38] indicate that quinapril and enalapril produce comparable reductions in blood pressure when given either once or twice daily in doses of 10 to 40 mg/day. In the treatment of mild to moderate hypertension, quinapril, 10 to 40 mg/day given in one or two doses, was comparable with captopril, 50 to 150 mg/day given two or three times daily.[39]

Schnaper[40] compared the efficacy and safety of quinapril and captopril administered concurrently with once-daily hydrochlorothiazide in 172 patients with moderate to severe hypertension. The results of this double-blind trial indicate that quinapril (20 to 80 mg twice daily) is significantly more effective at reducing blood pressure than captopril (50 to 200 mg twice daily). Throughout the course of the 6-week study, quinapril consistently showed efficacy superior to captopril despite faster captopril dose titration. In addition, black patients (n = 31) tended to respond better to quinapril therapy than to captopril therapy (72% and 54%, respectively).

In a 12-week, multicenter, open-label trial, Parra-Carrillo et al.[35] found that 81% of patients receiving quinapril monotherapy had a clinical response, defined as a reduction in sitting diastolic blood pressure to 90 mmHg or less.

Forette et al.[41] investigated the efficacy of quinapril in older patients (>65 years of age). After 4 weeks of treatment, 85% of patients were considered to have a clinical response (decrease in diastolic blood pressure ≥ 10 mmHg) to quinapril monotherapy.

In pooled data from the open-label extension phase of four double-blind trials (unpublished data, Medical Affairs Department, Parke-Davis), it was noted that of patients who initially responded to quinapril therapy, 86% continued to respond to this monotherapy after 12 months of treatment.

DOSE–RESPONSE RELATIONSHIP

An 8-week, placebo-controlled, multicenter, dose-response study involving 270 patients (median age, 50) assessed the efficacy and safety of quinapril, 5, 10, 40, and 80 mg/day given twice daily. The results of this study indicate that a positive dose-response relationship is shown for quinapril in doses of 5 to 80 mg, which is similar for both peak and trough effects. Although the incremental decreases in sitting diastolic blood pressure between 5 and 40 mg were not statistically significant, the dose-response relationship was statistically significant between 40 and 80 mg.[42]

Similar findings were reported by Maclean[33] in a double-blind, placebo-controlled trial of patients with mild to moderate essential hypertension. The author notes that as quinapril doses were increased from 20 to 40 to 80 mg/day (b.i.d. and q.d. regimens), there were corresponding decreases in diastolic blood pressure and increases in response rates. Reductions in sitting diastolic blood pressure ranged from 8 to 9 mmHg with quinapril 20 mg/day, 10 to 12 mmHg with quinapril 40 mg/day, and 12 to 13 mmHg with quinapril 80 mg/day. Response rates increased during the study as the dosage level increased, regardless

of regimen. The improved response was attributable to a dose effect.

DOSE TITRATION

Although the dosage of most antihypertensive drugs, including ACE inhibitors, is routinely titrated upward approximately every 2 weeks, Weir[43] suggested that a slower titration interval with quinapril (4 weeks) may be more effective with less drug in patients with moderate to severe hypertension receiving low-dose diuretic therapy.

Similar results were found in three optional-titration studies conducted in patients with mild to moderate hypertension. Quinapril was administered in daily doses of 10, 20, or 40 mg; titration intervals ranged from 2 to 4 weeks, and a diuretic could be added to nonresponders receiving quinapril at 40 mg/day. The percentages of patients receiving each dosage were determined, and it was demonstrated that most patients with hypertension were maintained on 10 mg/day to 40 mg/day as monotherapy. In a comparison of results from studies using once-daily dosing with rapid titration (every 2 weeks) versus slow titration (every 4 weeks), 60% of patients were maintained on 20 mg/day with slow titration, and only 35% were maintained with rapid titration (unpublished data, Medical Affairs Department, Parke-Davis).

THE ADOPT PROGRAM

The Accupril Decision on Pharmaco Therapy (ADOPT)[44] clinical trial program was designed to evaluate the single-agent, single-dose antihypertensive efficacy of quinapril in mildly to moderately hypertensive patients, including those generally considered to be at increased cardiovascular risk, such as blacks, diabetics, the elderly, and patients with multiple medical problems. Efficacy (control) was defined as a final diastolic blood pressure of 90 mmHg or less or a decrease of at least 10 mmHg from baseline.

In this large (n = 12,275), community-based trial, physicians were instructed to initiate quinapril therapy at 10 or 20 mg once daily. If blood pressure control was not achieved after 4 weeks of therapy, the dose was doubled for an additional 4 weeks. Overall, diastolic blood pressure was controlled in 81% of this diverse population; physicians who completed the global evaluation rated tolerability as "excellent" in 78% of the patients.

The ADOPT intent-to-treat population (n = 10,944) was divided by age into three groups: Group 1, 64 years or younger (n = 8005); Group 2, 65 to 74 years (n=2313); and Group 3, ≥ 75 years (n=599). Quinapril as a single agent produced the following control rates: Group 1—81%; Group 2—84%; and Group 3—86%.

The ADOPT intent-to-treat database contained information on 1467 black hypertensive patients (13.4% of the data). Seventy-three percent (73%) of these patients achieved single agent control with quinapril.

Both caucasian and black patients experienced an 11-mmHg decrease in diastolic blood pressure, however, the mean baseline and final visit pressures were greater in blacks (99 and 88 mmHg in blacks compared with 96 and 85 mmHg in caucasians). In general, the ADOPT results were in agreement with data found in the randomized, comparative, or placebo-controlled studies.

In patients with special medical conditions that required concomitant medication, quinapril demonstrated comparable single agent efficacy. Control rates for hypertensive patients with diabetes, hyperlipidemia, or arthritis were 80%, 81%, and 84%, respectively.

The frequency and severity of associated adverse events in this community-based population agreed with such data in previous trials. Neither age, race, nor gender had an effect on the distribution of these events. Most notable adverse events were cough (4.7%), headache (1.6%), dizziness (1.6%), asthenia (1.5%), nausea (0.6%), and rash (0.5%).

CLINICAL EFFICACY IN CONGESTIVE HEART FAILURE

ACE inhibitors are emerging as key agents in the treatment of CHF. Clinical trials have shown that ACE inhibitors produce favorable hemodynamic effects in CHF without the adverse effects of vasodilators.[45, 46] ACE inhibitors are being used extensively to achieve afterload reduction and relief of symptoms in patients with CHF. Quinapril given twice daily is the fourth ACE inhibitor approved for the treatment of CHF, joining captopril, enalapril, and lisinopril.

The efficacy of quinapril in the management of heart failure has been established in a number of controlled clinical trials. The primary measure of efficacy in these studies was maximal exercise tolerance. In addition, each study assessed several secondary end points, including changes in New York Heart Association (NYHA) functional class, signs and symptoms of heart failure, and quality of life (unpublished data, Medical Affairs Department, Parke-Davis).

One study showed a significant dose-response relationship for improvement in maximal exercise tolerance. Riegger[47] summarized the results of this double-blind trial consisting of 225 patients with CHF (NYHA classes III and IV). The author noted that treatment with quinapril in addition to maintenance therapy with digitalis, diuretics, or both produced a significant *dose-related* improvement in exercise time in addition to a significant improvement in NYHA functional class compared with placebo. This beneficial effect was also found after 12 months of therapy with quinapril. No serious side effects were recorded, particularly no symptomatic hypotension or deterioration of renal function. A subset of patients who entered the study and who were not receiving concomitant medications showed the same beneficial response following quinapril administration as was demonstrated for patients receiving concomitant therapy of diuretics alone, digitalis alone, or digitalis plus diuretics.

Several studies were conducted to evaluate the efficacy of quinapril administered once daily. Northridge et al.[48] compared the effects of quinapril (maximum daily dose 20 mg) given once daily versus twice daily in patients with mild CHF. Mean exercise time (the primary end point) was 65 seconds and 53 seconds longer in patients receiving quinapril once daily and twice daily, respectively, compared with placebo ($p < .01$). There was no significant difference between the two dosing regimens. Similar findings were reported in a multicenter trial (n = 62) comparing the efficacy and safety of 20 mg of quinapril administered once or twice daily in patients with CHF. Although the investigators noted a slightly more pronounced effect with the twice-daily regimen than with the once-daily regimen, the results were not statistically significant (unpublished data, Medical Affairs Department, Parke-Davis).

In a double-blind, multicenter trial, Gavazzi et al.[49] compared the efficacy and safety of quinapril once daily versus captopril twice daily in patients with mild to moderate CHF. Exercise tolerance improved in the quinapril and captopril groups by 22% and 16%, respectively ($p < .001$ versus baseline in each group). Results indicate that quinapril, 10 to 20 mg once daily, is as effective and as well tolerated as captopril 25 to 50 mg given twice daily.

The efficacy, safety, and clinical consequences of abrupt cessation of quinapril therapy in patients with NYHA class II or III CHF were also studied.[50] The investigators found that in patients who received quinapril for 2 to 3 months, continued therapy with quinapril for an additional 4 months maintained the clinical stability and exercise capacity of patients with heart failure. Withdrawal of quinapril in these patients resulted in a slow, progressive decline in clinical status.

SAFETY AND TOLERABILITY

Quinapril has been evaluated for safety in 4960 adult patients, including 655 patients 65 years of age or older, who participated in controlled clinical trials. More than 1400 of these patients have been evaluated for safety while treated for 1 year or more. Quinapril has been well tolerated by most patients in clinical trials.

In double-blind comparative studies of patients with mild, moderate, or severe hypertension or CHF, adverse events with quinapril were usually mild and transient, with an incidence of 12%; this was similar to captopril (16%) and enalapril (15%). The frequency of withdrawal due to adverse events was less with quinapril (3.7%) than with enalapril (8.0%) or captopril (6.4%); the placebo withdrawal rate was 2.3%. There was a slightly higher incidence of adverse events among patients with hypertension who were also receiving a diuretic.[32, 51]

Quinapril treatment is associated with a lower incidence of orthostatic hypotension than either enalapril or captopril (6.1% versus 8.6% and 9.4%, respectively). First occurrences of hypotension were also less frequent for quinapril (0.4%) than for either captopril (2.2%) or enalapril (1.5%).[52]

Gottlieb et al.[53] demonstrated that quinapril titrated to 10 mg twice daily in patients with NYHA class III or IV CHF was safe and effective with minimal risk of functional renal insufficiency. The glomerular filtration rate deteriorated in only 5 of 20 patients with quinapril therapy after initial treatment with digoxin and diuretics. Overall, the glomerular filtration rate increased after quinapril therapy from 49 ± 6 to 56 ± 7 ml/min/1.73 m^2. The authors concluded that initial poor renal function or low blood pressure does not increase the risk of renal deterioration with quinapril.

As part of the Accupril NDA, the relationship between quinapril dose and adverse events in 2338 patients with hypertension or CHF was analyzed. The analysis indicated that adverse events were unrelated to increasing quinapril daily doses of 10 to 80 mg with or without concomitant diuretics. Similar findings were reported by Maclean[33] in a double-blind, placebo-controlled trial of 270 patients with mild to moderate essential hypertension. The results of this study indicate that quinapril is well-tolerated. Reported adverse events were scarcely more frequent than in the placebo group, and as the dose increased, the number of patients reporting adverse events decreased.

An overall summary of all adverse events by total daily dose for two fixed-dose studies in patients with CHF (unpublished data, Medical Affairs Department, Parke-Davis) shows that increasing quinapril doses of up to 40 mg daily are not associated with statistically significant increases in the reporting of adverse events.

CONCLUSIONS

Quinapril is an ACE inhibitor approved for the treatment of hypertension and CHF that possesses increased affinity for binding to tissue ACE and an enhanced association with tissue ACE, once bound. These properties may explain why the drug has prolonged antihypertensive activity beyond its pharmacokinetic half-life. These pharmacologic properties may prove to be important in the management of diseases such as hypertension and CHF, in which cardiovascular remodeling and restructuring are involved, as more is learned about the therapeutic implications of antagonizing plasma and tissue-based ACE.

REFERENCES

1. Kaplan HR, Taylor DG, Olson SC, et al: Quinapril: A preclinical review of the pharmacology, pharmacokinetics, and toxicology. Angiology 40:335, 1989.
2. Olson SC, Horvath AM, Michniewicz BM, et al: The clinical pharmacokinetics of quinapril. Angiology 40:351, 1989.
3. Croog SH, Levine S, Testa MA, et al: The effects of antihyper-
tensive therapy on the quality of life. N Engl J Med 314:1657, 1986.
4. Williams GH: Converting-enzyme inhibitors in the treatment of hypertension. N Engl J Med 319:1517, 1988.
5. Packer M, Lee WH, Yushak M, et al: Comparison of captopril and enalapril in patients with severe chronic heart failure. N Engl J Med 315:847, 1986.
6. Johnston CI, Fabris B, Yamada H, et al: Comparative studies of tissue inhibition by angiotensin converting enzyme inhibitors. J Hypertens 7(Suppl 5):S11, 1990.
7. Fabris B, Chen B, Pupic V, et al: Inhibition of angiotensin-converting enzyme (ACE) in plasma and tissue. J Cardiovasc Pharmacol 15(Suppl 2):S6, 1990.
8. Ferry JJ, Horvath AM, Sedman AJ, et al: Influence of food on the pharmacokinetics of quinapril and its active diacid metabolite, CI-928. J Clin Pharmacol 27:397, 1987.
9. Halstenson CE, Opsahl JA, Rachael K, et al: The pharmacokinetics of quinapril and its active metabolite, quinaprilat, in patients with various degrees of renal function. J Clin Pharmacol 32:344, 1992.
10. Horvath AM, Olson SC, Ferry JJ, et al: Pharmacokinetics of quinapril and its active metabolite, quinaprilat, in patients with hepatic impairment. J Clin Pharmacol 28:917, 1988.
11. Wadworth AN, Brogden RN: Quinapril: A review of its pharmacological properties, and therapeutic efficacy in cardiovascular disorders. Drugs 41:378, 1991.
12. Dzau VJ: Tissue angiotensin II in myocardial hypertrophy and failure. Arch Intern Med 153:937, 1993.
13. Unger T, Gohlke P: Tissue renin-angiotensin systems in the heart and vasculature: Possible involvement in the cardiovascular actions of converting enzyme inhibitors. Am J Cardiol 65:31, 1990.
14. Dzau VJ: Implications of local angiotensin production in cardiovascular physiology and pharmacology. J Cardiovasc Pharmacol 10(Suppl 7):S9, 1987.
15. Johnston CI: Angiotensin II: A dual tissue and hormonal system for cardiovascular control. J Hypertens 10(Suppl 7):S13, 1992.
16. Reams GP: Angiotensin-converting enzyme in renal and cerebral tissue and implications for blood pressure management. Am J Cardiol 69:59C, 1991.
17. Steckelings U, Lebrum C, Qadri F, et al: Role of brain angiotensin in cardiovascular regulation. J Cardiovasc Pharmacol 19(Suppl 6):S72, 1992.
18. Lee MA, Martin P, Manfred B, et al: Effects of angiotensin-converting enzyme inhibitors on tissue renin-angiotensin systems. Am J Cardiol 70:12C, 1992.
19. Unger T, Ganten D, Lang RE, et al: Is tissue converting inhibition a determinant of the antihypertensive efficacy of converting enzyme inhibitors? J Cardiovasc Pharmacol 6:872, 1984.
20. Keuneke C, Yacullo R, Metzger R, et al: The role of tissue renin-angiotensin systems in hypertension and effects of chronic converting-enzyme inhibition. Eur Heart J 11(Suppl D):11, 1990.
21. Kromer E, Riegger G: Effects of long-term angiotensin-converting enzyme inhibition on myocardial hypertrophy in experimental aortic stenosis in the rat. Am J Cardiol 62:161, 1988.
22. Schunkert H, Jackson B, Tang SS, et al: Distribution and functional significance of cardiac angiotensin-converting enzyme in hypertrophied rat heart. Circulation 87:1328, 1993.
23. Dzau VA, Pratt RE: Tissue angiotensin II in experimental restenosis after vascular injury: Evidence for local activation. J Cardiovasc Pharmacol 20(Suppl B):S28, 1992.
24. Texter M, Lees RS, Pitt B, et al: The Quinapril Ischemic Event Trial (QUIET) design and methods: Evaluation of chronic ACE inhibitor therapy after coronary artery intervention. Cardiovasc Drugs Ther 7:273, 1993.
25. Dzau VJ: Worldwide clinical experience with ACE inhibitors: The role of quinapril [summary]. J Cardiovasc Pharmacol 15(Suppl 2):S62, 1990.
26. Lees KR, MacFadyen RJ, Reid JL: Tissue angiotensin-converting enzyme inhibition: Relevant to clinical practice? Am J Hypertens 3:266S, 1990.
27. Nash DT: Comparative properties of angiotensin-converting enzyme inhibitors: Relations with inhibition of tissue angiotensin-converting enzyme and potential clinical implications. Am J Cardiol 67:26C, 1992.

28. Kaplan HR, Cohen DM, Essenburg AD, et al: CI-906 and CI-907: New orally active nonsulfhydryl angiotensin-converting enzyme inhibitors. Fed Proc 43:1326, 1984.

29. Kinoshita A, Urata H, Bumpus FM, et al: Measurement of angiotensin I converting enzyme inhibition in the heart. Circ Res 73:51, 1993.

30. Nakajima T, Yamada T, Setoguchi M, et al: Prolonged inhibition of local angiotensin-converting enzyme after single or repeated treatment with quinapril in spontaneously hypertensive rats. J Cardiovasc Pharmacol 19:102, 1992.

31. Ondetti MA: Structural relationships of angiotensin converting-enzyme inhibitors to pharmacologic activity. Circulation 77(Suppl I):74, 1988.

32. Frank GJ, Knapp LE, Olson SC, et al: Overview of quinapril, a new ACE inhibitor. J Cardiovasc Pharmacol 15(Suppl 2):S14, 1990.

33. Maclean D: Quinapril: A double-blind, placebo-controlled trial in essential hypertension. Angiology 40:370, 1989.

34. Durante M, Yulde J, Crisostomo M, et al: A parallel-group, double-blind study of once daily quinapril versus enalapril in the treatment of mild-to-moderate essential hypertension. J Intern Med 29:173, 1991.

35. Parra-Carrillo JZ, Alcocer DBL, Olvera S, et al: Multicentric study of quinapril, an angiotensin-converting enzyme inhibitor, in the treatment of mild-to-moderate essential hypertension. Curr Ther Res 51:185, 1992.

36. Sedman AJ, Posvar E: Clinical pharmacology of quinapril in healthy volunteers and in patients with hypertension and congestive heart failure. Angiology 40(4 Part 2):360, 1989.

37. Taylor SH: A comparison of the efficacy and safety of quinapril with that of enalapril in the treatment of mild to moderate essential hypertension. Angiology 40:382, 1989.

38. Sanchez S, Luna A, Orozco R, et al: Quinapril versus enalapril in the treatment of mild-to-moderate essential hypertension. Clin Ther 13:651, 1991.

39. Taylor SH: The treatment of mild-to-moderate hypertension with ACE inhibitors. J Cardiovasc Pharmacol 15(Suppl 2): S24, 1990.

40. Schnaper HW: Comparison of the efficacy and safety of quinapril vs captopril in treatment of moderate to severe hypertension. Angiology 40(4 Part 2):389, 1989.

41. Forette B, Koen R, and Vicaut E: Efficacy and safety of quinapril in the elderly hypertensive patient. Am Heart J 123:1426, 1992.

42. Frank GJ, Knapp LE: Overview of the clinical development of quinapril. Choices in Cardiology 2(Suppl I):30, 1991.

43. Weir MR: Speed and duration of dose titration with the ACE inhibitor quinapril: Relationship with efficacy in patients with moderate-to-severe hypertension. J Hum Hypertens 8:725, 1994.

44. Dzau V, Julius S, Weber MA: ADOPT trial results: Comparison of response rates by age, race, medical history [abstract]. Am J Hypertens 7:123A, 1994.

45. The Consensus Trial Study Group: Effects of enalapril on mortality in severe congestive heart failure. N Engl J Med 316:1429, 1987.

46. The Captopril-Digoxin Multicenter Research Group: Comparative effects of therapy with captopril and digoxin in patients with mild to moderate heart failure. JAMA 259:539, 1988.

47. Riegger GAJ: The effects of ACE inhibitors on exercise capacity in the treatment of congestive heart failure. J Cardiovasc Pharmacol 15(Suppl 2):S41, 1990.

48. Northridge DB, Rose E, Raftery ED, et al: A multicentre, double-blind, placebo-controlled trial of quinapril in mild, chronic heart failure. Eur Heart J 14:403, 1993.

49. Gavazzi A, Marioni C, Campana C, Montemartini C: Comparative trial of quinopril versus captopril in moderate congestive heart failure. J Hypertens 12(Suppl 4):S89, 1994.

50. Pflugfelder PW, Baird MG, Tonkon MJ, et al: Clinical consequences of angiotensin-converting enzyme inhibitor withdrawal in chronic heart failure: A double-blind, placebo-controlled study of quinapril. J Am Coll Cardiol 22:1557, 1993.

51. Frank GJ, Knapp LE, McLain RW: Overall tolerance and safety of quinapril in clinical trials. Angiology 40:405, 1989.

52. Knapp LE, Frank GJ, McLain R, et al: The safety and tolerability of quinapril. J Cardiovasc Pharmacol 15(Suppl 2):S47, 1990.

53. Gottlieb SS, Robinson S, Weir MR, et al: Determinants of the renal response to ACE inhibition in patients with congestive heart failure. Am Heart J 124:131, 1992.

CHAPTER 85

Fosinopril

Domenic A. Sica, M.D.

HISTORY

A number of structurally distinct angiotensin-converting enzyme (ACE) inhibitors exist. ACE inhibitors are effective zinc ligands and thereby interrupt the conversion of angiotensin I to angiotensin II.[1] The zinc ion found in ACE is an important catalyst to the reaction with angiotensin I, because it intensifies polarization of the carboxyl group of peptide substrates such as angiotensin I, thereby rendering it more susceptible to nucleophilic attack and ensuing hydrolytic cleavage. The avidity of binding to the zinc ligand and the number of complementary binding sites determine the final degree of inhibitory activity and therefore the potency of an ACE inhibitor. Moreover, the size, conformation, and lipophilicity of an individual ACE inhibitor determines its metabolism, route of elimination, and tissue penetration.[2–3]

The first ACE inhibitor, captopril, was characterized by the presence of a sulfhydryl group, which served as its zinc ligand for ACE. Another group of ACE inhibitors, including benazepril, cilazapril, enalapril, lisinopril, quinapril, and ramipril, rely on a carboxyl (COOH) group for the formation of a ligand with zinc. More recently, a new compound, fosinopril, was developed. This compound is the first member of the ACE inhibitor drug class that depends on a phosphinyl group to incapacitate ACE by its zinc ligand relationship (Fig. 85–1).[4]

CHEMISTRY AND PHARMACOLOGY

The chemical structure of fosinopril, fosinoprilat, and their primary metabolites is given in Figure 85–2. Fosinopril sodium ([1,4S]-4-cyclohexyl-1-[[[2-methyl-1-(1-oxopropexy)propoxy] (4-phenylbutyl)phosphinyl]acetyl]-L-proline, monosodium salt) has a molecular weight of 585.65. It is a prodrug that is completely deesterified in the liver and gastrointestinal mucosa, either during or shortly after absorption, to form the

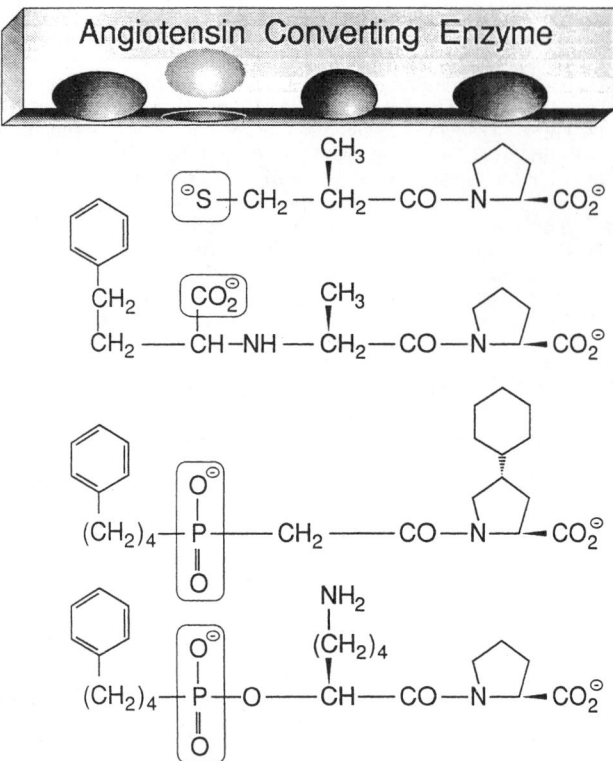

Figure 85–1. Structural differences of active moieties of ACE inhibitors.

tard angiotensin I conversion were 23 and 11 nM, respectively. Captopril and fosinopril have different half-lives, which explains the differing durations of action of these two compounds. For example, 24 hours after administration of placebo, captopril, or fosinopril to conscious rats, angiotensin I infusions have been shown to increase mean arterial pressure (MAP) 44 ± 1 mmHg in captopril-treated animals and only 22 ± 5 mmHg in fosinopril-treated animals. These differences dissipate in the presence of renal insufficiency.[8]

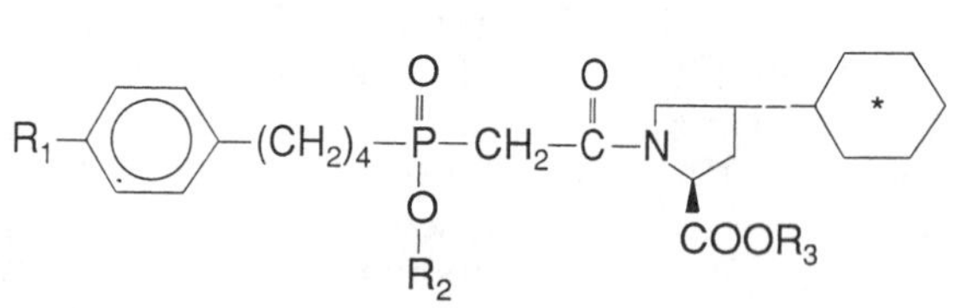

ACE inhibitors differ in their capacity to inhibit tissue specific ACE. An *ex vivo* study in spontaneously hypertensive rats compared the differences in distribution and degree of tissue ACE inhibition for several ACE inhibitors (captopril, enalapril, lisinopril, ramipril, zofenopril, and fosinopril) with individual drug doses normalized for differences in potency. Fosinopril was notable for prolonged and sustained ACE inhibitory activity in brain and myocardial tissues. In the kidney, fosinopril displayed weak and short-lived activity.[9] The latter observation might relate to the hepatobiliary elimination of this compound with "less drug" available for renal elimination/distribution.

PHARMACOKINETICS

Fosinopril is primarily absorbed from the jejunum and proximal ileum (60%), with the remaining fraction absorbed from more distal ileal segments (30%).[8, 10] Fosinopril pharmacokinetic data from healthy volunteers are available from two studies.[7, 11] After oral dosing, the average absorption of fosinopril is 36%. Protein binding ranges between 95% and 99% with minimal partitioning into the red blood cell compartment.[7] This high degree of protein binding for fosinopril is not unexpected, because within the ACE inhibitor class, the level of protein binding correlates strongly with lipophilicity.[3] Consistent with the extensive protein binding of this compound, the average steady-state volume of distribution was 9.8 L.[7] The plasma elimination half-life ($T_{1/2}$) of fosinopril in subjects with normal renal and hepatic function is approximately 12 hours;[7, 11] total, renal, and nonrenal clearances of fosinoprilat average 39, 17, and 22 ml/min, respectively.[7]

After oral administration, fosinopril undergoes rapid and extensive *hydrolysis*; compounds that predominate 1 to 24 hours after administration of a single radiolabeled dose of fosinopril are fosinoprilat (70% to 80%) and two metabolites of fosinoprilat, a β-glucuronide conjugate (15% to 20%) and a hydroxy analogue of the diacid (5%).[7] Neither metabolite has been extensively studied as to its antihypertensive potency.

Peak serum fosinoprilat concentration (C_{max}) and area under the serum fosinoprilat concentration-time curve ($AUC_{fosinoprilat}$) correlate with fosinopril dose in healthy volunteers. C_{max} values of fosinoprilat following single oral doses (10 to 640 mg) ranged from 131 to 5600 μg/L and occurred anywhere from 2.4 to

active diacid fosinoprilat.[5] Fosinoprilat is distinguished from most other ACE inhibitors[6] by having an almost equal total body clearance by both hepatic and renal routes.[7] The higher molecular weight and lipophilicity of fosinopril are possible explanations for its partial elimination by biliary excretion.[2–3]

In vitro inhibitory potency data for fosinoprilat are available from purified rabbit lung ACE and guinea pig ileum preparations.[8] IC_{50} (concentration of drug required for 50% inhibition of ACE activity) concentrations for captopril and fosinoprilat required to re-

Compound	R_1	R_2	R_3
Fosinopril	H	$(CH_3)_2-CH-O-C-C-C_2H_5$	Na
Fosinoprilat	H	H	H
p-Hydroxy fosinoprilat	–OH	H	H
Fosinoprilat glucuronide	H	H	COOH

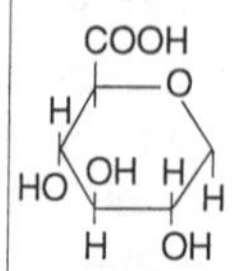

Figure 85–2. Chemical structures of fosinopril, fosinoprilat, and their primary metabolites. (Adapted from Sica DA, Gehr TW, Duchin K, et al: The pharmacology and pharmacokinetics of fosinopril. Rev Contemp Pharmacother 4:1, 1993.)

4.2 hours (T_{max}) after drug administration (Fig. 85–3). Steady-state C_{max} and T_{max} values for fosinoprilat following 2 weeks of dosing in healthy volunteers did not differ from those values found after an initial dose.[11]

The aging process per se does not modify any of the pharmacokinetic features of fosinopril or fosinoprilat.[12] This is in contrast to most other ACE inhibitors, wherein elimination is significantly delayed because of senescence-related renal insufficiency.[13] Renal insufficiency has considerably less of an effect on fosinoprilat elimination than it does on elimination of other ACE inhibitors.[6, 14] In a single-dose study of fosinoprilat elimination in graded renal insufficiency, although total body clearance (TBC) declined in parallel with the change in renal function, the constant and preserved hepatic elimination of fosinoprilat negated any clinically significant deterioration in its elimination profile.[15] The long-term dosing studies of Sica et al.[16] further substantiate the importance of hepatic elimination to the maintenance of "clinically normal" fosinoprilat kinetics. Ten-day treatment regimens with once-daily fosinopril, enalapril, or lisinopril were accompanied by accumulation indices ($AUC_{Day\ 10}$/$AUC_{Day\ 1}$) of 1.27, 1.77, and 2.62, respectively (Fig. 85–4).

Single-dose pharmacokinetic parameters for fosinoprilat in patients with end-stage renal disease maintained on either continuous ambulatory peritoneal dialysis[17] or hemodialysis[18] are similar to those values found in advanced renal insufficiency. Long-term dosing of fosinopril has not been examined in end-stage renal disease, but because dialytic clearance with either modality is negligible,[16, 17] single-dose kinetic parameters derived from advanced chronic renal failure studies probably could be extrapolated to this population.

Two studies have examined the pharmacokinetics of fosinopril in hepatic disease.[19, 20] In a single-dose study with radiolabeled fosinopril, the presence of cirrhosis modified the rate, but not the extent, of prodrug conversion to its active diacid form.[19] This observation is most readily explained by the fact that the deesterification of fosinopril occurs not only in the liver but also within gastrointestinal mucosa and perhaps other tissues. In this regard, *in vitro* hydrolysis studies of fosinopril sodium in canine tissues show the following order of esterase activity: liver = kidney > small intestine > blood and lung.[5] In patients with cirrhosis, dosing for 14 days with 10 mg/day of fosinopril resulted in modest and clinically insignificant increases in the $AUC_{fosinoprilat}$ whether examined after single or multiple doses.[20] This latter observation again stresses the importance of the dual route of elimination for fosinoprilat in curtailing drug accumulation when liver or renal disease is present.

EFFECTS ON PATHOPHYSIOLOGY

Single and multiple-dose fosinopril with[21–23, 25, 26] or without[23–28] concomitant diuretic therapy, effectively

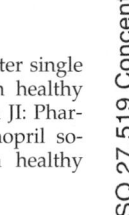

Figure 85–3. Mean serum concentration of fosinoprilat after single oral dose administration of fosinopril 10 to 640 mg in healthy volunteers. (Adapted from Duchin KL, Waclawski AP, Tu JI: Pharmacokinetics, safety and pharmacologic effects of fosinopril sodium, an angiotensin converting enzyme inhibitor in healthy subjects. J Clin Pharmacol 31:58, 1991.)

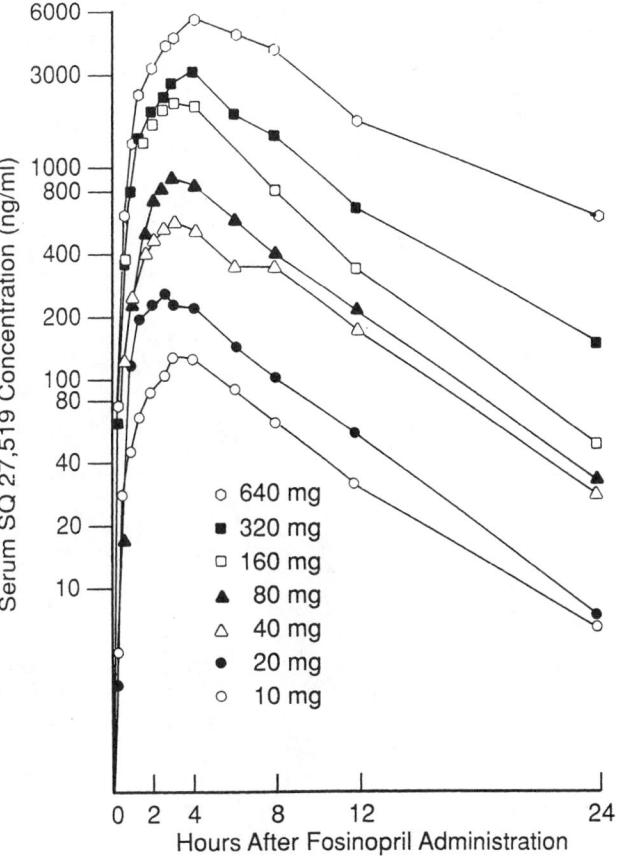

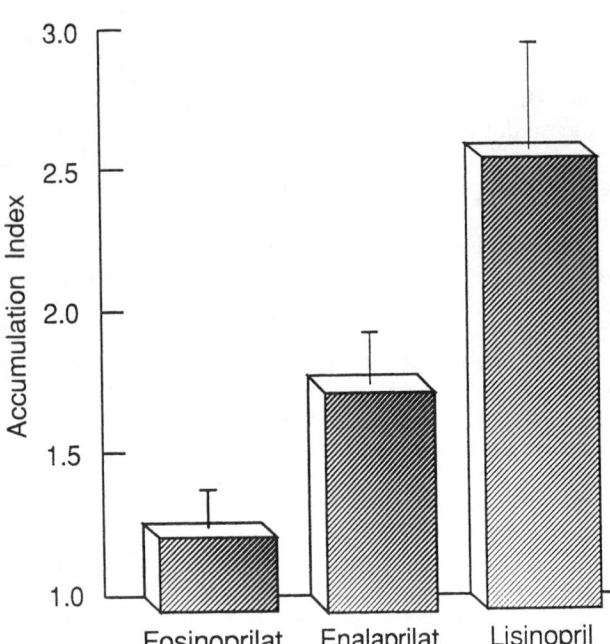

Figure 85–4. Accumulation indices (AUC day 10/AUC day 1) for fosinoprilat, enalaprilat, and lisinopril after administration of fosinopril 10 mg, enalapril 2.5 mg, or lisinopril 5 mg once daily for 10 days to a total of 35 patients with creatinine clearance values, 30 ml/min. Statistically significant enalaprilat versus fosinoprilat: $p < .05$; lisinopril versus fosinoprilat: $p < .001$. (Adapted from Sica DA, Cutler RE, Parmer RJ, et al: Comparison of the steady-state pharmacokinetics of fosinopril, lisinopril, and enalapril in patients with chronic renal insufficiency. Clin Pharmacokinet 20:420, 1991.)

lowers MAP in humans as well as in a number of animal models of hypertension[29, 30] (Table 85–1). The onset of action of fosinopril is gradual and sustained over 24 hours,[23, 27] and long-term treatment is not accompanied by tachyphylaxis.[23] The greatest reduction in blood pressure occurs within 3 to 6 hours after dosing[23] and approximates the time to peak blood levels of fosinoprilat.[11] The decline in MAP is accompanied by significant reductions in systemic[29–32] and renal vascular resistance[30, 31] (Table 85–2) and is not associated with reflex tachycardia in either normal volunteers[11] or treated hypertensives.[22, 27]

Fosinopril doses of approximately 20 mg/day achieve near-maximal reductions in MAP in responders with mild to moderate hypertension.[23, 25, 27] Insig-

nificant additional decrements in MAP occur at doses of 40 mg[23, 25] or 80 mg (Fig. 85–5).[23] When chlorthalidone or hydrochlorothiazide is added to fosinopril, blood pressure is reduced significantly more than with either chlorthalidone[21, 22] or fosinopril monotherapy.[25] In mild-to-moderate hypertension monotherapy, response rates for fosinopril are nearly identical to those achieved with enalapril[26] or sustained-release nifedipine.[24] In moderate-to-severe hypertension, the combination of fosinopril and chlorthalidone proved more effective than a combination of propranolol and chlorthalidone[22] (see Table 85–1). In these same studies, fewer patients receiving fosinopril required addition of prazosin to achieve goal blood pressure. When required, the addition of prazosin to the fosinopril

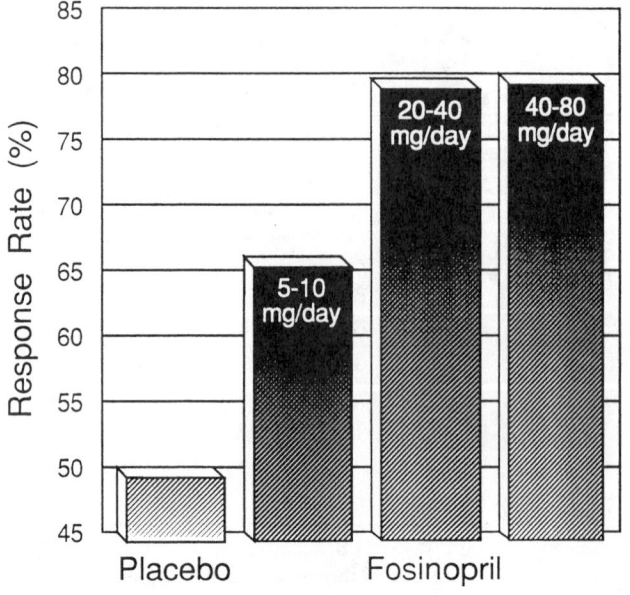

Figure 85–5. Response rates (percentage of patients with sitting diastolic blood pressure < 90 mmHg or a > 10% decrease in this parameter from baseline after 12 weeks' administration of fosinopril 5 to 80 mg once daily or placebo to a total of 380 patients with mild to moderate hypertension; initial dosages were doubled after 4 weeks therapy if sitting diastolic blood pressure remained > 90 mmHg. (Data from Pool JL: Antihypertensive effect of fosinopril, a new angiotensin converting enzyme inhibitor: Findings of the Fosinopril Study Group II. Clin Ther 12:520, 1990. Figure adapted from Murdoch D, McTavish D: Fosinopril: A review of its pharmacodynamic and pharmacokinetic properties, and therapeutic potential in essential hypertension. Drugs 43:123, 1992.)

Table 85–1. **Summary of Clinical Trials Assessing the Antihypertensive Efficacy of Several Fosinopril Regimens in Relation to Placebo, Enalapril, Hydrochlorothiazide, Propranolol, and Sustained-Release Nifedipine, in Patients with Essential Hypertension**

Reference	Study Design	Dosage (mg, once daily)	Number of Patients	Study Duration (weeks)	Position of Blood Pressure Measurement	Mean Percentage Reduction in Blood Pressure versus Baseline		
						SBP	DBP	% of Patients Responding[a]
Dose-ranging trials								
Anderson et al. (23)[b]	m, r, db, p	Placebo	54	8	Supine	7	11*	64
		10	55			10*	13*	76
		40	53			12*†	16*†	83
		80	58			16*	18*	92
	nb[c]	10–80	89	52		8–14*	11–17*	
Pool (25)[d]	m, r, db, p	Placebo	77	12	Sitting		9*	50
		5–10	74				14*	66
		10–20	71				15*	—
		20–40	79				16*	79†
		40–80	79				17*	80†
Ward et al. (21)[f]	m, r, db, p	Placebo	57	8	Sitting		6	50
		5	60				9‡	59†
		10	55				10‡	49
		20	56				12‡†	72‡†
Comparison with enalapril								
Goldstein et al. (26)[b]	m, r, db, p	FOS: 10–20	115	12	Sitting		9*	50
		ENA: 5–10	116				10*	52
Comparison with hydrochlorothiazide								
Forslund et al. (28)	db, p	FOS: 5–10	8	8	Not stated	5*	7*	
		HCTZ: 25–50	9			14*	10*	
Comparison with propranolol								
Miller et al. (22)[a, b, e, f]		FOS: 20–40	53	12	Sitting		16*	81
		PRO: 40–80 b.i.d.	53				16*	92
Comparison with sustained-release nifedipine								
Clementy (24)	m, r, db, p	FOS: 10	49	8	Supine	16*	17*	90
		SR, NIF: 20 b.i.d.	50			15*	18*	96

[a]Usual response = diastolic blood pressure ≤ 90 mmHg or a reduction in this parameter of ≥ 10% vs baseline. Data reported (% responders) include diuretic add-on where indicated.
[b]Concomitant chlorthalidone (≤ 25 mg/day) was administered if goal blood pressure was not achieved.
[c]Continuation of 8-week double-blind trial.
[d]Concomitant hydrochlorothiazide 25 mg/day was administered if goal blood pressure was not achieved. Data reported (% responsers) include diuretic add-on where indicated.
[e]Patients received chlorthalidone 25 mg/day throughout the trial.
[f]Prazosin 1 mg twice daily was added to the regimens if goal blood pressure was not achieved. Dose titration of prazosin was permitted.
Abbreviations: SBP, systolic blood pressure; DBP, diastolic blood pressure; m, multicenter; r, randomized; db, double-blind; p, parallel; nb, nonblind; bid, twice daily; FOS, fosinopril; ENA, enalapril; HCTZ, hydrochlorothiazide; PRO, propranolol; SR, NIF, sustained-release nifedipine.
Statistically significant difference versus baseline (*), versus placebo (‡), or versus other nonindicated regimens symbol (†); —, data not provided.
Adapted from Murdoch D, McTavish D: Fosinopril: A review of its pharmacodynamic and pharmacokinetic properties, and therapeutic potential in essential hypertension. Drugs 43:123, 1992.

and chlorthalidone treatment regimen resulted in an additional 8% decrement in seated diastolic blood pressure (Fig. 85–6).[22]

Fosinopril causes a significant reduction in left ventricular mass index and a modest improvement in left ventricular performance in patients with essential hypertension[30, 32, 33] (Tables 85–3 and 85–4). During monotherapy with captopril (113 ± 10 mg/day), lisinopril (52 ± 10 mg/day), or fosinopril (52 ± 6 mg/day) in further studies of patients with essential hypertension maintained at comparable levels of blood pressure control, only fosinopril significantly increased stroke volume and cardiac output.[32, 34] These changes were accompanied by an increase in the absolute value of the peak ejection rate and a decrease in the time to peak ejection rate; findings consistent with a favorable effect on cardiac systolic function. Fur-

thermore, the absolute value for peak filling rate[32, 34] increased in these studies, suggesting an improvement in diastolic function. This latter observation was unique to fosinopril and was tentatively attributed to the physicochemical and/or cardiophilic properties of the phosphinic acid–containing fosinopril.

Fosinopril has not been reported to adversely affect intracardiac conduction or coronary blood flow. Its effects on arteries and veins are likely to be similar to those of other ACE inhibitors, wherein arterial and venodilation occur and vascular compliance increases.[35] Blood pressure reduction with fosinopril does not precipitate either sodium[30, 31] or volume retention[24, 30] (see Table 85–2). In accordance with prior therapy with other ACE inhibitors, monotherapy with fosinopril can be accompanied by an increase in serum potassium and/or hyperkalemia.[36] Alternatively,

Table 85–2. **Short-term Effects of Fosinopril on Regional Hemodynamics and Urinary Electrolyte Excretion in Nine Patients**

	Baseline Values	Short-Term Effects
Splanchnic		
Plasma flow (ml/min)	343 ± 86	324 ± 73
Blood flow (ml/min)	558 ± 132	519 ± 115
Vascular resistance (U)	21 ± 5	21 ± 6
Renal		
Blood flow (ml/min)	896 ± 183	989 ± 288
Vascular resistance (U)	14 ± 4	12 ± 3*
Glomerular filtration rate (ml/min)	117 ± 25	123 ± 31
Filtration fraction (%)	25 ± 8	24 ± 7
Urine		
Sodium excretion (mEq/day)	175 ± 56	174 ± 64
Fractional sodium excretion (%)	1.0 ± 0.5	0.9 ± 0.2
Potassium excretion (mEq/day)	62 ± 32	69 ± 25
Fractional potassium excretion (%)	12 ± 5	13 ± 5

*$p < .05$ versus baseline.

Adapted from Oren S, Messerli F, Grossman E, et al: Immediate and short-term cardiovascular effects of fosinopril, a new angiotensin-converting enzyme inhibitor, in patients with essential hypertension. J Am Coll Cardiol 17:1183, 1991. Reprinted with permission from the American College of Cardiology.

when fosinopril is coadministered with a diuretic, diuretic-induced hypokalemia is attenuated.[21] The incidence of hyperkalemia in chronic renal failure, attributable to fosinopril, may be less than with other ACE inhibitors.[37] This observation, albeit preliminary, may be explained by the fact that fosinopril is

Table 85–3. **Short-term Systemic, Hemodynamic, and Fluid Volume Responses to Fosinopril in Nine Patients**

	Baseline Values	Short-Term Effects
Noninvasive arterial pressure (mmHg)		
Systolic	162 ± 17	144 ± 15*
Diastolic	93 ± 7	84 ± 6*
Mean	115 ± 10	104 ± 7*
Invasive arterial pressure (mmHg)		
Systolic	156 ± 16	142 ± 16‡
Diastolic	89 ± 6	81 ± 5*
Mean	111 ± 9	101 ± 8‡
Heart rate (beats/min)	68 ± 8	66 ± 8
Cardiac output (L/min)	5.5 ± 1.4	5.75 ± 1.2
Stroke volume (ml/beat)	79 ± 16	88 ± 17‡
Total peripheral resistance (U)	21 ± 4	18 ± 3*
Total blood volume (liters)	5.1 ± 1	4.9 ± 0.7
Plasma volume (liters)	3.1 ± 0.6	3.0 ± 0.4
Red cell mass (liters)	2.0 ± 0.5	1.9 ± 0.4
Central blood volume (liters)	2.8 ± 0.4	2.7 ± 0.8
Norepinephrine (pg/ml)	200 ± 67	190 ± 61
Epinephrine (pg/ml)	20 ± 8	30 ± 15
Dopamine (pg/ml)	13 ± 5	10.5 ± 1.0
Plasma renin activity (ng/ml/hr)	1.35 ± 0.49	4.26 ± 2†
Aldosterone (ng/dl)	7.49 ± 3.3	4.5 ± 1.8‡

*$p < .01$ versus baseline.
†$p < .001$ versus baseline.
‡$p < .05$ versus baseline.

Adapted from Oren S, Messerli F, Grossman E, et al: Immediate and short-term cardiovascular effects of fosinopril, a new angiotensin-converting enzyme inhibitor, in patients with essential hypertension. J Am Coll Cardiol 17:1183, 1991. Reprinted with permission from the American College of Cardiology.

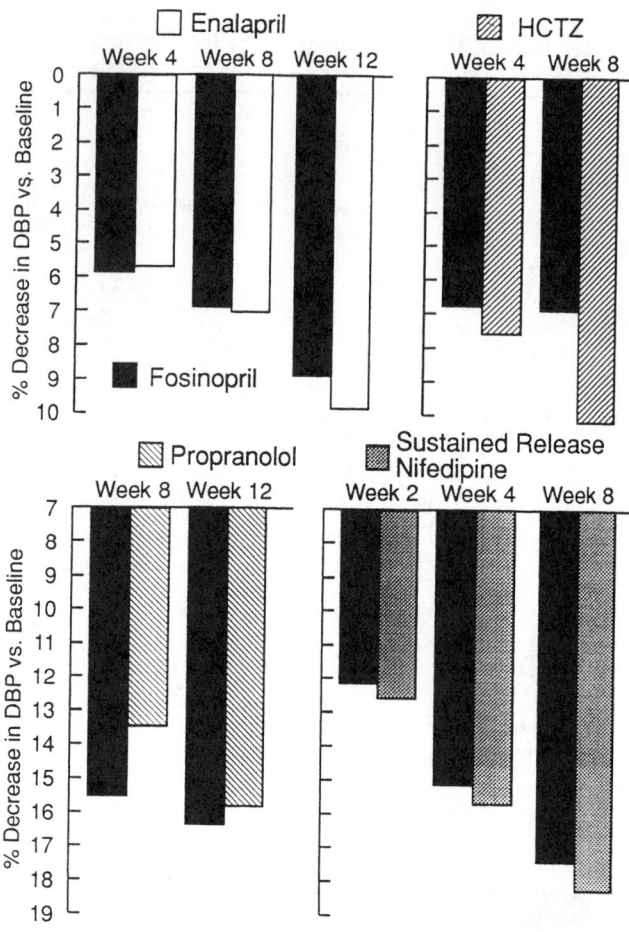

Figure 85–6. Percentage decreases in diastolic blood pressure (DBP) in four different 8- to 12-week double-blind trials comparing fosinopril 5 to 40 mg/day (n = 8 to 115) with enalapril 5 to 10 mg/day (n = 116; Goldstein et al.;[26] hydrochlorothiazide 25 to 50 mg/day (n = 9; Forslund et al.;[28] sustained-release nifedipine 40 mg/day (n = 50; Clementy et al.;[24] or propranolol 80 to 160 mg/day (n = 53; Miller et al.[22]) in patients with essential hypertension. All blood pressure reductions were statistically significant versus baseline; no significant differences were noted between fosinopril and comparator regimens. (Adapted from Murdoch D, McTavish D: Fosinopril: A review of its pharmacodynamic and pharmacokinetic properties, and therapeutic potential in essential hypertension. Drugs 43:123, 1992.)

"nonaccumulating" in chronic renal failure[16] and thereby reduces the likelihood of aldosterone secretion being suppressed.

As with other ACE inhibitors, fosinopril administration triggers a reactive rise in plasma renin activity[11, 16–18, 30, 37] and modest,[11, 16–18, 30] if not occasionally absent,[37, 38] suppression of plasma aldosterone. These findings are consistent with "non–angiotensin II" factors mediating aldosterone release. Short-term therapy for 12 weeks with fosinopril does not cause reflex sympathetic activation as evidenced by absence of change in plasma norepinephrine or epinephrine values[30] (see Table 85–3). In separate studies, 8 weeks of treatment with fosinopril did not alter atrial natriuretic peptide[28] or antidiuretic hormone concentrations.[28] Fosinopril is neutral with regard to lipoprotein and carbohydrate metabolism and may slightly enhance cellular glucose disposal.[39]

Table 85–4. Effects of Fosinopril on Hemodynamics and Cardiac Function in Patients with Essential Hypertension

Reference	Number of Patients	Dosage (mg/day)	Study Duration (weeks)	Patient Status	Statistically Significant Percentage Changes in Hemodynamic Parameters versus Baseline										
					MAP	SBP	DBP	HR	CO	SV	ESS	Vcf	PER	PFR	SVR
Nonblind studies															
Oren et al. (30)	10	10	sd	Rest (supine)	−14	−13	−15	±	±	±	±	±			−24
		10–40	12		−10	−11	−10	±	±	+11	−16	+17			−14
Waldemar et al. (47)	8	10–40[a]	4–12	Rest (supine)		−10	−13								
Zusman et al. (34)[b]	12	[not stated]	[not stated]	Rest		−14	−16	±	+10	+6			+18	+16	−27
				Exercise		−11	−12	±	+6	+11			±	±	−16
Double-blind studies															
Guller and Reeves (57)	12	FOS: 10–20 HCTZ: 25–50	8	Rest (sitting)			↓		↑[c]		↓	↑			↓
							↓		±[c]		±	±			±
Sullivan et al. (38)	11	20–40	8	Rest (supine)		−11	−17	±							
				Exercise		−3	−9	±							

[a] Patients received concomitant chlorthalidone 25 mg/day throughout the trial.
[b] Study design not stated; assumed to be nonblind.
[c] Cardiac index.
Abbreviations: FOS, fosinopril; HCTZ, hydrochlorothiazide; sd, single dose; MAP, mean arterial pressure; SBP, systolic blood pressure; DBP, diastolic blood pressure; HR, heart rate; CO, cardiac output; SV, stroke volume; ESS, left ventricular end-systolic wall stress; Vcf, left ventricular velocity of circumferential fiber shortening; PER, peak ejection rate; PFR, peak filling rate; SVR, systemic vascular resistance; ±, no statistically significant change versus baseline; ↑, statistically significant increase versus baseline (absolute value not stated); ↓, statistically significant decrease versus baseline (absolute value not stated).

The effects of fosinopril on renal function are similar to those observed with other ACE inhibitors. Fosinopril has a clearly evident antiproteinuric effect in either normotensive[40] or hypertensive[41] proteinuric subjects. It also either maintains or augments renal blood flow[16, 30, 42] and glomerular filtration rate[16, 30, 42] despite the decline in blood pressure in treated patients with essential hypertension. Long-term intervention studies designed to evaluate a "renal-preserving" effect for fosinopril are not available, but it is anticipated that results would be similar to those achieved with other ACE inhibitors, such as enalapril and captopril.[43] Reflective of a class effect, fosinopril therapy can diminish renal function in the presence of bilateral renal artery stenosis, moderate to severe volume depletion, and/or advanced congestive heart failure.[44]

In spontaneously hypertensive rats, oral fosinopril therapy markedly reduced the lower limit of cerebral blood flow with no effect on its upper limit (data on file, Bristol-Myers Squibb); alternatively, intravenously administered fosinoprilat significantly reduced both the upper and lower limits of autoregulation by as much as 20 mmHg.[45] This broadening of the autoregulatory plateau may maintain cerebral perfusion despite marked reductions in blood pressure and/or orthostatic effects. In accordance with these findings, patients treated with 25 mg of chlorthalidone and given fosinopril sodium in incremental doses (10 to 40 mg/day) sustained no drop in total cerebral blood flow or its regional distribution at peak and trough drug concentrations despite significant decrements in blood pressure.[46–47] The mechanisms whereby fosinopril maintains constant cerebral blood flow are incompletely elucidated, though there is strong presumptive evidence for large cerebral vessel dilatation. Inhibition of angiotensin II production in the luminal wall of these vessels may result in a compensatory constriction of smaller vessels, thereby preserving cerebral blood flow and expanding auto-regulatory capacity.[46] The prolonged inhibition of brain ACE following administration of fosinopril[9] may partly explain the observations of Waldemar et al.[47]

CLINICAL USE

Fosinopril is approved for the management of essential hypertension. As with other ACE inhibitors, fosinopril should be introduced cautiously to the treatment regimen of patients with secondary forms of hypertension associated with high plasma renin activity levels, volume depletion, high pretreatment blood pressure levels, or congestive heart failure. In each of these conditions, the risk of first-dose hypotension is considerably higher.[48] Administration of 20 mg of fosinopril was accompanied by an acute 16% reduction in seated diastolic blood pressure;[21] thus, it may be prudent to titrate therapy slowly when there are confounding factors for first-dose hypotension. Patients should be cautioned about the attendant risk of intercurrent volume depletion.

A number of the adverse events associated with fosinopril are common to the ACE inhibitor class. These include hyperkalemia, hypotension with or without associated reversible prerenal azotemia, chronic nonproductive cough, anemia, and angioedema. Cough may be somewhat reduced with fosinopril than with other ACE inhibitors,[24] which may relate to its structural dissimilarities[49] and/or its minimal accumulation in renal failure states.[50] Anemia occurs as a class effect with ACE inhibitors, though the degree of change in hemoglobin concentration is generally of little clinical significance.[21, 25] Headache, dizziness, fatigue, diarrhea, and nausea and vomiting can occur with fosinopril but with a frequency similar to or slightly greater than that of placebo.[26, 36] Fosinopril is contraindicated in bilateral renal artery stenosis,[51] renal artery stenosis in a solitary kidney,[51, 52] hypotension, the second and third trimesters of pregnancy,[53] and after ACE inhibitor-related angio-edema.[54, 55] Fosinoprilat is detectable in breast milk and should not be administered to nursing mothers (data on file, Bristol-Myers Squibb).

Fosinopril has not been reported to interfere with other drugs. Fosinopril is likely to have an additive effect with other non–ACE inhibitor antihypertensive compounds and synergy with antihypertensive compounds that promote release of plasma renin activity. Modest, clinically insignificant alterations in drug pharmacokinetics occur when fosinopril is administered with chlorthalidone, hydrochlorothiazide, furosemide, propranolol, or nifedipine.[14] As with many other orally administered compounds, antacids decrease the bioavailability of fosinoprilat by approximately 30%.[14, 56] If concomitant therapy with antacids is indicated, doses of each agent should be separated by at least 2 hours.

Unlike other ACE inhibitors that are exclusively eliminated by the kidneys[6] and require dose adjustment in the presence of renal insufficiency, fosinopril can be used without dose adjustment when therapy is initiated. The limited accumulation of fosinopril in the presence of renal[16] or hepatic insufficiency[19, 20] permits its use with considerably less concern about drug accumulation and extended physiologic effect, such as hypotension or possibly hyperkalemia. The patient populations most likely to respond to fosinopril are similar to those responding to monotherapy with other ACE inhibitors. Differences in efficacy between fosinopril and other ACE inhibitors are unlikely. Until formal dose-response relationships are derived in target populations, it is to be anticipated that conventional doses of fosinopril, in populations such as diabetic and African-American hypertensive patients, will be less successful in the monotherapeutic control of blood pressure. Fosinopril is distinguishable from several other ACE inhibitors in that it requires only once-daily administration and it undergoes systemic elimination by both renal and hepatic mechanisms. The recommended initial dose of fosinopril is 10 mg once daily, both as monotherapy and when the drug is added to a diuretic. Dosage should then be adjusted according to blood pressure response. The usual dosage required to achieve acceptable trough blood pressure readings is 20 to 40 mg/day. In some patients, blood pressure effect may wane by the end of a 24-hour dosing interval; in such persons, dividing the daily dose should be considered. Initiation doses for fosinopril in the presence of renal insufficiency are the same as for individuals with normal renal function. If patients are receiving multiple antihypertensive medications and fosinopril is to be added, diuretics should be continued, but the other antihypertensive agents should be tapered gradually and replaced by fosinopril.

SOCIOECONOMIC CONSIDERATIONS

Compliance with a fosinopril-based antihypertensive regimen is as good as, if not better than, other agents taken once daily. The cost of fosinopril is not dramatically different from that of other ACE inhibitors but, like the other recently released ACE inhibitors—ramipril, benazepril, and quinapril—it costs less on average than the older ACE inhibitors. The cost of therapy can be lessened by addition of a diuretic to an existing regimen. This maneuver is typically synergistic and permits reduction in fosinopril dose.

SUMMARY

Fosinopril is highly effective in the management of essential hypertension and is remarkably free of side effects. Like other ACE inhibitors, it has a high rate of success as monotherapy in unselected populations and therefore is becoming a drug of choice. Its unique, dual-metabolic elimination offers some advantage over other renally eliminated ACE inhibitors, but the true nature of this advantage still requires a better definition of concentration-effect relationships in patients with essential hypertension with or without renal insufficiency.

REFERENCES

1. Kostis JB: Angiotensin converting enzyme inhibitors: Emerging differences and new compounds. Am J Hypertens 2:57, 1989.
2. Ondetti MA: Structural relationships of angiotensin converting enzyme inhibitors to pharmacological activity. Circulation 1(Suppl):74, 1988.
3. Ranadive SA, Chen AX, Serajuddin ATM: Relative lipophilicities and structural-pharmacological considerations of various angiotensin-converting enzyme inhibitors. Pharm Res 9:1480, 1992.
4. Krapcho J, Turk C, Cushman DW, et al: Angiotensin-converting enzyme inhibitors: Mercaptan, carboxyalkyl dipeptide, and phosphinic acid inhibitors incorporating 4-substituted prolines. J Med Chem 31:1148, 1988.
5. Morrison RA, Singhvi SM, Peterson E, et al: Relative contribution of the gut, liver, and lung to the first-pass hydrolysis (bioactivation) of orally administered 14C-fosinopril sodium in dogs. Drug Metab Disp 18:253, 1990.
6. Sica DA: Kinetics of angiotensin-converting enzyme inhibitors in renal failure. J Cardiovasc Pharmacol 20(Suppl 10):S13, 1992.
7. Singhvi SM, Duchin KL, Morrison RA, et al: Disposition of fosinopril sodium in normal volunteers. Br J Clin Pharmacol 25:9, 1988.
8. DeForrest JM, Waldron TL, Harvey C, et al: Fosinopril, a phosphinic acid inhibitor of angiotensin I converting enzyme: In vitro and preclinical in vivo pharmacology. J Cardiovasc Pharmacol 14:730, 1989.
9. Cushman DW, Wang FL, Fung WC, et al: Differentiation of angiotensin converting enzyme inhibitors by their selective inhibition of ACE in physiologically important target organs. Am J Hypertens 2:294, 1989.
10. Creasey WA, Brennan J, McKinstry J, et al: Absorption of fosinopril from various sites within the gastrointestinal tract. Acta Pharmacol Toxicol 59(Suppl 5):83, 1986.
11. Duchin KL, Waclawski AP, Tu JI, et al: Pharmacokinetics, safety and pharmacologic effects of fosinopril sodium, an angiotensin converting enzyme inhibitor in healthy subjects. J Clin Pharmacol 31:58, 1991.
12. Levinson B, Sugerman AA, Couchman T, et al: Advanced age per se has no influence on the kinetics of the active diacid of fosinopril. J Clin Pharmacol 26:555, 1986.
13. Reid JL, MacDonald NJ, Lees KR, et al: Angiotensin-converting enzyme inhibitors in the elderly. Am Heart J 117:751, 1989.
14. Sica DA, Gehr TW, Duchin K: The pharmacology and pharmacokinetics of fosinopril. Rev Contemp Pharmacother 4:1, 1993.

15. Hui K, Duchin K, Kripalani KJ, et al: Pharmacokinetics of fosinopril in patients with various degrees of renal function. Clin Pharmacol Ther 49:457, 1991.
16. Sica DA, Cutler RE, Parmer RJ, et al: Comparison of the steady-state pharmacokinetics of fosinopril, lisinopril, and enalapril in patients with chronic renal insufficiency. Clin Pharmacokinet 20:420, 1991.
17. Gehr TWB, Sica DA, Grasela DM, et al: Fosinopril pharmacokinetics and pharmacodynamics in chronic ambulatory peritoneal dialysis. Eur J Clin Pharmacol 41:165, 1991.
18. Gehr TWB, Sica DA, Grasela DM, et al: The pharmacokinetics and pharmacodynamics of fosinopril in hemodialysis patients. Eur J Clin Pharmacol 45:431, 1993.
19. MacLeod CM, Bartley EA, Kripalani KJ, et al: Effect of hepatic function on disposition of fosinopril in humans. J Clin Pharmacol 30:839, 1990.
20. Ford NF, Lasseter KC, Hammett JL, et al: Single-dose and steady-state pharmacokinetics of fosinopril in patients with hepatic impairment. Am J Hypertens 5:123A, 1992.
21. Ward TD, et al: The additive effect of fosinopril in patients taking chlorthalidone for the treatment of mild-to-moderate essential hypertension. Drug Invest 3(Suppl 4):25, 1991.
22. Miller WE, et al: Randomized, double-blind, comparison of fosinopril and propranolol added to diuretic therapy for the treatment of moderate-to-severe hypertension. Drug Invest 3(Suppl 4):32, 1991.
23. Anderson RJ, Duchin KL, Gore RD, et al: Once-daily fosinopril in the treatment of hypertension. Hypertension 17:636, 1991.
24. Clementy J, et al: Double-blind, randomized study of fosinopril vs nifedipine SR in the treatment of mild-to-moderate hypertension in elderly patients. Drug Invest 3(Suppl 4):45, 1991.
25. Pool JL: Antihypertensive effect of fosinopril, a new angiotensin converting enzyme inhibitor: Findings of the Fosinopril Study Group II. Clin Ther 12:520, 1990.
26. Goldstein RJ, et al: A multicentre, randomized, double-blind, parallel comparison of fosinopril sodium and enalapril maleate for the treatment of mild-to-moderate essential hypertension. Drug Invest 3(Suppl 4):38, 1991.
27. Mallion JM, Vaisse B: The duration of action and efficacy of fosinopril in the treatment of mild-to-moderate hypertension [abstract]. Presented at the Second International Symposium on ACE Inhibition, London, February 17–19, 1991.
28. Forslund T, Franzen P, Backman R: Comparison of fosinopril and hydrochlorothiazide in patients with mild to moderate hypertension. J Intern Med 230:511, 1991.
29. Murdoch D, McTavish D: Fosinopril: A review of its pharmacodynamic and pharmacokinetic properties, and therapeutic potential in essential hypertension. Drugs 43:123, 1992.
30. Oren S, Messerli FH, Grossman E, et al: Immediate and short-term cardiovascular effects of fosinopril, a new angiotensin-converting enzyme inhibitor, in patients with essential hypertension. J Am Coll Cardiol 17:1183, 1991.
31. DeForrest JM, Waldron TL, Harvey C, et al: Blood pressure lowering and renal hemodynamic effects of fosinopril in conscious animal models. J Cardiovasc Pharmacol 16:139, 1990.
32. Zusman RM: Fosinopril and cardiac performance. Rev Contemp Pharmacother 4:25, 1993.
33. Gaudio C, Tanzilli G, Collatina S, et al: Effect of fosinopril on regression of left ventricular hypertrophy in essential hypertension as detected by magnetic resonance imaging. Am J Hypertens 6:119, 1993.
34. Zusman RM, Christensen DM, Higgins J, et al: Effects of fosinopril on cardiac function in patients with hypertension: Radionuclide assessment of left ventricular systolic and diastolic performance. Am J Hypertens 5:219, 1992.
35. Safar ME, Bouthier JA, Levenson JA, et al: Peripheral large arteries and the response to antihypertensive treatment. Hypertension 5(Suppl III):63, 1983.
36. Cooper M, Kong CL, Kahn SN, et al: The clinical efficacy of fosinopril. Rev Contemp Pharmacother 4:17, 1993.
37. Keilani T, Schleuter W, Molteni A, et al: Converting enzyme inhibition with fosinopril does not suppress plasma aldosterone and may not cause hyperkalemia despite moderate renal impairment. J Am Soc Nephrol 2:281, 1991.
38. Sullivan PA, Dineen M, Cervenka J, et al: Effects of fosinopril, a once-daily angiotensin converting enzyme inhibitor, on resting and exercise-induced changes of blood pressure, hormonal variables, and plasma potassium in essential hypertension. Am J Hypertens 1:280S, 1988.
39. Allemann Y, Baumann S, Jost M, et al: Insulin sensitivity in normotensive subjects during angiotensin converting enzyme inhibition with fosinopril. Eur J Clin Pharmacol 42:275, 1992.
40. Maschio G, Zucchelli P, Cagnoli L, et al: ACE inhibition reduces proteinuria in normotensive patients with IgA nephropathy. J Am Soc Nephrol 3:658, 1992.
41. Keilani T, Schlueter WA, Levin ML, et al: Improvement of lipid abnormalities associated with proteinuria using fosinopril, an angiotensin converting enzyme inhibitor. Ann Intern Med 118:246, 1993.
42. Toto RD, Mitchell HC, Fletcher ST, et al: Long-acting converting enzyme inhibitors (ACE inhibitors) lower blood pressure equally in blacks and whites with kidney disease and hypertension. Am J Hypertens 6:50, 1993.
43. Lebovitz H, Cnaan A, Wiegmann T, et al: Enalapril slows the progression of renal disease in NIDDM: Results of a 3-yr multicenter, randomized, prospective, double-blind study. J Am Soc Nephrol 3:335, 1992.
44. Keane WF, Anderson S, Aurell M, et al: Angiotensin converting enzyme inhibitors and progressive renal insufficiency. Ann Intern Med 111:503, 1989.
45. Paulson OB, Waldemar G, Andersen AR, et al: Role of angiotensin in autoregulation of cerebral blood flow. Circulation 77:1, 1988.
46. Paulson OB, Waldemar G, Strandgaard S: Fosinopril and cerebral blood flow. Rev Contemp Pharmacother 4:35, 1993.
47. Waldemar G, Ibsen H, Strandgaard S, et al: The effect of fosinopril sodium on cerebral blood flow in moderate essential hypertension. Am J Hypertens 3:464, 1990.
48. Hodsman GP, Isles CG, Murray GD, et al: Factors related to first dose hypotensive effect of captopril. Br Med J 286:832, 1983.
49. Germino FW, Lastra J, Pool P, et al: An open-label pilot study evaluating the cough profile of fosinopril sodium in hypertensive patients with documented cough associated with previous ACE inhibitor monotherapy. Am J Hypertens 6:113, 1993.
50. Sorooshian M, Eynon CA, Webb DJ, et al: Cough associated with angiotensin converting enzyme inhibitors: Increased frequency in renal failure. Eur J Int Med 2:15, 1991.
51. Hricik DE, Browning PJ, Kopelman R, et al: Captopril-induced functional renal insufficiency in patients with bilateral renal artery stenoses or renal artery stenosis in a solitary kidney. N Engl J Med 308:373, 1983.
52. Curtis JJ, Luke R, Whelchel JD, et al: Inhibition of angiotensin-converting enzyme in renal-transplant recipients with hypertension. N Engl J Med 308:377, 1983.
53. Piper JM, Ray WA, Rosa FW: Pregnancy outcome following exposure to angiotensin-converting enzyme inhibitors. Obstet Gynecol 80:429, 1992.
54. Slater EE, Merrill DD, Guess HA, et al: Clinical profile of angioedema associated with angiotensin converting-enzyme inhibition. JAMA 260:967, 1988.
55. Israili ZH, Hall WD: Cough and angioneurotic edema associated with angiotensin-converting enzyme inhibitor therapy. Ann Intern Med 117:234, 1992.
56. Moore L, Kramer A, Swites B, et al: Effect of cimetidine on the kinetics of the active diacid of fosinopril. J Clin Pharmacol 28:946, 1988.
57. Guller B, Reeves R: Short term hemodynamic effects of fosinopril and hydrochlorothiazide in hypertension [abstract no. 100]. J Clin Pharmacol 30:856, 1990.

CHAPTER 86

Cilazapril

Bernard Waeber, M.D., and Hans R. Brunner, M.D.

HISTORY

Angiotensin-converting enzyme (ACE) inhibitors are now well-established drugs for the treatment of hypertension and congestive heart failure.[1, 2] Cilazapril belongs to this class of agents.[3, 4] It blocks the renin-angiotensin system by interfering with the cleavage of angiotensin I to the active pressor peptide angiotensin II. Cilazapril is a prodrug that has to be hydrolyzed after oral absorption to its active form, the diacid cilazaprilat. This compound, unlike the first orally active ACE inhibitor captopril, is devoid of a sulfhydril group.

This chapter reviews the pharmacodynamic and pharmacokinetic properties of cilazapril. It also summarizes the experience with this new medication in the management of cardiovascular disorders.

PRECLINICAL STUDIES
In Vitro Experiments

Cilazaprilat [9(S)-[1(S)-(ethoxycarbonyl)-3-phenylpropylamino]octahydro-10-oxo-6H-pyradazo [1,2-a]-[1,2]diazepine-1-(S)-carboxylic acid] is a potent inhibitor of ACE in tissue preparations. Using the artificial substrate Hip-HisLeu for assessing ACE activity, the IC_{50} values of this compound in rabbit lung, human lung, and human plasma are 1.93, 1.39, and 0.61 nmol/L, respectively. In similar conditions, the corresponding values for captopril are 6.93, 13.05, and 15.70 nmol/L, and those of enalaprilat are 3.12, 2.93, and 1.66 nmol/L.[3] The greater potency of cilazaprilat relative to captopril and enalaprilat has been confirmed in rat plasma and tissues by means of radioinhibitory binding and displacement assays,[5] as well as in isolated guinea-pig ileum by determining the angiotensin I–induced contractions.[6] Cilazaprilat is tightly bound to ACE, with a Ki of 0.05 nmol/L[6] and has a high specificity for ACE.[7]

In Vivo Experiments

As expected in anesthetized rats, cilazaprilat causes a dose-dependent blockade of the angiotensin I–induced pressor response while it potentiates the vasodepressor effect of exogenous bradykinin.[6] Cilazapril lowers blood pressure in spontaneously hypertensive rats as well as in two-kidney renal hypertensive rats during both acute and chronic administration.[6, 8, 9] In rats with genetic hypertension, cilazapril, 10 mg/kg/day by mouth, is equally as effective in decreasing blood pressure as captopril, 100 mg/kg/day by mouth.[8] Cilazapril prevents the development of hypertension in spontaneously hypertensive rats as well

as in newly clipped two-kidney renal hypertensive rats.[10] It also reduces blood pressure in dogs made hypertensive by renal artery clipping on one side and encapsulation of the kidney controlaterally.[11] The antihypertensive efficacy of cilazapril is enhanced by salt depletion.[6, 11] In the spontaneously hypertensive rat, cilazapril lowers blood pressure without altering heart rate and cardiac output and leads to a preferential redistribution of blood flow to the kidney.[12] In these animals, cilazapril also prevents cardiac hypertrophy. In isolated perfused heart, it improves coronary reserve measured during maximal coronary vasodilation.[8] The regression of left ventricular hypertrophy resulting from cilazapril treatment is associated with recovery of a normal pattern of myosin isoenzymes in cardiac myofibrils.[13] The left ventricular pumping ability of spontaneously hypertensive rats is increased by cilazapril therapy.[14] Cilazapril can decrease the mortality of stroke-prone spontaneously hypertensive rats.[15] The cerebral vascular reserve, known to be impaired in genetically hypertensive rats,[16] is normalized during prolonged ACE inhibition with cilazapril.[17]

Acute ACE inhibition with cilazapril reduces plasma angiotensin II levels in spontaneously hypertensive rats while having no concurrent effect on circulating bradykinin concentrations.[9] Inhibition of vascular ACE activity persists longer than that of plasma ACE activity.[10] The media/lumen ratio of large- and small-resistance arteries is increased in hypertensive animals.[18] Factors other than the blood pressure level per se can promote vascular growth, including angiotensin II. Cilazapril makes it possible to normalize the arterial wall thickness of different types of arteries (coronary, renal, carotid, and mesenteric) in spontaneously hypertensive rats.[19] Moreover, it can correct the endothelial dysfunction associated with high blood pressure, restoring a normal vasodilatory response to acetylcholine.[20] There is some indication that cilazapril is more effective in preventing vascular remodeling than a pure arteriolar dilator such as hydralazine, a drug that activates the renin-angiotensin system when lowering blood pressure.[8, 21] Cilazapril markedly suppresses neointima formation in response to balloon catheter–induced vascular injury of the rat carotid artery.[22] Cilazapril also benefits intimal hyperplasia in injured arteries and vascular grafts in primates.[23]

CLINICAL STUDIES
Pharmacokinetic Properties

In healthy volunteers, cilazapril is rapidly absorbed and converted to cilazaprilat, which achieves peak plasma concentrations between 1.5 and 2 hours after single administration.[7] The bioavailability of cilazapril is about 60%[24] and is little affected by food intake.[25] Cilazaprilat is eliminated almost exclusively by renal excretion,[24] and a reduced dosage is recommended in patients with a creatinine clearance below 15 ml/min.[26] Cilazaprilat undergoes a biphasic elimination with a rapid initial half-life of approximately 1.5 hours and a prolonged terminal half-life of 30 to 50 hours.[24] The latter phase is probably due to a slow dissociation of cilazaprilat from ACE.[7] Cilazaprilat does not accumulate during repeated administration of cilazapril.[27] The pharmacokinetics of cilazapril in patients with hypertension or congestive heart failure are essentially the same as in healthy subjects.[28, 29] Cilazapril induces a dose-dependent inhibition of plasma ACE, which is still markedly suppressed by approximately 70% to 80% at 24 hours after intake of 1.25 to 10 mg of cilazapril.[27, 30] Following single oral doses of cilazapril, ACE activity is nearly completely blocked within 1 hour. The degree of inhibition is directly proportional to the circulating concentration of cilazaprilat. Angiotensin II practically disappears from plasma when ACE activity is maximally inhibited. Reactive hyperreninemia occurs as angiotensin II normally exerts a negative feedback action on renin secretion.[27, 30]

Pharmacodynamic Properties in Normotensive Volunteers

Cilazapril has no consistent blood pressure and heart effect in salt-replete normotensive subjects after both single and multiple administration,[27, 30] but it reduces blood pressure after salt depletion.[31] Acute ACE inhibition with this agent has no impact on cardiovascular reflexes.[32] Cilazapril slightly increases effective renal plasma flow in healthy subjects without altering glomerular filtration rate.[32] As anticipated, this inhibitor prevents the constrictor effect of angiotensin I as assessed in human dorsal hand veins *in situ*.[33]

Studies in Patients with Cardiovascular Disorders

Cilazapril is an effective and well-tolerated antihypertensive agent.[3, 4, 34] Single doses of cilazapril, 5, 10, and 20 mg, lower blood pressure of hypertensive patients to a similar extent, the response being practically maximal after 1 hour and lasting for at least 8 hours.[35] Even a dose of 1.25 mg can sustain reductions in blood pressure for up to 24 hours.[36] The duration of action of cilazapril is prolonged during chronic therapy, allowing a once-daily regimen.[37, 38] Cilazapril is significantly more effective at 5 than at 2.5 mg once a day; however, there is no clear-cut difference between 5 and 10 mg once a day.[39] The response rate of cilazapril monotherapy is between 40% and 65%.[34, 39] The efficacy of this agent can be enhanced by addition of a diuretic[31, 34, 37, 40] or a β-blocker.[41] Overall, cilazapril therapy is comparable, in terms of blood pressure–lowering action, to that of a diuretic or a β-blocker.[34, 42]

In double-blind studies, the incidence of adverse events observed during cilazapril treatment is very close to that seen with placebo, with no dose-dependent character.[34] Cough and angioedema may be caused by all ACE inhibitors, cilazapril included. During cilazapril monotherapy, cough was a problem in fewer than 2% of patients.[34] ACE inhibition with this agent is also effective and safe in elderly patients.[43] For an equivalent blood pressure reduction, patients receiving cilazapril and the β-blocker atenolol have a similar quality of life, whereas symptomatic complaints and discontinuation are more common during treatment with a slow-release formulation of the calcium antagonist nifedipine.[44]

Cilazapril lowers blood pressure generally without causing a reflex heart rate acceleration,[32, 45] and spectral analysis of heart period variability during ACE inhibition with this compound suggests a reduction in vasomotor sympathetic control.[45] The maximal exercise performance is not altered by cilazapril.[46] In hypertensive patients with sleep-related breathing disorders, cilazapril effectively reduced nocturnal blood pressure without disturbing the ratio of rapid eye movement (REM) to non-REM sleep, whereas the number of apneas per hour decreased significantly.[47]

Cilazapril lowers blood pressure without impairing renal function, and it can be administered safely in hypertensive patients with chronic renal failure with no major risk of hyperkalemia.[34, 48, 49] A favorable effect of cilazapril in hypertensive type II diabetics with chronic renal failure is its reduction of proteinuria and prevention of kidney function decline.[50] In diabetic subjects, cilazapril can reduce microalbuminuria even in the absence of modification of systemic blood pressure.[51]

Acute ACE inhibition with cilazapril increases coronary blood flow in renovascular hypertensive patients (i.e., patients with a generally overactive renin-angiotensin system).[52] Long-term treatment reduces left ventricular mass in patients with cardiac hypertrophy.[40] Patients with stable chronic congestive heart failure respond to cilazapril at doses of 2.5 to 5 mg/day with an increase in exercise capacity and functional improvement.[53, 54] The hemodynamic response is characterized by decreases in systemic blood pressure, in systemic vascular resistance, and in pulmonary capillary wedge pressure, whereas cardiac index increases at rest and during submaximal exercise.[53]

Treatment for 1 year with cilazapril leads to a regression of arteriolar hypertrophy as reflected by a reduction of the media/lumen ratio determined in subcutaneous resistance arteries obtained by gluteal biopsies.[55] The hypothesis that chronic ACE inhibition could prevent restenosis following percutaneous transluminal coronary angioplasty has been tested in humans.[56] Unfortunately, cilazapril does not appear to improve the outcome following the revascularization.

Like other ACE inhibitors, cilazapril has no effect on total cholesterol, high-density-lipoprotein cholesterol, low-density-lipoprotein cholesterol, and triglycerides.[57] Insulin resistance is found in a large fraction of patients with essential hypertension, dyslipidemias, and obesity. Cilazapril treatment has no significant effect on fasting plasma glucose and insulin, but it improves tolerance and heightens insulin response to oral glucose.[58]

CONCLUSIONS

The long-acting ACE inhibitor cilazapril is an effective and well-tolerated drug for the treatment of patients with hypertension and/or congestive heart failure. This agent can be used safely in patients with associated cardiovascular disorders and may even have beneficial effects beyond those one might expect from its blood pressure–lowering action.

REFERENCES

1. Williams GH: Converting-enzyme inhibitors in the treatment of hypertension. N Engl J Med 319:1517, 1989.
2. Deedwania PC: Angiotensin-converting enzyme inhibitors in congestive heart failure. Arch Intern Med 150:1798, 1990.
3. Natoff IL, Attwood MR, Eichler DA, et al: Cilazapril. Cardiovasc Drug Rev 8:1, 1990.
4. Deget F, Brogden RN: Cilazapril. A review of its pharmacodynamic and pharmacokinetic properties, and therapeutic potential in cardiovascular disease. Drugs 41:799, 1991.
5. Johnston CI, Cubela R, Jackson B: Relative inhibitory potency and plasma drug levels of angiotensin converting enzyme inhibitors in the rat. Clin Exp Pharmacol Physiol 15:123, 1988.
6. Natoff IL, Nixon JS, Francis RJ, et al: Biological properties of the angiotensin-converting enzyme inhibitor cilazapril. J Cardiovasc Pharmacol 7:569, 1985.
7. Francis RJ, Brown AN, Kler L, et al: Pharmacokinetics of the converting enzyme inhibitor cilazapril in normal volunteers and the relationship to enzyme inhibition: Development of a mathematical model. J Cardiovasc Pharmacol 9:32, 1987.
8. Clozel JP, Véniant M, Hess P, et al: Effects of two angiotensin converting enzyme inhibitors and hydralazine on coronary circulation in hypertensive rats. Hypertension 18(Suppl II):8, 1991.
9. Nakamura Y, Nakamura K, Matsukura T. Vascular angiotensin converting enzyme activity in spontaneously hypertensive rats and its inhibition with cilazapril. J Hypertens 6:105, 1988.
10. Hefti F, Fischli W, Gerold M: Cilazapril prevents hypertension in spontaneously hypertensive rats. J Cardiovasc Pharmacol 8:641, 1986.
11. Holck M, Fischli W, Hefti F, et al: Cardiovascular effects of the new angiotensin-converting-enzyme inhibitor, cilazapril, in anaesthetized and conscious dogs. J Cardiovasc Pharmacol 8:99, 1986.
12. Clozel JP: Effects of nitrendipine and cilazapril alone or in combination on hemodynamics and regional blood flows in conscious spontaneously hypertensive rats. J Cardiovasc Pharmacol 12:600, 1988.
13. Pirrelli AM, Ricci S, Vulpis V: Effect of cilazapril on isomyosin pattern in the spontaneously hypertensive rat. Am J Med 94(Suppl 4A):50, 1993.
14. Frohlich ED, Horinaka S: Cardiac and aortic effects of angiotensin converting enzyme inhibitors. Hypertension 18(Suppl II):2, 1991.
15. Véniant M, Clozel JP, Kuhn H, et al: Protective effect of cilazapril on the cerebral circulation. J Cardiovasc Pharmacol 19(Suppl 6):94, 1992.
16. Johansson BB, Nilsson B: Cerebral vasomotor reactivity in normotensive and spontaneously hypertensive rats. Stroke 10:572, 1979.
17. Clozel JP, Kuhn H, Hefty F: Effects of cilazapril on the cerebral circulation in spontaneously hypertensive rats. Hypertension 14:645, 1989.
18. Mulvany MJ: Control of vascular structure. Am J Med 94(Suppl 4A):20, 1994.
19. Clozel JP, Kuhn H, Hefti F: Decreases of vascular hypertrophy

in four different types of arteries in spontaneously hypertensive rats. Am J Med 94(Suppl 4A):92, 1994.
20. Clozel M: Mechanism of action of angiotensin converting enzyme inhibitors on endothelial function in hypertension. Hypertension 18(Suppl II):37, 1991.
21. Hajdu MA, Heistad DD, Ghoneim S, et al: Effects of antihypertensive treatment on composition of cerebral arterioles. Hypertension 18(Suppl II):15, 1991.
22. Osterrieder W, Müller RKM, Powell JS, et al: Role of angiotensin II in injury-induced neo-intima formation in rats. Hypersion 18(Suppl II):60, 1991.
23. Hanson SR, Powell JS, Dodson T, et al: Effects of angiotensin converting enzyme inhibition with cilazapril on intimal hyperplasia in injured arteries and vascular grafts in the baboon. Hypertension 18(Suppl II):70, 1991.
24. Williams PEO, Brown AN, Rajaguru S, et al: The pharmacokinetics and bioavailability of cilazapril in normal man. Br J Clin Pharmacol 27(Suppl II):181, 1989.
25. Massarella JW, De Feo TM, Brown AN, et al: The influence of food on the pharmacokinetics and ACE inhibition of cilazapril. Br J Clin Pharmacol 27(Suppl):205, 1989.
26. Fillastre JP, Moulin B, Godin M, et al: Pharmacokinetics of cilazapril in patients with renal failure. Br J Clin Pharmacol 27(Suppl):275, 1989.
27. Nussberger J, Fasanella d'Amore T, Porchet M, et al: Repeated administration of the converting enzyme inhibitor cilazapril to normal volunteers. J Cardiovasc Pharmacol 9:39, 1987.
28. Meredith PA, Elliot HL, Reid JL, et al: The pharmacokinetics and angiotensin converting enzyme inhibition dynamics of cilazapril in essential hypertension. Br J Clin Pharmacol 27(Suppl):263, 1989.
29. Rosenthal E, Francis RJ, Brown AN, et al: A pharmacokinetic study of cilazapril in patients with congestive heart failure. Br J Clin Pharmacol 27(Suppl II):267, 1989.
30. Fasanella d'Amore T, Bussien JP, Nussberger J, et al: Effects of single doses of the converting enzyme inhibitor cilazapril in normal volunteers. J Cardiovasc Pharmacol 9:26, 1987.
31. Nilsen OG, O Sellevold FM, Romfo OS, et al: Pharmacokinetics and effects on renal function following cilazapril and hydrochlorothiazide alone and in combination in healthy subjects and hypertensive patients. Br J Clin Pharmacol 2(Suppl II):323, 1989.
32. Elliott HL, Ajayi AA, Reid JL: The influence of cilazapril on indices of autonomic function in normotensives and hypertensives. Br J Clin Pharmacol 27(Suppl):303, 1989.
33. Belz GG, Beermann C, Schloss J, et al: The effect of oral cilazapril and prazosin on the constrictor effects of locally infused angiotensin I and noradrenaline in human dorsal hand veins. Br J Clin Pharmacol 28:608, 1989.
34. Kögler P: Cilazapril: A new non-thiol-containing angiotensin-converting enzyme inhibitor. Worldwide clinical experience in hypertension. Am J Med 87(Suppl 6B):50, 1989.
35. Ajayi AA, Elliott HL, Reid JL: The pharmacodynamics and dose-response relationships of the angiotensin converting enzyme inhibitor, cilazapril, in essential hypertension. Br J Clin Pharmacol 22:167, 1986.
36. Shionoiri H, Gotoh E, Sugimoto K, et al: Antihypertensive effects and pharmacokinetics of single and consecutive doses of cilazapril in hypertensive patients with normal or impaired renal function. Br J Clin Pharmacol 27(Suppl):285, 1989.
37. Waeber B, Wohler D, Lüscher TF, et al: Antihypertensive efficacy of cilazapril in general practice: Assessment by ambulatory blood pressure monitoring. Am J Med 94(4A):60, 1993.
38. Kobrin I, Güntzel P, Viskoper R, et al: Antihypertensive duration of action of cilazapril in patients with mild to moderate essential hypertension. Drugs 41(Suppl I):31, 1991.
39. Mroczek WY, Klein J, Burris JF: Dose-finding study of cilazapril (Inhibace) in patients with uncomplicated essential hypertension. Clin Exp Hypertens [A] 13:1415, 1991.
40. Sanchez RA, Traballi CA, Marco EJ, et al: Long-term evaluation of cilazapril in severe hypertension. Assessment of left ventricular and renal function. Am J Med 87(Suppl 6B):56, 1989.
41. Erb KA, Essig J, Breithaupt K, et al: Clinical pharmacodynamic studies with cilazapril and a combination of cilazapril and propranolol. Drugs 41(Suppl I):11, 1991.
42. Morgan TO, Multicentre Study Group: Efficacy of cilazapril

compared with hydrochlorothiazide in the treatment of mild-to-moderate essential hypertension. Am J Med 87(Suppl 6 B):37, 1989.

43. Kobrin I, Ben-Ishay D, Bompani R, et al: Efficacy and safety of cilazapril in elderly patients with essential hypertension. A multicenter study. Am J Med 87(Suppl 6B):33, 1989.

44. Fletcher AE, Bulpitt CJ, Chase DM, et al: Quality of life with three antihypertensive treatments: Cilazapril, atenolol, nifedipine. Hypertension 19:499, 1992.

45. Pagani M, Lucini D, Pizzinelli P, et al: Modulation of sympathetic vasomotor control with cilazapril in mild hypertension. Am J Med 94(Suppl 4A):54, 1993.

46. Derman WE, Ernotte D, Noakes TD: Comparative effects of cilazapril and atenolol on maximal and prolonged submaximal exercise performance in hypertensive males. Am J Med 94(Suppl 4A):69, 1993.

47. Mayer J, Peter JH: First experience with cilazapril in the treatment of sleep apnoea-related hypertension. Drugs 41(Suppl I):37, 1991.

48. Sanchez RA, Traballe CA, Marco EJ, et al: Effects of ACE inhibition on renal hemodynamics in essential hypertension and hypertension associated with chronic renal failure. Drugs 41(Suppl I):25, 1991.

49. Carlsen JE, Hansen FM, Jensen HA: Efficacy and safety of cilazapril in hypertensive patients with moderate to severe renal impairment. Am J Med 87(Suppl 6B):79, 1989.

50. Bursztyn M, Kobrin I, Fidel J, et al: Improved kidney function

51. Philipps PJ, Phillipou G, Bowen KM, et al: Diabetic microalbuminuria and cilazapril. Am J Med 94(Suppl 4A):59, 1993.

52. Magrini F, Reggiani P, Fratianni G, et al: Coronary blood flow in renovascular hypertension. Am J Med 94(Suppl 4A):45, 1994.

53. Kiowski W, Drexler H, Meinertz T, et al: Cilazapril in congestive heart failure. A pilot study. Drugs 41(Suppl I):54, 1991.

54. Dösseger L, Aldor E, Baird MG, et al: Influence of angiotensin converting enzyme inhibition on exercise performance and clinical symptoms in chronic heart failure: A multicentre, double-blind, placebo-controlled trial. Eur Heart J 14(Suppl C):18, 1993.

55. Schiffrin EL, Deng LY, Larochelle P: Effects of a beta-blocker or a converting enzyme inhibitor on resistance arteries in essential hypertension. Hypertension 23:83, 1994.

56. The Multicenter European Research Trial With Cilazapril After Angioplasty to Prevent Transluminal Coronary Obstruction and Restenosis (MERCATOR) Study Group: Does the new angiotensin converting enzyme inhibitor cilazapril prevent restenosis after percutaneous transluminal coronary angioplasty? Results of the MERCATOR study: A multicenter, randomized, double-blind placebo-controlled trial. Circulation 86:100, 1992.

57. Romo M, Auvinen J, Hirvonen H, et al: Effect of cilazapril on lipids. Am J Med 94(Suppl 4A):53, 1993.

58. Santoro D, Natali A, Palombo C, et al: Effects of chronic angiotensin converting enzyme inhibition on glucose tolerance and insulin sensitivity in essential hypertension. Hypertension 20:181, 1992.

CHAPTER 87

Moexipril

Michael Stimpel, M.D.

HISTORY

Angiotensin-converting enzyme (ACE) inhibitor therapy has become a valuable option in the treatment of hypertension and congestive heart failure, and in some situations it is considered a "first-line" therapeutic choice.[1] Moexipril is a new nonsulfhydryl, long-acting ACE inhibitor. In contrast with captopril, the first orally active ACE inhibitor,[2] moexipril is a prodrug that undergoes cleavage of the ester group to yield the pharmacologically active agent moexiprilat.

By April 1995, moexipril was approved in the United States and in Great Britain for the indication of primary hypertension. So far, more than 400 healthy volunteers and 3400 patients with mild, moderate, and severe hypertension have been studied in clinical trials performed in the United States and in different European countries. In approximately 500 hypertensive patients, treatment with moexipril lasted for 6 to 24 months (Investigator's brochure, June 22, 1993, Schwarz Pharma AG, Monheim, Germany).

CHEMISTRY AND PHARMACOLOGY

Moexipril hydrochloride, the hydrochloride salt of moexipril, has the empirical formula $C_{27}H_{35}N_2O_7Cl$ and a molecular weight of 535.04. It is chemically defined as 2-[2-[[(1(ethoxycarbonyl)-3-phenylpropyl]amino]-1-oxypropyl]-6,7-dimethoxy-1, 2, 3, 4-tetrahydroisoquinoline-3-carboxylic acid, hydrochloride (S, S, S).

Moexipril is a prodrug, which is bioactivated after oral administration by hydrolysis of the ethylester to moexiprilat, a highly active ACE inhibitor. ACE is a peptidyl dipeptidase that catalyzes the conversion of the inactive decapeptide angiotensin I to the vasoconstrictor substance angiotensin II. Angiotensin II is a potent peripheral vasoconstrictor that also stimulates aldosterone secretion by the adrenal cortex and provides negative feedback on renin secretion. ACE is identical to kininase II, an enzyme that degrades bradykinin, an endothelium-dependent vasodilator.[3] On the one hand, inhibition of ACE results in decreased angiotensin II formation, leading to decreased vasoconstriction, increased plasma renin activity, and decreased aldosterone secretion. On the other hand, it results in a decreased degradation of bradykinin, the vasodilating property of which is mainly mediated through the release of nitric oxide (NO) and prostacyclin (PGI_2) from the endothelium by activation of B_2-kinin receptors.[4, 5] It is unclear how much the inhibited degradation of bradykinin contributes to the antihypertensive and cardioprotective effects of ACE inhibitors,[6] which are presently thought to be primarily based on the inhibition of systemic and local angiotensin II formation.[7-9]

Moexiprilat is approximately 1000 times more potent than moexipril in inhibiting ACE and kininase II

(Study No. GIHBP-002-92, data on file, Schwarz Pharma AG, Monheim, Germany, 1990). Compared with ACE inhibition by enalaprilat, moexiprilat was approximately four times more potent *in vitro*.[10] No differences in ACE inhibition were observed when 10 mg/kg/day of moexipril or 10 mg/kg/day of enalapril were orally administered for 4 weeks in spontaneously hypertensive rats.[10] Inhibition of ACE resulted in an approximate 50% decrease in angiotensin II, and the area under the curve (AUC) was increased by almost 300% (data on file, Schwarz Pharma AG, Monheim, Germany, 1992).

PHARMACOKINETICS

Moexipril is relatively rapidly converted to its active metabolite moexiprilat. Both moexipril and moexiprilat are converted to diketopiperazine derivatives and unidentified metabolites. After oral administration, maximum plasma concentration of moexipril is reached after 1 hour, independently of dose. The time of peak plasma concentration (C_{max}) of moexiprilat is approximately 1.5 hours, and elimination half-life is estimated at 2 to 9 hours in various studies, the variability reflecting a complex elimination pattern that is not simply exponential. Like all ACE inhibitors, moexiprilat has a prolonged terminal elimination phase, presumably reflecting slow release of drug bound to the ACE. Accumulation of moexiprilat with repeated dosing is minimal, approximately 30%, compatible with a functional elimination half-life of approximately 12 hours. Over the dose range of 7.5 to 30 mg, pharmacokinetics are approximately dose-proportional (Study No. GHBA-628, data on file, Schwarz Pharma AG, Monheim, Germany, 1992).

As with benazepril (37%), fosinopril (32%), and lisinopril (30%),[11-13] moexipril has a low bioavailability of approximately 20%, reflecting a poor absorption with significant fecal excretion of moexiprilat. As has been reported for other ACE inhibitors,[14, 15] the bioavailability of moexipril was reduced by food. However, food did not significantly affect ACE inhibition 24 hours after oral administration of moexipril (Study No. PHAKI 867, data on file, Schwarz Pharma AG, Monheim, Germany, 1994).

After intravenous administration of moexipril, approximately 40% of the dose appears in urine as moexiprilat, and approximately 26% appears as moexipril, with small amounts of the metabolites; approximately 20% of the intravenous dose appears in feces, principally as moexiprilat. Only 1% of unchanged moexipril, approximately 7% of moexiprilat, and approximately 5% of other metabolites are excreted into the urine when the drug is given orally. Of a single oral dose, 52% is recovered in feces as moexiprilat and 1% is recovered as moexipril (Study No. GHBA-628, data on file, Schwarz Pharma AG, Monheim, Germany, 1992).

The effective half-lives of both moexipril and moexiprilat are increased with decreasing renal function. Data are too few to characterize this relationship fully, but at creatinine clearances in the range of 10 to 40

ml/min, the half-life of moexiprilat is increased by a factor of 3 to 4.

In patients with mild to moderate cirrhosis, given single 15-mg doses of moexipril, the C_{max} of moexipril was increased by approximately 50% and the AUC was increased by approximately 120%, whereas the C_{max} for moexiprilat was decreased by approximately 50% and the AUC was increased by almost 300% (Study No. GHBA-636, data on file, Schwarz Pharma AG, Monheim, Germany, 1992).

In elderly male subjects (65 to 80 years old) with clinically normal renal and hepatic function, the AUC and C_{max} of moexiprilat are approximately 30% greater than such values in younger subjects (18 to 39 years old) (Study No. GHBA-637, data on file, Schwarz Pharma AG, Monheim, Germany, 1992).

No clinically important pharmacokinetic interactions were observed when moexipril was administered concomitantly with hydrochlorothiazide, digoxin, cimetidin (Study Nos. PHAKI 751, GHBA-626 and -627, data on file, Schwarz Pharma AG, Monheim, Germany, 1992), and warfarin.[16]

Single and multiple doses of 15 mg or more of moexipril caused a sustained inhibition of plasma ACE activity of 80% to 90% 24 hours after dosing.

CLINICAL USE

All therapeutic trials of moexipril have involved either mild to moderate or moderate to severe essential hypertension. So far, no data are available on its therapeutic efficacy in indications that have generally been claimed for ACE inhibitors as a class (e.g., congestive heart failure).

Moexipril in Hypertension

Moexipril has been shown to be effective in patients with all degrees of essential hypertension. Its effectiveness was not influenced by patient age, gender, or weight. Like other ACE inhibitors,[17, 18] moexipril seems to be less effective in decreasing trough blood pressure in blacks than in nonblacks. However, the number of black patients studied on moexipril is still limited. In multiple clinical studies in the dose range of 7.5 to 30 mg once daily, moexipril lowered sitting diastolic and systolic blood pressure at trough more than placebo did by 3 to 6 mmHg and 4 to 11 mmHg, respectively. Moexipril controlled blood pressure in 40% to 60% of patients with mild to moderate hypertension.[19] Doses above 30 mg did not show any additional increase of antihypertensive efficacy (data on file, Schwarz Pharma AG, Monheim, Germany).

In a placebo-controlled study using continuous ambulatory blood pressure measurement, moexipril, 15 mg once daily, had significant antihypertensive activity for 24 hours following 8 weeks of therapy.[20, 21] The 7.5-mg dose of the drug showed antihypertensive activity for approximately 12 hours after dosing in this study, though in prior clinical studies, this lower dose was still effective at the end of a 24-hour dosing period even after 2 years of therapy.[22]

Compared with other standard antihypertensive agents, such as hydrochlorothiazide (once daily),[19] captopril (twice a day),[23] and verapamil (once daily),[24] moexipril taken once daily has proved to be about as efficacious in lowering blood pressure in mild to moderate hypertension. In elderly patients (≥ 65 years), the antihypertensive effect of 15 mg of moexipril (once daily) was comparable with that of 25 mg of hydrochlorothiazide (once daily).[25] In studies investigating the interaction of moexipril with other antihypertensive agents, such as hydrochlorothiazide,[26] nifedipine,[27] and verapamil,[28] the added effect of moexipril was similar to its effect as monotherapy. As add-on therapy in moderate to severe hypertensive patients, the combined treatment of hydrochlorothiazide and moexipril[26] or nifedipine and moexipril[27] was more effective than monotherapy with the diuretic or the calcium antagonist alone. Moexipril alone or in combination with hydrochlorothiazide has been used for up to 2 years in younger (≤ 65 years) and elderly (≥ 65 years) patients with mild to moderate hypertension without loss of antihypertensive efficacy.[22, 29, 30] No rebound effect was observed when moexipril was withdrawn after 12 weeks of treatment in patients with mild to moderate hypertension.[31]

Adverse Events

The safety profile of moexipril does not essentially differ from that reported for other ACE inhibitors. Experience on safety with moexipril is still restricted to data from clinical trials performed in approximately 3400 hypertensive patients and 400 healthy volunteers. More than 250 of these patients studied were treated with moexipril for 1 to 2 years. The overall incidence of reported adverse events was similar in patients treated with moexipril to that reported in patients treated with placebo. Reported adverse events were usually mild and transient, and there were no differences in adverse reaction rates related to gender, race, age, duration of therapy, or total daily dose within the range of 3.75 to 60 mg. Discontinuation of therapy because of adverse experiences was required in 3.4% of patients treated with moexipril and in 1.8% of patients treated with placebo. The most common reasons for discontinuation in patients treated with moexipril were cough (0.7%) and dizziness (0.4%). Table 87–1 shows all adverse experiences considered at least possibly related to treatment that ocurred at any dose in placebo-controlled trials in more than 1% of patients treated with moexipril alone and that were at least as frequent in the moexipril group as in the placebo group. Other adverse events occurring in more than 1% of patients on moexipril but that were at least as frequent in patients on placebo include headache, upper respiratory infection, rhinitis, dyspepsia, nausea, peripheral edema, sinusitis, chest pain, and urinary frequency. Other adverse events that have been reported with other ACE inhibitors have also been observed with moexipril: symptomatic hypotension (<1%), angioedema or facial edema (<0.5%), hyperkalemia (1.3%), and minor increases in blood urea nitrogen (BUN) or creatinine (1%). Increases of BUN or creatinine are more likely in patients receiving concomitant diuretics than in those on moexipril alone and in patients with compromised renal function. Although severe neutropenia did not occur in patients treated with moexipril, as with other ACE inhibitors, monitoring of white blood cell counts should be considered for patients who have collagen-vascular disease, especially if the disease is associated with impaired renal function. Available data from clinical trials of moexipril are insufficient to show that moexipril does not cause agranulocytosis at rates similar to those of captopril.[14]

Dosage and Administration

The recommended starting dose of moexipril for treatment of hypertension in patients not receiving diuretics is 7.5 mg once daily. Dosage should be adjusted according to blood pressure response. In some patients, the antihypertensive effect of moexipril may not persist throughout 24 hours. Blood pressure should, therefore, be measured just prior to dosing to determine whether blood pressure control is satisfactory. If not, increased dose or divided dosing can be tried. The recommended dose range is 7.5 to 15 mg daily, administered in one or two doses. Some patients will benefit from a further increase in dose to 30 mg. If goal blood pressure is not achieved with moexipril monotherapy, a thiazide diuretic or another antihypertensive drug may be added. An initial dosage of 3.75 mg once daily is recommended in patients

Table 87–1. **Adverse Events of Moexipril, Moexipril/HCTE, and HCTE in Placebo-Controlled Studies***

Adverse Event	Moexipril (n = 1355)	Moexipril/ HCTZ (n = 604)	HCTZ (n = 327)	Placebo (n = 417)
Headache	11	7	7	12
Upper respiratory infection	8	4	4	7
Cough	7	5	1	3
Vertigo	5	3	2	2
Pain	4	2	3	4
Diarrhea	4	3	2	1
Influenza syndrome	4	3	1	1
Rhinitis	4	1	1	4
Fatigue	3	4	2	1
Sinusitis	2	1	1	2
Pharyngitis	2	2	1	1
Back pain	2	1	1	3
Dyspepsia	2	1	0	1
Nausea	2	1	1	1
Peripheral edemas	2	1	0	2
Rash	2	1	1	1
Hypokalemia	< 1	2	1	0
Hyperuricemia	< 1	3	3	1

Figures represent percentages.
HCTZ, hydrochlorothiazide.
*Not necessarily judged to be related to the drug.

with a creatinine clearance of 40 ml/min/1.73 m² or less and in patients for whom a preexisting diuretic therapy cannot be discontinued.

Contraindications

The known contraindications for ACE inhibitors (e.g., bilateral renal artery stenoses, stenosis in the renal artery supplying a solitary kidney, marked volume depletion, pregnancy, lactation) also apply to moexipril.

REFERENCES

1. Opie LH: Preface. *In* Opie LH (ed): Angiotensin Converting Enzyme Inhibitors. Scientific Basis for Clinical Use. New York: Authors' Publishing House, 1992.
2. Ondetti MA, Rubin B, Cushman DW: Design of specific inhibitors of angiotensin-converting enzyme: A new class of orally active antihypertensive agents. Science 196:441, 1977.
3. Brunner HR, Waeber B, Nussberger J: Angiotensin-converting enzyme inhibitors in arterial hypertension. *In* Messerli FH (ed): Cardiovascular Drug Therapy, 2nd ed. Philadelphia: WB Saunders, 1995.
4. Douglas JG: Subpressor infusions of angiotensin II after glomerular binding, prostaglandin E₂, and cyclic AMP production. Hypertension 11(Suppl III):49, 1987.
5. Schini BV, Boulanger C, Regoli D, Vanhoutte PM: Bradykinin stimulates the production of cyclic GMP via activation of B₂-kinin receptors in cultured porcine aortic endothelial cells. J Pharmacol Exp Ther 252:581, 1990.
6. Waeber B, Juillerat-Jeanneret L, Aubert JF, et al: Involvement of the kallikrein kinin system in the antihypertensive effect of the angiotensin enzyme inhibitors. Br Clin Pharmacol 27:175S, 1989.
7. Campbell DJ: Circulating and tissue angiotensin systems. J Clin Invest 79:1, 1987.
8. Mac Fayden RJ, Lees KR, Reid JL: Tissue and plasma angiotensin converting enzyme and the response to ACE inhibitor drugs. Br J Clin Pharmacol 31:1, 1991.
9. Veltmar A, Gohlke P, Unger T: From tissue angiotensin converting enzyme inhibition to antihypertensive effect. Am J Hypertens 4:263s, 1991.
10. Edling O, Gohlke P, Bao G, Unger Th: In-vitro-und invivo Charakterisierung des neuen ACE-Hemmers Moexipril: Vergleich mit Enalapril. Hochdruck 12:49, 1993.
11. Waldmeier F, Kaiser G, Ackermann R, et al: The disposition of [14C]-labelled benazepril HCl in normal adult volunteers after single and repeated oral dose. Xenobiotica 21:251, 1991.
12. Singhvi SM, Duchin KL, Morrision RA, et al: Disposition of fosinopril sodium in healthy subjects. Br J Clin Pharmacol 25:9, 1988.
13. Lancaster SG, Todd PA: Lisinopril: A preliminary review of its pharmacodynamic and pharmacokinetic properties and therapeutic use in hypertension and congestive heart failure. Drugs 35:646, 1988.
14. Heel RC, Brogden RN, Speight TM, Avery GS: Captopril: A preliminary review of its pharmacological properties and therapeutic efficacy. Drugs 20:409, 1980.
15. Massarella IW, DeFeo TM, Brown AN, et al: The influence of food on the pharmacokinetics and ACE inhibition of cilazapril. Br J Clin Pharmacol 27:205S, 1989.
16. Van Hecken A, Verbesselt R, Depre M, et al: Moexipril does not alter the pharmacokinetics or pharmacodynamics of warfarin. Eur J Clin Pharmacol 45:291, 1993.
17. Saunders E, Weir MR, Kong W, et al: A comparison of the efficacy and safety of a β-blocker, a calcium channel blocker, and a converting enzyme inhibitor in hypertensive blacks. Arch Intern Med 15:1707, 1990.
18. Materson BJ, Reda DJ, Cushman WC, et al: Single-drug therapy for hypertension in men: A comparison of six antihypertensive agents with placebo. N Engl J Med 328:914, 1993.
19. Drayer JI, Stimpel M, Fox AAL, Weber MA: The antihypertensive properties of the angiotensin converting enzyme inhibitor moexipril given alone or in combination with a low dose of a diuretic. Am J Therap (In press).
20. White WB, Whelton A, Kaihlanen PM: Assessment of the efficacy and pharmacodynamics of moexipril by ambulatory blood pressure monitoring [abstract]. Am J Hypertens 6:102A, 1993.
21. White WB, Whelton A, Fox AAL, et al: Tri-center assessment of the efficacy and pharmacodynamics of the ACE inhibitor, moexipril, by ambulatory blood pressure monitoring. Clin Pharmacol Ther 35:233, 1995.
22. White WB, Fox AAL, Stimpel M: Long-term efficacy and safety of moexipril in the treatment of hypertension. J Hum Hypertens 8:917, 1994.
23. Stimpel M, Loh IK: Moexipril versus captopril in patients with mild to moderate hypertension. Am J Hypertens 8:183A, 1995.
24. Abernethy DR, Fox AL, Stimpel M: Moexipril in the treatment of mild to moderate essential hypertension: Comparision with sustained release verapamil. J Clin Pharmacol (In press).
25. Stimpel M, Koch B, Persson B: Treatment of hypertension in elderly patients: Comparison of moexipril to hydrochlorothiazide. Pharmacol Res (In press).
26. Dickstein K, Aarsland T, Ferrari P, et al: Comparison of the efficacy of three dose levels of moexipril versus placebo as add-on therapy to hydrochlorothiazide in patients with moderate hypertension. J Cardiovasc Pharmacol 24:247, 1994.
27. Persson B, Widgren BR, Fox AAL, Stimpel M: Antihypertensive effects of moexinew ACE inhibitor, as add on therapy to nifedipine in patients with essential hypertension. J Cardiovasc Pharmacol (In press).
28. Chrysant SG, Fox AAL, Stimpel M: Comparison of moexipril—A new ACE inhibitor—To verapamil-SR as add on therapy to low dose hydrochlorothiazide in hypertensive patients. Am J Hypertens 8:418, 1995.
29. Stimpel M, Weber MA: Moexipril, a new ACE inhibitor, as mono-therapy or in combination with hydrochlorothiazide in the long-term (two years) treatment of essential hypertension. Poster presentation, 9th Scientific Meeting of the American Society of Hypertension, New York, 1994.
30. White WB, Stimpel M: Long-term safety and efficacy of moexipril alone and in combination with hydrochlorothiazide in elderly patients with hypertension. J Hum Hypertens (In press).
31. Lucas CP, Darga LL, Fox AAL, Stimpel M: A study of the efficacy and safety of moexipril in mild to moderate hypertension. Am J Therap (In press).

IX.

Angiotensin Inhibitors

CHAPTER 88

Losartan

Michael A. Weber, M.D.

Losartan is the first nonpeptide antagonist of the angiotensin II receptor to be developed clinically. This agent works selectively at the AT_1 receptor and in clinical trials has been shown to be an effective antihypertensive agent. Although this agent has been widely studied in the research laboratory, its clinical development thus far has focused primarily on the prescribed clinical trials required to satisfy the regulatory requirements for marketing approval in the United States. Many of losartan's potentially interesting and important clinical effects on the heart, kidneys, and other relevant organs, as well as on important neurohumoral and metabolic mechanisms, are yet to be fully studied and described in humans. This chapter provides a preliminary appraisal of this drug, which was expected to become available for general clinical use during 1995.

HISTORICAL BACKGROUND

The development and availability of losartan can be seen as an inevitable consequence of a growing and continuing interest in the renin-angiotensin system that was triggered by the original work of Goldblatt with renovascular hypertension in 1934. The most important starting point for clinical physiology, however, was the creation and refinement of the renin thesis by Laragh et al.[1] in the early 1970s. This bold idea sought to bring a logical underpinning to the spectrum of so-called essential hypertension. In patients with high or medium renin levels, classified by use of an innovative renin-sodium nomogram, the renin-angiotensin system itself was considered to play a primary or substantive role in producing hypertension; in patients with low renin, sodium excess, renal changes, or other mechanisms are largely responsible for increasing the blood pressure. At the same time—well before the current techniques of molecular and cellular biology helped demonstrate proliferative and other potentially atherogenic actions of angiotensin II—Laragh and his colleagues accurately predicted the adverse prognostic implications of high-renin hypertension.[2]

Pharmacologic Probes

In retrospect, the story of losartan began with a totally different drug class, the β-blockers. It was with these agents that the renin hypothesis began to be defined. Specifically, the β-blocker propranolol, which has clear inhibitory effects on the secretion of renin from the juxtaglomerular cells of the kidney, was shown to decrease blood pressure most effectively in high-renin patients.[3] In contrast, propranolol produced only minimal effects in low-renin patients, or—perhaps as a result of unmasking of α-adrenergic tone—even produced a small pressor action.[4]

Two probes with greater selectivity further advanced this work. The first of these was saralasin, a peptide analogue of angiotensin II, which selectively displaced angiotensin II from its receptors. This agent played a major role in confirming the participation of the renin-angiotensin system in clinical hypertension.[5, 6] Unfortunately, saralasin had clear drawbacks as a clinical tool. It could be administered only intravenously and had a very brief duration of action; sudden discontinuation of treatment resulted in severe and rapid rebound increases in blood pressure. In addition, saralasin exhibited partial agonist properties. Although it decreased blood pressure in high-renin states, its blood pressure–lowering effects were only minimal in patients with medium-renin hypertension; in low-renin states, saralasin actually increased the blood pressure. Losartan, which chemically is completely unrelated to saralasin, now many years later represents the vindication of this pharmacologic approach.

The second innovative probe that, once and for all, verified the critical place of the renin axis in hypertension was the angiotensin-converting enzyme (ACE) inhibitor. Early experiences with the intravenously administered peptide agent teprotide confirmed the earlier work performed with the β-blockers and saralasin.[6, 7] Subsequent studies with orally administered ACE inhibitors demonstrated during long-term treatment that inhibition of the renin-angiotensin system represented a logical and effective approach to the management of hypertension.[8, 9] Of course, the ACE inhibitors can produce actions beyond their blockade of the renin-angiotensin system, creating possibilities that various other mechanisms of action may contribute to their antihypertensive efficacy.[10]

Finally, there has been recent interest in drugs that block the enzymatic action of renin on its substrate. These renin inhibitors typically have been dipeptides and have been shown to produce effects in hypertensive patients that are qualitatively similar to those observed with ACE inhibitors and angiotensin receptor blockers. Thus, they most effectively reduce blood pressure in high-renin patients or in individuals whose renin-angiotensin systems have been stimulated by the use of diuretic therapy.[11] Unfortunately, problems with adequate oral absorption of these agents, together with the complexity and high cost of their manufacture, have limited their further clinical development. The angiotensin receptor antagonists, therefore, currently appear to offer the greatest potential for development in this area.

THE DEVELOPMENT OF LOSARTAN

Despite the logic of using such peptide analogues of angiotensin II as saralasin to investigate the potential of angiotensin receptor blockade, long-term clinical therapy of hypertension clearly requires the use of long-acting oral agents. The series of advances that culminated in losartan are summarized in Figure 88–1.[12] The first tenable molecules were N-benzylimidazoles that were first evaluated by Takeda Chemical Industries of Osaka. These agents were found to be selective angiotensin receptor antagonists with a competitive action. They were relatively weak, however, and early testing revealed that it would be necessary to design more potent orally effective antagonists with selective affinity for this receptor.

Scientists at DuPont Merck Pharmaceutical Company, in pursuit of this goal, synthesized N-benzylimidazole phthalamic acid derivatives. Unfortunately, although these agents produced clear pharmacologic actions when given parenterally, they lacked activity when given by mouth. A major step forward came with the creation of biphenyl carboxylic acids. These agents represented an improvement over previous molecules in that they exhibited at least partial absorption after oral administration, although plasma concentrations were still inconsistent. In a systematic evaluation of methods to improve oral availability of these biphenyls, the investigators tested differing acidic groups as bioisosteric replacements for the carboxylic acid. Finally, the search for a receptor antagonist with consistent oral activity and a long duration of action led to the replacement of the carboxylic acid group with a tetrazole ring structure exhibiting increased lipophilic properties.

Losartan has been the first of these agents to enter systematic clinical trials, but other compounds produced by this team of investigators, some of which appear to exhibit very high potency and affinity for the angiotensin II receptor, continue to be evaluated and developed. A far more detailed account of this

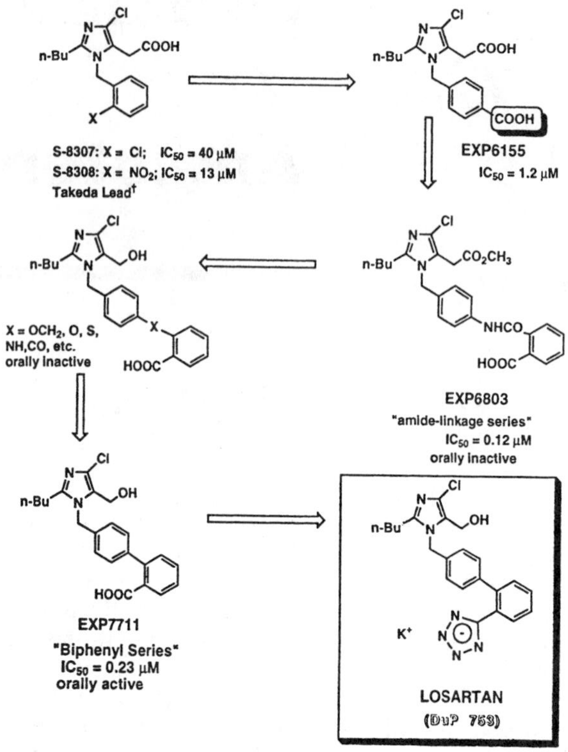

Figure 88–1. The evolution of the nonpeptide angiotensin II receptor antagonists, culminating in the synthesis of losartan. (Reprinted by permission of Elsevier Science Inc. from Wexler RR, Carini DJ, Duncia JV, et al: Rationale for the chemical development of angiotensin II receptor antagonists. Am J Hypertens 5:209S, 1992. Copyright 1992 by American Journal of Hypertension, Inc.)

interesting and exciting research program has been published previously.[12]

PHARMACOLOGIC ACTIONS

Preliminary studies have shown that losartan powerfully inhibits the specific binding of angiotensin II (as revealed by radiolabeled techniques) to smooth muscle preparations obtained from animals or humans[13-15] and also is able to inhibit angiotensin II binding to isolated adrenal cortical microsomes obtained from the rat.[13] Losartan clearly is a competitive antagonist and in classic fashion causes rightward shifts of the concentration-contractile response curve to angiotensin II.[13] Similar studies are summarized in Figure 88–2. This work, performed in the pithed rat,[16] demonstrates the ability of increasing doses of losartan (also referred to as DuP 753) to produce progressively greater rightward shifts of the diastolic pressor response to testing with angiotensin II. As shown in Figure 88–2, it is noteworthy that losartan has no effect on the pressor responses to norepinephrine, further confirming the selectivity of this drug for the angiotensin II receptor. Further evidence supporting the specificity of losartan's action has come from blood pressure studies performed in differing renin states: for example, in normotensive or DOCA salt-hypertensive rats, which is a model of low-renin hypertension, losartan did not decrease blood pressure;

however, in rats whose renin systems had been stimulated by furosemide pretreatment, losartan evoked a clear blood pressure–lowering response.[17]

In another renin-dependent model, the renal hypertensive rat, losartan also produced clear antihypertensive effects similar to those produced by ACE inhibition.[17] This action persisted for more than 24 hours, confirming the long duration of action of this compound.[17] This antihypertensive action was not associated with changes in heart rate. A further study demonstrated that whereas losartan was inactive hemodynamically in Wistar-Kyoto control rats, it was effective in decreasing blood pressure in the spontaneously hypertensive rat; of note, bilateral nephrectomy abolished this antihypertensive action of losartan.[18] Again, this action was similar to that observed with the ACE inhibitor captopril in this model of hypertension. In a study with an interesting historical

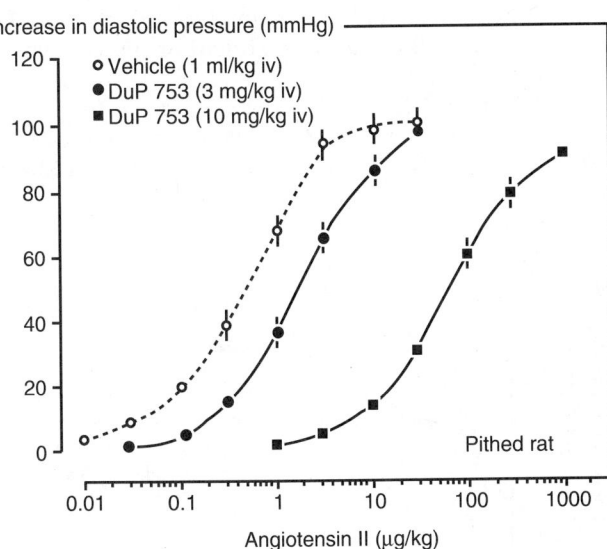

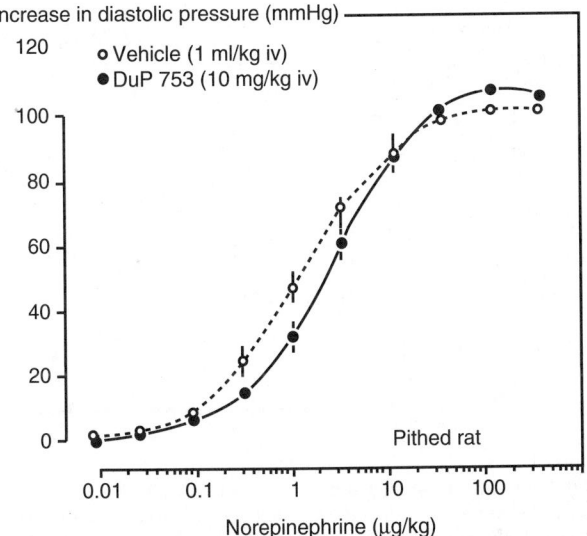

Figure 88–2. The effects of the angiotensin II-receptor antagonist losartan (DuP 753) on diastolic blood pressure responses to infusions of angiotensin II and norepinephrine in the pithed rat. (Data from Wong PC, Price WA, Chiu AT, et al: In vivo pharmacology of DuP 753. Am J Hypertens 5[Suppl]:288S, 1991.)

twist, losartan was able to prevent the pressor response produced by the angiotensin II peptide analogue saralasin.[19]

THE ACTIVE METABOLITE E-3174

Although losartan itself clearly has strong binding affinity for angiotensin II receptors and produces predictable pharmacologic and hemodynamic effects, there is strong evidence that its active metabolite—E-3174—has powerful and sustained effects. Experience in the rat has shown that this 5-carboxylic acid is a major metabolite of losartan[20] and that it binds specifically to angiotensin II receptor sites found in the adrenal cortex. It differs from losartan in that it might have noncompetitive antagonist properties at the receptor and can produce nonparallel rightward shifts of contractile responses to angiotensin II.

The importance of E-3174 has been shown by studies in which administration of losartan in conscious rats produces a biphasic inhibition of pressor responses to angiotensin II.[16] This also has been reported in renal hypertensive animals.[19] These findings suggest that the initial action against angiotensin II is produced by the parent compound losartan, whereas the later antagonism is produced by its metabolite. Studies with direct intravenous injections of E-3174 have shown that this compound is far more potent than losartan itself as an inhibitor of angiotensin II pressor responses.[21]

The action of this metabolite appears important in humans. In healthy volunteers after administration of losartan, concentrations of E-3174 actually reached higher plasma concentrations than the parent drug, and it was eliminated more slowly.[22] Moreover, the E-3174 plasma levels more closely paralleled effective blockade of angiotensin II pressor responses than did concentrations of losartan. It appears that conversion of losartan to E-3174 occurs readily in almost all patients, and that the efficiency of this metabolic step does not appear to be a determining factor in whether or not treatment with losartan is effective in individual patients. Studies of the pharmacokinetics of losartan and E-3174 have concluded that the principal long-term actions of the drug are most likely linked to the prolonged effects of the metabolite.[22]

RECEPTOR HETEROGENEITY

It is clear that there is more than one form of the angiotensin II receptor. There are two principal receptor classes that by radioligand binding studies have been labeled as AT_1 and AT_2 binding sites.[23] Most, if not all, of the known cardiovascular effects of angiotensin II appear to be linked to its actions at AT_1 receptors; the role of the AT_2 binding sites is not yet clear.[24] Table 88–1 lists the receptor subtypes associated with differing tissues and responses to angiotensin II.[25]

Cloning studies have identified cDNA and genes for each of two separate although closely similar isoforms of AT_1 receptors; these have been labeled $AT_{1}a$

Table 88–1. **Functional Responses to Angiotensin II**

Tissue	Response	Receptor Subtype
Blood vessels/vascular smooth muscle	Contraction	AT_1
	Hypertrophy	AT_1
	Angiogenesis	AT_1/AT_2
	Intimal hyperplasia	AT_1
Kidney	Proximal tubular ion transport	AT_1/AT_2
	Constriction of afferent/efferent arterioles	AT_1
Adrenal cortex	Aldosterone release	AT_1
Adrenal medulla	Catecholamine release	AT_1
Myocardium	Contractility	AT_1
	Hypertrophy	AT_1
	Inhibition of collagenase	AT_1/AT_2
Brain	Arginine vasopressin release	AT_1
	Thirst/drinking	AT_1
	Luteinizing hormone and prolactin	AT_1/AT_2
	"Behavior"	AT_1/AT_2
Reproductive organs	Myometrial contraction (from pregnant animals)	AT_1

Data from Timmermans P, Benfield P, Chiu AT, et al: Angiotensin II receptors and functional correlates. Am J Hypertens 5:221S, 1992.

and AT_1b.[26, 27] The clinical and therapeutic importance of these differing angiotensin II receptor classes is not yet clear. Losartan and the other angiotensin II receptor antagonists now in development all are selective for the AT_1 class. Another type of agent, exemplified by PD 123177, is selective for the AT_2 receptor. It has not been possible to clearly define any hemodynamic, neurohumoral, functional, or structural effects of this agent, although some interesting speculations have been advanced regarding such issues as growth.[28, 29] It should be emphasized, however, that the AT_1 receptors, which are blocked by losartan, appear to mediate

all of the known major angiotensin II physiologic effects, including vasoconstriction, stimulation of aldosterone, and enhancement of catecholamines.[25]

PRELIMINARY HUMAN STUDIES

The early studies with losartan used protocols in which differing doses of losartan were tested against standard pressor boluses of angiotensin in normal volunteers. The principal study used doses of angiotensin I that produced approximately 30-mmHg increases in systolic blood pressure. The blood pressure effects of losartan in this setting are shown in Figure 88–3.[30] When administered as single oral doses, losartan inhibits the pressor response to angiotensin in a dose-dependent manner. Moreover, as shown in Figure 88–3, all doses are different from placebo, and it is also evident that the effect lasts for 24 hours. This is most clearly the case for the dose of 40 mg, thus predicting that a daily dose in this range could be effective during long-term treatment of clinical hypertension.

The chief hormonal effects of losartan in this study are shown in Figure 88–4.[30] Plasma immunoreactive angiotensin II concentrations increased with losartan

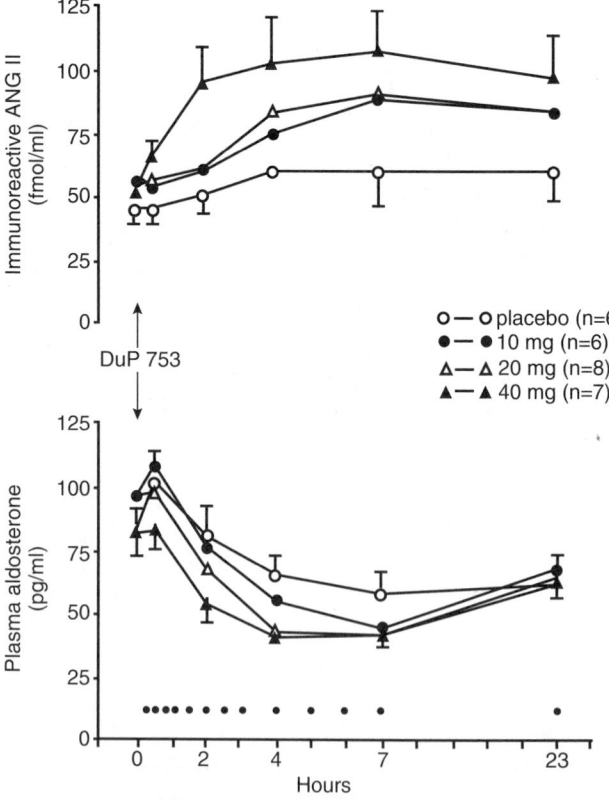

Figure 88–4. Effects of single doses of oral DuP 753 (10, 20, or 40 mg) or placebo on plasma aldosterone *(lower panel)* and immunoreactive angiotensin II (ANG II) *(upper panel)*. Bullets on abscissa, ANG I test-dose injections. Values are mean ± SEM. (Reproduced with permission from Christen Y, Waeber B, Nussberger J, et al: Oral administration of DuP 753, a specific angiotensin II receptor antagonist, to normal male volunteers. Circulation 83:1333, 1991. Copyright 1991, American Heart Association.)

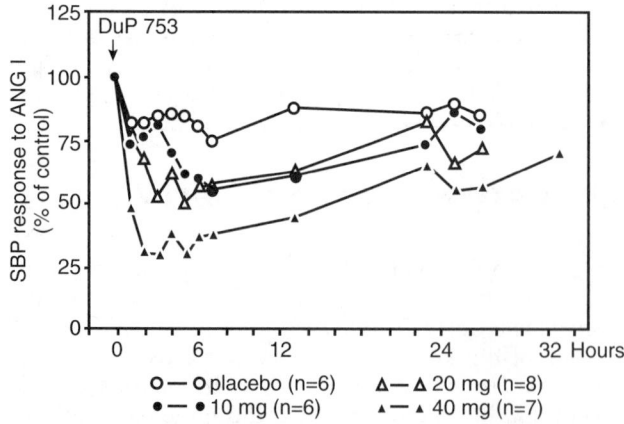

Figure 88–3. Plots of effects of single doses of oral DuP 753 (10, 20, or 40 mg) or placebo on systolic blood pressure (SBP) response (mean) to test doses of angiotensin I (ANG I) in healthy volunteers. (Reproduced with permission from Christen Y, Waeber B, Nussberger J, et al: Oral administration of DuP 753, a specific angiotensin II receptor antagonist, to normal male volunteers. Circulation 83:1333, 1991. Copyright 1991, American Heart Association.)

treatment, consistent with the pharmacologic action of this drug in blocking angiotensin II receptors. Plasma aldosterone concentrations also fell, but because of a similar reduction in the placebo group, the drug-induced changes with losartan were not significant. In general, it has been difficult to demonstrate consistent effects of losartan on aldosterone; presumably, despite inhibition of angiotensin II action, alternative pathways for aldosterone secretion appear to compensate for the drug's action.

In an extension of this work designed to determine whether losartan could inhibit pressor responses to angiotensin during repetitive dosing, normal volunteers were given daily doses of the drug during an 8-day period.[22] The investigators found that losartan significantly inhibited pressor responses to angiotensin II boluses throughout the study. Moreover, the highest dose of 40 mg inhibited the pressor action of angiotensin II 24 hours after drug dosing (trough effect) as well as at 6 hours after dosing (peak effect). Indeed, at peak, the 40-mg dose of losartan decreased the systolic blood pressure response to angiotensin II by 70%. As in the single-dose study, dose-dependent increases in plasma renin activity and plasma angiotensin II concentrations were observed.

Additional research examined doses of losartan of up to 120 mg daily and documented that the maximal effect—approximately an 80% inhibition of the pressor response to angiotensin II—occurred with a losartan dose of 80 mg daily.[22] In this work, it was also reported, as discussed earlier, that plasma concentrations of the metabolite E-3174 paralleled the profile of angiotensin II pressor inhibition more closely than did levels of losartan itself. The investigators noted that the concentration response curve of E-3174 tended to reach a plateau at a plasma concentration of about 200 ng/ml; this was the concentration of metabolite that corresponded to an oral losartan dose of 80 mg. As will be shown later, the conclusions of these studies by Brunner et al.[30, 31] were closely predictive of the major clinical trials of losartan that were subsequently carried out in hypertensive patients.

OTHER POTENTIAL ANTIHYPERTENSIVE MECHANISMS

It is likely that the principal antihypertensive action of losartan during acute and long-term antihypertensive therapy is mediated through antagonism of angiotensin II receptors. This is accomplished partly by losartan itself, but, as discussed earlier, the effects of the active metabolite E-3174 at the same receptor may be of even greater potency and duration.

Other mechanisms may also play a role. It is not known whether losartan has antihypertensive effects mediated in the central nervous system,[21, 32] but experimental work has shown that it binds to the presynaptic AT_1 receptors of sympathetic neurones, thereby decreasing norepinephrine secretion.[22] Additionally, losartan appears to stimulate the powerful vasodilator prostacyclin through an action at AT_1 receptors.[33] Finally, losartan has been shown to have antiprolifera-

tive actions on vascular smooth muscle,[34, 35] thus potentially counteracting the vascular wall hypertrophy that might predispose to heightened pressor reactivity in hypertension. It should be emphasized, however, that none of these mechanisms has yet been shown to contribute directly to the clinical antihypertensive actions of losartan.

CLINICAL EFFICACY

Losartan has undergone a rigorous clinical trial evaluation for a hypertension indication in the United States, and a New Drug Application has now been filed with the Food and Drug Administration. Because this work has been completed only recently, much of the appropriate data are still unpublished. However, two of the pivotal studies are described here.

Hospital Experience

The principal trial of losartan's antihypertensive efficacy in hospitalized patients is summarized in Table 88–2.[36] All patients had in-hospital diastolic blood pressure values of at least 95 mmHg immediately before treatment. The treatment in this dose-ranging study lasted for 5 full days. The patients were randomly allocated into five separate treatment groups, each with approximately 20 patients. Losartan was given once daily to three of these groups: one group was given 50 mg, a second group was given 100 mg, and the third was given 150 mg. There were two control groups. One received placebo throughout the study, whereas the other served as a positive control and was treated with the ACE inhibitor enalapril, 10 mg daily.

The effects of these treatments, as shown in Table 88–2, were measured by comparing the blood pressure values on day 5 with those recorded during the pretreatment baseline. Values are given at 6 hours after dosing, which represents the presumed peak effect of losartan, and 24 hours after dosing, defined as the trough effect at the end of the dosing interval. Compared with placebo, each of the three losartan groups, and also the enalapril group, experienced significantly greater decreases in systolic and diastolic

Table 88–2. **Losartan in Hospitalized White Hypertensive Patients (DBP $\geq$ 95 mmHg)**

	N	Decreases from Baseline in SBP/DBP on 5th Day of Treatment	
		6 hr Post Dose	*24 hr Post Dose*
Placebo	20	4.7/4.9	10.0/3.6
50 mg losartan	20	19.5/15.3	12.0/10.3
100 mg losartan	18	15.3/12.2	17.5/11.9
150 mg losartan	19	19.4/17.8	18.9/10.8
10 mg enalapril	18	18.2/16.1	15.3/10.3

*All treatment changes significantly different from placebo.
From Nelson E, Merrill D, Sweet C: Proceedings of the 5th European Meeting on Hypertension [Abstract 512]. Milan, Italy, 1991.

blood pressures both at peak and at trough. This relatively short-term inpatient experience established that losartan in doses of 50 mg, 100 mg, or 150 mg produced significant antihypertensive effects that were sustained for 24 hours when given once daily. There were no significant differences, however, among the four actively treated groups. Thus, the 50 mg losartan dose appeared to be as effective as the higher doses, and each of these doses appeared to produce antihypertensive effects similar to those found with enalapril.

Outpatient Experience

The findings from the first major outpatient study with losartan are summarized in Table 88–3.[37] This large-scale multicenter trial was performed in hypertensive patients, free of treatment for at least 3 weeks, whose supine diastolic blood pressures were at least 100 mmHg at the end of a placebo run-in. The average baseline blood pressure for these patients was 157/104 mmHg. As shown in Table 88–3, the patients were randomly allocated into seven separate groups with between 68 and 82 patients in each: five of the groups received losartan in doses of 10, 25, 50, 100, or 150 mg. One group received placebo, and the final group received the ACE inhibitor enalapril in a dose of 20 mg. All medications were administered as a single daily dose, and the period of active treatment lasted for 8 weeks.

The trough data indicate that neither the 10-mg nor the 25-mg dose of losartan produced blood pressure changes that were different from placebo. However, the 50-mg dose and the higher losartan doses all significantly decreased both systolic and diastolic blood pressures after 24 hours. Of interest, the reductions produced by the 50-mg losartan dose were at least equal to those produced by the higher doses. Thus, as with the in-hospital experience, losartan in a dose of 50 mg appears to define the upper end of the dose-response relationship for this drug.

The blood pressures measured at peak (6 hours after dosing) are also shown in Table 88–3. Unlike the trough effects, the 10-mg and 25-mg losartan doses produced significantly greater blood pressure decrements than placebo. However, the 50-mg dose appears to be more effective than either of the two low doses, although further dosage increases did not amplify the peak blood pressure changes. Enalapril 20 mg had similar antihypertensive effects to those found with the 50 mg or higher doses of losartan at both trough and peak.

It is noteworthy that the peak data appear to describe a clear dose-response curve in the range of 10 mg to 50 mg. This suggests that the low doses of losartan can produce hemodynamic effects but, presumably because of their pharmacokinetic characteristics, do not possess sufficient duration of action to have significant effects 24 hours after administration.

It is possible, however, that low doses given in a more frequent regimen, perhaps twice daily, could produce meaningful antihypertensive efficacy. In considering the trough data, it appears that the 50-mg losartan dose is pivotal in the antihypertensive action of this drug: lower doses seem ineffective, whereas higher doses offer relatively modest increases in efficacy. The effective duration of action of losartan in doses of 50 mg or higher is confirmed by the ratio of the trough and peak blood pressure effects. After subtraction of the placebo effects, the trough:peak ratios for the 50 mg, 100 mg, and 150 mg doses were 63%, 74%, and 52%, respectively. Thus, at least half of the drug's peak antihypertensive efficacy was still present at the end of the dosing interval. There was no meaningful difference between placebo and the active treatment with losartan in the incidence of adverse events during the 8 weeks of this study.

FURTHER EXPERIENCES

Additional studies to define the efficacy and clinical characteristics of losartan in the treatment of hypertension have been reported at clinical meetings and are now awaiting publication. For example, ambulatory blood pressure monitoring has been employed to further clarify appropriate dosing with losartan and to evaluate its efficacy throughout the 24-hour dosing interval. These studies have confirmed that a single daily dose of 50 mg produces meaningful efficacy that is sustained for 24 hours; a higher dose of 100 mg daily, given either as a single dose or as 50 mg twice daily, may offer increased efficacy in some patients.[38]

Other protocols have confirmed that losartan produces antihypertensive efficacy similar to that produced with other agents, including treatment with an ACE inhibitor, a β-blocker, or a diuretic. Importantly, losartan appears to be highly effective when combined with a low-dose diuretic. This finding, similar to that observed previously with ACE inhibitors, confirms the logic of using drugs that inhibit activity of the renin-angiotensin system in patients receiving diuretics. In summary, it is now well established that losartan, either as monotherapy or as part of com-

Table 88–3. Effects of Losartan on Outpatient Hypertensive Patients (Supine DPB ≥ 100 mmHg)

| | N | Decreases from Baseline in SBP/DBP After 8 Weeks' Treatment | |
		Trough	Peak
Placebo	69	3.9/5.7	1.1/4.9
10 mg losartan	71	7.3/7.3	9.1*/7.0
25 mg losartan	74	7.7/7.0	11.4*/9.8*
50 mg losartan	68	13.4*/10.5*	14.6*/12.1*
100 mg losartan	82	9.8*/10.1*	13.0*/10.6*
150 mg losartan	76	10.7*/9.8*	12.8*/12.4*
20 mg enalapril	71	13.7*/11.2*	17.8*/15.8*

Mean baseline: 157/104 mmHg.
*Significant.
Reprinted by permission of Elsevier Science Inc. from Nelson E, Arcuri K, Ikeda L, et al: Efficacy and safety of losartan in patients with essential hypertension. Am J Hypertens 5:19A, 1992. Copyright 1992 by American Journal of Hypertension, Inc.

bination treatment, is an effective antihypertensive agent.[38]

Side Effects

The clinical experience throughout the development of losartan has indicated that it is a well-tolerated drug with a favorable side effect profile similar to that observed with ACE inhibitors. Of importance, however, the problem of cough, which can occur in as many as 20% of patients treated with ACE inhibitors, does not occur more frequently with losartan than in patients treated with placebo. Pivotal studies designed to carefully evaluate the cough issue are still under way. Preliminary data obtained from the first of these major double-blind studies have indicated that in patients already known to exhibit cough responses to ACE inhibitors, treatment with losartan produces a cough incidence significantly lower than that with an ACE inhibitor and comparable with that observed during treatment with a diuretic.[38]

Metabolic Effects

Previous experience with ACE inhibitors indicated that those agents had some mildly beneficial effects on metabolic measurements. Perhaps because of their inhibition of angiotensin-stimulated aldosterone release, those agents have been shown to partly attenuate the potassium-wasting effects of diuretics. Similarly, experience with losartan has indicated a modest effect on potassium conservation during concomitant diuretic administration.[38] Likewise, there has been a slight tendency to ameliorate diuretic-induced increases in plasma glucose concentrations. In general, most other metabolic values, including lipid levels, renal function, and liver function all appear to be unaffected by losartan.

Of some interest, however, is the effect of losartan on plasma uric acid concentrations. Early studies have indicated that losartan possesses uricosuric properties,[39] which in turn result in modest decreases in plasma uric acid levels.[40] The clinical relevance of this action during long-term treatment with losartan in hypertensive patients is yet to be established.

OTHER CARDIOVASCULAR EFFECTS OF LOSARTAN

Vascular and circulatory effects, beyond reducing blood pressure, are emerging as critical properties of antihypertensive drugs. ACE inhibitors have already been widely evaluated in these areas. Thus, losartan and other potential angiotensin II (AII) receptor antagonists will be compared clinically with the ACE inhibitors in future studies, especially as these two drug classes work largely by blocking the renin-angiotensin system. Substantial and still growing experience with the ACE inhibitors has shown that these drugs have beneficial actions in critical organs such as the heart and kidneys. The ACE inhibitors have been shown to cause regression of left ventricular

hypertrophy and to improve both systolic and diastolic left ventricular function. They have also been shown to reduce renal glomerular hypertension, prevent nephropathy, and preserve renal function. Clearly, it is relevant to determine whether losartan also exhibits these important clinical attributes.

Although major clinical studies have not yet been undertaken with losartan, results from animal or *in vitro* research have produced some interesting findings. An important effect of losartan on renal physiology, shown in Figure 88–5, derives from a study that focused on the actions of the AII receptor antagonist on glomerular afferent and efferent arterioles in the isolated perfused hydronephrotic kidney.[41] As shown in Figure 88–5, AII produced marked vasocontrictor effects in these vessels, reducing their diameters by approximately one third. Losartan antagonized the vasocontrictor actions of AII and restored vascular diameter to baseline values in a dose-dependent fashion. This action of losartan appears to be analogous to the effects of ACE inhibitors in decreasing glomerular hypertension and protecting against renal dysfunction.[42]

Table 88–4 summarizes an important study comparing the effects of losartan and the ACE inhibitor captopril in the experimental postinfarct model of congestive heart failure in the Sprague-Dawley rat.[43] It is evident that losartan's effects on such key measurements as left ventricular end-diastolic pressure and volume index, as well as other hemodynamic variables, are virtually identical to those of captopril. Because captopril has proven clinical efficacy in the management of congestive heart failure, these early findings provide a clear incentive for studying losartan in patients with congestive heart failure.

Other investigational work with potential clinical relevance has been performed in the sodium-loaded Dahl S rat. This model becomes hypertensive and shows marked susceptibility to renal failure, strokes, and early death. As shown in Figure 88–6,[44] the rats

Table 88–4. **Post-Infarct CHF in the Sprague-Dawley Rat**

	Control	Captopril	100 mg Losartan Once Daily
Mean aortic pressure	107 ± 3	94 ± 5	97 ± 6
Right atrial pressure (mmHg)	2.3 ± 0.1	2.1 ± 0.4	1.9 ± 0.2
Left ventricular end-diastolic pressure (mmHg)	26.7 ± 1.5	15.8 ± 2.2*	14.2 ± 3.0*
End-diastolic volume index (ml/kg)	2.71 ± 0.10	2.18 ± 0.15*	2.03 ± 0.17*
Venous compliance (ml/mmHg/kg)	2.27 ± 0.06	3.02 ± 0.21*	2.80 ± 0.18*
N	9	9	10

Values are mean ± SEM
*Significantly different compared with control.
Reprinted by permission of Elsevier Science Inc. from Raya TE, Fonken SJ, Lee RW, et al: Hemodynamic effects of direct angiotensin II blockade compared to converting enzyme inhibition in rat model of heart failure. Am J Hypertens 4(Suppl):334S, 1991. Copyright 1991 by American Journal of Hypertension, Inc.

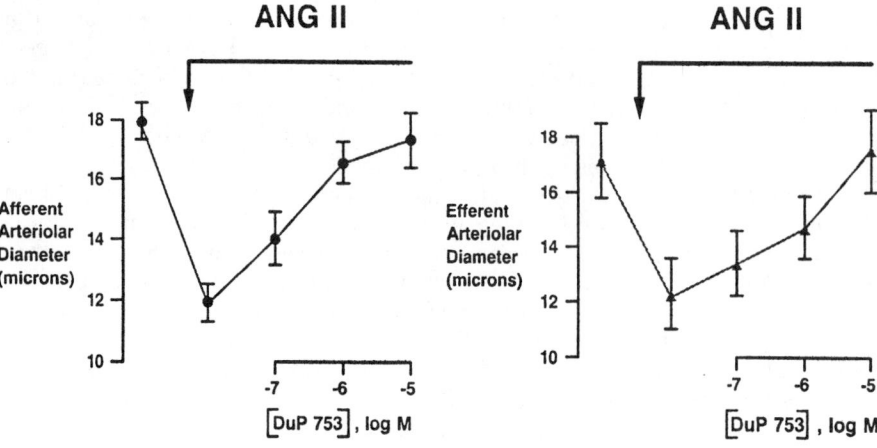

Figure 88–5. The effects of losartan (DuP 753) on renal afferent and efferent arteriolar diameters during angiotensin II infusion in isolated perfused hydronephrotic kidneys. (Data from Loutzenhiser R, Epstein M, Hayashi K, et al: Characterization of the renal microvascular effects of angiotensin II antagonist, DuP 753: Studies in isolated perfused hydronephrotic kidneys. Am J Hypertens 4[Suppl]:309S, 1991.)

treated with losartan during a 10-week study appeared to do much better than those receiving placebo. Indeed, approximately 70% of the losartan-treated rats were still alive at the end of the study, whereas only 30% of the rats in the control group were still alive.

A similar study has been performed in the spontaneously hypertensive rat, a model that also has an increased likelihood of strokes, renal failure, heart failure, and early death. After 12 weeks, more than 80% of the rats treated with losartan were still alive, whereas only approximately 20% of the group receiving a placebo had survived.[45]

SUMMARY AND COMMENT

The experience with losartan thus far shows it to be an effective and safe antihypertensive agent. Like the ACE inhibitors, it appears to work primarily by inhibiting activity of the renin-angiotensin system. Much remains to be learned about losartan and the other angiotensin receptor antagonists now in development. Beyond their antihypertensive properties, do they confer the same symptomatic and survival benefits that ACE inhibitors produce in congestive heart failure? Do they produce comparable beneficial effects on cardiac structure and function? Recently, ACE inhibitors have been shown to produce some novel and exciting actions: for example, they reduce clinical cardiac end points in patients who have suffered a myocardial infarction, and they can provide protection against renal failure and improve survival in patients with diabetic nephropathy. Physicians clearly will be eager to know whether the angiotensin II antagonists can rival—or hopefully exceed—this performance by the ACE inhibitors.

It could be tempting to assume that the two classes, ACE inhibitors and AT_1 antagonists, are fundamentally similar, perhaps only differing by virtue of the absence of cough during treatment with the AT_1 antagonists. Of course, this alone could be a strong incentive to develop and study this newer drug class; cough is a highly prevalent problem during ACE inhibitor treatment, especially in women patients, who in our aging population represent a rapidly growing and important part of our population with cardiovascular disease. But there may be more differences than just the presence or absence of the cough problem, and until appropriate comparative studies are performed, it would be incorrect to assume that the two classes are interchangeable. There are many relevant issues beyond the control of blood pressure itself, and creative research during the next few years will be of great interest in better defining the full potential role of losartan and the other AT_1 blockers in the full spectrum of cardiovascular disease.

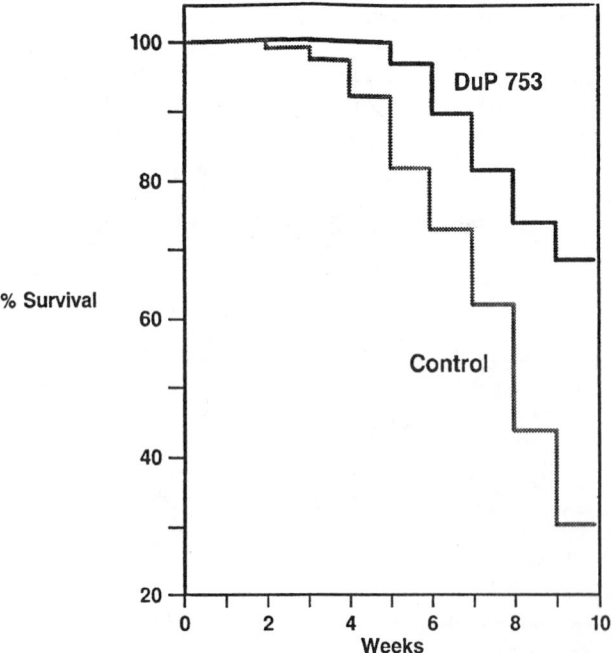

Figure 88–6. Survival of sodium-loaded Dahl S rats during treatment with losartan (DuP 753) or placebo. (Data from von Lutterotti N, Camargo JF, Mueller FB, et al: Angiotensin II receptor antagonist markedly reduces mortality in salt-loaded Dahl S rats. Am J Hypertens 4[Suppl]:346S, 1991.)

REFERENCES

1. Laragh JH, Baer L, Brunner HR, et al: Renin, angiotensin and aldosterone system in pathogenesis and management of hypertensive vascular disease. Am J Med 52:633, 1972.
2. Brunner HR, Laragh JH, Baer L, et al: Essential hypertension.

Renin and aldosterone, heart attack and stroke. N Engl J Med 286:441, 1972.

3. Buhler HR, Laragh JH, Baer L, et al: Propranolol inhibition of renin secretion. A specific approach to diagnosis and treatment of renin-dependent hypertensive diseases. N Engl J Med 187:1209, 1972.

4. Drayer JIM, Keim HR, Weber MA, et al: Unexpected pressor responses to propranolol in essential hypertension. Am J Med 60:897, 1976.

5. Streeten DHP, Anderson GH Jr, Dalakos TG: Angiotensin blockade: Its clinical significance. Am J Med 60:817, 1976.

6. Case DB, Wallace JM, Keim JH, et al: Estimating renin participation in hypertension. Superiority of converting enzyme inhibitor over saralasin. Am J Med 61:790, 1976.

7. Gavras H, Brunner HR, Laragh JH, et al: An angiotensin converting enzyme inhibitor to identify and treat vasoconstrictor and volume factors in hypertensive patients. N Engl J Med 291:817, 1974.

8. Case DB, Wallace JM, Laragh JH: Comparison between saralasin and converting enzyme inhibitor in hypertensive disease. Kidney Int 15(Suppl 9):S107, 1979.

9. Gavras H, Brunner HR, Turini GA, et al: Antihypertensive effect of the oral angiotensin converting enzyme inhibitor SQ 14225 in man. N Engl J Med 28:991, 1978.

10. Weber MA, Neutel JM, Smith DHG: Circulatory and extracirculatory effects of angiotensin-converting enzyme inhibition. Am Heart J 123:1414, 1992.

11. Weber MA, Neutel JM, Essinger I, et al: Assessment of renin dependency of hypertension with a dipeptide renin inhibitor. Circulation 81:1768, 1990.

12. Wexler RR, Carini DJ, Duncia JV, et al: Rationale for the chemical development of angiotensin II receptor antagonists. Am J Hypertens 5:209S, 1992.

13. Chiiu AT, McCall DE, Price WA, et al: Nonpeptide angiotensin II receptor antagonists. VII. Cellular and biochemical pharmacology of DuP 753, an orally active antihypertensive agent. J Pharmacol Exp Ther 252:711, 1990.

14. Timmermans PBMWM, Herblin WF, Ardecky RJ, et al: Angiotensin II Receptors. In Van Meel JCA, Doods H (eds): Receptor Data for Biological Experiments: A Guide to Specificity and Dosage. London: Ellis Horwood Ltd, 1991.

15. Chiu AT, McCall DE, Price WA, et al: In vitro pharmacology of DuP 753, a nonpeptide AII receptor antagonist. Am J Hypertens 4:282S, 1991.

16. Wong PC, Price WA, Chiu AT, et al: Nonpeptide angiotensin II receptor antagonists. VIII. Characterization of functional antagonism displayed by DuP 753, an orally active antihypertensive agent. J Pharmacol Exp Ther 252:719, 1990.

17. Wong PC, Price WA, Chiu AT, et al: Nonpeptide angiotensin II receptor antagonists. IX. Antihypertensive activity in rats of DuP 753, an orally active antihypertensive agent. J Pharmacol Exp Ther 252:726, 1990.

18. Wong PC, Price WA, Chiu AT, et al: Hypotensive action of DuP 753, an angiotensin II antagonist, in spontaneously hypertensive rats. Nonpeptide angiotensin II receptor antagonists: X. Hypertension 15:459, 1990.

19. Wong PC, Price WA, Chiu AT, et al: Nonpeptide angiotensin II receptor antagonists: Studies with EXP9270 and DuP 753. Hypertension 15:823, 1990.

20. Christ DD, Kilkson T, Wong N, et al: Formation and disposition of EXP3174, a pharmacologically active metabolite of the novel angiotensin II receptor antagonist DuP 753 [abstract 137]. International Society for the Study of Xenobiotica (ISSX), San Diego, CA, October 21–25, 1990.

21. Wong PC, Price WA, Chiu AT, et al: Nonpeptide angiotensin II receptor antagonists. XI. Pharmacology of EXP3174, an active metabolite of DuP 753—an orally active antihypertensive agent. J Pharmacol Exp Ther 255:211, 1990.

22. Munafo A, Christen Y, Nussberger J, et al: Drug concentration response relationships in normal volunteers after oral administration of losartan (DuP 753, MK 954), an angiotensin II receptor antagonist. Clin Pharmacol Ther 51:513, 1992.

23. Chiu AT, Herblin WF, McCall DE, et al: Identification of angio-

tensin II receptor subtypes. Biochem Biophys Res Commun 165:196, 1989.

24. Wong PC, Hart SD, Zaspel AM, et al: Functional studies of nonpeptide angiotensin II receptor subtype-specific ligands: DuP 753 (AII-l) and PD123177 (AII-2). J Pharmacol Exp Ther 255:584, 1990.

25. Timmermans P, Benfield P, Chiu AT, et al: Angiotensin II receptors and functional correlates. Am J Hypertens 5:221S, 1992.

26. Murphy TJ, Alexander RW, Griendling KK, et al: Isolation of a cDNA encoding the vascular type-1 angiotensin II receptor. Nature 351:233, 1991.

27. Sasamura H, Hein L, Krieger JE, et al: Cloning, characterization, and expression of two angiotensin receptor (AT-1) isoforms from the mouse genome. Biochem Biophys Res Commun 185:688, 1992.

28. Matsubara L, Brilla CG, Weber KT: Angiotensin II-mediated inhibition of collagenase activity in cultured cardiac fibroblasts [abstract]. FASEB J 6:A941, 1992.

29. Wong PC, Christ DD, Timmermans PB: Enhancement of losartan (DuP 753) induced angiotensin II receptor antagonism by PD123177 in rats. Eur J Pharmacol 220:267, 1992.

30. Christen Y, Waeber B, Nussberger J, et al: Oral administration of DuP 753, a specific angiotensin II receptor antagonist, to normal male volunteers. Circulation 83:1333, 1991.

31. Brunner HR, Christen Y, Munafo A, et al: Clinical experience with angiotensin II receptor antagonists. Am J Hypertens 5:243S, 1992.

32. Conway J, Johnston J, Coats A, et al: The use of ambulatory blood pressure monitoring to improve the accuracy and reduce the numbers of subjects in clinical trials of antihypertensive agents. J Hypertens 6:111, 1988.

33. Ohlstein EH, Gellai M, Brooks DP, et al: The antihypertensive effect of the angiotensin II receptor antagonist DuP 753 may not be due solely to angiotensin II receptor antagonism. J Pharmacol Exp Ther 262:595, 1992.

34. DePasquale MJ, Fossa AA, Holt WF, Mangiapane ML: Central DuP 753 does not lower blood pressure in spontaneously hypertensive rats. Hypertension 19:668, 1992.

35. Jaiswal N, Diz DI, Tallant EA, et al: Characterization of angiotensin receptors mediating prostaglandin synthesis in C6 glioma cells. Am J Physiol 260:1000, 1991.

36. Nelson E, Merrill D, Sweet C: Efficacy and safety of oral MK-954 (DuP 753), an angiotensin receptor antagonist, in essential hypertension. J Hypertens 9(Suppl 6):S468, 1991.

37. Nelson E, Arcuri K, Ikeda L, et al: Efficacy and safety of losartan in patients with essential hypertension. Am J Hypertens 5:19A, 1992.

38. Data on file, DuPont Merck Pharmaceutical Company.

39. Kauffman RF, Beans JS, Zimmerman KM, et al: Losartan, a nonpeptide angiotensin II (Ang II) receptor antagonist, inhibits neointima formation following balloon injury to rat carotid arteries. Life Sci 49:223, 1991.

40. Bui JD, Kimura B, Phillips MI: Losartan potassium, a nonpeptide antagonist of angiotensin II, chronically administered p.o. does not readily cross the blood-brain barrier. Eur J Pharmacol 219:147, 1992.

41. Loutzenhiser R, Epstein M, Hayashi K, et al: Characterization of the renal microvascular effects of angiotensin II antagonist, DuP 753: Studies in isolated perfused hydronephrotic kidneys. Am J Hypertens 4(Suppl):309S, 1991.

42. Bochicchio T, Sandoval G, Ron O, et al: Fosinopril prevents hyperfiltration and decreases proteinuria in post transplant hypertensives. Kidney Int 38:873, 1990.

43. Raya TE, Fonken SJ, Lee RW, et al: Hemodynamic effects of direct angiotensin II blockade compared to converting enzyme inhibition in rat model of heart failure. Am J Hypertens 4(Suppl):334S, 1991.

44. von Lutterotti N, Camargo MJ, Mueller FB, et al: Angiotensin II receptor antagonist markedly reduces mortality in salt-loaded Dahl S rats. Am J Hypertens 4(Suppl):346S, 1991.

45. Camargo MJ, von Lutterotti N, Pecker MS, et al: DuP 753 increases survival in spontaneously hypertensive stroke-prone rats fed a high sodium diet. Am J Hypertens 4(Suppl):341S, 1991.

X.

Arteriolar and Venous Vasodilators

Editors: Edward D. Frohlich and Bertram Pitt

A. Vasodilatation

CHAPTER 89

Principles and Practice of Vasodilatation

Michel E. Safar, M.D., Gérard M. London, M.D., and Jacques E. Chelly, M.D.

In animal experiments, vasodilating compounds are defined as drugs causing relaxation of arterial smooth muscle. Relaxation is usually demonstrated in *in vitro* experiments, which indicate that the tensile forces of prepared strips of arteries are diminished after the application of drugs.[1] For obvious practical reasons, large arteries are used predominantly in these animal experiments, and the most important questions of pharmacologists are related to the three main mechanisms of action of the different vasodilating drugs: receptor-dependent vasodilatation, channel blockade, and vasodilatation of unknown origin.

In clinical studies, the relaxant effect of the drug on arterial smooth muscle is much more difficult to evaluate. It is simply inferred from the geometric modifications of the vessels produced within the vascular system.[2-5] In other words, vasodilatation is assessed on the basis of a given increase in the diameter of the studied vessel(s). The situation *in vivo* is more complicated than it is *in vitro*, because the vascular system is studied in the presence of the accompanying pathophysiologic factors, in particular the pressure forces acting on the vessels and the counterregulatory mechanisms associated with vasodilatation. In addition, not only large arteries are involved in the cardiovascular system but also small arteries and veins. This latter point is particularly important to consider in view of the fact that relaxation of the vascular smooth muscle may have different functional consequences for the various vessels: resistive changes in small arteries, and capacitative changes in large arteries and veins.[2]

The purpose of the present review is to delineate the characteristics of vasodilatation in the different situations observed in human cardiovascular diseases. First, the conceptual framework of dilatation of small arteries, large arteries, and veins is discussed. Second, the different aspects of the counterregulatory mechanisms accompanying vasodilatation are examined in detail. Finally, three particular pathologic aspects are reviewed: congestive heart failure, hypertension, and arterial stenosis.

THE CONCEPTUAL FRAMEWORK
Small Arteries

Vasodilatation, which usually refers to an increase in the diameter and/or the number of small arteries, may be easily demonstrated under experimental conditions. In isolated organs, vasodilatation means either a decrease in perfusion pressure at a given flow or an increase in flow at a constant perfusion pressure.[4] Under these conditions, the Poiseuille law may be applied, accepting the assumption of a laminar flow in uniform vessels.[3] A linear relationship between pressure drop (Delta-P) and flow (F) through zero (Fig. 89–1) is assumed, so that

$$\text{Delta-P}/F = R = 8 \, nl/3.14 \, r^4$$

where R = resistance, l = length, r = internal radius of the vessel, and n = blood viscosity. Assuming l and n as constant, the change in resistance is proportional to the fourth power of the vessel radius and therefore serves predominantly to evaluate the caliber of the vessel and hence the degree of vasodilatation.

Although the Poiseuille law can be applied to isolated organs, several difficulties arise when this equation is applied *in vivo*, in either animals or human subjects. Vascular resistance is calculated simply from the ratio between mean arterial pressure and flow, although the basic hypothesis of the Poiseuille law cannot really be validated for several reasons.[1-5] First, the vessel length and blood viscosity must be assumed as constant in all situations. Second, nonlaminar flow frequently occurs in the body, especially if the blood vessel is stenotic. Finally, the pressure-flow relationship is probably not constantly linear through

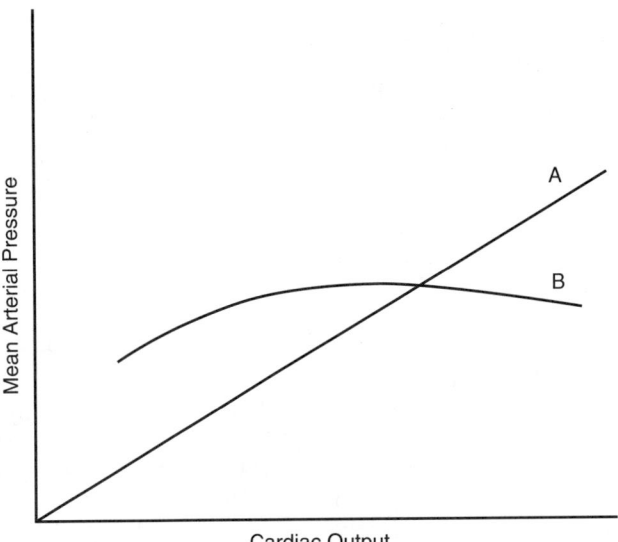

Figure 89–1. Schematized relation between mean arterial pressure and cardiac output.[3–5] The straight line through the origin (A) represents the Poiseuille law with a constant peripheral resistance. The curved line (B) is the pressure-flow relationship observed in the entire systemic bed of an intact dog. The main cause of the deviation from the straight line through the origin (as shown in B), leading to an almost constant pressure at various cardiac outputs, is the baroreceptor reflex.

zero because of the role of the neurohumoral control systems acting on the physiologic pressure range[3–5] and the large variations observed in the different regional circulations, a point that is explored in further detail later.

The factors that control regional blood flow can be grouped into two major categories: local and neurogenic. The latter refers to the sympathetic noradrenergic nerves and therefore to the control of flow via the baroreceptor areas. The former is invoked to explain the marked capacity for autoregulation displayed by certain organs under basal conditions. Autoregulation is defined as the phenomenon by which blood vessels alter their tone over a wide range of perfusion pressures to maintain constant organ or tissue blood flow through myogenic factors and metabolic factors (or the fractional oxygen requirement of a region to a fraction of the cardiac output delivered to this region).[6] With such measurements, different regional patterns may be observed. Under basal conditions, the heart uses 11% of systemic oxygen uptake but receives only 4% of the cardiac output, indicating that the major mechanism controlling blood flow is local and metabolic in nature. For the brain, there is a local control mechanism that is mainly myogenic for global flow and metabolic for regional flow. Renal flow is tightly autoregulated under basal circumstances by myogenic and other local mechanisms, and there is practically no capacity for vasodilatation. In contrast, the oxygen requirements of the skin are very low, and blood flow is almost entirely controlled by neurogenic mechanisms.[6]

Based on these classic assumptions about regional circulations, it now seems clear that calculation of

vascular resistance in the local systemic circulation may be a misleading index for the evaluation of vasodilatation in the whole body.[2–5] First, vascular resistance measures only the overall effect of changes in various parts of the circulation and does not rule out the possibility of dilatation of some vessels and constriction of others. Second, the calculation of resistance does not really differentiate between vasodilatation and the opening of previously closed vessels ("recruitment"). Finally, the resistance index does not identify the mechanism underlying the change in diameter of the vessels: an effect of the drug itself, but also a result of changes in neural stimuli, local metabolites, and transmural pressure. In other words, after drug administration, the calculation of resistance gives only a semiquantitative index of vasodilatation. It evaluates a net effect, that is, the algebraic sum of the action of the drug and the associated counterregulatory mechanisms.

Large Arteries

Although most animal studies showing arterial smooth muscle relaxation with drugs have been done on large arteries *in vitro*, most clinical investigations of vasodilatation are based on calculations of vascular resistance and hence on modifications in the status of small arteries. This is due to a methodologic approach favoring the calculation of vascular resistance, because the diameter of large arteries in human subjects is much more difficult to evaluate. Recently, noninvasive methods using echo-Doppler systems and echo-tracking techniques have been used in human subjects to determine the internal diameter of large vessels and their pulsatile changes.[7–9] Using this method, vasodilatation of large arteries may be more easily estimated.

For many years, large arteries have been considered as passive conduits, their diameter depending only on the mechanical factor of distending blood pressure. Thus, large arteries are expected to dilate passively when blood pressure is increased and to constrict when blood pressure decreases (see reviews in Noble,[3] Folkow,[4] and Westerhof and Huisman[5]). More recently, other independent mechanisms have been suggested to explain changes in the diameter of large arteries: (1) high flow per se may be responsible for arterial dilatation, the mechanism of which is partly endothelium dependent,[10–12] (2) large arteries in humans may respond actively to vasoactive substances and neurohumoral stimuli,[11–14] and (3) changes in the structure and function of endothelium may modify the vasodilating responses.[10, 12] For instance, Laurent et al.[13] have shown that, with subpressor doses of norepinephrine, brachial artery diameter is reduced more in hypertensive than in normal subjects. Also, after administration of nitrates, calcium antagonists, or converting enzyme inhibitors, brachial artery diameter increases significantly in hypertensive subjects, despite a concomitant reduction in blood pressure.[2] Surprisingly, for the same blood pressure reduction, dihydralazine tends rather to reduce brachial artery diameter.

Because of the active changes in large artery smooth muscle tone, both the conduit function of the large vessels (i.e., the capacity to drive blood flow) and their buffering function (i.e., the ability to modify the viscoelastic properties of the arterial system) may be modified.[2, 15] As far as the former is concerned, an active increase in brachial artery diameter may contribute to the increase in flow, as has been observed in the human hypertensive forearm after administration of calcium antagonists or converting enzyme inhibitors.[2, 15] On the other hand, in recent years, modifications in the viscoelastic properties of the arterial wall have been widely demonstrated after administration of antihypertensive drugs to hypertensive human beings. The viscoelastic properties of the arterial wall are usually evaluated in terms of compliance,[2, 15] that is, by measurement of the pressure-volume relationships within a vascular segment. Mathematically, compliance is the slope of the pressure-volume relationship at a specified point on the curve. For the same blood pressure reduction obtained with various antihypertensive drugs, arterial compliance may either be increased (nitrates, converting enzyme inhibitors, calcium antagonists) or remain unchanged (dihydralazine, propranolol),[2, 15] thus acting differently on arterial stiffness. Thus, depending on the kind of vasodilating agent, vasodilatation may have different effects on large and small arteries associated with two possible hemodynamic patterns: decreased vascular resistance and reduced arterial compliance (dihydralazine and derivatives, propranolol), or decreased vascular resistance and increased arterial compliance (nitrates, converting enzyme inhibitors, calcium antagonists). In recent years, it has been shown that, although evident at the site of the brachial artery, such changes may even differ substantially along the arterial tree, as a result of the large heterogeneity of the arterial system.[14]

In addition to compliance changes, arterial vasodilatation may induce significant changes in the timing of pressure wave reflections, which may contribute to modify per se the systolic blood pressure level and to alter the structure and function of the heart, a new chapter of vasodilatation that has been described very recently.[15]

Veins

In contrast with arteries, veins are an experimental model easier to use in the study of vascular smooth muscle relaxation in humans, because these structures are not exposed to the increased intraluminal pressure usually observed in most cardiovascular diseases.[16] However, venous vasodilatation is very difficult to assess for several reasons.[17] First, veins are usually not tubular in shape, making vasodilatation much more difficult to evaluate than in the case of small and large arteries. Second, the composition of veins is quite variable: whereas large veins contain a high percentage of collagen fibers, the muscular mass of

swollen veins exceeds that of collagen, especially in the lower limbs. Third, the degree of innervation of veins is less than that of resistance vessels, consisting mainly of sympathetic constrictor fibers. Fourth, because of the great variability in the structure and, therefore, the function of veins, generalizations are difficult. This observation is particularly true in human studies, which are usually restricted to the determination of venous compliance in the extremities.

In the physiologic pressure range, veins are more compliant than arteries. *In vivo* and *in vitro* studies of veins have revealed two types of pressure-volume (compliance) curves.[16, 17] One was described as curvilinear with convexity toward the volume axis, the other sigmoid. The latter is observed when the veins are in spasm or are constricted by neural or humoral stimuli. When the state of contraction is eliminated by warming, venodilator agents, or metabolic inhibitors, the curvilinear pressure-volume curve is observed. The sigmoid curve has been interpreted as a manifestation of the resistance to stretch of venous smooth muscle. The curvilinear curve with convexity toward the volume axis represents primarily the resistance to stretch of the connective tissue elements of the venous wall, the smooth muscle elements being in a state of relaxation. Under such conditions, it is very difficult to compare dilatation of veins with that of small and large arteries in clinical studies.

ENDOGENOUS HEMODYNAMIC AND NEUROHUMORAL RESPONSE TO VASODILATATION
Hemodynamic and Humoral Patterns

In normal and in hypertensive individuals, administration of vasodilator drugs not only produces direct peripheral vasodilatation but also activates counterregulatory mechanisms, which cause peripheral vasoconstriction, tachycardia, and an increase in cardiac output.[18, 19] The larger arteries and the venous system may also participate in the counterregulatory mechanisms.[3-5] The hemodynamic responses to drug treatment in such patients are the net result of these interacting forces, so that marked activation of reactive vasoconstrictor mechanism may greatly limit the magnitude of achievable peripheral vasodilatation and therapeutic hypotension. These vasoconstrictor forces become evident as rebound phenomena when, on abrupt discontinuation of short-acting vasodilators, drug-mediated vasodilatation rapidly disappears, leaving the reactive forces unopposed.[19] Such hemodynamic patterns are not limited to hypertensive patients. The occurrence of rebound hemodynamic events after the abrupt withdrawal of nitroprusside in patients with congestive heart failure suggests that similar reactive mechanisms may underlie the responses to vasodilator therapy in such patients as well, thereby limiting the magnitude of drug-mediated peripheral vasodilatation.[19] However, in congestive heart failure, circulatory reflexes are attenuated, the greatest attenuation being observed in individuals with the most marked left ventricular impairment.[19] The endogenous neurohumoral response seems capable not only of limiting the acute hemodynamic effects of drug therapy but also of modifying the benefits of long-term vasodilator administration. For example, with long-term therapy, neurohumoral response seems capable not only of limiting the acute hemodynamic effects of drug therapy but also of modifying the benefits of long-term vasodilator administration. For example, with long-term therapy, neurohumoral stimulation may result in significant salt and water retention that may further decrease the vascular responsiveness to vasodilator stimuli.[18]

The reactive vasoconstriction forces are the result mainly of vasodilatation-induced activation of the sympathetic nervous and renin-angiotensin systems.[18] For a long time, this activation has been attributed exclusively to baroreceptor mechanisms acting in the high-pressure system, with resulting simultaneous modifications in heart rate and vascular resistance.[3, 5, 15, 18] More recently, several examples of differential response of the cardiac and vascular effectors have been observed, suggesting that the heart rate and vascular controls may be affected differently. Indeed, the control of heart rate is influenced not only by sympathetic activity but also by changes in parasympathetic tone (as observed with dihydralazine).[18, 20] On the other hand, the control of vascular resistance is dependent not only on the cardiac mechanoreceptors in the high-pressure system but also in the low-pressure system.[21] The significant reduction in vascular resistance produced by dihydralazine is due not only to its pure arteriole-dilating effect but also to the drug-mediated increase in venous return. This prevents reflex arterial vasoconstriction via the cardiac mechanoreceptors.[22]

Intensity and Time Constant of the Neurohumoral Response

The intensity of the endogenous neurohumoral response is influenced not only by the kind of cardiovascular disease (hypertension, congestive heart failure) but also by the mechanism of action of each vasodilating drug. Sustained activation of the sympathetic nervous system is usually observed with direct vasodilators, such as dihydralazine, cadralazine, diazoxide, and minoxidil.[1] A transient baroreflex response is observed with the calcium antagonist nifedipine and also with other dihydropyridine derivatives.[1] In contrast, diltiazem and verapamil cause minimal changes in heart rate, except when a bolus injection is given.[1] Finally, with several antihypertensive agents, such as prazosin and its derivatives, nitrates (mainly in older subjects), and converting enzyme inhibitors, a heart rate response may not occur at all.[1]

Numerous explanations have been offered for the absence of tachycardia after administration of the latter vasodilators.[23] These include (1) a peripheral effect due to increased vagal parasympathetic tone; (2) a central venous effect on the modulation of afferent vagal and/or sympathetic outflow; (3) an action on baroreceptor reflex sensitivity or gain; (4) a peripheral sympathoinhibitory effect resulting from the pharmacologic action of the drug; and finally, (5) the specific effect of the drug on the vascular smooth muscle and, hence, on the tension of the large arteries.

Whatever the mechanisms may be, based on the clinical presence or absence of endogenous neurohumoral response, vasodilating drugs are often classified according to three hemodynamic patterns:[1] (1) predominant arteriolar dilatation (dihydralazine), which would be responsible for an important neurogenic response, an increase in cardiac output accompanying the decrease in vascular resistance; (2) predominant venous dilatation (nitrates), which would presumably be responsible for reduced venous return and cardiac output, and a small decrease in vascular resistance; and (3) combined venous and arteriolar dilatation (converting enzyme inhibitors), which would be compatible with an unchanged cardiac output and therefore a greater reduction in vascular resistance. Although this classification remains clinically useful, it underestimates the fact that the hemodynamic changes are the combined effects of the action of the vasodilating agent and of the countervailing baroreflex mechanisms that simultaneously cause peripheral vasoconstriction and tachycardia.

Influence of Age on the Neurohumoral Response

Aging may have an important influence on the neurohumoral and sympathetic responses. Indeed, the autonomic cardiac response is predominantly influenced by β_1-receptors, whereas the vascular response is influenced more by β_2- and α-receptors. Because the number and affinity of β-receptors are reduced with age, the heart rate baroreflex response also decreases significantly with aging.[24] On the other hand, the α-receptor-mediated vascular response may be exaggerated with age, as a result of unopposed α-vasoconstriction.[24] The vascular hyperresponsiveness is further favored by the increase in arterial and arteriolar vessel thickness usually observed with aging according to the concepts of Folkow.[4] For this reason, the general neurohumoral response to vasodilatation is greatly modified by aging. Although the increase in heart rate is attenuated with age, the vascular response may be preserved to a large extent, especially in the case of the hemodynamic response to orthostasis in hypertensive subjects.[20]

VASODILATATION AND CARDIOVASCULAR DISEASES

In this review, we have suggested that the hemodynamic and neurohumoral pattern of vasodilatation may differ according to the type of cardiovascular disease. Given this view, it should be remembered that, if the principal goal of vasodilatation is a decrease in cardiovascular morbidity and mortality, this goal may differ according to the type of cardiovascular disease: hypertension, congestive heart failure, or atherosclerosis, with or without stenotic arterial segment. In addition, as is emphasized in later chapters, changes in endothelial structure and function may modify greatly the extent of dilatation itself.[12]

Hypertension

Hypertension is characterized by normal systemic and regional blood flow in the presence of increased blood pressure. Renal blood flow alone may be reduced. Thus, the main problem is to obtain a significant blood pressure reduction with minor changes in blood flow, except perhaps in the case of the renal circulation. This therapeutic goal is important, because most antihypertensive drugs redistribute blood flow and even produce profuse circulation in some vascular areas without beneficial effect.[2]

Another important consideration is the hemodynamic mechanism of the drug's antihypertensive effect. Because blood pressure is the product of blood flow and vascular resistance, it is often believed that a given antihypertensive drug reduces blood pressure either through a decrease in blood flow or a decrease in vascular resistance, or both. This general concept implies that, in some cases, high blood pressure could be chronically reduced without any absolute or relative increase in the diameter of small arteries (see the first section of this chapter). Nevertheless, it should be remembered that resistance is calculated in hemodynamic studies; vasodilatation in hypertension may easily be demonstrated with classic vasodilating compounds, such as dihydralazine, calcium antagonists, or converting enzyme inhibitors. However, vasodilatation is often more difficult to demonstrate with drugs that cause an acute "increase in peripheral resistance," such as clonidine, diuretics, or β-blocking agents. However, in these latter cases, it has been shown that the onset of blood pressure reduction during long-term treatment with diuretics and different β-blockers is invariably associated with a fall in vascular resistance at any given level of cardiac output.[25] From this simple observation, it would appear not only that evaluation of vascular resistance may be a misleading approach in the assessment of arteriolar vasodilatation in hypertension but also that long-term blood pressure reduction in hypertension cannot be achieved without arteriolar vasodilatation.[2]

In hypertension, the goal of treatment is not per se to decrease blood pressure and to cause arteriolar vasodilatation. It is rather to decrease cardiovascular morbidity and mortality. Therapeutic trials have emphasized that antihypertensive drug treatment reduces significantly the incidence of stroke but causes fewer modifications in the incidence of ischemic heart disease.[26] For that reason, arterial vasodilatation, with its specific consequences on the buffering function of large arteries, should also be an important goal to consider in the treatment of hypertension.[2]

Another important aspect of vasodilatation in hypertension is the amplification of the vascular response in comparison with normotensive controls.[4, 5]

The relatively thick muscle coat surrounding the arteries and arterioles, the main effector organ in autoregulation, is affected in hypertension. This muscle coat hypertrophies as an adaptation to high intraluminal pressures, with consequent thickening of the arterial and arteriolar wall. This has been termed "structural autoregulation."[4] These adaptations function well at the local level, protecting the capillary bed against the effects of high blood pressure, without alteration in smooth muscle activity.[4] The generalized occurrence of the adaptation reinforces the pressure responses, because a given degree of muscle shortening gives rise to greater changes in vascular lumen, thus causing an amplification of the vasodilating response. In recent years, the concept has been developed in cardiovascular pharmacology. It is important to modify not only the "functional" aspect of vasodilatation (i.e., the diameter lumen) but also the structural aspect (i.e., the vessel hypertrophy). Based on some experimental and clinical studies,[27–29] the reversibility of structural vascular changes has been obtained at the site of arteries and, to a lesser extent, at the site of arterioles. Such differences between large and small arteries may be partly explained on the basis that vascular hypertrophy is influenced not only by the hemodynamic stimuli but also by specific growth factors.[12, 29]

Congestive Heart Failure

In contrast with hypertension, congestive heart failure is characterized by both an alteration of the pump function of the heart and a decrease in systemic and several regional blood flows. Therefore, one of the goals of therapy with vasodilators may be not only to improve cardiac performance through dilatation of peripheral arteries and veins but also to reduce ischemia in some regional circulations, particularly during exercise.[19]

Concerning the response to vasodilatation, the baseline hemodynamic and neurohumoral characteristics of patients with congestive heart failure are quite different from those of patients with hypertension.[30] This important aspect is described elsewhere, but it probably explains why, in congestive heart failure, pulmonary and systemic vasodilatation serve to increase cardiac output and reduce filling pressures with minimal pressure changes and tachycardia, a situation quite different from that of hypertension.[19]

Finally, the concept has been developed that the principal goal of vasodilatation in congestive heart failure should be not only to improve symptoms but also to reduce cardiovascular morbidity and mortality. This important aspect is described in the next chapters of this book, particularly for the use of converting enzyme inhibitors and various treatments of coronary artery disease.[31]

Atherosclerosis and Stenotic Arterial Segments

If the blood vessel is not uniform but contains a stenosis, Poiseuille's law can no longer be applied to

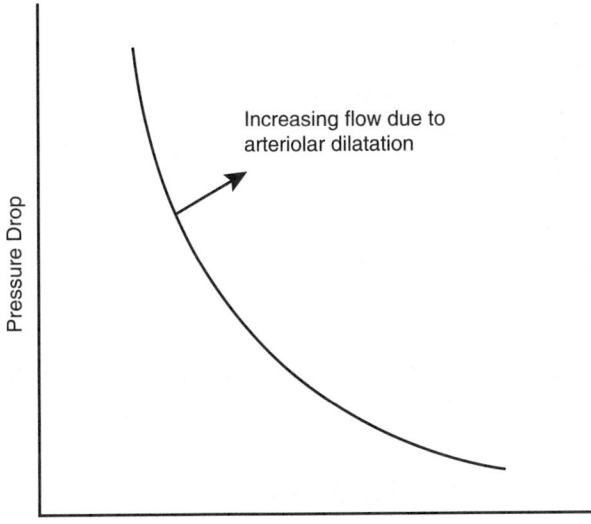

Figure 89–2. Pressure drop over an arterial stenosis as a function of the degree of stenosis (diagram represents decreasing degree of stenosis in abscissa and increasing values of pressure drop in ordinate).[5] At a higher flow (e.g., due to a vasodilator), the curve would move as indicated by the arrow, with the stenosis causing a greater drop in pressure.

evaluate vasodilatation (see the first section of this chapter). A more realistic approach to a stenosis must deal with the energy expenditure needed to make the flow enter the narrowing section, to form a laminar profile in the narrowed section, and to exit into the widening section.[5] As a clinical application of this general concept, it should be noted that all these energy losses have an approximately *quadratic relation to flow.* However, energy losses also depend on the shape of the stenosis.[5] Thus, for a constant stenosis, increases in flow produced by (poststenotic) arteriolar dilatation greatly increase pressure drop over the stenosis (Fig. 89–2), so that distal to the stenosis there would eventually be insufficient pressure left to perfuse the arterial segment. In other words, in subjects with arterial stenosis, it seems better to obtain a preferential dilatation of (prestenotic) large arteries rather than arterioles, in order to redistribute blood flow toward the impaired segments of the ischemic tissue.[32] This important topic has been extensively studied in the coronary circulation with nitrates[32] and is dealt with in more detail in other parts of this book.

CONCLUSION

The concept of vasodilatation has been oversimplified in clinical studies for many years. In the development of vasodilators, it is important to describe not only the arteriolar but also the arterial and venous effects. Both experimental and clinical cardiovascular pharmacology are involved if the goal of treatment of cardiovascular disease is not only to improve symptoms but also to reduce morbidity and mortality.

REFERENCES

1. Opie LH, Phil D: Drugs for the Heart, 2nd expanded ed. Orlando, FL: Grune & Stratton, 1987, pp 5–107.
2. Safar ME, Levy BI, Laurent S, London GM: Hypertension and the arterial system: Clinical and therapeutic aspects. J Hypertens 8(Suppl 7):S113, 1990.
3. Noble MIM: The Cardiac Cycle. Oxford: Blackwell, 1979, pp 141–209.
4. Folkow B: Physiological aspects of primary hypertension. Physiol Rev 62:347, 1982.
5. Westerhof N, Huisman RM: Arterial haemodynamics in hypertension. Clin Sci 72:391, 1987.
6. Zelis R: Nitrates: Mechanism of vasodilatation. *In* Cohn JN, Rittinghaussen R (eds): International Boehringer Mannheim Symposia. Berlin: Springer Verlag, 1984, pp 7–17.
7. Safar ME, Peronneau PP, Levenson JA, Simon A: Pulsed doppler: Diameter, velocity and flow of the brachial artery in sustained essential hypertension. Circulation 63:393, 1981.
8. Tardy Y, Meister JJ, Perret F, et al: Assessment of the elastic behaviour of peripheral arteries from a noninvasive measurement of their diameter-pressure curves. Clin Phys Physiol Meas 12:39, 1991.
9. Kawasaki T, Sasayama S, Yagi SI, et al: Noninvasive assessment of the age related changes in stiffness of major branches of the human arteries. Cardiovasc Res 21:678, 1987.
10. Pohl U, Holtz J, Busse R, et al: Crucial role of endothelium in the vasodilator response to increased flow in vivo. Hypertension 8:37, 1986.
11. London GM, Pannier BM, Laurent S, et al: Brachial artery diameter changes associated with cardiopulmonary baroreflex activation in humans. Am J Physiol 258(Heart Circ Physiol, 27):H773, 1990.
12. Vanhoutte PM (ed): Vasodilation. Vascular Smooth Muscle, Peptides, Autonomic Nerves, and Endothelium. New York: Raven Press, 1988, pp 401–550.
13. Laurent S, Juillerat L, London GM, et al: Increased response of brachial artery diameter to norepinephrine in hypertensive patients. Am J Physiol 255(Heart Circ Physiol 24):H36, 1988.
14. Arcaro G, Laurent S, Benetos A, et al: Heterogeneous effect of nitrates on large arteries of hypertensives. J Hypertens 9 (Suppl 6):42, 1991.
15. O'Rourke MF, Safar ME, Dzau VJ: Arterial vasodilation. Mechanisms and therapy. *In* Arnold E (ed): The Arterial System in Hypertension. London: Kluwer Academic Publishers, 1993, pp 50–116, 149–179, 200–219.
16. Simon G: Venous changes in renal hypertensive rats: The role of humoral factors. Blood Vessels 15:311, 1978.
17. Rothe CF: Venous system: Physiology of the capacitance vessels. *In* Shepherd JT, Abboud FM (eds): Handbook of Physiology. The Cardiovascular System: Peripheral Circulation and Organ Blood Flow, Vol III, Section 2. Bethesda, MD: American Physiological Society, 1983, pp 397–452.
18. Koch-Weser J: Vasodilator drugs in the treatment of hypertension. Arch Intern Med 113:1017, 1974.
19. Packer M, Le Jemtel TH: Physiologic and pharmacologic determinants of vasodilator response: A conceptual framework for rational drug therapy for chronic heart failure. Proc Cardiovasc Dis 24:275, 1982.
20. London GM, Weiss YA, Pannier BP, et al: Tilt test in essential hypertension: Differential responses in heart rate and vascular resistance. Hypertension 10:29, 1987.
21. Gauer OH: Mechanoreceptors in the intrathoracic circulation and plasma volume control. *In* Epstein M (ed): The Kidney in Liver Disease, Vol 1. New York: Elsevier, 1978, pp 3–19.
22. Shepherd AMM, Irvine NA: Differential hemodynamic and sympathoadrenal effects of sodium nitroprusside and hydralazine in hypertensive subjects. J Cardiovasc Pharmacol 8:527, 1986.
23. Millar JA, Sturani A, Rubin PC, et al: Attenuation of the antihypertensive effects of captopril by the opioid receptor antagonist naloxone. Clin Exp Pharmacol Physiol 10:253, 1983.
24. Bertel O, Buhler FR, Kiowski W, et al: Decreased beta-adrenoceptor responsiveness as related to age, blood pressure, and plasma catecholamines in patients with essential hypertension. Hypertension 2:130, 1980.
25. Man In't Veld AJ, Schalekamp MADH: Effects of 10 different beta-adrenoceptor antagonists on hemodynamics, plasma renin activity, and plasma norepinephrine in hypertension. The

key role of vascular resistance changes in relation to partial agonist activity. J Cardiovasc Pharmacol 5(Suppl 1):S30, 1983.

26. Freis ED: The veterans trial and sequelae. Br J Clin Pharmacol 13:67, 1982.
27. Levy BI, Michel JB, Salzmann JL, et al: Effects of chronic inhibition of converting enzyme on mechanical and structural properties of arteries in rat renovascular hypertension. Circ Res 63:227, 1988.
28. Asmar RG, Journo HJ, Lacolley PJ, et al: Treatment for one year with perindopril: Effect on cardiac mass and arterial compliance in essential hypertension. J Hypertens 6(Suppl 3):S33, 1988.

29. Heagerty AM, Aalkjaer C, Bund SJ, et al: Small artery structure in hypertension. Dual processes of remodeling and growth. Hypertension 21:391, 1993.
30. Packer M, Lee WH, Kessler PD, et al: Role of neurohormonal mechanisms in determining survival in patients with severe chronic heart failure. Circulation 75(Suppl IV):80, 1987.
31. Massie BM, Conway M: Survival of patients with congestive heart failure: Past, present, and future prospects. Circulation 75(Suppl IV):11, 1987.
32. Winbury MM: Proximal and distal coronary arteries. In Santamore WP, Bove AA (eds): Coronary Artery Disease. Baltimore: Urban & Schwartzenberg, 1983, pp 63–78.

CHAPTER 90

Endogenous and Therapeutic Nitrates

Thomas F. Lüscher, M.D., and Raghvendra K. Dubey, Ph.D.

The use of nitric oxide (NO) in cardiovascular therapy can be traced back to 1867, when Sir Thomas Lauder Brunton first used nitrate of amyl in a patient with angina pectoris,[1] although the mechanism remained unclear. Elucidation of the mechanism of action of nitrates has only evolved in the last decade, in particular with the discovery of endothelium-dependent vasorelaxation and its mediator, the endogenous nitrovasodilator, NO.[2, 3] Nitrovasodilators of different classes are extensively used in the medical treatment of angina pectoris, myocardial infarction, ischemic heart disease, and heart failure.[4–6] This chapter focuses on the current knowledge of (1) the mechanisms and vascular effects of the L-arginine NO pathway in normal vessels; (2) the role of NO in hypertension and atherosclerosis; (3) the mechanisms and actions of therapeutic nitrates as endogenous NO substitutes; and (4) the clinical implications of endogenous and nitrate-derived NO.

ENDOTHELIUM-DEPENDENT VASODILATION

Endothelium-dependent relaxation or vasodilation in response to physical/mechanical, chemical, and humoral stimuli occurs in blood vessels both *in vivo* and in isolated vessels *in vitro*.[2, 3, 7–10] Indeed, acetylcholine relaxes or dilates conduit and resistance arteries and increases local blood flow when infused intraarterially.[11, 12] In the human forearm circulation, intraarterial infusion of acetylcholine causes a pronounced increase in blood flow, unaffected by acetylsalicylic acid (which inhibits the formation of prostacyclin) or by phentolamine (which excludes a contribution by the prejunctional inhibitory effects of the muscarinic agonist on adrenergic neurotransmission).[12] Similarly, in sympathectomized animals, the vasodilator response to intraarterial acetylcholine is maintained,[13] thus indicating that the vasodilator effects of acetylcholine *in vivo* are not mediated by prostacyclin and are independent of the sympathetic nervous system. Further-

more, in the absence of endothelium (de-endothelized vessels), acetylcholine is unable to induce relaxation[2, 3] (Fig. 90–1). Finally, in the human forearm circulation, the vasorelaxant effects of acetylcholine are reduced

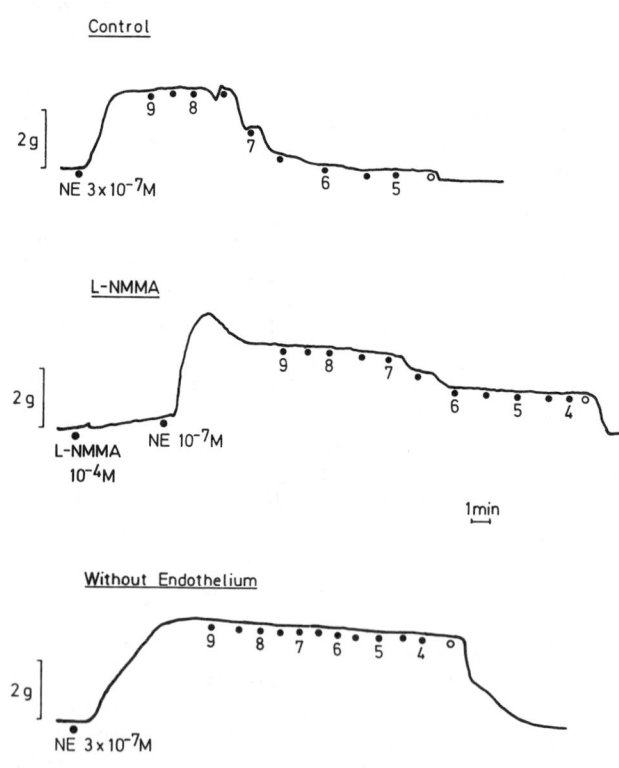

Figure 90–1. Influence of endothelium on acetylcholine-induced relaxation. Acetylcholine relaxed mammary arteries precontracted with norepinephrine (NE) in the presence, but not in the absence, of endothelium, implicating the presence of an endothelium-derived relaxing factor. In vessels with endothelium, acetylcholine-induced relaxations are partially reduced in the presence of L-N^G-monomethyl arginine (L-NMMA), an inhibitor for NO synthesis, suggesting that the relaxing factor generated by endothelium is NO.

by inhibitors of NO formation such as L-N^G-mono-methyl arginine (L-NMMA)[14] (Fig. 90–2).

NATURE OF ENDOTHELIUM-DERIVED RELAXING FACTOR (EDRF)

Interaction between the endothelium and vascular smooth muscle cells could occur either by direct cell-to-cell contact[15, 16] or by local mediators. In conduit arteries, the release of endothelium-derived relaxing factor(s) (EDRF) has been demonstrated using a "sandwich preparation" of the rabbit aorta[3] and confirmed with cascade-bioassay techniques using perfused blood vessels with endothelium or endothelial cells in culture as donor tissues.[17–22] Release of EDRF has also been demonstrated in resistance arteries *in vivo* using intravital microscopy and arteriography as well as *in vitro* using intraarteriolar perfusion and myographic techniques.[2, 23]

Endothelium-dependent relaxations occur in large (conduit) arteries and in resistance vessels of most mammalian species, including humans.[2, 7–10] EDRF release can occur both *in vitro* and *in vivo*.[2, 3, 10–12, 24–26] The release of EDRF can be demonstrated (1) under basal conditions; (2) in response to mechanical forces such as shear stress (exerted by the circulating blood);[27, 28] and (3) after activation of receptor operated mechanisms by acetylcholine, neurotransmitters, various local and circulating hormones, and substances derived from platelets and the coagulation system[10, 24–26] (Fig. 90–3). Because EDRF is a diffusible substance, experiments established to evaluate transit time between the donor segment with endothelium and the bioassay tissue without endothelium allowed the biologic half-life of EDRF to be estimated, which was found to be in the range of a few seconds.[3, 29] The scavenger of superoxide anions, superoxide dismutase, markedly stabilizes EDRF,[29] indicating that oxygen-derived free radical superoxide anion and hemoglobin inactivate the factor.[30] These observations and the stimulatory effects of EDRF on soluble guanylyl cyclase (with concomitant formation of cyclic guanosine 3',5'-monophosphate [cGMP]) led to the proposal[30, 31] that EDRF is the radical NO (see Fig. 90–3). Furthermore, antioxidants such as ascorbic acid, catecholamines, and phenidone inactivate EDRF or NO, demonstrating that the factor is an oxidized substance and that its oxidized state is essential for its biologic activity. Bradykinin releases NO from cultured endothelial cells, and the relaxations induced by exogenous nitric oxide are indistinguishable from those evoked by EDRF.[32] Furthermore, the amount of radical liberated in response to bradykinin (as measured by chemiluminescence) can explain the biologic activity of EDRF. Quantitative studies of NO levels have been difficult because of the labile nature of NO, although more recently intracellular recordings using a sensitive NO microsensor inserted into a single cell and one on the surface of adjacent endothelial cells demonstrated NO production by endothelial cells in response to bradykinin, with subsequent elevation of NO levels in underlying smooth muscle.[33] Hence, these findings, taken with the observations that chemical and biologic similarities exist between EDRF and NO in a variety of blood vessels[31, 32] and that NO is released in response to acetylcholine and the Ca^{2+} ionophore A23187 in rabbit aorta,[34] strongly indicate that the endothelium-derived nitric oxide (EDNO) has the same chemical characteristics as EDRF and is liberated in amounts sufficient to account for the vascular action of EDRF.[32] However, debate continues about whether NO is released as such or together with a carrier molecule (for instance the amino acid L-cysteine) to yield L-nitrocysteine.[35]

Vasodilator effects of NO are associated with an increase in intracellular cyclic 3',5'-guanosine monophosphate (cGMP) in vascular smooth muscle[36] (see Fig. 90–3). The inhibitor of soluble guanylyl cyclase, methylene blue, prevents the production of cGMP and inhibits endothelium-dependent relaxations.[36] Thus, EDNO causes relaxations by stimulating the enzyme and in turn the formation of cGMP (Fig. 90–4).[36] Soluble guanylyl cyclase is also present in platelets and activated by EDNO.[37–39] Increased levels of cGMP in platelets are associated with a reduced adhesion and aggregation (Fig. 90–5). Therefore, EDNO causes both vasodilation and platelet deactivation and thereby represents an important antispastic and antithrombotic feature of the endothelium.

FORMATION OF ENDOTHELIUM-DERIVED NITRIC OXIDE

In the presence of L-arginine, cultured porcine endothelial cells produce NO; when deprived of L-arginine, they lose their capability to generate NO, and upon restoration of L-arginine, their generating capability is restored.[40] It is now clear that EDNO is formed from L-arginine by oxidation of the guanidine-nitrogen terminal of L-arginine[40, 43, 44] (see Fig. 90–2). NO synthase has been cloned.[41] It is primarily a cytosolic enzyme requiring calmodulin, Ca^{2+}, and β-nico-

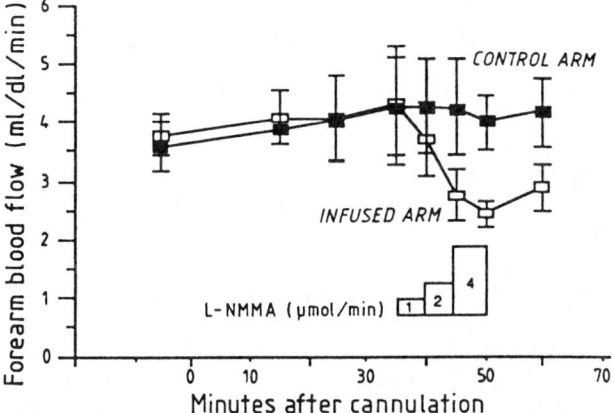

Figure 90–2. Effect of L-N^G-monomethyl arginine (L-NMMA) infusion into the brachial artery. L-NMMA (1 to 4 μmol/min) caused a dose-dependent decrease in basal forearm blood flow. (From Vallance P, Collier J, Moncada S: Effects of endothelium-derived nitric oxide on peripheral arteriolar tone in man. Lancet 2:997, 1989. © by The Lancet Ltd., 1989.)

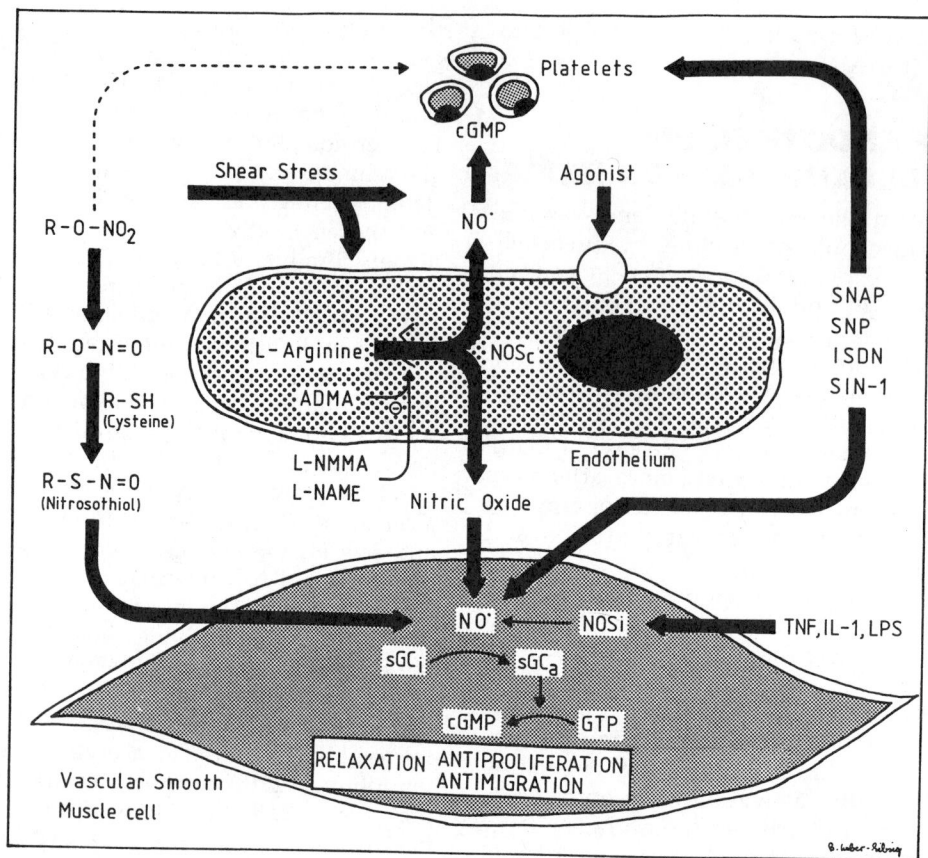

Figure 90–3. The L-arginine pathway in the blood vessel wall. Endothelial cells form nitric oxide (NO) from L-arginine via the activity of the constitutive nitric oxide synthase (NOS$_c$), which can be inhibited by analogues of the amino acid such as isometrical dymethyl arginine (ADMA), L-N^G-monomethyl arginine (L-NMMA), or L-nitroarginine methylester (L-NAME). Nitric oxide activates soluble guanylyl cyclase (sGC) in vascular smooth muscle and platelets, and it causes increases in cyclic 3',5'-guanosine monophosphate (cGMP), which mediates relaxation and platelet inhibition, respectively. Shear stress and receptor-operated agonists stimulate the release of nitric oxide. Vascular smooth muscle cells can form nitric oxide via the activity of an inducible (by tumor necrosis factor [TNF], interleukin-1 [IL-1], and lipopolysaccharide [LPS]) form of nitric oxide synthase (NOSi). Similar to endothelium, nitrovasodilators such as S-nitroso N-acetyl penicillamine (SNAP), sodium nitroprusside (SNP), isosorbide dinitrate (ISDN), and 3-morpholino-sydnonimine (SIN-1) can also generate NO and induce cGMP formation and induce vasorelaxation, antiproliferation, or antimigration effects on the smooth muscle and antiaggregatory effects on platelets. (Modified with permission from Lüscher TF, Vanhoutte PM: The Endothelium: Modulator of Cardiovascular Function. Boca Raton, FL: CRC Press, 1991, pp 1–215.)

tinamide adenine dinucleotide hydrogen phosphate (NADPH). It has similarities with cytochrome P-450 enzymes. Several isoforms of the enzyme occur not only in endothelial cells but also in platelets,[42] neutrophils,[43] macrophages,[44] vascular smooth muscle cells,[45–47] hepatocytes,[48] mesangial cells,[49] Kupffer cells,[50] kidney epithelial cells,[51] renal tubules,[52] neurons,[53] fibroblasts,[54] ovary,[55] and the brain.[56]

The NO synthase in endothelium (eNOS) appears to be expressed constitutively. NO formation in the blood vessels by eNOS is regulated by activation of Ca^{2+}, which binds to calmodulin, forming a complex that is a crucial cofactor for enzyme activity.[57, 58] This Ca^{2+} is made available through stimulation by agents such as acetylcholine and bradykinin that generate inositol 1,4,5-triphosphate (IP$_3$) production via the phosphoinositide second-messenger system. IP$_3$ elicits Ca^{2+} release from intracellular stores by binding to IP$_3$ receptors on the endoplasmic reticulum. Additionally, a portion of mobilized Ca^{2+} is thought to arise extracellularly. Alternatively, agonist-independent

NO release may also contribute to vascular tone. Both shear stress[27, 28] and deformation of vascular endothelium,[59] which accompanies pulsatile flow through blood vessels, stimulate NO release (through poorly defined mechanisms) and cause vasorelaxation by binding to the iron in the heme at the active site of guanylyl cyclase, thereby activating the enzyme to generate cGMP. cGMP may elicit muscle relaxation through influence on a Na^+-Ca^{2+} exchange, by stimulating the phosphorylation of poorly defined substrates by cGMP-dependent protein kinase, via direct action at a cGMP-gated channel, or as a consequence of cGMP-mediated activation or inhibition of phosphodiesterase.[60]

eNOS also has consensus sites for cyclic adenosine monophosphate (cAMP)–dependent phosphorylation.[61] Protein kinase C phosphorylation substantially diminishes NOS catalytic activity, whereas the effects of other types of phosphorylation are less apparent.[61] eNOS also contains a unique site that conceivably could account for the association of eNOS with mem-

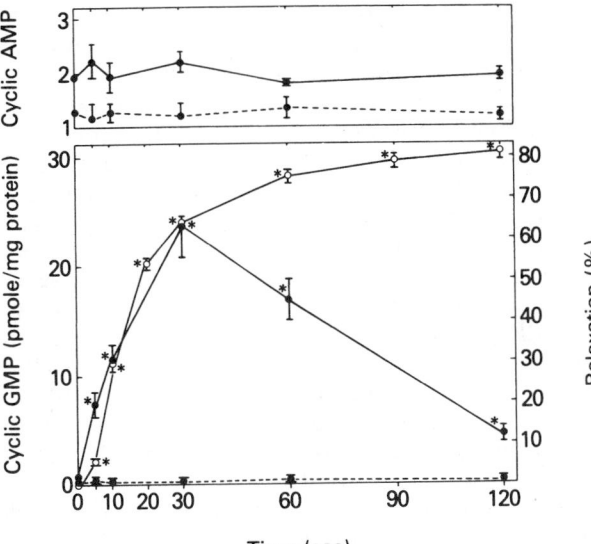

Figure 90–4. Time course and extent of the increase in cyclic 3',5'guanosine monophosphate (cyclic GMP) in the vascular smooth muscle cells of the rat aorta after stimulation with calcium ionophore A23187 (●). The increase in cyclic GMP is transient, whereas the relaxation of aortic rings is sustained (O). (*) Significantly different from control and (–) aortic rings without endothelium. (From Vanhoutte PM, Lüscher TF: In Tarazi RC, Zanchetti A [eds]: Handbook of Hypertension Vol. 8, Physiology and Pathophysiology of Hypertension-Regulatory Mechanisms. Amsterdam: Elsevier, 1986, pp 96–123.)

branes, whereas inducible NOS (found in smooth muscle cells) are cytoplasmic. Hence, the association of eNOS with cell membrane may direct delivery of NO both to underlying smooth muscle for efficient vasoregulation and to the blood-endothelial interface, where NO inhibits platelet aggregation.

In porcine coronary arteries, endothelium-dependent relaxations to serotonin are inhibited by analogues of L-arginine such as L-N^G-monomethyl arginine (L-NMMA) and are restored by L-arginine but not D-arginine.[62] In quiescent arteries, L-NMMA but not D-NMMA causes endothelium-dependent contractions.[63, 64] In intact organs such as the perfused porcine eye, L-nitro arginine methylester (L-NAME) markedly decreases local blood flow (Fig. 90–6).[65] When infused in rabbits, L-NMMA induces long-lasting increases in blood pressure that are reversed by L-arginine[66] (Fig. 90–7). This demonstrates that the vasculature is in a constant state of vasodilation as a result of the continuous basal release of NO from the endothelium. Of particular physiologic and pathophysiologic interest is the more recent discovery of an endogenous inhibitor of the L-arginine NO pathway, i.e., asymmetric dimethyl-arginine[67] (ADMA). This indicates that endogenously produced substances can regulate the activity of this pathway both locally and systemically, as it is also detected in plasma. Hence, an increased production and/or elimination of this endogenous inhibitor can profoundly affect the function of the cardiovascular system (e.g., in patients with renal failure).[67]

MECHANISM OF NITRIC OXIDE RELEASE AND ACTION

Release of NO from vascular endothelium is influenced by several factors that are constantly present in its immediate environment and include circulating neurohumoral factors, platelet-derived factors, and mechanical forces.

Neurohumoral Mediators

The endothelium releases NO in response to neurohumoral factors through the activation of specific endothelial receptors.[2] However, the signal transduction from the receptors to the release of NO differs. In the porcine and canine coronary artery, endothelium-dependent relaxations evoked by serotonin 5-hydroxytryptamine, α_2-adrenergic agonists, and leukotriene C_4 are abolished or reduced by pertussis toxin, which irreversibly ribosylates G_i proteins.[62, 68, 69] In

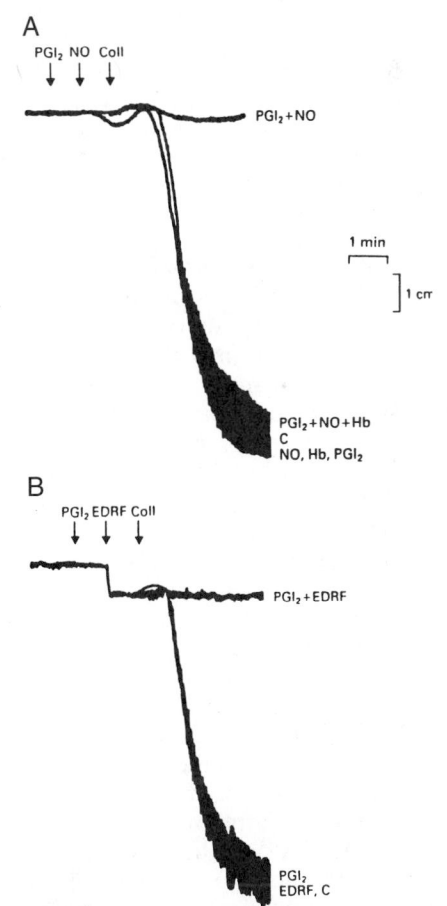

Figure 90–5. Effects of EDRF, NO, or prostacyclin (PGI$_2$) on the aggregation of human platelets in response to collagen (Coll). In the presence of hemoglobin (Hb), the combination of NO and PGI$_2$ cannot prevent aggregation and does not differ from control (C). In the absence of Hb, the same concentration of NO and PGI$_2$ completely inhibits platelet aggregation (*left panel*). Similar results are obtained if EDRF (released from porcine aortic endothelial cells in culture) is used instead of NO. (From Radomski MW, Palmer RMJ, Moncada S: Comparative pharmacology of endothelium-derived relaxing factor, nitric oxide and prostacyclin in platelets. Br J Pharmacol 92:181, 1987.)

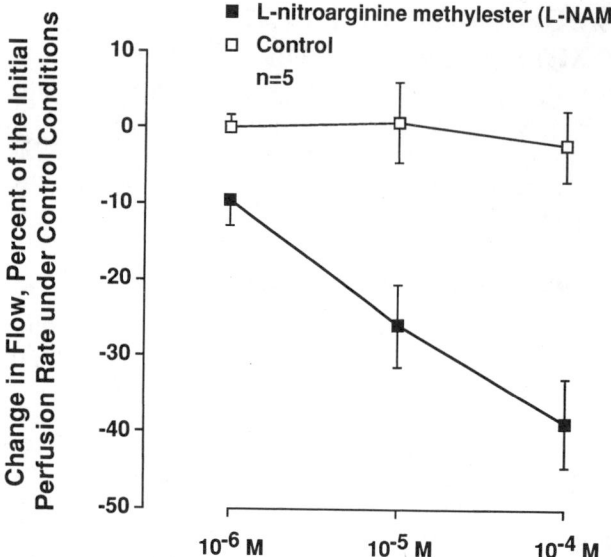

Figure 90–6. Effects of the inhibitor of NO production L-nitro arginine methylester (L-NAME) on ophthalmic flow in the intact perfused porcine eye. While flow in the time control remains constant, L-NAME causes a concentration-dependent potent inhibition of ophthalmic flow, indicating that the ophthalmic circulation is in a constant state of vasodilation as a result of the basal formation of NO. (From Meyer P, Flammer J, Lüscher TF: Endothelium-dependent regulation of the ophthalmic microcirculation in the perfused porcine eye: Role of nitric oxide and endothelins. Invest Ophthalmol Vis Sci 34:3614, 1993.)

release of EDRF.[58] Indeed, depletion of extracellular Ca^{2+} inhibits endothelium-dependent relaxation of muscarinic agonists but not those of the endothelium-independent vasodilator, sodium nitroprusside.[79–81] In addition, in cultured endothelial cells, stimulation of the release of EDRF by bradykinin, adenosine triphosphate (ATP), ADP, thrombin, and melitin is accompanied by an increase in cytoplasmic Ca^{2+} concentrations.[82–84] The contribution of the intracellular release of Ca^{2+} to the augmentation of the cytosolic level of the ion varies; however, the sustained release of EDRF requires the influx of extracellular Ca^{2+}, most likely through a receptor-operated Ca^{2+} channel.[84–89] Indeed, in isolated blood vessels, Ca^{2+} antagonists, such as verapamil or the dihydropyridines, do not prevent endothelium-dependent relaxation by acetylcholine[88–90] (although they may have some effect in perfused arteries[89]). Na^+–K^+ exchanges may also be important.[91] Additionally, intracellular alkalization induced by bradykinin sustains the activation of the constitutive NOS and the alterations in pHi independent of changes in $(Ca^{2+})i$, and represents a second intracellular mechanism for the regulation of cNOS activity in endothelial cells.

The production and/or release of EDRF requires oxygen, because anoxia prevents relaxation induced by acetylcholine but not that caused by endothelium-independent vasodilators.[92–94] In the rabbit aorta, endothelium-independent relaxation is reduced by

contrast, endothelium-dependent relaxation by bradykinin, by adenosine diphosphate (ADP), and particularly by the ionophore A23187 remain unaffected by the toxin.[62, 68–70] In intramyocardial coronary arteries, neither of the receptors is linked to a G_i protein.[63] Thus, at least two distinct biochemical pathways are involved in the release of NO. Loss of functional G_i proteins in regenerated endothelial cells causes a selective dysfunction of the serotonin-induced release of NO in porcine coronary arteries.[70]

In freshly harvested endothelial cells of the rabbit aorta, acetylcholine induces a transient hyperpolarization.[71] The importance of this change in membrane potential for the release of EDRF remains uncertain; however, as cultured endothelial cells preserve electrophysiologic responses, in particular hyperpolarization to acetylcholine,[72, 73] they lose their ability to release EDRF in response to the muscarinic agonist.

Bradykinin and histamine, but not the Ca^{2+} ionophore A23187, stimulate the metabolism of phosphoinositol in cultured endothelial cells,[74, 75] leading to the formation of inositol triphosphate, which induces intracellular Ca^{2+} mobilization.[76, 77] Phorbol esters (which downregulate protein kinase C) inhibit the release of EDRF evoked by acetylcholine or substance P but not that caused by Ca^{2+} ionophore A23187, indicating that diacylglycerol (which is concomitantly formed after activation of phospholipase C) is important in contributing to the release of the factor stimulated by certain receptor-operated agonists.[78]

Increases in intracellular Ca^{2+} in endothelial cells must play a crucial role in the production and/or

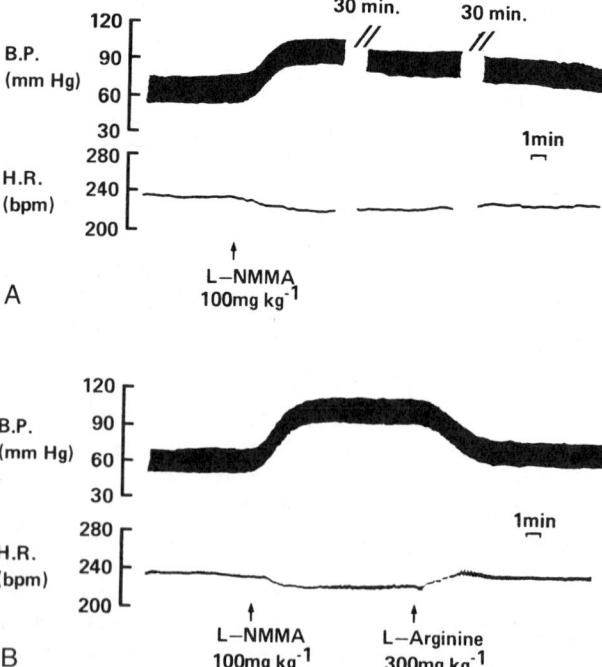

Figure 90–7. Effects of intravenous infusion of L-N^G-monomethyl arginine (L-NMMA) on blood pressure (BP) and heart rate (HR) in the intact rabbit. Infusion of L-NMMA causes a marked increase in systolic and diastolic blood pressure and a decrease in heart rate *(top panel).* This effect can be reversed by high dosages of L-arginine, which competes with L-NAME for the enzyme *(lower panel).* (From Rees DD, Palmer RMJ, Moncada S: The role of endothelium-derived nitric oxide in the regulation of blood pressure. Proc Natl Acad Sci USA 86:3375, 1989.)

agents that inhibit mitochondrial electron transport or that uncouple oxidative phosphorylation, suggesting that the production and/or release of the factor depends on mitochondrial synthesis of ATP.[94]

NO synthase has also been shown to have the capability to produce NO as well as superoxide,[95] and the effects of superoxide and its generation by endothelial cells are modulated by L-arginine, which is a substrate for NO generation, suggesting that NOS may participate in effects such as those involved in ischemia reperfusion.[96–98] Endothelial NO synthase also possesses sequence homology with mammalian cytochrome P-450 reductase enzyme,[41] which donates electrons for the cytochrome P-450–drug metabolizing enzymes. Interestingly, cytochrome P-450 reductase also donates electrons for heme oxygenase, which converts heme to biliverdin and carbon monoxide. Like NO, carbon monoxide stimulates cGMP formation and may thereby modulate vascular tone by relaxing smooth muscle of blood vessels.

NO may also act independent of cGMP. NO enhances ADP ribosylation of platelet proteins.[99] The target of the NO-stimulated ADP ribosylation is glyceraldehyde-3-phosphate-dehydrogenase (GADPH).[100, 101] GADPH is auto-ADP-ribosylated, a process that is stimulated by NO. Since ADP ribosylation involves the specific cysteine associated with NAD-dependent catalysis, ADP ribosylation involved inhibits GADPH activity. The decreased glycolysis associated with NO enhanced GADPH-ADP ribosylation could well mediate a number of actions of NO, such as myocardial stunning and hibernation, reperfusion injury, and neurotoxity. The physiologic relevance of NO-mediated ADP ribosylation awaits further investigation. Effects of NO on mitochondrial iron-sulfur enzymes may also mediate NO actions.[102]

More recently, endothelial NO synthase has been cloned,[44, 103–105] and it has been shown that NOS requires multiple oxidative cofactors that are associated with specific binding sites for oxidizing L-arginine to release NO. The cloned enzyme displays binding sites for NADPH, flavin adenine dinucleotide, and flavin mononucleotide. After treatment with carbon monoxide, NOS absorbs light at 450 nm, indicating properties of a cytochrome P-450 enzyme. NOS activity is also enhanced by tetrahydrobiopterin.[106, 107] The sequential transfer of electrons between the various cofactors facilitates catalytic function, culminating in heme directly donating the electrons that oxidize the guanidine moiety of arginine. All isoforms of NOS cloned thus far possess a recognition site for calmodulin.[108]

Mechanical Factors

Several mechanical factors, such as the shear forces acting on the endothelium as the blood flow is increased, can enhance the release of NO from the endothelial cells. Indeed both enhancement of flow[27, 28] and the onset of highly pulsatile flow with rhythmic dilations of the vascular wall have been shown to lead to increased release of EDRF (as observed by using detector vessels in the bioassay).[59, 108, 109] The magnitude of the contribution made by hyperpolarization due to shear stress and an increase in K+ conductivity has not yet been defined, although involvement of multiple K+ channels in mediating the release of NO in response to pulsatile and time-averaged shear stress has recently been reported.[110] Comparison of the effects of Ca^{2+} and calmodulin antagonists and protein kinase inhibitor H-7 on bradykinin and flow-mediated production of NO suggests that the initial laminar flow–stimulated NO production is very similar to bradykinin-mediated production and is Ca^{2+}- and calmodulin-dependent.[111] However, with continued exposure to flow, NO production was found to be a Ca^{2+}- and calmodulin-independent process that is shear stress and kinase dependent,[110] suggesting that the flow-mediated action of a kinase(s) on NOS may change the requirement of the enzyme for Ca^{2+} and calmodulin.[110, 111]

In vivo experiments using dogs have shown that chronic exercise stimulates the release of NO from coronary vascular endothelial cells and mediates the epicardial coronary artery dilation in response to brief occlusion and acetylcholine. Furthermore, NOS activity in the vasculature of exercising dogs was significantly increased after chronic exercise.[112]

ENDOTHELIAL EFFECTS OF NITRIC OXIDE

Endothelial cells contain soluble and particulate guanylyl cyclase and can form cGMP.[113] A number of stimuli that cause the release of EDRF, as well as nitrovasodilators and exogenous NO, augment the accumulation of cGMP by cultured endothelial cells.[113–115] The accumulation is inhibited by hemoglobin and methylene blue and augmented by superoxide dismutase.[114] The presence of the analogue of the cyclic nucleotide, 8-bromo cGMP, blunts relaxation evoked by acetylcholine and substance P, whereas ATP, A23187, and nitrovasodilators are unaffected.[116] One possible reason for the increase in cGMP is that EDRF feeds back in a negative fashion on its own release by activating the soluble guanyl cyclase of the endothelial cells.[113, 114–117]

NO itself can indeed affect the production of NO by endothelial cells by negative feedback mechanisms. It has recently been shown that treatment of purified eNOS as well as cultured endothelial cells with NO derived from NO-donor compounds or NO gas caused a marked inhibition of NO biosynthesis in response to both increased fluid shear stress and bradykinin.[117] More interestingly, human umbilical vein and arterial endothelial cells in culture synthesize an inhibitor of NO biosynthesis, N^G-dimethylarginine from L-arginine, as well as metabolize L-NMMA to citrulline and arginine and could possibly also metabolize ADMA through a similar pathway.[118] These results provide a potential mechanism for the physiologic and pathophysiologic regulation of NO synthesis within the endothelium.

Endothelium-derived NO can interact with endothelin production[119] (Fig. 90–8).[120] Indeed, production of the peptide from the endothelium of intact porcine aorta upon stimulation with thrombin is augmented in the presence of L-NMMA and methylene blue.[119] Because thrombin is known to cause endothelium-dependent relaxation in a variety of blood vessels, this indicates that the enzyme concomitantly activates the formation of NO and endothelin in the intima of intact blood vessels and that the former inhibits the production of the latter.[120, 121] In line with that observation, superoxide dismutase as well as the nonhydrolysable analogue of cGMP, 8-bromo cGMP, prevents the thrombin-induced formation of endothelin.[119] Similarly, nitrates such as 3-morpholino-sydnonimine (SIN-1) or nitroglycerin inhibit the production of endothelin induced by the enzyme[120] (see Fig. 90–8). Three inhibitory mechanisms regulating endothelin production have been delineated: (1) cGMP-dependent inhibition,[119, 122] (2) cAMP-dependent inhibition,[123] and (3) an inhibitory factor produced by vascular smooth muscle cells.[124] The cGMP-dependent mechanism can be activated by EDNO, nitroglycerin, SIN-1,[119, 120] and atrial natriuretic peptide (which activates particulate guanylyl cyclase).[2, 122] Thus, after inhibition of the endothelial L-arginine pathway, the thrombin-induced production of endothelin is augmented;[119] on the other hand, SIN-1 prevents the thrombin-induced endothelin release via a cGMP-dependent mechanism.[120] Endothelin can also release NO and prostacyclin from endothelial cells (via ET_B receptors),[125–127] which may represent a negative feedback mechanism.[128, 129] EDNO also interacts with the effects of endothelin at the level of vascular smooth muscle. Indeed, the contractions to the peptide are enhanced after endothelial removal, indicating that basal production of EDNO reduces its response.[130] Stimulation of the formation of EDNO by acetylcholine reverses endothelin-induced contractions in most blood vessels, although this mechanism appears to be less potent in veins.[130, 131]

Nitric Oxide and Renin-Angiotensin System

Indirect evidence also shows interaction between angiotensin II and EDNO. For example, part of the increases in arterial pressure during NO inhibition by L-NAME are suggested to be due to increases in angiotensin II concentrations. Indeed, plasma renin activity increases during L-NAME treatment in dogs[132] and rats.[133] Furthermore, angiotensin II antagonism with losartan attenuated the increase in arterial pressure,[133] although preliminary studies by Samsell et al.[134] suggest that acute losartan administration to rats on long-term oral L-NAME did not cause a decrease in arterial pressure.

Humoral Effects of Nitric Oxide

EDRF released from isolated blood vessels in the dog reduces the production of renin (demonstrated in slices of canine kidneys).[135] Anatomically, endothelial cells and juxtaglomerular cells are in close proximity in the wall of the preglomerular arterioles. Because endothelial cells can respond to shear stress, with an increased release of EDRF, modulation of renin release by the factor could link changes in perfusion pressure in the afferent arterioles with the release of renin enzyme. Hence, endothelial cells may act as the intrarenal baroreceptor.

HETEROGENEITY IN ENDOTHELIUM-DERIVED NITRIC OXIDE RELEASE

Hemodynamic and histologic studies provide evidence indicating functional and structural heterogeneity among endothelial cells of conduit and resistance vasculature as well as within the same vasculature.[2]

Large (Conduit) versus Resistance Arteries

Endothelial cells from conduit as well as resistance arteries are known to produce NO in response to acetylcholine;[2, 137] however, the amount of NO generated differs.[23, 136–138] Immunohistochemical localization of NOS demonstrated substantially lower amounts of NOS expression in small arteries,[139] sug-

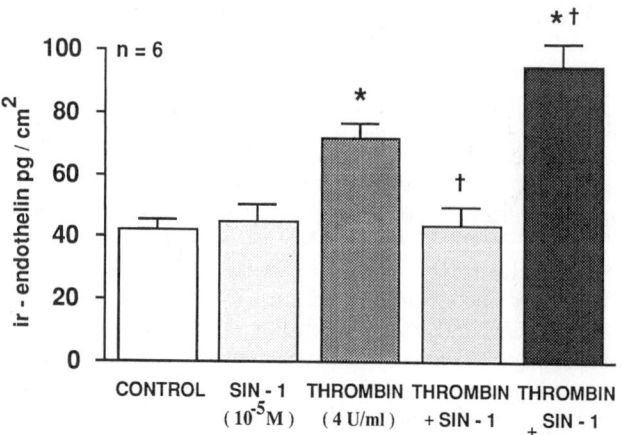

Figure 90–8. Effect of NO donor 3-morpholino-sydnonimine (SIN-1) on the production of endothelin induced by thrombin (4 IU/ml) in porcine aortas with endothelium. The amount of peptide produced is expressed as picograms immunoreactive (ir) endothelin released per square centimeter of intimal surface after 4 hours of incubation. Methylene blue (MB) was used to inhibit guanylyl cyclase. *$p < .05$ versus control; † $p < .05$ versus thrombin alone. (Reproduced with permission from Boulanger C, Lüscher TF: Hirudin and nitric oxide donors inhibit the thrombin-induced release of endothelin from the intact porcine aorta. Circ Res 68:1768, 1990. Copyright 1990, American Heart Association.)

gesting that the endothelial cells of resistance arteries may generate less NO and possibly more of a second factor, most likely EDHF.[2] Decreased release of NO within the renal arterioles was also demonstrated by Kon et al.,[139] who suggested that EDRF is mainly produced in conduit arteries and acts on downstream microcirculation. However, in contrast with their findings, several other groups have now successfully demonstrated the generation of NO within the renal microcirculation.[140] Nevertheless, it is possible that the amounts of NO generated may differ between the conduit and resistance beds. Arterioles in Dahl-S rats on 0.45% NaCl diet dilate in response to L-arginine,[23] suggesting that basal NO production in these vessels may be limited by the availability of endogenous substrate. L-Arginine also dilates arterioles in the rat cremaster muscle, and this response has been shown to be endothelium-dependent.[141] In addition, L-arginine decreases renal, mesenteric, and hind quarter vascular resistance in the rat,[142] suggesting that substrate availability may limit basal NO production in a number of organs. However, arterioles of hypertensive rats are unaffected by L-arginine at concentrations that cause vasodilation in normotensive DS rats, suggesting that in this model the absence of basal NO synthesis/release is not due to a lack of available substrate.[23]

Production, as well as action of agonist-induced endothelium-derived NO, may also vary within the same vessel. For example, in presence of either normal or abnormal endothelial function, acetylcholine and serotonin cause a preferentially distal constriction in the coronary artery.[138, 143] Furthermore, the differences in action tend to be extremely concentration dependent, and at selective stimulus concentrations opposite responses have been observed in different segments within the same coronary artery. For instance, acetylcholine tends to produce focal spasms of coronary arteries at the site of ergonovine-induced spasm.[144] Nevertheless, acetylcholine-induced vasodilation at the same sites have also been observed.[2] Hence, differences in release of NO in epicardial arteries and in resistance vessels could importantly contribute to the pathophysiology of hypertension and atherosclerosis.

Arteries versus Veins

Basal and stimulated release of NO is less pronounced in human veins than in arteries.[10, 64] This difference between human arteries and veins has also been demonstrated in vivo.[14, 145] In line with this observation, removal of the endothelium augments the contractile response to norepinephrine and serotonin in the mammary artery, but not in the saphenous vein.[64, 146] Furthermore, agonist-stimulated release of EDNO is much larger from arteries than from veins,[10, 64, 146, 147] and this heterogeneity of endothelium-dependent responses between arteries and veins is determined by different properties of the endothelium rather than those of the smooth muscle cells. Indeed, in general, veins respond better to NO or nitrovasodilators.[2]

SEX HORMONES AND ENDOTHELIUM-DERIVED NITRIC OXIDE

Increased cardiovascular risk in postmenopausal women[148] and lack of cardiovascular complications in normally ovulating women as compared with their age-matched men have led to the possibility that sex steroids could play an important role in this process. Similar to NO, estrogen inhibits smooth muscle cell migration and proliferation, increases blood flow, and modulates vascular tone, all processes importantly involved in the pathophysiology of hypertension and atherosclerosis.[149] Studies provide evidence that sex steroids can increase NO's expression by endothelial cells.[150] Sex steroids have been shown to be responsible for gender differences in EDRF/NO release from aorta of SHR.[151] Treatment of male and female gonadectomized SHR rats with estrogen and testosterone for 2 weeks showed that vasorelaxant effects due to EDRF/NO released in response to acetylcholine increased significantly in estrogen-treated male gonadectomized SHRs, whereas the same response was reduced in testosterone-treated female gonadectomized rats, suggesting that sex steroids modulate release of NO from endothelium and could be associated importantly with atherosclerotic vascular disease in postmenopausal women.[9] Estrogen treatment in vivo and in cultured bovine and porcine aortic endothelial cells significantly induced NOS activity in the heart and in cultured endothelial cells, respectively.[152] Although estrogen seems to be the most important regulator of NO synthesis, testosterone, follicle stimulating hormone, and progesterone have also been shown to modulate NO synthesis[153-155] and could individually, or in conjunction with other factors, importantly affect the basal release of NO and hence the vasculature.

RELEASE OF NITRIC OXIDE BY NONENDOTHELIAL CELLS

In addition to vascular endothelial cells, several other vascular as well as nonvascular cells are capable of generating NO either through the constitutive (i.e., endothelial cells, neurons, and platelets) or inducible form of NOS (i.e., macrophages, vascular smooth muscle cells [VSMC]).[2]

Several white blood cells such as leukocytes and monocytes/macrophages are able to produce NO, particularly if stimulated with cytokines and other substances, as they express the inducible form of NO synthase.[43, 44, 156, 157] The capacity of these cells to produce large amounts of NO if appropriately stimulated may contribute to local inflammatory responses of the microcirculation (in particular to the increased local tissue blood flow) as well as exerting a toxic effect important for immune responses.

RELEASE OF NITRIC OXIDE BY SMOOTH MUSCLE CELLS

Although vascular smooth muscles do not have any constitutive NO synthase, they do express inducible NO synthase when stimulated with cytokines such as interleukin-1β, tumor necrosis factor-alpha, and lipopolysaccharide[45–47] (see Fig. 90–3). The amounts of NO generated by smooth muscle cells in response to these agents is considerably higher and of longer duration than that generated by endothelial cells in response to various agonists. Hence, under pathologic situations, when the endothelium is damaged, the increased expression of cytokines at the site of injury may induce NO formation by the underlying smooth muscle cells and this could play an important role in the regulation of tone and growth, as well as platelet aggregation and adherence, at the site of injury.

VASCULAR EFFECTS OF ENDOTHELIUM-DERIVED NITRIC OXIDE

In blood vessels with endothelium, the relaxation induced by acetylcholine, histamine, and the Ca^{2+} ionophore A23187 .is associated with an increase in the intracellular concentration of cGMP in smooth muscle cells[36, 158] (see Fig. 90–4). The rise in cGMP in cells slightly precedes vascular relaxation. Removal of the endothelium prevents formation of cGMP induced by acetylcholine but not that evoked by sodium nitroprusside, nitroglycerin, or exogenous NO.[36] The inhibitor of soluble guanylyl cyclase, methylene blue, prevents or reverses endothelium-dependent relaxation by acetylcholine,[2, 10, 159] suggesting that the cyclic nucleotide mediates the vascular action of EDRF.

In quiescent aortas of rat and rabbit, the inhibitors of cGMP phosphodiesterase induce endothelium-dependent relaxation, suggesting that in intact blood vessels guanylyl cyclase is continuously activated.[160] Indeed, basal levels of cGMP are higher in preparations with, than those without, endothelium and are higher in cultured vascular smooth muscle grown in coculture with endothelial cells than in smooth muscle grown alone.[161]

Several mechanisms have been proposed to explain why cGMP induces vascular relaxation, including decreases in intracellular calcium and inhibitory effects on phosphoinositol metabolism and on protein kinases. Rat aortas with endothelium have a lower $^{45}Ca^{2+}$ content than those without endothelium, suggesting that EDRF released under basal conditions reduces Ca^{2+} influx, inhibits Ca^{2+} mobilization from intracellular stores, or augments the efflux of the ion.[162] In the rabbit aorta, endothelium-dependent relaxation evoked by acetylcholine is associated with a reduced Ca^{2+} influx.[163] Inhibitors of EDRF, such as phenidone, prevent the response, whereas sodium nitroprusside and 8-bromo-cGMP mimic it. Thus, EDRF induces relaxation in part by decreasing Ca^{2+} entry. Furthermore, cGMP, by activating protein kinase, stimulates cyclic 3′,5′-adenosine monophosphate–

dependent Ca^{2+} extrusion across the sarcolemma of vascular smooth muscle.[164]

cGMP inhibits the breakdown of phosphatidylinositol in vascular smooth muscle and in platelets,[76, 165, 166] but removal of the endothelium increases the hydrolysis of phosphatidylinositide with increased accumulation of inositol monophosphate in the aorta of the rat and rabbit.[76] Similar effects can be observed after the lysis of the endothelium or after inhibition of guanylyl cyclase.[76]

Finally, in the aorta, acetylcholine and sodium nitroprusside decrease the incorporation of labeled phosphate into myosin light chains.[36, 167, 168] Removal of the endothelium abolishes the effect of the muscarinic agonist but not that of the nitrovasodilator. Thus, EDRF may act through a cGMP-dependent protein kinase that controls the phosphorylation and dephosphorylation of myosin light chains.

ANTIPLATELET EFFECTS OF NITRIC OXIDE

Platelets also contain the enzyme soluble guanylyl cyclase and can form cGMP,[42, 169, 170] but increased production of cyclic nucleotide is associated with reduced platelet adhesion and aggregation. EDRF as well as exogenous NO inhibits platelet adhesion to the endothelium and platelet aggregation *in vitro* and *in vivo*[37–39, 42, 169–173] (see Fig. 90–5). Both also increase the content of cGMP and reduce the thrombin-induced rise in intracellular Ca^{2+}.[39, 174–178]

The potency of EDRF as an antiaggregant and disaggregant substance is comparable to prostacyclin.[33, 169] Prostacyclin and NO potentiate each other even at subthreshold concentrations in their antiaggregatory action.[33, 173] In the rabbit, intravenous infusions of the muscarinic agonist carbachol increase the platelet content in cGMP and inhibit aggregation induced by ADP.[172] Because both effects can be prevented by the simultaneous administration of either methylene blue or hemoglobin, EDRF is the most likely mediator.

Platelets are also able to stimulate NO[9, 24, 25] (see Fig. 90–8). Once released, platelet-derived NO can interact with the endothelium and vascular smooth muscle cells of the blood vessel wall. Interestingly, at the level of the endothelium, aggregating platelets release enough ATP and ADP to stimulate the release of endothelium-derived NO and cause endothelium-dependent relaxation in normal human arteries.[9, 25] ATP/ADP and, at least in certain arteries, serotonin can activate P_2-purinergic or $5HT_1$-serotonergic receptors, respectively, and both receptors, if present, are linked to the release of NO. Thus, release of EDRF in response to platelet-derived products may provide a negative feedback mechanism inhibiting adhesion and aggregation of the platelets at sites where they are activated. Hence, in intact blood vessels, aggregating platelets cause endothelium-dependent relaxations[9, 24, 25] even though they release potent vasoconstrictors such as thromboxane A_2 and serotonin.

In isolated vessels with intact endothelium, thrombin induces vasorelaxation through the generation of

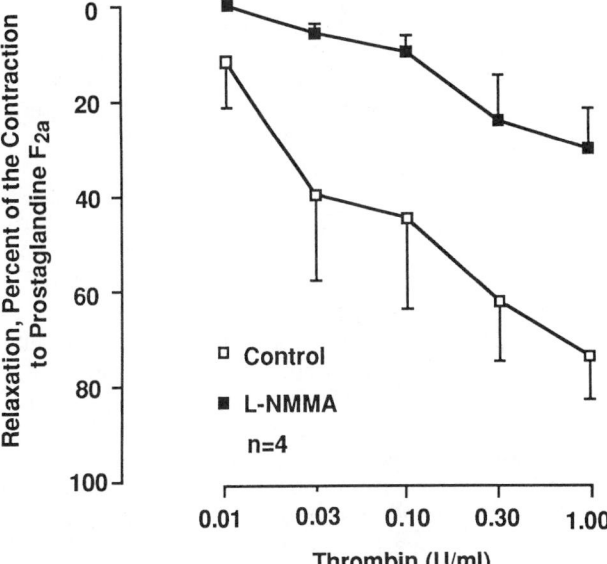

Figure 90–9. Thrombin induced endothelium-dependent relaxation of human coronary artery. Thrombin induced relaxation of mammary arteries precontracted with prostaglandin F_{2a}, an effect that was significantly reduced in the presence of NO synthesis inhibitor L-NMMA.

both NO and prostacyclin; this, in turn, also prevents platelet activation (Fig. 90–9). On the other hand, in vessels denuded of endothelium, thrombin induces profound platelet activation, and, in turn, the release of thromboxane A_2, which causes marked contraction and further platelet activation.[25, 179]

ANTIPROLIFERATIVE EFFECTS OF NITRIC OXIDE

Several vasoactive factors released from the endothelium have also been shown to influence growth of the underlying smooth muscle cells.[180] NO inhibits mitogenesis and cytokinesis of cultured vascular smooth muscle cells from both conduit as well as resistance arteries.[181–185] Whether endothelial cells generate enough NO to inhibit growth has not yet been demonstrated; however, NO released from cytokine-stimulated smooth muscle cells in cocultures has been shown to inhibit the growth of smooth muscle cells induced by fetal calf serum,[185] suggesting that endogenously generated NO is capable of inhibiting growth. Furthermore, several growth factors like platelet-derived growth factor (PDGF), basic fibroblast growth factor (bFGF), and epidermal growth factor (EGF) have been shown to induce growth of aortic smooth muscle cells (SMC) by modulating the release of NO.[185] Additionally, chemically derived NO (generated from vasodilators like S-nitroso N-acetyl penicillamine, sodium nitroprusside, and isosorbide dinitrate) inhibits fetal calf serum as well as angiotensin-induced growth of renal arteriolar smooth muscle cells[183] (Fig. 90–10). Because NO mediates its effect through the generation of cGMP, it has been shown that cGMP can also inhibit the growth of cultured smooth muscle cells.[183, 184] cGMP levels have been shown to increase in smooth muscle cells, mesangial cells, and cocultured endothelial cells and when treated with acetylcholine or bradykinin.[49, 113–115, 158, 161, 163] Additionally, more recently it has been shown that

heparin, a potent inhibitor of smooth muscle cell growth inhibitor generated by the endothelium, actually stimulates the release of NO from the endothelial cells,[186] which in turn could inhibit SMC growth. These observations would suggest that endothelial cells could also inhibit smooth muscle growth by generating NO.

In addition to smooth muscle cell proliferation, the abnormal vascular growth process in hypertension and atherosclerosis involves the migration of medial smooth muscle into the intima and consequently proliferation or rearrangement of migrated cells to form neointima.[187–189] These changes contribute importantly to the increased peripheral resistance observed

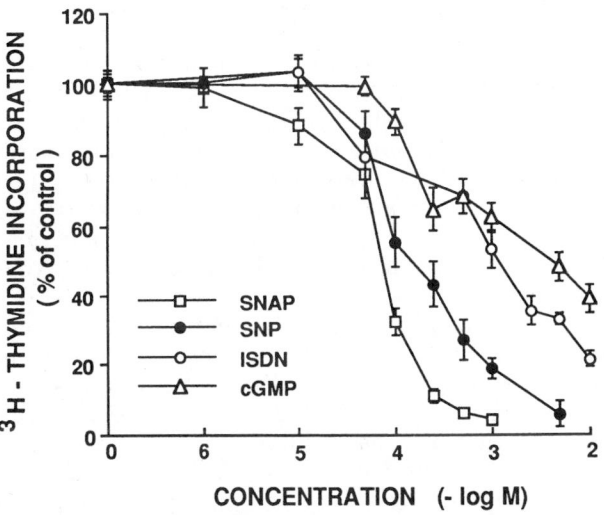

Figure 90–10. Inhibitory effects of nitrovasodilators {S-nitroso N-acetyl penicillamine (SNAP), sodium nitroprusside (SNP), isosorbide dinitrate (ISDN), and 8 bromo-cyclic 3',5'-guanosine monophosphate (cGMP) on fetal calf serum (FCS 5%) induced growth (DNA synthesis) of renal arteriolar smooth muscle cells. (From Dubey RK: Vasodilator-derived nitric oxide inhibits calf serum- and angiotensin-II-induced growth of renal arteriolar smooth muscle cells. J Pharm Exp Ther 269:402, 1994.)

in hypertension. PDGF, bFGF, and other growth factors known to increase at sites of endothelial injury in atherosclerosis (in conjunction with platelets and macrophages) are capable of inducing both proliferation and migration of smooth muscle cells. NO derived from nitrovasodilators and cytokine-stimulated smooth muscle cells inhibits fetal calf serum, PDGF, bFGF, EGF, and angiotensin II–induced growth of aortic and arteriolar smooth muscle cells.[180–185, 188] Additionally, we have shown that chemically derived NO, cGMP, and endogenous NO generated from interleukin-1β–stimulated smooth muscle cells inhibit angiotensin II–induced migration[181] and could play an important role in the remodeling aspect of the vessels during the pathogenesis of hypertension, atherosclerosis, and restenosis.[188] These findings suggest that NO generated from endothelium as well as from cytokine-stimulated smooth muscle cells (as could be the case when vascular injury occurs) can inhibit smooth muscle cell growth.

ENDOTHELIUM-DERIVED NITRIC OXIDE IN CLINICAL ARENA
Endothelium-Derived Nitric Oxide and Hypertension

Hypertension is associated with morphologic and functional alterations of the endothelium. In hypertensive blood vessels, endothelial cells have an increased volume and bulge into the lumen. The subintimal space exhibits structural changes with increased fibrin and cell disposition. Furthermore, the interaction of platelets and monocytes with the endothelium is increased as compared with normotensive controls.

Endothelium-dependent relaxations to acetylcholine are reduced in the aorta and the cerebral and peripheral microcirculation but not in the coronary circulation of hypertensive rats.[190–197] The vasodilator effects of acetylcholine in the human forearm of hypertensive subjects are blunted.[12, 198–200] However, not all the patients with hypertension appear to have endothelium dysfunction, at least not in the forearm circulation.[201] In contrast with the rat, in the human coronary circulation, impaired vasodilator responses occur in both epicardial and microvessels of hypertensive patients, in particular in the presence of left ventricular hypertrophy.[202–204]

In experimental animals, the degree of impairment of endothelium-dependent responses is positively correlated with the level of blood pressure and seems to become more pronounced as hypertension develops and with increased duration of hypertension.[205] This suggests that most, if not all, of the dysfunction of the endothelium occurring in hypertension is a consequence rather than a cause of hypertension. This could also explain why the degree of dysfunction differs in different studies, or may even be absent in early and/or mild hypertension. More recent data, however, demonstrated that already in pedigrees of hypertensive parents, endothelium-dependent vasodilation in the human forearm circulation may be impaired in the presence of normal blood pressure.[206] As under most circumstances, the response to the direct vasodilator sodium nitroprusside remains preserved; impaired responses to acetylcholine must be related to alterations in endothelial function.

Role of Endogenous Nitric Oxide in Hypertension

Endothelium-dependent responses of hypertensive arteries could be impaired as a result of (1) a decreased release of EDNO, (2) a decreased release of other endothelium-derived vasodilator substances such as EDHF or prostacyclin, (3) an impaired diffusion of these substances from the endothelium to the vascular smooth muscle cells, (4) a decreased responsiveness of the vascular smooth muscle cells to vasodilator substances, and/or (5) an augmented release of endothelium-derived contracting factors (Fig. 90–11).[207] Furthermore, the possibility has to be considered that at least under certain conditions the L-arginine/NO pathway is overactive as a compensatory mechanism in hypertension.

Formation of Nitric Oxide

The basal formation of NO (as assessed by the contractile effects of inhibitors of NO production) is reduced in established but not in early hypertension of spontaneously hypertensive rats (SHR), renovascular hypertensive rats (i.e., in mesenteric resistance arteries), and in the coronary arteries but not the aorta of ren-2 transgenic rats.[208, 209] Indeed, in the mesenteric resistance circulation, L-NMMA increases vasoconstrictor responses to norepinephrine more in Wistar-Kyoto rats than in the SHR.[209a] On the other hand, bioassay measurement EDRF in the aorta of the SHR revealed normal vasodilator effects.[210, 211] In the coronary arteries of ren-2 transgenic rats, endothelium-dependent contractions to L-NAME become markedly blunted as the duration of hypertension increases, whereas in the aorta the reverse is true.[209] Similarly, in patients with essential hypertension, infusion of L-NMMA into the brachial artery causes less vasoconstriction (or decreases in forearm blood flow) in hypertensive patients as compared with normotensive subjects, although the response to phenylephrine is comparable.[212] This suggests that the basal formation of NO is also reduced in patients with essential hypertension.

In an attempt to restore reduced endothelium-dependent vasodilation in patients with essential hypertension, Panza et al.[213] infused L-arginine, which augmented the vasodilation response to acetylcholine in normal subjects, whereas the responses to acetylcholine remained unchanged in subjects with essential hypertension. The ineffectiveness of L-arginine in improving endothelium-dependent vasodilation in hypertensive subjects could involve (1) reduced expression of muscarinic receptors (and possibly other endothelial receptors linked to L-arginine/NO pathway), (2) impaired signal transduction, (3) an altered

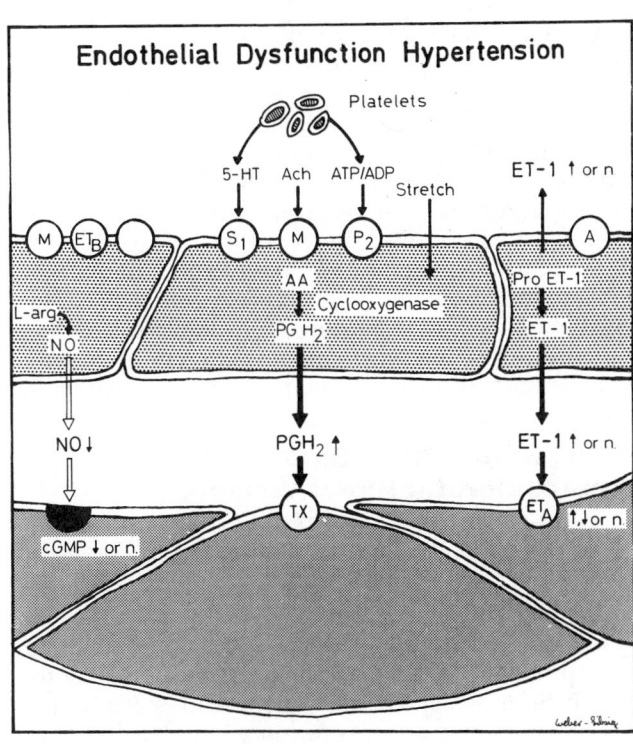

Figure 90–11. Endothelial dysfunction in hypertension. In hypertension, the basal formation of NO appears to be reduced under most conditions, whereas the stimulated formation of NO appears to be impaired in more advanced hypertension. In addition, the hypertensive endothelium can form cyclooxygenase-derived contracting factor (prostaglandin H_2; PGH_2). The effects of endothelin (ET-1) in hypertension are controversial. Increased, but mostly normal, circulating levels have been reported. The vascular responsiveness to endothelin can be reduced, normal, or increased. The concomitant reduced formation and responsiveness of vascular smooth muscle to endothelium-derived nitric oxide (NO) leads to an imbalance between NO and endothelium-derived contracting factors (EDCF), which may contribute to the increased peripheral vascular resistance and complications of hypertension. 5HT, serotonin; Ach, acetylcholine; L-arg, L-arginine; AA, arachidonic acid; cGMP, cyclic guanosine monophosphate. (Reproduced with permission from Lüscher TF, Boulanger CM, Dohi Y, et al: Endothelium-derived contracting factors [brief review]. Hypertension 19:117, 1992. Copyright 1992, American Heart Association.)

uptake mechanism of L-arginine into the endothelium, and/or (4) impaired activity of NO synthase. The possibility of a reduced responsiveness of hypertensive vascular smooth muscle to NO can be excluded, because the response to sodium nitroprusside was identical in normotensive and hypertensive subjects.[198–200] Quite a different explanation may be the possibility that an endothelium-derived contracting factor[196, 207] is formed in hypertensive patients as suggested by experimental work. This has also been observed in hypertensive patients in whom treatment with a cyclooxygenase inhibitor such as indomethacin improved endothelium-dependent vasodilation to acetylcholine.[200] However, because inhibition of cyclooxygenase-derived contracting factor (most likely prostaglandin H_2) does not normalize endothelium-dependent vasodilation in hypertensive subjects, this strongly suggests an additional defect that may, in fact, involve the L-arginine pathway, as discussed earlier.

In perfused mesenteric resistance arteries of the SHR, endothelium-dependent relaxations are reduced upon intraluminal but not extraluminal application of acetylcholine.[209a] This suggests that the intraluminal side of the endothelium, which is most exposed to blood pressure, is particularly prone to develop endothelial dysfunction.

However, not all hypertensive blood vessels and not all forms of hypertension are exhibiting alterations of the L-arginine/NO pathway. Indeed, in the coronary circulation of the SHR, very little endothelial dysfunction can be observed, even in very old rats.[197] Similarly, in the aorta of these animals, endothelium-dependent relaxations are normal in the presence of indomethacin[196] (to prevent the formation of vasocon-

strictor cyclooxygenase products; see Fig. 90–11). Also, bioassay experiments using the perfused SHR aorta revealed comparable amounts of biologically active NO.[210, 211] Bioassay experiments indicate that, at least in spontaneously hypertensive rats, luminal release of EDRF and prostacyclin induced by acetylcholine and histamine is normal or slightly increased.[210, 211] Furthermore, direct measurement of the L-arginine pathway in the aorta of the SHR revealed normal activity of NO synthase.[214] Hence, under certain conditions, the pathway may be augmented, presumably as a counter regulatory mechanism.

Impaired Response of Vascular Smooth Muscle Cell to Nitric Oxide

In contrast with the SHR, the Dahl rat aorta does not release a cyclooxygenase-dependent EDCF in response to acetylcholine, because indomethacin has no effect on the response to the muscarinic agonist.[205, 214a] Thus, it is likely that in this model, as in the aorta of DOCA-salt and renal hypertensive rats, a reduced responsiveness of the vascular smooth muscle to NO and possibly also an impaired diffusion of the factor from the endothelium to the vascular smooth muscle cells (as a result of extensive subendothelial thickening) are responsible for the blunted endothelium-dependent relaxations.[2]

To judge from experiments with sodium nitroprusside, which also induces relaxations by increasing cGMP,[36] the responsiveness of vascular smooth muscle cells to NO is normal in small mesenteric arteries and in the aorta of the SHR.[209a] Van de Voorde and Leusen[211] found normal relaxations to sodium nitroprusside in the aorta of DOCA-salt and renal hypertensive rats. This contrasts with findings of others in these forms of hypertension and in hypertensive Dahl rats in whom the relaxations to nitrovasodilators were found to be impaired.[214a] However, the relaxations were much less impaired than those to acetylcholine, and the maximal relaxation was not decreased. This would suggest that reduced responsiveness of hypertensive arteries to NO may not fully explain the blunted relaxations to acetylcholine. The different results published in the literature may be related to the duration of hypertension, as it appears that the response to NO becomes impaired as the hypertensive vascular changes become more pronounced.

Endogenous Nitric Oxide and Atherosclerotic Blood Vessels

Role of Endogenous Nitric Oxide in Hyperlipidemia

Morphologically, the endothelium remains intact in this prestage of atherogenesis.[215] Functionally, however, pronounced alterations occur, as far as both endothelium-dependent relaxations and the production of contracting factors are concerned. Particularly, oxidized low-density lipoproteins (OX-LDL) are present in human atherosclerotic lesions, and they may be important for the functional changes.[216]

Basal Release of Nitric Oxide

Chester et al.[217] examined the effect of L-NMMA on the basal tone and endothelium-dependent relaxation in atherosclerotic human epicardial coronary arteries. The basal release of nitric oxide was significantly lower in diseased than in normal arteries. Hence, atherosclerotic human coronary arteries lack an important protective mechanism that normally guards against vasospasm and thrombosis.

Endothelium-Dependent Relaxations

In isolated porcine coronary artery, OX-LDL inhibit endothelium-dependent relaxations to platelets, serotonin, and thrombin.[218-220] In contrast, relaxations to the NO donor linsidomine are well maintained, excluding a reduced responsiveness of vascular smooth muscle to EDNO. In the porcine coronary circulation, this inhibition is specific for OX-LDL, as it is not induced by comparable concentrations of native LDL.[218, 219] In the rabbit aorta, the effect of OX-LDL is mimicked by lysolecithin (a characteristic component of OX-LDL).[220] OX-LDL appear to activate an endothelial receptor distinct from the LDL receptor such as the scavenger receptor;[218] indeed, dextran sulfate, a competitive antagonist of modified LDL at this receptor,[218] prevents the endothelial effects of OX-LDL. The inhibitor of NO production L-NMMA exerts a similar inhibitory effect on endothelium-dependent relaxations as the modified lipoproteins, suggesting that OX-LDL specifically interfere with the L-arginine pathway. The activity of NO synthase, however, appears to remain unaffected, as L-arginine evokes a full relaxation in vessels treated with OX-LDL. Pretreatment with L-arginine restores the response to serotonin in vessels treated with OX-LDL. Furthermore, pretreatment of isolated vessels with L-arginine improves or restores the inhibited endothelium-dependent responses to serotonin. Thus, OX-LDL may interact with the intracellular signal transduction mechanisms (e.g., the function of G_i proteins)[221, 222] and/or the availability of L-arginine. This mechanism may also occur *in vivo*, as in hypercholesterolemic pigs; a similar inhibition of endothelium-dependent relaxation to serotonin occurs as in coronary arteries exposed to OX-LDL.[70, 222] In human subjects with hypercholesterolemia, L-arginine infusion augments the blunted increase in local blood flow in response to acetylcholine;[223-225] in contrast, the loss of endothelium-dependent vasodilation to acetylcholine in epicardial coronary arteries is unaffected by the amino acid, possibly because of the presence of fully developed atherosclerosis.[224]

In addition to their effect on the L-arginine pathway, both native and OX-LDL inactivate NO and cause endothelium-dependent[219] as well as endothelium-independent contraction.[219, 226]

Endothelium-Derived Nitric Oxide in Atherosclerosis

In contrast with hyperlipidemia, atherosclerosis is associated with more or less severe morphologic changes of the intima of large arteries (i.e., intimal thickening, accumulation and proliferation of smooth muscle cells and lipid containing macrophages).[215] Except at late stages, however, endothelial denudation does not occur.

Endothelium-Dependent Relaxations

In porcine coronary arteries, established atherosclerosis severely impairs endothelium-dependent relaxations to serotonin and also reduces endothelium-dependent relaxations to bradykinin, which are maintained in hypercholesterolemia.[70, 222, 227] However, endothelium-independent relaxations to nitrovasodilators remain preserved except in severely atherosclerotic arteries.[228] Similarly, in atherosclerotic coronary arteries of primates and humans, endothelium-dependent relaxations to acetylcholine, substance P, bradykinin, histamine, aggregating platelets, and calcium ionophore are attenuated,[8, 228-231] and *in vivo* acetylcholine as well as serotonin cause paradoxical vasoconstriction.[227]

Mechanism of Impaired Endothelium-Dependent Relaxation

Controversy exists as to the mechanism responsible for the marked impairment or loss of endothelium-dependent relaxations in atherosclerosis. Thus, bioassayable EDRF release in porcine coronary artery and rabbit with hypercholesterolemia and atherosclerosis clearly is reduced.[70, 232] Direct measurements of nitric oxide in the rabbit aorta, however, suggest an increased formation of NO with a concomitant massive breakdown of the endogenous nitrovasodilator (to the biologically inactive molecules nitrite and nitrate).[233] The latter observation would suggest an increased formation of superoxide radicals in the endothelium and other products inactivating NO and/or a decreased activity of superoxide dismutase in the blood vessel wall in atherosclerosis. It is conceivable that atherosclerosis in the more developed stages with marked invasion of monocytes and other blood cells induces NO synthase in the subintimal space and vascular smooth muscle cells. However, it is unknown whether similar alterations occur in human coronary arteries as they do in the rabbit aorta.

Role of Endogenous Nitric Oxide in Ischemia

NO synthase has also been shown to have the capability to produce NO as well as superoxide.[95] Superoxide is generated in the absence of arginine, whereas arginine addition reduces superoxide formation concomitant with enhanced production of NO. Endothelial superoxide has been implicated in myocardial and vascular damage after reperfusion,[2, 97, 98] and NOS may participate in such effects.[95, 96] However, it is unclear whether the low arginine levels associated with in vitro superoxide generation by NOS occur in intact cells in the microenvironment of NOS protein. It is notable that endothelium-dependent coronary dilation is impaired after ischemia reperfusion[97, 98] and that this impairment may be ameliorated by administration of L-arginine or pharmacologic donors of NO at doses not associated with vasodilation.[98] Thus, inactivation of superoxide radical by NO may be considered cardioprotective. Alternatively, because combinations of NO and superoxide generate toxic-free radicals (i.e., peroxynitrite), it is also conceivable that these molecules may be cytotoxic effectors associated with reperfusion injury.

Because endothelial NO synthase also possesses sequence homology with mammalian cytochrome P-450 reductase enzyme,[41] it donates electrons for the cytochrome P-450–drug metabolizing enzymes (as described earlier). Hence, NO may also act independently of cGMP, as NO enhances ADP ribosylation of platelet proteins and target glyceraldehyde-3-phosphate-dehydrogenase (as described above).[99, 100] There is decreased glycolysis associated with NO-enhanced GADPH-ADP ribosylation, and this could well mediate a number of actions of NO, such as myocardial stunning and hibernation, reperfusion injury, and neurotoxicity. The physiologic relevance of NO-mediated ADP ribosylation awaits further investigation.

ENDOTHELIUM-DERIVED NITRIC OXIDE AND THERAPEUTIC NITRATES

Similar to endothelium-derived NO, NO generated by nitroglycerin (converted in various steps yet to be identified) causes stimulation of smooth muscle soluble guanylyl cyclase activity and cGMP formation. Hence, as endothelium-derived NO, NO generated from organic nitrates causes vasodilation,[2] inhibits smooth muscle growth,[181–185] and prevents platelet activation and aggregation[37–39] (see Fig. 90–3). Thus, NO generated from vasodilators can be considered a substitute of endogenous NO.

Basal Nitric Oxide Release and Nitrates

Although therapeutic nitrates mediate their effects through the generation of NO, the vascular effects of exogenous nitrates are modulated by the presence of endothelium.[234–238] Indeed, in arteries with intact endothelial cells, the relaxing effects of sodium nitroprusside, nitroglycerin, or SIN-1 (the active metabolite of molsidomine) are reduced, compared with preparations without endothelium[236–238] (Fig. 90–12). As the basal formation of NO is smaller in veins as compared with arteries, this may also explain why nitrates have usually more pronounced effects in the venous as compared with the arterial circulation.[236] One interesting clinical implication of this phenomenon may be

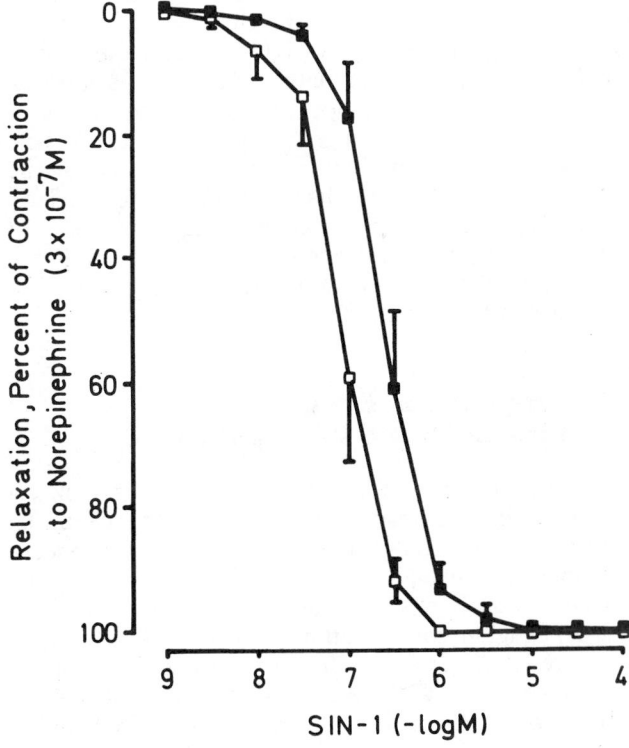

■ with endothelium (n=8)

□ w/o endothelium (n=6)

Figure 90–12. Effect of SIN-1 in human internal mammary arteries with (*solid squares*) and without (*open squares*) endothelium contracted with norepinephrine. SIN-1 evokes potent relaxations that are augmented in preparations without endothelium. (From Lüscher TF, Richard V, Yang Z: Interaction between endothelium-derived nitric oxide and SIN-1 in human and porcine blood vessels. J Cardiovasc Pharmacol 14(Suppl 11):76, 1990.)

the fact that nitrates preferentially dilate those vascular segments with dysfunctional endothelial cells.[239]

Nitrates can reduce endothelin production stimulated by thrombin via a cGMP-dependent mechanism,[119] which may provide a new vascular mechanism of action of nitrovasodilators such as SIN-1 and nitroglycerin.[120]

Effects of Nitrates in Diseased Vessels

In segments with defective or denuded endothelium, the vasodilator effects of nitroglycerin are stronger unless marked calcification of the vessel is present.[234-239] This finding also applies to other vasodilator substances, like cAMP-dependent ones, such as PGI_2 or papaverine, although less strongly. In fact, not only are uncalcified vascular segments with diminished endothelial function (achieved experimentally by endothelium denudation [see Fig. 90-6] or early arteriosclerosis) dilated by nitroglycerin, but the loss of endothelial function even enhances the effect of nitroglycerin. Indeed, coronary segments of patients that do not dilate to bradykinin (an endothelium-dependent vasodilator) are particularly responsive to nitroglycerin.[239] This surprising finding is probably explained by the fact that the presence of defects or functional disorders of the endothelium reduces the basal release of NO and thus the continued stimulation of guanylate cyclase (see earlier discussion). This, in turn, appears to increase the sensitivity of the underlying smooth vascular muscle to NO.[234-239] Hence, nitroglycerin is a "smart vasodilator" with particular effects in a diseased region. This may explain why even minimal doses of nitroglycerin, which did not cause any measurable venous pooling or reductions in blood pressure, can produce antiischemic effects.

Heterogeneous Effects of Nitrates in the Vasculature

Nitrates such as nitroglycerin can have different effects on different vascular segments;[240, 241] for example, the antiischemic effects of nitroglycerin at low concentrations are related only to dilation of the venous system (atrial pressure) and coronary vessels, and only at higher concentration does dilation of peripheral resistance vessels and in turn a decrease in afterload occur. Only at excessive concentrations are the myocardial resistance vessels dilated (presumably because small coronary vessels are not able to metabolize nitroglycerin and to release NO from its molecule). The therapeutic benefit of nitrovasodilators in treating ischemic heart disease lies in the fact that dilating effects are produced on the low-pressure system, together with a reduction in preload, and on the large coronary vessels even before there is a reduction in peripheral resistance as a consequence of arteriolar dilation, which would result in an undesirable decrease of coronary perfusion pressure.

NITRATE TOLERANCE

The loss of nitrovasodilator-induced drug action (nitrate tolerance) has been observed for more than 100 years.[242-251] This may affect both the intended drug action (i.e., vasodilation) as well as the side effects. Indeed, headache and flushing also tend to disappear in patients receiving chronic nitrate therapy. However, the mechanism by which nitrate tolerance comes into play still remains a mystery. The loss of nitrovasodilator-induced drug action may be based either on the specific loss of cGMP-dependent dilator effects at the vasculature ("true tolerance") or on the initiation of biologic counterregulatory processes ("pseudotolerance"), usually neurohormonal adaptations (i.e., activation of the renin-angiotensin system and sympathetic nervous system), that compensate for the reduction in vascular tone associated with the cGMP-dependent dilator effects.[243] Hence, multiple mechanisms may be involved in inducing nitrate tolerance.

In isolated blood vessels incubated with nitroglycerin (10^{-5} to 10^{-4} M) over a short period of time (up to an hour), the concentration-response curve to nitroglycerin and other nitrates is shifted to the right, indicating rapid occurrence of tolerance in vitro. In contrast with nitroglycerin, there is no loss of potency in vitro and in vivo to endogenous NO released from the endothelium, for instance, during flow-induced dilation.[244, 245] This also holds in large part true for NO-generating dilator substances, such as sodium nitroprusside and SIN-1,[245, 246] that release NO directly, already extracellularly, without there having to be an upstream conversion step in the vascular muscle cell, as with nitroglycerin.

The mechanisms for nitrate tolerance suggested to be involved include possible changes in the biotransformation of nitrates to NO; for example, organic nitrates may react with reduced sulfhydryl groups in vascular smooth muscle, leading to the formation of a disulfide linkage.[249, 250] This hypothesis is supported by numerous studies showing that an exogenous supply of free thiol can enhance nitrate potency and partially reverse tolerance both in vitro and in vivo.[250, 251] Some of these effects of thiol donor, however, may also be nonspecific.

Nitrates liberate NO either spontaneously (i.e., SNAP, SIN-1) or by enzymatic conversion within the blood vessels (i.e., SNP, ISDN).[248] The intermediary metabolites of nitrates generated in the process to liberate NO, which activate the enzyme-soluble guanylyl cyclase to produce cGMP and induce vasorelaxation, may indirectly cause nitrate tolerance by hindering the enzymatic conversion of these nitrates. Thus, another suggested mechanism for nitrate tolerance is that there is a reduction of vascular production of NO by nitrates such as nitroglycerin but not SNAP or SIN-1,[252-254] a decrease in the vascular metabolism to its dinitrate metabolites,[255, 256] an alteration of the cellular soluble guanylate cyclase,[257] or an increased enzymatic breakdown of the cGMP.

Although attractive, these nitrate tolerance mechanisms are only applicable to in vitro situations, and it remains uncertain whether these phenomena can explain *in vivo* tolerance, because isolated blood vessels are exposed to millimolar concentrations of nitroglycerin, whereas nanomolar concentrations of nitroglycerin are found in patients.[258] Tolerance develops within 30 minutes to 1 hour under *in vitro* conditions, whereas nitrate effects generally last for several hours before tolerance is evident in patients. Finally, a study by Watanabe et al.[259] suggests that nitrate tolerance involves both cellular and systemic events.

SUMMARY: IMPORTANCE OF ENDOGENOUS NITRIC OXIDE AND THERAPEUTIC NITRATES

The endothelium plays an important protective role in the circulation by releasing NO and prostacyclin as well as inhibitors of coagulation; these substances cause vasodilation, inhibit platelet adhesion, have antiproliferative properties, and inhibit platelet adhesion and aggregation. Substances released from aggregating platelets can evoke the release of NO and prostacyclin, coagulation, and growth. Thus, if platelets are activated in a blood vessel with intact endothelial cells, vasodilation and inhibition of platelet function occur. This would disaggregate and would flush away an evolving clot. In hypertension, endothelium-dependent relaxations are impaired under most conditions; in addition, the release of platelet-derived products, in particular serotonin, is enhanced. This may contribute to vascular complications and/or the increased peripheral resistance in hypertension. If, in hypertensive arteries, atherosclerotic vascular changes are superimposed, endothelium dysfunction becomes further reduced, an event that importantly contributes to the occurrence of myocardial infarction and stroke.

REFERENCES

1. Brunton TL: Use of nitrite of amyl in angina pectoris. Lancet 2:97, 1867.
2. Lüscher TF, Vanhoutte PM: The Endothelium: Modulator of Cardiovascular Function. Boca Raton, FL: CRC Press, 1991, pp 1–215.
3. Furchgott RF, Zawadzki JV: The obligatory role of endothelial cells in the relaxation of arterial smooth muscle by acetylcholine. Nature 299:373, 1980.
4. Parker JA: Nitrate therapy in stable angina pectoris. N Engl J Med 316:1635, 1987.
5. Jugdutt BJ, Warnica JW: Intravenous nitroglycerin therapy to limit myocardial infarct size, expansion, and complications. Circulation 314:906, 1988.
6. Cohn JN, Archibald DG, Ziesche S, et al: Effect of vasodilator therapy on mortality in chronic congestive heart failure. N Engl J Med 314:1547, 1986.
7. Furchgott RF, Vanhoutte PM: Endothelium-derived relaxing and contracting factors. FASEB J 3:2007, 1989.
8. Bossaller C, Habib GB, Yamamoto H, et al: Impaired muscarinic endothelium-dependent relaxation and cyclic guanosine 5'-monophosphate formation in atherosclerotic human coronary artery and rabbit aorta. J Clin Invest 79:170, 1987.
9. Förstermann U, Mügge A, Bode SM, et al: Response of human coronary arteries to aggregating platelets: Importance of endothelium-derived relaxing factor and prostanoids. Circ Res 63:306, 1988.
10. Lüscher TF, Diederich D, Siebenmann R, et al: Difference between endothelium-dependent relaxations in arterial and in venous coronary bypass grafts. N Engl J Med 319:462, 1988.
11. Ludmer PL, Selwyn AP, Shook TL, et al: Paradoxical vasoconstriction induced by acetylcholine in atherosclerotic coronary arteries. N Engl J Med 315:1046, 1986.
12. Linder L, Kiowski W, Bühler FR, et al: Indirect evidence for release of endothelium-derived relaxing factor in human forearm circulation in vivo: Blunted response in essential hypertension. Circulation 81:1762, 1990.
13. Webb RC, Vander AJ, Henry JP: Increased vasodilator responses to acetylcholine in psychosocial hypertensive mice. Hypertension 9:268, 1987.
14. Vallance P, Collier J, Moncada S: Effects of endothelium-derived nitric oxide on peripheral arteriolar tone in man. Lancet 2:997, 1989.
15. Davies PF, Ganz D, Diel PS: Reversible microcarrier-mediated junctional communication between endothelial cells and smooth muscle cell monolayers: An in vitro model of vascular cell interactions. Lab Invest 85:710, 1985.
16. Davies PF, Olesen S-P, Clapham DE, et al: Endothelial communication. Hypertension 11:563, 1988.
17. Boulanger C, Hendrickson H, Lorenz RR, et al: Release of different relaxing factors by cultured porcine endothelial cells. Circ Res 64:1070, 1989.
18. Cocks TM, Angus JA, Campbell JH, et al: Release and properties of endothelium-derived relaxing factor (EDRF) from endothelial cells in culture. J Cell Physiol 123:310, 1985.
19. Griffith TM, Edwards DH, Lewis MJ, et al: The nature of endothelium-derived vascular relaxant factor. Nature 308:645, 1984.
20. Gryglewski RJ, Palmer RMJ, Moncada S: Superoxide anion is involved in the breakdown of endothelium-derived vascular relaxing factor. Nature 320:454, 1986.
21. Lückhoff A, Busse R, Winter I, et al: Characterization of vascular relaxant factor released from cultured endothelial cells. Hypertension 9:295, 1987.
22. Rubanyi GM, Lorenz RR, Vanhoutte PM: Bioassay of endothelium-derived relaxing factor(s): Inactivation by catecholamines. Am J Physiol 249:H95, 1985.
23. Boegehold MA: Reduced influence of nitric oxide on arteriolar tone in hypertensive Dahl rats. Hypertension 19:290, 1992.
24. Cohen RA, Shepherd JT, Vanhoutte PM: Inhibitory role of the endothelium in the response of isolated coronary arteries to platelets. Science 221:273, 1983.
25. Yang Z, Stulz P, von Segesser L, et al: Different interactions of platelets with arterial and venous coronary bypass vessels. Lancet 337:939, 1991.
26. Vanhoutte PM, Lüscher TF: Peripheral mechanisms in cardiovascular regulation: Transmitters, receptors and the endothelium. *In* Tarazi RC, Zanchetti A (eds): Handbook of Hypertension Vol. 8, Physiology and Pathophysiology of Hypertension-Regulatory Mechanisms. Amsterdam: Elsevier, 1986, pp 96–123.
27. Rubanyi GM, Romero JC, Vanhoutte PM: Flow induced release of endothelium-derived relaxing factor. Am J Physiol 250:4145, 1986.
28. Pohl U, Holtz J, Busse R, et al: Crucial role of endothelium in the vasodilator response to increased flow in vivo. Hypertension 8:37, 1986.
29. Rubanyi GM, Vanhoutte PM: Superoxide anions and hyperoxia inactivate endothelium-derived relaxing factor. Am J Physiol 250:H822, 1986.
30. Ignarro LJ, Byrns RE, Buga GM, et al: Pharmacological evidence that endothelium-derived relaxing factor is nitric oxide: Use of pyrogallol and superoxide dismutase to study endothelium-dependent and nitric oxide-elicited vascular smooth muscle relaxation. J Pharmacol Exp Ther 244:181, 1988.
31. Furchgott RF: Studies on relaxation of rabbit aorta by sodium nitrite: The basis for the proposal that acid-activatable inhibitory factor from bovine retractor penis is inorganic nitrite and the endothelium-derived relaxing factor is nitric oxide. *In* Vanhoutte PM (ed): Vasodilatation: Vascular Smooth Muscle, Peptides, Autonomic Nerves and Endothelium. New York: Raven Press, 1988, pp 401–414.

32. Palmer RMJ, Ferrige AG, Moncada S: Nitric oxide release accounts for the biological activity of endothelium-derived relaxing factor. Nature 327:524, 1987.

33. Malinsiki T, Ziud T: Nitric oxide release from a single cell measured in-situ by a porphyrinic-based microsensor. Nature 358:676, 1992.

34. Chen W, Palmer RMJ, Moncada S: Release of nitric oxide from rabbit aorta. J Vasc Med Biol 1:2, 1989.

35. Meyers PR, Minor RL, Guerra R Jr, et al: Vasorelaxant properties of the endothelium-derived relaxing factor more closely resemble S-nitrosocysteine than nitric oxide. Nature 345:161, 1990.

36. Rapoport RM, Draznin MB, Murad F: Endothelium-dependent relaxation in rat aorta may be mediated through cyclic GMP-dependent protein phosphorylation. Nature 306:174, 1983.

37. Radomski MW, Palmer RMJ, Moncada S: Comparative pharmacology of endothelium-derived relaxing factor, nitric oxide and prostacyclin in platelets. Br J Pharmacol 92:181, 1987.

38. Radomski MW, Palmer RMJ, Moncada S: Endogenous nitric oxide inhibits human platelet adhesion to vascular endothelium. Lancet ii:1057, 1987.

39. Busse R, Lückhoff A, Bassenge E: Endothelium-derived relaxant factor inhibits platelet activation. Naunyn Schmiedebergs Arch Pharmacol 336:566, 1987.

40. Palmer RMJ, Ashton DS, Moncada S: Vascular endothelial cells synthesize nitric oxide from L-arginine. Nature 333:664, 1988.

41. Bredt DS, Hwang PM, Glatt CE, et al: Cloned and expressed nitric oxide synthase structurally resembles cytochrome P-450 reductase. Nature 351:714, 1991.

42. Radomski MW, Palmer RMJ, Moncada S: An L-arginine/nitric oxide pathway present in human platelets regulates aggregation. Proc Natl Acad Sci USA 87:5193, 1990.

43. McCall TB, Boughton-Smith NK, Palmer RMJ, et al: Synthesis of nitric oxide from L-arginine by neutrophils. Biochem J 261:293, 1989.

44. Hibbs JB, Taintor RR, Vavrin Z, et al: Nitric oxide: A cytotoxic activated macrophage effector molecule. Biochem Biophys Res Commun 157:87, 1988.

45. Bernhardt J, Tschudi MR, Dohi Y, et al: Release of nitric oxide from human vascular smooth muscle cells. Biochem Biophys Res Commun 180:907, 1991.

46. Julou-Schaeffer G, Gray GA, Fleming I, et al: Loss of vascular responsiveness induced by endotoxin involves L-arginine pathway. Am J Physiol 259:H-1038, 1990.

47. Beasely D, Schwartz JH, Brenner BM: Interleukin 1 induces prolonged L-arginine-dependent cyclic guanosine monophosphate and nitrite production in rat vascular smooth muscle cells. J Clin Invest 87:602, 1991.

48. Billiar D, Curran RD, Stuehr DJ, et al: Inducible cytosolic enzyme activity for the production of nitrogen oxides from L-arginine in hepatocytes. Biochem Biophys Res Commun 168:1034, 1990.

49. Marsden PA, Ballermann BJ: Tumor necrosis factor-alpha activates soluble guanylate cyclase in bovine glomerular mesangial cells via an L-arginine-dependent cyclic guanosine monophosphate and nitrite production in rat vascular smooth muscle cells. J Clin Invest 87:602, 1991.

50. Billiar TR, Curran RD, Steuhr DJ, et al: An L-arginine-dependent mechanism mediates Kupffer cell inhibition of hepatocyte protein synthesis in vitro. J Exp Med 169:1467, 1989.

51. Ishii KB, Chang B, Kerwin JF Jr, et al: Formation of endothelium-derived relaxing factor in porcine kidney epithelial LLC-PK1 cells: An intra and intercellular messenger for activation of soluble guanylate cyclase. J Pharmacol Exp Ther 256:38, 1991.

52. Markewitz BA, Michael JR, Kohan DE: Cytokine-induced expression of a nitric oxide synthase in rat renal tubule cells. J Clin Invest 91:2138, 1993.

53. Bredt DS, Hwang PM, Snyder SH: Localization of nitric oxide synthase indicating a neural role for nitric oxide. Nature 347:768, 1990.

54. Werner-Felmayer G, Werner ER, Fuchs D, et al: Tetrahydrobiopetrin-dependent formation of nitrite and nitrate in murine fibroblasts. J Exp Med 172:1599, 1990.

55. Ellman C, Corbett JA, Misko TP, et al: Nitric oxide mediates interleukin-1-induced cellular cytotoxicity in the rat ovary. A potential role for nitric oxide in the ovulatory process. J Clin Invest 92:3053, 1993.

56. Knowles RG, Palacios M, Palmer RMJ, et al: Formation of nitric oxide from L-arginine in the central nervous system: A transduction mechanism for stimulation of the soluble guanylate cyclase. Proc Natl Acad Sci 86:1, 1989.

57. Bredt DS, Snyder SH: Isolation of nitric oxide synthetase, a calmodulin requiring enzyme. Proc Natl Acad Sci USA 87:682, 1990.

58. Busse R, Mülsch A: Calcium-dependent nitric oxide synthesis in endothelial cytosol is mediated by calmodulin. FEBS Lett 265:133, 1990.

59. La Montagne D, Pohl U, Busse R: Mechanical deformation of vessel wall and shear stress determine the basal release of endothelium-derived relaxing factor in the intact rabbit coronary vascular bed. Circ Res 70:123, 1992.

60. Goy MF: cGMP: The wayward child of the cyclic nucleotide family. Trends Neurosci 74:293, 1991.

61. Bredt DS, Ferris CD, Snyder SH: Nitric oxide synthase regulatory sites: Phosphorylation by cyclic AMP dependent protein kinase, protein kinase C, and calcium/calmodulin protein kinase: Identification of flavin and calmodulin binding sites. J Biol Chem 267:10976, 1992.

62. Richard V, Tschudi MR, Lüscher TF: Differential activation of the endothelial L-arginine pathway by bradykinin, serotonin and clonidine in porcine coronary arteries. Am J Physiol 259:H-1433, 1990.

63. Tschudi M, Richard V, Bühler FR, et al: Importance of endothelium-derived nitric oxide in intramyocardial porcine coronary arteries. Am J Physiol 260:H13, 1990.

64. Yang Z, von Segesser L, Bauer E, et al: Differential activation of the endothelial L-arginine and cyclooxygenase pathway in the human internal mammary artery and saphenous vein. Circ Res 68:52, 1991.

65. Meyer P, Flammer J, Lüscher TF: Endothelium-dependent regulation of the ophthalmic microcirculation in the perfused porcine eye: Role of nitric oxide and endothelins. Invest Ophthalmol Vis Sci 34:3614, 1993.

66. Rees DD, Palmer RMJ, Moncada S: The role of endothelium-derived nitric oxide in the regulation of blood pressure. Proc Natl Acad Sci USA 86:3375, 1989.

67. Vallance P, Leone A, Calver A, et al: Accumulation of an endogenous inhibitor of nitric oxide synthesis in chronic renal failure. Lancet 339:572, 1992.

68. Flavanah NA, Shimokawa H, Vanhoutte PM: Pertussis toxin inhibits endothelium-dependent relaxations to certain agonists in porcine coronary arteries. J Physiol 408:549, 1989.

69. Flavahan NA, Vanhoutte PM: Pertussis toxin inhibits the basal and leukotriene C4-stimulated release of endothelium-derived relaxing factor(s). FASEB J 3/3:A533, 1989.

70. Shimokawa H, Flavahan NA, Vanhoutte PM: Natural course of the impairment of endothelium-dependent relaxations after balloon endothelium-removal in porcine coronary arteries. Circ Res 63:740, 1989.

71. Busse R, Fichtner H, Lückhoff A, et al: Hyperpolarization and increased free calcium in acetylcholine-stimulated endothelial cells. Am J Physiol 255:H965, 1988.

72. Olesen S-P, Clapham DE, Davies PF: Haemodynamic shear stress activates a K+ current in vascular endothelial cells. Nature 331:168, 1988.

73. Olesen S-P, Davies PF, Clapham DE: Muscarinic-activated K+ current in bovine aortic endothelial cells. Circ Res 62:1059, 1988.

74. Lambert TL, Kent RS, Whorton AR: Bradykinin stimulation of inositol polyphosphate production in porcine aortic endothelial cells. J Biol Chem 261:15288, 1986.

75. Loeb AI, Izzo NJ, Johnson RM, et al: Endothelium-derived relaxing factor release associated with increased endothelial cell inositol triphosphate and intracellular calcium. Am J Cardiol 62:36G, 1988.

76. Rapoport RM: Cyclic guanosine monophosphate inhibition of contraction may be mediated through inhibition of phosphatidyl-inositol hydrolysis in rat aorta. Circ Res 58:407, 1986.

77. Resink TJ, Grigorian GY, Moldabaeva AK, et al: Histamine-

induced phosphoinositide metabolism in cultured human umbilical vein endothelial cells. Association with thromboxane and prostacyclin release. Biochem Biophys Res Commun 144:438, 1987.

78. Lewis MJ, Hendersen AH: A phorbol ester inhibits the release of endothelium-derived relaxing factor. Eur J Pharmacol 137:167, 1987.

79. Long CJ, Stone TW: The release of endothelium derived relaxant factor is calcium dependent. Blood Vessels 22:205, 1985.

80. Singer HA, Peach MJ: Calcium and endothelial-mediated vascular smooth muscle cell relaxation in rabbit aorta. Hypertension 4(Suppl II):19, 1982.

81. Winquist RJ, Bunting PB, Schofield TL: Blockade of endothelium-dependent relaxation by the amiloride analog dichlorobenzamil: Possible role of Na + /Ca + + exchange in the release of endothelium-derived relaxing factor. J Pharmacol Exp Ther 235:644, 1985.

82. Johns A, Lategan TW, Lodge NJ, et al: Calcium entry through receptor-operated channels in bovine pulmonary artery endothelial cells. Tissue Cell 19:733, 1987.

83. Lodge NJ, Adams DJ, Johns A, et al: Calcium activation of endothelial cells. In Halpern W, Pegram BL, Brayden JE, et al (eds): The Proceedings of the Second International Symposium on Resistance Arteries. Ithaca, NY: Perinatology Press, 1988, p 152.

84. Lückhoff A, Busse R: Increased free calcium in endothelial cells under stimulation with adenine nucleotides. J Cell Physiol 126:414, 1986.

85. Lückhoff A, Pohl U, Mülsch A, et al: Differential role of extra- and intracellular calcium in the release of EDRF and prostacyclin from cultured endothelial cells. Br J Pharmacol 95:189, 1988.

86. Schilling WP, Ritchie AK, Navarro LT, et al: Bradykinin-stimulated calcium influx in cultured bovine aortic endothelial cells. Am J Physiol 255:H219, 1988.

87. Rubanyi GM, Schwartz A, Vanhoutte PM: The calcium agonist Bay K 8644 and (+) 202,791 stimulate the release of endothelial relaxing factor from canine femoral arteries. Eur J Pharmacol 117:143, 1985.

88. Rubanyi GM, Schwartz A, Vanhoutte PM: The effect of diltiazem and verapamil on endothelium-dependent responses in canine blood vessels. Pharmacologist 27:290, 1985.

89. Rubanyi GM, Schwartz A, Vanhoutte PM: Calcium transport mechanisms in endothelial cells regulating the synthesis and release of endothelium-derived relaxing factor. In Vanhoutte PM (ed): Relaxing and Contracting Factors: Biological and Clinical Research. Clifton, NJ: Humana Press, 1988, p 179.

90. Spedding M, Schini V, Schoeffter P, et al: Calcium channel activation does not increase release of endothelium-derived relaxant factors (EDRF) in rat aorta although release of EDRF may modulate calcium channel activity in smooth muscle. J Cardiovasc Pharmacol 8:1130, 1986.

91. De Mey JG, Vanhoutte PM: Interaction between Na + , K + exchanges and the direct inhibitory effect of acetylcholine on canine femoral arteries. Circ Res 46:826, 1980.

92. De Mey JG, Vanhoutte PM: Anoxia and endothelium dependent reactivity in canine femoral artery. J Physiol (London) 335:65, 1983.

93. Fürchgott RF: Role of the endothelium in responses of vascular smooth muscle. Circ Res 53:557, 1983.

94. Griffith TM, Edwards DH, Lewis MJ, et al: Production of endothelium-derived relaxant factor is dependent on oxidative phosphorylation and extracellular calcium. Cardiovasc Res 20:7, 1986.

95. Pou S, Surichamorn W, Bredt DS, et al: Generation of superoxide by purified brain nitric oxide synthase. J Biol Chem 267:24173, 1992.

96. Zweier JL, Kuppasamy P, Lutty GA: Measurement of endothelial cell free radical generation: Evidence for a central mechanism of free radical injury in post ischemic tissues. Proc Natl Acad Sci USA 85:4046, 1988.

97. VanBenthuysen KM, McMurtry IF, Horowitz LD: Reperfusion after acute coronary occlusion in dogs impairs endothelium-dependent relaxation to acetylcholine and augments contractile reactivity in vitro. J Clin Invest 79:265, 1987.

98. Weyrich AS, Ma XL, Lefer AM: The role of L-arginine in ameliorating reperfusion injury after myocardial ischemia in the cat. Circulation 86:279, 1992.

99. Brune B, Lapetina EG: Activation of a cytosolic ADP-ribosyltransferase by nitric oxide-generating agents. J Biol Chem 264:8455, 1989.

100. Zhang J, Snyder SH: Nitric oxide stimulates auto-ADP-ribosylation of glyceraldehyde-3-phosphate dehydrogenase in man. Proc Natl Acad Sci USA 89:9382, 1992.

101. Dimmeler S, Lottspeich F, Brune B: Nitric oxide causes ADP-ribosylation and inhibition of glyceraldehyde-3-phosphate dehydrogenase. J Biol Chem 267:16771, 1992.

102. Drapier J-C, Hibbs JB Jr: Differentiation of murine macrophages to express non-specific cytotoxicity for tumor cells results in L-arginine dependent inhibition of mitochondrial iron-sulfur enzymes in the macrophage effector cells. J Immunol 140:2829, 1988.

103. Sessa WC, Harrison JK, Barber CM, et al: Molecular cloning and expression of a cDNA encoding endothelial cell nitric oxide synthase. J Biol Chem 267:15274, 1992.

104. Lomas S, Marsden PA, Li GK, et al: Endothelial nitric oxide synthase: Molecular cloning and characterization of a distinct constitutive isoform. Proc Natl Acad Sci USA 89:6348, 1992.

105. Janssens SP, Shimouchi A, Quertermous T, et al: Cloning and expression of a cDNA encoding human endothelium derived relaxing factor/nitric oxide synthase. J Biol Chem 267:14519, 1992.

106. Tayeh MA, Marletta MA: Macrophage oxidation of L-arginine to nitric oxide, nitrite, and nitrate. J Biol Chem 264:19654, 1989.

107. Mülsch A, Busse R: Nitric oxide synthase in native and cultured endothelial cells: Calcium/calmodulin and tetrahydrobiopterin are cofactors. J Cardiovasc Pharmacol 17:552, 1991.

108. Dinerman JL, Lowenstein CJ, Snyder SH: Molecular mechanisms of nitric oxide regulation: Potential relevance to cardiovascular disease. Circ Res 73:217, 1993.

109. Pohl U, Busse R, Kuon E, et al: Pulsatile perfusion stimulates the release of endothelial autacoids. J Appl Cardiol 1:215, 1986.

110. Griffith TM, Hutcheson IR: Multiple K + channels mediate EDRF release to pulsatile and time-averaged stress [abstract 279]. Endothelium 1(Suppl):S71, 1993.

111. Kuchan MJ, Frangos JA: Differential role of calcium and calmodulin in the regulation of bradykinin- and flow-mediated nitric oxide production [abstract]. Endothelium 1(Suppl):S2, 1993.

112. Sessa WC, Pritchard K, Seyedi N, et al: Chronic exercise is a stimulus for coronary vascular NO production and endothelial cell nitric oxide synthase gene expression. Endothelium 1(Suppl):S1, 1993.

113. Martin W, White DG, Henderson AH: Endothelium-derived relaxing factor and atriopeptin-II elevate cyclic GMP levels in pig aortic endothelial cells. Br J Pharmacol 93:229, 1988.

114. Schini VB, Boulanger C, Regoli D, et al: Production of cGMP by kinins in cultured porcine aortic endothelial cells. FASEB J 3/3:A533, 1989.

115. Schini VB, Grant NJ, Miller RC, et al: Morphological characterization of cultured bovine aortic endothelial cells and the effects of atriopeptin II and sodium nitroprusside on cellular and extracellular accumulation of cyclic GMP. Eur J Cell Biol 47:53, 1988.

116. Evans HG, Smith JA, Lewis MJ: Release of endothelium-derived relaxing factor is inhibited by 8-bromo-cyclic guanosine monophosphate. J Cardiovasc Pharmacol 12:672, 1988.

117. Buga GM, Cohen G, Griscavage JM, et al: Negative feedback regulation of NO synthase and endothelial cell function by nitric oxide. Endothelium 1(Suppl):S19, 1993.

118. Fickling SA, Nussey SS, Vallance P, et al: Synthesis of Ng, Ng dimethylarginine from L-arginine by human endothelial cells. Endothelium 1(Suppl):S16, 1993.

119. Boulanger C, Lüscher TF: Release of endothelin from the porcine aorta: Inhibition by endothelium-derived nitric oxide. J Clin Invest 85:587, 1990.

120. Boulanger C, Lüscher TF: Hirudin and nitric oxide donors inhibit the thrombin-induced release of endothelin from the intact porcine aorta. Circ Res 68:1768, 1990.

121. Lüscher TF, Boulanger C, Yang Z, et al: Interaction between

endothelin and endothelium-derived relaxing factor(s). *In* Rubanyi GM (ed): Endothelin. Oxford, UK: Oxford University Press, 1991.

122. Saijonmaa O, Ristimäki A, Fyhrquist F: Atrial natriuretic peptide, nitroglycerine, and nitroprusside reduce basal and stimulated endothelin production from cultured endothelial cells. Biochem Biophys Res Commun 173:514, 1990.

123. Yokokawa K, Kohno M, Yasunari K, et al: Endothelin-3 regulates endothelin-1 production in cultured human endothelial cells. Hypertension 18:304, 1991.

124. Stewart DJ, Langleben D, Cernacek P, et al: Endothelin release is inhibited by coculture of endothelial cells with cells of vascular media. Am J Physiol 259:H1928, 1990.

125. Arai H, Hori S, Aramori I, et al: Cloning and expression of a cDNA encoding and endothelin receptor. Nature 348:730, 1990.

126. Sakurai T, Yanagisawa M, Takuwa Y, et al: Cloning of a cDNA encoding a non-isopeptide-selective subtype of the endothelin receptor. Nature 348:732, 1990.

127. Vane J: Endothelins come home to roost. Nature 348:673, 1990.

128. Dohi Y, Lüscher TF: Endothelin-1 in perfused hypertensive resistance arteries: Different intra- and extraluminal dysfunction. Hypertension 18:543, 1991.

129. Warner TD, Mitchell JA, de Nucci G, et al: Endothelin-1 and endothelin-3 release EDRF from isolated perfused arterial vessels of the rat and rabbit. J Cardiovasc Pharmacol 13(Suppl 5):85, 1989.

130. Lüscher TF, Yang Z, Tschudi M, et al: Interaction between endothelin-1 and endothelium-derived relaxing factor in human arteries and veins. Circ Res 66:1088, 1990.

131. Miller VM, Komori K, Burnett JC, et al: Differential sensitivity to endothelin in canine arteries and veins. Am J Physiol 257:H1127, 1989.

132. Salazar FJ, Pinilla JM, Lopez F, et al: Renal effects of prolonged synthesis inhibition of endothelium-derived nitric oxide. Hypertension 20:113, 1992.

133. Ribeiro MO, Antunes E, deNucci G, et al: Chronic inhibition of nitric oxide synthesis: A new model of arterial hypertension. Hypertension 20:298, 1992.

134. Samsell L, Engles K, Qui C, et al: Combined angiotensin type 1 receptor (AT$_1$) blockade with losartan (L) and alpha1-adrenoceptor blockade with prazosin (P) normalize BP in chronic endothelium derived relaxing factor (EDRF) blockade induced hypertension (EB-HT). J Am Soc Nephrol 3:551, 1992.

135. Vidal-Ragout MJ, Romero JC, Vanhoutte PM: Endothelium-derived relaxing factor inhibits renin release. Eur J Pharmacol 149:401, 1988.

136. Meyer E De, Feng XJ, Rampart M, et al: Thrombin induces nitric oxide production in porcine aortic valve endothelial cells. Endothelium 1(Suppl):S63, 1993.

137. Mulvany MJ, Aalkjaer C: Structure and function of small arteries. Physiol Rev 70:921, 1990.

138. Vogel RA: Endothelium-dependent vasoregulation of coronary artery diameter and blood flow. Circulation 88:325, 1993.

139. Kon V, Harris RC, Ichikawa I: A regulatory role of large vessels in organ circulation. J Clin Invest 85:1728, 1990.

140. DeNicole L, Blantz RC, Gabbai FB: NO and AII: Glomerular and tubular interaction in the rat. J Clin Invest 89:1248, 1992.

141. Nakamura T, Prewitt RL: Effect of Ng-monomethyl L-arginine on endothelium dependent relaxation in arterioles of one-kidney, one clip hypertensive rats. Hypertension 17:875, 1991.

142. Lacolley PJ, Lewis SJ, Brody MJ: Role of sympathetic nerve activity in the generation of vascular nitric oxide in urethane-anesthetized rats. Hypertension 17:881, 1991.

143. Lefroy DC, Crake T, Uren NG, et al: Effect of inhibition of nitric oxide synthesis on epicardial coronary artery caliber and coronary blood flow in humans. Circulation 88:43, 1993.

144. Suzuki Y, Tokunaga S, Ikeguchi S, et al: Induction of coronary artery spasm by intracoronary acetylcholine: Comparison with intracoronary ergonovine. Am Heart J 124:39, 1992.

145. Vallance P, Collier J, Moncada S: Nitric oxide synthesized from L-arginine mediates endothelium dependent dilation in human veins in vivo. Cardiovasc Res 23:1053, 1989.

146. Yang Z, Diederich D, Schneider K, et al: Endothelium-derived relaxing factor and protection against contractions induced by histamine and serotonin in the human internal mammary artery and in the saphenous vein. Circulation 80:1041, 1989.

147. Lüscher TF, Vanhoutte PM: Endothelium-dependent responses in human blood vessels. Trends Pharmacol Sci 9:181, 1988.

148. Lerner DJ, Kannel WB: Patterns of coronary heart disease morbidity and mortality in the sexes: A 26-year follow-up of the Framingham population. Am Heart J 111:383, 1986.

149. Foegh ML: Estradiol and myointimal proliferation. *In* Ramwell P, Rubyani G, Schillinger E (eds): Sex Steroids and the Cardiovascular System. Schering Foundation Workshop. Berlin, Springer-Verlag, 1992, p 129.

150. Schray-Utz B, Zeiher AM, Busse R: Expression of constitutive NO synthase in cultured endothelial cells is enhanced by 17β-estradiol. Circulation 88:I-80, 1993.

151. Kauser K, Rubyani GM: Gender differences in endothelial function of aortae from normotensive and spontaneously hypertensive rats. Endothelium 1(Suppl):S70, 1993.

152. Weiner C, Baylis S, Lizasoain I, et al: Regulation of NO-synthase by sex hormones. Endothelium 1(Suppl):S1, 1993.

153. Rubyani GM, Kauser K: Sexual steroid hormones are responsible for gender differences in EDRF/NO release from aorta of spontaneously hypertensive rats. Endothelium 1(Suppl):S1, 1993.

154. Weiner C, Lizasoain I, Snyder G, et al: Estradiol regulates pituitary follicle stimulating hormone release by an NO-dependent inhibitory pathway. Endothelium 1(Suppl):S6, 1993.

155. Miller VM, Vanhoutte PM: Progesterone and modulation of endothelium-dependent responses in canine coronary arteries. Am J Physiol 261:R1022, 1991.

156. Rimele TJ, Sturm RJ, Adams LM, et al: Interaction of neutrophils with vascular smooth muscle: Identification as a neutrophil-derived relaxing factor. J Pharmacol Exp Ther 245:102, 1988.

157. Hibbs JB Jr, Vavrin Z, Taintor RR: L-arginine is required for expression of the activated macrophage effector mechanism causing selective metabolic inhibition in target cells. J Immunol 138:550, 1987.

158. Förstermann U, Mülsch A, Böhme E, et al: Stimulation of soluble guanylate cyclase by an acetylcholine-induced endothelium derived factor from rabbit and canine arteries. Circ Res 58:531, 1986.

159. Martin W, Villani GM, Jothianandan D, et al: Selective blockade of endothelium-dependent and glyceryl trinitrate-induced relaxation by hemoglobin and by methylene blue in the rabbit aorta. J Pharmacol Exp Ther 232:708, 1985.

160. Martin W, Furchgott RF, Villani GM, et al: Phosphodiesterase inhibitors induce endothelium-dependent relaxation of rat and rabbit aorta by potentiating the effects of spontaneously released endothelium-derived relaxing factor (EDRF). J Pharmacol Exp Ther 237:539, 1986.

161. Ganz P, Davies PF, Leopold JA, et al: Short- and long-term interactions of endothelium and vascular smooth muscle in coculture: Effects of cyclic GMP production. Proc Natl Acad Sci USA 83:3552, 1986.

162. Godfraind T, Egleme C, Osachie IA: Role of endothelium in the contractile response of rat aorta alpha-adrenoceptor agonists. Clin Sci 68(Suppl 10):65, 1985.

163. Collins P, Lewis MJ, Henderson AH: Endothelium-derived factor relaxes vascular smooth muscle by cyclic-GMP mediated effects on calcium movements. *In* Vanhoutte PM (ed): Relaxing and Contracting Factors: Biological and Clinical Research. Clifton, NJ: Humana Press, 1988, p 267.

164. Popescu LM, Panoiu C, Hinescu M, et al: The mechanism of cGMP-induced relaxation in vascular smooth muscle. Eur J Pharmacol 107:393, 1980.

165. McNicol A, MacIntyre DE: Reversal of agonist induced phosphoinositide hydrolysis in human platelets by cAMP and cGMP and 1,2-diacylglycerol. Br J Pharmacol 61:159, 1991.

166. Takai Y, Karbuchi K, Matsubara T, et al: Inhibitory action of guanosine 3'5'-monophosphate on thrombin-induced phosphotidylinositol turnover and protein phosphorylation in human platelets. Biochem Biophys Res Commun 101:61, 1981.

167. Fiscus RR: Molecular mechanisms of endothelium mediated vasodilation. Semin Thromb Hemost 14(Suppl 1):12, 1988.

168. Fiscus RR, Rapoport RM, Murad F: Endothelium-dependent

and nitrovasodilator-induced activation of cyclic GMP-dependent protein kinase in rat aorta. J Cyclic Nucleotide Protein Phosphor Res 9:415, 1984.

169. Radomski MW, Palmer RMJ, Moncada S: The role of nitric oxide and cGMP in platelet adhesion to vascular endothelium. Biochem Biophys Res Comm 148:1482, 1987.

170. Alheid U, Frölich JC, Förstermann U: Endothelium-derived relaxing factor from cultured human endothelial cells inhibit aggregation of human platelets. Thromb Res 47:561, 1987.

171. Azuma H, Ishikawa M, Sekizaki S: Endothelium-dependent inhibition of platelet aggregation. Br J Pharmacol 88:441, 1986.

172. Hogan JC, Lewis MJ, Henderson AH: In vivo EDRF activity influences platelet function. Br J Pharmacol 94:1020, 1988.

173. MacDonald PS, Read MA, Dusting GJ: Synergistic inhibition of platelet aggregation by endothelium-derived relaxing factor and prostacyclin. Thromb Res 49:437, 1988.

174. Radomski MW, Palmer RMJ, Read NG, et al: Isolation and washing of human platelets with nitric oxide. Thromb Res 50:537, 1988.

175. Rae GA, Trybulec M, de Nucci G, et al: The anti-aggregating properties of vascular endothelium: Interactions between prostacyclin and nitric oxide. Br J Pharmacol 92:639, 1987.

176. Sneddon JM, Vane JR: Endothelium-derived relaxing factor reduces platelet adhesion to bovine endothelial cells. Proc Natl Acad Sci USA 85:2800, 1988.

177. Furlong B, Henderson AH, Lewis MJ, et al: endothelium-derived relaxing factor inhibits in vitro platelet aggregation. Br J Pharmacol 90:687, 1987.

178. Mellion BT, Ignarro LJ, Ohlstein EH, et al: Evidence for the inhibitory role of guanosine 3'5'-monophosphate in ADP-induced human platelet aggregation in the presence of nitric oxide and related vasodilators. Blood 57:946, 1981.

179. Yang Z, Arnet U, Bauer E, et al: Thrombin-induced endothelium dependent inhibition and direct activation of platelet vessel wall interaction: Role of nitric oxide, prostacyclin and thromboxane A$_2$. Circulation 89:2266, 1991.

180. Lüscher TF, Tanner FC: Endothelial regulation of vascular tone and growth. Am J Hypertens 6:283S, 1993.

181. Dubey RK, Ganten D, Lüscher TF: Enhanced migration of smooth muscle cells from Ren-2 transgenic rats in response to angiotensin II: Inhibition by nitric oxide. Hypertension 22:412, 1993.

182. Dubey RK, Overbeck HW: Culture of mesenteric arteriolar SMCs: Effect of PDGF, AII, and NO on growth. Cell Tissue Res 275:133, 1994.

183. Dubey RK: Vasodilator-derived nitric oxide inhibits fetal calf serum- and angiotensin-II-induced growth of renal arteriolar smooth muscle cells. J Pharmacol Exp Ther 269:402, 1994.

184. Garg UC, Hassid A: Nitric-oxide generating vasodilators and 8-bromo-cyclic guanosine monophosphate inhibit mitogenesis and proliferation of cultured rat vascular SMCs. J Clin Invest 83:1774, 1989.

185. Scott-Burden T, Schini VB, Elizondo E, et al: Platelet-derived growth factor suppresses and fibroblast growth factor enhances cytokine-induced production of NO by cultured aortic SMCs. Effects on cell proliferation. Circ Res 71:1088, 1992.

186. Yokokawa K, Tahara H, Kohno M, et al: Heparin regulates endothelin production through endothelium-derived nitric oxide in human endothelial cells. J Clin Invest 92:2080, 1993.

187. Jackson CL, Schwartz SM: Pharmacology of smooth muscle cell replication. Hypertension 20:713, 1992.

188. Dzau VJ, Gibbons GH: Vascular remodeling: Mechanisms and implications. J Cardiovasc Pharmacol 21(Suppl I):S1, 1993.

189. Casscells W: Migration of smooth muscle and endothelial cells: Critical events in restenosis. Circulation 86:723, 1992.

190. Konishi M, Su C: Role of endothelium in dilator responses of spontaneously hypertensive rat arteries. Hypertension 5:881, 1983.

191. Winquist RJ, Bunting PB, Baskin EP, et al: Decreased endothelium-dependent relaxation in New Zealand genetic hypertensive rats. J Hypertens 2:536, 1984.

192. De Mey JG, Gray SD: Endothelium-dependent reactivity in resistance vessels. Prog Appl Microcirc 88:181, 1985.

193. Lüscher TF, Vanhoutte PM: Endothelium-dependent responses to aggregating platelets and serotonin in spontaneously hypertensive rats. Hypertension 8(Suppl II):55, 1986.

194. Mayhan WG, Faraci FM, Heistad DD: Impairment of endothelium-dependent responses of cerebral arterioles in chronic hypertension. Am J Physiol 253:H1435, 1987.

195. Mayhan WG, Faraci FM, Heistad DD: Responses of cerebral arterioles to adenosine diphosphate, serotonin and the thromboxane analogue U-46619 during chronic hypertension. Hypertension 12(Suppl 6):556, 1989.

196. Lüscher TF, Vanhoutte PM: Endothelium-dependent contractions to acetylcholine in the aorta of the spontaneously hypertensive rat. Hypertension 8:344, 1986.

197. Tschudi MR, Criscione L, Lüscher TF: Effect of aging and hypertension on endothelial function of rat coronary arteries. J Hypertens 9(Suppl 6):164, 1991.

198. Panza JA, Quyyumi AA, Brush JE Jr, et al: Abnormal vascular endothelium-dependent vascular relaxation in patients with essential hypertension. N Engl J Med 323:22, 1990.

199. Creager MA, Roddy M-A, Coleman SM, et al: The effect of ACE inhibition on endothelium-dependent vasodilation in hypertension. J Vasc Res 29:97, 1992.

200. Taddei S, Virdis A, Mattei P, Salvetti A: Vasodilation to acetylcholine in primary and secondary forms of human hypertension. Hypertension 21(6 Pt 2):929, 1993.

201. Cockcroft JR, Chowienczyk PJ, Benjamin N, Ritter JM: Preserved endothelium-dependent vasodilatation in patients with essential hypertension. N Engl J Med 330:1036, 1994.

202. Treasure CB, Manoukian SV, Klein JL, et al: Epicardial coronary artery responses to acetylcholine are impaired in hypertensive patients. Circ Res 71:776, 1992.

203. Treasure CB, Klein JL, Vita JA, et al: Left ventricular hypertrophy secondary to hypertension is associated with impaired endothelium-mediated relaxation in the coronary microvessels. J Am Coll Cardiol 17:127A, 1991.

204. Zeiher AM, Drexler H, Saurbier B, et al: Endothelium-mediated coronary blood flow modulation in humans. Effects of age, atherosclerosis, hypercholesterolemia and hypertension. J Clin Invest 92:652, 1993.

205. Lüscher TF, Vanhoutte PM, Raij L: Antihypertensive therapy normalizes endothelium-dependent relaxations in salt-induced hypertension of the rat. Hypertension 9(Suppl III):193, 1987.

206. Taddei S, Virdis A, Mattei P, et al: Endothelium-dependent forearm vasodilation is reduced in normotensive with familial history of hypertension. J Vasc Res 29:389, 1992.

207. Lüscher TF, Boulanger CM, Dohi Y, et al: Endothelium-derived contracting factors [brief review]. Hypertension 19:117, 1992.

208. Dohi Y, Criscione L, Lüscher TF: Renovascular hypertension impairs formation of endothelium-derived relaxing factors and sensitivity to endothelin-1 in resistance arteries. Br J Pharmacol 104:349, 1991.

209. Tschudi MR, Noll G, Arnet U, et al: Specific reduction of basal formation of nitric oxide in coronary arteries of hypertensive Ren-2 transgenic rats. Circulation 89(6):2780, 1994.

209a. Dohi Y, Thiel M, Bühler FR, Lüscher TF: Activation of the endothelial L-arginine pathway in pressurized mesenteric resistance arteries: Effect of age and hypertension. Hypertension 15:170, 1990.

210. Lüscher TF, Romero JC, Vanhoutte PM: Bioassay of endothelium-derived vasoactive substances in the aorta of normotensive and spontaneously hypertensive rats. J Hypertens 4(Suppl 6):81, 1986.

211. Van de Voorde J, Leusen I: Endothelium-dependent and independent relaxation of aortic rings from hypertensive rats. Am J Physiol 250:H711, 1986.

212. Calver A, Collier J, Moncada S, et al: Effect of local intra-arterial N^G-monomethyl-L-arginine in patients with hypertension: The nitric oxide dilator mechanism appears abnormal. J Hypertens 10:1025, 1992.

213. Panza JA, Casino PR, Badar DM, et al: Effect of increased availability of endothelium-derived nitric oxide on endothelium-dependent vascular relaxation in normals and in patients with essential hypertension. Circulation 87:1475, 1993.

214. Nava E, Noll G, Lüscher TF: Increased cardiac activity of nitric oxide synthase in spontaneously hypertensive rats. Circulation 91:2310, 1995.

214a. Lüscher, Raij L, Vanhoutte PM: Endothelium-dependent responses in normotensive and hypertensive Dahl rats. Hypertension 9:157, 1987.

215. Ross R: The pathogenesis of atherosclerosis—an update. N Engl J Med 314:488, 1986.

216. Ylä-Herttuala S, Palinski W, Rosenfeld ME, et al: Evidence for the presence of oxidatively modified low-density lipoproteins in atherosclerotic lesions of rabbit and man. J Clin Invest 84:1086, 1989.

217. Chester AH, O'Neil GS, Moncada S, et al: Low basal and stimulated release of nitric oxide in atherosclerotic epicardial coronary arteries. Lancet 336:897, 1990.

218. Tanner FC, Noll G, Boulanger CM, et al: Oxidized low-density lipoproteins inhibit relaxations of porcine coronary arteries: Role of scavenger receptor and endothelium-derived nitric oxide. Circulation 83:2012, 1991.

219. Simon BC, Cunningham LD, Cohen RA: Oxidized low density lipoproteins cause contraction and inhibit endothelium-dependent relaxation in the pig coronary artery. J Clin Invest 86:75, 1990.

220. Kugiyama K, Kerns SA, Morrisett JD, et al: Impairment of endothelium-dependent arterial relaxation by lysolecithin in modified low-density lipoproteins. Nature 344:160, 1990.

221. Flavahan NA: Atherosclerosis or lipoprotein-induced endothelial dysfunction: Potential mechanisms underlying reduction in dysfunction in EDRF/nitric oxide activity. Circulation 85:1927, 1992.

222. Shimokawa H, Vanhoutte PM: Hypercholesterolemia causes generalized impairment of endothelium-dependent relaxation to aggregating platelets in porcine arteries. J Am Coll Cardiol 13:1402, 1989.

223. Creager MA, Cooke JP, Mendelsohn ME, et al: Impaired vasodilation of forearm resistance vessels in hypercholesterolemic humans. J Clin Invest 86:228, 1990.

224. Drexler H, Zeiher AM, Meinzer K, et al: Correction of endothelial dysfunction in coronary microcirculation of hypercholesterolemic patients by L-arginine. Lancet 338:1546, 1991.

225. Creager MA, Gallagher SH, Girerd XJ, et al: L-Arginine improves endothelium-dependent vasodilation in hypercholesterolemic humans. J Clin Invest 90:1248, 1992.

226. Galle J, Bassenge E, Busse R: Oxidized low-density lipoproteins potentiate vasoconstrictions to various agonists by direct interaction with vascular smooth muscle. Circ Res 66:1287, 1990.

227. Golino P, Piscione F, Willerson JT, et al: Divergent effects of serotonin on coronary-artery dimensions and blood flow in patients with coronary atherosclerosis and control patients. N Engl J Med 324:641, 1991.

228. Förstermann U, Mügge A, Alheid U, et al: Selective attenuation of endothelium-mediated vasodilation in atherosclerotic human coronary arteries. Circ Res 62:185, 1988.

229. Bossaller C, Yamamoto H, Lichtlen PR, et al: Impaired cholinergic vasodilation in the cholesterol-fed rabbit in vivo. Basic Res Cardiol 82:396, 1987.

230. Freimann PC, Mitchell GG, Heistad DD, et al: Atherosclerosis impairs endothelium-dependent vascular relaxation to acetylcholine and thrombin in primates. Circ Res 58:783, 1986.

231. Heistad DD, Mark AL, Marcus ML, et al: Dietary treatment of atherosclerosis abolishes hyperresponsiveness to serotonin: Implications to vasospasm. Circ Res 61:346, 1987.

232. Verbeuren TJ, Jordaens FH, Zonnekeyn LL, et al: Effect of hypercholesterolemia on vascular reactivity in the rabbit. I. Endothelium-dependent and endothelium-independent contractions and relaxations in isolated arteries of control and hypercholesterolemic rabbits. Circ Res 58:552, 1986.

233. Minor RL, Myers RR Jr, Guerra R Jr, et al: Diet-induced atherosclerosis increases the release of nitrogen oxides from rabbit aorta. J Clin Invest 86:2109, 1990.

234. Shirasaki T, Su C, Lee TJ-F, et al: Endothelial modulation of vascular relaxation to nitrovasodilators in aging and hypertension. J Pharmacol Exp Ther 239:861, 1986.

235. Diederich D, Yang Z, Bühler FR, et al: Impaired endothelium-dependent relaxations in hypertensive resistance arteries involve the cyclooxygenase pathway. Am J Physiol 258:H445, 1990.

236. Lüscher TF, Richard V, Yang Z: Interaction between endothelium-derived nitric oxide and SIN-1 in human and porcine blood vessels. J Cardiovasc Pharmacol 14(Suppl 11):76, 1990.

237. Moncada S, Rees DD, Schultz R, et al: Development and mechanism of a specific supersensitivity to nitrovasodilators after inhibition of vascular nitric oxide synthase in vivo. Proc Natl Acad Sci USA 88:2166, 1990.

238. Pohl U, Busse R: Endothelium-derived relaxant factor inhibits effects of nitrocompounds in isolated arteries. Am J Physiol 252:H307, 1987.

239. Rafflenbeul W, Bassenge E, Lichtlen PR: Competition between endothelium- and nitroglycerin-induced coronary vasodilation. Circulation 78(Suppl II):II-455, 1988.

240. Bassenge E, Stewart DJ: Effects of nitrates in various vascular sections and regions. Z Kardiol 75(Suppl 3):1, 1986.

241. Selke FW, Myers PR, Bates JN, et al: Influence of vessel size on the sensitivity of porcine microvessels to nitroglycerin. Am J Physiol 258:H515, 1990.

242. Stewart DD: Remarkable tolerance to nitroglycerin. Philadelphia Polyclinic 6:171, 1888.

243. Packer M: What causes tolerance to nitroglycerin? The 100 year old mystery continues. J Am Coll Cardiol 16:932, 1990.

244. Stewart DJ, Elsner D, Sommer O, et al: Altered spectrum of nitroglycerin action in long-term treatment: Nitroglycerin-specific venous tolerance with maintenance of arterial vasodepressor potency. Circulation 74:573, 1986.

245. Stewart DJ, Holtz J, Bassenge E: Long-term nitroglycerin treatment: Effect on direct and endothelium mediated large coronary artery dilation in conscious dogs. Circulation 75:847, 1987.

246. Berkenboom G, Fontaine J, Degre S: Persistence of the response to SIN1 on isolated coronary arteries rendered tolerant to nitroglycerin in vitro or in vivo. J Cardiovasc Pharmacol 12:345, 1988.

247. Mülsch A, Busse R, Bassenge E: Desensitization of guanylate cyclase in nitrate tolerance does not impair endothelium-dependent responses. Eur J Pharmacol 158:191, 1988.

248. Feelish M, Noak E: Correlation between nitric oxide formation during degradation of organic nitrates and activation of guanylate cyclase. Eur J Pharmacol 139:19, 1987.

249. Needleman P, Johnson EM Jr: Mechanisms of tolerance development to organic nitrates. J Pharmacol Exp Ther 184:709, 1973.

250. Fung HL, Chomg S, Kowluk E: Mechanisms of nitrate action and vascular tolerance. Eur Heart J 10(Suppl A):2, 1989.

251. Chung S-J, Fung H-L: Identification of the subcellular site for nitroglycerin metabolism to nitric oxide in bovine coronary smooth muscle cells. J Pharmacol Exp Ther 253:614, 1990.

252. Chung S-J, Fung H-L: A common enzyme may be responsible for the conversion of organic nitrates to nitric oxide in vascular microsomes. Biochem Biophys Res Commun 185:932, 1992.

253. Ignarro LJ, Lippton H, Edwards JC, et al: Mechanisms of vascular smooth muscle relaxation by organic nitrates, nitrites, nitroprusside and nitric oxide: Evidence for the involvement of S-nitrosothiols as active intermediates. J Pharmacol Exp Ther 218:739, 1981.

254. Chung S-J, Fung H-L: Relationship between nitroglycerin-induced vascular relaxation and nitric oxide production: Probes with inhibitors and tolerance development. Biochem Pharmacol 45:157, 1993.

255. Fung HL, Poliszczuk R: Nitrosothiol and nitrate tolerance. Z Kardiol 75(Suppl 3):25, 1986.

256. Slack CJ, McLaughlin BE, Brien JF, et al: Biotransformation of glyceryl trinitrate and isosorbide dinitrate in vascular smooth muscle made tolerant to organic nitrates. Can J Physiol Pharmacol 67:1381, 1989.

257. Waldman SA, Rapoport RM, Ginsburg R, et al: Desensitization to nitroglycerin in vascular smooth muscle from rat and human. Biochem Pharmacol 35:3525, 1986.

258. Fung H-L: Pharmacokinetics of nitroglycerin and long acting nitrate esters. Am J Med 74(Suppl 6B):13, 1983.

259. Watanabe H, Kakihana M, Ohtsuka S, et al: Platelet cyclic GMP: A potentially useful indicator to evaluate the effects of nitroglycerin and nitrate tolerance. Circulation 88:29, 1993.

B. Arteriolar Vasodilators

CHAPTER 91

Minoxidil

Vito M. Campese, M.D.

Minoxidil (2,4-diamino-6-piperidinopyrimidine-3-oxide) is the most potent oral vasodilator available; it acts directly on vascular smooth muscle cells, producing a decrease in peripheral vascular resistance and blood pressure. Because of significant side effects, the use of this drug is limited only to patients with hypertension refractory to other commonly used antihypertensive agents.

PHARMACOKINETICS

After oral administration, minoxidil is rapidly absorbed from the gastrointestinal tract, reaching maximal plasma concentration after approximately 1 hour.[1, 2] More than 95% of the drug is absorbed from the gastrointestinal tract. In patients with end-stage renal failure, the gastrointestinal absorption may be delayed.[3]

Because the drug concentrates in extravascular sites, such as arterial smooth muscle cells, and skeletal or myocardial muscle,[4] the volume of distribution exceeds that of water.[1, 5] The high affinity of minoxidil for vascular smooth muscle cells may explain its prolonged hypotensive action. Minoxidil is metabolized predominantly by the liver; 67% is conjugated with glucuronic acid to form a metabolite (minoxidil-*o*-glucuronide) with similar, albeit noticeably reduced, pharmacologic activity; 18% is converted into a totally polar compound; 2.5% is converted into 4-OH minoxidil. Twelve percent of the intact drug and most of its metabolites are excreted by the kidney,[1, 6] whereas only 1% to 3% is found in the feces.

The elimination half-life ranges between 2.8 and 4.2 hours, with an elimination constant of 0.16 to 0.29 hr^{-1}.[1-3, 5] Minoxidil has minimal protein binding and is readily dialysable across cuprophane membranes used for hemodialysis. At a blood flow of 200 ml/min, dialysis clearance is 48 ml/min, and an average of 32% of the drug is removed with a standard hemodialysis.[3] Thus, the drug should not be administered immediately before dialysis. The hypotensive action is linearly related to the log of the dose administered.[7, 8] However, there is no clear relationship between plasma levels and antihypertensive activity. Peak blood concentration of the drug occurs after 1 hour, whereas the peak hypotensive effect occurs only after 2 to 6 hours. Moreover, the hypotensive effect may endure for 12 to 72 hours, despite a half-life of only 2.8 to 4.2 hours.[1, 6]

PHARMACODYNAMIC PROPERTIES
Hypotensive Action

Minoxidil is a direct vasodilator and decreases peripheral vascular resistance.[7, 9, 10] A good correlation has been shown between oral dose and hypotensive activity[7, 8] and between degree of hypertension and hypotensive effect. The drug is effective irrespective of the degree of renal function or of the underlying renal disease (Fig. 91–1).[11]

After prolonged therapy, tachyphylaxis can occur as a consequence of fluid retention and stimulation of the sympathetic and renin-angiotensin-aldosterone systems.[12] The tachyphylaxis can be prevented by the concomitant administration of a diuretic and a β-blocker or a centrally acting antiadrenergic agent or a converting enzyme inhibitor.[3, 12, 13]

The precise mechanism for the vasodilator action of minoxidil is not known. The drug has no direct effect on the central nervous system or on adrenergic neural or receptor function.[9] Its activity is not inhibited by β-adrenergic, cholinergic, or histaminergic blockers.[7] It has been suggested that vasodilators may decrease blood pressure by interfering with calcium movements within the vascular smooth muscle cells.[14] Minoxidil and diazoxide block calcium uptake from the cell membrane, whereas nitroprusside inhibits intracellular release of calcium or the effects of calcium on contractile proteins.[14]

Hemodynamic Effects

Acutely, minoxidil decreases mean arterial pressure and systemic vascular resistance, whereas heart rate and cardiac index increase.[9, 15] Sannerstedt et al.[15] studied the acute effects of minoxidil given over 24 hours in doses of 15 to 45 mg. Blood pressure decreased, whereas heart rate and cardiac output increased. After prolonged treatment, cardiac output and heart rate usually return to pretreatment levels (Fig. 91–2).[12]

Like hydralazine and diazoxide, minoxidil dilates primarily arterioles but has little effect on capacitance vessels.[14] This results in decreased arteriolar resistance and increased venous return with a consequent rise in heart rate, cardiac output, cardiopulmonary blood volume, and pulmonary artery pressure. Conversely, vasodilators such as sodium nitroprusside and prazosin, which dilate both arterioles and veins, decrease the afterload as well as the preload to the heart, resulting in minimal changes in cardiac output and a decrease in pulmonary artery pressure.[16] The nitrates, on the other hand, dilate predominantly the veins, reducing the preload to the heart and decreasing cardiac output. Orthostatic hypotension is a feature of vasodilators acting on capacitance vessels as well as on resistance vessels but not of those vasodilators,

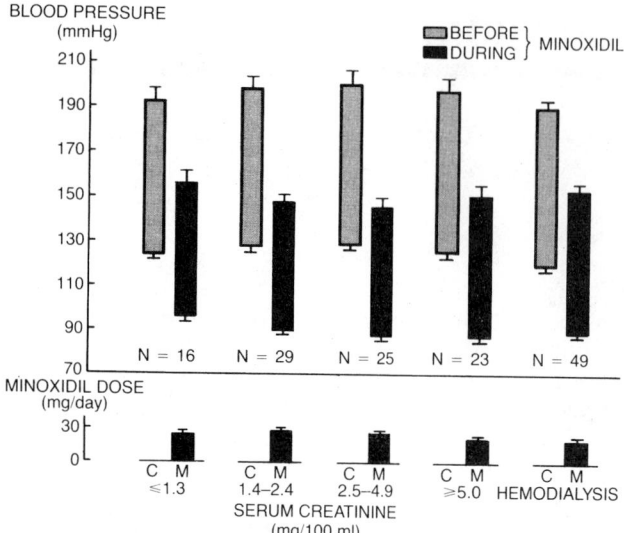

Figure 91–1. Effect of minoxidil on supine blood pressure in patients with refractory hypertension and various levels of renal function. Vertical brackets indicate 1 SE. C, period before minoxidil; M, period during minoxidil therapy; N, number of patients studied. (From Keusch GW, Weidmann P, Campese VM, et al: Minoxidil therapy in refractory hypertension. Analysis of 155 patients. Nephron 21:1, 1978. Reproduced with permission of S Karger AG, Basel.)

such as minoxidil, that act predominantly on resistance vessels. Minoxidil increases blood flow to the skeletal muscles, skin, gastrointestinal tract, pancreas, and coronary arteries but not to the spleen, liver, pituitary gland, and the central nervous system.[17, 18]

Effect on the Sympathetic Nervous System

Peripheral arteriolar vasodilation results in activation of the carotid and aortic baroreceptor reflex arc, stimulation on the sympathetic nervous system (SNS), and increased plasma and urinary norepinephrine

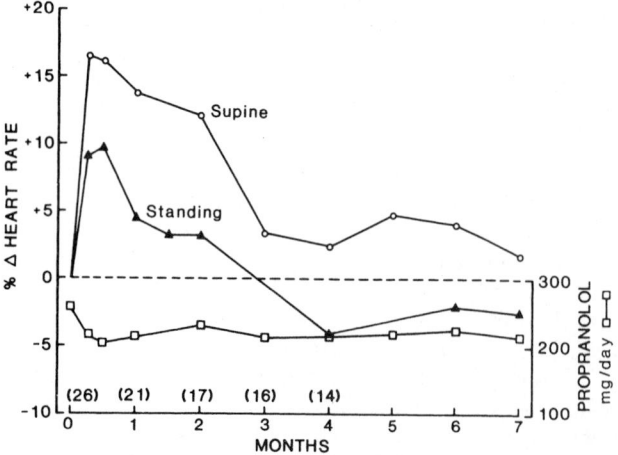

Figure 91–2. Changes in heart rate with duration of treatment. Figures in parentheses are the numbers of patients. (From Campese VM, Stein D, DeQuattro V: Treatment of severe hypertension with minoxidil: Advantages and limitations. J Clin Pharmacol 19:231, 1979.)

concentrations.[19, 20] After chronic administration, minimal or no significant changes in urinary norepinephrine excretion can be detected.[20, 22, 23]

Effect on the Renin-Angiotensin-Aldosterone System

Acute administration of minoxidil results in increased plasma renin activity (PRA)[1, 9, 20, 24–26] and plasma[24–27] and urinary[20–23] aldosterone levels. After prolonged administration, PRA levels remain elevated,[20, 22, 24] whereas plasma aldosterone levels usually normalize.[22, 25, 26] The increase in PRA is largely due to activation of the SNS, and it can be reduced by β-blocking agents; in part, it is due to direct activation of intrarenal baroreceptors,[28, 29] and this component is not suppressed by β-blockers.

The increase in plasma aldosterone level after acute administration of minoxidil is thought to be secondary to increased release of renin, but it cannot be blocked by saralasin or propranolol.[17] Enhanced hepatic metabolic clearance of aldosterone caused by hepatic vasodilation[30] may explain the dichotomy between PRA and plasma or urine aldosterone levels during chronic administration of the drug.

Effect on Renal Function

After acute administration, a decrease,[23, 31, 32] no change,[9] or an increase[33] in renal blood flow has been observed. In the normal dog, minoxidil does not modify effective renal blood flow or glomerular filtration rate (GFR),[34, 35] but it may shift blood flow from the outer to the inner cortex.[35]

The effects of prolonged minoxidil therapy on GFR are variable and may depend on the cause of the hypertension, the preexisting degree of renal function, and the presence or absence of malignant hypertension. Minoxidil does not produce any change in renal function in the majority (95%) of patients with essential hypertension and normal renal function. However, GFR decreased in 23% of patients with essential hypertension and a baseline creatinine of more than 1.5 mg/dl and in 52% of patients with renal parenchymal diseases and baseline serum creatinine levels higher than 1.5 mg/dl[9, 10, 12, 18–20, 23, 26, 36–47] (Table 91–1). In the latter two groups, the deterioration in renal function may be caused by inadequate blood pressure control or by the natural progression of the underlying renal parenchymal disease. In more than one third of patients with malignant hypertension, renal function improves. In patients with severe hypertension and advanced renal failure requiring dialysis,[2, 48] renal function can occasionally improve to a point at which dialysis may no longer be required.

THERAPEUTIC TRIALS

Several therapeutic trials have demonstrated the efficacy of minoxidil in the management of the most severe forms of hypertension. However, because of a significant incidence of serious side effects, the drug

Table 91–1. **Effect of Minoxidil on Serum Creatinine (SC) Levels**

| | | SC Concentration During Treatment | | |
Condition	Patients	Stable	Increase (≥20%)	Decrease (≥20%)
Essential hypertension (SC <1.5 mg/dl)	113	107 (95%)	4 (4%)	2 (2%)
Essential hypertension (SC >1.5 mg/dl)	153	101 (66%)	35 (23%)	17 (11%)
Renal parenchymal disease (SC >1.5 mg/dl)	36	12 (33%)	21 (59%)	3 (8%)
Malignant hypertension	57	34 (59%)	5 (9%)	18 (32%)

Includes data from the following articles: Andersson and Sivertsson[18]; Brunner et al.[20]; Bryan et al.[23]; Camel et al.[36]; Campese et al.[12]; Connor et al.[19]; Devine et al.[37]; Gilmore et al.[9]; Gottlieb et al.[26]; Hammond and Kirkendall[38]; Javier et al.[39]; Klotman et al.[40]; Larochelle et al.[41]; McChesney and Amend[42]; Mitchell et al.[43]; Mutterperl et al.[44]; Nawar et al.[45]; Ryan et al.[46]; Wilburn et al.[47]; Zacest et al.[10] Most patients were receiving minoxidil plus a diuretic and a β-blocker. None of the studies cited was controlled; comparative studies evaluating the effect on renal function of other drugs used under similar conditions would help clarify this issue further.

is currently used only in patients with severe hypertension refractory to other antihypertensive agents. Before the introduction of minoxidil, bilateral nephrectomy was considered inevitable in many patients with severe uncontrollable hypertension while receiving maintenance hemodialysis.[49–52] Minoxidil has been effectively used as a medical alternative to bilateral nephrectomy in most of these cases.[53] Some side effects can be overcome by the concomitant use of other antihypertensive agents, such as β-blockers, angiotensin-converting enzyme inhibitors, diuretics, or antiadrenergic agents. Inadequate response has been described only rarely or in patients with pheochromocytoma, transplant rejection, or acute cerebrovascular accidents.[54] When ineffective, the possibility of inadequate intestinal absorption has to be considered.[55]

Severe Hypertension in Children

Minoxidil in combination with antiadrenergic agents and diuretics has been effectively used in the acute and chronic management of children with severe hypertension and with the hemolytic uremic syndrome.[56, 57]

Hypertensive Urgencies and Emergencies

Minoxidil has been effectively used in the management of hypertensive urgencies.[58] However, because the onset of action occurs gradually over 2 to 4 hours, it should not be the drug of first choice for the management of hypertensive emergencies. In these circumstances, sodium nitroprusside, nifedipine, or intravenous labetalol should be used preferentially.

In Combination with Other Drugs

Propranolol in doses of 80 to 240 mg/day potentiates the hypotensive effect of minoxidil,[9] in part because it prevents the rise in cardiac output and in part because it inhibits renin secretion. Centrally acting agents, such as clonidine or methyldopa, may also potentiate the antihypertensive effect of minoxidil by reducing sympathetic hyperactivity and the increase

in plasma renin activity.[43, 55, 59, 60] Several studies have shown that a combination of minoxidil and angiotensin-converting enzyme inhibitors may also be very effective in patients with refractory hypertension.[61, 62]

SIDE EFFECTS

Significant side effects occur frequently in patients treated with minoxidil, limiting its use to the more severe cases of hypertension and occasionally requiring discontinuation of the drug. The most common side effects are sodium and fluid retention, tachycardia, and hypertrichosis.

Sodium and Fluid Retention

Minoxidil causes sodium and fluid retention, peripheral edema, and, in the most severe cases, congestive heart failure.[1, 9, 23, 38, 41, 63] The degree of sodium and water retention correlates with the dose and the degree of renal insufficiency.[46] Because chronic administration of minoxidil does not cause any consistent change in GFR, effective renal blood flow, or aldosterone secretion, the effects on sodium retention cannot be exclusively attributed to alterations in renal hemodynamics. Thus, a direct effect of minoxidil on sodium reabsorption in the renal tubules has been suggested.[35] The administration of diuretics, such as furosemide, is always necessary to prevent sodium retention. Patients with moderate to severe renal failure[41, 46, 54] or with severe obstructive cardiomyopathy[54] may become unresponsive to furosemide, and congestive heart failure may develop. In these cases, dialysis or discontinuation of the drug may be necessary. Anuric patients treated with minoxidil who are receiving maintenance hemodialysis may experience a greater increase in body weight during the interdialytic periods[11] (Fig. 91–3). Because these patients have no urine output, the increase in body weight has been attributed to increased thirst and sodium intake caused by reflex stimulation of the renin-angiotensin system.[64–66] The increase in thirst subsides with bilateral nephrectomy.[67]

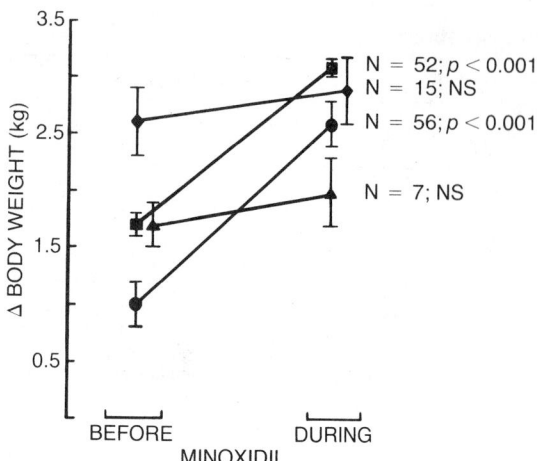

Figure 91–3. Weight gain between dialysis before and during minoxidil therapy for refractory hypertension in four patients. N, number of interdialysis periods. (From Keusch GW, Weidmann P, Campese VM, et al: Minoxidil therapy in refractory hypertension. Analysis of 155 patients. Nephron 21:1, 1978. Reproduced with permission of S Karger AG, Basel.)

Affecting the Cardiovascular System

Ischemic Heart Disease

Minoxidil causes tachycardia and palpitations as a result of reflex stimulation of the sympathetic nervous system. During the first 2 weeks of treatment, depression of ST segments and T-wave flattening or inversion can be seen in as many as 90% of patients.[4, 23, 41, 46, 68, 69] After 3 to 6 months of therapy, usually these abnormalities revert spontaneously; occasionally, they may persist for several years. Episodes of angina and/or myocardial infarction may also occur.[12, 37, 38, 70]

Pericardial Effusion

Minoxidil can cause or aggravate pericardial effusion, occasionally leading to cardiac tamponade and death.[10, 12, 19, 43, 47, 71] The incidence of pericardial effusion is difficult to estimate because many patients have renal insufficiency and no baseline echocardiogram before treatment. In a retrospective uncontrolled analysis of 1869 patients treated with minoxidil, 91 instances of clinically relevant pericardial effusion were found, 21 resulting in cardiac tamponade,[71] mainly among patients on dialysis. This incidence would not appear to be different from the 10% incidence of pericarditis ascribed to dialysis patients.[72] However, clinical experience and the fact that the effusion may occasionally recur when patients are rechallenged with minoxidil indicate a cause-effect relationship.

The mechanisms for the pericardial effusion are not clear, but several factors could play a role, including sodium retention, increased myocardial blood flow, or imbalance of Starling forces in the pericardial and superficial myocardial capillaries.

In patients with mild pericardial effusion, discontinuation of the drug may not be necessary. In the most severe cases, the drug should be discontinued or, alternatively, a pericardiectomy should be performed.

Pulmonary Hypertension

During treatment with minoxidil, some patients may have pulmonary hypertension,[31, 47, 73] but in two prospective studies, no changes in pulmonary artery pressure were observed when minoxidil was given in combination with propranolol.[40, 74] This has been attributed to a disproportionately large increase in cardiac output with a relatively small decrease in pulmonary vascular resistance.[31] In patients with congestive heart failure, pulmonary artery pressure may actually decrease, probably as a result of improved left ventricular function.[31] Tarazi et al.[16] have described two types of pulmonary hypertension associated with minoxidil therapy. The first (the congestive type) is characterized by marked fluid retention, a rise in pulmonary wedge pressure, and a decline in cardiac output. The second type (hyperkinetic pulmonary hypertension), more frequent than the first type, is characterized by a marked rise in cardiac output and a lesser increase in pulmonary wedge pressure and total blood volume. It usually improves with the administration of propranolol.

Elevated pulmonary artery pressure has been described in hypertensive patients treated with a vasodilator other than minoxidil,[75] such as hydralazine and diazoxide, and a direct correlation has been observed between systemic and pulmonary vascular resistance.[76] On the contrary, nitroprusside and glyceryl trinitrate (nitroglycerin) decrease pulmonary artery pressure.[16]

Hemorrhagic and Necrotic Myocardial Lesions

Hemorrhagic and degenerative lesions of the right atrium have been observed in dogs, but not in rats or monkeys, treated with minoxidil. Myocardial focal necrosis may also occur in the papillary muscles of the left ventricle in dogs or rats.[77] There is, however, no evidence that lesions in the right atrium occur in humans.[78]

Hypertrichosis

Hypertrichosis occurs in nearly all patients treated with minoxidil for more than 4 weeks.[37, 48, 56] The hair growth may involve the temples, forehead, face, pinna of the ear, eyebrows, forearm, and eventually all the hairy surfaces of the body. The hair growth appears to be of the intermediate type, with pigmentation and intermittent medullation and a normal shaft.[79] This seriously limits the use of this drug in women and has been responsible for reactive depression in some patients.

The hair growth is not due to hormonal imbalance, because serum levels of testosterone and urinary excretion of hydroxysteroids and ketosteroids remain unchanged,[46, 80] but it may be due to increased blood flow in the skin; other potent vasodilators, such as diazoxide, may also cause hypertrichosis.[81, 82] The hypertrichosis is reversible and disappears 1 to 2 months after discontinuation of the drug. For cosmetic purposes, it may be controlled with calcium thioglycolate depilatory.[80]

Other Side Effects

Minoxidil does not cause hepatic, renal, hematologic, or central nervous system toxicity. Pulsating headache can occasionally occur.[10, 41] Derangement of glucose metabolism has been described, but a causal relationship is dubious.[70, 76] Itching of the eyes has also been described.[77] Polymenorrhea has been reported in two patients.[41] Skin rashes, including pruritic bullous eruption, have occurred in some patients, often early in the course of therapy.

REFERENCES

1. Gottlieb TB, Thomas RC, Chidsey CA: Pharmacokinetic studies of minoxidil. Clin Pharmacol Ther 13:436, 1972.
2. Lowenthal DT, Onesti G, Mutterperl R, et al: Long-term clinical effects, bioavailablility and kinetics of minoxidil in relation to renal function. J Clin Pharmacol 18:500, 1978.
3. Bennett WM, Golper TA, Muther RS, et al: Efficacy of minoxidil in the treatment of severe hypertension in systemic disorders. J Cardiovasc Pharmacol 2(Suppl 2):142, 1980.
4. Pluss RG, Orcutt J, Chidsey CA: Tissue distribution and hypotensive effects of minoxidil in normotensive rats. J Lab Clin Med 79:639, 1972.
5. Lowenthal DT, Affrime MB: Pharmacology and pharmacokinetics of minoxidil. J Cardiovasc Pharmacol 2(Suppl 2):93, 1980.
6. Thomas RC, Harpootlian H: Metabolism of minoxidil, a new hypotensive agent. II. Biotransformation following oral administration to rats, dogs, and monkeys. J Pharmacol Sci 64:1366, 1975.
7. DuCharme DW, Freyburger WA, Graham BE, et al: Pharmacologic properties of minoxidil: A new hypotensive agent. J Pharmacol Exp Ther 184:662, 1973.
8. O'Malley K, McNay JL: A method for achieving blood pressure control expeditiously with oral minoxidil. Clin Pharmacol Ther 18:39, 1975.
9. Gilmore E, Weil J, Chidsey C: Treatment of essential hypertension with a new vasodilator in combination with beta-adrenergic blockade. N Engl J Med 282:521, 1970.
10. Zacest R, Frewin DB, Robinson MA, et al: Clinical and haemodynamic effects of minoxidil in refractory hypertension. Drug 11(Suppl 1):177, 1976.
11. Keusch GW, Weidmann P, Campese VM, et al: Minoxidil therapy in refractory hypertension. Analysis of 155 patients. Nephron 21:1, 1978.
12. Campese VM, Stein D, DeQuattro V: Treatment of severe hypertension with minoxidil: Advantages and limitations. J Clin Pharmacol 19:231, 1979.
13. Limas CJ, Freis ED: Minoxidil in severe hypertension with renal failure: Effect of its addition to conventional antihypertensive drugs. Am J Cardiol 31:355, 1973.
14. Chidsey CA, Gottlieb TB: The pharmacologic basis of antihypertensive therapy: The role of vasodilator drugs. Prog Cardiovasc Dis 27:99, 1974.
15. Sannerstedt R, Brorson L, Berglund G, et al: Minoxidil. Haemodynamic and clinical experiences with a new peripheral vasodilator. Acta Med Scand 197:409, 1975.
16. Tarazi RC, Dustan HP, Bravo EL, et al: Vasodilating drugs: Contrasting haemodynamic effects. Clin Sci Mol Med 51(Suppl):575, 1976.
17. Humphrey SJ, Wilson E, Zins GR: Whole body tissue blood flow in conscious dogs treated with minoxidil [abstract]. Fed Proc 33:583, 1974.
18. Andersson O, Sivertsson R: Renal function and vascular resistance during long-term minoxidil treatment of severe hypertension. J Cardiovasc Pharmacol 2(Suppl 2):123, 1980.
19. Connor G, Wilburn RL, Bennett CM: Double-blind comparison of minoxidil and hydralazine in severe hypertension. Clin Sci Mol Med 51:593, 1976.
20. Brunner HR, Jaeger P, Ferguson RK, et al: Need for beta-blockade in hypertension reduced with long-term minoxidil. Br Med J 2:385, 1978.
21. Mitchell HC, Pettinger WA: Long-term treatment of refractory hypertensive patients with minoxidil. JAMA 239:2131, 1978.
22. Meier A, Weidmann P, Ziegler WH: Catecholamines, renin, aldosterone, and blood volume during chronic minoxidil therapy. Klin Wochenschr 59:1231, 1981.
23. Bryan AK, Hoobler SW, Rosenzweig J, et al: Effect of minoxidil on blood pressure and hemodynamics in severe hypertension. Am J Cardiol 39:796, 1977.
24. Baer L, Radichevich I, Williams GS: Treatment of drug-resistant hypertension with minoxidil or angiotensin converting enzyme inhibitor: Blood pressure, renin aldosterone, and electrolyte responses. J Cardiovas Pharmacol 2(Suppl 2):206, 1980.
25. Grim CE, Luft FC, Grim CM, et al: Rapid blood pressure control with minoxidil: Acute and chronic effects on blood pressure, sodium excretion, and the renin-aldosterone system. Arch Intern Med 139:529, 1979.
26. Gottlieb TB, Katz FH, Chidsey CA: Combined therapy with vasodilator drugs and beta-adrenergic blockade in hypertension. Circulation 45:571, 1972.
27. Campbell WB, Pettenger WA, Keeton K, et al: Vasodilating antihypertensive drug-induced aldosterone. A study of endogenous angiotensin-mediated aldosterone release in the rat. J Pharmacol Exper Ther 193:166, 1975.
28. Pettinger WA, Keeton K: Altered renin releases and propranolol potentiation of vasodilatory drug hypotension. J Clin Invest 55:236, 1975.
29. O'Malley K, Velasco M, Wells J, et al: Control plasma renin activity and changes in sympathetic tone as determinants of minoxidil-induced increase in plasma renin activity. J Clin Invest 55:230, 1975.
30. Pratt JH, Grim CE, Parkinson CA: Minoxidil increases aldosterone metabolic clearance in hypertensive patients. J Clin Endocrinol Metab 49:834, 1979.
31. Hall D, Froer KL, Loracher C: Treatment of severe hypertension with minoxidil and its effects on systemic and pulmonary haemodynamics. Clin Sci Molec Med 51(Suppl):587, 1976.
32. Rosello S, O'Malley K, Boles M, et al: Impairment of renal autoregulation in hypertension with nephrosclerosis. Clin Res 22:301A, 1974.
33. Liebau G, Hayduk K, Bundschu HD: Klinische erfahrungen mit minoxidil, einen neuen antihypertonikum. Verh Dtsch Ges Inn Med 80:277, 1974.
34. Robie NW, McNay JL: Comparative splanchnic blood flow effects of various vasodilator compounds. Circ Shock 4:69, 1977.
35. Zins GR: Alterations in renal function during vasodilator therapy. In Fanelli GM, Wesson LG (eds): Recent Advances in Renal Physiology and Pharmacology. Baltimore: University Park Press, 1974, pp 165–186.
36. Camel GH, Carmody SE, Perry HMI: Use of minoxidil in the azotemic patient. J Cardiovasc Pharmacol 2(Suppl 2):173, 1980.
37. Devine BL, Fife R, Trust PM: Minoxidil in severe hypertension after failure of other hypotensive drugs. Br Med J 2:667, 1977.
38. Hammond JJ, Kirkendall WM: Minoxidil therapy for refractory hypertension and chronic renal failure. South Med J 72:1429, 1979.
39. Javier R, Dumler F, Park JH, et al: Long-term treatment with minoxidil in patients with severe renal failure. J Cardiovasc Pharmacol 2(Suppl 2):149, 1980.
40. Klotman PE, Grum CE, Weinberger KY, et al: The effects of minoxidil on pulmonary and systemic hemodynamics in hypertensive man. Circulation 55:394, 1977.
41. Larochelle P, Berniade V, Hamet P, et al: Minoxidil in severe hypertension. Eur J Clin Pharmacol 14:1, 1978.
42. McChesney JA, Amend WJC Jr: Minoxidil in the treatment of refractory hypertension due to a spectrum of causes. J Cardivoasc Pharmacol 2(Suppl 2):131, 1980.

43. Mitchell HC, Graham RM, Pettinger WA: Renal function during long-term treatment of hypertension with minoxidil. Comparison of benign and malignant hypertension. Ann Intern Med 93:676, 1980.

44. Mutterperl RE, Diamond FB, Lowenthal DT: Longterm effects of minoxidil in the treatment of malignant hypertension in chronic renal failure. J Clin Pharmacol 16:498, 1976.

45. Nawar T, Nolin L, Plante GE, et al: Long-term treatment of severe hypertension with minoxidil. Can Med Assoc J 19:1178, 1977.

46. Ryan JR, Jain AK, McMahon FG: Minoxidil treatment of severe hypertension. Curr Ther Res 17:55, 1975.

47. Wilburn RL, Blaufuss A, Bennett CM: Long-term treatment of severe hypertension with minoxidil, propranolol and furosemide. Circulation 52:706, 1975.

48. Campese VM: Minoxidil: A review of its pharmacological properties and therapeutic use. Drugs 22:257, 1981.

49. Lazarus JM, Hampers CL, Bennett AH, et al: Urgent bilateral nephrectomy for severe hypertension. Ann Intern Med 76:733, 1972.

50. Mahony JF, Gibson GR, Sheil AGR, et al: Bilateral nephrectomy for malignant hypertension. Lancet 1:1036, 1972.

51. Onesti G, Swartz C, Ramirez O, et al: Bilateral nephrectomy for control of hypertension in uremia. Trans Am Soc Artif Intern Organs 144:361, 1968.

52. Weidmann P, Maxwell MH, Lupu AN, et al: Plasma renin activity and blood pressure in terminal renal failure. N Engl J Med 285:757, 1971.

53. Pettinger WA: Minoxidil and the treatment of severe hypertension. N Engl J Med 303:922, 1980.

54. Wells JO: Unusual cases of resistance to minoxidil therapy. J Cardiovasc Pharmacol 2(Suppl 2):228, 1980.

55. Pettinger WA, Mitchell HC: Minoxidil—an alternative to nephrectomy for refractory hypertension. N Engl J Med 289:167, 1973.

56. Pennisi AJ, Takahashi M, Bernstein BH, et al: Minoxidil therapy in children with severe hypertension. J Pediatr 90:813, 1977.

57. Sinaiko AR, O'Dea RF, Mirkin BL: Clinical response of hypertensive children to long-term minoxidil therapy. J Cardiovasc Pharmacol 2(Suppl 2):181, 1980.

58. Bauer JH, Alpert MA: Rapid reduction of severe hypertension with minoxidil. J Cardiovasc Pharmacol 2(Suppl 2)189, 1980.

59. Pettinger WA, Mitchell HC, Gullner HG: Clonidine and the vasodilating beta blocker antihypertensive drug interaction. Clin Pharmacol Ther 22:164, 1977.

60. Velasco M, Silva H, Morillo J, et al: Cardiovascular hemodynamic interactions between clonidine and minoxidil in hypertensive patients. Chest 83(Suppl 2):360, 1983.

61. Traub YM, Levey BA: Combined treatment with minoxidil and captopril with refractory hypertension. Arch Intern Med 143:1142, 1983.

62. Seedat YK, Rawat R: Captopril combined with minoxidil, beta-blocker and furosemide in the treatment of refractory hypertension. Eur J Clin Pharmacol 25:9, 1983.

63. Pedersen OL: Long-term experiences with minoxidil in combi-nation treatment of severe arterial hypertension. Acta Cardiol 32:283, 1977.

64. Epstein AN, Fitzsimons JT, Rolls BJ: Drinking induced by injection of angiotensin into the brain of the rat. J Physiol (London) 210:457, 1970.

65. Fitzsimons JT: The physiological basis of thirst. Kidney Int 10:3, 1976.

66. Severs WB, Summmy-Long J, Taylor JS, et al: A central effect of angiotensin: Release of pituitary pressor material. J Pharmacol Exper Ther 174:27, 1970.

67. Rogers PW, Kurtzman NA: Renal failure, uncontrollable thirst, and hyperreninemia. Cessation of thirst with bilateral nephrectomy. JAMA 225:1236, 1973.

68. Jacomb RG, Brunnberg FJ: The use of minoxidil in the treatment of severe essential hypertension: A report on 100 patients. Clin Sci Mol Med 51(Suppl):577, 1976.

69. Hall D, Froer KL, Rudolph W: Serial electrocardiographic changes during long-term treatment of severe hypertension with minoxidil. J Cardiovasc Pharmacol 2(Suppl 2):200, 1980.

70. Traub YM, Redmond DP, Rosenfeld JB, et al: Treatment of severe hypertension with minoxidil. Isr J Med Sci 11:991, 1975.

71. Martin WB, Spodick DH, Zins GR: Pericardial disorders occurring during open-label study of 1,869 severely hypertensive patients treated with minoxidil. J Cardiovasc Pharmacol 2(Suppl 2):217, 1980.

72. Bailey GL, Hanapers CC, Hager EG, et al: Uremic pericarditis: Clinical features and management. Circulation 38:582, 1968.

73. Dormois JC, Young JL, Nies AS: Minoxidil in severe hypertension: Value when conventional drugs have failed. Am Heart J 90:360, 1975.

74. Alpert MA, Bauer JH, Parker BM, et al: Pulmonary hemodynamics in systemic hypertension—long-term effect of minoxidil. Chest 76:379, 1979.

75. Taylor SH, Donald KW, Bishop JM: Circulatory studies in hypertensive patients at rest and during exercise. Clin Sci 16:351, 1957.

76. Atkins JM, Mitchell HC, Pettinger WA: Increased pulmonary vascular resistance with systemic hypertension. Effect of minoxidil and other antihypertensive agents. Am J Cardiol 39:802, 1977.

77. Herman EH, Balazs T, Young R, et al: Acute cardiomyopathy induced by the vasodilating antihypertensive agent minoxidil. Toxicol Appl Pharmacol 47:493, 1979.

78. Sobota JT, Martin WB, Carlson RG, et al: Minoxidil: Right atrial cardiac pathology in animals and man. Circulation 62:376, 1980.

79. Burton JL, Marshall A: Hypertrichosis due to minoxidil. J Dermatol 101:593, 1979.

80. Earhart RN, Ball J, Nuss DD, et al: Minoxidil-induced hypertrichosis: Treatment with calcium thioglycolate depilatory. South Med J 70:442, 1977.

81. Muller SA: Hirsutism. Am J Med 46:803, 1969.

82. Nickerson M: Antihypertensive agents and the drug therapy of hypertension. *In* Goodman LS, Gilman AG (eds): The Pharmacological Basis of Therapeutics, 4th ed. New York: Macmillan, 1971, p 728.

C. Arteriolar and Venous Vasodilators

CHAPTER 92

Nitroprusside

Joseph Murphy, M.B., M.R.C.P.I., F.A.C.C., Carl J. Lavie, M.D., F.A.C.C., F.A.C.P., and Dennis R. Bresnahan, M.D., F.A.C.C., F.A.C.P.

Nitroprusside is a potent, rapidly acting, intravenously administered vasodilator that directly relaxes the smooth muscle of both arteriolar and venous vascular beds. This effect is balanced in that arteriolar and venous tone are reduced about equally. Nitroprusside is frequently classified as the prototypical vasodilator and has been used extensively in the treatment of hypertensive emergencies, acute valvular insufficiency, states of low cardiac output, and congestive myocardial failure. Its distinctive features include the ability to reduce arterial pressure to the desired level in most patients and its extremely short half-life. These properties make nitroprusside a valuable agent for the management of many emergency situations, particularly hypertensive crises, acute pulmonary edema, and acute aortic dissection.

BACKGROUND

Although the hypotensive effect of nitroprusside in animals was initially described in 1887 by Davidsohn,[1] it was not until 1974 that the drug was approved for clinical use. Since then, nitroprusside has become an integral part of the pharmacologic armamentarium for emergency medicine, critical care medicine, anesthesiology, and the treatment of cardiovascular diseases.

PHARMACOLOGY
Chemistry

Nitroprusside is chemically disodium pentacyanonitro-sylferrate(2-) dihydrate ($Na_2Fe(CN)_5NO \cdot 2H_2O$), a water-soluble, reddish-brown powder with a molecular weight of 297.95. It is an iron coordination complex compound that forms red, rhomboid, bipyramidal crystals. On spectrophotometry, nitroprusside has two absorptive peaks at 394 nm and 498 nm.[2]

Mechanism of Action

Nitroprusside is a potent, rapidly acting, intravenously administered hypotensive agent whose action is mediated by its nitroso group rather than by its metabolites. Nitroprusside, in common with a heterogeneous group of other pharmacologic agents, is classified as a nitrovasodilator. These agents share the property of producing their biologic effects via the release of nitric oxide.[3-5] Nitroprusside has an oxidation state of +3 and can release nitric oxide nonenzymatically by means of a one-electron reduction that occurs on exposure to even mild reducing agents or vascular smooth muscle membranes. Nitric oxide release is thought to be accompanied by cyanide release in small quantities. A large body of scientific literature has been published on the physiologic role of nitric oxide in the vascular wall and its close, if not identical, properties to endothelium-dependent relaxing factor.[6-15] A review of this subject is beyond the scope of this chapter.

In summary, nitric oxide is thought to react with the cytosolic enzyme, soluble guanylate cyclase, to activate it and thereby increase the intracellular concentrations of cyclic guanosine monophosphate (cGMP). This in turn inhibits activation of the phosphoinositol pathway, which is responsible for stimulating calcium influx across the sarcolemmal membrane and intracellular calcium release, leading to increased cytosolic free calcium. An increase in cGMP in vascular smooth muscle relaxes vascular smooth muscle tone, more specifically when this is increased by receptor-mediated stimulation.

Nitroprusside has no significant direct effect on intracellular cyclic adenosine monophosphate or adenosine triphosphate levels or on contractile proteins.[16] Although nitroprusside is strongly suspected of causing vasodilation via intracellular messenger cGMP, a definitive causal relationship has not been demonstrated.[16] By whatever mechanism, nitroprusside has a marked but balanced vasodilator effect on both resistance and capacitance vessels.

Metabolic Degradation

Nitroprusside is degraded by the nonenzymatic cleavage of the molecule, resulting in release of the cyanide group, which then reacts with circulating thiosulfate in the liver to form thiocyanate. This reaction is catalyzed by the enzyme rhodanese. The precise mechanism of nitroprusside cleavage in vivo has not been determined, but reactions with tissue compounds containing sulfhydryl groups (cysteine, methionine, and reduced glutathione) are probably involved.[17] It has also been postulated that a reaction between hemoglobin and nitroprusside may lead to cyanide release.[18] Although the principal method of cyanide deactivation is via its reaction with thiosulfate, alternative but quantitatively minor pathways of cyanide inactivation include reactions with methemoglobin to form cyanmethemoglobin and with hydroxycobalamin to form cyanocobalamin. Cyanate is selectively taken up by red blood cells, and free plasma cyanate is the principal determinant of toxicity. The rate-limiting factor for the inactivation of cyanide is the availability of thiosulfate. Administration of thiosulfate has been shown to protect against nitroprusside toxicity.[19] The liver is the principal site of inactivation of the cyanide group,[20] and liver failure sometimes leads to cyanide toxicity.

Clinical Administration

Nitroprusside (Nipride, Nitropress) is available solely as an intravenous preparation. The compound is light-sensitive and should be freshly prepared and used within 6 hours, if possible. Nitroprusside infusions have been shown to be stable for 12 hours from the time of preparation if protected from light. The infusion bottle should be wrapped in photoopaque aluminum foil or dark plastic to prevent degradation. Nitroprusside is available in 5-ml vials containing 50 mg of drug. The standard infusion of nitroprusside (100 μg/ml) is prepared by dissolving the contents of the vial in 3 ml of 5% dextrose in water and adding this solution to a further 250 or 500 ml of 5% dextrose in water. The fresh solution may have a faint brownish color. The infusion should be started at 0.2 μg/kg/min and increased by 0.2 μg/kg/min every 5 to 10 minutes to a maximal dosage of 10 μg/kg/min. The infusion rate is titrated against the blood pressure, which should be monitored continuously (often by intraarterial monitoring). If the maximal dosage of 10 µg/kg/min does not lead to an adequate hypotensive effect within 10 minutes, the infusion should be stopped and an alternative drug started. Tachyphylaxis has not been reported in human studies.

PATHOPHYSIOLOGY
Myocardial Blood Flow

Although most evidence indicates that nitroprusside increases total coronary blood flow, some experimental and clinical evidence suggests that nitroprusside may lead to a "coronary steal syndrome" by preferentially dilating coronary arterioles to nonischemic myocardium with a resultant decrease in blood flow to the ischemic zone. Chiariello et al.[21] compared the effects of nitroprusside and nitroglycerin on ischemic injury during acute myocardial infarction and reported that, although these agents had similar overall hemodynamic effects, nitroprusside increased whereas nitroglycerin decreased the sum of precordial ST-segment elevations. In addition, in contrast with nitroglycerin, nitroprusside decreased myocardial blood flow to the ischemic zones and decreased intercoronary collateral flow (Table 92–1). Mann et al.[22] reported that in patients with coronary angiographic evidence of collateral blood flow, nitroglycerin increased whereas nitroprusside decreased coronary blood flow to the ischemic zone. Gopal et al.[23] reported contradictory evidence following studies on nitroprusside's effect on myocardial blood flow in conscious dogs in which balloon-cuff occluders had been implanted around the left anterior descending coronary artery. In this study, nitroprusside decreased aortic mean and left ventricular diastolic pressures but increased blood flow to both ischemic and nonis-

chemic myocardial regions. The authors suggested that nitroprusside improved myocardial perfusion to acutely ischemic myocardial tissue, despite a fall in aortic pressure, by decreasing resistance to flow in coronary collateral vessels or decreasing myocardial tissue pressure. In summary, clinicians using nitroprusside must be aware that this agent can worsen myocardial ischemia in susceptible patients. However, nitroprusside is unlikely to be harmful in patients with significant hypertension and left ventricular dysfunction, especially if the pulmonary capillary wedge pressure is significantly elevated.

Saphenous Vein and Internal Mammary Artery Grafts

Jett et al.[24] studied the effect of nitroprusside and nitroglycerin on vascular ring segments of human internal mammary arteries *in vitro* and on experimental canine internal mammary artery and saphenous vein bypass grafts. Nitroprusside was more effective than nitroglycerin in inhibiting potassium- and norepinephrine-induced vascular ring contraction. Blood flow to saphenous vein bypass grafts increased with nitroprusside but decreased with nitroglycerin (see Table 92–1). The internal mammary artery grafts, however, responded differently, with a significant decrease in blood flow with nitroprusside and an increase with nitroglycerin.

Platelet Function

In human studies, nitroprusside has a dose-dependent inhibitory effect on platelet aggregation.[25] Inhibition by sodium nitroprusside of platelet aggregation and diminution of adenosine diphosphate–induced aggregation are also thought to be mediated by an increase in intracellular levels of cGMP.[26] However, the clinical significance of this platelet inhibition is uncertain.

CLINICAL INDICATIONS
Hypertensive Emergencies

Nitroprusside's rapid onset of action and ease of administration make it the agent of choice for the initial treatment of most hypertensive emergencies.[27] The onset of action following intravenous initiation of nitroprusside is 1 to 10 minutes. It is consistently effective in nearly all cases, and the dosage can be titrated to the desired arterial blood pressure. The drug has the disadvantage that it must be given intravenously, usually in an intensive care setting and often with intraarterial blood pressure monitoring. It ceases to act within minutes of cessation of the infusion. It has the added benefit, however, of preload and afterload reduction in patients with hypertension-induced left ventricular failure.

The choice of hypotensive agent depends on the cause of the hypertensive crisis.[28] In general, nitroprusside is the agent of choice in patients with left

Table 92–1. **Comparison of Nitroprusside and Nitroglycerin**

Variable	Nitroprusside	Nitroglycerin
Preload	↓ ↓	↓ ↓
Afterload	↓ ↓ ↓	↓
Mean arterial pressure	↓ ↓ ↓	↓
Ventricular wall stress	↓ ↓	↓
Ejection fraction	↔ ↑	↔
Cardiac output	↑ ↑	↑ ↓ ↔
Heart rate	↔ ↑	↑ ↓ ↔
Regurgitant fraction	↓ ↓	↓ ↔
Myocardial Perfusion		
Ischemic zone	↓ ↑ ↔	↑
Nonischemic zone	↑	↑
Collateral vessels	↔ ↓	↑
Saphenous vein grafts	↑	↓
Internal mammary grafts	↓	↑
Summary		
Severe hypertension	Agent of choice	Minimally useful
Congestive heart failure:		
Low output	Agent of choice	May be deleterious
Pulmonary congestion	Very useful	Very useful
Mitral regurgitation	Agent of choice	Useful
Acute myocardial ischemia	May be deleterious	Useful

↓, decreases; ↔, no change; ↑, increases.

ventricular failure, hypertensive encephalopathy, postoperative hypertension, and head injury or stroke. In myocardial ischemia, β-blockers and intravenously administered nitroglycerin are probably preferable. Phentolamine is the agent of choice in hypertensive crisis caused by catecholamine excess. In dissecting aortic aneurysm, trimethaphan or nitroprusside may be combined with a β-blocker.

Nitroprusside has been used successfully in the treatment of severe preeclampsia with drug-resistant hypertension,[29] severe hypertension due to clonidine withdrawal,[30] and phentolamine-resistant pheochromocytomas.[31] Although nitroprusside has been used successfully during pregnancy in selected cases, limited information is available regarding the risks of maternal and fetal toxicity; other hypotensive agents should be used wherever possible.

Acute Myocardial Ischemia and Infarction

The rationale for using nitroprusside in patients with acute myocardial infarction is based on the findings that improving myocardial perfusion by coronary vasodilatation and reducing cardiac work by reductions in preload, afterload, and left ventricular wall stress will improve the myocardial oxygen supply/demand ratio and thereby reduce infarct size. Nitroprusside has been shown to reduce left ventricular filling pressure and improve ventricular function in acute infarction.[32, 33] Nitroprusside may also have an additional beneficial effect in acute infarction by decreasing platelet aggregation and relieving coronary artery spasm.

The hemodynamic and clinical effects of nitroprusside have frequently been compared with those of nitroglycerin in patients with acute myocardial infarction. Both agents are potentially deleterious in this setting because they may lead to significant arterial hypotension with consequent reduction in diastolic coronary perfusion or reflex tachycardia with increased myocardial oxygen consumption. Several studies from both animal and clinical investigations suggest that nitroglycerin may be superior to nitroprusside in acute infarction because of its greater effect on increasing myocardial blood flow to ischemic zones and promoting intercoronary collateral blood flow.[21, 22, 34]

Three randomized trials have studied the effect of nitroprusside on survival in myocardial infarction.[35-37] These trials comprised 1190 patients, with reductions in mortality between control and treatment groups of 36% to 28% (not significant),[35] 12% to 6% ($p < .05$),[36] and 19% to 17% (not significant),[37] respectively. Pooled data from these studies showed an overall reduction in mortality from 106 of 595 patients (17.8%) in the control group to 85 of 595 patients (14.3%) treated with nitroprusside ($p < .10$).[38] Pooled data from seven nitroglycerin trials in acute myocardial infarction showed an overall reduction in mortality from 87 of 425 control patients (20.5%) to 51 of 426 patients (12%) treated with intravenously administered nitroglycerin ($p < .001$).[38] Although the overall mortality difference was of conventional statistical significance in the nitroglycerin trials but not in the nitroprusside trials, there was no evidence of significant heterogeneity of effect between the two active treatments.[38] In conclusion, the real benefit in mortality reduction was probably in the range of 10% to 30% for all trials in which patients were treated with either nitroglycerin or nitroprusside. Although it is difficult to directly compare these two agents, our current policy is to treat patients with acute myocardial infarction with intravenously administered nitroglycerin as the agent of choice (see Table 92–1).

Breisblatt et al.[39] compared the effects of intravenously administered nitroglycerin or nitroprusside in a randomized study of 40 patients with unstable angina. This study reported that intravenously administered nitroglycerin and nitroprusside had equal efficacy, and acute hemodynamics and left ventricular function improved substantially in most patients. Again, we believe that intravenously administered nitroglycerin is the agent of choice and that nitroprusside should be reserved for patients with unstable angina and concomitant hypertension with significant left ventricular dysfunction.

Congestive Cardiac Failure and Low-Output States

Impedance to left ventricular ejection has long been recognized as a major determinant of left ventricular function.[40, 41] In addition, venoconstriction occurs in patients with congestive heart failure, causing redistribution of blood from the capacitance vessels toward the central circulation.

Nitroprusside, because of its short half-life and mixed arteriolar and venodilator properties, is frequently the vasodilator of choice for the treatment of acute congestive heart failure. It is specifically indicated for the acute management of patients with left ventricular failure secondary to systemic hypertension, mitral or aortic valve incompetence, or acute myocardial infarction. From a hemodynamic point of view, it has a dual benefit for the patient, both by increasing cardiac output and by reducing pulmonary congestion. The use of nitroprusside in critically ill patients is not without risk; ideally, patients should be observed in an intensive care setting with invasive monitoring of systemic arterial pressure, pulmonary capillary wedge pressure, pulmonary artery pressure, and cardiac output. These indices allow accurate titration of the infusion rate against the fall in pulmonary capillary wedge pressure and the increase in cardiac output while avoiding an excessive reduction in arterial pressure. Nitroprusside is especially valuable in patients with elevated left ventricular filling pressures and blood pressures greater than 100 mmHg. It is contraindicated in the presence of systemic hypotension.

Congestive cardiac failure is associated with increased arteriolar and venous vasoconstriction mediated through increases in sympathetic tone, circulating catecholamines, increased vasopressin levels, and activation of the renin-angiotensin-aldosterone system. This vasoconstriction is counterproductive in many patients because of the drop in cardiac output associated with increased peripheral resistance. Venoconstriction raises right and left atrial filling pressures, leading to symptoms of pulmonary congestion. Vasodilators tend to antagonize these effects with a resultant increase in cardiac output, a decrease in pulmonary congestion, or both.

The hemodynamic effects of nitroprusside differ markedly in patients with and without cardiac failure. In patients with normal ventricles, the left ventricle operates on the steep portion of the Frank-Starling curve. Dilatation of the venous capacitance vessels by nitroprusside causes a reduction in preload, which results in a fall in cardiac output and stroke volume. Although aortic impedance is also reduced by nitroprusside, the stroke volume-impedance relationship is relatively flat in the normal patient, and the reduction of afterload does not compensate for the reduction in preload. Consequently, stroke volume and cardiac output fall. The fall in stroke volume results in hypotension and reflex tachycardia due to stimulation of baroreceptors.

In contrast, in patients with failing ventricles, the ventricles operate on the flat portion of the Frank-Starling curve and have relatively steep stroke volume-impedance relationships. In these patients, nitroprusside increases cardiac output primarily by increasing stroke volume as a result of lowered aortic impedance. The resultant fall in left ventricular filling pressure is due to a reduction in preload caused by dilation of the venous capacitance vessels and greater left ventricular systolic emptying. The response to vasodilator therapy in patients with heart failure is variable and depends on where the ventricle is operating on the Frank-Starling curve and on the shape of the ventricular function curve. Patients in whom cardiac output and stroke volume most dramatically improve are those with the lowest cardiac output and the highest systemic vascular resistance.[42]

Franciosa et al.[32] reported in 1972 that nitroprusside infusion improved left ventricular function in patients with myocardial infarction and low-output congestive heart failure. Systemic arterial pressure was only modestly reduced, because the increase in cardiac output usually balanced the vasodilation induced. Reflex tachycardia, which is commonly induced by nitroprusside in patients with normal ventricular function, does not occur in patients with heart failure. This may result from the already high basal sympathetic tone in heart failure and the counterbalancing effect of increased cardiac output on peripheral vasodilatation. Sudden cessation of nitroprusside infusion has been reported to lead to rebound hemodynamic deterioration in some patients.[43]

Nitroprusside reduces the regurgitant volume and increases the forward cardiac output in patients with mitral or aortic regurgitation.[44–46] Weiland et al.[45] showed that nitroprusside infusion produced a greater increase in cardiac output in patients with severe left-sided heart failure and secondary mitral incompetence than it did in a group of patients with heart failure but without significant mitral regurgitation.

Nitroprusside frequently has been combined with digoxin, diuretics, and dobutamine in the treatment of heart failure. Because nitroprusside possesses both arteriolar and venodilator properties, it is often not valuable to combine it with other vasodilators. However, we occasionally combine nitroprusside with nitroglycerin (orally, topically, or intravenously), especially in patients with myocardial ischemia and/or very elevated capillary wedge pressures.

A comparative study of nitroprusside and dobutamine in right ventricular dysfunction due to infarction showed that dobutamine resulted in a greater increase in cardiac output.[47] Compared with dobutamine, nitroprusside causes a greater reduction in pulmonary capillary wedge pressure for a similar increase in cardiac output.[48] Nitroprusside also causes a reduction in myocardial oxygen consumption in contrast with the increase caused by dobutamine. Sturm et al.[49] investigated the combined use of nitroprusside and dopamine in 10 patients who required intraaortic balloon pumping for weaning from cardiopulmonary bypass. They reported that nitroprusside alone significantly increased mean cardiac index and reduced systemic vascular resistance. The combination of dopamine and nitroprusside resulted in a further augmentation of the cardiac index and reduction of systemic vascular resistance. This study documented the efficacy of combination therapy with vasodilators and inotropic agents in the management of postcardiotomy, low-output states wherein the cardiac index was less than 2.0 L/min/m^2 and the systemic vascular resistance was greater than 2000 dyne/sec/cm^{-5}.

Aortic Dissection

Acute aortic dissection is a medical emergency with an annual prevalence in the United States of over 2000 cases.[50] The goal of medical therapy in this setting is to limit progression of the dissection by lowering systemic pressure and decreasing the velocity of left ventricular ejection (dV/dt). Trimethaphan (Arfonad), a ganglion-blocking agent, is considered by some authors to be the drug of choice for the reduction of blood pressure in aortic dissection, because it depresses dV/dt, in contrast with the increase in dV/dt observed with nitroprusside. However, in our experience, nitroprusside's ease of use and familiarity to both nursing and medical staff makes it the drug of choice in most cases of acute aortic dissection.

By reducing aortic impedance, nitroprusside can lead to an increase in the velocity of dV/dt, a significant determinant of aortic wall stress, and might lead to further propagation of the aortic dissection.[51] When used in this setting, the drug should be combined with an intravenously administered β-blocker (e.g., propranolol, metoprolol, atenolol, or esmolol), which reduces the force of left ventricular contraction, thereby decreasing dV/dt. In patients who are initially hypertensive, systolic arterial pressure should be lowered to 100 to 110 mmHg. In normotensive patients, the systolic pressure should be reduced by 20 to 30 mmHg. If chest or back pain continues, indicating continued propagation of the dissecting hematoma, blood pressure can be further reduced while the patient is monitored closely for evidence of tissue hypoperfusion. Hemodynamic monitoring of intraarterial blood pressure, pulmonary artery wedge pressure, and cardiac output, as well as continuous assessment of urinary output, are important in this setting, but hypotensive therapy should not be delayed pending placement of catheters for hemodynamic monitoring.

Congenital Heart Disease

Benitz et al.[52] reported the use of nitroprusside in 58 neonates with assorted conditions, including persistent pulmonary hypertension of the newborn, clinical shock, systemic hypertension, and pulmonary hypoplasia. Toxic effects were not observed, and the investigators concluded that nitroprusside was effective and safe during the neonatal period. Walsh et al.[53] studied the effects of nitroprusside on ductal blood flow and oxygen-induced ductus arteriosus closure in fetal lambs. They reported an increase in ductal blood flow and marked attenuation of oxygen-induced ductal closure. The clinical efficacy of nitroprusside in maintaining ductal patency is unproven.

Pulmonary Hypertension

The results of nitroprusside infusion in pulmonary hypertension vary. It has a direct effect on the pulmonary vascular smooth muscle and, in selected patients, may lead to a reduction in pulmonary artery pressure and pulmonary vascular resistance.[54] Pearl et al.[55] reported that nitroprusside did not significantly reduce pulmonary vascular resistance or mean pulmonary artery pressure in canine experiments with oleic acid–induced pulmonary hypertension. It also had no effect in the sepsis-induced pulmonary hypertension model in piglets.[56]

Hypotensive Anesthesia and Surgery

Nitroprusside has been used extensively for the controlled reduction of arterial blood pressure during surgery.[57] Tolerance to blood loss and hypovolemia during operations may be impaired because of impairment by nitroprusside of reflex vasoconstrictor activity. Pretreatment of patients with captopril has been shown to reduce the requirements for nitroprusside and lower the blood cyanide level in some patients undergoing hypotensive anesthesia.[58] Although nitroprusside inhibits platelet aggregation, patients undergoing cardiac surgery who were treated with nitroprusside experienced no increased need for blood products or acute mediastinal drainage when compared with control subjects.[59]

Other Indications

Nitroprusside has also been shown to be an effective treatment for arterial spasm due to severe ergotism.[60–62] In some studies, addition of nitroprusside to peritoneal dialysis solutions increased peritoneal clearances without a significant increase in serum thiocyanate or dialysate cell counts.[63, 64] Nitroprusside has been reported to be effective for the treatment of ergonovine-induced coronary artery spasm that is refractory to nitroglycerin.[65]

ADVERSE EFFECTS

As with most vasodilators, the most common untoward effect of nitroprusside is an exaggeration of the hypotensive effect, leading to coronary, cerebral, and systemic hypoperfusion. A rapid fall in arterial pressure with nitroprusside can lead to nausea, vomiting, palpitations, restlessness, and sweating, which can be relieved by slowing or temporarily stopping the infusion. Long-term infusion of nitroprusside may be associated with a decrease in blood arterial oxygen saturation and tension, which is probably mediated through ventilation/perfusion on mismatch secondary to pulmonary vascular vasodilation in areas of poor lung ventilation. As previously discussed, nitroprusside may also cause a "coronary steal syndrome."

Teratogenic effects have not been described with nitroprusside administration, but human data are extremely limited in this area. In experimental studies,[66] nitroprusside and its adenine complex have been shown to be nonmutagenic for induction of chromosome breaks and point mutations. In addition, prolonged administration of nitroprusside has rarely resulted in hypothyroidism.[67] As reviewed earlier, most prolonged toxicity with nitroprusside is related to excessive accumulation of metabolites, notably thiocyanate ion. Thiocyanate tends to accumulate with prolonged administration (over 72 hours), even when infusion rates are moderate (about 3 μg/min), but such accumulation is more marked with increased infusion rates and in patients in whom thiocyanate elimination is decreased because of renal insufficiency. Thiocyanate is relatively nontoxic and is removed by renal excretion; it has a half-life of 5 to 7 days. In the presence of renal failure, thiocyanate toxicity may occur with dyspnea, nausea, vomiting, convulsions, rigidity, tremor, disorientation, and psychotic behavior. Plasma thiocyanate levels over 5 to 10 mg/100 ml are associated with toxic symptoms. Thiocyanate is effectively removed by peritoneal dialysis.[68]

Table 92–2. **Contraindications to Nitroprusside Use**

Disorder	Reason
Hepatic failure	Inability to detoxify cyanide
Leber's optic atrophy	Disorder of cyanide metabolism
Tobacco amblyopia	Disorder of cyanide metabolism
Vitamin B_{12} deficiency	Abnormal cyanide metabolism
Hypothyroidism	May exacerbate hypothyroidism

Table 92–3. **Precautions with Nitroprusside Therapy**

Disorder	Reason
Renal failure	Inability to metabolize thiocyanate
Brain tumor/stroke	May increase intracranial pressure
Eclampsia	Effects on the fetus largely unknown
Aortic stenosis	Poor ability to increase cardiac output
Hypertrophic cardiomyopathy	May increase outflow tract gradient

Hemodynamic deterioration has been reported after cessation of nitroprusside infusion in patients with chronic congestive cardiac failure. This is considered to be the result of activation of vasoconstrictor compensatory mechanisms, including the renin-angiotensin system and sympathetic nervous system. Orally administered balanced venous and arterial vasodilators (e.g., hydralazine with long-acting nitrates, prazosin, or angiotensin-converting enzyme inhibitors) should be substituted following discontinuation of nitroprusside in order to achieve a continued response similar to that of nitroprusside.

Contraindications to nitroprusside use and conditions requiring special precautions are outlined in Tables 92–2 and 92–3, respectively.

Management of Cyanide Toxicity

Cyanide toxicity should be treated by discontinuation of the nitroprusside infusion and administration of sodium nitrite 3% solution at a rate of less than 2.5 to 5.0 ml/min to a total dose of 10 to 15 ml/min. This should be followed by the injection of sodium thiosulfate, 12.5 g in 50 ml of 5% dextrose in water, over a 10-minute period. The patient should then be watched closely, and if further signs of cyanide toxicity develop, sodium nitrite and sodium thiosulfate injections can be repeated at one half of the doses given. Sodium thiosulfate may also be given by continuous infusion.[69]

REFERENCES

1. Davidsohn K: Versuche uber die Wirkung des Nitroprussidnatriums. Thesis, Albertus-university, Konigsberg, Prussia, 1887. Cited by Kreye VAW: Sodium nitroprusside. In Scriabine A (ed): Pharmacology of Antihypertensive Drugs. New York: Raven Press, 1980, pp 373–396.
2. Frank JM, Johnson JB, Rubin SH: Spectrophotometric determination of sodium nitroprusside and its photodegradation products. J Pharm Sci 65:44, 1976.
3. Schror K, Woditsch I, Forster S: Generation of nitric oxide from organic nitrovasodilators during passage through the coronary vascular bed and its role in coronary vasodilatation and nitrate tolerence. Blood Vessels 28:62, 1991.
4. Marletta MA, Tayeh MA, Havel JM: Unravelling the biological significance of nitric oxide: Minireview. Biofactors 2:219, 1990.
5. Lowenstein CJ, Synder SH: Nitric oxide, a novel biological messenger. Cell 70:705, 1992.
6. Kelm M, Schrader J: Control of coronary vascular tone by nitric oxide. Circ Res 66:1561, 1990.
7. Ignarro LJ: Biological actions and properties of endothelium-derived nitric oxide formed and released from artery and vein. Circ Res 65:1, 1989.
8. Palmer RMJ, Ferrige AG, Moncada S: Nitric oxide release accounts for the biological activity of endothelium-derived relaxing factor. Nature 327:524, 1987.
9. Collins P, Henderson AH, Lang D, Lewis MJ: Endothelium-derived relaxing factor and nitroprusside compared in noradrenaline- and K+-contracted rabbit and rat aortae. J Physiol (Lond) 400:395, 1988.
10. Vita JA, Treasure CB, Nabel EG, et al: Coronary vasomotor response to acetylcholine relates to risk factors for coronary artery disease. Circulation 81:491, 1990.
11. Drexler H, Zeiher AM, Wollschlager H, et al: Flow-dependent coronary artery dilatation in humans. Circulation 80:466, 1989.
12. Gordon JB, Ganz P, Nabel EG, et al: Atherosclerosis influences the vasomotor response of epicardial coronary arteries to exercise. J Clin Invest 83:1946, 1989.
13. Nabel EG, Ganz P, Gordon JB, et al: Dilation of normal and constriction of atherosclerotic coronary arteries caused by the cold pressor test. Circulation 77:43, 1988.
14. Nabel EG, Selwyn AP, Ganz P: Paradoxical narrowing of atherosclerotic coronary arteries induced by increases in heart rate. Circulation 81:840, 1990.
15. Chilian WM, Dellsperger KC, Layne SM, et al: Effects of atherosclerosis on the coronary microcirculation. Am J Physiol 258:h529, 1990.
16. Kreye VAW: Sodium nitroprusside. In Scriabine A (ed): Pharmacology of Antihypertensive Drugs. New York: Raven Press, 1980, pp 373–396.
17. Nakamura S, Shin T, Hirokata Y, et al: Inhibition of mitochondrial respiration by sodium nitroprusside and the mechanism of cyanide liberation. Br J Anaesthesiol 49:1239, 1977.
18. Smith RP, Kruszyna H: Nitroprusside produces cyanide poisoning via a reaction with hemoglobin. J Pharmacol Exp Ther 191:557, 1974.
19. Michenfelder JD, Tinker JH: Cyanide toxicity and thiosulfate protection during chronic administration of sodium nitroprusside in the dog: Correlation with a human case. Anesthesiology 47:441, 1977.
20. Page IH, Corcoran AC, Dustan HP, et al: Cardiovascular actions of sodium nitroprusside in animals and hypertensive patients. Circulation 11:188, 1955.
21. Chiariello M, Gold HK, Lienbach RC, et al: Comparison between the effects of nitroprusside and nitroglycerin on ischemic injury during acute myocardial infarction. Circulation 54:766, 1976.
22. Mann T, Cohn PF, Holman BL, et al: Effect of nitroprusside on regional myocardial blood flow in coronary disease: Results in 25 patients and comparison with nitroglycerin. Circulation 57:732, 1978.
23. Gopal MA, Neill WA, Oxendine JM: Effect of nitroprusside on myocardial blood flow in acute regional coronary ischemia in conscious dogs with and without ventricular distension. Cardiovasc Res 17:267, 1983.
24. Jett GK, Arcici JM Jr, Hatcher CR Jr, et al: Vasodilator drug effects on internal mammary artery and saphenous vein grafts. J Am Coll Cardiol 11:1317, 1988.
25. Mehta J, Mehta P: Comparative effects of nitroprusside and nitroglycerin on platelet aggregation in patients with heart failure. J Cardiovasc Pharmacol 2:25, 1980.
26. Böhme E, Graf H, Schultz G: Effects of sodium nitroprusside and other smooth muscle relaxants on cyclic GMP formation in smooth muscle and platelets. Adv Cycl Nucl Res 9:131, 1978.
27. Ahern DJ, Grim CE: Treatment of malignant hypertension with sodium nitroprusside. Arch Intern Med 133:187, 1974.
28. Kaplan NM: Clinical Hypertension. Baltimore: Williams & Wilkins, 1986.
29. Paull J: Clinical report of the use of sodium nitroprusside in severe pre-eclampsia. Anaesth Intensive Care 3:72, 1975.
30. Brodsky JB, Bravo JJ: Acute postoperative clonidine withdrawal syndrome. Anesthesiology 44:519, 1976.
31. Nourok DS, Gwinup G, Hamwi GJ: Phentolamine-resistant pheochromocytomas treated with sodium nitroprusside. JAMA 183:841, 1963.
32. Franciosa JA, Gulha NH, Limas CJ, et al: Improved left ventricular function during nitroprusside infusion in acute myocardial infarction. Lancet 1:650, 1972.

33. Passamani ER: Nitroprusside in myocardial infarction. N Engl J Med 306:1168, 1982.

34. Lavie CJ, Gersh BJ: Acute myocardial infarction: Initial presentation, management and prognosis. Mayo Clin Proc 65:531, 1990.

35. Hockings BEF, Cope GD, Clarke GM, et al: Randomized controlled trial of vasodilator therapy after myocardial infarction. Am J Cardiol 48:345, 1981.

36. Durred JD, Lie KI, van Capelle FJL, et al: Effect of sodium nitroprusside on mortality in acute myocardial infarction. N Engl J Med 306:1121, 1982.

37. Cohn JN, Franciosa JA, Francis GS, et al: Effect of short-term infusion of sodium nitroprusside on mortality rate in myocardial infarction complicated by left ventricular failure. Results of VA cooperative study. N Engl J Med 306:1129, 1982.

38. Yusuf S, Collins R, MacMahon S, et al: Effect of intravenous nitrates on mortality in acute myocardial infarction: An overview of the randomized trials. Lancet 2:1088, 1988.

39. Breisblatt WM, Navratil DL, Burns MJ, et al: Comparable effects of intravenous nitroglycerin and intravenous nitroprusside in acute ischemia. Am Heart J 116:465, 1988.

40. Sonnenblick EH, Downing SE: Afterload as a primary determinant of ventricular performance. Am J Physiol 204:604, 1963.

41. Imperial ES, Levy MN, Zieske H Jr: Outflow resistance as an independent determinant of cardiac performance. Circ Res 9:1148, 1961.

42. Mookerjee S, Henion W, Warner R, et al: Sodium nitroprusside therapy in congestive cardiomyopathy. Variability in hemodynamic response. J Clin Pharmacol 18:67, 1978.

43. Packer M, Meller J, Medina N, et al: Rebound hemodynamic events after the abrupt withdrawal of nitroprusside in patients with severe chronic heart failure. N Engl J Med 301:1193, 1979.

44. Bolen JL, Alderman EL: Hemodynamic consequences of afterload reduction in patients with chronic aortic regurgitation. Circulation 53:879, 1976.

45. Weiland DS, Konstam MA, Salem DN, et al: Contribution of reduced mitral regurgitant volume to vasodilator effect in severe left ventricular failure secondary to coronary artery disease or idiopathic dilated cardiomyopathy. Am J Cardiol 58:1046, 1986.

46. Goodman DJ, Rossen RM, Holloway EL, et al: Effect of nitroprusside on left ventricular dynamics in mitral regurgitation. Circulation 50:1025, 1974.

47. Dell'Italia LJ, Starling MR, Blumhardt R, et al: Comparative effects of volume loading, dobutamine and nitroprusside in patients with predominant right ventricular infarction. Circulation 72:1327, 1985.

48. Pierpont G, Hale KA, Franciosa JA, et al: Effects of vasodilators on pulmonary hemodynamics and gas exchange in left ventricular failure. Am Heart J 99:208, 1980.

49. Sturm JT, Fuhrman TM, Sterling R, et al: Combined use of dopamine and nitroprusside therapy in conjunction with intra-aortic balloon pumping for the treatment of postcardiotomy low-output syndrome. J Thorac Cardiovasc Surg 82:13, 1981.

50. Doroghazi RM, Slater EE: Aortic Dissection. New York: McGraw-Hill, 1983.

51. Palmer RF, Lasseter KC: Nitroprusside and aortic dissecting aneurysm [letter]. N Engl J Med 294:1403, 1976.

52. Benitz WE, Malachowski N, Cohen RS, et al: Use of nitroprusside in neonates: Efficacy and safety. J Pediatr 106:102, 1985.

53. Walsh RS, Ely SW, Mentzer RM Jr: Response of lamb ductus arteriosus to nitroglycerin and nitroprusside. Surg Res 44:8, 1988.

54. Knapp E, Gmeiner R: Reduction of pulmonary hypertension by nitroprusside. Int J Clin Pharmacol Biopharm 15:75, 1977.

55. Pearl RG, Rosenthal MH, Ashton JP: Pulmonary vasodilator effects of nitroglycerin and sodium nitroprusside in canine oleic acid-induced pulmonary hypertension. Anesthesiology 58:514, 1983.

56. Rudinsky BF, Komar KJ, Strates E, et al: Neither nitroglycerin nor nitroprusside selectively reduces sepsis-induced pulmonary hypertension in piglets. Crit Care Med 15:1127, 1987.

57. Da Pian R, Pasqualin A, Scienza R, et al: Deep controlled hypotension with sodium nitroprusside in the surgical treatment of intracranial arterial aneurysms. J Neurosurg Sci 23:109, 1979.

58. Woodside J Jr, Garner L, Bedford RF, et al: Captopril reduces the dose requirements for sodium nitroprusside—induced hypotension. Anesthesiology 60:413, 1984.

59. Snow N, Lucas A, Gray LA Jr: Effect of nitroprusside on postoperative blood loss in the cardiac surgical patient. Crit Care Med 9:827, 1981.

60. Carliner NH, Denune DP, Finch CS Jr, et al: Sodium nitroprusside treatment of ergotamine-induced peripheral ischemia. JAMA 227:308, 1974.

61. Whitsett TL, Myers WS, Hartsuck JM: Nitroprusside reversal of ergotamine-induced ischemia [letter]. Am Heart J 96:700, 1978.

62. Skowronski GA, Tronson MD, Parkin WG: Successful treatment of ergotamine poisoning with sodium nitroprusside. Med J Aust 2:8, 1979.

63. Nolph KD, Ghods AJ, Brown PA, et al: Effects of intraperitoneal nitroprusside on peritoneal clearances in man with variations of dose, frequency of administration and dwell times. Nephron 24:114, 1979.

64. Nolph KD, Rubin J, Wiegman DL, et al: Peritoneal clearances with three types of commercially available peritoneal dialysis solutions. Effects of pH adjustment and intraperitoneal nitroprusside. Nephron 24:34, 1979.

65. Hastey CE, Erwin SW, Ramanathan KB: Ergonovine-induced coronary spasm refractory to intracoronary nitroglycerin but responsive to nitroprusside. Am Heart J 107:778, 1984.

66. Bodi Z, Antal K, Szabad J: Nonmutagenic activity of nitroprusside. Acta Biol Acad Sci Hung 32:61, 1981.

67. Noukok DS, Glassock RJ, Solomon DH, et al: Hypothyroidism following prolonged sodium nitroprusside therapy. Am J Med Sci 248:129, 1964.

68. Palmer RF, Lasseter KC: Drug therapy: Sodium nitroprusside. N Engl J Med 300:294, 1975.

69. Schulz V, Bonn R, Kammerer H, et al: Counteraction of cyanide poisoning by thiosulfate when administering sodium nitroprusside as a hypotensive treatment. Klin Wochenschr 57:905, 1979.

CHAPTER 93

Nitroglycerin

Richard L Mueller, M.D., and Stephen Scheidt, M.D.

HISTORY

Nitroglycerin has a long and fascinating history. One of the few drugs in the pharmacopeia discovered before the twentieth century, the explosive is also one of the few drugs adopted by regular physicians from homeopathic physicians. It was intimately involved in the establishment of the world's foremost prize honoring artistic, scientific, and political endeavors. Nitroglycerin was synthesized in 1846 by the Italian chemist Ascanio Sobrero during a systematic search for other explosives after Christian Schoenbein's synthesis of guncotton earlier that year. Guncotton was formed by mixing cotton with nitric and sulfuric acids; nitroglycerin was formed by mixing glycerin with the same acids.[1]

As an explosive, nitroglycerin quickly replaced the ancient blackpowder or gunpowder. In 1867, Swedish chemist-industrialist Alfred Nobel established the first factory for his improved explosive, dynamite, produced by adsorbing the dangerously unstable liquid nitroglycerin with diatomaceous earth. The resultant solid proved to be a safer and more efficient explosive, and in 1875, Nobel invented gelatinous nitroglycerin for underwater use by adding nitrocellulose to nitroglycerin. Modern dynamite contains nitroglycerin as well as inorganic and other organic nitrates. Alarmed by the carnage his products wrought, Nobel established his famed prizes with profits derived from nitroglycerin.

It is doubtful that an explosive would have ever been used medically were it not for the fervent adoption of nitroglycerin by homeopaths. By 1847, Constantine Hering, a German disciple of homeopathy's founder Samuel Hahnemann, advocated the therapeutic use of nitroglycerin (which he called *glonoine*) for headaches. Invoking homeopathy's doctrine of "like cures like" and its advocacy of testing the effects of all substances on human subjects, Hering and other homeopaths tasted the explosive and experienced violent headaches, palpitations, and tachycardia.[2] Homeopaths quickly used nitroglycerin for a score of conditions, with the notable exception of angina.

Although regular physicians scorned homeopaths and their drugs, the homeopaths eagerly tried to convert regular physicians to their remedies. Hering convinced William Jackson, a medical student, to conduct conventional animal studies with nitroglycerin in 1849, but Jackson was unable to find human volunteers who would brave the headaches it provoked. In 1858, Alfred Field of London tried glonoine at the urging of homeopaths and was the first to use nitroglycerin for angina in patients, although he is not usually credited with this. However, Harley and Fuller published negative accounts of this use the same year, and use by regular physicians remained rare. In 1864, Albers published the first documentation of nitroglycerin's vasodilator properties, which he and others attributed to the drug's effects on "vasomotor nerves" rather than on vessels directly.[1]

Meanwhile, amyl nitrite was synthesized by Antoine Balard in 1844. After studies by colleagues Guthrie, Richardson, and Gamgee at Edinburgh from 1859 to 1863, T. Lauder Brunton became the first to use amyl nitrite for angina in 1867. A 23-year-old medical intern at the time of his report,[3] Brunton never tried nitroglycerin on human subjects because it gave him violent headaches. Brunton also advocated the use of nitrates for congestive heart failure in 1888, and that year Fussel reported the treatment of acute pulmonary edema with hypodermically administered nitroglycerin.[4]

Field's earlier report notwithstanding, William Murrell of London is credited with being the first to use nitroglycerin for angina; he was only 26 years old at the time of his 1879 report.[5] Because Field, Brunton, and Murrell were all aware that homeopaths used nitroglycerin for headache, current cardiovascular therapeutics is greatly indebted to the field of homeopathy. Enthusiasm quickly grew for this use of nitroglycerin, though it would be years before the other remedies of the day—aconite, brandy, arsenic, strychnine, and terpentine—were abandoned. Improving on Murrell's oily preparation, Martindale prepared nitroglycerin tablets by 1880. Parke Davis and Company, still the largest manufacturer of nitroglycerin tablets, introduced their pills in 1882.[6]

No other drug is available in as many forms and routes of administration as nitroglycerin. Many formulations have been available for decades, including nitroglycerin subcutaneous injections and ointment since 1864, as well as orally administered nitroglycerin.[6] Newer, ingenious formulations include solution for intravenous use, approved in the United States since 1981, transdermal patches and buccal or transmucosal tablets since 1982, and translingual spray since 1986. The history of nitrates has continued its tumultuous and controversial course since the 1960s as the dictum that nitroglycerin is dangerous in acute myocardial infarction has given way to broad use of nitrates for indications such as congestive heart failure, unstable angina, and myocardial infarction. The history of nitrates continues to be written in the 1990s[2] as the many biologic roles of nitric oxide, the active principle of all nitrates, are revealed.

CHEMISTRY

The most commonly used nitrovasodilators, the organic nitrates and nitrites, are all synthetic alcohol esters of nitric acid and nitrous acid, respectively. Other nitrovasodilators include sodium nitroprusside, an inorganic nitrate; molsidomine, an organic, nitrogen-containing sydnonimine type of compound; and nicorandil, an organic nitrate compound that also stimulates the opening of potassium channels. The latter two compounds are not available in the United States. Chemically, the nitrates and nitrites are not truly nitro compounds, because they contain carbon-oxygen-nitrogen bonds rather than direct carbon-nitrogen bonds. Thus, the name nitroglycerin is actually a misnomer, glyceryl trinitrate being more accurate. All nitrovasodilators are prodrugs that act as replacement therapy for endogenous endothelial vasodilators such as nitric oxide or S-nitrosothiol compounds.

Nitroglycerin, chemically known as 1,2,3-propanetriol trinitrate, has a low molecular weight (227) and is lipophilic, allowing for rapid and complete absorption from skin and mucosa. Nitroglycerin is a white to yellow, oily, thick liquid that is volatile, flammable, and explosive; it is slightly soluble in water and readily soluble in alcohol and has a sweet, burning taste. Pure liquid nitroglycerin is very susceptible to heat or shock-induced explosion; it is rendered solid and nonexplosive by the addition of incipients such as sucrose, lactose, alcohol, polyethylene glycol, propylene glycol, or povidone. Amyl nitrite, an extremely volatile liquid with similar properties, is available in a crushable vial and remains extremely flammable and explosive as dispensed. Solid nitroglycerin in tablet form contains about 10% nitroglycerin by weight. The solid form, no longer explosive, is still extremely volatile as well as light-, moisture-, and heat-sensitive. Thus, tablets should be kept in their original brown glass bottles, and their tightly secured metal caps should be replaced quickly after opening. Tablets usually lose potency through volatilization within 3 to 4 months.[7]

Intravenously administered nitroglycerin is stabilized with the solvents propylene glycol and ethyl alcohol and is readily absorbed by polyvinyl chloride–type plastics. Practical consequences include the risk of alcohol intoxication at high doses, a controversial heparin resistance possibly induced by propylene glycol or more likely nitroglycerin itself, and the need to use only glass bottles and special polyethylene tubing to prevent loss of 40% to 50% of the active agent. Buccal nitroglycerin is adsorbed onto a special polymer matrix that forms a film over the buccal mucosa and releases nitroglycerin slowly; transdermal patches contain an active-drug reservoir, often containing a drug-absorbing polymer, that releases nitroglycerin into the skin through a semipermeable membrane. The rate-limiting determinant of active drug release is either the rate of release from the polymer in the reservoir or through the semipermeable membrane, depending on the formulation. Oral time-release preparations contain active drug adsorbed into granules.[7]

PHARMACOKINETICS

Nitroglycerin is quickly and completely absorbed through the skin and all mucosal surfaces, including those of the gastrointestinal tract and oral cavity. Absorption of mucosal or dermal nitroglycerin begins within minutes and continues for many hours, depending on the formulation. The volume of distribution is very large, and clearance is extensive and very rapid, even exceeding cardiac output; plasma nitroglycerin has a half-life of only 1 to 4 minutes. Nitroglycerin is approximately 60% bound by plasma proteins; the dinitrate active metabolites are 30% to 60% bound.[8] Nitroglycerin is a heavily tissue-bound drug, such that plasma stores account for less than 1% of the total body nitrate pool.[9] A plasma level greater than 1 ng/ml is the accepted minimal therapeutic value; nitroglycerin ointment reliably produces plasma levels of 4 to 6 ng/ml, and intravenous infusions may produce levels of more than 20 ng/ml. Nitroglycerin patches produce widely variable plasma levels, depending mainly on the surface area over which the nitroglycerin ointment or patch is applied, but also to some extent on the skin characteristics and interindividual variability in drug absorption, binding, distribution, and metabolism. The very low and highly fluctuating drug levels are the result of extensive tissue binding and metabolism. Sites of extraction in descending order of magnitude include vascular tissues, the liver, and red blood cells; more than 60% of plasma nitroglycerin is extracted across the arteriovenous vascular bed, such that arterial levels are four times greater than venous levels. Rapid liver degradation produces extensive first-pass clearance, is mediated by the enzyme glutathione organic nitrate reductase, and results in low bioavailability (less than 10%) when nitroglycerin is administered orally. Thus, bioavailability is much higher when the drug is given transmucosally by the sublingual, translingual (spray), transmucosal (buccal), or transdermal routes. However, high doses of orally administered nitroglycerin can overcome first-pass metabolism and achieve therapeutic concentrations.[10]

Much metabolism, especially first-pass conversion of ingested drug, occurs in the liver; nitrate reductase cleaves off nitrite ions, producing 1,2- and 1,3-dinitroglycerols. These dinitrates are less potent than the parent molecule by a factor of 10 to 14, but because their half-lives are 1 to 3 hours, they probably account for most of the prolonged activity of nitroglycerin. Further denitrification produces the 1- and 2-mononitroglycerols, which lack vasoactivity. These metabolites impair clearance of the parent drug, thereby increasing its concentration during long-term doses and resulting in dose- and time-dependent clearance. Complete metabolism eventually yields glycerol and carbon dioxide, as well as glucuronated mononitrates, which are eliminated by the kidneys.[8] In addition, substantial metabolism occurs within red blood cells and vascular tissue. Interaction with tissue sulfhydryl groups causes similar denitrification by poorly characterized enzymes of nitroglycerin via release of nitrite ion or nitric oxide. Unlike the hepatic nitrate reductase, the erythrocyte nitrate reductase is not glutathione-dependent.

Thus, the onset and duration of action of various nitroglycerin formulations depends largely on the route of administration as well as the rate and amount of absorption of active drug.

PHARMACODYNAMICS

The main site of action of all nitrovasodilators is the vascular smooth muscle cell. Actually, all smooth muscle cells, including those of the respiratory, gastrointestinal, and genitourinary tracts, relax in response to nitroglycerin; however, the drug's main therapeutic action occurs at vascular smooth muscle.[7] Considerable controversy continues about the exact sequence and sites of metabolism as well as about the identity of the metabolites within the vessel wall, but the following general model is widely accepted.

Nitrovasodilator agents all are prodrugs of some sort, releasing the active agents nitrite ion, nitric oxide, or S-nitrosothiols via either enzymatically or nonenzymatically mediated redox reactions.[11–16] Nitroglycerin and its dinitroglycerol active metabolites, as well as other nitrovasodilators, react with sulfhydryl donors such as cysteine and glutathione within the vascular wall, resulting in reduction of nitrate moieties and their release from the parent molecule as nitrite ion, as nitric oxide, as S-nitrosothiols such as S-nitrosocysteine, or even as thionitrates.[13] Several such pathways are probably operative at different sites; in the extracellular space surrounding the vascular smooth muscle cell, sulfhydryl donors react nonenzymatically with all nitrovasodilators to produce nitric oxide or S-nitrosothiols, which then diffuse into the smooth muscle cell for possible further metabolism. This is the only pathway for nitroprusside and molsidomine, which are designated "direct" donors of nitric oxide, whereas all other nitrovasodilators are prodrugs that provide nitric oxide indirectly, via enzymatic reactions.

For organic nitrates and nitrites, this extracellular pathway is likely less quantitatively important than their enzymatic redox reactions with at least two different metabolizing enzymes found within the smooth muscle sarcolemma.[13] The first is probably glutathione S-transferase, which likely cleaves nitrite ion from the parent molecule; nitrite then diffuses into the cell and may be converted in the cytoplasm to nitric oxide. The second is an as yet unnamed membrane-bound, nitrate-reducing enzyme that probably cleaves nitric oxide from the parent molecule; nitric oxide then diffuses into the cell. A third metabolizing enzyme that may be involved is cytochrome P-450. What is agreed on is that the organic nitrovasodilators react with sulfhydryl groups outside or inside the cell to release any or all of the following effectors: nitrite ion, nitric oxide, or S-nitrosothiols. Any particular scheme remains speculative at present, though several versions claim experimental support.

The next steps are also subject to controversy. Workers contending that nitrite ion is the mediator released from the parent molecule also report that it is then transformed within the smooth muscle cytoplasm into nitric oxide or S-nitrosothiols, either directly or via conversion first to nitrous acid.[17] Those supporting the direct release of nitric oxide from the parent molecule at the sarcolemma are still split into two camps, one believing that nitric oxide itself is identical to the endogenous nitrovasodilator, endothelium-derived relaxation factor (EDRF), and that EDRF is the active agent of exogenous nitrate prodrugs;[18] the other camp cites conflicting evidence supporting the conversion of nitric oxide to S-nitrosothiols, which many claim to be the actual EDRF.[19]

Regardless of whether nitric oxide or an S-nitrosothiol acts as the active derivative of nitrovasodilators and shares identity with EDRF, the putative active moiety effects smooth muscle relaxation by stimulating soluble, cytoplasmic guanylate cyclase by reacting with the ferrous ion of its heme prosthetic group. Similarly, nitric oxide is degraded mainly by inactivation by hemoglobin's ferrous ion. The effector, either the endogenous EDRF or nitric oxide/S-nitrosothiols derived from an exogenous nitrovasodilating drug, thus leads to production of cyclic guanosine monophosphate, which reduces intracellular calcium content by reducing calcium influx into the cell, by promoting its efflux, or both. The resultant reduction in intracellular calcium leads to smooth muscle relaxation and vasodilation, which underlies nearly all the vascular effects of EDRF and of the nitrovasodilator drugs.[20]

Endogenously or exogenously derived nitric oxide/S-nitrosothiol also produces antithrombotic effects by stimulating platelet guanylate cyclase, reducing intraplatelet calcium levels, and thus inhibiting platelet activation, adhesion, and aggregation.[17, 21] Leukocyte and macrophage adhesion to endothelium is likewise inhibited by nitric oxide.[22] Older theories invoking prostacyclin release as a mechanism of vasodilation remain controversial.[23]

Thus, nitrovasodilator drugs release the mediator nitric oxide/S-nitrosothiol, identical to EDRF, either directly or indirectly via metabolic intermediates, and either by enzymatic or by nonenzymatic redox reactions with tissue sulfhydryl groups. Vasorelaxation and platelet inhibition result when nitric oxide/S-nitrosothiol stimulates soluble guanylate cyclase. The ubiquity of endogenously produced nitric oxide and its involvement in not only vasoreactivity and thrombosis but also regulation of the central nervous system, erection, gastrointestinal and genitourinary function, and the immune system is currently intensely interesting and important.[20] As the biology of nitric oxide/EDRF has yielded to scientific inquiry, it has become clear that the venerable nitrovasodilators/explosives of the nineteenth century are merely prodrugs of this elegant endogenous system.

PHARMACOLOGY

The predominant therapeutic vascular effect of nitroglycerin is vasodilation; other important effects of possible but unproven therapeutic importance include its antiplatelet activity[17, 21] as well as the smooth muscle and cardiac myocyte antiproliferative effects of all nitrovasodilators and EDRF.[24] Nitroglycerin-induced vasodilation occurs as a direct effect on vascular smooth muscle, independent of reflex or neurohormonal vascular control systems. Nitroglycerin-induced vasodilation occurs throughout the vascular tree with a dose-related regional specificity. Low doses predominantly produce venodilation, especially of large-capacitance veins, whereas increasing doses produce large-conductance arterial dilation followed by resistance arterial dilation, such as in the coronary tree, and finally arteriolar dilation. This dose-related vasoselectivity is probably mediated by regional vascular variations in the activity of the nitrate-metabolizing membrane enzyme.[25]

Venodilation produces dramatic preload reduction, leading to a reduction in myocardial oxygen demand due to lessened ventricular wall stress via reduced chamber size and end-diastolic pressure. Also, oxygen supply is enhanced to subendocardial layers particularly susceptible to ischemia, because reduction in diastolic cavity pressure increases the perfusion gradient across a coronary artery stenosis. Preload reduction also has salutary effects on pulmonary and systemic venous congestion in acute or chronic heart failure. In patients without heart failure, preload reduction typically leads to reductions in stroke volume, which then often lead to baroreflex activation and reflex tachycardia and even arterial vasoconstriction to maintain blood pressure. In those with heart failure, preload reduction often leads to enhanced stroke volume as ventricular pressure-volume relationships become more optimal according to the Frank-Starling relationship.[26, 27]

At higher doses, nitroglycerin produces several coronary arterial effects practically ideal for those with atherosclerotic disease.[26, 27] Nitroglycerin at reasonable doses dilates large, epicardial coronary arteries without dilating small coronary arteriolar resistance vessels. This selectivity within the coronary tree ensures that steal phenomena are avoided; indeed, ischemic territories are selectively perfused, because epicardial coronary dilation and reduction of diastolic ventricular pressures increase the transtenotic perfusion pressure in diseased vessels. Arteriolar dilators such as dipyridamole, adenosine, and nitroprusside may provoke coronary steal (redistribution of coronary flow away from diseased territories); because arterioles distal to atheromata are already maximally dilated, drug-induced dilation of arterioles distal to undiseased segments increases flow through those arteries, presumably at the expense of the diseased territories.[28]

Other beneficial coronary artery effects of nitroglycerin include preferential dilation of stenotic segments, which are usually eccentrically diseased and thus still have a rim of normal, vasoresponsive smooth muscle;[29] dilation and even growth of collateral vessels;[30, 31] and prevention of coronary vasospasm, especially at the site of stenoses.[32, 33] All of these effects increase myocardial oxygen supply, as does the drug's antiplatelet effects. At slightly higher doses, conductance arterial dilation reduces arterial reflectance waves, leading to improved arterial compliance.[34, 35] At still higher doses, arteriolar dilation reduces afterload, thus reducing blood pressure as well as myocardial oxygen demand.[26, 27, 36] With afterload reduction, stroke volume usually increases, unless reflex vasoconstriction supervenes. Blood pressure may fall, but it may remain stable if unloading increases cardiac output or if reflex vasoconstriction occurs. Nitroglycerin has complex direct and indirect vascular, coronary, and cardiac effects that differ among patients and at different doses; thus, it is impossible to predict its exact effects on all hemodynamic parameters in a given patient. For example, myocardial oxygen demand may fall so low that coronary blood flow actually declines as supply matches low demand. However, the *ratio* of oxygen supply to demand is reliably increased.[26, 27]

Finally, new evidence indicates that nitric oxide exerts antiproliferative effects on vascular smooth muscle and cardiac myocytes,[24] which may inhibit atherosclerosis and vascular and myocardial remodeling as well as improve vascular and myocardial compliance. Ventricular unloading with nitroglycerin

soon after myocardial infarction prevents pathologic remodeling mediated by infarct expansion and extension.[37] Pulmonary artery and right atrial pressures are also reduced by nitroglycerin.[27] Nitroglycerin has no direct myocardial or conduction system effects.

ADVERSE EFFECTS

Given its potent cardiovascular effects, nitrovasodilator drugs are remarkably well-tolerated and free of serious side effects.[7] The most common adverse effects are headache and postural dizziness. Although headaches frequently disappear after several days to weeks of use, they occur in up to 40% of patients on oral or transdermal therapy and require discontinuation in about 10% of patients. Postural dizziness is common, especially in those with volume depletion, but is rarely serious except for the minority of patients who develop profound hypotension and paradoxic bradycardia or even asystole. This phenomenon is most common in patients with volume depletion or acute inferior myocardial infarction, especially if the right ventricle is involved. It is likely caused by ventricular underfilling due to venodilation, followed by activation of cardiopulmonary receptors, which trigger a vagal reflex arc.

Palpitations are common, either due to reflex tachycardia or due to increased stroke volume. Drug rash is rare with most forms of nitroglycerin, except for transdermal patches. Patch rashes are usually due to the adhesive, less commonly to nitroglycerin itself. Rare but alarming adverse events include electrical arcing and skin burns due to placement of cardioversion paddles on nitroglycerin ointment, as well as the explosion of a patch exposed to a microwave source. Nausea may also occur, and nitroglycerin may produce hypoxemia via worsening ventilation-perfusion mismatch through pulmonary vasodilation.[38]

Methemoglobinemia is a rare but potentially serious complication. Nitrite ions released during metabolism of nitroglycerin can oxidize hemoglobin to methemoglobin, impairing oxygen-carrying capacity of the blood. Although toxicity is rare in normal adults receiving large intravenous doses of nitroglycerin, those at risk are mainly infants, who have enhanced gastrointestinal conversion of unabsorbed nitrate to nitrite due to high gut pH, and patients with deficiencies of NADH methemoglobin reductase or cytochrome b5 reductase. Toxicity is diagnosed by documenting elevated methemoglobin levels or chocolate-brown blood with normal P_{O_2} and signs of inadequate oxygen delivery. Treatment consists of intravenous administration of methylene blue.[7] The ability of amyl and sodium nitrite to rapidly produce methemoglobinemia is exploited as part of the antidote for cyanide poisoning. Methemoglobin avidly draws cyanide ions from cytochrome iron-heme groups, producing cyanmethemoglobin, which reacts with intravenously administered thiosulfate to produce thiocyanate and methemoglobin. Thiocyanate, a less toxic ion, is excreted by the kidneys, and any excess methemoglobin can be cleared with methylene blue.

Nitrate dependence and rebound were documented decades ago in munitions workers who suffered headaches on Mondays, which abated during the week because of tolerance,[39] followed by cases of angina, myocardial infarction, and even sudden death on weekends during nitrate withdrawal.[40] Rebound is thought to be mediated by vasospasm; thus, if possible, nitrates should not be discontinued abruptly. Approximately 10% of angina patients, but a higher percentage of patients with heart failure, are resistant to even high doses of nitrates. This resistance phenomenon differs from tolerance because it occurs even at the onset of therapy. The mechanism is unclear but probably involves high levels of neurohormonal activation as well as edema of the vessel wall.[41, 42]

Nitrates are contraindicated in patients with severe aortic stenosis or hypertrophic cardiomyopathy with severe outflow tract obstruction. These patients may suffer fatal hypotension as a result of preload and afterload reduction in the face of a fixed ventricular outflow obstruction. In the past, nitroglycerin was thought to be contraindicated in patients with acute myocardial infarction or glaucoma; currently, nitroglycerin is believed to have no effects on glaucoma and is desirable in most infarction patients.[7]

Patients receiving high doses of intravenously administered nitroglycerin have occasionally suffered alcohol intoxication, Wernicke's encephalopathy, or gout due to the up to 5% ethanol content of these preparations.[7] Conflicting reports have raised the issue of possible heparin resistance in patients receiving intravenously administered nitroglycerin because of putative conformational changes in antithrombin III induced by nitroglycerin itself or by the solvent propylene glycol.[43–46] Nitroglycerin has been reported to decrease the bioavailability of tissue plasminogen activator because of enhanced hepatic blood flow and drug clearance, but the magnitude of this effect is uncertain.[47, 48]

There are no animal or human data regarding the safety of nitroglycerin during pregnancy and lactation or its effects on carcinogenesis, mutagenesis, or fertility.[7]

AVAILABLE PREPARATIONS
Short-Acting Delivery Systems

All short-acting nitroglycerin formulations are indicated for the short-term prophylaxis or treatment of anginal attacks; because of its longer duration of action, transmucosally administered nitroglycerin is also useful for long-term prophylaxis (up to 5 hours). Because of their brief presence in plasma, none of the short-acting preparations induces nitrate tolerance.

Sublingually Administered Nitroglycerin

Sublingual tablets, available in 0.15-, 0.3-, 0.4-, and 0.6-mg doses, rapidly produce therapeutic blood levels and are the treatment of choice for relief of acute anginal attacks. Onset of action is within 0.5 to 3 minutes, peak action is at 2 to 5 minutes, and duration of action is 10 to 30 minutes.[7, 10, 49] For acute anginal attacks, up to three sublingual tablets, 5 minutes apart, may be used before the patient should seek emergency care.

Translingually Administered Nitroglycerin

Nitroglycerin spray delivers 0.4 mg of nitroglycerin per metered dose. The spray acts as rapidly as sublingual tablets with a similarly brief duration of action.[7, 10, 49] Although it is more expensive per dose than sublingual tablets, the spray has a considerably longer shelf-life, is less fragile than the tablets, and may be more cost-effective than tablets for patients with infrequent angina. There was increased demand for the spray during the 1993 United States shortage of sublingual nitroglycerin tablets.

Transmucosally Administered Nitroglycerin

Buccal nitroglycerin is a sustained-release lozenge that becomes sealed to the oral mucosa, releasing the drug from a polymer base as the lozenge slowly dissolves. Available in 1-, 2-, and 3-mg doses, onset of action is as rapid as it is with sublingually or translingually administered formulations, because absorption is through the same systemic route that avoids hepatic clearance. However, because of the slow dissolution of the lozenge, duration of action is 3 to 5 hours; maximal effects are seen within a few minutes. Thus, buccal nitroglycerin is both short- and long-acting and may be used to abort an anginal attack or for prophylaxis before a protracted activity expected to cause angina. The patient may eat, drink, and talk during use. Disadvantages include the possibility of inadvertent dislodgment with unnoticed loss of protection and inadvertent chewing causing an undesired bolus effect.[7, 10, 49]

Long-Acting Delivery Systems

All long-acting nitroglycerin preparations share the promise of convenient dosing and several hours of angina prophylaxis due to their prolonged presence in plasma; however, they also share the threat of nitrate tolerance if poorly planned dosing leads to continuous nitrate exposure. Because of their relatively slow onset of action, none of these preparations is indicated for aborting anginal attacks, except for the immediately acting intravenous form. All are currently approved for long-term angina prophylaxis. However, in recognition of the lack of substantial data supporting their efficacy during long-term dosing and their propensity for inducing nitrate tolerance, the Cardiovascular and Renal Drugs Advisory Committee of the United States Food and Drug Administration (FDA) recommended in 1993 that labeling for most orally administered nitrates be changed. The new labeling would state that all orally administered nitrates not shown to be effective for long-term dosing should be used only for the short term or as single doses.

Orally Administered Nitroglycerin

Available in 2.5-, 6.5-, and 9-mg doses, orally administered nitroglycerin is usually used twice daily. Onset of action is 20 to 45 minutes, peak action is at 60 to 90 minutes, and duration is 2 to 8 hours. Limited data indicate that single doses improve exercise tolerance for up to 5 hours, but there are no data on the efficacy of long-term therapy.[7, 10, 49]

Nitroglycerin Ointment

Available in one 15 mg/inch, 2% strength, nitroglycerin ointment is given in doses of 0.5 to 3 inches. Onset of action is 20 to 60 minutes, peak action is at 1 to 2 hours, and duration of action is 3 to 8 hours. Ointment is usually used every 4 to 6 hours in hospitalized patients with acute ischemic syndromes or congestive heart failure, although tolerance occurs readily with such frequent dosing. To avoid tolerance, ointment should be used only two or three times a day; one 8- to 12-hour nitrate-free interval a day is advisable. Although doses are prescribed as a linear measurement, the ointment should be spread out thinly over an area of 2 × 3 to 4 × 5 inches, depending on the linear dose. Occlusion of the ointment enhances absorption by increasing skin hydration and prevents inadvertent removal of the ointment or exposure of hospital personnel to nitroglycerin if they touch the patient's area of drug application.[7, 10, 49]

Transdermal Patches

Available in 0.1-, 0.2-, 0.3-, 0.4-, 0.6-, and 0.8-mg/hr doses, transdermal patches deliver a steady dose of nitroglycerin. One patch contains a liquid nitroglycerin reservoir, with drug delivery regulated by a semipermeable membrane; other patches contain active drug bonded to a polymer, with drug delivery regulated by release from the polymer. Onset of action is at 30 to 60 minutes, steady-state levels occur within 2 hours, and duration of release is at least 24 hours. Although the patches release drug for up to 24 hours, tolerance develops within 24 hours of continuous use, so patches should be applied for only 10 to 12 hours per day to allow for a sufficient nitrate-free interval to avoid tolerance.[7, 10, 49]

Intravenously Administered Nitroglycerin

Available as 5- and 10-mg/ml solutions that are diluted with normal saline or 5% dextrose solutions to provide infusates of 50 to 100 mg nitroglycerin/250 ml, typical doses vary considerably, from starting doses of 5 µg/min up to 500 to 600 µg/min or even more. Onset of action is immediate, as is offset when the infusion is stopped. Plasma levels of over 20 ng/ml can be achieved with high doses.[50] Glass bottles and non–polyvinyl chloride plastic tubing must be used to avoid the loss of half the active drug via adsorption onto plastics. Usually used for critically ill patients with acute ischemic syndromes or congestive heart failure, intraarterial catheter monitoring and often catheter monitoring of the right side of the heart are generally advisable to detect life-threatening hypotension and to titrate dosages to desired hemodynamic end points.

Infusion rates are usually initiated at 5 to 10 µg/min, and titrated upward in stepwise fashion using 10- to 20-µg/min increments to predetermined end points such as a 10% fall in systolic or mean arterial blood pressure (but not below 90 or 80 mmHg, respectively) in normotensive patients, or a 30% fall in hypertensive patients. Infusion for only 12 hours a day has been shown to avert the tolerance that develops within 24 hours during continuous therapy.[7, 10, 37, 49]

INDICATIONS

Nitroglycerin and other nitrates are approved only for the treatment or prophylaxis of angina. It is noteworthy that, to date, the FDA has not approved any of the nitrates for the treatment of myocardial infarction or congestive heart failure, although substantial data support their use in these conditions.

Stable Angina Pectoris

Nitroglycerin, in its various formulations, is a cornerstone therapy for chronic stable angina. As discussed, nitroglycerin by various mechanisms reduces myocardial oxygen demand while improving oxygen supply, thereby ameliorating ischemia. In addition, nitroglycerin's antiplatelet activity and antiproliferative effects on smooth muscle cells and cardiac myocytes may have additional beneficial effects on coronary artery disease. In stable angina, nitroglycerin relieves pain and increases exercise capacity, allowing a greater workload to be achieved before ischemia supervenes.[51] The wide variety of nitroglycerin formulations allows practitioners to select different preparations with different pharmacokinetics in order to abort acute anginal attacks and provide short- and long-term prophylaxis against angina. Only nitrates provide rapid relief of angina within minutes.

Limitations of nitroglycerin for angina pectoris include possible reflex tachycardia, paradoxic bradycardia, or excessive hypotension, with attendant undesirable effects on myocardial oxygen energetics. However, combination therapy with β-blockers, calcium antagonists, or both generally prevents the reflex tachycardia often seen with nitrates; conversely, bradycardia induced by β-blockers can be offset by nitroglycerin. Additionally, nitroglycerin-induced reduction in ventricular wall stress, increase in myocardial contractility, and decrease in coronary resistance favorably offset the unfavorable effects of β-blockers on these determinants of ischemia. Thus, these agents usually complement nitroglycerin. Another major limitation is nitrate tolerance, but as will be discussed later, tolerance is readily avoided with intermittent dosing. The disadvantage of intermittent dosing is that, by definition, nitrate-free periods are created, during which patients are theoretically more prone to ischemia. Combination therapy with β-blockers, calcium antagonists, or both is useful as background therapy during nitrate-free periods.

Although nitrates are invaluable agents for treating and preventing anginal episodes, there are no randomized data addressing whether or not nitrates used for chronic coronary disease prevent myocardial infarction or alter survival.

Unstable Angina Pectoris

Although no randomized trials have assessed the effects of nitrates on myocardial infarction or death in unstable angina, they are mainstays of treatment for this disorder as well.[52] Numerous studies, usually employing nitroglycerin ointment or intravenous infusions, have documented dramatic symptomatic relief,[53, 54] reduction of narcotic analgesic requirements,[53, 54] reduction of ischemia,[55] and improvement in cardiac output, diastolic function, and left ventricular ejection fraction.[56] Although tolerance to continuous nitroglycerin is of concern in unstable angina, there are few data, because treatment is often brief. Nitroglycerin is also the treatment of choice, along with calcium antagonists, for rest angina due to coronary vasospasm.[57]

Myocardial Infarction

As recently as the 1970s, standard cardiology texts maintained that nitroglycerin was contraindicated in acute myocardial infarction. Concern centered around the possibility that excessive hypotension would lower coronary perfusion pressure, increase heart rate, and worsen ischemic injury; in addition, nitroglycerin was thought to possibly induce a coronary steal syndrome similar to that encountered with nitroprusside.[58] Although the latter fear is unfounded, indiscriminate and excessive nitroglycerin dosing can clearly lead to an increase in infarction size by producing hypotension.[59] It is now clear that use of nitroglycerin in acute infarction must be judicious, with strict attention paid to preventing excessive hypotension.

Clearly, all the beneficial effects of nitroglycerin in chronic angina are especially desirable in acute infarction and, as expected, not only limit infarct size[37, 60–62] but also prevent or treat left ventricular dysfunction.[63–66] Experimental studies documented limitation of ischemic injury when coronary perfusion pressure is maintained,[67] leading to 10 randomized clinical trials.[37, 60, 62, 68–74] A few of the trials, assessing nitroprusside[71] or nitroglycerin[37, 60] administered intravenously for up to 48 hours following acute myocardial infarction, appeared to document statistically significant mortality reductions, but sample sizes were small, and not all studies agreed. However, a 1988 meta-analysis of the three nitroprusside trials and the seven nitroglycerin trials,[75] all conducted without concomitant thrombolytics, reported a strong trend toward mortality reduction with nitroprusside and statistically significant mortality reductions of 49% with nitroglycerin and 35% in all 10 trials of nitrovasodilators combined. These trials avoided mean blood pressure reductions greater than 10% and documented mortality reductions for both inferior and anterior infarctions.

However, although meta-analysis is highly suggestive, it cannot substitute for large, randomized trials of sufficient power. Such trials were reported in 1994 and 1995; the GISSI-3 trial[75a] randomized more than 19,000 patients with acute infarction presenting within 24 hours of symptom onset to lisinopril, nitrates, or both. Nitrates consisted of intravenously administered nitroglycerin for the first 24 hours followed by 10 mg/day of transdermal nitroglycerin or 50 mg/day of controlled-release isosorbide-5-mononitrate. The trends toward reduction of mortality or mortality and severe ventricular dysfunction were insignificant with nitrates over 6 weeks, although the addition of nitrates to lisinopril provided an additional 6% reduction in either end point compared with lisinopril alone. The nitrates were very well tolerated with no evidence of any adverse effects on end points. Similar trends toward mortality reduction were reported at 5 weeks and at 1 year of follow-up by the ISIS-4 trial[75b] of more than 58,000 patients randomized to magnesium, captopril, and/or 60 mg/day of controlled-release isosorbide-5-mononitrate. Unlike with the GISSI-3 results, the ISIS-4 investigators found no additive benefit of nitrates with either treatment agent. Interestingly, mononitrate produced a significant mortality reduction during the first day that was later lost. However, it appears that although nitrates were safe and effective in reducing chest pain, there is at best only a mild mortality benefit, if any.

Although nitrates do not appear to dramatically improve overall mortality in infarction patients, they favorably influence many other end points. Chest pain is clearly and safely ameliorated, but additionally, left ventricular function is improved,[63–66] ischemic injury and infarct size are limited,[37, 60–62] remodeling of the left ventricle through infarct extension and expansion is prevented,[37, 68, 76, 77] and complications such as cardiogenic shock,[37] heart block,[37] heart failure,[37, 68, 78] and left ventricular aneurysm and thrombus[37] are significantly reduced by nitroglycerin. Thus, nitroglycerin remains a cornerstone of therapy for acute infarctions, especially those complicated by ventricular dysfunction or ongoing ischemia. Although overall mortality is likely insignificantly reduced by nitrate therapy, some patient subsets may derive more benefit; likewise, all patients appear to derive significant mortality benefit during the first day of treatment. Care must be taken to avoid excessive hypotension during treatment.

Congestive Heart Failure

Vasodilator therapy emerged in the 1980s as the treatment of choice for acute and chronic congestive heart failure. Nitrates clearly have salutory hemodynamic effects in acute heart failure, namely improvement of cardiac output, improvement of coronary perfusion, and reduction of ischemia as well as of ventricular filling and pulmonary artery pressures. Like arterial vasodilators, nitrates have been shown to improve symptoms, exercise tolerance,[79-81] and hemodynamics[82] during long-term administration to patients with chronic heart failure. Most studies have used isosorbide dinitrate. Given their powerful venodilating effects, nitrates are an attractive choice, and their use is particularly beneficial in patients with predominantly congestive symptoms due to high ventricular filling pressures. In large doses, nitrates may increase cardiac output, but this effect is secondary. Because venodilation occurs at low doses, reduction in filling pressures often can be achieved without substantial hypotension, an advantage in many patients with severe heart failure in whom hypotension may limit therapeutic options. Because a large proportion of patients with heart failure have ischemic heart disease as a causal or complicating factor, nitroglycerin's anti-ischemic properties are especially attractive. Nitroglycerin is particularly useful when combined with pure arterial vasodilators such as hydralazine, because such a combination leads to "balanced" venous and arterial vasodilation.

Relatively high doses of nitrates are often required in heart failure, probably because of the antagonistic effects of the activated neurohormonal state usually seen in these patients.[41, 42] In critically ill patients, intravenously administered nitroglycerin should be used in addition to invasive monitoring with arterial catheters and right-sided heart catheters to ensure safety and to titrate drug dosage to desired reductions (usually 10% to 30%) in right atrial and pulmonary capillary wedge pressures. In outpatients, relatively high doses of long-acting nitrates are used. However, nitrate tolerance also occurs in these patients, so intermittent dosing is mandatory to preserve efficacy.[83]

The only randomized trials addressing mortality effects of nitrates in chronic heart failure were the V-HeFT I and II studies.[84, 85] The first study documented a marginally statistically significant reduction in mortality compared with placebo or prazosin using hydralazine and isosorbide dinitrate given four times a day, even though this dosing regimen is known to induce rapid nitrate tolerance. In the second study, the hydralazine-isosorbide dinitrate combination led to a significantly higher mortality rate compared with enalapril while producing superior exercise tolerance and ventricular function. Future studies will examine the interesting suggestion that nitrates and converting enzyme inhibitors have complementary salutary effects in chronic heart failure.

TOLERANCE

The major practical drawback to therapy with all nitrovasodilators remains the phenomenon of tolerance, whereby a constant dose produces diminishing physiologic effects or an increasing dose is required to produce a similar effect.[40, 42, 86, 87] Tolerance was recognized decades ago in munitions workers exposed to nitroglycerin, who also demonstrated rebound phenomena. These workers developed Monday headaches, which abated during the week (tolerance), and some had ischemic events on weekends (rebound).[39, 40, 88, 89] Tolerance has subsequently been documented with all forms of nitrovasodilators (except for the "direct" nitric oxide donors) that are used continuously; only 24 hours is required to produce nearly complete tolerance, and cross-tolerance between different nitrates occurs. Furthermore, tolerance occurs whether long-acting nitrate preparations are used for chronic angina, unstable angina, myocardial infarction, or congestive heart failure. The only formulations not documented to induce tolerance are those that are short-acting and used infrequently, such as sublingual tablets and spray.[87] Although tolerance had been amply demonstrated for decades, it attracted little attention until it was "rediscovered" with the introduction of transdermal patches in 1982.[90] Initially touted as the first round-the-clock nitrate formulation, it became clear that continuous patch use produced near total tolerance within 24 hours of use.[91] Since then, nitrate tolerance has been an active area of research, but remains a frustrating limitation to the promises of nitrate therapy.

Nitrate tolerance becomes likely as dose increases and dosing interval decreases. Several mechanisms have been proposed to explain nitrate tolerance; although each has some support, evidence is often conflicting. It is likely that all contribute to tolerance, which may thus be a multifactorial phenomenon or may be due to differing mechanisms in different patients. Candidate mechanisms include depletion of sulfhydryl groups that release nitrite or nitric oxide from nitrates, neurohormonal activation of the sympathetic and renin systems, volume expansion induced by vasodilation and possibly by vasopressin activation, cytochrome P-450 inhibition, and down-regulation of soluble guanylate cyclase, which mediates the actions of nitric oxide/S-nitrosothiols.[40, 42, 86, 87, 90] Studies have attempted to circumvent tolerance by antagonizing some of the putative mechanisms, leading to mixed and generally disappointing results. Strategies have included administration of sulfhydryl donors, such as N-acetylcysteine, methionine, and captopril;[83, 86, 92-95] of angiotensin-converting enzyme inhibitors;[92, 96] and of diuretics.[97, 98] Others have shown that very high doses of nitrates can at least transiently overcome tolerance, which is rarely absolute.[99]

However, none of these strategies has yielded convincing or practical results. At present, the only effective strategy is prevention through prudent dosing regimens.[86, 87, 90] Tolerance is readily avoided by employing the lowest effective dose in an asymmetrically timed, intermittent schedule that provides for significant nitrate-free periods each day. The required daily nitrate-free period appears to be 8 to 12 hours. Thus, patches should be worn only for 12 hours a day,[100-103] ointment should be applied only two or three times daily rather than every 4 hours,[7] nitroglycerin should be infused intravenously only 12 hours a day,[7] and other nitrates should also incorporate 8- to 12-hour nitrate-free intervals.[86, 87, 90, 104]

The drawback of intermittent dosing, of course, is loss of protection or even nitrate rebound during nitrate-free intervals. This is especially problematic in the setting of acute heart failure or acute ischemic syndromes. Combination therapy is encouraged in order to minimize the risks of intermittent dosing. Fortunately, true nitrate rebound during intermittent therapy is rarely a clinical problem.[89] Further research on the biology of nitric oxide may lead to effective preventive strategies that will allow for continuous therapy. A deeper understanding of the enzymatic steps in the activation of prodrug nitrates to nitric oxide may allow for the circumvention of tolerance, because "direct" nitric oxide donors, such as molsidomine and nitroprusside, do not induce tolerance.

CONCLUSIONS

After a fascinating history marked by over a century of use, nitroglycerin remains a mainstay of therapy for acute and chronic ischemic heart disease as well as acute and chronic heart failure. Nitroglycerin's physiologic actions are complex, are mediated via the ubiquitous and powerful nitric oxide system, and are practically ideal for most patients with ischemic heart disease or heart failure. Serious adverse effects are remarkably uncommon. Tolerance remains the main obstacle to full exploitation of nitrate therapy; the mechanism is likely variable or multifactorial, and the only effective current strategy is prevention through intermittent dosing. Further research on nitric oxide should yield substantial advances in the use of its prodrugs, the nitrovasodilators.

REFERENCES

1. Fye WB: Vasodilator therapy for angina pectoris: The intersection of homeopathy and scientific medicine. J Hist Med Allied Sci 45:317, 1990.
2. Hering C: Glonoin or nitro glycerine. (Americanische Arzpneiprufungen, translated with additions.) History as proved and applied by C. Hering, Philadelphia, 1847–1851. N Engl Med Gaz 9:255, 1874.
3. Brunton TL: On the use of nitrite of amyl in angina pectoris. Lancet 2:97, 1867.
4. Fye WB: T. Lauder Brunton and amyl nitrite: A Victorian vasodilator. Circulation 74:222, 1986.
5. Murrell W: Nitro-glycerine as a remedy for angina pectoris. Lancet 1:113, 1879.
6. Fye WB: Nitroglycerin: A homeopathic remedy. Circulation 73:21, 1986.
7. American Hospital Formulary Service: Drug Information '93. Bethesda, MD: American Society of Hospital Pharmacists, 1993: 1093.
8. Physicians' Desk Reference. Montvale, NJ: Medical Economics Data Production, 1994, p 1764.
9. Fung H: Interpretation of nitroglycerin pharmacokinetics. Cardiovasc Rev Rep 5:426, 1984.
10. Frishman WH, Landau AJ: Pharmacology of contemporary nitrate therapy. Cardiol Board Rev 10:S(9)13, 1993.
11. Fung HL, Chung SJ, Bauer JA, et al: Biochemical mechanisms of organic nitrate action. Am J Cardiol 70:4B, 1992.
12. Ignarro LJ, Lippton H, Edwards JC, et al: Mechanism of vascular smooth muscle relaxation by organic nitrates, nitrites, nitroprusside and nitric oxide: Evidence for the involvement of S-nitrosothiols as active intermediates. J Pharmacol Exp Ther 218:739, 1981.
13. Harrison DG, Bates JN: The nitrovasodilators: New ideas about old drugs. Circulation 87:1461, 1993.
14. Chung SH, Fung HL: Identification of the subcellular site for nitroglycerin metabolism to nitric oxide in bovine coronary smooth muscle cells. J Pharmacol Exp Ther 253:614, 1990.
15. Feelisch M: The biochemical pathways of nitric oxide formation from nitrovasodilators: Appropriate choice of exogenous NO donors and aspects of preparation and handling of aqueous NO solutions. J Cardiovasc Pharmacol 17(Suppl 3):S25, 1991.
16. Feelisch M, Noack E: Nitric oxide (NO) formation from nitrovasodilators occurs independently of hemoglobin or nonheme iron. Eur J Pharmacol 142:465, 1987.
17. Stamler JS, Loscalzo J: The antiplatelet effects of organic nitrates and related nitroso compounds in vitro and in vivo and their relevance to cardiovascular disorders. J Am Coll Cardiol 18:1529, 1991.
18. Palmer RMJ, Ashton DS, Moncada S: Vascular endothelial cells synthesize nitric oxide from L-arginine. Nature 333:664, 1988.
19. Myers PR, Minor RL, Guerra R, et al: Vasorelaxant properties of the endothelium-derived relaxing factor more closely resemble S-nitrosocysteine than nitric oxide. Nature 345:161, 1990.
20. Moncada S, Higgs A: The L-arginine-nitric oxide pathway. N Engl J Med 329:2002, 1993.
21. Gerzer R, Karrenbrock W, Siess W, et al: Direct comparison of the effects of nitroprusside, SIN 1, and various nitrates on platelet aggregation and soluble guanylate cyclase activity. Thromb Res 52:11, 1988.
22. Kubes P, Suzuki M, Granger DN: Nitric oxide: An endogenous modulator of leukocyte adhesion. Proc Natl Acad Sci U S A 88:4651, 1991.
23. Schror K, Abland B, Weiss P, et al: Stimulation of coronary vascular PGI₂ by organic nitrates. Eur Heart J 9:25, 1988.
24. Garg UC, Hassid A: Nitric oxide-generating vasodilators and 8-bromo-cyclic guanosine monophosphate inhibit mitogenesis and proliferation of cultured rat vascular smooth muscle cells. J Clin Invest 83:1774, 1989.
25. Bassenge E, Zanzinger J: Nitrates in different vascular beds, nitrate tolerance, and interactions with endothelial function. Am J Cardiol 70:23B, 1992.
26. Cohn JN: Pharmacologic mechanisms of nitrates in myocardial ischemia. Am J Cardiol 70:38G, 1992.
27. Abrams J: Mechanisms of action of the organic nitrates in the treatment of myocardial ischemia. Am J Cardiol 70:30B, 1992.
28. Macho P, Vatner SF: Effects of nitroglycerin and nitroprusside on large and small coronary vessels in conscious dogs. Circulation 64:1101, 1981.
29. Brown BG, Bolson EL, Peterson RB, et al: The mechanisms of nitroglycerin action: Stenosis vasodilatation as a major component of drug response. Circulation 65:1089, 1981.
30. Cohen MV, Downey JM, Sonnenblick EH, et al: The effects of nitroglycerin on coronary collaterals and myocardial contractility. J Clin Invest 52:2836, 1973.
31. Feldman RL, Pepine CJ, Conti CR: Magnitude of dilatation of large and small coronary arteries by nitroglycerin. Circulation 64:324, 1980.
32. Lam JYT, Chesebro JH, Fuster V: Platelets, vasoconstriction and nitroglycerin during arterial wall injury. Circulation 78:212, 1988.
33. Gage JE, Hess OM, Murakami T, et al: Vasoconstriction of stenotic coronary arteries during dynamic exercise in patients with classic angina pectoris. Reversibility by nitroglycerin. Circulation 73:865, 1986.
34. Kelly RP, Gibbs HH, Morgan JJ, et al: Nitroglycerin has more favorable effects on left ventricular afterload than apparent from measurements of pressure in peripheral artery. Eur Heart J 11:138, 1990.
35. Simon AC, Levenson JA, Levy BY, et al: Effect of nitroglycerin on peripheral large arteries in hypertension. Br J Clin Pharmacol 14:241, 1982.

36. Ludbrook PA, Byme JD, Kurnick PB, et al: Influence of reduction of preload and afterload by nitroglycerin on left ventricular diastolic pressure-volume relations and relaxation in man. Circulation 56:937, 1966.

37. Jugdutt BI, Warnica JW: Intravenous nitroglycerin therapy to limit myocardial infarct size, expansion and complications. Effect of timing, dosage and infarct location. Circulation 78:906, 1988.

38. Hales CA, Westphal D: Hypoxemia following the administration of sublingual nitroglycerin. Am J Med 65:911, 1978.

39. McGuinness BW, Harris EL: "Monday head": An interesting occupational disorder. Br Med J 2:745, 1961.

40. Frishman WH: Tolerance, rebound and time zero effect of nitrate therapy. Am J Cardiol 70:43G, 1992.

41. Kulick D, Roth A, McIntosh N, et al: Resistance to isosorbide dinitrate in patients with severe chronic heart failure: Incidence and attempt at hemodynamic prediction. J Am Coll Cardiol 12:1023, 1988.

42. Elkayam U, Mehra A, Shotan A, et al: Nitrate resistance and tolerance: Potential limitations in the treatment of congestive heart failure. Am J Cardiol 70:98B, 1992.

43. Becker RC, Corrao JM, Bovill EG, et al: Intravenous nitroglycerin-induced heparin resistance: A qualitative antithrombin III abnormality. Am Heart J 119:1254, 1990.

44. Col J, ColDebeys C, Lavenne-Pardonge E, et al: Propylene-glycol-induced heparin resistance during nitroglycerin infusion. Am Heart J 110:171, 1985.

45. Lepor NE, Amin DK, Berberian L, et al: Does nitroglycerin induce heparin resistance? Clin Cardiol 12:432, 1989.

46. Berk SI, Grunwald A, Pal S, et al: Effect of intravenous nitroglycerin on heparin dosage requirements in coronary artery disease. Am J Cardiol 72:393, 1993.

47. Mehta JL, Nicolini FA, Nichols WW, et al: Concurrent nitroglycerin administration decreases thrombolytic potential of tissue-type plasminogen activator. J Am Coll Cardiol 17:805, 1991.

48. Eisenberg PR, Jaffe AS: Intravenous nitroglycerin does not decrease the efficacy of tPA in patients with acute myocardial infarction [abstract]. J Am Coll Cardiol 19:179, 1992.

49. Thadani U, Whitsett T, Hamilton SF: Nitrate therapy for anginal ischemic syndrome: Current perspectives including tolerance. Curr Probl Cardiol 13:731, 1988.

50. Elkayam U, Kulick D, McIntosh N, et al: Incidence of early tolerance to hemodynamic effects of continuous infusion of nitroglycerin patients with coronary artery disease and heart failure. Circulation 76:577, 1987.

51. Parker JO: Nitrate therapy in stable angina pectoris. N Engl J Med 316:1635, 1987.

52. Horowitz JD: Role of nitrates in unstable angina pectoris. Am J Cardiol 70:64B, 1992.

53. Kaplan K, Davison R, Parker M, et al: Intravenous nitroglycerin in the treatment of angina at rest unresponsive to standard nitrate therapy. Am J Cardiol 51:694, 1983.

54. Mikolich JR, Nicoloff NB, Robinson PH, et al: Relief of refractory angina with continuous intravenous nitroglycerin. Chest 77:375, 1980.

55. DePace NL, Herling IH, Kotler MN, et al: Intravenous nitroglycerin for rest angina. Potential pathophysiologic mechanism of action. Ann Intern Med 142:1806, 1982.

56. Breisblatt WM, Vita NA, Armuchastegui M, et al: Usefulness of serial radionuclide monitoring during graded nitroglycerin infusion for unstable angina pectoris for determining left ventricular function and individualized therapeutic dose. Am J Cardiol 61:685, 1988.

57. Ginsburg R, Lamb IH, Schroeder JS, et al: Randomized, double-blind comparison of nifedipine and isosorbide dinitrate therapy in variant angina pectoris due to coronary artery spasm. Am Heart J 103:44, 1982.

58. Come PC, Pitt B: Nitroglycerin induced severe hypotension and bradycardia in patients with acute myocardial infarction. Circulation 54:624, 1977.

59. Jugdutt BI, Becker CC, Hutchins GM, et al: Effect of intravenous nitroglycerin on collateral blood flow and infarct size in the conscious dog. Circulation 63:17, 1981.

60. Bussman WD, Passek D, Seidel W, et al: Reduction of CK and CK-MB indexes of infarct size by intravenous nitroglycerin. Circulation 63:615, 1981.

61. Jugdutt BI, Sussex BA, Warnica JW, et al: Persistent reduction in left ventricular asynergy in patients with acute myocardial infarction by intravenous infusion of nitroglycerin. Circulation 68:1264, 1983.

62. Jaffe AS, Geltman EM, Tiefenbrunn AJ, et al: Reduction of infarct size in patients with inferior infarction with intravenous glyceryl trinitrate. Br Heart J 49:452, 1983.

63. Gold HK, Leinbach RC, Sanders CA: Use of sublingual nitroglycerin in congestive heart failure following acute myocardial infarction. Circulation 46:839, 1972.

64. Flaherty JT, Reid PR, Kelly DT, et al: Intravenous nitroglycerin in acute myocardial infarction. Circulation 51:132, 1975.

65. Epstein SE, Kent KM, Goldstein RE, et al: Reduction of ischemic injury by nitroglycerin during acute myocardial infarction. N Engl J Med 292:29, 1975.

66. Armstrong PW, Walker DC, Burton JR, et al: Vasodilator therapy in acute myocardial infarction: A comparison of sodium nitroprusside and nitroglycerin. Circulation 52:1118, 1975.

67. Jugdutt BI: Myocardial salvage by intravenous nitroglycerin in conscious dogs: Loss of beneficial effect with marked nitroglycerin-induced hypotension. Circulation 72:907, 1985.

68. Flaherty JT, Becker LC, Bulkley BH: A randomized prospective trial of intravenous nitroglycerin in patients with acute myocardial infarction. Circulation 68:576, 1983.

69. Hockings BEF, Cope GD, Clarke GM, et al: Randomized controlled trial of vasodilator therapy after myocardial infarction. Am J Cardiol 48:345, 1981.

70. Durrer JD, Lie KI, Capelle FJL, et al: Effect of sodium nitroprusside on mortality in acute myocardial infarction. N Engl J Med 306:1121, 1982.

71. Cohn JN, Franciosa JA, Francis GS, et al: Effect of short-term infusion of sodium nitroprusside on mortality rate in acute myocardial infarction complicated by left ventricular failure: Results of a Veterans Administration Cooperative study. N Engl J Med 306:1129, 1982.

72. Chiche P, Baligadoo SJ, Derrida JP: A randomized trial of prolonged nitroglycerin infusion in acute myocardial infarction [abstract]. Circulation 59,60(Supp II):165, 1979.

73. Nelson GIC, Silke B, Ahuja RC, et al: Haemodynamic advantages of isosorbide dinitrate over furosemide in acute heart failure following myocardial infarction. Lancet 1:730, 1983.

74. Lis Y, Bennett D, Lambert G, et al: A preliminary double-blind study of intravenous nitroglycerin in acute myocardial infarction. Intensive Care Med 10:179, 1984.

75. Yusuf S, Collins R, MacMahon S, et al: Effect of intravenous nitrates on mortality in acute myocardial infarction: An overview of the randomized trials. Lancet 1:1088, 1988.

75a. Gruppo Italiano per lo Studio della Sopravvivenza nell'Infarto Miocardico: GISSI-3: Effects of lisinopril and transdermal glyceryl trinitrate singly and together on 6-week mortality and ventricular function after acute myocardial infarction. Lancet 343:1115, 1994.

75b. ISIS-4 (Fourth International Study of Infarct Survival) Collaborative Group: ISIS-4: A randomised factorial trial assessing early oral captopril, oral mononitrate, and intravenous magnesium sulphate in 58 050 patients with suspected acute myocardial infarction. Lancet 345:669, 1995.

76. Jugdutt BI: Delayed effects of early infarct-limiting therapies on healing after myocardial infarction. Circulation 72:907, 1985.

77. Michorowski BL, Senaratne MPJ, Jugdutt BI: Deterring myocardial infarct expansion. Cardiovasc Rev Rep 8:55, 1987.

78. Cohn JN: Mechanisms of action and efficacy of nitrates in heart failure. Am J Cardiol 70:88B, 1992.

79. Franciosa JA, Cohn JN: Effect of isosorbide dinitrate on response to submaximal and maximal exercise in patients with congestive heart failure. Am J Cardiol 43:1009, 1979.

80. Leier LV, Huss P, Magorien RD, et al: Improved exercise capacity and differing arterial and venous tolerance during chronic isosorbide dinitrate therapy for congestive heart failure. Circulation 67:817, 1983.

81. Franciosa JA, Goldsmith SR, Cohn JN: Contrasting immediate and long-term effects of isosorbide dinitrate on exercise capacity in congestive heart failure. Am J Med 69:559, 1980.

82. Franciosa JA, Cohn JN: Sustained hemodynamic effects without tolerance during long-term isosorbide dinitrate treatment of chronic left ventricular failure. Am J Cardiol 45:648, 1980.

83. Packer M, Lee WEI, Kessler PD, et al: Prevention and reversal of nitrate tolerance in patients with congestive heart failure. N Engl J Med 317:799, 1987.

84. Cohn JN, Archibald DG, Ziesche S, et al: Effect of vasodilator therapy on mortality in chronic congestive heart failure: Results of a Veterans Administration Cooperative study (V-HeFT). N Engl J Med 314:1547, 1986.

85. Cohn JN, Johnson G, Ziesche S, et al: A comparison of enalapril with hydralazine-isosorbide dinitrate in the treatment of chronic congestive heart failure. N Engl J Med 325:303, 1991.

86. Elkayam U: Tolerance to organic nitrates: Evidence, mechanisms, clinical relevance, and strategies for prevention. Ann Intern Med 14:667, 1991.

87. Amsterdam EA: Rationale for intermittent nitrate therapy. Am J Cardiol 70:55G, 1992.

88. Morton WE: Occupational habituation to aliphatic nitrates and the withdrawal hazards of coronary disease and hypertension. J Occup Med 19:197, 1977.

89. Lange RL, Reid MS, Tresch DD, et al: Nonatheromatous ischemic heart disease following withdrawal from chronic industrial nitroglycerin exposure. Circulation 46:666, 1972.

90. Abrams J: Designing nitrate regimens to avoid tolerance. Cardiol Board Rev 10(Suppl 9):24, 1993.

91. Transdermal Nitroglycerin Cooperative Study Steering Committee: Acute and chronic antianginal efficacy of continuous twenty-four-hour application of transdermal nitroglycerin. Am J Cardiol 58:1263, 1991.

92. Katz R, Levy WS, Buff L, et al: Prevention of nitrate tolerance with angiotensin converting enzyme inhibitors. Circulation 83:1271, 1991.

93. Horowitz JD, Antman EM, Lorell BH, et al: Potentiation of the cardiovascular effects of nitroglycerin by N-acetylcysteine. Circulation 68:1247, 1983.

94. Horowitz JD, Henry CA, Syrjanen ML, et al: Combined use of nitroglycerin and N-acetylcysteine in the management of unstable angina pectoris. Circulation 77:787, 1988.

95. Dupuis J, Lalonde G, Lemieux R, et al: Tolerance to intravenous nitroglycerin in patients with congestive heart failure: Role of increased intravascular volume, neurohumoral activation and lack of prevention with N-acetylcysteine. J Am Coll Cardiol 16:923, 1990.

96. Dakak N, Makhoul N, Flugelman MY, et al: Failure of captopril to prevent nitrate tolerance in congestive heart failure secondary to coronary artery disease. Am J Cardiol 66:608, 1990.

97. Parker JD, Farrell B, Fenton T, et al: Effects of diuretic therapy on the development of tolerance during continuous therapy with nitroglycerin. J Am Coll Cardiol 20:616, 1992.

98. Sussex BA, Campbell NR, Raiu MK: Nitrate tolerance is modified by diuretic treatment. Circulation 80(III):200, 1990.

99. Frishman W, Giles T, Greenberg S, et al: The high dose nitroglycerin patch in angina: a placebo-controlled, double-blind study [abstract]. Circulation 76(IV):127, 1987.

100. DeMots H, Glasser SP, on behalf of the Transderm-Nitro Trial Study Group: Intermittent transdermal nitroglycerin therapy in the treatment of chronic stable angina. J Am Coll Cardiol 13:786, 1989.

101. Cowan JC, Bourke JP, Reid DS, et al: Prevention of tolerance to nitroglycerin patches by overnight removal. Am J Cardiol 60:271, 1987.

102. Luke R, Sharpe N, Coxon R: Transdermal nitroglycerin in angina pectoris: Efficacy of intermittent application. J Am Coll Cardiol 10:642, 1987.

103. Sharpe N, Coxon R, Webster M, et al: Hemodynamic effects of intermittent transdermal nitroglycerin in chronic congestive heart failure. Am J Cardiol 59:895, 1987.

104. Parker JO, Farrell B, Lahey KA, et al: Effect of intervals between doses on the development of tolerance to isosorbide dinitrate. N Engl J Med 316:1440, 1987.

CHAPTER 94

Long-Acting Nitrates

Richard L. Mueller, M.D., and Stephen Scheidt, M.D.

This chapter reviews the nitrovasodilator drugs other than nitroglycerin that are available in the United States, including isosorbide dinitrate (ISDN), isosorbide-5-mononitrate (IS-5-MN), erythrityl tetranitrate (ET), and pentaerythritol tetranitrate (PET). Although certain formulations of isosorbide dinitrate and erythrityl tetranitrate are short-acting, the nonnitroglycerin nitrovasodilators are used predominantly as long-acting preparations; long-acting nitroglycerin formulations are covered in Chapter 93. Although the shortest-acting of all nitrovasodilators, amyl nitrite is included in this chapter for completeness. Molsidomine, a direct nitric oxide donor of the sydnonimine class of compounds, and nicorandil, a nitrate that also opens membrane potassium channels, are not reviewed because they are not currently available in the United States.

As with the long-acting preparations of nitroglycerin, the other long-acting nitrates share the promise of convenient dosing and many hours of angina prophylaxis due to their prolonged presence in plasma, but they also are subject to nitrate tolerance if poorly planned dosing leads to continuous nitrate exposure.

CHEMISTRY

ISDN, IS-5-MN, ET, and PET are all synthetic alcohol esters of nitric acid, whereas isoamyl nitrite is a synthetic mixture of isomers of an alcohol ester of nitrous acid. Amyl nitrite is an organic nitrite, whereas the others are organic nitrates.[1]

Amyl nitrite is an extremely volatile, highly flammable and explosive, yellow liquid that is minimally soluble in water and freely soluble in ethanol. Amyl nitrite has an ethereal, peculiar, fruity odor and a pungent, aromatic taste. Unlike other nitrates that are rendered unexplosive by dilution with inert incipients, commercial preparations of amyl nitrite remain flammable and explosive and must be handled with care. Amyl nitrite is dispensed in fragile glass vials covered with cloth; the vial is crushed, leaking the volatile liquid into the cloth, from which it is inhaled in the manner that smelling salts are used.

In contrast, the nitrates listed above are white, odorless, crystalline solids that are variably soluble in water and ethanol. They are nonvolatile, explosive in their pure state but nonexplosive after the addition of diluents. ISDN is sparingly soluble in water; IS-5-MN is freely soluble in water; ET and PET are insoluble in water. ISDN is known chemically as 1, 4:3, 6 dianhydro-sorbital-2, 5-dinitrate; IS-5-MN is 1, 4:3, 6-dianhydro-, D-glucitol 5-nitrate; ET is 1, 2, 3, 4-butanetetrol tetranitrate; and PET is 2, 2 bishydroxymethyl-1, 3 propanediol tetranitrate.[1]

PHARMACOKINETICS

The pharmacokinetics of all nitrovasodilators are complex and not fully defined. However, those of ISDN are considerably less complex and better defined than those of nitroglycerin. Compared with nitroglycerin, plasma levels of ISDN are easier to measure, because comparable doses result in plasma concentrations of ISDN at least an order of magnitude higher than those for nitroglycerin. Also, the high arteriovenous extraction of nitroglycerin, in some studies more than 60%, is far less for ISDN, eliminating the need for separate analyses of ISDN pharmacokinetics in the arterial and venous circulations.[2]

The bioavailability of orally administered ISDN varies from 17% to 48%, whereas it is 31% to 59% with the sublingual route. The terminal half-life of ISDN varies with the route of administration, for reasons not understood. The half-life is approximately 20 minutes, 60 minutes, and 4 hours after intravenous, sublingual, and oral administration, respectively. As with nitroglycerin, first-pass hepatic metabolism of ISDN is substantial, and unlike the case with nitroglycerin, accounts for nearly all of its metabolism. Like nitroglycerin, ISDN has a very large volume of distribution, but its systemic clearance is lower than that of nitroglycerin: greater than hepatic blood flow but less than the cardiac output. As noted, vascular tissue extraction is far less than for nitroglycerin or even absent. As with nitroglycerin, the clearance and metabolism of ISDN are decreased by its metabolites, isosorbide-5-mononitrate (IS-5-MN) and isosorbide-2-mononitrate (IS-2-MN), thereby raising the concentration of the parent molecule. Thus, ISDN's half-life depends on both the route of administration and the duration of treatment.[3]

These mononitrate metabolites are generated by hepatic denitrification of ISDN by the enzyme glutathione organic nitrate reductase, also described as glutathione S-transferase in many texts. The mononitrate metabolites are further metabolized to inorganic nitrite ion, isosorbide, the glucuronidated mononitrates, and at least five other metabolites. The mononitrates are also metabolized primarily by the same hepatic enzymes, but, unlike ISDN, are not subject to first-pass metabolism. The mononitrates are active metabolites; 2-ISMN has ⅓ to ⅙ the vasodilating potency of the parent molecule, whereas IS-5-MN has

⅟₃₀ to ⅟₁₀₀ its activity. However, because the half-lives of 2-ISMN and IS-5-MN are approximately 2.5 and 5 hours, respectively, the overall activity of IS-5-MN exceeds that of both 2-ISMN and ISDN itself. Thus, IS-5-MN is the predominant active metabolite of ISDN and accounts for most of the activity of the administered dose; fully 60% of ISDN is converted to IS-5-MN.[3]

Because the mononitrates are active metabolites accounting for most of the activity of ISDN, IS-5-MN itself has been developed as a therapeutic agent owing to several pharmacokinetic advantages over the parent molecule. In addition to its longer half-life compared with ISDN, the bioavailability of orally administered IS-5-MN is nearly 100% because of complete absorption and no hepatic first-pass metabolism, and its volume of distribution is lower. IS-5-MN is only 5% bound to plasma proteins, and maximal plasma concentrations are achieved within 30 to 60 minutes of oral dosing. Unlike ISDN and nitroglycerin, the half-life of IS-5-MN does not change with multiple dosing. Furthermore, the disposition of IS-5-MN does not vary with renal or hepatic insufficiency, cardiac failure, or advanced age; low body weight is the only clinical state that mandates dosage adjustment. Food decreases the rate but not the extent of absorption of IS-5-MN. Unlike ISDN, IS-5-MN does not require hepatic metabolism for expression of its full activity, because it is the main active metabolite of ISDN. Compared with other nitrates, IS-5-MN produces quite predictable plasma levels, with little inter- or intra-individual variability in therapeutic doses. Of the total orally administered dose of IS-5-MN, 96% is excreted in the urine, with only 1% found in the feces. About 2% of the dose is excreted as the unchanged drug, along with at least five inactive metabolites.[4]

Amyl nitrite is completely absorbed through respiratory mucosa, then metabolized by organic nitrate reductase to nitrite ion and isoamyl alcohol. ET and PET are approximately 50% bioavailable and undergo sequential denitrification to their respective trinitrate, dinitrate, and mononitrate metabolites, all of which are inactive, before undergoing terminal denitrification to their alcohol moieties.[1]

PHARMACODYNAMICS

(See Chapter 93.)

PHARMACOLOGY

Although nitrovasodilators relax all smooth muscle throughout the body, the predominant therapeutic effect is vasodilation. ISDN, IS-5-MN, ET, PET, and amyl nitrite produce dose-dependent vasodilation throughout the vascular tree similar to the way nitroglycerin does. With increasing doses, these nitrates and nitrites first produce venodilation, especially of large-capacitance veins, followed by arterial dilation of large-conductance vessels, followed by arterial dilation of coronary and other medium-sized vessels, followed by arteriolar dilation at very high doses.[5] For more details, see Chapter 93.

ADVERSE EFFECTS

ISDN, IS-5-MN, ET, PET, and amyl nitrite all share nitroglycerin's adverse effects (see Chapter 93). In summary, all nitrates and nitrites may produce headache, orthostatic hypotension and/or dizziness, syncope, paradoxic bradycardia, reflex tachycardia, methemoglobinemia, palpitations, nausea, rash, nitrate tolerance, or rebound vasospasm. All nitrates and nitrites and, indeed, all vasodilators of any type are contraindicated in patients with severe aortic stenosis or severe obstructive hypertrophic cardiomyopathy.[1] Several adverse effects unique to intravenously administered nitroglycerin, such as alcohol intoxication, gout, Wernicke's encephalopathy,[1] and heparin[6, 7] and/or t-PA resistance,[8, 9] are not seen with the nonparenterally administered nitrates. Overall, considering their potent vascular effects, the nitrovasodilators are surprisingly well tolerated, with only rare serious adverse effects. There are no data to evaluate the effects of any nitrovasodilator on pregnancy, nursing, carcinogenesis, mutagenesis, and fertility. Amyl nitrite has some unique adverse effects, including hemolytic anemia and the potential for patient diversion of the drug for recreational use as a sexual pleasure enhancer.[1]

AVAILABLE PREPARATIONS
Short-Acting Preparations

Short-acting nitrate or nitrite preparations are indicated for the treatment or short-term prophylaxis of angina pectoris as single doses. Because of their brief presence in plasma, they do not produce nitrate tolerance, but they are not effective for prolonged or chronic angina prophylaxis.

Amyl Nitrite

Available in 0.3-ml crushable vials, amyl nitrite has a very rapid onset of action on the order of 30 seconds. Likewise, duration of action is brief, lasting only up to 6 minutes. The rapid kinetics are mainly due to the rapid and brief absorption inherent in the inhalation of a volatile liquid. Care must be taken with the vials, which are flammable and potentially explosive. Amyl nitrite is such a powerful vasodilator that it is more potent than the largest sublingual nitroglycerin dose; syncope is a real concern, so doses should be administered with the patient in the supine or sitting position. Amyl nitrite may be used for the rare patient with unusually severe angina episodes that do not respond to maximal doses of sublingually administered nitroglycerin.[1]

Sublingually Administered and Chewable Isosorbide Dinitrate

Sublingually administered ISDN is available as 2.5-, 5-, and 10-mg tablets. Compared with sublingually administered nitroglycerin, the onset of action of sublingually administered ISDN is slower at 3 to 15 minutes, and the duration of action is longer at 1 to 2 hours. Chewable ISDN is available as 5- and 10-mg tablets; mainly because of transmucosal oral absorption, it possesses pharmacokinetics identical to that of sublingually administered ISDN.[1, 10, 11]

Sublingually Administered Erythrityl Tetranitrate

Available as 5- and 10-mg tablets, sublingually administered ET's onset of action within 3 to 15 minutes and 2-hour duration of action resemble those of sublingually administered and chewable ISDN.[1, 10, 11]

Long-Acting Preparations

As discussed in the previous chapter, long-acting nitrate preparations are indicated for prolonged prophylaxis of angina because of their prolonged presence in plasma; however, nitrate tolerance is likely if poorly planned dosing leads to continuous exposure. Because of their relatively slow onset of action, long-acting preparations are not indicated for aborting acute anginal episodes. In 1993, the Cardiovascular and Renal Drugs Advisory Committee of the United States Food and Drug Administration recommended a change in the labeling of all nitrates not shown to be effective for long-term use. The revised labeling would approve these agents only for single-dose or short-term use.

Orally Administered Isosorbide-5-Mononitrate, Immediate and Sustained Release

Orally administered IS-5-MN is available as 10- and 20-mg immediate-release and 60- and 120-mg sustained-release tablets. The immediate-release tablets have an onset and duration of action of 30 to 60 minutes and 7 hours, respectively, whereas the sustained-release tablets have an onset and duration of action of 1 to 2 hours and 12 hours, respectively. Regimens that avert nitrate tolerance include 5 to 20 mg of the immediate-release IS-5-MN given twice daily in asymmetric fashion, 7 hours apart, and 30 to 120 mg of the sustained-release formulation given once daily. As a newly introduced nitrate in the United States, the IS-5-MN preparations have been more extensively studied than any of the other nitrates for long-term use, along with nitroglycerin patches. Such regimens have been shown to avoid tolerance, maintain beneficial effects on exercise tolerance for at least 14 hours of the day over at least 2 to 6 weeks of long-term dosing, and produce no rebound exacerbation of angina during the nitrate-free interval. Because IS-5-MN has been amply demonstrated to retain efficacy with long-term use when dosed properly, the imminent Food and Drug Administration (FDA) relabeling of nitrates should not affect these new preparations.[10–12]

Orally Administered Erythrityl Tetranitrate

Available as 5- and 10-mg tablets, orally administered ET's onset and duration of action are 30 minutes and 3 to 6 hours, respectively. Data on efficacy as well as tolerance-averting dosing strategies are lacking, but an 8- to 12-hour daily nitrate-free interval is advisable.[1, 10, 11]

Orally Administered Pentaerythritol Tetranitrate, Immediate and Sustained Release

Orally administered, immediate-release PET is available as 8-, 10-, 20-, 40-, and 80-mg tablets, whereas sustained release PET is available as 30- and 45-mg capsules and 80-mg tablets. The onset and duration of action of immediate-release PET are similar to those of orally administered ET at 30 minutes and 3 to 6 hours, respectively. The onset and duration of action of sustained-release PET are 2 hours and 6 to 10 hours, respectively. Data on efficacy as well as tolerance-averting dosing strategies are lacking, but an 8- to 12-hour daily nitrate-free interval is advisable.[1, 10, 11]

Orally Administered Isosorbide Dinitrate, Immediate and Sustained Release

Orally administered ISDN is available as 5-, 10-, 20-, 30-, and 40-mg immediate-release tablets as well as 40-mg sustained-release tablets. The immediate-release tablets have an onset and duration of action of 15 to 30 minutes and 3 to 6 hours, respectively, whereas the sustained-release tablets have an onset and duration of action of 30 to 60 minutes and 6 to 10 hours, respectively. These pharmacokinetics roughly resemble those of nitroglycerin ointment and orally administered capsules. Regimens that avoid nitrate tolerance include immediate-release ISDN tablets administered two to three times daily, or sustained-release ISDN tablets once or twice daily. Either regimen should include asymmetric dosing times during the day in order to maximize nitrate-free intervals, with the last dose usually by 5 PM so that, allowing for a 6- to 8-hour duration of action, there remains at least an 8-hour nitrate-free interval after the last dose's plasma concentrations have fallen to very low or absent levels.[1, 10, 11]

INDICATIONS

As discussed in the previous chapter, the nitrates and nitrites are nearly ideal agents for the treatment of angina because of their salutory effects on both myocardial oxygen supply and demand. Although the clinical significance is still unclear, nitrovasodilators also inhibit platelet[13] and leukocyte[14] functions as well as vascular smooth muscle proliferation.[15] All nitrates are approved only for the treatment or prophylaxis of angina. Despite considerable evidence supporting their use, it is noteworthy that, to date, none of the nitrates are approved for use in myocardial infarction or congestive heart failure.[3] In addition to use for angina, amyl nitrite is used as a provocative, diagnostic agent in the clinical or laboratory evaluation of heart murmurs and as a component of the antidote for cyanide poisoning.[1]

Chapter 93 reviews the use of nitroglycerin in unstable angina, myocardial infarction, and congestive heart failure in detail. Other nitrates are theoretically also of benefit in these conditions, but not all preparations have been studied for all indications. Of note is that the ISIS-4 study,[15a] which assessed the effects of nitrates as well as captopril and magnesium in acute myocardial infarction, used sustained-release IS-5-MN (60 mg/day). The study found a statistically significant mortality reduction in the nitrate group only during the first day of treatment; thereafter, there was only a statistically nonsignificant trend toward a benefit up to 5 weeks. Orally administered nitrate treatment was very well tolerated and not associated with any adverse impact on any end points. Its contemporary study, the GISSI-3 trial,[15b] found similar results using 24 hours of intravenously administered nitroglycerin followed by 6 weeks of either a nitroglycerin patch or 50 mg/day of IS-5-MN. All other randomized trials of nitrates in acute myocardial infarction have used nitroprusside or nitroglycerin for brief periods following admission.[16, 17]

As for congestive heart failure therapy, the only randomized trials examining the effects of nitrates on survival, the V-HeFT I[18] and II[19] trials, both employed ISDN combined with hydralazine. The dose of ISDN was 40 mg four times daily in both trials. V-HeFT I compared mortality in placebo, prazosin, and hydralazine-ISDN groups, finding a statistically significant mortality reduction only with hydralazine-ISDN treatment. V-HeFT II found a statistically significant reduction in mortality with enalapril treatment compared with hydralazine-ISDN; however, the hydralazine-ISDN group had statistically significant superior left ventricular function and exercise capacity. As in the case of nitroglycerin, dosages of long-acting nitrates in congestive heart failure are frequently higher than for angina, given frequent relative nitrate resistance due to neurohormonal activation and its antagonism of nitrate-induced vasodilation.

ET, PET, and amyl nitrite have not been investigated in unstable angina, myocardial angina, or congestive heart failure.

TOLERANCE

As discussed in the previous chapter, poorly designed nitrate dosing regimens that produce continuous drug exposure will predictably result in tolerance, regardless of the preparation.[20-24] Only the short-acting nitrates do not induce tolerance, because of their brief presence in the plasma. Rebound increases in ischemia are also possible with continuous nitrate therapy.[25, 26] As with nitroglycerin,[27] tolerance to the long-acting nitrates is easily avoided by employing intermittent dosing and asymmetric timing of drug doses during the day. These simple strategies ensure an 8- to 12-hour daily nitrate-free interval, which has been shown to prevent tolerance, regardless of the nitrate preparation.[28] There are inadequate data on tolerance induction and avoidance with ET and PET, but an 8- to 12-hour nitrate-free interval is advisable.[29] Extensive data on ISDN have demonstrated that daily dosing four times a day (of the immediate-release preparation) will induce tolerance,[28, 30] whereas twice-daily dosing will not,[28] especially if the doses are asymmetrically timed during the waking hours. Studies in which ISDN is administered three times a day have yielded mixed results, with some showing rapid attenuation of effects.[30] However, other studies, especially those employing asymmetric dosing, have demonstrated avoidance of tolerance.[28] Several studies have established that once-daily sustained-release IS-5-MN or asymmetrically dosed, twice-daily immediate-release IS-5-MN retains clinical efficacy during long-term dosing without tolerance or rebound phenomena.[12, 29, 31–33] Pharmacologic efforts to prevent nitroglycerin tolerance, including administration of angiotensin-converting enzyme inhibitors, sulfhydryl group donors, and diuretics, have met with mixed results.[23] There are few data regarding these strategies for preventing tolerance to other nitrates; one study found no benefit to N-acetylcysteine coadministration with ISDN.[34]

CONCLUSIONS

The long-acting nitrates ISDN, IS-5-MN, ET, and PET share all the beneficial effects of nitroglycerin for the indications of chronic stable angina, unstable angina, myocardial infarction, and congestive heart failure. Although not all preparations have been studied for all indications, the varied pharmacokinetics and advantages of these nitrates expand the arsenal against coronary disease and heart failure. In particular, ISDN and IS-5-MN have been shown to be useful in congestive heart failure and myocardial infarction, respectively. As with nitroglycerin, poorly designed dosage strategies that produce continuous nitrate exposure will lead to nitrate tolerance. However, such tolerance is readily averted with asymmetrically timed, intermittent dosing that incorporates an adequate daily nitrate-free interval. IS-5-MN, recently introduced in the United States as immediate-release and sustained-release tablets, enjoys several pharmacokinetic advantages over other nitrates for long-term use, has been extensively evaluated, and has been shown to be effective with long-term use without incurring either tolerance or rebound phenomena. ET and PET are rarely used because they offer no advantages over similar nitrates and lack data substantiating their efficacy with long-term use. Amyl nitrite is a unique, ultra-short-acting nitrite of mostly historical interest. When used, it is more often as a diagnostic agent or cyanide antidote than as antianginal therapy.

REFERENCES

1. American Hospital Formulary Service: Drug Information 93. Bethesda, MD: American Society of Hospital Pharmacists, 1993, p 1093.
2. Needleman P, Lang S, Johnson EM: Organic nitrates: Relationship between biotransformation and rational angina pectoris therapy. J Pharmacol Exp Ther 181:489, 1972.
3. Physicians' Desk Reference. Montvale, NJ: Medical Economics Data Production, 1994, p 2549.
4. Abshagen UWP: Pharmacokinetics of isosorbide mononitrate. Am J Cardiol 70:61G, 1992.
5. Bassenge E, Zanzinger J: Nitrates in different vascular beds, nitrate tolerance, and interactions with endothelial function. Am J Cardiol 70:23B, 1992.
6. Becker RC, Corrao JM, Bovill EG, et al: Intravenous nitroglycerin-induced heparin resistance during nitroglycerin infusion. Am Heart J 110:171, 1985.
7. Berk SI, Grunwald A, Pal S, et al: Effect of intravenous nitroglycerin on heparin dosage requirements in coronary artery disease. Am J Cardiol 71:393, 1993.
8. Mehta JL, Nicolini FA, Nichols WW, et al: Concurrent nitroglycerin administration decreases thrombolytic potential of tissue-type plasminogen activator. J Am Coll Cardiol 17:805, 1991.
9. Eisenberg PR, Jaffe AS: Intravenous nitroglycerin does not decrease the efficacy of t-PA in patients with acute myocardial infarction [abstract]. J Am Coll Cardiol 19:179, 1992.
10. Frishman WH, Landau AJ: Pharmacology of contemporary nitrate therapy. Cardiol Board Rev 10:S13, 1993.
11. Fung HL: Pharmacokinetics of nitroglycerin and long-acting nitrate esters. Am J Med 74(6B):13, 1983.
12. Thadani U, de Vane PJ: Efficacy of isosorbide mononitrate in angina pectoris. Am J Cardiol 70:67G, 1992.
13. Stamler JS, Loscalzo J: The antiplatelet effects of organic nitrates and related nitroso compounds in vitro and in vivo and their relevance to cardiovascular disorders. J Am Coll Cardiol 18:1529, 1991.
14. Kubes P, Suzuki M, Granger DN: Nitric oxide: An endogenous modulator of leukocyte adhesion. Proc Natl Acad Sci U S A 88:4651, 1991.
15. Garg UC, Hassid A: Nitric oxide-generating vasodilators and 8-bromo-cyclic guanosine monophosphate inhibit mitogenesis and proliferation of cultured rat vascular smooth muscle cells. J Clin Invest 83:1774, 1989.
15a. ISIS-4 (Fourth International Study of Infarct Survival) Collaborative Group: ISIS-4: A randomised factorial trial assessing early oral captopril, oral mononitrate, and intravenous magnesium sulphate in 58 050 patients with suspected acute myocardial infarction. Lancet 345:669, 1995.
15b. Gruppo Italiano per lo Studio della Sopravvivenza nell'Infarto Miocardico: GISSI-3: Effects of lisinopril and transdermal glyceryl trinitrate singly and together on 6-week mortality and ventricular function after acute myocardial infarction. Lancet 343:1115, 1994.
16. Yusuf S, Collins R, MacMahon S, et al: Effect of intravenous nitrates on mortality in acute myocardial infarction: An overview of the randomized trials. Lancet 1:1088, 1988.
17. Jugdutt BI, Warnica JW: Intravenous nitroglycerin therapy to limit myocardial infarct size, expansion and complications. Effect of timing, dosage and infarct location. Circulation 78:906, 1988.
18. Cohn JN, Archibald DG, Ziesche S, et al: Effect of vasodilator therapy on mortality in chronic congestive heart failure: Results of a Veterans Administration Cooperative study (V-HeFT). N Engl J Med 314:1547, 1986.
19. Cohn JN, Johnson G, Ziesche S, et al: A comparison of enalapril with hydralazine-isosorbide dinitrate in the treatment of chronic congestive heart failure. N Engl J Med 325:303, 1991.
20. Elkayam U: Tolerance to organic nitrates: Evidence, mechanisms, clinical relevance, and strategies for prevention. Ann Intern Med 14:667, 1991.
21. Elkayam U, Mehra A, Shotan A, et al: Nitrate resistance and tolerance: Potential limitations in the treatment of congestive heart failure. Am J Cardiol 70:98B, 1992.
22. Amsterdam EA: Rationale for intermittent nitrate therapy. Am J Cardiol 70:55G, 1992.
23. Abrams J: Designing nitrate regimens to avoid tolerance. Cardiol Board Rev 10(S9):24, 1993.
24. Transdermal Nitroglycerin Cooperative Study Steering Committee: Acute and chronic antianginal efficacy of continuous

twenty-four hour application of transdermal nitroglycerin. Am J Cardiol 58:1263, 1991.

25. Morton WE: Occupational habituation to aliphatic nitrates and the withdrawal hazards of coronary disease and hypertension. J Occup Med 19:197, 1977.

26. Lange RL, Reid MS, Tresch DD, et al: Nonatheromatous ischemic heart disease following withdrawal from chronic industrial nitroglycerin exposure. Circulation 46:666, 1972.

27. DeMots H, Glasser SP, on behalf of the Transderm-Nitro Trial Study Group: Intermittent transdermal nitroglycerin therapy in the treatment of chronic stable angina. J Am Coll Cardiol 13:786, 1989.

28. Parker JO, Farrell B, Lahey KA, et al: Effect of intervals between doses on the development of tolerance to isosorbide dinitrate. N Engl J Med 316:1440, 1987.

29. Thadani U: Role of nitrates in angina pectoris. Am J Cardiol 70:43B, 1992.

30. Bassan MM: The daylong pattern of the antianginal effect of long-term three times daily administered isosorbide dinitrate. J Am Coll Cardiol 16:936, 1990.

31. Friedman G and the ISMN Study Group: Comparative clinical trial of isosorbide mononitrate and isosorbide dinitrate in patients with stable angina pectoris. J Invasive Cardiol 4:319, 1992.

32. Thadani U, Friedman R, Jones JP, et al: Nitrate tolerance: Eccentric versus concentric twice daily therapy with isosorbide-5-mononitrate in angina pectoris [abstract]. Circulation 80(II):216, 1989.

33. Thadani U and the IS-5-MN Study Group: Isosorbide-5-mononitrate (IS-5-MN) in angina pectoris: Efficacy of A.M. and P.M. doses, lack of tolerance and zero hour effect during eccentric BID therapy. Circulation 84(II):144, 1991.

34. Parker JO, Farrell B, Rose BF: Nitrate tolerance: The lack of effect of N-acetylcysteine. Circulation 76:572, 1987.

CHAPTER 95

Isosorbide Mononitrate

Udho Thadani, M.B.BS., M.R.C.P., F.R.C.P.C.

HISTORY

The conclusion of Needleman et al.[1] in the 1970s that orally administered organic nitrates, including isosorbide dinitrate (ISDN), were inactive because of their complete metabolic inactivation during their first passage through the liver led to extensive research in the pharmacokinetics and pharmacodynamics of ISDN and its metabolites.[2] It was already known that the isosorbide-5-mononitrate (IS-5-MN) was the main metabolite of ISDN,[3, 4] and subsequently in isolated organs 2 and 5 mononitrates were shown to exhibit nitrate-like vascular activity.[5, 6] IS-5-MN did not undergo first-pass hepatic inactivation and had no active metabolites. In patients with coronary artery disease, IS-5-MN exerted antianginal effects.[7, 8]

IS-5-MN was first introduced for clinical use in Germany under the trade name ISMO in November 1981; since then, the drug has been introduced in several other countries, including the United States in 1992.

CHEMISTRY

IS-5-MN (ISMO, Monoket) is 1,4:3,6-dianhydro-D-glucitol,5-nitrate ($C_6H_9NO_6$), an organic nitrate whose molecular weight is 191.14. IS-5-MN is a crystalline powder with a melting point of 89° to 91°C. It is readily soluble in water, methanol, ethanol, and acetone.

PHARMACOLOGY

IS-5-MN is the major active metabolite of ISDN,[5] and most of the clinical activity of ISDN is attributable to the mononitrate.[5]

The principal pharmacologic activity of IS-5-MN is relaxation of vascular smooth muscle and consequent dilation of the veins and large arteries at lower concentrations and dilation of the arterioles at higher concentrations.[6] The pronounced venodilation promotes venous pooling of blood and decreases the venous return to the heart, thereby reducing left ventricular end-diastolic pressure and pulmonary capillary wedge pressure (preload).[7] Afterload is also reduced by the reduction of peripheral vascular resistance and an increase in vessel distensibility.[8] Dilation of the coronary arteries, including stenosis dilation, also occurs, but the relative importance of preload reduction, afterload reduction, and coronary dilation remains undefined.[9]

Tolerance toward circulatory, antianginal, and anti-ischemic effects of IS-5-MN develops with three or four times daily dosing with 30 to 50 mg IS-5-MN.[10, 11] Tolerance can be avoided with a 20-mg dose administered in the morning and again 7 hours later (eccentric b.i.d. dosing), so that there is a gap of 17 hours between the second dose of each day and the first dose of the next day.[12–16] The dosing interval required to prevent tolerance with doses higher than 20 mg has not been defined.[17] Standard twice-daily treatment with 20 mg IS-5-MN is not effective throughout the dosing interval and produces partial tolerance.[18]

PHARMACOKINETICS

IS-5-MN is measured by gas chromatography with electron capture detection. The detection limit is 5 $\mu g/L^{-1}$.[19] In humans, IS-5-MN from ISMO and Monoket tablets is rapidly and completely absorbed from the gastrointestinal tract and is not subject to first-pass metabolism in the liver. The absolute bioavailability of IS-5-MN from ISMO and Monoket tablets is nearly 100%.[20, 21] Maximum serum concentrations of

IS-5-MN are achieved 30 to 60 minutes after oral ingestion.[20, 21]

The volume of distribution of IS-5-MN is approximately 0.6 L/kg, and less than 4% is bound to plasma proteins.[20, 21] It is cleared from the serum by denitration to isosorbide, glucuronidation to the mononitrate glucuronide, and denitration/hydration to sorbitol.[22, 23] None of these metabolites is vasoactive.[22, 23] Less than 1% of administered IS-5-MN is eliminated in the urine.

The alpha phase half-life is 8.6 minutes, and the beta phase half-life is approximately 4.2 hours and is not dose dependent.[20, 21] The rate of absorption is slowed by food, but overall bioavailability is unchanged.[24] It is quite possible that enterohepatic recirculation occurs. Kinetics are not significantly influenced by advancing age[22] or hepatic[25] or renal disease.[26]

There is good correlation between fall in blood pressure and plasma IS-5-MN levels after the first dose,[27] but this relationship is lost during sustained treatment as a result of development of tolerance.[28] There is a linear relationship between dose and plasma concentrations after single and multiple dosing.[23]

EFFECTS ON PATHOPHYSIOLOGY
Effects on Hemodynamics

IS-5-MN produces dose-dependent reduction in cardiac output secondary to a reduction in venous return due to venodilation.[29] There is a dose-dependent decrease in mean and systolic arterial blood pressure and right atrial pressure.[29] In dogs, the threshold dose for decrease in peripheral resistance and systolic blood pressure is between 0.1 and 0.3 mg/kg, whereas the threshold for the decrease in right atrial pressure is 10 times lower.[29]

IS-5-MN produces dilation of the epicardial coronary arteries but produces little change in mean coronary blood flow.[30, 31]

IS-5-MN has no effect on hepatic blood flow; whether portal pressure decreases remains unknown.[32]

At constant intravenous infusion of lower doses of IS-5-MN (12 μg/ml), reduction in blood pressure is not attenuated, and there is no blunting of response to nitroglycerin.[33] In contrast with high-dose infusion (26 μg/ml), a slightly reduced responsiveness to nitroglycerin is observed.[33] A reduced responsiveness occurs when IS-5-MN is given at shorter (frequent) intervals.[33]

In patients with coronary artery disease, initial dose of IS-5-MN produces a reduction in cardiac output and a fall in blood pressure and pulmonary arterial pressure at rest and during exercise.[34, 35] After 2 weeks of treatment with 20 mg four times a day, the blood pressure effects are attenuated, and there is also an attenuation of pulmonary arterial pressure decrease at rest as well as during exercise.[35] Similar observations have been reported with 50 mg t.i.d. treatment with IS-5-MN, but not with 20 mg t.i.d. treatment.[35]

In patients with heart failure, beneficial effects on hemodynamics have been reported after single-dose studies.[36, 37]

Effects on Ventricular Function and Structure

IS-5-MN reduces cardiac dimensions and improves cardiac contractility,[38] and this is especially pronounced in patients with congestive cardiac failure.[39] It is unknown whether any structural alterations occur.

Effects on Electrophysiology

IS-5-MN has no direct effects on conduction or refractory period of cardiac conduction tissue or the myocardium. Electrocardiographic PR, QRS, or QT intervals are not altered by IS-5-MN.

Effects on Coronary Blood Flow

Coronary blood flow is not significantly altered despite dilation of the epicardial coronary arteries.[30, 31] In patients with atherosclerotic coronary artery disease, stenosis dilation and improvement in flow to the ischemic areas occur after the initial doses of IS-5-MN. Effects on coronary blood flow during long-term treatment have not been well studied.

Effects on Arteries and Veins

There is preferential venodilation at lower doses and dilation of large conductance arteries.[6] As the dose is increased, dilation of muscular arteries and resistance vessels occurs[6] with a fall in peripheral vascular resistance.

Effects on Fluid Volume State and Electrolytes

Intravascular volume increases during long-term treatment as a result of a shift of fluid from extravascular space to intravascular space, but there is no alteration in serum electrolyte levels.

Endocrine and Metabolic Effects

In medium-term studies in humans, no endocrine or metabolic effects have been reported.

Effects on Renal Function

IS-5-MN has no adverse effects on renal function.

Effects on Fetus

The effects of IS-5-MN on fetus and newborn infants in humans have not been studied, and IS-5-MN should be avoided in pregnant females.

Effects on Central Nervous System

In therapeutic doses, no effects have been observed.

CLINICAL USE
Indications

The only approved indication is in patients with stable angina pectoris. In Europe, IS-5-MN is also used to treat heart failure, but the studies are inadequate to provide appropriate therapeutic guidance for this indication.

Stable Angina Pectoris

In patients with stable angina pectoris, first doses of IS-5-MN increase angina-free walking duration and decrease exercise-induced ST-segment depression.[27] Improvement in exercise duration on the treadmill or bicycle is observed within 30 minutes and persists for up to 6 to 8 hours after 20 and 40 mg doses.[17, 27] During chronic treatment with standard b.i.d., t.i.d., and q.i.d. regimens, tolerance develops and it is not possible to provide continuous antianginal and antiischemic prophylaxis with any of the doses or dosing regimens.[17] Tolerance can be avoided with eccentric b.i.d. dosing (Fig. 95–1) given in the morning and 7 hours later.[14–16] This dosing strategy improves exercise duration for 12 to 14 hours.[15, 16] Eccentric b.i.d. treatment with a 5-mg dose is not effective, and partial tolerance development leads to a reduction in duration of effects with 10-mg eccentric b.i.d. dosing with Monoket.[16]

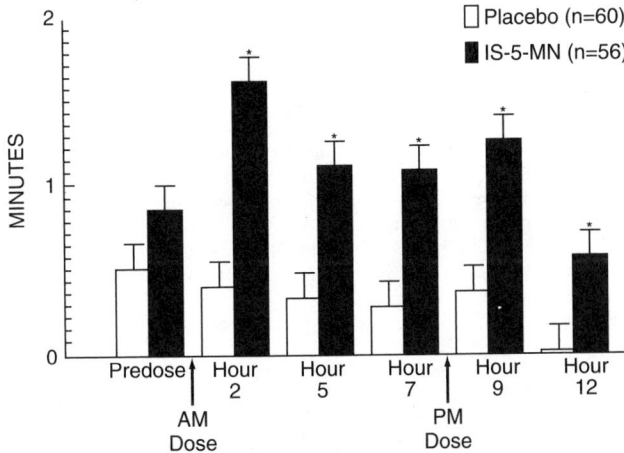

Figure 95–1. Change in exercise duration among patients receiving placebo and those receiving isosorbide-5-mononitrate therapy. Mean changes in total exercise duration from respective pretherapy baseline values after 0800-hour and 1500-hour doses of isosorbide-5-mononitrate (IS-5-MN) and placebo. Total exercise duration increased significantly ($p < .01$) with IS-5-MN compared with placebo at 2, 5, and 7 hours after the 0800-hour dose and at 2 and 5 hours after the 1500-hour dose (hours 9 and 12 after the 0800-hour dose). Exercise time before the 0800-hour dose did not change significantly. Mean values ± SE are shown by the vertical bars. *$p < .01$. (From Thadani U, Maranda C, Amsterdam E, et al: Lack of pharmacologic tolerance and rebound angina pectoris during twice daily therapy with isosorbide-5-mononitrate. Ann Intern Med 120:355, 1994.)

Eccentric b.i.d. treatment with a 20-mg dose avoids tolerance and is not associated with a rebound increase in nocturnal or early morning anginal attacks or a deterioration of exercise performance each morning before the administration of the morning dose compared with exercise performance before the initiation of treatment.[13, 15, 16]

PRECAUTIONS AND ADVERSE EFFECTS

Most adverse effects are dose related. Hypotension due to venodilation with reduced cardiac output may lead to dizziness.[40–42] Rarely bradycardia associated with hypotension may lead to syncope and collapse. This is usually reversed by placing the patient in the supine position or Trendelenburg's position. Nausea, vomiting, and urinary and fecal incontinence are uncommon.[40–42] Headaches are the most common adverse effect and have been reported in 32% to 38% of the patients in different studies.[15, 16] However, in the majority of patients, these are mild, and patients often get used to the headaches. In 2% to 3% of patients, headaches may be severe with or without associated nausea and necessitate withdrawal of treatment.[15] Apprehension, restlessness, weakness, vertigo, and dizziness may occur rarely. Tachycardia, palpitations, and orthostatic hypotension may also occur. Other adverse reactions reported in less than 1% of the patients are pruritus and rash, abdominal pain, diarrhea, dyspepsia, and vomiting; association with IS-5-MN is, however, uncertain.[41, 42]

ACUTE OVERDOSAGE

Overdose symptoms include hypotension; tachycardia; warm, flushed skin; headaches; palpitations; syncope; and increased intracranial pressure with confusion and neurologic deficits.[41, 42]

Gastric lavage should be performed or emesis induced followed by charcoal administration.[41–43] Hypotension is managed by elevating the legs and administering intravenous fluids. If necessary, an α-adrenergic agonist, e.g., methoxamine or phenylephrine, may be used.[41–43] Adrenaline and related β-agonists should be avoided.[41]

CONTRAINDICATIONS
Absolute

1. Allergic reactions to organic nitrates are extremely rare, but they do occur.[42, 43] IS-5-MN is contraindicated in patients who are allergic to it.
2. Obstructive hypertrophic cardiomyopathy: By reducing venous return, left ventricular outflow obstruction might increase.
3. Low cardiac output secondary to hypovolemia.
4. Inferior myocardial infarction with right ventricular involvement.
5. Raised intracranial pressure.
6. Cardiac tamponade.

7. Pregnant females: IS-5-MN should be avoided during pregnancy as there are no adequate data on the safety of IS-5-MN in humans during pregnancy.

Relative Contraindications

1. Arterial hypoxemia and cor pulmonale.
2. Mitral valve prolapse.
3. Glaucoma.

INTERFERENCE WITH OTHER DRUGS

IS-5-MN should be used with caution in combination with other antihypertensive drugs, phenothiazines, and tricyclic antidepressants.[41] Use with alcohol may produce severe hypotension and collapse.[41]

USE IN PATIENTS WITH IMPAIRED ORGAN FUNCTION

No dosage adjustment is necessary in patients with renal or hepatic impairment.[42, 43]

PLACE IN ANTIHYPERTENSIVE ARSENAL

IS-5-MN is not indicated for the treatment of hypertension.

DOSAGE AND ADMINISTRATION

The recommended regimen of ISMO tablets is 20 mg twice a day, with the two doses given 7 hours apart.[15, 42] For most patients, this can be achieved by taking the first dose on awakening and the second dose 7 hours later. Dosage adjustments are not necessary for elderly patients or patients with altered renal or hepatic function.[42]

The recommended dose for Monoket is 10 to 20 mg twice a day, with the two doses given 7 hours apart.[43] The 10-mg dose leads to development of tolerance and is less effective than the 20-mg dose.[16, 17]

COST

IS-5-MN is more expensive than generic ISDN, but in contrast with ISDN, which has variable inter- and intraindividual bioavailability after oral ingestion, IS-5-MN has predictable pharmacokinetics and dose adjustment is not necessary. This simplifies the clinical use of IS-5-MN.[44]

REFERENCES

1. Needleman P, Lang S, Johnson EM Jr: Organic nitrates: Relationship between biotransformation and rational angina pectoris therapy. J Pharmacol Exp Ther 181:485, 1972.
2. Abshagen U: Introductory remarks on the development of isosorbide-5-mononitrate. In Cohn JN, Rittinghausen R (eds): Mononitrates. Berlin: Springer-Verlag, 1985, pp 3–4.
3. Sisenwine SF, Ruelius HW: Plasma concentrations and urinary excretion of isosorbide dinitrate and its metabolites in the dog. J Pharmacol Exp Ther 176:296, 1971.
4. Down WH, Chasseaud LF, Grundy RK: Biotransformation of isosorbide dinitrate in humans. J Pharm Sci 63:1147, 1974.
5. Bogaert MG, Rosseel MT: Vascular effects of the dinitrate and mononitrate esters of isosorbide, isomannide and isoidide. Naunyn Schmiedebergs Arch Pharmacol 275:339, 1972.
6. Wendt RL: Systemic and coronary vascular effects of the 2- and the 5-mononitrate esters of isosorbide. J Pharmacol Exp Ther 180:732, 1992.
7. Stauch M, Grewe N, Nissen H: Die wirkung von 2- und 5-isosorbid mononitrat auf das belastungs—EKG von patienten mit koronariusuffizienz. Verh Dtsch Ges Kreislaufforsch 41:182, 1975.
8. Michel D: Der Einflub Von Metaboliten des isosorbiddinitrate anf das belastungs—EKG bei koronarinsuffizienz. Herz/Kreisl 8:444, 1976.
9. Abshagen U, Sporl-Radun S: First data on effects and pharmacokinetics of isosorbide-5-mononitrate in normal man. Eur J Clin Pharmacol 19:423, 1981.
10. Tauchert M, Jansen W, Osterspey A, et al: Dose dependence of tolerance during treatment with mononitrates. Z Kardiol 72(Suppl 3):218, 1983.
11. Rennhak U, Riebesel T, Biamino G: A double-blind cross-over study on the effectiveness and possible development of tolerance during long term therapy with isosorbide-5-mononitrate or isosorbide dinitrate slow release in coronary artery disease. In Cohn JN, Rittinghausen R (eds): Mononitrates. Berlin: Springer-Verlag, 1985, pp 147–153.
12. Thadani U, Bittar N: Effects of 8:00 am and 2:00 pm doses of isosorbide-5-mononitrate during twice daily therapy in stable angina pectoris. Am J Cardiol 70:286, 1992.
13. Thadani U, Friedman R, Jones JP, et al: Nitrate tolerance: Eccentric versus concentric twice daily therapy with isosorbide-5-mononitrate in angina pectoris [abstract]. Circulation II:216, 1989.
14. Thadani U, de Vane PJ: Efficacy of isosorbide mononitrate in angina pectoris. Am J Cardiol 70:67G, 1992.
15. Thadani U, Maranda C, Amsterdam E, et al: Lack of pharmacologic tolerance and rebound angina pectoris during twice daily therapy with isosorbide-5-mononitrate. Ann Intern Med 120:353, 1994.
16. Parker JO, and the Isosorbide-5-Mononitrate Study Group: Eccentric dosing with isosorbide-5-mononitrate in angina pectoris. Am J Cardiol 72:871, 1993.
17. Thadani U, Lipicky RJ: Short and long-acting oral nitrates for stable angina pectoris. Cardiovasc Drugs Ther 8:611, 1994.
18. Thadani U, Prasad R, Hamilton SF, et al: Usefulness of twice daily isosorbide-5-mononitrate in preventing development of tolerance in angina pectoris. Am J Cardiol 60:477, 1987.
19. Taylor T, Chasseaud LF, Major R, et al: Isosorbide-5-mononitrate pharmacokinetics in humans. Biopharm Drug Dispos 2:255, 1981.
20. Major RM, Taylor T, Chasseaud LF, et al: Isosorbide-5-mononitrate kinetics. Clin Pharmacol Ther 35:653, 1983.
21. Straehl P, Galeazzi RL, Soliva M: Isosorbide-5-mononitrate and isosorbide-2-mononitrate kinetics after intravenous and oral dosing. Clin Pharmacol Ther 36:485, 1984.
22. Mannebach H, Ohlmeier H, Möllendorff E, et al: Steady-state-Kinetic von Isosorbid-5-Mononitrat bei Patienten mit Koronarer herzkrankheit. Med Welt 32(14A):517, 1981.
23. Abshagen U: Pharmacokinetics of ISDN, sustained release ISDN, and IS-5-MN. In Cohn JN, Rittinghausen R (eds): Mononitrates. Berlin: Springer-Verlag 1985, pp 53–66.
24. Laufen H, Leitold M: The effect of food on the oral absorption of isosorbide-5-mononitrate. Br J Clin Pharmacol 18:967, 1984.
25. Akpan W, Endele R, Neugerauer G, et al: Pharmacokinetics of IS-5-MN after oral and intravenous administration in patients with hepatic failure. In Cohn JN, Rittinghausen R (eds): Mononitrates. Berlin: Springer-Verlag, 1985, pp 86–91.
26. Bogaert MG, Rosseel MT, Boelaert J, et al: Fate of isosorbide dinitrate and mononitrates in patients with renal failure. Eur J Clin Pharmacol 21:73, 1981.

27. Thadani U, Prasad R, Hamilton SF, et al: Isosorbide-5-mononitrates in angina pectoris: Plasma concentrations and duration of effects after acute therapy. Clin Pharmacol Ther 42:58, 1987.

28. Thadani U, Whitsett TL: Relationship of pharmacokinetic and pharmacodynamic properties of organic nitrates. Clin Pharmacokinet 15:32, 1988.

29. Strein K, Bossert F, Bartsh W, et al: Pharmacodynamics of organic nitrates—in vitro and in vivo studies. In Julian DG, Rittinghausen R, Uberbacher HJ (eds): Mononitrates II. Berlin: Springer-Verlag, 1987, pp 5–12.

30. Bassange E, Stewart DJ: Differential effects of isosorbide-5-mononitrates on epicardial coronary arteries and relevant hemodynamic parameters: Special aspects of nitrate action. In Julian DG, Rittinghausen R, Uberbacher HJ (eds): Mononitrates II. Berlin: Springer-Verlag, 1987, pp 13–19.

31. Gross GJ, Müller-Beckmann B: Effect of isosorbide-5-mononitrate on coronary collateral blood flow in dogs. In Julian DG, Rittinghausen R, Uberbacher HJ (eds): Mononitrates II. Berlin: Springer-Verlag, 1987, pp 20–27.

32. Hayes PC, Morrison L, Bouchier IAD: Effect of glyceryl trinitrate, isosorbide-5-mononitrate and propranolol on apparent liver blood flow. In Cohn JN, Rittinghausen R (eds): Mononitrates. Berlin: Springer-Verlag, 1985, pp 73–77.

33. Sponer G, Strein K: Development and disappearance of tolerance to organic nitrates in conscious dogs. In Cohn JN, Rittinghausen R (eds): Mononitrates. Berlin: Springer-Verlag, 1985, pp 101–106.

34. Ohlmeier H, Mertens HM, Mannebach H, et al: Tolerance and rebound phenomenon in nitrate therapy. In Cohn JN, Rittinghausen R (eds): Mononitrates. Berlin: Springer-Verlag, 1985, pp 107–123.

35. Jansen W, Tauchert M, Osterspey A, et al: Comparison of the hemodynamic effects of various doses of isosorbide-5-mononitrate following single-dose and long-term administration in patients with coronary heart disease. In Cohn JN, Rittinghausen R (eds): Mononitrates. Berlin: Springer-Verlag, 1985, pp 171–187.

36. Tronconi L, Raisaro A, Recusani F, et al: Efficacy of IS-5-MN (ISMO 20) in patients with coronary artery disease and impaired left ventricular function. In Cohn JN, Rittinghausen R (eds): Mononitrates. Berlin: Springer-Verlag, 1985, pp 306–310.

37. Shiavoni G, Marazzi M, Montenero AS, et al: Hemodynamic effects of IS-5-MN in patients with congestive heart failure. In Cohn JN, Rittinghausen R (eds): Mononitrates. Berlin: Springer-Verlag, 1985, pp 311–316.

38. Rubartelli P, Abbadessa F, Badano L, et al: Effects of isosorbide-5-mononitrates on hemodynamic parameters and left ventricular function in patients with coronary heart disease. In Julian DG, Rittinghausen R, Uberbacher HJ (eds): Mononitrates II. Berlin: Springer-Verlag, 1987, pp 129–132.

39. Lopez Sendon J, Mont JLI, Sanz I, et al: Hemodynamic effects of isosorbide-5-mononitrate in patients with heart failure following acute myocardial infarction. In Julian DG, Rittinghausen R, Uberbacher HJ (eds): Mononitrates II. Berlin: Springer-Verlag, 1987, pp 133–137.

40. Nyberg G: Current status of isosorbide-5-mononitrate. In Rezakovic DZE, Alpert JS (eds): Nitrate Therapy and Nitrate Tolerance: Current Concepts and Controversy. Basel: Karger, 1993, pp 358–396.

41. Thadani U, Whitsett TL: Isosorbide-5-mononitrate. In Dollery C (ed): Therapeutic Drugs. New York: Churchill Livingstone, 1991, pp I108–I111.

42. ISMO. In Physicians' Desk Reference. Montvale, NJ: Medical Economics Data Production, 1994, p 2548.

43. Monoket. In Physicians' Desk Reference. Montvale, NJ: Medical Economics Data Production, 1994, p 2183.

44. Larrat EP: Cost effectiveness study of nitrate therapy using a decision analysis methodology. Hosp Formul 29:277, 1994.

CHAPTER 96

Imdur

M. J. Kendall, M.D., F.R.C.P.

Imdur is a specific controlled-release formulation of isosorbide mononitrate developed to provide effective long-term nitrate therapy, which is potentially difficult because tolerance may develop rapidly to some nitrate regimens and renders them ineffective. The key aims of this chapter, therefore, are to review the problem of tolerance, demonstrate that tolerance does not develop when Imdur is taken once daily, and compare Imdur therapy with other methods used to provide long-term nitrate therapy. The development of an effective slow-release preparation has occurred in parallel with a marked increase in our understanding of the effects of nitrates, which in addition to their relatively well known hemodynamic effects also mimic the beneficial actions of endothelium-derived relaxing factor and have a positive impact on the underlying coronary artery disease.

PHARMACOKINETICS

The development of Imdur was based on the so-called Durules principle described by Sjogren.[1] The active substance, isosorbide-5-mononitrate (IS-5-MN), is contained in an inert matrix so that the drug close to the periphery is released relatively rapidly and that buried more deeply is released more slowly. The 60-mg tablet when given to 15 healthy male subjects as a single tablet or as two halves produces a plasma concentration curve as shown in Figure 96–1.[2] The plasma concentrations rise to 500 nmol/L in 30 minutes and reach a sustained peak approximately 4 hours after dosing of about 2000 to 3000 nmol/L. Toward the end of the 24-hour dosing interval, the plasma concentrations fall to subtherapeutic levels.

Several other studies[3–5] have confirmed the results shown in Figure 96–1, and the mean pharmacokinetic data from these studies are presented in Table 96–1. Plasma concentrations during long-term dosing are comparable to those after short-term dosing.[3] Furthermore, the pharmacokinetics of IS-5-MN are not influenced by the presence of heart failure[6] or renal[7] or hepatic insufficiency.[8] In addition, it has been shown that there is no interaction of Imdur with β-blockers, and the release of nitrate from the Imdur preparation is not affected by intestinal pH or the presence of food.[5]

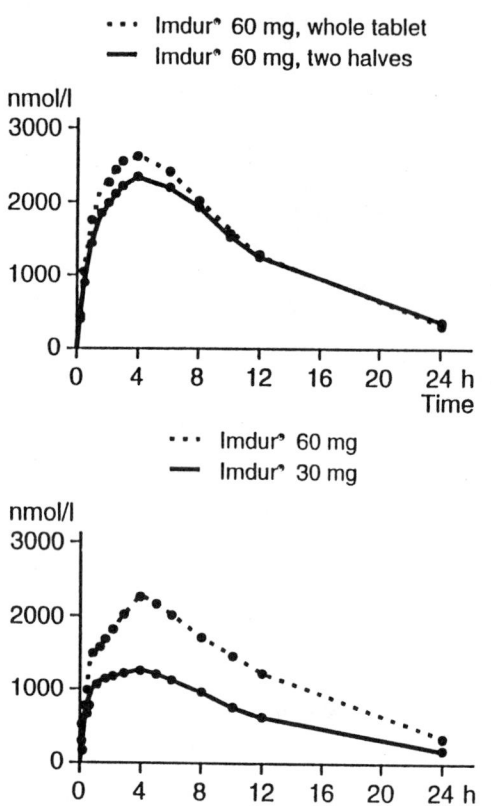

Figure 96–1. Plasma concentration time curves obtained after giving Imdur as one tablet or two halves[2] and as a whole and a half tablet.[3] (Adapted from Jonsson UE: Various administration forms of nitrate and their possibilities. Drugs 33[Suppl 4]:23, 1987; and Kendall MJ: Long-term therapeutic efficacy with once-daily isosorbide-5 mononitrate [Imdur]. J Clin Pharm Ther 15:169, 1990.)

CLINICAL USE
Indications

Long-acting nitrates may be used in the management of patients with angina pectoris, myocardial infarction, and heart failure. Of these, angina is the major indication.

Table 96–1. **Summary of Some Pharmacokinetic Variables from Different Single-dose Studies in Which Healthy Subjects Were Given Imdur 60 mg**

Pharmacokinetic Variable	Mean Value (± SE)		
	Study A (n = 15)	Study B (n = 8)	Study C (n = 8)
T_{max} (hr)	4.5 ± 0.3	3.6 ± 0.4	3.7 ± 0.2
C_{max} (nmol/L)	2430 ± 72	2218 ± 111	2258 ± 115
C_{12} (nmol/L)	1258 ± 56	1164 ± 88	1208 ± 76
C_{24} (nmol/L)	340 ± 23	289 ± 31	432 ± 32
AUC_{0-24} (nmol/L.hr)	31,337 ± 1065	28,039 ± 1482	29,844 ± 1867

Abbreviations: C_{max}, maximum plasma concentration; T_{max}, time to reach C_{max}; C_{12} and C_{24}, plasma concentrations at 12 and 24 hours, respectively; AUC_{0-24}, area under the plasma concentration time curve over 24 hours.

Adapted from Jonsson UE: Various administration forms of nitrate and their possibilities. Drugs 33(Suppl 4):23, 1987.

Angina Pectoris

Patients with angina are usually advised to take a sublingual glyceryl trinitrate (GTN) tablet to prevent an expected attack of pain or to abort an attack that has started. For the patient who suffers an anginal attack only infrequently, this may be all that is required. For those with more frequent episodes of angina, prophylactic therapy is needed, and long-acting nitrates, β-adrenoceptor blocking drugs (β-blockers), or calcium antagonists may be used. There is no agreement as to the order in which these drugs should be used, nor would it be easy to define three subgroups of angina sufferers for which each of the three prophylactic therapies might be considered most appropriate. Table 96–2 sets out some of the reasons for considering long-term nitrate therapy, in the form of Imdur, as a first choice.

The efficacy of nitrate therapy is not doubted, provided that steps are taken to prevent the development of tolerance. Long-term therapy with isosorbide dinitrate[9, 10] and nitrate patches[11, 12] has been shown to reduce pain and improve exercise tolerance. Isosorbide mononitrate (Imdur), given 60 or 120 mg once daily on rising in the morning, has also been shown to be effective.[13–15] A demonstration of the efficacy is shown in Figure 96–2.

Acute Myocardial Infarction

Because nitrates have been shown to reduce heart work and improve coronary blood flow, they might be expected to reduce pain, infarct size, and myocardial damage and thereby to improve the patient's prognosis. However, these theoretical gains have to be demonstrated, as there are theoretical risks and hazards resulting from hypotension and compensatory tachycardia.

In early studies on patients having an acute myocardial infarction (MI), nitrate infusions were shown to improve cardiac function by reducing both preload

Table 96–2. **Advantages of Imdur for Long-term Therapy of Angina**

1. It is effective.
2. It addresses both sides of the coronary blood flow:heart work imbalance, which causes angina by improving coronary blood flow and reducing heart work by decreasing venous return and thereby reducing cardiac output.
3. The regimen is simple—one tablet daily.
4. Tolerance does not develop.
5. Rebound angina is not a problem.
6. The efficacy of acute nitrate therapy has usually been demonstrated to both doctor and patient.
7. There are no contraindications. Nitrates are not contraindicated in patients with liver disease, renal impairment, or any other medical condition.
8. Nitrates do not cause any organ damage, and, in particular, they have **no** negative inotropic effects.
9. There are no adverse metabolic effects, i.e., cholesterol, glucose, and other biochemical parameters are not altered.
10. There are no long-term adverse effects.

Relevant references for all of the above are given in the text.

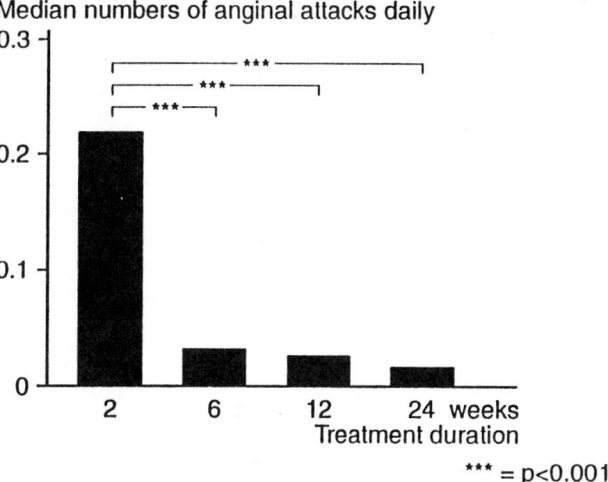

Median numbers of anginal attacks daily

*** = p<0.001

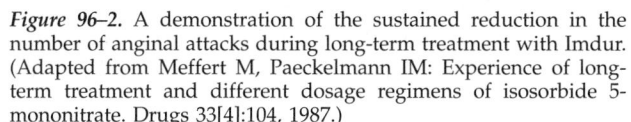

Figure 96–2. A demonstration of the sustained reduction in the number of anginal attacks during long-term treatment with Imdur. (Adapted from Meffert M, Paeckelmann IM: Experience of long-term treatment and different dosage regimens of isosorbide 5-mononitrate. Drugs 33[4]:104, 1987.)

and afterload.[16–18] The benefit was most obvious in those with some left ventricular dysfunction. Further, in addition to the peripheral effects, nitrate therapy reduced ischemic damage as shown by continuous ST-segment mapping.[19] In a subsequent randomized prospective trial, 104 patients with an acute MI were given intravenous nitroglycerin over 48 hours followed by nitrate ointment for 72 hours or placebo.[19] Patients treated within 10 hours of the onset of symptoms had a lower 3-month mortality (14%) than the late treatment and placebo-treated groups (mortality, 21% to 28%). This difference was not statistically significant, perhaps because of the small numbers studied. The results of four other studies[16, 20] confirmed the potential of nitrates to reduce myocardial damage if given at the time of infarction. In 1988, a meta-analysis of the trials of intravenous nitrate use in acute myocardial infarction was published in the *Lancet*.[21] It was based on 2000 patients included in 10 trials. The authors reported "These trials did demonstrate fairly consistent reductions in cardiac enzyme release with treatment, suggesting infarct size limitation. The mortality results, on the other hand, were not so clear-cut." Thus, it appeared that nitrates had a demonstrable beneficial effect on cardiac function and infarct size, although there was doubt as to whether nitrates would reduce mortality. Imdur was therefore included in ISIS 4, a study of three different treatments in 58,000 patients suffering an acute myocardial infarction.[22] This study showed that Imdur was safe and well tolerated, but its impact on mortality, 2 to 3 lives saved per 1000 patients treated, was not statistically significant.

In conclusion, there is good evidence that nitrates given early to a patient having a myocardial infarction decrease infarct size, reduce left ventricular dysfunction, and help prevent the subsequent development of left ventricular failure. The excellent review by Jugdutt[20] summarizes the extensive literature on this subject. The fact that the hemodynamically protective effects of nitrates do not produce a reduction in the early mortality from myocardial infarction should not preclude drugs like Imdur from having an important role in the management of the infarct patient. They may reduce left ventricular enlargement, cardiac failure, and late mortality.

Heart Failure

Nitrates may have a prophylactic role and a therapeutic role in the management of heart failure. Because most patients who have congestive cardiac failure have underlying ischemic heart disease, it follows that any measure that reduces ischemic damage may be expected to reduce the severity of any subsequent heart failure. Nitrates are known to be effective in angina, reducing the severity of an attack, and they may also reduce the frequency of clinically relevant but silent ST-segment changes.[23, 24] These effects may reduce ischemic damage in angina sufferers. In those having an infarct, there are a number of studies referred to previously that show that nitrate therapy reduces ischemic damage[16, 19, 20] and the subsequent damaging remodeling[17, 18, 20] that occurs after infarction. These later observations may be seen as analogous to the effects produced by an angiotensin-converting enzyme (ACE) inhibitor,[25] which have subsequently been shown to translate into reduced morbidity from heart failure after infarction.[26]

The improvement in the symptoms of paroxysmal nocturnal dyspnea in response to sublingual GTN was first reported by Johnson et al. in 1957.[27] Later, Cohn explored in detail the hemodynamic benefits of nitrate therapy in patients with left ventricular failure.[28] When it became clear that IS-5-MN was the most active metabolite, it was logical to assess its effect in patients with cardiac failure. Therefore, Murray and Gammage[29] gave this drug to 11 patients with acute left ventricular failure after a myocardial infarct. Pulmonary wedge pressure was reduced, cardiac output increased, and most, although not all, patients improved clinically. Data on the role of nitrates in the management of chronic cardiac failure are more limited. There are studies, such as that by Stephens et al.,[30] that have shown that IS-5-MN may help patients with "chronic left ventricular failure due to

Table 96–3. **Long-term Treatment Study, Adverse Reactions**

Treatment length (weeks)	2	6	12	24
Total number of patients	105	104	103	103
Number reporting symptoms	28	6	5	5
Number reporting headache	21*	3*	4	3

Number of patients reporting adverse effects during long-term treatment with IS-5-MN.

*$p<.001$

Adapted from Meffert M, Paeckelmann I-M: Experience of long-term treatment and different dosage regimens of isosorbide 5-mononitrate. Drugs 33(4):104, 1987.

ischemic heart disease or cardiomyopathy." In this study,[30] left and right ventricular filling pressures were reduced, and the hemodynamic benefits and improved exercise tolerance were still demonstrable after several weeks of treatment. Further studies on the role of Imdur in patients with chronic heart failure are needed.

Precautions, Adverse Effects, and Drug Interactions

The two problems associated with the use of nitrates are headaches and the development of tolerance. By comparison, other unwanted effects are infrequent and minor.

Because nitrates dilate both veins and arteries, they would be expected to cause headaches and hypotension. The latter may occur as mild dizziness or faintness that is rarely severe enough to require the patient to sit or lie down. Headache, on the other hand, is common (15% to 25%) and may be severe enough to prevent the patient's being able to tolerate the drug. Some patients are particularly sensitive to vasodilators, and this will usually have become apparent if they have ever taken sublingual GTN. A strategy for dealing with this adverse effect is therefore needed. The patient needs to be warned, should be started on a low dose, take analgesics as necessary, and be advised that the symptom usually persists for only 1 to 2 weeks. Several studies have confirmed that the number of patients with headache decreases rapidly with time (Tables 96–3 and 96–4).

Drug interactions are uncommon and rarely clinically relevant. Drugs that cause hypocalcemia, hypo-

Table 96–4. **Imdur Adverse Reactions**

Symptoms	Number of Patients	
	1st week	2nd week
• mild headache	5	3
• moderate headache	2	0
Total	7	3

Number of patients reporting headache in the first and second weeks of treatment with Imdur.

Adapted from Meffert M, Paeckelmann I-M: Experience of long-term treatment and different dosage regimens of isosorbide 5-mononitrate. Drugs 33(4):104, 1987.

tension, or brachycardia may make the patient more prone to suffer from lightheadedness and other symptoms associated with hypotension.

Special Patient Groups

Unlike with most other drugs, it is rarely necessary to be concerned about the patient's age, sex, coexisting disorders, or concomitant drug therapy when prescribing nitrates. In relation to the specific preparation, Imdur, adverse effects are uncommon. Headaches do occur, but because the rate of change in plasma concentrations and therefore vasodilatation occurs more slowly, headaches tend to be less frequent and less severe. If headache is a problem, the tablets can be halved without the loss of controlled-release properties. Other symptoms are infrequent (see Table 96–3).

In the recently completed ISIS-4 study,[22] approximately half the 58,000 patients took Imdur once daily. The drop-out rate was very low, and preliminary reports (American Heart Association, 1993) indicated that headache occurred in approximately 2.3% taking nitrates compared with 0.5% receiving placebo, whereas symptoms associated with hypotension (0.5% on Imdur and 0.4% on placebo) were less common. Other symptoms were not significantly more common in those taking Imdur, and very few patients withdrew because of the adverse effects of therapy. In this large study, Imdur was well tolerated.

Nitrates (Imdur) in Management

Angina

Long-acting nitrates are one of the options available to treat angina in patients whose disease is not adequately controlled with relatively infrequent doses of sublingual GTN. In this situation, there is no agreed strategy. However, the following might be suggested:

1. If the patient responds well to sublingual GTN but needs to use it two to three times per day, better control might be achieved by taking long-acting nitrates in addition.
2. If the patient had several attacks per day, then a β-blocker could be offered unless contraindicated or a calcium antagonist or a long-acting nitrate such as Imdur. The reasons for choosing Imdur in this situation are set out in Table 96–2.

Acute Myocardial Infarction

This is now a complex situation in which a number of different therapies, particularly thrombolysis and aspirin, are clearly indicated. In some instances, intravenous nitrates are used, particularly if the patient goes into heart failure. In the ISIS-4 trial,[22] Imdur had no impact on mortality, although it was found to be safe and well tolerated. Because nitrates are known to have a beneficial effect on hemodynamic measurements and to have the potential to reduce infarct size, it would seem sensible to administer nitrates to try to reduce the risk that the patient will go on to develop left ventricular failure at a later date. As Jugdutt[20] has suggested that it is desirable to give a low-dose regimen intravenously at the earliest opportunity, it may be reasonable to suggest that oral Imdur given when the patient is first seen may achieve the same beneficial effect. The ISIS 4 study confirmed that Imdur did not cause serious unwanted effects and could therefore be taken by patients well before they reach the protective environment of the hospital or its special care unit.

Heart Failure

The potential benefits of nitrate therapy in the management of acute cardiac failure are becoming well accepted. The role of oral therapy (in the form of Imdur, for example) in the treatment of chronic cardiac failure is less clear. On the basis of our knowledge of its hemodynamic actions, its use would seem logical. The trials that have been done show that nitrates are effective, but further studies are needed to establish the role of oral IS-5-MN in the management of chronic heart failure.

WHICH LONG-ACTING NITRATE REGIMEN?

The three main alternatives are the nitrate patch, eccentric dosing with either isosorbide mononitrate (ISMN) or isosorbide dinitrate (ISDN), or IS-5-MN in a controlled-release form (Imdur) orally once daily.

If the patch is removed after 12 to 14 hours and left off for 10 to 12 hours, tolerance is not likely to develop.[11, 12, 31] The disadvantages of this regimen are that the patient must remember to remove the patch and, once it is removed, the plasma nitrate concentrations fall fairly rapidly and protection is lost. In some instances,[12, 31] a rebound effect has occurred, and the patient has been at increased risk of having attacks of angina at night.

Asymmetric dosing (i.e., 8 AM and 3 PM) with ISDN or ISMN provides effective symptom control by day, and tolerance should not develop.

Unfortunately, if the doses are too close together, the patient spends most of the 24 hours on no therapy, and if they are spaced too widely, tolerance may develop. Furthermore, it is very difficult for the patient to remember to take the second tablet at the correct time unless it is at a convenient time (evening meal or bed time) or unless symptoms recur.[32, 33]

Imdur taken once daily is a simple alternative and encourages good compliance. It is effective approximately 30 minutes after ingestion and provides adequate plasma concentrations during the day, when the patient is active and at risk of suffering from angina. Thereafter, the concentrations fall slowly. A number of studies[13, 15] have confirmed that tolerance does not develop, efficacy is maintained, and rebound angina does not occur.[32]

REFERENCES

1. Sjogren J: Studies on a sustained release principle based on an inert plastic matrix. Acta Pharm Suec 1971, 8:153.
2. Jonsson UE: Various administration forms of nitrate and their possibilities. Drugs 33(Suppl 4):23, 1987.
3. Kendall MJ: Long-term therapeutic efficacy with once-daily isosorbide-5-mononitrate (Imdur). J Clin Pharm Ther 15:169, 1990.
4. Uusitalo A: Anti-anginal efficacy of a controlled-release formulation of isosorbide-5-mononitrate once daily in angina patients on chronic β-blockade. Acta Med Scand 223:219, 1988.
5. Jonsson UE: Development of long acting delivery systems. Eur J Clin Pharmacol 38(Suppl 1):S15, 1990.
6. Mannebach H, Ohlmeier H, Mollendorff EV, et al: Steady-state-kinetik von Isosorbid-5-Mononitrat bei Patienten mit koronarer Herzkrankheit. Med Welt 32:517, 1981.
7. Evers J, Krakamp B, Klimkait W, et al: Pharmacokinetics of isosorbide-5-nitrate in renal failure. Eur J Clin Pharmacol 30:349, 1986.
8. Akpan W, Endele R, Neugebauer G, et al: Pharmacokinetics of IS-5-MN after oral and intravenous administration and patients with hepatic failure. In Cohn JN, Rittinghausen R (eds): Mononitrates. Berlin: Springer-Verlag, 1985, pp 86–91.
9. Thadani U, Fung H-L, Darke AC, et al: Oral isosorbide dinitrate in angina pectoris: Comparison of duration of action and dose-response relation during acute and sustained therapy. Am J Cardiol 49:411, 1982.
10. Muller G, Hacker W, Schneider G: Intraindividual comparison of the action of equal doses of isosorbide-5-endomononitrate, slow release isosorbide dinitrate and placebo in patients with coronary heart disease. Klin Wochenschr 61:409, 1983.
11. Steering Committee, Transdermal Nitroglycerin Cooperative Study: Acute and Chronic antianginal efficacy of continuous twenty-four hour application of transdermal nitroglycerin. Am J Cardiol 1263, 1991.
12. Demots H, Glasser HP: Intermittent transdermal nitroglycerin therapy in the treatment of chronic stable angina. J Am Coll Cardiol 13:786, 1989.
13. Nyberg P, Carlens P, Lindstrom E, et al: The effect of isosorbide-5-mononitrate (5-ISMN) Durules on exercise tolerance in patients with exertional angina pectoris. A placebo controlled study. Eur Heart J 7:835, 1986.
14. Wisenberg G, Roks C, Nichol P, et al: Sustained effect of and lack of development of tolerance to controlled-release isosorbide-5-mononitrate in chronic stable angina pectoris. Am J Cardiol 15:569, 1989.
15. Meffert M, Paeckelmann I-M: Experience of long-term treatment and different dosage regimens of isosorbide 5-mononitrate. Drugs 33(4):104, 1987.
16. Flaherty JT: Role of nitrates in acute myocardial infarction. Am J Cardiol 70:73B, 1992.
17. Judgutt BI: Delayed effects of early infarct limiting therapies on healing after myocardial infarction. Circulation 72:907, 1985.
18. Judgutt BI: Effect of nitroglycerin and ibuprofen on left ventricular topography and rupture threshold during healing after myocardial infarction in the dog. Can J Physiol Pharmacol 66:385, 1988.
19. Flaherty JT, Come PC, Baird MG, et al: Effects of intravenous nitroglycerin on left ventricular function and ST segment changes in acute myocardial infarction. Br Heart J 38:612, 1976.
20. Judgutt BI: Effects of nitrate therapy on ventricular remodelling and function. Am J Cardiol 72:161 G, 1993.
21. Yusuf S, Collins R, Mac Mahon S, et al: Effect of intravenous nitrates on mortality in acute myocardial infarction: An overview of the randomized trials. Lancet 1:1088, 1988.
22. ISIS-4 Collaborative Group: ISIS-4: A randomised factorial trial assessing early oral captopril, oral mononitrate and intravenous magnesium sulphate in 58,050 patients with suspected acute myocardial infarction. Lancet 345:669, 1995.
23. Schang SJ, Pepine CJ: Transient asymptomatic ST segment depression during daily activity. Am J Cardiol 39:396, 1977.
24. Shell WE: Mechanisms and therapy of silent myocardial is-

chaemia and the effects of transdermal nitroglycerin. Am J Cardiol 56:231, 1985.

25. Pfeffer MA, Lamas GA, Vaughan DE, et al: Effect of captopril on progressive ventricular dilatation after anterior myocardial infarction. N Engl J Med 319:80, 1988.

26. Pfeffer MA, Braunwald E, Moye LA, et al: Effect of captopril on mortality and morbidity in patients with left ventricular dysfunction after myocardial infarction. Results of the Survival and Left Ventricular Enlargement Trial (SAVE). N Engl J Med 327:669, 1992.

27. Johnson JB, Fairley A, Carter C: Effects of sublingual nitroglycerin on pulmonary artery pressure in patients with failure of the left ventricle. N Engl J Med 257:1114, 1957.

28. Cohn J: Nitrates for congestive heart failure. Am J Cardiol 56:19A, 1985.

29. Murray RG, Gammage MD: Isosorbide-5-mononitrate in the treatment of left ventricular failure following acute myocardial infarction. Cardiology 74(Suppl 1):58, 1987.

30. Stephens JD, Marks C, Woodings D, Vandenburg NJ: Acute and chronic use of isosorbide-5-mononitrate in patients with heart failure. Cardiology 74(Suppl 1):69, 1987.

31. Ferratini M, Pirelli S, Merlini P, et al: Intermittent transdermal nitroglycerin monotherapy in stable exercise induced angina: A comparison with a continuous schedule. Eur Heart J 10:998, 1989.

32. Olsson G, Allgen J, Amtorp O, et al: Absence of pre-dose rebound phenomena with once daily 5-ISMN in a controlled-release formulation. Eur Heart J 13:814, 1992.

33. Lofdahl P: Compliance as a factor in the development of nitrate tolerance: A patient investigation. J Int Med Res 21:51, 1993.

XI.

Calcium Antagonists

Editors: Robert Roberts and Alberto Zanchetti

A. Principles and Practice of Calcium Antagonism

CHAPTER 97

Cardiovascular Uses of Calcium Antagonists*

William H. Frishman, M.D., and Edmund H. Sonnenblick, M.D.

The calcium antagonists are available in the United States for the treatment of patients with angina pectoris (diltiazem, nifedipine, amlodipine, nicardipine, verapamil, bepridil), for long-term treatment of systemic hypertension (verapamil, isradipine, diltiazem, amlodipine, nicardipine, felodipine), for the management of hypertensive emergencies and perioperative hypertension (intravenous nicardipine), for treatment and prophylaxis of supraventricular arrhythmias (diltiazem, verapamil), and for reducing morbidity and mortality in patients with subarachnoid hemorrhage (nimodipine). These drugs are also being evaluated for a multitude of other cardiovascular (Table 97–1) and noncardiovascular conditions. New agents (mibefradil, nisoldipine) and extended-release formulations (controlled-onset extended-release verapamil, coatcore nisoldipine) are also under investigation and about to be approved for clinical use.

ANGINA PECTORIS

The antianginal mechanisms of calcium antagonists are complex (Table 97–2).[1-7] The drugs exert vasodilator effects on the coronary and peripheral vessels and they have depressant effects on cardiac contractility and conduction, which are actions that may be important in mediating the antianginal effects of the drugs.[2-7] The drugs are only mild dilators of epicardial vessels not in spasm, but they markedly attenuate sympathetically mediated and ergonovine-induced coronary vasoconstriction; these actions provide a rational basis for the effectiveness of the drugs in vasospastic ischemic syndromes.[2, 3, 6] In patients with exertional angina pectoris, the peripheral vasodilator actions of diltiazem and verapamil and the inhibitory effects on the sinus node serve to atten-

uate the increases in double product (heart rate × systolic blood pressure) that normally accompany, and serve to limit, exercise.[3, 5]

Stable Angina Pectoris

Multiple double-blind, placebo-controlled studies have clearly confirmed the efficacy of diltiazem,[7-11] nifedipine,[12, 13] amlodipine, nicardipine, verapamil,[14-19] and bepridil[20, 21] in the management of stable angina pectoris, with patients showing a reduction in chest pain attacks and nitroglycerin consumption and improved exercise tolerance. Calcium antagonists for the most part appear to be as safe and effective as β-blockers and nitrates when used as monotherapy.[22-29] They can

Table 97–1. Cardiovascular Uses of Calcium Antagonists

Angina pectoris*
  Effort angina
  Rest angina
  Prinzmetal's variant
Arrhythmia treatment and prophylaxis* (acute and chronic): verapamil
Systemic hypertension*
Hypertensive emergencies*
Hypertrophic cardiomyopathy: verapamil
Congestive heart failure: nifedipine
Myocardial infarction(containing size of infarct)
Myocardial infarction (preventing Q-wave infarcts in non-Q-wave infarctions): diltiazem
Primary pulmonary hypertension: nifedipine
Peripheral vascular disease
  Raynaud's phenomenon
  Intermittent claudication
Cerebral arterial spasm† (subarachnoid hemorrhage): nimodipine
Stroke: nimodipine
Mesenteric insufficiency
Migraine headache prophylaxis: nimodipine
Deacceleration of atherosclerosis
Prevention of cardiomyopathy

*Use approved by the U.S. Food and Drug Administration.

Adapted in part with permission from Frishman WH, Sonnenblick EH: The calcium channel blockers. In Schlant RC, Alexander RW (eds): Hurst's The Heart, 8th ed. New York: McGraw Hill, 1994.

Table 97–2. **Hemodynamic Effects of the Calcium Antagonists on Myocardial Oxygen Supply and Demand**

	Verapamil	Nifedipine	Diltiazem	Nicardipine	Bepridil
Demand					
Wall tension	↑ ↔	↔ (Reflex)	↔	↔ (Reflex)	
Systolic blood pressure	↓	↓	↓	↓	↔
Ventricular volume	↑	↔	↔	↔	↑
Heart rate	↓*	↑ (Reflex)	↓ ↔	↑ (Reflex)	↓
Contractility	↓↓	↓	↓	↔ ↓	↔
Supply					
Coronary blood flow	↑	↑↑	↑	↑↑	↑
Coronary vascular resistance	↓	↓↓	↓	↓↓	↓
Spasm	↓	↓	↓	↓	↓
Diastolic perfusion time	↑	↓	↑ ↔	↓	↑
Collateral blood flow	↔	↑	↑	↑	↑

↑, Increase; ↓, decrease; ↔, no apparent effect.
*Heart rate may increase acutely but decreases with chronic use.

also be used as single-dose therapies in hypertensive patients with angina.[29, 30]

When choosing between a calcium antagonist and a β-adrenergic blocking drug in the management of patients with effort-related symptoms, it is apparent that some patients do better with one drug than with the other. Unfortunately, other than initiating a therapeutic trial, little can be done to predict with confidence which agent will perform better in the management of a specific patient. However, both verapamil and diltiazem can be used as effective alternatives in patients who remain symptomatic despite therapy with β-blockers and as first-time antianginal drugs in patients with contraindications to β-blockade; the use of nifedipine as a first-line drug in its original formulations was limited by the reflex tachycardia and potential aggravation of angina that accompanied its use.[8, 28, 31] However, this is probably not a problem with the sustained-delivery nifedipine (GITS) formulation.[32] Diltiazem is also approved as a once-daily treatment for angina pectoris in a sustained-delivery formulation.

Bepridil is available in doses of 200 to 400 mg once daily for use in patients with angina pectoris whose disease is refractory to other antianginal drug therapy.[21] Close monitoring of patients with this drug is necessary at the onset of therapy because a small percentage of patients can have a prolongation of the QT interval on electrocardiographic evaluation. Bepridil can be combined with a β-blocker if necessary.[33]

The effects of abrupt withdrawal of verapamil and propranolol in patients with angina pectoris have been compared.[34] Ten percent of patients with stable effort-related symptoms experienced a severe clinical exacerbation of the anginal syndrome upon withdrawal of propranolol; no patient experienced rebound symptoms when verapamil was abruptly discontinued.[34] There also appear to be no major withdrawal reactions with nifedipine and diltiazem.[8]

Angina at Rest

Angina at rest comprises a wide spectrum of disorders, ranging from variant angina (ST elevation) associated with angiographically normal coronary arteries to unstable angina with ST depression or elevation associated with multivessel coronary artery disease.[5, 7, 30] It has been suggested that coronary vasospasm or thrombosis plays a major role in the pathogenesis of ischemia in most patients with angina at rest, regardless of the coronary anatomy.[3] In clinical trials, calcium antagonists were effective in the treatment of this syndrome because of their ability to block spontaneous and drug-induced spasm.[35–42]

The comparative efficacy of verapamil and propranolol was assessed in a randomized, blinded crossover trial in patients with rest angina. Only verapamil reduced symptomatic and asymptomatic episodes of ischemia. These findings are consistent with the concept that coronary vasospasm plays a crucial role in patients with angina at rest; in contrast, rather than providing any benefit, propranolol may exacerbate vasospastic phenomena.[43]

Another study assessed the comparative efficacy of verapamil and nifedipine. Both verapamil and nifedipine proved equally effective, and neither drug depressed ventricular function in the subjects while they were at rest or exercising.[44] Accordingly, in the management of patients with variant angina, the choice of a calcium antagonist is likely to be determined not so much by which drug is more effective but by patient tolerance.

The usefulness of calcium antagonists in the long-term management of unstable angina was demonstrated in a double-blind randomized clinical trial showing that the administration of nifedipine to patients receiving nitrates and propranolol reduced the number of patients with unstable anginal syndromes who required surgery for relief of pain. The incidence of sudden death and myocardial infarction was similar in the two groups.[45] However, clinical benefits were largely confined to patients whose pain was accompanied by ST-segment elevation.

Combination Therapy

Therapy combining calcium antagonists with nitrates, β-blockers, or both may be more efficacious for the

Table 97–3. **Hemodynamic Effects of Calcium Antagonists, β-Blockers, and Combination Treatment**

	Calcium Antagonists	β-Blockers	Combination
Heart rate	↓ ↔ ↑ (Reflex)	↓	↓ ↔
Contractility	↓ ↔ (Reflex)	↓	↓ ↔
Wall tension	↓	↔	↓
Systolic blood pressure	↓	↓	↓
Left ventricular volume	↓ ↔	↑	↑ ↔
Coronary resistance	↓	↑ ↔	↓ ↔

↑, Increase; ↓, decrease; ↔, no apparent effect.
From Frishman WH: Beta-adrenergic blockade in the treatment of coronary artery disease. *In* Hurst JW (ed): Clinical Essays on the Heart, Vol 2. New York: McGraw-Hill, 1984, p. 48.

treatment of angina pectoris than one drug used alone.[5, 7, 24, 33, 46, 47] The hemodynamic effects of a calcium antagonist–β-blocker combination are shown in Table 97–3.[24] Because adverse effects can occur from this combination (heart block, severe bradycardia, congestive heart failure), patients should be carefully selected and observed.[48, 49] The hemodynamic effects of combined nitrate–calcium antagonist therapy are shown in Table 97–4. Hypotension should be avoided. Different calcium antagonists may also be combined (nifedipine with verapamil or diltiazem) with added benefit; however, side effects may be prohibitive compared with those seen in monotherapy.[8]

ARRHYTHMIAS
Atrial Fibrillation

Except in rare situations, verapamil is ineffective in converting acute and chronic atrial fibrillation to normal sinus rhythm (Table 97–5).[50] However, verapamil (oral and intravenous) is effective for decreasing and controlling ventricular rate during atrial fibrillation by prolonging atrioventricular (AV) nodal conduction and refractoriness and thereby increasing AV block.[50] Clinical trials with verapamil in patients with atrial

Table 97–4. **Hemodynamic Rationale for Combining Nitrates and Calcium Antagonists in Angina Pectoris**

	Nitrates	Calcium Antagonists	Combination
Heart rate	↑ (Reflex)	±	↑ (Reflex)
Blood pressure	↓	↓	↓ ↓
Heart size	↓ 0	± ↑	0
Contractility	↑ (Reflex)	↓	0
Venomotor tone	↓	0	↓
Peripheral resistance	↓	↓	↓ ↓ ?
Coronary resistance	↓	↓	↓ ↓ ?
Coronary blood flow	↑	↑	↑ ↑ ?
Collateral blood flow	↑	↑	↑ ↑ ?

↑, Increase; ↓, decrease; ↓ ↓, questionable additive effects; ±, inconsistent change; 0, no change.
From Frishman WH: Beta-adrenergic blockade in the treatment of coronary artery disease. *In* Hurst JW (ed): Clinical Essays on the Heart, Vol 2. New York: McGraw-Hill, 1984, p 48.

Table 97–5. **Effects of Verapamil in Treatment of Common Arrhythmias**

Effective
Supraventricular tachycardia
  AV nodal reentrant PSVT
  Accessory pathway reentrant PSVT
  SA nodal reentrant PSVT
  Atrial reentrant PSVT
Atrial flutter (ventricular rate decreased but arrhythmia will convert only occasionally)
Atrial fibrillation (ventricular rate decreases but arrhythmia will convert only occasionally)

Ineffective
Sinus tachycardia
Nonparoxysmal automatic atrial tachycardia
Atrial fibrillation and flutter in WPW syndrome (ventricular rate may not decrease)
Ventricular tachyarrhythmias*

AV, atrioventricular; PSVT, paroxysmal supraventricular tachycardia; SA, sinoatrial; WPW, Wolff-Parkinson-White.
*Only limited experience in this area.
From Frishman WH, LeJemtel T: Electropharmacology of calcium channel antagonists in cardiac arrhythmias. PACE 5:407, 1982. With permission of Futura Publishing Co.

fibrillation have shown that its ability to decrease ventricular rate appears to be unrelated to the chronicity of the arrhythmia, its cause, or the patient's age.[51–54] Verapamil appears to be more effective than digoxin in slowing the rapid ventricular rate in response to physical activity.[55] The drug can be used orally in combination with digoxin in treating acute and chronic atrial fibrillation and flutter.[50] Studies with intravenous diltiazem have shown it to be an effective agent for reducing rapid ventricular rates in patients with atrial fibrillation,[56] and the drug is now available for this indication in parenteral form for bolus or continuous infusion therapy.

Paroxysmal Supraventricular Tachycardia

Virtually all cases of supraventricular tachycardia resulting from intranodal reentry and those related to the circus-movement type of tachycardia in preexcitation respond promptly and predictably to intravenous verapamil or diltiazem, whereas only approximately two thirds of ectopic atrial tachycardias convert to sinus rhythm after adequate doses of the drug.[50, 56–58] Intravenous verapamil and diltiazem are highly efficacious in treating reentry paroxysmal supraventricular tachycardia regardless of cause or patient age.[50, 58]

The recommended dose range of verapamil for terminating paroxysmal supraventricular tachycardia in adults is 0.075 to 0.15 mg/kg infused over 1 to 3 minutes, repeated at 30 minutes.[55] In patients with myocardial dysfunction, the dose should be reduced. Children have been safely treated with a regimen of 0.075 to 0.15 mg/kg.[50] The recommended dose of diltiazem is 0.25 mg/kg infused over 2 minutes, repeated at 0.35 mg/kg after 15 minutes.[56]

There have been few clinical studies comparing intravenous verapamil and diltiazem with other standard regimens in the treatment of paroxysmal supraventricular tachycardia.[59] However, in a number of clinical situations verapamil and diltiazem may offer an advantage over either digitalis preparations or β-adrenergic blockers. For instance, in cases where there is an urgent need to terminate paroxysmal supraventricular tachycardia, verapamil would be preferable because it can produce therapeutic responses within 3 minutes of infusion, whereas the effects of digoxin are not evident for approximately 30 minutes.[50] Also, should drug therapy fail to produce normal sinus rhythm, the short durations of action of verapamil and diltiazem permit earlier cardioversion without some of the dangers that accompany electric cardioversion during digoxin therapy. Verapamil and diltiazem also offer distinct advantages over β-adrenergic blocking drugs in patients whose arrhythmias are associated with chronic obstructive lung disease or peripheral vascular disease.[50]

Oral verapamil has been approved for prophylaxis against paroxysmal supraventricular tachycardia in doses of 160 to 480 mg/day with favorable results.[60, 61] Diltiazem is not yet approved for use in oral form as an antiarrhythmic agent.

Atrial Flutter

In most patients, the immediate effect of intravenous verapamil and diltiazem in atrial flutter is an increase in AV block that slows the ventricular response; this is rarely followed by a return to sinus rhythm.[50, 54] In some, the response occurs through the development of atrial fibrillation with a controlled ventricular response.[50] A single intravenous dose of verapamil or diltiazem has been found to be of diagnostic value in differentiating rapid atrial flutter from paroxysmal supraventricular tachycardia when these two arrhythmias are indistinguishable on the electrocardiogram. In atrial flutter, AV block increases immediately, revealing the true nature of the arrhythmia.[52] Oral verapamil has also been used to convert paroxysmal atrial flutter and reduce the rapid ventricular rates associated with this arrhythmia.[61]

Preexcitation

Verapamil and diltiazem have been found to induce reversion of most cases of accessory pathway supraventricular tachycardia.[57] Using intracardiac recordings of electric activity during programmed electric stimulation of the heart, data have become available regarding the actions of verapamil on the electrophysiologic properties of the accessory pathway in overt cases of the Wolff-Parkinson-White (WPW) syndrome.[62, 63] The drug has a minimal effect on the antegrade and retrograde conduction times and on the refractory period.[50, 64, 65] Verapamil and diltiazem therefore terminate accessory pathway paroxysmal supraventricular tachycardia in the same manner as they do AV nodal reentrant paroxysmal supraventricular tachycardia; that is, by slowing AV nodal conduction and increasing refractoriness. Mini-

mal effects of verapamil and diltiazem on the electrophysiologic properties of the bypass tract are consistent with the observation that the drugs are ineffective in atrial fibrillation, complicating WPW syndrome in which fibrillatory impulses, as with digoxin, travel predominantly through the anomalous pathway.[52]

Ventricular Arrhythmias

Intravenous verapamil and diltiazem have no apparent benefit in the treatment of ventricular arrhythmias except in acute myocardial infarction.[64, 66] Oral verapamil has no demonstrated role in the management of ventricular tachyarrhythmias. However, bepridil, with its class-I antiarrhythmic activity, has been shown to be effective in the short-term and long-term control of ventricular arrhythmias.[20] The drug is not approved in the United States for use as an antiarrhythmic agent.

Precautions in Treating Arrhythmias

A diseased sinoatrial (SA) node is much more sensitive to slow-channel blockers and may be depressed to the point of atrial standstill.[67] Sinus arrest can also occur without overt evidence of "sick sinus syndrome."[50] Calcium channel blockade also may suppress potential AV nodal escape rhythms that need to arise if atrial standstill occurs.[50] In patients with the brady-tachy form of sick sinus syndrome, neither digoxin nor β-adrenoceptor blocking drugs should probably be combined with verapamil or diltiazem in the prophylaxis of tachyarrhythmias unless a demand ventricular pacemaker is inserted before drug therapy is started.[50]

SYSTEMIC HYPERTENSION

Calcium antagonists are effective in the treatment of systemic hypertension and hypertensive emergencies.[68–71] Their possible mechanisms of action include peripheral vasodilation, antiadrenergic effects, natriuretic effects, and direct negative inotropic effects. Calcium antagonists can be considered a potential first-line therapy for initiating treatment in some patients with chronic hypertension. A large experience in the United States has been collected evaluating diltiazem,[72, 73] nifedipine,[42, 74] amlodipine,[75] nicardipine,[76, 77] felodipine,[78] nisoldipine,[79] and isradipine[80] in patients with hypertension. Verapamil, nicardipine, nifedipine, felodipine, and diltiazem are available in the United States in both conventional and sustained-release oral formulations, allowing once-daily and twice-daily dosing.[81] Amlodipine is approved for once-daily use and isradipine for twice-daily use. Under investigation in hypertension are new sustained-release formulations of nisoldipine (coat-core)[79] and verapamil (controlled-onset extended-release)[82] and a new agent, mibefradil, a benzimidazolyl-substituted derivative that binds competitively at both verapamil and diltiazem binding sites.[5]

The calcium antagonists reduce both systolic and

diastolic pressures with a minimal amount of side effects, including orthostasis.[69, 70] They can cause left ventricular hypertrophy to regress in patients with hypertension.[83, 83a] These drugs may also exhibit antiadrenergic and natriuretic activities.[84] They can be combined with other antihypertensive drugs if necessary (β-blockers, angiotensin-converting enzyme inhibitors, and diuretics).[69, 70] They are equally effective in black and white patients[85] and in young and old patients.[69, 70] They do not lower the pressures of normotensive subjects.[69, 70] The drugs may be most useful in patients with low-renin, salt-dependent forms of hypertension.[86, 87]

Some of the calcium antagonists have also been shown to be beneficial and safe in patients with severe hypertension and hypertensive crisis.[69, 70, 88–90] Single oral, sublingual, and intravenous doses of these drugs have rapidly and smoothly reduced blood pressure in adults and children without causing significant untoward effects.[69, 70, 88–90] The absolute reduction in blood pressure with treatment appears to be inversely correlated with the height of the pretreatment blood pressure level, and few episodes of hypotension have been reported.[88] Continuous hemodynamic monitoring of patients does not seem necessary in most instances.[88] Intravenous nicardipine has been approved for clinical use in the treatment of hypertensive emergencies and perioperative hypertension. Its clinical utility compared with other parenteral treatments needs to be determined.[91, 92]

"SILENT" MYOCARDIAL ISCHEMIA

In addition to their favorable effects in relieving painful episodes of myocardial ischemia, the calcium antagonists are also effective in relieving transient myocardial ischemic episodes (detected by electrocardiographic evaluation) that are unrelated to symptoms ("silent" myocardial ischemia).[93, 94] Diltiazem,[8] nifedipine (low dose), and verapamil alone and in combination with β-blockers and nitrates all have been shown to be effective in reducing the number of ischemic episodes and their duration.[95] The prognostic importance of relieving silent myocardial ischemia with calcium antagonists and other treatments has been evaluated in a study sponsored by the National Heart, Lung, and Blood Institute.[96]

MYOCARDIAL INFARCTION

Several experimental studies have indicated that nifedipine, verapamil, and diltiazem can reduce the size of myocardial necrosis induced in experimental ischemia.[97–100] Ischemia can lead to diminished adenosine triphosphate (ATP) production, which can eventually affect the sodium and calcium ion pumps with the ultimate consequence of calcium ion accumulation in the cytoplasm and calcium overload in the mitochondria. Calcium antagonists can diminish myocardial oxygen consumption and inhibit the influx of calcium ions to the myofibrils and thus favorably influence the outcome of experimental coronary oc-

clusion.[98, 101] These experimental observations have suggested the use of calcium antagonists for reducing or containing the extent of myocardial infarction during acute coronary artery occlusions in humans and as an adjunct to cardioplegia during open heart surgery. However, there have been no adequate studies in human subjects to support these approaches.

Compared with the established protective actions of some β-blocking drugs used intravenously or orally in prolonging life and reducing the risk of nonfatal reinfarction in survivors of an acute myocardial infarction,[102] the results with calcium antagonists (diltiazem, lidoflazine, nifedipine, verapamil) have not been as favorable.[103–115] More than 17,000 patients have been studied in 11 randomized controlled trials. Eight of the 11 trials showed a small excess in mortality in the treated group (not statistically significant in any trial). Overall, there were 836 deaths among the 8678 patients randomized to the active treatment group (9.5%) compared with 830 deaths among the 8762 control subjects (9.1%).

The plausibility of these mortality results with calcium antagonists is supported by a failure to show a beneficial effect on infarct size, development of myocardial infarctions, or reinfarctions in most trials of patients with myocardial infarctions or unstable angina.[114, 116] A trial using diltiazem in patients with non-Q-wave infarction reported a reduction in recurrent myocardial infarction in the diltiazem-treated patients but no reduction in mortality.[109] In a larger trial with diltiazem in infarction survivors, no favorable effects on mortality were seen.[113] A subgroup of patients with left ventricular dysfunction did worse with diltiazem therapy than with a placebo; however, diltiazem therapy appeared effective in patients with relatively normal left ventricular function.[113] Similarly, a more recent study did show a benefit with verapamil compared with a placebo in infarction survivors, with less benefit observed in patients with left ventricular dysfunction.[117]

Prophylactic use of calcium antagonists to improve patient survival following myocardial infarction cannot be recommended as a first-line therapy unless there are specific indications for using these drugs.[103, 115, 118] However, in patients with contraindications to β-adrenergic blockade, the use of verapamil or diltiazem can be considered in survivors of myocardial infarction who have good ventricular function.[118]

HYPERTROPHIC CARDIOMYOPATHY

Propranolol remains the therapeutic agent of choice for symptomatic patients with hypertrophic cardiomyopathy. The beneficial effects produced by propranolol derive from its blocking sympathetic stimulation of the heart.[119]

Clinical studies have shown that the administration of verapamil can also improve exercise capacity and symptoms in many patients with hypertrophic cardiomyopathy.[120–122] The exact mechanism by which verapamil produces these beneficial effects is not known. Acute and chronic verapamil administration reduces left ventricular outflow obstruction, but examination of indices of left ventricular systolic function during chronic therapy shows that this effect does not result from a reduction in left ventricular hypercontractility.[119] Because patients with hypertrophic cardiomyopathy also exhibit abnormal diastolic function, improvement in diastolic filling may be responsible in part for the benefits of verapamil.[119] Enhanced early diastolic filling and improvement in the diastolic pressure-volume relationship might be expected to result in an increase in left ventricular end-diastolic volume, which would decrease the venturi forces that act to move the anterior mitral valve leaflet across the outflow tract toward the septum.[119] The decrease would cause a diminution of obstruction, reducing left ventricular pressure and myocardial wall stress and thus raising the threshold at which symptoms occur.[119]

In a large study[108] of patients with hypertrophic cardiomyopathy refractory to β-blockers, verapamil proved to be effective on a long-term basis, with almost 50% of patients showing either a significant improvement in exercise tolerance or in symptoms. Approximately 50% of patients who were considered to be candidates for surgery because of moderately severe symptoms unresponsive to propranolol showed significant improvement on verapamil, and surgery was no longer considered necessary.[119]

Other studies have reported that chronic administration of verapamil not only can improve symptoms in patients with hypertrophic cardiomyopathy but can reduce the left ventricular muscle mass and the ventricular septal thickness measured by echocardiographic and electrocardiographic analysis.[120] Verapamil and nifedipine were shown to improve the impaired left ventricular filling characteristics.[123, 124] This beneficial effect on left ventricular diastolic relaxation has not occurred after administration of propranolol.[123]

There may be serious and fatal complications of verapamil treatment in patients with hypertrophic cardiomyopathy.[119] These complications result from either the accentuated hemodynamic or the electrophysiologic effects of the drug. It is not clear whether the fatal complications occur as a result of verapamil-induced reduction in blood pressure with a resultant increase in left ventricular obstruction or the negative inotropic effects of the drug.[119] Verapamil probably should not be used in patients with clinically evident congestive heart failure. The loss of sequential atrial ventricular depolarization caused by the electrophysiologic effects of the drug could also compromise cardiac function. The adverse electrophysiologic effects are often transient; however, they could prevent the use of larger drug doses, which might provide better relief.[119]

If the calcium antagonist effects of verapamil are responsible for its therapeutic actions in hypertrophic cardiomyopathy, other drugs in this class also may be useful. However, the results of a double-blind trial comparing verapamil with nifedipine indicated that verapamil is more effective than nifedipine in improving exercise tolerance and clinical symptoms.[124, 125]

CONGESTIVE HEART FAILURE

The potent systemic vasodilatory actions of nifedipine and other dihydropyridine calcium antagonists make them potentially useful as afterload-reducing agents in patients with left ventricular failure.[126–128] Unlike other vasodilatory drugs, however, nifedipine also exerts a direct negative inotropic effect on the myocardium that is consistent with its ability to block transmembrane calcium transport in cardiac muscle cells.[126, 129] The successful use of nifedipine as a vasodilator in patients with left ventricular failure would be dependent on its ability to reduce ventricular afterload to a degree that exceeds its direct negative inotropic actions, thereby leading to an improvement in hemodynamics and forward flow.[130]

Studies evaluating the effect of nifedipine on hemodynamics in patients with heart failure have uniformly demonstrated significant reductions in systemic vascular resistance, usually associated with increases in cardiac output.[130] Our group[131] and others[132] have found that resting ejection fractions also rise with nifedipine therapy. Reflex increases in heart rate have been reported,[131] but most investigators have found heart rate to remain the same[132, 133] and, in isolated cases, to fall.[134] Left ventricular filling pressures usually decrease[132, 133] or do not change significantly,[130, 134] but there are instances of heart failure in which pulmonary capillary wedge pressures rise with the use of nifedipine.[135, 136] Patients with left ventricular dysfunction and nearly normal levels of left ventricular afterload, i.e., disproportionately low wall stress, and those with intrinsic fixed mechanical interference to forward flow, such as aortic stenosis, appear most likely to have unfavorable hemodynamic responses to nifedipine therapy.[127, 128] Most of the published data have dealt only with the acute hemodynamic effects of the agent after single sublingual dosing; little work has been done on the use of nifedipine as chronic oral therapy for left ventricular failure.

Total clinical experience with nifedipine and the new dihydropyridine calcium antagonists in chronic heart failure is limited.[127, 128] Therefore, the evidence at present would not support use of these drugs as a ventricular unloading agent of first choice because there are other vasodilators available that do not have negative inotropic activity.[128] Use of dihydropyridine calcium antagonists as acute vasodilator therapy in patients with left ventricular failure should be considered only if additional clinical reasons for its administration exist, i.e., angina pectoris and systemic hypertension, particularly if these conditions play important contributory roles in the development or exacerbation of left ventricular dysfunction. The drug should be administered only after careful assessment of the clinical situation and preferably with invasive monitoring of pulmonary artery or pulmonary capillary wedge pressure.[128] Additional clinical experience, including controlled clinical trials, will ultimately help define the precise role of calcium antagonists in the acute and chronic treatment of systolic heart failure. There is evidence to suggest that calcium antagonists may provide some benefit to patients with predominantly diastolic ventricular dysfunction, but more data are needed to substantiate this claim.

PRIMARY PULMONARY HYPERTENSION

Primary pulmonary hypertension is an entity characterized by excessive pulmonary vasoconstriction and increased pulmonary vascular resistance induced by unknown stimuli.[137] Typically, the affected patient is a young to middle-aged woman with fatigue, dyspnea, chest discomfort, or syncope. Despite many attempts, the results of drug treatment have been generally unsatisfactory, and the syndrome continues to bear a poor prognosis.[137]

Based on the data currently available, it may be concluded that some calcium antagonists provide beneficial responses in selected patients with pulmonary hypertension.[137-139] In general, patients with less severe pulmonary hypertension appear to respond better than do those with more advanced disease.[140] Furthermore, early treatment may serve to attenuate progression of the disease.

CEREBRAL ARTERIAL SPASM AND STROKE

A major complication of subarachnoid hemorrhage is cerebral arterial spasm, which may occur several days after the initial event.[141] Such a spasm may be a focal or diffuse narrowing of one or more of the larger cerebral vessels, which may cause additional ischemic neurologic deficits. Although the exact cause of this spasm is unknown, it is postulated that a combination of various blood constituents and neurotransmitters produces a milieu that enhances the reactivity of the cerebral vasculature.[141] The final pathway for the vasoconstriction, however, involves an increase in the free intracellular calcium concentration.[142] Accordingly, it is reasonable to postulate that the calcium antagonists may have a beneficial effect in reducing cerebral spasm.[143]

Although verapamil and nifedipine have been shown to prevent cerebral arterial spasm in experimental studies,[144, 145] nimodipine, a nifedipine analogue, has demonstrated a preferential cerebrovascular action in this disorder.[146] The lipid solubility of nimodipine enables it to cross the blood-brain barrier; this quality may account for its more potent cerebrovascular effects. In a recent multicenter placebo-controlled study involving 125 patients,[141] nimodipine significantly reduced the occurrence of severe neurologic deficits following angiographically demonstrated cerebral arterial spasm. All patients had a documented subarachnoid hemorrhage and a normal neurologic status within 96 hours of entry into the study. Whereas 8 of the 60 placebo-treated patients had a severe neurologic deficit, only 1 of 55 patients treated with nimodipine had such an outcome. Nimodipine is now approved for use in improving of neurologic outcome by reducing the incidence and severity of ischemic deficits in patients with subarachnoid hemorrhage from ruptured congenital aneurysms who are in good neurologic condition post-ictus. The recommended dose is 60 mg by mouth every 4 hours for 21 consecutive days.

Subsequent investigations have suggested that increased cellular calcium concentration may be implicated in neuronal death after ischemia.[147] Nimodipine administered to laboratory animals after global cerebral ischemia had a more favorable effect on neurologic outcome than did a placebo.[148] The results of a prospective, double-blind, placebo-controlled trial of oral nimodipine administered to 186 patients within 24 hours of an acute ischemic stroke showed a reduction in both mortality and neurologic deficit with active treatment. The benefit was confined predominantly to men.[147] Nimodipine was recently approved for use in oral form for reducing the risk of morbidity and mortality in patients with subarachnoid hemorrhage.

MIGRAINE AND DEMENTIA

Classic migraine is characterized by prodromal symptoms with transient neurologic deficits. Cerebral blood flow is reduced during these prodromes and then is increased during the subsequent vasodilatory phase, causing severe headache.[149] Because the entry of calcium ions into the smooth muscle cells is the final common pathway that controls vasomotor tone, calcium antagonists may prevent or ameliorate the initial focal cerebral vasoconstriction.[150]

Results from controlled studies have demonstrated that 80% to 90% of patients with vascular headaches benefit from nimodipine, confirming the selectivity of this agent for the cerebral blood vessels.[151] Verapamil and nifedipine also have been reported to be effective in the prophylaxis of migraine but are less selective for the cephalic blood vessels and thus cause more systemic side effects.[151, 152] Relief from the migraine prodrome usually began 10 to 14 days after initiation of the drugs but could be delayed 2 to 4 weeks.[153] Cerebral vascular resistance was decreased by all three established calcium antagonists, but only nimodipine reduced the cerebral vasoconstriction induced by inhalation of 100% oxygen.[151] None of the calcium antagonists is effective against muscle contraction or tension headache.

Multiple clinical trials are now being carried out examining the effects of calcium antagonists on the progression of dementing illness, both vascular and Alzheimer types. The results have been equivocal to date.

OTHER CARDIOVASCULAR USES

Calcium antagonists have been shown to be effective in some patients with Raynaud's phenomenon, mesenteric insufficiency, and intermittent claudication.[143, 144] They have also been shown in experimental studies to be effective in arresting the atherosclerotic process.[154, 155] However, studies using noninvasive indices of assessment to determine whether specific calcium antagonists can retard the progress of atherosclerosis in human subjects have revealed conflicting results.[156, 157] A recent report showed that diltiazem could retard the development of coronary artery disease in heart transplant recipients.[158]

Coronary artery vasospasm may be an important pathophysiologic mechanism in cardiomyopathy.[159] Verapamil treatment has been shown experimentally to reduce vasospasm in response to myocarditis and, by this mechanism, to prevent the development of cardiomyopathy.[160]

NONCARDIOVASCULAR APPLICATIONS

Calcium antagonists are being investigated for the treatment of bronchial asthma, nocturnal cramps, esophageal spasm, dysmenorrhea, and premature labor.[143, 161] The pathophysiology of these conditions may be influenced in part by abnormalities in calcium ion transport across cell membranes, thus explaining the potential application of calcium antagonist.

REFERENCES

1. Keefe D, Frishman WH: Clinical pharmacology of the calcium channel blocking drugs. In Packer M, Frishman WH (eds): Calcium Channel Antagonists in Cardiovascular Disease. Norwalk, CT: Appleton-Century-Crofts, 1984, p 3.
2. Braunwald E: Mechanism of action of calcium channel blocking agents. N Engl J Med 307:1618, 1983.
3. Weiner DA: Calcium channel blockers. Med Clin North Am 72:83, 1988.
4. Singh BN, Chew CYC, Josephson MA, et al: Hemodynamic mechanisms underlying the antianginal actions of verapamil. Am J Cardiol 50:886, 1982.
5. Frishman WH: Current status of calcium channel blockers. Curr Probl Cardiol 19(11):639, 1994.
6. Stone PH, Antman EM, Muller JE, et al: Calcium channel blocking agents in the treatment of cardiovascular disorders: Part II. Hemodynamic effects and clinical applications. Ann Intern Med 93:886, 1980.
7. Theroux P, Taeymans Y, Waters D: Calcium antagonists: Clinical use in the treatment of angina. Drugs 25:179, 1983.
8. Frishman WH, Charlap S, Kimmel B, et al: Diltiazem compared to nifedipine and combination treatment in patients with stable angina: Effects on angina, exercise tolerance and the ambulatory ECG. Circulation 77:774, 1988.
9. Hossack KF, Pool PE, Steele P: Efficacy of diltiazem in angina of effort—a multicenter trial. Am J Cardiol 49:457, 1982.
10. Strauss WE, McIntyre KM, Parisi AR, et al: Safety and efficacy of diltiazem hydrochloride for the treatment of stable angina pectoris—report of a cooperative trial. Am J Cardiol 49:560, 1982.
11. Weiner DA, Cutler SS, Klein MD: Efficacy and safety of sustained-release diltiazem in stable angina pectoris. Am J Cardiol 57:6, 1986.
12. Moskowitz RM, Piccini PA, Nacarelli GV, et al: Nifedipine therapy for stable angina pectoris: Preliminary results of effects on angina frequency and treadmill exercise response. Am J Cardiol 44:811, 1979.
13. Mueller HS, Chahine RA: Interim report of multicenter double-blind placebo-controlled studies of nifedipine in chronic stable angina. Am J Med 71:645, 1981.
14. Bala Subramanian V, Parmasivan R, Lahiri A, et al: Verapamil in chronic stable angina—a controlled study with computerized multistage treadmill exercise. Lancet 1:841, 1980.
15. Pine MB, Citron PD, Bailly DJ, et al: Verapamil versus placebo in relieving stable angina pectoris. Circulation 65(Suppl I):17, 1982.
16. Weiner DA, Klein MD: Verapamil therapy for stable exertional angina. Am J Cardiol 50:1153, 1982.
17. Frishman WH, Charlap S: Verapamil in the treatment of chronic stable angina. Arch Intern Med 143:1407, 1983.
18. Weiner DA, Klein MD, Cutler SS: Evaluation of sustained-release verapamil in chronic stable angina pectoris. Am J Cardiol 59:215, 1987.
19. Scheidt S, Frishman WH, Packer M, et al: Long-term effectiveness of verapamil in stable and unstable angina pectoris: One year follow-up of patients treated in placebo-controlled double-blind randomized clinical trials. Am J Cardiol 50:1185, 1982.
20. Shapiro W, DiBianco R, Thadani U, and other members of the Bepridil Collaborative Study Group: Comparative efficacy of 200, 300 and 400 mg of bepridil for chronic stable angina pectoris. Am J Cardiol 55:36C, 1985.
21. Singh BN for the Bepridil Collaborative Study Group: Comparative efficacy and safety of bepridil and diltiazem in chronic stable angina pectoris refractory to diltiazem. Am J Cardiol 68:306, 1991.
22. Livesley B, Catley PF, Campbell RC, et al: Double-blind evaluation of verapamil, propranolol and isosorbide dinitrate against placebo in the treatment of angina pectoris. Br Med J 1:375, 1973.
23. Frishman WH, Klein NA, Strom JA, et al: Superiority of verapamil to propranolol in stable angina pectoris—a double-blind randomized crossover trial. Circulation 65(Suppl I):51, 1982.
24. Frishman WH: Beta-adrenergic blockade in the treatment of coronary artery disease. In Hurst JW (ed): Clinical Essays on the Heart, Vol 2. New York: McGraw-Hill, 1984, p 25.
25. Lynch P, Darie H, Krikler S, et al: Objective assessment of antianginal treatment: A double-blind comparison of propranolol, nifedipine, and their combination. Br Med J 48:131, 1981.
26. Kenmure ACF, Scruton JH: A double-blind controlled trial of the anti-anginal efficacy of nifedipine compared with propranolol. Br J Clin Pract 8:49, 1980.
27. Bala Subramanian V, Bowles MJ, Davies AB, et al: Comparative effectiveness of verapamil and propranolol in angina of effort. Am J Cardiol 50:1158, 1982.
28. Bala Subramanian V, Bowles MJ, Khupml NS, et al: Comparative effectiveness of verapamil and nifedipine in stable angina pectoris. Am J Cardiol 50:1173, 1982.
29. Frishman WH, Klein N, Klein P, et al: Comparison of oral propranolol and verapamil for combined systemic hypertension and angina pectoris: A placebo-controlled double-blind randomized crossover trial. Am J Cardiol 50:1164, 1982.
30. Frishman WH, Charlap S: Calcium channel blockers for combined systemic hypertension and myocardial ischemia. Circulation 75:V154, 1988.
31. Boden WE, Korr KS, Bough EW: Nifedipine-induced hypotension and myocardial ischemia in refractory angina pectoris. JAMA 253:1131, 1985.
32. Frishman WH, Sherman D, Feinfeld DA: Innovative drug delivery systems in cardiovascular medicine: Nifedipine-GITS and clonidine-TTS. Cardiol Clin 5:703, 1987.
33. Frishman WH: Comparative efficacy and concomitant use of bepridil and beta blockers in the management of angina pectoris. Am J Cardiol 69: 50D, 1992.
34. Frishman WH, Klein N, Strom J, et al: Comparative effects of abrupt withdrawal of propranolol and verapamil in angina pectoris. Am J Cardiol 50:1180, 1982.
35. Johnson SM, Mauitson DR, Willerson JT, et al: A controlled trial of verapamil for Prinzmetal's variant angina. N Engl J Med 304(15):862, 1981.
36. Mehta J, Conti CR: Calcium channel antagonists in the treatment of unstable angina. Am J Cardiol 50:919, 1982.
37. Theroux P, Waters DD, Affaki GS, et al: Provocative testing with ergonovine to evaluate the efficacy of treatment with calcium antagonists in variant angina. Circulation 60:504, 1979.
38. Antman E, Muller JE, Goldberg S: Nifedipine therapy for coronary artery spasm experience in 127 patients. N Engl J Med 302:1269, 1980.

39. Schroeder JS, Feldman RL, Griles TD, et al: Multiclinic controlled trial diltiazem for Prinzmetal's angina. Am J Med 72:227, 1982.
40. Feldman RL, Pepine CJ, Whittle J, et al: Short- and long-term responses to diltiazem in patients with variant angina. Am J Cardiol 49:554, 1982.
41. Goldberg S, Reichek N, Wilson J, et al: Nifedipine in the treatment of Prinzmetal's (variant) angina. Am J Cardiol 44:804, 1979.
42. Prida XE, Gelman JS, Feldman RL, et al: Comparison of diltiazem alone and in combination in patients with coronary artery spasm. J Am Coll Cardiol 9:412, 1987.
43. Parodi O, Simonetti I, L'Abbate A, et al: Comparative effectiveness of verapamil and propranolol in angina at rest. Am J Cardiol 50:923, 1982.
44. Johnson SM, Mauritson DR, Willerson JT, et al: Comparison of verapamil and nifedipine in the treatment of variant angina pectoris—preliminary observations in 10 patients. Am J Cardiol 47:1295, 1981.
45. Gerstenblith G, Ouyang P, Achuff S, et al: Nifedipine in unstable angina: A double-blind randomized trial. N Engl J Med 306:885, 1982.
46. Subramanian B, Bowles MK, Davies AB, et al: Combined therapy with verapamil and propranolol in chronic stable angina. Am J Cardiol 49:125, 1982.
47. Dargie HJ, Lynch PG, Krikler DM, et al: Nifedipine and propranolol: A beneficial drug interaction. Am J Med 71:676, 1981.
48. Packer M, Leon MB, Bonow RO, et al: Hemodynamic and clinical effects of combined therapy with verapamil and propranolol in ischemic heart disease. Am J Cardiol 50:903, 1982.
49. Packer M, Frishman WH: Calcium channel antagonists in perspective. In Packer M, Frishman WH (eds): Calcium Channel Antagonists in Cardiovascular Disease. Norwalk, CT: Appleton-Century-Crofts, 1984, p XVII.
50. Frishman WH, LeJemtel T: Electropharmacology of calcium channel antagonists in cardiac arrhythmias. PACE 5:402, 1982.
51. Schamroth L, Krikler DM, Garrett C: Immediate effects of intravenous verapamil in cardiac arrhythmias. Br Med J 1:660, 1972.
52. Heng MK, Singh BN, Roche AHG, et al: Effects of intravenous verapamil on cardiac arrhythmias and on the electrocardiogram. Am Heart J 90:487, 1975.
53. Klein HO, Pauzner H, DiSegni E, et al: The beneficial effects of verapamil in chronic atrial fibrillation. Arch Intern Med 139:747, 1979.
54. Weiner I: Verapamil therapy for atrial flutter and fibrillation. In Packer M, Frishman WH (eds): Calcium Channel Antagonists in Cardiovascular Disease. Norwalk, CT: Appleton-Century-Crofts, 1984, p 257.
55. Klein HO, Kaplinsky E: Comparative effectiveness of verapamil and digoxin in atrial fibrillation. Am J Cardiol 50:894, 1982.
56. Ellenbogen KA, Dias VC, Plumb VJ, et al: A placebo-controlled trial of continuous intravenous diltiazem infusion for 24-hour heart rate control during atrial fibrillation and atrial flutter: A multicenter trial. J Am Coll Cardiol 18:891, 1991.
57. Krikler DM, Spurrel RAJ: Verapamil in the treatment of paroxysmal supraventricular tachycardia. Postgrad Med J 50:447, 1974.
58. Singh BN, Nademanee D, Baky S: Calcium antagonists: Uses in the treatment of cardiac arrhythmias. Drugs 25:125, 1983.
59. Hartel G, Hartikainen M: Comparison of verapamil and practolol in paroxysmal supraventricular tachycardia. Eur J Cardiol 4:87, 1976.
60. Tonkin AM, Aylward PE, Joel SE, et al: Verapamil in prophylaxis of paroxysmal atrioventricular nodal reentrant tachycardia. J Cardiovasc Pharmacol 2:473, 1980.
61. Mauritson DR, Winniford MD, Walker WS, et al: Oral verapamil for paroxysmal supraventricular tachycardia: A long-term, double-blind, randomized trial. Ann Intern Med 96:409, 1982.
62. Spurrell RAJ, Krikler DM, Sowton GE: The effect of verapamil on the electrophysiological properties of the anomalous atrioventricular connections in Wolff-Parkinson-White syndrome. Br Heart J 36:256, 1974.
63. Matsuyama E, Konishi T, Okazaki H, et al: Effects of verapamil on accessory pathway properties and induction of circus movement tachycardia in patients with the Wolff-Parkinson-White syndrome. J Cardiovasc Pharmacol 3:11, 1981.
64. Singh BN, Collet J, Chew CYC: New perspectives in the pharmacologic therapy of cardiac arrhythmias. Prog Cardiovasc Dis 22:243, 1980.
65. Shigenobu K, Schneider JA, Sperelakis N: Verapamil blockade of slow Na^+ and Ca^{++} responses in myocardial cells. J Pharmacol Exp Ther 190:280, 1974.
66. Gotsman M, Lewis B, Bakst A, et al: Verapamil in life-threatening tachyarrhythmias. S Afr Med J 46:2017, 1972.
67. Carrasco HA, Fuenmayor A, Barboza J, et al: Effect of verapamil on normal sino-atrial node dysfunction and on sick sinus syndrome. Am Heart J 96:760, 1978.
68. Frishman WH, Stroh JA, Greenberg SM, et al: Calcium Channel blockers in systemic hypertension. Curr Probl Cardiol 12:287, 1987.
69. Spivack C, Ocken S, Frishman WH: Calcium antagonists: Clinical use in treatment of systemic hypertension. Drugs 25:154, 1983.
70. Frishman WH, Stroh JA, Greenberg SM, et al: Calcium Channel blockers in systemic hypertension. Med Clin North Am 72:449, 1988.
71. Cummings DM, Amadio P, Nelson L, et al: The role of calcium channel blockers in the treatment of systemic hypertension. Arch Intern Med 151:250, 1991.
72. Frishman WH, Zawada ET, Smith LK, et al: A comparative study of diltiazem and hydrochlorothiazide as initial medical therapy for mild to moderate hypertension. Am J Cardiol 59:615, 1987.
73. Massie B, MacCarthy EP, Ramanathan KB, et al: Diltiazem and propranolol in mild to moderate essential hypertension as monotherapy or with hydrochlorothiazide. Ann Intern Med 107:150, 1987.
74. Ferlinz J: Nifedipine in myocardial ischemia, systemic hypertension and other cardiovascular disorders. Ann Intern Med 105:714, 1986.
75. Johnson BF, Frishman WH, Brobyn R, et al: A randomized placebo-controlled, double-blind comparison of amlodipine and atenolol in patients with essential hypertension. Am J Hypertens 5:727, 1992.
76. Charlap S, Kimmel B, Laifer L, et al: Twice daily nicardipine in the treatment of patients with mild to moderate hypertension. J Clin Hypertens 2:271, 1986.
77. Taylor SH, Frais MA, Lee P, et al: A study of the long term efficacy and tolerability of oral nicardipine in hypertensive patients. Br J Clin Pharmacol 20(Suppl 1):139S, 1985.
78. Todd PA, Faulds D: Felodipine: A review of the pharmacology and therapeutic use of the extended-release formulation in cardiovascular disorders. Drugs 44:251, 1992.
79. Lewis BS: Efficacy and safety of nisoldipine coat core in the management of angina pectoris, systemic hypertension, and ischemic ventricular dysfunction. Am J Cardiol 75(13):46E, 1995.
80. Hamilton BP: Treatment of essential hypertension with PN 200-110 (isradipine). Am J Cardiol 59:141, 1987.
81. Katz B, Rosenberg A, Frishman WH: Controlled release drug delivery systems in cardiovascular medicine. Am Heart J 129:359, 1995.
82. Cutler NR, Anders RJ, Jhee SS: Placebo-controlled evaluation of three doses of a controlled-onset, extended-release formulation of verapamil in the treatment of stable angina pectoris. Am J Cardiol 75:1102, 1995.
83. Hachamovitch R, Strom JA, Sonnenblick EH, et al: Left ventricular hypertrophy in hypertension and the effects of antihypertensive drug therapy. Curr Probl Cardiol 13(6):311, 1988.
83a. Frishman WH, Skolnick AE: Effects of calcium blockade on hypertension-induced left ventricular hypertrophy. Circulation 80(Suppl IV):151, 1989.
84. Buhler F, DeLeeuw PW, Doyle A, et al: Calcium metabolism and calcium channel blockers for understanding and treating hypertension. Am J Med 77(6B):1, 1984.
85. Cubeddu LX: Racial differences in response to antihypertensive drugs: A focus on verapamil. J Clin Hypertens 3:55S, 1986.

86. Buhler FR, Hulthen UL, Kiowski W, et al: Greater antihypertensive efficacy of the calcium channel inhibitor verapamil in older and low renin patients. Clin Sci 63:439S, 1982.

87. Erne P, Bolli P, Bertel O, et al: Antihypertensive monotherapy with calcium antagonists relates to older age, liver pretreatment renin and higher blood pressure: Comparison of nifedipine and verapamil. Hypertension 5(Suppl II):97, 1983.

88. Frishman WH, Weinberg P, Peled H, et al: Calcium entry blockers for the treatment of severe hypertension and hypertensive emergencies. Am J Med 77:35, 1984.

89. Beer N, Gallegos I, Cohen A, et al: Efficacy of sublingual nifedipine in the acute treatment of systemic hypertension. Chest 79:571, 1981.

90. Ellrodt AG, Ault M, Riedinger MS, et al: Efficacy of sublingual nifedipine in hypertensive emergencies. Am J Med 79:19, 1985.

91. Wallin JD, Fletcher E, Ram CV, et al: Intravenous nicardipine for the treatment of severe hypertension. Arch Intern Med 149(12):2662, 1989.

92. IV Nicardipine Study Group: Efficacy and safety of intravenous nicardipine in the control of postoperative hypertension. Chest 99:393, 1991.

93. Frishman WH, Teicher M: Antianginal drug therapy for silent myocardial ischemia. Med Clin North Am 72:185, 1988.

94. Deedwania PC, Carbajal EV: Silent myocardial ischemia: A clinical perspective. Arch Intern Med 151:2373, 1991.

95. Knatterud GL, Bourassa MG, Pepine CJ, et al, for ACIP Investigators: Effects of treatment strategies to suppress ischemia in coronary artery disease patients: 12 week results of the Asymptomatic Cardiac Ischemia Pilot (ACIP). J Am Coll Cardiol 24:11, 1994.

96. The ACIP Investigators: Asymptomatic Cardiac Ischemia Pilot Study (ACIP). Am J Cardiol 70:744, 1992.

97. Millard RW, Lathrop DA, Grupp G, et al: Differential cardiovascular effects of calcium channel blocking agents: Potential mechanisms. Am J Cardiol 49:499, 1982.

98. Nayler WG: Cardioprotective effects of calcium ion antagonists in myocardial ischemia. Clin Invest Med 3:91, 1980.

99. Selwyn AP, Welman E, Fox K, et al: The effects of nifedipine on acute experimental myocardial ischemia and infarction in dogs. Circ Res 44:16, 1979.

100. Maroko PR: Experimental infarction studies. Clin Invest Med 3:139, 1980.

101. Zsoter TT, Church JG: Calcium antagonists—pharmacodynamic effects and mechanism of action. Drugs 25:93, 1983.

102. Frishman WH, Furberg CD, Friedewald WT: β-Adrenergic blockade in survivors of acute myocardial infarction. N Engl J Med 310:830, 1984.

103. Yusuf S, Held P, Furberg CD: Update of effect of calcium antagonists in myocardial infarction or angina in light of the second Danish Verapamil Infarction Trial (DAVIT II) and other recent studies. Am J Cardiol 67:1295, 1991.

104. Crea F, Deanfield J, Crean P, et al: Effects of verapamil in preventing early post infarction angina and reinfarction. Am J Cardiol 55:900, 1985.

105. Gottlieb SO, Weiss JL, Flaherty JT, et al: Effect of nifedipine on clinical course and left ventricular function in low risk acute myocardial infarction: A double-blind randomized trial [abstract]. Circulation 70:257, 1984.

106. Sirnes PA, Overskeid K, Pedersen TR, et al: Evolution of infarct size during the early use of nifedipine in patients with acute myocardial infarction: The Norwegian Nifedipine Multicenter Trial. Circulation 70:638, 1984.

107. Wilcox RG, Hampton JR, Banks DC, et al: Trial of early nifedipine treatment in patients with suspected myocardial infarction (the TRENT Study) [abstract]. Br Med J 293:1204, 1986.

108. The Danish Study Group on Verapamil in Myocardial Infarction: Verapamil in acute myocardial infarction. Eur Heart J 5:516, 1984.

109. Gibson RS, Boden WE, Theroux P, et al: Diltiazem and reinfarction in patients with non-Q-wave myocardial infarction. N Engl J Med 315:423, 1986.

110. Muller JE, Morrison J, Stone PH, et al: Nifedipine therapy for patients with threatened and acute myocardial infarction: A randomized, double-blind, placebo-controlled comparison. Circulation 69:740, 1984.

111. Neufeld HN: Calcium antagonists in secondary prevention after acute myocardial infarction: The Secondary Prevention Reinfarction Nifedipine Trial (SPRINT). Eur Heart J 7(Suppl B):51, 1986.

112. de Geest, Kesteloot H, Piessens J: Secondary prevention of ischemic heart disease: A long-term controlled lidoflazine study. Acta Cardiol Suppl 24:7, 1979.

113. The Multicenter Diltiazem Postinfarction Trial Research Group: The effect of diltiazem on mortality and reinfarction after myocardial infarction. N Engl J Med 319:385, 1988.

114. Yusuf S, Furberg CD: Effects of calcium channel blockers on survival after myocardial infarction. Cardiovasc Drug Ther 1:343, 1987.

115. Messerli FH: "Cardioprotection"—not all calcium antagonists are created equal. Am J Cardiol 66:855, 1990.

116. Skolnick AE, Frishman WH: Calcium channel blockers in myocardial infarction. Arch Intern Med 149:1669, 1989.

117. The Danish Study on Verapamil in Myocardial Infarction: The effect of verapamil on mortality and major events after myocardial infarction: The Danish Verapamil Infarction Trial II (DAVIT II). Am J Cardiol 66:779, 1990.

118. Frishman WH, Skolnick AE, Miller KP: Secondary prevention post infarction: The role of β-adrenergic blockers, calcium channel blockers and aspirin. In Gersh BJ, Rahimtoola SH (eds): Management of Myocardial Infarction. New York: Elsevier Science Publishing, 1991, p 469.

119. Cohen LS, Braunwald E: Amelioration of angina pectoris in idiopathic hypertrophic subaortic stenosis with beta-adrenergic blockade. Circulation 35:847, 1967.

120. Rosing DR, Bonow RO, Packer M, et al: Verapamil therapy for the management of hypertrophic cardiomyopathy. In Packer M, Frishman WH (eds): Calcium Channel Antagonists in Cardiovascular Disease. Norwalk, CT: Appleton-Century-Crofts, 1984, p 313.

121. Rosing DR, Kent KM, Maron BJ, et al: Verapamil therapy—new approach to the pharmacologic treatment of hypertrophic cardiomyopathy: II. Effects on exercise capacity and symptomatic status. Circulation 60:1209, 1979.

122. Rosing DR, Kent KM, Borer JS, et al: Verapamil therapy—a new approach to the pharmacologic treatment of hypertrophic cardiomyopathy: I. Hemodynamic effects. Circulation 60:1201, 1979.

123. Bonow RO, Rosing DR, Bacharach SL, et al: Effects of verapamil on left ventricular systolic function and diastolic filling in patients with hypertrophic cardiomyopathy. Circulation 64:787, 1981.

124. Lorell BH, Paulus WJ, Grossman W, et al: Modification of abnormal left ventricular diastolic properties by nifedipine in patients with hypertrophic cardiomyopathy. Circulation 65:499, 1982.

125. Rosing DR, Cannon RO, Watson RM, et al: Comparison of verapamil and nifedipine effects on symptoms and exercise capacity in patients with hypertrophic cardiomyopathy [abstract]. Circulation 66(Suppl II):II24, 1982.

126. Henry PD, Borda L, Schuchleib R: Chronotropic and inotropic effects of vasodilators. In Lichtlen PR, Kmura E, Taira N (eds): International Adalat Panel Discussion: New Experimental and Clinical Results. Amsterdam: Excerpta Medica, 1979, p 14.

127. Charlap S, Kimmel B, Frishman WH: Calcium Channel blockers in heart failure. In Julian DG, Wenger NK (eds): Cardiology, Vol IV. London: Butterworths, 1986, p 179.

128. Landau AJ, Gentilucci M, Cavusoglu E, Frishman WH: Calcium antagonists for the treatment of congestive heart failure. Cor Art Dis 5:37, 1994.

129. Cohn JN, Franciosa JA: Vasodilator therapy of cardiac failure. N Engl J Med 297:27, 1977.

130. Elkayam U, Weber L, Torkan B, et al: Comparison of hemodynamic responses to nifedipine and nitroprusside in severe chronic congestive heart failure. Am J Cardiol 53:1321, 1984.

131. Losardo AA, Klein NA, Beer N, et al: Beneficial effects of sublingual nifedipine in patients with ischemic heart disease and depressed left ventricular function. Angiology 33:811, 1982.

132. Klugmann S, Salvi A, Camerini F: Haemodynamic effects of nifedipine in heart failure. Br Heart J 43:440, 1980.

133. Polese A, Fiorentini C, Olivari MT, et al: Clinical use of a calcium antagonistic agent (nifedipine) in acute pulmonary edema. Am J Med 66:825, 1979.

134. Fifer MA, Colucci WS, Lorell BH, et al: Comparison of hemodynamic responses to nifedipine in heart failure: Comparison with nitroprusside. J Am Coll Cardiol 5:731, 1985.

135. Brooks N, Cattell M, Pidgeon J, et al: Unpredictable response to nifedipine in severe heart failure. Br Med J 281:1324, 1980.

136. Elkayam U, Weber L, McKay C, et al: Spectrum of acute hemodynamic effects of nifedipine in severe congestive heart failure. Am J Cardiol 546:560, 1985.

137. Fein SA, Frishman WH: The pathophysiology and management of primary pulmonary hypertension. Cardiol Clin 5: 563, 1987.

138. Kambara H, Fujimoto K, Wakabayashi A, et al: Primary pulmonary hypertension: Beneficial therapy with diltiazem. Am Heart J 101:230, 1981.

139. DeFeyter PJ, Kerkkamp HJJ, deJong JP: Sustained beneficial effect of nifedipine in primary pulmonary hypertension. Am Heart J 105:333, 1983.

140. Packer M: Vasodilator therapy for primary pulmonary hypertension: Limitations and hazards. Ann Intern Med 103:258, 1985.

141. Allen GS, Ahn HS, Preziosi TJ, et al: Cerebral arterial spasm—a controlled trial of nimodipine in patients with subarachnoid hemorrhage. N Engl J Med 308:619, 1983.

142. Towart R: The pathophysiology of cerebral vasospasm and pharmacological approaches to its management. Acta Neurochir (Wien) 62:253, 1982.

143. Bussey HI, Talbert RL: Promising uses of calcium channel blocking agents. Pharmacotherapy 4:137, 1984.

144. Allen GS, Bahr AL: Cerebral arterial spasm: Part X. Reversal of acute and chronic spasm in dogs with orally administered nifedipine. Neurosurgery 4:43, 1979.

145. Allen GS, Banghart SB: Cerebral arterial spasm: Part IX. In vitro effects of nifedipine on serotonin, phenylephrine and potassium-induced contractions of canine basilar and femoral artery. Neurosurgery 4:37, 1979.

146. Kazda S, Towart R: Nimodipine: A new calcium antagonistic drug with a preferential cerebrovascular action. Acta Neurochir 63:259, 1982.

147. Gelmers HJ, Gorter K, DeWeerdt CJ, et al: A controlled trial of nimodipine in acute ischemic stroke. N Engl J Med 318:203, 1988.

148. Steen PA, Gisvold SE, Milde JH, et al: Nimodipine improves outcome when given after complete cerebral ischemia in primates. Anesthesiology 62:406, 1985.

149. Edmeads J: Cerebral blood flow in migraine. Headache 17:148, 1977.

150. Meyer JS: Calcium channel blockers in the prophylactic treatment of vascular headache. Ann Intern Med 102:395, 1985.

151. Meyer JS, Hardenberg J: Clinical effectiveness of calcium entry blockers in prophylactic treatment of migraine and cluster headaches. Headache 23:266, 1983.

152. Solomon GD, Steele JG, Spaccavento LJ: Verapamil prophylaxis of migraine: A double-blind placebo-controlled study. JAMA 250:2500, 1983.

153. Meyer JS, Dowell R, Mathew NJ, et al: Clinical and hemodynamic effects during treatment of vascular headaches with verapamil. Headache 24:313, 1984.

154. Ram CV: Antiatherosclerotic and vasculoprotective actions of calcium antagonists. Am J Cardiol 66:29I, 1990.

155. Fleckenstein A, Fleckenstein-Grun G: Protection by calcium antagonists against experimental arterial calcinosis. In Pyorala K, Rapaport E, Konig K, et al (eds): Secondary Prevention of Coronary Heart Disease. New York: Thieme-Stratton, 1983, p 511.

156. Borhani NO, Bond MG, Sowers JR, et al: The Multicenter Isradipine/Diuretic Atherosclerosis Study: A study of the antiatherogenic properties of isradipine in hypertensive patients. J Cardiovasc Pharmacol 18(Suppl 3):515, 1991.

157. McClellan K: Unexpected results from the MIDAS atherosclerosis [meeting report]. Inpharma 4:932, 1994.

158. Schroeder JS, Gao S-Z, Alderman EL, et al: A preliminary study of diltiazem in the prevention of coronary artery disease in heart transplant recipients. N Engl J Med 328:164, 1993.

159. Factor SM, Minase T, Cho S, et al: Microvascular spasm in the cardiomyopathic Syrian hamster: A preventable cause of focal myocardial necrosis. Circulation 66:342, 1982.

160. Factor SM, Sonnenblick EH: Microvascular spasm as a cause of cardiomyopathies. Cardiovasc Rev Rep 4:1177, 1983.

161. Schwartz ML, Rotmensch HH, Frishman WH, et al: Potential applications of calcium channel antagonists in the management of noncardiac disorders. In Packer M, Frishman WH (eds): Calcium Channel Antagonists in Cardiovascular Disease. Norwalk, CT: Appleton-Century-Crofts, 1984, p 371.

CHAPTER 98

Calcium Antagonists in the Prevention of Atherosclerosis

William W. Parmley, M.D.

Despite progress made in its prevention, recognition, and treatment, heart disease remains the number one cause of mortality in the United States. Atherosclerosis of the coronary arteries is the primary cause of heart disease and remains a major challenge because of its slow, asymptomatic development and its often sudden and catastrophic manifestations. Numerous studies on the causes of atherosclerosis have emphasized its multifactorial nature.[1] Major factors include genetic predisposition, male sex, cigarette smoking, hypertension, lipid abnormalities, and diabetes. Despite this knowledge of the factors that contribute to the development of coronary artery disease, we have much to learn in predicting its rate of development in an individual patient.

Hypertension is one of the most important factors contributing to the development of atherosclerosis. Because hypertension is frequently a lifelong problem, some form of pharmacologic therapy may be used for many years in individual patients. This necessity has raised considerable concern about the additional effects of a pharmacologic agent apart from its presumed beneficial effect in lowering blood pressure. For example, several studies[2] have noted that the β-blockers and thiazide diuretics can adversely affect lipid profiles, as characterized by a reduction in the high-density lipoprotein cholesterol concentration, a rise in the low-density lipoprotein (LDL) cholesterol concentration, or both. On the other hand, some drugs such as doxazosin can favorably affect the lipid profile in patients so treated.[3] Although it is unclear whether these modest changes necessarily influence either the potential for developing atherosclerosis or its time course, it seems preferable to use agents that favorably affect lipid profiles or, alternatively, that have been shown to reduce the rate at which atherosclerosis progresses.

As a class, the calcium antagonists have emerged as beneficial therapy for a wide variety of cardiovascular disorders. In particular, one of their greatest uses may be in the management of essential hypertension. Recent evidence has focused on the potential for calcium antagonists to retard the development of experimental atherosclerosis. The purpose of this chapter is to briefly summarize these results.

PATHOGENESIS OF ATHEROSCLEROSIS

Although agreement is incomplete on the processes that lead to the development of atherosclerosis, certain general facts and principles appear to be important.[4] The fatty streaks seen in the arteries of children are probable precursors of the atherosclerotic fibrous plaque that develops, but some controversy remains about this topic. The fatty streaks appear to be caused in part by the migration of monocytes or macrophages, and perhaps some smooth muscle cells, through the endothelial layer. These cells then take up lipid and are thereby transformed into foam cells; the lipid in these foam cells exists primarily in the form of cholesterol and cholesterol ester. Much of the lipid located within these fatty streaks undoubtedly comes from the plasma, but it may be hydrolyzed and reesterified once it enters the cells.

Central to most hypotheses describing atherosclerosis is the crucial role of the endothelium. Damage to the endothelium may be the initial precipitating event that sets in motion a sequence of events leading to atherosclerosis. Causes of endothelial damage could include, among others, such factors as mechanical injury from hypertension, hypercholesterolemia, homocystinemia, and immune injury. With endothelial damage, platelet attachment can occur, and the role of the platelets becomes pivotal in the development of atherosclerotic plaques. Following platelet aggregation, platelet-derived growth factor is released, which leads to the migration of smooth muscle cells from the media to the intima and subsequent mitosis of these cells. These smooth muscle cells subsequently secrete elastin, collagen, and glycosaminoglycans. These substances can bind LDL cholesterol, which may be crucial in the development of extracellular deposits of lipid and, in the late stage, leads to the formation of a fibrous plaque. The complex atherosclerotic plaque consists primarily of an accumulation of these smooth muscle cells laden with lipid, which is mostly cholesterol and cholesterol esters. The cells also exist in a matrix of lipid, collagen, elastic fibers, and glycosaminoglycans. The extracellular matrix, together with these cells, forms a fibrous cap that covers a large underlying deposit of cell debris and extracellular lipid. The late stage of this so-called complex plaque is characterized by cell necrosis, calcification, hemorrhage, and mural thrombosis.

CALCIUM AND ATHEROSCLEROSIS

Normally, there is about a 10,000-fold concentration gradient of calcium from the extracellular to the intracellular space. During any injury to cell membranes, there is a natural flow of calcium from the extracellular space into the cell, with subsequent cellular damage and death.[5] Much of this cellular damage may be produced by attachment of calcium to mitrochondria, which depresses their phosphorylation potential and levels of high-energy phosphates, thus impairing cellular structure and function. During cell damage or death, calcification is an invariable accompaniment, as witnessed by the calcification of damaged atherosclerotic tissue.

Calcium has been shown to be a cofactor in many of the steps involved in the pathogenesis of atherosclerosis, including aggregation of platelets, release of platelet-derived growth factor, smooth muscle cell mitosis, lipid binding to macromolecules, and protein synthesis. This role of calcium has led to the speculation that inhibition of calcium entry might retard or prevent the atherosclerotic process. The next sections summarize a few of the studies that have investigated the potential benefit of drugs that interfere with calcium entry in experimental atherosclerosis.

EFFECTS OF DRUGS ON EXPERIMENTAL ATHEROSCLEROSIS

Catecholamines appear to enhance the entry of calcium through the adenyl cyclase-cyclic adenosine monophosphate system. A potential role in retarding the development of atherosclerosis may therefore exist for agents that interfere with the catecholamine system. In an early study, Whittington-Coleman and Carrier[6] fed rabbits cholesterol and oral reserpine, a reserpine analogue, and guanethidine. They noted that calcium content, fat deposition, and the number of intimal lesions in the aorta were decreased and postulated that decreased calcium entry may have played a role. In this study, rabbits were fed a 2% (by weight) cholesterol diet for 10 weeks. In general, the drugs did not affect lipid levels, and a slight decrease in arterial pressure occurred. Additional studies by this same group[7] with propranolol showed a reduction in the calcium content of treated animals fed a high-lipid diet compared with control animals that did not receive the propranolol. The reduction in atherosclerosis in both of these studies suggests catecholamines or their subsequent effects on calcium entry play an important role.

A number of studies have evaluated a wide range of drugs that appear to share the common property of decreasing the amount of calcium in the aorta, even though they are otherwise quite different in their pharmacologic effects. Morrison et al.[8] gave young adult rats a high-lipid diet and excess vitamin D, which led to the development of severe lesions in the coronary arteries and aorta. The subsequent addition of chondroitin sulfate A showed a marked reduction in coronary lesions that contained lipid. No decrease occurred, however, in levels of either liver lipids or plasma lipids. The presumed mechanism of chondroitin sulfate A was to inhibit the deposition of calcium in connective tissue.

In another model employing hypervitaminosis D, nicotine, and a hypercholesterolemic diet, Rosenblum et al.[9] noted the effectiveness of EHDP (ethane-1-hydroxy-1,1-diphosphonate) in preventing atherosclerosis. An inhibition of arterial calcification and the development of plaques occurred but no major effect on serum lipid levels was noted. EHDP also inhibited vitamin D-induced hypercalcemia. In general, the diphosphonates appeared to be effective in inhibiting the pathologic calcification that occurs in this animal model.

Potokar and Schmidt-Dunker[10] showed that three diphosphonic compounds also inhibited vitamin D–induced calcification of aortas and kidneys in rats. It is of interest that these compounds were chosen because of *in vitro* effectiveness in preventing crystallization of hydroxyapatite.

Chan et al.[11] studied thiophene compounds. These compounds markedly reduce calcium and phosphorus levels in rats. In tissue, they can inhibit spontaneous and parathyroid-induced resorption of bone. The proposed mechanism of action is inhibition of calcium transfer out of bone. In rabbits fed high-lipid diets, several thiophene compounds reduced the increased calcium level to normal although there was no effect on cholesterol levels. A clear-cut reduction was seen in the development of atherosclerosis in these animals. A close correlation was noted between the amount of calcium deposition in the aorta and the atherosclerotic lesions. In a related study, Wartman et al.[12] noted that EDTA, the calcium chelator, also apparently inhibited plaque formation in rabbits fed high-lipid diets.

Kramsch and Chan[13] studied the effects of EHDP and colcemide in rabbits receiving a high-lipid diet. Both drugs were somewhat effective alone, but the combination was especially effective in preventing the development of atherosclerosis. Suggested mechanisms include the fact that colcemide binds to tubule subunits and disrupts the microtubular assembly. This action was believed to suppress proliferation and mobility in the cells as well as the ability of cells to secrete substances such as connective tissue proteins and glycosaminoglycans. Both drugs were shown to decrease both serum and lesion content of calcium in these animals.

Although many studies have been done with lipids fed to rabbits, this procedure creates mostly a foam cell model of atherosclerosis and does not approach the complex lesions seen in patients with atherosclerosis. Monkeys, however, appear to have lesions more comparable with those seen in humans. Kramsch et al.[14] extended these studies to monkeys and demonstrated that the agents discussed previously, as well as diphosphonates or lanthanum, a metallic element that occurs in rare earth minerals and has been shown to displace calcium from cell membranes, were effective in decreasing wall calcium and the degree of atherosclerosis. In these studies, the aortas removed from the treated animals had less collagen, elastin, cholesterol, calcium, and DNA than the aortas from untreated animals.

CALCIUM ANTAGONISTS AND EXPERIMENTAL ATHEROSCLEROSIS

The first study with a calcium antagonist was done by Henry and Bentley,[15] who studied the effects of nifedipine in rabbits fed a high-lipid diet. Forty milligrams per day was given in divided doses. Only transient changes occurred in arterial pressure, and these were thought not to play an important role in the protective effect demonstrated. Plasma cholesterol levels rose to just under 2000 mg/dl. In the animals on the diet only, 40% of the aorta was covered with lesions stained by Sudan 4, which indicates lipid deposition, whereas the rabbits treated with nifedipine had lesions over only 17% of the area. Similarly, a reduction occurred in the cholesterol concentration in the aortic tissue.

Other studies with the dihydropyridines have confirmed this protective effect against atherosclerosis. Willis et al.[16] used high-dose nifedipine and nicardipine in rabbits fed a high-cholesterol diet. They found that these two drugs reduced aortic lesions and both cholesterol and triglyceride levels in the aorta. There are a few clues as to the mechanism of action of the dihydropyridines. Nakao et al.[17] noted that nicardipine inhibited the migration of cultured vascular smooth muscle cells—an important step in the genesis of an atherosclerosis plaque. In another study, Etingin and Hajjar[18] showed that nifedipine increased cholesteryl ester hydrolysis, producing a 50 percent loss of cholesterol and cholesteryl esters from aortic cultured smooth muscle cells, which were filled with lipid.

The positive effects of diltiazem were demonstrated by Ginsburg et al.,[19] who also evaluated the effects of lanthanum and flunarizine on aortic and coronary atherosclerosis. Rabbits were fed a 2% cholesterol diet for 10 weeks, and all three drugs decreased lipid deposition in the aorta from 52% of the endothelial surface in the control group to about 37% in the treated group. These authors noted one interesting fact: there was no suppression of atherogenesis in the intramural coronary arteries.

Our own studies have primarily used verapamil as a calcium antagonist. In the initial study,[20] the use of lanthanum as well as of different doses of verapamil were evaluated. In rabbits fed a high-lipid diet for 10 weeks, cholesterol levels rose to about 2000 mg/dL. The animals treated with verapamil did not have a reduction in lipid levels. If anything, the levels may have been slightly higher. Figure 98–1 shows representative aortas from the different groups of rabbits.[21] A reduction occurred in the degree of lipid deposition in the animals treated with the high dose of vera-

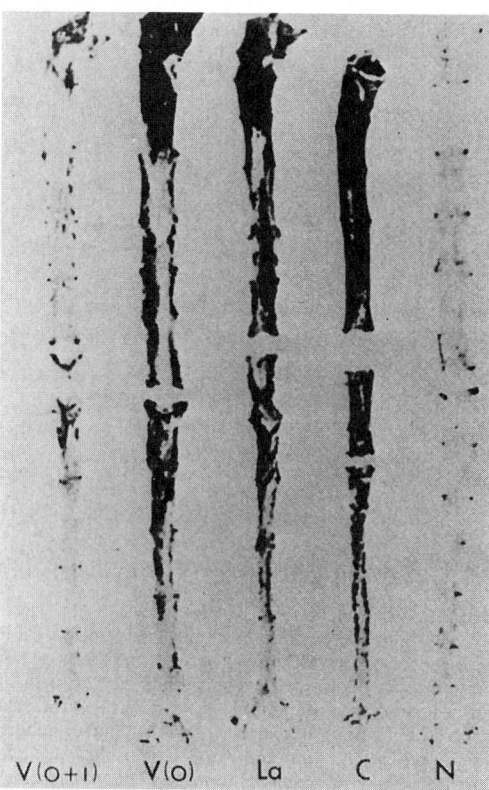

Figure 98–1. Representative aortas from different groups of rabbits showing the surface area (black) involved with atherosclerosis (Sudan 4 stain). From left to right, oral plus injected high-dose verapamil [V(o + i)], oral high-dose verapamil [V(o)], lanthanum (La), control (C) atherosclerotic, and normal (N) rabbits. (From Rouleau JL, Parmley WW, Stevens J, et al: Verapamil suppresses atherosclerosis in cholesterol-fed rabbits. J Am Coll Cardiol 1:1453, 1983.)

pamil. Despite this apparently high dose, however, serum levels of verapamil were low (12 ng/ml) compared with usual clinical levels, which may range from 100 to 200 ng/ml. It therefore appears that the high doses given in rabbits are compatible with the usual doses of calcium antagonists given to patients. Figure 98–2 shows the relationship of the percentage of aortic endothelial surface that was lipid-stained as a function of the serum cholesterol level. A slight but not statistically significant reduction in the amount of endothelial surface involved was noted in the lanthanum and low-dose verapamil groups, whereas the high-dose verapamil group showed a substantial reduction from 75% to 25%, even though there was a slight increase in the serum cholesterol level.

To determine whether verapamil might have been protective by lowering blood pressure, another study[22] was performed in which groups of animals were treated for 10 weeks with either verapamil, metoprolol, hydralazine, or a combination of metoprolol and hydralazine. The results of this study are shown in Figure 98–3. The percentage of aortic surface covered by plaque is shown as a function of the blood pressure throughout the study (obtained by an ear artery occlusion technique). In the control group approximately 50% of the aorta was covered by plaque. No protective effect was noted in the hydralazine

group, the metoprolol group, and the metoprolol-hydralazine combination group, despite a slight reduction in arterial pressure. The results in the group with undetectable levels of verapamil were similar to those in the control group, whereas there was a slight reduction in blood pressure but a more substantial reduction in plaque in the group with detectable serum levels of verapamil. Thus, although there was a slight reduction in blood pressure in all of the treated groups when compared with the control group, only the group with detectable serum levels of verapamil showed a reduction in the percentage of aortic surface covered by plaque. It therefore appeared that reduction of blood pressure was not a contributing factor to the protective effect of verapamil.

After demonstrating that the development of experimental atherosclerosis could be attenuated with verapamil, a study was designed to determine whether the atherosclerotic process in the rabbit model could be reversed with either verapamil or a combination of verapamil and a change in diet.[23] Rabbits were again placed on a high-lipid diet for various times during a 24-week period and treated with verapamil at various times to evaluate the role of verapamil in either preventing or causing a regression of atherosclerosis. Figure 98–4 demonstrates the percentage of surface area on the aorta covered by lipid for the different groups. Each black dot represents a 12-week period on a high-lipid diet, whereas an open circle represents 12 weeks on a normal diet. An additional outer circle represents treatment with verapamil dur-

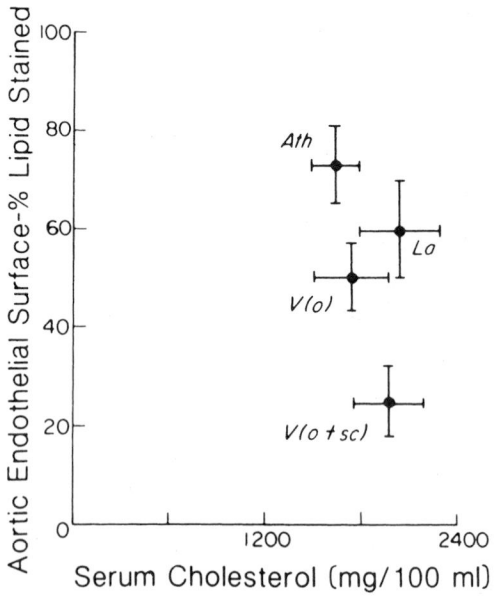

Figure 98–2. Relationship of the percentage of aortic surface involved with athersclerosis to the mean serum cholesterol concentration within each group of rabbits. The atherosclerotic control (Ath) animals are at the top. The rabbits treated with oral plus subcutaneous verapamil V(o + sc) had less surface area involved than the atherosclerotic (Ath) control subjects. V(o), rabbits treated with oral high-dose verapamil; La, rabbits treated with lanthanum. (From Rouleau JL, Parmley WW, Stevens J, et al: Verapamil suppresses atherosclerosis in cholesterol-fed rabbits. J Am Coll Cardiol 1:1453, 1983.)

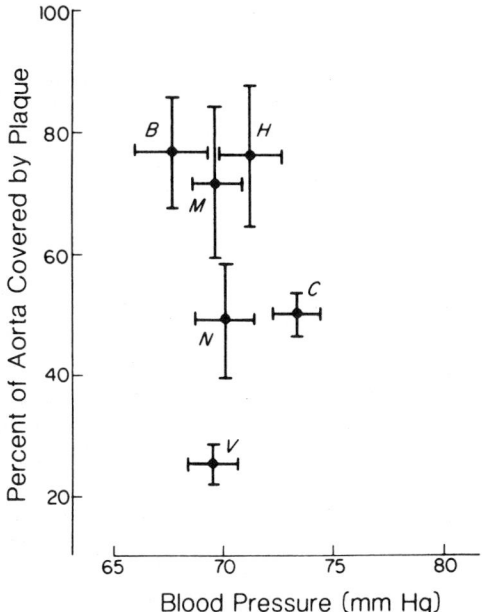

Figure 98–3. Average blood pressure in different groups of rabbits during the entire study plotted in relation to the percentage of aortic surface covered by plaque. C, control atherosclerotic group; M, metroprolol; H, hydralazine; B, hydralazine plus metoprolol; N, nondetectable serum levels of verapamil; V, detectable serum levels of verapamil. Note that all drug-related groups had a slightly lower blood pressure than control subjects. Only the group with detectable serum levels of verapamil (V), however, had a reduction in atherosclerotic plaque. (From Blumlein SL, Sievers R, Kidd P, et al: Mechanism of protection for atherosclerosis by verapamil in the cholesterol-fed rabbit. Am J Cardiol 54:884, 1984.)

normal diet halfway through the study apparently did not retard the development of atherosclerosis, indicating that a sequence of events had been set in motion that could not be easily reversed by diet alone at that point. Group IV comprises animals treated with verapamil and a high-lipid diet for all 24 weeks. These animals experienced a reduction in lipid deposition compared with the control group (group II). Group V was given verapamil only during the last 12 weeks and showed a slight but not statistically significant reduction in lipid deposition compared with the control group (group II). Of interest was group VI, which had a normal diet and which received verapamil during the last 12 weeks and showed significantly less atherosclerosis than the control groups (groups II and III). Thus, it appeared that a combination of verapamil and switching to a normal diet was required to retard the continued deposition of lipid. Group VI therefore was comparable with group I because both groups had received a high-lipid diet for the first 12 weeks.

It is clear that findings in this animal model, studied for a short time, may not have direct relevance to humans. Nevertheless, it appears that verapamil was far more effective in preventing atherosclerosis than it was in inducing its regression. If this principle has application to humans, it would suggest that the long-term application of calcium antagonists before the establishment of severe atherosclerosis may be more beneficial than the application of calcium antagonists during an established end stage of atherosclerosis. From the rabbit data, it appears that cessation of cholesterol feeding can cause regression of early aortic atherosclerotic lesions, whereas in several studies lesions induced by several months of cholesterol feeding did not undergo reduction in response to a change in diet alone.

Not all studies of calcium antagonists have yielded positive results. Stender et al.[24] reported no effect with high-dose nifedipine in rabbits fed cholesterol. The reason for this negative finding is not clear but may be related to the dose and route of administration.

ing that 12-week period. Groups I and II therefore represent the effects of 12 and 24 weeks, respectively, on the high-lipid diet. Note the progression of atherosclerosis from about 35% to 80%. This increase represents the natural progression of the deposition of lipid from 12 to 24 weeks. In group III (normal diet for the last 12 weeks), the percentage of lipid deposition was almost the same as that of rabbits on the high-lipid diet for all 24 weeks (group II). Thus, switching to a

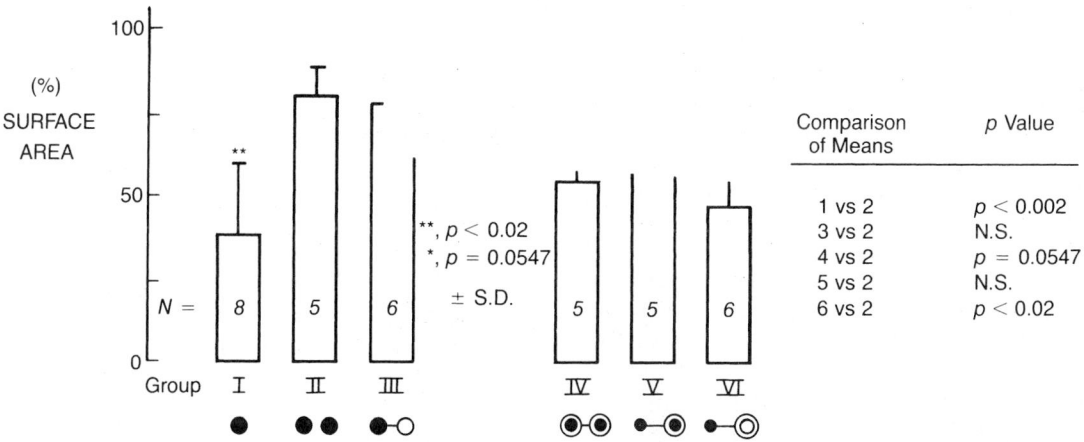

Figure 98–4. Percentage of aortic surface area covered by plaque for different groups of rabbits. ●, 12 weeks on a high-lipid diet; ○, 12 weeks on a normal diet; ◯, 12-week treatment with verapamil. See text for discussion. (From Sievers R, Rashid T, Garrett J, et al: Verapamil and diet halt progression of atherosclerosis in cholesterol-fed rabbits. Cardiovasc Drugs Ther 1:65, 1987.)

Because the nifedipine was given sublingually, it may have produced hypotension leading to a reflexive increase in sympathetic discharge. Increased catecholamine levels presumably contribute to atherosclerosis, because agents that interfere with catecholamines have had a protective effect against the development of experimental atherosclerosis. Therefore, in this study, reflexive sympathetic discharge may have countered any beneficial effects of nifedipine.

In another negative study, Naito et al.[25] found that nicardipine and diltiazem were ineffective in cholesterol-fed rabbits. Minimal aortic involvement, however, and wide variability in the results may have influenced the outcome of the study.

An interesting model of atherosclerosis is the Watanabe rabbit, which appears to lack LDL receptors and is therefore an animal model of familial hypercholesterolemia. In studies of such rabbits treated with verapamil[26] or nifedipine,[27] there was no protection against the development of atherosclerosis. Perhaps the insult of the hypercholesterolemia was too great or, alternatively, the presence of LDL receptors might be important in mediating the effects of verapamil. Stein and associates[28] concluded that verapamil worked by enhancing the uptake and disposal of LDL cholesterol by the LDL receptors. Thus, without any LDL receptors, verapamil would be ineffective. The drug captopril was effective in Watanabe rabbits in reducing the development of atherosclerosis.[29] Because ACE inhibitors reduce calcium influx by attenuating sympathetic outflow and reducing angiotensin-II levels, these data are consistent with the calcium hypothesis.

CLINICAL STUDIES

A number of clinical studies have addressed the question of the potential for calcium antagonists to attenuate the progression of atherosclerosis. Results from a few studies are described below.

Kober et al.[30] retrospectively evaluated 43 patients following bypass surgery or angioplasty, 26 of whom received verapamil and 17 of whom received no calcium antagonist. Over an average of 16 months there was a similar progression of coronary disease in both groups. Regression of high-grade lesions was more frequent in the verapamil-treated group than in the control group (41% versus 12%), and the development of new lesions was more frequent in the control group (10.9% versus 3.3%).

The International Nifedipine Trial on Atherosclerosis (INTACT)[31] randomized patients to nifedipine (steady-state dose of 20 mg qid) or a placebo. After an average follow-up of 2 years, there was no significant difference in lesion progression or regression. There were, however, fewer new lesions (0.59 versus 0.82) in the nifedipine-treated group.

In the Montreal Heart Institute Study,[32] patients were randomized to nicardipine versus placebo. As in the INTACT study, there was no difference in progression or regression between the two groups at 24 months. However, progression of low-grade lesions was less frequent in the nicardipine-treated group (9.0% versus 16.3%).

In a group of patients with new-onset angina, Loaldi et al.[33] randomized them to nifedipine, propranolol, or isosorbide dinitrate. With angiographic follow-up at 2 years, 31% of the nifedipine-treated patients had progression of lesions compared with 53% of those receiving propranolol and with 47% of those receiving isosorbide dinitrate.

A study by Schroeder et al.[34] suggested that diltiazem can attenuate the development of atherosclerosis in heart transplant recipients. Three additional trials will be reported soon. These are the Multicenter Isradipine Diuretic Atherosclerosis Study (MIDAS),[35] the Frankfurt Isoptin Progression Study (FIPS), and the Verapamil-Hypertension Atherosclerosis Study (VHAS).[36]

The significance of these clinical trials is difficult to judge. In general, these studies show no regression, with the exception of the Kober trial.[30] The most consistent effect is fewer new lesions in the patients treated with a calcium antagonist. This effect is very modest, although the average time interval is short (2 years). This result, however, is consistent with animal studies in which the usual effect is attenuation rather than regression of lesions. Perhaps this effect would be clinically significant in patients with hypertension who were treated for many years. It is important to appreciate that not all experimental studies have shown a positive result with calcium antagonists. In 44 such studies,[37] 31 demonstrated attenuation when the calcium antagonist was started early. In eight studies, no benefit was seen when the calcium antagonist was started late. This further emphasizes the principle that calcium antagonists may be better at primary rather than secondary prevention.

The potential mechanism or mechanisms whereby calcium antagonists attenuate atherosclerosis is still uncertain. They might affect any of the calcium-dependent processes in the development of atherosclerosis. This might include their effects on hydrolysis of cholesterol esters,[38] on lipoprotein uptake,[28] or on smooth muscle cell migration[39] and mitosis.[40] Whatever their principal effects, this potential benefit of calcium antagonists should be carefully considered by clinicians choosing long-term therapy for essential hypertension.

REFERENCES

1. Kannel WB: New perspectives on cardiovascular risk factors. Am Heart J 114:213, 1987.
2. Weidmann P, Vehlinger DE, Gerber A: Editorial review: Antihypertensive treatment and serum lipoproteins. J Hypertens 3:297, 1985.
3. Trost BN, Weidmann P, Reisen W, et al: Comparative effects of doxazosin and hydrochlorothiazide on serum lipids and blood pressure in essential hypertension. Am J Cardiol 59:99G, 1987.
4. Wissler RW: Principles of the pathogenesis of atherosclerosis. In Braunwald E (ed): Heart Disease, 2nd ed. Philadelphia: WB Saunders, 1984, p 1183.
5. McCall D, Walsh RA, Frohlich ED, et al: Calcium entry blocking drugs: Mechanisms of action, experimental studies and clinical uses. Curr Probl Cardiol 10:8, 1985.

6. Whittington-Coleman PJ, Carrier O Jr: Effects of agents altering vascular calcium in experimental atherosclerosis. Atherosclerosis 12:15, 1970.

7. Whittington-Coleman PJ, Carrier O Jr, Douglas BH: The effects of propranolol on cholesterol-induced atheromatous lesions. Atherosclerosis 18:337, 1973.

8. Morrison LM, Bajwa GS, Alfin-Slater RB, et al: Prevention of vascular lesions by chondroitin sulfate A in the coronary artery and aorta of rats induced by a hypervitaminosis D, cholesterol-containing diet. Atherosclerosis 16:105, 1972.

9. Rosenblum IY, Flora L, Eisenstein R: The effect of disodium ethane-1 hydroxyl-1,1-diphosphonate (EHDP) on rabbit model of atheroarteriosclerosis. Atherosclerosis 22:411, 1975.

10. Potokar M, Schmidt-Dunker M: The inhibitory effect of new diphosphonic acids on aortic and kidney calcification in vivo. Atherosclerosis 30:313, 1978.

11. Chan CT, Wells H, Kramsch DM: Suppression of calcific fibrous-fatty plaque formation in rabbits by agents not affecting elevated serum cholesterol levels. Circ Res 43:115, 1978.

12. Wartman A, Lampe TL, McCann DS, et al: Plaque reversal with Mg EDTA in experimental atherosclerosis: Elastin and collagen metabolism. J Atheroscler Res 7:331, 1967.

13. Kramsch DM, Chan CT: The effect of agents interfering with soft tissue calcification and cell proliferation on calcific fibrous-fatty plaques in rabbits. Circ Res 42:562, 1978.

14. Kramsch DM, Aspen AJ, Rozier LJ: Atherosclerosis: Prevention by agents not affecting abnormal levels of blood lipids. Science 213:1511, 1981.

15. Henry PD, Bentley KI: Suppression of atherosclerosis in cholesterol-fed rabbit treated with nifedipine. J Clin Invest 68:1366, 1981.

16. Willis AL, Nagel B, Churchill V, et al: Anti-atherosclerotic effects of nicardipine and nifedipine in cholesterol-fed rabbits. Arteriosclerosis 5:250, 1985.

17. Nakao J, Ito H, Oyama T, et al: Calcium dependency of aortic smooth muscle cell migration induced by 12-L-hydroxy-5,8,10,14-eicosatetraenoic acid—effects of A23187, nicardipine, and trifluorperazine. Atherosclerosis 46:309, 1983.

18. Etingin OR, Hajjar DP: Nifedipine increases cholesteryl ester hydrolytic activity in lipid-laden rabbit arterial smooth muscle cells: A possible mechanism for its anti-atherogenic effect. J Clin Invest 75:1554, 1985.

19. Ginsburg R, Davis K, Bristow MR, et al: Calcium antagonists suppress atherogenesis in aorta but not in the intramural coronary arteries of cholesterol-fed rabbits. Lab Invest 49:154, 1983.

20. Kramsch DM, Aspen AJ, Apstein CS: Suppression of experimental atherosclerosis by the Ca++-antagonist lanthanum. J Clin Invest 65:967, 1980.

21. Rouleau J-L, Parmley WW, Stevens J, et al: Verapamil suppresses atherosclerosis in cholesterol-fed rabbits. J Am Coll Cardiol 1:1453, 1983.

22. Blumlein SL, Sievers R, Kidd P, et al: Mechanism of protection for atherosclerosis by verapamil in the cholesterol-fed rabbit. Am J Cardiol 54:884, 1984.

23. Sievers R, Rashid T, Garrett J, et al: Verapamil and diet halt progression of atherosclerosis in cholesterol fed rabbits. Cardiovasc Drugs Ther 1:65, 1987.

24. Stender S, Stender I, Nordestgaard B, et al: No effect of nifedipine on atherogenesis in cholesterol-fed rabbits. Arteriosclerosis 4:389, 1984.

25. Naito M, Kuzuya F, Asai K, et al: Ineffectiveness of Ca²⁺-antagonists nicardipine and diltiazem on experimental atherosclerosis in cholesterol-fed rabbits. Angiology 35:622, 1984.

26. Tilton GD, Buja LM, Bilheimer DW, et al: Failure of a slow channel calcium antagonist, verapamil, to retard atherosclerosis in the Watanabe heritable hyperlipidemic rabbit: An animal model of familial hypercholesterolemia. J Am Coll Cardiol 6:141, 1985.

27. Va Niekerk JLM, Hendriks T, De Boer HHM, et al: Does nifedipine suppress atherogenesis in WHHL rabbits? Atherosclerosis 53:91, 1984.

28. Stein O, Leitersdorf E, Stein Y: Verapamil enhances receptor-mediated endocytosis of low density lipoproteins by aortic cells in culture. Arteriosclerosis 5:35, 1985.

29. Chobanian AV, Haudenschild CC, Nickerson C, et al: Antiatherogenic effect of captopril in the Wananabe heritable hyperlipidemic rabbit. Hypertension 15:327, 1990.

30. Kober G, Schneider W, Kaltenbach M: Can the progression of coronary sclerosis be influenced by calcium antagonists? J Cardiovasc Pharmacol 13(Suppl 4):S2, 1990.

31. Lichtlen PR, Hugenholtz PG, Rafflenbeul W, et al: Retardation of angiographic progression of coronary artery disease by nifedipine: Results of the International Nifedipine Trial on Anti-atherosclerotic Therapy (INTACT). Lancet 335:1109, 1990.

32. Waters D, Lesperance J, Francetich M, et al: A controlled clinical trial to assess the effect of a calcium channel blocker on the progression of coronary atherosclerosis. Circulation 82:1940, 1990.

33. Loaldi A, Polese A, Montorsi P, et al: Comparison of nifedipine, propranolol and isosorbide dinitrate on angiographic progression and regression of coronary arterial narrowings in angina pectoris. Am J Cardiol 64:433, 1989.

34. Schroeder JS, Gao SZ, Alderman EL, et al: A preliminary study of diltiazem in the prevention of coronary artery disease in heart transplant recipients. N Engl J Med 328:164, 1993.

35. The MIDAS Research Group, Furberg CD, Byington RP, et al: Multicenter Isradipine Diuretic Atherosclerosis Study (MIDAS). Am J Med 86(Suppl 4A):37, 1989.

36. Zanchetti A, Magnani B, Dal Pal'o C: Atherosclerosis and calcium antagonists: The Verapamil-Hypertension Atherosclerosis Study (VHAS). J Hum Hypertens 6(Suppl 2):545, 1992.

37. Jackson CL, Bush RC, Bowyer DE: Mechanism of antiatherogenic effect of calcium antagonists. Atherosclerosis 80:17, 1989.

38. Etingin OR, Hajjar DP: Nifedipine increases cholestryl ester hydrolytic activity in lipid-laden rabbit arterial smooth muscle cells: A possible mechanism for its antiatherogenic effect. J Clin Invest 75:1554, 1985.

39. Nakao J, Ito H, Ooyama T, et al: Calcium dependency of aortic smooth muscle cell migration induced by 12-L-hydroxy-5,8,10,14-eicosatetraenoic acid. Atherosclerosis 46:309, 1983.

40. Van Valen RG, Deacon RW, Farley C, et al: Antiproliferative effect of calcium channel blockers PN 200-110 and PY 108-068 in the rat carotid model of balloon catheterization [abstract]. Fed Proc 44:737, 1985.

CHAPTER 99

Cardiac Effects of Calcium Antagonists in Hypertension

Franz H. Messerli, M.D., and Franz C. Aepfelbacher, M.D.

Since Fleckenstein's pioneering observations that calcium antagonists have a "cardioprotective" effect against isoproterenol-induced myocardial necrosis,[1] a variety of other effects of calcium antagonists on the heart have been identified. In this context, it is important to differentiate between the direct and indirect cardiac effects of calcium antagonists.[2, 3] Thus, most calcium antagonists will exert negative inotropic and chronotropic effects in isolated myocyte preparations. In hypertensive patients, however, calcium antagonists, because of their powerful unloading effect, may acutely increase cardiac output and heart rate and thereby be perceived as positive inotropic and chronotropic agents.[4–7] Even verapamil has been shown to increase cardiac output and heart rate when given intravenously.[6] Analysis of the cardiac effects of calcium antagonists becomes even more difficult because normal and diseased myocardium may respond differently. In addition, the effects on afterload, left ventricular hypertrophy (LVH), coronary blood flow, left ventricular filling, contractility, and conduction vary from one calcium antagonist to another.[4–8] The following is an attempt to analyze the effects of calcium antagonists on cardiac function and structure in patients with hypertension.

EFFECTS ON ARTERIAL PRESSURE

All calcium antagonists lower arterial pressure when given acutely and with prolonged administration.[4–8] Although there are head-to-head comparisons of five different calcium antagonists, it seems that there is little if any difference in blood pressure-lowering potency among the various agents, provided that adequate doses are given.[4–8] The effect on arterial pressure seems to be somewhat more powerful in elderly or black patients, who are characterized by low activity of the renin-angiotensin system, than in young or white patients,[9, 10] although age and race dependency of the antihypertensive effects have not been documented by all studies.[9, 10] Conceivably the greater efficacy of calcium antagonists in elderly patients may depend on a higher pretreatment blood pressure and on decreased metabolic activity. At least in one study much of the correlation between age and antihypertensive response was lost when corrections for pretreatment pressures and plasma levels were made.[11]

EFFECTS ON HEART RATE

Calcium antagonists lower arterial pressure by decreasing total peripheral resistance. As a consequence, reflexive tachycardia and an increase in cardiac output are common.[4–8] Cardioacceleration occurs acutely with the first dose of most agents but becomes less pronounced with chronic administration.[4–6] However, with some of the dihydropyridine calcium antagonists, such as nifedipine and nitrendipine, even after months of administration a slight increase in heart rate has been documented in some studies. An increase in plasma catecholamine (and in plasma renin) activity usually accompanies this positive chronotropic effect, indicating a reflexive increase in activity of the sympathetic nervous system.[4–8] In contrast, chronic administration of drugs such as verapamil and, to a lesser extent, diltiazem and gallopamil has been shown to decrease heart rate and to lead to a fall in plasma catecholamine and angiotensin concentrations.[4, 6] Similarly, long-term administration of isradipine, felodipine, or amlodipine seems to have little if any effect on heart rate and seems not to activate the sympathetic nervous system or the renin-angiotensin system (Table 99–1).[5, 12] Conceivably, the direct effect of these drugs on the sinus nodes prevents the reflexive tachycardia seen with other dihydropyridine antagonists.[13, 14]

EFFECTS ON CORONARY BLOOD FLOW

All calcium antagonists are vasodilators and therefore increase coronary blood flow.[15–21] It must be emphasized that coronary blood flow is but one determinant of the myocardial oxygen supply-and-demand equilibrium.[22] Other determinants, such as heart rate, contractility, and arterial pressure, are also profoundly and variably affected by calcium antagonists. Thus, their overall effects on myocardial oxygenation will depend on an interplay of these mechanisms.[22–26] It therefore should not be surprising that, in certain clinical situations, some calcium antagonists may even have a detrimental effect on myocardial oxygenation. Thus, acute exacerbation of angina and even acute myocardial infarction were observed when arterial pressure was excessively lowered as a result of reflexive cardioacceleration and a paradoxical increase in myocardial oxygen demand.[27–30]

Calcium antagonists, however, generally improve myocardial oxygenation by unloading the heart, increasing coronary blood flow, and reducing myocardial energy consumption.[15–21] These properties have made them agents of choice in treating certain forms of angina pectoris, particularly when it is caused by vasospasm.[17–19] Agents that accelerate heart rate, such

Table 99–1. **Acute and Long-term Effects of Calcium Antagonists on Heart Rate, Contractility, and Plasma Catecholamine Levels**

	Acute Effects		Long-term Effects		
Drug	*Heart Rate*	*Contractility*	*Heart Rate*	*Contractility*	*Plasma Catecholamine Levels*
Verapamil	↑	↓ ↓	↓ ↓	↓ ↓	↔
Diltiazem	↑	↓ ↓	↓	↓ ↓	↔
Gallopamil	↑	↓ ↓	↓	↓ ↓	↔
Nifedipine	↑ ↑	↓	↑	↓	↑ (?)
Nitrendipine	↑ ↑	↓	↑	↓	↑ (?)
Nicardipine	↑ ↑	↔	↑	↓	↑ (?)
Isradipine	↑ ↑	↔	↔	↔	↔
Felodipine	↑	↔	↔	↔	↔
Amlodipine	↑	↔	↔	↔	↔

as most dihydropyridine calcium antagonists, evidently are somewhat less effective in improving myocardial oxygenation than agents that diminish heart rate. Effects of calcium antagonists on LVH and left ventricular filling that become evident only after prolonged administration also improve the equilibrium between myocardial oxygen supply and demand.[4–6, 8]

EFFECTS ON CARDIAC CONDUCTION

In pharmacologic doses, most calcium antagonists diminish the automaticity of the sinus node, slow conduction in the atrioventricular (AV) node, and have little if any effect on the automaticity of the myocytes.[31] These electrophysiologic properties, however, vary a great deal from one drug to another and also seem to depend upon the form of application.[31–33] Verapamil, when given intravenously, has a marked effect on the AV node that can be used therapeutically in patients with supraventricular tachycardia.[34–37] In fact, transient AV block is not an uncommon occurrence with intravenous verapamil.[31] In contrast, complete AV block is exceedingly rare with oral verapamil. A slight prolongation of the PR interval to about the same extent can be seen with both verapamil and diltiazem, provided that equipotent oral antihypertensive doses are used.[31] The dihydropyridine calcium antagonists generally have less effect on cardiac conduction than the nondihydropyridine calcium antagonists.[31]

EFFECTS ON CARDIAC CONTRACTILITY

By and large, calcium antagonists are negative inotropic agents and therefore are likely to impair cardiac pump function to some extent (see Table 99–1).[2, 3, 37–47] The most profound negative inotropic effect is seen with verapamil and diltiazem.[32, 34–38, 46] This direct effect is partially overridden by afterload reduction and its reflexive sympathetic drive elicited by most of the dihydropyridine derivates. Some of the newer agents, such as isradipine, felodipine, and amlodipine, seem to have little if any negative inotropic

effect. In fact, some of these drugs have been used successfully in patients with congestive heart failure caused by predominantly systolic dysfunction. Thus, favorable hemodynamic responses such as decreases in pulmonary wedge pressure and end-diastolic ventricular pressure were documented when these agents (isradipine, felodipine, and amlodipine) were given over a short period.[48] In contrast to other dihydropyridine calcium antagonists, little or no stimulation of the sympathetic nervous system or the renin-angiotensin system occurs with isradipine, felodipine, or amlodipine. In this context, it should be remembered that improvement of hemodynamics in patients with congestive heart failure does not necessarily parallel increased survival rate. Two placebo-controlled studies evaluating the effects of amlodipine and felodipine on morbidity and mortality in patients with congestive heart failure have been presented and seem to attest to the safety of these agents in certain patients with congestive heart failure. As a general rule, however, most calcium antagonists should be avoided in patients with congestive heart failure caused by systolic dysfunction.

EFFECTS ON LEFT VENTRICULAR FILLING

Considered simplistically, left ventricular filling consists of an early diastolic active relaxation phase and a late diastolic passive distensibility phase. Calcium antagonists have been documented to have a favorable effect on both.[49, 50] When given intravenously, they improve early diastolic relaxation,[50] which has been shown to be impaired very early in patients with essential hypertension.[50] This effect may be heart rate dependent and seems to be most pronounced with verapamil, less so with diltiazem, and even less so with the dihydropyridine calcium antagonists. With prolonged administration of most calcium antagonists, late diastolic distensibility is improved as well. This effect may be related to a decrease in left ventricular wall thickness resulting from prolonged administration.[51, 52] The clinical significance of decreased left ventricular filling in patients with hypertension, and of its improvement by calcium channel blockade, is unclear. However, certain patients with long-standing hypertension have been documented to have latent or overt congestive heart failure primarily as the result of impaired filling. In such patients, the nondihydropyridine calcium antagonists that lower heart rate, especially verapamil, are the drugs of choice because they not only lower arterial pressure but also improve ventricular filling.[53-62]

EFFECTS ON LEFT VENTRICULAR MASS

Left ventricular hypertrophy has been identified as one of the strongest pressure-independent risk factors for sudden death, acute myocardial infarction, congestive heart failure, and other cardiovascular morbidity and mortality.[53-62] In fact, LVH was identified as the most powerful cardiovascular risk factor known. These epidemiologic findings clearly abolish the concept that LVH is a benign adaptive process serving to compensate for the increased hemodynamic burden. Although it is unclear whether a reduction in LVH confers benefits over and above the benefit of lowering blood pressure, the effects that various antihypertensive agents have on LVH come under scrutiny. Most calcium antagonists tend to reduce left ventricular mass when given for a sustained period.[63] However, a meta-analysis[64] indicates that the dihydropyridine calcium antagonists have a less powerful effect on left ventricular mass than the nondihydropyridine calcium antagonists. Thus, for any given decrease in arterial pressure, verapamil and diltiazem have been shown to reduce left ventricular mass more than nifedipine, nitrendipine, or nicardipine. A limited number of studies are available with felodipine and isradipine, but all of them have been shown to decrease left ventricular mass (Table 99–2). The decrease in left ventricular mass documented with calcium antagonists is associated with improved ventricular filling, diminished ventricular ectopy, and preserved contractility.[4-6, 8, 52, 65-81] Thus, calcium antagonists reduce or prevent all pathophysiologic sequelae of LVH. For this reason, it seems a logical (also unproven) extrapolation that the "melting away" of a powerful risk factor, such as LVH, would be beneficial for a hypertensive patient.

REDUCTION IN REINFARCTION RATE—"CARDIOPROTECTION"

After an acute myocardial infarction, the intact myocardium is the Achilles heel for further ischemia or necrosis. The question of whether or not this Achilles heel is amenable to medical therapy becomes of utmost importance. A distinct therapeutic benefit in patients following myocardial infarction has been documented with aspirin, β-blockers, ACE inhibitors, and, to a lesser extent, warfarin. Calcium antagonists have yielded disappointing results in these patients. In a recent review in the *British Medical Journal*, Held et al., by analyzing all available trials,[82] came to the conclusion that "Channel blockers do not reduce the risk of initial or recurrent infarction or death when given to patients with acute myocardial infarction or unstable angina" (p 1187). Approximately 1 year after this meta-analysis, the second Danish Verapamil Infarction Trial (DAVIT II) showed for the first time that verapamil reduced the reinfarction rate when therapy was started one week after the acute event.[83] A decrease in the reinfarction rate was previously documented with diltiazem in patients with non-Q-wave infarction only.[84] In this and in previous studies, the effects of verapamil and diltiazem were more pronounced when patients with congestive heart failure were excluded.[85] In a pooling of all patients in the DAVIT I and DAVIT II studies who survived day 7 after acute myocardial infarction, significant decreases in mortality, major events, and reinfarction rate were noted in verapamil-treated patients when compared with those receiving a placebo.[86] The order of magnitude of these benefits was similar to that achieved in numerous β-blocker trials.

At present, calcium antagonists that lower heart rate should be reserved for post–myocardial infarction patients without congestive heart failure who cannot tolerate a β-blocker or in whom a β-blocker is contraindicated. No benefits have been shown for the dihydropyridine calcium antagonists in the patient having suffered a myocardial infarction.

ANTIATHEROMATOUS EFFECTS

A variety of experimental studies have documented that calcium antagonists can exert antiatheromatous effects in certain animal models, such as cholesterol-fed rabbits.[87-94] Again, not all calcium antagonists have been shown to be equipotent in this regard.[87-98] Although these findings are very provocative and have tremendous clinical appeal, they cannot be extrapolated directly to the clinical situation. Nevertheless some recent studies have shown that calcium antagonists may have a favorable influence on the progression of vascular disease in the coronary and carotid circulation (Table 99–3).[99-105]

CALCIUM ANTAGONISTS AND HYPERTENSIVE HEART DISEASE

Hypertensive heart disease is characterized by LVH and its pathophysiologic sequelae. Numerous studies have shown that the classic adaptation to a sustained increase in arterial pressure consists of concentric LVH, that is, thickening of the wall at the expense of chamber volume.[54, 58, 106, 107] Even before an increase in left ventricular mass can be identified, left ventricular filling (predominant in the early relaxation phase) becomes impaired.[108] With established LVH, late diastolic filling also diminishes. LVH also unfavorably influences the myocardial oxygen supply-and-demand equilibrium: Oxygen demand increases because of increased myocardial mass and increased hemodynamic burden; oxygen supply diminishes because of vascular rarification and microvascular and macrovascular coronary artery disease.[106, 107, 109-111] Ventricular ectopy is common in patients with LVH and has

Table 99–2. **Reduction of Left Ventricular Mass with Calcium Antagonists**

Author	Year	Drug	Duration (months)	Reduction (percent)	Number of Patients
Muiesan et al.[65]	1986	Verapamil	3	17	22
Schmieder et al.[6]	1987	Verapamil	3	6	7
Schulman et al.[66]	1990	Verapamil	6	18	15
Granier et al.[67]	1990	Verapamil	3	26	13
Amodeo et al.[4]	1986	Diltiazem	1	10	10
Weiss and Bent[68]	1987	Diltiazem	6	19	17
Szlachic et al.[52]	1989	Diltiazem	4	15	15
Senda et al.[69]	1990	Diltiazem	6	2*	9
Gottdiener et al.[70]	1991	Diltiazem	2	5	77
Ferrara et al.[71]	1984	Nifedipine	2	0*	10
Muiesan et al.[65]	1986	Nifedipine	3	13	19
Phillips et al.[133]	1991	Nifedipine	12	19	16
Totteri et al.[78]	1993	Nifedipine	12	19	10
Ferrara et al.[132]	1985	Nitrendipine	2	3*	20
Drayer et al.[72]	1986	Nitrendipine	12	3*	30
Giles et al.[73]	1987	Nitrendipine	2	10	7
Grossman et al.[8]	1988	Nitrendipine	3	13	17
Carr and Prisant[74]	1990	Isradipine	1	9	9†
Grossman et al.[5]	1991	Isradipine	3	10	10
Saragoca et al.[75]	1991	Isradipine	3	14	17
Vyssoulis et al.[79]	1993	Isradipine	6	14	45
Manolis et al.[80]	1993	Isradipine	6	17	15
Pringle et al.[77]	1989	Felodipine	6	24	14
Wetzchewald et al.[76]	1990	Felodipine	9	12	75
Leenen and Holliwell[81]	1992	Felodipine	12	9	20

*Nonsignificant.
†Responders only.

been shown to occur in patients with concentric, eccentric, and isolated septal hypertrophy as well.[59, 62, 106–117] Left ventricular contractility is usually well preserved in patients with LVH, although it has been shown to progressively decline as LVH progresses.[106, 118, 119] Thus, hypertensive heart disease is characterized by LVH and its pathophysiologic sequelae: ventricular ectopy, myocardial ischemia, and impaired left ventricular systolic and diastolic function.

Calcium antagonists have been shown to be particularly beneficial in patients with hypertensive heart disease. They not only diminish the hemodynamic burden and decrease left ventricular mass but also seem to confer a specific benefit, because they have been documented to diminish ventricular ectopy[120]

and improve myocardial oxygenation and left ventricular filling while conserving or improving contractile function. With regard to reduction of LVH, improvement of left ventricular filling, and reduction of ventricular dysrhythmias, verapamil and perhaps diltiazem seem to be somewhat preferable to other calcium antagonists. However, no head-to-head comparison between two different calcium antagonists has been done to document clinical differences in this regard.

EFFECT ON RENAL DISEASE

Most attention regarding calcium antagonists has focused on cardiac effects. The finding that this class of drugs has beneficial effects on kidney function has

Table 99–3. **Antiatheromatous Effects of Calcium Antagonists in Clinical Trials**

Year	Acronym	Drug	Target Circulation	Duration (months)	Results
1990	Montreal Heart Institute Trial[99]	Nicardipine	Coronary	24	No significant effect
1990	INTACT[100]	Nifedipine	Coronary	36	Decrease in new lesions, no change in established lesions
1990	VAS[101]	Verapamil	Coronary	24	Decrease of restenosis rate after PTCA
1993	Heart transplant recipients[104]	Diltiazem	Coronary	24	Prevention of reduction of coronary artery diameters
1994	MIDAS[102]	Isradipine	Carotid	36	Slowed progression after 6 months; no difference at end of study
1994	FIPS[105]	Verapamil	Coronary	36	Pending
1994	VHAS[103]	Verapamil	Carotid	36	Pending

PTCA, percutaneous transluminal coronary angioplasty.

been largely ignored. A variety of studies in different experimental models suggest that calcium antagonists primarily attenuate preglomerular (afferent) arteriolar vasoconstriction with variable results on the efferent arteriole.[121-123] Several clinical studies indicate that pretreatment with calcium antagonists may not only ameliorate acute cyclosporine-induced renal vasoconstriction and presumably nephrotoxicity,[124] but may also protect against the development of acute renal failure in the setting of cadaveric renal transplantation[125] and radiocontrast administration.[126]

The effects of calcium antagonists on progression of renal disease in patients with essential hypertension are still controversial. Theoretical considerations suggest that vasoactive agents that preferentially reduce the resistance of the afferent arteriole may lead to an increase in glomerular capillary pressure, thereby accelerating glomerulosclerosis.[127] However, clinical studies have indicated that long-term treatment with calcium antagonists in patients with chronic renal failure is associated with well maintained renal function;[128, 129] in fact, a study comparing captopril and nifedipine on progression of renal insufficiency found no difference in the renoprotective effects of the two drugs.[130] A possible explanation for these findings is that calcium antagonists may have additional renoprotective properties besides their microcirculatory effects, such as reduction of renal hypertrophy, modulation of mesangial traffic of macromolecules, attenuation of the mitogenic effects of growth factors, and decreased free radical formation.[127] However, additional studies will be required to determine the exact mechanisms and the specificity of the renoprotective effects of calcium antagonists. A review by Kilaru and Bakris has indicated that the renoprotective effects, as measured by microproteinuria in diabetic patients, are more pronounced with the nondihydropyridine drugs than with the dihydropyridine agents.[131]

CONCLUSIONS

By definition, all antihypertensive drugs, including calcium antagonists, lower arterial pressure. However, calcium antagonists, apart from lowering arterial pressure, have a variety of beneficial effects in patients with hypertensive heart disease: they reduce LVH and improve its sequelae, such as ventricular dysrhythmias, impaired filling and contractility, and myocardial ischemia. Certain calcium antagonists have been shown to reduce the reinfarction rate, others to be beneficial in patients with congestive heart failure, and all of them have the potential for decreasing atherogenesis. Although the efficacy with regard to some of these properties clearly varies from one calcium antagonist to the other, they are attractive first-choice agents for therapy in patients with essential hypertension, particularly those with cardiac involvement.

REFERENCES

1. Fleckenstein A: Specific inhibitors and promoters of calcium action in the excitation-contraction coupling of heart muscle and their role in the prevention of myocardial lesions. *In* Harris P, Opie L (eds): Calcium and the Heart: Proceedings of the Meeting of the European Section of the International Study Group for Research in Cardiac Metabolism. New York: Academic Press, 1970, pp 135–188.
2. Kohlhardt M, Fleckenstein A: Inhibition of the slow inward current by nifedipine in mammalian ventricular myocardium. Naunyn Schmeidebergs Arch Pharmacol 298:267, 1977.
3. Nayler WG, Szeto J: Effect of verapamil on contractility, oxygen utilization, and calcium exchangeability in mammalian heart muscle. Cardiovasc Res 6:120, 1972.
4. Amodeo C, Kobrin I, Ventura HO, et al: Immediate and short-term hemodynamic effects of diltiazem in patients with hypertension. Circulation 73:108, 1986.
5. Grossman E, Messerli FH, Oren S, et al: Cardiovascular effects of isradipine in essential hypertension. Am J Cardiol 68:65, 1991.
6. Schmieder RE, Messerli FH, Garavaglia GE, et al: Cardiovascular effects of verapamil in patients with essential hypertension. Circulation 75:1030, 1987.
7. Ventura HO, Messerli FH, Oigman W, et al: Immediate hemodynamic effects of a new calcium-blocking agent (nitrendipine) in essential hypertension. Am J Cardiol 51:783, 1983.
8. Grossman E, Oren S, Garavaglia GE, et al: Systemic and regional hemodynamic and humoral effects of nitrendipine in essential hypertension. Circulation 78:1394, 1988.
9. Buhler FR, Hulthen UL, Kiowski W, et al: Greater antihypertensive efficacy of the calcium channel inhibitor verapamil in older and low renin patients [abstract]. Clin Sci 82:S439, 1982.
10. Erne P, Bolli P, Bertel O, et al: Factors influencing the hypotensive effects of calcium antagonists. Hypertension 5(Suppl II):97, 1983.
11. Canadian Felodipine Study Group: A dose-response study of felodipine in patients remaining hypotensive on a beta-blocker. Drugs 34(Suppl 3):176, 1987.
12. Leonetti G, Gradnik R, Terzoli L, et al: Effects of single and repeated doses of the calcium antagonist felodipine in blood pressure, renal function, water balance and renin-angiotensin-aldosterone system in hypertensive patients. J Cardiovasc Pharmacol 8:1243, 1986.
13. Hossack KF: Conduction abnormalities due to diltiazem. N Engl J Med 307:953, 1982.
14. Taira N: Differences in cardiovascular profile among calcium antagonists. Am J Cardiol 59:24B, 1987.
15. Bache RJ, Tockman BA: Effect of nitroglycerin and nifedipine on subendocardial perfusion in the presence of flow-limiting coronary stenosis in the awake dog. Circ Res 50:678, 1982.
16. DeServi S, Farrario M, Ghio S, et al: Effects of diltiazem on regional coronary hemodynamics during atrial pacing in patients with stable exertional angina: Implications for mechanisms of action. Circulation 73:1253, 1986.
17. Emanuelsson H, Homberg S: Mechanisms of angina relief after nifedipine: A hemodynamic and myocardial metabolic study. Circulation 68:124, 1983.
18. Gunther S, Green L, Muller JE, et al: Prevention by nifedipine of abnormal coronary vasoconstriction in patients with coronary artery disease. Circulation 63:849, 1981.
19. Hossack KF, Brown RG, Stewart DK, et al: Diltiazem-induced blockade of sympathetically mediated constriction of normal and diseased coronary arteries: Lack of epicardial coronary dilatory effect in humans. Circulation 70:465, 1984.
20. Matsuzaki M, Gallagher KP, Patritti J, et al: Effects of a calcium-entry blocker (diltiazem) on regional myocardial flow and function during exercise in conscious dogs. Circulation 69:801, 1984.
21. Subramanian VB, Bowles MJ, Davies AB, et al: Calcium channel blockade as primary therapy for stable angina pectoris: A double-blind placebo-controlled comparison of verapamil and propanolol. Am J Cardiol 50:1158, 1982.
22. Maseri A: Pathogenetic mechanisms of angina pectoris: Expanding views. Br Heart J 43:648, 1980.
23. Brown BG, Bolson EL, Dodge HT: Dynamic mechanisms in human coronary stenosis. Circulation 70:917, 1984.
24. Connon RO III, Matson RM, Rosing DR, et al: Angina caused by reduced vasodilator reserve of the small coronary arteries. J Am Coll Cardiol 1:1359, 1983.
25. Epstein SL, Talbot TL: Dynamic coronary tone in precipitation,

exacerbation, and relief of angina pectoris. Am J Cardiol 48:797, 1980.

26. Stone PH, Muller JE, Turi ZG, et al: Efficacy of nifedipine therapy in patients with refractory angina pectoris: Significance of the presence of coronary vasospasm. Am Heart J 106:644, 1983.

27. Boden WE, Korr KS, Bough EW: Nifedipine-induced hypotension and myocardial ischemia in refractory angina pectoris. JAMA 253:1131, 1985.

28. Schanzenbacher P, Deeg P, Liebau G, et al: Paradoxical angina after nifedipine: Angiographic documentation. Am J Cardiol 53:345, 1984.

29. Schanzenbacher P, Liebau G, Deeg P, et al: Effect of intavenous and intracoronary nifedipine on coronary blood flow and myocardial oxygen consumption. Am J Cardiol 51:712, 1983.

30. Sias ST, MacDonald PS, Triester B, et al: Aggravation of myocardial ischemia by nifedipine. Med J Aust 142:48, 1985.

31. Singh BN, Nademanee K: Use of calcium antagonists for cardiac arrhythmias. Am J Cardiol 59:153B, 1987.

32. Angus JA, Richmond DR, Dhumma-Upakorn P, et al: Cardiovascular action of verapamil in the dog with particular reference to myocardial contractility and atrioventricular conduction. Cardiovasc Res 10:623, 1976.

33. Nakaya H, Schwartz A, Millard RW: Reflex chronotropic and inotropic effects of calcium channel-blocking agents in conscious dogs: Diltiazem, verapamil, and nifedipine compared. Circ Res 52:302, 1983.

34. Heng MK, Singh BN, Roche AHG, et al: Effects of intravenous verapamil on cardiac arrhythmias and on the electrocardiogram. Am Heart J 90:487, 1975.

35. Rinkenberger RL, Prystowsky EN, Heger JJ, et al: Effects of intravenous and chronic oral verapamil administration in patients with supraventricular tachyarrhythmias. Circulation 62:996, 1980.

36. Singh BN, Nademanee K, Baky S: Calcium antagonists: Clinical uses in treating arrhythmias. Drugs 25:125, 1983.

37. Sung RJ, Elser B, McAllister RG, Jr: Intravenous verapamil for termination of re-entrant supraventricular tachycardias: Intracardiac studies correlated with plasma verapamil concentrations. Ann Intern Med 93:682, 1980.

38. Bonow RO, Leon MB, Rosing DR, et al: Effects of verapamil and propanolol on left ventricular systolic function and diastolic filling in patients with coronary artery disease: Radionuclide angiographic studies at rest and during exercise. Circulation 63:1337, 1981.

39. Brooks N, Cattell M, Pidgeon J, et al: Unpredictable response to nifedipine in severe cardiac failure. Br Med J 281:1324, 1980.

40. Chew CY, Hecht HS, Collett HT, et al: Influence of severity of ventricular dysfunction on hemodynamic responses to intravenously administered verapamil in ischemic heart disease. Am J Cardiol 47:917, 1981.

41. De Buitleir M, Rowland E, Krikler DM, et al: Hemodynamic effects of nifedipine given alone or in combination with atenolol in patients with impaired left ventricular function. Am J Cardiol 55:15E, 1985.

42. Elkayam U, Weber L, McKay C, et al: Spectrum of acute hemodynamic effects of nifedipine in severe congestive heart failure. Am J Cardiol 56:560, 1985.

43. Ferlinz J, Easthope JL, Aronow WS: Effects of verapamil on myocardial performance in coronary disease. Circulation 68:124, 1983.

44. Klein HO, Ninio R, Oren V, et al: The acute hemodynamic effects of intravenous verapamil in coronary artery disease: Assessment by equilibrium-gated radionuclide ventriculography. Circulation 67:101, 1983.

45. Lamping KA, Gross GJ: Differential effects of intravenous vs intracoronary nifedipine on myocardial segment function in ischemic canine hearts. J Pharmacol Exp Ther 228:28, 1977.

46. Packer M, Lee WH, Medina N, et al: Comparative negative inotropic effects of nifedipine and diltiazem in patients with severe left ventricular dysfunction [abstract]. Circulation 72(Suppl III):275, 1985.

47. Serruys PW, Brower RW, Ten Katen HJ, et al: Regional wall motion from radiopaque markers after intravenous and intracoronary injections of nifedipine. Circulation 63:584, 1981.

48. Greenberg B, Siemienczuk D, Broudy D: Hemodynamic effects

of PN 200-110 (isradipine) in congestive heart failure. Am J Cardiol 59:70B, 1987.

49. Inoiye I, Massie B, Loge D, et al: Abnormal left ventricular filling: An early finding in mild to moderate systemic hypertension. Am J Cardiol 53:120, 1984.

50. Walsh RA, O'Rourke RA: Direct and indirect effects of calcium entry blocking agents on isovolumic left ventricular relaxation in conscious dogs. J Clin Invest 75:1426, 1985.

51. Smith VE, White WB, Meeran MK, et al: Improved left ventricular filling accompanies left ventricular mass during therapy of essential hypertension. J Am Coll Cardiol 8:1449, 1986.

52. Szlachic J, Tubau JF, Vollmer C, et al: Effects of diltiazem on left ventricular mass and diastolic filling in mild to moderate hypertension. Am J Cardiol 63:198, 1989.

53. Aronow WS, Koenigsberg M, Schwartz KS: Usefulness of echocardiographic left ventricular hypertrophy in predicting new coronary events and atherothrombotic brain infarction in patients over 62 years of age. Am J Cardiol 61:1130, 1988.

54. Casale BN, Devereux RB, Milner M, et al: Value of echocardiographic measurement of left ventricular mass in predicting cardiovascular morbid events in hypertensive men. Am J Hypertens 3:8, 1990.

55. Cooper RS, Simmons BE, Castaner A, et al: Left ventricular hypertrophy is associated with worse survival independent of ventricular function and the number of coronary arteries severely narrowed. Am J Cardiol 65:441, 1990.

56. Kannel WB: Prevalence and natural history of electrocardiographic left ventricular hypertrophy. Am J Med 75(Suppl 3a):4, 1983.

57. Kannel WB, Gordon T, Castelli WP, et al: Electrocardiographic left ventricular hypertrophy and risk of coronary heart disease: The Framingham Study. Ann Intern Med 72:813, 1970.

58. Koren MJ, Devereux RB, Casale PN, et al: Relation of left ventricular mass and geometry to morbidity and mortality in men and women with uncomplicated hypertension. Ann Intern Med 114:345, 1991.

59. Le Heuzey J-Y, Guize L: Cardiac prognosis in hypertensive patients: Incidence of sudden death and ventricular arrhythmias. Am J Med 84(Suppl 1B):65, 1988.

60. Levy D, Garrison RJ, Savage DD, et al: Left ventricular mass and incidence of coronary heart disease in an elderly cohort. Ann Intern Med 110:101, 1989.

61. Levy D, Garrison RJ, Savage DD, et al: Prognostic implications of echocardiographically determined left ventricular mass in the Framingham Heart Study. N Engl J Med 322:1561, 1990.

62. Messerli FH, Ventura HO, Elizardi DJ, et al: Hypertension and sudden death: Increased ventricular ectopy activity in left ventricular hypertrophy. Am J Med 77:18, 1984.

63. Pearson AC, Pasierski T, Labovitz AJ: Left ventricular hypertrophy: Diagnosis, prognosis, and management. Am Heart J 121:148, 1991.

64. Cruickshank JM, Lewis J, Moore V, et al: Reversibility of left ventricular hypertrophy by differing types of antihypertensive therapy. J Hum Hypertens 6:85, 1992.

65. Muiesan G, Agabiti-Rosei E, Romanelli G, et al: Adrenergic activity and left ventricular function during treatment with calcium antagonists in essential hypertension. Am J Cardiol 57:44D, 1986.

66. Schulman SP, Weiss JL, Becker LC, et al: The effects of antihypertensive therapy on left ventricular mass in elderly patients. N Engl J Med 322:1350, 1990.

67. Granier P, Douste-Blazy MY, Tredez P, et al: Improvement in left ventricular hypertrophy and left ventricular diastolic function following verapamil therapy in mild to moderate hypertension. Eur J Clin Pharmacol 39(Suppl 1):S45, 1990.

68. Weiss RJ, Bent B: Diltiazem-induced left ventricular mass regression in hypertensive patients. J Clin Hypertens 3:135, 1987.

69. Senda Y, Tohkai M, Shida Y, et al: ECG-gated cardiac scan and echocardiographic assessments of left ventricular hypertrophy: reversal by 6-month treatment with diltiazem. J Cardiovasc Pharmacol 16:298, 1990.

70. Gottdiener J, Reda D, Notargiacomo A, et al: Comparison of monotherapy on LV mass regression in mild-to-moderate hypertension: Echocardiographic results of a multicenter trial [abstract]. J Am Coll Cardiol 17(Suppl A):178A, 1991.

71. Ferrara LA, De Simone G, Mancini M, et al: Changes in left ventricular mass during a double-blind study with chlorthali-

done and slow-release nifedipine. Eur J Clin Pharmacol 27:525, 1984.

72. Drayer JI, Hall WD, Smith VE, et al: Effect of the calcium channel blocker nitrendipine on left ventricular mass in patients with essential hypertension. Clin Pharmacol Ther 40:697, 1986.

73. Giles TD, Sander GE, Roffidal LC, et al: Comparison of nitrendipine and hydrochlorthiazide for systemic hypertension. Am J Cardiol 60:103, 1987.

74. Carr AA, Prisant LM: The new calcium antagonist isradipine: Effect on blood pressure and the left ventricle in black hypertensive patients. Am J Hypertens 3:8, 1990.

75. Saragoca MD, Portella FE, Abreu P, et al: Regression of left ventricular hypertrophy in the short-term treatment of hypertension with isradipine. Am J Hypertens 4(2 Pt 2):188S, 1991.

76. Wetzchewald D, Klaus D, Garanin G, et al: Regression of left ventricular hypertrophy by felodipine or a combination of felodipine and metoprolol [abstract]. J Cardiovasc Pharmacol 15(Suppl 4):S48, 1990.

77. Pringle SD, Barbour M, Simpson IA, et al: Effect of felodipine on left ventricular mass and Doppler-derived hemodynamics in patients with essential hypertension [abstract]. In 4th International Symposium on Calcium Antagonists: Pharmacology and Clinical Research, Florence, Italy, 1989, p 174.

78. Totteri A, Scopelliti G, Bertini M, et al: Evaluation of regression of left ventricular hypertrophy after antihypertensive therapy: Comparative echo-Doppler study of ace-inhibitors and calcium-antagonists [Italian]. Minerva Cardioangiol 41:231, 1993.

79. Vyssoulis GP, Karpanou EA, Pitsavos LE, et al: Regression of left ventricular hypertrophy with isradipine antihypertensive therapy. Am J Hypertens 6(3 Pt 2):82S, 1993.

80. Manolis AJ, Kolovou G, Handanis S, et al: Regression of left ventricular hypertrophy with isradipine in previously untreated hypertensive patients. Am J Hypertens 6(3 Pt 2):86S, 1993.

81. Leenen FH, Holliwell DN: Antihypertensive effect of felodipine associated with persistent sympathetic activation and minimal regression of left ventricular hypertrophy. Am J Cardiol 69:639, 1992.

82. Held PH, Yusuf S, Furberg CD: Calcium channel blockers in acute myocardial infarction and unstable angina. An overview. Br Med J 299:1187, 1989.

83. The Danish Study Group on Verapamil in Myocardial Infarction: Effect of verapamil on mortality and major events after myocardial infarction (The Danish Verapamil Infarction Trial II—DAVIT II). Am J Cardiol 66:779, 1990.

84. Gibson RS, Boden WE, Theroux P, et al: Diltiazem and reinfarction in patients with non-Q-wave myocardial infarction: Results of a double-blind, randomized multicenter trial. N Engl J Med 315:423, 1986.

85. The Multicenter Diltiazem Postinfarction Trial Research Group: The effect of diltiazem on mortality and reinfarction after myocardial infarction. N Engl J Med 319:385, 1988.

86. Messerli FH: Cardioprotection—not all calcium antagonists are created equal. Am J Cardiol 66:855, 1990.

87. Blumlein SL, Sievers R, Kidd P, et al: Mechanism of protection from atherosclerosis by verapamil in the cholesterol-fed rabbit. Am J Cardiol 54:884, 1984.

88. Habib JB, Bossaller C, Wells S, et al: Preservation of endothelium-dependent vascular relaxation in cholesterol-fed rabbits by treatment with the calcium blocker PN 200 110. Circ Res 58:305, 1986.

89. Henry PD, Bentley KI: Suppression of atherogenesis in cholesterol-fed rabbits treated with nifedipine. J Clin Invest 68:1366, 1981.

90. Ohata I, Sakomoto N, Nagano K, et al: Low density lipoprotein-lowering and high density lipoprotein-elevating effects of nicardipine in rats. Biochem Pharmacol 33:2199, 1984.

91. Rouleau J-L, Parmley WW, Stevens J, et al: Verapamil suppresses atherosclerosis in cholesterol-fed rabbits. J Am Coll Cardiol 1:1453, 1983.

92. Sugano N, Nakashimo Y, Matsushima T, et al: Suppression of atherosclerosis in cholesterol-fed rabbits by diltiazem injection. Arteriosclerosis 6:237, 1986.

93. Walldius G: Effect of verapamil on serum lipoproteins in patients with angina pectoris. Acta Med Scand 681(Suppl):43, 1983.

94. Willis AL, Nagel B, Churchill V, et al: Antiatherosclerotic effects of nicardipine and nifedipine in cholesterol-fed rabbits. Arteriosclerosis 5:250, 1985.

95. Naito M, Kuzuya F, Asai K-I, et al: Ineffectiveness of Ca^{++}-antagonists nicardipine and diltiazem on experimental atherosclerosis in cholesterol-fed rabbits. Angiology 35:622, 1984.

96. Overturf ML, Smith SA: Failure of high therapeutic dosage of nifedipine to suppress atherosclerosis in cholesterol-fed rabbits [abstract]. Arteriosclerosis 2:408a, 1982.

97. Stender S, Stender I, Nordestgaard B, et al: No effect of nifedipine on atherogenesis in cholesterol-fed rabbits. Arteriosclerosis 4:389, 1984.

98. Van Niekerk JL, Hendricks T, De Boer HH, et al: Does nifedipine suppress atherogenesis in WHHL rabbits? Atherosclerosis 53:91, 1984.

99. Waters D, Lesperance J, Francetich M, et al: A controlled clinical trial to assess the effect of a calcium channel blocker on the progression of coronary atherosclerosis. Circulation 82:1940, 1990.

100. Lichtlen PR, Hugenholtz PG, Rafflenbeul W, et al: Retardation of angiographic progression of coronary artery disease by nifedipine. Lancet 335:1109, 1990.

101. Hoberg E, Schwarz F, Schoemig A, et al: Prevention of restenosis by verapamil. The Verapamil Angioplasty Study (VAS) [abstract]. Circulation 82(Suppl III):428, 1990.

102. Borhani NO, Bond MG, Sowers JR, et al: The multicenter isradipine/diuretic atherosclerosis study: A study of the antiatherogenetic properties of isradipine in hypertensive patients. J Cardiovasc Pharmacol 18(Suppl 3):S15, 1991. (Final results presented at the meeting of the International Society of Hypertension, Melbourne, Australia, March 1994.)

103. Zanchetti A, Magnani B, Dal Palu C, et al: Atherosclerosis and calcium antagonists: The VHAS. J Hum Hypertens 6(Suppl 2):S45, 1992.

104. Schroeder JS, Shao-Zhou G, Alderman EL, et al: A preliminary study of diltiazem in the prevention of coronary artery disease in heart-transplant recipients. N Engl J Med 328:164, 1993.

105. Schneider W, Kober G, Roebruck P, et al: Retardation of development and progression of coronary atherosclerosis: A new indication for calcium antagonists? Eur J Clin Pharmacol 39(Suppl 1):S17, 1990.

106. Folkow B: The fourth Volhard Lecture: Cardiovascular structural adaptation: Its role in the initiation and maintenance of primary hypertension. Clin Sci Mol Med 55(Suppl 4):3S, 1978.

107. Strauer BE: Ventricular function and coronary hemodynamics in hypertensive heart disease. Am J Cardiol 44:999, 1979.

108. Tubau FJ, Szlachic J, Braun S, et al: Impaired left ventricular functional reserve in hypertensive patients with left ventricular hypertrophy. Hypertension 14:1, 1989.

109. Marcus ML, Harrison DG, Chilian WM, et al: Alterations in the coronary circulation in hypertrophied ventricles. Circulation 75(I pt 2):I-19, 1987.

110. Opherk D, Mall G, Zebe H, et al: Reduction of coronary reserve: A mechanism for angina pectoris in patients with hypertension and normal coronary arteries. Circulation 69:1, 1984.

111. Schwarzkopff B, Frenzel H, Vogt M, et al: Myocardial structure in patients with reduced coronary reserve in hypertensive heart disease [abstract]. Circulation 80(Suppl II):II-839, 1989.

112. Levy D, Anderson KM, Savage DD, et al: Risk of ventricular arrhythmias in left ventricular hypertrophy: The Framingham Heart Study. Am J Cardiol 60:560, 1987.

113. Siegel D, Cheitlin MD, Black DM, et al: Risk of ventricular arrhythmias in hypertensive men with left ventricular hypertrophy. Am J Cardiol 65:742, 1990.

114. Widimsky J, Cifkova R: Hypertension and arrhythmias: A review. Cor Vasa 31:157, 1989.

115. Messerli FH, Nunez BD, Ventura HO, et al: Overweight and sudden death: Increased ventricular ectopy in cardiopathy of obesity. Arch Intern Med 147:1725, 1987.

116. Nunez BD, Messerli FH, Garavaglia GE, et al: Exaggerated atrial and ventricular excitability in hypertensive patients with isolated septal hypertrophy (ISH) [abstract]. J Am Coll Cardiol 9:225A, 1987.

117. Papademetriou V, Notagariacomo A, Heine D, et al: Ventricu-

lar arrhythmias in patients with essential hypertension [abstract]. J Am Coll Cardiol 13:105A, 1989.

118. Schmieder RE, Messerli FH: Reversal of left ventricular hypertrophy: A desirable therapeutic goal? J Cardiovasc Pharmacol 16(Suppl 6):S16, 1990.

119. Schmieder RE, Ruddel H, Grube E, et al: Depressed myocardial contractility in early left ventricular hypertrophy (LVH) [abstract]. Circulation 78(Suppl II): II-75, 1988.

120. Messerli FH, Nunez BD, Nunez MM: Hypertension and sudden death: Disparate effects of calcium entry blocker and diuretic therapy on cardiac dysrhythmias. Arch Intern Med 149:1263, 1989.

121. Yoshioka T, Shiraga H, Yoshida Y, et al: "Intact nephrons" as the primary origin of proteinuria in chronic renal disease: Study in the rat model of subtotal nephrectomy. J Clin Invest 82:1614, 1988.

122. Anderson S: Renal hemodynamic effects of calcium antagonists in rats with reduced renal mass. Hypertension 17:288, 1991.

123. Isshiki T, Amodeo C, Messerli FH, et al: Diltiazem maintains renal vasodilation without hyperfiltration in hypertension. Cardiovasc Drugs Ther 1:359, 1987.

124. Dawidson I, Rooth P, Fry WR, et al: Verapamil improves the outcome after cadaver renal transplantation. J Am Soc Nephrol 2:983, 1991.

125. Wagner K, Albrecht S, Neumayer H: Prevention of posttransplant acute tubular necrosis by the calcium antagonist diltiazem: A prospective randomized study. Am J Nephrol 7:287, 1987.

126. Russo D, Testa A, Della Volpe L, et al: Randomized prospective study on renal effects of two different contrast media in humans. Nephron 55:254, 1990.

127. Epstein M: Calcium antagonists and renal protection. Arch Intern Med 152:1573, 1992.

128. Kasiske BL, Kalil RS, Ma J, et al: Effect of anti-hypertensive therapy on the kidney in patients with diabetes: A meta-regression analysis. Ann Intern Med 118:129, 1993.

129. Slataper R, Vicknair N, Sadler R, et al: Comparative effects of different antihypertensive treatment on progression of diabetic renal disease. Arch Intern Med 153:973, 1993.

130. Zucchelli P, Zucchala A, Borghi M, et al: Long-term comparison between captopril and nifedipine in the progression of renal insufficiency. Kidney Int 42:452, 1992.

131. Kilaru P, Bakris GL: Microalbuminuria and progressive renal disease. J Hum Hypertens 8:809, 1994.

132. Ferrara LA, Fasano ML, de Simone G, et al: Antihypertensive and cardiovascular effects of nitrendipine: A controlled study vs. placebo. Clin Pharmacol Ther 38:434, 1985.

133. Phillips RA, Ardeljan M, Shimabukuro S, et al: Effect of nifedipine GITS on left ventricular mass and diastolic function in severe hypertension. J Cardiovasc Pharmacol 17(Suppl 2):S172, 1991.

B. Specific Calcium Antagonists

CHAPTER 100

Verapamil

Matthew R. Weir, M.D., and Prince K. Zachariah, M.D., Ph.D.

HISTORY

Verapamil was the first compound described with the property of selectively inhibiting the transmembrane flux of calcium ions in excitable tissues.[1] It was first synthesized in 1962 and initially was believed to be a β-adrenergic blocking drug.[2, 3]

For 20 years, verapamil has been used as a chemical probe in studies of excitation-contraction coupling in cardiac cells and has contributed to the understanding of the genesis of cardiac arrhythmias.[4] Verapamil has demonstrated clinical utility in the treatment of patients with supraventricular tachyarrhythmias,[5, 6] angina pectoris,[7–12] hypertrophic cardiomyopathy,[13] and hypertension.[14]

CHEMISTRY

The chemical structure of verapamil is similar to that of papaverine, yet it is structurally different from other paradigms of calcium antagonists (e.g., diltiazem and nifedipine). It has an asymmetric carbon and is optically active. The enantiomers of the racemic mixture have different electrophysiologic properties. The S- enantiomer is much more active in its ability to block the voltage-gated calcium channel compared with the less active R+ enantiomer.[15] Whether the pharmacokinetic properties of the two isomers differ has yet to be elucidated. Furthermore, neither the receptor-drug interaction nor the site of action of ve-

rapamil is fully understood. Although all calcium antagonists have structural analogues, each has its own characteristic pharmacologic profile.

PHARMACOKINETICS

Verapamil is a basic compound that is rapidly absorbed, and peak levels are attained at 30 to 90 minutes after dosing. Although more than 90% of the administered dose is absorbed, verapamil demonstrates a significant first-pass metabolism, which compromises bioavailability.[16] Of the three types of available calcium antagonists, verapamil is the least bioavailable agent, with about 10% to 20% of the administered drug reaching the systemic circulation after oral dosing. However, in patients with hepatic failure, the percentage increases to about 50%; thus, the dose must be reduced to one fourth or one third of normal.[16] In patients in renal failure, no differences in bioavailability have been documented.[17] The pharmacokinetic properties of verapamil are listed in Table 100-1.

Verapamil is widely distributed and has a high volume of distribution (3 to 6 L/kg). Limited experience shows that the drug has a redistribution phase after initial distribution of 18 to 35 minutes. After intravenous administration of verapamil, a short-lived maximal hemodynamic effect is noted at 5 minutes, whereas the peak negative dromotropic effect

Table 100–1. **Pharmacokinetics of Verapamil**

Absorption	>90%
Bioavailability	10%–20%
Protein binding	85%–95%
Therapeutic plasma core	80–300 ng/ml
Elimination half-life	
Acute	2–6 hr
Chronic	8–12 hr
Volume of distribution	4 L/kg
Clearance	13 ± 7 ml/min/kg
Metabolism	Demethylation: 85% first-pass metabolism
Active metabolite	Norverapamil
Recovery in urine	70%
Recovery in feces	15%

These are approximate estimates from various reports.

occurs at about 15 minutes and lasts as long as 6 hours. About 90% of the drug is bound by protein and it has an initial elimination half-life of 4 to 5 hours.

The therapeutic plasma concentration is 80 to 300 ng/ml. During long-term oral administration, nonlinear accumulation of the drug occurs with reduced clearance and prolongation of the half-life.[18, 19] This observation suggests that verapamil could be administered twice daily after reaching steady-state levels. Several sustained-release preparations of verapamil with prolonged duration of action are available, and the plasma peak concentration is reached at 3 to 5 hours after oral administration. The steady-state plasma levels remain in the therapeutic range for a prolonged period with this sustained-release preparation. After the steady state is reached, the half-life ranges between 4.5 and 12 hours.

Verapamil is extensively metabolized in the liver. Although several metabolites have been identified, only one, norverapamil (an *N*-demethylated form), is reported to have pharmacologic activities similar to those of the parent compound, but at only about 20% of the potency of verapamil. Although norverapamil is not seen in plasma after intravenous administration of verapamil, accumulation of this metabolite has been noted after chronic oral use. This factor might contribute to the enhancement of the efficacy of verapamil after prolonged use, especially for the treatment of hypertension. The enzyme system responsible for the metabolism of verapamil is dependent on cytochrome P-450 reductase and is inducible by other drugs including phenobarbital. The metabolism of verapamil is also dependent on hepatic blood flow. Drugs such as cimetidine can prolong the half-life of verapamil by inhibiting hepatic metabolism. Because of enterohepatic cycling, 70% of verapamil metabolites are recovered in the urine and 15% in the feces.

Chronobiologic Release

Numerous studies, including the classic Framingham study, have shown that sudden cardiac death, myocardial infarction, myocardial ischemia, angina, and ischemic stroke have a 70% greater risk of occurring between the hours of 7:00 A.M. and 9:00 A.M. than

throughout the remainder of the day.[19a] Increases in blood pressure and heart rate near the time of awakening are postulated to contribute to the increased risk of cardiovascular events observed in the early morning. Therefore, patients with hypertension, coronary artery disease (CAD), and/or ischemic heart disease (IHD) are most vulnerable to fatal cardiac events during these hours seemingly governed by the patient's natural body clock.

Covera-HS (verapamil hydrochloride) utilizes a novel delivery system, COER-24 (controlled-onset-extended-release), that was developed as a chronotherapeutic treatment for hypertension and angina. Taken once daily at bedtime, Covera-HS was specifically designed to synchronize verapamil release within the physiologic patterns of the human body's natural circadian rhythm of blood pressure and heart rate, providing peak concentrations coinciding with the rising blood pressure in the early waking hours. During evening hours and sleep, when blood pressure is at its lowest level, the extent of blood pressure reduction by Covera-HS is decreased.

PHARMACOLOGIC EFFECTS

Verapamil likely exerts its primary effect at the cellular level by blocking the transmembrane movement of calcium ions through calcium channels that are either voltage activated or receptor activated, which results in two major changes: alterations of the electrophysiologic properties of the cell membrane and decreases in the intracellular concentration of calcium.[20–22]

There is also evidence that verapamil and other calcium antagonists inhibit potassium efflux from certain types of cells,[23–25] an effect that is likely independent of their ability to block calcium influx, although there is some debate in this regard. Some investigators suspect that this effect may be as important or more important than the ability of the drugs to decrease calcium influx with regard to certain cellular functions, particularly cell growth.[23–25] This is of interest because the active and inactive enantiomers of verapamil are similarly capable of blocking proliferative responses of lymphocytes, mesangial cells, and vascular smooth muscle cells to various stimuli.[25–27] Calcium antagonists also inhibit cellular uptake of various precursor molecules necessary for cell growth (e.g., thymidine, leucine, uridine), an effect that may be linked to the ability of these drugs to inhibit potassium efflux from cells.[15]

Verapamil has also been demonstrated to block opiate, muscarinic, and both α_1- and α_2-adrenergic receptors in various tissues.[28] The clinical significance of these effects are unknown, but ultimately may be shown to be important in the regulation of cell function in some tissues.

Despite the diverse effects of verapamil and other calcium antagonists on transmembrane flux of various ions, an important effect of calcium antagonists is on the voltage-gated L-calcium channels. These channels have a slower time course, activation, and recovery than the sodium-dependent fast channels. The action potential of the cardiac cell is dependent on both fast-current and slow-current channels. However, the calcium current predominates in the sinoatrial (SA) and atrioventricular (AV) nodes as well as in ischemic myocardium. Because verapamil is a racemic mixture, the electrophysiologic effects vary with the enantiomers. The active calcium channel–blocking enantiomer depresses the maximal rate of rise of the action potential and has other electrophysiologic properties, including influencing the overall shape of the action potential.[29, 30] Furthermore, these effects are markedly enhanced by prolonged exposure to verapamil.[31] Because verapamil and diltiazem have a more pronounced effect on the SA and AV nodes, these two calcium antagonists decrease heart rate. Suppression of calcium influx during phase 2 of the action potential can result in a negative inotropic effect; however, this may be modified by the reflex response to the associated peripheral vasodilation and dose of drug used. The possibility of negative inotropic effect should be kept in mind with all calcium antagonists, especially verapamil and diltiazem. Furthermore, these drugs can also block the fast channel and thus prevent intracellular influx of sodium.

The role of calcium in the contraction of vascular smooth muscle is of similar importance to that in the contraction of cardiac muscle. An important action of verapamil on vascular smooth muscle cell is to limit calcium influx, and the mechanism is similar to that described in cardiac tissues. Inhibition of formation of actinomycin complex results in vasodilation, the extent of which varies in different vascular beds. When extracellular calcium enters the cell, it is bound to calmodulin; the calcium-calmodulin complex then stimulates an enzyme called myosin light-chain kinase, which phosphorylates myosin. This action is followed by the interaction of actin and myosin, resulting in smooth muscle contraction. Verapamil also inhibits other types of smooth muscle contraction, thus causing relaxation of the gastrointestinal tract and bronchi.[32, 33]

Preliminary data also show that calcium antagonists, including verapamil, inhibit the secretion of insulin;[34, 35] however, exocrine and endocrine secretions mediated by calcium (pancreatic secretion, insulin, adrenal corticosteroids, and testicular and ovarian hormones) may also be influenced by verapamil. Calcium antagonists have been shown to inhibit platelet aggregation *in vitro*. Release of platelet-aggregating factors such as adenosine diphosphate (ADP) involves calcium-mediated steps, and verapamil inhibits this mechanism of action.[36] Calcium antagonists also inhibit both ADP and epinephrine-mediated platelet aggregation.[37]

Calcium antagonists, including verapamil, also exhibit *in vitro* antiproliferative properties on human lymphocytes.[25] These effects require higher concentrations of drug than what is normally achieved clinically with chronic dosing. However, the drugs theoretically may support conventional immunosuppression such as that used in organ transplant recipients.[38]

EFFECTS ON PATHOPHYSIOLOGY
Hemodynamics

Verapamil can influence cardiovascular hemodynamics by three principal actions: coronary artery dilation, negative inotropic effect, and peripheral artery dilation. The effects of verapamil in animals and in humans are not comparable with those seen in isolated muscle preparations.[39, 40] In isolated cardiac tissues, verapamil exerts a marked negative inotropic effect and depressant effect on the SA and AV nodes. These effects can be antagonized competitively by calcium and by catecholamines.[41] The systemic vasodilator action of verapamil can activate reflex sympathetic responses, which seems to modify the negative effect on cardiac contractility and conduction. However, the depressant effects are more likely to be manifested in the presence of an intrinsic disorder of contractility or conduction or the inability to stimulate the sympathetic systems in the presence of verapamil.[42]

Extensive hemodynamic studies in subjects with stable coronary artery disease or rheumatic heart disease have been reported. In most reports, verapamil produced a moderate decrease in the mean arterial pressure consequent to a decline in vascular resistance without changing the cardiac and stroke volume indexes.[43–46] The hemodynamic effects after intravenous administration of 10 mg of verapamil in 20 patients are shown in Table 100–2.[47] Hemodynamic changes occurred within 3 to 5 minutes and disappeared within 10 minutes after infusion. Systolic, diastolic, and mean arterial pressures decreased; pulmonary artery pressure did not change; and left ventricular end-diastolic pressure increased. However, there was no significant increase in stroke volume, cardiac index, or heart rate. The hemodynamic response in the hypertensive patient after administration of verapamil is not significantly different.[48]

Although the actions of verapamil on resting left ventricular pump performance are well defined, data on hemodynamics during exercise are rare. In a limited study[49] of patients with coronary artery disease, verapamil was able to prevent an exercise-induced decline in the left ventricular ejection fraction and in electrocardiographic and segmental wall abnormalities induced by ambulatory exercise. Other studies[7, 8] also demonstrated a reduction in resting and exercise rate product with antianginal effects. All of these studies compared verapamil with propranolol for antianginal effect and rate product improvement; the exercise rate pressure product was less with verapamil despite a comparable antianginal effect. An excellent review of this was presented by Singh et al.[50]

Ventricular Function

Verapamil has been shown to decrease contractility in *in vitro* tissue preparations in a dose-dependent fash-

Table 100-2. **Hemodynamic Effects of Intravenous Administration of Verapamil in 20 Patients with Heart Disease**

	Group		
	*Before Verapamil**	*After Verapamil**	*Significance (p)*
Heart rate (beats/min)	74 ± 12	75 ± 12	NS
Mean arterial pressure (mmHg)	94 ± 17	82 ± 13	<.0005
Right ventricular end-diastolic pressure (mmHg)	4 ± 2	7 ± 2	<.0005
Left ventricular end-diastolic pressure (mmHg)	12 ± 4	14 ± 4	<.025
Cardiac index (L/min/m²)	2.8 ± 0.6	3.1 ± 0.7	<.0005
Stroke volume index (ml/m²)	57 ± 12	63 ± 13	<.025
Systemic vascular resistance (dyn-sec-cm^{-5})	1413 ± 429	1069 ± 235	<.0005
Ejection fraction (%)	55 ± 16	61 ± 18	<.01

NS, not significant.
*Values are mean ± standard deviation.
Reproduced with permission from Ferlinz J, Easthope JL, Aronow WS: Effects of verapamil on myocardial performance in coronary disease. Circulation 59:313, 1979. Copyright 1979, the American Heart Association.

ion. However, the dose of verapamil commonly used in coronary vasodilation has little effect on contractility; although slight decreases in contractility are reported with verapamil, such effects are not commonly associated with myocardial dysfunction.

In contrast to the experience in patients with adequate left ventricular function, verapamil may exert a significant cardiodepressant effect in patients with severely impaired left ventricular performance before therapy.[44] These data indicate that patients with impaired ventricular function are particularly susceptible to the negative inotropic effect of verapamil. Therefore, this drug can exacerbate clinical evidence of congestive heart failure, especially in patients with an ejection fraction of less than 30%.

Conduction System

The effects of verapamil on the SA and AV nodes were outlined earlier. The drug has both negative chronotropic and dromotropic effects. These actions are manifested with the therapeutic doses of verapamil used for angina, arrhythmias, and hypertension. Both SA and AV nodal cells in humans rely on the slow-channel system for impulse activation, and verapamil slows the response rate and is useful for treating arrhythmias in nodal tissue associated with a reentrant mechanism such as paroxysmal supraventricular tachycardia and paroxysmal atrial tachycardia. Thus, bradycardia and asystole are associated with enhancement of the SA and AV nodal actions of the slow-channel blockade by verapamil, because of excessive drug levels, patient sensitivity, or drug interaction. Verapamil has no direct effect on atrial or ventricular myocardial fibers.

The actions of verapamil are most evident in the proximal conduction system (SA and AV nodes) and may be manifested as a depressant effect on the rate of sinus node discharge (negative chronotropic effect) and institution of conduction velocity through the AV node (negative dromotropic effect). In clinical studies, verapamil prolongs the A–H interval.[51] Verapamil significantly prolongs the AV nodal effective and functional refractory period in humans.[51-53] Intravenous administration of verapamil shortened the refractory period of the accessory pathway and accelerated the ventricular response during atrial fibrillation in patients with Wolff-Parkinson-White syndrome.[54]

Coronary Blood Flow

The effect of verapamil on coronary hemodynamics demonstrates a marked increase in coronary blood flow in patients without coronary disease[55] but not in patients with diseased vessels. However, the coronary artery resistance in patients with coronary artery disease was reduced and the effect on blood flow and myocardial oxygen consumption was variable.[56-59] Compared with nitroglycerin and dipyridamole, verapamil exerts only a modest effect on coronary vascular resistance.[47, 60]

Renal Function, Electrolytes, and Endocrine Effects

No net effects on renal function have been shown in patients after short-term or long-term[48, 61-63] oral therapy with verapamil. No significant changes in renal blood flow, glomerular filtration rate (GFR), and filtration fraction have been noted. However, renal vascular resistance was reduced in parallel with the reduction in total peripheral resistance; the mechanism of reduction in renal vascular resistance is likely related to diffuse vasodilation throughout the kidney. The lack of change in GFR and filtration fraction suggests balanced preglomerular and postglomerular vasorelaxation. Long-term treatment with verapamil demonstrated no significant effect on plasma volume or body weight. However, verapamil, like other calcium antagonists, does facilitate sodium excretion, most likely through direct inhibition of renal tubular reabsorption of sodium.[64] Plasma renin activity was significantly increased after acute intravenous administration of verapamil, but no consistent findings have been reported after long-term oral administration in normal or hypertensive patients. There is no effect on plasma aldosterone levels, but the effects of intrarenal angiotensin II have been noted to be blocked after oral verapamil.[61, 62, 65]

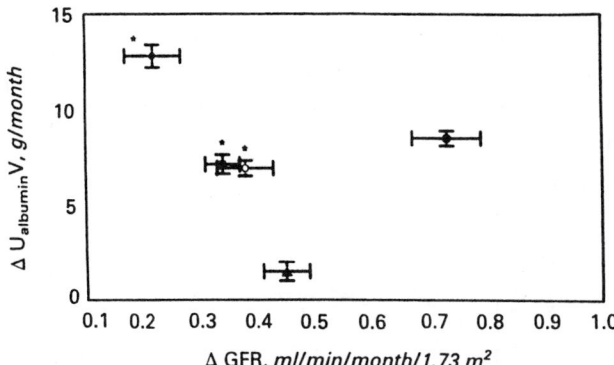

Figure 100–1. The relationship between the rate of loss of GFR and change in 24-hour urine albumin excretion over 1 year of study. Symbols are: (●) lisinopril alone, (■) verapamil SR (sustained-release) alone, (♦) lisinopril plus verapamil SR, (▲) hydrochlorothiazide plus guanfacine, (○) lisinopril alone corrected for initial decline in GFR. * $p < .05$, significantly slower rate of decline in GFR compared with hydrochlorothiazide and guanfacine group. (From Bakris GL, Barnhill BW, Sadler R: Treatment of arterial hypertension in diabetic humans: Importance of therapeutic selection. Kidney Int 41:912, 1992.)

Verapamil has also been demonstrated to possess antiproteinuric effects in macroproteinuric patients with adult onset diabetes mellitus and mild renal dysfunction.[66] These antiproteinuric effects are additive with those of angiotensin-converting enzyme (ACE) inhibitors, and are likely not only related to blood pressure reduction. In experimental studies, verapamil potentiates the efferent glomerular arteriolar dilation induced by ACE inhibition, and this property may facilitate improved glomerular capillary pressure reduction.[67] Verapamil also reduces efferent glomerular arteriolar tone and improves glomerular permselectivity to proteins.[68] These experimental observations likely explain the clinical antiproteinuric effects of the drug. The reduction in blood pressure and proteinuria with verapamil has been associated with a slowing in the rate of loss of renal function in hypertensive diabetics with mild renal dysfunction (Fig. 100–1). It remains to be seen whether patients with other forms of proteinuric renal diseases will benefit from this effect.

Central Nervous System

Calcium antagonists act to block the influx of calcium in cells in the myocardium and vascular smooth muscle and do not possess any adrenergic, cholinergic, or histaminergic effects. The central effects resulting from calcium channel blockade therefore are few and rare. However, vasospasm from subarachnoid hemorrhage has been reversed successfully with verapamil, but such clinical reports need to be further investigated.

CLINICAL USES

Because calcium antagonists were first introduced for the treatment of variant angina caused by coronary artery spasm, this group of drugs has become an important therapeutic agent for the management of several cardiovascular diseases. Other uses have been suggested but not clinically proved. Various suggested uses are listed in Table 100–3. This section elaborates on only the approved or accepted uses of verapamil.

Anginal Syndrome

Verapamil has been shown to decrease the frequency of angina attacks in patients with chronic stable angina and to improve exercise tolerance and decrease sublingual nitrate consumption.[69–71] During treadmill or bicycle exercise, verapamil increases the exercise time to ST-segment depression by electrocardiographic monitoring and prolongs the time to the development of angina or total exercise duration. The double product (heart rate × blood pressure) is lower at any workload with verapamil administration, which is an indication of lower myocardial oxygen demand. However, the peak of double product obtained during exercise shows no difference between patients receiving verapamil and those not receiving therapy, even though it occurs at higher exercise levels in patients receiving verapamil. The beneficial effect of verapamil in patients with chronic stable angina is likely from both reduction in myocardial oxygen demand and an improvement in coronary blood flow. However, the exact mechanism is controversial and not well understood. Verapamil, also with other calcium antagonists, provides an alternative or additive therapy to nitrates and β-adrenergic blockers for the treatment of chronic stable angina. Several studies have attempted to compare verapamil with a β-adrenergic blocker (propranolol) and long-acting nitrates. The results of these studies are variable and demonstrate that verapamil is more or equally effective for reducing the frequency of angina attacks and improving exercise tolerance.[7–9, 72] In some studies, combined therapy with a β-adrenergic blocker or a long-acting nitrate has been more efficacious than monotherapy. Neither tachyphylaxis nor partial tolerance has been reported with verapamil.[73]

Verapamil may also have clinical utility in limiting

Table 100–3. **Possible Uses of Verapamil**

Approved or Accepted
  Anginal syndrome
    Chronic stable angina
    Unstable angina
    Variant angina
  Post myocardial infarct
  Supraventricular arrhythmia
  Hypertrophic cardiomyopathy
  Hypertension
Not Approved or Not Accepted
  Pulmonary hypertension
  Asthma or other bronchospasm
  Subarachnoid hemorrhage
  Intermittent claudication
  Vasospastic disease (Raynaud's phenomenon)
  Migraine

ischemic myocardial damage. Experimental models have demonstrated that treatment with verapamil before an ischemic injury reduces infarct size.[74-77] When treatment is continued after coronary artery occlusion, the beneficial effect is maintained.[71, 78] Consequently, clinical trials have been performed to see if prophylactic treatment with verapamil would prevent or limit myocardial ischemic injury,[79-81] because verapamil has been demonstrated to be effective in prevention of ischemic episodes in patients with stable angina, unstable angina, vasospastic angina, and silent ischemia.[82-85] Verapamil also reduces the prevalence of ventricular ectopic beats[82] and prevents exercise-induced ventricular tachycardia.[86, 87] In the Danish Verapamil Infarction Trial II, long-term (18 months) treatment with verapamil after an acute myocardial infarction caused a significant reduction in major cardiac events (Fig. 100–2) and a reduction in mortality in those patients without systolic heart failure (Fig. 100–3).[88] These positive results may be related to both antiischemic and negative chronotropic effects of the drug to facilitate coronary perfusion.

Unstable Angina

Verapamil has been shown to improve rest angina.[89] An element of increased coronary spasm probably contributes to myocardial ischemia. Coronary spasm is more likely in patients with unstable angina than in those with stable angina. Therefore, drugs that produce coronary vasodilation (verapamil, other calcium antagonists, and nitrates) are likely to be more efficacious than β-adrenergic blockers.

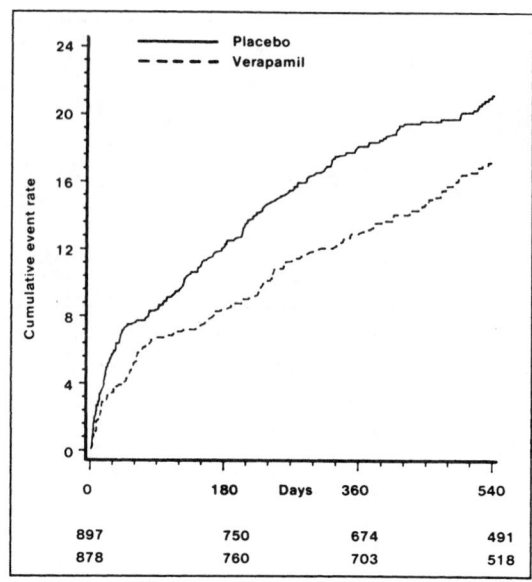

Figure 100–3. Cumulative major event rate with placebo or verapamil (p = .03). The number of patients at risk are shown at the bottom (placebo, n = 897; verapamil, n = 878). (Reprinted with permission from the Danish Study Group on Verapamil in Myocardial Infarction: Effect of verapamil on mortality and major events after acute myocardial infarction [The Danish Verapamil Infarction Trial II—DAVIT II]. Am J Cardiol 66:779, 1990.)

Variant Angina

On electrocardiograms, verapamil has demonstrated antiischemic effects by decreasing episodes of ST-segment elevation or depression resulting from coronary artery spasm.[12] Furthermore, verapamil has an ability to reduce, prevent, or reverse angiographically demonstrated coronary artery spasm. Long-acting nitrates and calcium antagonists are similar in their effectiveness for preventing recurrent episodes of coronary artery spasm. However, because of predictable pharmacokinetic properties and a smaller incidence of side effects, a calcium antagonist is more frequently prescribed.

Supraventricular Arrhythmias

Intravenous verapamil is effective for rapidly terminating reentrant paroxysmal supraventricular tachycardia, reverting some 90% of cases to sinus rhythm within minutes of administration.[6, 90, 91] With verapamil, the ventricular rate is slowed in atrial flutter and fibrillation.[92] Verapamil is contraindicated in patients with preexcitation syndrome who have atrial fibrillation with a rapid ventricular response because it can accentuate conduction through the bypass tract.[54] The effect of verapamil in multifocal atrial tachycardia is generally poor, and its role in ectopic atrial tachycardia is not well defined.

Hypertrophic Cardiomyopathy

Because hypertrophic cardiomyopathy is characterized by augmented systolic ventricular performance

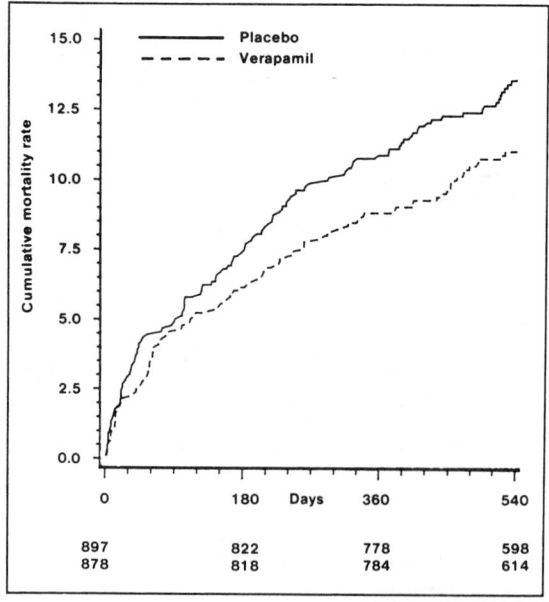

Figure 100–2. Cumulative mortality rate with placebo or verapamil (p = .11). The number of patients at risk are shown at the bottom (placebo, n = 897, verapamil, n = 878). (Reprinted with permission from the Danish Study Group on Verapamil in Myocardial Infarction: Effect of verapamil on mortality and major events after acute myocardial infarction [The Danish Verapamil Infarction Trial II—DAVIT II]. Am J Cardiol 66:779, 1990.)

and impaired diastolic function, verapamil and other calcium antagonists might be expected to normalize the hemodynamic abnormalities and to improve symptoms. The overall beneficial effects are similar to those found with β-blockers such as propranolol.[93]

Coronary artery disease and hypertension impair diastolic function because of ischemia and the net result is inadequate removal of calcium from the cytosol of cardiac myocytes during diastole, and as a consequence, incomplete dissociation of contractile proteins.[94] Thus, the myocytes maintain tension, even during the early relaxation phase of diastole, limiting the rate and extent of the filling of the ventricle and normal left ventricular diastolic pressure. Higher filling pressures are necessary to distend the ventricle, and forward flow during the subsequent systole may be compromised by reduced filling of the ventricle in diastole, because of less stroke volume available for the next systole.

The most appropriate drugs for diastolic heart failure are β-blockers, which slow the heart rate and give the ventricle more time to fill with blood, and calcium antagonists such as verapamil, which lower cytosol calcium and allow more complete dissociation of contractile proteins and thus tension release. Verapamil also reduces heart rate and ischemia and their contribution to impaired diastolic filling.

Studies performed at the National Institutes of Health have demonstrated that verapamil has a beneficial effect on left ventricular diastolic relaxation and compliance in patients with either hypertrophic cardiomyopathy or hypertension. Moreover, improved LV diastolic filling characteristics have been associated with increases in functional exercise capacity in such patients.[95–97] Attenuation of myocardial hypertrophy in hypertensive patients with verapamil has also been associated with a decreased incidence of ventricular arrhythmia and improved exercise tolerance.[98, 99]

Hypertension

Because the calcium antagonists are effective arterial vasodilators, it was speculated that alterations of calcium kinetics within vessel walls may be an important factor in the pathogenesis of hypertension. Clinical studies of the use of verapamil and other calcium antagonists indicate that the degree of blood pressure reduction is directly related to the magnitude of the pretreatment blood pressure. Therefore, normotensive subjects usually do not show any significant hypotensive response after oral administration of verapamil.

The antihypertensive effect of verapamil is evident during the first week of therapy, but the maximal response may not be achieved for at least 3 or 4 weeks. The hypotensive effect of verapamil is at least comparable with or better than that of other calcium antagonists or other classes of antihypertensive agents. Verapamil has demonstrated consistent antihypertensive activity independent of age, race, or salt intake. Some investigators even suggest that verapamil has a more potent antihypertensive effect with higher salt intake.[100–104] The combination of verapamil with a β-adrenergic blocker has generally been avoided because of common negative inotropic actions of these drugs. Some studies, however, have demonstrated an additive hypotensive effect of verapamil with thiazides or ACE inhibitors.

Several studies have shown that calcium antagonists not only maintain renal blood flow and glomerular filtration rate while lowering peripheral vascular resistance but also may increase renal blood flow and glomerular filtration rate in hypertensive patients. Verapamil has been shown to cause regression of left ventricular hypertrophy and to be useful for reversing diastolic dysfunction caused by hypertension. Elderly patients with hypertension are more apt to have concomitant peripheral vascular disease, left ventricular hypertrophy, diabetes mellitus, and chronic obstructive pulmonary disease. Verapamil therapy does not adversely affect these concomitant disease states. Calcium antagonists have proved to be equally effective in black patients with hypertension, unlike β-adrenergic blockers or ACE inhibitors. Patients who respond well to diuretic therapy are likely to respond to therapy with calcium antagonists. Verapamil and other calcium antagonists, in contrast to diuretics, do not affect blood glucose, potassium, magnesium, uric acid, or serum lipid levels.[105] Additionally, calcium antagonists do not have their antihypertensive effect offset by nonsteroidal antiinflammatory drugs (NSAIDs),[106, 107] which does occur with such drugs as diuretics, β-blockers, or ACE inhibitors. This is an important point in older hypertensive patients who frequently require both NSAIDs and antihypertensive medication.[108]

Coronary Artery Disease

Two recent studies, the Danish Verapamil Infarction Trial II (DAVIT II)[109] and the Angina Prognosis Study in Stockholm (APSIS),[110] attest to the benefits of verapamil in patients with coronary artery disease. In the DAVIT II study, a total of 1775 patients were randomized to either placebo or verapamil (360 mg/day) 7 to 15 days after suffering acute myocardial infarction (MI). The verapamil group had a 17% reduction in reinfarction and major event rates during a 12- to 18-month follow-up.

In patients without congestive heart failure, an impressive 36% reduction of mortality and 33% reduction of reinfarction rates were noted. These provocative findings make verapamil the drug of choice in the post-MI patient in whom a β-blocker is contraindicated or not tolerated. Of note, the beneficial effects were more pronounced in hypertensive than in normotensive patients.

The APSIS study was a primary prevention trial in more than 800 patients with stable angina pectoris. Patients were randomized to either metoprolol or verapamil. Both drugs were equally well tolerated and had the same effect on mortality, cardiovascular end points, and measures of quality of life. Importantly, patients concomitantly suffering from hypertension did better with verapamil than with metoprolol.

Both of these recent studies attest to the unique features of verapamil, which may be related to its negative chronotropic and/or inotropic effect. The DAVIT II and the APSIS data are in sharp contrast to the reports with the dihydropyridine calcium antagonists in which no effect or even an increase in mortality was documented in the patients with coronary artery disease.

ADVERSE REACTIONS

The risk of adverse reactions with verapamil will depend on the route of administration, the conditions being treated, dosage of the drug, and the presence of other drugs. The most concerning side effects, which infrequently occur, are negative inotropism and SA and AV nodal conduction disturbances. Chronic therapy with oral verapamil has shown first-degree AV block in some patients, but the development of advanced heart block is rare unless antecedent conduction system disease is present. Frank cardiac failure is detected only in patients with depressed left ventricular ejection fraction, and cardiac failure uncommonly is precipitated in the presence of normal left ventricular systolic function or mild dysfunction unless patients have been treated with β-adrenergic blockers. Side effects are reported in approximately 8% of patients, the most common of which is constipation; other occasionally reported side effects include headache, dizziness, nausea, and ankle edema (Table 100–4). An increase in the serum levels of hepatic enzymes has been reported, but frank toxicity is rare. Otherwise, the drug is well tolerated with effects on the quality of life comparable with those of other commonly used antihypertensive agents.[111]

After administration of intravenous verapamil, the pharmacologically expected side effect of a transient decrease in blood pressure has been noted. However, serious side effects such as persistent hypotension, bradycardia, and, rarely, ventricular asystole have also been reported.[112] In most cases, the patients had been receiving chronic therapy with a β-adrenergic blocker or digoxin or had hypokalemia before verapamil was administered. This tendency suggests that intravenous verapamil should be given with great caution in patients receiving any of the above-mentioned combination therapies or in the presence of hypokalemia. However, if such a serious adverse effect occurred in this setting, it might be reversed by intravenous atropine, isoproterenol, or calcium gluconate.[112] In cases of asystole, temporary ventricular pacemaker therapy may also be effective. Severe hypotension should be treated with norepinephrine. Verapamil is clearly contraindicated in patients with sick sinus syndrome, second-degree or third-degree heart block, Wolff-Parkinson-White syndrome, or left ventricular systolic dysfunction with an ejection fraction of less than 30%.

DRUG INTERACTION

Verapamil should be used cautiously in the presence of β-adrenergic blockers because of the potential for synergistic hypotension, bradycardia, and asystole, although no significant complications will occur in most patients with essential hypertension. Verapamil combined with antiarrhythmic agents such as quinidine, procainamide, or disopyramide potentially could induce hypotension and bradycardia; therefore, extreme vigilance should be exercised when prescribing these combinations so that potential problems can be detected and avoided. Oral verapamil has been shown to increase the half-life of digoxin, decrease digoxin clearance, and increase digoxin plasma levels. Thus, the plasma digoxin level should be monitored carefully when verapamil is used in combination with

Table 100–4. **Adverse Reactions to Calcium Antagonists**

Side Effect	Calcium Antagonists		
	Nifedipine	*Verapamil*	*Diltiazem*
Dizziness or light-headedness	10.0	3.6	Unk
Peripheral edema	10.0	1.7	2.4
Headache	10.0	1.8	2.0
Flushing or heat sensation	10.0	Unk	Unk
Transient hypotension	5.0	2.9	Unk
Nausea	10.0	1.6	2.7
AV block (third degree)	Unk	0.8	0.4
Bradycardia	Unk	1.1	2.0
Palpitations	2.0	Unk	Unk
Congestive heart failure	2.0	0.9	Unk
Constipation	Unk	6.3	Unk
Fatigue	Unk	1.1	1.1
Syncope	0.5	Unk	Unk
Rash	Unk	Unk	1.8
Overall incidence	17.0	8.0	4.0

Data are from 2100 patients with angina.
Unk, Incidence is unknown.
Adapted from McMahon FG: Management of Essential Hypertension: The New Low-Dose Era, 2nd ed. Mount Kisco, NY: Futura Publishing Company, 1984, pp 393–416.

digoxin; if indicated, the digoxin dose should be decreased by 50%, especially in the presence of renal dysfunction. Verapamil may lower serum lithium levels, increase carbamazepine concentrations, or potentiate the action of neuromuscular blocking agents and inhalation anesthetics. Rifampin therapy may markedly reduce the bioavailability of oral verapamil. Cimetidine may inhibit the metabolism of verapamil. Verapamil may also decrease metabolism of cyclosporine and raise its serum levels approximately 30%.

DOSAGE AND ADMINISTRATION

The dose of intravenous verapamil is 0.075 to 0.15 mg/kg infused over 1 to 3 minutes in children and adults. An approximate maintenance intravenous dose is 0.005 mg/kg/min or 5 to 10 mg every 30 minutes in adults. The recommended oral dose ranges from 120 to 480 mg/day. The frequency of administration is dependent on the condition for which treatment is prescribed. For patients with cardiac supraventricular arrhythmia and angina, it is recommended that the drug be given in three divided doses of the immediate-release form of verapamil. However, for patients with hypertension, a once-daily schedule with 180 mg is used with the sustained-release preparation. However, in certain cases, the dosage of a sustained-release verapamil could be decreased to 120 mg once daily. If a dose of 360 to 480 mg of sustained-release verapamil is to be prescribed, the dose then should be divided into 180 to 240 mg twice daily. These recommendations are only guidelines; the dosage and frequency should be individualized for each patient.

CONCLUSION

Verapamil is the first of the first-generation calcium antagonists. It has a variety of actions at the cellular level, some of which may be more important than others in the treatment of various disease states. The property of diminishing calcium entry into cardiac and smooth muscle cells results in therapeutic actions of coronary vasodilation and relief of angina, treatment of systemic hypertension, and prevention and treatment of supraventricular tachycardia. The drug is well absorbed in the gastrointestinal tract but is extensively metabolized by the liver. The sustained-release formulation is useful for prolonged action and improved compliance, and can be administered once daily for the treatment of hypertension. However, angina symptoms should be treated with at least a twice-daily dosage of the sustained-release preparation or with multiple divided doses of immediate-release formulation verapamil.

Several attributes of verapamil, including maintaining tissue and target organ perfusion, decreasing left ventricular mass and proteinuria, efficacy in a broad variety of hypertensive patients irrespective of age, race, or sodium intake, and absence of biochemical side effects, make it a desirable drug therapy. The side-effect profile is also attractive for the treatment of chronic conditions, especially hypertension, and has been well accepted by many patients. Extreme caution should be used when administering this drug to patients with left ventricular systolic dysfunction, a high degree (second- or third-degree) heart block, or sick sinus syndrome. Drug interaction, especially with digoxin, should be kept in mind when a combination of agents is used.

REFERENCES

1. Fleckenstein A, Tritthart H, Flackenstein B, et al: Eine neue Gruppe kompetitiver zweiwertiges Ca-Antagon-isten (Iproveratril, D 600, Prenylamin) mit starken Hemmeffekten auf die elektromechanische Koppelung im Warmblüter-Myokard. Pfluegers Arch 307:25, 1969.
2. Haas H, Härtfelder G: α-Isopropyl-α-[(N-methyl-N-homoveratryl)-γ-amino-propyl]-3,4-dimethoxyphenylacetonitril, eine Substanz mit coronargefässerweiternden Eigenschaften. Arzneimittelforschung 12:549, 1962.
3. Melville KI, Benfey BG: Coronary vasodilatory and cardiac adrenergic blocking effects of Iproveratril. Can J Physiol Pharmacol 43:339, 1965.
4. Schmid JR, Hanna C: A comparison of the antiarrhythmic actions of two new synthetic compounds, Iproveratril and MJ 1999, with quinidine and pronethalol. J Pharmacol Exp Ther 156:331, 1967.
5. Krikler DM, Spurrell RAJ: Verapamil in the treatment of paroxysmal supraventricular tachycardia. Postgrad Med J 50:447, 1974.
6. Sung RJ, Elser B, McAllister RG Jr: Intravenous verapamil for termination of re-entrant supraventricular tachycardias: Intracardiac studies correlated with plasma verapamil concentrations. Ann Intern Med 93:682, 1980.
7. Johnson SM, Mauritson DR, Corbett JR, et al: Double-blind, randomized, placebo-controlled comparison of propranolol and verapamil in the treatment of patients with stable angina pectoris. Am J Med 71:443, 1981.
8. Frishman WH, Klein NA, Strom JA, et al: Superiority of verapamil to propranolol in stable angina pectoris: A double-blind, randomized crossover trial. Circulation 65(Suppl I):I51, 1982.
9. Pine MB, Citron PD, Bailly DJ, et al: Verapamil versus placebo in relieving stable angina pectoris. Circulation 65:17, 1982.
10. Kimura E, Kishida H: Treatment of variant angina with drugs: A survey of 11 cardiology institutes in Japan. Circulation 63:844, 1981.
11. Waters DD, Théroux P, Szlachcic J, et al: Provocative testing with ergonovine to assess the efficacy of treatment with nifedipine, diltiazem and verapamil in variant angina. Am J Cardiol 48:123, 1981.
12. Johnson SM, Mauritson DR, Willerson JT, et al: A controlled trial of verapamil for Prinzmetal's variant angina. N Engl J Med 304:862, 1981.
13. Rosing DR, Kent KM, Maron BJ, et al: Verapamil therapy: A new approach to the pharmacologic treatment of hypertrophic cardiomyopathy: II. Effects on exercise capacity and symptomatic status. Circulation 60:1208, 1979.
14. Frishman WH, Strom JA, Greenberg SM, et al: Calcium-channel blockers in systemic hypertension. Curr Probl Cardiol 12:287, 1987.
15. Weir MR, Peppler R, Gomolka D, Handwerger BS: Evidence that the antiproliferative effect of verapamil on afferent and efferent immune responses is independent of calcium channel inhibition. Transplantation 54:681, 1992.
16. Somogyi A, Albrecht M, Kliems G, et al: Pharmacokinetics, bioavailability and ECG response of verapamil in patients with liver cirrhosis. Br J Clin Pharmacol 12:51, 1981.
17. Mooy J, Schols M, v Baak M, et al: Pharmacokinetics of verapamil in patients with renal failure. Eur J Clin Pharmacol 28:405, 1985.
18. Kates RE: Calcium antagonists: Pharmacokinetic properties. Drugs 25:113, 1983.

19. McAllister RG Jr, Hamann SR, Blouin RA: Pharmacokinetics of calcium-entry blockers. Am J Cardiol 55:30B, 1985.

19a. Willich SN, Levy D, Rocco MB, et al: Circadian variation in the increase of sudden cardiac death in the Framingham Heart Study population. Am J Cardiol 60:801, 1987.

20. Fleckenstein A: Specific inhibitors and promoters of calcium action in the excitation-contraction coupling of heart muscle and their role in prevention or production of myocardial lesions. In Harris P, Opie L (eds): Calcium and the Heart. London: Academic Press, 1971, p 135.

21. Nayler WG, Szeto J: Effect of verapamil on contractility, oxygen utilization, and calcium exchangeability in mammalian heart muscle. Cardiovasc Res 6:120, 1972.

22. Nayler WG, Krikler D: Verapamil and the myocardium. Postgrad Med J 50:441, 1974.

23. Chandy KG, DeCoursey TE, Cahalan MD, et al: Voltage-gated potassium channels are required for human T lymphocyte activation. J Exp Med 160:369, 1984.

24. Schell SR, Nelson DJ, Fozzard HA, et al: The inhibitory effects of K$^+$ channnel agents on T lymphocyte proliferation and lymphokine production are "non-specific." J Immunol 139:3224, 1987.

25. Weir MR, Gomolka D, Peppler R, Handwerger BS: Mechanisms responsible for inhibition of lymphocyte activation by agents which block membrane calcium or potassium channels. Transplant Proc 25:605, 1993.

26. Weir MR, Bhandaru S, Bakris GL: Inhibition of insulin-mediated mesangial cell proliferation is unrelated to blockade of the voltage-gated slow calcium channel. J Am Soc Nephrol 2:470, 1991.

27. Simpson LL, Standley PR, Zhang F, et al: Role of calcium in vascular smooth muscle proliferation: Anti-proliferative effect of verapamil enantiomers—independence from calcium channel blockade. Circulation Res (In press).

28. Simpson LL, Zhang F, Standley PR, et al: Antiproliferative effects of verapamil enantiomers in vascular smooth muscle cells. J Vasc Biol Med (In press).

29. Braunwald E: Mechanism of action of calcium-channel-blocking agents. N Engl J Med 307:1618, 1983.

30. Bayer R, Kalusche D, Kaufmann R, et al: Inotropic and electrophysiological actions of verapamil and D 600 in mammalian myocardium: III. Effects of the optical isomers on transmembrane action potentials. Naunyn Schmiedebergs Arch Pharmacol 290:81, 1975.

31. Ehara T, Daufmann R: The voltage- and time-dependent effects of (-)-verapamil on the slow inward current in isolated cat ventricular myocardium. J Pharmacol Exp Ther 207:49, 1978.

32. Patel KR: Calcium antagonists in exercise-induced asthma. Br Med J 282:932, 1981.

33. Cerrina J, Denjean A, Alexandre G, et al: Inhibition of exercise-induced asthma by a calcium antagonist, nifedipine. Am Rev Respir Dis 123:156, 1981.

34. Devis G, Somers G, Van Obberghen E, et al: Calcium antagonists and islet function: I. Inhibition of insulin release by verapamil. Diabetes 24:547, 1975.

35. Hermansen K, Iversen J: Effect of verapamil on pancreatic glucagon release from the isolated, perfused canine pancreas. Scand J Clin Lab Invest 37:139, 1977.

36. Chierchia S, Crea F, Bernini W, et al: Antiplatelet effects of verapamil in man [abstract]. Am J Cardiol 47:399, 1981.

37. Mehta D, Mehta J, Ostrowski N, Brigmon L: Inhibitory effects of diltiazem on platelet activation caused by ionophore A23187 plus ABP or epinephrine in subthreshold concentrations. J Lab Clin Med 102:332, 1983.

38. Weir MR: Therapeutic benefit of calcium channel blockers in cyclosporine-treated organ transplant recipients: Blood pressure control and immunosuppression. Am J Med 90(5A):325, 1992.

39. Ellrodt G, Chew CYC, Singh BN: Therapeutic implications of slow-channel blockade in cardiocirculatory disorders. Circulation 62:669, 1980.

40. Singh BN, Ellrodt G, Peter CT: Verapamil: A review of its pharmacological properties and therapeutic use. Drugs 15:169, 1978.

41. Singh BN, Williams EMV: A fourth class of anti-dysrhythmic action? Effect of verapamil on ouabain toxicity, on atrial and ventricular intracellular potentials, and on other features of cardiac function. Cardiovasc Res 6:109, 1972.

42. Singh BN, Hecht HS, Nademanee K, et al: Electrophysiologic and hemodynamic effects of slow-channel blocking drugs. Prog Cardiovasc Dis 25:103, 1982.

43. Singh BN, Roche AHG: Effects of intravenous verapamil on hemodynamics in patients with heart disease. Am Heart J 94:593, 1977.

44. Chew CYC, Hecht HS, Collett JT, et al: Influence of severity of ventricular dysfunction on hemodynamic responses to intravenously administered verapamil in ischemic heart disease. Am J Cardiol 47:917, 1981.

45. Lewis BS, Mitha AS, Gotsman MS: Immediate haemodynamic effects of verapamil in man. Cardiology 60:366, 1975.

46. Atterhög J-H, Ekelund L-G: Haemodynamic effects of intravenous verapamil at rest and during exercise in subjectively healthy middle-aged men. Eur J Clin Pharmacol 8:317, 1975.

47. Ferlinz J, Easthope JL, Aronow WS: Effects of verapamil on myocardial performance in coronary disease. Circulation 59:313, 1979.

48. Schmieder RE, Messerli FH, Garavaglia GE, et al: Cardiovascular effects of verapamil in patients with essential hypertension. Circulation 75:1030, 1987.

49. Josephson MA, Hecht HS, Hopkins JM, et al: Oral verapamil vs propranolol in coronary artery disease: Evaluation of left ventricular function by exercise radionuclide ventriculography [abstract]. Am J Cardiol 47:463, 1981.

50. Singh BN, Chew CYC, Josephson MA, et al: Pharmacologic and hemodynamic mechanisms underlying the antianginal actions of verapamil. Am J Cardiol 50:886, 1982.

51. Wellens HJJ, Tan SL, Bär FWH, et al: Effect of verapamil studied by programmed electrical stimulation of the heart in patients with paroxysmal re-entrant supraventricular tachycardia. Br Heart J 39:1058, 1977.

52. Rowland E, Evans T, Krikler D: Effect of nifedipine on atrioventricular conduction as compared with verapamil: Intracardiac electrophysiological study. Br Heart J 42:124, 1979.

53. Tonkin AM, Aylward PE, Joel SE, et al: Verapamil in prophylaxis of paroxysmal atrioventricular nodal reentrant tachycardia. J Cardiovasc Pharmacol 2:473, 1980.

54. Gulamhusein S, Ko P, Carruthers SG, et al: Acceleration of the ventricular response during atrial fibrillation in the Wolff-Parkinson-White syndrome after verapamil. Circulation 65:348, 1982.

55. Luebs ED, Cohen A, Zaleski EJ, et al: Effect of nitroglycerin, intensain, isoptin and papaverine on coronary blood flow in man: Measured by the coincidence counting technic and rubidium. Am J Cardiol 17:535, 1966.

56. Simonsen S: Pharmacological effects on coronary haemodynamics: A comparative study between atenolol, verapamil, nifedipine and carbocromen. Acta Med Scand (Suppl) 645:97, 1981.

57. Chew CYC, Brown BG, Wong M, et al: The effects of verapamil on coronary hemodynamics and vasomobility in patients with coronary artery disease [abstract]. Am J Cardiol 45:389, 1980.

58. Ferlinz J, Turbow ME: Antianginal and myocardial metabolic properties of verapamil in coronary artery disease. Am J Cardiol 46:1019, 1980.

59. Harder DR, Belardinelli L, Sperelakis N, et al: Differential effects of adenosine and nitroglycerin on the action potentials of large and small coronary arteries. Circ Res 44:176, 1979.

60. Brown BG, Josephson MA, Petersen RB, et al: Intravenous dipyridamole combined with isometric handgrip for near maximal acute increase in coronary flow in patients with coronary artery disease. Am J Cardiol 48:1077, 1981.

61. Sorensen SS, Thomsen O, Danielsen H, et al: Effect of verapamil on renal plasma flow, glomerular filtration rate and plasma angiotensin II, aldosterone and arginine vasopressin in essential hypertension. Eur J Clin Pharmacol 29:257, 1985.

62. Leonetti G, Cuspidi C, Sampieri L, et al: Comparison of cardiovascular, renal, and humoral effects of acute administration of two calcium channel blockers in normotensive and hypertensive subjects. J Cardiovasc Pharmacol 4:S319, 1982.

63. de Leeuw PW, Birkenhäger WH: Effects of verapamil in hypertensive patients. Acta Med Scand 681(Suppl):125, 1984.

64. Romero JC, Raij L, Granger JP, et al: Multiple effects of calcium

entry blockers on renal function in hypertension. Hypertension 10:140, 1987.

65. Bauer JH, Sunderrajan S, Reams G: Effects of calcium entry blockers on renin-angiotensin-aldosterone system, renal function and hemodynamics, salt and water excretion and body fluid composition. Am J Cardiol 56:62H, 1985.

66. Bakris GL, Barnhill BW, Sadler R: Treatment of arterial hypertension in diabetic humans: Importance of therapeutic selection. Kidney Int 41:912, 1992.

67. Carmines PK, Navar LG: Disparate effects of calcium channel blockade on afferent and efferent arteriolar responses to angiotensin II. Am J Physiol 256:F1015, 1989.

68. Yoshioka T, Shiraga H, Yoshida Y, et al: "Intact nephrons" as the primary origin of proteinuria in chronic renal disease. J Clin Invest 82:1614, 1988.

69. Tan ATH, Sadick N, Kelly DT, et al: Verapamil in stable effort angina: Effects on left ventricular function evaluated with exercise radionuclide ventriculography. Am J Cardiol 49:425, 1982.

70. Pepine CJ, Feldman RL, Hill JA, et al: Clinical outcome after treatment of rest angina with calcium blockers: Comparative experience during the initial year of therapy with diltiazem, nifedipine, and verapamil. Am Heart J 106:1341, 1983.

71. Przyklenk K, Kloner RA: Effect of verapamil on postischemic "stunned" myocardium: Importance of the timing of treatment. J Am Coll Cardiol 11:614, 1988.

72. Arnman K, Rydén L: Comparison of metoprolol and verapamil in the treatment of angina pectoris. Am J Cardiol 49:821, 1982.

73. Weiner DA, McCabe CH, Cutler SS, et al: Efficacy and safety of verapamil in patients with angina pectoris after 1 year of continuous, high-dose therapy. Am J Cardiol 51:1251, 1983.

74. Nayler WG: Calcium antagonists and the ischemic myocardium. Int J Cardiol 15:267, 1987.

75. Kloner RA, Braunwald E: Effects of calcium antagonist on infarcting myocardium. Am J Cardiol 59:84B, 1987.

76. Skolnick AE, Frishman WH: Calcium channel blockers in myocardial infarction. Arch Intern Med 49:1669, 1989.

77. Reimer KA, Jennings RB: Verapamil in two reperfusion models of myocardial infarction. Lab Invest 51:655, 1984.

78. Yellon DM, Hearse J, Maxwell MP, et al: Sustained limitation of myocardial necrosis 24 hours after coronary artery occlusion: Verapamil infusion in dogs with small myocardial infarcts. Am J Cardiol 51:1409, 1984.

79. Hansen JF, Sigurd B, Mennemgaard K, Lyngbye J: Verapamil in acute myocardial infarction. Dan Med Bull 27:105, 1980.

80. The Danish Study Group on Verapamil in Myocardial Infarction: Verapamil in acute myocardial infarction. Am J Cardiol 54:24E, 1984.

81. The Danish Study Group on Verapamil in Myocardial Infarction: The Danish studies on verapamil in myocardial infarction. Br J Clin Pharmacol 21:197S, 1986.

82. Subramanian VB, Bowles ML, Lahiri A, et al: Long-term antianginal action of verapamil assessed with quantitated serial treadmill stress testing. Am J Cardiol 48:529, 1981.

83. Mauritson DR, Johnson SM, Winniford MD, et al: Verapamil for unstable angina at rest: A short-term randomized, double-blind study. Am Heart J 106:652, 1983.

84. Mauri F, Mafrici A, Biraghi M, et al: Effectiveness of calcium antagonist drugs in patients with unstable angina and proven coronary artery disease. Eur Heart J 9:158, 1988.

85. Maseri A: Comparison of verapamil and propranolol therapy for angina at rest: A randomized, multiple crossover, controlled trial in the coronary care unit. Am J Cardiol 57:899, 1986.

86. Woelfel A, Foster JR, McAllister RG, et al: Efficacy of verapamil in exercise-induced ventricular tachycardia. Am J Cardiol 56:292, 1985.

87. Gülker H, Godejohann U, Dorsel T, et al: Prophylaxe belastungsinduzierter ventrikulärer Arrhythmien durch Verapamil. Z Kardiol 76:404, 1987.

88. The Danish Study Group on Verapamil in Myocardial Infarction: Effect of verapamil on mortality and major events after acute myocardial infarction (The Danish Verapamil Infarction Trial II—DAVIT II). Am J Cardiol 66:779, 1990.

89. Mehta J, Pepine CJ, Day M, et al: Short-term efficacy of oral verapamil in rest angina: A double-blind placebo controlled trial in CCU patients. Am J Med 71:977, 1981.

90. Mitchell LB, Schroeder JS, Mason JW: Comparative clinical electrophysiologic effects of diltiazem, verapamil and nifedipine: A review. Am J Cardiol 49:629, 1982.

91. Rozanski JJ, Zaman L, Castellanos A: Electrophysiologic effects of diltiazem hydrochloride on supraventricular tachycardia. Am J Cardiol 49:621, 1982.

92. Waxman HL, Myerburg RJ, Appel R, et al: Verapamil for control of ventricular rate in paroxysmal supraventricular tachycardia and atrial fibrillation or flutter: A double-blind randomized cross-over study. Ann Intern Med 94:1, 1981.

93. Kaltenbach M, Hopf R, Kober G, et al: Treatment of hypertrophic obstructive cardiomyopathy with verapamil. Br Heart J 42:35, 1979.

94. Cuocolo A, Sax FL, Brush JE, et al: Left ventricular hypertrophy and impaired diastolic filling in essential hypertension: Diastolic mechanisms for systolic dysfunction during exercise. Circulation 81:978, 1990.

95. Bonow RO, Dilsizian V, Rosing DR, et al: Verapamil-induced improvement in left ventricular diastolic filling and increased exercise tolerance in patients with hypertrophic cardiomyopathy: Short- and long-term effects. Circulation 72:853, 1985.

96. Brush JE, Udelson JE, Bachrach SL, et al: Comparative effects of verapamil and nitroprusside on left ventricular function in patients with hypertension. J Am Coll Cardiol 14:515, 1989.

97. Cody RJ, Kubo SH, Covit AB, et al: Exercise hemodynamics and oxygen delivery in human hypertension: Response to verapamil. Hypertension 8:3, 1986.

98. Messerli FH, Nunez BD, Nunez MM, et al: Hypertension and sudden death: Disparate effects of calcium entry blockers and diuretic therapy on cardiac dysrhythmias. Arch Intern Med 149:1263, 1989.

99. Schulman SP, Weiss JL, Becker LC, et al: The effects of antihypertensive therapy on left ventricular mass in elderly patients. N Engl J Med 322:1350, 1990.

100. Speders S, Sosna J, Schumacher A, et al: Efficacy and tolerability of isoptin SR in essential hypertension—results of a Phase IV study under practice conditions. Hochdruck 8:3, 1988.

101. Cox JP, O'Boyle CA, Mee F, et al: The antihypertensive efficacy of verapamil in the elderly evaluated by ambulatory BP measurement. J Hum Hypertens 2:410, 1988.

102. Saunders E, Weir MR, Kong BW, et al: A comparison of the efficacy and safety of a beta blocker, calcium channel blocker, and converting enzyme inhibitor in hypertensive blacks. Arch Intern Med 150:1707, 1990.

103. Weir MR: Impact of age, race, and obesity on hypertensive mechanisms and therapy. Am J Med 90(5A):39, 1991.

104. Nicholson JP, Resnick LM, Laragh JH: The antihypertensive effect of verapamil at extremes of dietary sodium intake. Ann Intern Med 107:329, 1987.

105. Midtbo K, Lauve O, Hals O: No metabolic side effects of longterm treatment with verapamil in hypertension. Angiology 39:1025, 1988.

106. Houston MC: Nonsteroidal anti-inflammatory drugs and antihypertensives. Am J Med 90(Suppl 5A):42S, 1991.

107. Klassen DK, Young DY, Peterson CA: Assessment of blood pressure during nonsteroidal anti-inflammatory drug therapy in hypertensive patients treated with calcium channel blockers. Arch Intern Med (In press).

108. Weir MR: Hypertension and arthritis: Coprevalence and implications for therapy. Comorbidity in Cardiovascular Disease 1:3, 1992.

109. The Danish Study Group on Verapamil in Myocardial Infarction: Effect of verapamil on mortality and major events after acute myocardial infarction (The Danish Verapamil Trial II–DAVIT II). Am J Cardiol 66:779, 1990.

110. Rehnqvist N, Hjemdahl P, Billing E, et al: Prevention of cardiac events in patients with angina pectoris. Results of the APSIS study [abstract]. Eur Heart J 16(Suppl H):18, 1995

111. Croog SH, Kong BW, Levine S, et al: Hypertensive black men and women: Quality of life and effects of antihypertensive medications. Arch Intern Med 150:1733, 1990.

112. Lewis JG: Adverse reactions to calcium antagonists. Drugs 25:196, 1983.

CHAPTER 101

Gallopamil

Roberto Ferrari, M.D., Ph.D.

HISTORY

Although gallopamil is generally considered a derivative of verapamil, the prototype of the phenylalkylamine class of calcium antagonists, its history is as old as that of verapamil. It was synthesized in 1968 by Ferdinand Dengel, the chief chemist of Knoll Company in Ludwigshafen, West Germany.[1] It was the 600th verapamil derivative tested in Dengel's laboratories. It was therefore called "D-600." It was found to be the second drug (after verapamil) that perfectly met the strict experimental criteria established by Fleckenstein for characterizing the action mechanism of highly specific calcium antagonists.[2-4]

CHEMISTRY

Gallopamil is a methoxy derivative of verapamil. The chemical structure of gallopamil is 5-[2-(3,4-dimethoxy) ethyl] methylaminol-2-isopropyl-2 (3,4,5-trimethoxy-phenyl) pentanenitrile hydrochlorate. Compared with verapamil, gallopamil has a methoxy group in the meta-position.

PHARMACOLOGY

Gallopamil, as the other calcium antagonists of its class, inhibits transmembrane calcium influx into myocardial, cardiac pacemaker, and vascular smooth muscle cells with the same intensity.[5] In papillary muscles and isolated myocytes, gallopamil reduces calcium-dependent adenosine triphosphate (ATP) splitting and contraction.[5,6] The use of patch-clamping techniques reveals that this effect is a result of inhibition of the slow calcium-dependent inward current, with no effect on the fast sodium current or outline potassium current. Beck et al.,[6] adding both gallopamil and D-890—a quaternary, permanently charged, highly hydrophilic derivative of gallopamil—externally or internally to isolated myocytes, showed that gallopamil rapidly penetrates into the cell, blocks the open channels, and dissociates from the receptor in diastole.

Further insight into the possible intracellular action of gallopamil on heart muscle comes from the finding that, at concentrations between 10 and 100 nM (within the therapeutic range in humans), gallopamil reduces calcium efflux through the calcium channels of the sarcoplasmic reticulum.[7] In addition, gallopamil inhibits calcium transport across the inner mitochondrial membrane.[8] The inhibition occurs over a wide range of free calcium concentrations but requires high doses of the drug (from 10^{-7} M).[8] Contrary to the effect exercised on sarcoplasmic reticulum, the effect on mitochondria is specific for gallopamil because verapamil and dihydropyridines in general fail to affect mitochondrial calcium transport.[9,10] Both of these intracellular actions are relevant in explaining the cardioprotection exerted by gallopamil,[8] and may contribute to its therapeutic action.

Although the primary site of action of gallopamil on the heart sarcolemma is the "L" type of ventricular calcium channels, it also acts on the "T" type of calcium channels located on the atria, thus influencing the transmembrane influx of calcium ions of sinoatrial and atrioventricular nodal cells. Electrophysiologic studies show that gallopamil suppresses the calcium-dependent subthreshold oscillations that occur at low nodal membrane potential and it decreases the slope of slow diastolic depolarization, thus retarding the initiation of propagated impulses.[10] Its potency on cardiac pacemaker cells, however, is at least 10 times less than that of verapamil.[10]

On vascular smooth muscle cells from different preparations, gallopamil is a powerful inhibitor of transmembrane calcium entry through the voltage-operated calcium channels.[5,11] Its potency is intermediate between that of verapamil and nifedipine.[12] Gallopamil in pig coronary vasculature and rabbit femoral artery suppresses the tonic and phasic contractile responses to acetylcholine, histamine, serotonin, and norepinephrine, suggesting that it is also active on the "receptors operating" calcium channels.[13] As phasic norepinephrine-induced contractions are exclusively initiated by calcium release from internal stores, the intracellular action of gallopamil is then relevant to this effect.[13]

MOLECULAR EFFECTS OF GALLOPAMIL CARDIOPROTECTION

Myocardial ischemia causes a series of metabolic, ionic, and neurohumoral changes that lead to reperfusion damage and loss of cell viability.[14] These include development of intracellular acidosis, decline of intracellular levels of high energy phosphates, calcium overload, excess production of oxygen free radicals, and leakage of intracellular enzymes and of noradrenaline.[15,16] Alterations of intracellular calcium are thought to play a central role in the sequence of metabolic disarrangements causing irreversibility of the ischemic damage.[17]

It is not surprising that, experimentally, calcium antagonists have been successfully utilized to protect the myocardium against ischemic and reperfusion damage.[18] In general, these drugs are cardioprotective when administered before or at the time of ischemia. They produce no effect when given several minutes after ischemia or during reperfusion.[19] Their main mechanism of action relates to their ability to reduce calcium influx and myocardial contractility before ischemia. This, in turn, results in ATP sparing with conservation of high energy stores and calcium homeostasis during ischemia, thus allowing full recovery of metabolism and function during reperfusion.

The cardioprotective effects of gallopamil have been tested in several animal models.[8, 19–21] Interestingly, gallopamil is the only calcium antagonist of its class able to provide protection even when administered on reperfusion although to a lesser degree compared with its effects if given before ischemia.[8] This unique action of gallopamil is most likely caused by the reduction of mitochondrial calcium accumulation, a process that is highly stimulated on reperfusion, which irreversibly impairs the ATP-producing capacity of the mitochondria.[17]

There are also other characteristics of gallopamil that might be important in its cardioprotective effect. Modification of the handling of calcium by the sarcolemma and sarcoplasmic reticulum is likely to maintain calcium homeostasis during ischemia.[7] Unexpectedly, gallopamil and other calcium antagonists of the phenylalkylamine type have been shown to modify ischemia and reperfusion-induced noradrenaline release via a mechanism not yet identified but thought to be different from blockade of calcium channels.[7, 22–24] Noradrenaline release on reperfusion plays an important role in promoting calcium entry and ventricular fibrillation.[23] Finally, microcirculatory changes resulting from repetitive induction of ischemia in rats also are attenuated by pretreatment with gallopamil.[25]

PHARMACOKINETICS

Gallopamil is administered as its racemate. S-Gallopamil is a more active enantiomer. Three assays are available for determining gallopamil concentrations in human plasma. These include high-performance liquid chromatography,[26] capillary gas chromatography,[27] and gas chromatography–mass spectrometry.[28]

In healthy subjects, intravenous administration of 2 mg of gallopamil results in a mean plasma concentration of 62 μg/L at the end of the injection.[29] Single-dose administration of gallopamil as conventional tablets of 50 and 100 mg results in mean maximum plasma concentrations of 31 and 50 μg/L, respectively. Single doses of sustained-release tablets (100 mg) provide maximum plasma concentrations of 13 μg/L, but the area under the plasma concentration–time curve increases from 67 to 162 μg/L·hr.[29] Because of extensive first-pass hepatic metabolism, the systemic availability of gallopamil is low (15% after a single dose and 23% after repeated doses). Approximately 93% of gallopamil binds to albumin, independently of drug concentration.[30] At a steady state, the distribution volume of gallopamil is 145 L, suggesting that it is widely distributed in the body.[29]

Gallopamil is eliminated by hepatic metabolization. The principal metabolite is norgallopamil, the N-desmethyl derivative, which is pharmacologically inactive.[29] Mean total plasma clearance is 70 L/hr after intravenous administration (2 mg) and 306 L/hr after repeated 50-mg oral doses.[29, 31] The mean terminal elimination half-life is between 4 to 8 hours.[32] In patients with liver cirrhosis, the elimination half-life of gallopamil (25-mg single oral dose) is prolonged to a mean of 11.6 hours, and the absolute bioavailability increases to 60%.[33] Therefore, in these patients, the gallopamil dosage should be reduced by 50% or even 75%. In patients with coronary artery disease (CAD), there is a relationship between plasma gallopamil concentration and the percentage increase in exercise time.[27, 34]

EFFECTS ON PATHOPHYSIOLOGY
Effects on Hemodynamics

When administered to CAD patients (at dosages of 50 mg three times daily in conventional tablets or of 100 mg twice daily in sustained-release form), gallopamil decreases peripheral resistance and systolic and diastolic blood pressure and causes little change in resting heart rate.[35–41] During exercise, gallopamil decreases the gain in heart rate relative to the baseline value.[41–44] The rate pressure product during exercise after therapeutic dosages of gallopamil, varies between the studies, generally being decreased or unchanged.[36, 37, 43, 45, 46] Gallopamil causes a slight reduction of pulmonary pressure during exercise.[47]

Effects on Ventricular Function

Several studies are available on the effects of orally or intravenously administered gallopamil in patients with CAD,[47–49] myocardial infarction,[50] and hypertrophic cardiomyopathy.[51] In general, despite its negative inotropic effect, gallopamil does not significantly influence normal or moderately impaired ventricular function, because left ventricular ejection fraction does not change or improve after its administration. This is most likely the result of the combined action of gallopamil on smooth and cardiac muscles so that the effect on peripheral resistance overrides the direct effect on the myocardium. In this way, ejection fraction improves despite the reduction in contractility, which, in turn, causes a reduction of myocardial oxygen consumption, in itself an effect of particular relevance in CAD patients. In patients with acute myocardial infarction, angina, and hypertrophic cardiomyopathy, gallopamil increases isovolumic relaxation time, reflecting improvement of left ventricular diastolic function.[48–51] This probably is a result of (1) the ATP-sparing effect on the myocytes, making available more energy for calcium extrusion during diastole, and (2) the effects of gallopamil on sarcoplasmic reticulum.

Effects on Electrophysiology

Surprisingly, there are only a few studies on the electrophysiologic effects of gallopamil. Neuss et al.,[52] studied 20 patients during diagnostic His bundle electrocardiography within 20 minutes of gallopamil administration. Programmed atrial and ventricular pacing was carried out before and after intravenous administration of gallopamil 0.06 mg/kg, while potentials from the upper right atrium, the His bundle region, and from the right ventricle were recorded. The study showed that gallopamil increases sinus rate, nodal conduction time, Wenckebach point, and the functional and refractory period of the atrioventricular node. Sinoatrial node recovery time, however, is prolonged only in those patients with sick sinus syndrome.

Effects on Coronary Blood Flow

Intracoronary administration of gallopamil in dogs causes a dose-related increase in vascular conductance and a reduction in perfusion pressure and contractility.[53] Similarly, in humans, intracoronary administration of gallopamil (1.5 and 3.0 µg/kg) produces a dose-related coronary dilation, a decrease in mean arterial pressure, and a reduction of myocardial oxygen consumption.[54, 55] Intracoronary administration of gallopamil (0.4 mg) in patients subjected to percutaneous transluminal coronary angioplasty reduces ST-segment deviations as well as the myocardial release of lactate and hypoxanthine.[55] Intravenous administration of gallopamil causes a dilation of the stenosed arteries (26%) of patients with CAD.[56] Scintigrams obtained in CAD patients suggest that gallopamil improves regional myocardial perfusion[57] as well as the myocardial microperfusion in previously ischemic areas of the left ventricle.[58]

Effects on Arteries and Veins

At rest or during exercise, therapeutic doses of gallopamil decrease systolic and diastolic blood pressure in CAD patients with a greater decrease in those who develop ischemia during exercise.[27, 37, 38, 42] Pulmonary pressure is slightly reduced (18%, $p < .001$) during exercise in gallopamil recipients.[47] When administered according to therapeutic dosage, gallopamil has no effect on veins.

CLINICAL USE
Indications

Gallopamil is indicated for the treatment of patients with ischemic heart disease. The majority of studies have been performed on patients with chronic stable angina pectoris. Usually efficacy was demonstrated by exercise testing in double-blind or single-blind short-term or long-term trials involving patients allocated at random to receive gallopamil or an alternative treatment. These studies showed that gallopamil, administered in conventional or sustained-release form, is more effective than a placebo for improving exercise time and tolerance and delaying the ischemic threshold. Gallopamil is also superior to placebo in

decreasing the extent of ST depression at comparable and maximum workload.[40, 46, 59-61]

The efficacy of gallopamil has been compared with that of nifedipine[43] or diltiazem[62, 63] and atenolol[64] in patients with "stable" or "mixed" angina pectoris. There was no statistically significant difference in the overall efficacy between gallopamil 50 mg three times daily and nifedipine (10 or 20 mg three times daily).[43] However, nifedipine 30 mg daily is considered a subtherapeutic dose.[44] Gallopamil 50 mg three times daily proves more effective than diltiazem 60 mg three times daily in improving exercise duration,[62] the extent of ST-segment depression,[62] and the frequency of anginal attacks.[62] At the same dose, gallopamil has efficacy similar to that of atenolol 100 mg once daily in improving exercise duration in patients with stable exertional angina.[64]

Long-term studies are available on a total of 600 patients with stable exertional angina who received gallopamil 50 mg three times daily for 2 years. The results indicate that the improvement in exercise duration and workload, the reduction in the maximum ST depression, the frequency of anginal attacks, and glycerol trinitrate consumption achieved in the first months were maintained for the entire duration of the study.[65-68] Administration of gallopamil during 24-hour ambulatory electrocardiographic monitoring reduces the mean incidence of spontaneous asymptomatic as well as exercise-induced symptomatic episodes of ischemia.[69, 70] The reduction in ischemia is more evident on symptomatic episodes.[69] No valid data are available on the efficacy of gallopamil in patients with acute myocardial infarction or unstable angina.

Precautions and Adverse Effects

Therapeutic doses of gallopamil are well tolerated by the majority of patients. A noncomparative clinical trial involving 31,537 patients showed that the most common adverse effects consist of gastrointestinal (including nausea, constipation, epigastric pain, and others, present in a total of 4.4% to 8.3% of patients) and circulatory symptoms (including hypotension, flushing, and peripheral edema, present in a total of 2% to 2.3% of patients).[70] Other cardiovascular complaints include bradycardia (0.5%), first-degree and second-degree atrioventricular (AV) block (0.3%), aggravation of congestive heart failure (0.03%), and palpitations (0.5%). Withdrawal of treatment because of these adverse effects was necessitated in 1.4% to 3% of the patients.[70] Sinn and Wolf[71] reported a mean increase of 10 msec in the duration of PQ intervals in a group of 25 patients as a result of gallopamil administration. Steinbeck[72] described asymptomatic single episodes of type 1 second-degree AV block in 4 of 13 patients treated with 100 mg sustained-release gallopamil twice daily.

The good tolerability of patients to gallopamil has also been confirmed by the double-blind and single-blind therapeutic trials versus placebo. In no study was the incidence of adverse effects because of gallopamil administration statistically different from that of the placebo. Finally, the tolerability of gallopamil appears to be better than that of nifedipine[41, 43] and comparable with that of diltiazem.[37, 63]

Contraindications

Gallopamil is contraindicated in patients with marked sinus bradycardia, previous AV block, and atrial fibrillation/flutter with coexistent preexcitation syndrome (e.g., Wolff-Parkinson-White [WPW] syndrome). Gallopamil should not be used in patients with any type of acute or chronic severe pump failure, such as dilatative cardiomyopathy with low output syndrome, cardiogenic shock, or acute myocardial infarction.

Because gallopamil is predominantly metabolized in the liver (demethylation), it should not be administered to patients with documented cirrhosis of the liver, where there is increased bioavailability caused by shunts.

Dosage and Administration

The usual dosages of gallopamil in the treatment of CAD patients are 50 mg three times daily as a conventional immediate-release preparation and 100 mg twice daily as a sustained-release preparation.

REFERENCES

1. Fleckenstein-Grün G: Gallopamil: Cardiovascular scope of action of a highly specific calcium antagonist. J Cardiovasc Pharmacol 20(Suppl 7):S1, 1992.
2. Fleckenstein A, Fleckenstein B, Spah F, et al: Gallopamil (D-600)—ein Kalziumantagonist von hoher Wirkungsstarke und Spezifitat. Effekte auf Myokard und Schrittmacher. In Kaltenbach M, Hopf R (eds): Gallopamil: Pharmacological and Clinical Profile of a Calcium Antagonist. Berlin: Springer-Verlag, 1984, pp 1–34.
3. Fleckenstein-Grün G, Fleckenstein A: Blockade of the calcium dependent bioelectrical automaticity and electromechanical coupling of smooth muscle cells by gallopamil (D600). In Kaltenbach M, Hopf R (eds): Gallopamil: Pharmacological and Clinical Profile of a Calcium Antagonist. Berlin: Springer-Verlag, 1984, pp 33–48.
4. Raschack M, Gries J, Bühler V, et al: Studies on the cardiovascular effects of gallopamil. In Kaltenbach M, Hopf R (eds): Gallopamil: Pharmacological and Clinical Profile of a Calcium Antagonist. Berlin: Springer-Verlag, 1984, pp 72–80.
5. Pang CCY, Sutter MC: Effect of chronic treatment of spontaneously hypertensive rats with D600. Hypertension 3:657, 1981.
6. Beck OA, Witt E, Lehmann HU, et al: Die Wirkung von Gallopamil (D600) auf die intrakardiale Erregungsleitung und Sinusknotenautomatie beim Menschen. Z Kardiol 67:522, 1978.
7. Zucchi R, Ronca-Testoni S, Limbruno U, et al: Effect of gallopamil on cardiac sarcoplasmic reticulum. J Cardiovasc Pharmacol 20(Suppl 7):S11, 1992.
8. Ferrari R, Boffa GM, Ceconi C, et al: Effect of D-600 on ischemic and reperfused rabbit myocardium: Relation with timing modality of administration. Basic Res Cardiol 84:606, 1989.
9. Ferrari R, Boraso A, Cargnoni A: Effects of anipamil on myocardial sarcolemmal and mitochondrial calcium transport, comparison with verapamil and nifedipine. Eur J Pharmacol 189:149, 1990.
10. Ferrari R, Curello S, Ceconi C, et al: Cardioprotection by nisoldipine: Role of timing of administration. Eur Heart J 14:1258, 1993.
11. Raddino R, Poli E, Pasini E, et al: Effects of the novel calcium channel blocker, anipamil, on the isolated rabbit heart. Comparison with verapamil and gallopamil. Naunyn Schmiedebergs Arch Pharmacol 346:339, 1992.
12. Fleckenstein-Grün G: Role of transmembrane calcium supply in phasic and tonic activation of vascular smooth muscle. Vasodilators efficacy of calcium antagonists. In Berman MC, Gevers W, Opie LH (eds): Membrane and Muscles (CSV Symposium Series, Vol 6). New York: IRL Press, 1985, pp 235–255.
13. Bolton TB: Mechanisms of action of transmitters and other substances on smooth muscle. Physiol Rev 59:607, 1979.
14. Ferrari R, Curello S, Cargnoni A, et al: Metabolic changes during post-ischemic reperfusion. J Mol Cell Cardiol 20:19, 1988.
15. Ferrari R, Ceconi C, Curello S, et al: Myocardial damage during ischemia and reperfusion. Eur Heart J 14(Suppl G):25, 1993.
16. Ferrari R: Myocardial response to reperfusion after a prolonged period of ischemia. In Parrat JR (ed): Myocardial Response to Acute Injury. New York: Macmillan, 1992, pp 201–222.
17. Ferrari R, Pedersini P, Bongrazio M, et al: Mitochondrial energy production and cation control in myocardial ischemia and reperfusion. Basic Res Cardiol 88:495, 1993.
18. Ferrari R, Visioli O: Protective effects of calcium antagonists against ischemia and reperfusion damage. Drugs 42:14, 1991.
19. Ferrari R, Visioli O: Calcium channel blockers and ischemic heart disease: Theoretical expectations and clinical experience. Eur Heart J 12:18, 1991.
20. Faria DB, Gonclaves FR, Maroko PR: Three-dimensional analysis of infarct size reduction after administration of gallopamil in dogs. Arzneimittelforschung 40:19, 1990.
21. Villari B, Ambrosio G, Gollino G, et al: The effects of calcium antagonist treatment and oxygen radical scavenging of infarct size and the no-reflow phenomenon in reperfused hearts. Am Heart J 125:11, 1993.
22. Gettes LS, Cascio WE, Johnson T, et al: Local myocardial biochemical and ionic alterations during myocardial ischemia and reperfusion. Drugs 42(Suppl 1):7, 1991.
23. Schömig A, Rehmert G, Kurz T, et al: Calcium antagonism and norepinephrine release in myocardial ischemia. J Cardiovasc Pharmacol 20(Suppl 7):S16, 1992.
24. Kirchengast M, Hergenröder S: Reperfusion arrhythmias in closed-chest rats: The effect of myocardial noradrenalin depletion and calcium-antagonism. Clin Exp Pharmacol Physiol 18:217, 1991.
25. Neumann FJ, Tiefenbacher C, Tillmanns H, et al: Protective effect of gallopamil in myocardial stunning by repetitive ischemia and reperfusion of the rat heart [abstract 330]. Cardiovasc Drugs Ther 5(Suppl 3):1, 1991.
26. Fieger H, Blaschke G: Direct determination of the enantiomeric ratio of verapamil, its major metabolite norverapamil and gallopamil in plasma by chiral high-performance liquid chromatography. J Chromatogr 575:255, 1992.
27. Rose EL, Lahiri A, Raftery EB: Antianginal efficacy of sustained release gallopamil. Drug Invest 5:212, 1993.
28. Kokatsu J, Jingu S, Suwa T: Determination of gallopamil in human plasma by selected ion monitoring. Chem Pharm Bull 39:123, 1991.
29. Stieren BV, Bühler V, Hege HG, et al: Pharmacokinetics and metabolism of gallopamil. In Kaltenbach M, Hopf R (eds): Gallopamil: Pharmacological and Clinical Profile of a Calcium Antagonist. Berlin: Springer-Verlag, 1984, pp 88–93.
30. Rutledge DR, Chong MT, Nelson MV: Interspecies differences in the effect of pH on gallopamil protein binding to albumin and α_1-acid glycoprotein. Eur J Clin Pharmacol 40:603, 1991.
31. Eichelbaum M: Pharmakokinetik und Metabolismus von Gallopamil. Z Kardiol 78(Suppl 5):20, 1989.
32. Gross AS, Borstel B, Eichelbaum M: Determination of gallopamil in serum by gas chromatography-mass spectrometry. J Chromatogr 525:183, 1990.
33. Kaim AAH, Farker K: Pharmacokinetics and pharmacodynamics of gallopamil in patients with liver cirrhosis [abstract 36]. Naunyn Schmiedebergs Arch Pharmacol 34(Suppl):R9, 1992.
34. Scrutinio D, Lagoia R, Mangini SG, et al: Objective evaluation of gallopamil in patients with chronic stable angina. Exercise testing Holter monitoring, cross-sectional echocardiography and plasma levels. Eur Heart J 10:168, 1989.

35. Sesto M, Ivancic R, Custovic F: The effect of gallopamil on the haemodynamics of patients with coronary heart disease. *In* Kaltenbach M, Hopf R (eds): Gallopamil: Pharmacological and Clinical Profile of a Calcium Antagonist. Berlin: Springer-Verlag, 1984, pp 94–98.

36. Tartagni F, Maiello L, Marchetti G, et al: Clinical and haemodynamic effects of long-term administration of gallopamil in patients with coronary artery disease and normal or impaired left ventricular function. Am J Cardiol 63:291, 1989.

37. Marraccini P, Orsini E, Brunelli C, et al: Gallopamil and diltiazem: A double-blind, randomised, cross-over trial in effort ischemia. Eur Heart J 13:404, 1992.

38. Musso P, Ottello B, Pinnavaia A, et al: Influenza del gallopamil sulla perfusione miocardica nell'angina da sforzo. Minerva Cardioangiol 40:97, 1992.

39. Cherchi A, Lai C, Onnis E, et al: Slow-release gallopamil in patients with stable effort angina. J Cardiovasc Pharmacol 20(Suppl 7):S75, 1992.

40. Kottkamp H, Gülker H, Emmerich K, et al: Efficacy and tolerability of slow-release gallopamil in patients with stable exercise-induced angina pectoris. J Cardiovasc Pharmacol 20(Suppl 7):S88, 1992.

41. Lazzeroni E, Morozzi L, Campana M, et al: Efficacy and tolerability of gallopamil in coronary heart disease: A double blind cross-over comparison with nifedipine. Eur Heart J 13:526, 1992.

42. Grossmann G, Stauch M, Schmidt A, et al: The effect of gallopamil p.o. on global and regional ventricular function in patients with coronary heart disease. *In* Bender F, Meesmann W (eds): Treatment with Gallopamil. Results of Recent Research on Calcium Antagonism. Darmstadt, Germany: Steinkopff Verlag, 1989, pp 103–116.

43. Rettig GF, Jakob M, Sen S, et al: Comparison of dihydropyridine and phenylalkylamine calcium antagonists in patients with coronary heart disease. Drugs 42(Suppl 1):37, 1991.

44. Subramanian VB: Gallopamil and six other calcium antagonists in stable angina pectoris and a within-patient comparison of gallopamil with diltiazem. *In* Bender F, Meesmann W (eds): Treatment with Gallopamil. Results of Recent Research on Calcium Antagonism. Darmstadt, Germany: Steinkopff Verlag, 1989, pp 187–191.

45. Terrosu P, Ibba GV, Pes R, et al: Exercise cardiovascular responses to gallopamil in ischemic heart disease. Int J Cardiol 33:75, 1991.

46. Zanolla L, Carbonieri E, Rossi L, et al: Gallopamil in chronic stable angina: Antianginal effect and mechanism of action. Cardiology 80:324, 1992.

47. Gassuer A: Die pulmonale Hypertonie bei chronioch obstrukhren Lungenerkrankugen. Alemio-Lungenkikh 11:S1, 1986.

48. Mazzone O, Trovato GM, Caruso G: Long term treatment with gallopamil in ischemic heart disease: Echocardiographic evaluation. Curr Ther Res 50:73, 1991.

49. Di Mario C, Iavernaro A, Cucchini F: Acute effects of gallopamil on left ventricular systolic and diastolic function in patients with ischemic heart disease. Eur Heart J 12:1006, 1991.

50. Natale E, Ricci R, Tubaro M, et al: Diastolic ventricular dysfunction in noncomplicated acute myocardial infarction: The influence of gallopamil. J Cardiovasc Pharmacol 20(Suppl 7):S48, 1992.

51. Olbrich HG, Hopf R, Klepzig, et al: Diastolische Ventrikelfunktion bei hypertropischer, obstruktiver und nichtobstruktiver Kardiomyopathie. Wirkung von Gallopamil. Z Kardiol 78(Suppl 5):29, 1989.

52. Neuss H, Mitrovic V, Mitrovic I, et al: Pharmacodynamics and electrophysiology of gallopamil. *In* Kaltenbach M, Hopf R (eds): Gallopamil: Pharmacological and Clinical Profile of a Calcium Antagonist. Berlin: Springer-Verlag, 1984, pp 99–106.

53. Kovach AGB, Dora E, Koller A: Antihypoxic effect of gallopamil in the brain. *In* Kaltenbach M, Hopf R (eds): Gallopamil: Pharmacological and Clinical Profile of a Calcium Antagonist. Berlin: Springer-Verlag, 1984, pp 81–87.

54. Vigorito C, Giordano A, De Caprio L, et al: Effects of intracoronary gallopamil on coronary hemodynamics and myocardial oxygen consumption in humans. J Cardiovasc Pharmacol 17:822, 1991.

55. Neumann FJ, Ott I, Richardt G, et al: Effect of gallopamil on neutrophil function: Experimental and clinical studies. J Cardiovasc Pharmacol 20(Suppl 7):S21, 1992.

56. Sebening H, Sauer E: Effect of gallopamil on coronary arteries and hemodynamics. *In* Kaltenbach M, Hopf R (eds): Gallopamil: Pharmacological and Clinical Profile of a Calcium Antagonist. Berlin: Springer-Verlag, 1984, pp 114–116.

57. Tillmanns H, Neumann FJ, Parekh N, et al: Pharmacologic effects on coronary microvessels during myocardial ischemia. Eur Heart J 11(Suppl B):10, 1990.

58. Eichstadt H, Danne O, Koch HP, et al: Effects of intravenous and oral treatment with calcium antagonists on myocardial microperfusion. *In* Bender F, Meesmann W (eds): Treatment with Gallopamil: Results of Recent Research on Calcium Antagonism. Darmstadt, Germany: Steinkopff Verlag, 1989, pp 143–150.

59. Specchia G, Cobelli F, Tavazzi L, et al: Assessment of gallopamil (D-600) in patients with chronic stable angina pectoris. Results of a placebo-controlled single-blind study. *In* Bender F, Meesmann W (eds): Treatment with Gallopamil: Results of Recent Research on Calcium Antagonism. Darmstadt, Germany: Steinkopff Verlag, 1989, pp 179–185.

60. Mitrovic V, Niemela L, Neuss H, et al: Anti-anginal effect of the calcium antagonist gallopamil. *In* Kaltenbach M, Hopf R (eds): Gallopamil: Pharmacological and Clinical Profile of a Calcium Antagonist. Berlin: Springer-Verlag, 1984, pp 107–113.

61. Loskot F, Novotny P, Sucic P, et al: Koronartherapeutische Wirksamkeit von Gallopamil retard nach wiederholte Gabe im vergleich zu Placebo. Z Kardiol 78(Suppl 5):89, 1989.

62. Zenker GD, Rodl S, Gender K: Randomisierter Vergleich zwischen Gallopamil und Diltiazem bei angiographisch gesicherter Koronarer Herzkrankheit. Z Kardiol 78(Suppl 5):94, 1989.

63. D'Ascia G, Picardi G, Cittadini A, et al: Gallopamil and diltiazem in the treatment of effort angina. Curr Ther Res 51:45, 1992.

64. Sangiorgio P, Rubboli A, Mezzetti N, et al: Advantage of calcium antagonists over beta-blockers used as monotherapy in patients with stable effort angina: Comparison between gallopamil and atenolol [abstract]. Presented at the 5th International Symposium on Calcium Antagonists, Houston, 1991.

65. Pazzola A, Tonolo G, Troffa C, et al: Effects of long-term gallopamil in ischemic heart disease. Curr Ther Res 48:1030, 1990.

66. Pupita G, Mattei O, Mazzara D, et al: Trattamento a lungo termine dell'angina pectoris stabile con gallopamil. G Ital Cardiol 22:1049, 1992.

67. Segre G: Rivelazione multicentrica ospedaliera dell'efficacia e tollerabilità di gallopamil nell'angina pectoris. Farmaci 15:1, 1991.

68. Sucic M, Schiemann J: Results of an open multicentre study with 455 patients with coronary heart disease, treated with gallopamil for 1 year. *In* Kaltenbach M, Hopf R (eds): Gallopamil: Pharmacological and Clinical Profile of a Calcium Antagonist. Berlin: Springer-Verlag, 1984, pp 132–135.

69. Zehender M, Kosschech U, Hohnloser S, et al: Exercise-induced symptomatic and asymptomatic myocardial ischemia in patients with severe coronary artery disease: Focus on the efficacy and safety of gallopamil. J Cardiovasc Pharmacol 20(Suppl 7):S57, 1992.

70. Wolf E: Wutzen und Risiko einer antinginosen Therapie und Gallopamil in der täglichen Praxis. Therapiewoche 37:2372, 1987.

71. Sinn R, Wolf R: Wirkung von gallopamil retard 75 mg bei belastungsinduzierter myokardischamie. Z Kardiol 78(Suppl 5):83, 1989.

72. Steinbeck G: Calcium antagonists and silent myocardial ischemia. Drugs 43(Suppl 1):15, 1992.

CHAPTER 102

Diltiazem

Peter E. Pool, M.D.

HISTORY

The earliest work on a group of drugs later to be known as calcium antagonists was begun in Germany in late 1963; by 1969, enough was known of the properties of verapamil, gallopamil (D600), nifedipine, and niludipine to announce the existence of this group of drugs.[1] In 1966 in Japan, the Tanabe Seiyaku Company began work on the synthesis of 1,5-benzothiazepine derivatives as central nervous system antidepressants (compare the benzodiazepine, diazepam).[2] In 1968, the company discovered and began development of a novel series of 1,5-benzothiazepines that were found to have potent coronary vasodilatory properties.[3, 4] The D-*cis* isomer of a group of DL-*cis* 3-acetoxy-2-(4-methoxy phenyl) derivatives was finally selected, named CRD-401, and further developed. This drug, known as diltiazem (DTZ), was approved by the Japanese equivalent of the United States Food and Drug Administration (FDA) for the treatment of angina in 1973 and of hypertension in 1982. This was the same year in which it (Cardizem, Marion Laboratories) was first approved in the United States for the treatment of angina following its licensing by Marion Laboratories in 1976. In the ensuing years, Tanabe licensed it throughout most of the world to a number of different pharmaceutical companies under a variety of trade names. In January 1989, a twice-daily sustained-release formulation of DTZ (Cardizem-SR, Marion Laboratories) was approved by the FDA for use in patients with hypertension. This was followed in 1991 by an injectable form (Cardizem Injectable, Marion Merrell Dow) for supraventricular arrhythmias and by a once-daily formulation (Cardizem-CD, Marion Merrell Dow) initially approved for hypertension and subsequently approved in 1992 for angina. Another once-daily formulation (Dilacor-XR, Rhône-Poulenc Rorer) was separately approved for hypertension in 1992[5] and angina in 1995.

CHEMISTRY

DTZ (Fig. 102–1), D-*cis* 3-acetoxy-2,3-dihydro-5-{2-(dimethylamino)ethyl}-2-(p-methoxyphenyl)-1, 5-benzothiazepin-4(5H)-one hydrochloride, has two asymmetric centers (asterisks in Fig. 102–1) and is capable of *cis-trans* isomerism at these carbon atoms. The *trans* compounds are essentially devoid of vasodilating properties. The L-*cis* enantiomer has a tenfold greater duration of action than D-*cis* (DTZ), but it has only weak action,[4, 6] perhaps because of a separate mechanism.[7] The synthesis of DTZ has been described in detail elsewhere.[8–12] The alkylaminoalkyl substitution at the N5 atom is essential for activity. Replacement of the acetoxy function at C3 with some substituents provides products with similar activity. In the non-condensed aromatic ring, only replacement of methoxy by *para*-methyl is tolerated without marked loss of activity.[6, 9] A few other active benzothiazepine derivatives have been synthesized.[13] The molecular weight of DTZ is 450.98. It is soluble in water to the extent of 56.6 g/100 ml; it is also soluble in methanol and chloroform. DTZ has a pK_a of 7.7. It is a white crystalline powder with a bitter taste.

PHARMACOKINETICS

The pharmacokinetics of DTZ have been reviewed in detail and compared with other calcium antagonists.[14–20] Sensitive assay methods have been developed for DTZ[21–27] and its metabolites.[23, 26–33] Frozen plasma samples appear to be stable for 5 to 8 weeks.[34–36] Because it is largely metabolized in the liver, DTZ undergoes a significant first-pass effect,[37] which leads to large differences from person to person in absolute bioavailability, plasma concentration, and clearance. The major metabolic pathways involve o-deacetylation or N-demethylation (via cytochrome P-450IIIA enzymes[38]) followed by o-demethylation[29] (Fig. 102–2), and finally, in some instances, glucuronide or sulfate conjugation. There is evidence that progressive metabolite accumulation may inhibit DTZ biotransformation, leading to nonlinear DTZ accumulation.[39] Because the major metabolite present in the serum, desacetyl-DTZ, represents only 15% to 35% of the DTZ present and has only 40% to 50% of the pharmacologic activity of DTZ,[40] the metabolic products of DTZ are not considered clinically important in humans (see later section, Platelet Aggregation, for discussion of a potential exception). In a group of hypertensive patients, the N-demethyl metabolite was predominant.[41]

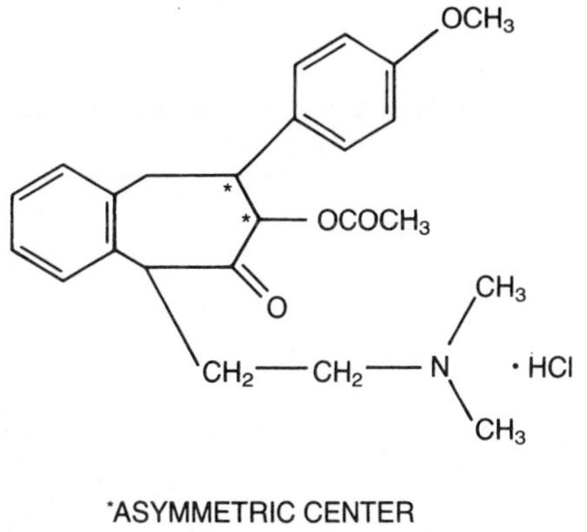

*ASYMMETRIC CENTER

Figure 102–1. Structure of diltiazem. The *asterisks* show the asymmetric centers.

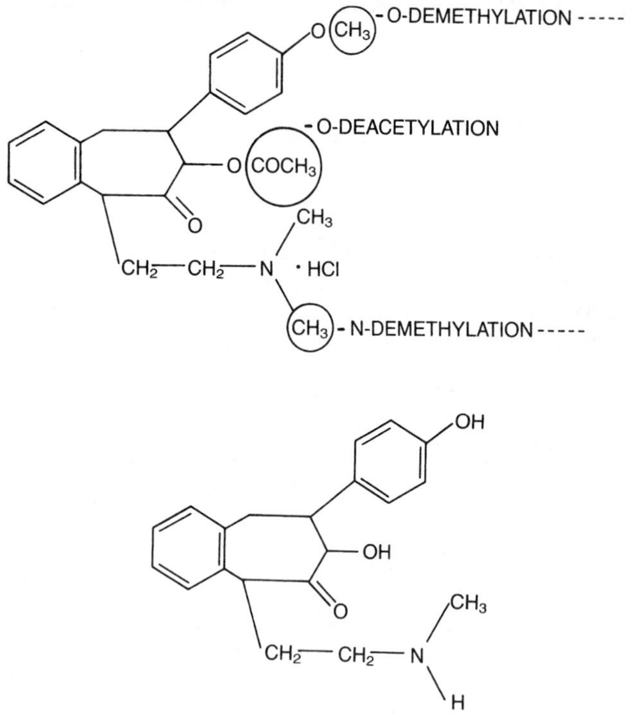

Figure 102–2. Structure and sites of metabolism of diltiazem and its final metabolized structure. Glucuronide or sulfate conjugation may take place at several points in the metabolic pathway.

The range of important pharmacokinetic parameters of the immediate-release tablet form of DTZ derived from a variety of sources[14–16, 19, 20, 42–44] is listed in Table 102–1. Sustained-release preparations for both twice-daily and once-daily use are now available, which have been achieved using various delivery systems.[45–50] When preparations of DTZ have been compared, strict bioequivalence has often not been found because of differences in time of onset, dissolution rate, C_{max}, and food effect.[51–53] The relevance of these differences cannot be evaluated because comparisons of clinical effects have not been published. Peak serum levels after use of a twice-daily preparation (Cardizem-SR) occur in 3 or 4 hours.[43, 44, 54] Steady-state DTZ levels are reached 2 or 3 days after initiation of oral dosing.[55] There is no food effect.[56] With once-daily preparations (Dilacor-XR, Cardizem-CD),

peak serum levels occur in the 4- to 6-hour and 10- to 14-hour range.[48, 49]

Although not found in one Japanese study,[20] it is generally accepted that saturation of first-pass metabolism is possible because DTZ kinetics are nonlinear and DTZ blood levels accumulate with long-term dosing.[57] In addition, absolute bioavailability increases with increasing dose because of saturation of the elimination pathway.[19, 43, 44, 58] This effect occurs with single doses, but apparently not with multiple dosing.[59, 60] Peak plasma concentrations were 72, 117, and 152 ng/cm³ after oral administration of single 60-, 90-, and 120-mg tablets.[43] In another study,[61] serum levels were 152 and 246 ng/ml with steady-state dosing at 240 and 360 mg/day.

DTZ is highly protein-bound (see Table 102–1). It is not displaced by desacetyl-DTZ, digoxin, phenylbutazone, propranolol, salicylic acid, or warfarin,[44, 62] nor does it displace warfarin.[63] However, DTZ has been reported to displace propranolol from serum proteins and raise propranolol free fractions significantly,[64] and it does inhibit warfarin disposition in humans in a stereospecific and regiospecific manner.[65] Finally, DTZ binds not only to albumin but even relatively more to lipoproteins[66] and α_1-acid glycoprotein,[66, 67] which is an acute phase reactant. Both lipoproteins and α_1-glycoprotein may be elevated in patients with acute coronary disease, a condition that could raise free DTZ levels. A number of drugs, such as lidocaine,[68] disopyramide, bupivacaine, and quinidine, decrease this binding, whereas myocardial infarction increases it.[69] Effects in myocardial infarction may be related to age, size, and left-sided failure.[70] During cardiopulmonary bypass, total DTZ is decreased but, because of decreased protein binding, free DTZ is unchanged.[71] Increased DTZ levels may be found during cardiopulmonary resuscitation (CPR).[72]

The hepatic clearance of DTZ is flow-dependent,[18] and, because hepatic flow declines with age, a decrease in hepatic clearance in the elderly would be expected. In fact, volume of distribution and total body clearance of DTZ were found to be decreased in the elderly.[73] In addition, peak plasma concentrations occurred later, and mean elimination half-life was longer (10.9 hours).[55] Absolute bioavailability, however, was unchanged.

Studies with intravenously administered DTZ[74, 75] have shown good correlations between changes in systemic vascular resistance, blood pressure, coronary flow, and serum concentrations of DTZ, with a minimum effective serum concentration calculated to be 96 to 100 ng/ml. This figure correlated well with studies in 53 patients monitored for angina control; a nonresponder group was identified in which plasma levels rarely exceeded 100 ng/ml, as opposed to the responders, in whom plasma levels were mostly higher than 100 ng/ml. In a study in dogs,[76] Wenckebach cycle length, basic conduction time, and atrioventricular (AV) nodal functional refractory period increased at mean minimum DTZ levels of 37, 83, and 175 ng/ml, with AV block developing between 379 and 1400 ng/ml.

Table 102–1. **Pharmacokinetic Properties of Diltiazem in Humans**

Absorption			90%
Absolute bioavailability (compared with intravenous dosing)			24–74%
T_{max} PO*			0.5–4.0 hours
Protein binding			77–86%
Elimination $T_{1/2}$			2–6 hours
Volume of distribution			3–8 L/kg
Peak plasma concentration:	IV	15 mg	80–100 ng/ml
	Oral	60 mg	31–246 ng/ml
	Oral	90 mg	44–274 ng/ml

*Time to peak plasma concentration after oral administration.

The effects of severe renal failure on the kinetics of DTZ have been evaluated in nine patients, of whom seven had inulin clearances of less than 50% of normal values.[77] The pharmacokinetic profile was similar to that of patients with normal renal function, as it was in another study in patients on continuous ambulatory peritoneal dialysis.[78] Because this study, as well as another,[79] was based on single doses of 120 mg, projections of long-term effects should not be based on it. In other patients with renal failure receiving intravenously administered DTZ, the extent and possibly the rate of its extravascular distribution was altered.[80]

The effect of calcium antagonists on the metabolism of other drugs has been studied with indocyanine green and antipyrine, marker compounds for liver blood flow and hepatic oxidative enzyme activity, respectively.[81] Although nifedipine and verapamil increase hepatic blood flow, DTZ does not.[82] On the other hand, DTZ and verapamil decrease antipyrine clearance, whereas nifedipine does not.[82] Propranolol levels have been observed to increase after DTZ administration as the result of inhibition of the oxidative metabolic pathway[83, 84] or displacement from proteins,[85-87] and probably not because of increased hepatic flow.[85] Hemodynamic effects of the change were minimal.[87] Conversely, propranolol reduced the oral clearance of DTZ and increased its bioavailability in one study,[88] whereas it increased desacetyl-DTZ in another study without affecting DTZ.[89] DTZ also has increased plasma levels of diazepam in dogs but not in humans,[90] apparently by inhibiting hepatic oxidative metabolism.[91] Long-term oral dosing with cimetidine lowered both systemic and oral clearance of DTZ.[92] Treatment with DTZ increases nifedipine bioavailability as well as decreases its clearance.[93-95] DTZ increases carbamazepine levels in rabbits[96] and has caused a neurotoxic reaction to carbamazepine in patients.[97-100] Amiodarone decreases total body clearance of DTZ and increases its area under the curve (AUC) value.[101] In rats, gentamycin nephrotoxicity is enhanced by DTZ.[102]

DTZ inhibits cytochrome P-450 reductase–dependent biotransformation of drugs[103] and reduces antipyrine clearance in humans (a measure of effects on drug oxidation).[104-108] Theophylline levels, however, were not affected[109] or were only minimally changed.[110] Smokers may experience a larger and possibly significant effect.[111]

DTZ has increased trough[112] and steady-state levels of digoxin[113-118] because of a prolonged elimination half-life. These findings have been associated with a nonsignificant decrease in renal clearance[115] and a decrease in extrarenal clearance.[113] The physiologic correlate has been lowered heart rate.[113, 115] In one study,[117] no change was noted after DTZ was withdrawn; in other studies,[119, 120] no change in digoxin levels or renal digoxin clearance[119] was found except when renal insufficiency was also present.[120] In general, it appears that DTZ has no effect on digoxin pharmacokinetics in healthy individuals,[121-123] but does modestly increase steady-state digoxin concentrations in patients with cardiac insufficiency[124, 125] by reducing extrarenal clearance of digoxin.[125] DTZ was associated with variable changes in plasma digitoxin level in one study.[126] In dogs, the acute positive inotropic and arterial constrictive effects of ouabain are attenuated by DTZ.[127]

PHARMACOLOGY
Cellular Effects

The general mechanisms of action of the calcium antagonists have been known for more than two decades,[1] but the details of this mechanism and the specificity enjoyed by each drug continue to be revealed. All calcium antagonists inhibit Ca^{2+} influx via voltage-operated channels and, to a lesser extent, receptor-operated channels, which may be of more than one type.[128] The voltage-operated channels open to Ca^{2+} transport with a lessening of the resting potential (electrical activation of the cell membrane, experimentally produced by K^+ depolarization). The receptor-operated channels respond to agonists such as norepinephrine. Other sites in the excitation–contraction coupling process involving Ca^{2+} include a sarcolemmal leak, Na^+-Ca^{2+} exchange, release of Ca^{2+} from the sarcoplasmic reticulum, mitochondrial Ca^{2+} transport, Ca^{2+} activation of calmodulin, and direct effects on the actin-myosin interaction.[129-133] At therapeutic concentrations, DTZ appears to inhibit extracellular Ca^{2+}-dependent increases in intracellular Ca^{2+} with no effects on the release of Ca^{2+} from intracellular storage sites or on Ca^{2+} sensitivity of the contractile elements.[134]

DTZ inhibits smooth muscle contraction in a dose-dependent manner and inhibits Ca^{2+} influx stimulated by α-adrenoreceptor activation (see later).[135] The interaction of DTZ with the calcium channel has been defined by a variety of studies[136-143] that indicate that there are channel-binding sites for at least DTZ, verapamil, and nifedipine and that these binding sites interact with one another allosterically. DTZ stimulates the binding of both ^{3}H-desmethoxyverapamil[136] and ^{3}H-nitrendipine,[138, 142] which identify the verapamil and nifedipine receptors, respectively, and DTZ may alter the number of binding sites and the characteristics of ^{3}H-isradipine binding.[144] These findings have been variably described for heart,[140, 143] brain,[136, 142] smooth muscle,[141] and skeletal muscle[137, 139] and have potential clinical implications, because DTZ potentiates the negative inotropy of nimodipine,[145] and nitrendipine potentiates the negative inotropy of DTZ,[146] presumably by this receptor interaction. A number of the physiologic specificities for the Ca^{2+} antagonists have also supported the concept of individual receptor sites as well as tissue selectivity. Effects on radioligand binding to calcium channels are highly stereospecific for the D-cis isomer.[147] Differential effects on chronotropy, inotropy,[148, 149] vasodilator activity,[150] conduction,[151] and vascular smooth muscle oxygen uptake[152] have supported individual receptor sites, whereas differing orders of potency for binding—as opposed to tissue response—have supported tissue selectivity.[153] The concentration dependence of block suggests that a single molecule of DTZ may be sufficient to block a channel,[154] and DTZ may bind to the outside as well as the inside of the membrane, at least in ventricular myocytes.[155] There is also spectroscopic evidence of the involvement of calcium in the interaction of DTZ with its membrane-bound receptor.[156] New classes of agents with binding properties distinct from DTZ have been found to bind to the benzothiazepine receptor complex.[157, 158] DTZ also affects cardiac sarcolemmal Na^+-Ca^{2+} exchange.[159]

An important feature distinguishing DTZ and verapamil from the dihydropyridine calcium antagonists is use dependence,[160, 161] a requirement for activation of the channel for blockade to take place. On activation, the channel goes from the resting state to the active state to the inactive state and back to the resting state. DTZ binds to the inactive channel[162, 163] with high affinity, and for the inactive state to be present (instead of the rest state), activation must have taken place. This quality may explain in part the predilection of DTZ as well as verapamil to AV nodal tissue (frequent activation) and of nifedipine, which is not use-dependent, to smooth muscle. It may also explain the different actions of DTZ in normal polarized cells as compared with ischemic depolarized cells.[164]

Whereas the classic actions of calcium antagonists are described in the preceding paragraphs, other studies have examined a variety of possible intracellular effects. DTZ does not readily penetrate smooth and skeletal muscle,[20, 165] but autoradiographic evidence of its uptake into mitochondria, at least in myocardial cells, has been presented.[91] This finding appears to be confirmed by studies showing the inhibition of caffeine-induced Ca^{2+} release from intracellular stores of skinned vascular muscle[166] or ventricular fibers;[167] inhibition by DTZ of Na^+-induced Ca^{2+} release from heart[168] and brain mitochondria,[169] but not uptake;[170] inhibition of Ca^{2+} transport in cardiac and skeletal sarcoplasmic reticulum;[171] and other intracellular processes,[172] including those of erythrocytes[173] and neutrophils.[174]

DTZ, unlike felodipine or bepridil, has no significant affinity for calmodulin,[175, 176] although one study[177] found an inhibition of arterial actomyosin superprecipitation, and another[178] identified an action on glycerinated dog heart muscle. DTZ may suppress tension independent of the inward Ca^{2+} current in frog ventricles, suggesting another mechanism of action.[179] Finally, DTZ blocks neurotransmission in the frog, possibly acting on the acetylcholine-activated channel as an open-channel blocker.[180]

A further effect of DTZ on cellular activity may be via a modulation of adrenergic activity. Both binding data[181] and other pharmacologic evidence[182] show that DTZ has no β-blocking activity. The effect of DTZ on the release of norepinephrine from nerve endings is contradictory, suggesting both inhibition[183, 184] and stimulation.[185, 186] α-Receptors, however, are affected.

The nature of the interaction of calcium antagonists with α-receptors has been confusing. Verapamil has been shown to have α-receptor blocking activity and has shown binding to $α_1$-receptors[187] and $α_2$-receptors.[188] However, because calcium antagonists generally inhibit the pressor response elicited by $α_2$-agonists and not those of $α_1$-agonists,[189] it was proposed that $α_2$-responses are mediated by translocation of extracellular calcium, whereas $α_1$-responses are mediated by mobilization of intracellular calcium.[190–193] Conversely, central $α_2$-receptor activity is not responsive to DTZ.[194] In some tissues, DTZ fails to inhibit any α-stimulation,[195] whereas in others, such as dog coronary arteries, which have both $α_1$- and $α_2$-receptors, DTZ is inhibitory.[196, 197] The issue does not revolve around the binding of DTZ to α-receptors, because this possibility has been disproved.[187, 188] Rather, the calcium influx that transduces the α-mediated signal is the target for DTZ. This question seems to have been resolved with the demonstration of $α_1$-receptor reserve.[198, 199] Noncompetitive blockade of calcium influx mediated by the $α_2$-receptor appears complete, but $α_1$-receptors appear to have a significant reserve population not blocked by DTZ and available for agonist action. When this reserve population is decreased by $α_1$-blockade, the remaining population, like the $α_2$-population, is susceptible to DTZ inhibition. Apparently, $α_1$-receptor reserve decreases with age, at least in rat aorta.[200]

Organ Effects

Hemodynamics and Regional Blood Flow

The effect of DTZ on hemodynamics in humans is complex, involving direct effects on the heart (both systolic and diastolic function), on the peripheral vessels, and on the reflexes that link them. In addition, the pretreatment circulatory status with respect to sympathetic tone and disease state conditions the response (e.g., vascular responsiveness is changed in patients with hypertension).[201] Whereas DTZ decreases overall peripheral vascular resistance, it has variable effects on regional flow[202, 203] and has selectivity for tissues (e.g., heart vs. blood vessels) different from that of other calcium antagonists.[204] For instance, when administered to open-chest cats, DTZ decreases heart rate and total peripheral resistance, increases cardiac output mildly, and increases coronary flow, brain flow, and kidney flow; however, it has negligible effects on skeletal muscle flow and a weak tendency to increase flow to the stomach and small intestine.[202, 203] The relative lack of increase in skeletal flow produced by DTZ at lower doses compared with the dihydropyridines explains in part why DTZ is relatively free of hemodynamic side effects at antianginal doses. In the renal circulation, DTZ enhances angiotensin II–induced prostacyclin synthesis.[205] In humans, DTZ appears to potentiate forearm blood flow responses to norepinephrine, possible by interfering with β-receptor–mediated vasorelaxing mechanisms.[206]

DTZ also attenuates baroreflex-induced tachycardia due to nitroglycerin administration and bradycardia due to phenylephrine infusion in humans,[207] but this is apparently not due to a direct effect on the baroreceptor.[208] In cats, baroreceptor sensitivity was increased by DTZ administration during evoked rises in pressure but depressed in response to vasodepressor challenges,[209] and in a study in six humans, DTZ enhanced baroreflex-mediated hypotension.[210]

Ventricular Function

Although the Ca^{2+} antagonists can depress ventricular function in vitro,[211] this effect is usually offset by sympathetic reflex effects in response to their vasodilating properties in vivo. Because of the pronounced vasodilating effects of the dihydropyridines, it often has appeared that DTZ, next to verapamil, had the greatest negative inotropic potential. In fact, despite many studies using DTZ in patients with serious ventricular dysfunction, evidence of adverse negative inotropy is unusual. In comparative in vitro studies with verapamil and nifedipine,[149] DTZ was by far the least negatively inotropic in guinea pig atria. A similar result was found in spontaneously beating cultured chick myocardial cells.[212] In electrically driven human papillary muscle strips obtained during cardiac surgery, the rank order of negative inotropism was verapamil > nifedipine > DTZ > isradipine.[213] In patients with coronary artery disease on long-term metoprolol treatment, intravenously administered DTZ (0.5 mg/ kg for 5 minutes followed by 15 mg/hr) increased contractility, decreased stroke work, and increased left ventricular (LV) compliance.[214]

In studies on both animals and humans, DTZ has had a beneficial effect in congestive heart failure by decreasing afterload,[215] restoring blood flow to impaired beds, and improving cardiac output. Intravenous injection of DTZ in unsedated dogs failed to reveal negative inotropy either before or after β-blockade with propranolol. Only intracoronary injection of DTZ revealed a small negative inotropic effect, substantially less than that caused by verapamil or nifedipine.[216] After equihypotensive doses of DTZ, verapamil, and nifedipine, contractility was increased by nifedipine, decreased by verapamil, and unchanged by DTZ.[217] Even after β-blockade, contractility was unchanged by DTZ.[134] In studies on papillary muscles from hearts with right ventricular pressure overload, DTZ had a greater negative inotropic effect than on muscles from normal hearts.[217] In studies on patients with depressed left ventricular (LV) function, intravenously administered DTZ improved ejection fraction (EF) and stroke volume index in a group with a mean EF of 29%[218] and improved EF, cardiac output, and fractional shortening in a group with a mean EF of 32%.[219] Orally administered DTZ improved stroke volume index but not LV stroke work index (LVSWI) in a group with a mean pretreatment value of 19 gm-m/m^2.[220] In the latter study, nifedipine was used as a comparative drug, and nifedipine significantly decreased LVSWI from 19 to 14 gm-m/m^2. Among coronary disease patients with an EF below 40%, intravenously administered DTZ was well tolerated,[221] but in

a study in which EF was stratified into three groups, a combination of intravenously administered DTZ and intravenously administered propranolol caused a rise in LV end-diastolic pressure in the lowest EF group (20% to 40%).[222] Intravenously administered DTZ reduced afterload and increased preload; the latter change was due to an increase in left atrial driving pressure, an improvement of ventricular relaxation, or both.[223] In a cineangiographic study in patients with coronary disease, DTZ had a mild negative inotropic effect, but global indices of systolic function were improved and area-EF improved in 53% of hypokinetic areas.[224] In conscious dogs with coronary artery occlusion treated with DTZ, there was no change in EF or peak diastolic filling rate.[225] In another study, coronary flow, ventricular function, and recovery improved,[226] and finally, in segments with the greatest ischemic dysfunction, DTZ-associated improvement in function was greatest.[227]

DTZ also has important effects on diastolic function. One study in awake dogs revealed impairment of LV relaxation,[228] and one study in 12 hypertensive patients found that DTZ had no consistent effect on diastolic filling.[229] Most studies in patients, however, report an improvement in diastolic function in those with hypertension,[230, 231] coronary disease,[232–234] or hypertrophic cardiomyopathy.[235–239] DTZ did not prevent the development of hypertension or LV hypertrophy (LVH) in rats made hypertensive, but it did inhibit the fibrosis characteristic of LVH in one study.[240] In another study in spontaneously hypertensive rats, DTZ prevented hypertrophy progression and normalized isomyosin composition.[241]

Electrophysiology

The sinoatrial (SA) and AV nodes depend on the slow Ca^{2+} channel for activation. The slow channel is also important in the plateau phase (phase 2) of the fast Na^+ channel–produced action potential, and it is probable that in disease states such as ischemia, in which the Na^+ channel is inactivated, the Ca^{2+} channel may predominate and form the basis for ventricular arrhythmias.[242] Characteristics of slow-channel–dependent tissues include low resting potentials, slow upstroke velocities (phase 0) that lead to slow conduction times, spontaneous pacemaker activity (phase 4 depolarization), and long refractory periods.[243] Slow-channel openings appear to occur in bursts, and less negative membrane potentials and β-receptor stimulation increase the probability that the channels will open. DTZ binds to the inactive state as opposed to the rested state (see section on cellular effects). As a consequence, the effects of DTZ are more prominent at faster pacing rates and at less negative resting membrane potentials.[244] This frequency dependence leads to increased depression of AV conduction during supraventricular arrhythmias.[245]

After intravenous administration, DTZ may acutely raise heart rate slightly because of reflex effects[246] and then return to control or a slightly slower rate. No significant changes in maximal corrected sinus node recovery time or SA conduction time were noted.[247-250] In patients with sinus node disease, however, sinus node recovery time and even sinus arrest may be prolonged.[250-252] Sinoatrial conduction velocity is decreased and may favor the occurrence of a sinus exit block.[253]

In the AV node, DTZ prolongs A-H conduction time and prolongs functional and effective refractory periods and AV nodal Wenckebach cycle length,[249, 250] but to a substantial degree less than verapamil does.[246, 254] No effect occurs in the bundle of His.[252]

The only electrocardiographic effect produced by DTZ in long-term oral treatment is slight prolongation of the PR interval.[255] In otherwise normal individuals with long PR intervals, DTZ may prolong the interval somewhat.[256] In a study of coronary artery disease patients younger than the age of 55, orally administered DTZ (180 mg/day), either alone or after β-blockade, did not adversely affect sinus node function or AV conduction.[257]

Coronary Flow and Myocardial Protection

Coronary dilatation is the best known action of the calcium antagonists. It began with the observation that potassium-constricted coronary arteries were dilated at low concentrations of nifedipine, verapamil, and DTZ.[258] Although not as potent as nifedipine, DTZ is more selective for coronary arteries.[2] In isolated coronary artery segments from many species including humans, DTZ has effectively inhibited spontaneous contractile activity or contractions induced by depolarization or a variety of stimulant substances, including prostaglandins,[259, 260] serotonin,[259] acetylcholine,[261] and KCl.[262] *In vivo* DTZ inhibited hand grip–induced sympathetic constriction in humans.[263] DTZ did not block leukotriene-induced coronary constriction in pigs, whereas verapamil did; however, it apparently did so by a non–calcium-mediated mechanism.[264] Thus, a variety of stimuli leading to coronary constriction appear to be mediated by calcium and blocked by DTZ and other calcium antagonists. In humans, intracoronary DTZ increases coronary flow without a change in heart rate or blood pressure equally after placebo or nitrate pretreatment[265] and does not depend on concomitant changes in hemodynamics.[266]

When ischemia is prolonged or when reperfusion occurs, calcium accumulates in the mitochondria of myocardial cells, and this condition as well as other factors leads to a variety of damaging processes, including loss of energy stores, cell disruption and death, and arrhythmias. This process is generally known as the *calcium paradox*. Because calcium is a substance common to both coronary flow regulation and the calcium paradox, the two processes have been closely related in research. In two early studies, in 1977[267] and 1979,[268] DTZ prevented adenosine triphosphate (ATP) depletion caused by isoproterenol or ischemia in rats and dogs. Subsequently, much literature has documented the cardioprotective effects of

DTZ either by effects on flow or flow redistribution or by effects on cellular structure and metabolism.

Examples of *in vitro* protective effects of DTZ include preservation of function of isolated rabbit[269] and rat heart mitochondria,[270] protection of isolated ventricular myocytes from a high K^+, N_2 environment independent of Na^+-Ca^{2+} exchange or the fast inactivating Ca^{2+} channel,[271] preservation of structure and function and inhibition of Ca^{2+} damage in rabbit papillary muscles treated with Ca^{2+}-containing solutions,[272] inhibition of leukocyte chemotaxis[273] or superoxide production,[274] and inhibition of ischemic injury in hearts isolated from hypertensive rats pretreated *in vivo* with DTZ.[275]

In models of prolonged myocardial ischemia or infarction in rats[276, 277] or dogs,[278, 279] DTZ has been shown in at least one study to limit infarct size acutely or, after 24 or 48 hours,[280-282] to decrease mortality,[280] increase myocardial and regional blood flow,[283] decrease premature ventricular contractions and ventricular fibrillation,[282, 283] improve LV segmental relaxation,[284] promote rapid recovery from ischemia[285] and decrease postischemic myocardial stunning,[278] and prevent ATP loss,[286-289] loss of mitochondrial function and calcium accumulation,[290] and loss of ultrastructure.[279] DTZ had no effect in one study,[225] and in another it was shown to salvage more myocardium when there was less of an area at risk for ischemia.[281]

In models of reperfusion in rats,[274, 291-301] guinea pigs,[302, 303] pigs,[304-306] rabbits,[307-309] cats,[310] and dogs,[311-326] DTZ protected mitochondria[297, 310] and preserved ATP[283, 297-299, 302, 326-328] even when administered after ischemia onset, provided that myocardial blood flow was sufficiently high.[326] DTZ also prevented structural damage,[291, 297, 307, 308, 312, 313, 319] decreased creatine kinase (CK) release,[293, 294, 327, 329] prevented Ca^{2+} accumulation,[293, 298, 310, 315, 318] prevented loss of function or preserved compliance,[298, 299, 303, 305, 310, 312, 317, 320, 321] inhibited derangements of regional myocardial blood flow,[315, 322, 330] decreased infarction size,[294, 304, 306, 311, 315, 318, 324, 331] but only when infused before occlusion,[325] improved survival,[316, 318] reduced ventricular fibrillation,[301] prevented norepinephrine depletion,[300, 332] prevented lipid peroxidation[309, 323] and neutrophil accumulation,[331] or prevented damage during hypothermia.[292, 295, 320, 321] DTZ failed to prevent norepinephrine depletion in one rat model in which nifedipine was effective[333] and, along with nifedipine and verapamil, failed to protect against the calcium paradox in another.[334] In a rabbit model, nifedipine and verapamil successfully prevented structural damage, whereas DTZ did not;[335] in a rat model, however, DTZ reduced the severity of ischemia with the least amount of cardiac depression among the three drugs.[336] The benefits of DTZ have been attributed to a decrease in energy demand and glycolysis rather than an improvement in energy substrate utilization.[337]

In dog studies, DTZ improved LV function[338] or cardiac output[339] or increased coronary blood flow or decreased oxygen demand[283] during cardiopulmonary resuscitation. In another study, norepinephrine-induced arrhythmias were suppressed.[340] In a study of resuscitation in pigs, DTZ enhanced cerebral blood flow and postarrest recovery of the electroencephalogram.[341]

Studies in dogs[320, 342] and rabbits[343] undergoing cardiopulmonary bypass with cardioplegic solutions containing DTZ have shown protection from the electron microscopic changes of the calcium paradox[342] and preservation of LV function[320] in some subjects, but no improvement in others.[343] Adenosine appears to be important in cardioprotection. In studies in whole blood from humans and rabbits, DTZ, along with other agents, inhibited adenosine uptake with the following series of potencies: dipyridamole > verapamil > DTZ > nifedipine > enalapril.[344]

Finally, in studies in humans, DTZ has been given during cardiopulmonary bypass for coronary[345–348] and valve surgery.[349] Among 40 patients undergoing crystalloid potassium cardioplegia—20 randomly assigned to receive DTZ and 20 to no added medication—tissue ATP and creatine phosphate levels were preserved better by DTZ. It also produced coronary vasodilation during cardioplegia and less reactive hyperemia during reperfusion. Postoperatively, however, systolic function was somewhat depressed.[345] In another study of 38 patients,[346] 25 with DTZ cardioplegia and 13 without, cardiac index increased significantly postoperatively only for patients treated with DTZ. In a study of 32 patients (16 randomly assigned to DTZ, 16 to placebo) with three-vessel coronary disease undergoing bypass with deep hypothermia,[347] DTZ lowered serum enzyme release and increased cardiac output and stroke work indices at equal levels of preload and afterload. In 62 patients (54 undergoing valve surgery and 8 undergoing other cardiac surgery), 31 received DTZ cardioplegia and 31 did not. CK release was significantly less with DTZ. The mortality rate was 2 of 31 in the group receiving DTZ and 4 of 31 in the other group, but this difference was not statistically significant.[349] In a study of 73 patients with anterior infarction treated in the first 6 hours with intravenously administered and then orally administered DTZ, there was a decrease in double-product of 7% ($p < .05$), in the frequency of ventricular tachycardia and fibrillation (0 vs. 8 patients, $p < .01$), and in mortality (0 vs. 4 patients, nonsignificant). Infarct size as measured by peak CK (-14%, nonsignificant), cumulative CK (-9%, nonsignificant), ischemic score (-12%, nonsignificant), and necrotic score (7%, nonsignificant) was also quantitatively less.[350] In 63 patients undergoing coronary bypass grafting, little benefit was noted using doses of DTZ ranging from 50 to 150 μg/kg.[348] In a randomized study during coronary angioplasty, DTZ (0.4 mg/kg bolus followed by an infusion of 15 mg/hr) reduced ATP breakdown as indicated by diminished hypoxanthine and urate production but did not attenuate ST elevation or lactate release.[351] Given to another 40 patients during coronary bypass surgery, DTZ led to no clear benefits and caused a greater need for catecholamine support and temporary pacemaker use.[352]

Thus, among the evidence for beneficial effects on coronary flow and cardioprotection, data support effects involving both Ca^{2+}-mediated and non–Ca^{2+}-mediated effects at the cellular level, effects on overall coronary flow, effects on systolic and diastolic function, and effects on redistribution of epicardial flow, endocardial flow, and ischemic zone flow.

Arteries, Atherosclerosis, and Veins

The effects of DTZ on arterial flow and resistance were discussed in the earlier section, Hemodynamics and Regional Blood Flow. Although the smooth muscle of the veins, like the arteries, is susceptible to DTZ's effects, little work has been done specifically on the venous effects of DTZ. In isolated spontaneously contracting rat portal vein, DTZ inhibits contractions at a concentration similar to that which is negatively inotropic in rat papillary muscle.[204] In isolated rabbit femoral artery and vein, DTZ inhibits norepinephrine-induced contractions equally in artery and vein at low concentrations ($<10^{-7}$ M), but contractions were greater in the artery at higher concentrations ($>10^{-7}$ M).[353] In dogs, DTZ dilates systemic capacitance beds at therapeutic concentrations.[354]

Work on DTZ as an antiatherogenic agent stemmed from the theoretical relationship between Ca^{2+} as a mediator of cell death and the role of intimal necrosis in the development of atheroma.[355] This led to several studies of the effect of DTZ and other calcium antagonists on animals fed cholesterol (although the atherosclerosis of cholesterol-fed animals and that of humans differ in many ways). A number of studies of verapamil and nifedipine have cited antiatherogenic effects.[355] DTZ suppressed aortic atherosclerosis but not that of intramural coronary arteries.[356] In this model, the subepicardial coronary arteries were not atherosclerotic, neither in the controls nor in DTZ-treated rabbits. In cholesterol-fed rabbits, DTZ lowered plasma low-density lipoprotein (LDL) cholesterol as well as aortic total and esterified cholesterol[357] and very significantly decreased the number of atheromatous lesions on the intimal surface of the aorta.[358] Another study showed no effect in the same model with DTZ or nicardipine.[359] DTZ was shown to retard progressive arterial calcinosis in spontaneously hypertensive rats[360] and to prevent vitamin D3–induced calcinosis of elastic fibers in arteries.[361] The latter study cited the results as evidence that Ca^{2+} antagonists also work on extracellular inexcitable tissue structures.

Other evidence has supported an antiatherogenic role for DTZ. DTZ suppressed the necrosis induced in cultured aortic smooth muscle cells by hyperlipidemic serum,[362] it suppressed intimal thickening and internal elastic lamina destruction in rabbit carotid artery induced by polystyrene tubing,[363] it stimulated LDL-receptor synthesis in human skin fibroblasts,[364] and it decreased apolipoprotein B secretion in rat hepatocytes.[365] DTZ has also been noted to inhibit the degradation of intracellular LDL, but this effect occurred only at higher concentrations of 50 to 100 μM[366] and, in another study, was related to the basic nature of DTZ rather than to its Ca^{2+} antagonistic effects.[367]

On the other hand, DTZ did not demonstrate protection against experimental atherogenesis in pigs[368] and did not exhibit the cytoprotective effects against oxidized LDL in lymphoid cells demonstrated for nifedipine.[369]

Platelet Aggregation

Calcium antagonists are known to inhibit platelet aggregation, and interest in their effects on platelets stems from the role of platelets in both the clotting process and vascular motility.[370] Platelet aggregation may be induced by adenosine diphosphate (ADP), thrombin, collagen, and other factors, but the response to ADP involves platelet shape changes, whereas the response to thrombin, collagen, and epinephrine does not.

In general, inhibition by DTZ and other calcium antagonists of platelet aggregation by a single inducing agent such as ADP requires supertherapeutic concentrations (>100 μM).[370-373] Conversely, aggregation induced by small amounts of many stimuli (probably closer to the *in vivo* situation) can be inhibited at 1 μM DTZ[370] and could be clinically significant.[374] DTZ also potentiates prostaglandin release from human umbilical veins,[375] which is both vasodilating and antiplatelet-aggregating.

Inhibition of platelet aggregation by DTZ correlates with changes in intracellular Ca^{2+} concentration as shown by studies using aequorin, an intracellular Ca^{2+} marker.[373]

The clinically important effects of DTZ on platelets in humans may be effects of DTZ metabolites, which are significantly more potent in inhibiting platelet aggregation than DTZ itself.[376] In studies of *in vivo* DTZ administration, antiaggregation effects on platelets were seen 24 hours after administration of a 120-mg oral dose in healthy volunteers[377] and after 2 days of oral dosing at 240 mg/day[378] in five normal men. In the latter study, no clinically relevant changes occurred in hemostasis despite the antiaggregating effect. In experimental coronary thrombosis in dogs, DTZ also had no effect.[379, 380] After DTZ administration, 180 mg/day for 4 weeks, 20 hypertensive patients had no changes in platelet aggregation after treadmill exercise,[381] although unexercised hypertensive patients in another study did experience an antiaggregatory effect.[382] On admission, the patients had hyperaggregable platelets, increased serum thromboxane B_2 and decreased 6-PGF. In patients receiving DTZ, the aggregation threshold increased ($p < .05$), thromboxane B_2 decreased ($p < .05$), and 6-PGF did not change. No changes were noted in the group receiving verapamil. DTZ also suppressed vasopressin-induced thromboxane B_2 synthesis.[383] In other studies, DTZ inhibited collagen- and thrombin-induced platelet aggregation[384] as well as thromboxane A_2 production[383, 385] from platelet-rich plasma. In pa-

tients with coronary artery disease, blood viscosity decreased significantly after 2 weeks of DTZ treatment, 180 mg/day,[386] and platelet aggregability and erythrocyte filtrability improved.[387]

Renal Function and Electrolytes

A major effect of DTZ on the kidney is to increase renal blood flow, glomerular filtration rate (GFR), and effective renal plasma flow while decreasing renal vascular resistance[388] and producing natriuresis. At the same time, renal autoregulation may be abolished.[389] The increase in renal blood flow could result from reversal of the vasoconstrictor effects of angiotensin II or norepinephrine. Evidence for the effects of angiotensin II has been demonstrated in dogs[390] and humans.[391] In perfused kidney of rats, DTZ appears to antagonize angiotensin II effects but not those of norepinephrine at doses of 10^{-7} to 10^{-6} M, and only to attenuate the effects of norepinephrine at greater than 10^{-5} M.[392] In another study on the same model, attenuation of norepinephrine effects was found at 5×10^{-6} M.[393] DTZ also causes greater increases in renal blood flow in first-degree relatives of patients with essential hypertension, in patients who are Na^+-restricted, and in the presence of angiotensin II.[394]

Evidence exists also for a direct diuretic effect of DTZ, independent of renal hemodynamic changes. In denervated kidneys of rats administered doses of DTZ that did not significantly alter hemodynamics, large increases were noted in salt and water excretion, which diminished at higher doses of DTZ when blood flow was decreased.[395] This finding indicated a direct tubular effect. In patients with congestive heart failure, DTZ produced a greater Na^+ excretion than it did in those without heart failure but without any significant effect on renal hemodynamics.[396]

The long-term renal effects of DTZ have been studied in 18 hypertensive patients given up to 480 mg/day for 6 months. There was no change in GFR, effective renal plasma flow, renal vascular resistance, or filtration fraction except in patients with low pretreatment GFR, in whom GFR and effective renal plasma flow were significantly improved.[397] In a comparison with captopril in Goldblatt-hypertensive rats, DTZ lowered afferent arteriolar resistance to a similar degree, but only captopril decreased efferent arteriolar resistance.[398] In contrast, studies by Isshiki et al. have demonstrated a fall in renal vascular resistance with a decrease in both afferent and efferent glomerular arterial pressure, with unchanged GFRs and filtration fractions in hypertensive humans and spontaneously hypertensive rats (SHRs) but not in normal Wistar-Kyoto (WKY) rats.[399] They found similar results with a DTZ congener, clentiazem.[400] Because those data were based on calculated glomerular hydrostatic pressure, they confirmed the results in the SHRs and in WKY rats using direct micropuncture measurements.[401] In diabetic rats, DTZ prevented albuminuria. The mechanism appeared to be preservation of glomerular heparan sulfate.[402] In dialysis-dependent patients with end-stage renal disease, DTZ reduced the interdialysis increase in plasma potassium.[403] In diabetic hypertensive patients, angiotensin-converting enzyme (ACE) inhibitors, verapamil, and DTZ,[404, 405] but not nifedipine,[405] appear to reduce microalbuminuria, whereas in hypertension alone, the mere lowering of blood pressure may be sufficient to decrease microalbuminuria.[406] In one study, 30 diabetics with renal disease were randomized to DTZ, lisinopril, or the combination of atenolol and furosemide and followed for 18 months. Given a similar level of arterial pressure control, both lisinopril and DTZ slowed progression of diabetic renal disease and reduced albuminuria to a greater extent than did the combination of a loop diuretic and β-adrenoreceptor antagonist.[407]

Endocrine and Metabolic Effects

Several studies have examined the relationship between DTZ administration and serum glucose and insulin levels. Glycemic control was preserved in both normal and diabetic rats receiving orally administered DTZ.[408] Twelve healthy volunteers treated with DTZ, 180 mg/day for 8 days, had no change in glucose, insulin, or glucagon levels,[409] and another group of 16 volunteers had no changes over 3 weeks in glucose, insulin, cortisol, or growth hormone levels compared with placebo.[410] In a study of 58 hypertensive patients, insulin-mediated glucose uptake measured by the euglycemic insulin clamp technique was unchanged by DTZ,[411] and no negative effect on diabetes control was noted in a placebo-controlled crossover study of 23 patients.[412] Thirteen adult-onset diabetics were classified with regard to glucose control before and after 3 months of treatment. The before treatment/after treatment classification was as follows: "good" 9/8, "fair" 2/2, "poor" 2/3.[413] In a group of 16 normal and 6 diabetic patients, DTZ had no effect on glucose tolerance or glucose-induced insulin secretion.[414] In a 30-month study in 26 diabetics (4 insulin, 9 sulfonylurea, 13 diet), no difference was found in glucose metabolism compared with a similar control group, but serum glucose level rose from 113 to 133 mg/dl.[415] The change in glucose level was not statistically significant, and there was no change in insulin levels. In a study of 97 hypertensive patients treated with DTZ for 6 months, average serum glucose level rose from 98 to 105 mg/dl.[416] Thus, although there may be a small long-term effect of DTZ on serum glucose levels, interference with diabetic management did not occur in these or other studies. Finally, in one patient with an inoperable insulinoma, blood glucose levels were normalized and remained so for 21 months on DTZ therapy.[417]

Because other antihypertensive and antianginal drugs adversely affect lipid metabolism, several investigators have examined DTZ for effects on serum lipid levels. Some speculation on possible beneficial lipid effects based on animal data led to the filing of a Belgian patent on DTZ as an antihyperlipidemic drug.[418] No changes were noted in serum cholesterol, LDL cholesterol, high-density lipoprotein (HDL) cholesterol, or triglyceride concentrations in healthy men;[318] in patients of various types over periods of 3 months,[419] 1 year, or 5 years;[420] or in 13 diabetic patients.[413] One study found no changes in 20 patients except for a fall in LDL cholesterol from 141 to 130 mg/dl ($p < .05$) over 8 weeks.[421] Another study found a fall in serum triglyceride concentration from 221 to 158 mg/dl in 27 patients over 6 weeks.[422] A third study during 29.5 weeks found changes only in HDL cholesterol level, which rose from 52 to 60 mg/dl ($p < .006$) accompanied by a fall in the cholesterol/HDL ratio of 4.7 to 4.2 ($p < .05$).[423] Thus, for serum lipids, there seems to be at most a small positive effect from treatment with DTZ.

DTZ lowered parathyroid hormone levels in a study of 30 subjects randomized to DTZ (120 to 360 mg/day) or hydralazine (75 to 150 mg/day),[424] and similar effects were found in isolated bovine parathyroid cells.[424] However, in a comparative study with felodipine in six healthy subjects, DTZ appeared to stimulate parathyroid hormone secretion, especially under hypocalcemic conditions.[425] Long-term treatment with DTZ did not alter pituitary hormone secretion in 12 cardiac patients.[426]

Effects on Other Organs and Other Uses

Apart from its cardiovascular effects, DTZ has effects on other organs via its relaxing action on smooth muscle. In studies of patients with asthma or obstructive airway disease, DTZ has not been particularly effective, perhaps because of the inability to attain adequate levels without side effects or because bronchial smooth muscle contraction depends on both internal and external Ca^{2+}.[427, 428] A combination of DTZ and nifedipine significantly[429] but weakly[430] antagonized methacholine-induced bronchoconstriction in asthmatics. DTZ also appears to inhibit the beneficial effects of theophylline on diaphragmatic contraction.[431]

DTZ was ineffective in patients with hypoxic pulmonary hypertension in dogs[432] and humans.[433] When DTZ was given intravenously to patients with pulmonary hypertension, it increased cardiac output and reduced pulmonary artery pressure at maximum exercise.[434] Vasodilator treatment for primary pulmonary hypertension is successful only occasionally.[435] In an isolated case report of a young woman with pulmonary artery pressure greater than systemic arterial pressure, orally administered DTZ conferred significant benefit.[436] In another series of five patients with precapillary pulmonary hypertension, four benefited from intravenous DTZ therapy.[437] In two patients with primary pulmonary hypertension, DTZ effectively controlled the disease and led to regression of right ventricular hypertrophy.[438] In a mixed group of eight patients with primary and secondary forms of pulmonary hypertension, DTZ lowered pulmonary artery pressure and pulmonary vascular resistance,[439] and high-dose DTZ (720 mg/day) has been effective.[440] In pulmonary hypertension secondary to chronic obstructive pulmonary disease, DTZ decreased pulmonary vascular resistance, but not as effectively as nifedipine.[441]

Because DTZ has produced decreased esophageal smooth muscle contraction in animals,[442] clinical studies were performed that showed a drop in lower esophageal sphincter pressure in normal volunteers[443] but no effect in patients with dysphagia.[444] In 14 patients with symptomatic strong esophageal contractions (9 with nutcracker esophagus), DTZ reduced both distal esophageal peristaltic pressure and chest pain scores,[445] but another study showed only marginal success.[446] DTZ improves blood flow in experimental intestinal ischemia in dogs[447] and demonstrated excellent control of proctalgia fugax in one case report.[448] Gastric emptying is not affected.[449] No major gastrointestinal antisecretory effects have been reported.[442]

DTZ has been effective in controlled studies in relieving the symptoms of primary Raynaud's phenomenon,[450, 451] but less so in Raynaud's phenomenon secondary to collagen-vascular disease.[451] It was effective in 65% of 17 patients with occupational Raynaud's syndrome (vibration disease).[452]

The inward Ca^{2+} current apparently plays no significant role in skeletal muscle activation.[453] DTZ has variably been found to have no effect,[453] mild depression of contractile force at probable supertherapeutic concentrations,[454] and potentiation of contraction at therapeutic concentrations.[455] However, during repetitive stimulation of skeletal muscle, DTZ enhanced the fatigue process.[456]

At therapeutic concentrations, DTZ antagonizes agonist-mediated tone in cerebral vessels but not intrinsic tone.[457, 458] DTZ has reduced cerebral vasospasm in cats in response to local administration of incubated blood[459] and in monkeys following subarachnoid hemorrhage.[460] A review of the efficacy of DTZ in treating migraine showed that the overall decrease in migraine frequency was 64%.[461] In another study, the success rate was 100%.[462] Daily intravenous followed by oral therapy has also seemed successful.[463] DTZ produces no increase in intracranial pressure after craniotomy.[464] DTZ has had no effect on tardive dyskinesia[465] and no benefit[466] or only a trend to benefit in Duchenne muscular dystrophy.[467]

In rats or mice, DTZ has had beneficial effects on endotoxin shock,[468, 469] restoring glucose and lactate with no adverse effect on mean arterial pressure;[470] in hemorrhagic shock, restoring gut absorptive capacity to normal;[471] reducing postischemic[472] and posthemorrhagic microcirculatory disturbances in kidney[473] and liver;[474, 475] and lowering blood viscosity[476] and improving immune responses[477] in hemorrhagic shock.

In renal transplantation patients, DTZ has increased the serum concentration of cyclosporine A, allowing doses of this immunosuppressant to be lowered, and at the same time has protected against both ischemic and drug-induced toxicity.[478–484] Not only is renal function improved, but medication costs are significantly reduced.[485, 486] In heart transplantation patients,

cyclosporine A cost can be reduced 38%[485] to 48%[486] with the concomitant use of low-dose DTZ. In a quantitative angiography study in heart transplantation patients, DTZ (52 patients) also reduced posttransplant coronary artery narrowing compared with no calcium antagonist treatment (54 patients).[487] DTZ also prevents posttransplant hypertension associated with cyclosporine A.[488] Finally, in lung transplantation patients, DTZ appears to limit the formation of pulmonary edema.[489]

Topical DTZ treatment transiently increased intraocular pressure in rabbits[490] and reduced contractility in extraocular muscles.[491] DTZ has inhibited contractions of isolated dog ureters.[492] DTZ also has inhibited uterine contractions[493] and exhibited some selectivity for uterine muscle.[494] During surgery for pheochromocytoma, DTZ has stabilized circulatory fluctuations;[495, 496] in untreated thyrotoxicosis, DTZ has improved symptoms.[497] DTZ also attenuates the hypertensive response to endotracheal intubation.[498–500]

A host of properties have been demonstrated for DTZ in single studies. DTZ decreases sperm motility[501] and relaxes detrusor muscle *in vitro*,[502] reduces postoperative adhesions[503] and improves skin flap survival,[504] potentiates the analgesic effects of morphine,[505] may reduce the progression of calcinosis in the CREST syndrome,[506] and inhibits experimental metastases of lymphosarcoma cells.[507]

Mechanism of Antiischemic Effect

The potential mechanisms of the antiischemic effect of DTZ are myriad. They relate to control of spontaneous or substance-mediated constriction of the coronaries at the level of both the conductance and resistance vessels: action on collateral flow;[508] inhibition of the action of constricting substances such as norepinephrine,[135] prostaglandins,[259] serotonin,[259] and acetylcholine;[261] redistribution of coronary flow by region, from epicardium to endocardium or into ischemic zones; or an effect on platelets.[370] Antiischemic effects also are explained by a decrease in myocardial energy demand caused by negative inotropy or a decrease in heart rate and blood pressure. The dose of calcium antagonist may also contribute to the mechanism of action, because too large a dose may decrease perfusion pressure and offset other effects.[509] The timing of treatment before or after ischemia will also define the mechanisms susceptible to calcium antagonist treatment. Finally, some mechanisms cited as important *in vitro* may not be relevant *in vivo* (e.g., negative inotropy is often cited as an important mechanism *in vitro* but is rarely expressed *in vivo*).[509]

Although one early paper[510] found no coronary dilating effect of DTZ in open-chest dogs, improvement in coronary flow has been demonstrated convincingly in further series in dogs. In comparative studies with nifedipine and verapamil, DTZ dilated both conductance and resistance coronary arteries, whereas nifedipine and verapamil affected only resistance arteries.[511] During ischemia, all three drugs increased flow to normal zones but not acutely to the severely ischemic zone.[512] DTZ did increase flow with chronic occlusion.[512] In marginal areas, DTZ increased flow where verapamil did not,[513] and DTZ redistributed flow to the subendocardium, whereas nifedipine increased subepicardial perfusion.[512] In other studies, DTZ increased subendocardial perfusion distal to a coronary stenosis,[514] increased perfusion of the ischemic area with no evidence of negative inotropy,[515] and improved myocardial blood flow to normal and ischemic border areas.[516]

DTZ has enhanced regional myocardial performance in ischemia, both alone[517] and in conjunction with atenolol;[518, 519] when DTZ was acting alone, the mechanism of its protective effect was not diminished contractility.[517] In fact, during pacing-induced ischemia in patients with coronary artery disease and either normal or impaired ventricular function, high-dose, intravenously administered DTZ improved coronary flow and LV pump function, particularly in those with previously impaired function.[520] In acute studies after brief ischemia, DTZ, along with nifedipine, blunted the hyperemic response.[521–523] This blunting may be beneficial, because the hyperemic response always exceeds the true flow debt and may be producing a coronary steal.[521] In addition, in dogs, DTZ prevents the early ischemic deterioration of cardiac function that occurs after a prior ischemic stress.[524] DTZ does not invalidate the diagnostic measurement of coronary flow reserve,[525] but it may suppress the myocardial ischemia following dipyridamole infusion.[526] In exercise studies in dogs, DTZ failed to improve function in the regional ischemic area because of a concomitant decrease in both heart rate and myocardial perfusion pressure, which were offsetting.[527]

Studies of the mechanism of coronary ischemia in humans have reached differing conclusions. Intravenously administered DTZ has dilated stenosed coronary arteries an average of 17% (diameter)[528] and has dilated coronary arteries in patients with coronary disease,[529–533] but overall coronary flow was not increased in one study.[531] Nitroglycerin may be additive to the effects of DTZ.[532, 533] The coronary dilating effects after acute intravenous infusion may be short-lived,[534, 535] and, citing pacing time to ischemia, other investigators have concluded that benefits are related solely to a decrease in energy demand.[536, 537] If so, the decrease in demand is probably not related to a depressant effect of LV function.[538] Of course, if demand is decreased, coronary flow must be maintained at a lowered systemic resistance for benefit to be achieved.[539]

The mechanism of action of DTZ during exercise in patients with myocardial ischemia was examined in a placebo-controlled crossover study that showed an increase in duration of exercise, a decrease in exercise ischemia, a decrease in ischemic myocardial risk area with thallium single photon emission computed tomography (SPECT), and a decrease in ST-segment depression of 24-hour ambulatory monitoring in patients receiving DTZ.[540] During routine living conditions, DTZ decreases frequency and severity of ST depression but less than propranolol,[541] and the effects of DTZ appear to be greatest on ischemic episodes preceded by an increase in heart rate.[542] Others have implicated an improvement in myocardial oxygen extraction[543] or a direct antiischemic effect on myocardial cells.[544] In studies comparing DTZ, nifedipine, and propranolol with placebo using exercise, angina symptoms, and ambulatory monitoring, it appears that the effects of these drugs are discordant.[545] All three drugs improved exercise slightly. Propranolol reduced the total number of ischemic episodes more than DTZ or nifedipine, and DTZ and propranolol reduced anginal symptoms more than nifedipine.

In patients with chronic coronary occlusion and collateral circulation, both DTZ and nifedipine have increased exercise duration via a reduction in myocardial oxygen consumption rather than an increase in collateral flow.[546] In collateral dependent areas, intravenously administered nitroglycerin has attenuated myocardial ischemia better than DTZ,[547] and in a few patients DTZ might cause a steal syndrome wherein collaterals supply a region distal to a coronary stenosis.[548]

Mechanism of Antihypertensive Effect

The antihypertensive effect of Ca^{2+} antagonists probably can be explained by direct inhibition of vascular smooth muscle constriction, of α-adrenergic activation, of activation by nonadrenergic mediators (e.g., serotonin or prostaglandins), or of processes that lead to diuresis.[549–551] However, in one study in rats, naloxone reversed the blood pressure but not the heart rate–lowering effects of DTZ, suggesting that central opioid mechanisms may modulate part of the blood pressure–lowering effect.[552]

Blood vessels of experimental hypertensive animals and hypertensive patients differ functionally and in their response to drugs from those in normal patients.[394, 553–557] In general, they are more responsive. Unlike the larger arteries that are controlled by voltage-operated channels more than receptor-operated channels, the resistance vessels have receptor-operated channels that are sensitive to the effects of DTZ.[558] In two studies in hypertensive humans,[559, 560] DTZ was shown to dilate both large and small arteries. DTZ may also regress structural changes of blood vessels associated with hypertension by its antimitogenic properties.[561]

In normal volunteers, intravenously administered DTZ briefly lowered blood pressure, which then returned to normal. After an infusion of norepinephrine or angiotensin II, DTZ attenuated the increase in blood pressure, and this attenuation was greater at higher levels of norepinephrine and angiotensin II.[562] Because DTZ also inhibits the vascular reactivity response to lower body negative pressure in hypertensive patients without affecting plasma norepinephrine response, it is likely that the effects of DTZ in reducing blood pressure are due at least in part to reduction in the postjunctional action of norepinephrine on vascular smooth muscle constriction.[562-565]

Some evidence suggests a direct diuretic effect of DTZ in rats[395] and in humans with congestive heart failure.[396] In mononuclear cells obtained from patients treated for 6 weeks with DTZ, intracellular potassium and magnesium levels are decreased.[566] In rats with renovascular hypertension and diabetes, DTZ ameliorates the development of cardiomyopathy, but the mechanism appears to be related simply to control of blood pressure.[567] In renal hypertensive rats, DTZ leads to a proportional regression of LVH and improvement of mechanical function even when blood pressure is not completely controlled.[568]

Mechanism of Antiarrhythmic Effect

In studies on patients with supraventricular tachycardias, intravenously administered and acute orally administered DTZ have effectively converted these rhythms to sinus rhythm in most cases, usually by block in the AV node after prolonging the functional and effective refractory period.[569-571] Not all studies had similarly good results.[572] When accessory pathways were involved, DTZ did not alter the antegrade or retrograde refractory periods of the accessory pathway, and conversion occurred via block in the AV node.[570] In one patient with preexcitation and atrial fibrillation, DTZ accelerated the ventricular rate.[570] Individuals vary significantly in terms of sensitivity of the AV node to DTZ.[573]

DTZ appears to slow the ventricular response in atrial fibrillation[574] by two mechanisms that increase concealed conduction: an increase in the atrial fibrillatory rate and a combination of an increase in rate with prolongation of the refractory period,[575] which increases with increasing ventricular rate because of DTZ's frequency-dependent effects.[576] This was clearly demonstrated in an electrophysiologic study in 25 patients in whom atrial pacing at various rates showed greater drug effects on the AV node at shorter cycle lengths and no effects by DTZ on sinus node recovery time, intraatrial conduction time, atrial effective refractory period, and HV interval.[577] Although a medium dose of DTZ reduces the ventricular response to atrial fibrillation more than a low dose, it also increases the degree of concealed conduction in the AV node and enhances the irregularity of the ventricular response.[578]

In AV reentrant tachycardias induced in dogs, both the degree of slowing and the rate of termination produced by DTZ increase at higher tachycardia rates,[579] although autonomic reflexes induced by DTZ may in part offset the rate effect.[580] The effect of DTZ in humans (12 patients, intravenously administered DTZ) results from depression of anterograde AV conduction.[581] In this study, there were no effects on refractoriness of the AV pathway.

DTZ has effectively suppressed triggered activity in dogs 1 day after infarction.[582] The mechanism of the reduction of ischemic arrhythmias has been hypothesized to involve a reduction in extracellular potassium electrode potential[583] with the resultant diminution of injury current across the ischemic border.[242] Another study has suggested that the protective effect against reperfusion-induced arrhythmias is mediated mainly by specific effects on the calcium channel with possible additional contributions from sodium channel blocking effects.[584] In canine Purkinje fibers, DTZ reduces the ischemia-induced increase in intracellular free Ca^{2+}.[585] Significant evidence in animal studies suggests that DTZ may have a role in the treatment of early ischemia-induced arrhythmias[586-591] but not late arrhythmias.[592] The effect of DTZ to reduce ischemia-induced conduction delay is independent of its effects on coronary flow and thus may be directly antiarrhythmic.[591, 593] In dogs, DTZ produced a flow-independent reduction of cellular depolarization during ischemia, which may explain its antifibrillatory effect.[594] In the absence of ischemia, DTZ appears to have little effect on preventing the induction of either atrial or ventricular fibrillation, but these investigators also found no effect after acute myocardial infarction.[595] Other investigators have also found no effect after myocardial infarction,[596] ischemia,[597] or reperfusion.[598] In a large study of dogs, intravenously administered DTZ corrected ischemia-induced electrical alternans of the ST segment.[599] In an electrophysiologic study in pigs at the onset of acute myocardial ischemia, intravenously administered DTZ (in direct contrast with lidocaine) reduced waveform delay and alternation and reduced ST elevation and negative T waves.[600] In dogs, DTZ improves the resuscitation rate from induced ventricular fibrillation when administered before or during early cardiopulmonary resuscitation.[601] Because naloxone, infused into the lateral cerebral ventricle of rats, may offset some of the ventricular arrhythmia–suppressant effects of DTZ, an endogenous opioid mechanism has been postulated to explain part of DTZ's effects.[602]

CLINICAL USE
Coronary Disease

The effects of DTZ have been studied in a variety of conditions associated with coronary heart disease. It has been studied in patients with angina, in those with silent ischemia, in those with ischemia secondary to interventional procedures such as percutaneous transluminal coronary angioplasty, and in patients after myocardial infarction. It is at least as effective in the black as in the nonblack population.[603] Because the angina of most patients in clinical practice is due to both excessive energy demand and transient impairment of supply,[604] it is somewhat artificial to divide these causes. In this review, symptomatic coronary disease is divided arbitrarily between studies of patients with chronic stable angina and studies of patients with variant, unstable, or progressive angina involving spasm or myocardial infarction. In patients with stable angina, intravenously administered DTZ has uniformly improved exercise performance alone[221, 605-607] and in combination with β-blockers[608, 609] or nitrates.[610]

Orally administered DTZ in doses of 180 mg/day or less in an aggregate of about 150 patients has uniformly improved exercise ability or decreased anginal episodes[611-618] even in diabetics,[415] and an exercise training effect could be achieved.[619] In oral doses up to 360 mg/day, improvement in exercise time was again achieved,[61, 620-635] with an increase in LV EF in some studies.[623, 625] In patients with an EF of 11% to 39%, no decrease was noted in LV function.[636] The distribution of cardiac output is not altered.[637] When both DTZ and nitroglycerin are given acutely before exercise, symptomatic hypotension may result.[638] A significant decrease in total ischemic time by Holter recording was noted,[639, 640] which was more pronounced in the morning when coronary tone is greatest.[639] Some of these studies were carried out using a twice-daily regimen with a sustained-release preparation (Cardizem SR).[61, 633, 640, 635] In other studies, this sustained-release preparation was equal in effect and longer acting than the immediate-release preparation.[641] In various studies, it was less effective than isosorbide dinitrate (ISDN),[642] more effective that isosorbide mononitrate[643] or metoprolol,[644] and, in combination with ISDN, more effective than the monotherapies.[642]

Studies in stable angina have compared DTZ with β-blockers,[645-654] other calcium antagonists,[646, 655-667] and nitrates[648, 668, 669] and found equivalent improvements in angina and exercise time for the most part, with dose proportions varying from study to study. In direct comparisons of DTZ and nifedipine, DTZ was consistently better-tolerated.[670, 671] In another study, DTZ was equivalent to amiodarone and better than nitroglycerin in antianginal properties.[669] In studies of DTZ compared with bepridil, bepridil was slightly more effective, but patients were chosen from a group resistant to maximum doses of DTZ.[664, 665] When LV function was evaluated, DTZ generally was preferred to propranolol, and DTZ was the best-tolerated drug in general.

DTZ has been used in combination with β-blockers (propranolol,[672-680] nadolol[681]), nitrates,[682] or other calcium antagonists (nifedipine,[683-686] felodipine[659]). In general, combination with a β-blocker has produced a greater antianginal effect, but SA and AV nodal problems as well as an occasional instance of heart failure have occurred if patients are not selected.[672] With exercise, DTZ added to long-term β-blockade produces a fall in systemic vascular resistance, a lesser increase in heart rate, and an increase in stroke volume.[687] The combination with nifedipine may yield more side effects.[685] All combinations of propranolol with DTZ, nifedipine, or verapamil have been equally effective in comparisons, but DTZ with propranolol was highly preferred and produced fewer side effects.[675] In combination with β-blockers, DTZ and nifedipine produced equal improvement with[662] or without[661] concomitant long-acting nitrates. ISDN did not improve the combined efficacy of DTZ and atenolol.[688]

About 300 patients with coronary spasm or variant angina have been studied. More are reported, but some of the patients appear in more than one report.[677, 678, 683, 689-709] Results have been good, with reduction in angina frequency averaging 94% in one large study,[689] with more pain-free days and less nitroglycerin used.[694] Long-term follow-up of 6 months,[689] 16 months,[692] and 20 months[690] has continued to show good results, but coronary events continue despite treatment. DTZ, nifedipine,[701] verapamil,[701] and bepridil[710] have been equally effective in reducing symptoms or in blocking ergotamine-stimulated spasm.[699, 711] The combination of DTZ and nifedipine has been more effective than either agent, but with significantly increased side effects.[708, 709] No withdrawal rebound was noted in one large crossover study.[696] The major difference noted in comparative studies was that patients receiving DTZ had the fewest side effects. Intravenously administered DTZ has also improved exercise performance and ischemia in syndrome X.[712]

Among patients hospitalized with unstable angina, DTZ was equal to propranolol in a 100-patient comparative study evaluating chest pain, death, infarction, and coronary bypass incidence.[713] Another study found DTZ more effective than propranolol in decreasing anginal pain.[714] In a third study, DTZ was effective[715] or tended to be effective[716] and was equal to bepridil.[715] A combination of DTZ and nifedipine has been successful in elderly patients with mixed angina.[717] Most patients treated with DTZ (360 mg/day) and amiodarone (600 to 1200 mg/day) did well at 6 months after admission for unstable angina except for occasional conduction problems.[718] Intravenously administered DTZ has also controlled unstable angina[719, 720] and was as effective as[721] or more effective[722] than intravenously administered nitroglycerin.

Among nearly 100 patients with stable coronary heart disease[723, 724] and over 50 patients after myocardial infarction,[725] DTZ has reduced the number of episodes of silent ischemia, improving LV function[725] and exercise test end points.[723]

In patients with acute myocardial infarction, intravenously administered DTZ has been well-tolerated except in those with significant ventricular function disorders.[726] This was also the case when DTZ was given sequentially with orally administered nifedipine.[727] In a study of 34 patients treated intravenously and then orally with DTZ, thallium SPECT showed significantly smaller perfusion defects and better ventricular function than in control patients despite normal CK and CK-MB indices.[728] The outcome of percutaneous transluminal coronary angioplasty in patients without variant angina was not affected by DTZ.[729] In a 45-patient study in which DTZ, 360 mg/day, was started within 6 hours of infarction and compared with placebo, ischemic and necrotic scores were lowered by DTZ.[730] The authors cautioned that the groups were not completely comparable.

DTZ has effectively reduced angina after myocardial infarction and ischemia[731-733] and, in a comparison with atenolol, produced a similar increase in exercise time but a lesser increase in time to ischemia.[734] DTZ is well tolerated hemodynamically after intravenous administration[735-737] and it has improved LV synergy and EF.[738] The first secondary prevention study in postinfarction patients compared the outcome of DTZ treatment with placebo in non–Q-wave infarction (Diltiazem Reinfarction Study). This multicenter study[739, 740] randomly assigned 287 patients to DTZ and 289 to placebo, initiating treatment 24 to 72 hours after the onset of symptoms. In the first 14 days, DTZ produced a reduction in cumulative life-table incidence of reinfarction of 51% ($p = .03$) and reduced the frequency of refractory postinfarction angina by 50% ($p = .03$). A follow-up analysis[741] showed a significant protective effect against early postinfarction angina associated with transient ST-T changes ($p = .01$). These latter changes were also highly correlated with reinfarction, peak CK-MB levels, and mortality. DTZ does not normalize the reduction in heart rate variability found after myocardial infarction.[742]

Subsequently, the Multicenter Diltiazem Postinfarction Trial (MDPIT) was designed to investigate the long-term effects of DTZ on mortality and cardiac event rates after myocardial infarction in 2466 patients from 38 hospitals in the United States and Canada who were begun on DTZ, 240 mg/day, 3 to 15 days after myocardial infarction and followed for 12 to 52 months (mean, 25).[743] DTZ had no overall effect, but this lack of overall effect resulted from an increase in event rate and mortality rate in a small number of patients (those with pulmonary congestion) and a significant decrease in events in most patients (those without pulmonary congestion).[744] DTZ appeared not to reduce either the incidence of post–myocardial infarction ventricular arrhythmias or sudden death during the first 3 months after myocardial infarction.[745] Because a prior short-term study with DTZ[739] had shown a reduction in cardiac event rate in non–Q-wave myocardial infarctions during a 14-day postinfarction period, a prespecified analysis of MDPIT was carried out and demonstrated a 40% reduction in 1-year mortality ($p < .03$) in patients with non–Q-wave myocardial infarction.[746, 747] These patients experienced parallel reductions in both mortality rate and cardiac event rate.[748] Although benefit was greatest in patients with a first infarction and without pulmonary congestion,[749] there was significant benefit irrespective of prior evidence of infarction[750] but only during the first 6 months after infarction and only preventing reinfarction in the same area.[751] The subgroup of patients with a history of hypertension also benefited from DTZ after myocardial infarction.[752]

A retrospective analysis of the non–Q-wave infarction patients from the prior Diltiazem Reinfarction Study examined the effect of high-dose (360 mg/day) DTZ on ventricular function and found no overall deterioration.[753] These data suggest that DTZ may be of value after myocardial infarction in patients with significant myocardium at risk, which may be spared, and not in those with more complete damage. Unfortunately, the complete explanation for the disparate effects of DTZ after myocardial infarction have never been forthcoming. The finding of beneficial effects of verapamil[754] but not of nifedipine[755] may suggest that

the heart rate–slowing calcium antagonists may provide an unidentified kind of protection, whereas other calcium antagonists do not. In view of the large number of agents that have demonstrated benefit in the post–myocardial infarction milieu (aspirin, β-blockers, ACE inhibitors), it is doubtful that calcium antagonists will find a role outside of symptom and ischemia protection unless new studies come to light.

In an animal model of failed coronary angioplasty (percutaneous transluminal coronary angioplasty [PTCA]), DTZ reduced myocardial injury.[756] In humans undergoing PTCA, DTZ delayed the time to ischemic ST alteration[757-759] and LV wall-motion abnormalities,[757] but it did not prevent restenosis or other late events.[760] Introduced directly into aortocoronary bypass grafts in 90 patients, DTZ increased graft flow by 64% without dropping perfusion pressure.[761]

The advantages of DTZ in the treatment of patients with coronary artery disease include efficacy against all areas of the disease, fixed stenosis, motility, and aggregation;[604] low side effects;[627-629] possible protective effects against ischemia,[713] reinfarction,[739] and reperfusion damage;[345] lack of significant negative inotropic effects;[762] and lack of adverse effects on coronary risk factors.[423]

Hypertension

Uncontrolled short-term[763-771] and long-term[420, 765, 772, 773] studies with DTZ in hypertensive patients formed the basis for the trials that followed. From these studies came evidence of twice-daily[767, 774-785] and once-daily[786-795] dosing efficacy and a reduction in LV mass.[768, 796, 797]

Several large multicenter trials have been conducted. In one study of 80 patients treated with DTZ, 90 to 270 mg/day, average blood pressure was reduced from 167/106 to 141/87 mmHg at 12 weeks. An improvement in exercise time was noted, and only five patients were eliminated from the study for intolerance.[798] Another study of 94 patients (49 DTZ, 45 placebo) used 180 mg/day for 6 weeks; mean blood pressure dropped by 15 mmHg in the group receiving DTZ ($p < .01$)[799] Antihypertensive monotherapy with the immediate-release tablet formulation of DTZ was effective when given every 8 hours, but if given every 12 hours, it did not provide 24-hour blood pressure control in some patients.[800]

Experience with the twice-a-day sustained-release formulation has shown it to maintain excellent effect throughout the 12-hour dosing period.[783, 801] There have been no effects on serum lipid levels, glucose, or electrolytes.[802] In a study involving 77 patients, 85% required a dose of 360 mg/day.[803] Blood pressure fell significantly from 156/100 to 145/90 mmHg over 12 weeks. Side effects were low, and no orthostatic blood pressure effects were produced.[803] In another study of 18 patients, mean arterial pressure fell from 121 to 108 mmHg, and there was a significant increase in GFR.[804] Long-term studies over 8 months showed no tachyphylaxis to treatment with sustained-release

DTZ, and there were no adverse effects on serum lipid levels.[423] The combination of DTZ and hydrochlorothiazide (HCTZ) was studied in a large factorial trial involving 297 patients,[778] in a subsequent dose-escalation trial in 298 patients,[775] and in a further parallel trial of 254 patients.[785] These studies established that the combination of DTZ and HCTZ produced an enhanced antihypertensive effect compared with the monotherapies.

Several once-a-day formulations have appeared around the world. It is not always possible to distinguish which long-acting formulation is being used in the studies in the literature. Twenty-four-hour efficacy has been demonstrated in studies of 127[795] and 107[789] patients and with ambulatory monitoring.[782, 792] In one of the ambulatory blood pressure studies, 300 mg/day but not 240 mg/day lowered blood pressure significantly.[782] In another study of 100 patients using placebo (240, 300, and 360 mg/day), there were significant antihypertensive differences between 240 and 300 mg/day but not between 300 and 360 mg/day.[791] A significant dose-response effect was found in studies of 275 patients[784] and 229 patients[793] with doses ranging from 90 to 540 mg/day. In other studies, 180 mg once daily was as effective as 90 mg twice daily,[788] but 240 mg once daily was not as effective as 120 mg twice daily.[786] In comparative studies, once-daily DTZ compared favorably with nitrendipine[787] and was more effective and better tolerated than HCTZ/triamterene in the elderly.[790] Among 96 patients treated in three parallel groups, a combination of DTZ (300 mg/day) and enalapril (20 mg/day) was equal in effect to monotherapy with DTZ, and both were more effective than enalapril.[794]

Although nifedipine is a more potent vasodilator than DTZ or verapamil, the three agents appear to have equal antihypertensive efficacy, with the major difference being a lower side effect profile for DTZ,[805] for which it has been preferred.[419] In terms of efficacy, DTZ has been as effective as HCTZ,[806-809] reserpine,[810] propranolol,[416, 811-814] metoprolol,[815-818] atenolol,[819, 820] captopril,[821, 822] enalapril,[774] isradipine,[823] nicardipine,[824] nitrendipine,[825] nifedipine,[421, 826-829] and verapamil.[830, 831] Although experience has been small, DTZ has been effective in the prevention and treatment of acute hypertensive events[832, 833] and the treatment of intraoperative[834] and postoperative[835] hypertension.

In combination studies, DTZ plus atenolol[820] and DTZ plus HCTZ/triamterene,[836] but not DTZ plus mefruside,[837] produce greater blood pressure lowering than the monotherapies; DTZ and HCTZ are equal in effect to metoprolol and HCTZ;[838] added transdermal clonidine improved control of DTZ-resistant hypertensives;[839] and in a case report, DTZ plus nifedipine successfully controlled severe hypertension.[840] When a combination of propranolol and HCTZ was replaced with sustained-release DTZ in patients with angina and hypertension, exercise performance was increased and equal blood pressure control was obtained in 74% of patients with DTZ monotherapy and in 100% with the addition of a diuretic.[841]

Equal or improved efficacy in blacks[842] and elderly people[777, 779, 780, 843-845] has been demonstrated, but age and renin activity have not been found to clinically predict antihypertensive response to DTZ.[776]

In other studies with hypertensive patients, exercise performance was generally improved[846] or unchanged with DTZ and was better in one respect or another than with propranolol[847] or atenolol.[848, 849] In these patients, the improvement in HDL cholesterol levels produced by exercise training was maintained with DTZ therapy but blunted with administration of propranolol.[850] In a similar comparison of exercise duration in young hypertensive patients receiving DTZ or atenolol, no difference was noted.[851] In another study by the same authors, however, DTZ was associated with no adverse effects in young hypertensives exposed to heat stress in a sauna, whereas systolic pressure fell significantly in subjects taking atenolol.[852] DTZ reduces catecholamine secretion in exercising hypertensives.[853] Treatment of hypertensive patients with DTZ leads to a reduction in LV mass[768, 796, 797, 812, 854] with an improvement in coronary reserve,[854] but it has no significant effect on LV systolic or diastolic function.[855]

The advantages of DTZ as an antihypertensive drug are equal efficacy to other popular treatments; near freedom from side effects;[773, 803, 807] lack of negative lipid effects or other laboratory abnormalities;[418, 423] lack of tachyphylaxis, orthostatic effects, or impairment of exercise performance;[423] ability to regress LV mass;[768, 796, 797, 812, 854] and good efficacy in blacks and the elderly population.[809, 843, 856] Twice-daily and once-daily sustained-release preparations have been effective.

Arrhythmias

Intravenously administered DTZ has been effective in converting paroxysmal supraventricular tachycardia (PSVT) to sinus rhythm. In an 87-patient study of induced SVT, four parallel doses of intravenously administered DTZ were compared with placebo. The conversion rates to sinus rhythm for doses of 0.05, 0.15, 0.25, and 0.45 mg/kg and placebo were 29%, 84%, 100%, 84%, and 25% respectively.[857] In 10 separate studies, DTZ, 0.25 mg/kg intravenously, converted PSVT in 125 of 167 patients (75%) to sinus rhythm.[246, 569, 570, 572, 858-863] DTZ, 0.15 mg/kg intravenously, was used with poor results, suggesting too low a dose.[864] In another study of varying intravenous doses, 6 of 10 patients had good results.[865] In a final study using a higher intravenous dose of 20 mg plus a second dose of 10 to 20 mg if necessary, the PSVT of 10 of 10 patients converted to sinus rhythm, and 35 of 35 patients with chronic paroxysmal atrial fibrillation or flutter converted to sinus rhythm or experienced a decreased in ventricular response to less than 100/min.[866] In 11 hyperthyroid patients, DTZ lowered heart rate and eliminated both supraventricular and ventricular arrhythmias.[867]

Orally administered DTZ has also been effective in treating patients with PSVT. In one study with electrophysiologic data, 10 of 16 patients with PSVT became uninducible with a dose of 270 mg/day. Clinical suppression was good in 12 of these patients during 6 months.[571] Among 36 patients with PSVT (24 AV reentry and 12 AV nodal reentry), a dose of 270 mg/day made 20 of 24 of the former and 8 of 12 of the latter uninducible. Thirteen of these patients had no attacks over the next 5 months.[868] Not every study, however, has demonstrated significant prevention of recurrence.[869] A placebo-controlled clinical study of acute oral conversion from PSVT to sinus rhythm was carried out in 15 patients with single oral doses of DTZ, 120 mg, plus propranolol, 160 mg. On placebo therapy, four patients converted to sinus rhythm, whereas on active treatment, 14 of 15 converted in an average of 27 minutes. Two patients experienced transient second-degree AV block on treatment. During long-term follow-up, the single-dose treatment converted 50 of 51 spontaneous episodes in an average of 21 minutes.[870] Individuals appear to vary significantly in terms of sensitivity of the AV node to DTZ.[573] Poor results have been reported using orally administered verapamil for conversion of PSVT to sinus rhythm (1 patient in 10). These results were shown to be due to low verapamil levels despite high doses because of prolonged gastric emptying time in patients with PSVT.[871] From the clinical trials of DTZ above, low DTZ levels are probably not a problem in the treatment of PSVT.

DTZ has not been effective in converting atrial fibrillation to sinus rhythm;[575, 872–875] however, intravenously[876–879] or orally at a higher dose of 360 mg/day as sole therapy,[875] it is effective in controlling the ventricular response, both at rest and during exercise.[880–882] Orally, the effect of DTZ on ventricular response is similar to that of propranolol[883] or verapamil.[881] Although DTZ reduces the heart rate response further when combined with propranolol, it does not increase exercise capacity further.[883] When DTZ was given intravenously with initial boluses of 20 mg, another 25 mg if necessary, and then infusions at 10 to 15 mg/hr, in three separate studies involving 189 patients, the DTZ response rate for significant slowing of ventricular response was 89%, whereas the placebo response rate was 9%.[574, 876, 879] Plasma DTZ concentration was strongly related to percentage of heart rate reduction, and DTZ metabolite concentrations were too low to have contributed to the effect.[877] In a separate study, nine patients with acute symptomatic congestive heart failure and rapid atrial fibrillation were treated with 2-minute infusions of 0.25 mg/kg followed, if necessary, by 0.35 mg/kg of DTZ. Rate was slowed in 8 of 9 patients with no clinical deterioration and some hemodynamic improvement.[878]

Orally administered DTZ in doses ranging from 180 to 360 mg/day have successfully reduced the ventricular response to atrial fibrillation.[884–886] The reduction of rate has been achieved without reduction in blood pressure or exercise capacity[884] and has been proportional to the baseline rate.[885] The mechanism for this effect has been demonstrated in canine experiments, which show a rate-dependent amplification of DTZ effects in atrial fibrillation[887] in line with its previously demonstrated frequency-dependent AV nodal conduction effects.[245] DTZ controls the exercise response better than digoxin.[886] The ventricular response was also controlled when DTZ was added to digoxin in patients in whom exercise ventricular response had been inadequate with digoxin.[888] Finally, evidence suggests that both intravenously administered and orally administered DTZ or verapamil may prolong the duration of episodes of electrically induced atrial fibrillation.[889] In patients with ventricular preexcitation, intravenously administered DTZ may increase the ventricular response when atrial fibrillation is present, which has been shown not to be the case with orally administered DTZ.[873]

DTZ has prevented arrhythmias in patients with Prinzmetal's angina,[890] but it has only modest efficacy in decreasing premature ventricular contractions. DTZ may suppress inducible ventricular tachycardia in some patients.[891] Experimental evidence suggests that DTZ may be effective in preventing ventricular fibrillation early in ischemic injury. These data are presented in the earlier section, Electrophysiology.

Congestive Heart Failure and Cardiomyopathy

Chronic DTZ administration has protected against disease progression in the cardiomyopathic hamster.[892] In 32 humans with hypertrophic cardiomyopathy, DTZ improved symptoms in 83% who had symptoms at baseline in one study[893] and improved abnormal measurements of diastolic function in 17 patients in another study.[894]

The negative inotropy of DTZ has often been misunderstood or overestimated. *In vitro* studies have indicated that of DTZ, nifedipine, and verapamil, DTZ is the least negatively inotropic.[149, 212, 213] In a study of 10 patients with chronic congestive heart failure, New York Heart Association (NYHA) class III or IV, with a mean EF of 22%, intravenously administered DTZ, 60 or 90 mg, caused no significant hemodynamic change.[895] In another study of 22 coronary heart disease patients given an average DTZ dose of 254 mg/day with an LV EF ranging from 11% to 39%, only one was withdrawn for progressive heart failure, and of those with a significant weight change, as many lost as gained weight.[636] When high-dose DTZ (0.4 mg/kg for 5 minutes followed by 0.4 mg/kg for 10 minutes) was administered to 23 coronary heart disease patients with an LV EF of less than 45%, coronary flow and LV function were improved.[520] In a study of 16 patients with NYHA class II heart failure, single doses of 90 and 180 mg of DTZ increased stroke volume and reduced heart rate.[896] However, in another study of 22 patients with chronic dilated cardiomyopathy, DTZ was added to conventional treatment with digoxin, diuretics, and vasodilators over an average period of more than 15 months.[897] This group was compared with a comparable historical control group with conventional treatment. The addition of DTZ produced a significant decrease in mortality (20% versus 0%, $p < .001$) and a significant increase in LV EF from 34% to 44% ($p < .001$), suggesting that DTZ may be useful in the treatment of patients with dilated cardiomyopathy. A retrospective analysis of the MDPIT study (cited earlier under Coronary Disease), however, questioned the conclusion that there was no consistent effect of new or worsened congestive heart failure during 12 to 52 months of follow-up. When patients with baseline low LV EF (<40%) were treated with DTZ, the incidence of late congestive heart failure was 21% compared with 12% in similar patients treated with placebo.[898] Thus, it is clear that DTZ administration is compatible with low LV EF, and may even improve it in some patients, but in others there is a late risk of congestive heart failure, and continuing observation is recommended.

Adverse Effects

DTZ was noted by one investigator who was experienced with DTZ and other cardiovascular drugs to be remarkably free from adverse effects.[899] The most common adverse reactions from DTZ in more than 2 million patient-years of experience were edema (2.4%), headache (2.1%), nausea (1.9%), dizziness (1.5%), rash (1.3%), and asthenia (1.2%).[900] Other reactions that might be predicted from its physiologic action are extensions of vasodilatation (flushing, edema, hypotension), negative inotropy (which is unusual), conduction disturbances, and smooth muscle relaxation (constipation, nausea).[713] A postmarketing surveillance study of 16,720 patients receiving DTZ in Great Britain revealed no previously unrecognized adverse reactions.[901]

Individual case reports and small series have reported a number of reactions, most idiosyncratic, to DTZ: a variety of skin rashes,[902–911] including one with thickening and sensory loss in the skin of the feet[903] and another with photosensitivity;[912] thrombocytopenia;[913, 914] one case of loss of smell and taste;[915] a poorly documented case of hyperosmolar nonketotic coma;[916] hyperplastic gingivitis;[917] myoclonus;[918] Lambert-Eaton myasthenic syndrome;[919] drug fever;[920] the induction of diabetes;[921] four instances of renal or hepatic toxicity;[922–925] irritability and hyperactivity[269] and psychosis[926] with lithium; akathisia (restlessness);[927, 928] precipitation of carbamazepine neurotoxicity;[929] pustular eruption reproduced on rechallenge;[930] rash and adenopathy;[931] increase in bleeding time in three patients;[932] AV conduction problems in seven patients;[933–935] cardiac arrest after intracoronary injection;[936] pulmonary edema in hypertrophic cardiomyopathy;[937] and hypotension or sinus bradycardia in combination with β-blockers.[938–942] The incidence of heart block has been reported at 0.2% overall and at 0.6% when used in conjunction with a β-blocker.[901] Although this incidence did not differ from that of the overall population, a relation to DTZ administration is implied.[901] There have also been a few elevations of hepatic enzymes (one severe), one case of

leukopenia, and rare erythema multiforme.[900] Many of these reactions have not been confirmed with rechallenge by drug.

A rebound in symptoms upon withdrawal of DTZ is not thought to occur. However, the possibility of a withdrawal syndrome in patients with angina was raised in a Holter study of 143 patients in which 3 patients receiving DTZ and 2 receiving verapamil were found to have significant increases in ischemic ST-segment abnormalities after withdrawal.[943] No rebound effect was found following DTZ withdrawal prior to coronary bypass surgery, nor was there any intraoperative effect when DTZ was given with high-dose fentanyl anesthesia.[944] Another uremic patient with normal coronary arteries suffered a myocardial infarction after DTZ withdrawal,[945] and 2 patients in whom DTZ was withdrawn prior to coronary bypass surgery had severe coronary spasm postoperatively.[946]

A survey of French poison centers revealed 134 cases of intentional or accidental overdose in children and adults ranging from 360 mg to 5400 mg.[947] The reactions were all predictable and included malaise and bradycardia in 16%, hypotension in 20%, cardiogenic shock in 4%, and cardiac arrest in 2.4%. Disorders of conduction included AV block of first degree (9%), second degree (2.4%), and third degree (9%). No patients died. A self-administered overdose of DTZ produces predictable effects (14 patients) that include hypotension, bradycardia, heart block,[948–959] and, in one case, asthenia and catatonia at a total ingested dose of 2640 mg.[948] The patient recovered within 48 hours. The dose in the other 13 patients was 9000, 7200, 6000, 5400, 4800, 4200, 1800 (4 patients), 1500, 1200, and 1250 mg, along with 500 mg of metoprolol in the last. All survived. Basic treatment was supportive with intravenous fluids, transvenous pacing, activated charcoal, and pharmacologic circulatory support. No evidence of negative inotropy was noted. Charcoal hemoperfusion was successful in reversing DTZ blood levels and promoting recovery in the patient who took both DTZ and metoprolol.[949] Another case manifested noncardiogenic pulmonary edema.[960] One patient experienced shock while receiving DTZ, metoprolol, propafenone, and sparteine because he was a poor metabolizer phenotype of sparteine/debrisoquine polymorphism, which occurs in 6.4% of the German population.[961] DTZ may potentiate bleeding after use of tissue-type plasminogen activator[962] and may potentiate the hypotensive reaction to contrast angiography.[963] Thus far, the highest recorded blood DTZ concentration with which the patient survived has been 6090 μg/L.[964] Only eight deaths have been reported with DTZ as the only cardioactive drug[965–969] with DTZ blood levels of 1500, 2500, 4000, 6700, 8000, 15,000, and 16,880 μg/L, as well as a final unknown level. A DTZ level of 8490 μg/L was reported in another death in conjunction with metoclopramide.[970]

Thus, DTZ has a mild side-effect profile, especially compared with other calcium antagonists and β-blockers. It has even compared favorably with placebo.[624]

Contraindications, Warnings, and Precautions

Studies of teratogenicity have revealed lethal effects of DTZ for mouse embryo (10 mg/kg) and rat embryo (200 mg/kg), teratogenic effects at 50 mg/kg for mouse and more than 600 mg/kg in rat, and maternal problems at 200 mg/kg.[971] Although not supported by human data, these findings have led to precautions for use in pregnant women, nursing mothers, and children.[900] In addition, there is a precaution for renal and hepatic dysfunction.[972]

Label warnings include AV conduction delays, congestive heart failure (although many patients with severely impaired LV function have done well on DTZ), hypotension, acute hepatic injury, and transient sinus pauses.[900]

Contraindications to DTZ include sick sinus syndrome, except with a functioning pacemaker, second- or third-degree AV block, hypotension (<90 mmHg systolic), and acute myocardial infarction with pulmonary congestion.[972]

Interference with Other Drugs

Potential interactions of DTZ with digoxin, propranolol, theophylline, quinidine, lidocaine, disopyramide, amiodarone, cimetidine, nifedipine, bupivacaine, carbamazepine, diazepam, and gentamycin are discussed under Pharmacokinetics. Nitrates occasionally produce hypotension when coadministered with DTZ.

Another potential interaction is that of DTZ with anesthetics, because halogenated anesthetics may themselves attenuate sympathetic reflexes and depress nodal function.[973] Experiments with pigs[974, 975] revealed significant blood pressure and conduction problems with DTZ and halothane. In experiments with DTZ and enflurane, isoflurane, or halothane anesthesia in isolated guinea pig hearts, combination treatment slowed atrial rates, prolonged AV conduction time, and depressed LV contractile function more than the individual agents did.[976, 977] In experiments with the same agents in dogs, very high serum levels of DTZ caused hypotension[978, 979] or, with sevoflurane, caused greater conduction changes and increased cardiac depressant effects.[980]

On the other hand, with halothane anesthesia, DTZ was found to decrease the effects of coronary occlusion,[981] to improve LV function,[982] to decrease epinephrine-induced arrhythmias,[983] and not to produce negative inotropy.[984] In a study comparing β-blockers and calcium antagonists with placebo in patients undergoing halothane anesthesia (29 control patients, 45 on calcium antagonists and β-blockers), heart block was not a significant problem, although it was expected to be, and the calcium antagonists alone had minimal effects.[973] In another study, one patient had AV conduction problems and another had sinus node conduction problems on DTZ and enflurane.[985] In combination with fentanyl anesthesia, DTZ produced hypotension in dogs[986] and lowered pressure in patients undergoing hip arthroplasty.[987] Bupivacaine toxicity was also increased twofold in dogs by DTZ.[988] Finally, the cardiostimulant effects of ketamine were not blocked by intravenously administered DTZ.[989] Thus, the interaction of DTZ with anesthetics is predictable from the pharmacologic actions of both classes of drugs.

DTZ interacts significantly with cyclosporine, inhibiting its metabolism,[990] inhibiting its cellular uptake,[991] or changing its volume of distribution.[992] It is commonly used in renal[993–995] and cardiac[486] transplantation patients (see Effects on Other Organs and Other Uses).

Use in Patients with Impaired Hepatic and Renal Function

Because DTZ is metabolized predominantly by the liver, its use in patients with acute hepatic disease cannot be recommended. Despite labeling precautions, however, DTZ has been used in patients with significant renal impairment, and, at least in those with hypertension or diabetes, it seems to be well tolerated and may even enhance function. In patients with hepatic cirrhosis, DTZ (90 mg/day) did not affect diuresis, natriuresis, arterial pressure, or the renin-angiotensin axis,[996] but elimination half-life is prolonged because of impaired oxidative metabolism of DTZ.[997]

Advantages and Disadvantages Compared with Similar Drugs

No similar drugs have a better side-effect profile than DTZ, which is probably its greatest single advantage.

In the treatment of patients with coronary disease, DTZ has a broader efficacy profile than the β-blockers because of its effect on coronary motility and perhaps platelet aggregation in addition to its effects on heart rate and blood pressure that limit energy demand. Compared with nifedipine, DTZ has disadvantages with respect to adverse effects on the SA and AV nodes, which, of course, may be an advantage if supraventricular arrhythmias are present. The side-effect profile of DTZ clearly is superior to those of both nifedipine and verapamil, and DTZ may be associated with fewer problems of sinus and AV node malfunction than is verapamil. Although evidence suggests a protective effect of DTZ in patients with myocardial infarction, DTZ is not considered preferable to β-blockers. For long-term treatment, lack of adverse lipid effects is a significant advantage.

In the treatment of hypertension, lack of adverse side effects and lipid effects may be even more important because of the long-term nature of treatment in this condition. Efficacy in black and elderly patients is an advantage over β-blockers, and lack of tachyphylaxis and fluid retention is an advantage over α-blockers. DTZ seems better tolerated than the ACE inhibitors because of the cough-related problems of the latter, and because ACE inhibitors have no antianginal properties. Effects on conduction are the major disadvantages compared with the ACE inhibitors.

In arrhythmias, the efficacy of orally administered DTZ may make it the drug of choice for conversion of PSVT to sinus rhythm, at least when the episodes are not frequent. Lack of adequate oral levels for verapamil in PSVT may give this advantage to DTZ.

Dosage and Administration

The common intravenous dose of DTZ for patients with PSVT is 0.25 mg/kg given over several minutes. A similar dose with an added infusion of 0.005 mg/kg/min to a total dose of 360 mg/day has been added in ischemic syndromes. In the American population, the common oral dose for the treatment of angina, either stable or variant, is 180 to 240 mg/day in a regimen of one to three doses per day, depending on the formulation. Doses half this size are used in many Asian populations. Doses of 360 mg/day and, rarely, up to 480 mg/day have been used with improved results in some patients. The oral dose for the treatment of hypertension is higher than that for angina, ranging from 240 to 480 mg/day in most patients.[845] At higher dose levels, one has to be cautious of saturating the elimination pathway, because serum levels

become disproportionately higher than the dose given. The sustained-release preparations are generally preferred.

SOCIOECONOMIC CONSIDERATIONS
Compliance with Regimen

Because of the mild side effect profile of DTZ, compliance with dosing has been excellent. In one study in which compliance was assessed and based on pill counts, patient compliance usually averaged 99% and never fell below 95%.[803] Once- or twice-daily dosing with various preparations aids compliance.

Cost

Cost of a treatment regimen is difficult to estimate because it must take into account not only the cost of the medication but also how difficult it is to titrate, how many physician visits are engendered by side effects, the possible need for laboratory monitoring, and the costs of laboratory tests themselves. On top of this figure is the undefined cost to the patient in terms of side effects, lifestyle, and possible progres-

Table 102–2. **Average Wholesale Price of Commonly Prescribed Anithypertensive and Antianginal Drugs**

Generic Name	Trade Name	Dose (mg)	1-Month Price ($)
prazosin	Minipress	5 t.i.d.	82.18
nifedipine	generic	20 t.i.d.	74.79
diltiazem	generic	90 t.i.d.	68.40
captopril	Capoten	50 b.i.d.	68.04
diltiazem	Cardizem SR	120 b.i.d.	66.15
nifedipine	Procardia XL	60/day	59.40
amlodipine	Norvasc	10/day	56.84
diltiazem	Cardizem CD	240/day	48.80
nifedipine	Adalat CC	60/day	43.65
metoprolol	Lopressor	100 b.i.d.	43.60
isradipine	Dynacirc	5 b.i.d.	43.02
enalapril	Vasotec	20/day	39.51
propranolol	Inderal LA	160/day	39.12
verapamil	Calan SR	240/day	35.90
verapamil	Isoptin SR	240/day	35.90
verapamil	Verelan	240/day	35.27
prazosin	generic	5 t.i.d.	29.93
diltiazem	Dilacor XR	240/day	28.26
doxazosin	Cardura	4/day	26.55
atenolol	Tenormin	100/day	25.02
atenolol	generic	100/day	20.07
propranolol	generic	40 t.i.d.	15.88
hydrochlorothiazide	Esidrix	50/day	5.29
hydrochlorothiazide	generic	50/day	1.11

Data from Red Book Update, Vol 12, October 1993. Montvale, NJ: Medical Economics Data, 1993.

sion or regression of both the condition being treated and any concomitant diseases.

The current average wholesale price[998] for 30 days of treatment with a representative effective dose of common orally administered antianginal and antihypertensive drugs is shown in descending order of price in Table 102–2. Of course, retail mark-up and dosing vary, making these prices only a rough index.

REFERENCES

1. Fleckenstein A: History of calcium antagonists. Circ Res 52:3, 1983.
2. Nagao T, Sato M, Nakajima H, et al: Studies on a new 1,5 benzothiazepine derivative (CRD-401). II. Vasodilator actions. Jpn J Pharmacol 22:1, 1972.
3. Nagao T, Narita H, Sato M, et al: Development of diltiazem, a calcium antagonist: Coronary vasodilating and antihypertensive actions. Clin Exp Hypertens [A] 4:285, 1982.
4. Sato M, Nagao T, Yamaguchi I, et al: Pharmacological studies on a new 1,5-benzothiazepine derivative (CRD-401). Arzneimittelforschung 21:1338, 1971.
5. Frishman WH: A new extended-release formulation of diltiazem HCl for the treatment of mild-to-moderate hypertension. J Clin Pharmacol 33:612, 1993.
6. Meyer H: Structural/activity relationships in calcium antagonists. *In* Opie LH (ed): Calcium Antagonists and Cardiovascular Disease. New York: Raven Press, 1984, pp 165–173.
7. Nasa Y, Ichihara K, Abiko Y: Both d-cis and l-cis-diltiazem have anti-ischemic action in the isolated, perfused working rat heart. J Pharmacol Exp Ther 255:680, 1990.
8. Kojic PB, Ruzic RZ, Sunjic V: Absolute conformation and configuration of (2S, 3S)-3-acetoxy-5-(dimethylaminoethyl)-2-(4-methoxyphenyl)-2,3-dihydro-1,5-benzothiazepin-4(5H)-one chloride (diltiazem hydrochloride). Helv Chim Acta 67:916, 1984.
9. Floyd D, Krapcho J: Benzothiazepine derivatives. US Patent 4,584,131, Apr 22, 1986.
10. Kugita H, Inoue H, Ikezaki M, et al: Synthesis of 1,5-benzothiazepine derivatives. Chem Pharm Bull 18:2028, 1970.
11. Li R, Farmer PS, Xie M, et al: Synthesis, characterization, and Ca(2+) antagonistic activity of diltiazem metabolites. J Med Chem 35:3246, 1992.
12. Schwartz A, Madan PB, Mohacsi E, et al: Enantioselective synthesis of calcium channel blockers of the diltiazem group. J Org Chem 57:851, 1992.
13. Yanagisawa H, Fujimoto K, Shimoji Y, et al: Synthesis and antihypertensive activity of 3-acetoxy-2,3-dihydro-5-[2-(dimethylamino)ethyl]-2-(4-methoxyphenyl)-1,5-benzothiazepin-4(5H)-one (diltiazem) derivatives having substituents at the 8 position. Chem Pharm Bull 40:2055, 1992.
14. Piepho RW: The calcium antagonists. Mechanisms of action and pharmacologic effects. Drug Ther 13:69, 1983.
15. McAllister RG, Hamann SR, Blouin RA: Pharmacokinetics of calcium-entry blockers. Am J Cardiol 55:30B, 1985.
16. Hermann P, Morselli PL: Pharmacokinetics of diltiazem and other calcium entry blockers. Acta Pharmacol Toxicol 57:10, 1985.
17. Anderssen KE: Calcium-entry blockers. A heterogeneous family of compounds. Acta Med Scand 694:142, 1985.
18. Piepho RW: Comparative clinical pharmacokinetics of the calcium antagonists. *In* Hoffman BF (ed): Calcium Antagonists: The State of the Art and Role in Cardiovascular Disease. Philadelphia: College of Physicians of Philadelphia, 1983, pp 159–174.
19. Smith MS, Verghese CP, Shand DG, et al: Pharmacokinetic and pharmacodynamic effects of diltiazem. Am J Cardiol 51:1369, 1983.
20. Etoh A, Kohno K, Takeuchi Y: Studies on diltiazem hydrochloride preparation (III). Its pharmacokinetics in man. Clin Rep 14:3082, 1980.
21. Rovei V, Mitchard M, Morselli P: Simple, sensitive and specific gas chromatographic method for the quantification of diltiazem in human body fluids. J Chromatogr 138:391, 1977.
22. Goebel KJ, Kolle EU: High-performance liquid chromatographic determination of diltiazem and four of its metabolites in plasma. Application to pharmacokinetics. J Chromatogr 345:355, 1985.
23. Abernethy DR, Schwartz JB, Todd EL: Diltiazem and desacetyldiltiazem analysis in human plasma using high-performance liquid chromatography: Improved sensitivity without derivatization. J Chromatogr 342:216, 1985.
24. Bonnefous JL, Boulieu R: Comparison of solid-phase extraction and liquid-liquid extraction methods for liquid chromatographic determination of diltiazem and its metabolites in plasma. J Liq Chromatogr 13:3799, 1990.
25. Nishi H, Fujimura N, Yamaguchi H, Fukuyama T: Direct enantiomeric separation of racemic precursors to diltiazem hydrochloride and clentiazem maleate by HPLC on a chiral ovomucoid column. Chromatographia 35:5, 1993.
26. Chaudhary RS, Gangwal SS, Avachat MK, et al: Determination of diltiazem hydrochloride in human serum by high-performance liquid chromatography. J Chromatogr Biomed Appl 614:261, 1993.
27. Zoest AR, Hung CT, Wanwimolruk S: Diltiazem: A sensitive HPLC assay and application to pharmacokinetic study. J Liq Chromatogr 15:1277, 1992.
28. Miyazaki M, Iwakuma T, Tanaka T: Synthesis of the metabolites and related compounds of diltiazem. Chem Pharm Bull 26:2889, 1978.
29. Sugihara J, Sugawara Y, Ando H, et al: Studies on the metabolism of diltiazem in man. J Pharmacobiodyn 7:24, 1984.
30. Yabana H, Nagao T, Sato M: Cardiovascular effects of the metabolites of diltiazem in dogs. J Cardiovasc Pharmacol 7:152, 1985.
31. Wiens RE, Runser DJ, Lacz JP, et al: Quantitation of diltiazem and desacetyldiltiazem in dog plasma by high-performance liquid chromatography. J Pharm Sci 73:688, 1984.
32. Yeung PKF, Montague TJ, Tsui B, McGregor C: High-performance liquid chromatographic assay of diltiazem and six of its metabolites in plasma: Application to a pharmacokinetic study in healthy volunteers. J Pharm Sci 78:592, 1989.
33. Delwar-Hussain M, Tam YK, Finegan BA, Coutts RT: Simple and sensitive high-performance liquid chromatographic method for the determination of diltiazem and six of its metabolites in human plasma. J Chromatogr Biomed Appl 582:1, 1992.
34. Bonnefous JL, Boulieu R, Lahet C: Stability of diltiazem and its metabolites in human blood samples. J Pharm Sci 81:341, 1992.
35. Caille G, Dube LM, Theoret Y, et al: Stability study of diltiazem and two of its metabolites using a high performance liquid chromatographic method. Biopharm Drug Dispos 10:107, 1989.
36. Yeung PKF, Mosher SJ, Klassen GA, McGilveray IJ: Stability of diltiazem and its metabolites in plasma during storage. Ther Drug Monit 13:369, 1991.
37. Ochs HR, Knuchel M: Pharmacokinetics and absolute bioavailability of diltiazem in humans. Klin Wochenschr 62:303, 1984.
38. Pichard L, Gillet G, Fabre I, et al: Identification of the rabbit and human cytochromes P-450IIIA as the major enzymes involved in the N-demethylation of diltiazem. Drug Metab Dispos 18:711, 1990.
39. Tsao SC, Dickinson TH, Abernethy DR: Metabolite inhibition of parent drug biotransformation. Studies of diltiazem. Drug Metab Dispos 18:180, 1990.
40. Rovei V, Gomeni R, Mitchard M, et al: Pharmacokinetics and metabolism of diltiazem in man. Acta Cardiol 35:35, 1980.
41. Montamat SC, Abernethy DR: N-monodesmethyldiltiazem is the predominant metabolite of diltiazem in the plasma of young and elderly hypertensives. Br J Clin Pharmacol 24:185, 1987.
42. Hermann P, Rodger SD, Remones G, et al: Pharmacokinetics of diltiazem after intravenous and oral administration. Eur J Clin Pharmacol 24:349, 1983.
43. Zelis RF, Kinney EL: The pharmacokinetics of diltiazem in healthy American men. Am J Cardiol 49:529, 1982.

44. Piepho RW, Bloedow DC, Lacz JP, et al: Pharmacokinetics of diltiazem in selected animal species and human beings. Am J Cardiol 49:525, 1982.

45. McClelland GA, Sutton SC, Engle K, Zentner GM: The solubility-modulated osmotic pump: In vitro/in vivo release of diltiazem hydrochloride. Pharm Res 8:88, 1991.

46. Murata K, Yamahara H, Kobayashi M, et al: Pharmacokinetics of an oral sustained-release diltiazem preparation. J Pharm Sci 78:960, 1989.

47. Wilding IR, Hardy JG, Maccari M, et al: Scintigraphic and pharmacokinetic assessment of a multiparticulate sustained release formulation of diltiazem. Int J Pharm 76:1, 1991.

48. Thiercelin JF, Necciari J, Caplain H, et al: Development and pharmacokinetics of a new sustained-release formulation of diltiazem. J Cardiovasc Pharmacol 16(Suppl 1):S31, 1990.

49. Ziemniak J, Colligon I, Head D: Steady-state dose proportionality of a once-a-day sustained-release diltiazem hydrochloride formulation in healthy subjects. Clin Ther 14:158, 1992.

50. Kelly JG, Devane JG, Geoghegan B: Pharmacokinetic properties and antihypertensive efficacy of once-daily diltiazem. J Cardiovasc Pharmacol 17:957, 1991.

51. Christrup LL, Bonde J, Rasmussen SN, et al: Single-dose and steady-state pharmacokinetics of diltiazem administered in two different tablet formulations. Pharmacol Toxicol 71:305, 1992.

52. De Bernardis E, Candido P, Lorefice R, et al: Comparative bioavailability of two tablet preparations of diltiazem in healthy volunteers. Arzneimittelforschung/Drug Res 42:25, 1992.

53. Joshi MV, Gokhale PC, Pohujani SM, et al: Bioinequivalence of marketed diltiazem preparations. Eur J Clin Pharmacol 39:189, 1990.

54. Kinney EL, Maskowitz RM, Zelis R: The pharmacokinetics and pharmacology of oral diltiazem in normal volunteers. J Clin Pharmacol 21:337, 1981.

55. Mitchard M, Durand A, Gomeni R, et al: Pharmacokinetics and metabolism of diltiazem in man (observations on healthy volunteers and angina pectoris patients). In Bing RJ (ed): New Drug Therapy with a Calcium Antagonist: Diltiazem. Hakone Symposium 1978. Amsterdam: Excerpta Medica, 1979, pp 152–167.

56. DuSouich P, Lery N, Lery L, et al: Influence of food on the bioavailability of diltiazem and two of its metabolites following the administration of conventional tablets and slow-release capsules. Biopharm Drug Dispos 11:137, 1990.

57. Hoglund P, Nilsson LG: Pharmacokinetics of diltiazem and its metabolites after single and multiple dosing in healthy volunteers. Ther Drug Monit 11:558, 1989.

58. Bianchetti G, Regazzi M, Rondanelli R, et al: Bioavailability of diltiazem as a function of the administered dose. Biopharm Drug Dispos 12:391, 1991.

59. Hoglund P, Nilsson LG: Pharmacokinetics of diltiazem and its metabolites after repeated multiple-dose treatments in healthy volunteers. Ther Drug Monit 11:543, 1989.

60. Hoglund P, Nilsson LG: Pharmacokinetics of diltiazem and its metabolites after repeated single dosing in healthy volunteers. Ther Drug Monit 11:551, 1989.

61. Weiner DA, Cutler SS, Klein MD: Efficacy and safety of sustained-release diltiazem in stable angina pectoris. Am J Cardiol 57:6, 1986.

62. Bloedow DC, Piepho RW, Nies AS, et al: Serum binding of diltiazem in humans. J Clin Pharmacol 22:201, 1982.

63. Mungall DR, Ludden TM, Hawkins DW, et al: Effect of diltiazem on warfarin plasma protein binding. J Clin Pharmacol 24:264, 1984.

64. Pieper JA: Diltiazem binding to human serum proteins [abstract 1-B]. Clin Pharmacol Ther 35:266, 1984.

65. Abernethy DR, Kaminsky LS, Dickinson TH: Selective inhibition of warfarin metabolism by diltiazem in humans. J Pharmacol Exp Ther 257:411, 1991.

66. Kwong TC, Sparks JD, Sparkd CE: Lipoprotein and protein binding of the calcium channel blocker diltiazem. Proc Soc Exp Biol Med 178:313, 1985.

67. Pieper JA: Diltiazem serum protein binding: Relationship to alpha 1 acid glycoprotein. Biopharm Pharmacokinet Eur Congr 2:360, 1984.

68. Kapur PA, Grogan DL, Fournier DJ: Cardiovascular interactions of lidocaine with verapamil or diltiazem in the dog. Anesthesiology 68:79, 1988.

69. Belpaire FM, Bogaert MG: Binding of diltiazem to albumin, alpha-1-acid glycoprotein and to serum in man. J Clin Pharmacol 30:311, 1990.

70. Nattel S, Talajic M, Goldstein RE, McCans J: Determinants and significance of diltiazem plasma concentrations after acute myocardial infarction. Am J Cardiol 66:1422, 1990.

71. Finegan BA, Hussain MD, Tam YK: Pharmacokinetics of diltiazem in patients undergoing coronary artery bypass grafting. Ther Drug Monit 14:485, 1992.

72. Capparelli EV, Zhao H, Hanyok JJ, et al: The effect of CPR on plasma diltiazem concentrations in dogs. Ann Emerg Med 20:1078, 1991.

73. Storstein L, Larsen A, Midtbo K, et al: Pharmacokinetics of calcium blockers in patients with renal insufficiency and in geriatric patients. Acta Med Scand 681:25, 1984.

74. Ellenbogen KA, Roark SF, Smith MS, et al: Effects of sustained intravenous diltiazem infusion in healthy persons. Am J Cardiol 58:1055, 1986.

75. Joyal M, Pieper J, Cremer K, et al: Pharmacodynamic aspects of intravenous diltiazem administration. Am Heart J 111:54, 1986.

76. Clozel JP, Billette J, Caille G, et al: Effects of diltiazem on atrioventricular conduction and arterial blood pressure: Correlation with plasma drug concentrations. Can J Physiol Pharmacol 62:1479, 1984.

77. Pozet N, Brazier JL, Hadj AA, et al: Pharmacokinetics of diltiazem in severe renal failure. Eur J Clin Pharmacol 24:635, 1983.

78. Grech-Belanger O, Langlois S, LeBoeuf E: Pharmacokinetics of diltiazem in patients undergoing continuous ambulatory peritoneal dialysis. J Clin Pharmacol 28:477, 1988.

79. Tawashi M, Marc-Aurele J, Bichet D, et al: Pharmacokinetics of oral diltiazem and five of its metabolites in patients with chronic renal failure. Biopharm Drug Dispos 12:95, 1991.

80. Tawashi M, Marc-Aurele J, Bichet D, et al: Pharmacokinetics of intravenous diltiazem and five of its metabolites in patients with chronic renal failure and in healthy volunteers. Biopharm Drug Dispos 12:105, 1991.

81. Hunt BA, Self TH, Lalonde RL, Bottorff MB: Calcium blockers as inhibitors of drug metabolism. Chest 96:393, 1989.

82. Bauer LA, Stenwall M, Horn JR, et al: Changes in antipyrine and indocyanine green kinetics during nifedipine, verapamil, and diltiazem therapy. Clin Pharmacol Ther 40:239, 1986.

83. Tateishi T, Nakashima H, Shitou T, et al: Effect of diltiazem on the pharmacokinetics of propranolol, metoprolol and atenolol. Eur J Clin Pharmacol 36:67, 1989.

84. Tateishi T, Ohashi K, Fujimura A, Ebihara A: The influence of diltiazem versus cimetidine on propranolol metabolism. J Clin Pharmacol 32:1099, 1992.

85. Etoh A, Yamakita H, Kohno K, et al: Studies on the drug interaction of diltiazem. III. Mechanism of the absorption enhancing effect of diltiazem on the co-administered propranolol [Japanese]. Yakugaku Zasshi 103:581, 1983.

86. Etoh A, Kohno K: Studies on the drug interaction of diltiazem. I. Effects of co-administered drugs and dosing conditions on the bioavailability of diltiazem. Yakugaku Zasshi 103:426, 1983.

87. Etoh A, Kohno K, Shimizu T: Studies on the drug interaction of diltiazem. II. Effect of co-administered diltiazem on the bioavailability of propranolol. Yakugaku Zasshi 103:434, 1983.

88. Maskasame C, Lankford SM, Bai SA: Effects of propranolol on the disposition and negative dromotropic activity of diltiazem in the dog during multiple dosing. Drug Metab Dispos 21:156, 1993.

89. Dimmitt DC, Yu DK, Elvin AT, Giesing DH: Pharmacokinetics of diltiazem and propranolol when administered alone and in combination. Biopharm Drug Dispos 12:515, 1991.

90. Etoh A, Kohno K: Studies on the drug interaction of diltiazem. IV. Relationship between first pass metabolism of various drugs and the absorption enhancing effect of diltiazem. Yakugaku Zasshi 103:581, 1983.

91. Ihara N, Kokufu T, Sugioka N, et al: Inhibitory effect of

diltiazem on diazepam metabolism in the mouse hepatic microsomes. Biol Pharm Bull 16:331, 1993.

92. Maskasame C, Lankford S, Bai SA: The effects of chronic oral diltiazem and cimetidine dosing on the pharmacokinetics and negative dromotropic action of intravenous and oral diltiazem in the dog. Biopharm Drug Dispos 13:521, 1992.

93. Ohashi K, Tateishi T, Sudo T, et al: Effects of diltiazem on the pharmacokinetics of nifedipine. J Cardiovasc Pharmacol 15:96, 1990.

94. Ohashi K, Sudo T, Sakamoto K, et al: The influence of pretreatment periods with diltiazem on nifedipine kinetics. J Clin Pharmacol 33:222, 1993.

95. Tateishi T, Ohashi K, Sudo T, et al: Dose dependent effect of diltiazem on the pharmacokinetics of nifedipine. J Clin Pharmacol 29:994, 1989.

96. Al-Humayyd MS: Elevation of carbamazepine plasma levels by diltiazem in rabbits: A potentially important drug interaction. Biopharm Drug Dispos 11:411, 1990.

97. Ahmad S: Diltiazem-carbamazepine interaction. Am Heart J 120:1485, 1990.

98. Gadde K, Calabrese JR: Diltiazem effect on carbamazepine levels in manic depression. J Clin Psychopharmacol 10:378, 1990.

99. Shaughnessy AF, Mosley MR: Elevated carbamazepine levels associated with diltiazem use. Neurology 42:937, 1992.

100. Maoz E, Grossman E, Thaler M, Rosenthal T: Carbamazepine neurotoxic reaction after administration of diltiazem. Arch Intern Med 152:2503, 1992.

101. David JB, Bialer M: Pharmacokinetic interaction between diltiazem and amiodarone in the dog. Biopharm Drug Dispos 10:423, 1989.

102. Gomez A, Martos F, Garcia R, et al: Diltiazem enhances gentamicin nephrotoxicity in rats. Pharmacol Toxicol 64:190, 1989.

103. Renton KW: Inhibition of hepatic microsomal drug metabolism by the calcium channel blockers diltiazem and verapamil. Biochem Pharmacol 34:2549, 1985.

104. Abernethy DR, Egan JM, Carrum G: Calcium antagonists inhibit oxidative drug biotransformation [abstract]. Clin Res 34:394A, 1986.

105. Carrum G, Egan JM, Abernethy DR: Diltiazem treatment impairs hepatic drug oxidation: Studies of antipyrine. Clin Pharmacol Ther 40:140, 1986.

106. Rocci M Jr, Vlasses PH, Lener ME, et al: Comparative evaluation of the effects of labetalol, verapamil and diltiazem on antipyrine and indocyanine green clearances. J Clin Pharmacol 29:891, 1989.

107. Klockowski PM, Lener ME, Sirgo MA, Rocci M Jr: Comparative evaluation of the effects of isradipine and diltiazem on antipyrine and indocyanine green clearances in elderly volunteers. Clin Pharmacol Ther 48:375, 1990.

108. Sakai H, Kobayashi S, Hamada K, et al: The effects of diltiazem on hepatic drug metabolizing enzymes in man using antipyrine, trimethadione and dibrisoquine as model substrates. Br J Clin Pharmacol 31:353, 1991.

109. Christopher MA, Harman E, Hendeles L: Clinical relevance of the interaction of theophylline with diltiazem or nifedipine. Chest 95:309, 1989.

110. Smith SR, Haffner CA, Kendall MJ: The influence of nifedipine and diltiazem on serum theophylline concentration-time profiles. J Clin Pharm Ther 14:403, 1989.

111. Nafziger AN, May JJ, Bertino JS Jr: Inhibition of theophylline elimination by diltiazem therapy. J Clin Pharmacol 27:862, 1987.

112. North DS, Mattern AL, Hiser WW: The influence of diltiazem hydrochloride on trough serum digoxin concentrations. Drug Intell Clin Pharm 20:500, 1986.

113. Sakai M, Ueda K, Takahashi T, et al: Comparison of the effects nifedipine and diltiazem have on serum digoxin concentration [Japanese]. Yakuri To Chiryo 11:318, 1983.

114. Rameis H, Magometschnigg D, Ganzinger U: The diltiazem-digoxin interaction. Clin Pharmacol Ther 36:183, 1984.

115. Oyama Y, Fujii S, Kanda K, et al: Digoxin-diltiazem interaction. Am J Cardiol 53:1480, 1984.

116. Fujii S, Akino E, Kimura T, et al: Diltiazem-digoxin interaction [abstract]. Jpn Circ J 47:877, 1983.

117. Gallet M, Aupetit JF, Lopez M, et al: Diltiazem and digoxin interaction: Development of digoxin plasma levels and electrocardiographic parameters in healthy subjects [French]. Arch Mal Coeur 79:1216, 1986.

118. Thiercelin JF, Hermann P, Warrington JP, et al: Interaction study between digoxin and calcium antagonists: Verapamil and diltiazem [abstract]. In World Conference on Clinical Pharmacology and Therapeutics. Washington, DC: 1983, p 47.

119. Elkayam U, Parikh K, Torkan B, et al: Effect of diltiazem on renal clearance and serum concentration of digoxin in patients with cardiac disease. Am J Cardiol 55:1393, 1985.

120. Pfeiffer VG: Glwichzeitige gabe von digoxin und diltiazem bei patienten mit herzinsuffizienz und koronarer herzerkrankung. Fortschr Med 103:699, 1985.

121. Boden WE, More G, Sharma S, et al: No increase in serum digoxin concentration with high-dose diltiazem. Am J Med 81:425, 1986.

122. Jones WN, Kern KB, Rindone JP, et al: Digoxin-diltiazem interaction: A pharmacokinetic evaluation. Eur J Clin Pharmacol 31:351, 1986.

123. Yoshida A, Fujita M, Kurosawa N, et al: Effects of diltiazem on plasma level and urinary excretion of digoxin in healthy subjects. Clin Pharmacol Ther 35:681, 1984.

124. Andrejak M, Hary L, Andrejak MT, Lesbre JPH: Diltiazem increases steady state digoxin serum levels in patients with cardiac disease. J Clin Pharmacol 27:967, 1987.

125. Kuhlmann J: Effects of nifedipine and diltiazem on plasma levels and renal excretion of beta-acetyldigoxin. Clin Pharmacol Ther 37:150, 1985.

126. Kuhlmann J: Effects of verapamil, diltiazem, and nifedipine on plasma levels and renal excretion of digitoxin. Clin Pharmacol Ther 38:667, 1985.

127. Watford WH, Walsh RA, O'Rourke RA: Diltiazem attenuates the inotropic and peripheral vascular effects of cardiac glycosides. Am Heart J 118:738, 1989.

128. Ratz PH, Flaim SF: Acetylcholine- and 5-hydroxytryptamine-stimulated contraction and calcium uptake in bovine coronary arteries: Evidence for two populations of receptor-operated channels. J Pharmacol Exp Ther 234:641, 1985.

129. Nayler WG, Dillon JS: Calcium antagonists and their mode of action: An historical overview. Br J Clin Pharmacol 21:97S, 1986.

130. Rimele TJ, Vanhoutte PM: Differential effects of calcium entry blockers on vascular smooth muscle. Int Angiol 3(Suppl):17, 1984.

131. Sperelakis N: Cyclic AMP and phosphorylation in regulation of Ca++ influx into myocardial cells and blockade by calcium antagonistic drugs. Am Heart J 107:347, 1984.

132. Schwartz A, Triggle DJ: Cellular action of calcium channel blocking drugs. Annu Rev Med 35:325, 1984.

133. Nayler WG: The heterogeneity of the slow channel blockers (calcium antagonists). Int J Cardiol 3:391, 1983.

134. Hirano K, Kanaide H, Abe S, Nakamura M: Effects of diltiazem on calcium concentrations in the cytosol and on force of contractions in porcine coronary arterial strips. Br J Pharmacol 101:273, 1990.

135. van Breemen C, Hwang O, Meisheri KD: The mechanism of inhibitory action of diltiazem on vascular smooth muscle contractility. J Pharmacol Exp Ther 218:459, 1981.

136. Ferry DR, Goll A, Gadow C, Glossmann H: (-)-3H-desmethoxyverapamil labelling of putative calcium channels in brain: Autoradiographic distribution and allosteric coupling to 1,4-dihydropyridine and diltiazem binding sites. Naunyn Schmiedebergs Arch Pharmacol 372:183, 1984.

137. Glossmann H, Ferry DR, Goll A, et al: Calcium channels: Basic properties as revealed by radioligand binding studies. J Cardiovasc Pharmacol 7:S20, 1985.

138. Glossmann H, Ferry DR, Goll A, Linn T: Molecular approach to the calcium channel. Adv Myocardiol 5:41, 1985.

139. Ferry DR, Glossmann H: Identification of putative calcium channels in skeletal muscle microsomes. FEBS Lett 148:331, 1982.

140. Balwierczak JL, Grupp IL, Grupp G, et al: Effects of bepridil and diltiazem on [3H]nitrendipine binding to canine cardiac sarcolemma. Potentiation of pharmacological effects of nitrendipine by bepridil. J Pharmacol Exp Ther 237:40, 1986.

141. Murphy K, Gould RJ, Largent BL, et al: A unitary mechanism of calcium antagonist drug action. Proc Natl Acad Sci U S A 80:860, 1983.
142. Yamamura HI, Schoemaker H, Boles RG, et al: Diltiazem enhancement of [3H]nitrendipine binding to calcium channel associated drug receptor sites in rat brain synaptosomes. Biochem Biophys Res Commun 108:640, 1982.
143. Ishii K, Taira N, Yanagisawa T: Differential antagonism by Bay k 8644, a dihydropyridine calcium agonist, of the negative inotropic effects of nifedipine, verapamil, diltiazem and manganese ions in canine ventricular muscle. Br J Pharmacol 84:577, 1985.
144. Miwa N, Kanaide H, Nishimura J, Nakamura M: Binding of [(3)H]-nitrendipine and [(3)H]-diltiazem to rat myocardial sarcolemma. Arzneimittelforschung/Drug Res 36:1059, 1986.
145. DePover A, Grupp IL, Grupp G, et al: Diltiazem potentiates the negative inotropic action of nimodipine in heart. Biochem Biophys Res Commun 114:922, 1983.
146. Garcia ML, King VF, Siegl P, et al: Binding of Ca++ entry blockers to cardiac sarcolemmal membrane vesicles. Characterization of diltiazem sites and their interaction with dihydropyridine and aralkylamine receptors. J Biol Chem 261:8146, 1986.
147. Ikeda S, Oka JI, Nagao T: Effects of four diltiazem stereoisomers on binding of d-cis-[(3)H]diltiazem and (+)-[(3)H]PN200-110 to rabbit T-tubule calcium channels. Eur J Pharmacol Mol Pharmacol 208:199, 1991.
148. Millard RW, Grupp G, Grupp IL, et al: Chronotropic, inotropic, and vasodilator actions of diltiazem, nifedipine, and verapamil. A comparative study of physiological responses and membrane receptor activity. Circ Res 52:I-29, 1983.
149. Perez JE, Borda L, Schuchleib R, et al: Inotropic and chronotropic effects of vasodilators. J Pharmacol Exp Ther 221:609, 1982.
150. Katz AM, Hager WD, Messineo FC, et al: Cellular actions and pharmacology of the calcium channel blocking drugs. Am J Med 77:2, 1984.
151. Lathrop DA, Valle-Aguilera JR, Millard RW, et al: Comparative electrophysiologic and coronary hemodynamic effects of diltiazem, nisoldipine and verapamil on myocardial tissue. Am J Cardiol 49:613, 1982.
152. Flaim SF, Irwin JM: Diltiazem, nifedipine, and verapamil: Evidence for dissimilar mechanisms of action in vascular smooth muscle (VSM) [abstract]. Fed Proc 40:624, 1981.
153. Bristow MR, Ginsburg R, Laser JA, et al: Tissue response selectivity of calcium antagonists is not due to heterogeneity of (3H)-nitrendipine binding sites. Br J Pharmacol 82:309, 1984.
154. Haynes LW: Block of the cyclic GMP-gated channel of vertebrate rod and cone photoreceptors by l-cis-diltiazem. J Gen Physiol 100:783, 1992.
155. Adachi-Akahane S, Amano Y, Okuyama R, Nagao T: Quaternary diltiazem can act from both sides of the membrane in ventricular myocytes. Jpn J Pharmacol 61:263, 1993.
156. Ananthanarayanan VS, Tetreault S, Saint-Jean A: Interaction of calcium channel antagonists with calcium: Spectroscopic and modeling studies on diltiazem and its Ca(2+) complex. J Med Chem 36:1324, 1993.
157. Felix JP, King VF, Shevell JL, et al: Bis(benzylisoquinoline) analogs of tetrandrine block L-type calcium channels: Evidence for interaction at the diltiazem-binding site. Biochemistry 31:11793, 1992.
158. Palfreyman MG, Dudley MW, Cheng HC, et al: Lactamides: A novel chemical class of calcium antagonists with diltiazem-like properties. Biochem Pharmacol 38:2459, 1989.
159. Takeo S, Elimban V, Dhalla NS: Modification of cardiac sarcolemmal Na+/Ca++ exchange by diltiazem and verapamil. Can J Cardiol 1:131, 1985.
160. Lee KS, Tsien RW: Mechanism of calcium channel blockade by verapamil, D600, diltiazem and nitrendipine in single dialysed heart cells. Nature 302:790, 1983.
161. Hirth C, Borchard U, Hafner D: Effects of the calcium antagonist diltiazem on action potentials, slow response and force of contraction in different cardiac tissues. J Mol Cell Cardiol 15:799, 1983.
162. Zahradnikova A, Zahradnik I: Interaction of diltiazem with single L-type calcium channels in guinea-pig ventricular myocytes. Gen Physiol Biophys 11:535, 1992.
163. Kanaya S, Arlock P, Katzung BG, et al: Diltiazem and verapamil preferentially block inactivated cardiac calcium channels. J Mol Cell Cardiol 15:145, 1983.
164. Lopez MG, Moro MA, Castillo CF, et al: Variable, voltage-dependent, blocking effects of nitrendipine, verapamil, diltiazem, cinnarizine and cadmium on adrenomedullary secretion. Br J Pharmacol 96:725, 1989.
165. Pang DC, Sperelakis N: Uptake of calcium antagonistic drugs into muscles as related to their lipid solubilities. Biochem Pharmacol 33:821, 1984.
166. Saida K, Van BC: Inhibiting effect of diltiazem on intracellular Ca++ release in vascular smooth muscle. Blood Vessels 20:105, 1983.
167. Asayama J, Tatsumi T, Miyazaki H, et al: Effect of diltiazem on spontaneous cyclic Ca(2+) release from sarcoplasmic reticulum. Eur J Pharmacol 175:309, 1990.
168. Vaghy PL, Johnson JD, Matlib MA, et al: Selective inhibition of Na+-induced Ca++ release from sarcoplasmic reticulum. Eur J Pharmacol 175:309, 1983.
169. Matlib MA, Schwartz A: Selective effects of diltiazem, a benzothiazepine calcium channel blocker, and diazepam, and other benzodiazepines on the Na+/Ca++ exchange carrier system of heart and brain mitochondria. Life Sci 32:2837, 1983.
170. Younes A, Schneider JM: Effects of bepridil on Ca2+ uptake by cardiac mitochondria. Biochem Pharmacol 33:1363, 1984.
171. Wang T, Tsai LI, Schwartz A: Effects of verapamil, diltiazem, nisoldipine and felodipine on sarcoplasmic reticulum. Eur J Pharmacol 100:253, 1984.
172. Raddino R, Poli E, Manca C, et al: Differenti siti di azione del diltiazem, nifedipina e verapamil sul miocardio e sulla muscolatura liscia aortica e coronarica. Cardiologia 31:47, 1986.
173. Khalil-Manesh F, Venkataraman K, Samant DR, Gadgil UG: Effects of diltiazem on cation transport across erythrocyte membranes of hypertensive humans. Hypertension 9:18, 1987.
174. Rosales C, Brown EJ: Calcium channel blockers nifedipine and diltiazem inhibit Ca(2+) release from intracellular stores in neutrophils. J Biol Chem 267:1443, 1992.
175. Etoh H, Tanaka T, Mitani Y, et al: The binding of the calcium channel blocker, bepridil, to calmodulin. Biochem Pharmacol 35:217, 1986.
176. Johnson JD, Vaghy PL, Crouch TH, et al: An hypothesis for the mechanism of action of some of the Ca++ antagonist drugs: Calmodulin as a receptor. In Yoshida H, Hagihara Y, Ebashi S (eds): Advances in Pharmacology and Therapeutics, Proceedings of the Eighth International Congress of Pharmacology, Tokyo, Vol 3. Oxford: Pergamon Press, 1982, pp 121–138.
177. Silver PJ, Dachiw J, Ambrose JM: Effects of calcium antagonists and vasodilators on arterial myosin phosphorylation and actin-myosin interactions. J Pharmacol Exp Ther 230:141, 1984.
178. Maruyama Y, Okayama H, Ishide N, et al: Effects of Ca antagonist on the contractile force in glycerinated dog heart muscles. Pflugers Arch 395:49, 1982.
179. Morad M, Tung L, Greenspan AM: Effect of diltiazem on calcium transport and development of tension in heart muscle. Am J Cardiol 49:595, 1982.
180. Kawagoe R, Mino H, Takeuchi A: Effects of organic CA antagonist, diltiazem, on neuromuscular transmission. Jpn J Physiol 40:325, 1990.
181. Flaim SF, Flaim KE, Zelis R: Diltiazem: Lack of myocardial beta-adrenergic receptor-binding capacity. Pharmacology 21:306, 1980.
182. Briley M, Cavero I, Langer SZ, et al: Evidence against beta-adrenoceptor blocking activity of diltiazem, a drug with calcium antagonist properties. Br J Pharmacol 69:669, 1980.
183. Tsuda K, Haneda T, Uejima K, et al: Effects of Ca-antagonists in noradrenaline release from sympathetic nerve endings [Japanese]. Yakuri To Chiryo 11:315, 1983.
184. Zelis R, Wichmann T, Starke K: Inhibition by diltiazem of norepinephrine release from sympathetic nerves in the rabbit pulmonary artery. Pharmacology 31:268, 1985.
185. Wolchinsky C, Zsoter TT: The effect of diltiazem on noradrenaline release. Br J Pharmacol 85:387, 1985.

186. Zsoter TT, Wolchinsky C: Effects of calcium antagonists on sympathetic nerve activity. Can J Cardiol 2:256, 1986.

187. Nayler WG, Thompson JE, Jarrott B: The interaction of calcium antagonists (slow channel blockers) with myocardial alpha adrenoceptors. J Mol Cell Cardiol 14:185, 1982.

188. Motulsky HJ, Snavely MD, Hughes RJ, et al: Interaction of verapamil and other calcium channel blockers with alpha-1 and alpha-2-adrenergic receptors. Circ Res 52:226, 1983.

189. Hicks PE, Tierney C, Langer SZ: Preferential antagonism by diltiazem of alpha-2-adrenoceptor mediated vasoconstrictor responses in perfused tail arteries of spontaneous hypertensive rats. Naunyn Schmiedebergs Arch Pharmacol 328:388, 1985.

190. van Zwieten PA, van Meel JCA, Timmermans PBMWM: Calcium antagonists and alpha-2-adrenoceptors: Possible role of extracellular calcium ions in alpha-2-adrenoceptor-mediated vasoconstriction. J Cardiovasc Pharmacol 4(Suppl 3):S273, 1982.

191. Timmermans PBMWM, van Meel JCA, van Zwieten PA: Calcium antagonists and alpha-receptors. Eur Heart J 4:11, 1983.

192. Langer SZ, Galzin AM: Effects of diltiazem and verapamil on presynaptic and postsynaptic actions mediated by alpha-1 and alpha-2-adrenoceptors. In Fleckenstein A, Hashimoto K, Herrmann M, et al (eds): New Calcium Antagonists: Recent Developments and Prospects, Diltiazem Workshop, Freiburg, Breisgau, May 1982. Stuttgart, Germany: Gustav Fisher, 1982, pp 131–136.

193. Cavero I, Shepperson N, Lefevre-Borg F, Langer SZ: Differential inhibition of vascular smooth muscle responses to alpha-1- and alpha-2-adrenoceptor agonists by diltiazem and verapamil. Circulation Res 52(Suppl I):69, 1983.

194. Galzin AM, Langer SZ: Presynaptic alpha-2-adrenoceptor antagonism by verapamil but not by diltiazem in rabbit hypothalamic slices. Br J Pharmacol 78:571, 1983.

195. Kappagoda T, Jayakody L, Senaratne M: The effect of diltiazem (dilt) and nicardipine (nic) on the contractile responses to alpha agonists in canine saphenous veins (csv) [abstract 7185]. Fed Proc 44:1639, 1985.

196. Toda N: Alpha-adrenoceptor subtypes and diltiazem actions in isolated human coronary arteries. Am J Physiol 250:H7118, 1986.

197. Rimele TJ, Rooke TW, Aarhus LL, et al: Alpha-1 adrenoceptors and calcium in isolated canine coronary arteries. J Pharmacol Exp Ther 226:668, 1983.

198. Ruffolo RR, Morgan EL, Messick K: Possible relationship between receptor reserve and the differential antagonism of alpha-1 and alpha-2 adrenoceptor-mediated pressor responses by calcium channel antagonists in the pithed rat. J Pharmacol Exp Ther 230:587, 1984.

199. Eskinder H, Gross GJ: Differential inhibition of alpha-1 vs. alpha-2 adrenoceptor-mediated responses in canine saphenous vein by nitroglycerin. J Pharmacol Exp Ther 238:515, 1986.

200. Wanstall JC, O'Donnell SR: Inhibition of norepinephrine contractions by diltiazem on aorta and pulmonary artery from young and aged rats: Influence of alpha-adrenoceptor reserve. J Pharmacol Exp Ther 245:1016, 1988.

201. Ekelund LG: Calcium channel blockade. Central hemodynamic effects. Acta Pharmacol Toxicol (Copenh) 58:59, 1986.

202. Hof RP: Patterns of regional blood flow changes induced by five different calcium antagonists. Prog Pharmacol 5:71, 1983.

203. Hof RP: Calcium antagonist and the peripheral circulation: Differences and similarities between PY 108-068, nicardipine, verapamil and diltiazem. Br J Pharmacol 78:375, 1983.

204. Kjellstedt A, Oreback B, Ljung B: Vascular and myocardial inhibition by felodipine, diltiazem and verapamil as related to drug concentration and time of exposure. Acta Physiol Scand 124:328, 1985.

205. Sharif MN, Kaushal RD, Iyer P, Wilson TW: Diltiazem potentiates angiotensin II-mediated renal prostacyclin synthesis. J Cardiovasc Pharmacol 20:638, 1992.

206. Pedrinelli R, Panarace G, Salvetti A: Calcium entry blockade and adrenergic vascular reactivity in hypertensives: Differences between nicardipine and diltiazem. Clin Pharmacol Ther 49:86, 1991.

207. Giudicelli JF, Berdeaux A, Edouard A, et al: Attenuation by diltiazem of arterial baroreflex sensitivity in man. Eur J Clin Pharmacol 26:675, 1984.

208. Kunze DL, Andersen MC, Torres LA: Do calcium antagonists act directly on calcium channels to alter baroreceptor function? J Pharmacol Exp Ther 239:303, 1986.

209. Abdel-Rahman AR, Ingenito AJ: Similarities and differences in the effects of verapamil, diltiazem and nifedipine on arterial baroreflexes of anesthetized cats. Arch Int Pharmacodyn Ther 275:33, 1985.

210. Kawashima S, Kogame T, Tateishi J, Iwasaki T: Baroreceptor reflex to neck suction and its modification by diltiazem in man. Jpn Heart J 30:343, 1989.

211. Henry PD: Comparative pharmacology of calcium antagonists: Nifedipine, verapamil and diltiazem. Am J Cardiol 46:1047, 1980.

212. Horowitz JD, Barry WH, Smith TW: Comparison of negative inotropic potency and reversibility of effects of six calcium channel blocker drugs in cultured myocardial cells. Circulation 66:II-139, 1982.

213. Schwinger RHG, Bohm M, Erdmann E: Negative inotropic properties of isradipine, nifedipine, diltiazem, and verapamil in diseased human myocardial tissue. J Cardiovasc Pharmacol 15:892, 1990.

214. Wiesfeld ACP, Remme WJ, Look MP, et al: Acute hemodynamic and electrophysiologic effects and safety of high-dose intravenous diltiazem in patients receiving metoprolol. Am J Cardiol 70:997, 1992.

215. Wong SS, Myerburg RJ, Ezrin AM, et al: Diltiazem and contraction in cat ventricular muscle during experimentally induced right ventricular systolic hypertension. Arch Int Pharmacodyn Ther 256:76, 1982.

216. Walsh RA, Badke FR, O'Rourke RA: Differential effects of systemic and intracoronary calcium channel blocking agents on global and regional left ventricular function in conscious dogs. Am Heart J 102:341, 1981.

217. Nakaya H, Schwartz A, Millard RW: Reflex chronotropic and inotropic effects of calcium channel-blocking agents in conscious dogs. Diltiazem, verapamil, and nifedipine compared. Circ Res 52:302, 1983.

218. Figulla HR, Kreuzer H, Luig H: Verapamil, diltiazem oder nifedipin bei schwerer linksventrikularer funktionsstorung? Eine vergleichsstudie der hamodynamischen akutwirkungen. Dtsch Med Wochenschr 111:11, 1986.

219. Maurer E, Nicoletti R, Brandt D, et al: Effect of calcium antagonists on cardiac performance in patients with dilatative cardiomyopathy evaluated by noninvasive methods. Clin Cardiol 6:399, 1983.

220. Packer M, Lee WH, Medina N, et al: Comparative negative inotropic effects of nifedipine and diltiazem in patients with severe left ventricular dysfunction [abstract 1099]. Circulation 72:III-275, 1985.

221. Materne P, Legrand V, Vandormael M, et al: Hemodynamic effects of intravenous diltiazem with impaired left ventricular function. Am J Cardiol 54:733, 1984.

222. Oesterle SN, Alderman EL, Beier SL, et al: Diltiazem and propranolol in combination: Hemodynamic effects following acute intravenous administration. Am Heart J 111:489, 1986.

223. Di Donato M, Maioli M, Marchionni N, et al: Effects of diltiazem on postextrasystolic potentiation in coronary heart disease patients. Eur Heart J 11:656, 1990.

224. Dash H, Copenhaver GL, Ensminger S: Improvement in regional wall motion and left ventricular relaxation after administration of diltiazem in patients with coronary artery disease. Circulation 72:353, 1985.

225. Urquhart J, Epstein SE, Patterson RE: Comparative effects of calcium-channel blocking agents on left ventricular function during acute ischemia in dogs with and without congestive heart failure. Am J Cardiol 55:10B, 1985.

226. Clozel JP, Theroux P, Bourassa MG: Effects of diltiazem on experimental myocardial ischemia and on left ventricular performance. Circulation Res 52(Suppl 1):120, 1983.

227. Taylor AL, Goglino P, Eckels R, et al: Differential enhancement of postischemic segmental systolic thickening by diltiazem. J Am Coll Cardiol 15:737, 1990.

228. Walsh RA, O'Rourke RA: Direct and indirect effects of calcium entry blocking agents on isovolumic left ventricular relaxation in conscious dogs. J Clin Invest 75:1426, 1985.

229. Inouye IK, Massie BM, Loge D, et al: Failure of antihypertensive therapy with diuretic, beta-blocking and calcium channel-blocking drugs to consistently reverse left ventricular diastolic filling abnormalities. Am J Cardiol 53:1583, 1984.

230. Isobe M, Kashida M, Isshiki T, et al: Effects of beta-blockers and Ca antagonists on diastolic function of the hypertrophied left ventricle: An echocardiographic study [Japanese]. J Cardiogr 12:939, 1982.

231. Matsumoto M, Nakjima S, Fukushima M, et al: Effect of diltiazem on diastolic performance of the hypertrophied left ventricle in patients with systemic hypertension and hypertrophic cardiomyopathy [Japanese]. J Cardiogr 13:905, 1983.

232. Takeuchi M, Fujitani K, Kurogane K, et al: Effects of diltiazem and nitroglycerin on left ventricular diastolic properties in patients with coronary artery disease. Jpn Heart J 26:509, 1985.

233. Brugger P, Lasser W, Klein G: Koronare Herzkrankheit. Wirkung von diltiazem auf die diastolische linksventrikulare funktion. Munch Med Wochenschr 126:996, 1984.

234. Murakami T, Hess OM, Krayenbuehl HP: Left ventricular function before and after diltiazem in patients with coronary artery disease. J Am Coll Cardiol 5:723, 1985.

235. Yazawa Y, Nagai T, Hayashi S, et al: Hemodynamic effects of diltiazem on hypertrophic cardiomyopathy [Japanese]. Yakuri To Chiryo 11:185, 1983.

236. Suwa M, Hirota Y, Kawamura K: Improvement in left ventricular diastolic function during intravenous and oral diltiazem therapy in patients with hypertrophic cardiomyopathy: An echocardiographic study. Am J Cardiol 54:1047, 1984.

237. Suwa M, Hirota Y, Kawamura K: Effects of diltiazem, nifedipine and propranolol on cardiac function in hypertrophic cardiomyopathy [Japanese]. Yakuri To Chiryo 11:217, 1983.

238. Nagao M, Yasue H, Omote S, et al: Diltiazem-induced decrease of exercise-elevated pulmonary arterial diastolic pressure in hypertrophic cardiomyopathy patients. Am Heart J 102:789, 1981.

239. Nagao M, Omote S, Takisawa A, et al: Effect of diltiazem on left ventricular isovolumic relaxation time in patients with hypertrophic cardiomyopathy. Jpn Circ J 47:54, 1983.

240. Baxter GF: Inhibition by diltiazem of left ventricle collagen proliferation during renovascular hypertension development in rats. J Pharm Pharmacol 44:277, 1992.

241. Tubau JF, Wikman-Coffelt J, Massie BM, et al: Diltiazem prevents hypertrophy progression, preserves systolic function, and normalises myocardial oxygen utilisation in the spontaneously hypertensive rat. Cardiovasc Res 21:606, 1987.

242. Clusin WT, Buchbinder M, Bristow MR, et al: Evidence for a role of calcium in the genesis of early ischemic cardiac arrhythmias. In Opie LH (ed): Calcium Antagonists and Cardiovascular Disease. New York: Raven Press, 1984, pp 293–302.

243. Mitchell LB, Schroeder JS, Mason JW: Comparative clinical electrophysiologic effects of diltiazem, verapamil and nifedipine: A review. Am J Cardiol 18:629, 1982.

244. Gilmour RF, Zipes DP: Slow inward current and cardiac arrhythmias. Am J Cardiol 55:89B, 1985.

245. Talajic M, Nattel S: Frequency-dependent effects of calcium antagonists on atrioventricular conduction and refractoriness: Demonstration and characterization in anesthetized dogs. Circulation 74:1156, 1986.

246. Rowland E, McKenna WJ, Guker H, et al: The comparative effects of diltiazem and verapamil on atrioventricular conduction and atrioventricular reentry tachycardia. Circulation Res 52:I-163, 1983.

247. Fujimoto T, Peter T, Mandel WJ: Electrophysiologic and hemodynamic actions of diltiazem: Disparate temporal effects shown by experimental dose-response studies. Am Heart J 101:403, 1981.

248. Kawai C, Konishi T, Matsuyama E, et al: Comparative effects of three calcium antagonists, diltiazem, verapamil and nifedipine, on the sinoatrial and atrioventricular nodes. Circulation 63:1035, 1981.

249. Mitchell LB, Jutzy KR, Lewis SJ, et al: Intracardiac electrophys-

iologic study of intravenous diltiazem and combined diltiazem-digoxin in patients. Am Heart J 103:57, 1982.

250. Sugimoto T, Ishikawa T, Kaseno K, et al: Electrophysiologic effects of diltiazem, a calcium antagonist, in patients with impaired sinus or atrio-ventricular mode function. Angiology 31:700, 1980.

251. Treese N, Kasper W, Pop T, et al: Depressive effect of diltiazem on sinus node function after autonomic blockage in man. In Fleckenstein A, Hashimoto K, Herrmann M, et al (eds): New Calcium Antagonists: Recent Developments and Prospects, Diltiazem Workshop, Freiburg, Breisgau, May 1982. Stuttgart, Germany: Gustav Fischer, 1983, pp 213–218.

252. Valette H, Barnay C, Lopez M, et al: Effects of intravenous diltiazem on sinus node function and atrioventricular conduction in patients. J Cardiovasc Pharmacol 5:62, 1983.

253. Kirchhof CJHJ, Bonke FIM, Allessie MA: Effects of verapamil, diltiazem and disopyramide on sinus function: A comparison with bepridil. Eur J Pharmacol 160:369, 1989.

254. Wellens HJJ, Tan SL, Bar FWH, et al: Effect of verapamil studied by programmed electrical stimulation of the heart in patients with paroxysmal re-entrant supraventricular tachycardia. Br Heart J 39:1058, 1977.

255. Ritterman JB, Hossack KF, Bruce RA: Acute and chronic effects of diltiazem on A-V conduction at rest and during exercise. J Electrocardiol 15:41, 1982.

256. Araki H, Hotokebuchi N, Ohta T, et al: Effects of diltiazem on PR intervals in healthy young adults. Clin Ther 8:196, 1986.

257. Kumar K, Bajaj R, Kaul U, Bahl VK: Electrophysiologic effects of oral diltiazem before and after beta blockade. Clin Cardiol 14:317, 1991.

258. Vanhoutte PM: Calcium entry blockers and vascular smooth muscle. Circulation 65(Suppl I):11, 1982.

259. Sato M, Ohashi M, Metz MZ, et al: Inhibitory effect of a calcium antagonist (diltiazem) on aortic and coronary contractions in rabbits. J Mol Cell Cardiol 14:741, 1982.

260. Kawasaki KI, Seki K, Miyazawa I, et al: Effects of diltiazem and nitroglycerin on prostaglandin F2 alpha-induced periodic contractions of isolated human coronary arteries. Jpn Circ J 49:145, 1985.

261. Taira N, Satoh K, Maruyama M, et al: Sustained coronary constriction and its antgonism by calcium-blocking agents in monkeys and baboons. Circ Res 52:I-40, 1983.

262. Ginsburg R, Bristow MR, Harrison DC, et al: Studies with isolated human coronary arteries. Some general observations, potential mediators of spasm, role of calcium antagonists. Chest 78:180, 1980.

263. Hossack KF, Brown BG, Stewart DK, et al: Diltiazem-induced blockade of sympathetically mediated constriction of normal and diseased coronary arteries: Lack of epicardial coronary dilatory effect in humans. Circulation 70:465, 1984.

264. Ezra D, Boyd LM, Goldstein RE, et al: Effects of calcium entry blockers on coronary constriction and myocardial ischemia due to leukotriene D41. J Pharmacol Exp Ther 233:229, 1985.

265. Vrolix MC, Sionis D, Piessens JH, et al: Coronary hemodynamics and coronary flow reserve after intracoronary diltiazem in humans. Am J Cardiol 68:1633, 1991.

266. Tsuiki K, Ohta I, Oh-Hara N, et al: Effect of diltiazem on coronary blood flow distribution in dog heart under ischemia. J Cardiovasc Pharmacol 14:268, 1989.

267. Takeo S, Takenaka F: Effects of diltiazem on high-energy phosphate contents reduced by isoproterenol in rat myocardium. Arch Int Pharmacodyn Ther 228:205, 1977.

268. Weishaar R, Ashikawa O, Bing RJ: Effect of diltiazem, a calcium antagonist, on myocardial ischemia. Am J Cardial 43:1137, 1979.

269. Valdiserri EV: A possible interaction between lithium and diltiazem: Case Report. J Clin Psychiatry 46:540, 1985.

270. Zografos P, Watts JA: Shifts in calcium in ischemic and reperfused rat hearts: A cytochemical and morphometric study of the effects of diltiazem. Am J Cardiovasc Pathol 3:155, 1990.

271. Miller LS, Barrett JN, Cameron J, et al: Differential effects of calcium antagonists on viability of adult rat ventricular myocytes. J Mol Cell Cardiol 17:1129, 1985.

272. Inoue K, Grupp I, Schwartz A, et al: X-ray microanalysis of rabbit heart papillary muscles treated with calcium containing

solutions before and after treatment with diltiazem [Japanese]. Jpn Pharmacol Ther 10:321, 1982.

273. Elferink JG, Deierkauf M: The effect of verapamil and other calcium antagonists on chemotaxis of polymorphonuclear leukocytes. Biochem Pharmacol 33:35, 1984.

274. Irita K, Fujita I, Takeshige K, et al: Calcium channel antagonist induced inhibition of superoxide production in human neutrophils. Biochem Pharmacol 35:3465, 1986.

275. Obata H, Tanaka H, Haneda T: Response of isolated perfused heart to ischemia after long-term treatment of spontaneously hypertensive rats with diltiazem. Jpn Circ J 54:89, 1990.

276. Hamm CW, Opie LH: Protection of infarcting myocardium by slow channel inhibitors: Comparative effects of verapamil, nifedipine, and diltiazem in the coronary-ligated, isolated working rat heart. Circ Res 52:I-129, 1983.

277. Hamm CW, Thandroyen FT, Opie LH: Protective effects on isolated hearts with developing infarction: Slow channel blockade by diltiazem versus beta-adrenoceptor antagonism by metoprolol. Am J Cardiol 50:857, 1982.

278. Nohara R, Kambara H, Okuda K, et al: Effect of diltiazem on stunned myocardium evaluated with (99m)Tc-pyrophosphate imaging in canine heart. Jpn Circ J 56:262, 1992.

279. Matsunaga H: The effect of diltiazem and dobutamine on myocardial ischemia. J Jpn Assoc Thorac Surg 37:68, 1989.

280. Zalewski A, Faria DB, Cheung Wm, et al: Comparative effects of five calcium antagonists on infarct size and mortality after coronary occlusion [abstract]. Circulation 66:II-66, 1982.

281. Zalewski A, Goldberg S, Faria DB, et al: Relation of myocardial salvage to size of myocardium at risk in dogs. Am J Cardiol 56:974, 1985.

282. Senda Y: Studies on relationships between changes in myocardial blood flow, electrocardiographic alterations and serum creatine kinase and histologic extent of myocardial infarction in conscious dogs with permanent coronary occlusion and effects of diltiazem hydrochloride on these variables [Japanese]. Fukuoka Igaku Zasshi 74:18, 1983.

283. Szekeres L, Udvary E, Vegh A: Importance of myocardial blood flow changes in the protective action of diltiazem in a new model of myocardial ischaemia. Br J Pharmacol 86:341, 1985.

284. Tilton GD, Bush LR, Apprill PG, et al: Effect of diltiazem and propranolol on left ventricular segmental relaxation during temporary coronary arterial occlusion and one month reperfusion in conscious dogs. Circulation 71:165, 1985.

285. Sasayama S, Takahashi M, Nakamura M, et al: Effect of diltiazem on pacing-induced ischemia in conscious dogs with coronary stenosis: Improvement of postpacing deterioration of ischemic myocardial function. Am J Cardiol 48:460, 1981.

286. Van Der Vusse GJ, Van Der Veen FH, Prinzen FW, et al: The effects of diltiazem on myocardial recovery after regional ischemia in dogs. Eur J Pharmacol 125:383, 1986.

287. De Jong JW, Harmsen E, De Tombe PP: Diltiazem administered before or during myocardial ischemia decreases adenine nucleotide catabolism. J Mol Cell Cardiol 16:363, 1984.

288. Ford DA, Sharp JA, Rovetto MJ: Erythrocyte adenosine transport: Effects of Ca^{++} channel antagonists and ions. Am J Physiol 248:H593, 1985.

289. Watts JA, Norris TA, London RE, et al: Effects of diltiazem on lactate, ATP, and cytosolic free calcium levels in ischemic hearts. J Cardiovasc Pharmacol 15:44, 1990.

290. Sato S, Tajika T, Kaga Y, et al: Effect of diltiazem on acute myocardial ischemia. Yakuri To Chiryo 13:1407, 1985.

291. Ashraf M, Onda M, Hirohata Y, et al: Therapeutic effect of diltiazem on myocardial cell injury during the calcium paradox. J Mol Cell Cardiol 14:323, 1982.

292. Baker JE, Hearse DJ: The temperature-sensitivity of slow channel calcium blockers in relation to their effect upon the calcium paradox. Eur Heart J 4:97, 1983.

293. Higgins AJ, Blackburn KJ: Prevention of reperfusion damage in working rat hearts by calcium antagonists and calmodulin antagonists. J Mol Cell Cardiol 16:427, 1984.

294. Flaim SF, Zelis R: Diltiazem pretreatment reduces experimental myocardial infarct size in rat. Pharmacology 23:281, 1981.

295. Piper HM, Hutter JF, Spieckermann PG: Temperature dependence of calcium antagonist action. Arzneimittelforschung 35:1495, 1985.

296. Rahusen FD, van GW, Robillard GT, Wildevuur C: Cardioprotection with the Ca-entry blocker, diltiazem. Monitoring of energy metabolism with 31P-NMR and assay of myocardial loss of nucleosides [abstract]. Pharm Weekbl (Sci) 7:234, 1985.

297. Rahamathulla PM, Ashraf M, Schwartz A, et al: Effects of diltiazem on anoxic injury in the isolated rat heart. J Am Coll Cardiol 1:1081, 1983.

298. Nayler WG, Gordon M, Stephens DJ, et al: The protective effect of prazosin on the ischaemic and reperfused myocardium. J Mol Cell Cardiol 17:685, 1985.

299. van Gilst WH, Boonstra PW, Terpstra JA, et al: Improved recovery of cardiac function after 24 h of hypothermic arrest in the isolated rat heart: Comparison of a prostacyclin analogue (ZK 36 374) and a calcium entry blocker (diltiazem). J Cardiovasc Pharmacol 7:520, 1985.

300. Nayler WG, Sturrock WJ: An inhibitory effect of verapamil and diltiazem on the release of noradrenaline from ischaemic and reperfused hearts. J Mol Cell Cardiol 16:331, 1984.

301. Baxter GF, Yellon DM: Attenuation of reperfusion-induced ventricular fibrillation in the rat isolated hypertrophied heart by preischemic diltiazem treatment. Cardiovasc Drugs Ther 7:225, 1993.

302. Jolly SR, Menahan LA, Gross GJ: Diltiazem in myocardial recovery from global ischemia and reperfusion. J Mol Cell Cardiol 13:359, 1981.

303. Narita H, Nagao T, Sato M, et al: Ischemia-reperfusion induced elevation of diastolic tension in the isolated guinea pig heart and the effects of calcium antagonists. Jpn Heart J 24:277, 1983.

304. Klein HH, Schubothe M, Nebendahl K, et al: The effect of two different diltiazem treatments on infarct size in ischemic, reperfused porcine hearts. Circulation 69:1000, 1984.

305. Cirino D, Signorini G, Mattioli R, et al: The cardioprotective effect of low-dose diltiazem in experimental acute heart ischemia. Cuore 9:513, 1992.

306. Klein HH, Pich S, Lindert S, et al: The effect of intracoronary diltiazem on regional myocardial function and development of infarcts in porcine hearts. Res Exp Med 189:15, 1989.

307. Cavero I, Boudot JP, Feuvray D: Diltiazem protects the isolated rabbit heart from the mechanical and ultrastructural damage produced by transient hypoxia, low-flow ischemia and exposure to Ca^{++}-free medium. J Pharmacol Exp Ther 226:258, 1983.

308. Tilton RG, Williamson EK, Cole PA, et al: Coronary vascular hemodynamic and permeability changes during reperfusion after no-flow ischemia in isolated, diltiazem-treated rabbit hearts. J Cardiovasc Pharmacol 7:424, 1985.

309. Koller PT, Bergmann SR: Reduction of lipid peroxidation in reperfused isolated rabbit hearts by diltiazem. Circ Res 65:838, 1989.

310. Bush LR, Li YP, Shlafer M, et al: Protective effects of diltiazem during myocardial ischemia in isolated cat hearts. J Pharmacol Exp Ther 218:653, 1981.

311. Knabb RM, Rosamond TL, Fox K, et al: Enhancement of salvage of reperfused ischemic myocardium by diltiazem. J Am Coll Cardiol 8:861, 1986.

312. Allen BS, Okamoto F, Buckberg GD, et al: Studies of controlled reperfusion after ischema. IX. Reperfusate composition: Benefits of marked hypocalcemia and diltiazem on regional recovery. J Thorac Cardiovasc Surg 92:564, 1986.

313. Allen BS, Okamoto F, Buckberg GD, et al: Studies of controlled reperfusion after ischema. IX. Effects of "duration" of reperfusate administration versus reperfusate "dose" on regional functional, biochemical, and histochemical recovery. J Thorac Cardiovasc Surg 92:594, 1986.

314. Kinoshita M, Takayama Y, Kato S, et al: Protection of coronary reperfusion injury by a calcium antagonist. Jpn Circ J 44:461, 1980.

315. Kinoshita M, Bito K, Mashiro I, et al: Beneficial effect of diltiazem on ischemia-reperfusion injury in the dog. Jpn Circ J 49:179, 1985.

316. Just H, Tschirkov A: Animal-experimental and clinical studies on myocardial protection with calcium antagonists in open heart surgery. In Fleckenstein A, Hashimoto K, Herrmann M, et al (eds): New Calcium Antagonists: Recent Developments

and Prospects, Diltiazem Workshop, Freiburg, Breisgau, May 1982. Stuttgart, Germany: Gustav Fischer, 1982, pp 151–164.

317. Bush LR, Maximilian DL, Tilton G, et al: Effects of propranolol and diltiazem alone and in combination on the recovery of left ventricular segmental function after temporary coronary occlusion and long-term reperfusion in conscious dogs. Circulation 72:413, 1985.

318. Bush LR, Romson JL, Ash JL, et al: Effects of diltiazem on extent of ultimate myocardial injury resulting from temporary coronary artery occlusion in dogs. J Cardiovasc Pharmacol 4:285, 1982.

319. Sashida H, Abiko Y: Protective effect of diltiazem on ultrastructural alterations induced by coronary occlusion and reperfusion in dog hearts. J Mol Cell Cardiol 18:401, 1986.

320. Vouhe PR, Helias J, Grondin CM: Myocardial protection through cold cardioplegia using diltiazem, a calcium channel blocker. Ann Thorac Surg 30:342, 1980.

321. Vouhe PR, Helias J, Robert P, et al: Myocardial protection through cold cardioplegia with potassium or diltiazem. Experimental evidence that diltiazem provides better protection even when coronary flow is impaired by a critical stenosis. Circulation 65:1078, 1982.

322. Acad BA, Kedem J, Weiss HR: Effect of diltiazem on regional oxygenation of reperfused myocardium. J Pharmacol Exp Ther 249:91, 1989.

323. Mak IT, Weglicki WB: Comparative antioxidant activities of propranolol, nifedipine, verapamil, and diltiazem against sarcolemmal membrane lipid peroxidation. Circ Res 66:1449, 1990.

324. Higginson L, Tang A, Knoll G, Calvin J: Effect of intracoronary diltiazem on infarct size and regional myocardial function in the ischemic reperfused canine heart. J Am Coll Cardiol 18:868, 1991.

325. Grover GJ, Sleph PG, Parham CS: Effect of diltiazem on infarct size, reperfusion flow and flow reserve: The effect of timing of treatment. J Pharmacol Exp Ther 246:263, 1988.

326. Itoh B, Matsubara T, Itoh K, et al: Effect of diltiazem on acute myocardial ischemia. Study of the relationship between regional myocardial blood flow and myocardial energy metabolism. Jpn Heart J 28:747, 1987.

327. Ashraf M, Onda M, Benedict JB, et al: Prevention of calcium paradox-related myocardial cell injury with diltiazem, a calcium channel blocking agent. Am J Cardiol 49:1675, 1982.

328. Kavanaugh KM, Aisen AM, Fechner KP, et al: Effects of diltiazem on phosphate metabolism in ischemic and reperfused myocardium using phosphorus(31) nuclear magnetic resonance spectroscopy in vivo. Am Heart J 118:1210, 1989.

329. Fitzpatrick DB, Karmazyn M: Comparative effects of calcium channel blocking agents and varying extracellular calcium concentration on hypoxia/reoxygenation and ischemia/reperfusion-induced cardiac injury. J Pharmacol Exp Ther 228:761, 1984.

330. Balderman SC, Chan AK, Gage AA: Verapamil cadioplegia: Improved myocardial preservation during global ischemia. J Thorac Cardiovasc Surg 88:57, 1984.

331. Rousseau G, St-Jean G, Latour JG, et al: Diltiazem at reperfusion reduces neutrophil accumulation and infarct size in dogs with ischaemic myocardium. Cardiovasc Res 25:319, 1991.

332. Nayler WG, Sturrock WJ: Calcium antagonists and the ischaemic myocardium. Eur Heart J 7:27, 1986.

333. Nayler WG, Sturrock WJ. Inhibitory effect of calcium antagonists on the depletion of cardiac norepinephrine during postischemic reperfusion. J Cardiovasc Pharmacol 7:581, 1985.

334. Ruigrok T, Slade AM, Nayler WG, et al: Calcium paradox and calcium entry blockers. Rev Cardiovasc Med 40:125, 1984.

335. Nayler WG: Cardioprotective effects of calcium ion antagonists in myocardial ischemia. Clin Invest Med 3:91, 1980.

336. Grover GJ, Sleph PG: Dissociation of cardiodepression from cardioprotection with calcium antagonists: Diltiazem protects ischemic rat myocardium with a lower functional cost as compared with verapamil or nifedipine. J Cardiovasc Pharmacol 14:331, 1989.

337. Lopaschuk GD, Barr R, Wambolt R: Effects of diltiazem on glycolysis and oxidative metabolism in the ischemic and ischemic/reperfused heart. J Pharmacol Exp Ther 260:1220, 1992.

338. Swenson RD, Emery MJ, Fellows CL, et al: Improved hemodynamics with diltiazem after resuscitation from cardiac arrest [abstract]. Crit Care Med 14:332, 1986.

339. Fellows CL, Weaver WD, Swenson RD, et al: Hemodynamic, electrocardiographic, and cellular effects of diltiazem treatment after cardiac arrest and resuscitation. J Crit Care 4:166, 1989.

340. Plambeck RD, Todd GL: Comparison of the protective effects of nifedipine with other calcium blockers (verapamil and diltiazem) on norepinephrine-induced myocardial necrosis [abstract]. Anat Rec 208:139A, 1984.

341. Lindner KH, Prengel AW, Ahnefeld FW, et al: Effects of diltiazem on oxygen delivery and consumption after asphyxial cardiac arrest and resuscitation. Crit Care Med 20:650, 1992.

342. Rebeyka IM, Axford-Gatley RA, Bush BG, et al: Calcium paradox in an in vivo model of multidose cardioplegia and moderate hypothermia. Prevention with diltiazem or trace calcium levels. J Thorac Cardiovasc Surg 99:475, 1990.

343. Murashita T, Hearse DJ, Avkiran M: Effects of diltiazem as an additive to St Thomas's Hospital cardioplegic solution in isolated neonatal and adult rabbit hearts. Cardiovasc Res 25:496, 1991.

344. Yeung PKF, Mosher SJ, Macrae DA, Klassen GA: Effect of diltiazem and its metabolites on the uptake of adenosine in blood: An in-vitro investigation. J Pharm Pharmacol 43:685, 1991.

345. Christakis GT, Fremes SE, Weisel RD, et al: Diltiazem cardioplegia. J Thorac Cardiovasc Surg 91:647, 1986.

346. Janosik DL, Barner HB, Schwartz MT, et al: Cardiac output one and five days following bypass surgery: Is it altered by the addition of diltiazem to the cardioplegic solution? [abstract]. Clin Res 33:197A, 1985.

347. Vouhe PR, Loisance DY, Aubry P, et al: Optimal myocardial preservation using diltiazem: Randomized clinical study. Abstr Cardiovasc Pharmacotherapy Int Symp 1985, p 181.

348. Barner HB, Swartz MT, Devine JE, et al: Diltiazem as an adjunct to cold blood potassium cardioplegia: A clinical assessment of dose and prospective randomization. Ann Thorac Surg 43:191, 1987.

349. Ueno Y, Tokunaga K, Kohda Y, et al: Myocardial protection with diltiazem in open heart surgery [Japanese]. Yakuri To Chiryo 11:345, 1983.

350. Lamaison D, Machecourt J, Cassagnes X, et al: Le diltiazem perfuse avant la 6eme heure d'un primo infarctus anterieur chez l'homme [abstract]. Arch Mal Coeur 79:560, 1986.

351. Bonnier JJRM, Huizer T, Troquay R, et al: Myocardial protection by intravenous diltiazem during angioplasty of single-vessel coronary artery disease. Am J Cardiol 66:145, 1990.

352. Kling D, Boldt J, Moosdorf R, et al: Hemodynamic effects of diltiazem in patients undergoing coronary artery bypass grafting. Anaesthesist 37:249, 1988.

353. Nakajima H, Nosaka K: A comparison of the effects of diltiazem and nitroglycerin on the norepinephrine-induced contractions in the isolated femoral artery and vein. Japan J Pharmacol 33:1282, 1983.

354. Abe C, Kotoo Y, Endo T, et al: Effects of four Ca++ antagonists on the systemic capacitance vessels and venous return curves in dogs. Jpn Circ J 48:934, 1984.

355. Henry PD: Atherosclerosis, calcium, and calcium antagonists. Circulation 72:456, 1985.

356. Ginsburg R, Davis K, Bristow M, et al: Calcium antagonists suppress atherogenesis in aorta but not in the intramural coronary arteries of cholesterol-fed rabbits. Lab Invest 49:154, 1983.

357. Sugano M, Nakashima Y, Tasaki H, et al: Effects of diltiazem on suppression and regression of experimental atherosclerosis. Br J Exp Pathol 69:515, 1988.

358. Sugano M, Nakashima Y, Matsushima T, et al: Suppression of atherosclerosis in cholesterol-fed rabbits by diltiazem injection. Arteriosclerosis 6:237, 1986.

359. Naito M, Kuzuya F, Asai K, et al: Ineffectiveness of Ca++ antagonists nicardipine and diltiazem on experimental atherosclerosis in cholesterol-fed rabbits. Angiology 35:622, 1984.

360. Frey M, Adelung C: Antihypertensive and anticalcinotic effects of calcium antagonists [abstract]. J Mol Cell Cardiol 17:167, 1985.

361. Zorn J, Fleckenstein A: Anticalcinotic effects of calcium antagonists in cardiac, renal, intestinal and vascular tissues [abstract 104]. Pfluegers Arch 403:R31, 1985.

362. Saito K, Birou H, Fukunaga H, et al: Diltiazem prevents the damage to cultured aortic smooth muscle cells induced by hyperlipidemic serum. Experientia 15:412, 1986.

363. Naito M, Asai K, Shibata K, et al: Anti-arteriosclerotic effect of diltiazem (III) [Japanese]. Yakuri To Chiryo 13:1545, 1985.

364. Filipovic I, Buddecke E: Calcium channel blockers stimulate LDL receptor synthesis in human skin fibroblasts. Biochem Biophys Res Commun 14:845, 1986.

365. Kwong TC, Sparks JD, Pryce DJ, et al: Inhibition of apolipoprotein B net synthesis and secretion from cultured rat hepatocytes by the calcium-channel blocker diltiazem. Biochem J 263:411, 1989.

366. Ranganathan S, Harmony J, Jackson RL: Effect of Ca++ blocking agents on the metabolism of low density lipoproteins in human skin fibroblasts. Biochem Biophys Res Commun 107:217, 1982.

367. Ranganathan S, Jackson RL: Effect of calcium-channel–blocking drugs on lysosomal function in human skin fibroblasts. Biochem Pharmacol 33:2377, 1984.

368. Sassen LMA, Lamers JMJ, Hartog JM, et al: Failure of diltiazem to suppress cholesterol-induced atherogenesis of endothelium-denatured arteries in pigs. Atherosclerosis 81:217, 1990.

369. Negre-Salvayre A, Salvayre R: Protection by Ca(2+) channel blockers (nifedipine, diltiazem and verapamil) against the toxicity of oxidized low density lipoprotein to cultured lymphoid cells. Br J Pharmacol 107:738, 1992.

370. Mehta JL: Influence of calcium-channel blockers on platelet function and arachidonic acid metabolism. Am J Cardiol 55:158B, 1985.

371. Onoda JM, Sloane BF, Honn KV: Antithrombogenic effects of calcium channel blockers: Synergism with prostacylin and thromboxane synthase inhibitors. Thromb Res 34:367, 1984.

372. Shinjo A, Sasaki Y, Inamasu M, et al: In vitro effect of the coronary vasodilator diltiazem on human and rabbit platelets. Thromb Res 13:941, 1978.

373. Ware JA, Johnson PC, Smith M, et al: Inhibition of human platelet aggregation and cytoplasmic calcium response by calcium antagonists: Studies with aequorin and quin2. Circ Res 59:39, 1986.

374. Salam SR, Saxena R, Saraya AK: Effect of calcium channel blocker (diltiazem) on platelet aggregation. Indian J Exp Biol 29:484, 1991.

375. Mehta J, Mehta P, Ostrowski N: Calcium blocker diltiazem inhibits platelet activation and stimulates vascular prostacyclin synthesis. Am J Med Sci 291:20, 1986.

376. Kiyomoto A, Sasaki Y, Odawara A, et al: Inhibition of platelet aggregation by diltiazem. Comparison with verapamil and nifedipine and inhibitory potencies of diltiazem metabolites. Circ Res 52:I-115, 1983.

377. Alusik S, Kubis M, Hrckova Y, et al: Antiagregacni ucinek diltiazemu. Vnitr Lek 31:877, 1985.

378. Cremer KF, Pieper JA, Joyal M, et al: Effects of diltiazem, dipyridamole, and their combination on hemostasis. Clin Pharmacol Ther 36:641, 1984.

379. Shea MJ, Bush LR, Romson JL, et al: The effect of diltiazem on coronary thrombosis in the conscious canine. Eur J Pharmacol 77:67, 1982.

380. Schumacher WA, Lucchesi BR: Effect of diltiazem on experimental coronary artery thrombosis in dogs. Pharmacology 41:16, 1990.

381. Yamaguchi K, Taniguchi N, Koide M, et al: Effects of diltiazem chloride on cardiovascular response, platelet aggregation and coagulating activity during exercise in hypertensive patients. Jpn Pharmacol Ther 10:381, 1982.

382. Pechan J, Okrucka A: Diltiazem inhibits the spontaneous platelet aggregation in essential hypertension. Cardiology 79:116, 1991.

383. Anfossi G, Mularoni E, Massucco P, et al: Calcium-channel blocking agents verapamil and diltiazem are inhibitors of vasopressin-induced human platelet activation. Clin Exp Pharmacol Physiol 18:767, 1991.

384. Anfossi G, Trovati M, Mularoni E, et al: Effects of diltiazem on thromboxane B-2 production from platelet-rich plasma and whole blood. Prostaglandins Leukot Essent Fatty Acids 44:149, 1991.

385. Ring ME, Corrigan J Jr, Fenster PE: Antiplatelet effects of oral diltiazem, propranolol, and their combination. Br J Clin Pharmacol 24:615, 1987.

386. Ernst E, Matrai A: Diltiazem alters blood rheology. Pharmatherapeutica 5:213, 1987.

387. Coppola L, Grassia A, Giunta R, et al: Effect of diltiazem on platelet aggregability, erythrocyte filtrability, and thromboelastographic pattern in normal and atherosclerotic subjects. Curr Ther Res Clin Exp 40:1090, 1986.

388. Ohmori F, Tamai J, Kawahara T, et al: Effect of diltiazem HCl on renal blood flow in humans. Doppler catheter analysis. Jpn Pharmacol Ther 13:147, 1990.

389. Ogawa N, Ono H: Different effects of various vasodilators on autoregulation of renal blood flow in anesthetized dogs. Jpn J Pharmacol 41:299, 1986.

390. Yamaguchi I, Ikezawa K, Nagao T, et al: Effects of diltiazem on renal blood flow and renal function during angiotensin II infusion in anesthetized dogs. J Pharmacobiodyn 9:257, 1986.

391. Anderson GH, Howland T, Domschek R, et al: Effect of sodium balance and calcium channel-blocking drugs on plasma aldosterone responses to infusion of angiotensin II in normal subjects and patients with essential hypertension. J Clin Endocrinol Metab 63:1126, 1986.

392. Jover B, Dupont M, Casellas D, et al: Comparative effects of nifedipine and diltiazem on vascular responses to norepinephrine and angiotensin II. Eur Heart J 4(Suppl G):21, 1983.

393. Steele TH, Challoner-Hue L: Renal interactions betwen norepinephrine and calcium antagonists. Kidney Int 26:719, 1984.

394. Blackshear JL, Garnic D, Williams GH, et al: Exaggerated renal vasodilator response to calcium entry blockade in first-degree relatives of essential hypertensive subjects. Hypertension 9:384, 1987.

395. Johns EJ: The influence of diltiazem and nifedipine on renal function in the rat. Br J Pharmacol 84:707, 1985.

396. Kinoshita M, Kuskawa R, Shimono Y, et al: The effect of diltiazem hydrochloride upon sodium diuresis and renal function in chronic congestive heart failure. Arzneimittelforschung 29:676, 1979.

397. Sunderrajan S, Reams G, Bauer JH: Long-term renal effects of diltiazem in essential hypertension. Am Heart J 114:383, 1987.

398. Frei U, Schindler R, Matthies C, Koch KM: Glomerular hemodynamics of the clipped kidney: Effects of captopril and diltiazem. J Pharmacol Exp Ther 263:938, 1992.

399. Isshiki T, Amodeo C, Messerli FH, et al: Diltiazem maintains renal vasodilation without hyperfiltration in hypertension: Studies in essential hypertensive man and the spontaneously hypertensive rat. Cardiovasc Drugs Ther 1:359, 1987.

400. Isshiki T, Pegram BL, Frohlich ED: Hemodynamic comparison of diltiazem and TA-3090 in spontaneously hypertensive and normal Wistar-Kyoto rats. Am J Cardiol 62:79G 1988.

401. Isshiki T, Nishikimi T, Uchino K, et al: Diltiazem reduces glomerular pressure in spontaneously hypertensive rats. Cardiovasc Drugs Ther 6:91, 1992.

402. Jyothirmayi GN, Reddi AS: Effect of diltiazem on glomerular heparan sulfate and albuminuria in diabetic rats. Hypertension 21:795, 1993.

403. Solomon R, Dubey A: Diltiazem enhances potassium disposal in subjects with end-stage renal disease. Am J Kidney Dis 19:420, 1992.

404. Bakris GL: Hypertension in diabetic patients. An overview of interventional studies to preserve renal function. Am J Hypertens 6(4 Suppl):140S, 1993.

405. Demarie BK, Bakris GL: Effects of different calcium antagonists on proteinuria associated with diabetes mellitus. Ann Intern Med 113:987, 1990.

406. Erley CM, Haefele U, Heyne N, et al: Microalbuminuria in essential hypertension. Reduction by differene antihypertensive drugs. Hypertension 21:810, 1993.

407. Slataper R, Vicknair N, Sadler R, Bakris GL: Comparative effects of different antihypertensive treatments on progression of diabetic renal disease. Arch Intern Med 153:973, 1993.

408. Salem HA, Abdel-Rahman MS, Dahab GM: Influence of diltiazem and/or propranolol on rat blood glucose levels in normal and diabetic animals. J Appl Toxicol 13:85, 1993.

409. Segrestaa JM, Caulin C, Dahan R, et al: Effect of diltiazem on plasma glucose, insulin and glucagon during and oral glucose tolerance test in healthy volunteers. Eur J Clin Pharmacol 26:481, 1984.

410. Kindermann W, Schmitt W, Wolfing A: Korperliche leistungsfahigkeit, metabolismus und hormonelles verhalten unter diltiazem. Z Kardiol 75:99, 1986.

411. Pollare T, Lithell H, Morlin C, et al: Metabolic effects of diltiazem and atenolol: Results from a randomized, double-blind study with parallel groups. J Hypertens 7:551, 1989.

412. Andren L, Hoglund P, Dotevall A, et al: Diltiazem in hypertensive patients with type II diabetes mellitus. Am J Cardiol 62:114G, 1988.

413. Ohneda A: Effect of diltiazem hydrochloride on glucose tolerance in diabetes mellitus. Jpn J Clin Exp Med 57:1, 1980.

414. Gasinska T, Prochaczek F, Beldzik A, et al: Carbohydrate tolerance and glucose-stimulated insulin secretion in patients treated with diltiazem. Pol Tyg Lek 41:335, 1986.

415. Oi K, Mizuno M, Hirata Y: Clincial experience with diltiazem hydrochloride (Herbesser) on ischemic heart diseases in diabetics. Clin Rep 14:4, 1980.

416. Massie BM, MacCarthy EP, Ramanathan KB, et al: Diltiazem and propranolol in mild to moderate essential hypertension as monotherapy or with hydrochlorothiazide. Ann Intern Med 107:150, 1987.

417. Vedrenne B, Grateau G, Escourolle H, et al: Inoperable insulinoma: Treatment with diltiazem. Ann Med Interne 142:380, 1991.

418. Tanabe Seiyaku Co Ltd: Antihyperlipidemia composition containing diltiazem [patent]. Belg 899867, 1984.

419. Wada S, Nakayama M, Masaki K: Effects of diltiazem hydrochloride on serum lipids: Comparison with beta-blockers. Clin Ther 5:163, 1982.

420. Sawai K: Effects of long-term administration of diltiazem hydrochloride in hypertensive patients. Clin Ther 5:422, 1983.

421. Schulte KL, Meyer SW, Haertenberger A, et al: Antihypertensive and metabolic effects of diltiazem and nifedipine. Hypertension 8:859, 1986.

422. Klein WW: Results of a study comparing nifedipine and diltiazem in essential arterial hypertension. In Bender F, Greeff K (eds): Calciumantagonisten zur Behandlung der Angina Pectoris, Hypertonie und Arrhythmie, First Dilzem Symposium, Copenhagen. Amsterdam: Excerpta Medica, 1982, pp 210–219.

423. Pool PE, Seagren SC, Salel AF: Effects of diltiazem on serum lipids, exercise performance and blood pressure: Randomized, double-blind, placebo-controlled evaluation for systemic hypertension. Am J Cardiol 56:86H, 1985.

424. Seely EW, Le-Boff MS, Brown EM, et al: The calcium channel blocker diltiazem lowers serum parathyroid hormone levels in vivo and in vitro. J Clin Endocrinol Metab 68:1007, 1989.

425. Villiger L, Casez JP, Takkinen R, Jaeger P: Diltiazem stimulates parathyroid hormone secretion in vivo whereas felodipine does not. J Clin Endocrinol Metab 76:890, 1993.

426. Velardo A, Ricci S, Zironi C, et al: Effects of prolonged treatment with diltiazem on pituitary secretion of luteinizing hormone, follicle-stimulating hormone, thyrotropin and prolactin. Horm Res 37:137, 1992.

427. McFadden ER: Calcium-channel blocking agents and asthma. Intern Med 95:232, 1981.

428. Ahmed T, Abraham WM: Role of calcium-channel blockers in obstructive airway disease. Chest 88:132S, 1985.

429. Kivity S, Brayer M, Topilsky M: Combined effect of nifedipine and diltiazem on methacholine-induced bronchoconstriction in asthmatic patients. Ann Allergy 68:175, 1992.

430. Ferrari M, Olivieri M, De-Gasperi M, Lechi A: Differential effects of nifedipine and diltiazem on methacholine-induced bronchospasm in allergic asthma. Ann Allergy 63:196, 1989.

431. Kolbeck RC, Speir WA: Diltiazem, verapamil, and nifedipine inhibit theophylline-enhanced diaphragmatic contractility. Am Rev Respir Dis 139:139, 1989.

432. Young TE, Lundquist LJ, Chesler E, et al: Comparative effects

433. of nifedipine, verapamil, and diltiazem on experimental pulmonary hypertension. Am J Cardiol 51:195, 1983.

433. Clozel JP, Delorme N, Battistella P, et al: Hemodynamic effects of intravenous diltiazem in hypoxic pulmonary hypertension. Chest 91:171, 1987.

434. Gassner A: Gunstige beeinflussung der pulmonalen hypertonie bei patienten mit chronischer obstruktiver atemwegerkuankung durch diltiazem. Schweiz Med Wochenschr 114:332, 1984.

435. McGoon MD, Vlietstra RE: Vasodilator therapy for primary pulmonary hypertension. Mayo Clin Proc 59:672, 1984.

436. Kambara H, Fujimoto K, Wakabayashi A, et al: Primary pulmonary hypertension: Beneficial therapy with diltiazem. Am Heart J 101:230, 1981.

437. Crevey BJ, Dantzker DR, Bower JS, et al: Hemodynamic and gas exchange effects of intravenous diltiazem in patients with pulmonary hypertension. Am J Cardiol 49:578, 1982.

438. Rich S, Brundage BH: High-dose calcium channel-blocking therapy for primary pulmonary hypertension: Evidence for long-term reduction in pulmonary arterial pressure and regression of right ventricular hypertrophy. Circulation 76:135, 1987.

439. Christman BW, McPherson CD, Newman JH, et al: An imbalance between the excretion of thromboxane and prostacyclin metabolites in pulmonary hypertension. N Engl J Med 327:70, 1992.

440. Rich S, Kaufmann E, Levy PS: The effect of high doses of calcium-channel blockers on survival in primary pulmonary hypertension. N Engl J Med 327:76, 1992.

441. Gassner A, Sommer G, Fridrich L, et al: Differential therapy with calcium antagonists in pulmonary hypertension secondary to COPD: Hemodynamic effects of nifedipine, diltiazem, and verapamil. Chest 98:829, 1990.

442. Castell DO: Calcium-channel blocking agents for gastrointestinal disorders. Am J Cardiol 55:210B, 1985.

443. Achem SR, Mendez-Vigo M, Stueben E, et al: Effects of diltiazem-isordil on esophageal motility in healthy controls. Gastroenterology 90:1320, 1986.

444. Frachtman RL, Botoman VA, Pope CE: A double-blind crossover trial of diltiazem show no benefit in patients with dysphagia and/or chest pain of esophageal origin. Gastroenterology 90:1420, 1986.

445. Cattau E Jr, Castell DO, Johnson DA, et al: Diltiazem therapy for symptoms associated with nutcracker esophagus. Am J Gastroenterol 86:272, 1991.

446. Drenth JPH, Bos LP, Engels LGJB: Efficacy of diltiazem in the treatment of diffuse oesophageal spasm. Aliment Pharmacol Ther 4:411, 1990.

447. Seemann WR, Mathias K, Roeren Th, et al: Adenosine and diltiazem. A new therapeutic concept in the treatment of intestinal ischemia. Invest Radiol 20:16, 1985.

448. Boquet J, Moore N, Lhuintre JP, et al: Diltiazem for proctalgia fugax [letter]. Lancet 1:1493, 1986.

449. Yavorski RT, Hallgren SE, Blue PW: Effects of verapamil and diltiazem on gastric emptying in normal subjects. Dig Dis Sci 36:1274, 1991.

450. Rhedda A, McCans J, Willan AR, et al: A double blind placebo controlled crossover randomized trial of diltiazem in Raynaud's phenomenon. J Rheumatol 12:724, 1985.

451. Kahan A, Amor B, Menkes CJ: A randomized double-blind trial of diltiazem in the treatment of Raynaud's phenomenon. Ann Rheum Dis 44:30, 1985.

452. Matoba T, Chiba M: Effects of diltiazem on occupational Raynaud's syndrome (vibration disease). Angiology 36:850, 1985.

453. Gonzalez-Serratos H, Valle-Aguilera R, Lathrop DA, et al: Slow inward calcium currents have no obvious role in muscle excitation-contraction coupling. Nature 298:292, 1982.

454. Gallant EM, Goettl VM: Effects of calcium antagonists on mechanical responses of mammalian skeletal muscles. Eur J Pharmacol 117:259, 1985.

455. Walsh KB, Bryant SH, Schwartz A: Diltiazem potentiates mechanical activity in mammalian skeletal muscle. Biochem Biophys Res Commun 122:1091, 1984.

456. Williams JH, Ward CH: Enhancement of skeletal muscle fa-

tigue by the calcium channel antagonist diltiazem. Res Commun Chem Pathol Pharmacol 69:107, 1990.

457. McCalden TA, Bevan JA: The effect of calcium withdrawal and calcium antagonists on cerebrovascular tone and responses to various agonists. *In* Heistad DD, Marcus ML (eds): Cerebral Blood Flow: Effects of Nerves and Neurotransmitters, Proceedings of a Symposium, Iowa City, June 1981. Developments in Neuroscience, Vol 14. New York: Elsevier/North Holland, 1981, pp 21–27.

458. Bevan JA: Selective action of diltiazem on cerebral vascular smooth muscle in the rabbit: Antagonism of extrinsic but not intrinsic maintained tone. Am J Cardiol 49:519, 1982.

459. Kyoi K, Yokoyama K, Tsukamoto M, et al: Experimental studies of the effect of diltiazem (Ca antagonist) on cerebral circulation and cerebral arterial spasm. No To Shinkei 34:1145, 1982.

460. Frazee JG, Bevan JA, Bevan RD, et al: Effect of diltiazem on experimental chronic cerebral vasospasm in the monkey. J Neurosurg 62:912, 1985.

461. Solomon GD: Comparative efficacy of calcium antagonist drugs in the prophylaxis of migraine. Headache 25:368, 1985.

462. Paterna S, Martino SG, Campisi D, et al: Evaluation of the effects of verapamil, flunarizine, diltiazem, nimodipine and placebo for migraine prophylaxis. A double-blind randomized cross-over study. Clin Ter 134:119, 1990.

463. D'Attoma G, D'Attoma A: Treatment of recalcitrant chronic migraine with i.v. infusion of diltiazem. Gazz Med Ital Arch Sci Med 148:313, 1989.

464. Kurokawa Y, Abiko S, Ikeyama Y, et al: Effect of diltiazem on intracranial pressure in patients after craniotomy. Jpn Pharmacol Ther 20:249, 1992.

465. Loonen AJM, Verwey HA, Roels PR, et al: Is diltiazem effective in treating the symptoms of (tardive) dyskinesia in chronic psychiatric inpatients? A negative, double-blind, placebo-controlled trial. J Clin Psychopharmacol 12:39, 1992.

466. Toifl K, Presterl E, Graninger W: Lack of effect of diltiazem in the treatment of Duchenne's muscular dystrophy: A double-blind placebo-controlled study. Wien Klin Wochenschr 103:232, 1991.

467. Bertorini TE, Palmieri GMA, Griffin JW, et al: Effect of chronic treatment with the calcium antagonist diltiazem in Duchenne muscular dystrophy. Neurology 38:609, 1988.

468. Goto M, Zeller WP, Lichtenberg RC, Hurley RM: Diltiazem treatment of endotoxic shock in suckling rats. J Lab Clin Med 120:465, 1992.

469. Maitra SR, Krikhely M, Dulchavsky SA, et al: Beneficial effects of diltiazem in hemorrhagic shock. Circ Shock 33:121, 1991.

470. Sayeed MM, Doroba A: Effects of diltiazem in the early phase of endotoxin shock in rats. Circ Shock 9:193, 1982.

471. Singh G, Chaudry KI, Chudler LC, Chaudry IH: Depressed gut absorptive capacity early after trauma-hemorrhagic shock: Restoration with diltiazem treatment. Ann Surg 214:712, 1991.

472. Petho A, Neumann T, Vetterlein F, Schmidt G: Influence of diltiazem on postischemic microcirculation and function in the rat kidney. Microvasc Res 38:223, 1989.

473. Wang P, Ba ZF, Meldrum DR, Chaudry IH: Diltiazem restores cardiac output and improves renal function after hemorrhagic shock and crystalloid resuscitation. Am J Physiol Heart Circ Physiol 262:H1435, 1992.

474. Wang P, Ba ZF, Dean RE, Chaudry IH: Diltiazem administration after crystalloid resuscitation restores active hepatocellular function and hepatic blood flow after severe hemorrhagic shock. Surgery 110:390, 1991.

475. Liang D, Thurman RG: Protective effects of the calcium antagonists diltiazem and TA3090 against hepatic injury due to hypoxia. Biochem Pharmacol 44:2207, 1992.

476. Singh G, Chaudry KI, Chaudry IH: Diltiazem reduces whole blood viscosity following trauma—Hemorrhagic shock and resuscitation. Circ Shock 39:231, 1993.

477. Meldrum DR, Ayala A, Perrin MM, et al: Diltiazem restores IL-2, IL-3, IL-6, and IFN-gamma synthesis and decreases host susceptibility to sepsis following hemorrhage. J Surg Res 51:158, 1991.

478. Ferguson CJ, Williams JD, Hillis AN, et al: Effects of the calcium channel blocker diltiazem on cyclosporin nephrotoxicity in renal transplant patients. Clin Transplant 6:391, 1992.

479. Guerin C, Berthoux P, Broyet C, Berthoux F: Effects of diltiazem on renal function and blood pressure after renal transplantation under cyclosporine A. Arch Mal Coeur Vaiss 82:1223, 1989.

480. Kunzendorf U, Walz G, Brockmoeller J, et al: Effects of diltiazem upon metabolism and immunosuppressive action of cyclosporine in kidney graft recipients. Transplantation 52:280, 1991.

481. Neumayer HH, Wagner K: Prevention of delayed graft function in cadaver kidney transplants by diltiazem: Outcome of two prospective, randomized clinical trials. J Cardiovasc Pharmacol 10:S170, 1987.

482. Neumayer HH, Kunzendorf U, Schreiber M: Protective effects of diltiazem and the prostacycline analogue iloprost in human renal transplantation. Renal Fail 14:289, 1992.

483. Wagner K, Albrecht S, Neumayer HH: Prevention of post-transplant acute tubular necrosis by the calcium antagonist diltiazem: A prospective randomized study. Am J Nephrol 7:287, 1987.

484. Puig JM, Lloveras J, Oliveras A, et al: Usefulness of diltiazem in reducing the incidence of acute tubular necrosis in Euro-Collins-preserved cadaveric renal grafts. Transplant Proc 23:2368, 1991.

485. Bourge RC, Kirklin JK, Naftel DC, et al: Diltiazem-cyclosporine interaction in cardiac transplant recipients: Impact on cyclosporine dose and medication costs. Am J Med 90:402, 1991.

486. Valantine H, Keogh A, McIntosh N, et al: Cost containment: Coadministration of diltiazem with cyclosporine after heart transplantation. J Heart Lung Transplant 11:1, 1992.

487. Schroeder JS, Gao SZ, Alderman EL, et al: A preliminary study of diltiazem in the prevention of coronary artery disease in heart-transplant recipients. N Engl J Med 328:164, 1993.

488. Macdonald P, Keogh A, Connell J, et al: Diltiazem co-administration reduces cyclosporine toxicity after heart transplantation: A prospective randomised study. Transplant Proc 24:2259, 1992.

489. Karck M, Haverich A: Nifedipine and diltiazem reduce pulmonary edema formation during postischemic reperfusion of the rabbit lung. Res Exp Med 192:137, 1992.

490. Beatty JF, Krupin T, Nichols PF, et al: Elevation of intraocular pressure by calcium channel blockers. Arch Ophthalmol 102:1072, 1984.

491. Jacoby J, Kahn DN, Pavlica MR, et al: Diltiazem reduces the contractility of extraocular muscles in vitro and in vivo. Invest Ophthalmol Visual Sci 31:569, 1990.

492. Sakanashi M, Kato T, Miyamoto Y, et al: Comparative effects of diltiazem and glycerol trinitrate on isolated ureter and coronary artery of the dog. Pharmacology 32:11, 1986.

493. Abel MH, Hollingsworth M: Comparison of nifedipine and diltiazem with salbutamol for prevention of preterm delivery in the ovariectomized, oestrogen-treated late pregnant rat. J Reprod Fertil 77:559, 1986.

494. Abel MH, Hollingsworth M: The potencies and selectivities four calcium antagonists as inhibitors of uterine contractions in the rat in vivo. Br J Pharmacol 85:263, 1985.

495. Fujiwara M, Zaha M, Odashiro M, et al: Use of diltiazem in the anesthetic management of epinephrine predominant pheochromocytoma. Jpn J Anesthesiol 41:1175, 1992.

496. Tokioka H, Takahashi T, Kosogabe Y, et al: Use of diltiazem to control circulatory fluctuations during resection of a phaeochromocytoma. Br J Anaesth 60:582, 1988.

497. Milner MR, Gelman KM, Phillips RA, et al: Double-blind crossover trial of diltiazem versus propranolol in the management of thyrotoxic symptoms. Pharmacotherapy 10:100, 1990.

498. Hasegawa J, Mitsuhata H, Matsumoto S, Enzan K: Attenuation of cardiovascular response to laryngoscopy and tracheal intubation with bolus injection diltiazem. Jpn J Anesthesiol 41:356, 1992.

499. Mikawa K, Ikegaki J, Maekawa N, et al: The effect of diltiazem on the cardiovascular response to tracheal intubation. Anaesthesia 45:289, 1990.

500. Shimada T, Mitsuhata H, Matsumoto S, et al: Effect of continuous infusion of diltiazem on cardiovascular responses to laryngoscopy and intubation. Jpn J Anesthesiol 40:1507, 1991.

501. Aaberg RA, Sauer MV, Sikka S, Rajfer J: Effects of extracellular ionized calcium, diltiazem and cAMP on motility of human spermatozoa. J Urol 141:1221, 1989.

502. Faustini S, Salvini A, Pizzi P, et al: Experimental study on the action of diltiazem on detrusor muscle and clinical evaluation in patients with detrusor hyperactivity. Arzneimittelforschung/Drug Res 39:899, 1989.

503. Steinleitner A, Lambert H, Montoro L, et al: Use of diltiazem for preventing postoperative adhesions. J Reprod Med Obstet Gynecol 33:891, 1988.

504. Kawabata H, Knight KR, Coe SA, et al: Experience with calcium antagonists nitrendipine, diltiazem, and verapamil and beta 2-agonist salbutamol in salvaging ischemic skin flaps in rabbits. Microsurgery 12:160, 1991.

505. Del Pozo E, Ruiz-Garcia C, Baeyens JM: Analgesic effects of diltiazem and verapamil after central and peripheral administration in the hot-plate test. Gen Pharmacol 21:681, 1990.

506. Farah MJ, Palmieri GMA, Sebes JI, et al: The effect of diltiazem on calcinosis in a patient with the CREST syndrome. Arthritis Rheum 33:1287, 1990.

507. Juraskova V, Sladek T: Antimetastatic action of diltiazem on LS/BL tumor cells in liver tumor-colony assay. Neoplasma 37:343, 1990.

508. Franklin D, Millard RW, Nagao T: Responses of coronary collateral flow and dependent myocardial mechanical function to the calcium antagonist, diltiazem. Chest 78:200, 1980.

509. de Leiris J, Richard V, Pestre S: Calcium antagonists and experimental myocardial ischemia and infarction. In Opie LH (ed): Calcium Antagonists and Cardiovascular Disease. Perspect Cardiovasc Res, Vol 9. New York: Raven Press, 1984, pp 103–109.

510. Saito D, Haraoka S, Hirano K, et al: Effect of diltiazem on coronary blood flow of the heart with experimental coronary sclerosis and on regional myocardial blood flow of the heart with acute myocardial ischemia. Arzneimittelforschung 27:1669, 1977.

511. Takeda K, Nakagawa Y, Katano Y, et al: Effects of coronary vasodilators on large and small coronary arteries of dogs. Jpn Heart J 18:92, 1977.

512. Zyvoloski MG, Brooks HL, Gross GJ, et al: Myocardial perfusion distal to an acute or chronic coronary artery occlusion: Effects of diltiazem and nifedipine. J Pharmacol Exp Ther 222:494, 1982.

513. Thuillez C, Maury M, Giudicelli JF: Differential effects of verapamil and diltiazem on regional blood flow and function in the canine normal and ischemic myocardium. J Cardiovasc Pharmacol 5:19, 1983.

514. Gross GJ, Warltier DC: Selective improvement in subendocardial perfusion distal to a flow-limiting coronary artery stenosis: Effects of the new calcium channel blocking agent, FR 34235, nifedipine and diltiazem. J Pharmacol Exp Ther 228:531, 1984.

515. Ohat I, Kaminishi T, Oh HN, et al: Direct effects of diltiazem on coronary blood flow distribution within ischemic left ventricle. Jpn Circ J 48:935, 1984.

516. Nakamura M, Kikuchi Y, Senda Y, et al: Myocardial blood flow following experimental coronary occlusion. Effects of diltiazem. Chest 78:205, 1980.

517. Perez JE, Sobel BE, Henry PD: Improved performance of ischemic canine myocardium in reponse to nifedipine and diltiazem. Am J Physiol 239:H658, 1980.

518. Guth BD, Tajimi T, Seitelberger R, et al: Experimental exercise-induced ischemia: Drug therapy can eliminate regional dysfunction and oxygen supply-demand imbalance. J Am Coll Cardiol 7:1036, 1986.

519. Matsuzaki M, Guth B, Tajimi T, et al: Effect of the combination of diltiazem and atenolol on exercise-induced regional myocardial ischemia in conscious dogs. Circulation 72:233, 1985.

520. Remme WJ, Krauss XH, Van Hoogenhuyze DCA, Kruyssen DACM: Hemodynamic tolerability and anti-ischemic efficacy of high dose intravenous diltiazem in patients with normal versus impaired ventricular function. J Am Coll Cardiol 21:709, 1993.

521. Dymek DJ, Bache RJ: Effects of nifedipine and diltiazem on coronary reactive hyperaemia. Cardiovasc Res 18:249, 1984.

522. Foult JM, Nitenberg A, Blanchet F, Zouioueche S: Effect of diltiazem on coronary reactive hyperemia in patients with flow-limiting coronary artery stenosis. Am Heart J 112:1232, 1986.

523. Bache RJ, Dymek DJ: Effect of diltiazem on myocardial blood flow. Circulation 65(Suppl I):19, 1982.

524. Saito T, Takagomi A, Kimura Y, et al: Single brief ischemia promotes altered myocardial response to subsequent ischemia characterized as ischemia-sensitized myocardium: Effects of anti-anginal drugs, diltiazem and nicorandil. Ther Res 13:89, 1992.

525. Rossen JD, Simonetti I, Marcus ML, et al: The effect of diltiazem on coronary flow reserve in humans. Circulation 80:1240, 1989.

526. Kubota I, Ikeda K, Igarashi H, et al: Inhibition of dipyridamole-induced myocardial ischemia by diltiazem in patients with coronary artery disease. J Cardiovasc Pharmacol 9:363, 1987.

527. Grohs JG, Fischer G, Raberger G: Cardiac and hemodynamic effects of diltiazem during exercise-induced myocardial dysfunction in dogs. J Cardiovasc Pharmacol 16:228, 1990.

528. Rafflenbeul W: Dilatation of coronary artery stenoses with diltiazem, IV. In Fleckenstein A, Hashimoto K, Herrmann M, et al (eds): New Calcium Antagonists: Recent Developments and Prospects, Diltiazem Workshop, Freiburg, Breisgau, May 1982. Stuttgart, Germany: Gustav Fischer, 1983, pp 181–182.

529. Bertrand ME, Dupuis BA, Lablanche JM, et al: Coronary hemodynamics following intravenous or intracoronary injection of diltiazem in man. J Cardiovasc Pharmacol 4:695, 1982.

530. Oeff M, Schroder R, Biamino G: Anderung der kontraktilitatsparameter, des koronarflusses und des mykardialen sauerstoffverbrauches nach diltiazem IV bei patienten mit koronarer herzkrankheit. Z Kardiol 73:717, 1984.

531. Serruys PW, Suryapranata H, Planellas J, et al: Effects of short-term intravenous administration of diltiazem on left ventricular function and coronary hemodynamics of patients with coronary artery disease. J Cardiovasc Pharmacol 7:1138, 1985.

532. Hess OM, Nonogi H, Bortone A, et al: Diltiazem alone and combined with nitroglycerin: Effect on normal and diseased human coronary arteries. Eur Heart J 10:142, 1989.

533. Nonogi H, Hess OM, Ritter M, et al: Prevention of coronary vasoconstriction by diltiazem during dynamic exercise in patients with coronary artery disease. J Am Coll Cardiol 12:892, 1988.

534. Bonzel T, Wollschlager H, Lollgen H, et al: Dilatation of epicardial coronary arteries by intravenous diltiazem in patients with coronary artery disease. Z Kardiol 74:238, 1985.

535. Remme WJ, Van Hoogenhuyze DCA, Hofman A, et al: Acute antiischaemic properties of high dosages of intravenous diltiazem in humans in relation to its coronary and systemic haemodynamic effects. Eur Heart J 8:965, 1987.

536. Servi SD, Perrario M, Ghio S, et al: Effects of diltiazem on regional coronary hemodynamics during atrial pacing in patients with stable exertional angina: Implications for mechanism of action. Circulation 73:1248, 1986.

537. Joyal M, Cremer K, Pieper J, et al: Effects of diltiazem during tachycardia-induced angina pectoris. Am J Cardiol 57:10, 1986.

538. Josephson MA, Hopkins J, Singh BN: Hemodynamic and metabolic effects of diltiazem during coronary sinus pacing with particular reference to left ventricular ejection fraction. Am J Cardiol 55:286, 1985.

539. Joyal M, Cremer KF, Pieper JA, et al: Systemic, left ventricular and coronary hemodynamic effects of intravenous diltiazem in coronary artery disease. Am J Cardiol 56:413, 1985.

540. Fell D, Goodman J, McLaughlin PR, et al: Modification of silent and exercise induced ischemia by diltiazem in stable coronary disease. Circulation 78:II-326, 1988.

541. Khurmi NS, O'Hara MJ, Bowles MJ, Raftery EB: Effect of diltiazem and propranolol on myocardial ischaemia during unrestricted daily life in patients with effort-induced chronic stable angina pectoris. Eur J Clin Pharmacol 32:443, 1987.

542. Takase B, Kurita A, Uehata A, et al: Effect of diltiazem on silent ischemic episodes, plasma bradykinin and prostaglandin metabolism. Int J Cardiol 37:177, 1992.

543. Kern MJ, Walsh RA, Barr WK, et al: Improved myocardial

oxygen utilization by diltiazem in patients. Am Heart J 110:986, 1985.

544. Kober G, Kastner R, Hopf R, et al: Die direkte myokardiale antiischamische wirkung von diltiazem beim menschen. Z Kardiol 75:386, 1986.

545. Borzak S, Fenton T, Glasser SP, et al: Discordance between effects of anti-ischemic therapy on ambulatory ischemia, exercise performance and anginal symptoms in patients with stable angina pectoris. J Am Coll Cardiol 21:1605, 1993.

546. Pupita G, Mazzara D, Centanni M, et al: Ischemia in collateral-dependent myocardium: Effects of nifedipine and diltiazem in man. Am Heart J 126:86, 1993.

547. Fujita M, Mikuniya A, McKown DP, et al: Effects of nitroglycerin and diltiazem on well-developed coronary collateral circulation in conscious dogs. Angiology 42:628, 1991.

548. Vigorito C, Giordano A, De Caprio L, et al: Regional coronary hemodynamic effects of diltiazem in man. Am Heart J 116:799, 1988.

549. Vanhoutte PM: Calcium-entry blockers, vascular smooth muscle and systemic hypertension. Am J Cardiol 55:17B, 1985.

550. van Zwieten PA, Timmermans PBMWM: Pharmacological basis of the antihypertensive action of calcium entry blockers. J Cardiovasc Pharmacol 7:S11, 1985.

551. van Breemen C, Lukeman S, Cauvin C: A theoretic consideration on the use of calcium antagonists in the treatment of hypertension. Am J Med 77:26, 1984.

552. Rabkin SW: Diltiazem and verapamil lower blood pressure in the unanaesthetized rat through CNS mechanisms involving endogenous opioids. Clin Exp Pharmacol Physiol 18:431, 1991.

553. Aoki K, Sato K, Kawaguchi Y: Increased cardiovascular responses of norepinephrine and calcium antagonists in essential hypertension compared with normotension in humans. J Cardiovasc Pharmacol 7:S182, 1985.

554. Zimmerman BG, Goering JL: Long-term renal and systemic effects of calcium entry blockers in normotensive and experimental hypertensive dogs. Am J Cardiol 56:47H, 1985.

555. Natsume T, Gallo AJ, Pegram BL, et al: Hemodynamic effects of prolonged treatment with diltiazem in conscious normotensive and spontaneously hypertensive rats. Clin Exp Hypertens [A] 7:1471, 1985.

556. Bohr DF, Webb RC: Vascular smooth muscle function and its changes in hypertension. Am J Med 77:3, 1984.

557. Blanstein MP, Hamlyn JM: Sodium transport inhibition, cell calcium and hypertension. Am J Med 77:45, 1985.

558. Cauvin C, Saida K, van Breemen C: Extracellular Ca dependence and diltiazem inhibition of contraction in rabbit conduit arteries and mesenteric resistance vessels. Blood Vessels 21:23, 1983.

559. Simon A, Safar ME, Levenson JA, et al: Action of vasodilating drugs on small and large arteries of hypertensive patients. J Cardiovasc Pharmacol 5:626, 1983.

560. Safar ME, Simon AC, Levenson JA, et al: Hemodynamic effects of diltiazem in hypertension. Circ Res 52:I-169, 1983.

561. Ko YD, Sachinidis A, Graack GH, et al: Inhibition of angiotensin II and platelet-derived growth factor-induced vascular smooth muscle cell proliferation by calcium entry blockers. Clin Invest 70:113, 1992.

562. Magometschnigg D, Hortnagl H, Rameis H: Diltiazem and verapamil: Functional antagonism of exogenous noradrenalin and angiotensin II in man. Eur J Clin Pharmacol 26:303, 1984.

563. Mohanty PK, Sowers JR, McNamara C, et al: Effects of diltiazem on hormonal and hemodynamic responses to lower body negative pressure and tilt in patients with mild to moderate systemic hypertension. Am J Cardiol 56:28H, 1985.

564. Mohanty PK, Sowers JR, Thames MD: Effects of hydrochlorothiazide and diltiazem on reflex vasoconstriction in hypertension. Hypertension 10:35, 1987.

565. Aoki K, Sato K: Pathophysiological background for the use of calcium antagonists. J Cardiovasc Pharmacol 7:S28, 1985.

566. Abraham AS, Brooks BA, Grafstein Y, et al: Effects of hydrochlorothiazide, diltiazem and enalapril on mononuclear cell sodium and magnesium levels in systemic hypertension. Am J Cardiol 68:1357, 1991.

567. Fein FS, Cho S, Malhotra A, et al: Beneficial effects of diltiazem on the natural history of hypertensive diabetic cardiomyopathy in rats. J Am Coll Cardiol 18:1406, 1991.

568. Grellet JP, Bonoron-Adele SM, Tariosse LJ, Besse PJ: Diltiazem and left ventricular hypertrophy in renovascular hypertensive rats. Hypertension 11:495, 1988.

569. Rozanski JJ, Zaman L, Castellanos A: Electrophysiologic effects of diltiazem hydrochloride on supraventricular tachycardia. Am J Cardiol 49:621, 1982.

570. Waleffe A, Hastir F, Kulbertus HE: Effects of intravenous diltiazem administration in patients with inducible tachycardia. Eur Heart J 6:882, 1985.

571. Yeh SJ, Fu M, Lin FC, et al: Serial electrophysiologic studies of the effects of oral diltiazem on paroxysmal supraventricular tachycardia. Chest 87:639, 1985.

572. Roy D, Marchand E, Chabot M, et al: Electrophysiologic effects of intravenous diltiazem in patients with recurrent supraventricular tachycardias. Can J Cardiol 1:302, 1985.

573. Fukuhara S, Echizen H, Naito M, et al: An interindividual variability in the sensitivity of atrioventricular node to diltiazem in patients with paroxysmal supraventricular tachycardia. J Clin Pharmacol 29:102, 1989.

574. Dias VC, Plumb VJ: Intravenous diltiazem in patients with atrial fibrillation/atrial flutter. A pilot dose-response study. Drug Invest 3:8, 1991.

575. Theisen K, Haufe M, Peters J, et al: Effect of the calcium antagonist diltiazem on atrioventricular conduction in chronic atrial fibrillation. Am J Cardiol 55:98, 1985.

576. Talajic M, Nayebpour M, Jing W, Nattel S: Frequency-dependent effects of diltiazem on the atrioventricular node during experimental atrial fibrillation. Circulation 80:380, 1989.

577. Talajic M, Lemery R, Roy D, et al: Rate-dependent effects of diltiazem on human atrioventricular nodal properties. Circulation 86:870, 1992.

578. Fujiki A, Mizumaki K, Tani M: Effects of diltiazem on concealed atrioventricular nodal conduction in relation to ventricular response during atrial fibrillation in anesthetized dogs. Am Heart J 125:1284, 1993.

579. Talajic M, Papadatos D, Villemaire C, et al: Antiarrhythmic actions of diltiazem during experimental atrioventricular reentrant tachycardias. Importance of use-dependent calcium channel-blocking properties. Circulation 81:334, 1990.

580. Nayebpour M, Talajic M, Jing W, Nattel S: Autonomic modulation of the frequency-dependent actions of diltiazem on the atrioventricular node in anesthetized dogs. J Pharmacol Exp Ther 253:353, 1990.

581. Frabetti L, Capucci A, Gerometta PS, et al: Intravenous diltiazem in patients with paroxysmal re-entrant supraventricular tachycardia. Int J Cardiol 23:215, 1989.

582. Gough WB, Zeiler RH, El-Sherif N: Effects of diltiazem on triggered activity in canine 1 day old infarction. Cardiovasc Res 18:339, 1984.

583. Blake K, Clusin WT: Effect of diltiazem on ischemic myocardial depolarization and extracellular K+ accumulation. Eur J Pharmacol 15:261, 1986.

584. Mitani A, Kinoshita K, Toshima Y, et al: The mechanism of protective effect of diltiazem on reperfusion-induced arrhythmias in isolated rat heart. Jpn Circ J 54:117, 1990.

585. Nanasi PP, Knilans TK, Varro A, et al: Active and passive electrical properties of isolated canine cardiac Purkinje fibers under conditions simulating ischaemia: Effect of diltiazem. Pharmacol Toxicol 71:52, 1992.

586. Opie LH, Thandroyen FT: Molecular and biochemical mechanisms underlying the role of calcium ions in malignant ventricular arrhythmias. Ann N Y Acad Sci 427:127, 1984.

587. Miyazaki T, Ogawa S, Sakurai K, et al: Ectopic ventricular tachycardia sensitive to calcium antagonists in acute myocardial infarction in dogs. Am J Cardiol 55:1085, 1985.

588. Schwartz PJ, Priori SG, Vanoli E, et al: Efficacy of diltiazem in two experimental feline models of sudden cardiac death. J Am Coll Cardiol 8:661, 1986.

589. Thandroyen FT: Protective action of calcium channel antagonist agents against ventricular fibrillation in the isolated perfused rat heart. J Mol Cell Cardiol 14:21, 1982.

590. Winslow E, Marshall RJ, Hope FG: Comparative effects of fast- and slow-ion channel blocking agents on reperfusion-induced arrhythmias in the isolated perfused rat heart. J Cardiovasc Pharmacol 5:928, 1983.

591. Fujimoto T, Peter T, Hamamoto H, Mandel WJ: Effects of diltiazem on conduction of premature impulses during acute myocardial ischemia and reperfusion. Am J Cardiol 48:851, 1981.

592. Thale J, Gulker H, Olbing B, et al: Antiarrhythmic and antifibrillatory action of diltiazem on early and late phase ventricular arrhythmias following coronary artery occlusion and on reperfusion ventricular arrhythmias. Pharmacology 33:1, 1986.

593. Nakaya H, Millard RW, Lathrop DA, et al: Flow-independent improvement by diltiazem of ischemia-induced conduction delay in porcine hearts. J Am Coll Cardiol 2:474, 1983.

594. Clusin WT, Buchbinder M, Ellis AK, et al: Reduction of ischemic depolarization by the calcium channel blocker diltiazem. Correlation with improvement of ventricular conduction and early arrhythmias in the dog. Circ Res 54:10, 1984.

595. Heuer H, Gulker H, Thale J, et al: Effects of diltiazem on vulnerability to atrial and ventricular reentrant arrhythmias in the normal and ischemic heart. Arzneimittelforschung 33:1113, 1983.

596. Yoshida S, Downey JM, Yellon DM, et al: Diltiazem reduced infarct size but not ventricular arrhythmias in 48 hour coronary embolized dogs. Can J Cardiol 1:346, 1985.

597. Opie LH, Thandroyen FT, Muller CA, et al: Calcium channel antagonists as antiarrhythmic agents: Contrasting properties of verapamil and diltiazem versus nifedipine. In Opie LH (ed): Calcium Antagonists and Cardiovascular Disease. New York: Raven Press, 1984, pp 303–311.

598. Sheehan FH, Epstein SE: Effects of calcium channel blocking agents on reperfusion arrhythmias. Am Heart J 103:973, 1982.

599. Hashimoto H, Suzuki K, Miyake S, Nakashima M: Effects of calcium antagonists on the electrical alternans of the ST segment and on associated mechanical alternans during acute coronary occlusion in dogs. Circulation 68:667, 1983.

600. Cardinal R, Carson L, Lambert C, et al: Opposite effects of lidocaine and diltiazem on electrophysiologic alterations in acutely ischemic porcine myocardium. Can J Physiol Pharmacol 67:697, 1989.

601. Capparelli EV, Hanyok JJ, Dipersio DM, et al: Diltiazem improves resuscitation from experimental ventricular fibrillation in dogs. Crit Care Med 20:1140, 1992.

602. Rabkin SW: The calcium antagonist diltiazem has antiarrhythmic effects which are mediated in the brain through endogenous opioids. Neuropharmacology 31:487, 1992.

603. DeVaughn-Belton E, Olaya PI Jr, Carryon P, et al: Surveillance study of diltiazem use in black and nonblack angina patients. J Natl Med Assoc 80:517, 1988.

604. Maseri A, Parodi O, Fox KM: Rational approach to the medical therapy of angina pectoris: The role of calcium antagonists. Prog Cardiovasc Dis 25:269, 1983.

605. Legrand V, Hastir F, Vandormael M, et al: Haemodynamic effects of intravenous diltiazem at rest and exercise in patients with coronary artery disease. Eur Heart J 5:456, 1984.

606. Schnellbacher K, Hirsch F, Roskamm H: Exercise hemodynamics in angina pectoris patients after intravenous application of diltiazem. In Fleckestein A, Hashimoto K, Herrmann M, et al (eds): New Calcium Antagonists: Recent Developments and Prospects, Diltiazem Workshop, Freiburg, Breisgau, May 1982. Stuttgart, Germany: Gustav Fischer, 1983, pp 175–179.

607. Puddu PE, Lanti M, Mangieri E, et al: Systemic hemodynamic effects of diltiazem at rest and during isometric exercise in patients with coronary artery disease. Cardiologia 30:121, 1985.

608. Kenny J, Daly K, Bergman G, et al: Beneficial effects of diltiazem combined with beta blockade in angina pectoris. Eur Heart J 6:418, 1985.

609. Rocha P, Baron B, Delestrain A, et al: Hemodynamic effects of intravenous diltiazem in patients treated chronically with propranolol. Am Heart J 111:62, 1986.

610. Pepine CJ, Joyal M, Cremer KF, et al: Hemodynamic effects of nitroglycerin combined with diltiazem in patients with coronary artery disease. Am J Med 76:47, 1984.

611. Oyama Y, Akutsu Y, Miyake N, et al: Experience with clinical use of CRD-401 in angina pectoris. Jpn J Clin Exp Med 49:1954, 1972.

612. Arce-Gomez E, Aspe y Rosas J, Barreiro LD: Efficacy of diltiazem hydrochloride in the treatment of chronic angina pectoris. Curr Ther Res 30:386, 1981.

613. De Backer G, Vincke J: Double-blind comparison of diltiazem and placebo in the treatment of exercise-inducible chronic stable angina pectoris. Acta Cardiol 37:245, 1982.

614. Kubota I, Watanabe Y, Ohyama T, et al: The beneficial effect of diltiazem on exercise-induced ST depression, measured by body surface mapping, in stable effort angina pectoris. Clin Ther 5:49, 1982.

615. Kubota I, Igarashi H, Ikeda K, et al: Attenuation of exercise-induced R wave increase after diltiazem in effort angina pectoris. Jpn Heart J 25:937, 1984.

616. Magometschnigg D: Unterschiede in der antanginosen wirkungsintensitat von diltiazem nach einmaliger und nach wiederholter verabreichung. Herz Kreislauf 14:342, 1982.

617. McCans JL: Dose response effects of diltiazem on treadmill tolerance in chronic stable angina: A randomized double-blind, placebo-controlled crossover trial. Can J Cardiol 1:17, 1985.

618. Wagniart P, Ferguson RJ, Chatman BR, et al: Increased exercise tolerance and reduced electrocardiographic ischemia with diltiazem in patients with stable angina pectoris. Circulation 66:23, 1982.

619. Chang K, Hossack KF: Effect of diltiazem on heart rate responses and respiratory variables during exercise: Implications for exercise prescription and cardiac rehabilitation. J Cardiac Rehab 2:326, 1982.

620. Strauss WE, McIntyre KM, Parisi AF, Shapiro W: Safety and efficacy of diltiazem hydrochloride for the treatment of stable angina pectoris: Report of a cooooperative clinical trial. Am J Cardiol 49:560, 1982.

621. Pool P, Seagren SC, Bonanno JA, et al: The treatment of exercise-inducible chronic stable angina with diltiazem. Chest 78:234, 1980.

622. Subramanian VB, Khurmi NS, Bowles MJ, et al: Objective evaluation of three dose levels of diltiazem in patients with chronic stable angina. J Am Coll Cardiol 1:1144, 1983.

623. Low RI, Takeda P, Lee G, et al: Effects of diltiazem-induced calcium blockage upon exercise capacity in effort angina due to chronic coronary artery disease. Am Heart J 101:713, 1981.

624. Hossack KF, Pool PE, Steele P, et al: Efficacy of diltiazem in angina on effort: A multicenter trial. Am J Cardiol 49:567, 1982.

625. Petru MA, Crawford MH, Sorensen SG, et al: Short- and long-term efficacy of high-dose oral diltiazem for angina due to coronary artery disease: A placebo-controlled, randomized, double-blind crossover study. Circulation 68:139, 1983.

626. Petru MA, Crawford MH, Kennedy GT, et al: Long-term efficacy of high-dose diltiazem for chronic stable angina pectoris: 16-month serial studies with placebo controls. Am Heart J 109:99, 1985.

627. Hossack KF, Pool PE, Seagren SC, et al: Long-term monotherapy of angina pectoris with diltiazem. Aust N Z J Med 15:221, 1985.

628. Lindenberg BS, Weiner DA, McCabe CH, et al: Efficacy and safety of incremental doses of diltiazem for the treatment of stable angina pectoris. J Am Coll Cardiol 2:1129, 1983.

629. Hossack KF, Kannagi T, Day B, et al: Long-term study of high-dose diltiazem in chronic stable exertional angina. Am Heart J 107:1215, 1984.

630. Go M, Hollenberg M: Improved efficacy of high-dose versus medium- and low-dose diltiazem therapy for chronic stable angina pectoris. Am J Cardiol 53:669, 1984.

631. Khurmi NS, Bowles MJ, O'Hara MJ, et al: Long-term efficacy of diltiazem assessed with multistage graded exercise tests in patients with chronic stable angina pectoris. Am J Cardiol 1:738, 1984.

632. Pool PE, Seagren SC: Long-term efficacy of diltiazem in chronic stable angina associated with atherosclerosis: Effect on treadmill exercise. Am J Cardiol 49:573, 1982.

633. Klinke WP, Juneau M, Grace M, et al: Usefulness of sustained-release diltiazem for stable angina pectoris. Am J Cardiol 64:1249, 1989.

634. Hossack KF, Bruce RA: Improved exercise performance in persons with stable angina pectoris receiving diltiazem. Am J Cardiol 47:95, 1981.

635. Klinke WP, Juneau M, Grace M, et al: Usefulness of sustained-release diltiazem for stable angina pectoris. Am J Cardiol 64:1249, 1989.

636. Zema MJ, Perlmutter S, Mankes S, Nikitopoulos C: Diltiazem treatment for the management of ischaemia in patients with poor left ventricular function: Safety of long term administration. Br Heart J 58:512, 1987.

637. Ogasawara S, Freedman SB, Ram J, Kelly DT: Effects of diltiazem and long-term beta-1-adrenergic blockade on hemodynamics and blood flow during exercise in patients with stable angina pectoris. J Am Coll Cardiol 15:184, 1990.

638. Bruce RA, Hossack KF, Kusumi F, et al: Excessive reduction in peripheral resistance during exercise and risk of orthostatic symptoms with sustained-release nitroglycerin and diltiazem treatment of angina. Am Heart J 109:1020, 1985.

639. Fazzini PF, Multino D, Zambaldi G: Diltiazem in spontaneous angina: Double-blind crossover study with Holter monitoring. G Ital Cardiol 15:1085, 1985.

640. Subramanian VB: Comparison of diltiazem and placebo. In Calcium Antagonists in Chronic Stable Angina Pectoris. Amsterdam: Elsevier, 1983, pp 161–173.

641. Vliegen HW, Van der Wall EE, Kragten JA, et al: Comparison of diltiazem standard formulation and diltiazem controlled release in patients with stable angina pectoris: A randomized, double-blind, cross-over, multicenter study. J Cardiovasc Pharmacol 21:552, 1993.

642. Lehmann G, Reiniger G, Haase HU, Rudolph W: Enhanced effectiveness of combined sustained-release forms of isosorbide dinitrate and diltiazem for stable angina pectoris. Am J Cardiol 68:983, 1991.

643. Emanuelsson H, Ake H, Kristi M, Arina R: Effects of diltiazem and isosorbide-5-mononitrate, alone and in combination, on patients with stable angina pectoris. Eur J Clin Pharmacol 36:561, 1989.

644. Posma JL, Van-Dijk RB, Lie KI: Sustained-release diltiazem versus metoprolol in stable angina pectoris. Eur Heart J 10:923, 1989.

645. O'Hara MJ, Khurmi NS, Bowles MJ, et al: Comparison of diltiazem at two dose levels with propranolol for treatment of stable angina pectoris. Am J Cardiol 54:477, 1984.

646. Subramanian VB: Comparative evaluation of four calcium antagonists and propranolol with placebo in patients with chronic stable angina. Cardiovasc Rev Rep 5:91, 1984.

647. Lagioia R, Mangini SG, Dibenedetto A, et al: Rapporto dose-effetto e durata d'azione del diltiazem nell'angina da sforzo stabile. Confronto con propranololo. Cardiologia 30:213, 1985.

648. Chaitman BR, Wagniart P, Pasternac A, et al: Improved exercise tolerance after propranolol, diltiazem or nifedipine in angina pectoris: Comparison at 1, 3, and 8 hours and correlation with plasma drug concentration. Am J Cardiol 53:1, 1984.

649. Anderson JL, Wagner JM, Datz FL, et al: Comparative effects of diltiazem, propranolol, and placebo on exercise performance using radionuclide ventriculography in patients with symptomatic coronary artery disease: Results of a double-blind, randomized, crossover study. Am Heart J 107:698, 1984.

650. Adamo L, Novo S, Bucca V, et al: Effects of calcium entry blockers and of beta-blockers on exercise tolerance in patients of different age suffering from angina pectoris. Eur Heart J 6:80, 1985.

651. Wheatley D: A comparison of diltiazem and atenolol in angina. Postgrad Med J 61:785, 1985.

652. Riley M, Elborn JS, Khan MM, et al: Comparative effects of epanolol and diltiazem on exercise performance and respiratory gas exchange in angina pectoris. Eur Heart J 13:1116, 1992.

653. Meyer EC, Makov UE, Palant A: Monotherapy of stable angina pectoris with bopindolol in comparison with diltiazem. Cardiology 78:179, 1991.

654. Merino A, Alegria E, Castello R, et al: Complementary mechanisms of atenolol and diltiazem in the clinical improvement of patients with stable angina. Angiology 40:626, 1989.

655. Kober G: Efficacy and tolerance of diltiazem in patients suffering from coronary insufficiency—double-blind crossover study versus nifedipine. In Diltiazem Kyoto Conference, I, Clinical Session, Kyoto. Kyoto, Japan: Tanabe Seiyaku, 1980, pp 132–144.

656. Klein W: Ergebnisse einer vergleichsuntersuchung zwischen nifedipin und diltiazm bei stabiler angina pectoris. In Bender F, Greeff K (eds): Calciumantagonisten zur Behandlung der Angina Pectoris, Hypertonie und Arrhythmie, First Dilzem Symposium, Copenhagen, June 1981. Amsterdam: Excerpta Medica, 1982, pp 115–125.

657. Frishman WH, Charlap S, Goldberger J, et al: Comparison of diltiazem and nifedipine for both angina pectoris and systemic hypertension. Am J Cardiol 56:41H, 1985.

658. Weiner DA, McCabe CH, Cutler SS, et al: The efficacy and safety of high-dose verapamil and diltiazem in the long-term treatment of stable exertional angina. Clin Cardiol 7:648, 1984.

659. Pucci PD, Pollavini G, Zerauscheck M, Fazzini P: Acute effects on exercise tolerance of felodipine and diltiazem, alone and in combination, in stable effort angina. Eur Heart J 12:55, 1991.

660. Schulz J, Lubnau E, Grossmann M, Ruck W: Double-blind randomized study of the anti-anginal and anti-ischaemic efficacy of fendiline and diltiazem in patients with coronary heart disease. Curr Med Res Opin 12:521, 1991.

661. Siu SC, Jacoby RM, Phillips RT, Nesto RW: Comparative efficacy of nifedipine gastrointestinal therapeutic system versus diltiazem when added to beta blockers in stable angina pectoris. Am J Cardiol 71:887, 1993.

662. Meluzin J, Zeman K, Stetka F, Simek P: Effects of nifedipine and diltiazem on myocardial ischemia in patients with severe stable angina pectoris treated with nitrates and beta-blockers. J Cardiovasc Pharmacol 20:864, 1992.

663. Caponnetto S, Canale C, Terrachini V, et al: Open comparative study to assess the efficacy and safety of two calcium antagonists: Amlodipine and diltiazem in the treatment of symptomatic myocardial ischemia. Postgrad Med J 67(Suppl 5):S54–S56, 1991.

664. Singh BN: Comparative efficacy and safety of bepridil and diltiazem in chronic stable angina pectoris refractory to diltiazem. Am J Cardiol 68:306, 1991.

665. DiBianco R: Bepridil treatment of chronic stable angina: A review of comparative studies versus placebo, nifedipine, and diltiazem. Am J Cardiol 69:56D, 1992.

666. Marraccini P, Orsini E, Brunelli C, et al: Gallopamil and diltiazem: A double-blind, randomized cross-over trial in effort ischaemia. Eur Heart J 13:404, 1992.

667. D'Ascia C, Picardi G, Cittadini A, et al: Gallopamil and diltiazem in the treatment of effort angina. Double-blind, crossover, randomized study. Curr Ther Res Clin Exp 51:145, 1992.

668. Hossack KF, Eldridge JE, Buckner K: Comparison of acute hemodynamic effects of nitroglycerin versus diltiazem and combined acute effects of both drugs in angina pectoris. Am J Cardiol 58:722, 1986.

669. Lesbre JP, Eloy JP: An open comparison of amiodarone with diltiazem and glyceryl trinitrate in patients with stable exertional angina. Drugs 29:31, 1985.

670. Wallace WA, Wellington KL, Murphy GW, Liang C: Comparison of antianginal efficacies and exercise hemodynamic effects of nifedipine and diltiazem in stable angina pectoris. Am J Cardiol 63:414, 1989.

671. Klinke WP, Kvill L, Dempsey EE, Grace M: A randomized double-blind comparison of diltiazem and nifedipine in stable angina. J Am Coll Cardiol 12:1562, 1988.

672. Leon MB, Rosing DR, Bonow RO, et al: Combination therapy with calcium-channel blockers and beta blockers for chronic stable angina pectoris. Am J Cardiol 55:69B, 1985.

673. Kenny J, Kiff P, Holmes J, et al: Beneficial effects of diltiazem and propranolol, alone and in combination, in patients with stable angina pectoris. Br Heart J 53:43, 1985.

674. Hung J, Lamb IH, Connolly SJ, et al: The effect of diltiazem and propranolol, alone and in combination, on exercise performance and left ventricular function in patients with stable effort angina: A double-blind, randomized, and placebo-controlled study. Circulation 68:560, 1983.

675. Johnston DL, Lesoway R, Humen DP, et al: Clinical and hemodynamic evaluation of propranolol in combination with verapamil, nifedipine and diltiazem in exertional angina pectoris: A placebo-controlled, double-blind, randomized, crossover study. Am J Cardiol 55:680, 1985.

676. Boden WE, Bough EW, Reichman MJ, et al: Beneficial effects

of high-dose diltiazem in patients with persistent effort angina on beta-blockers and nitrates: A randomized, double-blind, placebo-controlled crossover study. Circulation 71:1197, 1985.

677. Schroeder JS, Hung J, Lamb IH, et al: The effect of diltiazem and propranolol, alone and in combination, on exercise performance and left ventricular function in patients with stable exertional angina. In Proceedings of the 8th Asian Pacific Congress on Cardiology, Taipei, 1983, pp 115–123.

678. Strauss WE, Parisi AF: Superiority of combined diltiazem and propranolol therapy for angina pectoris. Circulation 71:951, 1985.

679. Morse JR: Comparison of combination nifedipine-propranolol and diltiazem-propranolol with high dose diltiazem monotherapy for stable angina pectoris. Am J Cardiol 62:1028, 1988.

680. Humen DP, O'Brien P, Purves P, et al: Effort angina with adequate beta-receptor blockade: Comparison with diltiazem alone and in combination. J Am Coll Cardiol 7:329, 1986.

681. Miller WE, Vittitoe J, O'Rourke RA, Crawford MH: Nadolol versus diltiazem and combination for preventing exercise-induced ischemia in severe angina pectoris. Am J Cardiol 62:372, 1988.

682. Abrams J, Hoekenga D: Failure of combination antianginal therapy with diltiazem and nitroglycerin: Are two drugs better than one? J Am Coll Cardiol 7:27A, 1986.

683. James WE, Leman RB, Assey ME: Use of combined calcium channel blockers for therapy of refractory angina pectoris. J Sci Med Assoc 82:65, 1986.

684. Toyosaki N, Toyo-Oka T, Natsume T, et al: Combination therapy with diltiazem and nifedipine in patients with effort angina pectoris. Circulation 77:1370, 1988.

685. Frishman W, Charlap S, Kimmel B, et al: Diltiazem, nifedipine, and their combination in patients with stable angina pectoris: Effects on angina, exercise tolerance, and the ambulatory electrocardiographic ST segment. Circulation 77:774, 1988.

686. De Caprio L, Acanfora D, Odierna L, et al: Acute effects of nifedipine, diltiazem and their combination in patients with chronic stable angina: A double-blind, randomized, cross-over, placebo-controlled study. Eur Heart J 14:416, 1993.

687. Silke B, Goldhammer E, Sharma SK, et al: An exercise hemodynamic comparison of verapamil, diltiazem, and amlodipine in coronary artery disease. Cardiovasc Drugs Ther 4:457, 1990.

688. El Tamimi H, Davies GJ, Kaski JC, et al: Effects of diltiazem alone or with isosorbide dinitrate or with atenolol both acutely and chronically for stable angina pectoris. Am J Cardiol 64:717, 1989.

689. Schroeder JS, Lamb IH, Ginsburg R, et al: Diltiazem for long-term therapy of coronary arterial spasm. Am J Cardiol 49:533, 1982.

690. Schroeder JS, Lamb IH, Bristow MR, et al: Prevention of cardiovascular events in variant angina by long-term diltiazem therapy. J Am Coll Cardiol 1:1507, 1983.

691. Nakamura M, Koiwaya Y: Beneficial effect of diltiazem, a new antianginal drug, on angina pectoris at rest. Jpn Heart J 20:613, 1979.

692. Feldman RL, Pepine CJ, Whittle J, et al: Short- and long-term responses to diltiazem in patients with variant angina. Am J Cardiol 49:554, 1982.

693. Pepine CJ, Feldman RL, Whittle J, et al: Effect of diltiazem in patients with variant angina: A randomized double-blind trial. Am Heart J 101:719, 1981.

694. Rosenthal SJ, Ginsburg R, Lamb IH, et al: Efficacy of diltiazem for control of symptoms of coronary arterial spasm. Am J Cardiol 46:1027, 1980.

695. Schroeder JS, Feldman RL, Giles TD, et al: Multiclinic controlled trial of diltiazem for Prinzmetal's angina. Am J Med 72:227, 1982.

696. Schroeder JS, Walker SD, Skalland ML, et al: Absence of rebound from diltiazem therapy in Prinzmetal's variant angina. J Am Coll Cardiol 6:174, 1985.

697. Walker SD, Skalland ML, Hemberger JA, et al: Lack of rebound with diltiazem. Chest 84:335, 1983.

698. Yasue H, Takizawa A, Nagao M, et al: Pathogenesis of angina pectoris in patients with one-vessel disease: Possible role of dynamic coronary obstruction. Am Heart J 112:263, 1986.

699. Malpartida F, de la Morena G, Barba J, et al: Asociacion de nifedipina y diltiacem en el espasmo coronario rebelde. Valoracion mediante pruebas de provocacion. Rev Esp Cardiol 38:170, 1985.

700. Shimamoto M, Shinozaki T, Chihara K, et al: Surgical treatment for variant angina—diltiazem drip infusion to prevent perioperative spasm. Kyobu Geka 35:399, 1983.

701. Pepine CJ, Feldman RL, Hill JA, et al: Clinical outcome after treatment of rest angina with calcium blockers: Comparative experience during the initial year of therapy with diltiazem. nifedipine, and verapamil. Am Heart J 106:1341, 1983.

702. Yasue H, Omote S, Takizawa A, et al: Exertional angina pectoris caused by coronary arterial spasm: Effects of various drugs. Am J Cardiol 43:647, 1979.

703. Ambrosio G: Calcium-channel blockers in vasospastic angina—A review. Postgrad Med J 59:26, 1983.

704. Ferrini D, Bugiardini R, Galvani M, et al: Effetti opposti del propranololo e del diltiazem sulla soglia d'angina durante test da sforzo in pazienti con sindrome. G Ital Cardiol 16:224, 1986.

705. Tilmant PY, Lablanche JM, Thieuleux FA, et al: Detrimental effect of propranolol in patients with coronary arterial spasm countered by combination with diltiazem. Am J Cardiol 52:230, 1983.

706. Carver JR, Spitzer S, Mason D, et al: Diltiazem, nifedipine combination in coronary artery spasm. Chest 5:296, 1984.

707. Bourmayan C, Artigou JY, Barrillon AG, et al: Prinzmetal's variant angina unresponsive to calcium channel-blocking drugs but responsive to combined calcium channel- and beta-blocking drugs. Am J Cardiol 51:1792, 1983.

708. Bory M, Joly P, Bonnet JL, Coutelen N: Combined nifedipine and diltiazem in the treatment of refractory spastic angina. Arch Mal Coeur Vaiss 82:581, 1989.

709. Prida XE, Gelman JS, Feldman RL, et al: Comparison of diltiazem and nifedipine alone and in combination in patients with coronary artery spasm. J Am Coll Cardiol 9:412, 1987.

710. Ducloux G, Manouvrier J, Bajolet A, Guermonprez JL: Comparison of the effects of bepridil and diltiazem in Prinzmetal's angina. A crossed, randomized double-blind study of 14 observations. Ann Cardiol Angeiol 35:167, 1986.

711. Waters DD, Theroux P, Szlachicic J, et al: Provocative testing with ergonovine to assess the efficacy of treatment with nifedipine, diltiazem and verapamil in variant angina. Am J Cardiol 48:123, 1981.

712. Fabietti F, Vizza CD, Sciomer S, et al: The efficacy of diltiazem in effort-induced ischemia in patient with syndrome X. Cuore 7:777, 1990.

713. Theroux P, Taeymans Y, Morissette D, et al: A randomized study comparing propranolol and diltiazem in the treatment of unstable angina. J Am Coll Cardiol 5:717, 1985.

714. Andre-Fouet X, Usdin JP, Gayet CH, et al: Comparison of short-term efficacy of diltiazem and propranolol in unstable angina at rest—A randomized trial in 70 patients. Eur Heart J 4:691, 1983.

715. Gibelin P, Leonetti J, Morand P: Etude comparee en double insu de deux calcibloqueurs dans l'angor instable (bepridil et diltiazem). Rev Med 24:1317, 1983.

716. Hagemeijer F, Schelling A, Marinissen K, et al: Impending myocardial infarction treated intravenously with diltiazem [abstract 314]. Abstracts Cardiovascular Pharmacotherapy International Symposium, 1985.

717. Dumitriu M, Hillebrand W, Wieser HX: Combined antianginal treatment with diltiazem and nifedipine in elderly patients with severe mixed angina. Herz Kreislauf 25:41, 1993.

718. Medvedowsky JL, Barnay C, Hanvic G: Le traitement de l'angine de poitrine instable par l'association amiodarone-diltiazem. Ann Cardiol Angeiol (Paris) 31:339, 1982.

719. Colombo G, Zucchella G, Planca E, et al: Intravenous diltiazem in the treatment of unstable angina: A study of efficacy and tolerance. Clin Ther 9:536, 1987.

720. Wernisch M, Suntinger A, Sterz H: Clinical experience with parenteral diltiazem in the treatment of angina pectoris. Ther Osterr 6:820, 1991.

721. Stephinger U: Comparison between i.v. Diltiazem versus i.v. Nitroglycerin in the treatment of unstable angina pectoris. Herz Kreislauf 20:54, 1988.

722. Fang ZY, Picart N, Abramowicz M, et al: Intravenous diltia-

zem versus nitroglycerin for silent and symptomatic myocardial ischemia in unstable angina pectoris. Am J Cardiol 68:42C, 1991.

723. Theroux P, Baird M, Juneau M, et al: Effect of diltiazem on symptomatic and asymptomatic episodes of ST segment depression occurring during daily life and during exercise. Circulation 84:15, 1991.

724. Zharov EI, Galichenko IV, Martynov AI, et al: Effect of diltiazem on silent myocardial ischemia. Kardiologiya 31:15, 1991.

725. Van der Wall EE, Cats VM, Blokland JAK, et al: The effects of diltiazem on cardiac function in silent ischemia after myocardial infarction. Am Heart J 118:655, 1989.

726. Gibelin P, Benoit Ph, Camous JP, et al: Tolerance clinique et hemodynamique du diltiazem intraveineux a la phase aigue de l'infarctus du myocarde. Ann Cardiol Angeiol (Paris) 34:263, 1985.

727. Sakai M, Ueda K, Nakahara K, et al: Comparative effects of three calcium antagonists (nifedipine, verapamil, diltiazem) on hemodynamics in recent myocardial infarction. Kokyu To Junkan 33:159, 1985.

728. Zannad F, Amor M, Karcher G, et al: Effect of diltiazem on myocardial infarct size estimated by enzyme release, serial thallium-201 single-photon emission computed tomography and radionuclide angiography. Am J Cardiol 61:1172, 1988.

729. Corcos T, David PR, Val PG, et al: Failure of diltiazem to prevent restenosis after percutaneous transluminal coronary angioplasty. Am Heart J 109:926, 1985.

730. Wolf JE (DTZ Multicentered French Study): Diltiazem may limit the extension of acute anterior myocardial infarction in man [abstract #338]. Abstracts Cardiovascular Pharmacotherapy International Symposium, 1985.

731. Schioppa M, Rengo F, De CL, et al: Valutazione clinica del diltiazem nell'angina post-infartuale. Cardiologia 30:375, 1985.

732. Nakamura M, Koiwaya Y: Effect of diltiazem on recurrent spontaneous angina after acute myocardial infarction. Circulation Res 52:I-158, 1983.

733. Koiwaya Y, Torii S, Takeshita A, et al: Postinfarction angina caused by coronary arterial spasm. Circulation 65:275, 1982.

734. Berthout P, Bassand J, Schipman C, et al: Activite anti-ischemique comparee de l'atenolol et du diltiazem. Rev Med Interne 6:259, 1985.

735. Ghio S, De Servi S, Ferrario M, et al: Acute haemodynamic effects of diltiazem in patients with recent Q-wave myocardial infarction. Eur Heart J 9:740, 1988.

736. Ogawa H, Yasue H, Nakamura N, et al: Hemodynamic effects of intravenous diltiazem in patients with acute myocardial infarction. Clin Cardiol 10:323, 1987.

737. Renard M, Sterling I, Van Camp G, et al: Comparison of the effects of intravenous diltiazem vs placebo on hemodynamics and blood gases in the acute phase of myocardial infarction. Ann Cardiol Angeiol 36:509, 1987.

738. Bostrom PA, Lilja B, Johansson BW, Meier K: The effect of oral diltiazem on left ventricular performance in postinfarction patients. Clin Cardiol 11:739, 1988.

739. Gibson RS, Boden WE, Theroux P, et al: Diltiazem and reinfarction in patients with non-Q-wave myocardial infarction. N Engl J Med 315:423, 1986.

740. Pratt CM, Gibson R, Boden W, et al: Design of a multicenter, double-blind study to assess the effects of prophylactic diltiazem on early reinfarction after non-Q-wave myocardial infarction: Diltiazem reinfarction study. Am J Cardiol 58:906, 1986.

741. Gibson RS, Young PM, Boden WE, et al: Prognostic significance and beneficial effect of diltiazem on the incidence of early recurrent ischemia after non-Q-wave myocardial infarction: Results from the multicenter diltiazem reinfarction study. Am J Cardiol 60:203, 1987.

742. Cook JR, Bigger J Jr, Kleiger RE, et al: Effect of atenolol and diltiazem on heart period variability in normal persons. J Am Coll Cardiol 17:480, 1991.

743. The Multicenter Diltiazem Postinfarction Trial Research Group: The effect of diltiazem on mortality and reinfarction after myocardial infarction. N Engl J Med 319:385, 1988.

744. Moss AJ, Oakes D, Benhorin J, Carleen E: The interaction between diltiazem and left ventricular function after myocardial infarction. Circulation 80(Suppl IV):102, 1989.

745. Bigger J Jr, Coromilas J, Rolnitzky LM, et al: Effect of diltiazem on cardiac rate and rhythm after myocardial infarction. Am J Cardiol 65:539, 1990.

746. Boden WE, Krone RJ, Kleiger RE, et al: Electrocardiographic subset analysis of diltiazem administration on long-term outcome after acute myocardial infarction. Am J Cardiol 67:335, 1991.

747. Boden WE: Management of non-Q-wave myocardial infarction: Role of diltiazem versus beta-blocker therapy. J Cardiovasc Pharmacol 6(Suppl):S55, 1990.

748. Boden WE, Kleiger RE, Miller JP, et al: Favorable effect of diltiazem on late mortality and reinfarction after non-Q-wave myocardial infarction: Multicenter Diltiazem Post-Infarction Trial (MDPIT). J Am Coll Cardiol 13:6A, 1989.

749. Krone RJ, Boden WE, Kleiger RE, et al: Prophylactic diltiazem benefits patients with non-Q-wave myocardial infarction without pulmonary congestion or prior MI. The Multicenter Diltiazem Postinfarction Trial (MDPIT). Circulation 78:II-258, 1988.

750. Boden WE, Greenberg H, Kleiger RE, et al: Role of electrocardiographic location on diltiazem treatment effect in non-Q wave myocardial infarction: Multicenter Diltiazem Post-Infarction Trial (MDPIT). J Am Coll Cardiol 13:6A, 1989.

751. Wong SC, Greenberg H, Hager WD, Dwyer Jr EM: Effects of diltiazem on recurrent myocardial infarction in patients with non-Q wave myocardial infarction. J Am Coll Cardiol 19:1421, 1992.

752. Moss AJ, Oakes D, Rubison M, et al: Effects of diltiazem on long-term outcome after acute myocardial infarction in patients with and without a history of systemic hypertension. Am J Cardiol 68:429, 1991.

753. Boden WE, Gibson RS, Bough EW, et al: Effect of high-dose diltiazem on global and regional left ventricular function during the early course of acute non-Q wave myocardial infarction. Am J Noninvasive Cardiol 2:1, 1988.

754. The Danish Study Group on Verapamil in Myocardial Infarction: Secondary prevention with verapamil after myocardial infarction. Am J Cardiol 66:33I, 1990.

755. Yusuf S, Held P, Furberg C: Update of effects of calcium antagonists in myocardial infarction or angina in light of the second Danish verapamil infarction trial (DAVIT-II) and other recent studies. Am J Cardiol 67:1295, 1991.

756. Rose GC, Jordan JC, Jolly SR: Intracoronary diltiazem limits infarct size during prolonged angioplasty balloon inflation. Drug Dev Res 28:460, 1993.

757. Kern MJ, Pearson A, Woodruff R, et al: Hemodynamic and echocardiographic assessment of the effects of diltiazem during transient occlusion of the left anterior descending coronary artery during percutaneous transluminal coronary angioplasty. Am J Cardiol 64:849, 1989.

758. Kern MJ, Deligonul U, Labovitz A: Effects of diltiazem and nifedipine on systemic and coronary hemodynamics and ischemic responses during transient coronary artery occlusion in patients. Am Heart J 119:47, 1990.

759. Piessens J, Brzostek T, Stammen F, et al: Effect of intravenous diltiazem on myocardial ischemia occurring during percutaneous transluminal coronary angioplasty. Am J Cardiol 64:1103, 1989.

760. O'Keefe J Jr, Giorgi LV, Hartzler GO, et al: Effects of diltiazem on complications and restenosis after coronary angioplasty. Am J Cardiol 67:373, 1991.

761. Elert O, Schanzenbacher P: Effect of nifedipine, diltiazem and sin-1A on regional myocardial perfusion after selective application into aortocoronary bypass grafts immediately following bypass surgery. Herz Kreislauf 22:362, 1990.

762. Ravazzi PA, Villa M, Martinelli V, et al: Valutazione delle modificazioni indotte dal diltiazem 120 mg, in pazienti affetti da cardiopatia ischemica, mediante test da sforzo al cicloergometro. Minerva Cardioangiol 34:493, 1986.

763. Abe T: Clinical trial of diltiazem hydrochloride in hypertension. Mod Clin Med 20:1255, 1978.

764. Akihama T, Mamiya S, Miura A, et al: Clincial effect of diltiazem hydrochloride (Herbesser) in hypertension. Mod Clin Med 20:1507, 1978.

765. Aoki K, Sato K, Kondo S, et al: Hypotensive effects of diltiazem to normals and essential hypertensives. Eur J Clin Pharmacol 25:475, 1983.

766. Akanabe H, Ishiguro M, Yagi Y, et al: Effect of diltiazem hydrochloride in essential hypertension. Int J Clin Pharmacol Ther Toxicol 23:63, 1985.

767. Lewis JE, Balfour DC, Brown SG, et al: Diltiazem in hypertension: A preliminary dose-finding and efficacy multicenter study. Curr Ther Res Clin Exp 37:566, 1985.

768. Amodeo C, Kobrin I, Ventura HO, et al: Immediate and short-term hemodynamic effects of diltiazem in patients with hypertension. Circulation 73:108, 1986.

769. Akahoshi M, Aoi W, Baba K, et al: Long term effects of diltiazem on renin-angiotensin system and hemodynamics in essential hypertension. Jpn Pharmacol Ther 10:389, 1982.

770. O'Rourke RA: Rationale for calcium entry-blocking drugs in systemic hypertension complicated by coronary artery disease. Am J Cardiol 56:34H, 1985.

771. Rosatti F, Cella PL, Fici F, et al: Diltiazem in the therapy of arterial hypertension: Polygraphic assessment of left ventricular performance. Curr Ther Res Clin Exp 36:701, 1984.

772. Ohta T: Long-term observation on clinical hypotensive effect of diltiazem hydrochloride. Clin Rep 12:2833, 1978.

773. Klein W: Long-term treatment of hypertension with the calcium channel blocker diltiazem. Clin Cardiol 10:358, 1987.

774. Weir MR, Haynie R, Vertes V, et al: A comparison of the efficacy and tolerability of enalapril and sustained-release diltiazem in mild to moderate essential hypertension. Clin Ther 12:473, 1990.

775. Weir MR, Weber MA, Punzi HA, et al: A dose escalation trial comparing the combination of diltiazem SR and hydrochlorothiazide with the monotherapies in patients with essential hypertension. J Hum Hypertens 6:133, 1992.

776. Shepherd AMM, LeForce C, Park GD, et al: The determinants of response to diltiazem in hypertension. Clin Pharmacol Ther 50:338, 1991.

777. Montamat SC, Abernethy DR: Calcium antagonists in geriatric patients: Diltiazem in elderly persons with hypertension. Clin Pharmacol Ther 45:682, 1989.

778. Burris JF, Weir MR, Oparil S, et al: An assessment of diltiazem and hydrochlorothiazide in hypertension: Application of factorial trial design to a multicenter clinical trial of combination therapy. JAMA 263:1507, 1990.

779. Elkik F, Claudel S, Carcone B, Grippon P: Demographic factors and response to hypertensive treatment. Diltiazem fixed dose study. Arch Mal Coeur Vaiss 82:1299, 1989.

780. Elkik F, Claudel S, Carcone B, Grippon P: Demographic factors and the antihypertensive effect of diltiazem. J Cardiovasc Pharmacol 17:685, 1991.

781. Massie B, MacCarthy EP, Ramanathan KB, et al: Diltiazem and propranolol in mild to moderate essential hypertension as monotherapy or with hydrochlorothiazide. Ann Intern Med 107:150, 1987.

782. Herpin D, Brion N, Debregeas B: Comparison of the antihypertensive effects of sustained-release diltiazem 240 and 300 mg in patients with mild to moderate hypertension with analysis of ambulatory blood pressure profiles. Curr Ther Res Clin Exp 47:328, 1990.

783. Pool PE, Salel AF: New antihypertensive agents: Part III. Sustained-release diltiazem in hypertension: Clinical safety and efficacy. Pract Cardiol 16:52, 1990.

784. Whelton A, Eff J, Magner DJ: Sustained antihypertensive activity of diltiazem SR: Double-blind, placebo-controlled study with 24-hour ambulatory blood pressure monitoring. J Clin Pharmacol 32:808, 1992.

785. Pool PE, Applegate WB, Woehler T, et al: A randomized, controlled trial comparing diltiazem SR, hydrochlorothiazide, or their combination in the therapy of essential hypertension. Pharmacotherapy 13:487, 1993.

786. Nikkila M, Inkovaara J, Heikkinen J: Once daily compared with twice daily administration of slow-release diltiazem as monotherapy for hypertension. Ann Med 23:141, 1991.

787. Schule KL: Comparison of antihypertensive efficacy and safety of the calcium channel-blockers diltiazem and nitrendipine at rest and during exercise under once-daily medication. Herz Kreislauf 25:154, 1993.

788. Schulte KL, Lenz T: Diltiazem 180 mg—effective blood pressure reduction with a daily single dosage in the therapy of essential hypertension? Herz Kreislauf 23:264, 1991.

789. Woehler TR, Eff J, Graney W, et al: Multicenter evaluation of the efficacy and safety of sustained-release diltiazem hydrochloride for the treatment of hypertension. Clin Ther 14:148, 1992.

790. Djian J, Roy M, Forette B, et al: Efficacy and tolerance of sustained-release diltiazem 300 mg and a diuretic in the elderly. J Cardiovasc Pharmacol 16(Suppl 1):S51, 1990.

791. Djian J, Ferme I, Zannad F, et al: Effects of sustained-release diltiazem on blood pressure and serum lipids: A multicenter, randomized, placebo-controlled study. J Cardiovasc Pharmacol 16(Suppl 1):S38, 1990.

792. Dupont AG, Coupez JM, Jensen P, et al: Twenty-four hour ambulatory blood pressure profile of a new slow-release formulation of diltiazem in mild to moderate hypertension. Cardiovasc Drugs Ther 5:701, 1991.

793. Felicetta JV, Serfer HM, Cutler NR, et al: A dose-response trial of once-daily diltiazem. Am Heart J 123:1022, 1992.

794. Ferme I, Djian J, Tcherdakoff P: Comparative study on monotherapy with sustained-release diltiazem 300 mg and enalapril 20 mg in mild to moderate arterial hypertension. J Cardiovasc Pharmacol 16(Suppl 1):S46, 1990.

795. Massie BM, Der E, Herman TS, et al: 24-Hour efficacy of once-daily diltiazem in essential hypertension. Clin Cardiol 15:365, 1992.

796. Senda Y, Tohkai H, Kimura M, et al: ECG-gated cardiac scan and echocardiographic assessment of left ventricular hypertrophy: Reversal by 6-month treatment with diltiazem. J Cardiovasc Pharmacol 16:298, 1990.

797. Szlachcic J, Tubau JF, Vollmer C, Massie BM: Effect of diltiazem on left ventricular mass and diastolic filling in mild to moderate hypertension. Am J Cardiol 63:198, 1989.

798. Giesecke HJ, Guckenbiehl W, Hagemann I: Ergebnisse einer multicenter-studie mit diltiazem bei hypertonie. In Bender F, Greeff K (eds): Calciumantagonisten zur Behandlung der Angina Pectoris, Hypertonie und Arrhythmie, First Dilzem Symposium, Copenhagen, June 1981. Amsterdam: Excerpta Medica, 1982, pp 220–226.

799. Ikeda M, Aoki K, Arakawa K, et al: Clinical effect of diltiazem (Herbesser) on essential hypertension—comparison with placebo by double-blind method. Med Prog 110:302, 1979.

800. Pool PE, Reeves RL, Weber MA, for the Multicenter Investigators: Antihypertensive monotherapy with tablet (prompt-release) diltiazem: Multicenter controlled trials. Cardiovasc Drug Ther 4:1089, 1990.

801. Pool PE, Herron JM, Rosenblatt S, et al: Sustained-release diltiazem: Duration of antihypertensive effect. J Clin Pharmacol 29:533, 1989.

802. Pool PE, Herron JM, Rosenblatt S, et al: Metabolic effects of antihypertensive therapy with a calcium antagonist. Am J Cardiol 62:109G, 1988.

803. Pool PE, Massie BM, Venkataraman K, et al: Diltiazem as monotherapy for systemic hypertension: A multicenter, randomized, placebo-controlled trial. Am J Cardiol 57:212, 1986.

804. Sunderrajan S, Reams G, Bauer JH: Renal effects of diltiazem in primary hypertension. Hypertension 8:238, 1986.

805. Frishman WH, Charlap S, Michelson EL: Calcium channel blockers in systemic hypertension. Am J Cardiol 58:157, 1986.

806. Inouye IK, Massie BM, Benowitz N, et al: Antihypertensive therapy with diltiazem and comparison with hydrochlorothiazide. Am J Cardiol 53:1588, 1984.

807. Frishman WH, Kirkendall W, Lunn J, et al: Diuretics versus calcium-channel blockers in systemic hypertension: A preliminary multicenter experience with hydrochlorothiazide and sustained-release diltiazem. Am J Cardiol 56:92H, 1985.

808. Zawada ET, Williams L, McClung DE, et al: Renal-metabolic consequences of antihypertensive therapy with diltiazem versus hydrochlorothiazide. Mineral Electrolyte Metab 13:72, 1987.

809. Frishman WH, Zawada ET, Smith LK, et al: Comparison of hydrochlorothiazide and sustained-release diltiazem for mild-to-moderate systemic hypertension. Am J Cardiol 59:615, 1987.

810. Ogawa K, Ban M, Ito N, et al: Diltiazem for treatment of essential hypertension: A double-blind controlled study with reserpine. Clin Ther 6:844, 1984.

811. Yamakado T, Oonishi N, Kondo S, et al: Effects of diltiazem

on cardiovascular responses during exercise in systemic hypertension and comparison with propranolol. Am J Cardiol 52:1023, 1983.

812. Weiss RJ, Bent B: Diltiazem-induced left ventricular mass regression in hypertensive patients. J Clin Hypertens 3:135, 1987.

813. Chellingsworth MC, Kendall MJ, Wright AD, et al: The effects of verapamil, diltiazem, nifedipine and propranolol on metabolic control in hypertensives with non-insulin dependent diabetes mellitus. J Hum Hypertens 3:35, 1989.

814. Boeijinga JK, Aghina-JCFM, Breimer DD: Diltiazem versus propranolol in borderline and mild hypertension. Efficacy and tolerance in a double-blind study. Curr Ther Res Clin Exp 47:184, 1990.

815. Trimarco B, DeLuca N, Ricciardelli B, et al: Diltiazem in the treatment of mild or moderate essential hypertension. Comparison with metoprolol in a crossover double-blind trial. J Clin Pharmacol 24:218, 1984.

816. Lacourciere Y, Poirier L, Boucher S, Spenard J: Comparative effects of diltiazem sustained-release formulation and metoprolol on ambulatory blood pressure and plasma lipoproteins. Clin Pharmacol Ther 48:318, 1990.

817. Hedner T, Thulin T, Gustafsson S, Olsson SO: A comparison of diltiazem and metoprolol in hypertension. Eur J Clin Pharmacol 39:427, 1990.

818. Dahlof C, Hedner T, Thulin T, et al: Effects of diltiazem and metoprolol on blood pressure, adverse symptoms and general well-being. Eur J Clin Pharmacol 40:453, 1991.

819. Weir MR, Josselson J, Giard MJ, et al: Sustained-release diltiazem compared with atenolol monotherapy for mild to moderate systemic hypertension. Am J Cardiol 60:36I, 1987.

820. Tonkin AL, Wing LMH, Russell AE, et al: Diltiazem and atenolol in essential hypertension: Additivity of effects on blood pressure and cardiac conduction with combination therapy. J Hypertens 8:1015, 1990.

821. Wolfson P, Abernathy D, DiPette DJ, Zusman R: Diltiazem and captopril alone or in combination for treatment of mild to moderate systemic hypertension. Am J Cardiol 62:103G, 1988.

822. Lacourciere Y, Poirier L, Boucher S, Spenard J: Comparative effects of diltiazem sustained-release and captopril on blood pressure control and plasma lipoproteins in primary hypertension: A randomized, double-blind, crossover study. J Hum Hypertens 4:553, 1990.

823. Black HR, Lewin AJ, Stein GH, et al: A comparison of the safety of therapeutically equivalent doses of isradipine and diltiazem for treatment of essential hypertension. Am J Hypertens 5:141, 1992.

824. Naukkarinen VA, Nieminen MS: Comparison of nicardipine and diltiazem in the treatment of mild and moderate hypertension. Curr Ther Res Clin Exp 51:582, 1992.

825. Heilmann E: Comparison between diltiazem and nitrendipine in essential hypertension. Z Allgemeinmed 68:642, 1992.

826. Frishman WH, Charlap S, Kimmel B, et al: Calcium-channel blockers for combined angina pectoris and systemic hypertension. Am J Cardiol 57:22D, 1986.

827. Klein WW: Treatment of hypertension with calcium channel blockers: European data. Am J Med 77:143, 1984.

828. Yamakado T, Oonishi N, Nakano T, et al: Effects of nifedipine and diltiazem on hemodynamic responses at rest and during exercise in hypertensive patients. Jpn Circ J 49:415, 1985.

829. Schulte KL, Meyer-Sabellek WA, Haertenberger A, et al: Effects of diltiazem and nifedipine on blood pressure, plasma catecholamines and serum lipoproteins in essential hypertension. J Hypertens 3:423, 1985.

830. Trimarco B, Volpe M, Ricciardelli B, et al: Valutazione clinica del diltiazem nel trattamento dell' ipertensione arteriosa essenziale. Confronto con il verapamil. Rass Int Clin Ter 62:1593, 1982.

831. Hollifield JW, Heusner JJ, DesChamps MK, Gray J: A double-blind, randomized, crossover comparison of equivalent (by weight) oral doses of verapamil and diltiazem in patients with mild to moderate hypertension. J Cardiovasc Pharmacol 4:S68, 1989.

832. Frishman WH, Weinberg P, Peled HB, et al: Calcium entry blockers for the treatment of severe hypertension and hypertensive crisis. Am J Med 77:35, 1984.

833. Retamal O, Coriat P, Pamela F, et al: Prevention des poussees hypertensives apres chirurgie carotidienne. Interet de la nifedipine et du diltiazem. Ann Fr Anesth Reanim 5:278, 1986.

834. Koh H, Hashimoto Y, Takagi H, et al: Clinical study of total intravenous anesthesia with droperidol, fentanyl and ketamine—effects of nicardipine, diltiazem and nifedipine on intraoperative hypertension. Jpn J Anesthesiol 42:217, 1993.

835. Mullen JC, Miller DR, Weisel RD, et al: A comparison of diltiazem, nifedipine, and nitroprusside. J Thorac Cardiovasc Surg 96:122, 1988.

836. Chockalingam A, Robitaille MN, Annable L, et al: Diltiazem and hydrochlorothiazide/triamterene as initial therapy for mild to moderate essential hypertension. A comparative study. Drug Invest 4:173, 1992.

837. Schulte KL, Meyer-Sabellek W, Rocker L, et al: Effects of diltiazem alone and combined with mefruside on cardiovascular response at rest and during exercise, carbohydrate metabolism and serum lipoproteins in patients with systemic hypertension. Am J Cardiol 60:826, 1987.

838. Thulin T, Hedner T, Gustafsson S, Olsson SO: Diltiazem compared with metoprolol as add-on therapies to diuretics in hypertension. J Hum Hypertens 5:107,1991.

839. Lueg MC, Herron J, Zellner S: Transdermal clonidine as an adjuvant to sustained-release diltiazem in the treatment of mild-to-moderate hypertension. Clin Ther 13:471, 1991.

840. Busse JC, De-Velasco RE, Pellegrini EL: Combined use of nifedipine and diltiazem for the treatment of severe hypertension. South Med J 84:502, 1991.

841. Kawanishi DT, Leman RB, Pratt CM, O'Rourke RA: Efficacy and safety of sustained-release diltiazem as replacement therapy for beta blockers and diuretics for stable angina pectoris and coexisting essential hypertension: A multicenter trial. Am J Cardiol 60:29, 1987.

842. Moser M, Lunn J, Materson BJ: Comparative effects of diltiazem and hydrochlorothiazide in blacks with systemic hypertension. Am J Cardiol 56:101H, 1985.

843. Schwartz JB, Abernathy DR: Responses to intravenous and oral diltiazem in elderly and younger patients with systemic hypertension. Am J Cardiol 59:1111, 1987.

844. Leehey DJ, Hartman E: Comparison of diltiazem and hydrochlorothiazide for treatment of patients 60 years of age or older with systemic hypertension. Am J Cardiol 62:1218, 1988.

845. Materson BJ, Reda DJ, Cushman WC, et al: Single-drug therapy for hypertension in men—A comparison of six antihypertensive agents with placebo. N Engl J Med 328:914, 1993.

846. Lund-Johansen P, Omvik P: Effect of long-term diltiazem treatment on central haemodynamics and exercise endurance in essential hypertension. Eur Heart J 11:543, 1990.

847. Szlachcic J, Hirsch AT, Tubau JF, et al: Diltiazem versus propranolol in essential hypertension: Responses of rest and exercise blood pressure and effects on exercise capacity. Am J Cardiol 59:393, 1987.

848. Myburgh DP, Gordon NF: Comparison of diltiazem and atenolol in young, physically active men with essential hypertension. Am J Cardiol 60:1092, 1987.

849. Cohen-Solal A, Baleynaud S, Laperche T, et al: Cardiopulmonary response during exercise of a beta-1-selective beta-blocker (atenolol) and a calcium-channel blocker (diltiazem) in untrained subjects with hypertension. J Cardiovasc Pharmacol 22:33, 1993.

850. Stewart KJ, Effron MB, Valenti SA, Kelemen MH: Exercise training versus exercise training with diltiazem or propranolol: Effects on lipids in men with mild hypertension. J Am Coll Cardiol 13:241A, 1989.

851. Luurila OJ, Gröhn P, Heikkilä J, et al: Exercise capacity and hemodynamics in persons aged 20 to 50 years with systemic hypertension treated with diltiazem and atenolol. Am J Cardiol 60:832, 1987.

852. Luurila OJ, Kohvakka A, Sundberg S: Comparison of blood pressure response to heat stress in sauna in young hypertensive patients treated with atenolol and diltiazem. Am J Cardiol 64:97, 1989.

853. Isojima K, Takase B, Arakawa K, et al: Effects of diltiazem on hemodynamics, plasma catecholamine and renin activity during exercise in hypertension. J Cardiol 21:383, 1991.

854. Motz W, Vogt M, Scheler S, et al: Prophylaxis with vascular-effective substances. Z Kardiol 81(Suppl 4): 199, 1992.
855. Ramanathan KB, Ratts TE, Griffin B, Sullivan JM: Comparative effects of propranolol and diltiazem on systolic and diastolic left ventricular function in essential hypertension. J Hum Hypertens 4:677, 1990.
856. Massie BM: Antihypertensive therapy with calcium-channel blockers: Comparison with beta blockers. Am J Cardiol 56:97H, 1985.
857. Dougherty AH, Jackman WM, Naccarelli GV, et al: Acute conversion of paroxysmal supraventricular tachycardia with intravenous diltiazem. Am J Cardiol 70:587, 1992.
858. Hung JS, Yeh SJ, Lin FC, et al: Usefulness of intravenous diltiazem in predicting subsequent electrophysiologic and clinical responses to oral diltiazem. Am J Cardiol 54:1259, 1984.
859. Ito R, Yamamoto S, Takagi S, et al: Electrophysiologic effects of diltiazem hydrochloride on supraventricular tachycardia. Yakuro to Chiryo 11:107, 1983.
860. Jauernig R, Gao TL, Rizos I, et al: Electrophysiological studies in assessment of diltiazem for paroxysmal supraventricular tachycardia: Clinical and experimental results. In Fleckenstein A, Hashimoto K, Herrmann M, et al (eds): New Calcium Antagonists: Recent Developments and Prospects, Diltiazem Workshop, Freiburg, Breisgau, May 1982. Stuttgart, Germany: Gustav Fischer, 1983, pp 221–223.
861. Betrui A, Chaitman BR, Bourassa MG, et al: Beneficial effect of intravenous diltiazem in the acute management of paroxysmal supraventricular tachyarrhythmias. Circulation 67:88, 1983.
862. Sternbach GL, Schroeder JS, Eliastam M, et al: Intravenous diltiazem for the treatment of supraventricular tachycardia. Clin Cardiol 9:145, 1986.
863. Huycke EC, Sung RJ, Dias VC, et al: Intravenous diltiazem for termination of reentrant supraventricular tachycardia: A placebo-controlled, randomized, double-blind, multicenter study. J Am Coll Cardiol 13:538, 1989.
864. Manz M, Steinbeck G, Luederitz B: Comments concerning the effect of diltiazem in supraventricular tachycardia [German]. In Bender F, Greeff K (eds): Calciumantagonisten zur Behandlung der Angina Pectoris, Hypertonie und Arrhythmie, First Dilzem Symposium, Copenhagen, June, 1981. Amsterdam: Excerpta Medica, 1982, pp 297–306.
865. Mitsuoka T, Yano K, Matsumoto Y, et al: The effects of intravenous diltiazem on supraventricular arrhythmias. Jpn Heart J 23:124, 1982.
866. Naito M, Mitani I, Masao I, et al: Beneficial effect of intravenous diltiazem on supraventricular tachyarrhythmias. J Am Coll Cardiol 5:481, 1985.
867. Roti E, Montermini M, Roti S, et al: The effect of diltiazem, a calcium channel-blocking drug, on cardiac rate and rhythm in hyperthyroid patients. Arch Intern Med 148:1919, 1988.
868. Yeh SJ, Kou HC, Lin FC, et al: Effects of oral diltiazem in paroxysmal supraventricular tachycardia. Am J Cardiol 52:271, 1983.
869. Clair WK, Wilkinson WE, McCarthy EA, Pritchett ELC: Treatment of paroxysmal supraventricular tachycardia with oral diltiazem. Clin Pharmacol Ther 51:562, 1992.
870. Yeh, SJ, Lin FC, Chou YY, et al: Termination of paroxysmal supraventricular tachycardia with a single oral dose of diltiazem and propranolol. Circulation 71:104, 1985.
871. Hamer A, Tanasescu DE, Marks JW, et al: Failure of episodic high-dose oral verapamil therapy to convert supraventricular tachycardia: A study of plasma verapamil levels and gastric motility. Am Heart J 114:334, 1987
872. Akino E, Fujii S, Kanda K, et al: Effect of diltiazem on serum digoxin concentration and diurnal changes of ventricular rate in patient with atrial fibrillation. Yakuri To Chiryo 11:307, 1983.
873. Shenasa M, Fromer M, Faugere G, et al: Efficacy and safety of intravenous and oral diltiazem for Wolff-Parkinson-White syndrome. Am J Cardiol 59:301, 1987.
874. Ochs HR, Anda L, Eichelbaum M, et al: Diltiazem, verapamil, and quinidine in patients with chronic atrial fibrillation. J Clin Pharmacol 25:204, 1985.
875. Roth A, Harrison E, Mitani G, et al: Efficacy and safety of medium- and high-dose diltiazem alone and in combination with digoxin for control of heart rate at rest and during exercise in patients with chronic atrial fibrillation. Circulation 73:316, 1986.
876. Ellenbogen KA, Dias VC, Plumb VJ, et al: A placebo-controlled trial of continuous intravenous diltiazem infusion for 24-hour heart rate control during atrial fibrillation and atrial flutter: A multicenter study. J Am Coll Cardiol 18:891, 1991.
877. Dias VC, Weir SJ, Ellenbogen KA: Pharmacokinetics and pharmacodynamics of intravenous diltiazem in patients with atrial fibrillation or atrial flutter. Circulation 86:1421, 1992.
878. Heywood JT, Graham B, Marais GE, Jutzy KR: Effects of intravenous diltiazem on rapid atrial fibrillation accompanied by congestive heart failure. Am J Cardiol 67:1150, 1991.
879. Salerno DM, Dias VC, Kleiger RE, et al: Efficacy and safety of intravenous diltiazem for treatment of atrial fibrillation and atrial flutter. Am J Cardiol 63:1046, 1989.
880. Maragno I, Santostasi G, Gaion RM, et al: Low- and medium-dose diltiazem in chronic atrial fibrillation: Comparison with digoxin and correlation with drug plasma levels. Am Heart J 116:385, 1988.
881. Lundstrom T, Ryden L: Ventricular rate control and exercise performance in chronic atrial fibrillation: Effects of diltiazem and verapamil. J Am Coll Cardiol 16:86, 1990.
882. Vitale P, Auricchio A, De Stefano R, et al: Efficacy of diltiazem to control heart rate and to improve exercise capacity in chronic atrial fibrillation. Double-blind cross-over study. Cardiologia 34:73, 1989.
883. Dahlstrom CG, Edvardsson N, Nasheng C, Olsson SB: Effects of diltiazem, propranolol, and their combination in the control of atrial fibrillation. Clin Cardiol 15:280, 1992.
884. Atwood JE, Myers JN, Sullivan MJ, et al: Diltiazem and exercise performance in patients with chronic atrial fibrillation. Chest 93:20, 1988.
885. Bischoff KO, Lueg L, Standop M: Negative-dromotropic effect of diltiazem in chronic atrial fibrillation at rest and during exercise. Herz Kreislauf 24:156, 1992.
886. Maragno I, Santostasi G, Alitto F, et al: Efficacy of diltiazem for control of ventricular rate in chronic atrial fibrillation. Cardiologia 32:1019, 1987.
887. Talajic M, Nayebpour M, Jing W, Nattel S: Amplification of diltiazem's effects on the AV node by rapid atrial input leads to selective actions during atrial fibrillation. J Am Coll Cardiol 13:164A, 1989.
888. Steinberg JS, Katz RJ, Bren GB, et al: Efficacy of oral diltiazem to control ventricular response in chronic atrial fibrillation at rest and during exercise. J Am Coll Cardiol 9:405, 1987.
889. Shenasa M, Kus T, Fromer M, et al: Effect of intravenous and oral calcium antagonists (diltiazem and verapamil) on sustenance of atrial fibrillation. Am J Cardiol 62:403, 1988.
890. Salerno JA, Previtali M, Panciroli C, et al: Ventricular arrhythmias during acute myocardial ischaemia in man. The role and significance of R-ST-T alternans and the prevention of ischaemic sudden death by medical treatment. Eur Heart J 7A:63, 1986.
891. Gill JS, Ward DE, Camm AJ: Comparison of verapamil and diltiazem in the suppression of idiopathic ventricular tachycardia. Pace 15:2122, 1992.
892. Weishaar RE, Burrows SD, Kim SN, et al: Protection of the failing heart: Comparative effects of chronic administration of digitalis and diltiazem on myocardial metabolism in the cardiomyopathic hamster. J Appl Cardiol 2:339, 1987.
893. Toshima H, Koga Y, Nagata H, et al: Comparable effects of oral diltiazem and verapamil in the treatment of hypertrophic cardiomyopathy. Double-blind crossover study. Jpn Heart J 27:701, 1986.
894. Iwase M, Sotobata I, Takagi S, et al: Effects of diltiazem on left ventricular diastolic behavior in patients with hypertrophic cardiomyopathy: Evaluation with exercise pulsed Doppler echocardiography. J Am Coll Cardiol 9:1099, 1987.
895. Kulick DL, McIntosh N, Campese VM, et al: Central and renal hemodynamic effects and hormonal response to diltiazem in severe congestive heart failure. Am J Cardiol 59:1138, 1987.
896. Halabi A, Linde M, Saathoff H, et al: Hemodynamic effects of diltiazem and nitrendipine assessed by noninvasive methods

in patients with congestive heart failure. Am J Noninvasive Cardiol 4:60, 1990.

897. Figulla HR, Rechenberg JV, Wiegand V, et al: Beneficial effects of long-term diltiazem treatment in dilated cardiomyopathy. J Am Coll Cardiol 13:653, 1989.

898. Goldstein RE, Boccuzzi SJ, Cruess D, et al: Diltiazem increases late-onset congestive heart failure in postinfarction patients with early reduction in ejection fraction. Circulation 83:52, 1991.

899. Subramanian VB: Adverse effects of calcium antagonists—A review of the literature. In Calcium Antagonists in Chronic Stable Angina Pectoris. Amsterdam: Elsevier, 1983, pp 217–229.

900. Quigley MA, White KL, McGraw BF: Interpretation and application of world-wide safety data on diltiazem. Acta Pharmacol Toxicol (Copenh) 57:61, 1985.

901. Waller PC, Pearce GL, Rawson NSB, et al: Post-marketing surveillance of diltiazem by prescription-event monitoring. Pharm Med 4:319, 1990.

902. Hammentgen R, Lutz G, Kohler U, Nitsch J: Maculopapular exanthema during diltiazem medication. Dtsch Med Wochenschr 113:1283, 1988.

903. Ilia R, Goldfarb B, Gueron M: Skin thickening and sensory loss of the feet during diltiazem therapy. Int J Cardiol 35:115, 1992.

904. Jones SK, Reynolds NJ, Crossley J, Kennedy CTC: Cutaneous reaction to diltiazem resulting in an exacerbation of angina. Clin Exp Dermatol 14:457, 1989.

905. Kanesashi M, Kitamura K, Oosawa J, et al: A case of diltiazem-induced eruption. Skin Res 34(Suppl 14):144, 1992.

906. Romano A, Pietrantonio F, Garcovich A, et al: Delayed hypersensitivity to diltiazem in two patients. Ann Allergy 69:31, 1992.

907. Schaller S: Drug eruption due to diltiazem provoked exanthema. Z Hautkr 67:920, 1992.

908. Sheehan-Dare RA, Goodfield MJD: Widespread cutaneous vasculitis associated with diltiazem. Postgrad Med J 64:467, 1988.

909. Wirebaugh SR, Geraets DR: Reports of erythematous macular skin eruptions associated with diltiazem therapy. DICP Ann Pharmacother 24:1046, 1990.

910. Taylor JW, Cleary JD, Atkinson RC: Stevens-Johnson syndrome associated with diltiazem. Clin Pharm 9:948, 1990.

911. Nishimura T, Yoshioka K, Katoh J, et al: Pustular drug eruption induced by diltiazem HCl. Skin Res 33(Suppl 10):251, 1991.

912. Young L, Shehade SA, Chalmers RJG: Cutaneous reactions to diltiazem. Clin Exp Dermatol 15:467, 1990.

913. Baggott LA: Diltiazem-associated immune thrombocytopenia. Mt Sinai J Med 54:500, 1987.

914. Kuo M, Winiarski N, Garella S: Nonthrombocytopenic purpura associated sequentially with nifedipine and diltiazem. Ann Pharmacother 26:1089, 1992.

915. Berman JL: Dysomia, dysgeusia, and diltiazem. Ann Intern Med 102:717, 1985.

916. Ahmad S: Diltiazem and hyperglycemia-coma. J Am Coll Cardiol 6:494, 1985.

917. Giustiniani S, Robustelli-della-Cuna F, Marieni M: Hyperplastic gingivitis during diltiazem therapy. Int J Cardiol 15:247, 1987.

918. Jeret JS, Somasundaram M, Asaikar S: Diltiazem-induced myoclonus. N Y State J Med 92:447, 1992.

919. Ueno S, Hara Y: Lambert-Eaton myasthenic syndrome without anti-calcium channel antibody: Adverse effect of calcium antagonist diltiazem. J Neurol Neurosurg Psychiatry 55:409, 1992.

920. Dominguez EA, Hamill RJ: Drug-induced fever due to diltiazem. Arch Intern Med 151:1869, 1869.

921. Iversen E, Jeppesen D, Steensgaard-Hansen F: Direct diabetogenic effect of diltiazem? J Intern Med 227:285, 1990.

922. Achenbach V, Rafelt M, Wagner K, et al: Acute renal failure due to diltiazem. Lancet 1:176, 1985.

923. Asorey A, Garcia-Alegria JJ, Jimenez LC, et al: Cholestatic hepatitis from diltiazem [1]. Eur J Intern Med 2:5, 1992.

924. Shallcross H, Padley-SPG, Glynn MJ, Gibbs DD: Fatal renal and hepatic toxicity after treatment with diltiazem. Br Med J 295:1236, 1987.

925. Toft E, Vyberg M, Therkelsen K: Diltiazem-induced granulomatous hepatitis. Histopathology 18:474, 1991.

926. Binder EF, Cayabyab L, Ritchie DJ, Birge SJ: Diltiazem-induced psychosis and a possible diltiazem-lithium interaction. Arch Intern Med 151:373, 1991.

927. Jacobs MB: Diltiazem and akathisia. Ann Intern Med 99:794, 1983.

928. Palat GK, Hooker EA, Movahed A: Secondary mania associated with diltiazem. Clin Cardiol 7:611, 1984.

929. Brodie MJ, MacPhee G: Carbamazepine neurotoxicity precipitated by diltiazem. Br Med J 292:1170, 1986.

930. Sugimoto K, Ichikawa S, Konishi K, et al: A case of pustular drug eruption due to diltiazem HCl. Skin Res 28:412, 1986.

931. Scolnick B, Brinberg D: Diltiazem and generalized lymphadenopathy. Ann Intern Med 102:558, 1985.

932. Saunders FW, Shedden PD: Possible hematologic complications. Surg Neurol 25:82, 1986.

933. Hossack KF: Conduction abnormalities due to diltiazem. N Engl J Med 307:953, 1982.

934. Ishikawa T, Imamura T, Koiwaya Y, et al: Atrioventricular dissociation and sinus arrest induced by oral diltiazem. N Engl J Med 309:1124, 1983.

935. Hartwell BL, Mark JB: Combinations of beta-blockers and calcium channel blockers: A cause of malignant preoperative conduction disturbances? Anesth Analg 65:905, 1986.

936. Allal J, Coisne D, Barraine R: Heart arrest after intracoronary injection of diltiazem. Presse Med 19:428, 1990.

937. Natarajan D, Sharma SC, Sharma VP: Pulmonary edema with diltiazem in hypertrophic obstructive cardiomyopathy. Am Heart J 120:229, 1990.

938. Reboud JP, Wolf JE, Machecourt J, et al: Accidents au cours de l'association diltiazem-beta-bloquants. Presse Med 26:1396, 1984.

939. Lamaison D, Vacher D, Berenfeld A, et al: Cardiogenic shock with sinus bradycardia or arrest in two patients with concomitant beta-blockers and slow-release diltiazem. Therapie 45:411, 1990.

940. Hassell AB, Creamer JE: Profound bradycardia after the addition of diltiazem to a beta blocker. Br Med J 298:675, 1989.

941. Sagie A, Strasberg B, Kusnieck J, Sclarovsky S: Symptomatic bradycardia induced by the combination of oral diltiazem and beta blockers. Clin Cardiol 14:314, 1991.

942. Yust I, Hoffman M, Aronson RJ: Life-threatening bradycardic reactions due to beta blocker-diltiazem interactions. Isr J Med Sci 28:292, 1992.

943. Subramanian VB, Bowles MJ, Khurmi NS, et al: Calcium antagonist withdrawal syndrome: Objective demonstraton with frequency-modulated ambulatory ST-segment monitoring. Br Med J 12:520, 1983.

944. Larach DR, Hensley F Jr, Pae WE, et al: Diltiazem withdrawal before coronary artery bypass surgery. J Cardiothorac Anesth 3:688, 1989.

945. Kozeny GA, Ragona BP, Bansal VK, et al: Myocardial infarction with normal results of coronary angiography following diltiazem withdrawal. Am J Med 80:1184, 1986.

946. Engelman RM, Hadji-Rousou I, Breyer RH, et al: Rebound vasospasm after coronary revascularization in association with calcium antagonist withdrawal. Ann Thorac Surg 37:469, 1984.

947. Lambert H, Weber M, Renaud D: Acute diltiazem poisoning: Survey of the French Poison Centers. J Toxicol Clin Exp 10:229, 1990.

948. Gibelin P, Maccario M, Lapalus P, et al: Voluntary diltiazem intoxication. Presse Med 13:745, 1984.

949. Anthony T, Jastremski M, Elliott W, et al: Charcoal hemoperfusion for the treatment of a combined diltiazem and metoprolol overdose. Ann Emerg Med 15:1344, 1986.

950. Buffet MOG, Raclot P: Clinetique du diltiazem au cours d'un surdosage volontaire. Presse Med 13:1338, 1984.

951. Jean Ph, Hayek LM: Acute poisoning with diltiazem: Report of a case. J Toxicol Clin Exp 23:447, 1985.

952. Rey JL, Lecuyer D, Bernaconi P, et al: Self-poisoning with diltiazem resulting in sinus failure and atrio-ventricular block. Presse Med 12:1873, 1983.

953. Snover SW, Bocchino V: Massive diltiazem overdose. Ann Emerg Med 15:1221, 1986.

954. Jaeger A, Sauder P, Bianchetti G, et al: Diltiazem acute poisoning: Hemodynamic and kinetic study. J Toxicol Clin Exp 10:243, 1990.

955. Henderson A, Stevenson N, Hackett LP, Pond SM: Diltiazem overdose in an elderly patient: Efficacy of adrenaline. Anaesth Intensive Care 20:507, 1992.

956. Garcia del Pozo JM, Siquier B, Vicens C: An attempt to commit suicide with diltiazem. Rev Esp Cardiol 44:355, 1991.

957. Erickson FC, Ling LJ, Grande GA, Anderson DL: Diltiazem overdose: Case report and review. J Emerg Med 9:357, 1991.

958. Beauvoir C, Passeron D, Du-Cailar G, Millet E: Haemodynamic aspects of diltiazem poisoning. Ann Fr Anesth Reanim 10:154, 1991.

959. Connolly DL, Nettleton MA, Bastow MD: Massive diltiazem overdose. Am J Cardiol 72:742, 1993.

960. Humbert V Jr, Munn NJ, Hawkins RF: Noncardiogenic pulmonary edema complicating massive diltiazem overdose. Chest 99:258, 1991.

961. Wagner F, Jahnchen E, Trenk D, et al: Severe complications of antianginal drug therapy in a patient identified as a poor metabolizer of metoprolol, propafenone, diltiazem, and sparteine. Klin Wochenschr 65:1164, 1987.

962. Becker RC, Caputo R, Ball S, et al: Hemorrhagic potential of combined diltiazem and recombinant tissue-type plasminogen activator administration. Am Heart J 126:11, 1993.

963. Morris DL, Wisneski JA, Gertz EW, et al: Potentiation by nifedipine and diltiazem of the hypotensive response after contrast angiography. J Am Coll Cardiol 6:785, 1985.

964. Ferner RE, Odemuyiwa O, Field AB, et al: Pharmacokinetics and toxic effects of diltiazem in massive overdose. Hum Toxicol 8:497, 1989.

965. Weise J, Dlug E, Schneider V, et al: Tödliche diltiazenvergiftung. Z Rechtsmed 100:271, 1988.

966. Roper TA, Sykes R, Gray C: Fatal diltiazem overdose: Report of four cases and review of the literature. Postgrad Med J 69:474, 1993.

967. Darmanaden R, Kienlen J, Rouve MB: One case of fatal poisoning by diltiazem [4]. Therapie 47:80, 1992.

968. Kaliciak HA, Huckin SN, Cave WS: Case report: A death attributed solely to diltiazem. J Anal Toxicol 16:102, 1992.

969. Holzbecher MD, Hutton CJ: A fatal case involving diltiazem. J Can Soc Forensic Sci 21:135, 1988.

970. Beno JM, Nemeth DR: Diltiazem and metoclopramide overdose. J Anal Toxicol 15:285, 1991.

971. Ariyuki F: Effects of diltiazem hydrochloride (CRD-401) on pre- and post-natal development of mice and rats. Clin Rep 8:3401, 1974.

972. Physicians' Desk Reference, 47th ed. Montvale, NJ: Medical Economics Data, 1993.

973. Henling CE, Slogoff S, Kodali SV, et al: Heart block after coronary artery bypass—effect of chronic administration of calcium-entry blockers and beta blockers. Anesth Analg 63:515, 1984.

974. Kates RA, Zaggy AP, Norfleet EA, et al: Comparative cardiovascular effects of verapamil, nifedipine, and diltiazem during halothane anesthesia in swine. Anesthesiology 61:10, 1984.

975. Pierrot M, Hugon S, Blaise F, et al: Interference hemodynamique entre l'halothane et le diltiazem etude experimentale chez le porc. Ann Fr Anesth Reanim 2:153, 1983.

976. Gallenberg LA, Stowe DF, Marijic J, et al: Depression of atrial rate, atrioventricular nodal conduction, and cardiac contraction by diltiazem and volatile anesthetics in isolated hearts. Anesthesiology 74:519, 1991.

977. Broadbent MP, Swan PC, Jones RM: Interactions between diltiazem and isoflurane. An in vitro investigation in isolated guinea pig atria. Br J Anaesth 57:1018, 1985.

978. Kapur PA, Campos JH, Buchea OC: Plasma diltiazem levels, cardiovascular function, and coronary hemodynamics during enflurane anesthesia in the dog. Anesth Analg 65:918, 1986.

979. Kapur PA, Campos JH, Tippit SE: Influence of diltiazem on cardiovascular function and coronary hemodynamics during isoflurane anesthesia in the dog: Correlation with plasma diltiazem levels. Anesth Analg 65:81, 1986.

980. Ookawa I, Manabe M, Yamaguchi T, et al: Interaction between diltiazem and sevoflurane in the canine blood-perfused papillary muscle and sinoatrial node preparations. Jpn J Anesthesiol 40:439, 1991.

981. Nagelhout JJ, Beuthin FC: The effect of diltiazem on myocardial ischemia during halothane anesthesia in dogs. Pharmacologist 26:242, 1984.

982. Nakata F, Kemmotsu O, Tanaka R: Hemodynamic interaction of calcium entry blockers and halothane with experimentally produced myocardial ischemia. Jpn J Pharmacol 36:138P, 1984.

983. Iwatsuki N, Katoh M, Ono K, et al: Antiarrhythmic effect of diltiazem during halothane anesthesia in dogs and humans. Anesth Analg 64:964, 1985.

984. Iwatsuki N, Amaha K: Inotropic interaction betwen diltiazem and halothane in isolated canine heart muscle. Masui 32:81, 1983.

985. Hantler CB, Wilton N, Learned DM, et al: Impaired myocardial conduction in patients receiving diltiazem therapy during enflurane anesthesia. Anesthesiology 67:94, 1987.

986. Griffin RM, Dimich I, Pratilas V, et al: Cardiovascular effects of diltiazem infusion during fentanyl anesthesia. Anesth Analg 64:223, 1985.

987. Bernard JM, Pinaud M, Carteau S, et al: Hypotensive actions of diltiazem and nitroprusside compared during fentanyl anaesthesia for total hip arthroplasty. Can Anaesth Soc J 33:308, 1986.

988. Finegan BA, Whiting RW, Tam YK, Clanachan AS: Enhancement of bupivacaine toxicity by diltiazem in anaesthetized dogs. Br J Anaesth 69:492, 1992.

989. Pierrot M, Hugon S, Blaise M, et al: Modifications by diltiazem of ketamine cardiovascular effects. Ann Fr Anesth Reanim 2:154, 1983.

990. Tjia JF, Back DJ, Breckenridge AM: Calcium channel antagonists and cyclosporine metabolism. Br J Clin Pharmacol 28:362, 1989.

991. Nagineni CN, Lee DBN, Misra BC, Yanagawa N: Cyclosporine-A transport in isolated renal proximal tubular cells: Inhibition by calcium channel blockers. Biochem Biophys Res Commun 157:1226, 1988.

992. Wagner K, Henkel M, Heinemeyer G, Neumayer H-H: Interaction of calcium blockers and cyclosporine. Transplant Proc 20:561, 1988.

993. Campistol JM, Oppenheimer F, Vilardell J, et al: Interaction between cyclosporin and diltiazem in renal transplant patients. Nephron 57:241, 1991.

994. Chrysostomou A, Walker RG, Russ GR, et al: Diltiazem in renal allograft recipients receiving cyclosporine. Transplantation 55:300, 1993.

995. Brockmoller J, Neumayer HH, Wagner K, et al: Pharmacokinetic interaction between cyclosporin and diltiazem. Eur J Clin Pharmacol 38:237, 1990.

996. Tozun N, Berkman K, Tankurt E, et al: Effect of diltiazem on renal function in patients with liver cirrhosis. Int J Clin Pharmacol Ther Toxicol 29:198, 1991.

997. Kurosawa S, Kurosawa N, Owada E, et al: Pharmacokinetics of diltiazem in patients with liver cirrhosis. Int J Clin Pharmacol Res 10:311, 1990.

998. Red Book Update, Vol 12, October 1993. Montvale, NJ: Medical Economics Data Production, 1993.

CHAPTER 103

Nifedipine

Leon Resnekov, M.D., F.R.C.P., Franz H. Messerli, M.D., and Franz C. Aepfelbacher, M.D.

Nifedipine is the first of the dihydropyridine drugs to be used clinically. Experimental and clinical differences between nifedipine, diltiazem, and verapamil have been studied by Kawai et al.[1] and reviewed by Braunwald.[2]

PHARMACOLOGY

Nifedipine, a yellow, crystalline substance, is soluble in ethanol but completely insoluble in water. As with the other calcium antagonists, nifedipine blocks the slow channel selectively in heart and vascular smooth muscle.

Approximately 95% of nifedipine is absorbed after an oral dose, and peak plasma levels are reached within approximately 30 to 45 minutes. The bioavailability of nifedipine is 65% to 75%. Ninety-five percent is protein bound, the elimination half-life is approximately 5 hours, and its effective plasma concentration is 25 to 100 ng/ml. It is metabolized to a nonactive acid metabolite by the liver and is excreted by both the kidneys (85%) and the gastrointestinal tract (15%).

Nifedipine was initially marketed as a 10-mg or 20-mg capsule that should be protected from light and moisture. A long-acting preparation has now become available—nifedipine XL. In this formulation, the liquid is encased in a push-pull osmotic pump control system that permits release of nifedipine at a constant rate over a 24-hour period.[3, 4]

Compared with verapamil and diltiazem, nifedipine has less first-pass metabolism and no active metabolites.

Also, unlike verapamil and diltiazem, nifedipine causes neither slowing of the heart (sinus node) nor lessening of atrioventricular nodal conduction in usual therapeutic doses.[1] Nifedipine, one of the most potent of the currently available calcium antagonists, increases cardiac output and heart rate as a reflex response to its intense peripheral vasodilation. The sympathetic response appears to be associated with the rate of nifedipine absorption. Kleinbloesem et al. showed that a slow infusion of nifedipine was associated with no heart rate changes and a smoother blood pressure response.[5] Therefore, the slow release of conventional nifedipine is not associated with clinically significant heart rate changes. The absence of slowing of the heart or of conduction across the atrioventricular node can be advantageous in the management of angina pectoris, when calcium antagonists are combined with β-adrenergic blocking drugs. However, the increase in heart rate that may occur when conventional nifedipine is given can lead to acute cardiac ischemia. Patients at risk should therefore be protected against such deleterious responses by combining nifedipine with a β-adrenergic blocking drug or by using a slow-release formulation.

Hemodynamic Effects

Nifedipine causes selective dilation of arterial resistance vessels with little effect on venous pooling.[6] A reflexive stimulation of sympathetic activity follows the fall in blood pressure, resulting in both increases in heart rate and a positive inotropic effect. However, it should be noted that *in vitro* nifedipine, like most other calcium antagonists, is negatively inotropic.[7] *In vivo*, however, vascular smooth muscle is relaxed by nifedipine at a lesser concentration than that needed to cause a direct depressant effect on the myocardium.[8, 9] Therefore, after a dose of conventional nifedipine, the overall effects are lowering of blood pressure, enhancement of cardiac contractility and segmental ventricular function, and a modest increase in both heart rate and cardiac output.[10]

Renal Hemodynamics

The effects of nifedipine depend on renal vascular tone.[11] With normal perfusion pressure, nifedipine has little effect on either the renal perfusate flow or the glomerular filtration rate of an isolated kidney preparation.[12] However, using a similar model, during ischemia precipitated by norepinephrine, nifedipine caused the reduced glomerular filtration rate to return to its previous level.[13] Nifedipine has been shown, therefore, to enhance the renal perfusate flow as well as the glomerular filtration rate in the presence of renal vasoconstriction. It seems, however, that the renal microvasculature has a varying response and sensitivity to nifedipine that depends on the underlying mechanism of renal vasoconstriction.[12] Conceivably, nifedipine modulates the activity of intrarenal angiotensin and prostanoids to bring about its effects.[11]

SIDE EFFECTS

Untoward effects resulting from nifedipine administration are caused most often by rapid and pronounced peripheral vasodilation.[14] Dizziness, hypotension, flushing, headache, and palpitations may occur. On rare occasion, precipitation or worsening of angina pectoris has been reported. Ankle edema is a fairly common adverse effect caused by precapillary dilation without accompanying venodilation. Very rarely is heart failure precipitated by nifedipine unless the condition is already incipient and/or β-adrenergic blocking drugs are concomitantly being given. The overall incidence of side effects is approximately 10% to 15%. Untoward effects can be lessened by swallowing capsules of nifedipine after meals to lessen the rate of absorption. The use of long-acting preparations of nifedipine has greatly improved the safety and tolerability of nifedipine and the previously mentioned side effects have become much rarer.

DRUG INTERACTIONS
Digoxin

Belz et al. initially reported a 45% increase in serum digoxin concentrations after nifedipine dosage.[15] Subsequently, Pedersen et al.[16] found little change in total body digoxin clearance after nifedipine dosage. Similarly, Zylber-Katz et al.[17] could find no significant change in digoxin half-life, the area under the time-concentration curve, or the volume of digoxin distribution during nifedipine therapy. Schwartz et al., who studied the effects of the coadministration of digoxin and nifedipine in healthy individuals and those with chest pain syndromes, could find no significant change in steady-state serum digoxin concentrations.[18, 19] It is important, however, to monitor both the serum digoxin concentration and the physiologic end points during initiation of nifedipine therapy in patients receiving digoxin. There is no current evidence, however, that, as a routine, digoxin dosage should be modified during therapy with nifedipine. In contrast with nifedipine, verapamil is known to increase serum digoxin levels,[20] and digoxin dosage should be adjusted when verapamil is added to the therapeutic regimen. The combination of diltiazem and digoxin can worsen sinus and atrioventricular nodal dysfunction, but diltiazem does not cause the level of serum digoxin to rise.[21, 22]

Cimetidine, Ranitidine, and Phenytoin

Cimetidine, ranitidine, and phenytoin[23, 24] may cause peak nifedipine plasma levels to rise significantly. This is more common with cimetidine and less so with ranitidine and phenytoin. Conceivably, cimetidine inhibits hepatic cytochrome (P-450), the enzyme system thought to be responsible for the first-pass metabolism of nifedipine. Thus, caution is needed when giving nifedipine to a patient who is already receiving one of these three drugs.

Coumarin Anticoagulants

Usually nifedipine causes little change in prothrombin time in patients maintained on chronic coumarin therapy.

β-Adrenergic Blocking Drugs, Diuretics, Nitrates, Aspirin, and Allopurinol

No important drug interactions occur when nifedipine is coadministered with these drugs. As previously documented, however, in patients in incipient heart failure, adding nifedipine to β-adrenergic blocking drugs may occasionally precipitate overt heart failure because of an inappropriate fall in blood pressure.

PREGNANCY

No adequate or well-controlled studies are available in pregnant women. Because nifedipine is teratogenic in rats given 30 times the maximal recommended human dose, and is embryotoxic as well, nifedipine should be used in pregnancy only if the potential benefit justifies the possible risk to the fetus.

CLINICAL USES OF NIFEDIPINE
Syndromes of Myocardial Ischemia

Thrombolytic therapy and heparin with or without concomitant aspirin are commonly used during the evolving stage of myocardial infarction.[25–27] Aspirin is prophylactically used to prevent myocardial ischemia in patients at risk. Nifedipine has also been shown to have antiplatelet actions[28] that might enhance its overall effect during acute myocardial ischemia.

A further potential use of nifedipine in the management of acute myocardial ischemia is to reduce myocardial damage. Because hypoxia causes considerable calcium overload,[29] a net influx of calcium ions into the myocardial cell occurs. Mitochondria take up an excess amount of the ion, a process requiring high-energy phosphate. Eventually, with the excess influx of calcium ions into mitochondria, energy production is lessened and the mitochondria may be irreparably harmed. Less adenosine triphosphate (ATP) is now available for pumping out calcium from the cell. With further increases in cytosolic calcium, the membrane of the cell becomes damaged, and permanent cell damage and death follow.[30–33]

Pioneering experimental work by Fleckenstein et al. has shown that calcium antagonists can decrease the degree of myocardial necrosis and preserve mitochondrial and cell membrane integrity.[34] The contractile function of the myocardial cell is thereby preserved, limiting the degree of ischemic myocardial damage.

Acute Myocardial Infarction

The previously mentioned theoretical considerations and experimental findings lead to a number of clinical trials evaluating the effects of nifedipine in patients with acute myocardial infarction. Muller et al. reported one of the first large studies;[35] however, the results were disappointing. Mean infarct size was unchanged and mortality was even greater in patients treated with nifedipine than in those given a placebo (8% versus 0%). Similar results were obtained in other studies, such as the Trial of Early Nifedipine Treatment (TRENT),[36] the Norwegian Nifedipine Multicenter Trial,[37] and the Secondary Prevention Reinfarction Israeli Nifedipine Trial (SPRINT).[38] In the SPRINT II trial,[39] which differed from the first trial mainly in the much earlier administration after myocardial infarction (as early as possible versus 7 to 21 days after the event), an interim analysis of the data demonstrated a significant excess mortality in the nifedipine group (15.8% versus 12.6%), and this difference was entirely due to an excess in mortality within the first 6 days of treatment. This study had to be discontinued as soon as this was known. A similar effect was seen in the International Nifedipine Trial on Antiatherosclerotic Therapy (INTACT),[40] a study in which the effect of nifedipine on progression of coronary artery disease was investigated. Although treatment with nifedipine led to a 28% reduction in the number of new lesions after 3 years as compared with placebo, it also increased cardiac mortality.

In contrast, Gottlieb et al.[41] reported that early infarct expansion was reduced with nifedipine in patients with an initial left ventricular ejection fraction of more than 35%, but no differences were observed in the clinical outcome. Because these results are without additional confirmation, the authors of this study advised caution in the interpretation of their findings.

It is probable that the failure of nifedipine to reduce the size of infarct in the vast majority of studies relates to the need for rapidly establishing myocardial perfusion if real benefit is to be achieved. Furthermore, nifedipine, because of its peripheral vasodilation, might cause hypotension and paradoxically reduce rather than enhance coronary perfusion. Similarly, tachycardia in association with the hypotension could result in an increased rather than decreased myocardial oxygen demand.

In summary, nifedipine has failed to show a beneficial effect on the progression of evolving myocardial infarction or the size of the infarct in those who already have developed myocardial damage. On the contrary, the available data seem to suggest a deleterious effect on clinical outcome, that is, a possible increased mortality in patients receiving nifedipine early during the course of acute myocardial infarction.

Unstable Angina Pectoris

Various clinical trials investigated the effect of nifedipine in unstable angina, and the results are quite inconsistent. In angina due to coronary vasospasms (Prinzmetal's angina), nifedipine has been shown to be of benefit,[42] as have several other calcium antagonists.[43, 44] In addition, several studies documented a beneficial effect of nifedipine in unstable angina. Antman et al., who studied 127 patients with unstable angina pectoris in most of whom maximal conventional therapy had failed to control rest angina, documented that in doses of 40 to 60 mg/day nifedipine eliminated spontaneous pain in 63% of patients, and in almost 90%, the frequency of episodes of spontaneous angina pectoris fell by at least one half.[45] Shick et al.[46] undertook a controlled double-blind study with

a withdrawal period and demonstrated the superior effectiveness of nifedipine versus placebo. Hugenholtz et al.[47] and Moses et al.[48] have also documented the effectiveness of nifedipine for treating unstable angina pectoris.

However, other clinical trials, such as the Holland Interuniversity Nifedipine/Metoprolol Trial (HINT) showed an increased risk for myocardial infarction in patients assigned to nifedipine alone, and the study had to be discontinued.[49] In addition, another more recent trial questioned the usefulness of nifedipine in the management of unstable angina[50] by showing an increase in the number and duration of ischemic episodes in patients with angina at rest.

In view of these results, it is therefore not surprising that health authorities in countries where nifedipine was an approved drug in the treatment of unstable angina, such as Germany, recently withdrew this indication[51] and recommend nifedipine and other 1,4-dihydropyridine calcium antagonists only for the treatment of hypertension and stable and vasospastic angina.

Stable Angina Pectoris

In contrast to the previously mentioned findings in unstable angina and evolving myocardial infarction, many studies have demonstrated the effectiveness of nifedipine in treating chronic stable angina pectoris. Even a single sublingual dose of 10 to 20 mg has been shown not only to reduce the frequency of episodes of angina by 23% to 100% but also to increase exercise tolerance by 20% to 70% compared with placebo during graded stress testing.[14] At any given exercise load, the tension time index is reduced. With more chronic usage, 60 mg of nifedipine in daily divided doses has been shown to be superior to a placebo.[52] Combining nifedipine with propranolol was more effective than either drug alone, and although adverse effects emerged, they were not unduly severe and were easily controllable.[53] Mueller and Chahine[54] have reported a multicenter, double-blind, placebo-controlled study of the effects of nifedipine in chronic stable angina pectoris, documenting the superiority of nifedipine over placebo. A similar benefit of nifedipine has been documented by Moskowitz et al.[55] Nifedipine XL is equally effective and has better safety and tolerability.

The dosage of nifedipine should be carefully titrated.[56] Too small a dose will not produce a clinical benefit; a dose that is inappropriately large may increase the heart rate and precipitate hypotension that could be deleterious. The latter can be prevented by adding a β-adrenergic blocking drug to the regimen.

Nifedipine XL, with or without β-adrenergic blockade, has also been shown to reduce early morning and late afternoon circadian peaks of myocardial ischemia in patients with chronic stable angina pectoris.[57] It is apparent that, at present, no single ideal antianginal medication exists. Nitrates when used long term have important side effects and limited duration of maximal effect and are prone to a relatively rapid development of tachyphylaxis. β-Adrenergic blocking drugs have certain potential advantages and are now available with cardioselectivity, but, unfortunately, at higher doses such selective effects are lost. However, β-adrenergic blocking drugs do not improve myocardial oxygen supply or coronary blood flow. In patients with insulin-dependent diabetes mellitus or bronchospasm, β-blockers can be used only with extreme caution, if at all; furthermore, they may be contraindicated should ventricular function be severely reduced or sinoatrial and atrioventricular node function be depressed. In contrast, nifedipine reduces any tendency to coronary vasoconstriction, enhances coronary flow, improves myocardial perfusion, and may reduce the abnormal diastolic stiffness of the ventricle during ischemic states. Furthermore, there is no evidence that tachyphylaxis emerges during prolonged nifedipine usage.

Concomitant Therapy

Many patients with myocardial ischemia are maintained on combined therapy with nifedipine, β-adrenergic blocking drugs, and chronically administered nitrates. Nesto et al.[58] studied the effects of adding nifedipine to maximal β-adrenergic blocking drug and nitrate therapy. They demonstrated an improvement in global left ventricular function at comparable workloads and in ejection fractions during exercise. Episodes of exercise-induced ischemia were reduced when nifedipine was added to maximal doses of β-adrenergic blocking drugs and nitrates, without any significant effect on myocardial oxygen demand. De Buitleir et al.,[59] who investigated the effects of nifedipine alone or in combination with atenolol in patients with impaired left ventricular function, concluded that removal of sympathetic nervous system support for the impaired ventricle by β-adrenergic blockade rather than nifedipine may be the decisive factor in precipitating hemodynamic deterioration in these patients. A further study of the effects of nifedipine and β-adrenergic blocking drug interaction[60] revealed no adverse effects on the electrophysiologic, hemodynamic, or left ventricular functional parameters in patients with normal left ventricular function at rest. Furthermore, depressed left ventricular segments appeared to improve after the addition of nifedipine.

From these studies, one can conclude that a combination of nifedipine, β-adrenergic blocking drugs, and chronic nitrate therapy ameliorates myocardial ischemia in association with left ventricular improvement.

Withdrawal of Nifedipine Therapy

It is known that when β-adrenergic blocking drugs are abruptly discontinued, a rebound anginal effect may emerge in certain patients. Until quite recently, investigators have been uncertain whether a similar effect occurs when calcium antagonists are withdrawn. Gottlieb et al.[61] studied the effects of acutely withdrawing nifedipine in 81 patients with angina at rest who were part of a double-blind, randomized trial of nifedipine versus placebo.[48] No untoward effects of acute nifedipine withdrawal either in patients undergoing coronary bypass surgery or in stable patients on long-term medical therapy were found. However, patients who continue with angina at rest may have episodes of early recurrent ischemia when nifedipine is withdrawn suddenly.[48]

Potential Deleterious Effects

A number of reports have documented the emergence of myocardial ischemia after nifedipine administration.[62] Several mechanisms have been postulated, including (1) reduction in coronary perfusion pressure and shortening of diastolic perfusion time because of a reflex increase in heart rate,[63] (2) pre- and poststenotic segment vasodilation resulting in more severe stenosis,[64] (3) narrowing of a stenotic coronary artery segment because of a decrease in intraluminal distending pressure,[65] and (4) dilation of intramural resistance vessels by nifedipine, causing a pressure decrease immediately beyond an atherosclerotic narrowing of the coronary artery and thereby greatly reducing effective flow down that vessel.

Diabetic patients being treated for angina pectoris with nifedipine should have blood glucose levels monitored if nifedipine is to be discontinued, because reports of sudden dangerous falls in blood glucose levels have been published.[66] Furthermore, normal volunteers taking nifedipine not infrequently have a rise in blood sugar levels. Because a delayed insulin response is associated with nifedipine administration, the management of diabetes may have to be adjusted.[67]

Hypertension

Nifedipine, like other calcium antagonists, reduces arterial pressure by diminishing arterial smooth muscle tone, thereby decreasing total peripheral resistance. Furthermore, nifedipine causes blood pressure to fall without changing sodium transport.[68] In fact, the antihypertensive effect of nifedipine XL is not blunted by high salt intake.

Although, in general, hypertension responds well to nifedipine treatment at any age, the patients who benefit most are the elderly, black patients, and those whose hypertension is associated with arteriosclerotic coronary artery disease or diabetes mellitus. Many patients with hypertension, particularly the elderly, concomitantly suffer from other diseases. These include coronary artery disease, heart failure, diabetes mellitus, obstructive lung disease, and peripheral vascular disease. In addition to lowering arterial pressure, nifedipine also may be beneficial in treating these associated diseases. Unlike many of the antihypertensive drugs, nifedipine does not usually impair sexual function or worsen lipid profiles. Its effects are not associated with biochemical change, mental depression, sedation, or sleep disturbances.[69–73] In elderly patients with hypertension, doses of nifedipine as low as 10 mg twice daily have been shown to be effective.[73] Often, monotherapy with nifedipine successfully reduces levels of blood pressure to an optimal range.[65] Prescribing nifedipine XL, a once-a-day therapy, greatly improves patient compliance.

Patients with hypertension can be characterized according to three interrelated factors: plasma renin activity, sensitivity to dietary salt intake, and calcium metabolism indices.[74, 75] When hypertensive patients were treated with nifedipine, those whose renin levels were initially low had a greater reduction in blood pressure, and vice versa. Furthermore, the greatest decrease in blood pressure was observed in patients with lower ionized calcium levels.[76] Another important aspect of antihypertensive therapy is its effect on hypertensive target-organ damage. It is now well established that nifedipine can effectively decrease left ventricular hypertrophy, and a recent report suggested that nifedipine has beneficial effects on renal function and 24-hour urinary protein excretion.[77]

Nifedipine should be used with caution in unstable hypertensive urgencies. Among possible side effects have been reports of myocardial ischemia or even infarction when nifedipine was used.[78] The usual cause is exaggerated hypotension with associated myocardial ischemia and even infarction. At the same time, hypotension is associated with reflexive activation of the sympathetic nervous system and increases in myocardial contractility and heart rate. Myocardial oxygen consumption is enhanced, causing worsening of myocardial ischemia.

Hypertrophic Cardiomyopathy

Although clinical experience in the management of hypertrophic cardiomyopathy has been greatest with verapamil, nifedipine has also been tried.[79] Both reduce sarcoplasmic calcium, thereby enhancing the very reduced diastolic relaxation of the condition. When combined with β-adrenergic blocking drugs, excessive myocardial contractility is lessened, reducing the likelihood of emergence of life-threatening dysrhythmias. Concomitant nifedipine and propranolol therapy has been reported as giving beneficial results, both short and long term.[79]

Patients being managed with such combination therapy require very careful follow-up to ensure that adverse effects do not emerge and that benefit is occurring and being maintained.

Diastolic Dysfunction

Increased stiffness of the myocardium occurs, and the relaxation time during diastole is prolonged. The cardiac output is maintained, therefore, at the expense of an elevated pulmonary venous pressure. Backward transmission to the lungs of the increased left ventricular diastolic pressure results in pulmonary congestion despite preservation of systolic contractile function.[80]

Diastolic dysfunction occurs particularly in conditions that cause hypertrophy—hypertension, aortic stenosis, and hypertrophic cardiomyopathy, as well as in chronic coronary artery disease and acute myocardial ischemia. Conditions associated with volume overload, such as valvar regurgitation or renal failure, also cause diastolic dysfunction. One of the most common precipitants is increased interstitial fibrosis of the heart and cross-linkage of collagen that occurs in old age.[81]

Nifedipine,[82] as well as other calcium antagonists,[83, 84] has been shown to improve diastolic relaxation time and to lessen diastolic dysfunction, including in the elderly.[85]

Pulmonary Hypertension

When pulmonary hypertension is present and is associated with a high pulmonary vascular resistance and hypertrophy of pulmonary arterioles, vasodilators are frequently of little use.[86] They are more effective on the systemic than the pulmonary circulation,[87] and any decline in pulmonary artery pressure may be secondary to peripheral arterial vasodilation and reduced cardiac output, rather than a reduction in pulmonary vascular resistance.

Nifedipine, in conventional doses, has been the most widely tested drug in patients with primary pulmonary hypertension.[88] Reports of both short-term[89, 90] and long-term benefits[91, 92] have followed. More recently, high-dose nifedipine, up to 240 mg/day, has been reported to be of moderate success in limited numbers of patients.[93]

Adverse effects including systemic hypotension, cardiogenic shock, pulmonary edema, and even death have been reported fairly frequently.[94–97] Curiously, no increased frequency of untoward responses emerged when high-dose nifedipine was given.[98] More recently, the use of adenosine has been tried and compared with nifedipine.[99]

Pulmonary hypertension associated with chronic obstructive lung disease and hypoxic vasoconstriction may respond to nifedipine, which can cause dilation of the bronchial airways and bring about clinical benefit.[100, 101]

Therefore, at least two conclusions seem appropriate. First, nifedipine, like other calcium antagonists, has selective effects for specific vascular beds, acting preferentially on vascular smooth muscle that is constricted, and less so on unaffected arteries and arterioles. Second, to date, no drug or drug combination has been uniformly successful, and the management of pulmonary hypertension remains a therapeutic challenge that is both complex and difficult.

Peripheral Vascular Disease

Nifedipine has been used in severe Raynaud's phenomenon in a dose of 20 mg three times daily and has been compared with a placebo after 1 week of either therapy, with a phase of crossover.[102] Patients in the nifedipine group showed significant improvement in digital blood flow after cold challenge, as demonstrated by improved skin-temperature recovery time.[102] Other groups of investigators have confirmed the benefit of nifedipine in patients with primary Raynaud's phenomenon.[103, 104]

Nifedipine is particularly effective for vasospastic peripheral vascular disorders such as primary Raynaud's phenomenon.[105] However, it is less effective for fixed peripheral vascular disease secondary to arteriosclerosis.

Noncardiovascular Uses

Nifedipine has been used in cerebrovascular disease, migraine, esophageal spasm, spastic conditions of the bowel, urinary urgency, dysmenorrhea, and precipitant labor. In all these conditions, the aim of such therapy has been to reduce spasms of smooth muscle, and variable degrees of success have been achieved. At present, nifedipine usage has been approved by the United States Food and Drug Administration only for vasospastic angina, chronic stable angina pectoris, and hypertension. Appropriately designed and conducted clinical trials are needed to document the effectiveness of nifedipine in noncardiovascular diseases as guidance for its therapeutic use.

SUMMARY

Nifedipine, the first of the dihydropyridine group of calcium antagonists, is one of the most potent of the calcium antagonists currently approved for clinical use in the United States. Nifedipine has a more powerful peripheral than cardiac effect and, in usual clinical doses, does not depress function of the sinoatrial or atrioventricular nodes. It is used in the prevention and management of symptomatic and asymptomatic syndromes of acute and chronic myocardial ischemia, with or without associated left ventricular dysfunction, as well as in the management of systemic hypertension, hypertensive emergencies, congestive heart failure, hypertrophic cardiomyopathy, pulmonary hypertension, and peripheral vascular disease. Side effects occur in 10% to 15% of patients being treated with conventional nifedipine, usually because of rapid and pronounced peripheral vasodilation that causes hypotension and associated increases in heart rate. Ankle edema may also occur. Side effects may be lessened by judicious choice of dosage and by lessening the rate of absorption by having the patient swallow the capsules after meals. A controlled-release preparation of nifedipine is now available that reduces still further the incidence of side effects and provides relatively constant delivery of nifedipine over 24 hours.

REFERENCES

1. Kawai C, Konishi T, Matsuyama E, et al: Comparative effects of three calcium antagonists, diltiazem, verapamil and nifedipine on the sinoatrial and atrioventricular nodes: Experimental and clinical studies. Circulation 63:1035, 1981.
2. Braunwald E: Mechanism of action of calcium-channel-blocking agents. N Engl J Med 307:1618, 1982.
3. Swanson DR, Barday BL, Wong PS, et al: Nifedipine gastrointestinal therapeutic system. Am J Med 83(Suppl 6B):3, 1987.
4. Frishman WH: An innovative approach to the management of hypertension [special report]. Postgrad Med Oct 1988, pp 52–56.
5. Kleinbloesem CH, Van Brummelen P, Danhof M, et al: Rate of increase in the plasma concentration of nifedipine as a major determinant of its hemodynamic effects in humans. Clin Pharmacol Ther 41:26, 1987.
6. Robinson BF, Dobbs RJ, Kelsey CR: Effects of nifedipine on resistant vessels, arteries and veins in man. Br J Clin Pharmacol 10:433, 1980.
7. Henry PD: Comparative pharmacology of calcium antagonists: Nifedipine, verapamil and diltiazem. Am J Cardiol 46:1047, 1980.
8. Antman EM, Stone PH, Muller JE, et al: Calcium-channel blocking agents in the treatment of cardiovascular disorders. Part I: Basic and clinical electrophysiologic effects. Ann Intern Med 93:875, 1980.
9. Ono H, Hashimoto K: In vitro tissue effects of calcium flux inhibition. In Stone PH, Antman EM (eds): Calcium Channel Blocking Agents in the Treatment of Cardiovascular Disorders. Mount Kisco, NY: Futura Publishing, 1983, pp 155–175.
10. Serruys PW, Brower RW, Ten Katen JH, et al: Regional wall motion from radiopaque markers after intravenous and intracoronary injections of nifedipine. Circulation 63:584, 1981.
11. Loutzenhiser R, Epstein M: Effects of calcium antagonists on renal hemodynamics. Am J Physiol 249(5 Pt 2):F619, 1985.
12. Loutzenhiser R, Epstein M, Horton C, et al: Reversal by the calcium antagonist nisoldipine of norepinephrine-induced reduction of GFR. Evidence for preferential antagonism of preglomerular vasoconstriction. J Pharmacol Exp Ther 232:382, 1985.
13. Loutzenhiser RD, Epstein M: Renal hemodynamic effects of calcium antagonists. Am J Med 82(Suppl 3B):23, 1987.
14. Stone PH, Antman EM, Muller JE, et al: Calcium channel blocking agents in the treatment of cardiovascular disorders. Part II. Hemodynamic effects and clinical applications. Ann Intern Med 93:886, 1980.
15. Belz GG, Aust PE, Munkes R: Digoxin plasma concentrations and nifedipine: Correspondence. Lancet 1:845, 1981.
16. Pedersen KE, Dorph-Pederson A, Hudt S, et al: Effect of nifedipine on digoxin kinetics in healthy subjects. Clin Pharmacol Ther 32:562, 1982.
17. Zylber-Katz E, Koren G, Levy M: Pharmacokinetic study of nifedipine co-administration [abstract]. Clin Pharmacol Ther 35:114, 1984.
18. Schwartz JB, Raizner A, Akers S: The effects of nifedipine on serum digoxin concentration and renal digoxin clearance. Am Heart J 107:669, 1984.
19. Schwartz JB, Migliore PJ: Effect of nifedipine on serum digoxin concentration and renal digoxin clearance. Clin Pharmacol Ther 36:19, 1984.
20. Lang R, Klein HO, Weiss E, et al: Effect of verapamil on blood level and renal clearance of digoxin [abstract]. Circulation 62(Suppl III):83, 1980.
21. Oyamar Y, Fuji S, Kana K, et al: Digoxin-diltiazem interaction. Am J Cardiol 53:1480, 1984.
22. Kuhlmann J: Effects of nifedipine and diltiazem on plasma levels and renal excretion of beta-acetyldigoxin. Clin Pharmacol Ther 37:150, 1985.
23. Ahmad S: Nifedipine-phenytoin interaction [letter]. J Am Coll Cardiol 3:1582, 1984.
24. Maseri A: The changing face of angina pectoris: Practical implications. Lancet 1:746, 1983.
25. TIMI Study Group: The thrombolysis in myocardial infarction (TIMI) trial: Phase I findings. N Engl J Med 312:932, 1985.
26. ISIS (International Studies of Infarct Survival) Pilot Study Investigators: Randomized factorial trial of high-dose intravenous streptokinase, of oral aspirin and of intravenous heparin in acute myocardial infarction. Eur Heart J 8:634, 1987.
27. Verstraete M, Bernard R, Bory M, et al: Randomized trial of intravenous recombinant tissue-type plasminogen activator versus intravenous streptokinase in acute myocardial infarction: Report from the European Cooperative Study Group for recombinant tissue-type plasminogen activator. Lancet 1:842, 1985.

28. Dale J, Laudmark KH, Myhre E: The effects of nifedipine, a calcium antagonist, on platelet function. Am Heart J 105:103, 1983.
29. Nayler WG, Poole-Wilson PA, Williams A: Hypoxia and calcium. J Mol Cell Cardiol 11:683, 1979.
30. Burton KB: Lanthanum probe studies of cellular pathophysiology induced by hypoxia in isolated cardiac muscle. J Clin Invest 60:1289, 1977.
31. Henry PD, Schuchleib R, Davis J, et al: Myocardial contraction and accumulation of mitochondrial calcium in ischemic rabbit heart. Am J Physiol 233:H667, 1977.
32. Henry PD, Schuchleib R, Bordas LJ, et al: Effects of nifedipine on myocardial perfusion and ischemic injury in dogs. Circ Res 43:372, 1978.
33. Wrogemenn RR, Pena SDJ: Mitochondrial calcium overload: A general mechanism for all necrosis in muscle diseases. Lancet 1:672, 1976.
34. Fleckenstein JA, Kammermeier H, Doring H, et al: Zum Wirkungs-Mechanismus neuartiger Koronardilalatoren mit gleichzeitig Sauerstoff-einsparenden, myokard-Effekten. Prenylamin und Iproveratril. Z Kreislaufforsch 56:716, 1967.
35. Muller JE, Morrison J, Stone PH, et al: Nifedipine therapy for patients with threatened and acute myocardial infarction: A randomized double-blind, placebo-controlled comparison. Circulation 69:740, 1984.
36. Wilcox RG, Hampton JR, Banks DC, et al: Trial of early nifedipine in acute myocardial infarction: The TRENT Study. Br Med J 293:1204, 1986.
37. Sirnes PA, Overskeid K, Pedersen TR, et al: Evolution of infarct size during the early use of nifedipine in patients with acute myocardial infarction: The Norwegian Multicenter Trial. Circulation 70:638, 1984.
38. The SPRINT Study Group: Secondary Prevention Reinfarction Israeli Nifedipine Trial (SPRINT). A randomized intervention trial of nifedipine in patients with acute myocardial infarction. Eur Heart J 9:354, 1988.
39. The SPRINT Study Group: SPRINT II: Results. Eur Heart J 9(Suppl 1):350A, 1988.
40. Lichtlen PR, Hugenholtz PG, Rafflenbeul W, et al: Retardation of angiographic progression of coronary artery disease by nifedipine: Results of the International Nifedipine Trial on Antiatherosclerotic Therapy (INTACT). Lancet 335:1109, 1990.
41. Gottlieb SO, Becker LC, Weiss JL, et al: Nifedipine in acute myocardial infarction: An assessment of left ventricular function, infarct size, and infarct expansion. Br Heart J 59:411, 1988.
42. Hill JA, Feldman RL, Pepine CJ, et al: Randomized double-blind comparison of nifedipine and isosorbide dinitrate in patients with coronary arterial spasm. Am J Cardiol 49:431, 1982.
43. Johnson SM, Mauritson DR, Willerson JT, et al: A controlled trial of verapamil for Prinzmetal's variant angina. N Engl J Med 304:862, 1980.
44. Schroeder JS, Feldman RL, Giles TD, et al: Multiclinic controlled trial of diltiazem for Prinzmetal's angina. Am J Med 72:227, 1982.
45. Antman E, Muller J, Goldberg S, et al: Nifedipine therapy for coronary artery spasm. N Engl J Med 302:1269, 1980.
46. Shick EC Jr, Liang C, Heupler FA Jr, et al: Randomized withdrawal from nifedipine: Placebo-controlled study in patients with coronary artery spasm. Am Heart J 104:690, 1982.
47. Hugenholtz PG, Michels HR, Surrys PW, et al: Nifedipine in the treatment of unstable angina, coronary spasm and myocardial ischemia. Am J Cardiol 47:163, 1981.
48. Moses JW, Wertheimer JH, Bodenheimer MM, et al: Efficacy of nifedipine in rest angina refractory to propranolol and nitrates in patients with obstructive coronary artery disease. Ann Intern Med 94:425, 1981.
49. The HINT Research Group: Early treatment of unstable angina in the coronary care unit: A randomized, double-blind, placebo-controlled comparison of recurrent ischemia in patients treated with nifedipine or metoprolol or both. Br Heart J 56:400, 1986.
50. Ardissino D, Savonitto S, Egstrup K, et al: Transient myocardial ischemia during daily life in rest and exertional angina pectoris, and comparison of the effectiveness of metoprolol vs nifedipine. Am J Cardiol 67:946, 1991.
51. Arzneimittelkommision der deutschen Ärzteschaft: Calciumkanal-Blocker der 1,4 Dihydropyridin-Klasse. Deutsches Ärzteblatt 91:A-2512, 1994.
52. Ekelund LG, Ono L: Antianginal efficiency of nifedipine with and without a beta-blocker, studied with exercise test: A double-blind randomized sub-acute study. Clin Cardiol 2:203, 1979.
53. Lynch L, Dargie H, Kirkler S, et al: Objective assessment of antianginal treatment: A double-blind comparison of propranolol, nifedipine and their combination. Br Med J 281:184, 1980.
54. Mueller HS, Chahine RA: Interim report of multicenter double-blind, placebo-controlled studies of nifedipine in chronic stable angina. Am J Med 71:645, 1981.
55. Moskowitz RM, Piccini PA, Nacarelli G, et al: Nifedipine therapy for stable angina pectoris: Preliminary results of effects on angina frequency and treadmill exercise response. Am J Cardiol 44:811, 1979.
56. Deanfield J, Wright C, Fox K: Treatment of angina pectoris with nifedipine: Importance of dose titration. Br Med J 286:1467, 1983.
57. Parmley WW, Nesto RW, Singh BN, et al: Attenuation of the circadian patterns of myocardial ischemia with nifedipine GITS in patients with chronic stable angina. J Am Coll Cardiol 19:1380, 1992.
58. Nesto RW, White HD, Ganz P, et al: Addition of nifedipine to maximal beta-blocker-nitrate therapy: Effects on exercise capacity and global left ventricular performance at rest and during exercise. Am J Cardiol 55:3E, 1985.
59. de Buitleir M, Rowland E, Krikler DM: Hemodynamic effects of nifedipine given alone and in combination with atenolol in patients with impaired left ventricular function. Am J Cardiol 55:15E, 1985.
60. Vetrovec GW, Parker VE: Acute electrophysiologic, hemodynamic and left ventricular effects of nifedipine and beta-blocker interactions: Maintenance of global and regional left ventricular wall motion. Am J Cardiol 55:21E, 1985.
61. Gottlieb SO, Ouyang P, Achuff SC, et al: Acute nifedipine withdrawal: Consequences of pre-operative and late cessation of therapy in patients with prior unstable angina. J Am Coll Cardiol 4:382, 1984.
62. Schanzenbaher P, Deeg P, Liebau G, et al: Paradoxical angina after nifedipine: Angiographic documentation. Am J Cardiol 53:345, 1984.
63. Schulz W, Kober G, Kram G, et al: Influence of intracoronary and intravenous nifedipine on diameters of coronary vessels and stenoses. In Rafflenbeul W, Lichtlen PR, Bakon R (eds): Unstable Angina Pectoris. Stuttgart, West Germany: George Thieme, 1981, pp 259–265.
64. Kreuzer W, Schenk WG: Effect of local vasodilation on blood flow through arterial stenosis. Eur Surg Res 5:233, 1973.
65. Santamore WP, Walinsky P: Altered coronary flow responses to vasoactive drugs in the presence of coronary arterial stenosis in the dog. Am J Cardiol 45:276, 1981.
66. Charles S, Ketel Slegers JM, Buysschaert M, et al: Hyperglycaemic effects of nifedipine. Br Med J 283:19, 1981.
67. Heagerty AM, Bing RF, Thurston H, et al: Calcium antagonists in hypertension: Relation to abnormal sodium transport. Br Med J 287:1405, 1983.
68. Chobanian AV: Treatment of the elderly hypertensive patient. Am J Med 77(Suppl 2B):22, 1984.
69. Vetrovec GW, Parker VE: Alternative medical treatment for patients with angina pectoris and adverse reactions to beta-blockers: Usefulness of nifedipine. Am J Med 81(Suppl 4A):20, 1986.
70. Muller FB, Bolli P, Erne P, et al: Use of calcium antagonists as monotherapy in the management of hypertension. Am J Med 77(Suppl 2B):2, 1984.
71. Stessman J, Leibel B, Yagil Y, et al: Nifedipine in the treatment of hypertension in the elderly. J Clin Pharmacol 25:193, 1985.
72. Landmark K: Long-term antihypertensive and metabolic effects of nifedipine slow-release tablets in elderly hypertensives. Acta Med Scand 714:187, 1986.
73. Nicita-Mauro V, Barbera N, Buemi M, et al: Nifedipine in the treatment of arterial hypertension in the elderly: Preliminary report. Gerontology 28:357, 1980.

74. Resnick LM, Laragh JH, Sealey JE, et al: Divalent cations in essential hypertension: Relations between serum ionized calcium, magnesium, and plasma renin activity. N Engl J Med 309:888, 1983.

75. Resnick LM, Muller FB, Laragh JH: Calcium-regulating hormones in essential hypertension: Relation to plasma renin activity and sodium metabolism. Ann Intern Med 105:649, 1986.

76. Resnick LM, Nicholson JP, Laragh JH: Calcium, the renin-angiotensin system, and the hypotensive response to nifedipine. Hypertension 10:254, 1987.

77. Wang L, Lee DP, Wu ZW, DeQuattro V: Nifedipine GITS and enalapril lower blood pressure and proteinuria effectively in elderly hypertensives [abstract]. Eur Heart J 15(Suppl):532, 1994.

78. O'Mailia JJ, Sandler GE, Giles TD: Nifedipine-associated myocardial ischemia or infarction in the treatment of hypertensive urgencies. Ann Intern Med 107:185, 1987.

79. Landmark K, Sire S, Thaulow E, et al: Haemodynamic effects of nifedipine and propranolol in patients with hypertrophic obstructive cardiomyopathy. Br Heart J 48:19, 1982.

80. Soufer R, Wohlegelernter D, Vita NA, et al: Intact systolic left ventricular function in clinical congestive heart failure. Am J Cardiol 55:10, 1992.

81. Wei JY: Age and the cardiovascular system. N Engl J Med 327:17, 1992.

82. Lorell BH, Paulus WJ, Grossman W, et al: Modification of abnormal left ventricular diastolic properties by nifedipine in patients with hypertrophic cardiomyopathy. Circulation 65:499, 1982.

83. Hanrath P, Mathey DG, Kremer P, et al: Effect of verapamil on left ventricular isovolumic relaxation time and regional left ventricular filling in hypertrophic cardiomyopathy. Am J Cardiol 45:1258, 1980.

84. Suwa M, Hirota Y, Kawamura K: Improvement in left ventricular diastolic function during intravenous diltiazem therapy in patients with hypertrophic cardiomyopathy: An echocardiographic study. Am J Cardiol 54:1047, 1984.

85. Wei JY: Use of calcium entry blockers in elderly patients: Special consideration. Circulation 80(Suppl):IV-171, 1989.

86. Packer MB, Greenberg B, Massie B, et al: Deleterious effects of hydralazine in patients with primary pulmonary hypertension. N Engl J Med 306:1326, 1982.

87. Rich S, Martinez J, Lam W, et al: A reassessment of the effects of vasodilator drugs in primary pulmonary hypertension. Guidelines for determining a pulmonary vasodilator response. Am Heart J 105:119, 1983.

88. Rich S: Primary pulmonary hypertension. Progr Cardiovasc Dis 31:205, 1988.

89. Camerini F, Alberti E, Klugman N, et al: Primary pulmonary hypertension: Effects of nifedipine. Br Heart J 44:352, 1980.

90. Wise JR: Nifedipine in the treatment of primary pulmonary hypertension. Am Heart J 105:693, 1983.

91. Saito D, Haraoka S, Yoshida H, et al: Primary pulmonary hypertension improved by long-term oral administration of nifedipine. Am Heart J 105:1041, 1983.

92. DeFeyter PJ, Kerkkamp MJJ, deJong JP: Sustained beneficial effects of nifedipine in primary pulmonary hypertension. Am Heart J 105:333, 1983.

93. Rich S, Brundage BH: High-dose calcium-blocking therapy for primary pulmonary hypertension: Evidence for long-term reduction in pulmonary arterial pressure and regression of right ventricular hypertrophy. Circulation 76:135, 1987.

94. Aramatorio GJ, Uretsky BF, Reddy PS: Hypotension and sinus arrest with nifedipine in pulmonary hypertension. Chest 87:265, 1985.

95. Packer M, Medina N, Yushak M: Adverse hemodynamic and clinical effects of calcium-channel blockade in pulmonary hypertension secondary to obliterative pulmonary vascular disease. J Am Coll Cardiol 4:890, 1984.

96. Batra AK, Segall PH, Ahmed T: Pulmonary edema with nifedipine in primary pulmonary hypertension. Respiration 47:161, 1985.

97. Farber HW, Karlinsky JB, Faling J: Fatal outcome following nifedipine for primary pulmonary hypertension. Chest 23:708, 1983.

98. Rich S, Kaufman E, Levy PS: The effect of high doses of calcium-channel blockers on survival in primary pulmonary hypertension. N Engl J Med 327:76, 1992.

99. Schrader BJ, Inbar S, Kaufman L, et al: Comparison of the effects of adenosine and nifedipine in pulmonary hypertension. J Am Coll Cardiol 19:1060, 1992.

100. Calcium-channel blockers and asthma [editorial]. Thorax 38:481, 1983.

101. Simmoneau G, Escourrou P, Duroux P, et al: Inhibition of hypoxic pulmonary vasoconstriction by nifedipine. N Engl J Med 304:1582, 1981.

102. White CJ, Phillips WA, Abrahams LA, et al: Objective benefit of nifedipine in the treatment of Raynaud's phenomenon. Am J Med 80:623, 1986.

103. Sarkozi J, Bookman AAM, Mahon W, et al: Nifedipine in the treatment of idiopathic Raynaud's syndrome. J Rheumatol 13:331, 1986.

104. Gjarup T, Kelboek H, Hartling OJ, et al: Controlled double-blind trial of the clinical effect of nifedipine in the treatment of idiopathic Raynaud's phenomenon. Am Heart J 3:742, 1986.

105. Banks AK, White CJ: Calcium-channel blockers in the treatment of peripheral vascular diseases. Prac Cardiol 14:31, 1987.

CHAPTER 104

Nicardipine

Charles R. Lambert, M.D., Ph.D., and Carl J. Pepine, M.D.

HISTORY

Nicardipine was first synthesized by Yamanouchi Pharmaceutical Co., Tokyo, Japan, in the early 1970s and introduced as a cerebral vasodilator in 1976.[1] Its vasodilating effect was first attributed to cyclic adenosine monophosphate (cAMP) phosphodiesterase inhibition.[1] Subsequently, it was repeatedly shown to inhibit transmembrane calcium influx into vascular smooth muscle.[2-5] Nicardipine has been marketed in Japan since 1981 as Perdipine (YC-93), and elsewhere as Vasonase, Cardene, Nicodel, Nerdipina, and Dacarel (RS-69216). The drug has been found to be of value for the management of patients with myocardial ischemia and systemic hypertension. It has also shown promise for use in other cardiovascular and some cerebrovascular disorders. Nicardipine is currently marketed in Mexico, Belgium, Denmark, and the United Kingdom for systemic hypertension and stable angina, and in Spain for cerebrovascular indications. The drug is approved in the United States for use in angina pectoris and systemic hypertension.

CHEMISTRY

Nicardipine is 2,6-dimethyl-4(3-nitrophenyl)-1,4 dihydropyridine-3,5-dicarboxylic acid 3-[2-(N-benzyl-N-methyl amino)] ethyl ester 5-methyl ester hydrochloride.[6] Nicardipine is supplied as an opaque white or white–to–opaque light blue powder in a hard gelatin capsule containing either 20 or 30 mg of nicardipine hydrochloride. The oral form is stable for at least 3 years. Nicardipine is also available in a sustained-release formulation (Cardene SR), which consists of a two-component hard gelatin capsule. A powder component contains 25% nicardipine hydrochloride, and a spherical granule component contains the remainder of the nicardipine dose. Nicardipine is water soluble; therefore, an intravenous preparation is also available. This preparation is stable under ordinary light and hospital conditions and does not require special infusion apparatus because absorption to plastic tubing has not been a problem. The pK_a of nicardipine is such that at physiologic pH in extracellular fluid the drug is 50% protonated.

PHARMACOKINETICS
Absorption

Studies in animals (mice, rats, and dogs) and in humans have shown that oral doses of ^{14}C-labeled nicardipine are rapidly and completely absorbed.[7] Nicardipine constitutes only a small fraction of the circulating compound–related activity that is detected in plasma. This is a result of extensive hepatic first-pass metabolism.

In humans, peak plasma concentrations of nicardipine are reached at approximately 1 hour after oral dosage as a capsule formulation (Fig. 104–1).[8-11] This rapid absorption is attributed to its high aqueous solubility. Maximal plasma concentrations of nicardipine in volunteers given oral doses of 10, 20, 30, and 40 mg to steady state (t.i.d. dosing for three days) are approximately 15, 35, 90, and 130 μg/L, respectively.[12] The systemic bioavailability of nicardipine averaged 35% after 30 mg at steady state. The plasma half-life of nicardipine at steady state averaged 8.6 hours. Thus, despite the fact that nicardipine is well absorbed after oral administration, its systemic bioavailability is low. This is apparently due to extensive presystemic metabolism.[13] Cardene SR administration results in detectable plasma levels within 20 minutes, with a broad peak between 1 and 4 hours. Cardene SR has somewhat lower bioavailability than the immediate-release formulation, except at the highest dose. Fluctuation in plasma levels may be further reduced when Cardene SR is given with meals.

Nicardipine is highly protein bound (> 95%) over a wide range of plasma concentrations. *In vivo* protein-binding studies using therapeutic concentrations of a variety of drugs, including digoxin, diuretics, and β-blockers, have shown that none significantly displaced nicardipine from protein-binding sites. However, the package insert in the United States advises

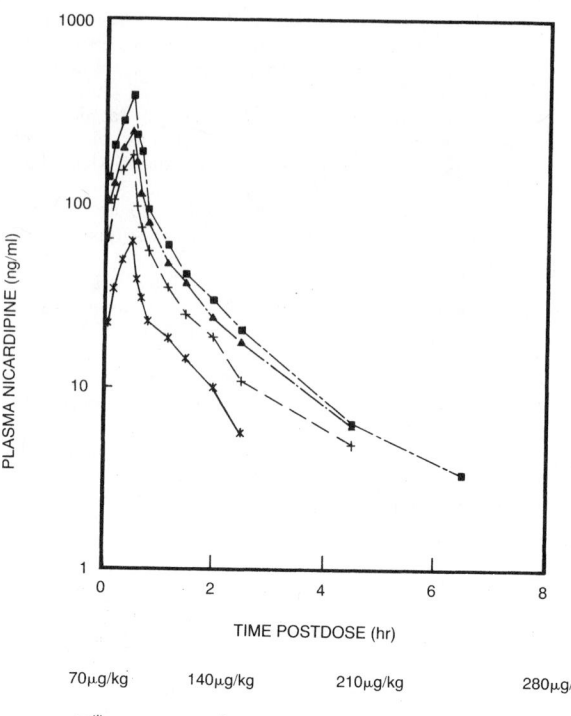

Figure 104–1. Plasma nicardipine levels, indicated after dose. (Unpublished data from ICM Study 1107, Syntex Corporation, Palo Alto, CA.)

monitoring serum digoxin levels after concomitant therapy with nicardipine is initiated.

Metabolism and Elimination

In four subjects given oral ^{14}C-labeled nicardipine, urinary and fecal excretion accounted for 60% and 35%, respectively, of the dose. Excretion was rapid: more than 90% of the urinary excretion occurred within 48 hours of dosing. Nicardipine is rapidly and extensively metabolized in human subjects. Less than 1% of the oral dose of nicardipine is detected in urine in any species.[7, 14-17] The vasodilating activity of all the metabolites of nicardipine is considerably less than 1% of that seen with the drug itself.[18, 19] Thus, the pharmacologic effects of the drug are attributable to nicardipine as a parent compound. Steady-state plasma levels of nicardipine are achieved on about day 3, using a regimen of 10, 20, and 30 mg three times daily (Unpublished data, Syntex Corporation, ICM Study 1107, Palo Alto, CA). Elimination half-life after intravenous administration ranges from approximately 50 to 70 minutes.[14, 20, 21] After single oral doses of 10 mg and 40 mg, the elimination half-life ranges from approximately 50 to 100 minutes.[11, 14] Less than 1% of the oral dose of intact nicardipine is detected in the urine of any species.

Patients with poor renal function associated with hypertension achieve higher maximal plasma concentrations when compared with healthy volunteers. This is associated with a decrease in overall clearance of the drug, although no evidence for significant drug accumulation has been presented.[8, 22] No significant differences in volume of distribution, protein binding, or hepatic function account for the reduction of nicardipine clearance in uremic patients.[23] The manufacturer suggests reducing the dose in patients with renal failure (Personal communication, Syntex Labs, Palo Alto, CA, November 1987). Hemodialysis does not appear to influence nicardipine kinetics. It has been concluded that patients with chronic renal failure with or without dialysis may use the drug safely with little change in dose or frequency of administration.

Nicardipine plasma levels were measured in patients with impaired hepatic function and in six healthy volunteers. Oral clearance in the patients (18 ml/min/kg) was reduced to almost one fifth of that in the volunteers (82 ml/min/kg). The terminal plasma half-life of nicardipine was prolonged 6.5-fold in patients compared with volunteers and appeared to be related to reduced total systemic clearance and increased volume of distribution.[24] It is suggested that lower doses of nicardipine be used to initiate therapy in patients with liver impairment or reduced hepatic blood flow. Studies in rats have shown significant concentrations of nicardipine in maternal milk after oral administration.

PHARMACOLOGY
In Vitro Pharmacology

Like other 1,4 dihydropyridines, nicardipine binds to membrane receptors linked to voltage-sensitive calcium channels. Nicardipine (pki 9.7) has a higher affinity for these receptors than nisoldipine (pki 9.6), nitrendipine (pki 9.2), nimodipine (pki 9.1), and nifedipine (pki 8.2). (Relative affinity constants for these compounds are in parentheses.[25]) Nicardipine has very weak affinity for muscarinic and α-adrenergic receptors.[26] The latter activity has been found to be partially responsible for the coronary artery dilation caused by two other closely related 1,4 dihydropyridine calcium antagonists[27] and is also likely to be operative with nicardipine. Some inhibition of cardiac sarcolemmal sodium-calcium exchange by nicardipine has also been observed,[28] and, as stated earlier, cAMP phosphodiesterase inhibition has been documented in cell-free preparations.[2] Kinetic studies support the existence of a nicardipine-binding site separate from the active site on calmodulin-dependent phosphodiesterase.[29] Further differences in binding characteristics of nicardipine and nifedipine have been described in frog heart ventricle strips.[30] These studies suggest that nicardipine interacts with one and nifedipine with two receptors on the dihydropyridine-binding complex. Furthermore, the binding energy for nifedipine varied with closed and open status of calcium channels, whereas the effect of nicardipine was irreversible. Nicardipine has very weak and probably insignificant calcium agonist activity. In the paper reporting this finding, only one dose was evaluated, and the apparent agonist effect could have been due to coronary vasodilation or improved perfusion.[31]

In vivo studies using various preparations all show effects secondary to inhibition of calcium flux by nicardipine. The calcium-dependent action potential seen in partially depolarized myocardium is blocked in a concentration-dependent fashion by nicardipine.[32] The relative potencies of various calcium antagonists have been compared in vitro by studying normalized responses of myocardial and vascular smooth muscle tissue. When potency is measured by the inhibitory concentration of the antagonist needed to cause a 50% reduction in maximal response (IC_{50}), nicardipine is the most potent of the dihydropyridines studied for vascular smooth muscle. In addition, it exhibits the highest degree of selectivity for vascular smooth muscle.[33] Nifedipine and nicardipine also have been compared with respect to selectivity for coronary and mesenteric vascular smooth muscle. The ratio of the negative log (IC_{50}) for these compounds in coronary/mesenteric vessels is 10.72 for nicardipine and 4.47 for nifedipine. Thus, nicardipine exhibits selectivity for coronary vascular smooth muscle, and nifedipine does not.[34] Similar findings have been reported using human arterial segments studied post mortem.[35]

In vitro studies show that nicardipine exhibits differences from other 1,4 dihydropyridines with respect to binding, relative coronary vascular smooth muscle specificity, and degree of myocardial depressant activity. Although nicardipine inhibits calcium-dependent action potential and depresses both spontaneous sinoatrial node rate and atrioventricular nodal conduction in vitro,[36] these effects are less prominent than those observed with other dihydropyridines.

Animal Pharmacology

When given to anesthetized dogs, nicardipine (0.001 to 0.01 mg/kg) produces a dose-dependent increase in coronary blood flow. This is accompanied by a decrease in both arterial pressure and coronary arteriovenous oxygen difference, an increase in cardiac output, and little change in myocardial oxygen consumption, heart rate, maximum dP/dt, and cardiac work.[37] In the same model, regional vascular reactivity to nicardipine ranked in the following order: vertebral > coronary > carotid > mesenteric = femoral > renal arteries. At higher doses (0.1 mg/kg intravenously), nicardipine produces further decreases in arterial pressure associated with reflex tachycardia and increased dP/dt. At even higher doses (0.3 mg/kg intravenously), nicardipine causes a slight decrease in dP/dt, no change in heart rate, and some prolongation of the PQ interval. If a β-adrenergic blocker is administered or bilateral vagotomy is performed, the increases in heart rate and dP/dt seen with intermediate doses of nicardipine are abolished. Similar effects are observed in conscious normotensive monkeys.[37]

The hemodynamic effects of nicardipine have been studied in spontaneous (SHR), renal (RHR), and salt retention (DOCA) hypertensive rat models. Nicardipine caused a dose-dependent fall in systolic pressure with associated tachycardia in all three models.[37] The hypotensive effect of the drug was significantly more pronounced in the hypertensive animals than in normotensive controls. Associated with the hypotensive effect was a significant increase in urine volume and excretion of sodium, potassium, and chloride in salt-loaded normotensive animals. Chronic treatment of hypertensive animals showed continued efficacy without associated tachycardia. Nicardipine has also been shown to reverse left ventricular and vascular hypertrophy in hypertensive rats, although minimal coronary vascular resistance remains elevated.[38-40] Similar hemodynamic and renal effects have been observed during oral nicardipine treatment of renal hypertensive dogs.[41] Intravenous administration of nicardipine to anesthetized dogs is associated with increased renin release and plasma renin activity.

Effects of intravenous nicardipine (1 to 10 µg/kg) in a model of myocardial ischemia produced by partial left anterior descending (LAD) coronary artery occlusion and atrial tachycardia (pacing) were studied by Alps et al.[42] Nicardipine attenuated indices of ischemia in this model without affecting intraatrial, atrioventricular, or intraventricular conduction. Dogs given nicardipine orally (1 to 2 mg/kg) for 16 weeks before LAD occlusion developed increased collateral flow when compared with control animals. Effects of three nicardipine treatment protocols on myocardial infarction size were studied in an acute 6-hour LAD occlusion model using baboons.[42] These protocols included acute preligation and postligation treatment, postligation treatment alone, and long-term (6 months) preligation treatment. Myocardial infarction size was significantly limited in all three nicardipine treatment groups when compared with nontreated controls.[42]

Myocardial protection with nicardipine was also documented in dogs that survived 3 months of LAD occlusion[42] and in a postligation baboon model. In contrast, no myocardial preservation was observed with postligation administration of nifedipine or verapamil in the baboon model.[43] Endo et al.[44] reported results of nicardipine treatment in canine myocardial infarction models. Again, pretreatment or early postocclusion therapy with nicardipine limited the infarct size. Sandhu and Biro[45] found no protective effect of postocclusion nicardipine administration in a canine model of myocardial infarction.

Mechanisms for possible myocardial protection during ischemia include prevention of calcium loading and the "oxygen paradox" by nicardipine.[46] Nicardipine may also offer protection from free radical injury[47] and from posthypoxic hepatic injury.[48] It offers myocardial preservation when added to cardioplegia solution.[49-51] Nicardipine has also been shown to be an inhibitor of angiogenesis in vitro[52] and to inhibit hyperplastic changes in venous bypass grafts.[53]

As stated earlier, nicardipine exhibits marked cerebrovascular vasodilator activity. This effect is approximately 50 to 330 times more potent than that caused by papaverine and other cerebrovascular reference drugs such as isoxsuprine and cinnarizine.[54, 55] The duration of cerebrovascular dilation after nicardipine is much longer than that seen with papaverine.[56] Nicardipine has been shown to prevent ischemia-related neuronal cell death in rats[57] and gerbils.[58] The protective effect of nicardipine in ischemic brain injury may be related to alterations in leukotriene C4 and prostaglandin E_2 levels.[59]

Applied Pharmacology

General

In normotensive volunteers without cardiovascular disease, intravenous administration of nicardipine produces decreases in arterial blood pressure and the pre-ejection period, whereas heart rate and left ventricular ejection time increase.[60] Hemodynamic studies in our laboratories[61, 62] show intravenous administration of nicardipine to be associated with decreased arterial pressure and systemic and coronary vascular resistance (Fig. 104–2). Coronary blood flow, cardiac output, heart rate, and indices of left ventricular contractile state increase. The augmented coronary blood flow persists even at the same heart rate using an atrial pacing model. These hemodynamic alterations are similar to those described in animal models and are a manifestation of intense vasodilation with little or no inotropic or chronotropic effects. The reflex increase in heart rate seen with acute intravenous nicardipine disappears with chronic oral administration, probably as a result of resetting of baroreceptors.[63] A convenient way to separate the direct cardiac effects of nicardipine from the peripheral effects is to use intracoronary injection (Fig. 104–3).[64, 65] Such studies show no direct or reflex chronotropic response and confirm that nicardipine is a potent coronary vasodilator causing minimal depression of systolic and diastolic myocardial function. Other investigators have used invasive and noninvasive methods to study the hemodynamic and myocardial effects of nicardipine in patients with left ventricular function ranging from normal to severely depressed.[66-70] A uniform finding is the lack of an important negative inotropic effect at clinically relevant doses.

Some investigations of the cardioprotective effect of nicardipine have been conducted in human subjects. In 10 patients with angina in whom ^{14}C-lactate was infused, left ventricular lactate extraction fraction increased more than the ^{14}C-lactate extraction ratio after intravenous nicardipine administration, indicating a reduction in left ventricular lactate production.[71, 72] Similarly, in a randomized double-blind parallel group of 35 patients with angina, myocardial lactate uptake decreased to a greater extent while they were receiving propranolol than while receiving nicardipine.[73] Decreased lactate production and release of hypoxanthine (indicating depletion of high-energy phosphate stores) have also been reported in 12 patients during percutaneous transluminal coronary angioplasty when balloon occlusion was preceded by intracoronary injection of nicardipine.[74] These reductions in left ventricular lactate production (i.e., improved lactate extraction) further support the

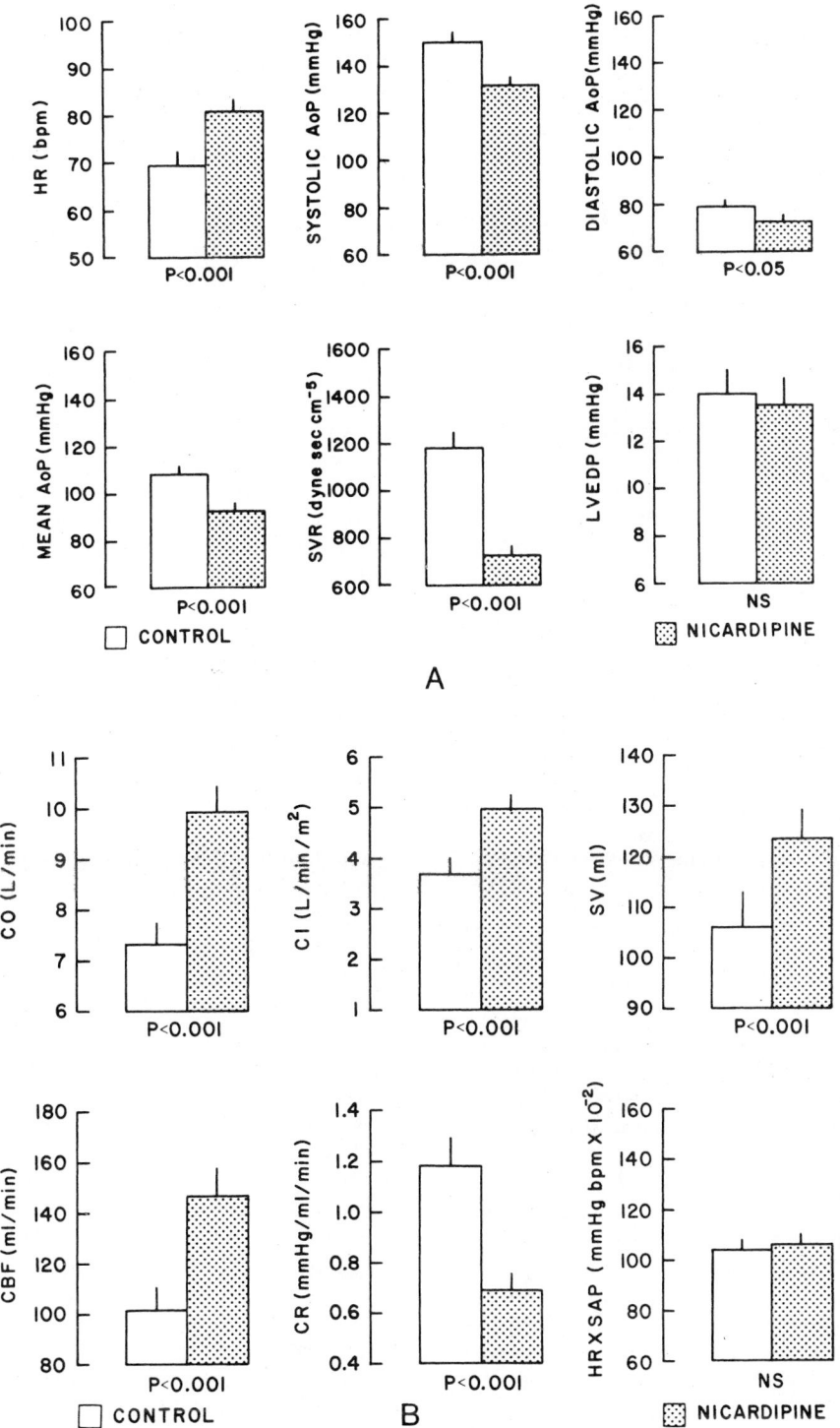

Figure 104–2. A, Summary data (mean + standard error of the mean) for 15 patients during the control period *(open bars)* and after 15 minutes of nicardipine infusion *(dotted bars)* as described in the text. AoP, aortic pressure; HR, heart rate; LVEDP, left ventricular end-diastolic pressure; NS, not significant; SVR, systemic vascular resistance.

B, Summary data (mean + standard error of the mean) for 15 patients during the control period and during a steady state with nicardipine infusion as described in the text. CBF, coronary blood flow; CI, cardiac index; CO, cardiac output; CR, coronary resistance; HR × SAP, product of heart rate and systolic aortic pressure; NS, not significant; SV, stroke volume. (From Lambert CR, Hill JA, Nichols WW, et al: Coronary and systemic hemodynamic effects of nicardipine. Am J Cardiol 55:652, 1985. Adapted with permission from American Journal of Cardiology.)

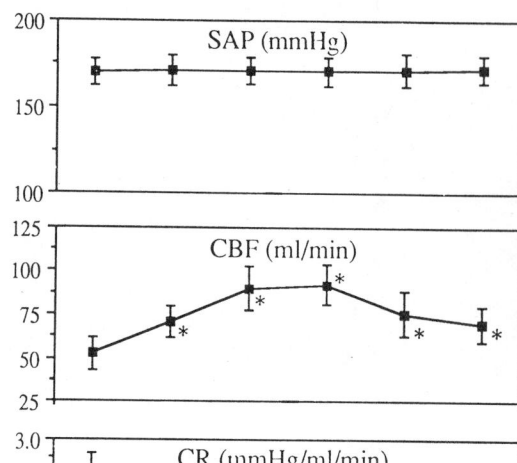

Figure 104–3. Effects of intracoronary nicardipine on coronary blood flow and resistance. Intracoronary nicardipine, administered as a 0.2-mg bolus diluted in 1 ml of blood directly into the left coronary artery, causes a prompt increase in coronary blood flow peaking approximately 60 seconds after infusion associated with a decline in coronary resistance; this effect begins to dissipate after approximately 90 seconds. No changes in arterial pressure or heart rate were observed. Data displayed for systolic aortic pressure (SAP, *top panel*), great cardiac vein flow (CBF, *mid panel*), and anterior regional coronary resistance (CR, *lower panel*) at various intervals after infusion. (Adapted from Lambert CR, Buss DD, Pepine CJ: Effects of nicardipine on myocardial function in vitro and in vivo. Circulation 81(Suppl III):III–145, 1990.)

hypothesis that nicardipine may improve perfusion and aerobic metabolism in chronically ischemic areas.[74, 75] This, along with increases in coronary flow induced by the drug, would allow enhanced oxygen utilization and reduced lactate production in under-perfused areas, potentially leading to improvements in ventricular function.[71–73] The effects of nicardipine in preventing stress-induced myocardial ischemia are discussed later.

Nicardipine has been shown to be a potent cerebrovascular dilator in patients after topical application[76] and oral administration.[77] Nicardipine has little effect on glucose and insulin dynamics in humans[78] and affects neither basal nor stimulated pituitary hormone release.[79] Nicardipine produces a mild natriuresis; however, no effect on adrenal responsiveness is seen.[80] Nicardipine has no significant effects on serum lipids or hormonal or metabolic responses to food and exercise.[81]

Myocardial Ischemia

Most of the data published to date indicate that calcium antagonists prevent myocardial ischemia largely by reducing myocardial oxygen demand for a given level of work.[82] In other patient subsets, particularly those with angina at rest, evidence suggests that calcium antagonists prevent coronary artery spasm and perhaps some less severe alterations in coronary

smooth muscle tone.[83] It is also likely that, in some patient subsets, calcium antagonists act by a combination of both of these mechanisms. However, the first-generation calcium antagonists (verapamil, nifedipine, and diltiazem) are a diverse group of compounds with different chemical structures and physiologic effects. Therefore, the precise mechanism responsible for prevention of ischemia is likely to differ for each drug and for each patient.

Studies in our laboratory were conducted to investigate the systemic and coronary hemodynamic effects of nicardipine in 15 patients with angina pectoris of effort.[61] Nicardipine was administered intravenously in a dose sufficient to decrease systolic blood pressure 10 to 20 mmHg. At this dose, nicardipine acutely increased both heart rate and cardiac output as systemic vascular resistance decreased. The divergent effects on heart rate and blood pressure resulted in no significant change in the double product. Thus, nicardipine administered at rest should have a very favorable antiischemic profile because of an increase in myocardial oxygen supply for the same oxygen demand. Left ventricular function improved as stroke volume increased significantly, and left ventricular end-diastolic pressure was unchanged. These findings suggest that the net effect of nicardipine on hemodynamic determinants of myocardial oxygen demand is to maintain these variables without significant depression of myocardial function. Relative to myocardial oxygen supply, coronary blood flow increased despite a decrease in blood pressure and hence coronary perfusion pressure. Further investigation revealed an increase in myocardial oxygen consumption of 18%, even though the product of heart rate and systolic pressure was unchanged.[62]

Examination of some determinants of myocardial oxygen consumption revealed that an increase in function in ischemic regions may account for some of the observed changes. With parenteral acute administration of nicardipine, this increase in myocardial function may also be, in part, reflex in origin.[71] Additional possibilities include a positive inotropic effect either by inhibiting cAMP phosphodiesterase or by dose-dependent calcium agonistic activity,[31] as described *in vitro.* If these latter two mechanisms were operative in patients, one would expect such actions to increase ischemia in patients with severe coronary disease if there were no additional effect to improve blood flow to ischemic regions. Indeed, we found a disproportionate increase of 41% in coronary blood flow when compared with one of 18% in myocardial oxygen consumption, resulting in a very favorable change in the estimated supply/demand ratio (Fig. 104–4).[84] The decrease in coronary resistance observed after nicardipine was greater than the decrease in systemic vascular resistance even when heart rate was controlled. This finding again suggests selectivity for the coronary circulation when compared with the systemic circulation.

In order to be uniformly beneficial as an antiischemic agent, a drug would have to cause no maldistribution of coronary blood flow, sometimes termed

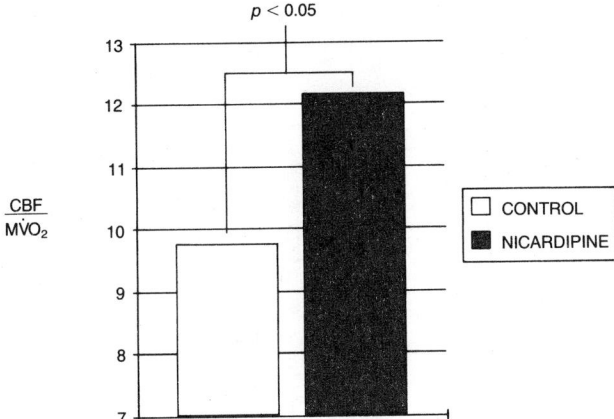

Figure 104–4. Effect of intravenous nicardipine on myocardial oxygen supply-consumption relationship. Myocardial oxygen supply reflected coronary blood flow (CBF) increases as oxygen demand, reflected in myocardial oxygen consumption (MV̇O₂), decreased, resulting in a significant increase in this relationship. (Reproduced with permission from Pepine CJ, Lambert CR: Usefulness of nicardipine for angina pectoris. Am J Cardiol 59:13J, 1987. Copyright 1987, American Heart Association.)

"coronary steal." We have seen only one patient in whom myocardial ischemia occurred during acute parenteral administration of nicardipine.[85] The mechanism responsible for ischemia in this case was failure of coronary flow to increase in a collateral-dependent region and not a coronary steal. As noted earlier, the increase in heart rate and the evidence for reflex sympathetic drive seen after acute parenteral nicardipine administration are not seen with chronic oral administration.[6, 63] A hemodynamic and quantitative coronary angiographic study of intravenous nicardipine and nitroglycerin revealed both drugs to be potent coronary dilators; however, nicardipine dilated small (<2 mm²) and large segments equally, whereas nitroglycerin had a proportionately greater effect on small vessels (Fig. 104–5).[86]

Overall, these observations made at rest in patients without ischemia suggest that nicardipine generally improves the relationship of myocardial oxygen supply to demand. Thus, nicardipine should have a favorable hemodynamic profile as an antiischemic agent and may be particularly effective in patients with dynamic coronary factors contributing to myocardial ischemia and poor left ventricular function.

To test this hypothesis, the authors performed studies designed to assess the effect of nicardipine on either exercise- or pacing-induced ischemia in patients with coronary artery disease.[75] Nicardipine significantly prolonged bicycle exercise duration and time to onset of 1 mm of ST-segment depression in these patients. Associated hemodynamic changes included decreased left ventricular end-diastolic pressure, decreased systemic and coronary vascular resistances, increased coronary blood flow and myocardial oxygen consumption, and no change in the double product (Fig. 104–6). During the stress of controlled tachycardia (i.e., atrial pacing), the heart rate threshold for myocardial ischemia was unchanged by nicar-

dipine despite improvement in the ratio of coronary blood flow to myocardial oxygen consumption and with hemodynamic changes otherwise similar to those seen during exercise. Although the paced heart rate threshold for angina did not change during nicardipine treatment, marked improvement in the myocardial metabolic state was observed as measured by lactate metabolism (Fig. 104–7). Similar salutary effects of nicardipine on lactate metabolism have been shown by other workers.[72, 87, 88] Improved diastolic function after nicardipine administration may be seen in patients with coronary artery disease.[69, 71] Early diastolic filling increased from 43% to 52% ($p < .05$) after 5 mg and from 35% to 52% ($p < .02$) after 10 mg of intravenous nicardipine. These changes were accompanied by a reduction in the time constant of isovolumic pressure fall, although this improvement did not reach statistical significance. Others have not observed significant load-independent effects of nicardipine on diastolic function.[67]

The mechanisms by which nicardipine may benefit patients with coronary disease include reduction in myocardial oxygen demand (decreased systolic pressure), increased myocardial oxygen delivery (increased coronary flow) that results in associated improvement in myocardial metabolic state (increased lactate extraction), and improved diastolic (reduced end-diastolic pressure) and systolic (increased stroke volume) myocardial function. The coronary vasodilator effect of nicardipine may be particularly important in patients with a vasomotor component to their myocardial ischemia.

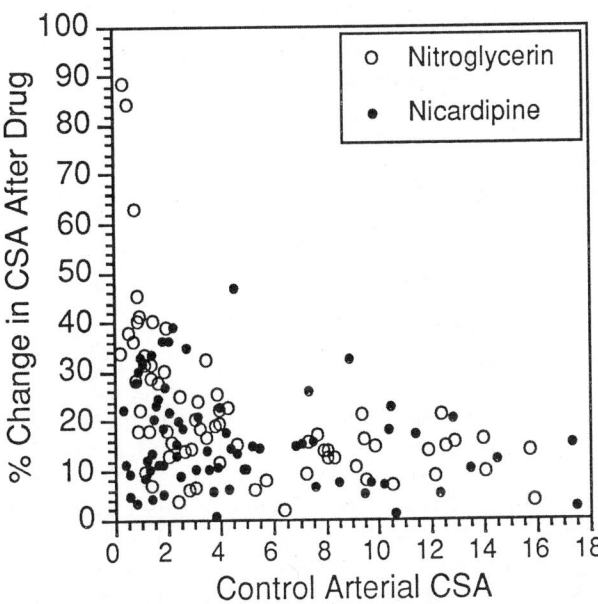

Figure 104–5. Quantitative angiographic comparison of the effects of intravenous (equihypotensive doses) nicardipine and nitroglycerin in patients at rest without ischemic heart disease. The percentage change in coronary artery cross-sectional area is compared with the control cross-sectional area. CSA, cross-sectional area. (Unpublished data from the investigation described in reference 86.)

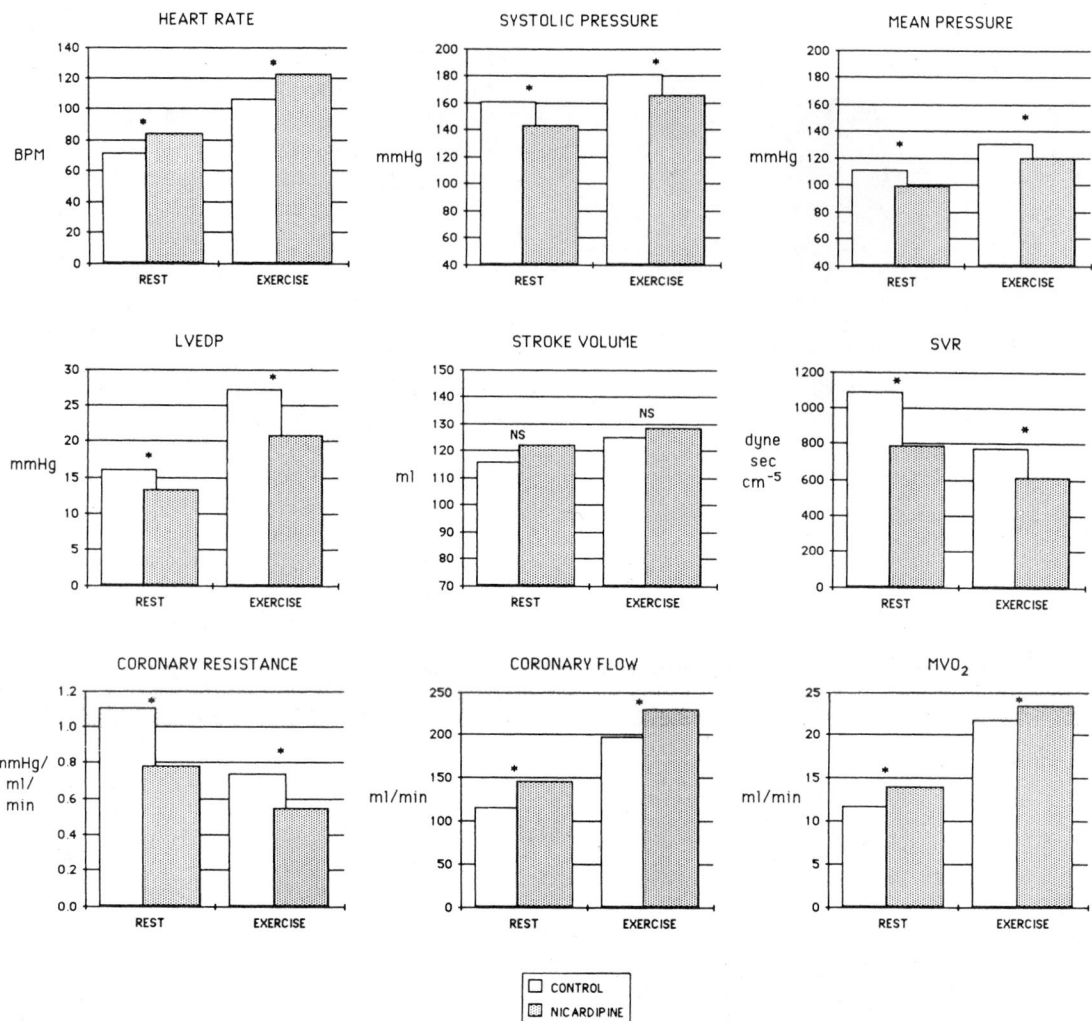

Figure 104–6. Effect of intravenous nicardipine administration on coronary and systemic hemodynamics as well as myocardial oxygen consumption at rest and during supine bicycle exercise to development of myocardial ischemia. *p < .05. LVEDP, left ventricular end-diastolic pressure; SVR, systemic vascular resistance. (From Lambert CR, Hill JA, Feldman RL, et al: Effects of nicardipine on exercise and pacing induced myocardial ischemia in angina pectoris. Am J Cardiol 60:471, 1987. Adapted with permission of the American Journal of Cardiology.)

CLINICAL USE
Effort-Induced Angina

Placebo-Controlled Studies

Deedwania et al.[89] treated 18 patients with chronic effort angina using doses of nicardipine up to 120 mg/day (mean dose, 98 mg daily). Treatment was continued for 1 to 4 months, and measurements were made during treadmill exercise at 2 and 4 months. After 4 months, the total exercise duration increased 22% compared with placebo, time to onset of angina increased 17%, and time to onset of 1 mm of ST-segment depression increased 26%. A reduction in frequency of angina of 50% and a decrease in nitroglycerin consumption of approximately 42% were also observed.

Four placebo-controlled double-blind trials[90–93] including 127 patients corroborate the findings of Deedwania et al.[89] The controlled trials employed doses ranging from 30 to 120 mg/day for a duration of 2 to

6 weeks. Overall, nicardipine increased exercise time approximately 20%, and time to onset of 1 mm ST-segment depression 29%, while decreasing angina frequency 50% and nitroglycerin consumption 41%. Average improvements in indices of myocardial ischemia observed in these clinical trials of oral nicardipine are illustrated in Table 104–1.[84] In two of these four studies,[90, 91] 21 patients were treated for 6 months or longer, and the antianginal effects of nicardipine were maintained without important adverse effects. These short- and long-term results are summarized in Table 104–1.[84]

Multicenter Study

Efficacy

The largest number of patients studied with nicardipine were reported from the multicenter trial by Scheidt et al.[92] Nicardipine was administered at a dose of 30 mg or 40 mg three times per day to

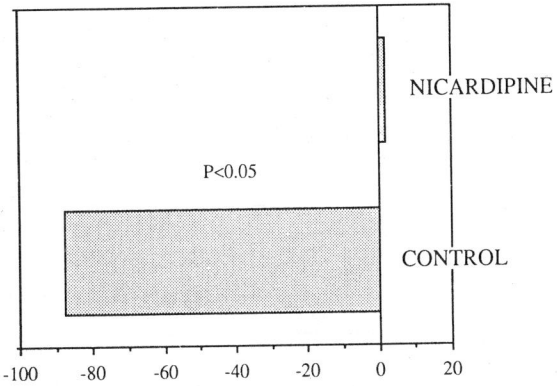

LACTATE EXTRACTION
% CHANGE FROM REST TO ISCHEMIA

Figure 104–7. Effects of intravenous nicardipine on myocardial lactate metabolism. Myocardial lactate extraction during tachycardia-induced (atrial pacing) ischemia. Before nicardipine (control), tachycardia stress resulted in an 88% decrease in myocardial lactate extraction. During nicardipine infusion (nicardipine), the same tachycardia stress resulted in an increase in myocardial lactate extraction. (From Lambert CR, Hill JA, Feldman RL, et al: Effects of nicardipine on exercise and pacing induced myocardial ischemia in angina pectoris. Am J Cardiol 60:471, 1987. Used with permission of the American Journal of Cardiology.)

patients with chronic stable angina on effort, using a randomized, double-blind crossover design. Of the 66 patients enrolled, two had insufficient angina during the placebo period and were withdrawn. Eight additional patients were withdrawn before crossover; therefore, 56 patients were included in the final analysis. Duration of exercise, cumulative oxygen consumption, and time to onset of angina and maximal ST-segment depression increased significantly with nicardipine. Although peak heart rate during exercise increased significantly with nicardipine, blood pressure at maximal workload decreased. Thus, the double product reached at maximal workload, or peak double product, was unchanged by nicardipine. The percentage of patients who stopped exercise because of ischemia (either angina or ST-segment depression) decreased from 100% with placebo to 70% with nicardipine.

Adverse Effects

Of the 63 patients evaluated for side effects in the multicenter study, eight (13%) reported adverse effects considered severe enough to discontinue study participation.[93] Seven of these patients were receiving nicardipine, and one was receiving placebo. One patient had exercise-induced hypotension while taking nicardipine and later was found to have triple-vessel disease with 80% narrowing of the left main coronary artery. Three others complained of increased angina, and two of these three also had lightheadedness and flushing. One other patient had headache and lightheadedness. Three patients sustained non–Q-wave myocardial infarctions during the trial, but only two were taking nicardipine. No significant difference was seen in new electrocardiographic abnormalities or noncardiovascular complaints on comparing nicardipine and placebo treatments. There were no significant changes in clinical hematology, chemistry, or urinalysis during the trial when nicardipine and placebo periods were compared. In general, side effects and adverse events with nicardipine are similar to other agents in the dihydropyridine class.

Comparison Studies

Three controlled studies[93–95] comparing nicardipine with other antianginal agents have been reported (Table 104–2).[84] McGill et al.[94] compared nicardipine (90 mg/day) with propranolol (120 mg/day). After a 2-week, single-blind placebo period, 25 patients with effort angina were randomized to receive either nicardipine or propranolol for 4 weeks and then crossed over to alternate therapy for 4 weeks after a 1-week "washout" period. Compared with placebo, both drugs improved exercise time to onset of 1 mm of ST-segment depression and all other indices of ischemia studied. Nicardipine, however, depressed neither resting heart rate nor maximal workload as did propranolol. Side effects were less frequent in nicardipine treatment periods compared with propranolol. DiPasquale et al.[93] compared nicardipine (80 mg/day) with nifedipine (40 mg/day) in 12 patients with chronic effort angina. Nicardipine, nifedipine, or placebo was

Table 104–1. Double-Blind, Placebo-Controlled Trials of Nicardipine in Chronic Stable Effort-Induced Angina

Author	Year	Patients	Dose (mg/day)	Duration (wk)	Exercise Time	Time to ≥1 mm ST ↓	Angina Frequency	NTG Use
					\multicolumn{4}{c}{% Change from Placebo to Optimal Dose}			
Khurmi et al.[90]	1984	20	30–120	2	+35	+50	−50	−20
		11*	120	26	+44			
DiPasquale et al.[93]	1984	12	80	3	+18	+20	−67	−77
Scheidt et al.[92]	1985	56	90–120	6	+8	+18	−15	−4
Gheorghiade et al.[91]	1985	20	90–120	2	+18	+28	−68	−63
		10*	90–120	26	+18	+10		
TOTAL								
Mean or range		108	30–120	2–6	(20)	(29)	(−50)	(−41)
*Long-term		21	90–120	26	(31)	(10)		

NTG, nitroglycerin; ST ↓, ST-segment depression; ( ), mean data.
From Pepine CJ, Lambert CR: Usefulness of nicardipine for angina pectoris. Am J Cardiol 59:15J, 1987.

Table 104–2. **Comparison-Controlled Trials of Nicardipine in Stable Effort-Induced Angina**

Author	Year	Patients	Drug (mg/day)	Duration (wk)	Comparison of Change*			
					Exercise Time	Time to ≥1 mm ST ↓	Angina Frequency	NTG Use
Bowles et al.[95]	1983	134	Nicardipine (120)	NA	p NS	NA	NA	NA
			Nifedipine (60)	NA	p NS	NA	NA	NA
DiPasquale et al.[93]	1984	12	Nicardipine (80)	3	p NS	p NS	p NS	p NS
			Nifedipine (40)	3	p NS	p NS	p NS	p NS
McGill et al.[94]	1986	25	Nicardipine (90)	4	p NS	p NS	p NS	p NS
			Propranolol (120)	4	p NS	p NS	p NS	p NS
TOTALS (Mean)		171		4–6	*Range of Change*			
Nicardipine					+18%–30%	+20%–35%	−51%–67%	−64%–77%
Nifedipine					+21%–39%	+36%	−56%	−38%
Propranolol					+14%	+32%	−55%	−39%

NA, data not available; NTG, nitroglycerin; p NS, p not significant; ST ↓, ST-segment depression.
*Nicardipine versus study drug.
From Pepine CJ, Lambert CR: Usefulness of nicardipine for angina pectoris. Am J Cardiol 59:16J, 1987.

each given for a 3-week period in a double-blind, randomized crossover fashion. Compared with placebo, both drugs lowered systolic pressure at rest and during submaximal exercise. Both agents improved exercise duration, time to onset of angina, and time to onset of 1.5 mm of ST-segment depression while decreasing the frequency of angina and nitroglycerin consumption. Thus, at the doses used, no significant differences were found comparing the antianginal effects or side effects of the two dihydropyridine drugs. Bowles et al.[95] found that nicardipine was generally comparable to nifedipine in prolonging exercise time and time to onset of ST-segment depression. However, details of the comparison of nicardipine with other agents were lacking.

Rest Angina

To our knowledge, published data on use in patients with rest angina due to coronary spasm are limited to a study done in our laboratory.[6] In this trial, the antiischemic effects and safety of nicardipine were assessed in 17 patients with angina at rest and documented coronary artery spasm. Eleven of these 17 patients had previously documented unsatisfactory results using long-acting nitrates or other calcium antagonists. The average daily dose of nicardipine for optimal relief of angina was 89 mg/day (range, 40 to 160 mg/day) identified during a single-blind treatment phase. During a double-blind crossover treatment phase, angina frequency was significantly decreased during 2 weeks of nicardipine treatment compared with placebo, from an average of 2.1 to 0.47 episodes per day. A similar decrease in nitroglycerin consumption was observed from 2.8 to 0.51 tablets per day.

Ambulatory monitoring during placebo periods revealed that 51 episodes of ischemic-type ST-segment shifts occurred during 482 hours of monitoring. Only 24% of these episodes were associated with pain; the remaining were silent. The change of silent episodes was from 10% to 3.1%. During nicardipine administration, only 15 episodes of ST-segment shifts oc-

curred during 489 hours of monitoring, and only two of these episodes (13%) were associated with angina. The remainder were silent.

Overall, the side effects observed were minimal, and there was no significant difference between the number of patients reporting adverse experiences when taking nicardipine compared with placebo. One patient developed a burning skin rash with nicardipine treatment, necessitating early termination of the study. We concluded that nicardipine was effective and safe in preventing symptomatic and asymptomatic ischemia in patients with coronary spasm. Our results suggest that nicardipine may be particularly beneficial in patients with rest angina who have had unsatisfactory responses to other therapy.

Hypertension

Applied Pharmacology

The pharmacologic principles defined earlier in animal models apply also to patients with hypertension. The primary mode of action of nicardipine in hypertension is arteriolar vasodilation, although the slight natriuretic effect may also play a role. The primary systemic vasodilator response to oral nicardipine was documented in patients with essential hypertension using simultaneous Doppler velocimetry and strain gauge plethysmography.[96] Mean, systolic, and diastolic pressures were significantly reduced, as was forearm vascular resistance during oral nicardipine therapy. An increase in brachial artery compliance and a decrease in characteristic impedance were documented after acute therapy, and these changes were maintained with long-term administration. Similarly, changes in brachial artery diameter, blood velocity, and blood flow were observed. Thus, nicardipine is effective in hypertension through dilation of both small and large peripheral arteries with only a transient acute increase in heart rate occurring with initiation of therapy in some patients. Others have also documented beneficial increases in large vessel compliance with nicardipine.[97] Nicardipine has been shown to attenuate the hemodynamic response to smoking in hypertensive patients[98] and to inhibit endothelin-1–induced constriction of systemic capacitance and resistance vessels.[99] Nicardipine but not diltiazem has been shown to antagonize the pressor response associated with adrenergic vascular reactivity in hypertensive patients.[100]

Clinical Use

The efficacy of nicardipine for hypertension was clearly illustrated by Jones et al.[101] using continuous 24-hour ambulatory blood pressure monitoring. Reduction in blood pressure was maintained throughout the monitoring period, which included dynamic exercise stress. The normal circadian variation in blood pressure was not suppressed.

Similar efficacy was demonstrated by Littler and Young[102] in patients with essential hypertension taking a single daily dose of 30-mg nicardipine. A controlled double-blind parallel group study of nicardipine in 50 patients with essential hypertension was reported by Asplund.[103] Nicardipine administered in a 30-mg dose three times daily was continued for 6 weeks. The nicardipine group had an average reduction in systolic/diastolic pressures of 21/15 mmHg, and no significant heart rate changes were observed. A mean increase in plasma renin activity of 52% was seen during nicardipine therapy.[104] In a double-blind trial, Forette et al.[9] studied the antihypertensive effects of nicardipine in 31 elderly patients. Dosage varied from 10 to 30 mg of nicardipine three times a day (average, 69 mg/day). Nicardipine produced significant sustained reductions in mean, systolic, and diastolic blood pressures. No problems with orthostasis and no changes in heart rate were observed. Taylor et al.[104] conducted a dose-titration study of nicardi-

pine in 54 patients with essential hypertension. All but three patients achieved the targeted reduction in blood pressure with either 10 or 20 mg of nicardipine three times daily. Only one patient required 40 mg and three required 30 mg three times a day. The long-term (1 year) efficacy and tolerability of nicardipine in 91 patients with essential hypertension were also studied by Taylor et al.[105] Dosage was adjusted for target blood pressure, and excellent control was achieved throughout the study. The most frequently reported side effects were peripheral edema and headaches, and these events were dose-related. Takabatake et al.[106] also found nicardipine to be effective additive therapy or monotherapy in patients with essential hypertension. Supine and erect blood pressure changes occurring after 6 weeks of treatment with nicardipine are summarized in Figure 104–8.[107] Nicardipine also has been shown to be safe and effective in patients with hypertension in association with severe chronic renal failure.[8]

Combination therapy with nicardipine and β-adrenergic blockade has been found to be effective in both short- and long-term studies in patients with ischemic heart disease with or without hypertension.[108] Nicardipine has also been shown to be an effective agent for use as a third drug in combination with diuretics and an angiotensin-converting enzyme inhibitor in patients with severe hypertension.[109] A randomized study of 43 patients with essential hypertension found nicardipine to be as or more effective than pindolol as second-line treatment.[110]

The efficacy profile of the sustained-release (SR) formulation of nicardipine is identical to that of the standard-release preparation.[111] Nicardipine therapy has been shown to produce regression of left ventricular hypertrophy in hypertension,[112] although conflict-

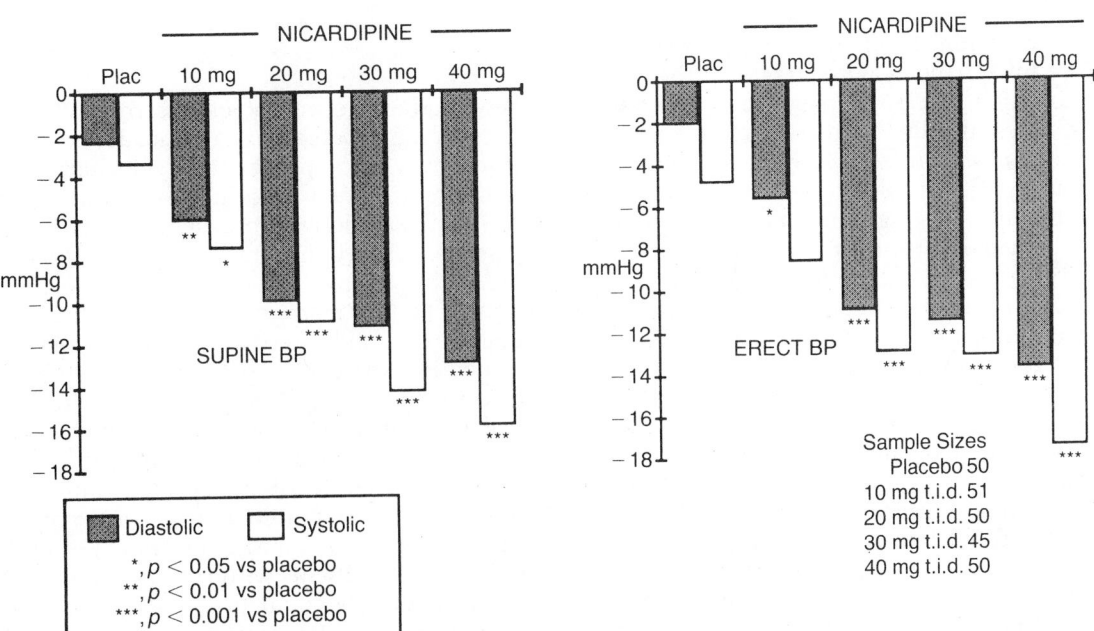

Figure 104–8. Average blood pressure changes from baseline after 6 weeks of treatment with four doses of nicardipine twice daily or with placebo. (Unpublished data from ICM Study 1025, Syntex Laboratories, Palo Alto, CA.)

ing data have been reported.[113] Nicardipine has also been shown to produce a better quality of life than propranolol[114] and does not affect performance in hypertensive athletes.[115] Comparative studies have shown nicardipine SR (b.i.d.) and nifedipine SR (b.i.d.) to be similar in antihypertensive efficacy.[116] Similar results were reported in a comparison of nicardipine SR and verapamil SR.[117] Nicardipine SR (40 mg b.i.d.) was reported to be superior to nitrendipine (20 mg q.d.) when antihypertensive efficacy was assessed by 24-hour ambulatory blood pressure monitoring.[118]

Both formulations of nicardipine have been shown to be effective in elderly hypertensive patients.[119-124] Although side effect profiles in these studies have been typical, dizziness may be a problem in elderly patients with concomitant diuretic-related hypovolemia.[125] Lipid profiles are generally unaffected by nicardipine.[126, 127]

Heart Failure

Applied Pharmacology

Several observations made earlier suggest that nicardipine may be useful in patients with congestive heart failure. Nicardipine possesses very little negative inotropic effect *in vitro* or *in vivo*. Although nicardipine may cause a shift of the end-systolic pressure volume ratio, indicating a negative inotropic effect in patients with severe left ventricular dysfunction, this may be associated with increase in net pump function as indexed by stroke volume.[66] The marked coronary and systemic vasodilatory effects of the drug should favorably affect hemodynamics, particularly in patients with ischemic cardiomyopathy.

Clinical Use

Lahiri et al.[128] administered 10 mg of nicardipine intravenously to 10 patients with class II-III (New York Heart Association [NYHA]) congestive heart failure. Acute responses included increased relative left ventricular ejection fraction (+23%), increased heart rate, and decreased systemic blood pressure. With continued oral therapy (40 mg three times daily) for 4 weeks, sustained improvement in systolic and diastolic indices of ventricular function were seen without an associated increase in heart rate. The sustained improvement in left ventricular ejection fraction documented in this study was substantial (+42%). Bellinetto and Lessem[129] conducted an 8-week open study using 20 to 40 mg of nicardipine three times daily in 15 patients with moderate congestive heart failure. These patients were withdrawn from digoxin and given a titrated nicardipine dose that was continued for 6 weeks. All but two patients showed improved functional class. Decreases in peripheral edema and mean body weight were also documented. Exercise duration and resting left ventricular ejection fraction increased in all but two patients.

Acute hemodynamic changes associated with higher (20 mg) doses of intravenous nicardipine in patients with chronic congestive heart failure were reported by Greenbaum et al.[130] Increases of 64% and 35% were seen in cardiac index and stroke volume index, respectively. Systemic blood pressure and vascular resistance decreased, as did pulmonary vascular resistance, although mean pulmonary and capillary wedge pressures remained constant.

Thus, preliminary studies support the use of nicardipine in patients with congestive heart failure. Before this therapy can be widely applied, larger, long-term, double-blind, placebo-controlled trials must be performed in more clearly defined and homogeneous patient groups. Only then will the specific place of nicardipine in the treatment of heart failure be defined.

Cerebrovascular Disease

Applied Pharmacology

Nicardipine administered intravenously has been shown to increase cerebral blood flow in healthy volunteers.[131] Human studies have also shown that 20 mg of nicardipine three times daily (oral) increases carotid artery diameter and carotid blood flow 10% to 35%.[77] As mentioned earlier, nicardipine promotes cerebral blood flow and abolishes cerebral arterial spasm.[54, 55, 76, 132]

Intravenous nicardipine given to surgical patients without intracranial pathology consistently increased cerebral spinal fluid pressure, but the increases were not clinically significant.[133] Furthermore, they were always accompanied by simultaneous decreases in arterial pressure, which resulted in reduction of cerebral perfusion pressure. Thus, in the absence of intracranial pathology, nicardipine appears not to cause potentially harmful intracranial effects.

Clinical Use

Few studies are available concerning the efficacy of nicardipine in cerebrovascular insufficiency. One such study by Vintro and Viaplana[134] included 41 patients with chronic cerebrovascular insufficiency in a double-blind parallel group design of nicardipine versus placebo. Nicardipine improved clinical status, as indexed by fatigue, anorexia, dizziness, mood, emotional state, memory, and initiative. Similarly, Fujiwara et al.[135] reported improvement in global evaluation indices in patients with cerebrovascular disease during oral nicardipine therapy. A drug surveillance study in 3150 outpatients with cerebrovascular disease found nicardipine to be safe and effective.[136] Handa et al.[137] reported improvement in cerebrovascular symptoms in a cohort of 32 patients treated with oral nicardipine. Handa et al.[138] also reported on 38 patients with ruptured aneurysms of the anterior cerebral circulation who appeared to benefit from nicardipine therapy. A randomized double-blind placebo-controlled trial of high-dose intravenous nicardipine included 449 treated and 457 placebo patients studied with angiographic data after subarachnoid hemorrhage.[139, 140] Fifty-one percent of placebo-treated patients had moderate to severe vasospasm compared with 33% of the nicardipine-treated patients. Forty-nine percent of placebo-treated patients having transcranial Doppler examination had middle cerebral artery flow velocity of more than 120 cm/sec compared with 23% of the nicardipine-treated patients. Despite these findings, the overall 3-month mortality and functional status were not different in the groups. Further studies of nicardipine in hemorrhagic and ischemic stroke are under way.[141]

Raynaud's Phenomenon

A multicenter placebo-controlled double-blind study of patients with primary Raynaud's phenomenon found a significant reduction in the number, but not intensity, of crises with nicardipine therapy.[142] The sustained-release preparation was also found to be effective in reducing both the number and severity of episodes, as well as the time to peak flow during postischemic reactive hyperemia.[143] A third study[144] of nicardipine in patients with Raynaud's phenomenon did not show efficacy; however, plasma concentrations of the drug tended to be low.

DOSAGE AND ADMINISTRATION

Based on data from controlled studies of patients with either myocardial ischemia or systemic hypertension, the recommended oral dose of nicardipine ranges from 20 to 40 mg three times daily. Treatment may be instituted at 20 mg twice daily and increased to optimal control of either angina or hypertension over several weeks. Low oral clearance of nicardipine in cirrhotic patients implies a need to decrease dosage. Nicardipine 20 mg b.i.d. for 1 week was well tolerated by 12 patients with liver cirrhosis.[24] The sustained-release formulation of nicardipine should be dosed beginning at 30 mg b.i.d. and may be adjusted to 45 and 60 mg b.i.d. as indicated. Although nicardipine has been used in hypertensive emergencies,[145–148] optimal dosing and route of administration may vary depending on the clinical scenario. The drug can be used intravenously in hospitalized patients with recurrent ischemia or hypertension who need immediate treatment or cannot take oral medication (e.g., perioperative state).

SUMMARY

Nicardipine is a new dihydropyridine calcium antagonist differing from other drugs in this class with respect to binding characteristics, chemistry, and relative vascular selectivity and subselectivity with regard to both the coronary and cerebral circulations. Nicardipine can be given parenterally or orally and is well tolerated. Efficacy and safety have been demonstrated for treatment of ischemic heart disease and systemic hypertension. Preliminary data also suggest possible use for treatment of heart failure and certain forms of cerebrovascular disease; however, further studies are needed in these areas.

REFERENCES

1. Takenaka T, Usuda S, Nomura T, et al: Vasodilator profile of a new 1,4-dihydropyridine derivative, 2,6-dimethyl-4(3-nitrophenyl)-1,4-dihydropyridine-3,5-dicarboxylic acid 3-[2-(N-benzyl-N-methyl amino)]-ethyl ester 5-methyl ester hydrochloride (YC-93). Arzneimittelforschung 26:2172, 1976.
2. Sakamoto N, Terai M, Takenaka T, et al: Inhibition of cyclic AMP phosphodiesterase by 2,6-dimethyl-4-(3-nitrophenyl)-1,4-dihydropyridine-3,5-dicarboxylic acid 3-[2-(N-benzyl-N-methyl amino)]-ethyl ester 5-methyl ester hydrochloride (YC-93), a potent vasodilator. Biochem Pharmacol 27:1269, 1978.
3. Terai M, Takenaka T, Maeno H: Inhibition of calcium influx in rabbit aorta by nicardipine hydrochloride (YC-93). Biochem Pharmacol 30:375, 1981.
4. Casteels R, Droogmans G: Exchange characteristics of the noradrenaline-sensitive calcium store in vascular smooth muscle cells of rabbit ear artery. J Physiol (Lond) 317:263, 1981.
5. Yamamoto M, Ohta T, Toda N: Mechanisms of relaxant action of nicardipine, a new Ca+ +-antagonist, on isolated dog cerebral and mesenteric arteries. Stroke 14:270, 1983.
6. Gelman JS, Feldman RL, Scott E, et al: Nicardipine for angina pectoris at rest and coronary arterial spasm. Am J Cardiol 56:232, 1985.
7. Higuchi S, Sasaki H, Shiobara Y, et al: Absorption, excretion and metabolism of a new dihydropyridine diester cerebral vasodilator in rats and dogs. Xenobiotica 7:469, 1977.
8. Clair F, Bellet M, Guerret M, et al: Hypotensive effect and pharmacokinetics of nicardipine in patients with severe renal failure. Curr Ther Res 38:74, 1985.
9. Forette F, Bellet M, Henry JF, et al: Effect of nicardipine in elderly hypertensive patients. Br J Clin Pharmacol 20(Suppl 1):125S, 1985.
10. Graham DJM, Freedman D, Dow RJ, et al: Pharmacokinetics of nicardipine following oral and intravenous administration in man. Postgrad Med J 60(Suppl 4):7, 1984.
11. Seki T, Takenaka T: Pharmacological evaluation of YC-93, a new vasodilator, in healthy volunteers. Int J Clin Pharmacol 15:267, 1977.
12. ICM Study 1057. Syntex Corporation, Palo Alto, CA.
13. Higuchi S, Shiobara Y: Metabolic fate of nicardipine hydrochloride, a new vasodilator, by various species in vitro. Xenobiotica 10:889, 1980.
14. Higuchi S, Shiobara Y: Comparative pharmacokinetics of nicardipine hydrochloride, a new vasodilatory in various species. Xenobiotica 10:447, 1980.
15. Higuchi S, Sasaki H, Seki T: Pharmacokinetic studies on nicardipine hydrochloride, a new vasodilator, after repeated administration to rats, dogs and humans. Xenobiotica 10:897, 1980.
16. Rush WR, Alexander O, Hall DJ, et al: The metabolism of nicardipine hydrochloride in healthy male volunteers. Xenobiotica 16:341, 1986.
17. Dow RJ, Graham DJM: A review of the human metabolism and pharmacokinetics of nicardipine hydrochloride. Br J Clin Pharmacol 22(Suppl):195S, 1986.
18. Higuchi S, Sasaki H, Takenaka T, et al: Nicardipine. Presented at the 95th annual meeting of the Pharmaceutical Society of Japan, Nishinomiya, April 4–6, 1975.
19. Shibanuma T, Iwanami M, Fujimoto M, et al: Synthesis of metabolites of 2-(N-benzyl-N-methylamino methyl-2,6-dimethyl-4-(3-nitrophenyl)-1,4-dihydropyridine-3,5-dicarboxy (nicardipine). Chem Pharmacol Bull 28:2809, 1980.
20. Campbell B, Kelman A, Sumner D, et al: Non-invasive measurement of the acute haemodynamic effects of a new calcium channel blocker, nicardipine. Br J Clin Pharmacol 17:188P, 1984.
21. Jamieson MJ, Jeffers TA, Dow R, et al: Nicardipine infusion: Pharmacokinetics, haemodynamics and effects on the systolic time intervals. Br J Clin Pharmacol 19:536P, 1985.
22. Lee AM, Williams R, Warnock D, et al: The effects of nicardi-

pine in hypertensive subjects with impaired renal function. Br J Clin Pharmacol 22(Suppl):297S, 1984.

23. Ahmed JH, Grant AC, Rodger RS, et al: Inhibitory effect of uraemia on the hepatic clearance and metabolism of nicardipine. Br J Clin Pharmacol 32(1):57, 1991.

24. D'Heygere F, Ling T, Waddell G, et al: Evaluation of steady state plasma levels of nicardipine in liver impaired patients [abstract]. Eur Heart J 8:144, 1987.

25. Whiting RL: Animal pharmacology of nicardipine and its clinical relevance. Am J Cardiol 59:3J, 1987.

26. Thayer SA, Welcome M, Chhabra A, Fairhurst SA: Effects of dihydropyridine calcium channel blocking drugs on rat brain muscarinic and alpha-adrenergic receptors. Biochem Pharmacol 34:175, 1985.

27. Knight DR, Vatner SF: Calcium channel blockers induce preferential coronary vasodilation by an α1-mechanism. Am J Physiol 253:H604, 1987.

28. Takeo S, Adachi K, Sakanashi M: The possible action of nicardipine on the cardiac sarcolemmal Na-Ca exchange. Biochem Pharmacol 34:2303, 1985.

29. Wu Z, Sharma RK, Wang JH: The mechanism of inhibition of calmodulin-dependent cyclic nucleotide phosphodiesterase by dihydropyridine calcium antagonists. Hua Hsi I Ko Ta Hsueh Hsueh Pao 23(1):17, 1992.

30. Velena AH, Dubur GJ, Vitolina RO, et al: Effect of ryodipine on electromechanical parameters of heart and vessels, cAMP phosphodiesterase activity and swelling-contraction cycle of mitochondria. Arzneimittelforschung 35:907, 1985.

31. Thomas G, Gross R, Schramm M: Calcium channel modulation: Ability to inhibit or promote calcium influx resides in the same dihydropyridine molecule. J Cardiovasc Pharmacol 6:1170, 1984.

32. Patmore L, Whiting RL: Selective calcium entry blocking properties of nicardipine. Proceedings of the 9th International Congress of Pharmacology, 880P, 1984.

33. Clarke B, Grant D, Patmore L: Comparative calcium entry blocking properties of nicardipine, nifedipine and Py-108068 on cardiac and vascular smooth muscle. Br J Pharmacol 79:333P, 1983.

34. Clarke B, Eglen RM, Patmore L: Cardioselective calcium entry blocking properties of a nicardipine metabolite. Br J Pharmacol 83:437P, 1984.

35. Miyazawa I: Coronary artery selectivity of nicardipine in human—implication of organ differences. Jpn Circ J 50:536, 1986.

36. Tamamura T, Konishi T, Matsuda H: Electrophysiological effects of nicardipine hydrochloride on isolated SA and AV nodes of the rabbit. J Mol Cell Cardiol 13:67, 1981.

37. Takenaka T, Asano M, Shiono K, et al: Cardiovascular pharmacology of nicardipine in animals. Br J Clin Pharmacol 20:7S, 1985.

38. Amenta F, Bronzetti E, Ferrante F: Nicardipine and vascular hypertrophy. Am Heart J 122(1 Pt 2):324, 1991.

39. Grellet J, Bonoron-Adele S, Stuyvers B, et al: Nicardipine and cardiac hypertrophy: Effects on left ventricular mass. Haemodynamics and mechanical performance in renovascular hypertensive rats. Cardiovasc Res 25(6):484, 1991.

40. Ferrante F, Bronzetti E, Ciriaco E, et al: Effect of nicardipine treatment upon cardiac hypertrophy in spontaneously hypertensive rats: A morphometric and ultrastructural study. J Hypertens 10(6):507, 1992.

41. Abe Y, Komori T, Miura K, et al: Effects of the calcium antagonist nicardipine on renal function and renin release in dogs. J Cardiovasc Pharmacol 5:254, 1983.

42. Alps BJ, Calder C, Wilson A: Nicardipine in models of myocardial infarction. Br J Clin Pharmacol 20:29S, 1985.

43. Alps BJ, Calder C, Wilson A: The beneficial effect of nicardipine compared with nifedipine and verapamil in limiting myocardial infarct size in baboons. Arzneimittelforschung 33:868, 1983.

44. Endo T, Nejima J, Fujita S, et al: Comparative effects of nicardipine, a new calcium antagonist, on size of myocardial infarction after coronary artery occlusion in dogs. Circulation 74:420, 1986.

45. Sandhu R, Biro GP: Changes in the myocardial area at risk,

infarct size, and collateral flow following nicardipine infusion in dogs. Can J Physiol Pharmacol 69(12):1789, 1991.

46. Hano O, Silverman HS, Blank PS, et al: Nicardipine prevents calcium loading and "oxygen paradox" in anoxic single rat myocytes by a mechanism independent of calcium channel blockade. Circ Res 69(6):1500, 1991.

47. Mak IT, Bodhme P, Weglicki WB: Antioxidant effects of calcium channel blockers against free radical injury in endothelial cells. Correlation of protection with preservation of glutathione levels. Circ Res 70(6):1099, 1992.

48. Fujita Y, Kimura K, Takaori M: Influence of nicardipine on post-hypoxic injury in the isolated perfused rat liver. Resuscitation 22(3):253, 1991.

49. Mitchell ME, De Boer DA, Crittenden MD, Clark RE: Nicardipine: Myocardial protection in isolated working hearts. Ann Thorac Surg 54(4):712, 1992.

50. Onoda K, Yada I, Murata T, et al: The enhancement of myocardial protection through an acalcemic storage solution containing nicardipine, a potent calcium channel blocker. A basic study using rat ventricular myocytes. Transplantation 51(5):1084, 1991.

51. Brown PS Jr, Parenteau GL, Holland FW, Clark RE: Pretreatment with nicardipine preserves ventricular function after hypothermic ischemic arrest. Ann Thorac Surg 51(5):739, 1991.

52. Kaneko T, Nagata I, Kikuchi H, et al: The effect of nicardipine on angiogenesis in vitro. Nippon Geka Hokan 61(2):150, 1992.

53. Gokce O, Gokce C, Gunel S, et al: Preventive effect of nicardipine on hyperplastic changes in venous bypass grafts. World J Surg 17(1):94, 1993.

54. Roca J, Balasch J: Effect of nicardipine on vertebral blood flow in dogs. Drugs Exp Clin Res 6:399, 1984.

55. Takenaka T: Effect on the cerebral circulation of 2,6-dimethyl-4-(3-nitrophenyl)-1,4-dihydropyridine-3,5-dicarboxylic acid 3-2-(N-benzyl-N-methylamino)-ethyl ester 5-methyl ester hydrochloride (YC-93). Clin Rep (Tokyo) 8:51, 1974.

56. Takenaka T, Handa J: Cerebrovascular effects of YC-93, a new vasodilator in dogs, monkeys and human patients. Int J Clin Pharmacol Biopharmacol 17:1, 1979.

57. Alps BJ, Haas W: The potential beneficial effect of nicardipine in a rat model of transient forebrain ischemia. Neurology 37:809, 1987.

58. Alps BJ, Calder C, Hass WK, et al: Comparative protective effects of nicardipine, flunarizine, lidoflazine, and nimodipine against ischaemic injury in the hippocampus of the Mongolian gerbil. Br J Pharmacol 93:877, 1988.

59. Aktan S, Aykut C, Oktay S, et al: Nicardipine reduces the levels of leukotriene C4 and prostaglandin E2, following different ischemic periods in rat brain tissue. Prostaglandins Leukot Essent Fatty Acids 45(3):223, 1992.

60. Campbell BC, Kelman AW, Hillis WS: Noninvasive assessment of the hemodynamic effects of nicardipine in normotensive subjects. Br J Clin Pharmacol 20:55S, 1985.

61. Lambert CR, Hill JA, Nichols WW, et al: Coronary and systemic hemodynamic effects of nicardipine. Am J Cardiol 55:652, 1985.

62. Lambert CR, Hill JA, Feldman RL, et al: Effects of nicardipine on left ventricular function and energetics in man. Int J Cardiol 10:237, 1986.

63. Young MA, Watson RD, Littler WA: Baroreflex setting and sensitivity after acute and chronic nicardipine therapy. Clin Sci 66:233, 1984.

64. Visser CA, Koolen JJ, Van Wezel HB: Effects of intracoronary nicardipine and nifedipine on left ventricular function and coronary sinus blood flow. Br J Clin Pharmacol 22:313S, 1986.

65. Lambert CR, Buss DD, Pepine CJ: Effects of nicardipine on myocardial function in vitro and in vivo. Circulation 81(Suppl III):III-139, 1990.

66. Aroney CN, Semigran MJ, Dec GW, et al: Inotropic effect of nicardipine in patients with heart failure: Assessment by left ventricular end-systolic pressure-volume analysis. J Am Coll Cardiol 14:1331, 1989.

67. Aroney CN, Semigran MJ, Dec GW, et al: Left ventricular diastolic function in patients with left ventricular systolic dysfunction due to coronary artery disease and effect of nicardipine. Am J Cardiol 67(9):823, 1991.

68. Borow KM, Neumann A, Lang RM, et al: Noninvasive assessment of the direct action of oral nifedipine and nicardipine on left ventricular contractile state in patients with systemic hypertension: Importance of reflex sympathetic responses. J Am Coll Cardiol 21(4):939, 1993.

69. Garcia-Barreto D, Franquiz J, Sanchez Catasus C, et al: The hemodynamics of oral nicardipine determined by radioisotope ventriculography in patients with ischemic cardiopathy. Arch Inst Cardiol Mex 61(1):21, 1991.

70. Ogawa T, Sekiguchi T, Ishii M, et al: Acute effects of intravenous nicardipine on hemodynamics and cardiac function in patients with a healed myocardial infarction and no evidence of congestive heart failure. Am J Cardiol 68(4):301, 1991.

71. Rousseau MF, Etienne J, Van Mechelen H, et al: Hemodynamic and cardiac effects of nicardipine in patients with coronary artery disease. J Cardiovasc Pharmacol 6:833, 1984.

72. Rousseau MF, Vincent MF, Cheron P, et al: Effects of nicardipine on coronary blood flow, left ventricular inotropic state and myocardial metabolism in patients with angina pectoris. Br J Clin Pharmacol 20:147S, 1985.

73. Rousseau MF, Hanet C, Lavenne-Pardonge E, et al: Changes in myocardial metabolism during therapy in chronic stable angina: A comparison of long-term dosing with propranolol or nicardipine. Circulation 73:1270, 1986.

74. Hanet C, Rousseau M, Vincent M, et al: Effects of nicardipine on myocardial metabolism and coronary haemodynamics: A review. Br J Clin Pharmacol 22:215S, 1986.

75. Lambert CR, Hill JA, Feldman RL, et al: Effects of nicardipine on exercise and pacing induced myocardial ischemia in angina pectoris. Am J Cardiol 60:471, 1987.

76. Gaab MR, Czech T, Korn A: Intracranial effects of nicardipine. Br J Clin Pharmacol 20:67S, 1985.

77. Thuillez C, Gueret M, Duhaze P, et al: Nicardipine: Pharmacokinetics and effects on carotid and brachial blood flows in normal volunteers. Br J Clin Pharmacol 18:837, 1984.

78. Dow RJ, Baty J, Isles TE: The effect of nicardipine on glucose and drug-stimulated insulin secretion in normal volunteers. Br J Clin Pharmacol 20:75S, 1985.

79. Isles TE, Baty J, Dow RJ: The effect of nicardipine on pituitary hormone release in normal volunteers. Br J Clin Pharmacol 20:84S, 1985.

80. Larochelle P: Renal tubular effects of calcium antagonists. Kidney Int Suppl 36:S49, 1992.

81. Ahmed JH, Elliott HL, Hosie J, et al: Effects of nicardipine on the metabolic responses to food and exercise. J Hum Hypertens 6(2):139, 1992.

82. Pepine CJ, Conti CR: Calcium blockers in coronary heart disease. Parts I and II. Mod Conc Cardiovasc Dis 50:61, 1981.

83. Pepine CJ, Feldman RL, Hill JA, et al: Clinical outcome after treatment of rest angina with calcium blockers: Comparative experience during the initial year of therapy with diltiazem, nifedipine, and verapamil. Am Heart J 106:1341, 1983.

84. Pepine CJ, Lambert CR: Usefulness of nicardipine for angina pectoris. Am J Cardiol 59:13J, 1987.

85. Lambert CR, Hill JA, Feldman RL, et al: Myocardial ischemia during intravenous nicardipine infusion. Am J Cardiol 55:844, 1985.

86. Lambert CR, Grady T, Hashimi W, et al: Hemodynamic and angiographic comparison of intravenous nitroglycerin and nicardipine mainly in subjects without coronary artery disease. Am J Cardiol 71(5):420, 1993.

87. Thomassen A, Bagger JP, Nielsen TT, et al: Metabolic and hemodynamic effects of nicardipine during pacing-induced angina pectoris. Am J Cardiol 59:219, 1987.

88. Rousseau MF, Renkin J, Lavenne-Pardonge E, et al: Myocardial protection by intracoronary injection of nicardipine during transluminal coronary angioplasty [abstract]. Circulation 72:III-400, 1985.

89. Deedwania PC, Thao TP, Andrew HT: Long-term efficacy of nicardipine, a new calcium channel blocker, in chronic stable angina [abstract]. Clin Res 33:20A, 1985.

90. Khurmi NS, Bowles MJ, Bala Subramanian V, et al: Short- and long-term efficacy of nicardipine, assessed by placebo-controlled single- and double-blind crossover trials in patients with chronic stable angina. J Am Coll Cardiol 4:908, 1984.

91. Gheorghiade M, St Clair C, St Clair J, et al: Short- and long-term treatment of stable effort angina with nicardipine, a new calcium channel blocker: A double-blind, placebo-controlled, randomised repeated cross-over study. Br J Clin Pharmacol 20(Suppl 1):195S, 1985.

92. Scheidt S, Lewinter MM, Hermanovich J, et al: Nicardipine for stable angina pectoris. Br J Clin Pharmacol 20(Suppl 1):178S, 1985.

93. DiPasquale G, Lusa AM, Manini GL, et al: Comparative efficacy of nicardipine, a new calcium antagonist, versus nifedipine in stable effort angina. Int J Cardiol 6:673, 1984.

94. McGill D, McKenzie W, McCredie M: Comparison of nicardipine and propranolol for chronic stable angina pectoris. Am J Cardiol 57:39, 1986.

95. Bowles MJ, Bala Subramanian V, O'Hara MJ, et al: Computer-assisted treadmill exercise testing in the evaluation of four calcium ion antagonists against propranolol in chronic stable angina [abstract A-915:283]. Proceedings of the VIIIth Asian Pacific Congress of Cardiology, Taipei, Taiwan, November 27–December 2, 1983.

96. Levenson J, Simon A, Bouthier J, et al: The effect of acute and chronic nicardipine therapy on forearm arterial haemodynamics in essential hypertension. Br J Clin Pharmacol 20(Suppl 1):107S, 1985.

97. De Cesaris R, Ranieri G, Filitti V, Andriani A: Large artery compliance in essential hypertension. Effects of calcium antagonism and beta-blocking. Am J Hypertens 5(9):624, 1992.

98. Fogari R, Zoppi A, Malamani GD, Corradi L: Effects of calcium channel blockers on cardiovascular responses to smoking in normotensive and hypertensive smokers. Int J Clin Pharmacol Res 12(2):81, 1992.

99. Takai K, Ito H, Nagata K, et al: Nicardipine inhibits the endothelin-1-induced constriction of systemic capacitance and resistance vessels. J Cardiovasc Pharmacol 17(Suppl 7):S305, 1991.

100. Pedrinelli R, Panarace G, Salvetti A: Calcium entry blockade and adrenergic vascular reactivity in hypertensives: Differences between nicardipine and diltiazem. Clin Pharmacol Ther 49(1):86, 1991.

101. Jones RI, Hornung RS, Sonecha T, et al: The effect of nicardipine on ambulatory blood pressure and the pressor response to static and dynamic exercise. Br J Clin Pharmacol 20(Suppl 1):114S, 1985.

102. Littler WA, Young MA: The effect of nicardipine on blood pressure, its variability and reflex cardiac control. Br J Clin Pharmacol 20(Suppl 1):115S, 1985.

103. Asplund J: Nicardipine hydrochloride in essential hypertension—a controlled study. Br J Clin Pharmacol 20(Suppl 1):120S, 1985.

104. Taylor SH, Frais MA, Lee P, et al: Anti-hypertensive dose-response effects of nicardipine in stable essential hypertension. Br J Clin Pharmacol 20(Suppl 1):135S, 1985.

105. Taylor SH, Frais MA, Lee P, et al: A study of the long-term efficacy and tolerability of oral nicardipine in hypertensive patients. Br J Clin Pharmacol 20(Suppl 1):139S, 1985.

106. Takabatake T, Ohta H, Yamamoto Y, et al: Antihypertensive effect of nicardipine hydrochloride in essential hypertension. Int J Clin Pharmacol Ther Toxicol 20:346, 1982.

107. ICM Study 1025. Syntex Laboratories, Palo Alto, CA.

108. Lambert CR: Combination therapy with nicardipine and beta-adrenergic blockade for angina pectoris. Clin Cardiol 15:231, 1992.

109. Lacourciere Y, Poirier L, Levesque C, Provencher P: Ambulatory blood pressure monitoring for the assessment of nicardipine as a third drug in severe essential hypertension. Eur J Clin Pharmacol 42(2):131, 1992.

110. Penttila O, Kannianinen E, Jounela A, Huikko M: A comparative study of nicardipine and pindolol as secondline treatments in essential hypertension. J Int Med Res 20(3):218, 1992.

111. Webster J, Petrie JC, Jeffers TA, et al: Nicardipine sustained release in hypertension. Br J Clin Pharmacol 32(4):433, 1991.

112. Dunn FG, Burns JM, Hornung RS: Left ventricular hypertrophy in hypertension. Am Heart J 122(1 Pt 2):312, 1991.

113. Dittrich HC, Adler J, Ong J, et al: Effects of sustained-release nicardipine on regression of left ventricular hypertrophy in systemic hypertension. Am J Cardiol 69(19):1559, 1992.

114. Weir MR, Josselson J, Ekelund LG, et al: Nicardipine as antihypertensive monotherapy: Positive effects on quality of life. J Hum Hypertens 5(3):205, 1991.

115. Marcadet DM, Blanc AS, Lopez AA, et al: Efficacy and tolerance of LA 50 mg nicardipine in hypertensive athletes. Arch Mal Coeur Vaiss 84(11):1569, 1991.

116. Maetzel FK, Teufel WE, Griebel A, Glocke MH: Double-blind, randomized comparative study of the antihypertensive effect of nicardipine slow-release and nifedipine slow-release in hypertensive patients with coronary heart disease. Cardiovasc Drugs Ther 5(3):647, 1991.

117. Gradman AH, Frishman WH, Kaihlanen PM, et al: Comparison of sustained-release formulations of nicardipine and verapamil for mild to moderate systemic hypertension. Am J Cardiol 70(20):1571, 1992.

118. Fogari R, Tettamanti F, Zoppi A, et al: Nitrendipine 20 mg once daily versus nicardipine slow release 40 mg twice daily in mild essential hypertension: Evaluation by 24-hour ambulatory blood pressure monitoring. Clin Exp Hypertens [A] 14(4):587, 1992.

119. Kuramoto K, Ikeda M, Kaneko Y, et al: Analysis of advancing age on the response to nicardipine among 467 adult hypertensive patients. J Hypertens 9(1):59, 1991.

120. Calvo Gomez C, Lado Lado FL, Cinos Ramos L, et al: The efficacy of nicardipine in treating arterial hypertension in elderly patients. A multicenter outpatient study. Ann Med Interna 9(4):170, 1992.

121. Antonicelli R, Pagelli P, Paciaroni E: Nicardipine retard in the therapy of elderly diabetic hypertensives: Final report of observational study. J Hypertens Suppl 10(2):S69, 1992.

122. Chen JW, Chen CH, Wang SP, Chang MS: Comparison of nicardipine and nifedipine in treatment of Chinese senile hypertension placebo-control, double-blind, randomized and crossover study. Chung Hua I Hsueh Tsa Chih (Taipei) 50(4):321, 1992.

123. Porchet HC, Loew F, Gauthey L, Dayer P: Serum concentration-effect relationship of (+/−)-nicardipine and nifedipine in elderly hypertensive patients. Eur J Clin Pharmacol 43(5):551, 1992.

124. Mancia G, Buoninconti R, Errico M, et al: Efficacy and tolerability of nicardipine retard and captopril in hypertension in the aged. Results of a multicenter study. Minerva Med 83(11):731, 1992.

125. Le Jeunne C, Hugues FC, Munera Y, Ozanne H: Dizziness in the elderly and calcium channel antagonists. Biomed Pharmacother 45(1):33, 1991.

126. Tariq AR, Maheendran K, Kamsiah J, Christina P: Dose requirement and effect of nicardipine on lipid profile in mild to moderate essential hypertensives. Med J Malaysia 47(3):182, 1992.

127. Pasanisi F, Marotta T, Ferrara LA, et al: Evaluation of lipid metabolism during antihypertensive treatment with nicardipine SR. Eur J Clin Pharmacol 43(3):225, 1992.

128. Lahiri A, Robinson CW, Tovey J, et al: Intravenous nicardipine in patients with chronic heart failure: A nuclear stethoscope study. Postgrad Med J 60(Suppl 4):35, 1984.

129. Bellinetto A, Lessem J: Effects of nicardipine hydrochloride in cardiac failure: A dose titration and tolerance study. Curr Ther Res 36:938, 1984.

130. Greenbaum RA, Wan S, Evans TR: The acute haemodynamic effects of nicardipine in patients with chronic left ventricular failure. Eur J Clin Pharmacol 30:383, 1986.

131. Savage I, James I: The effect of nicardipine hydrochloride on cerebral blood flow in normotensive volunteers. Br J Clin Pharmacol 21:591P, 1986.

132. Handa J: Cerebral vascular effects of a new derivative of 1,4 dihydropyridine (YC-93), with special reference to its effect on the experimental basilar artery spasm in cats. Nihon Geka Hokan 44:343, 1975.

133. Nishikawa T, Omote K, Namiki A, et al: The effects of nicardipine on cerebrospinal fluid pressure in humans. Anesth Analg 65:507, 1986.

134. Vintro MC, Viaplana JM: Double-blind clinical trial of nicardipine and a placebo in patients with chronic cerebral vascular insufficiency. Med Clin (Barc) 84:308, 1985.

135. Fujiwara T, Yamada N, Iwai N, et al: Clinical effect of nicardipine hydrochloride (YC-93) on cerebrovascular disorders. Jpn Arch Intern Med 27:327, 1980.

136. Lozano R, Balaguer A: Nicardipine in the treatment of outpatients with cerebrovascular disorders. Clin Ther 13(4):496, 1991.

137. Handa J, Koyama T, Tsuji H, et al: Clinical effect of a new 1,4 dihydropyridine derivative, YC-93, in patients with cerebrovascular diseases. Arch Jpn Chir 48:400, 1979.

138. Handa J, Matsuda M, Nakasu Y, et al: Early operation of aneurysmal subarachnoid hemorrhage—use of nicardipine, a calcium channel blocker. Arch Jpn Chir 53:619, 1984.

139. Haley EC Jr, Kassell NF, Torner JC: A randomized trial of nicardipine in subarachnoid hemorrhage: Angiographic and transcranial Doppler ultrasound results. A report of the Cooperative Aneurysm Study. J Neurosurg 78(4):548, 1993.

140. Haley EC Jr, Kassell NF, Torner JC: A randomized controlled trial of high-dose intravenous nicardipine in aneurysmal subarachnoid hemorrhage. A report of the Cooperative Aneurysm Study. J Neurosurg 78(4):537, 1993.

141. Rosenbaum D, Zabramski J, Frey J, et al: Early treatment of ischemic stroke with a calcium antagonist. Stroke 22(4):437, 1991.

142. Controlled multicenter double-blind trial of nicardipine in the treatment of primary Raynaud phenomenon. French cooperative multicenter group for Raynaud phenomenon, Paris, France. Am Heart J 122(1 Pt 2):352, 1991.

143. Ferri C, Cecchetti R, Cini G, et al: Slow-releasing nicardipine in the treatment of Raynaud's phenomena without underlying diseases. Clin Rheumatol 11(1):76,1992.

144. Wollersheim H, Thien T: Double-blind placebo-controlled crossover study of oral nicardipine in the treatment of Raynaud's phenomenon. J Cardiovasc Pharmacol 18(6):813, 1991.

145. Ram CV: Management of hypertensive emergencies: Changing therapeutic options. Am Heart J 122(1 Pt 2):356, 1991.

146. Tamburino C, Russo G, Di Paola R, Giuffrida G: Pulmonary edema during cardiac catheterization successfully treated with bolus administration of nicardipine. Cardiovasc Drugs Ther 5(2):495, 1991.

147. Savi L, Montebelli MR, D'Alonzo S, et al: Sublingual nicardipine versus nifedipine to treat hypertensive urgencies. Int J Clin Pharmacol Ther Toxicol 30(2):41, 1992.

148. Komsuoglu B, Sengun B, Bayram A, Komsuoglu SS: Treatment of hypertensive urgencies with oral nifedipine, nicardipine, and captopril. Angiology 2(6):447, 1991.

CHAPTER 105

Intravenous Nicardipine

J. David Wallin, M.D., and Constance F. Neely, M.D.

Nicardipine hydrochloride is a calcium ion flux inhibitor of the 1,4-dihydropyridine substituted class. Unlike nifedipine, the prototype drug of this class, nicardipine is water soluble and therefore suitable for intravenous administration. In addition, nicardipine has several properties, such as an absence of electrophysiologic effect on the heart and minimal negative inotropic properties, that make it a desirable agent for the parenteral management of severe hypertension.

CLINICAL PHARMACOLOGY, PHARMACOKINETICS, AND PHARMACODYNAMICS

Nicardipine inhibits transmembrane flux of calcium ions through voltage-dependent calcium channels into the cytoplasm of smooth muscle and cardiac muscle cells. Nicardipine is more selective to vascular smooth muscle compared with cardiac muscle. After infusion of varying doses for a 48-hour period into 37 patients with mild to moderate hypertension (Fig. 105–1), pharmacokinetics of nicardipine were determined and found to decrease triexponentially.[1] There

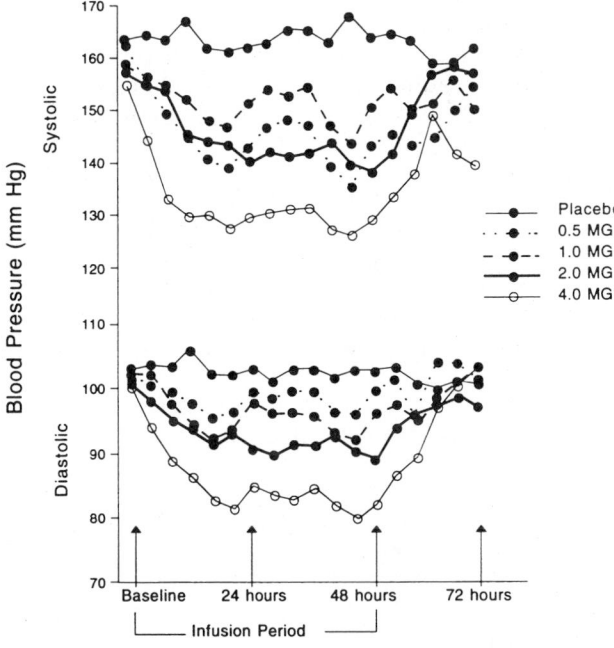

Figure 105–1. Mean systolic and diastolic blood pressures in millimeters of mercury are shown for each treatment group with mild to moderate hypertension for both the 48-hour constant-infusion period and the 24-hour follow-up period. (From Cook E, Clifton GG, Vargas R, et al: Pharmacokinetics, pharmacodynamics, and minimum effective clinical dose of intravenous nicardipine. Clin Pharmacol Ther 47:710, 1990.)

was a rapid early phase (α-half-life of 2.7 minutes), an intermediate phase (β-half-life of 44.8 minutes), and a slow terminal phase (γ-half-life of 14.4 hours) that was detected only after long-term infusions. Total plasma clearance was 0.4 L/kg·hr and the apparent volume of distribution was 8.3 L/kg. Plasma concentrations increased rapidly during the first 2 hours of infusion, increased at a slower rate after 2 hours, and approached steady state at 16 to 24 hours. In this study and in others, there was excellent correlation between plasma concentrations of nicardipine and blood pressure reduction.

EFFECTS ON PATHOPHYSIOLOGY

Lambert et al.[2] examined the effects of intravenously administered nicardipine on both coronary artery and systemic hemodynamics during cardiac catheterization in men being evaluated for exertional chest pain. When systolic blood pressure was reduced 10 to 20 mmHg, heart rate increased from 69 to 81 beats per minute, cardiac output increased from 7.3 to 9.9 L/min, and systemic vascular resistance fell from 1183 to 733 dyne cm^{-5}. Stroke volume increased and coronary blood flow increased 44%. This study demonstrated that coronary resistance decreased to a significantly greater extent than systemic resistance, suggesting a direct coronary vasodilatory effect. A second study by Pepine and Lambert[3] investigated direct effects after intracoronary injection of nicardipine and demonstrated an immediate increase in coronary blood flow without changes in systemic hemodynamic measurements. In these studies and others no effect on venous resistance was noted. Studies conducted in patients with acute myocardial infarction who received intravenous nicardipine demonstrated no evidence of depression of left ventricular pump performance.[4] Other studies have also shown minimal effects on cardiac performance.[5] As with other dihydropyridine calcium antagonists, there was no significant effect on sinus or atrioventricular nodes.

When given intravenously, nicardipine produces a mild natriuresis, which is an effect it has in common with other dihydropyridine calcium antagonists. This has not been quantified by metabolic balance studies for this drug given intravenously. No alterations in electrolytes or changes in endocrine or metabolic variables have been described. The effects of intravenous nicardipine on renal function have not been studied, but it is likely that they do not differ from those of orally administered nicardipine. With this agent, there is usually an increase in both glomerular filtration rate and renal blood flow associated with a decrease in renal vascular resistance. These effects on renal hemodynamics are believed to be primarily caused by a fall in afferent arteriolar resistance.

CLINICAL USE
Indications

Intravenous nicardipine is indicated for the short-term treatment of hypertension when oral therapy is not feasible or not desirable.

Precautions

Monitoring of blood pressure during administration is required. Intravenous nicardipine may produce symptomatic hypotension, and use in patients with strokes must be particularly meticulous to avoid hypotension. In patients who are hepatically challenged, the dose of nicardipine should be reduced. Similarly, in renally challenged patients, the area under the curve (AUC) in pharmacokinetic studies was observed to be higher and systemic clearance reduced. Careful dose titration is advised in both groups of patients.

Contraindications

Intravenous nicardipine is contraindicated in patients with a known hypersensitivity to the drug and in patients with hemodynamically significant aortic stenosis.

DRUG INTERACTIONS
Fentanyl Anesthesia

Hypotension has been reported during fentanyl anesthesia when a β-blocker and calcium antagonist were used concomitantly.

Cyclosporine

Nicardipine increases cyclosporine levels, making it necessary to carefully monitor cyclosporine levels when the drugs are used together.

PLACE IN ANTIHYPERTENSIVE ARSENAL

The agents that are currently in use to treat hypertension by a parenteral route are shown in Table 105–1. Table 105–2 lists important desirable features of drugs that are used to manage hypertension in critical care settings. Each agent listed in Table 105–1 has shown a general association between the dose used and therapeutic effect. However, only nicardipine has shown a close correlation between dose, blood level, and therapeutic effect. This has been demonstrated both in patients with mild to moderate hypertension and in severe hypertensive patients. Titratability is an important feature of medications used in the critical care environment. Diazoxide, enalaprilat, and labetalol are

Table 105–1. **Current Antihypertensive Agents Available for Parenteral Use**

Medication	Mechanism of Action
Diazoxide	Direct vasodilator
Enalaprilat	Angiotensin converting enzyme inhibitor
Esmolol	β-blocker
Labetalol	α-, β-blocker
Nitroprusside	Direct vasodilator
Nitroglycerin	Direct vasodilator
Nicardipine	Calcium antagonist

not titratable because of their length of action and slow offset of action. Once these drugs are administered, the effect of a given dose will be present for the length of action of the agent. Nitroprusside, nitroglycerin and nicardipine, and esmolol can be titrated to effect and have predictable offset of action should it be desirable to allow blood pressure to increase. Esmolol is a selective, β₁-adrenergic blocker that is used primarily for the treatment of supraventricular tachyarrhythmias; however, it may be used in combination with other drugs including nitroglycerin and nicardipine for blood pressure and heart rate control in patients with suspected coronary artery disease. There are significant risks of overdosing and hypotension, particularly with diazoxide and labetalol; these risks are less with enalapril, nitroprusside, nitroglycerin, and nicardipine. Diazoxide increases cardiac output and disrupts autoregulation of cerebral blood flow, making it unsuitable for clinical situations such as cerebral vascular accidents and dissecting aneurysms. All direct-acting vascular smooth muscle relaxants decrease cerebral vascular resistance, increase cerebral blood volume and intracranial pressure, inhibit hypoxic pulmonary vasoconstriction, and are associated with a reflex tachycardia. Enalaprilat, nitroprusside, and nitroglycerin dilate veins as well as arterioles, which is a desirable hemodynamic property in several clinical situations such as heart failure. Nitroprusside reacts with red blood cells, resulting in the release of cyanide, which is metabolized to thiocyanate in the liver. As opposed to nitroprusside, there are no toxic metabolites associated with nitroglycerin and nicardipine. Also, rebound hypertension can occur after the discontinuation of nitroprusside; this is not associated with the use of nicardipine. Nicardipine has minimal effects on myocardial con-

Table 105–2. **Desirable Properties of a Parenteral Antihypertensive Agent**

1. Predictable relationship between pharmacokinetic and hemodynamic properties.
2. Titratability.
3. Predictable offset of action.
4. Minimal risk of hypotension.
5. Minimal unwanted hemodynamic changes.
6. No cumulative effects or toxic metabolic products.
7. No tachyphylaxis.
8. Convenient transfer to oral medication.

tractility and does not produce coronary steal syndrome, which is reported to occur with nitroprusside. None of the agents listed in Table 105–1 have tachyphylaxis as a feature of therapy. Only enalapril, labetalol, and nicardipine have an oral form to allow convenient transfer to an oral agent. Overall, nicardipine, as the most recent addition to this list, appears to possess most if not all of the desirable properties of parenteral antihypertensive agents.

DOSAGE AND ADMINISTRATION

Clinical studies have examined the use of intravenous nicardipine in several clinical settings. The following information is presented for patients with moderate hypertension, patients with severe hypertension, and intraoperative and postoperative patients.

Patients with Moderate Hypertension

A patient with moderate hypertension is likely to be one who is in a critical care or emergency room setting, who cannot be given oral medications, and in whom it is desired to reduce blood pressure. The clinical study that is most relevant to this group is a study in which nicardipine in doses varying from 0.5 to 4 mg/hr was infused for a 48-hour period to a

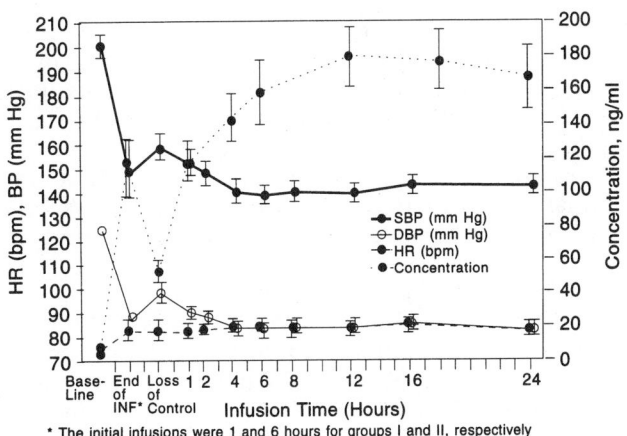

* The initial infusions were 1 and 6 hours for groups I and II, respectively

Figure 105–3. Mean (+ SE) values for supine systolic and diastolic blood pressures, heart rate, and plasma nicardipine concentrations (ng/ml) at various reference points during the administration of intravenous nicardipine for the treatment of severe hypertension. These data are cumulative for groups I and II in which there was an initial infusion period of 1 or 6 hours followed by a loss of control evaluation and then a second infusion of 24 hours' duration. Note: The early portion of the time scale is discontinuous. (From Wallin JD, Cook ME, Blanski L, et al: Intravenous nicardipine for the treatment of severe hypertension. Am J Med 85:335, 1988.)

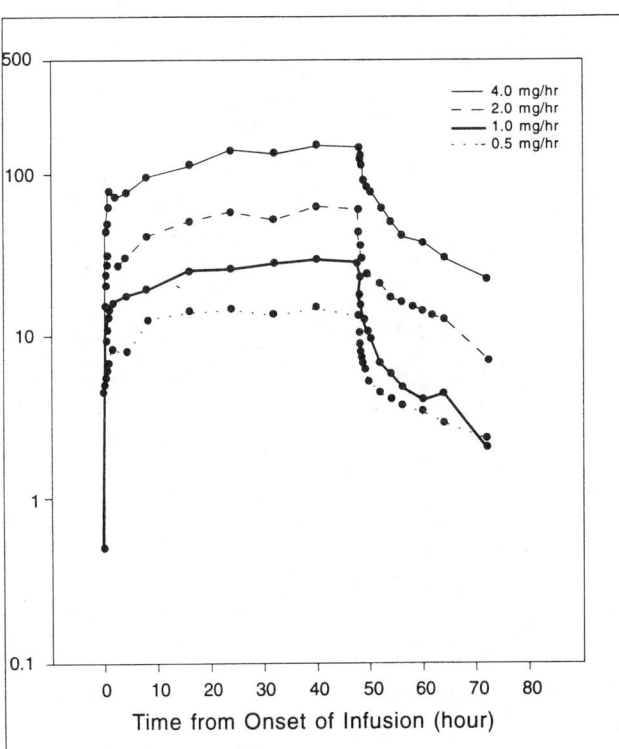

Figure 105–2. Mean plasma nicardipine concentrations in nanograms per milliliter are shown from groups of patients with mild to moderate hypertension receiving 0.5, 1, 2, or 4 mg/hr nicardipine during both the 48-hour constant-infusion period and the 24-hour follow-up period. (From Cook E, Clifton GG, Vargas R, et al: Pharmacokinetics, pharmacodynamics, and minimum effective clinical dose of intravenous nicardipine. Clin Pharmacol Ther 47:711, 1990.)

group of patients with mild and moderate hypertension.[1] The effects of these doses on blood pressure are shown in Figure 105–1. In the group that received 4 mg/hr, a significant decrease in blood pressure was noted in 20 minutes, with a continued fall but at a much slower rate during the first 120 minutes of infusion. With doses of 0.5 mg/hr, 1 mg/hr, and 2 mg/hr significant decreases in blood pressure were not seen until 90 minutes after the start of infusion. In this study, a dose-related fall in blood pressure with increasing doses of nicardipine was documented. After 12 to 15 hours, pharmacodynamic equilibrium was achieved with each dose. Figure 105–2 shows the plasma concentrations of nicardipine during these infusions. There is a rapid increase in plasma concentration with equilibrium reached in 12 to 16 hours. From a practical standpoint, a starting infusion rate of 3 to 4 mg/hr appears appropriate in patients with moderate hypertension in whom blood pressure control is desired within 1 to 2 hours. If faster reduction of blood pressure is indicated, a starting dose of 5 to 8 mg may be employed, or a small bolus of 2 to 3 mg may be given to achieve significant plasma levels and blood pressure reduction more rapidly.

Patients with Severe Hypertension

Several clinical studies offer insight into the use of nicardipine in patients with severe hypertension. A dose-ranging study was conducted[6] in which patients with diastolic blood pressure exceeding 120 mmHg received nicardipine at infusion rates varying from 4 to 15 mg/hr (Fig. 105–3). The time required to reach therapeutic goal (diastolic blood pressure [DBP] < 95 mmHg) was 1.11 hours for the 4-mg dose, 0.54 hour for the 5-mg dose, and 0.31 hour for the 15-mg dose. It should be noted that in many patients with severe hypertension, reduction of blood pressure to these levels at a relatively slow rate may be clinically desirable.

In order to assess the time of offset of action after initial stabilization of blood pressure, infusions were discontinued (see Fig. 105–3). The average period until blood pressure increased (>10 mmHg) was 21 minutes. The infusions were then restarted and continued for 24 hours in order to assess stability of effect. The mean infusion rate that achieved stable blood pressure control was 7.3 mg/hr in this study.

A second clinical study[7] that examined the effect of nicardipine in patients with severe hypertension was a placebo-controlled, double-blind multicenter trial in 123 patients with diastolic blood pressure greater than 120 mmHg. These patients were randomized to receive nicardipine or a placebo in a ratio of 3:2. They entered a first titration period in which nicardipine was infused at rates of 5, 7.5, 10, and 12. 5 mg/hr sequentially over four 15-minute intervals or equivalent rates of placebo were infused. If blood pressure was reduced to a DBP of less than 110 mmHg, the patient was classified as a titration responder and received a continued infusion of the initial solution in a blinded fashion for up to 6 hours or until a therapeutic response was achieved (DBP <95 mmHg for therapeutic responders). If the initial infusion did not reduce the DBP to lower than 110 mmHg, the patient was classified as a titration failure and received open-label nicardipine. Of the 73 patients who received nicardipine, 70 were titration responders (96%) and 69 patients eventually entered the maintenance phase of the study (95%). Of the 50 patients who received the placebo, there were seven titration responders and no therapeutic responders. Forty-three of the 50 patients responded to open-label nicardipine. The mean dose required for a therapeutic response was 8.7 mg/hr in this study. Figure 105–4 displays the effects of nicardipine and placebo on blood pressure and heart rate.

From these two studies and others in which the mean infusion rate for response was clustered tightly about 8 mg/hr, a patient with severe hypertension should initially be treated with an infusion rate of nicardipine of 5 mg/hr. Sequentially the infusion can be increased to 7.5, 10.0, and 12.5 mg/hr over 15-minute periods until the desired blood pressure is achieved. At that point, it is probably prudent to reduce the infusion rate to 7.5 to 10 mg/hr.

Postoperative Hypertension

A double-blind multicenter study[8] compared nicardipine with placebo in 121 patients who were recovering from either cardiac (16 patients) or noncardiac (105 patients) surgery. In this study, patients were randomized 3:2 to either nicardipine or placebo and were titrated with infusion rates of 10, 12.5, and 15 mg/hr over 5-, 5-, and 15-minute titration periods, respectively, until a therapeutic response (decrease of

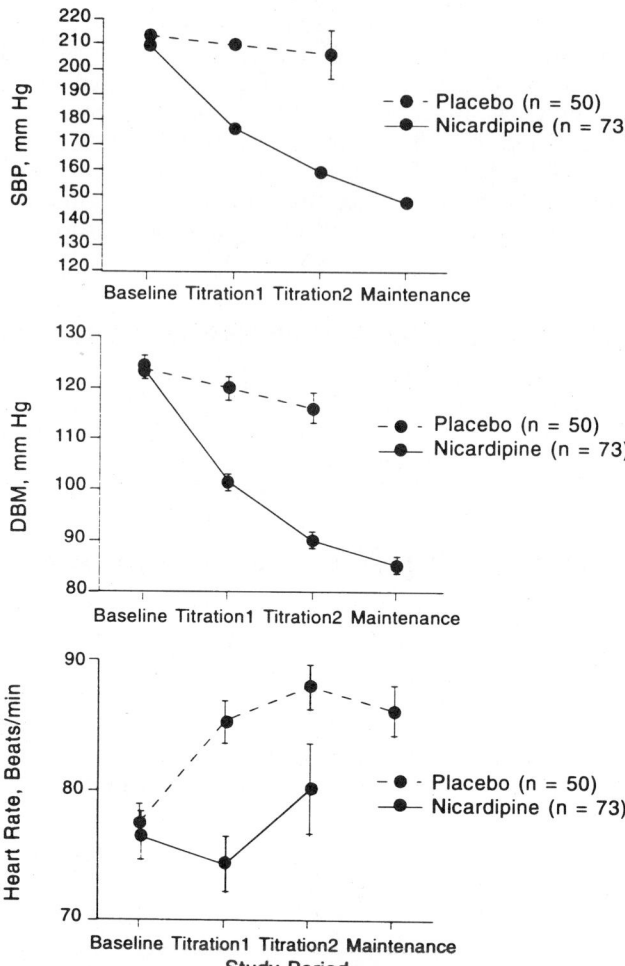

Figure 105–4. Effect of intravenous nicardipine versus placebo on systolic blood pressure (SBP), diastolic blood pressure (DBP), and heart rate. The percentage change from the baseline level is significantly different between the intravenous nicardipine- and placebo-treatment groups at the end of both titration periods. Also, in the nicardipine group, blood pressure and heart rate are significantly different at the end of the titration 1, titration 2, and maintenance periods compared with baseline values. (From Wallin JD, Fletcher E, Ram VS, et al: Intravenous nicardipine for the treatment of severe hypertension. Arch Intern Med 149:2667, 1989. Copyright 1989, American Medical Association.)

SBP or DBP by 15% from the baseline value) was achieved. In the responders, the infusion rate was decreased to 3 mg/hr to avoid hypotension. Nonresponders were unblinded and treated with open-label nicardipine. Of 71 patients randomized to nicardipine, 67 achieved a therapeutic response; of 50 patients who received the placebo, six were responders. The mean dose and mean time to a therapeutic response were 12.8 mg/hr and 11.5 minutes in randomized responders to nicardipine and 12.5 mg/hr and 10.3 minutes in the open-label responders. The plasma nicardipine level at therapeutic response was 84.6 ng/ml. At the end of the maintenance infusion (average, 6.8 hours), the nicardipine level was 61 ng/ml, and at offset (average, 17.5 minutes), it was 32.5 ng/ml. The mean maintenance infusion rate required to continue blood pressure control was 3 mg/hr. Of a total of 110 patients receiving nicardipine, adverse effects occurred in 19 (17%). Hypotension (4.5%), nausea and vomiting (4.5%), and tachycardia (2.7%) were the most common adverse effects; 4 of the 19 patients were removed from the study.

An open-label, prospective, randomized, multicenter study compared nicardipine with nitroprusside for the treatment of postoperative hypertension in patients recovering from cardiac and noncardiac surgery.[9] One hundred thirty-nine patients with postoperative hypertension received either nicardipine (71 patients) or nitroprusside (68 patients). Using dosing schedule as described in the placebo-controlled postoperative study, the average dose of nicardipine to achieve a therapeutic response (>15% reduction in blood pressure) was 13 to 14 mg/hr and the average maintenance dose was 2 to 3 mg/hr. Time to therapeutic response was approximately 14 minutes. Fewer dose changes were required during titration and maintenance of nicardipine than nitroprusside. Both nicardipine and nitroprusside were equally effective in controlling blood pressure in both cardiac and noncardiac surgical patients. The incidence of adverse effects was higher with nitroprusside (18% nitroprusside versus 7% nicardipine). The most common adverse effects were hypotension and tachycardia. Nine percent of the patients receiving nitroprusside versus none of the patients receiving nicardipine were removed from the study.

From these studies, it appears that the starting infusion rate of nicardipine in postoperative patients should be higher than in the medical patients. The purpose of this is to more rapidly achieve control of blood pressure. A safe and effective dosage appears to be 10 mg/hr, with fairly rapid (5-minute) titrations to 12.5 and 15 mg/hr. Once blood pressure is satisfactorily reduced, a smaller maintenance dose appears to be effective, which averaged 3 mg/hr.

ADVERSE REACTIONS

These studies demonstrated that adverse reactions were not uncommon but not severe. Most commonly seen were headache and nausea, averaging 27% and 10%, respectively. In the early studies several patients developed phlebitis at the site of infusion. It was determined that this was related to length of infusion, not concentration of nicardipine, and it never occurred prior to 15 hours of infusion. Accordingly, it is recommended that the infusion site be changed every 12 hours.

REFERENCES

1. Cook E, Clifton GG, Vargas R, et al: Pharmacokinetics, pharmacodynamics, and minimum effective clinical dose of intravenous nicardipine. Clin Pharmacol Ther 47:706, 1990.
2. Lambert CR, Hill JA, Nichols WW, et al: Coronary and systemic hemodynamic effects of nicardipine. Am J Cardiol 55:652, 1985.
3. Pepine CJ, Lambert CR: The effect of nicardipine on coronary blood flow. Am Heart J 116:248, 1988.
4. Silke B, Verma SP, Hafizullah M, et al: Hemodynamic effects of nicardipine in acute myocardial infarction. Postgrad Med J 60(4):29, 1984.
5. Aroney CN, Semigran MJ, Dec GW, et al: Inotropic effect of nicardipine in patients with heart failure: Assessment by left ventricular end-systolic pressure-volume analysis. J Am Coll Cardiol 14:1333, 1989.
6. Wallin JD, Cook ME, Blanski L, et al: Intravenous nicardipine for the treatment of severe hypertension. Am J Med 85:331, 1988.
7. Wallin JD, Fletcher E, Ram CV, et al: Intravenous nicardipine for the treatment of severe hypertension. Arch Intern Med 149:2662, 1989.
8. I. V. Nicardipine Study Group: Efficacy and safety of intravenous nicardipine in the control of postoperative hypertension. Chest 99(2):393, 1991.
9. Halpern NA, Goldberg M, Neely C, et al: Postoperative hypertension: A multicenter, prospective, randomized comparison between intravenous nicardipine and sodium nitroprusside. Crit Care Med 20(12):1637, 1992.

CHAPTER 106

Nitrendipine

Wolfgang Kiowski, M.D.

Nitrendipine is a dihydropyridine derivative[1] structurally related closely to its mother compound, nifedipine (Fig. 106–1). Like all calcium antagonists, its main action is derived primarily from the inhibition of transmembranous calcium influx into cells through an inhibition of voltage-dependent slow calcium channels in myocardial and vascular smooth muscle cells. Despite the structural similarity, nitrendipine is distinctly different from nifedipine and also from verapamil-type or diltiazem-type calcium antagonists. Clinically, it has been evaluated widely for the treatment of arterial hypertension; this chapter therefore focuses predominantly on its use in patients with hypertension, but some newer data also exist regarding its efficacy in patients with angina pectoris.

PHARMACOLOGY

Nitrendipine is readily absorbed from the gastrointestinal tract. Measurements using radiolabeled nitrendipine show that absorption of an oral dose given as a tablet was about 80% to 90%.[2, 3] After absorption, the drug undergoes extensive hepatic metabolization, resulting in a bioavailability of only some 20%.[2, 3] All five known metabolites are 1000 times less potent than the parent compound.[4] Peak plasma concentra-

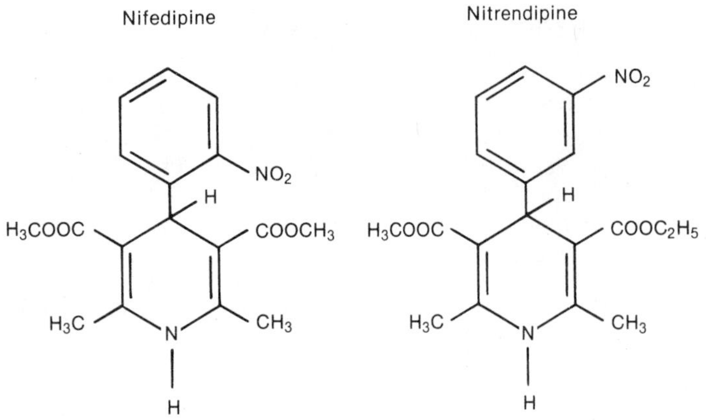

Nifedipine

Nitrendipine

Figure 106–1. The structure of nitrendipine and its mother compound, nifedipine.

tions are observed after 1 or 2 hours. Protein binding of nitrendipine is high (>95%).[3] Elimination occurs via renal excretion, and 41% of an oral dose can be recovered from the urine in the form of its major metabolites. Elimination half-life has been found to be approximately 8 hours but has been described to be approximately 20 hours when a more sensitive capillary gas chromatic procedure is used for analysis of plasma samples.[2]

No drug accumulation occurred when nitrendipine was given during 1 to 3 weeks,[4, 5] and there were no pharmacokinetic interactions after 1 week of therapy in which nitrendipine was combined with cimetidine, ranitidine, atenolol, metoprolol, acebutolol, digitoxin,[6] or with cyclosporine in hypertensive renal transplant recipients.[7] Grapefruit juice or other flavonoid-containing nutrients may inhibit the stereoselective cytochrome-P-450–dependent metabolism of nitrendipine.[8] In one study,[6] but not in another,[9] increased plasma digoxin concentrations were observed during simultaneous treatment with nitrendipine.

Available data suggest that in subjects with normal liver function hepatic enzymes responsible for the drug's extensive metabolism are not saturated at clinically used dosages.[5] If the metabolic capacity of the liver is reduced (e.g., in cirrhosis), bioavailability may be much higher than normal,[10] and dosages may require careful monitoring and adjustment according to the clinical effects in such patients. In contrast, impairment of renal function does not significantly influence the pharmacokinetics of nitrendipine.[11]

Pharmacokinetics subsequent to less effective hepatic metabolism also seem to be altered in older patients, and lower drug dosages than those administered in younger subjects may be needed for a comparable effect.[12] However, this finding is not unequivocal[13] and needs confirmation.

ELECTROPHYSIOLOGIC EFFECTS

The main electrophysiologic effect of nitrendipine is the blockade of calcium channels in myocardium and vascular smooth muscle.[14, 15] These effects lead to reduced intracellular free calcium concentration, diminished tension development, and reduction of vascular tone and cardiac contractile force. This effect is much

greater in vascular smooth muscle than in myocardium for all calcium antagonists, but, in clinical use, 1-4-dihydropyridine calcium antagonists in general have less effect on the myocardium than verapamil-type and diltiazem-type calcium antagonists. The reduction of calcium movement into cells can readily be shown *in vitro*, but a reduction in free cytosolic calcium concentration is also demonstrable, (e.g., in platelets from patients treated with oral nitrendipine for hypertension; Fig. 106–2). Nitrendipine differs from nifedipine in that for a given vascular effect, nitrendipine has less effect on the myocardium than nifedipine.[16] Nitrendipine therefore seems to have a certain vascular selectivity; this *in vitro* finding is also demonstrable in normal humans, in whom, with other cardiovascular effects being similar,[17] nitrendipine exhibits greater forearm vasodilation than nifedipine.

It is not clear why calcium antagonists have a greater effect in vascular smooth muscle than in myocardium and why, for example, nitrendipine seems to be more vasculoselective than nifedipine. The modulated receptor hypothesis,[18] as first proposed for local anesthetics, can explain many findings. Thus, calcium channels are presumably in equilibrium between a resting and an inactivated state. Nitrendipine would bind with high affinity to its binding site at the calcium channel when the calcium channel is in an inactivated state. The binding of nitrendipine supposedly leads to a proportional decrease of calcium channels in the resting state, which then are not available for

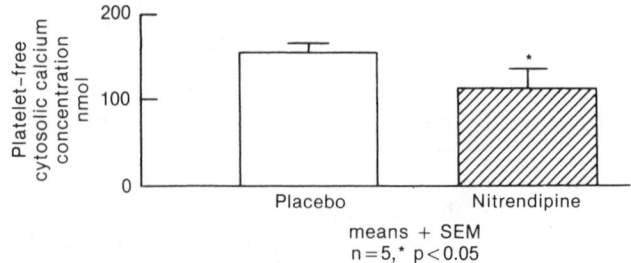

Figure 106–2. Platelet-free cytosolic calcium concentration before and after 6 weeks of treatment with nitrendipine (mean dose, 26 mg/day) in five patients with mild to moderate essential hypertension.

transmembraneous calcium influx during cell depolarization. Because transition from the resting to the inactivated state depends on membrane depolarization, and because resting potential in vascular smooth muscle is much less negative than in myocardium, a high proportion of calcium channels may be in the inactivated state and nitrendipine binds to them avidly. Because of the negative resting potential of myocardium, calcium channels in cardiac tissue presumably are predominantly in the resting state and nitrendipine does not bind to them easily. The relative vascular selectivity of nitrendipine may be due to the finding that, although it binds with high affinity to calcium channels in the inactivated state, it does so slowly. Thus, cardiac calcium channels that are briefly in the inactivated state during depolarization may not be affected by nitrendipine but may be affected by drugs such as verapamil, diltiazem, or nifedipine, which bind rapidly to the calcium channel in its inactivated state.

MECHANISMS OF ACTION

The electrophysiologic effects translate into a marked vasodilator activity not only *in vitro*[19] but also *in vivo*. When nitrendipine is infused into a brachial artery of patients with hypertension, the resulting vasodilatation is equivalent to metabolic vasodilatation after the release of 10 minutes of arterial occlusion (Fig. 106–3). After both acute[20] and chronic[21, 22] oral administration, hemodynamic measurements also show a reduction of total peripheral vascular resistance[22] with little if any effect on the venous circulation. A reflex increase of sympathetic activity leading to an increase in heart rate, cardiac output, and plasma renin activity occurs acutely, but most of these changes return to control values during long-term therapy,[22] which is a pattern similarly seen with the mother compound, nifedipine.[23]

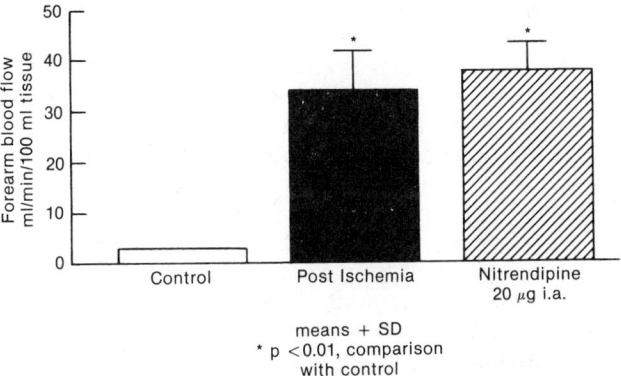

Figure 106–3. Forearm vasodilator response to nitrendipine in six patients with essential hypertension. Forearm blood flow (venous occlusion plethysmography) was measured under control conditions and immediately after 10 minutes of arterial occlusion (blood pressure cuff on upper arm inflated to 40 mmHg above systolic pressure). After return to control values, nitrendipine in a total dose of 20 µg was infused into a brachial artery over 2 minutes, and forearm blood flow was measured in the second minute of the infusion.

The lack of a negative inotropic effect *in vivo* is suggested by an upward left shift of the Frank-Starling curve in patients with severe congestive heart failure who are given oral nitrendipine.[24] This lends clinical support to the contention that the drug exhibits a high vascular selectivity.

The renal effects of nitrendipine also have received widespread attention. Acute administration of nitrendipine caused significant natriuresis and diuresis in healthy volunteers[25] and in patients with hypertension.[26] The mechanisms underlying this effect are not completely understood because nitrendipine does not seem to influence renal blood flow[27] or glomerular filtration rate.[22, 25–27] Possibly, a direct proximal tubular effect contributes to the diuretic and natriuretic effects,[25, 28] which may persist for at least 2 weeks after initiation of treatment.[28]

METABOLIC EFFECTS

Nitrendipine has been shown in most trials to be devoid of effects on either glucose or lipid metabolism. Thus, no changes were noted in the levels of fasting blood glucose, total cholesterol levels, total triglyceride concentrations, or high-density cholesterol levels in patients with essential hypertension who were treated with nitrendipine for 6 to 8 weeks.[29] Moreover, carbohydrate metabolism remained unchanged during long-term treatment in patients with diabetes mellitus and hypertension as assessed extensively by fasting blood glucose levels, urinary glucose excretion, serum insulin concentrations after a standard meal, and glycosylated hemoglobin A1.[30] A reduction of serum low-density lipoprotein levels[31] in patients with uncomplicated hypertension and an improved glucose tolerance in insulin-resistant obese hypertensive men have also been described.[32] Finally, some evidence suggests that nitrendipine also increases uric acid excretion and lowers plasma uric acid concentrations.[30] Thus, nitrendipine in clinically used dosages can be regarded as neutral or, in selected cases, potentially even as beneficial with respect to biochemical variables known to be associated with increased cardiovascular risk.

USE IN HYPERTENSION

Numerous studies have evaluated the effects of nitrendipine in patients with essential hypertension (compare Hulthen and Katzman[33]). All have found significant decreases of blood pressure without unwanted orthostatic effects when given in monotherapy. Although heart rate was elevated for as long as 3 weeks after initiation of treatment, no changes occurred during longer therapy. A typical example of the effects of nitrendipine monotherapy is given in Figure 106–4, showing an excellent and, as shown by others during follow-up for 1 to 5 years,[34] sustained antihypertensive effect in patients with uncomplicated mild to moderate hypertension. When nitrendipine is given alone, mild to moderate essential hypertension can be effectively controlled in 40% to 70% of an unselected

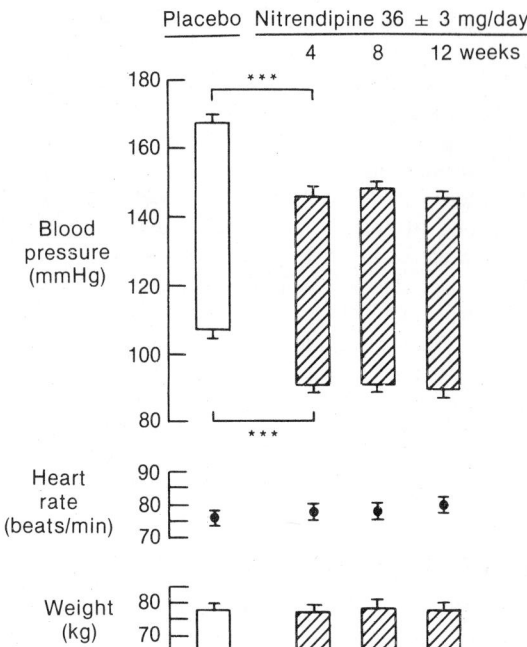

Placebo   Nitrendipine 36 ± 3 mg/day
                    4   8   12 weeks

Figure 106–4. Effects of nitrendipine monotherapy on blood pressure, heart rate, and weight in 46 patients with mild to moderate uncomplicated essential hypertension. Treatment had to be discontinued in two patients because of headaches and in one patient because of ankle edema.

patient population. Despite the fact that nitrendipine is a potent arteriolar vasodilator, it does not lead to volume retention,[22] a finding also borne out by unchanged body weight. This effect may well be related to its diuretic and natriuretic effects.

The antihypertensive efficacy of nitrendipine was compared with that of various other drugs, and overall it was found to be equally or more effective than diuretic therapy,[35, 36] β-blockade,[37] and angiotensin-converting enzyme (ACE) inhibition[38, 39] or other calcium antagonists such as diltiazem[40] or amlodipine.[41] Sodium intake does not seem to influence the blood pressure–lowering effect of nitrendipine.[42] Nitrendipine also reduces blood pressure during ergometric exercise[40, 43] and mental stress.[44] In particular, the hemodynamic response to mental stress was more physiologic after nitrendipine administration than after dosing with the β-blocker oxprenolol: in contrast with oxprenolol, nitrendipine allows systemic vascular resistance to fall into the range seen in normotensive subjects.[36]

Nitrendipine also has been used in combination with other antihypertensive agents. Additional decreases in blood pressure were observed when it was combined with β-blockers, diuretics, and ACE inhibitors. The use of nitrendipine with β-blockers[45–48] and diuretics[34, 46, 48] can control blood pressure effectively in some 60% to 80% of patients, and the combination with an ACE inhibitor has been reported to be as effective as or even more effective than the combination of an ACE inhibitor and a diuretic (e.g., a success rate of more than 90%).[49]

Because of the drug's comparatively long pharma-

cologic half-life, the possibility that it can control blood pressure with once-daily administration has been investigated. Satisfactory blood pressure control 24 hours after administration of a single dose of nitrendipine has been reported in a high percentage of patients (13 of 16 patients).[50] Of patients responding to monotherapy, 95% could be maintained chronically on a once-daily regimen,[51] but this does not seem to be a persistent finding. Thus, 20 mg of nitrendipine had no antihypertensive effect 24 hours after once-daily administration,[47] and 24-hour blood pressure monitoring indicated a lack of control of the early morning increase in blood pressure[52, 53] and a smaller effect during sleep[54, 55] using a once-daily regimen.[42] Although the importance of the early morning rise in blood pressure is not clear, the latter results indicate—not unexpectedly—that casual blood pressure recordings may not adequately reflect blood pressure response throughout the day. More precise assessments of blood pressure control therefore may be warranted in patients treated with a once-daily regimen.

A better antihypertensive response in older patients, often with low plasma renin activity, has been observed in some but not all studies with nitrendipine. Although many trials investigating this aspect were not double-blind trials, an age- and renin-dependent response pattern recently has also been found in black African patients in a double-blind comparative study with atenolol.[56] In addition, nitrendipine was more effective than methyldopa in hypertensive black African patients.[57] These findings lend support to the proposed better response of older patients and those with low renin and seems to parallel the pattern observed for other calcium antagonists, which also appear to be more efficacious in older and low-renin patients.[58]

Effects on Cardiac and Renal Function and Hypertensive Vascular Changes

Because nitrendipine effectively lowers blood pressure, it is not entirely surprising that a reduction of left ventricular mass is commonly seen during long-term therapy.[22, 59–61] The magnitude of this effect seems to be similar to that observed e.g., with the ACE inhibitor captopril.[61] Because of the known increase of cardiovascular risk associated with left ventricular hypertrophy, the reduction of left ventricular mass may reflect a benefit to the patient in addition to or independent from the associated blood pressure reduction. Furthermore, long-term treatment with nifedipine improved systolic and diastolic left ventricular function[22, 61] in hypertensive patients during long-term treatment. Moreover, minimal forearm vascular resistance, which is an indirect estimate of arteriolar structure, decreased during long-term nitrendipine therapy, indicating a regression of hypertensive vascular changes.[59]

Because experimental evidence also suggests a beneficial effect of calcium antagonists in hypertensive patients with impaired renal function with or without concomitant diabetes mellitus, this aspect has also been studied in humans using nitrendipine but the results are inconclusive. In one study, overall renal function improved in patients with hypertension and type I diabetes mellitus to a similar extent as with the ACE inhibitor enalapril,[62] whereas albuminuria, as an indirect estimate of a worsening of long-term renal function, increased in another.[63] Obviously, more data are needed in that respect.

USE IN ANGINA PECTORIS

Although studies with nitrendipine have concentrated on its antihypertensive effects, evidence also suggests that it is useful in patients with chronic ischemic heart disease and angina pectoris. Thus, nitrendipine monotherapy improved exercise tolerance time and reduced ischemic electrocardiographic (ECG) changes in patients with angina pectoris with[64] or without hypertension.[65] It was also markedly effective in patients with variant angina.[66] Nitrendipine was similarly effective compared with diltiazem in hypertensive patients with angina pectoris[67] and, interestingly, the combination of nitrendipine and diltiazem afforded an additional benefit in those patients whose symptoms were not controlled by the respective monotherapy.[67] Combination therapy with a long-acting nitrate also proved effective in hypertensive patients with angina pectoris.[68] Although the database related to antiischemic effects of nitrendipine is still small, it appears that nitrendipine leads to improved symptoms and a reduction of ischemic reactions during exercise.

SIDE EFFECTS

No serious unwanted effects have been observed, but those characteristic for 1-4-dihydropyridine calcium antagonists are also seen with nitrendipine. Thus, headaches, facial flushing, ankle edema, palpitations, tachycardia, and dizziness have been reported in various frequencies in different trials. When nitrendipine was compared with a placebo in controlled trials, only headaches and peripheral edema were significantly more frequent during nitrendipine therapy. Unwanted effects occur most frequently during the first 2 or 3 weeks of therapy and often diminish in severity or subside.[69] An exception to this pattern is ankle edema, which seems to become more pronounced with prolonged treatment but also subsides readily when therapy is withdrawn. In one of the largest long-term (>1 year) trials, only 8% of patients discontinued therapy because of unwanted effects.[34] Nitrendipine does not cause orthostatic hypotension and does not change indices of hematology, urinalysis, or chemistry (including serum glucose and blood lipid levels).

CONCLUSION

Nitrendipine is a member of the dihydropyridine family of calcium antagonists that shares many of the group properties with, for example, the mother compound nifedipine but nevertheless is sufficiently different to deserve a place in its own right. Nitrendipine is efficacious as monotherapy, and, because of its long elimination half-life, may be administered in selected patients on a once-daily basis, which is a factor of great importance in a usually asymptomatic disease in which drug compliance is inversely related to the number of tablets per day. Side effects are usually mild and transient, and the drug is generally neutral with respect to metabolic side effects. The drug's high selectivity for vascular smooth muscle over myocardium, and the lack of a demonstrable negative inotropic effect in patients with congestive heart failure, also make it safe for the treatment of patients with hypertension complicated by left ventricular failure or in combination with β-blockers. Although experience in patients with coronary artery disease is limited, reasonable evidence suggests that nitrendipine is also useful in patients with hypertension, coronary artery disease, or both. Thus, nitrendipine is well suited not only for first-line treatment of mild to moderate uncomplicated hypertension but also for patients in whom complications of longstanding hypertension (e.g., heart failure or coronary artery disease) have developed.

REFERENCES

1. Meyer H, Bossert F, Wehinger E, et al: Synthese und vergleichende pharmakologische Untersuchungen von 1,4-Dihydro-2,6-dimethyl-4-(3-nitrophenyl)pyridin-3,5-dicarbonsäureesiern mit nicht identischen Esterfunktionen. Arzneimittelforschung 31:407, 1981.
2. Krol GJ, Lettieri JT, Yeh SC, et al: Disposition and pharmocokinetics of 14-C-nitrendipine in healthy volunteers. J Cardiovasc Pharmacol 9(Suppl 4):122, 1987.
3. Mikus G, Eichelbaum M: Pharmacokinetics, bioavailability, metabolism, and hemodynamic effects of the calcium channel antagonist nitrendipine. J Cardiovasc Pharmacol 9(Suppl 4):140, 1987.
4. Raemsch KD, Sommer J: Pharmacokinetics and metabolism of nitrendipine. In Scriabine A, Vanov S., Deck, U. (eds): Nitrendipine. Baltimore: Urban and Schwarzenberg, 1984, pp 409–420.
5. Hansson L, Andren L, Oro L, et al: The antihypertensive effects of nitrendipine in patients with essential hypertension. J Cardiovasc Pharmacol 6(Suppl 7):933, 1984.
6. Kirch W, Hutt HJ, Heidemann H, et al: Drug interactions with nitrendipine. J Cardiovasc Pharmacol 6(Suppl 7):986, 1984.
7. Scholz DE, Lippert J, Gellert J, et al: Assessment of the effect of nitrendipine on blood pressure and renal function in hypertensive renal transplant recipients. Presented at the Second Generation Calcium Antagonists and the Treatment of Hypertension, Valencia, Spain, April, 1991.
8. Soons PA, Vogels BA, Roosemalen MC, et al: Grapefruit juice and cimetidine inhibit stereoselective metabolism of nitrendipine in humans. Clin Pharmacol Ther 50:394, 1991.
9. Ziegler R, Wingender W, Boehme K, et al: Study of pharmacokinetic and pharmacodynamic interaction between nitrendipine and digoxin. J Cardiovasc Pharmacol 9(Suppl 4):101, 1987.
10. Lasseter KC, Shamblen EC, Murdoch AA, et al: Steady state pharmacokinetics of nitrendipine in hepatic insufficiency. J Cardiovasc Pharmacol 6(Suppl 7):880, 1984.
11. Aronoff GR, Sloan RS: Nitrendipine kinetics in normal and impaired renal function. Clin Pharmacol Ther 38:212, 1985.
12. Lettieri J, Krol G, Yeh S, et al: Pharmocokinetics of nitrendipine in elderly and young healthy volunteers. J Cardiovasc Pharmacol 9(Suppl 4):142, 1987.

13. Kendall MJ, Lobo J, Jack DB, et al: The influence of age on the pharmocokinetics of nitrendipine. J Cardiovasc Pharmacol 9(Suppl 4):96, 1987.

14. Bean BP: Nitrendipine block of cardiac calcium channels: High-affinity binding to the inactivated state. Proc Natl Acad Sci USA 81:6388, 1984.

15. Bean BP, Sturek M, Puga A, et al: Calcium channels in muscle cells isolated from rat mesenteric arteries: Modulation by dihydropyridine drugs. Circ Res 59:229, 1986.

16. Katz AM, Leach MM: Differential effects of 1,4-dihydropyridine calcium channel blockers: Therapeutic implications. J Clin Pharmacol 11:825, 1987.

17. Graefe KH, Ziegler R, Wingender W, et al: Plasma level—effect relationships for some acute cardiovascular effects of nisoldipine and other dihydropyridine calcium antagonists. In Hugenholtz PG, Meyer J (eds): Nisoldipine. Berlin: Springer Verlag, 1987, pp 67–75.

18. Hille B: Local anaesthetics: Hydrophilic and hydrophobic pathways for the drug: Receptor interaction. J Gen Physiol 69:497, 1977.

19. Towart R, Stoepel K: The vascular mechanisms of action of Bay e 5009, a new calcium antagonist with a potent antihypertensive action. Naunyn Schmiedebergs Arch Pharmacol 308(Suppl):R18, 1979.

20. Ventura HO, Messerli FH, Oigman W, et al: Immediate hemodynamic effects of a new calcium channel blocking agent (nitrendipine) in essential hypertension. Am J Cardiol 51:783, 1983.

21. Fouad FM, Pedrinelli R, Bravo EL, et al: Clinical and systemic hemodynamic effects of nitrendipine. Clin Pharmacol Ther 35:768, 1984.

22. Grossman E, Oren S, Garavaglia GE, et al: Systemic and regional hemodynamic and humoral effects of nitrendipine in essential hypertension. Circulation 78:1394, 1988.

23. Kiowski W, Bertel O, Erne P, et al: Hemodynamic and reflex mechanisms of acute and chronic antihypertensive therapy with the calcium channel blocker nifedipine. Hypertension 5:170, 1983.

24. Cohn JN: Calcium antagonists and left ventricular function: Effects of nitrendipine in congestive heart failure. Am J Cardiol 58:27D, 1986.

25. Wallia R, Greenberg A, Puschett JB: Renal hemodynamic and tubular transport effects of nitrendipine. J Lab Clin Med 105:498, 1985.

26. Luft FC, Aronoff GR, Sloan RS, et al: Calcium channel blockade with nitrendipine: Effects on sodium homeostasis, the renin-angiotensin system and the sympathetic nervous system. Hypertension 7:438, 1985.

27. Pedrinelli R, Fouad FM, Tarazi RC, et al: Nitrendipine, a calcium blocker: Renal and humoral effects in human arterial hypertension. Arch Intern Med 146:62, 1986.

28. Lupinacci L, Palomino C, Greenberg A, et al: Chronic effects of nitrendipine on renal hemodynamics and tubular transport. Clin Pharmacol Ther 43:6, 1988.

29. Ferrara LA, Soro S, Fasano ML: Effects of nitrendipine on glucose and lipid serum concentrations. Curr Ther Res 37:614, 1985.

30. Trost BN, Weidmann P: Nitrendipine in patients with hypertension and diabetes mellitus. J Cardiovasc Pharmacol 9(Suppl 4):280, 1987.

31. Veroli C: The effects of nitrendipine on glycemia, uricemia, lipids, and body-mass index during long-term antihypertensive treatment. Curr Ther Res 50:449, 1991.

32. Beer NA, Jakubowicz DJ, Beer RM, et al: Effects of nitrendipine on glucose tolerance and serum insulin and dehydroepiandrosterone sulfate levels in insulin-resistant obese and hypertensive men. J Clin Endocrinol Metab 76:178, 1993.

33. Hulthen UL, Katzman PL: Review of long-term trials with nitrendipine. J Cardiovasc Pharmacol 12(Suppl 4):11, 1988.

34. Weber MA: Prolonged calcium channel blocker therapy of hypertension. J Cardiovasc Pharmacol 12(Suppl 4):16, 1988.

35. Morledge J, Brown RD, Byyny R, et al: Comparative study of the effects of nitrendipine and hydrochlorothiazide in hypertensive patients. J Cardiovasc Pharmacol 9(Suppl 4):224, 1987.

36. Giles TD, Sander GE, Roffidal LE, Mazzu A: Comparison of effects of nitrendipine vs hydrochlorothiazide on left ventricular structure and function and neurohumoral status in systemic hypertension. Am J Cardiol 65:1265, 1990.

37. McMahon FG, Brobyn R, Kann J, et al: A double blind comparative study of nitrendipine and propranolol in the treatment of hypertension. J Cardiovasc Pharmacol 9(Suppl 4):228, 1987.

38. Cennari C, Nami R, Bianchini C, et al: Nitrendipine and the angiotensin converting enzyme inhibitors in the treatment of hypertension. J Cardiovasc Pharmacol 9(Suppl 4):245, 1987.

39. Carlsen JE, Galloe A, Kober L, et al: Comparison of efficacy and tolerability of spirapril and nitrendipine in arterial hypertension. Drug Invest 3:172, 1991.

40. Gambini G, Valori C, Bianchi L, Bozza M: Acute and short-term effects of nitrendipine and diltiazem at rest and during exercise in hypertensive patients. Clin Ther 13:680, 1991.

41. Englert R, Beressem P, von Manteuffel E, et al: Amlodipine compared to nitrendipine for the treatment of mild-to-moderate hypertension. Postgrad Med J 67:35, 1991.

42. Salvetti A, Arzilli F, Innocenti P, et al: The antihypertensive effect of nitrendipine and its interaction with sodium intake: A multicenter crossover trial. J Hypertension 9:364, 1991.

43. Franz IW, Wievel D: Antihypertensive effects on blood pressure at rest and during exercise of calcium antagonist, beta-receptor blockers, and their combination in hypertensive patients. J Cardiovasc Pharmacol 6(Suppl 7):1045, 1986.

44. Schmieder R, Ruddel H, Neus H, et al: Disparate hemodynamic responses to mental challenge after antihypertensive therapy with beta blockers and calcium entry blockers. Am J Med 82:11, 1987.

45. Orö L, Ryman T: Combination of nitrendipine with metoprolol and a comparison with nifedipine in patients insufficiently treated with the beta-blocker alone. J Cardiovasc Pharmacol 9(Suppl 4):238, 1987.

46. Kirkendall WM, Adlin V, Canzanello V, et al: Comparative study of the safety and efficacy of nitrendipine, atenolol, and hydrochlorothiazide in combination in the treatment of hypertension. J Cardiovasc Pharmacol 9(Suppl 4):232, 1987.

47. McLean D, Mitchell ET, Lewis R, et al: Comparison of once daily atenolol, nitrendipine and their combination in mild to moderate essential hypertension. Br J Clin Pharmacol 29:455, 1990.

48. Zaeh D, Haider B, Brown P, Silas E: Efficacy and safety of combinations of nitrendipine, atenolol, and hydrochlorothiazide in black hypertensive patients. J Hum Hypertens 4:157, 1990.

49. Brouwer RML, Bolli P, Erne P, et al: Antihypertensive treatment using calcium antagonists in combination with captopril rather than diuretics. J Cardiovasc Pharmacol 7(Suppl 4):88, 1985.

50. Müller FB, Bolli P, Erne P, et al: Antihypertensive therapy with the long-acting calcium antagonist nitrendipine. J Cardiovasc Pharmacol 6:S1073, 1984.

51. Kiowski W, Bertel O, Braun H: Antihypertensive monotherapy with nitrendipine in general practice. J Cardiovasc Pharmacol 12(Suppl 4):149, 1988.

52. Meyer-Sabellek W, Schulte KL, Streitberg B, et al: 24-hour non-invasive oscillometric blood pressure monitoring: Evaluation of the antihypertensive circadian profile of nitrendipine. J Cardiovasc Pharmacol 12(Suppl 4):22, 1988.

53. Schrader J, Schoel G, Buhr-Schinner H, et al: Comparison of the antihypertensive efficiency of nitrendipine, metoprolol, mepindolol and analapril using ambulatory 24-hour blood-pressure monitoring. Am J Cardiol 66:967, 1990.

54. Uguccioni M, Mocini D, Dini FL, et al: Effect of nitrendipine once daily on 24-hour ambulatory blood pressure: A four-month follow-up. Curr Ther Res 50:702, 1991.

55. Asmar R, Benetos A, Brahimi M, et al: Arterial and antihypertensive effects of nitrendipine: A double-blind comparison versus placebo. J Cardiovasc Pharmacol 20:858, 1992.

56. M'Buyamba-Kabangu JR, Lepira B, Lijnen P, et al: Intracellular sodium and the response to nitrendipine or atenolol in African blacks. Hypertension 11:100, 1988.

57. Seedat YK: Nitrendipine in a fixed stepped-dose study compared with methyldopa in black and Indian hypertensive patients. Curr Ther Res 48:10, 1990.

58. Amery A, Bolli P, Dollery C, et al: Calcium antagonists alone

or in combination in today's antihypertensive therapy. A round-table discussion. J Cardiovasc Pharmacol 12(Suppl 4):101, 1988.

59. Agabiti-Rosei E, Muiesan ML, Rizzoni D, et al: Regression of cardiovascular structural changes after long-term antihypertensive treatment with the calcium antagonist nitrendipine. J Cardiovasc Pharmacol 18:5, 1992.

60. Modena MG, Mattioli AV, Parato VM, Mattioli G: Effect of antihypertensive treatment with nitrendipine on left ventricular mass and diastolic filling in patients with mild to moderate hypertension. J Cardiovasc Pharmacol 19:148, 1992.

61. Vogelsberg H, Curtius JM, Welslau R, Steffen M: Antihypertensive Therapie mit Captopril oder Nitrendipin: Einfluss auf die linksventrikuläre Muskelmasse unddie diastolische Funktion. Herz Kreislauf 23:256, 1991.

62. Jungmann E, Haak T, Malanyn M, et al: Effects of nitrendipine vs enalapril on microalbuminuria and alpha-1-microglobulin excretion in patients with type 1 diabetes mellitus. Eur J Clin Invest 23:A42, 1993.

63. Kloke HJ, Wetzels JF, van Hamersvelt HW, et al: Effects of nitrendipine and cilazapril on renal hemodynamics and albu-minuria in hypertensive patients with chronic renal failure. J Cardiovasc Pharmacol 16:924, 1990.

64. Schmoeckel M, Arendt RM, Hauck R, et al: Acute and chronic effects of nitrendipine on hemodynamics and myocardial ischemia in patients with combined angina pectoris and hypertension. J Cardiovasc Pharmacol 12(Suppl 4):170, 1988.

65. Ceyhan B, Oto A, Oram E, et al: Anti-ischemic effects of nitrendipine. Cuore e Vasi 6:399, 1989.

66. Kishida H, Kato K, Toyama S, et al: Clinical effects of nitrendipine on variant angina pectoris. Jpn Heart J 32:297, 1991.

67. Andreyev N, Bichkov I, Skutelis A, Andreyeva T: Comparison of diltiazem, nitrendipine, and their combination for systemic hypertension and stable angina pectoris. J Cardiovasc Pharmacol 18:73, 1991.

68. Dini FL, Iurato A: Nitrendipine plus long-acting nitrates combination therapy in hypertensive patients with ischaemic heart disease. Cuore e Vasi 8:675, 1991.

69. Stoepel K, Deck K, Corsing C, et al: Safety aspects of long-term nitrendipine therapy. J Cardiovasc Pharmacol 6(Suppl 7):1072, 1984.

CHAPTER 107

Nisoldipine

Philip A. Poole-Wilson, M.D., F.R.C.P.

HISTORY

Nisoldipine is a second-generation calcium antagonist with an increased potency for smooth muscle relative to cardiac muscle. Initial investigations of the pharmacology of nisoldipine took place in the early 1980s. Nisoldipine is now available for clinical use in some European countries.

CHEMISTRY

Nisoldipine is a 1,4-dihydropyridine with a structure similar to that of nifedipine. The complete chemical name for nisoldipine is 1,4-dihydro-2,6-dimethyl-4-(o-nitrophenyl)pyridine-3,5-dicarboxylic acid 3-isobutyl, 5-methyl ester. Nisoldipine differs from nifedipine only by the substitution of an isobutylic instead of a methyl group in one of the two ester groups. This minor structural difference leads to important changes in effect.

PHARMACOLOGY

The early pharmacology of nisoldipine has been reported in several substantial reviews on nisoldipine[1-5] in particular, and on calcium antagonists in general.[6,7] Only more recent references are included here. The effects of nisoldipine do not differ qualitatively from those of other dihydropyridine calcium antagonists such as nifedipine. The potency with regard to cardiac muscle is similar to nifedipine but the potency for relaxation of vascular smooth muscle is increased four to ten times. As with other calcium antagonists, any effect on the ischemic myocardium in animal experiments *in vitro* is best seen if the drug is given before the period of ischemia rather than at the time of reperfusion.[8] In animal studies and in humans, the major effect is vasodilatation with a reduction of systemic vascular resistance, an increase in cardiac index and stroke volume, a decrease in blood pressure, and tachycardia. The tachycardia can be prevented by the simultaneous administration of a β-blocker, suggesting that it is caused by sympathetic activation consequent upon a lowering of the blood pressure. Nisoldipine increases oxygen supply to ischemic myocardium and reduces anaerobic glycolysis. In animal studies, nisoldipine limits infarct size and reduces the incidence of reperfusion arrhythmias. However, the role of calcium antagonists is controversial.[9-11] Nisoldipine has only a minor, if any, effect on plasma lipid levels, a minor diuretic action, an inhibitory action on platelet aggregation *in vitro* and *in vivo*, and results in variable changes of plasma renin and aldosterone after long-term use.

PHARMACOKINETICS

The peak effect of nisoldipine occurs 2 hours after oral administration. The duration of action varies between 2 and 15 hours, with a likely duration of action in patients with minor disease of approximately 6 to 8 hours. The volume of distribution is approximately 5 L/kg, indicating that the drug is distributed extensively throughout the body. More than 99% of the drug is protein bound.

The drug is well absorbed regardless of food intake. There is substantial first-pass metabolism in the liver and gut wall, leading to the formation of many metabolites. Single doses of 2.5-, 5-, 10-, and 20-mg tablets reached C_{max} values of 0.4, 0.9, 1.4, and 3.4 mg/L. Labeling studies demonstrate that at least 80% of the radioactivity is eliminated by the kidneys and the remainder in the feces. Unchanged nisoldipine could not be detected in mice. Liver dysfunction increases the plasma concentration, whereas, not surprisingly, renal dysfunction appears to have little effect.

The oral daily dose is 10 to 20 mg given in two equally divided doses. Some patients require an increase to a maximum of 40 mg/day. The effects of the drug appear to last up to 7 hours.

A "coat-core" controlled-release preparation to enable once-daily administration is under development.[12] The 24-hour plasma profile of nisoldipine "coat-core" is plateau-shaped with little peak-trough fluctuation. A steady state is achieved quickly, usually with the second dose.

EFFECTS ON PATHOPHYSIOLOGY
Effects on Hemodynamics

Nisoldipine causes vasodilation and a reduction in the systemic vascular resistance. The change in resistance is accompanied by an increase in cardiac index and a fall of blood pressure. Heart rate increases as a result of reflex sympathetic stimulation. The reflex response can be inhibited by β-adrenoreceptor antagonists. In general, the pulmonary wedge pressure is unchanged or reduced slightly.

The administration of nisoldipine (2 μg/kg) intravenously to patients with acute myocardial infarction caused vasodilation, an increase in cardiac output, and an increase in heart rate that was judged to be sufficiently great to contraindicate nisoldipine in acute myocardial infarction.[13] Similar changes without an increase in pulmonary wedge pressure have been found in patients with chronic heart failure after nisoldipine 20 mg orally.[14] In a study over 3 months, many of these effects were not maintained, and neurohumoral changes were absent after chronic administration.[15]

Effects on Ventricular Function and Structure

As with other calcium antagonists, a possible harmful effect of nisoldipine is a negative inotropic effect in patients with preexisting left ventricular dysfunction. Calcium antagonists do not have a beneficial effect in heart failure, although some of the newer calcium antagonists such as amlodipine and felodipine are being tested in large clinical trials.[16, 17] Nisoldipine is similar in its pharmacologic effects to these calcium antagonists.

Nisoldipine orally (10 mg twice daily) improves diastolic function over 2 months in patients with ischemic left ventricular dysfunction, the effect being partly a result of improved coordination of ventricular contraction.[18] Estimation of ventricular volumes by radionuclide techniques showed no change with nisoldipine.[19] In the DEFIANT I study, 135 patients were followed up for 1 month.[20] Patients were included if they had sustained a recent myocardial infarction and had an ejection fraction below 50% with mild left ventricular dysfunction. Doppler indices of diastolic function improved, exercise time increased but ventricular volumes were unchanged. Similar results in terms of small and variable changes in volumes and ejection fraction have been reported by others.[21, 22] In 19 patients with heart failure of New York Heart Association classes 2 to 4 given 10 mg nisoldipine three times daily, no change in heart rate or ejection fraction measured by radionuclide methods was observed.[23] There was a small increase in exercise time. Nisoldipine has been shown to improve systolic and diastolic function in patients with hibernating myocardium.[24]

These results taken together demonstrate the expected results from administration of a drug with vasodilator properties. Reflex tachycardia is a problem for the use of nisoldipine in many ischemic syndromes. In general calcium antagonists have not been shown to be of benefit in the context of myocardial infarction.[25, 26] The use of calcium antagonists in patients after myocardial infarction without moderate ventricular impairment is being investigated in a large study of 550 patients (DEFIANT II).[27] The primary end point is exercise capacity. Benefit may accrue because of the ability of nisoldipine (coat-core) to increase regional blood flow and offset the consequences of myocardial hibernation.

Effects on Electrophysiology

In vitro studies in tissue preparations have shown that nisoldipine can prolong the atrioventricular conduction time and have a variety of other electrophysiologic effects.[28–30] These results were obtained at doses substantially higher than those that would be used in vivo. Animal experiments have not demonstrated any change in electrophysiologic variables except at very high concentrations. At such concentrations, the blood pressure is reduced and activation of the sympathetic system may lead to shortening of the atrioventricular conduction time.

Electrophysiologic studies in patients have failed to reveal any significant electrophysiologic effect. In nine patients with atrioventricular block, no reduction of conduction was shown after intravenous nisoldipine.[31] In this respect, the drug differs from other calcium antagonists such as diltiazem or verapamil.

Effects on Coronary Blood Flow

Coronary blood flow is dependent on blood pressure, autoregulation of coronary flow, and the presence of pathologic conditions within the coronary artery. Nisoldipine dilates coronary arteries, increases myocardial blood flow, and decreases coronary vascular resistance. These effects are dose dependent. Vasospasm of the coronary arteries can be reversed by nisoldipine.

Although calcium antagonists may delay the progression of the atheromatous process in animal models and humans with atheromatous obstructive coronary artery disease, no data are available on this effect with nisoldipine in humans. Several early studies showed that nisoldipine benefitted patients with angina pectoris.[4] These trials involved small numbers of patients. More recently, further studies have been reported. In 82 patients with angina randomized to nisoldipine 10 mg twice daily, all exercise variables were improved, but there was only a partial suppression of silent ischemia assessed by 72-hour monitoring of the electrocardiogram.[32] In a larger study of 185 patients given nisoldipine 2.5 to 10 mg twice daily, no overall benefit was observed, although there was a trend in favor of the drug.[33] At the higher dose, side effects were common. In 52 patients with angina, no reduction of silent ischemia was observed with a dose of 5 to 10 mg nisoldipine.[34]

Nisoldipine is probably as effective as nifedipine when combined with atenolol for the treatment of angina.[35] Nisoldipine can usefully be added to treatment with propranolol.[36] Any beneficial effect on angina may be explained by an increase of blood flow,[37] and nisoldipine seems to protect the myocardium in the context of short periods of ischemia as experienced during percutaneous coronary angioplasty.[38]

These findings with regard to the treatment of angina pectoris, although strongly suggestive of a benefit (which would be anticipated in the light of current knowledge of calcium antagonists), fall short of absolute proof. One reason for the variability may be the short duration of action and the powerful vasodilator action with an accompanying fall of blood pressure. It is possible that reduction of blood pressure could be excessive for part of the day and the patient be unexposed to drug at other times of the day with twice daily dosage. The use of the "coat-core" preparation may resolve these problems.

Effects on Arteries and Veins

Nisoldipine has greater effect on arteries than veins. Differential effects in different arterial beds have not been fully explored. Renal blood flow is not increased after prolonged exposure.

Nisoldipine has been widely investigated for the treatment of hypertension.[4] More recent studies have confirmed earlier findings.[12, 39] Twelve patients have been studied using 24-hour monitoring.[40] The advantageous use of nisoldipine for hypertension has been reported in hypertensive diabetics,[41] postpartum women,[42] and in the presence of β-adrenoceptor antagonists such as atenolol[42] and propranolol.[43]

Effects on Fluid Volume State and Electrolytes

Nisoldipine alone induces a mild diuresis. This effect does not persist after long-term treatment. In general, any effect on renal vascular resistance or blood flow is transient. Plasma electrolytes are not affected by nisoldipine.

Endocrine and Metabolic Effects

In normotensive persons, nisoldipine has no effect on plasma renin activity or on aldosterone concentrations when given orally. In hypertensive patients, there is a small increase in the plasma renin level although the aldosterone concentration is unchanged. After a period of 18 months, neither plasma renin activity nor the aldosterone concentration are affected. When used long term in heart failure, the renin-angiotensin system is not activated although there is considerable variability among patients.[14, 15] In congestive heart failure, the response to nisoldipine is complex and depends on the clinical circumstances relating to the severity of heart failure. One study found plasma renin levels but not aldosterone to be lowered after 4 weeks' treatment. Intravenous treatment may activate plasma renin activity. This is not unexpected in view of the lowering of blood pressure that may follow intravenous administration. A similar finding may pertain to some patients with heart failure in which excessive vasodilatation may activate the sympathetic system and the renal angiotensin system.

Effects on Renal Function

Nisoldipine has only minor effects on renal function. Blood flow, renal vascular resistance, and glomerular filtration rate remain largely unchanged. Nisoldipine can have a minor transient diuretic effect.

Effects on the Central Nervous System

Nisoldipine has no effects on the central nervous system other than to induce dizziness when the reduction of blood pressure is excessive.

CLINICAL USE
Indications

Nisoldipine is currently on the market in some countries in Europe. The treatment of hypertension is the best established indication. Nisoldipine would be expected to be advantageous in the treatment of angina pectoris, but the results of recent trials have been conflicting.

Calcium antagonists have not been demonstrated to have advantage in the management of acute myocardial infarction.[25, 26] In unstable angina, in general, these drugs are used as a last resort.

A review of the use of calcium antagonists in heart failure did not demonstrate that these drugs had an advantage.[16] Two calcium antagonists currently are being investigated for this indication in large mortality trials.

Post Myocardial Infarction

In the double-blind, multicenter DEFIANT II study, 542 patients who had suffered an acute myocardial infarction (MI) were randomized to either nisoldipine 40 mg/day or placebo. The patients had diminished ventricular function, as defined by an ejection fraction of 25% to 50%, although no symptoms or signs of congestive heart failure. Exercise tolerance after 6 months was similar in both groups. Clinical adverse events (death, angina, and myocardial infarction) were less common in the nisoldipine group, whereas the occurrence of congestive heart failure was not different from that in the placebo group. The authors concluded that treatment with nisoldipine can be considered safe in the post MI patient.

Adverse Effects

The adverse effect profile of nisoldipine is similar to other dihydropyridine receptor antagonists. The main side effects are dizziness and hypotension. A proportion of patients, possibly as high as 10%, develop ankle edema that reverses on cessation of the drug.

REFERENCES

1. New aspects of the treatment of ischemic heart disease with calcium antagonists. Proceedings of the International Nisoldipine Symposium. Dusseldorf, Germany, March 27–29, 1992. J Cardiovasc Pharmacol 20(Suppl 5):S1, 1992.
2. Proceedings: New aspects on nisoldipine. Stuttgart: Schattauer, 1990, pp 1–148.
3. Proceedings: Nisoldipine 1987. Berlin: Springer-Verlag, 1987, pp 1–348.
4. Friedel HA, Sorkin EM: Nisoldipine. A preliminary review of its pharmacodynamic and pharmacokinetic properties, and therapeutic efficacy in the treatment of angina pectoris, hypertension and related cardiovascular disorders. Drugs 36:682, 1988.
5. Mitchell J, Frishman W, Heiman M: Nisoldipine: A new dihydropyridine calcium-channel blocker. J Clin Pharmacol 33:46, 1993
6. Nayler WG: Second Generation of Calcium Antagonists. Berlin: Springer-Verlag, 1991.
7. Nayler WG: Calcium Antagonists. London: Academic Press, 1988.
8. Ehring T, Bohm M, Heusch G: The calcium antagonist nisoldipine improves the functional recovery of reperfused myocardium only when given before ischemia. J Cardiovasc Pharmacol 20:63, 1992.
9. Kloner RA, Braunwald E: Effects of calcium channel antagonists on infarcting myocardium. Am J Cardiol 59:84B, 1987.
10. Kloner R, Przyklenk K: Experimental infarct size reduction with calcium channel blockers. J Am Coll Cardiol 18:876, 1991.
11. Opie LH, Coetzee WA: Role of calcium ions in reperfusion arrhythmias. Relevance to pharmacological intervention. Cardiovasc Drugs Ther 2:623, 1991.
12. Chandler MH, Clifton GD, Lettieri JT, et al: Multiple dose pharmacokinetics of four different doses of nisoldipine in hypertensive patients. J Clin Pharmacol 32:571, 1992.
13. Wilson J, Commerford PJ, Millar RS, et al: Hemodynamic effects of nisoldipine, a highly specific calcium antagonist, in patients with acute myocardial infarction. Cardiovasc Drugs Ther 6:41, 1992.
14. Dei Cas L, Metra M, Ferrari R, et al: Acute and chronic effects of the dihydropyridine calcium antagonist nisoldipine on the resting and exercise hemodynamics, neurohumoral parameters, and functional capacity of patients with chronic heart failure. Cardiovasc Drugs Ther 7:103, 1993.
15. Schofer J, Hobuss M, Aschenberg W, et al: Acute and long-term haemodynamic and neurohumoral response to nisoldipine vs captopril in patients with heart failure: A randomized double-blind study [see comments]. Eur Heart J 11:712, 1990.
16. Parameshwar J, Poole-Wilson PA: The role of calcium antagonists in the treatment of chronic heart failure. Eur Heart J 14(Suppl A):38, 1993.
17. Packer M: Calcium channel blockers in chronic heart failure. Circulation 82:2254, 1990.
18. Pouleur H, van Eyll C, Gurne O, et al: Analysis of the mechanisms underlying the changes in left ventricular filling dynamics during oral nisoldipine therapy in patients with anterior myocardial infarction. Eur Heart J 13:952, 1992.
19. Tartagni F, Melandri G, De Tommaso I, et al: Effects of nisoldipine in coronary artery disease: A radioisotopic approach. J Cardiovasc Pharmacol 20(Suppl 5):S65, 1992.
20. The DEFIANT Research Group: Improved diastolic function with the calcium antagonist nisoldipine (coat-core) in patients post myocardial infarction: Results of the DEFIANT study. Doppler flow and ehocardiography in functional cardiac insufficiency: Assessment of nisoldipine therapy. Eur Heart J 13:1496, 1992.
21. de Cock CC, Visser FC, Peels KH, et al: Effects of nisoldipine on systolic and diastolic function in postinfarction patients with reduced left ventricular function: A randomized, double-blind, placebo-controlled study. Eur Heart J 12:1012, 1991.
22. Eichstaedt H: Effects of calcium antagonists in patients with coronary disease and heart failure: Left ventricular function following nisoldipine measured by radionuclide ventriculography. J Cardiovasc Pharmacol 20(Suppl 5):S50, 1992.
23. Lewis BS, Makhoul N, Merdler A, et al: Effect of nisoldipine on exercise performance in heart failure following myocardial infarction. Cardiology 79:39, 1991.
24. Pouleur H, van Eyll C, Gurne O, et al: Effects of prolonged nisoldipine administration on the "hibernating" myocardium. J Cardiovasc Pharmacol 20(Suppl 5):S73, 1992.
25. Yusuf S, Held P, Furberg C: Update of effects of calcium antagonists in myocardial infarction or angina in light of the second Danish Verapamil Infarction Trial (DAVIT-II) and other recent studies [editorial]. Am J Cardiol 67:1295, 1991.
26. Held PH, Yusuf S, Furberg CD: Calcium channel blockers in acute myocardial infarction and unstable angina: An overview. Br Med J 299:1187, 1989.
27. MacNeil AB, St John Sutton M, Poole-Wilson PA, et al: Doppler flow, echocardiography and functional improvement: Assessment of nisoldipine therapy (DEFIANT-II study). Objectives and design. Clin Trials Meta 28:267, 1993.
28. An RH, He RR: Rate- and voltage-dependent effects of m-nisoldipine on action potential of partially depolarized guinea pig papillary muscle. ChungKuo Yao Li Hsueh Pao/Acta Pharmacologica Sinica 13:118, 1992.
29. An RH, Fan ZZ, He RR: Effects of m-nisoldipine on transmembrane currents of guinea pig papillary muscles. Chung Kuo Yao Li Hsueh Pao/Acta Pharmacologica Sinica 13:341, 1992.
30. An RH, Fan ZZ, He RR: Effects of m-nisoldipine on delayed afterdepolarization of canine Purkinje fibers. Chung Kuo Yao Li Hsueh Pao/Acta Pharmacologica Sinica 13:23, 1992.
31. Klein HH: Clinical experience with nisoldipine in patients with atrio-ventricular blocks. Arzneimittelforschung 40:260, 1990.
32. Tzivoni D, Banai S, Botvin S, et al: Effects of nisoldipine on myocardial ischemia during exercise and during daily activity. Am J Cardiol 67:559, 1991.
33. Thadani U, Zellner SR, Glasser S, et al: Double-blind, dose-response, placebo-controlled multicenter study of nisoldipine. A new second-generation calcium channel blocker in angina pectoris [see comments]. Circulation 84:2398, 1991.
34. Fox K, Pool J, Vos J, et al: The effects of nisoldipine on the total ischaemic burden: The results of the ROCKET study. Eur Heart J 12:1283, 1991.
35. Donaldson KM, Dawkins KD, Waller DG: A comparison of nisoldipine and nifedipine, in combination with atenolol, in the management of myocardial ischaemia. Eur Heart J 14:534, 1993.
36. De Caprio L, Papa M, Acanfora D, et al: Acute effects of nisoldipine, propranolol, and their combination in patients with chronic stable angina: A double-blind, randomized, cross-over, placebo-controlled study. J Cardiovasc Pharmacol 16:325, 1990.
37. Yokota M, Miyahara T, Iwase M, et al: Hemodynamic mechanisms of antianginal action of calcium channel blocker nisoldipine in dynamic exercise-induced angina. Circulation 81:1887, 1990.
38. Amende I, Herrmann G, Simon R, et al: Intracoronary nisoldipine: Effects on acute myocardial ischemia during coronary angioplasty. Cardiovasc Drugs Ther 2:807, 1989.
39. Rosenfeld JB, Zabludowski J: The efficacy and tolerability of nifedipine (NIF) and nisoldipine (NIS) both alone and combined with a beta-blocker in patients with essential hypertension: A multicenter, parallel-group study. J Clin Pharmacol 29:1013, 1989.
40. Blau A, Herzog D, Shechter P, et al: Effect of nisoldipine on ambulatory blood pressure under 24-hour noninvasive monitoring. Isr J Med Sci 28:688, 1992.
41. Clarke CW, Kubik MM: Nifedipine and nisoldipine in hypertensive diabetics. J Hum Hypertens 5:517, 1991.
42. Belfort MA, Kirshon B: Nisoldipine—a new orally administered calcium antagonist used in the treatment of severe postpartum pregnancy-induced hypertension. Preliminary results. S Afr Med J 81:267, 1992.
43. Chamiec T, Bednarz B, Budaj A, et al: Efficacy and tolerance of nisoldipine vs propranolol in patients with essential hypertension. Mater Med Pol 22:188, 1990.

CHAPTER 108

Mibefradil The First L- and T-Calcium Antagonist

Jean-Paul Clozel, M.D., Robert Pordy, M.D., and Bertram Pitt, M.D.

DISCOVERY

Calcium antagonists are now widely used for the treatment of hypertension[1, 2] and angina pectoris.[3] However, the efficacy of the presently available calcium antagonists is limited by three main factors (Fig. 108–1): (1) Side effects such as headache, leg edema, or constipation occur before maximal effect is reached; (2) the plasma concentration is insufficient because of pharmacokinetic problems such as high first-pass metabolism or a half-life that is too short; and (3) cardiac reflexes oppose the therapeutic effects of the drug.

A screening program therefore was initiated at F. Hoffmann-La Roche Ltd. aimed at discovering a new calcium antagonist without the problems mentioned earlier. Several pharmacologic tests were set up to discard drugs that could have had the same problems as existing calcium antagonists. For example, an isolated perfused heart preparation was used to select a drug without negative inotropism. Intestinal transit time was measured in mice to avoid drugs inducing constipation. This program led to the discovery of mibefradil in 1986.

The main properties of mibefradil are:

- Chemically, mibefradil which is a single enantiomer, belongs to a new chemical class (tetralene derivatives).
- Mibefradil blocks both L- and T-voltage–operated calcium channels.
- Mibefradil has no negative inotropic properties at biologically relevant plasma concentrations, even on failing hearts.
- *In vivo*, mibefradil does not produce reflex tachycardia but rather decreases heart rate slightly.
- Mibefradil is selective for the coronary circulation versus the peripheral circulation.
- During long-term therapy in humans, mibefradil has an optimal pharmacokinetic profile with a half-life of 10 to 15 hours and nearly complete absorption because of a lack of first-pass metabolism.

Because of these pharmacologic properties, mibefradil is an extremely effective antihypertensive and antiischemic drug. In addition, because mibefradil lacks negative inotropic effects, it is presently being evaluated as a new treatment for heart failure. The drug is presently in phase III of clinical development. Therefore, this chapter will describe the experimental and clinical pharmacology of mibefradil as well as the results obtained in phase I and II of clinical development.

CHEMISTRY

The chemical name of Ro 40-5967 is (1S,2S)-2-[2-[[3-(2-benzimidazolyl)propyl]methylamino]ethyl]-6-fluoro-1,2,3,4-tetrahydro-1-isopropyl-2-naphthyl methoxyacetate dihydrochloride. It was synthesized by Dr. F. Marti at F. Hoffmann-La Roche Ltd., in Basel, Switzerland. The compound has a molecular weight of 568.56. It is an odorless white crystalline powder with a bitter taste. It is chemically stable, water soluble, and light insensitive. Its pK_a values are 4.8 and 5.5. It is noteworthy that Ro 40-5967 is a single enantiomer.

PHARMACOLOGY
Binding Studies

Several competitive binding studies have been performed.[4] They show that mibefradil can compete competitively with [3H] desmethoxyverapamil and [3H] SR 33557 and allosterically with diltiazem (Fig. 108–2). Mibefradil does not affect the specific binding of the dihydropyridine [³H] PN-200-110.[5] Thus, mibefradil has unique binding characteristics. Most likely it binds to sites different from those described

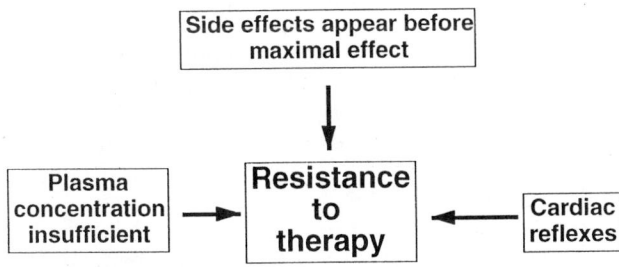

Figure 108–1. Factors limiting the efficacy of available calcium antagonists.

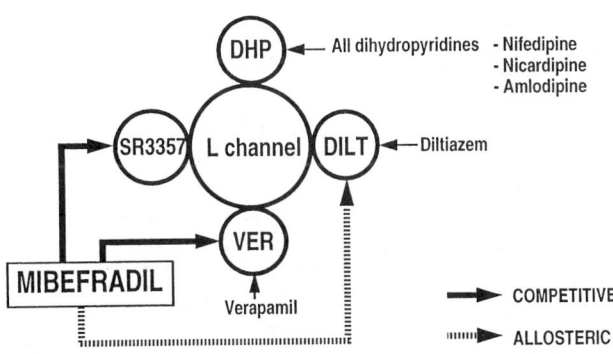

Figure 108–2. Binding characteristics of mibefradil on the L-channel. Mibefradil interacts either in a competitive or allosteric manner with the verapamil (VER), diltiazem (DILT), dihydropyridine (DHP), and fantofarone (SR3357) receptors.

for phenylalkylamines, dihydropyridine, or benzothiazepine calcium antagonists. This different binding site is also suggested by the fact that, in contrast to existing calcium antagonists, mibefradil is able to block T-channels at lower concentrations than those needed to block L-type voltage-operated calcium channels.[6]

Cellular Electrophysiology

The main characteristic of mibefradil is that it can block both L- and T-type calcium channels. As shown in Table 108–1, these two channels have distinct electrophysiologic properties.

Blockade of T-Type Voltage-Operated Calcium Channels

All commonly used calcium antagonists act primarily on L-type (long-lasting, high-voltage-activated) Ca^{2+} channels and not on T-type (transient, low-voltage-activated) Ca^{2+} channels. The precise physiologic role of these T-type channels present in smooth muscle cells[7] and sinus node cells[8] is not yet understood, mainly because no selective blocker of these channels is yet available. Voltage clamp experiments performed in primary cultures of vascular muscle cells have shown that mibefradil does selectively block these T-channels and was approximately 10 times more potent in blocking T-channels than L-channels.[6] In the same preparation, nisoldipine was completely unable to block T-channels. Selective blockade of the T-type calcium channels has also been observed in human medullary thyroid carcinoma cells.[9] In these cells, inhibition of the T-type calcium current was not voltage-dependent in contrast with the inhibition of the L-type calcium current.

Because blockade of these T-channels was observed at therapeutic concentrations, this blockade of the T-channel might contribute to the favorable pharmacodynamic profile of mibefradil, especially in patients with heart failure. T-channels have been shown to be overexpressed in failing hearts[10] and could be responsible for the high incidence of ventricular fibrillation observed in patients with heart failure.

Blockade of L-Type Voltage-Operated Calcium Channels

Mibefradil is able to block cardiac[11, 12] and vascular[13–15] L-type voltage-operated calcium channels.

Table 108–1. **Characteristics of the L- and T-Type Voltage-Operated Ca²⁺ Channels**

Characteristic	L	T
Conductance (ps)	25	8
Activation	High voltage	Low voltage
Inactivation	Slow	Transient
Selective blockers	All CCB	Mibefradil

CCB, calcium channel blockers.

Voltage clamp experiments performed on isolated myocytes from guinea pigs have shown that the IC_{50} of mibefradil is 0.2 μM. In this preparation, mibefradil is highly selective for the L-type calcium current versus the Na^+ current, which is blocked by mibefradil with an IC_{50} of 55 μM.[11]

A very interesting characteristic of the blockade of the L-type cardiac channel is the very high potential dependence of this blockade.[11] In isolated guinea pig cardiac myocytes, the IC_{50} of the calcium current shifts from 230 nM to 12,000 nM when the membrane holding potential is adjusted from −50 mV to −80 mV. This potential dependence is not as marked with mibefradil and might explain why mibefradil is not negatively inotropic at therapeutic concentrations. In contrast, in vascular smooth muscle cells, which have a higher membrane potential, mibefradil can effectively block calcium entry and produces a marked vasodilation.

Mibefradil also has distinct features compared with other calcium antagonists for blocking the vascular L-type calcium channel as shown by experiments performed in vascular smooth muscle cells cultured from dog coronary and saphenous arteries. Mibefradil acts on a wider range of voltages on both instantaneous and resting Ca^{2+} currents. It produces a more significant resting state block and it is selective for coronary over saphenous arteries.[15]

Experiments have also been performed on Chinese hamster ovary (CHO) cells transfected with either the smooth muscle α-1 subunit alone (CHOα1) or a combination of the smooth muscle α-1 subunit and the skeletal muscle β-1 subunit (CHOαβ1).[13] Experiments in CHOα1 showed that indeed mibefradil is able to block recombinant L-type channels.[13] This block was strongly voltage- and frequency-dependent. Surprisingly, results were different in CHOαβ1 cells, because in 60% of the cells, mibefradil inhibited the barium current. However, in 40% of the cells mibefradil activated the barium current, which shows that in this model, mibefradil can have partial agonistic effects.[13]

In Vitro Pharmacology

In vitro, mibefradil is characterized by its absence of negative inotropism at therapeutic concentrations and by its selectivity for the coronary versus the peripheral vasculature. Several *in vitro* preparations have been used to test the effects of mibefradil including isolated rat aortic rings, guinea pig left atrium, and guinea pig ileum. Mibefradil is markedly less potent than verapamil in decreasing contractions of the guinea pig left atrium despite a similar potency on the rat aorta.[5] This absence of negative inotropism is also observed in isolated blood-perfused rat hearts where the main effect of mibefradil is an increase of coronary blood flow.[5, 16, 17]

The vascular relaxation induced by mibefradil is partly mediated by a release of nitric oxide by the endothelium.[18] For example, relaxations evoked by mibefradil of arteries precontracted by phenylephrine

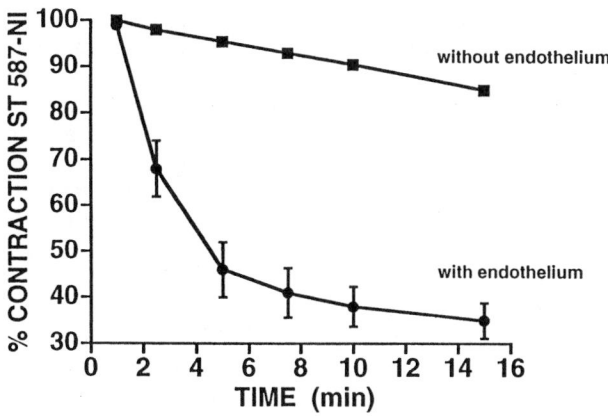

Figure 108–3. Influence of the relaxing effect of mibefradil on the endothelium in isolated rings of dog femoral artery. The artery was precontracted with ST 587 (10^{-5} M) and a dose of 10^{-5} M of mibefradil was administered on isolated rings with or without endothelin. (From Boulanger CM, Nakashima M, Olmos L, et al: Effects of the Ca^{2+} antagonist RO 40-5967 on endothelium-dependent responses of isolated arteries. J Cardiovasc Pharmacol 23:869, 1994.)

or ST 847 are markedly increased when endothelium is present (Fig. 108–3). To our knowledge, this endothelium-mediated relaxation is not observed with other commonly used calcium antagonists. Finally, an interesting *in vitro* property of mibefradil is its low potency to relax intestinal smooth muscle cells,[5] which most likely explains the absence of constipation induced by this drug.

In Vivo Hemodynamic Effects of Mibefradil

Several *in vivo* studies have confirmed the results obtained *in vitro* with mibefradil and have shown that mibefradil is devoid of negative inotropic effects at therapeutic concentrations. In conscious rats[17] and an-

esthetized dogs,[19, 20] the main effects of mibefradil are a coronary vasodilation, a peripheral vasodilation, and a decrease of heart rate. There is no decrease of cardiac contractility as shown by an absence of decrease of $LVdP/dt_{max}+$. In contrast, in the same models, drugs such as diltiazem or verapamil[20] have marked negative inotropic effects.

EFFECTS OF MIBEFRADIL IN EXPERIMENTAL MODELS OF HYPERTENSION
Efficacy in Several Experimental Models of Hypertension

The first experiments evaluating the antihypertensive effects of mibefradil were performed in rats with renovascular hypertension (2 kidneys/1 clip), spontaneous hypertension, or DOCA salt hypertension.[21] In the first two experimental models, the renin-angiotensin system is stimulated and in the third model the renin-angiotensin system is inhibited. In the three models, mibefradil was very active with a potency about three times higher than that of verapamil (Fig. 108–4) and with a duration of action about three times longer (Fig. 108–5). The antihypertensive effect of mibefradil was not associated with a reflex tachycardia but rather with a small decrease of heart rate. The antihypertensive effect of mibefradil was sustained when mibefradil was given long term, and no tachyphylaxis was observed during long-term administration.[21]

Effects of Mibefradil on End-Organ Damage

Hypertension is characterized by pathologic alterations of some organs such as the heart, the kidneys, and the endothelium. These alterations and their re-

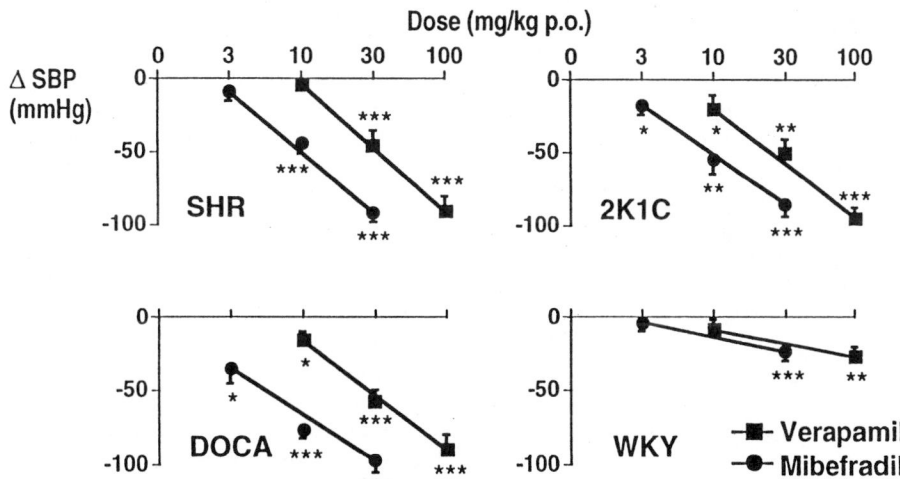

Figure 108–4. A comparison of the blood pressure lowering effects induced by verapamil or mibefradil in normotensive (WKY), spontaneously hypertensive (SHR), renal hypertensive (2K1C), or DOCA hypertensive rats. Both drugs were given orally. (From Hefti F, Clozel JP, Osterrieder W: Antihypertensive properties of the novel calcium antagonist (1S,2S)-2-[2-[[3-(2-benzimidazolyl)propyl]methylamino]ethyl]-6-fluoro-1,2,3,4-tetrahydro-1-isopropyl-2-naphthyl methoxyacetate dihydrochloride in rat models of hypertension. Arzneimittelforschung/Drug Res 40(I):417, 1990.)

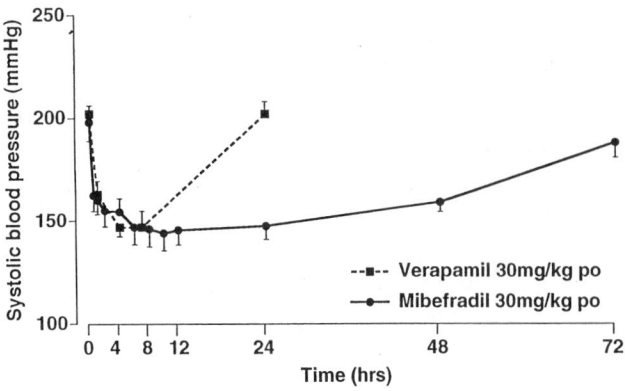

Figure 108–5. Duration of the antihypertensive effect of mibefradil and verapamil in spontaneously hypertensive rats. Both mibefradil and verapamil were given at equihypotensive doses. (From Hefti F, Clozel JP, Osterrieder W: Antihypertensive properties of the novel calcium antagonist (1S,2S)-2-[2-[[3-(2-benzimidazolyl)propyl]-methylamino]ethyl]-6-fluoro-1,2,3,4-tetrahydro-1-isopropyl-2-naphthyl methoxyacetate dihydrochloride in rat models of hypertension. Arzneimittelforschung/Drug Res 40(I):417, 1990.)

gression are not always parallel to the changes of arterial blood pressure. Drugs such as minoxidil or hydralazine can markedly decrease arterial pressure without decreasing cardiac hypertrophy.[22] We therefore evaluated the effects of mibefradil on end-organ damage.

In renovascular hypertensive rats, we tested the effects of long-term administration of mibefradil and compared them with those of enalapril.[23] Doses of mibefradil (30 mg/kg/day) and enalapril (3 mg/kg/day) were chosen in order to produce a similar decrease in arterial pressure. In the heart, both mibefradil and enalapril prevented the cardiac fibrosis secondary to hypertension, as shown by a decrease of perivascular collagen content.[23] Both drugs could also markedly improve coronary vascular reserve.[23] Enalapril was more efficient than mibefradil in decreasing cardiac hypertrophy.

In this model of renovascular hypertension, the renal effects of mibefradil and enalapril were different.[24] Mibefradil, in contrast with enalapril, could prevent the progressive increase in creatinine and urea levels observed in these rats. Both mibefradil and enalapril, to a smaller extent, could markedly prevent the vascular lesions present in the non-clipped kidney. However, like enalapril, mibefradil decreased the medullary surface area of the clipped kidney, most likely as a result of the decrease of renal perfusion pressure below the renal stenosis. In contrast with what has been described with other calcium antagonists such as nitrendipine,[25] mibefradil did not increase proteinuria. However, in this model, enalapril was more efficient than mibefradil in decreasing proteinuria.

Effect of Mibefradil on Endothelial Function

In spontaneously hypertensive rats, mibefradil was able to prevent the endothelial dysfunction and the subendothelial infiltration of monocytes and macro-

phages in the aorta.[26] Aortas of spontaneously hypertensive rats treated with mibefradil were more responsive to acetylcholine and the area of intima was markedly decreased.[26] Prevention of the infiltration of the aorta with monocytes might be important for the prevention of the progression of atherosclerosis, because these monocytes are slowly transformed into foam cells after loading with cholesterol. In salt-sensitive Dahl rats, mibefradil can also markedly improve endothelial function and increase endothelium-mediated relaxation to acetylcholine.[27] In this model, as in spontaneous hypertension,[26] relaxation to a nitric oxide (NO) donor is improved. Therefore, it is likely that mibefradil can also act by potentiating the intracellular effects of edothelium-derived relaxing factor (EDRF).

EFFECTS OF MIBEFRADIL IN EXPERIMENTAL MODELS OF CARDIAC ISCHEMIA

In humans, cardiac ischemia is associated with several pathologic conditions. Cardiac ischemia can be secondary to a decrease in coronary blood flow caused by a fixed coronary artery stenosis (stable angina pectoris), coronary artery spasm (Prinzmetal's angina), or a coronary thrombosis (myocardial infarction). The effects of mibefradil therefore have been tested in several experimental models reproducing these conditions.

The conditions of stable angina pectoris were mimicked in anesthetized dogs where coronary perfusion pressure was controlled by using an extracorporeal circulation.[19] By decreasing the coronary perfusion pressure, it was possible to induce cardiac ischemia. In this model, mibefradil could markedly prevent cardiac ischemia without decreasing cardiac contractility. In contrast, mibefradil could not improve cardiac function probably because its intrinsic negative inotropic effects were masking the beneficial antiischemic effects.

Mibefradil was also protective in another model of stable angina pectoris, in which cardiac ischemia was induced by exercising conscious dogs that had an aneroid constrictor implanted around the circumflex artery producing a slowly progressive stenosis.[28] In this model, the beneficial effect of mibefradil was also not associated with a negative inotropic effect. The effect of mibefradil was also tested in conscious dogs with a chronic left ventricular dysfunction caused by a myocardial infarction. In some of these dogs (sensitive dogs) exercise induces ventricular fibrillation requiring cardiac resuscitation with electric shock. In other dogs (resistant dogs) exercise alone is not able to induce ventricular fibrillation. However, injection of cocaine prior to exercise sensitized these dogs.[29] In both cases, mibefradil could also protect these dogs against the occurrence of this type of ventricular fibrillation.[30]

Mibefradil could also increase the threshold of ventricular fibrillation in pigs that had a 30-minute coronary ligation followed by reperfusion.[31] Finally, mibefradil was able to reduce infarct size in a dog model.[32] In both models, mibefradil was as efficient as verapamil in reducing infarct size but without its detrimental negative inotropic effects.

EFFECTS OF MIBEFRADIL IN EXPERIMENTAL MODELS OF HEART FAILURE

One of the main risks of calcium antagonists is the decrease of cardiac function resulting from their negative inotropism. It has been suggested that this negative inotropism, caused by the blockade of the L-type channels of the myocardial cells, is responsible for the excess of mortality observed for patients with myocardial infarction and heart failure treated with diltiazem.[33]

It therefore was important to experiment to determine if the absence of negative inotropism was observed not only in normal hearts but also in failing hearts. Thus, the effects of mibefradil were evaluated in three experimental models of heart failure:

1. A myocardial infarction model in rats[17]
2. A model in rabbits where heart failure was induced by the combination of pressure and volume overload[34]
3. A dog model of pacing-induced heart failure[35]

In rats with chronic congestive heart failure caused by myocardial infarction, mibefradil could decrease afterload without decreasing cardiac contractility.[17] In contrast, diltiazem was negatively inotropic at doses producing a similar afterload reduction. *In vitro*, in isolated perfused hearts from rats with heart failure, a similar difference was observed. Mibefradil, in contrast with diltiazem, had no negative inotropic effect.

A similar advantage of mibefradil was also observed in isolated perfused hearts from rabbits that had heart failure induced by a double pressure and volume overload. In these rabbits, mibefradil was less negatively inotropic than both verapamil and diltiazem.[34]

Finally, the effects of mibefradil were tested in a dog model where heart failure was induced by chronic left ventricular pacing at a rate of 240 or 260 beats/min.[35] In this model, mibefradil was less negatively inotropic than diltiazem despite a similar afterload reduction. In conscious dogs, diltiazem had no negative inotropic effect in normal conditions. Diltiazem was negatively inotropic only in dogs with heart failure. Mibefradil, in contrast with diltiazem, did not stimulate the renin-angiotensin system (as shown by the absence of a significant increase of plasma renin activity) or catecholamine production.

The mechanism explaining the lack of negative inotropic effects of mibefradil is still not understood. One factor could be the high voltage dependence of the blockade of the myocardial L-type channel.[11] The other factor might be a partial agonistic effect, which has been observed in Chinese hamster ovary cells expressing the α-1 subunit of the cardiac L-type calcium channels.[9] In any case, all these data indicate that mibefradil should be safe in patients with congestive heart failure.

OTHER INDICATIONS

Mibefradil has been shown to be effective in preventing pulmonary hypertension and cardiovascular remodeling occurring in rats with hypoxia.[36] Mibefradil is also effective in a model of acute lung edema caused by septic shock combined with hypoxia.[37] Thus, mibefradil might be useful in the treatment of pulmonary hypertension.

Mibefradil has also been tested in a model of vascular injury in rats. In this model, neointima formation occurs after deendothelialization of the carotid artery. This neointima might explain restenosis after vascular angioplasty. Calcium channel blockade with verapamil has already been shown to be ineffective in this model despite very high doses.[38] However, mibefradil can prevent neointima formation by approximately 50%.[39] This effect does not seem to be related to the blockade of L-type calcium channels. The ineffectiveness of verapamil could be a result of the blockade of the T-channels or one of the other cellular targets described previously.[40]

HUMAN PHARMACOKINETICS AND METABOLISM

Because the drug is given for chronic indications such as hypertension and angina pectoris, the most relevant pharmacokinetic information is obtained after multiple oral dosing. In this case, the drug is rapidly absorbed, with a C_{max} reached within 1 to 2 hours. The bioavailability after multiple dosing is greater than 90% in the therapeutic dose range. This high bioavailability is a result of the inhibition of the first-path metabolism during long-term dosing. The elimination half-life is between 10 and 15 hours, which explains why the drug can be given once a day and a steady state is reached within 3 to 4 days. The volume of distribution at steady state is larger than the plasma volume and ranges from 130 to 220 L. Systemic clearance does not depend on the dose and is around 200 ml/min. Elimination is mainly through metabolic inactivation by the liver. The alcohol derivative of mibefradil (Ro 40-5966) has been detected in the plasma of patients treated long-term with mibefradil. *In vivo*, this metabolite has a potency that is 10 times lower than that of mibefradil.

MAIN PHARMACODYNAMIC PROPERTIES IN CLINICAL TRIALS

Mibefradil has a unique hemodynamic profile associating (1) a decrease in peripheral vascular resistance, (2) a decrease in heart rate, and (3) an absence of negative inotropic effects. This hemodynamic profile has been observed in normal volunteers,[41] hypertensive patients,[42] and patients with angina pectoris.[42] The decrease of peripheral vascular resistance explains the decrease of arterial pressure, which is limited in normal volunteers and in normotensive patients with angina pectoris (5 mmHg) but is more marked in hypertensive patients (up to 15 mmHg depending on the dose).

Despite the decrease of arterial pressure and peripheral vascular resistance, mibefradil does not produce a reflex tachycardia, which is observed with dihydropyridine-type calcium antagonists. In contrast, mibefradil decreases heart rate up to 8 beats/min with a dose of 150 mg/kg.[42] This decrease of heart rate, associated with an increase of the PR interval is most likely a result of a direct effect of mibefradil on the sinus node and the atrioventricular conduction system. The decrease of heart rate induced by mibefradil seems more marked than the decrease induced by diltiazem or verapamil. This stronger effect might be caused by the blockade of the T-channels present in the sinus node cells.

The absence of negative inotropism has been demonstrated in normal volunteers where even extremely high doses (240 mg PO) did not decrease cardiac contractility indexes and increased cardiac output.[41] This absence of negative inotropism has also been shown in patients with stable angina pectoris where ejection fraction did not decrease even with a dose of 200 mg.[43]

Finally, invasive hemodynamic studies performed in patients with a normal cardiac function as well as in patients with severe heart failure[44] have shown that mibefradil does not alter the pressure-volume relationship in contrast with other calcium antagonists such as nicardipine.[45]

CLINICAL USE

Mibefradil has been evaluated for the treatment of hypertension, angina pectoris, and heart failure.

Hypertension

In a study performed on 64 hypertensive patients, mibefradil proved to be a potent antihypertensive drug.[42] This antihypertensive effect is long-lasting, justifying once-a-day dosing. The peak-trough ratio at the steady state is more than 80%. The extent of the antihypertensive effect is dose-dependent and reaches 25 mmHg for diastolic blood pressure (placebo corrected). Despite the large blood pressure reduction, there is no reflex tachycardia but rather a decrease of heart rate and no neurohormonal activation (no change of plasma renin, aldosterone, norepinephrine, or epinephrine activity).

In these hypertensive patients, mibefradil also prolonged the PQ time, but first-degree AV block did not appear with doses lower than 100 mg. In addition, the PQ time increase was also clearly dissociated from the decrease of arterial pressure.

The results of this first study have been confirmed in a larger study where the drug was given for 4 weeks to 200 hypertensive patients. This study also showed the prolonged antihypertensive effect of mibefradil. The therapeutic doses of mibefradil seem to be between 50 and 100 mg. For these doses, the drug is extremely well tolerated and does not produce high degree AV conduction disturbances.

Angina Pectoris

The antianginal effects of mibefradil were tested after single doses[43] or after two-week multiple dosing.[46] Both studies showed a marked antianginal effect. Mibefradil increased total exercise duration, time to onset of angina, and time to ST depression. There was also a dose-related decrease in the number and duration of silent ischemic episodes as determined by Holter monitoring. The active doses for this indication seem to be between 50 and 100 mg.

Heart Failure

Up to now, all clinical trials with mibefradil have shown no negative inotropism, confirming preclinical studies. Because ischemia might be involved in the progression of heart failure and because a decrease of afterload has been shown to be beneficial in heart failure, it is tempting to believe that mibefradil might be useful for the treatment of heart failure. In addition, mibefradil is also effective in preventing sudden death in an experimental model. Therefore, a large clinical program evaluating the effects of mibefradil on exercise capacity, quality of life, and mortality in patients with heart failure has been undertaken. The trial (called MACH I) will recruit 900 patients who will be followed up for 3 years.

CONCLUSION

Mibefradil is the first representative of a new class of calcium antagonists and the first T-channel blocker. It is too early to evaluate the possible clinical benefit of blocking T-channels with this drug. However, preliminary results obtained in head-to-head comparisons with other calcium antagonists seem to show a clear superior efficacy of mibefradil. Long-term effects need to be assessed as well as the potential of this drug in heart failure.

REFERENCES

1. Bühler FR, Kiowski W: Calcium antagonists in hypertension. J Hypertens 5(Suppl 3):S3, 1987.
2. Reid JL, Meredith PA, Pasanisi F: Clinical pharmacological aspects of calcium antagonists and their therapeutic role in hypertension. J Cardiovasc Pharmacol 7(Suppl 4):S18, 1985.
3. Oparil S, Calhoun DA: The calcium antagonists in the 1990s: An overview. Am J Hypertens 4:396, 1991.
4. Triggle D: Receptor binding of mibefradil. (Submitted for publication).
5. Osterrieder W, Holck M: In vitro pharmacologic profile of RO 40-5967, a novel Ca^{2+} channel blocker with potent vasodilator but weak inotropic action. J Cardiovasc Pharmacol 13:754, 1989.
6. Mishra SK, Hermsmeyer K: Selective inhibition of T-type Ca^{2+} channels by RO 40-5967. Circ Res 75:144, 1994.

7. Akaike N, Kanaide H, Kuga T, et al: Low-voltage-activated calcium current in rat aorta smooth muscle cells in primary culture. J Physiol 416:141, 1989.

8. Hagiwara N, Irisawa H, Kameyama M: Contribution of two types of calcium currents to the pacemaker potentials of rabbit sino-atrial node cells. J Physiol 395:233, 1988.

9. Mehrke G, Zong XG, Flockerzi V, et al: The Ca^{2+} channel blocker RO 40-5967 blocks differently T-type and L-type Ca^{2+} channels. (Submitted for publication).

10. Nuss BH, Houser SR: T-type Ca^{2+} current is expressed in hypertrophied adult feline left ventricular myocytes. Circ Res 73:777, 1993.

11. Fang L-M, Osterrieder W: Potential-dependent inhibition of cardiac Ca^{2+} inward currents by RO 40-5967 and verapamil: Relation to negative inotropy. Eur J Pharmacol 196:205, 1991.

12. Lacinova L, Welling A, Bosse E, et al: Interaction of RO 40-5967 with the stable expressed a1 subunit of the cardiac L-type calcium channel. (Submitted for publication).

13. Welling A, Donatin K, Bosse E et al: Voltage- and use-dependent block of the expressed L-type calcium channel by RO 40-5967. (Submitted for publication).

14. Mishra SK, Hermsmeyer K: Resting state block and use independence of rat vascular muscle Ca^{2+} channels by RO 40-5967. J Pharmacol Exp Ther 269(1):178, 1994.

15. Bian K, Hermsmeyer K: Ca^{2+} channel actions of the non-dihydropyridine Ca^{2+} channel antagonist RO 40-5967 in vascular muscle cells cultured from dog coronary and saphenous arteries. Naunyn Schmiedebergs Arch Pharmacol 348:191, 1993.

16. Clozel JP, Véniant M, Osterrieder W: The structurally novel Ca^{2+} channel blocker RO 40-5967, which binds to the [^{3}H] desmethoxyverapamil receptor, is devoid of the negative inotropic effects of verapamil in normal and failing rat hearts. Cardiovasc Drugs Ther 4:731, 1990.

17. Véniant M, Clozel JP, Hess P, et al: RO 40-5967, in contrast to diltiazem, does not reduce left ventricular contractility in rats with chronic myocardial infarction. J Cardiovasc Pharmacol 17:277, 1991.

18. Boulanger CM, Nakashima M, Olmos L, et al: Effects of the Ca^{2+} antagonist RO 40-5967 on endothelium-dependent responses of isolated arteries. J Cardiovasc Pharmacol 23:869, 1994.

19. Clozel JP, Banken L, Osterrieder W: Effects of RO 40-5967, a novel calcium antagonist, on myocardial function during ischemia induced by lowering coronary perfusion pressure in dogs: Comparison with verapamil. J Cardiovasc Pharmacol 14:713, 1989.

20. Orito K, Satoh K, Taira N: Cardiovascular profile of RO 40-5967, a new nondihydropyridine calcium antagonist, delineated in isolated, blood perfused dog hearts. J Cardiovasc Pharmacol 22:293, 1993.

21. Hefti F, Clozel JP, Osterrieder W: Antihypertensive properties of the novel calcium antagonist (1S,2S)-2-[2-[[3-(2-benzimidazolyl)propyl]methylamino]ethyl]-6-fluoro-1,2,3,4-tetrahydro-1-isopropyl-2-naphthyl methoxyacetate dihydrochloride in rat models of hypertension. Arzneimittelforschung/Drug Res 40(I)(4):417, 1990.

22. Sen S, Farazi RC, Khairallah PA, et al: Cardiac hypertrophy in spontaneously hypertensive rats. Cardiovasc Res 35:775, 1974.

23. Véniant M, Clozel JP, Heudes D, et al: Effects of RO 40-5967, a new calcium antagonist, and enalapril on cardiac remodeling in renal hypertensive rats. J Cardiovasc Pharmacol 21:544, 1993.

24. Véniant M, Heudes D, Clozel JP, et al: Calcium blockade versus ACE inhibition in clipped and unclipped kidneys of 2K1C rats. Kidney Int 46:421, 1994.

25. Wenzel UO, Troschau G, Schoeppe W, et al: Adverse effect of calcium channel blocker nitrendipine on nephrosclerosis in rats with renovascular hypertension. Hypertension 20:233, 1992.

26. Gray GA, Clozel M, Clozel JP, et al: Effects of calcium channel blockade on the aortic intima in spontaneously hypertensive rats. Hypertension 22:569, 1993.

27. Boulanger CM, Desta B, Clozel JP, et al: Chronic treatment with the Ca^{2+} channel inhibitor RO 40-5967 potentiates endothelium-dependent relaxations in the aorta of the hypertensive salt sensitive Dahl rat. Blood Pressure 3:193, 1994.

28. Guth BD: Reduction of exercise-induced contractile dysfunction in dogs using a novel calcium blocker (RO 40-5967). Cardiovasc Drugs Ther 6:167, 1992.

29. Billman GE: Effect of calcium channel antagonists on cocaine-induced malignant arrhythmias: Protection against ventricular fibrillation. J Pharmacol Exp Ther 266:407, 1993.

30. Billman GE: RO 40-5967 a novel calcium channel antagonist, protects against ventricular fibrillation. Eur J Pharmacol 229:179, 1992.

31. Muller CA, Opie LH, McCarthy J, et al: Antiarrhythmic effects of the calcium channel blocker RO 40-5967 in pigs with acute regional myocardial ischemia and reperfusion: A comparison with verapamil. J Pharmacol Exp Ther 1994, submitted.

32. Vander Heide RS, Schwartz LM, Reimer KA: The novel calcium channel antagonist, RO 40-5967, limits myocardial infarct size in dogs. Cardiovasc Res 28:1526, 1994.

33. The Multicenter Diltiazem Postinfarction Trial Research Group: The effect of diltiazem on mortality and reinfarction after myocardial infarction. N Engl J Med 319:385, 1988.

34. Ezzaher A, El Houda Bouanani N, Bo Su J, et al: Increased negative inotropic effect of calcium-channel blockers in hypertrophied and failing rabbit heart. J Pharmacol Exp Ther 257:466, 1991.

35. Su J, Renaud N, Carayon A, et al: Effects of the calcium channel blockers diltiazem and RO 40-5967 on systemic hemodynamics and plasma noradrenaline levels in conscious dogs with pacing-induced heart failure. Br J Pharmacol 113:395, 1994.

36. Ono S, Voelkel NF: Inflammation and pulmonary hypertension during hypoxia. *In* Ueda G (ed): High Altitude Medicine. Matsumoto, Japan: Shinshu University Press, 1992, p 347.

37. Ono S, Westcott JY, Chang SW, et al: Endotoxin priming followed by high altitude caused pulmonary edema in rats. J Appl Physiol 74:1534, 1993.

38. Powell JS, Clozel JP, Müller RKM, et al: Inhibitors of angiotensin-converting enzyme prevent myointimal proliferation after vascular injury. Science 245:186, 1989.

39. Schmitt R, Clozel JP, Bühler F: Effects of mibefradil on neointima formation. (Submitted for publication).

40. Zernig G: Widening potential for Ca^{2+} antagonists: Non-L-type Ca^{2+} channel interaction. Trends Pharmacol Sci 11:38, 1990.

41. Schmitt R, Kleinbloesem CH, Osterrieder W: RO 40-5967 a calcium antagonist of a new generation? Eur J Clin Pharmacol 36(Suppl):A336, 1989.

42. Schmitt R, Kleinbloesem CH, Belz GG: Hemodynamic and humoral effects of the novel calcium antagonist RO 40-5967 in patients with hypertension. Clin Pharmacol Ther 52:314, 1992.

43. Portegies MCM, Schmitt R, Kraaij CJ, et al: Lack of negative inotropic effects of the new calcium antagonist RO 40-5967 in patients with stable angina pectoris. J Cardiovasc Pharmacol 18:746, 1991.

44. Chapelie F, Stoleru L, et al: RO-40-5967, a new calcium antagonist profile: Bradycardia without myocardial depression. Circulation 90:I-28, 1994.

45. Aroney CN, Semigran MJ, Dec WG, et al: Inotropic effect of nicardipine in patients with heart failure: Assessment by left ventricular end-systolic pressure-volume analysis. J Am Coll Cardiol 14:1331, 1989.

46. Bakx AL, van der Wall EE, Braun S: Effects of a new calcium channel blocker in patients with stable angina pectoris [abstract]. J Am Coll Cardiol 23:416a, 1994.

CHAPTER 109

Isradipine

Ehud Grossman, M.D., Shmuel Oren, M.D., and Franz H. Messerli, M.D.

Calcium antagonists are a heterogeneous group of drugs with respect to structure, affinity, and activity in different tissues. Few calcium antagonists are available in the United States. Isradipine is a second-generation dihydropyridine derivative that is approved for the treatment of hypertension.

CHEMISTRY

Isradipine [3,5-pyridinedicarboxylic acid 4-(4-benzofurazonyl)-1,4 dihydro 2,6 dimethyl-methyl 1-methylethyl ester], with a molecular weight of 371.39, is a member of the dihydropyridine class. Its chemical structure is similar to that of nifedipine but with a benzofurazanyl group rather than a nitrophenyl group at position 4 of the pyridine. This substitution may impart to the drug its lesser negative inotropic effect compared with other calcium antagonists (Sandoz, data on file). Isradipine has a racemic form in which the (+)-[S]-enantiomer is 160 times more active than the (−)-[R]-enantiomer.[1]

PHARMACOLOGY

Isradipine is rapidly and almost completely absorbed after oral administration, and a dose-related decrease in blood pressure is obtained within 2 or 3 hours of oral intake.[2] The parent compound is approximately 95% bound to circulating plasma proteins at all concentrations encountered. It is converted to at least 15 metabolites that are excreted partly in the urine and partly via the biliary tract.[3, 4] The major metabolites of isradipine have been identified and tested for evidence of calcium channel blockade. None had a relevant calcium antagonistic activity *in vitro*. Thus, the pharmacodynamic effects of isradipine are attributed entirely to the drug itself.[4] The drug is fat-soluble and is known to cross the blood-brain barrier.[5] The elimination of isradipine is biphasic with a mean terminal half-life of 8.3 hours. Plasma clearance is 43.8 L/hr. In several experimental models, isradipine has had a long half-life. In spontaneously hypertensive rats, blood pressure was reduced as long as 48 hours after oral administration. However, the duration of action has been reported to differ from one effect to the other. One study in animals showed that the effects of isradipine on heart rate were of short duration, whereas cerebral vasodilatation persisted longer.[6]

PHARMACODYNAMICS
Cellular Effects

Isradipine has both a highly specific and a low nonspecific affinity to the dihydropyridine binding site of the L-type calcium channel.[7] Like other drugs acting selectively on slow channels, isradipine has little effect on the normal cardiac action potentials.[7] In an *in vitro* experiment on guinea pig papillary muscle, the only significant effect was a reduction of the action potential duration at 30% repolarization, as has been described for other calcium antagonists.[8] Isradipine is a remarkably potent antagonist of contraction induced by depolarization in vascular smooth muscle of various origins,[2] as has been described with other calcium antagonists.[9-12] Its potent activity has been shown in rabbit aorta,[7] in dog coronary arteries, and in cerebral vessels.[13] In spiral strips of human anterior cerebral arteries (obtained at autopsy) and in canine basilar arteries, isradipine was more potent than nimodipine or nifedipine in inhibiting depolarization-induced contraction.[13] In a similar study using streptokinase as a stimulator for the arterial contraction,[7] isradipine proved to be more potent than the other two antagonists. In contrast with its remarkable inhibitory effect on voltage-operated channels, isradipine had little effect on receptor-operated channels. Thus, isradipine did not alter contractions induced by noradrenaline and had only minimal effect on serotonin-induced contractions. Although in rabbit aorta many calcium antagonists exert a preferential blockade of potential-operated calcium channels over receptor-operated channels,[14] the isradipine's high selectivity is unusual. Despite its low specificity for receptor-operated channels in rabbit aorta, isradipine was a potent inhibitor of serotonin-induced contraction in dog basilar arteries.[14] This finding might suggest the existence of receptor-operated calcium channels with different structures or functional properties.

The effects of isradipine on the heart were investigated most extensively by Wada et al.,[15] who measured the effect of the drug concomitantly on coronary blood vessels, sinus node, atrioventricular conduction, and myocardium. According to their experiments, isradipine elicits effects on the heart that differ from those of other available calcium antagonists.[16, 17] Isradipine is predominantly a coronary vasodilator, as is nifedipine. However, isradipine inhibits the sinus node with little effect on atrioventricular conduction, and its negative inotropic effect is weak. A protective effect against ischemia has been shown for various calcium antagonists.[18-21] Similarly, isradipine has an antiischemic effect that is related mainly to its ability to preserve blood flow to the inner layers of the left ventricular wall.[22]

Animal Studies

Controlled studies in animals corroborated the results *in vitro*, indicating that isradipine produces its dominant effect on the vascular bed while affecting the heart to a lesser extent.[23-25] The selective activity of isradipine on the sinus node was reflected in conscious animals by attenuated reflex tachycardia in response to a decrease in blood pressure. The weak cardiodepressive effect that was described *in vitro* was not even documented *in vivo* because of the dose-limiting effect of vasodilatation. Isradipine preferentially dilates the vessels of the heart, brain, and skeletal muscles in experimental animals[26] and, like other calcium antagonists, has minimal effect on the venous system.[27-30] Its long-lasting effect on the cerebral circulation might be of clinical interest. In one study,[31] isradipine reduced the pathologic symptoms in the central nervous system caused by occlusion of the middle cerebral artery (cerebroprotection). In addition to improving the cerebral blood flow, isradipine, by reducing the excessive calcium influx occurring during ischemia, probably reduces the demands of the neurons for adenosine triphospate required to maintain intracellular calcium homeostasis.

Studies[32-35] indicate that calcium antagonists such as nifedipine, verapamil, nicardipine, and diltiazem may suppress atherogenesis in rabbits fed cholesterol. In a dosage that exerted no hypotensive effect, isradipine suppressed atherogenesis in rabbits fed cholesterol and reduced the impairment of endothelium-dependent relaxation evoked by acetylcholine.[24] These effects occurred without a decrease in plasma total cholesterol. Besides the antiatherosclerotic effect, Handley et al.[24] found that, at 1 hour and at 24 hours after balloon catheterization, isradipine had not reduced the extent of platelet deposition at the surface of the denuded vessels. This finding might indicate that the inhibition of lesion development is related to a diminished mitogenic response of smooth muscle cells in the damaged vessel wall rather than to an antiplatelet mechanism.

The antihypertensive effect of isradipine has been evaluated in spontaneously hypertensive rats.[2] Orally administered isradipine caused a significant decrease in blood pressure that lasted 6 hours when a low dose was used, and blood pressure remained significantly decreased 48 hours after the highest dose. The fall in blood pressure was accompanied by a brief decrease in heart rate; only the highest doses (50 mg/kg) caused a transient increase in heart rate. Similar experiments with subcutaneous administration of a tenfold smaller dose yielded comparable effects. Like other calcium antagonists,[36, 37] isradipine, in a dose of 1 mg/kg, has a natriuretic effect in rats. This effect is associated with an increase in water excretion and no significant effect on potassium excretion. The natriuretic effect is dose-dependent; however, the mechanism of the diuretic action is not fully understood.[2]

Calcium antagonists have a variable effect on renin secretion.[38] A fall in blood pressure induced by isradipine increased renin release in conscious rabbits to the same extent as with other vasodilators, such as nitroprusside and dihydrazine.[39] The magnitude of the pressure decrease, rather than vasodilatation or the direct effect, determined the degree of renin secre-

tion. A similar response has been shown with other dihydropyridine calcium antagonists.

DRUG INTERACTIONS

Some drug interactions with isradipine have been noted. β-Blockers with and without intrinsic sympathomimetic activity, such as pindolol and propranolol, change the hemodynamic response to isradipine. In one study,[40] both β-blockers blunted the positive inotropic effect of isradipine. In the same study, it was shown that verapamil decreased cardiac output and caused peripheral vasoconstriction in animals previously treated with propranolol. Unlike the effect on verapamil, pretreatment with propranolol only blunted the isradipine-induced increase in cardiac output and total peripheral conductance. In rabbits, pretreatment with a converting enzyme inhibitor, spirapril, blunted the effects of isradipine on central venous pressure, cardiac output, and the increase in flow to the heart, brain, and skeletal muscles.[41] The decrease in hepatic-arterial and pancreatic blood flow induced by isradipine was also prevented, and a similar tendency was observed in the spleen, stomach, small intestine, cecum, and arteriovenous shunt flow, indicating that the renin-angiotensin system is at least partially responsible for the hemodynamic effects of isradipine.[41] Unlike verapamil,[42] which substantially increases serum digoxin, and diltiazem,[43] and also appears to increase steady-state digoxin levels to a lesser extent, isradipine has no clinically relevant interactions with digoxin.[44] Isradipine in a dose of 5 mg twice a day does not impair theophyllin metabolism in normal volunteers[45] and does not affect the pharmacokinetics of cyclosporine in renal transplant patients.[46, 47] Unlike verapamil and diltiazem, which inhibit cytochrome P-450 reductase–dependent biotransformation of drugs,[48] isradipine does not affect hepatic enzyme activity in elderly volunteers.[49]

CLINICAL USE

Because of its hemodynamic properties of pronounced peripheral vasodilatation as well as its anti-ischemic effect with minimal cardiodepression, isradipine seems to be an ideal drug for the treatment of patients with hypertension, angina pectoris, and even congestive heart failure.

Hypertension

Isradipine, like other calcium antagonists, decreases arterial pressure through a decrease in total peripheral resistance[50] with only minimal increase in heart rate and plasma renin activity.[50] Many studies have demonstrated the effectiveness of isradipine in lowering blood pressure.[50-64] The response rate (diastolic blood pressure, <90 mmHg) with isradipine (2.5 to 10 mg twice a day) as monotherapy ranged between 52% and 78% in various studies.[53-61] The drug is well tolerated by most patients, and the rate of side effects is low. In the SWISS isradipine study, 1472 hypertensive patients with a mean age of 57 years were treated with isradipine (2.5 mg twice a day) for 4 weeks. Blood pressure decreased significantly from 168 ± 18/102 ± 8 mmHg to 151 ± 16/92 ± 9 mmHg. Only two patients withdrew because of lack of efficacy, and 94 patients withdrew because of side effects.[61]

The antihypertensive effect of isradipine is independent of age and race, indicating that the drug is also effective in young white hypertensive patients.[65] However, as with other calcium antagonists,[66] there is evidence that the drug is more effective in patients with low-renin hypertension.[67]

The initial recommended dose of isradipine is 1.25 mg twice a day, and the maximal dose is 10 mg twice a day. Using the regular formulation twice daily adequately controls blood pressure for 24 hours. Viskoper et al.,[68] in a placebo-controlled study, gave isradipine (1.25 to 2.5 mg twice a day) to 14 hypertensive patients for 8 weeks. Blood pressure was assessed by 24-hour ambulatory blood pressure monitoring. Isradipine decreased blood pressure significantly throughout the day when compared with placebo.

A slow-release formulation of isradipine (SRO) has been introduced. Several studies[53, 69–76] demonstrated that SRO is effective in a once-daily dose. Arzilli et al.[71] showed that the SRO compound gave a trough-to-peak ratio of 70%, supporting a once-daily administration. Christensen et al.[75] compared the antihypertensive effect of isradipine given twice daily in the regular formulation or given once daily in the SRO formulation in 32 hypertensive patients. Both groups received a total dose of 5 mg daily, and both treatments resulted in a satisfactory blood pressure reduction during 24 hours. Holmes et al.[72] also found that the SRO formulation had the same antihypertensive effect as the regular formula taken twice daily, with slightly fewer side effects.

The SRO compound had a similar effect on 24-hour blood pressure when it was given once daily in the morning or the evening,[70] and no adjustment in the total daily dose was necessary when switching from one form to the other.[69]

Our group evaluated the immediate and long-term hemodynamic effects of isradipine in 11 hypertensive patients.[50] Oral administration of 5 mg caused a significant decrease in blood pressure from 165 ± 19/88 ± 9 mmHg to 133 ± 9/72 ± 8 mmHg within 2.5 hours. The fall in arterial pressure was related to a significant decrease in the index of total peripheral resistance (43 ± 6 U to 27 ± 3 U) associated with a substantial increase in heart rate and cardiac output (Fig. 109–1). Because the stroke volume did not change, the increase in cardiac output was related mainly to higher pulse rate due to reflexive adrenergic stimulation.

After 3 months of oral treatment, arterial pressure remained significantly decreased as a result of low peripheral resistance. However, the activation of the sympathetic nervous system, which was responsible for elevated heart rate and cardiac output after the acute administration, abated after short-term treatment. Renal blood flow increased after oral therapy

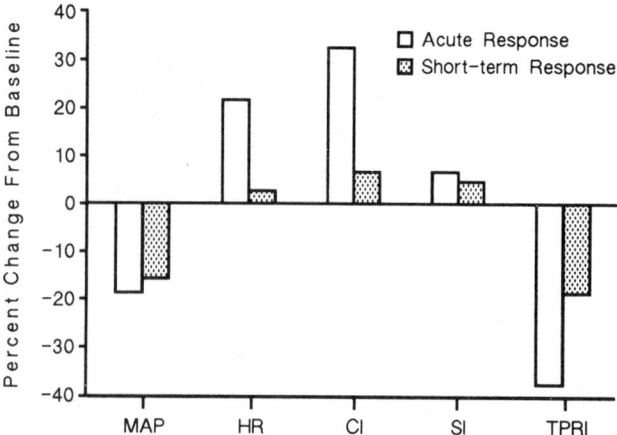

Figure 109–1. Hemodynamic response to isradipine. Acute and short-term effects. MAP, mean arterial pressure; HR, heart rate; CI, cardiac index; SI, stroke volume index; TPRI, total peripheral resistance index.

as a result of decreased renal vascular resistance. Splanchnic blood flow decreased slightly, which might support previous experimental results regarding the vasoconstrictive effect of isradipine on the splanchnic circulation. Like other calcium antagonists, isradipine induced diuretic and natriuretic effects.[77, 78] The diuretic and natriuretic effects of isradipine were observed within 1 to 3 hours after administration,[78] and the maximal diuretic and natriuretic effects were obtained with a subhypotensive dose of 2.5 mg daily.[77] The authors failed to observe a natriuretic effect despite a decrease in blood volume.[50] This lack may be due to the small number of patients in the study, all of whom were on an *ad libitum* sodium diet.

Hypertension with Associated Diseases

Isradipine is effective in diabetic hypertensive patients.[79, 80] In an open, noncomparative study, Parreira et al.[79] gave isradipine (2.5 to 10 mg daily) to 28 hypertensive diabetic patients for 24 weeks. Blood pressure decreased from 168.1 ± 9.3/102.7 ± 6 mmHg at baseline to 140.7 ± 11.9/81.6 ± 7.5 mmHg after 6 months of treatment. Blood pressure was controlled in all but one patient at the end of the study. Blood pressure control was achieved without any metabolic changes.

In a placebo-controlled, double-blind crossover study, Klause et al.[80] evaluated the effect of isradipine on glucose tolerance and insulin secretion. The systolic blood pressure was significantly lowered by isradipine compared with placebo. Fasting blood glucose, glucose levels, and basal and stimulated insulin during the oral glucose tolerance remained unchanged.

Isradipine has also been shown to be effective in patients with mild renal failure,[81] in cyclosporine-treated renal transplant recipients,[82] and in patients with cyclosporine-induced hypertension.[83]

Pregnancy-Induced Hypertension

The efficacy and safety of isradipine in pregnancy-induced hypertension were evaluated in some studies.[84-87] Preliminary results indicate the drug to be effective and safe in hypertensive pregnant women and their fetuses. Isradipine passed the placental barrier, but its concentration was considerably lower in the fetal compartment.[84] Isradipine given intravenously as a bolus dose (0.5 to 1.5 mg) decreased blood pressure in pregnant women with little effect on uterine activity and fetal heart rate.[85] In an open study, isradipine was given in a dose of 5 to 10 mg daily for 8 days to 27 women with pregnancy-induced hypertension.[86] The drug significantly reduced mean arterial pressure without affecting uteroplacental blood flow and pulsatility indices. In another open study, isradipine was given to nine pregnant women with hypertension from the 26th week of gestation until delivery.[87] A dose of 2.5 to 10 mg daily reduced blood pressure significantly with a slight increase in maternal heart rate. All measurements in the newborn were within normal ranges, and no malformations were detected.

Hypertensive Emergencies

Parenteral isradipine is useful in the treatment of hypertensive crisis and in intraoperative and perioperative hypertension.[88-92]

In 10 symptomatic patients with hypertensive crisis, intravenous administration of isradipine in a dose of 7.2 µg/kg/hr for 3 hours reduced mean arterial pressure significantly from 135.2 ± 4.4 mmHg to 116.2 ± 3.6 mmHg.[88] Sublingually administered isradipine at a dose of 1.25 to 5 mg was used in 27 patients with hypertensive crisis.[89] The onset of action occurred approximately 30 minutes after dosing and reached its maximum effect within 2 hours of administration. Mean arterial pressure decreased from 153.4 ± 4.3 to 120.0 ± 2.3 mmHg at 60 minutes and to 118.0 ± 2.1 mmHg at 2 hours after administration. Isradipine was administered intravenously to 21 patients with intraoperative hypertension during abdominal surgery.[90] Infusion of 0.5 mg (10 ml) over 5 minutes decreased mean arterial pressure by 40% within 2 minutes, and the blood pressure remained low for at least 45 minutes. The responder rate was 92% at 2 minutes and 100% after the fourth minute following infusion. Continuous intravenous infusion of isradipine in a dose of up to 0.9 µg/kg/min provided rapid blood pressure control in 10 patients who developed hypertension after aortocoronary bypass grafting.[91]

Effects on Left Ventricular Mass

Like other calcium antagonists,[93-96] isradipine decreases left ventricular hypertrophy.[50, 60, 97-102]

Vyssoulis et al.[99] gave isradipine (5 mg daily) to 45 hypertensive patients. After 6 months of therapy, interventricular septal thickness and posterior wall thickness decreased by 10.7% and 5.8%, respectively, resulting in a decrease of 13.4% in left ventricular mass index. Saragoca et al.[97] gave isradipine (5 mg daily) to 12 hypertensive patients with left ventricular hypertrophy. After 6 months of therapy, left ventricular mass index decreased significantly (from 184.2 ± 10.2 g/m² to 125.9 ± 6.4 g/m²) in association with a significant decrease in total ventricular extrasystoles (from 4035 ± 1461 beats/day to 421 ± 159 beats/day). The Lown and Wolf classification of ventricular arrhythmias improved in eight patients. Other investigators[60, 100, 101] have demonstrated that reduction in left ventricular mass index by isradipine is associated with improvement in left ventricular function.

Effects on Blood Vessels

Isradipine, in addition to its antihypertensive effect, may have some protective effects against thrombosis and atherosclerosis.[103-108]

Gleerup et al.[103] evaluated the fibrinolytic activity of isradipine (5 to 10 mg daily) for 14 days in hypertensive and normotensive subjects. Fibrinolytic activity was assessed by measuring euglobulin clot lysis time, tissue plasminogen activator activity, and its inhibition. Isradipine had no effect in controls but augmented fibrinolytic activity in the hypertensive patients. Fetkovska et al.[104] studied the effects of isradipine on platelet response to serotonin and low-density lipoprotein (LDL) in a controlled open study in 17 hypertensive patients. Following 4 weeks of treatment with isradipine (2.5 to 5 mg daily), both the serotonin-induced and the LDL-induced platelet aggregations were significantly decreased. A further decrease in these indices was observed after 12 weeks of treatment. Fitcha et al.[106] demonstrated a decrease in platelet aggregation in response to adenosine diphosphate, serum thromboxane B_2, and β-thromboglobulin. Slonim et al. also observed a reduction in blood viscosity with isradipine.[105, 108]

Isradipine slightly increased high-density lipoprotein (HDL) cholesterol levels without adversely affecting other lipids.[109-112] Stein et al.[112] evaluated the effect of isradipine on lipid profiles in elderly hypertensive patients during an open-label study. After 1 year of treatment, total cholesterol decreased by 7.5 mg/dl, and HDL cholesterol increased significantly by 3.9 mg/dl, resulting in a significant decrease in the ratio of total to HDL cholesterol. Experimentally, isradipine can be shown to have antiatheromatous effects that interfere with the main pathogenetic mechanisms of atherosclerosis.[113] These effects are mediated by the release of prostaglandin I_2 and endothelium-derived relaxing factor and the subsequent elevation of intracellular adenosine 3′,5′-cyclic phosphate and guanosine 3′,5′-monophosphate, respectively.

MIDAS

To establish the clinical relevance of isradipine on the arterial wall in hypertensive patients, a 3-year clinical trial was carried out in the United States.[114] This study included 800 hypertensive patients aged 40 and over and compared the efficacy of isradipine (2.5 to 5 mg twice a day) and hydrochlorothiazide (12.5 to 25 mg twice a day) in retarding atherosclerosis in the carotid arteries. The results, as reported at the meeting of the International Society of Hypertension in 1994, showed a decrease in carotid artery wall thickness in isradipine-treated patients when compared with the diuretic group after 6 months of therapy. For the remainder of the study period, no further difference was observed between the two treatment groups. Although the results of this study are promising and provocative, they fail to clearly document antiatheromatous effects of isradipine in hypertensive patients.

Comparison with Other Antihypertensive Agents

Few studies were designed to compare the safety and efficacy of isradipine with those of other antihypertensive agents.[58, 62, 115–127]

When compared with hydrochlorothiazide (HCTZ), isradipine (5 to 20 mg daily) lowered blood pressure as effectively as HCTZ (25 to 50 mg daily) but produced more side effects.[123] In another study, Holtzman et al.[121] showed that the rate of response was significantly higher with isradipine (5 to 15 mg daily) than with HCTZ (25 to 50 mg daily).

In comparison with β-blockers, isradipine (5 to 20 mg daily) was as effective as propranolol (120 to 480 mg daily) in the treatment of hypertension not controlled by HCTZ alone.[124] The efficacy of isradipine (5 to 20 mg daily) was similar to that of atenolol (50 to 100 mg daily) in lowering blood pressure.[125] In another study, isradipine (2.5 to 5 mg daily) was compared with metoprolol (100 to 200 mg daily) in hypertensive patients who were habitual snorers.[119] Isradipine was more suitable than metoprolol for the treatment of these patients.

Isradipine (5 to 20 mg daily) was more effective in lowering blood pressure than prazosin (4 to 16 mg daily).[122, 127]

When compared with converting enzyme inhibitors, isradipine (5 to 10 mg daily) was more effective in lowering blood pressure than enalapril (5 to 40 mg daily).[62] Both drugs were similarly well tolerated. In our experience, isradipine (5 to 20 mg daily) was more effective in lowering blood pressure than fosinopril (10 to 40 mg daily), but isradipine did not blunt pressure increase during isometric stress, whereas fosinopril did.[128] Isradipine was also compared with other calcium antagonists.[58, 115, 117, 118] It seems that isradipine is as potent as felodipine and nifedipine in lowering blood pressure but is superior to other dihydropyridines in terms of incidence of adverse effects.[115, 117, 118] When compared with diltiazem, isradipine at a mean dose of 13.7 mg daily was more potent in lowering blood pressure than diltiazem (293 mg daily) according to Vermeulen et al.,[126] whereas Black et al.[58] found both drugs to be equally potent. Isradipine can be safely and effectively combined with β-blockers, diuretics, and converting enzyme inhibitors.[120, 124, 125]

Adverse Effects

Adverse effects have been reported but seem to be few and minor. The main side effects are leg pains, palpitations, abdominal discomfort, flushing, disturbing dreams, headache, constipation, leg edema, noncardiac chest pain, dizziness, and fatigue. Headache usually appears early after drug initiation and diminishes substantially after a few days. Rarely, sinus tachycardia and first-degree atrioventricular block have been reported. Isradipine tends to increase glucose and cholesterol levels but to a minor extent.[3, 40, 52] Calcium antagonists mainly dilate the arterial tree, with minimal effect on the venous system; thus, as described,[125] orthostasis is not expected. However, in our study,[50] two patients developed asymptomatic postural hypotension that was documented during the upright tilt test.

Congestive Heart Failure

Unlike most other calcium antagonists that exert a negative inotropic effect,[130] isradipine has potent vasodilatory properties at doses much lower than those associated with a negative inotropic effect. Consequently, the drug may be of value in the management of patients with congestive heart failure.[29] By virtue of their ability to decrease afterload, vasodilators allow the failing heart to empty more efficiently. Thus, afterload reduction can improve cardiac performance in patients with congestive heart failure.[131] However, the efficacy of many available agents appears to be limited by pseudotolerance and multiple side effects. Among the calcium antagonists, isradipine, because of its specific and vasoselective activity, seems to be an ideal compound for patients with congestive heart failure. In a preliminary clinical study, a group of 12 patients with severe congestive heart failure were evaluated hemodynamically;[29] isradipine (15 mg given orally) caused a decrease in mean arterial pressure accompanied by an increase in stroke volume and cardiac index and a decrease in total peripheral resistance. The acute effect was not associated with a significant change in either heart rate or pulmonary wedge pressure. Six of seven patients who continued isradipine therapy showed impressive clinical improvement that was also reflected by a decrease in cardiothoracic ratio. No reflex tachycardia was observed in these patients, whereas significant increases followed acute administration of isradipine to our patients (with mild essential hypertension). Conceivably, the sympathetic responsiveness is exhausted in patients with congestive heart failure, and no further cardioacceleration will occur. Despite these encouraging hemodynamic results, isradipine should be used cautiously, if at all, in patients with congestive failure until a morbidity and mortality study has documented benefits.

Angina Pectoris

Because of their ability to dilate coronary arteries, calcium antagonists were introduced primarily as antianginal agents.[132] Isradipine has also been shown to have an antiischemic effect in experimental models.[22] This property was attributed predominantly to the ability of the drug to redistribute coronary flow preferentially to the endocardium. In a clinical study in which patients with exercise-induced stable angina pectoris were given a single dose of isradipine, the drug was well tolerated and exerted significant antianginal activity.[133] In a preliminary, double-blind, multicenter study,[134] the effectiveness of isradipine was compared with that of placebo, nifedipine, or isosorbide dinitrate. Isradipine exerted substantial antianginal effects in patients with exercise-induced angina pectoris resulting from coronary artery obstruction. Exercise time to the onset of anginal pain and time to development of more severe angina on the treadmill were substantially increased by isradipine, in parallel with the decrease in the number of anginal attacks and amount of glycerol trinitrate consumed. The antianginal effect of the drug was equal to that of nifedipine and better than that of isosorbide dinitrate. As judged from the electrocardiogram, the antiischemic effects of isradipine were similar to those of nifedipine.

SUMMARY

Many studies indicate that isradipine (2.5 to 10 mg twice daily) or the SRO compound (once daily) is effective in treating patients with arterial hypertension, angina pectoris, and congestive heart failure. Isradipine is at least as effective as other calcium antagonists in the treatment of hypertension and ischemic heart disease and may have fewer negative inotropic and chronotropic effects. Hemodynamically, it reduces systemic vascular resistance, preserves cardiac output, and improves renal and cerebral blood flow, and it reduces left ventricular mass. Short-term treatment with isradipine stimulates neither the adrenergic nor the renin-angiotensin systems and causes neither water nor sodium retention. Only a few side effects have been reported, and most of these abate during longer treatment. Unlike verapamil, isradipine can be used safely in combination with β-blockers and does not change plasma digoxin levels. Its long-acting effect allows twice-daily or even once-daily dosing. This, together with its promising antiatheromatous properties, makes isradipine an excellent first-line drug for the treatment of essential hypertension.

REFERENCES

1. Hof RP, Hof A, Ruegg UT, et al: Stereoselectivity at the calcium channel: Different profiles of hemodynamic activity of the enantiomers of dihydropyridine derivative PN-200-110. J Cardiovasc Pharmacol 8:221, 1986.
2. Hof RP, Salzmann R, Siegl H: Selective effects of PN 200-110 (isradipine) on the peripheral circulation and the heart. Am J Cardiol 59:30B, 1987.
3. Hamilton BP: Treatment of essential hypertension with PN 200-110 (isradipine). Am J Cardiol 59:141B, 1987.
4. Hof RP, Ruegg UT: Pharmacology of the new calcium antagonist isradipine and its metabolites. Am J Med 84:13, 1988.
5. Supavilai P, Karobath M: The interaction of PY108-068 and of PN200-110 with calcium channel binding sites in rat brain. J Neural Transplant 60:149, 1984.
6. Hof RP, Hof A, Scholtysik G, et al: Effects of the new calcium antagonist PN-200-110 on the myocardium and the regional peripheral circulation in anesthetized cats and dogs. J Cardiovasc Pharmacol 6:407, 1984.
7. Hof RP, Scholtysik G, Loutzenhiser R, et al: PN-200-110, a new calcium antagonist: Electrophysiological, inotropic, and chronotropic effects on guinea pig myocardial tissue and effects on contraction and calcium uptake of rabbit aorta. J Cardiovasc Pharmacol 6:399, 1984.
8. Bayer R, Kaufmann R, Rodenkincher R, et al: Die Winkungen von Calciumantagonisten auf isoliertes Myokardgewebe und ihre molekularen Winkungsmechanismen. Herz 7:203, 1982.
9. Lathrop DA, Valle-Aguilera JR, Millard RW, et al: Comparative electrophysiologic and coronary hemodynamic effects of diltiazem, nisoldipine, and verapamil on myocardial tissue. Am J Cardiol 49:613, 1982.
10. Nabata H: Effects of calcium antagonistic coronary vasodilators on myocardial contractility and membrane potentials. Jpn J Pharmacol 27:239, 1977.
11. Kohlhardt M, Fleckenstein A: Inhibition of the slow inward current by nifedipine in mammalian ventricular myocardium. Naunyn Schmiedebergs Arch Pharmacol 298:267, 1977.
12. Sholtysik G, Schaad A: Cardiac cellular electrophysiology as a tool to prove Ca^{2+} slow channel inhibition by PY 108—068. Triangle 21:49, 1983.
13. Muller-Schweinitzer E, Neumann P: In vitro effect of calcium antagonists Pn 200—110, nifedipine, and nimodipine on human and canine cerebral arteries. J Cereb Blood Flow Metabol 3:354, 1983.
14. Kazda S, Knorr A, Towart R: Common properties and differences between various calcium antagonists. Prog Pharmacol 5:83, 1983.
15. Wada Y, Satoh K, Taira N: Separation of the coronary vasodilator from the cardiac effects of PN-200-110, a new dihydropyridine calcium antagonist in dog heart. J Cardiovasc Pharmacol 7:190, 1985.
16. Moromura S, Tiara N: Differential effects of organic slow inward current inhibitors verapamil and nifedipine on rate of atrioventricular rhythm and supraventricular tachycardia in the canine isolated, blood perfused AV node preparation. Naunyn Schmiedebergs Arch Pharmacol 315:241, 1981.
17. Taira N, Kawada M, Satho K: Cardiac versus coronary vasodilator actions of KB-944, a new calcium antagonist, assessed in isolated, blood perfused heart preparations of dogs. J Cardiovasc Pharmacol 5:349, 1983.
18. Nayler WG: The pharmacological protection of the ischemic heart: The use of calcium and beta adrenoceptor antagonists. Eur Heart J 1(Suppl B):5, 1980.
19. Nayler WG, Ferrany R, Williams A: Protective effect of pretreatment with verapamil, nifedipine and propranolol on mitochondrial function in the ischemic and reperfused myocardium. Am J Cardiol 46:242, 1980.
20. Henry PD, Shuchleib R, Bonda LJ, et al: Effects of nifedipine on myocardial perfusion and ischemic injury in dogs. Circ Res 43:372, 1978.
21. Reimer KA, Jenning RB: Effects of calcium channel blockers on myocardial preservation during experimental acute myocardial infarction. Am J Cardiol 55:107B, 1985.
22. Cook NS, Hof RP: Cardioprotection by calcium antagonist PN-200-110 in the absence and presence of cardiodepression. Br J Pharmacol 86:181, 1985.
23. Habib JB, Bossaller C, Wells S, et al: Preservation of endothelium dependent vascular relaxation in cholesterol fed rabbit by treatment with calcium blocker PN 200—110. Circ Res 58:305, 1986.
24. Handley DA, Van Valen RG, Melden MK, et al: Suppression of rat carotid lesion development by the calcium channel blocker PN-200-110. Am J Pathol 124:88, 1986.
25. Hof RP: Comparison of cardiodepressant and vasodilator effects on PN 200—110 (isradipine), nifedipine, and diltiazem in anesthetized rabbits. Am J Cardiol 59:37B, 1987.
26. Hof RP: Analysis of peripheral vascular actions of the new calcium antagonist isradipine. Am J Med 84:18, 1988.

27. Hof RP: Calcium antagonists and the peripheral circulation: Differences and similarities between PY 108—68, nicardipine, verapamil and diltiazem. Br J Pharmacol 78:375, 1983.

28. Kurnik PB, Tiefenbrunn AJ, Ludbrock PA: The dependence of the cardiac effects of nifedipine on the responses of the peripheral vascular system. Circulation 69:963, 1984.

29. Greenberg B, Siemienczuk D, Broudy D: Hemodynamic effects of PN 200—110 (isradipine) in congestive heart failure. Am J Cardiol 59:70B, 1987.

30. Hof RP: Calcium antagonists, vasoconstrictors and the peripheral circulation. Gen Pharmacol 18:459, 1987.

31. Sauter A, Rudin M: Calcium antagonists reduce the extent of infarction in rat middle cerebral artery occlusion model as determined by quantitative magnetic resonance imaging. Stroke 17:1228, 1986.

32. Henry PD, Bentley KI: Suppression of atherogenesis in cholesterol fed rabbits treated with nifedipine. J Clin Invest 68:1366, 1981.

33. Rouleau J, Parmley WW, Stevens J, et al: Verapamil suppresses atherosclerosis in cholesterol-fed rabbits. J Am Coll Cardiol 1:1453, 1983.

34. Willis AL, Nagel B, Churchill V, et al: Antiatherosclerotic effects of nicardipine and nifedipine in cholesterol fed rabbits. Arteriosclerosis 5:250, 1985.

35. Ginsburg R, Davis K, Bristow MR, et al: Calcium antagonists suppress atherogenesis in aorta but not in the intramural coronary arteries of cholesterol fed rabbits. Lab Invest 49:154, 1983.

36. Johns EJ: The influence of diltiazem and nifedipine on renal function in the rat. Br J Pharmacol 84:707, 1985.

37. Loutzenhiser R, Epstein M: Effects of calcium antagonists on renal hemodynamics. Am J Physiol 249:F619, 1985.

38. Dietz JR, Davis JO, Freeman RH, et al: Effects of intrarenal infusion of calcium entry blockers in anesthetized dogs. Hypertension 5:482, 1983.

39. Hof RP, Evenou JP, Miyashita AH: Similar increase in circulating renin after equihypotensive doses of nitroprusside, dihydralazine or isradipine in conscious rabbits. Eur J Pharmacol 136:251, 1987.

40. Hof RP: Interaction between two calcium antagonists and two beta blockers in conscious rabbits: Hemodynamic consequences of differing cardiodepressant properties. Am J Cardiol 59:43B, 1987.

41. Hof RP, Hof A: The renin angiotensin system modulates the peripheral vascular effects of the calcium antagonist isradipine in anaesthetized rabbits. J Cardiovasc Pharmacol 12:233, 1988.

42. Belz GG, Doering W, Munkes R, et al: Interaction between digoxin and calcium antagonists and antiarrhythmic drugs. Clin Pharmacol Ther 33:410, 1983.

43. Yoshida A, Fujita M, Kurasawa N, et al: Effects of diltiazem on plasma level and urinary excretion of digoxin in healthy subjects. Clin Pharmacol Ther 35:681, 1984.

44. Johnson BF, Wilson J, Marawaha R, et al: The comparative effects of verapamil and a new dihydropyridine calcium channel blocker on digoxin pharmacokinetics. Clin Pharmacol Ther 42:66, 1987.

45. Perreault MM, Kazierad DJ, Wilton JH, et al: The effect of isradipine on theophylline pharmacokinetics in healthy volunteers. Pharmacotherapy 13(2):149, 1993.

46. Vernillet L, Bourbigot B, Codet JP, et al: Lack of effect of isradipine on cyclosporin pharmacokinetics. Fundam Clin Pharmacol 6(8—9):367, 1992.

47. Endersen L, Bergan S, Holdaas H, et al: Lack of effect of the calcium antagonist isradipine on cyclosporine pharmacokinetics in renal transplant patients. Ther Drug Monit 13(6):490, 1991.

48. Renton KW: Inhibition of hepatic microsomal drug metabolism by the calcium channel blockers diltiazem and verapamil. Biochem Pharmacol 34:2549, 1985.

49. Klockowski PM, Lener ME, Sirgo MA, et al: Comparative evaluation of the effects of isradipine and diltiazem on antipyrine and indocyanine green clearances in elderly volunteers. Clin Pharmacol Ther 48(4):375, 1990.

50. Grossman E, Messerli FH, Oren S, et al: Cardiovascular effects of isradipine in essential hypertension. Am J Cardiol 68(1):65, 1991.

51. Nelson EB, Pool JL, Taylor AA: Antihypertensive activity of isradipine in humans: A new dihydropyridine calcium channel antagonist. Clin Pharmacol Ther 40:694, 1986.

52. Winer N, Thys-Jacobs S, Kumar R, et al: Evaluation of isradipine (PN-200-110) in mild to moderate hypertension. Clin Pharmacol Ther 42:442, 1987.

53. Abarquez RF Jr, Sy RG, Castillo RR: Efficacy of slow release oral isradipine in moderate to severe hypertension with add on spirapril. Am J Hypertens 6:77S, 1993.

54. Yodfat Y, Cristal N: A multicenter, double-blind, randomized, placebo controlled study of isradipine and methyldopa as monotherapy or in combination with captopril in the treatment of hypertension. The LOMIR-MCT-IH Research Group. Am J Hypertens 6:57S, 1993.

55. Magometschnigg D: Isradipine in the treatment of mild to moderate hypertension. The Australian Multicenter Isradipine cum Spirapril Study (AMICUS). Am J Hypertens 6:49S, 1993.

56. Lüscher TF, Waeber B: Efficacy and safety of various combination therapies based on a calcium antagonist in essential hypertension: Results of a placebo controlled randomized trial. J Cardiovasc Pharmacol 21:305, 1993.

57. Luomanmaki K, Inkovaara J, Hartikainen M, et al: Efficacy and tolerability of isradipine and metoprolol in treatment of hypertension: The Finnish Isradipine Study in Hypertension (FISH). J Cardiovasc Pharmacol 20:296, 1992.

58. Black HR, Lewin AJ, Stein GH, et al: A comparison of the safety of therapeutically equivalent doses of isradipine and diltiazem for treatment of essential hypertension. Am J Hypertens 5:141, 1992.

59. Kirch W, Burger KJ, Weidinger G, et al: Efficacy and tolerability of the new calcium antagonist isradipine in essential hypertension. J Cardiovasc Pharmacol 15:(Suppl 1):S55, 1990.

60. Carr AA, Prisant LM: The new calcium antagonist isradipine. Effect on blood pressure and the left ventricle in black hypertensive patients. Am J Hypertens 3:8, 1990.

61. Lüscher TF, Waeber B: Calcium antagonists as first line therapy in hypertension results of the Swiss isradipine study. Swiss hypertension society. J Cardiovasc Pharmacol 18(Suppl 3):S1, 1991.

62. Eisner GM, Johnson BF, McMahon FG, et al: A multicenter comparison of the safety and efficacy of isradipine and enalapril in the treatment of hypertension. Am J Hypertens 4:154S, 1991.

63. Miller H: Isradipine: Overall clinical experience in hypertension in the United States. Am J Hypertens 4:135S, 1991.

64. Gomez G, Melgarejo E, Narvaez J, et al: Multicenter evaluation of efficacy, tolerability and safety of the new first line antihypertensive drug, isradipine, in a Latin American population. Am J Hypertens 4:128S, 1991.

65. Batlouni M, Armaganijan D, Ghorayeb N, et al: Clinical efficacy and tolerability of isradipine in the treatment of mild to moderate hypertension in young and elderly patients. J Cardiovasc Pharmacol 19(Suppl 3):S537, 1992.

66. Resnick LM, Laragh JH: Renin, calcium metabolism and the pathophysiologic basis of antihypertensive therapy. Am J Cardiol 56:68H, 1985.

67. Carr M, Prisant LM: The calcium antagonist isradipine and its effect on blood pressure related to plasma renin activity. Am J Hypertens 3:354, 1990.

68. Viskoper JR, Laszt A, Farragi D: The antihypertensive action of isradipine in mild essential hypertension. J Cardiovasc Pharmacol 18(Suppl 3):S9, 1991.

69. Holmes DG, Kutz K: Bioequivalence of a slow release and non retard formulation of isradipine. Am J Hypertens 6:70S, 1993.

70. Fogari R, Malacco E, Tettamanti F, et al: Evening vs morning isradipine sustained release in essential hypertension: A double blind study with 24 hour ambulatory monitoring. Br J Clin Pharmacol 35:51, 1993.

71. Arzilli F, Gandolfi E, Del-Prato C, et al: Antihypertensive effect of once daily sustained release isradipine: A placebo controlled cross over study. Eur J Clin Pharmacol 44:23, 1993.

72. Holmes D, Moullet C: Clinical equivalence of once daily administration of a modified release formulation of isradipine and twice daily administration of the standard formulation. Multicenter Study Group. J Cardiovasc Pharmacol 19(Suppl 3):S61, 1992.

73. Winer N, Kirkendall WM, Canosa FL, et al: Placebo controlled trial of once a day isradipine monotherapy in mild to moderately severe hypertension. J Clin Pharmacol 30:1006, 1990.

74. Lacourciere Y, Poirier L, Dion D, et al: Antihypertensive effect of isradipine administered once or twice daily on ambulatory blood pressure. Am J Cardiol 65:467, 1990.

75. Christensen HR, Kampmann JP, Simonsen K: A randomized comparison of isradipine slow release given once daily with isradipine twice daily on 24 hour blood pressure in hypertensive patients. J Hum Hypertens 5:121, 1991.

76. Diemont WL, Stegeman CJ, Beekman J, et al: Low dose isradipine once daily effectively controls 24-h blood pressure in essential hypertension. Am J Hypertens 4:163S, 1991.

77. Zanchetti A, Leonetti G: Natriuretic effects of calcium antagonists. Clinical implications. Drugs 40(Suppl 2):15, 1990.

78. Kramer BK, Haussler M, Ress KM, et al: Renal effects of the new calcium channel blocking drug isradipine. Eur J Clin Pharmacol 39:333, 1990.

79. Parreira JM, Correia LG, Pereira E, et al: Antihypertensive efficacy, safety, and tolerability of isradipine in hypertensive patients with diabetes. Am J Hypertens 6:104S, 1993.

80. Klauser R, Speiser P, Gisinger C, et al: Platelet aggregation and metabolic control are not affected by calcium antagonist treatment in type II diabetes mellitus. J Cardiovasc Pharmacol 15(Suppl 1):S93, 1990.

81. Wittenberg C, Rosenfeld JB: Long term antihypertensive and renal effects of isradipine in hypertensive patients with normal and reduced renal function. J Cardiovasc Pharmacol 19(Suppl 3):S93, 1992.

82. McCrea JB, Francos GF, Burke JF, et al: The beneficial effects of isradipine on renal hemodynamics in cyclosporine treated renal transplant recipients. Transplantation 55:672, 1993.

83. Berg KJ, Holdaas H, Endresen L, et al: Effects of isradipine on renal function in cyclosporin treated renal transplanted patients. Nephrol Dial Transplant 6:725, 1991.

84. Lunell NO, Bondesson U, Grunewald C, et al: Transplacental passage of isradipine in the treatment of pregnancy induced hypertension. Am J Hypertens 6:110S, 1993.

85. Wide-Swensson D, Ingemarsson I, Arulkumaran S, et al: Effects of isradipine, a new calcium antagonist, on maternal cardiovascular system and uterine activity in labour. Br J Obstet Gynaecol 97:945, 1990.

86. Lunell NO, Garoff L, Grunewald C, et al: Isradipine, a new calcium antagonist: Effects on maternal and fetal hemodynamics. J Cardiovasc Pharmacol 18(Suppl 3):S37, 1991.

87. Feiks A, Grunberger W, Meisner W: Influence of isradipine on the maternal and fetal cardiovascular system in hypertensive disorders in pregnancy. Am J Hypertens 4:200S, 1991.

88. Saragoca MA, Mulinari RA, Oliveira AF, et al: Parenteral isradipine reduces blood pressure in hypertensive crisis. Am J Hypertens 6:112S, 1993.

89. Saragoca MA, Portela JE, Plavnik F, et al: Isradipine in the treatment of hypertensive crisis in ambulatory patients. J Cardiovasc Pharmacol 19(Suppl 3):S76, 1992.

90. Edouard A, Dartayet B, Ruegg C, et al: The use of calcium antagonists to treat intra-operative hypertension—evaluation of efficacy and safety of a new dihydropyridine derivative, intravenous isradipine, during abdominal surgery. Eur J Anaesthesiol 8:351, 1991.

91. Lawrence CJ, Lestrade A, de Lange S: Isradipine, a calcium antagonist, in the control of hypertension following coronary artery bypass surgery. Am J Hypertens 4:207S, 1991.

92. Ruegg PC, Karmann U, Keller H: Management of perioperative hypertension using intravenous isradipine. Am J Hypertens 4:203S, 1991.

93. Schmieder RE, Messerli FH, Garavaglia GE, et al: Cardiovascular effects of verapamil in patients with essential hypertension. Circulation 75:1030, 1987.

94. Messerli FH, Oren S, Grossman E: Effects of calcium channel blockers on systemic hemodynamics in hypertension. Am J Med 84:8, 1988.

95. Grossman E, Oren S, Garavaglia GE, et al: Systemic and regional hemodynamic and humoral effects of nitrendipine in essential hypertension. Circulation 78:1394, 1988.

96. Messerli FH, Oren S, Grossman E: Left ventricular hypertrophy and antihypertensive therapy. Drugs 35(Suppl 5):27, 1988.

97. Saragoca MA, Cassiolatto JL, Vanetta AM, et al: Reversal of left ventricular hypertrophy with isradipine induces diminution of cardiac arrhythmias. Am J Hypertens 6:89S, 1993.

98. Manolis AJ, Kolovou G, Handanis S, et al: Regression of left ventricular hypertrophy with isradipine in previously untreated hypertensive patients. Am J Hypertens 6:86S 1993.

99. Vyssoulis GP, Karpanou EA, Pitsavos CE, et al: Regression of left ventricular hypertrophy with isradipine antihypertensive therapy. Am J Hypertens 6:82S, 1993.

100. Torok E, Borbas S, Lengyel M, et al: Regression of cardiac hypertrophy in hypertensive patients by long term treatment with isradipine. J Cardiovasc Pharmacol 19(Suppl 3):S79, 1992.

101. Bielen EC, Fagard RH, Lijnen PJ, et al: Comparison of the effects of isradipine and lisinopril on left ventricular structure and function in essential hypertension. Am J Cardiol 69:1200, 1992.

102. Saragoca MA, Portela JE, Abreu P, et al: Regression of left ventricular hypertrophy in the short term treatment of hypertension with isradipine. Am J Hypertens 4:188S, 1991.

103. Gleerup G, Hender T, Hjorting-Hansen E, et al: Does antihypertensive therapy affect the natural protection against thrombosis? J Cardiovasc Pharmacol 18(Suppl 3):S34, 1991.

104. Fetkovska N, Sebekova K, Fedelesova V, et al: Serotonin and platelet activation during treatment with isradipine. J Cardiovasc Pharmacol 18(Suppl 3):S31, 1991.

105. Slonim A, Cristal N: Cardiovascular diseases, blood rheology, and dihydropyridine calcium antagonists. J Cardiovasc Pharmacol 19(Suppl 3):S96, 1992.

106. Fitscha P, Virgolini I, Rauscha F, et al: Effects of isradipine on platelet function in hypertension at rest and during exercise. Am J Hypertens 4:178S, 1991.

107. Fetkovska N, Fedelesova V, Kozlovsky M, et al: Platelet activating effect of low density lipoprotein and its reversal by isradipine. Am J Hypertens 4:175S, 1991.

108. Slonim A, Paran E, Cristal N: Effect of isradipine on factors affecting blood viscosity. Am J Hypertens 4:172S, 1991.

109. Meric M, Goren T, Atilgan D, et al: Metabolic, hematological, and cardiac effects of long term isradipine treatment in mild to moderate essential hypertension. J Cardiovasc Pharmacol 19(Suppl 3):S58, 1992.

110. Ding YA, Han CL, Chou TC, et al: Effects of the calcium antagonist isradipine on 24-hour ambulatory blood pressure, platelet aggregation, and neutrophil oxygen free radicals in hypertension. J Cardiovasc Pharmacol 19(Suppl 3):S32, 1992.

111. Norgaard K, Jensen T, Feldt-Rasmussen B: Effects of isradipine in type 1 (insulin dependent) diabetic patients with albuminuria and normal blood pressure. J Hum Hypertens 6:145, 1992.

112. Stein GH, Matthews K, Bannatyne RE, et al: Long term lipid profiles with isradipine and hydrochlorothiazide treatment in elderly hypertensive patients. J Cardiovasc Pharmacol 15(Suppl 1):S90, 1990.

113. Sinzinger H, Fitscha P: Antiatherosclerotic actions of isradipine. J Cardiovasc Pharmacol 19(Suppl 3):S29, 1992.

114. Borhani NO, Miller ST, Brugger SB, et al: MIDAS: Hypertension and atherosclerosis. A trial of the effects of antihypertensive treatment on atherosclerosis. MIDAS Research Group. J Cardiovasc Pharmacol 19(Suppl 3):S16, 1992.

115. Cutler SA, Hammond JJ: A multicenter comparison of isradipine and felodipine in the treatment of mild to moderate hypertension. The physician's study group. Am J Hypertens 6:44S, 1993.

116. Gross P, Koppenhagen K, Wudel E, et al: Hemodynamic effects of isradipine and nifedipine in chronic sustained hypertension. J Cardiovasc Pharmacol 19(Suppl 3):S84, 1992.

117. Welzel D, Burger KJ: The calcium antagonist isradipine in the therapy of hypertension. A double blind crossover comparison with nifedipine. Drugs 40(Suppl 2):60, 1990.

118. Welzel D, Burger KJ, Weidinger G: Calcium antagonists as first line antihypertensive agents: A placebo controlled, comparative trial of isradipine and nifedipine. J Cardiovasc Pharmacol 15(Suppl 1):S70, 1990.

119. Kantola I, Rauhala E, Erkinjuntti M, et al: Sleep disturbances in hypertension: A double blind study between isradipine and metoprolol. J Cardiovasc Pharmacol 18(Suppl 3):S41, 1991.

120. Fitscha P, Meisner W, Hitzenberger G: Evaluation of isradipine

and captopril alone or in combination for the treatment of hypertension. J Cardiovasc Pharmacol 18(Suppl 3):S12, 1991.

121. Holtzman JL, Abrams A, Cutler R, et al: Multicenter comparison of once and twice daily isradipine to hydrochlorothiazide for the treatment of hypertension in elderly patients. Clin Pharmacol Ther 48:590, 1990.

122. Swartz SL, Gonasun LM, McAllister RG Jr, et al: A multicenter comparison of isradipine and prazosin for treatment of essential hypertension. Cardiovasc Drugs Ther 4:413, 1990.

123. Carlsen JE, Kober L: Blood pressure lowering effect and adverse events during treatment of arterial hypertension with isradipine and hydrochlorothiazide. Drug Invest 2:10, 1990.

124. Prisant LM, Carr M, Nelson EB, et al: Isradipine vs. propranolol in hydrochlorothiazide treated hypertensives: A multicenter evaluation. Arch Intern Med 149:2453, 1989.

125. A multicenter evaluation of the safety and efficacy of isradipine and atenolol in the treatment of hypertension. Am J Med 86(Suppl 4A):119, 1989.

126. Vermeulen A, Wester A, Willemse PFA, et al: Comparison of isradipine and diltiazem in the treatment of essential hypertension. Am J Med 84(Suppl 3B):42, 1988.

127. Kirkendall WM: Comparative assessment of first line agents for treatment of hypertension. Am J Med 84(Suppl 3B):32, 1988.

128. Grossman E, Messerli FH, Oren S, et al: Disparate cardiovascular response to stress tests during isradipine and fosinopril therapy. Am J Cardiol 72:574, 1993.

129. Midtbo K, Hats O, Vander Meer J: Verapamil compared with nifedipine in the treatment of essential hypertension. J Cardiovasc Pharmacol 4(Suppl 1):S363, 1982.

130. Lo RI, Takeda P, Mason DT, et al: The effects of calcium channel blocking agents on cardiovascular function. Am J Cardiol 62:669, 1982.

131. Cohn JN, Franciosa JA: Vasodilator therapy of heart failure. N Engl J Med 297:27, 1977.

132. Maseri A, Parodi O, Fox KM: Rational approach to the medical therapy of angina pectoris. The role of calcium antagonists. Prog Cardiovasc Dis 25:269, 1983.

133. Handler CE, Sowton E: Safety tolerability and efficacy of PN 200—110 a new calcium antagonist in patients with angina and coronary heart disease. Eur J Clin Pharmacol 27:415, 1984.

134. Taylor SH, Jackson NC, Allen J, et al: Efficacy of a new calcium antagonist PN-200-110 (isradipine) in angina pectoris. Am J Cardiol 59:123B, 1987.

CHAPTER 110

Amlodipine

William H. Frishman, M.D., and Dawn Hershman, M.D.

Amlodipine is a member of a new dihydropyridine subclass of calcium antagonists (prototypes felodipine, nicardipine, isradipine) and is approved for use in the treatment of patients with systemic hypertension and angina pectoris. The clinical usefulness of calcium channel blockade has been well established in the treatment of hypertension[1] and angina[2] and is being explored in a range of other disorders that are mediated by vasoconstrictor or vasospastic reactions. The newer dihydropyridine subclass of calcium antagonists represents an advance over agents of the other classes (verapamil, nifedipine, diltiazem, and others) in that the newer agents cause much less cardiac depression and fewer conduction disorders.

PHARMACODYNAMICS

In Vitro Activity and Mechanistic Studies

Amlodipine inhibited both calcium- and potassium-induced contractions in rat aorta. In contrast with nifedipine, the inhibitory effect of amlodipine develops very gradually, the peak effect being seen at about 3.5 hours (30 minutes for nifedipine). Kinetic analysis indicates that amlodipine associates with and dissociates from its receptor at least two orders of magnitude more slowly than related drugs are reported to do. Moreover, the potency of amlodipine was more than 10 times greater against Ca^{2+} responses than against K^+ responses.[3] Conventional concentration-response curves (Fig. 110–1) allowed for comparison of inhibitory concentration (IC_{50}) values (at the 3.4-hour time point) for amlodipine and nifedipine and confirmed the greater potency of amlodipine against Ca^{2+} responses (1.9 nM) compared with K^+ responses (19.4 nM); nifedipine, in contrast, was only slightly more potent against Ca^{2+} (4.1 nM) than against K^+ responses (7.1 nM). Determination of PA_2 values (negative log of the molar concentration of antagonist required to produce an agonist/dose ratio equal to 2) against Ca^{2+} responses in both rat aorta and dog coronary artery indicated that amlodipine was a competitive antagonist and slightly more potent than nifedipine (PA_2 values of 9.22 and 9.12 for amlodipine and nifedipine, respectively, in rat aorta);[4] both compounds were somewhat more potent (PA_2 values of 9.5 for both drugs) in dog coronary artery.

Matlib et al.[5] have shown that amlodipine is a potent inhibitor of potassium chloride–induced contractions of the coronary artery from both pigs and humans.

The greater potency of amlodipine (and difference from nifedipine) in antagonizing Ca^{2+} responses versus K^+ responses suggests the possibility that amlodipine may display greater voltage dependence than nifedipine. To examine this possibility, rat portal veins were exposed to various depolarizing concentrations of K^+. The inhibitory effects of various concentrations of either amlodipine or nifedipine were examined on contractions to added high-K^+ solution. Both drugs showed an increase in potency as membrane potential became increasingly negative, with amlodipine showing a greater change (60 times) than nifedipine (6.5

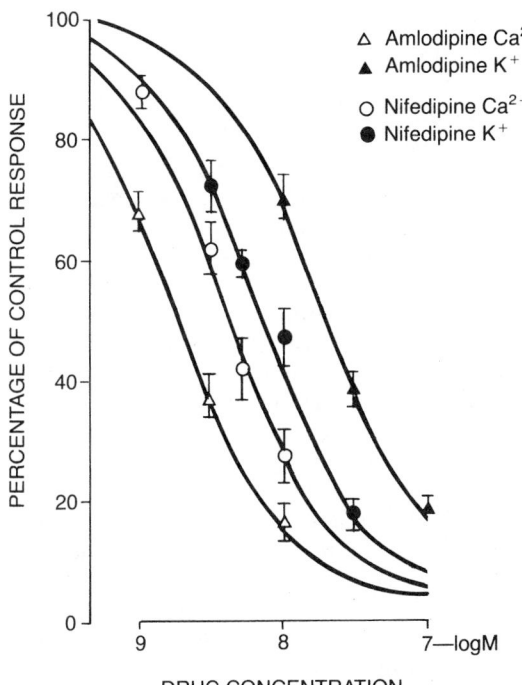

Figure 110–1. Concentration-response curves of amlodipine and nifedipine for the inhibition of Ca^{2+} responses and K^+ responses in rat aorta. Data were derived from the 3.5-hour values, fitted to a sigmoid relationship by a curve-fitting program. Slopes of the individual curves did not differ significantly from one another (*p* > .1), and a common slope was therefore adopted. Each curve differed significantly from the others with respect to their midpoints (*p* < .1001). *Bars* represent standard error of the mean.

times) over the examined range (−8 to −90 mV) of membrane potential.[6]

Phenylephrine-induced contractions of rat aorta were inhibited noncompetitively by both amlodipine and nifedipine, but only some 50% of the phenylephrine response was susceptible to calcium channel blockade. Comparison of IC_{50} values obtained in these experiments with those obtained against Ca^{2+}-induced responses in the same tissue does not suggest any difference in activity of either drug against receptor-operated as opposed to voltage-dependent calcium channels.[3]

In Langendorff-perfused guinea pig hearts, amlodipine and nifedipine showed similar negative inotropic activities; the concentrations producing a 50% inhibition of cardiac contraction were 10 times greater than for inhibition of vascular muscle contraction.[3] However, as in experiments in vascular muscle, amlodipine displayed a markedly longer time to maximal effect (150 to 180 minutes) than nifedipine (10 to 20 minutes). Both drugs displayed modest negative chronotropic effects (approximately 20%) at concentrations of 50 nM. Similar results were obtained in perfused rat hearts in which the measurement of coronary flow showed that amlodipine caused coronary vasodilation at low concentrations, but this effect was reversed at high concentrations because of the negative inotropic effect.[5]

Electrophysiologic experiments conducted using

isolated papillary muscles from guinea pig hearts confirmed that amlodipine is a highly selective Ca^{2+} channel blocker that inhibits cardiac slow action potentials in a non–use-dependent manner and with no effect on the fast Na^+ channel.[3]

Radioligand-binding experiments designed to characterize the interactions of amlodipine with calcium channel binding sites in bovine brain and in cardiac membranes from dog and rat showed that amlodipine interacts competitively and at high affinity with the dihydropyridine recognition site.[7] Thus, amlodipine displaced [3H]nitrendipine and [3H](+)isradipine with k_j values in the low nanomolar range; these effects were highly time-dependent, suggesting slow association of amlodipine. Experiments using [3H]amlodipine as the radioligand also supported high affinity binding to the dihydropyridine site, as shown by its complete displacement by nitrendipine (Fig. 110–2). Kinetic analysis of [3H]amlodipine binding confirmed its very slow association and dissociation with the receptor site. Verapamil caused partial displacement of [3H]amlodipine binding in accord with its reported effects on binding of other dihydropyridine radioligands.

However, the interactions of [3H]amlodipine with other calcium antagonist molecules were clearly more complex than those of other dihydropyridine radioli-

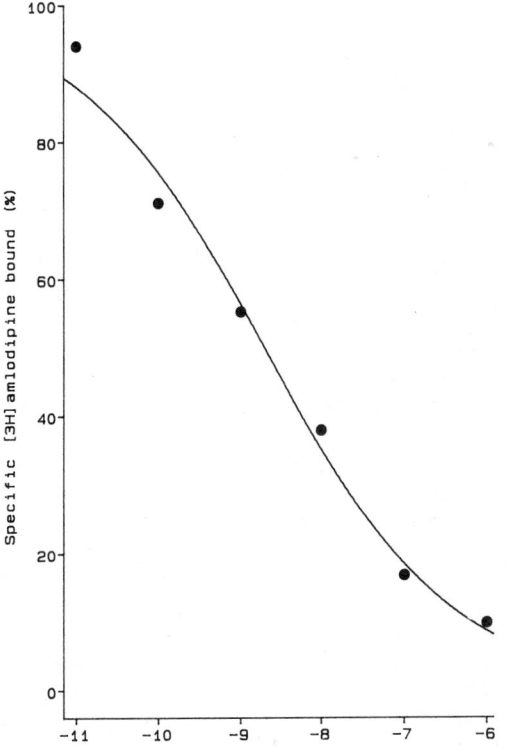

Figure 110–2. Displacement by nitrendipine of the specific binding of [3H]amlodipine to membranes from bovine brain. Membranes were incubated for 90 minutes at 25°C with [3H]amlodipine (30 to 60 Ci/mmol; concentration 0.2 nM) and varying concentrations of nitrendipine. Nonspecific binding was determined in the presence of a high concentration (10 μM) of unlabeled amlodipine. Results are means of triplicate determinations. The k for nitrendipine was 3.3 nM as calculated from this experiment.

gands.[7] [³H]Amlodipine labeled three times more binding sites in canine ventricular microsomes than did [³H](+)isradipine, and the displacement of [³H]amlodipine by dihydropyridines (nitrendipine, amlodipine itself) was characterized by slope factors of less than unity, suggesting multiple binding sites. Most surprisingly, diltiazem caused complete displacement of [³H]amlodipine in both bovine brain and dog cardiac membranes, suggesting interaction with a common binding site, in contrast with its allosteric stimulatory effect on the binding of other dihydropyridine radioligands. Experiments using [³H]diltiazem as the radioligand also indicated that amlodipine combines the effects of a dihydropyridine and a benzothiazepine; amlodipine caused complete displacement of binding at 25°C in rat cardiac membranes, whereas nitrendipine had little effect. At 37°C, amlodipine caused stimulation followed by displacement of [³H]diltiazem binding in both rat and dog cardiac membranes, whereas nitrendipine and isradipine caused only stimulation.[8] This possible direct action of amlodipine at the benzothiazepine receptor site is supported by molecular modeling, showing overlap between the three-dimensional structures of amlodipine and diltiazem.

Cardiovascular Effects

Cardiovascular Activity in Normotensive Animals

In anesthetized dogs, amlodipine is a potent coronary and peripheral vasodilator: ED_{50} values (effective dose) of 103 and 212 μg/kg for reductions of coronary and systemic vascular resistances, respectively. The reductions in vascular resistance are associated with corresponding increases in cardiac output, coronary flow, heart rate, and myocardial contractility.[4] In these respects, amlodipine is similar to nitrendipine; however, it differs markedly, because amlodipine possesses a slower onset of action, having minimal effect on blood pressure, and displays a long duration of action.[9] Amlodipine, like nitrendipine, causes slight, transient, negative inotropic responses only at very high doses (1600 and 128 μg/kg, respectively), in excess of those required to cause maximal vasodilation. Neither drug adversely affects cardiac conduction as assessed by PR interval.

In conscious dogs, intravenously administered amlodipine (250 to 1000 μg/kg) produces long-lasting (up to 4 hours) hemodynamic effects consistent with the actions of an arteriolar vasodilator.[9] After pretreatment with propranolol, the vasodilator effects of amlodipine (500 and 1000 μg/kg) were not changed but, as expected, increases in heart rate and hence cardiac output were attenuated, resulting in a greater lowering of blood pressure. In the presence of propranolol, a slight and transient depression of myocardial contractility occurred; no untoward effects on cardiac conduction were observed.

In conscious dogs in which autonomic nervous input to the heart was suppressed by concomitant administration of atropine and propranolol, intravenously administered amlodipine (250 to 500 μg/kg) was shown to produce modest negative inotropic and chronotropic effects similar in magnitude to those of nifedipine (Pfizer, data on file).

Oral administration of amlodipine (0.5 to 2.0 mg/kg) to conscious dogs produced dose-related reductions in systemic vascular resistance with reflex increases in heart rate, cardiac output, and myocardial contractility; maximum effects were achieved much later (3 to 5 hours) than after parenteral administration (5 to 30 minutes). Oral administration of 1 mg/kg for 13 days produced hemodynamic effects consistent with the acute observations, as well as some day-to-day carryover of response, but some nonprogressive attenuation of peak effect was evident (Pfizer, data on file).

Gross et al. investigated the potentially protective effects of amlodipine in myocardial ischemia.[10] In anesthetized dogs subjected to 45 minutes of coronary artery occlusion followed by 1 hour of reperfusion, intravenous pretreatment with amlodipine (200 μg/kg) markedly improved the recovery of myocardial segmental function in the ischemic and reperfused region and attenuated the loss of adenine nucleotides and the increase in tissue water. In addition, Nayler[11] has shown that amlodipine administration to rats 10 mg/kg/day in diet or 0.25 mg/kg intravenously, prior to removal of the hearts for perfusion, improved the functional recovery of hearts stunned by 10 minutes of ischemia and attenuated Ca^{2+} gain upon reperfusion after 30 or 60 minutes of ischemia.

The cardioprotective effects of amlodipine on ischemia and myocardial reperfusion were confirmed using two additional experimental models.[12] In feline hearts made globally ischemic for 60 minutes, followed by reperfusion for 60 minutes, pretreatment with amlodipine resulted in protection from depressed myocardial contractility, increased left ventricular end-diastolic activity, and a shift to the left in the pressure-volume curves. In addition, a trend was seen toward an increase in coronary blood flow following reperfusion in the amlodipine-treated group. In canine hearts, the induction of ischemia for 90 minutes, followed by 6 hours of reperfusion, resulted in a reduction of infarct size in the amlodipine group compared with placebo. In addition, a gradual reduction in coronary blood flow was prevented in the amlodipine group. In this study, amlodipine administration was begun 75 minutes following ischemia and 15 minutes prior to reperfusion. Infarct size was measured using both Evans-blue dye and triphenyltetrazolium chloride technique.

Amlodipine was not found to worsen ventricular function when 0.25 mg/kg of amlodipine was administered following ligation of the left anterior descending artery (LAD) in 40 dogs.[13] There was no difference in dP/dt, ejection fraction, or end-diastolic pressure between the amlodipine and placebo groups. There was, however, a nonsignificant trend toward less-functional infarct expansion in the amlodipine-treated group. Furthermore, in the amlodipine group, there was a mild reduction in diastolic pressure and a non-significant trend towards reduction in systolic pressure. The results suggested that amlodipine did not cause any negative inotropic effects during coronary occlusion or reperfusion.

One study suggests that the antiischemic effects seen with amlodipine pretreatment may result from amlodipine attenuating the increase in endothelin-1 binding site density normally observed with ischemia.[14] It is thought that the binding of endothelin-1 results in coronary vasoconstriction, positive inotropic activity, and increased cytosolic calcium. The decrease in endothelin-1 binding sites, therefore, can decrease the damage caused by myocardial infarction.

In contrast, Hagar et al.[15] could not find a decrease in myocardial infarct extent, infarct expansion, wall thinning, or left ventricular cavity dilation 21 days after infarction in amlodipine-treated rats. Drug treatment began 24 hours prior to occlusion of the LAD and continued 7 days following surgery. The three arms of this study consisted of a control group (n = 18), 0.25 mg/kg of amlodipine (n = 16), and 1.0 mg/kg of amlodipine (n = 16). In the high-dose group, mean values of scar thickness tended to be lower and left ventricular cavity size tended to be larger when compared with placebo; however, these differences were not statistically significant. Therefore, despite the effectiveness of angiotensin-converting enzyme (ACE) inhibitors and intravenous nitrates in reducing early infarct expansion, there is no evidence that calcium antagonist treatment with amlodipine can produce similar effects.

Antihypertensive Activity in Hypertensive Animals

Amlodipine produced dose-related reductions in blood pressure of spontaneously hypertensive Okamoto rats after oral administration (1, 3, and 10 mg/kg). In this respect, it was approximately twice as potent as nifedipine and had a considerably longer duration of action, with effects that were maintained for at least 6 hours after administration (Fig. 110–3). Indeed, Fleckenstein et al.[16] showed that amlodipine (10 and 30 mg/kg) was the most potent and longest-acting 1,4-dihydropyridine among a group of calcium antagonists evaluated in spontaneously hypertensive Okamoto rats. In young, spontaneously hypertensive Okamoto rats given amlodipine for 12 weeks in their diet (equivalent to 8 mg/kg/day), the normal age-dependent increase in blood pressure was attenuated with no change in heart rate, plasma renin activity, or ventricular weight.[17] In a similar study involving treatment for 30 weeks at a dose of 10 mg/kg/day, Nayler[11] showed that, in addition to causing a marked attenuation of the rise in blood pressure, amlodipine prevented the development of cardiac hypertrophy in these animals; the ratio of ventricular weight to body weight was reduced to a value similar to that of untreated, normotensive Wistar-Kyoto rats (which showed no blood pressure or cardiac weight response to amlodipine). In mature, spontaneously hypertensive Okamoto rats receiving amlodipine for 8 weeks (in-diet administration of 8 mg/kg/day), a marked antihypertensive effect was evident by day 2 that

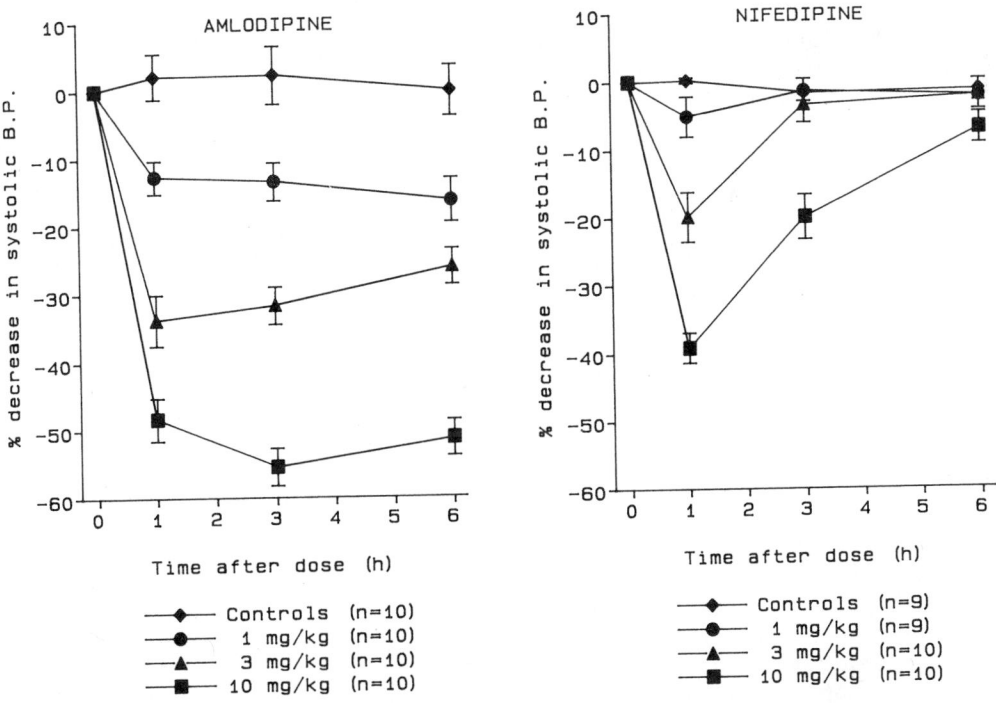

Figure 110–3. Acute oral antihypertensive efficacy of amlodipine and nifedipine in spontaneously hypertensive rats. Systolic blood pressure was recorded by an automated tail-cuff method before and at 1, 3, and 6 hours after oral gavage dosing with amlodipine, nifedipine, or their respective vehicles (distilled water or 25% polyethyleneglycol 200 in distilled water). Predose pressures for the two groups of animals were, respectively, 181 ± 3 and 190 ± 2 mmHg (mean ± standard error of the mean). The doses of amlodipine and nifedipine required to reduce blood pressure by 30% (ED$_{30}$) were calculated to be 2.5 and 5.6 mg/kg, respectively.

attained maximum effect by day 5.[17] This effect was maintained for the remaining treatment period with no change in heart rate. In addition, treated animals showed a small but statistically significant reduction in ventricular weight and a marked elevation in plasma renin activity.

In conscious renal hypertensive dogs, oral administration of amlodipine (0.5, 1, and 2 mg/kg) produced dose-related reductions in blood pressure, with maximum effects occurring between 3.5 and 7.0 hours after dose.[18] In contrast, nifedipine (0.05 to 0.25 mg/kg) caused rapid and relatively transient responses (recovery within 3 to 6 hours). Dose-related tachycardia accompanied the hypotensive effects of both compounds. In a separate comparative study, oral administration of nitrendipine (0.125 to 0.5 mg/kg) also produced rapid and short-lived antihypertensive effects; however, the degree of heart rate increase for similar decreases in blood pressure was greater for nitrendipine than for amlodipine (0.25 to 1 mg/kg) (Pfizer, data on file).

The slow onset and long-lasting antihypertensive effects of amlodipine were confirmed in conscious renal hypertensive dogs in which blood pressure was recorded continuously for 24 hours while the dogs were ranging freely within kennels. Thus, amlodipine (1 mg/kg by mouth) produced a maximal decrease in blood pressure 13 hours after dose, with antihypertensive efficacy maintained from 3 to at least 17 hours after dose. In contrast, 6 hourly oral doses of nitrendipine (1 mg/kg) over the same period produced discrete blood pressure reductions that were rapid in onset and that recovered within each 6-hour dosing interval (Pfizer, data on file).

In multiple-dose studies (14 days' duration) in conscious renal hypertensive dogs, orally administered amlodipine (0.025 and 0.05 mg/kg/day—doses that are ineffective acutely) produced progressive reductions in the daily resting predose blood pressure, which stabilized after 4 or 5 days and which gradually recovered to predose values during the 72 hours after cessation of treatment.[18] In a separate 10-day study at the higher dose, acute daily predose hypotensive responses were observed in addition to the gradual reduction in predose pressure. The minimum blood pressures achieved each day were similar, and tolerance did not develop. Heart rate was affected inconsistently, but anorexia and subcutaneous edema developed in the later stages of the high-dose study.

In a study designed to relate the antihypertensive efficacy of amlodipine to its pharmacokinetic profile, conscious renal hypertensive dogs received amlodipine (0.4 or 0.8 mg/kg/day) for 9 days. The results of this study indicated that the antihypertensive effect produced and the associated steady-state plasma concentrations were dose-related, well correlated, and consistent with the long half-life of the drug. In contrast with the other multiple-dose studies, however, plasma renin activity and plasma aldosterone concentration increased, which probably countered the anti-

hypertensive efficacy of amlodipine to some extent (Pfizer, data on file).

Amlodipine given intravenously (0.25, 0.5, and 1 mg/kg) to conscious renal hypertensive dogs produced dose-related reductions in blood pressure and increases in heart rate; maximum effects on blood pressure occurred 60 to 75 minutes after administration with no recovery after the higher doses during the 3-hour observation period. Although amlodipine (0.5 and 1 mg/kg) inhibited the normal maintenance of blood pressure during postural change in these dogs, the effect was less severe than that of agents known clinically to be associated with postural hypotension (Pfizer, data on file).

In a study designed to assess the hemodynamic effects of a combination of the calcium antagonist amlodipine (0.5 mg/kg) and the ACE inhibitor benazeprilat (10 mg/kg) in hypertensive rats, a greater reduction in blood pressure was elicited with combination therapy than was obtained with either therapy alone.[19] In addition, the accompanying tachycardia was no greater with combination therapy than that evoked by the same dose of amlodipine. The results of this study suggest that blood pressure control may be adequate with lower doses of each agent when given in combination, with a possible decrease in adverse events. Further studies are required to evaluate this hypothesis.

Cardiovascular Activity in Patients with Stable Angina

After intravenous infusion of amlodipine (four consecutive doses with a total cumulative dose of 20 mg) in patients with stable angina, systemic vascular resistance was decreased, thereby reducing left ventricular afterload and leading to an augmentation of cardiac performance.[20] In another study, after intravenous infusion of amlodipine (two consecutive doses with a total cumulative dose of 10 mg), pulmonary artery occlusion pressure (preload) and left ventricular filling pressure were decreased during constant load exercise (Pfizer, data on file). In a third study, after a single intravenously administered 10-mg dose of amlodipine and under nonpaced heart conditions, left ventricular dP/dt values increased. Under paced heart conditions after amlodipine infusion, blood pressure was reduced to a greater degree, and a higher level of pacing frequency and pacing time were required to elicit anginal symptoms. Coronary sinus oxygen saturation increased under nonpaced and paced heart conditions after amlodipine administration but, in general, myocardial metabolic indices (coronary sinus oxygen saturation, coronary sinus lactate, coronary sinus pyruvate, coronary sinus free fatty acid) showed little change.[21]

Effects on the Renal System

In normotensive rats and spontaneously hypertensive Okamoto rats, a single oral 10-mg/kg dose of amlodipine produced a substantial natriuretic effect with some increase in urine volume within a 24-hour period. These effects were greater than those produced by diltiazem (100 mg/kg by mouth) and were in marked contrast with the substantial antinatriuretic effect of the directly acting vasodilator, minoxidil. Normotensive rats also received a once-daily 10-mg/kg oral dose of amlodipine for 4 days, which produced marked natriuresis and diuresis in contrast with the smaller and inconsistent responses to twice-daily dosing with felodipine (10 mg/kg) or nitrendipine (30 mg/kg). In spontaneously hypertensive Okamoto rats receiving amlodipine in their diet (equivalent to 8 mg/kg/day), marked and sustained increases above control values in both urine volume and sodium excretion were seen over a 4-week period.[17]

Johns[22] has investigated the mechanism of the natriuretic effect of amlodipine in both normotensive rats and spontaneously hypertensive Okamoto rats. Intravenously administered amlodipine had little effect on renal hemodynamics despite a reduction in blood pressure, but glomerular filtration rate was modestly increased in spontaneously hypertensive Okamoto rats. However, amlodipine caused substantial increases in urine flow and in both absolute and fractional sodium excretion; these effects were found to be located in the distal portions of the renal tubule (including the loop of Henle), because absorption of fluid and sodium in the proximal nephron was unaffected. An additional study showed that amlodipine inhibited the ability of renal nerve stimulation to enhance tubular sodium reabsorption in spontaneously hypertensive Okamoto rats but not in normotensive rats,[23] which may translate to natriuretic effects of amlodipine in hypertensive patients.

In anesthetized saline-loaded dogs, bolus intravenous doses of amlodipine (up to 200 μg/kg) produced diuretic and natriuretic effects with up to a fourfold increase in sodium excretion; threshold effects were seen at a dose of 25 μg/kg. At doses higher than 400 μg/kg, these effects were reversed. In further experiments, a single intravenous dose of amlodipine (105 μg/kg), which produces half maximal coronary vasodilation, produced fourfold and twofold increases in sodium excretion and urine volume, respectively, over a 2-hour period; potassium excretion was only slightly elevated.[24]

In conscious normotensive dogs, a single 125 μg/kg intravenous dose of amlodipine approximately doubled the recovery of a previously administered saline load within a 3-hour period.[25]

After daily administration of amlodipine for 6 weeks (mean dose, 8.8 mg/day) to patients with essential hypertension, renal vascular resistance was significantly reduced compared with baseline values. This change was associated with a decrease in systemic arterial pressure and an increase in both glomerular filtration rate, as measured by insulin clearance, and effective renal plasma flow, as measured by paraaminohippurate clearance, compared with baseline levels.[26] There was a slight increase in plasma renin activity after acute administration of amlodipine

(15 mg), but this increase was not apparent after 6 weeks of amlodipine therapy.

PHARMACOKINETIC PROPERTIES

The half-life and oral bioavailability of amlodipine in humans are compared with other calcium antagonists in Table 110-1.[27-32]

Absorption

Amlodipine is well absorbed in animals as judged by the urinary excretion of drug-related material. Oral bioavailability of amlodipine ranges from about 30% in rabbits to 100% in rats. In humans, amlodipine appears to be completely absorbed after oral administration, because the amounts of radiolabel excreted into urine (approximately 60%) and feces (approximately 25%) are the same after oral and intravenous administration.[33] The absolute bioavailability of amlodipine in humans is 60% to 65%.

Food had no effect on the rate of absorption of amlodipine or the total amount of drug absorbed.[32, 34, 35]

Distribution

As for other dihydropyridine calcium antagonists,[36] plasma protein binding of amlodipine is high (rat: 95%, dog: 97%, human: 97%).

Tissue distribution studies have been conducted in rats (pregnant and nonpregnant), rabbits, and dogs; as expected from the large volume of distribution for the unchanged drug (20 to 40 L/kg), low levels of drug-related material were observed in blood, brain, and amniotic fluid. The highest concentrations were observed in the liver, lung, kidneys, and adrenal glands. In humans, amlodipine has an apparent volume of distribution of 21 L/kg.[32]

Metabolism and Excretion

After oral administration of [14C]amlodipine to humans, approximately 60% of the administered radiolabel is recovered in the urine, and 20% to 25% is ultimately recovered in the feces. Examination of urine shows that amlodipine is extensively metabolized, because only 10% of the urinary radioactivity consists of unchanged drug. The remaining radioactivity is distributed among nine inactive metabolites, all of which have been oxidized to the pyridine analogue.[33]

In animals and humans, amlodipine follows first-order elimination kinetics. The values for plasma half-life from single-dose intravenous studies range from 3 hours in rats to 35 hours in humans.[32] Because the volume of distribution for amlodipine in all species investigated is large (21 to 32 L/kg), the longer half-life in mice, dogs, and humans than in rats reflects lower rates of metabolic clearance. In animals and humans, plasma concentrations after oral dosing are generally more sustained than after intravenous dosing. This profile results from peak concentrations that

Table 110–1. **Pharmacokinetic Properties of Some Dihydropyridine Calcium Antagonists in Humans**

Reference	Compound	Dosage	Plasma Half-Life (hr)	Oral Bioavailability (%)
Kleinbloesem et al.[27]	Nifedipine	10 mg t.i.d.	1.7	56 (10–70)
Vinge et al.[28]	Nimodipine	45 mg q.i.d.	1.1	16 (3–40)
Graham et al.[29]	Nicardipine	10 mg t.i.d.	4.8	16 (11–21)
Raemsch and Sommer[30]	Nitrendipine	10 mg b.i.d.	3.7	29 (14–55)
Edgar et al.[31]	Felodipine	20 mg b.i.d.	2.8 (14*)	15 (6–22)
Faulkner et al.[32]	Amlodipine	10 mg o.d.	45.0	64 (52–88)

*Terminal phase

generally are achieved about 6 hours after administration, suggesting that the drug is absorbed slowly in all species.

The long plasma half-life (about 45 hours) of amlodipine in humans taking multiple oral doses is suitable for a once-daily dosage regimen.[32] The sustained duration of action of amlodipine, as well as its good bioavailability, are properties that set it apart from other dihydropyridine calcium antagonists (see Table 110–1).

The long plasma half-life of amlodipine in dogs and humans and its moderate half-life in mice leads to accumulation with multiple dosing until a steady state is achieved. In dogs and humans, the accumulation is twofold and threefold, with steady-state concentrations approached by the fourth and seventh doses, respectively. In each species investigated, plasma concentrations generally were proportional to the doses administered.

Plasma concentrations of amlodipine in elderly women (≥65 years) may be higher than those in young men (≤45 years). Although the time to maximum plasma concentration and the elimination half-life for elderly men (≥65 years) and women are within the range observed for young men, the area under the plasma concentration–time curves for young men after a 5-mg dose was 1.3 and 2 times that of elderly men and women, respectively. The mean maximum plasma concentration for elderly women was significantly greater than that observed in elderly men; the latter mean maximum plasma concentration was similar to that observed in young healthy men.[37]

The pharmacokinetics of amlodipine have been studied in elderly subjects with and without hypertension. Sixteen healthy elderly subjects consumed 5 mg of amlodipine in a single oral dose and were compared with 12 young subjects who consumed 10 mg of amlodipine in a single oral dose. Elimination half-life was more prolonged in the elderly patients (48 versus 35 hours).[38]

Similarly, after single intravenous doses of amlodipine were given to hypertensive subjects, elimination half-life was prolonged (64 versus 48 hours) and total clearance was decreased (309 versus 410 ml/min) in the elderly patients.[39–41]

Pharmacokinetics in Renal and Hepatic Impairment

In 27 patients with varying degrees of renal impairment, amlodipine (5 mg) was administered orally once daily for 14 days. Plasma concentrations in patients with mild and moderate renal impairment (creatinine clearance, 15 to 29 and 30 to 80 ml/min, respectively) were higher than in patients with severe renal impairment (creatinine clearance, <15 ml/min). Mean elimination half-lives and accumulations in all renally impaired patients were within the range observed in normal volunteers. The data also indicate that any changes in pharmacokinetic parameters (area under the plasma concentration–time curve, maximum plasma concentration, time to the first occurrence of maximum plasma concentration, and elimination half-life) in renally impaired patients would be limited to increases of twofold or less compared with normal volunteers.[42] Because the degree of renal impairment was not correlated with changes in amlodipine plasma concentration, upward titration of amlodipine should be carried out slowly and carefully.

During long-term oral dosing, there is a greater accumulation of amlodipine in patients with severe liver disease than in patients with normal hepatic function. Patients with cirrhosis had prolonged elimination half-lives after a single oral dose of 5 mg of amlodipine. Mean peak plasma concentrations were 2.4 ng/ml for cirrhotic patients and 2.94 ng/ml for controls (Pfizer, data on file).

THERAPEUTIC TRIALS
Studies in Systemic Hypertension

All patients who entered double-blind studies had diagnoses of essential hypertension with untreated diastolic pressure between 95 and 114 mmHg in both the standing and supine positions. Efficacy analyses were based on changes in predose (24 hours after previous dose) supine and standing blood pressure from the baseline value to the end of therapy value. For studies of upward titration, patients followed a protocol-specific titration sequence until goal blood pressure was achieved. Goal blood pressure was defined as a reduction in average supine and average standing diastolic blood pressure to less than 90 mmHg and by at least 10 mmHg (versus end of the placebo run-in period) as measured at the end of the dosing interval. Baseline was defined as the last blood pressure measurement during the placebo run-in period. Pulse rate (supine and standing) was analyzed similarly. In addition to the assessment of mean changes in blood pressure, response was quantitatively assessed. Response was defined as a reduction in supine diastolic pressure to less than 90 mmHg or a reduction of 10 mmHg or more from baseline.

Comparisons with Placebo

Data from two multicenter studies and one single center are presented here. The first multicenter study was a double-blind, 4-week, randomized, parallel-design, dose-response study. After a 4-week, single-blind, placebo run-in period, patients were randomized to receive 1.25 mg (40 patients), 2.5 mg (40 patients), 5 mg (44 patients), or 10 mg (40 patients) of amlodipine or placebo (39 patients). No dosage adjustment was permitted. Statistically significant reductions of at least 11 mmHg for all four blood pressure parameters were observed in the group receiving 10 mg of amlodipine compared with the group receiving placebo (Fig. 110–4). No statistically significant changes were found in pulse rate in any of the groups receiving amlodipine compared with the group receiving placebo. In addition, statistically significant reductions in diastolic pressure (both supine and standing) were observed at the 2.5- and 5-mg dosages of amlodipine compared with the placebo group. The responder rate was higher in each of the groups receiving amlodipine (48% to 63%) than in the group receiving placebo (33%) (Pfizer, data on file).

The second multicenter study was a double-blind, 8-week, randomized, parallel comparison of three doses of amlodipine and placebo, with the possibility of a single stepped-dose titration from 1.25 to 2.5, 2.5 to 5, or 5 to 10 mg after 4 weeks of double-blind

therapy if goal blood pressure was not attained. Randomization to double-blind treatment was preceded by a 4-week, single-blind, placebo run-in period. Two efficacy analyses were performed, one after 4 weeks of double-blind therapy and the second after 8 weeks of double-blind therapy. After 4 weeks of therapy, the difference in mean systolic and diastolic pressure changes between the group receiving 5 mg of amlodipine and the group taking placebo was statistically significant in both the supine and the standing positions (mean decrease, ≥8 mmHg). In the group taking 2.5 mg of amlodipine, supine blood pressure was reduced to a statistically significant degree (mean decrease, ≥6 mmHg) compared with the placebo group. No clinically important pulse rate changes were observed in any of the treatment groups in either the supine or standing positions. After 4 weeks of double-blind therapy, the amlodipine dosage was doubled for 44 of 47 patients in the 1.25- to 2.5-mg regimen, for 39 of 44 patients in the 2.5- to 5-mg regimen, and for 35 of 45 patients in the 5- to 10-mg regimen. The lowest dose for which there was a significant difference between groups receiving amlodipine and that receiving placebo for all four blood pressure measurements was the 2.5- to 5-mg regimen. No clinically important changes in pulse rate were recorded in any treatment groups in either the supine or the standing position. The responder rate was higher in all of the groups taking amlodipine (41% to 73%) than in that receiving placebo (25%). Mean decreases in supine and standing blood pressures of at least 10 mmHg were observed in the groups receiving 2.5 to 5 mg and 5 to 10 mg of amlodipine after 8 weeks of double-blind therapy.[43]

Several studies have evaluated the pattern of blood pressure control over 24 hours with a single dose of amlodipine. One single-center study was a double-blind, 4-week, randomized, parallel-design, fixed-dosage study. After a 4-week, single-blind, placebo run-in period, patients were randomized to receive either 5 mg of amlodipine (10 patients) or placebo (5 patients). Blood pressure was measured with a standard mercury sphygmomanometer 24 hours after administration. In addition, ambulatory blood pressure was measured for the entire 24 hours after administration at the end of the placebo run-in period and at the end of the study. Despite the small number of patients in this study, statistically significant reductions of at least 12 mmHg were noted in all four blood pressure parameters for the group receiving amlodipine compared to the group receiving placebo, with no statistically significant changes in pulse rate. The responder rate for the group taking amlodipine was considerably higher than that of the group receiving placebo (90% versus 10%). Generally, ambulatory diastolic blood pressure decreased to below 90 mmHg during the 24-hour measuring period in the group taking amlodipine, which indicated smooth blood pressure control during normal daily activity without affecting the normal diurnal pattern (Fig. 110–5). A similar pattern of time-effect relationships was observed for the mean ambulatory systolic blood pressures; the

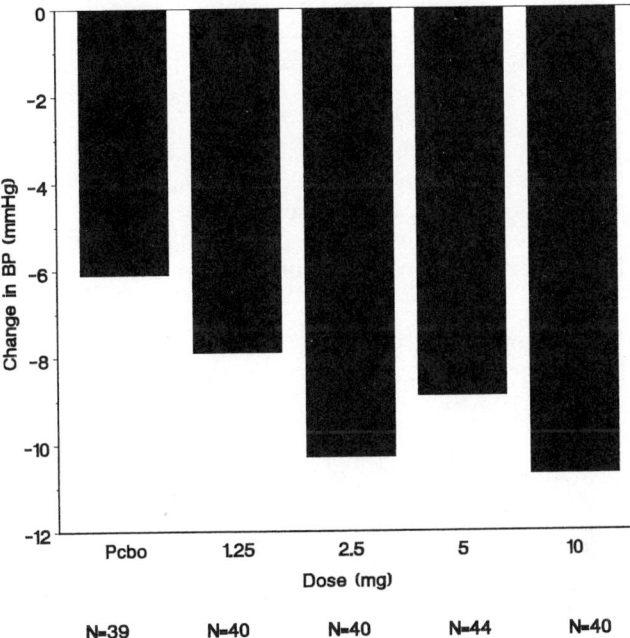

Amlodipine Dose Response

Change in Supine Diastolic Blood Pressure (mmHg)

N=39 N=40 N=40 N=44 N=40

Figure 110–4. Change in supine diastolic blood pressure after administration of amlodipine (1.25, 2.5, 5, or 10 mg) or placebo for 4 weeks.

Mean Ambulatory Diastolic BP (mmHg)
Amlodipine

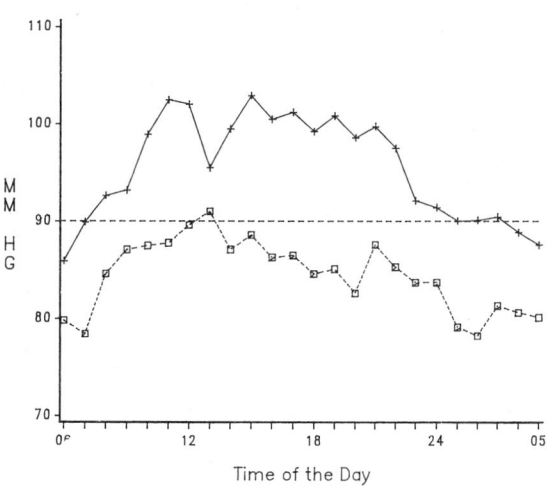

Time of the Day

Mean Ambulatory Diastolic BP (mmHg)
Placebo

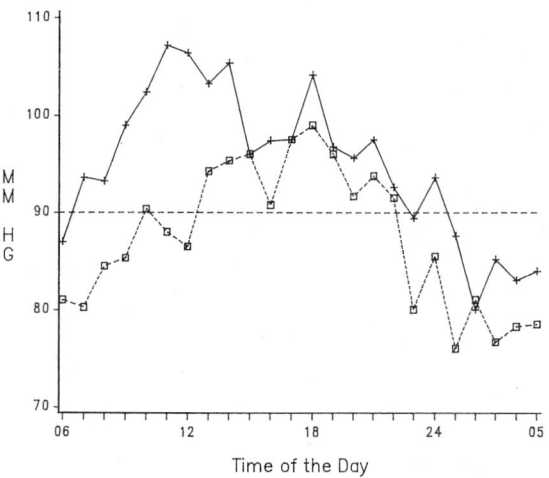

Time of the Day

Figure 110–5. Mean ambulatory diastolic blood pressure (BP) during the 24-hour dosing interval after 4 weeks of amlodipine therapy or placebo therapy.

baseline and final curves are clearly separated. In contrast, placebo-treated patients did not show clinically relevant sustained decreases in ambulatory blood pressure over the 24-hour interval but did show the expected diurnal blood pressure changes during this period.[44]

In a similar study,[45] the 24-hour effectiveness of amlodipine (5 to 10 mg once daily) was evaluated using continuous intraarterial blood pressure monitoring. Monitoring was performed at baseline and after 4 weeks of active treatment in 11 patients with mild to moderate hypertension. Mean blood pressure was significantly reduced during both daytime and nighttime measurements, with no change in heart rate.[45]

The long-term efficacy and tolerability of amlodipine has been evaluated in the Treatment of Mild

Hypertension Study, a double-blind, placebo-controlled, randomized trial that compared six antihypertensive interventions for the treatment of mild hypertension over the course of 4 years.[46] Hypertensive men and women (n = 902) with diastolic blood pressures of less than 100 mmHg were recruited for the study. All participants were advised to reduce weight, dietary sodium intake, and alcohol intake and to increase physical activity. In addition, participants were randomly selected to take placebo, chlorthalidone, acebutolol, doxazosin, amlodipine, or enalapril. For participants with diastolic blood pressures above 95 mmHg on three successive follow-up visits or above 105 mmHg at a single visit, medication dosage was doubled. Nutrition and exercise counseling alone (placebo group) reduced systolic blood pressure by an average of 9.1 ± 0.7 mmHg and diastolic blood pressure by 8.6 ± 0.4 mmHg. Amlodipine (5 mg) was associated with a mean decrease in systolic blood pressure of 15.6 ± 0.9 mmHg and a decrease in diastolic blood pressure of 12.9 ± 0.4 mmHg. There was no significant difference between the placebo and amlodipine treatment groups in relation to quality of life indices or side effect severity scores.

Amlodipine has been found to be safe and efficacious in the elderly and in both genders. Twenty-five patients with isolated systolic hypertension who were between the ages of 65 and 90 years were treated with amlodipine (5 to 10 mg) for 10 weeks in a single-blind, placebo-controlled study.[47] Amlodipine produced significant reduction in mean sitting diastolic and systolic blood pressures. There was no significant change in heart rate. The global efficacy of amlodipine was assessed as excellent or good for 84% of the patients. The toleration of amlodipine was assessed as excellent or good in 88% of patients.

In addition, results from the Amlodipine Cardiovascular Community Trial have shown amlodipine to be an effective and safe once-daily form of monotherapy for both male and female patients and both elderly and young patients.[48, 49] The results from this study in 491 patients were obtained after a 2-week placebo period, followed by a 4-week upward titration phase to achieve goal blood pressure (defined as sitting diastolic blood pressure <90 mmHg or a 10-mmHg reduction in sitting diastolic blood pressure), followed by a 12-week maintenance period.

Comparisons with Positive Control Subjects

Atenolol

One multicenter study was a double-blind, 8-week, randomized, parallel-design, three-way comparative dose-titration study of amlodipine versus atenolol versus placebo. After a 4-week placebo run-in period, patients were randomly assigned to receive once-daily administration of amlodipine (41 patients), atenolol (43 patients), or placebo (41 patients). Amlodipine dosage was doubled biweekly from a starting dose of 2.5 mg to a maximum dose of 10 mg or until goal blood pressure was achieved. Atenolol was similarly titrated from an initial dose of 50 mg up to 100 mg after 4 weeks of therapy. Statistically significant reductions of at least 10 mmHg in supine and standing systolic and diastolic pressures were observed in the amlodipine and atenolol groups when each was compared with placebo. No clinically significant differences were observed in blood pressure between the groups receiving amlodipine and atenolol. Atenolol produced statistically significant reductions of at least 9 beats/min in mean pulse rate in both positions compared with the group taking placebo and the group taking amlodipine, whereas there was no significant difference in supine or standing pulse rate in the amlodipine group compared with the placebo group. The responder rate for the group receiving amlodipine (61%) was comparable with that of the group taking atenolol (65%), and it was considerably higher for both groups than for patients taking placebo (11%).[50]

Verapamil

This multicenter study was a double-blind, 8-week, randomized, parallel-design, three-way comparative dose-titration study of amlodipine versus verapamil versus placebo.[51] After a 4-week, single-blind, placebo run-in period, patients were randomized to receive amlodipine (53 patients), verapamil (54 patients), or placebo (53 patients). Amlodipine was administered once daily, and verapamil and placebo were administered twice daily. Blood pressure was measured 24 hours after administration for the group taking amlodipine and 12 hours after administration for the groups receiving verapamil or placebo; the amlodipine-treated group received placebo as their second dose. Amlodipine dosage was doubled biweekly from a starting dose of 2.5 mg to a maximum dose of 10 mg or until goal blood pressure was achieved. Verapamil was similarly titrated from an initial daily dose of 160 mg to 320 mg after 4 weeks of therapy. Compared with placebo, both verapamil and amlodipine lowered supine and standing diastolic and systolic blood pressures to a statistically significant extent. For supine and standing diastolic blood pressures, amlodipine lowered blood pressure approximately 2.5 mmHg more than verapamil. This difference was found to be significant on a two-tailed test. No differences in mean pulse rate were recorded in any of the three treatment groups. The responder rate for the group taking amlodipine (72%) was higher than that of the group receiving verapamil (48%); the rate for both groups was higher than for the group taking placebo (31%).

Hydrochlorothiazide

A multicenter study compared the efficacy of amlodipine with that of hydrochlorothiazide after 12 weeks of double-blind therapy. After a 4-week, single-blind, placebo run-in period, patients were randomized to receive either amlodipine (78 patients) or hydrochlorothiazide (38 patients). Amlodipine dosage was doubled at monthly intervals from a starting dose of 2.5 mg once daily to a maximum dose of 10 mg once daily or until goal blood pressure was achieved. Hydrochlorothiazide dosage was doubled at monthly intervals from a starting dose of 25 mg to a maximum dose of 100 mg. Clinically significant decreases of at least 9 mmHg in all four blood pressure parameters were observed in both the group taking amlodipine and that receiving hydrochlorothiazide, with no statistically significant differences between the two groups. The responder rates for the two groups were comparable (62% versus 61%).[52]

Angiotensin-Converting Enzyme Inhibitors

Two studies compared the safety and efficacy of amlodipine to those of captopril and enalapril, respectively. The first study was a double-blind, parallel, comparative study of once-daily, orally administered amlodipine (5 to 10 mg daily) and twice-daily, orally administered captopril (25 to 50 mg twice daily) in adult patients with mild to moderate hypertension.[53] The data presented are the result of an interim analysis of data from 40 patients. After a 4-week placebo run-in period, patients were randomized for 10 weeks of active treatment. The dose of amlodipine (5 mg once daily) or captopril (25 mg twice daily) was doubled after 2 weeks if supine diastolic blood pressure remained above 90 mmHg. Blood pressure was assessed 24 hours after a dose of amlodipine and 12 hours after a second dose of captopril. Clinically significant decreases in blood pressure parameters were observed compared with placebo baseline in both the group receiving amlodipine and the group receiving captopril. The two groups showed no statistically significant differences in blood pressure parameters. A significant increase in standing heart rate was observed with captopril therapy. The response rate was highest in the amlodipine-treated group (90.3% versus 78.9%).

The second study was an observer-blind, randomized, parallel-group study comparing amlodipine and enalapril in the treatment of moderate to severe hypertension.[54] After a 2-week placebo run-in phase, 31 subjects were randomized to either amlodipine (5 mg once daily) or enalapril (5 mg once daily) for 8 weeks of treatment. The dose was doubled at week 2 or at week 4 if supine blood pressure exceeded 140/90 mmHg to a maximum of 20 mg of enalapril and 10 mg of amlodipine. Although both treatments were more effective than placebo, amlodipine yielded better results in terms of standing and supine diastolic blood pressures and a nearly significant difference in terms of supine systolic pressure. There was no significant change in heart rate in either treatment group. Data from home blood pressure recordings were analyzed in relation to mean area under the curve. The reduction in area under the curve for diastolic blood pressure was greater for amlodipine ($p = .04$). No difference was observed for systolic pressure.

Multiple Drug Comparisons

Amlodipine was compared with the β-blocker doxazosin, the ACE inhibitor enalapril, and placebo in a 4.4-year parallel design multicenter study of mild hypertension. Although this trial reported some differences in blood pressure control, side effects, quality of life, biochemical effects, and target organ damage, these differences did not present a pattern that consistently favored some drugs and not others.[55–57]

To test the hypothesis that some antihypertensive drugs affect patient outcomes more than others, amlodipine, doxazosin, and lisinopril are being compared to chlorthalidone in 40,000 subjects with mild hypertension (Antihypertensive and Lipid Lowering Treatment to Prevent Heart Attack [ALLHAT]). An attempt will be made in this multicenter, double-blind study to achieve comparable blood pressure control with each drug, to see whether a 20% reduction in coronary heart disease event rate can be observed with the three nondiuretic treatments compared with diuretic.

Combination Therapy

Several studies have evaluated the safety and efficacy of amlodipine (2.5 to 10 mg, once daily) added to ineffective monotherapy with other agents for the treatment of moderate to severe hypertension. In one multicenter, double-blind, parallel study,[58] amlodipine was compared with placebo as add-on therapy in 91 hypertensive patients inadequately controlled on hydrochlorothiazide (50 mg daily for 4 weeks). Clinically significant decreases in all standing and supine blood pressure parameters were observed in the group taking amlodipine. No differences were found between groups in terms of heart rate or electrocardiogram (ECG) changes. Peripheral edema was the only side effect that occurred more frequently in the amlodipine-treated group.

Similarly, in a computer-randomized, double-blind, two-way crossover study, amlodipine (10 mg) was compared with placebo as add-on therapy in 29 hypertensive patients in whom captopril had yielded inadequate blood pressure control (25 mg twice daily for 4 weeks).[59] Again, clinically significant decreases in blood pressure parameters were observed only in the group taking amlodipine. No differences were found between groups in terms of heart rate or ECG changes. Ankle swelling and flushing were the two most frequent amlodipine-related side effects.

Amlodipine has also been shown to be an effective add-on agent to the ACE inhibitor enalapril. In a study design identical to the one just cited, amlodipine (10 mg), when added to enalapril (10 mg), was shown to significantly reduce all blood pressure when compared with enalapril plus placebo.[60] There were no differences between treatment groups in terms of heart rate, ECG, or body weight.

The arterial vasodilator effects of sodium nitroprusside, amlodipine alone, and amlodipine with verapamil were compared in eight patients with mild to moderate hypertension.[61] Arterial vasodilation was assessed by measuring changes in forearm blood flow. Nitroprusside infusion resulted in a 449% increase in flow; amlodipine alone resulted in a 687% increase in flow. The maximal effect was seen using a dose of 45 μg/min/100 ml of amlodipine. The addition of verapamil (40 μg/min/100 ml) to the maximal dose of amlodipine resulted in a further increase in flow. The results confirm that like the other calcium antagonists, amlodipine is a powerful arterial vasodilator. Furthermore, the added vasodilator effect of verapamil suggests a different site of action for the two calcium antagonists. The mechanism of interaction, efficacy, tolerability, and safety need to be determined for this combination drug regimen.

Studies have been carried out examining the efficacy of combining low doses of calcium antagonists and ACE inhibitors as combination formulations in the treatment of hypertension. One such formulation is amlodipine 2.5 mg and benazepril 10 mg, which has been approved for use in hypertension (Lotrel). The combination formulation was shown to be more effective in lowering blood pressure than either component used alone, with a side effect profile similar to that for each monotherapy and placebo.[62]

Studies in Stable Angina

All patients who entered double-blind studies had diagnoses of stable exertional angina. Efficacy parameters included total exercise time, total workload, weekly angina attack rate, and weekly nitroglycerin consumption. Efficacy analyses for total exercise time and total workload were performed on changes from baseline value to end of therapy (24 hours after previous doses). Baseline values for total exercise time and total workload were determined from the last exercise test performed during the placebo run-in period. Baseline values for angina attack rate and nitroglycerin consumption were the number of angina attacks and the number of nitroglycerin tablets consumed during the last week of the placebo run-in period. In addition to these parameters of efficacy, the patients' self-assessments and the investigators' global evaluations were analyzed at the end of therapy and compared with baseline assessments. For all dose-titration studies, patients followed a prescribed titration sequence until optimal antianginal effect had been achieved. Optimal antianginal effect was defined as an abolition of anginal attacks and elimination of ischemic findings on any objective tests obtained in the 2 weeks before review. Total exercise time was measured using treadmill exercise testing according to the modified Bruce protocol[63] or using bicycle ergometry. Total workload in kilopondmeters was estimated after treadmill exercise testing and measured after bicycle exercise testing.

Comparisons with Placebo

Two multicenter, double-blind, 4-week, randomized, parallel-design, dose-response studies were conducted. After a 2-week, single-blind, placebo run-in period, patients were randomized to receive 1.25, 2.5, 5, or 10 mg of amlodipine or placebo. No dosage adjustment was permitted.

The first study involved 21 evaluable subjects in the 1.25-mg group, 25 in the 2.5-mg group, 24 in the 5-mg group, 28 in the 10-mg group, and 25 in the placebo group. At the highest dose level (10 mg/day), amlodipine produced a clinically and statistically significant increase compared with placebo in total treadmill exercise time (16% versus 1%) and total workload (32% versus 3%) (Fig. 110–6) and a significant decrease in angina attack rate (−50% versus −10%) and nitroglycerin consumption (−50% versus −20%). In addition, the total work performed was significantly increased (16%) in the 5-mg group. All other doses of amlodipine also significantly reduced angina attack rate (range, −33% to −43%). Some 70% of the patients taking amlodipine experienced improvement at the end of the study according to the investigators' global evaluations. In addition, the patients' self-ratings showed that amlodipine was associated with greater improvement than was placebo.[64]

The largest dose-response study done to date involved 136 patients with stable, exercise-induced angina pectoris.[65] Compared with placebo, all doses of amlodipine induced an increase in exercise capacity 24 hours after the first dose. Compared with placebo at the highest dose level (10 mg daily), amlodipine increased total exercise duration (31% versus −6%) and exercise time to angina onset (48% versus −8%),

and it decreased angina attack frequency (2.5 versus 1 attacks/week), angina symptoms (48% versus 25%), and nitroglycerin consumption (1.5 versus 0.5 tablets/week). These differences were statistically significant. The highest rate of patients becoming completely symptom-free occurred in the 5-mg amlodipine group (19%). The investigators' overall evaluation showed a significant improvement at each dose level of amlodipine compared with placebo.

The effects of amlodipine (10 mg daily) on both maximal and submaximal exercise performance were studied in 16 patients with chronic stable angina.[66] Consistent with other studies, when compared with placebo, amlodipine decreased both angina frequency and nitroglycerin consumption. At the same time, amlodipine was shown to produce a significant increase in peak oxygen consumption and endurance time during the submaximal exercise test without altering heart rate or double product. During the maximal exercise test, peak oxygen consumption was increased significantly, but total exercise time and other time-related variables were not significantly increased, although the trend was for amlodipine to prolong these values.

Comparisons with Positive Control Subjects

Nadolol

An ongoing multicenter, double-blind, 26-week, randomized dose-titration study compared the efficacy of amlodipine with that of nadolol. After a 2-week, single-blind, placebo run-in period, patients were randomized to receive either amlodipine (32 patients) or nadolol (29 patients). Amlodipine dosage was doubled at monthly intervals from a starting dose of 2.5 mg once daily to a maximum dose of 10 mg once daily or until optimal antianginal efficacy was attained. Nadolol dosage was doubled at monthly intervals from a starting dose of 40 mg once daily to a maximum dose of 160 mg once daily. An interim analysis showed that neither amlodipine nor nadolol had a significant effect on total treadmill exercise time (2% for amlodipine versus −3% for nadolol). However, amlodipine was associated with a 7% increase in total workload versus a 6% decrease with nadolol. Amlodipine was comparable with nadolol in effects on angina attack rate (−88% versus −83%) and was superior with respect to nitroglycerin consumption (−100% versus −50%) (Pfizer, data on file).

Diltiazem

An ongoing, double-blind, 8-week, randomized dose-titration study compared the efficacy of amlodipine with that of diltiazem.[67] After a 2-week, single-blind, placebo run-in period, patients were randomized to receive either amlodipine or diltiazem. Amlodipine was administered once daily, and diltiazem was administered three times daily. Bicycle ergometer testing was performed 24 hours after administration for the amlodipine-treated group and 12 hours after the final

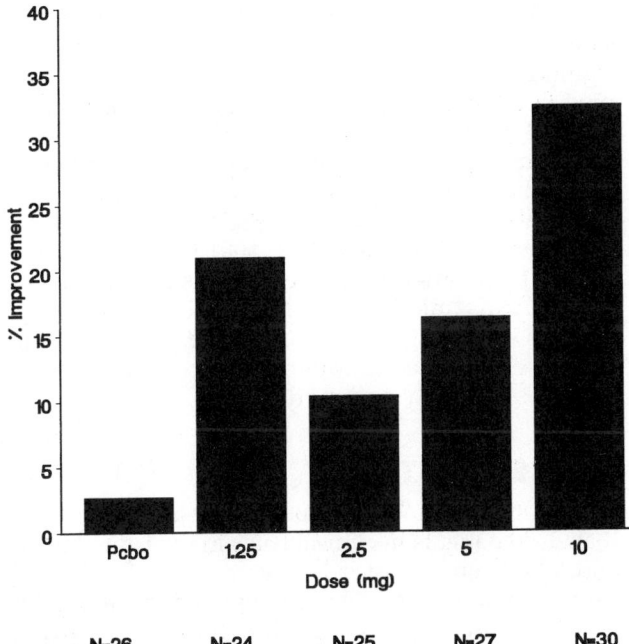

Figure 110–6. Percentage of improvement of total workload (geometric mean) after the administration of amlodipine (1.25, 2.5, 5, or 10 mg) or placebo for 4 weeks.

dose for the diltiazem-treated group. Amlodipine dosage was doubled biweekly from a starting dose of 2.5 mg to a maximum dose of 10 mg or until optimal antianginal effect was attained. Diltiazem was titrated from an initial daily dose of 180 mg to 360 mg after 4 weeks of therapy. The amlodipine group had non-significant increases in exercise time, duration to angina onset, and total work compared with the diltiazem group. Both groups showed a decrease in the mean number of angina attacks and nitroglycerin consumption, although the differences between the groups were not statistically significant. The investigators' overall evaluation of improvement was rated at 82% for the amlodipine group and 80% for the diltiazem group.

Combination Therapy with β-Adrenergic Blockers

In one multicenter, 4-week, double-blind, parallel, randomized study, amlodipine was compared with placebo as add-on therapy in 134 patients with chronic stable angina pectoris being maintained on various β-adrenergic blocking agents.[68] After a 2-week placebo period, patients were randomized to receive either amlodipine (2.5, 5, and 10 mg daily) or placebo compared with placebo plus β-blockade. Exercise capacity improved with β-blockers plus amlodipine at 5 and 10 mg daily. Similarly, total exertional work was significantly improved with 5 and 10 mg of amlodipine. The 10-mg dose of amlodipine increased time to 1-mm ST-segment depression. All three doses of amlodipine reduced angina frequency and nitroglycerin consumption, although the differences from placebo were not significant. No differences were observed in terms of rate-pressure product. The patients' self-assessment of angina severity revealed significant improvements in 40% to 50% of the patients taking 5 and 10 mg of amlodipine ($p < .01$).

Similar results were described from a European, multicenter, 8-week, double-blind, placebo-controlled, dose-titration study.[69] Amlodipine produced a significantly greater increase in the time to onset of angina compared with placebo as add-on therapy in patients inadequately treated with β-blockers. The total exercise time increased and angina attack frequency and nitroglycerin consumption rate decreased compared with placebo, but the results were not significant. Investigators' assessment of efficacy was 83% and 60% for the amlodipine and placebo groups, respectively.

Studies in Vasospastic Angina

In one multicenter, randomized, parallel, double-blind study,[70] amlodipine (10 mg daily) was compared with placebo in patients who had a history of angina at rest. In addition, the patients had either documentation of reversible ST-segment elevation on ECG or of spontaneous or ergonovine-induced coronary artery spasm during cardiac angiography that resulted in at least 70% luminal coronary narrowing and was accompanied by either ischemic chest pain or ST-

segment shifts. After a 3- to 14-day single-blind, placebo run-in, 52 patients were randomized to either 10 mg of amlodipine or placebo every morning for 4 weeks. After 4 weeks, patients were given the option of continuing on open-label year. The rate of anginal attacks decreased significantly during amlodipine therapy as compared with placebo. Nitroglycerin consumption decreased similarly during this time, although the results were not statistically significant. Amlodipine had no significant effect on heart rate or on systolic or diastolic blood pressure compared with placebo. Peripheral edema was the only side effect reported more frequently in the active treatment group. In the 20 patients who entered the open-label protocol, mean frequency of angina decreased from 1.6 to 0.1 episodes per day after 1 year. Similarly, nitroglycerin intake decreased from 1.3 to 0.2 tablets per week.

Studies in Congestive Heart Failure

Amlodipine has less of a negative effect than the dihydropyridine nifedipine.[71] It has been suggested that amlodipine might be a suitable adjunct to conventional therapy (diuretics, digitalis, ACE inhibitors) in patients with chronic congestive heart failure. A pilot, placebo-controlled study demonstrated the safety and efficacy of adding amlodipine to conventional heart failure treatments in patients with improvements in symptoms and exercise tolerance. Most recently the effects of amlodipine were assessed in a thorough, double-blind prospective study in patients with congestive heart failure. Eleven hundred and fifty-three patients with a left ventricular ejection fraction of less than 30% were randomized to receive either amlodipine or placebo in addition to conventional therapy with diuretic, digitalis, and ACE inhibitors. The amlodipine group had a reduction in all-cause mortality that did not quite reach statistical significance ($p < .07$). However, patients on amlodipine fared significantly better than those on placebo ($p < .03$) in the subgroup having dilated cardiomyopathy. Amlodipine was neither detrimental nor beneficial in the other subgroup with ischemic cardiomyopathy. All-cause mortality was 21.5% with amlodipine and 34.9% with placebo ($p < .001$) in patients with dilated cardiomyopathy. These data suggest that it is safe to add amlodipine to conventional therapy in patients with congestive heart failure, and in the subgroup with dilated cardiomyopathy amlodipine diminishes mortality and morbidity.

SIDE EFFECTS

The safety of amlodipine has been evaluated in more than 2500 patients in clinical trials in the United States and elsewhere. Most adverse reactions considered drug related during amlodipine therapy were mild or moderate. In controlled studies directly comparing amlodipine with placebo in the clinical development program, the rate of discontinuation of amlodipine was no different from that of placebo (only 0.5% of

Table 110–2. **Percentage Incidence of Side Effects: Placebo-Controlled Studies**

Adverse Effect	Amlodipine (n = 1438)	Placebo (n = 998)
Edema	3.1	0.3
Headache	1.8	0.7
Flushing	1.5	0
Nausea	0.8	0.3
Palpitations	0.6	0.1
Dizziness	0.5	0.5

patients). The most frequently reported side effects are listed in Table 110–2. No significant difference was observed between amlodipine and placebo in the incidence of side effects except for edema, flushing, and headache (Pfizer, data on file).

Amlodipine has not been associated with clinically significant changes in routine laboratory tests. No clinically relevant changes were noted in serum potassium, serum glucose, total triglycerides, total cholesterol, high-density lipoprotein (HDL) cholesterol, uric acid, blood urea nitrogen, creatinine, or liver function tests (Pfizer, data on file).

Unlike other drugs possessing diuretic properties that show upward trends in triglyceride and very-low-density lipoprotein cholesterol levels and downward trends in HDL cholesterol, amlodipine has been shown not to have significant effects on plasma lipid and lipoprotein levels after 12 weeks of treatment in hypertensive patients.[72] Studies have shown that amlodipine (5 mg daily) given to healthy young men does not change insulin sensitivity or secretion, nor does it change lipoprotein regulation.[73] In addition, amlodipine does not alter lipid fractions or glucose metabolism in patients with diabetes mellitus.[74]

Gingival overgrowth is an unwanted effect associated with use of calcium antagonists, especially dihydropyridines. Hyperplastic gingivitis was reported in three patients consuming 5 to 10 mg daily of amlodipine for 4 to 8 months.[75] The enlargement of gingival tissue began 2 to 3 months the medication was started. The concentration of amlodipine in the gingival crevicular fluid was more than 200 times higher than the increase observed with nifedipine.

In one study in well-compensated New York Heart Association (NYHA) classes II and III heart failure patients already receiving digoxin, diuretics, and ACE inhibitors, amlodipine did not lead to clinical deterioration as assessed by exercise tolerance, left ventricular ejection fraction, and clinical symptoms.[76] In fact, amlodipine treatment resulted in increased exercise time and improved symptoms compared with placebo. No studies have been performed in patients with NYHA class IV congestive symptoms. Amlodipine should be used with caution in treating patients with angina or hypertension who have coexisting congestive heart failure.

DRUG INTERACTIONS

The possible cardiovascular interactions between nitroglycerin and amlodipine were investigated in dogs anesthetized with pentobarbitone. The dogs were prepared so that aortic blood pressure, central venous pressure, heart rate, ECG (lead II), and respiration could be recorded and were subjected to a 2-minute, 90-degree, head-up tilt. There was no evidence of an exaggerated hemodynamic response or of impairment of the postural reflex response to tilt when nitroglycerin (5 µg/kg/min) was infused intravenously for 6 minutes in the presence of intravenously administered amlodipine (150 µg/kg).

One clinical study evaluated the influence of amlodipine on the steady-state pharmacokinetics of digoxin. Twenty-one male volunteers received daily 0.375-mg doses of digoxin for 2 weeks prior to the daily administration of either amlodipine (5 mg) or placebo for an additional 2 weeks. At the end of week 4, the groups were crossed over to the alternative regimen. No statistically significant differences were observed between the groups treated with amlodipine and placebo with respect to plasma digoxin concentrations and digoxin renal clearance.[77]

Another study addressed the effect of concomitant cimetidine therapy on the disposition of amlodipine. Twelve male volunteers were treated with cimetidine (400 mg twice daily) or placebo for 14 days. On the seventh day, the volunteers were challenged with a single oral dose of amlodipine (10 mg). After a 2-week period, the volunteers were subjected to the alternative treatment. No statistically significant changes in amlodipine pharmacokinetics (area under the plasma concentration–time curve, terminal elimination constant, peak plasma concentration, and time to their occurrence) were observed during cimetidine therapy compared with placebo (Pfizer, data on file).

The potential interaction between amlodipine and cyclosporine was evaluated in 10 hypertensive patients who had undergone kidney transplantation.[78] Patients were receiving cyclosporine for a mean period of 16 months. Amlodipine (5 mg) was administered for 12 weeks. Treatment with amlodipine had no effect on cyclosporine trough blood levels, creatinine, blood urea nitrogen, creatinine clearance, or urea clearance. In addition, amlodipine did not alter the time to reach the maximum concentration of cyclosporine in the blood.

Data on *in vitro* human plasma indicate that amlodipine has no effect on protein binding of digoxin, phenytoin, warfarin, or indomethacin (Pfizer, data on file).

DOSAGE AND ADMINISTRATION

In clinical studies of patients with mild to moderate essential hypertension or patients with stable exertional angina, most patients responded satisfactorily to amlodipine with doses of 5 or 10 mg daily. Thus, the usual initial oral dose of amlodipine is 5 mg daily with a one-step titration to 10 mg daily if necessary to achieve the desired reduction in blood pressure or decrease in the incidence of angina attacks.

Small, fragile, elderly individuals or patients with hepatic insufficiency may be started on 2.5 mg daily.

SUMMARY

Compared with other calcium antagonists, amlodipine offers certain unique benefits. It demonstrates marked coronary and peripheral vasodilator properties with no apparent change in heart rate and minimal depression of contraction or electrical conduction. It may also be administered with commonly used medications (e.g., digoxin, cimetidine) without danger of drug interaction. Thus, amlodipine is of particular value in patients with angina and compromised cardiac function or conduction abnormalities, as well as in patients taking multiple medications, including β-blockers. The long half-life (35 to 50 hours) and smooth onset of action of amlodipine allow for 24-hour therapeutic efficacy with once-daily administration without leading to reflex tachycardia. This simplified dosage regimen improves compliance, especially in many elderly patients on multiple drug regimens who require antianginal medication.

In patients with systemic hypertension, amlodipine is effective with once-daily dosage, acting on the primary pathophysiology of idiopathic hypertension-increased peripheral vascular resistance.[1] It appears to be at least as effective as atenolol, hydrochlorothiazide, verapamil, captopril, and enalapril, and it is as well tolerated as these agents. Amlodipine can provide even greater blood pressure control when combined with hydrochlorothiazide, enalapril, and captopril. Amlodipine appears to have no effects on plasma lipids, blood sugar, electrolytes, and uric acid. Its most common side effect is mild peripheral edema.

In summary, amlodipine is a calcium antagonist that, when given once daily, effectively treats stable angina[2] and hypertension.[1] Its efficacy in the treatment of angina is comparable with that of β-blockers and other calcium antagonists. As an antihypertensive, it is at least as effective as β-blockers, ACE inhibitors, diuretics, and other calcium antagonists. It may soon become available as adjunctive treatment in patients with congestive heart failure.[79]

REFERENCES

1. Burris JF, Allenby KS, Mroczek WJ: The effect of amlodipine on ambulatory blood pressure in hypertensive patients. Am J Cardiol 73:39A, 1994.
2. Taylor SH: Usefulness of amlodipine for angina pectoris. Am J Cardiol 73:28A, 1994.
3. Burges RA, Gardiner DG, Gwilt M, et al: Calcium channel blocking properties of amlodipine in vascular smooth muscle and cardiac muscle in vitro: Evidence for voltage modulation of vascular dihydropyridine receptors. J Cardiovasc Pharmacol 9:110, 1987.
4. Burges RA, Carter AJ, Gardiner DG, et al: Amlodipine, a new dihydropyridine calcium channel blocker with slow onset and long duration of action. Br J Pharmacol 85:281, 1985.
5. Matlib MA, French JF, Grupp IL, et al: Vasodilatory action of amlodipine on rat aorta, pig coronary artery, human coronary artery and on isolated Langendorff rat heart preparations. J Cardiovasc Pharmacol 12(Suppl 7):S50, 1988.
6. Burges RA, Dodd MG, Gardiner DG: Pharmacological profile of amlodipine. Am J Cardiol 64:101, 1989.
7. Rigby JW, Greengrass PM, Gardiner DG, et al: Interaction of amlodipine with calcium channel binding sites. Cardiovasc Drugs Ther 1:281, 1987.
8. Burges R, Maisey D: Unique pharmacologic properties of amlodipine. Am J Cardiol 73:2A, 1994.
9. Dodd MG, Gardiner DG, Carter AG, et al: The hemodynamic properties of amlodipine in anesthetized and conscious dogs: Comparison with nitrendipine and influence of beta-adrenergic blockade. Cardiovasc Drugs Ther 3(4):545, 1989.
10. Gross G, Farber NE, Pieper GM: Effect of amlodipine on myocardial function and metabolic recovery following coronary occlusion and reperfusion in dogs. FASEB J 2:1054, 1988.
11. Nayler WG: The effect of amlodipine on hypertension-induced hypertrophy and reperfusion induced calcium overload. J Cardiovasc Pharmacol 12(Suppl 7):S41, 1988.
12. Hoff PT, Tamura Y, Lucchesi BR: Cardioprotective effects of amlodipine on ischemia and reperfusion in two experimental models. Am J Cardiol 66l:10H, 1990.
13. Kloner RA, Hale SL, Alker KJ: Absence of hemodynamic deterioration in the presence of amlodipine following experimental myocardial infarction. J Cardiovasc Pharmacol 20:837, 1992.
14. Nayler WG, Ou RC, Gu XH, et al: Effect of amlodipine pretreatment on ischaemia-reperfusion-induced increase in cardiac endothelin-l binding site density. J Cardiovasc Pharmacol 20:416, 1992.
15. Hagar JM, Newman LG, Kloner RA: Effects of amlodipine on myocardial infarction, infarct expansion, and ventricular geometry in the rat. Am Heart J 124:571, 1992.
16. Fleckenstein A, Frey M, Zorn J, et al: Particular antihypertensive profile of amlodipine administered orally to Okamoto rats (SHRs) and NaCl-loaded salt-sensitive rats. J Cardiovasc Pharmacol 12(Suppl 7):S39, 1988.
17. Burges RA, Gardiner DG, Carter AJ, et al: Amlodipine: Long-term natriuretic and antihypertensive activity in spontaneously hypertensive rats with developing and established hypertension. Ann N Y Acad Sci 522:516, 1988.
18. Dodd MG, Machin I: Antihypertensive effects of amlodipine, a novel dihydropyridine calcium channel blocker. Br J Pharmacol 85:335, 1985.
19. Bazil MK, Webb RL: Hemodynamic effects of amlodipine and benazeprilat in spontaneously hypertensive rats. J Cardiovasc Pharmacol 21:405, 1993.
20. Frais MA, Silke B, Verma SP, et al: A haemodynamic dose finding study with a new slow-calcium channel blocker (amlodipine) in coronary artery disease. Herz 11:351, 1986.
21. Hogg KJ, Hornung RS, Hillis WS, et al: Pharmacodynamics of amlodipine: Hemodynamic effects and antianginal efficacy after atrial pacing. Am Heart J 118:1107, 1989.
22. Johns EJ: A study of the renal actions of amlodipine in the normotensive and spontaneously hypertensive rat. Br J Pharmacol 94:311, 1988.
23. Johns EJ: A study of the action of amlodipine on adrenergically regulated sodium handling by the kidney in normotensive and hypertensive rats. Br J Pharmacol 93:561, 1988.
24. Carter AJ, Gardiner DG, Burges RA: Natriuretic activity of amlodipine, diltiazem and nitrendipine in saline-loaded anesthetised dogs. J Cardiovasc Pharmacol 12(Suppl 7):S34, 1988.
25. Dodd MG, Machin I, Carter AJ, et al: Natriuretic properties of amlodipine in the dog. Cardiovasc Drugs Ther 1:229, 1987.
26. Bauer JH, Reams GP: Amlodipine monotherapy reverses renal vascular abnormalities in hypertension. Kidney Int 31:295, 1987.
27. Kleinbloesem CH, Van Brummelen P, Van de Linde J, et al: Nifedipine: Kinetics and dynamics in healthy subjects. Clin Pharmacol Ther 35:742, 1984.
28. Vinge E, Andersson KE, Brandt L, et al: Pharmacokinetics of nimodipine in patients with aneurysmal subarachnoid haemorrhage. Eur J Clin Pharmacol 30:421, 1986.
29. Graham DJM, Dow RJ, Freedman D, et al: Pharmacokinetics of nicardipine following oral and intravenous administration in man. Postgrad Med J 60(Suppl 4):7, 1984.

30. Raemsch KD, Sommer J: Pharmacokinetics and metabolism of nitrendipine. *In* Scriabine A, Vanov S, Deck D (eds): Nitrendipine. Baltimore: Urban & Schwarzenberg, 1984, pp 409–422.

31. Edgar B, Regardh CG, Johnsson G, et al: Felodipine kinetics in healthy man. Clin Pharmacol Ther 38:205, 1985.

32. Faulkner JK, McGibney D, Chasseaud LF, et al: The pharmacokinetics of amlodipine in healthy volunteers after single intravenous and oral doses and after 14 repeated oral doses given once daily. Br J Clin Pharmacol 22:21, 1986.

33. Beresford AP, McGibney D, Humphrey MJ, et al: Metabolism and kinetics of amlodipine in man. Xenobiotica 18:245, 1988.

34. Abernethy DR: An overview of the pharmacokinetics and pharmacodynamics of amlodipine in elderly persons with systemic hypertension. Am J Cardiol 73:10A, 1994.

35. Abernethy DR, Schwartz JB: Pharmacokinetics of calcium antagonists under development. Clin Pharmacokin 15:1, 1988.

36. Rosenkranz H, Schlossmann K, Scholtan W: The binding of 4-(2′-nitrophenyl)-2,6-dimethyl-1,4-dihydropyridine-3,5-dicarboxylic and dimethyl ester (nifedipine) and other coronary-active substances to serum proteins. Arzneimittelforschung 24:455, 1974.

37. Elliott HL, Meredith PA, Faulkner J, et al: A comparative evaluation of the disposition of amlodipine in young and elderly subjects. J Cardiovasc Pharmacol 12(Suppl 7):S64, 1988.

38. Abernethy DR, Gutkowska J, Lambert MD: Amlodipine in elderly hypertensive patients: Pharmacokinetics and pharmacodynamics. J Cardiovasc Pharmacol 12(Suppl 7):S60, 1988.

39. Elliot HL, Meredith PA, Reid JL, et al: A comparison of the disposition of single oral doses of amlodipine in young and elderly subjects. J Cardiovasc Pharmacol 39:799, 1988.

40. Burges RA, Dodd MG: Amlodipine. Cardiovasc Drug Rev 8(1):25, 1990.

41. Abernethy DR: The pharmacokinetic profile of amlodipine. Am Heart J 118:1100, 1989.

42. Laher MS, Kelly JG, Doyle GD, et al: Pharmacokinetics of amlodipine in renal impairment. J Cardiovasc Pharmacol 12(Suppl 7):S60, 1988.

43. Frick MH, McGibney D, Tyler HM: Amlodipine: A double-blind evaluation of the dose-response relationship in mild to moderate hypertension. J Cardiovasc Pharmacol 12(Suppl 7):S76, 1988.

44. Mroczek WJ, Burris JF, Allenby KS: A double-blind evaluation of the effect of amlodipine on ambulatory blood pressure in hypertensive patients. J Cardiovasc Pharmacol 12(Suppl 7):S79, 1988.

45. Haber ME, Brigden G, Al-Khawaja I, et al: Twenty-four hour blood pressure control with the once daily calcium antagonist amlodipine. Br J Clin Pharmacol 151:1413, 1989.

46. Neaton JD, Grimm RH Jr, Prinea RJ, et al: Treatment of mild hypertension study: Final results. JAMA 270(6):713, 1993.

47. Vandewoude MFJ, Lambert M, Vryens R: Open evaluation of amlodipine in the monotherapeutic treatment of systolic hypertension in the elderly. J Cardiovasc Pharmacol 17(1):S28, 1991.

48. Sowers JR, DiBona GF, Kloner RA, et al: Influence of age on the antihypertensive and metabolic effects of amlodipine in patients with essential hypertension [abstract]. J Am Soc Nephrol 3:537, 1992.

49. Sowers JR, DiBona GF, Kloner RA, et al: Influence of sex on the antihypertensive and metabolic effects of amlodipine in patients with essential hypertension [abstract]. J Am Soc Nephrol 3:538, 1992.

50. Frishman WH, Brobyn RD, Brown RD, et al: Amlodipine versus atenolol in essential hypertension. Am J Cardiol 73:50A, 1994.

51. Lorimer AR, Smedsrud T, Walker P, et al: A comparison of amlodipine, verapamil and placebo in the treatment of mild to moderate hypertension. J Hum Hypertens 3:191, 1989.

52. Burris JF, Ames RP, Applegate WB, et al: Double-blind comparison of amlodipine and hydrochlorothiazide in patients with mild to moderate hypertension. J Cardiovasc Pharmacol 12(Suppl 7):S98, 1988.

53. Velasco M, Urbina A, Silva H, et al: A double-blind, parallel, comparative evaluation of amlodipine versus captopril in the monotherapeutic treatment of mild to moderate essential hypertension. J Cardiovasc Pharmacol 17(1):Sl9, 1991.

54. Fowler F, Webster J, Lyons K, et al: A comparison of amlodipine with enalapril in the treatment of moderate/severe hypertension. Br J Clin Pharmacol 35:491, 1993.

55. The Treatment of Mild Hypertension Research Group: The Treatment of Mild Hypertension Study: A randomized, placebo-controlled trial of a nutritional-hygienic regimen along with various drug monotherapies. Arch Intern Med 151:1413, 1991.

56. Neaton JD, Grimm RH Jr, Prineas RJ, et al, for the Treatment of Mild Hypertension Study: Final results. JAMA 270:713, 1993.

57. Grimm RH: Antihypertensive treatment comparison trials: Quality of life effects. *In* Izzo JL, Black HR (eds): Hypertension Primer. Dallas, TX: American Heart Association, 1993, pp 202–204.

58. Glasser SP, Chrysant SG, Graves J, et al: Safety and efficacy of amlodipine added to hydrochlorothiazide therapy in essential hypertension. Am J Hypertens 2:154, 1989.

59. MacLean D, Mitchell ET, Wilcox RG, et al: Amlodipine and captopril in moderate-severe essential hypertension. J Hum Hypertens 2:127, 1988.

60. Jensen H, Garsdal P, Davies J: Amlodipine with enalapril therapy in moderate-severe essential hypertension. J Hum Hypertens 4:541, 1990.

61. Kiowski W, Erne P, Linder L, et al: Arterial vasodilator effects of the dihydropyridine calcium antagonist amlodipine alone and in combination with verapamil in systemic hypertension. Am J Cardiol 66:1496, 1990.

62. Frishman WH, Ram CVS, McMahon FG, et al, for the Benazepril/Amlodipine Study Group: Comparison of amlodipine and benazepril monotherapy to combination therapy in patients with systemic hypertension: A randomized, double-blind, placebo-controlled, parallel group study. J Clin Pharmacol (In press).

63. Bruce RA, Hornstein TR: Exercise stress testing in evaluation of patients with ischemic heart disease. Prog Cardiovasc Dis 11:371, 1969.

64. Thadani U: Amlodipine—a once a day calcium channel blocker in the treatment of angina pectoris: A parallel, dose response, placebo controlled study. J Cardiovasc Pharmacol 12(Suppl 7):S114, 1988.

65. Taylor SH, Lee P, Jackson N, et al: A double-blind, placebo-controlled, parallel dose-response study of amlodipine in stable exertional angina pectoris. J Cardiovasc Pharmacol 17(1):S46, 1991.

66. Kinnard DR, Harris M, Hossack KF: Amlodipine in angina pectoris: Effect on maximal and submaximal exercise performance. J Cardiovasc Pharmacol 12(Suppl 7):S110, 1988.

67. Bernink PJLM, Weerd P, Cate FJ, et al: An 8 week, double-blind study of amlodipine and diltiazem in patients with stable exertional angina pectoris. J Cardiovasc Pharmacol 17(1):S53, 1991.

68. DiBianco R, Schoomaker FW, Singh JB, et al: Amlodipine combined with beta blockade for chronic angina: Results of a multicenter, placebo-controlled, randomized, double-blind study. Clin Cardiol 15:519, 1992.

69. Klein W, Mitrovic V, Neuss H, et al: A 6 week, double-blind comparison of amlodipine and placebo in patients with stable exertional angina pectoris receiving concomitant beta blocker therapy. J Cardiovasc Pharmacol 17(1):S50, 1991.

70. Chahine RA, Feldman RL, Giles TD: Randomized placebo-controlled trial of amlodipine in vasospastic angina. J Am Coll Cardiol 21(6):1365, 1993.

71. Landau AJ, Gentilucci M, Cavusoglu E, et al: Calcium antagonists for the treatment of congestive heart failure. Coron Art Dis 5:37, 1994.

72. Ahaneku JE, Taylor GO, Agbedana EO, et al: Effects of amlodipine on plasma lipid and lipoprotein levels in hypertensive patients. J Intern Med 232:489, 1992.

73. Ferrari P, Giachino D, Weidmann P, et al: Unaltered insulin sensitivity during calcium channel blockade with amlodipine. Eur J Clin Pharmacol 41:109, 1991.

74. Beretta-Piccoli C, Zanetti-Elshater F, Riesen W, et al: Calcium antagonists for diabetic hypertension: Metabolic and renal effects of amlodipine [abstract]. Am J Hypertens 6(5):128, 1993.

75. Ellis JS, Seymour RA, Thomason JM, et al: Gingival sequestra-

tion of amlodipine and amlodipine-induced gingival over-growth [abstract]. Lancet 341:1102, 1993.
76. Packer M, Nicod P, Khandheria BR, et al: Randomized, multi-center, double-blind placebo-controlled evaluation of amlodipine in patients with mild to moderate heart failure [abstract]. J Am Coll Cardiol 17(2):274A, 1991.
77. Schwartz JE: The effects of amlodipine on steady-state digoxin

concentrations and renal digoxin clearance. J Cardiovasc Pharmacol 12:1, 1988.
78. Grezard O, Sharobeem R, Najjar AA, et al: Effect of amlodipine on cyclosporin pharmacokinetics [abstract]. Am J Hypertens 6(5):1038, 1993.
79. Frishman WH: Current Cardiovascular Drugs, 2nd ed. Philadelphia: Current Science, 1995.

CHAPTER 111

Felodipine

Margareta I. L. Nordlander, Ph.D., Franz H. Messerli, M.D., and Alberto Zanchetti, M.D.

Felodipine, a second-generation dihydropyridine calcium antagonist, exerts its potent antihypertensive effects by relaxing vascular smooth muscle, predominantly in the arteriolar resistance vessels.[1] In contrast with other calcium antagonists, felodipine has shown no direct effect on myocardial function.[2-5] Felodipine has been marketed in most countries worldwide for the treatment of hypertension. The drug was introduced internationally in an extended-release formulation, allowing once-daily administration.

CHEMISTRY

Felodipine, 4-(2,3-dichlorophenyl)-1,4-dihydro-2,6-dimethyl, 3,5-pyridinedicarboxylic acid ethyl methyl ester, is a member of the dihydropyridine class. The molecular formula is $C_{18}H_{19}Cl_2NO_4$. Felodipine has been shown to be highly lipophilic and is a weak base (pK_a, < 1), but for practical purposes it behaves as a neutral compound. The structural differences between felodipine and the related derivate, nifedipine, account for felodipine's comparatively more pronounced vascular versus myocardial activity.

PHARMACOLOGY

Felodipine exerts its main action by inhibition of contractility in the myogenically active vascular smooth muscle in arteriolar resistance vessels. In an *in vitro* model, the depression of myocardial contractility by 50% required a concentration of felodipine 118 times higher than that required to depress myogenically active vascular smooth muscle by 50%. Thus, felodipine has a vascular versus myocardial selectivity of 118. Corresponding values are 1 for verapamil and 17 for nifedipine.[2] Felodipine's vasodilatory abilities predominantly affect arteriolar resistance vessels, whereas it has no apparent effect on venous vessel tone.[6]

Like other calcium antagonists, felodipine also was reported to produce some degree of transient natriuresis/diuresis, presumably based on a direct tubular effect.[7] This effect was most pronounced during the first 6 or 12 hours and lost significance after 24 hours.

The effect on potassium excretion was small, and plasma concentrations of potassium were unchanged. According to micropuncture studies of the kidney in rats, all diuretic activity of felodipine was localized along the distal convoluted tubule and the collecting duct.[8] However, lithium clearance studies in healthy volunteers showed that an effect at the proximal tubule may contribute to the diuretic effect at higher doses.[9]

PHARMACOKINETICS
Absorption

After oral administration, felodipine is completely absorbed from the gastrointestinal tract.[10] Time to peak plasma concentration varies with the type of felodipine formulation used. With oral solutions, peak plasma concentration is reached within 15 to 90 minutes; with conventional tablets, it is reached after 1 to 2 hours; and when the extended-release formulation is given, plasma peak effect and maximal blood pressure effect are reached after 3 to 5 hours.[10] The mean oral bioavailability amounts to 15%, indicating significant presystemic elimination via the liver.[10] Felodipine undergoes no dose-dependent change in bioavailability.

Distribution and Metabolism

After administration, felodipine achieves a volume of distribution of 10 L/kg, and less than 1% of the drug remains in the blood plasma.[10] Felodipine is extensively (more than 99%) bound to plasma proteins.[10] Pharmacologic studies have shown that metabolites of felodipine all appear to be without vasodilating activity.[10] The first step in metabolism involves the oxidation of felodipine by the cytochrome P-450 system.[10] Thereafter, further metabolic processes result in at least 15 different metabolites.

Elimination

Felodipine is completely eliminated via its metabolites, and no parent drug appears in the urine. Within

72 hours of an intravenous dose of felodipine, about 70% was eliminated as metabolites by the kidneys.[11] Only 10% of the administered dose was excreted in the feces.[11] The mean terminal plasma half-life of felodipine in middle-aged hypertensive patients, regardless of the state of renal function, was around 24 hours.[10] A prolonged half-life and higher mean plasma concentrations were observed in elderly hypertensive patients, because clearance of felodipine decreased with age.[10, 12] Comparison with an age-matched control group showed that liver disease did not appear to affect felodipine plasma concentrations.[12]

EFFECTS ON PATHOPHYSIOLOGY

Felodipine's main effect has been identified as a direct and selective relaxation of vascular smooth muscle in the resistance vessels that results in specific hemodynamic changes. Therefore, we will focus first on the typical hemodynamic changes before examining other effects.

Hemodynamics

The potent vasodilatory effect of felodipine monotherapy in patients with essential hypertension has been documented to reduce mean arterial pressure by as much as 25% of pretreatment values.[13] Felodipine's vasodilatory efficacy *in vitro* was demonstrated to be stronger than that of nifedipine.[14] In hypertensive patients, an increase in heart rate was observed after an initial dose, apparently induced by sympathetic baroreflex activation.[15] However, heart rate returned to pretreatment values within 1 week's treatment with felodipine, possibly as a result of adaptive baroreceptor resetting.[16]

The hemodynamic effects of felodipine in hypertensive patients have been investigated both after a single dose and after 1 year of treatment. Acutely, the decrease in total peripheral resistance and blood pressure was accompanied by increases in heart rate, stroke volume, and cardiac output.[13, 15] During long-term treatment, however, the only persistent changes were a decreased peripheral resistance and blood pressure, whereas systemic flow and heart rate remained unchanged.[17] Felodipine lowered both systolic and diastolic pressures to a similar extent in the supine and upright postures.[18] The hemodynamic response to upright tilting was also unchanged.[19] The extended-release formulation provides 24-hour control of blood pressure with once-daily dosing.[20] After withdrawal, no rebound effect was observed, and blood pressure returned slowly to pretreatment values over several days.[21]

Effects on the Heart

Because felodipine is highly vascular-selective, cardiac contractility has not been reduced at therapeutic doses in clinical studies;[3, 5, 22] in fact, the possibility of a positive inotropic effect has been discussed.[23] Cheng et al. compared the inotropic effects of felodipine, nifedipine, and amlodipine in conscious dogs.[24] The authors were able to show that at doses that produced equivalent arterial dilatation, only felodipine increased contractile performance, whereas both nifedipine and amlodipine had a negative inotropic effect. Clinical studies confirm a higher vascular selectivity of felodipine compared with nifedipine. Studies have documented that cardiac contractility remains virtually unchanged after felodipine, whereas nifedipine produces a depressant effect.[3, 5] At a dose that produced similar coronary dilation, nifedipine when given by intracoronary injection depressed contractility, whereas felodipine did not.[3]

Several authors have studied the effects of felodipine on atrioventricular conduction. Ronn et al.[25] and Carruthers and Bailey[26] found no change in the PQ interval, even when felodipine was added to a β-blocker. In contrast, Been et al.[27] reported a significant prolongation of the atrio-His (A-H) interval after felodipine administration, using invasive electrophysiologic techniques in patients with some cardiac abnormalities. Although the degree of prolongation of the A-H interval was only one half that of verapamil,[27, 28] possible antiarrhythmic properties were suggested. However, in another invasive electrophysiologic study, Amlie et al.[29] found no effect of felodipine on sinus or AV-nodal function. Furthermore, it must be emphasized that electrocardiographic data collected from numerous clinical studies showed no clinically relevant prolongation of PR interval in patients with essential hypertension (Merck, Sharp & Dohme, data on file, 1989).

In the course of untreated hypertension, structural cardiovascular adaptation occurs, resulting in left ventricular hypertrophy and progressive thickening of the media in resistance vessels.[30] After felodipine treatment, a reduction of these cardiovascular structural changes was found in spontaneously hypertensive rats.[31] Several studies in hypertensive patients have demonstrated the ability of felodipine to cause reduction of left ventricular hypertrophy.[32-34] One study investigated 76 patients with untreated hypertension and echocardiographic evidence of left ventricular hypertrophy as judged by posterior wall thickness.[32] Long-term treatment with felodipine significantly reduced left ventricular mass by 20% in these patients.

Effects on Renal Function

In animal experiments, felodipine produced diuresis and natriuresis by directly affecting sodium and water reabsorption in the distal tubule and collecting duct.[8] Dose-related decreases in renal vascular resistance, causing increases in renal blood flow and glomerular filtration rate, were obtained in spontaneously hypertensive rats.[35]

In healthy normotensive subjects, felodipine has also been shown to exert acute natriuretic and diuretic effects.[7, 36] A distal tubular effect was demonstrated, and at higher dose levels, proximal reabsorption was inhibited.[8] In hypertensive patients, Leonetti et al.[21] reported that felodipine induced a marked increase in natriuresis and diuresis that occurred as early as during the first 6 hours after single-dose administration. On repeated administration, the increased natriuresis and diuresis seemed to disappear after the second day, although a negative sodium balance was maintained.[21] The acute natriuretic and diuretic effects of felodipine are accompanied by a significant increase in renal blood flow with no simultaneous change in glomerular filtration rate.[21, 37, 38] Renal blood flow was still increased after several days.[21]

However, renal blood flow has been reported to return to pretreatment values after 2 months of continued felodipine therapy.[38] In normotensive as well as in hypertensive subjects, the natriuretic effect of felodipine seems to be inversely related to dose.[39, 40] The natriuretic effect of felodipine seems to be evident at smaller doses, corresponding to those clinically employed, and to be less clear at higher doses.[39, 40] Increased plasma renin activity has been reported during short-term administration of felodipine. During long-term treatment, however, plasma renin activity returned to baseline values.[41]

Effects on the Central Nervous System

Felodipine is an extremely lipophilic agent and therefore can cross the blood-brain barrier. Several of felodipine's effects on the cerebral vasculature have been documented. Intravenous felodipine administration caused an increase in cortical blood flow in spontaneously hypertensive rats.[42] At a given change in arterial pressure, felodipine induced a greater increase in cortical perfusion than did nimodipine.[42] Felodipine reversed constriction of subarachnoid arteries induced by injection of serotonin.[43] In severely hypertensive patients, cerebral blood flow tended to increase during infusion of felodipine but was not affected during continued oral treatment.[44]

CLINICAL USE

The finding that felodipine is a potent arteriolar dilator with no adverse effect on heart function makes it suitable for the treatment of arterial hypertension. Patients with angina pectoris, congestive heart failure, or impaired renal function may also benefit from felodipine treatment.

In Hypertension

The antihypertensive efficacy of felodipine has been extensively demonstrated in various studies in which felodipine as monotherapy was compared with placebo or antihypertensive agents. Other studies have assessed felodipine in combination therapy. Finally, felodipine has been tested in special patient populations, such as in elderly hypertensive patients and in hypertensive patients with renal insufficiency.

As monotherapy, felodipine extended release (ER) at doses between 5 and 20 mg once daily has been shown to lower systolic and diastolic pressures significantly better than placebo.[20, 45, 46] In elderly patients, lower doses may be effective, and 2.5 mg once daily is sufficient in 30% to 50% of cases.[47, 48]

At doses of 5 to 10 mg once daily, felodipine ER was found to be as effective as amlodipine (5 to 10 mg once daily)[49] or atenolol (50 to 100 mg once daily)[50] but more effective than nifedipine sustained-release (SR) (10 to 20 mg twice a day)[51] or captopril (25 to 50 mg twice a day).[52] Felodipine ER (10 mg once daily) also had a better antihypertensive effect than enalapril (10 mg once daily)[53] or hydrochlorothiazide (25 mg once daily).[54] In a comparison of felodipine (5 mg once daily) and nifedipine SR (20 mg twice a day), treatments were equally effective, but only 1 of 37 patients treated with felodipine withdrew because of adverse events, compared with 5 of 40 patients in the nifedipine group.[55]

When added to treatment with a β-blocker, felodipine ER (5, 10, or 20 mg once daily) lowered arterial pressure significantly better than placebo.[56] In patients with unsatisfactory blood pressure control despite treatment with a β-blocker, felodipine ER (10 to 20 mg once daily) was found to be markedly more effective than nifedipine SR (20 to 40 mg twice a day).[57]

In previous trials using the conventional tablet formulation of felodipine (administered twice a day), addition of felodipine to a β-blocker lowered blood pressure significantly more than the addition of hydrochlorothiazide,[58, 59] hydralazine,[60] or prazosin.[61] The combination of felodipine and a β-blocker was also more effective than traditional triple therapy (β-blocker plus diuretic plus hydralazine).[62]

In long-term studies, the reduction in arterial pressure achieved shortly after beginning treatment with felodipine was maintained throughout an observation period of 6 to 48 months with no decrease in the antihypertensive response.[32, 33, 63, 64]

Felodipine has also been tested successfully in elderly hypertensive patients,[53, 65–67] including patients with isolated systolic hypertension.[68, 69] The greater efficacy of felodipine with increasing patient age seemed to depend on higher pretreatment blood pressures and decreased metabolic capacity of the liver: when corrections were made for initial blood pressure and plasma drug concentration, much of the positive correlation between age and fall in blood pressure was lost.[70]

In hypertensive patients with reduced renal function, felodipine administration resulted in successful long-term control of systolic and diastolic pressure. The average initial blood pressure value of 190/110 mmHg was reduced to 150/90 mmHg 6 months to 1 year after the beginning of treatment. In patients with stable renal function, this successful lowering of arterial pressure was accompanied by a mean increase in glomerular filtration rate from 55 to 70 ml/min. In five of the six patients with progressive renal disease, the rate of progression was reduced from 9 to 5 ml/min/year during felodipine treatment.[71] Larsson et al.[72] observed that felodipine had the same pharmacokinetic profile in hypertensive patients with impaired renal function as it did in healthy subjects. An observed accumulation of felodipine metabolites lacked clinical relevance, because all these metabolites are hemodynamically inactive.

Finally, Sluiter et al.[73] treated seven patients with intravenously administered felodipine during a hypertensive crisis and observed a rapid blood pressure reduction with improvement of symptoms and signs of hypertensive encephalopathy.

In Congestive Heart Failure

Calcium antagonists are known to improve left ventricular function in certain patients with chronic congestive heart failure.[74-78] However, because of their negative inotropic effect, calcium antagonists cannot be generally recommended in this situation. Calcium antagonists with higher vascular selectivity, such as felodipine, seem to have a reduced risk of depressing contractility and therefore appear promising in the treatment of congestive heart failure. Indeed, most study groups demonstrated an improvement in ventricular function characterized by an increase in cardiac output and a decrease in pulmonary wedge pressure after felodipine administration.[77-84]

Tan et al.[84] also observed an increase in cardiac output with felodipine, but did not find improved exercise capacity or decreased symptoms. However, in a double-blind, placebo-controlled, 8-week study of felodipine, Dunselman et al.[81] found a reduction in systemic vascular resistance and mean arterial pressure at rest, whereas stroke volume and cardiac output increased and pulmonary wedge pressure remained unchanged. In parallel, exercise tolerance increased by 26%, and other symptoms decreased after administration of felodipine. Similarly promising results have been found in other studies,[82, 83] and Kassis et al.[83] observed reduced levels of noradrenaline after 6 months of treatment with felodipine. These results are provocative, because plasma norepinephrine levels have been identified as a powerful determinant of mortality in congestive heart failure. The Vasodilator Heart Failure Trial (VHeFT III) was designed to determine whether felodipine ER, a vasoselective calcium antagonist, is a safe and effective vasodilator for use in heart failure. Patients had their therapy optimized using enalapril and diuretics with or without digoxin before being randomized to felodipine ER or placebo. The study included a total of 451 male patients in whom exercise tolerance, mortality, and morbidity data were assessed. The treatment groups were equivalent in terms of age, etiology, ejection fraction, and exercise treadmill time. During follow-up that averaged 540 days, 60 patients died (13% mortality). There was no difference between felodipine ER and placebo in overall mortality in subgroup analyses of patients with or without coronary artery disease. Other subgroup analyses of mortality provided numbers too small from which to draw any meaningful conclusions. Change in peak exercise capacity at 12 weeks and plasma norepinephrine levels were similar between the felodipine ER–

and placebo-treated patient groups. Plasma atrial natriuretic peptide was reduced by felodipine ER but not placebo.

In Angina Pectoris

The hemodynamic effects of felodipine in patients with angina pectoris are similar to those seen in hypertensive patients.[85] Arterial pressure is reduced, owing to a fall in total peripheral resistance, and there is a transient increase in heart rate. Coronary blood flow increases, because felodipine dilates coronary resistance vessels and increases the diameter of epicardial coronary arteries.[86]

The efficacy of felodipine in patients with stable effort angina has been demonstrated in studies lasting 1 day to 4 weeks, both when used as monotherapy and when given together with a β-blocker.[87-90] Exercise duration increased 10% to 60%, and anginal attack rate and consumption of nitroglycerine decreased. Schulte et al.[91] compared felodipine ER (10 mg once daily) with nifedipine retard (20 mg twice daily) in the treatment of stable angina pectoris. After 2 weeks of treatment, felodipine increased exercise time to onset of anginal symptoms and time to 1-mm ST-segment depression significantly more than nifedipine.

Calcium antagonists are generally considered highly effective drugs in the treatment of vasospastic angina. In a study by Ardissino et al.,[92] ST-segment elevation and chest pain could be provoked by hyperventilation in 11 of 13 patients during placebo treatment but could not be induced in any of the 13 patients during felodipine treatment. Another study by the same authors showed that felodipine, given once daily, was at least as effective as nifedipine capsules given four times daily.[93]

Adverse Effects

The most commonly observed adverse events after acute felodipine administration are headache and flushing, both of which are dose-dependent. Dizziness, fatigue, and palpitations after acute dosing have also been described. Dose-dependent peripheral edema due to precapillary vasodilatation and increased capillary pressure and filtration[94] is the most common adverse event during long-term treatment. Glucose tolerance and insulin release have been shown to remain practically unchanged.[95-98] Serum lipids[98-100] and serum potassium also remain unaltered.[38]

Interaction with Other Drugs

Interaction of felodipine administered as conventional tablets and digitalis has been observed when both drugs are given concomitantly to patients with congestive heart failure.[101, 102] Conventional tablets of felodipine (10 mg twice a day) caused an 11% increase in digoxin peak plasma levels,[103] although no interaction with digoxin occurred when the extended-release formulation was used.[103]

Felodipine's bioavailability has been reduced in patients on long-term anticonvulsant drugs, which induce the enzymes of the cytochrome P-450 system.[104] As a consequence of increased presystemic metabolism, the mean bioavailability of felodipine in treated epileptic patients was only 6.3% of that obtained in healthy volunteers.[104]

Because cimetidine can inhibit the enzymes of the P-450 system, which are involved in the initial step in felodipine metabolism, interaction between the two drugs appears to be probable. An experimental study found that felodipine plasma concentration increased by 50% during concomitant treatment with cimetidine.[105] Plasma concentrations of felodipine are moderately increased by grapefruit juice (as occurs with other dihydropyridines), because felodipine contains high levels of flavonoids, which inhibit cytochrome P-450.[106, 107] However, intake of flavonoid-containing food did not correlate with antihypertensive effect or tolerability of felodipine in a large clinical study of 286 patients.[108]

After concomitant therapy with metoprolol and felodipine, small increases were found in both the mean maximal plasma concentration and the 12-hour postdose area under the curve of metoprolol.[109] However, two studies did not find any influence of felodipine on metoprolol plasma concentrations.[110, 111]

Contraindications

Apart from hypersensitivity, the only existing contraindication for the use of felodipine is pregnancy. Safety and efficacy of felodipine have not been studied in pregnancy.

Dosage and Administration

Both conventional tablets and extended-release tablets of felodipine (5 mg or 10 mg) have been studied extensively. The extended-release tablets offer the advantage of once-daily administration and are the only formulation marketed. In addition, a felodipine solution for oral administration as well as an intravenous solution has been developed and used in clinical studies. However, only the intravenous solution may become available for clinical use.

Felodipine ER should be initiated at 5 mg once daily and titrated according to the patient's response. In general, felodipine (5 to 10 mg once daily) is effective as monotherapy. In rare cases of hypertension, the dose of felodipine has been 20 mg or higher.

SUMMARY

Felodipine is a dihydropyridine calcium antagonist that has specific vasoselective properties without a negative inotropic effect at clinically used doses. These characteristics make it especially suitable as monotherapy for arterial hypertension. Felodipine is remarkably effective and well tolerated and can be used in hypertensive patients with concomitant congestive heart failure, angina pectoris, and renal impairment, as well as in patients with diabetes or gout. The drug also appears promising in the treatment of elderly patients with hypertension. Conceivably, felodipine also may be used in patients who have angina pectoris without hypertension. A multicenter study is currently in progress to define the role of felodipine in congestive heart failure.

REFERENCES

1. Bostrom SL, Ljung B, Nordlander M, et al: Action of felodipine in vascular smooth muscle. In Hidaken H, Hartshorne D (eds): Calmodulin: Antagonists and Cellular Physiology. New York: Academic Press, 1984, p 273.
2. Ljung B: Vascular selectivity of felodipine. Drugs 29(Suppl 2):46, 1985.
3. Koolen JJ, Van Wezel HB, Piek J, et al: Effects of intracoronary felodipine versus nifedipine on left ventricular contractility and coronary sinus blood flow in stable angina pectoris. Am J Cardiol 74:730, 1994.
4. Nordlander M, Abrahamsson T, Akerblom B, Thalén P: Vascular versus myocardial selectivity of dihydropyridine calcium antagonists as studied in vivo and in vitro. Pharmacol Toxicol 76:56, 1995.
5. Redfield MM, Neumann A, Tajik AJ, et al: Effect of long acting oral felodipine and nifedipine on left ventricular contractility in patients with systemic hypertension: Differentiation between reflex sympathetic and direct contractile responses. J Am Coll Cardiol [Special issue]:348A, 1994.
6. Muir AL, Wathen CG, Hannan WJ: Effects of felodipine on resistance and capacitance vessels in patients with essential hypertension. Drugs 29(Suppl 2):59, 1985.
7. DiBona GF: Renal effects of felodipine: A review of experimental evidence and clinical data. J Cardiovasc Pharmacol 15(Suppl 4):S29, 1990.
8. DiBona GF, Sawin LL: Renal tubular site of action of felodipine. J Pharmacol Exp Ther 228:420, 1983.
9. Katzman PL, DiBona GF, Hokfelt B, Hulthen UL: Acute renal tubular and hemodynamic effects of the calcium antagonist felodipine in healthy volunteers. J Am Soc Nephrol 2:1000, 1991.
10. Dunselman PH, Edgar B: Felodipine clinical pharmacokinetics [review]. Clin Pharmacokinetics 21:418, 1991.
11. Edgar B, Regardh CG, Johnsson G, et al: Felodipine kinetics in healthy men. Clin Pharmacol Ther 38:205, 1985.
12. Blychert E: Felodipine pharmacokinetics and plasma concentration vs effect relationships. Blood Pressure 2(Suppl):1, 1992.
13. Andersson OK, Granerus G, Hedher T, Wysocki M: Systemic and renal hemodynamic effects of single oral doses of felodipine in patients with refractory hypertension receiving chronic therapy with beta-blockers and diuretics. J Cardiovasc Pharmacol 7:544, 1985.
14. Nyborg NCB, Mulvany MJ: Effect of felodipine, a new dihydropyridine vasodilator on contractile responses to potassium, noradrenaline, and calcium in mesenteric resistance vessels of the rat. J Cardiovasc Pharmacol 6:499, 1984.
15. Fagard R, Lijnen P, Moerman E, et al: Acute hemodynamic and humoral responses to felodipine and metoprolol in mild hypertension. Eur J Clin Pharmacol 32:71, 1987.
16. Smith SA, Mace PJ, Littler WA: Felodipine, blood pressure and cardiovascular reflexes in hypertensive humans. Hypertension 8:1172, 1986.
17. Lund-Johansen P, Omvik P: Chronic hemodynamic effects of tiapamil and felodipine in essential hypertension at rest and during exercise. J Cardiovasc Pharmacol 15(Suppl 4):S42, 1990.
18. Campbell LM, Cowen KJ, Cranfield FR, et al: Felodipine-ER once daily as monotherapy in hypertension. J Cardiovasc Pharmacol 15:569, 1990.
19. Mace PJ, Stallard TJ, Littler WA: Felodipine in hypertension. Eur J Clin Pharmacol 29:383, 1985.

20. Faison EP, Goldberg AL, Dobbins TW, et al: Felodipine ER ABPM Study Group. Dose response relationship and 24-hour efficacy were observed with once daily extended-release felodipine using 24-hour ambulatory blood pressure monitoring. Am J Hypertens 4:105A, 1991.

21. Leonetti G, Gradnik R, Terzoli L, et al: Effects of single and repeated doses of the calcium antagonist felodipine on blood pressure, renal function, electrolytes and water balance, and renin-angiotensin-aldosterone system in hypertensive patients. J Cardiovasc Pharmacol 8:1243, 1986.

22. Culling W, Ruttley MS, Sheridan DJ: Acute haemodynamic effects of felodipine during beta blockade in patients with coronary artery disease. Br Heart J 52:431, 1984.

23. Drake-Holland AJ, Pugh S, Noble MI, Mills C: Problem of measuring the positive inotropic property of a vasodilating drug: An illustration using felodipine. Cardiovasc Res 21:631, 1987.

24. Cheng CP, Noda T, Nordlander M, et al: Comparison of effects of dihydropyridine calcium antagonists on left ventricular systolic and diastolic performance. J Pharmacol Exp Ther 268:1232, 1994.

25. Ronn O, Bengtsson B, Edgar B, Raner S: Acute haemodynamic effects of felodipine and verapamil in man, singly and with metoprolol. Drugs 29(Suppl 2):16, 1985.

26. Carruthers SG, Bailey DG: Tolerance and cardiovascular effect of single dose felodipine/beta-blocker combinations in healthy subjects. J Cardiovasc Pharmacol 10(Suppl 1):S169, 1987.

27. Been M, Macfarlane PW, Hillis WS: Electrophysiological effects of felodipine. Drugs 29(Suppl 2):76, 1985.

28. Rowland E, Evans T, Kirkler D: Effect of nifedipine on atrioventricular conduction as compared with verapamil. Intracardiac electrophysiological study. Br Heart J 42:124, 1979.

29. Amlie JP, Endresen K, Sire S: The effect of felodipine on the sinus and atrioventricular nodes in patients with ischemic heart disease. J Cardiovasc Pharmacol 15(Suppl 4):S25, 1990.

30. Folkow B: Physiological aspects of primary hypertension [review]. Physiol Rev 62:347, 1982.

31. Lundin SA, Hallback-Nordlander MI: Regression of structural cardiovascular changes by antihypertensive therapy in spontaneously hypertensive rats. J Hypertens 2:11, 1984.

32. Wetzchewald D, Klaus D, Garanin G, et al: Regression of left ventricular hypertrophy during long-term antihypertensive treatment—a comparison between felodipine and the combination of felodipine and metoprolol. J Intern Med 231:303, 1992.

33. Cerasola G, Cottone S, Nardi E, et al: Reversal of cardiac hypertrophy and left ventricular function with the calcium antagonist felodipine in hypertensive patients. J Hum Hypertens 4:703, 1990.

34. Pringle SD, Barbou M, Simpson IA, et al: Effect of felodipine on left ventricular mass and Doppler-derived haemodynamics in patients with essential hypertension. In 4th International Symposium on Calcium Antagonists, Pharmacology and Clinical Research, Florence, May 25–27, 1989, p 174.

35. Nordlander M, DiBona G, Ljung B, et al: Renal and cardiovascular effects of acute and chronic administration of felodipine to SHR. Eur J Pharmacol 113:25, 1985.

36. Edgar B, Bengtsson B, Elmfeldt D, et al: Acute diuretic/natriuretic properties of felodipine in man. Drugs 29(Suppl 2):176, 1985.

37. Andersson OK, Hedner T, Granérus G: Felodipine in combination with a beta-blocker and a diuretic in chronic treatment of patients with refractory hypertension. Drugs 34(Suppl 3):156, 1984.

38. Hulthen UL, Katzman PL: Renal effects of acute and long-term treatment with felodipine in essential hypertension. J Hypertens 6:231, 1988.

39. Zanchetti A, Leonetti G: Discussion on the natriuretic effect of calcium antagonists [review]. J Cardiovasc Pharmacol 10(Suppl 1):S161, 1987.

40. Bengtsson-Hasselgren B, Edgar B, Ronn O: Dose-dependent effects of felodipine on diuresis and natriuresis in healthy subjects. J Cardiovasc Pharmacol 12:134, 1988.

41. Cerasola G, Cottone S, Mangano MT, et al: Effects of felodipine on natriuresis, atrial natriuretic factor, the renin-angiotensin-aldosterone system, and blood pressure in essential hypertension. Clin Ther 10:694, 1988.

42. Thoren P, Westling H, Skarphedinsson JO: Effect of calcium antagonists felodipine and nimodipine on cortical blood flow in the spontaneously hypertensive rat. J Hypertens 7(Suppl 4):S153, 1989.

43. Vallfors B, Ahlman H, Dalstrom A: The influence of felodipine or ketanserin on 5-HT-induced cerebrovascular spasm. In 5th International Symposium on Vascular Neuroeffector Mechanisms, Paris, August 6–8, 1984.

44. Thulin T, Fagher B, Grabowski M, et al: Cerebral blood flow in patients with severe hypertension, and acute and chronic effects of felodipine. J Hypertens 11:83, 1993.

45. Wester A, Lorimer AR, Westberg B: Felodipine extended release in mild to moderate hypertension. Curr Med Res Opin 12:275, 1991.

46. Weber MA, Goldberg AI, Faison EP, et al: Extended-release felodipine in patients with mild to moderate hypertension. Clin Pharmacol Ther 55:346, 1994.

47. Dunlay MC, Lipschutz KH, Nelson EB, et al: A multicenter study of felodipine ER and placebo in elderly and young hypertensive patients [abstract]. Am J Hypertens 4:25A, 1991.

48. Landahl SJ, Wiklund I: Quality of life and blood pressure control in the treatment of elderly hypertensive patients. A comparison between Plendil(R) and hydrochlorothiazide. Am J Hypertens 7:112A, 1994.

49. Koenig W, Multicentre Study Group: Efficacy and tolerability of felodipine and amlodipine in the treatment of mild to moderate hypertension. A randomized double-blind multicentre trial. Drug Invest 5:200, 1993.

50. Waite MA, Bone ME, Kubik MM, et al: A comparison of the efficacy and tolerability of felodipine ER and atenolol given as monotherapy in mild to moderate hypertension. Br J Clin Pharmacol 32:661P, 1991.

51. Goudie AW, Gupta OM, Gray PL, et al: A comparison of felodipine and nifedipine as monotherapy in patients with mild to moderate hypertension. Curr Ther Res 55:625, 1994.

52. Alberti A, Balice G, Gueli Aletti D, et al: A comparison between two different dosages of felodipine extended release and captopril in the treatment of mild to moderate hypertension. Curr Ther Res 50:333, 1991.

53. Morgan TO, Anderson A, Jones E: Comparison and interaction of low dose felodipine and enalapril in the treatment of essential hypertension in elderly subjects. Am J Hypertens 5:238, 1992.

54. Koenig W, Sund M, Binner L, et al: Comparison of once daily felodipine 10 mg ER and hydrochlorothiazide 25 mg in the treatment of mild to moderate hypertension. Eur J Clin Pharmacol 41:197, 1991.

55. Hosie J, Langan JJ, Scott M, et al: Effectiveness and tolerability of felodipine once daily and nifedipine twice daily as monotherapies for mild hypertension. J Drug Dev 5:129, 1992.

56. Brun J, Froberg L, Kronmann P, et al: The Swedish general practitioner felodipine study group. Optimal felodipine dose when combined with metoprolol in arterial hypertension: A Swedish multicenter study within primary health care. J Cardiovasc Pharmacol 15(Suppl 4):S60, 1990.

57. Littler WA: Control of blood pressure in hypertensive patients with felodipine extended release or nifedipine retard. Br J Clin Pharmacol 30:871, 1990.

58. Ibsen H, Westberg B: The efficacy and tolerability of long-term felodipine treatment in hypertension. The Scandinavian Multicenter Group. Cardiovasc Drugs Ther 4:641, 1990.

59. Groom P, Simpson RJ, Sing B, et al: A double-blind comparison of felodipine and hydrochlorothiazide added to metoprolol to control hypertension. Eur J Clin Pharmacol 34:21, 1988.

60. Hansson L, Dahlof B, Gudbrandsson T, et al: Antihypertensive effect of felodipine or hydralazine when added to beta-blocker therapy. J Cardiovasc Pharmacol 12:94, 1988.

61. Jackson B, Morgan TO, Gibson J, Anderson A: Felodipine versus prazosin as an addition to a beta-blocker in the treatment of essential hypertension. The Australian Multicentre Study. Drugs 34(Suppl 3):109, 1987.

62. Asplund J, Collste P, Danielsson M, et al: Can standard triple

treatment of hypertension be replaced by the combination of felodipine and a beta-blocker? The Swedish Multicentre Study Group. J Hypertens 4(Suppl 4):S446, 1986.

63. Collste P, Danielsson M, Elmfeldt D, et al: Long term experience of felodipine in combination with beta-blockade and diuretics in refractory hypertension. Drugs 29(Suppl 2):124, 1985.
64. Flygt G: Long-term treatment of hypertension with felodipine. J Cardiovasc Pharmacol 15(Suppl 4):S103, 1990.
65. Hosie J, Mulder AW, Westberg B: Binational MC Study Group. Felodipine once daily in elderly hypertensives. J Hum Hypertens 5:49, 1991.
66. Raveau-Landon C, Savier CH, Dewailly P, et al: Double-blind study of felodipine ER versus the hydrochlorothiazide-amiloride combination in elderly hypertensive patients. Semin Hop Paris 67:1785, 1991.
67. Dunlay MC, Lipschutz KH, Nelson EB, et al: Felodipine Study Group. A multicenter study of felodipine ER and placebo in elderly and young hypertensive patients. Am J Hypertens 4:25A, 1991.
68. Wing LM, Russell AE, Tonkin AL, et al: Felodipine, metoprolol and their combination compared with placebo in isolated systolic hypertension in the elderly. Blood Press 3:82, 1994.
69. Wing LMH, Russell AE, Tonkin AL, et al: Mono- and combination therapy with felodipine or enalapril in elderly patients with systolic hypertension. Blood Press 3:90, 1994.
70. Leenen FHH, Logan AG, Myers MG, et al: Canadian Felodipine Study Group. Antihypertensive efficacy of the calcium-antagonist felodipine in patients with persisting hypertension on beta-adrenoceptor blocker therapy. Br J Clin Pharmacol 26:535, 1988.
71. Herlitz H, Bjorck S, Nyberg G, et al: Clinical evaluation of felodipine in patients with refractory hypertension. Drugs 34(Suppl 3):151, 1987.
72. Larsson R, Karlberg BE, Gelin A, et al: Acute and steady-state pharmacokinetics and antihypertensive effects of felodipine in patients with normal and impaired renal function. J Clin Pharmacol 30:1020, 1990.
73. Sluiter HE, Huysmans T, Thiens TA, Koene RA: Hemodynamic effects of intravenous felodipine in normotensive and hypertensive subjects. Drugs 29(Suppl 2):144, 1985.
74. Colucci WS: Usefulness of calcium antagonists for congestive heart failure. Am J Cardiol 59:52B, 1987.
75. Polese A, Fiorentini C, Olivari MT, Guazzi MD: Clinical use of a calcium antagonist agent (nifedipine) in acute pulmonary edema. Am J Med 66:825, 1979.
76. Colucci WS, Fifer MA, Lorell BH, Wynne J: Calcium channel blockers in congestive heart failure: Theoretic considerations and clinical experience. Am J Med 78(Suppl 2B):9, 1985.
77. Emanuelsson H, Hjalmarson A, Holmberg S, Waagstein F: Acute haemodynamic effects of felodipine in congestive heart failure. Eur J Clin Pharmacol 28:489, 1985.
78. Tweddel AC, Hutton I: Felodipine in ventricular dysfunction. Eur Heart J 7:54, 1986.
79. Timmis AD, Campbell S, Monaghan MJ, et al: Acute haemodynamic and metabolic effects of felodipine in congestive heart failure. Br Heart J 51:445, 1984.
80. Timmis AD, Smyth P, Kenny JF, et al: Effects of vasodilator treatment with felodipine on haemodynamic responses to treadmill exercise in congestive heart failure. Br Heart J 52:314, 1984.
81. Dunselman PH, Kuntze CE, van Bruggen A, et al: Efficacy of felodipine in congestive heart failure. Eur Heart J 10:354, 1989.
82. Kassis E, Amtorp O, Waldorff S, Fitz-Hansen P: Efficacy of felodipine in chronic congestive heart failure: A placebo controlled haemodynamic study at rest and during exercise and orthostatic stress. Br Heart J 58:505, 1987.
83. Kassis E, Amtorp O: Long-term clinical, hemodynamic, angiographic, and neurohumoral responses to vasodilation with felodipine in patients with chronic congestive heart failure. J Cardiovasc Pharmacol 15:S347, 1990.
84. Tan LB, Murray RG, Littler WA: Felodipine in patients with chronic heart failure: Discrepant haemodynamic and clinical effects. Br Heart J 58:122, 1987.
85. Emanuelsson H, Holmberg S: No adverse effects from high

doses of felodipine to patients with coronary heart disease. Clin Cardiol 8:329, 1985.
86. Emanuelsson H, Ekstrom L, Hjalmarsson A, et al: Felodipine-induced dilatation of epicardial coronary arteries: A randomized, double-blind study. Angiology 37:1, 1986.
87. Scardi S, Pandullo C, Pivotti F, et al: Acute effects of felodipine in exertional angina pectoris. Am J Cardiol 61:691, 1988.
88. Verdecchia P, Gattesci C, Benemio G, et al: Increased exercise tolerance and reduced electrocardiographic ischaemia 3 and 12 hours after oral felodipine in effort angina. Eur Heart J 10:70, 1989.
89. Canale C, Terrachini V, Vallebona A, et al: Antiischaemic activity of two doses of felodipine in stable effort angina. Philipp J Cardiol 19(Suppl 1):1, 1990.
90. Lorimer AR, MacFarlane P, Pringle S, et al: The effects of felodipine in angina pectoris. Eur J Clin Pharmacol 38:415, 1990.
91. Schulte K-L: Felodipine, once daily, provides anti-anginal and anti-ischemic effects for 24 h—a double-blind comparison with nifedipine, twice daily, and placebo in patients with stable exercise induced angina pectoris. Eur Heart J (In press).
92. Ardissino D, Savonitto S, Zanini P, et al: Effect of felodipine on hyperventilation-induced ischemic attacks in variant angina pectoris. Am J Cardiol 63:104, 1989.
93. Ardissino D, Savonitto S, Mussini A, et al: Felodipine (once daily) versus nifedipine (four times daily) for Prinzmetal's angina pectoris. Am J Cardiol 68:1587, 1991.
94. Gustafsson D: Microvascular mechanisms involved in calcium antagonist edema formation. J Cardiovasc Pharmacol 10(Suppl 1):S121, 1987.
95. Hedner T, Elmfeldt D, Von Schenck H, et al: Glucose tolerance in hypertensive patients during treatment with the calcium antagonist felodipine. Br J Clin Pharmacol 24:145, 1987.
96. Katzman PL, Hulthén UL, Hökfelt B: Glucose tolerance and secretion and clearance of insulin during long term felodipine treatment. Drugs 34(Suppl 3):93, 1987.
97. Capewell S, Collier A, Matthews D, et al: A trial of the calcium antagonist felodipine in hypertensive type 2 diabetic patients. Diabet Med 6:809, 1989.
98. Scherstén BFE: Unchanged lipid and lipoprotein concentrations in hypertensive patients with Type II diabetes mellitus during one year of treatment with felodipine and nifedipine compared with placebo. Am J Hypertens 7:73A, 1994.
99. Nilsson-Ehle P: Felodipine does not affect plasma lipoprotein concentrations [abstract]. J Cardiovasc Pharmacol 12(Suppl 6):S183, 1988.
100. Nielsen MR, Winkel OP, Ahlstrom F, et al: Effects on plasma lipids during long-term antihypertensive treatment with felodipine. Drug Invest 4:361, 1992.
101. Dunselman PHJM, Scaf AHJ, Kuntze CEE, et al: Interaction between felodipine and digoxin in patients with congestive heart failure [abstract]. Cardiovasc Drug Ther 1:231, 1987.
102. Rehnqvist N, Billing E, Moberg L, et al: Pharmacokinetics of felodipine and effect on digoxin plasma levels in patients with heart failure. Drugs 34(Suppl 3):33, 1987.
103. Kirch W, Laskowski M, Ohnhaus EE, et al: Effects of felodipine on plasma digoxin levels and haemodynamics in patients with heart failure. J Intern Med 225:237, 1989.
104. Capewell S, Freestone S, Critchley JAJH, et al: Gross reduction in felodipine bioavailability in patients taking anticonvulsants. Br J Clin Pharmacol 24:243P, 1987.
105. Janzon K, Edgar B, Landborg P, et al: The influence of cimetidine and spironolactone on the pharmacokinetics and haemodynamic effects of felodipine in healthy subjects. Acta Pharmacol Toxicol 59(Suppl 1):98, 1986.
106. Bailey DG, Spence JD, Munoz C, Anold JM: Interaction of citrus juices with felodipine and nifedipine [see comments]. Lancet 337:268, 1991.
107. Edgar B, Bailey DG, Bergstrand R, et al: Formulation dependent interaction between felodipine and grapefruit juice [abstract]. Clin Pharmacol Ther 47:181, 1990.
108. Faison E, Edgar B, Dobbins T, et al: Influence of bioflavonoid intake on the antihypertensive effects of felodipine extended-release (FER). Clin Pharmacol Ther 49:191, 1991.
109. Smith SR, Wilkens MR, Jack DB, et al: Pharmacokinetic inter-

actions between felodipine and metoprolol. Eur J Clin Pharmacol 31:575, 1987.
110. Hoffman J, Fox Y, German Multicentre Study Group: Efficacy and tolerability of the fixed combination of felodipine 5 mg plus metoprolol 50 mg in comparison with the individual

components in the treatment of hypertension. J Drug Dev 3:201, 1991.
111. Dahlöf B, Jönsson L, Borgholst O, et al: Improved antihypertensive efficacy of the felodipine-metoprolol extended-release tablet compared with each drug alone. Blood Press 1:37, 1993.

CHAPTER 112

Lacidipine in the Treatment of Hypertension

Giuseppe Mancia, M.D., Arduino A. Mangoni, M.D., Stefano Carugo, M.D., Maria Luisa Stella, M.D., and Cristina Giannattasio, M.D., Ph.D.

Lacidipine is a dihydropyridine molecule that differs from the original dihydropyridine, nifedipine, in its spatial configuration (the aromatic group is perpendicular to the dihydropyridine ring), in the presence of a number of substituents in the molecule, and in the presence of a t-butyl group, which gives the drug a marked lipophylicity.[1]

Lacidipine was developed by Glaxo Italy Research Laboratories in 1984 and is now available as a once-a-day antihypertensive drug in a number of countries. This chapter briefly reviews the blood pressure–lowering and hemodynamic effects of lacidipine in animal preparations and hypertensive models. It then summarizes the pharmacokinetic properties of the drug. Finally, it addresses evidence of the clinical efficacy and tolerance profile of lacidipine in human hypertension.

ANIMAL STUDIES
In Vitro Studies

In vitro studies have shown that lacidipine (1) inhibits the contraction produced in the auricular artery of the rabbit by increasing doses of calcium chloride,[2] (2) causes a dose-dependent relaxation of the calcium-induced contraction of the rat aorta, with an effect comparable with that induced by nitrendipine but obtained at lower doses (i.e., at an IC_{50} value [the drug concentration capable of a 50% inhibition of smooth muscle contraction] of only 0.08 nmol/L),[3] and (3) has no influence on the rabbit auricular artery contraction induced by norepinephrine and thus on intracellular mobilization of calcium, even at high concentrations.[3] Thus, lacidipine acts as a powerful blocker of calcium entrance into the cells. Its mechanism of action is similar to that of other dihydropyridines; indeed, binding studies have observed a high affinity of the drug for the specific dihydropyridine receptor with a dissociation constant of approximately 1 nmol/L.[4]

In Vivo Studies

The effects of lacidipine *in vitro* have also been confirmed by studies in normotensive animals and in several hypertension models.[2] Lacidipine has been found to lower blood pressure in the normotensive rat (although at higher doses than in spontaneously hypertensive rats [SHRs]), the pithed rat, and the open-chest anesthetized dog. Lacidipine has shown a substantial blood pressure–lowering effect in the SHR, in the Dahl-S rat, in the stroke-prone hypertensive rat, and in the renovascular hypertensive dog (Goldblatt model).[2, 3, 5] In some of these studies, lacidipine showed not only a greater antihypertensive efficacy but also a less immediate, a more powerful, and a more prolonged action than that of nitrendipine. In the dog, for example, blood pressure was still significantly reduced 6 hours after an intravenous dose of lacidipine, whereas the effect of nitrendipine disappeared after 30 minutes.[4]

Vascular Selectivity

Animal studies have also provided data on the vascular effects of lacidipine associated with (and responsible for) the blood pressure fall. The most important findings are that, *in vivo*, the drug has been found to be highly vascular-selective, the ratio between the ability to reduce blood pressure by 25% and to exert a cardiodepressant effect (e.g., negative inotropic influence, heart rate slowing, A-V conduction slowing, inhibition of Purkinje cells, automatism) being much higher than that established in the same preparations for calcium antagonists, such as verapamil, diltiazem, nitrendipine, and amlodipine.[4, 5] It has also been found that in the isolated coronary artery preparation of the rat, the tonic contraction induced by high K^+ concentration (i.e., the contraction governed by calcium channels of the B-type) is more easily reduced by lacidipine than by nisoldipine and nifedipine, suggesting that lacidipine may be particularly effective on the coronary vessels.[6] Finally, in the anesthetized dog equipped with electromagnetic flow-probes, the more marked and prolonged blood pressure fall induced by lacidipine as compared with nitrendipine was accompanied by a marked and prolonged fall in systemic vascular resistance, and a rise in renal, coronary, and cerebral blood flow.[7] Thus, *in vivo*, the vascular effects of lacidipine predominate over the cardiac ones. These effects include all or most arterioles; in vital organs, the magnitude of these effects is so pronounced as to increase perfusion despite the reduction in pressure.

PHARMACOKINETIC PROPERTIES

The pharmacokinetics of lacidipine have been studied by traditional methods, first in several animal species and then in healthy volunteers and in hypertensive patients. The results obtained in humans can be summarized as follows:[4, 8] (1) Lacidipine is rapidly and extensively absorbed after oral administration and undergoes a marked first-pass effect in the liver. (2) The peak plasma concentration occurs after 1 hour, and the half-life of the drug in plasma is approximately 8 hours. (3) Lacidipine is mainly eliminated by the biliary route in the form of inactive metabolites. (4) The pharmacokinetic parameters are similar at the different doses of the drug employed clinically (discussed later) and after single and multiple administrations. These parameters are also similar in normal volunteers and hypertensive patients. (5) As expected from the elimination pattern, the pharmacokinetics of the drug are not altered in patients with severe kidney disease, whereas the drug's bioavailability is increased in elderly subjects, presumably because of a reduction in hepatic metabolic and excretory functions. Thus, the dose of lacidipine does not need to be different in hypertensive patients with or without renal insufficiency. It probably needs to be reduced in elderly hypertensive subjects and in patients with liver damage, although this reduction is presumably necessary only if the damage is severe.

Finally, the drug's pharmacokinetics support a treatment regimen based on once-a-day administration and ensures that, during long-term treatment, the drug does not accumulate. The rationale for once-a-day dosing is strengthened by the lipophylicity of lacidipine[9] and by its slow diffusion and deeper location into the cell membrane,[10] which accounts for the extended presence of the drug at the receptor compartment and perhaps also for its gentle action.[10]

ANTIHYPERTENSIVE EFFICACY IN HUMAN HYPERTENSION
Mild to Moderate Hypertension

To date, the antihypertensive efficacy of lacidipine has been tested in several thousand mild-to-moderate hypertensive patients, most of whom were recruited for studies with a double-blind, parallel-group design versus placebo or other antihypertensive drugs.

In all patients, lacidipine was given in a single daily dose, and blood pressure was measured 22 to 24 hours later (i.e., immediately before the next dose). The most frequent dose employed was 4 mg daily, but doses as low as 1 mg and as high as 8 mg daily were also tested. The results are as follows: (1) Lacidipine lowers systolic and diastolic blood pressure significantly more than placebo at the 7th day after its initial administration.[4, 11] (2) The antihypertensive effect becomes more evident when treatment is

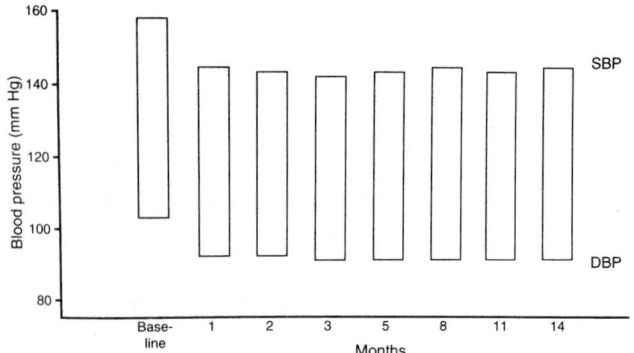

Figure 112–1. Systolic (SBP) and diastolic (DBP) blood pressure during long-term treatment with lacidipine (From Zanchetti A: Lacidipine: Pharmacological and clinical profile. Chester, England: Adis, 1991, pp 1–59.)

extended to 1 to 3 months.[11] (3) Prolongation of treatment to 1 year or more (open studies) does not cause any attenuation of the earlier antihypertensive effect (Fig. 112–1).[4] (4) The blood pressure–lowering effect of lacidipine is similar to that of hydrochlorothiazide (25 to 50 mg four times a day), atenolol (50 to 100 mg four times a day), and nifedipine SR (20 to 40 mg twice a day).[12–15] Its antihypertensive effect is also similar to that of the angiotensin-converting enzyme (ACE) inhibitors with regard to both diastolic and systolic blood pressures.[16] (5) The antihypertensive effect is obtained in some patients with 2 mg given once a day, but most patients respond to 4 to 6 mg given once a day, and a smaller additional number of patients respond to 8 mg given once a day (Fig. 112–2).[4] Thus, the recommended starting dose with lacidipine is 2.0 mg once daily, and the optimal dosage to control blood pressure is 4 mg once daily and continued with 6 mg daily if no satisfactory response is obtained. Monotherapy with lacidipine can be expected to effectively lower blood pressure (i.e., to reduce blood pressure values to <140/90 mmHg with

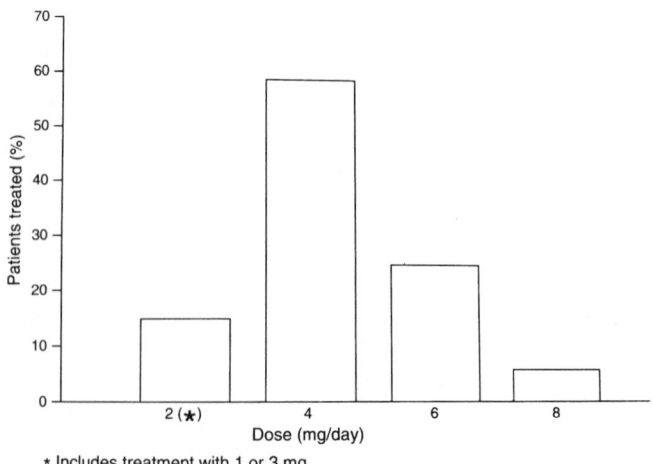

* Includes treatment with 1 or 3 mg

Figure 112–2. Doses used in clinical studies with lacidipine in 1400 patients. "Patients treated" refers to responders. (From Zanchetti A: Lacidipine: Pharmacological and clinical profile. Chester, England: Adis, 1991, pp 1–59.)

a fall of at least 10% from baseline values) in 50% to 60% of patients with mild to moderate hypertension. This number can increase substantially if the drug is given with other antihypertensive agents. There is evidence that lacidipine is effective when coadministered with atenolol or hydrochlorothiazide.[12–15] Lacidipine can also be given with an ACE inhibitor in line with the recommendations of the World Health Organization/International Society of Hypertension guidelines for treatment of mild hypertension.[17]

Hypertension in the Elderly

The antihypertensive effect of lacidipine in severe hypertension has not been studied, because investigators have focused on mild to moderate hypertension, the largely predominant condition.[18] However, lacidipine has been shown to be effective in diabetic hypertensive patients,[19] and a large database confirms that lacidipine is effective in elderly hypertensive patients as well. The doses employed in elderly patients have been similar to those employed in middle-aged hypertensive patients, and the antihypertensive effects have been as strong as those obtained in parallel groups treated with classic antihypertensive agents.[4, 20] Lacidipine has been shown to reduce blood pressure markedly in isolated systolic hypertension of the elderly. In a double-blind, parallel-group study, lacidipine (2 to 4 mg once a day) has been shown to lower systolic blood pressure significantly more than enalapril (10 to 20 mg once a day) and slightly, although not significantly, more than nitrendipine (10 to 20 mg once a day) (Fig. 112–3).[21] The use of lacidipine in isolated systolic hypertension of the elderly is being investigated in a large and long-term multicenter study[22] similar in design to the Systolic Hypertension in the Elderly Program (SHEP).[23]

Additional Blood Pressure Measurements

It has become customary to assess the efficacy of new antihypertensive drugs by means of blood pressure

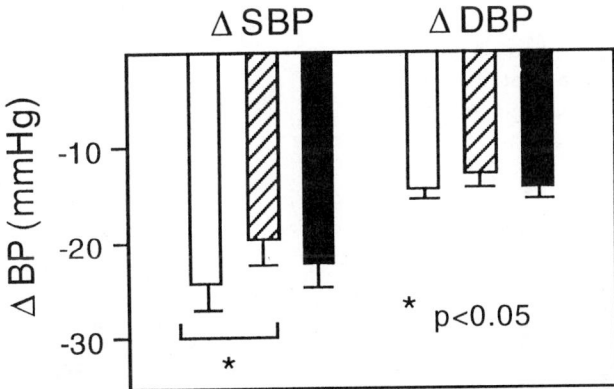

Figure 112–3. Mean (+SEM) decreases in systolic (SBP) and diastolic (DBP) blood pressure induced by 8-week treatment with lacidipine (□), nitrendipine (▨), and enalapril (■) in patients with isolated systolic hypertension. (From Chaignon MM, Mourad JJ, Guedon J: Comparative effects of antihypertensive drugs on systolic blood pressure. J Hypertens 11[Suppl 1]:S27, 1993.)

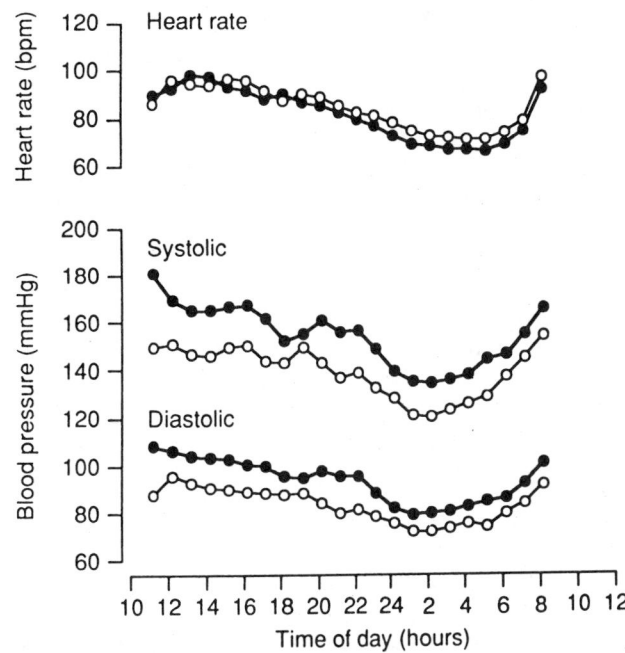

Figure 112–4. Circadian curves of intraarterial blood pressure and heart rate before and after treatment with lacidipine (4 to 8 mg q.i.d.) in hypertensive patients. (From Raftery EB: Lacidipine and circadian variations in blood pressure: Considerations for therapy. J Cardiovasc Pharmacol 17[Suppl 4]:S20, 1991.)

measurements other than "clinic" blood pressure. It has been thus shown that lacidipine can lower elevated blood pressure not only at rest but also when blood pressure is raised by exercise.[24] It has also been shown that the blood pressure–lowering effect of lacidipine is exerted over 24 hours (i.e., that the elevated daytime and the relatively low nighttime values are both reduced) (Fig. 112–4)[24–27] and that blood pressure variability is also reduced.[28] Finally, the 24-hour blood pressure data have shown that the drug has a trough-to-peak ratio of about 60% to 70%, which implies that, for the proposed once-daily regimen, its antihypertensive effect is well balanced throughout the between-dose interval.[29] A 24-hour blood pressure–lowering effect and an adequate trough-to-peak ratio have been demonstrated also in elderly hypertensive patients.[30] This is of clinical relevance because peak blood pressure values, 24-hour average blood pressure, daytime and nighttime mean blood pressures, blood pressure variability, and possibly trough-to-peak ratios of the antihypertensive effect have been shown to be associated with the organ damage of hypertension[31] and may thus be regarded as variables to be therapeutically addressed in the hypertensive patient.

EFFECTS ON HEMODYNAMIC AND HUMORAL PATTERNS

Acute administration of lacidipine is accompanied by only modest tachycardia, presumably because of the smooth action of the drug.[4] Furthermore, during prolonged administration of lacidipine, heart rate values are virtually identical to those observed before treatment (see Fig. 112–4), the disappearance of the modest initial tachycardia probably resulting from the downward resetting of the arterial baroreflex that occurs with calcium antagonist treatment of hypertension.[32]

Lack of any sustained tachycardia during lacidipine administration is accompanied by a cardiovascular pattern that resembles the one documented for dihydropyridines, perhaps with more obvious favorable changes:[33] (1) The blood pressure fall induced by lacidipine is accompanied by no increase or reduction in cardiac output, and it is thus entirely due to a reduction in systemic vascular resistance (i.e., the variable that, when increased, accounts for the blood pressure elevation in established hypertension).[34] (2) There is no evidence for a depressor effect on cardiac contraction, automatism, and conduction during long-term lacidipine administration.[4] (3) The reduction in blood pressure and systemic vascular resistance is accompanied by no change or by an increase in renal blood flow (paraaminohippurate clearance),[35] coronary blood flow (as determined by positron emission tomography [PET]),[36] and carotid artery blood flow (as determined by Doppler echocardiography).[37, 38] (4) Lacidipine does not change renal filtration rate and leads to diuresis and natriuresis.[39] Thus, in line with animal data, the lacidipine-dependent reduction in vascular resistance of vital organs is pronounced enough to more than offset the consequence of reduced pressure on tissue perfusion and prevent any (transient) renal dysfunction. Long-term administration of lacidipine does not change plasma norepinephrine, plasma renin activity, or plasma aldosterone levels,[40] indicating that any initial increase reflexively or directly triggered by the blood pressure fall disappears; thus, neural and humoral counter mechanisms are not likely to offset the antihypertensive effect. Plasma aldosterone modulation, pituitary hormone secretion, and baroreflex sensitivity[41–43] are unchanged during lacidipine administration, suggesting no deterioration of the endocrine and reflex mechanisms involved in circulatory control.

ADDITIONAL PROPERTIES

Antihypertensive treatment reduces cardiovascular morbidity and mortality, but the rate of coronary and other cardiovascular complications remains higher than that of normotensive subjects.[44] This has stimulated the search for properties of antihypertensive drugs that may protect the cardiovascular system, in addition to the protective effect on blood pressure–lowering per se. For calcium antagonists, one of these properties has been identified as prevention of calcium deposition in the cells, because in normal and ischemic tissues, such deposition accelerates tissue damage and death.[45] Calcium antagonists in general, and lacidipine in particular, however, also have other properties that may operate in this direction. One of them is regression of left ventricular hypertrophy, which in hypertensive patients increases the chance of cardiovascular complications and death.[46] This condition can be regressed with lacidipine treatment at the expense of no impairment of systolic and diastolic functions (Fig. 112–5).[47, 48] Another such property is the lack of unfavorable effects on risk factors often associated with hypertension (e.g., lipid profile, insulin resistance),[49] unlike classic antihypertensive drugs such as diuretics and β-blockers. Lacidipine exhibits a third group of potentially tissue-protective properties: (1) it reduces the platelet aggregation induced in hypertensive patients by adenosine diphosphate as nifedipine does,[4] (2) it has an antioxidant influence on rat cortical membranes more potent than that of other calcium antagonists,[4] and (3) it has an antiatherogenic effect, also more potent than that of other antihypertensive drugs.[50, 51] Although shown only in an animal model of atherosclerosis, the last effect appears to be so marked that the antiatherogenic properties of lacidipine are now being examined in a large-scale, double-blind study in which lacidipine and atenolol are being administered for 4 years to hypertensive patients with Doppler echocardiographic evidence of carotid atherosclerosis.[52]

Two other results possibly relevant to the protective

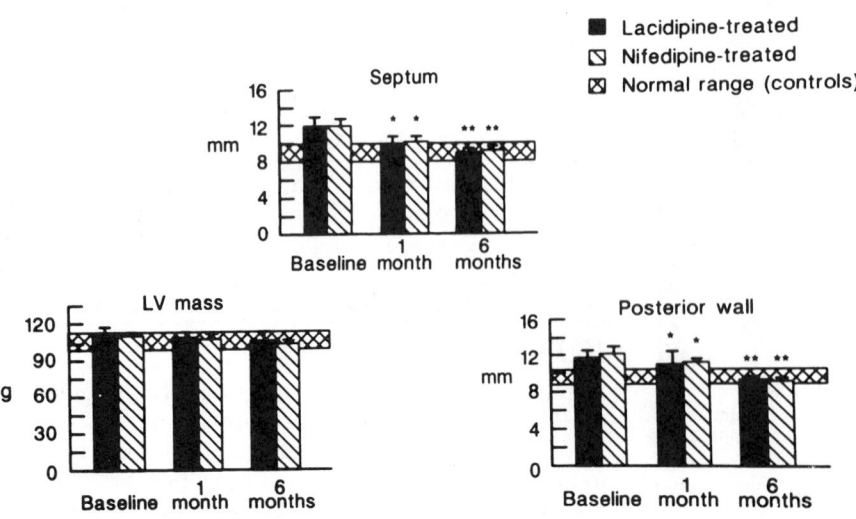

- ■ Lacidipine-treated
- ◨ Nifedipine-treated
- ⊠ Normal range (controls)

Figure 112–5. Left ventricular (LV) mass at baseline and after treatment with lacidipine and nifedipine in hypertensive patients. (From Sheiban I, Arosio E, Montesi G, et al: Remodeling of left ventricular geometry and function induced by lacidipine and nifedipine SR in mild-to-moderate hypertension. J Cardiovasc Pharmacol 17[Suppl 4]:S68, 1991.)

Table 112–1. **The Most Frequent Adverse Effects (%) Reported in Middle-Aged (n = 1372) and Elderly (<65 yrs, n = 334) Hypertensive Patients Treated with Lacidipine**

Event	Middle-Aged	Elderly
Headache	14.1	10.2
Flushing	10.4	7.5
Edema	7.3	9.9
Dizziness	5.7	6.6
Palpitations	5.2	4.2
Malaise/fatigue	3.6	2.4
Gastric disorder	2.7	3.0

effect of lacidipine on the cardiovascular system are worthy of mention: (1) The increase in coronary blood flow (PET measurements) obtained by dipyridamole in hypertensive patients is significantly more marked following prolonged treatment with lacidipine than it is before such treatment.[36] (2) Prolonged treatment with this drug also allows regression of the abnormality in radial artery compliance seen in mild to moderate hypertension.[53, 54] This suggests that not only cardiac structural alterations but also arteriolar and arterial structural alterations are favorably affected by lacidipine, which might thus aid both functional and anatomic cardiovascular normalization. Whether this means a greater degree of protection will have to be demonstrated. Lacidipine, however, has been shown to have a vasculoprotective effect in hypertensive animal models independent of its blood pressure–lowering effect.[55] It has also shown nephroprotective properties in the context of the nephrotoxicity produced by cyclosporine.[56]

TOLERANCE PROFILE

The large number of hypertensive patients studied with lacidipine provides a large database for evaluating the safety and the side effect profile of the drug. As shown in Table 112–1, the most common side effects of lacidipine are those typical of the dihydropiridine drugs (i.e., tibial edema, headache, flushing, palpitations, and dizziness). This is the case also in elderly subjects.[57] The type and mildness of side effects, however, lead to a treatment withdrawal rate comparable with or less than that of other agents and only moderately greater than that of placebo.[15, 20, 32] In many subjects, the side effect profile of lacidipine was similar to that of nifedipine SR administered twice daily. Interestingly, however, tibial edema was less frequent during both short-term and long-term (14 months) treatment. Further studies are needed to confirm this report and to clarify the possible mechanisms. Lacidipine has been shown to slightly improve the quality of life of elderly hypertensive subjects, with an overall effect comparable with that seen with captopril.[58]

CONCLUSIONS

Lacidipine is one of the newest dihydropiridines made available for the treatment of hypertension. It has been extensively studied in mild to moderate hypertension. It has shown a sustained antihypertensive effect when given once daily at doses of 4 to 6 mg with a favorable hemodynamic and side-effect profile. Its antihypertensive efficacy has been documented also in systodiastolic hypertension and in systolic hypertension of the elderly. Lacidipine also has a number of additional properties, among which is a pronounced antiatherogenic effect in animal models of atherosclerosis, possibly because of its pronounced lipophilicity and prolonged presence in the cell membranes. Ongoing studies will determine whether lacidipine has antiatherogenic and other tissue-protective properties in hypertensive patients.

REFERENCES

1. Gaviraghi G: Lacidipine, a new 1,4-dihydropiridine calcium channel antagonist possessing a potent and long lasting antihypertensive activity. In Van Der Groot H, Domany G, Pallos L, Timmerman H (eds): Trends in Medicinal Chemistry, 1988. Amsterdam: Elsevier, 1989, pp 675–690.
2. Godfraind T, Salomone S: Functional interaction of lacidipine with calcium channels in vascular smooth muscle. J Cardiovasc Pharmacol 18(Suppl 11):S1, 1991.
3. Micheli D, Collodel A, Semeraro C, et al: Lacidipine: A calcium antagonist with potent and long-lasting antihypertensive effect in animal studies. J Cardiovasc Pharmacol 15(4):666, 1990.
4. Zanchetti A: Lacidipine: Pharmacological and clinical profile. Chester, England: Adis, 1991.
5. Micheli D, Ratti E, Toson G, et al: Pharmacology of lacidipine, a vascular selective calcium antagonist. J Cardiovasc Pharmacol 17(Suppl 4):S1, 1991.
6. Van Zwieten PA, Pfaffendorf M: Similarities and differences between calcium antagonists: Pharmacological aspects. J Hypertens 11(Suppl 1):S3, 1993.
7. Micheli D, Tarter G, Cesarani R: Cardiovascular profile of lacidipine in anesthetized dogs. In IVth International Symposium on Calcium Antagonists, Pharmacology and Clinical Research, Florence, 1989, p 248.
8. Hall ST, Harding SM, Evans GL, et al: Clinical pharmacology of lacidipine. J Cardiovasc Pharmacol 17(Suppl 4):S9, 1991.
9. Van Zwieten PA, Pfaffendorf M: Pharmacology of dihydropyridine calcium antagonists: Relationship between lipophilicity and pharmacodynamic response. J Hypertens 2(Suppl 6):S3, 1993.
10. Herbette LG, Gaviraghi G, Tulenco T, et al: Molecular interaction between lacidipine and biological mechanisms. J Hypertens 2(Suppl 1):S13, 1993.
11. Perelman M: Selection of initial and maintenance dosage for lacidipine, a new once-daily calcium antagonist, for the treatment of hypertension. J Cardiovasc Pharmacol 17(Suppl 4):S14, 1991.
12. Chiariello M, for the Southern Italy Lacidipine Study Group: A double-blind comparison of the efficacy and safety of lacidipine and hydrochlorothiazide in essential hypertension. J Cardiovasc Pharmacol 17(Suppl 4):S35, 1991.
13. The United Kingdom Lacidipine Study Group: A double-blind comparison of the efficacy and safety of lacidipine with atenolol in the treatment of essential hypertension. J Cardiovasc Pharmacol 17(Suppl 4):S27, 1991.
14. Leonetti G, for the Northern Italian Study Group: Comparative study of lacidipine and nifedipine SR in the treatment of hypertension. An Italian multicenter study. J Cardiovasc Pharmacol 17(Suppl 4):S31, 1991.
15. Leonetti G: Clinical function of lacidipine, a new dihydropyridine calcium antagonist, in the treatment of hypertension. J Cardiovasc Pharmacol 18(Suppl 11):S18, 1991.
16. Guedon J, Herrero G, Salvi S: Assessment of lacidipine, a new long-acting 1,4 dihydropyridine calcium antagonist, for the pri-

mary care of elderly hypertensive patients. Cardiology in the Elderly 1:141, 1993.

17. 1993 Guidelines for the Management of Mild Hypertension: Memorandum from a World Health Organization/International Society of Hypertension meeting. Guidelines Sub-Committee. J Hypertens 11(9):905, 1993.

18. Kannel WB, Sorlie P: Hypertension in Framingham. In Paul O (ed): Epidemiology and Control of Hypertension. New York: Stratton, 1975, pp 553–592.

19. Galeone F, Giuntoli F, Fiore G, et al: Antihypertensive and metabolic effects of lacidipine in patients with NIDDM and/or hypertension. J Cardiovasc Pharmacol 23(Suppl 5):S105, 1994.

20. Rizzini P, Castello C, Salvi S, et al: Efficacy and safety of lacidipine, a new long-lasting calcium antagonist, in elderly hypertensive patients. J Cardiovasc Pharmacol 17(Suppl 4):S38, 1991.

21. Chaignon MM, Mourad JJ, Guedon J: Comparative effects of antihypertensive drugs on systolic blood pressure. J Hypertens 11(Suppl 1):S27, 1993.

22. Malacco E, Gnemmi AE, Romignoli A, et al: Systolic hypertension in the elderly: Long-term lacidipine treatment. J Cardiovasc Pharmacol 23(Suppl 5):S62, 1994.

23. SHEP Cooperative Research Group: Prevention of stroke by antihypertensive drug treatment in older persons with isolated systolic hypertension. Final results of the Systolic Hypertension in the Elderly Program. JAMA 265(24):3255, 1991.

24. Fariello R, Boni E, Corda L, et al: Exercise-induced modifications in cardiorespiratory parameters of hypertensive patients treated with calcium antagonists. J Hypertens 9(Suppl 3):S67, 1991.

25. Raftery EB: Lacidipine and circadian variations in blood pressure: Considerations for therapy. J Cardiovasc Pharmacol 17(Suppl 4):S20, 1991.

26. Palatini P, Penzo M, Guzzardi G, et al: Ambulatory blood pressure monitoring in the assessment of antihypertensive treatment: 24 hour blood pressure control with lacidipine once a day. J Hypertens 9(Suppl 3):S61, 1991.

27. Veglio F, Rabbia F, Molino P, et al: Analysis of 24-hour blood pressure profile by Fourier series during lacidipine therapy. J Cardiovasc Pharmacol 23(Suppl 5):S113, 1994.

28. Meredith PA: Duration of action and trough to peak ratios of calcium antagonists. Res Clin For 16(1):29, 1994.

29. Meredith PA, Elliot HL: FDA guidelines on trough:peak ratios in the evaluation of antihypertensive agents. J Cardiovasc Pharmacol 23(Suppl 5):S26, 1994.

30. Zito M, Abate G, Cervone C, et al: Effects of antihypertensive therapy with lacidipine on ambulatory blood pressure in the elderly. J Hypertens 9(Suppl 3):S79, 1991.

31. Mancia G, Di Rienzo M, Parati G: Clinical conference: Ambulatory blood pressure monitoring use in hypertension research in clinical practice. Hypertension 21(4):510, 1993.

32. Mancia G, Parati G, Grassi G, et al: Calcium antagonists and neural control of circulation in essential hypertension. J Hypertens 5(Suppl 4):S49, 1987.

33. Mancia G, Ferrari AU, Giannattasio C, et al: Vascular effects of lacidipine: A review of animal and human data. J Hypertens 11(Suppl 1):S39, 1993.

34. Folkow B: Physiological aspects of primary hypertension. Physiol Rev 62:347, 1982.

35. Rappelli A, Baldinelli A, Zingaretti O: The effects of antihypertensive therapy on renal function. J Hypertens 9(Suppl 3):S37, 1991.

36. Camici P, Palombo C, Gistri R, et al: Effect of lacidipine on coronary vasodilator reserve in hypertensive patients: A study with positron emission tomography. Am J Hypertens 4(Suppl):57A, 1991.

37. Safar ME: Effects of lacidipine on the carotid and cerebral circulations in essential hypertension. J Cardiovasc Pharmacol 17(Suppl 4):S51, 1991.

38. Kuriyama Y, Sawada T, Omae T: Antihypertensive drugs and cerebral circulation. In Omae T, Zanchetti A (eds): How Should Elderly Hypertensive Patients Be Treated? Tokyo: Springer-Verlag, 1989, pp 69–81.

39. Ruilope LM, Lahera V, Rodicio JL: Evaluation of the renal effect of calcium antagonist. J Cardiovasc Pharmacol 23(Suppl 5):S49, 1994.

40. Russo G, Tamburino C, Aiello R, et al: Effetti della somministrazione cronica di lacidipina in pazienti con scompenso cardiaco lieve-moderato. Risultati preliminari [abstract 85]. Cardiologia 38(Suppl 2-12):12, 1993.

41. Elliott HL: Calcium antagonism: Aldosterone and vascular responses to catecholamines and angiotensin II in man. J Hypertens 11(Suppl 6):S13, 1993.

42. Carpene G, Opocher G, Zanferrari G, et al: Effect of lacidipine on pituitary function in essential hypertension. J Cardiovasc Pharmacol 18(Suppl 11):S26, 1991.

43. Carretta R, Bardelli M, Fabris F, et al: Ultrasonographic assessment of baroreceptor sensitivity. A new method based on the measurement of pulsatile arterial diameter changes. High Blood Pressure 1:51, 1992.

44. Isles CG, Walker LM, Beevers GD, et al: Mortality of patients of the Glasgow Blood Pressure Clinic. J Hypertens 4:141, 1986.

45. Fleckenstein A, Frey M, Fleckenstein Grun G: Antihypertensive and arterial anticalcinotic effects of calcium antagonists. Am J Cardiol 57(7):1D, 1986.

46. Levy D, Garrison RJ, Savage DD, et al: Prognostic implications of echocardiographically determined left ventricular mass in the Framingham Heart Study. N Engl J Med 322(22):1561, 1990.

47. Sheiban I, Arosio E, Montesi G, et al: Remodeling of left ventricular geometry and function induced by lacidipine and nifedipine SR in mild-to-moderate hypertension. J Cardiovasc Pharmacol 17(Suppl 4):S68, 1991.

48. Betocchi S, Chiariello M: Effects of calcium antagonists on left ventricular structure and function. J Hypertens 11(Suppl 1):S33, 1993.

49. Crepaldi G, Pessina AC, Rahn KH: Effects of different antihypertensive agents on the overall cardiovascular risk profile. J Hypertens 11(Suppl 6):S37, 1993.

50. Bernini F, Corsini A, Raiteri M, et al: Effects of lacidipine on experimental models of atherosclerosis. J Hypertens 11(Suppl 1):S61, 1993.

51. Soma MR, Corsini A, Paoletti R, et al: Calcium antagonists in atherosclerosis: Focus on lacidipine. Res Clin For 16(1):43, 1994.

52. Bond G, Dal Palu C, Hansson L, et al: The ELSA trial: Protocol of a randomized trial to explore the differential effect of antihypertensive drugs on atherosclerosis in hypertension. J Cardiovasc Pharmacol 23(Suppl 5):S85, 1994.

53. Laurent S, Hayoz D, Trazzi S, et al: Isobaric compliance of the radial artery is increased in patients with essential hypertension. J Hypertens 11(1):89, 1993.

54. Trazzi S, Santucciu C, Mancia G: Radial artery compliance in essential hypertension: Effects of antihypertensive therapy with lacidipine. J Hypertens 11(Suppl 6):S17, 1993.

55. Cristofori P, Micheli D, Terron A, et al: Lacidipine: Experimental evidence of vasculoprotective properties. J Cardiovasc Pharmacol 23(Suppl 5):S90, 1994.

56. Rodicio JL, Morales JM, Ruilope LM: Lipophilic dihydropyridines provide renal protection from cyclosporin toxicity. J Hypertens 11(Suppl 6):S21, 1993.

57. Endersby CA, Brown EG, Perelman MS: Safety profile of lacidipine: A review of clinical data. J Cardiovasc Pharmacol 17(Suppl 4):S45, 1991.

58. Leonetti G, Comerio G, Cuspidi C: Evaluating quality of life in hypertensive patients. J Cardiovasc Pharmacol 23(Suppl 5):S54, 1994.

CHAPTER 113

Bepridil

Peter Schulman, M.D., F.A.C.C.

HISTORY

The discovery of bepridil and other calcium antagonists can ultimately be traced to the investigators who began unraveling the complexities of muscle energetics. Calcium's role in excitation-contraction coupling was first proposed by Alexander Sandow in 1952.[1] This important development led to the recognition of the central role of calcium in cardiac and vascular smooth muscle contraction and spawned the search for agents that could modulate the effects of cellular calcium for therapeutic use. In 1962, these efforts resulted in the development of the first clinically useful calcium antagonist, verapamil, ushering in an important new era in cardiovascular pharmacology. Dozens of additional calcium antagonists, most never approved, were tested in the late 1960s and early 1970s. Bepridil, an agent with additional properties beyond calcium channel blockade, was synthesized by scientists at the Centre Européen de Recherches Mauvernay (CERM) in Riom, France, in 1972. Numerous investigations in animals and humans have contributed to our knowledge of bepridil. And while our understanding of this agent's complex pharmacology is far from complete, bepridil has been of significant value in many patients with ischemic heart disease.

CHEMISTRY

Bepridil, or β-[(2-methylpropoxy)methyl]-*N*-phenyl-*N*-(phenylmethyl)-1-pyrrolidine-ethanamine monohydrochloride monohydrate, with a molecular weight of 366.5, is chemically unrelated to other calcium antagonists. The chemical structure of bepridil hydrochloride is shown in Figure 113–1. With its asymmetric carbon atom (see Fig. 113–1, asterisk), bepridil, like verapamil, is a racemate. But unlike verapamil, its two optical isomers have similar electrophysiologic properties,[2, 3] and the agent in clinical use is a racemic mixture.

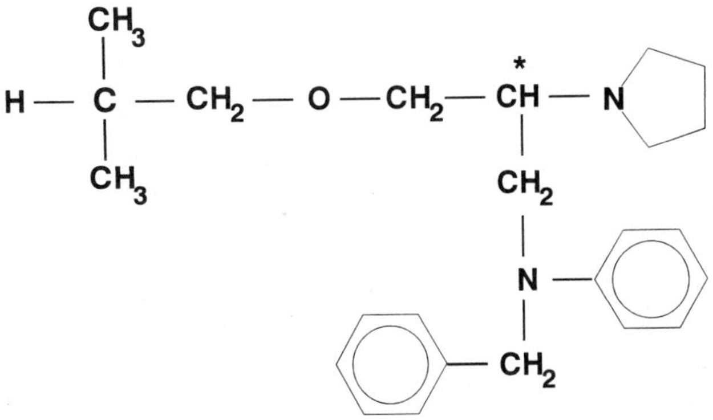

Bepridil hydrochloride is a crystalline white powder highly soluble in acetone. Unlike diltiazem and verapamil, it is only slightly soluble in water. Its high lipid solubility allows penetration of cell membranes, which contributes to its long half-life of elimination.

PHARMACOLOGY

The pharmacology of bepridil is complex not only because of its dual site of action at the cellular level but also because of its multitude of pharmacologic actions (Table 113–1). Bepridil acts both at the cell membrane and intracellularly. At the level of the cell membrane, bepridil, like other calcium antagonists, inhibits the movement of calcium ion influx through the "slow channels" during the action potential.[4] By inhibiting calcium ion influx through these channels, such agents inhibit sinoatrial automaticity and atrioventricular (AV) nodal conduction. In general, this results in a slowing of the heart rate and a prolongation of AV conduction. Yet, despite the common ability of calcium antagonists to inhibit calcium ion entry, their net effect on heart rate and AV nodal conduction can vary widely as a result of a multitude of confounding factors including (1) the mode of binding to the calcium channel, (2) the selectivity for cardiac or smooth muscle, (3) the use dependency (difference in effect as a function of the frequency and duration of stimulation), and (4) the pharmacologic effect at sites other than the cell membrane.

Bepridil inhibits both voltage-dependent and receptor-operated calcium channels.[4] Activity of the receptor-operated channels is modulated by receptors for agonists such as norepinephrine, serotonin, or angiotensin II. These channels not only regulate smooth muscle contraction, thereby determining vasomotor

Figure 113–1. Chemical structure of bepridil. Bepridil is a racemic mixture. The asterisk (*) indicates the asymmetric carbon atom.

Table 113–1. **Summary of Bepridil's Pharmacologic Effects**

Cell Membrane Effects
Inhibition of voltage-dependent Ca^{2+} channels
Inhibition of receptor-operated Ca^{2+} channels
Inhibition of fast Na^+ channels
Inhibition of outward depolarizing K^+ current

Intracellular Effects
Inhibition of calmodulin-calcium complexes in vascular smooth muscle cells
Inhibition of calmodulin-induced attenuation of myocardial contractility
Stimulation of calcium-dependent Mg^{2+} ATPase

tone, but may also promote smooth muscle proliferation, which contributes to atherosclerosis.[5] Blockade of these channels could theoretically result in retarded plaque formation. However, the ultimate clinical utility of bepridil and other calcium antagonists in preventing the atherosclerotic process is unknown.

At the cell membrane, in addition to its effects on the calcium channels, bepridil also inhibits the "fast" sodium channels.[6, 7] This results in a slowing of the rate of rise of the phase 0 action potential, conferring on bepridil the properties of a type I antiarrhythmic drug.

Bepridil exerts several additional pharmacologic properties at the cell membrane. It inhibits the outward potassium repolarizing current.[8, 9] This results in a prolongation of the cardiac action potential, leading to prolongation of the QT interval. Bepridil also inhibits the sodium-calcium exchange, which extrudes calcium in exchange for sodium and which is operative during depolarization. Prolongation of the action potential duration (and, thus, lengthening of the QT interval) occurs by this mechanism as well.

Bepridil differs from most other calcium antagonists in that it acts intracellularly as well as at the cell membrane. Intracellularly, it acts primarily as a calmodulin inhibitor.[10] Within vascular smooth muscle cells, where calmodulin promotes smooth muscle contraction (e.g., vasoconstriction), bepridil's inhibitory effect on calmodulin promotes vasodilation. On the other hand, in myocardial cells, where calmodulin attenuates contraction by inhibiting calcium release from the sarcoplasmic reticulum, bepridil's inhibition of calmodulin augments muscular shortening. In addition, Solaro et al. have shown that bepridil significantly increases intracellular adenosine triphosphatase (ATPase) activity in pig heart tissue, which also promotes increased force of contraction.[11] These intracellular effects that enhance contractility may account for the relative lack of clinically important negative inotropic effect and further distinguish bepridil from other calcium antagonists that only operate at the cell membrane.

PHARMACOKINETICS

Like the other calcium antagonists, bepridil is completely absorbed via the gastrointestinal tract.[12] After absorption, there is a substantial first-pass hepatic uptake, and as a result, 59% oral bioavailability is achieved. Peak plasma levels are achieved approximately 2 hours after ingestion of a single dose and 2 to 3 hours after ingestion during chronic dosing regimens.[13] Food in the stomach delays drug absorption slightly but does not reduce the extent of absorption.[14]

Bepridil's metabolic fate is complex. It undergoes extensive transformation in the liver via three principal metabolic pathways.[15] Overall, 17 metabolites have been identified. Although little is known about most of these, one has shown some pharmacologic activity similar to the parent compound in a guinea pig heart.[14] In healthy male volunteers, two thirds of

a radiolabeled dose was excreted in the urine within 10 days, but less than 0.1% was excreted unchanged.[14]

Bepridil is highly protein bound. In the usual therapeutic dose range, the fraction of free bepridil is only 0.23%.[16, 17] After a single oral dose, Benet found a terminal elimination half-life of 33 hours in healthy volunteers.[14] With chronic oral dosing, the half-life is extended to 42 hours in healthy normal individuals[13, 18] and up to 4.5 days in patients with angina.[19] Because a dose-response relationship is not well established, plasma drug levels are not considered helpful in individual patients.

PHYSIOLOGIC EFFECTS
Electrophysiologic and Electrocardiographic Effects

In addition to its antiischemic properties, discussed later, bepridil possesses substantial antiarrhythmic properties that fall into three of the categories in the commonly used classification system. The inhibition of the fast sodium channel classifies bepridil as a type IB drug. It also falls into the category of type III drugs because it blocks the potassium channel and prolongs refractoriness. Finally, bepridil belongs to the type IV drugs—those that block the calcium channels. These heterogeneous drug actions result in a multitude of effects on electrophysiologic and electrocardiographic parameters discussed here and summarized in Table 113–2.

Intravenous and oral doses of bepridil lengthen the refractory periods in the atrium and AV node, as well as in the His-Purkinje tissue and ventricle.[20] Lengthening of the refractory period in accessory pathways has also been shown.[21]

Through its inhibition of transmembrane ion transport, bepridil reduces atrial and ventricular automaticity and prolongs the action potential duration as well. The attenuation of atrial automaticity is due to calcium channel inhibition, whereas the prolongation of the action potential duration is due to its inhibitory effects on both the outward potassium current as well as on the sodium-calcium exchange mechanism.

At therapeutic doses, the surface electrocardiogram exhibits a slight slowing of the sinus rate of approximately 5% with little or no effect on the PR interval and no effect on the QRS interval. In United States trials, prolongation of the QT_c interval occurred in approximately 80% of angina patients with an overall

Table 113–2. **Summary of Bepridil's Electrophysiologic and Resulting Electrocardiographic Effects**

Parameter	Electrophysiologic Effect	Effect on ECG
Sinus node automaticity	Decreased	Heart rate ↓
AV node conduction	Decreased	PR unchanged or ↑
Action potential duration	Increased	QT ↑
Phase 0 upstroke velocity	Reduced	QRS unchanged
Repolarization	Modified	T waves flat, notched

average prolongation of 8%.[22] Only 5% of angina patients exhibited excessive QT_c prolongation of more than 25%[22]—which serves as a marker for proarrhythmia. The T waves in patients treated with bepridil often take on a characteristically flattened and notched appearance[20, 23] (Fig. 113–2).

Hemodynamic Effects

The hemodynamic profile of bepridil bears some similarity to that of other calcium antagonists. It is principally an arterial vasodilator. Yet, unlike other calcium antagonists, it produces far greater dilation of the coronary arteries than of the peripheral arteries. Remme et al.[24] studied the hemodynamics of intravenous bepridil in 2 patients with coronary artery disease and intact left ventricular function. Five-minute infusions of both low dose (2 mg/kg) and high dose (4 mg/kg) were evaluated. Coronary arterial resistance fell 23% and 41%, respectively, in the low- and high-dose groups, with a corresponding increase in

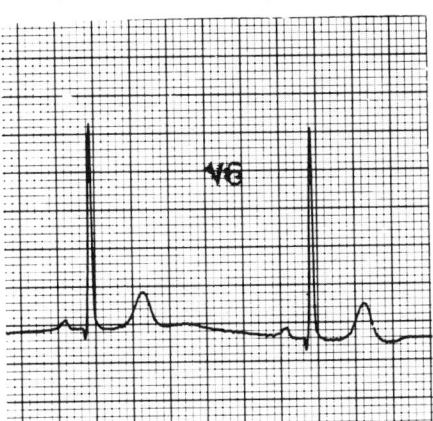

BASELINE

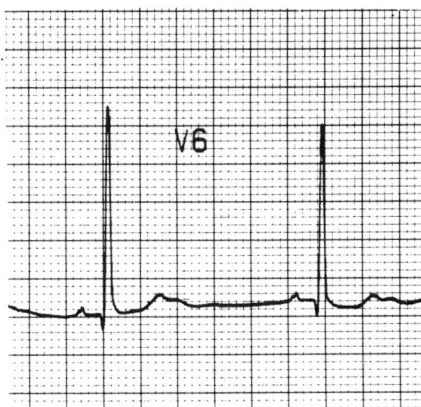

BEPRIDIL 200 mg/day

Figure 113–2. Electrocardiographic effects of bepridil. Baseline and post-treatment electrocardiographs from a 78-year-old woman with severe angina. During bepridil therapy (200 mg/day), the QT is prolonged, and there is characteristic notching of the T wave.

coronary blood flow of 17% and 47%. The fall in coronary resistance was accompanied by no change in systemic resistance with the low-dose infusion and only a 16% decline with the high-dose infusion.[24]

Both low- and high-dose intravenous bepridil resulted in an 8% to 9% decline in resting heart rate and an approximately 10% decline in systolic blood pressure, but only the high-dose infusion resulted in a transient elevation of the left ventricular end-diastolic pressure (LVEDP) from 11 to 15 mmHg, whereas the low dose had no significant effect on LVEDP.[24]

In patients with coronary artery disease and reduced left ventricular function, intravenous bepridil resulted in a mild reduction in resting left ventricular performance. Josephson et al.[25] studied 11 such patients. At a dose of 2 mg/kg infused over 15 minutes, bepridil reduced heart rate by 9%, reduced cardiac index by 14%, and reduced maximum left ventricular dP/dt by 16%.[25]

In contrast with acute intravenous dosing, chronic dosing with oral bepridil appears to have little or no negative inotropic effect, in patients both with normal or with impaired left ventricular function. Zusman et al.[26] evaluated resting left ventricular hemodynamics in 13 patients with angina and normal or nearly normal left ventricular systolic function. Resting left ventricular ejection fraction (LVEF) was 0.45 during placebo therapy and 0.49 after 4 weeks of oral bepridil, 400 mg/day. Cardiac output was 5.9 L/min with placebo and 6.0 with bepridil. The differences were not statistically significant.[26] Similarly, in a cohort of patients with coronary disease and reduced resting left ventricular function (mean LVEF, 0.33; range, 0.17 to 0.44), De Marco et al.[27] found no deleterious effect of chronic oral bepridil on resting cardiac performance. Furthermore, when these patients were stressed by rapid atrial pacing, bepridil ameliorated the rise in left ventricular filling pressure compared with control.[27]

Although many other calcium antagonists are useful in the treatment of hypertension, bepridil's antihypertensive effects do not appear to be clinically relevant. Intravenous infusions of low-dose and high-dose bepridil result in a drop in systolic blood pressure of approximately 15 mmHg, but blood pressure returns to normal after 5 minutes.[24] DiBianco found no significant change in systolic blood pressure after chronic oral monotherapy in standard dose ranges.[28] The lack of antihypertensive effect is likely due to the predominance of coronary rather than systemic vasodilation.

Effect on Angina

Bepridil possesses substantial antiischemic effects both as a single agent and in combination with other antianginal agents. In a double-blind, randomized, controlled trial, Shapiro et al. compared 200, 300, and 400 mg bepridil, given once daily, with placebo in patients with chronic stable angina.[29] Compared with placebo, active therapy was accompanied by a significant improvement in the anginal attack rate, the number of nitroglycerin tablets consumed, and the treadmill exercise testing parameters, including time to angina, time to 1-mm ST depression, and total exercise time. Higher doses of bepridil were associated with greater improvements compared with baseline.[29] Similar improvements in angina and exercise testing indices compared with placebo were found in other investigations.[30]

Data on head-to-head comparisons of bepridil monotherapy with other antianginal agents are limited. In a crossover study by Frishman et al.[31] of bepridil (200 to 400 mg once daily) and propranolol 80 to 320 mg in divided doses, these two drugs were similar in terms of clinical indicators of efficacy—anginal episodes and nitroglycerin consumption. However, bepridil was more effective in improving exercise testing parameters—time to onset of angina and total work performed.[31]

Katz et al.[32] compared bepridil and nifedipine monotherapy in 97 patients with chronic stable angina. Bepridil resulted in a statistically greater improvement in total treadmill exercise time and time to 1-mm ST segment depression as well as a greater reduction in the anginal attack rate. In addition, there were fewer dropouts as a result of adverse drug reactions in the bepridil group (8% versus 25%).[32]

Frishman[33] evaluated the effect of combination antianginal therapy with propranolol. Compared with propranolol alone (with placebo), the addition of bepridil was associated with an improvement in the anginal attack rate and the number of anginal attacks. Furthermore, there were statistically significant improvements in the following exercise testing parameters: total exercise time, time to onset of angina, time to 1-mm ST depression, and total work performed.[33]

Given the evidence of bepridil's effectiveness as monotherapy and in combination with other agents, it is likely that bepridil was on course to approval by the United States Food and Drug Administration for the treatment of angina in the mid 1980s. However, as reports surfaced from France of the occurrence of torsade de pointes in patients treated with bepridil,[34] especially in association with excessive QT_c prolongation, extensive testing of bepridil in the United States was temporarily halted. When investigations in the United States resumed in the late 1980s, the focus of bepridil investigations was redirected toward the treatment of patients with refractory angina.

In the first major report after the redirection of bepridil investigations, Singh et al.[35] studied 86 patients with severe stable angina. Study subjects remained symptomatic despite therapy with maximally tolerated doses of diltiazem along with nitrates and β-blockers if tolerated. While therapy with the other agents continued uninterrupted, patients were randomized to receive in a blinded fashion either bepridil, titrated stepwise from 200 to 400 mg/day, or their current dose of diltiazem. Compared with diltiazem, bepridil increased the time to onset of angina and time to 1-mm ST depression and was well tolerated, reflecting an improvement in the overall angina control.[35] Although the study design of this

trial does not allow a true head-to-head comparison of the two drugs in patients with severe or refractory stable angina, the results do suggest a possible advantage of bepridil in this setting. Our experience in the past 5 years supports such a role for bepridil, and in approximately 75 patients with unacceptable angina inadequately controlled with other available medical or surgical therapy, the addition of bepridil yielded substantial clinical improvement in the majority (P. Schulman, personal observations).

CLINICAL USE
Indications

Although it has been shown to be effective as angina monotherapy, bepridil is currently indicated in the United States only for patients with severe yet stable angina pectoris whose therapeutic response to other antianginal therapies is suboptimal or for patients intolerant to standard anginal therapy. Although these indications seem straightforward, in actuality they are imprecise and leave much to the physician's judgment to determine whether bepridil is indicated (Table 113–3).

First, physicians' interpretations of "suboptimal control" can be highly subjective. For example, most physicians would agree that a retired, relatively sedentary patient with one episode of mild angina per month during extreme exertion on current medical therapy is "optimally" controlled. On the other hand, whether an 80-year-old home-bound patient 10 years post bypass, on three antianginal drugs and having five episodes of angina per week on standard therapy, is optimally controlled is debatable.

In addition, physicians' enthusiasm to proceed to coronary angioplasty or coronary artery bypass is also highly variable, yet the decision whether to revascularize greatly affects the decision to prescribe bepridil. The increase in the number of revascularization procedures performed in the United States for the treatment of angina[36] has likely reduced the number of patients who would have otherwise received bepridil.

Physician views of "intolerance" to other anginal medications can also be highly variable. For example, although severe intolerance, such as a throbbing nitrate headache, is readily ascertained, the occurrence of reduced sexual function with β-blockers may go unreported and be unknown to the physician. Therefore, physicians who specifically ask their patients

Table 113–3. **Considerations in the Choice of Bepridil as an Antianginal Agent**

Frequency and severity of anginal attacks
Ease of precipitation of angina
Side effects (sometimes occult) of current medical regimen
Suitability of coronary artery revascularization: bypass surgery or angioplasty
Comorbid medical conditions
Contraindications to bepridil

taking β-blockers about sexual dysfunction are likely to find more patients who are intolerant of standard anginal therapy.

Despite the imprecision with respect to bepridil's stated indications, the following can be concluded about its use. Given its potential, however small, for precipitating rhythm disturbances and the need for more careful monitoring than with other agents, bepridil is not indicated as a first antianginal drug. However, it can be highly effective in many patients with severe stable angina whose condition would not otherwise be as well controlled.

In its current formulation and recommended dosing, bepridil is not well suited for the treatment of unstable angina. Unstable angina requires therapies that have a quick onset of action and that can be rapidly titrated. Oral bepridil has none of these properties. Furthermore, bepridil initiation generally requires discontinuation of some preexisting therapy if another calcium antagonist is being given, and the resulting therapeutic hiatus could result in worsening of myocardial ischemia until the effect of bepridil becomes manifest.

Future dosing regimens for unstable angina to surmount the problems associated with bepridil's slow onset of action may become available. For example, intravenous bepridil or combination intravenous and oral bepridil may prove beneficial in this setting. Finally, in a recent study of 208 patients with unstable angina,[37] investigators used a high-dose oral leading regimen of bepridil, 900 mg on the first day and 500 mg on the second and third days. When compared with a regimen of oral diltiazem, 360 mg/day, bepridil's efficacy was similar in terms of incidence of recurrent angina and myocardial infarction, total mortality, and adverse events.[37]

Dosing

Dosing guidelines for bepridil are shown in Table 113-4. The day before initiation of bepridil, all other calcium antagonists should be discontinued. A baseline serum potassium level should be measured and potassium given if needed to maintain the level in the high-normal range. A baseline electrocardiogram should be recorded, and the QT_c (QT divided by the square root of the R-R interval) should be measured to ensure that it is within the normal range (≤ 0.44 second).

Bepridil is generally initiated at a dose of 200 mg once daily. Because of the long half-life (42 hours), steady-state therapy will not be seen for several days, and hence a therapeutic effect will take time to develop. Thus, patients should be advised about the possible delay in efficacy. If 7 to 10 days have elapsed and a satisfactory response is not obtained, the dose can be upwardly titrated first to 300 mg daily and later to 400 mg daily with at least 10 to 14 days allowed between, to achieve a steady state for each new dose level. Before dose increase, an electrocardiogram should be recorded to ensure that the QT_c is within the acceptable limits (≤ 0.52 second on ther-

Table 113-4. Dosing Guidelines for Bepridil

Prior to beginning therapy:
1. Discontinue all calcium channel blockers and other drugs that prolong the QT. Measure the QT_c—do not introduce bepridil if the $QT_c > 0.44$ sec.
2. Determine the serum potassium level—do not initiate therapy if low.

Dosing:
1. Begin bepridil, 200 mg, once daily (in elderly patients, consider 100 mg/day).
2. After 10–14 days, reassess symptoms and repeat ECG to determine QT_c.
3. Reduce dose or discontinue bepridil if $QT_c > 0.52$ sec.
4. If a satisfactory response is not obtained, the dose can be increased by 100 mg increments every 10 to 14 days to a maximal dose of 400 mg/day if $QT_c \leq 0.52$ sec.
5. Recheck serum potassium level when clinically indicated, and replace potassium as needed to keep the level in the high-normal range.

Long-term follow-up:
1. Perform ECG periodically to recheck QT_c. (However, once on a steady-state dose, the QT_c is unlikely to change significantly.)
2. Perform serum potassium measurement when clinically indicated.
3. Caution patient to call when any new medications are introduced or when health status changes significantly.

apy). Once a stable dose is maintained, the frequency of monitoring of the serum potassium and QT_c depends on the individual patient. Those patients whose electrolytes are more likely to vary will require more frequent monitoring.

Bepridil is suitable for use in combination with β-blockers[33] and nitrates.[35] Because of its mild negative chronotropic effect, there is a potential for excessive heart rate slowing when bepridil is used in combination with β-blockers. The substitution of β-blocking agents with intrinsic sympathomimetic activity (ISA), such as pindolol, for non-ISA β-blockers can be useful in this setting. Bepridil can be added to other antianginal agents with the exception of other calcium antagonists.

Contraindications and Precautions

Because bepridil can precipitate torsade de pointes,[34, 38] it should be avoided in conditions that otherwise predispose to this life-threatening arrhythmia. Hypokalemia is a contraindication to bepridil. Potassium-wasting diuretics are to be avoided unless potassium replacement is given concomitantly. If a patient currently taking bepridil requires diuretics, potassium-sparing agents are preferable, and regular monitoring of the serum potassium level should be performed. Patients should be aware of the importance of potassium monitoring, because they are likely to encounter physicians unfamiliar with bepridil.

Retrospective evaluation from France of the overall experience with bepridil used for angina in the early 1980s indicates an incidence of torsade de pointes of approximately 0.11%.[34] As experience with bepridil increased and the importance of careful QT_c monitoring was recognized, the incidence of torsade de pointes has decreased. By 1989, the annual incidence had fallen to 0.0092% of patients treated.[38]

Bepridil should also be avoided with other conditions and drugs that increase the risk of torsade de pointes. These include a baseline prolonged QT_c (> 0.44 second), profound bradycardia, significant ventricular arrhythmias, and conduction disturbances. In addition, the tricyclic antidepressants and antiarrhythmic drugs should be avoided in combination with bepridil.

Although bepridil has not been expressly studied in the setting of acute myocardial infarction, because of the electrical instability that can occur, it should be avoided. In light of the results of Cardiac Arrhythmia Suppression Trial (CAST),[39, 40] in which treatment of patients with recent myocardial infarction with any of several antiarrhythmic drugs (mostly type IC) increased the risk of sudden death, bepridil should probably be avoided in such patients as well, until additional safety and efficacy data are available.

Bepridil's intracellular actions tend to mitigate the negative inotropic effect of calcium channel blockade at the cell membrane. Nonetheless, left ventricular function can deteriorate in some patients. As a result, it should be avoided in patients with markedly reduced systolic function at rest. Although there are no specific guidelines on an ejection fraction below which bepridil is contraindicated, in my experience, worsening of congestive heart failure rarely occurs in patients with ejection fractions higher than 0.35. Signs of congestive heart failure are somewhat more likely to occur in patients with ejection fractions between 0.25 and 0.35, but I have treated many such patients without adverse effect and without the need for added diuretics.

Two cases of severe leukopenia were reported during phase III clinical trials.[41] However, the relationship between the bepridil and the hematologic disorder in these two cases is uncertain. Nausea or abdominal discomfort occurs in approximately 15% of patients. Taking the drug with food can ameliorate this problem.

Interaction with Other Drugs

In general, bepridil should not be given with drugs that have like actions, such as calcium antagonists and antiarrhythmics. If bepridil is to replace another calcium antagonist, the other agent should not be given the day bepridil is started. However, because bepridil's therapeutic action does not take effect for several days, there may be a temporary worsening of angina during that period. Therefore, in some patients, we have successfully "overlapped" other calcium antagonists with bepridil for periods of up to 3 days to minimize the therapeutic hiatus. However, this regimen is not generally recommended.

Few significant interactions with other drugs have been found. Investigations on the concomitant administration of digoxin have yielded variable results.[14, 42] In clinical practice, it should be anticipated that serum digoxin levels on a stable dose will rise by approxi-

mately 30% after the introduction of bepridil therapy.[42]

Use in Elderly Patients and in Patients with Impaired Organ Systems

In a pharmacokinetic study in elderly patients, the elimination half-life of bepridil was more than doubled in comparison with younger subjects.[43] As a result, physicians should consider reducing the starting dose to 100 mg/day in patients older than 70 years.

Data are limited on the use of bepridil in patients with significant renal or hepatic impairment because, as with other therapeutic agents, clinical trials have excluded patients with significant renal or hepatic disease. However, because bepridil's principal metabolites are inactive and excreted unchanged in the urine, adjustment for mild to moderate renal impairment is probably not necessary.[14] On the other hand, because bepridil undergoes extensive hepatic metabolism, caution should be exercised in patients with significant hepatic impairment.

COST

Bepridil is expensive. In a survey of seven Hartford area retail pharmacies in late 1993, the retail price of bepridil ranged from $2.09 to $2.70 for a 200-mg tablet (in lots of 100 tablets). By comparison, the price of Cardizem CD ranged from $1.75 to $1.84 for a 360-mg tablet (S. Januska, unpublished data). Thus, in comparison with other standard antianginal medication, this drug is expensive. However, given its potential benefit in patients with refractory angina pectoris,[36] bepridil could potentially result in fewer doctor visits and hospital admissions.

SUMMARY AND CONCLUSIONS

Bepridil is a unique calcium antagonist with complex pharmacologic properties and metabolism. Although it has been shown to be effective in the general angina population, because of concerns about the development of cardiac arrhythmias, bepridil is currently indicated as a second-line agent for patients with angina who are not optimally controlled on standard therapy or for patients who are intolerant of standard therapy.

Among other precautions, the use of bepridil requires careful monitoring of the electrocardiogram and the serum potassium level. With appropriate diligence on the part of the physician, the risk of cardiac arrhythmias appears acceptably low.[38] Given its demonstrated efficacy[34] in a patient population severely limited by angina, it is likely that the use of bepridil will increase as physicians become more at ease with its monitoring requirements.

REFERENCES

1. Sandow A: Excitation-contraction coupling in muscular response. Yale J Biol Med 25:176, 1952.

2. Van Amsterdam FTM, Zaagsma J: Stereoisomers of calcium antagonists discriminate between coronary vascular and myocardial sites. Naunyn Schmiedebergs Arch Pharmacol 337:213, 1988.

3. Van Amsterdam FTM, Haas M, Zaagsma J: Dynamic and kinetic differences of the vascular and myocardial effects of calcium antagonists in the rat heart. J Cardiovasc Pharmacol 9:570, 1987.

4. Flaim SF, Ratz PH, Swigart SC, Gleason MM: Bepridil hydrochloride alters potential-dependent and receptor-operated calcium channels in vascular smooth muscle of rabbit aorta. J Pharmacol Exp Ther 234:63, 1985.

5. Gill A, Flaim SF, Damiano BP, et al: Pharmacology of bepridil. Am J Cardiol 69:11D, 1992.

6. Kane KA, Winslow E: Antidysrhythmic and electrophysiologic effects of a new antianginal agent, bepridil. J Cardiovasc Pharmacol 2:193, 1980.

7. Vogel S, Crampton R, Sperelakis N: Blockade of myocardial slow channels by bepridil (CERM 1978). J Pharmacol Exp Ther 210:378, 1979.

8. Stuart J, Ellory JC, Stone PCW: Rheological action of bepridil on normal and sickle erythrocytes. Clin Hemorheol 9:247, 1989.

9. Berger F, Borchard U, Hafner D: Effects of calcium entry blocker bepridil on repolarizing and pacemaker currents in sheep cardiac purkinje fibres. Naunyn Schmiedebergs Arch Pharmacol 339:638, 1989.

10. Ito H, Ishikawa T, Hidaka H: Effects on calmodulin of bepridil, an antianginal agent. J Pharmacol Exp Ther 230:737, 1984.

11. Solaro RJ, Bousquet P, Hohnson JD: Stimulation of cardiac myofiliment force, ATPase activity and troponin C Ca++ binding by bepridil. J Pharmacol Exp Ther 238:502, 1986.

12. Ng KT, Hills JF, Wu WN: The absorbtion, excretion and biotransformation of bepridil HCl (Bp) in man [abstract]. Fed Proc 43:655, 1984.

13. Desiraju RK, Gemzik B, Naya K, Esterling DE: Steady-state dose proportionality and pharmacokinetics of bepridil in healthy volunteers [abstract]. Clin Pharmacol Ther 35:234, 1984.

14. Benet LZ: Pharmacokinetics and metabolism of bepridil. Am J Cardiol 55:8C, 1985.

15. Zeller FP, Spinler SA: Bepridil: A new long-acting calcium channel blocking agent. Drug Intell Clin Pharm 21:487, 1987.

16. Albengres E, Urien S, Pognat J-F, Tillement J-P: Multiple binding of bepridil in human blood. Pharmacology 28:139, 1984.

17. Pritchard JF, McKown LA, Dvorchik BH, et al: Plasma protein binding of bepridil. J Clin Pharmacol 25:347, 1985.

18. Flaim SF, Cummings DM: Bepridil hydrochloride: A review of its pharmacologic properties. Curr Ther Res 39:568, 1986.

19. Marshall RJ, Winslow E, Lamar JC, Apoi E: Bepridil. In Scriarbine A (ed): New Drugs Annual: Cardiovascular Drugs, Vol 2. New York: Raven Press, 1984, pp 157–176.

20. Prystowsky EN: Electrophysiologic and antiarrhythmic properties of bepridil. Am J Cardiol 55:59C, 1985.

21. Rowland E, McKenna W, Krikler D: Electrophysiological and antiarrhythmic effects of bepridil in re-entry AV tachycardia—comparison with verapamil and ajmaline [abstract]. Circulation 68(Suppl III):311, 1983.

22. Prystowsky EN: Effects of bepridil on cardiac electrophysiologic properties. Am J Cardiol 69:63D, 1992.

23. Hill JA, Pepine CJ: Effects of bepridil on the resting electrocardiogram. Int J Cardiol 6:319, 1984.

24. Remme WJ, van Hoogenhuyze DCA, Krauss XH, et al: Dose related coronary and systemic haemodynamic effects of intravenous bepridil in patients with coronary artery disease. Eur Heart J 8:130, 1987.

25. Josephson MA, Mody T, Coyle K, Singh BN: Effects on hemodynamics and left ventricular ejection fraction of intravenous bepridil for impaired left ventricular function secondary to coronary artery disease. Am J Cardiol 60:44, 1987.

26. Zusman RM, Christensen DM, Kanarek DJ, et al: Evaluation of bepridil for the treatment of angina pectoris: Evidence for preservation of left ventricular function. Am J Cardiol 55:30C, 1985.

27. De Marco T, Deedwania P, Chatterjee K: Systemic and coronary hemodynamic efffects of bepridil in patients with depresssed left ventricular function. Am J Cardiol 69:31D, 1992.

28. DiBianco R: Bepridil treatment of chronic stable angina: A review of comparative studies versus placebo, nifedipine, and diltiazem. Am J Cardiol 69:56D, 1992.

29. Shapiro W, Di Bianco R, Thadani U, et al: Comparative efficacy of 200, 300 and 400 mg of bepridil for chronic stable angina pectoris. Am J Cardiol 55(Suppl):36C, 1985.

30. Narahara K: Hemodynamic effects of bepridil in patients with coronary artery disease. Am J Cardiol 69:17D, 1992.

31. Frishman WH, Charlap S, Farnham DJ, et al: Combination propranolol and bepridil therapy in stable angina pectoris. Am J Cardiol 55(Suppl):43C, 1985.

32. Katz RJ, Thadani U, and the Bepridil-Nifedipine Multicenter Group: Bepridil vs nifedipine for treatment of chronic stable angina. J Am Coll Cardiol 7(Suppl):231A, 1986.

33. Frishman WH: Comparative efficacy and concomitant use of bepridil and beta blockers in the management of angina pectoris. Am J Cardiol 69(Suppl):50D, 1992.

34. Rapport de Pharmacovigilance (code 800). Riom Cedex, France: L Riom Laboratories-CERM, 1985.

35. Singh BN, for the Bepridil Collaborative Study Group: Comparative efficacy and safety of bepridil and diltiazem in chronic stable angina pectoris refractory to diltiazem. Am J Cardiol 68:306, 1991.

36. 1993 Heart and Stroke Facts Statistics. Dallas, TX: American Heart Association, 1992.

37. Bory M, Quilliet L: Etude comparative de l' efficacité et de la tolérance du bépridil et du diltiazem dans l'angor instable. Ann Cardiol Angeiol 43:77, 1994.

38. Coumel P: Safety of bepridil: From review of the European data. Am J Cardiol 69(Suppl):75D, 1992.

39. Preliminary report: Effect of encainide and flecainide on mortality in a randomized trial of arrhythmia suppression after myocardial infarction. N Engl J Med 321:406, 1989.

40. Akiyama T, Pawitan Y, Greenberg H, et al: Increased risk of death and cardiac arrest from encainide and flecainide in patients after non-Q-wave acute myocardial infarction in the Cardiac Arrhythmia Suppression Trial. Am J Cardiol 68:1551,1991.

41. Physicians' Desk Reference 1992. Montvale, NJ: Medical Economics Data, 1992, pp 1383–1385.

42. Hollingshead LM, Faulds D, Fitton A: Bepridil: A review of its pharmacologic properties and therapeutic use in stable angina. Drugs 44:935, 1992.

43. Hakamaki T, Apoil E, Arstila M, et al: Bepridil in the elderly: A pharmacologic and clinical monitoring study. Curr Ther Res 44:752, 1988.

XII.

Lipid-Lowering Drugs

Editors: Antonio Gotto and Scott Grundy

CHAPTER 114

Nicotinic Acid

Carl J. Lavie, M.D., F.A.C.C., F.A.C.P., F.A.C.C.P., and Richard V. Milani, M.D., F.A.C.C.

The water-soluble B vitamin, nicotinic acid or niacin, was discovered to be an essential dietary component in the early 1900s. In the 1950s, because of the work of Altschul and Herman, it was found to have significant antihyperlipidemic effects.[1] Since that time, doses higher than 1 g/day have been shown to have quite significant effects on all aspects of the lipid profile by lowering levels of low-density lipoproteins (LDL) as well as very-low-density lipoproteins (VLDL) and at the same time raising levels of the cardioprotective high-density lipoproteins (HDL). Although somewhat limited by bothersome but non-life-threatening side effects, nicotinic acid has been shown to be a very efficacious, safe, and cost-effective agent for the treatment of most lipid disorders, and during the past two decades, several studies suggest that this agent is associated with a reduction in cardiac events, cardiac mortality, and all-cause mortality.

ABSORPTION, DISTRIBUTION, PHARMACOKINETICS, AND METABOLISM

Crystalline nicotinic acid is rapidly absorbed after an oral dose and is rapidly excreted in the urine. After a 1-g oral dose, peak serum levels are obtained in 30 to 60 minutes and reach 15 to 30 μg/ml; the plasma elimination half-life ranges from 20 to 40 minutes in humans.[2-4] Nicotinic acid accumulates in blood cells with a whole blood/plasma ratio of 110:1.[5] Less than one fifth of an oral dose is bound to the serum proteins in humans.[6]

The metabolism and the biotransformation of nicotinic acid follow two major routes. Dietary nicotinic acid (12 to 18 mg/day is needed for physiologic functions as a vitamin) is largely metabolized by the liver to nicotinamide and its derivatives.[2] Nicotinamide, which is also referred to as niacin, seems to have no effect on lipid metabolism and cannot be used instead of nicotinic acid. Clinically the names "nicotinic acid" and "niacin" are often used interchangeably when referring to this lipid medication. Nicotinamide, how-

ever, is an essential precursor of many important coenzymes critical to metabolic pathways; its derivatives are eventually secreted in the urine. In pharmacologic doses, nicotinic acid undergoes a detoxification process where a major byproduct is its glycerin conjugate, nicotinuric acid, which does have significant lipid activity.[2, 3, 7] This byproduct is detected in the urine in large quantities approximately 6 to 8 hours after a large oral dose of nicotinic acid. It is still debated whether the major active lipid-lowering agent is nicotinic acid or nicotinuric acid, which is secreted largely unchanged in the urine after large doses used to treat patients with hyperlipoproteinemia.

MECHANISM OF ACTION

The lipid-lowering effects of nicotinic acid are the result of declines in VLDL, LDL, and intermediate-density lipoproteins (IDL). A major mechanism of action seems to be its effects on decreasing hepatic VLDL synthesis and serum triglyceride levels by decreasing free fatty acids and possibly by decreasing insulin secretion.[2, 8] Some increase in VLDL elimination during processing to LDL has also been found. The falls in LDL and IDL seem to be secondary effects, because these lipoproteins are important sequential products of VLDL metabolism. Nicotinic acid also tends to normalize the type of VLDL particle found in many patients with hypertriglyceridemia by reducing the particle size of VLDL and decreasing the number of particles.[8-10] This may contribute to antiatherosclerotic effects, because large VLDL may promote atherosclerosis and increase the lipid content of macrophages.

In contrast with VLDL and LDL, HDL-C levels rise after administration of nicotinic acid, probably via decreasing the catabolic rate of HDL. Because HDL clearance is usually accelerated in patients with hypertriglyceridemia, reducing the elevated VLDL levels may cause a dramatic rise in HDL by correcting the abnormal rapid clearance.[2, 11]

Levels of the major protein components of VLDL

and LDL (e.g., apolipoproteins B, E, and C) fall significantly following administration of nicotinic acid, and levels of the major apolipoproteins of HDL (e.g., apolipoprotein A1) also increase because of reduced metabolism of HDL particles.[12] Another lipoprotein, lipoprotein(a) [or Lp(a)], is receiving considerable attention, since some studies indicate that elevated levels of Lp(a) may be the most prevalent lipid abnormality in patients with coronary artery disease (CAD). Thus far, most nonpharmacologic and drug treatment regimens have no significant effect on Lp(a), but nicotinic acid alone or in combination with neomycin has been shown to reduce this potentially atherogenic lipoprotein particle.[13, 14]

CLINICAL EFFICACY
Elevated LDL

Since its original recommendations in 1988, the National Cholesterol Education Program (NCEP) has emphasized reducing elevated levels of LDL-C for both the primary and secondary prevention of coronary heart disease (CHD).[15] After failure of nonpharmacologic therapy, the current recommendations from the NCEP are to institute drug therapy for most individuals with persistent LDL-C levels of 190 mg/dl or higher with a goal of LDL-C levels of less than 130 mg/dl for primary prevention and a goal of LDL-C levels of less than 100 mg/dl in patients with known vascular disease, particularly CHD.[16]

At usual daily doses of 1 to 6 g/day, nicotinic acid produces substantial reductions in levels of total cholesterol and LDL-C. With immediate-release crystalline nicotinic acid, daily doses of 1.5 g/day usually reduce LDL-C levels by 10% to 15%; reduction in LDL-C is in the range of 15% to 25% with daily doses of 3 g; and a reduction of 25% to 30% in LDL-C can be obtained with daily doses of 4 g/day.[12] As with other drugs, percentage reductions in LDL-C generally are higher in patients with higher baseline levels of LDL-C, and individuality in responses is considerable. Reductions in LDL-C with nicotinic acid, however, occur in patients with LDL-C elevations produced by heterozygous familial hypercholesterolemia or with polygenic disorders.

Elevated Triglycerides

Although the role of triglycerides as an independent CHD risk factor remains controversial, substantial data suggest that elevated triglycerides are strongly associated with increased risk of CHD and potentiate the risk associated with increased LDL-C and low HDL-C.[17] In fact, one meta-analysis suggests that triglycerides are an independent risk factor for CHD, even in models that contain HDL-C.[18]

Because nicotinic acid alters lipid levels by reducing the products of VLDL particles (usually 80% triglycerides), this leads to a significant lowering of VLDL levels and triglycerides. In general, patients with triglyceride levels of more than 1000 mg/dl or

persistent levels between 500 and 1000 mg/dl deserve drug treatment to reduce the risk of pancreatitis. Others with borderline triglyceride elevations (e.g., 200 to 500 mg/dl) often need drug therapy when this is accompanied by other dyslipidemias or in patients with known CHD. By reducing VLDL production, nicotinic acid often reduces plasma triglycerides by 40% to 70% with concomitant moderate increases in HDL-C.[12] Because VLDL particles are converted partially to LDL, inhibition of VLDL production by nicotinic acid also lowers LDL-C levels, particularly in patients with baseline hypertriglyceridemia.

Combined Hyperlipoproteinemia

In combined hyperlipoproteinemia, VLDL and LDL are both elevated in a given patient; at various times, an individual patient may experience various degrees of elevation of these two lipoproteins. Because nicotinic acid reduces both VLDL and LDL levels, it is often the drug of first choice in such patients, producing substantial reductions in levels of total cholesterol, LDL-C, and triglycerides, often with concomitant increases in HDL-C.

"Isolated" Low HDL-C

Although the original NCEP recommendations underemphasized the importance of HDL-C in their assessment and treatment guidelines,[15-17, 19-23] substantial data suggest that this may be the strongest lipid risk factor for CHD.[19-23] In fact, data from our institution and elsewhere suggest that low levels of HDL-C are considerably more prevalent than elevated LDL-C levels in both elderly and younger coronary patients,[20, 22, 24] and many patients with CHD have "isolated" low HDL-C (HDL-C < 35 mg/dl) with relatively normal levels of total cholesterol, LDL-C, and triglycerides.[24] The most recent guidelines from the NHLBI Consensus Conference on Triglycerides and HDL-C[25] and the NCEP II[15] have provided greater emphasis on the importance of HDL-C in both assessment and treatment.

Although nicotinic acid is known to increase levels of HDL-C by 10% to 35% in patients with elevated LDL-C levels or in patients with hypertriglyceridemia, very few data are available on the effects in patients with low levels of HDL-C (i.e., < 35 mg/dl), particularly in patients with isolated low HDL-C who are often considered to be very resistant to various treatment regimens. However, in 36 patients with CHD and very low levels of HDL-C (< 30 mg/dl), we demonstrated greater than 30% increases in HDL-C levels (+27% in patients with "isolated" low HDL-C and +41% in patients with low HDL-C and elevated triglycerides) in those treated with sustained-release nicotinic acid (average dose 2.4 g/day).[26] Other recent data demonstrated that higher doses of crystalline nicotinic acid (4.5 g/day) produced similar increases in HDL-C levels in patients with isolated low HDL-C, which were significantly greater than HDL-C improvements after either lovastatin or gemfibrozil therapy.[27] Although considerable controversy exists regarding exactly when to use drug therapy in patients with "isolated" low HDL-C, substantial epidemiologic data suggest that these patients are at considerable risk for CHD, particularly if other CHD risk factors are also present. At this time, we believe that nicotinic acid is the drug of first choice for most such patients who require pharmacologic treatment.

Elevated Lp(a)

At this time, despite data implicating Lp(a) as a strong lipid risk factor for CHD, no data are available regarding benefits of reducing levels of Lp(a) or regarding CAD risks in patients with "isolated" increases in Lp(a) and otherwise relatively normal lipid profiles.[17] Therefore, it is probably premature at this time for clinicians to place major emphasis on this lipoprotein fraction in the routine assessment and treatment of CAD. However, when measured, it is reasonable to consider that nicotinic acid is the only agent known to reduce levels of Lp(a). The use of nicotinic acid therefore could be more strongly considered in patients with elevated levels of Lp(a), particularly in patients with clinical and lipid profiles that are otherwise suitable for treatment with this agent.

Dysbetalipoproteinemia (Type III Hyperlipoproteinemia)

In the rare lipid disorder dysbetalipoproteinemia (type III hyperlipoproteinemia) in which there is abnormal processing of VLDL particles and accumulation of lipoprotein remnants, nicotinic acid produces reductions of more than 50% in both VLDL and IDL levels and is therefore probably the drug of first choice in the treatment of these patients.[12]

MAJOR STUDIES WITH NICOTINIC ACID
Coronary Drug Project

In the Coronary Drug Project,[28] more than 3900 men who had suffered a myocardial infarction (MI) were randomized to receive 3 g/day of crystalline nicotinic acid or a placebo. Despite a compliance rate of only approximately 50%, total cholesterol fell by 10% in drug-treated patients, with a 27% reduction in subsequent MI at the end of 5 years. Although total mortality was not affected by nicotinic acid therapy in the initial study, long-term follow-up of these patients demonstrated a significant 11% reduction in total mortality in the drug-treated patients, including significant reductions in CAD mortality. This study therefore suggests a potential long-term benefit from a relatively short course of therapy with nicotinic acid.

Stockholm Ischemic Heart Disease Study

In the Stockholm Ischemic Heart Disease Study,[29] 555 consecutive survivors of acute MI were randomized to a control group and a treatment group (clofibrate 1 g twice daily and 1 g three times daily of long-acting nicotinic acid). In the treatment group, 59% received at least 1.5 g/day of nicotinic acid. Compared with a placebo, total cholesterol and triglycerides were reduced by 13% and 19%, respectively, in patients receiving drug therapy. At the end of 5 years, significant reductions in total mortality and CHD mortality of 26% and 36%, respectively, were noted in the drug-treated patients.

Cholesterol-Lowering Atherosclerosis Study (CLAS)

In the Cholesterol-Lowering Atherosclerosis Study (CLAS),[30] 162 men with known CHD and saphenous vein grafts (SVG) were randomized to dietary therapy and a placebo versus a more stringent diet and combination drug therapy with colestipol (30 g/day) and nicotinic acid (average dose, 4 g/day). At the end of 2 years, total cholesterol, LDL-C, and LDL-C/HDL-C levels fell by 26%, 43%, and 57%, respectively, with a 37% increase in HDL-C levels in the drug-treated patients who also had less progression of CAD in both their native coronary arteries as well as the SVGs. Most impressively, after only 2 years of follow-up, disease regression was noted in 16% of the drug-treated patients versus only 2% of the control group. A four-year follow-up of this cohort has been published (CLAS-II), demonstrating even more marked benefits in the drug-treated patients, who had less progression and more regression of CAD, both in their native arteries as well as in the SVGs, compared with patients receiving the placebo.[31]

Familial Atherosclerosis Treatment Study (FATS)

In the Familial Atherosclerosis Treatment Study (FATS),[32] 120 patients with known CAD and elevated levels of apolipoprotein B (> 125 mg/dl) were randomized to a control group (no drug or colestipol at the discretion of the primary physician), lovastatin (40 mg/day) plus colestipol (30 g/day), or nicotinic acid (4 g/day) plus colestipol (30 g/day). In the nicotinic acid/colestipol group, LDL-C levels were reduced by 32% and HDL-C levels increased by 43%. Compared with the control group, both treatment groups had substantial increases in coronary lesion regression and had significant reductions in CAD progression. After only 3 years of follow-up, the drug-treated patients had threefold to fourfold reductions in major CHD events. Although LDL-C levels fell more impressively in the patients treated with lovastatin (−46% versus −32%), HDL-C levels increased considerably more in the patients treated with nicotinic acid (+43% versus +15%). Likewise, CAD regression and reductions in CHD events were somewhat more impressive in patients treated with nicotinic acid.

CLINICAL USE OF NICOTINIC ACID

The major problems associated with nicotinic acid therapy (discussed in detail later) are troublesome but usually non-life-threatening side effects (Table 114–1). Many of these effects can be minimized or eliminated by starting with very low doses (e.g., 100 to 200 mg), taking the drug with meals, premedication with a low dose of a cyclooxygenase inhibitor (e.g., 325 mg of aspirin) 30 minutes before each dose of nicotinic acid (particularly for the first daily dose and for the first month of therapy), and, possibly, using a sustained-released preparation (again, particularly during the first weeks or months of therapy). Most side effects diminish or disappear after 2 to 4 weeks of treatment.

Many physicians treating patients with lipid disorders frequently begin therapy with crystalline nicotinic acid, which should be started at low doses and given three to four times daily. A common schedule is to begin with 100-mg tablets with or following a meal and to double the dose at intervals of 5 to 10 days if side effects have abated or decreased. After

Table 114–1. Side Effects of Nicotinic Acid

Effect	Percentage of Patients
Minor	
Cutaneous	
Flushing	90%
Pruritus	10%–50%
Rash	10%–50%
Dry skin	10%–50%
Acanthosis nigricans	<5%
Gastrointestinal	
Upper abdominal discomfort	5%–20%
Nausea	5%–20%
Vomiting	1%–2%
Anorexia	<1%
Diarrhea	<1%
Abnormal chemistry values	
Uric acid	(see text)
Glucose	(see text)
Transaminase	(see text)
Major	
Elevated transaminase (threefold)	<10% (more with sustained release)
Elevated alkaline phosphatase	<1%
Peptic ulcer disease	Rare
Myopathy	Rare (more common with HMG-CoA reductase inhibitors)
Diabetes mellitus	Rare (more common with baseline insulin resistance)
Cardiac effects	Rare
Coagulopathy	Rare

HMG-CoA, hydroxylmethylglutaryl coenzyme A.

reaching a total daily dose of approximately 1.5 g/day, it is reasonable to allow the dose to stabilize for 4 to 6 weeks and then to reassess the lipid profile along with an assessment of plasma glucose levels, transaminase values, and possibly uric acid levels. If further lipid treatment is needed and there are no major adverse effects present, the dose can be increased to 2 g/day and eventually to 3 g/day. The patient should be monitored 6 to 12 weeks after each dose increase. Although we typically treat patients with moderate doses (e.g., 1.5 to 3.0 g/day of nicotinic acid), others have frequently used doses of 4.5 or 6 g/day.[12, 30–32] However, the incidence of systemic side effects (discussed later) markedly increased with doses higher than 3 g/day.

Despite the known increased propensity for producing hepatic toxicity, we frequently begin treatment with sustained-release preparations, which we feel are considerably better tolerated by most patients, unless either the patient or the referring physician expresses a preference for a short-acting form of nicotinic acid.[26, 33, 34] When using a sustained-release nicotinic acid (e.g., Slo-Niacin) preparation, we usually begin therapy at a dosage of 500 mg twice daily with meals; after 2 to 3 weeks, we increase the dosage to 1.5 to 2.0 g/day in two to three divided doses. After 2 to 3 months of treatment, chemistry results are again monitored. If these laboratory test findings are normal and further lipid treatment is desired, we often increase the dosage, particularly in patients with CHD or a high risk of CHD, to 2 to 3 g/day in two or three divided doses.

COMBINATION THERAPY

Nicotinic acid alone often produces satisfactory reductions in serum triglycerides and cholesterol with increases in HDL-C levels. However, many patients cannot tolerate high doses of nicotinic acid, and others continue to have dyslipidemia despite high doses of the drug. In such patients, the addition of a second lipid agent is needed. Alternatively, nicotinic acid can be added when other drug regimens produce beneficial, but less than desired, effects on lipid concentrations.

Nicotinic Acid and Gemfibrozil

Although nicotinic acid often produces dramatic improvements in triglyceride and HDL-C levels, some patients require additional treatment. In our experience, these drugs can be safely combined with synergistic effects on VLDL metabolism, thus producing marked additional improvements in patients with hypertriglyceridemia and low HDL-C levels, with mild additional lowering of LDL-C levels.

Nicotinic Acid and Bile Acid Sequestrant Resins

Several studies combined nicotinic acid and bile acid sequestrant resins, producing very marked reductions in LDL-C (30% to 50%) and LDL-C/HDL-C levels (approximately 60%).[12, 30–32] This regimen appears to be extremely safe and effective for patients with various lipid disorders, because nicotinic acid improves all aspects of the lipid profile and bile acid sequestrant resins, which are relatively contraindicated as monotherapy in patients with hypertriglyceridemia, are very effective in lowering LDL-C levels.[21] The major problem with this combination, however, is troublesome side effects from each individual agent.

In our experience, nicotinic acid can also be effectively and safely combined with soluble fiber (e.g., oat bran or psyllium) as a very inexpensive, well-tolerated alternative to prescription drug therapy.[35]

Nicotinic Acid and Hydroxylmethylglutaryl Coenzyme A (HMG-CoA) Reductase Inhibitors

Hydroxylmethylglutaryl coenzyme A (HMG-CoA) reductase inhibitors are extremely effective for reducing LDL-C levels, but produce only very minimal improvements in triglyceride and HDL-C levels, which can be greatly enhanced by the addition of nicotinic acid. The side effects of this regimen are mostly caused by nicotinic acid because, in our experience, the adverse effects of HMG-CoA reductase inhibitors are essentially equal to those of a placebo. The combination of these agents, however, has been associated with an increased risk of myopathy (reported to be up to a 1% to 2% risk when lovastatin is combined with $\geq$ 1.5 g/day of nicotinic acid).[21, 34] To our knowledge, the risk of myopathy is not increased when using lower doses of nicotinic acid. Theoretically, the more hydrophilic HMG-CoA reductase inhibitors (e.g., pravastatin and fluvastatin) should have a lower risk of myopathy in combination with nicotinic acid.

ADVERSE EFFECTS

The most frequent problems with nicotinic acid therapy are troublesome but non-life-threatening, relatively minor side effects (see Table 114–1).

Minor Effects

The most troublesome of the "minor" adverse effects include cutaneous flushing and upper abdominal discomfort. The skin effects include cutaneous flushing in as many as 90% of patients (much less common and less severe with the sustained-release preparations), pruritus in 10% to 50%, as well as rash, dry skin, and acanthosis nigricans (in well less than 5% of patients). Upper abdominal discomfort and nausea are also fairly common (5% to 20% of patients) and may be slightly less common and severe with the sustained-release preparations. A few patients may experience vomiting, anorexia, or diarrhea.

Many patients may experience mild but usually asymptomatic abnormalities in blood chemistry values, including elevations in uric acid, glucose, and transaminase values; these chemistry findings often remain in the "normal" range despite statistically significant increases compared with baseline values. In an occasional patient, gout, diabetes, or significant increases in liver enzymes (e.g., > 1.5- to 3-fold increases in transaminase values in 3% to 10%) may develop, necessitating a decrease in dosage or discontinuation of nicotinic acid.

Major Effects

Occasionally, major side effects from nicotinic acid may develop, often requiring discontinuation of therapy. In our experience, physician-recommended discontinuation of nicotinic acid therapy is most frequently a result of persistent, but asymptomatic, threefold elevations in transaminase values. This adverse effect is probably more common in patients treated with sustained-release preparations of nicotinic acid (particularly at doses > 2 g/day) and can sometimes be handled by changing to crystalline nicotinic acid or a reduction in the dose.[34] More rarely, frank hepatitis can occur, or elevations in alkaline phosphatase or serum bilirubin levels (probably less than 1% of patients), necessitating discontinuation of nicotinic acid therapy.[12, 34] Nicotinic acid frequently causes upper abdominal discomfort and the development of peptic ulcer disease, and gastrointestinal bleeding occasionally occurs; therefore, peptic ulcer disease is a fairly strong relative contraindication to the use of this agent.

Other less common but potentially serious adverse effects of nicotinic acid therapy include myopathy (well less than 1%, but may be more frequent when combined with HMG-CoA reductase inhibitors),[21, 34] precipitating frank diabetes mellitus (making this therapy relatively contraindicated in patients with known diabetes or significant insulin resistance),[12, 28] and cardiac effects, including increasing atrial tachyarrhythmias or possibly unstable ischemic syndromes.[28] Furthermore, we recently described seven retrospectively identified patients in whom clotting factor deficiency, protein deficiency, and coagulopathy (e.g., prothrombin time more than 1.5 times the control value) developed in conjunction with only minimal increases in transaminase values (1.5 to 2 times normal) associated with sustained-release nicotinic acid therapy.[33, 36, 37] This syndrome has recurred after rechallenge with sustained-release nicotinic acid but not with crystalline preparations of the drug. Despite these occurrences, as well as the increased liver function abnormalities seen with sustained-release nicotinic acid preparations, we feel that the adverse effects associated with sustained-release nicotinic acid are completely reversible and should not be life-threatening in closely monitored patients. We believe that the greater tolerability of the sustained-release preparation of nicotinic acid will likely outweigh its risk, particularly in patients with known CHD or a high risk for this disease.[19, 34, 37]

CONCLUSION

Despite the troublesome side effects with nicotinic acid, we feel that this agent has generally been under-

Table 114–2. **Summary of Nicotinic Acid**

Dose:	1–6 g/day (usually 1.5–3.0 g/day)
Types:	Crystalline (immediate release) and sustained-release preparations
Administration:	Two or three daily doses (with meals)
Lipid effects:	Reduces total cholesterol, triglyceride, and LDL-C levels, and increases HDL-C level. Also lowers Lp(a) levels
Side effects	
Minor:	Cutaneous flushing, upper abdominal discomfort
Major:	Liver function abnormalities, peptic ulcer disease, diabetes, cardiac arrhythmias, coagulopathy
Benefits:	One of a few lipid medications associated with significant reductions in cardiac events, cardiac mortality, and total mortality.

LDL-C, low-density lipoprotein cholesterol; HDL-C, high-density lipoprotein cholesterol; Lp(a), lipoprotein(a).

utilized for the treatment of lipid disorders. Nicotinic acid improves all aspects of the lipid profile and, with the exception of patients with diabetes, is extremely effective and safe for most patients at high risk for atherosclerotic cardiovascular disease. To our knowledge, nicotinic acid is one of the few lipid agents that has been associated with significant reductions in CHD events, CHD mortality, and all-cause mortality, and thus should be the drug of choice for many patients with known CHD or a high risk for CHD (Table 114–2).

Acknowledgments

We thank Angela Lorio and Lauren Oddo for their assistance in preparing the manuscript.

REFERENCES

1. Altschul R, Herman IH: Influence of oxygen inhalation on cholesterol metabolism. Arch Biochem Biophys 51:308, 1954.
2. Figge HL, Figge J, Souney PF, et al: Nicotinic acid: A review of its clinical use in the treatment of lipid disorders. Pharmacotherapy 8:287, 1988.
3. Miller HN, Hamilton JG, Goldsmith GA: Investigation of the mechanism of action of nicotinic acid on serum lipid levels in man. Am J Clin Nutr 8:480, 1960.
4. Carlson LA, Oro L, Ostman J: Effect of a single dose of nicotinic acid on plasma lipids in patients with hyperlipoproteinemia. Acta Med Scand 183:457, 1968.
5. Frank O, Baker H, Sobotka H: Blood and serum levels of water-soluble vitamins in man and animals. Nature 197:490, 1963.
6. Robinson WT, Cosyns L, Krami M: An automated method for the analysis of nicotinic acid in serum. Clin Chem 11:46, 1978.
7. Mrochec JE, Jolley RL, Young DS, Turner WJ: Metabolic response of humans to ingestion of nicotinic acid and nicotinamide. Clin Chem 22:1821, 1976.
8. Grundy SM, Mok HYI, Zeck L, Berman M: Influence of nicotinic acid on metabolism of cholesterol and triglycerides in man. J Lipid Res 22:24, 1981.
9. Packard CJ, Munro A, Lorimer AR, et al: Metabolism of apolipoprotein B in large triglyceride rich VLDL of normal and hypertriglyceridemic subjects. J Clin Invest 70:168, 1984.
10. Sacks FM, Breslow JL: Very low-density lipoproteins stimulate cholesterol ester formation in U937 macrophages. Heterogeneity and biologic variation among humans. Arteriosclerosis 7:35, 1987.
11. Shepard J, Packard CJ, Patsch JR, et al: Effects of nicotinic acid therapy on plasma high density subfraction and composition and on apolipoprotein A metabolism. J Clin Invest 63:858, 1979.
12. Brown WV, Howard WJ, Field L: Nicotinic acid and its derivatives. *In* Rifkind BM (ed): Drug Treatment and Hyperlipidemia. New York: Marcel Dekker, 1991, pp 189–213.
13. Carlson LA, Hamsten A, Asplund A: Pronounced lowering of serum levels of lipoprotein Lp(a) in hyperlipidemic subjects treated with nicotinic acid. J Intern Med 226:271, 1989.
14. Guvakav A, Hoeg JM, Kostner G, et al: Levels of lipoprotein Lp(a) decline with neomycin and niacin treatment. Atherosclerosis 57:293, 1985.
15. Report of the National Cholesterol Education Program Expert Panel on Detection, Evaluation, and Treatment of High Blood Cholesterol in Adults. Arch Intern Med 148:36, 1988.
16. Expert Panel on Detection, Evaluation and Treatment of High Blood Cholesterol in Adults: Summary of the Second Report of the National Cholesterol Education Program (NCEP) Expert Panel on Detection, Evaluation, and Treatment of High Blood Cholesterol in Adults (Adult Treatment Panel II). JAMA 269:3015, 1983.
17. Lavie CJ: Lipid and lipoprotein fractions and coronary artery disease [editorial]. Mayo Clin Proc 68:618, 1993.
18. Hokanson JE, Austin MA: Triglycerides is a risk factor for coronary disease in men and women: A meta-analysis of population-based studies [abstract]. Circulation 88 (Suppl I):I-510, 1993.
19. Lavie CJ, O'Keefe JH, Blonde L, Gau GT: High-density lipoprotein cholesterol: Recommendations for routine testing and treatment. Postgrad Med 87:36, 1990.
20. Lavie CJ, Milani RV: National Cholesterol Education Program's recommendations, and implications of "missing" high-density lipoprotein cholesterol in cardiac rehabilitation programs. Am J Cardiol 68:1087, 1991.
21. Lavie CJ, Gau GT, Squires RW, Kottke BA: Management of lipids in primary and secondary prevention of cardiovascular diseases. Mayo Clin Proc 63:605, 1988.
22. Mailander L, Lavie CJ, Milani RV, Gaudin D: Emphasis on high-density lipoprotein cholesterol in patients with coronary artery disease. South Med J 86:508, 1993.
23. Lavie CJ, Milani RV, Boykin C: High-density lipoprotein cholesterol is the strongest lipid risk factor in elderly coronary patients [abstract]. J Cardiopulm Rehab 13:334, 1993.
24. Milani RV, Lavie CJ: Benefits of vigorous nonpharmacologic therapy in patients with "isolated" low high-density lipoprotein cholesterol [abstract]. Circulation 86 (Suppl I):I63, 1992.
25. NIH Consensus Development Panel on Triglycerides, High-density Lipoprotein, and Coronary Heart Disease. JAMA 269:505, 1993.
26. Lavie CJ, Mailander L, Milani RV: Marked benefit with sustained-release niacin therapy in patients with "isolated" very low levels of high-density lipoprotein cholesterol and coronary artery disease. Am J Cardiol 69:1083, 1992.
27. Vega GL, Grundy SM: Lipoprotein responses to treatment with lovastatin, gemfibrozil, and nicotinic acid in normolipidemic patients with hypoalphalipoproteinemia. Arch Intern Med 154:73, 1994.
28. Coronary Drug Project Group: Clofibrate and niacin in coronary heart disease. JAMA 231:360, 1975.
29. Carlson LA, Rosenhamer G: Reduction in mortality in the Stockholm Ischaemic Heart Disease Secondary Prevention Study by combined treatment with clofibrate and nicotinic acid. Acta Med Scand 223:405, 1988.
30. Blankenhorn DH, Nessim SA, Johnson RL, et al: Beneficial effects of combined colestipol-niacin therapy on coronary atherosclerosis and coronary venous bypass grafts. JAMA 81:3233, 1987.
31. Cashin-Hemphil L, Mack W, Pogada JM, et al: Beneficial effects of colestipol-niacin on coronary atherosclerosis: A 4-year follow-up. J Am Coll Cardiol 264:3013, 1990.
32. Brown G, Albers J, Fisher L, et al: Regression of coronary artery

disease as a result of intensive lipid-lowering therapy in men with high levels of apolipoprotein B. N Engl J Med 323:1289, 1990.

33. Dearing BD, Lavie CJ, Lohmann TP, Genton E: Niacin-induced clotting factor synthesis deficiency with coagulopathy. Arch Intern Med 152:861, 1992.

34. Milani RV, Lavie CJ: Recommendations for managing patients with low HDL-cholesterol levels. Journal of Myocardial Ischemia 4:27, 1992.

35. O'Keefe Jr JH, Lavie CJ, O'Keefe JO: Dietary prevention of coronary artery disease: How to help patients modify eating habits and reduce cholesterol. Postgrad Med 85:243, 1989.

36. Dearing BD, Lavie CJ, Lohmann TP, Genton E: Clotting factor deficiency and coagulopathy induced by sustained-release niacin [abstract]. In Proceedings of the 14th Interamerican Congress of Cardiology, Orlando, FL, 1992, p 103.

37. Lavie CJ: Sustained-release niacin for low levels of high-density lipoprotein cholesterol. Mayo Clin Proc 68:201, 1993.

CHAPTER 115

Bile Acid Sequestrants: Cholestyramine and Colestipol

W. Virgil Brown, M.D., and Leah Colwell-Adams, Pharm.D.

HISTORY AND CHEMISTRY

The reduction of serum cholesterol and, most specifically, low-density lipoprotein cholesterol has become the focus of a major national effort to reduce the incidence of arteriosclerotic cardiovascular disease.[1] One of the most time-honored methods of lowering plasma cholesterol has been the use of drugs that increase the fecal excretion of cholesterol or its major breakdown products, the bile acids. The oral administration of granular ion exchange resins that bind bile acids has been used to treat elevated plasma low-density lipoprotein cholesterol (LDL-C) for more than 25 years.[2] There are two major commercial products available for prescription use, cholestyramine and colestipol.

The concept of chelating the highly negatively charged bile acids as a method of lowering cholesterol is believed to have originated with Siperstein et al., who noticed cholesterol reduction during the administration of iron salts to chickens.[3] Increased bile acid–iron chelates were found in the stool and subsequently other more easily tolerated agents for sequestering bile acids were sought. Certain polymeric ion exchange resins used in industry and in the chemistry laboratory for binding and separating negatively charged molecules were found to perform in this capacity when properly prepared for safe ingestion. These agents have also proved useful in reducing blood plasma bile acids that accumulate in the skin of patients with obstructive liver disease, giving symptomatic relief from the associated pruritus. Their major pharmacologic intent has been to reduce the progression of arteriosclerosis in patients with LDL-C elevations. The demonstrated efficacy in lowering LDL-C levels and in preventing coronary heart disease, as well as the low incidence of significant adverse reactions,[4] led the National Cholesterol Education Program (NCEP) to propose these agents as drugs of first choice for managing hypercholesterolemia in patients without concurrent hypertriglyceridemia.[1]

Cholestyramine (Fig. 115–1) is the copolymer of styrene and diphenyl benzene, which contains trimethylbenzylammonium groups that provide a strong positive charge. The pharmacologic preparation is the chloride salt of this basic ion exchange resin, which is hydrophilic but insoluble in water. It is provided as a finely granular powder consisting of fractured irregular particles, ranging from 45 to 225 μm in diameter.

Colestipol (see Fig. 115–1) is also a powdered basic ion exchange copolymer synthesized from diethylene triamine and 1-chloro-2,3-epoxy propane. Like cholestyramine, it has multiple protonated amine groups providing positive charges and is supplied as the chloride salt. Both agents are administered orally in quantities of several grams as a suspension in liquid. Neither is altered by digestive enzymes nor absorbed from the gastrointestinal tract. Colestipol powder consists of smooth, round beads ranging in size from 50 to 450 μm.[5]

PHARMACOLOGY

Bile acid sequestrants have been given in daily doses up to 48 g/day or more. The usual recommended total daily dose for cholestyramine is from 4 to 24 g, and colestipol, 5 to 30 g. For these agents to be effective, they must adsorb significant quantities of bile acids in the proximal portion of the small intestine and prevent their absorption into the body in the distal ilium.[6, 7] The binding capacity of these resins varies with the specific bile acid as well as the pH and the content of other salts or charged amphipathic molecules (fatty acids and phospholipids) in the solution. In water, cholestyramine has the capacity to bind up to 2 g of bile salts per gram of anhydrous resin.[8, 9] Binding studies suggest that, at higher concentrations, much of the binding capacity is dependent on the formation of micellar structures without a one-to-one ionic bonding. The sequestrants should, therefore, have a greater capacity for those bile acids with lower critical micellar concentrations. However, the observed increase in total daily fecal bile acid secretion

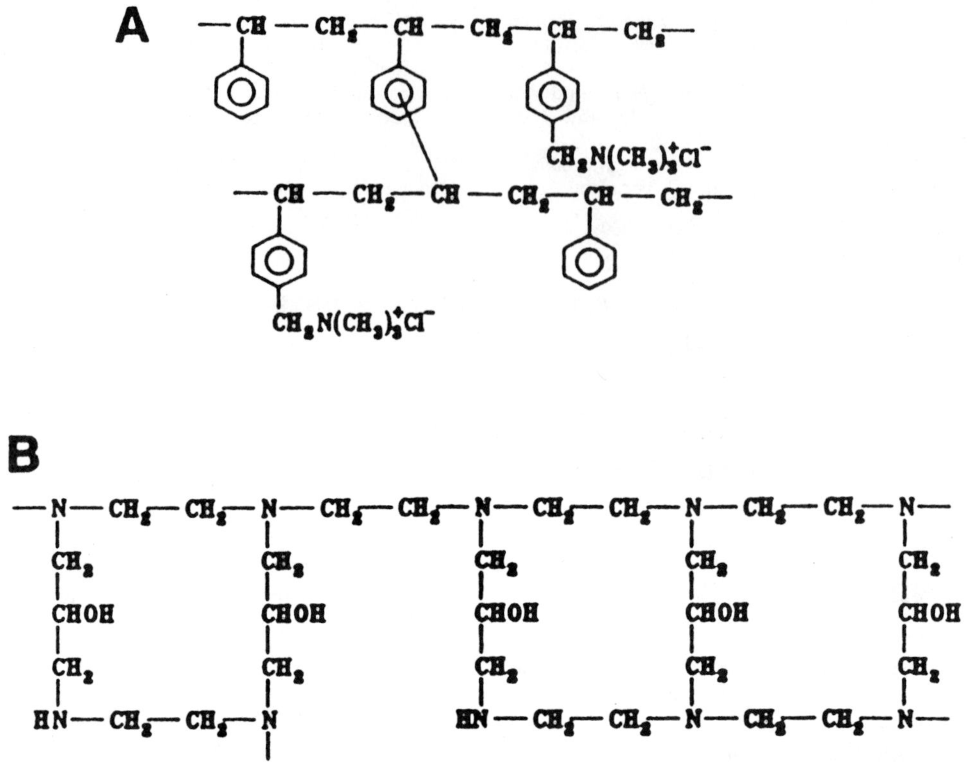

A —CH—CH$_2$—CH—CH$_2$—CH—CH$_2$—

CH$_2$N(CH$_3$)$_3^+$Cl$^-$

—CH—CH$_2$—CH—CH$_2$—CH—CH$_2$—

CH$_2$N(CH$_3$)$_3^+$Cl$^-$

B —N—CH$_2$—CH$_2$—N—CH$_2$—CH$_2$—N—CH$_2$—CH$_2$—N—CH$_2$—CH$_2$—N—

CH$_2$ CH$_2$ CH$_2$ CH$_2$ CH$_2$

CHOH   CHOH   CHOH   CHOH   CHOH

CH$_2$ CH$_2$ CH$_2$ CH$_2$ CH$_2$

HN—CH$_2$—CH$_2$—N   HN—CH$_2$—CH$_2$—N—CH$_2$—CH$_2$—N—

Figure 115–1. The chemical structures of cholestyramine resin *(A)* and colestipol hydrochloride *(B)*.

in association with a dose of 32 g of cholestyramine is usually less than 2 g/day,[10] less than 3% of the demonstrated capacity *in vitro*. In the laboratory, colestipol has a lower maximal capacity, binding approximately 0.5 g per gram of choleic acid. However, the *in vivo* effects of the two resins are only modestly different: a 5-g dose of colestipol is approximately equal to a 4-g dose of cholestyramine in accelerating bile acid loss from the intestine and in lowering plasma cholesterol concentrations.

The relative binding capacity for both cholestyramine and colestipol is greater for the deoxy bile salts such as choleic acid than for deoxycholic acid. The taurine conjugates of all bile acids have greater affinity than the glycine conjugates.[5] From *in vitro* experiments at physiologic concentrations of the bile acids, one would predict that they all would associate rapidly in the intestine with both colestipol and cholestyramine. The speed of uptake into the resin should not be a factor in limiting their potency. A more important mechanistic issue in determining the ability of these agents to promote excretion of bile acids from the gut may be the rates of disassociation. As the resin–bile acid complex passes through the distal ileum, the bile acids are absorbed and removed from the intestinal contents. The aqueous concentration is replenished by disassociation from the interstices of the granules. As a result, virtually all bile acids could be removed from the resin if the intestinal transit time is sufficiently slow. However, this may be a more complex process than simply separating an ionic bond, with lipophilic properties of the resin playing a role in reducing the rate of departure of the bile

acid. *In vitro* studies demonstrate that taurine and glycine conjugates of both chenodeoxycholate and deoxycholate are disassociated much more slowly (T½ > 1 hour) than those of the conjugates of choleic acid.[5] The release of the glycine derivatives is slightly more rapid than that of the taurine conjugates, and the disassociation rates from colestipol are more rapid than those from cholestyramine. These observations appear to explain the preferential increase in excretion of deoxy and chenodeoxy choleic acid and their conjugated derivatives and the relatively small change in choleic acid excretion during sequestrant treatment. These alterations in excretory patterns are also consistent with the observed change in gallbladder and serum bile acid composition—a relative rise in choleic acid and its conjugates and an increase in the ratio of total glycine to taurine conjugated bile acids.[11]

EFFECTS ON LIPIDS AND LIPOPROTEINS
Cholesterol and Bile Acid Metabolism

The excretion of cholesterol from the body is almost entirely a function of the hepatobiliary tree and the gastrointestinal tract. The sterol departs in the feces in the form of cholesterol itself or its major metabolic products, the bile acids. The liver excretes 200 to 600 mg of cholesterol daily. This joins with an equivalent amount from the diet of persons who habitually eat meat and other animal products.[12, 13] Approximately half of this total is absorbed in the small intestine.

The actual absorption may vary from 10% to 90% among individuals.[14] There may be a brief reduction of cholesterol absorption during the first few days of treatment at high doses of the sequestrants.[14] However, cholestyramine and colestipol appear to have little or no long-term effect on this pathway.

The total body content of bile acids is approximately 2 to 4 g, and this is continuously excreted into the duodenum as the gallbladder empties, providing a detergent-like solubilization of dietary fats for digestion. In the distal ileum, more than 95% of the secreted bile acids are reabsorbed. This hepato-biliary-intestinal cycle is repeated from 5 to 10 times daily. Under normal conditions, only approximately 200 to 600 mg of bile acids escape into the colon and are lost in the feces daily. When the bile acid sequestrants are introduced into the intestinal tract, bile acid excretion may increase by two- to tenfold.[10] Reduction in rate of return of bile acids to the liver causes a decrease in their concentration within the liver. The biosynthesis of bile acids is under constant feedback inhibition, and the decline in concentration in the hepatocyte activates the enzyme 7-alpha-hydroxylase.[15, 16] This enzyme catalyzes the formation of 7-alpha-hydroxy cholesterol from cholesterol, the first, and rate-limiting, step in the synthesis of both choleic and chenodeoxycholic acids. Experiments with the feeding of one of these two bile acids cause a suppression in the synthesis of both in concert.[17] As a result, a sustained increase in bile acid secretion produces a continued increase in the utilization of intracellular cholesterol for bile acid formation. The result in humans is a rapid restoration and maintenance of the total body pool of bile acids at near normal levels.[18] The liver microsomal cholesterol content declines slightly, and this has the important effect of stimulating increased cholesterol synthesis by inducing the enzyme hydroxymethylglutaryl coenzyme A (HMG-CoA) reductase.[19-21]

The reduction in hepatic microsomal cholesterol also induces the synthesis of low-density lipoprotein (LDL) receptors, which populate the hepatic cell membrane and increase the ability of the liver to bind, remove, and degrade LDL.[22] This effect is the major operative change causing a fall in plasma cholesterol, and it is the fall in LDL-C level that provides the major index of efficacy in using these drugs in the clinical setting.

Low-Density Lipoprotein Metabolism

Within hours to days of beginning pharmacologic doses of either cholestyramine or colestipol, there are measurable changes in the metabolism of all the lipoproteins: chylomicrons, very-low-density lipoproteins (VLDL), low-density lipoproteins (LDL), and high-density lipoproteins (HDL). The major effect of interest is the usual reduction of LDL cholesterol by 25% to 355 mg/dl within 3 to 4 weeks.[2] This is due to both a decrease in particle number, as indicated by a decline in the apolipoprotein B, as well as a decrease in the cholesterol content of LDL.[23] The decline in the number of LDL particles seems fully explained by the increased expression of LDL receptors and the resulting increase in the fractional clearance of LDL from the plasma space.[24] Evidence that this was due specifically to the LDL receptor and not other pathways of uptake has been provided by Shepherd et al.[25] This is consistent with the finding that patients who are genetically deficient in LDL receptors (homozygous familial hypercholesterolemia) show minimal responsiveness to resin therapy.[26]

Very-Low-Density Lipoprotein Metabolism

Bile acid sequestrants not only increase hepatic cholesterol synthesis but also triglyceride synthesis as well.[27] This is associated with accelerated triglyceride secretion from the liver, with increased VLDL formation and a rise in plasma VLDL triglyceride levels.[28, 29] The mechanism of increased hepatic triglyceride synthesis is not understood. It has been suggested that increased activity of a key regulatory enzyme, phosphatidic acid phosphatase, may be stimulated by a decreased chenodeoxycholic acid content of the liver cell.[30] This is consistent with the observation that feeding chenodeoxycholic acid has a significant hypotriglyceridemic effect.[31]

The increased VLDL production rate raises plasma triglyceride levels in normal individuals 10% to 50%. This is usually inconsequential if the baseline triglyceride levels are 250 mg/dl or less. It is of interest that the content of triglyceride per VLDL particle increases. This may be due to an increased uptake and degradation of smaller VLDL, which have a lower triglyceride-to-protein ratio.[22] These smaller VLDL are known to bind to the LDL receptor through either the apolipoprotein B-100 (apo B-100) or apolipoprotein E (apo E) on their surface.[32] Because LDL receptors are increased, the accelerated production of VLDL is partially balanced by increased VLDL uptake. Therefore, the change in VLDL synthesis is probably greater than indicated by the small rise in plasma concentrations when cholestyramine or colestipol is administered. This increase in plasma triglyceride clearance has been observed in subjects with normal plasma triglyceride concentrations but was not found in hypertriglyceridemic patients given cholestyramine.[28] This may help explain the marked increase in plasma triglycerides observed when patients with familial hypertriglyceridemia are treated with the bile sequestrants.[33] These individuals often have impaired VLDL clearance for reasons unrelated to LDL receptors, and therefore the availability of more LDL receptors may not ameliorate the accelerated synthesis. This is most clearly demonstrated in the disorder dysbetalipoproteinemia, in which a marked delay in the clearance of chylomicron and VLDL remnants results from a genetic defect in the structure of apo E making it a poor ligand for the LDL receptor.[34] Cholestyramine or colestipol therapy usually raises the triglyceride level severalfold in dysbetalipoproteinemia.[35]

High-Density Lipoprotein Metabolism

During cholestyramine treatment, HDL cholesterol levels have been found to rise from 2% to 8%. This appears to be due to a unique increase in the larger, more lipid-rich, HDL_2 fraction with no change in HDL_3.[36] There is also an increase in the major protein of HDL, apolipoprotein AI (apo AI), without a significant rise in apolipoprotein AII, the apparent result of a selective increase in production of apo AI.[37] In animals, approximately half of the apo AI is synthesized in the intestine,[38] and, when rats are fed cholestyramine in the fasting state, apo AI output into intestinal lymph is increased, whereas other lipoproteins are decreased.[39] HDL metabolism may be changed in yet another way. It has been observed that the enzyme lecithin-cholesterol acyltransferase (LCAT), which esterifies cholesterol with fatty acids in HDL, is increased with administration of bile acid sequestrants. LCAT is also increased in association with a rise in the plasma triglyceride levels.[40, 41] However, increased VLDL may lead to a transfer of cholesterol ester out of HDL into VLDL, and LCAT activity may increase in a secondary manner following removal of the product of the reaction from HDL, making it a better substrate for the esterification reaction. Whether there is a rise in HDL cholesterol could depend on the VLDL composition and concentration, because HDL often falls with the rise of triglyceride in hypertriglyceridemia.

DRUG FORMULATIONS

Cholestyramine is available as Questran. In each dose there are 4 g of anhydrous cholestyramine resin and 5 g of additives, which include sucrose, propylene glycol alginate, polysorbate 80, acacia, citric acid, and yellow dyes #10 and #6. This is available in single-dose, foil-wrapped packs or in cartons (378 g) that are provided with a scoop that dispenses a standard dose.

Questran Light is formulated as a dose of 4 g of cholestyramine resin with aspartame (containing phenylalanine) as the sweetener, yellow dye #10 and red dye #40, as well as flavoring agents such as citric acid. Propylene glycol alginate, colloidal silicon dioxide, and xanthin gum are additives. Single-dose, foil-wrapped packs and containers (210 g) are available.

Colestipol hydrochloride granules are supplied as Colestid, without additives other than small amounts of silicon dioxide. The standard dose is 5 g, which is available in foil-wrapped packets. Larger bulk containers (300 g and 500 g) are available with a scoop for dispensing the 5-g dose.

Colestipol is also available as Flavored Colestid, which contains sweetener and orange flavorings. A 7.5-g scoop or packet (one dose) contains 5 g of colestipol hydrochloride with additional ingredients including aspartame, beta-carotene, citric acid, flavor (both artificial and natural), glycerine, maltol, mannitol, and methylcellulose.

Colestid tablets contain 1 g of active drug, micronized colestipol hydrochloride. The tablets are light yellow in color and are tasteless and odorless. Other ingredients are cellulose acetate phthalate, glycerol triacetate, carnauba wax, hydroxypropyl methylcellulose, magnesium stearate, povidone, and silicon dioxide. The tablets should be swallowed whole and should not be cut, chewed, or crushed.

CLINICAL USE
Indications for Use

The only lipoprotein abnormality in which clinical benefit from the use of bile acid sequestrants has been demonstrated is elevated LDL-C. It is, therefore, important to document the LDL elevation and to monitor its response to dietary and other lifestyle changes before beginning drug therapy. Because the bile acid sequestrants increase plasma triglycerides and markedly worsen hypertriglyceridemia of several causes, it is important to measure the fasting triglyceride levels and to avoid these agents in anyone with concentrations of more than 300 mg/dl.[33] If triglyceride reductions are achieved with other treatment, use of cholestyramine or colestipol can be considered.

The increase in HDL-C is so small and variable, that a low HDL-C level is not an indication for using cholestyramine or colestipol. In one major study, cholestyramine significantly reduced the risk of heart disease only in those patients whose baseline HDL-C level was above average (45 mg/dl). The reason for this was not evident but did not appear to be related to a greater rise in triglycerides in the patients with low HDL-C.[42]

The National Cholesterol Education Program Guidelines suggest considering using bile sequestrants in middle-aged individuals whose LDL-C remains higher than 190 mg/dl after adequate dietary change has been made.[1] In diabetic patients or in persons with more than one major cardiovascular risk factor, such as high blood pressure, cigarette smoking, age older than 45 for men and older than 55 for women, such drug therapy is appropriate if the LDL-C is higher than 160 mg/dl. The patients with highest risk are those who already manifest arteriosclerotic cardiovascular disease. These individuals should be treated when their LDL values are 130 mg/dl or more. These treatment guidelines are outlined in Table 115–1. In most patients, the institution of diet, exercise, smoking cessation, and control of metabolic disorders such as diabetes should be attempted for several weeks before instituting drug therapy. This often allows use of a lower dose of drug in achieving a given therapeutic goal. It also provides for a new baseline of LDL values from which to judge the efficacy of the bile acid sequestrants. Documenting efficacy is particularly important because the treatment may be needed indefinitely at considerable cost.

Administration

Successful use of the bile acid sequestrants requires an artful approach by the physician. The need to

Table 115–1. **The National Cholesterol Education Program Guidelines for the Initiation of Treatment of Elevated LDL Cholesterol and Goals for LDL for Each Level of Risk**

Patient Category	Initiation Level	LDL Goal
Dietary Therapy		
No CVD, < two risk factors	≥160 mg/dl	<160 mg/dl
No CVD, ≥ two risk factors	≥130 mg/dl	<130 mg/dl
With CVD	>100 mg/dl	<100 mg/dl
Drug Treatment		
No CVD, < two risk factors	≥190 mg/dl	<160 mg/dl
No CVD, ≥ two risk factors	≥160 mg/dl	<130 mg/dl
With CVD	≥130 mg/dl	>100 mg/dl

Diet therapy should precede drug therapy. The lower risk patient is treated less aggressively. The highest risk patient is judged to be the person who has established cardiovascular disease (CVD).

From Grundy SM, Bilheimer D, Chait A, et al: Summary of the Second Report of the National Cholesterol Education Program (NCEP) Expert Panel on Detection, Evaluation, and Treatment of High Blood Cholesterol in Adults (Adult Treatment Panel II). JAMA 269:3015–3023, 1983.

dispense a powder and to suspend it in a liquid once or twice each day makes these agents less convenient than simply taking a tablet. Although tablets of colestipol are available, each contains only 1 g of active resin and at least four to five will be consumed per dose. The need to time the dose when taken with other drugs and the occurrence of constipation during the early course of therapy further impede good adherence to a prescribed regimen. Key elements in achieving compliance are (1) beginning with a low dose (4 to 10 g daily) and increasing only after 4 to 6 weeks, (2) explaining the adverse reactions and methods of avoiding them, (3) informing the patient of the proven efficacy and safety of these agents, and (4) selecting the patient without contraindications.

It is recommended that the initial total daily dose of bile acid sequestrants not exceed 10 g. The efficacy is similar if given as a single dose or twice daily with meals.[43–45] At this dose level, the mean reduction of LDL-C approaches 20%. After 4 to 6 weeks, the LDL-C and triglyceride levels should be reassessed. If there has been inadequate reduction in LDL-C and the patient has been without significant adverse reactions, the dose may be doubled and given in equal quantities twice daily (with meals). Further increases may be made at intervals of 4 to 6 weeks, with a total dose of 24 g daily of cholestyramine or 30 g daily of colestipol hydrochloride. An average reduction of 25% to 35% in LDL-C may be expected at maximal dosage. There is considerable individual variability in the reduction of LDL-C, and a rare patient may show a 50% reduction. When a minimal effect is found, it is often difficult to determine whether this is physiologic or a result of compliance problems. There is usually modest further reduction in cholesterol with doses of more than 16 to 20 g/day. At higher doses, adverse reactions grow more frequent, with their associated difficulties in adherence. If additional cholesterol reduction is needed, it may prove more efficacious and less expensive to add a second drug that works by a different mechanism.[46] Niacin or HMG-

CoA reductase inhibitors are often very effective in combination with the bile acid sequestrants.

The palatability of bile acid sequestrants was poor when they were initially introduced 30 years ago. However, modern agents have no unpleasant odor or taste, and the size of the resin beads has been reduced so that they are easily hidden by using fruit juice or other carriers in the suspending liquid. In taste tests, approximately 60% of patients find one or more of the preparations to be satisfactory in water as the only vehicle. An explanation that these agents can be mixed into any liquid or puréed food, such as applesauce, frappes, carbonated beverages, and fruit juices of any type, may give the patient a series of alternatives to deal with palatability problems. The only significant warning in this area is to avoid adding the resin before cooking because this may alter the beads and reduce their efficacy. Often a palatability problem can be solved by simply changing preparations, because there are differences in flavorings, additives, and texture. The reason for preference of one over the other is often difficult to define. The tablets may prove to be a better choice for those who need only a low dose and cannot tolerate the granularity of the suspended powder.

Adverse Reactions

Because the bile acid–binding resins are not absorbed, the adverse reactions are primarily related to the gastrointestinal tract. Adverse reactions that have been attributed to these agents are constipation, abdominal pain, eructation, heartburn, and increased gas. Diarrhea is occasionally observed. All of these are common human problems, and it is difficult to know whether they are caused by the drug in each instance. The Lipid Research Clinics Coronary Primary Prevention Trial provided the most extensive experience using a double-blind comparison to parallel placebo treatment in a total cohort of more than 3800 patients.[47] All treated patients in this trial were given 24 g of cholestyramine daily (12 g twice daily) as the initial dose and were followed up for at least 7 years. The frequency of complaints at the end of the first year and after 7 years are given in Table 115–2. Constipation was a complaint in 39%, compared with 10% in the placebo group, after 1 year, but this difference had almost disappeared after 7 years. Fiber-rich dietary supplements and other remedies had been prescribed. Heartburn, eructation, and nausea also seemed to have been increased during the early phase.

Constipation may be the result of reducing the concentrations of free bile acids in the colon, where they act as a normal stimulant. By beginning with 10 g or less daily and providing some initial advice, such as an increase in high-fiber foods or the addition of fiber supplements with increased water, the initial constipation can be reduced to a minimal problem for most patients. After a few weeks of adjustment, the dose commonly can be increased without significant problem. The use of foods or supplements enriched

Table 115–2. **Percentage of Participants (Total Cohort >3800) Reporting Moderate or Severe Side Effects with Cholestyramine**

Side Effect	Pretreatment		1st Year		7th Year	
	Placebo	*Resin*	*Placebo*	*Resin*	*Placebo*	*Resin*
Abdominal pain	5	5	11	15	7	7
Belching or bloating	10	10	16	27	6	9
Constipation	3	4	10	39	4	8
Diarrhea	6	5	11	10	8	4
Gas	22	22	26	32	12	12
Heartburn	10	10	10	27	7	12
Nausea	4	3	8	16	4	3
Vomiting	2	2	5	6	3	2
At least one gastrointestinal side effect	34	34	43	68	26	29

The adverse reactions reported during the Lipid Research Clinics Coronary Primary Prevention Trial at the end of the first year and seventh year of treatment are given. The resin-treated patients received diet and cholestyramine, 12 g twice daily for the entire period. The placebo patients received an inactive powder to be taken in identical fashion. The treatment was randomized and double-blind. Symptoms were treated according to protocol including the use of fiber supplements and laxatives as necessary.

From The Lipid Research Clinics Coronary Primary Prevention Trial Results: (I) Reduction in incidence of coronary heart disease; (II) The relationship of reduction in incidence of coronary heart disease to cholesterol lowering. JAMA 251:351–374, 1984.

with soluble fibers, such as pectin, guar, or psyllium, is particularly attractive because they also provide some cholesterol reduction in their own right.[48, 49] Adding 5 g (a heaping teaspoonful) of psyllium with the dose of resin provides sufficient stool softening to prevent constipation in the great majority of patients.[48] Increasing fluid intake and high-fiber foods is important to ensure normal bowel function while using the bile acid sequestrants.

With high doses, direct intestinal irritation (heartburn [27%], nausea, and rarely vomiting) occurs in as many as 30% of patients. Use of antacids or simethicone preparations during the early phases of treatment may relieve these symptoms. The flatulence and belching may result from air swallowing associated with the attempts to drink the material rapidly. It is primarily a problem early in treatment. Simply taking these agents with meals and beginning with low doses greatly reduce the incidence of these problems. Recent evidence that cholestyramine causes a release of cholecystokinin may explain some of these enteric effects, because this hormone causes increased gastrointestinal motility, relaxation of the lower esophageal sphincter,[50] and contraction of the gallbladder.[51]

At high dose levels, diarrhea has been observed and may be caused by the direct irritation of the colon, but in rare patients it is the result of an allergy to additives, such as dyes, and can be treated by simply changing to other preparations. In some patients with intrinsic bowel disease, cholecystokinin release may be a contributory factor.

Obtaining a careful history of bowel dysfunction with attention to preceding abdominal pain and colonic or anorectal disorders such as proctitis, hemorrhoids, constipation, or diarrhea may prepare the way for prophylactic care and in some cases the avoidance of these medications. Peptic ulcer disease may be exacerbated. Disorders such as regional ileitis or ulcerative colitis are considered contraindications.

In patients taking other drugs, the timing of doses must be given careful attention. The positively charged resins may adsorb a variety of other nega-

tively charged drugs. These include β-adrenergic blocking agents, hydrochlorothiazide, furosemide, tetracycline, penicillin G, gemfibrozil, digoxin, and thyroxine.[52] In general, it is best to assume that any drug may be adsorbed. Patients should be instructed to take oral medications at least 1 hour before or 4 hours after each dose of the sequestrant.

Chemical changes in the blood have been observed in long-term studies and are of unknown significance. To date, these have not been related to any adverse effects or clinical symptoms. Changes in these chemical measures include a small rise in alkaline phosphatase level, a drop in plasma beta-carotene level, and a rise in iron binding capacity.[53]

The demonstrated interference with thyroid hormone (T_4) absorption, when given exogenously, and the known enterohepatic circulation of T_4 raised the possibility of inducing changes in the homeostasis of the thyroid gland. When the possibility was investigated by Witztum et al., no change in T_4 or thyroid-stimulating hormone (TSH) levels was observed in a group of 17 patients over 9 weeks with colestipol administration of as much as 30 g/day.[54]

The bile acid sequestrants have been used in children with severe hypercholesterolemia with good results, with no evidence of retardation in growth or development.[55] Large doses (70 g daily) have been given to young pigs, and normal growth and weight gain were observed.[56] In very small children[57] and metabolically compromised adults, a hyperchloremic acidosis has been induced, but this is a very rare finding.[58]

There is also the possibility of long-term interference with the absorption of fat-soluble vitamins A, D, E, and K. This has not been a significant problem, even in large studies involving thousands of patients for several years. Although carotene levels have declined, this is thought to reflect the reduction in LDL, which is a major carrier of plasma carotenoids. However, case reports of vitamin K deficiency in patients with chronic liver disease have appeared, and the vitamin levels have been found to be slightly reduced compared with controls in some studies. It is advisable to prescribe vitamins A and D at the usual recommended daily dietary allowances.

MAJOR CLINICAL TRIALS

The Lipid Research Clinics Coronary Primary Prevention Trial (LRC-CPPT) was a study of 3806 men, aged 35 to 59, with primary hypercholesterolemia.[47] All patients were given a low-fat, low-cholesterol diet upon entering the study. One half of the randomized patients received placebo, while the other half was given cholestyramine (24 g/day). The primary end point of the study was fatal and nonfatal myocardial infarction (MI). At the end of 7.4 years of follow-up, a significant reduction of 17% was found for the primary end point. The cholestyramine group experienced reductions of 13.4% and 20.3%, respectively, for the total and LDL cholesterol. Additionally, the incidence of new positive exercise treadmill tests, angina, and coronary artery bypass operations was reduced by 25%, 20%, and 21%, respectively. The LRC-CPPT was one of the first large placebo-controlled, randomized double-blind trials to show that cholesterol reduction decreases the incidence of cardiovascular morbidity and mortality.

In 1987, results from the Cholesterol Lowering Atherosclerosis Study (CLAS) were reported.[59] This was a randomized, placebo-controlled angiographic study in 162 middle-aged men who had previously undergone coronary artery bypass grafting. These men were randomized to treatment with either 30 g of colestipol and 3 to 12 g of niacin daily or placebo. The treatment lasted 2 years and provided a decrease in the LDL-C level of 43% and an increase in the HDL-C level of 37%. A significant reduction was seen in the number of lesions that progressed, as well as the percentage of patients with new lesions in the colestipol/niacin–treated cohort. Regression of atherosclerotic lesions was seen in 16.2% of the colestipol/niacin–treated patients, whereas regression was seen in only 2.4% of the placebo-treated patients.[4]

Reduction in the progression of atherosclerotic lesions in the coronary arteries was confirmed in the Familial Atherosclerosis Treatment Study (FATS) in 1989.[60] Two active treatment groups were used in which patients were randomized to colestipol (30 g)/niacin (4 g), colestipol (30 g)/lovastatin (40 mg) daily, or placebo. The population of randomized patients consisted of 120 men, younger than 62 years of age, with a family history of early coronary disease, elevated apo B levels, and coronary disease previously diagnosed with angiography. At the end of 2.5 years, LDL-C level was reduced 32% in the colestipol/niacin–treated group, 46% in the lovastatin/niacin–treated group, and 7% in the group receiving placebo. HDL-C level increased by 43% in the colestipol/niacin–treated group, 15% in the lovastatin/colestipol–treated group, and 5% in the group receiving placebo. Evidence of regression was found in 39% of the patients randomized to colestipol/niacin, 32% of those randomized to lovastatin/niacin, and only 11% of the

placebo-treated patients. This study, along with the CLAS study, gives significant evidence that regression of established coronary lesions does occur but may require aggressive pharmacologic and lifestyle interventions.

REFERENCES

1. Grundy SM, Bilheimer D, Chait A, et al: Summary of the Second Report of the National Cholesterol Education Program (NCEP) Expert Panel on Detection, Evaluation, and Treatment of High Blood Cholesterol in Adults (Adult Treatment Panel II). JAMA 269:3015, 1983.
2. Levy RI, Frederickson DS, Stone NJ, et al: Cholestyramine in type II hyperlipoproteinemia. Ann Intern Med 79:51, 1983.
3. Siperstein MD, Nichols CW, Chaikoff IL: Effects of ferric chloride and bile on plasma cholesterol and atherosclerosis in cholesterol-fed bird. Science 117:386, 1953.
4. Rifkind BM (ed): Bile Acid Sequestrants: Drug Treatment of Hyperlipidemia. New York: Marcel Dekker, 1991.
5. Benson GM, Haynes C, Blanchard S, et al: In vitro studies to investigate the reasons for the low potency of cholestyramine and colestipol. J Pharm Sci 82:80, 1993.
6. Packard CJ, Shepherd J: The hepatobiliary axis and lipoprotein metabolism: Effects of bile acid sequestrants and ileal bypass surgery. J Lipid Res 23:1081, 1982
7. Shepherd J: Mechanism of action of bile acid sequestrants and other lipid lowering drugs. Cardiology 76(Suppl 1):65, 1989.
8. Bilicki CV, White JL, Hem SL, et al: Effect of anions on adsorption of bile salts by colestipol hydrochloride. Pharm Res 6:794, 1989.
9. Konechnik TJ, Kos R, White JL: In vitro adsorption of bile salts by colestipol hydrochloride. Pharm Res 6(7):619, 1989.
10. Miettinen TA: Effects of hypolipidemic drugs on bile acid metabolism in man. Adv Lipid Res 18:65, 1981.
11. Garbutt JT, Kenney TJ: Effect of cholestyramine on bile acid metabolism in normal man. J Clin Invest 51(11):2781, 1972.
12. Dietschy JM, Wilson JD: Regulation of cholesterol metabolism. N Engl J Med 282:1128, 1970.
13. Grundy SM: Dietary and drug regulation of cholesterol metabolism in man. In Paoletti R, Glueck CJ (eds): Lipid Pharmacology, Vol II. New York: Academic Press, 1976, pp 127–161.
14. McNamara DJ, Davidson NO, Samuel P, et al: Cholesterol absorption in man: Effect of administration of clofibrate and/or cholestyramine. J Lipid Res 21:1058, 1980.
15. Myant NB, Mitropoulos KA: Cholesterol 7 alpha-hydroxylase. J Lipid Res 18:135, 1977.
16. Hashim SA, Van Itallie TB: Cholestyramine resin therapy for hypercholesterolemia. JAMA 192:289, 1965.
17. Einarsson K, Hellstrom K, Kallner M: Effect of cholic acid feeding on bile acid kinetics and neutral fecal steroid excretion in hyperlipoproteinemia (types II and IV). Metabolism 23:863, 1974.
18. Grundy SM, Ahrens EH, Salen G: Interruption of the enterohepatic circulation of bile acids in man: Comparative effects of cholestyramine and ileal exclusion on cholesterol metabolism. J Lab Clin Med 78:94, 1971.
19. Schoenfield LS, Bonorris GG, Ganz P: Induced alterations in the rate-limiting enzymes of hepatic cholesterol and bile-acid synthesis in the hamster. J Lab Clin Med 82:858, 1973.
20. Kim DN, Rogers DH, Li JR, et al: Effects of cholestyramine on cholesterol balance parameters and hepatic HMG CoA reductase and cholesterol 7 alpha-hydroxylase activities in swine. Exp Mol Pathol 26:434, 1977.
21. Mitropoulos KA, Knight BL, Reeves BE: 3-Hydroxyl-3-methylglutaryl coenzyme A reductase. Biochem J 185:435, 1980.
22. Brown MS, Goldstein JL: A receptor-mediated pathway for cholesterol homeostasis. Science 232:34, 1986.
23. Witztum JL, Schonfeld G, Weidman SW, et al: Bile sequestrant therapy alters the composition of low density and high density lipoproteins. Metabolism 28:221, 1979.
24. Levy RI, Langer T: Hypolipidemic drugs and lipoprotein metabolism. Adv Exp Med Biol 26:155, 1972.

25. Shepherd J, Bicker S, Lorimer AR, et al: Receptor-mediated low density lipoprotein catabolism in man. J Lipid Res 20:999, 1979.

26. Breslow JL, Spaulding DR, Lux SE, et al: Homozygous familial hypercholesterolemia. N Engl J Med 293:900, 1975.

27. Angelin B, Einarsson K, Hellstrom K, et al: Bile acid kinetics in relation to endogenous triglyceride metabolism in various types of hyperlipoproteinemia. J Lipid Res 19:1004, 1978.

28. Angelin B, Einarsson K, Hellstrom K, et al: Effects of cholestyramine and chenodeoxycholic acid on the metabolism of endogenous triglyceride in hyperlipoproteinemia. J Lipid Res 19:1017, 1978.

29. Beil U, Crouse JR, Einarsson K, et al: Effect of interruption of the enterohepatic circulation of bile acids on the transport of very low density lipoprotein triglycerides. Metabolism 31:438, 1982.

30. Angelin B, Bjorkhem I, Einarsson K: Influence of bile acids on the soluble phosphatidic acid phosphatase in rat liver. Biochem Biophys Res Commun 100:606, 1981.

31. Update. Chenodeoxycholic acid and gallstones. JAMA 245:2378, 1981.

32. Russell DW, Brown MS, Goldstein JL: Different combinations of cysteine-rich repeats mediate binding of low density lipoprotein receptor to two different proteins. J Biol Chem 264:21682, 1989.

33. Crouse JR: Hypertriglyceridemia: A contraindication for use of bile acid resins. Am J Med 83:243, 1987.

34. Mahley RW, Rall SC: Type III hyperlipoproteinemia (dysbetalipoproteinemia): The role of apolipoprotein E in normal and abnormal lipoprotein metabolism. *In* Scriver CR, Beaudet AL, Sly WS, Valle D (eds): The Metabolic Basis of Inherited Disease, 6th Ed. New York: McGraw-Hill, 1989, pp 1195–1213.

35. Hoogwerf BJ, Peters JR, Frantz ID Jr, Hunninghake DB: Effect of clofibrate and colestipol singly and in combination on plasma lipids and lipoproteins in type III hyperlipoproteinemia. Metabolism 34:978, 1985.

36. Shepherd J, Packard CJ: Effects of drugs on high density lipoprotein metabolism. *In* Gotto AM, Smith LC, Allen B (eds): Atherosclerosis V. New York: Springer-Verlag, 1980, p 591.

37. Shepherd J, Packard CJ, Morgan J, et al: The effects of cholestyramine on high density lipoprotein metabolism. Atherosclerosis 33:433, 1979.

38. Wu AL, Windmueller HG: Relative contributions by liver and intestine to individual plasma apolipoproteins in the rat. J Biol Chem 254:7316, 1979.

39. Bearnot H, Riley J, Green P, et al: Effect of bile diversion on rat intestinal high density lipoprotein formation [abstract]. Circulation 62:III-17, 1980.

40. Miller JP: Lecithin-cholesterol acyl transferase activity and cholestyramine resin therapy in man. Eur J Clin Invest 6:471, 1976.

41. Wallentin L: Lecithin: cholesterol acyl transfer rate and high density lipoproteins in plasma during dietary and cholestyramine treatment of type IIa hyperlipoproteinemia. Eur J Clin Invest 8:383, 1978.

42. Gordon DJ, Knoke J, Probstfield JL, et al, for the Lipids Research Clinics Program: High-density lipoprotein cholesterol and coronary heart disease in hypercholesterolemic men: The Lipid Research Clinics Coronary Primary Prevention Trial. Circulation 74:1217, 1979.

43. Hunninghake DB, Peterson F, Swenson M, et al: Efficacy of once versus twice-a-day dosage of cholestyramine in Type IIa hyperlipoproteinemia [abstract]. Pharmacology 21:176, 1979.

44. Superko HR, Greenland P, Manchester RA, et al: Effectiveness of low dose colestipol therapy in patients with moderate hypercholesterolemia. Am J Cardiol 70:135, 1992.

45. Lyons D, Webster J, Fowler G, et al: Colestipol at varying dosage intervals in the treatment of moderate hypercholesterolemia. Br J Clin Pharmacol 37:59, 1994.

46. Schrott HG, Stein EA, Dujovne CA, et al: Enhanced low-density lipoprotein cholesterol reduction and cost-effectiveness by low-dose colestipol plus lovastatin combination therapy. Am J Cardiol 75:34, 1995.

47. The Lipid Research Clinics Coronary Primary Prevention Trial Results: (I) Reduction in incidence of coronary heart disease; (II) The relationship of reduction in incidence of coronary heart disease to cholesterol lowering. JAMA 251:351, 1984.

48. Miettinen TA: Dietary fiber and lipids. Am J Clin Nutr 45:1237, 1988.

49. Bell LP, Hectorne K, Reynolds H, et al: Cholesterol lowering effects of psyllium hydrophilic mucilloid. JAMA 261:3419, 1989.

50. Masclee AAM, Jansen JBMJ, Rovati LC, et al: Effect of cholestyramine and cholecystokinin receptor antagonist CR1505 (loxiglumide) on lower esophageal sphincter pressure in man. Dig Dis Sci 38:1889, 1993.

51. Palasciano G, Chiloiro M, Belfiore A, et al: Cholestyramine alters feedback mechanism of bile acids and cholecystokinin in the regulation of gallbladder motility in humans [abstract]. Hepatology 10:603, 1989.

52. Hunninghake DB: Resin therapy. Adverse effects and their management. *In* Fears J, Barcelona JR (eds): Pharmacological Control of Hyperlipidemia. Prous Science Publishers, SA, 1986, pp 67–89.

53. Brensike JF, Levy RI, Kelsey SF: Effects of therapy with cholestyramine on progression of coronary arteriosclerosis: Results of the NHLBI Type II Coronary Intervention Study. Circulation 69:213, 1984.

54. Witztum JL, Laurence SJ, Schonfeld G: Thyroid hormone and thyrotropin levels in patients placed on colestipol hydrochloride. J Clin Endocrinol Metab 46:838, 1978.

55. Stein EA: Treatment of familial hypercholesterolemia with drugs in children. Arteriosclerosis 9(Suppl I):I-145, 1989.

56. Schneider DL, Gallo DG, Sarett HP: Effect of cholestyramine on cholesterol metabolism in young adult swine. Proc Soc Exp Biol Med 121:1244, 1966.

57. Kleinman PK: Cholestyramine and metabolic acidosis. N Engl J Med 200(15):861, 1974.

58. Scheel PJ, Whelton A, Rossiter K, Watson A: Cholestyramine-induced hyperchloremic metabolic acidosis. J Clin Pharmacol 32:536, 1992.

59. Blankenhorn DH, Nessim SA, Johnson RL, et al: Beneficial effects of combined colestipol-niacin therapy on coronary atherosclerosis and coronary venous bypass grafts. JAMA 257(23):3233, 1987.

60. Brown G, Albers JJ, Fisher LD, et al: Regression of coronary artery disease as a result of intensive lipid lowering therapy in men with high levels of apolipoprotein B. N Engl J Med 323:1289, 1990.

CHAPTER 116

Clofibrate

Dennis R. Feller, Ph.D., Howard A.I. Newman, Ph.D.,
Larry M. Hagerman, B.S., and Donald T. Witiak, Ph.D.

HISTORY

With approval by the Food and Drug Administration (FDA) in 1966, clofibrate (Atromid-S) became the first fibrate introduced in the United States. Two clofibrate analogues, gemfibrozil (Lopid) and fenofibrate (Lipidil), subsequently received FDA approval in 1981[1] and 1993,[2] respectively. The initial work by Thorp and Waring[3] in 1962 established the efficacy of clofibrate in lowering serum lipid levels in rats. Because these early preclinical studies used clofibrate and androsterone in combination,[3, 4] this combination was also used in initial studies in humans.[5] However, when clofibrate alone was used in over 1300 patients,[6] serum cholesterol and triglyceride levels were lowered significantly, and use of androsterone combinations was discontinued. Many studies corroborate these original observations of reductions in serum triglyceride concentrations, but effects on cholesterol vary considerably and generally are of a small magnitude.[7]

Clofibrate became the most widely prescribed lipid-lowering drug in the mid-1970s. However, upon publication of the negative findings from two major clinical studies in 1975 and 1978, use of clofibrate decreased dramatically. The Coronary Drug Project[8] provided the first long-term study to test the efficacy of clofibrate with respect to reducing morbidity or mortality from coronary artery disease. In this study, 1000 men who had previously had a myocardial infarction took clofibrate for 6 years, whereas a control group of 3000 men took a placebo. At the conclusion of the study, there was no significant difference in the incidence of cardiovascular events (fatal or nonfatal) between the two groups. Subsequently, the World Health Organization (WHO) conducted a very large study in 5000 asymptomatic, hypercholesterolemic men given clofibrate for 5 years and compared the incidence of cardiovascular and noncardiovascular events with that in a control group of 5000 men given a placebo.[9] At the end of this study, the age-adjusted total mortality in the clofibrate-treated group was 44% higher than in the placebo group. Noncardiovascular causes, primarily malignancies involving the gastrointestinal tract, and an increased incidence of cholelithiasis and mortality from cholecystectomy produced the observed excess deaths. Although the clofibrate-treated group had a significant 25% reduction in nonfatal myocardial infarctions when compared with the placebo treatment, there was no difference in the incidence of fatal myocardial infarction.

Clofibrate is currently indicated for treatment of primary dysbetalipoproteinemia (type III hyperlipidemia) when there is an inadequate dietary response. Other uses may include the treatment of adult patients having hypertriglyceridemia (type IV and type V hyperlipidemias) with increased risk for abdominal pain and pancreatitis, and of patients with disfiguring xanthomata.

CHEMISTRY

Clofibrate [ethyl 2-(4-chlorophenoxy)-2-methylpropionic acid], the ethyl ester of clofibric acid (molecular weight, 242.5), is a nearly colorless or pale yellow oily liquid that is insoluble in water and miscible with many organic solvents.[10] 4-Chlorophenol, acetone, and chloroform are starting materials for the synthesis of clofibric acid, which is subsequently esterified with ethanol to yield clofibrate.[11] Originally, commercial preparations of clofibrate outside the United States contained trace amounts of 4-chlorophenol (a potential hepatotoxin), but this contaminant is now removed.[12-14] Atromid-S is prepared as orange, oblong, soft gelatin capsules containing 500 mg clofibrate and a mixture of FD&C yellow, blue, and red dyes. Because clofibrate is sensitive to light and oxygen, capsules of Atromid-S are stored in light-resistant containers. This drug should not be stored frozen or at high temperatures.

Clofibrate is rapidly hydrolyzed by plasma and tissue esterases *in vivo* to form the active metabolite clofibric acid (Fig. 116–1).[11] Clofibric acid, rather than the parent drug, provides the pharmacologic actions and toxicities associated with clofibrate therapy. Clofibric acid, an organic acid ($pK_a = 4.7$), ionizes

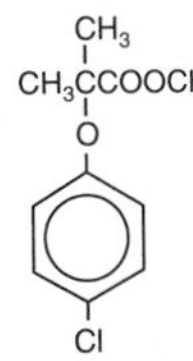

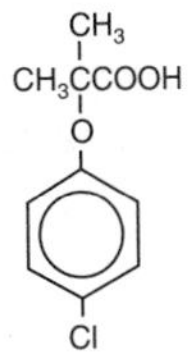

Figure 116–1. The chemical structures of clofibrate and clofibric acid.

at physiologic pH and is highly bound to plasma proteins.

PHARMACOLOGY
Effects on Blood Lipids and Lipoproteins

Clofibrate predominantly lowers serum triglyceride concentrations in patients with elevated very-low-density lipoproteins (VLDL) (type IV and type V hyperlipoproteinemias) and elevated intermediate-density lipoproteins (IDL) (type III hyperlipoproteinemia). The serum triglyceride lowering actions of clofibrate in humans with type III and type IV hyperlipidemias are primarily related to an increased intravascular catabolism of serum triglyceride-rich lipoproteins (VLDL and IDL). However, certain hypertriglyceridemic patient populations (type IV hyperlipidemia) may respond to clofibrate by mechanisms involving a decrease in hepatic triglyceride or VLDL synthesis and/or VLDL release from the liver.[15-19] The increased VLDL triglyceride hydrolysis of clofibrate is related to the activation of adipose tissue or muscle lipoprotein lipases, which accelerate the rate of intravascular catabolism of VLDL and IDL to produce low-density lipoprotein (LDL). Clofibrate-mediated increases in LDL cholesterol levels of hypertriglyceridemic patients (types IIb, IV, and V hyperlipemias) may result from the increased breakdown of VLDL and conversion to LDL.[15, 20-22]

Clofibrate treatment also inhibits peripheral mobilization of free fatty acids by blocking the activation of adenylate-cyclase–sensitive triglyceride lipase in adipose tissue and increasing enzyme activities involved in liver fatty acid metabolism.[7, 11, 23-26] The blockade of lipolysis reduces plasma fatty acid availability to the liver, which may indirectly decrease triglyceride biosynthesis.

The serum cholesterol– and LDL cholesterol–lowering effects of clofibrate are variable. The mechanism of hypocholesterolemia for clofibrate is unknown and may involve one or more of the following: (1) an inhibition of liver cholesterol biosynthesis at the level of conversion of 3-hydroxy-3-methylglutaryl coenzyme A (HMG-CoA) to mevalonic acid; (2) an increase in biliary neutral sterol excretion; or (3) an increase in tissue cholesterol mobilization. Serum cholesterol catabolism remains unchanged in humans after clofibrate treatment;[27] however, acidic and neutral sterol excretion into bile increases with clofibrate treatment.[27-29] The net loss of cholesterol into bile and subsequently into the feces presumably occurs by mobilization of cholesterol from extrahepatic tissues by clofibrate. This action explains the increased lithogenicity of bile, cholecystitis, and gallstone formation seen in patients during long-term administration.[11, 30, 31] The mechanism underlying cholesterol mobilization from extrahepatic tissues may involve elevations in HDL cholesterol concentrations by clofibrate,[20, 21, 32-34] thereby increasing peripheral cholesterol tissue removal to the liver for neutral sterol elimination into

bile. Thus, prolonged treatment with clofibrate may also benefit patients with xanthomata.

Effects on Apoproteins

In normocholesterolemic rats treated with clofibrate, both total serum cholesterol and triglyceride concentrations diminish. Reductions in levels of apoproteins (apo) A-I, B, and C-III also occur. Apoprotein E levels remain unchanged.[35] Cholesterol and apo B concentrations remain unchanged with clofibrate treatment in cholesterol-fed rats, but triglycerides increase. The apo A-I concentration also drops in drug-treated cholesterol-cholic acid–fed rats coupled with a reduction in apo A-IV. In VLDL and IDL apo C-III-0 declines and in HDL the same apoprotein increases.[36] Although no change takes place in apo E concentrations in normal rats,[35] a sharp increase takes place in VLDL apo E in cholesterol-fed rats.[36] These findings correspond with liver mRNA studies in rats where the expression of apo A-IV is reduced in rat liver but not in rat intestine.[37] Both fenofibrate and clofibrate also inhibit gene expression of apo A-I in rat liver, which reflects in a drop in apo A-I, A-II, and A-IV concentrations in serum. Apoprotein E levels also declined. Conversely, gemfibrozil increased cholesterol and apo E concentrations without increasing apo A-I or A-IV levels.[38] Other studies with cholesterol-fed rats show a small decrease in both apo B and cholesterol concentrations with fibrate administration. Gemfibrozil gives the greatest reduction in both apo B and cholesterol concentrations in cholesterol-fed rats, and when compared with the other fibrates, gemfibrozil gave the only reduction in apo E in this model.[39]

In human studies, somewhat different apolipoprotein changes result from treatment with clofibrate and the other fibrate analogues. Overall with treatment of type IIa,[40, 41] type IIb, type III,[42] and type IV[43] patients, total triglyceride and cholesterol levels are reduced. In type IV patients both the triglyceride and the cholesterol reductions occur in VLDL.[43] Except for type III patients, lowering of apo B levels occurs in all phenotypes. In type III patients apo E diminishes with clofibrate treatment with no changes in apo A-II, A-IV, C-II, or C-III.[42] With Hep 2G cells as a model for liver cells, the action of clofibrate induces decreased apo B secretion with no effect on apo A-I,[44] but fenofibrate with the same hepatoma cells demonstrates decreased triglycerides secretion with concomitant reductions in apo B secretion. Inversely, apo A-I secretion rises with fenofibrate treatment.[44] Ciprofibrate incubated with the Hep 2G model demonstrates inhibition of cholesterol biosynthesis from acetate and mevalonate.[45]

Combination with Other Lipid-Lowering Agents

The combination of clofibrate with other commercially available hypolipidemic agents has generally produced additive or synergistic effects in hyperlipidemic patients.[7, 46, 47] Lovastatin alone or in combination with clofibrate lowers total and LDL cholesterol and VLDL cholesterol concentrations in type III hyperlipoproteinemia.[48] Positive results are reported with clofibrate and colestipol,[49-55] cholestyramine,[7, 56] nicotinic acid and its prodrugs,[57-59] and Secholex (DEAE-Sephadex)[56, 60, 61] in hyperlipidemic patients. Combinations of nicotinic acid and fenofibrate[62, 63] and of colestipol and fenofibrate[64, 65] also are beneficial in lowering serum lipid and lipoprotein concentrations. A dramatic lowering of serum HDL-cholesterol concentrations may occur in hyperlipidemic patients receiving a combination of clofibrate and probucol;[66] such a deficiency in HDL may increase the risk for congestive heart disease in this patient population.

Clofibrate Analogues

Selected newer, commercially available hypolipidemic analogues of clofibrate that are being evaluated in humans or are currently used in Europe generally exhibit the same profile of hypotriglyceridemic activity (increased VLDL catabolism by stimulating lipoprotein lipase [LpL])[67] as clofibrate but may have advantages over clofibrate for certain phenotypes (IIa and IIb). These fibrates produce modest reductions in total and LDL cholesterol levels in type IIa hyperlipoproteinemia; produce less consistent reductions in LDL cholesterol and significant decreases in triglyceride levels in type IIb hyperlipoproteinemia; and significant reductions in VLDL and serum triglycerides in type IV hyperlipoproteinemia.[68] Ciprofibrate and fenofibrate reduce total cholesterol, LDL cholesterol VLDL cholesterol, and apo B concentrations and increase HDL cholesterol and apo A levels in type II hypercholesterolemic patients.[69] Ciprofibrate produces greater increases in HDL cholesterol and apo A levels than fenofibrate and possesses a long half-life, so that a single daily dose may be administered.

The clofibrate analogue bezafibrate reduces serum total cholesterol and triglyceride concentrations in diabetic patients as well as the triglycerides and cholesterol in VLDL. Concomitant reductions in apo B levels occur with increases in apo A-II and HDL cholesterol and an increase in the HDL_3/HDL_2 ratio.[70] In nondiabetic hypertriglyceridemic patients bezafibrate treatment also increases HDL cholesterol with a concomitant rise in apo A-I.[71] Hypercholesterolemic patients treated with bezafibrate also have reductions in both total and LDL cholesterol and total and VLDL triglyceride concentrations. Apoprotein B reductions parallel these changes in serum lipid concentrations. The HDL level rises concomitant with a rise in apo A-I and A-II.[72] In type II hyperlipoproteinemic patients a reduction in total cholesterol is accompanied by a reduced cholesterol content of both VLDL and LDL with a reduced total serum triglyceride concentration. In these patients HDL cholesterol remains unchanged with treatment. Overall these patients have a bezafibrate-induced increased receptor-mediated LDL catabolism,[73] which accounts for the observed reduction in apo B seen in bezafibrate-treated type IIa patients.[71] Ciprofibrate[69, 74, 75] and ethophylline clofibrate[76] dem-

onstrate generally comparable hypolipidemic properties to the other analogues. However, fenofibrate is more effective than ciprofibrate in raising HDL levels.[69] Ciprofibrate is able to convert atherogenic small dense LDL, which can readily oxidize to larger more benign particles.[77]

Effect on Hepatic Fatty Acid Metabolism and Peroxisomal Proliferation

Clofibrate and related fibrates belong to a group of compounds called hepatic peroxisomal proliferators, which represent a unique chemical class of nonmutagenic (genotoxic) carcinogens in rodent species.[78] Peroxisomes contain catalase, hydrogen peroxide–generating enzymes, and enzymes for the β-oxidation of long-chain fatty acids. Peroxisome proliferation is defined as a pronounced increase in the size and number of hepatic peroxisomes and in the activity of lipid-metabolizing enzymes of the peroxisomal fatty acid β-oxidation pathway, including acyl-CoA oxidase, which functions in the catabolism of long-chain fatty acids.[79]

Hepatic peroxisomal proliferation persists during long-term administration of clofibrate and related fibrate analogues including gemfibrozil (Lopid) and fenofibrate (Lipidil) to laboratory animals.[79, 80] An increased number of hepatocellular tumors and malignant neoplasms of the intestine, pancreas, and Leydig cells also occurs with a variety of agents structurally related to clofibrate (gemfibrozil, fenofibrate, bezafibrate, and ciprofibrate) known to cause hepatic peroxisomal proliferation in these rodent species.[79, 81-85] Fibrates are proposed to interact with a ligand-specific cytosolic receptor, called a peroxisome proliferator-activated receptor (PPAR), that belongs to the steroid hormone receptor superfamily.[86] Human and rodent isoforms of the PPAR are now known, and the mechanism of peroxisomal proliferation has been linked to a specific induction of peroxisome-containing enzymes of the long-chained fatty acid β-oxidation pathway. One theory proposes that an accumulation of hydrogen peroxide, formed as a side reaction of the enzyme acyl-CoA oxidase in peroxisomes, leads to the generation of free radical reactive oxygen species and subsequent cell damage, with putative formation of hydroxy adducts of DNA nucleotide bases. However, the mechanism of carcinogenic action for fibrates is unknown. The existence of a parallel phenomenon of peroxisome proliferation with fibrate treatment in higher species (monkeys) and humans and its relationship to carcinogenesis remains a controversial issue. In 1974, the FDA listed clofibrate as a potential tumorigen, and this agent, as well as related fibrate analogues, requires an assessment of risks to benefits in patients.

Fatty acid oxidation in isolated hepatocytes[26] or perfused liver[23, 24] increases with clofibrate. Fibrates, in rodent species, increase hepatic β-oxidation of fatty acids by peroxisomes and/or mitochondria.[87] Clofibrate and its analogues markedly stimulate the activity of peroxisomal acyl-CoA oxidase and other enzymes in this fatty acid β-oxidation pathway.[85, 88, 89] Increased hepatic FA oxidation will also reduce triglyceride and VLDL biosynthesis or release, and these two actions of clofibrate may explain part of the triglyceride-lowering response in animals.[7, 24, 90]

Apparently, clofibrate did not modify hepatic triglyceride synthesis or VLDL release in most human studies.[7, 15-19] However, the increased intravascular catabolism of VLDL to LDL by clofibrate may lead to an elevated fatty acid (FA) uptake in liver. If clofibrate treatment induces enzymes of pathways of hepatic β-oxidation of fatty acids in both mitochondria and peroxisomes, the incorporation of these fatty acids will be diminished. Thus, a reduction in the pool fatty acids as a result of the intravascular hydrolysis of VLDL-triglyceride may contribute in part to the antitriglyceridemic action of clofibrate.

Administration of clofibrate to animals produces a marked hepatomegaly associated with a proliferation of mitochondria, endoplasmic reticulum, and peroxisomes,[7, 11, 91, 92] and these hepatic effects usually reverse.[92] Liver enlargement in humans is related to an increase in mitochondria, endoplasmic reticulum, and either an increase or no change in peroxisomes.[11, 92, 93] Elevations in serum HDL cholesterol levels are associated with endoplasmic reticulum proliferation.[94, 95] This effect may explain the modest rise in serum HDL concentrations by clofibrate in hyperlipidemic patients.[20, 21, 34]

Effects on Platelet Function

Clofibrate may normalize thrombogenic potential in high-risk patient populations.[96] Clofibrate therapy decreases platelet sensitivity (adhesiveness) in type IIb patients,[97] prolongs platelet survival time,[98] and produces a benefit in patients with platelet hypersensitivity in the absence of a serum lipid–lowering effect.[99] The antiaggregatory effects of clofibrate in humans are variable.[7] In human platelet preparations,[7, 100-102] clofibric acid blocks the release of arachidonic acid from platelet membrane phospholipids and acts as an inhibitor of prostaglandin biosynthesis in vitro.[102] Analogues of clofibric acid also possess similar antiaggregatory profiles and are more potent inhibitors of platelet function.[102, 103] Plasma fibrinogen concentrations generally decrease upon initial therapy with a return toward normal, and plasma fibrinolysis usually increases in patients on clofibrate therapy.

PHARMACOKINETICS

Clofibrate, intact and as clofibric acid, undergoes rapid and complete absorption after oral administration. During intestinal absorption, clofibrate undergoes extensive hydrolysis to its active metabolite, clofibric acid.[4, 104-106] The mean absorptive half-life of clofibrate (1- to 2-g dose) in humans is 1.7 hours, and maximal serum concentrations of clofibric acid (100 to 180 μg/ml) occur within 3 to 6 hours. Unchanged clofibrate is not detected in plasma after oral adminis-

tration. Clofibric acid is highly plasma protein–bound (93% to 98%) and possesses a small volume of distribution (5 to 9 L). The elimination half-life of clofibric acid from plasma at therapeutic doses is between 13 and 17 hours, with variations of 6 to 24 hours.[105, 107] In patients with renal disorders, the elimination half-life of clofibric acid is increased, leading to marked elevations in drug concentration. A 1-g dosing regimen, twice daily, in humans is an appropriate dosing regimen that maintains steady-state concentrations of clofibric acid of 100 to 160 μg/ml.

Clofibric acid undergoes extensive conjugation in the liver to form the 1-O-acyl glucuronide as the major in vivo metabolite.[4, 104-107] Clofibric acid and its glucuronide metabolite are eliminated in the urine (>97% of the dose) within 72 hours. The 1-O-acyl glucuronide of clofibric acid in liver is secreted into bile and undergoes extensive enterohepatic circulation. This glucuronide metabolite is hydrolyzed by bacterial β-glucuronidases in the gastrointestinal tract, and liberated clofibric acid is reabsorbed into the bloodstream. Higher plasma levels of this glucuronide metabolite occur in patients with renal insufficiency or Gilbert's syndrome.[105, 107, 108]

Urinary isomeric 2-, 3-, and 4-O-acyl glucuronides of clofibric acid are reported in patients given clofibrate; their formation occurs by a nonenzymatic pH-dependent intramolecular migration of glucuronic acid from the 1-O-acyl glucuronide conjugate of clofibric acid.[109, 110] These isomeric ester glucuronides, unlike the 1-O-acyl glucuronide, do not undergo enzymatic hydrolysis by β-glucuronidase or enterohepatic circulation. The taurine conjugate of clofibric acid has been isolated in several species but not in humans.[111]

CLINICAL USE
Indications

Clofibrate is indicated for primary dysbetalipoproteinemia (type III hyperlipoproteinemia) that does not respond adequately to diet.[112] Clofibrate may be considered in severely hypertriglyceridemic patients (serum triglyceride levels, >1000 mg/dl) to reduce the risk of pancreatitis. Clofibrate is not useful in type I hypercholesterolemia where the hypertriglyceridemia is related to elevation of chylomicrons rather than VLDL.

Beneficial effects of clofibrate are found for the treatment of endogenous hypertriglyceridemias (types IV and V), of familial combined hyperlipidemia (types IIa, IIb, and IV), either alone or in drug combination, and in diabetic retinopathy.[113, 114] Clofibrate may be useful in type IIb, type IV, and type V hyperlipemias when diet and drug therapy with nicotinic acid (niacin) or gemfibrozil are not effective.[115]

Precautions and Adverse Effects

An increased incidence of non-CHD-related deaths in hyperlipidemic patients[31] is associated with a possible increase in morbidity and mortality after cholecystectomy and from malignancies of the liver, pancreas, and intestine of clofibrate-treated patients.[31] Liver tumorigenicity has been confirmed in animals.[79, 82, 83, 116] Gallstone enlargement and cholelithiasis and cholecystitis are also potentially adverse effects observed with the use of fibrates.[117] Clinicians have strongly advised the evaluation of benefits versus risks in patients undergoing clofibrate treatment,[31, 118] and the FDA issued a warning about the potential tumorigenicity associated with clofibrate therapy in humans.[119] Similar concerns exist for other fibrates such as fenofibrate and gemfibrozil.

Gastrointestinal symptoms (abdominal discomfort, diarrhea, and constipation) are the most common complaints associated with fibrate therapy.[120] Skin rashes, fatigue, headache, loss of libido, impotence, and insomnia occur less frequently. Clofibrate therapy induces flu-like symptoms that accompany myositis, myotonia, and myalgia in a small number of patients.[121, 122] Hepatotoxicity and severe liver dysfunctions (hepatitis) are infrequently reported with fibrate therapy.[123]

Skeletal muscle myopathies (myositis, myalgia) are observed in patients given fibrates. Myotonic excitability produced by clofibrate is related to a decrease in electrical threshold, which produces a prolonged contraction of skeletal muscle.[124] The myotonia-inducing potency of fibrates is correlated to a decreased chloride conductance in skeletal muscle fibers, whereas potassium currents are unaffected.[125] Clofibric acid and related fibrate analogues, as anions at physiologic pH, may directly act on a binding site that regulates the chloride channel in this tissue.[126]

Contraindications

To prevent risk to fetuses and infants, clofibrate is contraindicated in women during pregnancy, lactation, or of childbearing age not practicing birth control.[11, 15, 115] Clofibric acid accumulates in maternal breast milk and fetal serum, and embryotoxicities have been observed with clofibrate and other fibrates in animal studies at doses greater than those used therapeutically.[127]

Clofibrate is also contraindicated in patients with primary biliary cirrhosis or other significant hepatic and renal dysfunctions.[112] If drug therapy is instituted in patients with compromised liver or kidney function, the dosage of clofibrate should be reduced to minimize the adverse effects seen with elevated clofibric acid concentrations.

The use of fibrates is contraindicated in patients with preexisting skeletal muscle disorders.[127] In these patients, severe myopathy followed by rhabdomyolysis and acute renal failure may occur if drug therapy is not terminated.[128, 129] Hypothyroidism may accentuate these adverse effects.[122, 130] The extent of skeletal muscle damage by fibrates may be assessed by monitoring the activity of serum creatine kinase.

Similar to fibrates, patients taking statins may also complain of these skeletal muscle disorders. Thus, combination therapy of fibrates and statins (lovastatin, pravastatin, and simvastatin) is also contraindicated. Fulminant rhabdomyolysis has been seen as early as 3 weeks or after several months in patients given clofibrate and lovastatin therapy. The combination of fibrates and statins should be avoided.

Interference with Other Drugs

Clofibric acid binds extensively to plasma proteins and may displace the binding of acidic drugs (phenytoin, tolbutamide, and coumarin-type anticoagulants) to these sites, leading to an enhancement of the pharmacologic response and/or toxicity for such compounds.[15, 105] Combination therapy with clofibrate and coumarin-type drugs necessitates a frequent monitoring of prothrombin clotting times and may require a reduction in the dose of the anticoagulant by 50% or more.[15] Coadministration of rifampin and clofibrate to patients reduces serum clofibric acid concentrations and increases the dose of clofibrate required.[105]

Use in Patients with Impaired Organ Function

Adverse effects of clofibrate therapy including hepatotoxicity, cholelithiasis, renal disease, or skeletal muscle disorders may require cessation or a reduction in clofibrate dosage. Diseases of the kidney (nephrotic syndrome or renal insufficiency) and liver (including biliary cirrhosis) may produce elevations in the retention of clofibric acid so that plasma levels increase.[105, 107] Such patients may exhibit myositis and severe renal failure requiring a reduction or termination of fibrate (clofibrate, gemfibrozil, or ciprofibrate) therapy.[122, 131, 132]

The Place of Clofibrate in the Antilipidemic Arsenal

Clofibrate is no longer the primary drug for the treatment of hypercholesterolemias or hypertriglyceridemias and should be restricted to those hypertriglyceridemic patients who do not tolerate or are unresponsive to niacin or gemfibrozil therapy. However, clofibrate remains an appropriate drug for the treatment of type III (primary dysbetalipoproteinemia) patients who do not respond to diet alone. This drug should be discontinued if a significant lipid response is not observed after several months.

An assessment of risks and benefits for each patient is recommended. Severe adverse effects of clofibrate reported in clinical studies suggest that a drug other than clofibrate should be selected. Clofibrate produces malignant tumors in rodents, and patients are exposed to an increased risk of cholelithiasis during clofibrate treatment. Finally, no substantial evidence of a reduction in cardiovascular mortality in patients on clofibrate therapy is available.

Other drugs (statins and bile acid sequestrants) are generally the drugs of first choice for the treatment of hypercholesterolemias. Occasionally, a fibrate may be used when these first-line drugs are either not tolerated or the desired lipid response is not achieved. In patients with disorders of types IIa, IIb, or III who also have elevated serum VLDL-triglyceride concentrations (>250 mg/ml) and are not responsive to niacin, addition of a fibrate or probucol may provide a lowering of LDL-cholesterol levels. Coadministration of fibrates with a bile acid sequestrant (cholestyramine or colestipol) or probucol may produce an adequate response in lowering the serum cholesterol level; however, this combination is less effective than other combinations. The combination of fibrates with statins is generally avoided because the potentially life-threatening complications of myositis and rhabdomyolysis with or without severe renal failure are reported.

Dosage and Administration

Clofibrate is administered orally at 2 g/day in divided doses for initial and maintenance doses. Three grams daily may be needed to reach the desired response. Maximal serum lipid responses, particularly triglyceride lowering effects, are usually observed within 1 week of treatment, and return to original values in 2 or 3 weeks after cessation of therapy.

SOCIOECONOMIC CONSIDERATIONS
Compliance with Regimen

Adverse effects associated with oral clofibrate therapy are relatively few. Other than the requirement of multiple dosing (e.g., four capsules a day or two capsules twice a day), patient compliance is generally good.

Compliance was monitored by measurement of serum clofibric acid concentrations in type IV patients treated for one year.[133] Only one patient out of ten was noncompliant. Clofibrate blood levels were positively correlated with lowering of serum triglycerides, uric acid, and bilirubin in these patients.[133] Dosage adjustments may be necessary after several weeks of treatment in order to reach the desired lipid response, but this does not represent an inconvenience for patients.

Cost

Clofibrate (Atromid-S) is sold commercially under at least 80 trade names worldwide, and approximately 20 generic brands are currently available in the United States.[11] The average wholesale cost of Atromid-S (2 g daily, four 500-mg capsules) is approximately $2.88 per day; and is about two to four times more expensive than a generic clofibrate ($0.68 to $1.12 per day).* This recommended dosing regimen of Atromid-S is comparable with the cost of gemfibrozil (Lopid, two

600-mg tablets daily; $2.30 per day) and Nicolar (four 500-mg tablets daily; $2.24/day).* However, generic niacin (four 500-mg tablets) costs about $0.32 per day and is considerably less expensive than the Nicolar or timed-release Nicobid brands.

REFERENCES

1. Parke-Davis' Lopid gemfibrozil has been approved by FDA for use as a lipid regulating agent to combat 2 types of hyperlipoproteinemia. Medical World News 451:40, 1982.
2. Fournier seeking to finalize Lipidil marketing partnership; second half 1994 launch expected. F-D-C Reports—Prescription Pharmaceuticals and Biotechnology "The Pink Sheet" T&G 56(2):5, 1994.
3. Thorp JM, Waring WS: Modification of metabolism and distribution of lipids by ethyl chlorophenoxyisobutyrate. Nature 194:948, 1962.
4. Thorp JM: Experimental evaluation of an orally active combination of androsterone and ethyl chlorophenoxyisobutyrate. Lancet 1:1323, 1962.
5. Oliver MF: Reduction of serum-lipid and uric-acid levels by an orally active androsterone. Lancet 1:1321, 1962.
6. Pinter KG: Drugs and atherosclerosis. Annu Rev Pharmacol 6:251, 1966.
7. Witiak DT, Newman HAI, Feller DR: Clofibrate and Related Analogs, A Comprehensive Review. Medicinal Research Series, Vol 7. New York: Marcel Dekker, 1977.
8. The Coronary Drug Project Research Group: Clofibrate and niacin in coronary heart disease. JAMA 231:360, 1975.
9. Report from the Committee of Principal Investigators: A cooperative trial in the primary prevention of ischemic heart disease using clofibrate. Br Heart J 40:1069, 1978.
10. Merck Index, 10th ed. Rahway, NJ: Merck and Co., 1983.
11. World Health Organization: IARC Monograph on the Evaluation of Carcinogenic Risk of Chemicals (Some Pharmaceutical Drugs), Vol 24. Geneva, Switzerland: WHO, 1980, pp 39–58.
12. Koibuchi M, Ejima A: Determination of pharmaceutical preparations by gas chromatography. VI. Determination of p-chlorophenol in clofibrate capsule using flame photometric and flame thermionic detector. J Hyg Chem 25:301, 1979.
13. Phornchirasilp S, Patel ST, Hanson JM, et al: Pharmacologic effects of 4-chlorophenol in rats: Comparison to clofibrate. Proc Soc Exp Biol Med 191:139, 1989.
14. Phornchirasilp S, Victor DeSouza JJ, Feller DR: In vivo and in vitro studies of the hepatotoxic effects of 4-chlorophenol in mice. Biochem Pharmacol 38:961, 1989.
15. Levy FI: Drugs used in the treatment of hyperlipoproteinemias. In Gilman AG, Goodman LS, Gilman A (eds): The Pharmacological Basis of Therapeutics, 6th ed. New York: Macmillan, 1980, pp 834–847.
16. Nikkila EA, Huttunen JK, Ehnholm C: Effect of clofibrate on postheparin plasma triglyceride lipase activities in patients with hypertriglyceridemia. Metabolism 26:179, 1977.
17. Taylor KG, Holdsworth G, Galton DJ: Clofibrate increases lipoprotein-lipase activity in adipose tissue of hypertriglyceridaemic patients. Lancet 2:1106, 1977.
18. Lithell H, Boberg J, Hellsing K, et al: Increase of the lipoprotein lipase activity in human skeletal muscle during clofibrate administration. Eur J Clin Invest 8:67, 1978.
19. Kissebah AH, Adams PW, Harrigan P, et al: The mechanism of action of clofibrate and tetranicotinoylfructose (Bradilan) on the kinetics of plasma free fatty acid and triglyceride transport in type IV and type V hypertriglyceridaemia. Eur J Clin Invest 4:163, 1974.
20. Nestel PJ: Lipoprotein protein kinetics during lipid-lowering trials. In Fumagalli R, Kritchevsky D, Paoletti R (eds): Drugs Affecting Lipid Metabolism. Amsterdam: Elsevier/North Holland, 1980, p 159.

*Average wholesale values were taken from the Blue Book (American Druggist, 1992–1993) and 1993 Red Book (Drug Topics), based on purchase of 100 each of the 500-mg capsule.

*Average wholesale values were taken from the Blue Book (American Druggist, 1992–1993) and 1993 Red Book (Drug Topics), based on purchase of 100 each of the 500-mg capsule.

21. Carlson LA, Olsson G, Ballantyne D: On the rise in low density and high density lipoproteins in response to the treatment of hypertriglyceridaemias in type IV and type V hyperlipoproteinaemias. Atherosclerosis 26:603, 1977.

22. Pichardo R, Boulet L, Davignon J: Pharmacokinetics of clofibrate in familial hypercholesterolemia. Atherosclerosis 26:573, 1977.

23. MacKerer CR: Effect of subacute administration of clofibrate on the oxidation of fatty acids by liver mitochondria. Biochem Pharmacol 26:2225, 1977.

24. Laker ME, Mayes PA: The immediate and long term effects of clofibrate on the metabolism of the perfused rat liver. Biochem Pharmacol 28:2813, 1979.

25. Krishnakantha TP, Kurup CK: Increase in hepatic catalase and glycerol phosphate dehydrogenase activities on administration of clofibrate and clofenapate to the rat. Biochem J 130:167, 1972.

26. Kim J, Goldfischer S, Biempica L: Changes produced by clofibrate in hepatocytes of rats with sucrose-induced hyperlipidemia. Exp Mol Pathol 25:263, 1976.

27. Grundy SM, Ahrens EH Jr, Salen G, et al: Mechanisms of action of clofibrate on cholesterol metabolism in patients with hyperlipidemia. J Lipid Res 13:531, 1972.

28. Horlick L, Kudchodkar BJ, Sodhi HS: Mode of action of chlorophenoxyisobutyric acid on cholesterol metabolism in man. Circulation 43:299, 1971.

29. Nestel PJ, Hirsch EZ, Cousens EA: The effect of chlorophenoxyisobutyric acid and ethinyl estradiol on cholesterol turnover. J Clin Invest 44:891, 1965.

30. Bateson MC, Maclean D, Ross PE, Bouchier LA: Clofibrate therapy and gallstone induction. Am J Dig Dis 23:623, 1978.

31. Committee of Principal Investigators: WHO Cooperative Trial on Primary Prevention of Ischemic Heart Disease Using Clofibrate to Lower Serum Cholesterol: Mortality follow-up. Lancet 2:379, 1980.

32. Patsch JR, Yeshurun D, Jackson RL, et al: Effects of clofibrate, nicotinic acid and diet on the properties of the plasma lipoproteins in a subject with type III hyperlipoproteinemia. Am J Med 63:1001, 1977.

33. Hunningshake DB: Drug treatment of type II hyperlipoproteinemia. Effects on plasma lipid and lipoprotein levels. In Gotto AM, Smith LC, Allen B (eds): Atherosclerosis. New York: Springer-Verlag, 1980, p 74.

34. Falko JM, Witztum JL, Schonfeld G, et al: Type III hyperlipoproteinemia: Rise in high-density lipoprotein levels in response to therapy. Am J Med 66:303, 1979.

35. Dashti N, Ontko JA: Alterations in rat serum lipids and apolipoproteins following clofibrate treatment. Atherosclerosis 49:255, 1983.

36. Kamanna VS, Newman HA, Patel ST, et al: Serum lipoprotein and apoprotein concentrations in 4-(4-chlorophenyl)-2-hydroxytetronic acid and clofibrate-treated cholesterol and cholic acid-fed rats. Lipids 24:25, 1989.

37. Staels B, van Tol A, Verhoeven G, et al: Apolipoprotein A-IV messenger ribonucleic acid abundance is regulated in a tissue-specific manner. Endocrinology 126:2153, 1990.

38. Staels B, van Tol A, Andreau T, et al: Fibrates influence the expression of genes involved in lipoprotein metabolism in a tissue-selective manner in the rat. Arterioscler Thromb 12:286, 1992.

39. Krause BR, Newton RS: Gemfibrozil increases both apo A-1 and apo E concentrations. Comparison to other lipid regulators in cholesterol-fed rats. Atherosclerosis 59:95, 1986.

40. Mertz DP, Suermann I, Gohmann E: Influence of "prudent" diet and clofibrate upon apolipoprotein B in hyperlipoproteinemia type IIa. Med Klin 74:279, 1979.

41. Nestel PJ, Hunt D, Wahlqvist ML: Clofibrate raises plasma apoprotein A-1 and HDL-cholesterol concentrations. Atherosclerosis 37:625, 1980.

42. Ballantyne D, Ballantyne FC, Stromberg P, et al: Effect of clofibrate on the composition of very low and low density lipoprotein subfractions in type III hyperlipoproteinemia. Clin Chim Acta 83:117, 1978.

43. Naruszewicz M, Szostak WB, Cybulska C, et al: The influence of clofibrate on lipid and protein components of very low density lipoproteins in type IV hyperlipoproteinemia. Atherosclerosis 35:383, 1980.

44. Hahn SE, Goldberg DM: Modulation of lipoprotein production in Hep G2 cells by fenofibrate and clofibrate. Biochem Pharmacol 43:625, 1992.

45. Qin W, Infante J, Wang SR, et al: Regulation of HMG-CoA reductase, apoprotein-B and LDL receptor gene expression by the hypocholesterolemic drugs simvastatin and ciprofibrate in Hep G2, human and rat hepatocytes. Biochim Biophys Acta 1127:57, 1992.

46. Fears R: Drug treatment of hyperlipidaemia. Drugs of Today 20:257, 1984.

47. Hagerman LM, Newman HAI, Feller DR, et al: Antilipidemic agents. In Verderame M (ed): Handbook of Cardiovascular and Anti-inflammatory Agents. Boca Raton, FL: CRC Press, 1986, pp 225–260.

48. Illingworth DR, O'Malley JP: The hypolipidemic effects of lovastatin and clofibrate alone and in combination in patients with type III hyperlipoproteinemia. Metabolism 39:403, 1990.

49. Goodman DS, Noble RP, Dell RB: The effects of colestipol resin and of colestipol plus clofibrate on the turnover of plasma cholesterol in man. J Clin Invest 52:2646, 1973.

50. Fellin R, Baggio G, Briani G, et al: Long-term trial with colestipol plus clofibrate in familial hypercholesterolemia. Atherosclerosis 29:241, 1978.

51. Hunninghake DB, Probstfield JL, Crow LO: Effect of colestipol and clofibrate on plasma lipid and lipoproteins in type IIa hyperlipoproteinemia. Metabolism 30:605, 1981.

52. Kane JP, Malloy MJ, Tun P, et al: Normalization of low-density-lipoprotein levels in heterozygous familial hypercholesterolemia with a combined drug regimen. N Engl J Med 304:251, 1981.

53. Dujovne CA, Hurwitz A, Kauffman RE, et al: Colestipol and clofibrate in hypercholesterolemia. Clin Pharmacol Ther 16:291, 1974.

54. Nestel PJ, Miller NE, Clifton Bligh P: Effects of colestipol and clofibrate on cholesterol turnover. Aust N Z J Med 3:630, 1973.

55. Hoogwerf BJ, Peters JR, Frantz ID Jr, et al: Effect of clofibrate and colestipol singly and in combination on plasma lipids and lipoproteins in type III hyperlipoproteinemia. Metabolism 34:978, 1985.

56. Howard AN, Hyams DE: Combined use of clofibrate and cholestyramine or DEAE sephadex in hypercholesterolaemia. Br Med J 3:25, 1971.

57. Olsson AG, Oro L, Rossner S: Dose-response effect of single and combined clofibrate (Atromidin) and niceritrol (Perycit) treatment on serum lipids and lipoproteins in type II hyperlipoproteinaemia. Atherosclerosis 22:91, 1975.

58. Rosenhamer G, Carlson LA: Effect of combined clofibrate–nicotinic acid treatment in ischemic heart disease. Atherosclerosis 37:129, 1980.

59. Carlson LA, Rosenhamer G: Reduction of mortality in the Stockholm Ischemic Heart Disease Secondary Prevention Study by combined treatment with clofibrate and nicotinic acid. Acta Med Scand 223:405, 1988.

60. Evans RJ, Howard AN, Hyams DE: An effective treatment of hypercholesterolaemia using a combination of Secholex and clofibrate. Angiology 24:22, 1973.

61. Ritland S, Fausa O, Gjone E, et al: Effect of treatment with a bile-sequestering agent (Secholex) on intestinal absorption, duodenal bile acids, and plasma lipids. Scand J Gastroenterol 10:791, 1975.

62. Olsson AG, Carlson LA, Erikson U, et al: Regression of computer estimated femoral atherosclerosis after pronounced serum lipid lowering in patients with asymptomatic hyperlipidaemia [letter]. Lancet 1:1311, 1982.

63. Rossner S, Olsson AG: Effects of combined procetofene–nicotinic acid therapy in treatment of hypertriglyceridaemia. Atherosclerosis 35:413, 1980.

64. Heller FR, Desager JP, Harvengt C: Plasma lipid concentrations and lecithin: Cholesterol acyltransferase activity in normolipidemic subjects given fenofibrate and colestipol. Metabolism 30:67, 1981.

65. Lehtonen A, Viikari J: Fenofibrate and cholestyramine in type II hyperlipoproteinaemia. Artery 10:353, 1982.

66. Davignon J, Nestruck AC, Alaupovic P, et al: Severe hypo-alphalipoproteinemia induced by a combination of probucol and clofibrate. Adv Exp Med Biol 201:111, 1986.
67. Ginsberg HN: Changes in lipoprotein kinetics during therapy with fenofibrate and other fibric acid derivatives. Am J Med 83:66, 1987.
68. Hunninghake DB, Peters JR: Effect of fibric acid derivatives on blood lipid and lipoprotein levels. Am J Med 83:44, 1987.
69. Rouffy J, Chanu B, Bakir R, et al: Comparative evaluation of the effects of ciprofibrate and fenofibrate on lipids, lipoproteins and apoproteins A and B. Atherosclerosis 54:273, 1985.
70. Prager R, Schernthaner G, Kostner GM, et al: Effect of bezafibrate on plasma lipids, lipoproteins, apolipoproteins AI, AII and B and LCAT activity in hyperlipidemic, non-insulin-dependent diabetics. Atherosclerosis 43:291, 1982.
71. Wirth A, Middelhoff G, Braeuning C, et al: Treatment of familial hypercholesterolemia with a combination of bezafibrate and guar. Atherosclerosis 45:291, 1982.
72. Mordasini R, Riesen W, Oster P, et al: Reduced LDL- and increased HDL-apoproteins in patients with hypercholesterolaemia under treatment with bezafibrate. Atherosclerosis 40:153, 1981.
73. Stewart JM, Packard CJ, Lorimer AR, et al: Effects of bezafibrate on receptor-mediated and receptor-independent low density lipoprotein catabolism in type II hyperlipoproteinaemic subjects. Atherosclerosis 44:355, 1982.
74. Schwandt P, Weisweiler P: Effect of bezafibrate on the high-density lipoprotein subfractions HDL_2 and HDL_3 in primary hyperlipoproteinemia type IV. Artery 7:464, 1980.
75. Cattin L, Da Col PG, Feruglio FS, et al: Efficacy of ciprofibrate in primary type II and IV hyperlipidemia: The Italian multicenter study. Clin Ther 12:482, 1990.
76. Kollar J, Rozdobud'kova V, Koprovicova J, et al: Is Etolip suitable for treatment of various types of hyperlipoproteinemias? Vnitr Lek 37:470, 1991.
77. Bruckert E, Dejager S, Chapman MJ: Ciprofibrate therapy normalises the atherogenic low-density lipoprotein subspecies profile in combined hyperlipidemia. Atherosclerosis 100:91, 1993.
78. Reddy JK, Azarnoff DL, Hignite CE: Hypolipidaemic hepatic peroxisome proliferators form a novel class of chemical carcinogens. Nature 283(5745):397, 1980.
79. Reddy JK, Lalwani ND: Carcinogenesis by hepatic peroxisome proliferators: Evaluation of the risk of hypolipidemic drugs and industrial plasticizers to humans. Crit Rev Toxicol 12:1, 1983.
80. Moody DE, Reddy JK: Morphometric analysis of the ultrastructural changes in rat liver induced by the peroxisome proliferator SaH 42–348. J Cell Biol 71:768, 1976.
81. Reddy JK: Hepatic peroxisome proliferation and carcinogenic effects of hypolipidemic drugs. In Fumagalli R, Kritchevsky D, Paoletti R (eds): Drugs Affecting Lipid Metabolism. Amsterdam: Elsevier/North Holland, 1980, p 301.
82. Reddy JK, Qureshi SA: Tumorigenicity of the hypolipidaemic peroxisome proliferator ethyl-alpha-p-chlorophenoxyisobutyrate (clofibrate) in rats. Br J Cancer 40:476, 1979.
83. Svoboda DJ, Azarnoff DL: Tumors in male rats fed ethyl chlorophenoxyisobutyrate, a hypolipidemic drug. Cancer Res 39:3419, 1979.
84. Eacho PI, Feller DR: Hepatic peroxisome proliferation induced by hypolipidemic drugs and other chemicals. In Witiak DT, Newman HAI, Feller DR (eds): Antilipidemic Drugs. Pharmacochemistry Library, Vol 17. Amsterdam: Elsevier, 1991, p 375.
85. Lalwani ND, Reddy MK, Qureshi SA, et al: Evaluation of selected hypolipidemic agents for the induction of peroxisomal enzymes and peroxisome proliferation in the rat liver. Hum Toxicol 2:27, 1983.
86. Issemann I, Green S: Activation of a member of the steroid hormone receptor superfamily by peroxisome proliferators. Nature 347:645, 1990.
87. Lazarow PB, De Duve C: A fatty acyl-CoA oxidizing system in rat liver peroxisomes; enhancement by clofibrate, a hypolipidemic drug. Proc Natl Acad Sci U S A 73:2043, 1976.
88. Reddy JK, Krishnakantha TP: Hepatic peroxisome proliferation: Induction by two novel compounds structurally unrelated to clofibrate. Science 190:787, 1975.

89. Lazarow PB: Three hypolipidemic drugs increase hepatic palmitoyl-coenzyme A oxidation in the rat. Science 197:580, 1977.
90. Odonkor JM, Rogers MP: Effects of ethyl-CPIB (clofibrate) on tissue lipoprotein lipase and plasma post-heparin lipolytic activity in rats. Biochem Pharmacol 33:1337, 1984.
91. Hess R, Staubli W, Reiss W: Nature of the hepatomegalic effect produced by ethyl chlorophenoxyisobutyrate in the rat. Nature 208:856, 1965.
92. Svoboda DJ, Azarnoff DL: Effects of selected hypolipidemic drugs on cell ultrastructure. Fed Proc 30:841, 1971.
93. Hanefeld M, Kemmer C, Leonhardt W, et al: Effects of p-chlorophenoxyisobutyric acid (CPIB) on the human liver. Atherosclerosis 36:159, 1980.
94. Sirtori CR, Gomarasca P, D'Atri G, et al: Pharmacological profile of BR-931, a new hypolipidemic agent that increases high-density lipoproteins. Atherosclerosis 30:45, 1978.
95. Kaukola S, Manninen V, Neuvonen PJ, et al: Effect of phenytoin on serum lipoproteins in middle-aged men. J Cardiovasc Pharmacol 3:207, 1981.
96. Green KG, Heady A, Oliver MF: Blood pressure, cigarette smoking and heart attack in the WHO co-operative trial of clofibrate. Int J Epidemiol 18:355, 1989.
97. Colman RW, Calvalho A, Vaillancourt R, et al: Clofibrate reversal of platelet hypersensitivity in hyperlipoproteinemia. Stroke 5:299, 1974.
98. Gilbert JB, Mustard JF: Some effects of Atromid on platelet economy and blood coagulation in man. J Atheroscler 3:623, 1963.
99. Mustard JF, Packham MA, Moore S, et al: Thrombosis and atherosclerosis. In Schlettler G, Weizel A (eds): Atherosclerosis. Proceedings of the 3rd International Symposium. New York: Springer-Verlag, 1973, p 253.
100. Packham MA, Mustard JF: Pharmacology of platelet-affecting drugs. Circulation 62(6 Pt 2):V26, 1980.
101. Lin CY, Smith S: The effect of halofenate and clofibrate on aggregation and release of serotonin by human platelets. Life Sci 18:563, 1976.
102. Huzoor-Akbar, Patel S, Kokrady SS, et al: Effects of clofibrate and 6-substituted chroman analogs on human platelet function: Mechanism of inhibitory action. Biochem Pharmacol 30:2013, 1981.
103. Witiak DT, Kokrady SS, Patel ST, et al: Hypocholesterolemic and antiaggregatory properties of 2-hydroxytetronic acid redox analogues an their relationship to clofibric acid. J Med Chem 25:90, 1982.
104. Cayen MN, Ferdinandi ES, Greselin E, et al: Clofibrate and clofibric acid: Comparison of the metabolic disposition in rats and dogs. J Pharmacol Exp Ther 200:33, 1977.
105. Gugler R, Hartlapp J, Jensen C: Factors affecting the disposition of clofibrate. In Fumagalli R, Kritchevsky D, Paoletti R (eds): Drugs Affecting Lipid Metabolism. Amsterdam: Elsevier/North Holland, 1980, p 183.
106. Baldwin JR, Witiak DT, Feller DR: Disposition of clofibrate in the rat. Acute and chronic administration. Biochem Pharmacol 29:3143, 1980.
107. Cayen MN: Metabolic disposition of antihyperlipidemic agents in man and laboratory animals. Drug Metab Rev 11:291, 1980.
108. Kutz K, Schulte A, Jensen C, Gugler R: Impaired drug conjugation in subjects with Gilbert's syndrome (GS). Gastroenterology 73:A31, 1977.
109. Hignite CE, Tschanz C, Lemons S, et al: Glucuronic acid conjugates of clofibrate: Four isomeric structures. Life Sci 28:2077, 1981.
110. Sinclair KA, Caldwell J: The pH dependent intramolecular rearrangement of glucuronic-acid conjugates of xenobiotics. Biochem Soc Trans 9:215, 1981.
111. Caldwell J, Emudianughe TS, Smith RL: Species variation in the taurine conjugation of clofibric acid [proceedings]. Br J Pharmacol 66:421P, 1979.
112. Physicians' Desk Reference, 47th ed. Montvale, NJ: Medical Economics Data Production, 1993, pp 2547–2548.
113. Gavelli MS, Vitaliano E, Rossi FG, et al: Therapy of hypercholesterolemia and hypertriglyceridemia. Comparison of hypolipemic effects of lovastatin and gemfibrozil. Clin Ther 136:31, 1991.

114. Keen H, Lewis B, Miller NE, et al: Clofibrate and hyperlipidaemia [letter]. Lancet 2:1241, 1980.
115. Levy RI: Currently available drugs for treatment for hyperlipoproteinemia. *In* Lemberger L, Riedenberg MM (eds): Proceedings of the 2nd World Conference on Clinical Pharmacology. Bethesda, MD: ASPET, 1984, p 916.
116. Bentley P, Calder I, Elcombe C, et al: Hepatic peroxisome proliferation in rodents and its significance to humans. Food Chem Toxicol 31:857, 1993.
117. Brown WV: Potential use of fenofibrate and other fibric acid derivatives in the clinic. Am J Med 83:85, 1987.
118. Serious adverse effects with clofibrate. N Z Med J 92:315, 1980.
119. Clofibrate indication modified. Drug Therapy 9:16, 1979.
120. Blane GF: Comparative toxicity and safety profile of fenofibrate and other fibric acid derivatives. Am J Med 83:26, 1987.
121. Chauvin M, Zupan M, Brechenmacher C: Atypical muscular syndrome with myolysis during long term treatment with fibrates. Arch Mal Coeur 81:921, 1988.
122. Hattori N, Shimatsu A, Murabe H, et al: Clofibrate-induced myopathy in a patient with primary hypothyroidism. Jpn J Med 29:545, 1990.
123. Migneco G, Mascarella A, La-Ferla A, et al: Clofibrate hepatitis. A case report. Minerva Med 77:799, 1986.
124. Conte-Camerino D, Mambrini M, DeLuca A, et al: Enantiomers of clofibric acid analogs have opposite actions on rat skeletal muscle chloride channels. Pflugers Arch 413:105, 1988.
125. Kwiecinski H, Lehmann-Horn F, Rudel R: Drug-induced myotonia in human intercostal muscle. Muscle Nerve 11:576, 1988.
126. Conte-Camerino D, Tortorella V, Bettoni G, et al: A stereospecific binding site regulates the Cl$^-$ ion channel in rat skeletal muscle. Pharmacol Res Commun 20:1077, 1988.
127. Ujhazy E, Onderova E, Horakova M, et al: Teratological study of the hypolipidaemic drugs etofylline clofibrate (VULM) and fenofibrate in Swiss mice. Pharmacol Toxicol 64:286, 1989.
128. Margarian GJ, Lucas LM, Colley C: Gemfibrozil-induced myopathy. Arch Intern Med 151:1873, 1991.
129. Godoy JM, Nicaretta DH, Balassiano SL, et al: The importance of clinical diagnosis. Myopathies induced by clofibrate. Arq Neuropsiquiatr 50:123, 1992.
130. Rumpf KW, Quellhrost E, Scheler F: Diabetic nephropathy, hypothyroidism and clofibrate-induced myopathy. Med Klin 71:2023, 1976.
131. Pierce LR, Wysowski DK, Gross TP: Myopathy and rhabdomyolysis associated with lovastatin-gemfibrozil combination therapy. JAMA 264:71, 1990.
132. Baglin A, Lasserre N, Prinseau J, et al: Rhabdomyolysis under treatment by ciprofibrate in the nephrotic syndrome [letter]. Therapie 42:247, 1987.
133. Dujovne CA, Azarnoff DL, Huffman DH, et al: One-year trials with halofenate, clofibrate and placebo. Clin Pharmacol Ther 19:352, 1976.

CHAPTER 117

Fenofibrate

James Shepherd, Ph.D., F.R.C.Path., F.R.C.P., and Allan Gaw, M.B., Ph.D.

HISTORY

Clofibrate, the ethyl ester of *p*-chlorophenoxyisobutyric acid (CPIB) is one of the longest serving lipid-lowering agents still in clinical use. Development work started in 1947 and was originally aimed at producing a fatty acid analogue capable of interfering with lipid metabolism.[1] When it was brought to the marketplace in 1963, it continued to masquerade as a fatty acid synthesis inhibitor that inhibited fat metabolism via a hormonal mechanism.[2] Even now, although this concept is discredited, the detailed mechanism of action of the drug is still not completely understood.[3] During the 1970s clofibrate was adopted for use in a number of trials aimed at determining the effectiveness of lowering cholesterol levels in the treatment or prevention of coronary heart disease.[4-6] All showed benefit in terms of reduction in total coronary events in the treated groups, the reductions being greatest in those individuals with the highest risk (i.e., hypertensive smokers who showed significant decreases in cholesterol in response to therapy). The pharmaceutical industry was not slow to grasp the significance of these findings despite the qualifications that accompanied them (see later) and began to invest heavily in a search for new and potent analogues of clofibrate, a search that has led to the emergence of a family of fibrates (Fig. 117–1) with similar mechanisms of action but differing potencies and lipoprotein selectivities. Whereas clofibrate demonstrated greater effectiveness in triglyceride reduction, the new generation agents were chosen to offer a broader spectrum of lipid-lowering effects, reductions in triglyceride being accompanied by similar decrements in total and low-density lipoprotein (LDL) cholesterol and a rise in high-density lipoprotein (HDL) cholesterol. Such general purpose lipid-lowering agents therefore offer an attractive alternative to the statins in the treatment of hyperlipidemia. Fenofibrate (see Fig. 117–1) represents one of these new generation multipurpose compounds.

CHEMISTRY

Fenofibrate (isopropyl[4^1-(p-chlorobenzoyl)-2-phenoxy-2-methyl]propionate: $C_{20}H_{21}ClO_4$) is an off-white powder that is practically insoluble in water, which is a factor that influences (limits) its absorption and bioavailability. To overcome this problem, the compound has been comicronized with sodium lauryl sulfate, a process that reduces the size of the fenofibrate crystals, increases their wettability, prevents their aggregation in aqueous media, and, in consequence, improves their bioavailability and the predictability of their dissolution. As a consequence, a 200-mg single dose of the comicronized formulation is reported to produce the same plasma levels of fenofibric acid as the 100-mg standard capsule formulation given in three daily doses.

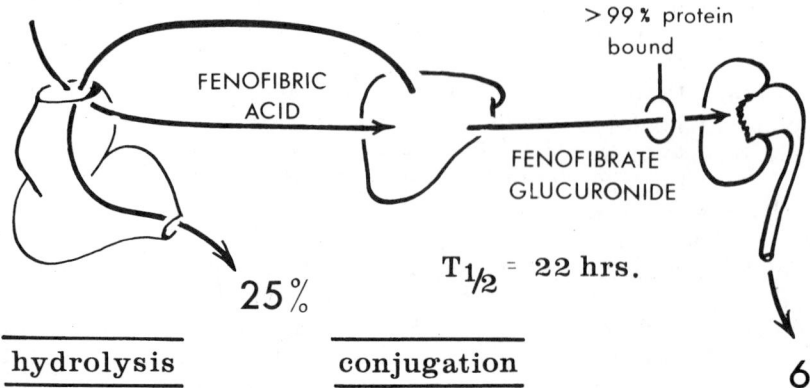

Figure 117–1. The structure of the fibrates.

PHARMACOLOGY

Fenofibrate is the only clofibrate derivative that, in common with its parent, must be hydrolyzed[7] in the intestine (Fig. 117–2) to release the active agent, fenofibric acid. The latter then circulates, albumin-bound, and is ultimately excreted, largely via the kidneys, following modification or hepatic conjugation with glucuronic acid.[8] Administration of the drug with a meal accelerates its absorption and in the 7 days[8] following a single postprandial oral dose, 60% is excreted in the urine and 25% in the feces. Interestingly, the plasma levels of the drug that are achieved following ingestion of single, incremental doses from 100 to 500 mg with meals do not demonstrate dose proportionality, suggesting that at higher dose levels the absorption of the drug is incomplete. The recommended therapeutic dose of the standard fenofibrate formulation, 100 mg administered three times daily with meals, results in the achievement of steady-state plasma levels by day 8, which is consistent with an elimination half-life of fenofibric acid of approximately 20 to 24 hours.[9]

Because the majority of excretion occurs via the kidneys, it is not surprising that plasma accumulation[10] occurs in patients with renal insufficiency. In this situation the drug should be given with caution and in reduced dosage. There is no predictable relationship between the elimination half-life of fenofibric acid and creatinine clearance. The pharmacokinetics and metabolism of fenofibrate in men and women are the same, and no special precautions need to be taken when administering the drug to elderly patients[11] as long as their renal function is competent.

As indicated earlier, comicronization of fenofibrate with sodium lauryl sulfate increases the predictability of its absorption and its bioavailability. Comparative studies with the standard and comicronized formulations (Table 117–1) indicate that 200 mg of the comicronized version given once a day is as efficacious as 300 mg of the standard formulation prescribed singly or in three divided doses. The time required to reach the concentration peak (T_{max}, see Table 117–1) is almost identical for the two preparations, as is the elimination half-life. Similarly, the quantity of drug absorbed, as indicated by the area under the plasma concentration curve (AUC, see Table 117–1) is virtu-

ORAL
FENOFIBRATE

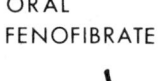

Figure 117–2. Fenofibrate pharmacology.

Table 117–1. **Comparative Bioavailabilities of a Capsule Containing 200 mg Comicronized Fenofibrate, a Capsule Containing 300 mg of the Standard Drug, and Three 100-mg Capsules of Standard Fenofibrate**

Variable	Comicronized Fenofibrate (200 mg)	Standard Fenofibrate (300 mg)	Standard Fenofibrate (3 × 100 mg)
T_{max} (hr)	5.9 ± 2.6	5.6 ± 1.7	6.0 ± 1.0
C_{max} (mg/L)	11.0 ± 2.6	10.7 ± 3.0	10.2 ± 3.7
$T\frac{1}{2}$ (hr)	15.4 ± 4.4	17.9 ± 8.1	22.0 ± 6.8
AUC (mg/L · hr)	176.7 ± 48.9	171.3 ± 56.0	180.0 ± 52.1

T_{max}, time required to reach concentration peak; C_{max}, maximum concentration recorded; $T\frac{1}{2}$, apparent elimination half-life; AUC, area under the concentration curve.

ally identical for the 300-mg standard preparation and the 200-mg comicronized version, reflecting the greater efficiency of uptake of the latter. The bioequivalence of the 200-mg comicronized formulation and the 300-mg standard preparation suggests that the comicronization increases the bioavailability of fenofibrate by approximately 30%.

The fibrates as a class are potent, broad-spectrum, lipid-lowering agents, capable of lowering both cholesterol and triglyceride levels in the plasma and raising HDL cholesterol concentrations. As is the case for any drug family, there is variability in responsiveness to the fibrates, which is in part a result of interindividual variation and partly of pharmacokinetic differences between the formulations.

LIPID-LOWERING EFFECTS AND CLINICAL POTENCY

The effectiveness of fenofibrate has been assessed in more than 150 trials worldwide, the majority of these using a daily dosage of 300 mg of the standard formulation. Combined analysis of 12 placebo-controlled trials of 2 to 3 months' duration done in Europe showed that standard fenofibrate produced on average a 20% to 25% reduction in the plasma cholesterol levels of hypercholesterolemic individuals and a 40% to 45% fall in hypertriglyceridemic triglyceride values. More specific information can be drawn from two double-blind placebo-controlled studies done in the United States.[12, 13] One of these[12] measured the clinical utility of 300 mg/day fenofibrate in 240 adults with hypercholesterolemia or combined hyperlipidemia. The results are presented in Table 117–2. All

treatment values were significantly different from those of controls ($p < .01$). Two other trials,[14, 15] which depended on angiography as the end point, merit special mention. The first,[14] conducted in 62 dyslipidemic patients, targeted changes in femoral atherosclerotic lesions after 12 months' treatment; the other was done in 42 dyslipidemic individuals with partial coronary occlusion. One half of the patients in the first study were given fenofibrate (200 mg b.i.d.) plus nicotinic acid (4 g/day); the other half received a placebo. Although the trialists did not claim major clinical benefits for the actively treated group, they did observe regression in five patients in this category with no change in the controls.

The second study[15] investigated 21 patients with coronary atherosclerosis who received a combination of diet and fenofibrate (200 to 400 mg/day) for an average of 21 months. Their results, in comparison with data collected from 21 control subjects, showed a trend toward regression in plaque area in the affected vessels. The numbers were too small to detect changes in clinical events.

EFFECTS ON LIPOPROTEIN METABOLISM

Fenofibrate, like other members of this class of drugs, has an effect on the circulating levels and metabolism of all plasma lipoproteins. Its putative mechanisms of action are outlined in Fig. 117–3.

Metabolism of Triglyceride-Rich Lipoproteins

The primary action of fenofibrate is to reduce plasma levels of triglyceride-rich lipoproteins. This is brought about by attacks on two fronts of triglyceride metabolism. First, there is a decrease in hepatic triglyceride synthesis, which is secondary to reduced peripheral lipolysis and diminished free fatty acid flux back to the liver. Second, very-low-density lipoprotein (VLDL) catabolism is enhanced as a result of a sustained rise[16] in lipoprotein lipase activity and consequently increased intravascular VLDL triglyceride lipolysis.

The fibrate-induced increase in lipoprotein lipase activity also provides an explanation for the fall in postprandial lipemia seen in both normocholesterolemic and hypercholesterolemic patients treated with

Table 117–2. **Effect of Fenofibrate (300 mg/day) on 240 Subjects with Hypercholesterolemia or Combined Hypercholesterolemia/Hypertriglyceridemia**

	Percentage Change in Treated versus Placebo	
	Hypercholesterolemic (type IIa) Subjects	Hypercholesterolemic/ Hypertriglyceridemic
Total cholesterol	−17.1	−20.4
Total triglyceride	−33.7	−66.9
LDL cholesterol	−20.7	−5.6
HDL cholesterol	+12.3	+18.8
LDL/HDL ratio	−25.2	−13.3

FIBRATES AND LIPOPROTEIN METABOLISM

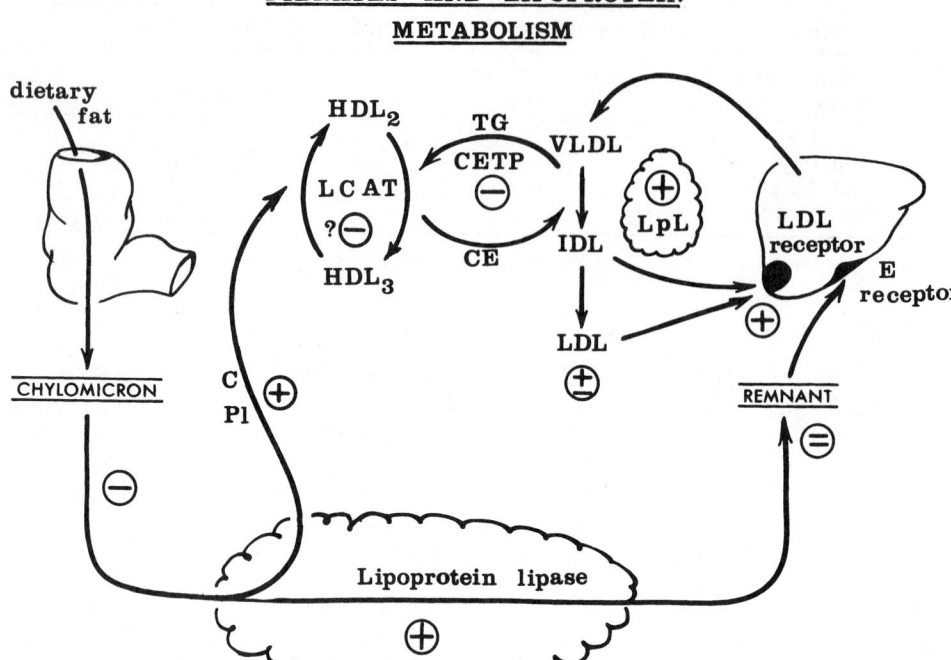

Figure 117–3. Putative mechanisms of action of fenofibrate. Dietary lipids are absorbed from the gut and packaged into large triglyceride-rich particles called chylomicrons. These particles undergo lipolysis by the endothelium-bound enzyme lipoprotein lipase (LpL) in the capillary beds of adipose tissue and skeletal muscle. This process yields smaller chylomicron remnant particles that are thought to be cleared from the circulation via the apo E receptor on hepatocytes. Redundant surface material containing cholesterol (C) and phospholipid (Pl) is also lost into the high-density lipoprotein (HDL) density interval. Very-low-density lipoprotein (VLDL) is continually secreted by the liver to carry endogenously produced lipid, and these particles also undergo lipolysis by the actions of LpL. As VLDL is delipidated by this enzyme, intermediate-density lipoproteins (IDL) and finally low-density lipoproteins (LDL) are formed. Both these products are removed from the plasma by the LDL receptor. The fibrates, by stimulating LpL activity, increase the clearance rate of chylomicrons and the delipidation rate of apo B–containing lipoproteins (VLDL, IDL). Because of the compositional changes that take place in the LDL interval, the fibrates stimulate an increase in receptor-mediated clearance of this lipoprotein, although the final level of LDL in the plasma is largely dictated by the phenotype of the patient prior to fibrate therapy (see text). Cholesteryl ester transfer protein (CETP) together with lecithin-cholesterol acyltransferase (LCAT) facilitate the intravascular remodeling of HDL, resulting in this lipoprotein becoming relatively triglyceride (TG) enriched and cholesterol ester (CE) depleted. The fibrates effectively reduce CETP activity by limiting the availability of triglyceride-rich substrates and in turn the net transfer of TG into HDL. A more direct inhibitory effect on LCAT activity has been proposed although this has yet to be confirmed in humans.

fenofibrate.[16] This change in chylomicron metabolism was associated with a highly significant increase in postheparin lipoprotein lipase activity (37%, $p < .001$), and only a marginal increment in that of hepatic lipase. Such an effect may be an important feature of the antiatherogenic potential of the fibrates, because postprandial lipemia is considered by many to be an additional risk factor for coronary heart disease (CHD).[17] The presence of CHD has also been associated with prolonged and exaggerated hypertriglyceridemia following a fat load. Such abnormal clearance of chylomicrons and their remnants seen in patients with CHD is corrected by fibrate therapy.[16] The fibrates therefore reduce levels of triglyceride-rich lipoproteins in a consistent and readily explicable fashion.

LDL Metabolism

The means by which the fibrates lower plasma low-density lipoprotein (LDL) cholesterol levels in patients with hypercholesterolemia has been a point of controversy.[3] The most recent hypothesis, suggested by our own group to explain the LDL-cholesterol–lowering effect of the fibrates,[18] has evolved from a series of *in vivo* human metabolic studies performed over the last decade. In a previous investigation[19] of the mechanism of action of bezafibrate in type II hyperlipoproteinemia, the LDL-lowering effect was ascribed to increased clearance of LDL via the LDL

receptor pathway as a result of stimulated receptor activity. In the light of present knowledge of the heterogeneity of LDL, it was pertinent to reexamine these findings and ask whether the enhanced receptor-mediated catabolism of LDL was caused by a change in the receptor or the ligand. Arguably, fibrate therapy may perturb the LDL subfraction distribution in a way that increases the affinity of circulating LDL particles for the LDL receptor. Evidence for such an effect was observed in a group of hypercholesterolemic subjects treated with fenofibrate.[18]

Early studies of LDL turnover and of the mechanism of action of fibrate therapy assumed LDL to be an homogeneous entity.[19, 20] However, more recently it has been demonstrated that LDL exists in the plasma of normal and hyperlipidemic subjects as a heterogeneous population of particles that can be divided into three subfractions on the basis of size and density.[21–23] Preliminary investigations have indicated that these fractions have distinct properties. LDL-I, the largest and most buoyant, is present in high concentrations in young women, whereas LDL-II is the major species in most individuals.[24, 25] LDL-III appears to be specifically elevated when plasma triglyceride levels are raised,[24, 26] and a predominance of small, dense LDL in combination with a raised triglyceride level and low levels of HDL has been associated with a threefold increase in the risk of myocardial infarction.[26] These changes have been collectively described as an atherogenic lipoprotein phenotype or ALP.[27] There is strong evidence to suggest that ALP, and more specifically the distribution of LDL subfractions, is influenced by a major gene.[28, 29] However, the profile is also significantly altered by the effects of diet and pharmacologic agents.[30]

Concurrent with these studies on the structure of LDL, there has been a reevaluation of its *in vivo* kinetic behavior and new multicompartmental models have been constructed to take account of LDL metabolic heterogeneity. In recent studies we have divided LDL into a pool A, which had a rapid clearance rate and proposed high affinity for LDL receptors, and a pool B, which had a slower catabolic rate and a proposed reduced level of receptor-mediated catabolism.[31]

Fibrates are believed to reduce the levels of triglyceride-rich lipoproteins in the circulation through two main mechanisms, decreased hepatic triglyceride synthesis secondary to diminished free fatty acid flux to the liver and enhanced chylomicron and VLDL clearance resulting from stimulated lipoprotein lipase activity.[3, 16, 32–34] Because VLDL and LDL are closely linked in a metabolic cascade, it is to be expected that changes in the turnover of the former will have consequences for the latter. This is indeed the case, but the perturbations are more subtle than would be predicted from a simple precursor-product relationship.

In our earlier investigations,[19] treatment with a fibrate increased the fractional catabolic rate (FCR) of LDL via its high affinity receptor, and this mechanism explained the reduction in plasma LDL protein and cholesterol concentrations. We postulated that the drug (bezafibrate) had activated receptors so that increased clearance of LDL was the result of altered intracellular cholesterol homeostasis in hepatocytes. This metabolic response was similar to that proposed previously for resins and for statins.[3] However, the more detailed kinetic analysis undertaken in our investigation with fenofibrate[18] suggested that the change in LDL metabolism was the result of a combination of two effects, an increase in LDL catabolism, which we attributed to stimulated receptor activity, and an alteration in the nature of circulating LDL, so that its ligand-binding properties were enhanced. Previously we have shown[35, 36] that the VLDL → LDL delipidation cascade contains parallel pathways that have the potential to give rise to LDL species with differing metabolic properties; large VLDL appear to be metabolized to slowly catabolized LDL, whereas smaller VLDL are converted to rapidly cleared LDL. Thus, we postulated that fibrate therapy, by diminishing the production of larger VLDL particles, reduces the formation of the slowly metabolized LDL. Furthermore, we suggest that this may be caused by a fibrate-induced suppression of triglyceride synthesis relative to hepatic apolipoprotein B production and hence the secretion of smaller VLDL precursor particles. Evidence to support this hypothesis comes from studies of type III and type IV hyperlipoproteinemic patients that show that fibrate therapy causes a reduc-

tion in the synthesis of large triglyceride-rich VLDL.[37] Furthermore, the association between pool B apo LDL synthetic rate and plasma triglyceride level is consistent across the studies we have performed.

It has been suggested that small, dense LDLs are metabolized more slowly that their larger counterparts because of their reduced affinity for the receptor pathway.[23] This mechanism would provide a structural basis for the pool A/pool B division in the model that was mentioned earlier. Most subjects with primary moderate hypercholesterolemia prior to therapy have relatively low LDL-III and high LDL-I concentrations, which is consistent with their low plasma triglyceride levels.[23, 26] A significant proportion of their LDL, we propose, would contribute to pool A. The exact physical designation of the apo LDL in pool B of our model is unclear. It does not appear to be synonymous with the dense LDL-III alone but rather with some combination of LDL-II and III. In summary, our kinetic analyses have revealed that fenofibrate increases LDL receptor-mediated clearance, at least in part, by promoting the synthesis of a more receptor-active LDL.

LDL Structure

When fibrates are given to hypertriglyceridemic subjects they correct an often initially low plasma LDL level. This change in the total LDL mass is accompanied by an alteration in LDL composition.[38] The particles become enriched in cholesteryl ester and relatively depleted in phospholipid and triglyceride, thereby increasing the lipid core-coat ratio. This change in lipid composition is consistent with an increase in LDL particle size, away from the small, dense LDL characteristic of hypertriglyceridemia.

In patients who are normotriglyceridemic yet hypercholesterolemic, fenofibrate therapy lowers the total LDL mass. This is predominantly a result of a significant decrease in the LDL subfraction of mid-density (LDL-II). The changes in the LDL subfractions of lower (LDL-I) and higher (LDL-III) density are inversely related, the most consistent finding being an increase in LDL-I and a decrease in LDL-III levels.[32] That is, the drug induces a shift in the LDL subfraction profile to lighter species in both normolipidemic and hypertriglyceridemic subjects. The larger, lighter LDL species were also found to be less susceptible to oxidative modification than their small, dense counterparts.[39] Gemfibrozil has been recently reported[40] to induce the same changes in LDL subfractions in type II hyperlipoproteinemia, in non-insulin-dependent diabetes mellitus, and in familial combined hyperlipidemia. Reports that ciprofibrate has the same effect reveal that this phenomenon must be viewed as a fibrate family trait. Thus, in several forms of hyperlipidemia, fenofibrate therapy induces a redistribution of LDL density and size toward lighter and larger particles, an LDL subfraction profile that has been associated with reduced coronary risk.

Cholesterol Synthesis

Besides their effects on triglyceride and apo B metabolism, the fibrates are also reputed to have an inhibitory effect on hepatic cholesterol synthesis. This action was first attributed to inhibition of hydroxymethylglutaryl coenzyme A (HMG-CoA) reductase, the rate-limiting enzyme of cholesterol biosynthesis. Early work by Berndt et al.[41] demonstrated both the inhibition of this enzyme by clofibrate and bezafibrate in rat liver microsomes in vitro, and a fall in its activity in liver microsomes isolated from fibrate-fed rats. Schneider et al.[42] have also demonstrated lowered activity of HMG-CoA reductase in freshly isolated mononuclear cells from patients treated with fenofibrate, but in other studies using bezafibrate, Stange et al.[43] reported no drug-induced effect on HMG-CoA reductase activity. McNamara et al.[44] also observed no change in the rate of cholesterol synthesis in mononuclear cells freshly isolated from patients receiving clofibrate therapy. Other recent studies have demonstrated fibrate-induced inhibition of the regulatory enzymes in cholesterol biosynthesis. Castillo et al.[45] observed reduced activity of the enzyme HMG-CoA reductase, both in vivo and in vitro, in chick liver in response to therapy, whereas Cosentini et al.[46] demonstrated in a total of 15 patients that bezafibrate reduced the incorporation of labeled acetate into nonsaponifiable lipids in freshly isolated blood mononuclear cells. Again, however, there is some equivocation in the literature[47] in that another fibrate, gemfibrozil, has been shown to increase hepatic sterol biosynthesis, but this time in rats.

Ciprofibrate was found to inhibit cholesterol synthesis from ^{14}C-labeled acetate in the human hepatoma cell line Hep G2, but this inhibition was not associated with any decrease in HMG-CoA reductase activity. Nor was there any ciprofibrate-associated change in either apo B secretion or apo B mRNA levels.[48] Hahn and Goldberg[49] supported these findings by examining fenofibrate and clofibrate in the same cell line. Pulse-chase studies revealed no change in apo B synthesis.

Belichard et al.[50] found that long-term fenofibrate therapy, in marked contrast to lovastatin, did not result in a fall in tissue ubiquinone levels in an animal model. This suggests that the fibrate probably does not inhibit the classical cholesterol synthesis pathway at a step proximal to geranyl transferase, which forms farnesyl pyrophosphate, the last common precursor of both cholesterol and ubiquinone. In our own studies[51] we have found that not only are 24-hour urinary mevalonate levels unaffected by fenofibrate therapy, but neither are plasma lathosterol levels. The latter is a more immediate cholesterol precursor that has been used as an indirect index of cholesterol biosynthetic rates. So, if fibrates suppress cholesterol synthesis, they must do so even more downstream than originally thought.

However, there have been a number of criticisms leveled at many studies in this field. First, just as there are differences between rodents and human subjects in the hepatic toxicology of the fibrates (see later), there also appear to be important species dissimilarities in the effect of the fibrates on the enzymes of cholesterol metabolism.[52]

Much of the published data have also been criticized either because of invalid methodology,[53] or the use of unrealistically high concentrations of drug in vitro. Newton and Krause[54] pointed out that many in vitro experiments may be flawed because the concentrations of fibrates used greatly exceed their potential concentration in vivo. Similar levels of HMG-CoA reductase inhibition were achieved by these workers when compactin was used as a positive control at in vitro levels 10,000-fold lower than that required of the fibrates. On this basis, they suggested that the observed inhibitory effect of the fibrates on HMG-CoA reductase in vitro may represent a nonspecific rather than a physiologic effect at a specific regulatory site on the enzyme. While there has been some equivocation in the literature from in vivo and in vitro experiments, the emerging consensus is that the fibrates do indeed inhibit cholesterol synthesis in humans but by some means other that the direct inhibition of the enzyme HMG-CoA reductase. Further work in this area will not only provide a more detailed model for the mechanism of action of fibrate therapy but will also afford us an opportunity to study the intracellular control of cholesterol synthesis, which is a topic still poorly understood.

HDL Metabolism

In hypercholesterolemia, fibrate-induced reductions in LDL cholesterol are commonly accompanied by increases in HDL cholesterol, leading to important changes in the calculated atherogenic risk index. In hypertriglyceridemic patients with a type V phenotype, fibrates commonly increase plasma HDL cholesterol and apo A-I and A-II. When the kinetic changes associated with these alterations in plasma levels were studied, it was found that they depended primarily on an increment in the rates of synthesis of the proteins.[55] In FH heterozygous patients, similar studies using fenofibrate also revealed increases in the synthetic rate of apo A-I.[56] Because the latter variable rose more than the clearance, the end result was again a fibrate-induced increase in plasma apo A-I.

Recently, apo A-I, A-II, and A-IV mRNA levels were found to be selectively reduced in the livers of fibrate-fed rats. This effect may be species-specific, for such a finding would be inconsistent with published kinetic studies if we assume that messenger levels can be equated with protein turnover rates. The intravascular remodeling of HDL is thought to depend on the activities of two enzymes, lecithin-cholesterol acyltransferase (LCAT), and cholesteryl ester transfer protein (CETP). LCAT plays a central role in the maturation of spheroidal HDL particles from discoidal precursors, whereas CETP facilitates the equimolar exchange of triglyceride to, and cholesteryl ester from, HDL. CETP activity therefore results in a shift from larger HDL_2 to smaller HDL_3, whereas

LCAT reverses this reaction. Because they reduce the availability of triglyceride-rich substrates, the fibrates should, in theory, inhibit the action of CETP. A potential effect of the fibrates on LCAT has only recently been defined. Staels et al.[57] reported that they induced a fall in LCAT mRNA levels associated with reduced plasma LCAT "activity." This effect was shown to be tissue-specific, LCAT mRNA levels being reduced in liver but not in testis and brain. Again, however, a caveat must be offered in that these studies were performed in rats and as yet they have not been confirmed in humans. If CETP and LCAT activities are both decreased by fibrate therapy in humans, the resultant effects on HDL composition and function will depend on the relative inhibition of each process, because each is thought to antagonize the other.

TOXICOLOGY
Hepatomegaly and Carcinogenicity

All fibrates, when given to rodents, have been shown to cause hepatomegaly and peroxisome proliferation.[58] The peroxisomal proliferation in rat liver induced by fibrates has recently been demonstrated to be a receptor-mediated process[59] with the fibrates acting as inducers of the so-called peroxisome proliferator activated receptor (PPAR). The apparent lack of a similar effect in human subjects in response to fibrate therapy was seen as evidence that humans do not possess this receptor. However, this hypothesis was refuted when the human homologue of the rodent PPAR was recently cloned.[60] The basis of the species specificity of this hepatic response therefore remains to be discovered. The waters were further muddied when Pill et al.[61] demonstrated that fibrate-induced peroxisomal proliferation was not only species-specific but also strain-dependent in rats. Consequently, these authors counsel caution in the "generalization and extrapolation from rodent studies."

Hepatocellular carcinomata have been observed in rodents receiving fibrate therapy but the carcinogenic dose of clofibrate, gemfibrozil, and fenofibrate per kilogram in these species appears to be at least 12 times higher than the recommended human therapeutic dose.[58] Moreover, this characteristic hepatic toxicity appears to be species-specific.[62] Studies in nonhuman primates and human liver biopsy specimens have shown no such hepatic changes.[62] Large clinical studies in human subjects bear this out, with no excess of neoplasms in the gemfibrozil treatment arm of the Helsinki Heart Study[63] and indeed no hepatic tumors at all.

Bile Lithogenicity

Clofibrate therapy has been shown to increase the biliary secretion of cholesterol and reduce that of bile acids.[64] These compositional changes in bile induce supersaturation leading to an increased risk of gallstone formation during long-term treatment with clofibrate. Subsequently a number of studies have hinted

at similar increases in biliary cholesterol secretion with the other fibrates. Although the increased bile lithogenicity associated with the fibrates has therefore been described as a class effect, there is evidence to suggest that fenofibrate does not significantly increase the relative concentration of cholesterol in the bile.[65] Certainly no excess risk of gallstone formation has been reported to date with the recommended clinical dose of fenofibrate,[62] the fibrate with which we have longest experience after clofibrate.

Fenofibrate should be used with caution, however, in patients with preexisting gallstones, because any increase in bile lithogenicity in such individuals may accelerate stone formation and precipitate the need for surgery. The evidence so far would suggest that the risk in patients who are initially free of gallbladder disease is too small to merit any contraindication on these grounds.

ADVERSE CLINICAL EFFECTS

The fibrates, in general, are well-tolerated drugs. The most common side effects in clinical practice are gastrointestinal disturbances such as dyspepsia, nausea, and flatulence. Skin rashes, particularly urticaria, are the usual cause of withdrawal of treatment, but such an eventuality occurs in less than 2% of treated patients. Table 117-3 cites those events that were reported by more than 1% of the patients involved in the two United States–based fenofibrate clinical trials mentioned earlier.[12, 13] Before beginning treatment, it is prudent to record a number of laboratory safety measurements including a full blood count and liver and kidney function tests, which, uncommonly, may show variation outside the acceptable reference values during therapy. Rarely is withdrawal of treatment

Table 117-3. **Adverse Events Recorded During Studies of Long-Term Standard Fenofibrate Therapy. Events Reported by More than 1% of Patients During the Conduct of Two United States Clinical Trials**

System	Adverse Event
General	Asthenia, infection, influenza, pains, headaches
Cardiovascular	Arrhythmia
Gastrointestinal tract	Dyspepsia, flatulence, nausea, eructation, vomiting, abdominal pain, constipation, diarrhea
Musculoskeletal	Arthralgia
Neurologic	Decreased libido, paresthesia, increased appetite, insomnia, dizziness
Respiratory	Cough, rhinitis, sinusitis
Dermatologic	Pruritus, rash
Urogenital	Polyuria, vaginitis
Sensory	Earache, vision disorder, conjunctivitis, ocular irritation

Treatment was withdrawn from 6% of patients receiving fenofibrate and 2% receiving placebo.

Data from Brown WV, Dujovne CA, Farquhar JW, et al: Effects of fenofibrate on plasma lipids. Double-blind, multicenter study in patients with type IIa or IIb hyperlipidemia. Arteriosclerosis 6:670, 1986; and Goldberg AC, Schonfeld G, Feldman EB, et al: Fenofibrate for the treatment of type IV and V hyperlipoproteinemias: A double-blind, placebo-controlled multicenter US study. Clin Ther 11:69, 1989.

necessary. Of course, pretreatment assessment of kidney function also serves to alert the prescriber to overdosage caused by drug accumulation in renal insufficiency. Fenofibrate should not be given to patients with severe renal disorders or with significant hepatic dysfunction or gallstones, even though, as reported previously, there is no evidence of an increased incidence of gallstones during therapy.

In patients receiving anticoagulant therapy, the dosage of anticoagulant should be reduced by about one third at the commencement of treatment and then gradually adjusted as required. No proven pharmacologic interactions between fenofibrate and other drugs have been recorded, although *in vitro* studies have suggested that it may displace phenylbutazone from plasma protein binding and as a consequence potentiate its action. Possible similar interactions with oral hypoglycemic agents should also be kept in mind.

There are no reports of ill effects from overdosage, nor are there any specific antidotes. Gastric lavage and general supportive measures should be instituted if indicated clinically.

USEFUL DRUG COMBINATIONS WITH FENOFIBRATE

Lipid-lowering drugs have been used in combined regimens with the expectation that two or more drugs may act synergistically to correct aberrant lipoprotein metabolism or that they may serve to offset each other's unwanted effects on the lipid profile. The prescription of fibrates in combined regimens with bile acid sequestrant resins was examined soon after the introduction of the resins.[66] This form of combination is now in wide use and raises an important question: does the joint administration of an anion exchange resin affect the absorption of a fibrate? When a combined regimen of a fibrate and colestipol was examined, the bioavailability of the fibrate was reduced by the coadministration of the two drugs.[67] However, separating the administration of the drugs by at least 2 hours obviates this interaction. In designing new combined regimens, an exciting possibility should be that of fibrate plus HMG-CoA reductase inhibitor. Enthusiasm for such a regimen was, however, curbed when reports of myopathy associated with lovastatin plus gemfibrozil therapy were published.[68] Despite this, and because the combination had shown such early promise, other studies have demonstrated the efficacy and safety of this regimen in different types of hyperlipoproteinemia.[69] However, caution is still urged by most investigators who suggest careful follow-up of these patients with serial creatine kinase measurements and liver function tests.

CONCLUSIONS

Fenofibrate is an important member of the fibrate drug family whose clinical utility is now well established. Its broad-spectrum activity facilitates the treatment of both hypercholesterolemia and hypertriglyceridemia, and in mixed hyperlipidemia the fibrates constitute the drugs of choice. Prevention trials of its clinical benefit in this area are long overdue. It offers a good safety profile, and recent studies suggest that it may not only lower the level of circulating lipoproteins but may also have an important influence on their quality.

Acknowledgments

We acknowledge the excellent secretarial help of Trina Bush. This work was completed during the tenure of grants from the British Heart Foundation (FS/92001 and FS/94001).

REFERENCES

1. Thorp JM: An experimental approach to the problem of disordered lipid metabolism. J Atheroscler Res 3:351, 1963.
2. Oliver MF: Reduction of serum lipid and uric acid levels by an orally active androsterone. Lancet 1:1321, 1962.
3. Gaw A, Shepherd J: Fibric acid derivatives. Curr Opin Lipidol 2:39, 1991.
4. Committee of Principal Investigators: A cooperative trial in the primary prevention of ischaemic heart disease using clofibrate. Br Heart J 10:1069, 1978.
5. Coronary Drug Project Research Group: Clofibrate and niacin in coronary heart disease. JAMA 231:360, 1975.
6. Group of Physicians of the Newcastle upon Tyne Region: Trial of clofibrate in the treatment of ischaemic heart disease. Br Med J 4:767, 1971.
7. Mainguy Y, Vidal R, Strolin-Benedetti M: Species differences in in vitro hydrolysis of fenofibrate by plasma and intestinal esterases. J Clin Pharm 4:59, 1985.
8. Strolin-Benedetti M, Guichard JP, Vidal R, et al: Kinetics and metabolic fate of ^{14}C-fenofibrate in human plasma. Acta Pharmacol Toxicol 59:167, 1986.
9. Desager JP, Harvengt C: Clinical pharmacokinetic study of procetofene, a new hypolipidemic drug in volunteers. Int J Clin Pharmacol 16:570, 1978.
10. Desager JP, Costermans J, Verbeckmoes R, et al: Effect of hemodialysis on plasma kinetics of fenofibrate in chronic renal failure. Nephron 31:51, 1982.
11. Guichard JP, Strolin-Benedetti M, Houin G, et al: Pharmacokinetics of fenofibrate in the elderly. *In* Paoletti R (ed): Drugs Affecting Lipid Metabolism. Berlin: Springer-Verlag, 1987, pp 328–332.
12. Brown WV, Dujovne CA, Farquhar JW, et al: Effects of fenofibrate on plasma lipids. Double-blind, multicenter study in patients with type IIa or IIb hyperlipidemia. Arteriosclerosis 6:670, 1986.
13. Goldberg AC, Schonfeld G, Feldman EB, et al: Fenofibrate for the treatment of type IV and V hyperlipoproteinemias: A double-blind, placebo-controlled multicenter US study. Clin Ther 11:69, 1989.
14. Erikson V, Helmius G, Hemmingsson A, et al: Repeat femoral arteriography in hyperlipidemic patients. A study of progression and regression of atherosclerosis. Acta Radiol 29:303, 1988.
15. Hahmann HW, Bunte T, Hellwig N, et al: Progression and regression of minor coronary arterial narrowings by quantitative angiography after fenofibrate therapy. Am J Cardiol 67:957, 1991.
16. Simpson HS, Williamson CM, Olivecrona T, et al: Prostprandial lipemia, fenofibrate and coronary artery disease. Atherosclerosis 85:193, 1990.
17. Zilversmit DB: Atherogenesis: A postprandial phenomenon. Circulation 60:473, 1979.
18. Caslake MJ, Packard CJ, Gaw A, et al: Fenofibrate and low density lipoprotein metabolic heterogeneity in hypercholesterolemia. Arterioscler Thromb 13:702, 1993.
19. Stewart JM, Packard CJ, Lorimer AR, et al: Effects of bezafibrate

on receptor-mediated and receptor-independent LDL catabolism in Type II hyperlipoproteinemic subjects. Atherosclerosis 44:355, 1982.

20. Langer T, Strober W, Levy RI: The metabolism of low density lipoprotein in familial type II hyperlipoproteinemia. J Clin Invest 51:1528, 1972.

21. Krauss RM, Burke DJ: Identification of multiple subclasses of plasma lipoproteins in normal humans. J Lipid Res 23:97, 1982.

22. Fisher WR: Heterogeneity of plasma low density lipoproteins. Manifestations of the physiologic phenomenon in man. Metabolism 32:283, 1983.

23. Thompson GR, Teng B, Sniderman AD: Kinetics of LDL subfractions. Am Heart J 113:514, 1987.

24. Griffin BA, Caslake MJ, Yip B, et al: Rapid isolation of low density lipoprotein (LDL) subfractions from plasma by density gradient ultracentrifugation. Atherosclerosis 83:59, 1990.

25. McNamara JR, Campos H, Ordovas J, et al: Effect of gender, age and lipid status on low density lipoprotein subfraction distribution. Arteriosclerosis 7:483, 1987.

26. Austin MA, Breslow JL, Hennekens CH, et al: Low density lipoprotein subclass patterns and risk of myocardial infarction. JAMA 260:1917, 1988.

27. Austin MA, King MC, Vranizan KM, et al: Atherogenic lipoprotein phenotype. A proposed genetic marker for coronary heart disease risk. Circulation 82:495, 1990.

28. Austin MA, Krauss RM: Genetic control of low density lipoprotein subclasses. Lancet 2:592, 1986.

29. Austin MA, Brunzell JD, Fitch WL, et al: Inheritance of low density lipoprotein subclass pattern in familial combined hyperlipoproteinemia. Arteriosclerosis 10:520, 1990.

30. Griffin BA, Caslake MJ, Gaw A, et al: Effects of cholestyramine and acipimox on subfractions of plasma low density lipoprotein. Studies in normolipidemic and hypercholesterolemic subjects. Eur J Clin Invest 22:383, 1992.

31. Caslake MJ, Packard CJ, Series JJ, et al: Plasma triglyceride and low density lipoprotein metabolism. Eur J Clin Invest 22:96, 1992.

32. Shepherd J, Griffin BA, Caslake MJ, et al: The influence of fibrates on lipoprotein metabolism. Atherosclerosis Rev 22:163, 1991.

33. Chan MK: Gemfibrozil improves abnormalities of lipid metabolism in patients on continuous ambulatory peritoneal dialysis: The role of postheparin lipases in the metabolism of high density lipoprotein subfractions. Metabolism 38:939, 1989.

34. Goldberg AP, Applebaum-Bowden DM, Bierman EL, et al: Increase in lipoprotein lipase during clofibrate treatment of hypertriglyceridemia in patients on hemodialysis. N Engl J Med 301:1073, 1979.

35. Packard CJ, Munro A, Lorimer A, et al: Metabolism of apolipoprotein B in large triglyceride-rich very low density lipoproteins of normal and hypertriglyceridemic subjects. J Clin Invest 74:2178, 1984.

36. Demant T, Bedford D, Packard CJ, et al: The influence of apolipoprotein E polymorphism on apolipoprotein B-100 metabolism in normolipemic subjects. J Clin Invest 88:1490, 1991.

37. Packard CJ, Clegg RJ, Dominiczak MH, et al: Effects of bezafibrate on apolipoprotein B metabolism in type III hyperlipoproteinemic subjects. J Lipid Res 27:930, 1986.

38. Shepherd J, Caslake MJ, Lorimer AR, et al: Fenofibrate reduces low density lipoprotein catabolism in hypertriglyceridemic subjects. Arteriosclerosis 5:162, 1985.

39. de Graaf J, Hendriks JC, Demacker PN, et al: Identification of multiple dense LDL subfractions with enhanced susceptibility to in vitro oxidation among hypertriglyceridemic subjects. Normalisation after clofibrate treatment. Arterioscler Thromb 13:712, 1993.

40. Tsai MY, Yuan J, Hunninghake DB: Effect of gemfibrozil on composition of lipoproteins and distribution of LDL subspecies. Atherosclerosis 95:35, 1992.

41. Berndt J, Gaumert R, Still J: Mode of action of the lipid lowering agents clofibrate and BM 15.075 on cholesterol biosynthesis in rat liver. Atherosclerosis 30:147, 1978.

42. Schneider A, Stange EF, Ditschuneit HH, et al: Fenofibrate treatment inhibits HMG CoA reductase activity in mononuclear cells from hyperlipoproteinemic patients. Atherosclerosis 56: 257, 1985.

43. Stange EF, Fruholz M, Osenburgge M, et al: Bezafibrate fails to directly modulate HMG CoA reductase or LDL catabolism in human mononuclear cells. Eur J Clin Pharmacol 40(Suppl 1):S37, 1991.

44. McNamara DJ, Davidson NO, Fernadez S: In vitro cholesterol synthesis in freshly isolated mononuclear cells of human blood: Effect of in vivo administration of clofibrate and/or cholestyramine. J Lipid Res 21:65, 1980.

45. Castillo M, Burgos C, Rodriguez-Vico F, et al: Effects of clofibrate on the main regulatory enzymes of cholesterogenesis. Life Sci 46:397, 1990.

46. Cosentini R, Blasi F, Trinchera M, et al: Inhibition of cholesterol biosynthesis in freshly isolated blood mononuclear cells from normolipidemic subjects and hypercholesterolemic patients treated with bezafibrate. Atherosclerosis 79:253, 1989.

47. Maxwell RE, Nawrocki JW, Uhlendorf PD: Some comparative effects of gemfibrozil, clofibrate, bezafibrate, cholestyramine and compactin on sterol metabolism in rats. Atherosclerosis 48:195, 1983.

48. Qin W, Infante J, Wang S-R, et al: Regulation of HMG CoA reductase, apoprotein B and LDL receptor gene expression by the hypocholesterolemic drugs simvastatin and ciprofibrate in Hep G2, human and rat hepatocytes. Biochim Biophys Acta 1127:57, 1992.

49. Hahn SE, Goldberg DM: Modulation of lipoprotein production in Hep G2 cells by fenofibrate and clofibrate. Biochem Pharmacol 43:625, 1992.

50. Belichard P, Pruneau D, Zhiri A: Effect of a long term treatment with lovastatin or fenofibrate on hepatic and cardiac ubiquinone levels in cardiomyopathic hamsters. Biochim Biophys Acta 1169:98, 1993.

51. Gaw A, Stewart JP, Pappu AS, et al: Urinary mevalonic acid and plasma lathosterol: Responses to fenofibrate therapy. In Halpern MK (ed): Molecular Biology of Atherosclerosis. London: John Libbey and Co, 1992, p 579.

52. Stahlberg D, Reihner E, Ewerth S, et al: Effects of bezafibrate on hepatic cholesterol metabolism. Eur J Clin Pharmacol 40(Suppl 1):S33, 1991.

53. Fears R: Pharmacological control of 3-hydroxy-3-methylglutaryl Coenzyme A reductase activity. In Sabine JR (ed): 3-Hydroxy-3-Methylglutaryl Coenzyme A Reductase. Boca Raton, FL: CRC Press, 1983, p 261.

54. Newton RS, Krause BR: Mechanisms of action of gemfibrozil: Comparison of studies in the rat to clinical efficacy. In Fears R, Levy RI, Shepherd J, et al (eds): Pharmacological Control of Hyperlipidemia. Barcelona: JR Prous, 1986, p 171.

55. Saku K, Gartside PS, Hynd BA: Mechanism of gemfibrozil action on lipoprotein metabolism. J Clin Invest 75:1702, 1985.

56. Malmendier CL, Delcroix D: Effects of fenofibrate on high and low density lipoprotein metabolism in heterozygous familial hypercholesterolemia. Atherosclerosis 55:161, 1985.

57. Staels B, van Tol A, Skretting G, et al: Lecithin: Cholesterol acyltransferase gene expression is regulated in a tissue-selective manner by fibrates. J Lipid Res 33:727, 1992.

58. Blane GF: Comparative toxicity and safety profile of fenofibrate and other fibric acid derivatives. Am J Med 83(Suppl 5B):26, 1987.

59. Gebel T, Arand M, Oesch F: Induction of the peroxisome proliferator activated receptor by fenofibrate in rat liver. FEBS Lett 309:37, 1992.

60. Sher T, Yi HF, McBride OW, et al: cDNA cloning, chromosomal mapping, and functional characterization of the human peroxisome proliferator activated receptor. Biochemistry 32:5598, 1993.

61. Pill J, Volkl A, Hartig F, et al: Differences in the response of Sprague-Dawley and Lewis rats to bezafibrate: The hypolipidemic effect and the induction of peroxisomal enzymes. Arch Toxicol 66:327, 1992.

62. Balfour JA, McTavish D, Hill RC: Fenofibrate. A review of its pharmacodynamic and pharmocokinetic properties and therapeutic use in dyslipidemia. Drugs 49:260, 1990.

63. Frick MH, Elo O, Haapa K, et al: Helsinki Heart Study: Primary prevention trial with gemfibrozil in middle-aged men with dyslipidemia. N Engl J Med 317:1237, 1987.

64. Grundy SM, Ahrens EH, Salen G: Mechanisms of action of

clofibrate on cholesterol metabolism in patients with hyperlipidemia. J Lipid Res 13:531, 1972.

65. Palmer RH: Effects of fibric acid derivatives on biliary lipid composition. Am J Med 83(Suppl 5B):37, 1987.

66. Goodman DS, Noble RP, Dell RB: The effects of colestipol resin and of colestipol plus clofibrate on the turnover of plasma cholesterol in man. J Clin Invest 52:2646, 1973.

67. Forland SC, Feng Y, Cutler RE: Apparent reduced absorption of gemfibrozil when given with colestipol. J Clin Pharmacol 30:29, 1990.

68. Pierce LR, Wysowski DK, Gross TP: Myopathy and rhabdomyolysis associated with lovastatin-gemfibrozil combination therapy. JAMA 264:71, 1990.

69. Shepherd J: Fibrates and statins in the treatment of hyperlipidaemia: An appraisal of their efficacy and safety. Eur Heart J 16:5, 1995.

CHAPTER 118

Ciprofibrate

Cesare R. Sirtori, M.D., Ph.D., and Luigi Colombo, M.D.

Ciprofibrate belongs to the series of aryloxyacetic acid derivatives generally defined as "fibric acids" or "fibrates." This series of chemicals, the prototype of which is clofibrate, has been successfully used in the management of hyperlipidemias. Fibric acids are one of the major classes of lipid-modifying agents. The others are anion exchange resins, nicotinic acid and derivatives, probucol, and hydroxymethylglutaryl coenzyme A (HMG-CoA) reductase inhibitors.[1]

Ciprofibrate, which shares many of the properties of fibrates, was developed in the United States in the mid 1970s.[2] Since then, this compound has been the object of numerous investigations of its pharmacologic and clinical properties but has been distributed in only a few countries, most recently the United Kingdom.[3] Ciprofibrate may have the advantages of very low dosage and extended kinetics,[4] with a potentially favorable profile in comparison with other currently available lipid-lowering medications.

CHEMISTRY

Ciprofibrate is the 2-[4-(2,2-dichlorocyclopropyl)phenoxy]-2-methylpropanoic acid. It is a white-yellow crystalline powder that is insoluble in water. The chemical structure is that of a classic aryloxyacetic acid derivative. Unlike clofibrate and fenofibrate, ciprofibrate is not in a prodrug form (i.e., it is not an ethyl ester), and it has the unique property, among fibric acids, of being a racemate. As indicated by the arrow in Figure 118–1, it has an asymmetric carbon atom leading to two stereoisomers. One of these, the

L (−) isomer has significantly different properties, including that of a shorter plasma kinetic half-life of 32 hours versus 139 hours for the D (+) isomer in humans and a somewhat different pharmacodynamic profile in animals (in particular a lesser stimulatory activity on peroxisomal β-oxidation). Possible clinical development of this new agent is pending (C. Hodel, personal communication, 1993).

Ciprofibrate is a weakly acidic drug that at physiologic pH is ionized and therefore relatively hydrophobic, thus likely to stay in the vascular compartment.

PHARMACOLOGY

Ciprofibrate, a fibric acid, shares with compounds such as clofibrate, bezafibrate, gemfibrozil, and others the property of activating liver catabolism of triglycerides, possibly by a mechanism involving the activation of a nuclear receptor (peroxisome proliferator associated receptor, PPAR).[5] Based on this mechanism, it was proposed recently that these compounds be named "fraudulent fatty acids."[6] In fact, unlike their dietary counterparts, fibric acids are converted to the thioester derivatives, activating the peroxisomal system. Thus, fibric acids dispose of fatty acids partly by a metabolic pathway different from mitochondria.[7]

A similar "fraudulent fatty acid" behavior is displayed by long chain n-3 fatty acids from fish oil and a large number of chemicals, including phthalates, MEDICA 16, acetylsalicylic acid, and others.[6] The sequence of events leading to the metabolism of these

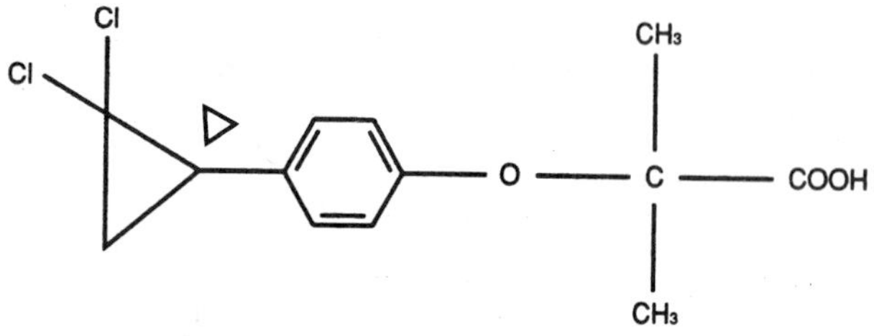

Figure 118–1. Structural formula of ciprofibrate. The arrowhead points to the asymmetric carbon atom.

$C_{13}H_{14}Cl_2O_3$ MW 289.2
White/yellow crystalline powder, insoluble in water

FRAUDULENT FATTY ACIDS

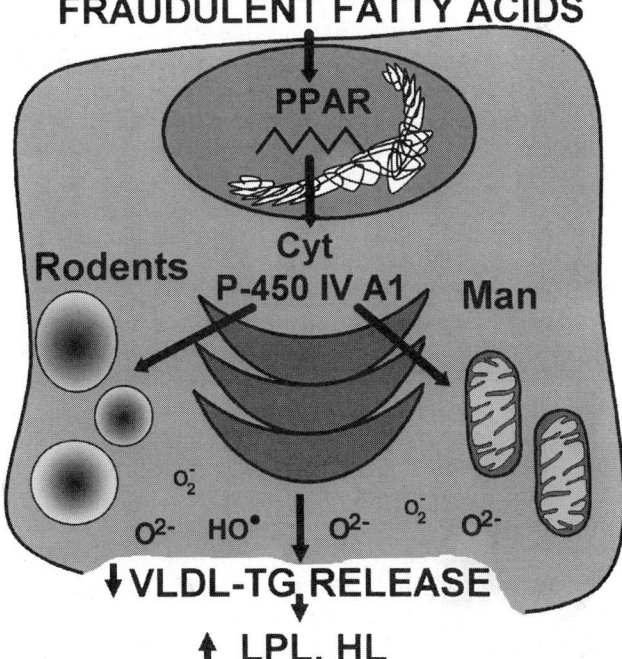

Figure 118-2. Cellular mechanisms of fraudulent fatty acids in exerting their catabolic activity on fatty acid metabolism. These molecules interact with a liver nuclear receptor (PPAR), in turn activating cytochrome P-450 IV A1. These cytochromes are directly responsible for the ω-hydroxylation of fatty acids, leading, through as yet unclear mechanisms (formation of peroxidative products?), to enhanced mitochondrial β-oxidation (in humans) or peroxisomal β-oxidation (in rodents). An alternative view is that the primary transformation is exerted by cytochrome P-450 IV A1, leading to the formation of dicarboxylic acids, these latter ultimately activating the PPAR.[9]

diverse chemicals involves stimulating (probably as a consequence of PPAR activation) a microsomal cytochrome system, P-450 IV A, catalyzing the ω-oxidation of fatty acids, and subsequently activating the peroxisomal/mitochondrial catabolic systems[8] (Fig. 118-2). The exact sequence of events is still incompletely understood, although it was recently hypothesized that dicarboxylic acids (the products of ω-oxidation) may be the ultimate PPAR activators.[9] In all circumstances, enhanced liver catabolism of endogenous or exogenous fatty acids occurs, resulting in a significant decrease in triglyceride secretion.

The consequence of enhanced fatty acid catabolism and reduced triglyceride production is activation in the periphery of plasma catabolic systems, including lipoprotein lipase (LPL) and hepatic lipase (HL).[10] This is the more direct and more easily detected consequence of ciprofibrate administration in humans.[11] Increased levels of LPL and HL, in turn, lead to enhanced breakdown of triglycerides circulating in very-low-density lipoproteins (VLDL), which reduces their concentrations in plasma. Enhanced VLDL catabolism also leads to an enhanced transfer of free cholesterol to the high-density lipoprotein (HDL) fraction, in turn resulting in increased circulating HDL-cholesterol (HDL-C) levels.

Although this mechanism certainly explains, to a large extent, the therapeutic activity of ciprofibrate, similar to that of other "fraudulent fatty acids," the activation of the PPAR system (in animals, particularly rodents) has been found to lead to distinct changes in liver morphology resulting in severe toxicity. Upon continued administration of ciprofibrate in food, the rodent liver develops a marked proliferation of peroxisomes with liver cell enlargement and, particularly when treatment starts in young animals, hepatocyte multiplication and eventually malignant tumors.[12] In some rodent strains, this sequence of events may also lead to distant metastases. Interestingly, this type of neoplastic transformation is not generally associated with reduction of the rodent's life span, and animals have a normal, active behavior up to the end of their lives. Withdrawal of the drug from food results in clear tumor regression.

Although these toxicologic findings are still the object of debate as far as their cellular mechanism is concerned, particularly because ciprofibrate, like other fibric acids, is apparently nongenotoxic, their direct transfer to humans or other higher species appears unlikely. In fact, in humans, peroxisomal proliferation is minimal or nonexistent, whereas, in this species, mitochondria are frequently found to be enlarged and apparently hyperactive after fibric acid treatment.[13] Thus, even if ciprofibrate, because of its high potency, also rates high as far as peroxisomal proliferation and tumor development are concerned,[14] these observations do not have to be transferred to humans. The long-term experience with the agent (see later discussion) has not given rise to any significant worry regarding possible carcinogenicity.

PHARMACOKINETICS

Absorption of oral ciprofibrate is rapid and extensive, leading to an 80% recovery of drug in the urine. The time to maximal levels in plasma (T_{max}) is approximately 1 hour. Bioavailability by the oral route is generally high, with minimal intersubject variation, as it relates to maximum concentration (C_{max}) and to area under the curve (AUC).[3] These data are also consistent with a minimal first-pass metabolism. Ingestion of the drug with food leads to very slight changes in either half-life or AUC.[3] On the other hand, C_{max} is reduced approximately 17.5% with a delayed T_{max}, up to 3 hours.[3]

Ciprofibrate, like most fibric acids (and thus sharing the property of physiologic fatty acids), is highy bound to albumin in the circulation (95% or more). The drug has a relatively reduced apparent volume of distribution (11.7 L) that is consistent with ionization at the physiologic pH, making it relatively hydrophobic.[15] On the other hand, clearance from plasma is definitely reduced (between 1.35 and 1.55 ml/kg/hr), with an elimination half-life calculated between 40 and 80 hours. As indicated previously, the two stereoisomers of the compound may show significantly different kinetic properties, both in humans and in rats (Table 118-1), so that the different handling of the two may lead to individually different

Table 118–1. **Pharmacokinetic Parameters for D (+) and L (−) Ciprofibrate Following a Single Oral Dose**

	Rat, 10 mg/kg		Man, 100 mg	
	D (+)	L (−)	D (+)	L (−)
C_{max} (μg/ml)	75.7	77.9	12.0	8.6
T½	159	27	139	32
AUC (μg/hr/ml)	7086	3114	1210	180

half-lives. Ciprofibrate, like most fibric acids, has a major route of elimination in the kidney, with minimal biliary excretion; unlike humans, rodents dispose of ciprofibrate primarily by the fecal route.

In view of the drug's elevated hydrophobicity, extensive glucuronidation is carried out in the liver, which leads to more than 70% clearance of the drug as the glucuronide conjugate. In addition, the presence of three minor unidentified metabolites has been described. There does not appear to be any significant interindividual variability in ciprofibrate metabolism-kinetics, and therefore no high-risk group has been identified.

CLINICAL USE
Indications

Ciprofibrate is indicated for the treatment of hyperlipoproteinemias that respond to fibric acid administration. It is generally agreed that all hyperlipoproteinemias respond to some extent to fibric acid treatment, but hypertriglyceridemias (types IV and V in the Fredrickson classification) are generally the most responsive and are the syndromes in which ciprofibrate provides the best therapeutic effect. In a long-term study in type IV patients, triglyceride reduction ranged between −33.9% and −50.7% in the course of 5 years of continued treatment.[16] In these patients, there was also a significant rise in HDL-C levels, predictable based on the mechanism of the drug. This biochemical change occurs in type IV and in other hyperlipoproteinemias.

An interesting feature of ciprofibrate is its remarkable activity in hypercholesterolemic patients, types IIA and IIB.[17, 18] In these patients, reductions of LDL-C, at times reaching 30% or more, have been described upon prolonged administration of ciprofibrate. These findings are observed in patients with familial type IIA hyperlipoproteinemia and in those with mixed type IIB. Apparently, the marked effect on LDL, described in uncontrolled trials, could also be ascertained in a placebo-controlled trial lasting 12 weeks, in which a 24% reduction in LDL-C levels was described (Fig. 118–3).[19]

Therefore, although ciprofibrate shares with other fibric acids a potent activity on plasma triglycerides (type IV and V hyperlipoproteinemias) and it is probably highly effective in type III hyperlipoproteinemias (although few specific data have been reported), it may also compete with HMG-CoA reductase inhibitors in the management of type II hyperlipoproteinemias. In this connection, however, one single comparative study has been made available.[20] In this study, 170 patients with type IIB hyperlipoproteinemia were randomized to receive either simvastatin (10 mg/day) or ciprofibrate (100 mg/day). As shown in Table 118–2, there was no significant difference after 8 weeks in the effect of the two drugs. Doses were thereafter raised in patients with unsatisfactory responses up to 20 and 200 mg/day, respectively. After 16 weeks in these subsamples of patients, the activity of simvastatin on either total cholesterol or LDL-C level was slightly better.

In addition to its activity on plasma lipids, ciprofibrate, like most of the other fibrates (but not gemfibrozil), lowers plasma fibrinogen levels.[21] Although this last property has as yet unexplained mechanisms, it offers an additional potentially useful tool for cardiovascular disease prevention. In a direct evaluation of ciprofibrate's activity on major clotting parameters in type IIA-IIB patients, a plasma fibrinogen reduction of approximately 20% was noted after 12 weeks of treatment with ciprofibrate 100 mg/day.[22] In these same patients, there were no significant alterations in platelet aggregability, but after 12 weeks of treatment, a 6% rise in percent antiplasmin activity and a 13.2% rise in fibrinolysis (fibrin plate assay) were noted.

Another potential mechanism recently described for ciprofibrate in the regulation of cholesterol metab-

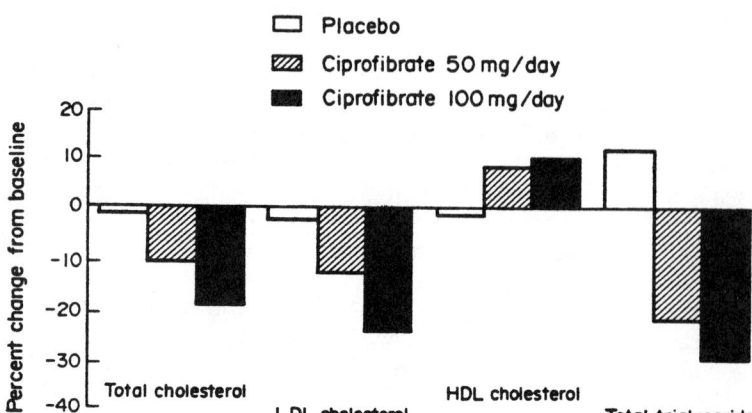

Figure 118–3. Effect of ciprofibrate treatment given for 12 weeks in a double-blind trial at low (50 mg) and standard (100 mg/day) doses in patients with type IIA hyperlipidemias.[19]

Table 118–2. **Mean values (±SD) of Cholesterol and Triglycerides in Type IIB Patients Treated with Either Simvastatin or Ciprofibrate**

	Total Cholesterol (mg/dl)			Triglyceride (mg/dl)		
	Week 0	*Week 8*	*Week 16*	*Week 0*	*Week 8*	*Week 16*
Simvastatin						
10 mg (n = 85)	304 ± 33	237 ± 34	—	240 ± 38	205 ± 48	—
20 mg* (n = 78)	303 ± 33	238 ± 34	213 ± 27	240 ± 38	207 ± 48	189 ± 47
Ciprofibrate						
100 mg (n = 84)	301 ± 35	241 ± 34	—	238 ± 38	159 ± 49	—
200 mg* (n = 63)	309 ± 35	254 ± 29	222 ± 25	239 ± 39	170 ± 50	143 ± 51

*Patients not fully responding to either 100 mg ciprofibrate or 10 mg simvastatin (LDL-cholesterol > 200 mg/dl after 8 weeks) received the higher dose (20 versus 200 mg/day) for a further 8 weeks. Their mean data at week 8 therefore relate to the lower daily dose.

From Farnier M, Truong-Tan N, Regy C: Comparative multicentre trial of the efficacy and tolerability of ciprofibrate and simvastatin in the treatment of mixed type IIB hyperlipoproteinaemias. J Drug Dev 5:13, 1992.

olism is the ability to directly inhibit liver acyl CoA–cholesterol acyltransferase activity.[23] The impact of this alteration on plasma cholesterol levels in humans cannot at present be estimated.

CAUTIONS AND ADVERSE EFFECTS (BY ORGAN SYSTEM)
Gastrointestinal

Ciprofibrate, like most fibric acids, is generally well tolerated by the gastrointestinal tract. In a French evaluation of the major side effects of fibric acids, no significant gastrointestinal disturbances were attributed to ciprofibrate, although there have been a small number of reports involving other fibrates.[24]

Liver

As with other fibrates, ciprofibrate treatment is associated with a significant reduction of plasma alkaline phosphatase (potentially a useful mechanism, in view of the apparent correlation between this alteration and a reduced thrombotic tendency).[25] In some cases, increases in transaminase are also described; in the long-term study, there was a mean rise of aspartate transaminase (AST) of 31% after 1 year and of alanine transaminase (ALT) of +26%.[16] However, the mean values remained stable thereafter, and no patient reached the pathologic range. Lactate dehydrogenase (LDH) levels also rose to a smaller extent (+9% after 1 year and +4.4% at year 10).[16] Again, these changes never reached the pathologic range. Albumin levels were somewhat reduced after 5 and 10 years of treatment, but it is difficult to judge whether such changes are related to treatment or to physiologic alterations in a group of patients with a mean age at entry of 56.7 years.[16]

In view of the potential for ciprofibrate or related compounds to lead to an enhanced risk of gallstones (presumably because of a higher secretion of free cholesterol by the biliary route during treatment), a specific study was carried out by Angelin et al.[26] These authors noted that, after 6 weeks of treatment, increased cholesterol saturation in the gallbladder bile

was present in 14 of 19 hyperlipoproteinemic patients treated with ciprofibrate (100 mg/day) in contrast with pathologic bile composition in only nine patients before treatment. Increased cholesterol saturation, consequent to a raised hepatic secretion of cholesterol (in the presence of unchanged rates of bile acid and phospholipid secretion), did not, however, appear to be a steady phenomenon. After 1 year of treatment, in contrast with a stabilization of serum lipids, biliary composition and cholesterol saturation had returned to pretreatment values in essentially all patients. Thus, apparently ciprofibrate, unlike clofibrate, exerts hypolipidemic activity without a consistent increase in the relative cholesterol concentration in bile.

Finally, liver biopsies taken 12 to 64 months after therapy were examined.[16] There was no evidence of peroxisomal proliferation, generally seen in the rodent, which confirms that these effects are species specific. In addition, no significant structural changes were noted in the livers of treated patients.

Hematologic and Other Side Effects

Careful evaluation of hematologic changes during the previously quoted long-term study[16] detected only a reduction of hemoglobin, statistically significant at years 1 and 5 and at the last value during treatment. Changes (−4.9% or less) appear to have minor clinical value, and it is difficult to evaluate whether the effect is directly related to drug treatment or just a consequence of aging.

Despite some isolated reports of myopathy during ciprofibrate treatment, similar to cases involving other fibric acids,[14] during the long-term study on this drug, creatine kinase (CK) levels were not associated with definite clinical symptoms and in no case reached pathologic levels, although they increased significantly (+65.3% at 1 year and +45.9% at the end of the study).

Other biochemical findings, such as a small rise in creatinine occurring during the first year and a transient glycemic drop at the same interval, were again small and of no apparent clinical interest.

An overall evaluation of ciprofibrate, compared with other fibric acids within a Pharmacovigilance

Table 118–3. Tolerability of Ciprofibrate

- Clinical and biologic tolerance is generally good.
- Mild and transient adverse effects: diarrhea, nausea and vomiting, headache, rash.
- Small increases (somewhat reversible with prolonged administration) of liver transaminase levels, fall in alkaline phosphatase level.
- Small increase in creatine phosphokinase level; rare reports of myopathy in patients with predisposing factors (kidney impairment, excessive doses).

program in France,[24] led to the observation of a small number of skin reactions, of erythematous type, and a few cases of clotting alterations (when used with oral anticoagulants) and of "general malaise," including impotence and weight loss (Table 118–3).

CONTRAINDICATIONS

At this time, there are apparently no definite contraindications to the use of ciprofibrate (as in general to the use of other fibric acids). Obviously, drugs with major activity in the liver should be used with caution in patients with clear-cut or presumable (high ethanol intake) liver abnormalities. This might also be the case of patients with preexisting gallstones (although no reports have indicated an increased risk of biliary colic in ciprofibrate-treated patients). As indicated, caution should be exercised in patients treated with oral anticoagulants, clearly potentiated by ciprofibrate or by other fibric acids.

DRUG INTERACTIONS

The most significant interaction of ciprofibrate and other fibrates is with oral anticoagulants. These agents are potentiated by fibrates, by as yet not fully explained mechanisms. It is unlikely that only a displacement interaction (from the very high binding of ciprofibrate) is in play. More likely, fibric acids affect warfarin and other oral anticoagulants by increasing their affinity for a postulated receptor system.[27] Whatever the case, combined treatment with ciprofibrate and oral vitamin K antagonists should be viewed with caution. When necessary, doses of the anticoagulant should be reduced.

Although the French Pharmacovigilance[24] report does not suggest any other undue side effects secondary to interactions with ciprofibrate, care should be given when ciprofibrate is administered with other drugs of potential use in other metabolic conditions. Such is the case of oral hypoglycemic sulphonylureas and, particularly, of HMG-CoA reductase inhibitors. In the latter case, the potential risk of myopathy associated with treatment should not be disregarded.[28] Although no clinical data are now available on such a potentially dangerous interaction between ciprofibrate and statins, its occurrence is not unlikely, and combined treatment should be avoided if possible.

USE IN PATIENTS WITH IMPAIRED ORGAN FUNCTION

The total dosage of ciprofibrate should be decreased in patients with renal failure, and intervals of administration should be prolonged concomitantly. Although no specific data are available, it may be presumed that glucuronide-conjugated ciprofibrate is eliminated by dialysis.

In view of the significant metabolic handling by the liver, ciprofibrate should be used with caution in all patients with liver impairment of a congenital or viral nature (Gilbert's disease, hepatitis) or secondary to ethanol intake. Blood level monitoring, with this or similar agents, is not generally helpful. Monitoring of liver enzymes and the use of good sense will help in preventing any potential liver toxicity.

PLACE IN THE LIPID-LOWERING ARSENAL

Ciprofibrate is the last of the major fibric acids to become widely available (after clofibrate, bezafibrate, fenofibrate, and gemfibrozil). Compared with, for example, gemfibrozil, availability of ciprofibrate is still restricted, not including some European countries and most of the American continent. Among fibric acids, ciprofibrate shows some appeal because of

- its very low daily dose (lowest among fibrates);
- its long half-life, necessitating once-daily administration (in some cases even skipping weekends);
- its apparent high efficacy on plasma LDL-C;
- its balanced activity against lipids/lipoproteins and also against some clotting parameters (not shared, in this last case, by gemfibrozil).

For these reasons, ciprofibrate may be an alternative to HMG-CoA reductase inhibitors in the management of type IIA hyperlipoproteinemia (in which the latter drugs are generally superior to fibrates) and probably is as effective as statins (because of the potent triglyceride-lowering activity) in mixed hyperlipoproteinemias (types IIB and III). Comparative data on simvastatin have been provided, indicating minimal or no differences in cholesterol-lowering potential.[20] In addition, no data are available on the potential activity on lipoprotein(a) [Lp(a)] levels, although it may be safely presumed that, as with other fibric acids, activity is minimal if it exists.[29] Large-scale trials evaluating ciprofibrate, also in comparison with other fibric acids, have underlined the excellent subjective tolerability of the compound, with a minimal incidence of gastrointestinal or other side effects.

DOSAGE AND ADMINISTRATION

Daily doses of ciprofibrate are 100 to 200 mg, given as single administrations (in view of the long half-life of the agent). Although no data are available on the effects of food on activity, the excellent absorption of the drug in fasting conditions would suggest that food in the gastroduodenal tract should not alter efficacy to a large extent.

Although a scheme for daily dose changes according to kidney impairment has not been made available, a standard policy (applicable also to other fibric acids) is to start with the lowest possible dose (50 mg if scored tablets are available) given on alternate days, for example, in patients on dialysis. Doses may be raised gradually thereafter until the expected effect is achieved. In type II patients, concomitant administration of an anion exchange resin markedly improves efficacy.

In resistant cases, a daily dose of 200 mg (in rare cases 300 mg) may be tested. Studies examining high doses showed that the 200-mg daily dose is more hypotriglyceridemic and hypocholesterolemic than the lower doses.[18, 20] In these studies, 200 mg/day of ciprofibrate led to significantly better total cholesterol and LDL-C reductions than 100 mg/day, leading in many cases to achievement of normal levels. The lack of a double-blind clinical protocol addressing this issue does not, however, allow one to consider this conclusion as final evidence. In the presence of good subjective tolerability and a lack of biochemical data suggesting liver or other parenchymal toxicity, it may be wise to raise the dosage to 200 mg/day or even higher in selected cases.

SOCIOECONOMIC CONSIDERATIONS

In spite of persisting negative views on lipid-lowering therapies, particularly in primary prevention,[30] there is no doubt that in high-risk patients (including classic cases of familial and nonfamilial hypercholesterolemias, but also patients with low HDL-C and the combination of high triglyceride and low HDL-C) drug treatment may offer an important therapeutic option. Recent data also indicate that hypolipidemic drugs have a 10- to 15-fold higher preventive power against reinfarctions and coronary deaths in secondary prevention than in primary prevention.[31]

Evaluation of ciprofibrate should consider as the reference drug gemfibrozil, the most widely used fibric acid derivative, which clearly exerted a powerful preventive activity in a primary prevention trial in Finland.[32] From this study, it could be established that subjects with high triglyceride and low HDL-C levels could benefit from a reduction of more than 70% in the risk of myocardial infarction.[33] Transfer of this type of information from one drug to another is always disputable, but ciprofibrate may carry some significant advantage over gemfibrozil. First, ciprofibrate can lower fibrinogen levels, and second, the total cholesterol– and LDL-C–lowering activities of ciprofibrate are apparently better than those of gemfibrozil, although a direct comparison is unavailable. From available data, it could also be suggested that ciprofibrate has a cholesterol-lowering potential similar to that exerted by HMG-CoA reductase inhibitors.

The combination of powerful cholesterol-lowering potential and classic traits of fibric acids, such as triglyceride-lowering and HDL-C–raising properties, may make ciprofibrate the first choice in numerous syndromes of hyperlipoproteinemia. Until now, the clinical use of ciprofibrate has not been extensive, and, in addition, animal toxicology data have caused concern. At present, a wider experience with ciprofibrate is advocated, in order to more properly classify this agent among lipid-lowering medications. The possible development of the L (−) enantiomer is also awaited with interest.

REFERENCES

1. O'Connor P, Freely J, Shepherd J: Lipid lowering drugs. Br Med J 300:667,1990.
2. Arnold A, McAuliff JP, Powers LG, et al: The results of animal studies with ciprofibrate, a new orally effective hypolipidemic drug. Atherosclerosis 32:155, 1979.
3. Betteridge DJ: Ciprofibrate—a profile. Postgrad Med J 69:S42, 1993.
4. Cayen MN: Disposition, metabolism and pharmacokinetics of antihyperlipidemic agents in laboratory animals and man. Pharmacol Ther 29:157, 1985.
5. Issemann I, Green S: Activation of a member of the steroid hormone receptor superfamily by peroxisome proliferators. Nature 347:645, 1990.
6. Sirtori CR, Galli C, Franceschini G: Fraudulent (and non fraudulent) fatty acids for human health. Eur J Clin Invest 23:686, 1993.
7. Latruffe N: Peroxisomes: Biochemistry, molecular biology and genetic disease. Biochimie 75:143,1993.
8. Dreyer C, Krey G, Heller H, et al: Control of the peroxisomal β-oxidation pathway by a novel family of nuclear hormone receptors. Cell 68:879,1992.
9. Kaikaus RM, Chan WK, Lysenko N, et al: Induction of peroxisomal fatty acid β-oxidation and liver fatty acid-binding protein by peroxisome proliferators. J Biol Chem 268:9593, 1993.
10. Sirtori CR, Franceschini G: Effects of fibrates on serum lipids and atherosclerosis. Pharmacol Res 37:167, 1988.
11. Shepherd J: Mechanism of action of fibrate. Postgrad Med J 69:34, 1993.
12. Reddy JK, Azarnoff DL, Hignite CE: Hypolipidaemic hepatic peroxisome proliferators form a novel class of chemical carcinogens. Nature 283:397, 1980.
13. Hanefeld M, Kemner C, Kadner E: Relationship between morphological changes and lipid-lowering action of p-chlorphenoxyisobutyric acid (CPIB) on hepatic mitochondria and peroxisomes in man. Atherosclerosis 46:239, 1983.
14. Sirtori CR, Calabresi L, Werba JP, et al: Tolerability of fibric acids. Comparative data and biochemical bases. Pharmacol Res 26:243, 1992.
15. Edelson J, Benziger DP, Arnold A, et al: Blood levels, tissue distribution and the duration of action in rats of ciprofibrate, a new hypolipidemic agent. Atherosclerosis 33:351, 1979.
16. Örö L, Carlson LA, Olsson A, et al: Long-term efficacy and safety of ciprofibrate in patients with primary hyperlipidemia. Curr Ther Res 51:750, 1992.
17. Rouffy J, Chanu B, Bakir R, et al: Comparative evaluation of the effects of ciprofibrate and fenofibrate on lipids, lipoproteins and apoprotein A and B. Atherosclerosis 54:273, 1985.
18. Olsson AG, Örö L: Dose-response study of the effect of ciprofibrate on serum lipoprotein concentrations in hyperlipoproteinaemia. Atherosclerosis 42:229, 1982.
19. Illingworth DR, Olsen GD, Cook SF, et al: Ciprofibrate in the therapy of type II hypercholesterolemia, a double blind trial. Atherosclerosis 44:211, 1982.
20. Farnier M, Truong-Tan N, Regy C: Comparative multicentre trial of the efficacy and tolerability of ciprofibrate and simvastatin in the treatment of mixed type IIB hyperlipoproteinaemias. J Drug Dev 5:13, 1992.
21. Sirtori CR, Colli S: Drugs affecting thrombosis and atherosclerosis. Cardiovasc Drug Ther 7:817, 1993.

22. Simpson IA, Lorimer AR, Walker ID, et al: Effect of ciprofibrate on platelet aggregation and fibrinolysis in patients with hypercholesterolemia. Thromb Haemost 54:442,1985.
23. Ståhlberg D, Angelin B, Einarsson K: Effects of treatment with clofibrate, bezafibrate, and ciprofibrate on the metabolism of cholesterol in rat liver microsomes. J Lipid Res 30:953,1989.
24. Sgro C, Escousse A: Effets indésirables des fibrates (hors foie et muscle). Therapie 46:351, 1991.
25. Iatridis SG, Ferguson JH, Iatridis PG: Intestinal alkaline phosphatase as a thrombogenic and platelet-altering factor in rabbits. Thromb Diath Haemorrh 24:191,1970.
26. Angelin B, Einarsson K, Leijd B: Effect of ciprofibrate treatment on biliary lipids in patients with hyperlipoproteinaemia. Eur J Clin Invest 14:73, 1984.
27. Bjornsson TD, Meffin PJ, Swezey SE, et al: Effects of clofibrate and warfarin alone and in combination on the disposition of vitamin K. J Pharmacol Exp Ther 210:322, 1979.
28. Tobert JA: Efficacy and long term adverse effect pattern of lovastatin. Am J Cardiol 62:28J, 1988.
29. Werba JP, Safa O, Gianfranceschi G, et al: Plasma triglycerides and lipoprotein (a): Inverse relationship in a hyperlipidemic Italian population. Atherosclerosis 101:203, 1993.
30. Davey Smith G, Pekkanen J: Should there be a moratorium on the use of cholesterol lowering drugs? Br Med J 304:431, 1992.
31. Silberberg JS, Henry DA: The benefits of reducing cholesterol levels: The need to distinguish primary from secondary prevention. Med J Aust 155:665, 1991.
32. Frick MH, Elo O, Haapa K, et al: Helsinki Heart Study: Primary prevention trial with gemfibrozil in middle-aged men with dyslipidemia. Safety of treatment, changes in risk factors, and incidence of coronary heart disease. N Engl J Med 317:1237, 1987.
33. Huttunen JK, Manninen V, Manttari M, et al: The Helsinki Heart Study: Central findings and clinical implications. Ann Med 23:155, 1991.

CHAPTER 119

Gemfibrozil

Richard V. Milani, M.D., F.A.C.C., and Carl J. Lavie, M.D., F.A.C.C., F.A.C.P., F.A.C.C.P.

In 1962, Thorp and Waring discovered that aryloxyisobutyric acids reduced plasma triglycerides and cholesterol concentrations in rats.[1] These experiments led to the development of a class of new agents directed toward reducing triglycerides and cholesterol, the fibric acids. This class includes clofibrate, gemfibrozil, fenofibrate, ciprofibrate, and bezafibrate. Currently, the most widely used fibric acid in the United States and Europe is gemfibrozil (Lopid), which was introduced as a congener of clofibrate and has been approved for clinical use in the United States since 1982.

CHEMISTRY AND PHARMACOKINETICS

Gemfibrozil is a nonhalogenated phenoxypentanoic acid and resembles its parent drug, clofibrate, pharmacologically. It differs from clofibrate in its aliphatic chain and in the presence of two methyl groups in place of a chlorine atom on the phenoxy group (Fig. 119–1).

It is a white compound with a molecular weight of 250.35 that is stable under ordinary conditions. Its solubility in water and acid is 0.0019% and in dilute base is more than 1%. Gemfibrozil is absorbed from the intestine and is bound to plasma proteins. Its plasma half-life is 1.5 hours; it undergoes enterohepatic circulation and readily passes the placenta. Seventy percent of an administered dose of gemfibrozil is excreted in the urine, primarily as unchanged drug.[2] Six percent of an administered dose of gemfibrozil can be accounted for in the feces. The liver, however, modifies some of the drug at the methyl functions to hydroxymethyl or carboxyl derivatives and some of the compound to a quinol. Peak serum levels for gemfibrozil occur 1 to 2 hours after dosing. Plasma levels are proportional to dose and do not show accumulation after multiple doses of gemfibrozil.

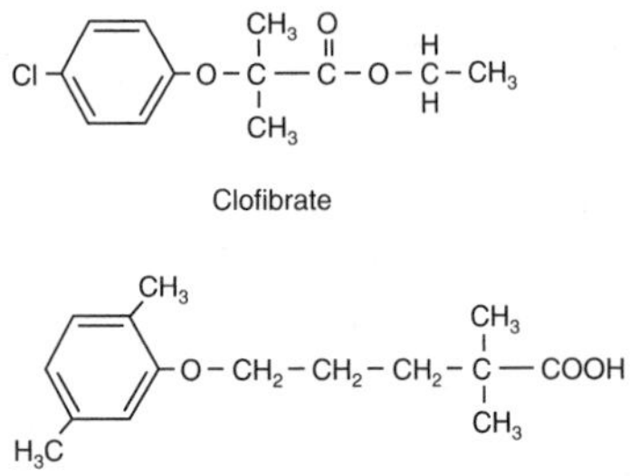

MECHANISM OF ACTION

Gemfibrozil is an antihyperlipidemic agent similar to clofibrate. In patients with hyperlipidemia, gemfibrozil has been shown to decrease low-density lipoprotein (LDL) levels as well as very-low-density lipoprotein (VLDL) levels, with substantial increases in high-density lipoprotein (HDL).[3] It appears to reduce incorporation of long-chain fatty acids into newly formed triglycerides, thus reducing VLDL synthesis and release from the liver.[4, 5] Gemfibrozil also appears to potentiate lipoprotein lipase (LPL) activity.[4, 6]

Gemfibrozil is quite effective in elevating HDL_2 cholesterol. It appears to increase synthetic rates of apolipoprotein (apo) A-I and apo A-II without changing the fractional catabolic rates.[3, 6–8] This effect on HDL can be, in part, due to the reduction in VLDL, because a reciprocal relationship exists between the two lipoproteins.

The mechanism by which gemfibrozil and other

Figure 119–1. Chemical structures for clofibrate and gemfibrozil.

fibric acids lower LDL cholesterol is not known. After administration of gemfibrozil, there is a modest but significant decrease in LDL level, which likely involves enhanced hepatic clearance of VLDL and intermediate-density lipoprotein (IDL), which would reduce the production of LDL.[3, 4, 9] In some patients taking gemfibrozil, LDL levels may not decrease and occasionally may even increase, but usually not to the abnormal range.

Gemfibrozil characteristically decreases plasma triglycerides by 40% to 55%. The maximal effect is generally achieved within 3 to 4 weeks after administration. VLDL cholesterol concentrations are also lowered to a comparable degree. HDL cholesterol levels may rise as much as 10% to 25%, and LDL cholesterol levels could be expected to be reduced by as much as 10% in hypercholesterolemic patients.[10, 11]

CLINICAL TRIALS

By far, the largest trial involving gemfibrozil is the Helsinki Heart Study, which was a primary prevention trial with gemfibrozil in middle-aged men with dyslipidemia. This randomized, 5-year, double-blind, placebo-controlled trial enrolled 4081 Finnish men between the ages of 40 and 55 who had dyslipidemia consisting of a serum concentration of non–HDL cholesterol (LDL cholesterol plus VLDL cholesterol) exceeding 5.2 mmol/L (200 mg/dl). Subjects with symptoms or signs of coronary heart disease (CHD) or other major diseases were excluded. Over the entire study period, gemfibrozil therapy reduced total cholesterol levels by 10%, LDL cholesterol levels by 11%, and triglyceride levels by 35% and raised HDL cholesterol levels by 11%, compared with placebo. These favorable lipid changes resulted in a 34% reduction in the incidence of definite CHD events (cardiac end points defined as cardiac death and fatal or nonfatal myocardial infarction) in those on active therapy (Fig. 119–2).[11–13]

In those patients with HDL cholesterol levels less than 35 mg/dl, gemfibrozil therapy resulted in a 62% reduction in CHD end points.[11] Although changes in HDL cholesterol levels were similar in all Fredrickson types, the effect on concentrations of total cholesterol and LDL cholesterol was largest in type IIA and on LDL minimal in type IV. The reduction of CHD incidence over placebo was largest in type IIB and smallest in type IIA.[11] When risk factors for CHD including age, blood pressure, smoking, drinking habits, baseline lipid levels, exercise, and relative weight were controlled by applying the Cox proportional hazards model, the changes in serum HDL and LDL cholesterol levels were both statistically significantly associated with the decline in CHD incidence within the gemfibrozil-treated group. Moreover, for every 1% increase in HDL cholesterol, there was a 3% reduction in the risk of CHD.[11]

In a more recent analysis of patients with different lipid subtypes in the Helsinki Heart Study, Manninen et al. reported that those individuals having an LDL/HDL ratio of more than 5 with triglyceride levels

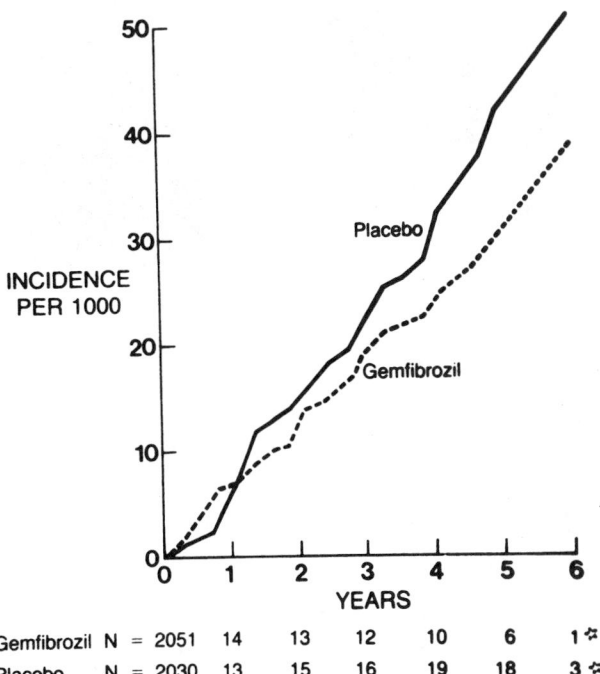

Figure 119–2. Kaplan-Meier cumulative incidence (per 1000) and annual number of cardiac end points, according to treatment group and time. Data for the 6th year were derived from 305 person-years of observation for gemfibrozil and from 316 person-years of observation for placebo. (Reprinted by permission from Frick MH, Elo O, Haapa K, et al: Helsinki Heart Study: Primary-prevention trial with gemfibrozil in middle-aged men with dyslipidemia: Safety of treatment, changes in risk factors, and incidence of coronary heart disease. N Engl J Med 317:1237, 1987. Copyright 1987, Massachusetts Medical Society.)

more than 200 mg/dl revealed a high-risk subgroup exhibiting a 3.8-fold increase in risk of CHD events within the 5-year study period.[14] The subgroup demonstrating this "lipid triad" exhibited a marked benefit from treatment with gemfibrozil, with a 71% lower incidence of CHD events than the corresponding placebo subgroup. This risk reduction is dramatic when compared with the significant 34% reduction in CHD incidence for the entire cohort and demonstrates the marked benefit of lipid therapy for individuals exhibiting this "lipid triad" (Fig. 119–3).

To date, there has been no large lipid intervention trial specifically designed for patients with type II diabetes. The largest body of data to date examining the impact of lipid-altering therapy in patients with type II diabetes exists within the Helsinki Heart Study.[15] Although this trial was not designed to examine the effect of lipid-lowering therapy in diabetic patients, type II diabetics were not excluded from enrollment. Of the 4081 men participating in the trial, 135 had type II diabetes at entry. Baseline parameters between diabetic and nondiabetic subjects are characteristic and shown in Table 119–1.

The overall incidence of myocardial infarction and cardiac death was more than double in diabetic participants when compared with their nondiabetic counterparts (7.4% versus 3.3%, respectively, $p < .02$). Although there is not enough statistical power to

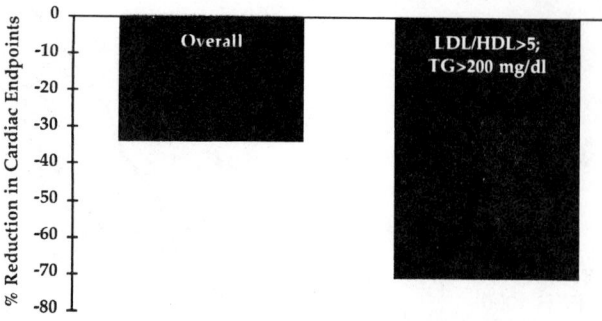

Figure 119–3. Helsinki Heart Study analysis: Reduction in incidence of cardiac events after treatment with gemfibrozil. LDL/HDL, low-density lipoprotein to high-density lipoprotein ratio; TG, triglycerides. (Data from Manninen V, Tenkanen L, Koskinen P, et al: Joint effects of serum triglyceride and LDL cholesterol and HDL cholesterol concentrations on coronary heart disease risk in the Helsinki Heart Study. Implications for treatment [see comments]. Circulation 85:37, 1992; and Manninen V, Elo M, Frick H, et al: Lipid alterations and decline in the incidence of coronary heart disease in the Helsinki Heart Study. JAMA 260:641, 1988.)

possibly demonstrate any significant therapeutic advantage in gemfibrozil-treated diabetic patients, the incidence of CHD events in the gemfibrozil-treated diabetic men was only 3.4% compared with 10.5% in the placebo group (NS), a risk reduction of 68% (Fig. 119–4).

Although this marked reduction in CHD events in the gemfibrozil-treated diabetic patients was not statistically significant (nor could it be by design), it does demonstrate the importance of lipid therapy in dyslipidemic diabetics and the potential role of gemfibrozil in these patients. Because the typical lipid disturbance in diabetes is an elevation of triglyceride levels and a reduced HDL cholesterol level, gemfibrozil is a well-suited agent for diabetic dyslipidemia.[15, 16]

In January 1993, the American Diabetes Association met to develop guidelines for treatment for dyslipidemia in diabetes.[17] Based on data from Helsinki and other studies, gemfibrozil is indicated as a first-line treatment in diabetic patients exhibiting elevation of triglycerides and/or reductions in HDL cholesterol levels. For diabetic patients with primarily elevations of LDL cholesterol, treatment with a hydroxymethylglutaryl coenzyme A (HMG-CoA) reductase inhibitor should be considered.

COMBINATION THERAPY

Gemfibrozil can be used safely in combination with bile acid resins and niacin. Studies with gemfibrozil and lovastatin (an HMG-CoA reductase inhibitor) have demonstrated an increased incidence of myopathy of approximately 5%.[18] Rhabdomyolysis and acute tubular necrosis have also been reported in patients receiving this combination.[19] Wiklund et al. reported the impact of combining gemfibrozil with pravastatin, a hydrophilic HMG-CoA reductase inhibitor, which was theoretically less likely to cause myalgia owing to its hydrophilicity.[20] In this study, 290 patients were randomized to treatment with pravastatin 40 mg once daily, gemfibrozil 600 mg twice daily, combination therapy with pravastatin and gemfibrozil, or placebo. Adverse events and clinical laboratory abnormalities were generally mild and transient in all groups, although creatine kinase levels tended to be higher with combination therapy. Severe myopathy was not observed with combination therapy. This combination significantly reduced levels of total cholesterol (29%), LDL cholesterol (37.1%), and VLDL cholesterol (49.4%) and increased HDL cholesterol levels (16.8%). It also resulted in a reduction of total cholesterol/HDL cholesterol (39.3%) and LDL/HDL cholesterol (45.8%). Further studies are needed to verify the safety of this combination therapy as well as to determine its impact over a longer period of time.

ADVERSE REACTIONS AND PRECAUTIONS

Gemfibrozil is quite well tolerated. The most frequent side effects noted are gastrointestinal disturbances

Table 119–1. **Mean Pretreatment Characteristics of Helsinki Heart Study Patients**

	NIDDM (n = 135)	Other (n = 3946)	*p*
Age (yr)	49.2	47.2	<.001
Hypertensive (%)	30	14	<.001
Smoker (%)	27	36	=.04
BMI (kg/m²)	28.5	26.6	<.001
TC (mg/dl)	291.6	289.2	=.41
LDL-C (mg/dl)	201.5	206.5	=.03
HDL-C (mg/dl)	45.6	48.7	<.001
LDL/HDL ratio	4.7	4.5	=.08
TG (mg/dl)	238.3	181.6	<.0001

BMI, body mass index; TC, total cholesterol; LDL-C, low-density lipoprotein cholesterol; HDL-C, high-density lipoprotein cholesterol; LDL/HDL, low-density lipoprotein/high-density lipoprotein; TG, triglyceride; NIDDM, non-insulin-dependent diabetes mellitus.
From Koskinen P, Mänttäri M, Manninen V, et al: Coronary heart disease incidence in NIDDM patients in the Helsinki Heart Study. Diabetes 15(7):820, 1992.

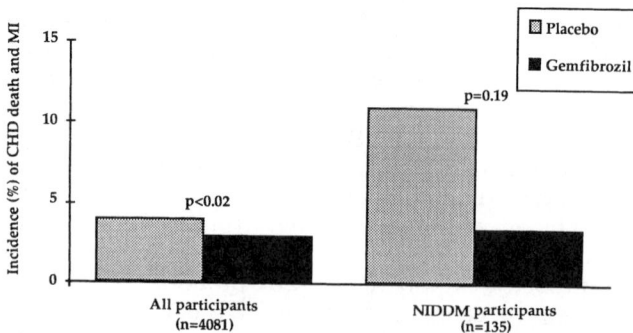

Figure 119–4. NIDDM in Helsinki Heart Study: 5-year incidence of CHD death and MI. NIDDM, non-insulin-dependent diabetes mellitus; CHD, coronary heart disease; MI, myocardial infarction. (Data from Frick MH, Elo O, Haapa K, et al: Helsinki Heart Study: Primary-prevention trial with gemfibrozil in middle-aged men with dyslipidemia: Safety of treatment, changes in risk factors, and incidence of coronary heart disease. N Engl J Med 317:1237, 1987; and Koskinen P, Mänttäri M, Manninen V, et al: Coronary heart disease incidence in NIDDM patients in the Helsinki Heart Study. Diabetes Care 15[7]:820, 1992.)

(nausea, abdominal pain, diarrhea), which were the only side effects noted of significance in the Helsinki Heart Study.[11, 12] Additionally, skin rashes and myalgia have been described. High levels of transaminase or serum alkaline phosphatase have been reported.[21] A few patients showed decreases in white blood cell count or hematocrit.

Gemfibrozil potentiates the action of warfarin or indandione anticoagulants. Frequent determinations of prothrombin time are advised if gemfibrozil and warfarin are given concomitantly. Doses of warfarin may need reduction during therapy with gemfibrozil.

The fibric acids, including gemfibrozil, increase the lithogenicity of bile, and they have been associated with an increased incidence of cholelithiasis and cholecystitis. Several studies in patients who were treated for longer than 1 year have shown a 1% to 1.5% incidence of new or enlarged gallstones, a frequency that is slightly higher than in untreated control subjects. The drugs promote gallstone formation by increasing the hepatic secretion of cholesterol into the bile and by decreasing the conversion of cholesterol into bile acids in the liver. Both these changes increase the saturation or lithogenicity of bile. As a result, gemfibrozil is contraindicated in patients with preexisting gallbladder disease. Gemfibrozil is also contraindicated in patients with severe renal dysfunction or hepatic disease, including primary biliary cirrhosis. The safety and effectiveness of gemfibrozil in children has not been established. Gemfibrozil is classified in the United States Food and Drug Administration (FDA) pregnancy category B.

INDICATIONS

The FDA has indicated gemfibrozil therapy in the following circumstances:

1. For the treatment of patients with very high serum triglyceride levels (types IV and V hyperlipidemia) who present a risk of developing pancreatitis.

2. For reducing the risk of developing CHD only in type IIB patients without a history of or symptoms of existing CHD in whom other measures, including diet, have failed and who have the following triad of lipid abnormalities: low HDL level with elevated LDL and triglyceride levels.

Although these recommendations are quite restrictive according to the FDA, most lipidologists feel gemfibrozil has a broader range of applications. Based on the American Diabetes Association guidelines for treatment of type II diabetics with dyslipidemia, gemfibrozil is indicated as a first-line therapy for diabetic patients with and without evidence of cardiovascular disease who exhibit elevations of triglyceride and/or reductions in HDL cholesterol levels.[17]

Additionally, although gemfibrozil has not been studied in a large secondary prevention trial, most experts agree that lipid alteration in dyslipidemic patients with CHD is appropriate therapy. Because gemfibrozil has been shown to alter lipids favorably and

reduce cardiac events in a large primary prevention trial, and because it does not have any unique hazards in patients with CHD, most lipid experts regularly use gemfibrozil in CHD patients with appropriate dyslipidemias requiring drug therapy.

REFERENCES

1. Thorp JM, Waring WS: Modification and distribution of lipids by ethyl chlorophenoxyisobutyrate. Nature 194:948, 1962.
2. Drug Evaluation Monographs, Vol 78. Denver, CO: Micromedex Inc., 1974–1993.
3. Saku K, Gartside P, Hynd B, Kashyap ML: Mechanism of action of gemfibrozil on lipoprotein metabolism. J Clin Invest 75:1702, 1985.
4. Lewis B: Session IV: Mode of action of gemfibrozil. Proc R Soc Med 69(Suppl 2):94, 1976.
5. Kissebah AH, Alfarsi S, Adams PW, et al: Transport kinetics of plasma free fatty acid, very low density lipoprotein triglycerides and apoprotein in patients with endogenous hypertriglyceridaemia: Effects of 2,2-dimethyl 5(2,5-xyloxy) valeric acid therapy. Atherosclerosis 24:199, 1976.
6. Saku K, Hynd BA, Gartside PS, Kashyap ML: Mechanisms of action of gemfibrozil in patients with subnormal high density lipoproteins and hypertriglyceridemia. Arteriosclerosis 3(5):484a, 1983.
7. Saku K, Hynd BA, Gartside PS, Kashyap ML: Mechanism of action of gemfibrozil in increasing HDL and lowering triglycerides [abstract]. Adv Exp Med Biol 183:449, 1985.
8. Gnasso A, Lehner B, Haberbosch W, et al: Effect of gemfibrozil on lipids, apoproteins, and postheparin lipolytic activities in normolipidemic subjects. Metabolism 35(5):387, 1986.
9. Carlson LA: Gemfibrozil: Effect on serum lipids, lipoproteins, postheparin plasma lipase activities and glucose tolerance in primary hypertriglyceridaemia. Proc R Soc Med 69(Suppl 2):58, 1976.
10. Grundy SM, Vega GL: Fibric acids: Effects on lipids and lipoprotein metabolism [review]. Am J Med 83(Suppl 5B):9, 1987.
11. Manninen V, Elo M, Frick H, et al: Lipid alterations and decline in the incidence of coronary heart disease in the Helsinki Heart Study. JAMA 260:641, 1988.
12. Frick MH, Elo O, Haapa K, et al: Helsinki Heart Study: Primary-prevention trial with gemfibrozil in middle-aged men with dyslipidemia: Safety of treatment, changes in risk factors, and incidence of coronary heart disease. N Engl J Med 317:1237, 1987.
13. Manninen V, Huttunen J, Heinonen O, et al: Relation between baseline lipid and lipoprotein values and the incidence of coronary heart disease in the Helsinki Heart Study. Am J Cardiol 63:42H, 1989.
14. Manninen V, Tenkanen L, Koskinen P, et al: Joint effects of serum triglyceride and LDL cholesterol and HDL cholesterol concentrations on coronary heart disease risk in the Helsinki Heart Study: Implications for treatment. Reprint. Dallas, TX: American Heart Association, 1988, pp 260–651.
15. Koskinen P, Mänttäri M, Manninen V, et al: Coronary heart disease incidence in NIDDM patients in the Helsinki Heart Study. Diabetes Care 15(7):820, 1992.
16. Vinik A, Colwell J: Effects of gemfibrozil on triglyceride levels in patients with NIDDM. Diabetes Care 16(1):37, 1993.
17. American Diabetes Association: Detection and management of lipid disorders in diabetes. Diabetes Care 16(5):828, 1993.
18. Pierce LR, Wysowski DK, Gross TP: Myopathy and rhabdomyolysis associated with lovastatin-gemfibrozil combination therapy [see comments]. JAMA 264:2991, 1990.
19. Marais GE, Larson KK: Rhabdomyolysis and acute renal failure induced by combination lovastatin and gemfibrozil therapy. Ann Intern Med 112:228, 1990.
20. Wiklund O, Angelin B, Bergman M, et al: Pravastatin and gemfibrozil alone and in combination for the treatment of hypercholesterolemia [see comments]. Am J Med 94:13, 1993.
21. McEvoy GK, et al (eds): AHFS Drug Information. Bethesda, MD: American Society of Hospital Pharmacists, 1990, p 894.

CHAPTER 120

Probucol

Masafumi Kuzuya, M.D., Ph.D., Akihisa Iguchi, M.D., Ph.D., and Carl J. Lavie, M.D.

Atherosclerotic plaques are the substrate for most cases of thrombotic arterial occlusions and therefore a major cause of cardiovascular mortality and morbidity. The importance of high serum cholesterol and low-density lipoprotein (LDL) levels as risk factors for cardiovascular disease and the benefit of lowering cholesterol and LDL levels for reducing risk are generally accepted.[1-4] Recently, increased attention has been focused on the hypothesis that oxidative modification of LDL may influence the development of atherosclerosis.[5] The oxidative modification of LDL alters its biologic properties *in vitro*, resulting in monocyte chemotaxis,[6] foam cell formation through scavenger receptors,[7] and the cytotoxicity of a variety of cultured cells.[8, 9] The presence of oxidized LDL in rabbit[10] or human[11] atherosclerotic lesions and the existence of autoantibodies that react with various forms of oxidized LDL suggest that oxidized LDL is indeed generated *in vivo*.[12]

Probucol, 4,4'-(isopropylidenedithio)bis(2,6-di-tert-butylphenol), originally introduced for clinical use as a hypocholesterolemic drug,[13] has been shown to possess potent antioxidant properties and to prevent oxidative modification of LDL.[14] In this chapter, we focus on probucol's antioxidant properties that may be related to its antiatherogenic effect.

ACTIONS BEYOND SERUM CHOLESTEROL LOWERING

Probucol therapy has consistently reduced total and LDL cholesterol levels by approximately 15% and 10%, respectively,[15-17] although the mechanism for its cholesterol lowering is not fully understood. There have been many reports of its preventive effect on the development of atherosclerotic lesions. Probucol reduced diet-induced aortic atherosclerotic lesions in rabbits,[18, 19] and its administration to hyperlipidemic patients was reported to cause the regression of tendinous or cutaneous xanthomas, a hallmark of atherosclerosis in homozygous familial hypercholesterolemic patients.[20, 21] In these early studies, these beneficial effects of probucol were believed to be involved in its cholesterol-lowering effect.

Yamamoto et al.[22] reported that probucol treatment in heterozygous or homozygous familial hypercholesterolemia caused the regression of both cutaneous xanthomas and tendon xanthomas. The xanthoma regressions were not correlated with the degree of cholesterol lowering observed. These findings provided initial evidence that probucol acts by other mechanisms in addition to cholesterol lowering. Wissler and

Vesselinovitch[23] reported probucol's beneficial effects on atherogenic diet-induced aortic lesions in nonhuman primates after 1 year of an atherogenic diet. They observed the effects of probucol alone, cholestyramine (another cholesterol-lowering drug) alone, and their combination on the serum cholesterol level and the regression of atherosclerotic lesions. Cholestyramine treatment or the combination of cholestyramine and probucol sharply lowered the serum cholesterol levels compared with probucol treatment alone; probucol alone or in combination with cholestyramine significantly increased lesion regression compared with cholestyramine alone. These results also indicate that probucol-induced regression may be independent of cholesterol lowering.

EFFECT ON OXIDATIVE MODIFICATION OF LDL

In 1986, Parthasarathy et al.[24] reported that probucol inhibited both cell-mediated and copper-catalyzed oxidative modification of LDL. In addition, the LDL isolated from the plasma of patients treated with probucol was also resistant to oxidative modification. More recently, the results of Parthasarathy et al. were confirmed by others,[25] who showed that probucol therapy inhibited copper-catalyzed oxidation of LDL as part of a substudy during the open prerandomization phase of the Probucol Quantitative Regression Swedish Trial (PQRST).[26] Parthasarathy et al.'s report focused attention on investigations of the action of probucol as an antioxidant instead of an agent for lowering cholesterol.

In 1987, two laboratories reported independently that probucol reduced the formation of atherosclerotic lesions in Watanabe heritable hyperlipidemic (WHHL) rabbits, an animal model for familial hypercholesterolemia. Kita et al.[27] observed that probucol prevented the progression of atherosclerosis in WHHL rabbits more than expected by the degree of plasma cholesterol level lowering. Carew et al.[28] also showed that, when probucol and lovastatin were administered independently to WHHL rabbits at doses designed to keep their cholesterol levels comparable, probucol more effectively reduced atherosclerotic lesion development. These observations suggest that there are additional antiatherogenic mechanisms for probucol other than simple cholesterol lowering. They proposed that probucol's antiatherogenic effect was related to limited LDL oxidation. Kita et al.[27] showed that LDL from control rabbits had a 10-fold increase in thiobarbituric acid–reactive substances, an indica-

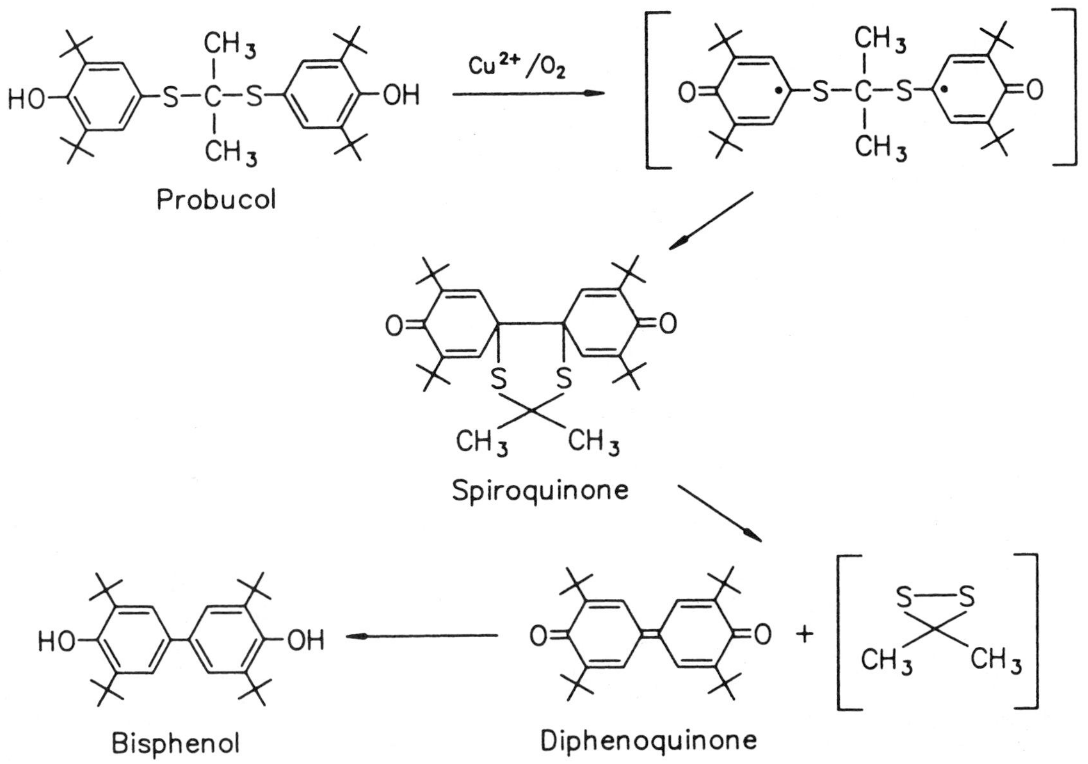

Figure 120–1. Proposed pathway for the Cu²⁺-induced degradation of probucol. (From Barnhart RL, Busch SJ, Jackson RL: Concentration-dependent antioxidant activity of probucol in low-density lipoproteins in vitro: Probucol degradation precedes lipoprotein oxidation. J Lipid Res 30:1703, 1989.)

tor of lipid peroxide, compared with that from probucol-treated rabbits. In addition, LDL in the control group was 7.4-fold more susceptible to copper-induced oxidative modification than LDL from probucol-treated rabbits. Carew et al.[28] reported that probucol treatment reduced the rate of injected labeled native LDL degradation in the macrophage-rich fatty-streak lesions of WHHL rabbits. They concluded that the inhibition of LDL degradation by probucol was due to inhibiting LDL oxidative modification to a form taken up and degraded by macrophages.

Mao et al.[29] prepared several probucol analogues that are not cholesterol lowering but have antioxidant activity. When these probucol analogues were administered to WHHL rabbits, the decrease in copper-catalyzed LDL lipid peroxidation was directly related to the serum concentration of the probucol analogues and was correlated with the inhibition of aortic atherosclerosis. Reports from different laboratories minimized the evidence that probucol's antiatherogenic effect on heritable hyperlipidemic rabbits was due to its cholesterol-lowering action and supported indirect and circumstantial evidence that its antiatherogenic effect was related to its antioxidant properties. More recently, several groups observed that probucol reduced neointimal thickening after balloon injury in rabbits[30] and swine[31] through its antioxidant properties.

Probucol was suspected to have antioxidant activity based on its structure. Probucol consists of two butylated hydroxytoluene moieties, with known hy-drophobic antioxidant activity connected by a sulfur-carbon-sulfur bridge. Pryor et al.[32] examined the efficiency of probucol in linoleic acid micelles containing sodium dodecyl sulfate. Probucol scavenged the peroxyl radical from this micellar system. Probucol may prevent the peroxidation of LDL lipid through scavenging peroxyl radicals by the two phenolic groups of probucol. Probucol phenoxyl radical has been observed during oxidation of LDL-containing probucol.[33] Barnhart et al.[34] showed that probucol in LDL was oxidized and converted to spiroquinone and then to diphenoquinone before LDL oxidation could be measured (Fig. 120–1). These probucol metabolites have been detected in the serum of probucol-administered modified WHHL rabbits.[35]

INCORPORATION INTO THE CELLULAR MEMBRANE

Probucol is a lipophilic compound that likely incorporates into cellular membrane. Relatively high concentrations of probucol were detected in the hearts of probucol-treated monkeys.[36] When probucol was incubated with erythrocyte suspensions containing lipoproteins, it was distributed in both the erythrocytes and the lipoproteins.[37] Our group[38] reported that the pretreatment of cultured vascular endothelial cells with probucol prevented cellular injury induced by organic hydroperoxide and oxidized LDL to the same extent as pretreatment with α-tocopherol (Fig. 120–2). In addition, the extent of cellular injury was inversely

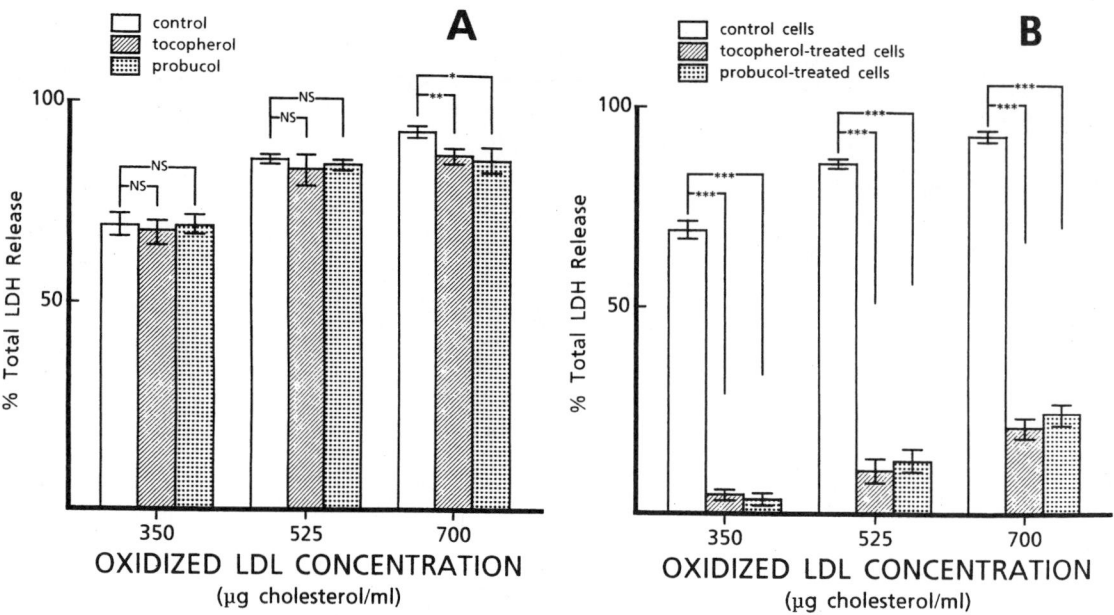

Figure 120–2. Effect of oxidized LDL on lactate dehydrogenase (LDH) release from endothelial cells (EC). *A,* EC at confluence in 24-well plates were incubated with oxidized LDL in the presence or absence of tocopherol or probucol for 8 hours. *B,* EC pretreated with tocopherol or probucol for 16 hours were incubated with oxidized LDL for 8 hours. Then LDH activity in the medium was determined. Values represent the means ± SD of triplicate wells: *$p < .05$; **$p < .01$; ***$p < .001$; NS, not significant. (From Kuzuya M, Naito M, Funaki C, et al: Probucol prevents oxidative injury to endothelial cells. J Lipid Res 32:197, 1991.)

related to the duration of the probucol incubation time and to the cellular content of probucol. Interestingly, the addition of probucol directly to medium containing hydroperoxide and oxidized LDL did not prevent endothelial cell toxicity (see Fig. 120–2). These results suggested that it was necessary for probucol to be incorporated into the cellular membrane to prevent cellular injury from hydroperoxide and oxidized LDL. When endothelial cells were treated with serum from patients who had had probucol administered, the endothelial cells absorbed the probucol from the serum.[38] Because serum probucol is carried predominantly in the lipoprotein fractions including LDL, these results may indicate that probucol can be transferred from lipoproteins to the endothelial cell layer during clinical administration. These observations indicate that probucol may prevent endothelial cell injury induced by various oxidative stresses in the same manner as membrane-associated vitamin E, a major lipid-soluble antioxidant present in cellular membranes.[39]

OTHER ACTIONS OF PROBUCOL

Although the antiatherogenic effect of probucol may be attributed to both its antioxidant action and its cholesterol-lowering action, as described earlier, there might be other actions of probucol. O'Brien et al.[40] observed that although probucol reduced the formation of the atherosclerotic lesion in WHHL rabbits, probucol did not suppress the presence of oxidized LDL in those lesions. These findings raise the possibility that probucol's antioxidant properties alone do not fully account for its antiatherogenic effect.

Ku et al.[41] found that probucol inhibited interleukin-1 (IL-1) secretion from lipopolysaccharide-stimulated macrophages. IL-1 is a potentially important cytokine in atherogenesis. Probucol also has an inhibitory effect on monocyte adhesion to endothelium in cholesterol-fed rabbits by a mechanism that is unrelated to its hypocholesterolemic effect.[42] Probucol has been shown to interact with the LDL particle and markedly affect the LDL structure.[43] Probucol completely protected LDL surface structure but did not completely prevent peroxidation of LDL lipids. It has been proposed that probucol prevents a secondary event that, in its absence, results in modification of lysine groups on the surface of LDL, leading to altered interactions with receptors.

Probucol is known to reduce not only LDL but also high-density lipoprotein (HDL) levels.[44] Its HDL-lowering effect has limited its therapeutic use in the United States. Matsuzawa et al.[45] showed that 6-year probucol treatment of patients with heterozygous familial hypercholesterolemia resulted in the improvement of stenosis in their coronary angiograms in spite of the reduction of HDL level. They concluded that the HDL reduction during probucol treatment was not an unfavorable change in lipoprotein metabolism. Furthermore, based on the results of probucol treatment in familial hyperalphalipoproteinemia, they proposed that probucol may act to reverse cholesterol transfer from peripheral tissues. This stimulatory effect of probucol on cholesterol ester transfer from HDL to lower-density lipoproteins was also found by others in hypercholesterolemic patients treated with probucol.[46, 47] Probucol also enhanced HDL-induced cellular cholesterol efflux in fibroblasts.[48] These obser-

Table 120–1. **Antiatherogenic Probucol Action**

Cholesterol lowering
Inhibition of lipoprotein oxidation
Prevention of cellular injury induced by oxidative stress
Promotion of reverse cholesterol transfer
Effect of LDL structure
Suppression of interleukin-1 secretion from macrophage
Inhibition of monocyte adhesion to endothelium
Unknown action(?)

vations raise the possibility that probucol may help reduce accumulation of cholesterol in peripheral tissue by enhancing its removal from cells.

Probucol incorporated into endothelial cells and monocytes/macrophages may prevent the oxidative modification of LDL by those cells by suppressing the production and release of oxygen radicals from those cells or by decreasing the lipoxygenase activity in a manner similar to that of vitamin E.[49–51]

The probucol actions thought to be related to its antiatherogenic effect are summarized in Table 120–1.

PHARMACOKINETICS, MECHANISM OF ACTION, AND ADVERSE EFFECTS

Most information regarding the pharmacokinetics and mechanism of action of probucol is related to its use as a hypolipidemic agent. The drug is typically administered in 250 mg or 500 mg doses twice daily. Drug absorption is limited to approximately 10%, but peak blood levels are higher when probucol is administered with food. In addition, blood levels typically gradually increase over the first 3 to 4 months of therapy with long-term oral administration, and then blood levels remain relatively constant over time. However, there does not seem to be a strong correlation between blood levels of probucol and its hypocholesterolemic action. This fat-soluble agent accumulates slowly in adipose tissues, and the major site of excretion is via the biliary system into the feces.[52]

Probucol typically lowers total cholesterol by 10% to 15%, by producing significant reductions in LDL cholesterol by as much as 25% in some studies.[17] Its major mode of action as a hypolipidemic agent is to reduce the fractional rate of LDL catabolism, by increasing excretion of bile acids, and it may inhibit some early steps in cholesterol biosynthesis. In addition, it may slightly reduce dietary cholesterol absorption. However, probucol does not seem to primarily affect the LDL receptors. In addition, it does not seem to reduce triglycerides or affect metabolism of very-low-density lipoproteins. Probucol reduces the synthesis of apolipoproteins A-I and A-II and may markedly reduce the levels of HDL cholesterol, thus increasing the LDL cholesterol/HDL cholesterol ratio.[52] As mentioned earlier, the clinical significance of this effect is uncertain.

The most common adverse effects of probucol are fairly minor gastrointestinal disturbances, particularly

diarrhea. The most serious adverse effect, however, seems to be drug-induced prolongation of the QT interval on the electrocardiogram, which has increased the propensity for serious dysrhythmias in both animals and humans. Therefore, probucol is not advocated in patients with baseline QT prolongation or in patients with known ventricular arrhythmias or with high risk of major dysrhythmias, as well as in patients using antiarrhythmic drugs (particularly type IA or type IC) for supraventricular arrhythmias.[17, 52, 53] Until further studies of its efficacy and safety are performed, these potential adverse effects on ventricular arrhythmias will likely limit the use of probucol as an antioxidant agent for both primary and secondary prevention of atherosclerosis.

SUMMARY

Clinical studies[54–56] have shown an inverse relationship between atherosclerotic disease and nonpharmacologic antioxidants such as vitamins C and E, carotene, or ubiquinone, suggesting that LDL oxidation may be a risk factor of atherosclerotic disease. The beneficial effect of probucol on atherosclerotic lesions of the WHHL rabbits has been reported in various laboratories, and there are indications that probucol may be useful in preventing atherosclerosis in human subjects. Further clinical studies are warranted, however, to examine the role of probucol in more detail in the development of atherosclerosis. A double-blind placebo-controlled trial (the Probucol Quantitative Regression Swedish Trial, PQRST)[26, 57] was concluded in December 1992. The aim of the PQRST is to determine whether probucol can retard the development of atherosclerosis or induce regression of atherosclerosis in hypercholesterolemic individuals. Unfortunately, the final result of the PQRST has not yet been published. In addition, the safety of this agent in patients with atherosclerosis, who may be at increased risk for ventricular dysrhythmias, is not yet fully established.

REFERENCES

1. Lipid Research Clinics Program: The lipid research clinics coronary primary prevention trial results: I. Reduction in incidence of coronary heart disease. JAMA 251:351, 1984.
2. Lowering blood cholesterol to prevent heart disease. JAMA 253:2080, 1985.
3. The Expert Panel: Report of the National Cholesterol Education Program Expert Panel on Detection, Evaluation, and Treatment of High Blood Cholesterol in Adults. Arch Intern Med 148:36, 1988.
4. The Expert Panel on Detection, Evaluation, and Treatment of High Blood Cholesterol in Adults: Summary of the Second Report of the National Cholesterol Education Program (NCEP) Expert Panel on Detection, Evaluation, and Treatment of High Blood Cholesterol in Adults (Adult Treatment Panel II). JAMA 269:3015, 1993.
5. Steinberg D, Parthasarathy S, Carew TE, et al: Beyond cholesterol: Modification of low-density lipoprotein that increases its atherogenicity [see comments]. N Engl J Med 320:915, 1989.
6. Quinn MT, Parthasarathy S, Fong LG, et al: Oxidatively modified low density lipoproteins: A potential role in recruitment

and retention of monocyte/macrophages during atherogenesis. Proc Natl Acad Sci U S A 84:2995, 1987.

7. Sparrow CP, Parthasarathy S, Steinberg D: A macrophage receptor that recognizes oxidized low density lipoprotein but not acetylated low density lipoprotein. J Biol Chem 264:2599, 1989.

8. Hessler JR, Morel DW, Lewis LJ, et al: Lipoprotein oxidation and lipoprotein-induced cytotoxicity. Arteriosclerosis 3:215, 1983.

9. Kuzuya M, Naito M, Funaki C, et al: Lipid peroxide and transition metals are required for the toxicity of oxidized low density lipoprotein to cultured endothelial cells. Biochim Biophys Acta 1096:155, 1991.

10. Rosenfeld ME, Palinski W, Yla-Herttuala S, et al: Distribution of oxidation specific lipid-protein adducts and apolipoprotein B in atherosclerotic lesions of varying severity from WHHL rabbits. Arteriosclerosis 10:336, 1990.

11. Yla-Herttuala S, Palinski W, Rosenfeld ME, et al: Evidence for the presence of oxidatively modified low density lipoprotein in atherosclerotic lesions of rabbit and man. J Clin Invest 84:1086, 1989.

12. Palinski W, Rosenfeld ME, Yla-Herttuala S, et al: Low density lipoprotein undergoes oxidative modification in vivo. Proc Natl Acad Sci U S A 86:1372, 1989.

13. Barnhart JW, Sefranka JA, McIntosh DD: Hypocholesterolemic effect of 4,4′(isopropylidenedithio)-bis(2,6-di-t-butylphenol) (probucol). Am J Clin Nutr 23:1229, 1970.

14. Kuzuya M, Kuzuya F: Probucol as an antioxidant and antiatherogenic drug [review]. Free Rad Biol Med 14:67, 1993.

15. McCaughan D: The long-term effects of probucol on serum lipid levels. Arch Intern Med 141:1428, 1981.

16. Tedeschi RE, Martz BL, Taylor HA, et al: Safety and effectiveness of probucol as a cholesterol lowering agent. Artery 10:22, 1982.

17. Lavie CJ, Gau GT, Squires RW, Kottke BA: Management of lipids in primary HDL and secondary prevention of cardiovascular diseases. Mayo Clin Proc 63:605, 1988.

18. Kritchevsky D, Kim HK, Tepper SA: Influence of 4,4′-(isopropylidenedithio)bis(2,6-di-t-butylphenol) (DH-581) on experimental atherosclerosis in rabbits. Proc Soc Exp Biol Med 136:1216, 1971.

19. Tawara K, Ishihara M, Ogawa H, Tomikawa M: Effect of probucol, pantethine and their combinations on serum lipoprotein metabolism and on the incidence of atheromatous lesions in the rabbit. Jpn J Pharmacol 41:211, 1986.

20. Harris RS Jr, Glimore HR III, Bricker LA, et al: Long-term oral administration of probucol [4,4′-(isopropylidenedithio)bis(2,6-di-butylphenol)] (DH-581) in the management of hypercholesterolemia. J Am Geriatr Soc 22:167, 1974.

21. Barker SG, Joffe BI, Mendelsohn D, et al: Treatment of homozygous familial hypercholesterolaemia with probucol. S Afr Med J 62:7, 1982.

22. Yamamoto A, Matsuzawa Y, Yokoyama S, et al: Effects of probucol on xanthomata regression in familial hypercholesterolemia. Am J Cardiol 57:29H, 1986.

23. Wissler RW, Vesselinovitch D: Combined effects of cholestyramine and probucol on regression of atherosclerosis in Rhesus monkey aortas. Appl Pathol 1:89, 1983.

24. Parthasarathy S, Young SG, Witztum JL, et al: Probucol inhibits oxidative modification of low density lipoprotein. J Clin Invest 77:641, 1986.

25. Regnström J, Walldius G, Carlson LA, et al: Effect of probucol treatment on the susceptibility of low density lipoprotein isolated from hypercholesterolemic patients to become oxidatively modified in vitro. Atherosclerosis 82:43, 1990.

26. Walldius G, Carlson LA, Erikson U, et al: Development of femoral atherosclerosis in hypercholesterolemic patients during treatment with cholestyramine and probucol/placebo: Probucol Quantitative Regression Swedish Trial (PQRST): A status report. Am J Cardiol 62:37B, 1988.

27. Kita T, Nagano Y, Yokode M, et al: Probucol prevents the progression of atherosclerosis in Watanabe heritable hyperlipidemic rabbit, an animal model for familial hypercholesterolemia. Proc Natl Acad Sci U S A 84:5928, 1987.

28. Carew TE, Schwenke DC, Steinberg D: Antiatherogenic effect of probucol unrelated to its hypocholesterolemic effect: Evidence that antioxidants in vivo can selectively inhibit low density lipoprotein degradation in macrophage-rich fatty streaks and slow the progression of atherosclerosis in the Watanabe heritable hyperlipidemic rabbit. Proc Natl Acad Sci U S A 84:7725, 1987.

29. Mao SJT, Yates MT, Rechtin AE, et al: Antioxidant activity of probucol and its analogues in hypercholesterolemic Watanabe rabbits. J Med Chem 34:298, 1991.

30. Ferns GA, Forster L, Stewart-Lee A, et al: Probucol inhibits neointimal thickening and macrophage accumulation after balloon injury in the cholesterol-fed rabbit. Proc Natl Acad Sci U S A 89:11312, 1992.

31. Schneider JE, Berk BC, Gravanis MB, et al: Probucol decreases neointimal formation in a swine model of coronary artery balloon injury: A possible role for antioxidants in restenosis. Circulation 88:628, 1993.

32. Pryor WA, Strickland T, Church DF: Comparison of the efficiencies of several natural and synthetic antioxidants in aqueous sodium dodecyl sulfate micelle solutions. J Am Chem Soc 110:2224, 1988.

33. Kalyanaraman B, Darley-Usmar VM, Wood J, et al: Synergistic interaction between the probucol phenoxyl radical and ascorbic acid in inhibiting the oxidation of low density lipoprotein. J Biol Chem 267:6789, 1992.

34. Barnhart RL, Busch SJ, Jackson RL: Concentration-dependent antioxidant activity of probucol in low density lipoproteins in vitro: Probucol degradation precedes lipoprotein oxidation. J Lipid Res 30:1703, 1989.

35. Mao SJ, Yates MT, Parker RA, et al: Attenuation of atherosclerosis in a modified strain of hypercholesterolemic Watanabe rabbits with use of a probucol analogue (MDL 29,311) that does not lower serum cholesterol. Arterioscler Thromb 11:1266, 1991.

36. Marshall FN: Pharmacology and toxicology of probucol [review]. Artery 10:7, 1982.

37. Urien S, Riant P, Albengres E, et al: In vitro studies on the distribution of probucol among human plasma lipoproteins. Mol Pharmacol 26:322, 1984.

38. Kuzuya M, Naito M, Funaki C, et al: Probucol prevents oxidative injury to endothelial cells. J Lipid Res 32:197, 1991.

39. Machlin LT, Bendich A: Free radical tissue damage: Protective role of antioxidant nutrients [review]. FASEB J 1:441, 1987.

40. O'Brien K, Nagano Y, Gown A, et al: Probucol treatment affects the cellular composition but not anti-oxidized low density lipoprotein immunoreactivity of plaques from Watanabe heritable hyperlipidemic rabbits. Arterioscler Thromb 11:751, 1991.

41. Ku G, Doherty NS, Schmidt LF, et al: Ex vivo lipopolysaccharide-induced interleukin-1 secretion from murine peritoneal macrophages inhibited by probucol, a hypocholesterolemic agent with antioxidant properties. FASEB J 4:1645, 1990.

42. Ferns GAA, Forster L, Stewart-Lee A, et al: Probucol inhibits mononuclear cell adhesion to vascular endothelium in the cholesterol-fed rabbit. Atherosclerosis 100:171, 1993.

43. McLean LR, Hagaman KA: Effect of probucol on the physical properties of low-density lipoproteins oxidized by copper. Biochemistry 28:321, 1989.

44. Riesen WF, Keller M, Mordasini R: Probucol in hypercholesterolemia: A double blind study. Atherosclerosis 36:201, 1980.

45. Matsuzawa Y, Yamashita S, Funahashi T, et al: Selective reduction of cholesterol in HDL2 fraction by probucol in familial hypercholesterolemia and hyperHDL2 cholesterolemia with abnormal cholesteryl ester transfer. Am J Cardiol 62:66B, 1988.

46. Sirtori CR, Sirtori M, Calabresi L, et al: Changes in high-density lipoprotein subfraction distribution and increased cholesteryl ester transfer after probucol. Am J Cardiol 62:73B, 1988.

47. Franceschini G, Sirtori M, Vaccarino V, et al: Mechanisms of HDL reduction after probucol: Changes in HDL subfractions and increased cholesteryl ester transfer. Arteriosclerosis 9:462, 1989.

48. Goldberg RB, Mendez A: Probucol enhances cholesterol efflux from cultured human skin fibroblasts. Am J Cardiol 62:57B, 1988.

49. Leb L, Beatson P, Fortier N, et al: Modulation of mononuclear phagocyte cytotoxicity by alpha-tocopherol (vitamin E). J Leukoc Biol 37:449, 1985.

50. Reddanna P, Rao MK, Reddy CC: Inhibition of 5-lipoxygenase by vitamin E. FEBS Lett 193:39, 1985.

51. Parthasarathy S: Evidence for an additional intracellular site of action of probucol in the prevention of oxidative modification of low density lipoprotein. J Clin Invest 89:1618, 1992.
52. Drug Evaluations Annual. American Medical Association, distributed by WB Saunders, Philadelphia, 1994, pp 2319–2320.
53. Physicians' Desk Reference, 48th ed. Montvale, NJ: Medical Economics Data Production, 1994, pp 1304–1306.
54. Riemersma RA, Wood DA, Macintyre CCA, et al: Risk of angina pectoris and plasma concentrations of vitamins A, C, and E and carotene [see comments]. Lancet 337:1, 1991.
55. Hanaki Y, Sugiyama S, Ozawa T, et al: Ratio of low-density lipoprotein cholesterol to ubiquinone as a coronary risk factor. N Engl J Med 325:814, 1991.
56. Gey KF, Puska P: Plasma vitamins E and A inversely correlated to mortality from ischemic heart disease in cross-cultural epidemiology. Ann N Y Acad Sci 570:267, 1989.
57. Walldius G, Regnstrom J, Nilsson J: The role of lipids and antioxidative factors for development of atherosclerosis: The Probucol Quantitative Regression Swedish Trial (PQRST). Am J Cardiol 71:15B, 1993.

CHAPTER 121

Lovastatin

Evan A. Stein, M.D., Ph.D., and Jonathan L. Isaacsohn, M.D.

HISTORY

Lovastatin is the first member of a new class of potent cholesterol-lowering drugs that work by reversibly inhibiting the rate-limiting enzyme in cholesterol biosynthesis, 3-hydroxy-3-methylglutaryl coenzyme A (HMG-CoA) reductase, to be approved by the United States Food and Drug Administration (FDA) and be marketed. It represents the culmination of a systematic drug discovery program aimed at safe and effective plasma cholesterol reduction. Like other first-generation HMG-CoA reductase inhibitors, lovastatin is a fungal metabolite that was initially isolated from two species, *Monascus ruber*[1] and *Aspergillus terreus*,[2] in 1980 and 1976, respectively.

Lovastatin and its associated class of compounds, pravastatin, simvastatin, and fluvastatin, over the last few years since their release for general clinical use, have revolutionized the management of hypercholesterolemia and provided the basis for implementation of new aggressive therapeutic guidelines promulgated by the National Cholesterol Education Program (NCEP) in the United States[3] and the European Atherosclerosis Society.[4]

Lovastatin has also been widely evaluated in clinical trials with atherosclerotic and cardiovascular end points[5-7] that have demonstrated its beneficial effect on the underlying atherosclerotic process.

CHEMISTRY

Lovastatin is the inactive lactone or prodrug form of 1', 2', 6', 7', 8', 8a'-hexahydro-3,5-dihydroxy-2',6'-dimethyl-8' (2'-methyl-1-oxybutoxy)-1'-naphthalene hexanoic acid (Fig. 121–1). The open-acid, hydroxy-acid component (see Fig. 121–1) is similar in structure to the intermediate step in the conversion of HMG-CoA to mevalonate (Fig. 121–2) and thus acts as a competitive, but reversible, inhibitor of the HMG-CoA reductase enzyme.

Lovastatin is an optically active crystalline solid, white to off-white in appearance, with a molecular formula of $C_{24}H_{36}O_5$ and a molecular weight of 404.55.

No polymorphic or solvate forms have been described, and the compound is nonhygroscopic. It is freely soluble in chloroform, soluble in methanol and acetone, poorly soluble in ethanol, and insoluble in water, 0.44×10^{-3} mg/ml at room temperature.[8]

PHARMACOLOGY

Approximately 80% of cholesterol in human beings is derived from endogenous synthesis starting with acetyl CoA (Fig. 121–3). Although the intestine and liver are the primary sites of synthesis, virtually all cells evaluated have the ability to produce cholesterol *de novo*. The major site of production is the liver, where nearly 80% of cholesterol synthesis occurs. Of the nearly 25 steps in cholesterol synthesis, only a few are considered rate limiting and the focus for attempting to control hepatic cholesterol production. Two of these steps, HMG-CoA reduction to mevalonate and farnesyl pyrophosphate to squalene, are considered the most optimal to inhibit in subjects with hypercholesterolemia. Both these rate-limiting steps, modulated by HMG-CoA reductase and squalene synthetase, respectively, occur before cyclization, after which metabolites that may accumulate are not easily recycled and may produce toxicity. Inhibition of HMG-CoA reductase, one of the earliest committed steps in cholesterol biosynthesis, results in accumulation of water-soluble HMG-CoA, which is readily catabolized to safe and less complex molecules.

The inhibition of HMG-CoA reductase by lovastatin not only reduces intracellular hepatic cholesterol synthesis and lipoprotein release but also results in a decrease in sterol-mediated low-density lipoprotein (LDL)-receptor suppression,[9] which in turn increases LDL-receptor activity and plasma LDL uptake and removal. In order to regulate the cholesterol content of the cell, cholesterol and other sterols appear to interact with sterol regulatory elements that are part of the promotor region of the 5' flanking region of the LDL-receptor gene. Suppression of cholesterol biosynthesis reduces available cholesterol, resulting

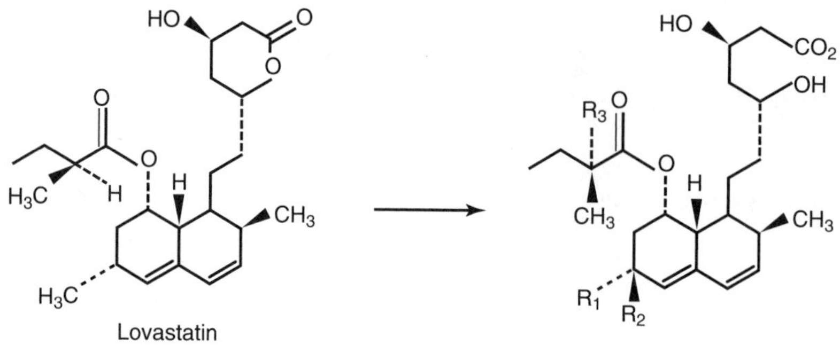

Lovastatin

(Lactone Form)

Figure 121–1. Structure of lactone and open-acid forms of lovastatin.

R_1	R_2	R_3		
H	H	H	Mevastatin	
CH_3	H	H	Lovastatin	Open Forms
CH_3	H	CH_3	Simvastatin	
H	OH	H	Pravastatin	

in decreased sterol binding and an increase in transcription of the LDL-receptor. A similar inhibitory mechanism appears to control production of the rate-limiting enzymes HMG-CoA reductase and HMG-CoA synthase, and thus lovastatin and other HMG-CoA reductase inhibitors result in an increase in the amounts of these two enzymes.[9]

When these reductase inhibitors are assayed in a bioassay system as the open-acid forms, the relative inhibitory activity of lovastatin to other reductase inhibitors is shown in Table 121–1;[10] it is approximately one third that of simvastatin but is threefold that of pravastatin. The latter may be due to assay conditions, because pravastatin is less lipid soluble, which may result in lower intracellular concentrations in the bioassay system.

PHARMACOKINETICS

Based on indirect studies using radioactively labeled lovastatin in both lactone and hydroxy-acid forms

and extrapolation from animal studies, absorption rates for lovastatin appear to be approximately 30%.[11] Sixty percent to 70% of the prodrug is extracted by the liver during first pass and is then activated to the hydroxy-acid form in the liver, where it exerts its desired effect. Metabolites, which do not possess reductase activity, are promptly excreted, mostly by the liver, with 80% to 90% recoverable in the feces and less than 10% in the urine. The other major organs in which lovastatin is found after administration are the spleen, testes, and adrenal glands, although the amount is 20 to 50 times lower than the levels found in hepatic tissue.

When lovastatin is administered to healthy human male subjects, the T_{max} occurs at 2 to 3 hours after dose.[12] Similar studies done on young and elderly males and females[13] showed differences in both absorption and metabolism that were related to both sex and age. The C_{max} in both young and elderly female subjects was approximately 50% higher than in their corresponding male groups. In the elderly,

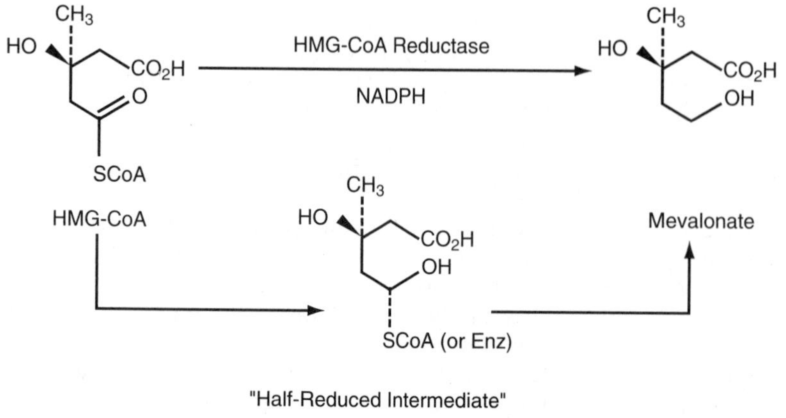

Figure 121–2. HMG-CoA reduction reaction.

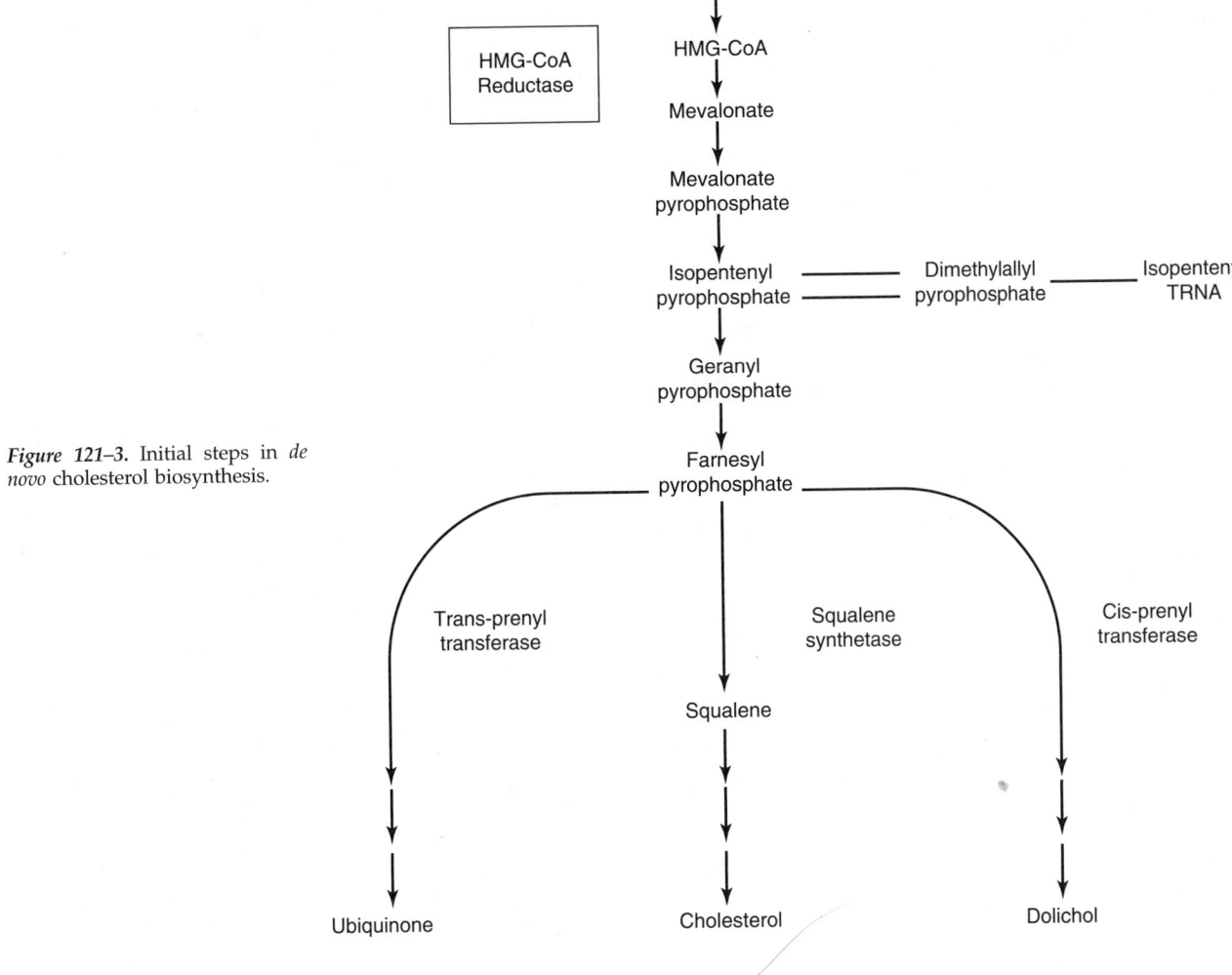

Figure 121–3. Initial steps in *de novo* cholesterol biosynthesis.

irrespective of sex, the C_{max} was 20% to 30% higher than in their respective younger counterparts.

The T_{max} in both sexes and both age groups was similar, at between 1.6 and 1.9 hours. The total amount of lovastatin (lactone and open-acid forms) in peripheral blood as judged by the area under the curve (AUC) showed the same differences between male and female subjects and between the young and the elderly as that found for C_{max}. Female subjects of both age groups had higher AUCs than their corresponding male subjects, and the elderly had higher AUCs than their younger counterparts.[13] Repetitive dosing of lovastatin over a period of 17 days resulted in a steady state in postdose plasma inhibitory levels

after 5 days. Because hepatic enzymes responsible for drug metabolism do not appear to decrease with age, the differences found in the elderly were thought most likely to be caused by the reduced hepatic size and blood flow that are known to occur with aging. It is unlikely that decreased renal function is important, because lovastatin is tightly bound to albumin and minimally available for clearance by the kidney. Similar differences in hepatic size and blood flow may also account for gender differences. However, these differences do not appear to necessitate differences in dosage recommendations.

Although lovastatin is lipid-soluble and can therefore cross cell membranes, including the blood-brain barrier, approximately 95% of the drug in plasma is tightly bound to albumin and is thus only minimally available, probably less than 5% of systemic concentration, for transcellular movement. The open-acid reductase inhibitor, pravastatin, although far less lipid soluble, is less tightly bound to albumin (approximately 50%) and has a higher T_{max}[12] than lovastatin; thus, there is most likely little difference in nonhepatic tissue concentration between the two agents.

Table 121–1. **Inhibitory Constant of Various HMG-CoA Reductase Inhibitors, Assayed as Open-Acid Forms**

Compound	K (M)	Reference
Simvastatin	0.6×10^{-9}	8
Mevastatin	1.4×10^{-9}	10
Pravastatin	2.2×10^{-9}	10

K, inhibitor constant; M, mol/L.

EFFECTS ON PATHOPHYSIOLOGY
Effects on Endocrine Function

Lovastatin is found in extrahepatic tissues, where it can reduce intracellular cholesterol synthesis and thus theoretically might reduce steroid hormone production, particularly the adrenocortical and gonadal hormones. Clinical studies in nonhomozygous familial hypercholesterolemic subjects have demonstrated that lovastatin does not reduce basal plasma cortisol levels or adrenocortical reserve.[14] There also have been no effects on testicular steroidogenesis.[15] The overall effect on male fertility has not been evaluated, although in clinical practice it has not emerged as a problem. The effects of lovastatin on gonadal hormones in premenopausal women have not been evaluated.

Effects on Coronary Atherosclerosis

In the Familial Atherosclerosis Treatment Study (FATS),[5] treatment with lovastatin or niacin in combination with a bile acid sequestrant for 2½ years resulted in a significantly reduced frequency of progression and increased frequency of regression of coronary atherosclerosis as assessed by quantitative coronary angiography. Furthermore, in the treated patients compared with the control patients, there was a significant reduction in cardiac events, including fatal and nonfatal myocardial infarction and the need for coronary bypass surgery, angioplasty, or peripheral vascular procedures.

In the Monitored Atherosclerosis Regression Study (MARS),[7] patients treated with 80 mg/day of lovastatin did not demonstrate significant differences in angiographic progression when assessed by computerized quantitative angiography. However, when assessed by a consensus opinion of expert angiographers, significant reductions were reported in the number of patients undergoing progression and significant increases in those patients undergoing regression. In the Canadian Coronary Atherosclerosis Intervention Trial (CCAIT),[6] patients treated with lovastatin at increasing doses to achieve a low-density lipoprotein cholesterol (LDL-C) level of less than 130 mg/dl demonstrated a significant slowing of progression of coronary atherosclerosis, more pronounced in the milder lesions. Furthermore, there was a significant inhibition in the development of new coronary lesions compared with the placebo-treated patients.

Effects on Endothelial Function

Normal functioning of the endothelium is disturbed by the presence of an atherosclerotic plaque.[16] Furthermore, it is now established that endothelial dysfunction is present in the setting of a number of risk factors for atherosclerosis, even if the arteries appear angiographically normal. Hypercholesterolemia, hypertension, and cigarette smoking all have been associated with endothelial dysfunction.[17]

It has been shown that cholesterol lowering with lovastatin,[18] pravastatin,[19] or cholestyramine[20] restores endothelial function, and paradoxic vasoconstriction, the hallmark of endothelial dysfunction, is reduced. In a study evaluating myocardial perfusion using dipyridamole positron emission scanning, vigorous cholesterol lowering over a 90-day period with lovastatin, cholestyramine, and a low-fat diet resulted in improved myocardial perfusion.[21] It is postulated that this very rapid effect was due to improved epicardial artery vasodilation as a result of improved endothelial function. In the setting of endothelial dysfunction, plasminogen activator inhibitor-1 (PAI-1) levels are elevated. In a study in hypercholesterolemic patients, 6 months of lovastatin therapy resulted in a reduction in PAI-1 levels, possibly reflecting restoration of endothelial function.[22]

CLINICAL USE
Indications

The major effect of lovastatin is a dose-dependent reduction of plasma LDL-C levels. In the Expanded Clinical Evaluation of Lovastatin (EXCEL) Study,[23] comprising more than 8000 patients, using dosages from 20 mg to 80 mg/day, LDL-C was reduced by 24% and 40%, respectively. In addition, triglycerides were reduced by 10% and 19%, and high-density lipoprotein cholesterol (HDL-C) levels were increased by 6.6% and 9.5%. These lipid effects were maintained during the 1-year study and in a subset of 977 patients who were followed up for 2 years.[24] In the lovastatin 5-year safety and efficacy study,[25] in 745 patients with severe hypercholesterolemia (mean total cholesterol of 360 mg/dl), using a dose titration protocol from 20 mg to 80 mg to achieve a goal LDL-C of less than 140 mg/dl, mean LDL-C levels were reduced by 40% and HDL-C levels increased by 12%. Most patients (77%) were treated at the 80-mg dose.

Lovastatin, either alone or in combination with other lipid-lowering drugs, has been evaluated in a number of secondary prevention trials, including the Familial Atherosclerosis Treatment Study (FATS),[5] UCSF-SCOR[26] study, Canadian Coronary Atherosclerosis Intervention Trial (CCAIT),[6] and the Monitored Atherosclerosis Regression Study (MARS).[7] Overall the angiographic evaluations demonstrated slowing of progression and greater regression in the treated patients compared with the control patients. Furthermore, significant reductions in cardiac event rates were achieved. Primary prevention studies using lovastatin are currently under way; however, no results are yet known.

The NCEP ATP II guidelines have established levels below which LDL-C should be reduced.[3] These levels depend on whether treatment is for primary or secondary prevention. Individuals targeted for primary prevention are divided into two subgroups. In the low-risk group, defined as fewer than two risk factors for coronary heart disease (CHD), the target LDL-C is less than 160 mg/dl. In the high-risk group, with two or more risk factors for CHD, the target LDL-C is less than 130 mg/dl. In patients with clinical atherosclerotic vascular disease, the target LDL-C is less than 100 mg/dl.

If target LDL-C levels have not been reached with dietary modification, lovastatin and the other HMG-CoA reductase inhibitors can be used as the drug of first choice. If lesser LDL-C reductions are required to achieve target LDL-C levels, drug therapy with a bile-acid resin may be initiated rather than starting with the HMG-CoA reductase inhibitor.

Lovastatin therapy is effective in patients with heterozygous familial hypercholesterolemia[27] and polygenic hypercholesterolemia as well as the nonfamilial forms of hypercholesterolemia.[28] It is also effective in the secondary forms of hypercholesterolemia, including diabetes[29] and the nephrotic syndrome.

Precautions and Adverse Effects

Lovastatin is generally a well-tolerated drug. In clinical trials with lovastatin, the overall frequency of patients withdrawn from the various studies because of an adverse experience has been very similar to the withdrawal rate in placebo patients. In some studies, there has been a slightly increased incidence of gastrointestinal symptoms, including constipation, flatulence and abdominal discomfort, rash, and myalgias.

Hepatotoxicity is the most common adverse effect. Elevations in the transaminase levels occurred in the EXCEL study in a dose-dependent manner.[23] During the first year of this study of more than 8000 patients, transaminase elevations more than three times the upper limits of normal occurred with a frequency of 0.1% at the 20-mg dose, 0.9% at the 40-mg dose, and 1.5% at the 80-mg dose. Of the 977 patients who were followed up into the second year of the trial, only one additional patient had transaminase elevations to three times the upper limits of normal.[24] Few episodes of transaminase elevation occurred in the first 4 months of therapy, with 87% occurring between the fourth and twelfth months. The 2-year follow-up study confirms that, after the first year of therapy, significant transaminase elevations are relatively uncommon. In the lovastatin 5-year safety and efficacy study, 80% of the significant transaminase elevations occurred during the first year of therapy.[25]

The majority of transaminase elevations are mild and transient (less than three times the upper limits of normal). This degree of transaminase elevation occurs in approximately 5% of lovastatin-treated patients and does not require termination of therapy. Mild baseline transaminase elevations are not absolute contraindications to lovastatin use, but closer observation and frequent monitoring should be done. In patients whose transaminase levels reach three times the upper limits of normal, lovastatin therapy should be terminated. The transaminase levels return to pretreatment levels within a few weeks. Rechallenge with an HMG-CoA reductase inhibitor can be considered if the clinical situation is appropriate. Patients who have transaminase elevations to levels less than three times the upper limits of normal can be

continued on therapy, but measurements of transaminase levels should be repeated more frequently.

In the majority of transaminase elevations, it is the alanine aminotransferase (SGPT) that reaches three times the upper limits of normal, with aspartate aminotransferase (SGOT) usually not increasing to the same degree, and results of other liver function tests, such as bilirubin and alkaline phosphatase, generally remaining unchanged. Gamma glutamyl transpeptidase is a poor index for monitoring these agents, because it is often elevated as a result of lovastatin catabolism inducing the microsomal drug metabolism system. In none of the patients in these studies was clinical hepatitis diagnosed, and to date no evidence of permanent liver damage has been documented. The cause of the transaminase elevation is not well established but is thought to be associated with the pharmacologic mechanism of HMG-CoA reductase inhibition. In a study in rabbits, lovastatin-induced hepatotoxicity could be prevented by pretreatment with mevalonate.[30]

Transient elevations of creatine kinase (CK) levels above the usual laboratory reference range with or without muscle symptoms occurred with equal frequency in the lovastatin-treated and placebo-treated patients in the EXCEL study.[23] Muscle symptoms with a CK level of more than 10 times the upper limits of normal occurred at a frequency of 0.1% at the 40-mg dose and 0.2% at the 80-mg dose. Rhabdomyolysis with renal failure was not observed during the 2-year trial. Thus, the incidence of myopathy is rare when lovastatin is used alone. The risk of myopathy is mildly increased when lovastatin is used in combination with gemfibrozil ($\pm 5\%$) or niacin ($\pm 2\%$) and substantially increased to approximately 30% when used with cyclosporine.[31] It has also been described with the concomitant use of erythromycin. Some of the affected patients had preexisting renal disease, often as a result of long-standing diabetes. If lovastatin therapy is used in conjunction with niacin, gemfibrozil, or cyclosporine, careful monitoring of the symptoms of muscle pain, tenderness, or weakness should be done as well as more frequent evaluations of CK levels. Lovastatin should not be used with these drugs in the setting of renal dysfunction. In the transplant patient receiving cyclosporine, lovastatin therapy should be withheld in any situation that might predispose the development of renal failure or if a systemic antifungal agent (azol derivative) is used. These situations appear to increase the risk of myositis and rhabdomyolysis in this group of patients.

Preclinical studies with high doses of lovastatin given for prolonged periods produced cataracts in beagle dogs, and there was initial concern that this might also occur in humans. However, in multiple studies, including the EXCEL study,[32] the 5-year lovastatin safety and efficacy study,[25] and a study using sophisticated photographic techniques to quantify changes in the lens,[33] there has not been a greater incidence of cataracts in lovastatin-treated patients compared with either placebo-treated or age-matched controls. As a result, an earlier recommendation for annual slit-lamp examinations has been removed from the package circular. Some initial noncontrolled studies suggested that lovastatin, by virtue of its lipid solubility, might cause insomnia. However, in controlled sleep laboratory studies, no such effect has been observed.[34, 35] In the 8000-patient EXCEL study, insomnia occurred at the same frequency in the lovastatin- and placebo-treated groups.[23]

Although the 5-year lovastatin safety and efficacy study was not a controlled study, the number of cancer cases was not more than expected based on the National Cancer Institute cancer incidence rates for the general United States population.[25]

Contraindications

As lovastatin exerts its major effect in, and is catabolized and excreted by, the liver, subjects with significant preexisting liver disease should not be administered lovastatin or other HMG-CoA reductase inhibitors. In patients with severe renal insufficiency (creatinine clearance, < 30 ml/min), the dose of lovastatin should probably not exceed 20 mg/day. In patients with this degree of renal dysfunction, plasma concentrations of the drug are increased. Lovastatin is contraindicated in pregnant or lactating women. It should be given to women of childbearing age with the understanding that the woman has no plans to get pregnant. If the woman should become pregnant while receiving treatment with lovastatin, it should be discontinued immediately. The safety and efficacy of lovastatin has not yet been established in children or adolescents, and thus treatment with HMG-CoA reductase inhibitors in these age groups is not generally recommended.

Drug Interactions

Clinical trials have not shown reduced LDL efficacy when lovastatin is coadministered with a bile acid sequestrant. However, optimally, the bile acid sequestrant should be given with the evening meal and lovastatin given at bedtime.

Propranolol has been demonstrated to reduce the systemic bioavailability of lovastatin most likely by slowing hepatic blood flow. This may result in an increased first-pass hepatic extraction of lovastatin. Whether this has any impact on lovastatin's lipid-lowering effect has not been established.[36] In patients receiving warfarin, lovastatin produced no effect on prothrombin times. However, with simvastatin, another HMG-CoA reductase inhibitor, slight increases in prothrombin times have been reported. In patients taking anticoagulants, prothrombin times should be measured after initiation of lovastatin therapy. There are no known interactions with digoxin, oral hypoglycemic agents, calcium antagonists, diuretics, and nonsteroidal antiinflammatory drugs.

No known interference with other agents has been reported.

Combination with Other Lipid-Lowering Agents

With the current NCEP guidelines recommending more vigorous control of LDL-C levels, it is often necessary to use more than one lipid-lowering agent simultaneously. Therapy should always commence with monotherapy before progressing to two- and finally three-drug combinations. Combination drug therapy may be advantageous for combined hyperlipidemias when hypercholesterolemia is present in addition to hypertriglyceridemia and/or a low HDL-C level. Often, adequate lipid control can be achieved using two or more drugs at lower doses, if intolerable side effects are present at higher doses of lovastatin alone.

For additional LDL-C lowering, a bile acid sequestrant or niacin, or both, can be added to lovastatin or other HMG-CoA reductase inhibitors. Triple therapy with these three drug classes is often necessary to treat patients with familial hypercholesterolemia, in whom baseline LDL-C levels are often higher than 250 mg/dl. For combination hyperlipidemias, lovastatin can be combined with immediate-release niacin or lower-dose fibrates. The combination of these medications with the increased risk of myositis should be carefully considered, especially because no controlled trials have yet demonstrated clinical benefit. If the combination is used, it is recommended that reduced doses of one or both agents are appropriate and that clinical symptoms, liver function, and CK levels be carefully monitored.

Dosage and Administration

In patients with no contraindications to lovastatin, treatment is usually started with 20 mg/day and, if necessary, is increased at 4- to 8-week intervals to a maximum of 80 mg/day. At the 40-mg and 80-mg doses, the drug is minimally more effective given in divided dosages.[23, 37] However, this slight benefit is outweighed by the inconvenience, and adequate efficacy can be achieved using lovastatin once a day. When given once a day, it is more effective when taken in the evening. This might be due to the diurnal variation in cholesterol synthesis, with more HMG-CoA reductase activity occurring during the nighttime hours. Higher plasma concentrations of the drug are achieved when lovastatin is given with meals. However, in clinical practice this benefit is minimal, and lovastatin can be taken without food if it is more convenient. The LDL-C–lowering effect of lovastatin is additive to a low-fat diet. In the diet lovastatin study,[38] 20 mg of lovastatin given in conjunction with a low-fat diet lowered LDL-C by 32%, whereas the same dose in the same group of patients lowered LDL-C by 23% when given with a high-fat diet.

As with all the other HMG-CoA reductase inhibitors, lovastatin demonstrates a decreasing dose-response curve. Thus, more LDL-C lowering per milligram of drug is achieved at the lower doses. The LDL-C–lowering effects are manifest within 2 weeks, with maximal reduction apparent 4 to 6 weeks after beginning therapy.

The drug is supplied as 10-mg, 20-mg, or 40-mg tablets. The usual starting dose is 20 mg; however, in some patients in whom metabolism may be compromised or the baseline LDL-C is only mildly elevated, the 10-mg dose may be more appropriate. In patients receiving concomitant cyclosporine therapy, plasma drug levels of lovastatin are increased,[22] predisposing to the development of myositis, rhabdomyolysis, and renal failure. In these situations, the 10-mg dose of lovastatin is the preferable dose.

SOCIOECONOMIC CONSIDERATIONS
Compliance

Lovastatin is extremely well tolerated, and all clinical studies have demonstrated compliance to dosage schedules in excess of 90%. Although there is slightly more LDL-C reduction with b.i.d. versus q.p.m. dosing of the same daily total dose, the added inconvenience is not considered clinically important. Thus, in clinical practice, single dosing (preferably with the evening meal) is recommended. Postmarketing studies have been conducted that have been at variance with long-term controlled studies in terms of continued adherence to therapy. In the 5-year lovastatin safety and efficacy study,[25] approximately 80% of subjects were still taking their prescribed dose of lovastatin. This contrasts with postmarketing observations that, 1 year after lovastatin or other HMG-CoA reductase inhibitors were prescribed, fewer than 50% of subjects continued to take these agents. As described previously, the side effects associated with lovastatin are relatively few, and other causes for poor compliance may be important. These include poor understanding by the patient of the need for long-term therapy, failure of the physician to schedule follow-up or provide feedback as to response, and the cost of continued therapy.

Cost

The cost of therapy is related to dose. The most common dose used, 20 mg daily, which is prescribed to approximately 60% of lovastatin-treated subjects, costs approximately $45.00 per month. The 40-mg daily dose prescribed to a further 30% of treated subjects costs approximately $90.00 per month, irrespective of whether one 40-mg or two 20-mg tablets are taken. For severely affected hypercholesterolemic subjects, such as those with heterozygous familial hypercholesterolemia (FH) who require 80 mg a day of lovastatin, the cost approaches $180.00 monthly. For these subjects, as much, or more, LDL-C lowering can be achieved with 40 mg a day of simvastatin, a chemically modified lovastatin molecule, for less than half the cost.

In order to provide the most cost-effective LDL-C–lowering therapy, it is recommended that lower doses of lovastatin, such as 20 mg daily, be combined with low-dose bile acid sequestrant (cholestyramine, 4 or 8 g, or colestipol, 5 or 10 g daily). Clinical studies indicate that not only more actual LDL-C reduction is produced but also the cost per mg/dl LDL-C reduction is lower than with high-dose HMG-CoA reductase inhibitor therapy.[39]

REFERENCES

1. Alberts AW, Chen J, Kuron G, et al: Mevinolin: A highly potent competitive inhibitor of hydroxy methyl glutaryl coenzyme A reductase and a cholesterol lowering agent. Proc Natl Acad Sci 77:3957, 1980.
2. Endo A, Kuroda M, Tanzawa K: Competitive inhibition of 3 hydroxy 3 methyl glutaryl coenzyme A reductase by ML-236A and ML-236B fungal metabolites having hypocholesterolemic activity. FEBS Lett 72:323, 1976.
3. National Cholesterol Education Program: Second report of the Expert Panel on Detection, Evaluation, and Treatment of High Blood Cholesterol (Adult Treatment Panel II). Circulation 89:1329, 1994.
4. Prevention of coronary heart disease: Scientific background and new clinical guidelines: Recommendations of the European Atherosclerosis Society prepared by the International Task Force for Prevention of Coronary Heart Disease. Nutr Metab Cardiovasc Dis 2:113, 1992.
5. Brown GE, Albers JJ, Fisher LD, et al: Niacin or lovastatin combined with colestipol regresses coronary atherosclerosis and prevents clinical events in men with evaluated apolipoprotein B. N Engl J Med 323:1289, 1990.
6. Waters D, Higginson L, Gladstone P, et al: Effects of monotherapy with an HMG-CoA reductase inhibitor on the progression of coronary atherosclerosis as assessed by serial quantitative arteriography. Circulation 89:959, 1994.
7. Blankenhorn DH, Azen SP, Kramsch DM, et al: Coronary angiographic changes with lovastatin therapy: The Monitored Atherosclerosis Regression Study (MARS). Ann Intern Med 119:969, 1993.
8. Alberts AW: HMG-CoA reductase inhibitors—the development. Atherosclerosis Rev 18:123, 1988.
9. Goldstein JL, Brown MS: Progress in understanding the LDL receptor and HMG-CoA reductase, two membrane proteins that regulate the plasma cholesterol. J Lipid Res 25:1450, 1984.
10. Haruyama H, Kuwano H, Kinoshita T, et al: Structure elucidation of the bioactive metabolites of ML-236B (mevastatin) isolated from dog urine. Chem Pharm Bull 34:1459, 1986.
11. Duggan DE, Chen HN, Bayne WF, et al: The physiological disposition of lovastatin. Drug Metab Dispos 17:166, 1989.
12. Pentikainon PJ, Saraheimo M, Schwartz JI, et al: Comparative pharmacokinetics of lovastatin, simvastatin, and pravastatin in humans. J Clin Pharmacol 32:136, 1992.
13. Cheng H, Rogers JD, Sweany AE, et al: Influence of age and gender on the plasma profiles of 3 hydroxy 3 methyl glutaryl coenzyme A (HMG-CoA) reductase inhibitory activity following multiple doses of lovastatin and simvastatin. Pharm Res 9:1629, 1992.
14. Illingworth DR, Corbin D: The influence of mevinolin on the adrenal cortical response to corticotropin in heterozygote familial hypercholesterolemia. Proc Natl Acad Sci U S A 82:6291, 1985.
15. Farnsworth WH, Hoeg JM, Maher M, et al: Testicular function in type II hyperlipoproteinemic patients treated with lovastatin (mevinolin) or neomycin. J Clin Endocrinol Metab 65:546, 1987.
16. Healy B: Endothelial cell dysfunction: An emerging endocrinology linked to coronary disease. J Am Coll Cardiol 16:357, 1990.
17. Celemajer DS, Sornen KE, Gooch VM, et al: Non-invasive detection of endothelial dysfunction in children and adults at risk of atherosclerosis. Lancet 340:1111, 1992.
18. Anderson TJ, Meredith IT, Yeung AL, et al: Cholesterol-lowering therapy improves endothelial function in patient with coronary atherosclerosis [abstract]. Circulation 88:I-368, 1993.
19. Egashira K, Hirooka Y, Kai H, et al: Reduction in serum choles-

terol with pravastatin improves endothelial dependent coronary vasomotion in patients with hypercholesterolemia. Circulation 89:2519, 1994.

20. Leung WH, Lau CP, Wong CK: Beneficial effect of cholesterol-lowering therapy on coronary endothelium-dependent relaxation in hypercholesterolemic patients. Lancet 341:1496, 1993.

21. Gould KL, Martucci JP, Goldberg DI, et al: Short-term cholesterol-lowering decreases size and severity of perfusion abnormalities by positron emission tomography after dipyridamole in patients with coronary artery disease. Circulation 89:1530, 1994.

22. Isaacsohn JL, Setaro JF, Nicholas C, et al: Effects of lovastatin therapy on plasminogen activator inhibitor-1 antigen levels. Am J Cardiol 74:735, 1994.

23. Bradford RH, Shear CL, Chremos AN, et al: Expanded Clinical Evaluation of Lovastatin (EXCEL) Study results. Arch Intern Med 151:43, 1991.

24. Bradford RH, Shear CL, Chremos AN, et al: Expanded Clinical Evaluation of Lovastatin (EXCEL) Study results: Two year efficacy and safety follow-up. Am J Cardiol 74:667, 1994.

25. Lovastatin Study Group I through IV: Lovastatin 5-year safety and efficacy study. Arch Intern Med 153:1079, 1993.

26. Kane JP, Malloy MJ, Ports TA, et al: Regression of coronary atherosclerosis during treatment of familial hypercholesterolemia with combined drug regimens. JAMA 264:3007, 1990.

27. Havel RJ, Hunninghake DB, Illingworth DR, et al: Lovastatin (mevinolin) in the treatment of heterozygous familial hypercholesterolemia. Ann Intern Med 107:609, 1987.

28. Lovastatin Study Group II: Therapeutic response to lovastatin (mevinolin) in non-familial hypercholesterolemia. JAMA 256:2829, 1986.

29. Garg A, Grundy SM: Lovastatin lowering cholesterol levels in non-insulin dependent diabetes mellitus. N Engl J Med 318:81, 1988.

30. Kornbrust DJ, MacDonald JS, Peter CP, et al: Toxicity of the HMG-CoA reductase inhibitor, lovastatin, to rabbits. J Pharmacol Exp Ther 248:498, 1989.

31. Tobert JA: Letter. N Engl J Med 318:48, 1988.

32. Laties AM, Shear LL, Lippa EA, et al: Expanded Clinical Evaluation of Lovastatin (EXCEL) Sudy: Results II. Assessment of human lens after 48 weeks of treatment with lovastatin. Am J Cardiol 67:447, 1991.

33. Friend J, Chylack LT, Khu P, et al: Lack of human cataractogenic potential of lovastatin: Results of 3-year study [abstract]. Invest Ophthalmol Vis Sci 33:1301, 1992.

34. Vgontzas AN, Kales A, Bixler EO, et al: Effects of lovastatin and pravastatin on sleep efficiency and sleep stages. Clin Pharmacol Ther 50:730, 1991.

35. Black DM, Lamkin G, Olivera EH, et al: Sleep disturbances and HMG-CoA reductase inhibitors [letter]. JAMA 264:1105, 1990.

36. Pan HY, Triscari J, DeVault AR, et al: Pharmacokinetic interaction between propranolol and the HMG-CoA reductase inhibitors pravastatin and lovastatin. Br J Clin Pharmacol 31:605, 1991.

37. Illingworth DR: Comparative efficacy of once versus twice daily mevinolin in the therapy of familial hypercholesterolemia. Clin Pharmacol Ther 40:338, 1986.

38. Hunninghake DB, Stein EA, Dujovne CA, et al: The efficacy of intensive dietary therapy alone or combined with lovastatin in outpatients with hypercholesterolemia. N Engl J Med 328:1213, 1993.

39. Schrott HG, Stein EA, Dujovne CA, et al: Enhanced low-density lipoprotein cholesterol reduction and cost effectiveness by low-dose colestipol plus lovastatin combination therapy. Am J Cardiol 75:34, 1995.

CHAPTER 122

Simvastatin*

M. Lytken Larsen, M.D., and D. Roger Illingworth, M.D., Ph.D.

HISTORY

Simvastatin is a recently developed competitive inhibitor of 3-hydroxy-3-methylglutaryl coenzyme A (HMG-CoA) reductase, the rate-limiting enzyme in cholesterol biosynthesis. The first compound of this type, mevastatin (originally called compactin), was isolated from extracts of *Penicillium citrinum* in 1976 by Endo et al.[1] An analogue of mevastatin called lovastatin (originally called mevinolin) was isolated from the soil fungus *Aspergillus terreus*. Simvastatin is a methylated derivative of lovastatin and differs structurally from mevastatin by two additional methyl groups and from lovastatin by one (Fig. 122–1). Simvastatin was first approved for prescription use in Sweden in 1988 and has been available in the United States since 1991. It is marketed under the trade name Zocor (Merck & Co.).

CHEMISTRY

Simvastatin is chemically [lS-[1α,3α,7β,8β(2S*,4S*), 8αβ]]-1,2,3,7,8,8a-hexahydro-3,7-dimethyl-8-[2-(tetra-hydro-4-hydroxy-6-oxo-2H-pyran-2-yl)ethyl]-1-naphtalenyl 2,2-dimethylbutanoate. The empirical formula of simvastatin is $C_{25}H_{38}O_5$, and its molecular weight is 418.57. The structural formula is shown in Figure 122–1.

PHARMACOLOGY

The conversion of HMG-CoA to mevalonate is an early step in the biosynthetic pathway of cholesterol and is catalyzed by the enzyme HMG-CoA reductase. Simvastatin is a specific competitive inhibitor of HMG-CoA reductase with an extremely high affinity for the enzyme.[2] Inhibition of HMG-CoA reductase reduces the conversion of HMG-CoA to mevalonic acid and ultimately leads to a reduction in the biosynthesis of cholesterol. Simvastatin acts primarily in the liver, where this inhibition of cholesterol biosynthesis results in an increased expression of high-affinity low-density lipoprotein (LDL) receptors present on hepatocyte membranes and, concurrently, a reduction in the biosynthesis of very-low-density lipoproteins (VLDL). This results in a reduction in the plasma concentrations of LDL, which is attributable to both

This work was supported in part by National Institutes of Health Grant RR334 from the General Clinical Research Centers Program and by a grant from the Danish Heart Foundation.

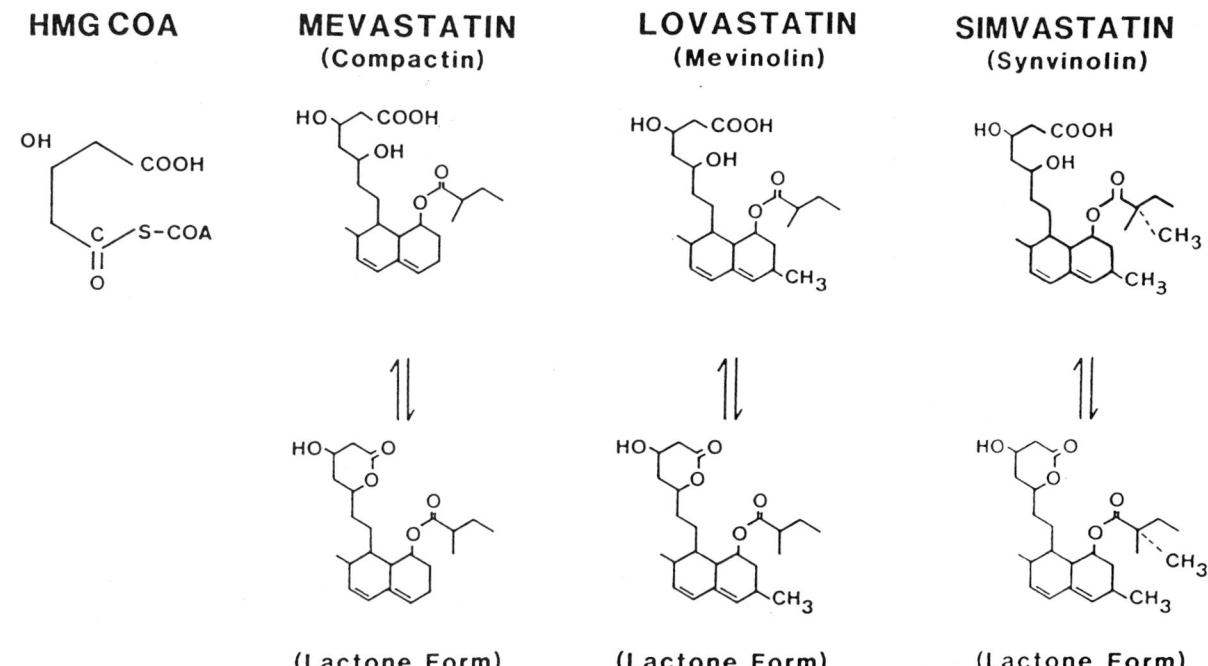

Figure 122–1. The structures of simvastatin and related HMG-CoA reductase inhibitors and the structure of HMG-CoA. Simvastatin is administered as the lactone form, and conversion to the active inhibitor occurs primarily in the liver (see text).

an increase in LDL catabolism, mediated by the increased expression of LDL receptors, and a concurrent reduction in VLDL and LDL synthesis.[3]

PHARMACOKINETICS

Very little information has been published in the literature that addresses the pharmacokinetics of simvastatin,[4] and most of the currently available data come from the manufacturer. Simvastatin is a prodrug with an inactive lactone ring; after oral administration, it is well absorbed from the gastrointestinal tract and is efficiently extracted by the liver, where hydrolysis of the lactone ring produces the active inhibitor (open acid) form of the drug (see Fig. 122–1). Hagemenas et al.[5] determined the time course of appearance of ^{14}C-simvastatin and metabolites in the plasma of four patients with heterozygous familial hypercholesterolemia each of whom received a single oral dose of 100 mg simvastatin (Fig. 122–2). ^{14}C-simvastatin (and metabolite) concentrations increased rapidly in plasma after oral administration of simvastatin, and peak levels occurred after 4 hours.[5] Simvastatin seems to reach the liver very quickly; in dogs, only 7% of the oral dose reached the general circulation.[6] In the liver, simvastatin is metabolized by the cytochrome P-450 system[7] and converted to several active metabolites. The metabolites are concentrated primarily in the liver, and, on the basis of animal studies,[6, 8] only a very small proportion of them leave the liver and are distributed to other organs. Simvastatin metabolites are mainly eliminated via biliary excretion and subsequent fecal elimination; after an oral dose of ^{14}C-labeled simvastatin in humans, 13% of the dose was excreted in the urine and 60% in the feces (manufacturer's information).

EFFECTS OF PATHOPHYSIOLOGY: ENDOCRINE AND METABOLIC EFFECTS
Effects on Lipid Metabolism

At clinically effective doses (10 to 40 mg/day), simvastatin has been shown to reduce the rate of formation of mevalonic acid by 25% to 35%.[5] Reduced formation of mevalonic acid leads to a corresponding decrease in hepatic cholesterol synthesis and a reduction in the cellular pool of cholesterol. This leads to a compensatory increase in the number of high-affinity LDL receptors expressed on the cell surface that, in turn, stimulate an increase in receptor-mediated catabolism of VLDL remnants, chylomicron remnants, and LDL.[5, 9, 10] Hepatic synthesis of VLDL and LDL may be reduced concurrently in response to therapy with an HMG-CoA reductase inhibitor.[11, 12] Treatment with simvastatin does not reduce plasma concentrations of lipoprotein(a), whereas recent studies indicate that this drug may reduce the oxidizability of LDL by altering its composition.[13, 14]

Other Metabolic Effects

Simvastatin interferes with cholesterol synthesis and could, theoretically, impair the adrenal and gonadal production of steroid hormones. Clinical studies have clearly demonstrated, however, that at the maximum dose (40 mg/day) simvastatin does not reduce basal

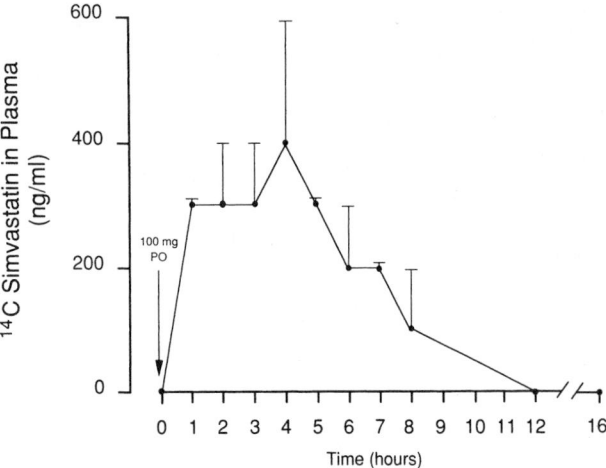

Figure 122–2. Time course of appearance of ¹⁴C-labeled simvastatin in plasma after oral administration. Data are mean ± S.E. values from four patients with familial hypercholesterolemia who each received a single oral dose of 100 mg ¹⁴C-labeled simvastatin at 8:00 AM after an overnight fast. All four patients had normal renal and hepatic function, and none was taking simvastatin on a chronic basis at the time of this pharmacokinetic study. (From Hagemenas FC, Pappu AS, Illingworth DR: The effects of simvastatin on plasma lipoproteins and cholesterol homeostasis in patients with heterozygous familial hypercholesterolemia. Eur J Clin Invest 20:150, 1990.)

plasma concentrations of cortisol or testosterone or impair the adrenal response to prolonged (24-hour) adrenocorticotropic hormone (ACTH) stimulation.[15, 16] The effects of simvastatin on fibrinogen levels have been variable; whereas one study showed a small decrease during treatment with simvastatin,[17] another report found an insignificant decrease (from 315 mg/dl to 289 mg/dl) in 23 patients treated with this drug.[18] Changes in glucose metabolism in nondiabetics have not been reported, and the drug does not influence insulin needs in patients with diabetes.

CLINICAL USE
Indications

Dietary modification, with restriction of saturated fats and cholesterol, represents the initial therapy for all patients with primary causes of hyperlipidemia, including those who will eventually require drug therapy. The recently published revised guidelines from the National Cholesterol Education Program[19] continue to identify LDL cholesterol as the primary target for hypolipidemic drug therapy to reduce the risk of premature coronary artery disease in the primary prevention setting or, in patients with established disease, potentially promote regression and prevent further progression of the atherosclerotic process. Treatment with simvastatin has been demonstrated recently to retard progression of atherosclerosis assessed angiographically at 2 and 4 years after institution of therapy in the Multicentre Antiatheroma Study (MAAS)[19a] and, in a landmark study, the Scandinavian Simvastatin Survival Study, to reduce total and cardiovascular mortality.[19b] In the MAAS Study,[19a]

treatment with simvastatin at a dose of 20 mg/day reduced LDL cholesterol concentations by 31%, and, compared with patients receiving a matched placebo, treatment with simvastatin was associated with a reduced rate of formation of new coronary lesions and resulted in retardation of progression or, in some patients, regression of coronary atherosclerosis assessed by sequential quantitative coronary angiography. In the most definitive study to address the benefits of cholesterol-lowering therapy (the Scandinavian Simvastatin Survival Study), treatment with simvastatin at doses of 20 or 40 mg/day in 2221 patients with known coronary artery disease was found to reduce total mortality by 30% during a mean treatment period of 5.4 years as compared with a group of similar patients treated with diet and placebo.[19b] This benefit in total mortality was attributable to a 42% reduction in deaths from coronary heart disease, and this reduction in total mortality was paralleled by reductions in all cardiovascular end points in the patients treated with simvastatin. In this study, mean concentrations of LDL cholesterol were reduced by 35%, and there was no increase in noncardiovascular causes of death or other unexpected side effects. The benefit of treatment became greater with increasing duration of therapy, and benefit was seen in both men and women as well as in subjects of different ages and, most importantly, across a wide range of cholesterol concentations (from 212 to 309 mg/dl). On the basis of this study, drug treatment with simvastatin in addition to diet can be advocated for patients with known coronary artery disease who also have increased plasma concentrations of LDL cholesterol, either in isolation or in the presence of mild hypertriglyceridemia. Simvastatin, as the most effective of the currently available HMG-CoA reductase inhibitors, can also be recommended as the drug of choice for patients with severe primary hypercholesterolemia in the absence of concurrent coronary artery disease.

Primary Hypercholesterolemia

The hypolipidemic effects of simvastatin are dose dependent, and proportionally greater decreases in the concentration of total and LDL cholesterol per milligram of drug administered are observed in response to the first 5 to 10 mg/day.

In patients with familial hypercholesterolemia, simvastatin at doses of 10, 20, and 40 mg/day has been shown to reduce plasma concentrations of LDL cholesterol by 28%, 30%, and 37%, respectively.[20] Other studies[18, 20–24] have shown similar or somewhat greater efficacy but confirm the view that at the maximal approved dose of simvastatin (40 mg/day) mean reductions of 35% to 45% in the plasma concentration of LDL cholesterol can be obtained. The reduction in LDL cholesterol is generally associated with a 10% to 30% decrease in plasma triglycerides and an overall tendency for HDL cholesterol to increase by 2% to 15% in patients with heterozygous familial hypercholesterolemia, familial combined hyperlipidemia, familial defective apolipoprotein B-100, and other less well characterized disorders.[18, 20-24] In adult patients with severe hypercholesterolemia, particularly those with heterozygous familial hypercholesterolemia, the combination of simvastatin and a bile acid sequestrant (e.g., cholestyramine) enhances the hypolipidemic effects seen with simvastatin as monotherapy, and this combination has been reported to reduce LDL concentrations by 54% to 64% in this patient population.[25, 26] This combination is physiologically attractive and combines one systemically acting drug with a nonabsorbable anion exchange resin. Combined therapy with simvastatin and other cholesterol-lowering drugs cannot be generally recommended, and such therapy should be undertaken only for highly selected patients who are likely to be seen and monitored by consultants or in centers specializing in disorders of lipid metabolism. This caution is based on the increased risk of toxicity associated with combinations that use simvastatin with either fibrates or nicotinic acid.[27]

Combined Hyperlipidemia

Simvastatin has proved useful in the treatment of patients with combined hyperlipidemia (e.g., due to familial combined hyperlipidemia) in which plasma concentrations of VLDL and LDL are increased or in patients with type III hyperlipidemia, in whom VLDL remnant particles accumulate in plasma. The effects of simvastatin have been investigated in patients with combined hyperlipidemia, and the drug has been shown to reduce plasma concentrations of LDL cholesterol by 25% to 45%; these changes have been accompanied by a decrease in plasma triglycerides of 30% to 50% and an increase in HDL cholesterol of 5% to 10%.[28, 29] The efficacy of simvastatin in patients with type III hyperlipidemia was evaluated by Feussner et al.;[30] in this study, plasma concentrations of cholesterol and triglycerides were reduced by 39.3% and 41.8%, respectively, in 19 patients treated with simvastatin at a dose of 20 mg/day. These changes were accompanied by a reduction in the plasma concentrations of VLDL and LDL; when a subset of the patients were treated with 40 mg/day of simvastatin, a further reduction of 22% in the concentration of LDL cholesterol was observed. These studies indicate that simvastatin is the drug of choice in patients with combined hyperlipidemia and exerts favorable changes on the plasma concentrations of individual lipoproteins.

Secondary Dyslipidemia

One of the most common secondary causes of dyslipidemia is by diabetes. Simvastatin has been shown to be useful in the treatment of selected patients with hyperlipidemia associated with diabetes mellitus in whom LDL concentrations were increased. Reductions of 25% to 40% in the plasma concentrations of LDL cholesterol have been reported in both insulin-dependent and non-insulin-dependent diabetics with or without diabetic nephropathy.[31-34]

Another secondary dyslipidemia is that observed in patients with renal insufficiency or nephrotic syndrome and those on hemodialysis. These patients also respond to treatment with simvastatin.[35]

PRECAUTIONS AND ADVERSE EFFECTS

Before initiation of therapy with any hypolipidemic drug, including simvastatin, secondary causes for hyperlipidemia (e.g., poorly controlled diabetes, hypothyroidism, nephrotic syndrome, dysproteinemias, obstructive liver disease, other drug therapy, or alcoholism) should be excluded. Long-term experience with simvastatin now extends from 5 to 7 years and continues to indicate that it is an efficacious and well-tolerated drug (Table 122–1) with few significant adverse effects.[22, 23] These include nausea, fatigue, insomnia, myalgias, headaches, changes in bowel function, and skin rashes. Less common but clinically important side effects include myopathy[36, 37] and elevations in liver enzyme levels. Myopathy is uncommon ($<0.1\%$) during monotherapy but appears to be dose dependent and is more common in combination therapy with cyclosporine, nicotinic acid, fibrates, or erythromycin. Dose-dependent elevations in liver enzymes to values greater than three times the upper limit of normal have been reported in 1% of patients taking simvastatin,[22] but these increases are usually transient and asymptomatic. It is, however, recommended that liver function tests and, if indicated, creatine kinase measurements be monitored at 6- to 8-week intervals during the first 6 to 12 months of therapy and three to four times yearly thereafter. The initial concerns that simvastatin may cause cataracts in humans necessitated regular slit-lamp examinations of the lens to monitor patients maintained on this drug; fortunately, no increased frequency of lenticular opacities has been demonstrated,[22] and annual slit-lamp examinations are no longer advised for patients treated with HMG-CoA reductase inhibitors.

Table 122–1. **Plasma Lipids and Lipoproteins at Baseline (on Diet) and After 7 Years of Treatment with Simvastatin Alone or in Combination with a Second Lipid-Lowering Drug**

	Baseline	Drug Treatment	Change	p
Total cholesterol (mg/dL)	351 ± 59	248 ± 44	−29%	<.001
LDL cholesterol (mg/dL)	265 ± 64	154 ± 45	−42%	<.001
HDL cholesterol (mg/dL)	53 ± 14	56 ± 17	+6%	ns
Triglycerides (mg/dL)	157 ± 83	184 ± 92	+17%	ns

Results are mean ± SD. ns, not significant.
The results are from 19 patients with primary hypercholesterolemia treated with simvastatin alone (n = 14) or in combination with a bile acid sequestrant (n = 3) or niacin (n = 2).

CONTRAINDICATIONS

Simvastatin is contraindicated in patients who are pregnant, those with known hypersensitivity to the drug, and those with cholestasis or other disorders associated with a potential impairment in the hepatic metabolism and excretion of simvastatin. The drug should be regarded as relatively contraindicated in patients with preexisting elevations in hepatic transaminase levels. Therapy should temporarily be withheld from any patient experiencing an acute or serious condition predisposing to the development of renal failure (e.g., sepsis; hypotension; major surgery; trauma; severe metabolic, endocrine, or electrolyte disorder; or uncontrolled epilepsy). Data on the safety of simvastatin during pregnancy and lactation are not available, and simvastatin should be administered to women of childbearing potential only when they are highly unlikely to conceive, and the drug should be promptly discontinued in any woman who conceives while taking it. Data on the safety and efficacy of simvastatin in pediatric patients with hypercholesterolemia are meager; use of this drug in the pediatric population should be regarded as investigational and cannot be generally recommended.

INTERFERENCE WITH OTHER DRUGS

Because simvastatin is metabolized by the cytochrome P-450 system, a potential for interactions with many other drugs may exist.[7] To date, however, very few drug interactions with simvastatin have been reported. Elevated concentrations of reductase inhibitors have been observed when this class of drugs, including simvastatin, has been administered concurrently with cyclosporine. Evidence indicates that the plasma concentrations of reductase inhibitors are increased approximately fourfold in this situation; this indicates that, in patients receiving simvastatin, the maximal dose should be 10 mg/day. An initial starting dose of simvastatin of 2.5 or 5 mg/day is recommended in patients who are already receiving cyclosporine. A combination of simvastatin and warfarin therapy has been associated with enhanced warfarin activity.[38] Administration of a single dose of digoxin to healthy male volunteers receiving simvastatin resulted in a slight elevation (<0.3 ng/ml) in digoxin concentrations in plasma; consequently, patients taking digoxin should be monitored appropriately when therapy with simvastatin is initiated.[38]

DOSAGE AND ADMINISTRATION

The magnitude of LDL reduction observed in individual patients treated with the same dose of simvastatin varies quite widely. It is therefore reasonable to start with a fairly low dose of the drug with the prospect that, in severely hypercholesterolemic patients, the dose will have to be increased during the course of therapeutic monitoring. In patients with normal renal and hepatic function, an initial dose of 5 to 20 mg of simvastatin once daily in the evening is recommended; for maintenance, the range is from 5 to no more than 40 mg/day. The daily dose can be given all at once,[20–22] but a significantly greater cholesterol reduction was observed when the single dose was given in the evening rather than in the morning.[39]

Information from controlled trials with the available HMG-CoA reductase inhibitors shows the dose-dependent effect of these drugs. These data also indicate that on a milligram-for-milligram basis lovastatin and pravastatin are of approximately equal efficacy in their ability to reduce concentrations of LDL cholesterol, whereas simvastatin is twice as potent (Table 122–2).[20, 40–45]

In patients with renal insufficiency, the recommended starting dose of simvastatin is 5 mg/day. Pharmacokinetic or pharmacodynamic studies of this dosage, however, have not been reported in this patient population.[4] In a group of cardiac transplant patients receiving cyclosporine and simvastatin (10 mg/day), no cases of renal toxicity or myotoxicity were observed during 8 months of follow-up.[46]

SOCIOECONOMIC CONSIDERATIONS

The decision to use drugs in the treatment of hyperlipidemia normally is a long-term, potentially lifelong commitment. To be effective, the goals of such therapy should be clear to both the physician and the patient before the initiation of treatment. In the expe-

Table 122–2. **Comparative Hypolipidemic Effects of HMG-CoA Reductase Inhibitors* in Patients with Heterozygous Familial Hypercholesterolemia**

| Daily Dose (mg) | Percentage Decrease in LDL Cholesterol | | | | | |
| | Lovastatin | | Simvastatin | | Pravastatin | |
	a	b	c	d	e	f
10	20 (13)	17 (20)	28 (8)	ND	ND	ND
20	28 (13)	25 (20)	30 (40)	38 (10)	21 (40)	ND
40	35 (13)	31 (20)	37 (7)	44 (10)	28 (40)	30 (43)
80	38 (13)	40 (20)	—	—	—	—

*Drugs were given twice daily.
HMG-CoA, hydroxymethylglutaryl coenzyme A; LDL, low-density lipoprotein; ND, not determined.
a, Illingworth and Sexton[41]; b, Havel et al.[42]; c, Mol et al[20]; d, Illingworth and Bacon[43]; e, Wiklund et al.[44]; f, Betteridge et al.[45] The numbers in parentheses refer to the number of patients studied on each dose of drug.

rience of the authors, patient compliance with simvastatin is excellent, and the drug has a remarkable profile of clinical efficacy and a low incidence of side effects.

REFERENCES

1. Endo A, Kuroda M, Tsujita Y: ML-236A, ML-236B, and ML-236C, new inhibitors of cholesterogenesis produced by Penicillium citrinum. J Antibiot 29:1346, 1976.
2. Hoffman WF, Alberts AW, Anderson PS, et al: 3-Hydroxy-3-methylglutaryl coenzyme A reductase inhibitors: 4. Side chain ester derivatives of mevinolin. J Med Chem 28:849, 1986.
3. Grundy SM: HMG-CoA reductase inhibitors: Clinical applications and therapeutical potential. In Rifkind BM (ed): Drug Treatment of Hyperlipidemia. New York: Marcel Dekker, 1991, pp 139–168.
4. Mauro VF: Clinical pharmacokinetics and practical applications of simvastatin. Clin Pharmakokinet 24:195, 1993.
5. Hagemenas FC, Pappu AS, Illingworth DR: The effects of simvastatin on plasma lipoproteins and cholesterol homeostasis in patients with heterozygous familial hypercholesterolaemia. Eur J Clin Invest 20:150, 1990.
6. Vickers S, Duncan CA, Chen I, et al: Metabolic disposition studies on simvastatin, a cholesterol-lowering prodrug. Drug Metab Dispos 18:138, 1990.
7. Vyas KP, Kari PH, Pitzenberger SM: Regioselectivity and stereoselectivity in the metabolism of HMG-CoA reductase inhibitors. Biochem Biophys Res Commun 166:1155, 1990.
8. Germershausen JI, Hunt VM, Bostedor RG, et al: Tissue selectivity of the cholesterol-lowering agents lovastatin, simvastatin and pravastatin in rats in vivo. Biochem Biophys Res Commun 158:667, 1989.
9. Brown MS, Goldstein JL: A receptor mediated pathway for cholesterol homeostasis. Science 232:34, 1986.
10. Cabezas MC, de Bruin TW, Kock LA, et al: Simvastatin improves chylomicron remnant removal in familial combined hyperlipidemia without changing chylomicron conversion. Metabolism 42:497, 1993.
11. Ginsberg HN, Le NA, Short MP, et al: Suppression of apolipoprotein B production during treatment of cholesteryl ester storage disease with lovastatin: Implications for regulation of apolipoprotein B synthesis. J Clin Invest 80:1692, 1987.
12. Reihne E, Rudling M, Stalberg D, et al: Influence of pravastatin, a specific inhibitor of HMG-CoA reductase, on hepatic metabolism of cholesterol. N Engl J Med 323:224, 1990.
13. Kleinveld HA, Demacker PNM, De Haan AFJ, et al: Decreased in vitro oxidizability of low-density lipoprotein in hypercholesterolaemic patients treated with 3-hydroxy-3-methylglutaryl-CoA reductase inhibitors. Eur J Clin Invest 23:289, 1993.
14. Giroux LM, Davignon J, Naruszzewicz M: Simvastatin inhibits the oxidation of low-density lipoproteins by activated human monocyte-derived macrophages. Biochim Biophys Acta 1165:335, 1993.
15. Prihoda JS, Pappu AS, Smith FE, Illingworth DR: The influence of simvastatin on adrenal corticosteroid production and urinary mevalonate during adrenocorticotropin stimulation in patients with heterozygous familial hypercholesterolemia. J Clin Endocrinol Metab 72:567, 1991.
16. Azzarito C, Boiardi L, Zini M, et al: Long-term therapy with high-dose simvastatin does not affect adrenocortical and gonadal hormones in hypercholesterolemic patients. Metabolism 41:148, 1992.
17. McDowell IF, Smye M, Trinick T, et al: Simvastatin in severe hypercholesterolaemia: A placebo controlled trial. Br J Clin Pharmacol 31:340, 1991.
18. Illingworth DR, Bacon S, Pappu AS, Sexton GJ: Comparative hypolipidemic effects of lovastatin and simvastatin in patients with heterozygous familial hypercholesterolemia. Atherosclerosis 96:53, 1992.
19. Summary of the second report of the National Cholesterol Education Program (NCEP) Expert Panel on Detection, Evaluation, and Treatment of High Blood Cholesterol in Adults (Adult Treatment Panel II). JAMA 269:3015, 1993.
19a. MAAS Investigators: Effect of simvastatin on coronary atheroma: The Multicentre Antiatheroma Study (MAAS). Lancet 344:633, 1994.
19b. Scandinavian Simvastatin Survival Study Group: Randomized trial of cholesterol-lowering in 4444 patients with coronary heart disease. The Scandinavian Simvastatin Survival Study (4S). Lancet 344:1383, 1994.
20. Mol MJ, Erkelens DW, Gevers Leuven JA, et al: Simvastatin (MK-733): A potent cholesterol synthesis inhibitor in heterozygous familial hypercholesterolaemia. Atherosclerosis 69:131, 1988.
21. Stein E, Kreisberg R, Miller V, et al: Effects of simvastatin and cholestyramine in familial and non-familial hypercholesterolemia. Arch Intern Med 150:341, 1990.
22. Boccuzzi SJ, Bocanegra TS, Walker JF, et al: Long-term safety and efficacy profile of simvastatin. Am J Cardiol 68:1127, 1991.
23. Molgaard J, Lundh BL, von Schenck H, Olsson AG: Long-term efficacy and safety of simvastatin alone and in combination therapy in treatment of hypercholesterolaemia. Atherosclerosis 91:S21, 1991.
24. Maher VM, Gallagher JJ, Thompson GR, et al: Response to cholesterol-lowering drugs in familial defective apolipoprotein B-100. Atherosclerosis 91:73, 1991.
25. Lintott CJ, Scott RS, Nye ER, et al: Simvastatin (MK 733): An effective treatment for hypercholesterolemia. Aust N Z J Med 19:317, 1989.
26. Molgaard J, von Schenck H, Olsson AG: Comparative effects of simvastatin and cholestyramine in treatment of patients with hypercholesterolaemia. Eur J Clin Pharmacol 36:455, 1989.
27. Betteridge DJ: Combination drug therapy for dyslipidaemia. Curr Opin Lipidol 4:49, 1993.
28. Ytre-Arne K, Nordoy A: Simvastatin and cholestyramine in the long-term treatment of hypercholesterolemia. J Intern Med 226:285, 1989.
29. Tikkanen MJ, Bocanegra TS, Walker JF, Cook T: Comparison of low dose simvastatin and gemfibrozil in the treatment of elevated plasma cholesterol—a multicenter study. Am J Med 87:47s, 1989.
30. Feussner G, Eichinger M, Ziegler R: The influence of simvastatin alone or in combination with gemfibrozil on plasma lipids and lipoproteins in patients with type III hyperlipoproteinemia. Clin Investig 70:1027-1035, 1992.
31. Kjaer K, Hangaard J, Petersen NE, et al: Effect of simvastatin in patients with type I (insulin-dependent) diabetes mellitus and hypercholesterolemia. Acta Endocrinol 126:229, 1992.
32. Owens D, Stinson J, Collins P, et al: Improvement in the regulation of cellular cholesterologenesis in diabetes: The effect of reduction in serum cholesterol by simvastatin. Diabet Med 8:151, 1991.
33. Paolisso G, Sgambato S, De-Riu S, et al: Simvastatin reduces plasma lipid levels and improves insulin action in elderly, non-insulin dependent diabetics. Eur J Clin Pharmacol 40:27, 1991.
34. Hommel E, Andersen P, Gall MA, et al: Plasma lipoproteins and renal function during simvastatin treatment in diabetic nephropathy. Diabetologia 35:447, 1992.
35. Wanner C, Horl WH, Luley CH, et al: Effects of HMG-CoA reductase inhibitors in hypercholesterolemic patients on hemodialysis. Kidney Int 39:754, 1991.
36. Bizzaro N, Bagolin E, Milani L, et al: Massive rhabdomyolysis and simvastatin. Clin Chem 38:1504, 1992.
37. Chariot P, Abadia R, Agnus D, et al: Simvastatin induced rhabdomyolysis followed by a MELAS syndrome. Am J Med 94:109, 1993.
38. Walker JF: Simvastatin: The clinical profile. Am J Med 87(Suppl 4a):44s, 1989.
39. Saito Y, Yoshida S, Nakaya N, et al: Comparison between morning and evening doses of simvastatin in hyperlipidemic subjects: A double-blind comparative study. Arterioscler Thromb 11:816, 1991.
40. Larsen ML, Illingworth DR: Drug treatment of dyslipoproteinemia. Med Clin North Am 78:225, 1994.
41. Illingworth DR, Sexton GJ: Hypocholesterolemic effects of mevinolin in patients with heterozygous familial hypercholesterolemia. J Clin Invest 74:1972, 1984.
42. Havel RJ, Hunninghake DB, Illingworth DR, et al: Lovastatin

(mevinolin) in the treatment of heterozygous famimal hypercholesterolemia: A multicenter study. Ann Intern Med 107:609, 1987.

43. Illingworth DR, Bacon SP: Treatment of heterozygous familial hypercholesterolemia with lipid-lowering drugs. Arteriosclerosis 9(1):1212, 1989.

44. Wiklund O, Angelin B, Fager G, et al: Treatment of familial hypercholesterolaemia: A controlled trial of the effects of pravastatin or cholestyramine therapy on lipoprotein and apolipoprotein levels. J Intern Med 228:241, 1990.

45. Betteridge DJ, Bhatnager D, Bing RF, et al: Treatment of familial hypercholesterolemia—United Kingdom Lipid Clinics Study of pravastatin and cholestyramine. Br Med J 304:1335, 1992.

46. Babir M, Rose M, Kushwaha S, et al: Low-dose simvastatin for the treatment of hypercholesterolaemia in recipients of cardiac transplantation. Int J Cardiol 33:241, 1991.

CHAPTER 123

Pravastatin

Jacques D. Barth, M.D., Ph.D, and G. B. John Mancini, M.D.

HISTORY

Pravastatin (formerly CS-514, SQ 31,000, RMS-415, eptastatin) is a competitive inhibitor of 3-hydroxy-3-methylglutaryl coenzyme A (HMG-CoA) reductase, the rate-limiting enzyme in cholesterol biosynthesis. This enzyme catalyzes the conversion of HMG-CoA reductase to mevalonic acid and has been considered the prime target for pharmacologic intervention for several decades. Several inhibiting compounds have been isolated from the fungal metabolite of *Aspergillus terreus*. The first report of inhibition of this enzyme was published in 1976.[1] Mevastatin (compactin) was the first HMG-CoA reductase inhibitor used in humans.[2] As a result of adverse and toxic effects in animal studies, development of this effective low-density lipoprotein cholesterol (LDL-C)–lowering compound was discontinued. Lovastatin (mevinolin) has become the first and reference HMG-CoA compound of the second generation.[3] Lovastatin decreases cholesterol biosynthesis and secondarily serum apolipoprotein B-100 concentrations without significant adverse effects in the cholesterol pathway.[4] A decrease in plasma triglyceride levels and modest increase in high-density lipoprotein cholesterol (HDL-C) concentrations have been established. Pravastatin is a potent competitive inhibitor of HMG-CoA reductase and was discovered as a minor metabolite of mevastatin. It was produced by microbial transformation of mevastatin using *Nocardia autotrophica*.[5]

CHEMISTRY

Pravastatin, like other HMG-CoA reductase inhibitors, competitively inhibits the rate-limiting enzyme in the cholesterol biosynthetic pathway. Although structurally related, only pravastatin has a hydroxy substituent on the hexahydronaphthalene nucleus, whereas lovastatin, mevastatin, and simvastatin differ from each other in the number of methyl substituents in the nucleus or in the ester side chain. The molecules exist as active hydroxy acids or as prodrug lactones. Pravastatin is administered in its active form as the hydroxy acid sodium salt. Lovastatin and simvastatin are administered as prodrug lactones and are

converted to their respective hydroxy acid forms *in vivo*.[6] Inferred from its chemical structure, it is apparent that the hydroxyl group makes pravastatin lactone more than 100 times more soluble in water than any of the other three lactones mentioned.

PRECLINICAL STUDIES ON EFFICACY, PHARMACOKINETICS, AND ANIMAL TOXICOLOGY

Pravastatin is a powerful competitive inhibitor of HMG-CoA reductase. Animal studies demonstrated that pravastatin is a tissue-selective inhibitor of HMG-CoA reductase. In freshly isolated rat hepatocytes, pravastatin inhibits acetate incorporation into sterols as effectively as does mevastatin or lovastatin[7, 8] (Fig. 123–1). However, in nonhepatic cell lines and types (e.g., adrenal and ovarian cell lines), pravastatin is 200- to 500-fold less potent than the other two inhibitors[5] (Fig. 123–2). Because the major site of cholesterol synthesis is the liver, this tissue-selective property of pravastatin may be a desirable clinical feature.

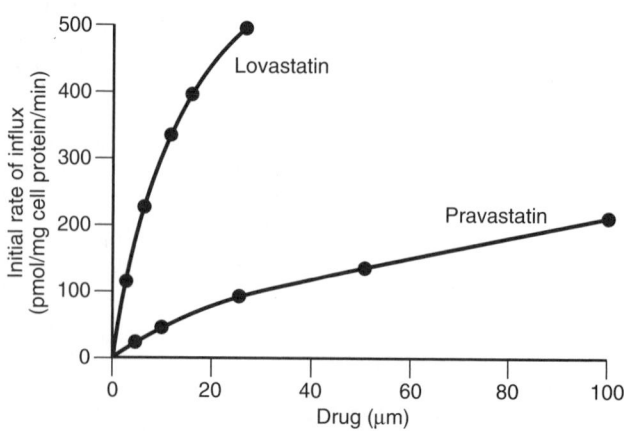

Figure 123–1. Transport of pravastatin and lovastatin into rat hepatocytes. (Adapted from Scott W: Hydrophilicity and the differential pharmacology of pravastatin. *In* Wood C (ed): Lipid Management: Pravastatin and the Differential Pharmacology of HMG-CoA Reductase Inhibitors. London: Royal Society of Medicine Services, Round Table Series, 1990, pp 17–28.)

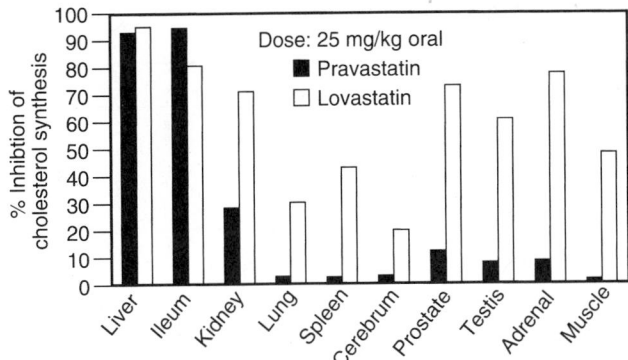

Figure 123–2. Inhibition of cholesterol synthesis in different tissues of rats orally dosed with 25 mg/kg pravastatin. (Adapted from Tsujita Y, Kuroda M, Shimada Y, et al: CS-514, a competitive inhibitor of 3-hydroxy-3-methylglutaryl-coenzyme A reductase: Tissue selective inhibitor of sterol synthesis and hypolipidemic effect on various animal species. Biochim Biophys Acta 877:50, 1986.)

Nevertheless, additional long-term safety studies of pravastatin and other HMG-CoA reductase inhibitors are required before definite conclusions can be reached.

In addition, pravastatin has been studied extensively in laboratory animals.[9] Oral LD$_{50}$ values in mice and rats ranged from approximately 9 g/kg to 12 g/kg or more. Intravenous LD$_{50}$ values in mice and rats were approximately 2000 mg/kg and 450 mg/kg, respectively. In subacute and chronic oral toxicologic studies, pravastatin was given daily to monkeys at doses of 24 to 800 mg/kg. One of four monkeys given 200 mg/kg and most monkeys given 400 mg/kg died or were sacrificed in moribund condition after approximately 2 weeks of dosing. Findings in these monkeys included vomiting and diarrhea and increases in levels of aspartate aminotransferase (ASAT), alanine aminotransferase (ALAT), lactate dehydrogenase (LDH), alkaline phosphatase, total bilirubin, creatinine, and blood urea nitrogen. Prolongations of activated partial thromboplastin time (APTT) and prothrombin time (PT) and elevated total white blood cell counts (owing mainly to neutrophils) were also observed in some animals. Pathologic examinations revealed hepatocellular damage and degenerative changes in the kidney affecting primarily the proximal tubules. Similar findings were noted in one of four animals given 100 mg/kg. No clear drug-induced abnormalities occurred in monkeys that received 50 mg/kg for 26 weeks or 25 mg/kg for 52 weeks.

Pravastatin was administered orally to rats at daily doses of 0.8 to 1000 mg/kg in several toxicologic studies (2 to 52 weeks). Although hepatic effects (generally mild) were observed at doses of 40 mg/kg or more in these studies, a dose of 500 mg/kg given for 52 weeks was generally well tolerated.

Although the cholesterol-lowering mechanism of pravastatin has not been fully elucidated, a reduction in LDL-C production and an increase in the fractional catabolic rate for LDL are likely.

HUMAN STUDIES

Pharmacokinetic studies in healthy subjects after an oral dose indicated that 34% of the dose is absorbed and the absolute bioavailability in the systemic circulation is 17%.[10, 11] The elimination half-life is from 1.5 to 2.0 hours. Protein binding ranges from 55% to 60%, and urinary excretion of unchanged drug is from 5% to 7% of the dose given. After a radiolabeled dose, 20% of total radioactivity was excreted in the urine, which includes pravastatin and its metabolites. The renal clearance accounts for 47% of total body clearance, and nonrenal clearance accounts for 53% of total body clearance. The hepatic extraction ratio, which gives an indication of the first-pass biotransformation, is 0.7 and suggests that pravastatin is heavily extracted in the liver and undergoes first-pass metabolism.

In a human pharmacokinetics study (12 healthy male volunteers) comparing pravastatin, lovastatin, and simvastatin, a significantly higher plasma concentration of HMG-CoA reductase inhibitory activity was found in favor of pravastatin.[12] This suggests that pravastatin-related inhibitory activity in peripheral tissues may be greater.

CLINICAL USE
Indications

Pravastatin is indicated as an adjunct to diet in the treatment of elevated LDL-C levels. Its use may be considered when, despite dietary measures, the LDL-C level exceeds 190 mg/dl (4.92 mmol/L), or when it exceeds 160 mg/dl (4.14 mmol/L) in individuals with at least two cardiovascular risk factors or when it exceeds 130 mg/dl (3.37 mmol/L) in individuals with established coronary heart disease (CHD).[13]

According to these Adult Treatment Panel II guidelines, a more specific goal is to be attained by lipid lowering. In primary prevention, low-dose bile acids sequestrants should be considered as first line of treatment when nonpharmacologic approaches have not been able to reduce CHD risk significantly, especially in men. The low-dose combination of a resin and a statin may be considered as an alternative.

In secondary cardiovascular prevention, drug therapy generally is indicated in patients with established CHD or other atherosclerotic disease if LDL-C levels are 130 mg/dl (3.4 mmol/L) or higher. Pravastatin has been shown to be effective in treatment of severe forms of hypercholesterolemia and for effective lowering of LDL-C levels in secondary prevention (Table 123–1). Long-term safety remains to be demonstrated.

Efficacy in Monotherapy

Pravastatin and Placebo

In a dose-response study of pravastatin, 306 patients with primary hypercholesterolemia received twice-daily doses of 5 mg, 10 mg, 20 mg pravastatin or placebo for 12 weeks.[14] Pravastatin treatment resulted in significant ($p < .0001$) dose-dependent mean reductions from baseline in LDL-C of 17.5%, 22.9%, and

Table 123–1. **Overview of Published Clinical Studies with Pravastatin**
(Percentage Decrease of LDL-Cholesterol Level)

Author	n	Type	Period	20 mg/day	40 mg/day
Pan[11]	11	Mixed	4 wk	−23%*	
Hunninghake et al.[14]	306	Mixed	12 wk	−23%	−31%
Rubenfire et al.[15]	82	Mixed	16 wk	−28%	−31%
Jones et al.[16]	150	Mixed	8 wk	−32%	−34%
Pearson et al.[17]	1062	Mixed	52 wk	−26%	
Simons et al.[18]	46	Mixed	3 yr		
Betteridge et al.[19]	128	FH	12 wk		−30%
Bard et al.[20]	24	Mixed	12 wk		−35%
Ditschuneit et al.[21]	23	Mixed	6 mo	−26%	−28%
Stalenhoef et al.[22]	48	FH	6 wk		−33%
Simvastatin Pravastatin Study Group[23]	550	Mixed	18 wk		−27%
McPherson et al.[24]	217	Mixed	8 wk	−28%	
The European Study Group[25]	145	Mixed		−22%*	
Wiklund et al.[26]	290	Mixed	12 wk		−33%
Crepaldi et al.[27]	192	Mixed	24 wk		−30%
Hoogerbrugge et al.[28]	20	FH	8 wk		−33%
Vanhanen and Miettinen[29]	7	FH	4 wk		−36%
Pravastatin Multicenter Study Group II[30]	311	Mixed	8 wk		−31%
Jacob et al.[31]	13	FH	52 wk		−39%
Contacos et al.[32]	32	Combined	6 wk		−26%
Mabuchi et al.[55]	13	FH		−33%	
Carmena et al.[56]	60	FH	52 wk		−26%
Yamamoto et al.[57]	369	Mixed	78 wk		−27%
Lovastatin/Pravastatin Study Group[58]	672	Mixed	18 wk		−27%

*Pravastatin 10 mg/day.
FH, familial hypercholesterolemia.

30.8%, respectively, for the three dosages tested. The reduction of LDL-C was log linear with respect to the dose. Maximum lipid-lowering effects occurred at 4 weeks and were sustained for the duration of the trial. Triglyceride levels decreased by as much as 15%, and HDL-C levels increased by a maximum of 7%. These latter effects did not appear to be dose dependent.

In another double-blind placebo-controlled study, 82 patients with primary hypercholesterolemia were studied for 16 weeks.[15] Results indicate that patients receiving 10 mg pravastatin twice a day for 8 weeks experienced a significant ($p < .01$) LDL-C reduction of 28%. At 20 mg twice a day for an additional 8 weeks, pravastatin reduced LDL-C by 31%. During this study, HDL-C increased, respectively, 9% and 11%, and triglyceride levels decreased slightly. This study revealed that sex was a possible independent predictor of response to pravastatin; men showed a more distinct response as compared with women. Pravastatin was well tolerated, and no serious toxic reactions were encountered.

A study assessing dose response in primary hypercholesterolemic patients resulted in a dose-dependent reduction of LDL-C[16] (Fig. 123–3). Pravastatin in 5, 10, 20, 40 mg or placebo was administered at bedtime in 150 patients. After 8 weeks, LDL-C had decreased by 32% with 20 mg and by 34% with 40 mg pravastatin. HDL-C increased 2% and 12%, respectively, whereas triglyceride levels decreased 11% and 24%, respectively. Few side effects were noted. It was concluded that pravastatin is an effective and well-tolerated lipid-lowering regimen for patients with hypercholesterolemia.

In a recently completed large multicenter study of 1062 hypercholesterolemic patients, 20 mg pravastatin was administered for 52 weeks.[17] This study confirmed findings of LDL-C change (−26%), HDL-C increase (+7%), and triglyceride decrease of 12% with 20 mg pravastatin. In addition, this trial is the first one to show that a rapid lipid lowering is also associated with a significant reduction of serious cardiovascular events (1 case in the pravastatin group versus 13 cases in the placebo group; $p < .001$) and for total serious events (6 cases in the pravastatin group versus 26 in the placebo group; $p < .001$).

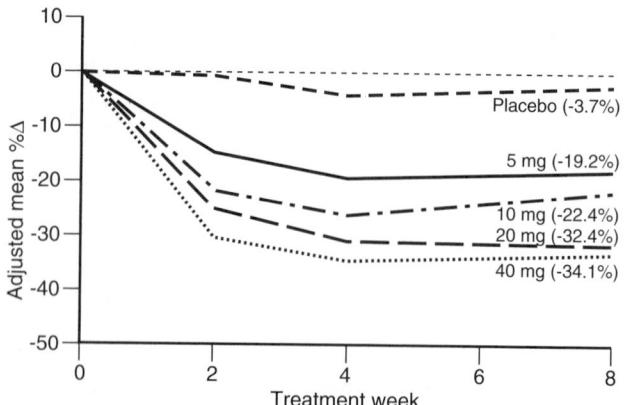

Figure 123–3. Time dose response of once-daily (evening dose) pravastatin and placebo on LDL-C in patients with primary hypercholesterolemia. (Adapted from Jones PH, Farmer JA, Cressman MD, et al: Once daily pravastatin in patients with primary hypercholesterolemia: A dose response study. Clin Cardiol 14:146, 1991. Copyrighted by and reprinted with the permission of Clinical Cardiology Publishing Company, Inc., and/or the Foundation for Advances in Medicine and Science, Inc., Mahwah, NJ 07430-0832, USA.)

Pravastatin and Other Lipid-Lowering Drugs

An Australian study assessing the intermediate term effects of pravastatin on patients with mixed hyperlipidemia was performed over 3 years.[18] Forty-six completed the study after being randomized to pravastatin 20 mg, pravastatin 40 mg, or cholestyramine 16 g/day. At 12 weeks, LDL-C was reduced by 26%, 30%, and 34%, respectively, in the pravastatin 20 mg, pravastatin 40 mg, and resin groups. HDL-C was increased in all regimens by 8% to 18%. Pravastatin 40 mg was the only regimen to decrease triglyceride levels. Side effects were minor, and compliance to therapy remained high during the 3-year period.

In a carefully designed study comparing the effects of pravastatin and cholestyramine in 128 patients with heterozygous familial hypercholesterolemia, the following results were found.[19] Pravastatin 40 mg/day was compared with cholestyramine 24 g/day in a double-blind, double-dummy, placebo-controlled study. LDL-C levels decreased 30% in the pravastatin group, and cholestyramine induced a 31% decrease. All patients tolerated cholestyramine in this trial.

In a 12-week study in 24 mixed hypercholesterolemic patients, cholestyramine (16 g/day) was compared with pravastatin (40 mg/day). An assessment of change in lipoprotein level and composition was made.[20] Results indicate that pravastatin lowered LDL-C by 35%, and cholestyramine lowered LDL-C by 31% at 12 weeks. No significant side effects occurred during the trial.

In a three-way comparative study of 84 patients on simvastatin (40 mg), 42 patients on lovastatin (40 mg), and 23 patients on pravastatin (40 mg) during 6 months' follow-up, the following results were obtained.[21] LDL-C decreased by 30%, 26%, and 28%, respectively. Triglyceride levels were lowered by 20%, 17%, and 6%. HDL-C increased 23%, 10%, and 8% on the three compounds. No significant difference in efficacy was established. In addition, no significant side effect was found. In the simvastatin group, four patients showed silent creatine kinase (CK) increases.

In a comparative study in the Netherlands, 48 patients with primary hypercholesterolemia were randomized to receive either pravastatin 40 mg or simvastatin 40 mg.[22] LDL-C was measured after 6 weeks and showed a decrease of 33% on pravastatin and 43% on simvastatin. Both drugs decreased triglyceride levels significantly by 10% and 15%, respectively. No serious side effects were reported.

Efficacy and safety were studied in patients with primary hypercholesterolemia comparing pravastatin with simvastatin.[23] This multicenter study in 550 patients with primary hypercholesterolemia lasted 18 weeks. Results indicated that the recommended maximal dosage (simvastatin 40 mg/day or pravastatin 40 mg/day) caused a decrease of LDL-C by 38% and 27%, respectively, and 18% and 14% for triglycerides. Both drugs were well tolerated and did not cause any serious side effect.

In a short-term study, efficacy of pravastatin and lovastatin in the management of primary hypercho-

lesterolemia was assessed.[24] In 217 patients with primary hypercholesterolemia treated for 8 weeks, lovastatin 20 mg/day, pravastatin 10 mg/day, and pravastatin 20 mg/day were compared. Both pravastatin 20 mg/day and lovastatin 20 mg/day resulted in a 28% reduction of LDL-C. Pravastatin 10 mg/day after 4 weeks was significantly more effective in lowering LDL-C than lovastatin. The frequency of side effects, including elevations in CK and liver function enzyme levels, was similar and low in all groups.

Pravastatin, 10 mg (n = 146), and simvastatin, 10 mg (n = 145), were tested in patients with primary hypercholesterolemia for 6 weeks.[25] LDL-C was reduced 32% by simvastatin and 22% by pravastatin. HDL-C increased by 7% and 5% with simvastatin and pravastatin, respectively. Triglyceride levels decreased by 13% and 6%, respectively. Both drugs were well tolerated, and few side effects occurred.

Efficacy in Combination Therapy with Other Lipid-Lowering Drugs

In a study assessing the effects of pravastatin and gemfibrozil alone or in combination, 290 patients were analyzed for 12 weeks.[26] LDL-C was lowered by 33% on pravastatin alone and 17% by gemfibrozil alone. HDL-C was increased by 15% and 6%, respectively, whereas triglyceride values declined 42% on gemfibrozil and 22% on pravastatin. The combination therapy lowered LDL-C by 20% and increased HDL-C by 17%. Triglyceride values were lowered by 49%. Adverse effects were generally mild, and only two patients showed asymptomatic CK elevation. It may be inferred from this study that the two drugs may be safely combined in selected cases.

Pravastatin was also studied and compared with gemfibrozil in a large Italian multicenter trial.[27] A total of 385 patients were randomly assigned to either 40 mg of pravastatin or 1200 mg gemfibrozil. After 24 weeks, LDL-C was reduced by 30% in the pravastatin group, whereas gemfibrozil reduced LDL-C by 17%. HDL-C increased 5% on pravastatin, whereas gemfibrozil led to a 17% increase. Serum triglyceride levels decreased 5% on pravastatin and 37% on gemfibrozil. In this mixed population, the incidence of side effects was low in both groups. Pravastatin was more effective in lowering LDL-C.

When pravastatin was compared in familial hypercholesterolemia alone and in combination with bile acid–binding resins, the following results were found.[28] In 40 patients who received 40 mg pravastatin, decreases of LDL-C of 33%, increases of HDL-C of 8%, and decreases of triglycerides of 14% were observed. After 8 weeks, 30 patients showed an additional 12% decrease in LDL-C when three packs a day of resins were added at 24 weeks. Resins alone in 22 patients resulted in a decrease in LDL-C of 22%. All three regimens were safe and effective.

In another study, the lipid-lowering effects of pravastatin and lovastatin in patients with familial hypercholesterolemia were assessed.[29] Administration of pravastatin 40 mg/day and lovastatin 40 mg/day was separated by a 3-month washout period. The reduction of LDL-C after 1, 2, and 4 weeks was 23%, 32%, and 32% for pravastatin. For lovastatin, the reduction was 23%, 30%, and 31%. The reductions in serum levels of the cholesterol precursor sterols, delta 8-cholesterol, desosterol, and lathosterol, were not significantly different after either drug.

Severe hypercholesterolemia often requires high-dose therapy with an HMG-CoA reductase inhibitor alone or in combination with a bile acid sequestrant. In a multicenter trial, pravastatin alone and in combination with cholestyramine was studied in hypercholesterolemic patients.[30] Results after 8 weeks in 311 patients showed a reduction of LDL-C by 31% with 20 mg pravastatin twice daily, whereas 40 mg twice daily reduced LDL-C by 38%. Cholestyramine (24 g) alone reduced LDL-C by 32%. Cholestyramine in combination with 40 mg/day pravastatin reduced LDL-C by 51%. HDL-C increased by 5% regardless of the regimen. All drug regimens were effective and well tolerated and did not show a tendency to increase CK.

In another study, the short and medium effects of pravastatin alone and in combination with cholestyramine on serum lipids in primary hypercholesterolemia were assessed.[31] Thirteen patients on 40 mg pravastatin and 8 g cholestyramine showed a decrease of LDL-C of 39% after 12 months of treatment. In 12 patients with identical baseline lipoprotein values, lovastatin 80 mg plus 8 g cholestyramine resulted in a 40% decrease in LDL-C.

The effect of fish oil in combination with pravastatin was studied in 32 patients with combined hyperlipidemia.[32] Pravastatin 40 mg/day reduced LDL-C by 30% ($p < .001$). Fish oil (3 g/day omega-3 fatty acids) reduced triglycerides by 30% ($p < .05$). Fish oil decreased the concentration of very-low-density lipoprotein (VLDL) by 37% ($p < .05$). The combined therapy proved to be safe and effective in lowering atherogenic intermediate-density lipoprotein (IDL) and VLDL particles by 35% ($p < .01$).

Safety and Side Effects

Elevation of Transaminases

Liver function disturbances are the most frequently noted side effects in the HMG-CoA reductase inhibitors. As pravastatin is more prevalent in the liver than the other HMG-CoA reductase inhibitors, a higher prevalence of liver function problems seemed possible. A study to assess this was done comparing pravastatin with simvastatin.[33] During the 6-month follow-up in the 100 simvastatin-treated and the 90 pravastatin-treated patients, the incidence of liver toxicity was 5% and 4.5%, respectively.

Creatine Kinase Elevations and Myopathy

In accordance with the pravastatin monograph product labeling, CK elevations, mostly transient, occurred in 1.6% of cases. This was only slightly higher than the rate in the placebo control population. The incidence of myopathy was found to be less than 0.1% in controlled clinical trials.

Lens

Cholesterol biosynthesis of the ocular lens is fragile and in prior studies was shown to be susceptible to a critical interference by HMG-CoA reductase inhibitors. Studies in dogs suggest that inhibition of cholesterol synthesis is responsible for cataract formation. Two studies comparing lovastatin versus pravastatin[34] and simvastatin versus pravastatin[35] in human lens cultures are important. Experiments in the human lens organ culture system showed lovastatin to be 100-fold more potent than pravastatin in inhibiting the cholesterol biosynthesis.

In Wistar rats, doses of 50 or 100 mg/kg lovastatin chow caused a reduction of 20% of lenticular cholesterol content. Pravastatin had no measurable effect.

When simvastatin was compared with pravastatin in the human lens, cholesterol synthesis was 100-fold greater with simvastatin than pravastatin using a radiolabeled [^{14}C]-cholesterol and [^{14}C]-fatty acid method.

Central Nervous System Effects

Lipophilic drugs like simvastatin and lovastatin may cross the blood-brain barrier. Hydrophilic agents like pravastatin are less likely to do so. Accordingly, there has been special interest in studying the influence on central nervous system (CNS) function.

In a comparative study, the effects of lovastatin and pravastatin on nighttime sleep and daytime performance quality and quantity of sleep were assessed in healthy volunteers.[36] Divided attention and vigilance as well as global performance were significantly affected in the lovastatin cases. No significant effect was observed in the pravastatin patients. An initial report in patients with established coronary artery disease[37] indicated that sleep pattern might deteriorate when simvastatin, a lipophilic HMG-CoA reductase, was used.

In another study, effects on sleep in 12 healthy volunteers given 40 mg lovastatin and 40 mg pravastatin were compared.[38] A markedly increased wake time after sleep onset and stage 1 sleep compared with baseline was found while the subjects were taking lovastatin. Pravastatin was not associated with these sleep disturbances. The clinical relevance of these findings remains to be determined.

Rash

When all side effects were assessed, dermatologic rash was significantly more prevalent in the pravastatin group as compared with placebo.

Steroid Metabolism

Because cholesterol plays a crucial part in steroid metabolism, changes may have an effect on the formation of steroid hormones and related metabolite formation. Mean decreases in plasma levels of testosterone within the normal range occurred in some patients receiving pravastatin; the magnitude of the decreases was small and was not different from that observed in a control population receiving cholestyramine, which has been proved safe in long-term use.

Although some effects of HMG-CoA reductase inhibitors on steroid metabolism have been reported, clinical implications are unclear.[39]

In a study comparing the effects of pravastatin and simvastatin on CoQ10, the following was recently reported.[40] CoQ10 is essential for the production of energy and also antioxidative properties. A diminution of CoQ10 availability could lead to membrane alterations with subsequent cellular damage. Simvastatin 20 mg/day was compared with pravastatin 20 mg/day for 3 months in two groups of five healthy volunteers. Data show that treatment with pravastatin and simvastatin lower LDL-C and CoQ10 significantly by about 40%. Longer-term studies are necessary to determine a possible long-term impact. The clinical relevance of these effects has not been determined.

Other possible adverse clinical effects have been trivial and nonspecific, occurring with equal frequency in pravastatin and control groups, and have not generally led to discontinuation of drug. The drug has been well tolerated. The only adverse event that occurred more commonly in pravastatin-treated patients than in those receiving placebo was rash. Increases in hepatic transaminases to more than three times the upper limit of normal leading to discontinuation of the drug have occurred in approximately 0.5% of patients. This was reversible on discontinuation of the drug.

There was no clear evidence of drug-induced myositis syndrome (myalgias associated with marked elevation of CK levels). One patient with baseline elevation of CK developed muscle aches and a marked elevation of CK during pravastatin therapy. Other patients on pravastatin or placebo have had marked elevations of CK without symptoms or with symptoms attributed to concomitant exercise programs. The CK elevations have resolved without withdrawal of study medication (pravastatin or placebo).

Interactions with Other Drugs

Drug-drug pharmacokinetic interaction studies indicate that bioavailability of pravastatin is diminished when it is combined with cholestyramine and colestipol. Antacids decrease pravastatin's bioavailability slightly, whereas H$_2$ blockers (cimetidine) increase this. Aspirin, nicotinic acid, gemfibrozil, probucol, warfarin, and digoxin do not change bioavailability of the pravastatin.

Dosage and Administration

Pravastatin is most effective when administered as a single dose in the evening or as a twice-daily regimen. A single dose in the morning is less effective.[41] Tablets are available containing 10 mg, 20 mg, and 40 mg pravastatin.

Changes in lifestyle and dietary therapy remain the cornerstone of lipid-lowering treatment. Some studies leave the impression that cholesterol-lowering agents negatively influence adherence to dietary prescription,[42] whereas other studies negate this.[43] The preferred recommended dose to start with is 10 mg pravastatin, and if the expected result remains below expectation, a doubling after 6 weeks to 20 mg/day pravastatin taken in the evening is indicated. The addition of low doses of bile acid sequestrants (colestipol 10 g/day or cholestyramine 8 g/day) is preferred to an increase in the pravastatin dose.

Use in Patients with Concomitant Diseases

Secondary hyperlipidemia in diseases like nephrotic syndrome remains a difficult treatment challenge. The hyperlipidemia of the nephrotic syndrome is characterized by an elevation of total cholesterol, LDL-C, and triglycerides, while HDL-C remains low or lowered. In a lipid-lowering study using pravastatin,[44] after dietary modification, 13 patients received pravastatin and 8 received placebo. The trial lasted 24 weeks and showed that 20 mg pravastatin reduced LDL-C by 28% from baseline. An increase in dosage did not result in an additional LDL-C decrease. Pravastatin was efficacious and safe in this population. Insufficient data are presently available to prescribe pravastatin safely in patients suffering from liver disease.

In patients with non-insulin-dependent diabetes mellitus, pravastatin reduced LDL-C effectively without causing significant side effects.[45]

Administration in the Elderly

Because elderly have a different and sometimes slower metabolism, dosage adjustment and incidence of side effects may be an issue. In a 48-week study in 13 elderly (65 to 75 years) hypercholesterolemic patients, these aspects were assessed in response to pravastatin therapy.[46] Results indicate that LDL-C decreased by 38% after 48 weeks with 20 mg/day pravastatin. The drug was well tolerated without significant side effects. In an overview article, data from 1800 hypercholesterolemic patients were pooled and then analyzed to compare the safety and efficacy in the elderly and the nonelderly.[47] Pravastatin 20 or 40 mg daily lowered LDL-C 25% to 33% and triglycerides 14% to 23%; HDL-C increased 5% to 10%. Short-term studies indicate that medication had to be withdrawn in 1% of cases, whereas in longer-term treatment, 0.4% of patients had to discontinue medication. Thus, pravastatin appears to be safe and effective in elderly patients with hypercholesterolemia.

Special Features

Lipoprotein(a) [Lp(a)] has emerged as an additional and independent atherogenic factor in the development of atherosclerosis. Pravastatin was studied in 306 participants in a phase II dose ranging study.[48] During the open-label study, LDL-C and triglycerides decreased significantly ($p < .01$), 33.6% and 19.9%

respectively. HDL-C increased significantly ($p < .01$). Lp(a) did not change during the intervention.

CONCLUSIONS

Pravastatin is an HMG-CoA reductase inhibitor, a new class of cholesterol-lowering agents. It has been shown to be efficacious, safe, and well tolerated in different populations. It has been reported to lower total cholesterol and LDL-C levels in patients with familial and nonfamilial hypercholesterolemia. It has not been shown to complicate metabolism or interact adversely in a significant way with other specific cardiovascular/lipid-lowering drugs. A multicenter, multinational study has indicated that the rapid cholesterol lowering induced by pravastatin may reduce serious cardiovascular events.

In addition, preliminary data indicate that it may cause a possible regression and/or deceleration of the atherosclerotic process.

Several trials with pravastatin have been completed. In the PLAC I, more than 400 patients with moderate hypercholesterolemia and evidence of coronary artery disease received either pravastatin 40 mg/day or placebo.[49] After a 3-year follow-up, progression of atherosclerosis slowed 40% to 50% based on the lumen diameter on the coronary angiograms (primary end points). The pravastatin group also showed a 60% reduction in nonfatal and fatal myocardial infarctions.

In the PLAC II study, there was a 35% slowing of the progression of atherosclerosis in the common carotid artery ($p < .03$) and an 80% reduction in nonfatal and fatal myocardial infarctions ($p = .03$) in the pravastatin group.[50]

REGRESS evaluated the effects of pravastatin on the progression of coronary atherosclerosis in a 2-year, double-blind, randomized, placebo-controlled trial of 885 men with moderate hypercholesterolemia and at least one coronary artery stenosis of more than 50%.[51] In the pravastatin group, there was a 40% to 66% slowing of progression of atherosclerosis based on mean obstruction diameter and minimum obstruction diameter. Similar to the previous studies, overall serious adverse cardiovascular events (myocardial infarction, sudden death, percutaneous transluminal coronary angioplasty [PTCA], stroke) were reduced 42%.

In the Kuopio Atherosclerosis Study (KAPS), a 45% slowing of the progression of carotid atherosclerosis and a 66% slowing of the progression of atherosclerosis in the common carotid artery were observed.[52]

The pooled analysis of the clinical events in the previously mentioned four studies (PLAC I, PLAC II, REGRESS, and KAPS)[53] comprised a total of 1891 patients randomized to either pravastatin or placebo. Overall reduction was 62% in nonfatal/fatal myocardial infarctions ($p < .001$), 62% in strokes ($p = .054$), and 46% in total mortality ($p = .168$).

Finally, in The West of Scotland Coronary Prevention Study a total of 6595 men with hypercholesterolemia (average cholesterol 272 ± 23 mg/dl) were randomly assigned to receive pravastatin 40 mg/day or placebo and followed up for an average of 4.9 years.[54]

Pravastatin lowered plasma cholesterol levels by 20% and LDL cholesterol levels by 25%. This fall in cholesterol was associated with a relative reduction in risk of definite coronary events (nonfatal myocardial infarction or death from coronary heart disease) by 31% ($p > .001$). Death from all cardiovascular causes was reduced by 32%. The authors concluded that treatment with pravastatin significantly reduced the incidence of myocardial infarction and death from cardiovascular causes without adversely affecting the risk of death from noncardiovascular causes in men with moderate hypercholesterolemia.

REFERENCES

 1. Endo A, Kuroda M, Tsujita Y: ML-236A, ML-236B and ML-236C, new inhibitors of cholesterol genesis produced by Penicillium citrinum. J Antibiot (Tokyo) 29:1346, 1976.
 2. Mabuchi H, Haba T, Tatami R, et al: Effect of an inhibitor of 3-hydroxy-3-methylglutaryl coenzyme A reductase on serum lipoproteins and ubiquinone-10 levels in patients with familial hypercholesterolemia. N Engl J Med 305:478, 1981.
 3. Alberts AW, Chen J, Kuron G, et al: Mevinolin: A highly potent competitive inhibitor of 3-hydroxy-3-methylglutaryl co-enzyme A reductase and a cholesterol lowering agent. Proc Natl Acad Sci USA 77:3957, 1980.
 4. Havel RJ, Hunninghake DB, Illingworth RD, et al: Lovastatin (mevinolin) in the treatment of heterozygous familial hypercholesterolemia. Ann Intern Med 107:609, 1987.
 5. Tsujita Y, Kuroda M, Shimada Y, et al: CS-514, a competitive inhibitor of 3-hydroxy-3-methylglutaryl-coenzyme A reductase: Tissue selective inhibitor of sterol synthesis and hypolipidemic effect on various animal species. Biochim Biophys Acta 877:50, 1986.
 6. Serajuddin ATM, Ranadive SA, Mahoney EM: Relative lipophilicities, solubilities, and structure-pharmacological considerations of 3-hydroxy-3-methylglutaryl-coenzyme A (HMG-CoA) reductase inhibitors pravastatin, lovastatin, mevastatin and simvastatin. J Pharm Sci 80:830, 1991.
 7. Scott W: Hydrophilicity and the differential pharmacology of pravastatin. *In* Wood C (ed): Lipid Management: Pravastatin and the Differential Pharmacology of HMG-CoA Reductase Inhibitors. London: Royal Society of Medicine Services, Round Table Series, 1990, pp 17–28.
 8. Komai T, Shigehara E, Tokui T, et al: Carrier mediated uptake of pravastatin by rat hepatocytes in primary culture. Biochem Pharmacol 43:667, 1992.
 9. Product monograph of Pravachol (Pravastatin). Princeton, NJ: Bristol-Myers Squibb Inc., 1992.
10. Pan HY, DeVault AR, Wang-Iverson D, et al: Comparative pharmacokinetics and pharmacodynamics of pravastatin and lovastatin. J Clin Pharmacol 12:1128, 1990.
11. Pan HY: Clinical pharmacology of pravastatin, a selective inhibitor of HMG-CoA reductase. Eur J Clin Pharmacol 40(Suppl 1):S15, 1991.
12. Pentikainen PJ, Saraheimo M, Schwartz JI, et al: Comparative pharmacokinetics of lovastatin, simvastatin and pravastatin in humans. J Clin Pharmacol 32:136, 1992.
13. Expert Panel on Detection, Evaluation and Treatment of High Cholesterol in Adults: Summary of the second report of the National Cholesterol Education Program Expert Panel on Detection, Evaluation and Treatment of High Blood Cholesterol in Adults (ATPII). JAMA 269:3015, 1993.
14. Hunninghake DB, Knopp RH, Schonfeld G, et al: Efficacy and safety of pravastatin in patients with primary hypercholesterolemia. Atherosclerosis 85:81, 1990.
15. Rubenfire M, Maciejko JJ, Blevins RD, et al: The effect of pravastatin on plasma lipoprotein and apolipoprotein levels in primary hypercholesterolemia. Arch Intern Med 151:2234, 1991.
16. Jones PH, Farmer JA, Cressman MD, et al: Once daily pravastatin in patients with primary hypercholesterolemia: A dose response study. Clin Cardiol 14:146, 1991.

17. Pearson ThA, Marx HJ, The Pravastatin Multinational Study Group for Cardiac Risk Patients: Effects of pravastatin in patients with serum total cholesterol levels from 5.2 to 7.8 mmol/L plus two additional atherosclerotic risk factors. Am J Cardiol 72:1031, 1993.

18. Simons LA, Nestel PJ, Clifton P, et al: Treatment of primary hypercholesterolemia with pravastatin: Efficacy and safety over three years. Med J Aust 157:584, 1992.

19. Betteridge DJ, Bhatnager D, Bing RF, et al: Treatment of familial hypercholesterolemia: United Kingdom Lipid Clinics Study of pravastatin and cholestyramine. Br Med J 304:1335, 1992.

20. Bard JM, Parra HJ, Douste-Blazy P, Fruchart JC: Effect of pravastatin, an HMG-CoA reductase inhibitor, and cholestyramine, a bile acid sequestrant, on lipoprotein particles defined by their apolipoprotein composition. Metabolism 39:269, 1990.

21. Ditschuneit HH, Kuhn K, Dischuneit H: Comparison of different HMG-CoA reductase inhibitors. Eur J Clin Pharmacol 40(Suppl 1):S27, 1991.

22. Stalenhoef AF, Lansberg PJ, Kroon AA, et al: Treatment of primary hypercholesterolemia. Short term efficacy and safety of increasing doses of simvastatin and pravastatin: A double blind comparative study. J Intern Med 234:77, 1993.

23. The Simvastatin Pravastatin Study Group: Comparison of the effcacy, safety and tolerability of simvastatin and pravastatin for hypercholesterolemia. Am J Cardiol 71:1408, 1993.

24. McPherson R, Bedard J, Connelly P, et al: Comparison of the short term efficacy and tolerability of lovastatin and pravastatin in the management of primary hypercholesterolemia. Clin Ther 14:276, 1992.

25. The European Study Group: Efficacy and tolerability of simvastatin and pravastatin in patients with primary hypercholesterolemia. Am J Cardiol 70:1281, 1992.

26. Wiklund O, Angelin B, Bergman M, et al: Pravastatin and gemfibrozil alone and in combination for the treatment of hypercholesterolemia. Am J Med 94:13, 1993.

27. Crepaldi G, Baggio G, Arca M, et al: Pravastatin vs gemfibrozil in the treatment of primary hypercholesterolemia: The Italian Multicentre Pravastatin Study. Arch Intern Med 151:146, 1991.

28. Hoogerbrugge N, Mol MJ, Van Dormaal JJ, et al: The efficacy and safety of pravastatin, compared to and in combination with bile acid binding resins, in familial hypercholesterolemia. J Intern Med 228:201, 1990.

29. Vanhanen H, Miettinen TA: Pravastatin and lovastatin similarly reduce serum cholesterol and its precursor levels in familial hypercholesterolemia. Eur J Clin Pharmacol 42:127, 1992.

30. Pravastatin Multicenter Study Group II: Comparative efficacy and safety of pravastatin and cholestyramine alone and combined in patients with hypercholesterolemia. Arch Intern Med 153:1321, 1993.

31. Jacob BG, Mohrle W, Richter WO, et al: Short- and long-term effects of lovastatin and pravastatin alone and in combination with cholestyramine on serum lipids, lipoproteins and apolipoproteins in primary hypercholesterolemia. Eur J Clin Pharmacol 42:353, 1992.

32. Contacos CH, Barter PHJ, Sullivan DR: Effect of pravastatin and omega-3 fatty acids on plasma lipids and lipoproteins in patients with combined hyperlipidemia. Arterioscler Thromb 13:1755, 1993.

33. Ballaré M, Campanini M, Airoldi G, et al: Hepatotoxicity of hydroxy-methylglutaryl coenzyme A reductase inhibitors. Minerva Gastroenterol Dietol 38:41, 1992.

34. de Vries AC, Cohen LH: Different effects of hypolipidemic drugs pravastatin and lovastatin on the cholesterol biosynthesis of the human ocular lens in organ culture and on the cholesterol content of the rat lens in vivo. Biochim Biophys Acta 1167:63, 1993.

35. de Vries AC, Vermeer MA, Bloemendal H, Cohen LH: Pravastatin and simvastatin differently inhibit cholesterol biosynthesis in human lens. Invest Ophthalmol Vis Sci 34:377, 1993.

36. Roth TH, Richardson GR, Sullivan JP, et al: Comparative effects of pravastatin and lovastatin on nighttime sleep and daytime performance. Clin Cardiol 15:426, 1992.

37. Barth JD, Kruisbrink OAE, Van Dijk AL: Inhibitors of hydroxy-methylglutaryl coenzyme A reductase for hypercholesterolemia. Br Med J 301:669, 1990.

38. Vgontzas AN, Kales A, Bixler EO, et al: Effects of lovastatin and pravastatin on sleep efficiency and sleep stages. Clin Pharmacol Ther 50:730, 1991.

39. Smals AGH, Weusten JJAM, Benraad TJ, et al: The HMG-CoA reductase inhibitor simvastatin suppresses human testosterone synthesis in vitro by a selective inhibitory effect on 17-ketosteroid-oxidoreductase enzyme activity. J Steroid Biochem Mol Biol 38:465, 1991.

40. Ghirlanda G, Oradei A, Manto A, et al: Evidence of plasma CoQ10 lowering effect of HMG-CoA reductase inhibitors: A double blind, placebo controlled study. J Clin Pharmacol 33:226, 1993.

41. Hunninghake DB: HMG-CoA reductase inhibitors. Curr Opin Lipidol 3:22, 1992.

42. Barth JD: Clinical comparison of the bile acid sequestrant colestipol and the HMG-CoA reductase inhibitor simvastatin in familial hyperlipidaemia—another perspective. Today's Therapeutic Trends 11:1, 1993.

43. Dobs AS, Sarma PS, Wilder L: Lipid lowering diets in patients taking pravastatin, a new HMG-CoA reductase inhibitor: Compliance and adequacy. Am J Clin Nutr 54:696, 1991.

44. Spitalewitz S, Porush JG, Cattran D, Wright N: Treatment of hyperlipidemia in the nephrotic syndrome: The effects of pravastatin therapy. Am J Kidney Dis 22:143, 1993.

45. Yoshino G, Kazumi T, Iwai M, et al: Long term treatment of hypercholesterolemic noninsulin dependent diabetics (NIDDM) with pravastatin (CS-514). Atherosclerosis 75:67, 1988.

46. Pernigotti MBL, Pedrazzini LPV, Gottero FBM, et al: One year experience in the treatment of elderly hypercholesterolemic patients with pravastatin. Curr Ther Res 50:151, 1991.

47. Mellies MJ, DeVault AR, Kassler-Taub K, et al: Pravastatin experience in elderly and non-elderly patients. Atherosclerosis 101:97, 1993.

48. Hunninghake DB, Stein EA, Mellies MJ: Effects of one year of treatment with pravastatin, an HMG-CoA reductase inhibitor, on lipoprotein A. J Clin Pharmacol 33:574, 1993.

49. Pitt B, Mancini BJ, Ellis SG, et al: Pravastatin limitation of atherosclerosis in the coronary arteries (PLAC I): Reduction in atherosclerosis progression and clinical events. J Am Coll Cardiol 26:1133, 1995.

50. Crouse JR III, Byington RP, Bond MG, et al: Pravastatin, lipids, and atherosclerosis in the carotid arteries (PLAC-II). Am J Cardiol 75:455, 1995 [published erratum appears in Am J Cardiol 75:862, 1995].

51. Jukema JW, Bruschke AVG, Van Boven AJ, et al: Effects of lipid lowering by pravastatin on progression and regression of coronary artery disease in symptomatic men with normal to moderately elevated serum cholesterol levels. The Regression Growth Evaluation Statin Study (REGRESS). Circulation 91:2528, 1995.

52. Salonen R, Nyyssonen K, Porkkala E, et al: Kuopio Atherosclerosis Prevention Study (KAPS). A population-based primary preventive trial of the effect of LDL lowering on atherosclerotic progression in carotid and femoral arteries. Circulation 92:1758, 1995.

53. Byington RP, Jukema JW, Salonen JT, et al: Reduction in cardiovascular events during pravastatin therapy. Pooled analysis of clinical events of the Pravastatin Atherosclerosis Intervention Program. Circulation 92:2419, 1995.

54. Shepherd J, Cobbe SM, Ford I, et al: Prevention of coronary heart disease with pravastatin in men with hypercholesterolemia. N Engl J Med 333:1301, 1995.

55. Mabuchi H, Kamon N, Fujita H, et al: Effects of CS-514 on lipoprotein lipid and apoprotein levels in patients with familial hypercholesterolemia. Metabolism 36:475, 1987.

56. Carmena R, De Oya M, Franco M, et al: Treatment of heterozygous familial hypercholesterolemia with pravastatin and/or cholestyramine: The Spanish Multicentre Pravastatin Study. In Crepaldi G, Gotto AM, Manzato E, Baggio G (eds): Atherosclerosis VIII. New York: Elsevier, 1989, pp 757–760.

57. Yamamoto A, Yokohama S, Yamamura T: Escape phenomenon occurs by lowering cholesterol with hydroxy-methylglutaryl coenzyme A (HMG-CoA) reductase inhibitor in patients with familial hypercholesterolemia. Atherosclerosis 71:257, 1988.

58. The Lovastatin Pravastatin Study Group: A multicenter comparative trial of lovastatin and pravastatin in the treatment of hypercholesterolemia. Am J Cardiol 71:810, 1993.

CHAPTER 124

Fluvastatin

Conrad B. Blum, M.D.

HISTORY

Fluvastatin was synthesized by Kathawala and others at Sandoz Research Institute in 1983;[1] the chemical synthesis program that led to the development of fluvastatin was initiated in 1979. It is the first totally synthetic inhibitor of 3-hydroxy-3-methylglutaryl coenzyme A (HMG-CoA) reductase, the rate-limiting enzyme of cholesterol biosynthesis. It is structurally distinct from previous HMG-CoA reductase inhibitors. All previous HMG-CoA reductase inhibitors have been closely related to one another and have been derived from fungal broths. Clinical studies with fluvastatin were initiated in 1986, and large-scale phase III clinical trials began in 1989. A total of 97 clinical studies involving more than 6300 subjects have been conducted or are currently under way. At the time of this writing (May 1994), the drug has been approved for marketing in the United Kingdom, United States, Canada, and Switzerland.

CHEMISTRY

The design of a series of synthetic HMG-CoA reductase inhibitors was guided by the assumption that the active site of HMG-CoA reductase contains two regions, one that recognizes the five-carbon unit of beta-hydroxy-beta-methylglutaryl CoA and a second region that is occupied by the CoA portion of HMG-CoA.[1] It was, therefore, hoped that it might be possible to prepare interesting synthetic inhibitors of HMG-CoA reductase utilizing a general structure with substituents that would mimic those two portions of HMG-CoA. The choices of substituents to occupy a CoA recognition site of the enzyme were made after considering the structural elements of CoA and the ring portion of compactin, the first HMG-CoA reductase inhibitor to have been developed. Fluvastatin is the monosodium salt of a fluorophenylated-indolic C3,C5 dihydroxy carboxylic acid.

Fluvastatin, a racemate, is [R*, S*-(E)]-(±)-3,5-dihydroxy-7-[3-(4-fluorophenyl)-1-(1-methylethyl)-1H-indol-2-yl]-6-heptenoic acid, monosodium salt. Its molecular weight is 433.5. It is a white–to–pale yellow, water-soluble powder.

PRECLINICAL STUDIES OF EFFICACY

Fluvastatin is a potent competitive inhibitor of HMG-CoA reductase,[1, 2] and this is the basis for its ability to reduce low-density lipoprotein (LDL) cholesterol levels in plasma. In a rat liver microsome assay system, fluvastatin has approximately 144 times the potency of compactin and 103 times the potency of lovastatin. In rats, it is five times more potent than lovastatin in inhibiting cholesterol synthesis.[1]

The hypocholesterolemic effects of fluvastatin have been studied in rats, dogs, rhesus monkeys, and cholesterol-fed hamsters.[2, 3] In a 5-week study in rats, the concentration of VLDL + LDL (very-low-density lipoprotein + low-density lipoprotein) cholesterol fell promptly and remained below baseline for the duration of the study. With a fluvastatin dose of 28.8 mg/kg, VLDL + LDL cholesterol had fallen by 50% after 1 week of treatment. In rats, there is a substantial increase in HMG-CoA reductase mass in response to treatment with inhibitors of this enzyme; consequently, the incorporation of ^{14}C-acetate into cholesterol more than doubled. Despite this, a 9% reduction in VLDL + LDL cholesterol remained after 5 weeks of treatment. These results suggested that increased clearance of lipoproteins from the circulation was responsible for the reduced plasma concentrations.

In male beagle dogs, fluvastatin administered orally in a dose of 1 mg/kg reduced LDL cholesterol by 25%. At this dose, a modest 15% reduction in high-density lipoprotein (HDL) cholesterol occurred; this is not surprising, because HDL carries most of the plasma cholesterol in the beagle. Similar reductions in HDL have also been reported in dogs treated with the HMG-CoA reductase inhibitors compactin and lovastatin, but this has not been found in humans.

In rhesus monkeys, after 4 weeks of treatment with fluvastatin in a dose of 30 mg/kg/day PO, LDL cholesterol was reduced 22% compared with controls.

Studies were conducted with the cholesterol-saturated fat-fed hamster because its lipoprotein metabolism has close similarities to that of humans.[4] In this model, fluvastatin in a dose of 13 mg/kg/day was found to be slightly more effective than a similar dose of lovastatin in reducing VLDL + LDL cholesterol (80% reduction with fluvastatin, 60% reduction with lovastatin). The reduction in plasma LDL cholesterol was associated with an increased fractional rate of clearance of LDL from plasma and an increased LDL receptor active in hepatocyte membranes.

PHARMACOKINETICS AND DRUG METABOLISM

Studies of the pharmacokinetics and metabolism of fluvastatin have given generally similar results in the mouse, rat, dog, monkey, and humans.[5, 6] Absorption of the drug is complete and rapid. In humans, peak blood levels occurred 0.5 hour after ingestion of fluvastatin (Fig. 124–1), and absorption was measured

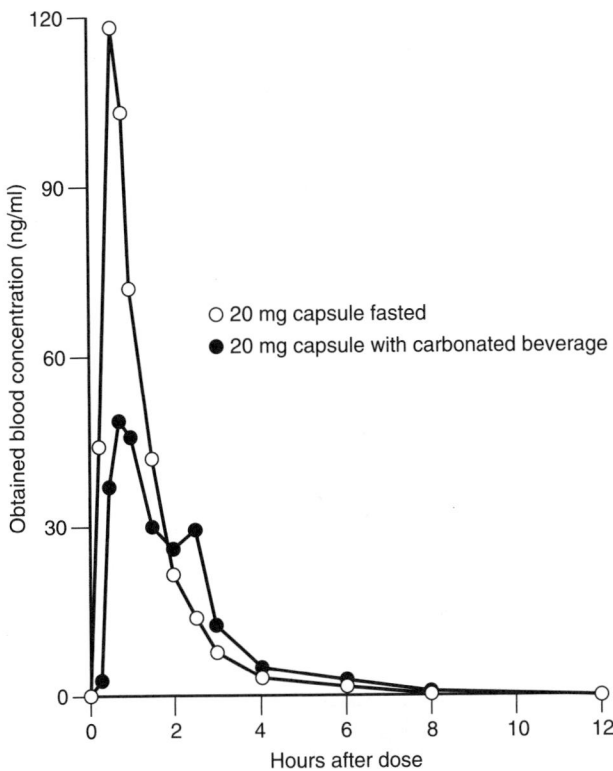

Figure 124–1. Fluvastatin blood concentrations in humans (n = 20 subjects).

as 98% of the administered oral dose. When fluvastatin is administered with food, absorption is slightly slower; the slowed absorption would be expected to increase first-pass hepatic metabolism of the drug, and in keeping with this expectation, a modest 25% reduction in bioavailability is seen when fluvastatin is taken with food. Because fluvastatin is unstable in acid environments, absorption is reduced when it is coadministered with an acidic carbonated beverage. Age does not appear to influence the metabolism of fluvastatin, nor does gender.[7]

Fluvastatin undergoes a saturable first-pass metabolism in the liver, and metabolites representing 95% of an orally administered dose enter the gastrointestinal tract through the biliary route and are excreted in the feces. The first-pass hepatic metabolism of fluvastatin results in an absolute bioavailability of 24% for an orally administered dose. In humans, saturation of first-pass hepatic metabolism is seen only at doses exceeding 20 mg, and this saturation results in 30% to 40% more bioavailability for a 40-mg dose than would be predicted from the response to 20 mg of fluvastatin. The first-pass saturation is minimized when the absorption of fluvastatin is reduced by administration of the drug with meals or at bedtime as recommended. This dosing regimen should, therefore, minimize the potential for side effects linked to peak concentration of the drug.[6] Hepatic insufficiency results in increased peak plasma concentrations and increased absolute bioavailability of orally administered fluvastatin. This observation warrants caution

when fluvastatin is considered for patients with hepatic insufficiency.[7]

For practical purposes, no active metabolites of fluvastatin are present in systemic plasma. Trivial amounts of fluvastatin lactone, which has 28% the activity of native fluvastatin, are present in systemic plasma. The plasma HMG-CoA reductase inhibitory activity associated with the lactone after oral dosing with fluvastatin is equivalent to 1.7% of the administered dose.[1, 8, 9]

Studies of the tissue distribution of fluvastatin show that it is highly targeted to the liver. When radiolabeled fluvastatin was given to rodents, vastly more radioactivity was seen in the liver than in any other organ (Fig. 124–2). Furthermore, after oral administration, fluvastatin is rapidly cleared from the systemic circulation (see Fig. 124–1); the effective elimination half-life ranges from 0.5 to 3.1 hours.[2] *In vitro* and *in vivo* experiments in the rat indicate that there is no significant transfer of fluvastatin through the blood-brain barrier.[10]

ANIMAL TOXICOLOGY

Preclinical studies performed in the rat, mouse, dog, and monkey have shown the following organs to be the major targets of toxic effects of fluvastatin: ocular lens, heart, nonglandular forestomach, liver, thyroid, and gallbladder.

Cataracts have occurred in the dog in doses of at least 16 mg/kg/day. As with other HMG-CoA reductase inhibitors, cataracts have not been induced in other species.[11]

Cardiac myofibrillar degeneration has occurred in pregnant rats treated with very high doses of fluvastatin (6 mg/kg/day) around the time of parturition. Detailed study indicates that this is a result of the combination of stress associated with endocrine and physiologic changes of late pregnancy and an exaggerated pharmacologic effect of fluvastatin.[2] This concept is supported by the observation that the toxicity was prevented by treatment with mevalonate.

Hyperkeratosis and hyperplasia of the nonglandular forestomach have occurred in the rat and mouse. The data suggest that the hyperkeratosis and hyperplasia are due to a local irritant action of fluvastatin; no forestomach effects are seen after intravenous dosing. The nonglandular forestomach, which is lined with squamous epithelium, is present only in rodents; in no species have abnormalities of the esophagus or stomach been seen. Thus, this side effect does not seem relevant to human beings.[2]

Fluvastatin is similar to other HMG-CoA reductase inhibitors in its ability to cause hepatocellular injury. This has been seen in rats, dogs, and monkeys treated with high doses of fluvastatin. This effect of fluvastatin is seen only with the active enantiomer, suggesting that it is related to the mechanism of action of the drug, inhibition of HMG-CoA reductase.[2]

In the rat, but not in other species, fluvastatin has caused increased weight of the thyroid gland and an increase in the number of follicular adenomas and

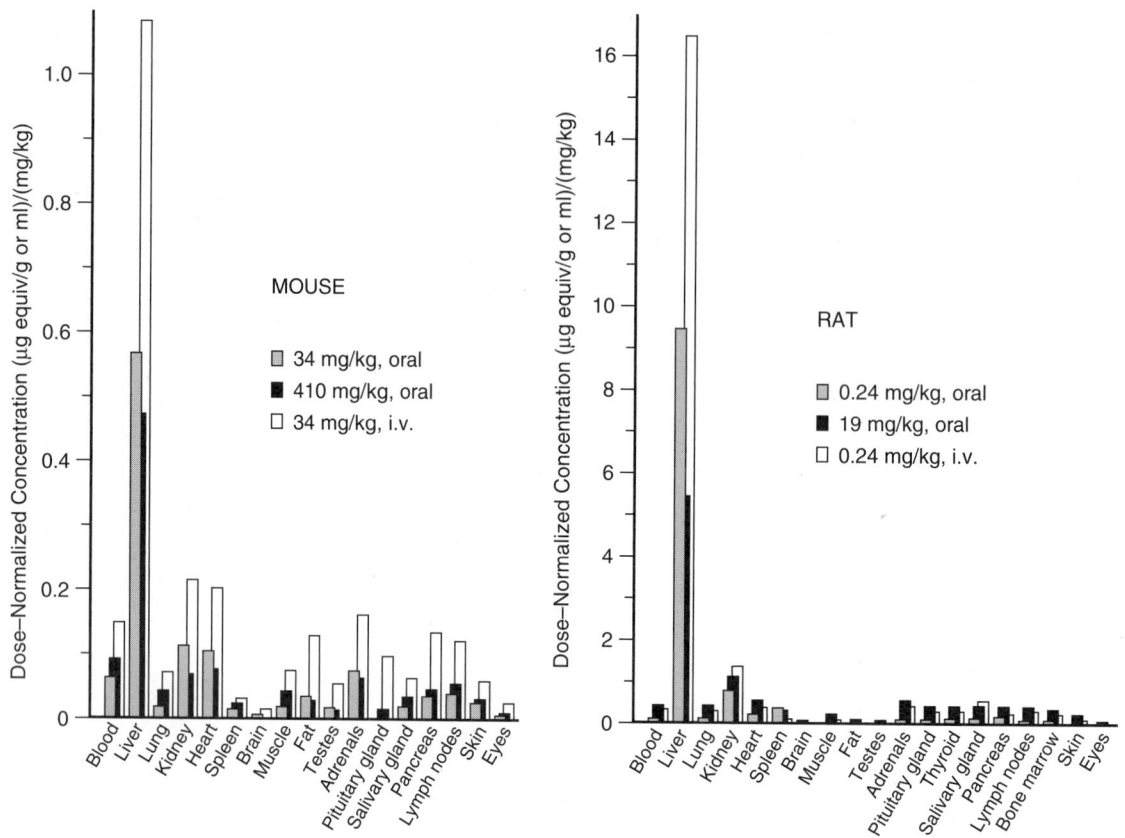

Figure 124–2. Organ distribution of radioactivity after a single or multiple oral dose of radiolabeled fluvastatin in the mouse and rat.

carcinomas. Similar thyroid changes have been reported in rats treated with simvastatin[12] and many other structurally diverse chemicals.[13] These abnormalities are probably related to increased clearance of thyroxine, and they are restricted to rodents. Treatment with thyroxine has prevented these abnormalities, suggesting that they are caused by increased stimulation of the thyroid by thyroid-stimulating hormone (TSH). In human studies, no statistically significant changes in TSH levels were associated with the use of fluvastatin. Thus, the data suggest that the thyroid abnormalities found in rodents bear no relevance for human beings.[2]

Gallbladder hemorrhages were seen in dogs treated with overtly toxic doses of fluvastatin (24 mg/kg/day). Gallblader hyperplasia was seen in dogs and in monkeys treated with extremely high doses of fluvastatin (8 to 12 mg/kg/day). These findings may relate to the large portion (70%) of unaltered fluvastatin that is excreted in the bile in these species. In humans, no parent drug is excreted in bile.[2]

In vitro studies have not shown fluvastatin to have any potential for mutagenicity. Furthermore, in contrast with other HMG-CoA reductase inhibitors, fluvastatin has not produced liver tumors or lung tumors in any species.[2]

The studies in animals have shown fluvastatin in doses of 8 mg/kg to have no effect on fasting serum glucose level in rats, no effect on blood pressure or heart rate in conscious normotensive rats, and no

effect on autonomic responses in anesthetized dogs. Furthermore, there were no overt changes in behavior and no increase in mortality in rats treated with fluvastatin 40 mg/kg.[2]

CLINICAL USE
Indications

Fluvastatin is used as an adjunct to diet in the treatment of elevated levels of LDL cholesterol. In accord with the recommendations of the National Cholesterol Education Program, its use may be considered when, despite dietary measures, LDL cholesterol exceeds 190 mg/dl, or when it exceeds 160 mg/dl in individuals with at least two risk factors for coronary heart disease (CHD), or when it exceeds 130 mg/dl in individuals who already have CHD.[14]

Efficacy in Monotherapy

Two large phase II double-blind trials of efficacy have been performed in the United States, one for dose ranging and the other to assess the effects of dose frequency. The results of the dose ranging study are shown in Figure 124–3. A total of 424 subjects with LDL cholesterol at least 160 mg/dl were assigned to treatment with placebo or fluvastatin in a dose of 5 mg, 15 mg, 30 mg, or 40 mg daily. The results shown are for the 412 subjects who completed this study.

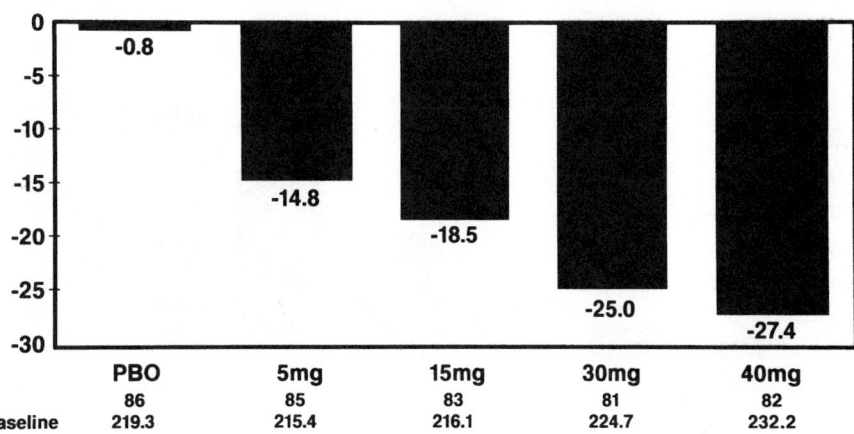

% Change in LDL-C

	PBO	5mg	15mg	30mg	40mg
N	86	85	83	81	82
Baseline LDL-C (mg/dL)	219.3	215.4	216.1	224.7	232.2

Figure 124–3. Fluvastatin dose response study. Percentage change in LDL-C. PBO designates placebo. Fluvastatin was given as a single evening dose in the amounts shown.

The period of double-blind treatment was 6 weeks. A progressively increasing effect was seen as the dose was increased, so that a 27.4% reduction in LDL cholesterol was associated with a 40-mg daily dose of fluvastatin.[2]

In a double-blind, placebo-controlled dose frequency study with 204 subjects, fluvastatin 20 mg each evening was compared with a dose of 10 mg twice daily.[15] The two dosing regimens gave very similar results for LDL reduction: 22.2% reduction for once-daily dosing, and 22.7% reduction for twice-daily dosing. Thus, fluvastatin may be used with a once-daily dosing regimen.

In phase III of clinical development, four large placebo-controlled studies investigated the effects of fluvastatin 20 mg daily. For three of the studies, baseline LDL cholesterol was restricted to at least 160 mg/dl. The fourth study involved subjects with familial hypercholesterolemia (FH), so baseline LDL cholesterol was required to be at least 200 mg/dl. Pooled results of these United States phase III studies, involving 1125 subjects treated with placebo or fluvastatin 20 mg daily are shown in Table 124–1. Six hundred forty-eight subjects were randomized to fluvastatin, and 477 to placebo; 58% were men, and 42% were

women. Fluvastatin 20 mg daily caused a 20.3% reduction in LDL cholesterol compared with the change in placebo. There was a small 2.2% increase in HDL cholesterol and a 9.3% reduction in the plasma triglyceride level. All of these changes were statistically highly significant.[2, 16]

A categorical analysis of the results (Fig. 124–4) showed that 67% of subjects treated with fluvastatin (20 mg daily) sustained an LDL reduction exceeding 15%. Fifty-three percent of subjects had more than a 20% reduction in LDL cholesterol. Thirty-three percent of subjects sustained more than a 25% reduction in LDL cholesterol, and 17% of subjects sustained more than a 30% reduction in LDL cholesterol.[2]

Subgroup analyses suggested that fluvastatin (20 mg daily) may be slightly more effective in reducing LDL cholesterol in women (mean reduction compared with placebo, 21.8%) than in men (mean reduction, 19.1%) ($p = .049$). Furthermore, there was slightly greater reduction of LDL among older subjects (19.7% for those younger than 65 years of age, and 22.8% for those at least 65 years of age) ($p = .0511$). Although the women enrolled in these studies did tend to weigh less than the men, the difference in weight did not account for the slightly greater LDL reduction seen in women. Dietary restriction of cholesterol and saturated fats was not related to the extent of the fluvastatin-induced reduction in LDL cholesterol. Furthermore, there did not appear to be any racial difference in responsiveness to fluvastatin. However, the number of blacks enrolled was small (n = 39), so the question of racial differences was not addressed with great statistical power in these studies.[2, 16]

Doses of 40 mg daily were tested in 210 subjects in the FH study. A mean 24.0% reduction in LDL cholesterol was seen with the 40-mg dose in this population (22.5% reduction for dosing with 40 mg each evening, and 25.4% for dosing with 20 mg twice daily). An LDL reduction exceeding 15% was achieved by 77% of patients taking fluvastatin 40 mg each evening and by 85% of those taking 20 mg twice daily.[2]

An 80-mg daily dosage has been studied in a small

Table 124–1. **Effects of Fluvastatin 20 mg Daily on Plasma Lipids and Lipoproteins**

		Baseline (mg/dl)	% Change
Cholesterol	Fluvastatin	297	−15.4
	Placebo	299	−0.2
LDL cholesterol*	Fluvastatin	215	−20.5
	Placebo	218	−0.2
HDL cholesterol†	Fluvastatin	50.7	2.4
	Placebo	50.3	0.2
Triglyceride*	Fluvastatin	153	−7.1
	Placebo	151	2.2

Pooled data from placebo-controlled United States phase III studies involving 1125 subjects.
*$p<.001$
†$p<.01$

Percent of Subjects

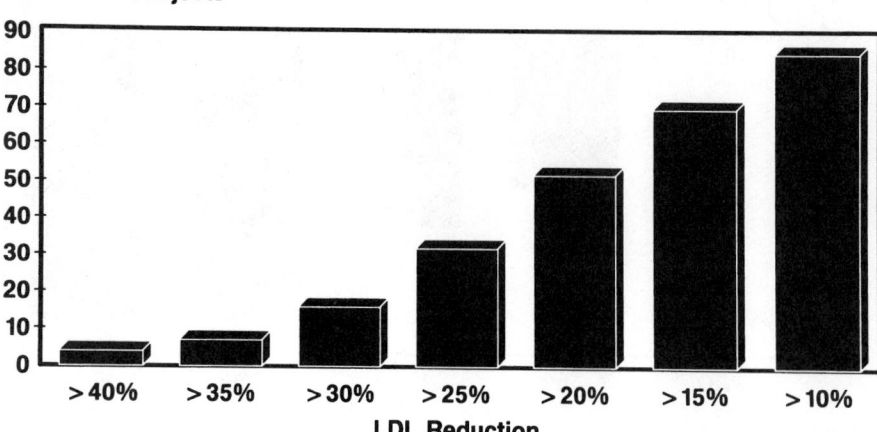

Figure 124–4. Categorical analysis of LDL-C response to 20 mg fluvastatin. Pooled results of placebo-controlled phase III trials, n = 1125. Graph indicates percentage of subjects with LDL-C reduction exceeding the amount shown.

pilot study of 40 FH patients. LDL cholesterol was reduced by 18.2% in those receiving fluvastatin 20 mg daily, by 27.1% in those receiving fluvastatin 40 mg each evening, and by 34.4% in those receiving 40 mg twice daily.[2]

The interindividual variability in responsiveness to fluvastatin has been examined in some detail using patients with FH.[17] It was found that patients characterized as having Sephardic and Lithuanian mutations demonstrated lesser responsiveness to fluvastatin 40 mg daily than did those with Lebanese or other haplotypes (16% to 18% LDL reduction versus 25% to 30% LDL reduction). Several genetic factors explained much of the variability in LDL response. These included LDL receptor haplotype, apolipoprotein E phenotype, and apolipoprotein(a) isoform.

Efficacy in Combination Therapy with Other Lipid-Lowering Drugs

Fluvastatin and cholestyramine have additive effects on LDL reduction when used concomitantly. This combination has been investigated in two short-term pharmacokinetic studies and in one longer study focusing on efficacy. The bioavailability of fluvastatin is reduced by nearly 90% when it is taken simultaneously with cholestyramine.[7] The reduction in bioavailability was limited to 43% when fluvastatin was administered 4 hours after an 8-g dose of cholestyramine. Despite this moderate reduction in bioavailability, there is an additive effect on LDL reduction when fluvastatin and cholestyramine are used together. In a 24-week placebo-controlled, parallel group study (Table 124–2), fluvastatin 20 mg daily (n = 38) yielded a 19.0% reduction in LDL cholesterol, cholestyramine 4 g twice daily (n = 36) resulted in a 13.6% reduction in LDL cholesterol, and fluvastatin 20 mg daily plus cholestyramine 4 g twice daily (n = 35) resulted in a 30.6% reduction in LDL cholesterol. The addition of cholestyramine did not substantially alter the small increases in HDL cholesterol seen with fluvastatin monotherapy. In this study, cholestyramine was taken twice daily with meals, and fluvastatin was taken at bedtime.[2, 7]

The combination of fluvastatin with nicotinic acid also caused additive reductions in LDL cholesterol. This combination was evaluated in a randomized, 73-subject, placebo-controlled, parallel group study. Fluvastatin (n = 38) or placebo (n = 35) was given for an initial 6 weeks; during the final portion of the study, all subjects were given nicotinic acid 1 g three times daily in addition to fluvastatin or placebo. Compliance to fluvastatin exceeded 95%; compliance to nicotinic acid was 88%. Fluvastatin 20 mg daily resulted in a 20.8% reduction in LDL cholesterol. When fluvastatin and nicotinic acid were used together, LDL cholesterol fell to 40.1% below the untreated baseline level. Nicotinic acid alone was associated with a 25.4% reduction in LDL cholesterol. LDL cholesterol fell by more than 50% in one third of subjects taking the combination of fluvastatin with nicotinic acid. HDL cholesterol increased modestly (4.5%) with fluvastatin alone, but the combination of fluvastatin plus niacin increased HDL much the same as niacin alone (33.1% versus 41.5%; $p < .10$). Treatment with fluvastatin alone did not influence the plasma level of lipoprotein(a) [Lp(a)], but with the addition of niacin, Lp(a) fell by 38%.[2]

Adverse Effects

The safety of fluvastatin has been studied in clinical trials involving approximately 6300 subjects worldwide. Approximately 4000 subjects in these trials were

Table 124–2. **Efficacy of Fluvastatin 20 mg Daily and Cholestyramine 4 g Twice Daily Alone and in Combination**

	Placebo (n = 37)	Fluvastatin (n = 38)	Cholestyramine (n = 36)	Fluvastatin Plus Cholestyramine (n = 35)
Cholesterol	−1.1	−14.5	−7.9	−21.5
LDL cholesterol	1.2	−19.0	−13.6	−30.6
HDL cholesterol	−1.7	4.2	4.3	3.2
Triglyceride	1.6	−10.5	11.4	11.4

Mean percent change from baseline in lipids and lipoproteins is shown for each randomization group.

treated with fluvastatin. Some individuals participated in more than one study, and some received placebo or an active control rather than fluvastatin. Thus, a total of 1881 unique subjects in North America were exposed to fluvastatin in clinical trials of the efficacy and safety of this drug. These subjects were exposed to fluvastatin for an average of 51 weeks each. More than 500 subjects have undergone at least 2 years of treatment with fluvastatin in a dose of 20 mg daily or more.[2]

Fluvastatin is similar to other HMG-CoA reductase inhibitors in having the ability to produce biochemical abnormalities of liver function. This property is the most important demonstrated toxicity of fluvastatin. Abnormalities of liver function, however, occurred uncommonly; notable increases in serum transaminases to values exceeding three times the upper limit of normal have occurred in 1.0% of fluvastatin-treated subjects in controlled clinical trials and in 0.4% of placebo-treated subjects. Sixty percent of these events have occurred during the first 13 weeks of treatment. Long-term open-label experience with fluvastatin in doses up to 40 mg twice daily also suggests that the development of notable transaminase elevation is quite uncommon after the initial 4 months of treatment. Patients demonstrating these abnormalities have generally been free of symptoms. On discontinuation of the medication, the biochemical abnormalities have usually returned to normal within 2 weeks. Baseline abnormalities in transaminases predict an increased risk of more severe abnormalities developing during treatment with fluvastatin; 42% of subjects having transaminase elevations beyond three times the upper limit of normal while taking fluvastatin had some abnormality at baseline.[2, 16]

Because skeletal muscle toxicity has been reported to occur with other HMG-CoA reductase inhibitors, it is of note that fluvastatin has not been associated with a single case of rhabdomyolysis. Only one case of myopathy (creatine kinase [CK] at least 10 times the upper limit of normal with myalgias or weakness) has occurred in association with fluvastatin, but in this case a recent increase in physical activity (pruning trees) provided an alternative explanation for muscular injury; one case of myopathy also occurred in a patient receiving placebo. In the placebo-controlled trials, myalgias have occurred with similar frequency in patients treated with fluvastatin (4.4%) and in those treated with placebo (4.5%). Similarly, the rate of marked CK elevations (>10 times the upper limit of normal) has been identical in the fluvastatin and placebo groups (0.4%); thus, the experience with fluvastatin does not suggest a drug-related effect on marked CK elevation.[2]

Abnormalities in the ocular lens were examined in controlled clinical trials because of the finding that fluvastatin can produce cataracts in dogs. In 1430 subjects who underwent slit-lamp examinations, newly occurring or worsening lenticular abnormalities were found in virtually identical frequency among those treated with fluvastatin (13.6%) and those treated with placebo (13.1%). Thus, the controlled studies in human subjects do not indicate any potential of fluvastatin to produce abnormalities in the lens.[2]

As noted earlier, hemorrhage has occurred in the gallbladders of dogs given lethal doses of fluvastatin (24 to 48 mg/kg/day), and minimal epithelial hyperplasia of gallbladder epithelium has been seen in nonhuman primates. With this background, gallbladder ultrasound examinations were performed in 166 subjects in two placebo-controlled clinical trials. The examinations were performed after 6 months of treatment. In a subset of the population, a repeat examination was performed after 1 year. These studies provided no corroboration of the preclinical findings of gallbladder hyperplasia. The frequency of new abnormalities in the gallbladder was slightly higher among the subjects not being treated with fluvastatin; this difference is probably a chance phenomenon.[2]

Abdominal pain and dyspepsia occurred more frequently among fluvastatin-treated subjects (15.1%) than with placebo (9.3%). The intensity of these symptoms has been relatively mild as they did not generally necessitate discontinuation of treatment. Both these symptoms occurred more commonly when fluvastatin was dosed as 40 mg each evening than with 20 mg once or twice daily.[2]

Fluvastatin is well tolerated in doses up to 40 mg twice daily. Not one of the 325 patients taking this dosage in a long-term extension study has discontinued treatment because of an adverse effect of the drug. In the controlled trials, it was found that compliance to treatment with fluvastatin was as high as with placebo; this was approximately 95%.[2]

Interactions with Other Drugs

Because fluvastatin is very highly bound to albumin, the potential for interaction with other protein-bound medications was studied. At therapeutic concentrations, this binding is not influenced by the presence of warfarin, aspirin, or glyburide.[5] Fluvastatin also does not influence the protein binding of these other drugs in undiluted plasma.

The pharmacokinetic interaction of fluvastatin with cholestyramine and the cholesterol-reducing efficacy of this combination have been described in a previous section. Treatment with cholestyramine alone often causes mild increases in transaminase levels. However, in a 27-week study, the combination of cholestyramine with fluvastatin did not result in more frequent transaminase elevation (17.4% for SGOT, 30.4% for SGPT; n = 205) than did the combination of cholestyramine with placebo (19.5% for aspartate transaminase [SGOT], 35.5% for alanine transaminase [SGPT]; n = 169). Thus, combination treatment with fluvastatin and cholestyramine does not appear to pose an increased threat of hepatotoxicity.[2]

The interaction of fluvastatin with nicotinic acid was investigated both pharmacokinetically and in a blinded clinical trial. Treatment with nicotinic acid 1 g three times daily did not alter the pharmacokinetics of fluvastatin; when a single 20-mg dose of fluvastatin was given, concurrent treatment with nicotinic acid caused only a trivial 2% change in the measured area under the curve (AUC) and C_{max} and a 6% change in T_{max}.[7]

The safety of the combination of fluvastatin with nicotinic acid was of concern because both of these drugs can be hepatotoxic and because the combination of the HMG-CoA reductase inhibitor lovastatin with nicotinic acid has been reported to be associated with an increased risk of myopathy. Combination treatment with fluvastatin and nicotinic acid was investigated in a double-blind, placebo-controlled study involving 73 subjects. The subjects were allocated to treatment for 6 weeks with either (1) the combination of fluvastatin 20 mg daily plus nicotinic acid 1 g three times daily or (2) the combination of placebo plus nicotinic acid. Although there was a greater incidence of SGOT elevations in the fluvastatin plus nicotinic acid group than in the placebo plus niacin group (23.7% versus 9.7%), this was not found with SGPT. The transaminase elevations that did occur were generally of a borderline nature; only one patient treated with fluvastatin plus nicotinic acid had a transaminase level exceeding twice the upper limit of normal, and he was matched by a patient with a similar transaminase elevation in the placebo plus nicotinic acid group. No cases of myopathy occurred, and the incidence of abnormal CK level was not elevated by the combination therapy. Thus, pharmacokinetic and clinical studies do not suggest that undue risk is associated with the combination of fluvastatin with nicotinic acid.[2]

Single-dose pharmacokinetic studies were performed to determine the effects on fluvastatin's pharmacokinetics of ongoing treatment with propranolol, cimetidine, ranitidine, omeprazole, and rifampicin. Propranolol was of interest because of its ability to influence hepatic blood flow. Cimetidine, ranitidine, and omeprazole were of interest because they inhibit gastric acid production; and fluvastatin is unstable in acid environments. Furthermore, these studies were intended to indicate whether dose adjustments may be needed when fluvastatin was administered along with drugs known to be potent mixed-function oxidase inducers (e.g., rifampicin) or with drugs known to be mixed-function oxidase inhibitors (e.g., cimetidine). Small but statistically significant increases in bioavailability occurred with cimetidine, ranitidine, and omeprazole. This increased bioavailability of fluvastatin probably results from reduced acid-catalyzed degradation of the drug as well as from reduced first-pass hepatic clearance consequent to the increased absorption rate. In the case of cimetidine, inhibition of cytochrome P-450 may also play a role. Pretreatment with the enzyme inducer rifampicin resulted in a 50% reduction in the major parameters of bioavailability, AUC and C_{max}.[2]

Fluvastatin has been demonstrated to have no effect on the pharmacokinetics of digoxin.[18]

Use in Patients with Impaired Organs

Because the metabolism of fluvastatin is reduced in patients with hepatic failure, the administration of this drug to patients with liver failure should usually be avoided. Because renal clearance of fluvastatin is very limited, there is no need for reduction in dose in patients with mild-to-moderate degrees of renal failure.[7]

Dosage and Administration

Treatment with fluvastatin should begin with a dose of 20 mg daily given at bedtime. The dose range is 20 to 40 mg daily. Splitting the 40-mg dosage into a twice-daily regimen produces a modest improvement in LDL reduction. A dose of 40 mg twice daily is currently under investigation, but there is not yet sufficient experience for this dose to be recommended.

When fluvastatin is used concomitantly with a bile acid sequestrant (cholestyramine or colestipol), it should be administered at least 2 hours after the bile acid sequestrant.[7]

COST

At the time of its initial marketing in the United States, the "ex-factory" price of fluvastatin was $0.85 per 20-mg capsule and $0.95 per 40-mg capsule. This price was substantially less than that for doses of other HMG-CoA reductase inhibitors providing similar reduction in LDL cholesterol.

SUMMARY

Fluvastatin is the first totally synthetic HMG-CoA reductase inhibitor. In doses of 20 and 40 mg daily, it reduced LDL cholesterol by an average of 20.5% and 24.0%, respectively. As with other HMG-CoA reductase inhibitors, transaminase elevations can occur with fluvastatin. However, this is quite uncommon, as the incidence of notable elevations of transaminases with fluvastatin is only 0.6% greater than with placebo. Although myopathy and rhabdomyolysis have been reported as rare side effects of other HMG-CoA reductase inhibitors, rhabdomyolysis has not occurred in association with fluvastatin, and there has been no case of myopathy clearly due to this drug. Fluvastatin is very well tolerated, and in controlled studies, compliance to treatment, approximately 95%, was as high for fluvastatin as for placebo.

Acknowledgments

The author is grateful to Drs. Leonard Gonasun, Leonard Jokubaitis, and David Weinstein, of Sandoz Research Institute, and to Dr. James Fattu, formerly of Sandoz Research Institute, for their assistance.

REFERENCES

1. Kathawala FG: HMG-CoA reductase inhibitors: An exciting development in the treatment of hyperlipoproteinemia. Med Res Rev 11:121, 1991.
2. Data on file: Sandoz Research Institute, East Hanover, NJ.
3. Engstrom RG, Weinstein DB, Kathawala FG, et al: Hypolipo-

proteinemic effects of a potent HMG-CoA reductase inhibitor. *In* Ninth International Symposium on Drugs Affecting Lipid Metabolism, Florence (Italy), 22–25 October, 1986 (Series, Lorenzini Foundation Symposium, No. 159). Milan: Fondazione Giovanni Lorenzini, 1986, p 26.

4. Dietschy JM, Spady DK, Stange EF: Quantitative importance of different organs for cholesterol synthesis and low-density-lipoprotein degradation. Biochem Soc Trans 11:639, 1983.
5. Tse FLS, Smith HT, Ballard FH, et al: Disposition of fluvastatin, an inhibitor of HMG-CoA reductase in mouse, rat, dog, and monkey. Biopharm Drug Dispos 11:519, 1990.
6. Tse FLS, Jaffe JM, Troendle A: Pharmacokinetics of fluvastatin after single and multiple doses in normal volunteers. J Clin Pharmacol 32:630, 1992.
7. Smith HT, Jokubaitis LA, Troendle AJ, et al: Pharmacokinetics of fluvastatin and specific drug interactions. Am J Hypertens 6:1S, 1993.
8. Dain JG, Gorski J, Nicoleti J, et al: Biotransformation of fluvastatin sodium in humans. Drug Metab Dispos 21:567, 1993.
9. Tse FLS, Nickerson DF, Yardley WS: Blood and plasma protein binding of fluvastatin. Int J Clin Pharmacol Ther Toxicol 30:305, 1992.
10. Guillot F, Misslin P, Lemaire M: Comparison of fluvastatin and lovastatin blood-brain barrier transfer using in vitro and in vivo methods. J Cardiovasc Pharmacol 21:339, 1993.
11. Hockwin O, Evans M, Roberts SA, et al: Post-mortem biochemistry of beagle dog lenses after treatment with fluvastatin (Sandoz) for two years at different dose levels. Lens and Eye Toxicity Research 7:563, 1990.
12. Smith PF, Grossman SJ, Gerson RJ, et al: Studies on the mechanism of simvastatin-induced thyroid hypertrophy and follicular cell adenoma in the rat. Toxicol Pathol 19:197, 1991.
13. Curran PG, DeGroot LJ: The effect of hepatic enzyme-inducing drugs on thyroid hormones and the thyroid gland. Endocr Rev 12:135, 1991.
14. Expert Panel on Detection, Evaluation, and Treatment of High Blood Cholesterol in Adults: Summary of the second report of the National Cholesterol Education Program (NCEP) Expert Panel on Detection, Evaluation, and Treatment of High Blood Cholesterol in Adults (Adult Treatment Panel II). JAMA 269:3015, 1993.
15. Keilson L, Dujovne C, Hunninghake D, et al: Efficacy of synthetic HMG-CoA reductase inhibitor fluvastatin. Arteriosclerosis 10:856a, 1990.
16. Jokubaitis LA, Troendle AJ, Fattu JM, et al: Clinical experience with fluvastatin, the first synthetic HMG-CoA reductase inhibitor. *In* Catapano AL, Gotto AM Jr, Smith LC, Paoletti R (eds): Drugs Affecting Lipid Metabolism. Boston: Kluwer Academic Publishers, 1993, pp 269–276.
17. Leitersdorf E, Eisenberg S, Eliav O, et al: Genetic determinants of responsiveness to the HMG-CoA reductase inhibitor fluvastatin in patients with molecularly defined heterozygous familial hypercholesterolemia. Circulation 87(Suppl III):III, 1993.
18. Garnett WR, Venitz J, Wilkens R, et al: Double-blind evaluation to determine the influence of fluvastatin in a patient population chronically receiving digoxin. Pharm Res 8(Suppl):S63, 1991.

XIII.
Positive Inotropic Agents

Editors: Jay N. Cohn and Wilson S. Colucci

A. Digitalization

CHAPTER 125

Principles and Practice of Digitalis

Kelly Anne Spratt, D.O., and James E. Doherty, M.D.

Digitalis glycosides are among the most frequently prescribed drugs in the United States. Annually, over 23 million prescriptions are filled at a cost of over 107 million dollars.[1] Although these drugs offer a unique advantage in the treatment of arrhythmias and heart failure, their narrow therapeutic window can precipitate toxicity, insidiously or rapidly, without warning. In the United States, digoxin is the most commonly used glycoside and is the focus of this chapter, with brief attention given to the less frequently used drug, digitoxin. Understanding the mechanism of action, clinical use, and drug interactions can guide clinicians in the prudent use of digitalis. This chapter also discusses the clinical manifestations of digitalis toxicity and provides an algorithm for treating this potentially lethal situation.

HISTORICAL PERSPECTIVE

The earliest use of cardiac glycosides can be traced to the ancient Egyptians and Romans, who used the digitalis-like substance "squill" as a heart tonic.[2] In the 1500s, foxglove was botanically categorized as *Digitalis purpurea*. In 1785, William Withering discussed the diuretic effects of this plant for "dropsy" (edema) in his famous treatise.[3] However, it was not until 1799 that the primary cardiac effect of digitalis was recognized, with the diuretic benefit a secondary phenomenon. In the early 20th century, the use of digitalis specifically for atrial fibrillation became widely accepted.

Only recently has it been recognized that the positive inotropic effect of digitalis makes this drug a valuable agent for the treatment of heart failure. Even today, mechanisms responsible for the therapeutic and toxic effects of digitalis continue to be investigated, accounting for the cyclical popularity of this drug for heart failure.

CHEMISTRY

Cardiac glycosides are formed through the combination of an aglycon and one to four sugar molecules

attached to a lactone ring. Pharmacologic properties are primarily a result of the aglycon, which is chemically related to bile acids, sterols, and steroid hormones. The sugar molecules influence pharmacokinetic properties. Hydroxyl groups attached to the sugar moiety further modify properties such as solubility. Digitoxin and digoxin differ by only one hydroxyl group, yet this hydroxyl group confers aqueous solubility for digoxin versus lipid solubility for digitoxin.

MECHANISM OF ACTION

The clinical benefits of digitalis are produced through a network of direct and indirect interactions upon the myocardium, vasculature, and autonomic nervous system. These interactions are responsible for a continuum of clinical effects ranging from the beneficial to the potentially lethal.

Digitalis directly inhibits sodium-potassium–activated adenosine triphosphatase (Na^+,K^+-ATPase), the so-called Na^+-K^+ pump.[4] As a result of this inhibition, the active process of exchanging intracellular sodium for extracellular potassium to maintain ionic equilibrium is inhibited (Fig. 125–1). This inhibition also increases intracellular calcium via two mechanisms. First there is an increased influx of calcium via modulation of the slow calcium channels. Second, as intracellular sodium accumulates, the sodium-calcium exchange pump is affected so that the usual exchange of extracellular sodium for intracellular calcium is decreased. This reduces the efflux of calcium and thus contributes to an increase in intracellular calcium. With each action potential, a greater amount of calcium remains available to the contractile apparatus. This increase in intracellular sodium and subsequent increase in intracellular calcium is considered to be responsible for the positive inotropic effect of digitalis.[5] Inhibition of Na^+,K^+-ATPase may yield an increase in extracellular potassium, warranting close monitoring of serum electrolytes of patients on this

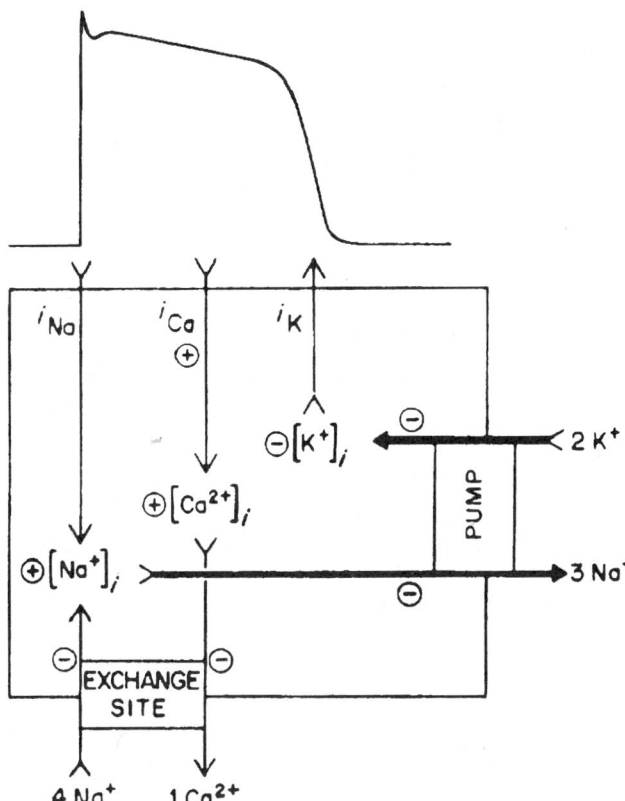

Figure 125–1. Usual fluxes of sodium (Na$^+$), potassium (K$^+$), and calcium (Ca^{2+}) across the cardiac cell membrane and the promotion (+) or inhibition (−) of these fluxes by digitalis. (From Hoffman BF, Bigger JT Jr: Digitalis and allied cardiac glycosides. *In* Gilman AG, Rall TW, Nies AS, Taylor P [eds]: Goodman and Gilman's The Pharmacological Basis of Therapeutics, 8th ed. New York: Pergamon Press, 1990, p 817. Reproduced with permission of The McGraw-Hill Companies.)

medication. Refractory hyperkalemia may become a serious consequence of digitalis toxicity.

The ability of digitalis to affect the electrical system of the heart occurs as a result of a direct depressant effect on the atrioventricular (AV) node and, more importantly, through modification of autonomic neural activity. Digitalis effectively increases vagal activity and reduces both sympathetic activity and catecholamine sensitivity. An increased sensitivity to acetylcholine within the AV node delays recovery of excitability and contributes to a slowing of conduction through the node. The increase in vagal activity also shortens the refractory period of atrial muscle, which may manifest itself clinically as conversion of atrial flutter to atrial fibrillation.

A clinically important direct effect of digitalis involves an increase in automaticity of usually quiescent myocardial tissue. By enhancing the slope of phase four (spontaneous depolarization) of the action potential, atrial tissue and Purkinje fibers have the potential to become automatic. Additionally, the increase in intracellular calcium may lead to propagation of delayed afterdepolarizations. It is important for clinicians to remember these effects when evaluating a patient on digitalis who is experiencing rhythm abnormalities such as atrial tachycardia or ventricular ectopy.

PHARMACOKINETICS (DIGOXIN)

Pharmacokinetics means drug movement and metabolism, and understanding the absorption, binding, distribution, and excretion of a drug is critical to its proper use.

Absorption

Absorption of digoxin occurs from the stomach and the upper small bowel. The usual tablet formulation is 60% to 80% absorbed; variability does occur, especially with generic formulations. Food may interfere with absorption and the medication should be taken on an empty stomach. A variety of medications that influence gastrointestinal motility can increase or decrease absorption of digoxin. One formulation of digoxin, similar to the digoxin elixir used for infant dosage, has been incorporated into a gelatin capsule, demonstrating improved absorption over the tablet form of the drug.[6] It is important to remember that, because of increased absorption, doses about 20% lower than conventional doses are recommended when using the gelatin capsule. Since this formulation of digoxin solution is 90% to 100% absorbed, its use may be advantageous in patients receiving long-term antibiotic therapy or those with delayed gastric emptying or malabsorption syndromes.

Figure 125–2 illustrates the early portion of the digoxin-turnover curves when the drug is given by different routes of administration. Absorption of digoxin by any route of administration is followed by

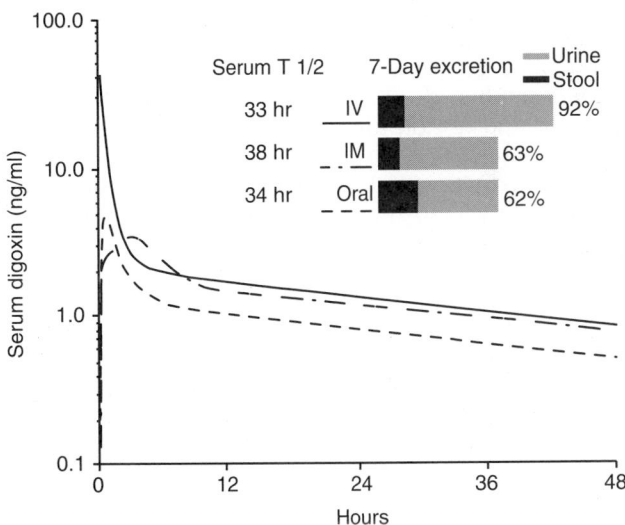

Figure 125–2. Serum turnover and 7-day excretion of tritiated digoxin in human subjects after intravenous (12 patients), intramuscular (10 patients), and oral (12 patients) administration. Note the important differences in pharmacokinetics in the early portions of the serum curves in different routes of administration. Seven-day excretion rates are plotted on the upper right and indicate that the kidney is the major organ of excretion by any route of administration. Although there is a slight difference in the serum half-time (T½) between the routes of administration, these are insignificant. The mean serum T½ is approximately 36 hours by any route of administration. (From Doherty JE: Determinants of digitalis dosage. J Ark Med Soc 66:121, 1969.)

an early rise in the serum concentration. Approximately 12 hours after this early distribution phase, equilibration of serum and tissue levels occurs. Absorption of the tablet form of digoxin is slightly less than the oral dosage depicted in this figure, which depicts absorption from the elixir dissolved on a sugar cube. The highest initial serum levels of digoxin occur after intravenous administration, followed by intramuscular administration and then the oral route. For clinical use, intramuscular administration is not recommended because of the local pain caused by the solvent, erratic absorption, and inadequate bioavailability. The mean dominant half-life of digoxin, regardless of route of administration, is 34 hours in subjects with normal renal function.[7-9]

The recent demonstration that 10% of patients may partially metabolize digoxin to the noncardioactive dihydrodigoxin before absorption from the gut has been shown to be clinically relevant. Such patients often require larger doses of oral drug to establish a therapeutic effect. The production of dihydrodigoxin seems to be a result of metabolism of the drug in the bowel by *Eubacterium lentum*, a microorganism present as a normal inhabitant in some patients. Antibiotics, especially erythromycin and tetracycline, may eliminate this organism, producing increased absorption of the drug.[10] For patients on a prolonged course of antibiotics, a concomitant reduction of oral digoxin dosage may prevent a sudden increase in serum digoxin levels.

Dosing Regimens

Several dosing regimens are outlined in Table 125–1. Initial dosing of digoxin is often empiric, based on clinical variables such as age, body mass, renal function, and concomitant medications. For digoxin, a water-soluble drug, dose is based on lean body weight and not on total body weight. Obese patients require the same dose of digoxin before and after weight reduction. Subsequent serum level monitoring is used to establish a maintenance level of 1.0 to 1.5 ng/ml.

Values outside this range may be appropriate for individuals who require more, or less, digoxin to achieve the desired therapeutic effect. If a clinical situation requires rapid onset of action, intravenous digoxin is preferred, usually given as a total of 1.0 to 1.5 mg intravenously over a 24-hour period. Smaller doses may be required in some patients. Dosing inter-

vals for initial digitalization may be as brief as every 2 hours for intravenous digoxin.

Oral digoxin may be initiated with either a single daily maintenance dose or a digitalizing loading dose regimen as outlined in Table 125–1. In many cases, a loading dose is not necessary and a daily maintenance dose of 0.125 to 0.25 (occasionally 0.50) mg orally may be given. Because steady-state concentrations occur after approximately five half-lives, full digitalization will be obtained in approximately 1 week. In patients with congestive heart failure, for whom digoxin is used frequently, renal perfusion may be diminished, prolonging the half-life and increasing the risk of toxicity.

Serum Digoxin Levels

Since 1969, the ability to measure serum digoxin levels by radioimmunoassay[11] has produced a better clinical standard for safe digoxin use. Although radioimmunoassay is a valuable and widely used test, errors caused both by the assay system itself and by laboratory technique may alter the recorded serum digoxin level.

Radioimmunoassay has low specificity and can cross-react with endogenous digitalis-like immunoreactive substances that may be present in renal failure, hepatic failure, pregnancy, newborns, some forms of hypertension, and congestive heart failure.[12-16] Further studies are required to determine the clinical significance of these substances. However, they may alter the reported serum digoxin level by as much as 50%. In some clinical situations, it is prudent to obtain a baseline serum digoxin level before initiating therapy to determine if such substances are present in the patient.

Failure to wait for the equilibration period, which may take up to 12 hours to occur after an oral dose, produces a major source of error in interpreting digoxin assays. Figure 125–2 underscores the importance of obtaining a serum sample for a digoxin level at the appropriate time after administration of the drug by any route. To obtain a serum level that corresponds to the concentration present in the myocardium, one must wait until the equilibration plateau is reached to obtain samples for digoxin assay: 2 to 4 hours after an intravenous dose, 8 to 10 hours after an intramuscular dose, and about 12 hours after an oral dose. Serum levels of digoxin of between 0.5 and 2.0 ng/ml are considered to be in the "therapeutic"

Table 125–1. **Recommended Oral Doses of Digitalis Glycosides**

Drug	Rapid Digitalization (24 hr)	Slow Digitalization	Maintenance	Parenteral
Digoxin	0.5 mg, then 0.25 mg every 4 hours × 4 if necessary (not to exceed 2 mg)	0.125–0.50 mg daily × 7	0.125–0.25 mg daily	1.0–1.5 mg in divided doses over 24 hours
Digoxin gelatin capsule	0.4 mg, then 0.2 mg hourly × 4 (not to exceed 1.6 mg)	0.1–0.4 mg daily × 7	0.1–0.4 mg daily	
Digitoxin	1.2–1.6 mg in divided doses	0.15 mg daily × 30	0.15 mg daily	1.0–1.6 mg in divided doses over 24 hours

range, although toxic symptoms may occur even in this range. Standardization of both dosing and serum collection times (such as evening dosing and morning serum collection) reduces this costly source of error.

Physical activity has been shown to decrease serum digoxin concentration[17] and, because of this phenomenon, at least 1 hour of supine rest is considered optimal prior to obtaining a specimen.[18] It is particularly important to remember this fact in the outpatient setting, especially before increasing a maintenance dose based upon a "subtherapeutic" serum digoxin level.

Poor understanding of digoxin pharmacokinetics and its prolonged half-life often results in incorrectly obtained specimens, unnecessary laboratory testing, and, occasionally, prolonged hospitalization representing considerable medical cost. Most important, because considerable overlap exists between therapeutic and toxic levels, clinical and electrocardiographic monitoring are essential correlates for establishing dosing schedules in individual patients.

Excretion

Figure 125–2 shows the excretion of tritiated digoxin after administration by several routes. Regardless of the route of administration, the major organ of excretion is the kidney—most digoxin is recovered unchanged in the urine. The larger amount present in the urine after intravenous administration is because larger amounts are excreted in the first 24 hours after the dose, when serum levels are highest after intravenous use. After a single dose of tracer-labeled digoxin, approximately 10% to 20% may be recovered from the stool, depending on the route of administration.[19]

DIGITOXIN
Absorption

Digitoxin is found in both *Digitalis purpurea* and *Digitalis lanata* and is available in all parts of the world. It is approximately 90% to 100% absorbed by the oral route of administration. Because digitoxin is lipid-soluble, dosages should be based on total body weight rather than lean body weight, which is an important point to recall in treatment of obese patients.

After absorption from the stomach, duodenum, and proximal jejunum, digitoxin is avidly (90% to 97%) bound to serum albumin. This property probably accounts for the higher recorded blood levels of digitoxin than digoxin, the latter being only approximately 20% protein bound. Serum levels of digitoxin are usually 20 to 25 ng/ml in a well-digitalized patient.

Excretion

Unlike digoxin, digitoxin is largely metabolized by the liver to inactive products. These cardioinactive metabolites are then eliminated by the kidneys. A smaller amount appears in the stool. Although the fraction of digitoxin enterohepatically recycled in dogs is approximately 27%, this value has not yet been measured in human subjects but may approach a similar figure.[20] Important features of this drug include nearly complete absorption and metabolic degradation for excretion. Digitoxin has a half-life of 5 to 7 days.

THERAPEUTIC USES OF DIGOXIN
Atrial Fibrillation

For years, treatment of atrial fibrillation (AF) has been synonymous with digoxin therapy. It is only recently, with increased understanding of the electrophysiologic benefits and limitations of digoxin as well as the spectrum of clinical syndromes that encompass AF, that the role of digoxin is undergoing reassessment.

The primary mechanism by which digoxin is effective in AF is through enhancement of vagal tone, resulting in prolonged atrioventricular (AV) nodal refractoriness with slowing of AV nodal conduction.[21] This response to digoxin is not seen in completely denervated hearts,[22] emphasizing the importance of the autonomic nervous system for clinical effect. On the other hand, efficacy of digoxin is reduced in clinical states of catecholamine excess such as exercise and fever, with breakthrough episodes of AF manifested as dyspnea or palpitations.[23]

Paroxysmal

The use of digoxin for either ventricular rate control or prevention of paroxysmal AF cannot be advocated. Recent data confirm the lack of beneficial effects of digoxin for either controlling the ventricular response during these paroxysms or preventing their occurrence.[24] In fact, the patients taking digoxin had more prolonged (more than 30 minutes) episodes of AF than patients not taking digoxin. This is attributed to the ability of digoxin to shorten the atrial refractory period.

Acute

Digoxin remains a reasonable therapeutic choice for ventricular rate control in patients with acute, new onset AF, especially if associated with impaired left ventricular function. Rapid intravenous digitalization results in high serum drug concentrations, with an initial clinical response often seen within 1 hour. If the patient's clinical situation is more tenuous, however, the use of intravenous calcium antagonists results in a clinical response (rate control) in 94% of patients in less than 5 minutes.[25] Although it was previously believed that digoxin facilitated conversion to normal sinus rhythm in acute AF, similar rates of cardioversion within 96 hours have occurred in studies comparing digoxin with a placebo.[26] Furthermore, preliminary data suggest that digoxin as monotherapy remains ineffective as a long-term antiarrhythmic medication for maintaining sinus rhythm following electrical cardioversion.[27]

Chronic

Digoxin is most commonly used for ventricular rate control in patients with chronic AF. For patients with more sedentary lifestyles, such as the very elderly or those with limiting comorbidities, this often provides adequate ventricular rate control therapy. However, several studies have demonstrated that while digoxin maintains ventricular rate control at rest, it is less effective during even mild exercise, when sympathetic tone is elevated. Monotherapy with β-adrenergic blocking agents or calcium antagonists has been shown to be more effective in this respect than has digoxin. There may be an advantage, however, to combination therapy with digoxin and either a β-blocker or a calcium antagonist, because combination therapy permits smaller doses of both drugs with equal efficacy.

The cost effectiveness of digoxin in AF has been addressed by several studies. The cost of 100 0.25-mg tablets averaged $9.40, whereas 100 tablets of either a calcium antagonist or a β-blocker ranged from $39.54 to $100.31.[28] This fails, however, to acknowledge the ineffectiveness of digoxin monotherapy in preventing recurrence of AF or the need for more frequent laboratory monitoring with digoxin. In one study of in-hospital digitalization for AF, the use of digoxin was associated with a more prolonged time to achieve ventricular rate control, resulting in prolonged hospital stay and increased costs.[29]

Heart Failure

The basic therapeutic regimen for treatment of heart failure includes digoxin, diuretics, and vasodilators. The role of digoxin in this triad is now firmly established. Digoxin is the only oral positive inotropic agent that has been demonstrated to produce a decrease in symptoms and improved exercise tolerance without a concurrent increase in mortality.[30, 31] In addition, digoxin has been shown to be cost effective in patients with heart failure by decreasing both emergency room visits and hospitalizations.[32] Finally, these benefits have been demonstrated in patients with heart failure who remain in AF as well as those in sinus rhythm.

Although digoxin is known to exert a positive inotropic effect on the myocardium, data suggest that, in heart failure, its primary benefit is via modulation of the maladaptive neurohumoral responses to decreasing cardiac output. The initial response to low cardiac output is an outpouring of sympathetic mediators.[33] Norepinephrine, aldosterone, and the renin-angiotensin system serve to increase heart rate, contractility, vasoconstriction, and sodium and water retention.[34] In an acute situation these counterregulatory responses are beneficial, sometimes life-saving, adaptations. However, chronically elevated catecholamine levels result in impaired β-adrenergic baroreceptor

function and baroreflex responsiveness.[35, 36] Preliminary evidence suggests that this resetting of baroreceptors may be mediated via the Na^+,K^+-ATPase pump.[37] By inhibiting this pump, digitalis may increase baroreceptor sensitivity and function.

Progression of heart failure is thought to be mediated through chronic unopposed excessive activation of the sympathetic nervous system.[38] Elevation of serum catecholamine levels precedes development of overt congestive heart failure in patients with mild left ventricular dysfunction.[39] Digitalis, via a direct sympathoinhibitory effect, acutely decreases serum norepinephrine levels.[40] The level of norepinephrine has been shown to have prognostic implications in heart failure.[41]

Two trials in patients in sinus rhythm with heart failure treated with digoxin have demonstrated a worsening of symptoms following withdrawal of digoxin therapy.[42, 43] In one of these studies, digoxin was shown to have additional benefit even in patients already receiving angiotensin-converting enzyme inhibitors.[43] Based on this information, digoxin should be standard therapy in any medical regimen for heart failure unless specifically contraindicated.

Despite the many benefits attributed to digoxin, actual demonstration of a survival benefit has yet to be shown. This is now being addressed by the prospective, placebo-controlled Digitalis Investigators Group (DIG) trial, sponsored by the National Heart, Lung, and Blood Institute of the National Institutes of Health. This trial will also address deterioration of symptoms and quality-of-life issues. More than 8000 patients have already been enrolled, and results were anticipated in 1995.

PRECAUTIONARY USES AND CONTRAINDICATIONS
After Recent Myocardial Infarction

The role of digoxin in the setting of acute myocardial infarction is controversial. In this setting it has been suggested that an increase in wall tension, contractility, and myocardial oxygen demand which may occur with digitalis may actually increase morbidity and mortality, possibly by increasing infarction size.[44, 45] Other data, however, suggest that this result more likely reflects the fact that older, weaker patients often require the inotropic support of digitalis and that, in fact, there is no digitalis-related increase in mortality if similar patient populations are compared.[46, 47] More rapidly acting intravenous inotropic agents are available for treatment of congestive heart failure associated with myocardial infarction. Although digoxin may be considered for some patients with supraventricular arrhythmias after infarction, antiischemic agents such as β-adrenergic blocking agents are often safer and more effective, providing that they do not precipitate congestive heart failure. Thus, in the setting of myocardial infarction, digoxin should be used with extreme caution and reserved only for those patients with a combination of supraventricular arrhythmia, especially AF, and congestive heart failure resulting from left ventricular dysfunction.

Prophylactic Use Before Cardiothoracic Surgery

Because AF and flutter may occur in as many as 50% of patients after cardiothoracic operations,[48] prophylactic use of digoxin has been suggested. However, two meta-analyses of all randomized controlled studies have failed to demonstrate the benefit of digoxin in this clinical situation.[49, 50] Although a slight decrease in ventricular rate was reported in those patients who did have supraventricular arrhythmias and had been given digoxin before surgery, it did not significantly alter the clinical outcome, and therefore the prophylactic use of digoxin before cardiothoracic operations cannot be recommended.

Renal Failure

Digoxin is excreted primarily in the urine, and the dosage must be reduced in the presence of decreased renal function.[51] Although digitoxin is metabolized in part to digoxin, excretion is not significantly impaired in renal insufficiency because of compensatory hepatic clearance.[52]

The best clinical index of digoxin excretion remains the creatinine clearance: the lower the creatinine clearance, the less digoxin will be cleared by the kidneys. Other indices of renal impairment such as a blood urea nitrogen level higher than 50 mg/dl should prompt reevaluation of digoxin dosing. In an anuric patient, the half-life of digoxin is prolonged to 4 to 6 days. Dosing in these patients is based on the creatinine clearance and may be as low as 0.125 mg orally every other day.

As use of peritoneal dialysis and hemodialysis has become widespread in the management of renal failure and drug intoxication, the effect of dialysis on digoxin kinetics has become important. A minimal amount of digoxin is cleared across the artificial kidney, with only 2% of the administered dose recovered in the dialysate bath. Findings are similar for peritoneal dialysis. Dialysis therefore is not an effective means for promoting excretion of digoxin, does not change dosage requirements of the drug, and is not effective in the management of digitalis toxicity.

Thyroid Disease

Thyroid hormone stimulates Na^+,K^+-ATPase activity and increases the number of these receptors.[53] In hypothyroidism this activity is depressed, and lower doses of digoxin are clinically effective. In the hyperthyroid state, thyroid hormone overdrives the sodium pump, and there is a relative refractoriness to the inhibitory effect of digoxin on this pump. In patients given the same dose of digoxin, those with hypothyroidism had a much higher serum digoxin level than those with hyperthyroidism.[54] Changes in maintenance dosing are necessary in patients in whom thy-

roid disorders develop, and evaluation of thyroid function is warranted in a stable patient who suddenly becomes resistant to digoxin or in whom digoxin toxicity develops.

Pregnancy

Digoxin is not teratogenic and may be used during pregnancy and lactation for controlling ventricular rate in AF or symptoms of mild congestive heart failure.[55] Serum digoxin levels often decrease by approximately 50% during pregnancy because of the normal increase in volume of distribution and glomerular filtration rate. Transplacental transfer of digoxin occurs, and digoxin levels in the fetus are similar to those in the mother. This phenomenon has been successfully used for intrauterine management of fetal supraventricular tachycardia.[56]

Pulmonary Disease

Patients with chronic obstructive pulmonary disease (COPD) appear to have heightened sensitivity to digitalis toxicity. These patients are often hypokalemic, hypoxic, and taking β-adrenergic agonists, each of which increases the potential for digitalis-related automatic ectopic pacemaker activity. The use of digitalis for isolated right ventricular failure and cor pulmonale is less well defined.[57] Although digoxin has been reported to increase diaphragmatic muscle contraction,[58, 59] this effect is controversial. Digoxin is not recommended in patients with COPD and isolated right ventricular dysfunction because of the increased risk of toxicity and lack of clear benefit.

DRUG INTERACTIONS

The serum level of digoxin may be dramatically influenced by other medications, including over-the-counter drugs. These interactions may produce pharmacokinetic changes and alter absorption, distribution, or excretion. Changes in the homeostatic milieu because of hypokalemia or a change in sympathetic tone, which may be caused by other drugs, may influence the bioavailability of digoxin. Some of these interactions are discussed later, but many other agents (Table 125–2) directly or indirectly alter digitalis levels, necessitating frequent review of medications.

Antiarrhythmic Drugs

Quinidine

The interaction of digoxin and quinidine is well documented.[60, 61] In more than 90% of patients receiving this drug combination, the serum digoxin levels increase twofold to threefold, often producing toxic effects, including lethal arrhythmias. Initially, quinidine displaces digoxin from binding sites in tissues, effectively leading to a redistribution of digoxin "on board." However, the increased steady-state concentration of digoxin is predominantly a result of a de-

Table 125–2. **Drugs Altering Digoxin Levels**

Drugs Increasing Serum Digoxin Levels	
• Antifungals	• Nonsteroidal antiinflammatory agents
• Angiotensin-converting enzyme inhibitors	• Succinylcholine
• Amiodarone*	• Propafenone
• Cyclosporine*	• Calcium antagonists*
• Benzodiazepines*	• Erythromycin*
• Quinidine/quinine*	• Disopyramide
• Reserpine	• Flecainide
	• Tetracycline

Drugs Decreasing Serum Digoxin Levels	
• Antacids	• Sulfonamides
• Chemotherapeutic agents	• Kaolin pectin
• Rifampin	• Colestipol
• Cholestyramine resins	• Metoclopramide
• Sucralfate	• Dietary fiber

*Marked increases in digoxin level.

crease in renal clearance of this drug as a result of quinidine. This dual mechanism warrants that the digoxin dose be decreased by half beginning several days before quinidine therapy is initiated.

Amiodarone

Amiodarone has been reported to increase digoxin levels by over 70% in adults[62] and even more in pediatric patients. This is the result of alteration in both renal and nonrenal clearance and a change in digoxin binding. Close monitoring of serum digoxin levels therefore is necessary both immediately and as long as 3 weeks after initiation of amiodarone therapy. In addition, because amiodarone has potent AV nodal blocking properties, this combination may lead to complete heart block.

Calcium Antagonists

The calcium antagonists variably increase serum digoxin levels. While nifedipine, isradipine, and felodipine are less likely to produce a clinically significant effect, both diltiazem and verapamil may increase levels to toxic ranges.[63, 64] The interaction of digoxin and verapamil has reportedly resulted in fatal arrhythmias.[65] Thus, all patients receiving both digoxin and calcium antagonists should have a concomitant reduction in digoxin dosage and frequent monitoring until a steady state of both drugs is achieved.

β-Adrenergic Blocking Agents

Although β-adrenergic blocking agents have not been shown to increase serum digoxin levels, it may be prudent to use lower doses of both drugs, because their additive effect may result in significant AV block.

Drugs Producing Electrolyte Abnormalities

Electrolyte abnormalities are common undesirable effects of diuretic agents, producing hypokalemia or hypomagnesemia, thereby enhancing digitalis action and increasing the risk of digitalis toxicity. Other drugs such as antifungal agents or cyclosporine may also produce hypomagnesemia, and close monitoring of serum digoxin levels is warranted.

Hypolipidemic Drugs

The bile acid sequestrant agents readily bind with digoxin and digitoxin, producing decreased absorption of both of these drugs.[66] Likewise, dietary fiber such as bran products also decreases absorption of digitalis.[67] Digoxin should be given at least 2 hours before these agents. The 3-hydroxy-3-methylglutaryl coenzyme A (HMG-CoA) reductase inhibitors, such as lovastatin or pravastatin, have not been shown to influence serum digoxin levels.

Antibiotics

Approximately 10% of the population partially metabolizes digoxin to inactive metabolites by the mechanism described previously. In these patients, use of erythromycin or tetracycline can alter bacterial flora in the bowel, causing a marked increase in the bioavailability of digoxin and a precipitous increase in the serum digoxin concentration by 50% to 100%.

DIGITALIS INTOXICATION

The reported incidence of digoxin toxicity has varied from a high of 20% in studies performed in the early 1970s[68, 69] to 5% suggested by more current data.[70] Authorities attribute this decline to the prescribing of lower doses of digoxin, a greater understanding of the conditions that predispose a patient to digoxin toxicity (Table 125–3), and the use of serum digoxin determinations to guide therapy.

In Older Patients

The incidence of digoxin toxicity in the elderly population appears to be higher than in the general population but this may not be a result of age alone. A combination of factors makes this group of patients especially vulnerable to this clinical problem. As the population ages, the incidence of both heart failure and AF increases, with the result that more elderly patients are given digoxin therapy. Changes associated with the usual aging process such as decreased body mass and thus volume of distribution, decrease

Table 125–3. **Factors Predisposing to Digitalis Toxicity**

- Electrolyte imbalance (hypokalemia, hypomagnesemia, hypercalcemia)
- Renal insufficiency
- Type and severity of underlying cardiac disease
- Hypoxemia
- Older age
- Hypothyroidism
- Drug interactions

in renal function, and hypoalbuminemia contribute to an increase in serum digoxin level.[71, 72] Sclerodegenerative changes within the cardiac conduction system may lead to increased AV block with much smaller doses of digoxin. The polypharmacy ubiquitous to elderly patients can lead to multiple drug interactions resulting in widely fluctuating digoxin availability. Finally, the symptoms of digoxin toxicity in elderly patients are often more insidious and nonspecific and, if unrecognized, lead to life-threatening initial presentations.[73]

Clinical Manifestations

Cardiac

Among the earliest and most frequent signs of digitalis toxicity are disorders of cardiac rhythm. Any change in the baseline electrocardiogram, such as a regularization of the ventricular response in AF, reflecting increased AV nodal block and enhanced junctional automaticity, should raise suspicion that the serum digitalis level is elevated. Rhythm disturbances reflect the ability of digoxin to increase automaticity, propagate spontaneous ventricular early afterdepolarizations, markedly enhance vagal tone, and depress AV nodal conduction. Although many rhythms may be associated with digoxin intoxication, certain disturbances such as atrial tachycardia with AV block, nonparoxysmal junctional tachycardia, and bidirectional ventricular tachycardia are closely associated with digoxin toxicity, and this diagnosis should be considered even in patients with such arrhythmias who have a "normal" serum digoxin level. However, the most common cardiac manifestation of digoxin toxicity is the development of ventricular extrasystoles, which may be multiform or occur in a pattern of bigeminy or trigeminy. One caveat remains, however, that patients receiving digoxin often have impaired ventricular function or ischemic heart disease; these ventricular extrasystoles may therefore be reflective of underlying cardiac disease and not necessarily digoxin toxicity. If the situation is unclear, digoxin should be withheld and the patient reassessed for clinical improvement, which will confirm the diagnosis of digitalis toxicity.

Extracardiac

More than half of patients with even a mildly elevated serum digoxin level have gastrointestinal discomfort including anorexia, nausea, and vomiting. These effects are thought to be mediated via the action of digoxin on the area postrema, a portion of the medulla unprotected by the blood-brain barrier.[74] Diarrhea, salivation, and abdominal pain may also be part of this syndrome because of increased vagal activity.

Various neuropsychologic syndromes have been associated with digoxin intoxication and are especially common initial complaints in older patients.[75–77] Although fatigue, malaise, and dizziness may represent early digoxin toxicity, these symptoms may be associated with the underlying cardiac disorder. Visual and auditory hallucinations, paranoid ideation, and depression may be seen with digoxin toxicity and could explain a change in mental status, especially in an older patient. Subtle clouding or blurring of vision is more common than the classically described change in color perception.

Hyperkalemia represents a life-threatening result of digoxin toxicity. Because digitalis essentially paralyzes the Na^+,K^+-ATPase pump, potassium may accumulate extracellularly, resulting in refractory hyperkalemia, a situation that further exacerbates cardiac arrhythmias. On the other hand, patients concomitantly taking diuretics may have hypokalemia that also is arrhythmogenic. Cautious replacement of potassium intravenously in hypokalemic patients should be part of the initial therapy in suspected digitalis toxicity.

Management

The diagnosis of digoxin toxicity is often a clinical one. A serum digoxin level greater than 2.0 ng/ml is highly supportive of digoxin toxicity, but levels that are within the "normal" range should not dissuade the clinician from pursuing this diagnosis in a symptomatic patient. The diagnosis is confirmed by symptomatic relief following drug withdrawal.

The management of digoxin toxicity is dependent upon the severity of the clinical situation. For most patients with mild symptoms, including arrhythmias that are not hemodynamically compromising, withdrawal of digoxin, cardiac monitoring, and supportive care are effective. For all patients, a pharmacologic algorithm for the management of digoxin toxicity should include correction of electrolyte abnormalities, amelioration of heart block, control of arrhythmias and, in severe cases, removal of cardioactive digoxin via use of digoxin immune Fab (ovine) antibody.

Electrolytes

Assessment of electrolytes, especially potassium and magnesium, is imperative. However, a normal serum potassium level may not reflect the potential intracellular potassium depletion that may occur because of inhibition of the Na^+-K^+ pump. Patients taking

Table 125–4. **Approximate Digibind Dose (in Number of Vials) for Reversal of a Single Large Digitalis Overdose**

Number of Digoxin Tablets or Capsules Ingested	Digibind Dose (Number of Vials)
25	9
50	17
75	25
100	34
150	50
200	67

Dose (in number of vials) = total digitalis body load in mg/0.6 mg digitalis bound per vial.

Table 125–5. **Approximate Adult Dose of Digibind (in Number of Vials) from a Steady-State Known Serum Digoxin Concentration**

Patient Weight (kg)	Number of Vials per Serum Digoxin Concentration						
	1 mg/ml	2 mg/ml	4 mg/ml	8 mg/ml	12 mg/ml	16 mg/ml	20 mg/ml
40	0.5	1	2	3	5	7	8
60	0.5	1	3	5	7	10	12
70	1	2	3	6	9	11	14
80	1	2	3	7	10	13	16
100	1	2	4	8	12	16	20

Dose (in number of vials) = (Serum digoxin concentration in ng/ml)(weight in kg)/100.

diuretics may have both hypokalemia and hypomagnesemia as predisposing factors for digoxin toxicity. Magnesium, which possesses natural rhythm-stabilizing properties, should be given empirically in a dose of 2 to 4 g intravenously to all patients not in overt renal failure.[78] Serum potassium ideally should be repleted to a level of 4.5 mEq/L, because this may be helpful in patients with ventricular extrasystoles or atrial tachycardia with block. Caution is required, however, because hyperkalemia may increase heart block or even precipitate asystole.

Heart Block

Atropine, a vagolytic, is the initial drug of choice for symptomatic bradyarrhythmias. Initial dosing is 0.5 to 1.0 mg intravenously with caution in patients at risk for glaucoma or urinary retention. For patients with hemodynamically compromising heart block or asystole, a transvenous right ventricular endocardial pacemaker electrode may be necessary. Care should be exercised during this procedure because these patients are at risk for refractory ventricular arrhythmias as a result of hyperexcitable myocardium.

Ventricular Arrhythmias

Lidocaine is the drug of choice for treatment of ventricular arrhythmias secondary to digoxin toxicity. Its advantages over procainamide or quinidine include a lack of effect on the AV node, lack of myocardial depression, and minimal effect on the infranodal conduction system. It also has a short half-life, and thus any adverse effects will be dissipated within 15 to 20 minutes after a single bolus. Lidocaine is given as a 50- to 100-mg intravenous bolus and then maintained as an intravenous infusion at 2 to 4 mg/min.

Phenytoin is a useful but infrequently used agent for ventricular arrhythmias associated with digoxin toxicity. Intravenous phenytoin may produce transient depression of myocardial function or hypotension, although less often than other antiarrhythmic agents. The use of phenytoin has declined with the advent of digoxin-specific antibodies for patients with digitalis-induced ventricular arrhythmias.

Digoxin-Specific Antibodies (Digibind)

Digoxin-specific antibody fragments are the treatment of choice for arrhythmias caused by digoxin toxicity that are associated with threatened or actual hemodynamic compromise.[79] Refractory hyperkalemia is also an indication for this therapy. These antibodies are effective at reversing toxicity from both digoxin and digitoxin. Although this therapy is initially expensive, it is cost effective, reducing length of hospital stay and use of procedures such as temporary pacemaker implantation.[80] Adverse effects are uncommon but include allergic reactions, exacerbation of heart failure because of withdrawal of digoxin, and recrudescence of digoxin toxicity in patients given an inadequate dose. A guide for calculating the recommended dose of digoxin antibody is illustrated in Tables 125–4 and 125–5. Use of antibody rapidly reduces the percentage of unbound (cardioactive) digoxin in the serum from between 75% and 90% to between 0% and 5% in minutes. The bound complex is renally excreted, which is an important management issue for patients with end-stage renal disease who may require repeat dosing. The routinely used serum assays cannot distinguish the antibody bound, cardioinactive digoxin from active drug. Thus, serum digoxin levels following administration of digoxin antibody are often markedly elevated, reflecting the extraction of digoxin from the tissues and into the serum as an inactive complex.[81] Monitoring of a therapeutic response ideally occurs through clinical improvement. However, in patients demonstrating little clinical change and for whom determination of an exact digoxin level is necessary, a free serum digoxin level may be obtained using a rapid ultrafiltration assay.[82]

Acknowledgments

We gratefully acknowledge Drs. Joseph R. DiPalma, Leonard S. Dreifus, Steven P. Kutalek, and Vincent Zarro for their thoughtful review of the manuscript and J. Christopher Bare and Arthur J. D'Adamo for technical assistance.

REFERENCES

1. Simonsen LL: What are pharmacists dispensing most often? Pharm Times 42:42, 1990.
2. Hoffman BF, Bigger JT Jr: Digitalis and allied cardiac glycosides. *In* Gilman AG, Rall TW, Nies AS, Taylor P (eds): Goodman and Gilman's The Pharmacological Basis of Therapeutics, 8th ed. New York: Pergamon Press, 1990, pp 814–839.
3. Withering W: An account of the foxglove and some of its medical uses, with practical remarks on dropsy and other diseases. *In* Willius FA, TE Keys (eds): Classics of Cardiology. New York: Henry Schuman, 1941, pp 231–252.

4. Rasmussen HH, Okita GT, Hartz RS, Ten Eick RE: Inhibition of electrogenic sodium pumping in isolated atrial tissue from patients treated with digoxin. J Pharmacol Exp Ther 252:60, 1990.
5. Smith TW: Digitalis: Mechanisms of action and clinical use. N Engl J Med 318:358, 1988.
6. Doherty JE, Marcus FI, Binnion PF: A multicenter evaluation of the absolute bioavailability of digoxin dosage forms. Curr Ther Res 35:301, 1984.
7. Doherty JE, Perkins WH, Mitchell GK: Tritiated digoxin studies in human subjects. Arch Intern Med 108:531, 1961.
8. Doherty JE, Perkins WH: Studies with tritiated digoxin in human subjects and intravenous administration. Am Heart J 63:528, 1962.
9. Doherty JE, Perkins WH, Gammil J, et al: Studies following intramuscular tritiated digoxin in human subjects. Am J Cardiol 15:170, 1965.
10. Lindenbaum J, Rund DG, Butler VP Jr, et al: Inactivation of digoxin by the gut flora: Reversal by antibiotic therapy. N Engl J Med 305:789, 1981.
11. Smith TW, Butler VP Jr, Haber E: Determination of therapeutic and toxic serum digoxin concentrations by radioimmunoassay. N Engl J Med 281:1212, 1969.
12. Graves SW, Brown B, Valdes R: An endogenous digoxin-like substance in patients with renal impairment. Ann Intern Med 99:604, 1983.
13. Nanji AA, Greenway DC: Falsely raised plasma digoxin concentrations in liver disease. Br Med J 287:432, 1985.
14. Stone J, Bentur Y, Zalstein E, et al: Effect of endogenous digoxin-like substances on the interpretation of high concentrations of digoxin in children. J Pediatr 117:321, 1990.
15. Graves SW, Valdes R, Brown BA, et al: Endogenous digoxin immunoreactive substance in human pregnancy. J Clin Endocrinol Metab 58:748, 1984.
16. Shilo L, Adawi A, Solomo G, Shenkman L: Endogenous digoxin like immunoreactivity in congestive heart failure. Br Med J 295:415, 1987.
17. Jogestrand T: Influence of everyday physical activity on the serum digoxin concentration in digoxin-treated patients. Clin Physiol 1:209, 1981.
18. Jogestrand T, Edner M, Haverling M: Clinical value of serum digoxin assays in outpatients: Improvement by the standardization of blood sampling. Am Heart J 117:1076, 1989.
19. Doherty JE: Determinants of digitalis dosage. J Ark Med Soc 66:121, 1969.
20. Perrier D, Mayersohn M, Marcus FI: Clinical pharmacokinetics of digitoxin. Clin Pharmacokinet 2:292, 1977.
21. Watanabe AM: Digitalis and the autonomic nervous system. J Am Coll Cardiol 5:35A, 1985.
22. Goodman W, Rossen RM, Cannom DS, et al: Effect of digoxin on atrioventricular conduction studies in patients with and without cardiac autonomic innervation. Circulation 75:251, 1975.
23. Falk RH, Leavitt JI: Digoxin for atrial fibrillation: A drug whose time has gone? Ann Intern Med 114:573, 1991.
24. Rawles JM, Metcalfe MJ, Jennings K: Time of occurrence, duration, and ventricular rate of paroxysmal atrial fibrillation: The effect of digoxin. Br Heart J 63:225, 1990.
25. Salerno DM, Dias VC, Kleiger RE, et al: Efficacy and safety of intravenous diltiazem for treatment of atrial fibrillation and flutter. Am J Cardiol 63:1046, 1989.
26. Falk RH, Knowlton AA, Bernard SA, et al: Digoxin for converting recent-onset atrial fibrillation to sinus rhythm: A randomized, double-blinded trial. Ann Intern Med 106:503, 1987.
27. Grande P, Sonne B, Pedersen A: A controlled study of digoxin and quinidine in patients DC reverted from atrial fibrillation to sinus rhythm. Circulation 74:II, 1986.
28. Zarowitz BJ, Gheorghiade M: Optimal heart rate for patients with chronic atrial fibrillation: Are pharmacologic choices truly changing? Am Heart J 123:1401, 1992.
29. Roberts SA, Diaz C, Nolan PE, et al: Effectiveness and costs of digoxin treatment for atrial fibrillation and flutter. Am J Cardiol 72:567, 1993.
30. Packer M, Carver JR, Rodeheffer RJ, et al: Effect of oral milrinone on mortality in severe chronic heart failure. N Engl J Med 325:1468, 1991.
31. Uretsky BF, Jessup M, Konstam MA, et al: Multicenter trial of enoximone in patients with moderate to moderately severe congestive heart failure: Lack of benefit compared with placebo. Circulation 82:774, 1990.
32. Captopril-Digoxin Multicenter Research Group: Comparative effects of therapy with captopril and digoxin in patients with mild to moderate heart failure. JAMA 259:539, 1988.
33. Ferguson DW, Berg WJ, Sanders JS: Clinical and hemodynamic correlates of sympathetic neural activity in normal humans and patients with heart failure: Evidence from direct microneurographic recordings. J Am Coll Cardiol 16:1125, 1990.
34. Creager MA, Faxon DP, Cutler SS, et al: Contribution of vasopressin to vasoconstriction in patients with congestive heart failure: Comparison with the renin-angiotensin system and sympathetic nervous system. J Am Coll Cardiol 7:758, 1986.
35. Hirsch AT, Dzau VJ, Creager MA: Baroreceptor function in congestive heart failure: Effect on neurohumoral activation and regional vascular resistance. Circulation 75(Suppl IV):IV36, 1987.
36. Bristow MR: Changes in myocardial and vascular receptors in heart failure. J Am Coll Cardiol 22(Suppl A):61A, 1993.
37. Heesch CM, Abboud FM, Thames MD: Acute resetting of carotid sinus baroreceptors: Possible involvement of electrogenic Na+ pump. Am J Physiol 247:H833, 1984.
38. Swedberg K: Protagonist's viewpoint: Is neurohormonal activation deleterious to the long-term outcome of patients with congestive heart failure? J Am Coll Cardiol 12:547, 1988.
39. Francis GS, Benedict C, Johnstone DE, et al, for the SOLVD Investigators: Comparison of neuroendocrine activation in patients with left ventricular dysfunction with and without congestive heart failure: A substudy of the studies of left ventricular dysfunction. Circulation 82:1724, 1990.
40. Gheorghiade M, Hall V, Lakier JB, et al: Comparative hemodynamic and neurohormonal effects of intravenous captopril and digoxin and their combination in patients with severe heart failure. J Am Coll Cardiol 13:134, 1989.
41. Cohn JN, Levine TB, Olivari MT, et al: Plasma norepinephrine as a guide to prognosis in patients with chronic congestive heart failure. N Engl J Med 311:819, 1984.
42. Uretsky BF, Young JB, Shahidi FE, et al: Randomized study assessing the effect of digoxin withdrawal in patients with mild to moderate chronic congestive heart failure: Results of the PROVED trial. J Am Coll Cardiol 22:955, 1993.
43. Packer M, Gheorghiade M, Young JB, et al: Withdrawal of digoxin from patients with chronic heart failure treated with angiotensin converting-enzyme inhibitors. N Engl J Med 329:1, 1993.
44. Bigger JT, Fleiss JL, Rolnitzky LM, et al: Effect of digitalis treatment on survival after myocardial infarction. Am J Cardiol 55:623, 1985.
45. Kober L, Torp-Pedersen C, Gadsboll N, et al: Is digoxin an independent risk factor for long-term mortality after acute myocardial infarction? Eur Heart J 15:382, 1994.
46. Ryan TJ, Bailey KR, McCabe CH, et al: The effect of digitalis on survival in high risk patients with coronary artery disease: The coronary artery surgery study. Circulation 67:735, 1983.
47. Madsen EB, Gilpin E, Henning H, et al: Prognostic importance of digitalis after acute myocardial infarction. J Am Coll Cardiol 3:681, 1984.
48. Lauer MS, Eagle KA, Buckley MJ, DeSanctis RW: Atrial fibrillation following coronary artery bypass surgery. Prog Cardiovasc Dis 31:367, 1989.
49. Andrews TC, Reimold SC, Berlin JA, Antman EM: Prevention of supraventricular arrhythmias after coronary artery bypass surgery: A meta-analysis of randomized controlled trials. Circulation 84(Suppl III):III-236, 1991.
50. Kowey PR, Taylor JE, Rials SJ, Marinchak RA: Meta-analysis of the effectiveness of prophylactic drug therapy in preventing supraventricular arrhythmias early after coronary artery bypass grafting. Am J Cardiol 69:963, 1992.
51. Doherty JE, Perkins WH, Wilson MC, et al: Studies with tritiated digoxin in renal failure. Am J Med 37:536, 1964.
52. Storstein L: The influence of renal function on the renal excretion of digitoxin and its cardioactive metabolites. Clin Pharmacol Ther 16:25, 1974.

53. Curfman GD, Crowley TJ, Smith TW: Thyroid-induced alteration in myocardial sodium- and potassium-activated adenosine triphosphatase, monovalent cation active transport and cardiac glycoside binding. J Clin Invest 59:586, 1977.
54. Doherty JE, Perkins WH: Digoxin metabolism in hypo- and hyperthyroidism: Studies with tritiated digoxin in thyroid disease. Ann Intern Med 64:489, 1966.
55. Brinkman CR, Woods JR: Effects of cardiovascular drugs during pregnancy. Cardiovasc Med 1:231, 1976.
56. Azancot-Benisty A, Jacqz-Algrain E, Guirgis NM, et al: Clinical and pharmacologic study of fetal supraventricular tachyarrhythmias. J Pediatr 121:608, 1992.
57. Mathur PN, Powles P, Pugsley SO, et al: Effect of digoxin on right ventricular function in severe chronic airflow obstruction. Ann Intern Med 95:283, 1981.
58. Aubier M, Viires N, Murciano D, et al: Effects of digoxin on diaphragmatic strength generation. J Appl Physiol 61:1767, 1986.
59. Aubier M, Murciano D, Viires N, et al: Effects of digoxin on diaphragmatic strength generation in patients with chronic obstructive pulmonary disease during acute respiratory failure. Am Rev Respir Dis 135:544, 1987.
60. Leahey EB Jr, Reiffel JA, Heissenbuttel RH, et al: Interaction between quinidine and digoxin. JAMA 240:533, 1978.
61. Bigger JT Jr: Quinidine-digoxin interaction. Int J Cardiol 1:109, 1981.
62. Nademanee K, Kannan R, Hendrickson J, et al: Amiodarone-digoxin interaction: Clinical significance, time course of development, potential pharmacokinetic mechanisms and therapeutic implications. J Am Coll Cardiol 4:111, 1984.
63. Klein HO, Lang R, DiSegni E, et al: Verapamil-digoxin interaction. N Engl J Med 303:160, 1980.
64. Rameis H, Magometschnigg D, Ganzinger U: The diltiazem-digoxin interaction. Clin Pharmacol Ther 36:183, 184.
65. Zatuchni J: Verapamil-digoxin interaction. Am Heart J 108:412, 1984.
66. Brown DD, Juhl RP, Warner SL: Decreased bioavailability of digoxin due to hypocholesterolemic interventions. Circulation 58:164, 1978.
67. Floyd RA: Digoxin interaction with bran and higher fiber foods. Am J Hosp Pharm 35:660, 1978.
68. Hurwitz N, Wade OL: Intensive hospital monitoring of adverse reaction to drugs. Br Med J 1:531, 1969.
69. Beller GA, Smith TW, Abelmann WH, et al: Digitalis intoxication: A prospective clinical study with serum level correlations. N Engl J Med 284:989, 1971.
70. Mahdyoon H, Battilana G, Rosman H, et al: The evolving pattern of digoxin intoxication: Observations at a large urban hospital from 1980–1988. Am Heart J 120:1189, 1990.
71. Ewy GA, Kapadia GG, Yao L, et al: Digoxin metabolism in the elderly. Circulation 39:449, 1969.
72. Guggenheim R, Reidenberg MM: Serum digoxin concentration and age. J Am Geriatr Soc 28:553, 1980.
73. Wofford JL, Ettinger WH: Risk factors and manifestations of digoxin toxicity in the elderly. Am J Emerg Med 9(Suppl 1):11, 1991.
74. Lely AH, van Enter CHJ: Non-cardiac symptoms of digitalis intoxication. Am Heart J 83:149, 1972.
75. Lyon AF, Degraff AC: The neurotoxic effects of digitalis. Am Heart J 65:839, 1963.
76. Portnoi VA: Digitalis delirium in elderly patients. J Clin Pharmacol 19:747, 1979.
77. Eisendrath SJ, Sweeney MA: Toxic neuropsychiatric effects of digoxin at therapeutic serum concentrations. Am J Psychiatry 144:506, 1987.
78. Cohen L, Kitzes R: Magnesium sulfate and digitalis-toxic arrhythmias. JAMA 249:2808, 1983.
79. Antman EM, Wenger TL, Butler VP Jr, et al: Treatment of 150 cases of life-threatening digitalis intoxication with digoxin specific Fab antibody fragments: Final report of a multicenter study. Circulation 81:1744, 1990.
80. Mauskopf JA, Wenger TL: Cost-effectiveness analysis of the use of digoxin immune Fab (ovine) for treatment of digoxin toxicity. Am J Cardiol 68:1709, 1991.
81. Rainey PM: Effects of digoxin immune Fab (ovine) on digoxin immunoassays. Am J Clin Pathol 92:779, 1989.
82. Ujhelyi MR, Colucci RD, Cummings DM, et al: Monitoring serum digoxin concentrations during digoxin immune Fab therapy. DICP 25:1047, 1991.

B. Inotropic Therapy

CHAPTER 126

Principles and Practice of Inotropic Therapy

Wilson S. Colucci, M.D.

GOALS OF THERAPY AND PATIENT SELECTION

By definition, a positive inotropic agent is one that causes an increase in the force of myocardial contraction. Clinically, this positive inotropic effect results in an improvement in left ventricular pump function such that the stroke work performed at any given filling pressure is increased. Theoretically, positive inotropic agents can be used to improve hemodynamic status when the syndrome of congestive heart failure is a result of reduced myocardial systolic function, a condition that most often is caused by ischemic myocardial injury, hypertension, myocarditis, or one of a large number of cardiomyopathic conditions that affect systolic function. Such patients frequently have dilated hearts characterized hemodynamically by decreases in left ventricular ejection fraction, stroke volume, and stroke work and by increases in left ventricular end-diastolic volume and filling pressure.

It is important to distinguish patients with systolic heart failure from those who have congestive heart failure resulting from conditions that result primarily in impairment of diastolic ventricular filling, such as restrictive or hypertrophic cardiomyopathy, mitral stenosis, or constrictive pericarditis. Because systolic function is not the predominant abnormality leading to the clinical syndrome in these latter conditions, the use of positive inotropic agents generally is not helpful, and it may even lead to a worsening of symptoms.

The goal of positive inotropic therapy is related closely to the clinical circumstances. In general, it is convenient to distinguish patients with acute, hemodynamically unstable congestive heart failure from those with more chronic, stable conditions. Although clinically useful, such a distinction is arbitrary, because patients with chronic stable syndromes can decompensate acutely, whereas patients with heart failure of recent onset may be relatively stable. Acute, hemodynamically unstable heart failure occurs most often in the setting of myocardial infarction and typically involves a substantial amount of myocardium. Patients with acute myocarditis or the recent onset of a rapidly progressive myocardial disease may also have rapid clinical onset and unstable hemodynamics, and it is not unusual for patients with long-standing myocardial dysfunction to seek treatment for acute hemodynamic deterioration. In approaching the treatment of such patients, a fundamental goal is to determine the role of myocardial failure, as opposed to other causes of hemodynamic instability such as hypovolemia, sepsis, and high output states.

After the presence of myocardial failure has been established, a number of additional questions must be addressed. First, if congestive heart failure occurs in the setting of an ischemic event, the role of ongoing ischemia must be considered, because primary therapy may best be directed at reduction of ischemia. Second, it must be considered to what extent a decrease in diastolic function, as may occur in the setting of acute ischemia, is contributing to the overall syndrome of congestive heart failure. Again, relief of ischemia may be of primary importance, and reduction of filling pressures may be more useful than the administration of a positive inotropic drug. Third, it should be determined whether the filling pressure is optimal. This determination may be accomplished by a therapeutic trial of volume infusion, but it should be performed under careful invasive monitoring in less stable patients.

In general, the goal of positive inotropic therapy in the acute setting is to achieve an improvement in forward cardiac output and thus improve perfusion to vital organs, including the central nervous system, kidneys, and heart. Arterial blood pressure may be increased in response to an increase in cardiac output; however, with positive inotropic agents, this effect is generally mild. Therefore, if hypotension caused by low cardiac output is profound, it may be necessary to administer a positive inotropic agent and a vasoconstrictor concomitantly. Likewise, if a reduction in systolic myocardial performance is not the fundamental problem, a pure vasoconstrictor agent may be a more effective method of increasing arterial pressure. The increase in perfusion of vital organs in response to a positive inotropic agent is relatively nonselective. If a selective increase in renal blood flow is desired, dopamine, a positive inotropic agent with selective renal dilator actions, or a converting enzyme inhibitor may be preferred.

In contrast to the goal of stabilizing hemodynamic function in the acute setting, the goal of therapy in an ambulatory patient with chronic stable congestive heart failure is to improve functional capacity, the quality of life, and survival. As with the acute use of positive inotropic agents, the primary hemodynamic effect is to increase cardiac output. There may also be a reduction in left ventricular filling pressure in response to improved pump function. However, the primary measure of the effectiveness of inotropic therapy in ambulatory patients is the degree to which exercise capacity, functional status, quality of life, and survival are improved.

MECHANISMS OF POSITIVE INOTROPIC ACTION

In myocardial tissue, the development of contractile force is the result of the interaction of the contractile proteins, actin and myosin.[1] This interaction is energy-dependent, requiring adenosine triphosphate, and is under the control of a group of regulatory proteins collectively referred to as tropomyosin. Tropomyosin in turn is regulated by the level of free cytosolic calcium, so that increases in cytosolic calcium are paralleled by an increase in the force developed by actin and myosin. The rhythmic contraction and relaxation of myocardium are the result of cyclic increases and decreases in free cytosolic calcium. The major source of this activator Ca^{2+} is the sarcoplasmic tubular system. However, it appears that release of this large Ca^{2+} store is "triggered" by the influx of a smaller amount of Ca^{2+} through voltage-dependent Ca^{2+}-influx channels that are under the regulation of membrane potential, such that membrane depolarization leads to an increase in Ca^{2+} influx (and hence an increase in $[Ca^{2+}]_i$) during systole.

Most positive inotropic agents act by increasing the delivery of Ca^{2+}. The digitalis glycosides inhibit Na^+,K^+-ATPase, which in turn favors Ca^{2+} influx by way of the Na^+-Ca^{2+} exchanger. The β-adrenergic agonists act on cell surface receptors that are coupled to adenylate cyclase and thus result in increased generation of cyclic adenosine monophosphate (cAMP). cAMP exerts a positive inotropic action by causing an increase in the influx of Ca^{2+} through voltage-dependent channels. The phosphodiesterase inhibitors also act to increase cAMP, but they do so more distally in the pathway by inhibiting degradation.

Myocardium from patients with severe heart failure has a relatively selective attenuation in its responsiveness to β-adrenergic stimulation but apparently normal responsiveness to Ca^{2+} and cAMP.[1–5] This reduced β-adrenergic responsiveness reflects one or more abnormalities in the pathway coupling the receptor to cAMP generation and may be a result of increased adrenergic tone, which is a common occurrence in patients with heart failure.[1, 6, 7] Exposure of β-adrenergic receptors to persistent stimulation by agonists results in a further downregulation or loss of β-adrenergic responsiveness that may be associated with decreases or even total loss of the hemodynamic response to β-adrenergic agonists. This tendency has been most evident for orally administered agonists such as pirbuterol and prenalterol[8–10] and it may occur to a lesser extent with dobutamine.[11] The functional consequences of β-adrenergic downregulation are more profound with partial agonists, such as pirbuterol and prenalterol (resulting in complete loss of response), than with full agonists, such as isoproterenol and dobutamine (resulting primarily in a rightward shift in the dose-response curve).[10] In practice, it generally is possible to maintain the desired hemodynamic response to full agonists, such as dobutamine, although higher infusion rates may be required as the treatment proceeds.

Several new positive inotropic agents have mechanisms of action in addition to phosphodiesterase inhibition. Some of these agents, such as pimobendan,[12] may act in part by increasing the Ca^{2+} sensitivity of contractile regulatory proteins. Vesnarinone,[13] and its intravenous counterpart, OPC-18,790,[14] have multiple mechanisms of action that may contribute to a positive inotropic effect, including inhibition of potassium currents, stimulation of inward sodium current, and phosphodiesterase inhibition.

POSITIVE INOTROPIC AGENTS AVAILABLE
β-Adrenergic Agonists

Several β-adrenergic agonists are available for intravenous administration. Although all of these agents exert a positive inotropic action through stimulation of myocardial β-adrenergic receptors, they differ substantially with regard to other pharmacologic actions. For instance, in addition to stimulation of myocardial β-adrenergic receptors, dopamine stimulates dopaminergic receptors (resulting in renal arterial dilation at low infusion rates) and α-adrenergic receptors (resulting in significant peripheral vasoconstriction at moderate and high infusion rates). In contrast, dobutamine has no net effect to stimulate vascular α-adrenergic receptors and therefore causes no increase, or even a small decrease, in peripheral vascular resistance; dobutamine causes no stimulation of dopamine receptors even at high doses.

As discussed above, the hemodynamic responses to oral β-adrenergic agonists frequently are not sustained during long-term therapy. The major role of β-adrenergic agonists at this time, therefore, is restricted to short-term hemodynamic management.

Phosphodiesterase Inhibitors

Several phosphodiesterase inhibitors are currently under active investigation as intravenous or oral treatment for congestive heart failure.[1] These agents share a relative selectivity for peak-III phosphodiesterase, the prevalent isoform found in myocardial and vascular tissues, and therefore differ from commonly used phosphodiesterase inhibitors such as aminophylline. Amrinone was the first phosphodiesterase inhibitor to be evaluated intensively for the treatment of heart failure.[1, 15, 16] It was approved by the United States Food and Drug Administration as an intravenous agent for the treatment of patients with severe congestive heart failure. Investigation of the oral formulation of amrinone was discontinued because it was found

that the ratio of therapeutic to adverse effects was not favorable for clinical use.

Milrinone, an analogue of amrinone, has also been approved by the FDA for intravenous use.[17, 18] Although there is evidence that oral milrinone is efficacious with regard to exercise capacity, milrinone caused a significant increase in mortality in patients with severe congestive heart failure[19] and was removed from further development as an oral agent. Oral pimobendan, a phosphodiesterase inhibitor that increases the myocardial responsiveness to calcium *in vitro*, has been shown to improve exercise capacity and quality of life[12] but has not been evaluated with regard to survival. Theoretically, because of its multiple mechanisms of action, pimobendan may have a more benign adverse effect profile than pure phosphodiesterase inhibitors.

The phosphodiesterase inhibitors exert *both* positive inotropic and direct vasodilator actions in patients with congestive heart failure, and it appears that the *net* hemodynamic effect of these agents is the result of significant contributions from both actions. For instance, it can be shown that the improvement in left ventricular pump function caused by intracoronary milrinone infusion (reflecting only the positive inotropic action of the drug on the myocardium) accounts for a significant component of the improvement caused by intravenous drug administration (which reflects both myocardial and vasodilator drug actions).[20] The effect of this vasodilator action is illustrated by a comparison of the hemodynamic effects caused by milrinone and dobutamine.[21] Although both agents cause marked increases in cardiac output, milrinone results in substantially greater decreases in left and right ventricular filling pressures and arterial pressure.

VESNARINONE

Vesnarinone[13] is an orally active positive inotropic agent with multiple pharmacologic mechanisms, including inhibition of the delayed outward and inward rectifying potassium currents, increased opening of sodium channels, and mild inhibition of phosphodiesterase. Although the relative contribution of each of these mechanisms to the net effect of vesnarinone is not known, this agent causes a fall in heart rate and has little or no vasodilator activity, whereas pure phosphodiesterase inhibitors are potent vasodilators and tend to increase heart rate. OPC-18,790,[14] an analogue of vesnarinone, is under development as an intravenous agent. Unlike vesnarinone, OPC-18,790 exerts a notable direct vasodilating action that contributes to its hemodynamic effect.

ACUTE POSITIVE INOTROPIC THERAPY

The selection of the appropriate positive inotropic agent for the acute management of a patient with hemodynamic abnormalities caused by myocardial failure depends to a large extent on the pattern of

Table 126–1. Hemodynamic Effects of Several Parenteral Positive Inotropic, Vasodilator, or Vasoconstrictor Agents

Effect	ISO	NE	DOPA$_{low}$	DOPA$_{high}$	DOB	AM/MIL	NP	EN
Positive inotropic	+	+		+	+	+		
Vasoconstriction		+		+				
Vasodilation (systemic)	+		+				+	+
Vasodilation (renal)			+					+

AM/MIL, amrinone or milrinone; DOB, dobutamine; DOPA$_{high}$, high-dose (5–14 μg/kg/min) dopamine; DOPA$_{low}$, low-dose (1–4 μg/kg/min) dopamine; EN, enalaprilat; ISO, isoproterenol; NE, norepinephrine; NP, nitroprusside.

hemodynamic compromise and the therapeutic goal. From the foregoing discussion, it is apparent that one can conveniently categorize the commonly used positive inotropic agents according to the presence or absence of vascular effects (Table 126–1). If a therapeutic priority is to increase arterial pressure to achieve a critical minimum level necessary to stabilize perfusion of vital organs, a concomitant vasoconstrictor action may be important. At the other extreme, if arterial pressure is excessive and insufficient perfusion of vital organs is due to left ventricular systolic failure, it may be preferable to employ a pure vasodilator (e.g., nitroprusside), a positive inotropic agent with vasodilator properties (e.g., amrinone), or a positive inotropic agent in combination with a vasodilator agent (e.g., dobutamine and nitroprusside together).

The use of low-dose dopamine to improve renal blood flow selectively is discussed in detail in Chapter 128. Numerous other combinations of agents may be used successfully (Table 126–2). For instance, the combination of dopamine and nitroprusside may be used to take advantage of both the renal dilatory and positive inotropic effects of dopamine without incurring an obligatory increase in systemic vascular resistance that may contribute to further decreases in left ventricular systolic function. Likewise, the combination of dobutamine and dopamine may be used to achieve a vasoconstrictor response (high-dose dopamine) or an increase in renal blood flow (low-dose dopamine) in the presence of maximal (or easily titrated) positive inotropic stimulation. Finally, because dobutamine and amrinone act by different pharmacologic mechanisms (e.g., β-adrenergic stimulation and phosphodiesterase inhibition, respectively), they may

be combined to achieve a greater positive inotropic response than is possible with either agent alone.[22]

In general, the best approach balances simplicity and flexibility. One should avoid redundant or antagonistic combinations. For instance, dobutamine alone may be preferable to the combination of high-dose dopamine and nitroprusside, if the only purpose of nitroprusside in this combination is to prevent the vasoconstrictor action of dopamine. Whether one should prefer the combination of dobutamine plus nitroprusside to monotherapy with amrinone is less clear. If the hemodynamic situation is likely to change over a short time, the increased flexibility of two short-acting agents may allow more precise minute-to-minute alterations in the regimen. Alternatively, when the hemodynamic pattern is likely to be stable, it may prove more convenient to titrate only a single agent such as amrinone or milrinone.

ORAL POSITIVE INOTROPIC AGENTS

Other than the digitalis glycosides, no positive inotropic agent is approved by the FDA for long-term oral use in patients with congestive heart failure. Parallel with the development of potent new positive inotropic agents, concern has grown that such agents might have deleterious effects if administered over long periods.[23, 24] There have been three major areas of concern: (1) that positive inotropic stimulation might have an adverse effect on myocardial energetics, such that myocardial cell death would be hastened or induced because of increased energy expenditure; (2) that these agents would provoke lethal arrhythmias through their effects of cAMP and Ca^{2+}; and (3) that these agents might cause impairment of myocardial relaxation, and thus a worsening of diastolic cardiac performance.[23, 24]

Whether these concerns, which are valid in a theoretical sense, will be reflected by significant adverse effects on patient survival or clinical course is unknown and can be addressed only through prospective, controlled trials. However, the results of the PROMISE trial,[19] which indicated that oral milrinone increased mortality in patients with severe congestive heart failure, have lent credence to these concerns. Prior chronic trials with milrinone did not show a significant adverse effect on survival at periods of up to 6 months.[25, 26] These efficacy trials differed from the

Table 126–2. Useful Combinations That Exert a Positive Inotropic Effect

Hemodynamic Goal	Combination
INO + VC	DOB + DOPA$_{high}$
INO + VC$_{renal}$	DOB + DOPA$_{low}$
INO + VD$_{sys}$	DOB + NP
max INO + VD$_{sys}$	DOB + AM/MIL
INO + VC/VD	DOPA$_{high}$ + NP

AM/MIL, amrinone or milrinone; DOB, dobutamine; DOPA$_{high}$, high-dose (5–14 μg/kg/min) dopamine; DOPA$_{low}$, low-dose (1–4 μg/kg/min) dopamine; INO, positive inotropy; NP, nitroprusside; VC, vasoconstriction; VC/VD, vasoconstriction or vasodilation (depending on NP dose); VD$_{renal}$, renal vasodilation; VD$_{sys}$, systemic vasodilation.

PROMISE trial in that they generally enrolled patients with relatively stable, moderate-to-severe congestive heart failure, whereas the PROMISE trial focused primarily on patients with severe, decompensated heart failure. Interestingly, an adverse effect on survival in the PROMISE trial occurred only in patients with class IV congestive heart failure and was not evident in class III patients. These observations raise the possibility that patients with more severe congestive heart failure may be more sensitive to the adverse survival effect of milrinone, perhaps because of an intrinsic increase in sensitivity to the agent or a decrease in the ability to metabolize the drug.

Because significant pharmacologic differences may exist among various positive inotropic agents, even within the same class, it is not possible to extrapolate results from one agent to another. This point is well illustrated by the results of the vesnarinone survival trial. This positive inotropic agent caused a 62% decrease in mortality in patients with moderate to severe congestive heart failure who were already receiving maximal conventional therapy, including converting enzyme inhibitors.[13] The mechanism by which vesnarinone caused an improvement in survival in this trial is not yet clear. Nevertheless, the impressive beneficial effect of vesnarinone suggests that oral positive inotropic agents may still play a significant role in the treatment of heart failure.[27]

An important issue yet to be addressed is the proper position of these new positive inotropic agents in the pharmacologic therapy of patients with chronic heart failure. Because vasodilators, particularly converting enzyme inhibitors, have been shown to improve survival in patients with congestive heart failure,[28–30] new positive inotropic agents most likely will be used in combination with converting enzyme inhibitors. Important questions remain regarding potential interactions between positive inotropic agents, converting enzyme inhibitors, digitalis, and other commonly used therapeutic agents. There is some evidence that pure phosphodiesterase inhibitors such as milrinone do not provide an additive exercise benefit when combined with digitalis.[25] On the other hand, it appears that milrinone may exert a further beneficial effect on exercise capacity in the presence of converting enzyme inhibitors.[26] The beneficial effects of vesnarinone on survival occurred in the presence of both digitalis and converting enzyme inhibitors.[13]

It is now apparent that generalizations regarding oral positive inotropic agents cannot be made. Whereas these agents have the ability to improve hemodynamic performance, exercise capacity, and survival, they also have the potential to induce serious arrhythmias and increase mortality. Difficulties in achieving good long-term results with pure phosphodiesterase inhibitors may be related, in part, to the relatively high doses of these drugs that have been employed. Newer agents combining additional mechanisms of action offer theoretical benefits and, in some cases (e.g., vesnarinone), seem to offer a real clinical advantage.

REFERENCES

1. Colucci WS, Wright RF, Braunwald E: New positive agents in the treatment of congestive heart failure. N Engl J Med 314:290, 349, 1986.
2. Bristow MR, Ginsberg R, Minole M, et al: Decreased catecholamine sensitivity and beta-adrenergic receptor density in failing human hearts. N Engl J Med 307:205, 1982.
3. Fowler MB, Laser JA, Hopkins GL, et al: Assessment of the beta-adrenergic receptor pathway in intact failing human heart: Progressive receptor down-regulation and subsensitivity to agonist response. Circulation 74:1290, 1986.
4. Colucci WS, Leatherman GF, Ludmer PL, et al: Beta-adrenergic inotropic responsiveness of patients with heart failure: Studies with intracoronary dobutamine infusion. Circ Res 61(Suppl I):I-82, 1987.
5. Feldman MD, Copelas L, Gwathmey JK, et al: Deficient production of cyclic AMP: Pharmacologic evidence of an important cause of contractile dysfunction in patients with end-stage heart failure. Circulation 75:331, 1987.
6. Levine TB, Francis GS, Goldsmith SR, et al: Activity of the sympathetic nervous system and renin-angiotensin system assessed by plasma hormone levels and their relation to hemodynamic abnormalities in congestive heart failure. Am J Cardiol 49:1659, 1982.
7. Cohn JN, Levine TB, Olivari MT, et al: Plasma norepinephrine as a guide to prognosis in patients with chronic congestive heart failure. N Engl J Med 311:819, 1984.
8. Colucci WS, Alexander RW, Williams GH, et al: Decreased lymphocyte beta-adrenergic receptor density in patients with heart failure and tolerance to the beta-adrenergic agonist pirbuterol. N Engl J Med 305:185, 1981.
9. Lambertz H, Meyer J, Erbel R: Long-term hemodynamic effects of prenalterol in patients with severe congestive heart failure. Circulation 69:298, 1984.
10. Kenakin TP, Ferris RM: Effects of in vivo B-adrenoceptor down-regulation on cardiac responses to prenalterol and pirbuterol. J Cardiovasc Pharmacol 5:90, 1984.
11. Unverferth DV, Blanford M, Kates RE, et al: Tolerance to dobutamine after a 72-hour continuous infusion. Am J Med 69:262, 1980.
12. Kubo SH, Gollub SB, Bourge R, et al: Beneficial effects of pimobendan on exercise tolerance and quality of life in patients with heart failure: Results of a multicenter trial. Circulation 85:942, 1992.
13. Feldman AM, Bristow MR, Parmley WW, et al, for the Vesnarinone Study Group: Effects of vesnarinone on morbidity and mortality in patients with heart failure. N Engl J Med 329:149, 1993.
14. Cody RJ, Leier CV, Bristow MR, et al: OPC-18790 produces titratable hemodynamic benefit in hospitalized patients with severe congestive heart failure [abstract]. Circulation 88:I-300, 1993.
15. Benotti JR, Grossman W, Braunwald E, et al: Hemodynamic assessment of amrinone: A new inotropic agent. N Engl J Med 299:1373, 1978.
16. LeJemtel TH, Keung E, Sonnenblick EH, et al: Amrinone: A new non-glycoside, non-adrenergic agent effective in the treatment of intractable myocardial failure in man. Circulation 59:1097, 1979.
17. Baim DS, McDowell AV, Cherniles J, et al: Evaluation of a new bipyridine inotropic agent—milrinone—in patients with severe congestive heart failure. N Engl J Med 309:748, 1983.
18. Maskin CS, Sinoway L, Chadwick B, et al: Sustained hemodynamic and clinical effects of a new cardiotonic agent, WIN 47203, in patients with severe congestive heart failure. Circulation 67:1065, 1983.
19. Packer M, Carver JR, Rodeheffer RJ, et al, on behalf of the PROMISE Study Research Group: Effect of oral milrinone on mortality in severe chronic heart failure. N Engl J Med 325:1468, 1991.
20. Ludmer PL, Wright RF, Arnold JMO, et al: Separation of the direct myocardial and vasodilator actions of milrinone: Studies utilizing an intracoronary infusion technique. Circulation 73:130, 1986.

21. Colucci WS, Wright RF, Jaski BE, et al: Milrinone and dobutamine in severe heart failure: Differing hemodynamic effects and individual patient responsiveness. Circulation 73(Suppl III):III-175, 1986.
22. Gage J, Rutman H, Lucido D, et al: Additive effects of dobutamine and amrinone on myocardial contractility and ventricular performance in patients with severe heart failure. Circulation 74:367, 1986.
23. Katz AM: Potential deleterious effects of inotropic agents in the therapy of chronic heart failure. Circulation 73(Suppl III):III-184, 1986.
24. Packer M, Medina N, Yushak M: Hemodynamic and clinical limitations of long-term inotropic therapy with amrinone in patients with severe chronic heart failure. Circulation 70:1038, 1984.
25. DiBianco R, Shabetai R, Kostuk W, et al: A comparison of oral milrinone, digoxin, and their combination in the treatment of patients with chronic heart failure. N Engl J Med 320:677, 1989.
26. Colucci WS, Sonnenblick EH, Adams KF, et al: Efficacy of phosphodiesterase inhibition with milrinone in combination with converting enzyme inhibitors in patients with heart failure: The Milrinone Trials Investigators. J Am Coll Cardiol 22:113A, 1993.
27. Colucci WS: What is the role of positive inotropic agents in the treatment of congestive heart failure? Heart Failure 9:126, 1993.
28. Cohn JN, Archibald DG, Ziesche S, et al: Effect of vasodilator therapy on mortality in chronic congestive heart failure. N Engl J Med 314:1547, 1986.
29. Cohn JN, Johnson G, Ziesche S, et al: A comparison of enalapril with hydralazine-isosorbide dinitrate in the treatment of chronic congestive heart failure. N Engl J Med 325:303, 1991.
30. The SOLVD Investigators: Effect of enalapril on survival in patients with reduced left ventricular ejection fractions and congestive heart failure. N Engl J Med 325:293, 1991.

C. Specific Positive Inotropic Agents

CHAPTER 127

Dobutamine

Andrea Hastillo, M.D., David O. Taylor, M.D., and Michael L. Hess, M.D.

HISTORY

During the early 1970s, Tuttle and Mills at the Lilly Research Laboratories began systematically modifying the chemical structure of isoproterenol[1] in an attempt to find a better inotropic agent. They found that removal of the side-chain β-hydroxyl group of isoproterenol decreased its automaticity and increased its contractility.[1] They then substituted various alkyl and aralkyl groups on the terminal nitrogen substituent and selected the derivative with the optimal combination of maximum contractility, minimum automaticity, and minimal blood pressure effects. The chemical name of this derivative with the best profile of effects is (±)-4-[2-[[3-(p-hydroxyphenyl)-1-methylpropyl]amino]ethyl]-pyrocatechol hydrochloride and its common name is dobutamine, and it has become a cornerstone in the treatment of acute congestive heart failure.

PHARMACOLOGY

Dobutamine mediates its effects via β₁-, β₂-, and α-receptor stimulation. Unlike dopamine, dobutamine does not mediate its effects by release of intramyocardial norepinephrine.[1-3] Tuttle suggested that this quality may be partially responsible for the less arrhythmogenic nature of the drug. Norepinephrine release in the myocardium may have deleterious effects by causing oxygen wasting in mitochondria and calcium accumulation within myocardial cells.[4, 5] Furthermore, Waldenstrom et al.[6] showed that myocardial cell damage can be caused by small doses of norepinephrine. Thus, because dobutamine does not mediate its effects through norepinephrine, it may be more beneficial in conditions of myocardial catecholamine depletion, such as chronic congestive heart failure or the use of norepinephrine-depleting antihypertensive drugs.[1]

Many investigators have shown that dobutamine increases contractility, thus increasing stroke volume and cardiac output with minimal effect on heart rate.[1, 7-13] The effect on contractility was originally thought to be exclusively β-receptor mediated,[1, 8, 11] but recent studies have pointed out the contribution of α-receptor stimulation to the inotropic selectivity.[14-18] Whether these α-receptors are purely myocardial or simply mediate a reflex modulation of heart rate is still in debate. Several researchers have shown the potent α₁-agonist activity of dobutamine. In phentolamine-treated cats, Kenakin and Johnson[18] showed that dobutamine did not demonstrate inotropic selectivity and exhibited a response that was not significantly different from isoproterenol. In addition, phentolamine did not change the effects of isoproterenol on inotropy. Schumann and other investigators[15, 18-21] have provided evidence that α₁-receptors in the myocardium cause positive inotropic changes with minimal increases in heart rate. This inotropic selectivity is decreased by vagotomy,[11, 13] ganglionic blockade,[10, 13] and α-adrenergic antagonists.[14, 18] Peripheral α-receptor activity to dobutamine has been demonstrated by several investigators using β-blocking drugs.[9, 11, 18]

Much of what is known of the individual receptor activity of dobutamine stems from the work of Ruffolo and his associates.[14, 16, 17] They showed that the (−)-enantiomer (levo) of dobutamine is mainly responsible for the α-receptor activity that produces increases in cardiac output, stroke volume, total peripheral resistance, and mean arterial pressure, but not heart rate. The (+) or dextro-enantiomer possesses mainly β₂- activity, causing increases in heart rate and thus cardiac output but not stroke volume. Other significant β-receptor–mediated effects are decreases in total peripheral resistance and mean arterial blood pressure.[14, 16, 17] Binkley et al.[22] studied the vascular effects of dobutamine in calves using the Jarvik heart model and infusing 6 to 24 μg/kg/min of racemic dobutamine. They concluded that the levo-isomer's activation of postsynaptic α-adrenergic receptors led to a decrease in the venous capacitance, an increase in venous flow, and thus an increase in central blood flow. β-Stimulation by the dextro-isomer led to a decrease in systemic vascular resistance, which resulted in an increase in both aortic and central blood flow. The commercial form of dobutamine is racemic. Owing to the competing α-β-activity stimulated by dobutamine, the net result is a significantly increased cardiac output and an increased stroke volume but usually no change in mean arterial pressure, because total peripheral vascular resistance falls significantly. The pulmonary vascular resistance falls insignificantly, and the heart rate does not change. Thus, dobutamine significantly improves left ventricular performance independently of direct myocardial stimulation.[22]

PHARMACOKINETICS

Dobutamine is available in intravenous form only and is administered by constant intravenous infusion. Pharmacokinetic studies reveal a disappearance half-life of 2.37 minutes in patients with heart failure[23] and a half-life of 1 or 2 minutes in normal dogs.[24] Steady-state levels are usually attained within 10 minutes.[23, 24] Because of its short half-life, dobutamine can be given only by continuous infusion. Kates and Leier[23] showed a volume of distribution of 0.202 ± 0.084 L/kg in seven patients with severe congestive heart failure and found a linear relationship between the volume of distribution and the extent of peripheral edema. The total body clearance of dobutamine averaged 2.35 L/min/m^2. The clearance appears to be related to its distribution into tissues rather than elimination or metabolism, because total body clearance was greater than cardiac output.[23]

Plasma levels increase linearly with infusion rates as shown by Leier et al.[25] Cardiac output and stroke volume increased linearly with plasma levels, whereas pulmonary capillary wedge pressure, systemic vascular resistance, and total vascular resistance decreased linearly. They used infusion rates of 2.5, 5, 7.5, and 10 μg/kg/min and did not test doses higher than 10 μg/kg/min because of their prior experience with undesired side effects occurring above this dose.[25] Vatner et al.[9] found that in conscious dogs cardiac output and stroke volume increased up to doses as high as 40 μg/kg/min, but significant tachycardia occurred at doses higher than 15 μg/kg/min.

Murphy et al.[24] examined the disposition of the drug in dogs, using dobutamine labeled with ^{14}C. They found that the major metabolite was 3-O-methyldobutamine and that it is inactive. The half-life of the degradation products was 1.9 hours by ^{14}C trac-

ing. Peak levels of dobutamine and its metabolites occur in 3 or 4 hours. Excretion of ^{14}C metabolites was 67% in urine and 30% to 35% in bile, with 20% in the stool, showing some enterohepatic circulation of these inactive metabolites.

Although plasma levels remain fairly constant after steady-state levels are reached, hemodynamic effects reach a maximum at 2 hours and then decrease thereafter, losing 33% of the maximum effect by 72 hours.[26] This effect can usually be overcome by simply increasing the maintenance infusion, although this is less likely to occur in older patients.[27] One possible mechanism for this tolerance involves downregulation of the adrenoreceptors. "Full sensitivity to beta-agonist drugs is restored seven to 10 days after discontinuation of therapy."[26]

EFFECTS ON HEMODYNAMICS

The hemodynamic effects of dobutamine have been studied extensively in various clinical settings, including chronic ischemic and idiopathic cardiomyopathies, acute ventricular failure from myocardial infarction, sepsis, pulmonary embolism, postcardiopulmonary bypass, and various animal models.

The most significant hemodynamic effect is the increase in cardiac output, which is almost entirely secondary to an increase in stroke volume. Stroke volume and cardiac output increase from 33% to 80% in various studies, with most showing an increase of 45% to 55% at doses between 5 and 15 μg/kg/min.[3, 7, 9, 28–56] Heart rate increases slightly with doses lower than 15 μg/kg/min. Some studies found increases as high as 25% to 38%,[9, 36, 53, 56] but most found increases from 0% to 15%.* Mean arterial blood pressure has been noted to increase slightly,[35] decrease slightly,[32, 47] or remain unchanged.[28, 29, 31, 38, 43, 48, 56] Systemic vascular resistance decreases 5% to 50%.† Central α-adrenergic withdrawal secondary to the increased cardiac output is probably more responsible for the decrease in systemic vascular resistance than direct β-stimulation.[58] Pulmonary vascular resistance also decreases 10% to 70%.[9, 29, 31, 34, 36, 50] Dobutamine has been found to inhibit the pulmonary vasoconstrictor response to hypoxia.[59–61]

Pediatric Patients

Dobutamine has been tested and used extensively in adults, but several studies have found equal efficacy in the pediatric population. Driscoll et al.[62] administered dobutamine at 2 and 7.75 μg/kg/min to 12 pediatric patients undergoing cardiac catheterization for investigation of congenital heart disease. They found increases in cardiac index and stroke volume and decreases in pulmonary capillary wedge pressure much as in adults. They found no change in total vascular resistance or heart rate but found a significant increase in both mean and systolic blood pres-

---

*References 7, 28, 29, 31–33, 37, 38, 41, 43, 44, 47, 48, 52.
†References 7, 28, 31, 34, 36, 40, 43, 44, 50, 52, 53, 56, 57.

sures. Schranz et al.[63] studied dobutamine in children with cardiovascular failure of various causes and found similar changes in cardiac index, stroke volume, mean arterial pressure, and heart rate but found significant decreases in systemic vascular resistance. In these patients, the increase in cardiac output was greater than the reflex decrease in vascular resistance; thus, mean blood pressure increased. Jose et al.[64] examined dobutamine therapy after congenital defect repairs in children and found that doses of 10 to 15 μg/kg/min were needed to allow adequate increases in cardiac index, but Bohn et al.[65] found the optimal dose in their series of children who underwent cardiopulmonary bypass was 7.5 μg/kg/min. Other studies in children have used doses of 2 to 15 μg/kg/min with good hemodynamic results.[62, 63, 66] Thus, it appears that in children, just as in adults, the optimal dose range must be individualized for each patient.

Geriatric Patients

Dobutamine appears to be less effective in the elderly population whether the individual is healthy[67] or has congestive heart failure. Rich et al.[27] compared a small group of younger individuals (≤70 years; mean, 55 years) with a small group of older patients (≥80 years; mean, 83 years) who had decompensated congestive heart failure. The hemodynamic response, as measured by cardiac output and stroke volume, to lower-dose dobutamine (5 μg/kg/min) was two times greater in the younger compared with the older group. In addition, when the dobutamine infusion was increased to 10 μg/kg/min, the younger group demonstrated a further increase in the hemodynamic measurements, whereas the elderly did not. The reason for this attenuated response to dobutamine and the lack of increased responsiveness to increasing doses in the elderly has not yet been explained.[27]

EFFECTS ON ELECTROPHYSIOLOGY

Dobutamine has slightly less arrhythmogenicity than dopamine and much less than epinephrine, norepinephrine, and isoproterenol.[7, 9, 31, 37] Dobutamine has a greater effect on ventricular adrenoreceptors than on the sinoatrial node.[11, 68] It also increases atrioventricular nodal conduction and may increase the ventricular rate in patients with atrial fibrillation or flutter;[69] therefore, digoxin may be needed to control the ventricular rate.

EFFECTS ON CORONARY AND PERIPHERAL BLOOD FLOW

Dobutamine increases blood flow to most vascular beds primarily as a result of an increase in cardiac output rather than its peripheral vasoactive effects. The increase in blood flow is greater in the iliac and femoral vessels and the skeletal and coronary beds than in renal and mesenteric beds, where blood flow is only slightly increased.[9, 40, 44, 56] Most investigators agree that the increase in coronary blood flow is secondary to decreased coronary vascular resistance, which appears to be mediated by local autoregulatory effects from the increased myocardial oxygen consumption caused by dobutamine rather than direct effects of the drug on the vascular tone.[4, 40, 41, 48, 51, 55, 70] However, Dubois-Randé et al.[71] designed a study in which dobutamine was infused into the left main coronary artery in nine patients with idiopathic dilated cardiomyopathy without effecting a major change in the heart rate and load conditions of the heart. Infusion of dobutamine led to an increase in the oxygen content of the coronary sinus blood flow, an increase in the coronary sinus blood flow, a decrease in the coronary sinus lactate concentration, and no change in the myocardial oxygen consumption. These results suggest that dobutamine does have a direct coronary vasculature dilatory effect.[71]

EFFECTS ON RENAL FUNCTION

Studies in patients with severe congestive heart failure have shown that dobutamine increases urine output between 0.25 and 2.5 ml/min and sodium excretion by 10 to 20 mEq/L.[7, 28, 33] This effect is primarily the result of the increase in cardiac output because dobutamine has minimal direct effects on renal vasculature in normal controls. Good et al.,[72] however, concluded that dobutamine, via its direct stimulation of β_1-receptors, accounts at least for the increased urinary sodium excretion they documented in patients with congestive heart failure undergoing a diuresis. Patients receiving the lower dose dobutamine failed to demonstrate an increase in urinary volume or sodium excretion whereas those receiving the high dose dobutamine showed increases in both variables.[72] Westman and Järnberg[73] studied dobutamine in healthy volunteers and found a decrease in glomerular filtration rate, no change in renal blood flow, and a decrease in both urine output and free water clearance. This agrees with other data on the β-agonist effect on renal function, which may be mediated through vasopressin.[67, 74] Robie and Goldberg[56] studied dobutamine and dopamine in anesthetized normal dogs and found no change in renal blood flow or renovascular resistance with dobutamine, whereas dopamine increased renal blood flow significantly because of its direct venodilatory effect. Dobutamine increases renin secretion,[54, 73, 75] most likely because of its β-agonist activity, which is similar to that of other β-agonists, which are known to stimulate renin release.[76]

CLINICAL USES
Chronic Congestive Heart Failure

Much of what is known about dobutamine's hemodynamic effects stems from clinical trials in patients with chronic congestive heart failure. Dobutamine increases stroke volume and cardiac output, decreases pulmonary capillary wedge pressure and systemic vascular resistance, and has only modest influence on heart rate and blood pressure in doses lower than 12 to 15 µg/kg/min.[7, 29, 30, 42, 43, 47] Its effect is, at least in an idiopathic dilated cardiomyopathic heart, attenuated by decreases in β-receptor concentration when dobutamine is infused via the intracoronary route.[77] This assumes particular importance when coupled to the discovery of Townend et al.[78] that 16 weeks of therapy with angiotensin-converting enzyme (ACE) inhibitors upregulates lymphocyte β-adrenoreceptors in heart failure. In this study, dobutamine infusion before and after the 16 weeks of ACE-inhibitor therapy was associated with increased cardiac index, stroke volume, and cardiac power output following the 16-week ACE-inhibitor course.[78] Gilbert et al. also were able to demonstrate an increase in β-adrenergic receptor density following treatment of an ACE inhibitor in patients with heart failure.[79]

Dobutamine is equivalent to or better than dopamine in its ability to increase cardiac output and offers a distinct advantage over dopamine in its ability to lower left ventricular filling pressures and systemic vascular resistance in patients with heart failure.[32, 56, 73] In patients with low cardiac output, high filling pressure, and acceptable blood pressures, dobutamine is the preferred inotropic agent. Patients with marked hypotension and normal or mildly increased filling pressures may benefit more from dopamine initially. Because of its renal and mesenteric vasodilating effects, the addition of low-dose dopamine may be the best option in patients with low cardiac output states and severe prerenal azotemia or bowel ischemia.

Loeb et al.[80] compared isoproterenol with dobutamine in patients with chronic congestive heart failure and found both equally effective in increasing cardiac output and decreasing filling pressure and vascular resistance. However, isoproterenol caused a significantly greater increase in heart rate, which may be detrimental in situations in which diastolic filling time or myocardial oxygen consumption are of concern.

Comparison with the newer inotropic agents milrinone, amrinone, and enoximone has found comparable increases in cardiac output and stroke volume, but the newer agents cause greater decreases in filling pressures and systemic vascular resistance and less effect on heart rate than dobutamine.[30, 32, 40, 43, 81, 82] In addition, amrinone does not seem to show attenuation of effect seen with dobutamine.[26, 83] Variation has been reported, however. Marcus et al.[84] demonstrated that 48-hour infusions of dobutamine or amrinone could achieve similar effects on the pulmonary capillary wedge pressure, cardiac index, mean arterial blood pressure, and systemic vascular resistance. The effect of amrinone on lowering right atrial pressure was greater and associated with a greater increase in heart rate (presumably because of baroreceptor activation) than dobutamine. Amrinone more predictably led to a decrease in pulmonary capillary wedge pressure (91% of patients) compared with dobutamine (65%) and more consistently produced a negative fluid balance at 48 hours compared with dobutamine (100% versus 78%). No significant adverse effects occurred at the doses used (maximum of 20 µg/kg/min for amrinone, 15 µg/kg/min for dobutamine). The dose of amrinone necessary to achieve predetermined hemodynamic measurements was more predictable than that of dobutamine and may make amrinone the best choice if right heart catheterization is relatively contraindicated during inotropic infusion.[84] Another benefit of the newer inotropic agents is their ability to decrease myocardial oxygen consumption in contrast with the increase caused by dobutamine.[40, 48, 79] Two studies have shown benefit using combinations of dobutamine and amrinone to produce improved hemodynamic effects than either agent alone and spare the adrenergic side effects of higher-dose dobutamine.[75, 85] One of these studies,[75] however, found that the addition of amrinone to dobutamine increased heart rate significantly and caused a decrease in cardiac output in 3 of 10 patients. They also found that adding amrinone to dobutamine caused a further increase in the elevated renin activity induced by dobutamine. Although optimistic about the improved short-term hemodynamic improvements in most of their patients, the authors suggested caution with the use of this combination because of its increase in heart rate, variable effect on cardiac index, and marked activation of the renin-angiotensin system.[75] In contrast, however, a later study in which nine patients with severe idiopathic dilated cardiomyopathy received dobutamine alone and then a combination of dobutamine and amrinone led to the conclusion that such a combination could be used safely at the bedside. These patients all improved their cardiac index with the addition of dobutamine (mean of 1.47 to 2.89 L/min/m²). The addition of amrinone increased the cardiac index even further to a mean of 3.64 L/min/m², although two patients demonstrated a decrease in cardiac index from 4.92 and 4.25 L/min/m² on dobutamine to 4.71 and 3.84 L/min/m², respectively. But even these two levels were higher than the baseline cardiac indices (1.48 and 1.97 L/min/m², respectively). In this study, dobutamine did not significantly increase the heart rate and, although the addition of amrinone did increase heart rate, there was no increase in coronary sinus lactate efflux. Myocardial oxygen consumption remained invariant. Thus, in a failing heart with its downregulated β-receptors, there is still potential for improvement in ventricular performance with the addition of a phosphodiesterase inhibitor, which may be accomplished without an increase in energy expenditure and with an increase in myocardial efficiency.[86] Such differences in mechanism of action and the presence of downregulation of myocardial β-receptors in cardiac failure may account for the observation of Dubois-Randé et al.[87] They found that in 34 patients who failed to respond to betamimetic drugs, 30 responded to enoximone.

When compared with dobutamine, nitroprusside caused similar increases in cardiac output primarily by its ability to decrease afterload. Nitroprusside causes a greater decrease in systemic vascular resistance than dobutamine, and dobutamine a greater increase in stroke volume than nitroprusside.[58, 88] Nitroprusside causes a greater decrease in left ventricular filling pressure than dobutamine but also significantly lowers arterial pressure.[58, 88] Nitroprusside also does not increase myocardial oxygen consumption.[89] Thus, nitroprusside is less useful in patients with marked hypotension but may be more beneficial than dobutamine in patients with adequate blood pressures and high filling pressure. The combination of dobutamine and nitroprusside is especially beneficial in patients with hypotension, low cardiac output, high filling pressure, and significant coronary artery stenosis.[58]

Use of outpatient dobutamine infusion, either intermittent or continuous, is being studied as an important method to improve the quality of life for patients as well as to save huge amounts of resources, including financial. Liang et al.[42] found that in patients with chronic congestive heart failure, 72-hour infusions of dobutamine improved functional class, left ventricular ejection fractions, and resting hemodynamics for up to 4 weeks. It has been postulated that dobutamine produces its long-term effect by altering the ultrastructure of the myocardial cells and thus perhaps improving cellular function.[90] Early but uncontrolled trials with outpatient dobutamine administered via portable infusion devices initially had optimistic results,[91, 92] but two later studies were disappointing. One such study[93] was an uncontrolled trial of 13 patients who received weekly, 48-hour infusions of dobutamine. The investigators found that all 13 patients had at least a 25% increase in cardiac output, but only seven improved in functional class. More disconcerting was the occurrence of sudden death in six patients. Only three patients survived the 26-week study period. One multicenter, randomized trial compared intermittent dobutamine (48 hr/wk) with a placebo but was discontinued prematurely when 15 of the 20 deaths occurred in groups assigned or crossed-over to dobutamine.[94] The high incidence of sudden death in these two studies raised the concern that dobutamine may be inducing or lowering the threshold to malignant ventricular arrhythmias. It is interesting to note that two of the three survivors in the first study were on amiodarone compared with none in the group of patients who died.[93] Presently in an uncontrolled trial at the Medical College of Virginia in which all patients receive outpatient dobutamine, there has been only one sudden death in the ten eligible for long-term follow-up (>3 months). This patient was the only one of the 10 not receiving amiodarone.

More recently, Miller et al.[95] reported their experiences with 11 patients with refractory class IV congestive heart failure who were not cardiac transplant candidates but who were dependent on dobutamine. All were treated as outpatients with either continuous or intermittent infusion of dobutamine via an indwelling central line. While on dobutamine, the functional class of the patients improved by 1.5 functional class units. Seven of the 11 patients were able to be weaned from dobutamine an average of 3.2 months after starting outpatient therapy. These seven were manageable with oral medications and were in functional class II congestive heart failure. Six who were weaned were alive throughout the follow-up period, which averaged 29 months. One died 2½ years following discontinuation of the dobutamine after developing recurrent heart failure. Four patients did not respond to the dobutamine infusion and these four died. Two died of progressive heart failure, one of progressive pulmonary sarcoidosis, and the last of pneumonia and sepsis. No patient died of cardiac dysrhythmias. Of note is that 5 of the 11 patients were taking amiodarone at the time of the dobutamine infusion for dysrhythmia control.[95] Currently, many centers in the United States are offering outpatient dobutamine as an alternative to in-hospital infusion.

Left Ventricular Failure

As with other sympathomimetic inotropic drugs, the dobutamine-induced increase in contractility and stroke volume is at the expense of increased myocardial oxygen consumption.[34, 40, 41, 48, 51, 55] This may seem counterproductive in cases where the goal is to decrease myocardial oxygen consumption, such as in myocardial failure secondary to acute infarction or ischemia. Inotropic agents can extend infarct size and exacerbate ischemia in patients with minimal ventricular dysfunction by further increasing myocardial oxygen demand and consumption.[49] The decreases in left ventricular filling pressures and afterload (wall tension) and the increases in cardiac output and coronary flow seen with dobutamine offset this increase in myocardial oxygen consumption in most situations. Several studies have found that although myocardial oxygen consumption increases, coronary blood flow increases accordingly and lactate extraction does not change, implying that ischemia is not produced.[40, 41, 50] Vatner and Baig[55] found that in dogs with acute coronary occlusion, dobutamine increased blood flow to normal and moderately ischemic tissues; however, if significant tachycardia occurred, a decrease in blood flow and deterioration of contractile function in ischemic zones was seen. Kupper et al.[41] also found that, in 3 of 15 patients with coronary artery disease who had significant increases in heart rate at higher doses of dobutamine, myocardial lactate extraction decreased and signs of ischemia developed. Pozen et al.[50] found that 4 of 18 patients with coronary artery disease and heart failure on maximally tolerated doses of dobutamine (7.5 to 15 µg/kg/min) developed abnormal lactate metabolism and angina, whereas seven patients with primary cardiomyopathy had no change in lactate metabolism. Therefore, heart rate must be closely monitored in patients with coronary disease receiving dobutamine.

Dobutamine has been used successfully in patients with left ventricular dysfunction resulting from acute myocardial infarction or ischemia without evidence of infarct extension or increases in ventricular ectopy.[28, 31, 35, 37, 41, 49, 50, 52] In an experimental infarction model, Maekawa et al.[44] found that dobutamine increased collateral blood flow to the ischemic myocardium, enhanced ventricular performance, and reduced infarct size compared with dopamine, which did none of these things. The authors believed that the release of norepinephrine by dopamine was responsible for its deleterious effects. Dell'Italia et al.[35] found that dobutamine increased cardiac index, stroke volume, and right ventricular ejection fraction much greater than volume loading or nitroprusside in patients with predominantly right ventricular myocardial infarction.

Vasodilators such as nitroglycerin and nitroprusside have added benefits in the treatment of ventricular dysfunction associated with coronary insufficiency with their ability to decrease preload and afterload and reduce myocardial oxygen consumption. Combination therapy with dobutamine and vasodilators is extremely useful in situations in which severe ventricular dysfunction after acute myocardial infarction is associated with mild hypotension and elevated filling pressures.[31, 58, 89]

Low Cardiac Output States After Cardiac Surgery

Inotropic agents have become a significant part of the treatment of ventricular dysfunction after cardiac surgery. A comparison between dobutamine, dopamine, and norepinephrine plus phentolamine in patients after revascularization or valve replacement found dobutamine to be superior because it produced the least tachycardia and vasoconstriction and the greatest increase in cardiac output.[96] DiSesa et al.[97] compared dobutamine with dopamine after revascularization or valve replacement and found that the two agents caused the same increases in cardiac output and heart rate, but dobutamine caused a decrease in systemic vascular resistance and left atrial pressure. Salomon found that dobutamine was superior to dopamine in postoperative cardiac dysfunction because of its "consistent dose-related increases in cardiac index without increases in heart rate, mean arterial pressure, pulmonary capillary wedge pressure."[98] Jaccard et al.[99] found that dobutamine was less effective than isoprenaline in increasing cardiac index in patients after surgical correction of tetralogy of Fallot. This seems to be because of the small left ventricle found in these patients and thus the smaller contribution of stroke volume to cardiac index when compared with heart rate.

After cardiac transplantation, recipients may develop immediate postoperative low cardiac output syndromes, which are usually treated with isoproterenol because of the need for inotropic as well as chronotropic support. Many case reports indicate the usefulness of dobutamine during episodes of heart failure caused by rejection. DeBroux et al.[100] studied dogs that were transplanted, developed low output failure immediately postoperatively, survived, and then developed acute cardiac allograft rejection and

heart failure. They demonstrated that during both periods of heart failure the infusion of 5 µg/kg/min of dobutamine led to an increase in cardiac index of 97% in the early postoperative period but only 35% during rejection. Increasing the infusion dose increased the cardiac index further in the rejecting dog heart. Thus, dobutamine appears to be useful in treatment of the rejecting heart, although the dose needs to be increased.[100]

Myocardial Failure from Other Causes

Molloy et al.[101] compared dobutamine and dopamine in eight patients with acute respiratory failure on mechanical ventilation. These drugs led to similar increases in cardiac index and stroke volume. Dobutamine, however, decreased pulmonary capillary wedge pressure, whereas dopamine increased it. The authors concluded that this effect on left ventricular filling pressures may be important in patients with respiratory failure from conditions causing increased capillary permeability because small changes in filling pressure can cause large changes in alveolar fluid accumulation.[101] Dobutamine has been used successfully in patients with pulmonary embolism and shock[102] and is better than dopamine in improving cardiac output in patients during severe acidosis.[103] Dobutamine increases cardiac index and stroke volume in both septic shock[104, 105] and toxic shock,[106] but dopamine remains the inotropic agent of choice in these situations because of its ability to increase blood pressure and systemic vascular resistance, which are both usually markedly depressed in patients with sepsis.[104, 105] Dobutamine may be useful in these situations when blood pressure is not significantly low, filling pressures are high, or the need for an additional inotropic agent arises.

Dobutamine and Deconditioning

One interesting effect of dobutamine is its apparent ability to prevent physical deconditioning induced by prolonged bed rest. Sullivan et al.[107] took 24 healthy men and assigned them to bed rest and randomly assigned them to 2 hours of daily exercise, dobutamine, or saline. They found that dobutamine prevented most of the physiologic manifestations of bed rest–induced deconditioning. This feature may prove useful in preventing the deconditioning associated with prolonged hospitalization from fractures, paralysis, other severe illness, and in the deconditioning associated with prolonged space travel.

Dobutamine and Diagnostic Studies

Although not approved by the Food and Drug Administration as a pharmacologic stress agent, dobutamine has been used as a stressor in various techniques used in the assessment of coronary artery disease. Mannering et al.[108] compared symptom-limited treadmill exercise testing with graded dobutamine infusion stress testing in 50 patients 3 weeks after myocardial infarction. The development of ST-segment depression was comparable by these two methods (concordance 88%), and the ST-segment depression sites were the same in all cases.

Mason, Freeman, and colleagues[109, 110] compared dobutamine with bicycle-exercise radionuclide ventriculography and examined the use of dobutamine as the stressor for thallium scintigraphy for the detection of coronary artery disease. They infused dobutamine in increasing doses of 5 to 20 µg/kg/min with scanning performed at the maximum tolerated dose and found it to be equivalent to bicycle exercise in detecting coronary artery disease. In their application to thallium scintigraphy, they found a sensitivity of 94% and a specificity of 87% for detecting coronary disease.[110] Although they did not compare dobutamine thallium with exercise or dipyridamole thallium scintigraphy in their study, it compares favorably with the sensitivities and specificities found in other series.[111, 112] The experience of Pennell et al.[113] with 50 patients undergoing dobutamine-thallium testing was similar—97% sensitivity and 80% specificity. They also established a significant relationship between the mean number of segments with abnormal perfusion and the number of diseased coronary arteries. There also appeared to be a relationship between the maximum dobutamine infusion tolerated and the treadmill exercise time. Six of the 50 patients had asthma, and all tolerated the dobutamine infusion.[113] Using dobutamine infusion and monitoring echocardiographic change, Segar et al. also demonstrated that dobutamine exercise can potentially provide information on the severity of the coronary artery disease.[114] Hays et al.[115] used incremental dobutamine infusion to a maximum of 40 µg/kg/min to demonstrate that although side effects are common, dobutamine–thallium-201 tomography is well tolerated; the overall sensitivity is 86% (100% for three-vessel disease), and the specificity is 90% for patients and 86% for individual vessels. Side effects included the development of typical chest pain in 26% and atypical chest pain in 5% of patients. Twenty-nine percent developed palpitations. However, 75% of patients tolerated an infusion up to 40 µg/kg/min and 97% tolerated an infusion rate of 30 µg/kg/min.

Berthe et al.[116] administered dobutamine and performed two-dimensional (2-D) echocardiography on 30 patients 5 to 10 days after acute myocardial infarction and found sensitivities and specificities of 85% and 88%, respectively, for detecting multivessel coronary artery disease. The overall accuracy was 87%. They concluded that the dobutamine stress test was a useful, cost-effective, and easily administered method for detecting multivessel disease after acute infarction. Mazeika et al.[117] evaluated 51 symptomatic patients with dobutamine-echocardiography and then followed them up for 24 ± 4 months, monitoring cardiac events (angioplasty, coronary grafts, unstable angina, acute myocardial infarction). Of the 23 patients with cardiac events, 74% had transient asynergy with dobutamine-echocardiography whereas 29% of patients without events had transient asynergy. They concluded that this test may be useful in selecting which patient should undergo further invasive evaluation for coronary artery disease.

A study by Marwick et al.[118] was developed to compare the sensitivity and specificity of two techniques to determine ischemic regional wall motion abnormality or abnormal myocardial perfusion using the same patients under the same conditions. Adenosine and dobutamine were infused and 2-D echocardiography and single photon emission computed tomography were selected to determine wall motion and perfusion. Adenosine stress echocardiography was the least sensitive and least accurate technique. They concluded that wall motion abnormalities and perfusion may be assessed with the dobutamine techniques and adenosine perfusion scintigraphy is equal to dobutamine perfusion scintigraphy. Functional evidence of regional ischemia should not be sought with adenosine echocardiography.

In an attempt to develop a mechanism to assess functional capacity of the failing heart and determine prognosis, Tan et al.[119] compared bicycle ergometry and incremental infusion of dobutamine on the pumping capability of stressed hearts. These two methods were similarly effective, although dobutamine infusion is more widely applicable in patients who cannot exercise adequately. Coupled with noninvasive Doppler echocardiography, incremental infusion of dobutamine may become valuable in determining the prognosis of patients with heart failure.

Hwang et al.[120] found dobutamine useful in assessing the severity of mitral stenosis during cardiac catheterization. It offers certain advantages over the more commonly used interventions. It has a lower incidence of arrhythmias than isoproterenol and is much easier to administer than exercise, which requires one or more free limbs and good patient cooperation.

Dobutamine is an ideal agent for these diagnostic applications because of its short half-life, its ability to be safely given from peripheral veins, and its relatively low incidence of adverse effects. It is the best pharmacologic agent available in detecting functional ischemia and may provide information on coronary artery disease severity and prognosis in heart failure. It can be used in patients not able or not inclined to exercise. It may be used in patients with asthma or severe chronic obstructive pulmonary disease provided they are free of dobutamine and sulfite allergy. Because most cardiologists and internists have experience with the use of dobutamine, it may have wider application than dipyridamole or atrial pacing.

PRECAUTIONS AND ADVERSE EFFECTS

As with any potent inotropic agent, continuous blood pressure and electrocardiographic monitoring should be performed. Although dobutamine can be safely used without invasive hemodynamic monitoring, balloon flotation pulmonary artery catheterization is recommended for optimal management of patients requiring dobutamine for prolonged periods (longer than 12 to 24 hours). The use of dobutamine without pulmonary artery catheterization may be appropriate for some patients with chronic class IV heart failure and known hemodynamics who require low to middle doses of dobutamine for inotropic support but are otherwise stable. Studies of the use of dobutamine in human pregnancy are lacking, and it is not known whether dobutamine crosses the placenta.[121]

Dobutamine should be used with caution in patients with severe dysrhythmias because it can induce or exacerbate these conditions, especially at higher doses. Adverse reactions include tachycardia, worsening of hypertension, and increases in ventricular ectopy, which are usually dose related. Presumably because of its direct β_2-receptor stimulation, dobutamine may cause reversible hypokalemia. In a study of 13 patients with severe dilated congestive heart failure, it was demonstrated that infusion of 10 ± 1 µg/kg/min of dobutamine, the plasma potassium decreased from 4.6 to 4.2 mEq/L. Although three patients developed worsening of dysrhythmias (one developed ventricular tachycardia that required cardioversion), no cause-and-effect relationship was documented.[122] Good et al. also demonstrated that dobutamine as well as dopamine infusion at higher levels led to significant decreases in serum potassium. High-dose dobutamine infusion also led to significant decreases in serum magnesium.[72] Because the usual patient with congestive heart failure already has a propensity for dysrhythmias, these patients should be carefully monitored for rhythm abnormalities while receiving dobutamine, especially if they are concomitantly receiving diuretics or digitalis. Goldenberg's study indicated that the effect on plasma potassium may persist after 45 minutes of discontinuation of the dobutamine infusion.[122]

Other miscellaneous adverse effects reported in 1% to 3% of patients include nausea, headache, anginal pain, palpitations, and shortness of breath (package insert). Eli Lilly and Company reports that no abnormal laboratory values have been attributed to dobutamine (package insert). Various other adverse effects include skin rash, eosinophilia, and bronchospasm.

CONTRAINDICATIONS

Dobutamine is contraindicated in patients with idiopathic hypertrophic subaortic stenosis and other obstructive hypertrophic cardiomyopathies. Although not absolutely contraindicated, dobutamine has little benefit in patients with severe aortic stenosis because it may induce or exacerbate ischemia without increasing cardiac output. Dobutamine is contraindicated in patients who have shown a prior hypersensitivity to the drug. Because the preparation contains sodium bisulfite, a history of sulfite allergy should be sought.[121] Allergic reactions to sulfite include anaphylaxis and bronchospasm.

DOSAGE AND ADMINISTRATION

The formulation of Dobutrex (Lilly) is supplied in a sterile lyophilized form for intravenous use only.

Dobutamine can be administered safely by peripheral vein; however, one case of dermal necrosis has been reported.[123] Each vial contains 250 mg of dobutamine plus a small amount of sodium bisulfite. Hydrochloric acid, sodium hydroxide, or both may be added to adjust the pH. Dobutamine is stable for 24 hours following preparation depending on the diluent used. Commonly used diluents include 5% dextrose, 0.45% and 0.9% normal saline, and lactated Ringer's solutions.[124] Dobutamine is incompatible with alkaline solutions, including 5% sodium bicarbonate. Dobutamine forms a precipitate and is thus incompatible directly mixed with furosemide, aminophylline, phenytoin, insulin, diazepam, bumetamide, and calcium gluconate. Depending on whether the additive drug is given via y-site injection or directly mixed, depending on the manufacturer of the additive drug, and the type of diluent used, a variety of drugs may be compatible with dobutamine, although the duration of activity and compatibility may vary. Drugs that have been found to be compatible with dobutamine under various circumstances include amiodarone, amrinone, atropine, bretyllium, calcium chloride, dopamine, epinephrine, heparin, isoproterenol, lidocaine, meperidine, magnesium, morphine, nitroglycerin, phenylephrine, potassium chloride, procainamide, propranolol, and verapamil.[124]

Because dobutamine is metabolized by virtually all tissues, no dosage adjustment is needed for renal, hepatic, or other organ impairment. The usual optimal dosage of dobutamine is from 2.5 to 15 µg/kg/min. It should be given only by continuous infusion. Dosages up to 40 µg/kg/min have been used in certain situations, but dose-related tachycardia usually limits dosages higher than 15 to 20 µg/kg/min. The optimal dose must be determined for each patient based on the response of the cardiac output, heart rate, blood pressure, and other hemodynamic variables.

SUMMARY

Dobutamine is an extremely effective inotropic agent directly increasing cardiac output, decreasing left ventricular filling pressures, and indirectly decreasing peripheral vascular resistance without significantly increasing heart rate or arrhythmogenicity. Dobutamine is useful in treating patients with chronic congestive heart failure as well as acute ventricular dysfunction from myocardial infarction, ischemia, and pulmonary embolism, as well as in adults and children after cardiac surgery. It also offers diagnostic alternatives in assessing coronary artery and valvular heart disease. It is assuming a greater role in the outpatient treatment of patients with chronic congestive heart failure and is a viable substitute for exercise in some diagnostic cardiac procedures. All of these factors, coupled with its relative ease of administration and paucity of serious side effects, make it an excellent and resilient member of the inotropic family.

Acknowledgment

We acknowledge the secretarial help of Mandy Hess.

REFERENCES

1. Tuttle RR, Mills J: Dobutamine: Development of a new catecholamine to selectively increase cardiac contractility. Circ Res 36:185, 1975.
2. Kawashima S, Combes J, Liang C-S, et al: Contrasting effects of dopamine and dobutamine on myocardial release of norepinephrine during acute myocardial infarction. Jpn Heart J 26:975, 1985.
3. Chiba S, Watanabe H, Kobayashi M, et al: Cardiovascular effects of dobutamine, dopamine and isoproterenol on the whole animal and isolated cross-perfused atrium in dogs. Jpn J Pharmacol 33:113, 1983.
4. Ceremuzynski L: Hormonal and metabolic reactions evoked by acute myocardial infarction. Circ Res 48:767, 1981.
5. Opie LH: Myocardial infarct size. Part I. Basic considerations. Am Heart J 100:355, 1980.
6. Waldenstrom AP, Hjalmarson AC, Thornell L: A possible role of noradrenaline in the development of myocardial infarction. An experimental study in the isolated rat heart. Am Heart J 95:43, 1978.
7. Leier CV, Heban P, Huss P, et al: Comparative systemic and regional hemodynamic effects of dopamine and dobutamine in patients with cardiomyopathic heart failure. Circulation 58:466, 1978.
8. Sonnenblick EH, Frishman WH, LeJemtel TH: Dobutamine: A new synthetic cardioactive sympathetic amine. N Engl J Med 300:17, 1979.
9. Vatner SF, McRitchie RJ, Braunwald E: Effects of dobutamine on left ventricular performance, coronary dynamics and distribution of cardiac output in conscious dogs. J Clin Invest 53:1265, 1974.
10. Liang CS, Hood WB: Dobutamine infusion in conscious dogs with and without autonomic nervous system inhibition: Effects on systemic hemodynamics, regional blood flow and cardiac metabolism. J Pharmacol Exp Ther 2:698, 1979.
11. Robie NW, Nutter DO, Moody C, et al: In vivo analysis of adrenergic receptor activity of dobutamine. Circ Res 34:663, 1974.
12. Lumley P, Broadley KJ, Levy GP: Analysis of the inotropic:chronotropic selectivity of dobutamine and dopamine in anesthetized dogs and guinea-pig isolated atria. Cardiovasc Res 11:17, 1977.
13. Gorczynski RJ, Wroble RW: Cardiovascular pharmacology of ASL-702. II. Mechanisms of inotropic selectivity. J Pharmacol Exp Ther 223:12, 1982.
14. Ruffolo RR, Messick K: Systemic hemodynamic effects of dopamine, ($\pm$) dobutamine and the ($+$) and ($-$)-enantiomers of dobutamine in anesthetized normotensive rats. Eur J Pharmacol 109:173, 1985.
15. Kenakin TP: An in-vitro quantitative analysis of the alpha-adrenoceptor partial agonist activity of dobutamine and its relevance to inotropic selectivity. J Pharmacol Exp Ther 216:210, 1981.
16. Ruffolo RR, Yaden EL: Vascular effects of the stereoisomers of dobutamine. J Pharmacol Exp Ther 224:46, 1983.
17. Ruffolo RR, Spradlin TA, Pollock GD, et al: Alpha- and beta-adrenergic effects of the stereoisomers of dobutamine. J Pharmacol Exp Ther 219:447, 1981.
18. Kenakin TP, Johnson SF: The importance of the alpha-adrenoceptor agonist activity of dobutamine to inotropic selectivity in the anaesthetized cat. Eur J Pharmacol 111:347, 1985.
19. Schumann HJ: Are there alpha-receptors in mammalian heart? Trends Pharmacol Sci 1:195, 1979.
20. Schumann HJ, Endoh M: Alpha-adrenoceptors in the ventricular myocardium: Clonidine, naphazoline, and methoxamine as partial alpha-agonists exerting a competetive dualism in action to phenylephrine. Eur J Pharmacol 36:413, 1976.
21. Schumann HJ, Wagner J, Knorr A, et al: Demonstration in human atrial preparations of alpha-adrenoceptors mediating positive inotropic effects. Naunyn Schmiedebergs Arch Pharmacol 302:333, 1978.
22. Binkley PF, Murray KD, Watson KM, et al: Dobutamine increases cardiac output of the total artificial heart. Circulation 84:1210, 1991.
23. Kates RE, Leier CV: Dobutamine pharmacokinetics in severe heart failure. Clin Pharmacol Ther 24:537, 1978.
24. Murphy PJ, Williams TL, Kau DL: Disposition of dobutamine in the dog. J Pharmacol Exp Ther 199:423, 1976.
25. Leier CV, Unverferth DV, Kates RE: The relationship between plasma dobutamine concentrations and cardiovascular responses in cardiac failure. Am J Med 66:238, 1979.
26. Unverferth DV, Blanford M, Kates RE, et al: Tolerance to dobutamine after a 72-hour continuous infusion. Am J Med 69:262, 1980.
27. Rich MW, Imburgia A: Inotropic response to dobutamine in elderly patients with decompensated congestive heart failure. Am J Cardiol 65:519, 1990.
28. El Allaf D, Cremers S, D'Orio V, et al: Combined haemodynamic effects of low doses of dopamine and dobutamine in patients with acute infarction and cardiac failure. Arch Int Physiol Biochim 92:S49, 1984.
29. Akhtar N, Mikulic E, Cohn J, et al: Hemodynamic effect of dobutamine in patients with severe heart failure. Am J Cardiol 36:202, 1975.
30. Amin DK, Shah PK, Shellock FG, et al: Comparative hemodynamic effects of intravenous dobutamine and MDL-17043, a new cardioactive drug, in severe congestive heart failure. Am Heart J 109:91, 1985.
31. Awan NA, Evenson MK, Needham KE, et al: Effects of combined nitroglycerin and dobutamine infusion in left ventricular dysfunction. Am Heart J 106:35, 1983.
32. Benotti JR, McCue JE, Alpert JS: Comparative vasoactive therapy for heart failure. Am J Cardiol 56:19B, 1985.
33. Beregovich J, Bianchi C, D'Angelo R, et al: Haemodynamic effects of a new inotropic agent (dobutamine) in chronic cardiac failure. Br Heart J 37:629, 1975.
34. Chatterjee K, Bendersky R, Parmley WW: Dobutamine in heart failure. Eur Heart J 3(Suppl D):107, 1982.
35. Dell'Italia LJ, Starling MR, Blumhardt R, et al: Comparative effects of volume loading, dobutamine and nitroprusside in patients with predominant right ventricular infarction. Circulation 72:1327, 1985.
36. DiSesa VJ, Brown E, Mudge GH, et al: Hemodynamic comparison of dopamine and dobutamine in the post-operative volume-loaded, pressure-loaded, and normal ventricle. J Thorac Cardiovasc Surg 83:256, 1982.
37. Gillespie TA, Ambos HD, Sobel BE, et al: Effects of dobutamine in patients with acute myocardial infarction. Am J Cardiol 39:588, 1977.
38. Goldstein RA, Passamani ER, Roberts R: A comparison of digoxin and dobutamine in patients with acute infarction and cardiac failure. N Engl J Med 303:846, 1980.
39. Graham R, Skoog C, Macedo W, et al: Dopamine, dobutamine and phentolamine effects on pulmonary vascular mechanics. J Appl Physiol 54:1277, 1983.
40. Gross R, Strain J, Greenberg M, et al: Systemic and coronary effects of intravenous milrinone and dobutamine in congestive heart failure. J Am Coll Cardiol 7:1107, 1986.
41. Kupper W, Waller D, Hanrath P, et al: Hemodynamic and cardiac metabolic effects of inotropic stimulation with dobutamine in patients with coronary artery disease. Eur Heart J 3:29, 1982.
42. Liang C-S, Sherman LG, Doherty JU, et al: Sustained improvement of cardiac function in patients with congestive heart failure after short-term infusion of dobutamine. Circulation 69:113, 1984.
43. Likoff MJ, Ulrich S, Hakki AH, et al: Comparison of acute hemodynamic response to dobutamine and intravenous MDL-17043 (enoximone) in severe congestive heart failure secondary to ischemic cardiomyopathy or idiopathic dilated cardiomyopathy. Am J Cardiol 57:1328, 1986.
44. Maekawa K, Liang C-S, Hood WB: Comparison of dobutamine and dopamine in acute myocardial infarction: Effects of systemic hemodynamics, plasma catecholamines, blood flows and infarct size. Circulation 67:750, 1983.

45. MacCannell KL, Giraud GD, Hamilton PL, et al: Haemodynamic responses to dopamine and dobutamine infusions as a function of duration of infusion. Pharmacology 26:29, 1983.

46. Makabali C, Weil MH, Henning RJ: Dobutamine and other sympathomimetic drugs for the treatment of low cardiac output failure. Semin Anesthesiol 1:63, 1982.

47. Maskin CS, Forman EH, Sonnenblick EH, et al: Failure of dobutamine to increase exercise capacity despite hemodynamic improvement in severe chronic heart failure. Am J Cardiol 51:177, 1983.

48. Monrad ES, Baim DS, Smith HS, et al: Milrinone, dobutamine, and nitroprusside: Comparative effects on hemodynamics and myocardial energetics in patients with severe congestive heart failure. Circulation 73(Suppl III):III-168, 1986.

49. Pacold I, Kleinman B, Gunnar R, et al: Effects of low-dose dobutamine on coronary hemodynamics, myocardial metabolism and anginal threshold in patients with coronary artery disease. Circulation 68:1044, 1983.

50. Pozen RG, DiBianco R, Katz RJ, et al: Myocardial metabolic and hemodynamic effects of dobutamine in heart failure complicating coronary artery disease. Circulation 63:1279, 1981.

51. Pouleur H, Marechel G, Balasim H, et al: Effects of dobutamine and sulmazol (AR-L115BS) on myocardial metabolism and coronary, femoral, and renal blood flow: A comparative study in normal dogs and in dogs with chronic volume overload. J Cardiovasc Pharmacol 5:861, 1983.

52. Richard C, Ricome JL, Rimailho A, et al: Combined hemodynamic effects of dopamine and dobutamine in cardiogenic shock. Circulation 67:620, 1983.

53. Tyden H, Nystrom SO: Dopamine versus dobutamine after open-heart surgery. Acta Anaesthesiol Scand 27:193, 1983.

54. Uretsky BF, Generalovich T, Verbalis JG, et al: Comparative hemodynamic and hormonal response of enoximone and dobutamine in severe congestive heart failure. Am J Cardiol 58:110, 1986.

55. Vatner SF, Baig H: Importance of heart rate in determining the effects of sympathomimetic amines on regional myocardial function and blood flow in conscious dogs with acute myocardial ischemia. Circ Res 45:793, 1979.

56. Robie NW, Goldberg LI: Comparative systemic and regional hemodynamic effects of dopamine and dobutamine. Am Heart J 90:340, 1975.

57. Vainionpaa V, Nuutinen L, Kairaluoma M, et al: Haemodynamic comparison of dopamine and dobutamine in normovolaemic and hypovolaemic dogs. Acta Anaesthesiol Scand 27:490, 1983.

58. Mikulic E, Cohn JN, Franciosa JA: Comparative hemodynamic effects of inotropic and vasodilator drugs in severe heart failure. Circulation 56:528, 1977.

59. Lejeune P, Leeman M, Deloof T, et al: Pulmonary hemodynamic response to dopamine and dobutamine in hyperoxic and in hypoxic dogs. Anesthesiology 66:49, 1987.

60. Furman WR, Summer WR, Kennedy TP, et al: Comparison of the effects of dobutamine, dopamine and isoproterenol on hypoxic pulmonary vasoconstriction in the pig. Crit Care Med 10:371, 1982.

61. McFarlane PA, Mortimer AJ, Ryder WA, et al: Effects of dopamine and dobutamine on the distribution of pulmonary blood flow during lobar ventilation hypoxia and lobar collapse in dogs. Eur J Clin Invest 15:53, 1985.

62. Driscoll DJ, Gillette PC, Duff DF, et al: Hemodynamic effects of dobutamine in children. Am J Cardiol 43:581, 1979.

63. Schranz D, Stopfkuchen H, Jungst BK, et al: Hemodynamic effects of dobutamine in children with cardiovascular failure. Eur J Pediatr 139:4, 1982.

64. Jose AB, Niguidula F, Botros S, et al: Hemodynamic effects of dobutamine in children [abstract]. Anesthesiology 55:3A, 1981.

65. Bohn DJ, Poirier CS, Edmonds JF, et al: Hemodynamic effects of dobutamine after cardiopulmonary bypass in children. Crit Care Med 8:367, 1980.

66. Berner M, Rouge JC, Friedli B: The hemodynamic effect of phentolamine and dobutamine after open-heart operations in children: Influence of the underlying heart defect. Ann Thorac Surg 35:643, 1983.

67. Kyriakides ZS, Kelesides K, Melanidis J, et al: Systolic function response of normal older and younger adult left ventricles to dobutamine. Am J Cardiol 58:816, 1986.

68. Lehr D, Mallow J, Krukowski M: Copious drinking and simultaneous inhibition of urine flow elicited by beta adrenergic stimulation and contrary effect of alpha adrenergic stimulation. J Pharmacol Exp Ther 158:150, 1967.

69. Masoni A, Alboni P, Malacarne C, et al: Effects of dobutamine on electrophysiological properties of the specialized conduction system in man. J Electrocardiol 12:361, 1979.

70. Gertz EW, Wisniski JA, Niese R, et al: Myocardial lactate extraction: Multidetermined metabolic function. Circulation 61:256, 1980.

71. Dubois-Randé JL, Merlet P, Duval-Moulin AM, et al: Coronary vasodilating action of dobutamine in patients with idiopathic dilated cardiomyopathy. Am Heart J 125:1329, 1993.

72. Good J, Frost G, Oakley CM, et al: The renal effects of dopamine and dobutamine in stable chronic heart failure. Postgrad Med J 68(Suppl 2):S7, 1992.

73. Westman L, Järnberg P-O: Effect of dobutamine on renal function in normal man. Acta Anaesthesiol Scand 30:72, 1986.

74. Schrier RW, Liebermann R, Ufferman R: Mechanisms of antidiuretic effects of beta-adrenergic stimulation. J Clin Invest 51:97, 1972.

75. Uretsky BF, Lawless CE, Verbalis JG, et al: Combined therapy with dobutamine and amrinone in severe heart failure: Improved hemodynamics and increased activation of the renin-angiotensin system with combined intravenous therapy. Chest 92:657, 1987.

76. Keeton TK, Campbell WB: The pharmacologic alteration of renin-release. Pharmacol Rev 32:82, 1980.

77. Merlet P, Delforge J, Syrota A, et al: Positron emission tomography with ¹¹C CGP-177 to assess β-adrenergic receptor concentration in idiopathic dilated cardiomyopathy. Circulation 87:1169, 1993.

78. Townend JN, Virk SJS, Qiang FX, et al: Lymphocyte beta adrenoceptor upregulation and improved cardiac response to adrenergic stimulation following converting enzyme inhibition in congestive heart failure. Eur Heart J 14:243, 1993.

79. Gilbert EM, Sandoval A, Larrabee P, et al: Effect of lisinopril on cardiac adrenergic drive and myocardial 13-receptor density in heart failure. Circulation 78(Suppl 11):576, 1988.

80. Loeb HS, Khan M, Saudaye A, et al: Acute hemodynamic effects of dobutamine and isoproterenol in patients with low output cardiac failure. Circ Shock 3:55, 1976.

81. Colucci WS, Wright RF, Jaski BE, et al: Milrinone and dobutamine in severe heart failure: Differing hemodynamic effects and individual patient responsiveness. Circulation 73(Suppl III):III-175, 1986.

82. Borow KM, Neumann A, Lang RM: Milrinone versus dobutamine: Contribution of altered myocardial mechanics and augmented inotropic state to improve left ventricular performance. Circulation 73(Suppl III):III-153, 1986.

83. Klein NA, Siskind SJ, Frishman WH: Hemodynamic comparison of intravenous amrinone and dobutamine in patients with chronic congestive heart failure. Am J Cardiol 48:170, 1981.

84. Marcus RH, Raw K, Patel J, et al: Comparison of intravenous amrinone and dobutamine in congestive heart failure due to idiopathic dilated cardiomyopathy. Am J Cardiol 66:1107, 1990.

85. Gage J, Rutman H, Lucido D, et al: Additive effects of dobutamine and amrinone on myocardial contractility and ventricular performance in patients with severe heart failure. Circulation 74:367, 1986.

86. Sundram P, Reddy HK, McElroy PA, et al: Myocardial energetics and efficiency in patients with idiopathic cardiomyopathy: Response to dobutamine and amrinone. Am Heart J 119:891, 1990.

87. Dubois-Randé JL, Loisance D, Benvenuti C, et al: Medical strategy in patients awaiting emergency heart transplantation. Arch Mal Coeur Vaiss 83:103, 1990.

88. Berkowitz C, McKeever L, Croke RP, et al: Comparative responses to dobutamine and nitroprusside in patients with chronic low output cardiac failure. Circulation 56:918, 1977.

89. Franciosa JA, Notargiacomo AV, Cohn JN: Comparative haemodynamic and metabolic effects of vasodilator and ino-

tropic agents in experimental myocardial infarction. Cardiovasc Res 12:254, 1978.

90. Unverferth DV, Leier CV, Magorien RD, et al: Improvement of human myocardial mitochrondria after dobutamine: A quantitative ultrastructural study. J Pharmacol Exp Ther 215:527, 1980.

91. Roffman DS, Applefeld MM, Grove WR, et al: Intermittent dobutamine hydrochloride infusions in outpatients with chronic congestive heart failure. Clin Pharm 4:195, 1985.

92. Applefeld MM, Newman KA, Grove WR, et al: Intermittent continuous outpatient dobutamine infusion in the management of congestive heart failure. Am J Cardiol 51:455, 1983.

93. Krell MJ, Kline EM, Bates ER, et al: Intermittent, ambulatory dobutamine infusions in patients with severe congestive heart failure. Am Heart J 112:787, 1986.

94. Dies F, Krell MJ, Whitlow P, et al: Intermittent dobutamine in ambulatory outpatients with chronic cardiac failure [abstract]. Circulation 74(Suppl II):II-11, 1986.

95. Miller LW, Merkle EJ, Herrmann V: Outpatient dobutamine for end-stage congestive heart failure. Crit Care Med 18:S30, 1990.

96. Gray R, Shah P, Singh B, et al: Low cardiac output states after open heart surgery: comparative hemodynamic effects of dobutamine, dopamine and norepinephrine plus phentolamine. Chest 80:16, 1981.

97. DiSesa VJ, Gold JA, Shemin RJ, et al: Comparison of dopamine and dobutamine in patients requiring postoperative circulatory support. Clin Cardiol 9:253, 1986.

98. Salomon NW, Plachetka JR, Copeland JG: Comparison of dopamine and dobutamine following coronary artery bypass grafting. Ann Thorac Surg 33:48, 1982.

99. Jaccard C, Berner M, Rouge JC, et al: Hemodynamic effect of isoprenaline and dobutamine immediately after correction of tetralogy of Fallot. J Thorac Cardiovasc Surg 87:862, 1984.

100. DeBroux ED, Lagace G, Dumont L, et al: Efficacy of dobutamine in the failing transplanted heart. J Heart Lung Transplant 11:1133, 1992.

101. Molloy DW, Ducas J, Dobson K, et al: Hemodynamic management in clinical acute hypoxemic respiratory failure: Dopamine vs. dobutamine. Chest 89:636, 1986.

102. Jardin F, Genevray B, Brun-Ney D, et al: Dobutamine: A hemodynamic evaluation in pulmonary embolism shock. Crit Care Med 13:1009, 1985.

103. Kosugi I, Tajimi K: Effects of dopamine and dobutamine on hemodynamics and plasma catecholamine levels during severe lactic acid acidosis. Circ Shock 17:95, 1985.

104. Regnier B, Safran D, Carlet J, et al: Comparative hemodynamic effects of dopamine and dobutamine in septic shock. Intensive Care Med 5:115, 1979.

105. Jardin F, Sportiche M, Bazine M, et al: Dobutamine: A hemodynamic evaluation in septic shock. Crit Care Med 9:329, 1981.

106. Fisher CJ, Horowitz BZ, Albertson TE: Cardiorespiratory failure in toxic shock syndrome: Effect of dobutamine. Crit Care Med 13:160, 1985.

107. Sullivan MJ, Binkley PF, Unverferth DV, et al: Prevention of bedrest-induced physical deconditioning by daily dobutamine infusions. J Clin Invest 76:1632, 1985.

108. Mannering D, Cripps T, Leech G, et al: The dobutamine stress test as an alternative exercise testing after acute myocardial infarction. Br Heart J 59:521, 1988.

109. Freeman ML, Palac R, Mason J, et al: A comparison of dobutamine infusion and supine bicycle exercise for radionuclide cardiac stress testing. Clin Nucl Med 9:251, 1984.

110. Mason JR, Palac RT, Freeman ML, et al: Thallium scintigraphy during dobutamine infusion: Non-exercise-dependent screening test for coronary disease. Am Heart J 107:481, 1984.

111. Francisco DA, Collins SM, Go RT, et al: Tomographic thallium-201 myocardial perfusion scintigrams after maximal coronary artery vasodilation with intravenous dipyridamole. Circulation 66:370, 1982.

112. Bodenheimer MM, Vidya SB, Fooshee CM, et al: Comparative sensitivity of the exercise electrocardiogram, thallium imaging and stress radionuclide angiography to detect the presence and severity of coronary heart disease. Circulation 60:1270, 1979.

113. Pennell DJ, Underwood SR, Swanton RH, et al: Dobutamine thallium myocardial perfusion tomography. J Am Coll Cardiol 18:1471, 1991.

114. Segar DS, Sawada SG, Brown SE, et al: Dobutamine stress echocardiography: Correlation of dose responsiveness and quantitative angiography. J Am Coll Cardiol 15:234A, 1990.

115. Hays JT, Mahmarian JJ, Cochran AJ, et al: Dobutamine thallium-201 tomography for evaluating patients with suspected coronary artery disease unable to undergo exercise or vasodilator pharmacologic stress testing. J Am Coll Cardiol 21:1583, 1993.

116. Berthe C, Pierard LA, Hiernaux M, et al: Predicting the extent and location of coronary artery disease in acute myocardial infarction by echocardiography during dobutamine infusion. Am J Cardiol 58:1167, 1986.

117. Mazeika PK, Nadazdin A, Oakley CM: Prognostic value of dobutamine echocardiography in patients with high pretest likelihood of coronary artery disease. Am J Cardiol 71:33, 1993.

118. Marwick T, Willemart B, D'Hondt A, et al: Selection of the optimal nonexercise stress for the evaluation of ischemic regional myocardial dysfunction and malperfusion. Comparison of dobutamine and adenosine using echocardiography and 99mTc-MIBI single photon emission computed tomography. Circulation 87:345, 1993.

119. Tan LB, Bain RJ, Littler WA: Assessing cardiac pumping capability by exercise testing and inotropic stimulation. Br Heart J 62:20, 1989.

120. Hwang MH, Pacold I, Piao ZE, et al: The usefulness of dobutamine in the assessment of the severity of mitral stenosis. Am Heart J 111:312, 1986.

121. Dobutamine. In McEvay GK (ed): AHFS Drug Information. Bethesda, MD: American Society of Hospital Pharmacists, 1993, pp 717–718.

122. Goldenberg IF, Olivari MT, Levine TB, et al: Effect of dobutamine on plasma potassium in congestive heart failure secondary to idiopathic or ischemic cardiomyopathy. Am J Cardiol 63:843, 1989.

123. Hoff JV, Beatty PA, Wade JL: Dermal necrosis from dobutamine [letter]. N Engl J Med 300:1280, 1979.

124. Dobutamine HCl. In Trissel LA (ed): Handbook on Injectable Drugs, 7th ed. Bethesda, MD: American Society of Hospital Pharmacists, 1992, pp 309–316.

CHAPTER 128

Dopamine

Michael B. Murphy, M.D., and Carl J. Vaughan, M.B.

HISTORICAL PERSPECTIVE

Dopamine (DA) is an endogenous catecholamine that was first synthesized in 1910 simultaneously by Barger and Ewins at the Wellcome Laboratories and in Germany by Mannich and Jacobsohn. Early workers recognized its similarities with other sympathomimetic amines, but it was Holtz who first suggested that it might have hypotensive effects in the guinea pig model. DA was introduced for the treatment of heart failure and shock in the 1960s and became widely available for clinical use in the 1970s.

CHEMISTRY

DA is formed *in vivo* from L-dopa by the action of dopa-decarboxylase. DA is metabolized in the kidneys, liver, and plasma by monoamine oxidase (MAO) and catechol-O-methyltransferase to 3-methoxy-4-hydroxyphenylacetic acid and 3,4-dihydroxyphenylacetic acid, which are both excreted in urine. Less than 10% of an administered dose is recovered unchanged in urine.

PHARMACOLOGY

Extensive pharmacologic studies have demonstrated that DA differs from all other available sympathomimetic amines.[1] DA acts on two DA receptor subtypes, DA1 and DA2.[2, 3] DA1 receptors are located postsynaptically and subserve vasodilation in renal, mesenteric, coronary, and cerebral arterial blood vessels (Fig. 128–1). DA1-induced vasodilation is observed in other vascular beds, but the responses are usually less prominent and may differ among species. For example, it appears that more DA1 receptors are in the human skeletal muscle vascular bed than in that of the dog.[2, 4]

DA2 receptors are located on postganglionic sympathetic nerves and autonomic ganglia (see Fig. 128–1). These receptors inhibit release of norepinephrine from sympathetic nerve storage sites. DA2 receptors are also located in the anterior lobe of the pituitary gland to inhibit prolactin release and in the emetic center of the medulla, where they induce nausea and vomiting. Complete separation of these two receptor subtypes is evidenced not only by diverse function but also by distinctly different chemical structure activity relationships and selective antagonists.[5] Among the most selective and specific DA1 antagonist is SCH 23390, and the most selective DA2 antagonist is LY 17155.

DA also acts on β- and α-adrenoceptors. DA increases cardiac contractile force, heart rate, and atrioventricular conduction by action on β_1-adrenoreceptors. DA acts on β_1-adrenoreceptors to directly stimulate β_1-adrenoreceptors and indirectly by releasing norepinephrine from myocardial sympathetic nerves. Although patients with severe congestive heart failure often experience marked reductions in myocardial norepinephrine stores, DA still can stimulate the myocardium by direct β_1-action.[6] DA has little or no action on β_2-adrenoreceptors.[2, 3]

DA also acts on α_1- and α_2-adrenoreceptors.[3] Both α-adrenoreceptor subtypes cause vasoconstriction in arterial and venous vascular beds. In general, cerebral and coronary blood vessels are constricted less than

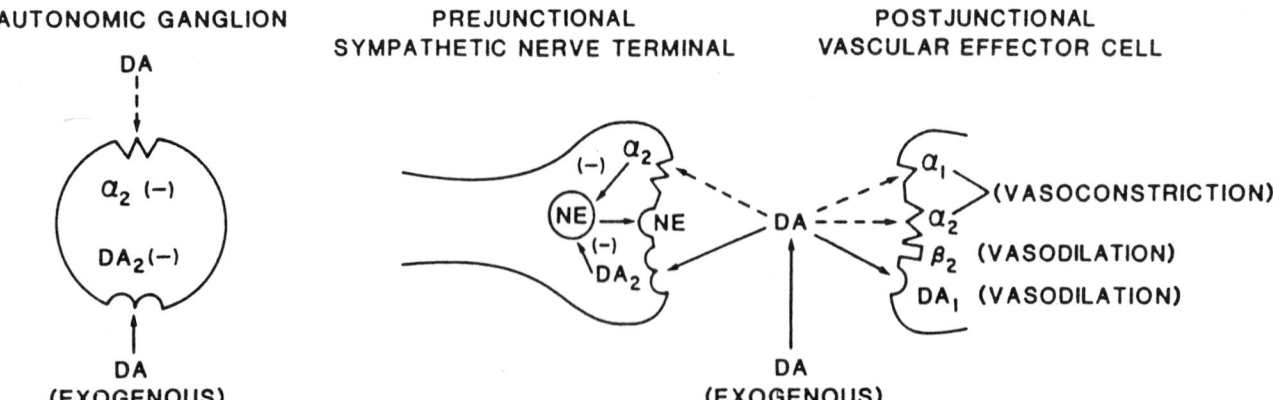

Figure 128–1. Location of α_2- and DA2-receptors on the autonomic ganglion and prejunctional sympathetic nerve terminal to inhibit release of norepinephrine. α_1-Receptors and α_2-receptors are located on the postjunctional vascular effector cell to cause vasoconstriction. DA1-receptors and β_2-adrenoreceptors also are located on the postjunctional vascular effector cell and induce vasodilation. When DA is injected exogenously, it acts on DA1 and DA2 receptors at lower doses and on α_1- and α_2-adrenoreceptors at higher doses. DA has little or no action on β_2-adrenoreceptors. DA also acts on β_1-adrenoreceptors on myocardial cells to increase cardiac contractility. NE, norepinephrine.

those of the skeletal muscle, mesentery, and kidneys. α_2-Adrenoreceptors serve similar functions as DA2 receptors in that, when activated, they inhibit release of norepinephrine from sympathetic storage sites (see Fig. 128–1).

In addition to these cardiovascular and neuronal effects, DA increases electrolyte excretion, especially sodium.[7] Although natriuresis could be entirely due to increments in renal blood flow,[8] there is growing evidence that DA also has a tubular effect that causes natriuresis.[9, 10]

CLINICAL APPLICATIONS

DA produces markedly different hemodynamic and renal effects in three general infusion ranges that can only be approximately called low, medium, and high infusion rates.[11] Because of extreme variations in doses required to activate these receptors in normal subjects and patients, it is impossible to predict the infusion rate required for an individual patient. Accordingly, with the exception of hypotensive emergencies in which perfusion pressure must be rapidly increased, the initial infusion rate should be begun at a low range (about 0.5 to 1 µg/kg/min), and the dose should be carefully titrated to produce the desired effects. For hypotensive emergencies, the rate can be doubled every 5 to 10 minutes until perfusion pressure is adequate.

Low Dose Range

DA2 receptors are activated at the lowest dose of DA.[1] At a slightly higher dose, DA1 receptors are recruited and hemodynamic effects may be observed.[7, 12, 13] Blood pressure may decrease slightly, but there is usually no change in heart rate, or heart rate may decrease. These effects are due to the DA1-mediated vasodilation and inhibition of the sympathetic nervous system. Diuresis and natriuresis usually occur in this dosage range, and renal blood flow increases.

Low-dose DA is frequently used to improve reduced renal perfusion and institute diuresis in furosemide-resistant patients.[14–18] In addition, low-dose DA is often used during procedures that compromise renal blood flow, including renal and hepatic transplantation.[19] The surgical literature suggests that prophylactic DA use preserves renal function in some patients, but this effect varies considerably and is still controversial.[20]

Medium Dose Range

This dose range of DA is used for the treatment of heart failure.[2, 7, 12] The infusion rate must be maintained at a level that does not cause vasoconstriction and thus impose increased afterload. Cardiac output usually increases, and there is a further increment in renal blood flow. Systemic vascular resistance decreases. Heart rate may be unchanged, increased, or decreased, depending on the predominance of DA2

and β_1-adrenoreceptor effects in individual patients. Pulmonary wedge pressure usually does not decrease.

Because intravenous infusions of DA do not dilate the capacitance bed and may increase venous tone,[21] DA frequently is administered with vasodilators such as nitroprusside or nitroglycerin, which dilate the venous beds.[22–24] DA also frequently is used in combination with dobutamine.[25, 26] Dobutamine does not act on DA1 receptors, but has a mixture of β- and α-adrenoreceptor actions, which permit greater increments in cardiac output than DA does. The infusion rates of the two sympathomimetic amines must be titrated carefully for the desired hemodynamic and renal actions.

The most serious adverse effects of medium-dose DA are cardiac arrhythmias and excessive tachycardia due to β_1-adrenoreceptor stimulation. In the event of serious arrhythmias, the dose must be reduced or the infusion discontinued.

Highest Dose Range

At the highest dose range, α_1- and α_2-adrenoreceptors are recruited, and blood pressure and systemic vascular resistance increase. The dose range to elevate blood pressure with DA varies extremely. Increments in blood pressure occur in normal subjects at infusion rates ranging from 2 to 10 µg/kg/min,[27] whereas some patients in shock may require more than 50 µg/kg/min.[28] Plasma volume deficits must be corrected before starting DA therapy for the treatment of hypotension and shock. Otherwise, because of poor venous return, cardiac output and renal blood flow would not increase, and excessive vasoconstriction and peripheral necrosis and gangrene could occur. In the event of extravasation of DA, phentolamine should be infiltrated throughout the ischemic area. In some patients, adequate perfusion pressure cannot be maintained with DA, and norepinephrine must be added to or substituted for DA.[29, 30]

PRECAUTIONS

Peripheral circulation must be monitored carefully to avoid gangrene and necrosis. These adverse effects usually occur only in patients in whom very large doses of DA must be administered to maintain perfusion pressure. Care must be used when DA is administered to patients with a history of occlusive vascular disease. Patients should be monitored closely for any change in color or temperature of the skin and extremities that may indicate compromised circulation. Neonates, children,[31] and the elderly should be carefully monitored for signs of peripheral ischemia. DA is contraindicated in patients with pheochromocytoma.

DRUG INTERACTIONS

The most common interactions result from concomitant administration of DA and other cardiovascular drugs. Excessive hypotension can occur when vasodilators, calcium antagonists, and α-adrenoreceptor blocking agents are administered. When β-adrenoreceptor blocking agents are administered, the cardiac effects of DA will be blocked, and peripheral resistance will increase excessively. Concomitant use of DA with cyclopropane or halogenated hydrocarbon anesthetics may cause ventricular arrhythmias.

Prior administration of MAO inhibitors may intensify and prolong the effects of DA, especially on arterial blood pressure.[32] In patients who receive MAO inhibitors 2 or 3 weeks before DA administration, the initial dose should be reduced to at least one tenth of the usual initial dose. DA should not be used in patients receiving ergot alkaloids unless absolutely necessary because of the possibility of peripheral vasoconstriction. Concurrent administration of a large dose of metoclopramide and other DA antagonists such as chlorpromazine and haloperidol could attenuate the renal effects of DA. DA2 receptors are blocked at much lower doses of these antagonists, possibly resulting in enhanced tachycardia and elevations in blood pressure when DA is infused.

TREATMENT OF CONGESTIVE HEART FAILURE

Two DA agonists have been studied in patients with congestive heart failure. With propylbutyl DA (PBDA), DA2 activity is more pronounced than DA1 activity compared with DA, and PBDA has no β_1-adrenoreceptor activity.[33] PBDA is a weak α-adrenoreceptor agonist. Thus, DA1 and DA2 receptors are activated without stimulating the heart or causing vasoconstriction. Fennell et al.[34] administered PBDA to 11 patients with congestive heart failure at rates of 5, 10, and 20 μg/kg/min and reported dose-dependent reductions in mean arterial pressure. Left ventricular filling pressure and pulmonary and systemic vascular resistance also were reduced. Cardiac index increased without changing either stroke work or heart rate. The major adverse effects of PBDA are nausea and vomiting. These effects were not observed with infusion rates of 20 μg/kg/min, the dose expected to be most useful for treating congestive heart failure. However, when the rate of infusion was increased to 40 μg/kg/min, emesis was observed in two of three normal volunteers and one of three patients with congestive heart failure.

Dopexamine, like DA, acts on DA1 and DA2 receptors. It differs from DA in that it is a potent β_2-adrenoreceptor agonist with little or no α- and β_1-adrenoreceptor activity.[35, 36] Dopexamine also has the unusual effect of preventing the uptake of exogenous and endogenous norepinephrine into sympathetic nerve terminals.[37]

Dose-related increments in cardiac index, stroke volume index, and heart rate and reductions in systolic and pulmonary vascular resistance have been reported in patients with congestive heart failure in whom dopexamine was infused at rates of 1 to 6 μg/kg/min.[38–41] Because of the complex actions of dopexamine, it is not known whether the hemodynamic effects of dopexamine are entirely the result of its vasodilating actions or whether a direct positive inotropic effect also occurs. Two possible mechanisms have been postulated. One is that dopexamine exerts an effect on myocardial β_2-adrenoreceptors to increase cardiac contractile force and heart rate. This concept is controversial because β_1- and not β_2-adrenoreceptors traditionally have been believed to mediate cardiac contractility.[40] The second is that inhibition of uptake of norepinephrine by sympathetic nerves may produce a greater increment in cardiac contractility and heart rate in patients with congestive heart failure than in normal subjects.[37] High levels of circulating norepinephrine are commonly found in patients with congestive heart failure. Dopexamine may provide higher concentrations of norepinephrine at the synapse by preventing uptake of the catecholamine. Hypotension and excessive increase in heart rate may limit dopexamine use in some patients. Dopexamine and PBDA are available for intravenous use. Finally, fenoldopam, a selective DA1 agonist, also has been found to increase cardiac output and to decrease systemic resistance in patients with congestive heart failure when administered orally.[42]

PRODRUGS

The bioavailability of orally administered DA is poor; therefore, DA must be administered intravenously. This deficiency limits the use of DA for long-term therapy.

L-Dopa

Levodopa (L-dopa) is the immediate biochemical precursor of DA. L-Dopa is decarboxylated by the enzyme, aromatic amino acid decarboxylase, to yield DA.

The background for L-dopa as therapy for heart failure began in the early 1970s in studies of patients with Parkinson's disease. In the first investigation, the β_1-adrenoreceptor activities of L-dopa were evaluated by noninvasive, systolic time-interval measurements. Single oral doses of L-dopa of 1 and 1.5 g produced about the same shortening of systolic time intervals as 2- and 4-μg/kg/min infusions of DA. These effects were clearly the result of β_1-adrenoreceptor activation, because they were completely blocked by propranolol.[43] The second study involved determination of renal plasma flow, inulin clearance, and sodium excretion in a separate series of patients with Parkinson's disease. Again, L-dopa increased these values to a similar extent as did 2- to 4-μg/kg/min infusions of DA.[44]

L-Dopa was first used in the treatment of congestive heart failure in a patient with severe failure. The patient had an excellent response to DA and nitroprusside but could not be weaned from these drugs. L-Dopa was administered with isosorbide dinitrate, and DA and nitroprusside were discontinued. The patient survived for 2 years with L-dopa as part of his regimen.[2]

This experience led to a more controlled invasive study of L-dopa in 10 patients with New York Heart Association class III and IV congestive heart failure.[45] In doses of 1.5 and 2 g, L-dopa produced significant increments in cardiac index and stroke volume index, as well as reductions in systemic vascular resistance. Mean arterial pressure, heart rate, left ventricular filling pressure, and mean right atrial pressure did not change. Five patients were treated for periods ranging from 3 to 12 months, and invasive studies were repeated. Similar cardiovascular changes occurred during the second study. In a more recent study, sustained hemodynamic improvement was documented in 12 additional patients treated for 12 weeks.[46]

Nausea and vomiting are common adverse effects of L-dopa.[47] These side effects can be reduced by gradual increments in dosage. Accordingly, patients receiving L-dopa for congestive heart failure usually are started at a dose of 250 mg four times a day, and the dose is gradually increased to 1 or 2 g over a 5- to 7-day period. In addition, 50 mg of piridoxine is administered to increase peripheral decarboxylation of L-dopa. It is important to emphasize that the peripheral, not the central, actions of DA are desired. Therefore, Sinemet must never be substituted for L-dopa, because it contains carbidopa, a decarboxylase inhibitor that blocks peripheral decarboxylation.

Ibopamine

Ibopamine is the diisobutyric ester of N-methyl DA (epinine). Epinine is released from ibopamine by plasma esterases after oral ingestion.[48] Epinine is a DA1 agonist that produces greater α-adrenoreceptor actions than DA; in addition, it is a potent β_1-adrenoreceptor agonist.

Ibopamine has been studied extensively for the treatment of congestive heart failure in Europe and is currently available in Italy for clinical use.[48] Many invasive studies have shown that oral ingestion of 50 to 300 mg of ibopamine increases cardiac index and decreases systemic vascular resistance.[48-52] One report suggested that, with continuing therapy, the hemodynamic effects of ibopamine are attenuated,[52] but attenuation has not been reported in other investigations.[37] Several studies also have reported diuretic and natriuretic effects.

Unlike L-dopa, ibopamine does not cause nausea and vomiting, apparently because ibopamine does not penetrate the chemoreceptor trigger zone in the area postrema. Ibopamine may cause heartburn. Large doses of ibopamine have been shown to produce transient elevations of pulmonary wedge pressure in some patients with severe congestive heart failure,[53] but this effect does not appear to be a serious problem with smaller doses.[37]

Dopamine and Hypertension

Because activation of DA1 and DA2 receptors decreases blood pressure, the possibility of using DA agonists as antihypertensive agents has been recognized for many years.[1] DA is not useful as an antihypertensive agent because of its α-adrenoreceptor activity. However, extensive studies in experimental animals and a few investigations in patients with hypertension have demonstrated that, after administration of α-adrenoreceptor blocking agents, arterial pressure is decreased with maintenance or improvement of renal blood flow.[1] Conducted in 1966, the first human study[54] demonstrated that infusion rates of DA of 1 to 1.5 µg/kg/min increased mean blood pressure an average of 10 mmHg in five patients with severe hypertension. After administration of phenoxybenzamine, 1 mg/kg, the same infusion rates of DA decreased blood pressure by an average of 37 mmHg. Creatinine clearance remained unchanged despite a pronounced reduction in blood pressure. More recently, investigations with the selective DA1 agonist fenoldopam and with relatively selective DA2 agonists have confirmed that activation of DA1 and DA2 receptors represents a new approach to the treatment of hypertension. Reviews and publications have discussed in detail the clinical use of DA1 and DA2 agonists in patients with hypertension.[55-58] (Fenoldopam is discussed in a separate chapter in this text.)

In addition to its therapeutic use, DA may be involved physiologically in the genesis or maintenance of hypertension. Supportive data for this hypothesis have been reviewed extensively.[59-61]

REFERENCES

1. Goldberg LI: Cardiovascular and renal actions of dopamine: Potential clinical applications. Pharmacol Rev 241:1, 1972.
2. Goldberg LI, Hsieh YY, Resnekov L: Newer catecholamines for treatment of heart failure and shock: An update on dopamine and a first look at dobutamine. Prog Cardiovasc Dis 4:327, 1977.
3. Goldberg LI, Rajfer SI: Dopamine receptors: Applications in clinical cardiology. Circulation 72:245, 1985.
4. Hughes AD, Thom SA, Woodall NM, et al: Dopamine produces forearm vasodilatation following alpha-adrenoceptor blockade by an action on vascular dopamine (DA1) receptors in man. J Hypertens 5:337, 1987.
5. Kohli JD, Goldberg LI: Functional models for and characteristics of DA1 and DA2 dopamine receptors in the periphery. In Hieble JP (ed): Cardiovascular Function of Peripheral Dopamine Receptors. New York: Marcel Dekker (In press).
6. Carroll JD, Lang RM, Neumann AL, et al: The differential effects of positive inotropic and vasodilator therapy on diastolic properties in patients with congestive cardiomyopathy. Circulation 74:815, 1986.
7. McDonald RH Jr, Goldberg LI, McNay JL, et al: Effects of dopamine in man: Augmentation of sodium excretion, glomerular filtration rate and renal plasma flow. J Clin Invest 43:1116, 1964.
8. Frederickson ED, Bradley TJ, Goldberg LI: Blockade of the renal effects of dopamine in the dog by the DA1 antagonist, SCH 23390. Am J Physiol 249:F236, 1985.
9. Felder RA, Blecher M, Calcagno PL, et al: Dopamine receptors in the proximal tubule of the rabbit. Am J Physiol 247:F499, 1984.
10. Bello-Reuss E, Higashi Y, Kanega Y: Dopamine decreases fluid reabsorption in straight portions of rabbit proximal tubule. Am J Physiol 242:F634, 1982.
11. Levinson PD, Goldstein DS, Munson PJ, et al: Endocrine, renal, and hemodynamic responses to graded dopamine infusions in normal men. J Clin Endocrinol Metab 60:821, 1985.
12. Beregovich J, Bianchi C, Rubler S, et al: Dose-related hemody-

namic and renal effects of dopamine in congestive heart failure. Am Heart J 87:550, 1974.

13. D'Orio V, El Allaf D, Juchmes J, et al: The use of low doses of dopamine in intensive care medicine. Arch Int Physiol Biochim Biophys 92:S11, 1986.

14. Henderson IS, Beattie TJ, Kennedy AC: Dopamine hydrochloride in oliguric states. Lancet 2:827, 1980.

15. Lindner A: Synergism of dopamine and furosemide in diuretic-resistant, oliguric acute renal failure. Nephron 33:121, 1983.

16. Hilberman M, Maseda J, Stinson EB, et al: The diuretic properties of dopamine in patients after open-heart operation. Anesthesiology 61:489, 1984.

17. Parker S, Carlon GC, Isaacs M, et al: Dopamine administration in oliguria and oliguric renal failure. Crit Care Med 9:630, 1981.

18. Mann HJ, Fuhs DW, Hemstrom CA: Acute renal failure. Drug Intell Clin Pharm 20:421, 1986.

19. Polson RJ, Park GR, Lindop MJ, et al: The prevention of renal impairment in patients undergoing orthotopic liver grafting by infusion of low dose dopamine. Anaesthesia 42:15, 1987.

20. Paul MD, Mazer CD, Byrick RJ, et al: Influence of mannitol and dopamine on renal function during elective intrarenal aortic clamping in man. Am J Nephrol 6:427, 1986.

21. Butterworth JF, Austin JC, Johnson MD, et al: Effect of total spinal anesthesia on arterial and venous responses to dopamine and dobutamine. Anesth Analg 66:209, 1987.

22. Miller RR, Awan NA, Joye JA, et al: Combined dopamine and nitroprusside therapy in congestive heart failure. Circulation 55:881, 1977.

23. Keung EC, Ribner HS, Schwartz W, et al: Effects of combined dopamine and nitroprusside therapy in patients with severe pump failure and hypotension complicating acute myocardial infarction. J Cardiovasc Pharmacol 2:113, 1980.

24. Loeb HS, Ostrenga JP, Gaul W, et al: Beneficial effects of dopamine combined with intravenous nitroglycerin on hemodynamics in patients with severe left ventricular failure. Circulation 68:813, 1983.

25. Richard C, Ricome JL, Rimailho JA, et al: Combined hemodynamic effects of dopamine and dobutamine in cardiogenic shock. Circulation 67:620, 1983.

26. Pedersen JE, Mortensen SA: Haemodynamic steady state via combined infusion of dobutamine and dopamine in the pretransplant phase. Acta Cardiol 42:295, 1987.

27. Horwitz D, Fox SM, Goldberg LI: Effects of dopamine in man. Circ Res 10:237, 1962.

28. Sprung CL, Caralis PV, Marcial EH, et al: The effects of high-dose corticosteroids in patients with septic shock. N Engl J Med 311:1137, 1984.

29. Goldberg LI, Talley RC, McNay JL: The potential role of dopamine in the treatment of shock. Prog Cardiovasc Dis 12:40, 1969.

30. Schaer GL, Fink MP, Parrillo JE: Norepinephrine alone versus norepinephrine plus low-dose dopamine: Enhanced renal blood flow with combination pressor therapy. Crit Care Med 13:492, 1985.

31. Zaritsky A, Chernow B: Use of catecholamines in pediatrics. J Pediatrics 105:341, 1984.

32. Horwitz D, Goldberg LI, Sjoerdsma A: Increased blood pressure responses to dopamine and norepinephrine produced by monoamine oxidase inhibitors in man. J Lab Clin Med 56:747, 1960.

33. Kohli JD, Weder AB, Goldberg LI, et al: Structure activity relationships of N-substituted dopamine derivatives as agonists of the dopamine vascular and other cardiovascular receptors. J Pharmacol Exp Ther 213:370, 1980.

34. Fennell WH, Taylor AA, Young JB, et al: Propylbutyldopamine: Hemodynamic effects in conscious dogs, normal human volunteers, and patients with heart failure. Circulation 67:829, 1983.

35. Brown RA, Dixon J, Farmer JB, et al: Dopexamine: A novel agonist at peripheral dopamine receptors and beta2-adrenoceptors. Br J Pharmacol 85:599, 1985.

36. Brown RA, Farmer JB, Hall JC, et al: The effects of dopexamine on the cardiovascular system of the dog. Br J Pharmacol 85:609, 1985.

37. Bass AS, Kohli JD, Lubbers NL, et al: Cardiovascular evaluation of dopexamine, an unusual dopamine receptor agonist. Clin Res 34:941A, 1986.

38. Dawson JR, Thompson DS, Signy M, et al: Acute haemodynamic and metabolic effects of dopexamine, a new dopaminergic receptor agonist, in patients with chronic heart failure. Br Heart J 54:313, 1985.

39. Svensson G, Sjogren A, Erhardt L: Short-term haemodynamic effects of dopexamine in patients with chronic congestive heart failure. Eur Heart J 7:697, 1986.

40. Bayliss J, Thomas L, Poole-Wilson P: Acute hemodynamic and neuroendocrine effects of dopexamine, a new vasodilator for the treatment of heart failure: Comparison with dobutamine, captopril, and nitrate. J Cardiovasc Pharmacol 9:551, 1987.

41. Tan LB, Littler WA, Murray RG: Beneficial haemodynamic effects of intravenous dopexamine in patients with low-output heart failure. J Cardiovasc Pharmacol 10:280, 1987.

42. Young JB, Leon CA, Pratt CM, et al: Hemodynamic effects of an oral dopamine receptor agonist (fenoldopam) in patients with congestive heart failure. J Am Coll Cardiol 6:792, 1985.

43. Whitsett TL, Goldberg LI: Effects of levodopa on systolic pre-ejection period, blood pressure, and heart rate during acute and chronic treatment of Parkinson's disease. Circulation 45:97, 1972.

44. Finlay GD, Whitsett TL, Cucinell EA, et al: Augmentation of sodium and potassium excretion, glomerular filtration rate, and renal plasma flow by levodopa. N Engl J Med 284:865, 1971.

45. Rajfer SI, Anton AH, Rossen J, et al: Beneficial hemodynamic effects of oral levodopa in heart failure: Relationship to the generation of dopamine. N Engl J Med 310:1357, 1984.

46. Rajfer SI, Rossen JD, Nemanich JW, et al: Sustained hemodynamic improvement during long-term therapy with levodopa in heart failure: Role of plasma catecholamines. J Am Coll Cardiol 10:1286, 1987.

47. Rinne UK, Molsa P: Levodopa with benserazide or carbidopa in Parkinson disease. Neurology 29:1584, 1979.

48. Classen HG, Schramm V (eds): Ibopamine. Arzneimittelforschung 36:285, 1986.

49. Itoh H, Kohli JD, Rajfer SI, et al: Comparison of the cardiovascular actions of dopamine and epinine in the dog. J Pharmacol Exp Ther 233:87, 1985.

50. Dei Cas L, Bolognesi R, Cucchini F, et al: Hemodynamic effects of ibopamine in patients with idiopathic congestive cardiomyopathy. J Cardiovasc Pharmacol 5:249, 1983.

51. Nakano T, Morimoto Y, Kakuta Y, et al: Acute effects of ibopamine hydrochloride on hemodynamics, plasma catecholamine levels, renin activity, aldosterone, metabolism and blood gas in patients with severe congestive heart failure. Arzneimittelforschung 36:1829, 1986.

52. Rajfer SI, Rossen JD, Douglas FL, et al: Effects of long-term therapy with oral ibopamine on resting hemodynamics and exercise capacity in patients with heart failure: Relationship to the generation of N-methyldopamine and to plasma norepinephrine levels. Circulation 73:740, 1986.

53. Ren JH, Unverferth DV, Leier CV: The dopamine congener, ibopamine, in congestive heart failure. J Cardiovasc Pharmacol 6:748, 1984.

54. McNay JL, MacCannell KL, Meyer MB, et al: Hypotensive effects of dopamine in dogs and hypertensive patients after phenoxybenzamine. J Clin Invest 45:1045, 1966.

55. Goldberg LI: Dopamine receptors and hypertension. Physiologic and pharmacologic implications. Am J Med 77:37, 1984.

56. Goldberg LI: Dopamine receptor subtypes and hypertension. Clin Exp Hypertens A9(5, 6):833, 1987.

57. Murphy MB, McCoy CE, Weber RR, et al: Augmentation of renal blood flow and sodium excretion in hypertensive patients during blood pressure reduction by intravenous administration of the dopamine 1 agonist fenoldopam. Circulation 76:1312, 1987.

58. Gluck Z, Jossen L, Weidman P, et al: Cardiovascular and renal profile of acute peripheral dopamine 1-receptor agonism with fenoldopam. Hypertension 10:43, 1987.

59. Kuchel O, Buu NT, Unger T: Dopamine-sodium relationship, is a part of the endogenous natriuretic system. Contrib Nephrol 13:17, 1978.

60. Lee MR: Dopamine and the kidney. Clin Sci 62:439, 1982.

61. Lee MR: Dopamine and the kidney. In Lote CJ (ed): Advances in Renal Physiology. New York: Alan R Liss, 1986, pp 218–246.

CHAPTER 129

Amrinone

Michael C. Kontos, M.D., Mark A. Wood, M.D., and Michael L. Hess, M.D.

HISTORY

The release of amrinone by the U.S. Food and Drug Administration in 1984 provided the first useful alternative to digitalis glycosides and catecholamines for the inotropic support of congestive heart failure. In patients with severe heart failure, amrinone increases cardiac output while reducing left ventricular filling pressure and systemic vascular resistance (SVR) through a mechanism of action distinct from that of the sympathomimetic amines or cardiac glycosides. This mechanism is believed to be related to amrinone's ability to increase intracellular levels of cyclic adenosine monophosphate (cAMP) through selective inhibition of phosphodiesterase F-III (PDEF-III). Amrinone was developed at the Sterling Winthrop Research Institute in Rensselaer, New York; its cardiotonic properties were first reported by Farah and Alousi[1] in 1978, and its peripheral vasodilatory activity was demonstrated soon afterward.[2] Intense clinical interest in amrinone established its utility in the treatment of congestive heart failure with a low incidence of side effects. Although initially available in intravenous and oral preparations, the orally administered drug has been withdrawn from use because of its high incidence of side effects[3] and lack of efficacy in ameliorating symptoms and improving exercise tolerance in carefully controlled, blinded, long-term clinical trials.[4, 5]

CHEMISTRY

Amrinone—chemically, S-amino-(3,4'-bipyridine)-6(1H)-1—is structurally unrelated to any previously known inotropic agent. It was known in the early literature as WIN40680. It has the trade name Inocor (Winthrop). A bipyridine derivative with the empiric formula $C_{10}H_9N_3O$ and molecular weight of 187.07, amrinone is structurally distinct from cardiac glycosides, catecholamines, and imidazolone derivatives. It is insoluble in water but miscible in ethanol, lactic, and hydrochloric acids. The drug is available as amrinone lactate in water at pH 3.2 to 4.0. Each milliliter of solution contains 5 mg of amrinone lactate and 0.25 mg of sodium metabisulfite. The drug is light-sensitive and also suffers loss of activity in dextrose solutions over time.[6]

PHARMACOLOGY

In patients with congestive heart failure, amrinone increases cardiac output, decreases ventricular filling pressures, and reduces SVR through direct cardio-tonic and vasodilatory properties. The drug's mechanism of action is well understood and is unrelated to those of the cardiac glycosides or sympathomimetic amines. Current theory focuses on its ability to raise intracellular levels of cAMP through selective inhibition of PDEF-III, the predominant cAMP-specific phosphodiesterase in cardiac tissue.[7-10] Several lines of evidence support these concepts. First, the effects of amrinone are unaffected by propranolol, reserpine, atropine, phenoxybenzamine, metiamide (an H_1- and H_2-blocker), chlorisondamine (a ganglionic blocker),[11, 12] or dantrolene.[13] The calcium antagonist verapamil produces partial antagonism of the drug's inotropic properties, but may be overridden by increased dosages of amrinone.[13] Second, the inotropic response to amrinone appears additive to that of the cardiac glycosides. Work by Schwartz et al.[14] has shown that amrinone has no effect on purified canine Na,K$^+$-ATPase or isolated sarcoplasmic reticulum (SR) Ca^{2+} transport and ATPase activity. Third, a considerable body of data correlates elevations in intracellular cAMP concentrations with the drug's inotropic and vasodilatory properties.[15-18] In contrast with early reports,[1] more recent work has shown that amrinone elevates intracellular concentrations of cAMP in guinea pig papillary muscles[17] and canine right ventricular muscle.[18] Amrinone inhibits the cAMP phosphodiesterase purified from canine myocardium (IC_{50} = 3 to 4 × 10^{-5} M) without altering cyclic guanosine monophosphate (cGMP) levels.[18] Adenylate cyclase activity in guinea pig myocardium is unaffected by amrinone.[14] The elevation of cAMP in canine myocardium is dose-dependent and correlates closely (r = 0.703) with the improvements in contractility.[18] Finally carbachol, an adenylate cyclase inhibitor, has been shown to attenuate the increase in intracellular cAMP in canine myocardium in response to amrinone and to block the inotropic effects of amrinone.[18]

As may be expected with a mechanism of action such as enzyme inhibition, myocardial sensitivity to amrinone varies among species. Adult human myocardium appears most sensitive, whereas the rat heart appears to be unresponsive or insensitive to amrinone.[19]

There are four proposed mechanisms by which amrinone may enhance myocardial contractility through increased intracellular concentrations of cAMP. Modulation of intracellular calcium is central to most theories:

1. Elevated intracellular concentrations of cAMP augment the influx of Ca^{2+} through sarcolemmal slow Ca^{2+} channels.[20] In isolated rabbit myocytes, amrinone, 100 µg/ml, stimulated a 50% increased uptake

of $^{45}Ca^{2+}$ within 30 seconds of treatment.[21] The enhanced uptake was blocked by the Ca^{2+} antagonist lanthanum chloride ($LaCl_3$). At steady state, amrinone produced higher intracellular concentrations of the radiolabel. Alousi et al.[13] demonstrated that the contractile response to amrinone declined with decreasing concentrations of Ca^{2+} superfusing guinea pig papillary muscles. Verapamil also partially antagonized the inotropic activity of amrinone. This enhanced conductivity through Ca^{2+} slow channels can be stimulated by phosphorylation of a sarcolemmal protein kinase by cAMP.[22] Alternatively, a direct effect on sodium-dependent Ca^{2+} conduction is suggested by the amrinone-enhanced Ca^{2+} influx into dog erythrocytes, which contain little or no PDEF-III activity.[12, 23]

2. Increased intracellular levels of cAMP in myocytes facilitate Ca^{2+} uptake and sequestration by the SR, thus releasing more Ca^{2+} to the contractile apparatus with each depolarization. cAMP phosphorylates the SR protein, phospholamban, which then stimulates Ca^{2+} transport. In cat atrial tissues and papillary muscles, the SR Ca^{2+} antagonist, ryanodine, completely blocked the cardiotonic effects of amrinone.[24]

3. Elevated levels of intramyocardial cAMP cause phosphorylation of some components of the molecular contractile apparatus, thus enhancing contractility.[25] Phosphorylation of troponin I decreases the affinity of actin-myosin complex for Ca^{2+}, effecting more rapid myocardial relaxation and decreasing the cross-bridging duration of actin and myosin.[25] Reversible phosphorylation of myosin is reported, but the effects of this phosphorylation are undefined.[26]

4. cAMP may block myocardial receptors for adenosine, an endogenous negative inotropic agent.[27]

Amrinone also increases metabolism of palmitic acid labeled with radioactive carbon (^{14}C) by 60% in isolated rabbit myocytes.[21] This effect is sensitive to the presence of Ca^{2+} and may serve to augment myocardial energy supplies. Glucose metabolism is unaltered. Because amrinone inhibits cAMP degradation, it should act synergistically or additively with inotropic agents that stimulate adenylate cyclase. This has been shown for dobutamine,[28] isoproterenol, and histamine.[12]

The vasodilatory mechanism of amrinone is also believed to be related to its effects on smooth muscle cAMP concentrations. In isolated rabbit aorta, a 70% increase in cAMP levels has accompanied amrinone-mediated vascular relaxation.[16] cAMP may enhance SR Ca^{2+} sequestration by phosphorylation of an SR Ca^{2+}-dependent ATPase. This Ca^{2+} can be extruded extracellularly. Amrinone also inhibits smooth muscle Ca^{2+} uptake stimulated by norepinephrine.[16] In addition, phosphorylation of myosin kinase in smooth muscle by cAMP inhibits formation of a myokinase-calmodulin-Ca^{2+} complex needed to activate myosin for cross-bridging with actin.[26] This inhibition of actin-myosin cross-bridging also results in smooth muscle relaxation. A nonspecific or multifaceted subcellular mechanism has also been suggested.[15, 16, 19]

PHARMOCOKINETICS

After rapid intravenous administration, amrinone undergoes biexponential clearance from the plasma.[29] In patients with New York Heart Association (NYHA) class III and IV heart failure, the rapid (α) distribution phase follows first-order kinetics with a half-life of 1.4 ± 0.13 minutes.[30] This phase represents equilibration of the drug into a volume of distribution estimated to be 41.2 ± 8.9 ml/kg, or about equal to the plasma volume. The terminal volume of distribution is much higher, 1.2 to 1.6 L/kg,[31, 32] consistent with a two-compartment, open-body model. Binding to plasma proteins is reported to be 10% to 49% by the manufacturer[33] and others.[34] In children less than 4 weeks old, the half-life was 22.2 ± 5.6 hours with a volume of distribution of 1.8 L/kg, which decreased to 6.8 ± 2.4 hours and 1.6 L/kg in children older than 4 weeks.[35]

Studies in normal human volunteers given amrinone, in doses from 0.8 to 2.2 mg/kg intravenously, roughly estimated the plasma half-life to be 2.6 ± 1.4 hours.[36] This figure follows first-order kinetics, and oral administration studies suggest that this value may be dose-dependent. In patients with severe congestive heart failure, the terminal plasma half-life is longer, averaging 5 to 8 hours, and is more variable, with a range of 3 to 15 hours,[30] possibly related to diminished renal clearance, hepatic dysfunction, or both. This does not appear to be different in patients with heart failure who have undergone bypass surgery, in whom the half-life of amrinone administered intravenously ranged from 2.9 to 4.6 hours.[34] Acetylator status influences clearance of the drug in healthy men.[29] In rapid acetylators (as determined by the isoniazid method), the mean plasma half-life was 2 hours, compared with 4.4 hours for slow acetylators. As expected, total body clearance rates were significantly greater for rapid acetylators.

There is a highly significant dose-response relationship between improvement in cardiac index and plasma amrinone concentration.[30, 37] Edelson et al.[30] demonstrated an excellent dose-response relationship in 14 patients with severe congestive heart failure. Following intravenous dosages of 0.75 to 3.5 mg/kg, plasma amrinone concentrations from 1 to 8 μg/ml were linearly related to percentage of improvement in cardiac index (r = .81). A plasma level of 3.7 μg/ml corresponded well with a 50% increase in cardiac index.

After an intravenous bolus is administered, hemodynamic effects are noticeable within 2 to 15 minutes,[38] with maximal hemodynamic effects usually observed within 10 minutes. Amrinone's duration of action after a single bolus, the biologic half-life, is extended to 60 to 90 minutes in patients with congestive heart failure.[39] The biologic half-life in normal volunteers is 5 to 30 minutes.[38] Thus, a continuous intravenous infusion is required for sustained effects.

Though some patients have been treated for prolonged periods intravenously with amrinone without a significant deterioration in their hemodynamic status,[40] there is some evidence that prolonged treatment may result in tolerance. This was first seen in patients treated with orally administered amrinone, in whom sustained improvement in symptoms and hemodynamics was not seen.[5, 41] Maisel et al.[42] monitored 11 patients who were treated with intravenously administered amrinone, which was held at a constant dose. Despite an initial significant improvement, pulmonary capillary wedge pressure, SVR, and cardiac output returned nearly to baseline after 72 hours of treatment. This was associated with a decrease in the number of β-adrenergic receptors on lymphocytes. This downregulation of β-receptors was associated with a rise in plasma catecholamines and may account for the development of tolerance. In contrast, cardiac output and pulmonary capillary wedge pressure improved and were sustained in 23 patients treated with amrinone for 48 hours.[43] However, it is unknown if the amrinone infusion was held constant.

The kidney is the primary route of excretion for amrinone and its metabolites. Within 96 hours after administration of ^{14}C-labeled amrinone to normal volunteers, 63% is recovered in the urine and 18% in the feces.[33] Although extensively metabolized through saturable addition pathways, free amrinone is the major form in urine, representing 10% to 40% of the initial dose excreted in the first 24 hours,[36] although renal clearance seems to vary substantially within and among patients.[32]

Six major metabolites have been identified in animals and man: N-glycoyl, N-acetate, O-glucuronide, N-glucuronide, S-glutathionyl, and 2-S-cysteine metabolites. The 2-S-cysteine and N-glucuronide forms are the major metabolites, constituting 13% and 12% of the initial dose, respectively.[19] It is unclear whether any of these metabolites exerts pharmacologic effects.[44]

EFFECTS ON PATHOPHYSIOLOGY
Effects on Congestive Heart Failure

Several properties make amrinone an attractive agent for treating acute congestive heart failure. It often has a profound influence on cardiac index through positive inotropy and salutary effects on preload and afterload. It is a direct pulmonary and peripheral vasodilator. It acts in concert with cardiac glycosides and sympathomimetics. Short-term intravenous amrinone therapy is remarkably free from side effects and, significantly, amrinone may *reduce* myocardial oxygen consumption despite improved contractility and augmented cardiac indices.

The efficacy of amrinone as a positive inotropic agent in animal studies is well established. Amrinone has significantly increased left ventricular positive and negative dP/dt$_{max}$ in isolated rabbit hearts under microcomputer-controlled loading conditions[45] and has enhanced ventricular contractility by 35% in open-chest dogs as measured directly with myocardial Walton-Brodie gauges.[46] In animals, amrinone reverses or improves experimental heart failure caused by verapamil, pentobarbital, propranolol, procainamide, acute cardiac tamponade, aortic balloon occlusion, and multiple coronary artery occlusions.[19, 24, 46-49]

Isolated human atrial tissue and ventricular muscle obtained from NYHA class I and II patients exhibit dose-related improvements in contractility in response to amrinone.[50, 51] The myocardium of class II patients showed a 12.9% to 56.1% increase in twitch tension. In 20 normal human volunteers given 1.8 to 2.2 mg/kg of amrinone intravenously, de Guzman et al.[38] demonstrated dose-related decreases in corrected preejection periods, left ventricular ejection periods, and total electromechanical systole. The effect of amrinone on the newborn myocardium is unclear. Some studies have suggested that it may depress myocardial force development in the neonatal period.[52-54] A later study demonstrated that this may be related to the use of lower doses, because higher doses resulted in a positive inotropic effect in papillary muscles from newborn rabbits.[55]

Amrinone is similarly effective in cardiac failure in human subjects resulting from coronary artery disease, ischemic and idiopathic cardiomyopathies, hypertensive cardiomyopathy, aortic regurgitation, mitral regurgitation or stenosis, acute myocardial infarction, or open heart surgery.[39, 56-61] Patients with restrictive cardiac disease may respond poorly to amrinone because of excessive preload reduction.[56]

The acute hemodynamic responses to intravenously administered amrinone in human subjects are consistent: few patients fail to respond, and these responses are sometimes dramatic. LeJemtel et al.,[39] using 0.25- to 3-mg/kg boluses in eight NYHA class III and IV patients, recorded mean increases of 49% in cardiac index (1.84 ± 0.32 L/min/m² to 2.74 ± 0.44 L/min/m²) with a 24% decrease in left ventricular filling pressure (25.8 ± 6.2 mmHg to 19.5 ± 6.8 mmHg). SVR and pulmonary vascular resistance fell by 29% and 39%, respectively. Similarly, Benotti et al.[58] found that in NYHA class III and IV patients, amrinone in repeated 0.5-mg/kg boluses improved mean cardiac output by 44%, increased left ventricular dP/dt by 42%, decreased pulmonary capillary wedge pressure by 42%, and lowered SVR by 32%. Stroke work index increased 54%. Cardiac index increased an average 69% (1.3 ± 0.04 L/min/m² to 2.2 ± 0.07 L/min/m²) in another study using nine patients with coronary artery disease.[60] Other authors report similar experiences with amrinone.[57, 61-64]

Similar results have also been seen when a constant infusion was used in patients with severe congestive heart failure. Klein et al.[65] observed a 50% increase in cardiac index (1.6 to 2.4 L/mm/m²) with a 23% decrease in wedge pressure and a concomitant 19% decrease in SVR after a 24-hour infusion of amrinone. Marcus et al.[43] found similar results with a 52% decrease in wedge pressure (from 25 to 12 mmHg) associated with a 50% increase in cardiac index (1.8 to 2.7 L/min) and a 26% decrease in SVR after a 48-hour infusion.

In most reports, mean systemic arterial pressures and heart rates are unchanged or minimally affected by amrinone; however, individual responses can vary.[64] Mild to moderate accelerations in heart rates have been reported,[65–67] with high-dose therapy more consistently associated with a chronotropic effect.[59] In one study,[65] increases in heart rate correlated with decreases in right atrial and pulmonary capillary wedge pressures, suggesting a baroreceptor response to decreased preload. Systemic blood pressure remains unaltered or is mildly decreased by amrinone administration. Exceptions are reported, with hypotension most commonly occurring with high-dose therapy[59, 68] as well as in patients with mitral stenosis and pulmonary hypertension,[68] in patients in whom the drug is started 24 hours after open heart surgery,[61] and in patients with restrictive cardiomyopathy due to amyloidosis.[56] Drug-induced hypotension is generally short-lived (resolving within 5 minutes in some studies),[67] is responsive to intravenous fluid administration,[3] and probably is secondary to peripheral vasodilation.

Attempts to document directly the positive inotropic effect of amrinone *in vivo* in human subjects have produced mixed results, leading some authors to conclude that effects on contractility are due solely to therapeutic reductions in ventricular preload and afterload or are due to catecholamine release.[64] Direct hemodynamic measurements of left ventricular dP/dt or calculated indices of left ventricular contractility (stroke volume index or stroke work index) are increased in some studies[58, 66] but unchanged in others.[56, 61] Left ventricular ejection fraction usually is increased by amrinone when measured by hemodynamics,[56] echocardiography,[69] or radionuclide ventriculography.[70] In support of a cardiotonic effect, Modena et al.[69] recorded significant increases in mean fractional shortening ($16.4 \pm 5.2\%$ to $21.5 \pm 5.3\%$) with decreased mean end-systolic volume (6.8 ± 0.8 cm to 6.45 ± 1 cm) and end-diastolic volume (5.8 ± 1 cm to 5.2 ± 1 cm) in 14 patients with NYHA class III and IV heart failure. Modification of afterload with methoxamine produced parallel shifts in the regression lines of fractional shortening and end-systolic stress in some patients, indicating an inotropic response.

In contrast, studies using intracoronary amrinone infusions, 0.5 mg/min, failed to demonstrate improvements in cardiac output, left ventricular pressures or volumes, dP/dt maximum or minimum, or the ratio of left ventricular end-diastolic pressure to left ventricular volume[71] during 2- to 15-minute infusion periods. Therapeutic coronary sinus plasma drug levels were documented in this study. However, these patients did respond to intravenously administered amrinone.

Finally, attempts to mimic the hemodynamic effects of amrinone in patients using pure vasodilators have also produced disparate results. Konstam et al.[70] found that amrinone produced a different relationship between arterial end-systolic pressure and left ventricular end-systolic volume from that of nitroprusside. They concluded the disparity was the result of an improvement in ventricular contractility by am-

rinone. Wilmshurst et al.,[64] however, found no enhancement of left ventricular dP/dt, left ventricular end-diastolic pressure, or cardiac output by amrinone compared with nitroprusside. Thus, with some exceptions, it is currently believed that amrinone possesses cardiotonic activity when administered to human subjects, but that the extent of this activity varies among patients and is synergistic with the vasodilatory effects of the drug. The vasodilatory effects appear to predominate at lower doses, whereas the positive inotropic effects become apparent when higher doses are used. The effects on right ventricular function are similar to the effects on left ventricular function, with the improvement in function related primarily to a reduction in right ventricular afterload.[72]

Remarkably, amrinone-mediated increases in cardiac output and contractility are usually associated with an unaltered or decreased myocardial oxygen consumption.[73, 74] This effect has been documented by calculation of rate-pressure products[60, 64, 66] and by decreases in myocardial arterial-to-venous oxygen differences. Myocardial oxygen consumption, calculated by the Fick method, decreased by 30% in one study.[60] The increased oxygen demand expected from augmented cardiac contractility appears to be offset or exceeded by the effects of reduced wall stress attending amrinone therapy in patients with congestive heart failure.[75, 76] This sparing effect on myocardial oxygen consumption may not be seen in nonfailing experimental heart models.[49]

Effects on Coronary Blood Flow

Amrinone can enhance coronary blood flow by several mechanisms, including direct vasodilation or by a secondary effect related to increased metabolic demand. A direct coronary vasodilatory effect is evident in isolated porcine coronary artery strips[46] and in guinea pig heart Langendorff preparations.[19] In the latter study, amrinone enhanced coronary flow more than did isoproterenol or ouabain. Microsphere studies in anesthetized dogs revealed a 25% increase in blood flow to all layers of the myocardium.[77] In studies on awake dogs, preferential subepicardial flow was suggested. Increased coronary flow may result from coronary vasodilation and enhanced cardiac output. Furthermore, reduction in left ventricular filling pressure without change in aortic pressure widens the pressure gradient in favor of increased coronary blood flow. However, enhanced coronary blood flow in human subjects has been difficult to document. Benotti et al.[60] reported a 17% decrease in coronary blood flow that accompanied a 30% decrease in myocardial oxygen consumption in nine patients with class III or IV heart failure. Intracoronary infusions of amrinone, 0.5 mg/min, had no effect on coronary artery resistance in another study.[78] Sundram et al.[74] reported an insignificant increase in coronary flow, associated with no change in myocardial oxygen consumption in nine patients with idiopathic cardiomyopathy.

Noncoronary Vasomotor Effects

A major therapeutic effect of amrinone results from its actions on the pulmonary and systemic vasculature. Intraarterially administered amrinone produces dose-related vasodilation in isolated perfused dog hind-limb preparations.[2] This vasodilation is unaffected by denervation, prostaglandin synthetase inhibition, and blockade of cholinergic, adrenergic, H_1-, or H_2-receptors. In isolated canine arterial tissue, amrinone relaxes contractions due to norepinephrine, electrical stimulation, prostaglandin F_2 (PGF_2), or Ca^{2+}.[79] In arterial strips precontracted with PGF_2, amrinone potentiates the vasodilatory response to adenosine but not to angiotensin II. It does not inhibit vascular P_1-purinoreceptors.[80] Amrinone mediates a dose-related relaxation of isolated human umbilical artery.[51] Similarly, amrinone relaxes isolated bovine pulmonary artery contracted with potassium chloride or phenylephrine.[81] Pretreatment with propranolol, atropine, or indomethacin has no inhibitory effects on amrinone-induced relaxation. Using a double-flow probe preparation in conscious newborn lambs, a direct pulmonary vasodilatory effect was demonstrated by Mammel et al.[82] in both hypoxic and nonhypoxic animals. Vasoactive threshold doses were smaller for pulmonary responses (0.3 mg/kg) than for systemic responses (1 mg/kg), suggesting disparate sensitivities.

In patients with congestive heart failure, amrinone produces marked reductions in SVR and pulmonary vascular resistances, whereas heart rate and blood pressure are usually unaffected because of commensurate increases in cardiac output. Systemically, afterload reduction may predominate.[72] Some trials report reductions of up to 50% in SVR[61] and pulmonary vascular resistance.[64, 83] Amrinone reduced pulmonary vascular resistance by 33% to 50% in 12 patients with pulmonary hypertension due to mitral stenosis.[67] Mean pulmonary artery pressure fell from 33 to 27 mmHg. Pulmonary shunt fraction increased modestly from 8% to 12%. The effects of amrinone on the pulmonary circulation were evaluated in children 2 months to 8.3 years old with one or more left-to-right shunts.[84] In patients with pulmonary artery hypertension, amrinone significantly reduced pulmonary artery pressure and pulmonary artery resistance.[84] In contrast, in a study of adults, only one of seven patients with primary pulmonary hypertension responded to amrinone therapy.[85] Although a direct pulmonary and systemic vasodilatory action is presumed to be the major action, improved hemodynamics with a consequent reduction of sympathetic vascular tone may also contribute.

Microsphere studies in dogs suggest selective enhancement of systemic blood flow to the left ventricle and renal cortices by 25% to 30% and 16% to 20%, respectively, even when cardiac output is not increased.[77, 86] One dog study[77] found that splenic and hepatic blood flow increased 5 minutes after amrinone infusion, but only splenic flow was elevated at 60 minutes. The drug decreased flow to the intestine, stomach, gall bladder, skeletal muscles, and central nervous system by 12% to 39%.

In human subjects with congestive heart failure, amrinone increased glomerular filtration rates from 82.2 ± 14.9 ml/min to 110 ± 20.6 ml/min and renal plasma flow from 186 ± 72.0 ml/min to 231 ± 88.8 ml/min.[87] Additional information on differential distribution of blood flow in humans is not available.

Effects on Electrophysiology

The electrophysiologic effects of amrinone are limited primarily to acceleration of heart rate at high doses and enhancement of atrioventricular nodal conduction. In animal studies, amrinone increases the intrinsic firing rate of rabbit sinus node pacemaker cells, perhaps by enhancing slow inward Ca^{2+} or inward Na^+ currents.[88] In canine Purkinje fibers, amrinone had no effect on resting membrane potential, action potential amplitude, maximal upstroke, or conduction velocity.[89] No oscillatory after-potentials or after-conductions were produced in depolarized Purkinje cells.[89] The drug does not enhance the toxicity of arrhythmogenic doses of ouabain in dogs.[90] Amrinone does reduce the functional refractory period of the atrioventricular node and A_2H_2 interval in canine hearts in a dose-related manner, whereas the A_2V_2 interval is unchanged.[91] Amrinone increased the amplitude of oscillatory after-potentials in digitalis-treated canine myocardial tissue[92] and partially reversed depressed atrioventricular conduction produced by verapamil, propanolol, and ouabain in dogs.[91] Amrinone did not enhance ventricular fibrillation occurring on reperfusion of occluded coronary arteries,[93] but it increased atrial and ventricular rates in dogs with circus flutter arrhythmias.

Few studies have investigated the electrophysiologic effects of amrinone in humans. Naccarelli et al.[94] studied 15 patients with severe congestive heart failure treated with intravenously administered amrinone, 10 to 20 μg/kg/min. No changes in electrocardiographic intervals accompanied increased cardiac indices. The maximal corrected sinus node recovery time and atrioventricular nodal and ventricular refractory periods were unaffected. The average maximal 1:1 atrioventricular nodal conduction rate was increased as the mean conduction interval fell from 371 ± 46 msec to 334 ± 47 msec. Amrinone did not exacerbate preexisting HV prolongations or the frequency of inducible ventricular arrhythmias. In contrast, ventricular ectopic activity increased in 2 of 11 patients treated with intravenously administered amrinone.[63] In patients on short-term oral amrinone therapy, no changes were reported in the number of premature ventricular contractions in 24 hours or runs of ventricular tachycardia per 24 hours recorded on Holter monitoring, but ventricular couplets per 24 hours were increased. One other study using long-term oral amrinone therapy also reported a proarrhythmic effect.[5] Amrinone may also accelerate preexisting supraventricular tachycardias.[94]

Metabolic Effects

Renal

Amrinone has no known specific effects on renal function except for an enhancement of cortical blood flow. In dogs, amrinone (30 µg/kg/min) produced no change in urinary volume; inulin clearance; Na^+, K^+, or Cl^- clearance; or plasma Na^+, K^+, or Cl^- levels.[24] With doses sufficient to reduce blood pressure, plasma renin increases as anticipated and urine volume and sodium excretion decrease.

Hepatic

Evidence suggests that amrinone may further depress already compromised hepatic microsomal metabolic capacity in patients with heart failure. Manzione et al.[95] demonstrated a 62% reduction in the aminopyrine breath test score in NYHA class III and IV patients given orally administered amrinone. The patients otherwise had normal serum levels of bilirubin, alkaline phosphatase, and serum glutamic-oxaloacetic transaminase.

Pulmonary

Amrinone relaxes isolated guinea pig pulmonary smooth muscle contracted by carbachol, histamine, or barium; in anesthetized dogs, amrinone inhibits histamine-induced bronchospasm in a dose-related manner.[96] Decreased intracellular availability of Ca^{2+} is suggested as the mechanism of action. The significance of this effect in humans is unknown. Acute reversible reductions in Pa_{O_2} occurred in patients given amrinone after cardiac surgery in two separate studies.[61, 93] The mechanism is unknown but may relate to an increased shunt fraction.[97]

Biochemical Effects

Amrinone has reduced arterial lactate concentrations by 24% without altering total body oxygen consumption.[60] Some studies report increased arterial and coronary sinus glucose levels.[64] In dogs and rabbits, amrinone is a thromboxane synthetase inhibitor, and it decreases thromboxane β_2 production in human blood in a dose-related fashion.[98] 6-Ketoprostaglandin F_1 levels are not affected. Amrinone is reported to inhibit platelet aggregation,[99, 100] possibly resulting from its effects on thromboxane synthesis and alterations in intracellular levels of cAMP and calcium. In some patients, the average plasma levels of epinephrine and norepinephrine may increase modestly,[101, 102] whereas in others, increases may exceed 100%.[42] Plasma renin activity was increased when amrinone was added to dobutamine in patients with congestive heart failure.[102] Increased levels of plasma free fatty acids have been reported in response to amrinone therapy.[64]

CLINICAL USE
Indications

Amrinone is approved for short-term intravenous use in adults with severe congestive heart failure of all causes but should be used with caution in patients with restrictive myocardial diseases. Amrinone appears to be safe and effective in patients with heart failure during the acute stages of myocardial infarction.[59, 66, 68] Amrinone has been administered to patients with documented myocardial infarctions within 4 to 18 hours of the onset of symptoms. In these patients, amrinone effectively increased cardiac output by 10% to 26%, reduced pulmonary capillary wedge pressure up to 38%, and decreased SVR 10% to 33%, whereas it increased heart rate by only 7% in one study[66] and lowered diastolic pressure in two studies.[59, 68] The rate-pressure products were unchanged.[66] Even at doses of 3600 µg/kg/min for 30 minutes,[68] no evidence was found of enhanced ischemia or precipitation of angina. Amrinone was shown not to increase the infarct size in a canine model of coronary occlusion and reperfusion.[103] The lowest effective doses are recommended to minimize accelerating heart rates, which would increase myocardial oxygen consumption.

Amrinone is effective in low output syndrome after coronary artery bypass. In one study, the addition of amrinone to maximal treatment, which included catecholamine and intraaortic balloon placement, resulted in an improvement in mean arterial pressure, cardiac index, and pulmonary capillary wedge pressure, allowing successful weaning from cardiopulmonary bypass.[104] Dupuis et al.[105] compared dobutamine with amrinone in 30 patients as a primary treatment of low cardiac output syndrome after bypass operations. Cardiac outputs exceeded 2.4 L/min in 11 of 15 patients given amrinone, whereas this occurred in only 6 of 15 patients treated with dobutamine. There was a similar incidence of myocardial ischemia (36% versus 33%) as detected by Holter monitor. Others[61, 106] have also shown amrinone to be of benefit in patients who are in cardiogenic shock despite treatment with adrenergic agonists or intraaortic balloon pumps.

Deeb et al.[107] found long-term intravenous amrinone treatment to be effective in 22 patients awaiting cardiac transplantation. Pulmonary artery pressure, pulmonary vascular resistance, and wedge pressure were reduced significantly along with an increase in cardiac output, without a decrease in mean arterial pressure. However, platelet counts decreased to below 30,000 in 2 of the 22 patients, necessitating platelet transfusion.

Pulmonary hypertension with a transpulmonic A gradient greater than 15 mmHg and a pulmonary vascular resistance exceeding 5 Woods units has been shown to result in an increase in the perioperative mortality rate in patients undergoing orthotic heart transplantation. Amrinone has been shown to be particularly effective in reversing pulmonary hypertension in these patients. In one study, pulmonary vascular resistance was reduced to less than 5 Woods units in 19 (86%) of 22 potential transplantation candidates with pulmonary hypertension treated with amrinone.[108]

Amrinone has also shown promise in experimental doxorubicin-[109] and anesthesia-related[110] myocardial depression, in weaning catecholamine-dependent patients,[111] and in counteracting severe verapamil[112, 113] and chloroquine intoxication.[114]

Precautions and Contraindications

Amrinone is contraindicated in patients known to show hypersensitivity reactions to the drug itself or to sodium metabisulfites. Like any inotropic agent, amrinone may worsen hemodynamics in hypertrophic obstructive cardiomyopathy. The drug can enhance atrioventricular nodal conduction and thus accelerate ventricular response to supraventricular tachyarrhythmias.[94]

Marked hypotension has been reported in a patient receiving disopyramide and amrinone; thus, this combination of drugs should be avoided.[115] Amrinone has been used safely in neonates, but it should be used cautiously in this population until more information is available.[35]

Amrinone should be used with caution in patients with hypotension, thrombocytopenia, and restrictive cardiomyopathies. Altered metabolism and clearance of the drug may occur in patients with impaired hepatic or renal function. In such instances, amrinone should be avoided or used only under intensive hemodynamic monitoring.

Adverse Reactions

Short-term intravenous administration of amrinone carries a low incidence of adverse reactions.[115] Dose-related, reversible thrombocytopenia occurs in about 2.4% of patients after short-term intravenous treatment.[115] Platelet levels are usually reduced modestly (to 50,000 to 100,000/mm^3) with long-term treatment but can be severely depressed (as low as 30,000/mm^3),[100, 107] and transfusions have been necessary in some amrinone-dependent patients.[107] The effect was related to the log-plasma amrinone concentration.[100] Platelet survival is reduced, and aggregation to arachidonate, collagen, adenosine diphosphate, and ristocetin may be abnormal in some patients.[100] Results of bone marrow examinations are normal or show increased megakaryocytes. A nonimmunologic mechanism appears to be involved, and clinical hemorrhage is rare. Development of mild thrombocytopenia does not necessarily require discontinuation of the drug. In some patients, platelet counts have returned to normal despite continuation of amrinone infusion.[116] Transient hypotension may occur in about 2% of patients intravenously receiving amrinone.[3, 58] This effect appears to be dose-related and responsive to either reduced rates of infusion or intravenous administration of fluids.[3]

A 0.5% to 2% incidence of gastrointestinal complaints attends intravenous amrinone therapy. These complaints most commonly are nausea (1.7%), vomiting (0.95%), abdominal pain (0.4%), and anorexia (0.4%).[115] Fewer than 1% to 2% of patients have elevated plasma hepatic enzymes when receiving intravenously administered amrinone.[115, 117] In a case report, lactate dehydrogenase (LDH), aspartate aminotransferase and alanine aminotransferase were elevated in one patient with normal total bilirubin.[117] Other studies report isolated LDH elevations.[118] A drug-induced hypersensitivity reaction has been suggested.[117] A proarrhythmic effect appears to be uncommon except for acceleration of ventricular responses to supraventricular dysrhythmias. Other infrequent side effects of intravenous use include local pain at the infusion site (0.2%),[115] chest pain (0.2%),[108] and eosinophilia.[117] True anaphylactic reactions to amrinone are rare.

Comparison with Other Drugs

Dobutamine

In a study by Klein et al. using NYHA class III and IV patients, amrinone and dobutamine similarly enhanced cardiac index and reduced SVR without changing myocardial oxygen consumption.[65] Pulmonary capillary wedge pressure was decreased by both drugs; however, these hemodynamic changes were attenuated after 8 hours of dobutamine but not amrinone therapy. In a randomized, double-blind study, Marcus et al.[43] compared dobutamine with amrinone in 46 consecutive patients with idiopathic dilated cardiomyopathy during a 48-hour infusion. In both sets of patients, a cardiac index increased significantly (2.1 to 3.0 L/min/m^2 with dobutamine versus 1.8 to 2.7 L/min/m^2 with amrinone), although pulmonary capillary wedge pressure was reduced to a greater extent with amrinone (50% versus 33%). Amrinone was associated with an increase in heart rate (102 beats/min to 110 beats/min); there was a decrease with dobutamine (103 beats/min to 98 beats/min). A negative fluid balance was more common in the amrinone group (23 of 23 patients—100%) than in the dobutamine group (18 of 23 patients—78%).

Sundram et al.[74] looked at the addition of amrinone (15 μg/kg/min) to dobutamine (15 μg/kg/min) in nine patients with idiopathic dilated cardiomyopathy. The cardiac index rose from a baseline of 1.47 ± 0.44 L/min/m^2 to 2.89 ± 1.1 L/min/m^2 with dobutamine and to 3.64 ± 1.05 L/min/m^2 when amrinone was added, with a further decrease in wedge pressure (28 ± 7 mmHg to 26 ± 8 mmHg to 20 ± 6 mmHg). There was no increase in myocardial oxygen consumption when amrinone was added. Uretsky et al.[102] found similar results when a bolus of amrinone was given to patients already being treated with dobutamine. Cardiac output increased further, and wedge pressure decreased. However, three patients had a significant decrease in their mean arterial pressure that was associated with a decrease in cardiac output.

In patients with acute myocardial infarction complicated by heart failure, Tanaka et al.[66] showed amrinone to have the greater effect on pulmonary capillary wedge pressure, but dobutamine effected larger increments in cardiac index. SVR was similarly reduced by both drugs. Amrinone elevated heart rate, whereas dobutamine did not. It would appear from these studies that amrinone and dobutamine produce comparable hemodynamic changes. Amrinone may be the more potent vasodilator, be better tolerated, and at higher doses spare myocardial oxygen consumption to a greater degree.

One randomized study compared dobutamine with amrinone in patients after myocardial infarction. In that study, amrinone decreased wedge pressure to a greater degree than dobutamine, despite a smaller increase in cardiac output.[119]

Dopamine

Dopamine has shown little effect on pulmonary capillary wedge pressure in patients with heart failure with or without acute myocardial infarction.[62, 66] Both drugs elevated cardiac output and reduced SVR in these studies. Blood pressure was elevated[62] or unchanged[66] by dopamine. Neither drug elevated the rate pressure product in Tanaka's study.[66] Given its effects on pulmonary capillary wedge pressure and its tendency to reduce rather than elevate blood pressure, amrinone may be preferable to dopamine, except in hypotensive patients.

Isoproterenol

Studying 10 patients with moderate congestive heart failure, Firth et al.[83] found that amrinone enhanced cardiac output only in patients with the most severe ventricular dysfunction. Amrinone did not decrease SVR or alter left ventricular dP/dt maximum or minimum. Heart rate, pulmonary capillary wedge pressure, and blood pressure were unchanged or minimally affected. In contrast, isoproterenol elevated cardiac output consistently and increased both left ventricular dP/dt_{max} aortic pressure and heart rate while decreasing SVR.

Nitroprusside

Not surprisingly, the comparative effects of the potent vasodilators amrinone and nitroprusside are similar. Konstam et al.[70] found that both drugs decreased SVR, pulmonary capillary wedge pressure, pulmonary artery pressure, and left ventricular end-diastolic volume and similarly increased cardiac index in nine NYHA class III and IV patients. Nitroprusside reduced end-systolic blood pressure more than amrinone did. The drugs showed different relationships of arterial end-systolic pressure to left ventricular end-systolic volume, however, suggesting a cardiotonic effect of amrinone. Wilmshurst et al.[64] found similar average responses to amrinone and nitroprusside in 14 patients but detected no inotropic effects of amrinone.

Cardiac Glycosides

No studies have compared amrinone with the cardiac glycosides in human subjects. However, the effects of amrinone appear to be additive to those of digitalis and are manifested in cases refractory to digitalis.

Milrinone

As a structural analogue of amrinone, milrinone elicits similar hemodynamic effects in patients with congestive heart failure but is about 30 times more potent.[120] Milrinone appears to produce a lower incidence of thrombocytopenia and may be less arrhythmogenic than amrinone.

Dosage and Administration

Treatment with amrinone is usually initiated with an intravenous bolus of 0.75 mg/kg over 2 to 3 minutes followed by a continuous infusion of 5 to 10 µg/kg/min. A second 0.75-mg/kg bolus may be given after 30 minutes if necessary. When the drug is being used to separate a patient from cardiopulmonary bypass, a larger initial bolus dose of 1.5 mg/kg may be needed. Amrinone should be diluted to 1 to 3 mg/ml in normal or half-normal saline. Amrinone loses activity with exposure to light or when mixed with solutions containing dextrose. All diluted solutions should be used within 24 hours. The risk of hypotension can be reduced by either loading it over a longer period (1.5 mg/kg over 5 to 10 min), which may prevent higher peak concentrations, or initiating therapy as a 40-µg/kg/min infusion for 1 hour followed by the appropriate maintenance rate. The maximal recommended cumulative dose is 10 mg/kg/24 hr; however, some patients have required up to 18 mg/kg/24 hr.[33] The rate of maintenance infusion depends on the patient's hemodynamic response. Changes in infusion rates should be made at least 1 hour apart to allow for possible accumulation of the drug in severely ill patients. Furosemide injected into amrinone intravenous lines forms a precipitate. No other drug should be given through amrinone lines.

CONCLUSIONS

Amrinone, a bipyridine derivative, is effective as an adjunct or an alternative to cardiac glycosides and sympathomimetic amines in the short-term management of severe congestive heart failure. In such patients, amrinone increases cardiac output, reduces left ventricular filling pressures, and decreases systemic and pulmonary vascular resistance while effecting little or no change in heart rate or systemic pressure. These salutary effects result from amrinone's cardiotonic and vasodilatory properties, but the relative contributions of these properties are debated. Renal hemodynamics are improved with an increase in cortical blood flow and, in therapeutic doses, result in no change in glomerular or tubular function. Hepatic function is rarely affected by long-term amrinone infusion. Amrinone's mechanism of action is uncertain but is probably related to elevations in intracellular cAMP levels secondary to selective inhibition of PDEF-III. Amrinone is well-tolerated intravenously. The most common side effects are thrombocytopenia, hypotension, and gastrointestinal complaints, but they are relatively infrequent. Remarkably, amrinone actually may reduce myocardial oxygen consumption in the failing heart because of beneficial effects on ventricular wall stress—effects not consistently attributed to the sympathomimetic amines. Amrinone also appears to be minimally arrhythmogenic and free from short-term tachyphylaxis. Thus, amrinone is a valuable agent for the treatment of severe congestive heart failure.

REFERENCES

1. Farah AE, Alousi AA: New cardiotonic agents: A search for a digitalis substitute. Life Sci 22:1139, 1978.
2. Alousi A, Helstrosky A: Amrinone: A positive inotropic agent with a direct vasodilative activity in the canine perfused hind limb preparation [abstract]. Fed Proc 39:855, 1980.
3. Wilmshurst PT, Webb-Peploe MM: Side effects of amrinone therapy. Br Heart J 49:447, 1983.
4. Massie B, Bourassa M, DiBianco R, et al: Long-term oral administration of amrinone for congestive heart failure: Lack of efficacy in a multicenter controlled trial. Circulation 71:963, 1985.
5. Packer M, Medina N, Yushak M: Hemodynamic and clinical limitations of longterm inotropic therapy with amrinone in patients with severe chronic heart failure. Circulation 70:1038, 1984.
6. Bottoroff MD, Ruttledge DR, Pieper JA: Evaluation of intravenous amrinone: The first of a new class of positive inotropic agents with vasodilator properties. Pharmacotherapy 5:227, 1985.
7. Evans DB: Modulation of cAMP: Mechanism for positive inotropic action. J Cardiovasc Pharmacol 8(Suppl 9):522, 1986.
8. Colucci WS, Wright RF, Braunwald E: New positive inotropic agents in the treatment of congestive heart failure. N Engl J Med 314:349, 1986.
9. Carpendo F, Floreani M, Cargnelli G: Competitive inhibition of phosphodiesterase activity by amrinone: Its implications in the cardiac effect of the drug. Pharmacol Res Comm 16:969, 1984.
10. Scholz H, Meyer W: Phosphodiesterase-inhibiting properties of newer inotropic agents. Circulation 73(Suppl III):90, 1986.
11. Alousi AA, Farah AE, Lesher GY, et al: Cardiotonic activity of amrinone (WIN 40680): 5-amino-3,4'-bipyridin-6(1H)-one. Circ Res 45:666, 1979.
12. Mancini D, LeJemtel T, Sonnenblick E: Intravenous use of amrinone for the treatment of the failing heart. Am J Cardiol 56:8B, 1985.
13. Alousi AA, Stankus GP, Stuart JC: The physiologic role of ions in the inotropic response to amrinone. Circulation 66(Suppl II):309, 1982.
14. Schwartz A, Grupp I, Grupp G, et al: Amrinone: A new inotropic agent, studies on organelle systems [abstract]. Circulation 59/60(Suppl 2):6, 1979.
15. Morgan JP, Gwathmey JK, DeFeo TT, et al: The effects of amrinone and related drugs on intracellular calcium in isolated mammalian cardiac and vascular smooth muscle. Circulation 73(Suppl III):65, 1986.
16. Meisheri KD, Palmer RF, Van Breemen C: The effects of amrinone on contractility, Ca^{2+} uptake and cAMP in smooth muscle. Eur J Pharmacol 61:159, 1980.
17. Honerjager P, Schafer-Korting M, Reiter M: Involvement of cyclic AMP in the direct inotropic action of amrinone. Arch Pharmacol 318:112, 1981.
18. Endoh M, Yamashita S, Taira N: Positive inotropic effect of amrinone in relation to cyclic nucleotide metabolism in the canine ventricular muscle. J Pharmacol Exp Ther 221:775, 1982.
19. Alousi AA, Dobreck HP: Amrinon. In Scriabine A (ed): New Drugs Annual: Cardiovascular Drugs. New York: Raven Press, 1983, pp 259–276.
20. Katz AM, Tada M, Kirchberger MA: Control of calcium transport in the myocardium by the cyclic-AMP-protein kinase system. In Drummond GI, Greengard P, Robison GA (eds): Advances in Cyclic Nucleotide Research, Vol 5. New York: Raven Press, 1975, p 453.
21. Frangakis CJ, Lasher KP, Alousi AA: Physiological and biochemical effects of amrinone on cardiac myocytes [abstract]. Circulation 66:II57, 1982.
22. Tsien RW: Cyclic AMP and contractile activity in heart. In Greengard P, Robison GA (eds): Advances in Cyclic Nucleotide Research, Vol 8. New York: Raven Press, 1977, pp 363–420.
23. Parker JC, Harper JR Jr: Effects of amrinone, a cardiotonic drug on calcium movement in dog erythrocytes. J Clin Invest 66:254, 1980.
24. Alousi AA, Edelson J: Amrinone. In Goldberg ME (ed): Pharmacological and Biochemical Properties of Drug Substances, Vol 3. Washington, DC: American Pharmaceutical Association, 1981, p 120.
25. England PJ, Pask HT, Mulk D: Cyclic AMP–dependent phosphorylation of contractile proteins. In Greengard P (ed): Advances in Cyclic Nucleotide Research, Vol 17. New York: Raven Press, 1984, p 383.
26. Adelstein RS, Pato MD, Conti MA: The role of phosphorylation in regulating contractile proteins. In Dummont JE, Greengard P, Robinson GA (eds): Advances in Cyclic Nucleotide Research, Vol 14. New York: Raven Press, 1981, p 373.
27. Scholz H: Inotropic drugs and their mechanisms of action. J Am Coll Cardiol 4:389, 1984.
28. Guimond JG, Matuschak GM, Meyers F, et al: Augmentation of cardiac function in end-stage heart failure by combined use of dobutamine and amrinone. Chest 90:302, 1986.
29. Hamilton RA, Kowalsky SF, Wright EM, et al: Effects of acetylator phenotype on amrinone pharmacokinetics. Clin Pharmacol Ther 40:615, 1986.
30. Edelson J, LeJemtel TH, Alousi AA, et al: Relations between amrinone plasma concentration and cardiac index. Clin Pharmacol Ther 29:723, 1981.
31. DiBianco R: The bipyridine derivatives: Amrinone and milrinone: In Leier C (ed): Cardiotonic Drugs: A Clinical Survey. New York: Marcel Dekker, 1986, p 199.
32. Rocci ML Jr, Wilson H, Likoff M, et al: Pharmacokinetics after single and steady state doses in patients with chronic cardiac failure [abstract]. Clin Pharmacol Ther 33:260, 1983.
33. Winthrop Breon Laboratories: FDA approved package insert—Inocor lactate injection—Brand of amrinone lactate. New York, 1984.
34. Bailey JM, Levy JH, Rogers HG, et al: Pharmacokinetics of amrinone during cardiac surgery. Anesthesiology 75:961, 1991.
35. Lawless S, Burckart G, Diven W, et al: Amrinone pharmacokinetics in neonates and infants. J Clin Pharmacol 28:283, 1933.
36. Kullberg MP, Freeman GB, Biddlecome C, et al: Amrinone metabolism. Clin Pharmacol Ther 29:394, 1981.
37. Benotti JR, Lesko LJ, McCue JE: Acute pharmacodynamics and pharmacokinetics of oral amrinone. J Clin Pharmacol 22:425, 1982.
38. de Guzman NT, Munoz O, Palmer RF, et al: Clinical evaluation of amrinone—A new inotropic agent [abstract]. Circulation 58(Suppl II):183, 1978.
39. LeJemtel TH, Keung E, Sonnenblick EH, et al: Amrinone: A new non-glycosidic, non-adrenergic cardiotonic agent effective in the treatment of intractable myocardial failure in man. Circulation 59:1098, 1979.
40. Bolling SF, Deeb DC, Crowley MM, et al: Prolonged amrinone therapy prior to orthotopic cardiac transplantation in patients with pulmonary hypertension. Transplantation Proceedings 20:753, 1988.
41. Corbolan R, Casanegra P, Mezzano D, et al: Effect and complications of chronic amrinone therapy in patients with dilated cardiomyopathy. J Am Coll Cardiol 3:471, 1984.

42. Maisel AS, Wright CM, Carter SM, et al: Tachyphylaxis with amrinone therapy: Association with sequestration and down-regulation of lymphocyte beta adrenergic receptors. Ann Intern Med 110:195, 1989.
43. Marcus RH, Raw K, Patel J, et al: Comparison of intravenous amrinone and dobutamine in congestive heart failure due to idiopathic dilated cardiomyopathy. Am J Cardiol 66:1107, 1990.
44. Rocci ML, Wilson H: The pharmacokinetics and pharmacodynamics of newer inotropic agents. Clin Pharmacokinet 13:91, 1987.
45. Haleen SJ, Evans DB, Kaplan HR: Microcomputer-controlled isolated working rabbit heart preparation. Comparison of amrinone, ouabain and isoproterenol [abstract]. Pharmacologist 22:268, 1980.
46. Millard RW, Dub G, Grupp G, et al: Direct vasodilation and positive inotropic actions of amrinone. J Mol Cell Cardiol 12:647, 1980.
47. Millard RW, Fowler NO, Gabel M: Hemodynamic and regional blood flow distribution responses to dextran, hydralazine, isoproterenol and amrinone during experimental cardiac tamponade. J Am Coll Cardiol 1:1461, 1983.
48. Fowler NO, Millard RW, Gabel M, et al: Cardiac tamponade: Relief by volume expansion, augmented inotropism and peripheral vasodilation [abstract]. Circulation 62(Suppl III):318, 1980.
49. Rude RE, Kloner RA, Maroko PR, et al: Effects of amrinone on experimental acute myocardial ischaemic injury. Cardiovasc Res 14:419, 1980.
50. Alousi AA, Palmer RF, Fullem L: Comparative inotropic activity of amrinone in isolated human atria and cat atria and papillary muscle [abstract]. J Mol Cell Cardiol 11(Suppl 1):2, 1979.
51. Wilmshurst PT, Walker JM, Fry CH, et al: Inotropic and vasodilator effects of amrinone on isolated human tissue. Cardiovasc Res 18:302, 1984.
52. Binah O, Legato MJ, Danilo P Jr, et al: Developmental changes in the cardiac effects of amrinone in the dog. Circ Res 52:747, 1983.
53. Binah O, Sodowich B, Vulliemoz Y, et al: The inotropic effects of amrinone and milrinone on neonatal and young canine cardiac muscle. Circulation 73(Suppl III):46, 1986.
54. Ross-Ascuitto N, Ascuitto R, Chen V, et al: Negative inotropic effects of amrinone in the neonatal piglet heart. Circ Res 61:847, 1987.
55. Klitzner TS, Shapir Y, Ravin R, et al: The biphasic effect of amrinone on tension development in newborn mammalian myocardium. Pediatr Res 27:144, 1990.
56. Wilmshurst PT, Thompson DS, Jenkins BS, et al: The hemodynamic effects of intravenous amrinone in patients with impaired left ventricular function. Br Heart J 49:77, 1983.
57. Siskind SJ, Sonnenblick EH, Forman R, et al: Acute sustained benefit of inotropic therapy with amrinone in exercise hemodynamics and metabolism in severe congestive heart failure. Circulation 64:966, 1981.
58. Benotti JR, Grossman W, Braunwald E, et al: Hemodynamic assessment of amrinone—A new inotropic agent. N Engl J Med 299:1373, 1978.
59. Verma SP, Silke B, Reynolds GW, et al: Hemodynamic dose-response effects of intravenous amrinone in left ventricular failure complicating acute myocardial infarction. J Cardiovasc Pharmacol 7:1101, 1985.
60. Benotti JR, Grossman W, Braunwald E, et al: Effects of amrinone on myocardial energy metabolism and hemodynamics in patients with severe congestive heart failure due to coronary artery disease. Circulation 62:28, 1980.
61. Goenen M, Pedemonte O, Baele P, et al: Amrinone in the management of low cardiac output after open heart surgery. Am J Cardiol 53:33B, 1986.
62. Benotti JR, McCue J, Love D, et al: Comparative inotropic therapy in heart failure patients [abstract]. Circulation 68(Suppl 3):510, 1983.
63. Weber KT, Andrews V, Janicki JS, et al: Amrinone and exercise performance in patients with chronic heart failure. Am J Cardiol 48:164, 1981.
64. Wilmshurst PT, Thompson DS, Juul SM, et al: Comparison of the effects of amrinone and sodium nitroprusside on hemodynamics, contractility, and myocardial metabolism in patients with cardiac failure due to coronary artery disease and dilated cardiomyopathy. Br Heart J 52:38, 1984.
65. Klein NA, Siskind SJ, Frishman WH, et al: Hemodynamic comparison of intravenous amrinone and dobutamine in patients with chronic congestive heart failure. Am J Cardiol 48:170, 1981.
66. Tanaka K, Takano T, Seino Y: Effects of intravenous amrinone on heart failure complicated by acute myocardial infarction: Comparative study with dopamine and dobutamine. Jpn Circ J 50:652, 1986.
67. Hess W, Arnold B, Veit S: The hemodynamic effects of amrinone in patients with mitral stenosis and pulmonary hypertension. Eur Heart J 7:800, 1986.
68. Taylor SH, Verma SP, Hussain M, et al: Intravenous amrinone in left ventricular failure complicated by acute myocardial infarction. Am J Cardiol 56:29B, 1985.
69. Modena MG, Benassi A, Mattioli G: Echocardiographic evaluation of cardiovascular effects of amrinone. Clin Cardiol 7:593, 1984.
70. Konstam MA, Cohen SR, Weiland DS, et al: Relative contributions of inotropic and vasodilation effects to amrinone-induced haemodynamic improvement in congestive heart failure. Am J Cardiol 54:242, 1986.
71. Wilmshurst PT, Thompson DS, Dittrich HC, et al: Effects of intravenous and intracoronary amrinone in congestive cardiac failure [abstract]. Circulation 66(Suppl 2):137, 1982.
72. Konstam MA, Cohen SR, Salem DN, et al: Effect of amrinone on right ventricular function: Predominance of afterload reduction. Circulation 74:359, 1986.
73. Baim DS: Effects of amrinone on myocardial energetics in severe congestive heart failure. Am J Cardiol 56:16B, 1985.
74. Sundram P, Reddy HK, McElroy PA, et al: Myocardial energetics and efficiency in patients with idiopathic cardiomyopathy: Response to dobutamine and amrinone. Am Heart J 119:891, 1990.
75. Goldstein RA: Clinical effects of intravenous amrinone in patients with congestive heart failure. Circulation 73(Suppl III):191, 1986.
76. Jentzer JH, LeJemtel TH, Sonnenblick EH, et al: Beneficial effects of amrinone on myocardial oxygen consumption during acute left ventricular failure in dogs. Am J Cardiol 48:75, 1981.
77. Einzig S, Rao GHR, Pierpont ME, et al: Effects of amrinone on regional myocardial and systemic blood flow distribution in the dog. Can J Physiol Pharmacol 60:811, 1982.
78. Wilmshurst PT, Thompson DS, Juul SM, et al: Effects of intracoronary and intravenous amrinone infusions in patients with cardiac failure and patients with near normal cardiac function. Br Heart J 53:493, 1985.
79. Toda N, Nakajima M, Nishimura K, et al: Responses of isolated dog arteries to amrinone. Cardiovasc Res 18:174, 1984.
80. Burnstock G: Cholinergic and purinergic regulation of blood vessels. In Bohr DF, Somlyo AP, Sparks HV Jr (eds): Vascular Smooth Muscle: The Cardiovascular System. Baltimore: Williams & Wilkins, 1980, pp 567–612.
81. Harbison RG, Lippton HL, Hyman AL, et al: Pulmonary vascular actions of amrinone and milrinone [abstract]. Circulation 70(Suppl II):728, 1984.
82. Mammel MC, Einzig S, Kulik TJ, et al: Pulmonary vascular effects of amrinone in conscious lambs. Pediatr Res 17:720, 1983.
83. Firth BG, Ratner AV, Grassman ED, et al: Assessment of the inotropic and vasodilation effects of amrinone versus isoproterenol. Am J Cardiol 54:1331, 1984.
84. Robinson BW, Gelband H, Mas MS: Selective pulmonary and systemic vasodilator effects of amrinone in children: New therapeutic implications. J Am Coll Cardiol 21:1461, 1993.
85. Rich S, Ganz R, Levy PS: Comparative actions of hydralazine, nifedipine and amrinone in primary pulmonary hypertension. Am J Cardiol 52:1104, 1983.
86. Einzig S, Pierpont ME: Acute effects of intravenous amrinone (5-amino-3,4'bipyridine-6,1H-one) on systemic blood flow distribution [abstract]. Am J Cardiol 47:491, 1981.

87. Schneeweiss A: Drug Therapy in Cardiovascular Diseases. Philadelphia: Lea & Febiger, 1986.
88. Kodama I, Kondo N, Shibata S: Effects of amrinone on the transmembrane action potential of rabbit sinus node pacemaker cells. Br J Pharmacol 80:511, 1983.
89. Piwonka RW, Canniff PC, Farah AE: In vitro electrophysiologic properties of amrinone in mammalian cardiac tissue. J Cardiovasc Pharmacol 5:1058, 1983.
90. Alousi AA, Fort D: The inotropic efficacy and safety of amrinone in the presence of other cardiovascular drugs in dogs [abstract]. Circulation 59/60(Suppl II):6, 1979.
91. Nusrat A, Tepper D, Hertzberg J, et al: Effects of amrinone on atrioventricular conduction in the intact canine heart. J Clin Pharmacol 23:257, 1983.
92. Rosenthal JE, Ferrier GR: Inotropic and electrophysiologic effects of amrinone in untreated and digitalized ventricular tissues. J Pharmacol Exp Ther 221:188, 1982.
93. Piwonka RW, Healey JF, Canniff PC, et al: Electrophysiological actions of amrinone in dogs with cardiac lesions. J Cardiovasc Pharmacol 5:1052, 1983.
94. Naccarelli GV, Gray EL, Dougherty AH, et al: Amrinone: Acute electrophysiologic and hemodynamic effects in patients with congestive heart failure. Am J Cardiol 54:600, 1984.
95. Manzione NC, Goldfarb JP, LeJemtel TH, et al: The effects of two new inotropic agents on microsomal liver function in patients with congestive heart failure. Am J Med Sci 291:88, 1986.
96. Mielens ZE, Buck DC: Relaxant effects of amrinone upon pulmonary smooth muscle. Pharmacology 25:262, 1982.
97. Prielipp RC, Butterworth JF, Zaloga GP, et al: Effects of amrinone on cardiac index, venous oxygen saturation and venous admixture in patients recovering from cardiac surgery. Chest 99:820, 1991.
98. Pattison A, Eason CT, Bonner FW: The in vitro effect of amrinone on thromboxane B2 synthesis in human whole blood. Thromb Res 42:817, 1986.
99. Grazer JM, Horowitz PM, McNamara DB, et al: Effects of amrinone on platelet aggregation and cyclic nucleotide levels. Fed Proc 43:980, 1984.
100. Wilmshurst PT, Al-Hasan SFA, Semple M, et al: The effects of amrinone on platelet count, survival and function in patients with congestive heart failure. Br J Clin Pharmacol 17:317, 1984.
101. Saborowski F, Griebenow R, Sirinyan G, et al: Metabolische und hamodynamische Befunde nache Gabe von Amrinone bei Patienten mit koronarer Herzkrankheit. Z Kardiol 7(Suppl 1):81, 1983.
102. Uretsky BF, Lawless CE, Verbalis JG, et al: Combined therapy with dobutamine and amrinone in severe heart failure. Chest 92:657, 1987.
103. Campbell CA, Mehta PM, Wynne J, et al: The cardiotonic agent amrinone does not increase anatomic infarct size. J Cardiovasc Pharmacol 9:225, 1986.
104. Fita G, Gomar C, Jimenez MJ, et al: Amrinone in perioperative low cardiac output syndrome. Acta Anaesthesiol Scand 34:482, 1990.
105. Dupuis JY, Bondy R, Cattran C, et al: Amrinone and dobutamine as primary treatment of low cardiac output syndrome following coronary artery surgery: A comparison of their effects on hemodynamics and outcome. J Cardiothorac Vasc Anesth 6:542, 1992.
106. Olsen KH, Kluger J, Fieldman A: Combination high dose amrinone and dopamine in the management of moribund cardiogenic shock after open heart surgery. Chest 94:503, 1988.
107. Deeb GM, Bolling SF, Guynn TP, et al: Amrinone versus conventional therapy in pulmonary hypertensive patients awaiting cardiac transplantation. Ann Thorac Surg 48:665, 1989.
108. Deeb GM, Bolling SF: The role of amrinone in potential heart transplant patients with pulmonary hypertension. J Cardiothorac Anesth 3:33, 1989.
109. Bernardini C, Del-Tacca M, Danesi R, et al: The influence of amrinone on cardiac toxicity induced by adriamycin in rats. Arch Int Pharmacodyn Ther 283:243, 1986.
110. Makela VH, Kopur PA: Amrinone blunts cardiac depression caused by enflurane and isoflurane anesthesia in the dog. Anesth Analg 66:215, 1987.
111. Levene D, Secter RA: Amrinone: A weaning agent in catecholamine dependence. Clin Cardiol 7:563, 1984.
112. Goenen M, Col J, Compere A, et al: Treatment of severe verapamil poisoning with combined amrinone-isoproterenol therapy. Am J Cardiol 58:1142, 1986.
113. Wolf LR, Spadafora MP, Otten EJ: Use of amrinone and glucagon in a case of calcium channel blocker overdose. Ann Emerg Med 22:1225, 1993.
114. Hantson PH, Ronveau JL, De Conick D, et al: Amrinone for refractory cardiogenic shock following chloroquine poisoning. Intensive Care Med 17:430, 1991.
115. Treadway G: Clinical safety of intravenous amrinone—A review. Am J Cardiol 56:39B, 1985.
116. Ansell J, Tiarks C, McCue J, et al: Amrinone-induced thrombocytopenia. Arch Intern Med 144:949, 1984.
117. Gilman ME, Margolis SC: Amrinone induced hepatoxicity. Clin Pharm 3:422, 1984.
118. Dunkman WB, Wilen MM, Franciosa JA: Adverse effects of long term amrinone administration in congestive heart failure. Am Heart J 105:861, 1983.
119. Silke B, Verma SP, Midtbo KA, et al: Comparative haemodynamic dose-response effects of dobutamine and amrinone in left ventricular failure complicating acute myocardial infarction. J Cardiovasc Pharm 9:19, 1987.
120. Alousi AA, Johnson DC: Pharmacology of the bipyridines: Amrinone and milrinone. Circulation 73(Suppl III):10, 1986.

CHAPTER 130

Milrinone

Marvin A. Konstam, M.D., and Carey D. Kimmelstiel, M.D.

Peak III phosphodiesterase (PDE-III) inhibitors are a recent addition to the pharmacologic armamentarium for achieving hemodynamic improvement in patients with acute congestive heart failure (CHF). Milrinone is the second PDE-III inhibitor approved for intravenous use; it is approximately 30 times more potent than its progenitor, amrinone.[1]

PHARMACOLOGY

The hemodynamic and clinical actions of milrinone in patients with heart failure result from a combination of inotropic and vasodilating properties. The improvement in indices of left ventricular relaxation and compliance reported with milrinone administration likely results from a combination of effects on myocardial relaxation and on loading characteristics, and it contributes to the drug's salutary hemodynamic effects.[2-4]

Milrinone's inotropic effect is thought to be mediated via cyclic adenosine monophosphate (cAMP). Milrinone inhibits PDE-III, the predominant phosphodiesterase in myocardium, resulting in increased concentrations of cAMP (Fig. 130–1).[4-6] cAMP activates protein kinases, resulting in phosphorylation of proteins involved in the control of voltage-dependent calcium channels of the plasma membrane and of the sarcoplasmic reticulum. Thus, increased myocyte contractility results from increased calcium delivery, along concentration gradients, to the contractile elements.[4, 5, 7] In addition to effects on membrane permeability and calcium flux during myocyte depolarization, cAMP activates phospholamban, which in turn stimulates energy-dependent calcium reuptake by the sarcoplasmic reticulum during repolarization.[6] Thus, milrinone, through phosphodiesterase inhibition and increased intracellular concentrations of cAMP, may accelerate calcium reuptake and myocardial diastolic relaxation. Although not established, it is likely that the vasodilator effects of milrinone are derived from phosphodiesterase inhibition, with resulting increases in cAMP concentration within vascular smooth muscle cells.[4, 8]

In addition to phosphodiesterase inhibition, it has been postulated that a portion of milrinone's physiologic actions are mediated via inhibition of the inhibitory guanine nucleotide binding protein (G_i-protein).[9] G_i inhibits the action of the β-adrenergic agonist-receptor complex on adenylate cyclase. Downregulation of this modulating protein would result in inotropic augmentation, increased sensitivity to β-adrenergic stimulation, and potential synergy between milrinone and β-adrenergic agonists.[9]

PHARMACOKINETICS

Intravenous bolus doses of 10 μg/kg and 125 μg/kg achieve serum milrinone concentrations of approximately 63 ng/ml and 639 ng/ml, respectively. The plasma elimination half-life of milrinone in healthy subjects is approximately 50 minutes.[10] Milrinone is primarily eliminated by renal excretion, with 80% to 85% recovered unchanged in the urine within 24 hours following intravenous administration to normal subjects. Renal clearance exceeds the glomerular filtration rate, suggesting that tubular secretion is involved.[1]

The pharmacokinetics of milrinone are altered in patients with heart failure.[11] In patients with moderate to severe heart failure (New York Heart Association [NYHA] functional class III to IV), intravenous bolus doses ranging from 12.5 to 75 μg/kg resulted in milrinone concentrations (measured 5 minutes after administration) that were linearly related to dose and ranged from approximately 80 to 450 ng/ml. Plasma elimination half-life was approximately double that seen in healthy subjects, averaging 1.7 hours.[10]

EFFECTS ON PATHOPHYSIOLOGY
Effects on Hemodynamics

In patients with heart failure, milrinone increases cardiac output, reduces left and right ventricular filling pressures, and reduces systemic and pulmonary vas-

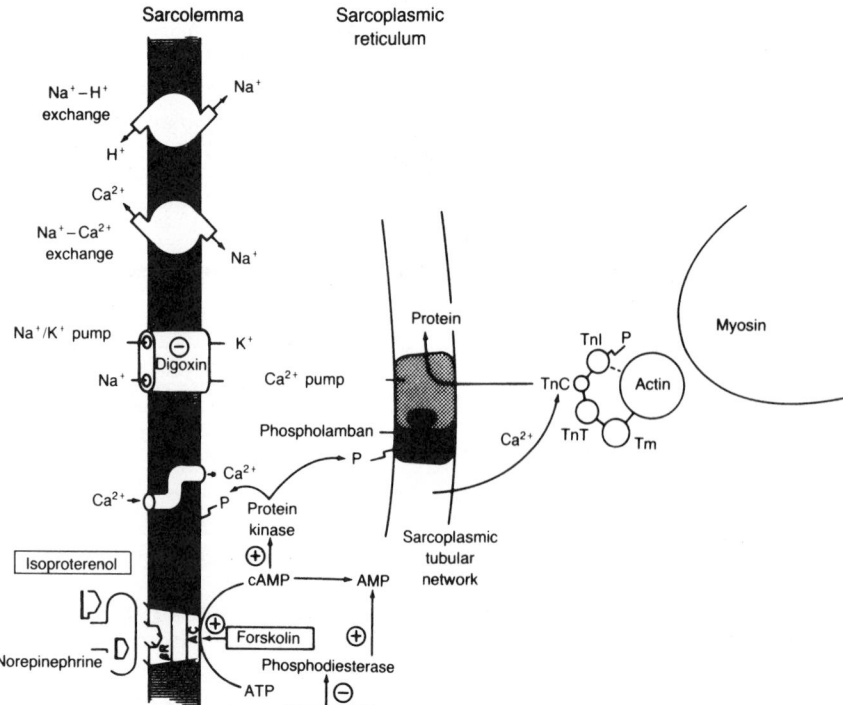

Figure 130–1. Role of cyclic adenosine monophosphate (cAMP) in myocardial contraction and mechanism of action of inotropic drugs. AC, adenylate cyclase; AMP, adenosine monophosphate; ATP, adenosine triphosphate; βR, beta-adrenergic receptor; P, phosphorylation; TnI, TnC, TnT, Tm, troponin-tropomyosin complex. (Adapted from Morgan JP: Abnormal intracellular modulation of calcium as a major cause of cardiac contractile dysfunction. N Engl J Med 325:625, 1991. Reprinted by permission of the New England Journal of Medicine.)

cular resistances.[7, 12–14] In the presence of a dilated left ventricle and elevated pulmonary artery wedge pressure, milrinone tends to cause a slight reduction in blood pressure; however, the blood pressure may be more markedly reduced in the presence of a nondilated left ventricle or reduced preload (pulmonary artery wedge pressure < 15 mmHg). Milrinone tends to increase heart rate slightly.

Hemodynamic responses to a range of intravenous doses of milrinone were evaluated in 189 patients with stable heart failure (NYHA functional class III or IV) in whom reduced ejection fraction was due to either ischemic heart disease or dilated cardiomyopathy.[15] Enrollment required a cardiac index of 2.5 L/min/M[2] or less or a pulmonary artery wedge pressure of at least 15 mmHg. A loading dose was administered over 10 minutes, followed by a 48-hour infusion. Doses were 37.5 µg/kg bolus, 0.375 µg/kg/min infusion; 50 µg/kg bolus, 0.50 µg/kg/min infusion; and 75 µg/kg bolus, 0.75 µg/kg/min infusion. Fifteen minutes after initiation of low-dose, medium-dose, and high-dose infusion, the mean cardiac output increased by 33%, 48%, and 56%, respectively (Fig. 130–2), and mean stroke work index increased by 33%, 60%, and 54%, respectively. Mean pulmonary artery wedge pressure and systemic vascular resistance decreased by 24% to 33% (Fig. 130–3) and 15% to 31%, respectively (Fig. 130–4). Mean arterial pressure decreased by 2% to 6% during milrinone infusion at low and moderate doses and by 8% to 16% during high-

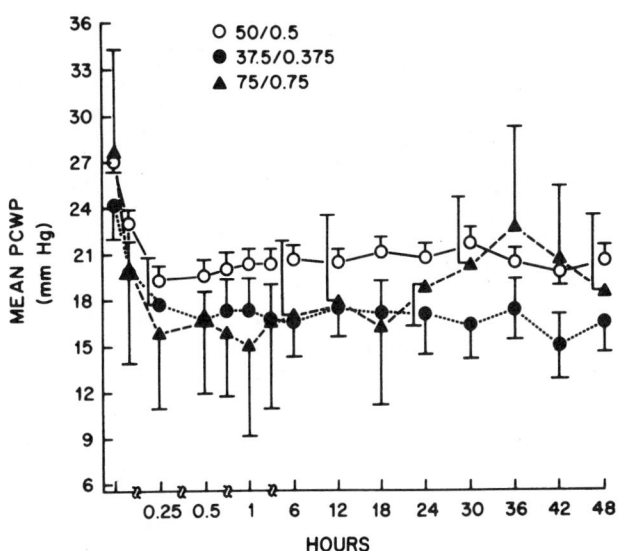

Figure 130–3. Mean pulmonary capillary wedge pressure (PCWP) over a 48-hour milrinone infusion period for different doses. "75/0.75" refers to patients who received a 75-µg/kg loading dose followed by an infusion of 0.75 µg/kg/min; "50/0.5" refers to patients who received a 50-µg/kg loading dose followed by an infusion of 0.50 µg/kg/min; and "37.5/0.375" refers to patients who received a 37-µg/kg loading dose followed by an infusion of 0.375 µg/kg/min. (Adapted from Anderson JL, Baim DS, Fein SA, et al: Efficacy and safety of sustained [48-hour] intravenous infusions of milrinone in patients with severe congestive heart failure: A multicenter study. J Am Coll Cardiol 9:711, 1987. Reprinted with permission from the American College of Cardiology.)

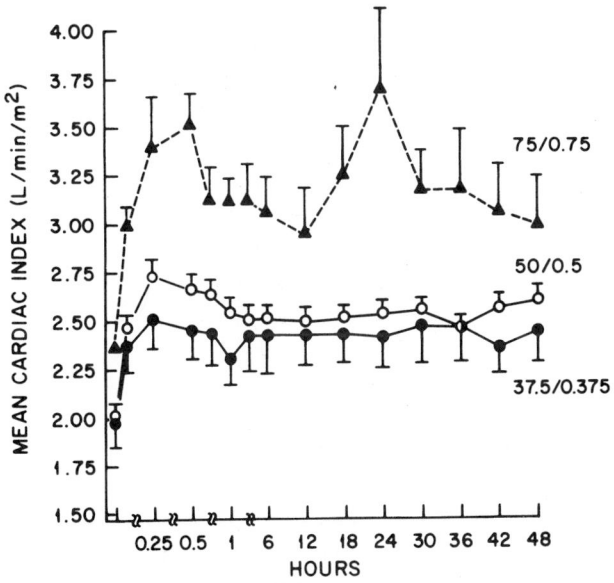

Figure 130–2. Mean cardiac index over a 48-hour milrinone infusion period. "75/0.75" refers to patients who received a 75-µg/kg loading dose followed by an infusion of 0.75 µg/kg/min; "50/0.5" refers to patients who received a 50-µg/kg loading dose followed by an infusion of 0.50 µg/kg/min; and "37.5/0.375" refers to patients who received a 37-µg/kg loading dose followed by an infusion of 0.375 µg/kg/min. (Adapted from Anderson JL, Baim DS, Fein SA, et al: Efficacy and safety of sustained [48-hour] intravenous infusions of milrinone in patients with severe congestive heart failure: A multicenter study. J Am Coll Cardiol 9:711, 1987. Reprinted with permission from the American College of Cardiology.)

dose infusion. Heart rate tended to increase slightly at all doses. Hemodynamic effects tended to remain fairly stable during the 48-hour infusion (see Figs. 130–2 to 130–5).

A similar study enrolled 105 patients with NYHA functional class III or class IV heart failure but administered only a single-dose regimen: a 50 µg/kg loading dose over 10 minutes, followed by a 48-hour infusion of 0.50 µg/kg/min.[16] Fifteen minutes after initiation of infusion, cardiac output increased by an average of 38%, stroke volume increased by 34%, pulmonary artery wedge pressure decreased by 28%, and mean systemic vascular resistance decreased by 23%. These hemodynamic effects remained fairly stable during the 48-hour infusion. Heart rate increased gradually during the period of infusion, reaching a maximum of 12% above baseline.

Hemodynamic effects of intravenous milrinone and dobutamine were compared in 82 patients with stable heart failure (NYHA functional class III to IV).[17] Most of the patients randomized to milrinone received a loading dose of 50 µg/kg over 10 minutes followed by an infusion of 0.50 µg/kg/min for 48 hours. The infusion rate could be increased to 0.62 µg/kg/min at 24 hours, based on hemodynamic effect. Patients randomized to dobutamine were titrated from an initial infusion rate of 2.5 µg/kg/min to a maximum of 15 µg/kg/min until hemodynamic benefit or adverse effect was observed, with infusions continuing for 48 hours. Both drugs increased cardiac output and stroke

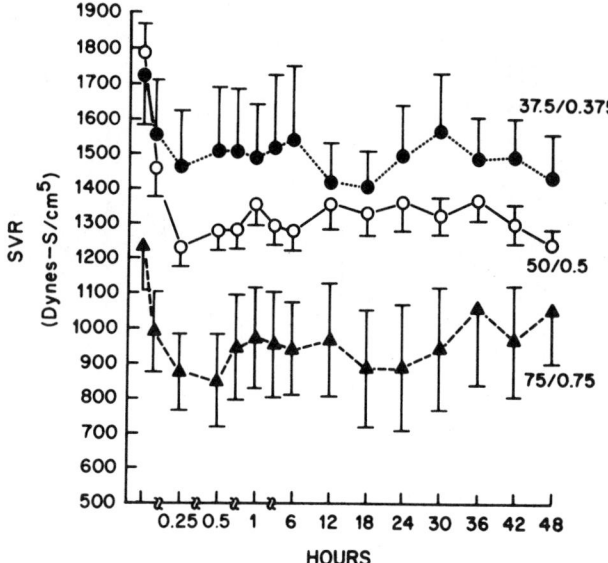

Figure 130–4. Systemic vascular resistance (SVR) over a 48-hour milrinone infusion period for different doses. "75/0.75" refers to patients who received a 75-μg/kg loading dose followed by an infusion of 0.75 μg/kg/min; "50/0.5" refers to patients who received a 50-μg/kg loading dose followed by an infusion of 0.50 μg/kg/min; and "37.5/0.375" refers to patients who received a 37-μg/kg loading dose followed by an infusion of 0.375 μg/kg/min. (Adapted from Anderson JL, Baim DS, Fein SA, et al: Efficacy and safety of sustained [48-hour] intravenous infusions of milrinone in patients with severe congestive heart failure: A multicenter study. J Am Coll Cardiol 9:711, 1987. Reprinted with permission from the American College of Cardiology.)

volume while reducing pulmonary artery wedge pressure and systemic vascular resistance. The hemodynamic benefits remained stable for the entire 48 hours.

The two drugs showed few differences. At 3 hours, heart rate was higher in dobutamine-treated patients than in milrinone-treated patients; thereafter, heart rates were similar. Blood pressure was reduced slightly in patients receiving milrinone and not in those receiving dobutamine; this difference was evident primarily during the early hours of the infusion, and tended to disappear by the second day. Pulmonary capillary wedge pressure decreased more in patients receiving milrinone; again, this difference was most evident early into the infusion.

In another trial,[18] 15 patients with NYHA functional class III or IV heart failure received increasing sequential doses of dobutamine (up to 14 μg/kg/min) and milrinone (up to 75 μg/kg). The two drugs induced comparable increases in cardiac index, stroke volume index, stroke work index, and heart rate, but milrinone induced greater reduction in mean arterial pressure, systemic vascular resistance, and left- and right-sided heart filling pressures. The peak rate of left ventricular pressure rise (dP/dt) increased more with dobutamine.

Thus, administration of milrinone to patients with heart failure, a dilated left ventricle, and elevated left ventricular filling pressure results in augmentation of

cardiac output and a reduction in ventricular filling pressures with a slight reduction in blood pressure and a slight increase in heart rate.

EFFECTS ON VENTRICULAR FUNCTION
Inotropic Actions

Evidence for clinically relevant positive inotropic action by milrinone in patients with heart failure comes from studies comparing the hemodynamic effects of milrinone and nitroprusside and from observations during direct intracoronary infusion of milrinone. Doses sufficient to produce equivalent decreases in mean arterial pressure in 11 patients resulted in significant increases in peak positive left ventricular dP/dt by intravenous milrinone but not by nitroprusside.[12] In a study designed to test the inotropic action of milrinone, independent of peripheral vasodilation, intracoronary milrinone was administered to 11 patients with NYHA functional class III or class IV heart failure.[19] Infusion at a rate of 6 μg/min resulted in significant increases in peak positive left ventricular dP/dt, whereas doses of approximately 200 μg/min

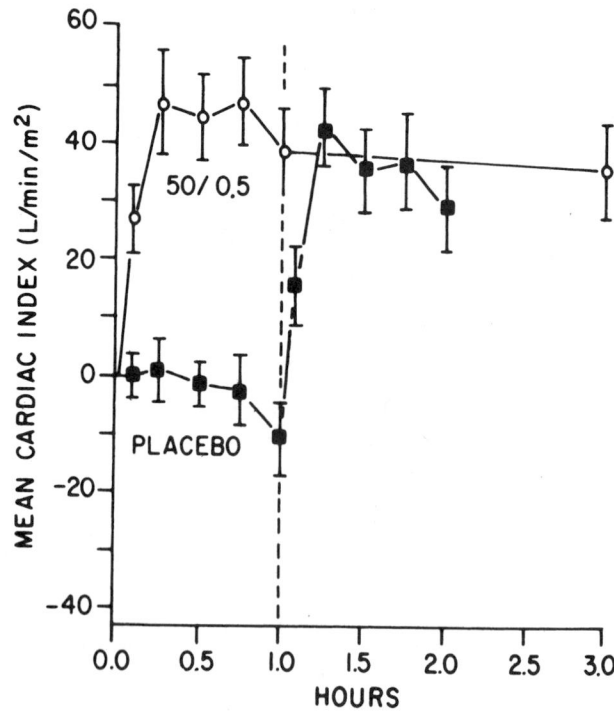

Figure 130–5. Mean cardiac index in patients receiving either milrinone or placebo infusion. Cardiac index increased in patients who received a milrinone loading dose of 50 μg/kg followed by a continuous infusion of 0.50 μg/kg/min but did not change during a placebo infusion; it also increased in patients (*dashed line*) who initially received placebo after they were switched to milrinone. (Adapted from Anderson JL, Baim DS, Fein SA, et al: Efficacy and safety of sustained [48-hour] intravenous infusions of milrinone in patients with severe congestive heart failure: A multicenter study. J Am Coll Cardiol 9:711, 1987. Reprinted with permission from the American College of Cardiology.)

were needed to induce significant reduction in systemic and pulmonary vascular resistances.

Effects on Diastolic Function

In 17 patients with heart failure,[20] incremental doses of milrinone up to 75 μg/kg increased peak negative left ventricular dP/dt by an average of 18% and significantly shortened the time constants of left ventricular relaxation. The maximal left ventricular filling rate increased by an average of 42%, whereas the pulmonary artery wedge pressure decreased. Individual diastolic pressure-volume curves were shifted downward, with reduction in left ventricular end-diastolic pressure by approximately 31%. The downward shifts appeared to be parallel, with little, if any, change in the pressure-volume slope. Thus, milrinone appears to directly augment myocardial relaxation, presumably through increases in intracellular cAMP. Changes in late-diastolic pressure-volume relationships may reflect an effect of milrinone on myocardial compliance, but are more likely to result from changes in extramyocardial factors, particularly relief of constraint by the right side of the heart.

Effects on the Right Ventricle

Milrinone has been found to augment right ventricular systolic performance in patients with left-sided heart failure, with augmentation in ejection fraction, and with reduced radionuclide-derived right ventricular end-systolic volume, as well as end-diastolic volume.[21] These effects are primarily related to a simultaneous reduction in right ventricular afterload and preload due to systemic and pulmonary vasodilation and to reduction in pulmonary venous pressure, with a modest contribution of augmented right ventricular contractility.

EFFECTS ON ELECTROPHYSIOLOGY AND CARDIAC RHYTHM

In 10 patients with NYHA functional class III or IV heart failure,[22] intravenously administered milrinone (50 μg/kg loading dose and 0.5 μg/kg/min infusion for 18 hours) had little effect on most electrophysiologic parameters (Table 130–1). Maximal 1:1 atrioventricular conduction time decreased by 6.1%.

A number of clinical investigations have indicated that milrinone, administered in therapeutic doses in patients with heart failure, may induce or aggravate ventricular arrhythmias. Comparison of Holter recordings before and after initiation of intravenous milrinone treatment in 12 patients with heart failure[23] revealed an increase in the average number of premature ventricular contractions from 62 to 123 per hour, an increase in couplets from 2 to 8 per hour, and in runs of ventricular tachycardia from 0.3 to 2.6 per hour. Published criteria[24–26] were used to identify a proarrhythmic effect in 2 of the 12 patients.

Table 130–1. **Electrophysiologic Measurements Before and After Intravenous Milrinone Administration (n = 10)**

Measurement	Control	Milrinone	p Value
Spontaneous cycle length	654 ± 135	643 ± 131	NS
PR interval	192 ± 37	188 ± 42	NS
QRS duration	141 ± 32	135 ± 27	NS
Corrected QT interval	448 ± 38	460 ± 46	NS
AH interval	97 ± 59	101 ± 69	NS
HV interval	59 ± 11	56 ± 8	NS
Atrial ERP	241 ± 47	236 ± 35	NS
Atrial FRP	282 ± 59	274 ± 27	NS
Atrioventricular ERP	293 ± 78	279 ± 44	NS
Atrioventricular FRP	365 ± 26	362 ± 63	NS
1:1 maximal atrioventricular conduction time	399 ± 133	374 ± 121	.01
1:1 maximal ventriculoatrial conduction time	470 ± 110	453 ± 78	NS
Ventricular ERP	246 ± 19	246 ± 24	NS
Ventricular FRP	267 ± 22	267 ± 32	NS
Maximal corrected sinus node recovery time	264 ± 103	190 ± 78	NS

All values listed in milliseconds (mean ± standard deviation).
ERP, effective refractory period; FRP, functional refractory period; NS, not significant.
Adapted with permission from Geraci SA, Gray EL, Goldstein RA, et al: Electrophysiologic effects of milrinone in patients with congestive heart failure. Am J Cardiol 57:624, 1986.

In another study of 47 patients,[16] milrinone treatment was associated with an increase in the number of premature ventricular contractions from 33 to 85 per hour, an increase in the frequency of ventricular tachycardia from 2.3 to 8.9 runs per hour, and an increase in the mean number of couplets per hour from 2 to 6.5 during the 48-hour milrinone infusion. Published criteria[24–26] were used to establish a proarrhythmic effect of milrinone in 10 (21%) of the patients. These results are similar to those of another study in which the frequency of premature ventricular contractions, episodes of ventricular tachycardia, frequency of ventricular couplets, and total repetitive forms were increased compared with such parameters in premilrinone therapy.[27] Eight patients met proarrhythmic criteria in this trial.

In a randomized, comparative trial of 48 hours of infusion of either milrinone or dobutamine in patients with heart failure,[17] in doses achieving comparable effect on cardiac output, there was no identifiable difference between the two agents regarding the induction of ventricular arrhythmia. The incidence of arrhythmias that were considered to represent adverse events was low with both drugs. Since these findings were based on routine cardiac rhythm monitoring, rather than on Holter recordings, they cannot be taken as the definitive word regarding the relative arrhythmogenicity of milrinone and dobutamine.

In summary, milrinone, administered in therapeutic doses for treatment of heart failure, appears to induce or aggravate ventricular arrhythmias in some patients. Most patients do not manifest rigorous criteria for proarrhythmia, and cessation of therapy or cardioversion for life-threatening arrhythmia is unusual during infusion of milrinone for hours to days. Monitoring of cardiac rhythm during drug administration is warranted.

Effects on Myocardial Energetics

When administered systemically to patients with heart failure, milrinone may effect a slight increase in myocardial oxygen consumption.[28] However, in doses of milrinone and dobutamine achieving comparable augmentation in cardiac output, only dobutamine was found to increase myocardial oxygen consumption.[13, 29] The potential for increased oxygen demand related to milrinone's inotropic effect was presumably offset by reduction in wall stress. Milrinone tends to reduce coronary vascular resistance. With intravenous administration, the effect on resistance is partially offset by the mild reduction in coronary perfusion pressure, resulting in no change or a slight increase in coronary blood flow and no change or a slight reduction in coronary arterial-venous difference in oxygen content.[28–30]

Effects on the Vasculature

The direct vasodilator effect of milrinone has been documented in human subjects during infusion into the brachial artery of 13 patients with chronic CHF.[31] With infusion rates that did not produce therapeutic systemic concentrations or detectible changes in systemic hemodynamics, milrinone reduced forearm vascular resistance and increased forearm blood flow. The clinical relevance of these findings is suggested by the observation that, in doses of milrinone and dobutamine that achieve comparable augmentation in cardiac output in patients with heart failure, milrinone tends to induce a greater reduction in mean arterial pressure and in ventricular filling pressure.[17]

Effects on Renal Function

As detailed previously, the clinical utility of milrinone is due both to its positive inotropism and to vasodilatory actions. *Ex vivo* studies in human renal arteries have shown potent vasodilation in response to milrinone.[32] Given these effects, one might expect improvement in parameters reflective of renal function in response to milrinone administration, especially considering the disproportionate shunting of blood away from the kidney in CHF patients.[33]

In a comparison of milrinone and captopril, both drugs induced an increase in renal blood flow (RBF), although the response was greater with captopril.[34] Increases in RBF were observed in response to single oral doses of both agents, an effect that tended to be greater with captopril. When milrinone was administered intravenously following captopril administration, RBF was not further augmented despite improvement in cardiac performance. Most patients studied in this trial were in a postprandial state that may, by itself, induce augmentation in RBF.[35]

In 13 CHF patients treated with orally administered milrinone for 1 month, there were no changes in RBF,

renal vascular resistance, or glomerular filtration rate (GFR) compared with prestudy baseline values.[36] However, patients whose cardiac index increased by more than 30% experienced uniform augmentation in GFR and were more likely to evidence elevation in RBF. The lack of a more profound benefit of milrinone on renal function in this study may variably be due to stimulation of renin production by milrinone,[33] tolerance to its effects, cAMP-induced reduction in GFR,[37] or other factors.

In summary, milrinone appears to have a salutary acute effect on RBF. Milrinone-induced augmentation of RBF may not translate into an equivalent improvement in GFR because vasodilation could interfere with glomerular autoregulation.[33] The limited available data relating to long-term administration suggest that milrinone therapy produces no consistent benefit to renal function.

CLINICAL USE
Indications

Intravenously administered milrinone is indicated for the treatment of patients with exacerbation of heart failure associated with reduced systolic performance to increase cardiac output and peripheral perfusion, to reduce left- and right-sided heart filling pressures, or both. It has been shown to be effective for a minimum of 48 hours, and in the absence of demonstrable tachyphylaxis, it is likely to maintain these effects for more prolonged periods of administration.

In addition to exacerbations of established heart failure, milrinone is likely to be effective in operative and perioperative management of patients with ventricular dysfunction and in patients with hemodynamic compromise related to acute myocardial infarction. However, at the time of this writing, the efficacy and safety of milrinone in these settings had not been adequately evaluated, and these indications had not been recognized by the Food and Drug Administration. Prolonged administration (weeks) may be warranted in some individuals, particularly severely immunocompromised patients awaiting cardiac transplantation.

Investigation of the use of milrinone in primary valvular heart disease has been limited. Milrinone is likely to improve hemodynamics in patients with heart failure and dilated left ventricles due to aortic regurgitation or mitral regurgitation.

Precautions and Adverse Effects

Although short-term infusion has not been associated with a substantial incidence of arrhythmias requiring specific treatment, the potential for proarrhythmia indicates the need for continuous monitoring of cardiac rhythm during milrinone infusion. Although a relationship between milrinone-induced proarrhythmia and electrolyte imbalance has not been identified, it appears prudent to monitor and attempt to normalize potassium and magnesium levels during treatment.

In most patients with heart failure, milrinone induces only a modest reduction in blood pressure. However, significant hypotension may occur, particularly in patients with baseline pulmonary artery wedge pressures below 15 mmHg. Therefore, if the presence of elevation in left ventricular filling pressure cannot be ascertained clinically, insertion of a pulmonary artery catheter is indicated prior to institution of milrinone therapy.

Milrinone's mild capacity to increase heart rate seldom constitutes a substantial clinical limitation.[8, 13, 16, 17] However, care should be exercised in instituting milrinone treatment in patients with atrial fibrillation or other supraventricular arrhythmias in whom ventricular response is poorly controlled.

Milrinone is reported to be associated with a small incidence of thrombocytopenia (approximately 2%). This incidence is considerably lower than that reported with amrinone, and may be more closely related to associated conditions or concomitant medications than to the medication itself. Adverse events associated wtih the use of amrinone are summarized in Table 130–2.

Interest in the long-term use of orally administered milrinone was lost following the observation of a 28% excess mortality rate, over 1 year, among patients with severe heart failure randomized to long-term oral milrinone therapy compared with patients randomized to placebo.[38] It is not certain whether this finding is related to milrinone's arrhythmogenic potential, an effect of long-term administration on cardiac structure or function, or a combination of these factors.

Contraindications

As discussed earlier, the use of milrinone in patients with normal or low left ventricular filling pressures may be associated with significant hypotension and should be avoided.

Table 130–2. **Adverse Events with Intravenous Milrinone in 189 Patients Enrolled in the U.S. Multicenter Trial**

Adverse Event	Number of Patients (%)
Angina	1 (0.5)
Chest pain	1 (0.5)
Headache	7 (3.7)
Hypotension	4 (2.1)
Nausea	1 (0.5)
Diarrhea	1 (0.5)
Hypokalemia	2 (1.1)
Oliguria	1 (0.5)
Pulmonary edema	1 (0.5)
Somnolence	1 (0.5)
Thrombocytopenia	4 (2.2)
Tremor	1 (0.5)

Adapted from Anderson JL, Baim DS, Fein SA, et al: Efficacy and safety of sustained (48-hour) intravenous infusions of milrinone in patients with severe congestive heart failure: A multicenter study. J Am Coll Cardiol 9:711, 1987. Reprinted with permission from the American College of Cardiology.

Little or no experience exists with use of the drug in patients with heart failure associated with preserved systolic function, including those with hypertrophic myopathy. Although milrinone may augment the rate of myocardial relaxation and could therefore benefit the impairment of diastolic performance in such patients, the absence of left ventricular dilation is likely to render them excessively sensitive to milrinone's vasodilator effects—that is, to induce hypotension out of proportion to any increase in cardiac output. Therefore, until this use has been investigated, milrinone should be avoided or used with extreme caution in such patients. Similar cautions apply to patients with aortic stenosis.

Use in Patients with Impaired Renal Function

The predominant route of milrinone excretion is renal, with active tubular secretion.[1] Severe renal impairment results in a prolonged half-life of milrinone, necessitating dose reduction in this clinical setting (see later section, Dosage and Administration).

Place in the Arsenal for Treatment of Acute Heart Failure

The hemodynamic profile of milrinone is similar to that of dobutamine. Compared with dobutamine, milrinone's relatively greater direct vasodilator effect tends to result in slightly greater reduction in ventricular filling pressures and slightly greater reduction in blood pressure in doses achieving the same augmentation in cardiac output. Milrinone is a rational first-line agent in patients in whom the goal is to achieve both reduction of left ventricular filling pressure and augmentation of cardiac output. If blood pressure is marginal, it is reasonable to consider initiation of treatment with dobutamine and to add milrinone as needed for additional hemodynamic benefit. In patients with adequate blood pressure, the combination of milrinone and pure vasodilators, such as nitroglycerin or nitroprusside, is an effective regimen.

The likelihood of a contribution of direct pulmonary vasodilator effect to milrinone's actions make it an effective choice for patients with evidence of significant right-sided heart failure. Milrinone alone or combined with pure vasodilators, dobutamine, or low-dose dopamine may be expected to augment renal perfusion and facilitate diuresis.

Dosage and Administration

Typically, intravenous milrinone therapy is initiated with a bolus of 50 µg/kg, administered over 10 minutes, followed by a continuous infusion at 0.50 µg/kg/min. In patients with a creatinine clearance of 0 to 30 ml/min/1.73 m², the infusion rate should be diminished to 0.20 to 0.33 µg/kg/min.

CONCLUSIONS

The present role for intravenous milrinone therapy is in the short-term management of acute heart failure. In this setting, the most appropriate therapeutic regimen is dictated by the specific hemodynamic profile at presentation.[39, 40]

Milrinone may rationally be used to augment cardiac output, to reduce pulmonary capillary wedge pressure, or both. These goals can be achieved without adversely affecting myocardial oxygen demand. The hemodynamic benefits are derived through inotropic and vasodilating effects and possibly by effects on myocardial relaxation. Milrinone may be combined with other inotropes such as dobutamine and other vasodilators such as nitroprusside or nitroglycerin.

Compared with milrinone, dobutamine has less vasodilatory potency; thus, for a given degree of augmentation in cardiac output, milrinone can produce a greater reduction in left- and right-sided heart filling pressures and in blood pressure.[18, 29] It has been suggested that the inotropic potency of dobutamine may be diminished in patients with high circulating concentrations of catecholamines, a common finding in patients with acute heart failure. However, the clinical significance of this finding is uncertain. The inotropic potency of milrinone should not be similarly affected.[18] In contrast with milrinone, dobutamine has been found to induce slight increases in myocardial oxygen consumption.[13, 29] The plasma elimination half-life of milrinone is longer than that of dobutamine, and therefore milrinone's effects persist longer than those of dobutamine. The longer plasma half-life also necessitates the use of loading doses prior to initiating continuous infusions. Because the salutary effects of nitroprusside are solely mediated via vasodilation, augmented cardiac output and reduced filling pressures are likely to be associated with greater reductions in blood pressure compared with milrinone. Thus, considering hemodynamic effects, milrinone can be viewed as combining the pharmacologic effects of dobutamine and nitroprusside.

REFERENCES

1. Alousi AA, Fabian RJ, Baker JF, Stroshane RM: Milrinone. *In* Scriabine A (ed): New Drugs Annual: Cardiovascular Drugs, Vol 3. New York: Raven Press, 1985, pp 245–283.
2. Chatterjee K: Newer oral inotropic agents: Phosphodiesterase inhibitors. Crit Care Med 18:S34, 1990.
3. Grossman W: Diastolic dysfunction and congestive heart failure. Circulation 81(Suppl 3):1, 1990.
4. Colucci WS: Cardiovascular effects of milrinone. Am Heart J 121:1945, 1991.
5. Sanders MR, Kostis JB, Frishman WH: The use of inotropic agents in acute and chronic congestive heart failure. Med Clin North Am 73:283, 1989.
6. Morgan JP: Abnormal intracellular modulation of calcium as a major cause of cardiac contractile dysfunction. N Engl J Med 325:625, 1991.
7. Colucci WS, Wright RF, Braunwald E: New positive inotropic agents in the treatment of congestive heart failure: mechanisms of action and recent clinical developments (second of two parts). N Engl J Med 314:349, 1986.
8. LeJemtel TH, Scortichini D, Levitt B, Sonnenblick EH: Effects of phosphodiesterase inhibition on skeletal muscle vasculature. Am J Cardiol 63:27A, 1989.
9. Stiles GL: Adrenergic receptor responsiveness and congestive heart failure. Am J Cardiol 67:13C, 1991.
10. Stroshane RM, Koss RF, Biddlecome CE, et al: Oral and intravenous pharmacokinetics of milrinone in human volunteers. J Pharm Sci 73:1438, 1984.
11. Benotti JR, Lesko LJ, McCue JE, Alpert JS: Pharmacokinetics and pharmacodynamics of milrinone in chronic congestive heart failure. Am J Cardiol 56:685, 1985.
12. Jaski BE, Fifer MA, Wright RF, et al: Positive inotropic and vasodilator actions of milrinone in patients with severe congestive heart failure: Dose-response relationships and comparison to nitroprusside. J Clin Invest 75:643, 1985.
13. Monrad ES, Baim DS, Smith HS, Lanoue AS: Milrinone, dobutamine, and nitroprusside: Comparative effects on hemodynamics and myocardial energetics in patients with severe congestive heart failure. Circulation 73(Suppl 3):168, 1986.
14. Baim DS, McDowell AV, Cherniles J, et al: Evaluation of a new bipyridine inotropic agent—milrinone—in patients with severe congestive heart failure. N Engl J Med 309:748, 1983.
15. Anderson JL, Baim DS, Fein SA, et al: Efficacy and safety of sustained (48-hour) intravenous infusions of milrinone in patients with severe congestive heart failure: A multicenter study. J Am Coll Cardiol 9:711, 1987.
16. Pflugfelder PW, O'Neill BJ, Ogilvie RI, et al: A Canadian multicentre study of a 48-h infusion of milrinone in patients with severe heart failure. Can J Cardiol 7:5, 1991.
17. Biddle TL, Benotti JR, Creager MA, et al: Comparison of intravenous milrinone and dobutamine for congestive heart failure secondary to either ischemic or dilated cardiomyopathy. Am J Cardiol 59:1345, 1987.
18. Colucci WS, Wright RF, Jaski BE, et al: Milrinone and dobutamine in severe heart failure: Differing hemodynamic effects and individual patient responsiveness. Circulation 73(Suppl 3):175, 1986.
19. Ludmer PL, Wright RF, Arnold JMO, et al: Separation of the direct myocardial and vasodilator actions of milrinone administered by an intracoronary infusion technique. Circulation, 73:130, 1986.
20. Monrad ES, McKay RG, Baim DS, et al: Improvement in indexes of diastolic performance in patients with congestive heart failure treated with milrinone. Circulation 70:1030, 1984.
21. Eichhorn EJ, Konstam MA, Weiland DS, et al: Differential effects of milrinone and dobutamine on right ventricular preload, afterload and systolic performance in congestive heart failure secondary to ischemic or idiopathic dilated cardiomyopathy. Am J Cardiol 60:1329, 1987.
22. Goldstein RA, Geraci SA, Gray EL, et al: Electrophysiologic effects of milrinone in patients with congestive heart failure. Am J Cardiol 57:624, 1986.
23. Anderson JL, Askins JC, Gilbert EM, et al: Occurrence of ventricular arrhythmias in patients receiving acute and chronic infusions of milrinone. Am Heart J 111:466, 1986.
24. Velebit V, Podrid P, Lown B, et al: Aggravation and provocation of ventricular arrhythmias by antiarrhythmic drugs. Circulation 65:886, 1982.
25. Morganroth J, Horowitz LN: Flecainide: Its proarrhythmic effect and expected changes on the surface electrocardiogram. Am J Cardiol 53:89b, 1984.
26. The CAPS Investigators: The cardiac arrhythmia pilot study. Am J Cardiol 57:91, 1986.
27. Ferrick KJ, Fein SA, Ferrick AM, Doyle JT: Effect of milrinone on ventricular arrhythmias in congestive heart failure. Am J Cardiol 66:431, 1990.
28. Baim DS, Monrad ES, McDowell AV, et al: Milrinone therapy in patients with severe congestive heart failure: Initial hemodynamic and clinical observations. *In* Braunwald E, Sonnenblick EH, Chakrin LW, Schwarz RP (eds): Milrinone. Investigation of New Inotropic Therapy for Congestive Heart Failure. New York: 1984, pp 143–153.
29. Grose R, Strain J, Greenberg M, LeJemtel TH: Systemic and coronary effects of intravenous milrinone and dobutamine in congestive heart failure. J Am Coll Cardiol 7:1107, 1986.

30. Baim DS: Effect of phosphodiesterase inhibition on myocardial oxygen consumption and coronary blood flow. Am J Cardiol 63:23a, 1989.
31. Cody RJ, Müller FB, Kubo SH, et al: Identification of the direct vasodilator effect of milrinone with an isolated limb preparation in patients with chronic congestive heart failure. Circulation 73:124, 1986.
32. Lindgren S, Andersson K-E: Effects of selective phosphodiesterase inhibitors on isolated coronary, lung and renal arteries from man and rat. Acta Physiol Scand 142:77, 1991.
33. Cody RJ: Renal and hormonal effects of phosphodiesterase III inhibition in congestive heart failure. Am J Cardiol 63:31a, 1989.
34. LeJemtel TH, Maskin CS, Mancini D, et al: Systemic and regional hemodynamic effects of captopril and milrinone administered alone and concomitantly in patients with heart failure. Circulation 72:364, 1985.
35. King AJ, Levey AS: Dietary protein and renal function. J Am Soc Nephrol 3:1723, 1993.
36. Cody RJ, Kubo SH, Covit AB, et al: Regional blood flow and neurohormonal responses to milrinone in congestive heart failure. Clin Pharmacol Ther 39:128, 1986.
37. Dworkin LD, Ichikawa I, Brenner BM: Hormonal modulation of glomerular function. Am J Physiol 244:f95, 1983.
38. Packer M, Carver JR, Rodeheffer RJ, et al: Effect of oral milrinone on mortality in severe chronic heart failure. N Engl J Med 325:1468, 1991.
39. Roberts R: Inotropic therapy for cardiac failure associated with acute myocardial infarction. Chest 93(Suppl):22s, 1988.
40. Weber KT, Janicki JS, Maskin CS: Pathophysiology of cardiac failure. Am J Cardiol 56:3b, 1985.

CHAPTER 131

Vesnarinone

Michael L. Hess, M.D., Joshua B. Shipley, M.D., Ph.D., and David E. Tolman, M.D.

Vesnarinone (OPC-8212) is a synthetic quinolinone that represents a very promising new drug being developed for treatment of patients with congestive heart failure.

Both *in vitro* and *in vivo* studies in a variety of animal species have demonstrated a direct positive inotropic effect of vesnarinone.[1] In intact animals, the drug significantly increases myocardial contractility with only minimal effects on blood pressure and no direct positive chronotropic effect. Paradoxically, in isolated tissue preparations, vesnarinone produces a direct negative chronotropic effect. Further, while producing a positive inotropic effect, there is only minimal peripheral vasodilation, thus making the drug's action distinctly different from angiotensin-converting enzyme (ACE) inhibitors and phosphodiesterase (PDE) inhibitors. Indeed, vesnarinone's action is unlike most other current inotropic agents. It is not a digoxin-like compound, for it has no effect on Na^+,K^+-ATPase and is not analogous to either catecholamine agonists or antagonist because it has no effect on the β-receptor. Likewise, vesnarinone is not a calcium antagonist. Like the nonglycoside cardiotonic agents amrinone and milrinone, vesnarinone is a specific inhibitor of PDE and produces an increase in intracellular cyclic adenosine monophosphate (cAMP). However, this mechanism cannot explain the observed negative chronotropic effects of vesnarinone or the increase in action potential duration reminiscent of class III antiarrhythmic agents.

The clinical effects of vesnarinone are unique as well. Like other cardiotonic agents, when the drug is administered at levels that produce measurable hemodynamic response, patients experience a decrease in symptoms but mortality may actually increase. When the drug is administered at lower doses, however, there is still symptomatic improvement but

mortality may be decreased. Thus, it appears that vesnarinone acts by multiple mechanisms that make the drug unique among the various agents available for the treatment of congestive heart failure.

PHYSICOCHEMICAL PROPERTIES

Vesnarinone was first synthesized by Otsuka Pharmaceuticals in 1983 and has the chemical name 3,4-dihydro-6-[4-(3,4-dimethoxybenzoyl)-1-piperazinyl]-2(1H)-quinolinone. The physicochemical properties of this agent were described in detail by Shimizu et al.[2] The compound occurs as a pale yellow crystalline powder that is both odorless and tasteless. The drug is highly lipophilic with only slight solubility in aqueous solutions. Vesnarinone is chemically stable and does not demonstrate significant photosensitivity. The molecular weight is 395.46, and the molecular formula is $C_{22}H_{25}N_3O_4$.

Pharmacology

Vesnarinone has a distinct pharmacologic profile and may affect myocardial contractility via several mechanisms. Not only does the drug inhibit PDE in a manner similar to the bipyridine agents amrinone and milrinone, but it also shows electrophysiologic properties that reflect type III antiarrhythmic actions. A completely novel action of the drug, inhibition of cytokine production by leukocytes, has also been identified. Each of these effects is discussed in detail.

Electrophysiologic Effects

Recent work has shown that one of the mechanisms underlying the pharmacologic actions of vesnarinone may be a direct augmentation of transmembrane ion channel activity.[3] Vesnarinone has been shown to decrease the delayed and the inward rectifier potassium currents without interfering with the inward Ca^{2+} current.[4] Indeed, vesnarinone may increase the Ca^{2+} inward flux. This latter effect is related to increased intracellular cAMP from inhibition of cyclic PDE. In addition, vesnarinone has been demonstrated to increase the action potential duration in isolated Purkinje fibers and ventricular myocytes.[5] These same authors were able to demonstrate that the mechanism of action potential prolongation was related to an increased open time of myocyte Na^+ channels leading to increased intracellular Na^+ activity and an increase in intracellular free Ca^{2+} via the Na^+/Ca^{2+} exchanger.[6] It has also been shown that vesnarinone produces rate-dependent effects on action potential duration and the effective refractory period without affecting the maximum rate of depolarization (V_{max}) in a manner similar to class III antiarrhythmics.[7]

The fact that vesnarinone increases intracellular cAMP via inhibition of PDE seems at odds with the observations that the drug has no positive chronotropic effect and demonstrates little vasodilating action. In fact, other cardiotonic agents such as the bipyridines amrinone and milrinone, which are potent PDE inhibitors, demonstrate profound peripheral vasodilating actions. In a study by Itoh et al., however, vesnarinone was shown to induce mild vasodilation not by PDE inhibition but, rather, by inhibiting the receptor-mediated Ca^{2+} channel and not the voltage-dependent Ca^{2+} channel of smooth muscle cells.[8] The concentration of drug required to decrease cytosolic Ca^{2+} in smooth muscle cells was considerably higher than that required to produce a positive inotropic response in isolated myocytes, which may explain the observed positive inotropy without concomitant vasodilation at therapeutic drug levels.

Another explanation of the unique hemodynamic profile demonstrated by vesnarinone may lie in its selective inhibition of cardiocyte PDE isoforms. In a study by Masuoka et al., vesnarinone was found to inhibit the cyclic guanosine monophosphate (cGMP)–inhibited PDE from myocytes 10 times more effectively than the cGMP-inhibited PDE from aorta.[9] These authors also found that the kinetics of inhibition by vesnarinone were of the mixed type, not the competitive type observed with amrinone or milrinone.

Immunomodulating Effects

In vitro, vesnarinone is capable of reducing the level of interleukin-6 (IL-6) and tumor necrosis factor (TNFα) secreted by mitogenically stimulated human peripheral lymphocytes. The level of cytokine production in stimulated cells is suppressed such that IL-6 and TNFα levels may fall to approach the level produced by nonstimulated cells. Other cytokines (IL-1αβ, ILNβ) produced by activated monocytes are not inhibited. This action points to a fairly specific inhibition of IL-6 and TNFα and has been observed in animal models of cytokine production *in vivo*.[10]

This anticytokine action directed against the proinflammatory cytokines IL-6 and TNFα may have very important ramifications in patients with congestive heart failure. The proinflammatory action of these cytokines may make a significant contribution to the pathogenesis of decompensated heart failure. It has now been shown that increases in both IL-6 and TNFα are associated with advanced heart failure. TNFα produces a reversible negative inotropic effect and experimentally is able to produce congestive failure with pulmonary edema. TNFα is also capable of producing a cardiomyopathy characterized by ventricular remodeling and ventricular dilation.[11] Further, it has been shown that the cardiomyopathic heart is quite capable of producing TNFα.[12]

The systemic effects of TNFα, including fever, cachexia, and muscle wasting, are well known. Further, the muscle wasting and negative nitrogen balance of advanced heart failure are well appreciated. This taken together with the negative inotropic effects of TNFα makes it interesting to speculate that TNFα plays an important role in the pathogenesis of decompensated congestive heart failure, and a very beneficial action of vesnarinone may be the inhibition of IL-6 and TNFα production.

It has been demonstrated that in a murine model of acute viral myocarditis both animal mortality and the extent of myocardial damage were limited by treatment with vesnarinone.[13] The beneficial effects of vesnarinone were shown to be related to the inhibition of natural killer cell activity. Interestingly, when animals were treated with amrinone, which also inhibits TNFα production but not natural killer cell activity, there was no reduction in myocardial damage.

Taken in aggregate, the selective inhibition of cytokine production by vesnarinone may prove to be more important than the acute hemodynamic effects of the drug in improving survival in patients with decompensated congestive heart failure.

PHARMACOKINETICS

The pharmacokinetics of vesnarinone have been studied in both animal models and humans. The drug may be administered either orally or intravenously, with a majority of the data on oral administration. The limited solubility of the drug in aqueous solution greatly limits the utility of intravenous (IV) administration because of the large amount of a cosolvent such as sulfolane required to administer even minimally effective doses. The hemodynamic effects of the drug are linearly related to the serum concentration, with measurable hemodynamic response occurring at serum concentrations starting at 10^{-9} M.[14] Because of the limited solubility of the compound, investigators were unable to find a dose that gave maximal response. In animal studies, however, vesnarinone was shown to be equipotent with amrinone in terms of positive inotropy but showed decreased vasodilation and decreased positive chronotropy when the drugs were administered at similar doses.[15]

Pharmacokinetic parameters for vesnarinone were determined by Miyamoto and Sasabe in several animal species.[16] When radiolabeled vesnarinone was given orally at a dose of 10 mg/kg, the drug was found to reach peak serum concentrations 3 to 4 hours after administration. The half-life of the drug was found to vary from 3 to 4 hours as well, depending on the animal species. The drug showed good oral bioavailability of approximately 30% in all species studied except beagle dogs, in which availability was somewhat lower at approximately 10%. After a 10 mg/kg oral dose in rats, 30% of the radioactivity was excreted in the urine and 60% in the feces in the first 72 hours. Tissue distribution of the drug was widespread, with a notable ninefold increased distribution to the liver when compared with blood, and a fivefold increase in the adrenal glands after 72 hours. Penetration into the central nervous system was low, with levels only 5% to 10% of that in blood. Studies on protein binding revealed that vesnarinone is approximately 80% protein bound in the serum. In studies on repeated dosing, no change in elimination kinetics or tissue distribution was noted after daily oral dosing in rats for 3 weeks. The biliary excretion of the drug was found to be high, approximately 22% of the administered dose at 48 hours, suggesting the existence of enterohepatic circulation. The time course of serum concentration of unchanged drug was consistent with a two-compartment open model, and data were analyzed yielding the pharmacokinetic parameters shown in Table 131–1. The differences from species to species were felt to be due to differences in the rate of metabolic clearance by the liver, which is the major site of drug elimination.

In humans, phase I studies have been thoroughly evaluated in Europe and Japan. Human doses between 30 and 480 mg have been administered to healthy volunteers with no adverse effects reported except headache (doses proposed for the treatment of heart failure range from 30 to 60 mg/day). Plasma elimination half-life is approximately 4.5 hours. Peak plasma concentrations in healthy volunteers who were orally administered 60 mg of vesnarinone range between 3.1 and 4.9 µg/ml. Time to peak plasma concentration in the orally administered dose is 4.17 to 7.4 hours. Terminal elimination half-life ($t_{1/2}$) is between 40.7 and 49.4 hours, with a plasma clearance of 0.234 to 0.254 L/hr every 4 hours.

ADVERSE REACTIONS

Small animal studies have demonstrated an increased incidence of thyroid tumors at doses of 500 mg/kg after 104 weeks of chronic administration. A testosterone-dependent increase in the incidence of benign skin tumors and malignant pilosebaceous tumors was observed in male rats at doses of 50 mg/kg or more. Based on this information, thyroid function studies have been measured in all clinical trials with vesnarinone, but no adverse thyroid effects have yet to be identified. There is a weak suggestion that vesnarinone may be associated with hyperglycemia and aggravation of diabetes. However, in a controlled trial in the United States, there was a 0.8% incidence of diabetes-related events in patients administered 60 mg of vesnarinone. Thus, this does not appear to be a very significant problem.

The major toxicity problem associated with vesnarinone therapy appears to be idiosyncratic neutropenia with an incidence of 2.0%. Further, when it occurs, absolute neutropenia (<500 granulocytes/mm³) is observed in a majority of these patients. In trials outside Japan when absolute neutropenia (<1000 granulocytes/mm³) occurred, it was associated with a 16% in-hospital mortality rate. The mechanism of the agranulocytoses is not understood. However, in spite of the low incidence, any patient begun on vesnarinone should have the granulocyte count monitored weekly for the first 16 weeks of therapy. If granulocytopenia develops (<2000/mm³), the drug should be withdrawn. To date, no patients have been rechallenged.

Clinical Trials

The clinical need for another safe and effective oral inotropic agent for use in patients with congestive heart failure cannot be overemphasized. Initial attempts to develop oral forms of inotropic agents using compounds that increase cAMP levels have met with disappointing results. Although providing short-term benefit by improving quality of life, oral forms of catecholamines such as L-dopa, pirbuterol, and prenalterol have unfortunately been associated with an increase in sudden death or no long-term benefit.[17–19] Another group of drugs that possess PDE inhibitor activity and thus inhibit the degradation of cAMP has also been similarly plagued by problems. Both milrinone and enoximone initially appeared beneficial, but they too were associated with a significant increase in sudden death.[20, 21] The only oral inotropic agent that has remained effective and safe to date is digoxin. Several clinical studies using vesnarinone show a great deal of promise for this newest oral inotrope.

Initial small, randomized clinical trials by Feldman et al.[10, 22] (Table 131–2) using vesnarinone demonstrated safe clinical improvement in heart failure

Table 131–1. **Pharmacokinetic Parameters for Vesnarinone***

Variable	RAT	Rabbit	Dog
C$_o$ (ng/ml)	5436	14,243	4983
Kel (L/hr)	0.99	0.66	0.18
T$_{1/2}$ (hr)	1.6	1.79	4.9
Vd (L/kg)	1.25	0.36	0.96
Tcl (L/kg/hr)	0.54	0.14	0.11
TUC (ng/hr/ml)	5508	21,495	27,306

*C$_o$, peak serum concentration; Kel, elimination rate constant; T$_{1/2}$, elimination half-life; Vd, volume of distribution; Tcl, total body clearance; TUC, total area under the concentration time curve.

From Miyamoto G, Sasabe H: Pharmacokinetics of a new positive inotropic agent, OPC-8212, in rat, rabbit, beagle dog and rhesus monkey. Arzneimittelforschung/Drug Res 34(1):394, 1984.

Table 131–2. **Summary of Clinical Trials Employing Vesnarinone**

Study	Dose	Inotropy	QLI	Mortality
Asanoi et al.[24]	60 mg	+	+ +	N/A
Feldman et al.[10]	60 mg	+	+ +	Decreased
Feldman et al.[23]	120 mg	+ +	+ +	Increased
	60 mg	±	+ +	Decreased

QLI, quality of life index.
±, no change.
+, modest increase.
+ +, intermediate response.

symptoms. These early trials randomized patients to vesnarinone 60 mg/day or placebo. In both of these small trials, Feldman was able to demonstrate a significant increase in peak oxygen uptake and improved quality of life while decreasing the frequency of premature ventricular contractions without an increase in heart rate. These promising findings led to the only large multicenter randomized trial of vesnarinone to be completed thus far (see Table 130–2).[23]

In this trial, patients with ejection fractions less than or equal to 30% were randomized to 120 mg/day of vesnarinone, 60 mg/day of vesnarinone, or placebo. Relatively early in the enrollment period there was found to be a significant increase in mortality in the 120 mg/day group, necessitating the termination of this arm of the study. Ultimately 477 patients were randomized to receive either 60 mg/day of vesnarinone or placebo for 6 months. There were no significant differences in clinical characteristics of the study patients. In both groups, the majority (70%) of patients had New York Heart Association (NYHA) class III congestive heart failure symptoms. Of these patients, 90% were on ACE inhibitor and digoxin. At the end of 6 months, investigators were able to demonstrate that 60 mg/day of vesnarinone led to a 50% decrease in the risk of worsening heart failure or death from any cause compared with placebo. At the end of the 6-month study period, there was a 6% mortality in the vesnarinone arm compared with 17% in the placebo arm. Importantly, the cause of death in the two groups was not statistically significant. Of those patients who died, 54% of the deaths were attributable to worsening heart failure in both the placebo and vesnarinone arms of the study. Forty-five percent of the deaths were sudden in the placebo group compared with 38% in the vesnarinone group. Overall, there was a 62% reduction in the risk of

death. The vesnarinone group also demonstrated a significant improvement in quality of life compared with placebo as assessed by the Sickness Impact Profile. Interestingly, these improvements in overall survival and quality of life existed despite no significant improvement in NYHA class or ejection fraction. The only significant deleterious side effect detected during the study was neutropenia. The development of neutropenia always occurred between 4 and 16 weeks of vesnarinone therapy and was reversible in each case. The overall incidence of developing neutropenia was 2.5%. There are ongoing studies comparing 30 mg/day versus 60 mg/day of vesnarinone and placebo.

CONCLUSIONS

Table 131–3 compares the hemodynamic and immunologic parameters of vesnarinone and the three major inotropic agents: dobutamine, the phosphodiesterase inhibitors amrinone and milrinone, and digoxin. Vesnarinone does not increase heart rate or lower arterial pressure. With its positive inotropic action, cardiac output increases, and in the patient with congestive heart failure, arterial pressure may even increase. The immunomodulating effects all are beneficial with inhibition of TNFα, IL-6, and natural killer cell activity. The hemodynamic effects of dobutamine are well known, with its potential increase in heart rate, decrease in arterial pressure, and increase in cardiac output. Unfortunately, there is no information in the immunomodulating effects of dobutamine. The hemodynamic profile of the PDE inhibitors are also well known, and they decrease TNFα but have no effect on IL-6. Likewise, for digoxin, the hemodynamic parameters are well characterized, but there are no data on its potential immunomodulating ability.

Therefore, the combination of various mechanisms by which vesnarinone has its effect sets it apart from previously studied oral inotropic agents. Not only do patients benefit from the positive inotropic effects of the drug, but the antiarrhythmic and immunomodulating actions may also significantly contribute to the observed improved clinical outcome in treatment groups. Indeed, these latter actions may prove to be more important than the positive inotropic effects of vesnarinone in reducing morbidity and mortality. It is this unique quality and what appears to be a safe and effective clinical profile which give vesnarinone the possibility of one day becoming part of the conventional therapeutic regimen for treating congestive heart failure.

Table 131–3. **Comparison of Inotropic Agents on Both Hemodynamic and Immunomodulating Parameters**

	HR	BP	CO	TNFα	IL-6	NK
Vesnarinone	→	→	↑	↓	↓	↓
Dobutamine	↑	→↓	↑	?	?	?
Amrinone/Milrinone	↑	↓	↑	↓	→	→
Digoxin	→↓	→	→↑	?	?	?

HR, heart rate; BP, blood pressure; CO, cardiac output; TNFα, tumor necrosis factor; IL-6, interleukin-6; NK, natural killer cell activity.

REFERENCES

1. Taira N, Endoh M, Iijima T, et al: Mode and mechanism of action of 3,4 Dihydro-6-[4-(3,4 dimethoxybenzoyl)-1-piperazinyl]-2(1H)-quinolinone (OPC-8212), a novel positive inotropic drug, on the dog heart. Arzneimittel forschung 34(3A):347, 1984.
2. Shimizu T, Osumi T, Niimi K, Nakayawa K: Physicochemical properties and stabilities of a new positive inotropic agent 3,4-dihydro-6-[4-(3,4-dimethoxybenzoyl)-1-piperazinyl]-2(1H)-quinolinone. Arzneimittelforschung/Drug Res 34(1):334, 1984.
3. Toshihiko I, Taira N: Membrane current changes responsible

for the positive inotropic effect of OPC-8212, a new positive inotropic agent, in single ventricular cells of the guinea heart. J Pharmacol Exp Ther 240(2):657, 1987.

4. Satoh H, Hashimoto K: Effect of OPC-8212 on the membrane currents of rabbit sino-atrial node cells. Arzneimittelforschung/Drug Res 34(1):376, 1984.

5. Lathrop DA, Schwartz A: Electromechanical effects of OPC-8212, a new positive inotropic agent. Arzneimittelforschung/Drug Res 34(1):371.

6. Lathrop DA, Schwartz A: Evidence for possible increase in Na channel open tissue and involvement of Na/Ca exchange by a new positive inotropic drug OPC-8212. Eur J Pharmacol 117:391, 1985.

7. Lathrop DA, Varro A, Schwartz A: Rate-dependent electrophysiological effects of OPC-8212: Comparison to sotalol. Eur J Pharmacol 164:487, 1989.

8. Itoh H, Kusayawa M, Shimamurra A, et al: Ca^{2+}-dependent and Ca^{2+}-independent vasorelaxation induced by cardiotonic PDE inhibitors. Eur J Pharmacol 240:57, 1993.

9. Masuoka H, Ito M, Sugioka M, et al: Two isoforms of cGMP-inhibited cyclic nucleotide phosphodiesterases in human tissues distinguished by their responses to vesnarinone, a new cardiotonic agent. Biochem Biophys Res Commun 190(2):412, 1993.

10. Feldman AM, Baughman KL, Lee WK, et al: Usefulness of OPC-8212, a quinolinone derivative, for chronic congestive heart failure in patients with ischemic heart disease for idiopathic dilated cardiomyopathy. Am J Cardiol 68:1203, 1991.

11. Levine B, Kalman J, Mayer L, et al: Elevated circulating levels of tumor necrosis factor in severe chronic heart failure. N Engl J Med 323:236, 1990.

12. Matsumari A, Shioi T, Yamada T, et al: Vesnarinone, a new inotropic agent, inhibits cytokine production by stimulated human blood from patients with heart failure. Circulation 89(3):955, 1994.

13. Sasayama DS: Treatment of virus-induced myocardial injury with a novel immunomodulating agent, vesnarinone. J Clin Invest 94:1212, 1994.

14. Miyazaki S, Sasayama S, Nukamura Y, et al: Acute hemodynamic effects of a new positive inotropic agent, OPC-8212, in conscious and anesthetized dogs. J Cardiovasc Pharmacol 8:14, 1986.

15. Yamashika S, Hosokawa T, Kojima M, et al: In vitro and in vivo studies of OPC-8212, a novel positive inotropic drug in various animals. Arzneimittelforschung/Drug Res 34(1):342, 1984.

16. Miyamoto G, Sasabe H: Pharmacokinetics of a new positive inotropic agent, OPC-8212, in rat, rabbit, beagle dog and rhesus monkey. Arzneimittelforschung/Drug Res 34(1):394, 1984.

17. Raifa SF, Anton AH, Rossen JD, Goldberg LI: Beneficial hemodynamic effects of oral levodopa in heart failure. N Engl J Med 310:1357, 1984.

18. Weber KT, Andrews V, Janicki JS, et al: Pirbuterol, an oral beta-adrenergic receptor agonist in the treatment of chronic cardiac failure. Circulation 66:1262, 1982.

19. Lambertz H, Meyer J, Erbel R: Long-term hemodynamic effects of prenalterol in patients with congestive heart failure. Circulation 69:298, 1984.

20. Packer M, Carvei JR, Rodeheffer RJ, et al: PROMISE Study Research Group: Effect of oral milrinone on mortality in severe chronic heart failure. N Engl J Med 325:1468, 1991.

21. Vretsky BF, Jessup M, Konstam MA, et al, for the Enoximone Multicenter Trial Group: Multicenter trial of oral enoximone in patients with moderate to moderately severe congestive heart failure. Circulation 82:774, 1990.

22. Feldman AM, Becker LC, Llewellyn MP, Baughman KL: Evaluation of a new inotropic agent, OPC-8212, in patients with dilated cardiomyopathy and heart failure. Am Heart J 116:771, 1988.

23. Feldman AM, Bristow MR, Parmley WW, et al, for the Vesnarinone Study Group: Effects of vesnarinone on morbidity and mortality in patients with heart failure. N Engl J Med 329:149, 1993.

24. Asanoi H, Sasyama S, Kameyama T, et al: Sustained inotropic effects of a new cardiotonic agent OPC-8212 in patients with chronic heart failure. Clin Cardiol 12:133, 1989.

CHAPTER 132

Carmoxirole

Robert M. Carey, M.D., and John H. Laragh, M.D.

HISTORY

In the 1970s, two distinct classes of dopamine (DA) receptors (DA1 and DA2) were identified and characterized as important in the regulation of the cardiovascular system.[1-3] DA1 receptors were localized postsynaptically in the medial layer of arterial blood vessels, including the renal, splanchnic, coronary, and cerebral circulations.[1-3] Stimulation of vascular DA1 receptors resulted in vasodilation. DA1 receptors also were found in the renal proximal tubules and cortical collecting ducts, activation of which engendered natriuresis and diuresis by decreasing tubular sodium reabsorption.[4, 5]

The DA2 receptor was located in presynaptic nerve terminals of the adrenergic nervous system and in sympathetic ganglia.[6-8] Stimulation of the presynaptic DA2 receptor attenuated norepinephrine release from sympathetic nerve endings, resulting in decreased vascular resistance. Activation of ganglionic DA2 receptors inhibited neurotransmission. Postsynaptic

DA2 receptors also have been described in the pituitary gland, kidney, and adrenal cortex. In the pituitary, DA2 receptor activation leads to inhibition of prolactin release from lactotroph cells.[9] In the kidney, DA2 receptors are present in the renal vasculature, glomerulus, and tubules, but little is known about the physiologic role of these receptors.[4, 5, 10] In the adrenal cortex, postsynaptic DA2 receptors are found in the zona glomerulosa, where they inhibit aldosterone secretion.[11, 12] DA2 receptors also have been identified in the chemoreceptor trigger zone in the central nervous system. Table 132–1 lists the location and physiologic role of DA2 receptors outside the blood-brain barrier.

Experimental and clinical studies have suggested that DA receptor stimulation might be effective in the treatment of hypertension.[1-3, 6-8] Selective postsynaptic DA1 receptor stimulation was shown to decrease blood pressure in patients with essential hypertension.[13] The bioavailability of the DA1 agonist, fenoldopam, was too low to provide an effective antihyper-

Table 132–1. **DA2 Receptors Outside the Blood-Brain Barrier**

Location	Physiologic Response
Peripheral adrenergic nerve terminals (presynaptic or prejunctional dopamine receptors)	Inhibition of noradrenaline release
Adrenal cortex	Inhibition of aldosterone secretion
Sympathetic ganglia	Inhibition of ganglionic transmission
Pituitary gland	Inhibition of prolactin release
Chemoreceptor trigger zone (CNS)	Emesis

tensive agent. However, these observations focused attention on the potential clinical usefulness of DA agonists in hypertension.

CHEMISTRY

Carmoxirole (EMD45609) is an indole derivative with the chemical name 3-(4-(4-phenyl 1,2,3,6-tetrahydro-1-pyridinyl)-butyl)-indol-acid hydrochloride.

Carmoxirole has a molecular weight of 410.95. The compound is sparingly soluble in water and is micronized to give a white powder. Carmoxirole is a nonhygroscopic compound that is not sensitive to heat, humidity, or oxygen exposure. It is sensitive to light, particularly in the solid state.

PHARMACOLOGY

Peripheral adrenergic nerve terminals are endowed with a large variety of receptors, as shown in Figure 132–1. These receptors are located on presynaptic ad-

renergic nerve varicosities and are important in the control of norepinephrine release. When stimulated, some of these receptors (facilitatory presynaptic receptors) augment norepinephrine release, whereas others (inhibitory presynaptic receptors) abrogate norepinephrine release. Inhibitory presynaptic receptors include α_2-adrenergic, adenosine, muscarinic, opiate, prostaglandin, and DA2 receptors.[14–20]

The pharmacologic mechanism of action of agonists at the presynaptic receptor differ fundamentally from those of other sympatholytic drugs. First, presynaptic receptor agonists do not deplete the adrenergic nerve terminals of their norepinephrine stores as do many of the available adrenergic neuron blocking agents.[21–23] Second, presynaptic receptor agonists inhibit norepinephrine release preferentially at low rates of impulse flow in sympathetic neurons.[14, 16, 24] Other adrenergic neuron blocking agents inhibit norepinephrine release over the entire frequency range of nerve discharge.[24] The presynaptic agonists lose their ability to inhibit norepinephrine release at an electrical nerve stimulation rate of 2 to 4 Hz. At higher rates of nerve stimulation, the quantity of norepinephrine release per action potential returns to normal. These two differences in the mechanism of action of presynaptic agonists as compared with adrenergic neuron blocking agents might aid the treatment of hypertension. Theoretically, blood pressure should be lowered at rest, but the sympathetic nervous system should still respond to a requirement for increased drive, as with exercise or stress. However, the question remains as to whether inhibition of norepinephrine release in the resting state is sufficient to lower blood pressure, or whether the noradrenergic burst rate in hypertension will be too high for effective noradrenergic blockade.

Carmoxirole is a potent selective agonist at the central nervous system DA2 receptor.[25, 26] Studies of

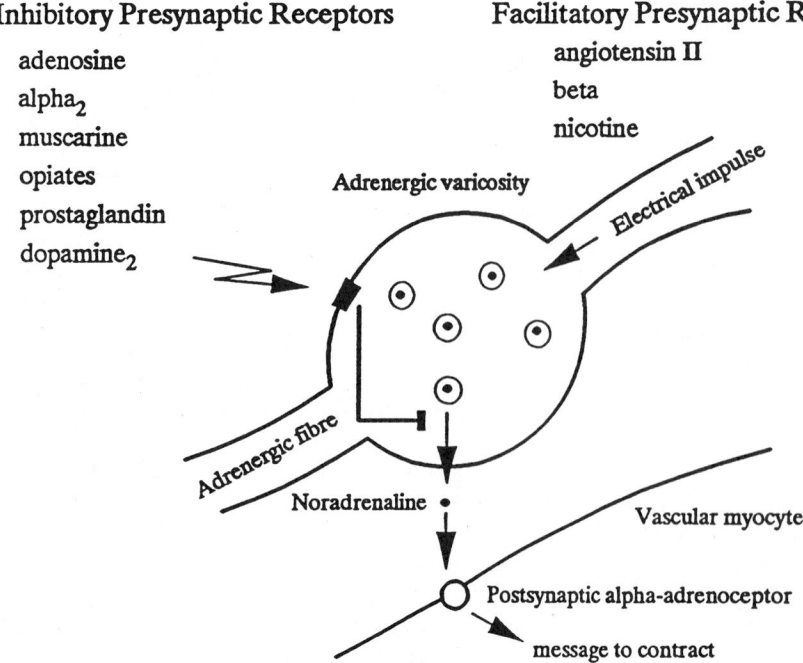

Inhibitory Presynaptic Receptors

adenosine
alpha$_2$
muscarine
opiates
prostaglandin
dopamine$_2$

Facilitatory Presynaptic Receptors

angiotensin II
beta
nicotine

Adrenergic varicosity

Electrical impulse

Adrenergic fibre

Noradrenaline

Vascular myocyte

Postsynaptic alpha-adrenoceptor

message to contract

Figure 132–1. Schematic representation of an adrenergic nerve varicosity at the terminal region of a peripheral sympathetic neuron. The membrane of the varicosity possesses various types of receptors (presynaptic receptors). Some of these receptors excite and some inhibit the release of the neurotransmitter, norepinephrine. The presynaptic dopamine receptor belongs to the DA2 receptor subtype. DA2 agonist-induced activity at the DA2 presynaptic receptor inhibits the amount of norepinephrine released per action potential.

Table 132–2. *In-Vitro* Binding of Carmoxirole on Plasma Membrane Preparations of Rat Brain Tissue

Ligand	Receptor Subtype	Carmoxirole	Quinpirole IC_{50} (mol/L)	Pergolide
ADTN	DA1	4×10^{-6}	1×10^{-5}	5×10^{-9}
ADTN	DA2	4×10^{-9}	7×10^{-8}	5×10^{-9}
Prazosin	α_1	1×10^{-7}	$>1 \times 10^{-5}$	7×10^{-6}
Idazoxan	α_2	6×10^{-7}	7×10^{-6}	5×10^{-7}
Rauwolscine	α_2	4×10^{-8}	3×10^{-6}	1×10^{-7}
DHA	β	$>1 \times 10^{-5}$	$>1 \times 10^{-5}$	ND
8-OH-DPAT	$5HT_{1A}$	2×10^{-8}	1×10^{-6}	7×10^{-8}
Ketanserin	$5HT_2$	2×10^{-6}	$>1 \times 10^{-5}$	3×10^{-7}
QNB	M_1/M_2	$>1 \times 10^{-5}$	ND	$>1 \times 10^{-5}$

ADTN, amino-6,7-dihydroxy-1,2,3,4-tetrahydronaphthalene; DHA, dihydroalprenolol; 8-OH-DPAT, 8-hydroxy-2(di-N-propylamino) tetralin; QNB, quinuclidinyl-benzilate; ND, not determined.

ligand binding to plasma membrane preparations of rat brain demonstrate a 1000-fold higher affinity of carmoxirole for the DA2 receptor class than the DA1 receptor subtype (Table 132–2). Carmoxirole has some binding affinity for the 5-HT$_{1A}$ receptor and for the α_2-adrenoceptor. Affinity for other receptors, including α_1- and β-adrenoceptors, 5HT$_2$ receptors, and muscarinic receptors, is negligible.[27] Studies characterizing carmoxirole have been limited to brain tissue, because the density of peripheral DA receptors is low and difficult to measure.[5] It is possible, although highly unlikely, that carmoxirole might exhibit different binding characteristics in plasma membranes of peripheral tissues. Although the central and peripheral DA receptors correspond pharmacologically, it remains uncertain whether the molecular and chemical sequences of these receptors differ.[28, 29]

In the rabbit ear artery, carmoxirole at concentrations as low as 10^{-9} M inhibited ^{3}H-norepinephrine release in response to electrical stimulation at a low frequency (0.5 Hz). Maximum effective concentration was 10^{-7} M. At 10^{-6} M, carmoxirole either had no (0.5 Hz) effect or increased ^{3}H-norepinephrine release because of its α_2-antagonist properties when frequency of stimulation was increased (2 Hz). The inhibitory effect of carmoxirole on electrically stimulated norepinephrine release was abolished by L-sulpiride, a selective DA2 antagonist. In pithed spontaneously hypertensive rats (SHRs), carmoxirole (0.1 mg/kg given intravenously) inhibited the pressure response to electrical stimulation of total sympathetic outflow. This response also was inhibited by L-sulpiride (0.1 mg/kg given intravenously). Carmoxirole also was shown to inhibit cardioaccelerator nerve–stimulated tachycardia in a dose-dependent manner in the anesthetized, vagotomized cat. Responses *in vivo* were observed only at low (1 to 2 Hz) rates of nerve stimulation. Thus, both *in vitro* and *in vivo* evidence show that the effects of carmoxirole are mediated at presynaptic DA2 receptors.

PHARMACOKINETICS

The pharmacokinetic profile of carmoxirole in humans has been reported by Meyer et al.[30] A single oral dose of ^{14}C-labeled carmoxirole (1 mg) was absorbed rapidly and almost completely (80%). The maximum concentration of the compound (8 ng/ml) was reached after 2 to 3 hours. Unchanged carmoxirole represented 60% and 50% of the total radioactivity in plasma at peak concentration and at 12 hours post dose, respectively. The major plasma and urinary metabolite was an ester-type glucuronide. Elimination of radioactivity in plasma followed a biphasic curve with an initial half-life of 5.5 ± 1.0 hours, probably reflecting the half-life of the unchanged substance. A small fraction of the compound is eliminated with a longer half-life (12.2 ± 2.3 hours), probably reflecting enterohepatic circulation of carmoxirole. The drug and metabolites are predominantly excreted by the kidneys.

Table 132–3 summarizes pharmacokinetic studies with the unlabeled compound (0.5 and 1.0 mg). Additional studies have shown that the rate of absorption is delayed by food, but the extent of absorption and the bioavailability are not affected by food.

Table 132–3. Pharmacokinetic Profile of Carmoxirole in 12 Healthy Male Subjects After Oral Administration of Single Doses of 0.5 mg and 1.0 mg

Parameter	0.5 mg Carmoxirole Mean (SD) n = 12	1.0 mg Carmoxirole Mean (SD) n = 12
C_{max} (ng $\cdot$ ml^{-1})	2.51 (0.47)	4.65 (1.28)
T_{max} (hr)	2.83 (0.99)	2.75 (1.16)
$T\frac{1}{2}$ (hr)	5.52 (1.96)	4.44 (1.60)
AUC$_{(0–12 hr)}$ (hr $\cdot$ ng $\cdot$ ml^{-1})	15.6 (4.4)	28.4 (7.2)
AUC$_{(0–20)}$ (hr $\cdot$ ng $\cdot$ ml^{-1})	21.1 (7.9)	36.0 (7.8)
CL/f (ml $\cdot$ min^{-1})*	427.7 (102.9)	493.3 (155.7)
CL/f (L $\cdot$ hr^{-1})	25.7 (6.2)	29.6 (9.3)
U$_{(0–24 hr)}$ (μg)	213 (17)	421 (46)
(% of the dose)	42.5 (3.3)	42.1 (4.6)

*Assuming f = 1.0.
C_{max}, maximum plasma concentration after single administration; t$_{max}$, time to attain maximum plasma concentration after administration; T$\frac{1}{2}$, plasma elimination half-life; AUC, area under concentration time curve; CL, clearance; U, renal excretion (sum of carmoxirole and its glucuronide).
From Meyer W, Bühring KU, Steiner K, et al: Pharmacokinetics and first clinical experiences with an antihypertensive dopamine DA-2 agonist. Eur Heart J 13(Suppl D):121, 1992.

EFFECTS ON PATHOPHYSIOLOGY
Effects on Hemodynamics

Carmoxirole is a potent and efficacious antihypertensive agent. In the SHR, carmoxirole engendered a dose-dependent decrease in blood pressure over a dose range of 0.1 to 10 mg/kg administered orally (Fig. 132–2). In renal hypertensive dogs, carmoxirole also was potent in decreasing blood pressure in a dose range of 0.005 to 0.05 mg/kg administered orally. In both of these models, the decrease in blood pressure was due to a decrease in peripheral vascular resistance. The antihypertensive effect of carmoxirole was blocked by the DA2 antagonists, L-sulpiride, or domperidone, but not by blockade of the 5-HT$_{1A}$ receptor. The decrease in blood pressure was associated with no change or a slight increase in renal blood flow, a reduction in splanchnic flow, and a marked increase in lower aortic blood flow. Thus, the arterial circulation to skeletal muscle is especially responsive to carmoxirole.

Studies also have been conducted in humans. In normal subjects, carmoxirole did not alter supine blood pressure. In patients with essential hypertension, a single oral dose of carmoxirole decreased blood pressure for at least 8 hours, but pressure had returned to baseline values at 24 hours. Figure 132–3 depicts decrements of systolic and diastolic blood pressure in patients with essential hypertension in the supine position in response to a single oral dose of carmoxirole. Heart rate did not change in response to

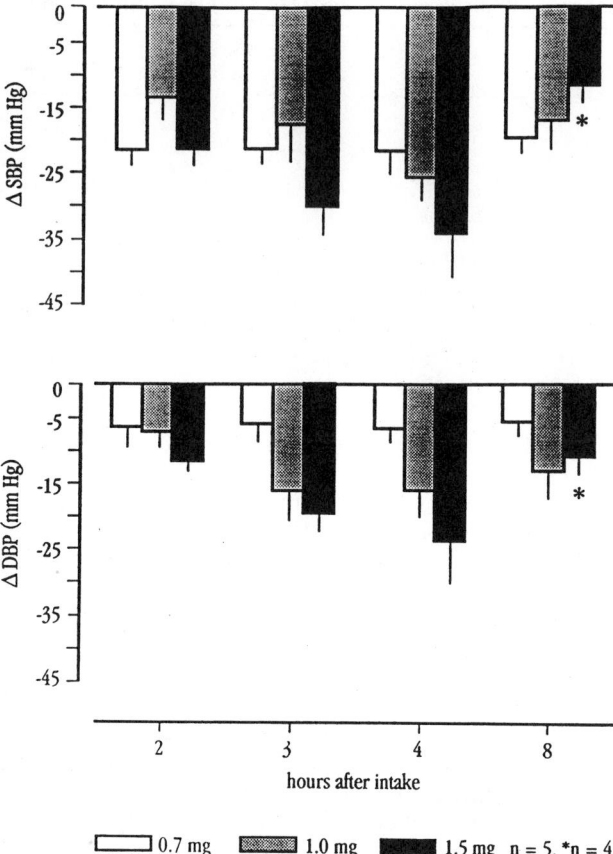

Figure 132–3. Decrements (mean ± ISE) of systolic blood pressure (SBP, *upper panel*) and diastolic blood pressure (DBP, *lower panel*) in patients with essential hypertension in response to a single oral dose of carmoxirole (0.7, 1.0, or 1.5 mg). Values are compared with those 24 hours after placebo administration in the same subjects.

carmoxirole. Blood pressure responses to carmoxirole were not effected by body position. Figure 132–4 demonstrates the hypotensive effect of carmoxirole in patients with essential hypertension in the supine and standing positions. No orthostatic hypotension or tachycardia was observed. After repeated administration for several weeks, carmoxirole reduced blood pressure at both 12 and 24 hours after drug administration. Figure 132–5 demonstrates that administration of carmoxirole in increasing doses (0.5, 1.0, and 2.0 mg) for a period of 2 weeks led to a dose-dependent decrease in blood pressure. Carmoxirole also reduced blood pressure of hypertensive patients engaged in exercise, but the effect was quantitatively less than under resting conditions. Thus, carmoxirole use apparently maintains exercise capacity and may prevent dangerous increases in blood pressure.

Endocrine and Metabolic Effects

After 6 weeks of therapy, carmoxirole has been shown to decrease plasma renin activity in patients with essential hypertension. This effect may be due to intrarenal inhibition of norepinephrine release. Carmoxirole also decreases serum prolactin concentrations, an effect mediated by stimulation of DA2 receptors

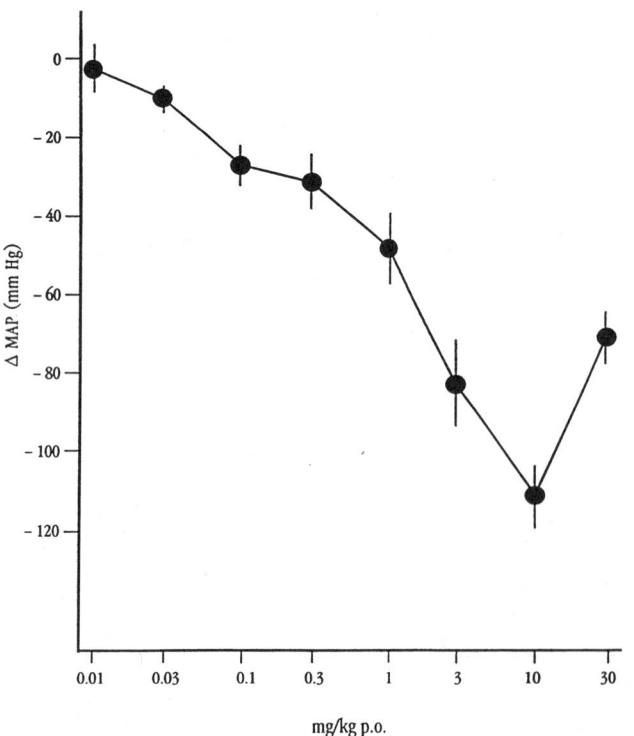

Figure 132–2. Lowering of mean arterial pressure (MAP) by carmoxirole in conscious spontaneously hypertensive rats. Results (mean ± ISE, n = 6–8) constitute changes from pretreatment values corrected for the vehicle effect.

on cell membranes of pituitary lactotrophs. Effects on aldosterone secretion have not been reported.

Effects on the Central Nervous System

In animal studies, carmoxirole was rapidly distributed but barely penetrated the blood-brain barrier. This was indicated by the results of experiments with measurement of striatal dopa accumulation in rats pretreated with reserpine and a dopa decarboxylase inhibitor. Inhibitory effects were observed only at doses beyond those sufficient to control blood pressure. This was confirmed in studies of rotational behavior in rats with unilateral lesions of the nigrostriatal pathway and by autoradiographic studies of carmoxirole accumulation in the brain. The fact that carmoxirole *does not cross the blood-brain barrier* allows for peripheral DA2 receptor stimulation without untoward effects at the central DA2 receptor.

CLINICAL USE

Carmoxirole is an experimental antihypertensive agent that is presently undergoing phase II clinical trials. Little or no information is available on the effects of carmoxirole on cardiac structure and function, electrophysiology, coronary blood flow, venous

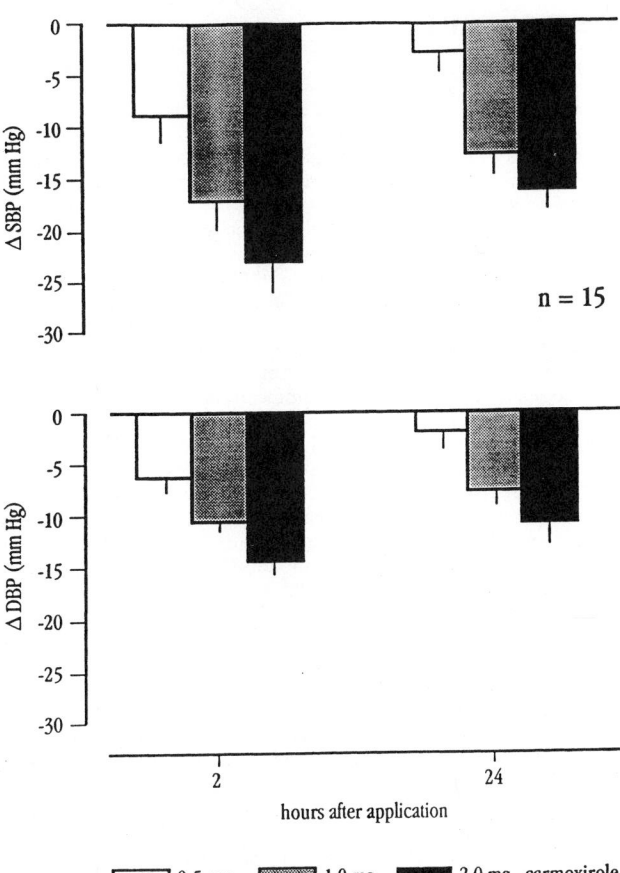

Figure 132–5. Decrements (mean ± ISE) of systolic blood pressure (SBP, *upper panel*) and diastolic blood pressure (DBP, *lower panel*) at the end of 2-week treatment periods with carmoxirole at 0.5, 1.0, and 2.0 mg given orally each day. Values are compared with corresponding values at the end of placebo prephase.

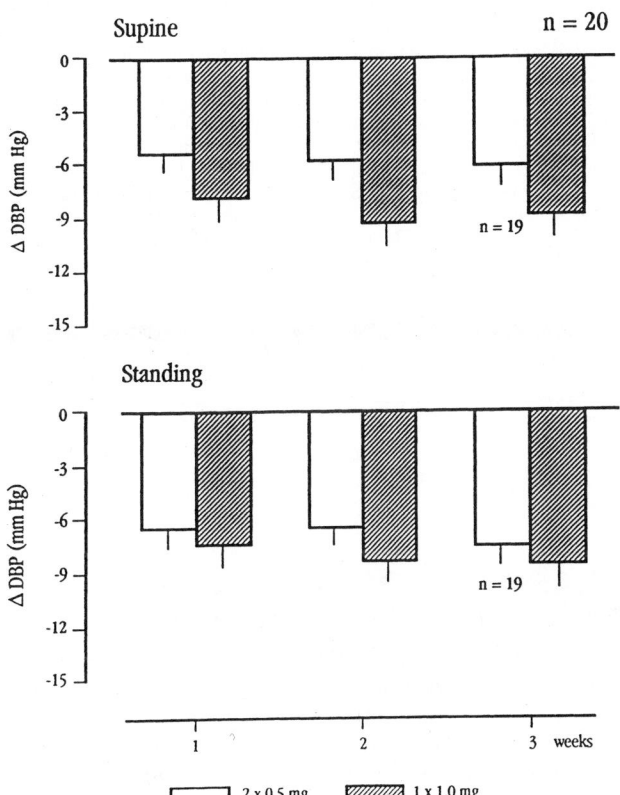

Figure 132–4. Decrements (mean ± ISE) of diastolic blood pressure (DBP) in patients with essential hypertension in the supine (*upper panel*) and standing (*lower panel*) positions after treatment with carmoxirole in two different dose regimens for 1, 2, and 3 weeks. Blood pressure was measured 12 hours (2 × 0.5 mg group) or 24 hours (1 × 1.0 mg group) after medication.

flow, fluid volume state, or renal function. Because of its unique mechanism of action, it is anticipated that carmoxirole will be appropriate for the long-term treatment of hypertension. In limited clinical studies, the drug has effectively lowered blood pressure in patients with essential hypertension. In clinical trials thus far reported, the rate of adverse events has been minimal. The major reported adverse events have been headache, dizziness, tiredness, nausea, pressure in the gastric area, and nasal congestion. It is interesting that nausea and vomiting have not been prominent adverse effects, because the emesis center is located in the area postrema, which lies outside the blood-brain barrier and should be exposed to carmoxirole. Nausea, vomiting, other gastric effects, and nasal congestion could be due to DA2 stimulation outside the central nervous system.

It is anticipated that carmoxirole will be effective in a once-daily oral regimen in the range of 1.0 to 1.5 mg daily. Theoretically, therefore, carmoxirole could be employed as a single antihypertensive agent. There is no reason to suspect that carmoxirole administration will result in sodium or fluid retention, but the relative effectiveness of combination with a diuretic agent will have to await results of future studies.

REFERENCES

1. Goldberg LI: Cardiovascular and renal actions of dopamine: Potential clinical applications. Pharmacol Rev 24:1, 1972.
2. Goldberg LI, Kohli JD: Peripheral dopamine receptors: A classification based on potency series and specific antagonism. TIPS 5:64, 1983.
3. Stoof JC, Kebabian JW: Two dopamine receptors: Biochemistry, physiology and pharmacology. Life Sci 35:2281, 1984.
4. Felder RA, Blecher M, Eisner GM, et al: Cortical tubular and glomerular dopamine receptors in the rat kidney. Am J Physiol 246:F557, 1984.
5. Felder RA, Felder CC, Eisner GM, et al: The dopamine receptor in adult and maturing kidney. Am J Physiol 257:F315, 1989.
6. Goldberg LI, Rajfer SI: Dopamine receptors: Applications to clinical cardiology. Circulation 72:245, 1985.
7. Lokhandwala MF, Barrett RJ: Dopamine receptor agonists in cardiovascular therapy. Drug Dev Res 3:299, 1983.
8. Hahn RA: Development of selective dopamine receptor agonists as novel cardiovascular drugs. Drug Dev Res 4:285, 1984.
9. Foord SM, Peters JR, Dieguez C, et al: Dopamine receptors on intact anterior pituitary cells in culture: Functional association with the inhibition of prolactin and thyrotropin. Endocrinol 112:1567, 1983.
10. Carey RM, Siragy HM, Ragsdale NV, et al: Dopamine-1 and dopamine-2 mechanisms in the control of renal function. Am J Hypertens 3:595, 1990.
11. Missale C, Lombardi C, De Cotiis R, et al: Dopaminergic receptor mechanisms modulating the renin-angiotensin system and aldosterone secretion: An overview. J Cardiovasc Pharmacol 14(Suppl 8):S29, 1989.
12. Carey RM: Dopaminergic control of aldosterone secretion. In Hieble JP (ed): Cardiovascular Function of Peripheral Dopamine Receptors. New York: Marcel Dekker, 1989, pp 297–314.
13. Carey RM, Stote RM, Dubb LW, et al: Selective peripheral dopamine-1 receptor stimulation with fenoldopam in human essential hypertension. J Clin Invest 74:2198, 1984.
14. Langer SZ: Presynaptic regulation of release of catecholamines. Pharmacol Rev 32:337, 1981.
15. Starke K: Presynaptic receptors. Ann Rev Pharmac Toxicol 21:7, 1981.
16. Starke K, Gothert M, Kilbinger H. Modulation of neurotransmitter release by presynaptic autoreceptors. Physiol Rev 69:864, 1989.
17. Lokhandwala MF: Presynaptic receptor systems on cardiac sympathetic nerves. Life Sci 24:1823, 1979.
18. Dahlof C: Studies on β-adrenoceptor mediated facilitation of sympathetic neurotransmission. Acta Physiol Scand 500(Suppl):1, 1981.
19. Long JP, Heintz S, Cannon JG, et al: Inhibition of the sympathetic nervous system by 5,6-dihydroxy-2-dimethyl-aminotetralin(M-7), apomorphine and dopamine. J Pharmacol Exp Ther 192:336, 1975.
20. Wilffert B, Smit G, deJonge A, et al: Inhibitory dopamine receptors on sympathetic neurons innervating the cardiovascular system of the pithed rat. Characterization and role in relation to presynaptic a₂-adrenoceptors. Naunyn Schmiedebergs Arch Pharmacol 326:91, 1984.
21. Brodie BB, Chang CC, Costa E: On the mechanism of action of guanethidine and bretylium. Br J Pharmacol 25:171, 1965.
22. Haeusler G, Haefely W, Huerlimann A: On the mechanism of adrenergic nerve blocking action of bretylium. Naunyn Schmiedebergs Arch Pharmacol 265:260, 1969.
23. Haeusler G, Haefely W: Modification of release by adrenergic neuron-blocking agents and agents that alter the action potential. In Paton DM (ed): The Release of Catecholamines from Adrenergic Neurons. Oxford: Pergamon Press, 1979, pp 185–216.
24. Illes P: Mechanisms of receptor-mediated modulation of transmitter release in noradrenergic, cholinergic and sensory neurons. Neuroscience 17:909, 1986.
25. Schelling P, Bergmann R, Böttcher H, et al: A new dopamine agonist selective for DA₂ receptors as an antihypertensive drug. Naunyn Schmiedebergs Arch Pharmacol 337(Suppl):R71, 1988.
26. Haase AF, Greiner HE, Seyfried CA: Neurochemical profile of EMD 45609 (carmoxirole), a dopamine DA₂-receptor agonist. Naunyn-Schmiedeberg's Arch Pharmacol 343:588, 1991.
27. Haeusler G, Lues I, Minck KO, et al: Pharmacological basis for antihypertensive therapy with a novel dopamine agonist. Eur Heart J 13(Suppl D):129, 1992.
28. Willems JL, Buylaert WA, Lefebvre RA, et al: Neuronal dopamine receptors on autonomic ganglia and sympathetic nerves and dopamine receptors in the gastrointestinal system. Pharmacol Rev 37:165, 1985.
29. Semeraro C, Ferrini R, Allievi L, et al: Peripheral vascular and neuronal effects of dopamine receptor agonists. A comparison with receptor binding studies in rat striatum. Naunyn Schmiedebergs Arch Pharmacol 342:539, 1990.
30. Meyer W, Bühring KU, Steiner K, et al: Pharmacokinetics and first clinical experiences with an antihypertensive dopamine DA-2 agonist. Eur Heart J 13(Suppl D):121, 1992.

CHAPTER 133

Ibopamine

Marco Metra, M.D., and Livio Dei Cas, M.D.

Despite advances obtained with the introduction of vasodilators and converting enzyme inhibitors, patients with chronic heart failure (HF) still have a poor prognosis and are often severely limited in their functional capacity. Therefore, new drugs that can become a part of standard therapy for HF are still needed.

Dopamine (DA) presents many features useful for the treatment of HF;[1-4] however, it is not active after oral administration. Research has therefore focused on the development of DA derivatives that can be administered orally.[5, 6] Ibopamine has emerged as one of the most interesting compounds and is the most widely studied DA derivative for the treatment of patients with chronic HF.

PHARMACOLOGIC BASIS AND CHEMICAL STRUCTURE

Two distinct peripheral DA receptors have been identified:[1-4] DA1 receptors are located postsynaptically and mediate vasodilation in renal, mesenteric, coronary, and cerebral blood vessels; DA2 receptors are located on postganglionic sympathetic nerve endings and sympathetic ganglia and inhibit norepinephrine (NE) release[1-4] and sympathetic transmission.[7] Other DA2 receptors are located in the adrenal cortex, where they inhibit aldosterone secretion induced by angiotensin II stimulation;[8] in the emetic center of the area postrema of the central nervous system, where they induce emesis; and in the anterior lobe of the pituitary gland, where they inhibit prolactin secretion.[1-4]

DA, infused intravenously at low doses (0.5 to 2 μg/kg/min), acts selectively on DA1 and DA2 receptors, inducing a decline in peripheral vascular resistance with an increase in renal blood flow, diuresis, and sodium excretion. At higher infusion rates, it also activates β1-receptors and induces NE release from storage sites in the sympathetic nerve endings with an increase in myocardial contractility and cardiac output. Lastly, at infusion rates higher than 4 μg/kg/min, it stimulates α-receptors with a consequent increase in peripheral vascular resistance and blood pressure; at these doses, excessive stimulation of β1-receptors can also lead to tachycardia and/or ventricular arrhythmias.[1-3]

Studies of phenylethylamine derivatives showed that the structural requirements for activation of DA vascular receptors are very strict and that, among these agents, only N-methyl DA (epinine) and N,N-di-propyl DA were identified as DA vascular receptor agonists.[9, 10] N,N-Di-propyl DA is, however, less potent, with a mean effective dose (ED50) that is approximately 30 times the ED50 values of DA and epinine.[11]

Animal Pharmacology

Epinine, like DA, is not active after oral administration because it undergoes extensive sulfate conjugation in the gut. Its 3,4-O-disobutyric ester, ibopamine, is its orally active prodrug. It is rapidly and extensively absorbed in the gut and is then rapidly hydrolyzed to epinine by plasma and tissue esterases (Fig. 133–1).

The first studies of the pharmacologic properties of

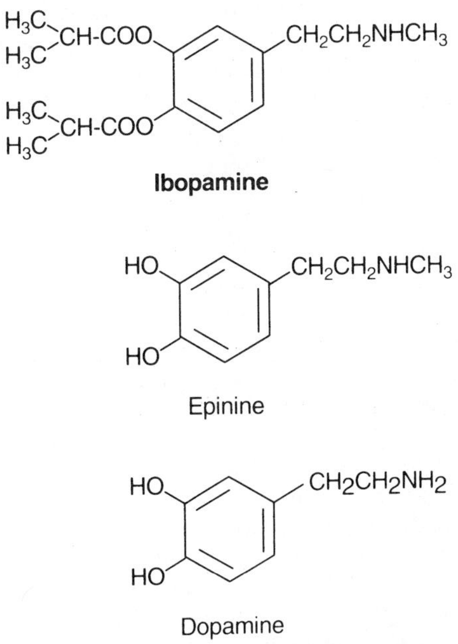

Figure 133–1. Chemical structures of dopamine, epinine and ibopamine. (From Spencer C, Faulds D, Fitton A: Ibopamine. A review of its pharmacodynamic and pharmacokinetic properties, and therapeutic use in congestive heart failure. Drugs Aging 3:556, 1993.)

ibopamine were performed in the anesthetized dog. Like intravenously administered DA, ibopamine, administered intraduodenally, induced an increase in renal blood flow with a concomitant reduction of renal vascular resistance. These changes became significant at the lowest dose of 0.8 mg/kg, with dose-dependent increments up to the dose of 24 mg/kg.[12] Urine flow also increased after doses of 4 to 8 mg/kg.[13] As with DA, the lowest doses of ibopamine increased renal flow without significant changes in other hemodynamic parameters. Starting with a dose of 8 mg/kg, intraduodenally administered ibopamine led to significant and dose-dependent improvement in indexes of myocardial contractility and relaxation alongside a concomitant, weaker increase of myocardial oxygen consumption and coronary blood flow.[12-15]

The effects on renal blood flow were mediated by DA receptor stimulation, whereas those on myocardial contractility were mediated by β-receptors, as shown by their selective inhibition by D-sulpiride and levomoprolol, respectively.[12-14]

Pulmonary pressures and left ventricular end-diastolic pressure were not significantly changed;[12, 13, 15] one study noted a biphasic response similar to the one described in HF patients.[15]

Because ibopamine does not pass through the blood-brain barrier, peripheral administration led to no significant effect on the central nervous system.[14, 16]

MECHANISM OF ACTION

N-Methyl-dopamine (epinine) is equipotent with DA at DA receptors with a weaker action on adrenergic receptors.[3, 5, 9, 10, 16-22] Its order of potency is DA1 = DA2 > β2 > β1 > α.[16-22]

Stimulation of DA receptors induces vasodilation both directly—through DA1 receptors, in the renal, mesenteric, cerebral, and coronary vascular beds[1-4]—and indirectly, through the inhibition of NE release induced by DA2 receptor stimulation. Natriuresis may occur as a result of an increase in renal blood flow and through direct stimulation of renal tubular DA1 receptors. Stimulation of DA2 receptors decreases sympathetic activity and inhibits angiotensin II–induced aldosterone secretion.[1-4, 7, 8] Activation of vascular β2-receptors may contribute to induce peripheral vasodilation, whereas stimulation of myocardial β-receptors may increase myocardial contractility.

At the doses used in clinical practice, ibopamine acts mainly through DA receptor stimulation with peripheral vasodilation, inhibition of the sympathetic and renin-angiotensin-aldosterone systems, and possibly increased natriuresis. Its actions on myocardial contractility are generally very weak[23] or absent.[24] There are three possible explanations for this phenomenon. First, the effect of epinine on myocardial contractility may be considered the algebraic sum of the decrease of sympathetic drive caused by DA2 receptor stimulation, which should decrease contractility, and by myocardial β-receptor stimulation, which should increase it. Second, the number and sensitivity of β_1-receptors, and thus the response to β_1-agonists, are reduced in patients with HF.[25, 26] Third, and most important, epinine stimulates β-receptors at doses 10 times[12, 21] to 1000 times higher than the ones active on DA receptors.[12–14, 18–22, 27] In one series of experiments, relaxation of vascular smooth muscle was obtained with epinine concentrations ranging from 10^{-10} to 10^{-7} M, whereas the inotropic effect became evident starting with concentrations of 10^{-5} M.[27] In the experiments performed after intraduodenal administration of ibopamine to anesthetized dogs, this drug induced a significant reduction of renal vascular resistance starting at a dose of 0.8 mg/kg, whereas myocardial dP/dt started to increase after a dose of 6 mg/kg.[12, 13] These data are further supported by the lack of desensitization of β- and α-adrenergic receptors after long-term administration of ibopamine (100 mg three times a day) to normal subjects.[28]

PHARMACOKINETICS

Ibopamine, after oral ingestion, is rapidly and extensively absorbed in the gut, and then, within a few minutes, undergoes hydrolysis by plasma and tissue esterases to epinine. Epinine can be detected in plasma within 5 to 10 minutes after ibopamine ingestion.[29] Peak plasma concentrations of free epinine are achieved 0.5 to 1 hour after ingestion, with a rapid decline to minimal levels within 2 hours. Epinine is partially conjugated to plasma proteins; the pharmacokinetics of conjugated epinine are slower—it reaches peak concentrations at 2 hours after ibopamine ingestion and has a half-life ranging from 1.5 to 4.5 hours.[29, 30]

Epinine is excreted mainly through kidneys after being either sulfoconjugated or hydrolyzed to dihydroxyphenilacetic acid (DOPAC) or homovanillic acid (HVA).[29]

The pharmacokinetics of ibopamine are not significantly modified in HF,[31, 32] except for a slight prolongation of the half-life of conjugated epinine.[31] In a study performed in patients with chronic HF, plasma levels of epinine peaked 0.5 hour after ingestion, with minimal levels detected after 4 and 8 hours. Peak epinine plasma concentrations averaged 26 ± 5, 20 ± 6, and 15 ± 4 ng/ml after oral ingestion of 300, 200, and 100 mg, respectively.[33]

Ibopamine pharmacokinetics are not modified by long-term therapy.[31] Even frequent administrations (e.g., every 3 to 4 hours) to patients with advanced HF did not significantly modify free epinine plasma levels.[34] These data show that enzymatic pathways involved in ibopamine metabolism do not become saturated after prolonged treatments or frequent daily administrations.

Higher levels of free and conjugated epinine with a longer half-life were observed in elderly HF patients, patients with liver cirrhosis,[30] and patients with advanced renal failure.[35] Epinine pharmacokinetic changes in elderly patients are related to the age-dependent decline of renal function.[30, 35]

The administration of ibopamine with, or shortly after, a meal reduced both the rate of appearance and the peak plasma levels of epinine with a concomitant blunting of its hemodynamic effects.[36, 37] Ibopamine thus should be administered in fasting conditions.

No correlation has been found between epinine pharmacokinetics and ibopamine pharmacodynamic effects. Ibopamine hemodynamic effects may last up to 4 to 8 hours after oral ingestion, when plasma levels of epinine are often not detectable.[33, 38] This discrepancy can be explained by a selective uptake of epinine by peripheral tissues, such as sympathetic nerve endings, so that plasma levels do not reflect epinine activity at the receptorial level.

CLINICAL EFFECTS
Hemodynamics

Acute hemodynamic effects of ibopamine have been widely studied using both open[33, 38–43] and placebo-controlled protocols.[23, 44] Ibopamine was orally administered at a dose of 100 mg in most of the studies;[23, 33, 40–44] doses of 200[23, 33, 38] and 300 mg[23, 33] were also tested (Table 133–1).

Ibopamine administration induced a significant increase in cardiac index, stroke volume, and stroke work indexes with a concomitant reduction in systemic vascular resistance (see Table 133–1) and no significant change of mean arterial pressure and heart rate.[23, 33, 38, 40–45] Peak hemodynamic changes generally occurred at about 1 to 2 hours with, in many studies, persistent changes up to 6 hours after drug ingestion.[23, 33, 39]

One study found a significant correlation between epinine plasma levels and the hemodynamic changes,[46] but another did not.[38] Similarly, the increase in cardiac index was greater after the dose of 200 mg than after that of 100 mg in one study[23] but not in another;[33] in both studies, the dose of 300 mg led to no significant improvement compared with the lower doses.[23, 33] The dose of ibopamine can, however, influence its duration of action, with a longer duration of action after doses of 200 and 300 mg.[33]

Pulmonary pressures and right atrial pressure were not significantly changed by ibopamine administration in most studies (see Table 133–1). In some studies, a biphasic response of mean right atrial pressure, pulmonary arterial pressure, and pulmonary wedge pressure was noted. This response consists of a transient, generally asymptomatic rise occurring 15 to 30 minutes after ibopamine ingestion, followed by a return to basal or lower values in the next 30 minutes.[23, 33, 47–50] Thereafter, filling pressures remain similar to basal values or tend to decrease below them.[23, 33, 49] The transient increase of filling pressures is dose-related, being evident above all with single doses of 200 to 300 mg;[23, 33] this increase also persists after repeated drug administrations[49] and, except in a few patients,[47, 48] has not been associated with adverse symptoms.[23, 33, 46] A lack of change and, in some patients, an increase of pulmonary pressures has been

Table 133–1. **Percentage of Hemodynamic Changes Induced by a Single Oral Dose of Ibopamine in Patients with Chronic Heart Failure**

Reference	Patients (n)	Ibopamine Dose (mg)	Mean Change (%)				
			CI	SVI	SWI	SVR	PWP
Dei Cas et al. (1983)[39]	10	150	31	30	31	−20	−22
Ren et al. (1984)[23]	10	100	—	13	—	−15	0
		200	20	13	—	−19	0
		300	20	16	—	−19	0
De Vita et al. (1986)[38]	11	200	35	37	48	−29	0
Rajfer et al. (1986)[33]	15	100	19	16	—	−14	− 7
		200	16	11	—	−12	−12
		300	25	19	—	−14	−10
Reffo et al. (1988)[40]	15	100	18	—	15	−15	−12
van Veldhuisen et al. (1990)[41]	13	100	33	35	40	−17	−11
van Veldhuisen et al. (1991)[42]	12	100	32	34	40	−20	−13
Itoh et al. (1992)[43]	10	100	15	11	—	−17	0
Dei Cas et al. (1992)[44]	11	100	32	25	39	−23	− 3
Mean		100–150	23	23	33	−17	− 9
Patient number			96	82	59	94	94
Mean		200	23	20	—	−19	—
Patient number			36	36	—	36	—
Mean		300	23	18	—	−16	—
Patient number			25	25	—	25	—

Percentages were calculated as changes from baseline values at peak hemodynamic effect.
CI, cardiac index; SVI, stroke volume index; SWI, stroke work index; SVR, systemic vascular resistance; PWP, pulmonary wedge pressure.

observed also after DA[51, 52] and levodopa administration.[53] This increase of pulmonary pressures can be prevented by the combination of either DA[52, 54] or ibopamine[44, 48, 55] with other vasodilators.

Comparative studies have shown that the hemodynamic changes following ibopamine administration (100 to 200 mg) are similar to those of an infusion of 2 to 4 μg/kg/min of DA;[23, 33, 38, 45] however, the percentage of hemodynamic changes observed after ibopamine administration has not been significantly correlated with different doses of DA.[45, 56] This may be explained by differences in the receptorial activity and neuroendocrine effects of the two drugs. In fact, plasma NE levels were reduced by ibopamine ingestion, whereas they increased during DA infusion[45] because of its tyramine-like activity.[1, 4]

Orally administered ibopamine has been successfully used as a substitute for intravenously administered DA in patients with unstable, severe HF who could not tolerate DA withdrawal and conventional oral therapy.[34, 57] In some of these patients, frequent daily administrations have been needed (up to 100 mg every 3 to 4 hours).[34]

Ibopamine hemodynamic effects are maintained also when it is administered with other vasodilators such as intravenously administered nitroprusside[55] and orally administered nifedipine,[58] enalapril,[44, 59] or captopril.[44, 60] As already noted, these associations may prevent the early rise of ventricular filling pressures after ibopamine administration.

The resting hemodynamic effects of ibopamine are maintained also during maximal bicycle exercise[44, 61]

and after long-term therapy (Fig. 133–2).[22, 34, 43, 44, 61, 62] This is important, because it is known that sympathomimetic agents lose their efficacy during long-term therapy because of the progressive downregulation of myocardial β1-receptors.[25, 26, 63] In contrast, persistence of the hemodynamic changes induced by the acute administration of ibopamine has been shown both in open, uncontrolled trials[12, 34, 43, 62] and in a double-blind, placebo-controlled study in which the resting and exercise hemodynamic changes induced by acute and long-term administration of ibopamine (100 mg three times a day) or placebo were compared.[44] In this study, ibopamine induced a significant increase of both resting and peak exercise cardiac indexes, stroke volume index, and stroke work index with a concomitant reduction of systemic vascular resistance. The results obtained after acute drug ingestion did not differ significantly from those obtained after readministration during long-term therapy (see Fig. 133–2).[44] In contrast, another study, in which higher doses of ibopamine were administered over the long term, noted partial attenuation of the early hemodynamic response to ibopamine.[33] It is possible that, at doses exceeding 200 mg three times a day, ibopamine also acts on myocardial β-receptors, with their consequent downregulation during long-term therapy.

Mechanism of the Hemodynamic Effects

The hemodynamic improvement observed after ibopamine administration can be mainly ascribed to the

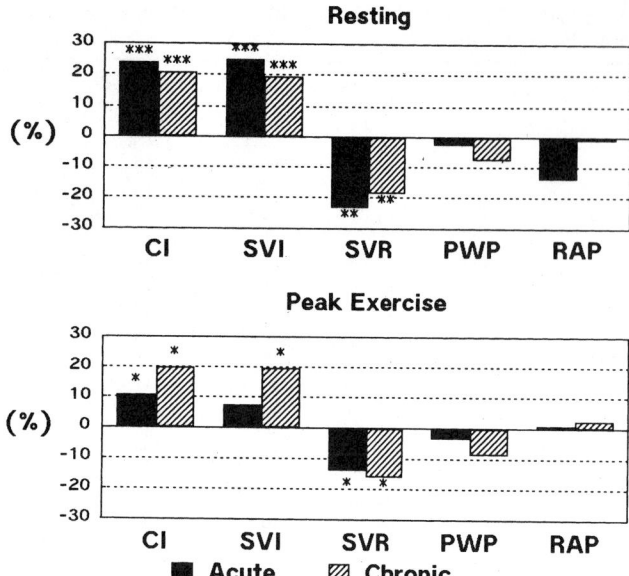

Figure 133–2. Changes of resting and exercise hemodynamics (%) after acute (*black bars*) and chronic (*hatched bars*) ibopamine administration (100 mg t.i.d.) to patients with chronic heart failure. CI, cardiac index; PWP, pulmonary wedge pressure; RAP, right atrial pressure; SVI, stroke volume index; SVR, systemic vascular resistance; ***, **, * = $p < .001$, .01, and .05, respectively, versus placebo (not reported). (From Dei Cas L, Metra M, Visioli O: Effects of acute and chronic ibopamine administration on resting and exercise hemodynamics, plasma catecholamines and functional capacity of patients with chronic congestive heart failure. Am J Cardiol 70:629, 1992.)

arterial vasodilation induced directly by stimulation of DA1 receptors and, to a lesser extent, postsynaptic β₂-receptors, and indirectly by the inhibition of NE release caused by DA2 receptor stimulation. Accordingly, peripheral vasodilatory activity of ibopamine, in HF patients, is significantly inhibited by the DA receptor antagonist sulpiride.[64]

Reduction of left ventricular afterload seems, therefore, the main determinant of the hemodynamic effects of ibopamine. A second mechanism may be the activation of myocardial β-receptors with an increase of myocardial contractility. However, the number and sensitivity of myocardial β₁-receptors are reduced in dilated cardiomyopathy,[25, 26] and both experimental[22, 27] and clinical data[23, 24] show that ibopamine, at a dose of 100 mg, has a very weak action on myocardial contractility. It may also be that the weak action of ibopamine on myocardial β-receptors is offset by the reduced sympathetic drive secondary to DA2 receptor stimulation.[45]

Systolic time intervals have been widely used to assess the inotropic activity of ibopamine. With this method, a decrease in preejection period and in the ratio of the preejection period to left ventricular ejection time, consistent with positive inotropic activity, has been found after ibopamine administration.[23, 65–69] The results obtained in patients with HF,[23] however, have been far less dramatic than those obtained in normal subjects[65, 67] and suggest that the inotropic

activity of ibopamine is mild, short-lived, and generally present only with doses exceeding 200 mg.[23]

In another study, the acute hemodynamic effects of intravenously administered epinine at doses of 0.5 and 1 μg/kg/min, yielding plasma levels comparable with those achieved after ingestion of 100 and 200 mg of ibopamine, were evaluated using right- and left-sided heart catheterization (Fig. 133–3).[24] Epinine infusion induced a significant reduction in systemic vascular resistance accompanied, at the dose of 1 μg/kg/min, by a significant increase in stroke volume index and left ventricular ejection fraction. Epinine infusion did not significantly change indexes of left ventricular contractility and isovolumetric relaxation, which are known to be improved by β-adrenergic stimulation (see Fig. 133–3).[24] These data further support the hypothesis that peripheral vasodilation is the main hemodynamic effect of ibopamine in patients with HF.

The slight activity of ibopamine on myocardial β₁-receptors is also shown by the results of long-term studies that showed the lack of tolerance development during long-term therapy.[34, 43, 44, 61, 62] Tolerance is known to develop during long-term administration of β-adrenergic agonists because of receptor downregulation.[63] Ibopamine's hemodynamic effects have been partially attenuated only in a study in which relatively high doses, probably able to also stimulate myocardial β-receptors, were used (300 mg three times a day in five patients, 200 mg three times a day in four patients, and 100 mg three times a day in only one patient).[33] Other studies found no evidence of tolerance development using the dose of 100 mg three

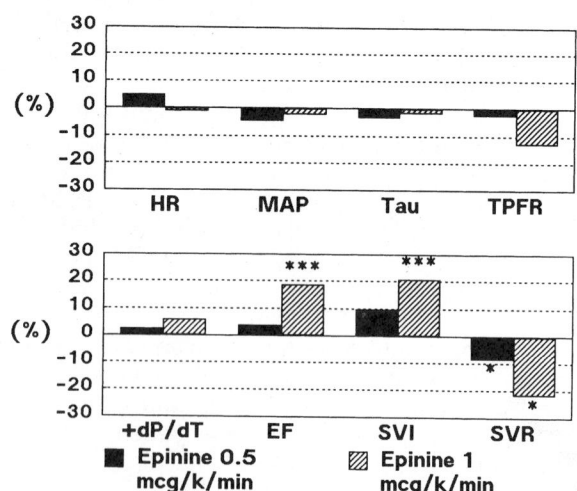

Figure 133–3. Change of indexes of left ventricular function (%) after intravenous epinine at doses of 0.5 μg/kg/min (*black bars*) and 1 μg/kg/min (*hatched bars*), in patients with chronic heart failure. +dP/dt, peak positive dP/dt; EF, ejection fraction; HR, heart rate; MAP, mean arterial pressure; SVI, stroke volume index; TAU, time constant of isovolumetric relaxation; TPFR, time to peak filling rate; ***, * = $p < .001$ and .05, respectively, versus placebo (not reported). (From Rousseau MF, Raigoso J, Van Eyll C, et al: Effects of intravenous epinine administration on left ventricular systolic performance, coronary hemodynamics and circulating catecholamines in patients with heart failure. J Cardiovasc Pharmacol 19:155, 1992.)

times a day.[43, 44, 62] At these doses, therefore, ibopamine does not seem to be active on myocardial β-receptors.

The mechanism of the transient increase of left ventricular filling pressures after ibopamine ingestion is still controversial. It is probably caused by stimulation of postsynaptic α_2-receptors in venous vascular bed. Venoconstriction may increase venous return and right ventricular preload, which, because of the diastolic interaction between the right and left ventricles, will shift upward the left ventricular diastolic pressure-volume curve.[24, 33] Postsynaptic α_2-receptors are known to present a greater density in several venous beds compared with the arterial tissues.[70-72] Thus, epinine plasma levels achieved after relatively high oral doses of ibopamine might induce vasodilation in the arterial bed through DA and β_2-receptor stimulation and, simultaneously, cause a transient increase of venous return through α_2-receptor activation.

Another potential mechanism of the transient increase of pulmonary pressures after ibopamine administration is pulmonary vessel constriction induced by α-adrenergic stimulation and partially offset by concomitant DA and β_2-receptor activation. This hypothesis has been experimentally demonstrated.[73, 74] However, pulmonary arteriolar vasoconstriction does not explain the concomitant rise of pulmonary wedge pressures.

Electrophysiology

Sympathetic stimulation, through its action on myocardial β-receptors, is known to induce potentially lethal ventricular tachyarrhythmias in patients with HF.[75] The arrhythmogenic potential of ibopamine has been, therefore, widely studied. This drug might increase the incidence of ventricular arrhythmias through its action on myocardial β-receptors, but it might also decrease it through the decrease of the cardiac sympathetic drive induced by presynaptic DA2 and, maybe, α_2-receptor stimulation.

Long-term therapy with ibopamine, 100 mg three times a day, did not significantly change electrocardiographic parameters and the frequency and complexity of ventricular and supraventricular tachyarrhythmias as measured with Holter monitoring in two placebo-controlled studies of 45 patients[76] and 97 patients[77] with moderate, chronic HF. Holter studies detected no significant proarrhythmic effect of ibopamine; in some studies, the frequency of ventricular premature beats was slightly, but significantly, decreased by ibopamine.[62, 76]

Ibopamine did not significantly change atrioventricular and intraventricular conduction times in invasive electrophysiologic studies performed both in healthy volunteers[78] and in HF patients with episodes of ventricular tachycardia.[42] In these patients, ibopamine, 100 mg orally, did not change the ventricular refractory period and had no proarrhythmic effect at programmed ventricular stimulation.[42]

These data further show that ibopamine, at least at the dose of 100 mg, is weakly active, or not active at all, on myocardial β-receptors, whereas its effects on DA receptors, with a decrease of cardiac sympathetic drive, predominate.

Renal Function

In the anesthetized dog, intraduodenally administered ibopamine has been shown to induce an increase in renal blood flow, diuresis, and natriuresis mediated by stimulation of DA receptors.[12, 13] However, concomitant stimulation of α-adrenergic receptors may counteract the vasodilating activity of epinine so that no significant change of renal blood flow was noted in other experiments.[16] Lastly, the direct effects of dopaminergic agents on glomerular filtration rate are still controversial.[79]

In healthy subjects, ibopamine ingestion induced a significant increase of creatinine clearance in some studies[80, 81] but not in others.[82] In one study, ibopamine (100 mg) did not change renal blood flow and led to a significant 10% rise of glomerular filtration rate, inhibited by the relatively selective DA2 antagonist metoclopramide.[83] In this same study, natriuresis increased mildly.[83] Results of other studies have been conflicting.[81, 82]

Ibopamine administration to patients with HF has induced a significant rise of renal blood flow, glomerular filtration rate, and natriuresis.[66, 84] In one study, the increases of renal blood flow and glomerular filtration rate averaged 15% and 11%, respectively, with a significant improvement 2 and 3 hours after ibopamine ingestion (100 mg).[84] Filtration fraction is not significantly changed by ibopamine, which is consistent with an effect mainly mediated by renal vasodilation, with similar effects on the afferent and efferent glomerular arterioles.[84] In contrast with these data, renal function was not significantly changed in another study in which patients with milder HF were studied and ibopamine was administered at a dose of 200 mg.[85] It is possible that when ibopamine doses exceed 200 mg, stimulation of α-receptors offsets the effects of DA receptor stimulation.[16] The improvement in renal perfusion and function after ibopamine might be clinically relevant and might increase the response to diuretic therapy and/or allow a reduction of the diuretic dose in patients with HF.[86]

Studies in patients with chronic renal failure have shown an increase of diuresis, renal blood flow, creatinine clearance, and electrolyte excretion[22, 87] with a slower progression of renal impairment[88] during ibopamine administration. Similarly, urine output, glomerular filtration rate, and sodium excretion have increased in patients with liver cirrhosis and normal sodium excretion but not in those with sodium retention at baseline.[89]

Neurohumoral System

In patients with chronic HF, activation of the sympathoadrenergic and renin angiotensin systems is associated with a poor prognosis. Angiotensin-converting enzyme (ACE) inhibitors have been shown to significantly improve survival and outcome, and β-blockers,

Table 133–2. **Percentage of Changes of Plasma Catecholamines Induced by Ibopamine in Patients with Chronic Heart Failure**

Reference	Patients (n)	Duration of Study	Drug	Mean Change % NE	EPI
Rajfer et al. (1986)[33]	15	Acute	Ibop	−51†	—
Nakano et al. (1986)[96]	11	Acute	Ibop	−24†	—
Caponetto et al. (1986)[111]*	30	6 months	Ibop	−35†	—
van Veldhuisen et al. (1991)[42]	12	1 week	Ibop	−23†	−20
Pizzorni et al. (1991)[98]	20	Acute	Ibop	−14†	−27†
	8	3 months	Plac	−11	+12
	9	3 months	Ibop	+15	+39
Dei Cas et al. (1992)[44]	12	Acute	Plac	—	—
	11		Ibop	−40†	—
	12	2 months	Plac	—	—
	11		Ibop	−26†	—
van Veldhuisen et al. (1993)[100]	11	1 month	Ibop	−29†	—
van Veldhuisen et al. (1993)[101]	53	6 months	Plac	+15	—
	53		Ibop	− 3†	—
	55		Dig	−24†	—
Girbes et al. (1993)[84]	10	Acute	Ibop	−12	−11
Rousseau et al. (1994)[102]	10	4–6 weeks	Plac	+22	—
	9		Ibop	−24†	—

Percentages were calculated as changes from baseline values at peak hemodynamic effect.
*Urinary norepinephrine was used in this study.
†*p* <.05 in comparison with baseline or, when present, placebo.
Plac, placebo; Ibop, ibopamine; Dig, digoxin.

in contrast with sympathoadrenergic agonists, seem to be able to improve clinical conditions and slow the progression of the disease. These data are consistent with the hypothesis that neurohumoral activation is one of the main determinants of the progression of HF.[90, 91] Therefore, the actions of ibopamine on some neurohumoral mechanisms may be useful for the long-term treatment of this syndrome.[92, 93]

Plasma NE is related to sympathoadrenergic activation[94] and is an independent prognostic indicator in patients with HF.[95] Many studies have shown that ibopamine administration can induce a significant reduction of plasma NE in patients with HF (Table 133–2).[33, 42, 44, 96–102] Ibopamine also blunted the sympathetic response to exercise as shown by the significant reduction of both resting and peak exercise plasma NE.[44, 99, 100]

Reduction of plasma NE is maintained also during long-term therapy (see Table 133–2).[44, 100–102] In a study, the hemodynamic and neurohumoral effects of ibopamine or placebo administration were evaluated before and after 2 months of long-term therapy.[44] Plasma NE levels averaged 733 ± 245 pg/ml at baseline, were significantly reduced by acute ibopamine administration, and remained decreased to 544 ± 227 pg/ml after long-term therapy, 12 hours after the last drug administration, with a further decline to 384 ± 145 pg/ml after the next ibopamine ingestion. The placebo group experienced no significant change.[44] In another study, plasma NE decreased from 516 ± 241 to 391 ± 208 pg/ml after long-term ibopamine ther-

apy, whereas plasma NE increased from 500 ± 257 to 611 ± 329 pg/ml with placebo.[102] It is interesting to note that both these studies were performed in patients also treated with ACE inhibitors, thus showing that neurohumoral activation remains in a significant proportion of these patients and that further inhibition of the sympathetic nervous system may be possible. In another large multicenter trial, plasma NE declined by 16 pg/ml after 6 months of ibopamine therapy, whereas it increased by 62 pg/ml in the placebo group.[101] Although the change after ibopamine was smaller than the one observed in a group of patients treated with digitalis, it was still significant compared with placebo.[101]

Reduction of plasma NE levels after ibopamine is likely caused by its action on presynaptic DA2 receptors, and possibly also α_2-receptors, with a consequent inhibition of NE release from its storage sites in the sympathetic nerve terminals.[1–4] Hemodynamic improvement induced by ibopamine might also reduce sympathoadrenergic activity. However, DA and levodopa, whose hemodynamic effects are similar to those of ibopamine, tend to increase plasma NE because of their tyramine-like activity.[45, 103, 104] In contrast, administration of DA2 agonists has caused a reduction of plasma NE similar to that observed after ibopamine administration, independent of any significant hemodynamic change.[45]

Some studies also showed a reduction of plasma epinephrine after ibopamine therapy;[97, 98] others did not confirm these data.[42, 44, 100, 102] It is known, however, that plasma epinephrine is mainly derived from the adrenal medulla and is therefore less related to sympathetic drive than plasma NE is.

Plasma aldosterone levels were significantly decreased by ibopamine administration in some studies[80, 105, 106] but not in others.[83, 84, 96, 98, 101] These discrepancies may be explained by the peculiar action of dopaminergic drugs on aldosterone secretion. In fact, these agents, through their action on DA2 receptors, selectively inhibit aldosterone secretion induced by angiotensin II without any influence on basal aldosterone secretion or on its secretion induced by other stimuli (e.g., adrenocorticotropic hormone).[8] Accordingly, 100 mg of ibopamine significantly reduced aldosterone only in HF patients with high baseline levels of this hormone.[45, 107] In this study, the relatively selective DA2 antagonist dihydroergotoxine had effects on plasma NE and aldosterone similar to those of ibopamine, further showing that the neuroendocrine actions of ibopamine are mainly mediated by DA2 receptors.[107]

Data regarding ibopamine effects on renin activity are conflicting, with some studies showing a decrease of plasma renin[96, 101, 108] and others no change.[45, 80, 83, 84, 102, 107] However, DA seems to have rather weak and divergent effects on renin secretion.[8] The reduction of plasma renin activity observed in some studies after ibopamine administration may be caused by the hemodynamic improvement or by reduced sympathetic stimulation of the juxtaglomerular cells rather than by a direct effect of this agent.

Plasma prolactin levels were reduced by ibopamine in normal subjects.[106] Plasma concentrations of endothelin I, angiotensin II, atrial natriuretic factor, and arginine vasopressin were not significantly affected by long-term ibopamine administration to HF patients in one study.[102]

CLINICAL EFFICACY

Many trials have investigated the effects of long-term ibopamine therapy on clinical symptoms, functional capacity, and quality of life of patients with HF (Tables 133–3 and 133–4).[44, 86, 98, 101, 102, 109–124] However, some important limits must be pointed out. First,

many of the placebo-controlled studies included only relatively small numbers of patients. Second, the various trials show important differences in HF severity and concomitant therapy: some studies included only patients with NYHA class I to II HF who did not need any other cardiovascular drug;[98, 117, 118] others included patients with advanced HF, still symptomatic despite maximal tolerated doses of digitalis, furosemide, and vasodilators.[44, 102, 114] Third, administration of ACE inhibitors may currently be considered warranted in every HF patient who can tolerate them because of their clear-cut beneficial effects on survival and disease progression;[91, 125, 126] digitalis glycosides, too, seem to be able to improve symptoms and functional capacity and stabilize the clinical course of HF patients.[127] It thus seems rational that every new drug proposed for the treatment of HF be first used in addition to diuretics, ACE inhibitors and, possibly, digitalis.[125, 126] Unfortunately, these principles were less clear when most of the studies of the clinical efficacy of ibopamine were projected; therefore, ibopamine has been often tested as an alternative to digitalis,[101, 115, 116, 118, 120, 121] diuretics,[117, 122] or ACE inhibitors,[59, 60, 119] and only a few studies have evaluated the clinical utility of ibopamine's association with these agents compared with placebo.[44, 102]

Clinical Symptoms

As already stated, ibopamine maintains its acute hemodynamic and neurohumoral effects after long-term administration without leading to tolerance.[34, 40, 43, 44, 62] Long-term ibopamine therapy has been shown to significantly improve symptoms, NYHA functional class, and clinical signs of HF in patients with severe,[34, 57] moderate,[41–44, 59–62, 86, 109–116, 119] and mild HF.[98, 117, 118, 120–122]

Unfortunately, the largest studies were not controlled with placebo and double-blinded.[121, 123] In one study, 544 HF patients were followed for 1 year during long-term ibopamine therapy associated with conventional treatment of HF.[123] Ibopamine significantly improved clinical symptoms, NYHA class, and Doppler parameters in most patients; the annual mortality

Table 133–3. **Placebo-Controlled Trials Regarding Clinical Efficacy of Ibopamine in Patients with Chronic Heart Failure**

Reference	Patients (*n*)	Ibopamine Dose (mg)	Protocol Design	Associated Drugs	Therapy Duration
Dei Cas et al. (1986)[109]	25	100 t.i.d.	Crossover single-blind	Dig + Diur	1 week
Gronda et al. (1986)[110]	8	100 b.i.d.–t.i.d.	Crossover double-blind	Dig + Diur	2 weeks
Caponetto et al. (1986)[111]	42	100 t.i.d.	Crossover double-blind	Dig + Diur	10 days
Trinchero et al. (1988)[112]	20	100 t.i.d.	Crossover single-blind	Dig + Diur + Vas	1 month
Condorelli et al. (1989)[113]	84	100 t.i.d.	Parallel double-blind	Dig + Fur	3 months
Dalla Volta et al. (1991)[86]	78	2.5/kg t.i.d.	Parallel double-blind	Fur	6 weeks
Pizzorni et al. (1991)[98]	40	100 t.i.d.	Parallel double-blind	None	3 months
Kayanakis et al. (1991)[114]	111	200 t.i.d.	Parallel double-blind	Dig + Fur + IDN	6 months
Dei Cas et al. (1992)[44]	23	100 t.i.d.	Parallel double-blind	Dig + Fur + ACEI	2 months
Rousseau et al. (1994)[102]	19	100 t.i.d.	Parallel double-blind	Dig + Fur + ACEI	4–6 weeks

Dig, digitalis glycosides; Diur, diuretics; Fur, furosemide; Vas, vasodilators; IDN, isosorbide dinitrate; ACEI, angiotensin-converting enzyme inhibitor.

Table 133–4. Placebo-Controlled Comparative Trials Regarding Clinical Efficacy of Ibopamine in Patients with Chronic Heart Failure

Reference	Patients (n)	Ibopamine Dose (mg)	Protocol Design	Associated Drugs	Therapy Duration
Ibopamine versus digoxin					
Cadel et al. (1986)[115]	14	50 t.i.d.	Crossover single-blind	Fur Vas	1 month
Alicandri et al. (1989)[116]	10	100 t.i.d.	Crossover double-blind	Diur	10 days
Kleber et al. (1990)[117]	60	200 b.i.d.	Parallel double-blind	None	1 month
van Veldhuisen et al. (1993)[101]	161	100 t.i.d.	Parallel double-blind	Fur	6 months
Ibopamine versus diuretics					
Kleber and Thyroff-Friesinger (1990)[118]	247	200 b.i.d.	Parallel double-blind	None	2 months
Ibopamine versus ACE inhibitor					
Barabino et al. (1991)[119]	150	50–100 t.i.d.	Parallel double-blind	Fur	6 months

Diur, diuretics; Fur, furosemide; Vas, vasodilators.

rate was 12.5%, which compares favorably with the mortality rates observed in similar study groups.[123]

In two relatively large multicenter, placebo-controlled, double-blind trials, clinical symptoms, NYHA class, and exercise duration improved significantly compared with placebo after 3 months of ibopamine therapy at a dose of 100 mg three times a day[113] or 200 mg three times a day.[114] Some studies have reported a reduction in the furosemide dose in patients treated with ibopamine,[86] but others have not.[101]

Many studies show that functional capacity was significantly improved by ibopamine as evaluated by the maximal exercise test.[98, 111–114, 116] Similar to what was observed with ACE inhibitors,[128] a significant improvement of functional capacity required at least 3 months of ibopamine therapy in some trials.[113, 114] Ibopamine did not lead to a significant improvement of exercise capacity in two other studies.[44, 101] In one of these studies, however, the study group was small, and follow-up duration was relatively short (2 months).[44] In the other trial, digoxin, but not ibopamine, improved maximal exercise capacity compared with placebo at intention-to-treat analysis, although not when only the 128 patients who completed the trial were analyzed, and ibopamine, but not digoxin, significantly increased exercise tolerance in the patients with milder left ventricular dysfunction.[101] However, it must be noted that scores of clinical symptoms were significantly improved by ibopamine, but not by digoxin or placebo, in this same study.[101]

In other comparative trials (see Table 133–4), ibopamine was at least as effective as digoxin,[115, 116, 118, 120] thiazide diuretics,[117, 122] captopril,[60, 119] or enalapril.[59]

Generally, improvement was greater when ibopamine was combined with these agents rather than used as monotherapy.[59, 60, 117] We believe that, except in patients who cannot tolerate them, ACE inhibitors should be used in all patients with HF because of their beneficial effects on mortality and progression of HF; therefore, the additive benefits of ibopamine combined with ACE inhibitors, diuretics (when necessary), and, possibly, digitalis should be more thoroughly assessed.

Mortality

Despite the benefits of ACE inhibitor therapy, the prognosis of patients with HF is still poor, and improvement of survival still remains the most important goal of therapy.[125, 126, 129] Assessment of the effects on survival of a new drug for the treatment of HF requires large study groups with a relatively long follow-up.[129] Up to now, no trial regarding ibopamine in HF satisfies these requirements; it is therefore impossible to draw any definite conclusion.

Hemodynamic improvement and, above all, inhibition of sympathoadrenergic activation and angiotensin II–induced aldosterone secretion are mechanisms that might improve survival of patients with HF.[90, 91] Mortality data given in the placebo-controlled trials of ibopamine in patients with HF are summarized in Table 133–5. According to these data, ibopamine, unlike inotropic drugs and sympathomimetic agents,[125, 126, 130] does not seem to worsen survival of HF patients. On the contrary, some data seem to suggest that it may improve prognosis (see Table 133–5). The prob-

Table 133–5. Cardiac Mortality in Placebo-Controlled Trials Regarding Clinical Efficacy of Ibopamine in Patients with NYHA Class II–III Heart Failure

Reference	Patients (n)	Ibopamine Dose (mg)	Mean Follow-Up Duration	Placebo	Ibopamine
Dalla Volta et al. (1991)[86]	78	2.5/kg t.i.d.	6 weeks	0/42 (0%)	0/36 (0%)
Pizzorni et al. (1991)[98]	40	100 t.i.d.	3 months	2/20 (10%)	0/20 (0%)
Kayanakis et al. (1991)[114]	80	200 t.i.d.	6 months	3/44 (7%)	1/36 (3%)
Dei Cas et al. (1992)[44]	23	100 t.i.d.	2 months	0/12 (0%)	0/11 (0%)
van Veldhuisen et al. (1993)[101]	161	100 t.i.d.	6 months	2/53 (4%)	1/53 (2%)
Barabino et al. (1991)[119]	150	50–100 t.i.d.	18 months	18/45 (40%)	11/42 (26%)

lem with these data is that, with only one exception,[44] they were collected from patients who were not treated with ACE inhibitors. Therefore, it is mandatory that the effects of long-term ibopamine on mortality be evaluated in a large, placebo-controlled, double-blind study in patients also treated with ACE inhibitors. Such a study, named PRIME II, is currently under way.

TOLERABILITY

All the main trials have shown that ibopamine is well tolerated in patients with HF. Its administration is associated with a low incidence of adverse effects that, in most controlled studies, is not significantly different from that of patients treated with placebo.[44, 101, 113–115, 117, 119]

Gastrointestinal symptoms are the adverse effects that seem to be more frequently associated with ibopamine;[110, 118] they appear, however, in no more than 3% of treated patients and do not generally cause discontinuation of treatment.[131] They include nausea, epigastric distress, heartburn, and, less frequently, vomiting, loose stools, abdominal pain, and diarrhea.[131]

Cardiovascular symptoms, such as chest pain, dyspnea, and palpitations, have been reported during ibopamine therapy.[117–119, 123, 124] However, their incidence is not significantly different from that in patients on placebo, and they were never interpreted as causally related to ibopamine.[111, 113–115, 117–120] A transient, early increase of pulmonary pressures after ibopamine ingestion has not been associated with any symptom; patients sporadically complain of epigastric discomfort and/or chest pain, sweating, and dyspnea during this pulmonary pressures rise.[47] These symptoms, however, have been generally reported after the first administration of relatively high doses of ibopamine (2.05 and 2.34 mg/kg, respectively, in two patients described in one study).[47]

As stated earlier, ibopamine does not seem to have proarrhythmic activity.[22, 62, 76–78, 101, 106, 115] In some studies, ventricular beats became less frequent during ibopamine treatment.[62, 76, 106] Sporadic cases of arrhythmias, possibly related to ibopamine, have been described, however.[60, 114, 120, 122] For example, ibopamine administration to one subject was associated with asymptomatic episodes of accelerated idioventricular rhythm, which disappeared after concomitant metoclopramide administration.[78]

Other adverse events reported in sporadic cases, and possibly related to ibopamine therapy, include tinnitus,[117] sweating,[117] itching,[121] and transaminases elevation.[114, 122] A case of reversible leukopenia has been reported in a patient after 2 days of ibopamine administration at 100 mg three times a day.[132]

In conclusion, ibopamine has excellent tolerability with hemodynamic, renal, and, above all, neurohumoral effects that make it potentially useful as an additive therapy for HF. This drug therefore warrants larger trials that will determine whether it may further improve quality of life and survival in patients with HF.

REFERENCES

1. Goldberg LI: Cardiovascular and renal actions of dopamine: Potential clinical applications. Pharmacol Rev 241:1, 1972.
2. Goldberg LI, Hsieh YY, Resnekov L: Newer catecholamines for treatment of heart failure and shock: An update on dopamine and a first look at dobutamine. Progr Cardiovasc Dis 19:327, 1977.
3. Goldberg LI, Rajfer SI: Dopamine receptors: Applications in clinical cardiology. Circulation 72:245, 1985.
4. Goldberg LI: The role of dopamine receptors in the treatment of congestive heart failure. J Cardiovasc Pharmacol 14(Suppl 5):S19, 1989.
5. Kohli JD, Weder AB, Goldberg LI, et al: Structure activity relationships of N-substituted dopamine derivatives as agonists of the dopamine vascular and other cardiovascular receptors. J Pharmacol Exp Ther 213:370, 1980.
6. Casagrande C, Santangelo F, Saini C, et al: Synthesis and chemical properties of ibopamine and of related esters of N-substituted dopamines—synthesis of ibopamine metabolites. Arzneimittelforschung 36:291, 1986.
7. Kohli JD, Metra M, Satoh Y, Goldberg LI: Dopamine receptors in the stellate ganglion of the dog. Eur J Pharmacol 164:265, 1989.
8. Missale C, Lombardi C, De Cotiis R, et al: Dopaminergic receptor mechanisms modulating the renin-angiotensin system and aldosterone secretion: An overview. J Cardiovasc Pharmacol 14(Suppl 8):S29, 1989.
9. Goldberg LI, Sonneville PF, McKay JL: An investigation of the structural requirements for dopamine-like renal vasodilation: Phenylethylamines and apomorphine. J Pharmacol Exp Ther 163:188, 1968.
10. Goldberg LI, Volkman PH, Kohli JD: A comparison of the vascular dopamine receptor with other dopamine receptors. Ann Rev Pharmacol Toxicol 18:57, 1978.
11. Volkman PH, Kohli JD, Goldberg LI, et al: Dipropyl-dopamine, a qualitatively different dopamine (DA) agonist. Fed Proc 36:1049, 1977.
12. Merlo L, Ghirardi P, Brusoni B, et al: Effects of ibopamine on systemic, pulmonary and regional hemodynamics. Experimental investigations in anesthetized dogs. Arzneimittelforschung 36:304, 1986.
13. Casagrande C, Merlo L, Ferrini R, et al: Cardiovascular and renal action of dopaminergic prodrugs. J Cardiovasc Pharmacol 14(Suppl 8):S40, 1989.
14. Bernardi L, Perlini S, Soffiantino F, et al: Acute hemodynamic effects of ibopamine and dopamine on isovolumic relaxation. Eur J Pharmacol 164:415, 1989.
15. Casagrande C, Metra M: Animal pharmacology. In Casagrande C, Metra M (eds): Ibopamine 1992: A Comprehensive, Updated Review. Milan: CNM Bresso, 1992, pp 20–50.
16. Itoh H, Kohli JD, Rajfer SI, Goldberg LI: Comparison of the cardiovascular actions of dopamine and epinine in the dog. J Pharmacol Exp Ther 233:87, 1985.
17. Nichols AJ, Ruffolo RR: Evaluation of the alpha and beta-adrenoceptor mediated activities of the novel, orally active inotropic agent, ibopamine, in the cardiovascular system of the pithed rat. Comparison with epinine and dopamine. J Pharmacol Exp Ther 242:455, 1987.
18. Bravo G, Ghysel Burton J, Jaumin P, Godfraind T: A comparison of the inotropic effects of dopamine and epinine in human isolated cardiac preparations. J Pharmacol Exp Ther 257:439, 1991.
19. Borchard U: Pharmakologische Grundlagen. Z Kardiol 80(Suppl 8):63, 1991.
20. Deighton NM, Motomura S, Bals S, et al: Characterization of the beta adrenoceptor subtype(s) mediating the positive inotropic effects of epinine, dopamine, dobutamine, denopamine and xamoterol in isolated human right atrium. J Pharmacol Exp Ther 262:532, 1992.
21. Schwinger RHG, Bohm M, Schulz C, et al: Cardiac inotropic

as well as coronary and pulmonary actions of epinine in human isolated tissues. J Pharmacol Exp Ther 265:346, 1993.

22. Spencer C, Faulds D, Fitton A: Ibopamine. A review of its pharmacodynamic and pharmacokinetic properties, and therapeutic use in congestive heart failure. Drugs Aging 3:556, 1993.

23. Ren JH, Unverferth DV, Leier CV: The dopamine congener, ibopamine, in congestive heart failure. J Cardiovasc Pharmacol 6:748, 1984.

24. Rousseau MF, Raigoso J, Van Eyll C, et al: Effects of intravenous epinine administration on left ventricular systolic performance, coronary hemodynamics and circulating catecholamines in patients with heart failure. J Cardiovasc Pharmacol 19:155, 1992.

25. Bristow MR, Hershberger RE, Port JD, et al: Beta-adrenergic pathways in nonfailing and failing human ventricular myocardium. Circulation 82(Suppl I):12, 1990.

26. Bristow MR: Changes in myocardial and vascular receptors in heart failure. J Am Coll Cardiol 22(Suppl A):61A, 1993.

27. Holubarsch C, Walde T, Hasenfuss G, Just H: Concentration-dependent separation between vasodilating and positive inotropic effect of dopamine/ibopamine [abstract]. Eur Heart J 12:183, 1991.

28. Brodde OE, Klusmann I, Wojcik M, et al: Lack of desensitization of alpha- and beta-adrenoceptor function during chronic treatment of healthy volunteers with ibopamine, an orally active dopamine receptor agonist. Eur J Clin Pharmacol 44:283, 1993.

29. Lodola E, Borgia M, Longo A, et al: Ibopamine kinetics after a single oral dose in healthy volunteers. Arzneimittelforschung 36:345, 1986.

30. Casagrande C, Metra M: Clinical pharmacokinetics. In Casagrande C, Metra M (eds): Ibopamine 1992: A Comprehensive, Updated Review. Milan: CNM Bresso, 1992, pp 76–88.

31. Azzolini F, De Caro L, Longo A, et al: Ibopamine kinetics after single and multiple dosing in patients with congestive heart failure. Int J Clin Pharmacol Ther Toxicol 26:544, 1988.

32. Azzolini F, Cattò G, Iacuitti G, et al: Ibopamine kinetics after a single oral dose in patients with congestive heart failure. Int J Clin Pharmacol Ther Toxicol 26:105, 1988.

33. Rajfer SI, Rossen JD, Douglas FL, et al: Effects of long-term therapy with oral ibopamine on resting hemodynamics and exercise capacity in patients with heart failure: Relationship to the generation of N-methyldopamine and to plasma norepinephrine levels. Circulation 73:740, 1986.

34. Dei Cas L, Metra M, Nodari S, Visioli O: Efficacy of ibopamine treatment in patients with advanced heart failure: Purpose of a new therapeutic scheme with multiple daily administrations. J Cardiovasc Pharmacol 14(Suppl 8):S111, 1989.

35. Salvadeo A, Villa G, Bovio G, et al: Pharmacokinetics of ibopamine in patients with renal impairment. Int J Clin Pharmacol Ther Toxicol 26:98, 1988.

36. De Mey C, Enterling D, Meineke I: Pharmacokinetic and pharmacodynamic interactions between single doses of ibopamine and food in normal man. Arzneimittelforschung 39:1138, 1989.

37. Scott SC, Locke-Haydon J, Pready NS, et al: Ibopamine (SKF 100168) pharmacokinetics in relation to the timing of meals. Br J Clin Pharmacol 23:585, 1987.

38. De Vita C, Triulzi E, Devizzi S, et al: Evaluation of acute hemodynamic effects and pharmacokinetic behaviour of ibopamine in patients with severe heart failure. Arzneimittelforschung 36:349, 1986.

39. Dei Cas L, Bolognesi R, Cucchini F, et al: Hemodynamic effects of ibopamine in patients with idiopathic congestive cardiomyopathy. J Cardiovasc Pharmacol 5:249, 1983.

40. Reffo GC, Gabellini A, Forattini C, et al: Double-blind acute hemodynamic invasive evaluation in congestive heart failure before and after open sustained treatment with ibopamine. Curr Ther Res 44:723, 1988.

41. van Veldhuisen DJ, Girbes AR, Crijns HJ, et al: Efficacy and safety of ibopamine in congestive heart failure. J Auton Pharmacol 10(Suppl 1):S115, 1990.

42. van Veldhuisen DJ, Crijns HJ, Girbes AR, et al: Electrophysiologic profile of ibopamine in patients with congestive heart failure and ventricular tachycardia and relation to its effects

43. Itoh H, Taniguchi K, Tsujibayashi T, et al: Hemodynamic effects and pharmacokinetics of long-term therapy with ibopamine in patients with chronic heart failure. Cardiology 80:356, 1992.

44. Dei Cas L, Metra M, Visioli O. Effects of acute and chronic ibopamine administration on resting and exercise hemodynamics, plasma catecholamines and functional capacity of patients with chronic congestive heart failure. Am J Cardiol 70:629, 1992.

45. Metra M, Missale C, Spano PF, Dei Cas L: Dopaminergic drugs in congestive heart failure. Hemodynamic and neuroendocrine responses to ibopamine, dopamine and dihydroergotoxine. J Cardiovasc Pharmacol 25:732, 1995.

46. Ghirardi P, Brusoni B, Mangiavacchi M, et al: Acute hemodynamic effects of ibopamine in patients with severe congestive heart failure. Br J Clin Pharmacol 19:613, 1985.

47. Humar F, Morgera T, Maras P, Camerini F: Hemodynamic evaluation of ibopamine in patients with refractory congestive heart failure. Arzneimittelforschung 36:360, 1986.

48. Marchionni N, Conti A, De Alfieri W, et al: Ibopamine in congestive heart failure refractory to digitalis, diuretics, and captopril. J Clin Pharmacol 26:74, 1986.

49. Hogg KJ, Hornung RS, Howie CA, Hillis WS: Early cardiovascular changes with ibopamine: Evidence for a biphasic hemodynamic action. Br J Pharmacol 24:435, 1987.

50. Di Mario C, Compostella L, Iavernaro A, et al: Onset of cardiovascular action after oral ibopamine. Early hemodynamic effects of single and repeated doses in patients with idiopathic dilated myocardiopathy. Arzneimittelforschung 40:661, 1990.

51. Loeb HS, Winslow EBJ, Rahimtoola SH, et al: Acute hemodynamic effects of dopamine in patients with shock. Circulation 44:163, 1971.

52. Stemple DR, Kleiman JH, Harrison DC: Combined nitroprusside-dopamine therapy in severe congestive heart failure: Dose related hemodynamic advantages over single drug infusions. Am J Cardiol 42:267, 1978.

53. Shah PK, Amin DK, Horn E: Adverse clinical and hemodynamic effects of oral levodopa in chronic congestive heart failure. Am Heart J 110:488, 1985.

54. Miller RR, Awan NA, Joye JA, et al: Combined dopamine and nitroprusside therapy in congestive heart failure. Greater augmentation of cardiac performance by addition of inotropic stimulation to afterload reduction. Circulation 55:881, 1977.

55. Dei Cas L, Fappani A, Riva S, et al: Hemodynamic advantage of combined administration of oral ibopamine and nitroprusside in patients with ischemic and idiopathic congestive cardiomyopathy. Clin Cardiol 8:427, 1985.

56. Dei Cas L, Metra M, Visioli O: Clinical pharmacology of inodilators. J Cardiovasc Pharmacol 14(Suppl 8):S60, 1989.

57. Kleber FX, Sabin GV, Thyroff-Friesinger U, et al: Ibopamine as a valuable adjunct and substitute for dopamine in bridging therapy before heart transplantation. Cardiology 81:121, 1992.

58. Munger MA, Nara AR, Pospisil RA, et al: Invasive pharmacodynamic characterization of combined ibopamine and calcium blocker therapy for heart failure. Pharmacotherapy 13:218, 1993.

59. Terrachini V, Canale C, Pastorino L, et al: Comparison between ibopamine, enalapril, and their association in the treatment of congestive heart failure. Curr Ther Res 50:753, 1991.

60. Ghiringhelli S, Glisenti F, Straneo G, Licciardello L: Ibopamine-captopril combination for the treatment of congestive heart failure in the elderly. A pilot study. Curr Ther Res 48:96, 1990.

61. Gavazzi A, Mussini A, Bramucci E: Hemodynamic evaluation during exercise test after acute and chronic ibopamine treatment in patients with congestive heart failure. Arzneimittelforschung 36:366, 1986.

62. Dei Cas L, Metra M, Nodari S, et al: Lack of tolerance development during chronic ibopamine administration to patients with congestive heart failure. Cardiovasc Drugs Ther 2:221, 1988.

63. Colucci WS, Alexander RW, Williams GH, et al: Decreased

lymphocyte beta-adrenergic receptor density in patients with heart failure and tolerance to the beta adrenergic agonist pirbuterol. N Engl J Med 305:185, 1981.

64. Longhini C, Ansani L, Musacci GF, et al: Peripheral hemodynamic effects of ibopamine in patients with congestive heart failure. A placebo-controlled, double-blind study. Cardiovasc Drugs Ther 3:199, 1989.

65. Dei Cas L, Manca C, Vasini G, et al: Noninvasive evaluation of left ventricular function through systolic time intervals following oral administration of SB 7505 in man. Arzneimittelforschung 36:498, 1980.

66. Dei Cas L, Manca C, Bernardini B, et al: Non invasive evaluation of the effects of oral ibopamine (SB7505) on cardiac and renal function in patients with congestive heart failure. J Cardiovasc Pharmacol 4:436, 1982.

67. Ren JH, Leithe ME, Huss P, et al: The effects of ibopamine on cardiovascular and renal function in normal human subjects. Curr Ther Res 34:667, 1983.

68. Ladelli L, Pezzano A, Sala G, et al: Studio ecocardiografico e poligrafico degli effetti acuti dell'ibopamina sulla performance cardiaca. G Ital Cardiol 13:239, 1983.

69. Stoddard MF, Chaitman BR, Byers SL, et al: Noninvasive assessment of diastolic and systolic properties of ibopamine in patients with congestive heart failure. Am Heart J 117:395, 1989.

70. Itoh H, Kohli JD, Rajfer SI: Alpha-adrenoceptor subtypes in canine mesenteric arteries and veins. Fed Proc 43:353, 1984.

71. De Mey J, Vanhoutte PM: Uneven distribution of postjunctional alpha1- and alpha2-adrenoceptors in canine arterial and venous smooth muscle. Circ Res 48:875, 1981.

72. Constantine JW, Lebel W, Archer R: Functional postsynaptic alpha2 but not alpha1 adrenoceptors in dog saphenous vein exposed to phenoxybenzamine. Eur J Pharmacol 85:325, 1982.

73. Shebuski RJ, Fujita T, Ruffolo RR Jr: Comparison of the alpha adrenoceptor activity of dopamine, ibopamine and epinine in the pulmonary circulation of the dog. J Pharmacol Exp Ther 241:6, 1987.

74. Shebuski RJ, Smith JM, Ruffolo RR Jr: Effect of dopamine, ibopamine and epinine on alpha and beta adrenoceptors in canine pulmonary circulation. Fundam Clin Pharmacol 3:211, 1989.

75. Podrid PJ, Fuchs T, Candinas R: Role of the sympathetic nervous system in the genesis of ventricular arrhythmia. Circulation 82(Suppl I):1103, 1990.

76. Caponetto S, Terrachini V, Canale C, et al: Absence of proarrhythmic effects of ibopamine in patients with congestive heart failure. J Cardiovasc Pharmacol 14(Suppl 8):S104, 1989.

77. Furlanello F, Aguglia C, Brusoni B, et al: Influence of ibopamine on heart rate and arrhythmic pattern in patients with congestive heart failure. A double-blind multicentre study. G Ital Cardiol 19:71, 1989.

78. van Veldhuisen DJ, Girbes AR, Crijns HJ, et al: The oral dopamine agonist, ibopamine, in normal man: Effects on rhythm, heart rate, blood pressure and catecholamines. Int J Clin Pharmacol Res 11:159, 1991.

79. Felder RA, Felder CC, Eisner GM, Jose PA: The dopamine receptor in adult and maturing kidney. Am J Physiol 257:F315, 1989.

80. Incerti PL, Badalamenti S, Lorenzano E, et al: Humoral and renal effects of ibopamine in normal subjects. Arzneimittelforschung 36:405, 1986.

81. Stefoni S, Coli L, Mosconi G, Prandini R: Ibopamine (SB 7505) in normal subjects and in chronic renal failure: A preliminary report. Br J Clin Pharamacol 11:69, 1981.

82. Harvey JN, Worth DP, Brown J, Lee MR: Lack of effect of ibopamine, a dopamine pro-drug, on renal function in normal subjects. Br J Clin Pharmacol 17:671, 1984.

83. Girbes AR, van Veldhuisen DJ, Smit AJ, et al: Renal and neurohumoral effects of ibopamine and metoclopramide in normal man. Br J Clin Pharmacol 31:701, 1991.

84. Girbes AR, Kalisvaart CJ, van Veldhuisen DJ, et al: Effects of ibopamine on renal haemodynamics in patients with severe congestive heart failure. Eur Heart J 14:279, 1993.

85. Kasmer RJ, Cutler RE, Munger MA, et al: Single-dose effects of ibopamine hydrochloride on renal function in patients with congestive heart failure. Br J Clin Pharmacol 30:485, 1990.

86. Dalla Volta S, Razzolini R, Roshan-Ali Y: Clinical efficacy of ibopamine in heart failure. Results of a double-blind clinical study. Am J Noninvas Cardiol 5(Suppl 1):15, 1991.

87. Russo GE, Scarpellini MG, Spaziani M: The effects of ibopamine on chronic renal insufficiency: A long term trial. Curr Ther Res 48:912, 1990.

88. Stefoni S, Mosconi G, Bonomini M, et al: The use of ibopamine in chronic renal failure: Long term results. Contrib Nephrol 81:264, 1990.

89. Salerno F, Incerti P, Badalamenti S, et al: Renal and humoral effects of ibopamine, a dopamine agonist, in patients with liver cirrhosis. Arch Intern Med 150:65, 1990.

90. Francis GS, Goldsmith SR, Levine TB, et al: The neurohumoral axis in congestive heart failure. Ann Intern Med 101:370, 1984.

91. Packer M: The neurohumoral hypothesis: A theory to explain the mechanism of disease progression in heart failure. J Am Coll Cardiol 20:248, 1992.

92. Taylor SH, Cicchetti V: Efficacy of ibopamine in the treatment of heart failure. Am Heart J 120:1583, 1990.

93. Lopez-Sendon J: Ibopamine in chronic congestive heart failure: Hemodynamic and neurohumoral effects. Am J Med 90(Suppl 5B):43S, 1991.

94. Leimbach WN, Wallin BG, Victor RG, et al: Direct evidence from intraneural recordings for increased central sympathetic outflow in patients with heart failure. Circulation 73:913, 1986.

95. Cohn JN, Johnson GR, Shabetai R, et al: Ejection fraction, peak exercise oxygen consumption, cardiothoracic ratio, and plasma norepinephrine as determinants of prognosis in heart failure. Circulation 87(Suppl VI):5, 1993.

96. Nakano T, Morimoto Y, Kakuta Y, et al: Acute effects of ibopamine hydrochloride on hemodynamics, plasma catecholamine levels, renin activity, aldosterone, metabolism and blood gas in patients with severe congestive heart failure. Arzneimittelforschung 36:1829, 1986.

97. Musso NR, Vergassola C, Pende A, Lotti G: Epinine kinetics and plasma catecholamine changes following oral administration of the prodrug ibopamine in patients with chronic heart failure. J Liquid Chromatogr 14:3707, 1991.

98. Pizzorni C, Barabino A, Di Benedetto G, et al: Neurohumoral evaluation and long-term treatment of mild congestive heart failure in elderly patients with ibopamine: A double-blind, placebo-controlled study. Am J Noninvas Cardiol 5(Suppl 1):23, 1991.

99. Girbes ARJ, van Veldhuisen DJ, Grevink RG, et al: Effects of ibopamine on exercise-induced increase in norepinephrine in normal men. J Cardiovasc Pharmacol 19:371, 1992.

100. van Veldhuisen DJ, Girbes ARJ, van den Broek SAJ, et al: Effects of ibopamine on the increase in plasma norepinephrine levels during exercise in congestive heart failure. Am J Cardiol 71:992, 1993.

101. van Veldhuisen DJ, Man in't Veld AJ, Dunselman PHJM, et al: Double-blind placebo-controlled study of ibopamine and digoxin in patients with mild to moderate heart failure: Results of the Dutch Ibopamine Multicenter Trial (DIMT). J Am Coll Cardiol 22:1564, 1993.

102. Rousseau MF, Konstam MA, Benedict CR, et al: Progression of left ventricular dysfunction secondary to coronary artery disease, sustained neurohumoral activation and effects of ibopamine therapy during long-term therapy with angiotensin-converting enzyme inhibitor. Am J Cardiol 73:488, 1994.

103. Rajfer SI, Rossen JD, Nemanich JW, et al: Sustained hemodynamic improvement during long-term therapy with levodopa in heart failure: Role of plasma catecholamines. J Am Coll Cardiol 10:1286, 1987.

104. Pouleur H, Raigoso J, Rousseau MF: Dopaminergic drugs in the management of chronic heart failure. Eur Heart J 12(Suppl C):29, 1991.

104. Rolandi E, Marchetti G, Franceschini R, et al: Inhibition of prolactin and aldosterone secretion by the dopamine derivative ibopamine. Eur J Clin Pharmacol 29:629, 1986.

106. Caponetto S, Terrachini V, Canale C, et al: Long term treatment of congestive heart failure with oral ibopamine. Effects on rhythm disorders and neurohumoral alterations. Cardiology 77(Suppl 5):43, 1990.

107. Missale C, Metra M, Sigala S, et al: Inhibition of aldosterone

secretion by dopamine, ibopamine, and dihydroergotoxine in patients with congestive heart failure. J Cardiovasc Pharmacol 14(Suppl 8):S72, 1989.

108. Wehling M, Zimmermann J, Theisen K: Extracardial effects of oral ibopamine versus furosemide in patients with mild to moderate heart failure. A double-blind, randomized trial. Cardiology 77(Suppl 5):81, 1990.

109. Dei Cas L, Barilli AC, Metra M, et al: Multicenter study on the clinical efficacy of chronic ibopamine administration. Arzneimittelforschung 36:383, 1986.

110. Gronda E, Brusoni B, Inglese E, et al: Effects of ibopamine on heart performance: A radionuclide ventriculography study in patients with idiopathic dilatative cardiomyopathy. Arzneimittelforschung 36:371, 1986.

111. Caponetto S, Allegro A, Belotti G, et al: Positive inotropic effect of ibopamine in patients with congestive heart failure. A multicenter investigation. Arzneimittelforschung 36:386, 1986.

112. Trinchero R, Ghisio A, Moratti M, et al: The effects of ibopamine on exercise capacity in patients with severe left ventricular dysfunction. Curr Ther Res 43:271, 1988.

113. Condorelli M, Bonaduce A, Montemurro A, et al: The long-term efficacy of ibopamine in treating patients with severe heart failure: A multicenter investigation. J Cardiovasc Pharmacol 14(Suppl 8):S83, 1989.

114. Kayanakis JG and The European Ibopamine Study Group: Six-month treatment of congestive heart failure with ibopamine: A double-blind randomized, placebo-controlled multicenter trial. Am J Noninvas Cardiol 5(Suppl 1):32, 1991.

115. Cadel A, Brusoni B, Pirelli P, et al: Effects of digoxin, placebo and ibopamine on exercise tolerance and cardiac rhythm of patients with chronic post-infarct left ventricular failure. Arzneimittelforschung 36:376, 1986.

116. Alicandri C, Fariello R, Boni E, et al: Ibopamine vs. Digoxin in chronic heart failure: A double-blind, crossover study. J Cardiovasc Pharmacol 14(Suppl 8):S77, 1989.

117. Kleber FX, Thyroff-Friesinger U: Treatment of mild chronic congestive heart failure with ibopamine, hydrochlothiazide, ibopamine plus hydrochlorothiazide or placebo. Cardiology 77(Suppl 5):67, 1990.

118. Kleber FX, Thyroff-Friesinger U: Ibopamine versus digoxin in the treatment of mild congestive heart failure. Cardiology 77(Suppl 5):75, 1990.

119. Barabino A, Galbariggi G, Pizzorni C, Lotti G: Comparative effects of long-term therapy with captopril and ibopamine in chronic congestive heart failure in old patients. Cardiology 78:243, 1991.

120. Cavalli A, Riva E, Schleman M, et al: Ibopamine as a substitute for digitalis in patients with congestive heart failure on chronic digoxin therapy. Int J Cardiol 22:381, 1989.

121. Sher D, Licciardello L, Ferrari V, et al: Safety of ibopamine therapy in congestive heart failure. Ibopamine cohort study: Baseline and 1-year results. Arzneimittelforschung 41:402, 1991.

122. Abbondati G, Cavalli A, Fucella LM, et al: Ibopamine versus hydrochlorothiazide/amiloride in patients with mild congestive heart failure. Cardiovasc Drugs Ther 3:897, 1989.

123. Rolandi E, Sabino F, Cantoni V, et al: Long-term therapy of chronic congestive heart failure with ibopamine: a multicenter trial. J Cardiovasc Pharmacol 14(Suppl 8):S93, 1989.

124. Fonseca C, Gouveia R, Ceia F, et al: A ibopamina no tratamento da insuficiencia cardiaca congestiva. Estudo multicentrico prolongado. Rev Port Cardiol 11:515, 1992.

125. Swedberg K: Reduction of mortality by pharmacological therapy in congestive heart failure. Circulation 87(Suppl IV):126, 1993.

126. Armstrong PW, Moe GW: Medical advances in the treatment of congestive heart failure. Circulation 88:2941, 1994.

127. Kelly RA, Smith TW: Digoxin in heart failure: Implications of recent trials. J Am Coll Cardiol 22(Suppl A):107A, 1993.

128. Drexler H, Banhardt U, Meinertz T, et al: Contrasting peripheral short-term and long-term effects of converting enzyme inhibition in patients with congestive heart failure: A double-blind, placebo-controlled trial. Circulation 79:491, 1989.

129. Yusuf S, Garg R: Design, results, and interpretation of randomized, controlled trials in congestive heart failure and left ventricular dysfunction. Circulation 87(Suppl VII):115, 1993.

130. Packer M: The development of positive inotropic agents for chronic heart failure: How have we gone astray? J Am Coll Cardiol 22(Suppl A):119A, 1993.

131. Casagrande C, Metra M: Safety profile of ibopamine. In Casagrande C, Metra M (eds): Ibopamine 1992: A Comprehensive, Updated Review. Milan: CNM Bresso, 1992, pp 212–219.

132. Said SAM, Bucx JJJ, Dankbaar H, et al: Ibopamine-induced reversible leukopenia during treatment for congestive heart failure. Eur Heart J 14:999, 1993.

XIV.
Antiarrhythmic Drugs

Editors: Douglas Zipes and A. John Camm

A. Principles and Practice of Antiarrhythmic Therapy

CHAPTER 134

Supraventricular Arrhythmias

Eric N. Prystowsky, M.D.

A clinical classification of supraventricular tachycardias is outlined in Table 134–1. These arrhythmias can be subdivided into three broad categories—sinus tachycardia, atrioventricular (AV) node–independent arrhythmias, and AV node–dependent arrhythmias.[1] Sinus tachycardia can be physiologic or nonphysiologic. AV node–independent arrhythmias are atrial tachyarrhythmias that are unaffected by AV node conduction block. AV node–dependent arrhythmias require conduction in the AV node or automaticity in the AV junction for maintenance of tachycardia.

SINUS TACHYCARDIA

Sinus tachycardia may be physiologic or nonphysiologic. Physiologic sinus tachycardia occurs as a response to certain stressful states, for example, exercise, hypoxia, fever, and hyperthyroidism. Sinus tachycardia is associated with increased sympathetic and decreased parasympathetic tone on the sinus node. By definition, the heart rate is 100 beats/min or more. Typically, the P wave closely resembles the

Table 134–1. Clinical Classification of Supraventricular Tachycardia

I. Sinus tachycardia
  A. Physiologic
  B. Nonphysiologic
    Paroxysmal sinus node reentry tachycardia
    Nonparoxysmal inappropriate sinus tachycardia
II. AV node–independent tachycardia
  A. Atrial fibrillation
  B. Atrial flutter
  C. Atrial tachycardia
  D. Premature atrial complexes
III. AV node–dependent tachycardia
  A. AV reentry
  B. AV node reentry
  C. Nonparoxysmal junctional tachycardia

AV, atrioventricular.

P wave that occurs during regular sinus rhythm. In some instances, a slight shift in the sinus node exit site may produce a slightly different P wave compared with sinus rhythm. Efforts to increase vagal tone, such as the Valsalva maneuver and carotid sinus massage, transiently slow the sinus rate, which quickly accelerates back to its previous rate.

Treatment of sinus tachycardia is directed at the causes of this rhythm. Correction of hypoxemia or other pathophysiologic states should lead to a slowing of the sinus rate.

Two types of nonphysiologic sinus tachycardia may occur. One is paroxysmal sinus node reentry,[2, 3] and the other is nonparoxysmal inappropriate sinus tachycardia.[4] Paroxysmal sinus node reentry tachycardia (SANRT) typically starts with a premature atrial complex, and the rate is usually 150 beats/min or less. It occurs more commonly in older patients with organic heart disease. SANRT is usually not a significant clinical problem and frequently terminates spontaneously after a few minutes. The P waves are very similar to those recorded during normal sinus rhythm, but if the rate is fast enough, the P waves may merge into the preceding T wave. Increased parasympathetic tone, intravenous adenosine, or verapamil usually terminates SANRT. It is helpful to record multiple electrocardiographic (ECG) leads during attempts to terminate tachycardia. Typically, the rate slows somewhat prior to termination, and P-wave morphology can be observed as the P wave emerges from the T wave. If treatment is necessary, β-adrenergic blockers, calcium antagonists, and digitalis may be useful to prevent recurrences of SANRT.[1]

Nonparoxysmal inappropriate sinus tachycardia can be a very troublesome arrhythmia that often occurs in younger individuals. The tachycardia is indistinguishable from sinus tachycardia by electrocardiographic criteria. However, the resting sinus rate is inappropriate for the physiologic state of the patient. In other words, these individuals frequently have si-

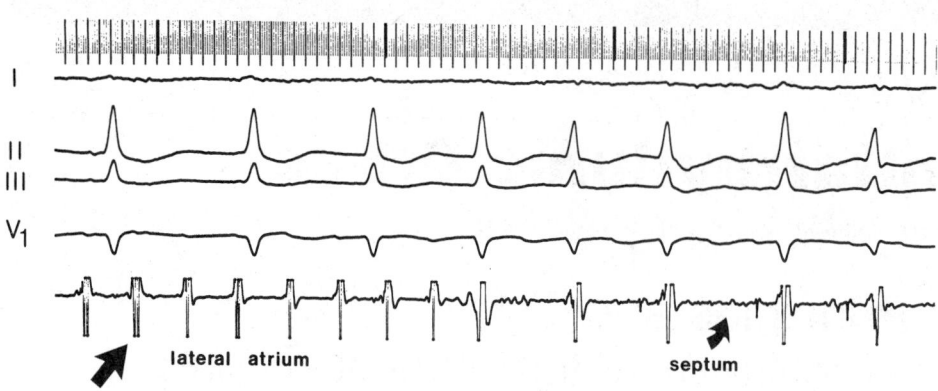

Figure 134–1. Atrial fibrillation with intracardiac recording from the right atrium demonstrating atrial electrograms that occur at regular and grossly irregular intervals. Simultaneous recordings were made from ECG leads I, II, III, and V_1 with an intracardiac recording from the right atrium. The lateral atrium demonstrates atrial electrograms occurring at relatively regular intervals (*straight arrow*). The anterior interatrial septal area shows grossly irregular low-amplitude fibrillatory electrograms (*curved arrow*). Note the His bundle depolarization prior to each QRS complex in the interatrial septal area.

nus rates of more than 100 beats/min during rest in the absence of any obvious conditions that would increase sinus automaticity. The mechanism of tachycardia appears to be enhanced automaticity, and it usually is affected by changes in autonomic tone. Thus, a 24-hour ECG recording shows diurnal variations in sinus rate, with slower rates in the evening than daytime, but overall the sinus rate is inappropriately high. In my experience, β-adrenergic blockers are the treatment of choice and often quite successful.[1] Slow-channel blockers also may be useful. Very uncommonly, drugs such as propafenone or flecainide may be necessary alone or in combination with β-blockers to suppress this arrhythmia. It may be nearly impossible to differentiate inappropriate sinus tachycardia from an atrial tachycardia originating very near the sinus node. Preliminary data suggest that radiofrequency endocardial catheter ablation of the sinus nodal area may be useful to cure inappropriate sinus tachycardia in some patients. Radiofrequency catheter ablation of the AV junction (see later) with insertion of a permanent pacemaker has also been used to treat refractory cases. In my opinion, this should be a treatment of last resort.

ATRIOVENTRICULAR NODE–INDEPENDENT ARRHYTHMIAS
Atrial Fibrillation

Atrial fibrillation (AF) is a paradigm of an AV node–independent supraventricular tachycardia. AF originates in the atria, and conduction through the AV node is not necessary for maintenance of tachycardia. Figure 134–1 is an ECG recording from a patient with AF. Note the irregular QRS complexes and no discernible P-wave activity in the ECG leads, although in leads I and V_1 there appear to be some fibrillatory waves. An intracardiac recording was obtained from two portions of the right atrium. This was done by moving the catheter from the lateral right atrium to the anterior interatrial septum near the His bundle recording site. Note the relatively

regular atrial activity in the lateral right atrium, but typical fibrillatory waves in the septal area. Thus, even though the surface electrocardiogram demonstrates AF, intracardiac tracings frequently record islands of regular atrial activity. In some patients, this often gives the appearance of atrial fibrillation/atrial flutter on the surface ECG. This arrhythmia should be considered AF for purposes of treatment.

There are three therapeutic tracks for the treatment of AF—drugs to depress AV nodal conduction and decrease the ventricular response; antiarrhythmic

A. Control

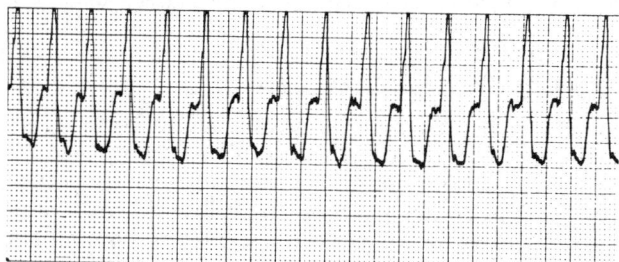

B. After RF Ablation of AVJ

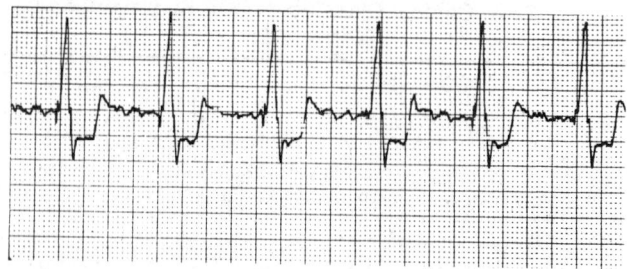

Figure 134–2. Rapid atrial fibrillation/flutter treated with radiofrequency catheter ablation of the atrioventricular junction to create heart block. *A,* Prior to ablation, there is a rapid ventricular response during atrial fibrillation/flutter. *B,* Radiofrequency (RF) ablation of the AV junction (AVJ) caused complete heart block, and a rate-responsive ventricular (VVIR) pacemaker was inserted that maintained a stable rhythm.

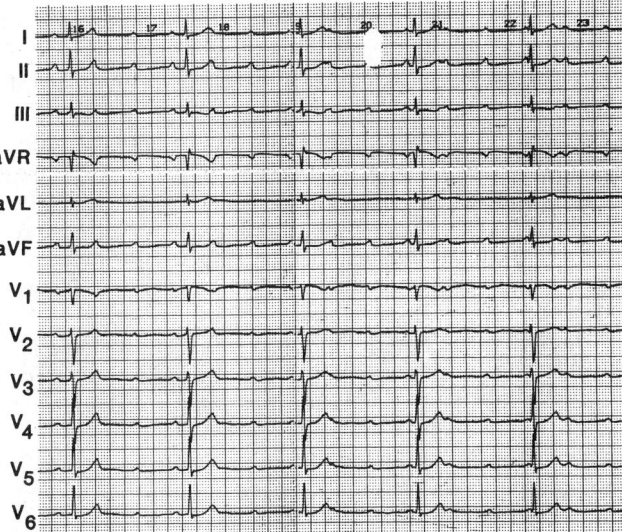

Figure 134–3. Simultaneous 12-lead electrocardiogram in a patient with complete heart block and junctional rhythm after radiofrequency ablation of AV junction.

agents to prevent recurrences of AF; and anticoagulation when appropriate.[1, 5-8] Because AV nodal conduction is not necessary to maintain AF, drugs that depress AV nodal conduction slow the ventricular response but do not generally restore sinus rhythm. Intravenous adenosine is therefore not useful in AF. I prefer to use verapamil or diltiazem if the patient can tolerate them. These agents produce substantial slowing of the ventricular response. Further, the negative dromotropic effect of these drugs is not reversed as much as it is with digitalis, with increases in sympathetic and decreases in parasympathetic tone. β-Adrenergic blockers are also useful to slow the ventricular response. After the ventricular response has been stabilized, antiarrhythmic drugs that affect atrial tissue may be used to restore sinus rhythm and prevent recurrences of atrial fibrillation. The choices are quinidine, procainamide, disopyramide, propafenone, flecainide, sotalol, and amiodarone. Preliminary data suggest moricizine may be useful to treat AF. Most of these drugs have not been approved by the Food and Drug Administration for treatment of supraventricular tachycardia. The choice of a particular agent should be individualized, selecting a drug least likely to cause significant side effects for that patient. Few data have demonstrated superiority of one drug over another. When appropriate, anticoagulation should be given.

Endocardial catheter ablation may be used to treat patients with recalcitrant AF or those individuals who prefer a nonpharmacologic approach.[9-11] At present, catheter ablation techniques to cure AF are under investigation. However, ablation can be directed at the AV junction to create complete heart block with subsequent pacemaker insertion (Fig. 134–2). In most patients, an ablation site can be chosen that will result in a stable junctional rhythm (Fig. 134–3). Regardless, we still recommend pacemaker insertion. Ablation can also be used to modify AV node conduction without heart block and without pacemaker insertion.

Atrial Flutter

Atrial flutter (AFl) as a "pure" arrhythmia occurs far less frequently than AF. As with AF, conduction through the AV node is not necessary to maintain AFl, and drugs or maneuvers that depress AV node conduction merely increase the AV conduction ratio (Fig. 134–4). Atrial flutter typically has a "saw-tooth" pattern of flutter waves that is seen best in ECG leads II, III, and aV_F. The AV conduction ratio is usually 2:1, and the ventricular rate is 150 beats/min because the atrial rate typically is 300 beats/min. However, variations both in atrial rate as well as in AV conduction ratio can occur (see Fig. 134–4). Atrial flutter most commonly occurs in patients with heart disease.

The pharmacologic approach involves calcium an-

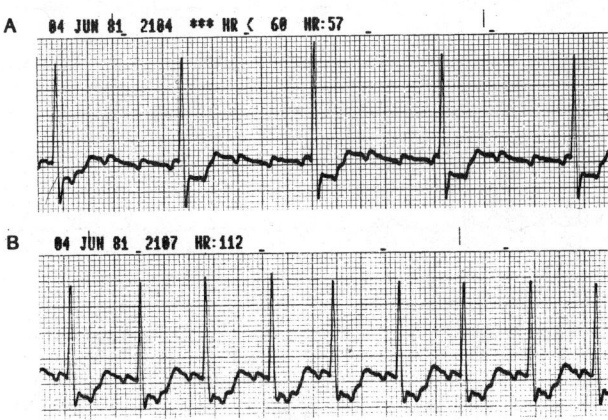

Figure 134–4. Effects of autonomic tone on atrial to ventricular conduction ratio in a patient with atrial flutter. This patient was undergoing antiarrhythmic drug treatment that resulted in slowing of the atrial flutter rate. *A,* The atrial to ventricular conduction ratio is 4:1; *B,* the atrial to ventricular conduction ratio is 2:1. Note that both tracings occurred during evening hours and only 3 minutes apart. It is presumed that changes in autonomic tone caused the variation in AV conduction ratio because no medicines were being given at this time. Clearly, AV conduction is irrelevant to maintenance of this tachycardia.

tagonists, β-adrenergic blockers, or digitalis to decrease the ventricular response, and the same agents that were suggested for AF to prevent recurrences of AFl.[1] As a rule, it is more difficult to slow the ventricular rate in AFl compared with AF. In general, after administering drugs to slow the ventricular response, I use nonpharmacologic methods to terminate the arrhythmia. Esophageal or right atrial pacing may restore sinus rhythm. Alternatively, transthoracic direct current cardioversion with 20 to 40 watts may be used.

Maintenance drug therapy for AFl is similar to that for AF, except anticoagulation is not usually required. Endocardial catheter ablation has been used to treat atrial flutter by two different approaches.[9, 12, 13] Ablation of sites in the posterior right atrium can cure AFl in some patients, and preliminary data are encouraging. Alternatively, one can ablate the AV junction and insert a permanent pacemaker as described for AF. With increasing advances in catheter design and energy delivery sources, endocardial catheter ablation may become the treatment of choice for patients with AFl.

Atrial Tachycardia

Atrial tachycardia (AT) may occur at various areas in the right and left atria, and P-wave morphology will depend on the origin of tachycardia. Atrial rates are quite variable, although usually stable in a particular patient. Approach to therapy may be pharmacologic or nonpharmacologic. In an acute situation, adenosine may be given for diagnostic and therapeutic reasons. AT is responsive to adenosine in many patients and may be terminated. In most cases, AV block precedes termination (Fig. 134–5).

This is a key observation because it documents that the tachycardia is an AV node–independent arrhythmia. Less commonly, AT may end with a QRS complex without prior AV block. This leads to a differential diagnosis between AT and AV node–dependent arrhythmias, which usually requires electrophysiologic testing. In many patients, adenosine and other drugs that block AV conduction will merely increase the AV conduction ratio and not terminate tachycardia. Nonpharmacologic therapy such as atrial pacing and cardioversion are often necessary to restore sinus rhythm.

Maintenance therapy is similar to that recommended for AFl. Radiofrequency catheter ablation can often cure AT, and this approach is gaining in popularity for long-term therapy.[14, 15]

ATRIOVENTRICULAR NODE–DEPENDENT TACHYCARDIAS

AV node–dependent tachycardias depend on AV node conduction or automaticity for maintenance of the tachycardia.[1] Nonparoxysmal junctional tachycardia is an exceedingly uncommon arrhythmia that is discussed elsewhere.[16, 17] The two most common forms of AV node–dependent tachycardia are atrioventricular reentry (AVRT) and AV node reentry (AVNRT). These are demonstrated schematically in Figure 134–6. The tachycardia circuit in AVNRT uses the AV node for anterograde conduction, and retrograde conduction most likely includes both AV nodal and atrial tissue (see Fig. 134–6A). Because anterograde

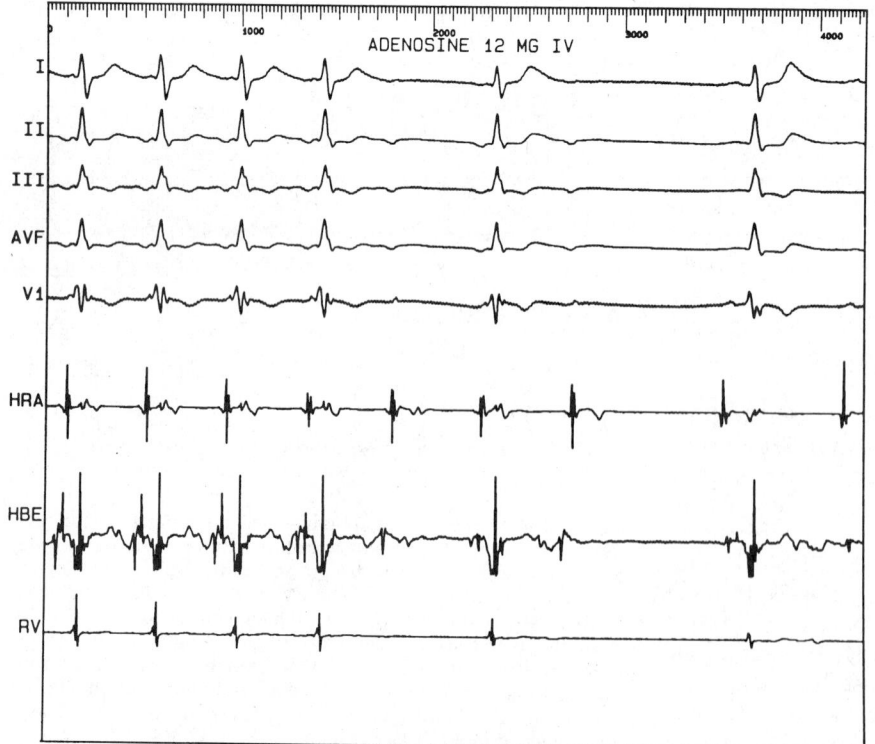

Figure 134–5. Effect of adenosine to terminate atrial tachycardia. Simultaneous tracings are ECG leads I, II, III, aV$_F$, and V$_1$, and intracardiac leads from the high right atrium (HRA), His bundle area (HBE), and right ventricle (RV). Adenosine 12 mg was given. Note that tachycardia terminates, but 2:1 AV block occurred before termination of tachycardia.

A. AVNRT

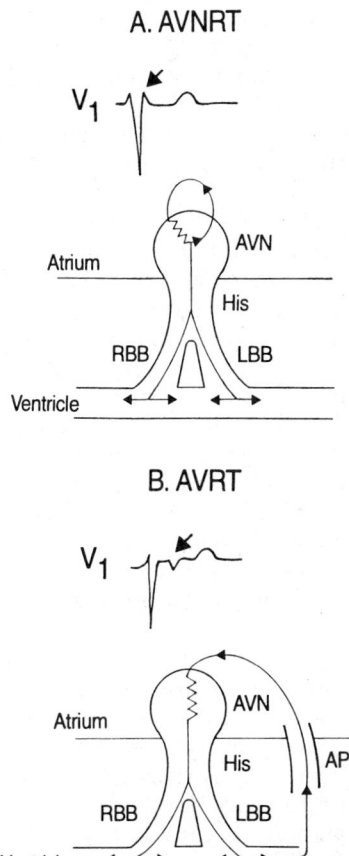

B. AVRT

Figure 134–6. Schematic of AV node reentry tachycardia (AVNRT) and AV reentry tachycardia (AVRT). *A*, V$_1$ is shown with the schematic of the reentrant circuit. There is relatively slow anterograde conduction over the AV node with nearly simultaneous activity of the atrium and ventricle. This leads to P-wave activity within or at the end of the QRS complex. The arrow points to a pseudo r-prime in V$_1$, which represents P-wave activity during tachycardia. *B*, In AV reentry, the tachycardia circuit is macroreentrant. Anterograde conduction occurs over the AV node/His-Purkinje system to activate the ventricle. Retrograde conduction proceeds from the ventricle over the accessory pathway to activate the atrium. There is a requisite amount of time necessary from ventricular activation to atrial activation. This usually allows sufficient time for P-wave activity to be noted in the early ST segment (*arrow* in V$_1$). Abbreviations: AVN, AV node; RBB, right bundle branch; LBB, left bundle branch; AP, accessory pathway.

conduct only in the retrograde direction. In the latter situation, the electrocardiogram during sinus rhythm does not have a delta wave. In AVRT, there is usually a substantial amount of time after the impulse activates the ventricle before the electrical wave front returns to the atrium over the accessory pathway. Thus, typically one can identify retrograde P-wave

A. Sinus

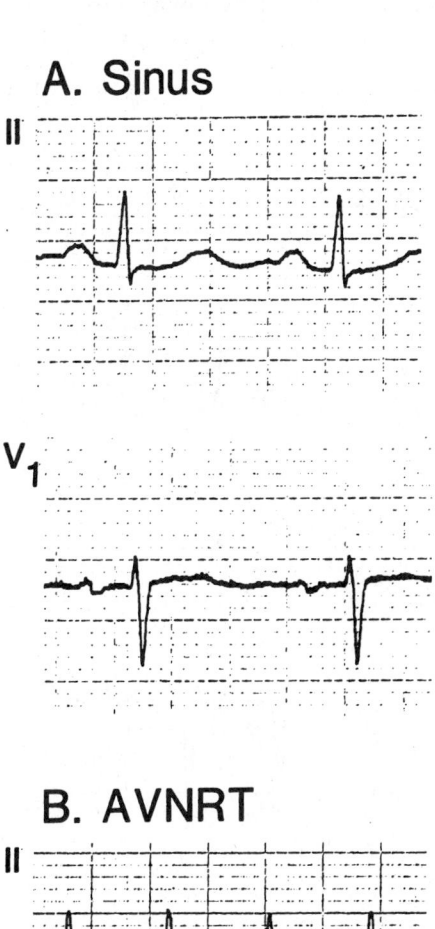

B. AVNRT

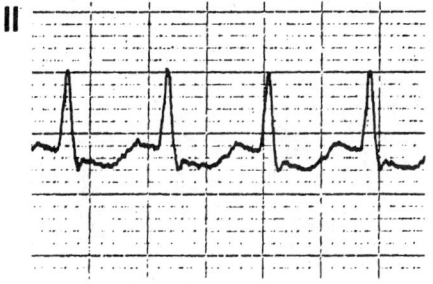

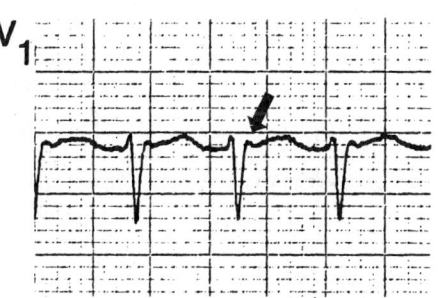

Figure 134–7. Electrocardiographic leads II and V$_1$ in sinus rhythm *(A)* and AV node reentrant tachycardia *(B)*. The *arrow* points to the pseudo r-prime noted during AV node reentry, which is absent during sinus rhythm.

conduction is relatively slow and retrograde conduction relatively fast, the atrium and ventricle are activated nearly simultaneously. Thus, clearly definable P-wave activity after the end of the QRS complex is distinctly unusual in the typical form of AVNRT. In ECG lead V$_1$, there is often a pseudo r-prime (see Fig. 134–6A). This excellent ECG sign strongly suggests AVNRT as the mechanism of tachycardia in a regular narrow QRS tachycardia.[18] The pseudo r-prime represents atrial activity at the end of the QRS complex, which is not present during sinus rhythm (Fig. 134–7).

Atrioventricular reentry uses the AV node for anterograde conduction and an accessory pathway for retrograde conduction. Patients with Wolff-Parkinson-White syndrome may have ventricular preexcitation, or the accessory pathway may be concealed, that is, activity in the early ST segment after the end of the QRS complex (Fig. 134–8). In summary, AVRT and AVNRT can often be differentiated electrocardiographically by a pseudo r-prime in V_1 during AVNRT and by retrograde P-wave activity in the early ST segment during AVRT.

Acute and long-term therapy for AVRT and AVNRT are similar. Both arrhythmias are AV node–dependent, and initial treatment is given to block AV node conduction and terminate tachycardia. An example of this is shown in Figure 134–9. This patient

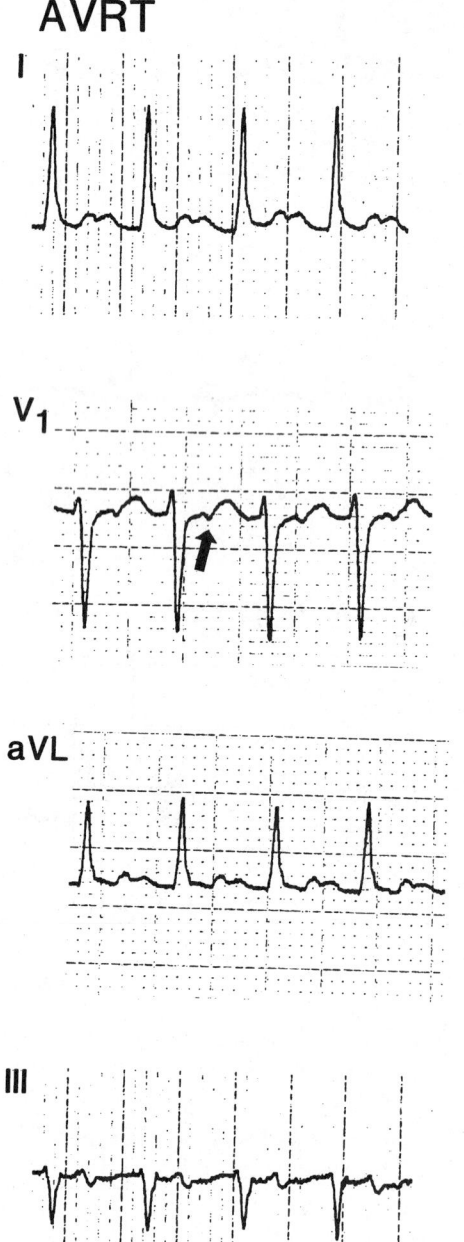

AVRT

Figure 134–8. Atrioventricular reentry tachycardia with retrograde P-wave activity (arrow) in the early ST segment.

with AVNRT was given 12 mg of intravenous adenosine. Note that AV node block occurs (atrial electrogram without His deflection) and coincides with termination of tachycardia, because AV nodal conduction is a requisite for maintenance of tachycardia. Although I prefer adenosine, intravenous verapamil or diltiazem is also very effective in terminating these arrhythmias. Alternatively, one should initially perform maneuvers to enhance vagal tone, for example, carotid sinus massage or the Valsalva maneuver, because these will often stop tachycardia. The patient should be supine and in a rested state to enhance vagal activity.

Radiofrequency catheter ablation has markedly altered the approach to long-term therapy for AVNRT and AVRT.[1, 19–23] I currently recommend ablation as first line treatment for adult patients with recurrent symptomatic tachycardia. Success rates are $\geq 90\%$ for both arrhythmias in most experienced laboratories, and the complication rate is relatively low. An example of radiofrequency ablation of AVRT is shown in Figure 134–10.

Pharmacologic therapy is also very effective for these arrhythmias. In patients with AVNRT, β-adrenergic blockers are often successful in preventing tachycardia. Alternatively, verapamil, diltiazem, and digitalis may be tried. Antiarrhythmic drugs that primarily affect retrograde conduction, such as disopyramide, propafenone, flecainide, sotalol and others, are also very useful. Unless militating circumstances are present, radiofrequency catheter ablation is recommended over the use of these latter agents for long-term therapy of this arrhythmia. In patients with AVRT without ventricular preexcitation, similar drug therapy can be recommended. If the electrocardiogram during sinus rhythm demonstrates ventricular preexcitation, digitalis should not be given unless the accessory pathway has documented poor anterograde conduction. In general, therapy should be directed at the accessory pathway because some of these patients can have AF with a rapid preexcited ventricular response. I prefer controlled-release disopyramide and flecainide because they can be given twice daily, but other agents are also effective.

Long RP Tachycardia

There are several varieties of supraventricular tachycardia that have an electrocardiographic finding of an RP interval equal to or longer than a PR interval during tachycardia.[1] Several mechanisms may be present as demonstrated in Figure 134–11. The patient can have an AT with a relatively short PR interval (Fig. 134–12). If the tachycardia rate is slow enough, the RP interval is longer than the PR interval. In this instance, ventricular activation is unrelated to the mechanism of tachycardia, and the RP-PR relationship is purely mathematical. Another mechanism is AVRT, which uses a slowly conducting accessory pathway for retrograde conduction. The third mechanism involves an unusual or atypical variety of AVNRT. In this instance, the tachycardia circuit is

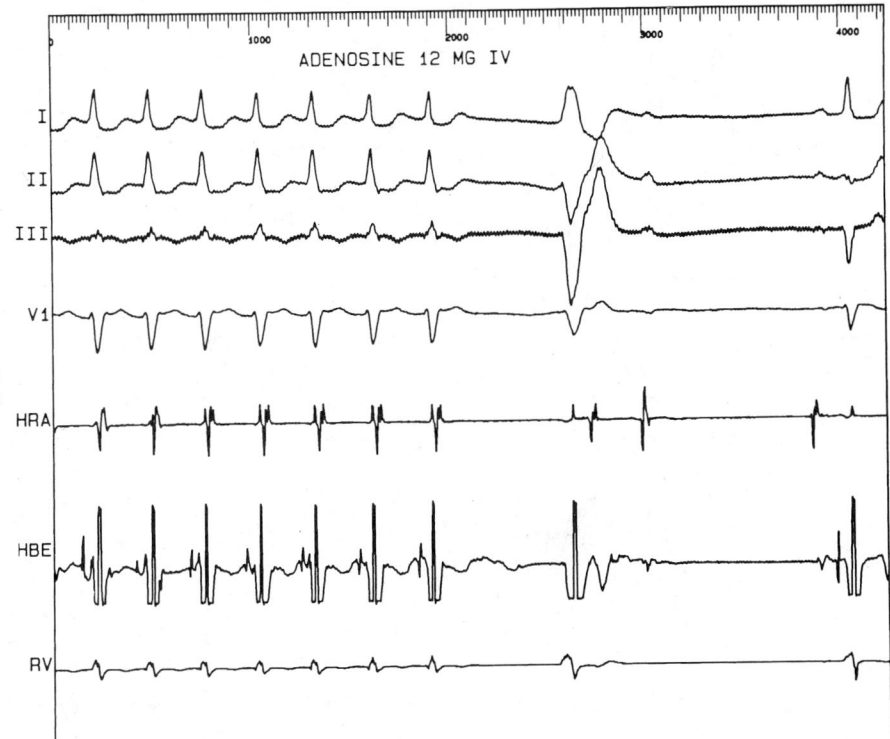

Figure 134–9. AV node reentry tachycardia terminated with intravenous adenosine with block anterograde in the AV node.

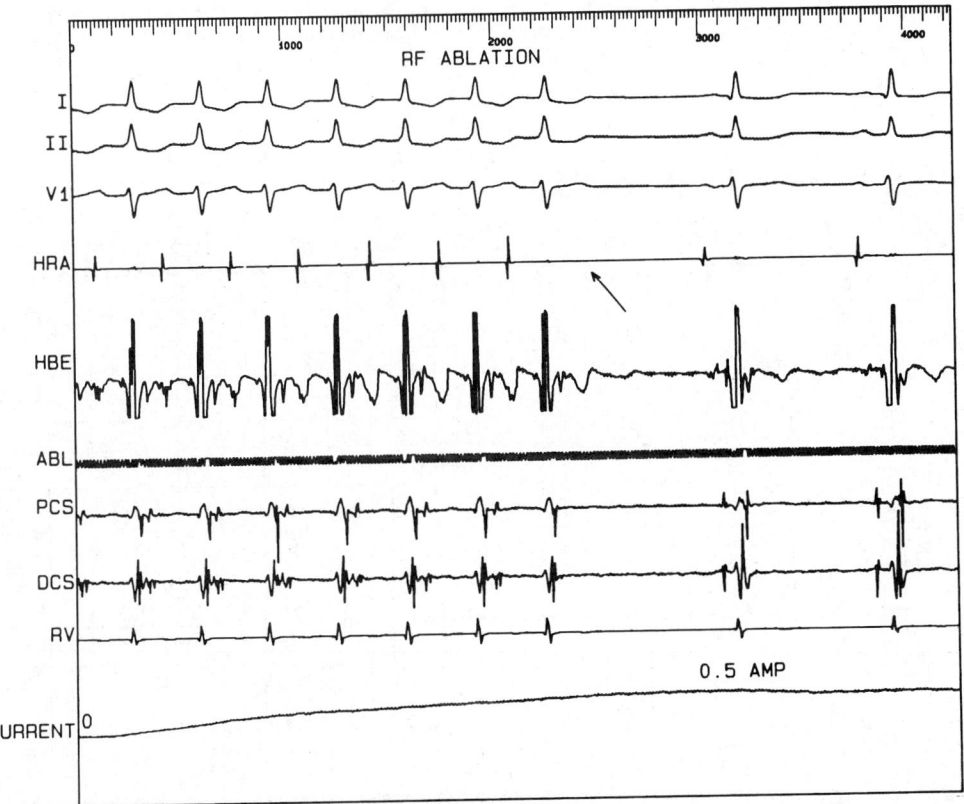

Figure 134–10. Radiofrequency (RF) ablation of AV reentry tachycardia. Simultaneously recorded tracings are ECG leads I, II, and V_1, and intracardiac tracings from the high right atrium (HRA), His bundle area (HBE), ablation (ABL) lead, proximal (PCS) and distal (DCS) coronary sinus leads, right ventricle (RV), and radiofrequency current. Note that within seconds after onset of current there is termination of tachycardia in the retrograde limb as shown by an absent A wave at the *arrow*. The ablation catheter was positioned at the site of the accessory pathway, and current was applied during tachycardia. Tachycardia terminated after the accessory pathway was ablated, and this prevented retrograde conduction.

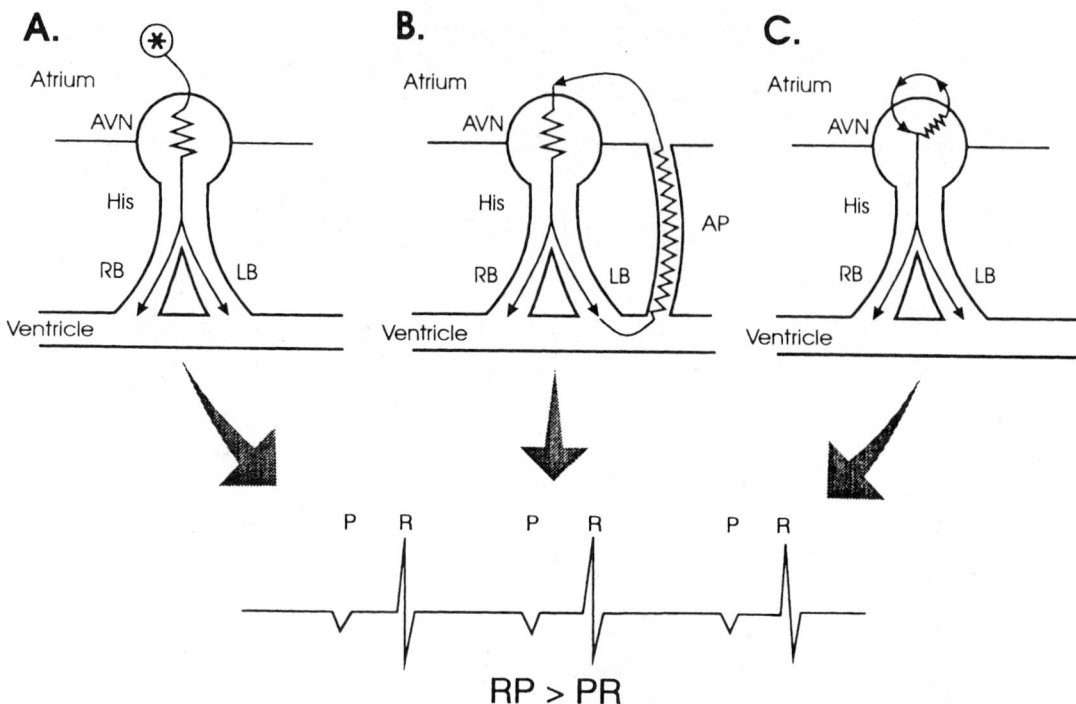

Figure 134–11. The mechanisms for long RP tachycardia include atrial tachycardia *(A)*, AV reentry tachycardia with slow retrograde conduction *(B)*, and the unusual variety of AV node reentry tachycardia *(C)*. See text for details.

Supraventricular Tachycardia

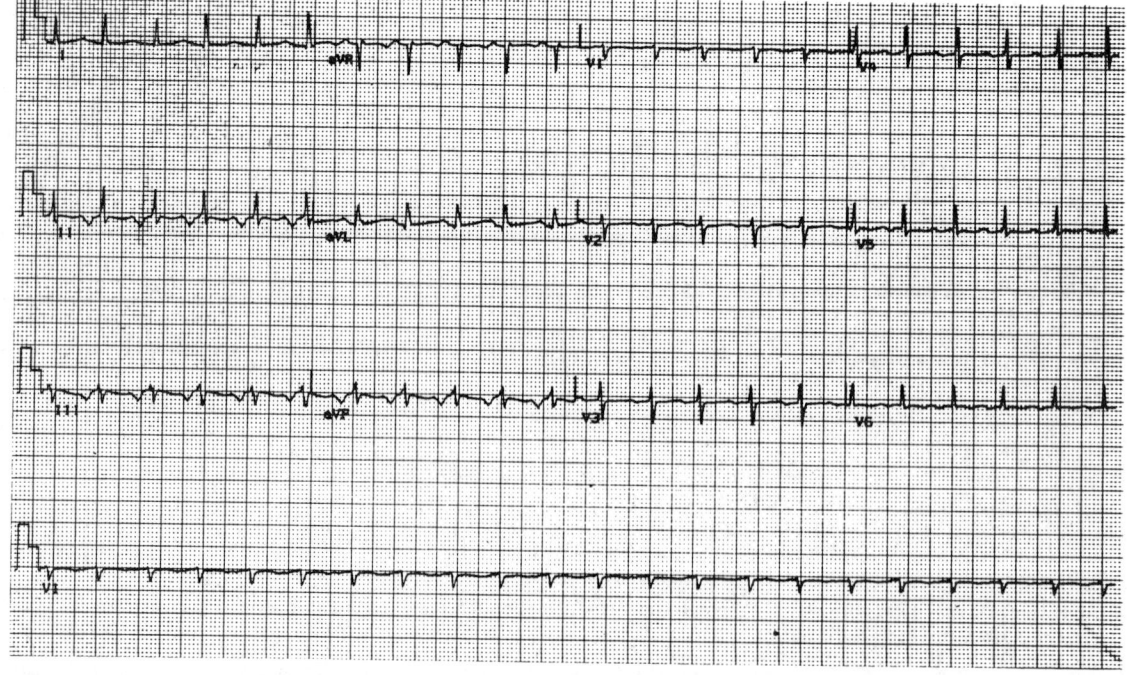

Figure 134–12. Atrial tachycardia with a short PR and long RP interval.

reversed from that shown in Figure 134–6. Antero-grade conduction is relatively fast and retrograde conduction slow.

Therapy for these arrhythmias ultimately depends on the tachycardia mechanism identified at electrophysiologic study. Acutely, I prefer intravenous adenosine to help differentiate mechanisms. In many cases of AT, the arrhythmia either continues with AV block, which eliminates AVRT from consideration and effectively rules out AVNRT, or terminates after some demonstration of preceding AV block. The demonstration of AV node independence allows one to follow the treatment course outlined earlier for AT. If tachycardia terminates without AV block, then electrophysiologic study is necessary to determine the mechanism of the arrhythmia. Long-term therapy depends on the identified mechanism of tachycardia.

REFERENCES

1. Prystowsky EN, Klein G: Cardiac Arrhythmias: An Integrated Approach for the Clinician. New York: McGraw-Hill, 1994.
2. Curry PVL, Krikler DM: Paroxysmal reciprocating sinus tachycardia. In Kulbertus HE (ed): Reentrant Arrhythmias: Mechanism and Treatment. Lancaster, PA: MTP, 1977, pp 39–62.
3. Gomes JA, Hariman RJ, Kang PS, et al: Sustained symptomatic sinus node reentrant tachycardia: Incidence, clinical significance, electrophysiologic observations and the effects of antiarrhythmic agents. J Am Coll Cardiol 5:45, 1985.
4. Bauernfeind RA, Amat-Y-Leon F, Dhingra RC, et al: Chronic nonparoxysmal sinus tachycardia in otherwise healthy persons. Ann Intern Med 91:702, 1979.
5. Prystowsky EN, Wharton JM, Page RL: Atrial fibrillation. In Rakel RE (ed): Conn's Current Therapy. Philadelphia: WB Saunders, 1993, pp 245–247.
6. Petersen P, Boysen G, Godtfredsen J, et al: Placebo-controlled, randomized trial of warfarin and aspirin for prevention of thromboembolic complications in chronic atrial fibrillation: The Copenhagen AFASAK study. Lancet 1:175, 1989.
7. The Stroke Prevention in Atrial Fibrillation Investigators: The stroke prevention in atrial fibrillation trial: Final results. Circulation 84:527, 1991.
8. The Boston Area Anticoagulation Trial for Atrial Fibrillation Investigators: The effect of low-dose warfarin on the risk of stroke in patients with nonrheumatic atrial fibrillation. N Engl J Med 323:1505, 1990.
9. Scheinman MM: Catheter ablation: Present role and projected impact on health care for patients with cardiac arrhythmias. Circulation 83:1489, 1991.
10. Scheinman MM, Morady E, Hess DS, et al: Catheter-induced ablation of the atrioventricular junction to control refractory supraventricular arrhythmias. JAMA 248:851, 1982.
11. Gallagher JJ, Svenson RH, Kasell JH, et al: Catheter technique for closed-chest ablation of the atrioventricular conduction system: A therapeutic alternative for the treatment of refractory supraventricular tachycardia. N Engl J Med 306:194, 1982.
12. Saoudi N, Attallah G, Kirkorian G, Touboul P: Catheter ablation of the atrial myocardium in human type I atrial flutter. Circulation 81:762, 1990.
13. Feld GK, Fleck P, Chen P-S, et al: Radiofrequency catheter ablation of human type 1 atrial flutter: Identification of a critical zone in the reentrant circuit by endocardial mapping techniques. Circulation 86:1233, 1992.
14. Kay GN, Chong F, Epstein AE, et al: Radiofrequency ablation for treatment of primary atrial tachycardias. J Am Coll Cardiol 21:901, 1993.
15. Tracy CM, Swartz JF, Fletcher RD, et al: Radiofrequency catheter ablation of ectopic atrial tachycardia using paced activation sequence mapping. J Am Coll Cardiol 21:910, 1993.
16. Pick A, Dominquez P: Nonparoxysmal AV nodal tachycardia. Circulation 16:1022, 1967.
17. Rosen KM: Junctional tachycardia: Mechanisms, diagnosis, differential diagnosis and management. Circulation 67:654, 1973.
18. Wellens HJJ, Gorgels APM, Rodriquez LM, et al: Supraventricular tachycardias: Mechanisms, electrocardiographic manifestations, and clinical aspects. In Josephson ME, Wellens HJJ (eds): Tachycardias: Mechanisms and Management. Mount Kisco, NY: Futura Publishing, 1993, pp 121–147.
19. Jackman WM, Wang X, Friday KJ, et al: Catheter ablation of accessory atrioventricular pathways (Wolff-Parkinson-White syndrome) by radiofrequency current. N Engl J Med 324:1605, 1991.
20. Kuck KH, Schluter M, Geiger M, et al: Radiofrequency current catheter ablation of accessory atrioventricular pathways. Lancet 337:1557, 1991.
21. Kay GN, Epstein AE, Dailey SM, et al: Selective radiofrequency ablation of the slow pathway for the treatment of atrioventricular nodal reentrant tachycardia. Evidence for involvement of perinodal myocardium within the reentrant circuit. Circulation 85:1675, 1992.
22. Jackman WM, Beckman KJ, McClelland JH, et al: Treatment of supraventricular tachycardia due to atrioventricular nodal reentry by radiofrequency catheter ablation of slow-pathway conduction. N Engl J Med 327:313, 1992.
23. Jazayeri MR, Hempe SL, Sra JS, et al: Selective transcatheter ablation of the fast and slow pathways using radiofrequency energy in patients with atrioventricular nodal reentrant tachycardia. Circulation 85:1318, 1992.

CHAPTER 135

Ventricular Arrhythmias

Peter R. Kowey, M.D., Ted D. Friehling, M.D., and Roger A. Marinchak, M.D.

Management of patients with ventricular arrhythmia is one of the most common, but still most difficult, problems in clinical medicine.[1] Ventricular arrhythmia is ubiquitous in any population examined, including individuals with little or no structural heart disease.[2] Nevertheless, the finding of ventricular arrhythmia in patients with any form of structural heart disease implies a worse prognosis than if ectopy is absent.[3] In addition to having a higher overall mortality, we now know that many of these high-risk individuals die of sustained ventricular arrhythmia.[4] These facts compel physicians to take ventricular arrhythmia very seriously indeed and to treat many individuals with antiarrhythmic drugs with the expectation that such a tactic will improve their outcome. Unfortunately, wholesale treatment of patients with ventricular arrhythmia is not warranted. Abolition of ventricular arrhythmia has not been proved to improve prognosis in most subgroups. In fact, many studies, most notably the Cardiac Arrhythmia Suppression Trial (CAST), have indicated that drug therapy may be associated with a worse prognosis. This is undoubtedly because the drugs themselves have an inherent toxicity.[5] For these reasons, it is important to target therapy for those at highest risk. For example, there is little controversy that patients who have suffered an episode of sustained ventricular tachycardia (VT) or ventricular fibrillation (VF) in the absence of a myocardial infarction must be treated, because the risk of a lethal recurrence is extraordinarily high in the years following the initial episode.[6, 7] Abolishing even simple ventricular ectopy in this group, if done compulsively and completely, confers protection against recurrence.[8] Conversely, patients with simple ventricular premature depolarizations (VPDs) who have never had a documented, sustained arrhythmic event, especially those with minimal or no heart disease, have an excellent prognosis and rarely require therapy.[9] In fact, the only indication for therapy in this large group is intolerable symptoms of palpitations.

For most other patient groups, the situation is much less clear. Patients with a myocardial infarction who have repetitive VPDs on predischarge ambulatory monitoring may have a sixfold greater chance of having a cardiac death within 6 months of the infarction compared with those without complex ectopic rhythm.[10] How to select those at highest risk in whom the toxicity of drug therapy is warranted is the object of intense research interest. One principle delineated by several investigators is that the extent of left ventricular dysfunction may be an important discriminator. Risk of sudden death in patients with ejection fractions of less than 35% to 40% and complex ventricular ectopy is raised severalfold over what it would be with either finding alone.[11] Use of multiple clinical characteristics and testing modalities for risk profiling has great promise for selection of patients in intermediate-risk groups who must be treated. This is the subject of several contemporary clinical trials.[12–17] However, it should be emphasized that the clinical endpoint for these trials includes all-cause cardiac mortality as well as sudden death. Distinguishing these outcomes is important in trying to understand the relative value of arrhythmia suppression versus other measures.

The purpose of this chapter is to review the many clinical problems, such as selection of patients for therapy, that we confront daily. This introduction should serve as a framework for the discussion of individual agents for the treatment of ventricular arrhythmia provided in later chapters by our distinguished colleagues. Most important, we hope that all these contributions place the problem of drug therapy for ventricular arrhythmia in perspective and thus facilitate the care of patients with this very common clinical problem.

PRINCIPLES OF DRUG MANAGEMENT

A physician may elect to use one of several forms of therapy for the treatment of patients with ventricular arrhythmia. However, in many cases, arrhythmia can be abolished simply by correcting an underlying condition. Our service is consulted occasionally to see patients, especially those in intensive care units, in whom hypoxia, electrolyte shifts, use of sympathomimetic drugs, or bradyarrhythmias are responsible for ventricular arrhythmia that is then vigorously treated with antiarrhythmic agents, frequently to no avail. In fact, ignorance of possible precipitating causes is particularly dangerous, since the toxicity of antiarrhythmic drugs is multiplied severalfold in the presence of such problems.[18–23] Hypokalemia provides an excellent example of sensitization of the ventricular myocardium to circulating catecholamines.[24] Under these circumstances, potassium repletion itself may abolish arrhythmia or may render the patient responsive to previously ineffective antiarrhythmic drugs. Other factors such as bradycardia may also predispose a patient to a tachyarrhythmia. Figure 135–1 depicts electrocardiograms obtained on a 78-year-old woman with bradycardia-associated torsade de pointes who was successfully treated with a permanent cardiac pacemaker, with no need for antiarrhythmic drug therapy.

If no easily correctable abnormality can be identified, patients may be treated with antiarrhythmic drugs, antitachycardia devices, or arrhythmia surgery. The majority of patients, even those with malignant ventricular arrhythmia, are amenable to drug treatment, which forms the linchpin of antiarrhythmic therapy. Previously, the risk and expense of nonpharmacologic therapies rendered them less useful for many patients. However, the advent of non-thoracotomy lead systems and tiered antitachycardia devices has increased their applicability and made them more

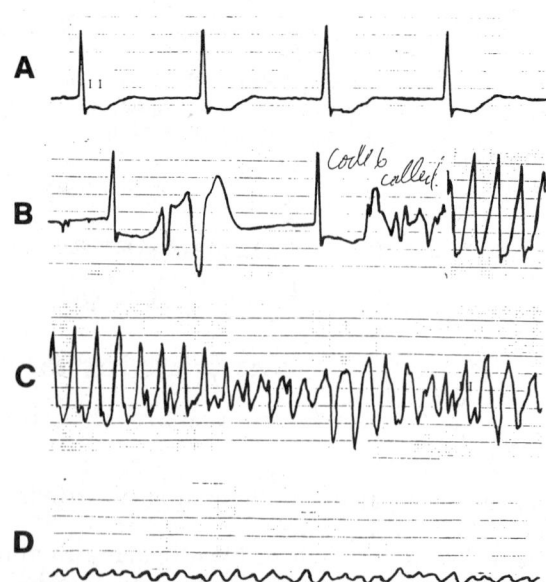

Figure 135–1. Torsade de pointes in a woman with bradycardia-tachycardia syndrome. *A,* Junctional rhythm at a rate of 40 beats/ min. *B,* Two ventricular beats cause a "long-short" sequence that initiates a polymorphic ventricular tachycardia. *C,* Sinusoidal pattern of torsade de pointes. *D,* Degeneration to ventricular fibrillation.

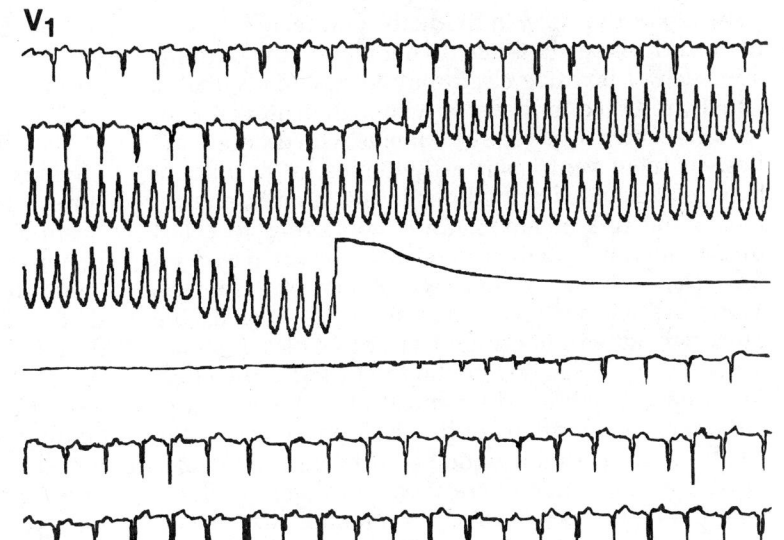

Figure 135–2. Ambulatory electrocardiogram depicting spontaneous initiation of sustained ventricular tachycardia at a rate of 200 beats/min in a patient with an automatic implantable cardioverter/defibrillator (AICD). Several seconds after onset of tachycardia, the AICD correctly senses the arrhythmia and terminates it, followed by a period of signal loss. A number of such AICD discharges occurred in the month after implantation until an antiarrhythmic drug was prescribed, which suppressed most of the episodes but had no deleterious effect on defibrillation thresholds.

practical for implementation earlier in the course of therapy.[25–29] Nevertheless, patients who undergo device implantation or extirpative surgery frequently require concomitant drug therapy after the procedure, in many cases to suppress arrhythmia that may cause the device to discharge frequently or to render the arrhythmia more responsive to antitachycardia pacing therapies before resorting to uncomfortable cardioverting shocks.[30–33] Figure 135–2 is an ambulatory electrocardiogram obtained on a 57-year-old man whose arrhythmia was successfully treated with an implantable cardioverter-defibrillator (ICD) but who also required treatment with a drug to prevent frequent firing of the device.

The process of selecting a drug is very complicated indeed and is predicated on several important principles. First, there is no such thing as a "first-line" antiarrhythmic drug. Therapy must be individualized to the patient, taking into account underlying conditions that might be aggravated by particular agents, drug history (including prior response to similar agents), and adverse effects. Second, response or lack of response to an agent in an antiarrhythmic drug class may not always be predictive of response to another agent of the same class, nor does it necessarily aid in selecting patients whose arrhythmias will be refractory to all medications.[34, 35] The selection of drug therapy is highly empirical, and success must be judged by a careful comparison of the levels of arrhythmia observed before and after drug treatment. Third, there are few large scale comparative trials of antiarrhythmic drug efficacy or potency. An exception is ESVEM (electrocardiographic study versus electrocardiographic monitoring), in which drugs were compared, although not blindly or in a controlled fashion.[36, 37] Therefore, most physicians select drugs based on the relative likelihood of an adverse effect. As part of this analysis, the physician must be absolutely convinced that the benefit of intervention outweighs the substantive risk of using an antiarrhythmic drug. Fourth, the physician must clearly establish an end-

point for therapy that is attainable and meaningful. Extinguishing ventricular ectopy in a patient without symptoms or a history of sustained arrhythmia may be unnecessary.[38] Similarly, the expectation that abolishing VPDs in a patient after myocardial infarction will reduce the chances of sudden death may not be reasonable.[39, 40] However, abolishing VPDs in a patient with intractable palpitations is clearly a reasonable endpoint. Fifth, the physician should have a clear idea of how much arrhythmia suppression is desirable. For most purposes, complete suppression of all ventricular arrhythmias is impractical and may be unnecessary to protect the patient from arrhythmia recurrence. However, suppression of all or most repetitive forms appears to be associated with a good outcome in patients with prior sustained arrhythmia.[8] Finally, the physician must determine the aggressiveness with which therapy should be pursued. Patients with recurrent, malignant arrhythmias require an intensive evaluation that only a hospital setting can provide. Use of complex and potentially dangerous antiarrhythmic drugs in such patients mandates in-hospital therapy with on-line electrocardiographic monitoring. Patients with minimal heart disease and symptomatic ventricular ectopy may be treated as outpatients using serial ambulatory monitoring to guide therapy, especially if drugs with less potential toxicity are selected.

The synthesis of all this information is a complex task that requires familiarity with a patient and his or her condition, testing procedures, and several of the available chemical entities. Once a decision is made to treat a patient with any antiarrhythmic drug, the next step is a definitive demonstration of drug effect by one of several testing techniques.

ANTIARRHYTHMIC DRUG TESTING
Methods of Drug Selection

Like the drug chosen, the method used for the evaluation of drug therapy should be individualized to the patient. For example, individuals with relatively simple ventricular arrhythmia do not require the rigorous approach of invasive electrophysiologic study that is usually reserved for patients with malignant ventricular arrhythmia. Conversely, patients who do not manifest frequent ventricular arrhythmias in the interim between sustained arrhythmic events are not amenable to the use of ambulatory monitoring to select proper therapy. Methods are also chosen based on physician familiarity and availability of resources. These are reasonable considerations as long as the physician adheres to certain basic principles. No matter which is chosen, the method to evaluate the effect of an antiarrhythmic drug must allow for a control period of observation with which to compare the results of drug administration. Any change in therapy must be accompanied by a repeat evaluation. Vigorous follow-up is required to monitor for breakthrough, the occurrence of adverse effects, or both. Aggressive therapy of any intercurrent condition is necessary.

The simplest method for evaluation of antiarrhythmic effect is symptom monitoring. That is, the patient quantitates the frequency of symptoms or "arrhythmia-free" intervals before and then after drug therapy.[41] If the former is reduced or the latter is prolonged significantly, it is reasonable to assume that the drug had a salutary effect. This approach has been advocated for the treatment of and applied to non-life-threatening supraventricular and ventricular arrhythmias that are perfectly sensed by the patient. Unfortunately, it is not feasible in the management of most patients with ventricular arrhythmias that either are not sensed or cause hemodynamic collapse. In the latter case, recurrent symptoms may be fatal.

Monitoring antiarrhythmic drug levels to maintain a "target" or therapeutic drug concentration has been advocated by some as a useful method of ensuring antiarrhythmic efficacy;[42] that is, maintenance of a "target" blood level could serve as a surrogate endpoint for arrhythmia monitoring. This tactic assumes that the reason for recurrence is a subtherapeutic blood level, a fact not verified in several studies. In fact, this approach has not been advocated by most investigators.

For most patients with malignant arrhythmia, the choice of tests to assess antiarrhythmic drug efficacy is either ambulatory monitoring and exercise testing (noninvasive) or electrophysiologic study (invasive). The former approach uses suppression of ambient ventricular ectopy exposed by ambulatory monitoring or exercise testing to predict the efficacy of drug therapy.[43] This approach assumes that the observed ectopic rhythm is a "trigger" for a sustained arrhythmia. Patients typically undergo 48 hours of ambulatory monitoring and exercise testing in a drug-free state. A drug is administered acutely or chronically, during which time a careful reevaluation is carried out. If at least 90% of repetitive VPDs are suppressed, the drug is considered beneficial, and the patient is discharged. If the drug is not successful, an alternative agent or a combination of agents is selected, and

testing is continued. Patients in whom an adequate program is identified have an excellent prognosis compared with those in whom no such program is found.[8, 44]

The advantages of the "noninvasive" approach are obvious. Patients need not undergo invasive procedures. The tests can be carried out in nearly any hospital, so referral to a center with invasive facilities is not necessary. Unfortunately, not all patients have sufficient ambient or exercise-induced arrhythmias that can be used to gauge drug efficacy, but they do have sporadic arrhythmic episodes that are quite severe.[45] In addition, the "formula" for noninvasive testing must be rigorously applied. Exercise testing is an important component of the testing procedure, especially because it may uncover an otherwise undetected poor response.[46] Omission of any component may preclude any conclusions regarding the value of the technique. Older studies suggested that the noninvasive approach might not be as effective as invasive testing in protecting patients against recurrent arrhythmias, although overall survival was comparable.[47] More recent evidence has contradicted these conclusions and purports to indicate that comparable reductions in mortality and events can be achieved with either method.[48]

The noninvasive approach is labor-intensive and applicable only to a minority of patients. Most clinicians prefer to use invasive techniques in patients who require antiarrhythmic drugs for the treatment of life-threatening ventricular arrhythmias.[49] Again, a baseline evaluation is required in which programmed electrical stimulation is used to induce clinical arrhythmias in the electrophysiology laboratory. An example of VT initiation is shown in Figure 135–3. Once the arrhythmia is reproducibly induced, an antiarrhythmic drug is administered, and testing is repeated. The inability to reinitiate the arrhythmia implies a direct antiarrhythmic effect of the drug and a greatly decreased likelihood that the arrhythmia will recur.[50] Continued inducibility, especially without any effect on the tachycardia rate, augurs poorly and usually prompts a search for alternative therapy with another drug, drug combination, device, or surgery.

As with the other methods, invasive testing has distinct advantages and disadvantages. Arrhythmias can be produced "on demand" using a technique that has few associated risks.[51] Consequently, it allows for a definitive demonstration of drug effect even in patients who have sporadic arrhythmias. It also permits precise delineation of the mechanism and location of arrhythmia, which is essential to the use of antiarrhythmic devices or surgery.[52] Unfortunately, the limitations of the technique are substantial. Programmed stimulation may provoke a "nonclinical" arrhythmia even in patients without significant structural heart disease.[53] Which induced arrhythmias should be treated is controversial. This is a particularly difficult problem in those cases in which the initial arrhythmia was never or was inadequately recorded. An example is a patient undergoing invasive testing for evaluation of syncope in whom polymor-

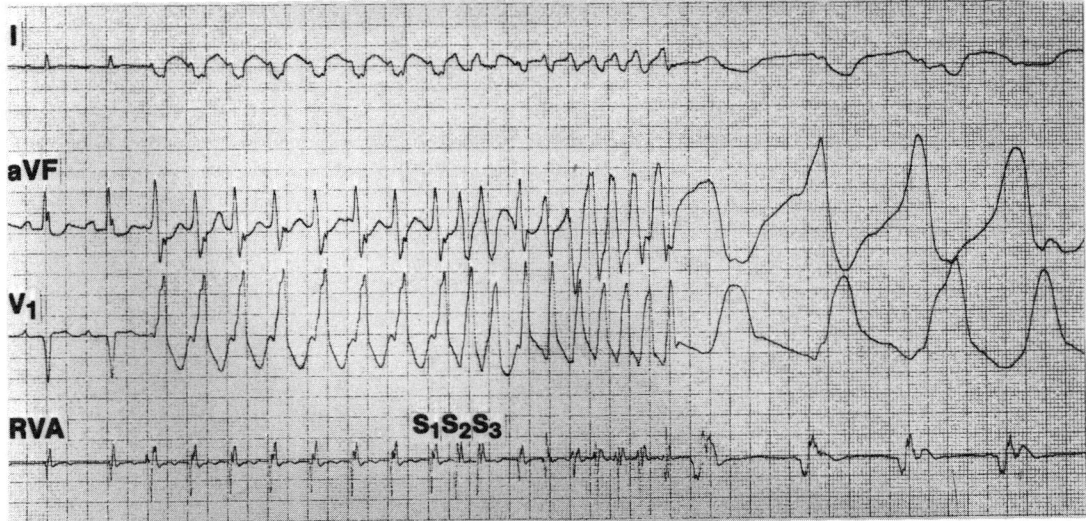

Figure 135–3. Induction of sustained ventricular tachycardia in a patient with a history of several spontaneous occurrences of the same arrhythmia. Surface electrocardiograms are shown together with one recorded from the right ventricular apex (RVA). Following eight drive beats (S1), two premature extrastimuli are delivered at coupling intervals of 240 and 230 msec (S2, S3). These initiate a monomorphic ventricular tachycardia (rate 230 beats/min). Note that the recording speed was increased from 25 to 100 mm/sec following initiation of the tachycardia.

phous sustained VT is induced in the electrophysiology laboratory.[54] What also remains controversial is the approach to patients in whom no arrhythmia can be provoked, or in whom arrhythmia induction cannot be reproduced, such as patients with nonischemic heart disease.[55] The value of invasive testing in patients without documented sustained arrhythmias is still unknown.[56, 57] Finally, there is no consensus regarding the relative value of endpoints less significant than noninducibility. Slowing of induced arrhythmia to hemodynamic tolerance has a salutary effect in most studies, but the recurrence rate of tachycardias slowed in this manner remains controversial.[58]

Even with all these limitations, invasive electrophysiologic testing is a useful way of evaluating patients with malignant arrhythmias, especially for the selection of appropriate antiarrhythmic therapy. While we look forward to the development of alternative methods, such as recording of late potentials by surface recording (which may be successfully combined with some of the more conventional methods of drug evaluation), these techniques now must be considered investigational.[59] An example of a signal-averaged electrocardiogram in a patient with sustained ventricular tachycardia is shown in Figure 135–4.

Procedures

Drug testing should not be viewed as an isolated event but as one that extends over a period of time in a patient's care. The first exposure of a patient to drug therapy frequently occurs in an acute-care setting, when the patient acutely receives the drug as a treatment for tachycardia. The fact that a drug effectively aborts a tachycardia in progress does not necessarily imply that it will be useful for prophylaxis

against recurrence of tachycardia. In addition, one should never assume that a related compound administered orally will have the same salutary effect as its intravenous cousin. This point is well illustrated in the case of intravenous lidocaine and oral tocainide, the responses to which are not always concordant.[60]

Drugs may be evaluated acutely, using large intravenous or oral doses.[61] This technique is feasible only if a usually therapeutic plasma-tissue concentration can be attained in a very brief period of time. Poor oral absorption or the need for repeated intravenous dosing precludes this approach. When drug testing is done successfully, either using ambulatory monitoring or invasive testing, the physician can gain valuable information regarding the relative likelihood of a beneficial drug effect.[8, 62]

Because the results of acute drug testing do not always guarantee a lasting therapeutic benefit, acute drug testing is frequently followed by a period of subacute dosing, lasting from 2 to several days, depending on the kinetics of the drug under study. This approach is also recommended for drugs such as flecainide, in which acute loading is not feasible and may even be dangerous. Subacute testing is particularly valuable, because here is an excellent correlation between a successful test in this phase and long-term prophylaxis.[8, 63]

Patients with serious ventricular arrhythmia treated with antiarrhythmic drugs require careful and comprehensive long-term surveillance. Maintenance of adequate plasma concentrations of an effective agent is required to guarantee long arrhythmia-free intervals. Any changes in concomitant medication may influence the response to an antiarrhythmic drug by pharmacologic or pharmacodynamic interactions.[64] Changes in associated or underlying conditions may also complicate drug therapy by rendering the patient

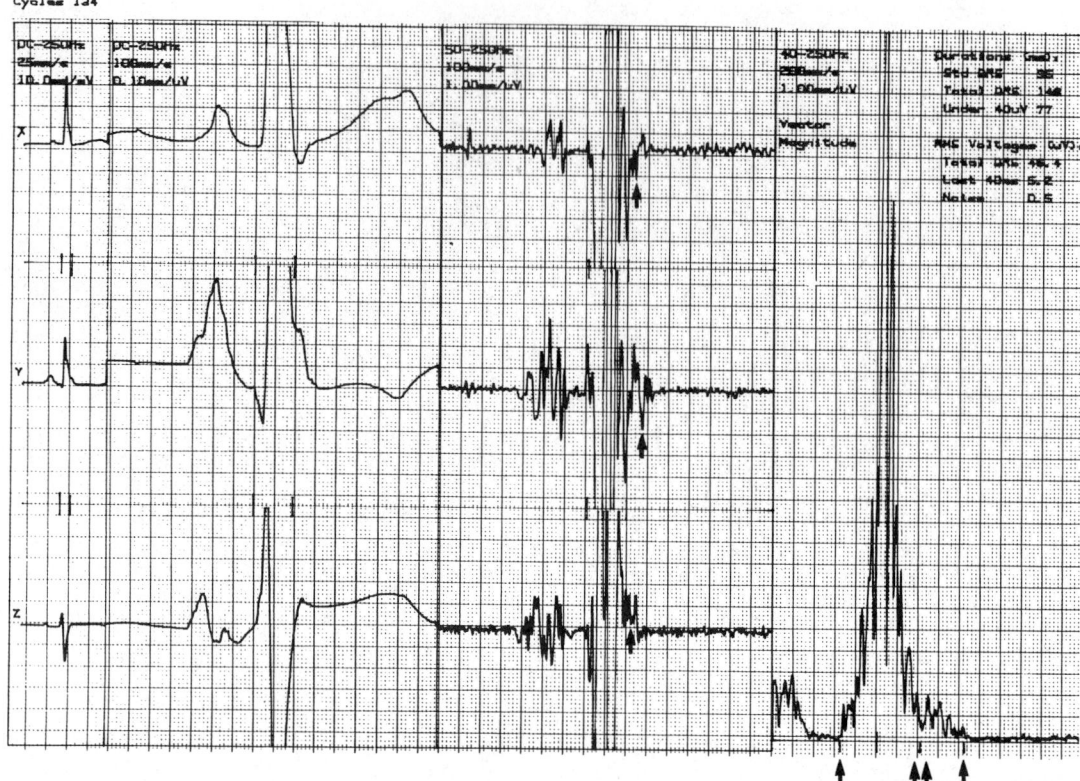

Figure 135–4. Detection of late potentials (LPs) in a patient with chronic recurrent ventricular tachycardia. *Column 1,* Orthogonal leads X, Y, and Z recorded in standard fashion. *Column 2,* Leads X, Y, and Z recorded using a fourfold increase in paper speed and tenfold amplification. *Column 3,* Leads X, Y, and Z recorded with a 100-fold increase in amplitude and with an increase in high-pass filter to 50 Hz. Note the low-amplitude, high-frequency LPs in the terminal portion of the QRS *(arrows). Column 4,* Time domain analysis of the LPs. Total QRS duration (between *large arrows*) is 148 msec. Of this, only 95 msec is the standard QRS duration (between *first large single and small double arrows*). LPs constitute the final 77 msec of the QRS, and the majority of these occur within the terminal 55 msec (between *small double and second large single arrow*).

more resistant to therapy.[65] Alternatively, improvement in some element of heart disease may render drug therapy unnecessary, a determination that can be made only if periodic reevaluations are carried out.[66]

We advocate close physician supervision and intermittent monitoring during the course of antiarrhythmic drug administration, regardless of indication for therapy or agent. This follow-up should be with the prescribing physician or a designate well acquainted with the facts of the case, especially the indications for therapy. The supervising physician should also have extensive experience in the use of antiarrhythmic drugs and should be well versed in adverse effects and their management. Strong consideration should be given to intermittent drug withdrawal whenever it is feasible, with repeat testing to assess the efficacy of the treatment program.

CLINICAL CONSIDERATIONS IN THE USE OF ANTIARRHYTHMIC DRUGS
Antiarrhythmic Drug Classification

The drug classification system, devised by Vaughn Williams and displayed in simple form in Table 135–1, has greatly influenced contemporary thought regard-

ing the electrophysiologic properties of old and new antiarrhythmic agents.[67, 68] In this schema, drugs that predominantly affect sodium channels are dubbed type I drugs and then are subclassified based on the relative potency of their effects on conduction velocity (type IC>IA>IB) and the presence or absence of a concomitant effect on repolarization (possessed only

Table 135–1. **Classification of Antiarrhythmic Drugs**

Class of Action	Examples
Class I: Blockade of sodium channels	
A. Moderate prolongation of conduction and repolarization	Quinidine Procainamide Disopyramide
B. Minimal effect on conduction and repolarization	Lidocaine Tocainide Mexiletine
C. Marked prolongation of conduction	Flecainide Encainide Propafenone
Class II: Blockade of β-adrenergic receptors	Propranolol Acebutolol
Class III: Prolongation of repolarization	Amiodarone Bretylium Sotalol
Class IV: Blockade of calcium channels	Verapamil Diltiazem

by type IA agents).[69] Type III drugs are those that are devoid of any effect on the sodium channel but that have as their action, prolongation of the plateau phase of the action potential because of potassium-channel modulation.[70] Drugs that block the β-adrenergic receptor and calcium channel are types II and IV, respectively.

This classification has been used as a kind of short-hand device for intelligent discussion, especially in new drug development. To the extent that antiarrhythmic drugs can influence one or another portion of the action potential, or selectively modulate ion flux or adrenergic tone, the classification system is workable. Unfortunately, the framers of the classification could never have anticipated that new antiarrhythmic drugs would cut across class distinctions, defying precise placement within the system. The most prominent example is amiodarone, which appears to have characteristics of all four major classes.[71]

Perhaps the most disturbing feature of the classification system is that it tempts one to draw clinical inferences. That is, physicians may assume that a patient's failure to respond to a drug of a given type implies that other drugs in the same class will not be effective. Likewise, the efficacy of a drug may prompt an unwitting physician to empirically prescribe another drug of the same class without subjecting the substitute agent to rigorous testing. The classification system simply does not have sufficient precision to meet these demands. Antiarrhythmic drug therapy remains an empirical art rather than a precise science. Therefore, even though response or nonresponse to a related compound may change the odds of a response, testing will always be required to prove the point.

In an effort to improve the classification of antiarrhythmic drugs, new schema have been proposed. Perhaps the most publicized has been the "Sicilian Gambit" in which the kinetics of drug action, receptor interaction, and various other pharmacologic effects have been incorporated.[72] This classification affords a more comprehensive summary of each drug class and allows a better understanding of how specific drugs might be used in clinical situation. Its disadvantage is its complexity, which makes it less appealing to practicing clinicians.

Antiarrhythmic Drug Monitoring

Chronic administration of antiarrhythmic drugs requires fairly detailed knowledge of the pharmacology of the agents used and how best to monitor them for biologic effects. Measurement of blood levels forms the mainstay of monitoring for most agents, especially because a therapeutic plasma concentration can be determined during acute and subacute drug trials.[73] Blood levels may vary during long-term therapy, influenced by administration of drugs that interact or by changes in hepatic or renal handling of the parent compound or metabolite.[74]

For several reasons, measurement of plasma levels for many antiarrhythmic drugs is not feasible or advisable. First, assays may not be available or may not routinely measure all active metabolites.[75] Second, patients may exhibit a good clinical response to a drug but do so over a very wide range of plasma blood concentrations. This obviates any firm recommendation regarding "target" blood levels. Third, blood levels, which can rise relatively rapidly after acute drug administration, may not reflect myocardial tissue concentration.[76] The most publicized example of this phenomenon is amiodarone.[77] Months of dosing may be required to obtain an antiarrhythmic effect that does not necessarily correlate with serum levels. In this case, investigators have attempted to identify one of several possible biologic markers of adequate amiodarone blood level, such as reverse T3 levels, corneal microdeposits, red blood cell concentration, and prolongation of QT intervals.[78–80]

In most cases, there is no good substitute for close clinical observation during antiarrhythmic therapy. For patients who undergo therapy guided by noninvasive testing, serial ambulatory monitoring and exercise testing are warranted.[81] When invasive testing has been used, blood level determination and measurement of electrocardiographic intervals may be used when possible. Symptom assessment is very important. Any suggestion of recurrent arrhythmia should prompt a reevaluation of the drug program, using the same invasive protocol used at the inception of therapy.[82]

Drug Metabolism

Several antiarrhythmic drugs are metabolized by the liver to forms that themselves are active electrophysiologically.[83] The extent of metabolism, the concentration of metabolites, and their relative activity compared with the parent compound must be taken into account when these drugs are used. The situation is rendered even more complicated by the fact that there may be marked heterogeneity among patients in their metabolism of antiarrhythmic drugs. Precise measurement of major, active metabolites is a requirement when using extensively metabolized drugs, or alternatively, there should be some method of measuring their composite electrophysiologic effects. Procainamide provides a good example of this problem. N-acetylprocainamide (NAPA), the major metabolite of procainamide, prolongs repolarization and refractoriness but, unlike procainamide, does not reduce conduction velocity.[84] Accumulation of NAPA, which can occur in patients with rapid hepatic acetylation and poor renal function (NAPA is primarily renally excreted), would not necessarily augment the antiarrhythmic effect of procainamide but could unpredictably increase the QT interval, predisposing the patient to the development of torsade de pointes. While this metabolic pathway is relatively well recognized, some newer antiarrhythmic drugs such as moricizine have multiple metabolites that are more difficult to measure and that have a multitude of electrophysiologic effects and pharmacokinetics that make clinical dosing more hazardous.[85] As will be discussed, other drugs may interact with antiarrhythmic compounds by changing the degree or extent of drug metabolism, perhaps in an unpredictable fashion.

Drug Interactions

The problem of drug interactions is not unique to antiarrhythmic compounds. Antiarrhythmic drug concentrations can be influenced by a variety of other agents and can themselves interfere with or potentiate drugs of other classes.[86] Many of these interactions are caused by changes in metabolism or excretion, whereas others involve displacement from protein or tissue binding sites, changes in volume of distribution, and end-organ competition.[87] The increase in digoxin levels by quinidine represents one of the first clinically important interactions described in the literature.[88] We have since learned that this interaction is complex indeed, since the increased digoxin levels caused by quinidine are not necessarily associated with an increased digoxin effect, perhaps because of altered binding of drug at the receptor.[89] The advent of new antiarrhythmic drugs will mandate careful monitoring of serum levels and biologic effects of concomitant medication, especially whenever any change is made in a chronic drug program.

The increasing use of devices to treat cardiac arrhythmia has occasioned another kind of interaction, drugs with devices.[31–33] Drugs may interact with a device in one of several ways. If an antiarrhythmic drug slows the heart rate and causes symptoms because of inadequate cardiac output, pacemaker support may be required.[90] A drug could be used to diminish the frequency of device activation, such as in patients with an ICD. However, the same drug could interfere with proper functioning of the ICD by reducing the rate of tachycardia to a point below the lower rate cut-off of the sensing algorithm.[91] The advent of tiered ICD has permitted use of initially less aggressive treatments such as antitachycardia pacing before employment of cardioversion defibrillation shocks.[26] With these devices, drugs may be beneficial in slowing tachycardia to rates at which pace termination might be more feasible.[32, 33] Antiarrhythmic drugs can also change pacing or defibrillation thresholds, increasing them by many times.[32, 33, 92] When this occurs, loss of pacemaker capture may occur, or worse, the stored defibrillation energy of an ICD may become inadequate. Tiered ICDs can also be used to perform noninvasive EP testing to assess chronic drug efficacy or changes in VT rate.[25–27] Finally, pacemakers may be used in concert with antiarrhythmic drugs to improve the efficacy of treatment of certain arrhythmia syndromes. For example, patients with congenital forms of the prolonged QT-interval syndrome may require a β-adrenergic blocking drug together with permanent pacemaker therapy.[93] Figure 135–5 depicts electrocardiograms from a patient in whom a tiered ICD was used to pace terminate a ventricular tachycardia that had been rendered slow and well tolerated using propafenone. During extended follow-up, the device was used several times to terminate spontaneous episodes of ventricular tachycardia.

Adverse Effects

All antiarrhythmic agents have associated adverse effects. Therefore, a particularly important component of the care of patients who receive these drugs is surveillance for side effects that may require dose attenuation or drug discontinuation.[94] When the antiarrhythmic drug was initiated for a lethal or potentially lethal arrhythmia, patients may be asked to persevere with therapy despite annoying side effects. The physician may also attempt to treat a side effect such as arthritis or hypothyroidism if the antiarrhythmic drug is absolutely necessary to prevent a lethal arrhythmia, especially if the condition has proved refractory to other drugs. The treating physician may be more inclined to stop therapy when the arrhythmia is not serious or when an alternative therapy, such as an antitachycardia device, is readily available.

Side effects can be divided into those that affect cardiovascular function and those that affect other organ systems. Cardiovascular side effects are predominantly hemodynamic or electrophysiologic. Several antiarrhythmic drugs depress pump performance or change systemic resistance in such a way as to

---

Figure 135–5. A, Induction of sustained ventricular tachycardia (VT) using the noninvasive programmed stimulation (NIPS) feature of a tiered, implantable cardioverter-defibrillator (ICD) during electrophysiologic (EP) testing before ICD implantation. The patient had suffered repeated episodes of hypotensive sustained VT that were refractory to antiarrhythmic drug therapy. ECG leads I, II, III, aVF, and V_1 are displayed. After the first sinus rhythm QRS complex on the left side of the tracing, eight paced QRS complexes with a cycle length of 400 msec (150 bpm) are followed by two ventricular extrastimuli delivered from the ICD that is functioning as a noninvasive stimulator. Monomorphic sustained VT with a right bundle branch block, right superior axis QRS morphology is induced and with a cycle length of 360 msec (167 bpm).

B, Detecting 24 QRS complexes of sustained VT at a cycle length of 400 msec the ICD automatically delivers eight automatic antitachycardia pacing (ATP) stimuli at a cycle length of 340 msec. These are followed by two ventricular ectopic complexes, termination of VT, and restoration of sinus rhythm. This VT and that depicted in (A) were induced from the same patient but exhibit slightly different QRS morphologies and rates.

C, A third monomorphic VT is induced in the same patient and is identical in rate and morphology to that induced in (A). Only leads I, II, and III are shown with continuous recordings from the top to bottom strips. After 20 sensed VT QRS complexes, the ICD automatically delivers two sequential ATP attempts that fail to terminate the VT. Following the second attempt, the ICD automatically escalates the aggressiveness of therapy by charging its capacitors and delivering a synchronous, 20-J shock 10 seconds later that restores sinus bradycardia. Postshock bradycardia pacing at a rate of 50 bpm is programmed to begin 3 seconds after the shock. The lack of consistent capture of the burst trains probably explains why this ATP attempt failed.

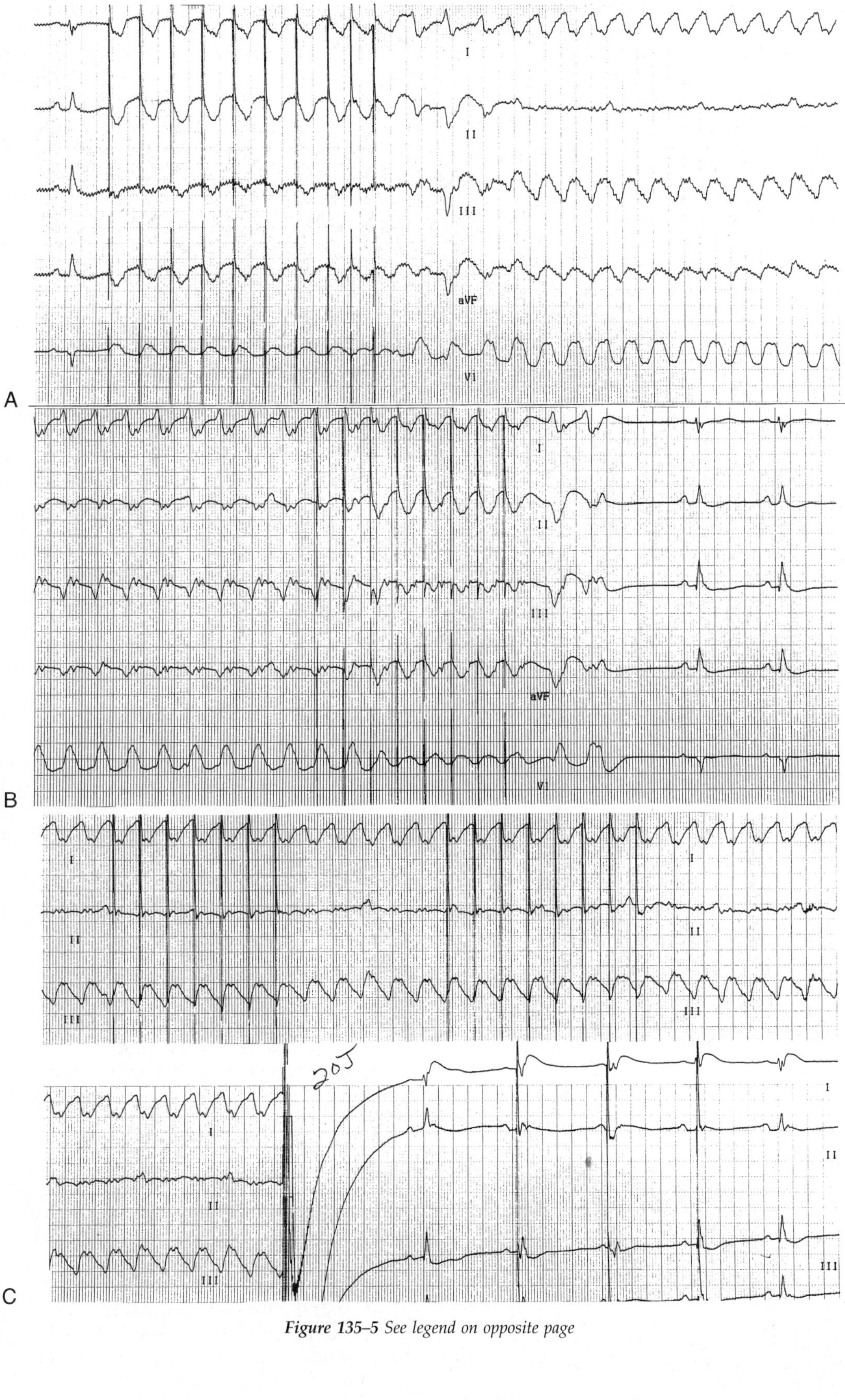

A

B

C

Figure 135–5 See legend on opposite page

increase filling pressures, and they selectively diminish output in patients with already impaired left ventricular function.[95] Since individuals who require aggressive therapy with potent antiarrhythmic drugs have baseline impairment of left ventricular function, the physician must monitor patients very carefully during loading and maintenance phases of therapy for the development of heart failure.[96] Use of some drugs, such as disopyramide and flecainide, is completely interdicted in patients with very severe left ventricular dysfunction.

The electrophysiologic effects of antiarrhythmic drugs may be considered a double-edged sword. The same drugs that quell the electrophysiologic disturbance that generates a cardiac arrhythmia also depress conduction and prolong repolarization in normal tissue. While this is usually of little consequence in patients with normal conduction systems, many patients have preexisting abnormalities that may be made worse by drug therapy and may then require pacemaker therapy.[97] Figure 135–6 illustrates a case of progressive atrioventricular block caused by procainamide that had been used to suppress inducible ventricular tachycardia.

Antiarrhythmic drugs have a propensity to aggravate ventricular arrhythmia, either by worsening preexisting arrhythmia or by generating a new arrhythmia, especially in patients with structurally abnormal hearts.[98] This aggravation may be the result of slowing of conduction, which may perpetuate a tachycardia circuit, or of prolongation of repolarization, which predisposes susceptible individuals to polymorphic ventricular tachycardia.[99, 100] Because paradoxic aggravation of arrhythmia may occur in 10% to 15% of

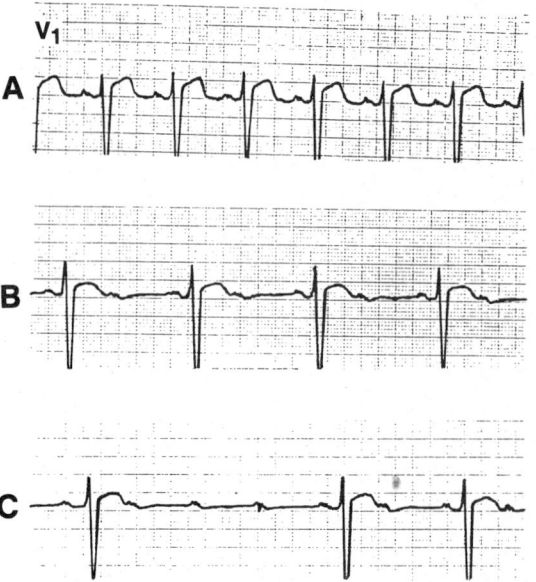

Figure 135–6. Development of atrioventricular block in a patient receiving procainamide for sustained ventricular tachycardia. *A,* Baseline tracing demonstrates QRS duration of 0.12 second, and a PR interval of 0.20 second. *B,* Development of 2:1 atrioventricular block. *C,* High-grade, second-degree atrioventricular block that prompted insertion of a permanent pacemaker to allow safe continuation of antiarrhythmic therapy.

drug exposures (depending on the agent used),[5] it represents a significant problem in the care of patients with arrhythmia, as discussed in Chapter 136.

Antiarrhythmic drugs are responsible for a number of noncardiac side effects, many annoying, some lethal. The spectrum of side effects for any individual agent, which is quite variable, is covered in a comprehensive fashion in chapters dealing with each agent. The most important principle to remember is that the physician who uses a particular agent must be intimately acquainted with all the potential adverse effects, must watch for them, and must intervene quickly and definitively when they occur. A delay in diagnosis or approach may have dire consequences, especially with the more potent membrane-stabilizing agents.

New and Investigational Antiarrhythmic Drugs

The adverse outcome of patients treated with class IC antiarrhythmic drugs in the CAST and other trials has led to a diminished use of these agents for ventricular indications.[39, 101] The medical community and industry have shown considerable interest in drugs with alternative electrophysiologic effects. The class III agents have been particularly popular in this regard, especially since the first class III approved for oral use, amiodarone, has proved to be one of the most effective drugs in the treatment of patients who have severe ventricular arrhythmias, even in those with very poor left ventricular function. The commonality of the class is the ability to extend the repolarization time, usually, but not exclusively, by blockade of one of the many potassium channels. By prolonging the time to the recovery of excitability, it is thought that these drugs make establishment of reentry less likely. As a class, these agents may be less potent as suppressants of spontaneous ventricular arrhythmia.[102]

Sotalol is the newest drug of this class to gain approval by the Food and Drug Adminstration for treatment of patients with life-threatening arrhythmia. Its efficacy in the electrophysiology arm of the ESVEM study was superior to the other drugs used, although comparisons were neither randomized nor blinded.[37] It is not clear how much of the efficacy of sotalol is contributed to by its β-blocking properties. It is known that it has the liability of causing torsade de pointes, an arrhythmia more commonly seen in patients who develop QT prolongation in concert with bradycardia.[103]

A number of new class III drugs are under active investigation. Unlike amiodarone and sotalol, which have one or more other electrophysiologic actions that could contribute to their efficacy, most of the new class III drugs simply prolong the action potential duration. The d-isomer of sotalol is an example of such a compound. Whether these drugs have better efficacy and tolerance compared with drugs already available remains to be seen, but that question is being studied in properly designed prospective clinical trials.[102] Many of these new agents, like sotalol, have a reverse use-dependent effect, meaning that they cause more QT prolongation at lower heart rates, increasing the likelihood of proarrhythmia during periods of bradycardia.[104] It is worth noting that these drugs may have some distinct advantages for modern clinical use. They do not appear to depress left ventricular function and may be safe in patients who have a history of heart failure. This is particularly important because so many patients with the most serious and resistant ventricular arrhythmias have left ventricular dysfunction. In addition, unlike drugs that have sodium channel blocking properties, class III drugs do not appear to cause an increase in the amount of current necessary to convert ventricular fibrillation (defibrillation threshold).[105] Hence, they may be of particular importance in patients who have an implantable device and require concomitant antiarrhythmic drug therapy. Finally, the frequency of organ toxic side effects may be less than with more conventional antiarrhythmic drugs, improving their applicability in patients with multiple-system disease states, which is also a common problem in patients with life-threatening ventricular arrhythmias.

Combination Therapy

What should be the approach to a patient who fails to respond to single antiarrhythmic drugs? Many investigators who propound combination drug trials have produced convincing evidence that dual therapy can be successful when single therapy fails.[106] Furthermore, use of two drugs at lower doses may obviate some of the dose-related side effects that occur when either is used in higher concentrations.[107] The decision to embark on combination testing depends in large measure on what therapeutic options are available should the patient fail drug therapy.

The choice of antiarrhythmic combinations is empirical. Choosing combinations is made particularly difficult because the number of drugs available is virtually infinite, limited only by the imagination of the treating physician. Certain combinations have achieved notoriety mainly because of previously published reports of their effectiveness. The most popular regimens are those that combine either a type IA or a type III drug with a type IB drug or a β-adrenergic blocker.[108, 109] No matter which combination is selected, that mixture should be considered a "new" drug for that patient and should be tested as rigorously as a single drug, even if both components have been safe and partially effective in earlier trials. This is especially true because antiarrhythmic drugs may interact with each other, exposing the patient to a toxicity not seen when either drug is used alone.

Issues in Long-Term Therapy

Initiation of antiarrhythmic therapy implies a long-term commitment on the part of a patient and his or her physician. If the drug is prescribed for malignant arrhythmia, all parties should recognize the seriousness of the commitment and the consequences of poor compliance. The physician should not assume that patients will necessarily comply with a program because they have a serious ventricular arrhythmia. In a recent report, 75% of 98 patients treated for ventricular arrhythmias had subtherapeutic blood levels of antiarrhythmic drugs during long-term follow-up.[110]

Several steps can be taken to mitigate the burden of antiarrhythmic drug therapy and to facilitate long-term cooperation. First, a patient should have a good psychological outlook on his or her situation. If the drug program is regarded as a handicap, the patient may attempt, perhaps subconsciously, to avoid treatment. The patient must share the physician's optimism that he or she will do well in the long term and that the drug program is merely insurance that this goal will occur. It is frequently useful to enlist the help of the spouse or significant other in an effort to make the medical program less imposing. This is especially important when prescribing drugs to impaired patients who may not fully understand or cannot implement drug dosing instructions.

The medical program must be simple. Combinations should be used only when absolutely necessary and when they have been proved effective. Once-daily or twice-daily dosing is preferred. Dosing should be planned carefully, so as not to interfere with the activities of daily living. Dosage that coincides with regular events such as meals will help. For patients with sporadic and well-tolerated arrhythmia, "cocktail therapy" may be warranted.[111] At arrhythmia onset, the patient ingests a large oral dose of a well-absorbed, rapidly acting antiarrhythmic drug, conclusively proven to reliably terminate the tachycardia.[112] This tactic obviously improves patient compliance and reduces side effects and cost but can only be implemented in carefully selected patients who have good hemodynamic tolerance of arrhythmia.

The price of drug therapy should be carefully considered. Many new antiarrhythmic drugs are very expensive indeed, and their use can easily deplete the resources of all except the very wealthy or those with a prescription plan. No matter how well intentioned they are, patients cannot be expected to take drugs that they cannot afford to purchase. The issue should be addressed even before the patient undergoes drug trials in the hospital.

Finally, patients are appropriately concerned about proposed duration of therapy. Unfortunately, information regarding drug discontinuation and changes in arrhythmia substrate is meager.[113] This is probably because physicians and patients alike are loath to discontinue an effective and well-tolerated drug program when that would require readmission to a hospital and another battery of tests. Where it has been tested, most patients retain an electrophysiologic lesion that favors an arrhythmia recurrence.[114] Therefore, for the majority of patients, therapy will be required for life. That is not to say that the physician may not take an opportunity to repeat baseline testing when the occasion permits, such as when a program causes intolerable side effects. In select cases, therapy may no longer be required and the patient may be spared the problems of chronic drug therapy.

CONCLUSION

The overriding feature in the use of drugs for the treatment of ventricular arrhythmia is a precise delineation of the benefit-risk equation. To make the point, one can construct clinical scenarios at either end of a spectrum. A patient with simple and asymptomatic ventricular ectopic rhythm and no or little structural heart disease can gain little benefit from drug therapy. Use of a drug with *any* risk in this situation is not warranted, because it would violate the principle of benefit outweighing risk. Conversely, a patient with a severe ischemic cardiomyopathy who has highly refractory, recurrent, sustained VT will require aggressive drug testing. Under these circumstances, use of a drug with a potential for severe toxic side effects may be warranted. In fact, many physicians would advocate implantation of a device in order to treat such a highly malignant arrhythmia or even a surgical procedure that carries a relatively high operative or in-hospital mortality. In any case, the risk of intervention can be escalated because of the immense clinical benefit that can be derived from preventing the recurrence of arrhythmia.

Samuel Levine may have captured the essence of the problem in his now-famous quote regarding high-dose quinidine therapy, then the only practical oral, ventricular antiarrhythmic agent.[115] To rationalize the attendant toxicity of the drug, Levine stated, "In the treatment of ventricular tachycardia, these matters (adverse effects) are of very little importance as the condition is already critical and fatal if uncontrolled. . . . The fact that the patient becomes nauseated, dizzy, weak, or develops diarrhea or ringing of the ears should not discourage the physician from persisting with this therapy, when the alternative is likely to be a fatal termination." With this philosophy of therapy, the careful physician will continue to treat patients who have serious and malignant ventricular arrhythmias with potentially toxic antiarrhythmic drugs to confer the greater benefit of life without imposing the liability of adverse effects.

Acknowledgment

The authors would like to thank Ms. Rose Marie Wells for her help in manuscript preparation.

REFERENCES

1. Lown B: Sudden cardiac death: The major challenge confronting contemporary cardiology. Am J Cardiol 43:313, 1979.
2. Brodsky M, Wu D, Denes P, et al: Arrhythmias documented by 24-hour continuous electrocardiographic monitoring in 50 male medical students without apparent heart disease. Am J Cardiol 39:390, 1977.
3. Ruberman W, Weinblatt E, Goldberg J, et al: Ventricular premature complexes and sudden death after myocardial infarction. Circulation 64:297, 1981.
4. Josephson ME, Horowitz LN, Spielman SR, et al: Electrophysiologic and hemodynamic studies in patients resuscitated from cardiac arrest. Am J Cardiol 44:948, 1980.
5. Velebit V, Podrid P, Lown B: Aggravation and provocation of ventricular arrhythmias by antiarrhythmic drugs. Circulation 65:886, 1982.
6. Ruskin JN, DiMarco JP, Garan H: Out-of-hospital cardiac arrest. Electrophysiologic observations and selection of long-term antiarrhythmic therapy. N Engl J Med 303:607, 1980.
7. Myerburg RJ, Kesserl KM, Castellanos A: Sudden cardiac death. Structure, function, and time-dependence of risk. Circulation 85:I-2, 1992.
8. Graboys T, Lown B, Podrid P, et al: Long-term survival of patients with malignant ventricular arrhythmia treated with antiarrhythmic drugs. Am J Cardiol 50:437, 1982.
9. Kennedy HL, Whitlock JA, Sprague MK: Long-term follow-up of asymptomatic healthy subjects with frequent and complex ventricular ectopy. N Engl J Med 312:193, 1985.
10. Bigger JT, Fleiss JL, Rolintzky LM, et al: Prevalence, characteristics, and significance of ventricular tachycardia detected by 24-hour continuous electrocardiographic recordings in the late hospital phase of acute myocardial infarction. Am J Cardiol 58:1151, 1986.
11. Bigger J, Fleiss J, Kleiger R, et al: The relationship among ventricular arrhythmias, left ventricular dysfunction and mortality in the two years after myocardial infarction. Circulation 69:250, 1984.
12. Gomes JA, Winters SL, Martinson M, et al: The prognostic significance of quantitative signal-averaged variables relative to clinical variables, site of myocardial infarction, ejection fraction and ventricular premature beats. A prospective study. J Am Coll Cardiol 13:377, 1989.
13. Cripps T, Bennett ED, Camm AJ, Ward DE: Inducibility of sustained monomorphic ventricular tachycardia as a prognostic indicator in survivors of recent myocaridal infarction: A prospective evaluation in relation to other prognostic variables. J Am Coll Cardiol 14:289, 1989.
14. LaRovere MT, Specchia G, Mortara A, Schwartz PJ: Baroreflex sensitivity, clinical correlates, and cardiovascular mortality among patients with a first myocardial infarction. A prospective study. Circulation 78:816, 1988.
15. Gomes JA, Winters SL, Stewart D, et al: New noninvasive index to predict sustained ventricular tachycardia and sudden death in the first year after myocardial infarction: Based on signal-averaged electrocardiogram, radionuclide ejection fraction and Holter monitoring. J Am Coll Cardiol 10:349, 1987.
16. Kleiger RE, Miller JP, Bigger JT Jr, Moss AJ, for the Multicenter Postinfarction Research Group: Decreased heart rate variability and its association with increased mortality after acute myocardial infarction. Am J Cardiol 59:256, 1987.
17. Kadish A, Schmaltz S, Calkins H, Morady F: Management of non-sustained ventricular tachycardia guided by electrophysiological testing. PACE 16:1037, 1993.
18. Pratt CM, Eaton T, Francis M, et al: The inverse relationship between baseline left ventricular ejection fraction and outcome of antiarrhythmic therapy: A dangerous imbalance in the risk-benefit ratio. Am Heart J 118:433, 1989.
19. Woosley RL: Pharmacokinetics and pharmacodynamics of antiarrhythmic agents in patients with congestive heart failure. Am Heart J 114:1280, 1987.
20. Echt DS, Liebson PR, Mitchell LB, et al: Mortality and morbidity in patients receiving encainide, flecainide, or placebo. The Cardiac Arrhythmia Suppression Trial. N Engl J Med 324:781, 1991.
21. Nattel S, Pederson DH, Zipes DP: Alterations in regional myocardial distribution and arrhythmogenic effects of aprindine produced by coronary artery occlusion in the dog. Cardiovasc Res 15:80, 1981.
22. Zerin NZ: Crime, misdemeanor, and arrhythmia. Decoding CAST. J Clin Pharmacol 31:1044, 1991.
23. Siddoway LA: Initial dosage selection of antiarrhythmic therapy. Am J Cardiol 62:2H, 1988.
24. Papametriou V: Diuretics, hypokalemia, and cardiac arrhythmias: A critical analysis. Am Heart J 111:1217, 1986.
25. Callans DJ, Josephson ME: Future developments in im-

plantable cardioverter defibrillators: The optimal device. Prog Cardiovasc Dis 36:227, 1993.

26. Leitch JW, Gillis AM, Wyse DG, et al: Reduction in defibrillator shocks with an implantable device combining antitachycardia pacing and shock therapy. J Am Coll Cardiol 18:145, 1991.

27. Bardy GH, Troutman C, Poole JE, et al: Clinical experience with a tiered-therapy, multiprogrammable antiarrhythmia device. Circulation 85:1689, 1992.

28. Yee R, Klein GJ, Leitch JW, et al: A permanent transvenous lead system for an implantable pacemaker cardioverter-defibrillator. Circulation 85:196, 1992.

29. Bardy GH, Hofer B, Johnson G, et al: Implantable transvenous cardioverter-defibrillators. Circulation 87:1152, 1993.

30. Josephson M, Harken A, Horowitz L: Long-term results of endocardial resection for sustained ventricular tachycardia in coronary disease patients. Am Heart J 104:51, 1982.

31. Reiffel T, Coromilas J, Zimmerman JM: Drug-device interactions: Clinical considerations. PACE 8:369, 1985.

32. Singer I, Guarnieri T, Kupersmith J: Implanted automatic defibrillators: Effects of drugs and pacemakers. PACE 11:2250, 1988.

33. Singer I, Kupersmith J: AICD Therapy: Drug/pacemaker interactions and future directions. Prim Cardiol 16:67, 1990.

34. Swiryn S, Baurenfeind R, Strasberg B, et al: Prediction of response to Class I antiarrhythmic drugs during electrophysiologic study of ventricular tachycardia. Am Heart J 104:43, 1982.

35. Kudenchuk PJ, Halperin B, Kron J, et al: Serial electropharmacologic studies in patients with ischemic heart disease and sustained ventricular tachyarrhythmias: When is drug testing sufficient? Am J Cardiol 72:1400, 1993.

36. Salerno DM, Gillingham KJ, Berry DA, Hodges M: A comparison of antiarrhythmic drugs for the suppression of ventricular ectopic depolarizations: A meta-analysis. Am Heart J 120:340, 1990.

37. Mason JW: A comparison of seven antiarrhythmic drugs in patients with ventricular tachyarrhythmias. N Engl J Med 329:452, 1993.

38. Kennedy HL, Whitlock JA, Sprague MK, et al: Long-term follow-up of asymptomatic healthy subjects with frequent and complex ventricular ectopy. N Engl J Med 312:193, 1985.

39. The Cardiac Arrhythmia Suppression Trial (CAST) Investigators: Preliminary report: Effect of encainide and flecainide on mortality in a randomized trial of arrhythmia suppression after myocardial infarction. N Engl J Med 321:406, 1989.

40. The Cardiac Arrhythmia Suppression Trial II Investigators: Effect of the antiarrhythmic agent moricizine on survival after myocardial infarction. N Engl J Med 327:227, 1992.

41. Marinchak RA, Friehling TD, Kowey PR: A clinician's approach to diagnosing supraventricular tachycardia. J Crit Illness 3:39, 1988.

42. Myerburg RJ, Conde C, Sheps DS: Antiarrhythmic drug therapy in survivors of prehospital cardiac arrest: Comparison of effects of chronic ventricular arrhythmias and recurrent cardiac arrest. Circulation 59:855, 1979.

43. Kim S: The management of patients with life-threatening ventricular tachyarrhythmias: Programmed stimulation or Holter monitoring (either or both)? Circulation 76:1, 1987.

44. Fisher J: Ventricular tachycardia—practical and provocative electrophysiology. Circulation 58:1000, 1978.

45. Bigger JT Jr, Reiffel JA: Holter versus electrophysiologic studies in the management of malignant ventricular arrhythmias. Am J Cardiol 51:1464, 1983.

46. Jelinek M, Lown B: Exercise stress testing for exposure of cardiac arrhythmias. Prog Cardiovasc Dis 16:497, 1974.

47. Mitchell L, Duff H, Manyari D, et al: A randomized clinical trial of the noninvasive and invasive approaches to drug therapy of ventricular tachycardia. N Engl J Med 317:1681, 1987.

48. Mason JW: A comparison of electrophysiologic testing with Holter monitoring to predict antiarrhythmic-drug efficacy for ventricular tachyarrhythmias. N Engl J Med 329:445, 1993.

49. Skale BT, Miles WM, Heher JJ, et al: Survivors of cardiac arrest: Prevention of recurrence by drug therapy as predicted by electrophysiologic testing or electrocardiographic monitoring. Am J Cardiol 57:113, 1986.

50. Waller TJ, Kay HR, Spielman SR, et al: Reduction in sudden death and total mortality by antiarrhythmic therapy evaluated by electrophysiologic drug testing: Criteria of efficacy in patients with sustained ventricular tachyarrhythmia. J Am Coll Cardiol 10:83, 1987.

51. Horowitz LN, Kay HR, Kutalek SP, et al: Risks and complications of clinical electrophysiologic studies: A prospective analysis of 1000 consecutive patients. J Am Coll Cardiol 9:1261, 1987.

52. Doherty JU, Josephson ME: Role of electrophysiologic testing in the therapy of ventricular arrhythmias. PACE 6:1070, 1983.

53. Brugada P, Abdollah H, Heddle B, et al: Results of a ventricular stimulation protocol using a maximum of 4 premature stimuli in patients without documented or suspected ventricular arrhythmias. Am J Cardiol 52:1214, 1983.

54. Akhtar M: Clinical spectrum of ventricular tachycardia. Circulation 5:1561, 1990.

55. Naccarelli GV, Prystowsky EN, Jackman WM, et al: Role of electrophysiologic testing in managing patients who have ventricular tachycardia unrelated to coronary artery disease. Am J Cardiol 50:165, 1982.

56. Sulpizi AM, Friehling TD, Kowey PR: Value of electrophysiologic testing in patients with nonsustained ventricular tachycardia. Am J Cardiol 59:841, 1987.

57. Buxton AE, Fisher JD, Josephson ME, et al: Prevention of sudden death in patients with coronary artery disease: The Multicenter Unsustained Tachycardia Trial (MUSTT). Prog Cardiovasc Dis 36:215, 1993.

58. Kim S, Seiden S, Felder S, et al: Is programmed stimulation of value in predicting the long-term success of antiarrhythmic therapy for ventricular tachycardia? N Engl J Med 315:356, 1986.

59. Wilber DJ, Kopp D, Olshansky B, et al. Nonsustained ventricular tachycardia and other high-risk predictors following myocardial infarction: Implications for prophylactic automatic implantable cardioverter-defibrillator use. Prog Cardiovasc Dis 36:179, 1993.

60. Hohnloser SH, Lange H, Raeder EA, et al: Short- and long-term therapy with tocainide for malignant ventricular arrhythmia. Circulation 73:143, 1986.

61. Kelliher GJ, Kowey PR, Engel TR, et al: Clinical pharmacology of antiarrhythmic agents. Cardiovasc Clin 16:287, 1985.

62. Horowitz LN, Josephson ME, Farshidi A, et al: Recurrent sustained ventricular tachycardia: Role of the electrophysiologic study in the selection of antiarrhythmic regimens. Circulation 58:986, 1978.

63. Josephson ME, Horowitz LN: Electrophysiologic approach to therapy of recurrent sustained ventricular tachycardia. Am J Cardiol 43:631, 1979.

64. Bigger JT: Perspectives on the current treatment of cardiac arrhythmias. Am J Cardiol 54:2B, 1984.

65. Kowey PR, Friehling TD, Marinchak RA, et al: The case for explantation of the automatic implantable cardioverter-defibrillator. Am J Cardiol 59:1210, 1987.

66. Garan H, Ruskin J, DiMarco J, et al: Electrophysiologic studies before and after myocardial revascularization in patients with life-threatening ventricular arrhythmias. Am J Cardiol 51:519, 1983.

67. Vaughan Williams EM: Classification of antiarrhythmic drugs. *In* Sandoe E, Flensted-Jensen E, Olesen KH (eds): Symposium on Cardiac Arrhythmias. Sweden: Astra, 1970, pp 449–472.

68. Vaughan Williams EM: A classification of antiarrhythmic actions reassessed after a decade of new drugs. J Clin Pharmacol 24:129, 1984.

69. Hoffman BF, Bigger JT: Antiarrhythmic drugs. *In* DiPalma JR (ed): Drill's Pharmacology in Medicine. New York: McGraw-Hill, 1971, pp 824–851.

70. Singh B, Nademanee K, Ikeda N, et al: Antiarrhythmic actions of compounds that prolong the action potential duration of cardiac muscle. *In* Lucchesi BR, Dingell JV, Schwartz PR Jr (eds): Clinical Pharmacology of Antiarrhythmic Therapy. New York: Raven Press, 1984, pp 105–126.

71. Morady F, DiCarlo LA, Krol RB, et al: Acute and chronic effects of amiodarone on ventricular refractoriness, intraventricular conduction and ventricular tachycardia induction. J Am Coll Cardiol 7:148, 1986.

72. Task Force of the Working Group on Arrhythmias of the European Society of Cardiology: The Sicilian Gambit. A new approach to the classification of antiarrhythmic drugs based on their actions on arrhythmogenic mechanisms. Circulation 84:1831, 1991.

73. Brown JE, Shand DG: Therapeutic drug monitoring of antiarrhythmic agents. Clin Pharmacokinet 7:125, 1982.

74. Woosley RI, Shand DG: Pharmacokinetics of antiarrhythmic drugs. Am J Cardiol 41:986, 1978.

75. Anderson JL, Stewart JR, Johnson TA, et al: Response to encainide of refractory ventricular tachycardia: Clinical application of assays for parent drug and metabolites. J Cardiovasc Pharmacol 4:812, 1982.

76. Ikeda N, Nademanee K, Singh B, et al: Electrophysiologic effects of amiodarone: Experimental and clinical observations relative to serum and tissue drug concentrations. Am Heart J 108:890, 1984.

77. Zipes DP, Prystowsky EN, Heger JT: Amiodarone: Electrophysiologic action, pharmacokinetics and clinical effects. J Am Coll Cardiol 3:1059, 1984.

78. Nademanee K, Singh BN, Henrickson JA, et al: Pharmacokinetic significance of serum reverse T3 levels during amiodarone treatment: A potential method for monitoring chronic drug therapy. Circulation 66:202, 1982.

79. Kaplan L, Cappaert W: Amiodarone keratopathy: Correlation to dosage and duration. Arch Ophthalmol 100:601, 1982.

80. Kowey P, Friehling T, Marinchak R, et al: Safety and efficacy of amiodarone: The low-dose perspective. Chest 93:54, 1988.

81. Lown B, Podrid P, DeSilva R, et al: Sudden cardiac death: Management of the patient at risk. Curr Prob Cardiol 4:1, 1980.

82. Kowey P, Friehling T: Uses and limitations of electrophysiology studies for the selection of antiarrhythmic therapy. PACE 9:231, 1986.

83. Kates R: Role of metabolites of antiarrhythmic drugs. Clin Pharmacol Antiarrhyth Ther 10:175, 1984.

84. Jaillon P, Winkle R: Electrophysiologic comparative study of procainamide and N-acetyl procainamide in anesthetized dogs. Concentration-response relationships. Circulation 60:1385, 1975.

85. Woosley RL, Morganroth J, Fogoros RN, et al: Pharmacokinetics of moricizine HCl. Am J Cardiol 60:35f, 1987.

86. Nestico P, Morganroth J: Cardiac arrhythmias in the elderly: Antiarrhythmic drug treatment. Cardiol Clin (Geriatric Cardiology) 9:285, 1986.

87. Oates J, Roden D, Wilkinson G, et al: The clinical pharmacology of new antiarrhythmic drugs: An overview. Clin Pharmacol Antiarrhyth Ther 10:157, 1984.

88. Bigger JT: The quinidine-digoxin interaction. Int J Cardiol 1:109, 1981.

89. Kim D, Akeva T, Brody T: Interaction between quinidine and cardiac glycosides involving binding sites in the guinea pig. J Pharmacol Exp Ther 218:108, 1981.

90. Friehling T, Marinchak R, Kowey P: Role of permanent pacemakers in the pharmacologic therapy of patients with reentrant tachyarrhythmias. PACE 11:83, 1988.

91. Winkle RA, Stinson E, Echt D, et al: Practical aspects of automatic cardioverter/defibrillator implantation. Am Heart J 108:1335, 1984.

92. Marinchak R, Friehling T, Kline R, et al: Effect of antiarrhythmic drugs on defibrillation threshold: Case report of an adverse effect of mexiletine and review of the literature. PACE 11:7, 1988.

93. Eldar M, Griffin JC, Abbott JA, et al: Permanent cardiac pacing in patients with the long QT syndrome. J Am Coll Cardiol 10:600, 1987.

94. Nygaard TW, Sellers TD, Cook TS, et al: Adverse reactions to antiarrhythmic drugs during therapy for ventricular arrhythmias. JAMA 256:55, 1986.

95. Kowey PR, Friedman PL, Podrid PJ, et al: Use of radionuclide ventriculography for assessment of changes in myocardial performance induced by disopyramide phosphate. Am Heart J 104:769, 1982.

96. Brodsky MA, Allen BJ: Ventricular tachycardia in patients with impaired left ventricular function: The role of propafenone. Clin Prog Electrophysiol Pacing 4:546, 1986.

97. Kowey PR, Engel TR: Overdrive pacing for ventricular tachyarrhythmias: A reassessment. Ann Intern Med 99:651, 1983.

98. Ruskin JN, McGovern B, Garan H, et al: Antiarrhythmic drugs: A possible cause of out-of-hospital cardiac arrest. N Engl J Med 309:1302, 1983.

99. Jackman WM, Friday KJ, Anderson JL, et al: The long QT syndromes: A critical review, new clinical observations and a unifying hypothesis. Prog Cardiovasc Dis 31:115, 1988.

100. Starmer CF, Lastra AA, Nesterenko VV, Grant AO: Proarrhythmic response to sodium channel blockade. Theoretic model and numerical experiments. Circulation 84:1364, 1991.

101. Hine LK, Laird NM, Hewitt P, Chalmers TC: Meta-analysis of empirical long-term antiarrhythmic therapy after myocardial infarction. JAMA 262:3037, 1989.

102. Singh BN, Singh SN, eds. A symposium: Controlling cardiac arrhythmias by lengthening repolarization: Emerging perspectives. Am J Cardiol 72:1f, 1993.

103. Ruffy R: Sotalol. J Cardiovasc Electrophysiol 4:81, 1993.

104. Hondeghem LM, Snyders DJ: Class III antiarrhythmic agents have a lot of potential but a long way to go. Reduced effectiveness and dangers of reverse use dependence. Circulation 81:686, 1990.

105. Wang M, Dorian P: DL and D sotalol decrease defibrillation energy requirements. PACE 12:1522, 1989.

106. Greenspan AM, Spielman SR, Webb CR, et al: Efficacy of combination therapy with mexiletine and a Type IA agent for inducible ventricular tachyarrhythmias secondary to coronary artery disease. Am J Cardiol 56:277, 1985.

107. Kim SG, Sieden S, Matos JA, et al: Combination of procainamide and quinidine for better tolerance and additive effects for ventricular arrhythmias. Am J Cardiol 56:84, 1985.

108. Marchlinski FE, Buxton AE, Miller JM, et al: Amiodarone versus amiodarone and a Type IA agent for treatment of patients with rapid ventricular tachycardia. Circulation 74:1037, 1986.

109. Berman ND, Loukides JE: The cellular electropharmacology of the simultaneous administration of propranolol and mexiletine: A class I and II antiarrhythmic drug combination. J Electrocardiol 20:297, 1987.

110. Squire A, Goldman ME, Kuppersmith J, et al: Long-term antiarrhythmic therapy. Problem of low drug levels and patient noncompliance. Am J Med 77:1035, 1984.

111. Margolis B, DeSilva RA, Lown B: Episodic drug treatment of paroxysmal arrhythmias. Am J Cardiol 45:621, 1980.

112. Benson DW, Dunnigan A, Green TP, et al: Periodic procainamide for paroxysmal tachycardia. Circulation 72:147, 1985.

113. McComb JM, Gold HK, Leinbach RC, et al: Reproducibility of the results of programmed ventricular stimulation early and late after myocardial infarction [abstract]. J Am Coll Cardiol 7:129A, 1986.

114. Schoenfeld MH, McGovern B, Garan H, et al: Long-term reproducibility of responses to programmed cardiac stimulation in spontaneous ventricular tachyarrhythmias. Am J Cardiol 54:564, 1984.

115. Armbrust CA, Levine SA: Paroxysmal ventricular tachycardia: A study of one hundred and seven cases. Circulation 1:28, 1950.

CHAPTER 136

Aggravation of Arrhythmia by Antiarrhythmic Drugs

Philip J. Podrid, M.D.

Over the past few years, many new antiarrhythmic agents have undergone clinical evaluation, and several have recently been approved for use in the United States.[1] The availability of these newer agents and the growing recognition that ventricular arrhythmia is an important and independent risk factor for sudden cardiac death[2, 3] have led to the widespread use of this class of drugs. While the antiarrhythmic agents are effective for suppressing spontaneous arrhythmia or preventing arrhythmia induction, side effects are frequent and limit the usefulness of these drugs.[1] Each agent is associated with a number of side effects, most of which are dose related and generally predictable. However, there are others that are unrelated to dose or serum blood level and are thus unpredictable. One of the most serious problems common to all these drugs is the potential to aggravate arrhythmia.[4] This toxic side effect was initially described with quinidine, but over the past few years it has become apparent that it is a complication associated with antiarrhythmic drug therapy in general. Although aggravation is well recognized as a serious adverse effect of drug therapy, the definitions of aggravation, its incidence, and prediction of patients at risk are still uncertain.

DEFINITION OF ARRHYTHMIA AGGRAVATION

Table 136–1 lists the different types of arrhythmia aggravation in patients with ventricular arrhythmia. For many years it has been recognized that quinidine

Table 136–1. **Types of Aggravation of Ventricular Arrhythmia**

Worsening of existing arrhythmia
- Increase in number of VPBs or repetitive forms (complete or nonsustained VT)
- Conversion of nonsustained VT or sustained VT
- Increase in the frequency of episodes of sustained VT
- Increase in the duration of VT episodes
- An arrhythmia more difficult or impossible to terminate (incessant)

Occurrence of a new arrhythmia
- SVT
- Polymorphic VT
- Torsade de pointes
- VF

Development of a bradyarrhythmia
- Sinus bradycardia, sinus arrest, or sinoatrial block
- Atrioventricular block

SVT, Supraventricular tachycardia; VF, ventricular fibrillation; VPB, ventricular premature beats; VT, ventricular tachycardia.

may cause syncope documented to be the result of a polymorphic ventricular tachycardia (VT) or nonsustained ventricular fibrillation (VF)[5] (Fig. 136–1). This event was only rarely observed and usually occurred in patients receiving quinidine and digoxin for therapy of atrial fibrillation. Although syncope was initially thought to be the result of an interaction with digoxin, quinidine has been established as the cause.[6] Polymorphic VT occurred in association with QT prolongation and often when quinidine blood levels were low and hypokalemia was present. This arrhythmia is now known as torsade de pointes,[7] and it is only one of several recognized types of arrhythmia aggravation.

In the first report of arrhythmia aggravation due to antiarrhythmic drugs, Velebit et al.[4] proposed the following definition for this complication when noninvasive methods are used to evaluate drug effect in patients with ventricular arrhythmia:

1. A fourfold increase in the frequency of ventricular premature beats (VPBs) compared with the baseline value;
2. A tenfold increase in the number of repetitive forms (couplets or runs of VT) compared with the baseline value (Fig. 136–2); or
3. The occurrence of a sustained VT not present during the control period (Fig. 136–3).

In a follow-up study involving electrophysiologic testing, Poser et al.[8] proposed the following criteria for drug-induced aggravation when invasive techniques are utilized for evaluation of drug effect in patients with ventricular arrhythmia:

1. Arrhythmia that is more easily provocable (i.e., requires fewer extrastimuli) compared with the control study;
2. The conversion of nonsustained VT to a sustained tachyarrhythmia when the same or fewer extrastimuli are used (Fig. 136–4); or
3. The induction of VT with a faster rate.

In these two studies, the baseline arrhythmia was well characterized, and random variability of spontaneous or induced arrhythmia was considered. Each patient underwent 48 hours of ambulatory monitoring or two control electrophysiologic studies before drug therapy. The criteria for arrhythmia aggravation were based on observations in patients with a history of serious VT in whom baseline arrhythmia (spontaneous or inducible) was consistently present and highly reproducible.

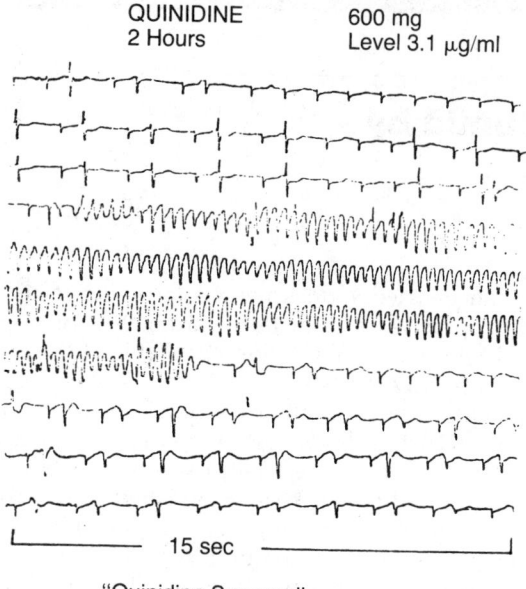

QUINIDINE　600 mg
2 Hours　Level 3.1 µg/ml

⊢——————— 15 sec ———————⊣

"Quinidine Syncope"
Nonsustained VF

Figure 136–1. Example of quinidine syncope. The patient had mitral stenosis and paroxysmal atrial fibrillation (AF). The patient was given 600 mg of quinidine in an attempt to revert the AF. Two hours after the drug was administered, nonsustained ventricular fibrillation (VF) or torsade de pointes occurred.

In patients who have never experienced serious arrhythmias, baseline arrhythmia has been observed to be highly variable from hour to hour[9] and day to day.[10] However, Morganroth et al.[10] reported that

Table 136–2. **Baseline VPBs/Hour Increase Necessary to Establish Arrhythmia Aggravation**

10–50	10×
51–100	5×
101–300	4×
>300	3×

VPB, ventricular premature beats.

variability was related to arrhythmia frequency. Patients who had a high density of spontaneous arrhythmia demonstrated less variability, and arrhythmia frequency was very reproducible. To account for the relationship between density, variability, and criteria for aggravation, Morganroth and Horowitz[11] defined aggravation as (1) the occurrence of a new tachyarrhythmia, and (2) increased frequency of VPBs according to the scheme expressed in Table 136–2. Additional forms of aggravation include an arrhythmia that is difficult to terminate or one that is incessant and cannot be terminated.[12]

Arrhythmia aggravation is usually primary, is unrelated to blood level or electrocardiographic changes, and occurs in the absence of provocating factors. Therefore, it is considered idiosyncratic. However, this complication may also be induced by a number of factors that can alter the action of antiarrhythmic drugs. Thus, high or toxic plasma drug concentrations, other medications, electrolyte abnormalities, ischemia, and catecholamines may affect the activity of these drugs and may result in arrhythmia aggrava-

CONTROL

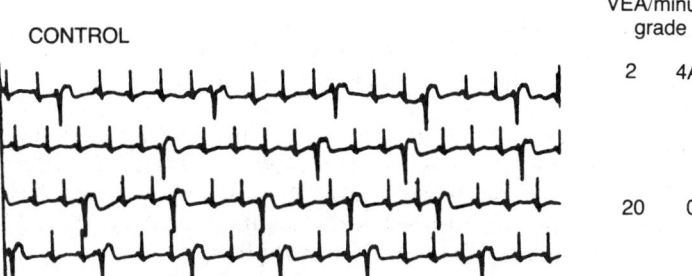

PROPAFENONE

⊢——————— 15 sec ———————⊣

VEA/minute grade

	2	4A	4B
	20	0	0
	9	25	2

Figure 136–2. An example of increased repetitive arrhythmia from antiarrhythmic drugs. The patient had frequent symptomatic ventricular premature beats (VPBs) documented on the monitor. There were as many as 20 VPBs per hour (grade 2). No couplets (grade 4A) or runs of ventricular tachycardia (VT, grade 4B) were seen. During therapy with propafenone, the patient developed couplets (grade 4A) for the first time, with up to 25 episodes per hour. Runs of VT (grade 4B), with up to two runs per hour, also occurred. The repetitive forms abated when drug therapy was discontinued. VEA, ventricular ectopic activity.

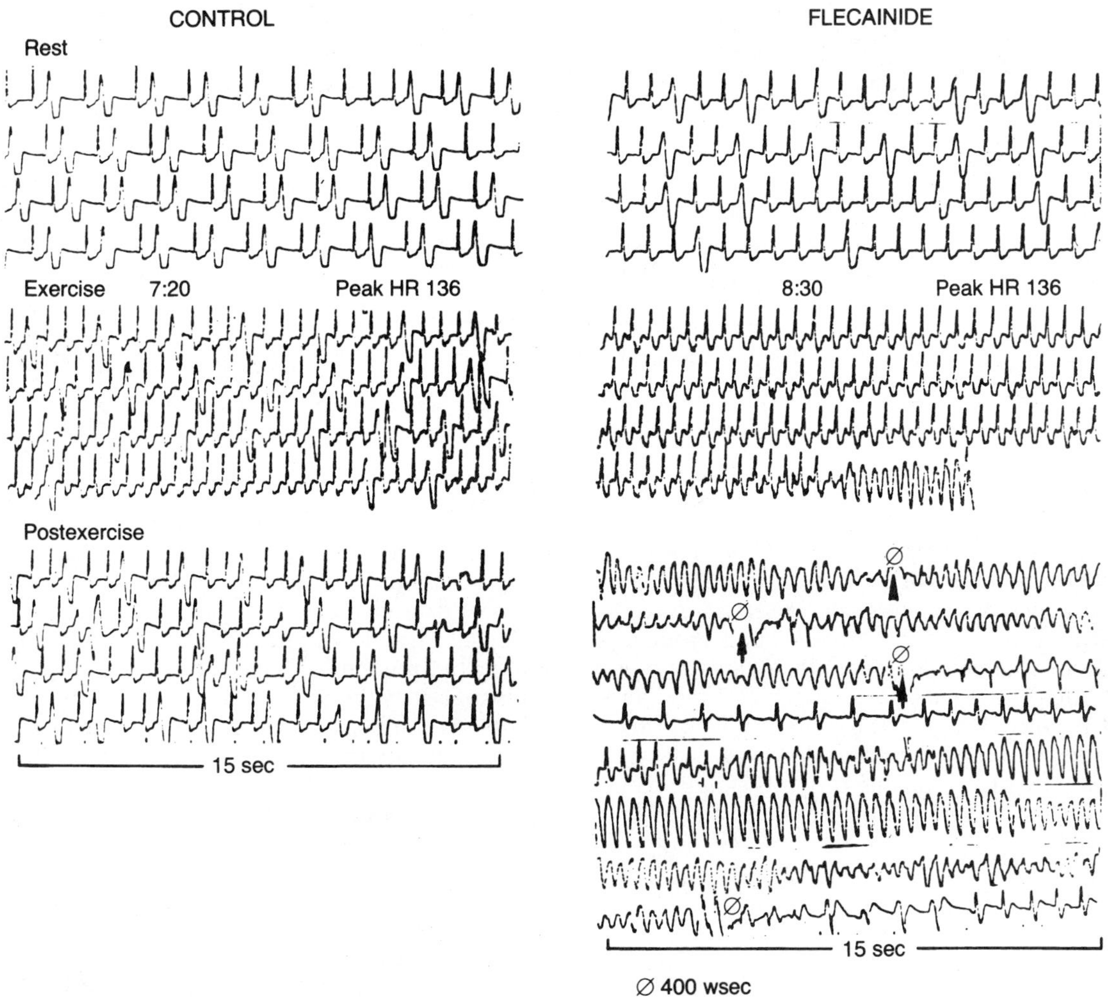

CONTROL   FLECAINIDE

Rest

Exercise   7:20   Peak HR 136   8:30   Peak HR 136

Postexercise

|— 15 sec —|

Ø 400 wsec

Figure 136–3. An example of drug-induced sustained ventricular tachycardia (VT). Before receiving the drug, the patient had frequent ventricular premature beats (VPBs) and an occasional episode of nonsustained VT that were induced by exercise. After 6 days of flecainide (150 mg b.i.d.), arrhythmia on monitoring was markedly suppressed. However, during exercise, sustained VT with syncope occurred and required four attempts at defibrillation before sinus rhythm was restored.

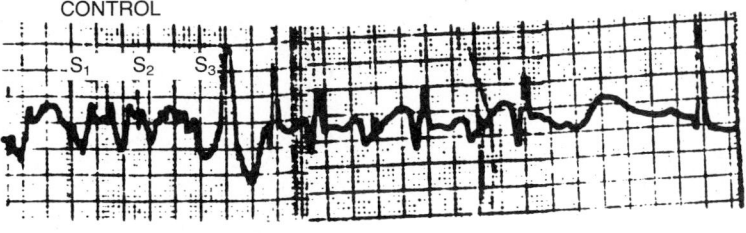

CONTROL

S₁   S₂   S₃

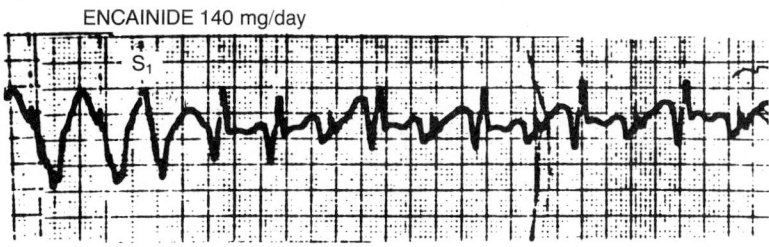

ENCAINIDE 140 mg/day

S₁

Figure 136–4. Aggravation of arrhythmia during electrophysiologic testing. During the initial study, three extrastimuli (S1, S2, S3) induced nonsustained ventricular tachycardia (VT). During therapy with encainide, one extrastimulus (S1) induced sustained VT.

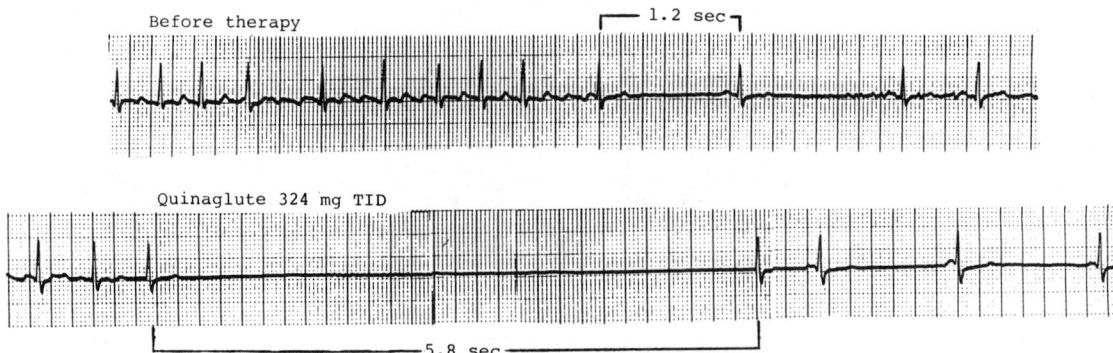

Figure 136–5. Sinus node dysfunction resulting from antiarrhythmic drug therapy. After spontaneous termination of paroxysmal atrial fibrillation (AF), sinus rhythm resumed after a 1.2-second pause. During therapy with quinidine gluconate, spontaneous termination of AF resulted in a 5.8-second pause, a result of sinus node depressions. The pause is ended by a junctional escape beat. Sinus node depression resolved after the drug was discontinued.

tion.[13] In general, correcting these abnormalities is effective therapy and will prevent further problems.

A major concern is whether the observed exacerbation of arrhythmia is truly a drug-related problem or only reflects spontaneous changes in the frequency of arrhythmia.[10] Although this question often can be resolved by rechallenging the patient, this approach is hazardous and not advisable. However, a drug can be implicated with reasonable certainty if aggravation involves a new arrhythmia or if there is a significant

change in the frequency of an existing arrhythmia that occurs in close temporal relationship to the initiation of drug therapy or a change in dose.[14]

Last, it should be remembered that any aggravation of arrhythmia may have different clinical implications. It may be a statistical but asymptomatic increase in VPBs, the clinical importance of which is uncertain; an increase in VPBs or repetitive forms that are symptomatic; or a sustained arrhythmia that results in a severe or life-threatening situation. While

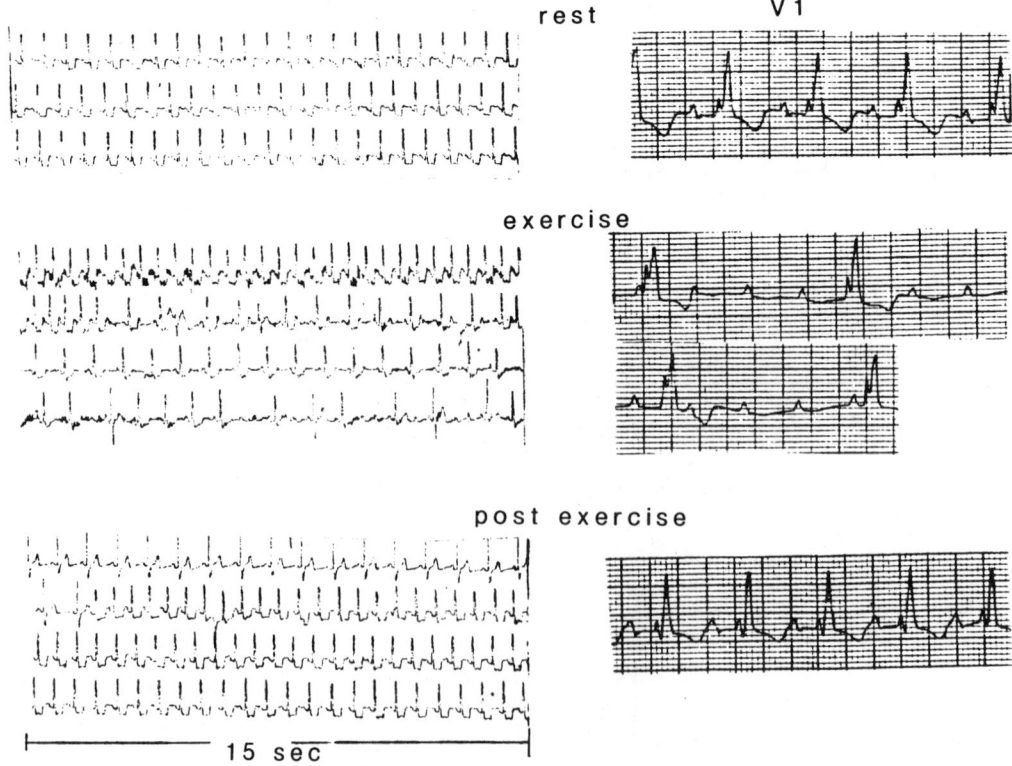

Figure 136–6. Example of AV nodal block caused by an antiarrhythmic drug. In baseline, the patient had a right bundle branch block and intact AV nodal conduction both at rest and during exercise. During treatment with an antiarrhythmic drug, an increase in sinus rate with exercise resulted in complete heart block. This is a result of the use-dependent effects of the drug on AV nodal conduction. As the sinus rate slowed in recovery, normal AV conduction was restored.

the clinical consequence of aggravation may vary, the recognition of this potentially serious complication remains most important.

BRADYARRHYTHMIA

While the most frequently described arrhythmia aggravation is ventricular, antiarrhythmic drugs can affect sinus and atrioventricular (AV) nodal function and result in serious or symptomatic bradyarrhythmias. Some of the antiarrhythmic drugs have a depressive effect on sinus node automaticity. While this is more commonly seen with the β-blockers, which block sympathetic inputs into the sinus node, or the calcium channel blockers, which have a direct effect on impulse formation, the membrane stabilizing antiarrhythmic agents may also impair sinus node automaticity (Fig. 136–5). Perhaps more commonly seen with antiarrhythmic drug therapy is depression of AV nodal function resulting in high grade (2-degree or 3-degree) AV block. The β-blockers and calcium channel blockers have frequently been implicated, but other antiarrhythmic drugs may also impair AV nodal conduction. While this effect may not be obvious in a resting state, it may become exposed at higher heart rates, such as during exercise testing (Fig. 136–6). This is because the membrane stabilizing drugs have a property of "use dependency," i.e., their depressive effect on impulse conduction becomes progressively more profound as the heart rate increases.[15] Hence, with a higher atrial rate, conduction through the AV node may be blocked. While not certain, it is possible that AV nodal block secondary to antiarrhythmic drugs is more common in patients with severe underlying heart disease.

SUPRAVENTRICULAR ARRHYTHMIAS

While not commonly appreciated, it is now well established that antiarrhythmic drugs may provoke or exacerbate supraventricular arrhythmias. This may occur in patients being treated for ventricular arrhythmias or those receiving drug therapy to treat a supraventricular tachyarrhythmia. While less frequently reported than aggravation of ventricular arrhythmia, several types have been observed (Table 136–3). One

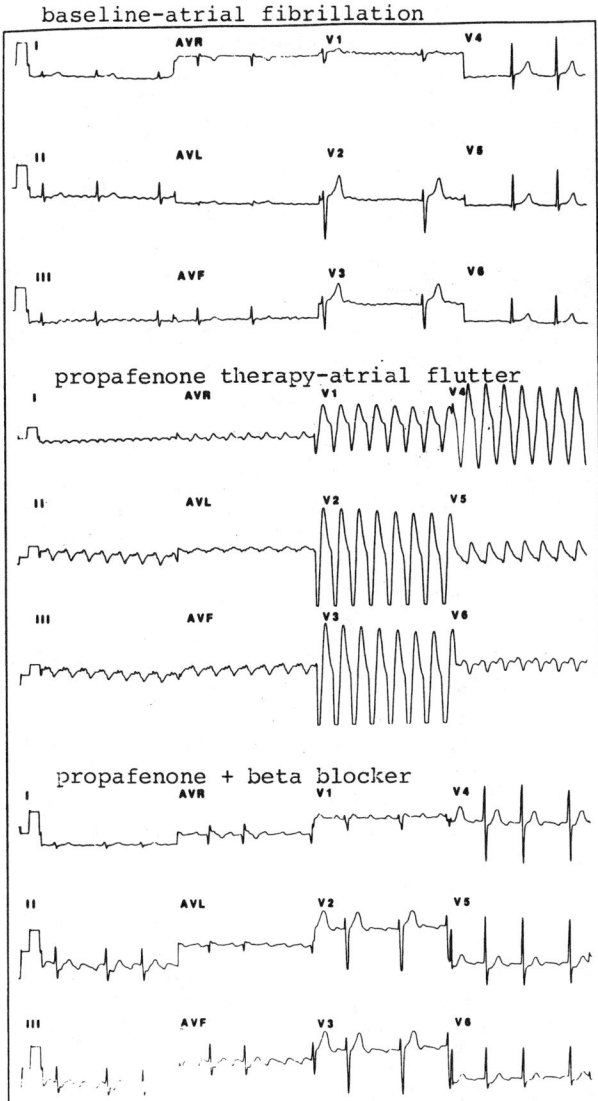

Figure 136–7. Aggravation of atrial arrhythmias during propafenone drug therapy given for reversion of atrial fibrillation. As a result of the drug, atrial fibrillation reverted to atrial flutter. Because of the slower atrial rate and a decrease in concealed AV nodal conduction, the ventricular rate increased. This was associated with a left bundle branch block due to the use-dependent effect of propafenone. The addition of a β-blocker slowed the ventricular response rate, normalized ventricular conduction, and exposed the atrial flutter. (From Murdock CJ, Kyles AE, Young-Lai-Wah JA, Vordeburgge S, Kerr CA: Atrial flutter in patients treated with propafenone. Am J Cardiol 66:755, 1990.)

Table 136–3. **Types of Proarrhythmia Involving Supraventricular Arrhythmia**

Atrial tachycardia with or without AV nodal block (as from digoxin)
Conversion of paroxysmal to sustained atrial fibrillation
Increased frequency of the supraventricular arrhythmia
Supraventricular tachyarrhythmia that becomes incessant
Acceleration of ventricular rate during a supraventricular tachyarrhythmia
    Slowing of atrial rate (for example, AF converted to atrial flutter or slowing of atrial flutter rate) decreasing concealed AV nodal conduction
    Preferential conduction down an accessory pathway

that has been well established is atrial tachycardia with or without AV nodal block that results from digoxin toxicity[16] Reported with the class IC antiarrhythmic drugs has been the conversion of atrial fibrillation to atrial flutter and an acceleration of the ventricular rate due to a decrease in concealed AV nodal conduction (Fig. 136–7).[17, 18] Not infrequently, the accelerated ventricular rate results in aberration of the QRS morphology (a result of the use-dependent effects of these drugs) and a misdiagnosis of VT.

Complicating the diagnosis of aggravation of supraventricular arrhythmia is the known variability and unpredictability of supraventricular tachyarrhythmia. Although similar to the concern with ventricular arrhythmias, the random variability of supraventricular arrhythmia has not been well studied and is largely unknown. Hence establishing this complication often becomes very difficult and may be overlooked, perhaps accounting for the infrequency with which the complication is reported.

INCIDENCE OF ARRHYTHMIA AGGRAVATION

In order to establish the overall frequency of arrhythmia aggravation and its incidence with individual drugs, a systematic approach to arrhythmia management is essential. There are two methods available for evaluating the effect of an antiarrhythmic drug. A noninvasive approach uses ambulatory monitoring and exercise testing, with drug efficacy based on the suppression of spontaneous arrhythmia.[19, 20] Invasive electrophysiology involves the induction of the clinical arrhythmia using programmed premature stimulation, and efficacy is defined as the inability to reinduce the arrhythmia.[20, 21] Despite the differences in these two approaches, the selection of a drug for long-term therapy requires establishment of the baseline level of arrhythmia, careful titration of drug dose, and careful evaluation of its effect on arrhythmia. Because there are no guidelines for predicting the response to a drug, it must be administered for a period of time, with efficacy evaluated invasively or noninvasively.

In a review of 1287 single-drug studies involving 400 patients performed using noninvasive methods for evaluation, aggravation of arrhythmia, as previously defined,[4] was observed in 117 studies, or 9% (see Table 136–3), and involved 34% of patients.[22] The incidence for individual drugs ranged from 5% to 19%. The type of aggravation that occurred was a fourfold increase in VPBs in 5% of studies, a 10-fold increase in repetitive form in 30% of studies, and sustained tachyarrhythmia that required intervention for termination in 65% of studies. When electrophysiologic testing is used to judge drug efficacy, the incidence of worsening of arrhythmia is higher. Invasive testing was employed in 52 patients who underwent 248 single-drug studies.[22] Aggravation of arrhythmia occurred in 45 studies, or 18%, ranging from 5% to 37% for individual agents. Tachyarrhythmia was more easily induced in 25%. VT at a faster rate was induced in 5%, while conversion from nonsustained VT to a sustained episode occurred in 70% of studies. Thus, the most frequent type of aggravation observed during invasive or noninvasive analysis was the most serious one (i.e., the provocation of sustained tachyarrhythmia).

Only a few other studies have reported arrhythmia aggravation with different antiarrhythmic agents. Rinkenberger et al.[23] reported aggravation of arrhythmia in 11 of 83 patients (13%) undergoing electrophysiologic testing. In this study, arrhythmia aggravation involved the conversion of nonsustained VT to sustained tachyarrhythmia. The drugs implicated included disopyramide, encainide, aprindine, amiodarone, and quinidine administered singly as well as in combination. However, the authors did not comment on the frequency of this complication with individual agents.

In an electrophysiologic study involving 121 patients who underwent 478 single-drug studies, Torres and associates[24] reported arrhythmia aggravation in 63 tests (12%) involving 43 patients (23%). The incidence of this complication ranged from 8% with procainamide and bepridil to 28% with ethmozine (Table 136–4). In a review of their overall experience with patients documented to have VT or VF who underwent electrophysiologic testing, Horowitz et al.[25] reported worsening of arrhythmia in 51 of 160 patients (32%) involving 68 of 432 single-drug and combination-drug trials (16%) (see Table 136–3). However, the incidence of this complication with most of the individual drugs used was not identified.

Rae and coworkers[26] reported on 314 patients who underwent 801 drug studies evaluated by electrophysiologic study. Overall, 122 patients (39%) experienced 193 episodes of proarrhythmia (24% of drug trials). The type of arrhythmia aggravation observed was conversion of nonsustained to sustained VT in 18% of studies, VT more difficult to terminate in 71%, VT more easily induced in 20%, and spontaneous VT or VF in 11%. Au et al.[27] reported on 24 patients without a history of VT who were treated with a class IA drug for suppression of VPBs. Electrophysiology studies were performed and arrhythmia aggravation occurred in 11% of studies involving 25% of patients. A study by Stanton et al.[28] involved 506 patients who underwent 1268 drug trials. Arrhythmia aggravation occurred in 6.9% of patients in 343 (3.4%) drug trials. The incidence with individual drugs varied from 0 to 12%. The most frequent type was incessant VT (23 of 43 events). Arrhythmia aggravation was most commonly seen among patients with sustained VT (10.3%), while only 6.8% of those with nonsustained ventricular tachycardia (NSVT) and 2.3% of patients with VF had this complication. Although only a few studies have reported the overall incidence of this complication, a number using individual drugs report worsening of arrhythmia and allow an estimate of the rate of occurrence.

Quinidine is most often implicated as the cause of arrhythmia aggravation. The first report was in 1921 by Kerr and Bender,[29] and since then, a number of reports of quinidine syncope have appeared.[5, 6, 30, 31] The majority of patients involved were receiving quinidine for therapy of atrial arrhythmia, and most were also receiving digitalis drugs. For example, in a review of 61 patients with quinidine syncope reported by Reynolds and VanderArk,[32] 59 were receiving digoxin. In contrast, Koster and Wellens[6] reported this complication in patients not receiving digitalis drugs. Arrhythmia aggravation has also occurred in patients receiving quinidine for treatment of VT. In each of the previous reports of arrhythmia aggravation resulting from quinidine therapy, the blood levels of quinidine were in the therapeutic range and occasionally they

Table 136–4. **Incidence of Arrhythmia Aggravation (%)**

Drug	Podrid et al.[20] (Noninvasive)	Stanton et al.[28] (Noninvasive)	Podrid et al.[20] (Invasive)	Horowitz et al.[25] (Invasive)	Rae et al.[26] (Invasive)	Torres et al.[24] (Invasive)
Amiodarone*	4*	4	—	—	30	—
Bepridil	—	—	—	—	—	8
Bethanidine	—	—	—	—	—	22
Cibenzoline	—	9	—	—	—	21
Disopyramide	6	1	5	—	—	—
Encainide	15	12	37	—	—	28
Ethmozine	11	10	14	—	33	15
Flecainide	12	4	—	—	37	—
Indecainide	19					16
Lidocaine	—	—	—	—	—	9
Lorcainide	8	—	24	—	—	—
Mexiletine	7	1	20	5	19	—
Procainamide	9	0	21	7	19	8
Propafenone	8	5	15	—	15	10
Quinidine	15	1	20	5	15	—
Tocainide	8	0	5	—	—	—
Verapamil	—	—	—	—	—	18
Overall	9	3†	18	16†	24†	13†

*Amiodarone data are from studies reported in literature.
†Data are incomplete, accounting for disparity of overall incidence as aggravation also occurred with combination therapy.

were subtherapeutic, but marked QT prolongation was present on the electrocardiogram. The type of drug-induced aggravation that presents with polymorphic VT and QT prolongation is termed torsade de pointes. This arrhythmic complication has also been reported with other antiarrhythmic drugs that prolong the QT interval (i.e., disopyramide[33, 34] and procainamide[35]). Although torsade de pointes is a recognized complication of these agents, it has been estimated to occur in only 1% to 2% of patients receiving quinidine. However, it may be more frequent in those who have underlying heart disease and in whom hypokalemia is present. Conceivably, drug-induced torsade de pointes or VF is a cause of out-of-hospital sudden death. Ruskin and coworkers[36] reported on six patients who experienced cardiac arrest during therapy with a type-1A drug, primarily quinidine. After drug withdrawal, electrophysiologic testing failed to induce any arrhythmia, while during therapy with the offending agent, sustained tachyarrhythmia was easily induced.

While torsade de pointes is the most commonly reported arrhythmic complication from quinidine therapy, other types do occur. Morganroth and Horowitz,[37] reviewing monitoring data in 360 patients with benign arrhythmia who received quinidine as part of outpatient comparative drug trials, reported six patients (2.1%) with a fourfold increase in VPBs and a 10-fold increase in repetitive forms. No serious arrhythmias were observed. In another review of 153 patients who had no history of serious ventricular arrhythmias, Morganroth et al.[38] reported a 2.6% incidence of aggravation with quinidine. The report of Velebit and associates[4] involved patients with a history of serious arrhythmias, and the incidence of aggravation resulting from quinidine was 15%.

Other antiarrhythmic drugs have been implicated in this complication. In an electrophysiologic study, Stavens et al.[39] reported that 3 of 15 patients (20%)

treated with propafenone developed incessant VT. In a review of the experience with flecainide in the United States, Morganroth and Horowitz[11] reported arrhythmia aggravation in 30 of 254 patients (12%) with a history of VT or VF who underwent electrophysiologic testing and in 4% of patients who underwent monitoring. Reid and coworkers[40] reported that 6 of 31 patients (19%) treated with flecainide developed incessant VT or VF that was more difficult to revert or that could not be terminated and resulted in death. Encainide aggravated arrhythmia in 11% of patients studied by Winkle et al.[41] and in 28% of patients reported by DiBianco et al.[42] There are also isolated reports of arrhythmia aggravation with other antiarrhythmic agents.

While the incidence of ventricular proarrhythmia in patients with a history of ventricular arrhythmia has been reported by a number of investigators, the incidence of proarrhythmia in patients receiving drug therapy for suppression of a supraventricular arrhythmia is unknown, but likely to be low as the majority of patients do not have significant heart disease. In reported series of patients with supraventricular tachyarrhythmia being treated with a class IC drug, the incidence of a new ventricular arrhythmia is low (<3%) and most often it is observed in those with underlying heart disease.[43, 44] However, Falk[45] reported that among 12 patients without heart disease being treated with flecainide for AF, three had VT or VF during exercise testing. The original reports of torsade de pointes involved quinidine therapy for prevention of AF[5, 29, 30] and certainly this is a well-established complication of the class IA and class III antiarrhythmic agents that can prolong the QT interval.[7, 46, 47] The occurrence of torsade de pointes is independent of the type of arrhythmia being treated, although it may be more common in patients with heart disease. The incidence of proarrhythmia as a result of a bradycardia or supraventricular tachyarrhythmia is also unknown and there have been only anecdotal reports of these complications.[17, 18, 48]

PREDICTORS OF RISK FOR AGGRAVATION

Although it is now well established that antiarrhythmic drugs can exacerbate arrhythmia, predicting patients at risk for this complication remains an important concern. Although QT prolongation may be a marker for the potential of torsade de pointes with quinidine, procainamide, disopyramide, and sotalol, QT prolongation is not generally observed with other agents. QT prolongation is frequently seen with amiodarone while torsade de pointes from this drug is rare. Moreover, in a number of studies, QT prolongation was not associated with other forms of arrhythmia aggravation.[4, 22] Additionally, QRS widening, which can occur during therapy with flecainide, encainide, and propafenone, is not a predictor of risk. Widening of electrocardiographic interval and aggravation of arrhythmia may occur when blood levels of these drugs exceed therapeutic values. However, aggravation has been reported to occur when blood levels were therapeutic and QRS widening was not present.[4, 14, 22] In the opinion of most investigators, this complication must therefore be considered an idiosyncratic reaction to antiarrhythmic drugs.

To establish whether there are any predictors for this complication, 51 patients who had arrhythmia aggravation with at least one of three drugs representing the three subclasses (quinidine, IA; mexiletine, IB; and encainide, IC) were compared with 102 patients who did not experience this complication with any agent tested, including the three study drugs.[22, 49] Variables examined include age, sex, type and extent of underlying heart disease, left ventricular ejection fraction (LVEF), presence of congestive heart failure, contraction abnormalities, baseline electrocardiographic intervals, electrocardiographic intervals during drug therapy, drug dose, blood level, density of arrhythmia during baseline studies, and nature of presenting arrhythmia. The only variables associated with the risk of drug-induced aggravation were the nature of the presenting arrhythmia and the presence of congestive heart failure due to left ventricular (LV) systolic dysfunction (Table 136–5). Patients with sustained VT or VF had a three- to fourfold greater risk of this complication than patients with only VPBs or nonsustained VT ($p = .01$). The average LV ejection fraction in patients with aggravation was 37%, compared with 43% in those without aggravation ($p = .08$). Patients with congestive heart failure and an LV ejection fraction less than 35% had a two- to threefold greater chance of arrhythmia aggravation compared with those with an LV ejection fraction greater than 35% ($p = .04$). Serum blood level, average drug dose, and electrocardiographic intervals were not helpful in predicting patients at risk.

The lack of association between aggravation and electrocardiographic intervals was also observed by Zipes[14] and Horowitz et al.[25] Likewise, the baseline

Table 136–5. **Predictors of Drug-Induced Aggravation**

Parameter	p
Age	NS
Sex	NS
Type of heart disease	NS
Presenting arrhythmia*	.01
Cardiomegaly	NS
History of CHF	NS
Diuretic use	NS
Ejection fraction	.08
EF <35%; vs. EF >35%	.04
Angina pectoris	NS
Anterior MI	NS
LV aneurysm	NS
Exercise duration	NS
Maximum ST depression	NS
Number of diseased vessels	NS
Baseline QRS, PR, QT intervals	NS
Interval changes on drug	NS
Density of baseline arrhythmia	NS
Daily dose of drug	NS
Drug serum level	NS

*Patients with ventricular premature beats or nonsustained ventricular tachycardia versus those with sustained ventricular tachycardia or fibrillation.

Data from Slater W, Lampert S, Podrid PJ, et al: Clinical predictors of arrhythmia worsening by antiarrhythmic drugs. Am J Cardiol 61:349, 1988.

density of VPBs, couplets, and runs of VT were of no value for prediction.[22, 49] Aggravation with one drug did not predict aggravation with any other antiarrhythmic drug, including those of the same class. Of 25 patients who had arrhythmia aggravation with quinidine, only four patients experienced aggravation while being treated with either procainamide or disopyramide. Thirteen patients with aggravation of arrhythmia due to mexiletine also received tocainide, and only three had experienced worsening arrhythmia with this drug. Of the 22 patients who had aggravated arrhythmia with encainide, 16 also had received flecainide, but only four had aggravation of arrhythmia with this drug. Last, more than one third of the episodes of aggravation were induced during exercise testing at a time when monitoring demonstrated complete suppression of arrhythmia. Therefore, exercise testing is an important tool for exposing this reaction (see Fig. 136–3).

The association between the type of presenting arrhythmia and the risk of aggravation has been observed by others. In the study by Winkle et al.[41] involving encainide, 10% of 90 patients with a history of a sustained VT or VF had aggravation, in contrast to only 1 of 47 patients (2%) being treated for VPBs. In the report by DiBianco et al.,[42] encainide caused aggravation in 28% of those with sustained VT or VF, compared with 15% in those with VPBs. A similar association was reported by Morganroth,[50] who reviewed the data on 245 patients involved in trials with encainide. The incidence of aggravation was 8% in those with VPBs or nonsustained VT and 11% in those with sustained arrhythmias. If only serious arrhythmic complications such as sustained VT, VF, or torsade de pointes were considered, the incidence fell to 4.2% and 8.5%, respectively. Aggravation occurred in 10% of patients with structural heart disease, compared with 3% in those without heart disease.

A similar relationship was observed during flecainide therapy.[11] Of 334 patients with VPBs or nonsustained VT, aggravation occurred in 4%, in contrast to a 12% incidence among the 254 patients who underwent electrophysiologic testing because of a history of sustained tachyarrhythmia. In an update of this experience involving 1330 patients, Morganroth[50] reported an overall worsening of arrhythmia in 3% of patients being treated for VPBs or nonsustained VT, compared with 16% in those with a sustained tachyarrhythmia. However, serious events were observed in only 0.4% and 7%, respectively. The incidence was 3% in those with structural heart disease and 0.4% in those without cardiac pathologic conditions. No association between LV function and aggravation was reported in either study by Morganroth. In the review of outpatient therapy with quinidine for therapy of benign VPBs, arrhythmic aggravation was observed in only 2%,[37] whereas in patients with serious arrhythmia, the reported incidence is 5% to 20% (see Table 136–4).

An association between congestive heart failure, LV dysfunction, and proarrhythmia has been less frequently reported.[22, 49] Pratt et al.[51] retrospectively reviewed data in 246 patients with complex ventricular arrhythmia receiving antiarrhythmic drug therapy. The incidence of cardiac toxicity, which included proarrhythmic as well as congestive heart failure, was 15% in patients with a LVEF of less than 30% and 2.1% in those with a LVEF of more than 30% ($p = .0005$). Moreover, life-threatening cardiac toxicity was seven times more frequent in those with NSVT and LVEF less than 30% compared with patients with NSVT and LVEF more than 30% (18% versus 2.3%, $p = .003$). While arrhythmia aggravation is more common in patients with a history of VT or VF who have congestive heart failure due to systolic dysfunction, the results of the Cardiac Arrhythmia Suppression Trial (CAST)[52] suggest that there are other factors that are associated with an increased risk. This study involved patients with a recent myocardial infarction who did not have a history of sustained VT or VF and did not have congestive heart failure and significant LV dysfunction. Sudden death was increased three- to fourfold in patients receiving encainide or flecainide when compared with those on a placebo. The mechanism for sudden death was presumed to be arrhythmia aggravation. An additional concern was that sudden death or proarrhythmia from the drug was observed throughout the trial and was not only an early event, i.e., occurring within the first few days of instituting antiarrhythmic drug therapy. This is in contrast to previous reports involving serious arrhythmia in whom arrhythmia aggravation was observed within a few days of starting therapy.[4, 53]

The results of CAST suggest that there are other factors responsible for proarrhythmia. Most important is the presence of ischemia, which may be overt or silent. The occurrence of ischemia and the associated metabolic and electrophysiologic changes can interact with antiarrhythmic drugs, altering their actions and perhaps potentiating proarrhythmia (Fig. 136–8).[54]

ETIOLOGY OF ARRHYTHMIA AGGRAVATION

The mechanism for aggravation of arrhythmia is unknown. The greater frequency of occurrence in patients with a history of serious arrhythmia who have LV dysfunction suggests that it results from interaction between structural disease of the myocardium, underlying electrical instability, and the expected pharmacologic and electrophysiologic actions of antiarrhythmic drugs. However, this does not explain why one drug may cause this complication while a drug with the same electrophysiologic properties is well tolerated and may even suppress arrhythmia. The frequent provocation of this complication during exercise testing suggests that in some situations other variable factors such as ischemia, metabolic changes, and catecholamines play a role in providing a trigger for arrhythmia (see Fig. 136–8). In the presence of an electrically "unstable" myocardium, the very properties of the drug that are associated with its antiar-

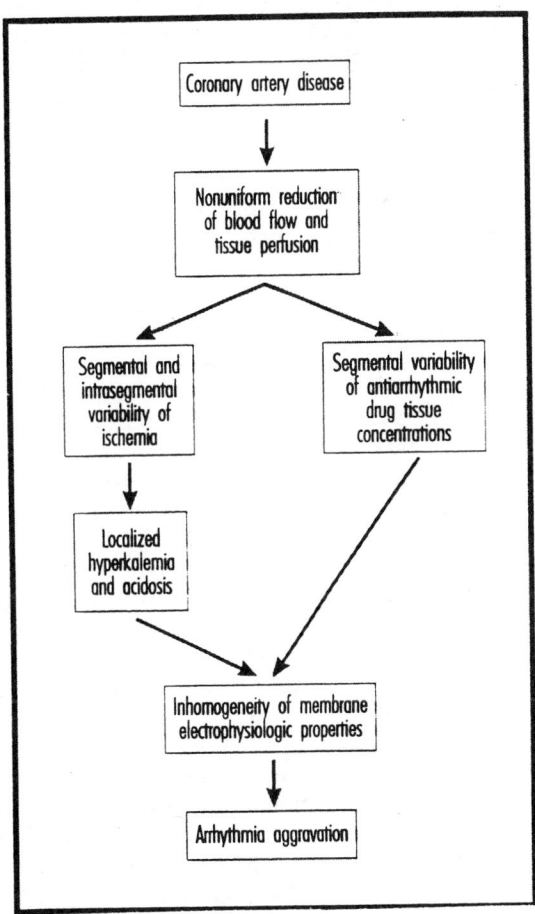

Figure 136–8. Proposed mechanism for the interaction between antiarrhythmic drugs and ischemia that may result in arrhythmia aggravation.

rhythmic effects may, in a vulnerable patient, alter the substrate unpredictably and enhance arrhythmogenesis. The important electrophysiologic effects produced by these drugs include alteration of myocardial conductivity and refractoriness, and it is possible that a change in either or both of these variables can result in an exacerbation of reentry and hence arrhythmia.

Antiarrhythmic drug action is different in normal and diseased myocardium, and therefore these agents alone, or in concert with other factors, may enhance the underlying inhomogeneity and the ability of the myocardium to generate and sustain arrhythmia. Moreover, in a diseased heart, there is marked variation in the blood flow to different regions of the myocardium, which results in differences in tissue and receptor concentration of drug. Such differences may be further augmented by a variability in tissue binding between normal and abnormal tissue. Since the degree of electrophysiologic changes and antiarrhythmic effect are related to tissue concentration, these inequalities may also exacerbate arrhythmia.

Also, other important factors, such as electrolyte fluxes, ischemia, pH changes, circulating catecholamines, and changes in autonomic tone may negate or enhance antiarrhythmic drug action or, by acting in concert with the underlying properties of the myocardium, exacerbate underlying inhomogeneity.

It is well established that antiarrhythmic drugs work by reducing membrane conductivity, excitability, and automaticity. In contrast, catecholamines enhance membrane conductivity, excitability, and automaticity. Thus, they can negate the electrophysiologic effects of these drugs.[55, 56] In some cases the changes in drug action that result from catecholamines may actually enhance the potential for proarrhythmia.

Sympathetic stimulation and catecholamines, in addition to many other factors, can produce myocardial ischemia in patients with heart disease. As a result of ischemia, there is an increase in extracellular potassium levels and the development of acidosis or a reduced pH.[57, 58] These metabolic alterations are heterogeneous because ischemia is nonuniform. These changes can modify the action of antiarrhythmic drugs, often intensifying their membrane effects.[59] Such changes are heterogeneous and foster the potential for arrhythmia aggravation (see Fig. 136–8).

In conclusion, aggravation of arrhythmia by antiarrhythmic drugs is a potentially serious and frequent complication common to all antiarrhythmic agents. Although the criteria for aggravation are uncertain, the possibility of this complication must be borne in mind when using these drugs. The incidence of arrhythmia worsening depends on the patient population studied and the definition of aggravation used. Although this complication is more common in patients with a history of serious arrhythmias who have LV dysfunction and in the presence of ischemia, its occurrence is unpredictable, and there are no helpful factors or variables that will identify a patient at risk. Cautious use of all antiarrhythmic drugs is therefore essential.

REFERENCES

1. Podrid PJ: Antiarrhythmic drug therapy: Benefits and hazards. Chest 88:618, 1985.
2. Ruberman W, Weinblatt T, Goldberg JD, et al: Ventricular premature beats and mortality after myocardial infarction. N Engl J Med 297:750, 1977.
3. Bigger JT, Weld F, Ronitzky LM: Prevalence, characteristics, and significance of ventricular tachycardia detected with ambulatory ECG recording in the late hospital phase of acute myocardial infarction. Am J Cardiol 48:815, 1981.
4. Velebit V, Podrid PJ, Lown B, et al: Aggravation and provocation of ventricular arrhythmias by antiarrhythmic drugs. Circulation 65:886, 1982.
5. Seltzer A, Wray HW: Quinidine syncope and paroxysmal ventricular fibrillation occurring during treatment of chronic atrial arrhythmias. Circulation 30:17, 1964.
6. Koster RW, Wellens HJJ: Quinidine-induced ventricular flutter and fibrillation without digitalis therapy. Am J Cardiol 38:519, 1976.
7. Keren A, Tzivoni D, Gavish D, et al: Etiology, warning signs and therapy of torsade de pointes. Circulation 64:1167, 1981.
8. Poser RF, Podrid PJ, Lombardi F, et al: Aggravation of arrhythmias induced with antiarrhythmic drugs during electrophysiologic testing. Am Heart J 110:4, 1985.
9. Winkle RA: Spontaneous variability of ventricular ectopics frequently mimics antiarrhythmic drug effect. Circulation 57:1116, 1978.
10. Morganroth J, Michelson EL, Horowitz LN, et al: Limitations of routine long-term electrocardiographic monitoring to assess ventricular ectopic frequency. Circulation 58:408, 1978.
11. Morganroth J, Horowitz LN: Flecainide—its proarrhythmic effect and expected changes in the surface electrocardiogram. Am J Cardiol 53:893, 1984.
12. Bigger JT, Jahar DI: Clinical types of proarrhythmic response to antiarrhythmic drugs. Am J Cardiol 59:2E, 1987.
13. Woosley RL, Roden DM: Pharmacologic causes of arrhythmogenic actions of antiarrhythmic drugs. Am J Cardiol 59:14E, 1987.
14. Zipes DP: Proarrhythmic effects of antiarrhythmic drugs. Am J Cardiol 59:26E, 1987.
15. Ranger S, Talajic M, Lemery R, et al: Amplification of flecainide-induced ventricular conduction during flecainide therapy. Circulation 79:1000, 1989.
16. Fisch C, Knoebel SB: Digitalis cardiotoxicity. J Am Coll Cardiol 5:91A, 1985.
17. Murdock CJ, Kyles AE, Young-Lai-Wah JA, et al: Atrial flutter in patients treated with propafenone. Am J Cardiol 66:755, 1990.
18. Feld GK, Chen PS, Nicod P, et al: Possible atrial proarrhythmia effects of class 1C antiarrhythmic agents. Am J Cardiol 60:378, 1990.
19. Graboys TB, Lown B, Podrid PJ, et al: Long-term survival of patients with malignant ventricular arrhythmia treated with antiarrhythmic drugs. Am J Cardiol 50:437, 1982.
20. Podrid PJ: Treatment of ventricular arrhythmia: Noninvasive versus invasive approach—applications and limitations. Chest 88:121, 1985.
21. Ruskin JN, DiMarco J, Garan N: Out-of-hospital cardiac arrest: Electrophysiologic observation and selection of long-term antiarrhythmic therapy. N Engl J Med 303:607, 1980.
22. Podrid PJ, Lampert J, Graboys TB, et al: Aggravation of arrhythmia by antiarrhythmic drugs—incidence and predictors. Am J Cardiol 59:38E, 1987.
23. Rinkenberger RL, Prystowsky EN, Jackman WN, et al: Drug conversion of nonsustained ventricular tachycardia to sustained ventricular tachycardia during serial electrophysiologic studies; identification of drugs that exacerbate tachycardia and potential mechanisms. Am Heart J 103:177, 1982.
24. Torres V, Flowers D, Somberg JC: The arrhythmogenicity of antiarrhythmic agents. Am Heart J 104:1040, 1985.
25. Horowitz LN, Greenspan AM, Rae AP, et al: Proarrhythmic responses during electrophysiologic testing. Am J Cardiol 59:45E, 1987.
26. Rae AP, Kay HR, Horowitz LN, et al: Proarrhythmia effects of antiarrhythmic drugs in patients with malignant ventricular

arrhythmia evaluated by electrophysiologic testing. J Am Coll Cardiol 12:131, 1988.

27. Au PK, Bhandari AE, Bream R, et al: Proarrhythmic effects of antiarrhythmic drugs during programmed ventricular stimulation in patients without ventricular tachycardia. J Am Coll Cardiol 9:389, 1987.

28. Stanton MS, Prystowsky EN, Fineberg NS, et al: Arrhythmogenic effects of antiarrhythmic drugs: A study of 506 patients treated for ventricular tachycardia or fibrillation. J Am Coll Cardiol 14:209, 1989.

29. Kerr WJ, Bender WL: Paroxysmal ventricular fibrillation with cardiac recovery in a case of auricular fibrillation and complete heart block while under quinidine sulfate therapy. Heart 9:269, 1921.

30. Rokseth R, Storstein O: Quinidine therapy of chronic auricular fibrillation. Occurrence and mechanism of syncope. Arch Intern Med 111:102, 1963.

31. Davies P, Leak D, Oran J: Quinidine-induced syncope. Br Med J 2:517, 1965.

32. Reynolds EW, VanderArk LR: Quinidine syncope and the delayed repolarization syndromes. Mod Concepts Cardiovasc Dis 54:117, 1976.

33. Frieden J: Quinidine effects due to disopyramide. N Engl J Med 298:97J, 1978.

34. Meltzer RS, Robert EW, McMorrow M, et al: Atypical ventricular tachycardia as a manifestation of disopyramide toxicity. Am J Cardiol 42:1044, 1978.

35. Castellanos A, Salhanick L: Electrocardiographic patterns of procainamide cardiotoxicity. Am J Med Sci 253:52, 1967.

36. Ruskin JN, McGovern B, Gavan H, et al: Antiarrhythmic drugs: A possible cause of out-of-hospital cardiac arrest. N Engl J Med 309:1302, 1983.

37. Morganroth J, Horowitz LN: Incidence of proarrhythmic effects from quinidine in the outpatient treatment of benign or potentially lethal ventricular arrhythmias. Am J Cardiol 56:585, 1985.

38. Morganroth J, Somberg JC, Pool PE, et al, for the Encainide-Quinidine Research Group: Comparative study of encainide and quinidine in the treatment of ventricular arrhythmia. J Am Coll Cardiol 7:9, 1986.

39. Stavens CS, McGovern B, Garan H, et al: Aggravation of electrically provoked ventricular tachycardia during treatment with propafenone. Am Heart J 110:24, 1985.

40. Reid PR, Griffith LSC, Platia EV, et al: Evaluation of flecainide acetate in the management of patients at high risk of sudden cardiac death. Am J Cardiol 53:108B, 1984.

41. Winkle RA, Mason JW, Griffin JC, et al: Malignant ventricular tachycardia associated with the use of encainide. Am Heart J 102:857, 1981.

42. DiBianco R, Fletcher RD, Cohen AZ, et al: Treatment of frequent ventricular arrhythmia with encainide. Assessment using serial ambulatory electrocardiograms, intracardiac electrophysiologic studies, treadmill exercise tests, and radionuclide cineangiographic studies. Circulation 105:1134, 1982.

43. Berns E, Rinkenberger RL, Jeany M, et al: Clinical efficacy and safety of flecainide acetate in the treatment of primary atrial tachycardias. Am J Cardiol 59:1337, 1987.

44. Pritchett ELC, Wikinson WE: Mortality in patients treated with flecainide and encainide for supraventricular arrhythmias. Am J Cardiol 67:976, 1991.

45. Falk RH: Flecainide-induced ventricular tachycardia and fibrillation in patients treated for atrial fibrillation. Ann Intern Med 111:107, 1989.

46. Kuck KH, Kunze KP, Bleifeld W: Sotalol-induced torsade de pointes. Am Heart J 109:174, 1984.

47. Jackman WM, Friday KJ, Anderson JL, Aliot EM: The long QT syndromes: A critical review of new clinical observations unifying hypothesis. Prog Cardiovasc Dis 31:15, 1988.

48. Marcus FI: The hazards of using type 1C antiarrhythmic drugs for the treatment of paroxysmal atrial fibrillation. Am J Cardiol 66:366, 1990.

49. Slater W, Lampert S, Podrid PJ, et al: Clinical predictors of arrhythmia worsening by antiarrhythmic drugs. Am J Cardiol 61:349, 1988.

50. Morganroth J: Risk factors for the development of proarrhythmic events. Am J Cardiol 59:132E, 1987.

51. Pratt CM, Eaton T, Frances M, et al: The inverse relationship between baseline left ventricular ejection fraction and outcome of antiarrhythmic drug therapy: A dangerous imbalance in the risk-benefit ratio. Am Heart J 118:433, 1989.

52. CAST Investigators: Preliminary report: Effect of encainide and flecainide on mortality in a randomized trial of arrhythmia suppression after myocardial infarction. N Engl J Med 321:406, 1989.

53. Minardo JD, Heger JJ, Miles WM, et al: Clinical characteristics of patients with ventricular fibrillation during antiarrhythmic drug therapy. N Engl J Med 319:257, 1988.

54. Podrid PJ, Fogel RI: Aggravation of arrhythmia by antiarrhythmic drugs, and the important role of underlying ischemia. Am J Cardiol 70:100, 1992.

55. Jazayeri MR, Wyhe G, Avitall B, et al: Isoproterenol reversal of antiarrhythmic effects in patients with inducible sustained ventricular tachyarrhythmias. J Am Coll Cardiol 14:705, 1989.

56. Morady F, Kou WH, Kadish AH, et al: Antagonism of flecainide electrophysiologic effect by epinephrine in patients with ventricular tachycardia. J Am Coll Cardiol 12:388, 1988.

57. Kagiyama Y, Hill JL, Gettes LS: Interaction of acidosis and increased extracellular potassium on action potential characteristics and conduction in guinea pig ventricular muscle. Circ Res 51:614, 1982.

58. Watanabe I, Johnson TA, Buchanan J, et al: Effect of graded coronary flow reduction on ionic, electrical and mechanical indices of ischemia in the pig. Circulation 76:1127, 1987.

59. Nattel S, Pederson DH, Zipes DP: Alternations in regional myocardial distribution and arrhythmogenic effects of aprindine produced by coronary artery occlusion in the dog. Cardiovasc Res 15:80, 1981.

B. Specific Antiarrhythmic Drugs

CHAPTER 137

Intravenous Adenosine as an Antiarrhythmic Agent

Clifford J. Garratt, D.M., and A. John Camm, M.D., F.R.C.P., F.A.C.C.

Adenosine is an endogenous nucleoside that is capable of causing transient atrioventricular (AV) nodal conduction block in humans.[1] It is this property that has stimulated its use for the diagnosis and treatment of cardiac arrhythmias. It was introduced for widespread clinical use in 1990, and at that time it was predicted that the agent would revolutionize the approach to acute management of broad-complex tachycardia.[2] In the space of 5 years, use of the agent has expanded dramatically and in many centers has become the first-line therapy for both narrow-complex and wide-complex tachycardia. The aim of this review is to examine the basis for the use of adenosine in these clinical situations and to provide an update on the effects of the agent on the spectrum of cardiac arrhythmias.

FORMATION, METABOLISM, AND FUNCTION OF ENDOGENOUS ADENOSINE

Adenosine is present in all cells of the body and is formed as a product of the enzymatic breakdown of adenosine triphosphate (ATP) via adenosine monophosphate (AMP) and S-adenosylhomocysteine via at least three enzymatic pathways, the relative importance of which depends upon the degree of tissue oxygenation. In the presence of hypoxia, adenosine production by cardiac myocytes is increased, the major route of adenosine production being the hydrolysis of AMP by 5-nucleotidases located in the cytosol and on the cell membrane.[3] It has been suggested that this increased production in response to hypoxia is a homeostatic response, adenosine acting as an antihypoxic substance[4, 5] by virtue of its vasodilatory and antiadrenergic[6, 7] properties. If endogenous adenosine does indeed have such a homeostatic role, it is likely to be almost exclusively at a local level, since the substance has a half-life in plasma of 0.6 to 1.5 seconds[8] because of deamination to inosine and uptake by red cells. The extent to which endogenous adenosine has a role in maintaining heart rate and conduction properties of normal or diseased hearts is unknown at present. Certainly, augmentation of endogenous adenosine levels by inhibition of breakdown (using dipyridamole) has detectable effects on AV nodal conduction,[9] although this of course does not prove a role for adenosine in "normal" concentrations. An overproduction of or hypersensitivity to adenosine in atrial tissue is an attractive potential mechanism of sick sinus syndrome,[10] and indeed there is some evidence of benefit in this syndrome with methylxanthine therapy (see later).

MECHANISM OF ACTION OF ADENOSINE

The cellular electrophysiologic effects of adenosine are competitively and reversibly antagonized by methylxanthines (but not by atropine) and are thought to be mediated by the specific A1 adenosine receptor. Stimulation of the A1 receptor on the cell surface is thought to influence (1) adenosine sensitive potassium channels, and (2) cyclic AMP (cAMP) production by means of an inhibitory guanine nucleotide-binding protein (Gi).[11]

Adenosine stimulates a specific time-independent outward potassium current in the sinus node, atrium, and AV node that appears to be identical to that stimulated by acetylcholine.[12, 13] The effect of this stimulation is to cause hyperpolarization of atrial myocytes, a decrease in atrial action potential duration,[14] and a decrease in the diastolic depolarization (phase 4) of the pacemaker cells of the sinus and AV nodes[15, 16] (Fig. 137–1). Although the agent does not produce depression of the upstroke (phase 0) of the action potential of sinus node cells, the upstroke of the action potential of the AV nodal "N" cells is depressed and may provide the basis for its AV nodal blocking action.[17] The ionic mechanism for this latter effect is not known.[18]

Adenosine-sensitive potassium channels are absent in ventricular myocytes and, in the absence of catecholamine stimulation, the agent has no effect on the ventricular action potential.[19] Ventricular myocardium is sensitive to adenosine, however, in the presence of catecholamines: adenosine inhibits catecholamine-induced inward calcium current, possibly via inhibition of cAMP production.[20]

CLINICAL EFFECTS OF INTRAVENOUS ADENOSINE
Intravenous Bolus Dose

DiMarco et al.[21] systematically evaluated the clinical electrophysiologic effects of adenosine in 15 patients in sinus rhythm who were undergoing diagnostic electrophysiologic study. The intravenous agent (mean dose, 179 μg/kg in 2 to 3 seconds via a peripheral vein) produced an initial sinus bradycardia lasting less than 10 seconds, which was followed by sinus tachycardia. The initial sinus bradycardia was accompanied by progressive AH prolongation and atrioventricular block, the HV interval remaining unaffected. Neither of these initial effects was influenced by the prior administration of atropine. More recent studies have shown that the effect of adenosine on the sinus and AV nodes is increased in duration and severity by dipyridamole[22] (a nucleoside-transport blocker) and abolished by aminophylline, suggesting that these effects are mediated by adenosine receptors. It is of interest that, in the presence of autonomic dysfunction, bolus adenosine causes sinus bradycardia but not the delayed sinus tachycardia,[23] suggesting that this is an autonomically mediated phenomenon. Sympathetic stimulation is the most likely mechanism, because it has been demonstrated that adenosine-induced sinus tachycardia is associated with an increase in plasma catecholamines and sympathetic nerve traffic.[24]

An intravenous bolus of adenosine causes a biphasic blood pressure response, with an initial increase in both systolic and diastolic blood pressure (simultaneous with AV conduction delay) followed by a decrease at the time of the secondary tachycardia.[23] Bolus doses are associated with dose-related symptoms of dyspnea, flushing, and chest discomfort or pain (starting at the time of AV conduction delay[25]). In general, the symptoms associated with bolus doses of adenosine are well tolerated by patients with arrhythmias, but less well by normal subjects. All effects are short-lived, lasting 15 to 20 seconds.

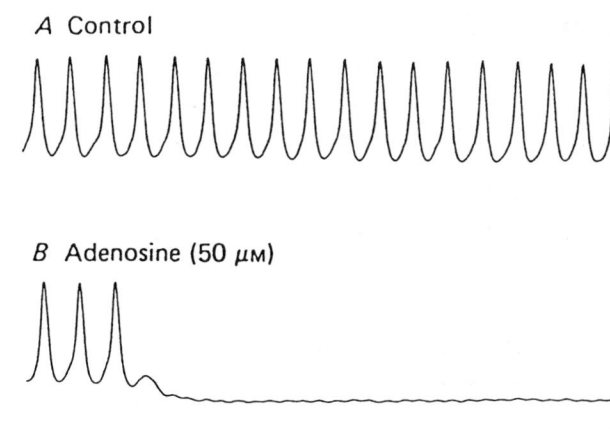

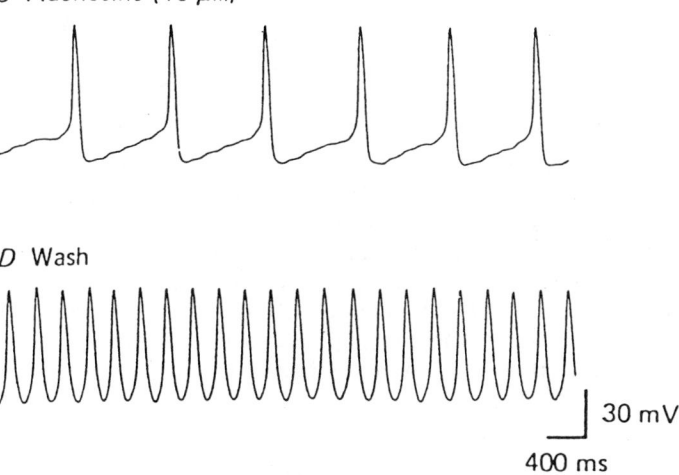

Figure 137–1. The effect of adenosine on pacemaker cells of the sinus node of a rabbit. (From Belardinelli L, Giles UR, West A: Ionic mechanisms of adenosine actions in pacemaker cells from rabbit hearts. J Physiol 405:615, 1988.)

Intravenous Infusion

Administration of adenosine as a continuous intravenous infusion results in a dose-dependent sinus tachycardia, AV nodal conduction being unaffected. Presumably this difference is related to a lower local concentration of adenosine at the AV node using the continuous infusion. As a consequence, adenosine is ineffective in the management of arrhythmias involving the AV node when given as a continuous infusion.

EFFECT OF ADENOSINE ON CARDIAC ARRHYTHMIAS
Atrial Fibrillation

Atrial fibrillation is not terminated by adenosine, but ventricular rate is transiently slowed because of the AV nodal blocking action of the drug. Studies of atrial activation frequency during atrial fibrillation have shown a marked increase in frequency after administration of adenosine, particularly in the right atrium.[26] This increase in frequency is spatially and temporally inhomogeneous and is likely to favor continuation of atrial fibrillation rather than termination.

Atrial Flutter and Intra-atrial Reentrant Tachycardia

Atrial flutter and intra-atrial reentrant tachycardia are caused by abnormal reentrant circuits within atrial myocardium. In nearly all cases the atrium is structurally abnormal, either as a result of ischemic heart disease or as a consequence of valvular or pulmonary vascular disease. The reentrant circuits do not involve adenosine-sensitive tissue and these arrhythmias are not adenosine-sensitive[27] (Fig. 137–2). Ventricular rate may transiently be slowed because of AV nodal block, but the tachycardia will continue unabated. In some cases ventricular rate may actually increase as a result of the secondary sympathetic activation associated with bolus doses of adenosine[28] (see later). Only occasionally will adenosine terminate atrial flutter, and then only following conversion of the flutter to fibrillation.

Sinoatrial Reentrant Tachycardia

Sinoatrial reentrant tachycardia is a relatively unusual cause of sustained, symptomatic arrhythmia and is thought to result from an abnormal reentrant circuit involving the sinus node, the perinodal atrial myocar-

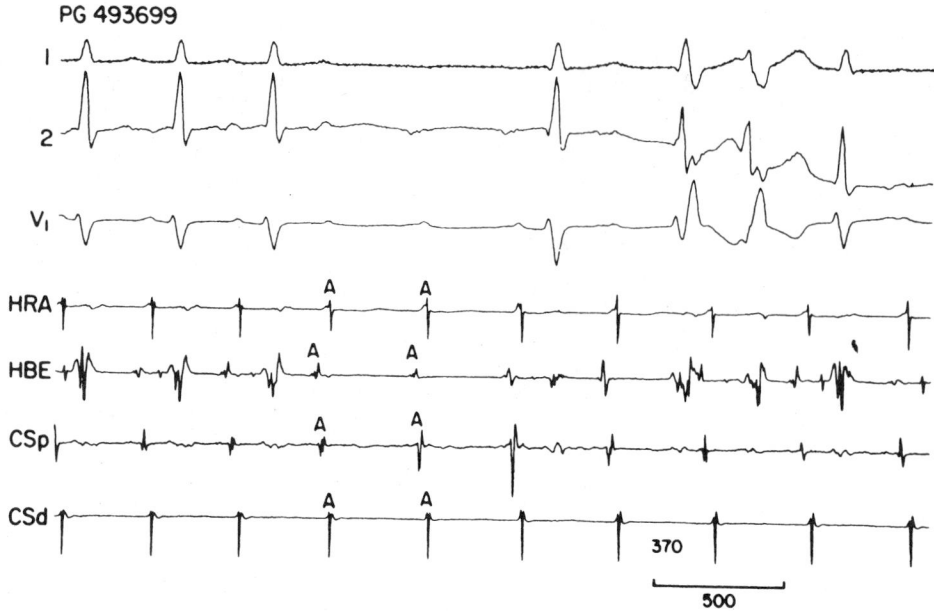

Figure 137–2. Effect of adenosine on intra-atrial reentrant tachycardia. The tachycardia is not terminated but transient AV block occurs. (From Wathen MS, Klein GJ, Yee R, Natale A: Classification and terminology of supraventricular tachycardia. Cardiol Clin 11:109, 1993.)

dium, or both. This arrhythmia is terminated by vagal maneuvers and also by adenosine,[29] usually with doses less than those required to terminate junctional tachycardias. This response to adenosine is, of course, compatible with the known effect of the agent on sinus node tissue and can distinguish these arrhythmias from other intra-atrial reentrant tachycardias described earlier.

Automatic Atrial Tachycardia

Automatic atrial tachycardia, a relatively uncommon arrhythmia, differs from intra-atrial reentrant tachycardia in that it is usually incessant and is not terminated by atrial premature beats. It is thought to have an automatic rather than reentrant mechanism and is adenosine- and ATP-sensitive.[30]

Nonpreexcited Junctional Tachycardias (Atrioventricular Nodal Reentrant Tachycardia and Atrioventricular Reentrant Tachycardia)

Non-preexcited junctional tachycardias form the great majority of narrow-complex regular tachycardias that come to medical attention and are often referred to by the more collective title of paroxysmal supraventricular tachycardia. Antegrade conduction (atrium-to-ventricle) occurs via the AV node, and retrograde conduction occurs either via an accessory connection (atrioventricular reentrant tachycardia, associated with the Wolff-Parkinson-White syndrome) or by a separate "fast pathway" within the AV node (atrioventricular nodal reentrant tachycardia). Adenosine is very effective in terminating both of these forms of arrhythmia by blocking antegrade conduction via the AV node[31–33] (Fig. 137–3). The efficacy of sequential doses of adenosine in terminating paroxysmal supraventricular tachycardia has been assessed in a pla-

cebo-controlled, multicenter trial of 163 patients.[34] The effects of sequential doses of 3, 6, 9, and 12 mg of adenosine administered through a peripheral vein were compared with those of corresponding volumes of normal saline. The cumulative success rates were 35%, 62%, 80%, and 91%, respectively. The final cumulative response to the placebo was 16%. The minimal effective dose varies between patients and also depends on the route of administration, the mean effective dose being significantly lower when administered via a central vein.

Before the introduction of adenosine into widespread clinical use, intravenous verapamil was the most widely used agent for terminating nonpreexcited junctional tachycardias. Direct comparisons of the two agents have found little difference in terms of efficacy or significant side effects,[32, 34] and in patients with no contraindications to adenosine or verapamil, there is little to choose between the drugs. Contraindications to the use of verapamil include a history suggestive of ventricular dysfunction, concomitant treatment with β-blocking agents, or very young age. Adenosine should be used with caution in patients suspected of having reversible airways obstruction and avoided in those with a clear diagnosis of asthma.[35, 36] The longer half-life of verapamil may be advantageous if tachycardia recurs shortly after it has been terminated with adenosine.

Preexcited Junctional Tachycardias

Preexcited junctional tachycardias can be defined as reentrant arrhythmias that involve accessory connections conducting in an antegrade direction (atrium-to-ventricle) and the AV node or occasionally other accessory connections conducting in a retrograde (ventricle-to-atrium) direction (antidromic tachycardia). They form the minority of arrhythmias occurring in patients with the Wolff-Parkinson-White syndrome, but are particularly important because of their association with an increased risk of multiple accessory pathways and sudden death. Accessory pathways that form the antegrade limb of these tachycardias are more likely than other accessory pathways to conduct with rapid ventricular rates in the event of atrial fibrillation.[37] As might be expected, adenosine will terminate a high proportion of antidromic tachycardias by blocking retrograde conduction via the AV node.[38] Administration of the agent, however, may be associated with acceleration of tachycardia or development of atrial arrhythmias that may cause further hemodynamic deterioration. For this reason adenosine is not considered as first-line therapy for acute management of these arrhythmias. If an antidromic tachycardia is the suspected diagnosis, agents with class 1a or 1c activity are probably the best initial therapy.

Mahaim-type tachycardias form a special subgroup of preexcited junctional tachycardia. In these arrhythmias the antegrade limb of the reentrant tachycardia is formed by a slowly conducting accessory connection that in most cases originates from the anterior or anterolateral right atrium and inserts onto the right bundle branch. As a consequence, these arrhythmias have an appearance similar to typical left-bundle-branch block on the surface electrocardiogram. Retrograde conduction is usually via the AV node. The connections involved in antegrade conduction are best called atriodextrofascicular fibers rather than Mahaim fibers. Mahaim's original description was of a fiber originating in the AV node rather than the right atrium. Adenosine is almost universally successful in terminating arrhythmias involving atriodextrofascicular fibers, because conduction within such fibers is relatively easily blocked by adenosine.[38]

His Bundle Tachycardia

His bundle tachycardia or junctional ectopic tachycardia (JET) is an arrhythmia that occurs principally in children. The diagnosis is made from the demonstration of atrioventricular dissociation and a narrow QRS complex tachycardia. These features are thought to represent an automatic tachycardia arising from an ectopic focus situated in the His bundle above the bifurcation. The etiology is unknown, but it is most often seen after cardiac surgery and its presence suggests a poor prognosis. His bundle tachycardia may be transiently slowed by adenosine but termination is unusual.

Fascicular Tachycardia

Fascicular tachycardia is the term usually given to ventricular tachycardia that arises from the inferoapical left ventricular septum, having a superior axis morphology resembling right-bundle-branch block on the surface electrocardiogram.[39] The arrhythmia is usually associated with a structurally normal heart and is thought to have a reentrant mechanism involving the posterior fascicle of the left ventricle.[40, 41] The tachycardia is unusual in that it is sensitive to verapamil, making it difficult to distinguish from a junctional tachycardia with aberrant conduction to the ventricles. It differs from the latter arrhythmia, however, in that it is insensitive to adenosine.[42]

Right Ventricular Outflow Tract Tachycardia

Right ventricular outflow tract tachycardia is, along with fascicular tachycardia described above, one of the two principal forms of ventricular tachycardia

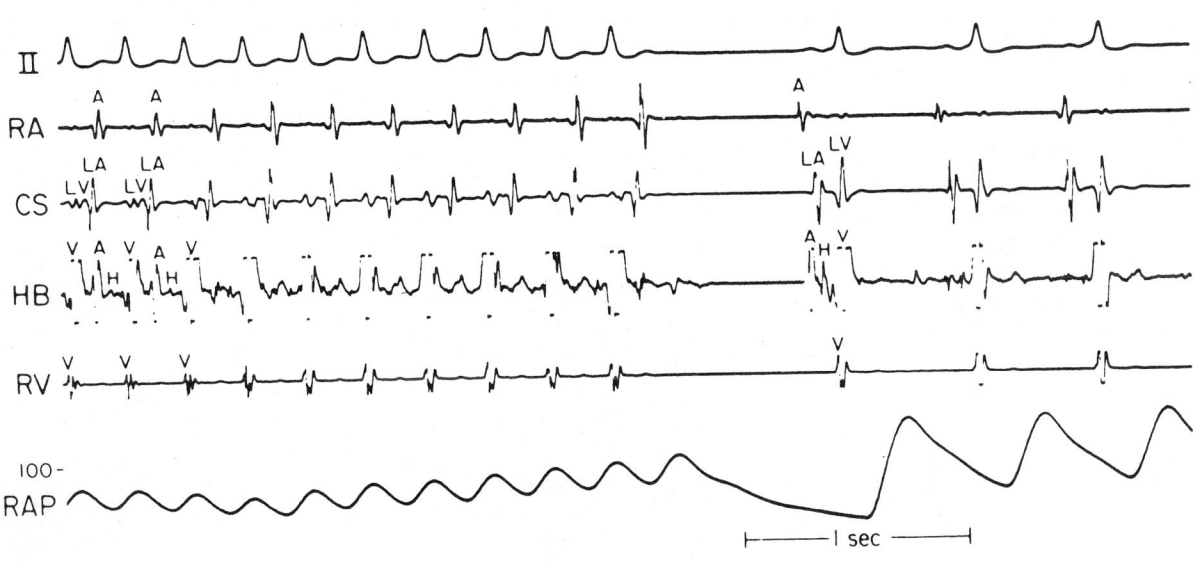

Figure 137–3. Termination of atrioventricular reentrant tachycardia by adenosine. Termination occurs at the level of the AV node in the antegrade direction. (From DiMarco JP, Sellers TD, Lerman BB, et al: Diagnostic and therapeutic use of adenosine in patients with supraventricular tachyarrhythmias. J Am Coll Cardiol 6:417, 1985. Reprinted with permission from the American College of Cardiology.)

Following intravenous adenosine (0.20mg/kg)

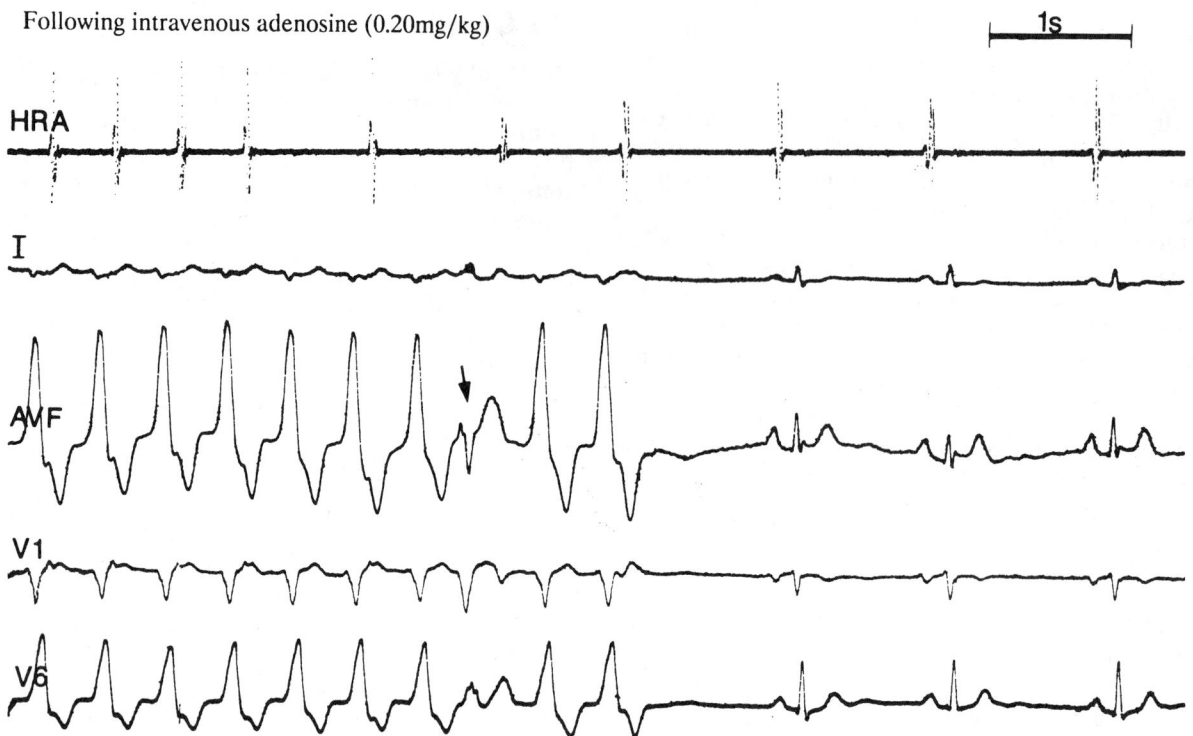

Figure 137–4. Termination of right ventricular outflow tract tachycardia by adenosine. Termination of tachycardia is preceded by retrograde ventriculoatrial block and a premature ventricular complex, both of which are markers of the action of adenosine. (From Griffith MJ, Garratt CJ, Rowland E, et al: The effects of adenosine on idiopathic ventricular tachycardia. Am J Cardiol 73:759, 1994.)

associated with a structurally normal heart. It is thought to be caused by triggered activity (a phenomenon exhibited by individual myocytes) rather than by a reentrant mechanism. As the name suggests, this tachycardia originates in the outflow tract of the right ventricle and has an inferior axis morphology resembling left-bundle-branch block on the surface electrocardiogram. This form of ventricular tachycardia is unique in that it is nearly always adenosine-sensitive (Fig. 137–4), giving rise to speculation that the triggered activity is cAMP-mediated.[43] This tachycardia should be differentiated from ventricular tachycardia

associated with right ventricular dysplasia, which is not adenosine-sensitive.

Ventricular Tachycardia Associated with Ischemic Heart Disease or Dilated Cardiomyopathy

The most common form of ventricular tachycardia is that associated with previous myocardial infarction. It arises from a reentrant circuit involving peri-infarction tissue and is not adenosine-sensitive.[43, 44] Ven-

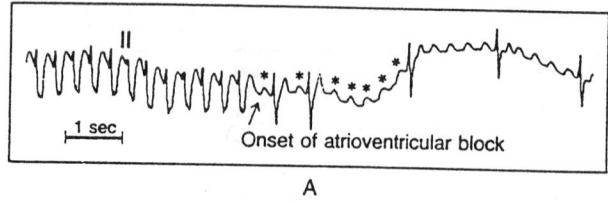

A

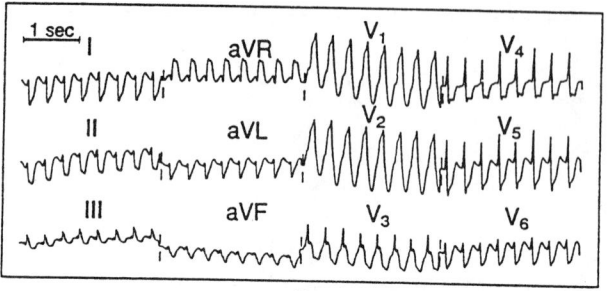

B

Figure 137–5. A, The unmasking of atrial flutter by IV adenosine in a 32-year-old man with dilated cardiomyopathy and a spontaneous episode of wide-complex regular tachycardia. Fifteen seconds after the administration of adenosine, the ventricular rate slowed, revealing flutter waves *(asterisks)* occurring at a rate identical to that of the original wide-complex tachycardia. *B,* In the same patient, the 12-lead electrocardiogram of the arrhythmia that would be considered diagnostic of ventricular tachycardia according to standard criteria, with an RS interval of more than 100 msec in V1 and V2 and an R-to-S ratio of less than 1 in V6. (From Camm AJ, Garratt CJ: Adenosine and supraventricular tachycardia. N Engl J Med 325:1621, 1991.)

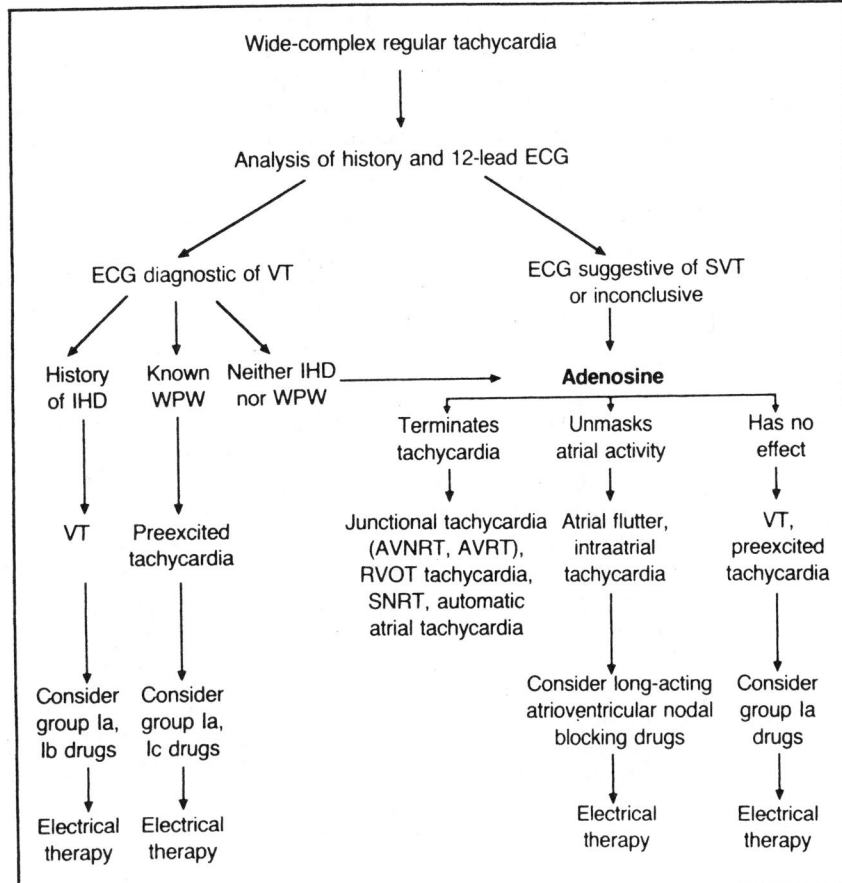

Figure 137–6. An approach to the management of wide-complex, regular tachycardia. (From Camm AJ, Garratt CJ: Adenosine and supraventricular tachycardia. N Engl J Med 325:1921, 1991.)

tricular tachycardia associated with dilated cardiomyopathy is also adenosine-insensitive.

ADVERSE EFFECTS OF ADENOSINE WHEN ADMINISTERED TO PATIENTS WITH CARDIAC ARRHYTHMIAS
Tachycardia Acceleration Due to Secondary Sympathetic Effects

Tachycardia acceleration due to secondary sympathetic effects is a form of the proarrhythmic effect of adenosine that has been reported with atrial flutter[28] in particular and also with atrial fibrillation.[45] It may be particularly likely if the atrial arrhythmia is conducted to the ventricles via an accessory pathway, since adenosine itself may shorten accessory pathway refractoriness.[46] Although these effects are transient and only occasionally cause clinical deterioration, they can be avoided if the correct diagnosis can be made from the surface electrocardiogram and adenosine therapy withheld if the rhythm is irregular or if flutter waves are clearly seen.

Induction of New Arrhythmias

The most common arrhythmia induced by adenosine is atrial fibrillation,[47] which is probably a result of the decrease in atrial refractoriness induced by the

agent.[48] This is particularly relevant to those patients with rapidly conducting accessory pathways, such as those with antidromic tachycardia, and adenosine should not be first-line therapy for these arrhythmias.

Bronchospasm

Intravenous adenosine is contraindicated in patients with asthma because bronchospasm may be induced.

ADENOSINE IN THE DIAGNOSIS OF WIDE COMPLEX TACHYCARDIA

Misdiagnosis of broad-complex tachycardia is frequent and the consequences of such a misdiagnosis are serious. Patients with ventricular tachycardia or preexcited atrial arrhythmias are frequently assumed to have supraventricular tachycardia with aberrant conduction and are treated with intravenous verapamil.[49, 50] The tachycardias will not be terminated and the additional hemodynamic compromise induced by verapamil (through direct negative inotropic and vasodilator effects) may lead to circulatory collapse and death. It can be argued that the principal problem leading to such a scenario is one of electrocardiographic recognition rather than an intrinsic problem with verapamil. Nevertheless, from a practical viewpoint, the availability of an AV nodal blocking agent without the problems of verapamil is obviously an advantage, particularly because the majority of patients with acute arrhythmias are seen by physicians with relatively little individual experience of arrhythmia management. Adenosine has been proposed as a safe alternative to verapamil for the termination of broad-complex tachycardias that are thought to be junctional in origin. More recently, adenosine has been proposed as a diagnostic agent in its own right, terminating junctional tachycardias, having no effect on ventricular tachycardia, and revealing atrial tachycardias (Fig. 137–5). Three studies have investigated the role of adenosine or ATP in the diagnosis of broad complex regular tachycardia. Griffith et al.[44] used adenosine in a regimen of incremental doses (0.05 to 0.25 mg/kg), as did Rankin et al.[33] (2.5 to 20 mg). Sharma et al.[30] used a standard 20-mg bolus dose. A total of 99 patients were studied, the majority during electrophysiologic testing. Twenty-nine had junctional tachycardia, 45 had ventricular tachycardia, and 25 had atrial arrhythmias. As a diagnostic test for reentrant junctional arrhythmias involving the atrioventricular node, adenosine-induced termination had a sensitivity of 90%, a specificity of 93%, and a positive predictive value of 92%. This compared favorably with the results of standard electrocardiographic criteria in the two studies in which this information was given. No patient with ventricular tachycardia had hemodynamic deterioration after the administration of adenosine or ATP, and all the effects were short-lasting and well tolerated.

Despite the excellent diagnostic ability of adenosine in broad-complex tachycardia demonstrated above, it is not appropriate to administer the agent to all patients presenting in this manner. In those patients with a history of myocardial infarction and an electrocardiogram that is typical of ventricular tachycardia, adenosine will be of no additional diagnostic value and will result in the patient's experiencing the side effects of the agent for no reason. Adenosine should be reserved for those patients whose electrocardiogram results suggest supraventricular tachycardia or are inconclusive[2] (Fig. 137–6). Obviously this decision is dependent to a degree on the ability of the clinician to interpret the electrocardiogram: an experienced arrhythmia specialist would use relatively little adenosine compared with an emergency room resident. The primary aim in the management of acute arrhythmia is to ensure patient safety, and adenosine has played a major role in achieving this.

REFERENCES

1. Honey RM, Ritchie WT, Thomson WAR: The action of adenosine upon the human heart. Q J Med 23:485, 1930.
2. Camm AJ, Garratt CJ: Adenosine and supraventricular tachycardia. N Engl J Med 325:162, 1991.
3. Sparks HV, Bardenheuer H: Regulation of adenosine formation by the heart. Circ Res 58:193, 1986.
4. Berne RM: Cardiac nucleotides in hypoxia: Possible role in regulation of coronary blood flow. Am J Physiol 204:31, 1963.
5. Newby AC: Adenosine and the concept of "retaliatory metabolites." Trends Biochem Sci 9:42, 1984.
6. Schrader J, Bauman G, Gerlach E: Adenosine as an inhibitor of
myocardial effects of catecholamines. Pflugers Arch 372:29, 1977.
7. Dobson JG: Mechanism of adenosine inhibition of catecholamine-induced responses in the heart. Circ Res 52:151, 1983.
8. Moser GH, Schrader J, Deussen A: Turnover of adenosine in plasma of human and dog blood. Am J Physiol 256:C799, 1989.
9. Lerman BB, Wesley RC, Belardinelli L: Electrophysiologic effects of dipyridamole on atrioventricular nodal conduction and supraventricular tachycardia: Role of endogenous adenosine. Circulation 80:1536, 1989.
10. Watt AH: Sick sinus syndrome: An adenosine-mediated disease. Lancet 1:786, 1985.
11. Kurachi Y, Nakajima T, Sugimoto T: On the mechanism of activation of muscarinic K+ channels by adenosine in isolated atrial cells: Involvement of GTP-binding proteins. Pflugers Arch 407:264, 1986.
12. Belardinelli L, Giles WR, West A: Ionic mechanisms of adenosine actions in pacemaker cells from rabbit heart. J Physiol 405:615, 1988.
13. Belardinelli L, Isenberg G: Isolated atrial myocytes: Adenosine and acetylcholine increase potassium conductance. Am J Physiol 244:H734, 1983.
14. Johnson EA, McKinnon Mg: Effect of acetylcholine and adenosine on cardiac cellular potentials. Nature 178:1174, 1956.
15. West GA, Belardinelli L: Correlation of sinus slowing and hyperpolarisation caused by adenosine in sinus node. Pflugers Arch 403:75, 1985.
16. Martynyuk A, Kane KA, Rankin AC, Cobbe SM: Adenosine increases potassium conductance in isolated rabbit atrioventricular nodal myocytes. Br Heart J 71:29, 1994.
17. Clemo HF, Belardinelli L: Effect of adenosine on atrioventricular conduction: Site and characterisation of adenosine action in the guinea pig atrioventricular node. Circ Res 59:427, 1986.
18. Belardinelli L, Linden J, Berne RM: The cardiac effects of adenosine. Prog Cardiovasc Dis 32:73, 1989.
19. Belardinelli L, Isenberg G: Actions of adenosine and isoproterenol on isolated mammalian ventricular myocytes. Circ Res 53:287, 1983.
20. Isenberg G, Belardinelli L: Ionic basis for the antagonism between adenosine and isoproterenol on isolated mammalian ventricular myocytes. Circ Res 55:309, 1984.
21. DiMarco JP, Sellers TD, Berne RM, et al: Adenosine: Electrophysiologic effects and therapeutic use for termination of paroxysmal supraventricular tachycardia. Circulation 68:1254, 1983.
22. Sylven C, Beerman B, Jonzon B, Brandt R: Angina pectoris-like pain provoked by intravenous adenosine in healthy volunteers. Br Med J 293:227, 1986.
23. Biaggioni I, Olafsson B, Robertson RM, et al: Cardiovascular and respiratory effects of adenosine in conscious man: Evidence for chemoreceptor activation. Circ Res 61:779, 1987.
24. Biaggioni I, Killian TJ, Mosqeda-Garcia R, et al: Adenosine increases sympathetic nerve traffic in humans. Circulation 83:1668, 1991.
25. Sylven C, Jonson B, Brandt R, Beerman B: Adenosine-provoked angina pectoris type pain: Time characteristics, influence of autonomic blockade and naloxone. Eur Heart J 8:738, 1987.
26. Botteron GW, Smith JM: Spatial and temporal inhomogeneity of adenosine's effect on atrial refractoriness in humans: Using atrial fibrillation to probe atrial refractoriness. J Cardiovasc Electrophysiol 5:477, 1994.
27. Haines DE, DiMarco JP: Sustained intra-atrial reentrant tachycardia: Clinical, electrocardiographic and electrophysiological characteristics and long-term follow up. J Am Coll Cardiol 15:1345, 1990.
28. Slade A, Garratt CJ: Proarrhythmic effect of adenosine in a patient with atrial flutter. Br Heart J 70:91, 1993.
29. Griffith MJ, Garratt CJ, Ward DE, Camm AJ: The effects of adenosine on sinus node reentrant tachycardia. Clin Cardiol 12:409, 1989.
30. Sharma AD, Klein GJ, Yee R: Intravenous adenosine triphosphate during wide QRS complex tachycardia: Safety, therapeutic efficacy and diagnostic utility. Am J Med 88:337, 1990.
31. DiMarco JP, Sellers TD, Lerman BB, et al: Diagnostic and therapeutic use of adenosine in patients with supraventricular tachyarrhythmias. J Am Coll Cardiol 6:417, 1985.

32. Garratt CJ, Linker NJ, Griffith MJ, et al: Comparison of adenosine and verapamil for termination of paroxysmal junctional tachycardia. Am J Cardiol 64:1310, 1989.
33. Rankin AC, Oldroyd KG, Chong E, et al: Value and limitations of adenosine in the diagnosis and treatment of narrow and broad complex tachycardias. Br Heart J 62:195, 1989.
34. DiMarco JP, Miles W, Akhtar M, et al: Adenosine for paroxysmal supraventricular tachycardia: Dose ranging and comparison with verapamil. Ann Intern Med 113:104, 1990.
35. Cushley MJ, Tattersfield AE, Holgate ST: Inhaled adenosine and guanosine on airway resistance in normal and asthmatic subjects. Br J Clin Pharmacol 15:161, 1983.
36. Cushley MJ, Tattersfield AE, Holgate ST: Adenosine-induced bronchoconstriction in asthma: Antagonism by inhaled theophylline. Am Rev Respir Dis 129:380, 1984.
37. Packer DL, Gallagher JJ, Prystowsky EN: Physiological substrate for antidromic reciprocating tachycardia. Circulation 85:574, 1992.
38. Garratt CJ, O'Nunain S, Griffith MJ, et al: The effects of intravenous adenosine on preexcited junctional tachycardias: Efficacy and proarrhythmic effects. Am J Cardiol 74:401, 1994.
39. Ward DE, Nathan AW, Camm AJ: Fascicular tachycardia sensitive to calcium antagonists. Eur Heart J 5:896, 1984.
40. Lin FC, Finley CD, Rahimtoola SH, Wu D: Idiopathic paroxysmal ventricular tachycardia with a QRS pattern of right bundle branch block and left axis deviation: A unique clinical entity with specific properties. Am J Cardiol 52:95, 1983.
41. Ohe T, Shimomura K, Aihara N, et al: Idiopathic sustained left ventricular tachycardia: Clinical and electrophysiological characteristics. Circulation 77:560, 1988.
42. Griffith MJ, Garratt CJ, Rowland E, et al: The effects of intravenous adenosine on idiopathic ventricular tachycardia. Am J Cardiol 73:759, 1994.
43. Lerman BB, Belardinelli L, West GA, et al: Adenosine-sensitive ventricular tachycardia: Evidence suggesting cyclic AMP-mediated triggered activity. Circulation 74;270, 1986.
44. Griffith MJ, Linker NJ, Ward DE, Camm AJ: Adenosine in the diagnosis of broad complex tachycardias. Lancet 1:672, 1988.
45. White RD: Acceleration of the ventricular response in paroxysmal lone atrial fibrillation following the injection of adenosine. Am J Emerg Med 11:245, 1993.
46. Garratt CJ, Griffith MJ, O'Nunain S, et al: The effects of intravenous adenosine on antegrade refractoriness of accessory atrioventricular connections. Circulation 84:1962, 1991.
47. Belhassen B, Viskin S, Laniado S: Sustained atrial fibrillation after conversion of paroxysmal reciprocating junctional tachycardia by intravenous verapamil. Am J Cardiol 62:835, 1988.
48. O'Nunain S, Garratt C, Paul V, et al: Effect of intravenous adenosine on human atrial and ventricular repolarisation. Cardiovasc Res 26:939, 1992.
49. Garratt CJ, Antoniou A, Ward DE, Camm AJ: Misuse of verapamil in preexcited atrial fibrillation. Lancet 1:367, 1989.
50. Rankin AC, Rae AP, Cobbe SM: Misuse of intravenous verapamil in patients with ventricular tachycardia. Lancet 1:472, 1987.

CHAPTER 138

Amiodarone

Charles R. Kerr, M.D., Mauricio B. Rosenbaum, M.D., and Pablo A. Chiale, M.D.

In December 1985, amiodarone was approved in the United States for the treatment of life-threatening arrhythmias only when other drugs were ineffective.[1] Because about ten drugs are used for the treatment of ventricular arrhythmias, once these have failed, chances are that the patient is very sick and the arrhythmias nearly intractable. Thus, large amounts of amiodarone are prescribed in doses as enormously high as 6000 mg/day,[2] and side effects are common and often serious. Because of these side effects, the use of amiodarone in the United States has been much restricted. In such circumstances, a full evaluation of the therapeutic options provided by the drug is nearly impossible or is likely to be heavily biased. This chapter reflects experience using amiodarone with no restrictions since 1970. We will emphasize the usefulness of low (600 to 1000 mg/wk) or moderate (2000 mg/wk) doses for the management of a wide variety of cardiac disorders, and the control of some life-threatening arrhythmias with doses no higher than 400 mg/day. Under such conditions, side effects are less common and not often serious.

HISTORY

Amiodarone was selected from a large series of benzofuran derivatives because of its highly relaxing effect on the coronary vascular bed.[3] It was synthesized in Belgium with the use of the benzofuran moiety present in khellin, a coronary dilator. The first report on its antianginal effect appeared in 1967.[4] Its antiarrhythmic activity in animals was reported in 1969,[5] the earliest attempts to elucidate its electrophysiologic properties were reported in 1970,[6] and the first clinical experience on its antiarrhythmic action after intravenous administration was published in 1970.[7] The current widespread use of the oral preparation as an extremely potent and versatile antiarrhythmic agent emanates from two clinical papers published in 1974[8] and 1976.[9]

CHEMISTRY

Figure 138–1 illustrates the chemical structure of amiodarone together with that of its natural (khellin) and synthetic (benzarone and benziodarone) precursors. Benziodarone was found to cause jaundice[10] and was discarded. The addition of two iodine atoms in the molecule, which was thought to enhance the coronary dilation effect, proved later to be essential for sustaining the antiarrhythmic activity of amiodarone. Attempts to replace the iodine atoms by bromine or hydrogen[11] failed to yield an effective antiarrhythmic compound, although iodine itself has none of the properties of amiodarone.[6]

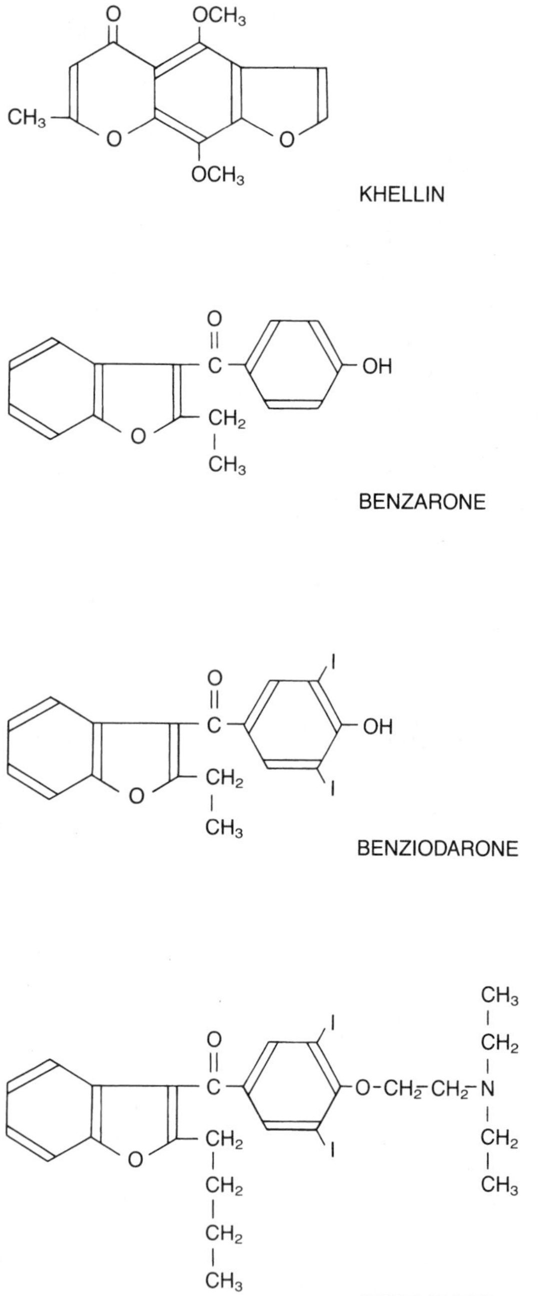

Figure 138–1. Chemical structures of amiodarone and its precursors, khellin, benzarone, and benziodarone.

GENERAL PHARMACOLOGIC EFFECTS

Charlier, the father of amiodarone, following a large series of studies,[12-27] defined a biological profile that was held responsible for the antianginal action[18] and that consists of (1) a long-lasting reduction in the heart rate, (2) a moderate and transient decrease in systemic blood pressure, (3) a reduction in myocardial oxygen consumption, (4) a marked increase in myocardial blood flow, and (5) a partial inhibition of the effects of catecholamines. However, these actions do not seem to account for the antiarrhythmic effects of

the drug. New chemical compounds sharing the same profile and a similar antianginal efficacy[28, 29] failed to show the antiarrhythmic properties of amiodarone.

Amiodarone has been shown to be a noncompetitive inhibitor of various α- and β-adrenergic cardiovascular phenomena.[18, 30, 31] Unlike β-blockers, it does not bind to the catecholamine recognition site of the β-receptor but appears to induce a significant decrease in the number of β-adrenoreceptors.[32-34]* Amiodarone also appeared to inhibit the stimulation of cardiac adenylate cyclase mediated by activation of different receptors.[33] Thus, the noncompetitive β-antagonistic properties of amiodarone appear to be a result of inhibition of the coupling of β-receptors with the regulatory unit of the adenylate cyclase complex, a result of a decrease in the number of receptors at the myocardial cell surface, or both. Amiodarone causes striking changes of cardiac metabolism.[15, 16, 23] The myocardial lactate/pyruvate ratio increases owing to a strong reduction in pyruvate, suggesting that oxidative metabolism is slowed in the cytoplasm. The energetic reserves tend to increase as shown by an increment of the ratio of high-energy compounds to phosphate acceptors (ATP-ADP; phosphocreatine/creatine). Amiodarone also inhibits the myocardial depletion of glycogen induced by epinephrine, theophylline, and dinitrophenol. The last kind of protection is also provoked by propranolol.[21] Unlike those of propranolol, not all the peripheral effects of catecholamines are inhibited by amiodarone. Thus, the antiadrenergic actions of amiodarone appear to be organ specific and practically restricted to the heart.

The previously described effects provide the rational basis for the use of amiodarone in patients with angina pectoris.[37-44] Amiodarone is an effective antianginal drug at oral doses of 1000 to 1400 mg/week. It is useful in patients who do not respond to β-blockers or who require excessively high (and not well-tolerated) doses. It is remarkably efficacious in aged patients with decubitus angina. Administered intravenously as a slow infusion of 1200 mg over 24 hours, it may be life-saving in patients with recurrent prolonged episodes of anginal pain who cannot undergo surgery. Furthermore, a "protective" action against the deleterious consequences of ischemia has been demonstrated under different experimental conditions,[45] including a substantial reduction in infarct size.[46]

EFFECTS ON MYOCARDIAL CONTRACTILITY AND CARDIAC PERFORMANCE

In animals, intravenous amiodarone caused a dose-related decrease in contractile force (well apparent with 10 mg/kg) and left ventricular dP/dt.[47] However, cardiac output increased because of the concom-

---

*Long-term treatment with β-blockers induces a significant increase in the number of β-adrenoreceptors,[35, 36] which may explain the hyperadrenergic state frequently observed following abrupt drug withdrawal. Obviously, amiodarone cannot be expected to induce this untoward effect.

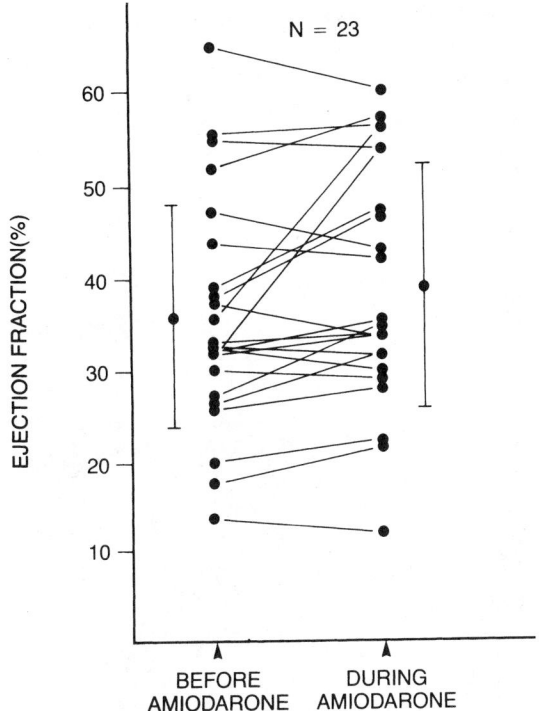

Figure 138–2. Effects of chronic amiodarone administration on left ventricular ejection fraction in 23 patients with refractory ventricular tachyarrhythmias. Amiodarone did not depress left ventricular ejection fraction even when the basal ejection fraction was severely reduced. (From Singh BN: Amiodarone: Historical development and pharmacologic profile. Am Heart J 106:788, 1983.)

itant reduction of systemic vascular resistance, and stroke volume increased even more because of the slowing of the heart rate.[12, 26, 27] A similar response was observed in patients with normal left ventricular function.[37, 39, 48, 49] In one study,[50] amiodarone was administered intravenously (5 mg/kg infused over 20 minutes) to 18 patients with depressed left ventricular function. Two developed severe hypotension. In the remaining 16 patients, the heart rate linearly decreased during the 60 minutes of observation; cardiac index and left ventricular stroke work index showed a transient decrease at 10 minutes, returning to control values by 60 minutes, and there was a tendency to higher pulmonary wedge pressure at 10 minutes, suggesting a transient depression of left ventricular function. When the ejection fraction was greater than 30%, cardiac index and stroke volume index remained virtually unchanged. Similar observations have been reported by others.[38, 51, 52] Furthermore, this mild and transient negative inotropic effect is restricted to rapid intravenous administration and does not occur during chronic oral therapy. In an early study,[53] amiodarone did not alter cardiac output after 30 days of treatment with 600 mg/day. In two later studies[54, 55] in which ejection fraction was measured by radionuclide ventriculography before and during protracted amiodarone therapy, there were no significant changes even in patients with ejection fractions as low as 15% to 20% (Fig. 138–2). These observations are in line with the knowledge that cardiac failure is rarely ag-

gravated by amiodarone,[56–58] even in patients with advanced cardiomyopathy.[59]

ELECTROPHYSIOLOGIC EFFECTS

Singh and Vaughan Williams[6] reported that amiodarone administered intraperitoneally in rabbits (20 mg/kg/day for 6 weeks) caused a progressive prolongation of the action potential duration (APD) in atrial and ventricular muscle. On this basis, the drug was classified as possessing a class III antiarrhythmic action.[60, 61] We were able to confirm that the oral chronic administration of amiodarone prolonged the APD in ventricular muscle of rabbit hearts and, to a lesser extent, in Purkinje fibers,[9] whereas in canine hearts, this effect was less marked in ventricular muscle and absent in Purkinje fibers.[62] In other studies,[63–65] amiodarone was found to actually shorten the APD in Purkinje tissue. Clinically, amiodarone greatly prolongs the monophasic action potential in the human right atrium[66] as well as the duration of the QT interval,[67–71] suggesting that it does indeed prolong the APD in human atrial and ventricular muscle. However, its antiarrhythmic actions may not only be a result of prolongation of the APD.[72] Other drugs or conditions that prolong the APD may be more arrhythmogenic than antiarrhythmic or may fail to show similar antiarrhythmic potency.

Lidocainelike (Class I) Effects of Amiodarone

In rabbit hearts,[9] high doses of amiodarone caused depression of membrane responsiveness in ventricular muscle and, to a lesser extent, in Purkinje fibers (Fig. 138–3). Amiodarone does indeed block sodium channels in neural[73] and cardiac tissue[63, 64, 74–76] and therefore possesses a class I antiarrhythmic action. Unlike quinidine, which primarily blocks open chan-

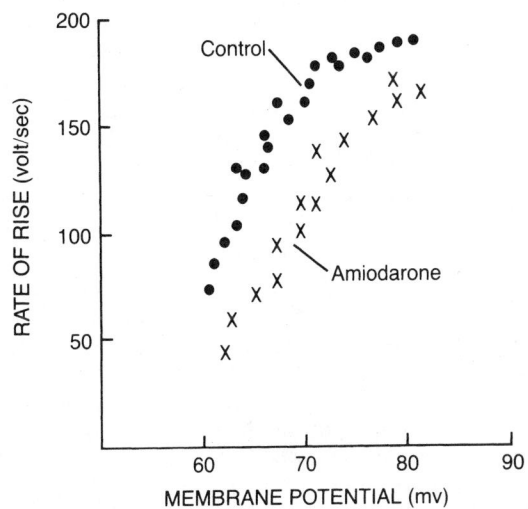

Figure 138–3. Effects of amiodarone on membrane responsiveness of ventricular fibers of rabbit hearts. Compared with controls, animals pretreated with amiodarone for several weeks demonstrated depressed membrane responsiveness.

nels, and closer to lidocaine, which blocks both open and inactivated channels,[75] amiodarone has a selective affinity for inactivated channels.

In practical terms, this means that the depressing effects of amiodarone on the rate of rise of action potential (V_{max}) and conduction velocity are greater at fast heart rates than at slow rates (use- or frequency-dependent effect), and in depolarized (injured) tissues. Through its well-known effect in slowing the heart rate, amiodarone may "deactivate" its sodium-channel effect during sinus rhythm. In fact, in one study,[63] amiodarone failed to cause any significant effect on V_{max} at a pacing rate of 60 beats/min (a rate commonly seen in chronically treated patients). However, the effect will be "in store" to be used only or mostly "on demand," when activated by a tachyarrhythmia or by premature beats.

Effects on Refractoriness and Conduction Velocity

In a study by Elizari et al.,[62] amiodarone was found to prolong the effective refractory period (ERP) of ventricular and Purkinje fibers of the canine heart, with a shortening of the relative RP and an increase of the ERP/APD ratio (Fig. 138–4). The take-off potential at which the earliest propagated responses did occur was shifted in a negative direction, and such responses showed an increase in V_{max} and conduction velocity, as has also been shown to occur with lidocaine.[77] These effects may prove to be highly antiarrhythmogenic by preventing the occurrence of slowly propagated premature responses. Clinically, amiodarone has been shown to prolong refractoriness in the atria, ventricles, AV node, His-Purkinje system, and accessory pathways.[78–82] This uniform effect on all cardiac tissues is probably the main reason for its antiarrhythmic versatility. From the selective affinity of amiodarone for inactivated sodium channels, it would be expected that its effects on injured (depolarized) cardiac tissues are "potentiated," as is well known to occur with lidocaine.[83] A clinical model was developed that makes it possible to test this hypothesis.[84–87] The basic principle of the model is as follows: if a patient has intermittent bundle branch block, the longest cycle length at which conduction becomes abnormal measures the duration of refractoriness in the affected fascicle, which can thus be estimated before and after drug administration (Fig. 138–5). A series of observations similar to that illustrated in Figure 138–5 showed that in humans, amiodarone did indeed cause depression of conduction and prolongation of refractoriness in diseased conducting fascicles.[88]

While therapeutic doses or slight overdosing of most class I antiarrhythmic drugs may cause manifest QRS widening, this is unlikely to occur with amiodarone even at extremely high doses. In eight patients, very high doses of amiodarone increased the mean QRS duration (during ventricular pacing at a cycle length of 600 msec) from 157 to 191 msec.[89] Under such conditions, this is not unexpected but cannot be

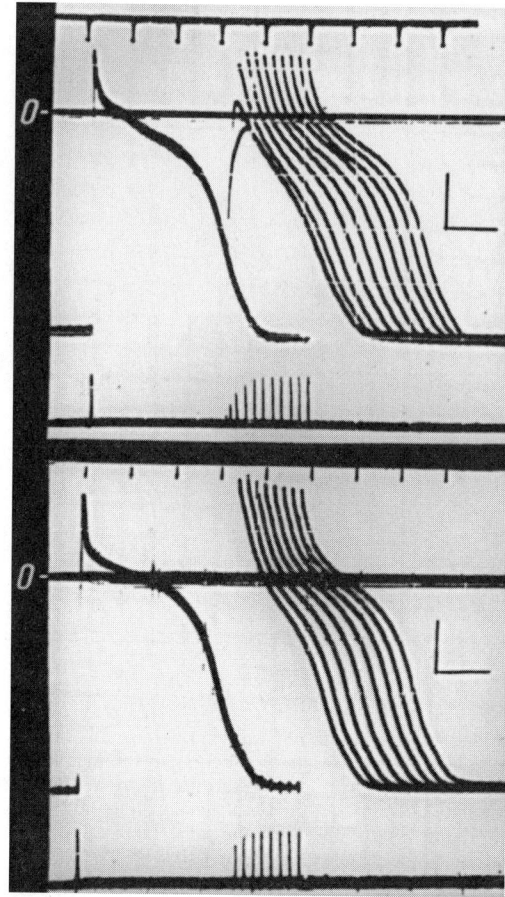

Figure 138–4. Effects of premature stimulation on the action potential of canine Purkinje fibers in a control animal *(top)* and in another dog pretreated with oral amiodarone (20 mg/kg during a month) *(bottom)*. In the control animal, the most premature responses were elicited at relatively reduced membrane potentials (about −60 mV) and showed low amplitude and slow rate of rise of the action potential. In this preparation, a clear relative refractory period could be identified. Conversely, the earliest responses in the Purkinje fibers under the effect of amiodarone occurred at significantly more negative membrane potentials, showing clearly normal upstroke velocity and normal amplitude. Thus, the relative refractory period may be assumed to be greatly reduced. Amiodarone also increased the overshoot of the action potential in the first premature responses.

extrapolated to the resting ECG during sinus rhythm. While most class I antiarrhythmic drugs cause moderate but consistent prolongation of the HV interval,[90, 91] amiodarone causes smaller or inconstant prolongation.[78–81, 92, 93] Therefore, amiodarone does not appear to cause any clinically meaningful depression of conduction in the normal heart. In this regard, amiodarone is again much closer to lidocaine than to any other class I antiarrhythmic agent[94] (unpublished observations).

Effects on Sinus Node Automaticity and AV Nodal Conduction

Amiodarone causes a persistent slowing of the sinoatrial rate[59, 69] and restrains the maximal increase in rate induced by exercise. This may be related to a partial inhibition of the sympathetic drive on the sinus node. However, in dogs treated with maximal doses of propranolol, amiodarone caused an additional slowing,[29, 95] suggesting a direct depressing effect that has been attributed to a decrease in slow inward current.[7, 96, 97] A depressing effect on sinoatrial conduction has also been suggested.[98, 99] The depressant effects of amiodarone on AV nodal conduction and refractoriness[78, 98, 100–105] may also be related in part to its antisympathetic action and in part to inhibition of the slow inward current.[97, 106–108]

Other Electrophysiologic Effects

Amiodarone was found to consistently inhibit depolarization-induced automaticity in guinea pig ventricular muscle[75] and to depress delayed afterdepolarization and triggered activity induced by low potassium in rabbit ventricular myocardium.[109] The mechanism by which amiodarone is effective in suppressing these potential sources of ventricular arrhythmias remains unclear. However, several studies have demonstrated that amiodarone blocks calcium channels and this may account for some of the observed antiarrhythmic effects.[106–115]

Amiodarone is a remarkably strong antifibrillatory drug, as shown by its ability to prevent ventricular fibrillation induced by coronary artery ligation (or after reperfusion) in a wide variety of experimental conditions.[9, 115, 116] The occurrence of atrial fibrillation induced by topical application of aconitine was also prevented by the previous administration of amiodarone.[117]

PHARMACOKINETICS

As early as 1969, Broekhuysen et al.,[20] using amiodarone labeled with the radioactive isotope of iodine, ^{131}I, were able to show that the drug is slowly absorbed but avidly retained within the body. Ten days after a single dose, body radioactivity remained constant and ^{131}I elimination (by the urine) was no greater than 1%. After administration of a single oral dose to six patients who had been under chronic treatment, the elimination of ^{131}I was shown to occur in two distinct phases. A relatively rapid phase was followed by a slow phase. The elimination half-life was estimated to be 18 to 40 days (mean, 28 days). In another study based on determinations of serum nonhormonal iodine,[118] the half-life was estimated to be 36 to 100 days (mean, 60 days). In cases in which an autopsy was performed, it was found that iodine accumulated in practically all body tissues.[20] According to tissue volume, the greatest reservoir was in skeletal muscle and fatty tissue. A noniodinated analogue (labeled with tritium) was also shown to have a very slow rate of elimination, but the presence of iodine further slowed renal elimination, thus partially contributing to the accumulation of the drug.

The development of a selective, high-performance liquid chromatographic method for the measurement of amiodarone[119–121] led to a series of new pharmacokinetic studies. However, the overall picture was not much changed. Absorption of amiodarone is slow, and bioavailability is low and variable.[122–124] In the circulation, it is almost completely bound to proteins.[125] There is a clear delay between the appearance of amiodarone in the plasma and its uptake by the myocardium[126–128] in which a concentration develops that reaches 10 to 50 times that in plasma. In adipose, liver, and pulmonary tissue, concentrations are 100 to 1000 times as high as those in plasma.[129–133] Renal excretion is negligible,[134–137] and amiodarone is not removed by hemodialysis.[137, 138] It is thought to be metabolized in the liver and the gut wall,[124] and the existence of enterohepatic recirculation is controversial.[134–139] From several studies, the terminal elimination half-life has been estimated to be 8 to 107 days.[121, 129, 131, 132, 134–136, 140–143] It was also confirmed that elimination of amiodarone is biphasic.[121] This was attributed to an initial, relatively rapid elimination from a central compartment that might include the heart, followed by a much slower clearance from a poorly perfused peripheral compartment composed largely of fat.[121, 144]

When the administration of amiodarone was discontinued after several weeks or months of successful therapy, persistence of the antiarrhythmic protection was shown to last from several days or weeks to several months.[9, 145] This property contributes greatly

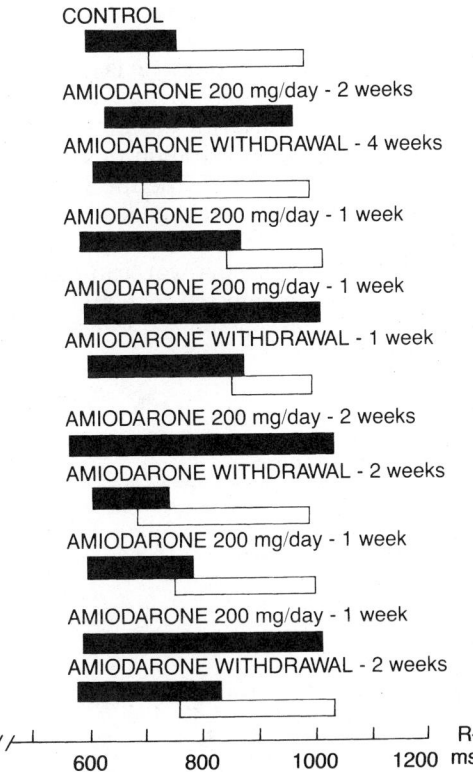

CONTROL

AMIODARONE 200 mg/day - 2 weeks

AMIODARONE WITHDRAWAL - 4 weeks

AMIODARONE 200 mg/day - 1 week

AMIODARONE 200 mg/day - 1 week

AMIODARONE WITHDRAWAL - 1 week

AMIODARONE 200 mg/day - 2 weeks

AMIODARONE WITHDRAWAL - 2 weeks

AMIODARONE 200 mg/day - 1 week

AMIODARONE 200 mg/day - 1 week

AMIODARONE WITHDRAWAL - 2 weeks

0   600   800   1000   1200   R-R msec

Figure 138–5. Effects of chronic amiodarone administration on intraventricular conduction in a patient with "tachycardia-dependent" or "phase 3" right bundle branch block (BBB). Black bars represent right BBB; white bars indicate normal conduction. R-R intervals are in milliseconds. Conduction over the damaged bundle branch was significantly impaired by amiodarone.

and perhaps decisively to the clinical usefulness of the drug. It liberates patients from the annoyance of a rigid hourly schedule and provides them with a more sustained antiarrhythmic protection. Dosage regimes in which the drug is discontinued 2 days every week are feasible.[9] However, the antiarrhythmic effects of amiodarone may take several days or weeks of treatment,[9] and this is obviously a disadvantage. Thus, there is a therapeutic "latency,"[145] the approximate duration of which is indicated in Table 138–1. Furthermore, although a large reduction of arrhythmias may occur after 5 to 15 days of treatment, the maximal steady-state effect of amiodarone is attained only at 3 to 5 months.[145] To shorten the latency, high oral loading doses or intravenous administration have been used.[2, 9, 52, 55, 128, 146–152] Even so, there appears to be a time lag that varies between a few hours and several days. It has been assumed that the delay in onset and offset of amiodarone effects is related solely to the extensive extracardiac storage of the drug.[75, 144] However, this leaves unexplained the time lag and the fact that the electrophysiologic effects of amiodarone persist for hours in preparations in which the Tyrode solution bathing the tissue of pretreated animals contains no drug ("no washout phenomenon").[62] Some additional, still undefined mechanisms are probably implicated.

The unusually large volume of distribution of amiodarone and the complicated kinetics of its elimination. as well as the poorly known interactions of the drug with its cardiac receptors, greatly limit the value of plasma concentrations in guiding antiarrhythmic therapy.[55, 132, 153] A major metabolite of amiodarone, desethylamiodarone, has been found to exist in high concentrations in humans,[121, 133, 137, 154–156] and to exert some relevant electrophysiologic effects.[64, 107, 109, 157–160] Desethylamiodarone was also shown to partially saturate nuclear thyroid hormone receptors in various tissues, including the heart.[161] The elimination half-life of desethylamiodarone is longer than that of amiodarone. A second metabolite, didesethylamiodarone, has been detected in dogs.[162]

INTERACTIONS WITH OTHER DRUGS

Amiodarone alters the pharmacokinetics of many drugs, acts synergistically with some, and antagonizes (and may be antagonized by) the effects of catecholamines. Some of these interactions may be useful in enhancing therapeutic effects, but many may imply a threat of adverse reactions. When amiodarone is added to a maintenance digoxin regime, the serum digoxin concentration rises linearly for 6 to 7 days until a plateau is reached,[163–165] and this may result in cardiac, gastrointestinal, and neurologic manifestations. Sinus node dysfunction, AV nodal block, or both are the most common cardiac consequences of this interaction,[166, 167] which depends not only on high serum digoxin levels but also on the additive effects of both drugs. Synergistic action on AV nodal conduction may be useful in slowing the ventricular rate in patients with atrial fibrillation in whom digoxin alone is ineffective, with the additional advantage that the arrhythmogenic effects of digoxin may be prevented. The combined administration of amiodarone and digoxin also appears to be highly effective in cases of incessant supraventricular tachycardia.[168] The mechanisms underlying interactions between amiodarone and digoxin are still unclear. An increase in digoxin bioavailability,[169] a reduction in its renal and extrarenal clearance,[164, 165] and displacement of digoxin from its storage sites[170] have been proposed to explain the increase in serum concentration. Since the serum digoxin level is usually doubled, the dose of digoxin should be halved when amiodarone is given concomitantly.

In patients taking warfarin, the prothrombin time is prolonged by the administration of amiodarone,[171] and bleeding may occur.[172, 173] The mechanism of this interaction has not been elucidated. It is not caused by displacement of warfarin from its plasma protein binding.[125, 171, 174] Since plasma warfarin concentration increases, it has been suggested that amiodarone may interfere with warfarin metabolism.[170] It has also been

Table 138–1. **Amiodarone: Dose-Response Relationships**

Type of Arrhythmia	Amiodarone Loading Dose (mg/day)	Treatment Maintenance Dose (mg/day)	Therapeutic Latency (days)	Persistence of Effect (days)
Recurrent SVT	600 (8–15 days)	100–300	5–10	30–150
Recurrent AF or AFL	600–800 (15–30 days)	200–400	10–20	15–90
PMVA in ischemic heart disease	600–800 (10–20 days)	400–600	20–30	30–40
PMVA in chronic chagasic myocarditis	800–1000 (30–60 days)	600–800	30–60	28–45
SRS VT and/or VF	600–1000 (15–30 days)	700	5–30	10–30

AF, Atrial fibrillation; AFL, atrial flutter; SRS, sustained recurrent symptomatic; SVT, supraventricular tachycardia; VF, ventricular fibrillation; VT, ventricular tachycardia.

reported that amiodarone directly depresses vitamin K-dependent clotting cofactors, thus enhancing the anticoagulant effect of warfarin.[172, 174] The dose of warfarin should be reduced by one third to one half when amiodarone is administered simultaneously.

Amiodarone develops strong interactions with other antiarrhythmic drugs. Good results have been obtained by combining amiodarone with quinidine[175] and mexiletine.[176] However, amiodarone was found to increase plasma concentrations of quinidine,[125, 177] procainamide,[177] flecainide,[178] aprindine,[179] and phenytoin.[180, 181] The higher plasma level plus the synergistic effect with drugs that also prolong repolarization may result in marked lengthening of the QT interval[177, 182, 183] and provocation of torsade de pointes. Until more is learned about these interactions, great caution is recommended when amiodarone is used in combination with any other antiarrhythmic drug.

The combination of amiodarone and β-blockers causes marked depressant effects on sinus node activity and AV nodal conduction, and sinus arrest or advanced AV block may occur.[184] A similar interaction may occur with diltiazem.[185] However, a combination of amiodarone and calcium blockers may be useful in treating patients with incessant supraventricular tachycardia.[186] The antagonistic effects of amiodarone on sympathetic activity have been discussed. In contrast, the administration of isoproterenol considerably reduces the prolongation of refractoriness induced by amiodarone in the accessory pathway of patients with Wolff-Parkinson-White (WPW) syndrome,[187, 188] implying that the antiarrhythmic action may be neutralized, at least partially. The extent to which catecholamines may antagonize other effects of amiodarone is not known.

INDICATIONS

Chronically administered oral amiodarone has proved to be remarkably effective in treating a wide variety of cardiac arrhythmias. This should be contrasted with the modest usefulness of intravenous amiodarone.

Intravenous Amiodarone

The most consistent electrophysiologic effect caused by intravenous amiodarone is slowing of conduction and prolongation of refractoriness in the AV node.[89, 107, 127, 189–191] Accordingly, intravenous amiodarone has been shown to be useful in terminating episodes of supraventricular tachycardia[192, 193] as well as in slowing the ventricular rate in atrial fibrillation (AF) or flutter (AFl).[93, 194, 195] However, similar effects are more consistently caused by intravenous verapamil. A continuous infusion of amiodarone has been reported to reduce ventricular ectopic rhythm in patients with complex ventricular arrhythmias,[147] but these results were much less impressive than those obtained during chronic oral therapy.[59, 196] Furthermore, intravenous amiodarone was scarcely effective in suppressing ventricular premature beats (VPBs), ventricular couplets (VCs), and runs of ventricular tachycardia (VT) in patients with chagasic heart disease.[197] Studies have emphasized the usefulness of intravenous amiodarone in the acute management of sustained VT,[52, 147, 198–202] ventricular fibrillation (VF) occurring after cardiac surgery,[195, 199, 200] as well as out-of-hospital cardiac arrest.[203] In atrial and ventricular tachyarrhythmias, intravenous amiodarone may be considered as an alternative in cases in which currently used drugs fail or are contraindicated. Intravenous amiodarone has no role in the treatment of torsade de pointes. The drug may be the first choice to treat recurrences of VT in patients under chronic treatment in whom an insufficient oral dose was the cause of recurrence. Currently, the main use of intravenous amiodarone is in shortening the latency when treatment is initiated for recurrent VT, VF, or both.[52, 55, 147, 148, 151, 199, 204]

Oral Amiodarone

Table 138–1 describes the loading and maintenance doses, the duration of the latency, and the persistence of antiarrhythmic protection in various arrhythmias in which amiodarone is most useful.

Paroxysmal Supraventricular Tachycardia (PSVT)

In our initial experience,[9] amiodarone provided total control of recurrent PSVT in 96% of 59 patients and in 100% of 20 patients with WPW syndrome. These impressive results were essentially confirmed by many other studies.[150, 188, 205–209] Amiodarone appears to be far superior to quinidine, β-blockers, digitalis, and verapamil in preventing PSVT related to an accessory pathway.[210] Although amiodarone is useful in controlling AV nodal reentrant tachycardias, verapamil and digitalis appear to be equally or more effective.[210] In the highly refractory, "incessant" type of PSVT, the combined use of amiodarone with small doses of digitalis may be needed to provide pharmacologic control of the arrhythmia.[168] The role of amiodarone in PSVT caused by sinoatrial reentry or by enhanced atrial or junctional automaticity has not been evaluated. Regardless of the underlying mechanism, recurrent PSVT may be readily prevented in most patients with low doses of amiodarone (100 to 300 mg/day) with a very low incidence of limiting side effects. However, the advent of catheter ablation, with an opportunity to cure these arrhythmias, will decrease the role of amiodarone.

Paroxysmal Atrial Fibrillation and Atrial Flutter

Amiodarone was found to be extremely effective for the control of recurrent AF and AFl. Episodes were prevented in 87.2% of 172 cases from six reported studies.[9, 150, 205–208]

Amiodarone is particularly effective for the prevention of AF in patients with accessory pathways, as well as for the treatment of the "vagal" type of AF.[211] In contrast, amiodarone is relatively ineffective in the "sympathetic" variety of AF[211] in which long-acting β-blockers may be more useful. The maintenance doses required to prevent AF or AFl were originally considered to be moderately high (300 to 400 mg/day).[212–217] However, several recent studies have emphasized the efficacy of low dose amiodarone to prevent recurrence of atrial fibrillation. Most of these data are from large retrospective studies that demonstrated successful maintenance of sinus rhythm in 53% to 79% of patients over follow-up periods ranging from 16 to 27 months. Doses of amiodarone ranged from 200 to 400 mg daily. Randomized studies have compared low-dose amiodarone with conventional drugs.

Martin et al.[216] compared amiodarone with disopyramide over a follow-up of 16 months, with successful maintenance of sinus rhythm in 79% with amiodarone and 55% with disopyramide. Furthermore, the side effects were significantly less with amiodarone. In another study, Vitolo et al.[217] compared amiodarone with quinidine, with maintenance of sinus rhythm at 6 months in 79% and 46% of patients, respectively.

Amiodarone is relatively ineffective in its oral form in converting chronic atrial fibrillation to sinus rhythm. However, intravenous amiodarone appears to be moderately successful. In a randomized study, intravenous amiodarone (1200 mg/day) restored sinus rhythm in 12 of 20 patients (60%) compared with 25% of patients with quinidine alone.[218] Oral amiodarone therapy may be given 2 to 3 weeks prior to DC cardioversion to prevent early redevelopment of atrial fibrillation. In summary, low-dose amiodarone appears to be effective in preventing atrial fibrillation with a low incidence of significant side effects.

Prevention of Sudden Cardiac Death in Patients After Myocardial Infarction and in Patients with Congestive Heart Failure

In patients who have survived myocardial infarction, ventricular ectopy and poor left ventricular function are predictors of a higher risk of sudden cardiac death.[219–221] The data showing that as few as 10 VPBs per hour was an independent predictor of sudden death led to the idea that suppression of these VPBs by antiarrhythmic drugs could improve survival. A number of trials investigated type I antiarrhythmic drugs. Most of these studies were too small to demonstrate any effect. Finally, the Cardiac Arrhythmia Suppression Trial (CAST) was designed to assess the efficacy of drugs that were potent for suppressing of VPBs (encainide, flecainide, and moricizine) compared with a placebo in patients after myocardial infarction.[222, 223] Encainide and flecainide significantly increased the mortality rate[222] and moricizine increased the early incidence of sudden cardiac death and was ineffective over the long term.[223] This study markedly altered the understanding of the use of type I antiarrhythmic drugs following myocardial infarction and heightened the awareness of the potential proarrhythmic effect of these drugs, particularly combined with recurrent ischemia.[224]

Amiodarone, by contrast, may be a safer and more potent agent. The calcium channel blocking effects and antiadrenergic effects, coupled with class III antiarrhythmic effects, may provide true protection against malignant arrhythmias in patients at risk. Furthermore, the absence of significant negative inotropic effect permits its use in patients with moderately to severely impaired ventricular function.

Amiodarone has been shown to be very potent in its suppression of complex ventricular arrhythmias.[55–59, 146, 196, 225–232] Studies have demonstrated amiodarone's ability to reduce runs of nonsustained ventricular tachycardia and reduce ventricular premature depolarization in a variety of clinical situations. Furthermore, amiodarone appears to have a low potential for proarrhythmic effect when compared with class I and other class III antiarrhythmic drugs.[232–234]

An emerging body of evidence suggests that amiodarone may be effective in preventing sudden death and the results of several large studies should soon be available that will definitively define the role of amiodarone in the patient population following MI. In a randomized, double-blind study, Ceremuzynski et al.[235] compared amiodarone with a placebo in their effects on mortality, ventricular arrhythmias, and clinical complications over a 1-year period following myocardial infarction. The population study was limited to patients at high risk who were not candidates for β-blocker therapy. They did not necessarily manifest complex ventricular arrhythmias. Patients with amiodarone had a significantly decreased incidence of death (6.9% versus 10.7%). There was also a significant difference in cardiac death favoring amiodarone, with the majority of deaths in both groups being sudden. The majority of deaths occurred within the first 6 months. Amiodarone, however, did not decrease the incidence of recurrent myocardial infarction.

In the Basel Antiarrhythmic Study of Infarct Survival (BASIS),[236] 312 patients following myocardial infarction who had complex ventricular arrhythmias on Holter monitoring, were randomized to treatment with individualized antiarrhythmic drugs, low-dose amiodarone (200 mg/day), or a placebo. After 1 year of follow-up, there was a significant reduction in mortality with amiodarone from 13% in the control group and 10% in patients treated by individualized antiarrhythmic drugs to 5% in patients treated with amiodarone. Amiodarone was discontinued after 1 year and long-term follow-up showed that the beneficial effect seen in the amiodarone-treated group persisted for up to 84 months ($p < .024$).[237] This suggests that the beneficial effects of amiodarone during the period of highest potential mortality results in improved long-term survival. There appears to be no rebound following the discontinuation of amiodarone.

The pilot study of the Canadian Amiodarone Myocardial Infarction Trial (CAMIAT) showed a trend favoring the use of amiodarone. Furthermore, it demonstrated the safety of low-dose amiodarone with few significant side effects.[238]

Two large scale trials should be completed in 1995.[239] The CAMIAT study will recruit 1200 patients with at least 10 ventricular premature depolarizations per hour on ambulatory ECG who will be randomized to receive either a placebo or amiodarone. The European Myocardial Infarction Arrhythmia Trial (EMIAT) will enroll 1500 patients with ejection fractions of less than 40% who will be randomized to amiodarone or a placebo. These patients will undergo ambulatory monitoring, but there is no arrhythmia criteria for entry. The completion of these two large multicenter trials should provide definitive evidence for assessing the potential efficacy of amiodarone in patients at risk following myocardial infarction.

Patients with congestive heart failure, both ischemic and nonischemic in cause, have a high incidence of sudden death.[240] In the Congestive Heart Failure: Survival Trial of Antiarrhythmic Therapy (CHF STAT) patients with class III or class IV heart failure and 10 or more ventricular premature beats per hour are being randomized to receive amiodarone or a placebo.[241] Six hundred seventy-four patients are to be enrolled in this multicenter Veterans Administration study and will be followed for 2 years. The sample size will permit analysis for a significant decrease in mortality.

In preliminary studies, therefore, amiodarone appears to have a beneficial effect in reducing sudden death in patients at high risk of lethal ventricular arrhythmias. Large scale clinical trials are currently under way which should provide definitive information on the role of amiodarone in these high-risk patients.

Sustained Recurrent Symptomatic Ventricular Tachycardia and Ventricular Fibrillation

The impact of amiodarone therapy on the survival of patients with sustained recurrent symptomatic (SRS) VT or VF is still only partly defined. The results of initial studies were encouraging. Thus, recurrences were abolished in 53% to 83% of patients in five studies[55, 151, 230, 232, 242] during mean follow-up periods of 10.1 to 21.5 months. However, in other reports,[80, 243] control of the arrhythmias occurred only in 28% and 48% of patients. In all studies, the doses of amiodarone required to prevent recurrences were much higher than those commonly utilized for other arrhythmias. In another study,[151] the mean loading dose was approximately 1000 mg/day and the mean maintenance dose was 700 mg/day, with striking interpatient variations, including patients who did well with 400 mg/day or even less and patients whose conditions were not controlled even with 1000 mg/day. Obviously, higher doses are likely to be associated with more frequent and adverse side effects. In spite of these limitations, amiodarone has several qualities that make it well suited for the treatment of SRS-VT/VF. First, as previously discussed, the antiarrhythmic efficacy of amiodarone is greater than that of other antiarrhythmic drugs. In fact, in all reported series, even those in which results were less spectacular, amiodarone often provided control of SRS-VT/VF previously refractory to several other drugs.[244, 245] Second, the arrhythmogenic potential of amiodarone

is extremely low[1, 229, 232–234] particularly in comparison with other drugs.[246] Third, amiodarone is practically devoid of negative inotropic effects and can be safely used in patients with any degree of ventricular dysfunction. Thus, it is difficult to endorse the recommendation that amiodarone be used only as a drug of last resort, particularly in patients with poor ventricular function, low likelihood of control with other drugs, or no means of assessing drug efficacy. The fear of dangerous side effects, of which no other extremely active antiarrhythmic agent is free, should not justify withholding amiodarone in many clinical conditions.

The separation of responders from nonresponders and the determination of the minimal effective dose of amiodarone would greatly improve the management of SRS-VT/VF, but both problems have proved to be elusive. Results of electrophysiologic testing were conflicting and rather discouraging. Thus, according to some studies,[56, 79, 242, 247–250] the efficacy of amiodarone cannot be predicted with clinical electrophysiologic studies, whereas according to others,[251–261] the electrophysiologic assessment does have some predictive value. From these studies, it appears that a group of patients who will probably remain free of arrhythmia while receiving amiodarone treatment can be identified (those in whom VT is no longer inducible), but this group is relatively small. Additional cases can be identified in which the chances of severe recurrences can be predicted depending on the character of a still-inducible VT (sustained, with severe hemodynamic consequences and a short cycle length). Nonetheless, electrophysiologic testing regarding efficacy of amiodarone seems to have less predictive value than it does with other drugs.[251] Data provided by Holter monitoring are also conflicting.[233, 254, 255, 262–266] In one study,[265] abolition of salvos of VT in patients with SRS-VT who had nonsustained VT during baseline Holter monitoring was a good predictor of long-term efficacy of amiodarone, but other investigators[254, 255] have reported a poor predictive value. As in the case of electrophysiologic testing, the wide variability of data among different laboratories is disturbing but not surprising. If full agreement is not reached regarding the dose of amiodarone and the duration of treatment (among other variables), uniform results can hardly be expected.

The minimal maintenance dose of amiodarone required to keep patients with SRS-VT/VF free from recurrences varies widely (from 200 to 1000 mg/day). Clearly, objective measurement of the minimal maintenance dose would be of the utmost importance, but so far, it has not been achieved. Neither measurement of plasma levels of the drug[55, 132, 153] nor monitoring of reversed T3 levels[58] has proved helpful. Until more reliable predictors of long-term efficacy of amiodarone evolve, treatment of SRS-VT/VF is bound to remain largely empirical.[151]

Sophisticated antitachycardia/defibrillator devices (implantable cardioverter-defibrillator [ICD]) have provided a strong alternative to the treatment of life-threatening ventricular arrhythmias. Recent generation devices have the capability of antitachycardia pacing, low energy cardioversion, and defibrillation. Nonrandomized retrospective analyses have demonstrated a high degree of efficacy in resuscitating patients from sudden death utilizing these devices.

The comparative efficacy of ICD implantation versus amiodarone is currently being explored in the Canadian Implantable Defibrillator Study (CIDS). Patients with ventricular tachycardia or ventricular fibrillation are being randomized to treatment with amiodarone or an ICD. Such a randomized study is required to assess the relative benefits of these two forms of therapy. Until such data are available, either form of therapy appears to be valuable and appropriate in patients with life-threatening ventricular arrhythmias.

Arrhythmias in Children

Amiodarone is remarkably effective for the treatment of pediatric arrhythmias, even in critical cases resistant to other antiarrhythmic agents.[209, 267-270] The complete control of arrhythmias was reported to range between 60% and 95% of patients, irrespective of mechanism, location, and previous response to other drugs. Although mostly used for supraventricular arrhythmias, amiodarone was also found to be effective in refractory, life-threatening VT.[271] In most studies, the loading dose was 10 mg/kg/day and the maintenance dose was approximately 5 mg/kg/day. The latency as well as the duration of antiarrhythmic protection was found to be shorter in children than in adults.[209] The incidence of side effects was remarkably low, and no side effects occurred in children younger than 10 years of age.[269] Amiodarone (in conjunction with digoxin) was successfully used to treat a patient with refractory fetal tachycardia.[272] Amiodarone crosses the placenta and is excreted in breast milk.[273, 274]

SIDE EFFECTS

Amiodarone causes a variety of side effects of which pulmonary toxicity is of greatest concern.

Pulmonary Toxicity

Amiodarone-induced pneumonitis is a diffuse, infiltrative process characterized by interstitial fibrosis and intraalveolar accumulation of foamy macrophages, inflammatory cells, and type II pneumocytes.[275-280] There is some evidence suggesting an immunologically mediated mechanism.[278, 281-283] However, a lipid-storage disorder[133, 276, 284-286] caused by inhibition of the lysosomal phospholipase[287] might also lead to secondary inflammation and fibrosis.[280] Dyspnea, nonproductive cough, chest pain, and fever are the main symptoms. Rales and, rarely, a pleuritic friction rub may be heard. Leukocytosis is common,[280] and blood eosinophilia has been reported in a few cases.[288] Chest x-ray films revealed diffuse bilateral interstitial or patchy alveolar infiltrates, without predilection toward either apical or basilar lung sites.[280, 289] Pulmonary function tests show a restrictive pattern,[275, 280, 290-292] with impairment of gas transfer marked by arterial hypoxemia, hypocapnia, and a reduction in total lung capacity (TLC) and hemoglobin-corrected diffusing capacity (DLCO). Transbronchial or open lung biopsy shows the histologic features previously mentioned. Preexistent lung abnormalities (interstitial densities on chest x-ray films; reduced TLC or DLCO) are predisposing factors.[290] One recent study of 70 patients that specifically excluded those with preexistent abnormalities in TLC or DLCO supported the predictive value of such tests, in that none of the patients developed pneumonitis during amiodarone therapy.[293] However, this has not been supported by others.[294] Treatment of amiodarone-induced pneumonitis involves reduction of the dose in milder cases,[280] or drug withdrawal, with corticosteroids in the more fulminant cases.[280, 295] Some patients who recovered from pneumonitis tolerated a low-dose rechallenge,[290, 294, 296] whereas others did not.[291, 297] An early diagnosis is essential in avoiding fatalities or residual effects, and in this regard repeated chest x-ray films and pulmonary function tests[291] may be useful. The value of computed tomographic scanning of the chest[298] and gallium scanning of the lungs[299-301] is doubtful. Although pneumonitis has been reported to occur as early as 14 days after commencement of treatment,[299] most cases occur after 3 to 12 months and even much later.[277]

The incidence of overt pneumonitis has been estimated to range between 0.07% and 13%[280] of patients receiving amiodarone treatment, while fatalities occurred in 0% to 3.9% in various series.[280] These disparate figures reflect differences in clinical characteristics of treated patients and especially in amiodarone dosage. Although some cases of amiodarone-induced pneumonitis were reported to occur during low-dose therapy,[302] most cases occur in patients receiving high doses, commonly no less than 600 to 800 mg/day.[276, 295, 303] This should be contrasted to the experience in Great Britain,[304] in which only a single case of pneumonitis occurred among 140 patients treated with a mean daily dose of 360 mg during an average follow-up of 2 years, and with the experience in Israel, in which Rotmensch et al.[305] (the first to report a case of pulmonary toxicity) saw this complication in only one patient of more than 400 patients they treated.[303] Furthermore, in most European countries, where amiodarone is extensively used at doses of 200 to 400 mg/day, pneumonitis is certainly uncommon. Placebo-controlled studies confirm that the incidence of pulmonary toxicity is low in patients after myocardial infarction who are treated with low-dose amiodarone.[235-238] Therefore, the much higher incidence reported from some centers in the United States (obviously depending on high doses given to extremely sick patients) has been overemphasized and should not be extrapolated to the general use of amiodarone in all its possible indications.

Using the smallest maintenance dose of amiodarone that allows for control of arrhythmias[25] and avoiding excessively high loading doses are prudent recommendations. As previously suggested,[294, 305] it would be inappropriate to withhold amiodarone from patients with life-threatening arrhythmias for fear of pulmonary toxicity. Kudenchuk et al.[280] suggest that, by patient prescreening and compulsive follow-up, morbidity and mortality from pulmonary toxicity can be substantially reduced.

Thyroid Dysfunction

Amiodarone alters the blood tests used to assess thyroid function: T4, reverse T3, and TSH serum levels are increased, whereas T3 levels are decreased.[306, 307] This seems to be caused by inhibition of the outer ring monodeiodination of T4, which impedes peripheral conversion of T4 into T3. However, the incidence of either hypothyroidism or hyperthyroidism is relatively low.[69, 308, 309] Changes in hormone indexes make the diagnosis of true thyroid dysfunction difficult. Judicious use of sensitive TSH assays, coupled, where necessary, with T4 and T3 assays, will result in appropriate assessment of thyroid function.[307] The following criteria were suggested: TSH level over 26 μU for hypothyroidism, and T4 over 2 mg/dl or T3 over 200 mg/dl for hyperthyroidism. Old age and preexisting thyroid disease seem to be risks for amiodarone-induced hypothyroidism.[304, 306, 310] Hyperthyroidism should be suspected even in the absence of typical symptoms in patients whose arrhythmias reappear or are reaggravated after a successful response to amiodarone.[59] Amiodarone withdrawal may suffice to slowly normalize thyroid function. However, in cases with severe clinical repercussions, thyroid hormone must be given to correct hypothyroidism (while amiodarone can still be administered), whereas antithyroid drugs must be used to treat hyperthyroidism.[311]

Ocular Effects

Dose-dependent corneal microdeposits are found on slit-lamp examination in up to 100% of patients (except children) under chronic amiodarone treatment.[312] After drug withdrawal, the changes regress in 3 to 7 months. Only 1.4% to 6% of patients complain of photophobia, colored halos, or blurring vision.[304, 312] No diminution of visual acuity, color vision defects, or intraocular pressure changes are caused by amiodarone.[312]

Neurologic Findings

A fine tremor of the hands and sleep disturbances are not uncommon. Proximal muscle weakness is seen only during administration of high loading doses.[304] A peripheral neuropathy and extrapyramidal process may also develop.[313–315] Most of these complications respond to a reduction in dose, and discontinuation of therapy is seldom necessary.[304]

Cardiac Effects

Amiodarone may greatly depress sinus node activity, particularly in the presence of overt or latent sinus node dysfunction,[59, 226] as well as during combined treatment with digoxin, β-blockers, or calcium antagonists.[184, 185, 316, 317] The occurrence of bundle branch block has been reported.[226] The proarrhythmic potential of amiodarone is low among antiarrhythmic agents with proven efficacy against ventricular arrhythmias,[1, 229, 232] but cases of polymorphous VT have been reported.[318, 319] However, the role of concomitant class I drugs or hypokalemia should be excluded.[320]

Dermatologic Findings

Skin photosensitivity is common, varying from an increased propensity toward suntan to erythema and edema of sun-exposed areas.[304, 321] These reactions may be attenuated by sunscreen barrier creams.[322] A slate-gray pigmentation affecting predominantly sun-exposed areas of the face[304, 323] may occur after 1 to 3 years of treatment. Skin discoloration may fade over a prolonged period, but it may only partially disappear after drug discontinuation.

Gastrointestinal and Hepatic Effects

Loss of appetite and nausea may occur during administration of high loading doses,[304] and constipation is frequent during chronic therapy. Biochemical alterations in hepatic function are common[79, 304] in patients receiving high doses of amiodarone, but clinically significant hepatic dysfunction is rare. However, death resulting from amiodarone-induced hepatitis has been reported.[324]

Summary

Most side effects experienced during amiodarone therapy appear to be dose or dose-duration dependent and can be corrected (or prevented) by a reduction in the dose.[304] With the exception of pulmonary toxicity, most side effects are tolerable, reversible, and seldom severe. In more than 2000 patients over the last 15 years, discontinuation of the drug because of intolerable side effects was approximately 5%; similar figures were reported by others in the United States[145] when similar doses were utilized. Patients receiving continuous treatment with amiodarone for 10 to 12 years are common. Despite some bothersome side effects, many patients are content to continue with the medication because of excellent control of the rhythm disorder.[145]

CONTRAINDICATIONS

There are few contraindications to the clinical use of amiodarone. It is not contraindicated in congestive heart failure or in patients with dilated cardiomyopathy in whom other drugs are highly arrhythmogenic. It is not contraindicated in patients with ischemic heart disease, coronary spasm, or both. It can be used carefully in patients with intraventricular conduction delay. If this is not the case, amiodarone should be given only after pacemaker implantation, as is also done in patients with second-degree AV block and severe sinus node dysfunction. Amiodarone is not contraindicated in patients with diabetes, bronchial asthma, or renal failure, but it should not be used in patients with overt or latent hepatic insufficiency.

REFERENCES

1. Mason JW: Amiodarone. N Engl J Med 316:455, 1987.
2. Mostow ND, Vrobel TR, Noon D, et al: Rapid suppression of complex ventricular arrhythmias with high-dose oral amiodarone. Circulation 73:1231, 1986.
3. Charlier R, Deltour G, Tondeur R, et al: Recherches dans la serie des benzofurannes. Etude pharmacologique preliminaire du butyl-2(diiodo-3',5'-N-diethilamine-ethoxy-4' benzoyl)-3 benzofuranne. Arch Int Pharmacodyn 89:255, 1962.
4. Vastesaeger M, Gillot P, Rasson G: Etude clinique d'une nouvelle medication anti-angoreuse. Acta Cardiol 22:483, 1967.
5. Charlier R, Delaunois G, Bauthier J, et al: Recherches dans la serie des benzofurannes. XL. Proprietes antiarrhythmiques de l'amiodarone. Cardiologia 54:82, 1969.
6. Singh BN, Vaughan Williams EM: The effect of amiodarone—a new anti-anginal drug—on cardiac muscle. Br J Pharmacol 39:657, 1970.
7. Van Schepdael J, Solvay H: Etude clinique de l'amiodarone dans les troubles du rhythme cardiaque. Presse Med 78:1849, 1970.
8. Rosenbaum MB, Chiale PA, Ryba D, et al: Control of tachyarrhythmias associated with Wolff-Parkinson-White syndrome with amiodarone hydrochloride. Am J Cardiol 34:215, 1974.
9. Rosenbaum MB, Chiale PA, Halpern MS, et al: Clinical efficacy of amiodarone 3S an antiarrhythmic agent. Am J Cardiol 38:934, 1976.
10. Cahal DA: Jaundice and "Cardivix." Lancet 2:754, 1964.
11. Vaughan Williams EM, Polster P: The effect on cardiac muscle of two drugs related to amiodarone, L 8040 and L 8462. Eur J Pharmacol 25:241, 1974.
12. Charlier R, Baudine A, Chailtet F: Recerehes dans la serie des benzofurannes. XXV. Effets hemodynamiques de l'amiodarone chez le chien. Acta Cardiol 22:323, 1967.
13. Charlier R, Baudine A, Chaillet F: Recherches dans la serie des benzofurannes. XXXII. Mode d'aetion de l'amiodarone sur le systeme cardiovasculaire. Arch Int Physiol Biochim 75:787, 1967.
14. Charlier R, Deltour G, Baudine A, et al: Recherches dans la serie des benzofurannes. XXVII. Antagonisme de l'amiodarone vis-à-vis de certains effets cardiovasculaires et metaboliques des catecholamines chez le chien. Arch Int Physiol Biochim 75:82, 1967.
15. Broekhuysen J, Laruel R, Debruck Laruel A: Recherches dans la serie des benzofurannes. XXVIII. Influence de l'amiodarone sur les reserves energetiques du myocarde chez le rat. Biochem Pharmacol 16:2069, 1967.
16. Broekhuysen J, Deltour G, Gislain M: Recherches dans la serie des benzofurannes. XXIX. Influence de l'amiodarone sur le metabolism du coeur chez le chien. Biochem Pharmacol 16:2077, 1967.
17. Baudine A, Chaillet F, Charlier R: Recherches dans la serie des benzofurannes. XXVI. Effets pharmacologiques generaux de l'amiodarone. Arch Int Pharmacodyn 169:469, 1967.
18. Charlier R, Deltour G, Baudine A: Pharmacology of amiodarone, an antianginal drug with a new biological profile. Arzneimittelforschung 18:1408, 1968.
19. Deltour G: Derives hydroxybenzoylbenzofuranniques d'interet pharmacologique et therapeutique. Actualites Pharmacologiques. 21 serie, Paris: Masson, 1968, pp 117–155.
20. Broekhuysen J, Laurel R, Sion R: Recherches dans la serie des benzofurannes. XXXVII. Etude comparée du transit et du metabolisme de l'amiodarone chez diverses especes animales et chez l'homme. Arch Int Pharmacodyn 177:340, 1969.
21. Broekhuysen J, Deltour G, Chislain M: Some biochemical effects of amiodarone. Arzneimittelforschung 19:1850, 1969.
22. Delaunois G, Bauthier J, Charlier R: Effets hemodynamiques de l'amiodarone chez l'animal euthyroide. Arch Int Pharmacodyn 187:265, 1970.
23. Deltour G, Broekhuysen J, Charlier R: Etude du mechanism biochimique d'action d'un agent antiangoreux: L'amiodarone. J Pharmacol (Paris) 1:39, 1970.
24. Petta JM, Zaccheo J: Comparative profile of W3428 and other antianginal agents on cardiac hemodynamic. J Pharmacol Ther 176:328, 1971.
25. Charlier R: Antianginal Drugs. Berlin: Springer-Verlag, 1971.
26. Charlier R, Delaunois G, Bauthier J: Caracteristiques et mechanismes de l'action de l'amiodarone sur le debit cardiaque et systolique chez le chien. Arzneimittelforschung 22:1698, 1972.
27. Charlier R, Delaunois G, Bauthier J: Incidence de l'amiodarone et des quelques agents bloquants sur la contractilite du ventricle gauche chez le chien. J Pharmacol (Paris) 4:57, 1973.
28. Gubin J, Rosseels G, Peiren M: Recherches—de proprietes antiangineuses en serie (dialkylaminoalcoxy-4) benzoyl-l ou-3 indolizines. Eur J Med Chem 12:345, 1977.
29. Charlier R, Richard JC, Bauthier JA: Amiodarone-like haemodynamic and non-competitive adrenergic properties of a benzoyl-indolizine. Arzneimittelforschung 27:1445, 1977.
30. Polster P, Broekhuysen J: The adrenergic antagonism of amiodarone. Biochem Pharmacol 25:131, 1976.
31. Bauthier J, Broekhuysen J, Charlier R: Nature of the inhibition by amiodarone of isoproterenol-induced tachycardia in the dog. Arch Int Pharmacodyn 219:45, 1976.
32. Nokin P, Clinet M, Schoenfeld P: Cardiac-adrenoceptor modulation by amiodarone. Biochem Pharmacol 32:2473, 1983.
33. Gagnol JP, Devos C, Clinet M: Amiodarone. Biochemical aspects and haemodynamic effects. Drugs 29(Suppl 3):1, 1985.
34. Sharma AD, Corr PB: Modulation by amiodarone of cardiac adrenergic receptors and their electrophysiologic responsivity to catecholamines [abstract]. Circulation 68(Suppl 3):99, 1983.
35. Glaubiger G, Lefkowitz RJ: Elevated beta-adrenergic receptor number after chronic propranolol treatment. Biochem Biophys Res Commun 78:720, 1977.
36. Aarons RD, Molinoff OB: Changes in the density of beta-adrenergic receptors in rat Lymphocytes, heart and lungs after chronic treatment with propranolol. J Pharmacol Exp Ther 221:439, 1982.
37. Cote P, Bourassa MG, Delaye J: Effects of amiodarone on cardiac and coronary hemodynamics and on myocardial metabolism in patients with coronary artery disease. Circulation 59:1165, 1979.
38. Remme WJ, Diederik CA, van Hoogenhuyze DCA: Amiodarone. Haemodynamic profile during intravenous administration and effect on pacing-induced ischaemia in man. Drugs 29(Suppl 3):11, 1985.
39. Remme WJ, van Hoogenhuyze DCA, Krauss XH: Acute hemodynamic and antiischemic effects of intravenous amiodarone. Am J Cardiol 55:639, 1985.
40. Kosinski EJ, Albin JB, Young E: Hemodynamic effects of intravenous amiodarone. J Am Coll Cardiol 4:565, 1984.
41. Pfisterer M, Burjart F, Muller-Brand J: Important differences between short- and long-term hemodynamic effects of amiodarone in patients with chronic ischemic heart disease at rest and during ischemia-induced left ventricular dysfunction. J Am Coll Cardiol 5:1205, 1985.
42. Pfisterer M, Burkart F: Effect of short- and long-term administration of amiodarone on ischemia-induced left ventricular dysfunction. Implications for combined antianginal drug therapy. Drugs 29(Suppl 3):23, 1985.
43. Rutizky B, Girotti AL, Rosenbaum MB: Efficacy of chronic amiodarone therapy in patients with variant angina pectoris and inhibition of ergonovine coronary constriction. Am Heart J 103:38, 1982.
44. Lesbre JP, Eloy JP: An open comparison of amiodarone with diltiazem and glyceryl trinitrate in patients with stable exertional angina. Drugs 29(Suppl 3):31. 1985.
45. Nokin P, Jungbluth L, Mouton L: Protective effects of amiodarone pretreatment on mitochondrial function and high energy phosphates in ischemic rat heart. J Mol Cell Cardiol 19:603, 1987.
46. DeBoer LWV, Nosta JJ, Kloner RA: Studies of amiodarone

during experimental myocardial infarction: Beneficial effects on hemodynamics and infarct size. Circulation 65:508, 1982.

47. Singh BN, Jewitt DE, Downey JM: Effects of amiodarone and L8040, novel antianginal and antiarrhythmic drugs, on cardiac and coronary hemodynamics and on cardiac intracellular potentials. Clin Exp Pharmacol Physiol 3:427, 1976

48. Ourbark P, Roeher R, Aziza JP: Effets hemodynamiques de l'injection intraveineuse de chlorhydrate d'amiodarone chez le sujet normal et le coronarien. Arch Mal Coeur 69:293, 1976.

49. Sicart M, Besse P, Chossat A: Action hemodynamique de l'amiodarone chez l'homme. Arch Mal Coeur 70:219, 1977.

50. Schwartz A, Shen E, Morady F: Hemodynamic effects of intravenous amiodarone in patients with depressed left ventricular function and recurrent ventricular tachycardia. Am Heart J 106:848, 1983.

51. van Hoogenhuyze D, van der Burgh P, de Wilde A: Acute effects of intravenous amiodarone in patients with complex ventricular dysrhythmias [abstract]. Am J Cardiol 49:1001, 1982.

52. Morady F, Scheinman MM, Shen E: Intravenous amiodarone in the acute treatment of recurrent symptomatic ventricular tachycardia. Am J Cardiol 51:156, 1983.

53. Barzin J, Freson A: Essais cliniques de l'amiodarone das les affections coronariennes. Bruxelles-Medicale 49:105, 1969.

54. Singh BN: Amiodarone: Historical development and pharmacologic profile. Am Heart J 106:788, 1983.

55. Haffagee CI, Love JC, Alpert JS: Efficacy and safety of long-term amiodarone in treatment of cardiac arrhythmias: Dosage experience. Am Heart J 106:935, 1983.

56. Nademanee K, Hendrickson JA, Kannan R, et al: Antiarrhythmic efficacy and electrophysiologic actions of amiodarone in patients with life-threatening ventricular arrhythmias: Potent suppression of spontaneously occurring tachyarrhythmias versus inconsistent abolition of induced ventricular tachycardia. Am Heart J 103:9S0, 1982.

57. Nademanee K, Hendrickson JA, Cannon DS: Control of refractory life-threatening ventricular arrhythmias by amiodarone. Am Heart 1 101:759, 1981.

58. Nademanee K, Singh BN, Hendrickson JAT: Pharmacokinetic significance of serum reverse 13 levels during amiodarone treatment: A potential method for monitoring chronic drug therapy. Circulation 66:202, 1982.

59. Chialo PA, Halpern MS, Nau GJ, et al: Efficacy of amiodarone during long-term treatment of malignant ventricular arrhythmias in patients with chronic chagasic myocarditis. Am Heart J 107:656, 1984.

60. Singh BN, Vaughan Williams EM: A third class of antiarrhythmic action. Effects on atrial and ventricular intracellular potentials, and other pharmacologic actions on cardiac muscle, of MJ 1999 and AH 3474. Br J Pharmacol 39:675, 1970.

61. Vaughan Williams EM: Classification of anti-arrhythmic drugs. In Sandoe E, Flensted-Jensen E, Olesen KH, et al (eds): Symposium on Cardiac Arrhythmias. Sodertalje, Sweden: Astra 1970, pp 449–469.

62. Elizari MV, Levi RJ, Novakosky A, et al: Cellular effects of antiarrhythmic drugs, remarks on methodology. In Symposium on Antiarrhythmic and Antianginal Drugs with Cumulative Effects. Paris: Sanofi Pharma International Ed., 1980, pp 9–23.

63. Yabek SM, Kato R, Singh BN: Acute effects of amiodarone on the electrophysiologic properties of isolated neonatal and adult cardiac fibers. J Am Coll Cardiol 5:1109, 1985.

64. Yabek SM, Kato R, Singh BN: Effects of amiodarone and its metabolite, desethylamiodarone, on the electrophysiologic properties of isolated cardiac muscle. J Cardiovasc Pharmacol 8:197, 1986.

65. Aomine M, McCullough J, Mayuga R, et al: Cellular electrophysiologic effects of acute exposure to amiodarone on canine cardiac Purkinje fibers [abstract]. Fed Proc 43:961, 1984.

66. Olsson SB, Brorson L, Varnauskas E: Class 3 antiarrhythmic action in man. Observations from monophasic action potential recordings and amiodarone treatment. Br Heart J 35:1255, 1973.

67. Facquet J, Nivet M, Grosgogeat Y, et al: L'influence de l'amiodarone sur le rythme cardiaque et l'electrocardiogramme. Therapie 25:335, 1970.

68. Friart J, Rasson G: Etude des modifications de l'electro-

cardiogramme provoquees par l'amiodarone. Arzneimittelforschung 21:1535, 1971.

69. Pritchard DA, Singh BN, Hurley PJ: Effects of amiodarone on thyroid function in patients with ischemic heart disease. Br Heart J 37:856. 1975.

70. Torres D, Tepper D, Flowers D, et al: QT prolongation and the antiarrhythmic efficacy of amiodarone. J Am Coll Cardiol 7:142, 1986.

71. Debbas NMG, du Cailar C, Bexton RS, et al: The QT interval: A predictor of the plasma and myocardial concentrations of amiodarone. Br Heart J 51:316, 1984.

72. Polikar R, Goy JJ, Schlapter J, et al: Effect of triiodothyronine substitution during amiodarone treatment for arrhythmia [abstract]. J Am Coll Cardiol 7:92A, 1986.

73. Revenko SV, Khodorov BI, Avrutskii MY: Blocking of inactivated sodium channels by the antiarrhythmic Cordarone. Biull Eksp Biol Med 89:702, 1980.

74. Mason JW, Hondeghem LM, Katzung BG: Amiodarone blocks inactivated cardiac sodium channels, Pflugers Arch 396:79, 1983.

75. Mason IW, Hondeghem LM, Katzung BG: Block of inactivated sodium channels and of depolarization-induced automaticity in guinea pig papillary muscle by amiodarone. Circulation Res 55:277, 1984.

76. Varro A, Nakaya Y, Elharrar V, et al: Use-dependent effects of amiodarone on Vmax in cardiac Purkinje and ventricular muscle fibers, Eur Pharmacol 112:419, 1985.

77. Rosen MR, Merker C, Pippenger CE: The effects of lidocaine on the canine ECG and electrophysiologic properties of Purkinje fibers. Am Heart J 91:191, 1976.

78. Wellens HJJ, Lie KI, Bar FW, et al: Effect of amiodarone in the Wolff-Parkinson-White syndrome. Am J Cardiol 38:189, 1976.

79. Heger JJ, Prystowsky EN, Jackman WM, et al: Amiodarone. Clinical efficacy and electrophysiology during long-term therapy for recurrent ventricular tachycardia or ventricular fibrillation. N Engl J Med 305:539, 1981.

80. Waxman HL, Groh WC, Marchlinski FE, et al: Amiodarone for control of sustained ventricular tachyarrhythmias: Clinical and electrophysiologic effects in 51 patients. Am J Cardiol 50:1066, 1982.

81. Shenasa M, Denker S, Mahrnud R, et al: Effect of amiodarone on conduction and refractoriness of the His-Purkinje system in the human heart. J Am Coll Cardiol 4:10S, 1984.

82. Reddy CP, Kuo CS: Effect of amiodarone on retrograde conduction and refractoriness of the His-Purkinje system in man. Br Heart J S1:648, 1984.

83. Kupersmith J, Antman EM, Hoffman BF: In vivo electrophysiological effects of lidocaine in canine acute myocardial infarction. Circ Res 36:84, 1975.

84. Rosenbaum MB: A new clinical and experimental model for studying the effects of antiarrhythmic drugs upon automaticity and conduction. Acta Cardiol Suppl 18:289, 1974.

85. Rosenbaum MB, Elizari MV, Chiale PA, et al: Relationships between increased automaticity and depressed conduction in the main intraventricular conducting fascicles of the human and canine heart. Circulation 49:818, 1974.

86. Chiale PA, Levi RJ, Halpern MS, et al: Effecto de diferentes drogas antiarritmicas sobre un caso de bloqueo de rama intermitente. Medicina (Buenos Aires) 35:1, 1975.

87. Chiale PA, Halpern MS, Nau GJ, et al: Drogas antiarritmicas de fuerte efecto acumulativo en la prevencion de la muerte subita. Rev Latina Cardiol 1:26, 1980.

88. Chiale PA, Halpern MS, Przybylski J, et al: Efectos del amiodarone sobre la conduccion intraventricular en casos clinicos de bloqueo de rama intermitente [abstract]. Presented at the XVI Congreso de la Cardiologia Argentina, Buenos Aires, 1977, p 48.

89. Morady F, Di Carlo LA, Krol RB, et al: Acute and chronic effects of amiodarone on ventricular refractoriness, intraventricular conduction and ventricular tachycardia induction. J Am Coll Cardiol 7:148, 1986.

90. Damato AN, Caracta AR, Akhtar M, et al: The effects of commonly used cardiovascular drugs on AV conduction and refractoriness. In Narula OS (ed): His Bundle Electrocardiography and Electrophysiology. Philadelphia: FA Davis, 1975, pp 105–125.

91. Knippel M, Pioselli D, Rovelli F: Antiarrhythmic drugs and

atrioventricular conduction. *In* Gensini GG (ed): Concepts on the Mechanism and Treatment of Arrhythmias. Mount Kisco, NY: Futura, 1974, pp 163–181.

92. Touboul P, Porte J, Huerta F, et al: Effets electrophysiotogiques de l'amiodarone dans de syndrome de Wolff-Parkinson-White. Arch Mal Coeur 69:855, 1976.

93. Benaim R, Denizeau JP, Melon J, et al: Les effets antiarythmiques de l'amiodarone injectable. A propos de 100 cas. Arch Mal Coeur 69:513, 1976.

94. Morady F, Di Carlo LA, Baerman JM, et al: Rate-dependent effects of intravenous lidocaine, procainamide and amiodarone on intraventricular conduction. J Am Coll Cardiol 6:179, 1985.

95. Charlier R: Cardiac actions in the dog of a new antagonist of adrenergic excitation which does not produce competitive blockade of adrenoceptors. Br J Pharmacol 39:668, 1970.

96. Goupil N, Lenfant J: The effects of amiodarone on the sinus node activity of the rabbit heart. Eur J Pharmacol 39:23, 1976.

97. Gloor MD, Urthaler F, James TN: Acute effects of amiodarone upon the canine sinus node and atrioventricular junctional region. J Clin Invest 71:1457, 1983.

98. Touboul P, Atallah G, Gressard A, et al: Effects of amiodarone on sinus node in man. Br Heart J 42:573, 1979.

99. Castillo-Fenoy A, Valere PE, Tricot R: Identification du potentiel sinusal chez le chien par electrocardiographie epicardique. Arch Mal Coeur 71:334, 1978.

100. Neus H, Nowak FG, Schlepper M, et al: The effects of antianginal drugs on AV-conduction in normal subjects. Arzneimittelforschung 24:213, 1974.

101. Marcus FI, Fontaine GH, Frank R, et al: Clinical pharmacology and therapeutic applications of the antiarrhythmic agent amiodarone. Am Heart J 101:480, 1981.

102. Coutte R, Fontaine G, Frank R, et al: Etude electrocardiologique des effets de l'amiodarone sur la conduction intracardiaque de l'homme. Ann Cardiol Angeiol 25:543, 1976.

103. Touboul P, Huerta F, Porte J, et al: Bases electrophysiologiques de l'action antiarythmique de l'amiodarone chez l'homme. Arch Mal Coeur 69:845, 1976.

104. Waleffe A, Bruninx P, Kulbertus HE: Effects of amiodarone studied by programmed electrical stimulation of the heart in patients with paroxysmal reentrant supraventricular tachycardia. J Electrocardiol 11:253, 1978.

105. Cabasson J, Puech P, Mellet IM: Analyse des effets electrophysiologiques de l'amiodarone par l'enregistrement simultane des potentiels d'action monophasiques et du faisceau de His. Arch Mal Coeur 69:691, 1976.

106. De Roode MR, Talajic M, Quantz M, et al: Amiodarone—a use-dependent calcium channel blocker? [abstract]. Clin Invest Med 9(Suppl B):63, 1986.

107. Talajic M, De Roode MR, Nattel S: Comparative electrophysiologic effects of intravenous amiodarone and desethylamiodarone in dogs: Evidence for clinically relevant activity of the metabolite, Circulation 75:265, 1987.

108. Nattel S, Talajic M, Quantz M, et al: Frequency-dependent effects of amiodarone on atrioventricular nodal function and slow-channel action potentials: Evidence for calcium channel-blocking activity. Circulation 76:442, 1987.

109. Ohta M, Karagueuzian HS, Mandel WJ, et al: Acute and chronic effects of amiodarone on delayed after- depolarization and triggered automaticity in rabbit ventricular myocardium. Am Heart J 113:289, 1987.

110. Mentrard O, Vassort G, Ventura-Clapier R: Effects of antiarrhythmic agents on the Ca conductance and the Na-Ca exchange in frog heart cells [abstract]. J Physiol (Lond) 353:76P, 1984.

111. Nishimura M, Follmer CH, Cigan AL, et al: Amiodarone blocks Ca^{++} current in guinea pig ventricular myocytes [abstract]. Circulation 74(Suppl II):169, 1986.

112. Nokin P, Clinet M, Swillens S, et al: Allosteric modulation of (3H) Nitrendipine binding to cardiac and cerebral cortex membranes by amiodarone. J Cardiovasc Pharmacol 8:1051, 1986.

113. Nishimura M, Follmer CH, Singer DH: Amiodarone blocks calcium current in single guinea pig ventricular myocytes. J Pharmacol Exp Ther 251:650, 1989.

114. Valenzuela C, Bennett PB: Voltage- and use-dependent modulation of calcium current in guinea pig ventricular cells by amiodarone and des-oxo-amiodarone. J Cardiovasc Pharmacol 17:894, 1991.

115. Patterson E, Eller BT, Abrams GD, et al: Ventricular fibrillation in a conscious canine preparation of sudden coronary death—prevention by short- and long-term amiodarone administration. Circulation 68:857, 1983.

116. Lubbe WF, McFayden ML, Muller CA, et al: Protective action of amiodarone against ventricular fibrillation in the isolated perfused rat heart. Am J Cardiol 43:533, 1979.

117. Winslow E: Hemodynamic and arrhythmogenic effects of aconitine applied to the left atria of anesthetized cats. Effects of amiodarone and atropine. J Cardiovasc Pharmacol 3:87, 1981.

118. Massin JP, Thomopoulos P, Karam J, et al: Le risque thyroidien d'un nouveau coronaro-dilatateur iode: L'amiodarone (Cordarone). Ann Endocrinol 32:438, 1971.

119. Flanagan RJ, Storey GCA, Holt DW: Rapid high-performance liquid chromatographic method for the measurement of amiodarone in blood plasma or serum at the concentrations attained during therapy. J Chromatogr 187:391, 1980.

120. Storey GCA, Holt DW: High-performance liquid chromatographic measurement of amiodarone and its desethyl metabolite in plasma or serum at the concentrations attained following a single 400-mg dose. J Chromatogr 245:377, 1982.

121. Holt DW, Tucker GT, Jackson PR, et al: Amiodarone pharmacokinetics. Am Heart J 106:840, 1983.

122. Pourbaix S, Berger Y, Desager JP: Absolute bioavailability of amiodarone in normal subjects. Clin Pharmacol Ther 37:118, 1985.

123. Berdeaux A, Roche A, Labaile T, et al: Tissue extraction of amiodarone and N-desethylamiodarone in man after a single oral dose. Br J Clin Pharmacol 18:759, 1984.

124. Barbey JT, Woosley RL: Pharmacokinetic approach to amiodarone dosage selection. Clin Prog Electrophysiol Pacing 4:310, 1986.

125. Lalloz MRA, Byfield PGH, Greenwood RM, et al: Binding of amiodarone by serum proteins and the effect of drugs, hormones and other interacting ligands. J Pharm Pharmacol 36:366, 1984.

126. Latiny R, Connolly SJ, Kates RE: Myocardial deposition of amiodarone in the dog. J Pharmacol Exp Ther 224:603, 1983.

127. Connolly SJ, Latiny R, Kates RE: Pharmacodynamics of intravenous amiodarone in the dog. J Cardiovasc Pharmacol 6:531, 1984.

128. Escoubet B, Coumel P, Poirier JM, et al: Suppression of arrhythmias within hours after a single oral dose of amiodarone and relation to plasma myocardial concentrations. Am J Cardiol 55:696, 1985.

129. Haffagee CI, Lov JC, Canada AT, et al: Clinical pharmacokinetics and efficacy of amiodarone for refractory tachyarrhythmias. Circulation 67:1347, 1983.

130. Maggioni AP, Maggi A, Volpi A, et al: Amiodarone distribution in human tissues after sudden death during Holter recording. Am J Cardiol 52:217, 1983.

131. Plomp TA, Van Rossum JM, Robles de Medina EO, et al: Pharmacokinetics and body distribution of amiodarone in man. Arzneimittelforschung 34:513, 1984.

132. Latini R, Tognoni G, Kates RE: Clinical pharmacokinetics of amiodarone. Clin Pharmacokinet 9:136, 1984.

133. Adams PC, Holt DW, Storey GCA, et al: Amiodarone and its desethyl metabolite: Tissue distribution and morphologic changes during long-term therapy. Circulation 72:1064, 1985.

134. Andreasen F, Agerback H, Bjerregaard P, et al: Pharmacokinetics of amiodarone after intravenous and oral administration. J Clin Pharmacol 19:293, 1981.

135. Anastasiou-Nana M, Levis GM, Moulopoulos S: Pharmacokinetics of amiodarone after intravenous and oral administration. Int Clin Pharmacol Ther Toxicol 20:S24, 1982.

136. Riva E, Gerna M, Latini R, et al: Pharmacokinetics of amiodarone in man. J Cardiovasc Pharmacol 4:264, 1982.

137. Harris L, Hind CRK, McKenna WJ, et al: Renal elimination of amiodarone and its desethyl metabolite. Postgrad Med J 59:440, 1983.

138. Bonati M, Gallet F, Volpi A, et al: Amiodarone in patients on long-term dialysis. N Engl J Med 308:906, 1983.

139. Fruncillo RJ, Bernhard R, Rocci ML: The biliary disposition of

amiodarone in the rat: Evidence against enterohepatic recirculation [abstract]. Clin Res 32:671A, 1984.

140. Kannan R, Nademanee D, Hendrickson JA, et al: Amiodarone kinetics after oral doses. Clin Pharmacol Ther 31:438, 1982.

141. Canada AT, Lesko JL, Haffajee CI: Disposition of amiodarone in patients with tachyarrhythmias. Curr Ther Res 30:968, 1981.

142. Staubli M, Bircher J, Galeazzi RL, et al: Serum concentrations of amiodarone during long-term therapy: Relation to dose, efficacy and toxicity. Eur J Clin Pharmacol 24:485, 1983.

143. Wilkinson PR, Rees JR, Storey JCA, et al: Amiodarone: Prolonged elimination following cessation of chronic therapy. Am Heart J 107:787, 1984.

144. Siddoway LA, McAllister B, Wilkinson GR, et al: Amiodarone dosing: A proposal based on its pharmacokinetics. Am Heart J 106:951, 1983.

145. Rosenbaum MB, Chiale PA, Haedo A, et al: Ten years of experience with amiodarone. Am Heart J 106:957, 1983.

146. Rakita L, Sobol M: Amiodarone in the treatment of refractory ventricular arrhythmias: Importance and safety of initial high-dose therapy. JAMA 250:1293, 1983.

147. Mostow ND, Rakita L, Vrobel TR: Amiodarone: Intravenous loading for rapid suppression of complex ventricular arrhythmias. J Am Coll Cardiol 4:97, 1984.

148. Kerin NZ, Blevins RD, Frumin H, et al: Intravenous and oral loading versus oral loading alone with amiodarone for chronic refractory ventricular arrhythmias. Am J Cardiol 5:89, 1985.

149. Rakita L, Sobol SM: Amiodarone treatment in refractory arrhythmias: Dose-ranging and importance of high initial dosage. Circulation 64(Suppl 4):263, 1981.

150. Ward DE, Comm AJ, Spurrel RAJ: Clinical antiarrhythmic effects of amiodarone in patients with paroxysmal tachycardia. Br Heart J 44:91, 1980.

151. Kaski JC, Girotti LA, Messuti H, et al: Long-term management of sustained, recurrent, symptomatic ventricular tachycardia with amiodarone. Circulation 64:273, 1981.

152. Holt P, Curry P, Way B, et al: Intravenous amiodarone: An effective antiarrhythmic agent. Am J Cardiol 49:1001, 1982.

153. Boppana VK, Greenspan A, Swanson BN, et al: Clinical efficacy and serum concentrations of amiodarone. Clin Pharmacol 33:209, 1983.

154. Rotmensch HH, Belhassen B, Swanson BN, et al: Steady-state serum amiodarone concentrations: Relationships with antiarrhythmic efficacy and toxicity. Ann Intern Med 101:462, 1984.

155. Heger JJ, Solow EB, Prystowsky EN, et al: Plasma and red blood cell concentrations of amiodarone during chronic therapy. Am J Cardiol 53:912–917, 1984.

156. Heger JJ, Prystowsky EN, Zipes DP: Relationships between amiodarone dosage, drug concentrations, and adverse side effects. Am Heart J 106:931, 1983.

157. Kannan R, Ikeda N, Wagner R, et al: Serum and myocardial kinetics of amiodarone and its desethyl metabolite after intravenous administration in rabbits. J Pharmacol Sci 73:1208, 1984.

158. Lambert C, Vermeulen M, Cardinal R, et al: Effect of the induction of amiodarone biotransformation on ventricular refractory periods in rats. J Pharmacol Exp Ther 238:307, 1986.

159. Nattel S: Pharmacodynamic studies of amiodarone and its active N-desethyl metabolite. J Cardiovasc Pharmacol 8:771, 1986.

160. Abdollah H, Brennan FJ, Brien JF: Effect of intravenous desethylamiodarone in dogs with myocardial infarction and inducible ventricular arrhythmias [abstract]. J Am Coll Cardiol 7:82A, 1986.

161. Latham KR, Sellitti DF, Goldstein RE: Interaction of amiodarone and desethyl-amiodarone with solubilized nuclear thyroid hormone receptors. J Am Coll Cardiol 9:872, 1987.

162. Latini R, Reginato R, Burlingame AL, et al: High-performance liquid chromatographic isolation and fast atom bombardment mass spectometric identification of N-desethylamiodarone, a new metabolite of amiodarone in the dog. Biomed Mass Spectrom 11:466, 1984.

163. Moysey JO, Jaggarao NSV, Grundy EN, et al: Amiodarone increases plasma digoxin concentration. Br Med J 282:272, 1981.

164. Nademanee K, Kannan R, Hendrickson J, et al: Amiodarone-digoxin interactions: Clinical significance, time course of de-

velopment, potential pharmacokinetic mechanisms and therapeutic implications. J Am Coll Cardiol 4:111, 1984.

165. Fenster PE, White NW Jr, Hanson CD: Pharmacokinetic evaluation of the digoxin-amiodarone interaction. J Am Coll Cardiol 5:108, 1985.

166. Oetgen WJ, Sobel SM, Tri TB, et al: Amiodarone-digoxin interaction: Clinical and experimental observations [abstract]. Circulation 66:382, 1982.

167. Nademanee K, Kannan R, Hendrickson JA, et al: Amiodarone-digoxin interaction during treatment of resistant cardiac arrhythmias [abstract]. Am J Cardiol 49:1026, 1982.

168. Wellens HJJ, Brugada P, Farre J, et al: Diagnosis and treatment of concealed accessory pathways in patients suffering from paroxysmal AV junctional tachycardia. In Rosenbaum MB, Elizardi MV (eds): Frontiers of Cardiac Electrophysiology. The Hague: Martinus Nijhoff, 1983, pp 773–797.

169. Maragno I, Sanostasi G, Gaion RM, et al: Influence of amiodarone on oral digoxin bioavailability in healthy volunteers. Int J Clin Pharmacol Res 4:149, 1984.

170. Marcus FI: Drug interactions with amiodarone. Am Heart J 106:924, 1983.

171. Serlin MJ, Sibeon RG, Green GJ: Dangers of amiodarone and anticoagulant treatment. Br Med J 283:57, 1981.

172. Hamer A, Peter T, Mandel WJ, et al: The potentiation of warfarin anticoagulation by amiodarone. Circulation 65:1025, 1982.

173. Rees A, Dalal JJ, Reid PG, et al: Dangers of amiodarone and anticoagulant treatment. Br Med J 282:1756, 1981.

174. Neyroz P, Bonati M: In vitro amiodarone protein binding and its interaction with warfarin. Experientia 41:361, 1985.

175. Belhassen A, Pelleg A, Miller HT, et al: Serial electrophysiological studies in a young patient with recurrent ventricular fibrillation. PACE 4:92, 1981.

176. Waleffe A, Mary-Rabine L, Legrand V, et al: Combined mexiletine and amiodarone treatment of refractory ventricular tachycardia. Am Heart J 100:188. 1980.

177. Saal AK, Werner JA, Greene HL, et al: Effect of amiodarone on serum quinidine and procainamide levels. Am J Cardiol 53:1264, 1984.

178. Shea P, Lal R, Kim SS, et al: Flecainide and amiodarone interaction. J Am Coll Cardiol 7:1127, 1986.

179. Southworth W, Friday KF, Ruffy R: Possible amiodarone-aprindine interaction. Am Heart J 104:323, 1982.

180. Gore JM, Haffajee CI, Alpert JS: Interaction of amiodarone and diphenylhydantoin. Am J Cardiol 54: 1145, 1984.

181. McGovern B, Geer VR, LaRaia PF, et al: Possible interaction between amiodarone and phenytoin. Ann Intern Med 101:650, 1984.

182. Tartini R, Kappenberger L, Steibrum W, et al: Dangerous interaction between amiodarone and quinidine. Lancet 1:1327, 1982.

183. Tartini R, Kappenberger L, Steibrum W: Gefahrliche interaktion zwischen amiodaron und antiarrhythmika der klasse I. Schweiz Med Wochenschr 112:1585, 1982.

184. Derrida JP, Ollagnier J, Benaim R, et al: Amiodarone et propranolol: Une association dangereuse. Nouv Presse Med 8:1429, 1979.

185. Lee TH, Friedman PL, Goldman L, et al: Sinus arrest and hypotension with combined amiodarone diltiazem therapy. Am Heart J 109:163, 1985.

186. Coumel P, Atuel P: Which arrhythmias are specifically susceptible to calcium antagonists? In Rosenbaum MB, Elizari MV (eds): Frontiers of Cardiac Electrophysiology. The Hague: Martinus Nijhoff, 1983, pp 340–348.

187. Przybylski J, Chiale PA, Halpern MS, et al: Unmasking of ventricular preexcitation by vagal stimulation or isoproterenol administration. Circulation 61:1030, 1980.

188. Wellens HJJ, Brugada P, Abdollah H: Effect of amiodarone in paroxysmal supraventricular tachycardia with or without Wolff-Parkinson-White syndrome. Am Heart J 106:876, 1983.

189. Coumel P, Bouvrain Y: Etude clinique des effets pharmacodynamiques et antiarrhythmiques de l'amiodarone. J Agreges 6:69, 1973.

190. Wellens HJJ, Brugada P, Abdollah H, et al: A comparison of the electrophysiologic effects of intravenous and oral amiodarone in the same patients. Circulation 69:120, 1984.

191. Ikeda N, Nademanee K, Kannan R, et al: Electrophysiologic

effects of amiodarone: Experimental and clinical observations relative to serum and tissue drug concentration. Am Heart J 108:890, 1984.

192. Gomes JAC, Kang PS, Hariman RJ, et al: Electrophysiologic effects and mechanisms of termination of supraventricular tachycardia by intravenous amiodarone. Am Heart J 107:214, 1984.

193. Alboni P, Shanta N, Pirani R: Effects of amiodarone on supraventricular tachycardia involving bypass tracts. Am J Cardiol 53:93, 1984.

194. Benaim R, Uzan C: Les effets antiarrhythmiques de l'amiodarone injectable. Rev Med 19:1959, 1978.

195. Installe E, Schoevaerdts JC, Gaddiseux PH: Intravenous amiodarone in the treatment of various arrhythmias following cardiac operations. J Thorac Cardiovasc Surg 81:302, 1981.

196. Kaski JC, Girotti LA, Elizari MV, et al: Efficacy of amiodarone during long-term treatment of potentially dangerous ventricular arrhythmias in patients with chronic stable ischemic heart disease. Am Heart J 107:648, 1984.

197. Acunzo RS, Elizari MV: Efectos comparativos de la 17 MCAA, mexiletina y amiodarona por via intravenosa en las arritmias ventriculares de la miocarditis cronica chagasica [abstract]. Rev Argent Cardiol 95:554, 1987.

198. Klein RC, Machell C: Efficacy of intravenous amiodarone for refractory ventricular tachycardia [abstract]. J Am Coll Cardiol 7:90A, 1986.

199. Mostow ND, Vrobel TR, Noon D, et al: Intravenous amiodarone hemodynamics, pharmacokinetics, electrophysiology and clinical utility. Clin Prog Electrophysiol Pacing 4:342, 1986.

200. Nalos PC, Ismail Y, Pappas JM, et al: Intravenous amiodarone for short-term treatment of refractory ventricular tachycardia or fibrillation. Am Heart J 122:1629, 1991.

201. Kowey PR, Marinchak RA, Rials SJ, et al: Electrophysiologic testing in patients who respond acutely to intravenous amiodarone for incessant ventricular tachyarrhythmias. Am Heart J 125:1628, 1993.

202. Perry JC, Knilans TK, Marlow D, et al: Intravenous amiodarone for life-threatening tachycarrhythmias in children and young adults. J Am Coll Cardiol 22:95, 1993.

203. Kentsch M, Kunze K, Bleifel W: Effect of intravenous amiodarone on ventricular fibrillation during out-of-hospital cardiac arrest [abstract]. J Am Coll Cardiol 7:82A, 1986.

204. Nademanee K, Feld G, Hendrickson JA: Does intravenous amiodarone shorten the latency of the onset of antiarrhythmic action of oral amiodarone in ventricular disrrhythmias? [abstract]. J Am Coll Cardiol 1:630, 1983.

205. Graboys TB, Podrid JP, Lown B: Efficacy of amiodarone for refractory supraventricular tachyarrhythmias. Am Heart J 106:870, 1983.

206. Leak D, Eydt J: Control of refractory cardiac arrhythmias with amiodarone. Arch Intern Med 139:425, 1979.

207. Lubbe W, Mercer C, Roche A, Lowe JB: Amiodarone in long-term management of refractory cardiac tachyarrhythmias. N Z Med J 93:31, 1981.

208. Whecker P, Puritz R, Ingram D, et al: Amiodarone in the treatment of refractory supraventricular and ventricular arrhythmias. Postgrad Med J 55:1, 1979.

209. Coumel P, Fidelle S: Amiodarone in the treatment of cardiac arrhythmias in children: One hundred thirty five cases. Am Heart J 100:1063, 1980.

210. Leelerq JF, Coumel P: The role of the AV node in supraventricular tachycardias. In Rosenbaum MB, Elizari MV (eds): Frontiers of Cardiac Electrophysiology. The Hague: Martinus Nijhoff, 1983, pp 376–396.

211. Coumel P, Leclerq JF: Role of the autonomie nervous system in the genesis of clinical arrhythmias. In Rosenbaum MB, Elizari MV (eds): Frontiers of Cardiac Electrophysiology. The Hague: Martinus Nijhoff, 1983, pp 552–581.

212. Crijns HJ, Van Gelder IC, Van Gilst WH, et al: Serial antiarrhythmic drug treatment to maintain sinus rhythm after electrical cardioversion for chronic atrial fibrillation or atrial flutter. Am J Cardiol 68:335, 1991.

213. Gosselink TM, Crijns HJGM, Van Gelder IC, et al: Low-dose amiodarone for maintenance of sinus rhythm after cardioversion of atrial fibrillation or flutter. JAMA 267:3289, 1992.

214. Estes NAM: Evolving strategies for the management of atrial fibrillation. The role of amiodarone. JAMA 267:3332, 1992.

215. Middlekauff HR, Wiener I, Saxon LA, Stevenson WG: Low-dose amiodarone for atrial fibrillation: Time for a prospective study? Ann Intern Med 116:1017, 1992.

216. Martin A, Benbow LJ, Leach C, Bailey RJ: Comparison of amiodarone and disopyramide in the control of paroxysmal atrial fibrillation and flutter [interim report]. Br J Clin Pract Symp Suppl 44:52, 1986.

217. Vitolo E, Tronci M, Larovere MT, et al: Amiodarone versus quinidine in the prophylaxis of atrial fibrillation. Acta Cardiol 36:431, 1981.

218. Zehender M, Hohnloser S, Muller B, et al: Effects of amiodarone versus quinidine and verapamil in patients with chronic atrial fibrillation: Results of a comparative study and a 2-year follow-up. J Am Coll Cardiol 19:1054, 1992.

219. Bigger JR Jr: Identification of patients at high risk for sudden cardiac death. Am J Cardiol 54:3, 1984.

220. The Multicenter Post-Infarction Research Group: Risk stratification and survival after myocardial infarction. N Engl J Med 309:332, 1983.

221. Bigger JT, Fleiss JL, Kleiger R, et al: The relationship among ventricular arrhythmias, left ventricular dysfunction, and mortality in the 2 years after myocardial infarction. Circulation 69:250, 1984.

222. Echt DS, Liebson PR, Mitchell BR, et al: Mortality and morbidity in patients receiving encainide, flecainide, or placebo: The Cardiac Arrhythmia Suppression Trial. N Engl J Med 324:781, 1991.

223. The Cardiac Arrhythmia Suppression Trial II Investigators. Effect of the anti-arrhythmic agent moricizine on survival after myocardial infarction. N Engl J Med 327:727, 1991.

224. Task Force of the Working Group on Arrhythmias of the European Society of Cardiology: CAST and beyond: Implication of the Cardiac Arrhythmia Suppression Trial. Circulation 81:1123, 1990.

225. Schmidt G, Goedel Meinen L, Jahns G, et al: Long-term efficacy of class I antiarrhythmic agents and amiodarone in patients with malignant ventricular arrhythmias. Drugs 29(Suppl 3):37, 1985.

226. Haedo AH, Chiale PA, Bandieri JD, et al: Comparative antiarrhythmic efficacy of verapamil. 17-monochloracetylajmaline, mexyletine and amiodarone in patients with severe chagasic myocarditis: Relation with the underlying arrhythmogenic mechanism. J Am Coll Cardiol 7:1114, 1986.

227. Neri R, Mestroni L, Salvi A, et al: Ventricular arrhythmias in dilated cardiomyopathy: Efficacy of amiodarone. Am Heart J 13:707, 1987.

228. McKenna WJ, Harris L, Rowland E, et al: Amiodarone for long-term treatment of patients with hypertrophic cardiomyopathy. Am J Cardiol 54:802, 1984.

229. Carrasco HA, Vicuna AV, Molina C: Effect of low oral doses of disopyramide and amiodarone on ventricular and atrial arrhythmias of chagasic patients with advanced myocardial damage. Int J Cardiol 9:425, 1985.

230. Nademanee K, Singh BN, Cannon DS, et al: Control of sudden recurrent arrhythmic deaths: Role of amiodarone. Am Heart J 106:895, 1983.

231. McKenna WJ: Does treatment influence the natural history of patients with hypertrophic cardiomyopathy? Drugs 29(Suppl 3):53, 1985.

232. Peter T, Hamer A, Mandel WJ, et al: Evaluation of amiodarone therapy in the management of drug-resistant cardiac arrhythmias: Long-term follow-up. Am Heart J 106:943, 1983.

233. Nademanee K, Singh BN, Hendrickson JA, et al: Amiodarone in refractory life-threatening ventricular arrhythmias. Ann Intern Med 98:577, 1983.

234. Harris L, McKenna WJ, Rowland E, et al: Side effect of long-term amiodarone therapy. Circulation 67:45, 1982.

235. Ceremuzynski L, Kieczar E, Kryeminska-Pakula M, et al: Effect of amiodarone on mortality after myocardial infarction: A double-blind, placebo-controlled study. J Am Coll Cardiol 20:1056, 1992.

236. Burkart F, Pfisterer M, Kiowski W, et al: Effect of antiarrhythmic therapy on mortality in survivors of myocardial infarction with asymptomatic ventricular arrhythmias: Basel Anti-arrhythmic Study of Infarct Survival (BASIS). J Am Coll Cardiol 16:1711, 1990.

237. Pfisterer ME, Kiowski W, Brunner H, et al: Long-term benefit

of l-year amiodarone treatment for persistent complex ventricular arrhythmias after myocardial infarction. Circulation 87:309, 1993.

238. Cairns JA, Connolly SJ, Gent M, Roberts R: Postmyocardial infarction mortality in patients with ventricular premature depolarizations: Canadian Amiodarone Myocardial Infarction Arrhythmia Trial Pilot Study. Circulation 84:550, 1991.

239. Cairns JA, Connolly SJ, Roberts R, Gent M: Amiodarone for patients with ventricular premature depolarizations after myocardial infarction. Circulation 87:637, 1993.

240. Singh SN, Bennett BH: Ventricular arrhythmias associated with congestive heart failure: The role for amiodarone. J Clin Pharmacol 31:1109, 1991.

241. Singh S, Fletcher RD, Fisher S, et al: Congestive heart failure: Survival trial of antiarrhythmic therapy (CHF STAT) Controlled Clin Trials 13:339, 1992.

242. Heger JJ, Prystowsky EN, Zipes DP: Clinical efficacy of amiodarone in treatment of recurrent ventricular tachycardia and ventricular fibrillation. Am Heart J 106:887, 1983.

243. Di Carlo A, Morady F, Sauve MJ, et al: Cardiac arrest and sudden death in patients treated with amiodarone for sustained ventricular tachycardia or ventricular fibrillation: Risk stratification based on clinical variables. Am J Cardiol 55:372, 1985.

244. Kim SG, Mannino MM, Chou R, et al: Rapid suppression of spontaneous ventricular arrhythmia during oral amiodarone loading. Ann Intern Med 117:197, 1992.

245. Weinberg BA, Miles WM, Klein LS, et al: Five year follow-up of 589 patients treated with amiodarone. Am Heart J 125:109, 1993.

246. Nguyen PT, Scheinman MM, Seger J: Polymorphous ventricular tachycardia: Clinical characterization. Therapy and the QT interval. Circulation 74:340, 1986.

247. Waxman HL: Efficacy of amiodarone for ventricular arrhythmias cannot be predicted with clinical electrophysiological studies. Int J Cardiol 3:76, 1983.

248. Hamer AW, Finerman WB Jr, Peter T, et al: Disparity between the clinical and electrophysiologic effects of amiodarone in treatment of recurrent ventricular tachyarrhythmias. Am Heart J 102:992, 1981.

249. Veltri EP, Reid PR, Platia EV, et al: Results of late programmed electrical stimulation and long-term electrophysiologic effects of amiodarone therapy in patients with refractory ventricular tachycardia. Am J Cardiol 55:375, 1985.

250. Kim SG, Fisher JD, Matos J: Poor predictive value of ventricular tachycardia induced by programmed stimulation in patients taking amiodarone. PACE 5:305, 1982.

251. McGovern B, Ruskin JN: The efficacy of amiodarone for ventricular arrhythmias can be predicted by clinical electrophysiological studies. Int J Cardiol 3:71, 1983.

252. McGovern B, Garan H, Malacoff RF, et al: Long-term treatment clinical outcom eof ventricular tachycardia or fibrillation treated with amiodarone. Am J Cardiol 53:1558, 1984.

253. Horowitz LN, Spielman SR, Greenspan AM, et al: Ventricular arrhythmias: Use of electrophysiologic studies. Am Heart J 106:881, 1983.

254. Horowitz LN, Greenspan AM, Spielman SR, et al: Usefulness of electrophysiologic testing in evaluation of amiodarone therapy for sustained ventricular tachyarrhythmias associated with coronary artery disease. Am J Cardiol 55:367, 1985.

255. Nacarelli GV, Fineberg NS, Zipes DP, et al: Amiodarone: Risk factors for recurrence of symptomatic ventricular tachycardia identified at electrophysiologic study. J Am Coll Cardiol 6:814, 1985.

256. Sokoloff NM, Horowitz LN: Amiodarone: The role of electrophysiologic testing. Clin Prog Electrophysiol Pacing 4:318, 1986.

257. Yazaki Y, Haffajee CI, Gold RL, et al: Electrophysiologic predictors of long-term clinical outcome with amiodarone for refractory ventricular tachycardia secondary to coronary artery disease. Am J Cardiol 60:293, 1987.

258. Schmitt C, Braehman J, Waldeeker B, et al: Amiodarone in patients with recurrent sustained ventricular tachyarrhythmias: Results of programmed electrical stimulation and long-term clinical outcome chronic treatment. Am Heart J 114:279, 1987.

259. Shannon JA, Hammill SC, Gersch BJ: Predictive value of early electrophysiologic testing in determining long-term outcome with amiodarone in patients with sustained ventricular tachycardia. Mayo Clin Proc 66:1114, 1991.

260. Rosenheck S, Sousa J, Calkins H, et al: Comparison of the results of electrophysiologic testing after short term and long-term treatment with amiodarone in patients with ventricular tachycardia. Am Heart J 121:1693, 1991.

261. Fananapaziv L, Epstein SE: Value of electrophysiologic studies in hypertrophic cardiomyopathy treated with amiodarone. Am J Cardiol 67:175, 1991.

262. Morady F, Scheinman MM, Hess DS: Amiodarone in the treatment of patients with ventricular tachycardia and ventricular fibrillation. PACE 6:609, 1983.

263. Marchlinski FE, Buxton AE, Flores BT, et al: Value of Holter monitoring in identifying risk for sustained ventricular arrhythmias recurrence on amiodarone. Am J Cardiol 55:709, 1985.

264. Veltri EP, Reid PR, Platia EV, et al: Amiodarone in the treatment of life-threatening ventricular tachycardia: Role of Holter monitoring in predicting long-term clinical efficacy. J Am Coll Cardiol 6:806, 1985.

265. Veltri EP, Griffith LSC, Platia EV, et al: The use of ambulatory monitoring in the prognostic evaluation of patients with sustained ventricular tachycardia treated with amiodarone. Circulation 74:1053, 1986.

266. Sokoloff NH, Spielman SR, Greenspan AM, et al: Utility of ambulatory electrocardiographic monitoring for predicting recurrence of sustained ventricular tachyarrhythmias in patient receiving amiodarone. J Am Coll Cardiol 7:938, 1986.

267. Kreutzer E, Zarlenga B, Roman MI, et al: Eficacia clinica de la amiodarona como antiarritmico en pediatria. Infancia 1:37, 1979.

268. Garson A, Gillete PC, McVey P, et al: Amiodarone treatment of critical arrhythmias in children and young adults. J Am Coll Cardiol 4:749, 1984.

269. Keeton BR, Bucknall CA, Curry PVL, et al: Use of amiodarone in childhood. Br J Clin Pract 40(Suppl 44):109, 1986.

270. Gillete PC, Zeigler V, Ross BA: Amiodarone in children. Clin Prog Electrophysiol Pacing 4:328, 1986.

271. Coumel P, Fidelle JE, Lucet V, et al: Catecholamine-induced severe ventricular arrhythmias in children: Report of four cases. Br Heart J 15:28, 1978.

272. Arnoux P, Seyral P, Llurens M, et al: Amiodarone and digoxin for refractory fetal tachycardia. Am J Cardiol 59:166, 1987.

273. McKenna WJ, Harris L, Rowland E, et al: Amiodarone therapy during pregnancy. Am J Cardiol 51:1231, 1983.

274. Peen IM, Barrett PA, Pannikote V, et al: Amiodarone in pregnancy. Am J Cardiol 56:196, 1985.

275. Sobol SM, Rakita L: Pneumonitis and pulmonary fibrosis associated with amiodarone treatment: A possible complication of a new antiarrhythmic drug. Circulation 65:819, 1982.

276. Marchlinski FE, Gansler TS, Waxman HL, et al: Amiodarone pulmonary toxicity. Ann Intern Med 97:839, 1982.

277. Suarez LD, Poderoso JJ, Elsner B, et al: Subacute pneumopathy during amiodarone therapy. Chest 83:566, 1983.

278. Russell DC, Paton L, Douglas AC: Amiodarone associated alveolitis and polyarthropathy: Treatment by plasma exchange. Br Heart J 50:491, 1983.

279. Butland RJA, Millard FJC: Fibrosing alveolitis associated with amiodarone. Eur J Respir Dis 65:616, 1984.

280. Kudenchuk PJ, Pierson DJ, Greene HL: Amiodarone pulmonary toxicity: Manifestations, pathophysiology and management. Clin Prog Electrophysiol Pacing 4:358, 1986.

281. Venet A, Caubarrere I, Bonan G: Five cases of immune-mediated amiodarone pneumonitis. Lancet 1:962, 1984.

282. Cantor JO, Osman M, Cerreta JM, et al: Amiodarone-induced pulmonary fibrosis in hamsters. Exp Lung Resp 6:1, 1984.

283. Akoum GM, Gauthier-Rahman S, Milleron B, et al: Amiodarone-induced hypersensitivity pneumonitis: Evidence of an immunological cell-mediated mechanism. Chest 85:133, 1984.

284. Costa-Jussa FR, Corrin B, Jacobs JM: Amiodarone lung toxicity: A human and experimental study. J Pathol 144:73, 1984.

285. Colgan T, Simon GT, Kay JM, et al: Amiodarone pulmonary toxicity. Ultrastruc Pathol 6:199, 1984.

286. Dake MD, Madison JM, Montgomery CK, et al: Electron microscopic demonstration of lysosomal inclusion bodies in lung, liver, lymph nodes and blood leukocytes of patients with amiodarone pulmonary toxicity. Am J Med 78:506, 1985.

287. Downar E, Shaikh N, Butany J: Amiodarone—a potent phospholipase inhibitor [abstract]. J Am Coll Cardiol 3:604, 1984.
288. Darmanata JI, Zandwikj NV, Duren DR, et al: Amiodarone pneumonitis: Three further cases with a review of published reports. Thorax 39:57, 1984.
289. Koslin DB, Chapman P, Youker JE, et al: Amiodarone-induced pulmonary toxicity. J Can Assoc Radiol 35:195, 1984.
290. Kudenchuk PJ, Pierson DJ, Greene HL, et al: Prospective evaluation of amiodarone pulmonary toxicity. Chest 86:541, 1984.
291. Veltri VP, Reid PR: Amiodarone pulmonary toxicity: Early changes in pulmonary function tests during amiodarone rechallenge. J Am Coll Cardiol 6:802, 1985.
292. Liu FLW, Cohen RD, Downar E, et al: Amiodarone pulmonary toxicity: Functional and ultrastructural evaluation. Thorax 41:100, 1986.
293. Finnegan MJ, Faragher EB: Amiodarone and chronic lung fibrosis. Postgrad Med 25:497, 1985.
294. Rakita L, Sobol SM, Mostow N, et al: Amiodarone pulmonary toxicity. Am Heart J 106:906, 1983.
295. Wood DL, Osborn J, Rook J, et al: Amiodarone pulmonary toxicity: Report of two cases associated with rapidly progressive fatal adult respiratory distress syndrome after pulmonary angiography. Mayo Clin Proc 60:601, 1985.
296. Zaher C, Hamer A, Peter T, et al: Low-dose steroid therapy for prophylaxis of amiodarone-induced pulmonary infiltrates. N Engl J Med 398:779, 1983.
297. Raeder EA, Podrid PJ, Lown B: Side effects and complications of amiodarone therapy. Am Heart J 109:975, 1985.
298. Standerstskjöld-Nordenstam CG, Wandtke JC, Hood WB Jr, et al: Amiodarone pulmonary toxicity. Chest radiography and CT in asymptomatic patients. Chest 88:143, 1985.
299. Zipes DP, Prystowsky EN, Heger JJ: Amiodarone: Electrophysiologic actions, pharmacokinetics and clinical effects. J Am Coll Cardiol 3:1059, 1984.
300. Dake MD, Hattner R, Warnock ML, et al: Gallium-67 lung uptake associated with amiodarone pulmonary toxicity. Am Heart J 109:1114, 1985.
301. van Rooij WJ, van der Meer SC, van Royen EA, et al: Pulmonary gallium-67 uptake in amiodarone pneumonitis. J Nucl Med 25:211, 1984.
302. Pozzi E, Sada E, Luisetti M, et al: Interstitial pneumopathy and low-dosage amiodarone. Eur J Respir Dis 65:620, 1984.
303. Rotmensch HH, Belhassen B, Ferguson RK: Amiodarone—benefits and risks in perspective. Am Heart J 104:1117, 1982.
304. Harris L, McKenna WJ, Rowland E, et al: Side effects and possible contraindications of amiodarone use. Am Heart J 106:916, 1983.
305. Rotmensch HH, Liron M, Tupilsky M, et al: Possible association of pneumonitis with amiodarone therapy [letter]. Am Heart J 100:412, 1980.

306. Amico JA, Richardson V, Alpert B, et al: Clinical and chemical assessment of thyroid function during therapy with amiodarone. Arch Intern Med 144:487, 1984.
307. Nademanee K, Singh BN, Callahan B, et al: Amiodarone, thyroid hormone indexes and altered thyroid function: Long-term serial effects in patients with cardiac arrhythmias. Am J Cardiol 58:981, 1986.
308. Sanmarti A, Permanyer M, Castellanos JM, et al: Chronic administration of amiodarone and thyroid function: A follow-up study. Am Heart J 103:1262, 1984.
309. Borowsky GD, Carofano CD, Rose LL, et al: Effect of long-term amiodarone therapy on thyroid hormone levels and thyroid function. Am J Med 78:443, 1985.
310. Weissel M, Weber H: Risk factor for development of amiodarone-induced thyroid dysfunction [letter]. J Am Coll Cardiol 10:717, 1987.
311. Abalovich MS, Gutierrez S, Aszenmil G, et al: Hipertiroidismo e hipotiroidismo inducidos por amiodarona. Medicina (Buenos Aires) 46:9, 1986.
312. Ingram DV: Ocular effects in long-term amiodarone therapy. Am Heart J 106:902, 1983.
313. Fischer C, Bady B, Trillet M, et al: Deux cas de neuropathie peripherique a l'amiodarone. Nouv Presse Med 6:3645, 1977.
314. Duboureau J, Jackquemier JM, Mazieres B, et al: Neuropathie a l'amiodarone d'apparition tardive. Presse Med 12:2766, 1983.
315. Werneau J, Montagne B, Grass E, et al: Atteintes neurologiques lors de traitements a l'amiodarone. IARC Medicale 6:23, 1986.
316. McGovern B, Caran H, Ruskin JN: Sinus arrest during treatment with amiodarone. Br Med J 284:160, 1982.
317. Alboni P, Fischer DM: Blocco sinoatriale in corso di terapia con amiodarone. G Ital Cardiol 3:288, 1973.
318. Sclarovsky S, Lewin RF, Kracoff O, et al: Amiodarone-induced polymorphous ventricular tachycardia. Am Heart J 105:6, 1983.
319. Westveer DC, Gadowski GA, Gordon S, et al: Amiodarone-induced ventricular tachycardia. Ann Intern Med 97:561, 1982.
320. Santinelli V, Chiariello M, Santinelli C, et al: Ventricular tachyarrhythmias complicating amiodarone therapy in the presence of hypokalemia. Am J Cardiol 53:1462, 1984.
321. Walter JF, Bradner H, Curtis GP: Amiodarone photosensitivity. Arch Dermatol 120:1591, 1984.
322. Ferguson J: Amiodarone: A study of cutaneous photosensitivity. Br J Clin Pract 40(Suppl 44):63, 1986.
323. Weiss SR, Lim HW, Curtis G: Slate-gray pigmentation of sun-exposed skin induced by amiodarone. J Am Acad Dermatol 11:898, 1984.
324. Lim PK, Trewby PN, Storey GCA, et al: Neuropathy and fatal hepatitis in a patient receiving amiodarone. Br Med J 288:1638, 1984.

CHAPTER 139

Bretylium Tosylate

Jeffrey L. Anderson, M.D.

HISTORY

Bretylium was introduced for the treatment of hypertension in 1959 but soon became obsolete for this indication because of its erratic absorption and the fact that patients developed rapid tolerance to its antihypertensive effects.[1, 2] Several years later, Bacaner[3] discovered that bretylium protected against induction of ventricular fibrillation in experimental cardiac preparations. Bretylium was subsequently used as an antiarrhythmic agent,[4] but understanding and acceptance of its clinical therapeutic potential was gradual. Marketing approval finally came in 1978.[5] Despite over 25 years of laboratory and clinical evaluation, the mechanisms of bretylium's antiarrhythmic actions and its role in clinical antiarrhythmic therapy continue to be debated.

CHEMISTRY

Bretylium possesses a unique quaternary ammonium structure. Because of its ionic structure, bretylium is highly soluble in water but is taken up poorly by lipid-rich cell membranes.

PHARMACOLOGY

Bretylium tosylate is the prototype of adrenergic neuron—blocking drugs possessing antiarrhythmic activity. Bretylium is a first-line agent for prophylaxis of and therapy for ventricular fibrillation and is a second-line agent for treatment of other life-threatening ventricular arrhythmias. Bretylium has complex pharmacologic actions, including indirect effects through its interactions with adrenergic neurons and direct (cardiac membrane) effects. Its interactions with adrenergic neurons include early sympathomimetic activity caused by norepinephrine release and subsequent adrenergic neuronal blockade. Bretylium's prominent effects on sympathetic neurons are a consequence of selective accumulation in sympathetic ganglionic and postganglionic adrenergic neurons, where it acts to inhibit norepinephrine release by depressing adrenergic neuronal excitability, inducing a chemical sympathectomy.

The proportionate lengthening of Purkinje fiber and ventricular muscle action potentials and refractory period duration are the electrophysiologic hallmarks of its direct (class III) cardiac electrophysiologic effects. The importance of the indirect versus the direct effects of bretylium on its clinical actions continues to be debated. It now appears that its indirect actions may be more important in its initial antifibrillatory activity and that its direct actions are more crucial in its delayed antiarrhythmic effects.

Bretylium is eliminated almost entirely as the intact molecule by the kidneys. No metabolites have been identified in laboratory animals or human subjects.

PHARMACOKINETICS

The development of high performance chromatographic assays for bretylium in recent years has allowed a reasonable assessment of plasma levels and pharmacokinetics.[6–8] After intravenous injection of bretylium in open-chest and intact dogs, serum concentrations decrease in a biexponential fashion, whereas myocardial concentrations increase for up to 6 hours; the ratio of myocardium-to-serum drug concentrations is maximal at about 12 hours.[9] Thereafter, parallel elimination of the drug from myocardium and serum is parallel with a half-life of 10.5 hours (Fig. 139–1).

In human volunteers, intravenous injection of bretylium leads to serum concentrations 10-fold higher or more than those occurring after oral administration.[10] Calculated oral bioavailability is low (averaging about 20% to 25%) and variable.[10–13] Elimination by both routes follows a biexponential curve, accounted for entirely by renal clearance (Table 139–1; Fig. 139–2). In one study,[10] the terminal elimination half-life averaged 13.5 hours after intravenous injection and 6 hours after oral dosing. Similar kinetics applied to cardiac patients after intravenous injection, which was entirely accounted for by renal elimination (averaging 400 ml/min); terminal elimination half-life averaged 13.5 hours.[11] In another study, plasma elimina-

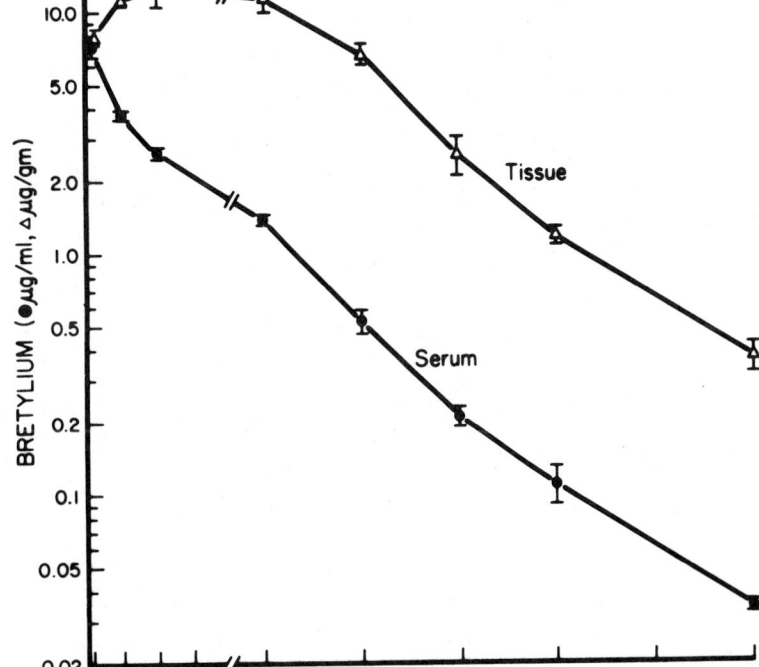

Figure 139–1. Kinetics of canine bretylium accumulation and elimination from myocardial tissue and serum after a 6 mg/kg intravenous injection. (Adapted with permission from Anderson JL, Patterson E, Conlon M, et al: Kinetics of antifibrillatory effects of bretylium: Correlation with myocardial drug concentrations. Am J Cardiol 46:583, 1980.)

Table 139–1. **Summary of Pharmacokinetic Variables**

1. Indications	Ventricular fibrillation and related rhythms
2. Administration	Parenteral (IV preferred, or IM)
3. How supplied	10-ml ampule containing 500 mg of bretylium tosylate in water
4. Bioavailability (oral drug)	20–25% (range, 10%–40%)
5. Dosing (see text for details)	IV Loading: 5–10 mg/kg IV Maintenance: 1–2 mg/min infusion or 5–10 mg/kg every 6 hours
6. Clearance (almost entirely renal) (ml/min/kg)	5–10
7. Volume of distribution at steady state (L/kg)	3–7
8. Elimination half-life (hours)	9–13
9. Percentage excreted unchanged in urine	90–100
10. Protein binding	<5%

IV, Intravenous; IM, intramuscular.

tion of bretylium was thought to be triexponential, with a terminal half-life of 9 hours.[12] Again, renal clearance exceeded the glomerular filtration rate, averaging from 620 to 730 ml/min for oral, intramuscular, and intravenous administration. The volumes of distribution appeared to be very high (450 to 590 L). In still other studies, a terminal half-life of from 7 to 11 hours was reported following oral, intramuscular, and intravenous administration, with renal clearance of 600 ml/min.[13]

Bretylium is negligibly bound to plasma proteins, has no known metabolites, and is not known to interact with other drugs.[10–13] Because of poor oral ab-

sorption and low steady-state drug concentrations (averaging about 200 ng/ml) during therapy,[11] oral administration of bretylium for maintenance therapy has generally been abandoned.

EFFECTS ON PATHOPHYSIOLOGY
Effects on Hemodynamics

Injections of bretylium cause a biphasic cardiovascular response.[14–16] Initially, norepinephrine is released from adrenergic nerve endings, which is accompanied by increases in heart rate and blood pressure. Competitive inhibition of acetylcholinesterase may be one mechanism for induction of norepinephrine release.[17] This is followed within 15 to 30 minutes by reductions in vascular resistance, heart rate, and blood pressure, which are manifestations of sympathetic neuronal blockade. Sympathetic ganglionic blockade is caused by interference with release, but not depletion, of stores of neurotransmitters. Bretylium also interferes with norepinephrine reuptake, without affecting postganglionic adrenergic receptor function.[14, 15]

In patients who had recently suffered a myocardial infarction, bretylium caused average initial rises (at 5 to 10 minutes) in systolic and diastolic blood pressures of 10 mmHg and in heart rate of 24 beats/min.[16] Later (within 1 hour), these measures fell below control values, by 26/14 mmHg for blood pressure and 6 to 14 beat/min for heart rate. No significant changes in right atrial, pulmonary artery, and pulmonary capillary wedge pressures; cardiac index; and stroke-work index were observed.

Effects on Ventricular Function

The effects of bretylium on cardiac function differ from those of most other antiarrhythmic drugs.[18, 19]

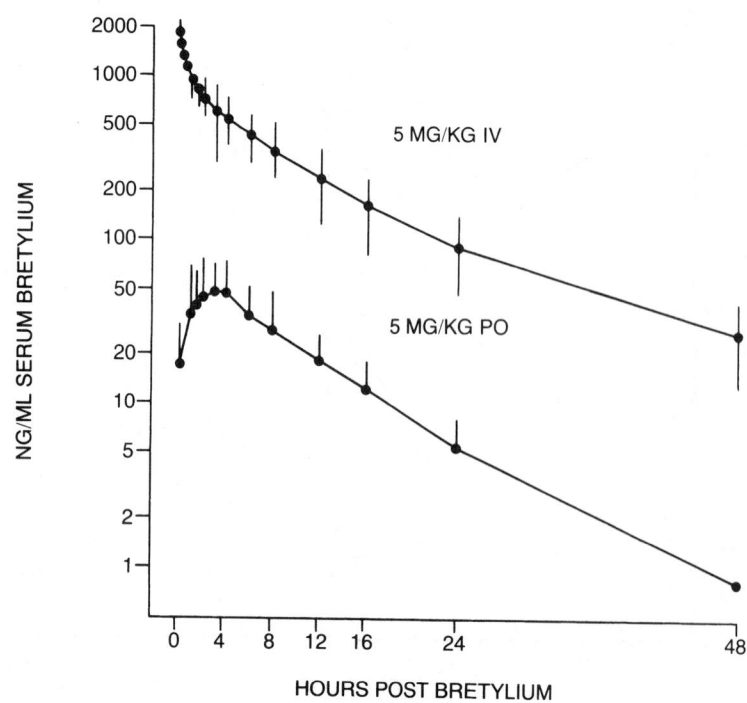

Figure 139–2. Serum concentration—time curves for bretylium (5 mg/kg) given intravenously and orally to 10 normal subjects. (From Anderson JL, Patterson E, Wagner JG, et al: Oral and intravenous bretylium disposition. Clin Pharmacol Ther 28:468, 1980.)

Bretylium leads to an initial positive inotropic effect, ascribed to norepinephrine release and abolished by β-receptor blockade. Later, contractility returns to control levels, but negative inotropic effects are generally not observed in experimental and clinical studies. However, a recent canine study[20] reported a deleterious effect of bretylium on hemodynamic recovery from ventricular fibrillation, which was thought to relate to bretylium's effects on function of the sympathetic nervous system. In contrast, in another experimental model of cardiac arrest, both bretylium and lidocaine preserved cardiac function 5 minutes after conversion, whereas function deteriorated after saline.[21] Bretylium alone prevented ventricular tachycardia or recurrence of fibrillation in all animals.

Effects on Electrophysiology

Bretylium causes electrophysiologic effects that are complex (indirect and direct) and time dependent. Early adrenergic stimulant activity may be important to acute antifibrillatory effects. Later, direct effects, such as lengthening of action potential duration and refractory period,[22, 23] appear in the setting of antiadrenergic activity. Direct effects are important to chronic antiarrhythmic activity and form the basis of bretylium's assignment to Vaughan Williams' antiarrhythmic class III.[24, 25]

Bretylium's direct activity does not affect membrane resting (diastolic) potential, rate or amplitude of depolarization (phase 0), membrane responsiveness, or conduction velocity.[26–31] Spontaneous Purkinje fiber automaticity may be affected by the indirect but not by the direct action of bretylium. However, bretylium characteristically lengthens duration of action potential and effective refractory period proportionately in Purkinje, ventricular, and also atrial fibers,[32–34] primarily by lengthening the plateau (phase 2) of the action potential.[26–31] The ionic basis for this electrophysiologic activity appears to be blockade of cardiac membrane potassium channels.[35] Bretylium also inhibits Na,K-ATPase, although the importance of this to antiarrhythmic and inotropic effects is unknown.[36]

The consistent effect of bretylium on recovery in Purkinje and ventricular myofibers contrasts with the often disparate effects on action potential duration at these two sites by class-I drugs. This may also be one explanation for the arrhythmogenic activity of some of these latter agents.[31]

In an alternative drug classification,[37] bretylium served as a prototype of agents with indirect, adrenergic neuronal activity. The early sympathetic stimulant activity of bretylium increases Purkinje fiber automaticity and may transiently return depressed membrane responsiveness toward normal (hyperpolarization).[38]

Electrophysiologic Actions in Infarcting and Hypoxic Myocardium

In a canine model of coronary occlusion and reperfusion,[39] bretylium limited the early decrease in ventricular refractory period caused by acute coronary occlusion and prevented the abrupt overshoot in refractory period duration that normally occurred with reperfusion. Effects were more pronounced after chronic (1 day) than acute (1 hour) bretylium therapy, suggesting a delayed, direct drug effect in reducing the dispersion of cardiac refractory periods between normal and ischemic (occluded/reperfused) tissues.

The effects of bretylium on conduction of premature impulses during acute ischemia and reperfusion have been studied in an anesthetized dog model.[40] Bretylium caused no further change in the delayed conduction of premature impulses in ischemic myocardium but did delay premature impulse conduction in normal zones, thus lessening the conduction time disparity between the two zones. The conduction of impulses across the boundaries between normal and ischemic zones was also delayed. Increases in the excitability threshold induced by ischemia were largely prevented.

Cardinal and Sasyniuk[41] studied the differential effects of bretylium in normal versus infarcted regions of Purkinje tissue and ventricular muscle in canine endocardial preparations. Infarction prolonged the action potential in the surviving Purkinje network, a condition favoring reentrant arrhythmia. Bretylium reduced this disparity by causing greater prolongation in action potential duration in normal than in infarcted tissue. Maximal effects were delayed for 1 hour, suggesting a direct rather than an adrenergic (indirect) action. Because these and other studies[39–42] have demonstrated the ability of bretylium to reduce the disparity in refractory period and conduction between normal and ischemic tissue, testing of bretylium for the treatment of serious, ischemia-related arrhythmias appears rational.

The beneficial potential of bretylium-induced catecholamine release in hypoxic myocardium has also been suggested.[38] In hypoxic canine Purkinje fibers, bretylium was shown to antagonize the hypoxia-related decreases in action potential duration and amplitude, membrane diastolic potential, and rate of depolarization. Hypoxic changes in fibers pretreated with reserpine (which depletes endogenous catecholamines) were not reversed by bretylium, except that, as in normal myocardium, action potential was prolonged. Thus, the catecholamine release accompanying bretylium injections resulted in membrane hyperpolarization.

Clinical Electrophysiologic Effects

Serial measurements of electrophysiologic variables have been made over a period of 90 minutes in patients undergoing cardiac catheterization or electrophysiologic study (Table 139–2).[43, 44] Small but significant shortening, rather than prolongation, of the ventricular refractory period was observed.[43] This suggests that the indirect (adrenergic) effects of bretylium may be of clinical importance in the early treatment effects on ventricular fibrillation, which typically responds to therapy within 10 to 15 minutes.

Table 139–2. **Early Serial Effects of Bretylium on Clinical Electrophysiology and Hemodynamics***

Measure (n = 10)	Control (0 Min)	Bretylium†	
		Early (15–30 Min)	*Late (75–90 Min)*
Heart rate (beats/min)	69 ± 11	82 ± 19‡	83 ± 13‡
Mean blood pressure (mmHg)	94 ± 11	121 ± 16‡	101 ± 19
PR interval (msec)	174 ± 22	172 ± 28	178 ± 24
QRS interval (msec)	88 ± 10	88 ± 13	87 ± 12
QTc interval (msec)	426 ± 32	418 ± 34	415 ± 29
Corrected sinus node recovery time (msec)	258 ± 105	269 ± 125	281 ± 84
Effective refractory periods (msec)			
Atrial	260 ± 23	248 ± 23	239 ± 25
AV nodal	≤344 ± 85	≤342 ± 148	≤308 ± 70§
Right ventricular	262 ± 21	246 ± 22	249 ± 21‡
Functional refractory period (msec)			
AV nodal	450 ± 76	436 ± 133	419 ± 77§

Data shown as means ± SD.
*In ten stable cardiac patients.
Changes in intracardiac (PA, AH, HV) and surface ECG intervals (PR, QRS, QTc) were not significant.
†5 mg/kg/15 min (load), then 1.5 mg/min (maintenance).
‡$p<.01$ versus control.
§$p<.05$ versus control.
Data from Anderson JL, Brodine WN, Patterson E, et al: Electrophysiologic effects of bretylium in man. Correlation with plasma bretylium concentrations. J Cardiovasc Pharmacol 4:871–882, 1982.

Effects on Ventricular Fibrillation Threshold

The observation that bretylium can dramatically increase the electrical threshold for induction of ventricular fibrillation (VF) in both normal and ischemic myocardium was the primary stimulus for its initial development as an antiarrhythmic agent.[3, 45–47] The effects of bretylium on ventricular fibrillation threshold have been shown to depend on the drug dose, the time, and the model.[9, 48, 49] After low doses of bretylium (2 mg/kg), canine ventricular fibrillation threshold increased gradually, in parallel with the ventricular effective refractory period, to peak at 3 hours.[9] In contrast, after higher drug doses (6 mg/kg), marked effects were evident within 2 minutes and persisted for 6 to 12 hours.[9] Three subsequent studies have shown the importance of adrenergic neuronal interaction to the early increases in the ventricular fibrillation threshold after bretylium administration.[48–50]

When the access of bretylium to adrenergic neurons was prevented in these studies by antagonism of the presynaptic amine transport pump with desipramine or nortriptyline, the early increase in the ventricular fibrillation threshold was prevented or attenuated.[49, 50] Treatment with 6-hydroxydopamine, causing chemical sympathectomy, or *d*-amphetamine, reversing blockade of adrenergic neurotransmission, also reduced the antifibrillatory effects.[49] The demonstration that β-blockers elevate the ventricular fibrillation threshold[51] provides additional supportive evidence for an antiadrenergic basis for at least some of the antifibrillatory effects seen after bretylium administration.[48]

In a canine model of cardiopulmonary resuscitation, lidocaine and bretylium were compared.[52] The ventricular fibrillation threshold increased transiently within 5 minutes of high-dose lidocaine administration and more gradually (within 5 to 10 minutes), but persistently, after bretylium (5 mg/kg).

Chronic (3 hours to 3 days) but not acute administration of bretylium reduced or prevented the induction of ventricular tachycardia by programmed electrical stimulation in a canine chronic infarction model.[53, 54] The slowly developing (direct) drug effects were thus beneficial, and the early or prosympathetic effects detrimental, on postinfarction, electrically inducible ventricular tachycardia.

Bretylium has also been shown to be effective in a conscious canine model of sudden ischemic cardiac death.[55, 56] In this model, ischemia induced by coronary thrombosis in conscious dogs with previous myocardial infarction resulted in ventricular fibrillation in 9 of 10 untreated versus 4 of 10 chronically treated animals ($p < .03$) (Fig. 139–3).[56] In the same model,[23] amiodarone and β-blockers, but not class-I agents, were also effective. In other studies, bretylium

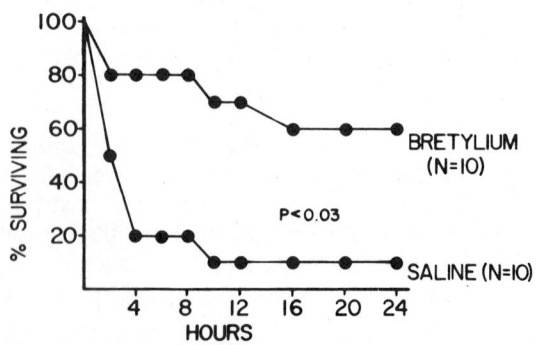

Figure 139–3. Effect of bretylium on survival in a canine model of sudden coronary death (ischemic ventricular fibrillation). Bretylium given as 10 mg/kg every 12 hours for four doses. (From Holland K, Patterson E, Lucchesi BR: Prevention of ventricular fibrillation by bretylium in a conscious canine model of sudden coronary death. Am Heart J 105:711, 1983.)

has been shown to reduce the risk of ventricular fibrillation during reperfusion.[57, 58] The effects of bretylium and amiodarone on reperfusion arrhythmias were compared in a Harris two-stage canine coronary artery ligation model.[58] Cardioversion was required in 4 of 9 dogs in the bretylium group versus 0 of 9 in the amiodarone group ($p < .05$).

Bretylium does not adversely affect internal or external (transthoracic) thresholds for electrical defibrillation, based on experimental studies.[59-62] By comparison, class I antiarrhythmic agents (quinidine, lidocaine) cause either no change or an increase in thresholds necessary for defibrillation.[59-62]

Other Pathophysiologic Effects

The effects of bretylium on coronary blood flow have not been carefully studied. The peripheral vascular effects of bretylium are explained by its adrenergic neuron—blocking activity that results in reductions in peripheral vascular resistance and blood pressure, an effect augmented by upright posture. These vascular effects of bretylium (chemical sympathectomy) may result in dependent pooling of intravascular volume. Otherwise, fluid volume status and electrolytes are unchanged. Bretylium causes no endocrine or metabolic effects and usually does not directly affect renal function. The specific actions of bretylium on renal blood flow have not been studied separately from its general neurovascular effects. Because of its charged structure, bretylium is effectively excluded from the central nervous system by the blood-brain barrier, and it does not usually cause clinically important central nervous system effects. Bretylium's prominent effects on peripheral (sympathetic) neuronal function have been described earlier.

CLINICAL USE
Clinical Experience and Drug Indications

Bretylium is considered a first-line agent for the treatment of ventricular fibrillation, especially following myocardial infarction.[5] It is also indicated for other life-threatening ventricular arrhythmias (i.e., ventricular tachycardia) that have not responded to lidocaine or other first-line agents. Bretylium is not recommended as a first-line drug for the suppression of ventricular ectopic rhythm.[63] It has not been tested clinically for use in acute supraventricular arrhythmias, although it shows activity in experimental models of atrial flutter and fibrillation.[32-34]

Most clinical reports of bretylium usage have involved patients with drug-refractory, life-threatening ventricular arrhythmia, in which it has often been used as a treatment of last resort for ventricular fibrillation.[22, 64-72] These mostly uncontrolled observations have suggested a beneficial effect of bretylium in 60% to 70% of patients.[68] In these studies, antifibrillatory effects have occurred within 10 to 15 minutes,[68] although maximal antiarrhythmic activity (suppression of ventricular ectopic rhythm or tachycardia) may be delayed for several hours.[63-73] Bretylium has shown less satisfactory activity when used for chronic ventricular arrhythmias, including ventricular tachycardia[74, 75] and ventricular ectopic beats.[63, 73]

Controlled Observations

In 27 consecutive cases of resistant ventricular fibrillation attended by a hospital cardiac arrest team, bretylium allowed successful termination by direct-current shock in 20 cases within 9 to 12 minutes.[69] Twelve patients (44%) survived to discharge. In a controlled emergency ward study in 59 patients with cardiopulmonary arrest, bretylium therapy was associated with survival in 35%, compared with 6% of patients treated with other resuscitative measures (including lidocaine) alone.[76] In another report, the outcome with bretylium treatment was inversely related to the time from cardiac arrest to therapy.[77]

In a Seattle Heart Watch study,[78] bretylium was compared with lidocaine in a controlled study in out-of-hospital patients experiencing ventricular fibrillation (n = 146). No significant difference was observed in the percentage of patients converting to an organized rhythm (about 90%), the proportion of patients successfully resuscitated (about 60%), and the percentage surviving to hospital discharge (25 of 74 = 35% of bretylium-treated versus 19 of 72 = 26% of lidocaine-treated patients). A similar randomized study was performed by the Milwaukee County Paramedic System in 91 patients with refractory ventricular fibrillation.[79] Conversion to an organized rhythm was slightly higher in lidocaine-treated than in bretylium-treated patients (81% versus 74%); obtaining a rhythm with a pulse was achieved in 56% versus 35%; survival to the emergency room was 23% versus 23%; and survival to discharge was 10% versus 5%. In studies by the Seattle Heart Watch group,[80, 81] the time to first successful cardioversion, rather than other measures, correlated with survival. Delays to and between shocks, but not absence of antiarrhythmic drug therapy, were associated with a poor outcome.

These and other observations are reflected in revised recommendations for Adult Advanced Cardiac Life Support.[82] Rapid and (if necessary) repeated electrical shock is considered the treatment of choice for ventricular fibrillation. Epinephrine is recommended as the first adjunctive medical therapy in cardioversion-resistant patients. Lidocaine is recommended as the first antiarrhythmic drug of choice in managing ventricular fibrillation and tachycardia because it appears to be as efficacious as bretylium but is safer. Bretylium is recommended for ventricular fibrillation and pulseless ventricular tachycardia when arrhythmia persists despite epinephrine and lidocaine administration and repeated cardioversions.

Other Indications

Torsade de pointes ventricular tachycardia is an unusual ventricular arrhythmia associated with heterogeneous, delayed repolarization and a prolonged QT interval that may lead to syncope or sudden death.[83, 84] The effects of bretylium on disparate recovery periods and catecholamine release might be beneficial. In this setting, bretylium has been successful in many but not in all cases and may be considered a second-line drug in selected cases of torsade de pointes. Bretylium protects the hypothermic ventricle with delayed repolarization in some models of experimentally induced ventricular fibrillation,[85–88] but it has not been well-studied in clinical trials for this indication.

Limited information from a few clinical trials[63, 73] suggests that bretylium is a relatively weak agent for suppression of ventricular ectopic activity and is generally not indicated for ventricular ectopic beats except when prevention of ventricular fibrillation is the primary therapeutic goal.

Bretylium has been tested as prophylactic therapy against ventricular fibrillation in acute myocardial infarction.[89–91] Although associated with a low incidence of ventricular fibrillation in observational studies,[89] its use has been associated with a higher incidence of clinically significant hypotension than that reported with either lidocaine or no therapy.[90, 91] For this reason, lidocaine rather than bretylium is currently preferred when prophylactic therapy for ventricular fibrillation is given to a patient experiencing acute myocardial infarction.

Bretylium was among several agents tested against polymorphous ventricular tachycardia associated with acute myocardial infarction in 11 patients.[92] This arrhythmia proved generally resistant to lidocaine, procainamide, and bretylium (none of five responded), although four responded to intravenous amiodarone. Bretylium was compared with lidocaine and saline in the prevention of ventricular fibrillation after aortic cross-clamp release in coronary artery bypass surgery.[93] The incidence of ventricular fibrillation among 33 randomized patients was 91% after saline, 64% after lidocaine, but only 36% after bretylium ($p < .01$).

Adverse Effects, Precautions, and Contraindications

The precautions regarding and adverse effects of bretylium are related primarily to its modification of adrenergic function. Initial catecholamine release may be associated with transient increases in heart rate and blood pressure that are usually mild but variable.[10, 16] A transient increase in ventricular ectopic beats may occur, and, rarely, sustained ventricular tachycardia or fibrillation has appeared shortly after drug administration.[94] Anxiety, excitement, flushing, substernal pressure, headache, and angina pectoris are other symptoms occasionally associated with catecholamine release.

Hypotension and postural hypotension often accompany bretylium therapy and may begin within 15 minutes. Hypotension has required drug discontinuation in about 10% of patients.[5, 64, 91] Because bretylium regularly causes postural hypotension, patients should remain supine during and after administration of the drug until blood pressure stabilizes. Bradycardia may also result from sympathetic blockade after bretylium. Tolerance may occur to a variable degree after several days. Supine hypotension is less severe but occurs to some extent in at least one half of patients. Asymptomatic hypotension is generally untreated unless severe (i.e., systolic pressure <80 mmHg). In patients who are relatively hypovolemic, volume replacement should be given. If supine systolic pressure falls below 75 mmHg, an infusion of dopamine or norepinephrine may be required to raise blood pressure. Cautious dosing with pressors should be performed because bretylium may enhance pressor response in a manner suggesting postdenervation hypersensitivity.

Partial pharmacologic reversal of hypotension has been accomplished with protriptyline, a secondary amine antidepressant.[95] Protriptyline, 5 to 10 mg every 6 to 8 hours, may be given to symptomatic hypotensive patients requiring continued bretylium therapy.[11, 95]

A patient with a fixed cardiac output caused by severe aortic stenosis or pulmonary hypertension may be unable to compensate for the peripheral vasodilatation caused by bretylium. In this situation, bretylium should be avoided, if possible, or should be given with vasoconstrictor amines, if needed, to support blood pressure. Ominous hypotension and circulatory failure may rarely develop in patients with severely compromised cardiac function or shock, in whom blood pressure is dependent on sympathetic stimulation.[91]

The initial release of norepinephrine caused by bretylium may aggravate digitalis toxicity and should be avoided in arrhythmias potentially related to digitalis intoxication. However, in an animal model of digitalis cardiotoxicity, bretylium exerted a beneficial effect ascribed to its antiadrenergic action.[96] Case reports of the beneficial effects of bretylium use in patients have also appeared.[97]

Nausea, vomiting, or retching have been reported in about 10% of patients. These effects are usually related to excessively rapid intravenous injections (<8 minutes).

Because bretylium is principally excreted via the kidneys, accumulation may occur in patients with advanced renal failure.[98, 99] In these patients, maintenance dosage should be reduced, and maintenance intervals should be increased.[99]

Intramuscular bretylium may cause irritation at injection sites, which should be rotated if this route is used. The safety of bretylium in children and during pregnancy has not been established. In one case, pregnancy, delivery, and breast-feeding were uncomplicated in a woman with long QT syndrome receiving long-term oral bretylium, and no side effects were observed in the infant.[100]

Additional adverse reactions occasionally to rarely reported after bretylium administration include diarrhea, flushing, anxiety, dyspnea, diaphoresis, conjunctivitis, and nasal stuffiness.[10] Renal dysfunction, emotional lability, lethargy, and macular rash have also been reported, but the relationship of bretylium to these reactions has not been clearly established. There are no absolute contraindications to the use of bretylium in the treatment of ventricular fibrillation or refractory, life-threatening ventricular arrhythmias.

Interference with Other Drugs

Bretylium is not metabolized and not significantly bound to plasma proteins.[10–13] Not surprisingly, pharmacologic interactions with other drugs have not been described. However, electrophysiologic interactions may occur, based on the indirect and direct effects of bretylium. For example, bretylium may enhance the response to catecholamine infusions, potentially exacerbate digitalis-induced arrhythmias, and interact electrophysiologically with other agents, such as quinidine.[101] Because bretylium is eliminated intact by active renal excretion, accumulation may occur in patients with advanced renal failure (especially when creatinine clearance is less than 25 ml/min).[98, 99] If prolonged administration is required, maintenance dosing should be reduced when infusions are given, or injection intervals should be increased. Dialysis increases bretylium clearance twofold. Hepatic dysfunction and heart failure are not known to change the pharmacokinetics of bretylium except to the extent that renal clearance is changed.

Dosage, Administration, and Cost

Bretylium is commercially supplied as either a trade-name drug (Bretylol, Dupont Critical Care) or a generic drug in 10-ml ampules containing 500 mg of bretylium tosylate in water for intravenous or intramuscular injection. One ampule contains a dose of 5 to 10 mg/kg body weight for a typical patient. The hospital pharmacy cost of Bretylol is approximately $6.00 per ampule. Other sources now supply bretylium for as little as $2.00 per dose.

Bretylium should be administered in a monitored, critical-care setting. For ventricular fibrillation and hemodynamically unstable ventricular tachycardia, an initial dose of 5 mg/kg is given undiluted by rapid intravenous injection together with other resuscitative measures. If ventricular fibrillation persists, the dosage may be increased to 10 mg/kg and repeated, together with other measures. There is comparatively little experience with total doses of higher than 30 mg/kg.

When hemodynamically stable ventricular arrhythmias require therapy, one ampule of bretylium is diluted at least fourfold with 5% dextrose or physiologic sodium chloride, to a minimum of 50 ml. The diluted solution should be administered to a dose of 5 to 10 mg/kg body weight over a period of at least 8 minutes (preferably, 15 to 30 minutes) to prevent nausea and vomiting. Subsequent doses may be given at 1- to 2-hour intervals if the arrhythmia persists.

For maintenance therapy, a diluted solution of bre-

tylium may be administered at a constant infusion at a rate of 1 to 2 or 3 mg/min. Alternatively, a dose of 5 to 10 mg/kg may be administered by slow injection (i.e., over 10 to 30 minutes) every 6 hours.

Intravenous therapy is preferred whenever possible. If intramuscular therapy is necessary, 5 to 10 mg/kg is given as an undiluted dose. Injection sites should be rotated, and major nerve territories should be avoided.

REFERENCES

1. Boura ALA, Green AF, McCoubrey A, et al: Darenthin: Hypotensive agent of a new type. Lancet 1:17, 1959.
2. Dollery CT, Emslie-Smith D, McMichael J: Bretylium tosylate in the treatment of hypertension. Lancet 2:296, 1960.
3. Bacaner MB: Bretylium tosylate for suppression of induced ventricular fibrillation. Am J Cardiol 17:528, 1966.
4. Bacaner MB: Treatment of ventricular fibrillation and other acute arrhythmias with bretylium tosylate. Am J Cardiol 21:530, 1968.
5. Bretylium (Bretylol) for ventricular arrhythmias [editorial review]. Med Lett 20:105, 1978.
6. Patterson E, Stetson P, Lucchesi BR: Sensitive gas chromatographic assay for the quantitation of bretylium in plasma, urine, and myocardial tissue. J Chromatogr 181:33, 1980.
7. Lai CM, Kamath BL, Carter JE, et al: GLC determination of bretylium in biological fluids. J Pharmacol Sci 69:681, 1980.
8. Théôret Y, Varin F: Simple, rapid and selective method using high-performance liquid chromatography for the determination of bretylium in plasma. J Chromatogr 575:162, 1992.
9. Anderson JL, Patterson E, Conlon M, et al: Kinetics of antifibrillatory effects of bretylium: Correlation with myocardial drug concentrations. Am J Cardiol 46:583, 1980.
10. Anderson JL, Patterson E, Wagner JG, et al: Oral and intravenous bretylium disposition. Clin Pharmacol Ther 28:468, 1980.
11. Anderson JL, Patterson E, Wagner JG, et al: Clinical pharmacokinetics of intravenous and oral bretylium tosylate in survivors of ventricular tachycardia or fibrillation. J Cardiovasc Pharmacol 3:485, 1981.
12. Garrett ER, Green JR Jr, Bialer M: Bretylium pharmacokinetics and bioavailabilities in man with various doses and modes of administration. Biopharm Drug Dispos 3:129, 1982.
13. Rapeport WG: Clinical pharmacokinetics of bretylium. Clin Pharmacokinet 10:248, 1985.
14. Boura ALA, Green AF: The actions of bretylium: Adrenergic neurone blocking and other effects. Br J Pharmacol 14:536, 1959.
15. Gokhale SD, Gulati OD, Kelkar VV: Mechanism of the initial adrenergic effects of bretylium and guanethidine. Br J Pharmacol 20:362, 1963.
16. Chatterjee K, Mandel WJ, Vyden JK, et al: Cardiovascular effects of bretylium tosylate in acute myocardial infarction. JAMA 223:757, 1973.
17. Schreiber G, Sokolovsky M: Competitive inhibition of acetylcholinesterase by bretylium: Possible mechanism for its induction of norepinephrine release. J Cardiovasc Pharmacol 7:1065, 1985.
18. Markis JE, Koch-Weser J: Characteristics and mechanism of inotropic and chronotropic actions of bretylium tosylate. J Pharmacol Exp Ther 178:94, 1978.
19. Hammermeister KE, Boerth RC, Warbasse JR: The comparative inotropic effects of six clinically used antiarrhythmic agents. Am Heart J 84:643, 1972.
20. Euler DE, Zeman TW, Wallock ME, et al: Deleterious effects of bretylium on hemodynamic recovery from ventricular fibrillation. Am Heart J 112:25, 1986.
21. Vachiery JL, Reuse C, Blecic S, et al: Bretylium tosylate versus lidocaine in experimental cardiac arrest. Am J Emerg Med 8:492, 1990.
22. Heissenbuttel RH, Bigger JT: Bretylium tosylate: A newly

available antiarrhythmic drug for ventricular arrhythmias. Ann Intern Med 91:229, 1979.

23. Patterson E, Lucchesi BR: Bretylium: A prototype for future development of antidysrhythmic agents. Am Heart J 106:426, 1983.

24. Vaughan-Williams EM: A classification of antiarrhythmic actions reassessed after a decade of new drugs. J Clin Pharmacol 24:129, 1984.

25. Anderson JL: Adrenergic neurone—blocking drugs as class III antiarrhythmic agents: Focus on bretylium. *In* Singh BN (ed): Control of Cardiac Arrhythmias by Lengthening Repolarization. Mount Kisco, NY: Futura Press, 1988, pp 315–351.

26. Bigger JT Jr, Jaffe CC: The effect of bretylium tosylate on the electrophysiologic properties of ventricular muscle and Purkinje fibers. Am J Cardiol 27:82, 1971.

27. Wit AL, Steiner C, Damato AN: Electrophysiologic effects of bretylium tosylate on single fibers of the canine specialized conducting system and ventricle. J Pharmacol Exp Ther 173:344, 1970.

28. Cervoni P, Ellis CH, Maxwell RA: The antiarrhythmic action of bretylium in normal, reserpine-pretreated, and chronically denervated dog hearts. Arch Int Pharmacodyn Ther 190:91, 1971.

29. Waxman MB, Wallace AG: Electrophysiologic mechanisms of bretylium tosylate on the heart. J Pharmacol Exp Ther 183:264, 1972.

30. Namm DH, Wang CM, Sayad S, et al: Effects of bretylium on rat cardiac muscle: The electrophysiological effects and its uptake and binding in normal and immunosympathectomized rat hearts. J Pharmacol Exp Ther 193:194, 1974.

31. Varro A, Nakaya Y, Elharrar V, et al: Effect of antiarrhythmic drugs on the cycle length—dependent action potential duration in dog Purkinje and ventricular muscle fibers. J Cardiovasc Pharmacol 8:178, 1986.

32. Mirro MJ, Webel RR, Kelly KJ, et al: Electrophysiologic properties of bretylium tosylate on atrial myocardium. J Cardiovasc Pharmacol 3:1312, 1981.

33. Boyden PA: Effects of pharmacologic agents on induced atrial flutter in dogs with right atrial enlargement. J Cardiovasc Pharmacol 8:170, 1986.

34. Goldberger AL, Pavelec RS: Vagally mediated atrial fibrillation in dogs: Conversion with bretylium tosylate. Int J Cardiol 13:47, 1986.

35. Bacaner MB, Clay JR, Shrier A, et al: Potassium channel blockade: A mechanism for suppressing ventricular fibrillation. Proc Natl Acad Sci USA 83:2223, 1986.

36. Tiku PE, Nowell PT: Selective inhibition of K(+)-stimulation of Na, K-ATPase by bretylium. Br J Pharmacol 104:895, 1991.

37. Goldberger AL, Curtis GP: An autonomic classification of antiarrhythmic drugs. J Electrocardiol 15:397, 1982.

38. Nishimura M, Watanabe Y: Membrane action and catecholamine release action of bretylium tosylate in normoxic and hypoxic canine Purkinje fibers. J Am Coll Cardiol 2:287, 1983.

39. Gibson JK, Stewart JR, Li YP, et al: Electrophysiologic effects of bretylium tosylate on the canine heart during coronary artery occlusion and reperfusion. J Cardiovasc Pharmacol 5:517, 1983.

40. Fujimoto T, Hamamoto H, Peter T, et al: Electrophysiologic effects of bretylium on canine ventricular muscle during acute ischemia and reperfusion. Am Heart J 105:966, 1983.

41. Cardinal R, Sasyniuk BI: Electrophysiological effects of bretylium tosylate on subendocardial Purkinje fibers from infarcted canine hearts. J Pharmacol Exp Ther 204:159, 1978.

42. Inoue H, Toda I, Nozaki A, et al: Effects of bretylium tosylate on inhomogeneity of refractoriness and ventricular fibrillation threshold in canine heart with quinidine-induced long QT interval. Cardiovasc Res 19:655, 1985.

43. Anderson JL, Brodine WN, Patterson E, et al: Electrophysiologic effects of bretylium in man. Correlation with plasma bretylium concentrations. J Cardiovasc Pharmacol 4:871, 1982.

44. Touboul P, Porte J, Huerta F, et al: Etude des proprietes electrophysiologiques du tosylate de bretylium chez l'homme. Arch Mal Coeur Vaiss 69:503, 1976.

45. Bacaner MB: Quantitative comparison of bretylium with other antifibrillatory drugs. Am J Cardiol 21:504, 1968.

46. Bacaner MB, Schrienemachers D: Bretylium tosylate for suppression of ventricular fibrillation after experimental myocardial infarction. Nature 220:494, 1968.

47. Kniffen FJ, Lomas TE, Counsell RE, et al: The antiarrhythmic and antifibrillatory actions of bretylium and its o-iodobenzyl trimethyl ammonium analog, UM 360. J Pharmacol Exp Ther 192:120, 1975.

48. Euler DE, Scanlon PJ: Mechanism of the effect of bretylium on the ventricular fibrillation threshold in dogs. Am J Cardiol 55:1396, 1985.

49. Frame VB, Wang HH: Importance of interaction with adrenergic neurons for antifibrillatory action of bretylium in the dog. J Cardiovasc Pharmacol 8:336, 1986.

50. Kopia GA, Lucchesi BR: Antifibrillatory action of bretylium: Role of the sympathetic nervous system. Pharmacology 34:37, 1987.

51. Anderson JL, Rodier HE, Green LS: Comparative effects of beta-adrenergic blocking drugs on experimental ventricular fibrillation threshold. Am J Cardiol 51:1196, 1983.

52. Chow MS, Kluger J, DiPersio DM, et al: Antifibrillatory effects of lidocaine and bretylium immediately postcardiopulmonary resuscitation. Am Heart J 110:938, 1985.

53. Patterson E, Gibson JK, Lucchesi BR: Prevention of chronic canine ventricular tachyarrhythmias with bretylium tosylate. Circulation 64:1045, 1981.

54. Patterson E, Gibson JK, Lucchesi BR: Postmyocardial infarction reentrant ventricular arrhythmias in conscious dogs: Suppression by bretylium tosylate. J Pharmacol Exp Ther 216:453, 1981.

55. Patterson E, Holland K, Eller BT, et al: Ventricular fibrillation resulting from ischemia at a site remote from previous myocardial infarction. A conscious canine model of sudden coronary death. Am J Cardiol 50:1414, 1982.

56. Holland K, Patterson E, Lucchesi BR: Prevention of ventricular fibrillation by bretylium in a conscious canine model of sudden coronary death. Am Heart J 105:711, 1983.

57. Wenger TL, Lederman L, Starmer CF, et al: A method for quantitating antifibrillatory effects of drugs after coronary reperfusion in dogs: Improved outcome with bretylium. Circulation 69:142, 1984.

58. Rosalion A, Snow NJ, Horrigan TP, et al: Amiodarone versus bretylium for suppression of reperfusion arrhythmias in dogs. Ann Thorac Surg 51:85, 1991.

59. Babbs DF, Yim GKW, Whistler SJ, et al: Elevation of ventricular defibrillation threshold in dogs by antiarrhythmic drugs. Am Heart J 98:345, 1979.

60. Koo CC, Allen JD, Pantridge JF: Lack of effect of bretylium tosylate on electrical ventricular defibrillation in a controlled study. Cardiovasc Res 18:762, 1984.

61. Kerber RE, Pandian NG, Jensen SR, et al: Effect of lidocaine and bretylium on energy requirements for transthoracic defibrillation: Experimental studies. J Am Coll Cardiol 7:397, 1986.

62. Dorian P, Fain ES, Davy JM, et al: Effect of quinidine and bretylium on defibrillation energy requirements. Am Heart J 112:19, 1986.

63. Duff HJ, Roden DM, Yacobi A, et al: Bretylium: Relations between plasma concentrations and pharmacologic actions in high-frequency ventricular arrhythmias. Am J Cardiol 55:395, 1985.

64. Koch-Weser J: Drug therapy: Bretylium. N Engl J Med 300:473, 1979.

65. Dhurandhar RW, Teasdale SJ, Mahon WA: Bretylium tosylate in the management of refractory ventricular fibrillation. Can Med Assoc J 105:161, 1971.

66. Sanna G, Archidiacono R: Chemical ventricular defibrillation of the human heart with bretylium tosylate. Am J Cardiol 32:982, 1973.

67. Terry G, Vellani CW, Higgins MR, et al: Bretylium tosylate in the treatment of refractory ventricular fibrillation complicating myocardial infarction. Br Heart J 32:21, 1970.

68. Dhurandhar RW, Pickron J, Goldman AM: Bretylium tosylate in the management of recurrent ventricular fibrillation complicating acute myocardial infarction. Heart Lung 9:265, 1980.

69. Holder DA, Sniderman AD, Fraser G, et al: Experience with bretylium tosylate by a hospital cardiac arrest team. Circulation 55:541, 1966.

70. Castaneda AR, Bacaner MB: Effect of bretylium tosylate on the prevention and treatment of postoperative arrhythmias. Am J Cardiol 25:461, 1970.
71. Day HW, Bacaner MB: Use of bretylium tosylate in the management of acute myocardial infarction. Am J Cardiol 21:530, 1968.
72. Bernstein JG, Koch-Weser J: Effectiveness of bretylium tosylate against refractory ventricular arrhythmias. Circulation 45:1024, 1972.
73. Romhilt DW, Bloomfield SS, Lipicky RJ, et al: Evaluation of bretylium tosylate for the treatment of premature ventricular contractions. Circulation 45:800, 1972.
74. Bauernfeind RH, Hoff JV, Swiryn S, et al: Electrophysiologic testing of bretylium tosylate in sustained ventricular tachycardia. Am Heart J 105:973, 1983.
75. Greene HL, Werner JA, Gross BW, et al: Failure of bretylium to suppress inducible ventricular tachycardia. Am Heart J 105:717, 1983.
76. Nowak RM, Bodnar TJ, Dronen S, et al: Bretylium tosylate as initial treatment for cardiopulmonary arrest: Randomized comparison with placebo. Ann Emerg Med 10:8, 1981.
77. Harrison BE, Amey BD: The use of bretylium in prehospital ventricular fibrillation. Am J Emerg Med 1:1, 1983.
78. Haynes RE, Chinn RL, Copass MK, et al: Comparison of bretylium tosylate and lidocaine in management of out-of-hospital ventricular fibrillation: A randomized clinical trial. Am J Cardiol 48:353, 1981.
79. Olson DW, Thompson BM, Darin JC, et al: A randomized comparison study of bretylium tosylate and lidocaine in resuscitation of patients from out-of-hospital ventricular fibrillation in a paramedic system. Ann Emerg Med 13:807, 1984.
80. Weaver WD, Fahrenbruch CE, Dennis D, et al: Efficacy of epinephrine and lidocaine for persistent ventricular fibrillation [abstract]. Circulation 72:III-8, 1985.
81. Weaver WD, Cobb LA, Hallstrom AP, et al: Factors influencing survival after out-of-hospital cardiac arrest. J Am Coll Cardiol 7:752, 1986.
82. Adult Advanced Cardiac Life Support. Part III. JAMA 268:2199, 1992.
83. Reynolds EW, Vander Ark CR: Quinidine syncope and the delayed repolarization syndromes. Mod Concepts Cardiovasc Dis 45:117, 1976.
84. Smith WM, Gallagher JJ: "Les torsades de pointes": An unusual ventricular arrhythmia. Ann Intern Med 93:578, 1980.
85. Nielson KC, Owman C: Control of ventricular fibrillation during induced hypothermia in cats after blocking the adrenergic neurons with bretylium. Life Sci 7:159, 1958.
86. Murphy K, Nowak RM, Tomlanovich MC: Use of bretylium tosylate as prophylaxis and treatment in hypothermic ventricular fibrillation in the canine model. Ann Emerg Med 15:1160, 1986.
87. Elenbaas RM, Mattson K, Cole H, et al: Bretylium in hypothermia-induced ventricular fibrillation in dogs. Ann Emerg Med 13:994, 1984.
88. Orts A, Alcavaz C, Delaney KA, et al: Bretylium tosylate and electrically induced cardiac arrhythmias during hypothermia in dogs. Am J Emerg Med 10:311, 1992.
89. Puddu PE, Jouve R, Saadjian A, et al: Experimental and clinical pharmacology of bretylium tosylate in acute myocardial infarction: A 15-year journey. J Pharmacol 17:223, 1986.
90. Taylor SH, Saxton C, Davies PS, et al: Bretylium tosylate in prevention of cardiac dysrhythmias after myocardial infarction. Br Heart J 32:326, 1970.
91. Luomanmaki K, Heikkila J, Hartel G: Bretylium tosylate: Adverse effects in acute myocardial infarction. Arch Intern Med 135:515, 1975.
92. Wolfe CL, Nibley C, Bhandari A, et al: Polymorphous ventricular tachycardia associated with acute myocardial infarction. Circulation 84:1543, 1991.
93. Kirlangitis J, Middaugh R, Knight R, et al: Comparison of bretylium and lidocaine in the prevention of ventricular fibrillation after aortic cross-clamp release in coronary artery bypass surgery. J Cardiothorac Anesth 4:582, 1990.
94. Anderson JL, Popat K, Pitt B: Paradoxical ventricular tachycardia and fibrillation after intravenous bretylium therapy. Arch Intern Med 141:801, 1981.
95. Woosley RL, Reele SB, Roden DM, et al: Pharmacologic reversal of the hypotensive effect that complicates antiarrhythmic therapy with bretylium. Clin Pharmacol Ther 32:313, 1982.
96. Lathers CM, Gerard-Ciminera JL, Baskin SI, et al: The action of reserpine, 6-hydroxydopamine, and bretylium on digitalis-induced cardiotoxicity. Eur J Pharmacol 76:371, 1981.
97. Vincent JL, Dufaye P, Berre J, et al: Bretylium in severe ventricular arrhythmias associated with digitalis intoxication. Am J Emerg Med 2:504, 1984.
98. Narang PK, Adir J, Josselson J, et al: Pharmacokinetics of bretylium in man after intravenous administration. J Pharmacokinet Biopharm 8:363, 1980.
99. Adir J, Narang PK, Josselson J: Nomogram for bretylium dosing in renal impairment. Ther Drug Monit 7:265, 1985.
100. Gutgesell M, Overholt E, Boyle R: Oral bretylium tosylate use during pregnancy and subsequent breast-feeding: A case report. Am J Perinatol 7:144, 1990.
101. Deazevedo IM, Watanabe Y, Dreifus LS: Electrophysiologic antagonism of quinidine and bretylium tosylate. Am J Cardiol 33:633, 1974.

CHAPTER 140

Disopyramide*

J. Marcus Wharton, M.D., John N. Hill, M.B., F.R.A.C.P., D.D.U., Nahum A. Freedberg, M.D., and Eric N. Prystowsky, M.D.

Disopyramide, or 4-(diisopropylamino)-2-phenyl-2-(2-pyridyl)butyramide (Fig. 140–1), is a synthetic antiarrhythmic agent that is chemically unlike quinidine or procainamide but has electrophysiologic properties similar to the other type IA antiarrhythmic agents. It was selected from more than 500 compounds developed in a research program to produce a new antiarrhythmic agent.[1] In 1962, Mokler and Van Arman[2] first demonstrated in animal models that disopyramide was an effective antiarrhythmic agent. In comparison with quinidine, disopyramide was equally or more effective for the pharmacologic conversion of electrically induced or aconitine-induced atrial flutter or fibrillation and of ischemia- or ouabain-induced ventricular arrhythmias.[2] Since that time, disopyramide has been shown to be an effective antiarrhythmic agent for the treatment of a number of clinical arrhythmias and has become a useful addition to the

*Supported in part by NIH Grant HLP-07063.

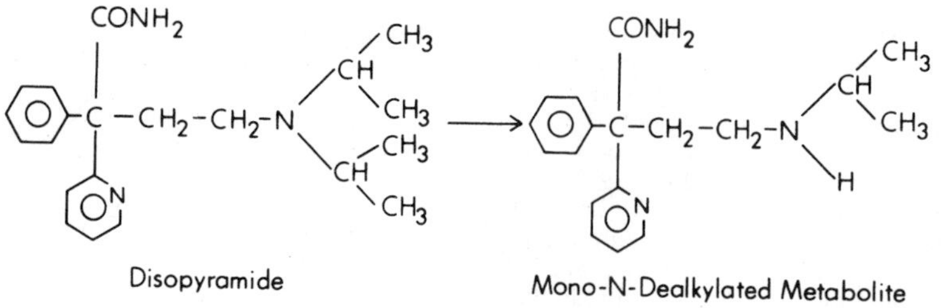

Figure 140–1. Chemical structure of disopyramide and its major metabolite, mono-N-dealkylated disopyramide (MND).

antiarrhythmic drug armamentarium. It was approved for use for ventricular arrhythmias by the United States Food and Drug Administration in 1977.

ELECTROPHYSIOLOGIC EFFECTS
Effects *In Vitro*

The cellular electrophysiologic effects of disopyramide as determined by studies *in vitro* are similar to those found for the other type IA antiarrhythmic agents, quinidine and procainamide. In normal His-Purkinje preparations, disopyramide (1) decreases action potential amplitude, (2) decreases the rate of rise of phase 0 ($\dot{V}_{max}$), (3) increases the action potential duration at all pacing cycle lengths, and (4) decreases the slope of phase 4 depolarization (spontaneous depolarization).[3, 4] All of these effects are concentration dependent. Maximum diastolic potential is typically unaltered or minimally decreased by disopyramide in concentrations of 2 to 5 µg/ml. Hypokalemic superfusates ($[K^+]_o$ = 2 mM) attenuate the effect of disopyramide on action potential amplitude, but there is still a significant decrease in $\dot{V}_{max}$ and an increase in action potential duration (APD).[4]

The decrease in $\dot{V}_{max}$ results in an anticipated decrease in His-Purkinje conduction time *in vitro*.[3, 4] Kus and Sasyniuk[3] noted a 5.9 ± 1.4% decrease in conduction velocity in a canine Purkinje fiber preparation exposed to 5 µg/ml of disopyramide (from 1.70 ± 0.21 m/sec to 1.63 ± 0.72 m/sec [SE]). In addition to decreasing the magnitude of $\dot{V}_{max}$, disopyramide produces a concentration-dependent shift to the right in the membrane responsiveness curve (the relation comparing $\dot{V}_{max}$ with resting membrane potential), indicating a decreased ability to depolarize myocardium with progressively premature stimuli.[3, 4] Thus, disopyramide increases the effective refractory period of His-Purkinje fibers in a concentration-dependent manner.

Disopyramide prolongs the APD in His-Purkinje preparations. The effect on the action potential waveform characteristically shows a steeper decline in the phase 2 plateau with a more gradual recovery during phase 3 (Fig. 140–2). The latter characteristic increases the APD, paralleling the increase in the effective refractory period (ERP) of the tissue. However, the changes in APD are always greater than the changes in ERP.[3, 4] In canine Purkinje fibers,[5] a biphasic response of APD to disopyramide has been observed: low doses prolonged APD, particularly at low stimulus frequencies, whereas the APD decreased below control values as the dose was increased. However, the decrements of APD at higher doses of disopyramide were not statistically significant.

The different optical isomers of disopyramide have divergent effects on repolarization. In the study by Mirro et al.,[6] the electrophysiologic effects of D-, L-, and DL- (racemic) stereoisomers of disopyramide were studied in a canine Purkinje preparation.

Both D- and DL-disopyramide prolonged APD90, whereas L-disopyramide shortened APD90. All of the stereoisomers had similar effects on $\dot{V}_{max}$, conduction time, and depolarization threshold. The differing effects of optical isomers of disopyramide on APD suggest stereospecific binding of disopyramide to the receptor systems modulating APD. Stereoisomers of the major metabolite of disopyramide, mono-N-dealkylated disopyramide (MND), appear to be three times less potent in their effects on $\dot{V}_{max}$ in guinea pig papillary muscle than their respective disopyramide parent stereoisomers.[7]

The effect of disopyramide on refractory periods may not be the same at all points along the His-Purkinje network. Myerburg et al.[8] have shown that the APD of the Purkinje fiber progressively increases from the proximal bundle of His to reach a maximum at distal points prior to termination of the Purkinje fibers in the ventricular myocardium. Beyond the distal point of maximal APD in the Purkinje fiber, the APD becomes shorter. The point of maximal APD in the distal Purkinje fibers serves as a gate of conduction across the fiber and determines the functional refractory period of the His-Purkinje system. It has been suggested that this disparity in APDs may play a role in the genesis of ventricular reentrant rhythms.[9, 10]

Kus and Sasyniuk[3] showed that at the 90% level of repolarization, disopyramide increased the APD of Purkinje fibers both in the gate region and in regions proximal and distal to this gate. However, the mean prolongation of APD90 was greater in the nongate cells. At APD50, disopyramide decreased the APD of Purkinje fibers in the gate region but increased it in Purkinje fibers located proximal or distal to the gate region. The net effect of these changes is a greater homogeneity of the APDs along the course of the Purkinje strand (see Fig. 140–2). This lessening of dispersion of refractory periods in the His-Purkinje network is particularly obvious at APD50 and APD75. It is possible that, in some patients, the antiarrhythmic action of disopyramide may be due to its ability to decrease the disparity of refractory periods in the His-Purkinje network, thus reducing the substrate for reentrant rhythms.[3]

Although less well studied, effects similar to those found in Purkinje fibers are also seen in atrial and ventricular myocardia.[3, 11, 12] In both, a concentration-dependent decrease occurs in the amplitude and rate of rise of the upstroke of the action potential and an increase in the APD at both APD50 and APD90.[3, 12] The resting membrane potential remains unchanged.

In one canine infarct model, the APD in the infarct

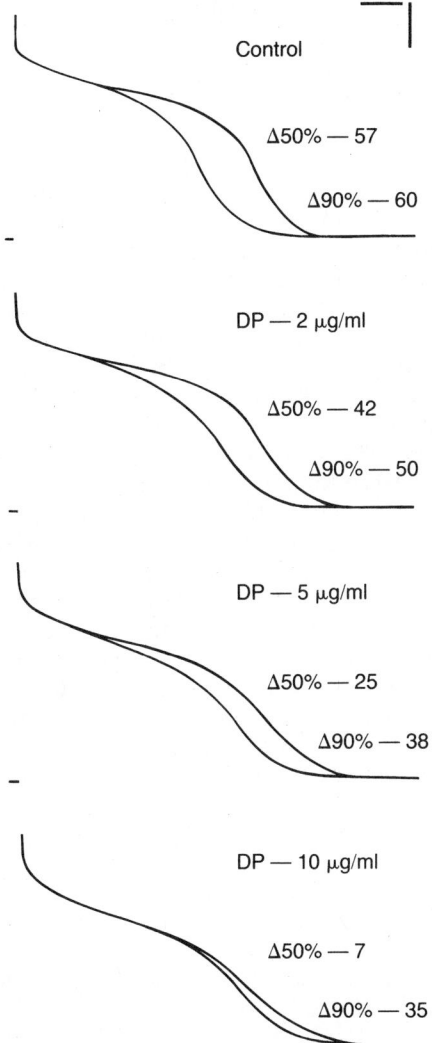

Figure 140–2. Superimposed action potentials recorded from Purkinje fibers proximal to, and at, the gate region are shown. The proximal action potential recordings have a shorter duration than those at the gate. The four consecutive panels illustrate the differential effects of disopyramide phosphate (DP) on repolarization in the different regions at concentrations of 2, 5, and 10 μg/ml compared with the control state. Δ50% and Δ90% refer to differences in the number of milliseconds indicated between action potential durations at the 50% and 90% level of repolarization, respectively. The horizontal and vertical calibrations in the upper right hand corner of the figure denote 50 msec and 25 mV, respectively. Note the increase in the action potential duration, the steeper slope of phase 2, the more gradual slope of phase 3, and the decreasing degree of dispersion of refractoriness between the two regions as the concentration of disopyramide is increased in the perfusate. See text for discussion. (Reproduced with permission from Kus T, Sasyniuk BI: Electrophysiological actions of disopyramide phosphate on canine ventricular muscle and Purkinje fibers. Circ Res 37:844, 1975. Copyright 1975, American Heart Association.)

zone was much longer than in normal regions.[13] Disopyramide minimally prolonged the APD in the infarct zone compared with the normal zone, suggesting that the antiarrhythmic efficacy of disopyramide in this infarct model may be related in part to a decrease in the dispersion of refractory periods induced by ischemia. However, in sheep Purkinje fibers superfused with hypoxic, hyperkalemic, acidotic but otherwise physiologic salt solution, disopyramide at high concentration could significantly prolong the APD90.[14] The effects of disopyramide on $\dot{V}_{max}$ in ischemic myocardia show significant differences among species.[14–16]

Katoh et al.[12] studied isolated rabbit sinus node preparations and noted no change in maximum diastolic potential or estimated takeoff potential of sinus node action potentials. There was significant prolongation of both APD50 and APD100. All of these findings held regardless of the level of cholinergic tone. However, the effect of disopyramide on the slope of phase 4 of the sinus node potential was dependent on the level of cholinergic tone (see later discussion). In the presence of cholinergic blockade with atropine, disopyramide decreased the slope of phase 4 and the spontaneous sinus cycle length.[11, 12] Disopyramide had no significant effect on corrected sinus node recovery time or on directly or indirectly measured sinoatrial conduction times, either at control or with cholinergic blockade or stimulation.[12]

Disopyramide affects the action potential of atrioventricular (AV) nodal pacemaker cells in a manner similar to that in the sinoatrial (SA) node.[17, 18] Spontaneously beating AV nodal pacemakers in rabbits also slow with the addition of disopyramide, but this effect appears to be due predominantly to an increase in APD rather than a decrease in rate of diastolic depolarization.[18] Atropine does not affect significantly the action potential characteristics and spontaneous rate changes induced by disopyramide in the AV node.[17]

As with other type IA agents, the effect of disopyramide on decreasing $\dot{V}_{max}$ and conduction velocity appears to be due to blockade of fast sodium channels. Yatani and Akaike[19] showed concentration-dependent inhibition of the fast sodium current during voltage clamping studies in isolated rat ventricle cells. The kinetics of this blocking effect suggests 1:1 binding between disopyramide and the sodium channel. This blockade tends to be enhanced by repetitive depolarization, that is, it shows frequency dependence.[20–22] Grant et al.[23] have further demonstrated that the open or closed state of the sodium channel is a critical determinant of the binding and unbinding kinetics of disopyramide. Gruber and Carmeliet[24] showed that disopyramide preferentially blocks the sodium channel in its open state.

Varro et al.[20] studied the frequency-dependent effects of several type I agents, including disopyramide in a concentration of 3.1 μg/ml, at both constant pacing cycle lengths and after abrupt changes in pacing cycle length in canine Purkinje fibers. Tonic block could not be shown because spontaneous diastolic depolarization interfered with the measurement of $\dot{V}_{max}$ at intervals greater than approximately 4 or 5 seconds. At these intervals, $\dot{V}_{max}$ had not recovered for disopyramide. At different stable pacing cycle lengths, there was a gradual decrease in $\dot{V}_{max}$ with decreasing pacing cycle lengths. The percentage of block was similar for procainamide and disopyramide at each pacing cycle length, but block was substantially greater with quinidine (Fig. 140–3). After abrupt changes in cycle length, the time course of recovery of $\dot{V}_{max}$ was 37.9 ± 9.4 seconds for disopyramide compared with 4.4 ± 0.8 seconds for procainamide and 8.3 ± 1.2 seconds for quinidine.[20] Thus, the time course of recovery for disopyramide appears to be substantially greater than that of either procainamide or quinidine after abrupt changes in cycle length.

In Purkinje preparations treated with tetraethylammonium in which slow response action potentials are generated, disopyramide has little effect on the maximum diastolic potential, APD, or APD50.[4] This study would suggest that disopyramide has little effect on the slow inward sodium current I_{si}. However, other workers have shown an effect of disopyramide on this current,[25] which tends to shorten APD. Prolongation of APD, mediated by effect of disopyramide on the ATP-sensitive delayed-rectifying outward potassium channel $I_{K.ATP}$, has been well documented.[6, 26, 27] The opposing effects of blockade of two channels affecting APD may account for the apparent inconsistencies in studies of disopyramide on APD in different cellular environments, including ischemia, and for the biphasic response of APD to dosage of disopyramide.[5, 14]

Mirro[28] provided evidence to suggest that disopyramide, as well as quinidine and procainamide, decreases cyclic adenosine monophosphate (cAMP) content of guinea pig atria in a concentration-dependent fashion. This decrease was associated with a decrease in the spontaneous rate of contraction and may in part explain the decrease in automaticity induced by the drug apart from its membrane-stabilizing properties. The mechanism by which disopyramide decreases cAMP was not explored, but disopyramide does not block the β-adrenergic receptor.[29]

Mokler and Van Arman[2] demonstrated that disopyramide blocked the bradycardia induced by stimulation of the right vagus nerve in dogs or by the addition of acetylcholine to the perfusate of the isolated rabbit heart. Comparison of the ability of atropine or disopyramide to block acetylcholine-induced spasm of isolated segments of rabbit ileum revealed that disopyramide had 0.5% of the anticholinergic effects of atropine.[2] Unlike quinidine, disopyramide does not appear to have any sympatholytic effect.[2] Mirro et al.[29] showed that disopyramide had greater anticholinergic effects than quinidine or procainamide, but much less than atropine, in blocking the negative chronotropic action of physostigmine on guinea pig right atria. These anticholinergic properties of disopyramide were substantially greater with D-disopyramide than with L-stereoisomer. This stereoselectivity was not seen with quinidine.[29] Further studies have shown that disopyramide competitively inhibits the binding of [³H] quinuclidinyl benzilate ([³HQNB]), a radiolabeled muscarinic receptor antagonist, to the muscarinic receptor of crude homogenates of guinea pig right atria or membrane vesicles of canine ventricle. Again, the D-disopyramide was much more effective in blocking [³HQNB] than was the L-stereoisomer.[29] Thus, the anticholinergic action of disopyramide appears to be due to a stereoselective drug interaction with muscarinic receptors. Investigation of the action of disopyramide on intestinal smooth muscle in the guinea pig[17] suggests that its

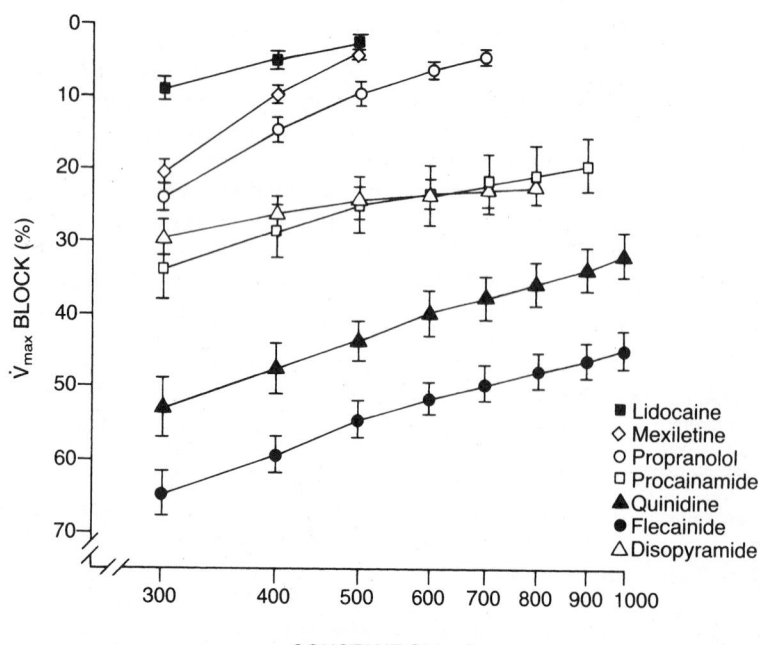

Figure 140–3. The effect of disopyramide and six other antiarrhythmic agents on the percentage of block in $\dot{V}_{max}$ between steady-state $\dot{V}_{max}$ and $\dot{V}_{max}$ in the presence of drug at various constant pacing cycle lengths (CL) from 300 to 1000 msec. The steady-state values represent drug-free $\dot{V}_{max}$ for disopyramide, procainamide, quinidine, and flecainide and during tonic block for lidocaine, mexiletine, and propranolol. Note that the percentage of block gradually increases for each of the antiarrhythmic agents at faster pacing rates (shorter pacing cycle lengths). Further, note that disopyramide *(open triangle)* and procainamide *(open square)* have similar use dependence compared with the other type IA agent quinidine *(solid triangle)*. (From Varro A, Elharrar V, Surawicz B: Frequency-dependent effects of several class I antiarrhythmic drugs on Vmax on action potential upstroke in canine cardiac Purkinje fibers. J Cardiovasc Pharmacol 7:482, 1985.)

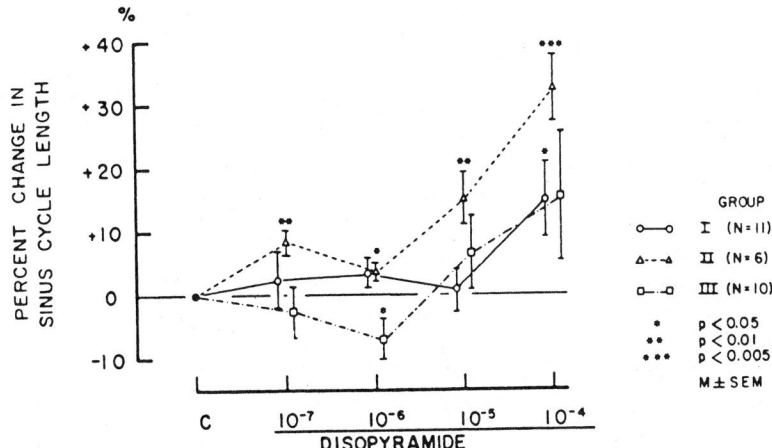

Figure 140–4. Variable concentration-dependent effect of disopyramide on the percentage change in spontaneous sinus cycle length in an isolated rabbit sinus node preparation. Group I *(open circle)* represents the control group, whereas preparations in Group II *(open triangle)* have been pretreated with atropine (1×10^{-6} M) and preparations in Group III have been pretreated with carbamylcholine (1×10^{-9} M). Note that under control conditions there is little change in the spontaneous sinus cycle length except at very high concentrations of disopyramide (10^{-4} M); however, during cholinergic blockade with atropine, there is a concentration-dependent increase in spontaneous sinus cycle length, reflecting the membrane-stabilizing properties of disopyramide. However, during cholinergic stimulation with carbamylcholine, there is a decrease in spontaneous sinus cycle length with lower concentrations of disopyramide (10^{-7} to 10^{-6} M), representing the anticholinergic effects of this agent. (Reproduced with permission from Katoh T, Karagueuzian HS, Jordan J, et al: The cellular electrophysiologic mechanism of the dual actions of disopyramide on rabbit sinus node function. Circulation 66:1216, 1982. Copyright 1982, American Heart Association.)

effects on M2 muscarinic receptors are approximately three times greater than effects on M1 receptors. It has been suggested[30, 31] that the major metabolite of disopyramide, MND, has significantly greater anticholinergic action than disopyramide and may be important in determining anticholinergic effects *in vivo*, but this issue is controversial.[32–35]

Mirro et al.[36] also studied the effect of underlying cholinergic tone on determining the electrophysiologic effects of disopyramide in guinea pig atria and canine Purkinje fibers. In atrial tissues, disopyramide administered in the control condition elicited a negative chronotropic response; however, after the addition of physostigmine to simulate increased cholinergic tone, disopyramide produced a positive chronotropic response.[36] In rabbit sinus node preparations, Katoh et al.[12] showed that disopyramide had no effect on spontaneous sinoatrial rate or phase 4 slope at baseline, decreased both after cholinergic blockade with atropine, and increased both at low concentrations of disopyramide (10^{-7} to 10^{-6} M) in the presence of carbamyl choline, but both decreased at high concentrations (10^{-5} to 10^{-4} M) (Fig. 140–4). The results of these experiments suggest that the effects of disopyramide on SA nodal automaticity depend on a complex interaction of its membrane-stabilizing and anticholinergic effects, with the negative chronotropic action of the drug potentially overridden by the anticholinergic actions in the presence of high cholinergic tone.

Similar complexities are seen in His-Purkinje preparations. Disopyramide superfused over Purkinje fibers prolonged the APD over control, but, in the presence of isoproterenol and acetylcholine, disopyramide shortened the APD.[36] Thus, disopyramide appeared to shorten the APD in the setting of adrenergic-cholinergic stimulation. Similar responses were

found for quinidine but not for procainamide.[36] Thus, the anticholinergic effects of disopyramide and its interaction with the degree of sympathetic and parasympathetic stimulation of the animal play an important role in determining its electrophysiologic effects and may help explain the variability in electrophysiologic effects seen *in vivo*.

Effects *In Vivo*

Animal Studies

Disopyramide has been shown in animal models to be an effective antiarrhythmic agent for both supraventricular and ventricular arrhythmias. Mokler and Van Arman[2] demonstrated that disopyramide was more effective than quinidine in the pharmacologic conversion of electrically induced or aconitine-induced atrial flutter and fibrillation or in ventricular arrhythmias induced by ischemia and ouabain.

Further studies have shown the efficacy of disopyramide in the prevention of ischemia-related ventricular arrhythmias. Chagnac et al.[37] showed that disopyramide could prevent the occurrence of both occlusion and reperfusion ventricular arrhythmias in a canine model. In comparison with placebo, disopyramide decreased the incidence of occlusion arrhythmias from 52% to 14% and of reperfusion arrhythmias from 33% to 8%, both of which were significant. Another study has shown that pretreatment of perfused rat hearts with disopyramide[38] could enhance postischemic contractile and metabolic recovery. The pronounced contractile recovery was associated with suppression of both the tissue ion derangements and the release of creatine kinase and purines induced by reperfusion. Disopyramide has also been noted to increase the ventricular fibrillation threshold in dogs with acute myocardial infarction (AMI), possibly to a greater degree than lidocaine.[39]

In dogs several days after infarction, disopyramide has a variable effect on suppression of inducible ventricular tachyarrhythmias. In a study by Cobbe et al.[40] in conscious dogs 3 to 8 days after infarction, intravenous disopyramide given in a dose to obtain mean serum levels of 3.7 ± 1.6 μg/ml was successful in suppressing inducible sustained ventricular tachycardia in 25% of animals and in suppressing inducible nonsustained ventricular tachycardia in 43% of animals.[40] The cycle length of inducible ventricular tachycardia was noted to increase in approximately a third of the animals. Patterson et al.[41] showed that the ability of disopyramide to suppress ventricular tachycardia induction in dogs 2 to 4 days after myocardial infarction was highly dependent on the steady-state plasma disopyramide concentration. In dogs with low plasma disopyramide concentrations of approximately 1 μg/ml, inducible ventricular tachycardia had a relatively rapid rate and long duration, and the zone of vulnerability for initiation of ventricular tachycardia was broader. Increasing the plasma concentration to approximately 2 or 4 μg/ml succeeded only in slowing the rate of induced ventricular tachycardia without decreasing its inducibility or duration. Only concentrations of disopyramide of more than 7 μg/ml succeeded in suppressing the inducibility of ventricular tachycardia. The most effective plasma concentration for preventing initiation of ventricular tachycardia in this canine model was higher than the concentrations usually recommended in humans. This difference suggests that it is probably better to give as much drug as tolerated to patients with serious ventricular arrhythmias rather than to target a specific plasma concentration end point.

As suggested by models *in vitro*, disopyramide appears to decrease the dispersion of refractory periods between ischemic and nonischemic zones in animal models. In a study by Levites and Anderson,[42] occlusion of the left anterior descending coronary artery produced a significant decrease in the effective refractory period in ischemic compared with nonischemic myocardium (Fig. 140–5). After administration of 3 mg/kg of intravenous disopyramide, the effective refractory periods in both zones increased, but there was a much greater increase in the ischemic zone. This resulted in the two refractory periods being similar, suggesting an overall decrease in the dispersion of refractory periods induced by ischemia. However, this effect was less obvious 15 and 30 minutes after infusion of disopyramide. This finding has been further confirmed in the works of others.[41]

One study of canine ventricular arrhythmias induced by coronary ligation and by digoxin[43] showed that the combination of low-dose mexiletine with disopyramide could enhance the antiarrhythmic effect of disopyramide.

Using a monophasic action potential (MAP) catheter, Edwards et al.[44] showed that disopyramide infu-

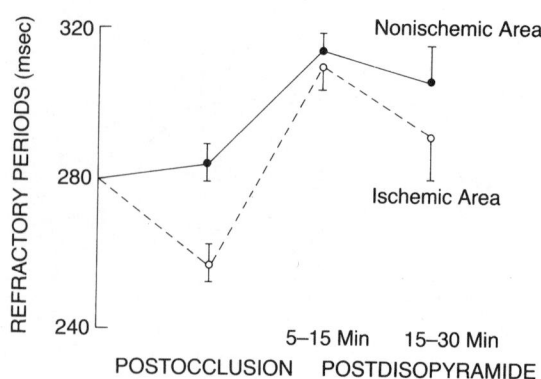

Figure 140–5. Effect of disopyramide on decreasing dispersion of refractoriness between ischemic and nonischemic areas in a canine model of myocardial ischemia. The refractory period is shown during the control period, following ligation of the left anterior descending coronary artery, and at 5 to 15 minutes and 15 to 30 minutes after a single intravenous dose of disopyramide, 3 mg/kg. Note that, during the control state, the refractory period of the two recording sites are the same (280 msec). After coronary artery occlusion, the refractory period in the nonischemic zone remains essentially unchanged, whereas that in the ischemic zone decreases significantly. Infusion of disopyramide increases the refractory period in both the ischemic and the nonischemic zones but more so in the ischemic zones such that the refractory periods are nearly equivalent in the two areas immediately after infusion of the drug. (From Levites R, Anderson GJ: Electrophysiological effects of disopyramide phosphate during experimental myocardial ischemia. Am Heart J 98:339, 1979.)

sion decreased the slope of phase 0 and prolonged the duration of the MAP of ventricular muscle primarily by decreasing the slope of phase 3 repolarization. An intravenous bolus of disopyramide also was noted to decrease the overall amplitude of the MAP, but this finding was not observed during continuous infusion. These findings of MAP parallel those changes noted by intracellular techniques measuring the transmembrane potential. In autonomically intact dogs, the atrial MAP duration changed insignificantly with disopyramide.[45]

Human Studies

The electrophysiologic effects of disopyramide have been studied extensively in humans and have been somewhat variable[46–62] (Table 140–1). As anticipated for a type IA agent, disopyramide typically prolongs the QT_c interval; the PR and QRS intervals are not affected or prolonged.[46–48, 56, 58, 59, 61] Spontaneous sinus cycle length typically does not change, but it may occasionally decrease[55, 57, 59] and has been noted to increase in patients given atropine.[60] In patients with normal SA nodal function, the sinus node recovery time and SA conduction time typically are not altered, but they may occasionally be increased in patients with intrinsic sinus node disease.[55, 56] In the study by LaBarre et al.,[56] patients with sick sinus syndrome and sinus arrest, SA exit block, or secondary pauses after termination of rapid atrial pacing were especially prone to have dramatic increases in spontaneous sinus cycle lengths and sinus node recovery times (up to 91% in the former and 544% with the latter).

This would indicate caution when using disopyramide in these individuals. However, Holter monitoring data in similar patients[63] suggested less sinus node suppression than predicted by electrophysiologic testing.

These variable effects of disopyramide in patients appear to be contradictory to what would be anticipated solely by its membrane-stabilizing properties. However, as shown with preparations *in vitro*, the anticholinergic effects of disopyramide can markedly alter its effects *in vivo* on conduction and spontaneous automaticity.

The AH interval typically remains unchanged, even in the setting of baseline AV nodal dysfunction.[58] The HV interval usually increases[52, 54, 56, 58, 59, 64] but has been reported to be unchanged by some;[49–51, 53] this finding may be influenced particularly by the presence of preexistent intraventricular conduction disturbances. Disopyramide may precipitate high-grade AV block in some patients with bifascicular block,[64, 65] but this is a rare event. Atrial and ventricular refractory periods are typically increased. AV nodal effective and functional refractory periods are usually unchanged, although the AV nodal ERP may be slightly decreased[49, 53, 58] and AV nodal functional refractory period (FRP) increased.[54, 60, 61]

Anticipated membrane-stabilizing effects on spontaneous automaticity and conduction are seen in patients pretreated with atropine and in transplanted denervated hearts.[60, 61] In the study by Birkhead and Vaughan Williams,[60] pretreatment with atropine uncovered the depressant effects of disopyramide: basic cycle length, sinus node recovery time, AH interval, AV nodal FRP, and atrial ERP were increased. In a study by Bexton et al.[61] on the electrophysiologic effects of disopyramide, 2 mg/kg IV, administered to heart transplant recipients, the spontaneous cycle length of the denervated donor right atrium increased from 626 ± 129 msec to 716 ± 148 msec, whereas that of the innervated residual recipient atrium decreased from 846 ± 195 msec to 659 ± 99 msec. There were also small insignificant increases in the sinus node recovery time of the donor atrium compared with small insignificant decreases in the sinus node recovery time of the recipient atrium. Likewise, SA conduction times in the donor sinus node increased in all patients except for one, whereas there were inconsistent effects on the recipient sinus node. The AH interval, HV interval, QRS duration, and QT interval all significantly increased in the transplanted human heart after administration of disopyramide. No significant changes were noted in the effective refractory period of the atrium or ventricle or of the AV node, but the functional refractory period of the AV node was noted to increase significantly.[61] This study in the denervated heart illustrates the expected membrane-stabilizing electrophysiologic effects of disopyramide. In the innervated heart, the depressant effects of diso-

Table 140–1. **Comparison of Electrophysiologic Effects of Disopyramide in Humans**

Reference	Patients	IV Dose (mg/kg)	Sinus Node			AV Conduction				Myocardial		
			SCL	SNRT	SACT	AH	AVERP	AVFRP	HV	AERP	AFRP	VERP
Josephson et al.[49]	12	1.0–2.0	0	—	—	0	↓	0	0	↑	—	—
Befeler et al.[50]	10	2.0	0	↓	—	0	0	0 (↑)	0	0	0	↑
Spurrell et al.[51]	10	2.0	—	—	—	0	0	0	0	↑	—	↑
Marrott et al.[52]	12	1.5	0	—	—	0	0	0	↑	↑	—	—
Caracta[53]	12	1.0–2.0	0	—	—	0	↓	—	0	↑	—	—
Kashani et al.[54]	14	2.0	0	—	—	0	↑	↑	↑	↑	↑	—
Reid and Williams[55]												
Sick sinus syndrome	12	2.0	0	↑	0 (↑)	—	—	—	—	—	—	—
Normal patients	6	2.0	0 (↓)	0 (↓)	0 (↓)	—	—	0	↑	—	↑	—
LaBarre et al.[56] (sick sinus syndrome)	16	2.0	0	0	0	0	—	0	↑	—	↑	—
Tsuchioka et al.[57] (sick sinus syndrome)	26	1.5	0 (↓)	0 (↑)	0	0	0	0	↑	↑	↑	0
Wilkinson et al.[58] (AV node dysfunction)	17	1.0–1.25	0	0	—	0	↓	—	—	0	—	—
Desai et al.[59] (patients with LBBB and RBBB)	22	2.0	↓	0	—	0	0	0	↑	↑	↑	↑
Birkhead and Vaughan Williams[60] (patients given atropine)	14	2.0	↑	↑	—	↑	—	↑	0	↑	—	—
Bexton et al.[61]												
Heart transplants	8	2.0										
Atrial remnant of recipient	8	2.0										
Donor			↑	↑	0 (↑)	↑	0	↑	↑	0 (↑)	—	↑
Recipients			↓	0 (↓)	0	—	—	—	—	—	—	—

AH, conduction time through AV node; AERP, atrial effective refractory period; AFRP, atrial functional refractory period; AV, atrioventricular; HV, conduction time between His bundle and earliest ventricular activation; LBBB, left bundle branch block; RBBB, right bundle branch block; SACT, sinoatrial conduction time; SCL, cycle length of sinus rhythm; SNRT, sinus node recovery time; VERP, ventricular effective refractory period; 0, no significant change; ↑, significant increase; ↓, significant decrease; 0 (↑ *or* ↓), no significant change but trend in the direction of the arrow; —, not available.

pyramide are typically altered by its anticholinergic effect, and the result depends on the level of baseline autonomic activity.

HEMODYNAMICS

Disopyramide has significant negative inotropic properties both *in vitro* and *in vivo* that are substantially greater than with either quinidine or procainamide. Mokler and Van Arman[2] originally showed a decrease in the force of contraction in isolated rabbit heart preparations in their original description of the pharmacologic effects of disopyramide. Nayler,[66] using isolated trabecular muscle preparations from guinea pigs and rabbits and papillary muscle preparations from humans, showed a concentration-dependent decrease in the peak developed tension that correlated with the decrease in superficially located, lanthanum-displaceable calcium stores.[66] Tissue adenosine triphosphate and creatine phosphate were not decreased. At high concentrations in guinea pig papillary muscles,[12] disopyramide could inhibit influx through slow calcium channels, but at low concentrations it had greater effect on contractility via inhibition of the sodium-calcium exchange mechanism. In another study, no frequency dependence of the negative inotropic effect of disopyramide could be identified.[67] Thus, the cellular mechanism by which disopyramide exerts its negative inotropic action remains poorly defined.

Disopyramide has been shown to be a potent negative inotropic agent *in vivo* in both anesthetized and unanesthetized animal preparations. In a study by Walsh and Horwitz,[68] unanesthetized, chronically instrumented dogs were given 1 mg/kg of intravenous disopyramide, which demonstrated its hemodynamic effects within 1 minute after infusion. They noticed a 34% increase in heart rate with a 16% decrease in stroke volume, resulting in no net change in overall cardiac output. Left ventricular dP/dt was noted to be decreased by 18%, and the systemic vascular resistance was increased by 33%. Mean aortic pressure was also noted to be increased by 22%. The administration of phenoxybenzamine did not block the vasoconstrictor effect of disopyramide.[68] Mathur[69] also demonstrated that disopyramide in doses of 1 to 3 mg/kg decreased coronary blood flow by 15% to 37%. In both studies, disopyramide was shown to be a much more potent negative inotropic agent than quinidine, perhaps because the vasodilatory response of quinidine partially attentuates the negative inotropic action of this drug. In a study using anesthetized rats,[70] disopyramide had more negative inotropic properties than either quinidine or flecainide.

Hemodynamic studies in humans after intravenously administered disopyramide show a decrease in the cardiac index and an increase in systemic vascular resistance.[7, 71–75] Heart rate typically is unchanged, and the blood pressure response is variable. Pulmonary capillary wedge pressure or left ventricular end-diastolic pressures are usually increased.[7, 73–75] However, the extent of these changes depends on the

degree of resting left ventricular dysfunction in the individuals studied.[75] In particular, in patients with poor left ventricular function, the decreases in cardiac output and the increases in left ventricular filling pressures can be dramatic. The effect on systemic blood pressure also depends on the degree of underlying left ventricular dysfunction; patients with normal left ventricular function typically have increases in systemic pressure, whereas patients with underlying left ventricular dysfunction typically have decreases in pressure. Kotter et al.,[72] in a hemodynamic study of patients with coronary artery disease given 2 mg/kg of intravenous disopyramide, showed that, in addition to increasing systemic vascular resistance, disopyramide also acutely caused a significant decrease in coronary artery blood flow with an increase in coronary vascular resistance, despite an overall increase in myocardial oxygen demand that normally would tend to result in coronary vasodilation. However, the increased myocardial oxygen demand overrode the vasoconstrictor response to disopyramide 30 minutes after infusion of the drug. Despite the acute response of an increased myocardial oxygen demand with a coronary vasoconstrictor response, these investigators noticed no precipitation of spontaneous angina or increase in myocardial lactate production.[72] Thus, the clinical significance of disopyramide's coronary vasoconstrictor effect is unknown.

Gottdiener et al.[76] showed that the radionuclide angiographic left ventricular ejection fraction of patients with coronary artery disease and idiopathic dilated cardiomyopathy receiving disopyramide for suppression of ventricular ectopic beats decreased significantly from 40 ± 15% to 33 ± 11% after oral loading of disopyramide to obtain a mean serum level of 3.6 ± 1.3 μg/ml (Fig. 140–6). Importantly, on chronic therapy with a mean serum level of 2.5 ± 0.5 μg/ml, no significant depression in ejection fraction during either rest or exercise could be found.[76] Thus, depression of left ventricular function could be documented by radionuclide techniques only during oral loading with disopyramide and at higher doses of the drug. Wisenberg et al.[77] compared the effects on left ventricular ejection fraction measured by radionuclide angiography between disopyramide, procainamide, and quinidine given orally. These investigators could find no significant difference in mean rest or exercise ejection fractions between the control state or therapy with disopyramide, procainamide, or quinidine, although their mean control ejection fraction was 60 ± 13%, representing a group with excellent left ventricular function who would be unlikely to have a dramatic negative inotropic response to disopyramide. In an invasive hemodynamic study comparing intravenous lidocaine, flecainide, and disopyramide in patients with uncomplicated myocardial infarction, disopyramide had the greatest negative inotropic action and lidocaine the least.[7]

Pollick et al.[78] showed that the negative inotropic effects of disopyramide were not stereoisomer dependent. They showed a 28.1 ± 11.8% mean maximum reduction in the fractional shortening of left ventricu-

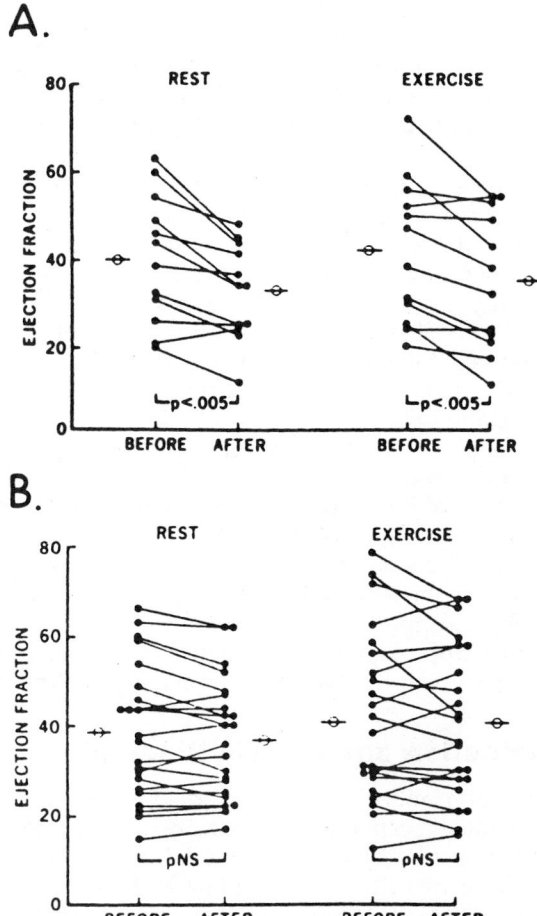

Figure 140–6. A, Rest and exercise ejection fractions obtained by radionuclide cineangiography before and after a single 300-mg oral dose of disopyramide in patients with coronary artery disease and idiopathic dilated cardiomyopathy. There is a significant decrease in the mean ejection fraction both at rest and with exercise after the single dose of disopyramide. *B*, Rest and exercise ejection fractions obtained 5 to 10 days after starting maintenance disopyramide at a dose of 600 mg/day. The mean rest and exercise ejection fractions on this chronic dose of disopyramide are not significantly different from the means obtained prior to initiation of therapy. (Adapted with permission from Gottdiener JS, Dibianco R, Bates R, et al: Effects of disopyramide on left ventricular function: Assessment by radionuclide cineangiography. Am J Cardiol 51:1554, 1983.)

lar dimension on echocardiography performed in six healthy volunteers regardless of whether D-, L-, or DL- (racemic) disopyramide was used. In addition, they showed a 28.6 ± 24.1% mean maximum reduction in peak left ventricular filling rates, suggesting a change in diastolic filling properties of the ventricle, a finding not seen in invasive hemodynamic studies.[67] Because the D- (and DL-) stereoisomer of disopyramide caused significant QT_c prolongation and the L-stereoisomer did not, the study suggests that the mechanism responsible for disopyramide's negative inotropic effects may be different from that responsible for its electrophysiologic properties in the ventricle. A more recent study found conflicting results, with the D-stereoisomer having fewer negative inotropic effects than the L-isomer.[79]

Multiple cases of disopyramide-induced hypotension, congestive heart failure, and electromechanical dissociation have been reported, typically in patients with severe underlying left ventricular dysfunction at the time of disopyramide administration.[80–82] Given the results of hemodynamic studies and these case reports, the authors believe that disopyramide is contraindicated in patients with severe left ventricular dysfunction or histories of congestive heart failure. In a study of 100 patients receiving short- or long-term disopyramide therapy for treatment of symptomatic ventricular arrhythmia,[83] 16 developed acute congestive heart failure thought to be secondary to disopyramide therapy. Three of these patients developed acute exacerbation of heart failure within 48 hours of initiation of disopyramide therapy. Fourteen of the 16 patients had evidence of left ventricular dysfunction. Of the 22 patients in this study who had histories of congestive heart failure, 55% developed clinically evident heart failure secondary to disopyramide. However, only 2 of the remaining 78 patients with no history of congestive heart failure developed this complication when given disopyramide.[83] This study substantiates the approach of not administering disopyramide in patients with histories of congestive heart failure. Conversely, these data demonstrate the relative safety of disopyramide regarding the occurrence of congestive heart failure in patients without histories of congestive heart failure, regardless of left ventricular ejection fraction. Another study has shown that if a clinical effect of disopyramide on left ventricular function occurs, it does so most commonly during the first week of use.[83] Thus, the clinical history of congestive heart failure is the best guide to the use of disopyramide in patients with abnormal left ventricular function. Interestingly, the combination of disopyramide and propranolol appears to have neither additive nor synergistic negative inotropic activity in normal individuals as assessed by noninvasive means.[84]

PHARMACOKINETICS

Disopyramide is a white crystalline racemic compound that is readily soluble in water and is available either as disopyramide base (Rythmodan) or disopyramide phosphate (Norpace). Disopyramide base composes 77.6% by weight of disopyramide phosphate. Only the phosphate preparation is available in the United States and is marketed as 100- and 150-mg capsules, with the dose being the amount of disopyramide base, rather than phosphate, available. In addition, both immediate- and controlled-release preparations are marketed commercially.

Absorption

Both disopyramide base and phosphate are rapidly and nearly completely absorbed. Studies *in vitro* revealed that, with the immediate-release form, 98% of the compound is released within 20 minutes compared with 10 hours for the controlled-release preparation.[85] After administration of a single dose of disopyramide-C[14], approximately 90% is absorbed in normal volunteers.[63] With the immediate-release preparation, a peak serum concentration is obtained within 0.5 to 2 hours after the oral dose is delivered. However, with the controlled-release preparation, peak serum concentration occurs approximately 3 or 4 hours after the initial dose (Fig. 140–7).[86]

Several studies have failed to reveal a significant difference in the bioavailability of disopyramide phosphate compared with disopyramide base. In a study by Bryson et al.,[87] the bioavailabilities were 82% and 68%, respectively, and, in a study by Dubetz et al.,[88] the bioavailabilities were 91% and 83%, respectively. The bioavailability of the immediate- and controlled-release preparations is also similar, with the controlled-release preparation having 91% of the bioavailability of the immediate-release preparation in one study.[86]

Disopyramide can also be given intravenously, but it may be associated with the development of marked hypotension, high-grade AV block, and increased heart failure. In the study by Sbarbaro et al.,[89] disopyramide infusion in patients with ventricular arrhythmias with and without AMI revealed the development of drug-induced complication in 9 of 33 trials (27%).[89] Complications included hypotension, complete heart block, heart failure, and proarrhythmia. More recent infusion regimens are associated with a lower incidence of side effects in selected patients.[65, 90, 91] Thus, it appears that intravenous disopyramide can be given safely to patients without preexistent left ventricular dysfunction or high-grade conduction disturbances, but it is not available in the United States for this route of administration.

Other routes of administration of disopyramide have also been investigated. Ashford et al.[92] gave disopyramide phosphate intramuscularly to eight patients and noted that it was well tolerated and that

detectable plasma levels were obtained within 5 minutes, with therapeutic levels obtained within 10 minutes. Bryson et al.[93] also investigated the intramuscular route of administration of disopyramide in seven patients with ischemic heart disease. They noted that therapeutic levels were obtained within 12 minutes in all patients and that a therapeutic level was maintained for a mean of 5.5 hours. However, the rate constant of absorption and the duration of a maintained therapeutic level showed significant individual variability. Thus, the intramuscular injection of disopyramide is also an effective route of administration that is well tolerated and obtains therapeutic levels relatively quickly. This route is not approved for use in the United States.

Duchateau et al.[94] have evaluated the bioavailability of disopyramide phosphate given rectally. The bioavailability of disopyramide phosphate suppositories given per rectum was 47% to 73% of that given orally. The authors concluded that therapeutic levels can be obtained by the rectal administration of disopyramide phosphate suppositories, but that the dose should be increased approximately 35% higher than that of the oral dose, given the more limited bioavailability.[94]

Distribution and Protein Binding

Distribution and elimination of disopyramide given intravenously can be described by a two-compartment, open pharmacokinetic model with a distribution phase half-life of 0.043 hour and a disposition phase half-life of 3.98 hours.[95] This rapid distribution half-life of approximately 3 minutes[87] is prolonged to approximately 15 minutes in patients with AMI.[96] Disopyramide, which is heavily protein-bound in serum, has a volume of distribution of 0.4 to 0.6 L/kg for the total amount of drug and 1.3 to 1.7 L/kg for the unbound drug.[95, 97, 98] After administration of the drug, disopyramide levels several times that of the

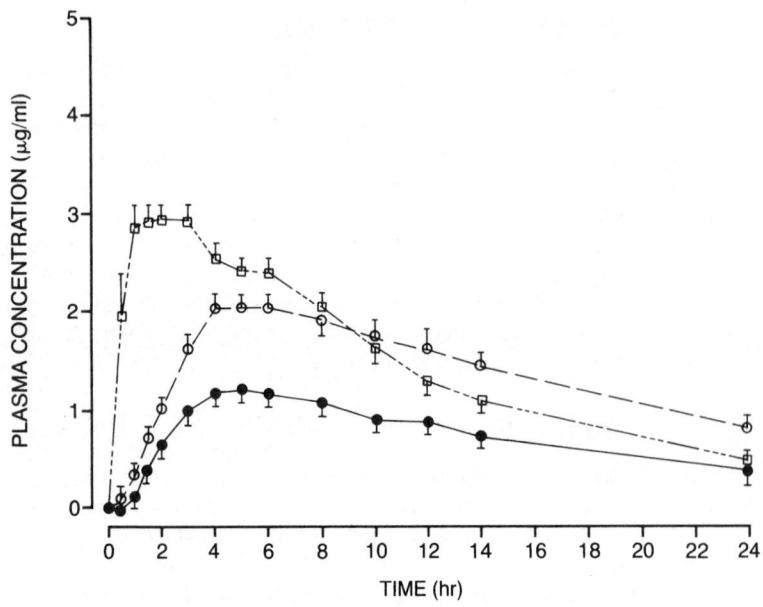

Figure 140–7. Mean ± SEM disopyramide plasma concentrations plotted as a function of the number of hours after a single oral dose. Concentration-time curves are shown for (1) a single oral dose of 300 mg of disopyramide phosphate given as two 150-mg immediate-release capsules *(open squares)*; (2) 300 mg of disopyramide phosphate given as two 150-mg controlled-release capsules *(open circles)*; and (3) 150 mg of disopyramide phosphate given as one 150-mg controlled-release capsule *(solid circles)*. Note the delayed and decreased peak plasma concentration of disopyramide obtained with the controlled-release preparation. (From Karim A, Schubert EN, Burns TS, et al: Disopyramide plasma concentrations following single and multiple doses of the immediate- and controlled-release capsules. Angiology 34:375, 1983. Reproduced with permission of the copyright owner, Westminster Publications, Inc., Roslyn, New York. All rights reserved.)

serum can be found in fat, liver, spleen, heart, and placenta.[94, 99] Relatively high concentrations of disopyramide in cord blood and breast milk, approximately 40% to 50% of the maternal level, have been found, indicating that a fetus or nursing infant may obtain appreciable levels of the drug.[100, 101] However, infant levels obtained do not appear to have clinical effects.[100, 101]

Disopyramide levels can be measured by a number of means, including spectrofluorometry, spectrophotometry, gas liquid chromatography, high-pressure liquid chromatography, and enzyme immunoassay.[95, 102] The latter three methods are reliable and adequate for monitoring drug levels. Stereospecific high-performance liquid chromatography can determine levels of disopyramide and MND stereoisomers simultaneously in either serum or urine.[11, 31] A reasonable serum drug level that is often associated with drug efficacy is typically in the range of 2 to 5 µg/ml. Supraventricular arrhythmias can typically be treated in the lower end of this serum range, whereas ventricular arrhythmias frequently require higher levels up to 7.5 µg/ml.[46] Unfortunately, a direct relationship exists between serum level and frequency of adverse reactions, and levels higher than 5 µg/ml generally are not well tolerated. Controlled-release disopyramide provides less interdose variation in unbound drug levels than the immediate-release formulation.[103] Regarding therapy for a particular patient, the authors use noninvasive or invasive methods to evaluate drug efficacy and rely on serum drug levels more as a guide to patient compliance or to determine unusual responses to common dosages of disopyramide.

Disopyramide and its major metabolite, MND, are both highly bound to α_1-acid glycoprotein (α_{1A}Gp).[104] Interestingly, this protein binding to α_{1A}Gp shows nonlinear (saturable) kinetics within the therapeutic range of disopyramide.[104-106] Thus, as serum disopyramide levels increase, small increases in the dose of disopyramide may result in marked increases in the amount of unbound drug, which is responsible for its pharmacologic effects. Both disopyramide and MND appear to bind competitively to the same site on α_{1A}Gp; thus, increases in the serum level of MND decrease the amount of bound disopyramide and increase the amount of free drug.[106, 107]

α_{1A}Gp is an acute-phase reactant, and fluctuations in its serum concentration result in significant interindividual and intraindividual variability in the amount of free and bound disopyramide. α_{1A}Gp is increased in patients with acute inflammatory and infectious processes, AMI, chronic renal failure requiring dialysis, and renal transplantation. Therefore, patients with these conditions have decreased amounts of unbound disopyramide that may attenuate the overall pharmacologic effect of the drug.[108, 109] In addition, α_{1A}Gp levels are generally higher in elderly individuals; however, the effect of this increase in α_{1A}Gp on decreasing amounts of free drug is probably attenuated by the typically decreased elimination kinetics of the geriatric population.[110] Chinese patients have lower α_{1A}Gp levels than Caucasian patients.[32] There-

fore, Chinese patients may require lower dosages of disopyramide to achieve a similar clinical effect.

Metabolism and Excretion

Disopyramide is excreted primarily unchanged in the urine. After a single dose of disopyramide, 80% is excreted predominantly as disopyramide in the urine and an additional 10% is excreted in feces.[63] Renal insufficiency requires dosage reduction. Karim et al.[95] found the mean elimination half-life to be 7.3 hours (range, 4 to 10 hours) in normal individuals. Sustained-release preparations have elimination half-lives of approximately 11 hours. Systemic clearance in children has been reported to be at least twice as fast as in normal adults;[75] in a small number of pediatric patients, half-life of disopyramide was reported to be 3.2 ± 0.6 hours.[111]

Both disopyramide and MND are excreted by the kidney, and renal clearances for either are approximately 170 to 180 ml/min in normal volunteers.[105] The increase in renal clearance above the glomerular filtration rate suggests that both glomerular filtration and tubular secretion are involved in renal clearance of the drug. This renal clearance is proportional to the amount of free drug available; thus, renal clearance is higher at higher drug levels because of the saturation of binding sites of α_{1A}Gp.[105] Haughey and Lima[105] noted that, at high dosages of disopyramide in some individuals, renal clearance starts to decrease, presumably secondary to saturation of the tubular mechanism of secretion of the drug. Despite the fact that disopyramide is a basic compound, alterations in urine pH do not appear to significantly alter the rate of renal excretion of disopyramide.[112]

Normally, most of the disopyramide is excreted unchanged in the urine, but approximately 15% to 25% of the dose is metabolized to MND[31] (see Fig. 140–1). Baines et al.[30] reported that MND had 24 times the anticholinergic properties of disopyramide in isolated guinea pig ileum. However, their finding of increased anticholinergic effects of MND suggested that this metabolite might be the major determinant of anticholinergic side effects in humans, particularly in individuals who are rapid metabolizers of disopyramide. Because MND is less protein bound than disopyramide, it is more rapidly cleared, and, typically, the serum level of MND is approximately 30% that of disopyramide.[63, 113, 114] However, renal clearance of MND tends to saturate at higher concentrations.[70] In the setting of renal impairment, the proportion of MND increases to approximately 50% of the disopyramide level. Renal clearance of disopyramide seems not to be stereospecific.[55]

In contrast, the metabolism of racemic disopyramide is stereospecific. The D-stereoisomer is metabolized more extensively than the L-isomer.[115] Thus, lower levels of the D-isomer are present in the body. This increased hepatic metabolism of the D-isomer does not appear to be the result of protein binding, because the D-isomer is more tightly protein bound, making free D-isomer less available for hepatic clearance.[116] Although the D-isomer has been shown *in vitro* to have greater anticholinergic properties than the L-isomer,[29] its effect is attenuated by the greater metabolism of the D-isomer and thus lower resultant serum activity.[33]

PHARMACOKINETICS IN DISEASE STATES

Because disopyramide and MND both are cleared primarily by the kidneys, chronic renal failure causes significant reduction in clearance of the drug, necessitating dosage reduction. In a study by Shen et al.,[117] a linear relationship was noted between the elimination rate constant and the endogenous creatinine clearance when the creatinine clearance was reduced below 40 ml/min. A decrease in the elimination rate constant was not observed until the creatinine clearance was reduced below this level. In addition, the plasma elimination half-life significantly increased when the creatinine clearance was less than 30 ml/min.[117] These findings have been confirmed by others.[118] The volume of distribution appears to be only modestly decreased.[117, 118] The results of these studies suggest that, in patients with creatinine clearances of more than 40 ml/min, no dose adjustment is needed. However, in patients whose creatinine clearance is less than 40 ml/min, the loading and maintenance doses of disopyramide should be reduced. Table 140–2 lists suggested initial dosing schedules for patients with mild to severe chronic renal impairment.[95]

Hemodialysis has little effect on the elimination half-life of disopyramide. In a study by Sevka et al.,[119] the mean elimination half-life was 16.8 ± 11.9 hours in patients on dialysis, compared with 16.1 ± 5.2 hours in patients not receiving dialysis. Less than 2.4% of a disopyramide dose was dialyzed in a 2-hour period. These results suggest that there is no need for a dose adjustment in patients undergoing hemodialysis.[119] Charcoal hemoperfusion removed no more than 5% of ingested disopyramide.[120] However, disopyramide is readily removed by hemoperfusion over Ambulite XAD 4 resin, and there is one case report of a patient with a disopyramide overdose who was treated with hemoperfusion with this agent.[34]

Therapy with disopyramide in patients with chronic renal failure, patients undergoing hemodialysis, and renal transplant recipients is further compli-

cated by the fact that serum α_{1A}Gp concentrations may vary by up to 10-fold between individuals with these conditions, compared with approximately two-fold in normal individuals.[108] Because higher α_{1A}Gp concentrations result in less unbound disopyramide, marked interindividual variability exists in the pharmacologic effect of disopyramide in patients with these renal conditions. Because of this variability, patients with renal insufficiency should be treated carefully initially with low dosages that are advanced slowly to higher dosages until a pharmacologic effect or toxicity occurs.[110]

During the acute phase of myocardial infarction, serum disopyramide levels may be relatively low when the drug is given orally. Ward and Kinghorn[121] showed that, after a single oral dose, the serum level in patients in the acute phase of myocardial infarction was approximately half that of normal individuals. This finding has been confirmed subsequently by others and has been ascribed by most investigators to be secondary to decreased absorption.[111, 122] These effects appear to attenuate in the later phase of recovery from AMI. Although previous investigators have not shown a change in elimination kinetics, one study[123] revealed that disopyramide given intravenously in the setting of AMI was still associated with lower serum levels. These authors found increased plasma clearance of the drug compared with historical control subjects, suggesting the possibility of altered pharmacokinetics in the acute phase of myocardial infarction. However, other investigators have not found any change in clearance of the drug.[111, 122] Another complicating factor in the setting of AMI is the fact that α_{1A}Gp levels increase, further decreasing the amount of free drug available.[109] Because increased dosages of disopyramide may need to be given in the first days after myocardial infarction, before normalization of the bioavailability of disopyramide in the later postinfarction setting, the patient must be monitored closely for the development of disopyramide-related toxicity, and the dosage should be decreased with time.

It is unusual to require initiation of any oral antiarrhythmic therapy in the first few days after myocardial infarction, and the most prudent course is to delay initiation of oral disopyramide until a few days after myocardial infarction. In the setting of congestive heart failure, a decrease in the plasma clearance of disopyramide occurs, presumably related to decreased renal perfusion and decreased hepatic conversion; a decrease also occurs in the apparent volume of distribution.[124] In the setting of mild to moderate congestive heart failure, these effects are probably minimal.[110] Because congestive heart failure is a relative contraindication to the use of disopyramide, these considerations rarely have to be entertained clinically.

In patients with hepatic dysfunction, conversion of disopyramide to MND is decreased. In a study by Bonde et al.,[125] significant reduction occurred in the clearance of unbound disopyramide and in its total volume of distribution and half-life in the setting of hepatic dysfunction. There was, however, no differ-

Table 140–2. **Starting Disopyramide Dosage in Renal Failure**

Creatinine Clearance (ml/min)	Dose (mg)	Dosing Interval
>40	100	Every 6 hr
30–40	100	Every 8 hr
15–30	100	Every 12 hr
<15	100	Every 24 hr

Adapted from Karim A, Nissen C, Azarnoff DL: Clinical pharmacokinetics of disopyramide. J Pharmacokinet Biopharm 10:465, 1982.

ence in the total elimination clearance. In patients with histologically verified cirrhosis of the liver, the serum concentration of $\alpha_{1A}Gp$ was significantly decreased, resulting in a higher unbound disopyramide fraction compared with a group of patients with ischemic heart disease.[125] Given these considerations, the dose of disopyramide should be decreased in patients with hepatic dysfunction.

DRUG INTERACTIONS

The administration of disopyramide in patients receiving digoxin causes no change in the serum digoxin level.[126] Likewise, there is probably not a significant interaction between disopyramide and warfarin,[127] although Haworth and Burrows reported one patient in whom the prothrombin time decreased after administration of disopyramide.[128] The addition of quinidine to disopyramide (or vice versa) results in a 10% to 15% increase in the minimum and maximum disopyramide (or quinidine) concentration.[95] Karim et al.[95] were unable to show any effect of propranolol or diazepam on disopyramide levels. However, Bonde et al.[129] demonstrated that atenolol decreased the clearance of disopyramide from 1.9 ± 0.71 ml/kg/min to 1.59 ± 0.68 ml/kg/min without affecting plasma half-life, concentration of metabolite, or volume of distribution of the drug. The exact nature of this interaction was not defined and requires confirmation. In general, when disopyramide is used in combination with other antiarrhythmic drugs, careful monitoring of electrophysiologic parameters and use of lower dosages of disopyramide as well as the combination agent(s) are recommended, because the results of interactions may be unpredictable in an individual patient.[96]

Significant interactions with disopyramide occur with drugs that induce hepatic enzymes. Several investigators showed that rifampin, phenytoin, and barbituates, which are known hepatic enzyme inducers, markedly increase the serum level of MND relative to disopyramide and may increase the incidence of anticholinergic side effects.[114, 130-132] Because of this risk of increased adverse reactions, patients taking these agents should be started on lower initial dosages of disopyramide and monitored closely for side effects as the dose is increased.

Erythromycin and other macrolide antibiotics have been shown to inhibit potently metabolism of disopyramide to MND.[133] In two elderly patients,[134] life-threatening arrhythmic complications may have resulted from this type of interaction.

ADVERSE REACTIONS

The most common adverse effects encountered with the administration of disopyramide relate to its anticholinergic properties. Side effects, which are usually dose related (e.g., visual blurring, dryness of the mouth, difficulty urinating, constipation, and abdominal discomfort), occur commonly, but only approximately 10% to 20% of patients have side effects severe

enough to necessitate discontinuation of the drug.[135-138] Disopyramide has been reported to cause acute urinary retention in elderly male patients with underlying benign prostatic hypertrophy,[139] and the drug has also been reported to precipitate closed-angle glaucoma.[140] Mild anticholinergic side effects typically attenuate with time and frequently do not require discontinuation of the medication. There is conflicting evidence concerning the degree of anticholinergic side effects when controlled-release and standard formulations are compared.[2, 86] Recently, Teichman et al.[138, 141] reported that sustained-release pyridostigmine bromide in dosages of 90 to 180 mg every 8 to 12 hours prevented the occurrence of anticholinergic side effects in patients started on disopyramide therapy, eliminated these side effects after they had developed, and allowed administration of higher dosages of disopyramide. The use of non-sustained-release pyridostigmine can result in cholinergic side effects and should be avoided. Pyridostigmine did not appear to decrease the overall antiarrhythmic efficacy of disopyramide.[138, 141] Thus, anticholinergic side effects with disopyramide frequently can be eliminated by the use of either controlled-release disopyramide or concomitantly administered sustained-release pyridostigmine.

Disopyramide, like other antiarrhythmic agents, can also be associated with gastrointestinal side effects such as nausea, vomiting, or diarrhea, and much less often with symptoms such as general fatigue or headache. The gastrointestinal side effects appear to be much less frequent than with quinidine in equivalent dosages. In a double-blind comparison study of quinidine sulfate, 1300 mg/day, and disopyramide, 600 mg/day, the discontinuation rate due to side effects was 36% with quinidine but only 10% with disopyramide.[135] Most side effects experienced with disopyramide therapy were secondary to anticholinergic properties and could theoretically be reversed, as mentioned previously. Thus, disopyramide appears to be better tolerated than quinidine in terms of noncardiac side effects. In fact, one of the attractive properties of disopyramide is good patient compliance for long-term therapy without the late development of new side effects.

Less common noncardiac side effects experienced with disopyramide include cholestatic jaundice,[142] laryngospasm,[143] acute psychosis,[144, 145] premature uterine contraction,[146] impotence,[147] and hypoglycemia.[148, 149] Strathman et al.[149] reviewed patient experience with disopyramide over approximately 4 million patient-months based on reports to G. D. Searle and Company up to 1980, and these investigators identified only 32 cases of hypoglycemia. Apparent risk factors for the development of hypoglycemia included older age and decreased hepatic or renal function. In a study in normal individuals, disopyramide decreased measured glucose in the fasting and fed state by 6.3% to 6.9% compared with the control state.[149] No significant changes were noted in either insulin or glucagon levels. The conclusion was that disopyramide has a small but clinically insignificant glucose-lowering effect in normal individuals but may rarely precipitate symptomatic hypoglycemia in the risk group identified here.[149] However, induction of severe hypoglycemia has been reported.[58] The mechanism for its hypoglycemic effect is thought to be secretion of endogenous insulin,[122] mediated by the effect of disopyramide on the ATP-sensitive potassium channel $I_{K,ATP}$,[26, 27] with inadequate counterregulatory hormonal response.

Disopyramide has a number of potentially adverse effects on the heart, including depression of left ventricular function,[7, 70–83] induction of heart block,[64, 65] prolongation of the QT interval,[83, 150] and generation or aggravation of tachyarrhythmias.[150–153] As mentioned earlier, disopyramide has significant negative inotropic effects and has been noted to cause profound hypotension, acute congestive heart failure, and electromechanical dissociation, typically in individuals with markedly depressed left ventricular function and history of congestive heart failure.[80–83] The drug is therefore contraindicated in this group of patients. Disopyramide has also been reported to precipitate high-grade AV block in patients with pre-existing bifascicular bundle branch block.[64, 65] The ability of disopyramide to stress further the conduction system to precipitate high grades of AV block has actually been used by some investigators, as has procainamide, to assess patients with bilateral bundle branch disease and syncope.[65] In the authors' experience, disopyramide, quinidine, or procainamide rarely cause Mobitz type II second-degree AV block in patients with bifascicular block in whom therapy is given for tachyarrhythmias.

Profound QT-interval prolongation occurs in approximately 7% of individuals given disopyramide,[83] and cases of disopyramide-induced torsade de pointes[139] and "disopyramide syncope"[58] have been reported. However, the overall frequency of proarrhythmic complications, quoted at 1% to 6% with disopyramide,[151, 152, 154] may be less than with either procainamide or quinidine. Proarrhythmia occurs more commonly in patients with lower left ventricular ejection fractions and in patients treated for sustained ventricular tachycardia.[153] Other conditions increasing the risk of proarrhythmia for any antiarrhythmic agent are preexisting repolarization abnormalities, including prolonged QT interval, electrolyte imbalance, particularly of potassium and magnesium, and rapid upward titration of dose.[96, 155] Women may be at higher risk of drug-related torsade de pointes.[156]

There is little experience with disopyramide in lactating women, and thus the overall safety of the drug in this situation is unknown, as it is with most agents. In pregnancy, there is good evidence that disopyramide may induce premature contractions and precipitate delivery.[16] The teratogenic effects of disopyramide are unknown. Although disopyramide may be found in significant concentrations in breast milk, the amount obtained by the infant typically is not clinically significant.[101]

Intentional or accidental overdosages of disopyramide may result in profound hypotension and circulatory arrest. In the study by Jaeger et al.[120] of 106 patients with disopyramide overdose, 23% developed cardiogenic shock and 16% developed circulatory arrest. High-grade conduction disturbances occurred in 8% and bradycardia in 22%. Roughly one quarter of the patients initially had anticholinergic side effects, and approximately half lost consciousness. Ventricular tachyarrhythmias occurred in 14%, and overall mortality was 12%. A toxic dose of disopyramide appeared to be higher than 1.5 g, with the average lethal dose being more than 2.8 g.[120]

Therapy for overdosages is simply supportive in nature. Charcoal hemoperfusion removed no more than 5% of the ingested dose, although, as noted before, hemoperfusion over Ambulite XAD 4 resin can be much more effective.[34, 120] Alkalinization of the urine appeared to have little effect on enhancing excretion of the drug.[112] Administration of sodium lactate, however, may improve intraventricular conduction.[120]

CLINICAL EFFICACY

Premature Ventricular Complexes and Nonsustained Ventricular Tachycardia

Disopyramide is an effective agent for suppression of premature ventricular complexes and nonsustained ventricular tachycardia. The overall efficacy has varied from 22% to 85% in suppressing ventricular ectopy by more than 80%.[14, 26, 27, 35, 135, 157–159] Most studies report an efficacy rate of approximately 60% to 80%. Disopyramide is even more effective in suppressing complex ventricular ectopy, with success rates ranging typically from 80% to 98%. Disopyramide appears to be as effective as the other type IA antiarrhythmic agents.[14, 26, 135] In a double-blind study comparing the efficacy of quinidine and disopyramide in 124 patients studied for 18 weeks, no significant difference was noted in efficacy between the two drugs.[135] However, the rate of withdrawal of patients for adverse reactions was greater for quinidine (36%) than for disopyramide (10%). Disopyramide may be more effective in suppressing both simple and complex ventricular ectopy than the class IB agents,[27, 157] but conflicting results have been reported.[158, 159] In one study, disopyramide, 600 mg daily, caused more than 80% suppression of simple and complex ventricular ectopy in 87% of patients, compared with mexiletine, 600 mg daily, which was effective in only 53% of patients. However, when mexiletine was given to a small cohort of patients at a much higher dose, 1000 mg daily, it was as efficacious as disopyramide.[27] In the authors' experience, it is rare for a patient to tolerate mexiletine at such a high dose. Combination therapy of disopyramide and mexiletine has also been tried and has been shown to be more effective than either disopyramide or mexiletine alone.[157]

In comparison with type IC agents, disopyramide, like other type IA agents, is not as effective in suppressing ventricular ectopy.[35, 160–163]

In a randomized, double-blind, crossover trial of flecainide and disopyramide, flecainide was effective for suppression of ventricular ectopy in 92% of patients compared with 39% of patients given disopyramide.[35] In addition, flecainide appears to be more effective than disopyramide for suppressing complex ventricular ectopy, and the incidence and severity of side effects were equivalent for the two medications. Encainide and propafenone, likewise, appear to be more effective in suppression of ventricular ectopy than disopyramide.[161-163] Disopyramide appears to be more effective than β-blockers in suppressing premature ventricular contractions. A study of controlled-release disopyramide compared with long-acting propranolol showed a greater than 80% suppression in premature ventricular contractions in 58% of patients treated with disopyramide compared with 17% treated with propranolol.[164] It is important to remember that there may be no clinical difference between suppression of approximately 90% versus approximately 60% of premature ventricular complexes in a given patient.

Sustained Ventricular Tachycardia

Disopyramide also has been shown to be effective in suppressing sustained ventricular tachycardia.[38, 45, 156, 165-167] Disopyramide has been effective in preventing the induction of ventricular tachycardia by programmed electrical stimulation in 4% to 34% of individuals.[48, 166, 167] In the study by Lerman et al.[48] of 50 patients with inducible sustained ventricular tachycardia, the arrhythmia could not be induced in 17 patients (34%) with a mean disopyramide plasma level of 3.6 ± 1.2 μg/ml. They noted that success of therapy was not significantly related to the plasma level,[48] which contradicts the findings of others.[46] They did note, however, that patients in whom ventricular tachycardia was no longer inducible had

shorter ventricular tachycardia cycle lengths than those who did not respond (225 ± 51 msec versus 281 ± 70 msec). In patients whose tachycardia was still inducible, the cycle length of tachycardia increased from 281 ± 70 msec to 347 ± 64 msec.[48] Of the 17 patients who were treated successfully with disopyramide, 11 were discharged from the hospital and followed up for a mean of 9 months, and 9 of these patients remained free of ventricular tachycardia.[48] Disopyramide, alone or in combination therapy, controlled sustained ventricular tachycardia in 19 of 25 patients who commenced disopyramide after publication of the Cardiac Arrhythmia Suppression Trial (CAST) preliminary report in August 1989.[96, 168] Only 3 of these 25 patients had a left ventricular ejection fraction measured at less than 30%. Disopyramide continues to be an effective agent for the treatment of sustained ventricular tachycardia.

Disopyramide is generally believed to be as effective as quinidine and procainamide.[156, 167] In the study of Wyse et al.[156] comparing disopyramide, quinidine, and procainamide in suppressing sustained ventricular tachycardia as assessed by programmed electrical stimulation, complete response rates were 19%, 28%, and 16%, and partial response rates were 19%, 19%, and 19%, respectively. Thus, the three type IA agents were not significantly different in overall efficacy.

In the study by Swiryn et al.,[38] the concordance rate (percentage of patients responding or not responding to both drugs) was 83% with procainamide and quinidine compared with 71% with procainamide and disopyramide and 67% with quinidine and disopyramide (Fig. 140–8). Nine patients had a discordant response to procainamide and disopyramide, and six of these did not respond to procainamide but responded to disopyramide. Similarly, nine patients had a discordant response with quinidine and disopyr-

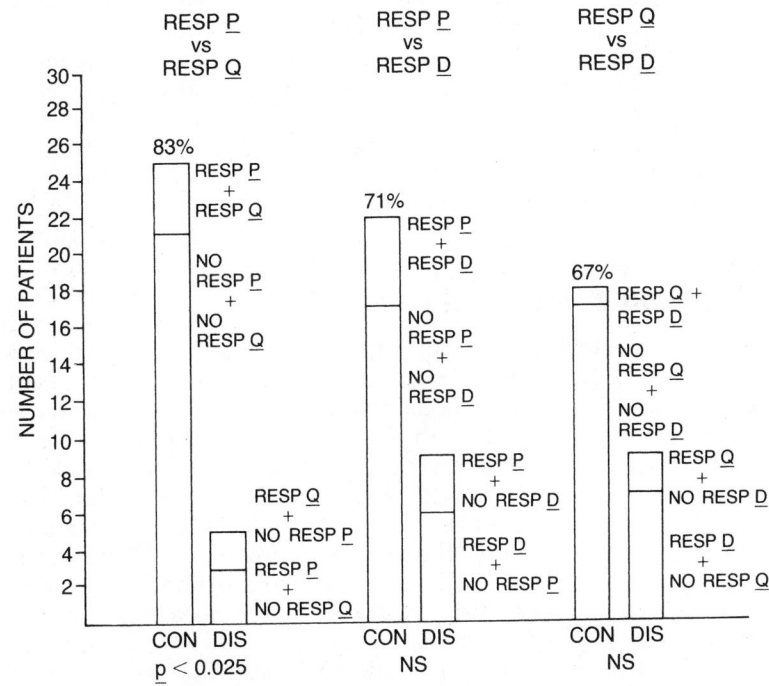

Figure 140–8. Bar graph illustrating concordant (CON) and discordant (DIS) responses (RESP) in patients with ventricular tachycardia treated with at least two of the following: disopyramide (D), procainamide (P), and quinidine (Q). Note that discordant responses were much more likely to occur between disopyramide and procainamide or disopyramide and quinidine than they were to occur between procainamide and quinidine. (From Swiryn S, Bauernfeind RA, Strasberg B, et al: Prediction of response to class I antiarrhythmic drugs during electrophysiologic study of ventricular tachycardia. Am Heart J 104:43, 1982.)

amide, and eight of these did not respond to quinidine but responded to disopyramide. Similar discordant responses were found by Wyse et al.[156] These data clearly demonstrate that inefficacy of quinidine or procainamide should not preclude a clinical trial of disopyramide in patients in whom this agent can be administered safely. The type IC agents appear to be more effective than disopyramide in suppressing ventricular tachycardia as assessed by noninvasive methods,[35, 162, 163] but few data are available on relative efficacy with programmed ventricular stimulation. Little information is available on combination therapy with disopyramide and other agents.[5, 43, 169]

Prevention of Sudden Death After Myocardial Infarction

An early study[170] suggested that disopyramide was effective in preventing ventricular arrhythmias and mortality after myocardial infarction. Although disopyramide prevents warning arrhythmias, four prospective placebo-controlled trials with disopyramide given to patients after admission for myocardial infarction have not shown a significant difference in mortality between treatment and placebo groups.[171–174] In addition, treatment with disopyramide was more often associated with the development of side effects necessitating its discontinuation than was placebo.[172, 174] In a placebo-controlled trial comparing oxprenolol with disopyramide, no significant difference was noted in 6-week mortality with placebo, oxprenolol, or disopyramide when these agents were compared by intention-to-treat analysis.[172] In patients with documented infarction, there was a trend toward decreased mortality in patients who were able to continue either of the antiarrhythmic agents, but these differences were not statistically significant when compared with placebo.[172] All studies attempting to assess the effect of disopyramide on long-term mortality and arrhythmic events after myocardial infarction have been hindered by relatively small numbers of patients. The ability of any antiarrhythmic agent to decrease mortality after myocardial infarction should be reassessed in light of changes in acute care (e.g., thrombolytic therapy) of patients with myocardial infarction.

Atrioventricular Nodal Reentrant Tachycardia

Studies have shown that both intravenous and oral disopyramide are effective in treating reciprocating tachycardia using dual AV nodal pathways.[47, 103, 175, 176] In studies using serial electrophysiologic testing, disopyramide given either intravenously or orally prevented reinduction of AV nodal reentrant tachycardia in 60% to 73% of patients.[103, 175, 176] As with other patient population groups, the electrophysiologic effects of disopyramide on anterograde conduction over the AV node were variable, as assessed by measurement of the AH interval and anterograde AV nodal effective and functional refractory periods.[103,] [175, 176] In general, the atrial myocardial effective and functional refractory periods increased. However, the effect on retrograde conduction, presumably over the fast conducting pathway, was more uniform with typical prolongation of the retrograde AV nodal effective refractory period.[103, 175, 176] The effectiveness of disopyramide in terminating and preventing AV nodal reciprocating tachycardia depends on a delicate interplay between alterations in refractory periods and conduction velocities of the tissues involved in the tachycardia circuit, which may be altered by either its membrane-stabilizing or anticholinergic properties. In a study by Brugada and Wellens,[103] AV nodal reciprocating tachycardia was prevented by four possible mechanisms: (1) sole prolongation of refractory periods of the fast conducting retrograde pathway; (2) shortening of anterograde conduction over the slow conducting pathway, so that the return cycle still found the fast retrograde pathway refractory; (3) shortening of anterograde refractory period, so that dual AV nodal physiology could not be demonstrated owing to the limitations of programmed stimulation by atrial refractory period; and (4) the combination of increasing retrograde refractory periods across the fast pathway and decreasing anterograde conduction across the slow pathway. Thus, disopyramide appears to be an effective agent for treatment of AV nodal reciprocating tachycardia. Furthermore, in the authors' experience, use of the controlled-release formulation makes this an excellent drug of early choice.

Atrioventricular Reciprocating Tachycardia (Wolff-Parkinson-White Syndrome)

Disopyramide is also effective in treating reciprocating tachycardia involving accessory bypass pathways as well as in decreasing the rate of anterograde conduction over the accessory pathway during atrial fibrillation or flutter.[43, 51, 175, 177, 178] Oral disopyramide prevents the induction of reciprocating tachycardia by programmed electrical stimulation in 0% to 70% of patients with Wolff-Parkinson-White syndrome.[175,] [178, 179] However, disopyramide increases the cycle length of induced reciprocating tachycardia by a mean of approximately 50 msec, primarily by increasing retrograde conduction time over the accessory pathway.[51, 175, 178, 179] A study by Kerr et al.[178] showed that disopyramide was effective in depressing accessory pathway conduction in patients with accessory pathways with short refractory periods.

Patients who have accessory pathways capable of rapid anterograde conduction are at greatest risk for the development of ventricular fibrillation. Disopyramide has been shown to depress anterograde conduction over the accessory pathway.[51, 175, 179] Combination of mexiletine with disopyramide can cause at least additive depression of anterograde accessory pathway conduction.[138]

In the study by Kerr et al.,[178] the shortest RR interval measured during atrial fibrillation increased from 169 ± 28 msec to 226 ± 24 msec, and the mean RR interval during atrial fibrillation increased from 255 ± 58 msec to 329 ± 62 msec (Fig. 140–9). Combination with mexiletine can lengthen the shortest and mean preexcited RR intervals during atrial fibrillation more than disopyramide alone.[138] Because disopyramide can cause a significant decrease in the ventricular response during atrial fibrillation, its use in this situation seems preferable to quinidine or procainamide.[177, 180] Whether disopyramide is as effective as type IC agents in this group of patients is unknown. Furthermore, whether any of these agents reduces the risk of sudden cardiac death is unclear, and our current approach to patients with rapid preexcited ventricular responses during spontaneous or induced atrial fibrillation is to recommend surgical ablation of the accessory pathway. Kerr et al.[178] also noted that the episodes of atrial fibrillation induced on oral disopyramide therapy in their patients with Wolff-Parkinson-White syndrome were both shorter and self-terminating after administration of the drug.

Atrial Fibrillation and Flutter

Disopyramide is also effective in the treatment of atrial fibrillation and flutter in patients without preexcitation syndromes when it is used in conjunction with drugs that slow AV nodal conduction. Efficacy rates range from 37% to 72% for the conversion to and maintenance of sinus rhythm.[181–188] In the study

by Hartel et al.,[181] disopyramide was compared with placebo in facilitating electric cardioversion of atrial fibrillation and in maintaining sinus rhythm after successful cardioversion. Cardioversion was successful in 83% of patients in the placebo group and in 75% of patients in the disopyramide group. Of patients who successfully underwent cardioversion, 72% remained in sinus rhythm at 3 months of follow-up in the disopyramide group, compared with only 30% in patients given placebo.[181] In another placebo-controlled study, 50% to 60% of patients taking disopyramide remained in sinus rhythm 1 year after cardioversion.[189]

Disopyramide also facilitates conversion of atrial flutter to sinus rhythm by overdrive pacing.[188] Like flecainide, disopyramide has been shown to cause preferential delay at the zone of slow conduction in the reentrant circuit of canine atrial flutter.[90]

In patients developing atrial tachyarrhythmias after cardiac surgery, disopyramide plus digoxin has been shown to be more effective than digoxin alone in returning patients to sinus rhythm.[182] Disopyramide and quinidine are equally effective in maintaining sinus rhythm after cardioversion.[184] In a comparison study of disopyramide versus a combination of quinidine and verapamil for the conversion of patients with atrial fibrillation and flutter, sinus rhythm was obtained in 37% of patients with disopyramide, compared with 50% of patients using the combination

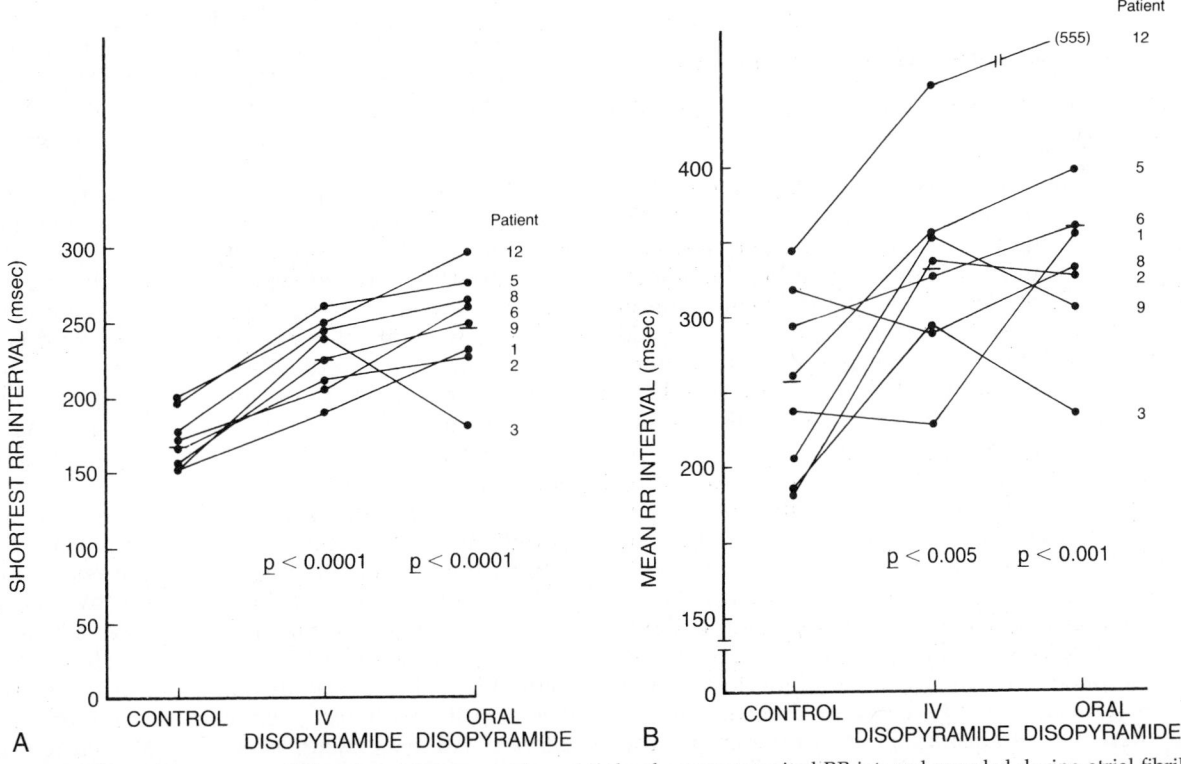

Figure 140–9. Effect of intravenous (IV) and oral disopyramide on (A) the shortest preexcited RR interval recorded during atrial fibrillation and (B) the mean RR interval recorded during atrial fibrillation in patients with the Wolff-Parkinson-White syndrome. Mean values are shown as horizontal bars. Note that both intravenous and oral disopyramide doses significantly increase the shortest and mean RR intervals during atrial fibrillation, regardless of the value of these parameters during the control state. (Reproduced with permission from Kerr CR, Prystowsky EN, Smith WM, et al: Electrophysiologic effects of disopyramide phosphate in patients with Wolff-Parkinson-White syndrome. Circulation 65:869, 1982. Copyright 1982, American Heart Association.)

of quinidine and verapamil.[183] The combination of disopyramide and digoxin was found to be as effective as intravenous sotalol in the conversion of atrial fibrillation after open heart surgery.[186] Disopyramide is less effective than low-dose amiodarone for treatment of paroxysmal atrial fibrillation.[187] However, in the authors' experience, no drug is as effective as amiodarone in the treatment of atrial fibrillation, especially in refractory patients. Studies comparing disopyramide with type IC agents in the treatment of atrial fibrillation and flutter are not available. Thus, disopyramide is an effective drug for treatment of patients with atrial fibrillation or flutter. However, the use of disopyramide alone is relatively contraindicated in patients with atrial flutter (as are quinidine or procainamide alone), because disopyramide may provoke 1:1 AV conduction during atrial flutter. This presumably is due to both the effect of disopyramide on slowing the rate of atrial flutter as well as enhancing AV nodal conduction with its anticholinergic properties.[191]

Other Atrial Arrhythmias

Disopyramide is also successful in suppressing symptomatic premature atrial complexes and other atrial tachyarrhythmias. However, little quantitative information is available as to the efficacy of this drug in these situations or the relative benefit of disopyramide versus other antiarrhythmic agents for the treatment of these conditions.

Other Clinical Uses of Disopyramide

Evaluation of the His-Purkinje System in Patients with Syncope

Recently, Bergfeldt et al.[65] suggested that the electrophysiologic properties of disopyramide are ideally suited for stressing the His-Purkinje system in evaluating patients with chronic bifascicular bundle branch block and syncope. The membrane-stabilizing effects of the medication would further impair His-Purkinje conduction, and the anticholinergic effects theoretically would facilitate conduction over the AV node to provide a greater stress on the His-Purkinje system. They gave disopyramide, 2 mg/kg IV, to three groups of patients: (1) patients with prior second- or third-degree AV block after myocardial infarction, (2) patients with bifascicular block after infarction but with no clinical histories of syncope or documented second- or third-degree AV block, and (3) patients with chronic bifascicular block and syncope but without documented second- or third-degree AV block. These authors defined a positive disopyramide test as the spontaneous induction of second- or third-degree AV block after the administration of disopyramide, the development of intra- or infra-Hisian block during atrial pacing or after rapid ventricular pacing, or a 50% increase in the baseline HV interval. The test was positive in 80% of patients known to have high-grade AV block, indicating that this test is reasonably sensi-

tive. The test was positive in only 10% of patients with chronic asymptomatic bifascicular block, which suggests an approximate specificity of 90% given the fact that this group is at relatively low risk for the development of subsequent high-grade AV block. In the group with chronic bifascicular block and syncope, the predictive value of the test was 80%.[65] If prolongation of the HV interval by 50% or more was excluded from this analysis, the sensitivity, specificity, and predictive value of a positive disopyramide test were 100%, 90%, and 83%, respectively.[65] A significant adverse reaction (hypotension) occurred in only 1 of the 27 patients studied. Although the results of this test indicate that disopyramide may be a useful adjunct in assessing patients with chronic bifascicular block and syncope, the number of patients used in this study was small, and a large-scale prospective study should be performed to confirm the usefulness of disopyramide in this situation. Of note, similar efforts to stress the His-Purkinje system have been made using intravenous procainamide.[190]

Vasovagal Syncope

In theory, disopyramide appears useful for the prevention of neurally mediated syncope. The anticholinergic properties of disopyramide would be anticipated to antagonize vagally mediated bradycardia. The negative inotropic properties of disopyramide may attenuate orthostatically induced cardiac hypercontractility, chamber obliteration, and increase in vagal tone. In addition, the vasoconstrictor properties of disopyramide may further support or maintain systemic pressure, decreasing the need for increased peripheral catecholamines, which are in part responsible for the increased contractility.

Milstein et al.[192] have suggested that low-dose oral disopyramide may be effective in preventing inducible and spontaneous neurally mediated syncope in humans. They studied seven patients with recurrent vasovagal syncope by provocation with upright tilt alone or with tilt plus isoproterenol infusion. Hypotension and bradycardia were induced in all patients with tilt or with tilt and isoproterenol infusion in the baseline state. However, 48 hours after starting oral disopyramide therapy at a dose of 450 mg/day to obtain a mean disopyramide level of 3.0 ± 0.25 mg/ml, all patients tolerated more than 10 minutes of upright tilt and upright tilt plus isoproterenol infusion without the development of symptoms, hypotension, or bradycardia. During follow-up over a mean 9-month period, all patients remained asymptomatic.[192] In another study, an even lower dose of disopyramide, 300 mg/day, resulted in normalization of prior positive tilt test results in six out of six patients.[162] All six patients were free of recurrent syncope during a median follow-up period of 16 months. However, Kelly et al.[193] reported that in their study all patients who were given 450 mg/day of disopyramide developed syncope at repeat tilt testing. These investigators found that higher doses (600 to 1200

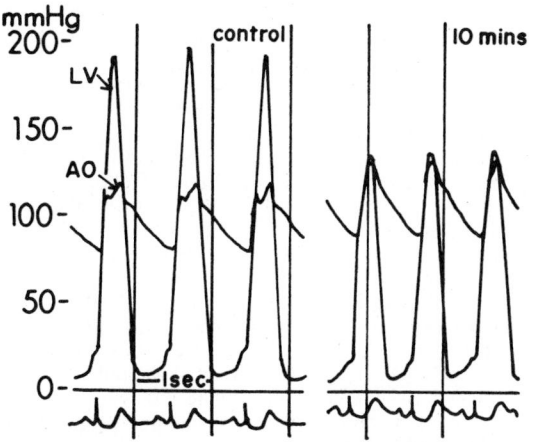

Figure 140–10. Simultaneous aortic (AO) and left ventricular (LV) pressures and electrocardiograms obtained at control and 10 minutes after intravenous infusion of disopyramide (100 mg) in a patient with a large left ventricular outflow tract gradient at rest due to HOCM. Note that, after intravenous infusion of disopyramide, the resting outflow tract gradient is nearly totally abolished. (From Pollick C: Muscular subaortic stenosis: Hemodynamic and clinical improvement after disopyramide. N Engl J Med 307:997, 1982.)

mg/day) may be necessary for effective prevention of syncope at tilt testing.

Finally, in a placebo-controlled, double-blind, randomized trial[166] involving 22 patients with two or more successive positive tilt test responses, intravenous disopyramide did not prevent neurally mediated syncope provoked by tilt testing, and the effects of oral disopyramide were overshadowed by a striking decrease in the incidence of positive test results regardless of therapy. Likewise, recurrence of syncope over long-term follow-up was infrequent, regardless of therapy. The authors concluded that the response to serial tilt testing in the assessment of efficacy of therapy should be interpreted with caution.

Hypertrophic Obstructive Cardiomyopathy

Pollick[194] used the negative inotropic properties of disopyramide to treat five patients with hypertrophic obstructive cardiomyopathy (HOCM). He noted that the basal pressure gradient across the subaortic stenosis was abolished (Fig. 140–10) and that the provokable gradient decreased in all four patients who had a baseline hemodynamic evaluation. In addition, two of these patients had a decrease in left ventricular end-diastolic pressure with disopyramide. In the three patients who were treated chronically, all had an increase in exercise capacity and a decrease in symptomatology, and one patient who had associated atrial tachycardia had a decrease in frequency of this rhythm.[194] In another study of 25 adults, Kimball et al.[195] showed that intravenous disopyramide could cause substantial acute reductions in both resting and postextrasystolic left ventricular outflow tract obstruction, without causing significant electrocardiographic changes. After long-term treatment of HOCM

patients with disopyramide, significant decreases have been shown in resting ejection fraction, peak ejection rate, and peak filling rate, measured by radionuclide ventriculography.[131] Rapid improvement in clinical signs and nearly complete abolition of severe left ventricular outflow tract obstruction have been documented in two children with HOCM who were given oral disopyramide.[89] The reduced outflow obstruction caused by disopyramide in HOCM seems to be due mainly to its negative inotropic effect and peripheral vasoconstrictive action. Improvements in Doppler echocardiographic parameters implying better left ventricular diastolic filling, comparable to those seen with diltiazem, have been documented after administration of disopyramide in one study,[125] but there is conflicting opinion about the effect of disopyramide on diastolic ventricular function.[131] Thus, disopyramide appears to be effective in treating symptoms and ameliorating hemodynamic abnormalities associated with HOCM and may be particularly effective in patients with associated rhythm disturbances such as atrial fibrillation.

SUMMARY

Disopyramide is a type IA agent with a unique combination of membrane-stabilizing properties as well as anticholinergic effects. The anticholinergic properties of disopyramide may alter its expected electrophysiologic responses *in vivo*. Disopyramide has been found to be useful in a number of clinical conditions, including treatment of premature atrial and ventricular complexes, atrial flutter and fibrillation, paroxysmal AV nodal and AV reentrant tachycardia, and sustained ventricular tachycardia and ventricular fibrillation. It has theoretical benefits and some apparent utility in the treatment of vasovagal syncope, and it has shown promise in the management of HOCM. The side effect profile of disopyramide is predictable and includes anticholinergic side effects, which may be attenuated by the concomitant administration of sustained-release pyridostigmine, and significant depression of left ventricular function.

REFERENCES

1. Vaughan Williams EM: Disopyramide. Ann N Y Acad Sci 432:189, 1984.
2. Mokler C, Van Arman C: Pharmacology of a new antiarrhythmic agent, diisopropylamino phenyl (2-pyridyl)-butyramide (SC-7031). J Pharmacol Exp Ther 136:114, 1962.
3. Kus T, Sasyniuk BI: Electrophysiological actions of disopyramide phosphate on canine ventricular muscle and Purkinje fibers. Circ Res 37:844, 1975.
4. Danilo P Jr, Hordof AJ, Rosen MR: Effects of disopyramide on electrophysiologic properties of canine Purkinje fibers. J Pharmacol Exp Ther 201:701, 1977.
5. James MA, Papouchado M, Vann Jones J: Combined therapy with disopyramide and amiodarone: A report of 11 cases. Int J Cardiol 13:248, 1986.
6. Mirro MJ, Watanabe AM, Bailey JC: Electrophysiologic effects of the optical isomers of disopyramide and quinidine in the dog. Dependence on stereochemistry. Circ Res 48:867, 1981.
7. Silke B, Frais MA, Verma SP, et al: Comparative haemody-

namic effects of intravenous lignocaine, disopyramide, and flecainide in uncomplicated myocardial infarction. Br J Clin Pharmacol 22:707, 1986.

8. Myerburg RJ, Stewart JW, Hoffman BF: Electrophysiological properties of the canine peripheral AV conducting system. Circ Res 26:361, 1970.

9. Wittig J, Harrison LA, Wallace AG: Electrophysiological effects of lidocaine on distal Purkinje fibers of canine heart. Am Heart J 86:69, 1973.

10. Rosen MR, Merker C, Gelband H, et al: Effects of procainamide on the electrophysiologic properties of canine ventricular conducting system. J Pharmacol Exp Ther 185:438, 1973.

11. Sekiya A, Vaughan Williams EM: A comparison of the antifibrillatory action and effects on intracellular cardiac potentials of pronethalol, disopyramide and quinidine. Br J Pharmacol 21:475, 1963.

12. Katoh T, Karagueuzian HS, Jordan J, et al: The cellular electrophysiologic mechanism of the dual actions of disopyramide on rabbit sinus node function. Circulation 66:1216, 1982.

13. Sasyniak BI, Kus T: Cellular electrophysiologic changes induced by disopyramide phosphate in normal and infarcted hearts. J Int Med Res 4(Suppl 1):20, 1976.

14. Newman R, Fonda D, Skoien A, et al: A comparison of disopyramide and quinidine in the suppression of ventricular arrhythmias in ambulatory patients. Aust N Z J Med 11:455, 1981.

15. Matsuda H, Konishi T, Tamamura T, et al: Electrophysiological effects of disopyramide on hypoxic rabbit ventricular muscle. Jpn Circ J 46:663, 1982.

16. Yamada S, Nishimura M, Watanabe Y: Electrophysiologic effects of disopyramide studied in a hypoxic canine Purkinje fiber model. J Electrocardiogr 15:31, 1982.

17. Nishimura M, Yamada S, Watanabe Y: Electrophysiologic effects of disopyramide phosphate on the spontaneous action potential and membrane current systems of the rabbit atrioventricular node [abstract]. Am J Cardiol 49:921, 1982.

18. Watanabe Y, Nishimura M, Yamada S: Significance of a combination of different experimental approaches. Lake Kawaguchi Conference of Cardiology, Japan. Heart 16:513, 1984.

19. Yatani A, Akaike N: Blockage of the sodium current in isolated single cells from rat ventricle with mexiletine and disopyramide. J Mol Cell Cardiol 17:467, 1985.

20. Varro A, Elharrar V, Surawicz B: Frequency-dependent effects of several class I antiarrhythmic drugs on Vmax of action potential upstroke in canine cardiac Purkinje fibers. J Cardiovasc Pharmacol 7:482, 1985.

21. Kojima M, Ban T, Sada H: Effects of disopyramide on the maximum rates of rise of action potential (Vmax) in guinea pig papillary muscles. Jpn J Pharmacol 32:91, 1982.

22. Yeh JZ, TenEick RE: Molecular and structural basis of reacting and use-dependent block of sodium current defined using disopyramide analogues. Biophys J 51:123, 1987.

23. Grant AM, Marshall RJ, Ankier SI: Some effects of disopyramide and its N-dealkylated metabolite on isolated nerve and cardiac muscle. Eur J Pharmacol 49:389, 1978.

24. Gruber R, Carmeliet E: The activation gate of the sodium channel controls blockade and deblockade by disopyramide in rabbit Purkinje fibres. Br J Pharmacol 97:41, 1989.

25. Coraboeuf E, Deroubaix E, Escande D, Coulombe A: Comparative effects of three class 1 antiarrhythmic drugs on plateau and pacemaker currents of sheep cardiac Purkinje fibres. Cardiovasc Res 22:375, 1988.

26. Chiariello M, Indolfi C, Bigazzi C, et al: Prajmalium bitartrate in chronic ventricular arrhythmias: Comparison with disopyramide. Eur J Clin Pharmacol 24:35, 1983.

27. Breithardt G, Seipel L, Lersmacher J, et al: Comparative study of the antiarrhythmic efficacy of mexiletine and disopyramide in patients with chronic ventricular arrhythmias. J Cardiovasc Pharmacol 4:276, 1982.

28. Mirro MJ: Effects of quinidine, procainamide and disopyramide on automaticity and cyclic AMP content of guinea pig atria. J Mol Cell Cardiol 13:641, 1981.

29. Mirro MJ, Manalan AS, Bailey JC, et al: Anticholinergic effects of disopyramide and quinidine on guinea pig myocardium. Mediation by direct muscarinic receptor blockade. Circ Res 47:855, 1980.

30. Baines MW, Davies JE, Kellet DN, et al: Some pharmacologic effects of disopyramide and a metabolite. J Int Med Res 4(Suppl):5, 1976.

31. Kates RE: Metabolites of cardiac antiarrhythmic drugs: Their clinical role. Ann N Y Acad Sci 432:75, 1984.

32. Sanner JH, Novotney RL, Schulze RH, et al: Anticholinergic properties of disopyramide phosphate and its mono-N-dealkylated metabolites [abstract]. Tokyo: Eighth International Congress of Pharmacology, July 19–24, 1981, p 506.

33. Iisalo E, Aatonen L: Anticholinergic activity in the serum of patients receiving maintenance disopyramide therapy. Br J Clin Pharmacol 17:325, 1984.

34. Gosselin B, Mathieu D, Chopin C, et al: Acute intoxication with disopyramide: Clinical and experimental study by hemoperfusion on Amberlite XAD 4 resin. Clin Toxicol 17:439, 1980.

35. Kjekshus J, Bathen J, Orning OM, et al: A double-blind, crossover comparison of flecainide acetate and disopyramide phosphate in the treatment of ventricular premature complexes. Am J Cardiol 53:72B, 1984.

36. Mirro MJ, Watanabe AM, Bailey JC: Electrophysiological effects of disopyramide and quinidine on guinea pig atria and canine cardiac Purkinje fibers. Dependence on underlying cholinergic tone. Circ Res 46:660, 1980.

37. Chagnac A, Pelleg A, Belhassen B, et al: Effects of disopyramide on reperfusion arrhythmias in dogs. J Cardiovasc Pharmacol 4:994, 1982.

38. Swiryn S, Bauernfeind RA, Strasberg B, et al: Prediction of response to class I antiarrhythmic drugs during electrophysiologic study of ventricular tachycardia. Am Heart J 104:43, 1982.

39. Hori Y, Okamoto R, Hatani M, et al: Studies on the preventive method of lowered ventricular fibrillation threshold during experimental acute myocardial infarction. A comparison between disopyramide phosphate and lidocaine. Jpn Heart J 22:801, 1981.

40. Cobbe SM, Hoffmann E, Ritzenhoff A, et al: Actions of disopyramide on potential reentrant pathways and ventricular tachyarrhythmias in conscious dogs during the late post-myocardial infarction phase. Am J Cardiol 53:1712, 1984.

41. Patterson E, Gibson JK, Lucchesi BR: Electrophysiologic effects of disopyramide phosphate on reentrant ventricular arrhythmias in conscious dogs after myocardial infarction. Am J Cardiol 46:792, 1980.

42. Levites R, Anderson GJ: Electrophysiological effects of disopyramide phosphate during experimental myocardial ischemia. Am Heart J 98:339, 1979.

43. Tajima T, Dohi Y: Electrophysiological effects of intravenous disopyramide phosphate on the Wolff-Parkinson-White syndrome. PACE 5:741, 1982.

44. Edwards IR, Martin JF, Ward JW: The effect of disopyramide in vivo measurement of monophasic action potential in canine heart muscle. J Int Med Res 4(Suppl 1):26, 1976.

45. Guimond C, Vasseur D, Godin B, et al: Intracardiac electrophysiological study of disopyramide in intact and chemically sympathectomized dogs. Eur Heart J 3:553, 1982.

46. Niarchos AP: Disopyramide: Serum level and arrhythmia conversion. Am Heart J 92:57, 1976.

47. DeBacker M, Stoupel E, Kahn RJ: Efficacy of intravenous disopyramide in acute cardiac arrhythmias. Eur J Clin Pharmacol 19:11, 1981.

48. Lerman BB, Waxman HL, Buxton AE, Josephson ME: Disopyramide: Evaluation of electrophysiologic effects and clinical efficacy in patients with sustained ventricular tachycardia or ventricular fibrillation. Am J Cardiol 51:759, 1983.

49. Josephson ME, Caracta AR, Lau SH, et al: Electrophysiological evaluation of disopyramide in man. Am Heart J 86:771, 1973.

50. Befeler B, Castellanos A, Wells DE, et al: Electrophysiologic effects of the antiarrhythmic agent disopyramide phosphate. Am J Cardiol 35:282, 1975.

51. Spurrell RAJ, Thorburn CS, Camm J, et al: Effects of disopyramide on electrophysiological properties of specialized conduction system in man and on accessory atrioventricular pathway in Wolff-Parkinson-White syndrome. Br Heart J 37:861, 1975.

52. Marrott PK, Ruttley MST, Winterbottom JT, et al: A study of

the acute electrophysiological and cardiovascular action of disopyramide in man. Eur J Cardiol 4:303, 1976.

53. Caracta A: The electrophysiology of Norpace (part III). Angiology 26:120, 1975.

54. Kashani IA, Shakibi JG, Siassi B: Electrophysiologic effects of disopyramide in children. Jpn Heart J 21:491, 1980.

55. Reid DC, Williams DO: Disopyramide and sinoatrial node function. Proceedings of the Disopyramide (Rhythmodan) Seminar, St. Johns College, Cambridge, England, March 1977, p 31.

56. LaBarre A, Strauss HC, Scheinman MM, et al: Electrophysiologic effects of disopyramide phosphate on sinus node function in patients with sinus node dysfunction. Circulation 59:226, 1979.

57. Tsuchioka Y, Mitsuda H, Eno S, et al: Electrophysiologic effects of disopyramide phosphate in patients with sinus node dysfunction. Jpn Circ J 46:693, 1982.

58. Wilkinson PR, Desai J, Hollister J, et al: Electrophysiologic effects of disopyramide in patients with atrioventricular nodal dysfunction. Circulation 66:1211, 1982.

59. Desai JM, Scheinman M, Peters RW, et al: Electrophysiological effects of disopyramide in patients with bundle branch block. Circulation 59:215, 1979.

60. Birkhead JS, Vaughan Williams EM: Dual effect of disopyramide on atrial and atrioventicular conduction and refractory periods. Br Heart J 39:657, 1977.

61. Bexton RS, Hellestrand KJ, Cory-Pearce R, et al: The direct electrophysiologic effects of disopyramide phosphate in the transplanted human heart. Circulation 67:38, 1983.

62. Prystowsky EN, Lloyd EA, Fineberg N, et al: A comparison of electrophysiologic effects of antiarrhythmic agents in humans. In Brugada P, Wellens HJJ (eds): Cardiac Arrhythmias: Where Do We Go From Here? Mt. Kisco, NY: Futura Publishing, 1987, pp 495–504.

63. Karim A: The pharmacokinetics of Norpace. Angiology 26(Suppl 1):85, 1975.

64. Timmis BI, Gutman JA, Haft JI: Disopyramide-induced heart block. Chest 79:477, 1981.

65. Bergfeldt L, Rosenqvist M, Vallin H, et al: Disopyramide induced second and third degree atrioventricular block in patients with bifascicular block. Br Heart J 53:328, 1985.

66. Nayler WG: The pharmacology of disopyramide. J Int Med Res 4(Suppl 1):8, 1976.

67. Garthwaite SM, McDonald SJ, Stickney JL: Effects of disopyramide, quinidine and lidocaine on cardiac muscle excitability and inotropy [abstract]. Fed Proc 43:960, 1984.

68. Walsh RA, Horwitz LD: Adverse hemodynamic effects of intravenous disopyramide compared with quinidine in conscious dogs. Circulation 60:1053, 1979.

69. Mathur PP: Cardiovascular effects of a newer antiarrhythmic agent, disopyramide phosphate. Am Heart J 84:764, 1972.

70. Hoffmeister HM, Hepp A, Seipel L: Negative inotropic effect of class-I antiarrhythmic drugs: Comparison of flecainide with disopyramide and quinidine. Eur Heart J 8:1126, 1987.

71. Leach AJ, Brown JE, Armstrong PW: Cardiac depression by intravenous disopyramide in patients with left ventricular dysfunction. Am J Med 68:839, 1980.

72. Kotter V, Linderer T, Schroder R: Effects of disopyramide on systemic and coronary hemodynamics and myocardial metabolism in patients with coronary artery disease: Comparison with lidocaine. Am J Cardiol 46:469, 1980.

73. Cameron J, Stafford W, Pritchard D, et al: Intravenous disopyramide in acute myocardial infarction: A haemodynamic and pharmacokinetic study. J Cardiovasc Pharmacol 6:126, 1984.

74. Thadani U, Manyari D, Gregor P, et al: Hemodynamic effects of disopyramide at rest and during exercise in normal subjects. Cathet Cardiovasc Diagn 7:27, 1981.

75. Block PJ, Winkle RA: Hemodynamic effects of antiarrhythmic drugs. Am J Cardiol 52:14C, 1983.

76. Gottdiener JS, Dibianco R, Bates R, et al: Effects of disopyramide on left ventricular function: Assessment by radionuclide cineangiography. Am J Cardiol 51:1554, 1983.

77. Wisenberg G, Zawadowski AG, Gebhardt VA, et al: Effects on ventricular function of disopyramide, procainamide and quinidine as determined by radionuclide angiography. Am J Cardiol 53:1292, 1984.

78. Pollick C, Giacomini KM, Blaschke TF, et al: The cardiac effects of d- and l-disopyramide in normal subjects: A noninvasive study. Circulation 66:447, 1982.

79. Lima JJ, Boudoulas H: Stereoselective effects of disopyramide enantiomers in humans. J Cardiovasc Pharmacol 9:594, 1987.

80. Desai JM, Scheinman MM, Hirschfield D, et al: Cardiovascular collapse associated with disopyramide therapy. Chest 79:545, 1981.

81. Story JR, Abdulla AM, Frank MJ: Cardiogenic shock and disopyramide phosphate. JAMA 242:654, 1979.

82. Bauman DJ: Myocardial depression with disopyramide. Ann Intern Med 94:411, 1981.

83. Podrid PJ, Schoenberger A, Lown B: Congestive heart failure caused by oral disopyramide. N Engl J Med 302:614, 1980.

84. Cathcart-Rake WF, Coker JE, Atkins FL, et al: The effect of concurrent oral administration of propranolol and disopyramide on cardiac function in healthy men. Circulation 61:938, 1980.

85. Nyquist O: The pharmacokinetic evaluation of controlled-release disopyramide tablets. Br J Clin Pract Symp 62(Suppl): 11, 1981.

86. Karim A, Schubert EN, Burns TS, et al: Disopyramide plasma concentrations following single and multiple doses of the immediate- and controlled-release capsules. Angiology 34:375, 1983.

87. Bryson SM, Whiting B, Lawrence JR: Disopyramide serum and pharmacologic effect kinetics applied to the assessment of bioavailability. Br J Clin Pharmacol 6:409, 1978.

88. Dubetz DK, Brown NN, Hooper WD, et al: Disopyramide pharmacokinetics and bioavailability [correspondence]. Br J Clin Pharmacol 6:279, 1978.

89. Sbarbaro JA, Rawling DA, Fozzard HA: Suppression of ventricular arrhythmias with intravenous disopyramide and lidocaine: Efficacy comparison in a randomized trial. Am J Cardiol 44:513, 1979.

90. Simpson RJ, Foster JR, Benge C, et al: Safety of multiple bolus loading of intravenous disopyramide. Am Heart J 106:505, 1983.

91. Reddy CP, Benes J, Beck B: Intravenous disopyramide: Safety and efficacy of a new dosage regimen. Clin Pharmacol Ther 35:610, 1984.

92. Ashford JJ, Carmichael D, Kidner PH: Pharmacokinetics of disopyramide administered by intramuscular, intravenous and oral routes to normal volunteers. Br J Pharmacol 66(Suppl):442, 1979.

93. Bryson SM, Kelman AW, Thomson AH, et al: The pharmacokinetics of intramuscular disopyramide phosphate. J Pharm Pharmacol 34(Suppl):94, 1982.

94. Duchateau AMJA, Merkus FWHM, Wilming R: Biofarmaceutische en farmacokinetische Aspecten van Disopyramide. Pharm Weekbl (Sci) 112:145, 1977.

95. Karim A, Nissen C, Azarnoff DL: Clinical pharmacokinetics of disopyramide. J Pharmacokinet Biopharm 10:465, 1982.

96. Rangno RE, Warnica W, Ogilvie RI, et al: Correlation of disopyramide pharmacokinetics with efficacy in ventricular tachyarrhythmia. J Int Med Res 4(Suppl 1):54, 1976.

97. Giacomini KM, Swezey SE, Turner-Tamiyasu K, et al: The effect of saturable binding to plasma proteins on the pharmacokinetic properties of disopyramide. J Pharmacokinet Biopharm 10:1, 1982.

98. Lima JJ, Haughey DB, Leier CV: Disopyramide pharmacokinetics and bioavailability following the simultaneous administration of disopyramide and C-disopyramide. J Pharmacokinet Biopharm 12:289, 1984.

99. Patterson E, Stetson P, Lucchesi BR: Disopyramide plasma and myocardial tissue concentrations as they relate to antiarrhythmic activity. J Cardiovasc Pharmacol 1:541, 1979.

100. Rotmensch HH, Elkayam U, Frishman W: Antiarrhythmic drug therapy during pregnancy. Ann Intern Med 98:487, 1983.

101. Hoppu K, Neuvonen PJ, Korte T: Disopyramide and breast feeding. Br J Clin Pharmacol 21:553, 1986.

102. Duchateau AMJA, Hollander JMR: Disopyramide: Analytical and pharmacokinetic review. Excerpta Med Intl Congress Ser 501:162, 1980.

103. Brugada P, Wellens HJJ: Effects of intravenous and oral diso-

pyramide on paroxysmal atrioventricular nodal tachycardia. Am J Cardiol 53:88, 1984.

104. Bredesen JE, Kierulf P: Relationship between alpha-1-acid glycoprotein and plasma binding of disopyramide and mono-N-dealkyldisopyramide. Br J Clin Pharmacol 18:779, 1984.

105. Haughey DB, Lima JJ: Influence of concentration-dependent protein binding on serum concentrations and urinary excretion of disopyramide and its metabolite following oral administration. Biopharm Drug Dispos 4:103, 1983.

106. Hinderling PH, Bres J, Garrett ER: Protein binding and erythrocyte partitioning of disopyramide and its monodealkylated metabolite. J Pharm Sci 63:1684, 1974.

107. Bredsen JE, Pike E, Lunde PKM: Plasma binding of disopyramide and mono-N-dealkyldisopyramide. Br J Clin Pharmacol 14:673, 1982.

108. Haughey DB, Kraft CJ, Matzke GR, et al: Protein binding of disopyramide and elevated alpha-1-acid glycoprotein concentrations in serum obtained from dialysis patients and renal transplant recipients. Am J Nephrol 5:35, 1985.

109. Piafsky KM, Sellers EM, Strauss H, et al: Plasma binding of lidocaine, disopyramide and propranolol in acute myocardial infarction [abstract no. 0346]. In Turner P, Padgham C (eds): World Conference on Clinical Pharmacology and Therapeutics. London: Macmillan, 1980.

110. Siddoway LA, Woosley RL: Clinical pharmacokinetics of disopyramide. Clin Pharmacokinet 11:214, 1986.

111. Pentikainen PJ, Huikuri H, Jounela AJ, et al: Disopyramide pharmacokinetics in patients with acute myocardial infarction. Eur J Clin Pharmacol 28:45, 1985.

112. Cunningham JL, Shen DD, Shudo I, et al: The effect of urine pH and plasma protein binding on renal clearance of disopyramide. Clin Pharmacokinet 2:373, 1977.

113. Hinderling PH, Garrett ER: Pharmacokinetics of the antiarrhythmic disopyramide in healthy humans. J Pharmacokinet Biopharm 4:199, 1976.

114. Aitio M, Mansury L, Tala E, et al: The effect of enzyme induction on the metabolism of disopyramide in man. Br J Clin Pharmacol 11:279, 1981.

115. Cook CS, Karim A, Sollman P: Stereoselectivity in the metabolism of disopyramide enantiomers in rat and dog. Drug Metab Dispos 10:116, 1982.

116. Lima JJ, Jungbluth GL, Devine T, et al: Stereoselective binding of disopyramide to human plasma protein. Life Sci 35:835, 1984.

117. Shen DD, Cunningham JL, Shudo I, et al: Disposition kinetics of disopyramide in patients with renal insufficiency. Biopharm Drug Dispos 1:133, 1980.

118. Francois B, Mallein R, Rondelet J, et al: Pharmacokinetics of disopyramide in patients with chronic renal failure. Eur J Drug Metab Pharmacokinet 8:85, 1983.

119. Sevka MJ, Matthews SJ, Nightingale CH, et al: Disopyramide hemodialysis and kinetics in patients requiring long-term hemodialysis. Clin Pharmacol Ther 29:322, 1981.

120. Jaeger A, Sauder JD, Tempe JM, Mantz JM: Intoxications aiguës par le disopyramide. Nouv Presse Med 10:2883, 1981.

121. Ward JW, Kinghorn GR: The pharmacokinetics of disopyramide following myocardial infarction with special reference to oral and intravenous dose regimens. J Int Med Res 4(Suppl 1):49, 1976.

122. Kumana CR, Rambihar VS, Willis K, et al: Absorption and antidysrhythmic activity of oral disopyramide phosphate after acute myocardial infarction. Br J Clin Pharmacol 14:529, 1982.

123. Elliott HL, Thomson AH, Bryson SM: Disopyramide in acute myocardial infarction: Problems with changing pharmacokinetics. Eur J Pharmacol 30:345, 1986.

124. Landmark K, Bredsen JE, Thaulow S, et al: Pharmacokinetics of disopyramide in patients with imminent to moderate cardiac failure. Eur J Clin Pharmacol 19:187, 1981.

125. Bonde J, Graudal NA, Pedersen LE, et al: Kinetics of disopyramide in decreased hepatic function. Eur J Clin Pharmacol 31:73, 1986.

126. Leahey EB, Feiffel JA, Giardina E-GV, et al: The effect of quinidine and other oral antiarrhythmic drugs on serum digoxin. Ann Intern Med 92:605, 1980.

127. Davis LJ, Cupit GC, Shimomura SK: Warfarin-disopyramide interaction? Drug Intell Clin Pharmacol 13:386, 1979.

128. Haworth E, Burroughs AK: Disopyramide and warfarin interaction. Br Med J 2:866, 1977.

129. Bonde J, Bodtker S, Angelo HR, et al: Atenolol inhibits the elimination of disopyramide. Eur J Clin Pharmacol 28:41, 1985.

130. Aitio M-L, Vuorenmaa T: Enhanced metabolism and diminished efficacy of disopyramide by enzyme induction? Br J Clin Pharm 9:149, 1980.

131. Nightingale J, Nappi JM: Effect of phenytoin on serum disopyramide concentrations. Clin Pharm 6:46, 1987.

132. Kapil RP, Axelson JE, Mansfield IL, et al: Disopyramide pharmacokinetics and metabolism: Effect of inducers. Br J Clin Pharmacol 24:781, 1987.

133. Wellens HJJ, Bar FW, Dassen WRM, et al: Effect of drugs in the Wolff-Parkinson-White syndrome. Am J Cardiol 46:665, 1980.

134. Ragosta M, Weihl A, Rosenfeld L: Potentially fatal interaction between erythromycin and disopyramide. Am J Med 86:465,1989.

135. Arif M, Laidlaw JC, Oshrain C, et al: A randomized, double-blind, parallel group comparison of disopyramide phosphate and quinidine in patients with cardiac arrhythmias. Angiology 34:393, 1983.

136. Bauman JL, Gallastegui J, Strasberg B, et al: Long-term therapy with disopyramide phosphate: Side effects and effectiveness. Am Heart J 111:654, 1986.

137. Ronnevik T, Gundersen T, Abrahamsen AM: Tolerability and antiarrhythmic efficacy of disopyramide compared to lignocaine in selected patients with suspected acute myocardial infarction. Eur Heart J 8:19, 1987.

138. Teichman SL, Ferrick A, Kim SG, et al: Disopyramide-pyridostigmine interaction: Selective reversal of anticholinergic symptoms with preservation of antiarrhythmic effect. J Am Coll Cardiol 10:633, 1987.

139. Danziger LH, Horn JR: Disopyramide-induced urinary retention. Report of nine cases and a review of the literature. Arch Intern Med 143:1683, 1983.

140. Trope GE, Hind VMD: Closed-angle glaucoma in patients on disopyramide [letter]. Lancet 1:329, 1978.

141. Teichman SL, Fisher JD, Matos JA, et al: Disopyramide-pyridostigmine: Report of a beneficial drug interaction. J Cardiovasc Pharmacol 7:108, 1985.

142. Craxi A, Gatto G, Maringhini A, et al: Disopyramide and cholestasis [letter]. Ann Intern Med 93:150, 1980.

143. Porterfield JG, Antman EM, Lown B: Respiratory difficulty after use of disopyramide. N Engl J Med 303:584, 1980.

144. Falk RH, Nisbet PA, Gray TJ: Mental distress in patients on disopyramide [letter]. Lancet 1:858, 1977.

145. Padheid PL, Smith DA, Fitzsimmons EJ, et al: Disopyramide and acute psychosis [letter]. Lancet 1:1152, 1977.

146. Leonard RF, Braun TE, Levy AM: Initiation of uterine contractions by disopyramide during pregnancy. N Engl J Med 299:84, 1978.

147. Drugs that cause sexual dysfunction. Med Letter 25:73, 1983.

148. Goldberg IJ, Brown LK, Rayfield EJ: Disopyramide (Norpace)-induced hypoglycemia. Am J Med 69:463, 1980.

149. Strathman I, Schubert EN, Cohen A, et al: Hypoglycemia in patients receiving disopyramide phosphate. Drug Intell Clin Pharm 17:635, 1983.

150. Riccioni N, Castiglioni M, Bartolomei C: Disopyramide-induced QT prolongation and ventricular tachyarrhythmias. Am Heart J 105:870, 1983.

151. Velebit V, Podrid P, Lown B, et al: Aggravation and provocation of ventricular arrhythmias by antiarrhythmic drugs. Circulation 65:886, 1982.

152. Stanton MS, Prystowsky EN, Fineberg NS, et al: Arrhythmogenic effects of antiarrhythmic drugs: A study of 506 patients treated for ventricular tachycardia or fibrillation. J Am Coll Cardiol 14:209, 1989.

153. Minardo JD, Heger JJ, Miles WM, et al: Drug associated ventricular fibrillation: Analysis of clinical and electrocardiographic features. N Engl J Med 319:257, 1988.

154. Podrid P: Aggravation of arrhythmia: A potential complication of therapy. Prim Cardiol 9:75, 1983.

155. Morganroth J, Horowitz LN: Incidence of proarrhythmic effects from quinidine in the outpatient treatment of benign or potentially lethal arrhythmia. Am J Cardiol 56:585, 1985.

156. Wyse DG, Mitchell LB, Duff HJ: Procainamide, disopyramide and quinidine: Discordant antiarrhythmic effects during crossover comparison in patients with inducible ventricular tachycardia. J Am Coll Cardiol 9:882, 1987.

157. Kim SG, Mercando AD, Fisher JD: Combination of disopyramide and mexiletine for additive efficacy for ventricular arrhythmias without additive side effects [abstract]. Circulation 76(Suppl IV):512, 1987.

158. McLaran CJ, Hossack KF, Neilson GH, et al: Oral tocainide versus disopyramide: A double-blind, randomized, crossover study of outpatients with stable ventricular premature beats. J Cardiovasc Pharmacol 6:657, 1984.

159. Allen-Narker AC, Roberts CJC, Marshall AJ, et al: Prophylaxis against ventricular arrhythmias in suspected acute myocardial infarction: A comparison of tocainide and disopyramide. Br J Clin Pharmacol 18:725, 1984.

160. Trosser A, Khan F, Jewitt DE: Evidence that flecainide is superior to disopyramide in suppressing chronic ventricular premature complexes. Br Heart J 54:644, 1985.

161. Caron JF, Libersa CC, Kher AR, et al: Comparative study of encainide and disopyramide in chronic ventricular arrhythmias: A double-blind placebo-controlled crossover study. J Am Coll Cardiol 5:1457, 1985.

162. Naccarella F, Bracchetti D, Palmieri M, et al: Comparison of propafenone and disopyramide for treatment of chronic ventricular arrhythmias: Placebo-controlled, double-blind, randomized crossover study. Am Heart J 109:833, 1985.

163. Jonason T, Ringqvist I, Bandh S, et al: Propafenone versus disopyramide for treatment of chronic symptomatic ventricular arrhythmias. Acta Med Scand 223:515, 1988.

164. Fechter P, Ha HR, Follath F, et al: The antiarrhythmic effects of controlled release disopyramide phosphate and long acting propranolol in patients with ventricular arrhythmias. Eur J Clin Pharmacol 25:729, 1983.

165. Vismara LA, Vera Z, Miller RR, et al: Efficacy of disopyramide phosphate in the treatment of refractory ventricular tachycardia. Am J Cardiol 39:1027, 1977.

166. Manz M, Steinbeck G, Nitsch J, et al: Treatment of recurrent sustained ventricular tachycardia with mexiletine and disopyramide. Br Heart J 49:222, 1983.

167. Rizos I, Brachmann J, Lengfelder W, et al: Effects of intravenous disopyramide and quinidine on normal myocardium and on the characteristics of arrhythmias: Intraindividual comparison in patients with sustained ventricular tachycardia. Eur Heart J 8:154, 1987.

168. The Cardiac Arrhythmia Suppression Trial (CAST) Investigators: Preliminary report: Effect of encainide and flecainide on mortality in a randomized trial of arrhythmia suppression after myocardial infarction. N Engl J Med 321:406, 1989.

169. Breithardt G, Seipel L, Abendroth RR: Comparison of the antiarrhythmic efficacy of disopyramide and mexiletine against stimulus-induced ventricular tachycardia. J Cardiovasc Pharmacol 3:1026, 1981.

170. Zainal N, Griffiths JW, Carmichael DJS, et al: Oral disopyramide for the prevention of arrhythmias in patients with acute myocardial infarction admitted to open wards. Lancet 2:887, 1977.

171. Jennings G, Jones MBS, Besterman EMM, et al: Oral disopyramide in prophylaxis of arrhythmias following myocardial infarction. Lancet 1:51, 1976.

172. Wilcox RG, Hampton JR, Rowley JM, et al: Randomised placebo-controlled trial comparing oxprenolol with disopyramide phosphate in immediate treatment of suspected myocardial infarction. Lancet 2:765, 1980.

173. Nicholls DP, Haybyrne T, Barnes PC: Intravenous and oral disopyramide after myocardial infarction. Lancet 2:936, 1980.

174. Kumana CR, Rambihar VS, Tanser PH, et al: A placebo-controlled study to determine the efficacy of oral disopyramide phosphate for the prophylaxis of ventricular dysrhythmias after acute myocardial infarction. Br J Clin Pharmacol 14:519, 1982.

175. Swiryn S, Bauernfeind RA, Wyndham CRC, et al: Effects of oral disopyramide phosphate on induction of paroxysmal supraventricular tachycardia. Circulation 64:169, 1981.

176. Sethi KK, Jaishankar S, Khalilullah M, Gupta MP: Selective blockade of retrograde fast pathway by intravenous disopyramide in paroxysmal supraventricular tachycardia mediated by dual atrioventricular nodal pathways. Br Heart J 49:532, 1983.

177. Bennett DH: Disopyramide in patients with the Wolff-Parkinson-White syndrome and atrial fibrillation. Chest 74:624, 1978.

178. Kerr CR, Prystowsky EN, Smith WM, et al: Electrophysiologic effects of disopyramide phosphate in patients with Wolff-Parkinson-White syndrome. Circulation 65:869, 1982.

179. Kou H-C, Hung J-S, Lee Y-S, et al: Effects of oral disopyramide phosphate on induction and sustenance of atrioventricular reentrant tachycardia incorporating retrograde accessory pathway conduction. Circulation 66:454, 1982.

180. Fujimura O, Klein GJ, Sharma AD, et al: Acute effect of disopyramide on atrial fibrillation in the Wolff-Parkinson-White Syndrome. J Am Coll Cardiol 13:1133, 1989.

181. Hartel G, Louhija A, Konttinen A: Disopyramide in the prevention of recurrence of atrial fibrillation after electroconversion. Clin Pharmacol Ther 15:551, 1974.

182. Campbell TJ, Morgan JJ: Treatment of atrial arrhythmias after cardiac surgery with intravenous disopyramide. Aust N Z J Med 10:644, 1980.

183. Beck OA, Gunther R, Hochrein H: Konversionsbehandlung von chronischem Vorhofflimmern und-flattern mit Disopyramid und einer Verapamil-Chinidin-Kombination: Vergleichende untersuchungen. Dtsch Med Wochenschr 107:1419, 1982.

184. Lloyd EA, Gersh BJ, Forman R: The efficacy of quinidine and disopyramide in the maintenance of sinus rhythm after electroconversion from atrial fibrillation. S Afr Med J 65:367, 1984.

185. Stewart DE, Ikram H: The use of intravenous disopyramide for the conversion of supraventricular tachyarrhythmias. N Z Med J 97:148, 1984.

186. Campbell TJ, Gavaghan TP, Morgan JJ: Intravenous sotalol for the treatment of atrial fibrillation and flutter after cardiopulmonary bypass. Comparison with disopyramide and digoxin in a randomised trial. Br Heart J 54:86, 1985.

187. Martin A, Benbow LJ, Leach C, et al: Comparison of amiodarone and disopyramide in the control of paroxysmal atrial fibrillation and atrial flutter [interim report]. Br J Clin Pract 44(Suppl):52, 1986.

188. Bella PD, Tondo C, Marenzi G, et al: Facilitating influence of disopyramide on atrial flutter termination by overdrive pacing. Am J Cardiol 61:1046, 1988.

189. Karlson B, Torstensson I, Abjurn C, et al: Disopyramide in the maintenance of sinus rhythm after electroconversion of atrial fibrillation—a one-year follow-up study. Eur Heart J 9:284, 1988.

190. Otero-Cagide M, Masterson ML, Wilkoff BL, et al: Syncope of undetermined etiology: Value of procainamide administration during a nondiagnostic cardiac electrophysiologic study. J Electrophysiol 2:437, 1988.

191. Robertson CE, Miller HC: Extreme tachycardia complicating the use of disopyramide in atrial flutter. Br Heart J 44:602, 1980.

192. Milstein S, Beutikofer J, Lesser J, et al: Disopyramide reversal of induced hypotension-bradycardia in neurally mediated syncope [abstract]. Circulation 76(Suppl):IV-175, 1987.

193. Kelly PA, Mann DE, Adler SW, et al: Low dose disopyramide often fails to prevent neurogenic syncope during head-up tilt testing. PACE 17(4 Pt 1):573, 1994.

194. Pollick C: Muscular subaortic stenosis: Hemodynamic and clinical improvement after disopyramide. N Engl J Med 307:997, 1982.

195. Kimball BP, Bui S, Wigle ED: Acute dose-response effects of intravenous disopyramide in hypertrophic obstructive cardiomyopathy. Am Heart J 125(6):1691, 1993.

CHAPTER 141

Dofetilide

T. Friedrich, M.D., D. J. Nichols, Ph.D., C. T. Alabaster, Ph.D., and D. M. Roden, M.D.

Dofetilide (code number UK-68,798) is the product of a synthetic drug program aimed at identifying a potent class III antiarrhythmic agent devoid of additional pharmacologic activity.[1] Dofetilide is a bis (aryl-alkyl) amine derived by synthetic modification around the sotalol structure. Preclinical and clinical profiles suggest that it may prove useful in the treatment of many reentrant type clinical dysrhythmias. Trials currently under way will help determine dofetilide's efficacy and safety.

PRECLINICAL STUDIES
Mechanism of Action

Voltage clamp measurements in isolated myocytes from guinea pigs and rabbits[2, 3] have shown that dofetilide prolongs repolarization of cardiac action potentials by inhibition of the rapidly activating/rapidly deactivating delayed rectifier, repolarizing potassium current (I_{Kr}). It is highly potent with K_D for block in rabbit myocytes of 3.9 nM with a Hill coefficient of 2.[2] Block of the current occurs during depolarization, i.e., when the channel is open and is voltage dependent such that block increases with depolarization.[2] The block induced by dofetilide is independent of frequency in the range of 0.5- to 5.0-second stimulus intervals when measured under steady-state conditions.[2] This has been attributed to slow dissociation of dofetilide from the channel.[4]

Dofetilide, at concentrations in excess of 1000 times the K_D for I_{Kr} block, has no activity on other cardiac repolarizing potassium currents studied.[2, 3, 5, 6] Thus, the transient outward current I_{to}, background inwardly rectifying current I_{K1}, the slowly activating/slowly deactivating voltage- and time-dependent current I_{KS}, and adenosine triphosphate (ATP)–dependent potassium channels all are unaffected. The proportion of repolarizing current carried by I_{Kr} appears to vary both among species[7] and with differences in pacing frequency.[5] Consequently, block of this current by dofetilide may lead to species- or rate-dependent differences in the magnitude of effect of dofetilide in prolonging action potential repolarization time (and hence action potential duration).

In ligand binding studies, dofetilide (10 μM) displays little affinity for adrenergic receptors (α_1, α_2, β), adenosine (A1), dopamine (D2), 5-hydroxytryptamine (5HT$_2$), muscarinic (M1), dihydropyridine, or opioid receptors.[8, 9] ³H-Dofetilide binds with relatively high affinity to a single population of noninteracting sites (K_D = 23 nM, B_{MAX} = 150 fmol/mg protein) in guinea pig membranes. It is displaced from this binding site

by a range of other class III agents with a rank order of potency for displacement that correlates closely to the rank order for prolongation of action potential duration (APD).[8] These studies have been confirmed more recently in guinea pig myocyte studies[10] and suggest a common binding site for dofetilide.

Pharmacologic Profile

Tissue Studies

Consistent with a selective action on I_{Kr}, dofetilide prolongs APD and effective refractory period (ERP) in a concentration-dependent manner in a variety of cardiac preparations (muscle, Purkinje fiber, and sinoatrial nodal cells)[3, 11, 12] (Fig. 141–1), including human myocardium.[13] In one study, sensitivity was greater in Purkinje fiber than in muscle both in terms

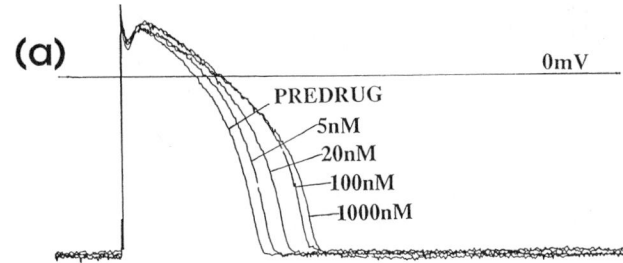

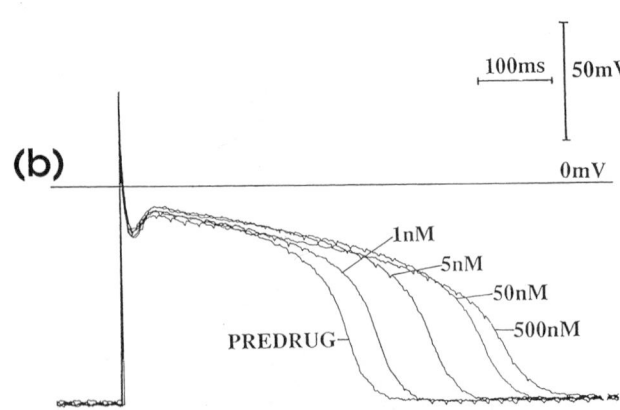

Figure 141–1. Influence of increasing concentrations of dofetilide on action potentials recorded from a single preparation of canine ventricular muscle (*a*) and Purkinje fiber (*b*), before and 20 minutes after superfusion with dofetilide at the final concentration indicated. (From Gwilt M, Arrowsmith JE, Blackburn KJ, et al: UK-68,798: A novel, potent and highly selective Class III antiarrhythmic agent which blocks potassium channels in cardiac cells. J Pharmacol Exp Ther 256:318, 1991. Copyright Williams & Wilkins, 1991.)

of threshold dose (1 versus 5 nM) and maximal effect (80% increase at 500 nM in Purkinje fiber versus 50% at 1 μM in muscle). No effect was observed on the resting membrane potential or on the amplitude of the action potential. The effect on APD plateaus at higher concentrations is consistent with block of a single current contributing to repolarization. Dofetilide prolongs APD in fetal rat but not adult rat myocardial tissue.[14, 15]

Several studies have shown that dofetilide at concentrations up to 1 μM does not depress the maximum rate of phase 0 depolarization as recorded from canine Purkinje fiber; guinea pig, canine, and ferret ventricular muscle; and rabbit sinoatrial node.[3, 11, 12, 16] This supports the concept that dofetilide lacks effect on the fast sodium channels, which is supported by an absence of depression of conduction velocity even at 1 μM.[3]

The effects of dofetilide have also been assessed in studies in which the *in vitro* conditions have been modified to simulate pathologic conditions. Simulated metabolic acidosis, a major component of myocardial ischemia, does not attenuate the class III actions of dofetilide.[17] However, alterations in external potassium concentration, designed to simulate hypokalemia or ischemia, have been variously described to modulate[18] or not[19] the APD-prolonging effects of dofetilide. Similarly, hypoxia has been seen to cause attenuation[20] or not[21] of the APD/ERP effects of dofetilide.

Many pharmacologic maneuvers that prolong APD have been reported to result in positive inotropic action.[22] Consistent with these observations, dofetilide produces concentration-related (and thus APD-related) increases in the developed tension, the rate of tension development, and the rate of relaxation without effect on the time to peak tension and only slightly prolonging the time to 50% relaxation of ferret papillary muscle.[16] Similar results are found in guinea pig papillary muscle preparations.[15] This is in contrast with commonly described negative inotropic effects of class I, II, and IV antiarrhythmic agents.

In guinea pig atria,[23] guinea pig Langendorff,[24] and rabbit sinus node preparations,[12] dofetilide exerts a modest negative chronotropic effect, slowing rate by approximately 20% at 100 nM, with no further effect on concentration up to 10 μM. This effect is not due to β-blockade[23] and parallels the increase in sinoatrial action potential duration.[12] Action potential prolongation in the sinus node may itself be expected to produce a slight decrease in rate; this is presumably the mechanism underlying dofetilide's effects in these experimental preparations.

As described earlier, variation in the contribution of I_{Kr} to the total repolarizing potassium current may vary with stimulation frequency. Thus, I_{Kr} may become the dominant delayed rectifier current at higher frequencies[5] and may account for the experimental observations of reduced class III effect of many potassium channel blockers (with the possible exception of amiodarone) at high, steady-state pacing frequencies. This property of negative or reverse rate dependency has also been reported for dofetilide.[11, 14, 18] These experimental observations have led some authors to suggest that efficacy would be lost during tachycardia.[25] However, other *in vitro* data suggest that dofetilide does not alter the time course of restitution and that the APD-prolonging effects are conserved during abrupt changes in pacing rate.[11] The concept that dofetilide retains pharmacologic activity during tachycardia is also supported by beneficial effects in animal models of tachycardia, fibrillation, heterogeneity of repolarization, and defibrillation energy (described later). During stimulation at slow rates, blockage of I_{Kr} may cause APD to be prolonged to the extent that early afterdepolarizations may occur[15] (see section on proarrhythmia).

Dofetilide appears to cause few actions in noncardiac tissues. Augmentation of phasic contractile tension in spontaneously active rat portal veins, at concentrations relevant to class III actions, is observed.[26] However, no effect is observed on quiescent aortic ring preparations or in those precontracted by spasmogens.

Whole Animal Studies

The electrophysiologic and hemodynamic profile of dofetilide in experimental animals is that predicted from the *in vitro* studies: In both anesthetized and conscious dogs, dofetilide increases the QT interval, QT_c interval, ventricular ERP, and atrial ERP without affecting the indices of conduction such as PR interval or QRS duration.[27–31] The compound is highly potent with clear activity after doses as low as 1 μg/kg IV and 12.5 μg/kg orally. The absence of effect of dofetilide on the electrocardiograph (ECG) of rats after intravenous doses of up to 1 mg/kg is consistent with the lack of I_{Kr} in this species.[32] In both guinea pigs[32] and dogs,[28] the attainment of finite maximum increases of QT interval of between 25% and 30% is again consistent with *in vitro* data. Hemodynamically the compound produces a mild degree of positive inotropic activity, correlated to its class III activity,[28, 30] and does not induce or aggravate depression of cardiac performance even in models of left ventricular dysfunction.[33]

In pentobarbitone-anesthetized dogs, dofetilide causes a small (<20%) reduction in heart rate.[28] This is not seen in chloralose-anesthetized or conscious dogs.[27, 30] The reason for this is unclear, but dofetilide appears to be capable of reducing rapid, but not normal, resting heart rate. However, dofetilide appears not to prevent exercise-induced elevation of sinus rate in dogs with myocardial ischemia undergoing exercise testing.[34] These studies have not detected any effect on blood pressure of dofetilide at doses below 300 μg/kg IV. At this dose and at 1 mg/kg, a small rise is seen.[30]

Studies in Models of Arrhythmia

Consistent with the concept that prolongation of ERP will terminate reentrant arrhythmias, several studies in a number of animal models have shown antiarrhythmic actions of dofetilide. In one study, dofetilide prevented the induction of ventricular tachycardia by programmed electrical stimulation in six of seven dogs with myocardial infarction.[31] Three-dimensional mapping suggested this effect was attributable to prolongation of ERP in the epicardial region of the infarct. No effect on conduction velocity was observed. In anesthetized dogs, the induction of ventricular fibrillation by 50 or 60 Hz electrical stimulation was made more difficult by administration of dofetilide.[28, 29] Spontaneous conversion from fibrillation to sinus rhythm occurred frequently in treated animals but not at all in untreated ones. Again these effects occurred at doses of 10 to 100 μg/kg, over which ERP is prolonged. Similarly, in a pilot study of atrial flutter (sterile pericarditis model), dofetilide terminated the arrhythmia in all four dogs.[35] An analysis of two-dimensional maps showed this to be attributable to a prolongation of ERP, particularly in areas of tissue exhibiting slowed conduction.

Coronary occlusion in the anesthetized pig leads to ventricular fibrillation (VF) in 80% of animals. In a randomized, placebo-controlled study of 32 animals, dofetilide (25 μg/kg + maintenance infusion) reduced the incidence of VF by half[36] (Fig. 141–2). This dose was associated with a 20% increase in QT_c interval. Coronary occlusion in the conscious dog with previous myocardial infarction also causes VF in 83% of animals. This too was reduced by dofetilide (to 33%), but the dose used (900 μg/kg) was very high.[37] Antiarrhythmic effects observed in the rat at higher doses[6, 38] still have been attributed to an effect on I_{KATP} channels.[6]

The antiarrhythmic efficacy of dofetilide in these studies is consistently associated with drug-induced prolongation of ERP with no effect on conduction velocity. However, a further possible mechanism of benefit is suggested by studies in anesthetized dogs in which dofetilide reduced the heterogeneity of repolarization interval induced by ventricular pacing near the maximal following frequency.[39] Increased heterogeneity of repolarization has been suggested as a substrate for ventricular fibrillation,[40] and the reduction seen by dofetilide in these studies may be relevant to its antifibrillatory activity. In contrast with the effects of dofetilide, quinidine was observed to increase the heterogeneity of repolarization.[39]

Proarrhythmia

Dofetilide, like other agents that prolong APD, can produce bradycardia-related arrhythmia. Early afterdepolarizations have been observed to occur *in vitro*, in guinea pig atria paced at 0.5 Hz, and in fetal rat heart, in the presence of 1 μM dofetilide.[14, 15] Anesthetized rabbits, pretreated with the α_1 adrenoceptor agonist methoxamine, consistently have torsade de pointes when administered dofetilide and other class III agents intravenously.[41]

CLINICAL STUDIES
Pharmacokinetics
Healthy Volunteers and Patients

Dofetilide is well absorbed, with a systemic bioavailability in excess of 90% (Fig. 141–3).[42] Mean maximal plasma concentrations (C_{max}) are achieved approximately 2 hours (range, 1 to 4 hours) after oral administration, and the elimination half-life from plasma is approximately 9.5 hours (range, 6 to 14 hours; Fig. 141–4).[42, 43] More than 60% of the drug is excreted unchanged in the urine; the remainder is metabolized in the liver. In a 10-day, double-blind, placebo-controlled, multiple-dose study, the accumulation ratio after twice-daily dosing was 1.5, and the peak trough plasma concentration ratio was 2.9.[44] After intravenous administration, the clearance (4.7 ml/min/kg) and volume of distribution (3.9 L/kg) are independent of dose and show low intra- and intersubject variability.[44] The dose-plasma concentration relationship is linear within the dose range studied (Fig. 141–5).[42–44] After oral administration, prolongation of the QT_c interval was directly proportional to the plasma concentration.

Interaction studies with digoxin, propranolol, and warfarin[44] have been conducted in healthy volunteers. No pharmacokinetic or pharmacodynamic interactions were observed.

Pharmacokinetic parameters in patients with ischemic heart disease are very similar to those described in normal healthy volunteers.[45]

Pharmacodynamics

Using the QT interval as a noninvasive measure for the influence of the drug on ventricular repolarization

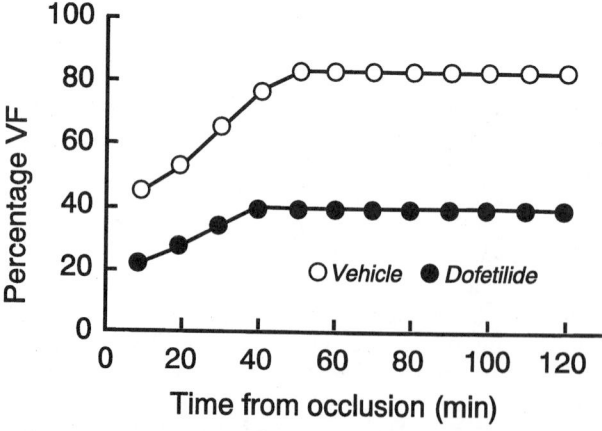

Figure 141–2. Effect of dofetilide on ventricular fibrillation (VF) in anesthetized pigs consequent to balloon occlusion of the left anterior descending coronary artery. The study was randomized with 16 animals in each group. Dofetilide was administered intravenously as a loading infusion of 25 μg/kg over 10 minutes prior to occlusion, followed by a maintenance infusion of 12.5 μg/kg/hr throughout the remaining time. (Data from Andersen HR, Wiggers HS, Knudsen LL, et al: Dofetilide suppresses ventricular fibrillation during acute myocardial ischemia, a randomized study in pigs. Circulation 86[Suppl I]: 301, 1992.)

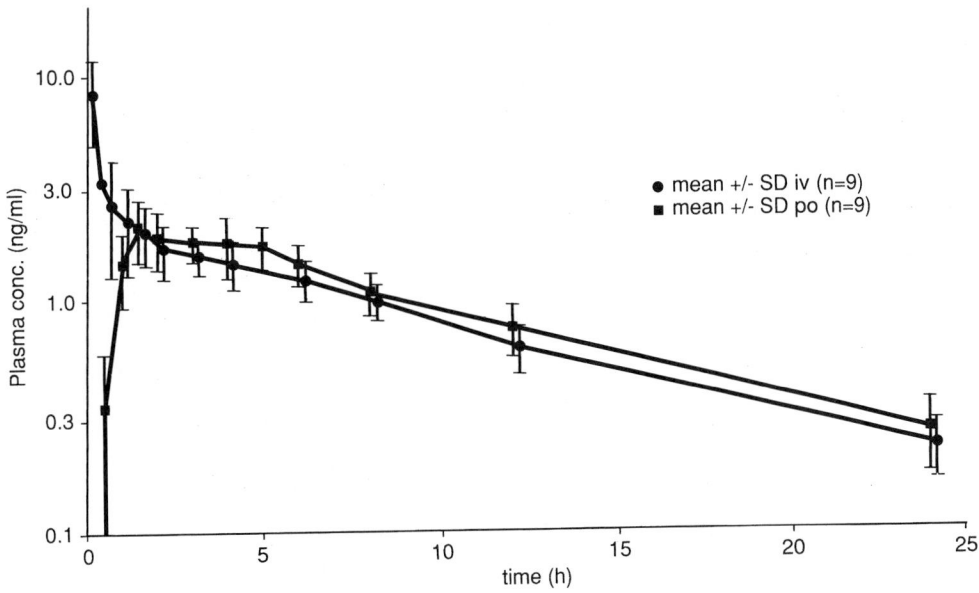

Figure 141–3. Mean plasma concentrations of dofetilide (ng/ml) versus time in human volunteers after single intravenous and oral doses of 0.5 mg.

and an indicator of electrophysiologic activity, the minimal active dose in volunteers is approximately 2 μg/kg intravenously[43] and approximately 10 μg/kg orally.[44] A total daily dose of 2.5 mg, administered twice daily for a 5-day period, resulted in mean prolongations of the QT_c interval of between 30 msec (at trough) and 100 msec (at peak), corresponding to a 10% to 30% increase from baseline.

Healthy Volunteers

After intravenous administration of the compound, prolongations of the QT_c interval of up to a 200-msec increase from baseline have been observed.[42–44]

Maximal effect is attained 10 to 20 minutes after completion of an intravenous infusion, indicating a rapid equilibration between plasma and ventricular myocardium. Even at high doses, there has been no evidence to suggest that dofetilide influences ECG variables other than the QT and QT_c interval; no effects have been observed on the RR or PR intervals or the QRS width. This supports the preclinical evidence that dofetilide selectively affects repolarization without any influence on conduction time in the myocardium (i.e., exerts a highly selective class III action).

No influence of dofetilide on blood pressure or heart rate has been observed in studies in healthy volunteers.[44]

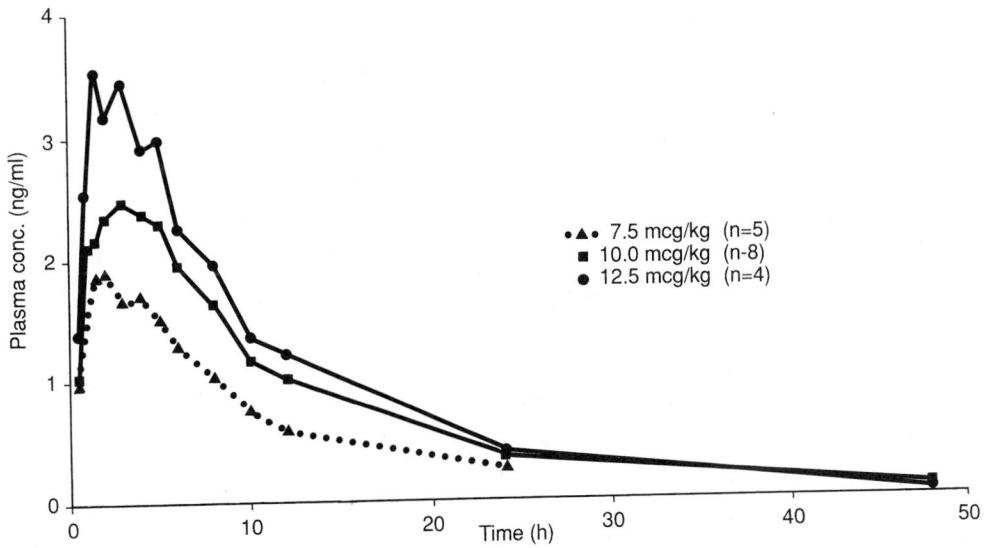

Figure 141–4. Mean plasma concentrations of dofetilide (ng/ml) versus time after single oral doses of 7.5 to 12.5 μg/kg.

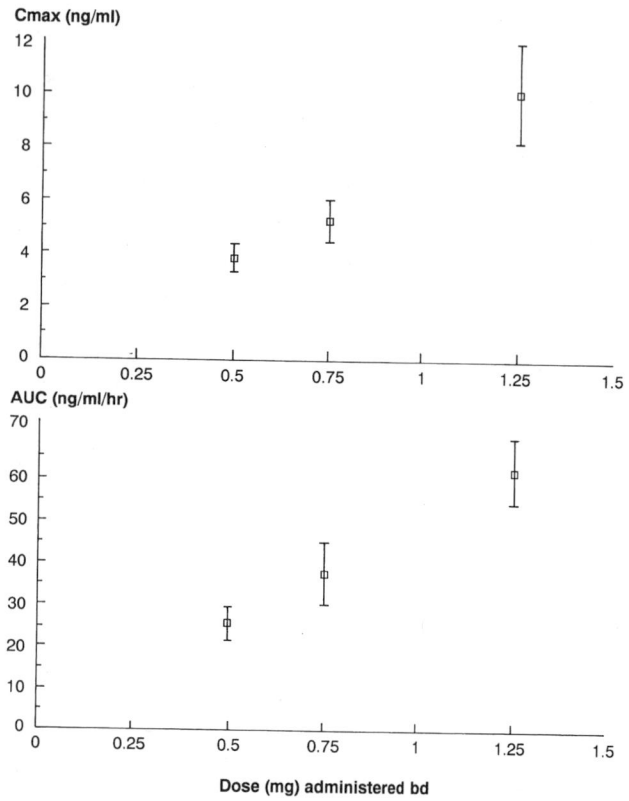

Figure 141–5. Maximal plasma concentrations (Cmax) and interdose area under the plasma concentration curve (AUC) versus dose at steady state (day 5) after administration of dofetilide 0.5 mg, 0.75 mg, and 1.25 mg b.i.d. Results are means + S.E.M. from seven subjects.

Patients

Intravenous administration of dofetilide to patients with ischemic heart disease[45] resulted in dose-dependent prolongations of the QT_c interval; doses of 1.5, 3.0, and 4.5 µg/kg resulted in mean peak prolongations of between 40 and 80 msec (10% to 20% increase from baseline). All changes were statistically significant ($p < .01$). A comparison of plasma drug concentration and change in QT_c from baseline, excluding the value at the end of the 10-minute infusion, revealed a linear correlation ($r = 0.81, p < .0001$).

The influence of dofetilide on cardiac electrophysiology has been evaluated in several studies.[45–49] In an open study in patients with supraventricular arrhythmias, Butrous et al.[46] found that dofetilide significantly increased effective refractory periods and monophasic action potentials (MAP) in the atria (AERP) and ventricles (VERP). Those findings were confirmed by Sedgwick et al.,[47] who in a double-blind, placebo-controlled study in patients with ischemic heart disease and stable angina pectoris reported dose-dependent increases in effective refractive periods in atria, ventricles, AV node, and the His-Purkinje system (Fig. 141–6). No changes were observed in RR, PR, PA, AH, or HV intervals or sinus node recovery time.

The same group also evaluated the influence of dofetilide on dispersion of ventricular repolarization

by MAP recordings from different ventricular sites as well as by surface interlead QT measurements.[43] They concluded that in this patient population dofetilide did not increase dispersion of repolarization.

The phenomenon of reverse use dependency was also studied by Sedgwick. MAPs were measured in atria and ventricles at drive cycle lengths ranging from 800 to 500 msec. Even at fast pacing rates, dofetilide appeared to retain the ability to increase action potential duration.[48] This was confirmed by Bailey et al.[49] in patients with congestive heart failure, severely reduced left ventricular ejection fraction (<30%), and life-threatening ventricular arrhythmias, evaluating the influence of dofetilide on MAPs at drive cycle lengths from 600 to 300 msec.

The same study also showed that in this patient population dofetilide (0.75 mg total daily dose) did not show any negative inotropic effect. If anything, dofetilide was associated with a small (nonsignificant) improvement in cardiac contractility as estimated from measurements of pulmonary capillary wedge pressure (PCWP), left ventricular dP/dt, and stroke work index.[49]

The efficacy of dofetilide in the prevention of ventricular tachycardia (VT) induction was studied using the intravenous formulation[50, 51] and oral formulation.[52] These dose-ranging studies explored doses from 0.6 to 15 µg/kg intravenously and from 0.25 to 1.0 mg b.i.d. orally, demonstrating that dofetilide at the higher dosages prevented reinduction of sustained VT/VF in the electrophysiologic laboratory in 40% to 60% of the patients. No dose-response correlation was detected in any of these studies owing to the relatively small numbers of patients in each dose group. The minimal effective dose in the intravenous studies was approximately 3.0 µg/kg; in the oral study, it was approximately 0.25 mg b.i.d. Increases in doses to higher than 1 mg total daily dose orally and 8.0 µg/kg intravenously did not increase response rates, but did increase the likelihood of excessive QT_c prolongation. In 75% of the patients who continued in the extension studies on long-term oral dofetilide, VT/VF remained well controlled.

The ability of dofetilide to convert atrial fibrillation (AF) or atrial flutter (AFl) to normal sinus rhythm (SR) was studied in an open study of 24 patients with a history of AF/AFl lasting less than 6 months before inclusion into the trial. Mean duration of the arrhythmia prior to inclusion into the study was 42 days (range, 1 to 150 days). Dofetilide was given intravenously during a 15-minute period; if conversion did not occur within 15 minutes after completion of the first infusion, a second infusion was given. At the lowest dose (2.5 + 2.5 µg/kg), four of eight patients converted to SR within 3 hours after completion of the second infusion. At the higher dose (4.0 + 4.5 µg/kg), 11 of 15 converted to SR.[53]

Dofetilide was also evaluated in patients with atrioventricular nodal reentrant tachycardia (AVNRT)[54] and in patients with atrioventricular reentrant tachycardia (AVRT).[55] Both studies were open dose-ranging studies in which five different dose levels of intrave-

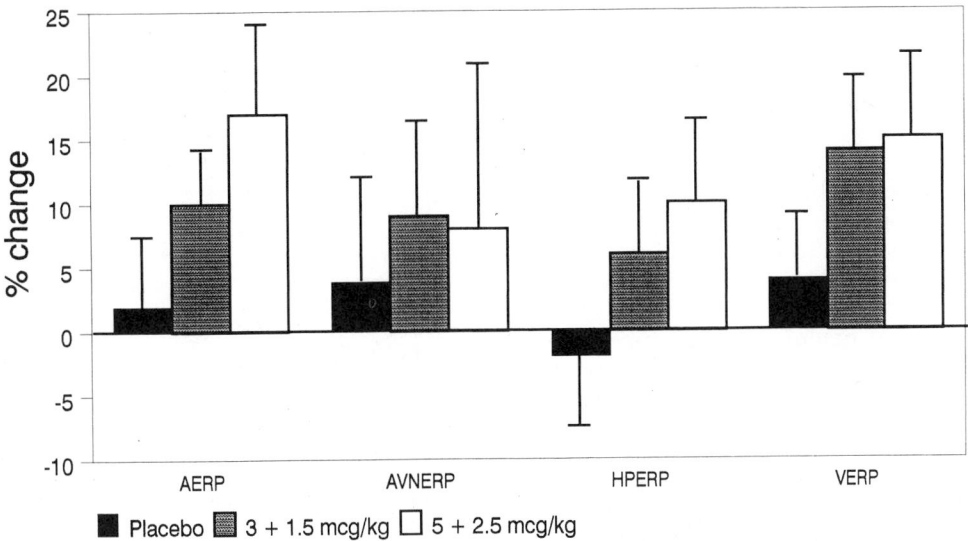

Figure 141–6. Mean percentage change from baseline after intravenous administration of placebo or dofetilide (low and high dose, respectively) in atrial effective refractory period (AERP), AV nodal effective refractory period (AVNERP), His-Purkinje system effective refractory period (HPERP), and ventricular effective refractory period (VERP). Values are means + S.E.M. from six patients per group.

nous dofetilide were evaluated (ranging from 1.5 to 15 µg/kg). Dofetilide was administered as a 15-minute loading infusion, followed by a 45-minute maintenance infusion; efficacy was assessed by programmed electrical stimulation at baseline and halfway through the maintenance infusion. Dose-dependent suppression of arrhythmia inducibility was detected in both studies. Four of five patients with AVNRT were rendered noninducible at the highest dose level (15 µg/kg), whereas four of nine of the patients with AVRT were rendered noninducible.

Gremillion et al.[56] evaluated the effect of dofetilide on defibrillation energy requirements in patients undergoing implantation of an implantable cardioverter-defibrillator (ICD). Defibrillation thresholds (DFTs) were determined before and after dofetilide infusion. DFTs decreased significantly from 6.9 ± 3.7 joules at baseline to 4.6 ± 2.6 joules during dofetilide infusion ($p < .05$), indicating that dofetilide in contrast with class I agents such as lidocaine or procainamide does not elevate DFTs and, in fact, reduces DFTs in patients receiving ICDs.[57]

SAFETY AND TOLERATION

Torsade de pointes is the major side effect of dofetilide, and other cardiovascular or noncardiovascular side effects appear to be virtually absent. The overall incidence of torsade de pointes has ranged from 1.3% in intravenous studies to 1.6% in oral studies. In healthy volunteers and in individuals with structurally normal hearts, even very high doses of dofetilide have not produced torsade de pointes. On the other hand, in patients with ventricular tachycardia, the incidence appears dose-related and is approximately 3% within the dose range used in phase III clinical trials. Some torsade de pointes cases have occurred

in the setting of electrophysiologic (EP) laboratories, where the relationship with medication or pacing is difficult to establish. Outside the EP laboratory, torsade de pointes cases after dofetilide treatment have generally occurred within minutes of intravenous infusion or within the initial days of starting oral treatment. Most cases seem to occur in association with predisposing factors such as pacemakers that are not functioning optimally, hypokalemia, concomitant medication with other drugs prolonging repolarization (tricyclic antidepressants, other class III antiarrhythmic drugs, etc.), or inherent prolonged QT interval. Other side effects have been reported (e.g., headache, sinus tachycardia, muscle cramps) that were generally mild and transient in nature and occurred with similar frequencies in the placebo-treated and the dofetilide-treated groups.

Laboratory safety test abnormalities outside the normal range have been observed after treatment with dofetilide. These abnormalities have occurred with similar frequencies in control groups (patients receiving placebo). No indications of a causal relationship with dofetilide, in both the healthy volunteer studies or in the patient studies, have been observed so far.

SUMMARY

Dofetilide is a potent and selective class III antiarrhythmic agent, which is under development for the treatment of reentrant tachyarrhythmias, including ventricular tachycardia, ventricular fibrillation, atrial fibrillation, atrial flutter, and paroxysmal supraventricular tachycardia. In preclinical studies, dofetilide shows the profile of a highly selective class III antiarrhythmic agent, increasing both the effective refractory period and the duration of the action potential without affecting the fast inward sodium current or calcium currents. Dofetilide does not influence conduction velocity within the His-Purkinje system or within the myocardium, nor does it impair cardiac contractility.

The pharmacokinetic profile of dofetilide in healthy volunteers and patients exhibits a linear dose–plasma concentration relationship and in healthy volunteers a linear plasma concentration–QT$_c$ relationship. The terminal plasma elimination half-life is 9 to 10 hours, and the systemic bioavailability is in excess of 90%. More than 60% of the parent compound is excreted unchanged via the kidneys, and the remainder is metabolized in the liver to inactive metabolites.

Pharmacodynamic data demonstrate dose- and concentration-dependent effects on myocardial repolarization, evidenced by significant prolongations of the effective and functional refractory periods, monophasic action potential duration, and QT$_c$ interval. No effects on sinus node function, conduction parameters, or cardiac contractility have been detected so far, supporting *in vitro* data showing that dofetilide is a highly selective class III antiarrhythmic agent.

Dofetilide has been administered to healthy volunteers and patients with ischemic heart disease without arrhythmias, as well as to patients with life-threatening ventricular arrhythmias, paroxysmal supraventricular tachycardia, and atrial fibrillation/flutter. Proarrhythmia (predominantly torsade de pointes) has occurred with an overall incidence of less than 2%. The drug has been well tolerated. Side effects have generally been transient and mild, not different from those that occurred in placebo-treated subjects. No clinically significant changes in laboratory safety tests have been detected.

Dofetilide appears to be effective in the acute termination of atrial fibrillation/flutter and in the prevention of induction of sustained VT/VF as well as atrioventricular reentrant tachycardia (AVRT) and atrioventricular nodal reentrant tachycardia (AVNRT).

Acknowledgments

We are indebted to Ms. Jenine Haniak for her excellent secretarial assistance; we are also grateful to our early clinical research group who provided data on pharmacokinetic and pharmacodynamic interactions.

REFERENCES

1. Cross PE, Arrowsmith JE, Thomas GN, et al: Selective Class III antiarrhythmic agents. 1. Bis(arylalkyl)amines. J Med Chem 33:1151, 1990.
2. Carmeliet E: Voltage- and time-dependent block of the delayed K$^+$ current in cardiac myocytes by dofetilide. J Pharmacol Exp Ther 262:809, 1992.
3. Gwilt M, Arrowsmith JE, Blackburn KJ, et al: UK-68,798: A novel, potent and highly selective Class III antiarrhythmic agent which blocks potassium channels in cardiac cells. J Pharmacol Exp Ther 256:318, 1991.
4. Carmeliet E: Use-dependent block and use-dependent unblock of the delayed K$^+$ current in cardiac cells. Circulation 86(Suppl I):615, 1992.
5. Jurkiewicz NK, Sanguinetti MC: Rate-dependent prolongation

6. Bril A, Faivre JF, Landais L, et al: Defibrillatory actions of dofetilide and glibenclamide on reperfusion arrhythmias in the rat; blockade of the ATP sensitive potassium channel as a common mechanism. J Mol Cell Cardiol 24(Suppl V):S68, 1992.
7. Colatsky TJ, Follmer CH, Starmer CF: Channel specificity in antiarrhythmic drug action. Mechanism of potassium channel block and its role in suppressing and aggravating cardiac arrhythmias. Circulation 82:2235, 1990.
8. Greengrass PM, Sanders FL, Wyllie MG: 3H-UK-68,798 (dofetilide) binds to a K$^+$-channel in guinea-pig cardiac tissue. Fundam Clin Pharmacol 5:408, 1991.
9. Pong SF, Kinney CM, Moorhead TJ: Receptor binding profiles of Class III antiarrhythmic agents. FASEB J 5:1215, 1991.
10. Chadwick CC, Ezrin AM, O'Connor B, et al: Identification of a specific radioligand for the cardiac rapidly activating delayed rectifier K$^+$ channel. Circ Res 72:707, 1992.
11. Knilans T, Lathrop DA, Nanasi PB, et al: Rate and concentration-dependent effects of UK-68,798, a potent new Class III antiarrhythmic agent, on canine Purkinje fibre action potential duration and Vmax. Br J Pharmacol 103:1568, 1991.
12. Montero M, Beyer T, Brachmann J, et al: Electrophysiological effects of a new Class III antiarrhythmic agent UK-68,798 in isolated sinus node and atrium of rabbits. Z Kardiol 80(Suppl 3):55, 1991.
13. Montero M, Schmitt C, Beyer T, et al: Effects of a new Class III antiarrhythmic agent, UK-68,798, on intracellular action potentials of human myocardium. Z Kardiol 81(Suppl I):22, 1992.
14. Abrahamsson C, Carlson L, Duker G: Action potential prolongation and early after depolarization induced by Class III antiarrhythmic agents in the fetal, but not the adult rat heart. J Mol Cell Cardiol 24(Suppl V):533, 1992.
15. Tande PM, Bjomstad H, Refsum H: Rate dependent Class III antiarrhythmic action, negative chronotropy and positive inotropy of a novel I$_K$ blocking drug UK-68,798. Potent in guinea pig but no effect in rat myocardium. J Cardiovasc Pharmacol 16:401, 1990.
16. Baskin EP, Serik MC, Wallace AA, et al: Effects of new and potent methanesuphonanilide class III antiarrhythmic agents in myocardial refractoriness and contractility in isolated cardiac muscle. J Cardiovasc Pharmacol 18:406, 1993.
17. Yang T, Tande PM, Refsum H: Electromechanical action of dofetilide and d-sotalol during stimulated metabolic acidosis in isolated guinea-pig ventricular muscle. J Cardiovasc Pharmacol 20:889, 1992.
18. Beyer T, Marschang W, Kuebler W, et al: Reverse "use dependent" Class III effects of UK-68,798 in relation to extracellular potassium concentration. Eur Heart J 13(Suppl):303, 1992.
19. Yang T, Tande PM, Lathrop DA, et al: Effects of altered extracellular potassium and pacing cycle length on the class III antirhythmic actions of dofetilide (UK-68,798) in guinea-pig papillary muscle. Cardiovasc Drugs Ther 6:429, 1992.
20. Forest MC, Cheval B, Bril A: Effects of dofetilide and glibenclamide on shortening of action potential and reduction of contractile force in guinea-pig ischemic papillary muscle. J Mol Cell Cardiol 24(Suppl VI):540, 1992.
21. Yang T, Tande PM, Lathrop DA, et al: Class III antiarrhythmic action by potassium channel blockade: Dofetilide attenuates hypoxia-induced electromechanical changes. Cardiovasc Res 26:1109, 1992.
22. Platou ES, Refsum H, Hotvedt R: Class III antiarrhythmic activity linked with positive inotropy: Electrophysiological and hemodynamic effects of the sea anemone polypeptide ATX II in the dog heart in situ. J Cardiovasc Pharmacol 8:459, 1986.
23. Yang T, Tande PM, Refsum H: Negative chronotropic effect of a novel class III antiarrhythmic drug, UK-68,798, devoid of β blocking action on isolated guinea pig atria. Br J Pharmacol 103:1417, 1991.
24. Miller KE, Carpenter JF, Brooks RR: Beta adrenergic receptor response of guinea pig heart in the presence of Class III antiarrhythmics. FASEB J 5:A1216, 1991.
25. Hondeghem LM, Snyders DJ: Class III antiarrhythmic agents have a lot of potential but a long way to go: Reduced effectiveness and dangers of reverse use dependence. Circulation 81:686, 1990.

26. Baskin E, Serik C, Wallace A, et al: Vascular effects of class III antiarrhythmic agents. Drug Development Research 26:481, 1992.

27. Dalrymple HW, Butler P, Dodd MG: Electrocardiographic and hemodynamic effects in conscious dogs of UK-68,798, a new Class III antiarrhythmic agent. Eur Heart J 10:395, 1989.

28. Gwilt M, Blackburn KJ, Burges RA, et al: Electropharmacology of dofetilide, a new class III agent, in anaesthetized dogs. Eur J Pharmacol 215:137, 1992.

29. Spinelli W, Parsons RW, Colatsky TJ: Effects of WAY-123,398, a new Class III antiarrhythmic agent, on cardiac refractoriness and ventricular fibrillation threshold in anaesthetized dogs: A comparison with UK-68,798, E-4031, and dl-sotalol. J Cardiovasc Pharmacol 20:913, 1992.

30. Wallace AA, Stupienski RF, Brooks LM, et al: Cardiac electrophysiology and inotropic actions of new and potent methane-sulphonanilide Class III antiarrhythmic agents in anaesthetized dogs. J Cardiovasc Pharmacol 18:687, 1991.

31. Zuanetti G, Corr PB: Antiarrhythmic efficacy of a new Class III agent, UK-68,798, during myocardial infarction: Evaluation using three-dimensional mapping. J Pharmacol Exp Ther 256:325, 1991.

32. Beatch GN, MacLeod BA, Abraham S, et al: The in vivo electrophysiological actions of the new potassium channel blocker, tedisamil and UK-68,798. Proc West Pharmacol Soc 33:5, 1990.

33. Mortensen E, Yang T, Refsum H: Class III antiarrhythmic action and inotropy: Effects of dofetilide in acute ischemic heart failure in dogs. J Cardiovasc Pharmacol 19:216, 1992.

34. Gout B, Jean J, Bril A: Comparative effects of a potassium channel blocking drug UK-68,798 and a specific bradycardiac agent, UL-FS49, on exercise induced ischemia in the dog: Significance of diastolic time on ischemic cardiac function. J Pharmacol Exp Ther 262:987, l992.

35. Schoels W, Offner B, Freigang K, et al: Termination of experimental atrial fibrillation by dofetilide: Differential effects on normal and slow conducting tissue. Z Kardiol 82(Suppl 1):175, 1993.

36. Andersen HR, Wiggers HS, Knudsen LL, et al: Dofetilide suppresses ventricular fibrillation during acute myocardial ischemia, a randomized study in pigs. Circulation 86(Suppl I):301, 1992.

37. Black SC, Chi L, Mu DX, et al: The antifibrillatory actions of UK-68,798, a class III antiarrhythmic agent. J Pharmacol Exp Ther 258:416, 1991.

38. Maynard AE, Carpenter JF, Decker GE, et al: Efficacy of d-sotalol, sematilide and UK-68,798 in the rat coronary artery ligation-reperfusion model of cardiac arrhythmia. FASEB J 5:A1216, 1991.

39. Gwilt M, King RC, Milne AA, et al: Dofetilide, a new class III antiarrhythmic agent reduces pacing-induced heterogeneity of repolarization in vivo. Cardiovasc Res 26:1102, 1992.

40. Moore EN, Spear JF: Ventricular fibrillation threshold. Its physiological and pharmacological importance. Arch Intern Med 135:446, 1975.

41. Carlsson L, Almgren O, Duker G: QTU-prolongation and torsades de pointes induced by putative Class III antiarrhythmic agents in the rabbit: Etiology and interventions. J Cardiovasc Pharmacol 16:276, 1990.

42. Tham TCK, MacLennan BA, Harron DWG, et al: Pharmacodynamics and pharmacokinetics of the novel Class III antiarrhythmic drug UK-68,798 in man. Br J Clin Pharmacol 31(Suppl II):243, 1991.

43. Gemmill JD, Howie CA, Meredith PA, et al: A dose-ranging study of UK68,798, a novel class III antiarrhythmic agent in normal volunteers. Br J Clin Pharmacol 32:429, 1991.

44. Rasmussen HS, Allen MJ, Blackburn KJ, et al: Dofetilide, a novel class III antiarrhythmic agent. J Cardiovasc Pharmacol 20(2):96, 1992.

45. Sedgwick M, Rasmussen HS, Walker D, et al: Pharmacokinetic and pharmacodynamic effects of UK-68,798, a new potential class III antiarrhythmic drug. Br J Clin Pharmacol 31:515, 1991.

46. Butrous GS, O'Nunain S, Ward J, et al: Clinical electrophysiologic profile of UK-68,798, a new class III antiarrhythmic agent. PACE 14(Suppl II):744, 1991.

47. Sedgwick M, Rasmussen HS, Cobbe SM: Clinical and electrophysiological effects of intravenous dofetilide (UK-68,798), a new class III antiarrhythmic agent in patients with angina pectoris. Am J Cardiol 69:513, 1992.

48. Sedgwick M, Rasmussen HS, Cobbe SM: Effects of the Class III antiarrhythmic drug dofetilide, on ventricular monophasic action potential duration and QT internal dispersion in stable angina pectoris. Am J Cardiol 70:1932, 1992.

49. Bailey WM, Nadamanee K, Edwards J, et al: Electrophysiologic and hemodynamic effects of dofetilide in patients with severe left ventricular dysfunction. Circulation 86(Suppl):I-265, 1992.

50. Echt DS, Lee JT, Murray KT, et al: A randomized, double-blind, placebo-controlled dose-ranging study of intravenous UK-68,798 (dofetilide) in patients with inducible sustained ventricular tachyarrhythmias. Circulation 84(Suppl II):II-714, 1991.

51. Thomsen PEB, Bashir Y, Kingma JH, et al: Dofetilide in the treatment of sustained monomorphic ventricular tachycardia. Eur Heart J 18(Suppl):304, 1992.

52. Brachmann J, Haverkamp W, Johns J, et al: The efficacy and safety of oral dofetilide in patients with sustained ventricular tachycardia. Circulation 86(Suppl):I-265, 1992.

53. Suttorp MJ, Polak PE, van't Hof A, et al: Efficacy and safety of a new class III antiarrhythmic agent, dofetilide, in patients with paroxysmal atrial fibrillation or atrial flutter. Am J Cardiol 69:417, 1992.

54. Conelly DT, Thomsen PEB, Camm AJ, et al: Efficacy and safety of dofetilide, a novel class III antiarrhythmic agent, in atrioventricular nodal reentrant tachycardia. Eur Heart J 18(Suppl): 304, 1992.

55. Wong CKY, Heald S, Thomsen PEB, et al: Electrophysiology, safety and efficacy of dofetilide in patients with atrioventricular reentrant tachycardia. A dose range study. Eur Heart J 18(Suppl):211, 1992.

56. Gremillion ST, Echt DS, Smith NA, et al: Beneficial effects of intravenous dofetilide in patients undergoing ventricular defibrillation testing. Circulation 86(Suppl):I264, 1992.

57. Echt DS, Gremillion ST, Lee JT, et al: Effects of procainamide and lidocaine on defibrillation energy requirements in patients receiving implantable cardioverter defibrillator devices. J Cardiovasc Electrophysiol 5(9):752, 1994.

CHAPTER 142

Flecainide

*Mark D. Carlson, M.D., Richard W. Henthorn, M.D.,
and Albert L. Waldo, M.D.*

Increased understanding of anatomic, physiologic, and biochemical mechanisms of arrhythmias has allowed investigators to develop several new and potentially more effective antiarrhythmic drugs in recent years. One of these drugs, flecainide, was developed by 3M Riker Laboratories, Inc., in the early 1970s and was the first type IC antiarrhythmic agent approved by the United States Food and Drug Administration (FDA) for treatment of ventricular arrhythmias. In the short period since its clinical introduction, flecainide has been shown to be safe and effective for treatment of life-threatening ventricular and supraventricular arrhythmias in patients without structural heart disease. It offers several clinical advantages over many other antiarrhythmic agents, including low incidence of organ toxicity, twice-daily dosing to achieve therapeutic efficacy, and measurable plasma levels that correlate with therapeutic efficacy and safety.

HISTORY

Flecainide acetate is a fluorinated aromatic hydrocarbon, first synthesized in 1972. The molecule is the product of a 3M Company program initiated in 1966 to develop new anesthetic drugs by adding fluorine to organic molecules.[1] Substitution of fluorine for hydrogen often imparts several beneficial properties to drug molecules. Fluorinated compounds often have greater lipid solubility, a characteristic that may improve absorption and distribution. The carbon–fluorine bond is stronger than the carbon–hydrogen bond (116 kcal/M versus 99 kcal/M), resulting in a metabolically more stable compound. Fluorine, the most electronegative element known, alters molecular electronic patterns and thus their interaction with nearby molecules. Finally, addition of fluorine, the radius of which is only slightly larger than that of hydrogen, does not significantly change the size or shape of the molecule.

Early attempts to fluorinate procainamide yielded several molecules with local anesthetic properties. These compounds differed from procainamide in that one or more trifluoroethoxy group side chains, rather than a single amino side chain, were attached to the benzene ring. A 3M pharmacologist, Jack Schmid, realizing that the two properties are related, suggested that compounds with local anesthetic properties should be evaluated for antiarrhythmic activity.

Studies in mice and dogs demonstrated that the 2,5-trifluoroethoxy isomer most effectively protected against ventricular fibrillation.[2] Modifications of the amide side chain then were investigated. Compounds with branching at the site of the amide nitrogen atom were found to be most potent, possibly because of protection from deactivation due to N-dealkylation in the liver. Thus, molecules with ring side chains incorporating the amide nitrogen atom were also investigated. The most potent of these, flecainide acetate, was synthesized by Elden Banitt in 1972.

In 1975, flecainide was tested clinically in healthy human volunteers for the first time. Results of acute phase II trials indicated that flecainide suppressed ventricular premature contractions (VPCs).[3, 4] Because of this finding and the expanding antiarrhythmic market, 3M developed a clinical plan in 1979 to evaluate flecainide for suppression of ventricular arrhythmias. Based on efficacy determined in dose-ranging studies by Hodges et al.,[5] Duff et al.,[6] and Anderson et al.,[7] the FDA assigned the drug a IB status (a new molecule representing a moderate advance over currently marketed drugs for similar indications). Because of the new status, 3M moved up the new drug application date, originally scheduled for 1984, to 1982. To meet this deadline, the oral form of flecainide was developed to the exclusion of the intravenous form.

PHARMACOKINETICS
Absorption

One of the distinct advantages of flecainide is that it is well absorbed. The drug may be administered orally in either tablet or capsule form. Mean time to peak plasma level is 3 hours after tablet ingestion and 4 hours after capsule ingestion.[8–12] Because extent of absorption is similar, the difference in absorption rate between capsule and tablet forms is of no consequence during steady-state dosing. Flecainide absorption rate does not change when the drug is administered with food or with aluminum hydroxide antacids.[8] In healthy subjects, more than 90% of an oral dose is delivered to the systemic circulation as unchanged flecainide.[8, 9] Thus, flecainide is well absorbed and does not undergo significant presystemic biotransformation (first-pass effect). Extent of absorption for solution and for both solid forms is similar.[8]

Plasma flecainide levels are related linearly to and are proportional to dose levels over a wide range.[9] Extent of absorption, like rate, is similar when the drug is administered with or without food. Antacids do not alter the extent of flecainide absorption. In separate studies of patients with heart failure and patients with renal insufficiency, extent and rate of flecainide absorption were similar to those of healthy subjects.[10, 13]

Half-Life and Plasma Clearance

During multiple oral dosing, flecainide accumulates to a steady plasma level within 3 or 4 days. After 7 days of twice-daily oral administration in 16 subjects, mean flecainide half-life and plasma clearance were 16 hours (range, 9 to 23 hours) and 6.9 ml/min/kg (range, 4.1 to 14.5 ml/min/kg), respectively.[8] After the initial dose in these individuals, the plasma half-life was 13 hours (range, 9 to 19 hours) and clearance was 7.3 ml/min/kg (range, 4.1 to 11.7 ml/min/kg). Plasma half-life, therefore, was moderately prolonged, but plasma clearance was virtually unchanged after multiple doses of the drug. No induction or inhibition of drug elimination was noted. Steady-state plasma levels demonstrated linear pharmacokinetics without unexpected drug accumulation during oral dosage regimens of 1.1 to 2.8 mg/kg twice daily.

During efficacy studies, the plasma half-life in 48 patients receiving flecainide for ventricular premature complexes ranged from 12 to 30 hours (mean, 20 hours).[7, 8, 14, 15] Plasma clearance in 11 of these patients was 6.2 ml/min/kg. Older age and depressed left ventricular function were thought to contribute to the reduced rate of elimination.

Volume of Distribution

Flecainide's volume of distribution after intravenous and oral administration (mean, 8.7 and 10.0 L/kg, respectively) reflects extensive distribution of the drug from plasma to most tissues other than brain.[8, 9] Cardiac tissue levels are 11- to 12-fold higher than plasma levels, but decrease at the same rate.[16] Plasma drug levels, therefore, accurately reflect flecainide cardiac tissue concentration. In rats, dogs, and monkeys, flecainide is retained only in the pigmented ocular tissues.[8, 16, 17] However, long-term studies of rats, dogs, baboons, and humans have not revealed evidence of ocular toxicity.

Metabolism

Flecainide is the acetate salt of N-(2-piperidylmethyl)-2,5-bis(2,2,2,-trifluoroethoxy)benzamide. In humans, flecainide undergoes meta-O-dealkylation, piperidine ring oxidation, and phenolic conjugation (Fig 142–1). Two major metabolites, meta-O-dealkylated flecainide and the meta-O-dealkylated lactam of flecainide, are found in urine and plasma. Both metabolites are present in free form or are conjugated as a glucuronide or sulfate. In canine models, the effect of meta-O-dealkylated flecainide on atrial conduction, the atrioventricular (AV) nodal refractory period, and the ventricular refractory period is similar to that of flecainide.[11] However, meta-O-dealkylated flecainide is at best 50% as potent as unchanged flecainide. The meta-O-dealkylated lactam of flecainide has less electro-physiologic effect and only 10% the potency of unchanged flecainide. Only meta-O-dealkylated flecainide has detectable antiarrhythmic activity (20% relative to unchanged flecainide).[8, 12] However, because plasma meta-O-dealkylated flecainide concentration is only 5% to 10% that of unchanged flecainide, the antiarrhythmic effect of the metabolite is of little clinical consequence.

Excretion

In healthy subjects, 81% to 90% of an oral flecainide dose is excreted in the urine, 10% to 50% as unchanged drug.[8, 12] Significant quantities of the two major metabolites are also found in the urine, mostly in the conjugated form. Only 4% to 6% of a single oral dose is found in the feces. Most is excreted within 24 hours. Under alkaline conditions (urine pH > 8), however, urinary unchanged flecainide concentration and plasma elimination decrease.

Flecainide excretion has been studied in patients with heart failure and renal insufficiency. Franciosa et al.[10] compared flecainide plasma elimination in 10 patients with heart failure (nine with New York Heart Association [NYHA] functional class III, one with class II) and nine healthy, age- and weight-matched subjects.[10] Plasma half-life was longer in patients with heart failure than in healthy subjects (19 versus 14 hours, $p < .05$). Plasma clearance, however, did not differ significantly between the two groups, nor did urinary excretion or renal clearance of unchanged flecainide 72 hours after dosing. These data suggest that heart failure prolongs flecainide plasma half-life but does not affect urinary excretion after a single dose. Importantly, during long-term administration, patients with heart failure may require a lower daily flecainide dose.

As expected, renal function impairment prolongs plasma half-life and decreases flecainide urinary excretion. Relative to unchanged drug, excretion of flecainide metabolites is more severely impaired in patients with renal dysfunction. Plasma and renal flecainide clearance correlate with urinary creatinine clearance in these patients ($p < .01$).[8] In patients undergoing dialysis, only 1% of a single oral dose is found in dialysate 24 hours after flecainide administration. The drug's large volume of distribution probably accounts for this small extent of removal.

Plasma Protein Binding

Flecainide plasma protein binding (mean, 40%) is independent of total drug concentration over a wide range (15 to 3400 ng/ml) exceeding therapeutic levels (200 to 1000 ng/ml).[18] Thus, at therapeutic and supratherapeutic levels, free and total flecainide concentrations are proportional. Plasma protein binding of flecainide in vitro has been assessed in the presence of 10 other drugs: digoxin, propranolol, practolol, quinidine, procainamide, disopyramide, diazepam, phenytoin, lidocaine, and furosemide.[8] At therapeutic concentrations of each of these drugs, flecainide protein

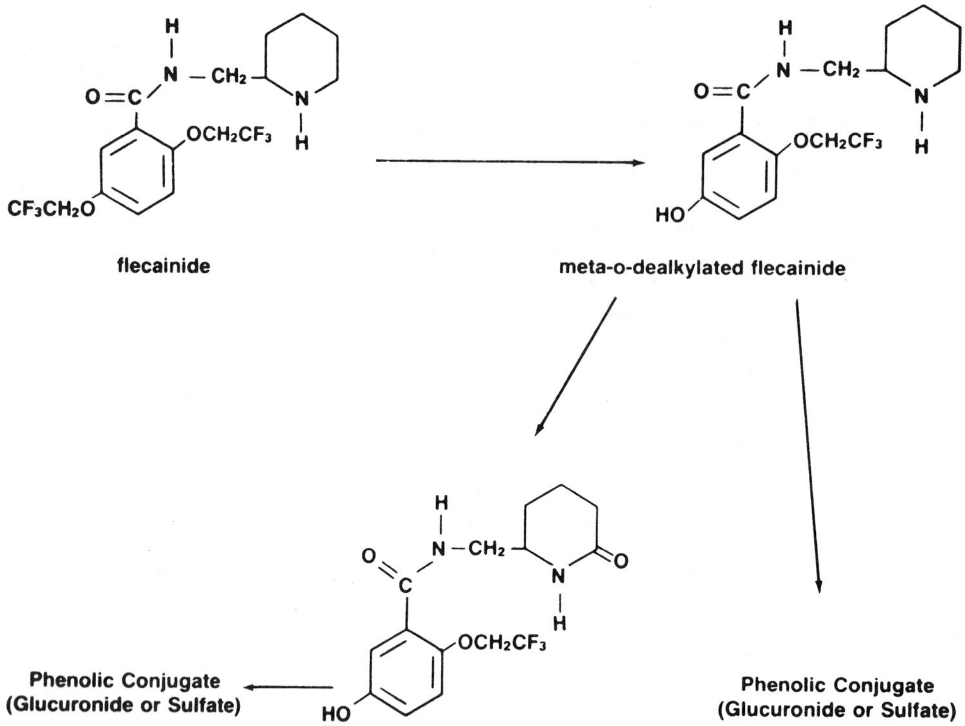

Figure 142–1. Major pathways of flecainide biotransformation in humans. (Adapted with permission from Conrad GJ, Ober RE: Metabolism of flecainide. Am J Cardiol 53:41B, 1984.)

binding was similar to that of controls. At threefold therapeutic concentrations of lidocaine and phenytoin, flecainide protein binding was approximately 15% less than the control. Thus, none of the drugs tested significantly affected flecainide plasma protein binding. Similarly, because it is not extensively bound to plasma protein, flecainide is not likely to displace significantly other protein-bound drugs.

α_1-Acid glycoprotein, a major determinant of basic drug protein binding, increases after myocardial infarction. In 10 patients studied for 5 days after myocardial infarction, flecainide plasma protein transiently increased and free drug decreased by 25%.[19] The clinical significance of these transient changes is unknown.

EFFECTS ON PATHOPHYSIOLOGY
Electrophysiologic Effects

Studies *In Vitro*

Electrophysiologic effects of flecainide have been demonstrated in isolated rabbit and canine myocardial tissue preparations. In Purkinje fibers and ventricular muscle, flecainide decreased maximal rate of rise ($\dot{V}_{max}$) of the action potential, action potential amplitude, and action potential overshoot.[20–22] These effects were use and concentration dependent. In ventricular muscle, flecainide increased the ventricular effective refractory period (ERP) and, to a lesser extent, the action potential duration (APD). In Purkinje fibers, APD decreased as flecainide concentration increased. The ERP of Purkinje fibers decreased at low

concentrations but returned to baseline at high flecainide concentrations.

Like other class I drugs, in addition to its use-dependent effects on action potential $\dot{V}_{max}$, flecainide shifted membrane responsiveness in the hyperpolarized direction. Flecainide decreased automaticity in isolated rabbit sinoatrial (SA) nodes and decreased isoproterenol-enhanced automaticity in canine Purkinje fibers. Flecainide had little effect on calcium-dependent slow-channel action potentials.[20–22]

These findings suggest that flecainide slows conduction by prolonging sodium-mediated, time-dependent refractoriness in cardiac tissues. Because it restricts the fast sodium current, Harrison classifies flecainide as a class IC antiarrhythmic drug.[23]

Studies *In Vivo*

In open-chest dogs, Hodess et al.[24] showed that, at clinically relevant plasma levels (400 to 700 ng/ml), flecainide slowed cardiac conduction globally.[24] The drug increased intraatrial conduction time, atrioventricular (AV) nodal conduction time, His-Purkinje conduction time, and ventricular activation time. Flecainide also increased the atrial effective refractory period and both the AV nodal functional and effective refractory periods. The magnitude of these effects was concentration dependent. The drug did not slow sinus or AV junctional pacemaker rate, but it did slow ectopic atrial and ventricular pacemakers.

Effects on Sinus Node and Atria

In humans, flecainide has variable effects on impulse formation, dependent on dose and underlying cardiac disease. In patients with apparently normal sinus node function, flecainide either slows or does not affect sinus rate.[7, 25-30] However, there are reports of dose-related asymptomatic sinus pauses and of prolongation of the sinus node recovery time.[31] In 11 patients with symptomatic sinus node dysfunction, corrected sinus node recovery time increased from 875 ± 181 msec to 1727 ± 507 msec after intravenous administration of flecainide.[32] Spontaneous sinus cycle length did not change. In contrast, in patients studied because of syncope or presyncope, Hellestrand et al.[33] demonstrated a small increase in heart rate after intravenous flecainide (65 to 69 beats/min, $p < .01$). Changes in corrected and uncorrected sinus node recovery time were not significant. In another study, the same authors showed that atrial conduction time, as measured by the PA interval, increased from 41 ± 13 msec to 50 ± 13 msec (22%) when patients took flecainide.[29] The ERP of the atria increased from 213 ± 32 msec to 219 ± 28 msec ($p = $ NS) in these patients. In patients with sinus nodal dysfunction, the atrial ERP increased from 267 ± 16 msec to 298 ± 19 msec ($p < .01$) on flecainide.[32]

Effects on Specialized Atrioventricular Conduction System

Several studies have shown that intravenous flecainide prolongs AV conduction. Percentage increases in the HV interval exceeded those in the AH interval (mean, 27% to 47% versus 15% to 22%)[26, 29, 30, 32] (Table 142–1). Increases in AH interval were greater in patients who had AH interval prolongation at baseline (>120 msec). Patients with normal AH intervals rarely developed abnormal AH intervals on flecainide therapy. The HV interval increased in 37 of 39 patients studied by Hellestrand et al.[29] HV prolongation to more than 55 msec occurred in 70% of these patients. Complete AH block and infranodal block have been reported in one patient with previously documented AV Wenckebach block and in four patients with pre-existing bundle branch block.[26, 29]

Effects on Ventricles

Flecainide also slows intraventricular conduction and prolongs the ventricular refractory periods in humans. Studies using monophasic action potential recordings have demonstrated that flecainide prolongs

right ventricular basal conduction time (time from pacemaker artifact to monophasic action potential upstroke) by 17%.[34] In a separate study, flecainide prolonged the time from onset of the surface electrocardiogram to the right ventricular apex electrocardiogram by 23%.[32] During ventricular pacing, flecainide increased monophasic APD by 9.6%.[5] In patients taking flecainide, the right ventricular ERP measured at the apex and outflow tracts was prolonged by 5% and 10%, respectively.[34]

Summary of Electrophysiologic Effects

In humans, flecainide slows conduction in all myocardial tissue, particularly in the His-Purkinje system (HV interval) and in the ventricles. Significant effects on refractory periods have been observed only in the ventricles. Sinus node recovery times are somewhat prolonged, an effect that may be clinically significant in patients with sinus node dysfunction.

Electrocardiographic Effects

Electrocardiographic studies in humans receiving flecainide are consistent with invasive electrophysiologic studies. In 7 of 10 studies, the PR interval increased (17% to 29%) after flecainide administration.[5-7, 26, 28, 34-36] Eleven of 13 studies demonstrated QRS complex prolongation of 11% to 27% after administration of the drug.[3, 5-7, 28-30, 32, 33-35] QT duration increased slightly (4% to 13%) in six studies[3, 6, 26, 28, 32, 36] and remained unchanged in four.[25, 26, 34, 35] QT prolongation during flecainide therapy results from QRS complex prolongation and is less than that observed in patients taking other class I antiarrhythmic drugs.[26] The JT (QT-QRS) interval, an index of ventricular repolarization that controls for QT lengthening secondary to QRS complex prolongation (i.e., secondary to prolongation of ventricular depolarization), was prolonged slightly in two studies,[28, 35] but it was significantly shortened in a third study.[29] Thus, data obtained from intracardiac and surface electrocardiograms show that flecainide prolongs ventricular conduction time but has little effect on repolarization.

Antiarrhythmic Effects

Ventricular Arrhythmias

Antiarrhythmic effects of flecainide were first studied in intact animals. During product development, flecainide and several other drugs were evaluated for potential antiarrhythmic activity. Mice pretreated with these drugs were exposed to chloroform until respiration ceased and ventricular fibrillation occurred. In this model, flecainide prevented ventricular fibrillation at lower concentrations than did quinidine, procainamide, lidocaine, or any of the other experimental fluorinated drugs.[1, 22]

Flecainide was then compared with these drugs in four canine arrhythmia models: (1) hydrocarbon-epinephrine–induced ventricular arrhythmias, (2)

Table 142–1. **Effects of Flecainide on Atrioventricular Conduction System**

Reference	AH Interval (msec)		HV Interval (msec)	
	Baseline	Flecainide	Baseline	Flecainide
Hellestrand et al.[29]	67 ± 21*	81 ± 33*	44 ± 9*	61 ± 12*
Seipel et al.[30]	89 ± 11*	103 ± 16*	51 ± 13*	59 ± 15*
Vik-Mo et al.[32]	124 ± 9†	143 ± 8†	41 ± 3†	52 ± 4†

*Standard deviation.
†Standard error of the mean.

ouabain-induced ectopic ventricular arrhythmias, (3) coronary artery ligation–induced ventricular arrhythmias, and (4) aconitine-induced atrial arrhythmias. Flecainide prevented or converted arrhythmias equally as well or more effectively than each of the other drugs tested. In another canine study, flecainide suppressed ouabain-induced ventricular arrhythmias more effectively than disopyramide, encainide, tocainide, mexiletine, or lidocaine. In one conscious canine model, however, neither intravenous loading nor maintenance flecainide prevented ventricular tachyarrhythmias during the early postinfarction period.[37]

In open-chest canine studies, flecainide increased the ventricular fibrillation threshold by as much as 122%. Increases in ventricular fibrillation threshold occurred most frequently at plasma flecainide concentrations of more than 1000 ng/ml and were maximal at 9300 ng/ml.[38] In humans, plasma flecainide concentrations higher than 1000 ng/ml are considered supratherapeutic.

Human studies of flecainide efficacy are complicated by differing end points or definitions, differences in underlying heart disease, and, in many cases, lack of appropriate control groups. In one study, flecainide suppressed at least 80% of VPCs in 30 of 35 patients; mean VPC suppression was 96%.[39] Complex ventricular ectopy (couplets, triplets, nonsustained ventricular tachycardia) decreased by 95%. In the Cardiac Arrhythmia Suppression Trial (CAST), flecainide suppressed VPCs by 80% or more and nonsustained ventricular tachycardia by 90% or more in 84% of patients taking 100 mg every 12 hours and in 16% of patients taking 150 mg every 12 hours.[40]

Anderson et al.[41, 42] evaluated flecainide efficacy in patients with spontaneous and inducible ventricular tachyarrhythmias. In patients receiving flecainide, ventricular tachyarrhythmias could not be induced in 9 of 15 patients. An outpatient trial of flecainide was attempted in 10 patients. At follow-up (median, 13.5 months), eight patients were still taking flecainide without recurrent ventricular tachycardia. In two patients, one with progressive heart failure and recurrent ventricular tachycardia and one with recurrent slower ventricular tachycardia, drug therapy was stopped.

Reid et al.[43] administered flecainide to 36 patients who had ventricular tachycardia (at least 3 consecutive beats at a rate of at least 120 beats/min) on 24-hour Holter monitoring. On average, therapy with 3.9 ± 1.0 antiarrhythmic drugs had failed with each patient. Flecainide eliminated ventricular tachycardia from the 24-hour Holter electrocardiographic recording in 32 of 36 patients. However, in 10 of these 32 patients, ventricular tachycardia was still induced at electrophysiologic study. Flecainide was discontinued in 29 of 36 patients for a variety of reasons (ineffective, 12 patients; noncardiac side effects, 2 patients; proarrhythmia, 2 patients; new conduction defects, 3 patients; unspecified, 10 patients). Ten patients died while taking flecainide, six suddenly. Of these six sudden deaths, five occurred within 5 days of initiating therapy and were observed to be due to

ventricular tachycardia. Patients who died had lower left ventricular ejection fractions (0.24 ± 0.1 versus 0.45 ± 0.2, $p < .05$) and were taking higher doses of flecainide (350 ± 85 mg versus 276 ± 59 mg, $p < .05$) than those who survived.

In a separate study, the same investigators found that 15 of 17 patients who had sustained or nonsustained ventricular tachycardia induced at baseline electrophysiologic study had ventricular tachycardia induced while taking flecainide.[44] This disparity between the studies of Anderson et al. and Reid et al. may be explained by differences in severity of heart failure. In the two studies, underlying heart disease, presenting arrhythmia, and number of previous antiarrhythmic drug trials were similar. However, Anderson et al. excluded patients with NYHA functional class III or IV heart failure, whereas Reid et al. did not.

In a study by Lal et al.,[45] 18 of 38 patients with sustained ventricular tachycardia or sudden cardiac death qualified for long-term treatment with flecainide. Twenty patients did not receive flecainide, because they failed electrophysiologic study with the drug (14 patients), had spontaneous recurrence (3 patients), had a proarrhythmic effect (2 patients), or had an automatic defibrillator implanted (1 patient). Of the 18 patients treated with flecainide, 15 (40%) were alive at follow-up (mean, 11 ± 3 months). Of the three deaths in the group treated with flecainide, only one was thought to be due to an arrhythmia.[45]

Webb et al.[46] administered oral flecainide to 24 patients with inducible, sustained, monomorphic ventricular tachycardia and remote myocardial infarction. The dose of flecainide was titrated to eliminate ventricular tachycardia and to reduce VPCs by 80% on 24-hour Holter monitoring. Of 18 patients undergoing repeat electrophysiologic testing on flecainide, 14 still had inducible ventricular tachycardia. In contrast with the baseline study, tachycardia cycle length increased by more than 100 msec, and symptoms during tachycardia were eliminated in 10 of 14 patients. During 16 ± 7 months' follow-up, no death or spontaneous arrhythmic event occurred in patients with no inducible ventricular tachycardia on flecainide. Ventricular tachycardia recurred in 4 of 10 patients, and sudden cardiac death occurred in 1 of 10 patients who continued to have inducible ventricular tachycardia and who were discharged on flecainide.

These data suggest that electrophysiologic testing improves risk stratification for recurrent ventricular tachyarrhythmias in patients taking flecainide after myocardial infarction. Patients in whom flecainide eliminates spontaneous ventricular tachycardia on 24-hour Holter monitoring but who continue to have inducible ventricular tachycardia (regardless of cycle length) remain at increased risk for recurrent ventricular tachycardia and sudden cardiac death.

Wynn et al.[47] determined whether suppression of inducible ventricular tachyarrhythmias with flecainide predicted efficacy of other antiarrhythmic drugs. In 26 of 29 patients in whom flecainide suppressed ventricular tachycardia, induction of ventricular tachycardia was also suppressed by other antiarrhythmic agents.[47] However, induction of ventricular tachycardia was suppressed by another drug in 15 of 26 patients in whom ventricular tachycardia was induced while on flecainide therapy. Thus, suppression of ventricular tachycardia at electrophysiologic study by flecainide predicts efficacy of other antiarrhythmic drugs; failure to suppress ventricular tachycardia, however, does not predict response to other drugs.

Comparison with Other Drugs

Several studies have compared flecainide with other antiarrhythmic drugs. One multicenter trial compared flecainide with quinidine in 233 patients with chronic ventricular ectopy.[35] Patients received placebo during weeks 1 and 4 and were assigned randomly to receive either quinidine or flecainide during weeks 2 and 3 of the study. VPCs were 95% suppressed in 75% of patients taking flecainide and 34% of patients taking quinidine. Ventricular couplets were 95% suppressed in 85% of patients on flecainide and 60% of patients taking quinidine ($p < .0001$). Nonsustained ventricular tachycardia was completely suppressed in 79% of patients taking flecainide compared with 60% of those receiving quinidine. Sixty-eight percent of patients taking flecainide versus 33% of patients taking quinidine had 80% suppression of VPCs and complete suppression of couplets and ventricular tachycardia ($p < .0001$).

Flecainide and disopyramide were compared in a randomized double-blind crossover study of 25 patients with VPCs.[48] Drug treatment periods were preceded and followed by placebo treatment. Median VPC suppression was 92% in patients taking flecainide and 39% in those taking disopyramide ($p < .01$).

Flecainide was compared with amiodarone in a randomized crossover study of 10 patients with frequent VPCs.[49] Patients took each drug for 12 days at gradually increasing doses or until therapeutic efficacy was achieved. Study periods were separated by a 30-day placebo period. VPC suppression during therapy with each of the drugs was similar (99.4% for patients receiving flecainide versus 96% for those taking amiodarone). These study results should be interpreted with caution because of the small study population, because 30 days may not be adequate to wash out amiodarone, and because 12 days may not be sufficient for amiodarone to achieve a therapeutic effect.

The Cardiac Arrhythmia Pilot Study (CAPS) compared the antiarrhythmic efficacy (>70% suppression of VPCs, >90% reduction in ventricular tachycardia) of flecainide, encainide, moricizine, imipramine, and placebo[50] in patients who had experienced acute myocardial infarctions 6 to 60 days before onset of therapy. Flecainide and encainide suppressed ventricular ectopy more effectively (83% and 79%, respectively) than moricizine (66%), imipramine (52%), and placebo (33%; $p < .0001$). Adverse effects were similar in patients taking flecainide and encainide. However,

adverse effects tended to occur less frequently while patients were taking flecainide or encainide than when they were receiving moricizine, imipramine, or placebo.

Because of its use-dependent properties, flecainide may prolong tachycardia cycle length and the duration of the QRS complex at high heart rates. Kidwell et al.[51] showed that use-dependent block of cardiac sodium channels increased ventricular tachycardia cycle length to a greater extent during flecainide therapy (increase of 82 ± 34 msec, $p < .0001$) than during therapy with procainamide (increase of 12 ± 15 msec) or lidocaine (increase of 8 ± 8 msec). The time constant for the onset of use-dependent ventricular tachycardia cycle length prolongation was slower for flecainide than for either procainamide or lidocaine (12.5 $\pm$ 5, 4.0 $\pm$ 1.3, and 0.52 $\pm$ 0.51 seconds).

In summary, flecainide is an effective drug when used to suppress VPCs and nonsustained ventricular tachycardia. Available data suggest that flecainide suppresses ventricular ectopy more effectively than quinidine, disopyramide, moricizine, or imipramine and is as effective as amiodarone. Long-term studies suggest that flecainide suppresses spontaneous sustained ventricular tachycardia as effectively as antiarrhythmic drugs other than amiodarone. Of note, flecainide has not been compared with sotalol for the treatment of ventricular arrhythmias. Patients with a history of sustained ventricular tachycardia whose ventricular ectopy is suppressed on Holter monitoring may still have sustained ventricular tachycardia induced at electrophysiologic study.

Supraventricular Arrhythmias

Although the FDA originally approved flecainide only for ventricular arrhythmias, cardiac electrophysiologists recognized that flecainide might be used effectively to treat supraventricular arrhythmias as well. The drug prolongs the ERP of the atria, AV node, and accessory AV connections. These characteristics suggested that flecainide might effectively treat ectopic and reentrant atrial arrhythmias, AV nodal reentrant tachycardia, and AV reciprocating tachycardia involving an accessory AV connection.

In October 1991, the FDA approved flecainide for the prevention of paroxysmal supraventricular tachycardia, atrial fibrillation, and atrial flutter in patients without structural heart disease. Several studies, both before and since this approval, have shown that the drug is effective for conversion and suppression of a variety of supraventricular arrhythmias. This is of particular note because this approval came well after the results of the Cardiac Arrhythmia Suppression Trial (CAST) were published.[52] Thus, despite the adverse effects of flecainide in patients with ventricular ectopy after myocardial infarction, it was recognized that the drug could be used safely and effectively in patients without structural heart disease.

Two groups have reviewed the literature regarding flecainide therapy for supraventricular tachyarrhythmias. Hohnloser and Zabel reviewed 60 studies in which flecainide was administered for a variety of supraventricular tachyarrhythmias.[53] Short-term flecainide administration terminated atrial fibrillation or atrial flutter in 65% and 28% of attempts, respectively. In 49% of patients, the drug was effective for long-term suppression of atrial fibrillation. In patients with paroxysmal atrial fibrillation, the drug reduced the number of attacks, prolonged the time between attacks, and improved quality of life. The latter criteria seem the appropriate measure of drug efficacy, as virtually all studies have shown that these arrhythmias tend to recur (at least once per year in 50% of patients) in spite of antiarrhythmic drug therapy. Flecainide terminated atrioventricular nodal reentrant tachycardia in 83% of patients and suppressed the arrhythmia during long-term therapy in 78% of patients. Acute and long-term efficacy for atrioventricular reentrant tachycardia was 74% and 69%, respectively. Atrial tachycardia terminated in 86% of patients and was suppressed in 95% of patients.

Anderson et al.[54] reviewed 80 articles or published abstracts concerning flecainide therapy for supraventricular tachyarrhythmias. Flecainide reportedly terminated 81% of AV nodal reentrant tachycardias, 88% of AV reciprocating tachycardias, and 100% of atrial tachycardias. The drug terminated atrial fibrillation or flutter in 62% and arrhythmias associated with Wolff-Parkinson-White syndrome in 73% of reported cases. Long-term oral flecainide controlled AV nodal reentrant tachycardia in 74%, AV reciprocating tachycardia in 81%, and ectopic atrial tachycardia in 83% of reported cases. Oral therapy controlled atrial flutter or fibrillation in 61% of reported cases. Because adverse effects were reported only in studies that included less than 60% of the patients reviewed, quantitation was difficult. In studies that reported adverse effects, cardiac side effects occurred in 6.9%, and noncardiac adverse effects occurred in 19.0% of patients. Proarrhythmic effects occurred in 4%, and heart failure occurred in less than 1% of these patients. Thus, flecainide is an effective drug and is well tolerated for the treatment of patients with a variety of supraventricular tachycardias.

Atrial Fibrillation and Atrial Flutter

The use of flecainide for treatment of atrial fibrillation has been studied more than it has for any other supraventricular arrhythmia. These studies indicate that the drug converts atrial fibrillation to sinus rhythm as effectively or more effectively than other antiarrhythmic drugs tested.[55-59] Furthermore, the drug effectively suppresses the arrhythmia when administered long term.

Conversion to Sinus Rhythm

In a study of 102 patients, intravenous flecainide converted acute atrial fibrillation to sinus rhythm more often than placebo (67% versus 35%, $p < .003$).[58] Suttorp et al.[59] found that intravenous flecainide (2 mg/kg) converts atrial fibrillation to sinus rhythm more often than does intravenous propafenone (2 mg/kg) (18/20, 90%, versus 11/20, 55%; $p = .02$). Capucci et al.[60] demonstrated that 300 mg of flecainide, administered as a single oral dose, converted atrial fibrillation to normal sinus rhythm (20/22 patients, 91%) more often than either intravenous amiodarone (5 mg/kg) (7/19, 37%, $p < .001$ versus flecainide) or placebo (10/21, 48%, $p < .01$).

Borgeat et al. were able to convert atrial fibrillation to sinus rhythm in 71% of patients after administration of oral flecainide.[57] They compared quinidine with flecainide for conversion of atrial fibrillation to sinus rhythm. Flecainide converted recent-onset atrial fibrillation (<10 days) to sinus rhythm as effectively as quinidine (86% versus 80%). Quinidine converted long-standing atrial fibrillation to sinus rhythm better than flecainide (40% versus 22%). However, in neither case was the difference between flecainide and quinidine statistically significant.

Hellestrand[61] administered intravenous flecainide to 128 patients with a variety of inducible and/or spontaneous supraventricular tachyarrhythmias. Flecainide increased atrial flutter cycle length by 52% ($p < .01$), but it terminated the rhythm in only two of nine patients. However, flecainide prevented induction in eight of nine patients with previously inducible nonsustained atrial flutter. The drug terminated atrial fibrillation in 9 of 11 patients. Before conversion to sinus rhythm, the mean ventricular response rate slowed from 156 to 120 beats/min ($p < .02$). Flecainide terminated ectopic atrial tachycardia in five of seven patients, preventing reinitiation as well in four of these five.

Suppression of Atrial Fibrillation

Flecainide has been extensively studied and its efficacy for suppressing atrial fibrillation compared with that of other drugs. The Danish-Norwegian Flecainide Multicenter Study Group[62] reported that flecainide suppressed paroxysmal atrial fibrillation better than did placebo ($p < .002$). The arrhythmia was completely suppressed in 12 of 24 (50%) patients who took the drug for 3 months. Clementy et al.[63] reported that flecainide (100 mg every 12 hours) prevented atrial fibrillation in 65% of 755 patients during 9 months' follow-up. Leclercq et al.[64] reported that flecainide, or flecainide combined with amiodarone, suppressed atrial fibrillation in 73% of patients in whom the arrhythmia was unresponsive to quinidine and/or amiodarone.

Chouty and Coumel[65] administered oral flecainide to 40 patients with frequent symptomatic atrial fibrillation refractory to antiarrhythmic drug therapy including, in most cases, amiodarone. Flecainide or flecainide combined with amiodarone controlled atrial fibrillation in 32 of 40 patients (80%).

The efficacy of flecainide for preventing atrial fibrillation in patients with the Wolff-Parkinson-White syndrome appears to be similar to that in patients without the syndrome. Kim et al.[66] studied 15 patients with atrial fibrillation and rapid ventricular response due to conduction across an accessory AV connection. Administration of intravenous flecainide prevented induction of atrial fibrillation in four of nine patients and eliminated anterograde accessory AV connection conduction in 9 of 16 patients. In five patients with continued ventricular preexcitation and in whom atrial fibrillation could still be induced, the mean shortest RR interval increased from 185 ± 29 msec to 281 ± 46 msec ($p < .01$). Seven of 14 patients who took oral flecainide (mean, 21 months) had no recurrent atrial fibrillation, and four reported rare palpitation. Two patients developed proarrhythmic effects: one patient with severe biventricular dysfunction developed new ventricular tachycardia, and one developed incessant atrial flutter. Flecainide was discontinued in a third patient because of headaches.

Pietersen et al. reported two sudden cardiac deaths in a long-term study of 26 patients with atrial fibrillation and the Wolff-Parkinson-White syndrome.[67] Thus, although flecainide may decrease the incidence of recurrent atrial fibrillation, it is not clear that it decreases the incidence of sudden cardiac death due to recurrent atrial fibrillation in patients with the syndrome.

Atrioventricular Reentrant Tachycardia

Several studies have shown that flecainide terminates, prevents reinduction of, and suppresses spontaneous AV reentrant tachycardia.[55, 61, 66, 68, 69] The drug appears to act primarily on retrograde conduction across the accessory connection.

Hellestrand and associates administered intravenous flecainide to 41 patients with AV accessory connections.[61] Flecainide terminated orthodromic AV reentrant tachycardia in 32 of 38 patients. In 31 patients, the tachycardia terminated owing to retrograde accessory connection conduction block. Flecainide abolished retrograde accessory AV connection conduction in 20 patients and prolonged retrograde conduction by more than 65 msec in 5 patients. Prolongation of retrograde AV conduction time by less than 50 msec correlated with the ability to reinduce AV reentrant tachycardia (14 of 16 patients).

The same investigators[33] demonstrated that flecainide has more profound effects on retrograde than on anterograde AV accessory connection conduction. Accessory connection conduction times and effective refractory periods were prolonged to a greater extent in the retrograde than the anterograde direction. Tachycardia cycle length increased in all patients, principally because of slower retrograde ventriculoatrial conduction times. AV reentrant tachycardia terminated via retrograde accessory connection conduction block in 11 of 12 patients.

Intravenous flecainide prevented induction of AV reentrant tachycardia in 11 of 18 patients studied by Zee-Cheng et al.[68] In the remaining seven patients, the induced tachycardia cycle length increased from 334 ± 45 msec to 399 ± 58 msec ($p < .005$), principally because of slowed retrograde conduction. The drug had more profound effects on retrograde than on anterograde accessory connection conduction. During follow-up (mean, 18.5 months), recurrent tachycardia occurred in three of five patients whose tachycardia was induced and in 2 of 10 patients whose tachycardia was suppressed during the electrophysiologic study on flecainide.[68]

Crozier[69] reported that intravenous flecainide terminated AVRT in more than 80% of cases. When administered orally, the drug suppressed atrioventricular reentrant tachycardia in more than 60% of patients but occasionally resulted in incessant tachycardia. Long-term success of the drug was predicted by abolition of accessory connection conduction and/or prevention of tachycardia induction during electrophysiologic testing. Concomitant administration of a β-adrenergic blocking drug improved long-term efficacy.

Atrioventricular Nodal Reentrant Tachycardia

Flecainide terminates, prevents induction of, and suppresses AV nodal reentrant tachycardia by slowing or blocking retrograde fast-pathway conduction.[53, 61] Flecainide was administered to 40 patients with AV nodal reentrant tachycardia (34 sustained, 6 nonsustained).[61] The drug terminated AV nodal reentrant tachycardia in 30 of 34 patients and prevented reinitiation of the arrhythmia in 19. In 29 patients, tachycardia terminated owing to retrograde fast-pathway conduction block. Flecainide abolished retrograde (fast pathway) conduction in 18 patients and prolonged the retrograde fast-pathway ERP in another 10. Retrograde fast-pathway ERP prolongation of less than 65 msec was associated with the ability to reinduce the arrhythmia in 8 of 12 patients.

O'Hara et al.[70] showed in dogs that flecainide attenuates action potential accommodation to heart rate, causing tachycardia-dependent action potential prolongation that accounts for most of the rate-dependent increase in atrial effective refractory period. The drug had a greater effect on retrograde than anterograde atrioventricular nodal conduction; Wenckebach cycle length increased to a greater extent during retrograde than anterograde conduction. Finally, the effects on atrioventricular nodal conduction were also rate dependent; the AH interval increased to a greater extent at higher heart rates.

In a study reported by Henthorn et al.,[71] 31 patients were randomly assigned and completed a double-blind, placebo-controlled, crossover trial of flecainide for paroxysmal supraventricular tachycardia. Fewer patients (6 versus 26, $p < .001$) had recurrence of supraventricular tachycardia while taking flecainide. The mean time to first recurrence and time between episodes were longer on flecainide therapy (54 days versus 11 days and 55 days versus 11 days, respectively; $p < .001$).

Hemodynamic Effects and Effects on Left Ventricular Function

Hemodynamic effects of flecainide have been studied most extensively in patients with coronary artery disease. LeGrand et al.[36] performed left ventricular cineangiography and measured hemodynamic parameters in 10 patients before and after intravenous flecainide infusion (2 mg/kg). Each patient had experienced a recent inferior myocardial infarction. Pulmonary capillary wedge pressure and mean pulmonary artery pressure increased after flecainide infusion (10 ± 3 mmHg to 13 ± 4 mmHg, $p < .01$, and 17.5 ± 2.5 to 20 mmHg ± 4 mmHg, $p < .001$, respectively). Mean systemic arterial pressure, systemic vascular resistance, and pulmonary vascular resistance did not change significantly. Left ventricular end-diastolic volume did not change, but end-systolic volume increased slightly, causing stroke index and ejection fraction to decrease.

Cohen et al.[72] measured hemodynamic parameters in 10 patients with uncomplicated myocardial infarction at 15-minute intervals for 1-hour and for 2-hour intervals, thereafter for 12 hours after intravenous flecainide infusion, 2 mg/kg. Mean pulmonary artery pressure increased from 15 ± 4 mmHg to 19 ± 3 mmHg ($p < .001$) and remained elevated for 6 hours. Mean pulmonary capillary wedge pressure increased from 9.5 ± 4 mmHg to 12 ± 2.5 mmHg ($p < .005$) and remained increased at 12 hours after infusion. Mean arterial pressure and systemic vascular resistance did not change. Cardiac index decreased from 2.8 ± 0.6 L/min/m^2 to 2.6 ± 0.6 L/min/m^2 ($p < .001$) but returned to baseline 2 hours after flecainide infusion. Left ventricular stroke volume index and stroke work index decreased transiently after flecainide infusion.

Josephson et al.[73] reported similar findings after intravenous flecainide infusion. Maximal hemodynamic effects were noted 5 to 10 minutes after drug infusion. However, within 30 minutes, hemodynamic variables were not significantly different than those measured before flecainide infusion. Although magnitude of decrease in left ventricular ejection fraction was independent of baseline ejection fraction, the percentage of decrease in ejection fraction was greatest in patients in whom baseline ejection fractions were reduced.

The same group demonstrated a concentration-dependent reduction in contractile force when isolated rabbit papillary muscle was superfused with flecainide.[74] The negative inotropic effect was reversed when calcium ion concentration was increased.

De Paola et al.[75] determined the effect of flecainide on left ventricular ejection fraction in 62 patients with heart disease of various causes. Radionuclide angiography was performed at baseline and on steady-state oral flecainide. Left ventricular ejection fraction decreased from 0.34 ± 13 to 0.32 ± 13 on oral flecainide

therapy. No patient with baseline left ventricular ejection fraction of more than 0.30 developed heart failure when receiving flecainide. In contrast, 7 of 33 (21%) patients with baseline ejection fractions of 0.30 or less had new or more severe heart failure on flecainide therapy. Seven of 12 patients with New York Heart Association (NYHA) functional class III or IV heart failure had left ventricular ejection fractions less than 0.30. Of these seven patients, five had worse heart failure and three died (two of heart failure) while taking flecainide.

These data suggest that flecainide is unlikely to cause or aggravate heart failure in patients with left ventricular ejection fractions of more than 0.30 or whose NYHA functional class is I or II. Patients with left ventricular ejection fractions of 0.30 or less are at risk for new or worsening heart failure when taking flecainide. History of NYHA functional class III or IV heart failure increases this risk.

Adverse Effects

Adverse effects of flecainide may be classified as cardiac and noncardiac. Noncardiac side effects include dizziness, blurred vision, disturbances of the central and peripheral nervous system, and gastrointestinal disturbances.[76] Noncardiac adverse effects are dose related; 30% of patients taking more than 400 mg/day report visual disturbances.[5-7, 35, 42, 77] Nausea occurs in 5% to 10% of patients taking high doses. Fewer than 5% of patients report flushing, chest pain, tremor, parasthesias, fatigue, and metallic taste.

Adverse cardiac effects may occur as a result of slowed conduction, slowed repolarization, increased pacing threshold, or myocardial inotropic depression. Like noncardiac adverse effects, cardiac side effects are dose related.

In a study by Hellestrand et al., flecainide increased right ventricular pacing voltage thresholds in chronically and newly implanted pacemakers by more than 30% and 100%, respectively.[33, 78] In five patients taking oral flecainide, mean threshold pulse duration increased by 160% to 200% after 3 weeks on the drug. Thresholds returned to normal 10 days after flecainide was stopped. Flecainide-induced failure to capture ventricular myocardium was reported in one patient who had a permanent pacemaker.[79]

Like all antiarrhythmic medicines, flecainide may cause or aggravate arrhythmias; the reported incidence is 3% to 12% of patients.[76] Because criteria for proarrhythmia have varied from study to study, these effects are difficult to quantitate. In addition, the significance of proarrhythmia may vary. Increased frequency of VPCs may be of no consequence; a slow incessant tachycardia without associated hypotension may be less important than an acute rapid tachycardia associated with hemodynamic collapse.

Nathan et al.[80] reported proarrhythmia in 7 of 152 (4.6%) patients taking the drug for a variety of arrhythmias. Of the seven patients, two had atrioventricular reciprocating tachycardia, one had atrioventricular nodal reentrant tachycardia, and three had ventricular tachycardia.

In 1982, 16 hospitalized patients who died of cardiac arrest while taking flecainide were examined.[81] Serum flecainide concentration was more than 1000 ng/ml in seven of the eight patients in whom levels were available. In the 13 for whom data were available, the left ventricular ejection fractions were less than 0.35. Nathan et al.[80] noted elevated serum flecainide concentrations in two of seven patients with proarrhythmic effects. Both studies suggested that concomitant antiarrhythmic therapy might increase the risk for proarrhythmia.

Fish et al.[82] reported on proarrhythmia experience from 36 institutions in 472 young patients (mean age, 9.9 years; range, 4 days to 26 years) taking flecainide. Proarrhythmia, using the criteria of Velebit et al.,[83] occurred in 7.4% of patients. Cardiac arrest and death occurred in 2.3% and 2.1% of patients, respectively, principally in the presence of underlying heart disease.

Flecainide has little or no effect on myocardial repolarization. Nonetheless, several investigators have reported cases of flecainide-induced QT prolongation and ventricular tachycardia.[84-86] Crijns et al. reported on one patient with marked flecainide intoxication (serum concentration, 2500 ng/ml) who developed giant inverted T waves without evidence of ventricular arrhythmias.[87] Torsade de pointes was reported in one patient who received intravenous drug for conversion of atrial fibrillation.[58] However, this arrhythmia has not been reported in patients taking the oral preparation.

Morganroth et al.[88] reported proarrhythmia in 7% of 1330 patients taking flecainide (2.3% serious, 1% lethal) for a variety of ventricular arrhythmias. Serious nonlethal proarrhythmias occurred in 6.6% of patients treated for sustained ventricular tachycardia, 0.9% with nonsustained ventricular tachycardia, and 0% with VPCs. Proarrhythmic death occurred in 3.1% of patients treated for sustained ventricular tachycardia, 0.2% with nonsustained ventricular tachycardia, and 0% with VPCs. Significant proarrhythmia and death occurred more commonly in patients with organic heart disease than in those without organic heart disease (2.6% versus 0.4% and 1.2% versus 0%, respectively).

In 1983, 3M Laboratories surveyed 57 investigators about 592 patients who were enrolled in studies of flecainide and ventricular ectopy.[76] In 44 of 588 (7%) patients evaluated, flecainide had proarrhythmic effects. In 37 patients, new or more severe ventricular tachycardia occurred during flecainide therapy. Patients with hemodynamically significant ventricular tachycardia or ventricular fibrillation at enrollment were more likely to have proarrhythmias than those who had nonhemodynamically significant ventricular ectopy (12% versus 4%). Ten of the 44 patients experienced proarrhythmic events within 2 days and 21 patients within 7 days of a change in flecainide dosage. Of the 44 patients with proarrhythmias, 52% had heart failure and a history of ventricular tachycardia.

Of 500 patients without proarrhythmia, only 18 had ventricular tachycardia and a history of heart failure.

In the Cardiac Arrhythmia Pilot Study (CAPS),[50] the incidence of proarrhythmia in patients taking flecainide (3%) was equal to that of patients taking placebo (Table 142–2). Although proarrhythmia tended to occur less frequently in patients taking imipramine, moricizine, or encainide (1%), no statistically significant differences were noted among treatment groups.

In 1989, the CAST investigators[52] reported that flecainide, administered for asymptomatic or minimally symptomatic ventricular ectopy, was associated with an increased risk for arrhythmic death and total cardiac mortality. CAST was designed to determine whether suppression of asymptomatic or minimally symptomatic ventricular ectopy after myocardial infarction improves survival. Patients were randomly assigned to receive one of three drugs (flecainide, encainide, or moricizine) or placebo after it was demonstrated that the drug suppressed ventricular ectopy ($\geq 80\%$ suppression of VPCs; $\geq 90\%$ suppression of nonsustained ventricular tachycardia). Of the 1498 patients enrolled, 641 received flecainide or its placebo and 857 received encainide or its placebo. After a mean follow-up of 10 months, 89 patients had died: 59 of arrhythmia (43 receiving drug versus 16 receiving placebo; $p = .0004$), 22 of nonarrhythmic cardiac causes (17 receiving drug versus 5 receiving placebo; $p = .01$), and 8 of noncardiac causes (3 receiving drug versus 5 receiving placebo; $p = $ NS). Thus, an excess of cardiac deaths, both arrhythmic and nonarrhythmic, occurred in patients receiving drug. The risk ratio for cardiac mortality when receiving either encainide or flecainide was 2.4:1, and for arrhythmic death it was 2.8:1. The results were similar when the drugs were analyzed individually. Based on these findings, the CAST data safety and monitoring board recommended that the study be terminated early for flecainide and encainide.

Falk[89] reported that 3 of 14 patients with atrial fibrillation developed ventricular arrhythmias (2) or experienced sudden cardiac death (1) while taking flecainide. Two patients, one with a prosthetic mitral valve and one with a structurally normal heart, developed ventricular arrhythmias during exercise. One patient with asymmetric ventricular septal hypertrophy experienced sudden death while waiting for a bus.

Several investigators have attempted to determine

Table 142–2. **Post–Myocardial Infarction Study of 502 Patients**

Drug	Initial Efficacy (%)	Intolerance (%)	Proarrhythmia (%)
Placebo	37	3	3
Flecainide	83	5	3
Encainide	79	3	1
Moricizine	66	5	1
Imipramine	52	26	1

the mechanism of flecainide-induced proarrhythmia. Suggested mechanisms include drug-induced heterogeneity of refractoriness, induction of new arrhythmia circuits, and adverse interactions of the drug with ischemic myocardium.

Using a Langendorff-perfused rabbit heart model of reentrant ventricular tachycardia, Brugada et al.[90] showed that intravenous flecainide facilitated induction of reentrant ventricular arrhythmias and was associated with multiple rather than a single reentrant circuit.

Krishman and Antzelevitch,[91] using an isolated muscle preparation, showed that flecainide shortened or markedly prolonged epicardial action potential duration but had little effect on endocardial action potential duration. 4-Aminopyridine, a transient outward current blocker, reversed flecainide-induced action potential shortening and reentrant activity. The authors concluded that flecainide was associated with a prominent epicardial transient outward current that was responsible for heterogeneity of refractoriness between the epicardium and the endocardium.

Most relevent to the CAST results, Kou et al.[37] evaluated the antiarrhythmic and antifibrillatory effects of flecainide during the early postinfarction period in a conscious canine model of sudden cardiac death. After an intravenous loading dose of 2 mg/kg, a maintenance intravenous infusion (1.0 mg/kg/hr) was given for 4 hours. The subsequent initiation of acute posterolateral ischemia resulted in the development of ventricular fibrillation in 3 of 17 dogs that had not had inducible ventricular tachyarrhythmias prior to "prophylactic" drug treatment. Two of three arrhythmic deaths occurred very shortly after the cessation of the flecainide maintenance infusion; the third was a late death. Further analysis of the CAST data by Echt et al.[52] and Akiyama et al.[92] provided strong indirect evidence that ischemia in combination with either flecainide or encainide mediated the increased risk for arrhythmic death associated with these drugs. Studies such as these have led to the strong recommendation that class IC antiarrhythmic agents should be avoided in patients with underlying coronary artery disease except perhaps to suppress supraventricular arrhythmias.[93]

The use-dependent channel-blocking characteristics of flecainide may facilitate the drug's antiarrhythmic effects but, in certain cases, may also result in proarrhythmia. Use-dependent induced QRS complex prolongation, particularly at high heart rates, may also mimic ventricular proarrhythmia. Crijns et al.[94] reported that 6 of 79 patients who received intravenous flecainide for the treatment of supraventricular tachycardias developed QRS complex prolongation during supraventricular tachycardia that mimicked ventricular tachycardia.

Thus, flecainide-induced proarrhythmia occurs in 3% to 12% of patients taking the drug for atrial, AV reentrant, or ventricular tachycardia. Severity of proarrhythmia correlates with severity of the presenting arrhythmia, severity of left ventricular dysfunction, plasma flecainide level (particularly if

> 1000 ng/ml), and the presence of myocardial ischemia. The use-dependent properties of flecainide may cause significant QRS complex prolongation, particularly at high heart rates, that can mimic ventricular tachycardia.

CLINICAL USE
Indications

Ventricular Arrhythmias

The FDA has approved flecainide for the prevention of documented ventricular arrhythmias, such as sustained ventricular tachycardia, that in the judgment of the physician are life-threatening. When used for sustained ventricular tachycardia, the drug should be started in a monitored setting in the hospital. Flecainide is not recommended for treatment of less severe ventricular arrhythmias, even if the arrhythmias are associated with symptoms.

Although flecainide suppresses VPCs, ventricular couplets, and nonsustained ventricular tachycardia more effectively than procainamide, quinidine, and disopyramide and is equally as effective as amiodarone, the drug should not be administered for these arrhythmias alone.

Patients in whom induced ventricular arrhythmias are suppressed at follow-up electrophysiologic study on flecainide are at decreased risk for recurrent ventricular arrhythmias or sudden cardiac death.[41, 43] Reduced ventricular ectopy during Holter monitoring of patients receiving flecainide less accurately predicts a favorable prognosis.[43]

Although the drug may be effective in patients with a variety of heart disease causes, it has been studied most extensively in patients with coronary artery disease. The best results can be expected in patients whose left ventricular ejection fractions are more than 0.30 and who do not have a history of NYHA class III or IV congestive heart failure.

The authors prescribe flecainide for sustained ventricular tachycardia only when the drug has been shown to suppress induction of the arrhythmia during an electrophysiology study and almost exclusively in patients with normal or only mildly impaired left ventricular dysfunction.

Supraventricular Arrhythmias

The FDA has also approved flecainide for the prevention of paroxysmal supraventricular tachycardia, atrial fibrillation, and atrial flutter associated with disabling symptoms in patients without structural heart disease. Indeed, many studies have shown that the drug is very effective in terminating, slowing, preventing induction of, and suppressing a variety of supraventricular tachyarrhythmias. Of note, many of the patients' arrhythmias in these studies had not responded to several previous antiarrhythmic medications. The authors use the drug as a first- or second-line therapy for patients with atrial tachyarrhythmias and structurally normal hearts as well as for patients with AV reentrant tachycardia who do not undergo or fail radiofrequency ablation of their AV accessory connection.

Precautions

The CAST results clearly indicate that flecainide should not be prescribed for the treatment of premature ventricular beats or asymptomatic nonsustained ventricular tachycardia in patients with a prior myocardial infarction.[40]

Because it may cause pauses or block, flecainide should be used cautiously in patients with sinus node dysfunction, AV conduction abnormalities, or bundle branch block. PR interval and QRS complex prolongation occur in many patients and, by themselves, do not warrant discontinuing therapy. Flecainide should be discontinued, however, in most patients who develop symptomatic bradycardia, pauses, or AV block. It can, of course, be used in these conditions in conjunction with an implanted pacemaker system.

Caution should be used when prescribing flecainide to patients who are taking other drugs that cause pauses or slow conduction (digoxin, verapamil, β-blockers, amiodarone). Flecainide was administered to 15 healthy men who had been taking digoxin for 10 days.[95] Plasma digoxin concentration was measured before dosing and 6 hours after administration of digoxin 3 and 5 days after flecainide was started (Table 142–3). Plasma digoxin levels on days 3 and 5 of flecainide therapy increased by 24% ± 35% before and 13% ± 19% after the digoxin dose. However, at 9 and 12 days after initiation of flecainide, plasma digoxin levels were similar to those measured before flecainide. McQuinn et al.[96] reported that flecainide did not affect serum digoxin concentration in 10 patients with heart failure. Thus, serum digoxin levels should be monitored until stable in patients taking both flecainide and digoxin.

Reports of cardiac decompensation and proarrhythmia have caused some investigators to suspect an interaction of amiodarone and flecainide.[97, 98] In seven patients taking oral flecainide, the dose-adjusted

Table 142–3. Dosage Recommendations for Oral Flecainide Therapy

Usual dosage:	100–400 mg/day
Usual initial dose:	50–100 mg
Initial maintenance dose:	50–100 mg every 12 hr
Dose increments:	50 mg every 12 hr every 4 days as needed
Usual effective regimens:	50, 100, 150, and 200 mg every 12 hr
Alternative:	50 or 100 mg every 8 hr; 50 mg every 8 to 12 hr in children
Maximum dosage:	300 mg every 12 hr (600 mg/day)

Conditions of altered dosage:
1. Decrease dosage in patients with end-stage renal disease (creatinine clearance ≤20 ml/min/m²)
2. Decrease or avoid in presence of marked left ventricular dysfunction (NYHA class III or IV congestive heart failure or left ventricular ejection fraction <0.30)
3. Decrease if given concomitantly with amiodarone

Therapeutic plasma level: 200–1000 mg/ml

plasma flecainide level increased when amiodarone was added to the regimen.[99] These data, and the observations of Coumel and Fontaine,[97, 98] suggest that the flecainide dose may be decreased by 33% to 50% when amiodarone is added to the regimen.

Although magnesium- and aluminum-based antacids do not affect flecainide absorption, cimetidine may interfere with flecainide elimination. Oral flecainide, 200 mg, was administered to eight male volunteers before and with cimetidine therapy.[100] Cimetidine increased plasma flecainide concentration by 9% to 28% and reduced renal clearance by 7% to 11%.

Flecainide should also be used cautiously in patients taking drugs that have a negative inotropic effect. The negative inotropic effects of propranolol and flecainide are additive.[95] Thus, patients who might otherwise tolerate flecainide may develop heart failure when the drug is administered with propranolol or another myocardial depressant.

Because it may increase pacing thresholds, flecainide should be used carefully in patients who have permanent or temporary cardiac pacemakers. Unless the patient is monitored continuously, pacemakers should be programmed to stimulus strengths appropriately higher than threshold before flecainide therapy is started. When steady-state serum levels are achieved, thresholds should again be determined, and, if necessary, the stimulus strength should be reprogrammed.

Because flecainide may increase defibrillation thresholds, it should be prescribed carefully in patients who have an automatic implantable cardioverter-defibrillator, particularly in patients who high baseline defibrillation thresholds.[38] Because the effect is concentration dependent, decreasing the flecainide dose may improve the defibrillation threshold while maintaining an antiarrhythmic effect.

Flecainide can be used safely in patients with NYHA functional class I or II heart failure. Flecainide plasma half-life increases by 25% in these patients.[11, 77] Flecainide is not recommended in patients whose left ventricular ejection fractions are less than 0.30 because it may aggravate heart failure. In addition, the authors do not recommend that the drug be used in patients with NYHA functional class III or IV heart failure.

Flecainide urinary excretion, mildly decreased in patients with moderate renal dysfunction, is markedly decreased in patients with end-stage renal disease.[8, 79] In these patients, the flecainide dose must be adjusted carefully to yield therapeutic levels and to avoid adverse effects.

Plasma Concentrations

The accepted plasma flecainide level therapeutic range is from 200 to 1000 ng/ml (mean, 500 ng/ml).[77, 80, 81, 101] In early efficacy studies of multiple oral doses performed in patients with VPCs, the minimal plasma flecainide level associated with efficacy (>95% suppression) was between 200 and 400 ng/ml.[15] During drug washout, return of VPCs (to >10% of baseline and >30/hr) occurred at a mean plasma flecainide concentration of 500 ng/ml.[5-7]

Trough plasma levels between 300 and 1600 ng/ml were efficacious and were not associated with side effects in patients taking flecainide to suppress VPCs. In patients with more serious cardiac disease, adverse effects have occurred at plasma flecainide levels as low as 700 ng/ml.[8] In patients who have organic heart disease, adverse effects occur more frequently at plasma flecainide concentrations of more than 1000 to 1500 ng/ml.[75-77]

Dosage and Administration

Flecainide is supplied in tablets of 50 mg, 100 mg, and 150 mg. Efficacy studies have confirmed that flecainide can be administered twice daily.[5-7] Ventricular ectopy was suppressed in 73% of patients taking 100 to 200 mg twice daily, and in an additional 23% who took 250 to 300 mg twice daily.[39] In a long-term study, flecainide suppressed ventricular ectopy in 9 of 14 patients at 100 mg twice daily, 3 of 14 patients at 150 mg twice daily, and 2 of 14 patients at 200 mg twice daily.[101]

Flecainide can be started with a loading dose of 200 mg. The authors recommend an initial maintenance dose of 50 to 100 mg every 12 hours (see Table 142–3). Because of the long half-life (up to 20 hours), the dose should be increased by 50- to 100-mg increments every 4 days until efficacy is achieved or until a maximum dose of 600 mg daily is reached (see Table 142–3). The usual effective regimen is 100 to 200 mg every 12 hours. However, in some patients, 100 mg may be given every 8 hours. Extreme caution should be exercised when administering more than 400 mg/day. The maximum dose is 300 mg every 12 hours (600 mg/day) (see Table 142–3).

Pritchett and Wilkinson[102] reported on the dose response characteristics of flecainide when the drug is administered for supraventricular tachycardia, atrial fibrillation, or atrial flutter. These investigators recommended that flecainide be started at 50 mg twice daily for supraventricular arrhythmias. Higher doses, up to 150 mg twice daily, were associated with increased efficacy but also increasing frequency of side effects. However, for paroxysmal supraventricular tachycardia (AVRT and AVNRT), a starting dose as high as 150 mg twice daily has been recommended.

CONCLUSIONS

Flecainide is an effective and well-tolerated drug for treating ventricular arrhythmias. The drug suppresses spontaneous ventricular ectopy and nonsustained ventricular tachycardia as effectively as amiodarone and better than other available antiarrhythmic drugs. The suppression rate of sustained ventricular tachycardia by flecainide is similar to that of other antiarrhythmic medicines. The patients in whom flecainide suppresses ventricular ectopy on 24-hour Holter monitoring may still be at risk for sustained ventricular tachycardia. In patients with a history of sustained

ventricular tachycardia, electrophysiologic studies accurately predict flecainide efficacy. Flecainide effectively suppresses or modulates the incidence of a variety of supraventricular tachyarrhythmias as well.

Flecainide is well absorbed, undergoes little clinically important metabolic transformation, is well distributed to tissues other than brain, and is excreted preferentially in the urine. The plasma half-life (mean, 16 hours) allows for twice-daily dosing (50 to 200 mg b.i.d.). Plasma levels correlate well with tissue levels, clinical efficacy (200 to 1000 ng/ml), and intoxication (>1000 ng/ml).

Flecainide is well tolerated, with little organ toxicity. Adverse effects (cardiac and noncardiac) occur more frequently at high doses (>400 mg/day). Proarrhythmia occurs in 3% to 12% of patients. Serious proarrhythmia occurs most often in patients who have sustained ventricular arrhythmias and left ventricular dysfunction. In patients with left ventricular dysfunction, flecainide may cause or aggravate heart failure. Therefore, the drug should not be used in patients who have left ventricular ejection fractions of less than 0.30 or NYHA functional class III or IV heart failure. Because of potential adverse interactions, flecainide should be administered cautiously to patients taking amiodarone, digoxin, cimetidine, propranolol, or any medications that depress myocardial contractility.

REFERENCES

1. Hudak JM, Banitt EH, Schmid JR: Discovery and development of flecainide. Am J Cardiol 53:17B, 1984.
2. Banitt EH, Coyne WE, Schmid JR, et al: Antiarrhythmics. N-(aminoalkylene)trifluoroethoxybenzamides and N-(aminoalkylene)trifluoroethoxynaphthamides. J Med Chem 18:1130, 1975.
3. Hoback J, Hodges M, Francis GS, et al: Flecainide (R-818), a new antiarrhythmic agent: Effects on ventricular premature beats. Circulation 58:II246, 1978.
4. Somani R: Antiarrhythmic effects of flecainide. Clin Pharmacol Ther 27:464, 1980.
5. Hodges M, Haugland JM, Granrud GJ, et al: Suppression of ventricular ectopic repolarizations by flecainide acetate, a new antiarrhythmic agent. Circulation 65:879, 1982.
6. Duff HS, Roden DM, Maffucci RJ, et al: Suppression of resistant ventricular arrhythmias by twice daily dosing with flecainide. Am J Cardiol 48:1133, 1981.
7. Anderson JL, Stewart JR, Perry BA, et al: Oral flecainide acetate for the treatment of ventricular arrhythmias. N Engl J Med 305:473, 1981.
8. Conard GJ, Ober RE: Metabolism of flecainide. Am J Cardiol 53:41B, 1984.
9. Conard GJ, Carlson GL, Frost JW, et al: Human plasma pharmacokinetics of flecainide acetate (R-818), a new antiarrhythmic, following single oral and intravenous doses. Clin Pharmacol Ther 25:218, 1979.
10. Franciosa JA, Wilen M, Weeks CE, et al: Pharmacokinetics and hemodynamic effects of flecainide in patients with chronic low output heart failure. J Am Coll Cardiol 1:699, 1983.
11. Guehler J, Gocnich CC, Lobler G, et al: Electrophysiologic effects of flecainide acetate and its major metabolites in the canine heart. Am J Cardiol 55:807, 1985.
12. McQuinn RL, Quarforth GJ, Johnson JA, et al: Biotransformation and elimination of 14C-flecainide acetate in humans. Drug Metab Dispos 12:414, 1984.
13. Forland SC, Burgess E, Blair AD, et al: Oral flecainide pharma-

cokinetics in patients with impaired renal function. J Clin Pharmacol 3:259, 1988.

14. Klempt HW, Nayebagha A, Fabry E: Antiarrhythmic efficacy of mexiletine, propafenone and flecainide in ventricular premature beats: A comparative study in patients after myocardial infarction. Z Kardiol 71:340, 1982.

15. Conard GJ, Cronheim GE, Klempt HW: Relationship between plasma concentrations and suppression of ventricular extrasystoles by flecainide acetate (R-818), a new antiarrhythmic, in patients. Arzneimittelforschung 32:155, 1982.

16. Conard GJ, Jernberg MJ, Carlson GL, et al: Metabolism of R-818, an antiarrhythmic candidate, in rats. Pharmacologist 17:194, 1975.

17. Conard GJ, Carlson GL, Jernberg MJ, et al: Metabolism of R-818, a new antiarrhythmic, in dogs. Academy of Pharmaceutical Sciences, 19th National Meeting, 1975, p 119.

18. Conard GJ, Carlson GL, Ober RE: Binding of flecainide acetate (R-818) to human plasma proteins in vitro. Academy of Pharmaceutical Sciences, 31st National Meeting, 1981, p 82.

19. Caplin JL, Johnston A, Hamer J, et al: Serum protein binding of disopyramide and flecainide after acute myocardial infarction. Circulation 68(Suppl III):III, 1983.

20. Yabek SM, Kato R, Ikeda N, et al: Effects of flecainide on the cellular electrophysiology of neonatal and adult cardiac fibers. Am Heart J 113:70, 1987.

21. Ikeda N, Singh BN, Davis LD, et al: Effects of flecainide on the electrophysiologic properties of isolated canine and rabbit myocardial fibers. J Am Coll Cardiol 5:303, 1985.

22. Kvam DC, Banitt EH, Schmid JR: Antiarrhythmic and electrophysiologic actions of flecainide in animal models. Am J Cardiol 53:22B, 1984.

23. Harrison DC: Antiarrhythmic drug classification: New science and practical applications. Am J Cardiol 56:185, 1985.

24. Hodess AB, Follansbee WP, Speer JF, et al: Electrophysiological effects of a new antiarrhythmic agent, flecainide, on the intact canine heart. J Cardiovasc Pharmacol 1:427, 1979.

25. Abitbol H, Califano JE, Abate C, et al: Use of flecainide acetate in the treatment of premature ventricular contractions. Am Heart J 105:227, 1983.

26. Estes III NAM, Garan H, Ruskin JN: Electrophysiologic properties of flecainide acetate. Am J Cardiol 53:26B, 1984.

27. Somani R: Antiarrhythmic effects of flecainide. Clin Pharmacol Ther 27:464, 1980.

28. Granrud G, Salerno D, Hodges M, et al: Long term flecainide is effective and well tolerated. Circulation 66:II69, 1982.

29. Hellestrand KJ, Bexton RS, Nathan AW, et al: Acute electrophysiologic effects of flecainide acetate on cardiac conduction and refractoriness in man. Br Heart J 48:140, 1982.

30. Seipel A, Abendroth RR, Breithardt G: Electrophysiologic effects of flecainide (R-818) in man. Circulation 62(Suppl III):III, 1980.

31. Wang T, Duff HJ, Roden DM, et al: Suppression of refractory arrhythmias with flecainide. Circulation 66(Suppl II):II, 1982.

32. Vik-Mo H, Ohm OJ, Lund-Johansen P: Electrophysiologic effects of flecainide acetate in patients with sinus nodal dysfunction. Am J Cardiol 50:1090, 1982.

33. Hellestrand KJ, Nathan AW, Bexton RS, et al: Electrophysiologic effects of flecainide acetate on sinus node function, anomalous atrioventricular connections, and pacemaker thresholds. Am J Cardiol 53:30B, 1984.

34. Olsson SB, Edvardsson N: Clinical electrophysiologic study of antiarrhythmic properties of flecainide: Acute intraventricular delayed conduction and prolonged repolarization in regular spaced and premature beats using intracardiac monophasic action potential with programmed stimulation. Am Heart J 102:864, 1981.

35. Flecainide-Quinidine Research Group: Flecainide versus quinidine for treatment of chronic ventricular arrhythmias: A multicenter trial. Circulation 67:1117, 1983.

36. LeGrand V, Vandormael M, Collignon P: Hemodynamic effects of a new antiarrhythmic agent, flecainide (R-818) in coronary artery disease. Am J Cardiol 51:422, 1983.

37. Kou WH, Nelson MD, Lynch JJ, et al: Effect of flecainide acetate on prevention of electrical induction of ventricular tachycardia and occurrence of ischemic ventricular fibrillation

during the early postmyocardial infarction period: Evaluation in a conscious canine model of sudden death. J Am Coll Cardiol 9:359, 1987.

38. Hodess AB, Follansbee WP, Spear JF, et al: Electrophysiological effects of a new antiarrhythmic agent, flecainide, on the intact canine heart. J Cardiovasc Pharmacol 1:427, 1979.

39. Woosley RL, Siddoway L, Duff HJ, et al: Flecainide dose-response relations in stable ventricular arrhythmias. Am J Cardiol 53:59B, 1984.

40. The Cardiac Arrhythmia Suppression Trial (CAST) Investigators: Effect of encainide and flecainide on mortality in a randomized trial of arrhythmia suppression after myocardial infarction. N Engl J Med 321:406, 1989.

41. Anderson JL, Lutz JR, Allison SB: Electrophysiologic and antiarrhythmic effects of oral flecainide in patients with inducible ventricular tachycardia. J Am Coll Cardiol 2:105, 1983.

42. Anderson JL: Experience with electrophysiologically guided therapy of ventricular tachycardia with flecainide: Summary of long term follow-up. Am J Cardiol 53:79B, 1984.

43. Reid PR, Griffith LSC, Platia EV, et al: Evaluation of flecainide acetate in the management of patients at high risk of sudden cardiac death. Am J Cardiol 53:108B, 1984.

44. Platia EV, Estes M, Heine DL, et al: Flecainide: Electrophysiologic and antiarrhythmic properties in refractory ventricular tachycardia. Am J Cardiol 55:956, 1985.

45. Lal R, Chapman PD, Naccarrelli GV, et al: Short- and long-term experience with flecainide acetate in the management of life-threatening ventricular arrhythmias. J Am Coll Cardiol 6:772, 1985.

46. Webb CR, Morganroth J, Senior S, et al: Flecainide: Steady state electrophysiologic effects in patients with remote myocardial infarction and inducible sustained ventricular arrhythmia. J Am Coll Cardiol 8:214, 1986.

47. Wynn J, Torres V, Flowers D, et al: Antiarrhythmic drug efficacy at electrophysiology testing: Predictive effectiveness of procainamide and flecainide. Am Heart J 111:632, 1986.

48. Kjekshus J, Bathen J, Orning OM, et al: A double blind, cross-over comparison of flecainide acetate and disopyramide phosphate in the treatment of ventricular premature complexes. Am J Cardiol 53:72B, 1984.

49. Dubner SJ, Elencwajg MD, Palma S, et al: Efficacy of flecainide in the management of ventricular arrhythmias: Comparative study with amiodarone. Am Heart J 109:523, 1985.

50. The Cardiac Arrhythmia Pilot Study Investigators: Effects of encainide, flecainide, imipramine, and moricizine on ventricular arrhythmias during the year after acute myocardial infarction: The CAPS. Am J Cardiol 61:501, 1988.

51. Kidwell GA, Greenspon AJ, Greenberg RM, et al: Use-dependent prolongation of ventricular tachycardia cycle length by type I antiarrhythmic drugs in humans. Circulation 87:118, 1993.

52. Echt DS, Liebson PR, Mitchell LB, et al: Mortality and morbidity in patients receiving encainide, flecainide, or placebo. N Engl J Med 324:781, 1991.

53. Hohnloser SH, Zabel M: Short- and long-term efficacy and safety of flecainide acetate for supraventricular arrhythmias. Am J Cardiol 70:3A, 1992.

54. Anderson JL, Jolivette DM, Fredell PA: Summary of efficacy and safety of flecainide for supraventricular arrhythmias. Am J Cardiol 62:62D, 1988.

55. Neuss H, Schlepper M: Long-term efficacy and safety of flecainide for supraventricular tachycardia. Am J Cardiol 62:56D, 1988.

56. Goy JJ, Kaufmann V, Kappenberger L, et al: Restoration of sinus rhythm with flecainide in patients with atrial fibrillation. Am J Cardiol 62:38D, 1988.

57. Borgeat A, Goy JJ, Maendly R, et al: Flecainide versus quinidine for conversion of atrial fibrillation to sinus rhythm. Am J Cardiol 58:496, 1986.

58. Donovan KD, Dobb GJ, Coombs LJ, et al: Efficacy of flecainide for the reversion of acute onset atrial fibrillation. Am J Cardiol 70:50A, 1992.

59. Suttorp MJ, Kingma JH, Jessurun ER, et al: The value of class IC antiarrhythmic drugs for acute conversion of paroxysmal atrial fibrillation or flutter to sinus rhythm. Am J Coll Cardiol 16:1722, 1990.

60. Capucci A, Lenzi T, Boriani G, et al: Effectiveness of loading oral flecainide for converting recent-onset atrial fibrillation to sinus rhythm in patients without organic heart disease or with only systemic hypertension. Am J Cardiol 70:69, 1992.

61. Hellestrand KJ: Intravenous flecainide acetate for supraventricular tachycardias. Am J Cardiol 62:16D, 1988.

62. Pietersen AH, Helleman H, for the Danish-Norwegian Flecainide Multicenter Study Group: Usefulness of flecainide for prevention of paroxysmal atrial fibrillation and flutter. Am J Cardiol 67:713, 1991.

63. Clementy J, Dulhoste MN, Laiter C, et al: Flecainide acetate in the prevention of paroxysmal atrial fibrillation: A nine-month follow-up of more than 500 patients. Am J Cardiol 70:44A, 1992.

64. Leclercq JF, Chouty F, Denjoy I, et al: Flecainide in quinidine-resistant atrial fibrillation. Am J Cardiol 70:62A, 1992.

65. Chouty F, Coumel P: Oral flecainide for prophylaxis of paroxysmal atrial fibrillation. Am J Cardiol 62:35D, 1988.

66. Kim SS, Smith P, Ruffy R: Treatment of atrial tachyarrhythmias and preexcitation syndrome with flecainide acetate. Am J Cardiol 62:29D, 1988.

67. Pietersen AH, Andersen ED, Sandoe E: Atrial fibrillation in the Wolff-Parkinson-White syndrome. Am J Cardiol 70:38A, 1992.

68. Zee-Cheng C, Kim SS, Ruffy R: Flecainide acetate for treatment of bypass tract mediated reentrant tachycardia. Am J Cardiol 62:23D, 1988.

69. Crozier I: Flecainide in the Wolff-Parkinson-White syndrome. Am J Cardiol 70:26A, 1992.

70. O'Hara G, Villemaire C, Talajic M, Nattel S: Effects of flecainide on the rate dependence of atrial refractoriness, atrial repolarization and atioventricular node conduction in anesthetized dogs. J Am Coll Cardiol 19:1335, 1992.

71. Henthorn RW, Waldo AL, Anderson JL, et al, and the Flecainide Supraventricular Tachycardia Study Group: Flecainide acetate prevents recurrence of symptomatic paroxysmal supraventricular tachycardia. Circulation 83:119, 1991.

72. Cohen AA, Daru V, Covelle G, et al: Hemodynamic effects of intravenous flecainide in acute noncomplicated myocardial infarction. Am Heart J 110:1193, 1985.

73. Josephson MA, Kaul J, Hopkins J, et al: Hemodynamic effects of intravenous flecainide relative to the level of ventricular function in patients with coronary disease. Am Heart J 109:41, 1985.

74. Josephson MA, Iheda N, Singh B: Effects of flecainide on ventricular function: Clinical and experimental correlations. Am J Cardiol 53:95B, 1984.

75. De Paola AA, Horowitz LN, Morganroth J, et al: Influence of left ventricular dysfunction on flecainide therapy. J Am Coll Cardiol 9:163, 1987.

76. Gentzkow GD, Sullivan JY: Extracardiac adverse effects of flecainide. Am J Cardiol 53:101B, 1984.

77. Anderson JL, Stewart JR, Crevey B: A proposal for the clinical use of flecainide. Am J Cardiol 53:112B, 1983.

78. Hellestrand KJ, Burnett PJ, Milne JR, et al: Effect of the antiarrhythmic agent flecainide acetate on acute and chronic pacing thresholds. PACE 6:892, 1983.

79. Walker PR, Panouchado M, James MA, et al: Pacing failure due to flecainide acetate. PACE 8:900, 1985.

80. Nathan AW, Hellestrand KJ, Bexton RS, et al: Proarrhythmic effects of the new antiarrhythmic agent flecainide acetate. Am Heart J 107:222, 1984.

81. Morganroth J, Horowitz LN: Flecainide: Its proarrhythmic effect and expected changes on the surface electrocardiogram. Am J Cardiol 53:89B, 1984.

82. Fish FA, Gillette PC, Benson DW Jr, for the Pediatric Electrophysiology Group: Proarrhythmia, cardiac arrest and death in young patients receiving encainide and flecainide. J Am Coll Cardiol 18:356, 1991.

83. Velebit V, Podrid P, Lown B, et al: Aggravation and provocation of ventricular arrhythmias by antiarrhythmic drugs. Circulation 65:886, 1982.

84. Lui HK, Garrett L, Dietrich P, et al: Flecainide-induced QT prolongation and ventricular tachycardia. Am Heart J 103:567, 1982.

85. Wehr M, Noll B, Krappe J: Flecainide induced aggravation of ventricular arrhythmias. Am J Cardiol 55:1643, 1985.

86. Spivak C, Gottlieb S, Miura DS, et al: Flecainide toxicity. Am J Cardiol 53:329, 1984.

87. Crijns HJ, Kingma JH, Viersma JW, Lie KI: Transient giant inverted T wave during flecainide intoxication. Am Heart J 113:214, 1987.

88. Morganroth J, Anderson JL, Gentzkow GP: Classification by type of ventricular arrhythmia predicts frequency of adverse cardiac events from flecainide. J Am Coll Cardiol 8:607, 1986.

89. Falk RH: Flecainide-induced ventricular tachycardia and fibrillation in patients treated for atrial fibrillation. Ann Intern Med 111:107, 1989.

90. Brugada J, Boersma L, Kirchhof C, et al: Proarrhythmic effects of flecainide. Experimental evidence for increased susceptibility to reentrant arrhythmias. Circulation 84:1808, 1991.

91. Krishman SC, Antzelevitch C: Flecainide-induced arrhythmia in canine ventricular epicardium. Phase 2 reentry? Circulation 87:562, 1993.

92. Akiyama T, Pawitan Y, Greenberg H, et al: Increased risk of death and cardiac arrest from encainide and flecainide in patients after non-Q-wave acute myocardial infarction in the Cardiac Arrhythmia Suppression Trial. Am J Cardiol 68:1551, 1991.

93. Waldo AL, Henthorn RW, Carlson MD: A perspective on ventricular arrhythmias: Patient assessment for therapy and outcome [review]. Am J Cardiol 65:30B, 1990.

94. Crijns HJ, VanGelder IS, Lie KI: Supraventricular tachycardia mimicking ventricular tachycardia during flecainide treatment. Am J Cardiol 62:1303, 1988.

95. Lewis GP, Holtzman JL: Interaction of flecainide with digoxin and propranolol. Am J Cardiol 53:52B, 1984.

96. McQuinn RL, Kvam DC, Parrish SL, et al: Digoxin (D) levels in patients with congestive heart failure (CHF) are not altered by flecainide (F) [abstract]. Clin Pharmacol Ther 43:150, 1988.

97. Fontaine G, Frank R, Ponet JL: Association amiodarone-flecainide dans le traitement des troubles du rythme ventriculaires graves. Arch Mal Coeur 77:1421, 1984.

98. Leclerq JF, Coumel P: La flecainide: Un nouvel antiarythmique. Arch Mal Coeur 76:1218, 1983.

99. Shea P, Lal R, Kim SS, et al: Flecainide and amiodarone interaction. J Am Coll Cardiol 7:1127, 1986.

100. Tjandra Mata TB, Verbesselt R, Van Hecken A, et al: Oral flecainide elimination kinetics: Effects of cimetidine. Circulation 68(Suppl III):III, 1983.

101. Meinertz T, Zehender MK, Geibel A, et al: Long-term antiarrhythmic therapy with flecainide. Am J Cardiol 54:91, 1984.

102. Pritchett ELC, Wilkinson WE: Mortality in patients treated with flecainide and encainide for supraventricular arrhythmias. Am J Cardiol 67:976, 1991.

CHAPTER 143

Mexiletine

Philip J. Podrid, M.D.

Mexiletine is structurally similar to lidocaine and has similar electrophysiologic effects. Unlike lidocaine, however, it can be administered orally because of a long half-life. Along with lidocaine and tocainide, mexiletine is a class IB agent as defined by the Vaughan Williams classification.[1] Mexiletine is an oral lidocaine congener that is effective for suppressing all forms of ventricular arrhythmias that occur acutely or are chronically present.

ELECTROPHYSIOLOGY

Animal studies *in vitro* have demonstrated that mexiletine possesses electrophysiologic activity typical of the class I agents, which are known as local anesthetics or membrane-stabilizing drugs.[2, 3] Mexiletine exerts effects on the ventricular muscle and Purkinje fibers but not on atrial tissue. As expected, it has no role in the treatment of atrial arrhythmias. The effects of mexiletine on the rapid inward sodium current have been studied in isolated ventricular preparations and are typical of this class of antiarrhythmic drugs.[4] When the tissue is treated with 50 μM concentrations of mexiletine, there is a 70% reduction in inward sodium current. In addition, a use-dependent block can be observed when lower concentrations of drug are used (i.e., 10 to 30 μM). The depressant effect on sodium ion influx is more profound at faster rates of stimulation, similar to what is observed with lidocaine. Additionally, there is rapid onset and offset of drug action. These findings suggest a voltage-dependent binding of mexiletine to sodium channels. As a result of mexiletine therapy, the maximal upstroke velocity of phase 0 of the action potential ($\dot{V}_{max}$) is slowed. This slowing produces a slowing of impulse conduction.

In isolated Purkinje fiber preparations, concentrations of mexiletine similar to those achieved with clinical use result in a significant shortening of action potential duration, a reduction in the action potential amplitude (phase 1), and slowing of $\dot{V}_{max}$ of phase 0 upstroke.[2] Mexiletine has no effect on normal phase 4 diastolic depolarization or spontaneous automaticity. In hypokalemic or isoproterenol-perfused tissues, an apparent shift of activation voltage occurs, which results in a suppression of automaticity.[3] These findings are not observed in atrial tissue even when therapeutic concentrations of mexiletine are achieved.[3]

In vivo, mexiletine demonstrates many of the same electrophysiologic properties as lidocaine.[5] In a comparison of lidocaine and mexiletine in several experimental arrhythmia models in animals, it was observed that both drugs markedly increase the ventricular fibrillation threshold of ischemic and non-ischemic hearts; both decrease the frequency of ventricular arrhythmias after acute coronary artery occlusion; and both abolish ouabain-induced arrhythmias. In the canine model, the mean concentrations of mexiletine required to suppress arrhythmias induced by an infusion of ouabain or catecholamines and during ischemia were 0.9 to 2.2 μg/ml, similar to levels obtained clinically.[6]

Several reports of the electrophysiologic effects of mexiletine on the human heart have been published. The cardiac electrophysiologic effects of mexiletine in patients are minimal. No consistent effects on atrial refractory period, sinus node function, or ventricular refractory period in normal cardiac tissue have been reported.[7, 8] Atrioventricular (AV) nodal refractory period is also unaltered, but the conduction time and pacing rate at which Wenckebach block develops are lengthened.[7] Although the effective refractory period of ventricular muscle is unaltered by mexiletine administration, the relative and effective refractory periods of the His-Purkinje system are prolonged,[8, 9] which reduce membrane excitability. The HV interval generally has been reported to be slightly prolonged or unchanged.[7, 8] As a result, the QRS interval on the electrocardiogram generally is unaltered. Because action potential duration and repolarization time are not changed, the QT interval is unaffected.

Although the electrophysiologic effects of mexiletine in normal persons are minimal, patients with heart disease who have underlying conduction system abnormalities can manifest significant effects. Sinus bradycardia, prolonged HV intervals, and abnormal sinus node recovery times have been reported.[8]

PHARMACOKINETICS

The pharmacologic profile of mexiletine has been studied extensively, and, because of its properties (Table 143–1), mexiletine is useful as an oral antiarrhythmic agent. Although mexiletine is similar to lidocaine, lidocaine has a short half-life because it undergoes extensive first-pass metabolism to deethylated compounds, which possess only weak antiarrhythmic effects but which are associated with toxicity. Mexiletine does not undergo this extensive first-pass metabolism, and, because of a longer half-life, it can be used orally.

The pharmacokinetics and bioavailability of mexiletine have been established in normal subjects.[10, 11] In healthy subjects, the bioavailability of the drug after a single oral dose is reported to be 88%, with peak plasma levels occurring 2 to 4 hours after drug administration.[10, 11] The mean half-life of elimination after oral administration of a single dose varies be-

Table 143–1. **Mexiletine Profile**

Mode of Action
Membrane stabilizer
Local anesthetic
 Reduces upstroke velocity phase 0; decreases conductivity
 Prolongs refractory period; decreases membrane excitability
 Reduces automaticity

Hemodynamics
No significant clinical effects

ECG
No significant changes

Pharmacology
Dosage
 Oral: 200–400 mg t.i.d.
 IV: loading; 10 mg/min up to 300–400 mg; maintenance;
  600–1200 mg over 24 hr
Half-life: 8–14 hr (mean, 11 hr)
Therapeutic blood level: 0.7–1.6 μg/ml
Minimal protein binding
Metabolism
 Hepatic, 85%—inactive metabolites
 Renal, 15%—unchanged drug (percentage changes with urinary
  pH)

tween 6.3 and 9.7 hours,[10, 11] with a total volume of distribution of approximately 5.5 L/kg. Intravenously administered mexiletine undergoes rapid distribution into this large total volume of distribution, probably as a result of rapid uptake by well-perfused tissues.[10] The therapeutic blood level in human subjects is reported to be 0.7 to 1.6 μg/ml.

In patients with coronary artery disease who have ventricular arrhythmias, the half-life of elimination of mexiletine during long-term therapy is more prolonged, with values of 11.3 to 14.7 hours being reported.[10, 12] In addition, the volume of distribution is also larger in patients with coronary artery disease.

Patients with an acute myocardial infarction (AMI) display altered mexiletine pharmacokinetics.[13] In the setting of AMI, the terminal half-life is longer, approximately 14.7 hours, compared with 11.3 hours when the same intravenous dose of mexiletine is given to patients 2 weeks after AMI. In addition, the total volume of distribution is increased (578 L versus 415 L) during the acute illness. Plasma protein binding, total plasma clearance, renal clearance, and mexiletine recovery in the urine, however, are unchanged when compared with what is observed when the drug is administered to patients 2 weeks after infarction. When mexiletine is administered by the oral route, there is a delay in gastrointestinal absorption in patients with an AMI compared with normal individuals.[14] Mexiletine is eliminated primarily by liver metabolism, and 85% is metabolized to inactive metabolites (e.g., parahydroxymexiletine, hydroxymethylmexiletine).[12, 15] Approximately 15% is excreted unchanged in the urine, and the urinary pH affects the percentage of mexiletine cleared by the kidney.[16, 17] In the presence of alkaline urine, the proportion of unchanged mexiletine resorbed by the tubules increases and renal excretion decreases, resulting in higher mexiletine blood levels and prolongation of

the half-life of mexiletine. In the presence of acidic urine, mexiletine elimination is increased, and half-life can be reduced. However, in the physiologic range of urinary pH, this effect is minimal.

Because the major route of metabolism for mexiletine is hepatic, renal insufficiency does not significantly affect the plasma kinetics for mexiletine as long as creatinine clearance is more than 10 ml/min.[16, 17] When creatinine clearance is less than 10 ml/min, the clearance of unmetabolized mexiletine is reduced and blood levels are increased.[18, 19] Therefore, in patients with severe renal insufficiency who have creatinine clearance rates of less than 10 ml/min, reduction of mexiletine dose and monitoring of plasma levels are appropriate. Furthermore, mexiletine is not dialyzable, eliminating the need for supplemental doses in patients receiving chronic hemodialysis. Antacids administered concomitantly with a dose of mexiletine have no effect on absorption or elimination of mexiletine.[20] Antacids do prevent the direct effect of these drugs on the gastrointestinal tract and decrease gastrointestinal toxicity.

Several drugs have been reported to alter the metabolism of mexiletine. Rifampicin has been demonstrated to increase nonrenal elimination of mexiletine by enhancing hepatic metabolism of the drug, resulting in a decrease in the elimination half-life.[21] Phenytoin has been reported to enhance mexiletine metabolism by induction of the hepatic monooxidase system, resulting in a shorter elimination half-life.[22] By increasing the conjugation of mexiletine with glucuronic acid, cigarette smoking also enhances the elimination of mexiletine.[23] Cimetidine, morphine sulfate, and atropine have been demonstrated to delay the absorption of mexiletine from the gastrointestinal tract by decreasing gastric motility, but they do not alter drug bioavailability, whereas metoclopramide speeds absorption.[24, 25] These drugs interfere with drug absorption, but maximal blood levels and the half-life are unchanged.

HEMODYNAMICS

Lidocaine possesses only slight negative inotropic effects and has been shown to produce minimal hemodynamic changes even in patients with far-advanced structural heart disease and substantial left ventricular dysfunction. It is expected that mexiletine also will have minor negative inotropic effects. Evaluation of mexiletine in animal models, normal volunteers, and patients with structural heart disease has demonstrated that the drug causes slight hemodynamic effects; the magnitude of these changes, however, is small and not clinically significant.

The relationship between the dose of mexiletine and its hemodynamic effects has been studied in anesthetized dogs.[26] Dogs were treated with incrementally increased doses of mexiletine, and frequent hemodynamic measurements were obtained. These measurements included pulmonary artery pressure, left atrial pressure, left ventricular pressure, left ventricular contractility or rate of pressure increase (dP/

dt), and aortic pressure. Boluses of mexiletine, 1.5 or 3 mg/kg, were given, and dosing was repeated every 5 minutes until death. These investigators noted a decline in left ventricular dP/dt after the first 1.5-mg/kg dose of mexiletine was given. This negative inotropic effect was associated with a decrease in pulmonary vascular resistance, but there was no reduction in arterial pressure or cardiac output. After infusion of the first dose of 3 mg/kg, there was also a reduction in pulmonary artery vascular resistance, associated with a decrease in left ventricular dP/dt of approximately 8%. As a larger dose of mexiletine was given, there was a further significant reduction in contractility (dP/dt). However, because of peripheral vasodilation and afterload reduction, there was no decline in cardiac output.

The hemodynamic effects of mexiletine also have been evaluated in anesthetized rats.[27] Wistar rats anesthetized with sodium pentobarbital were given either oral or intravenous mexiletine prior to or after induced ischemia. When intravenous mexiletine, 1 mg/kg, was given after the production of ischemia, there was a significant decrease in systolic pressure, diastolic pressure, and left ventricular contractility, or dP/dt. However, in animals pretreated with oral mexiletine, ischemia caused no significant differences in blood pressure, contractility, or heart rate.

In conscious rabbits, mexiletine also has been shown to decrease left ventricular dP/dt.[28] However, a marked arterial vasodilatory effect occurred, which resulted in a reduction in mean arterial pressure and no change in cardiac output. The reduction in dP/dt was substantial (41%) when a dose of 3.5 mg/kg was administered. This dose of mexiletine resulted in a serum level of 1.23 ± 0.16 µg/ml, which is comparable to the levels attained clinically in human subjects. In the same model, the administration of lidocaine and disopyramide in clinically comparable doses reduced dP/dt by 26% and 53%, respectively. However, like mexiletine, lidocaine produced a reduction in peripheral vascular resistance of afterload, and cardiac output was unaffected. Disopyramide, however, resulted in a 23% reduction in cardiac output because of a reflex increase of peripheral vascular resistance and afterload. In conclusion, mexiletine possesses negative inotropic activity and directly decreases left ventricular contractility. However, the drug also has effects on peripheral vascular resistance and, by reducing afterload, maintains stroke volume and cardiac output.

Several studies in humans have reported the effects of mexiletine on cardiac hemodynamics. In one study, the effects of a 1.5-mg/kg bolus injection of mexiletine were evaluated in a group of patients with coronary artery disease.[29] Seven of the 10 patients in this study had previously sustained a myocardial infarction and had underlying abnormalities of left ventricular wall motion. Mexiletine produced a small but significant increase in left ventricular end-diastolic pressure, heart rate, and systolic pressure. No effect on left ventricular inotropy or calculated dP/dt, stroke volume, or cardiac output was observed. In

another study by Saunamaki,[30] mexiletine did not change stroke volume, cardiac output, peripheral vascular resistance, or pulmonary capillary wedge pressure. In contrast, some studies have reported a small but significant rise in peripheral vascular resistance when the intravenous drug is infused.[31]

The hemodynamic effects of mexiletine were evaluated in a group of 24 patients with a variety of heart diseases who had ventricular, as well as supraventricular, arrhythmias.[32] Little or no change occurred in stroke volume, cardiac output, pulmonary end-diastolic pressure, or heart rate after 1- to 2-mg/kg bolus injections were given. Likewise, the drug caused no hemodynamic alterations after 400 to 600 mg of drug was infused over approximately 30 minutes. In patients with valvular heart disease, intravenous and oral mexiletine produced no effect on any measured hemodynamic parameter.[33, 34]

In these studies, mexiletine was evaluated in patients with intact left ventricular function. Data about the effect of oral mexiletine on left ventricular function in patients with reduced ejection fractions are sparse. Nevertheless, in this group of patients, any antiarrhythmic drug is likely to precipitate congestive heart failure. In patients with reduced left ventricular function, Stein et al.[35] evaluated the effect of oral mexiletine on resting ejection fractions as determined by radionuclide ventriculography. They observed no significant effect on left or right ventricular ejection fractions when doses of 200 to 400 mg three times a day were given and when a mean plasma level of 1.7 ± 0.9 µg/ml was achieved (Fig. 143–1). In addition, no effect on exercise tolerance was determined by exercise testing on a treadmill. Therefore, in patients with reduced ventricular function, there is no measurable effect on ejection fraction. Indeed, congestive heart failure is reported only infrequently as a complication of therapy with mexiletine.

CLINICAL EXPERIENCE WITH MEXILETINE
Noninvasive Evaluation

Although mexiletine was first introduced as an anticonvulsant agent,[36] its principal role has been in the treatment of ventricular arrhythmia (Table 143–2).[12, 37–50] Early clinical trials in patients with frequent ventricular premature complexes (VPCs) suggested that mexiletine was an effective therapy for suppression. However, most of these studies involved patients who did not have complex or sustained arrhythmia and who generally had minimal or no heart disease. Moreover, evaluation of efficacy depended on electrocardiographic rhythm strips rather than extended periods of ambulatory monitoring. Therefore, drug efficacy was uncertain as judged by these studies.

One of the first trials of mexiletine was reported by Talbot et al.[51] in 1973. The authors administered a single dose of intravenous mexiletine to 79 patients, and they observed complete suppression of VPCs in 72% documented by continuous bedside monitoring.

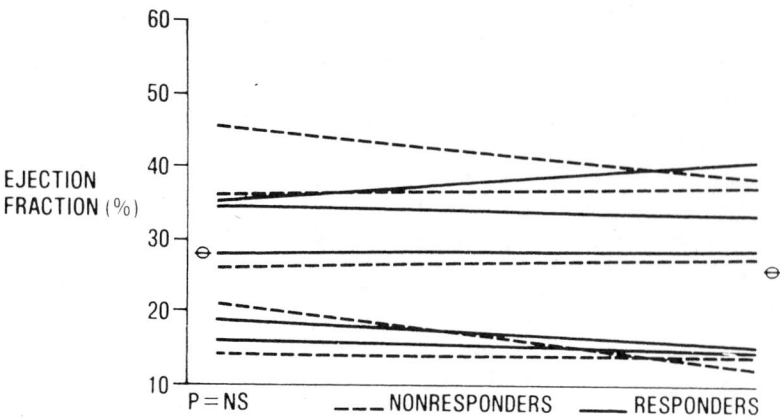

Figure 143–1. Effects of mexiletine on left ventricular ejection fraction (LVEF) in 10 patients with impaired LV function. Before administration of mexiletine, the average LVEF was 29%, and this was unaltered by the drug (28%). Although one patient did have a reduction in LVEF, no congestive heart failure occurred.

In several subsequent studies using oral mexiletine, Talbot et al.[37, 38] reported that the drug was of equivalent efficacy when administered to patients with AMI or chronic coronary artery disease or to those with no heart disease. However, one third of patients had side effects, limiting the usefulness of the drug. Similar confirmatory results with intravenous and oral drug were reported by Esser and Kikis,[39] Waleffe and Kulbertus,[40] and Campbell et al.[12]

One of the first studies with mexiletine that used ambulatory monitoring was reported in 1979 by Abinader and Cooper,[41] who administered oral mexiletine, 200 to 250 mg three times a day, to 10 patients with VPCs refractory to intravenous lidocaine and procainamide. As evaluated with 10 hours of continuous recording by ambulatory monitoring, six patients had complete suppression of VPCs, and an additional two had more than 75% reduction. VPC suppression was maintained during long-term therapy as determined by periodic 10-hour ambulatory monitoring.

Mehta and Conti[52] randomly administered mexiletine or placebo to 12 patients with frequent VPCs in a double-blind, crossover study. The doses used were 100 to 400 mg three times a day, and they reported that mexiletine significantly reduced the number of VPCs by 66% compared with only a 5% decrease with placebo ($p < .03$). Meoli et al.[42] administered oral mexiletine, up to 1000 mg/day, to 20 patients, most of whom had coronary artery disease. As evaluated with 24-hour ambulatory monitoring, the group as a whole had a 68% reduction in VPCs, and 11 patients had a 90% decrease. Similar efficacy was reported by Masotti et al.[43] in a group of 26 patients.

There have been reports in which intravenous mexiletine was administered to patients with sustained ventricular tachycardia (VT). In a report by Santinelli et al.,[44] six of seven patients in sustained VT responded to the drug with termination of VT and resumption of normal sinus rhythm. Wang et al.[45] reported efficacy (defined as termination of sustained VT) in six of eight patients. Long-term therapy with oral medication was continued in the six patients, five of whom remained free of recurrence during the follow-up period.

Mexiletine has also been reported to be effective in some patients with ventricular arrhythmia refractory to other drug therapy. Fenster and Kern[46] administered oral mexiletine to 22 patients with a history of sustained VT or ventricular fibrillation (VF) and to six with nonsustained VT. Each patient had arrhythmia

Table 143–2. **Studies of Mexiletine Efficacy Using Noninvasive Techniques**

Reference	Patients	Mode of Administration	Type of Arrhythmia	Efficacy (%)
Talbot[37]	59	IV	VPCs	72
Talbot et al.[38]	49	Oral	VPCs	90
Esser and Kikis[39]	39	Oral	VPCs	97
Waleffe and Kulbertus[40]	12	IV	VPCs, repetitive forms	75
Campbell et al.[12]	108	IV	VPCs	72
	48	Oral	VPCs	50
Abinader and Cooper[41]	10	Oral	VPCs	80
Meoli et al.[42]	20	Oral	VPCs	55
Masotti et al.[43]	24	Oral	VPCs	79
Santinelli et al.[44]	7	IV	Sustained VT	86
Wang et al.[45]	6	Oral	Sustained VT	83
Fenster and Kern[46]	22	Oral	Sustained VT and VF	29
Podrid and Lown[47]	107	Oral	Sustained VT, NSVT, and VF	60
Flaker et al.[48]	22	Oral	VPCs	27
Poole et al.[49]	51	Oral	Sustained VT, NSVT, and VF	12
Rutledge et al.[50]	58	Oral	VPCs	33

NSVT, nonsustained ventricular tachycardia; VF, ventricular fibrillation; VPCs, ventricular premature contractions; VT, ventricular tachycardia.

refractory to previous antiarrhythmic therapy, including quinidine, disopyramide, and procainamide. In six patients, side effects necessitated drug discontinuation, but 22 patients continued receiving therapy and were evaluated. Of these, 12 responded to mexiletine; however, side effects caused early discontinuation in four patients. Therefore, the drug was clinically useful in only 8 of 28 patients (29%).

Podrid and Lown[47] reported their experience with mexiletine in 108 patients with refractory ventricular tachyarrhythmias, including sustained VT or VF in 63 patients, nonsustained VT in 20, and only frequent VPCs in 25 patients. Efficacy was evaluated noninvasively with monitoring and exercise testing. Overall, 60% of patients had arrhythmia suppression, defined as total elimination of VT runs, more than 90% reduction of couplets, and more than 50% decrease in VPCs. Long-term therapy with mexiletine administered as monotherapy was continued in 38 patients, seven of whom discontinued therapy because of side effects. During an average follow-up of 13 months (3 to 27 months), the remaining 31 patients continued receiving the drug, free of recurrence or side effects.

In a follow-up study, Stein et al.[53] reviewed their experience with mexiletine in 313 patients, of whom 78 had drug-refractory VT or VF and 134 had refractory nonsustained VT associated with symptoms. The percentage of patients responding to the drug was similar to that previously reported by this group. In this study, no relationship was seen among the underlying heart disease, nature of the presenting arrhythmia, and response to mexiletine. Long-term therapy with mexiletine was continued in 107 patients who responded to the agent and were free of side effects during the brief period of maintenance therapy in the hospital. During a mean follow-up of 23 months (range, 1 to 70 months), the annual rate of sudden death was 3.6%, and recurrence of nonfatal arrhythmia was 4.9% a year. Side effects during the follow-up period necessitated drug discontinuation in 13 patients, and two patients died of progressive congestive heart failure. Mexiletine therapy was continued in 61 patients (67%) who remained free of arrhythmia and side effects.

Invasive Evaluation

Mexiletine was one of seven antiarrhythmic drugs used in the Electrophysiologic Study versus Electrocardiographic Monitoring Trial (ESVEM).[54] In this controlled trial, patients with a history of a sustained ventricular tachyarrhythmia were randomized to therapy selected by either electrophysiologic testing or ambulatory monitoring. Drugs used in this trial were imipramine, mexiletine, pirmenol, procainamide, propafenone, quinidine, and sotalol. In patients randomized to evaluation with ambulatory monitoring, mexiletine was effective for suppressing spontaneous ectopy in 67%. Unfortunately, the outcome in follow-up of patients in this trial receiving long-term therapy with mexiletine is not yet known.

Invasive electrophysiologic testing has also been used to evaluate the efficacy of mexiletine in patients with serious, sustained ventricular tachyarrhythmia (Table 143–3).[9, 47, 48, 55–59] DiMarco et al.[55] studied 35 patients with a history of sustained VT inducible during electrophysiologic testing in a drug-free state. Mexiletine alone or in combination with another previously ineffective drug prevented VT induction in 13 patients (37%), while 7 others had partial response. Six additional patients were managed noninvasively, and five responded with suppression of spontaneous arrhythmia. Long-term therapy was continued in 24 patients. Of the 17 with complete suppression of arrhythmia—five evaluated noninvasively and 12 who underwent electrophysiologic testing—only one had recurrence of arrhythmia after 12.6 months, whereas two of seven with a partial effect had recurrent arrhythmias after an average follow-up of 6.7 months. Of interest was an association between the response to mexiletine and the rate of VT. In 21 patients with induced, sustained VT recurring with a rate of more than 185 beats/min, a complete or partial response occurred in 15 (71%). In contrast, only three of eight patients (38%) with VT at a rate less than 185 beats/min responded to the drug ($p < .01$).

In an update of this initial experience, Schoenfeld et al.[56] reported on 140 patients with a history of VT or VF whose arrhythmias were inducible during baseline electrophysiologic testing. Mexiletine as monotherapy was effective in 23 patients (15%), whereas arrhythmias in an additional 30 patients (20%) were rendered noninducible when a second drug was added as adjunctive therapy. A partial response, defined as arrhythmia that was more difficult to induce or induced VT that had a slower rate, was observed in 19 patients (13%). Long-term therapy was continued in 83 patients. After an average follow-up of 14 months, there were 10 sudden deaths (12%) and six (7%) nonfatal recurrences of arrhythmias. Of note, 31 of the 83 patients who continued mexiletine therapy had arrhythmias that were still inducible while taking mexiletine, but most remained free of arrhythmia during follow-up. In this study,[56] it was observed that mexiletine was more effective in patients with VF or nonsustained VT, of whom 51% responded, compared with a 24% efficacy rate in patients with sustained VT. Unpublished data from Podrid in-

Table 143–3. **Studies of Mexiletine Efficacy Using Invasive Technique**

Reference	Patients	Efficacy (%)
DiMarco et al[55]	35	37*
Schoenfeld et al.[56]	140	15 monotherapy; 20 combination therapy
Podrid and Lown[47]	45	36
Flaker et al[48]	10	10
Manz et al[57]	30	10
Waspe et al[9]	33	24
Palileo et al[58]	17	6†
Kim et al.[59]	30	23

*Includes responders to monotherapy and combinations.
†Partial efficacy only.

volved 45 patients with drug-refractory, sustained VT or VF who underwent electrophysiologic testing. Of these, 16 (36%) had arrhythmias that were rendered noninducible while receiving mexiletine alone. After a follow-up of 30 months, there have been no deaths and only two nonfatal recurrences of arrhythmias.

Despite these reports of a good response to mexiletine, the experiences of other investigators have not demonstrated mexiletine to be an effective agent. In a study of Flaker et al.,[48] only 1 of 10 patients with VT who underwent electrophysiologic testing responded to the drug; and Manz et al.[57] reported success in only 3 of 30 patients with VT evaluated with electrophysiologic testing. In a study involving 51 patients with VF, sustained VT, or nonsustained VT who were evaluated invasively and discharged receiving mexiletine therapy, Poole et al.[49] reported that, after a mean follow-up of 10.4 months, 21 patients (41%) had arrhythmia recurrence, and the drug was discontinued in 17 patients (33%) because of side effects. Only six patients (12%) continued to receive the drug for chronic suppressive therapy. Waspe et al.[9] reported a good response to mexiletine in only 8 of 33 patients (24%) with a sustained ventricular tachyarrhythmia who underwent electrophysiologic testing, but in the nonresponders whose arrhythmias were still inducible, the drug altered neither mode of induction nor ventricular refractory periods. Palileo et al.[58] studied 17 patients with inducible sustained VT. Prior to repeat study on mexiletine, one patient discontinued the therapy because of side effects, and five patients had spontaneous VT. Of the remaining 11 patients, 10 continued to have inducible arrhythmias, and one patient's sustained VT was converted to a nonsustained episode. As has been noted by others, the cycle length of induced VT in the nonresponders was lengthened by the drug.

In ESVEM,[54] mexiletine was effective for preventing the induction of arrhythmia during electrophysiologic study in 12% of patients. A major concern is the role of electrophysiologic testing for predicting long-term outcome with mexiletine. Unfortunately, ESVEM did not report such data with individual agents. As with other drugs, it is well established that when patients' arrhythmias are rendered noninducible, they remain free of recurrence. However, continued inducibility does not always correlate with recurrent arrhythmia. In the study of Schoenfeld et al.,[56] 31 patients were discharged receiving mexiletine despite continued inducibility during therapy, but recurrence was infrequent in this group. Saksena and Craelius[60] discharged nine patients on long-term mexiletine, three of whom continued to have inducible arrhythmias. No recurrences happened during follow-up. Kim et al.[59] reported that a marked disparity in efficacy of mexiletine exists when invasive techniques are used, compared with the results during a noninvasive evaluation. These authors studied 30 patients with histories of VT or VF. Each patient had frequent VPCs on ambulatory monitoring, and 22 had runs of VT. Additionally, sustained VT was inducible in each patient during electrophysiologic testing. When mexile-

tine therapy was evaluated by electrophysiologic testing, only 23% of patients' arrhythmias were rendered noninducible, whereas almost 60% responded with suppression of spontaneous arrhythmia as determined by ambulatory monitoring. The results of these two techniques were discordant in 67% of patients, primarily as a result of greater efficacy when monitoring was used. However, the predictive accuracy of the two techniques was equivalent.

In conclusion, mexiletine is an effective antiarrhythmic drug. When evaluated noninvasively, 50% to 80% of patients respond with suppression of spontaneous arrhythmia, whereas with electrophysiologic testing, a favorable response—noninduction of VT—is observed in only 12% to 30% of patients. This disparity in efficacy rates has also been observed with each of the other antiarrhythmic agents.

Efficacy After Myocardial Infarction

An important group of patients often treated with antiarrhythmic drugs are those who have recently experienced AMI, in whom there is a greater risk of sudden cardiac death during the ensuing 6 to 12 months. Several studies have reported the use of mexiletine, often compared with placebo, in such patients (Table 142–4).[61–64] However, in most of these studies, efficacy was evaluated by electrocardiogram (ECG) rhythm strips, duration of therapy was short, and the drug dose was not titrated based on arrhythmia suppression because there was no attempt made to suppress arrhythmia. Rather, patients were randomly assigned to receive drug or placebo and were continued on this program regardless of the presence of arrhythmia.

Campbell et al.[61] administered mexiletine, 600 to 900 mg/day, to 48 patients with recent AMI. The median duration of therapy was only 3 months, but 25 patients continued for 6 months. In eight patients, the drug was discontinued because of side effects, and seven patients did not respond, so the drug was withdrawn. The authors concluded that the drug was effective for suppressing arrhythmia in patients after AMI, but they did not comment on mortality.

In a second study, Campbell et al.[62] randomly assigned 97 post-AMI patients to placebo or mexiletine at a dose of 250 mg three times a day. In this study, 24-hour ambulatory monitoring was used to evaluate efficacy, but therapy was continued for only 48 hours.

Table 143–4. **Mexiletine Therapy for Patients After Myocardial Infarction**

Reference	Patients	Dose (mg/day)	Duration of Therapy	Compared with Placebo (p value)
Campbell et al.[61]	48	600–900	3 mo	—
Campbell et al.[62]	97	750	48 hr	NS
Campbell et al.[63]	60	600–900	10 days	NS
IMPACT[64]	630	520*	12 mo	NS

*Long-acting mexiletine.

Mexiletine effectively suppressed all forms of ventricular arrhythmia, especially runs of VT. However, VF was rare in both groups, and no conclusion about the role of mexiletine in preventing sudden death was possible. In a comparison between lidocaine and intravenous mexiletine, mexiletine was more effective for suppressing complex forms, but, as with the Campbell study, duration was brief and efficacy was evaluated only by ECG rhythm strips.[65]

In a post-AMI trial comparing mexiletine with placebo and procainamide, the drugs were equally effective for suppressing arrhythmias, but, as with other similar studies, the duration of therapy was brief (10 days).[63] The most recent study was a double-blind, multicenter trial (IMPACT) that randomly assigned 630 patients after AMI to receive placebo or long-acting mexiletine, 260 mg twice daily.[64] Patients with more than 30 VPCs in any two sequential periods of monitoring in the cardiac care unit were entered, and the effects of therapy were evaluated with 24-hour monitoring at 1, 4, and 12 months. At all points of observation, the number of patients exhibiting frequent or complex arrhythmias was the same in the placebo and treatment groups. After a 1-year follow-up, the rates of sudden death were statistically the same: 7.6% in the group receiving mexiletine, and 4.8% in the group taking placebo. As with other studies of drug therapy after AMI, mexiletine failed to prevent sudden death. However, similar to other studies, many problems render the results inconclusive. Therapy was not based on the density or type of arrhythmia present, so patients with low-density arrhythmias were entered into the study; daily reproducibility of arrhythmias was not assessed; and dosage was not guided by arrhythmia suppression. The drug therapy was continued even if ineffective. The similarity in outcome between groups treated with drugs and groups taking placebo may be related to the same degree of arrhythmia suppression in both groups. Therefore, such studies do not provide valid conclusions about the role of mexiletine or other antiarrhythmic drugs for preventing sudden death after AMI.

Comparison with Other Antiarrhythmic Agents

A number of studies have compared mexiletine with other antiarrhythmic agents (Table 142–5).[66–73] Singh et al.[66] evaluated quinidine or mexiletine in 51 patients using ambulatory monitoring. After 12 weeks of therapy, they reported that the two drugs were of equivalent efficacy, defined as more than 70% reduction in VPCs. In another study comparing quinidine and mexiletine in 26 patients, Fenster and Hanson[67] also observed that these drugs were of equivalent efficacy for VPC suppression, but neither drug consistently reduced repetitive forms.

Studies comparing procainamide and mexiletine have reported that these agents are equally effective for suppressing all forms of arrhythmia, but side effects are far more common with procainamide.[68, 69]

Table 143–5. **Comparative Studies of Mexiletine**

Reference	Patients	Comparison Drug	Efficacy (%) Mexiletine	Other Drug
Singh et al.[66]	51	Quinidine	69	70
Fenster and Hanson[67]	26	Quinidine	54	62
Arakawa et al.[68]	55	Procainamide	88	85
Jewitt et al.[69]	25	Procainamide	52	60
Myburgh and Goldman[70]	27	Disopyramide	41	48
Trimarco et al.[71]	40	Disopyramide	95	80
Breithardt et al.[72]	12	Disopyramide	58	58*
Hession et al.[73]	79	Tocainide	38	32

*Complete and partial efficacy.

Four studies have compared mexiletine with disopyramide. Myburgh and Goldman[70] evaluated the two agents in 27 patients with recent AMI and reported equivalent efficacy. In a study involving 15 patients, Breithardt et al.[74] reported that low-dose mexiletine, 200 mg three times a day, was less effective than disopyramide, 150 mg three times a day, but the two drugs were of equivalent efficacy when a higher dose of mexiletine was used. In a study by Trimarco et al.[71] involving 40 patients treated with either disopyramide or mexiletine for 3 weeks, the two drugs had equal effect as evaluated with ambulatory monitoring. In a study using electrophysiologic testing, Breithardt et al.[72] administered mexiletine and disopyramide in random sequence to 12 patients with inducible VT. During therapy with each drug, arrhythmias in seven patients were rendered noninducible or were more difficult to induce.

Hession et al.[73] compared the efficacy of mexiletine with that of the other lidocaine congener, tocainide, in 79 patients (Fig. 142–2). The two drugs were of equivalent efficacy, with 38% of patients responding to each agent, but the response of one drug did not predict that of the other. Concordant responses were observed in only 53% of patients (p = NS). This lack of predictability was irrespective of the method of drug evaluation, nature of the underlying heart disease, type of presenting arrhythmia, or left ventricular ejection fraction. This confirms that, although these two agents are structurally similar and share the same electrophysiologic properties, they have different clinical effects.

Although not designed as a drug comparison trial, ESVEM did report the efficacy of the seven antiarrhythmic agents used. As seen in Table 142–6, the antiarrhythmic drugs used in this trial were of equal efficacy when evaluated noninvasively. When electrophysiologic testing was used, each of the agents was less effective, but the response rate was statistically similar for all of the drugs except for sotalol, which was more effective than the other agents (p < .001). The number of patients with side effects varied among the agents, but mexiletine had the lowest incidence of cardiovascular side effects.

It can be concluded that mexiletine is as effective as quinidine, procainamide, and disopyramide for

Mexiletine

		Effective	Ineffective	
Tocainide	Effective	12	19	31
	Ineffective	18	30	48
		30	49	79

Figure 143–2. Comparison between mexiletine and tocainide. Both drugs were evaluated either noninvasively or invasively in 79 patients. Although the drugs were of equal efficacy, concordant responses occurred in only 53% of patients.

Concordance 42/79 = 53%
Discordance 37/79 = 47%
p = NS

suppression of arrhythmia. Although mexiletine and tocainide are of equivalent efficacy, their clinical effects are different, and the response to one does not predict the effect of the other; therefore, they are not necessarily interchangeable.

Drug Interactions

Like other drugs, a number of important drug interactions are associated with mexiletine (Table 142–7). Such interactions are of two types. Pharmacokinetic interactions involve alterations in the absorption, distribution, or metabolism of one drug by another. Pharmacodynamic interactions involve a change in the pharmacologic effects of one drug by another agent. Because patients who are treated with mexiletine are likely to receive other agents, a review of known and possible drug interactions is important.

Pharmacokinetic Interactions

Because mexiletine has a high pK_a, it is in an ionized form in the acidic stomach and thus is poorly absorbed there.[10] However, antacids or sodium bicarbonate may alter the pH of the stomach and cause an increase in gastric absorption of the drug.[75] In most clinical situations gastric pH does not become basic, and absorption of mexiletine is not affected significantly.[20] Nevertheless, because antacids are often administered with mexiletine, it is an important concern.

The principal site of absorption of the drug is the small intestine, where a basic milieu exists. In addition to the potential for a change in absorption due to pH alteration, a delay in gastric emptying—such as occurs with antacids containing aluminum,[20] narcotics, sedatives, or anticholinergic ganglionic blockers[25]—causes a reduction in the rate of mexiletine absorption and time to peak levels, even though the amount ultimately absorbed and peak level achieved are not affected. Cimetidine, a drug commonly prescribed, also delays mexiletine absorption and the time to peak levels, but the amount of drug absorbed is not affected.[24]

Although not well studied, changes in the distribution of mexiletine may affect plasma levels of the drug and its antiarrhythmic action. Mexiletine has a large volume of distribution because of extensive tissue binding.[10] Any hemodynamic alterations, such as occurs in congestive heart failure or with use of drugs such as β-blockers or calcium antagonists, may change the volume of distribution of mexiletine and increase its plasma levels. Likewise, changes in hepatic blood flow may affect mexiletine metabolism and thus plasma levels.

A large amount of mexiletine exists in a free state in plasma, not protein-bound. Drugs such as warfarin that are tightly protein-bound are not displaced by mexiletine, and no important interactions have been described.[76] Because mexiletine is metabolized extensively by the liver, drugs that enhance liver metabo-

Table 143–6. **Results with Antiarrhythmic Drugs in ESVEM**

Drug	No. Patients Tested	Efficacy (%)		Adverse Effects (%)			
				Short-term		Long-term	
		Holter	EP Study	ALL	CV	ALL	CV
Imipramine	71	45	10	43	25	13	7
Mexiletine	**162**	**67**	**12**	**27**	**8**	**19**	**2**
Pirmenol	84	55	19	23	16	7	7
Procainamide	116	50	26	24	6	31	3
Propafenone	160	48	14	26	24	13	11
Quinidine	116	59	16	24	13	32	8
Sotalol	190	56	35	16	14	7	6

ESVEM, Electrophysiologic Study versus Electrocardiographic Monitoring; EP, electrophysiologic; CV, cardiovascular.
Adapted from Mason JW, for the Electrophysiologic Study versus Electrocardiographic Monitoring Investigators: A comparison of seven antiarrhythmic drugs in patients with ventricular tachyarrhythmias. N Engl J Med 329:452, 1993.

Table 143–7. Drug Interactions with Mexiletine

Pharmacokinetic
Delayed absorption (prolonged onset of peak values): antacids, narcotics, sedatives, anticholinergic ganglionic blockers, cimetidine.
Altered distribution (reduced tissue binding, increased plasma levels): as caused by β-blockers, calcium antagonists, or congestive heart failure.
Altered hepatic metabolism (increased metabolism, lower plasma levels): rifampin, phenytoin, barbiturates.
Changes in renal secretion by alkalinization of urine (increased plasma levels): sodium bicarbonate, diuretics.

Pharmacodynamic
Enhanced antiarrhythmic effect
  Combinations with β-blockers
  Combinations with other membrane-stabilizing drugs
No digoxin interaction

lism theoretically can increase nonrenal clearance of the drug and reduce its half-life. Rifampin[21] and phenytoin[22] have been reported to increase mexiletine metabolism, and drugs such as phenobarbital may also enhance metabolism and reduce the half-life of the drug.

Although most mexiletine (85%) is metabolized by the liver, some 10% to 15% is excreted unchanged in urine.[10] Renal excretion of drug is pH-dependent, and, in the presence of alkaline urine, tubular resorption of the nonmetabolized drug is increased, resulting in an increase in plasma mexiletine concentration.[18, 19] This increase has been observed when sodium bicarbonate or diuretics are used. When the urinary pH is within a physiologic range, the interaction is of little clinical importance. However, if urinary pH becomes significantly alkaline, it may be an important concern.

Pharmacodynamic Interactions

Digoxin and Mexiletine

A number of pharmacodynamic drug interactions have been described with antiarrhythmic agents. One of the most often observed is an interaction with digoxin, reported to occur with quinidine,[77] amiodarone,[78] and verapamil.[79] In a study by Leahy et al.,[80] mexiletine was administered to elderly patients with heart disease who received a stable dose of digoxin. No change in digoxin blood levels was observed. This finding was confirmed by Sales et al.,[81] who studied the combination in a young, healthy population. The patients were given digitalis and a stable dose of digoxin. The addition of mexiletine did not affect digoxin levels.

Combined Use with β-Blockers

Antiarrhythmic efficacy can be enhanced by the administration of antiarrhythmic drugs in combination. One of the most frequently used combinations is a β-blocking agent and a membrane-active drug such as mexiletine. In a report by Leahy et al.,[82] four patients in whom mexiletine was only partially effective had complete suppression of arrhythmias when propranolol was added. In a review of experience with mexiletine in the United States, Bigger[83] reported that only 14% of 185 patients taking low-dose mexiletine (200 mg t.i.d.) responded to the drug with at least a 70% reduction in VPCs. However, in 44 patients, the combined use at the same dose of mexiletine and a β-blocker resulted in a 30% efficacy rate ($p < .01$). This beneficial effect was also reported by Pacholke et al.,[84] who compared the efficacy of therapy with low-dose mexiletine or propranolol with the results achieved when the combination was administered. As judged by both monitoring and exercise testing, the combination was more effective than monotherapy with either drug. The beneficial effect of β-blocking agents as adjunctive therapy was also reported by Hirsowitz et al.[85] in a study involving 54 patients in whom membrane-active drugs alone were only partially effective. In 18 patients, the membrane drug used was mexiletine. The addition of a β-blocker, primarily metoprolol or propranolol, significantly reduced the number of VPCs, couplets, and runs of VT on ambulatory monitoring ($p < .05$) and exercise testing ($p < .001$). Of importance, monotherapy with β-blockers did not significantly reduce the frequency of couplets or runs of VT as evaluated by monitoring and exercise testing. These studies strongly suggest that the antiarrhythmic effect of mexiletine can be enhanced by concomitant administration of a β-blocking agent. In addition, it has been reported that, when these drugs are combined, the doses of the individual drugs can be reduced, decreasing the incidence of toxic side effects.

Combined Use with Another Membrane-Active Drug

Mexiletine is a type IB drug and therefore exerts only a weak effect on membrane conductivity and refractory periods. As a result, the ECG intervals, primarily the QRS and QT intervals, are unaffected, which suggests that the drug can be combined safely with other antiarrhythmic agents to enhance antiarrhythmic efficacy. Duff et al.[86] reported on 17 patients who did not respond to quinidine or in whom side effects from this drug occurred. The patients were treated with mexiletine, and the dose was titrated upward until side effects occurred. At the maximally tolerated dose, VPCs were reduced by only 63% and VT by 41% with mexiletine, whereas with quinidine the decrease was 59% and 35%, respectively. However, when mexiletine and quinidine were administered in combination, using doses less than those used when monotherapy was employed, an 85% reduction in VPCs and a marked (94%) suppression of repetitive forms were observed. Of importance, the incidence of all side effects was lower with combination therapy compared with monotherapy, largely because the doses used were smaller. With mexiletine monotherapy, 82% of patients had gastrointestinal or neurologic side effects, but these toxic reactions were reported by only 6% of patients during combination therapy. Additionally, the incidence of quinidine-induced side effects was reduced from 65% to 6%. Giardina and

Wechsler[87] evaluated low doses of drugs (quinidine, 200 mg q8h; mexiletine 146 mg q8h) and also reported an increased efficacy, i.e., 33% of patients responded to therapy with quinidine alone, but 93% responded to the combination.

Greenspan et al.[88] reported on 23 patients whose arrhythmias remained inducible despite therapy with mexiletine and quinidine administered separately. When the combination was used, arrhythmias in eight patients (35%) became noninducible, and the rate of the VT was significantly slowed in the remaining 15. Similar results were reported by Whitford et al.,[89] who combined quinidine or disopyramide with mexiletine in 80 patients undergoing electrophysiologic testing for management of ventricular tachycardia. Disopyramide has also been evaluated in combination with mexiletine, and, as with quinidine, efficacy is enhanced. Kim et al.[90] reported on 20 patients with spontaneous ectopy evaluated with ambulatory monitoring. Disopyramide used alone was effective in 20%, mexiletine in 5%, and the combination in 60%. In a study by Whitford et al.[89] involving electrophysiologic testing, this combination enhanced efficacy when compared with monotherapy. In contrast, Poole et al.[49] found no improvement in antiarrhythmic efficacy or outcome when mexiletine was combined with another agent. Of 51 patients, 25 received mexiletine in combination with quinidine, procainamide, or disopyramide. Recurrence of arrhythmia was observed in 12 patients (48%). Of 26 patients receiving therapy with only mexiletine, arrhythmia recurred in nine (35%) (p = NS).

Class IC agents have also been combined with mexiletine, although the data are limited. In a report by Mendes et al.,[91] 14 patients with sustained VT induced in the electrophysiology laboratory were treated with a class IC agent. VT remained inducible in each patient, although the cycle length of the VT increased from 260 to 340 msec (p < .05). With the addition of mexiletine to the IC agent, VT remained inducible; however, there was a further prolongation in the cycle length of the VT to 392 msec (p < .001). Additionally, the refractory period, which was not significantly altered by the class IC agent, was significantly prolonged with the combination (255 msec versus 267 msec, p < .05). Nine patients were discharged receiving the combination of a IC agent and mexiletine, and, after a 22-month follow-up, seven patients remained free of recurrent arrhythmia and side effects. Similar results were reported by Yeung-Lai-Weh et al.[92] in a study involving 16 patients who had VT induced despite procainamide and propafenone therapy. When mexiletine was added to propafenone, three patients (19%) no longer had VT induced; in the remaining patients, the cycle length of the VT compared with baseline increased from 262 to 350 msec with propafenone and to 390 msec when the combination was administered (p < .0001).

Drugs of other classes have also been combined with mexiletine. Waleffe et al.[93] reported a beneficial effect of a combination of mexiletine and amiodarone in nine patients. Three patients had frequent spontaneous episodes of VT. Although they responded to mexiletine, the necessary dose produced disturbing side effects. The remaining six patients had continued inducible arrhythmias during electrophysiologic testing despite mexiletine therapy. All nine received 3 days of intravenous mexiletine and intravenous amiodarone. At the end of 3 days, the three patients with spontaneous VT were free of arrhythmia, and the six patients undergoing electrophysiologic testing had noninducible arrhythmias. Although this suggests a beneficial effect from the combination, it is unclear whether amiodarone alone was responsible for the antiarrhythmic effects observed.

Adverse Effects

A problem common to all antiarrhythmic drugs is that their usefulness is limited by the occurrence of side effects (Table 142–8). The incidence of side effects of mexiletine has been reported to be as high as 80% in some series.[9, 37, 47, 52, 53, 57, 61, 66] The occurrence and frequency of side effects are related in part to the dose of drug used, the duration of therapy, the nature and extent of the underlying heart disease, and the type of arrhythmia being treated. In the series reported by Stein et al.[53] involving 313 patients with serious arrhythmia, the overall incidence of mexiletine toxicity was 24%. In this study, the blood level achieved did not correlate with side effects, and there was much overlap in levels between patients with and without mexiletine toxicity. Nevertheless, for an individual patient, there may be a relationship between occurrence of some side effects and the dose of drug and blood level achieved. In ESVEM,[54] adverse effects occurred in 27% of patients during short-term therapy, whereas with long-term therapy, 19% had adverse effects. Although the nature of side effects was not specified, cardiovascular toxicity was infrequent, occurring in 8% during short-term therapy and in 2% during long-term follow-up.

The most common adverse reactions are those involving the central nervous system, reported by 14% to 50% of patients. In the U. S. Emergency Program,[94]

Table 143–8. **Side Effects from Mexiletine**

Neurologic (14%–50%)	Gastrointestinal (9%–25%)
Dose-related	Nausea
Dizziness	Vomiting
Lightheadedness	Anorexia
Speech disorder	Constipation
Ataxia	Diarrhea
Tremor	
Not dose-related	**Cardiovascular (5%–10%)**
Behavior changes	Congestive heart failure
Memory impairment	Conduction abnormalities
Altered personality	Arrhythmia aggravation
Sleep disturbance	Hypotension
Psychological problems	**Other (>1%)**
	Urinary retention
	Rash
	Laboratory abnormalities
	(liver function tests; ANA)

ANA, antinuclear antibody.

the incidence of neurologic complaints was 33%. The most common complaints—which include dizziness, lightheadedness, paresthesias, ataxia, tremor, and speech disturbance—are usually related to the dose administered and the blood level achieved. A reduction in dose often diminishes the side effect, but drug discontinuation frequently is necessary. Other neurologic complaints are not dose-related but are a direct effect of the drug. These complaints include memory impairment, altered personality, changes in behavior, sleep disturbances, psychological problems, and, rarely, seizures. Many neurologic toxic reactions are similar to those occurring with lidocaine. Therefore, to avoid the precipitation of adverse neurologic reactions, lidocaine must be administered cautiously to patients being treated with mexiletine.

The next most common side effects, those involving the gastrointestinal tract, were reported in almost 25% of patients entered into the U. S. Emergency Program[94] and in 9% of patients reported by Stein et al.[53] Complaints included nausea, vomiting, anorexia, and abdominal discomfort. These side effects usually are due to a direct effect of the drug on the stomach and can be avoided or treated with antacids or coadministration of the drug with food. In general, there is no relationship to dose or blood levels. Other infrequent gastrointestinal side effects are diarrhea and constipation.

The most serious side effects involve the cardiovascular system and are reported to occur in 2% to 10% of patients.[53, 54] AV nodal block, bradycardia, and hypotension are unusual, but each occurs in approximately 1% of patients. In general, these complications are not dose-related. The occurrence of congestive heart failure is infrequent, reported in 0.9% of patients. However, it is more common in patients with a prior history of heart failure due to systolic dysfunction (2%).[95] Aggravation of arrhythmia, a problem common to all antiarrhythmic drugs, was observed in some 8% of patients.[96] This complication is unrelated to dose, blood level, or changes on the ECG and represents an idiosyncratic reaction. However, it is more common in patients with a history of sustained VT or VF and in those with poor LV function and congestive heart failure.

Other side effects are infrequent, each being reported in fewer than 1% of patients. These effects include urinary retention, rash, musculoskeletal complaints, and asymptomatic laboratory abnormalities such as neutropenia and elevated liver function test results. A positive antinuclear antibody develops in as many as 8% of patients,[47] but levels usually are low and change little over time, and no symptoms develop.

Although side effects from mexiletine are common, most are mild and abate when the dose is reduced or the drug discontinued.

CONCLUSION

Mexiletine is an effective antiarrhythmic drug that suppresses spontaneous arrhythmia in almost 60% of patients, and 15% to 30% of patients respond when electrophysiologic testing is used. Drug efficacy can be enhanced when combinations of mexiletine with β-blockers or other membrane drugs are administered. Although mexiletine rarely causes serious cardiovascular toxicity, disturbing side effects, primarily neurologic and gastrointestinal, are common and often limit the usefulness of this agent.

REFERENCES

1. Vaughan Williams EM: Subdivision of Class 1 drugs. In Reiser HJ, Horowitz LN (eds): Mechanism and Treatment of Cardiac Arrhythmias, Relevance of Basic Studies to Clinical Management. Baltimore: Urban & Schwartzenberg, 1985, pp 165–172.
2. Weld FM, Bigger JT Jr, Swistel D, et al: Electrophysiological effects of mexiletine (KÖ1173) on ovine cardiac Purkinje fibers. J Pharmacol Exp Ther 210:222, 1979.
3. Yamaguchi I, Singh BN, Mandel WJ: Electrophysiological actions of mexiletine on isolated rabbit atria and canine ventricular muscle and Purkinje fibres. Cardiovasc Res 13:288, 1979.
4. Hering S, Bodewei R, Wollenberger A: Sodium current in freshly isolated and in cultured single rat myocardial cells: Frequency and voltage-dependent block by mexiletine. J Mol Cell Cardiol 15:431, 1983.
5. Allan DJ, Kelly JG, James RGG, et al: Comparison of the effects of lidocaine and mexiletine on experimental ventricular arrhythmias. Postgrad Med J 53(Suppl 1):30, 1977.
6. Hashimoto K, Ishii M, Lomori S: Antiarrhythmic plasma concentrations of mexiletine on canine ventricular arrhythmias. J Cardiovasc Pharmacol 6:213, 1984.
7. McComish M, Robinson C, Kitson D, et al: Clinical electrophysiological effects of mexiletine. Postgrad Med J 53(Suppl 1):85, 1977.
8. Roos JC, Paalman DCA, Dunning AJ: Electrophysiological effects of mexiletine in man. Postgrad Med J 53(Suppl 1):92, 1977.
9. Waspe LE, Waxman HL, Buxton AE, et al: Mexiletine for control of drug-resistant ventricular tachycardia: Clinical electrophysiologic results in 44 patients. Am J Cardiol 51:1175, 1983.
10. Prescott LF, Clements JA, Pottage A: Absorption, distribution and elimination of mexiletine. Postgrad Med J 53(Suppl 1):50, 1977.
11. Haselbarth V, Doevendans JE, Wolf M: Kinetics and bioavailability of mexiletine in healthy subjects. Clin Pharmacol Ther 29:729, 1981.
12. Campbell NPS, Kelly JG, Adgey AAJ, et al: The clinical pharmacology of mexiletine. Br J Clin Pharmacol 6:103, 1978.
13. Pentikainen PJ, Halinen MO, Helin MJ: Pharmacokinetics of intravenous mexiletine in patients with acute myocardial infarction. J Cardiovasc Pharmacol 6:1, 1984.
14. Pentikainen PJ, Halinen MO, Helin MJ: Pharmacokinetics of oral mexiletine in patients with acute myocardial infarction. Eur J Clin Pharmacol 25:773, 1983.
15. Woolsey RL, Wang T, Stone W, et al: Pharmacology, electrophysiology and pharmacokinetics of mexiletine. Am Heart J 107:1058, 1984.
16. Kiddie MA, Kaye CM, Turner P: The influence of urinary pH on the elimination of mexiletine. Br J Clin Pharmacol 1:229, 1974.
17. Johnston A, Burgess CD, Warrington SJ, et al: The effect of spontaneous changes in urinary pH on mexiletine plasma concentrations and excretion during chronic administration to healthy volunteers. Br J Clin Pharmacol 8:349, 1979.
18. El Allaf D, Henrard L, Crochelet L, et al: Pharmacokinetics of mexiletine in renal insufficiency. Br J Clin Pharmacol 14:431, 1982.
19. Wang T, Wuellner D, Woolsey RL, et al: Pharmacokinetics and dialyzability of mexiletine in renal failure. Clin Pharmacol Ther 37:649, 1985.
20. Herzog P, Holtermuller KH, Kasper W, et al: Absorption of mexiletine after treatment with gastric antacids. Br J Clin Pharmacol 8:349, 1979.
21. Pentikainen PJ, Koivula IH, Hilunen HA: Effect of rifampicin

treatment on the kinetics of mexiletine. Eur J Clin Pharmacol 23:261, 1982.

22. Begg EJ, Chinwah PM, Webb C, et al: Enhanced metabolism of mexiletine after phenytoin administration. Br J Clin Pharmacol 14:219, 1982.

23. Grech-Belanger O, Gilbert M, Turgeon J, et al: Effect of cigarette smoking on mexiletine kinetics. Clin Pharmacol Ther 37:638, 1985.

24. Klein A, Sami M, Selinger K: Mexiletine kinetics in healthy subjects taking cimetidine. Clin Pharmacol Ther 37:669, 1985.

25. Wing LMH, Meffin PH, Grygeil JJ, et al: The effect of metoclopramide and atropine on the absorption of orally administered mexiletine. Br J Clin Pharmacol 9:505, 1980.

26. Carlier J: Hemodynamic, electrocardiographic, and toxic effects of the intravenous administration of increasing doses of mexiletine in the dog. Comparison with similar effects produced by other antiarrhythmics. Acta Cardiol (Brux) 25(Suppl):81, 1980.

27. Marshall RJ, Muir AW, Winslow E: Comparative antidysrhythmic and haemodynamic effects of orally or intravenously administered mexiletine and ORG 6001 in the anaesthetized rat. Br J Pharmacol 74:381, 1981.

28. Beltrame J, Aylward PE, McRitchie RJ, et al: Comparative haemodynamic effects of lidocaine, mexiletine, and disopyramide. J Cardiovasc Pharmacol 6:483, 1984.

29. Banin S, DaSilva A, Stone G, et al: Observations of the haemodynamics of mexiletine. Postgrad Med J 53:74, 1987.

30. Saunamaki KI: Haemodynamic effects of a new anti-arrhythmic agent, mexiletine (KO 1173), in ischaemic heart disease. Cardiovasc Res 9:788, 1975.

31. Henard L, Carlier J: Hemodynamic effects of an intravenous injection of mexiletine in patients hospitalized in intensive care units. Acta Cardiol (Brux) 25:101, 1980.

32. Pozenel H: Haemodynamic studies on mexiletine—a new antiarrhythmic agent. Postgrad Med J 53:78, 1977.

33. Campbell NPS, Zaidi SA, Adgey AAJ, et al: Observations on the hemodynamic effects of mexiletine. Br Heart J 41:182, 1979.

34. Kuhn P, Klicpera M, Kroiss A, et al: Antiarrhythmic and hemodynamic effects of mexiletine. Postgrad Med J 53(Suppl 1):81, 1977.

35. Stein J, Podrid P, Lown B: Effects of oral mexiletine on left and right ventricular function. Am J Cardiol 54:575, 1984.

36. Allen JD, Kofi Ekui M, Shanks RG, et al: The effect of KO 1173, new anticonvulsant agent, on experimental cardiac arrhythmias. Br J Pharmacol 45:561, 1972.

37. Talbot RG: Mexiletine. Am Heart J 89:537, 1975.

38. Talbot RG, Julian DG, Prescott LF: Long-term treatment of ventricular arrhythmia with oral mexiletine. Am Heart J 91:58, 1976.

39. Esser H, Kikis D: Behandlung von Rhythmusstorungen ventrikularin ayprungs mit KO 1173 (Mexiletine). Med Klin 72:1386, 1972.

40. Waleffe A, Kulbertus HE: The efficacy of intravenous mexiletine in ventricular ectopic activity. Acta Cardiol (Brux) 32:269, 1977.

41. Abinader EG, Cooper M: Mexiletine use in control of drug resistant ventricular arrhythmia. JAMA 242:337, 1979.

42. Meoli P, Sanna GP, Rovelli F: Studio clinico controllato con Holter e con livelli emtici della mexieltina nelle aritmie ventricolai. G Ital Cardiol 12:115, 1982.

43. Masotti G, Marettini A, Casolo GC, et al: Efficacy of mexiletine in the medium term treatment of ventricular arrhythmias: A randomized, double blind crossover trial against placebo in ambulatory patients. J Int Med Res 12:73, 1984.

44. Santinelli V, Chiariello M, Stanislao M, et al: Efficacia del mixiletine nel trattamento delle tachicardia ventricolori resistenti alla lidocaina: Resulti preliminari. G Ital Cardiol 12:454, 1982.

45. Wang RYC, Lu PK, Wong KL, et al: Mexiletine in the treatment of recurrent ventricular tachycardia. Prediction of long-term arrhythmia suppression from acute and short-term response. Clin Pharmacol 23:89, 1983.

46. Fenster PE, Kern KB: Mexiletine for refractory ventricular arrhythmia. Clin Pharmacol Ther 34:777, 1983.

47. Podrid PJ, Lown B: Mexiletine for ventricular arrhythmias. Am J Cardiol 47:895, 1981.

48. Flaker GC, Madigan NP, Alpert MA, et al: Mexiletine for recur-
ring ventricular arrhythmias. Assessment by long-term electrocardiographic recordings and sequential electrophysiologic studies. Am Heart J 108:490, 1984.

49. Poole JE, Werner JA, Bardy GH, et al: Intolerance and ineffectiveness of mexiletine in patients with serious ventricular arrhythmias. Am Heart J 112:322, 1986.

50. Rutledge JC, Harris F, Amsterdam TA: Clinical evaluation of oral mexiletine therapy in the treatment of ventricular arrhythmias. J Am Coll Cardiol 6:780, 1985.

51. Talbot RG, Clark RA, Nimmo J, et al: Treatment of ventricular arrhythmias with mexiletine (KO 1173). Lancet 2:399, 1973.

52. Mehta J, Conti LR: Mexiletine, a new antiarrhythmic agent for treatment of ventricular premature complexes. Am J Cardiol 49:455, 1982.

53. Stein J, Podrid PJ, Lampert J, et al: Long-term mexiletine for ventricular arrhythmia. Am Heart J 107:1091, 1984.

54. Mason JW, for the Electrophysiologic Study versus Electrocardiographic Monitoring Investigators: A comparison of seven antiarrhythmic drugs in patients with ventricular tachyarrhythmias. N Engl J Med 329:452, 1993.

55. DiMarco JP, Goran H, Ruskin JN: Mexiletine for refractory ventricular arrhythmias: Results using serial electrophysiologic testing. Am J Cardiol 47:131, 1981.

56. Schoenfeld MH, Whitford E, McGovern B, et al: Oral mexiletine in the treatment of refractory ventricular arrhythmias. The role of electrophysiologic techniques. Am Heart J 107:1071, 1984.

57. Manz M, Steinbeck G, Nitsch J, et al: Treatment of occurring sustained ventricular tachycardia with mexiletine disopyramide control by programmed ventricular stimulation. Br Heart J 49:222, 1983.

58. Palileo EV, Welch W, Hoff J, et al: Lack of effectiveness of oral mexiletine in patients with drug refractory paroxysmal sustained ventricular tachycardia. Am J Cardiol 50:1075, 1982.

59. Kim SG, Seiden SW, Matos JA, et al: Discordance between ambulatory monitoring and programmed stimulation in assessing efficacy of mexiletine in patients with ventricular tachycardia. Am Heart J 112:14, 1986.

60. Saksena A, Craelius W: The electropharmacology and therapeutic role of mexiletine. Clin Prog Pacing Electrophysiol 1:122, 1983.

61. Campbell NPS, Shanks RG, Tilly JG, et al: Long term oral antiarrhythmic therapy with mexiletine. Postgrad Med J 53(Suppl 1):143, 1977.

62. Campbell RWF, Achuff SC, Pottage A, et al: Mexiletine in prophylaxis of ventricular arrhythmia during acute myocardial infarction. J Cardiovasc Pharmacol 1:43, 1979.

63. Campbell RWF, Dolder MA, Prescott LF, et al: Comparison of procainamide and mexiletine in the prevention of ventricular arrhythmias after acute myocardial infarction. Lancet 1:1257, 1975.

64. IMPACT Research Group: International mexiletine and placebo antiarrhythmic coronary trial. 1. Report on arrhythmia and other findings. J Am Coll Cardiol 4:1148, 1984.

65. Horowitz JD, Anaveker JN, Morris PM, et al: Comparative trial of mexiletine and lidocaine on the treatment of early ventricular tachyarrhythmias after acute myocardial infarction. J Cardiovasc Pharmacol 3:409, 1981.

66. Singh JB, Rasul AM, Shah A, et al: Efficacy of mexiletine in chronic ventricular arrhythmia compared with quinidine. A single blind randomized trial. Am J Cardiol 53:84, 1984.

67. Fenster PE, Hanson CD: Mexiletine and quinidine in ventricular ectopy. Clin Pharmacol Ther 34:136, 1983.

68. Arakawa K, Doi Y, Hashiba K, et al: Well controlled comparative study of the clinical effectiveness of intravenous mexiletine and procainamide on premature ventricular contractions. Jpn Heart J 25:357, 1984.

69. Jewitt DE, Jackson G, McCornish M: Comparative antiarrhythmic efficacy of mexiletine, procainamide and tolamolol in patients with symptomatic arrhythmias. Postgrad Med J 53(Suppl 1):158, 1977.

70. Myburgh DP, Goldman AP: The antiarrhythmic efficacy of perhexiline maleate, disopyramide and mexiletine in ventricular ectopic activity. S Afr Med J 54:1053, 1978.

71. Trimarco B, Volpe M, Ricciardelli B, et al: Disopyramide and mexiletine: Which is the agent of choice on the long term

oral treatment of lidocaine responsive arrhythmias? Efficacy comparison on a randomized trial. Arch Int Pharmacodyn Ther 248:251, 1980.

72. Breithardt G, Seipel L, Abendroth RR: Comparison of the antiarrhythmic efficacy of disopyramide and mexiletine against stimulus induced ventricular tachycardia. J Cardiovasc Pharmacol 3:1027, 1981.

73. Hession M, Blum R, Podrid PJ, et al: Mexiletine and tocainide: Does response to one predict response to the other? J Am Coll Cardiol 7:338, 1986.

74. Breithardt G, Seipel L, Lersmacher J, et al: Comparative study of the antiarrhythmic efficacy of mexiletine and disopyramide in patients with chronic ventricular arrhythmias. J Cardiovasc Pharmacol 4:276, 1982.

75. Hurwitz A: Antacid therapy and drug kinetics. Clin Pharmacokinet 2:269, 1977.

76. Jerlin MJ, Breckenridge AM: Drug interactions with warfarin. Drugs 25:610, 1983.

77. Leahy EB, Bigger JT, Butler VD, et al: Quinidine-digoxin interaction: Time course and pharmacokinetics. Am J Cardiol 48:1141, 1981.

78. Moysey JO, Jaggarao NJU, Grundy EN, et al: Amiodarone increases plasma digoxin concentrations. Br Med J 182:272, 1981.

79. Klein HO, Lang R, Weiss E, et al: The influence of verapamil on serum digoxin concentrations. Circulation 65:998, 1982.

80. Leahy EB, Reiffel JA, Giardina E, et al: The effect of quinidine and other oral antiarrhythmic drugs on serum digoxin. A prospective study. Ann Intern Med 92:605, 1980.

81. Sales SD, Lowenthal DT, Affrime MB: Steady state digoxin concentration during oral mexiletine administration. Curr Ther Res 34:662, 1983.

82. Leahy EB, Heissenbuttil RH, Giardina E, et al: Combined mexiletine and propranolol treatment of refractory ventricular tachycardia. Br Med J 281:375, 1980.

83. Bigger JT: The interaction of mexiletine with other cardiovascular drugs. Am Heart J 107:1079, 1984.

84. Pacholke H, Back DA, Hochrein H: Antiarrhythmische Wirkungsverstarkung durch kombinerte Andwendung von Mexiletin and Propranolol. Dtsch Med Wochenschr 109:330, 1984.

85. Hirsowitz G, Podrid PJ, Lampert J, et al: The role of beta blocking agents as adjunct therapy to membrane stabilizing drugs in malignant ventricular arrhythmia. Am Heart J 111:852, 1986.

86. Duff HJ, Roden D, Primme EK, et al: Mexiletine in the treatment of resistant ventricular arrhythmias: Enhancement of efficacy and reduction of dose related side effects by combination with quinidine. Circulation 67:1124, 1983.

87. Giardina EGV, Wechsler ME: Low dose quinidine-mexiletine combination therapy versus quinidine monotherapy for treatment of ventricular arrhythmia. J Am Coll Cardiol 15:1138, 1990.

88. Greenspan AM, Speilman JR, Webb CR, et al: Efficacy of combination therapy with mexiletine and a type 1A agent for inducible ventricular tachyarrhythmias secondary to coronary artery disease. Am J Cardiol 56:277, 1985.

89. Whitford EG, McGovern B, Ruskin JN: Long-term efficacy of mexiletine alone and in combination with class 1A antiarrhythmic drugs for refractory ventricular arrhythmias. Am Heart J 115:360, 1988.

90. Kim SG, Mercando AD, Tam S, Fisher JD: Combination of disopyramide and mexiletine for better tolerance and additive effects for treatment of ventricular arrhythmias. J Am Coll Cardiol 13:659, 1989.

91. Mendes L, Podrid PJ, Fuchs T, Franklin S: Role of combination therapy with a class lC antiarrhythmic agent and mexiletine for ventricular tachycardia. J Am Coll Cardiol 17:1396, 1991.

92. Yeung-Lai-Wah JA, Murdock CJ, Borne J, Kerr CR: Propafenone mexiletine combination for the treatment of sustained ventricular tachycardia. J Am Coll Cardiol 20:547, 1992.

93. Waleffe A, Mary-Rabin L, Legrand D, et al: Combined mexiletine and amiodarone treatment of refractory recurrent ventricular tachycardia. Am Heart J 100:788, 1980.

94. Data on file. Boehringer Ingelfield, Ridgefield, CT, 1981.

95. Podrid PJ, Lampert S, Graboys JB, et al: Aggravation of arrhythmias by antiarrhythmic drugs: Incidence and predictors. Am J Cardiol 59:38E, 1987.

96. Ravid S, Podrid PJ, Lampert S, Lown B: Congestive heart failure induced by six of the newer antiarrhythmia drugs. J Am Coll Cardiol 14:1326, 1989.

CHAPTER 144

Moricizine

Joel Morganroth, M.D., and Freddy Abi-Samra, M.D.

HISTORY

Moricizine hydrochloride was synthesized in 1964 by Gritsenko et al.[1] at the Institute for Pharmacology of the Academy of Medical Sciences of the Soviet Union. In the past, the compound was called Ethmozin, Ethmosine, or Etmozin, and only later has its generic name been changed to moricizine and its trade name to Ethmozine.

The clinical development of moricizine as an orally administered antiarrhythmic agent spans a 21-year period from 1966 to 1987. Clinical trials conducted in the Soviet Union[2] from 1966 to 1971 led to its general use there in 1971. The drug was administered in daily doses of 10 to 75 mg three times a day. Studies conducted in the United States began in June 1976. As a result, the total daily dosage recommendations were increased to 600 to 900 mg, administered in three divided doses every 8 hours. The clinical develop-

ment was interrupted on two occasions because of preclinical findings. The first interruption in 1978 was due to unexplained monkey deaths, which were later found to be the result of a dosing error. The second, in 1982, was due to proliferative rat liver changes that were later classified as hyperplastic nodules. Nevertheless, after further trials were conducted in the United States,[3-9] it was approved by the United States Food and Drug Administration (FDA) in June 1990 to treat documented life-threatening ventricular arrhythmias. Moricizine along with encainide and flecainide was evaluated in post–myocardial infarction patients with asymptomatic ventricular ectopic beats in the Cardiac Arrhythmia Suppression Trial (CAST). Although adequate suppression of ventricular ectopic activity (VEA) could be achieved, mortality was increased with the use of encainide and flecainide and not significantly modified by the use of moricizine.

CAST II,[10] comparing moricizine with placebo, was terminated because of a low probability of a long-term survival benefit from the use of moricizine and because it enhanced mortality in the first 2 weeks of its use when compared with placebo.

After CAST II, plans for multicenter trials investigating the usefulness of moricizine for the treatment of paroxysmal supraventricular tachycardia (PSVT) and of atrial fibrillation were scrubbed.

CHEMISTRY

Structurally, moricizine is composed of a phenothiazine nucleus and two side chains. It is a white to off-white powder with the chemical name 10-(3-morpholinopropionyl)phenothiazine-2-carbamic acid ethyl ester hydrochloride.[11, 12] The morpholino side chain appears to be necessary for its antiarrhythmic activity. Moricizine has a lower pK_a (6.4) than other phenothiazines, which may account in part for its lesser degree of central nervous system effects.

PHARMACOLOGY
Clinical

After oral administration of conventional or radiolabeled moricizine to humans, both absorption and metabolism occur rapidly, as evidenced by peak plasma concentrations at 1 to 3 hours for both parent drug and total radioactivity.[13, 14] Although it is virtually completely absorbed from the gastrointestinal tract, moricizine has an absolute oral bioavailability in patients of only 38%, presumably because of first-pass metabolism.[15] Relative bioavailability (tablet versus solution) is 100%, and the presence of food delays absorption and slightly diminishes peak concentrations.[13]

Moricizine, like other phenothiazines, is extensively metabolized (>99%); between 20 and 30 proposed metabolites are found in human urine. No single confirmed or putative metabolite represents more than 1% of the administered dose.[13] It is unlikely that moricizine metabolism is under the same genetic control inherent in the oxidative metabolism of drugs such as debrisoquine or propranolol.[16] The extensive metabolism of moricizine, together with the fact that its systemic clearance approaches a theoretical limiting value of hepatic blood or plasma flow, suggests that moricizine has intermediate to high hepatic clearance.[14, 17]

After administration of a radiolabeled oral dose of moricizine to volunteers, 39% of the dose was found in urine and 57% in feces. Urinary excretion of radioactivity was complete within 48 hours, whereas fecal excretion persisted for up to 5 days.[14]

After a single intravenous bolus of moricizine was administered to patients, plasma clearance was 1.3 L/min, and the apparent volume of distribution was 210 L, resulting in an elimination half-life of 1.9 hours.[18] However, the elimination half-life in patients after oral administration is longer, ranging from 2 to 12 hours. A positive linear relationship exists between the dose in milligrams and both peak concentrations and area under the plasma concentration time curve. In contrast with single doses, multiple-dose pharmacokinetics suggest some nonlinearity in oral clearance. It is possible that with repeated administration of moricizine, hepatic enzyme induction occurs, accounting for an enhanced clearance.[13]

Although moricizine is distributed extensively (the oral distribution ranges from 200 to 600 L and is independent of body weight),[13] it has a high affinity for plasma proteins (approximately 93% bound). Thus, minor changes in protein binding (perhaps by displacement of moricizine by its metabolites or other drugs, or changes in binding capacity due to disease processes) potentially can transiently increase the free fraction and possibly the concentration of free moricizine as well. The fraction of moricizine bound to protein remains constant for doses in the therapeutic dosage.

Although steady-state trough plasma levels in patients who respond to moricizine therapy are significantly higher than in those who do not respond, monitoring of therapeutic concentrations is not useful clinically because of the drug's complex metabolism and the possible presence of active metabolites.[13, 17]

Clinical studies have been conducted in humans using a dosage regimen of every 8 hours. Data from patients with ventricular arrhythmias suggest that moricizine can be administered safely and effectively every 12 hours.[19, 20]

Drug Interactions

Cimetidine inhibits hepatic microsomal enzymes and thus decreases the clearance of many drugs.[21] When administered in combination, cimetidine decreases the clearance of moricizine by 48%, increases its mean plasma elimination half-life by 35%, and increases plasma concentrations by 40%.[21, 22] However, concomitant cimetidine administration did not result in further prolongation of PR and QRS intervals as induced by moricizine. In contrast with cimetidine, ranitidine does not alter moricizine metabolism.[23] Drugs that decrease hepatic blood flow, such as β-blockers like propranolol,[24] also may decrease the clearance of moricizine. Conversely, moricizine does not affect the pharmacokinetics of digoxin.[25, 26] Moricizine increases the plasma concentration of theophylline by 46% to 68% and decreases its elimination half-life by 20% to 34%.[23] Therefore, plasma theophylline concentrations should be monitored when moricizine is added. Although moricizine may slightly shorten the elimination half-life of warfarin,[23] neither the prothrombin time nor the warfarin dosage changes significantly after administration of moricizine is begun.

Electrophysiology

Moricizine is a class I antiarrhythmic drug. In preclinical studies it produces a dose-dependent decrease in maximal rate of phase 0 depolarization,[19] speeds repolarization of phases 2 and 3, decreases action potential duration (APD), and shortens effective refractory period (ERP) in canine Purkinje fibers. It does not affect the slope of phase 4 depolarization[19] but depresses both normal and abnormal automaticity by increasing transmembrane threshold voltage. In addition, it suppresses both early and delayed afterdepolarizations and triggered activity.

In humans, a single oral dose of 5.2 to 10.3 mg/kg has no significant effect on intracardiac conduction intervals or refractory periods.[27] Atrial and ventricular refractory periods and the corrected QT (QT_c) interval are not affected significantly.[28] The administration of multiple oral doses of moricizine to humans is associated with significant increases in the duration of the PR, AH, HV, QRS, and QT_c intervals. The increase in the QT_c interval is due to prolongation of the QRS interval, because the JT interval actually is shortened.[11] The clinical electrophysiologic properties of moricizine are summarized in Table 144–1.

Sinus node function in dogs appears not to be altered by moricizine as studied by direct perfusion into the sinus node artery.[29] Moricizine produces a larger increase of the PR, AH, and HV intervals when these baseline intervals are abnormal than when they are normal. Conversely, in patients with sinus node dysfunction at rest, a significant depression is likely to be demonstrated, including development of sinus bradycardia, lengthening of sinus node recovery time, and induction of second-degree or complete sinoatrial block. Therefore, like other antiarrhythmic agents, moricizine should be used with caution in patients with overt sinus node disease.[30]

Also, moricizine abolishes antegrade conduction over the accessory pathway (7 of 15 patients) and blocks retrograde conduction (5 of 27 patients), depressing conduction and prolonging the refractory periods of the accessory pathway.[30] However, in another study, electrophysiologic data indicated that infranodal conduction was prolonged but refractory periods were not consistently affected.[31] Limited data are available regarding the effects of moricizine on defibrillation energy requirements. Ujhelyi et al. showed that moricizine minimally increased defibrillation threshold (DFT) in dogs. However, when ad-

ministered in combination with lidocaine, it resulted in an 84% rise in DFT. This may have detrimental clinical implications.[32] There is some confusion with the classification of moricizine by the Vaughan Williams system. Much of the confusion is due to differences in concept about the key features used to classify the antiarrhythmic actions of drugs. Drugs with class I antiarrhythmic action bind to molecules in the Na^+ channel, impeding the inward surge of I_{Na} during activation. This translates into slowing of phase 0 of the action potential and slowing of the conduction, especially of premature impulses or those arising at low levels of transmembrane voltage.

Most pharmacologists subclassify drugs by their intensity of action in blocking the Na^+ channel: IB, weakest; IA, intermediate; and IC, the strongest.[33]

The Harrison modification of the Vaughan Williams classification featured effects on repolarization.[34] Class IA drugs tend to prolong APD in ventricular tissues. Class IB drugs tend to shorten the APD, whereas IC drugs have very little effect on repolarization.

Clearly, when classified by intensity of effect on the Na^+ channel, moricizine has type IA action. However, it also shortens APD (IB) and markedly depresses AV nodal, His purkinje, and ventricular conduction. Both the onset and offset kinetics of moricizine are slow (IC).[35]

Left Ventricular Function and Hemodynamics

The effects of moricizine on left ventricular function have been studied using echocardiographic, hemodynamic, and radionuclide assessments. Left ventricular performance is not affected by moricizine, even in patients with baseline left ventricular dysfunction. In patients with left ventricular ejection fractions of more than 30%, moricizine is well tolerated, but clinical deterioration of left ventricular function has been observed.[36] When data from patients' first exposures to moricizine were compared with baseline values, no statistically significant changes were observed in stroke volume, left ventricular ejection fraction, cardiac index, systemic vascular resistance, mean pulmonary artery pressure, pulmonary artery wedge pressure, and pulmonary vascular resistance. Small but statistically significant increases in mean arterial pressure, systolic blood pressure, and heart rate were seen, the causes of which are unknown. None of the changes in the heart rate or blood pressure was of clinical significance.[13]

In one placebo-controlled study,[37] left ventricular functions during rest and exercise were measured during right-sided catheterization in 20 patients with ventricular tachycardia. Moricizine was hemodynamically well tolerated in all but three patients. The latter could be identified by their inability to increase stroke volume during exercise. Furthermore, the hemodynamic response to moricizine during exercise appeared to predict the antiarrhythmic response to the drug. A depressed response to exercise was associated with an unfavorable antiarrhythmic overcome.

Table 144–1. **Effect of Moricizine on Clinical Electrophysiologic Variables**

Variable	No. of Patients	Control Values (msec)	Change with Moricizine	
			msec	*%*
Sinus cycle length	37	807	−64	−8*
PR interval	43	177	+36	+20†
AH interval	39	87	+15	+17†
HV interval	45	56	+14	+26
QRS interval	47	114	+21	+19†
QT_c interval	40	428	+20	+5
JT interval	43	265	−14	−5
RV ERP	22	246	+10	+4*

*$p <.05$.
†$p <.01$.
ERP, effective refractory period.

Of the 1072 patients in whom moricizine was used in uncontrolled trials in the United States,[38] 467 (44%) had a clinical history of congestive heart failure (CHF) and 71 (15%) had exacerbation of their heart failure. In the remaining 605 patients (56%) without previous CHF, symptoms of heart failure developed in 5 (0.8%). CHF was judged to be definitely related to moricizine in 12 patients (1%), whereas it was possibly due to the drug in another 12 patients (1%). CHF occurred within 2 weeks in 39 of 76 patients and within a year in 74 patients. The drug was discontinued in only 33 patients.

Overall, moricizine is relatively well tolerated by patients with left ventricular dysfunction and/or CHF, but its efficacy in preventing sustained ventricular arrhythmia decreased in those patients.[38]

EFFICACY

Measuring the efficacy of any antiarrhythmic drug is at best a difficult task. The ability of a drug to reduce the frequency of premature ventricular complexes and nonsustained ventricular tachycardia during ambulatory monitoring is often different from its ability to suppress inducibility of ventricular tachycardia by exercise or electrophysiologic testing. Furthermore, efficacy (as measured by any technique) is intimately related to the left ventricular ejection fraction, presence or absence of CHF, and the type of underlying heart disease. Finally and most importantly, laboratory efficacy may not accurately predict clinical benefits. In fact, the CAST study, for instance, showed a dissociation between the suppression of ventricular premature complex and the incidence of sudden cardiac death.

Efficacy of moricizine has been demonstrated in patients with benign or potentially lethal ventricular arrhythmias.[4-6, 19, 39-43] The effects of moricizine have also been documented in patients with lethal or malignant ventricular arrhythmias.[7, 8, 28, 30, 31, 44, 45] Drug efficacy was assessed by Holter monitoring, programmed electrical stimulation, and exercise tolerance tests (Table 144–2).[13]

Effect on Premature Ventricular Complexes and Nonsustained Ventricular Tachycardia

Holter monitoring data demonstrated that the onset of efficacy generally occurred within the first 24 hours

Table 144–2. **Summary of Efficacy Results in Patients with Ventricular Ectopy**

| Method | Patients with Efficacy | | |
	Controlled Studies	Compassionate Use	All Patients*
Holter	361/535 (76%)	34/55 (62%)	390/583 (67%)
PES	23/67 (34%)	11/50 (22%)	34/117 (29%)
ETT	26/34 (76%)	5/7 (71%)	31/41 (76%)
Global	—	121/254 (48%)	121/254 (48%)

PES, programmed electrical stimulation; ETT, exercise tolerance test.
*Patients evaluated both in controlled studies and in a compassionate use trial are counted only once.
From DuPont Pharmaceuticals, New Drug Application. Clinical Summary. Wilmington, DE, September, 1987. Used with permission.

of therapy, and patients who responded to moricizine did so within 3 to 5 days. Loading-dose regimens indicated that, although a greater suppression of ventricular ectopy was obtained in the first 7 hours of therapy, the time to achieve continuous suppression of ventricular arrhythmia was not significantly shortened relative to the usual dosage regimen, and these regimens have demonstrated potential for higher toxicity.[13]

In controlled clinical trials, approximately 20% of patients who received initial dosages of only 300 or 450 mg daily responded with a 75% or more reduction in mean hourly frequency of total ventricular complexes. Although the number of patients who received these doses was small, data suggest that initiation of therapy at this level would produce inappropriate delay in determining an effective dose in most instances. Efficacy of the drug was demonstrated in approximately half of patients who received 600 mg daily (200 mg every 8 hours). Efficacy was also shown with 750 and 900 mg; few additional patients achieved efficacy at doses exceeding 900 mg/day (Fig. 144–1). However, some patients have responded to moricizine using as much as 1350 mg/day.[11]

Approximately 50% of patients with lethal ventricular arrhythmias were judged to have efficacious responses to moricizine, compared with 70% of patients with potentially lethal or benign ventricular arrhythmias.[13] In patients with benign or potentially lethal ventricular arrhythmias, moricizine may be efficacious when given every 12 hours.[20]

Approximately 60% of patients in controlled trials with nonsustained ventricular tachycardia had abolition of ventricular tachycardia after 2 weeks of moricizine therapy. Response rates for total ventricular premature complexes (VPCs) or nonsustained ventricular tachycardia abolishment were not affected by age and only minimally affected by left ventricular ejection fraction. At the recommended total daily dosage of 600 to 900 mg, moricizine was more efficacious in patients with baseline left ventricular ejection fractions of at least 30% (approximately 58% responders) than in patients with left ventricular ejection fractions of less than 30% (51% responders).[13]

Comparative Studies

Moricizine also has been compared with other antiarrhythmic agents, including disopyramide, propranolol, and quinidine. In comparison studies, moricizine was more effective than disopyramide or propranolol.[43] In pooled analysis of the quinidine comparison studies, moricizine and quinidine generally were found to be equally effective depending on the total daily dose administered (Table 144–3). Moricizine always was more efficacious than quinidine in abolishment of ventricular tachycardia. Comparative data from CAPS evaluating moricizine versus encainide, flecainide, imipramine, and placebo (using a parallel design) indicated that moricizine was efficacious in 66% of patients, whereas 37% of patients responded

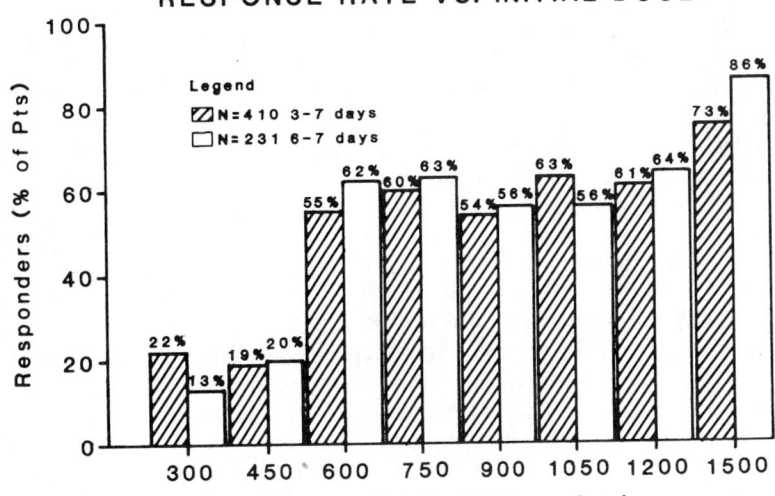

Figure 144–1. Response rate versus initial dose. (DuPont Pharmaceuticals, New Drug Application, clinical summary. Wilmington, DE, September 1987. Used with permission.)

to placebo. These patients were at high risk of sudden death because they had recently experienced myocardial infarction and had at least 10 VPCs an hour. In comparison, 52% of patients responded to imipramine, 79% to encainide, and 83% to flecainide.[13]

In CAPS, 52% of patients receiving 600 mg daily of moricizine responded; an additional 14% had efficacy when the total daily dose was increased to 750 mg daily. Moricizine was effective in 71% of patients with normal resting left ventricular function, in 67% of those with moderate decreases in ejection fraction at baseline (30% to 45%), and in 55% of those with low ejection fractions (22% to 29%).[13]

The effect of the suppression of ventricular ectopic activity by moricizine on subsequent mortality was examined in the CAST II study, which involved the randomization of patients with recent myocardial infarctions, asymptomatic or mildly symptomatic VPCs, and left ventricular ejection fraction of less than 40%.[46] During the initial 14-day exposure phase, 1325 patients were randomly assigned to receive placebo or moricizine. In this 2-week phase, treatment with moricizine was associated with an excess mortality (17 of 665 patients versus 3 of 660 patients given placebo; $p < .01$). In the long-term phase of the trial, there were

49 deaths among the 581 patients treated with moricizine as compared with 42 deaths among 574 patients receiving placebo ($p = .46$). The trial was discontinued because it was unlikely that a survival benefit would be achieved upon completion of the intended follow-up.

Effect on Sustained Ventricular Arrhythmias

In patients with a history of sustained ventricular tachycardia or fibrillation resistant to other antiarrhythmic drugs, short-term therapy with moricizine suppresses the induction of ventricular tachycardia as determined by electrophysiologic evaluation in 10% to 30% of patients.[7, 9, 28, 31] This is similar to other antiarrhythmic drugs.[47] In small studies of patients with reduced left ventricular ejection fraction, out-of-hospital cardiac arrest, or symptomatic ventricular tachycardia, who were also found to have inducible sustained ventricular arrhythmias, the arrhythmias remained inducible on follow-up electrophysiologic testing in 63% to 88% of patients after 1 to 37 days of treatment with oral moricizine at a dose of 10 to 15 mg/kg/day.[7, 28, 31] The tachycardia was slowed in one

Table 144–3. **Moricizine Versus Quinidine**

| | | | VPBs/hr | | | VT | |
| | | | | Patients with | | | Patients with |
Study	Drug	Mean Dose (mg/day)	Total Patients	≥75% Reduction	Mean Reduction	Total Patients	100% Reduction
N-10	Moricizine	767	17	7 (41%)	71%	15	15 (100%)
	Quinidine	1600	18	13 (72%)	90%	14	12 (86%)
N-26 and N-46	Moricizine	875	17	10 (59%)	84%	7	4 (57%)
	Quinidine	1288	13	5 (38%)	75%	4	2 (50%)
Post-MI Program*	Moricizine	788	17	6 (35%)	81%	12	11 (92%)
	Quinidine	1394	17	10 (59%)	78%	12	6 (50%)

MI, myocardial infarction; VPB, ventricular premature beats; VT, ventricular tachycardia.
*Interim analysis.

of these studies; ventricular tachycardia cycle length increased from 250 to 326 msec ($p < .001$).[28]

Programmed electrical stimulation studies were performed in 117 patients; this population consisted of 99 men and 18 women, with a mean age of 59.7 years. All 117 patients had cardiovascular disease, most commonly ischemic cardiomyopathy. Ejection fractions measured at baseline were obtained in 30 of the 117 patients, of whom 15 had ejection fractions of 30% or less and 24 had ejection fractions of 40% or less. Of the 117 patients, the investigators classified 34 (29%) as responders. Of these, 28 continued moricizine therapy for a mean of 203 days. Seventy-five of the 117 patients with paired electrophysiologic studies had sustained ventricular tachycardia inducible at baseline. In 25% of these patients given an average daily dose of 936 mg moricizine (12 mg/kg/day), sustained ventricular tachycardia was not inducible.[13]

Supraventricular Arrhythmias

Few data have been accumulated in patients with supraventricular arrhythmias, but an efficacious response has been demonstrated in patients with paroxysmal supraventricular tachycardia, frequent atrial premature complexes, and preexcitation syndrome.[48] Of particular interest is the apparent efficacy of moricizine in the treatment of ectopic atrial tachycardia, a frequently life-threatening arrhythmia in children and adolescents.[49, 50] In a small randomized study, we have found that when administered to patients with chronic atrial fibrillation, moricizine and quinidine were equally effective in maintaining normal sinus rhythm. Moricizine was, however, much better tolerated.

ADVERSE EFFECTS

Most adverse effects are reported during the first 2 weeks of drug therapy. Only 66 of the 1071 patients (6.2%) and subjects in moricizine trials discontinued the drug because of an adverse reaction. The most frequent adverse reactions requiring dosage reduction, particularly for individuals receiving 1200 to 1500 mg/day, were changes in electrocardiographic intervals, dizziness, and gastrointestinal complaints. Headache, hyperesthesia, and dizziness were the most frequently reported side effects in patients younger than 65 years of age, whereas cardiovascular events were more frequent in the geriatric group. Nausea and fatigue were also reported.[13]

Moricizine, like all other antiarrhythmic agents, can cause proarrhythmia. Of 908 patients with ventricular arrhythmias, 42 (3.2%) had a proarrhythmic episode. Of these, 19 (2.1%) died or experienced serious events such as the development of sustained ventricular tachycardia. Ten (1.1%) experienced less serious events, such as an increased frequency of nonsustained ventricular tachycardia beats or total VPCs. No difference was noted in the rate of serious proarrhythmias between patients with potentially lethal or lethal ventricular dysfunction. This finding suggests that proarrhythmia may be associated with moricizine less frequently than with other antiarrhythmic drugs (such as encainide or flecainide) in patients with malignant ventricular arrhythmias. Patients with lower left ventricular ejection fractions and more severe structural heart disease developed proarrhythmia more commonly than those with less-significant ventricular dysfunction. Proarrhythmia was not observed in patients with benign ventricular arrhythmias. No relationship was found between the daily dosage of moricizine and the incidence of proarrhythmia.[13]

Overall, fewer than 1% of patients with ventricular arrhythmias experienced congestive heart failure that may have been drug related. All events occurred in patients with prior histories of congestive heart failure or left ventricular dysfunction. Twelve patients experienced a 20% or greater decrease in left ventricular ejection fraction or cardiac index, but none discontinued moricizine or developed any clinical signs or symptoms of worsening congestive heart failure.[13]

In controlled clinical trials, patients taking moricizine had a slight increase (average, approximately 3 to 4 mmHg) in mean supine systolic blood pressure and a slight increase (2 to 5 beats/min) in heart rate compared with baseline measurements. No consistent change was observed in mean supine diastolic blood pressure. No patients were withdrawn from moricizine therapy because of these changes in vital signs.[13]

Consistent with the electrophysiologic findings noted previously, the 12-lead electrocardiographic (ECG) analysis indicated that moricizine was commonly associated with a slight increase in the PR (+12%), QRS (+14%), and QT_c (+2.1%) intervals. Again, the effect on the QT_c interval was due to the widening of the QRS complex, with shortening of the JT interval of 5%. Of 920 patients, only 10 had ECG changes of sufficient severity to warrant discontinuing moricizine treatment: 2 of 10 had AV block, 2 of 10 had junctional rhythms, 5 of 10 had marked intraventricular conduction defects, and 1 of 10 had frequent sinus pauses.[13]

Unlike other neuroleptic phenothiazines, moricizine has not been associated with any adverse reactions on the endocrine system related to dopaminergic antagonistic effects. There were no clinically significant effects on serum prolactin concentrations, and no patient developed galactorrhea or gynecomastia. Extrapyramidal effects such as dystonias or parkinsonian symptoms did not occur during moricizine therapy. Other neurologic side effects reported were sedation or drowsiness, insomnia, restlessness, anxiety, euphoria, agitation, depression, weakness, and headache.[13]

Moricizine was better tolerated than quinidine in crossover comparison studies. Gastrointestinal adverse reactions were more frequent during quinidine therapy (36% versus 3%), and the percentage of discontinuations was higher in the quinidine group (15% versus 4%).[13]

Six patients developed clinically significant elevations in serum liver enzymes that possibly were due to moricizine. The drug was not associated with anti-

Table 144–4. Adverse Effects Confirmed by Drug Washout: Drug/Dose Selection Phase in CAPS

Adverse Effect	Incidence of Adverse Effects (%)	
	Moricizine (n = 98)	Placebo (n = 100)
Proarrhythmia	1	3
Disqualifying VT	2	6
Conduction abnormalities	3	0
Congestive heart failure	0	0
Other adverse effects causing discontinuation	6	3

CAPS, Cardiac Arrhythmia Pilot Study; VT, ventricular tachycardia.
From DuPont Pharmaceuticals, New Drug Application, clinical summary. Wilmington, DE, September 1987. Used with permission.

nuclear antibody formation, and no new onset of the systemic lupus-like syndrome occurred in any patient receiving moricizine. Two patients (0.3% of those with evaluations) developed unexplained thrombocytopenia that may have been moricizine-related.[13] No ophthalmologic abnormalities were attributed to moricizine.[11]

For patients with potentially lethal ventricular arrhythmias, CAPS provides the best parallel placebo-controlled data on moricizine regarding comparative adverse effects. The adverse effects on 98 patients randomly assigned moricizine therapy were confirmed by drug washout and, when compared with placebo (Table 144–4), indicate a high rate of safety. During the long-term follow-up phase, tolerance of moricizine was comparable to that of placebo. The discontinuation rate due to adverse effects was 6% for patients taking moricizine versus 7% for those receiving placebo during this portion of the trial. Proarrhythmia, death, and cardiac arrest occurred more frequently in patients receiving placebo than those taking moricizine.[13]

CONCLUSION

Overall, moricizine has a relatively favorable toxicity profile; however, its effectiveness and safety in treating patients with varying arrhythmias have not yet been established.

Results from CAST II suggest that moricizine should not be given to post–myocardial infarction patients with left ventricular dysfunction and minimally symptomatic complex ventricular ectopy. There is currently no evidence that moricizine would be of any benefit in patients with dilated cardiomyopathy and ventricular ectopy. Although moricizine was highly effective in suppressing symptomatic (including syncope) ventricular ectopy in patients with mitral valve prolapse,[42] its effect on prevention of sudden cardiac death in this condition is unknown. Moricizine is useful as adjunctive therapy to suppress frequent nonsustained ventricular tachycardia in patients equipped with an internal cardioverter-defibrillator device. It is also useful in selected patients with inducible sustained ventricular tachycardia and

in young patients with ectopic atrial tachycardia. Moricizine may have a role in atrial fibrillation, particularly in patients with normal left ventricular ejection fraction (and therefore with a weak propensity toward proarrhythmia), but adequate supportive data are still lacking and may never become available.

REFERENCES

1. Gritsenko AN, Ermkova ZI, Zhuravlev SV: Synthesis of Ethmozine—a new drug with antiarrhythmic action. Khim Farm Zh 6:17, 1972.
2. Kaverina NV, Senova ZP, Mitrofanov VS, et al: Pharmacology of Ethmozine. Farmakol Toksikol 2:182, 1972.
3. The CAPS Investigators: The cardiac arrhythmia pilot study. Am J Cardiol 57:91, 1986.
4. Singh SN, DiBianco R, Gottdiener JS, et al: Effect of moricizine hydrochloride in reducing chronic high frequency ventricular arrhythmia: Results of a prospective, controlled trial. Am J Cardiol 53:745, 1984.
5. Pratt CM, Young JB, Francis MJ, et al: Comparative effect of disopyramide and ethmozine in suppressing complex ventricular arrhythmias by use of a double-blind, placebo controlled, longitudinal crossover design. Circulation 69:288, 1984.
6. Morganroth J, Pratt CM, Kennedy HL, et al: Efficacy and tolerance of Ethmozine (moricizine HCl) in placebo controlled trials. Am J Cardiol 60:48F, 1987.
7. Miura D, Wynn J, Torres V, et al: Antiarrhythmic efficacy of Ethmozine in patients with ventricular tachycardia as determined by programmed electrical stimulation. Am Heart J 111:661, 1986.
8. Pratt CM, Wierman A, Seals AA, et al: Efficacy and safety of moricizine in patients with ventricular tachycardia: Results of a placebo controlled prospective long-term clinical trial. Circulation 73:718, 1986.
9. Horowitz LN: Efficacy of moricizine in malignant ventricular arrhythmias. Am J Cardiol 65:41D, 1990.
10. The Cardiac Arrhythmia Suppression Trial II Investigators: Effect of the antiarrhythmic agent moricizine on survival after myocardial infarction. N Engl J Med 327:227, 1992.
11. Moricizine. In Merck Index, 10th ed. West Point, PA: Merck and Company, 1983.
12. Whitney CC, Weinstein SH, Gaylord JC: High performance liquid chromatographic determination of ethmozin in plasma. J Pharm Sci 70:462, 1981.
13. New Drug Application. DuPont Pharmaceuticals, Wilmington, DE, September 1987.
14. Howrie DL, Pieniaszek HJ, Fogoros RN, et al: Disposition of moricizine (Ethmozine) in healthy subjects after oral administration of radiolabeled drug. Eur J Clin Pharcacol 32:607, 1987.
15. Piotrovskii VK, Romina NN, Merkulova IN, et al: Bioavailability of Ethmozine with oral administration. Khim Farm Zh 221:912, 1983.
16. Alvan G, Von Bahr C, Seidman P, et al: High plasma concentration of β receptor blocking drugs and deficient debrisoquine hydroxylation. Lancet 1:333, 1982.
17. Woosley RL, Morganroth J, Fogoros R, et al: Pharmacokinetics of moricizine HCl. Am J Cardiol 60:35F, 1987.
18. Piotrovskii VK, Merkulova IN, Romina NN, Metelitsa VI: Pharmacokinetics of Ethmozine after a single intravenous injection. Kardiologiia 22:62, 1982.
19. Morganroth J, Pearlman AS, Dunkman WB, et al: Ethmozine: A new antiarrhythmic agent developed in the USSR. Efficacy and tolerance. Am Heart J 98:621, 1979.
20. Morganroth J: Safety and efficacy of a twice daily dosing regimen for moricizine (Ethmozine). Am Heart J 110:1188, 1985.
21. Powell JR, Donn KH: Histamine H2-antagonist drug interactions in perspective: Mechanistic concepts and clinical implications. Am J Med 77(5B):57, 1984.
22. Biollaz J, Shaheen O, Wood AJJ: Cimetidine inhibition of Ethmozine metabolism. Clin Pharmacol Ther 37:665, 1985.
23. Siddoway LA, Schwartz SL, Barbey JT, et al: Clinical pharmacokinetics of moricizine. Am J Cardiol 65:15D, 1990.

24. Bax NDS, Tucker GT, Lennard MS, et al: The impairment of lignocaine clearance by propranolol—major contribution from enzyme inhibition. Br J Clin Pharmacol 19:597, 1985.
25. MacFarland RT, Moeller VR, Pieniaszek HJ, et al: Assessment of the potential pharmacokinetic interaction between digoxin and Ethmozine. J Clin Pharmacol 25:138, 1985.
26. Kennedy HL, Sprague MK, Redd RM, et al: Serum digoxin concentrations during Ethmozine antiarrhythmic therapy. Am Heart J 111:667, 1986.
27. Morganroth J, Michelson EL, Kitchen JG, et al: Ethmozine: Electrophysiologic effects in man [abstract]. Circulation 64(Suppl IV):263, 1981.
28. Mann DE, Luck JC, Herre JM, et al: Electrophysiologic effects of Ethmozine in patients with ventricular tachycardia. Am Heart J 107:674, 1984.
29. Ruffy R, Rozenshtraukh LV, Elharrar V, et al: Electrophysiological effects of Ethmozine on canine myocardium. Cardiovascular Res 13:354, 1979.
30. Smetnev AS, Shugushev KK, Rosenshtraukh LV: Clinical, electrophysiologic and antiarrhythmic efficacy of moricizine HCl. Am J Cardiol 60:40F, 1987.
31. Dorian P, Echt DS, Mead RH, et al: Ethmozine: Electrophysiology, hemodynamics, and antiarrhythmic efficacy in patients with life-threatening ventricular arrhythmias. Am Heart J 112:327, 1986.
32. Ujhelyi MR, O'Raugers EA, Kluger J, et al: Defibrillation energy requirements during moricizine and moricizine-lidocaine therapy. J Cardiovasc Pharmacol 20:932, 1992.
33. Vaughan Williams EM: A classification of antiarrhythmic actions reassessed after a decade of new drugs. J Clin Pharmacol 24:129, 1984.
34. Harrison DC: Antiarrhythmic drug classification: New science and practical applications. Am J Cardiol 56:185, 1985.
35. Vaughan Williams EM: The relevance of cellular to clinical electrophysiology in classifying antiarrhythmic actions. J Cardiovasc Pharmacol 20(Suppl 2):S1, 1992.
36. Pratt CM, Podrid PJ, Seals AA, et al: Effects of Ethmozine (moricizine HCl) on ventricular function using echocardiographic, hemodynamic and radionuclide assessments. Am J Cardiol 60:73F, 1987.
37. Seals AA, English LD, Leon CA, et al: Hemodynamic effects of moricizine at rest and during supine bicycle exercise: Results in patients with ventricular tachycardia and left ventricular dysfunction. Am Heart J 112:36, 1985.
38. Podrid PJ, Beau SL: Antiarrhythmic drug therapy for congestive heart failure with focus on moricizine. Am J Cardiol 65:56D, 1990.
39. Podrid PJ, Lyakishev A, Lown B, Mazur N: Ethmozine, a new antiarrhythmic drug for suppressing ventricular premature complexes. Circulation 61:450, 1980.
40. Gear K, Marcus FI, Huang SK, et al: Ethmozine for ventricular premature complexes. Am J Cardiol 57:947, 1986.
41. Pratt CM, Yepsen SC, Taylor AA, et al: Ethmozine suppression of single and repetitive ventricular premature depolarizations during therapy: Documentation of efficacy and long-term safety. Am Heart J 106:85, 1983.
42. Pratt CM, Young JB, Wierman AM, et al: Complex ventricular arrhythmias associated with the mitral valve prolapse syndrome. Effectiveness of moricizine (ethmozine) in patients resistant to conventional antiarrhythmics. Am J Med 80:626, 1986.
43. Pratt CM, Butnam SM, Young JB, et al: Antiarrhythmic efficacy of Ethmozine (moricizine HCl) compared with disopyramide and propranolol. Am J Cardiol 60:52F, 1987.
44. Wyndham CRC, Pratt CM, Mann DE, et al: Electrophysiology of Ethmozine (moricizine HCl) for ventricular tachycardia. Am J Cardiol 60:67F, 1987.
45. Hession MJ, Lampert S, Podrid PJ, et al: Ethmozine (moricizine HCl) therapy for complex ventricular arrhythmias. Am J Cardiol 60:59F, 1987.
46. The Cardiac Arrhythmia Suppression Trial (CAST) Investigators: Preliminary report: Effect of encainide and flecainide on mortality in a randomized trial of arrhythmia suppression after myocardial infarctions. N Engl J Med 321:406, 1989.
47. Waxman HL, Buxton AE, Sadowski LM, et al: The response to procainamide during electrophysiologic study for sustained ventricular tachyarrhythmias predicts the response to other medications. Circulation 87:30, 1983.
48. Chazov EI, Shugusheu KK, Rosenshtraukh LV: Ethmozin I. Effects of intravenous drug administration on paroxysmal supraventricular tachycardia in the ventricular preexcitation syndrome. Am Heart J 108:475, 1984.
49. Evans VL, Garson A Jr, Smith RT, et al: Ethmozine (moricizine HCl): A providing drug for "automatic" atrial ectopic tachycardia. Am J Cardiol 60:83F, 1987.
50. Moak JP, Smith RT, Garson A Jr: Newer antiarrhythmic drugs in children. Am Heart J 113:179, 1986.

CHAPTER 145

Phenytoin

Richard N. Fogoros, M.D.

HISTORY

Phenytoin was first synthesized in 1908, and it has been used as an effective anticonvulsant since 1938. It was not until the early 1950s, however, that phenytoin was suggested as an antiarrhythmic agent. In 1958, the first such clinical use of phenytoin was reported. Leonard[1] successfully used the drug to suppress ventricular tachycardia in a patient whose arrhythmias had not responded to either quinidine or procainamide. The popularity of phenytoin as an antiarrhythmic agent appears to have peaked during the 1960s, a decade in which many reports describe its efficacy in treating ventricular arrhythmias.[2-4] However, in the 1970s, the United States Food and Drug Administration ruled that data were insufficient for formal approval of phenytoin for the treatment of cardiac arrhythmias. This ruling, and the subsequent approval of several newer antiarrhythmic drugs, caused phenytoin to largely fall out of favor as a treatment for arrhythmias. The use of phenytoin as an antiarrhythmic agent remains somewhat controversial. Some authorities simply do not consider the drug to be an effective agent against cardiac arrhythmias, except in very rare circumstances. Others have found it to be quite useful in several clinical situations.

PHARMACOLOGY

When administered orally, phenytoin is absorbed slowly and somewhat erratically, and variations in absorption can be compounded with use of different preparations of the drug. Thus, serum concentrations can peak at any time from 3 to 12 hours after an oral dose. Intramuscular administration is not recommended, because the drug precipitates in the tissues and absorption is slow. Phenytoin can be delivered rapidly to target tissues with intravenous administration, although the intravenous preparation of the drug is very alkaline, and phlebitis is common. Phlebitis can be minimized by giving the drug in intermittent injections rather than by continuous infusion and by injecting into a central vein. Phenytoin is extensively protein-bound. It is rapidly distributed to all tissues once absorption occurs.

Phenytoin is extensively metabolized by the liver to several inactive compounds; less than 5% of the administered drug is excreted unchanged in the urine. Phenytoin has biphasic elimination kinetics. At plasma concentrations of less than approximately 10 $\mu g/ml$, elimination is exponential, and the half-life is 6 to 12 hours. At higher plasma concentrations, elimination is dose-dependent, and plasma levels thus increase disproportionately with increases in dosage. This latter phenomenon is probably due to saturation of hepatic microsomal enzymes at higher plasma levels.[5]

For the treatment of ventricular arrhythmias, the therapeutic concentration of phenytoin is similar to that for treating seizures, 10 to 20 $\mu g/ml$.

ANTIARRHYTHMIC PROPERTIES OF PHENYTOIN

At least four properties of phenytoin render the drug potentially useful for the treatment of ventricular arrhythmias.

Class I Antiarrhythmic Effects

As summarized by Witt et al.,[6] phenytoin has a lidocaine-like effect on ion transport, resulting in a decrease in action potential duration and thus tissue refractoriness. Therefore, phenytoin is generally considered a class IB drug. In ischemic tissue, phenytoin can have a quinidine-like (class IA) effect on excitability; however, this is a property of other class IB drugs as well.[7]

Suppression of Automaticity

In animal models, phenytoin has been shown to suppress phase 4 activity[6] and therefore spontaneous diastolic depolarization.

Suppression of Triggered Activity

In animal models, phenytoin can suppress the afterdepolarizations thought to be responsible for digitalis-induced ventricular arrhythmias.[8]

Suppression of Sympathetic Tone

Phenytoin suppresses the sympathetic centers of the central nervous system, thus decreasing sympathetic activity in the cardiac nerves.[9-11]

CLINICAL USE OF PHENYTOIN IN THE TREATMENT OF CARDIAC ARRHYTHMIAS
Digitalis Toxicity

The least controversial use of phenytoin as an antiarrhythmic agent is in the treatment of digitalis-mediated tachyarrhythmias. The ability of phenytoin to suppress both atrial and ventricular arrhythmias associated with toxic levels of digitalis has been widely recognized since the early 1960s (digitalis toxicity is the only clinical setting in which phenytoin reliably treats atrial tachyarrhythmias). The drug's efficacy is thought to be due to its ability to suppress the afterdepolarizations seen with digitalis toxicity, although there may be a centrally mediated effect as well,[10] because intrathecally mediated phenytoin has been shown to be effective in treating these arrhythmias in dogs. When used in this clinical setting, phenytoin is generally administered intravenously, and the clinical response is usually quite rapid. Phenytoin is generally considered the antiarrhythmic drug of choice in the management of digitalis-mediated arrhythmias.

Ventricular Arrhythmias in Acutely Ill Patients

Several published reports in the 1960s pointed out the usefulness of phenytoin in managing ventricular arrhythmias in patients being treated in the intensive care setting. The drug was felt to be particularly effective in managing the arrhythmias seen with acute myocardial infarction, with the administration of general anesthesia, and during the early postoperative period. Although phenytoin largely has been supplanted by lidocaine in these settings, it is nonetheless occasionally helpful. Because arrhythmias occurring in the intensive care setting are generally not reentrant, the effect of phenytoin in these circumstances is probably a result of its suppression of automaticity and/or suppression of afterdepolarizations. In 1991, Hayashi et al.[11] reported that the suppressive effect of phenytoin on the epinephrine-induced arrhythmias in halothane-anesthetized dogs is centrally mediated. When used in acutely ill patients, phenytoin is generally administered intravenously. In our center, intravenously administered phenytoin is commonly used (usually after lidocaine has failed) in the management of postoperative ventricular arrhythmias, especially after cardiac surgery.

Ventricular Arrhythmias After Surgery for Congenital Heart Disease

Several reports since the 1970s have suggested that phenytoin may be particularly useful in the treatment of the chronic complex ventricular ectopy associated with surgical repair of congenital heart disease.[12-14] Such arrhythmias have been considered difficult to suppress, and orally administered phenytoin offers a relatively attractive alternative, because the drug has been used for decades in young people for the treatment of epilepsy and is generally well tolerated. It is not clear, however, that phenytoin reduces the subsequent risk of sudden death among patients with congenital heart disease, nor is the mechanism of action of phenytoin at all clear in this clinical setting.

Torsade de Pointes

Phenytoin is listed among the multitude of drugs that have been reported to be effective in the management of torsade de pointes.[15, 16] Presumably, both its effect on suppressing afterdepolarizations and its effect on lowering centrally mediated sympathetic tone play a role in treating these arrhythmias. Overdrive atrial or ventricular pacing, magnesium sulfate, and isoproterenol have been more reliably effective than phenytoin in this clinical setting. When used for torsade de pointes, phenytoin is administered intravenously.

Reentrant Ventricular Tachyarrhythmias

The use of phenytoin for reentrant ventricular arrhythmias has been less common and more controversial than the use of the drug for nonreentrant arrhythmias. Nonetheless, phenytoin undeniably has properties that allow it to be classified as a class I antiarrhythmic agent, and therefore some activity against reentrant arrhythmias should be expected. El-Sherif and Lazarra[17] stopped reentrant arrhythmias in dogs with phenytoin and confirmed the drug's ability to depress conduction in ischemic tissue. Dhatt et al.[18] used phenytoin to abolish His-Purkinje reentry in nonischemic human hearts. Two reports describe the systematic examination of phenytoin in suppressing inducible ventricular tachycardia. Epstein et al.[19] reported that phenytoin was effective in 11% of patients with inducible arrhythmias and concluded that it is therefore not very effective for human reentrant ventricular tachyarrhythmias. On the other hand, our group[20] reported similar efficacy (13%) but concluded that the drug is worth testing. This conclusion was based on the relative efficacies of quinidine (11%) and procainamide (14%) in the same population of patients. The long-term outcome of patients treated with phenytoin in our series was also similar to the outcome of patients treated with other agents. Because long-term therapy with phenytoin has been well tolerated by hundreds of thousands of patients over the last 50 years, we consider the drug an attractive option for patients with inducible ventricular tachyarrhythmias. Accordingly, we continue routine testing of phenytoin in such patients.

ADVERSE EFFECTS

When given acutely or over the long term, phenytoin is relatively well tolerated in comparison with many other antiarrhythmic agents.

Acute administration of phenytoin is most commonly associated with adverse effects related to the central nervous system (CNS). When loaded rapidly to the therapeutic range, vertigo and drowsiness are common. When plasma concentrations are above 20 μg/ml, ataxia and overt nystagmus are common. Most antiarrhythmic effects of the drug are seen with concentrations under 20 μg/ml. Thus, if ataxia or overt nystagmus occurs and the target arrhythmia has not yet responded, further administration of phenytoin is unlikely to help.

With long-term oral administration of phenytoin, similar adverse effects related to the CNS occur but are less common. Gastrointestinal side effects occur with orally administered phenytoin, most commonly nausea, vomiting, heartburn, and anorexia. These side effects can usually be controlled by administering the drug in divided doses.

Gingival hyperplasia occurs in up to 20% of children and young adults on long-term therapy but appears to be uncommon in older patients. This side effect is probably related to poor oral hygiene.

Several relatively rare complications of therapy with phenytoin include osteomalacia from interference with vitamin D metabolism, megaloblastic anemia from interference with folate metabolism, and hypersensitivity reactions. Very rare cases of lupus, hepatic necrosis, hematologic reactions, and pseudolymphoma have been reported.

INTERFERENCE WITH OTHER DRUGS

Plasma concentrations of phenytoin have increased during concomitant therapy with cimetidine, dicumarol, isoniazid, sulfonamides, and amiodarone. Plasma concentrations of phenytoin can be reduced when patients also receive carbamazepine or theophylline preparations; theophylline concentrations are also reduced by phenytoin. Phenytoin has been reported to increase the metabolism of oral contraceptives, thus decreasing their effectiveness.

DOSAGE AND ADMINISTRATION

Intravenous administration of phenytoin is most commonly used for treating digitalis-toxic arrhythmias, ventricular arrhythmias in the intensive care setting, torsade de pointes, and acute testing of the drug in the electrophysiology laboratory. Because the drug is highly alkaline, intermittent injection should be used, preferably via a central vein. Therapeutic concentrations can usually be obtained by administering a total of 7.5 to 10 mg/kg. No more than 50 mg/min of phenytoin should be given, and careful monitoring for adverse effects is warranted between injections. Intravenously administered phenytoin can cause transient hypotension, so blood pressure should be monitored during administration. If hypotension occurs, injections should be made less frequently (every 5 or 10 minutes). The onset of sustained lateral-gaze nystagmus has proven to be a reliable early indicator that adequate plasma levels have been achieved (i.e.,

10 µg/ml), and testing for lateral-gaze nystagmus before each injection can be helpful in titration during intravenous loading. The onset of ataxia or overt nystagmus (nystagmus while gazing straight ahead) indicates that levels are approximately 20 µg/ml; administration of the drug should be stopped if these signs are present.

When prescribing long-term therapy with phenytoin, the physician should consider the slow and potentially erratic absorption and the relatively long and dose-dependent half-life of the drug. A loading regimen is often used when initiating therapy, especially if therapeutic levels are desired within 24 hours. Oral loading of phenytoin can be achieved by giving 15 mg/kg on the first day, followed by 7.5 mg/kg on the second day in divided doses. Maintenance doses are approximately 5 mg/kg/day (usually 300 to 500 mg/day). Daily doses are usually given as two or three divided doses. In the therapeutic range, the elimination of phenytoin is generally dose-dependent, so long-term doses of the drug should be changed no more often than every 10 to 14 days. Patients should be cautioned against changing preparations of phenytoin, because absorption of the drug can change with different preparations.

SOCIOECONOMIC CONSIDERATIONS

As antiarrhythmic drugs go, phenytoin is among the least expensive. It is often profoundly less expensive than most of the newer antiarrhythmic agents. Compliance with phenytoin administration has been historically favorable, both in patients with seizure disorders and in patients with arrhythmias. Compliance can be judged by measuring plasma levels.

REFERENCES

1. Leonard WA: The use of diphenylhydantoin (Dilantin) sodium in the treatment of ventricular tachycardia. Arch Intern Med 101:714, 1958.
2. Mercer EN, Osborne JA: The current status of diphenylhydantoin in heart disease. Ann Intern Med 67:1084, 1967.
3. Helfant RH, Seuffert GW, Patton RD: The clinical use of diphenylhydantoin (Dilantin) in the treatment and prevention of cardiac arrhythmias. Am Heart J 77:315, 1969.
4. Dreifus LS, Watanabe Y: Current status of diphenylhydantoin. Am Heart J 80:709, 1970.
5. Witt AL, Rosen MR, Hoffman BF: Electrophysiology and pharmacology of cardiac arrhythmias. VIII. Cardiac effects of diphenylhydantoin. A. Am Heart J 90:265, 1975.
6. Witt AL, Rosen MR, Hoffman BF: Electrophysiology and pharmacology of cardiac arrhythmias. VIII. Cardiac effects of diphenylhydantoin. B. Am Heart J 90:397, 1975.
7. Hondeghem LM: Effects of lidocaine, phenytoin, and quinidine on the ischemic canine myocardium. J Electrocardiol 9:203, 1976.
8. Wasserstrom JA, Ferrier GR: Effects of phenytoin and quinidine on digitalis-induced oscillatory afterpotentials, aftercontractions, and inotropy in canine ventricular tissues. J Mol Cell Cardiol 14:725, 1982.
9. Moore SJ: Digitalis toxicity and treatment with phenytoin: a neurologic mechanism of action. Heart Lung 6:1035, 1977.
10. Garan H, Ruskin JN, Powell WJ Jr: Centrally mediated effect of phenytoin on digoxin-mediated ventricular arrhythmias. Am J Physiol 241:H67, 1981.
11. Hayashi Y, Kamibyashi T, Sumikawa K, et al: Phenytoin prevents epinephrine-induced arrhythmias through central nervous system in halothane-anesthetized dogs. Research Communications in Chemical Pathology and Pharmacology 74:59, 1991.
12. Garson A, Kugler JD, Gillette PC, et al: Control of late postoperative ventricular arrhythmias with phenytoin in young patients. Am J Cardiol 46:290, 1980.
13. Kavey REW, Blackman MS, Sondheimer HM: Phenytoin therapy for ventricular arrhythmias occurring late after surgery for congenital heart disease. Am Heart J 104:794, 1982.
14. Kugler JD, Pinsky WW, Cheatham JP, et al: Sustained ventricular tachycardia after repair of tetralogy of Fallot: New electrophysiologic findings. Am J Cardiol 51:1137, 1983.
15. Uhl JA: Phenytoin, the drug of choice in TCA overdose. Ann Emerg Med 10:270, 1981.
16. Vukmir RB, Stein KL: Torsades de pointes therapy with phenytoin. Ann Emerg Med 20:198, 1991.
17. El-Sherif N, Lazzara R: Re-entrant ventricular arrhythmias in the late myocardial infarction period 5. Mechanism of action of diphenylhydantoin. Circulation 57:465, 1978.
18. Dhatt MS, Akhtar M, Reddy CP, et al: Modification and abolition of re-entry within the His-Purkinje system in man by diphenylhydantoin. Circulation 56:720, 1977.
19. Epstein AE, Plumb VJ, Henthorn RW, et al: Phenytoin in the treatment of inducible ventricular tachycardia: Results of electrophysiologic testing and long-term follow-up. PACE 10:1049, 1987.
20. Fogoros RN, Fiedler SB, Elson JJ: Efficacy of phenytoin in suppressing inducible ventricular tachyarrhythmias. Cardiovasc Drugs Ther 2:171, 1988.

CHAPTER 146

Procainamide

Frank C. McGeehin, III, M.D., and Eric L. Michelson, M.D.

HISTORY

The antiarrhythmic effects of procaine were first described by Mautz in 1936.[1] Most noteworthy was procaine's ability to reduce the susceptibility of ventricular tissue to fibrillation when the compound was applied directly to the myocardium. This benefit of an increased threshold of ventricular muscle to fibrillation was severely limited by procaine's short duration of action. It was not until the 1950s that procainamide, a more stable derivative, was used in the clinical therapy of arrhythmias.[2] In either its oral or its parenteral form, procainamide has been one of the more commonly prescribed antiarrhythmic agents in the United States. The subsequent development of sustained-release preparations has enhanced the practicality of this drug for outpatient arrhythmia control.[3, 4]

CHEMISTRY

Procainamide is the amide analogue of procaine hydrochloride. The chemical name is p-amino-N-[2-(diethylamino)ethyl]benzamide monohydrochloride. It is a white to off-white, odorless crystal soluble in water and routinely administered physiologic solutions. The sustained-release preparations contain procainamide in a wax or cellulose matrix designed for prolonged release in the gastrointestinal tract. Following release of the drug, the nonabsorbed wax tablet matrix (or "ghost") may be detected in the stool.

PHARMACOLOGY

Procainamide is a prototypal class IA antiarrhythmic drug. It depresses phase 0 of the action potential, prolongs conduction, and slows repolarization. In the normal heart, procainamide will decrease atrial and ventricular excitability. This effect appears to be exaggerated in abnormal cardiac tissue. Typical of class IA agents, procainamide has a moderate use-dependent effect on the fast inward sodium channels to decrease the influx of sodium ions and thus diminish the maximum upstroke velocity of the action potential. The action potential amplitude is also diminished by procainamide. The plateau phase is shortened, but the repolarization phase appears to be prolonged. In normal cardiac tissue, the effective refractory period is increased more than the action potential duration (APD). In abnormal myocardium, refractory periods may be more markedly prolonged.[5]

Because membrane responsiveness is diminished by procainamide, the maximum rate of phase 0 depolarization is decreased at any given transmembrane potential. Conduction is slowed at any given resting membrane potential, with perhaps more pronounced results at less negative potentials. Consequently, conduction velocity through most cardiac tissues is reduced. This includes the atria, the infranodal conduction system, and ventricular tissue. It also includes, although to a much lesser extent, the atrioventricular (AV) node. The indirect vagolytic effects of procainamide are much less pronounced than those of either quinidine or disopyramide (other class IA agents); therefore, paradoxic enhancement of AV nodal conduction or the sinus rate is not usually apparent clinically.

Procainamide may also cause suppression of phase 4 depolarization, affecting both normal and abnormal automaticity. This may affect arrhythmias due to enhanced automaticity but, in susceptible patients, may also depress sinus node or escape pacemaker activity. Class IA drugs also increase the threshold voltage.

The electrophysiologic properties of procainamide have dose-related effects on the surface electrocardiogram. Most commonly, these are manifested as increases in the QRS and QT intervals.

In addition to procainamide, its active metabolite, N-acetylprocainamide (NAPA), also has electrophysiologic properties; however, these properties are quite distinct from those of the parent compound. NAPA has so-called class III activity, characteristic of amiodarone, sotalol, and bretylium as well. That is, the APD can be prolonged by NAPA without significant changes in maximum upstroke velocity.[6-8] Structural analogues of NAPA, such as sematilide, are currently under development as potential antiarrhythmic agents.[9]

PHARMACOKINETICS

The absorption of orally administered procainamide is relatively rapid; this also includes the sustained-release preparation. However, with the latter, less drug is available for immediate absorption, and the amount of drug presented to the gastrointestinal mucosa is more constant over time. Bioavailability via the oral route is in the range of 75% to 85% compared with that of intravenous administration for both the conventional and the sustained-release preparations. Procainamide usually reaches a peak blood level approximately 1 to 2 hours after ingestion and is minimally protein-bound. Following intramuscular injection (100 mg/ml or 500 mg/ml), procainamide reaches peak blood levels in approximately 15 to 60 minutes. To date, there has been no definite evidence of altered absorption when procainamide or its sustained-release preparation is taken with other medications or with meals. The half-life of procainamide hydrochloride is 3 to 4 hours (Table 146-1). The half-life of the sustained-release preparation is 5 to 7 hours. Both preparations are metabolized in part by the liver using first-order kinetics, although a large fraction (40% to 70%) is excreted unchanged by the kidneys by active tubular secretion and glomerular filtration. Approximately 16% to 33% of procainamide, as well as the slow-release form of this drug, is acetylated predominantly by the hepatic polymorphic N-acetyltransferases forming NAPA[10, 11] (approximately 16% to 21% in slow acetylators, 24% to 33% in rapid acetylators). NAPA is excreted via the kidneys and undergoes more limited metabolism, including some deacetylation to procainamide. For that reason, it is customary to measure serum levels of not only procainamide but also NAPA when monitoring blood levels in patients. The therapeutic activity in some patients may be based on the sum of the effects and levels of procainamide and NAPA. In some cases, these additive effects may be beneficial; in other cases, they are potentially deleterious. Procainamide and NAPA can be removed by hemodialysis but not by peritoneal dialysis. Dosage adjustments must be considered in patients with advanced hepatic or renal disease and in older patients. In addition, cardiac failure may markedly impair absorption, distribution, and clearance of procainamide, necessitating dosage modification.[12]

Table 146–1. **Pharmacology of Procainamide**

Form	Administration	Half-Life	Metabolism	Loading Dose	Maintenance Dose	Side Effects
Sustained-release procainamide	Oral	5–7 hours	Renal, ½; hepatic, ½	750–1500 mg	500–1000 mg q6 hours	Gastrointestinal; central nervous system; lupus-like syndrome; torsade de pointes; neutropenia
Procainamide	Oral	3–4 hours	Renal, ½; hepatic, ½	750–1500 mg	250–750 mg q3–4 hours	For oral and intravenous administration: gastrointestinal; central nervous system; lupus-like syndrome; torsade de pointes; neutropenia
	Intravenous	3–4 hours	Renal, ½; hepatic, ½	750–1500 mg	2–6 mg/min	For intravenous administration: hypotension; QRS widening

The NAPA/procainamide ratio in any given patient is based on the phenotypically determined rate of acetylation. It is estimated that approximately 40% of the North American population are rapid acetylators, and approximately 40% are slow acetylators. The slow acetylator phenotype is inherited in a Mendelian autosomal recessive pattern, whereas the rapid acetylator phenotype may be either homozygous or heterozygous for the dominant allele. The remaining 20% of patients fall into an intermediate range. The rapid acetylators will have a high NAPA/procainamide ratio.

The slow acetylators will have a low NAPA/procainamide ratio.[10, 11] The "therapeutic" blood level of procainamide is usually given independent of the NAPA level and is in the range of 4 to 12 μg/ml. This determination should be obtained at a trough level. As with all antiarrhythmic drugs, the dosage should achieve the desired antiarrhythmic response. The therapeutic drug level serves only as a rough guide for dosage. Low levels of procainamide may adequately suppress ventricular couplets and short runs of nonsustained ventricular tachycardia. However, they may be insufficient to abolish all ventricular ectopic rhythms or to treat sustained ventricular tachycardia.

EFFECTS ON PATHOPHYSIOLOGY
Effects on Hemodynamics

Intravenous administration of procainamide, especially rapid administration, can cause a fall in blood pressure partly mediated by peripheral vasodilation. Cardiac contractility in the normal heart is usually depressed minimally by this medication, and cardiac output is most often well maintained.

With oral dosage, it is uncommon for hemodynamics to be adversely affected or for this to be the major dose-limiting factor. However, caution is still needed when using this drug in patients with a markedly depressed ejection fraction or compromised ventricular function.

Systemic Effects

The systemic effects of procainamide on the functions of most other organs, including hepatic, renal, endocrine, and metabolic functions, are generally negligible. However, the side effects of procainamide can be multisystemic, including gastrointestinal or neurologic symptoms and the diffuse immunologic-mediated spectra of alterations constituting the "lupus-like syndrome" (see later sections, Hematologic Side Effects and Rheumatologic Side Effects).

CLINICAL USE: INDICATIONS
Ventricular Arrhythmias

Suppression of life-threatening ventricular arrhythmias is the principal therapeutic use for procainamide. This drug has been shown to decrease the frequency and severity of most ventricular arrhythmias, including sustained ventricular tachycardia, nonsustained ventricular tachycardia, ventricular couplets, isolated beats, multiform beats, and the "R on T" phenomenon. Procainamide has also been shown to be effective in approximately 20% to 30% of patients with recurrent sustained ventricular tachycardia guided by invasive electrophysiologic testing, predominantly in patients with coronary artery disease. In such patients, the results of acute electrophysiologic drug testing have generally been highly predictive of clinical outcome.[13–16] However, the successful suppression of ventricular ectopic rhythm on ambulatory monitoring has not always correlated with a reduction in mortality from ventricular tachycardia or fibrillation, as highlighted by the Cardiac Arrhythmia Suppression Trial with the drugs encainide, flecainide, and moricizine.[17] In addition, questions still remain about the use of either ambulatory monitoring or electrophysiologic testing, or both, to optimize therapy with all drugs, including procainamide.[18] These questions include criteria for efficacy, dosage, and the timing of serial studies, as well as methods of testing. Frequently, induction of ventricular tachycardia in the laboratory cannot be abolished, although the rate will be somewhat slower after intravenous administration of procainamide. The potential benefit of this effect is unclear.

One of the most important uses of intravenously administered procainamide has been in the acute suppression of ventricular arrhythmias in patients unresponsive to other intravenously administered antiarrhythmic medication such as lidocaine. In addition, procainamide can also be used as a first-line agent. In general experience, it has been found to be more likely to be effective than lidocaine in the acute treatment of recurrent sustained ventricular tachycardia occurring outside the setting of acute infarction. Procainamide has also been used in combination with other antiarrhythmic drugs in patients with refractory ventricular arrhythmias. However, such combinations, using either intravenously or orally administered procainamide, must be approached cautiously, because adverse effects—including sinus node suppression, conduction block, and hemodynamic compromise—may also be additive. Procainamide is frequently used postoperatively, when atrial and ventricular tachyarrhythmias may be a problem. It can be used as a first-line drug in elderly patients, who are more susceptible to the neurologic toxicity associated with lidocaine. One major advantage with procainamide is the availability of both parenteral and oral formulations and the ease of conversion from one to the other. In treating patients with life-threatening ventricular arrhythmias, therapy is usually initiated in the hospital. Procainamide can also be used to decrease the frequency of recurrence of sustained ventricular tachyarrhythmias in patients with implanted antiarrhythmic devices.

Supraventricular Arrhythmias and Wolff-Parkinson-White Syndrome

Procainamide has also been used to treat a variety of supraventricular tachyarrhythmias, although this indication is no longer included in the Food and Drug Administration (FDA)–approved labeling.

Procainamide can suppress episodes of atrial flutter and of paroxysmal atrial tachycardia, and it can be helpful in multifocal atrial tachycardia. It appears to be less effective in converting atrial fibrillation to normal sinus rhythm than quinidine. Procainamide has also been used acutely and prophylactically in patients with paroxysmal reentrant tachycardias confined to the AV node or involving a bypass tract (AV reciprocating tachycardias). The combination of procainamide with digoxin, a β-blocker, or a calcium antagonist also may help to suppress supraventricular tachyarrhythmias in patients who may not be candidates for definitive ablative therapy.

Procainamide can suppress anterograde and retrograde conduction over an AV bypass tract in some patients with Wolff-Parkinson-White (WPW) syndrome who may be susceptible to atrial fibrillation. This probably reflects prolongation of the refractory period as well as slowing of conduction velocity in atrial, ventricular, and accessory pathway tissue. The ability of an intravenous bolus of procainamide (e.g., 10 mg/kg over 5 minutes) to abolish all evidence of ventricular preexcitation on the electrocardiogram (short PR interval, delta wave, wide QRS complex, and repolarization abnormalities) has been used to identify the patients least likely to have rapid anterograde AV conduction if atrial fibrillation or flutter were to occur. Conversely, procainamide is generally least protective in patients with the most rapidly conducting bypass tracts.[19, 20]

CAUTIONS AND ADVERSE EFFECTS (BY ORGAN SYSTEMS)
Cardiovascular Side Effects

Intravenously administered procainamide may cause hypotension and reduced cardiac output, presumably because of peripheral vasodilatation, some direct depression of contractility, and, in part, the indirect effects of conduction slowing. This can usually be minimized if the intravenous dose is administered slowly. The drug should generally not be given in doses greater than 50 mg/min; a more typical dose is 100 mg every 5 minutes, especially in patients with left ventricular dysfunction. The negative inotropic effects of procainamide are minimal when contrasted with those of flecainide or disopyramide and are infrequently evident with oral administration.

Ventricular arrhythmias may be aggravated by any antiarrhythmic drug, including procainamide. Arrhythmia aggravation, or the so-called proarrhythmic effect, may be idiosyncratic or dose-related.[21] Patients with poor left ventricular function, underlying electrolyte derangements, and prolonged QT intervals prior to therapy are apparently at increased risk. Minor prolongation of the QT interval is an expected consequence of procainamide therapy. However, QT prolongation can be associated with a malignant polymorphic form of ventricular tachycardia known as torsade de pointes.[22] If torsade de pointes occurs with any class IA agent, many cardiologists think that all other class IA agents are also contraindicated. It is important to note that polymorphic ventricular tachycardia may also occur without noticeable prolongation of the QT interval. In such a case, it is prudent to discontinue procainamide therapy rather than increase the dose. It becomes paramount to monitor the QT interval during therapy with procainamide. Once the QT or QTc exceeds 500 msec, caution must be exercised, independent of the serum level. On the other hand, should polymorphic ventricular tachycardia occur in the setting of a normal QT interval in a patient not receiving an antiarrhythmic drug, procainamide may be considered a therapeutic option.[22]

Procainamide causes a mild dose-related widening of the QRS complex. Less commonly, it causes prolongation of the PR interval. No marked ST-segment changes have been ascribed to procainamide therapy. With intravenous administration, it is particularly prudent to monitor the electrocardiogram as well as blood pressure; one must be cautious not to exceed

25% widening of either the QRS or the QT, or both, with 50% prolongation considered an absolute contraindication to further dosing.

Gastrointestinal Side Effects

Gastrointestinal side effects are among the most common adverse reactions in patients receiving procainamide. They include nausea, vomiting, anorexia, and, less commonly, diarrhea. These side effects resolve spontaneously with cessation of therapy.

Hematologic Side Effects

Procainamide can produce serious hematologic disorders (0.5% of patients), particularly leukopenia or agranulocytosis (sometimes fatal), and less commonly bone marrow depression, hypoplastic anemia, and thrombocytopenia.[23-25] Because these effects have been noted most often during the first 12 weeks of therapy, the 1995 package insert recommends that complete blood counts be performed more frequently during this period. If clinical events or laboratory findings suggest a hematologic disorder, procainamide should be discontinued. Blood counts usually return to normal within 1 month of discontinuation. Susceptible patients with preexisting cytopenia should avoid the drug. A 1984 report suggested that patients receiving sustained-release procainamide after open heart surgery may be more susceptible to neutropenia.[24] However, these patients had other potentially confounding variables, and a subsequent study[25] failed to confirm these observations. Nevertheless, it would be prudent to monitor white blood cell counts more frequently in such patients, at least initially. Thrombocytopenia or positive Coombs test results and immune hemolytic anemias are uncommon, although red blood cell autoimmune phenomena can be detected in many more patients.[26]

Rheumatologic Side Effects

The most well known of the procainamide side effects is the "lupus-like syndrome" (LLS). Antinuclear antibody (ANA) test results will be positive in a substantial portion of patients receiving procainamide, usually in a homogeneous pattern. This may occur in 30% to 83% of patients receiving procainamide or a sustained-release preparation for longer than 6 months.[27] Only a small minority of patients who develop positive ANA test results will go on to develop symptoms of polyarthralgias or myalgias or a constellation of symptoms including headache, weakness, and fever; other possibilities are abnormal liver function test results, elevated serum amylase, or hematologic changes. The finding of pleural pericarditis associated with LLS is even less common. Of note is the observation that the findings of pleural pericarditis and many other aspects of LLS seem to be more common in phenotypically slow acetylators.[11] A major distinction between systemic lupus erythematosus (SLE) and drug-induced lupus is the absence of renal involvement in the latter.[28] This contrasts with a 40% to 45% incidence of renal involvement in patients with SLE. In addition, the central nervous system is not involved in drug-induced lupus, although procainamide can cause central nervous system side effects, including confusion, psychosis, and infrequently convulsions. Dermatologic findings that are common (70%) in SLE are uncommon (5% to 18%) in procainamide-associated disease, as is the development of joint deformities. In drug-induced lupus, symptoms ordinarily resolve rapidly over days to weeks after discontinuation of procainamide, even without specific therapy. Drug-induced lupus tends to be a milder disease than SLE.[28]

The development of both positive ANA test results and LLS is influenced by hepatic N-acetyltransferase activity. The slow acetylator patient develops positive ANA test results more rapidly and with lower total drug dosage than the rapid acetylator patient.[11] It has also been shown that patients treated with NAPA develop positive ANA test results less frequently than do those receiving procainamide. Thus, it appears that acetylation may inactivate the autoimmunity-inducing capacity of procainamide.

The spectra of serologic and laboratory findings in procainamide-induced LLS also differ from those of SLE.[28] Antibodies in LLS tend to be directed predominantly against a histone-DNA complex, single-stranded DNA (sDNA), and ribonucleoprotein.[29] Antinuclear antibodies associated with SLE such as those to native DNA, Smith (Sm) antigen, and Sjögren's syndrome antigen (SS-A) have not, with few exceptions, been described in LLS. Also, the hypocomplementemia frequently found in SLE is rare in LLS. Thus, for distinguishing between LLS and SLE in a particular patient, measurements of anti-DNA antibodies (common in SLE, rare in LLS) and serum complement levels (often low in SLE, normal in LLS) are usually the most helpful commercially available serologic tests.

ANA monitoring is recommended for patients taking procainamide. However, many question its utility, because positive ANA test results will develop in most such patients, whereas symptoms will develop only in a minority. Therefore, much research has been directed toward the discovery of a serologic parameter that could be used as a predictor of high risk for the development of clinical manifestations of LLS or as an objective marker for the presence of disease in patients who have equivocal symptoms. Immunoglobulin G antibodies directed against the H2A-H2B histone complex[30] and antiguanosine ANAs[31] have been suggested as possible serologic markers for procainamide-associated LLS. Until these or other serologic markers have been confirmed as predictors of LLS, positive ANA test results should not preclude further therapy with procainamide in asymptomatic patients. However, in patients with positive ANA test results and bothersome symptoms attributable to LLS, procainamide therapy should be discontinued unless the patient suffers from recurrent, life-threatening arrhythmia not controllable by other antiarrhythmic agents. Further clinical evaluation is warranted if these symptoms persist after cessation of procainamide therapy.

Neurologic Side Effects

Dizziness, fatigue, psychosis with hallucinations, and ataxia have been associated with procainamide therapy. Other reported side effects include depression, confusion, convulsions, giddiness, and taste disturbances.

Other Side Effects

As with nearly all drugs, allergic skin reactions, including various eruptions such as maculopapular rashes and, rarely, angioneurotic edema, have been associated with procainamide therapy. Other hypersensitivity reactions include eosinophilia, hypergammaglobulinemia, fever, and, rarely, respiratory insufficiency.

Contraindications

Previous allergic reactions or hypersensitivity to procainamide is a contraindication to its use. Possible cross-reactivity to other procaine-related drugs must be considered. Procainamide is also contraindicated in patients with advanced AV conduction block (e.g., Mobitz II or third-degree block) unless a functional electric pacemaker is in place. Procainamide also should be avoided in patients with myasthenia gravis because of its procaine-like effect on reducing acetylcholine release at motor nerve endings, which may even induce respiratory failure. In administering procainamide, particularly intravenously, QRS and/or QT prolongation by more than 25% indicates caution, and 50% prolongation is a contraindication to further dosage. Procainamide is probably also contraindicated in patients with a history of ventricular proarrhythmia associated with QT prolongation while they are receiving any class IA drug, and procainamide should not be used for the treatment of arrhythmias in patients with marked baseline QT prolongation. Procainamide should be used with caution in patients with preexisting cytopenia or bone marrow failure. According to the package insert, procainamide is a pregnancy category C drug and its "safety and effectiveness in children have not been established."

Drug Interactions

A number of drug interactions with procainamide have been recognized, in addition to the obvious potential for interaction with other drugs having antiarrhythmic or electrophysiologic properties (e.g., tricyclic antidepressants), drugs affecting cardiac hemodynamics, hypotensive agents, or drugs affecting electrolytes. For example, diuretics producing hypokalemia, hypomagnesemia, or both not only may neutralize the antiarrhythmic efficacy of procainamide

(and other antiarrhythmics) but also may potentiate proarrhythmia. Similarly, a host of drugs and toxins that prolong the QT interval may precipitate adverse effects in this regard.[22]

Other potential interactions include additive effects with anticholinergic agents; antagonism of anticholinesterases, thereby aggravating paralysis in myasthenia gravis; reduced clearance of procainamide and NAPA by cimetidine;[32] and potentiation of skeletal muscle relaxants such as succinylcholine. Procainamide may also enhance or prolong the neuromuscular blocking activity of drugs such as bacitracin and the aminoglycosides, producing respiratory depression. Furthermore, the addition of either amiodarone[33] or quinidine[34] to procainamide may result in increased procainamide blood levels and requires monitoring to facilitate dosage adjustments.

Use in Patients with Impaired Organ Function

The total dosage of procainamide should be decreased in patients with renal failure. Both procainamide and NAPA may accumulate excessively in these patients. Therefore, serum levels (peak, trough, or both, depending on the circumstances) should be monitored following the initiation of therapy, after subsequent dosage adjustments, or when renal function changes. Some dialysis patients with chronic renal failure should be considered candidates for an alternative antiarrhythmic agent if adverse effects (including excessive QT prolongation) result from accumulation of high levels of NAPA.

Because a portion of procainamide is metabolized by the liver, severe hepatic dysfunction would necessitate a reduction in procainamide therapy. Again, serum and trough levels would serve as a guide to dosing regimens in this instance. Underlying cardiac dysfunction and advancing age should also be considered factors in decreasing dosage.

PLACE IN THE ANTIARRHYTHMIC ARSENAL

Procainamide is a first-line drug for the suppression and prophylactic treatment of ventricular tachyarrhythmias. Its efficacy profile is generally comparable with that of the other available class IA agents, quinidine and disopyramide, from which it is chemically distinct. However, of these three agents, it is the only one available for intravenous (and intramuscular) administration, thus facilitating its use in acute care, emergency, and electrophysiologic laboratory settings. Consequently, it has also become the prototypal class IA agent for acute drug testing in the electrophysiologic laboratory, although the crossover rate among individual class IA agents may be only 60% to 90% or less.[16, 35–37] Conversion from intravenous to oral therapy with procainamide is usually straightforward. Because noncardiovascular side effects are relatively common with each of the class IA agents, direct efficacy comparisons are often limited by dose, individual tolerance, and patient selection, as well as by efficacy criteria. In short-term use, procainamide may be better tolerated than quinidine or disopyramide, but with long-term administration, LLS becomes a more common problem. However, procainamide can be used in patients with advanced structural heart disease and reduced ejection fractions, an advantage over disopyramide, and may be less likely to precipitate polymorphic ventricular tachycardia than quinidine, although this has not been subjected to rigorous study. Unlike quinidine, procainamide does not increase serum digoxin levels.

Comparisons with drugs of other classes are even more limited, although some studies have addressed this issue, usually in selected patients with fixed drug dosages, often using 24-hour ambulatory electrocardiographic recordings and sometimes using invasive electrophysiologic testing.[18] Generally, the percentage of patients in whom frequent and complex ventricular ectopic rhythm (e.g., couplets, nonsustained tachycardia) is effectively suppressed is greater with procainamide than with the class IB drugs (e.g., mexiletine, tocainide) or with the β-blockers, and a substantial number of patients experience bothersome side effects with doses of these alternative drugs necessary to effectively suppress ambient ectopic rhythm. In comparison, the class IC drugs (e.g., flecainide, encainide) are effective in a larger percentage of patients and are more likely to abolish nearly all ectopic rhythm, although neither of these attributes necessarily translates into more effective prevention of sudden cardiac death. In fact, to the contrary, in the preliminary data from the Cardiac Arrhythmia Suppression Trial, the use of encainide, flecainide, or moricizine was associated with a marked increase in cardiac mortality and sudden cardiac death/cardiac arrest in postmyocardial infarction patients with apparent suppression of ventricular ectopic beats and short runs of ectopic beats.[17]

To date, in patients surviving an acute myocardial infarction and at apparently increased risk for sudden death, none of the traditional, first-line "antiarrhythmic" agents has shown efficacy in this regard. However, emerging data on amiodarone and possibly sotalol are more promising, and data for several β-blockers are compelling.[38] Presumably, the latter were effective via multiple mechanisms. Proarrhythmia is even more problematic with the class IC agents in patients with compromised left ventricular function. Also, the potential for depressing cardiac function and precipitating heart failure in patients with limited reserve appears to be greater with encainide, and particularly with flecainide, than with procainamide, quinidine, or the class IB agents. In most series of patients with refractory, recurrent, and/or inducible sustained ventricular tachyarrhythmias, class IB and β-blocking drugs[39] are effective in only a small percentage of patients as monotherapy but are much more effective when combined with class IA agents, including procainamide. In the United States, the class III drug amiodarone has generally been reserved

for patients refractory to or intolerant of other conventional agents. However, its use has been more liberal in other countries, particularly at lower dosages, and emerging data support its use in various high-risk populations. In addition, in the Electrophysiologic Study Versus Electrocardiographic Monitoring trial,[18] sotalol was especially promising and is gaining favor as a first-line agent for the treatment of ventricular arrhythmias. The other approved class III drug, bretylium (administered intravenously), is a potentially effective alternative to either lidocaine or procainamide in the management of severe, immediately life-threatening ventricular tachyarrhythmias in the acute care setting. Perhaps most important, therapy must be individualized with respect to both drug(s) and dosage, considering the specific arrhythmia, the goals of therapy, concomitant diseases and medications (e.g., digoxin interacting with quinidine), and the nature and extent of cardiac dysfunction.

In the management of supraventricular arrhythmias and the WPW syndrome arrhythmias, procainamide again offers the advantage of both intravenous and oral formulations in those situations for which and in patients for whom a class IA drug would be indicated. Intravenously administered procainamide can be useful in controlling multifocal and ectopic atrial tachycardias and may convert atrial flutter or fibrillation to sinus rhythm. Although not studied definitively, orally administered procainamide has been considered second-line to quinidine or disopyramide in converting atrial fibrillation or preventing its recurrence. In this regard, some of the newer, more "potent" drugs, such as the class IC agent flecainide, may be alternatives in patients without compromised cardiac function. There may be less potential for inadvertent ventricular rate acceleration with procainamide than with either quinidine or disopyramide, because it is less vagolytic; however, monitoring is advised, particularly in patients with atrial flutter. To slow AV nodal conduction and control ventricular rate, digoxin, verapamil, or a β-blocker such as esmolol or propranolol usually is administered initially or concomitantly. With the class IC drugs, preliminary investigational data suggest that accelerated AV conduction may be less likely and that conversion to sinus rhythm may be at least as likely as with conventional agents. Emerging data on class III agents such as sotalol and amiodarone also are promising. Moreover, conduction is also slowed effectively in many patients with AV bypass tracts. The risk of embolization complicating conversion to sinus rhythm is presumably comparable with each of these drugs.

In the acute pharmacologic management of paroxysmal supraventricular tachycardias involving the AV node, verapamil has been the drug of choice for many patients; adenosine has been advocated more recently, and diltiazem is also available. Exceptions to the use of verapamil or diltiazem are patients with the WPW syndrome in whom accelerated AV conduction during atrial fibrillation is possible and patients with sick sinus syndrome who are at risk for profound secondary bradycardia.

DOSAGE AND ADMINISTRATION

The intravenous loading dose of procainamide is usually 750 to 1500 mg administered as 100 mg every 5 minutes, followed by a maintenance infusion of 2 to 6 mg/min. As noted previously, intravenous administration of procainamide should generally not exceed 50 mg/min because of the possibility of hypotension and, occasionally, profound QRS widening. Both blood pressure and electrocardiogram should be carefully monitored during intravenous infusion of procainamide, particularly during drug loading. Conversion of the intravenous administration of procainamide to an oral preparation can be calculated using the 24-hour total dosage of this drug, because procainamide is well absorbed and highly bioavailable. Therefore, if procainamide is being infused at a rate of 2 mg/min, the total daily dose is 2880 mg/day. The patient could be treated with a sustained-release preparation of procainamide in doses of 750 mg every 6 hours. An alternative but less desirable dosage schedule would be (conventional) procainamide given as 375 to 500 mg every 3 to 4 hours. The oral loading dose is essentially the same as the intravenous loading dose. However, gastrointestinal upset may preclude a large oral dose initially. Therefore, with the realization that it will take a longer time to reach therapeutic levels, it may be easier to begin with a maintenance dose. For example, with sustained-release procainamide given every 6 hours, it will take approximately five doses to achieve a steady-state level. The usual maintenance doses are as follows: for conventional procainamide, 250 to 750 mg every 3 to 4 hours; for the sustained-release preparation, 500 to 1000 mg every 6 hours using the same total daily dosage.

Each patient's dosage must be determined individually. Moreover, patients should be advised not to break, bite, crush, or chew the sustained-release tablets, because this may interfere with their designed dissolution characteristics. Furthermore, dosage may have to be adjusted downward in elderly patients or those with hepatic or renal disease. The bioavailability and mean drug concentrations of both procainamide and NAPA are approximately the same in patients treated with either preparation. However, there is an advantage with the sustained-release preparations: the peak levels may be slightly lower and the trough levels somewhat higher when compared with administration of standard procainamide every 3 hours.[4] Thus, drug levels are more uniform. This may be of some importance in limiting toxicity and maintaining efficacy. Blood levels are readily available for procainamide and NAPA and may be helpful in individual patients to document compliance, efficacy, inefficacy, or adverse effects.

NAPA has been the subject of active investigation to determine its spectrum of efficacy, safety, and tolerability as a distinct class III antiarrhythmic agent.[6]

SOCIOECONOMIC CONSIDERATIONS

Several issues relevant to the use of antiarrhythmic drugs are taking on ever-increasing importance in the present climate of medical practice in which considerations of cost-effectiveness, medical-legal implications, quality of life, and documentation of outcome are being mandated. Conventional procainamide is a relatively inexpensive antiarrhythmic drug when indicated but requires frequent dosage on a schedule nearly precluding compliance. The sustained-release preparations facilitate better compliance at somewhat increased cost. The costs of treatment must also take into consideration the costs of laboratory testing and related medical care. New formulations are currently under development that should make twice-daily administration a reality.

Finally, the goals of therapy must be clearly defined for each individual patient and the outcome must be monitored in order to maximize benefits and minimize potential untoward consequences.

Acknowledgments

We gratefully acknowledge the secretarial assistance of Eileen Allison with the preparation of this chapter.

REFERENCES

1. Mautz FR: The reduction of cardiac irritability by the epicardial and systemic administration of drugs as a protection in cardiac surgery. J Thorac Surg 5:612, 1936.
2. Mark LC, Kayden JJ, Steele JM, et al: The physiological disposition and cardiac effects of procainamide. J Pharmacol Exp Ther 102:5, 1951.
3. Giardina EGV, Fenster PE, Bigger JT, et al: Efficacy, plasma concentrations and adverse effects of a new sustained-release procainamide preparation. Am J Cardiol 40:855, 1980.
4. Michelson EL, Dreifus LS: Sustained-release and immediate-release procainamide: Comparative efficacy and bioequivalency in ambulatory patients with frequent premature ventricular contractions. Vasc Med 2:155, 1984.
5. Michelson EL, Spear JF, Moore EN: Effects of procainamide on strength-interval relations in normal and chronically infarcted canine myocardium. Am J Cardiol 47:1223, 1987.
6. Singh BN, Feld G, Nademanee K: Arrhythmia control by selective lengthening of cardiac repolarization: Role of N-acetylprocainamide, active metabolite of procainamide. Angiology 37:930, 1986.
7. Steinberg MI, Michelson EL: Cardiac electrophysiologic effects of specific class III substances. *In* Reiser HJ, Horowitz LN (eds): Mechanisms and Treatment of Cardiac Arrhythmias: Relevance of Basic Studies to Clinical Management. Baltimore: Urban and Schwarzenberg, 1985, pp 263–281.
8. Haffajee CI: Clinical effects of class III antiarrhythmic agents. *In* Reiser HJ, Horowitz LN (eds): Mechanisms and Treatment of Cardiac Arrhythmias: Relevance of Basic Studies to Clinical Management. Baltimore: Urban and Schwarzenberg, 1985, pp 283–294.
9. Wong W, Pavlou HN, Birgersdotter UM, et al: Pharmacology of the class III antiarrhythmic agent sematilide in patients with arrhythmias. Am J Cardiol 69:206, 1992.
10. Reidenberg MM, Drayer DE, Levy M: Polymorphic acetylation of procainamide in man. Clin Pharmacol Ther 17:722, 1975.
11. Woosley RL, Drayer DE, Reidenberg MM, et al: Effect of acetylator phenotype on the rate at which procainamide induces antinuclear antibodies and the lupus syndrome. N Engl J Med 298:1157, 1978.
12. Kessler KM, Kayden DS, Estes DM, et al: Procainamide phar-

macokinetics in patients with acute myocardial infarction or congestive heart failure. J Am Coll Cardiol 7:1131, 1986.

13. Horowitz LN, Josephson ME, Farshidi A, et al: Recurrent sustained ventricular tachycardia. 3. Role of the electrophysiologic study in selection of antiarrhythmic regimens. Circulation 58:986, 1978.

14. Greenspan AM, Horowitz LN, Spielman SR, et al: Large-dose procainamide therapy for ventricular tachyarrhythmia. Am J Cardiol 46:453, 1980.

15. Marchlinski FE, Buxton AE, Vassallo JA, et al: Comparative electrophysiologic effects of intravenous and oral procainamide in patients with sustained ventricular arrhythmias. J Am Coll Cardiol 4:1247, 1984.

16. Oseran DS, Gang ES, Rosenthal ME, et al: Electropharmacologic testing in sustained ventricular tachycardia associated with coronary heart disease: Value of the response to intravenous procainamide in predicting the response to oral procainamide and oral quinidine treatments. Am J Cardiol 56:883, 1985.

17. Epstein AE, Hallstrom AP, Rogers WJ, et al: Mortality following ventricular arrhythmia suppression by encainide, flecainide, and moricizine after myocardial infarction. The original design concept of the Cardiac Arrhythmia Suppression Trial (CAST). JAMA 270:2451, 1993.

18. Mason JW, for the Electrophysiologic Study Versus Electrocardiographic Monitoring Investigators: A comparison of electrophysiologic testing with Holter monitoring to predict antiarrhythmic-drug efficacy for ventricular tachyarrhythmias. N Engl J Med 329:445, 1993.

19. Wellens HJJ, Braat S, Brugada P, et al: Use of procainamide in patients with the Wolff-Parkinson-White syndrome to disclose a short refractory period of the accessory pathway. Am J Cardiol 50:1087, 1982.

20. Boahene KA, Klein GJ, Sharma AD, et al: Value of a revised procainamide test in the Woff-Parkinson-White syndrome. Am J Cardiol 65:195, 1990.

21. Velebit V, Podrid P, Lown B, et al: Aggravation and provocation of ventricular arrhythmias by antiarrhythmic drugs. Circulation 65:886, 1982.

22. Soffer J, Dreifus LS, Michelson EL: Polymorphous ventricular tachycardia associated with normal and long QT intervals. Am J Cardiol 49:2021, 1982.

23. Berger BE, Hauser DJ: Agranulocytosis due to new sustained-release procainamide. Am Heart J 105:1035, 1983.

24. Ellrodt AG, Murata GH, Riedinger MS, et al: Severe neutropenia associated with sustained-release procainamide. Ann Intern Med 100:197, 1984.

25. Meyers DG, Gonzalez ER, Peters LL, et al: Severe neutropenia associated with procainamide: Comparison of sustained-release and conventional preparations. Am Heart J 109:1393, 1985.

26. Kleinman S, Nelson R, Smith L, et al: Positive direct antiglobulin tests and immune hemolytic anemia in patients receiving procainamide. N Engl J Med 311:809, 1984.

27. Mongey AB, Donovan-Brand R, Thomas TJ, et al: Serologic evaluation of patients receiving procainamide. Arthrit Rheum 35:219, 1992.

28. Harmon C, Portanova J: Drug-induced lupus: Clinical and serological studies. Clin Rheumatol 8:121, 1982.

29. Lahita R, Kluger J, Drayer DE, et al: Antibodies to nuclear antigens in patients treated with procainamide or acetylprocainamide. N Engl J Med 301:1382, 1979.

30. Rubin R, McNally EM, Nufinow SR, et al: IgG antibodies to the histone complex H2A-H2B characterize procainamide-induced lupus. Clin Immunol Immunopathol 36:49, 1985.

31. Weisbort RH, Yee WS, Colburn KK, et al: Antiguanosine antibodies: A new marker for procainamide-induced systemic lupus erythematosus. Ann Intern Med 104:310, 1986.

32. Bauer LA, Black D, Gensler A: Procainamide-cimetidine drug interaction in elderly male patients. J Am Geriatr Soc 38:467, 1990.

33. Saal AK, Werner JA, Greene HL, et al: Effect of amiodarone on serum quinidine and procainamide levels. Am J Cardiol 53:1264, 1974.

34. Hughes B, Dyer JE, Schwartz AB: Increased procainamide plasma concentrations caused by quinidine: A new drug interaction. Am Heart J 114:908, 1987.

35. Waxman HL, Burton AE, Sadowski LM, et al: The response to procainamide during electrophysiologic study for sustained ventricular tachyarrhythmias predicts the response to other medications. Circulation 67:30, 1983.

36. Rae AP, Sokoloff NM, Webb CR, et al: Limitations of failure of procainamide during electrophysiologic testing to predict response to other medical therapy. J Am Coll Cardiol 6:410, 1985.

37. Wyse DG, Mitchell LB, Duff HJ: Procainamide, disopyramide and quinidine: Discordant antiarrhythmic effects during cross-over comparison in patients with inducible ventricular tachycardia. J Am Coll Cardiol 9:882, 1987.

38. Teo KK, Yusuf S, Furberg CD, et al: Effects of prophylactic antiarrhythmic drug therapy in acute myocardial infarction. An overview of results from randomized controlled trials. JAMA 270:1589, 1993.

39. Steinbeck G, Andresen D, Bach P, et al: A comparison of electrophysiologically guided antiarrhythmic drug therapy with beta-blocker therapy in patients with symptomatic, sustained ventricular tachyarrhythmias. N Engl J Med 327:987, 1992.

CHAPTER 147

Propafenone

James A. Reiffel, M.D., Katherine T. Murray, M.D., and Eric N. Prystowsky, M.D.

Propafenone is an antiarrhythmic agent that was originally synthesized in 1970. The drug has been marketed in West Germany since 1977 by Knoll A.G. and in the United States since 1990. Its primary action is the block of transmembrane sodium channels with prominent slowing of conduction throughout the heart. Because its effects on action potential duration (APD) and effective refractory period (ERP) are more modest, it has been classified as a class IC antiarrhythmic agent. The chemical structure of propafenone (2'-[2-hydroxy-3(propylamino)propoxy]-3-phenylpropiophen-[cfl]one hydrochloride) resembles that of β-adrenoreceptor blockers, and the drug possesses weak β-adrenergic and calcium antagonist activity. As with many β-adrenoreceptor blockers, the commercial preparation is a racemic mixture of r- and s-stereoisomers. Published data demonstrate that propafenone is effective for the treatment of both supraventricular and ventricular tachyarrhythmias, with a relatively low incidence of side effects. In the United States, propafenone is approved by the Food and Drug Administration (FDA) for the treatment of life-threatening ventricular arrhythmias, and it has been submitted for a supraventricular tachyarrhythmic indication.

BASIC ELECTROPHYSIOLOGY

Propafenone produces a number of concentration-dependent electrophysiologic effects *in vitro*. Its principal action is potent depression of the maximal rate of rise of phase 0 ($\dot{V}_{max}$) of the transmembrane action potential in atrial and ventricular muscle as well as in Purkinje fibers without a change in resting membrane potential.[1-6] This effect results from block of transmembrane sodium channels and appears to be most pronounced in ischemic tissue with reduced transmembrane resting potential.[5] Dose-ranging experiments in canine Purkinje fibers show that propafenone can depress $\dot{V}_{max}$ in fast-channel tissue at concentrations as low as 0.1 μM.[7] As with all local anesthetic agents,[8] reduction of $\dot{V}_{max}$ by propafenone is frequency- or use-dependent, with greater decrease in $\dot{V}_{max}$ at more rapid rates. Recovery from $\dot{V}_{max}$ depression or block is usually monoexponential; for propafenone, this process has a time constant for recovery of 4 to 15 seconds.[1, 4, 7] Dissociation of propafenone from the sodium channel is slower than for agents such as quinidine. This may account for the greater degree of conduction slowing as reflected in QRS prolongation during normal sinus rhythm with propafenone and similar antiarrhythmic drugs such as flecainide and encainide.[9] During use-dependent block, propafenone may have preferential affinity for the inactivated state of the sodium channel,[4] though some binding may occur during the activated state.[10] At concentrations of 10 μM or higher, propafenone produces tonic block of $\dot{V}_{max}$ in addition to its frequency-dependent effects and causes the resting membrane potential to rise to more positive values.[3, 4]

In addition to its effects on $\dot{V}_{max}$, propafenone may affect APD. Shortening of the plateau, or phase 2, of the action potential in both ventricular muscle and Purkinje fibers has been reported at concentrations as low as 1 μM.[1-3, 5, 7] However, unaltered, lengthened, and shortened APD have all been seen,[1, 10-14] perhaps related to cell type and experimental conditions. Shortening is most common in Purkinje fibers, and lengthening is more common in myocytes. Alterations in the ERP generally parallel the change in APD,[14] but the ERP usually remains greater than the APD. Thus, the ratio of the ERP to the APD remains greater than 1, a property of many antiarrhythmic drugs. Because its primary action is potent sodium-channel blockade with less of an effect on APD and ERP, propafenone has been classified as a class IC antiarrhythmic agent.

At concentrations greater than 1 μM, propafenone also decreases automaticity as evidenced by a reduction in the slope of phase 4 depolarization in various tissues, including atrial muscle, Purkinje fibers,[2, 3] and rabbit sinoatrial (SA) nodal cells.[14a] After coronary occlusion in dogs, propafenone suppresses delayed afterdepolarizations arising from ischemic endocardium.[5] At high concentrations, propafenone can inhibit the slow inward current.[2, 11, 15] In this respect, it is 100 times less potent than verapamil. This property appears to reside in the active metabolite, 5-OH-propafenone, rather than in the parent compound. The clinical significance of this effect is unclear. Propafenone may also prolong APD in the sinus node.[11] In diseased human myocardium, propafenone can suppress the spontaneous activity observed in cells with abnormally elevated resting transmembrane potential.[6]

Propafenone possesses stereoselective β-adrenoreceptor blocking activity as demonstrated in various animal models and in human subjects,[2, 11, 16-18] which is not surprising given its structural resemblance to propranolol. This property resides primarily in the s-enantiomer of the parent compound.[19, 20] In anesthetized dogs[17] as well as in isolated guinea pig[2] and rabbit[11] atrial preparations, propafenone antagonized the chronotropic and inotropic effects of isoproterenol. McLeod et al.[18] investigated the β-adrenoreceptor blocking actions of propafenone using numerous techniques. In human subjects, propafenone was one fortieth as potent as propranolol in producing β-adrenergic blockade as assessed by heart rate response to isoproterenol administration. The drug also modestly suppressed exercise-induced tachycardia. When a competitive binding assay was used with ^{125}I-iodocyanopindolol in human cardiac and rat lung membranes, propafenone was one fiftieth as potent as propranolol in its affinity for the β-adrenoreceptor. According to its effects on isoproterenol-stimulated adenylate cyclase activity in frog erythrocyte membranes, the drug appeared to be a nonselective β-adrenergic blocker without intrinsic sympathomimetic activity. The authors[18] concluded that some degree of β-adrenoreceptor blockade would be expected at the dosages of propafenone used clinically. Because propafenone has nonlinear kinetics, at a dose of 900 mg/day, the plasma levels are significant, and the β-blockade may be substantial. This may be particularly true for slow metabolizers and may explain the side effect of asthma in some of these patients.

ELECTROPHYSIOLOGIC EFFECTS *IN VIVO*

Consistent with its potent effects on $\dot{V}_{max}$, propafenone slows conduction throughout the heart in a dose-dependent fashion. Oral therapy is generally associated with prolongation of the PR and QRS intervals[19-28] on the order of 15% to 20% at doses of 600 to 900 mg/day. Usually, no change occurs in the QT$_c$ interval. When the QT interval lengthens, it generally is because of widening of the QRS interval with minimal or no change in the JT interval. After intravenous administration of 1 to 2 mg/kg of propafenone, these electrophysiologic effects are somewhat less pronounced, with a significant increase occurring primarily in the QRS interval.[29-31] In some series, an increase in the PR interval has correlated with propafenone plasma concentration,[32, 33] but one study found no such correlation in 30 patients with sustained ventricular tachyarrhythmias,[28] probably because active metabolites (see later) contribute to the clinical effects. Changes in QRS duration have also varied, but such changes have correlated with plasma propafenone concentration in some series.[34, 35] In the isolated perfused rabbit heart model, propafenone myocardial levels correlated highly ($r = .96$) with increase in the QRS interval.[36]

Parameters measured during programmed electrical stimulation (PES) using intracardiac catheters demonstrate alterations of conduction and refractory periods throughout the heart during treatment with propafenone. Intraatrial conduction time increases, as do AH and HV intervals; the refractory periods of the right atrium, right ventricle, and atrioventricular (AV) node; and the atrial pacing cycle length producing Wenckebach block during oral therapy.[21, 30, 37] Typically, the cycle length of sustained ventricular tachycardia, if inducible, is also prolonged during drug therapy. Similar changes are observed following intravenous administration.[29-31, 38-40] Concentration-response data for changes in intracardiac parameters as measured during PES are lacking. Also, corrected sinus nodal recovery time and SA conduction time may be prolonged after oral or intravenous administration,[21, 30, 41] but some investigators have found these parameters to be unchanged with propafenone therapy.[29] In one study of 17 patients,[42] corrected sinus nodal recovery time did not change after intravenous administration of propafenone, 1.5 to 2 mg/kg, but SA conduction time was minimally prolonged. SA entrance block during pacing may explain the limited effect on sinus recovery time in such patients. After autonomic blockade with atropine and propranolol, both parameters increased significantly.

In patients with AV accessory pathways, propafenone lengthens the ERP of the accessory pathway in both anterograde and retrograde directions, and complete block can occur in either direction.[30, 39, 40, 43-46] As expected, propafenone also lengthens the shortest pacing cycle length that yields 1:1 conduction over the accessory pathway in both anterograde and retrograde directions. The shortest preexcited RR interval during atrial fibrillation is significantly prolonged with slowing of the ventricular rate. In patients with dual AV nodal physiology and supraventricular tachycardia, propafenone prolongs the refractory period of the AV node in both fast and slow pathways, anterograde and retrograde. It may cause block in the slow pathways[39, 40, 43] anterograde or retrograde, or in the fast pathways retrograde.

Preliminary data indicate that in both dogs[47, 48] and human subjects,[49-52] ventricular propafenone elevates pacing thresholds. The mean change following a single oral dose of 450 mg is 46%.[49] In addition, the sensing threshold can be reduced by an average of 15%. Elevations in the defibrillation threshold have also been reported, though a decrease has been reported in pigs under specific experimental conditions.[53]

HEMODYNAMIC EFFECTS

The administration of propafenone in animal models and in human subjects may be associated with negative inotropic effects. In general, therapy by either the oral or intravenous route is not associated with a change in resting blood pressure[21-23, 27, 29, 51] though decreases have been reported, even with a single 150-mg dose.[19, 54-57] In anesthetized, closed-chest dogs, intravenously administered propafenone, 4 mg/kg, produced a drop in pulmonary arterial and aortic systolic pressures with a reduction in cardiac output from 4.5 ± 1.0 L/min to 3.8 ± 0.7 L/min during atrial pacing.[47] In 28 patients with ventricular tachycardia undergoing PES, intravenously administered propafenone, 2 mg/kg, followed by a 1- to 2-mg/min infusion, was given during hemodynamic monitoring.[29] Right atrial, pulmonary arterial, and pulmonary capillary wedge pressures increased significantly, with a rise in systemic and pulmonary vascular resistances and a drop in cardiac index from 2.6 ± 0.8 L/min/m^2 to 2.3 ± 0.7 L/min/m^2 during sinus rhythm.

In another group of 60 patients with ventricular tachycardia,[58] ejection fraction in sinus rhythm as measured by M-mode echocardiography was unchanged during oral propafenone therapy when the baseline ejection fraction was greater than 50%. However, in patients whose baseline ejection fraction was less than 50%, ejection fraction in sinus rhythm significantly dropped from 34% to 29%, with 3 of 21 patients giving evidence of congestive heart failure (CHF). Conversely, Brodsky et al.[59] observed 10 patients with ventricular arrhythmias and symptomatic CHF orally taking propafenone, 900 mg/day, as outpatients. In eight of the patients, the left ventricular ejection fraction was measured by radionuclide ventriculography and was less than 40% in each case. The mean ejection fraction for the group was unchanged during treatment, but two patients experienced drops of at least 5%, whereas another had an apparent increase of 14%, making interpretation of the data difficult. In 1 of the 10 patients, propafenone was discontinued because of clinical worsening of heart failure. The same laboratory published similar results in a larger series in 1987.[60]

Some investigators have suggested a dose-related effect. This may relate to pharmacodynamics determined by metabolic pattern. In patients without historical or clinical evidence of CHF, oral propafenone therapy at a mean dose of 879 mg/day caused a drop in ejection fraction from 52% to 48% as measured by radionuclide ventriculography; a second group of patients with a history of CHF and baseline ejection fraction less than 45% experienced no change in ejection fraction at a mean oral dose of 600 mg/day.[61] From this evidence, one might conclude that propafenone will usually be tolerated by patients with left ventricular dysfunction but that worsening or new congestive symptoms can be precipitated.

Cautious observation and/or slower dosing increments would be prudent if propafenone is to be used in patients with a history of CHF.

As stated earlier, propafenone therapy probably produces some degree of β-adrenoreceptor blockade, particularly at higher doses. After single oral doses of 300 mg or during therapy with 300 mg every 8 hours, the peak heart rate during exercise testing has been reduced compared with baseline in several studies.[18, 28, 51] This may be one mechanism underlying the hemodynamic observations.

PHARMACOKINETICS

After oral administration, propafenone is absorbed rapidly and completely, with peak levels in 2 or 3 hours.[32, 62] Because of extensive first-pass metabolism in most patients, oral bioavailability is low and appears to increase with increasing dosage. In a group of normal volunteers, bioavailability was 5% after oral administration of 150 mg of propafenone and 12% after 300 mg.[62] This finding suggests that the process of presystemic hepatic clearance may be a saturable one, with a disproportionate nonlinear rise in plasma concentration as daily dosage is increased (e.g., as occurs with phenytoin). Evidence for this quality was also reported by Connolly et al.[21] during treatment of 13 patients with frequent ventricular ectopy. After a threefold increase in dosage, plasma drug concentration increased by 10 times. Bioavailability is enhanced significantly during concomitant food intake, with high levels achieved in most patients.[63]

After intravenous administration of propafenone, elimination kinetics indicate that propafenone distribution follows a two-compartment model in most patients.[34, 62, 64, 65] Total volume of distribution at steady state ranges from 1.9 to 3.6 L/kg, reflecting not only extensive protein binding (95%) but also uptake in tissues. In the isolated perfused rabbit heart model, myocardial concentrations were estimated to exceed those in the perfusate by more than 100 times. Autopsy of one patient receiving long-term propafenone therapy showed drug accumulation in various tissues with highest concentrations in the liver and lung, but plasma concentration was not measured.[66]

In more than 90% of patients, propafenone is metabolized rapidly and extensively in the liver.[35, 67, 68] Metabolic products of glucuronide and sulfate conjugates constitute the principal form of propafenone excretion in the feces and urine.[34, 67] The primary metabolites seen in plasma are 5-hydroxypropafenone and N-depropylpropafenone,[66, 69] but numerous other metabolites have been reported.[67] In fewer than 10% of patients, a principal hepatic cytochrome P-450 enzyme responsible for propafenone metabolism appears to be either deficient or absent.[35, 68] These patients may experience β-blocking actions even at low doses rather than only at doses that exceed saturation of hepatic clearance.[70] This metabolic defect is a genetic trait and is coinherited with a similar defect in

the biotransformation of the antihypertensive drug debrisoquin to its principal metabolite, 4-hydroxydebrisoquine.[71] The metabolism of debrisoquin demonstrates bimodal distribution with two distinct patient populations—extensive and poor metabolizers. The responsible enzyme appears to play a similar and important role in the biotransformation of numerous other compounds.[72] In patients who are poor metabolizers of debrisoquin and propafenone, 5-hydroxypropafenone is present in plasma in small amounts or not at all. In addition, these patients demonstrate marked reduction in propafenone clearance, with increases in elimination half-life and in the plasma concentration generated per milligram of dose administered.[35] These patients are also more likely to experience central nervous system side effects and greater β-blocking effects owing to the higher plasma concentrations of the parent compound obtained during therapy. However, propafenone appears to be equally antiarrhythmic in extensive and in poor metabolizers. Available data indicate that the enzyme involved converts propafenone to 5-hydroxypropafenone, which also possesses class IC actions.[73]

During long-term oral therapy with propafenone, the plasma concentrations of 5-hydroxypropafenone and N-depropylpropafenone vary. Ratios of total metabolite plasma concentration at steady state can range from 9% to 27% (mean 18%) for N-depropylpropafenone and from 6% to 73% (mean, 23%) for 5-hydroxypropafenone. As stated, some of this variability may relate to genetically determined differences in metabolic capabilities. The elimination half-life of these metabolites is probably longer than the elimination half-life of propafenone.[69] In humans, it appears that 5-hydroxypropafenone can accumulate in tissues at concentrations similar to propafenone concentrations.[66] In canine Purkinje fibers, the electrophysiologic characteristics and potency of 5-hydroxypropafenone are similar to those of propafenone, whereas those of N-depropylpropafenone are somewhat less.[7] Protein binding in plasma for both metabolites is less extensive than with the parent compound. This information suggests that these metabolites contribute to the antiarrhythmic or toxic effects of propafenone therapy in human subjects.

At steady-state dosing, a wide range of values has been reported for the elimination half-life of propafenone. Salerno et al.[74] reported values of 1.8 to 17.2 hours in patients with frequent ventricular ectopy, whereas Connolly et al.,[21] in similar patient populations, reported a range of 2.4 to 11.8 hours, and Siddoway et al.[34, 35] found values of 1.8 to 32.3 hours. With long-term administration, the half-life has been reported to be twice as long as that following the first dose.[75] In general, the elimination half-life for extensive metabolizers of propafenone ranges from 2 to 10 hours (mean 5.5 hours); for poor metabolizers, it ranges from 10 to 32 hours (mean 17.2 hours). Given this information, as well as the fact that the title course for drug accumulation is simply a reflection of that for elimination,[76] we can expect steady-state parent and metabolite plasma concentrations in all patients after 3 or 4 days of oral therapy with a given dose of propafenone.

As with elimination half-life, the propafenone plasma concentrations associated with suppression of ventricular arrhythmias vary greatly among individuals. In several studies of patients with frequent ventricular ectopy, effective plasma concentrations ranged from 42 to 3271 ng/ml,[19, 20, 23, 34, 35] and, in general, plasma concentration did not correlate with antiarrhythmic response. In patients with sustained ventricular tachyarrhythmias in whom therapy was guided by noninvasive or invasive testing, effective plasma concentrations ranged from 314 to 1627 ng/ml.[28] The genetic differences in metabolism that lead to variable accumulation of active propafenone metabolites probably account in large part for the unpredictable concentration-response relationship of this drug. In a group of 28 patients with frequent ventricular ectopy, effective plasma concentrations were 42 to 1356 ng/ml (mean 334 ng/ml) for extensive metabolizers and 1408 to 1801 ng/ml (mean 1579 ng/ml) for poor metabolizers.[35] (Similar variability has been reported in patients with supraventricular tachycardias.[70]) In these 28 patients, most adverse effects to the central nervous system occurred at plasma concentrations above 1000 ng/ml, with greater overlap for poor metabolizers between toxic and effective plasma concentrations. Therefore, the therapeutic range for propafenone varies and depends on the patient's metabolic phenotype. It is emphasized that the therapeutic range refers only to retrospective data, which yield ranges of plasma concentrations associated with antiarrhythmic and toxic effects.[77] For an individual patient, drug effect should be detected by electrocardiographic parameters, and drug efficacy should be assessed by noninvasive or invasive parameters rather than by drug plasma concentrations.

Although propafenone can be administered orally or intravenously, only the tablet form is available in the United States. In general, the initial dosage is 150 mg every 8 hours. The total daily dosage is increased every 3 or 4 days to a maximum of 900 mg/day by mouth as necessary for antiarrhythmic response. Although dosages of 1200 mg/day and higher have been used, the safety of these higher doses is not well established. During oral propafenone therapy in most adult patients, dosages of 600 to 900 mg/day are required for effective treatment of ventricular arrhythmias.[19, 23, 26–28, 51, 78] In slow metabolizers, twice-a-day dosing is sometimes effective, though most patients require a three-times-a-day (q8h) regimen. Because of the disproportionately large increase in plasma concentration that can occur with increasing dosage, it is suggested that each dosage increment be no greater than 50% of the previous dose.

Information on dosage in children is limited. However, in children given propafenone to treat junctional ectopic tachycardia after cardiac surgery,[79] the average loading dose required to achieve appropriate slowing of the rate of tachycardia was 1.7 mg/kg administered intravenously in 0.2-mg/kg increments every 10 to 15 minutes.[78] This therapeutic effect was maintained using an infusion regimen of 0.004 mg/kg/min after the loading dose. In 58 patients aged 2 days to 16 years with a variety of arrhythmias, Reimer et al.[80] used 1.5 mg/kg administered intravenously followed by 308 mg/m² or 16.8 mg/kg administered orally. Similarly, in 24 pediatric patients with paroxysmal supraventricular tachycardia (PSVT), Musto et al.[56] used 1.5 mg/kg administered intravenously during a protocol in the electrophysiology laboratory, and Guccione et al.[81] used 8 to 15 mg/kg/day administered orally in 57 children with a variety of arrhythmias with an overall efficacy of 30% to 50%.

MODIFICATIONS IN DISEASE STATES

Severe hepatic dysfunction can significantly influence the pharmacokinetics of propafenone. In this situation, oral dosing is associated with a variable increase in bioavailability, a reduction in clearance, and decreased protein binding with an increase in free plasma concentrations of propafenone.[82] Consequently, it is recommended that the dose be reduced by 50% in patients with renal insufficiency; no change in propafenone clearance or half-life has been reported, though the disposition of active metabolites may be altered.[83, 84] Although no specific data are available on dosing modifications in patients with renal insufficiency or CHF, the drug should be administered cautiously to such patients, because 19% to 38% of propafenone metabolites are excreted in the urine over a 48-hour period.[67]

DRUG INTERACTIONS

Oral therapy with propafenone produces a dose-dependent increase in digoxin plasma concentrations in human subjects. At a dose of 450 mg/day, digoxin plasma concentrations may rise by 34% to 40%,[85, 86] whereas oral therapy with 900 mg/day can cause an increase of 57% to 136% (mean 83%).[20] This effect appears to be long-lasting during long-term therapy. Interindividual variation is reported. Propafenone probably displaces digoxin from tissue-binding sites, because renal clearance of a single oral dose of digoxin was unchanged by concomitant therapy with propafenone.[86] Based on this information, the authors suggest that the dose of digoxin be reduced an average of 50% should therapy with propafenone be started. Digoxin plasma concentration should be measured when steady state is reached, and the dose of digoxin should be adjusted accordingly. Additionally, the additive pharmacodynamic effects of digoxin and β-blocker actions on nodal tissue need to be considered and monitored.

Propafenone can also potentiate the effects of warfarin therapy.[87, 88] In normal volunteers, propafenone therapy during long-term warfarin treatment is associated with a 38% rise in warfarin levels and often an increase in prothrombin time. The mechanism of this effect is probably an alteration in warfarin metabolism. Caution should be used, and the prothrombin time should be monitored carefully when patients taking warfarin are given propafenone.

Given the inhibitory effects of cimetidine on hepatic enzymes, it is not surprising that this drug might raise plasma concentrations of propafenone somewhat. In a study of normal volunteers,[89] administration of cimetidine combined with propafenone caused a rise of 23% in propafenone plasma concentrations. When poor metabolizers of propafenone were excluded, this elevation was about 31%. Small but significant increases in the QRS interval occurred from 98 ± 4 msec during propafenone therapy to 103 ± 3 msec during concomitant therapy with propafenone and cimetidine. Elimination half-life was also increased by 14% or by 21% when poor metabolizers were excluded.

Because of the potential for additive electrophysiologic and hemodynamic effects, propafenone should be used with great caution in combination with calcium antagonists or β-adrenoreceptor blockers. Data indicate the addition of propafenone to therapy with either metoprolol or propranolol[90, 91] causes a significant increase in plasma concentration of the β-adrenoreceptor blocker. This effect is associated with a greater degree of β-adrenoreceptor antagonism during combination therapy than with either metoprolol or propranolol alone. The mechanism of these drug interactions is unclear, but it may involve inhibition of systemic clearance of the β-adrenoreceptor blocker by propafenone. Few data are available regarding combination therapy with other antiarrhythmic agents. Quinidine has been found to be a potent inhibitor of the cytochrome P-450 enzyme that oxidizes debrisoquin to 4-hydroxydebrisoquin.[92] In patients taking debrisoquin, concomitant administration of quinidine leads to a reduction in debrisoquin metabolism with elevated levels of parent drug.[93] Similarly, administration of quinidine and propafenone together inhibits propafenone metabolism somewhat, with a subsequent rise in parent plasma drug concentration and a reduction in metabolites.[94] In general, during combination therapy with antiarrhythmic drugs, doses of each individual agent should be decreased initially. Lastly, rifampin may reduce propafenone levels,[95] whereas propafenone may increase plasma levels of cyclosporine, desipramine, and theophylline.[96–98]

ADVERSE EFFECTS

During oral therapy with propafenone, noncardiovascular side effects are usually mild and often transient.[99–102] Their incidence appears to be dose-dependent. Symptoms most commonly encountered include a bitter or metallic taste, dry mouth, constipation, nausea or vomiting, and dizziness. Diplopia, paresthesia, fatigue, and headache also occur. These side effects lead to discontinuation of therapy in 5% to 10% of patients (range 0% to 22%).[19, 20, 23–26, 30, 37, 51, 103] During intravenous administration of 1 or 2 mg/

kg of propafenone, minimal side effects have been reported.[39, 40, 43] In a comparative study, the incidence of side effects with propafenone during dose ranging was lower than with disopyramide.[104] The incidence has been similar to or less than that seen with quinidine[27, 105] and was similar to that of sotalol in one trial (7% vs. 8%).[106] Infrequent adverse reactions include positive antinuclear antibodies,[22, 29] with one case of a systemic lupus-like syndrome,[107] elevated liver function tests,[19] cholestatic jaundice,[108] reduced potency and spermatogenesis,[109] psychosis,[110] and aggravation of seizures[29] or myasthenia gravis. Bronchospasm has also been seen, which is thought to be related to β-adrenergic blockade. This adverse effect has been documented in asthmatic patients both clinically and during pulmonary function testing, and caution should be used in treating such patients with propafenone.[111]

Important cardiovascular side effects of propafenone include the precipitation or exacerbation of CHF, conduction disturbances, and aggravation of arrhythmia. In some series of patients with a history of heart failure symptoms, the drug was well tolerated,[59, 78] whereas in others, precipitation of heart failure occasionally resulted in discontinuation of therapy.[58, 59] In a study of 60 patients with ventricular arrhythmias treated with propafenone, CHF developed in 3 patients.[61] All had reduced ejection fractions, with a mean value of 22%. In another group of patients with ejection fractions of less than 40%, two had increasing dyspnea, one of whom had definite evidence of CHF.[59] In a multicenter study of 774 patients,[99] 3.4% had new or worsened CHF. Therefore, propafenone should be given cautiously with low initial dosages and careful dose escalation in patients with compensated CHF. In patients with overt clinical evidence of heart failure, the drug probably should be avoided.

Because of its potent electrophysiologic effects, propafenone can depress intracardiac conduction as well as SA and AV nodal function. During oral therapy, first-degree AV block is common[22, 61, 112] but does not necessitate discontinuation of the drug. Second-degree AV block and complete heart block also have been described.[19, 58, 110] Widening of the QRS complex has been manifested by intraventricular conduction disturbances or by bundle branch block, which occurs with an incidence of 4% to 8%.[20, 25, 27] Sinus bradycardia, SA block, and sinus arrest occasionally are reported.[25, 41, 58] In the setting of second- or third-degree AV block or significant sinus node dysfunction, propafenone should not be given in the absence of a functioning electronic pacemaker.

The incidence of aggravation of arrhythmia during propafenone therapy varies widely, from 2% to 19%.[19, 21, 23, 58, 110, 112–115] In a series of 774 patients, it was 5.3%.[99] This variation is due in part to different definitions of proarrhythmia as well as to the wide spectrum of patient populations that have been treated. Such aggravation is more likely in patients with a history of sustained ventricular tachyarrhythmia, ischemia, and/or ventricular disease or dysfunction. Incessant tachycardia sometimes occurs. Stanton et al.,[114, 116] defining proarrhythmia as a new symptomatic or worsened established ventricular arrhythmia, documented that propafenone caused proarrhythmia in 5% to 6% of patients, but none died and no episodes of ventricular fibrillation or torsade de pointes occurred. Rare cases of torsade de pointes have been reported, however, when propafenone was combined with amiodarone or when the drug produced bradycardia.[117, 118] As with class IA and other class IC agents, propafenone may provoke sustained atrial flutter in patients treated for atrial fibrillation.[119] The low incidence of ventricular proarrhythmia in the absence of structural heart disease or ventricular arrhythmias favors propafenone as a first-line drug in patients with symptomatic supraventricular tachyarrhythmias and normal hearts. Conversely, its proarrhythmic profile suggests that it is a second-line drug in patients with ventricular arrhythmias and organic heart disease.

The ingestion of large doses of propafenone can be life-threatening, with symptoms that include coma, seizures, respiratory depression, hypotension, sinus bradycardia and sinus arrest, conduction disturbances, and ventricular tachycardia. Generally, supportive measures are recommended, because the drug is poorly removed by hemodialysis.[120]

CLINICAL EFFICACY
Ventricular Ectopy

In several double-blind, placebo-controlled trials, propafenone has been found to suppress chronic, high-frequency ventricular ectopic depolarizations and nonsustained ventricular tachycardia.[19, 20, 22, 51] During the dose-ranging phase of these trials, in which maximal doses of 900 to 1200 mg/day were used, the antiarrhythmic response was satisfactory in 67% to 87% of patients, usually defined as an 80% or greater reduction in baseline ventricular ectopy with elimination of complex forms. These results have been confirmed in other studies with less-rigid investigational protocols.[23, 26, 79, 110] The ventricular arrhythmias of many patients treated with propafenone in these trials had been refractory to a number of Class IA and/or IB antiarrhythmic drugs. In several studies, efficacy was confirmed during long-term outpatient follow-up. Nonsustained ventricular tachycardia (NSVT) is usually reduced more than total ventricular premature depolarizations (VPDs) are.[74] VPD reductions (similar to the conduction effects) are dose-dependent.[121]

A number of studies have compared the effectiveness of propafenone with that of other antiarrhythmic agents in suppression of chronic, stable ventricular arrhythmias. In a comparison between disopyramide, 600 mg/day, and propafenone, 900 mg/day, in 12 patients with frequent ventricular ectopic depolarizations, arrhythmia was suppressed in 6 of 12 patients taking disopyramide and in 6 of 12 taking propafenone.[122] In another study using a similar patient population, propafenone, 450 mg/day, and disopyramide,

300 mg/day, effectively suppressed ventricular arrhythmias in 4 of 10 and 1 of 10 patients, respectively.[123] Also, higher-dose propafenone, 900 mg/day, was effective in six of nine patients, whereas higher-dose disopyramide, 600 mg/day, was successful in four of seven patients. The authors concluded that propafenone was a more effective antiarrhythmic agent in this group of patients; it was also better tolerated. Another study that compared propafenone, 450 mg/day, with disopyramide, 600 mg/day, found the two agents to have comparable efficacy at the doses administered.[124] In 25 patients with frequent ventricular ectopy, propafenone was more effective than quinidine in achieving satisfactory suppression of ventricular arrhythmias using a range of dosages.[27] Episodes of nonsustained ventricular tachycardia were similarly reduced by both agents. In a crossover trial of propafenone, 300 mg twice a day, and slow-release quinidine, 800 mg twice a day, efficacy rates were identical, although 2 of 12 patients responded to only propafenone and 2 of 12 to only quinidine.[105] In yet another comparison in 105 patients randomized to either quinidine or propafenone, response rates were identical (with a trend favoring propafenone).[125] Discontinuation was higher on quinidine. In 12 patients with coronary artery disease and frequent ventricular ectopic depolarizations, suppression of ventricular arrhythmia was 94% with flecainide, 80% with propafenone, and only 53% with mexiletine.[126] Propafenone at an intravenous dose of 1 mg/kg was similar in efficacy to lidocaine in suppressing frequent ventricular ectopy in patients admitted to coronary care units because of chest pain.[127] Finally in a multidrug comparison, Salerno et al.[74] reported similar NSVT reductions for flecainide, encainide, and propafenone (>92%); slightly higher VPD reduction for flecainide than for propafenone (93% versus 77%); and greater efficacy for all three of these agents than for moricizine. Two-year withdrawal rates were highest for moricizine and slightly higher for propafenone than for flecainide. Facchini et al.[128] reported similar efficacy with flecainide and propafenone, which exceeded that for disopyramide, mexiletine, tocainide, and propranolol (in that order). Single-dose responses to flecainide and propafenone had an 89% correlation with steady-state responses.

Ventricular Tachycardia and Fibrillation

As is true with most available antiarrhythmic agents, propafenone is less effective in suppressing sustained than in suppressing nonsustained ventricular tachyarrhythmias. Connolly et al.[21] examined the efficacy of propafenone in suppressing recurrent ventricular tachycardia and ventricular fibrillation in 16 patients, of whom 14 had sustained clinical arrhythmias. During PES after oral treatment with propafenone, only one patient was found to be "noninducible"; ventricular tachycardia became nonsustained in another. Of the patients who had sustained arrhythmias induced while taking propafenone, induction was more difficult in two; in two other patients, the ventricular rate was less than 125 beats/min. After hospital discharge, arrhythmias recurred in the patient who was noninducible and in those with slower ventricular tachycardia, whereas the patient whose ventricular tachycardia had become nonsustained and whose arrhythmias had become harder to induce experienced no recurrence.

More definitive information comes from Chilson et al.,[37] who examined the effects of oral propafenone therapy in 25 patients with recurrent ventricular tachycardia and ventricular fibrillation. In 14 of these patients, the presenting arrhythmia was sustained; in 15 patients, therapy was guided by PES. While taking propafenone, three patients, one of whom had sustained arrhythmia at baseline, were found to be noninducible and experienced no recurrence of their arrhythmias over some 11 months of follow-up. Seven others with inducible arrhythmias that were slow and well tolerated were discharged on propafenone therapy. Two of these patients who had sustained ventricular tachycardia at baseline had recurrent arrhythmias, whereas five patients, including two with sustained ventricular tachyarrhythmias at baseline, did not.

The same laboratory[103] reported a study of 129 patients with recurrent ventricular tachycardia or ventricular fibrillation who were also treated with propafenone. Seventy-three patients had histories of either sustained ventricular tachycardia (50 patients) or cardiac arrest (23 patients) at baseline. Fifty-three patients were discharged taking propafenone, and follow-up averaged 26.8 months. A total of 35 patients remained asymptomatic without recurrent arrhythmias, including 11 of 15 patients with a history of sustained ventricular tachycardia and four of seven with a history of cardiac arrest. PES was performed in 31 patients before and during propafenone therapy. All nine patients who were noninducible on the drug did well during outpatient follow-up. Of the 22 patients with ventricular tachycardia inducible during treatment with propafenone, 17 remained asymptomatic. Patients in whom arrhythmia recurred had easier modes of induction (fewer extra stimuli) at drug study compared with asymptomatic patients. The authors concluded that noninducibility while taking propafenone predicted a good outcome with treatment, whereas an easier mode of induction predicted recurrence of arrhythmia. The correlation of noninducibility (achieved in 26% of 50 patients) with good outcome was also reported by Podczeck et al.[129] and by Budde et al.[130] The latter group noted that noninducibility with propafenone was more likely in patients with faster baseline ventricular tachycardia (VT), higher left ventricular ejection fraction, or lower left ventricular end-diastolic pressure.

The utility of noninvasive and invasive testing was examined in still another 30 patients treated with orally administered propafenone, all of whom had sustained ventricular tachycardia or ventricular fibrillation at baseline.[28] Therapy was thought to be successful in 16 patients as judged by 24-hour ambulatory electrocardiographic monitoring and exercise treadmill testing. In a group of patients who also underwent PES, the results of therapy guided in this fashion were concordant with the results of noninvasive evaluation. Overall, 10 patients experienced no recurrence of arrhythmias during long-term follow-up for about 10 months. Similarly, Kowey et al.[131] reported good outcome (only one sudden cardiac death [SCD] and three recurrent VTs) in 20 patients discharged with good responses to Holter or electrophysiologic monitoring.

One might conclude from the findings in these somewhat complex series that in patients with sustained VT and in patients who are inducible when not taking the drug but noninducible when taking propafenone, long-term freedom from arrhythmia and drug tolerance are good. It may also be reasonable to use propafenone for long-term therapy if the arrhythmia induced while receiving drug therapy is hemodynamically tolerable. These results are similar to conclusions drawn for some other drugs. Whether Holter-guided therapy is as predictive of outcome as EPS with propafenone seems less settled.

Like oral propafenone treatment, treatment with intravenous propafenone has yielded variable clinical results in patients with sustained ventricular tachyarrhythmias. In 14 patients with sustained ventricular tachycardia, Doherty et al.[31] reported little success in suppressing arrhythmias induced by PES and intravenously administered propafenone. After treatment with a variety of dosage regimens, only one patient became noninducible, and six demonstrated new morphologies of ventricular tachycardia. In one patient, the arrhythmia became incessant after treatment with propafenone; in another patient, more rapid ventricular tachycardia, which was poorly tolerated, was induced. Shen et al.[29] examined the results of intravenously administered propafenone, 2 mg/kg, followed by infusions of 1 to 2 mg/min in 28 patients with recurrent ventricular tachycardias. It is unclear how many of these patients had a history of sustained arrhythmias at baseline. In patients treated with an infusion of 1 mg/min after the loading dose of propafenone, one of nine become noninducible, with a mean plasma concentration of 934 ng/ml. In the group treated with an infusion of 2 mg/min after intravenous loading, 3 of 11 patients became noninducible, with a mean plasma concentration of 1447 ng/ml. Preliminary data suggest that response to intravenously administered propafenone or intravenously administered procainamide may predict response to orally administered propafenone.[132]

With respect to refractory ventricular arrhythmias, early data suggest that combination therapy of propafenone with other antiarrhythmic agents may be useful. In two studies reported by Klein et al.,[133, 134] the addition of propafenone to either quinidine or procainamide in patients with frequent ventricular ectopy led to improved antiarrhythmic efficacy and a reduction in and lower incidence of side effects. The combination of propafenone and amiodarone has also been efficacious in resistant patients.[135] These drugs have not been found to alter each other's serum concentration.[135] We have also found propafenone and mexiletine to be occasionally useful in combination.

Supraventricular Arrhythmias

Although propafenone has not received approval from the FDA for use in patients with supraventricular tachycardia, data show that it is effective against a wide variety of supraventricular arrhythmias, including AV nodal reentry, AV reentry (Wolff-Parkinson-White syndrome), and atrial flutter and fibrillation. Most reported clinical trials have been performed in Europe.

Propafenone is effective in the treatment of reciprocating tachycardia resulting from AV nodal reentry, both acutely and during long-term management.[39, 40, 43, 136, 137] Waleffe et al.,[39] using an intravenous dose of 2 mg/kg, terminated tachycardia in four of five patients, all by block in the retrograde fast pathway. In three patients, the arrhythmia was no longer inducible. Shen et al.[43] obtained similar results when three patients with AV nodal reentry converted to normal sinus rhythm and were subsequently noninducible. Two of these patients also had retrograde block in the fast pathway of the AV node. In another small series, Allen et al.[137] showed a 40% long-term efficacy with orally administered propafenone in five patients with AV nodal reentrant tachycardia (AVNRT). Santinelli et al. noted slightly lower oral efficacy (6 of 11 patients) in patients with AVNRT or AVRT (450 to 900 mg/day) compared with intravenous efficacy (9 of 11 patients) using 1.5 to 2.0 mg/kg.[136] Larger trials confirm these results. In 24 patients with reciprocating tachycardia resulting from either AV nodal reentry or AV reentry reported by Manz et al., 10 of 20 patients whose arrhythmias were inducible by PES were rendered noninducible after intravenous propafenone therapy.[43] Four additional patients became noninducible after oral therapy. After hospital discharge, six of seven patients who were noninducible had no further recurrence of arrhythmias, whereas five of seven patients who remained inducible had breakthrough arrhythmias.

Propafenone is a useful agent in the treatment of AV reentry. In six patients with orthodromic reciprocating tachycardia reported by Waleffe et al.,[39] arrhythmia was terminated in five patients with intravenously administered propafenone, 2 mg/kg. In three patients, termination resulted from retrograde block in the accessory pathway. Only one patient was noninducible after arrhythmia termination. In the series of Shen et al.,[43] 9 of 14 patients with AV reentry converted to sinus rhythm after intravenous propafenone therapy by block of retrograde conduction in the accessory pathway in each case. A lower intravenous dose of propafenone, 1.0 to 1.5 mg/kg, terminated AV reentry in two of seven patients reported by Disertori et al.[45] Breithardt et al.[30] reported the results of propafenone therapy in 47 patients with AV accessory pathways. Twenty-three of these patients underwent PES before and after therapy with either intravenously or orally administered drug. Recipro-

cating tachycardia could be induced in 14 patients at baseline. Following treatment, three patients were noninducible; in three other patients, however, the tachycardia became nonsustained. During follow-up of 2 or 3 years, 40% of patients were asymptomatic, and another 42% reported only rare, slow, self-terminating episodes and continued treatment with propafenone. Frank et al.[44] reported that two of seven patients with orthodromic reciprocating tachycardia at baseline PES were rendered noninducible after treatment with propafenone at a daily oral dose of 900 mg. In addition, in three of five patients, atrial fibrillation could no longer be induced. After a mean follow-up of about 12 months, eight patients remained asymptomatic. Similarly, Sethi et al.[138] reported an efficacy of 89% (eight of nine patients) for orally administered propafenone (300 mg three times a day) in preventing inducible AVRT in patients who were inducible at baseline EPS. They also reported complete antegrade accessory pathway block in four of five patients with manifested Wolff-Parkinson-White syndrome and retrograde accessory pathway block in six of nine patients studied. Santinelli et al.[136] reported that orally administered propafenone was effective in four of seven patients with Wolff-Parkinson-White syndrome and AVRT following doses of more than 600 mg/day. Thus, propafenone appears to be effective treatment in patients with either AV nodal reentry or AV reentry.

Substantial data suggest that propafenone is also useful in the treatment of other atrial arrhythmias. In three patients with supraventricular tachycardia due to intraatrial reentry, intravenous propafenone therapy successfully terminated tachycardia, but a nonsustained form of the arrhythmia could be induced subsequently.[43]

Propafenone is useful in the treatment of a variety of supraventricular arrhythmias in children, but the long-term safety of its use in this situation is unknown. Musto et al.[139] reported that propafenone was effective in the acute termination and long-term prophylaxis of reciprocating tachycardias related to both AV nodal reentry and AV reentry. In addition, the drug effectively slowed the tachycardia rate of rapid junctional ectopic tachycardia following surgical repair of congenital heart disease.[79]

Propafenone also is useful in both the termination and the prophylaxis of atrial flutter and atrial fibrillation. In a group of patients with chronic arrhythmias of this nature reported by Beck et al.,[140] propafenone, in daily oral doses of up to 1800 mg, converted 17 of 41 patients to normal sinus rhythm. Similarly, Porterfield and Porterfield[141] reported conversion of chronic atrial fibrillation to normal sinus rhythm by propafenone in 17 of 26 patients. Long-term atrial fibrillation recurred in 3 of 20 patients converted by drug or DC energy (mean dose 840 mg/day). Only 19% discontinued the drug for side effects despite the high doses. Kerr et al.[142] reported complete or partial long-term efficacy in 40 of 53 patients with previously drug-refractory atrial fibrillation. Seven had underlying heart disease. The dose range was 300 to 1200 mg/day. Efficacy was also reported in 30 of 47 patients by Hammill et al.;[143] episodes of paroxysmal atrial fibrillation were reduced by more than 90% in 25 patients, including 17 with total suppression over 1½ years. Five patients, however, noticed an increase in frequency of atrial fibrillation with propafenone. Long-term efficacy in a larger and perhaps more clearly characterized series of patients has also been reported by Antman et al.[144] Propafenone was used in a stepped-care approach (propafenone followed by sotalol followed by amiodarone) and in a randomized trial (propafenone vs. sotalol); in both cases, propafenone performed in patients with either drug-refractory paroxysmal atrial fibrillation (PAF) or cardioverted chronic atrial fibrillation refractory to class IA agents. These authors showed approximately 40% 6-month and 30% long-term efficacy, despite the history of prior drug resistance. Doses were 450 to 900 mg/day. Efficacy was similar to that of dl-sotalol. Drug discontinuation rates for side effects were less than 10% with both agents. Perhaps more importantly, two well-performed controlled clinical trials of propafenone versus placebo demonstrated the drug's efficacy in atrial fibrillation and flutter.[145, 146] Connolly and Hoffert,[145] using a dose-finding phase followed by a randomized, double-blind, placebo-controlled, crossover phase in 18 patients, demonstrated a reduction in PAF by propafenone. Pritchett et al.[146] also confirmed propafenone's efficacy in 17 patients, as judged by abolition of PAF, reduction in frequency of episodes, or prolongation of interepisode interval. Additional relevant observations come from a multicenter study of 2146 patients with supraventricular arrhythmias wherein open-label drug showed "very good" or "good" efficacy in 54% and 25%, respectively.[147] Even when propafenone does not abolish atrial fibrillation, it may be beneficial. Santinelli et al.,[148] for example, demonstrated clinically important prolongation of shortest RR intervals (from 190–270 to 320–420 msec) in patients with Wolff-Parkinson-White syndrome and atrial fibrillation.

These data show that propafenone is effective in the therapy of a variety of supraventricular tachyarrhythmias. In oral doses, it can reduce or prevent AV nodal reentrant tachycardia, AV reciprocating tachycardia, atrial fibrillation and flutter, and a variety of other supraventricular arrhythmias. The dose requirements may be higher in patients with atrial fibrillation, in whom the incidence of side effects leading to discontinuation is both dose-related and, at commonly used doses (450 to 900 mg/day), seems to be substantially less frequent than has been reported for quinidine. Propafenone may decrease the ventricular response in atrial fibrillation over the AV node, especially in patients with prominent β-blocking effects (slow metabolizers or high doses) and over bypass tracts, wherein antegrade conduction block and/or prolonged bypass tract refractoriness can be effected. Because atrial fibrillation can be converted to slower flutter with an increased ventricular response, propafenone should not be used in patients with atrial fibrillation flutter in the absence of ventricular rate control (usually with concomitant AV nodal blocking agents).

CONCLUSIONS

Propafenone is a potent antiarrhythmic agent that blocks inward sodium current. At clinically used dosages, the drug probably also causes some β-adrenoreceptor blockade. The PR and QRS intervals often are significantly prolonged during oral therapy. The effective oral dose usually ranges from 450 to 900 mg/day, and the elimination half-life varies in a genetically determined fashion. The drug is usually administered three times daily, though occasionally twice a day, and is generally well tolerated, with a low incidence of noncardiac side effects. It appears to be effective against a wide spectrum of both atrial and ventricular arrhythmias and compares favorably with standard antiarrhythmic therapy. Although data from the Cardiac Arrhythmia Suppression Trial (CAST)[149] have affected the indications for which propafenone (as well as other agents) is approved in the United States (in CAST, mortality in patients within 2 years of an acute myocardial infarction with asymptomatic nonsustained ventricular arrhythmias was greater during treatment with encainide and flecainide, agents with actions similar to that of propafenone, than during treatment with placebo), it should be remembered that although propafenone is classified as a IC agent because of its electrophysiologic properties at a cellular level, its β-blocking properties, binding kinetics, and pharmacologic effects *in vivo* are not identical to the effects of encainide and flecainide.

REFERENCES

1. Kohlardt M, Seifert C: Inhibition of ($\dot{V}_{max}$) of the action potential by propafenone and its voltage-, time-, and pH-dependence in mammalian ventricular myocardium. Naunyn Schmiedebergs Arch Pharmacol 315:55, 1980.
2. Ledda F, Mantelli L, Manzini S, et al: Electrophysiologic and antiarrhythmic properties of propafenone in isolated cardiac preparations. J Cardiovasc Pharmacol 3:1162, 1981.
3. Karagueuzian HS, Kato T, Sugi K, et al: Electrophysiologic effects of propafenone, a new antiarrhythmic drug, on isolated cardiac tissue. Circulation 66(Suppl II):379, 1982.
4. Kohlhardt M, Seifert C: Tonic and phasic INa blockade by antiarrhythmics: Different properties of drug binding to fast sodium channels as judged from ($\dot{V}_{max}$) studies with propafenone and derivatives in mammalian ventricular myocardium. Pflugers Arch 396:199, 1983.
5. Zeiler RH, Gough WB, El-Sherif N: Electrophysiologic effects of propafenone on canine ischemic cardiac cells. Am J Cardiol 54:424, 1984.
6. McCullough JR, Chua WT, Cohn MJ, et al: Electrophysiologic actions of propafenone in diseased human myocardium. Fed Proc 41:1107, 1982.
7. Thompson KA, Iansmith DH, Siddoway LA, et al: Potent electrophysiologic effects of the major metabolites of propafenone in canine Purkinje fibers. J Pharmacol Exp Ther 244(3):950, 1988.
8. Grant AO, Starmer CF, Strauss HC: Antiarrhythmic drug action: Blockade of the inward sodium current. Circ Res 55:427, 1984.

9. Roden DM, Woosley RL: Flecainide. N Engl J Med 315:36, 1986.

10. Hunjo H, Watanabe T, Kamiya K, et al: Effects of propafenone on electrical and mechanical activities of single ventricular myocytes isolated from guinea pig hearts. Br J Pharmacol 97:731, 1989.

11. Dukes ID, Vaughan Williams EM: The multiple modes of action of propafenone. Eur Heart J 5:115, 1984.

12. Katoh T, Karagueuzian HS, Sugi K, et al: Effects of propafenone on sinus nodal and ventricular automaticity: In vitro and in vivo correlation. Am Heart J 113:941, 1987.

13. Rouet R, Libersa CC, Broly F, et al: Comparative electrophysiological effects of propafenone, 5-hydroxypropafenone, and N-depropylpropfenone on guinea pig ventricular muscle fibers. J Cardiovascular Pharmacol 14:577, 1989.

14. Winslow E, Campbell JK: Comparative frequency-dependent effects of three class Ic agents, Org 7797, flecainide and propafenone, on ventricular action potential duration. J Cardiovascular Pharmacol 18:911, 1991.

14a. Satoh H, Hashimoto K: Effect of propafenone on the membrane currents of rabbit sinoatrial node cells. Eur J Pharmacol 99:185, 1984.

15. Kohlhardt M: Der Einflub von Propafenon auf den Transmembranaren Na;^{Pl} und Ca;$^{PI\cdot Pl}$ Strom der Warmbluter-Myokardfaser-Membran. Drug Dev Eval 1:35, 1977.

16. Paietta E, Poch G, Kukovetz WR: Analyse der Blockerwirkung von Propafenone (SA 79). Drug Dev Eval 1:20, 1977.

17. Brown NL, Worcel M, Zanirato J: Beta-adrenoreceptor antagonist activity of propafenone in the anaesthetized dog. Br J Clin Pharmacol 88:289P, 1986.

18. McLeod AA, Stiles GL, Shand DG: Demonstration of beta adrenoreceptor blockade by propafenone hydrochloride: Clinical pharmacologic, radioligand binding and adenylate cyclase activation studies. J Pharmacol Exp Ther 228:461, 1984.

19. Stoschietzky K, Klein W, Stark G, et al: Different stereoselective effects of R- and S-propafenone: Clinical pharmacology, electrophysiologic, and radioligand binding studies. Clinic Pharmacol Therapy 47:740, 1990.

20. Hii JT, Duff JH, Burgess ED: Clinical pharmacokinetics of propafenone. Clinical Pharmacokinet 21:1, 1991.

21. Connolly SJ, Kates RE, Lebsack CS, et al: Clinical efficacy and electrophysiology of oral propafenone for ventricular tachycardia. Am J Cardiol 52:1208, 1983.

22. De Soyza N, Terry L, Murphy ML, et al: Effect of propafenone in patients with stable ventricular arrhythmias. Am Heart J 108:285, 1984.

23. Hammill SC, Sorenson PB, Wood DL, et al: Propafenone for the treatment of refractory complex ventricular ectopic activity. Mayo Clin Proc 61:98, 1986.

24. Prystowsky EN, Heger JJ, Chilson DA, et al: Antiarrhythmic and electrophysiologic effects of oral propafenone. Am J Cardiol 54:26D, 1984.

25. Coumel P, Leclercq J, Assayag P: European experience with the antiarrhythmic efficacy of propafenone for supraventricular and ventricular arrhythmias. Am J Cardiol 54:60D, 1984.

26. Schamroth L, Myburgh DP, Schamroth CL, et al: Oral propafenone in the suppression of chronic stable ventricular arrhythmias. Chest 87:448, 1985.

27. Dinh H, Murphy ML, Baker BJ, et al: Efficacy of propafenone compared with quinidine in chronic ventricular arrhythmia. Am J Cardiol 55:1520, 1985.

28. Podrid PJ, Lown B: Propafenone: A new agent for ventricular arrhythmia. J Am Coll Cardiol 4:117, 1984.

29. Shen EN, Sung RY, Morady F, et al: Electrophysiologic and hemodynamic effects of intravenous propafenone in patients with recurrent ventricular tachycardia. J Am Coll Cardiol 3:1291, 1984.

30. Breithardt G, Borggrefe M, Wiebringhaus E, et al: Effect of propafenone in the Wolff-Parkinson-White syndrome: Electrophysiologic findings and long-term follow-up. Am J Cardiol 54:29D, 1984.

31. Doherty JU, Wayman HL, Kienzle MG, et al: Limited role of intravenous propafenone hydrocholoride in the treatment of sustained ventricular tachycardia: Electrophysiologic effects and results of programmed ventricular stimulation. J Am Coll Cardiol 4:378, 1984.

32. Keller K, Meyer-Estorf G, Beck OA, et al: Correlation between serum concentration and pharmacologic effect on atrioventricular conduction time of the antiarrhythmic drug propafenone. Eur J Clin Pharmacol 13:17, 1978.

33. Blanke H, Aschbrenner B, Karsch KR, et al: Plasmaspiegel Wirkungs-Beziehung und Organverteilung von Propafenon. Dtsch Med Wochenschr 104:587, 1979.

34. Siddoway LA, Roden DM, Woosley RL: Clinical pharmacology of propafenone: Pharmacokinetics, metabolism and concentration-response relations. Am J Cardiol 54:9D, 1984.

35. Siddoway LA, Thompson KA, McAllister CB, et al: Polymorphism of propafenone metabolism and disposition in man: Clinical and pharmacokinetic consequences. Circulation 75:785, 1987.

36. Gillis AM, Kates RE: Myocardial uptake kinetics and pharmacodynamics of propafenone in the isolated perfused rabbit heart. J Pharmacol Exp Ther 237:708, 1987.

37. Chilson DA, Heger JJ, Zipes DP, et al: Electrophysiologic effects and clinical efficacy of oral propafenone therapy in patients with ventricular tachycardia. J Am Coll Cardiol 5:1407, 1985.

38. Seipel L, Breithardt G, Both A: Elekrophysiologische Effekt der Antiarrhythmika Disopyramid und Propafenon auf das menschliche Reizleitungssystem. Z Kardiol 64:731, 1975.

39. Waleffe A, Mary-Rabine L, de Rijbel R, et al: Electrophysiologic effects of propafenone studied with programmed electrical stimulation of the heart in patients with recurrent paroxysmal supraventricular tachycardia. Eur Heart J 2:345, 1981.

40. Manz M, Steinbeck G, Luderitz B: Usefulness of programmed stimulation in predicting efficacy of propafenone in long-term antiarrhythmic therapy for paroxysmal supraventricular tachycardia. Am J Cardiol 56:593, 1985.

41. Alboni P, Filippi L, Pirani R, et al: Effetti elettrofisiologici del propafenone in pazienti con dis funzione del nodo sinusale. G Ital Cardiol 14:297, 1984.

42. Alboni P, Pirani R, Paparella N, et al: A method for evaluating different modes of action of an antiarrhythmic drug in man: The effects of propafenone on sinus nodal functions. Int J Cardiol 7:255, 1985.

43. Shen EN, Keung E, Huycke E, et al: Intravenous propafenone for termination of reentrant supraventricular tachycardia: A placebo-controlled, randomized, double-blind, crossover study. Ann Intern Med 105:655, 1986.

44. Frank R, Tonet JL, Lacroix H, et al: Electrophysiologic effects and efficacy of oral propafenone in the Wolff-Parkinson-White Syndrome. Circulation 70(Suppl II):442, 1984.

45. Disertori M, Vergara G, Inama G, et al: Studio degli effetti elettrofisiologici del propafenone in pazienti con preeccitazione cardiaca. Boll Soc Ital Cardiol 26:1725, 1981.

46. Clementy J, Sourdille N, Pedeboscq C, et al: Etude electrophysiologique de la propafenone dans le syndrome de Wolff-Parkinson-White. Ann Cardiol Angeiol (Paris) 31:351, 1982.

47. Karagueuzian HSJ, Katoh TJ, McCullen A, et al: Electrophysiologic and hemodynamic effects of propafenone, a new antiarrhythmic agent, on the anesthetized, closed-chest dog: Comparative study with lidocaine. Am Heart J 107:418, 1984.

48. Karagueuzian HSJ, Fujimoto TJ, Katoh TJ, et al: Suppression of ventricular arrhythmias by propafenone, a new antiarrhythmic agent, during acute myocardial infarction in the conscious dog: A comparative study with lidocaine. Circulation 66:1190, 1982.

49. Kafka WJ, Hildebrand U, Delius W: Effect of antiarrhythmic agents on chronic pacing and sensing thresholds. Circulation 72(Suppl III):173, 1985.

50. Diewitz MJ, Anton D: Auswirkungen von Propafenone. HCl auf die myokardial Reizschwelle des Menschen bei intrevenoser und oraler Verabreichung. Drug Dev Eval 1:56, 1977.

51. Nigro PJ, Ganci BJ, Piccone IJ, et al: Variations in ventricular pacing threshold and in paced QRS width in patients treated with flecainide and propafenone. New Trends in Arrhythmia 6:405, 1990.

52. Montefoschi NJ, Boccadamo R: Propafenone-induced acute variation of chronic atrial pacing threshold: A case report. PACE 13:480, 1990.

53. Pavri BBJ, Reiffel JA: Postoperative management of the ICD

patient. *In* Spotnitz HM (ed): Research Frontiers in Implantable Defibrillator Surgery. Austin: RG Landes, 1992, p 41.

54. Bianconi L, Boccadamo R, Pappalardo A, et al: Effectiveness of intravenous propafenone for conversion of atrial fibrillation and flutter of recent onset. Am J Cardiol 64:335, 1989.

55. Connolly SJH, Mulji ASJ, Hoffert RNJ, et al: Randomized placebo-controlled trial of propafenone for treatment of atrial tachyarrhythmias after cardiac surgery. J Am Coll Cardiol 10:1145, 1987.

56. Musto B, D'Onofrio A, Cavallaro CJ, et al: Electrophysiological effects and clinical efficacy of propafenone in children with recurrent paroxysmal supraventricular tachycardia. Circulation 78:863, 1988.

57. Touboul PJ, Moleur PJ, Mathieu MPJ, et al: A comparative evaluation of the effects of propafenone and lidocaine on early ventricular arrhythmias after acute myocardial infarction. Eur Heart J 9:1188, 1988.

58. Podrid PJ, Cytryn RJ, Lown B: Propafenone: Noninvasive evaluation of efficacy. Am J Cardiol 54:53D, 1984.

59. Brodsky MA, Allen BJ, Abata D, et al: Propafenone therapy for ventricular tachycardia in the setting of congestive heart failure. Am Heart J 110:794, 1985.

60. Baker BJ, Brodsky MA, Dinh HA, et al: Hemodynamic effect of propafenone and the experience in patients with congestive heart failure. J Electrophysiol 1:527, 1987.

61. Baker BJ, Dinh H, Kroskey D, et al: Effect of propafenone on left ventricular ejection fraction. Am J Cardiol 54:20D, 1984.

62. Hollmann M, Vrode E, Hotz D, et al: Investigations on the pharmacokinetics of propafenone in man. Arneimmittel-forschung 33:763, 1983.

63. Axelson JE, Chan GL-Y, Kirsten EB, et al: Food increases the bioavailability of propafenone. Br J Clin Pharmacol 23:735, 1987.

64. Seipel L, Breithardt G: Propafenone—a new antiarrhythmic drug. Eur Heart J 1:309, 1980.

65. Connolly S, Lebsack C, Winkle RA, et al: Propafenone disposition kinetics in cardiac arrhythmia. Clin Pharmacol Ther 36:163, 1984.

66. Latini R, Marchi S, Riva E, et al: Distribution of propafenone and its active metabolite, 5-hydroxypropafenone, in human tissues. Am Heart J 113:843, 1987.

67. Hege HG, Hollmann M, Kaumeier S, et al: The metabolic fate of 2H-labelled propafenone in man. Eur J Drug Metab Pharmacokinet 9:41, 1984.

68. Siddoway LA, McAllister CB, Want T, et al: Polymorphic oxidative metabolism of propafenone in man. Circulation 68(Suppl III):64, 1983.

69. Kates RE, Yee YG, Winkle RA: Metabolite cumulation during chronic propafenone dosing in arrhythmia. Clin Pharmacol Ther 37:610, 1985.

70. Lee JT, Kroemer HK, Silberstein DJ, et al: The role of genetically determined polymorphic drug metabolism in the betablockade produced by propafenone. N Engl J Med 322:1764, 1990.

71. Boriani G, Strocchi E, Capucci A, et al: Relationships between debrisoquine hydroxylation and propafenone pharmacokinetcs. Drug Invest 2:114, l990.

72. Roden DM, Want T, Woosely RL, et al: Pharmacokinetic and pharmacologic aspects of polymorphic drug oxidation in man. *In* Benet LZ, Levy G, Ferraiolo BJ (eds): Pharmacokinetics: A Modern View. New York: Plenum, 1984, pp 217–234.

73. Haefeli EW, Vozeh S, Ha HR, Fallath F: Comparison of the pharmacodynamic effects of intravenous and oral propafenone. Clin Pharmacol Ther 48(3):245, l990.

74. Salerno DM, Fifield J, Hodges M: Antiarrhythmic drug therapy for suppression of ventricular arrhythmia: Experience with 122 patients treated for two years. J Clin Pharmacol 30:226, 1990.

75. Giani P, Landolina M, Giudici V, et al: Pharmacokinetics and pharmacodynamics of propafenone during acute and chronic administration. Eur J Clin Pharmacol 34:187, 1988.

76. Woosley RL, Shand DG: Pharmacokinetics of antiarrhythmic drugs. Am J Cardiol 41:986, 1978.

77. Steurer G, Weber H, Schmidinger H, et al: Plasma propafenone concentration in the evaluation of antiarrhythmic efficacy. Eur Heart J 12:526, 1991.

78. Naccarella R, Bracchetti D, Palmieri M, et al: Propafenone for refractory ventricular arrhythmias: Correlation with drug plasma levels during long-term treatment. Am J Cardiol 54:1008, 1984.

79. Garson A, Moak JP, Smith RT, et al: Usefulness of intravenous propafenone for control of postoperative junctional ectopic tachycardia. Am J Cardiol 59:1422, 1987.

80. Reimer A, Paul T, Kallfel HC: Efficacy and safety of intravenous and oral propafenone in pediatric cardiac dysrhythmias. Am J Cardiol 68:741, 1991.

81. Guccione P, Drago F, Di Donato R, et al: Oral propafenone therapy for children with arrhythmias: Efficacy and adverse effects in midterm follow-up. Am Heart J 122:1022, 1991.

82. Lee JT, Yee Y-G, Dorian P, et al: Influence of hepatic dysfunction on the pharmacokinetics of propafenone. J Clin Pharmacol 27:384, 1987.

83. Burgess E, Duff H, Wilkes P: Propafenone disposition in renal insufficiency and renal failure. J Clin Pharmacol 29:112, 1989.

84. Botsch S, Evers J, Hardtmann E, et al: Steady state pharmacokinetics of propafenone in patients with renal failure. Naunyn Schmiedbergs Arch Pharmacol 345(Suppl):R3, 1992.

85. Belz GG, Matthews J, Doering W, et al: Digoxin and antiarrhythmics: Pharmacodynamic and pharmacokinetic studies with quinidine, propafenone, and verapamil. Clin Pharmacol Ther 31:202, 1982.

86. Cardaioli P, Compostella L, De Domenica R, et al: Influenza del propafenone sulla farmacocinetica della digossina somministrata per via orale: Studio su volontari sani. G Ital Cardiol 16:237, 1986.

87. Steinback K, Frohner K, Meisl F, et al: Interaction between propafenone and other drugs. *In* Schlepper M, Olsson B (eds): Cardiac Arrhythmias: Diagnosis, Prognosis, Therapy. Proceedings of the First International Rytmonorm Congress. New York: Springer-Verlag, 1983, pp 141–147.

88. Kates RE, Yee Y-G, Kirsten EB: Interaction between warfarin and propafenone in healthy volunteer subjects. Clin Pharmacol Ther 42:305, 1987.

89. Pritchett ELC, Smith WM, Kirsten EB: Pharmacokinetic and pharmacodynamic interactions of propafenone and cimetidine. J Clin Pharmacol 28:619, 1988.

90. Kowey PR, Kirsten RB, Chau-Hwei JR, et al: Interaction between propranolol and propafenone in healthy volunteers. J Clin Pharmacol 29:512, 1989.

91. Wagner F, Kalusche D, Trenk DJ, et al: Drug interaction between propafenone and metoprolol. Br J Clin Pharmacol 24:213, 1987.

92. Inaba TJ, Nakano M, Otton SV, et al: A human cytochrome p-450 characterized by inhibition studies as the spartein-debrisoquine monooxygenase. Can J Physiol Pharmacol 62:860, 1984.

93. Inaba T, Tyndale RE, Mahon WA: Quinidine: Potent inhibition of sparteine and debrisoquine oxidation *in vivo*. Br J Clin Pharmacol 22:199, 1986.

94. Funck-Brentano C, Kroemer HK, Pavlou H, et al: Genetically determined interaction between propafenone and low dose. Quinidine: Role of active metabolites in modulating net drug effect. Br J Clinical Pharmacol 27:435J, 1989.

95. Castel JM, Cappiello E, Leopaldi D, et al: Rifamipicin lowers plasma concentrations of propafenone and its antiarrhythmic effect. Br J Clin Pharmacol 36:155, 1990.

96. Katz MR: Raised serum levels of desipiramine with the antiarrhythmic propafenone. Correspondence. J Clin Psychol 52:432, 1991.

97. Lee BL, Dohrmann ML: Theophylline toxicity after propafenone treatment: Evidence for drug interaction. Clin Pharmacol Ther 51:353, 1992.

98. Spes CHJ, Angermann CE, Horn KJ, et al: Ciclosporin-propafenone interaction. Klin Wochenschr 68:872, l990.

99. Ravid S, Podrid PJ, Novrit B: Safety of long-term propafenone therapy for cardiac arrhythmia—experience with 774 patients. J Electrophysiol 1:580, 1987.

100. Cueni L, Podrid PJ: Propafenone therapy in patients with serious ventricular arrhythmia—noninvasive evaluation of efficacy. J Electrophysiol 1:548, 1987.

101. Dinh H, Baker BJ, de Soyza N, et al: Sustained therapeutic efficacy and safety of oral propafenone for treatment of chronic ventricular arrhythmias: A 2-year experience. Am Heart J 115:92, 1988.

102. Geibel A, Meinertz T, Zehender M, et al: Antiarrhythmic efficacy and tolerance of oral propafenone in patients with frequent ventricular arrhythmias: Experience of a multicentre study. Eur Heart J 10(Suppl E):81, 1989.

103. Minardo JD, Miles WM, Heger JJ, et al: Propafenone therapy for ventricular arrhythmias—role of electrophysiologic testing. Circulation 74(Suppl II):312, 1986.

104. Naccarella F, Bracchetti D, Palmieri M, et al: Comparison of propafenone and disopyramide for treatment of chronic ventricular arrhythmias: Placebo-controlled, double-blind, randomized crossover study. Am Heart J 109:833, 1985.

105. Nielsen H, Sorum C, Rasmussen V, et al: Propafenone versus quinidine slow-release for the treatment of chronic ventricular arrhythmias. Acta Cardiol 45:359, 1990.

106. Reimold SC, Cantillon CO, Friedman PL, et al: Propafenone versus sotalol for suppression of recurrent symptomatic atrial fibrillation. Am J Cardiol 71:558, 1993.

107. Guindo J, de la Serna AR, Borja J, et al: Propafenone and syndrome of the lupus erythematosus type. Ann Intern Med 104:589, 1986.

108. Schuff-Werner P, Kaiser D: Cholestatische Hepatitis nach antiarrhythmischer Therapie mit Propafenon. Dtsch Med Wochenschr 105(4):137, 1980.

109. Korst HA, Brandes J-W, Littmann K-P: Potenz-und spermiogenesestorungen durch propafenon. Dtsch Med Wochenschr 105(34):1187, 1980.

110. Siddoway LA, Thompson KA, Bergstrand RH, et al: Safety and efficacy of propafenone in treatment of refractory ventricular arrhythmias. J Am Coll Cardiol 3:474, 1984.

111. Hill MR, Gotz VP, Harman E, et al: Evaluation of the asthmogenicity of propafenone, a new antiarrhythmic drug. Chest 90:698, 1986.

112. Stavens CS, McGovern B, Garan H, et al: Aggravation of electrically provoked ventricular tachycardia during treatment with propafenone. Am Heart J 110:24, 1985.

113. Farre J, Grande A, Albo PS, et al: Arrhythmogenic effects of antiarrhythmic drugs in patients with an old myocardial infarction and asymptomatic ventricular ectopic activity as studied by programmed electrical stimulation. Eur Heart J 8(Suppl A):113, 1987.

114. Stanton MS, Prystowsky EN, Fineberg NS, et al: Arrhythmic effects of antiarrhythmic drugs: A study of 506 patients treated for ventricular tachycardia or fibrillation. J Am Coll Cardiol 14:209, 1989.

115. Buss J, Neuss H, Bilgin Y, et al: Malignant ventricular tachyarrhythmias in association with propafenone treatment. Eur Heart J 6:424, 1985.

116. Stanton MS, Prystowsky EN, Fineberg NS, et al: The incidence of ventricular tachycardia or ventricular fibrillation as proarrhythmic effects during drug treatment of ventricular arrhythmia. J Am Coll Cardiol 9:245A, 1987.

117. Marcus FI: Drug interactions with amiodarone. Am Heart J 106:924, 1986.

118. Hii JT, Wyse DG, Gillis AM, et al: Propafenone-induced torsades de pointes: Cross-reactivity with quinidine. PACE 14:1568, 1991.

119. Murdock CJ, Kyles AE, Yeung-Lai-Wah JA, et al: Atrial flutter in patients treated for atrial fibrillation with propafenone. Am J Cardiol 66:755, 1990.

120. Budde T, Beyer M, Breithardt G, et al: Therapie der schweren Propafenonintoxikation-Eliminationsversuch Mittels Hamoperfusion. Z Kardiol 75:764, 1986.

121. Singh BN, Kaplinsky E, Kirsten E, et al: Effects of propafenone on ventricular arrhythmias: Double-blind, parallel, randomized, placebo-controlled dose-ranging study. Am Heart J 116:1542, 1988.

122. Naccarella F, Palmieri M, del Corso P, et al: Comparison of the efficacy of propafenone versus disopyramide for complex premature ventricular contractions: Evaluation with long-term monitoring. Arzneimittelforschung 32:547, 1982.

123. Clementy J, Callocchio M, Briacaud H: Comparative study of the therapeutic effect of propafenone and disopyramide in the oral treatment of chronic ventricular premature beats. In Schlepper M, Olsson B (eds): Cardiac Arrhythmias: Diagnosis, Prognosis, Therapy. Proceedings of the First International Rytmonorm Congress. New York: Springer-Verlag, 1983, pp 159–169.

124. Neuss H, Schlepper M: Clinical pharmacology of propafenone. In Schlepper M, Olsson B (eds): Cardiac Arrhythmias: Diagnosis, Prognosis, Therapy. Proceedings of the First International Rytmonorm Congress. New York: Springer-Verlag, 1983, pp 113–124.

125. Hodges M: Role of propafenone in the treatment of ventricular premature beats. J Electrophysiol 1:536, 1987.

126. Klempt H-W, Nayebagha A: Propafenone, flecainide and mexiletine in the treatment of stable ventricular premature beats. In Schlepper M, Olsson B (eds): Cardiac Arrhythmias: Diagnosis, Prognosis, Therapy. Proceedings of the First International Rytmonorm Congress. New York: Springer-Verlag, 1983, pp 171–178.

127. Rehnqvist N, Sjorgren A, Svensson G, et al: Comparative investigation of the antiarrhythmic effect of propafenone and lidocaine in patients with ventricular arrhythmias during acute myocardial infarction. Eur Heart J 5(Suppl B):129, 1984.

128. Facchini M, Bonazzi O, Priori SG, et al: Multiple comparison of several antiarrhythmic agents by acute oral drug testing in patients with chronic ventricular arrhythmias. Eur Heart J 9:462, 1988.

129. Podczeck A, Frohner K, Hief C, et al: Acute and long-term efficacy of propafenone in patients with sustained ventricular tachyarrhythmias: Assessment with programmed ventricular stimulation. Eur Heart J 12:796, 1991.

130. Budde T, Borggrefe M, Podczeck A, et al: Acute and long-term efficacy of oral propafenone in patients with ventricular tachyarrhythmias. J Cardiovasc Pharmacol 18:254, 1991.

131. Kowey P, Stohler JL, Friehling TD: Propafenone in the treatment of patients with malignant ventricular tachyarrhythmias. Can J Cardiol 71:175, 1991.

132. Katz RJ, Bren GB, Varghese PJ, et al: Oral propafenone for refractory ventricular arrhythmias—predictors of efficacy. Circulation 68(Suppl III):271, 1983.

133. Klein RC, Huang SK, Marcus FI, et al: Enhanced antiarrhythmic efficacy of propafenone when used in combination with procainamide or quinidine. Am Heart J 114:551, 1987.

134. Klein RC, Marcus FI: Efficacy of propafenone when used in combination antiarrhythmic therapy. J Electrophysiol 1:575, 1987.

135. Morgera T, Dreas L, Humar F, et al: The use of associated propafenone in patients with amiodarone-resistant ventricular tachycardia. Int J Cardiol 31:187, 1991.

136. Santinelli V, de Paola M, Turco P, et al: Paroxysmal supraventricular tachycardia: Experience with propafenone. Angiology 40:563, 1989.

137. Allen BJ, Brodsky MA, Doria R, et al: Oral propafenone therapy for patients with paroxysmal supraventricular tachyarrhythmia. Chest 94:853, 1988.

138. Sethi KK, Prasad R, Mohan JC, et al: Electrophysiologic effects of oral propafenone in Wolff-Parkinson-White syndrome studied by programmed electrical stimulation. Ind Heart J 43:5, 1991.

139. Musto B, D'Onofrio A, Musto A, et al: Effetti elettrofisiologici ed efficacia cliica del propafenone in pazienti di eta pediatrica con tachicadia parossisticca reciprocante sopraventricolare. G Ital Cardiol 16:336, 1986.

140. Beck OA, Lehmann H-U, Hochrein H: Propafenon und Lidoflazin bei chronischem vorhofflimmern und-flattern. Dtsch Med Wochenschr 103:1068, 1978.

141. Porterfield JG, Porterfield LM: Therapeutic efficacy and safety of oral propafenone for atrial fibrillation. Am J Cardiol 63:114, 1989.

142. Kerr CR, Klein GJ, Axelson JE, et al: Propafenone for prevention of recurrent atrial fibrillation. Am J Cardiol 61:914, 1988.

143. Hammill SC, Wood DL, Gersh BJ, et al: Propafenone for paroxysmal atrial fibrillation. Am J Cardiol 61:473, 1988.

144. Antman EM, Beamer AD, Cantillon C, et al: Therapy of refractory symptomatic atrial fibrillation and atrial flutter: A staged care approach with new antiarrhythmic drugs. J Am Coll Cardiol 15:698, 1990.
145. Connolly SJ, Hoffert DL: Usefulness of propafenone for recurrent paroxysmal atrial fibrillation. Am J Cardiol 63:817, 1989.
146. Pritchett ELC, McCarthy EA, Wilkinson WE: Propafenone treatment of symptomatic paroxysmal supraventricular arrhythmias. Ann Intern Med 114:539, 1991.
147. Clementy J, Coate P, Metzinger M: Etude de L'efficacite et de la tolerance de la propafenone dans le traitement des troubles du rythme cardiaque. Ann De Cardiologie et D'Angeiology 4:207J, 1987.
148. Santinelli V, Turco PJ, De Paola M, et al: Propafenone in Wolff-Parkinson-White syndrome at risk. Cardiovasc Drugs Ther 4:686, 1990.
149. The Cardiac Arrhythmia Suppression Trial (CAST) Investigators: Effects of encainide and flecainide on mortality in a randomized trial of arrhythmia suppression after myocardial infarction. N Engl J Med 321:406, 1989.

CHAPTER 148

Quinidine

Jean M. Nappi, Pharm.D., and Jay W. Mason, M.D.

HISTORY

Quinidine is one of many naturally occurring alkaloids that are derived from the bark of the cinchona tree. Quinidine is believed to have been first used clinically in 1749 by the French physician Jean Baptiste de Senac in a patient with atrial fibrillation.[1] In this century, it has been used widely in the management of supraventricular and ventricular arrhythmias, and it is the prototypical antiarrhythmic agent to which others are compared. Despite the availability of numerous antiarrhythmic agents, quinidine maintains a prominent place in the management of rhythm disorders.

PHARMACOLOGY

Quinidine is the dextro stereoisomer of quinine. Quinidine is a weak base and is available as the sulfate, gluconate, and polygalacturonate salts, which respectively contain 83%, 62%, and 60% of active drug (Table 148–1). The predominant electrophysiologic effects of quinidine are typical of a drug that blocks the fast inward sodium channel. The pharmacologic effects of quinidine are complex because of its anticholinergic (indirect) properties. Quinidine's direct effects are to slow the rate of rise of phase 0 of the action potential, lengthen the effective refractory period to a greater degree than it lengthens the duration of action potential, and decrease the rate of diastolic depolarization. Clinically, this should lead to a decrease in heart rate, prolonged atrioventricular (AV) nodal and His-Purkinje conduction, prolonged atrial and ventricular effective refractory periods, and an increase in the QRS complex and the QT interval. In intact humans, the indirect or vagolytic properties of quinidine may predominate in the sinus and AV nodes, resulting in an increase in heart rate and an increase in conduction through the AV node.[2] Because of the latter action, it is prudent to first administer digoxin (or another drug that will slow conduction through the AV node) in patients with atrial fibrillation or atrial flutter who are going to receive quinidine. This will avoid the potential complication of accelerated ventricular rates due to the enhanced AV nodal conduction that follows administration of quinidine. The His-Purkinje system is minimally affected by vagal tone, and thus the expected direct effects of quinidine occur unopposed. Many electrophysiologic effects of quinidine are more marked under conditions of ischemia, hypoxia, and tachycardia.

The hemodynamic effects of quinidine are somewhat misunderstood. One may commonly hear reference to the "myocardial depressant" effects of quinidine. However, Mason et al.[3] evaluated three indices of myocardial function in cardiac transplant recipients who received intravenous infusions of quinidine. Cardiac transplant patients were used in the study so that the cardiac autonomic effects and the reflex effects induced by the peripheral vascular action of quinidine were eliminated. Quinidine in therapeutic concentrations did not significantly change mean circumferential velocity, mean segmental shortening, or ejection fraction. Preload and afterload were not controlled in this study, and although systemic vascular

Table 148–1. **Quinidine Salts**

Available Salt	Product Description	Percent (%) Quinidine Base	Amount of Active Drug
Quinidine sulfate	200-mg tablet	83	166 mg
	300-mg tablet	83	249 mg
Quinidine gluconate	324-mg tablet	62	200 mg
	80 mg/ml (solution)	62	50 mg/ml
Quinidine polygalacturonate	275-mg tablet	60	165 mg

resistance did not change, preload was decreased. As a result, end-systolic, end-diastolic, and stroke volumes were decreased. Quinidine is known to affect both resistance and capacitance vessels, resulting in decreases in systemic arterial pressure and cardiac output. To avoid deleterious hemodynamic effects, care in the intravenous use of quinidine is necessary.

Because of the drug's electrophysiologic properties, one can expect to see widening of the QRS complex and the QT interval. These effects can be just as useful as plasma concentrations in monitoring quinidine therapy. Quinidine excess is suggested when the QRS duration increases 30% or more beyond baseline values regardless of plasma concentration or dose. Other untoward effects related to high plasma concentrations include sinus arrest, high-grade AV block, and abnormal automaticity.[4]

PHARMACOKINETICS

After quinidine is orally administered, its bioavailability is about 70% to 80% but may vary widely in different patients. Because quinidine is a weak base, it is absorbed primarily in the small intestine. The peak plasma concentration is generally reached within 1 to 3 hours after the ingestion of quinidine sulfate tablets. The time to peak plasma concentration of the sustained-release preparations is slower and more protracted. Except for aluminum hydroxide gel, the absorption of orally administered quinidine may be decreased by some antacid or antidiarrheal preparations that are given to alleviate the diarrhea associated with quinidine. The rate but not the extent of absorption of quinidine may be reduced in patients with congestive heart failure.[5, 6] Absorption following intramuscular administration is erratic and incomplete. Intramuscular absorption of quinidine may be associated with pain and muscle damage.

The distribution of quinidine is best described by a two-compartment model with an overall volume of distribution of 3 L/kg.[7] This volume may be reduced in patients with congestive heart failure[5] but increased in patients with cirrhosis.[8] Seventy percent to 90% of quinidine is bound to plasma proteins, primarily albumin and α_1 acid glycoprotein.[9] The plasma protein binding of quinidine appears to be diminished in patients with liver disease, whereas binding has been shown to be increased following trauma, surgery, cardiac arrest, or myocardial infarction.[10-12]

Quinidine is eliminated from the body primarily via metabolism by the mixed-function oxidase system in the liver. The mean elimination half-life of quinidine is 6 to 7 hours; however, this value varies considerably among patients. There are conflicting data regarding the relationship between dose and plasma concentrations of quinidine. It is unknown whether the disposition kinetics of quinidine are dose-dependent. The metabolites that have been identified include 3-hydroxyquinidine, 2-oxoquinidione, quinidine-N-oxide, quinidine 10,11-dihydroldiol, and O-desmethyl-quinidine.[13] The 3-hydroxyquinidine and 2-oxoquinidione metabolites are considered the prin-

cipal products of metabolism and are believed to possess antiarrhythmic activity. Vozeh et al.[14] reported a significant correlation between the serum concentration of 3-hydroxyquinidine and changes in the QT interval. They also reported additive effects when the metabolite was studied in combination with quinidine.[14] Renal excretion of unchanged drug accounts for 10% to 20% of a given dose.[7] Renal excretion occurs by glomerular filtration and depends on the pH of the urine. Renal clearance of quinidine may diminish with increased urine pH.[15] Renal clearance of quinidine is positively correlated with creatinine clearance and is therefore lower in the elderly population.[16] Quinidine is not significantly removed by peritoneal dialysis or hemodialysis.[17-19]

Dosage and Administration

Quinidine dosage requirements vary considerably among patients because of variations in pharmacokinetic parameters, presence of active metabolites, changes in the amount of quinidine bound to plasma proteins, and pharmacodynamic differences relating to the type of arrhythmia being treated. In addition, the prescriber should keep in mind that each of the quinidine salts contains a different amount of quinidine base. A conservative starting dose is approximately 12.5 mg/kg/day of quinidine base. This converts to an oral starting dose of 15 mg/kg/day of quinidine sulfate, or 20 mg/kg/day of quinidine gluconate. Generally, conventional quinidine sulfate is given every 6 hours. Sustained-release preparations can be given every 8 hours. The dosage regimen should be individualized for each patient according to serum concentrations and therapeutic response.

An oral loading dose may be given for rapid control of arrhythmia. As much as 600 mg of quinidine sulfate has been given safely.[20] However, doses in the range of 200 to 300 mg of quinidine sulfate every 3 to 4 hours (up to a total of 1000 to 1200 mg) are more common. Intolerance to gastrointestinal side effects usually limits the amount of quinidine one can administer.

Quinidine gluconate may also be administered intravenously. A slow intravenous diluted infusion of quinidine gluconate, 0.4 to 0.5 mg/kg/min (equivalent to 0.25 to 0.31 mg/kg/min of quinidine base) has been shown to be safe and effective.[21] Torres et al.[22] have also administered intermittent boluses of 80 mg of quinidine gluconate every 5 minutes to a total dose of 800 mg. Hemodynamically significant hypotension occurred in approximately 10% of patients in these two studies but was successfully treated with saline infusion and a reduced rate of drug administration.

Generally, patients in congestive heart failure require smaller doses of quinidine because of their smaller volumes of distribution.[23] In patients with cirrhosis, the drug has a prolonged half-life; therefore, these patients require less frequent dosing or smaller doses.[8] Quinidine may be used safely in patients with these disorders, but careful monitoring is necessary.

Drug Interactions

Quinidine is known to have clinically significant interactions with a number of other commonly used cardiovascular agents. The most common interaction is between quinidine and digoxin. Although these two drugs have been combined for decades, this interaction was first described in 1978.[24] In a retrospective chart review, Leahey et al.[24] found that digoxin levels rose substantially (twofold) in 25 of 27 patients. This interaction has since been described in detail.[25, 26] Quinidine reduces the renal and nonrenal clearance of digoxin and displaces digoxin from tissue binding sites. The magnitude of this interaction appears to depend on serum concentrations of quinidine. The volume of distribution of digoxin may be reduced by 30% to 40%, and the reduction in digoxin clearance may be reduced by 30% to 50%. Serum digoxin concentrations begin to increase soon after quinidine therapy is initiated, but a new steady-state serum concentration of digoxin is not reached for at least 5 days and, in some cases, for much longer. Recommendations to decrease the digoxin dose by one half and to follow the serum digoxin levels closely when initiating quinidine therapy have been made,[27] although some would argue that displacement of digoxin from its cardiac binding sites by quinidine may result in a decrease in the inotropic effect of the drug.[28]

Quinidine has also been reported to affect the elimination but not the volume of distribution of digitoxin.[29, 30] Quinidine may produce a 40% to 50% increase in serum digitoxin concentrations, whereas digoxin produces a twofold increase. Serum concentrations of quinidine have been reported to be affected in other drug interactions as well. Verapamil was reported to increase the serum quinidine concentration in one patient,[31] whereas nifedipine was reported to lower this concentration.[32, 33] Other clinically important interactions of quinidine are listed in Table 148-2.[34, 35]

CLINICAL USE

For many clinicians, quinidine remains the antiarrhythmic agent of first choice. It has proven efficacy for both supraventricular and ventricular arrhythmias. Quinidine can be used to convert atrial fibrillation or flutter to normal sinus rhythm. For reasons listed previously, in these situations most clinicians administer digoxin before quinidine. Quinidine is also used on a long-term basis to maintain normal sinus rhythm in these patients and is useful in managing supraventricular tachyarrhythmias associated with Wolff-Parkinson-White syndrome. Quinidine may interrupt the reentrant circuit by acting directly on the accessory pathway to slow conduction and prolong the refractory period.[36, 37] Additionally, quinidine has been shown to be effective in the suppression of acute ventricular ectopy and ventricular tachycardia, and it is often given for maintenance therapy.

SIDE EFFECTS

Much has been written about quinidine syncope, which is believed to result from ventricular tachyarrhythmias, often in the face of usual or even low plasma quinidine concentrations.[38] Commonly one sees torsade de pointes (twisting of the points) on the electrocardiogram. Although one expects to see some increase in the QT interval of patients receiving quinidine, marked prolongation precedes torsade de pointes. Many cases of quinidine syncope have been reported in patients who were taking the drug in an attempt to control atrial arrhythmias. As a result, patients usually were also taking digitalis. Undoubtedly, some cases of "quinidine syncope" have been a result of digitalis-induced arrhythmias. However, quinidine syncope occurs in the absence of digitalis therapy[39] and with serum digoxin concentrations within the therapeutic range.[40] The most effective form of treatment for quinidine-induced ventricular arrhythmias is ventricular overdrive pacing.[41] Direct current countershock and various agents (isoproterenol, lidocaine, bretylium, magnesium sulfate, calcium gluconate, and atropine) whose effectiveness has not been well established[38, 42] have also been tried. The serum potassium and magnesium concentrations should be brought into the normal range if they are low.

As mentioned previously, quinidine is known to affect the vasculature. Quinidine has direct vasodilating properties as well as the ability to oppose α-adrenergic receptors.[43] Hypotension may be a problem when quinidine is administered too quickly via the intravenous route. Additionally, caution should be used when quinidine is administered concomitantly with other agents known to affect the vasculature. Hypotension has been reported with the combination of quinidine and verapamil.[44]

Unfortunately, many patients are unable to tolerate the drug on a long-term basis. Gastrointestinal symptoms consisting of nausea, anorexia, vomiting, cramping, and diarrhea are the most common adverse effects reported with the use of quinidine.[45] Though tolerance to these symptoms may develop, they remain the most frequent reason for discontinuation of the drug. The less-common syndrome of cinchonism consists of impaired hearing, tinnitus, light-headedness, blurred vision, flushing, and tremor. In most individuals, gastrointestinal side effects and cinchonism are dose- and concentration-dependent.

Hypersensitivity reactions to quinidine may include fever, skin rash, angioneurotic edema, thrombocytopenia, hemolytic anemia, agranulocytosis, respiratory depression, hepatitis, and lupus erythematosus.[46-48] The liver involvement described by Geltner et al.[47] commenced in most patients within 2 weeks of initiation of quinidine, and liver biopsies showed granulomatous foci in the parenchyma consisting of lymphocytes, histiocytes, and sometimes eosinophils.

Quinidine is not recommended in patients with intraventricular conduction defects or AV block. Ab-

Table 148–2. **Drug Interactions with Quinidine**

Drug	Mechanism	Result
Acetazolamide, sodium bicarbonate	Alkalinize the urine	Renal reabsorption of quinidine is increased
Amiodarone	Inhibits hepatic metabolism	Higher serum quinidine concentrations
Antacids	Possible alkalinization	Renal reabsorption of quinidine is increased
Antacids (excluding Al OH₃)	Decrease GI absorption	Lower serum quinidine concentrations
Anticoagulants	Additive hypothrombinemic effects	Increased effect of anticoagulant
Barbiturates	Enhance hepatic metabolism	Lower serum quinidine concentrations
β-Blockers (atenolol, metoprolol, propranolol, timolol)	Inhibit metabolism in extensive metabolizers	Higher serum concentrations of beta blocker
Cholinergic drugs	Quinidine has anticholinergic properties	Decreased effect of cholinergic drugs
Cimetidine	Inhibits hepatic metabolism	Higher serum quinidine concentrations
Codeine	Inhibits hepatic metabolism to morphine	Decreased analgesic effect
Digoxin	Decreases clearance	Higher serum digoxin concentrations
Kaolin-pectin	Decreases GI absorption	Lower serum quinidine concentrations
Ketoconazole	Inhibits hepatic metabolism	Higher serum quinidine concentrations
Neuromuscular blocking agents	Quinidine depresses cholinesterase activity	Increased effect of neuromuscular blocking agent
Phenytoin	Enhances hepatic metabolism	Lower serum quinidine concentrations
Rifampin	Enhances hepatic metabolism	Lower serum quinidine concentrations
Tricyclic antidepressants	Inhibit hepatic metabolism	Higher imipramine, desipramine serum concentrations
Verapamil	Inhibits hepatic metabolism	Higher serum quinidine concentrations

Data from Hansten PD, Horn JR: Drug Interactions and Updates. Vancouver, WA: Applied Therapeutics, 1993; and Tatro DS: Drug Interaction Facts. St. Louis: Facts and Comparisons, 1993.

normal rhythms and aberrant impulses due to escape mechanisms should not be treated with quinidine. Patients with severe congestive heart failure and renal dysfunction as well as the elderly should be carefully observed for signs of toxicity.

COMPARATIVE TRIALS

New antiarrhythmic agents are often compared with quinidine in efficacy and safety studies (Table 148–3). In a randomized, double-blind, multicenter, parallel-design trial comparing disopyramide with quinidine,

the two drugs showed similar efficacy, but disopyramide was better tolerated.[49] Quinidine was compared with tocainide[50] in a double-blind, parallel trial involving 133 patients with ventricular arrhythmias. Thirty-two patients were withdrawn because of adverse effects or administrative reasons. In the remaining 101 patients, 12 of 54 (22%) randomized to tocainide and 18 of 47 (38%) randomized to quinidine had at least a 75% reduction in premature ventricular contractions (PVCs). Ventricular tachycardia was completely abolished in 8 of 38 patients (21%) on tocainide and in 10 of 28 patients (36%) on quinidine.

Table 148–3. **Comparative Efficacy of Quinidine with Other Antiarrhythmic Agents**

Reference	Study Design	Type of Arrhythmia	No. of Patients	Results (% of Patients Responding)	Intolerable Side Effects
49	DB, parallel	Ventricular	124	61% disopyramide 69% quinidine	10% disopyramide 35% quinidine
50	DB, parallel	Ventricular	133	37% tocainide 50% quinidine	27% tocainide 24% quinidine
51	SB, parallel	Ventricular	51	69% mexiletine 70% quinidine	8% mexiletine 13% quinidine
52	DB, parallel	Ventricular	26	54% mexiletine 62% quinidine	38% mexiletine 54% quinidine
53	DB, parallel	Ventricular	280	85% flecainide 57% quinidine	13% flecainide 15% quinidine
54	DB, crossover	Ventricular	226	48% sotalol 59% quinidine	5% sotalol 4% quinidine
55	Parallel	Ventricular	74	43% sotalol 33% quinidine	7% sotalol 32% quinidine
56	Not stated	Atrial fibrillation	60	67% flecainide 60% quinidine	7% flecainide 27% quinidine
57	Open, parallel	Atrial fibrillation prophylaxis	183	52% sotalol 48% quinidine	11% sotalol 26% quinidine

DB, double-blind; SB, single-blind.

There was no statistically significant difference between the two groups in regard to efficacy of the drug. Fifty-one percent of patients receiving tocainide and 64% of patients receiving quinidine reported adverse reactions. The most commonly reported side effects were diarrhea (with quinidine) and dizziness (with tocainide). Twenty-seven percent of patients receiving tocainide and 24% of patients receiving quinidine discontinued their medication because of adverse effects.

In a similar study comparing mexiletine and quinidine, PVCs were reduced by at least 70% in 16 of 23 patients (70%) in the quinidine group and 18 of 26 patients (69%) in the mexiletine group.[51] Two patients in each group had to discontinue the drug because of intolerable side effects. There was no significant difference between the two groups in terms of efficacy for suppression of PVCs, ventricular couplets, or ventricular tachycardia. In a double-blind study with 26 patients, comparing mexiletine to quinidine, ventricular ectopy was suppressed by 70% in 54% of patients receiving mexiletine and 62% receiving quinidine.[52]

One of the largest trials done to date compared flecainide with quinidine in a double-blind, parallel group design.[53] In this study, there was a statistically significant difference between the two treatment groups. PVCs were suppressed by at least 80% in 85% of patients receiving flecainide versus 57% of patients receiving quinidine. Couplets and ventricular tachycardia were completely suppressed in 68% of patients treated with flecainide compared with 33% of patients treated with quinidine. There was no difference in the number of patients who discontinued the drug because of adverse effects. Two patients in the quinidine group and none in the flecainide group met criteria for arrhythmia exacerbation.

Hanyok and MacNeil described a randomized crossover comparison of quinidine and sotalol.[54] Patients receiving quinidine had a slightly greater reduction in the hourly PVC rate: 87% for quinidine versus 78% for sotalol ($p < .04$). The target reduction in PVCs of 75% was reached in 59% of the quinidine patients versus 48% of sotalol patients ($p = .13$). Gastrointestinal side effects were common in the quinidine patients (33%), whereas the sotalol patients were more likely to report dyspnea (11%) and bradycardia (4%). Four patients receiving sotalol developed new or worsening heart failure.

The concern over the proarrhythmic effects of quinidine and other antiarrhythmic agents has intensified since the publication of the Cardiac Arrhythmia Suppression Trial.[55] Morganroth and Goin published the results of a meta-analysis of quinidine and four other antiarrhythmic agents (flecainide, tocainide, mexiletine, and propafenone) in patients with benign or potentially lethal ventricular arrhythmias.[56] The authors examined the data from four randomized, double-blind, active controlled, parallel design trials. Over 1000 patients were enrolled in these four trials. The combined risk of dying on quinidine was significantly higher compared with the other four drugs, with a risk difference of 1.6%. They concluded that

quinidine may increase mortality as compared with other class I antiarrhythmic agents. These meta-analyses do not provide rigorously controlled comparisons and thus are suggestive rather than definitive. Nevertheless, the use of class I antiarrhythmic agents in patients with benign or potentially lethal arrhythmia must be carefully weighed against the risk.

In the ESVEM trial, several antiarrhythmic agents, including quinidine, were evaluated in patients with lethal ventricular arrhythmias. ESVEM was a multicenter trial evaluating electrophysiologic study versus electrocardiographic (Holter) monitoring in patients with spontaneous ventricular tachycardia, aborted sudden death, or unmonitored syncope.[57] Patients were randomized to one of six drugs (mexiletine, quinidine, procainamide, sotalol, propafenone, or imipramine, which was replaced with pirmenol) and serial assessments were performed until one was found to be effective. Among the 296 responders who received long-term therapy, patients who received sotalol, compared with the pooled results of the other agents, had the lowest actuarial probability for arrhythmia recurrence ($p < .001$), death from any cause ($p = .004$), death from a cardiac cause ($p = .02$), and death from arrhythmia ($p = .04$). After 1 year of treatment, patients receiving quinidine had a $40 \pm 9\%$ chance of probability of arrhythmia recurrence, compared with a $21 \pm 4\%$ chance if they were receiving sotalol.[58]

Quinidine has also been used for many years in the management of atrial fibrillation. Flecainide was compared with quinidine[59] in 60 patients who had atrial fibrillation of variable duration. Overall, the incidence of conversion to normal sinus rhythm was similar in the two groups (60% in the quinidine group versus 67% in the flecainide group). If atrial fibrillation had been present for less than 10 days, there was a higher incidence of conversion to normal sinus rhythm in both groups. If atrial fibrillation had been present for more than 10 days, quinidine was more effective in converting the rhythm to normal sinus (40% vs. 22%). Adverse effects were more frequent but less severe in the patients receiving quinidine.

Quinidine has also been compared with sotalol for the maintenance of sinus rhythm following cardioversion of atrial fibrillation.[60] In a multicenter Swedish study, 52% of patients receiving sotalol versus 48% of patients receiving quinidine remained in normal sinus rhythm following cardioversion. Of those who relapsed, the patients receiving quinidine were more symptomatic. More patients receiving quinidine (26%) than patients receiving sotalol (11%) were withdrawn from the study because of side effects.

Coplen et al. conducted a meta-analysis to evaluate the quinidine-related mortality in patients with atrial fibrillation.[61] The analysis included six trials involving over 800 patients. Patients either received quinidine or were in a control group and followed for a minimum of 3 months following cardioversion to assess the efficacy and safety of quinidine in maintaining sinus rhythm. The proportion of patients remaining in normal sinus rhythm at 3, 6, and 12 months following

Table 148–4. **Cost Comparison of Antiarrhythmic Agents**

Drug	Average Daily Dose	Approximate Daily Cost ($)*
Quinidine sulfate tablets (generic)	800 mg	0.37
Quinidine gluconate tablets (generic)	972 mg	0.86
Procainamide capsules (generic)	2000 mg	0.31
Procainamide SR+ tablets (generic)	2000 mg	1.34
Disopyramide capsules (generic)	400 mg	0.60
Disopyramide SR+ (generic)	300 mg	0.74
Norpace CR (disopyramide)	300 mg	1.44
Tonocard (tocainide)	1200 mg	2.35
Mexitil (mexiletine)	600 mg	2.55
Tambocor (flecainide)	200 mg	2.00
Rythmol (propafenone)	450 mg	2.34
Ethmozine (moricizine)	600 mg	1.99
Cordarone (amiodarone)	400 mg	5.06
Betapace (sotalol)	320 mg	4.35

*Cost was based on the lowest average wholesale price (AWP) to a pharmacy. Patients will pay approximately 30% more than AWP.
Prices were obtained from the 1993 Redbook. When more than one product was available, the lowest price was used.
SR+, sustained release.

cardioversion were 69%, 58%, and 50% for quinidine and 45%, 33%, and 25% for the control group. However, the unadjusted mortality rate in the quinidine-treated group was 2.9% versus 0.8% for the control group. This brings into question the risk/benefit ratio of using quinidine in these patients.

Quinidine was combined with a number of other antiarrhythmic agents in an attempt to enhance efficacy and decrease toxicity. Duff et al.[62] reported that in 17 patients who had partial responses or dose-limiting side effects to both quinidine and mexiletine, enhanced antiarrhythmic activity and fewer side effects occurred when lower than maximal doses of the two drugs were combined. In a study using electrophysiologic testing, Greenspan et al.[63] found that the combination of mexiletine and either quinidine or procainamide was again more effective than either agent used alone. Klein et al.[64] evaluated the addition of propafenone in patients receiving either quinidine or procainamide. Combination therapy resulted in significantly more suppression of PVCs and complex arrhythmias than could be achieved with monotherapy.

Duffy et al.[65] tested quinidine or disopyramide alone and in combination with procainamide in nine patients undergoing electrophysiologic study for documented ventricular tachycardia or fibrillation. Although tachycardia cycle length was increased with the combinations of drugs, induction of tachycardia was also easier with the combination in 9 of 13 tests in which this was assessed. Kim et al.[66] found that the combination of procainamide and quinidine was more effective than the maximal tolerated dose of either agent alone when given to patients with frequent PVCs.

SUMMARY

Although several new antiarrhythmic agents are available and more are under investigation, quinidine still holds a prominent place among drugs used in the management of patients with cardiac rhythm dis-

orders. This is due to quinidine's wide spectrum of antiarrhythmic activity, the availability of oral and parenteral forms, and the fact that physicians are generally familiar with the drug as a result of its use for many years. Quinidine is the agent least expensive to the patient. Unfortunately, most patients must take conventional quinidine sulfate tablets at least four times daily. The sustained-release preparations may offer a more convenient dosage schedule but are more expensive (Table 148–4). Many patients treated with quinidine experience gastrointestinal side effects, which in a minority are intolerable.

When quinidine is used, it is helpful to monitor serum concentrations. The drug should be used carefully in patients who may have changes in volume of distribution, protein binding, or elimination. Because quinidine leads to quinidine syncope and other forms of arrhythmia exacerbation in a substantial minority of patients, it is safest to initiate therapy under in-hospital monitoring. The use of quinidine as well as other class I antiarrhythmic agents may be associated with increases in mortality. The risk must be carefully weighed against the potential benefit for each patient.

REFERENCES

1. Willus FA, Keys TE: Cardiac Clinics XCIV: A remarkable early reference to the use of cinchona in cardiac arrhythmia. Mayo Clin Proc 17:294, 1942.
2. Mason JW, Winkle RA, Rider AK, et al: The electrophysiologic effects of quinidine in the transplanted human heart. J Clin Invest 59:481, 1977.
3. Mason JW, Winkle RA, Ingels NB, et al: Hemodynamic effects of intravenously administered quinidine on the transplanted human heart. Am J Cardiol 40:99, 1977.
4. Bigger JT, Hoffman BF: Antiarrhythmic drugs. In Gilman AG, Goodman LS, Rall TW, et al (eds): Goodman and Gilman's The Pharmacological Basis of Therapeutics. New York: Macmillan, 1985, pp 756–762.
5. Crouthamel WG: The effect of congestive heart failure on quinidine pharmacokinetics. Am Heart J 90:335, 1975.
6. Ueda CT, Dzindzio BS: Bioavailability of quinidine in congestive heart failure. Br J Clin Pharmacol 11:571, 1981.
7. Ueda CT, Hirschfeld DS, Scheinman MM, et al: Disposition kinetics of quinidine. Clin Pharmacol Ther 19:30, 1976.

8. Kessler KM, Humphries WC, Black M, et al: Quinidine pharma-cokinetics in patients with cirrhosis or receiving propranolol. Am Heart J 96:627, 1978.
9. Edwards DJ, Axelson JE, Slaughter RL, et al: Factors affecting quinidine protein binding in humans. J Pharmacol Sci 73:1264, 1984.
10. Fremstad D, Bergerud K, Haffner JF, et al: Increased plasma binding of quinidine after surgery: A preliminary report. Eur J Clin Pharmacol 10:441, 1976.
11. Kessler KM, Lisker B, Conde C, et al: Abnormal quinidine binding in survivors of prehospital cardiac arrest. Am Heart J 107:665, 1984.
12. Garfinkel D, Mamelok RD, Blaschke TF: Altered therapeutic range for quinidine after myocardial infarction and cardiac surgery. Ann Intern Med 107:48, 1987.
13. Rakhit A, Holford NHG, Guentert TW, et al: Pharmacokinetics of quinidine and three of its metabolites in man. J Pharmacokinet Biopharm 12:1, 1984.
14. Vozeh S, Bindschedler M, Ha H, et al: Pharmacodynamics of 3-hydroxyquinidine alone and in combination with quinidine in healthy persons. Am J Cardiol 59:681, 1987.
15. Gerhardt RE, Knouss RF, Thyrum PT, et al: Quinidine excretion in aciduria and alkaluria. Ann Intern Med 71:927, 1969.
16. Ochs HR, Greenblatt DJ, Woo E, et al: Reduced quinidine clearance in elderly patients. Am J Cardiol 42:481, 1978.
17. Chin TWF, Pancorbo S, Comty C, et al: Quinidine pharmacoki-netics in continuous ambulatory peritoneal dialysis. Clin Exp Dialysis Apheresis 5:391, 1981.
18. Hall K, Meatherall B, Krahn J, et al: Clearance of quinidine during peritoneal dialysis. Am Heart J 104:646, 1982.
19. Gibson TP: Dialyzability of common therapeutic agents. Dial-ysis Transplant 8:24, 1979.
20. Gaughan CE, Lown B, Lanigan J, et al: Acute oral testing for determining antiarrhythmic drug efficacy. Am J Cardiol 38:677, 1976.
21. Swerdlow CD, Yu JO, Jacobson E, et al: Safety and efficacy of intravenous quinidine. Am J Med 75:36, 1983.
22. Torres V, Flowers D, Miura D, et al: Intravenous quinidine by intermittent bolus for electrophysiologic studies in patients with ventricular tachycardia. Am Heart J 108:1437, 1984.
23. Ueda CT, Dzindzio BS: Quinidine kinetics in congestive heart failure. Clin Pharmacol Ther 23:158, 1978.
24. Leahey EB, Reiffel JA, Drusin RE, et al: Interaction between quinidine and digoxin. JAMA 240:533, 1978.
25. Bussey HI: The influence of quinidine and other agents on digitalis glycosides. Am Heart J 104:289, 1982.
26. Bussey HI: Update on the influence of quinidine and other agents on digitalis glycosides. Am Heart J 107:143, 1984.
27. Bigger JT: The quinidine-digoxin interaction: What do we know about it? N Engl J Med 301:779, 1979.
28. Hirsh PD, Weiner HJ, North RL: Further insights into digoxin-quinidine interaction: Lack of correlation between serum di-goxin concentration and inotropic state of the heart. Am J Cardiol 46:863, 1980.
29. Garty M, Sood P, Rollins DE: Digitoxin elimination reduced during quinidine therapy. Ann Intern Med 94:35, 1981.
30. Fenster PE, Powell JR, Graves PE, et al: Digitoxin-quinidine interaction: Pharmacokinetic evaluation. Ann Intern Med 93:698, 1980.
31. Trohman RG, Estes DM, Castellanos A, et al: Increased quini-dine plasma concentrations during administration of ver-apamil: A new quinidine-verapamil interaction. Am J Cardiol 57:706, 1986.
32. Green JA, Clementi WA, Porter C, et al: Nifedipine-quinidine interaction. Clin Pharmacol 2:461, 1983.
33. Farringer JA, Green JA, O'Rourke RA, et al: Nifedipine-induced alterations in serum quinidine concentrations. Am Heart J 108:1570, 1984.
34. Hansten PD, Horn JR: Drug Interactions and Updates. Vancou-ver, WA: Applied Therapeutics, 1993.
35. Tatro DS: Drug Interaction Facts. St. Louis: Facts and Compari-sons, 1993.
36. Wellens HJJ, Drurer D: Effect of procainamide, quinidine and ajmaline in the Wolff-Parkinson-White syndrome. Circulation 50:114, 1974.

37. Sellers TD, Campbell RWF, Bashore TM, et al: Effects of pro-cainamide and quinidine sulfate in the Wolff-Parkinson-White syndrome. Circulation 55:15, 1977.
38. Roden DM, Woosley RL, Primm RK: Incidence and clinical features of the quinidine-associated long QT syndrome: Impli-cations for patient care. Am Heart J 111:1088, 1986.
39. Koster RW, Wellens HJJ: Quinidine-induced ventricular flutter and fibrillation without digitalis therapy. Am J Cardiol 38:519, 1976.
40. Bauman JI, Bauernfeind RA, Hoff JV, et al: Torsades de pointes due to quinidine: Observations in 31 patients. Am Heart J 107:425, 1984.
41. Anderson JL, Mason JW: Successful treatment by overdrive pacing of recurrent quinidine syncope due to ventricular tachy-cardia. Am J Med 64:715, 1978.
42. Stratmann HG, Kennedy HL: Torsades de pointes associated with drugs and toxins: Recognition and management. Am Heart J 113:1470, 1987.
43. Schmid PG, Nelson LD, Mark AL, et al: Inhibition of adrenergic vasoconstriction by quinidine. J Pharmacol Exp Ther 188:124, 1974.
44. Maisel AS, Molutsky HJ, Insel PA: Hypotension after quinidine plus verapamil. N Engl J Med 312:167, 1985.
45. Cohen IS, Jick H, Cohen SI: Adverse reactions to quinidine in hospitalized patients: Findings based on data from the Boston Collaborative Drug Surveillance Program. Prog Cardiovasc Dis 20:151, 1977.
46. Eisner EV, Carr RM, MacKinney AA: Quinidine-induced agran-ulocytosis. JAMA 238:884, 1977.
47. Geltner D, Chajek T, Rubinger D, et al: Quinidine hypersensi-tivity and liver involvement. Gastroenterology 70:650, 1976.
48. West AG, McMahon M, Portanova JP: Quinidine-induced lupus erythematosus. Ann Intern Med 100:840, 1984.
49. Arif M, Laidlaw JC, Oshrain C, et al: A randomized double-blind parallel group comparison of disopyramide phosphate and quinidine in patients with cardiac arrhythmias. Angiology 34:393, 1983.
50. Morganroth J, Oshrain C, Steele PP: Comparative efficacy and safety of oral tocainide and quinidine for benign and poten-tially lethal ventricular arrhythmias. Am J Cardiol 56:581, 1985.
51. Singh JB, Rasul AM, Shah A, et al: Efficacy of mexiletine in chronic ventricular arrhythmias compared with quinidine: A single-blind, randomized trial. Am J Cardiol 53:84, 1984.
52. Fenster PE, Hanson CD: Mexiletine and quinidine in ventricu-lar ectopy. Clin Pharmacol Ther 34:136, 1983.
53. The Flecainide-Quinidine Research Group: Flecainide versus quinidine for treatment of chronic ventricular arrhythmias. Cir-culation 67:1117, 1983.
54. Hanyok JJ, MacNeil DJ: Sotalol versus class I and II antiarrhyth-mic agents. Cardiovasc Drugs Ther 4:603, 1990.
55. The Cardiac Arrhythmia Suppression Trial (CAST) Investiga-tors: Preliminary Report: Effect of encainide and flecainide on mortality in a randomized trial of arrhythmia suppression after myocardial infarction. N Engl J Med 321:406, 1989.
56. Morganroth J, Goin JE: Quinidine-related mortality in the short-to-medium term treatment of ventricular arrhythmias: A meta-analysis. Circulation 84:1977, 1991.
57. The ESVEM Investigators: The ESVEM Trial. Electrophysiologic study versus electrocardiographic monitoring for selection of antiarrhythmic therapy of ventricular arrhythmias. Circulation 79:1354, 1989.
58. Mason JW: A comparison of seven antiarrhythmic drugs in patients with ventricular arrhythmias. N Engl J Med 329:452, 1993.
59. Borgeat A, Goy J, Maendly R, et al: Flecainide versus quinidine for conversion of atrial fibrillation to sinus rhythm. Am J Cardiol 58:496, 1986.
60. Juul-Möller S, Edvardsson N, Rehnqvist-Ahlberg N: Sotalol versus quinidine for the maintenance of sinus rhythm after direct current conversion of atrial fibrillation. Circulation 82;1932, 1990.
61. Coplen SE, Antman E, Berlin JA, et al: Efficacy and safety of quinidine therapy for maintenance of sinus rhythm after cardioversion: A meta-analysis of randomized controlled trials. Circulation 82:1106, 1990.

62. Duff HJ, Roden D, Primm RK, et al: Mexiletine in the treatment of resistant ventricular arrhythmias: Enhancement of efficacy and reduction of dose-related side effects by the combination of quinidine. Circulation 67:1124, 1983.
63. Greenspan AM, Spielman SR, Webb CR, et al: Efficacy of combination therapy with mexiletine and a type IA agent for inducible ventricular tachyarrhythmias secondary to coronary artery disease. Am J Cardiol 56:277, 1985.
64. Klein RC, Huang SK, Marcus Fl, et al: Enhanced efficacy of propafenone when used in combination with procainamide or quinidine. Am Heart J 114:551, 1987.
65. Duffy CE, Swiryn S, Bauernfeind RA, et al: Inducible sustained ventricular tachycardia refractory to individual class I drugs: Effect of adding a second class I drug. Am Heart J 106:450, 1983.
66. Kim SG, Seiden SW, Matos JA, et al: Combination of procainamide and quinidine for better tolerance and additive effects for ventricular arrhythmias. Am J Cardiol 56:84, 1985.

CHAPTER 149

Sotalol

Bramah N. Singh, M.D., Ph.D.

Although sotalol has been the prototype of the so-called class III antiarrhythmic compounds and its unique electrophysiologic properties were described in 1970,[1] only recently has it drawn widespread attention as an agent for controlling cardiac arrhythmias.[2-5] There are several reasons. The CAST trials[6,7] and various meta-analytic studies of different electrophysiologic classes of compounds have indicated the potentially lethal propensity of sodium-channel blockers when they are used for arrhythmia control in patients with structural heart disease.[8,9] Extensive experience with the drug amiodarone, which is widely perceived as acting principally via lengthening cardiac repolarization and by adrenergic inhibition, has contributed to the increasing shift from the use of class I to class III agents.[10,11] This chapter presents the evolving role of dl-sotalol as an antiarrhythmic drug relative to its pharmacodynamic actions. The nonantiarrhythmic effects of the drug such as its utility in controlling hypertension, ischemic heart disease, and other β-blocker indications are not discussed herein. Such indications are similar to the overall spectrum of therapeutic activity of β-blockade, which is discussed elsewhere in this volume. The focus here is on the role of sotalol in treating ventricular and supraventricular arrhythmias.

PHARMACOLOGIC CONSIDERATIONS

The pharmacologic effects of sotalol are dominated by its dual propensity to competitively block β-receptors without a predilection for β_1- or β_2-receptors and by the property for prolonging the myocardial action potential duration (APD) associated with the corresponding increases in cardiac refractoriness consistent with a class III electrophysiologic action.[12] Structurally, sotalol is 4'-(2 isopropylamino-1-hydroxyethyl)-methylsulfonamide; it is a racemate of d- and l-isomers, both of which have equal class III activity; only the l-isomer has significant β-adrenoceptor blocking activity.[12]

β-Blocking Actions

Sotalol is a selective β-adrenoceptor blocking drug with little or no sodium-channel blocking actions; it has no measurable intrinsic sympathomimetic activity. An interesting feature of the drug's pharmacologic effect is that it does exhibit nonadrenergically mediated positive inotropic activity,[13,14] which may be related to its potency for prolonging the cardiac action potential duration. On a molar basis, the potency of sotalol as a β-blocker is approximately one third that of the reference β-blocker, propranolol.[15] Sotalol produces competitive blockade of both β_1- and β_2-adrenoceptors in *in vitro* and *in vivo* experimental models.[16] The large differences in the *in vitro* and *in vivo* potencies of sotalol compared with propranolol are undoubtedly related to the oral bioavailability of sotalol compared with the poor bioavailability of propranolol.

Electrophysiologic Actions

In 1970, Singh and Vaughan Williams[1] found that sotalol markedly prolonged action potential duration (APD) in isolated atrial and ventricular multicellular preparations. Such an effect was not found with conventional β-blockers. Sotalol did not exhibit any effect on conduction velocity, but as might be expected because of its β-blocking property, it slows the sinus node frequency by depressing phase 4 depolarization. Strauss et al.[17] also found that sotalol increased action potential duration as well as refractory period in both canine ventricular muscle and Purkinje fibers; however, the effects on Purkinje fibers were more sensitive and of a greater magnitude. In addition, these authors showed that the effect of sotalol to increase APD was directly related to cycle length and that this effect was also much more dramatic in Purkinje fibers relative to that in ventricular muscle. Since these original reports, many other investigators have confirmed the ability of sotalol to increase APD. Such an effect of frequency of stimulation on the APD has subsequently been termed "reversed" rate dependency.[18] These effects have been shown to reside equally in the d-isomer of sotalol as well, and are not a result of β-adrenoceptor antagonism. Both d- and l-sotalol enantiomers increase action potential duration primarily by blocking the time-dependent outward delayed rectifier K$^+$ current (I$_k$). Carmeliet[19] showed that both d- and dl-sotalol decreased I$_k$ in a concentration-related manner. There is a lesser effect on the inward rectifying potassium current. Under certain conditions such as bradycardia and hypokalemia, the lengthening of the QT interval produced by sotalol may lead to the development of the polymorphic ventricular tachycardia designated torsade de pointes, which may develop in a proportion of patients.

The clinical electrophysiologic effects of sotalol can be predicted from the drug's effects in isolated tissues as well as in experimental animals.[19-21] Thus, sotalol prolongs the QT and QT$_c$ intervals without any significant effect on QRS or PR intervals.[12] These QT-prolonging effects are also demonstrable when heart rates are maintained constant by pacing. As might be expected, sotalol has no effect on atrial (PA interval), His-Purkinje (HV interval) or ventricular (QRS interval) conduction velocity, but it significantly slows atrioventricular (AV) nodal conduction[20] and increases the sinus cycle lengths as a consequence of both β-adrenoceptor blockade and QT$_c$ prolongation. Substantially higher concentrations of sotalol are required for measurable class III actions of sotalol than for its β-blocking effect. These effects are readily distinguished from those of conventional β-antagonists, which increase only the PR interval and AV nodal refractoriness because of β-adrenoceptor blocking actions on the AV node.[20] In contrast, sotalol increases the voltage-dependent refractoriness in the atria and ventricles. Furthermore, sotalol, unlike conventional β-blockers, reduces defibrillation threshold.

HEMODYNAMIC EFFECTS OF SOTALOL
Inotropic Correlates of Prolonged Cardiac Repolarization

As indicated, in contrast to conventional β-blockers, sotalol increases the time course of cardiac repolarization.[22] This has two consequences. The first is the corresponding increase in the effective refractory period and, second, in isolated tissues the lengthening of the action potential duration is associated with a positive inotropic effect.[23-25] In whole animals and in humans such a positive inotropic effect is not always translated into an improvement in ventricular performance, since in the *in vivo* setting the indices of contractility are modulated by the associated β-blocking properties of the drug. However, in most patients the positive inotropic effect of sotalol is not completely negated by β-blockade. Nevertheless, in comparison to the conventional β-blockers, the negative inotropic effect of sotalol is less.[22]

Hemodynamic Effects in Humans

The hemodynamic effects of sotalol in humans are likely to be variable compared with those of conventional β-blockers. For example, Thumala et al.[26] showed that a single 0.1- to 0.5-mg/kg dose of intravenous sotalol given into the pulmonary artery produced no measurable depressant hemodynamic effects at rest or during exercise. A depressant effect became evident, however, during constant right ventricular pacing. There were decreases in LV dP/dt, cardiac index, and stroke index with an increase in the arteriovenous oxygen difference. Hutton et al.[27] reported similar findings. On the other hand, Brooks et al.[28] and Frankl and Soloff[29] noted neither negative nor positive effects on hemodynamic variables during chronic oral administration in doses up to 0.6 mg/kg despite the fact that a subset of their patients had advanced degrees of heart failure. Their data raise the possibility that during chronic oral sotalol administration, the positive inotropic effects resulting from lengthened repolarization and the depressant effects resulting from β-blockade in the case of sotalol are neutralized. Thus, the depressant effect on sotalol on systemic hemodynamic functions might be expected to be less than those of conventional β-blockers, which often induce cardiac decompensation in patients with compromised left ventricular function. Nevertheless, sotalol may still induce cardiac failure or exacerbate it when there is an imbalance between the positive and negative inotropic effects of the drug. It has been found that chronic sotalol administration might increase left ventricular systolic function at rest and with exercise as noted by Mahmarian et al.[30] in a series of patients being studied for the suppression of PVCs. They found measurable increases in the left ventricular ejection fraction; in two of their patients with markedly depressed ventricular ejection fraction sotalol worsened cardiac failure. In two others, cardiac arrest and torsade de pointes developed, respectively, suggesting the need for caution in the use of sotalol in patients in cardiac failure or in those with markedly lowered ejection fraction even though the drug is often well tolerated in the subset of patients with ventricular tachycardia or fibrillation.[2, 3] Heart failure may be aggravated by the drug in situations in which cardiac performance is critically dependent on augmented adrenergic drive.

PHARMACOKINETICS OF SOTALOL

The pharmacokinetics of sotalol conform to an open two-compartment model in which its absorption, distribution, and elimination are by a first-order kinetics.[31, 32] The d-isomer and the dl-sotalol have similar kinetics in humans[33] and the pharmacokinetics of sotalol is not changed during long-term drug administration. It is unique among β-adrenoceptor antagonists insofar as the drug is nearly 100% bioavailable after oral administration; it is completely absorbed and is not metabolized. There is no first-pass effect. The peak plasma concentration is reached between 2 and 4 hours after an oral dose. Co-ingestion with food leads to a modest reduction in bioavailability. Sotalol is very hydrophilic and does not bind to plasma proteins. In addition, sotalol does not accumulate in the brain, and consequently clinical central nervous system side effects are rare.[32]

Since the drug is fully bioavailable, is not metabolized, and is not bound to plasma proteins, fluctuations in serum concentrations are small, the plasma half-life is long (10 to 15 hours), and plasma levels are linearly related to dose. The clinical pharmacokinetic profile of sotalol is summarized in Table 149–1. Because sotalol is largely excreted by the kidneys in an unchanged form, the plasma concentrations of the drug will vary linearly with creatinine clearance. Therefore, dose adjustment is necessary in proportion to the degree of renal dysfunction present. For creatinine clearance greater than 60 ml/min, 12-hour dosing intervals are appropriate. This may be increased to 12 to 24 hours when the creatinine clearance is between 30 and 69 ml/min, and to 36 to 48 hours for patients with the clearance of 10 to 30 ml/min. For even lower levels of creatinine clearance, dosage needs to be determined on an individual basis with careful clinical monitoring. It should be emphasized that sotalol clearance is also reduced in elderly patients, in whom lower doses should be used.

Sotalol does not produce pharmacokinetic drug interactions when it is given together with antacids, digoxin, hydrochlorothiazide diuretics, cholestyramine, or warfarin. However, numerous pharmacodynamic interactions with numerous cardioactive compounds are likely. This is especially so in the case of other antiadrenergic drugs (verapamil, diltiazem, amiodarone) and other QT prolonging agents (class III agents including amiodarone, tricyclic antidepressants, phenothiazines, terfenadine). Coadministration with erythromycin may also be imprudent.

CONTROLLING CARDIAC ARRHYTHMIAS WITH SOTALOL

It is likely that the net antiarrhythmic effects of sotalol stem from its combined β-blocking actions and its property for consistently inducing prolonged cardiac

Table 149–1. **Clinical Pharmacokinetic Profile of Sotalol**

Absorption rate	T_{MAX} 2–3 hours
Extent of absorption	>90% of dose
Extent of bioavailability	~100% of dose
Binding to plasma protein	0%
Approximate volume of distribution	1.6–2.4 L/kg
Elimination	
Renal (unchanged)	~90%
Biotransformation	0
Approximate plasma half-life	15 (7–18) hours
Pattern of elimination kinetics	First order
Kinetic model applicable	Open two compartment
Metabolites	None detected
Steady state/dose ratio	Two-fold variation
Special features	Accumulation in renal failure, kinetics not affected by liver function

From Sundquist H: Basic review and comparison of β-blocker pharmacokinetics. Curr Ther Res 28(Suppl):38S, 1980.

repolarization as manifested by the long QT/QT_c intervals on the surface electrocardiogram.[22] However, the relative importance of the two components of the drug's action in this regard is not clear. It is likely to vary with the arrhythmia under treatment, the nature of the cardiac disease that forms the substrate for the arrhythmia, and the modulating factors (e.g., electrolyte disturbances) that might be present. Clearly, in patients with ischemic heart disease, the β-blocking actions of the drug are likely to be of paramount importance.

Numerous experimental and clinical reports document a broad range of antiarrhythmic effects in the case of dl-sotalol. For the most part, the clinical results are in accord with those documented in a wide variety of experimental models in which the antifibrillatory effects of dl-sotalol and d-sotalol have been studied extensively.[34-40] The spectrum of dl-sotalol effects in arrhythmias is wider than that of conventional β-blockers.[22] It is likely to exceed that of d-sotalol, being a composite of the β-blocking effects as well as the voltage-dependent refractory period effects of d-sotalol.[12] This issue is discussed in the chapter devoted to d-sotalol in this volume.

SOTALOL IN SUPRAVENTRICULAR TACHYARRHYTHMIAS

The overall effects of sotalol (as is the case with any other pharmacologic agent now being introduced) in supraventricular arrhythmias should be viewed in relation to the changes that have occurred recently in the electrode catheter ablation of paroxysmal supraventricular tachycardias (PSVTs) with or without accessory tracts in the heart and some cases of atrial flutter.[3] Because these newer approaches carry an extremely high frequency of success with prospects for cure, prophylactic drug therapy of PSVTs is likely to be used much less often than previously in areas where ablative techniques are available.

Because sotalol is a β-blocker and a class III agent, it is likely to be as effective as conventional β-blockers in reducing atrial extrasystoles and other ectopic atrial tachycardias. The drug will also be effective in slowing sinus tachycardia and the ventricular response in atrial flutter and fibrillation, in terminating reentrant supraventricular tachycardia, and in controlling the recurrence of a proportion of such arrhythmias during prophylactic drug administration.[4, 41-44] In the acute conversion of reentrant paroxysmal supraventricular tachycardias, the precise role of the drug is uncertain since no blinded comparative studies against established therapy (e.g., intravenous verapamil or adenosine) have been carried out. A recent paper[42] summarized the findings of seven open trials using intravenous sotalol (0.4 to 1.5 mg/kg) in the acute management of patients with PSVT. Of the 106 patients studied in these trials, 47 (44%) patients experienced conversion to sinus rhythm. The results of electrophysiologic studies in six clinical trials demonstrated that administration of intravenous sotalol (0.6 to 2.75 mg/kg) prevented reinduction of sustained

PSVT in 44 of 75 (59%) patients. However, the predictive accuracy of the acute response for the long-term effects of the drug remains unclear. The antifibrillatory effects of sotalol because of its class III[40, 44] action are likely to make it more effective in maintaining sinus rhythm in patients with atrial fibrillation and flutter following cardioversion. Of these various situations, in which the drug is likely to be effective, that of the greatest potential utility is the role the drug might have in maintaining the stability of sinus rhythm after cardioversion of atrial fibrillation or flutter. The drug's role in the acute termination of PSVT is only of theoretical interest in light of the fact that intravenous diltiazem, verapamil, and especially adenosine are highly effective and generally safer in most instances. Therefore, the efficacy of sotalol in this setting will not be discussed here.

Atrial Flutter and Fibrillation

There is an electrophysiologic rationale for the potential utility of sotalol or d-sotalol for the acute conversion of atrial flutter and fibrillation to sinus rhythm and for maintaining stability of sinus rhythm during chronic drug prophylaxis.[38] The precise efficacy of the drug on both counts remains unclear, however. The published studies have not been adequately controlled, nor have they employed adequate techniques to study dose-response relationships. Acute conversion rates have been variable, but a slowing of the ventricular rates has been consistent as might be expected for a β-blocker. The conversion rate may be up to 40% to 50% in selected patients, which compares favorably with intravenous procainamide, and possibly with intravenously administered newer class III agents or class IC agents such as flecainide. The maintenance of sinus rhythm after conversion is potentially of greater practical importance. Here, too, there have been no placebo-controlled studies.

Antman et al.[44] evaluated 74 patients with symptomatic chronic recurrent atrial fibrillation unresponsive to conventional class I antiarrhythmic agents (one to five drugs, with a median of two). The study design was such that the effects of "stepped care" treatment with propafenone, sotalol, and amiodarone was evaluated in alleviating the symptoms by controlling ventricular rate and/or conversion to sinus rhythm. Sotalol was highly effective (72% success rate) in maintaining sinus rhythm in patients with chronic atrial fibrillation previously refractory to class IA antiarrhythmic agents. Although at 6 months of follow-up, only 41% of the 74 patients were free of atrial fibrillation while receiving propafenone, 72% of patients receiving sotalol remained free of atrial fibrillation. However, these figures cannot be accepted in place of those acquired in randomized, blinded, controlled studies.

The maintenance of sinus rhythm after DC conversion by sotalol was recently compared with quinidine in a Swedish multicenter clinical trial.[45] In this study, 183 patients with chronic atrial fibrillation were randomized to receive sotalol (98 patients) or quinidine (85 patients) 2 hours after conversion to sinus rhythm with DC conversion. Patients randomized to sotalol initially received 80 mg b.i.d. for 1 week, after which, if needed, the dose could be increased to 160 mg twice daily. For patients assigned to quinidine, slow-release preparation of quinidine sulfate was administered in 600 mg b.i.d. dosage. At the end of the 6-month study period, 49 (52%) of 95 evaluable patients randomized to sotalol were still in sinus rhythm compared with 38 (48%) of 79 patients receiving quinidine. Although some patients were receiving digitalis, the presence or absence of digitalis therapy did not significantly alter the success rate in the two groups of patients. At 1 month, 39 patients were receiving a dose of sotalol of 80 mg twice daily and 50 patients received 160 mg twice daily. Sixty-four percent of patients on the 80-mg dosage and 50% of the patients on the 160-mg dosage were in sinus rhythm at 6 months. In patients with relapse into atrial fibrillation while on treatment with sotalol and digitalis, the ventricular rate decreased from 80 to 68 beats/min ($p < .03$) compared with the baseline recording before DC conversion. In patients treated with digitalis in the quinidine group, the ventricular rate increased from 80 to 109 beats/min ($p < .02$) compared with the baseline. Compared with sotalol, significantly greater numbers of patients receiving quinidine experienced overall adverse drug reactions as well as the need to withdraw from the study because of intolerable side effects. In patients treated with sotalol, 27 of 97 patients (28%) reported side effects compared with 43 of 86 patients (50%) in the group treated with quinidine ($p < .01$). The overall withdrawal rate for intolerable side effects or recurrence of atrial fibrillation was 11% for sotalol patients compared with 27% for patients treatment with quinidine ($p < .03$). Two patients (one in each treatment group) had proarrhythmic events in the early phase of treatment while patients were still in the hospital.

The results of this prospective clinical trial are important for several reasons. First, the results demonstrated no significant differences between the numbers of patients maintained in sinus rhythm after 6 months of sotalol or quinidine treatment given after successful DC cardioversion. Second, the patients treated with quinidine had significantly greater adverse drug experiences and a large percentage (27%) were withdrawn because of intolerable side effects or recurrence of atrial fibrillation. Finally, during recurrence of atrial fibrillation, patients treated with sotalol and digitalis maintained a slow ventricular response, whereas those receiving quinidine and digitalis had an increase in their ventricular response during the recurrence. These findings clearly suggest that sotalol is not only equally effective in maintaining sinus rhythm after DC conversion in patients with chronic atrial fibrillation, but it is also better tolerated than quinidine in the chronic treatment of these patients. These results are particularly noteworthy in view of the recent findings from a meta-analysis performed by Coplen et al.,[46] which indicated that in patients with atrial fibrillation, chronic therapy with quinidine is associated with increased mortality. Although not fully established, it is thought that the increased mortality is most likely secondary to the proarrhythmic effects of quinidine. In the study by Juul-Moller et al.,[45] the effects of sotalol or quinidine on cardiac mortality could not be evaluated because there was no placebo group. However, there was only one death in each treatment limb. The overall efficacy of sotalol in maintaining sinus rhythm compared with low-dose amiodarone is not known. From uncontrolled studies, it is becoming increasingly felt that low-dose amiodarone[9] is currently the most effective agent in this context. However, this is merely an impression from uncontrolled small and noncomparative studies. A direct comparison in a randomized study will be necessary for valid conclusions.

Sotalol in Atrial Fibrillation/Flutter Complicating Pre-excitation

Manz et al.[47] studied the effects of intravenous sotalol (80 mg) in 11 patients with the WPW syndrome and in 9 patients with AV nodal reentrant PSVT. Sotalol prolonged the ERP of the right atrium and ventricle with a delay in conduction in the AV node and bypass tracts in the anterograde as well as retrograde directions. The tachycardia rate was slowed from 182 to 153 beats/min and the ventricular rate during atrial fibrillation slowed from 148 to 112 beats/min. Sotalol exerted a depressant effect in all parts of the reentrant circuit including the atrium, ventricle, AV node, and bypass tracts. Thus, the data indicate that the drug is likely to be effective in preventing the rapid ventricular response to atrial fibrillation in patients with the WPW syndrome as well as in preventing reciprocating tachycardias. In a recent study[48] of 22 patients with the WPW syndrome resistant to multiple conventional drugs, the effects of sotalol were evaluated during electrophysiologic study as well as long-term prophylactic therapy. Sustained reciprocating tachycardia was rendered noninducible in 13 of 18 patients with inducible tachycardia during the electrophysiologic evaluation. The anterograde as well as retrograde effective periods of accessory pathways were significantly prolonged by 20% and 28%, respectively. The long-term therapy during a follow-up period ranging from 1 to 47 months revealed a 77% success rate in controlling symptomatic tachycardia. Again, these salutary effects of the drug need to be considered in light of the emerging data on electrode catheter ablation of these arrhythmias, a technique that is highly effective in providing a cure in the majority of cases of reentrant PSVT with or without bypass tracts, although the long-term effects of the invasive procedure require continued surveillance.

Sotalol in Supraventricular Tachyarrhythmias After Coronary Artery Bypass Surgery

Supraventricular arrhythmias may complicate the postoperative course of about 33% of patients undergoing cardiac surgery, especially myocardial revascularization.[49] These arrhythmias are significantly reduced by the prophylactic administration of β-blockers but not by digoxin or calcium antagonists such as verapamil.[50] Suttorp et al.[51] compared the effects of propranolol and sotalol in preventing the occurrence of supraventricular arrhythmias in patients undergoing coronary artery bypass grafting (CABG) in 450 patients who did not have severely depressed left ventricular function or had contraindications to β-blockade. Four treatment regimens were used: low-dose sotalol (40 mg t.i.d.), low-dose propranolol (10 mg q.i.d.), high-dose sotalol (80 mg t.i.d.) or high-dose propranolol (20 mg q.i.d.). The drug administration was initiated within 4 to 6 hours after the completion of CABG and continued for 6 postoperative days. The results showed that both agents markedly reduced the postoperative incidence of supraventricular arrhythmias compared with historical controls and there was no significant further effect by doubling the dose of the two β-blockers. In a subsequent study,[52] the authors conducted a double-blind, placebo-controlled randomized study in which 40 mg of sotalol or a matching placebo was given every 6 hours beginning 6 hours after surgery and continued to the sixth postoperative day. The sample size was 300 consecutive post-CABG patients. There was treatment failure in 49 (33%) of 150 of the placebo-treated patients and in 24 (16%) of the 150 patients treated with sotalol ($p < .005$). Of interest, atrial fibrillation was the only arrhythmia seen in the sotalol group, but in the placebo-controlled group there was atrial fibrillation in 42 cases, atrial flutter in three, atrial tachycardia in three, and sinus tachycardia in one. These data indicate that sotalol is effective in reducing the incidence of postoperative supraventricular arrhythmias in patients undergoing CABG, but they do not indicate whether the beneficial effect is mediated primarily via β-blockade or the drug's class III actions. In this regard, the effects of d-sotalol in the post-CABG patients will be of interest.

SOTALOL IN VENTRICULAR ARRHYTHMIAS

The spectrum of ventricular arrhythmias amenable to therapy with sotalol needs to be considered relative to the β-blocking properties of the drug along with its clearly demonstrated class III actions.[22] The relative significance of the two actions might be gauged by directly comparing the therapeutic effects of dl-sotalol with those of d-sotalol. Such studies have not been performed. In treating ventricular arrhythmias, it is clearly important to define whether therapy is being administered for relief of symptoms or for prolonging survival by reducing arrhythmia mortality. In recent years, sotalol has drawn increasing attention as an agent that might be superior to class I agents, especially for the treatment of VT/VF and survivors of cardiac arrest in patients with significant cardiac disease. However, as is the case with all other major antiarrhythmic agents (barring β-blockers), there are no stringently controlled clinical trials that have un-equivocally established that the drug does indeed prolong survival by controlling ventricular arrhythmias.

Suppressant Effects on Premature Ventricular Contractions

Sotalol decreases premature ventricular contractions (PVCs) in about 50% of the patients.[53-55] Anderson[53] reported sotalol to be effective in 59% of the patients versus 11% in placebo. Liddell et al.[54] found that 67% of patients responded to sotalol (in doses up to 640 mg/day) compared with 39% responding to procainamide in a multicenter crossover design protocol. Deedwania[55] found a higher degree of PVC suppression by sotalol compared with propranolol for the same degree of β-blockade. The clinical utility of the PVC-suppressant effect of sotalol remains uncertain in light of the dichotomy between suppression of PVCs and mortality noted in the CAST trials[6, 7] albeit with an entirely different electrophysiologic class of compounds. However, as in the case of other antiarrhythmic agents, which have the potential to suppress PVCs and nonsustained ventricular tachycardia, sotalol may be used for relief of symptoms associated with extra systoles; its choice for such an indication will be a matter of individualized therapy in selected patients. Whether suppression of PVCs or nonsustained ventricular tachycardia will lead to a reduction in sudden death (in line with "the PVC hypothesis") and arrhythmia mortality remains as yet an unproven hypothesis as it is in the case of other anti-ectopic agents.

Sotalol in Patients After Myocardial Infarction (MI)

Because sotalol is a potent β-blocker and has a powerful antifibrillatory effect by virtue of prolonging the action potential duration, the drug might be expected to reduce sudden death and prolong survival in post-MI patients. Only one controlled trial has been performed with the drug and the data have been positive but indecisive. It is known that prophylactic β-blockade after the index infarct has been found to reduce mortality at 1 year by 18% to 47% in different trials.[8] The beneficial effect correlated with the degree of reduction of heart rate;[56] sotalol reduces heart rate but its effect on mortality was less striking.[57] In this placebo-controlled, double-blind, multicenter study, 1456 patients were randomized to sotalol (320 mg sotalol given once daily) and to a placebo. Therapy was started between 5 and 14 days after myocardial infarction. At the end of 12 months, the mortality rate was 8.9% for the placebo group and 7.3% for the sotalol group. This 18% mortality reduction effected by sotalol did not reach statistical significance. The reason for the less than expected benefit remains unclear. A number of factors might have contributed. The trial design used a 60:40 randomization scheme; the dose of the drug was fixed, and it is possible

that a number of patients had been given potassium-wasting diuretics in the early stages of the trial. Indeed, the survival curves indicated a slight excess in deaths during the early phases of the study, suggesting a proarrhythmic (? torsade de pointes) reaction to the drug. Finally, the patients were not selected for high risk on the basis of ambient arrhythmias in which the class III action of the drug might have exerted a greater beneficial effect. Clearly, these are speculations, and it is unlikely that a trial with sotalol in infarct survivors will be repeated. In a small randomized but not placebo-controlled trial, a 320-mg dose of sotalol given twice daily (a high dose) was compared with timolol and encainide in high-risk survivors of acute infarction.[58] This study was terminated prematurely because of the findings of a higher incidence of sudden death in the group treated with sotalol compared with those treated with encainide or timolol. Thus, the available data to date neither negate nor support the use of sotalol for *routine* secondary prevention in the survivors of myocardial infarction.

Sotalol in Patients with Symptomatic VT/VF and/or Aborted Sudden Death

Recent data have suggested that sotalol might have a major role in the prophylactic treatment of patients with these arrhythmia syndromes. The role of the drug in these patients began to be determined in the early 1980s.[2, 3]

A number of studies[2, 3, 59-72] have reported on the use sotalol in controlling VT/VF and in survivors of sudden death. Most of the studies have utilized programmed electrical stimulation (PES) as a technique for guiding therapy of VT/VF and sudden death when sotalol was used as a test agent. The rate of prevention of inducible VT/VF varied between 28% and 79%, and the decision to include the patients for long-term therapy was based on a positive response to sotalol during acute testing. The stimulation protocol for PES as well as the period of follow-up have been variable in the earlier studies. The percentage of patients at the end of the follow-up period receiving the drug varied between 19% and 69%. The incidence of arrhythmia recurrences in "responders" ranged between 0% and 27% at the end of the observation period. Only a few of the recurrences were fatal.

Despite the limitations and variability of protocol used in different laboratories, the effects of sotalol on the prevention of inducibility of VT/VF have been consistently higher than those reported for class I agents as a class. The average effectiveness for preventing reinduciblity of VT/VF for most class I agents has been reported to be about 20%.[73-78] The reported response rate for sotalol is variable but numerically higher[64] than that for procainamide. The use of triple extra stimuli reported by Singh et al.[64] in a multicenter study comparing sotalol and procainamide gave the response rates of 30% for sotalol and 20%

for procainamide. Of note, Nademanee et al.[3] found a reasonably concordant predictive accuracy of Holter monitoring and PES. For this reason, the outcome of a study designed to compare the predictive accuracy of the techniques is of much clinical importance. It has a major bearing on how therapy with sotalol in VT/VF may reasonably be designed and monitored.

Significance of the Electrophysiologic Versus Electrocardiographic Monitoring Study

For judging effectiveness of sotalol in the control of VT/VF, ESVEM is a landmark study.[70, 72, 79] The findings of ESVEM have been the subject of much controversy, understandably so since they are at variance with long-entrenched clinical practice. However, it is the only controlled clinical study of its kind, and it seems unreasonable to examine its flaws relative to the results of uncontrolled previous studies. In ESVEM, the relative merits of the two techniques in predicting long-term drug responses in patients with symptomatic VT/VF and those surviving cardiac arrests were determined.[79] From 2103 patients screened, 486 patients satisfied the predetermined entry criteria. They were randomized to Holter-guided therapy (n = 244) and to PES-guided therapy (n = 242). The drug therapy tested in a randomized fashion was six class I agents and sotalol; drug trials were positive in 14% of the PES groups and 38% in the Holter limb. Of the responders (n = 297) 45% eventually had their therapy selected by PES and 77% by Holter. The patients were followed for 6 years. ESVEM yielded two important findings. The first indicated no statistically significant difference between PES and Holter monitoring in predicting the occurrence of sudden death, arrhythmia recurrence, cardiac or total mortality. Second, sotalol was found to be a more effective antiarrhythmic agent than six class I agents when considered individually or collectively.[70, 72] At 1 year, arrhythmia recurrence was found in 44% of patients given class I agents and 21% (Fig. 149–1) in those given sotalol ($p < .0007$), a low predictive accuracy. In fact, the recurrence of VT in 44% of the patients given class I agents guided by Holter or PES appears too low for a predictive technique to be of clinical utility. Nevertheless, in the case of responders, Holter monitoring yielded a higher rate of complete efficacy compared with PES. For this reason, the ESVEM investigators concluded that "in patients with clinical characteristics similar to those of our study population, if antiarrhythmic drug therapy is to be used to prevent the recurrence of ventricular tachyarrhythmias, treatment with sotalol and assessment of its potential efficacy by Holter monitoring is a reasonable initial strategy."[72] A number of other conclusions of a practical nature can be drawn from the ESVEM results. The ESVEM findings should also raise the issue regarding the validity of "guided therapy" per se in the sense that neither Holter monitoring nor PES has ever been validated against an inherently valid tech-

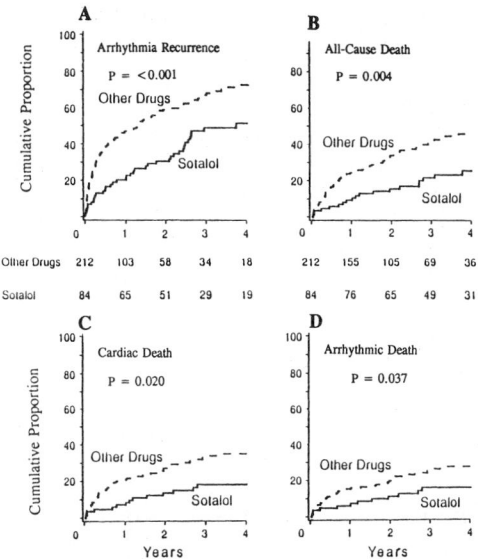

Figure 149–1. Actuarial probability of events in patients on class I agents and sotalol during long-term therapy after selection of agents with guided therapy at serial testing (either programmed electrical stimulation for Holter monitoring). Cumulative arrhythmia recurrence *(A)*, all-cause mortality *(B)*, cardiac death *(C)*, and arrhythmic death *(D)* for sotalol compared with six class I agents collectively in patients who received a drug efficacy prediction are shown. The *p* values are determined by multivariate Cox regression. (From Mason JW and the ESVEM Investigators: A comparison of seven antiarrhythmic drugs in patients with ventricular tachyarrhythmias. N Engl J Med 329:452, 1993.)

nique. As indicated elsewhere,[80] the guided approach may merely differentiate "responders" from "nonresponders" with inherently different prognosis. It appears that the responses demonstrated in ESVEM might be interpreted as *drug-specific* rather than *technique-specific*, sotalol being more effective than class I agents because of its unique pharmacologic properties, combining as it does β-blocking properties and class III actions. However, from these studies it cannot be concluded that class I agents are superior to no treatment or to placebo, since ESVEM could not address this fundamental issue. Indeed, in the absence of a concurrent control, the same criticism may apply to the results with sotalol. On the other hand, sotalol produces β-blockade, which per se in virtually all subsets of patients produces a beneficial effect on mortality. It is also noteworthy that a recent study has indicated that β-blockade with metoprolol given empirically produced effects no different from therapy guided by PES in patients with inducible monomorphic ventricular tachycardia in the setting of clinically symptomatic arrhythmias.[81] At least in one albeit uncontrolled study, responders and nonresponders to PES-guided therapy had identical clinical outcome with respect to arrhythmia recurrence.[82] Sotalol was significantly more effective than class I agents in ESVEM. When this is considered in light of the overall data on class I agents, it will become increasingly difficult to justify the continued use of sodium-channel blockers in the prophylactic treatment of VT/VF. The data also support the use of sotalol guided either by Holter monitoring or PES. Whether the drug can be used empirically as is the case of amiodarone remains to be clarified.[83] An unresolved issue is the comparative efficacy of sotalol versus amiodarone in patients with VT/VF and survivors of cardiac arrest. There are no controlled studies comparing the effects of the two drugs. However, in a small, open randomized study,[84] no difference was found between the two treatment groups at the end of 1 year. However, the numbers of patients enrolled were small, and the short observation period seriously limited the significance of the study.

Thus, for the present, it is reasonable to consider using sotalol and amiodarone (ahead of class I agents) as first line therapy for symptomatic VT/VF and for survivors of cardiac arrest. The role of pure class III agents remains unclear. Whether sotalol and/or amiodarone will prove equal or superior in efficacy to implantable cardioverter defibrillators (ICDs) in controlling VT/VF or preventing recurrences of sudden death is the subject of a number of ongoing controlled clinical trials. It is likely that in the case of many patients these agents will be used in conjunction with ICDs.

ADVERSE REACTIONS WITH SOTALOL

The adverse reactions that develop during intravenous or oral therapy with sotalol stem from its β-blocking actions and its propensity to lengthen repolarization. Adverse reactions to β-blockade include tiredness, lassitude, impotence, depression, headache, and cardiac effects such as aggravation of heart failure. These are similar to those induced by other β-antagonists. Barring the occurrence of torsade de pointes (see later), the cardiovascular effects are predictable on the basis of the drug's propensity to block β-receptors. However, uncontrolled clinical data suggest that the proclivity of the drug to induce or exacerbate congestive heart failure is less than that with conventional β-blockers. As mentioned above, it may be related to the class III actions of the drug tending to negate the intrinsic depressant effects of β-blockade.[22]

In the Julian trial[57] in which over 1400 patients were randomized either to a placebo or to sotalol, at the end of 1 year of treatment 25% of the drug-treated subjects versus 21% of those taking the placebo had to stop taking the drug because of adverse reactions. In a large data base of the sponsor of sotalol (Bristol-Myers-Squibb), the reported incidence of adverse reactions requiring drug discontinuation in a population of 1288 patients from 12 randomized studies was 16% (exclusive of torsade de pointes—see later). That sotalol is generally well tolerated was indicated by the study from Sweden on atrial fibrillation[45] and by the results of the ESVEM trial in which the drug caused fewer side effects than all the six class I agents used in the trial.[70, 72, 79]

Like all β-blockers, sotalol has been found to produce sinus arrest, atrioventricular block (generally intranodal), and severe bradycardia which, on occasion, may require the implantation of an artificial pacemaker. Similarly, as is the case with all drugs that prolong ventricular repolarization, sotalol may induce torsade de pointes but not to the same extent for a given degree of QT lengthening.[85] A number of cases of torsade de pointes have been reported occurring with therapeutic doses of drugs as well as with overdosage.

With sotalol, torsade de pointes may develop both with intravenous as well as with short-term and long-term drug administration. The occurrence of torsade de pointes is especially likely in the setting of renal failure, hypokalemia, and bradycardia at high drug concentrations. The proarrhythmia is also likely in situations where there is preexisting lengthening of the QT$_c$ interval.[86-96] Neuvonen et al.[92, 93] have reported a correlation between the serum sotalol concentration and prolongation of the QT$_c$ interval.

Severe ventricular arrhythmias, including ventricular tachycardia and fibrillation, were initially reported in five of six cases of sotalol poisoning and correlated with the prolongation of the QT$_c$ interval and serum sotalol concentration.[92, 93] Most other cases of torsade de pointes following sotalol therapy have also been observed with overdosage,[86, 89, 91, 95, 96] although a case was reported in the context of so-called therapeutic serum concentration; this patient, however, was using an additional inappropriate concomitant medication.[88] McKibbin et al.[92] reported a series of 13 patients who developed syncope and prolonged QT interval while taking therapeutic doses of sotalol. Polymorphous ventricular tachycardia was observed in 12 patients, and criteria typical of torsade of pointes were present in 10 patients. Interestingly, 12 of 13 patients in this series had been treated with a combination of sotalol and hydrochlorothiazide without adequate potassium supplementation, which results in reduced serum potassium concentration. Four patients were also taking other drugs (three on disopyramide and two on tricyclic antidepressants) known to cause prolongation of QT interval. The QT interval returned to normal in all patients after withdrawal of the drugs and the correction of the hypokalemia. Sotalol can induce life-threatening ventricular arrhythmias, particularly when given in combination with hydrochlorothiazide without potassium supplementation. However, when the dose of the drug is kept low and the patient's electrolyte (especially potassium) status is monitored carefully, the incidence of torsade de pointes is low.[2, 3] The use of sotalol in the setting of renal failure or with concomitant therapy with drugs known to prolong the QT interval (e.g., quinidine, disopyramide, phenothiazines, or tri- and tetracyclic depressants) is not advisable because of the greater risk of proarrhythmia, and when absolutely necessary it should only be done under close medical supervision.

The risk of torsade de pointes in patients with ventricular arrhythmia has been described in several recent studies.[97, 98] In the study by Kehoe et al.[97] 236 patients with sustained ventricular tachyarrhythmias were treated acutely with sotalol and 151 received long-term oral sotalol therapy. Seventeen of the 18 (7%) patients who developed proarrhythmia did so during the acute phase, only one during long-term drug administration. Eleven patients had torsade de pointes, and most proarrhythmic events occurred within 7 days of therapy. From the data in 181 clinical studies that enrolled 5856 patients, 1288 patients with ventricular arrhythmias were examined by Soyka et al.[98] for arrhythmogenic effects. The overall incidence of proarrhythmic events in these patients was 4.3% (56 patients) and 24 of the 56 patients had torsade de pointes. Although no universal relationship was found with previously described factors such as bradycardia, hypokalemia, and long QT interval, the patients with proarrhythmic events had longer mean QT_c interval at baseline as well at 1 week during therapy with sotalol. The results of available studies also indicated that the overall risk of proarrhythmic events including torsade de pointes was greater in patients with sustained ventricular tachyarrhythmias, left ventricular dysfunction, marked bradycardia, and prolonged QT interval. Because most of the proarrhythmic events occurred within the first 7 days and in general responded to reduction in dosage or discontinuation of sotalol, it is advisable that high-risk patients be hospitalized and given sotalol therapy under close supervision and continuous ECG monitoring.

AN APPROACH TO OPTIMAL DOSING WITH SOTALOL

Sotalol is a relatively simple compound pharmacokinetically. Intravenously, it is given in a dosage of 0.2 to 1.5 mg/kg of dl-sotalol over 2 to 3 minutes under electrocardiographic and hemodynamic control. Although a dose of 80 to 960 mg/day has been used in the past, it is clear that the higher doses are rarely necessary and may be associated with a greater incidence of torsade de pointes, heart failure, or severe bradycardia. Monitoring of electrolyte disturbances during sotalol therapy is imperative, and the drug is best avoided in patients who need significant concomitant diuretic therapy.

CONCLUSIONS

The recent focus on sotalol as a broad-spectrum antiarrhythmic compound for the control of supraventricular and ventricular arrhythmias appears justified. Expanding evidence indicates that sotalol is a unique antiarrhythmic agent combining potent nonselective β-blocking properties and a propensity to increase the action potential duration. The negative inotropic effect caused by β-blockade is attenuated but not abolished by its action potential lengthening effect. The drug's pharmacokinetics are simple with an elimination half-life of 10 to 15 hours. Sotalol prevents inducible VT/VF in approximately 30% of patients with a higher figure for the suppression of spontaneously occurring arrhythmias documented on Holter recordings. Therapy in VT/VF can be guided by either

technique, although the possibility is not excluded that empiric therapy might be equally valid. Studies involving a placebo comparison in patients with ICDs will be necessary to validate such an approach. Sotalol exerts a potent antifibrillatory action modulated by its antiadrenergic effects. The compound therefore exerts broad spectrum antiarrhythmic actions in supraventricular and ventricular arrhythmias. Sotalol is superior to class I agents, especially in VT/VF and in survivors of cardiac arrest, but the antiarrhythmic efficacy of sotalol compared with that of amiodarone is not known. In recent years, sotalol has emerged as a major antifibrillatory compound for the control of life-threatening ventricular arrhythmias as the main indication, but it may also have a significant role in maintaining the stability of sinus rhythm in patients with atrial fibrillation and flutter after electrical conversion.

Acknowledgments

I am indebted to Diane Gertschen for help in the preparation of this chapter. In writing it I have relied somewhat on the material that appears in a chapter that is jointly authored by myself and Michael Antonaccio on a similar subject and published in Cardiovascular Pharmacology & Therapeutics *edited by B.N. Singh, V.J. Dzau, P.M. Vanhoutte, and R.L. Woosley and published by Churchill Livingstone, New York, 1994.*

REFERENCES

1. Singh BN, Vaughan Williams EM: A third class of antiarrhythmic action: Effects on atrial and ventricular intracellular potentials, and other pharmacological actions on cardiac muscle of MJ 1999 and AH 3474. Br J Pharmacol 39:675, 1970.
2. Senges J, Lengfelder W, Jauernig R, et al: Electrophysiologic testing of therapy with sotalol for sustained ventricular tachycardia. Circulation 69:577, 1984.
3. Nademanee K, Feld G, Hendrickson JA, et al: Electrophysiologic and antiarrhythmic effects of sotalol in patients with life-threatening ventricular tachyarrhythmias. Circulation 72:555, 1985.
4. Singh BN: A symposium: Controlling cardiac arrhythmias with sotalol, a broad-spectrum antiarrhythmic with beta-blocking effects and class III activity. Am J Cardiol 65:1A, 1990.
5. Singh BN, Aliot E, Lazzara R: Class III antiarrhythmic drugs: Potential impact on antiarrhythmic therapy. Eur Heart J 14(H):1, 1993.
6. The Cardiac Arrhythmia Suppression Trial (CAST) Investigators: Preliminary report: Effect of encainide and flecainide on mortality in a randomized trial of arrhythmia suppression after myocardial infarction. N Engl J Med 321:406, 1989.
7. The Cardiac Arrhythmia Suppression Trial II Investigators: Effect of the anti-arrhythmic agent moricizine on survival after myocardial infarction. N Engl J Med 327:227, 1992.
8. Yusuf S, Teo KK: Approaches to prevention of sudden death: Need for fundamental reevaluation. J Cardiovasc Electrophysiol 2:S233, 1991.
9. Ahmed R, Singh BN: Anti-arrhythmic drugs. Curr Opin Cardiol 8:10, 1993.
10. Anderson JL: Sotalol in life-threatening ventricular arrhythmias: A unique class III antiarrhythmic. Am J Cardiol 72:1A, 1993.
11. Singh BN, Singh SN: A symposium: Controlling cardiac arrhythmias by lengthening repolarization: Emerging perspectives. Am J Cardiol 72:1F, 1993.
12. Singh BN: Antiarrhythmic action of dl-sotalol in ventricular

and supraventricular arrhythmias. J Cardiovasc Pharmacol 2:590, 1992.

13. Antonaccio MJ, Gomoll AW: Sotalol: Pharmacological and anti-arrhythmic effects. Cardiovasc Drug Rev 6:239, 1988.
14. Antonaccio MJ, Gomoll AW: Pharmacology, pharmacodynamics and pharmacokinetics of sotalol. Am J Cardiol 65:12A, 1990.
15. Blinks JR: Evaluation of the cardiac effects of several β-adrenergic blocking agents. Ann NY Acad Sci 139:673, 1967.
16. Antonaccio MJ, Gomoll AW: Pharmacologic basis for the antiarrhythmic and hemodynamic effects of sotalol. Am J Cardiol 72(4):27A, 1993.
17. Strauss HC, Bigger JT Jr, Hoffman BF: Electrophysiological and β-receptor blocking effects of MJ 1999 on dog and rabbit cardiac tissue. Circ Res 26:461, 1970.
18. Hondeghem LM, Snyders DJ: Class III anti-arrhythmic agents have a lot of potential but a long way to go: Reduced effectiveness and dangers of reverse use dependence. Circulation 81:686, 1990.
19. Carmeliet E: Electrophysiologic and voltage clamp analysis of the effects of sotalol on isolated cardiac muscle and Purkinje fibers. J Pharmacol Exp Ther 232:817, 1985.
20. Gomoll AW, Bartek MJ: Comparative β-blocking activities and electrophysiologic actions of racemic sotalol and its optical isomers in anesthetized dogs. Eur Pharmacol 132:123, 1986.
21. Lathrop DA: Electromechanical characterization of the effects of racemic sotalol and its optical isomers on isolated canine ventricular trabecular muscles and Purkinje strands. Can J Physiol Pharmacol 673:1506, 1985.
22. Singh BN: Historical development of the concept of controlling cardiac arrhythmias by lengthening repolarization: Particular reference to sotalol. Am J Cardiol 65(Suppl):3A, 1990.
23. Gomoll AW, Braunwald E: Comparative effects of sotalol and propranolol on myocardial contractility. Arch Int Pharmacodyn Ther 205:3438, 1973.
24. Tande PM, Refsum H: Class III antiarrhythmic action linked with positive inotropy: Effects of the d- and l-isomer of sotalol on isolated rat atria and threshold and suprathreshold stimulation. Pharmacol Toxicol 62:272, 1988.
25. Singh BN, Nademanee K: Control of cardiac arrhythmias by selective lengthening of repolarization: Theoretical considerations and clinical observations. Am Heart J 109:421, 1985.
26. Thumala A, Hammermeister K, Campbell WB, et al: Hemodynamic studies with sotalol in man, performed at rest, during exercise, and during right ventricular pacing. Am Heart J 82:439, 1971.
27. Hutton I, Lorimer AR, Hillis WE, et al: Hemodynamics and myocardial infarction after sotalol. Br Heart J 34:787, 1972.
28. Brooks H, Banas J, Mesieter S, et al: Sotalol-induced beta-blockade in cardiac patients. Circulation 42:99, 1970.
29. Frankl WS, Soloff LA: Sotalol: A new safe adrenergic receptor blocking agent. Am J Cardiol 22:266, 1968.
30. Mahmarian JJ, Verani MS, Hohman T, et al: The hemodynamic effects of sotalol and quinidine: Analysis of the use of rest and exercise gated radionuclide angiography. Circulation 76:324, 1987.
31. Ritschel WA: Compilation of pharmacokinetic parameters of beta-adrenergic blocking agents. Drug Intell Clin Phamacol 14:746, 1980.
32. Sundquist H: Basic review of beta-blocker pharmacokinetics. Curr Ther Res 28(Suppl):38S, 1980.
33. Poirier JM, Jallon P, Lecocq V, et al: The pharmacokinetics of d-sotalol and dl-sotalol in healthy volunteers. Eur J Clin Pharmacol 19:557, 1990.
34. Lynch JL, Wilber DJ, Montgomery DG, et al: Antiarrhythmic and antifibrillatory actions of the levo- and dextrorotatory isomers of sotalol. J Cardiovasc Pharmacol 6:1132, 1984.
35. Patterson E, Lynch JL, Lucchesi BR: Antiarrhythmic and anti-fibrillatory actions of the beta-adrenergic antagonist, dl-sotalol. J Pharmacol Exp Ther 230:519, 1984.
36. Lynch JL, Coskey LA, Montgomery DG, et al: Prevention of ventricular fibrillation by dextrorotatory sotalol in a conscious canine model of sudden coronary death. Am Heart J 109:949, 1985.
37. Lucchesi B, Lynch JJ: Preclinical studies on the antifibrillatory effects of sotalol and its optical isomers. *In* Singh B (ed): Control

of Cardiac Arrhythmias by Lengthening Repolarization. Mount Kisco, NY: Futura Publishing, 1988, p 245.
38. Feld GK, Venkatesh N, Singh BN: Pharmacologic conversion and suppression of experimental and canine atrial flutter: Differing effects of d-sotalol, quinidine, and lidocaine and significance of changes in refractoriness and conduction. Circulation 74:197, 1986.
39. Spinelli W, Hoffman BF: Mechanisms of termination of reentrant atrial arrhythmias by Class I and Class III antiarrhythmic agents. Circ Res 65:1565, 1989.
40. Bertrix L, Timour-Chah Q, Lang J, et al: Protection against ventricular and atrial fibrillation by sotalol. Cardiovasc Res 20:358, 1986.
41. Teo KK, Harte M, Horgan JH: Sotalol infusion in the treatment of supraventricular tachyarrhythmias. Chest 87:113, 1985.
42. Camm AJ, Paul V: Sotalol for paroxysmal supraventricular tachycardias. Am J Cardiol 100:921, 1990.
43. Brugada P, Smeets JLRM, Brugada J, et al: Mechanism of action in supraventricular arrhythmias. Cardiovasc Drugs Ther 4:619, 1990.
44. Antman EM, Beamer AD, Cantillon C, et al: Therapy of refractory symptomatic atrial fibrillation and flutter: A staged care approach with new antiarrhythmic drugs. J Am Coll Cardiol 15:698, 1990.
45. Juul-Möller S, Edvardsson N, Rehnqvist-Ahlberg NR: Sotalol versus quinidine for the maintenance of sinus rhythm after direct current conversion of atrial fibrillation. Circulation 82:1932, 1990.
46. Coplen SE, Antman EM, Berlin JA, et al: Efficacy and safety of quinidine therapy for maintenance of sinus rhythm after cardioversion: A meta-analysis of randomized control trials. Circulation 82:1108, 1990.
47. Manz M, Kuhl AJ, Luderitz B: Sotalol dei supraventricularer tachycardie elektrophysiologische Messungen bein Wolff-Parkinson-White Syndrom und AV-Knotenreentrytachykardie. Kardiologie 74:500, 1985.
48. Millar RN: Efficacy of sotalol in controlling reentrant supraventricular tachycardias. Cardiovasc Drugs Ther 4:625, 1990.
49. Vecht RJ, Nicholaides EP, Ikweuke JK, et al: Incidence and prevention of supraventricular tachyarrhythmias early after coronary artery bypass surgery. Int J Cardiol 13:125, 1986.
50. Andrews RC, Reinold SC, Berlin KA, Antman EM: Prevention of supraventricular arrhythmias after coronary artery bypass surgery: A meta-analysis of randomized control clinical trials. Circulation 84(III):236, 1991.
51. Suttorp MJ, Kingma JH, Tjon Joe Gin RM, et al: Efficacy and safety of low- and high-dose sotalol versus propranolol in the prevention of supraventricular tachyarrhythmias early after coronary artery bypass operations. J Thorac Cardiovasc Surg 100:921, 1990.
52. Suttorp MJ, Kingma JH, Peels HO, Koomen EM: Effectiveness of sotalol in preventing supraventricular tachyarrhythmias shortly after coronary artery bypass grafting. Am J Cardiol 68:1163, 1991.
53. Anderson JL: Effectiveness of sotalol for therapy of complex ventricular arrhythmias and comparisons with placebo and Class I antiarrhythmic drugs. Am J Cardiol 65:37A, 1990.
54. Lidell C, Rehnqvist N, Sjogren A, et al: Comparative efficacy of oral sotalol and procainamide in patients with chronic ventricular arrhythmias: A multicenter study. Am Heart J 109:970, 1985.
55. Deedwania PK: Suppressant effects of conventional beta-blockers and sotalol on complex and repetitive ventricular premature complexes. Am J Cardiol 65:43A, 1990.
56. Kjekshus J: Importance of heart rate determining beta-blocker efficacy in acute and longterm myocardial infarction interventional trials. Am J Cardiol 57:43F, 1986.
57. Julian DG, Jackson FS, Prescott RJ, et al: Control trial of sotalol for one year after myocardial infarction. Lancet 1:1142, 1982.
58. Spielman SR, Kay HR, Morganroth J, et al: Drug therapy in high risk patients following acute myocardial infarction: The results of the timolol, encainide and sotalol trial. Circulation 72(Suppl III):15, 1985.
59. Gonzalez R, Scheinman MM, Herre JM, et al: Usefulness of sotalol for drug-refractory malignant ventricular arrhythmias. J Am Coll Cardiol 13:1435, 1988.

60. Singh S: Sotalol for refractory sustained ventricular tachycardia and non-fatal cardiac arrest. Am J Cardiol 62:399, 1988.
61. Steinbeck G, Bach P, Haberi R: Electrophysiologic and antirrhythmic efficacy of oral sotalol for sustained ventricular tachyarrhythmias: Evaluation by programmed stimulation and ambulatory electrocardiogram. J Am Coll Cardiol 8:949, 1986.
62. Ruder MA, Ellis T, Lebsack C, et al: Clinical experience with sotalol in patients with drug-refractory ventricular arrhythmias. J Am Coll Cardiol 13:145, 1989.
63. Kienzle MG, Martin JB, Wendt DJ, et al: Enhanced efficacy of oral sotalol for sustained ventricular tachycardia refractory to type I antiarrhythmic drugs. Am J Cardiol 61:1012, 1988.
64. Singh BN, Kehoe R, Woosley RL, et al: Multicenter trial of sotalol compared with procainamide in the suppression of ventricular tachycardia induced by programmed electrical stimulation: A double-blind randomized study, parallel evaluation. Am Heart J 129:87, 1995.
65. Kus T, Campa MA, Nadeau R, et al: Efficacy and electrophysiologic effects of oral sotalol in patients with sustained ventricular tachycardia caused by coronary artery disease. Am Heart J 123:82, 1992.
66. Jordaens LJ, Palmer A, Clement DL: Low-dose oral sotalol for monomorphic ventricular tachycardia: Effects during programmed electrical stimulation and follow-up. Eur Heart J 10:218, 1989.
67. Kuchar DL, Garan H, Vendittie FJ, et al: Usefulness of sotalol in suppressing ventricular tachycardia or ventricular fibrillation in patients with healed myocardial infarcts. Am J Cardiol 64:33, 1989.
68. Ruffy R: Sotalol. J Cardiovasc Electrophysiol 4:81, 1993.
69. Kopelman HA, Woosley RL, Lee JT, et al: Electrophysiologic effects of intravenous and oral sotalol for sustained ventricular tachycardia secondary to coronary artery disease. Am J Cardiol 61:1006, 1988.
70. Klein RC and the ESVEM Investigators: Comparative efficacy of sotalol and Class I anti-arrhythmic agents in patients with ventricular tachycardia and fibrillation: Results of the electrophysiology study versus electrocardiographic monitoring (ESVEM) trial. Eur Heart J 14(Suppl H):78, 1993.
71. Singh SN, Cohen A, Chen Y, et al: Sotalol for refractory sustained ventricular tachycardia and nonfatal cardiac arrest. Am J Cardiol 62:399, 1988.
72. Mason JW and the ESVEM Investigators: A comparison of seven antiarrhythmic drugs in patients with ventricular tachyarrhythmias. N Engl J Med 329:452, 1993.
73. Marchlinski FE, Buxton AE, Vassalle JA, et al: Comparative electrophysiologic effects of intravenous and oral procainamide in patients with sustained ventricular arrhythmias. J Am Coll Cardiol 4:1247, 1984.
74. Singh BN, Deedwania P, Nademanee K, et al: Sotalol: A review of its pharmacodynamic and pharmacokinetic properties, and therapeutic use. Drugs 34:311, 1987.
75. Manz M, Steinbeck G, Nitsch J, et al: Treatment of recurrent sustained ventricular tachycardia with mexiletine and disopyramide. Br Heart J 49:222, 1983.
76. Horowitz LN: Encainide in lethal ventricular arrhythmias evaluated by electrophysiologic testing and decrease in symptoms. Am J Cardiol 58:83C, 1986.
77. Flecainide Ventricular Tachycardia Study Group: Treatment of resistant ventricular tachycardia with flecainide acetate. Am J Cardiol 57:1299, 1986.
78. Chilson DA, Heger JJ, Zipes DP, et al: Electrophysiologic effects and clinical efficacy of oral propafenone therapy in patients with ventricular tachycardia. J Am Coll Cardiol 5:1407, 1985.
79. Mason JW and the ESVEM Investigators: A randomized comparison of electrophysiologic study and electrocardiographic monitoring for prediction of antiarrhythmic drug efficacy in patients with ventricular tachyarrhythmias. N Engl J Med 329:445, 1993.
80. Singh BN: Choice and chance in drug therapy of cardiac arrhythmias: Technique versus drug-specific responses in evaluation of efficacy. Am J Cardiol 72:114F, 1993.
81. Steinbeck G, Andersen D, Bach P, et al: A comparison of electrophysiologically-guided antiarrhythmic therapy with betablocker in patients with symptomatic sustained ventricular tachyarrhythmias. N Engl J Med 327:987, 1992.
82. Kehoe RF, McNeil DJ, Zheutlin TA, et al: Safety and efficacy of oral sotalol for sustained ventricular tachyarrhythmias refractory to other antiarrhythmic agents. Am J Cardiol 72:56A, 1993.
83. Nora M, Zipes DP: Empiric use of amiodarone and sotalol. Am J Cardiol 72:62F, 1993.
84. Amiodarone vs. Sotalol Study Group: Multi-centre randomized trial of sotalol versus amiodarone for chronic ventricular tachyarrhythmias. Eur Heart J 1:685, 1989.
85. Singh BN: When is QT prolongation anti-arrhythmic and when is it pro-arrhythmic? Am J Cardiol 63:867, 1989.
86. Elonen E, Neuvonen PH, Tarssanen L, et al: Sotalol intoxication with prolonged QT interval and severe tachyarrhythmias. Br J Med 1:1184, 1979.
87. Kontopoulos A, Filindris A, Manoudis F, et al: Sotalol induced torsade de pointes. Postgrad Med 57:321, 1981.
88. Krapf R, Gertsch M: Torsade de pointes induced by sotalol despite therapeutic concentrations. Br Med J 290:1784, 1985.
89. Laakso M, Pentikainen PH, Lampainen E: Sotalol, prolonged Q-T interval, and ventricular tachyarrhythmias. Ann Clin Res 13:439, 1981.
90. Laakso M, Pentikainen PH, Pyrola K, Neuvonen PJ: Prolongation of the Q-T interval caused by sotalol—possible association with ventricular tachyarrhythmias. Eur Heart J 2:355, 1981.
91. Laakso M, Pentikainen PJ, Pyorala K: Sotalol and QTc interval. Lancet 2:1168, 1981.
92. McKibbin JK, Pocock WA, Barlow JB, et al: Sotalol hypokalemia, syncope and torsade de pointes. Br Heart J 51:157, 1984.
93. Neuvonen PJ, Elonen E, Vuorenmass T, Laakso M: Prolonged QT interval and severe tachyarrhythmia, common features of sotalol intoxication. Eur J Clin Pharmacol 20(2):85, 1981.
94. Neuvonen PH, Elonen E, Tanskanen A, et al: Sotalol prolongation of the QTc interval in hypertensive patients. Clin Pharmacol Ther 7:25, 1982.
95. Benton P, Sheriden J, Mulcahy R: A case of sotalol poisoning. Ir J Med Sci 151:126, 1982.
96. Montagna M, Groppi A: Fatal sotalol poisoning. Arch Toxicol 43:221, 1980.
97. Kehoe R, Zheutlin T, Dunnington C, et al: Safety and efficacy of sotalol in patients with drug-refractory sustained ventricular tachyarrhythmias. Am J Cardiol 65:58A, 1990.
98. Soyka LF, Wirz C, Spangenburg RB: Clinical safety profile of sotalol in patients with arrhythmias. Am J Cardiol 65:74A, 1990.

d-Sotalol

Bramah N. Singh, M.D., Ph.D.

In recent years, sotalol hydrochloride has emerged as an important antifibrillatory agent that combines the dual properties of blocking β-adrenoceptors and of prolonging the duration of the cardiac action potential.[1-5] Sotalol is a racemic mixture of dextro- and levo-isomers, which have an identical potency for lengthening the action potential duration (APD) but have a large difference in their β-blocking propensities.[6] The separation of the two isomers as pure chemical entities has therefore provided the opportunity for determining the relative importance of β-blocking activity versus that of prolonged APD in the control of cardiac arrhythmias. The rationale for the development of d-sotalol as a therapeutic agent for arrhythmic control stems from its reduced β-blocking actions. For this reason, d-sotalol is likely to induce fewer β-blocker-related side effects, with a lower incidence of bronchospasm, and a lower induction of heart failure and torsade de pointes because of a lower bradycardiac effect.

Numerous experimental studies have shown that racemic sotalol and the l-isomer are 10 to 12 and 14 to 50 times more potent, respectively, on a milligram basis than d-sotalol in antagonizing isoprenaline-induced relaxation of smooth muscle in the trachea.[7] In isolated mammalian atria, sotalol has been reported to be 32 to 40 times and dl-sotalol 11 times more potent than the d-isomer as a β-antagonist.[8] In intact animals, dl-sotalol appears to be 10 to 15 times as potent as d-sotalol in antagonizing heart rate increases induced by isoprenaline.[7] These differences are also found in humans.

ELECTROPHYSIOLOGIC ACTIONS
In Isolated Tissue Preparations

The major electrophysiologic effect of d-sotalol and the racemate is to prolong the duration of the action potential and the corresponding effective refractory period,[6, 9, 10] a property that is unrelated to β-blockade. For example, Kato et al.[6] found that equimolar concentrations of d- and l-isomers exerted an identical effect on the duration of the action potential in canine ventricular muscle or Purkinje fibers. Similar observations were made by Campbell,[11] who found no evidence for block in sodium-channel activity. Concentrations of 1 to 50 μM d- and dl-sotalol greatly increased the APD in isolated preparations of guinea pig and human (biopsy specimen) atria. Campbell[11] also determined the time course of repolarization in guinea-pig sinus nodes; he found that d-sotalol, in concentrations that had no effect on the slope of phase 4 depolarization, prolonged the APD to the extent

that it significantly increased the sinus cycle length (Fig. 150–1). The data suggested that d-sotalol had the ability to reduce sinus frequency without affecting phase 4 depolarization, i.e., without the mediation of an antiadrenergic effect. These data may account for the observation that d-sotalol reduces heart rate more than might be expected from its weak β-blocking actions. As in the case of the racemate, d-sotalol does not exhibit a significant effect on the resting membrane potential nor on the maximal rate of depolarization.[9, 11] As in the case of dl-sotalol, the effect of the d-isomer on the APD is frequency-dependent with the effect becoming progressively attenuated at high rate stimulation ("reversed" or use dependency).[12] Carmeliet[13] showed that both d- and dl-sotalol decreased I_K in a concentration-related manner, the IC_{50} being obtained at 10^{-5} M and total inhibition at 10^{-4} M, a concentration range consistent with the ability of sotalol to prolong APD. Neither d- nor dl-sotalol changed activation kinetics, and the effect on the APD

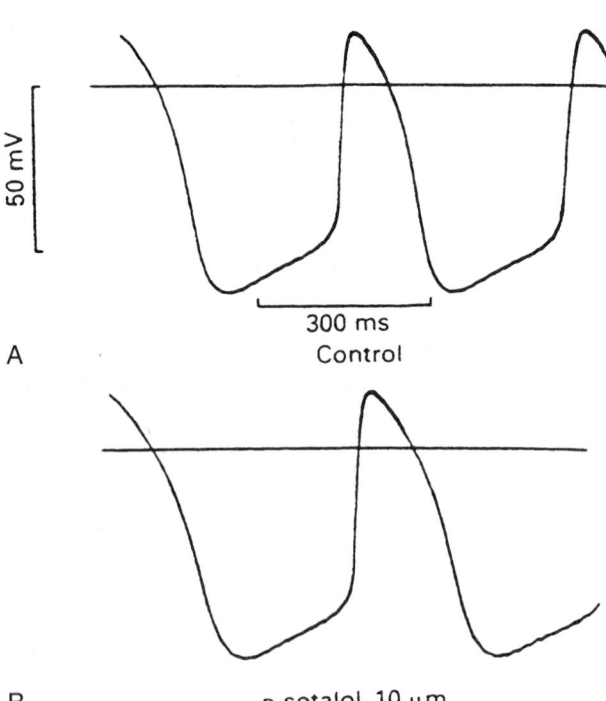

Figure 150–1. Action potentials recorded from the same guinea pig sinoatrial node cell before *(A)* and 30 minutes after *(B)* exposure to d-sotalol, 10 μM. The spontaneous cycle length is prolonged, and this effect is almost entirely a result of the slowing of repolarization. Thus, the slowing of sinus frequency by d-sotalol is largely independent of β-blockade. (From Campbell TH: Cellular electrophysiological effects of d- and dl-sotalol in guinea-pig sinoatrial node atrium and ventricle and human atrium: Differential tissue sensitivity. Br J Pharmacol 90:593, 1987.)

was related to β-adrenoreceptor antagonism; it was not entirely accounted for by a reduction in the number of conducting I_K channels, single-channel conductance, or the mean open time. It is known that the I_K results from the activation of two separate outward K^+ currents, namely, a very rapid current, I_{Kr}, and a slowly activating current I_{KS}.[14] Class III antiarrhythmic agents, including d-sotalol, inactivate I_{Kr} but not I_{KS}.[14] Both d- and dl-sotalol, especially at high concentrations, may also inhibit the background or inward rectifying K^+ current (I_{KI}).

In Human Subjects *In Vivo*

The effects in conscious animals and in human subjects are similar for d- and dl-sotalol except for the influence on those variables that are affected by adrenergic stimulation. These are not altered by d-sotalol. For example, d-sotalol has little or no effect on atrioventricular nodal refractoriness or conduction, but both agents increase the defibrillation threshold and increase the ventricular fibrillation threshold. The effects of d- and dl-sotalol on prolonging the QT and QT_c intervals are equivalent; neither affects the QRS or PR intervals.[15, 16] Both compounds exert a similar effect on the effective refractory period in the atria, ventricles, bypass tracts, and His-Purkinje systems.[17] These effects on the refractory period result from prolongation of the APD in these tissues. In human subjects, the overall effects[18-20] are evident during infusions of d-sotalol (1 to 2 mg/kg) or dl-sotalol (1 mg/kg). Furthermore, RR intervals were more potently lengthened by dl-sotalol compared with d-sotalol, consistent with the data from experimental animals. d-Sotalol does, however, produce a modest reduction in heart rate, an effect that is in part a result of the prolongation of the APD in the sinus node.

The effects of d- and dl-sotalol on the APD have been confirmed in humans by monophasic action potential recordings in the ventricle.[19, 20] Huikuri[21] recently reported on the effects of intravenous d-sotalol (2 mg/kg) on the frequency-dependent effects on the APD in the human ventricle obtained by monophasic action potential recordings. They compared the effects of chronic amiodarone administration in a similar subset of patients. As might be expected from observations in animal models, d-sotalol demonstrated a significant reverse use-dependent effect on the human ventricular APD (Fig. 150-2A), whereas amiodarone had an equal effect in prolonging the ventricular APD at fast and slow heart rates (Fig. 150-2B).

The overall electrophysiologic properties of d-sotalol are identical to those of dl-sotalol except for the additional properties that the racemate has by virtue of its β-blocking activity. d-Sotalol might therefore function as a pure class III agent.[17] In Table 150-1, the electrophysiologic effects of prototypical and newer class III agents relative to their potential antiarrhythmic and proarrhythmic actions are summarized. It therefore appears reasonable to examine the potential antiarrhythmic and proarrhythmic actions of d-sotalol within the framework of the known electropharmaco-

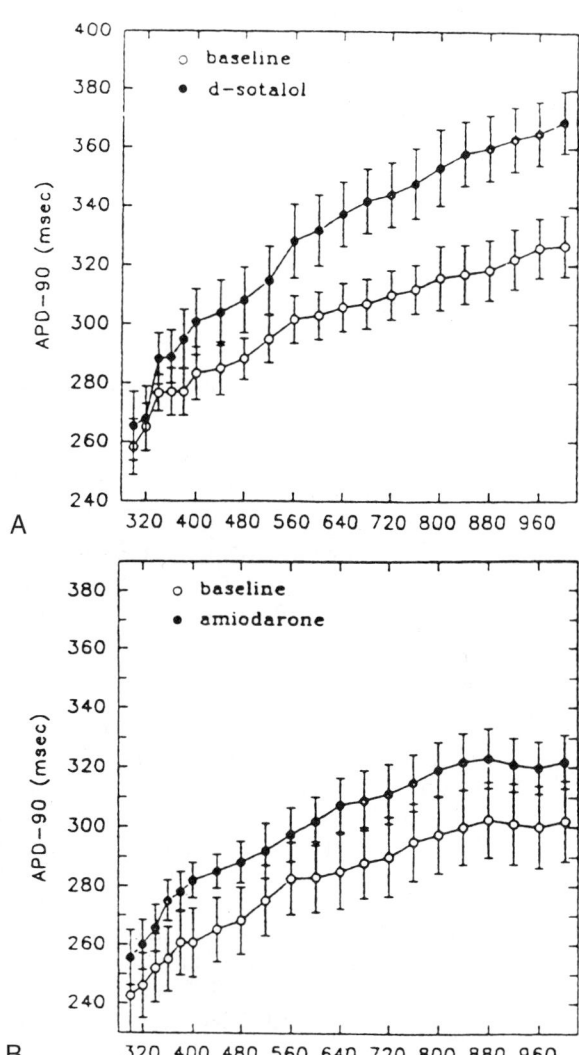

Figure 150–2. Effects of intravenous d-sotalol *(A)* and chronic oral amiodarone *(B)* treatment on the action potential restitution curve. APD, action potential duration at 90% repolarization. The data shown are means ± SEMs from patients in whom monophasic action potential recordings were obtained before and after drug treatment. (From Huikuri HV, Yli-Mäyry S: Frequency-dependent effects of d-sotalol and amiodarone on the action potential duration of the human right ventricle. PACE Pacing Clin Electrophysiol 15(11 Pt 2):2103, 1992.)

logic and clinical effects of dl-sotalol, amiodarone, and the pure class III agents. Since the antiarrhythmic and proarrhythmic actions of these compounds can be placed in perspective only in relation to their effects on ventricular function, their inotropic and hemodynamic properties are clearly important. These aspects of d-sotalol will therefore be examined before discussing its potential therapeutic utility as an antiarrhythmic compound.

INOTROPIC AND HEMODYNAMIC EFFECTS

The inotropic and hemodynamic effects of d-sotalol are of much interest in light of the link between

Table 150–1. **Electrophysiologic Effects of Prototypical and Newer Class-III Agents**

Parameter	dl-Sotalol	Amiodarone	d-Sotalol	New Class-III Agents
Bradycardia	+ + + +	+ + +	+	+
PR interval	↑ + +	↑ + +	0	0
AH	↑ + +	↑ + +	0	0
QT	↑ + + +	↑ + + + +	↑ + + +	↑ + + +
HV interval	0	↑ + +	0	0
QRS	±	+	±	±
AERP	↑ + + +	↑ + + + +	↑ + + +	↑ + + +
AV nodal ERP	↑ + + +	↑ + + +	0	0
VERP	↑ + + +	↑ + + + +	↑ + + +	↑ + + +
Bypass tract ERP	↑ + + +	↑ + + + +	↑ + + +	↑ + + +
Reverse use-dependency	Present	Absent	Present	Present
Suppression of PVCs	60%	80%–90%	?	?
Inducibility of VT/VF	30% or higher	8%–10%	30% or higher	20%–30%
Torsade de pointes	3%–5%	<1%	1.5%	? 3%–8%

APD and tension development in cardiac muscle.[22–24] Prolongation of the APD is associated with a positive inotropic effect,[22] demonstrated most consistently in isolated cardiac muscle.[23] In the case of dl-sotalol, changes in the indices of contractility are modulated by the associated β-blocking properties of the drug.[9] On the other hand, d-sotalol is likely to function more as a "pure" class II agent with minimal β-blocking activity. It might be expected to exert little or no negative inotropic effect. There are limited clinical data, but a number of experimental studies indicate that d-sotalol may have a modest positive inotropic effect, rarely producing a negative inotropic effect.[9, 17]

Tande and Refsum[23] studied the effects of d- and l-isomers of sotalol on refractoriness and inotropy in isolated rat atria over a wide range of drug concentrations. They found the two isomers had similar effects on refractoriness. However, the d-isomer *increased* isometric contractile force by 10%, whereas the l-isomer had no effect when the atria were stimulated at threshold values. Mortensen et al.[24] found that after β-blockade d-sotalol in anesthetized dogs exerted cardiodepressant effects in doses that produced significant prolongation of the QT_c interval. The same authors[25] found that in dogs with acute ischemic heart failure d-sotalol was devoid of cardiodepressant effects. In contrast, Hoffmeister et al.[26] reported that d-sotalol may produce a variable spectrum of negative inotropic effect in ischemic and nonischemic animal models especially at high doses of the drug. They suggested that at the higher dose range, d-sotalol may exert a significant β-blocking action which may outweigh the potential positive inotropic effects of the drug resulting from its class III actions. Clearly, clinical data in patients with varying levels of ventricular function will be necessary to define the precise hemodynamic profile of d-sotalol. It is, however, reasonable to assume that the d-isomer is likely to produce less depressant effects than the l-isomer or the racemate. Preliminary data in human subjects with low ejection fractions are in line with these considerations,[27] and the drug was found to be hemodynamically tolerated in a small group of patients when it was given as an infusion (1.5 to 2.75 mg/kg) in the course of electrophysiologic studies for supraventricular tachyarrhythmias.

PHARMACOKINETICS

The pharmacokinetic profile of d-sotalol is similar to that of the racemate,[28] which has been discussed at length in this volume. Data that deal specifically with the pharmacokinetics of d-sotalol are still limited. Poirier et al.[29] investigated the pharmacokinetic features of d-sotalol in six healthy volunteers given single intravenous doses of 0.25, 0.50, 1, and 2 mg/kg and one 100-mg oral dose in comparison with the kinetics of 1 mg/kg IV dl-sotalol. They found no significant differences in the disposition of d- and dl-sotalol. The elimination half-life was 7.2 hours and the kinetics were linear. The renal clearance of d-sotalol was 56% to 77% of total clearance, and the absolute bioavailability of the drug was nearly 100% with an elimination half-life of 7.5 hours. There was no first-pass effect. It is reasonable to assume that the overall pharmacokinetic profile of the d-isomer is similar to that of dl-sotalol and that the drug is not metabolized nor is it protein bound. As in the case of dl-sotalol, the dose of d-sotalol requires adjustment in accordance with renal function. However, the precise range of clinical doses relevant to the control of cardiac arrhythmias remains to be defined.

ANTIARRHYTHMIC EFFECTS

The potential clinical utility of d-sotalol as an antiarrhythmic compound needs to be placed within a perspective that allows for the overall shift away from the use of class I agents in controlling supraventricular and ventricular arrhythmias in patients with significant structural heart disease.[30–38] Such a trend has stemmed from the outcome of the CAST Trials,[30, 31] the growing evidence of the deleterious effects of class I agents as suggested from meta-analysis of randomized clinical trials of patients after myocardial infarction,[32] and from recent controls comparing sotalol and amiodarone to guided therapy with class I agents.[36–38] These lines of evidence have favored the increasing use of β-blockers, amiodarone, and dl-sota-lol in the treatment of patients at high risk for sudden death.[38]

The spectrum of dl-sotalol effects in arrhythmias is wider than that of conventional β-blockers;[17] the effects of d-sotalol are poorly defined but are under intensive investigation. Preliminary data will be discussed to draw some tentative conclusions about the potential role of the drug in controlling supraventricular and ventricular arrhythmias. To what extent the β-blocking actions of dl-sotalol contribute to its net antiarrhythmic actions relative to the drug's class III properties may indicate the overall spectrum of action of d-sotalol. To date, no direct controlled comparisons between d- and dl-sotalol in human subjects have been reported. In recent years, there has been a major change in the role of drug therapy of cardiac arrhythmias,[30-38] and further changes are imminent. The focus is on newer class III agents for two major indications: (1) atrial fibrillation and flutter for acute conversion and maintenance of sinus rhythm, and (2) the prophylactic treatment of ventricular tachycardia and ventricular fibrillation (VT/VF). They may also be used as treatment for recurrence of sudden arrhythmia with the ultimate aim of reducing arrhythmia and total mortality. The overall utility of d-sotalol or other newer class III agents needs to be examined within this framework.

SUPRAVENTRICULAR ARRHYTHMIAS

As a result of the introduction of adenosine, verapamil, and diltiazem for acute conversions and of catheter ablation of paroxysmal supraventricular tachycardias (PSVTs) and certain cases of atrial flutter, the role of drug therapy for the acute conversion and the maintenance of sinus rhythm in patients with various supraventricular tachyarrhythmias is undergoing a major change. Thus, reorientation is necessary. The potential role of d-sotalol is in conversion of atrial flutter and fibrillation and the maintenance of sinus rhythm long-term.

The rationale for the effectiveness of d-sotalol for converting atrial flutter and fibrillation to sinus rhythm and maintaining its stability is somewhat compelling. Using a canine model of atrial flutter and quinidine, d-sotalol, and lidocaine, Feld et al.[39] found that d-sotalol was significantly more effective than quinidine or lidocaine (which was virtually ineffective) in terminating inducible atrial flutter or in preventing its reinducibility. d-Sotalol restored sinus rhythm in 14 of 15 (93%) dogs with atrial flutter (induced by an intercaval crush and rapid atrial pacing), whereas quinidine was effective in 9 of 15 (60%), and lidocaine in 2 of 10 (20%). d-Sotalol also prevented flutter reinduction in 8 of 15 (53%), whereas quinidine was effective in 4 of 15 (27%) and lidocaine in none. Prolongation of atrial refractoriness was the crucial determinant of both conversion and prevention of reinduction of atrial flutter.

In another dog model of atrial flutter,[40] several class I agents (disopyramide, flecainide, propafenone) were very effective in terminating the arrhythmia, as was d-sotalol. However, the class I agents acted by markedly increasing cycle length, whereas d-sotalol prolonged refractoriness.[40] Of particular interest are some observations on dl-sotalol, the electrophysiologic effects of which in the atria are likely to be similar to those of d-sotalol. Bertrix et al.[41] measured the fibrillation threshold in canine ventricles and atria concurrently with the amplitude and duration of the monophasic action potential, effective refractory period, the conduction time in the contractile fibers, and the fibrillation rate once fibrillation had been triggered. Sotalol increased the fibrillation threshold in association with an increase in the duration of the action potential and the effective refractory period. The fibrillation rate slowed but conduction time did not change. In atria in which vulnerability to fibrillation had been enhanced by acetylcholine (presumably by reversing the cholinergically mediated shortening of the APD and refractoriness, the overall changes were more striking than in the ventricles. Sotalol antagonized the changes induced by acetylcholine. The data for d-sotalol are likely to be similar but clinical experience is limited. The difference between the effects of the d-isomer and those of the racemate, however, can be found in cases of persisting atrial fibrillation and flutter. In these cases the d-sotalol will be less effective than the dl-sotalol in controlling the ventricular response.

VENTRICULAR ARRHYTHMIAS

There is now much experimental evidence substantiating the antiarrhythmic potential of d-sotalol. As with dl-sotalol, d-sotalol decreases the defibrillation energy requirements in dogs anesthetized with pentobarbital, enflurane, and pentanyl.[42] Such an action is associated with an increase in the ventricular effective refractory period and in the ventricular fibrillation threshold. As also might be expected, d-sotalol, like the racemate, exerts similar beneficial action in experimental ischemia models produced by acute or chronic coronary artery ligation.[43] For example, dl-sotalol and d-sotalol have been found to be highly effective in preventing the induction of reentrant ventricular tachyarrhythmias in the Lucchesi canine infarct-ischemia model in which a variety of agents have been compared. However, enough clinical data to permit conclusions regarding the ultimate role of the d-isomer in the control of ventricular tachycardia and fibrillation are not yet available.

One of the earliest clinical studies of the treatment of VT/VF with d-sotalol was that of Schwartz et al.[27] They performed programmed electrical stimulation (PES) in 28 men and 10 women, mean age 67 years and a mean ejection fraction of 37%. All had inducible VT/VF. d-Sotalol (2 mg/kg given as an infusion over 15 minutes) did not affect the QRS or PR intervals but the RR interval was increased. d-Sotalol prevented reinduction of VT/VF in 18 of 38 (47%) patients; 17 patients were tested with procainamide and only four responded. d-Sotalol prevented reinduction in 7 of these 17 patients. Eleven responders on d-sotalol were discharged home taking oral d-sotalol (100 to 400 mg b.i.d.). One patient died after acute myocardial infarction one month after discharge from the hospital and another patient had cardiac arrest but survived. He was given amiodarone. The nine patients who continued on d-sotalol had remained well at a mean follow-up of 14 months. The authors concluded that d-sotalol is an effective, well-tolerated antiarrhythmic drug.

The most extensive experience with d-sotalol in the treatment of VT/VF has been reported by Brachmann et al.[44, 45] In 84 patients with a history of sustained VT/VF, Brachmann et al.[44, 45] evaluated the effectiveness of d-sotalol by PES before and after intravenous administration of 1.5 to 2.5 mg/kg d-sotalol. An additional 29 patients were tested in a similar manner after the oral administration of 400 to 600 mg/day d-sotalol. Effectiveness was defined as the suppression of inducible VT/VF. After intravenous d-sotalol, in 38% the inducible VT/VF became noninducible after a mean of 4.3 other drugs had proved ineffective. A 82.5% effectiveness for suppression (33 of 40) was found in those in whom oral d-sotalol was given before reassessment. During 12 months of follow-up, only 16% of those in whom the arrhythmias were suppressed after the drug had a recurrence of the arrhythmia, whereas 43% of those in whom the arrhythmia was not suppressed had a recurrence. This difference was statistically significant ($p < .05$). There was one case of torsade de pointes. The estimated survival rate of successfully treated patients was 95% after 1 year and 88% after 2 years of continuous therapy. Only 5 of 56 patients taking d-sotalol had to discontinue therapy because of adverse drug reactions. The authors concluded that the effectiveness of d-sotalol is comparable with that reported for dl-sotalol, which, in the ESVEM study,[37] was found to be superior to six class I agents. A number of studies are in progress in this subset of patients. It should be emphasized that the PES data reviewed herein need to be interpreted in the light of the fact that, like all previous studies with other antiarrhythmic agents, including dl-sotalol, there have been no concomitant control subjects and the comparison has always been between responders and nonresponders. Thus, it is not completely clear whether there is an impact on mortality in absolute terms. To demonstrate this, a prospective study should be done in which the test drug is compared with placebo in patients with implanted intracardiac defibrillators (ICDs) in both treatment limbs. Such trials with d-sotalol are ongoing.

It should also be stressed that the effects of d-sotalol in high-risk postinfarct patients remain uncertain, but a double-blind, placebo-controlled study—Survival with Oral D-Sotalol (SWORD)—involving high-risk patients after myocardial infarction was recently prematurely terminated.[46] This study was designed to enroll 6400 patients to test the hypothesis that d-sotalol would reduce total mortality in patients older than 18 years of age with a left ventricular ejection fraction less than 40%; two subsets of patients were enrolled into the study. In the first were patients who had sustained myocardial infarction within 42 days of the acute event, and in the second subset were those who had incurred myocardial infarction after 42 days at the time of entry into the study. The latter group were required to have had a documented history of cardiac failure (New York Heart Association class II or III). Patients satisfying the entry criteria were randomized to placebo or to d-sotalol 100 mg b.i.d., which was increased to 200 mg b.i.d. if tolerated. The trial was stopped (because the boundary for harm was crossed) when 3119 patients had been enrolled (mean follow-up about 156 days). It was noteworthy that 42 (2.7%) died in the placebo group and 71 (4.6%) died in the group given d-sotalol ($p = .005$). There were no significant differences between the two groups in any of the baseline characteristics, the mean left ventricular ejection fractions for both groups being approximately 30%; 29.2% of the patients enrolled into the study had recent myocardial infarction, and 70.8% had remote infarcts. It was also of note that the trend for mortality for both groups was similar for the remote as well as those with recent infarcts, with an increasing divergence of the survival curves as a function of time.

CONCLUSIONS

Whether the clinical properties and the overall utility of d-sotalol approximate those of "pure" class III agents or those of dl-sotalol will require further studies in various subsets of patients with cardiac arrhythmias. However, theoretical considerations permit certain tentative conclusions. For example, the drug exerts minimal β-blocking activity and exhibits little or no negative inotropic actions. Thus, it is likely to be safer in patients with congestive heart failure dependent on sympathetic stimulation for compensation. Another important advantage of d-sotalol is its lack of so-called β-blocker side effects. Similarly, because it produces less bradycardia (which may be due to markedly attenuated β-blocking actions and/or the direct effects on the sinus node by prolonging the APD), d-sotalol is likely to induce a lower rate of torsade de pointes. These clearly beneficial effects may need to be balanced against the possibility that the loss of β-blocking actions in the dextro-isomer may be associated with some reduction in the overall efficacy as an antifibrillatory agent. However, graded doses of β-blockers may be added to attain a particular therapeutic effect as indicated in individual patients. These all are critical issues which can be addressed only by controlled comparisons with dl-sotalol. The discontinuation of the SWORD study and a major VT/VF trial has led to the drug's being abandoned from further studies. The impact of such a step on the development of other "pure" class agents remains unclear.

REFERENCES

1. Senges J, Lengfelder W, Jauernig R, et al: Electrophysiologic testing of therapy with sotalol for sustained ventricular tachycardia. Circulation 69:577, 1984.
2. Nademanee K, Feld G, Hendrickson JA, et al: Electrophysiologic and antiarrhythmic effects of sotalol in patients with life-threatening ventricular tachyarrhythmias. Circulation 72:555, 1985.
3. Singh BN: A symposium: Controlling cardiac arrhythmias with sotalol, a broad-spectrum antiarrhythmic with beta-blocking effects and class III activity. Am J Cardiol 65:1A, 1990.
4. Singh BN, Aliot E, Lazzara R: Class III antiarrhythmic drugs: Potential impact on antiarrhythmic therapy. Eur Heart J 14(H):1, 1993.
5. Singh BN: Antiarrhythmic action of dl-sotalol in ventricular and supraventricular arrhythmias. J Cardiovasc Pharmacol 2:590, 1992.
6. Kato R, Ikeda N, Yabek R, et al: Electrophysiologic effects of the levo- and dextro-rotatory isomers of sotalol in isolated cardiac muscle and their in vivo pharmacokinetics. J Am Coll Cardiol 7:116, 1986.
7. Gomoll AW, Bartek MJ: Comparative beta-blocking activities and electrophysiologic actions of racemic sotalol and its optical isomers in anesthetized dogs. Eur J Pharamacol 132:123, 1986.
8. Levy JV, Richard V: Inotropic and chronotropic effects of a series of beta-adrenergic blocking drugs: Some structure-activity relationships. Proc Soc Exp Biol Med 122:373, 1966.
9. Lathrop DA: Electromechanical characterization of the effects of racemic sotalol and its optical isomers on isolated canine ventricular trabecular muscles and Purkinje strands. Can J Physiol Pharmacol 673:1506, 1985.
10. Singh BN: Historical development of the concept of controlling cardiac arrhythmias by lengthening repolarization: Particular reference to sotalol. Am J Cardiol 65(Suppl):3A, 1990.
11. Campbell TH: Cellular electrophysiological effects of d- and dl-sotalol in guinea-pig sino-atrial node, atrium and ventricle and human atrium: Differential tissue sensitivity. Br J Pharmacol 90:593, 1987.
12. Hondeghem LM, Snyders DJ: Class III anti-arrhythmic agents have a lot of potential but a long way to go. Reduced effectiveness and dangers of reverse use dependence. Circulation 81:686, 1990.
13. Carmeliet E: Electrophysiologic and voltage clamp analysis of the effects of sotalol on isolated cardiac muscle and Purkinje fibers. J Pharmacol Exp Ther 232:817, 1985.
14. Sanguinetti M, Jurkiewicz NK: Two components of cardiac delayed rectifier K+ current. J Gen Physiol 96:195, 1990.
15. Lynch JL, Wilber DJ, Montgomery DG, et al: Antiarrhythmic and antifibrillatory actions of the levo- and dextrorotatory isomers of sotalol. J Cardiovasc Pharmacol 6:1132, 1984.
16. Lynch JL, Coskey LA, Montgomery DG, et al: Prevention of ventricular fibrillation by dextrorotatory sotalol in conscious canine model of sudden coronary death. Am Heart J 109:949, 1985.
17. Singh BN: Arrhythmia control by prolonging repolarization: The concept and its potential therapeutic impact. Eur Heart J 14(Suppl H):14, 1993.
18. McComb JM, McGovern B, McGowan JB, et al: Electrophysiological effects of d-sotalol in humans. J Am Coll Cardiol 10:211, 1987.
19. Echt DS, Bert LE, Clusin WT, et al: Prolongation of human cardiac monophasic action potential by sotalol. Am J Cardiol 50:108, 1982.
20. Haywood RP, Taggart P: Effect of sotalol on human atrial action potential duration and refractoriness: Cycle length dependency of Class III activity. Cardiovasc Res 20:100, 1986.
21. Huikuri HV, Yli-Mäyry S: Frequency-dependent effects of d-sotalol and amiodarone on the action potential duration of the human right ventricle. PACE Pacing Clin Electrophysiol 15(11 Pt 2):2103, 1992.
22. Singh BN, Nademanee K: Control of cardiac arrhythmias by selective lengthening of repolarization: Theoretical considerations and clinical observations. Am Heart J 109:421, 1985.
23. Tande PM, Refsum H: Class III antiarrhythmic action linked with positive inotropy: Effects of the d- and l-isomer of sotalol on isolated rat atria and threshold and suprathreshold stimulation. Pharmacol Toxicol 62:272, 1988.
24. Mortensen E, Tande PM, Klow NE, et al: Plasma concentrations and hemodynamic effects of d-sotalol after beta-blockade. Pharmacol Toxicol 67:420, 1990.
25. Mortensen E, Tande PM, Klow NE, et al: Inotropy and class III antiarrhythmic activity: d-sotalol in experimental heart failure. J Mol Cell Cardiol 21(Suppl 4):S51, 1992.
26. Hoffmeister HM, Muller S, Seipel L: Effect of new class II antiarrhythmic agent d-sotalol on contractile function of postischemic myocardium. J Cardiovasc Pharmacol 17:1027, 1991.
27. Schwartz J, Crocker K, Wynn J, et al: The antiarrhythmic effects of d-sotalol. Am Heart J 111:539, 1987.
28. Funck-Brentano C: Pharmacokinetic and pharmacodynamic profiles of d-sotalol and dl-sotalol. Eur Heart J 14(Suppl H):30, 1993.
29. Poirier JM, Jaillon P, Lecocq V, et al: The pharmacokinetics of d-sotalol and dl-sotalol in healthy volunteers. Eur J Clin Pharmacol 38:579, 1990.
30. The Cardiac Arrhythmia Suppression Trial (CAST) Investigators: Preliminary report: Effect of encainide and flecainide on mortality in a randomized trial of arrhythmia suppression after myocardial infarction. N Engl J Med 321:40, 1989.
31. The Cardiac Arrhythmia Suppression Trial II Investigators: Effect of the anti-arrhythmic agent moricizine on survival after myocardial infarction. N Engl J Med 327:227, 1992.
32. Yusuf S, Teo KK: Approaches to prevention of sudden death: Need for fundamental reevaluation. J Cardiovasc Electrophysiol 2:S233, 1991.
33. Ahmed R, Singh BN: Anti-arrhythmic drugs. Curr Opin Cardiol 8:10, 1993.
34. Anderson JL: Sotalol in life-threatening ventricular arrhythmias: A unique class III antiarrhythmic. Am J Cardiol 72:1A, 1093.
35. Singh BN, Singh SN: A symposium: Controlling cardiac arrhythmias by lengthening repolarization: Emerging perspectives. Am J Cardiol 72:1F, 1993.
36. The CASCADE Investigators: The Cascade Study—Randomized antiarrhythmic drug therapy in survivors of cardiac arrest in Seattle. Am J Cardiol 72:280, 1993.
37. Mason JW, on Behalf of the ESVEM Investigators: A comparison of seven antiarrhythmic drugs in patients with ventricular tachyarrhythmias. N Engl J Med 329:452, 1993.
38. Singh BN: Choice and chance in drug therapy of cardiac arrhythmias: Technique versus drug-specific responses in evaluation of efficacy. Am J Cardiol 72:114F, 1993.
39. Feld GK, Venkatesh N, Singh BN: Pharmacologic conversion and suppression of experimental and canine atrial flutter: Differing effects of d-sotalol, quinidine, and lidocaine and significance of changes in refractoriness and conduction. Circulation 74:197, 1986.
40. Boyden PA, Graziano JN: Multiple models of termination of re-entrant excitation around an anatomic barrier in the canine atrium during the action of d-sotalol. Br Heart J 14(Suppl H):41, 1993.
41. Bertrix I, Timour-Chah Q, Lang J, et al: Protection against ventricular and atrial fibrillation by sotalol. Cardiovasc Res 20:358, 1986.
42. Wang M, Dorian P: Dl- and d-Sotalol decrease defibrillation energy requirements. PACE Pacing Clin Electrophysiol 12:1522, 1989.
43. Lucchesi B, Lynch JJ: Preclinical studies on the antifibrillatory effects of sotalol and its optical isomers. In Singh B (ed): Control of Cardiac Arrhythmias by Lengthening Repolarization. Mount Kisco, NY: Futura Publishing Company, 1988, p 245.
44. Brachmann J, Beyer T, Schmitt C: Electrophysiologic and antiarrhythmic effects of d-sotalol. J Cardiovasc Pharmacol 20:S91, 1992.
45. Brachmann J, Schols W, Beyer T, et al: Acute and chronic antiarrhythmic efficacy of d-sotalol in patients with sustained ventricular tachyarrhythmias. Eur Heart J 14(Suppl H):85, 1993.
46. Waldo AL, Camm AJ, De Ruyter H, et al: Preliminary results from the Survival with Oral D-Sotalol (SWORD) Trial [abstract]. J Am Coll Cardiol 25:15A, 1995.

C. Sinus Node Inhibitors

CHAPTER 151

Sinus Node Inhibitors: Zatebradine and Other Agents

James D. Murphy, M.D., and Carl J. Pepine, M.D.

INTRODUCTION AND TERMINOLOGY

The concept of manipulating heart rate independent of other cardiocirculatory actions represents a relatively new approach to the treatment of cardiovascular disorders. Several pharmacologic agents, termed *sinus node inhibitors*, reduce heart rate in subjects both at rest and during exercise as their primary mechanism of action. Some of them formerly were called "bradycardic agents." However, because bradycardia at rest is difficult to define and may be caused by a number of mechanisms (e.g., heart block, β-adrenergic blockers, and so on), the term *sinus node inhibitor* is preferred because it more specifically denotes the mechanism by which these agents may be beneficial. Before discussing the pharmacology of these agents, it is helpful to review the importance of heart rate in circulatory function and disease states.

RATIONALE FOR DEVELOPMENT

Importance of Heart Rate in Cardiac and Circulatory Function

The physiologic role of heart rate is crucial in both circulatory and cardiac functions. In terms of circulatory dynamics, changes in heart rate are the principal means of providing the rapid adjustments in cardiac output that are required to meet the body's continually changing demands for blood flow. An increase in heart rate results in an increase in the force of myocardial contraction (Bowditch effect). An increase in heart rate and rate-related inotropy are important considerations in both myocardial ischemia and hypertension related to high cardiac output.[1] In other clinical states such as postoperative tachycardia and hypertension, the acute phase of myocardial infarction, thyrotoxicosis, mitral valve stenosis, tetralogy of Fallot, and hypertrophic cardiomyopathy, the rise in heart rate may be deleterious to circulatory function.

Myocardial oxygen consumption (MVO_2) serves as an estimate of total energy utilization of the heart under steady-state conditions.[2] Under clinical conditions that place a restraint on coronary flow and hence a ceiling on the availability of oxygen to the myocardium, MVO_2 becomes a primary determinant of myocardial ischemia. Heart rate, in addition to intramyocardial tension, contractile state of myocardium, basal

metabolism, and external work (energy associated with shortening against a load) determine MVO_2.[2]

Heart rate is the principal determinant of MVO_2 and is also a determinant of the volume and distribution of blood flow to the myocardium. The latter relates particularly to the smaller vessels that supply the subendocardium. However, the diastolic myocardial perfusion time, which is largely determined by heart rate, becomes paramount in maintaining blood flow even in the larger arteries.[3-5] In the presence of a flow-limiting coronary stenosis, an increase in heart rate results in a linear reduction in coronary flow and a redistribution of blood flow toward the epicardium.[6, 7] Slowing heart rate has an antiischemic effect by reducing myocardial oxygen demand and increasing myocardial oxygen delivery by prolonging the time available for diastolic myocardial perfusion.[3, 4, 8-13]

Increases in heart rate have long been known to be an important cause of myocardial ischemia during physical or emotional stress or tachyarrhythmias. Many episodes of nocturnal and daytime ischemia are associated with a prior heart rate increase.[14]

Heart Rate as a Predictor of Adverse Outcome

Increased heart rate has been associated with increased risk for adverse outcomes in many reports. A heart rate of more than 90 beats/min is predictive of early mortality after acute myocardial infarction.[15] The maximal heart rate recorded at any time during initial hospitalization for information is an important positive predictor of 1 year mortality.[16] Conversely, in the first 24 hours of hospitalization, bradycardia is negatively associated with 1 year mortality.[16] Several workers have demonstrated that the circadian variation in hourly frequency of myocardial infarction approximates the time (hours) when heart rate and systolic blood pressure are rising, suggesting common triggering mechanisms.[17, 18] Data from the Framingham Study have shown that heart rate at entry is an important predictor of death in normotensive and hypertensive subjects over long-term follow-up.[19]

Pharmacologic Reduction in Heart Rate

Agents that reduce heart rate or limit its rise in response to stress are effective antiischemic agents. Heart rate slowing agents may induce an antiischemic effect by decreasing or limiting MVO_2 and increasing diastolic perfusion time, thereby increasing blood flow to the subendocardium.

β-Blockers were the first major heart rate–slowing agents to be used as antiischemic agents. These agents decrease MVO$_2$ through a reduction of heart rate, systolic pressure, and myocardial contractility. The heart rate reduction effect of β-blockers also increases coronary flow by prolonging diastolic perfusion time. Studies on exercising dogs with experimental coronary artery narrowing show that either propranolol or atenolol improves blood flow to ischemic subendocardium.[20–24] Studies in which hearts were paced to rates seen prior to β-blocker administration show little to no antiischemic effects.[23] Other authors have reported similar findings in patients with coronary artery disease.[25, 26] There is a reduced incidence of myocardial infarction in patients taking β-adrenergic blocking agents that blunt or eliminate the morning rise in heart rate.[17] Mulcahy et al. found a decrease in the frequency of silent ischemia episodes in patients treated with β-blockade but not in patients treated with an agent that increases heart rate (e.g., nifedipine).[18] It is clear that the heart-rate-reducing effect of β-blockade is a primary determinant in the antiischemic effect.

Studies employing β-blockers in patients with acute myocardial infarction have shown a reduction in early and late mortality,[27] reduced infarction size,[28] improved exercise tolerance,[29, 30] increased exercise time to ST depression,[29, 30] decreased length of hospitalization,[31] and decreased incidence of atrial and ventricular arrhythmias.[32] β-Blockers also reduce angina frequency, severity, and duration of both asymptomatic and symptomatic ischemia.[30, 33, 34] Several studies have related these beneficial outcomes to a reduction in heart rate. A close relationship between magnitude of heart rate suppression and magnitude of infarct size limitation[28] and also magnitude of reduction in mortality has been demonstrated.

Despite the clinical benefit of β-blockers, there is a reluctance to use them even in conditions such as acute myocardial infarction. Clinical surveys show that less than 30% of postmyocardial infarction patients are receiving β-blockers in the United States. This reluctance is largely related to concern about tolerability in specific populations, such as patients with asthma, chronic obstructive pulmonary disease, hypotension, or depressed left ventricular function. In addition, they may cause other side effects (e.g., atrioventricular [AV] block, fatigue, impotence, depression) in any population.

Some calcium antagonists, such as verapamil and diltiazem, also reduce heart rate. These agents also decrease blood pressure and increase or redistribute blood flow to ischemic myocardium. But in some patients these agents cause significant AV block, profound bradycardia, or congestive heart failure. Furthermore, there are some data that suggest that in the early postmyocardial infarction period patients with evidence of heart failure treated with these agents may have an increase in mortality.

Background of Specific Bradycardic Agents

The new class of bradycardic agents known as sinus node inhibitors were developed to selectively decrease heart rate with little or no effect on cardiac conduction, contractility, or vascular smooth muscle tone. Recognizing the potential clinical utility of a "specific bradycardic agent" in the early 1970s, a verapamil derivative, AQ-A 39, that met these criteria was developed.[35] Around the same time, alinidine (ST 567) was derived from clonidine.[35] Despite similar bradycardia activity, AQ-A 39 was found to have significant class III antiarrhythmic properties and therefore did not undergo further clinical study.[36] Another agent derived from verapamil was zatebradine (UL-FS 49). Zatebradine had desirable heart rate–slowing effects without important class III antiarrhythmic properties. Because these agents inhibit heart rate in proportion to the level of heart rate, greater inhibitor effects are seen during stress when heart rate was high. Thus, they do not necessarily produce bradycardia at rest. Since their specific mechanism of action on the sinus node was identified, these drugs have become known as sinus node inhibitors. Most recently, ZD7288 (Zeneca) has been added to this clinically promising class of drugs that all share the same or very similar mechanism(s) of action.

While alinidine was the first extensively studied drug within this group, it no longer is under clinical investigation because of clonidine-like side effects including dry mouth, hypotension, and drowsiness.[24] The initial clinical studies, however, did demonstrate significant heart rate slowing without significant effects on cardiac conduction or contractility.[36, 37] Animal studies confirmed its ability to reduce heart rate to result in antiischemic effects.[38, 39] Because most of the subsequent work has focused on zatebradine, we will detail its pharmacologic properties.

ZATEBRADINE
Chemistry

Zatebradine has the chemical name 1,3,4,5-tetrahydro-7,8-dimethoxy-3[3-[[2-(3,4-dimenthoxyphenyl)-ethyl]-methylamino]propyl]-2H-3-benzazepin-2-one-hydrochloride with the molecular formula ($C_{26}H_{36}N_2O_5$ HCl). Its molecular weight is 493.05. It is soluble in water and methanol and is sparingly soluble in 96% ethanol. It is available in 1.25 mg, 2.5 mg, 5.0 mg, and 7.5 mg tablets. It is also available in injectable form.

Pharmacodynamics

Zatebradine reduces heart rate by slowing the spontaneous diastolic depolarization of sinoatrial node pacemaker cells. This is achieved by blocking the I_f current in sinoatrial node pacemaker cells.[40, 41] This mechanism of action is different from that of β-blockers and calcium antagonists in that, at the doses studied, zatebradine works directly on the I_f current without other significant effects.[40–42] The I_f current is a hyperpolarizing activated current, carried by sodium and potassium, that is particularly important in modulating the slow diastolic depolarization necessary to maintain sinus node pacemaker activity.[43] Zatebradine has been shown to act intracellularly in a positively charged form.[41, 44] Van Bogaert has proposed a mechanism by which zatebradine causes a selective, "use-dependent" and reversible blockade of I_f currents[41, 44–46] without a shift in the activation curve. At hyperpolarized potentials, unblocking of the I_f current occurs.[45] Alinidine and its derivatives, on the other hand, primarily shift the activation curve of the I_f current to more hyperpolarized potentials and therefore cause a tonic block of the I_f current at high concentrations.[45] The clinical significance of this is that in states with high levels of sympathetic stimulation, such as angina pectoris, an increase in heart rate is realized in part by a shift of the I_f current activation range to polarized levels. By blocking the I_f current, zatebradine has the potential to reduce heart rate and prevent harmful effects of increased heart rate on myocardial oxygen balance. A frequency-dependent reduction in the heart rate may provide a reduced chronotropic response to β-catecholamines without causing severe bradycardia at rest.[45] Blockade of I_f channels is voltage-dependent and use-dependent and thereby is consistent with a slow onset of action and slow washout.

In contrast with calcium antagonists, clinically relevant concentrations of zatebradine have little effect on L-type calcium channels.[45] There also is evidence that zatebradine may interact with calcium antagonists. Blockade of calcium L-type channels is also rate-dependent. The T-type calcium channels are only modestly influenced by relatively high concentrations of zatebradine.

In healthy volunteers, single oral doses of zatebradine ranging from 2.5 mg to 40 mg produced a bradycardic effect, with an onset of action in 1 to 3 hours and a maximal effect in 3 to 6 hours.[47] The greatest decrement in heart rate occurred with the 40-mg dose and resulted in a 20-beat/min decrement, or about 32%. The maximal tolerated single oral dose in healthy, young volunteers was determined to be 40 mg with associated maximal plasma levels of 150 to 250 ng/ml.[47] The duration of heart rate effect ranged from 12 to 16 hours.[47] Effects of zatebradine on heart rate at the end of a 6-minute bicycle ergometry exercise test were similar to effects on resting heart rate.[48–52] The heart rate slowing effect was dose related, with maximal reduction occurring between 3 and 6 hours after administration. Overall, the reduction in heart rate was greater following exercise than at rest. Stroke volume was increased after 4 days of treatment, and resting heart rate remained reduced, resulting in no change in cardiac output.[52]

Pharmacokinetics

Several hundred volunteers have received zatebradine in multiple phase 1 clinical trials with both short- and long-term oral administration. Pharmacokinetics were determined after oral and intravenous administration of 25 mg of zatebradine to healthy volunteers.[53]

Approximately 78% of the parent drug is absorbed after oral administration.[53] Absolute bioavailability, however, is only approximately 44% because of first-pass effect. Steady-state plasma levels are achieved approximately 36 hours after twice-daily oral dosing.[54] Dose proportionality is seen between oral twice-daily doses of 2, 5, and 10 mg.[54] Maximum plasma concentrations are reached 1.5 hours after administration.[53]

Total body clearance is 600 to 700 ml/min,[48, 53, 55] of which 44 ml/min is renal and the remainder nonrenal. Elimination half-life is between 2 and 3 hours. Dissociation between half-life and duration of action is thought to be a result of active tissue binding. Decreased clearance in the elderly has been documented and is thought to be due to decreased hepatic flow and decreased liver weight.[54, 56, 57]

Animal Studies

The hemodynamic effects of zatebradine have been extensively studied in both normal animals and models with chronic ischemia, left ventricular failure, left ventricular hypertrophy, and animals undergoing isoflurane-induced anesthesia. Zatebradine has a consistent dose-response effect reducing heart rate in dogs,[58, 59] pigs,[8, 60] rats, cats,[60] and rabbits.[61] It is a highly specific sinus node inhibitor that has little or no effect on left ventricular dP/dt, mean arterial pressure, left ventricular relaxation, coronary vascular tone, end-diastolic pressure, and end-systolic pressure in normal animals when corrected for the degree of tachycardia.[58, 62, 63] One study suggested that in normal exercising dogs, zatebradine actually may have a positive inotropic effect in that it increased positive dP/dt.[64]

In a study of isolated, blood-perfused, canine hearts, zatebradine decreased myocardial oxygen consumption by a bradycardic mechanism and not by decreasing contractility.[65] Zatebradine prolonged diastole without affecting coronary resistance, therefore increasing myocardial oxygen supply.[66] In a study of conscious dogs with chronic single-vessel coronary stenosis, zatebradine attenuated exercise-induced ischemia-related myocardial dysfunction and improved perfusion to ischemic myocardium without compromising contractile function of nonischemic myocardium.[9, 10] β-Blockers, while they improved blood flow and the contractile state of ischemic myocardium, caused contractile dysfunction of nonischemic myocardium in the same animal model.[66, 67] In an exercise study of normal dogs, propranolol caused a greater decrease in dP/dt, left ventricular work, and left ventricular power than was caused by zatebradine.[64]

In a model of variable coronary occlusion in anesthetized swine, marked improvement in subendocardial blood flow and contractile function occurred when zatebradine was infused to slow heart rate.[8]

Furthermore, there were separate relationships between coronary flow per minute and contractile function at different heart rates. This would imply that other factors may contribute to the antiischemic effect of zatebradine. These include increased blood flow, decreased (MVO_2) secondary to a decreased number of contractions per minute, and increased diastolic perfusion time.[8]

In studies involving isolated guinea pig atria,[68] anesthetized dogs,[10] and anesthetized pigs,[62] zatebradine induced bradycardia without altering contractility. Furthermore, its bradycardic effect was preserved in the presence of therapeutic doses of isoproterenol,[62, 63] dobutamine,[69] and epinephrine.[70]

These studies demonstrate a persistent bradycardic effect, with a significant increase in dP/dt, left ventricular pressure, and contractility.[62, 68-70] Based on these animal studies, zatebradine, as an adjunctive therapy to β-adrenergic agonists, may be useful in the treatment of heart failure. Zatebradine has been shown to prevent the adverse effect of tachycardia on the lower limit of subendocardial autoregulation. This mechanism would be useful in the setting of chronic heart failure. Van Woerkins et al.,[71] using a conscious pig model, evaluated zatebradine in the setting of chronic mild left ventricular dysfunction secondary to myocardial infarction. Here, zatebradine reduced heart rate without causing a significant change in the duration of left ventricular systole, but it caused a significant increase in the duration of diastole.[71] In doses up to 100 μg/kg, zatebradine did not influence blood pressure; whereas there was a 10% reduction in left ventricular dP/dt and cardiac output.[71]

The electrophysiologic effects of zatebradine have been studied in rabbits,[61] dogs,[59] and cats.[60] In anesthetized rabbits with coronary artery occlusion, verapamil and zatebradine were compared with respect to prevention of ventricular fibrillation during ischemia. Verapamil was more effective than zatebradine in preventing ischemia-related ventricular fibrillation.[61] Zatebradine, however, did prevent ventricular fibrillation, and this effect was directly related to its bradycardic effect.[61] In a canine Purkinje fiber model, zatebradine had markedly less calcium channel blocking effect than verapamil.[59] There was no change in action potential amplitude or resting membrane potential after therapeutic doses of zatebradine.[59] Zatebradine was further studied to evaluate effects on T-type or L-type calcium channels.[72] It was found to have minimal effects on both of these channels in single isolated guinea pig myocytes, but the effect was thought to be clinically insignificant.[72] In anesthetized cats, zatebradine caused prolongation of the QT interval and the effective refractory period of 29% and 24%, respectively.[60] Zatebradine increased cycle length by approximately 50% with little or no change in blood pressure or electrocardiographic PQ or QRS intervals.[60]

Zatebradine has been found to be more efficacious than propranolol in decreasing the tachycardiac response to isoflurane anesthesia.[73] As expected, zatebradine did not block the hemodynamic response to isoproterenol.[73] In another study, zatebradine was evaluated with respect to its effect on diastolic function during isoflurane anesthesia in normal dogs, dogs with physiologic left ventricular hypertrophy and bradycardia, and dogs with pressure overload–induced left ventricular hypertrophy.[74] There was a significant decrease in heart rate in normal dogs and in dogs with pathologic but not physiologic left ventricular hypertrophy. There was no effect on diastolic function or other hemodynamic findings in any of these dogs.[74]

Clinical Studies

Four unpublished, double-blind, placebo-controlled European trials have been done in patients with chronic stable angina.[75-78] The first two studies were done with oral regimens and the latter two with intravenous zatebradine. In these trials, zatebradine caused a reduction in heart rate both at rest and with exercise, although a clear dose-response relationship was not established. Zatebradine also increased exercise tolerance and time to onset of ST segment depression in patients with chronic stable angina.[76, 78] In two studies, nitroglycerin consumption significantly decreased.[76, 78] In one study, the number and severity of anginal attacks also decreased during long-term administration.

These trials demonstrated that there was no significant effect on cardiac output or diastolic blood pressure. On the other hand, one study suggested a lowering of systolic blood pressure.[76] In that study, however, the patients were borderline hypertensive, and the degree of heart rate reduction was more prominent than in the other studies. Dose-dependent reductions in heart rate have been shown, with the greatest magnitude occurring in the 10 mg/day regimen (5 mg oral twice daily).[78] Treatment with 5 mg/day also showed clinically relevant improvement at 2 and 10 hours after administration, although there was no statistically significant difference compared with the placebo. The 2.5 mg/day regimen was not significantly different compared with the placebo.

In the two intravenous dosing trials, all variables were measured 15 minutes after administration. Knowing that the peak heart rate slowing effect of zatebradine does not occur until 1 to 3 hours after administration, these trials may have shown more significance if they had made heart rate response measurements later. These trials are useful to document lack of significant negative inotropic effect but are inadequate to evaluate possible efficacy in hypertension.

One recent study demonstrated maximal heart rate reduction 80 to 90 minutes after the infusion of zatebradine was started.[79] Another study[80] evaluated a 45-minute zatebradine infusion and found no significant change in AH interval, AV node effective refractive period, right ventricular effective refractory period, or VA conduction time, although there was a slight increase in the Wenckebach rate. It should be noted, however, that in two patients given the drug who had a baseline prolonged HV interval, there was significant prolongation of the HV interval when compared with the placebo.

Adverse Effects

Doses of zatebradine that significantly reduce heart rate (5 to 40 mg/day) are generally well tolerated in healthy volunteers and in patients with chronic stable angina, whether the drug is administered as a single oral or intravenous dose or administered as a long-term oral regimen. The most commonly occurring adverse effects attributable to zatebradine include visual symptoms, fatigue, headache, and dizziness. The visual phenomena occur in a dose-related manner and generally are described as photopsia (e.g., light flashes, flickering in peripheral vision), optical preservations, and nonspecific visual disturbances. Visual disturbances were experienced by 18 of 21 of those receiving 30 mg.[51, 52, 54-56, 81] At lower doses, the effects generally occurred 2 to 3 days after treatment, and the effects were transient and resolved spontaneously while therapy continued. Of 344 patients who received zatebradine, 14.5% reported visual phenomena. In a study of 24 volunteers receiving 7.5 to 30 mg/day for 7 days, there were no pathologic findings despite extensive ophthalmologic examination. The visual disturbance, while annoying, does not seem to interfere with activities.

One study of patients with borderline hypertension initially showed a significant reduction in diastolic and systolic blood pressure.[76] However, a change in diastolic blood pressure was the only significant change in blood pressure variables seen in other studies. It is thought that the decline in diastolic pressure is attributable to the increase in diastolic time. No study patients or healthy volunteers experienced symptomatic bradycardia or hypotension. Some also have raised the possibility of change in QRS, PR, and QT_c intervals.[76]

One patient in study 140.16 had a 40-beat run of ventricular tachycardia (VT).[78] Two patients in the 5 mg/day study developed symptomatic atrial fibrillation. There was no knowledge of whether or not these patients had previous ventricular or atrial arrhythmias. Four patients in the 140.16 study demonstrated isolated increases in hepatic enzymes.[78] One patient who received a single dose of zatebradine had significant elevation of creatine phosphokinase and aldolase levels. Retrial 30 days later in the same man did not show a similar response.

In summary, oral doses of 2.5, 5.0, and 7.5 mg twice daily appear to be efficacious in patients with stable, chronic ischemic heart disease. However, because of the small number of patients studied, it is not clear whether this agent will have a clinically significant effect on hepatic enzymes, measured electrocardiographic variables, or cardiac conduction.

Toxicology

After acute oral toxicity was studied in rats[82] and dogs,[83] and after intravenous administration, toxicity was studied in rabbits.[84] Central venous system effects, including sedation, tremor, and convulsions, were seen in rats and rabbits; ataxia and lethargy were seen in dogs. Necropsy demonstrated congestive hyperemia in the livers and kidneys of animals that died.

In high doses, zatebradine caused salivation, convulsions, emesis, and ataxia in all species tested. Miosis also was seen in rabbit trials. Death was caused by acute cardiac failure. At high doses, zatebradine caused respiratory sinus arrhythmias, extrasystoles, and second-degree atrioventricular block. Administration of 300 mg/kg to rats resulted in toxic cardiac effects including increased heart weight and fibrotic intracardiac lesions. The fibrotic intramyocardial lesions underwent partial remission during the 6-week recovery period.

High doses also led to consistent reductions in systolic blood pressure. Increased diastolic blood pressure was seen in control and low-dose groups. There were increases in SGPT, AP, and GDH in 52-week oral[85, 86] and 4-week IV dog studies,[87, 88] suggesting a possible hepatic effect at high doses (25 and 5 mg/kg, respectively). These changes correlate with centrilobar fatty change and an increase in liver weights. There was no dose-related impairment of fertility or reproduction following oral zatebradine of up to 300 mg/kg/day in the male animals and 80 mg/kg/day in the female animals. Weak teratogenicity was seen in doses of 100 mg/kg. Rabbits showed no teratogenicity in doses of 100 mg/kg. There was no demonstrable mutagenicity shown in testing of zatebradine.

ZENECA (ZD7288)

Several other agents have shown promise as sinus node inhibitors. One such agent, Zeneca (ZD7288), is in clinical trial.

Chemistry

ZD7288 has the chemical name of 4-(N-ethyl-N-phenylamino)-1,2-dimethyl-6-(methylamino) pyrimidinium chloride, with the molecular formula $C_{14}H_{21}N_4Cl$. It is available as a round, biconvex, white, film-coated tablet containing 2.5 mg, 10 mg, or 50 mg. The injectable form consists of 5 ml of a clear, colorless, sterile isotonic solution of ZD7288, in a concentration of 1 mg/ml.

Pharmacodynamics

Zeneca (ZD7288) is a calcium antagonist derivative with the properties of a sinus node inhibitor, and it produces its effect by blocking diastolic depolarization of sinus node pacemaker cells. Unlike zatebradine, however, its mechanism of action is not use-dependent.[89] Its mechanism of action has been shown to be devoid of cholinergic, β-adrenergic, or histaminergic activity.[90] There is a slight electrophysiologic difference between ZD7288 and other heart rate slowing agents in that ZD7288 has much less effect on the

Ik current and therefore does not produce prolongation of action potential duration to the extent observed with alinidine and zatebradine.[91, 92]

In animal studies, ZD7288 has been shown to decrease heart rate without causing depression of myocardial contractility, blood pressure, atrioventricular conduction time, cardiac output, or total peripheral resistance that was not attributed to the reduction in heart rate alone.[93-97] In conscious animals with exercise-induced tachycardia, heart rate was reduced, but the exercise-associated increase in cardiac output was maintained unless tachycardia was reduced by more than 30%.[97]

Pharmacokinetics

Initial pharmacokinetic studies in human volunteers[98, 99] have demonstrated that systemic exposure of the drug increases linearly with the increased oral doses. There was wide intervolunteer variation in data of plasma concentration, presumably because of variable absorption and/or extensive first-pass metabolism. ZD7288 appeared to be rapidly absorbed at all doses, with peak plasma concentrations occurring 1 to 3 hours postdose. Maximal plasma concentrations of approximately 19.8 ± 12.3 mg/ml were obtained after a single dose of 29.5 mg of ZD7288. No significant accumulation would be expected with once-daily dosing. Plasma elimination profiles were biphasic, with a rapid initial elimination phase extending out to approximately 12 hours followed by a slower terminal phase.

Five studies were conducted in the United Kingdom in healthy male volunteers. A study of safety and tolerance of single doses ascending up to 29.5 mg demonstrated that this dosage was well tolerated with no serious adverse events.[98] In a single-dose isoprenaline challenge study,[100] doses of 20 mg and 30 mg were both found to be efficacious in producing heart rate reduction while preserving the positive inotropic effect of isoprenaline. The 2.5- and 10-mg doses were not effective.[100] In a single-dose study that included exercise 2 hours after a dose, heart rate at the highest common workload was significantly reduced with ZD7288 compared with the placebo. With the 10-mg, 20-mg, and 30-mg doses, exercise heart rate declined by 5 beats/min, 9.5 beats/min, and 13.6 beats/min, respectively.[101] In a multiple-dose, placebo-controlled, crossover study, 30 mg once daily was given for 8 days. On days 1 and 8 during exercise tests, there were significant reductions in heart rate 2 and 8 hours postdosing. The drug was well tolerated, with no withdrawal symptoms or serious adverse events.[102]

In a series of drug interaction studies, the ability of ZD7288 to reduce heart rate was unaffected when subjects were pretreated with therapeutic doses of heparin, nitrendipine, verapamil, atenolol, trinitroglycerin, digitalis, mexiletine, and disopyramide. Conversely, the cardiac effects of these drugs were unaffected by coadministration with ZD7288 with the exception that reflex tachycardia caused by the vasodilators was abolished.

ZD7288 was considered to have no biologically significant effects other than those related to its known mechanism of action on autonomic or neuromuscular function in vitro. Single oral doses of ZD7288 reduced gastric emptying. This was not seen after intravenous administration; therefore, the effect was thought to be a local effect. The same effect was seen in studies of alinidine and zatebradine, implying some common mechanism of action. The clinical relevance of this remains to be seen, since there were no effects seen in human drug studies. In summary, human volunteer data indicate that ZD7288 is an effective and safe agent that is well tolerated in single and multiple dosing intervals. It is effective in reducing heart rate response to exercise as well as in the presence of intravenously administered β-adrenergic agonists. It not only is effective at reducing heart rate response but also preserves the inotropic effects of both exogenously administered catecholamines and those released as a result of exercise.

CLINICAL USES

Several ongoing multicenter clinical trials are evaluating zatebradine and ZD7288 as specific sinus node inhibitors to treat patients with myocardial ischemia. Additionally, these agents could be beneficial in patients with heart failure, acute myocardial infarction, perioperative sinus tachycardia, and perhaps mild systemic hypertension. As yet, none of these promising new agents is approved for clinical use.

SUMMARY

Studies of sinus node inhibitors have emphasized their efficacy in the treatment of patients with chronic stable angina caused by coronary artery disease. Investigators are also exploring their use as short-term treatments in a number of other settings. Short-term use may prove beneficial in acute or unstable ischemic syndromes such as myocardial infarction and unstable angina, perioperative tachycardia, and myocardial ischemia during coronary intervention. Furthermore, they may prove useful in controlling the unwanted tachycardia induced by anesthetic and inotropic agents. The latter indication may be of particular use in the treatment of acute decompensation of congestive heart failure.

CONCLUSIONS

Sinus node inhibitors are a new class of drugs that reduce heart rate by a direct effect on the sinus node and have the potential to reduce or prevent myocardial ischemia. Lack of effect on blood pressure and contractility sets them apart from traditional antiischemic agents such as β-blockers and calcium antagonists. Zatebradine remains the most intensively studied and potentially useful agent in this new class of drugs.

REFERENCES

1. Frohlich ED: Hyperdynamic circulation and hypertension. Postgrad Med 5:64, 1972.
2. Sonnenblick EH, Ross J, Braunwald E: Oxygen consumption of the heart. Am J Cardiol 22:328, 1968.
3. Gout B, Jean J, Bril A: Comparative effects of a potassium channel blocking drug, UK-768, 798, and a specific bradycardic agent, UL-FS 49, on exercise-induced ischemia in the dog: Significance of diastolic time on ischemic cardiac function. J Pharmacol Exp Ther 262:987, 1992.
4. Ferro G, Spinelli L, Duilio C, et al: Diastolic perfusion time at ischemic threshold in patients with stress-induced ischemia. Circulation 84:49, 1991.
5. Weintraub W, Hattori S, Agarwal JB, et al: The relationship between myocardial blood flow and contraction by myocardial layer in the canine left ventricle during ischemia. Circ Res 48:430, 1981.
6. Ball RM, Bache R: Distribution of myocardial blood flow in the exercising dog with restricted coronary artery inflow. Circ Res 38:60, 1976.
7. Canty JM, Giglia J, Kandath D: Effect of tachycardia on regional function and transmural myocardial perfusion during graded coronary pressure reduction in conscious dogs. Circulation 82:1815, 1990.
8. Indolfi C, Guth BD, Miura T, et al: Mechanisms of improved ischemic regional dysfunction by bradycardia. Circulation 80:983, 1989.
9. Guth BD, Heusch G, Seitelberger R, et al: Elimination of exercise-induced regional myocardial dysfunction by a bradycardic agent in dogs with chronic coronary stenosis. Circulation 75:661, 1987.
10. Guth BD, Heusch G, Seitelberger R, et al: Role of heart rate reduction in the treatment of exercise-induced myocardial ischemia. Eur Heart J 8(Suppl L):61, 1987.
11. O'Brien P, Drage D, Saeian K, et al: Regional redistribution of myocardial perfusion by UL-FS 49, a selective bradycardic agent. Am Heart J 123:566, 1992.
12. Nabel EG, Selwyn AP, Ganz P: Paradoxical narrowing of atherosclerotic coronary arteries induced by increases in heart rate. Circulation 81:850, 1990.
13. Indolfi C, Guth BD, Shunichi M, et al: Heart rate reduction improves myocardial ischemia in swine: Role of interventricular blood flow redistribution. Am J Physiol 261:H910, 1991.
14. Quyyumi AA, Wright CA, Mockus LJ, Fox KM: Mechanisms of nocturnal angina pectoris: Importance of increased myocardial oxygen demand in patients with severe coronary artery disease. Lancet 1:1207, 1984.
15. Henning H, Gilpin EA, Covell JW, et al: Prognosis after acute myocardial infarction: A multivariate analysis of mortality and survival. Circulation 59:1124, 1979.
16. Madsen EB, Gilpin E, Henning H, et al: Prediction of late mortality after myocardial infarction from variables measured at different times during hospitalization. Am J Cardiol 53:47, 1984.
17. Pepine CJ: B-blockers or calcium antagonists in silent ischemia? Eur Heart J 14(F):7, 1993.
18. Mulcahy D, Keegan J, Cunningham D, et al: Circadian variation of total ischaemic burden and its alteration with antianginal agents. Lancet 2:755, 1988.
19. Gillman MW, Kannel WB, Belanger A, et al: Influence of heart rate on mortality among persons with hypertension: The Framingham Study. Am Heart J 125:1148, 1993.
20. Guth BD, Heusch G, Seitelberger R, et al: Mechanism of beneficial effect of B-adrenergic blockade on exercise-induced myocardial ischemia in conscious dogs. Circ Res 60:738, 1987.
21. Gross GJ, Buck JD, Warltier DC, et al: Role of autoregulation in the beneficial action of propranolol on ischemic blood flow distribution and stenosis severity in the canine myocardium. J Pharmacol Exp Ther 222:635, 1982.
22. Matsuzaki M, Patritti J, Tajimi T, et al: Effects of B-blockade on regional myocardial flow and function during exercise. Am J Physiol 247:H52, 1984.
23. Buck JD, Hardman JF, Warltier DC, et al: Changes in ischemic blood flow distribution and dynamic severity of a coronary stenosis induced by beta blockade in the canine heart. Circulation 64:708, 1981.
24. Shanks RG: The clinical pharmacology of alinidine and its side-effects. Eur Heart J 8(Suppl L):83, 1987.
25. Schang SJ, Pepine CJ: Coronary and myocardial metabolic effects of combined glyceryl trinitrate and propranolol administration. Observations in patients with and without coronary disease. Br Heart J 40:1221, 1978.
26. Schang SJ, Pepine CJ: Effects of propranolol on coronary hemodynamic and metabolic responses to tachycardia stress in patients with and without coronary disease. Cathet Cardiovasc Diagn 3:47, 1977.
27. β-Blocker Heart Attack Trial Research Group: A randomized trial of propranolol in patients with acute myocardial infarction. JAMA 247:1707, 1982.
28. Kjekshus JK: Importance of heart rate in determining beta-blocker efficacy in acute and long-term acute myocardial infarction intervention trials. Am J Cardiol 57:43F, 1986.
29. Harris FJ, Low RI, Paumer L, et al: Antianginal efficacy and improved exercise performance with timolol. Am J Cardiol 51:13, 1983.
30. Stone PH, Gibson RS, Glasser SP, et al: Comparison of propranolol, diltiazem, and nifedipine in the treatment of ambulatory ischemia in patients with stable angina. Circulation 82:1962, 1990.
31. Herlitz J, Hartford M, Pennert K, et al: Goteborg Metoprolol trial: Clinical observations. Am J Cardiol 53:37D, 1984.
32. Hjalmarsor A: Metoprolol in acute myocardial infarction (MIAMI). Am J Cardiol 56:1G, 1985.
33. Theroux P, Taeymans Y, Morissette D, et al: A randomized study comparing propranolol and diltiazem in the treatment of unstable angina. J Am Coll Cardiol 5:717, 1985.
34. Gottlieb SO, Weisfeldt ML, Ouyang P, et al: Effect of the addition of propranolol to therapy with nifedipine for unstable angina pectoris: A randomized, double-blind, placebo-controlled trial. Circulation 73:331, 1986.
35. Kobinger W: History of specific bradycardic agents [editorial]. Eur Heart J 8(Suppl L):5, 1987.
36. Beyer T: Differential electrophysiological effects of AQ-A39 on normal and infarcted canine cardiac Purkinje fibers [abstract #216]. Naunyn Schmiedebergs Arch Pharmacol 335(Suppl): R54, 1987.
37. Kobinger W, Lillie C: Specific bradycardic agents—a novel pharmacological class? Eur Heart J 8(Suppl L):7, 1987.
38. Wiegand V, Kreuzer H: Acute haemodynamic effects of a specific bradycardic agent in patients with coronary heart disease and impaired left ventricular function. Eur Heart J 8(Suppl L):105, 1987.
39. Schamhardt HC, Verdouw PD, Saxena PR: Improvement of perfusion and function of ischemic porcine myocardium after reduction of heart rate by alinidine. J Cardiovasc Pharmacol 3:728, 1981.
40. Ginneken ACG, Bouman LN, Jongsma HJ, et al: Alinidine as a model of the mode of action of specific bradycardic agents on SA node activity. Eur Heart J 8(Suppl L):25, 1987.
41. van Bogaert PP, Goethals M: Blockade of the pacemaker current by intracellular application UF UL-FS 49 and UL-AH 99 in sheep cardiac Purkinje fibers. Eur J Pharmacol 229:55, 1992.
42. Lillie L, Kobinger W: Differentiation between specific bradycardic agents on calcium channel inhibitors by means of BaCl$_2$ automaticity [abstract #217]. Naunyn Schmiedebergs Arch Pharmacol 335 (Suppl):R55, 1987.
43. DiFrancesco D: The pacemaker current in the sinus node. Eur Heart J 8(Suppl L):19, 1987.
44. van Bogaert PP: Proceedings of the Physiological Society. J Physiol 446:342P, 1992.
45. Goethals M, Raes A, van Bogaert PP: Use-dependent block of the pacemaker current I$_f$ in rabbit sinoatrial node cells by zatebradine (UL-FS 49). Circulation 88(Pt 1):2389, 1993.
46. van Bogaert PP, Goethals M, Simoens C: Use- and frequency-dependent blockade by UL-FS 49 of the I$_f$ pacemaker current in sheep cardiac Purkinje fibers. Eur J Pharmacol 187:241, 1990.
47. Narjes H: Tolerability and pharmacokinetics after a single oral administration of 20, 30, 40 and 50 mg UL-FS 49 CL in healthy volunteers. Bl Deutschland, No. 140.53, Unpublished report, Draft/UL-FS 49, July 20, 1992.

48. Duong N: First use in man, dose-finding, single oral dose, tolerance and pharmacokinetics. Dr. Karl Thomae GmbH, Study No. 140.1, Unpublished report MD-8703/UL-FS 49 (U88-0599), October 11, 1985.

49. Duong N: Dose-effect trial with 5 and 10 mg UL-FS 49 p.o., tolerance and pharmacokinetics in healthy volunteers. Dr. Karl Thomae GmbH, Study No. 140.2, Unpublished report DM-9001/UL-FS 49 (U85-0863), November 25, 1985.

50. Cornelissen PJG, Duong N, van Tol RGL: Placebo-controlled single-dose tolerability, pharmacodynamic and pharmacokinetic study of UL-FS 49 CL in healthy volunteers, administered by infusion (during 20 Minutes) and in increasing doses (1, 2, 5, 10 and 15 mg). Dr. Karl Thomae GmbH, Study No. 140.3, Unpublished report DM-8908/UL-FS 49 (U88-0391), April 15, 1988.

51. Seiberling M: Comparative tolerance, pharmacodynamic and pharmacokinetic study after 7 days oral administration of multiple doses of 2.5, 5 and 10 mg UL-FS 49 CL in healthy volunteers. Biodesign GmbH, Study No. 140.4, Unpublished report MD-8701/UL-FS 49 (U87-0222), November 29, 1986.

52. Duong N: Tolerability, efficacy and pharmacokinetics of 7.5 mg UL-FS 49 CL b.i.d. p.o. for 7 Days in healthy volunteers. Dr. Karl Thomae GmbH, Study No. 140.5, Unpublished report MD-8803/UL-FS 49 (U87-1056), November 4, 1987.

53. Cornelissen PJG, Duong N, van Tol RGL: Single dose pharmacokinetics of [^{14}C]-labelled UL-FS 49 CL: Investigations into blood/plasma level, excretion and metabolite pattern in healthy volunteers following intravenous and oral administration of 7.5 mg UL-FS 49. Dr. Karl Thomae GmbH, Study No. 140.19, Unpublished report MD-9001/UL-FS 49 (U89-0654), November 9, 1989.

54. Brickl R: Steady state kinetics and dose dependency of a tablet formulation of UL-FS 49 CL in healthy volunteers, 2.5, 5 and 10 mg b.i.d. over 4 days. Bl Deutschland No. 140.23, Unpublished report U92-0166/UL-FS 49, March 13, 1992.

55. Duong N: Determination of adrenaline, noradrenaline, renin, angiotensin II and aldosterone during a pilot study with 7.5 mg UL-FS 49 b.i.d. for 3 days in healthy volunteers. Dr. Karl Thomae GmbH, Study No. 140.13, Unpublished report MD-8801/UL-FS 49 (U87-1059), February 22, 1987.

56. Brickl R: Steady state kinetics of a tablet formulation in healthy elderly volunteers: 5 mg UL-FS 49 CL b.i.d. over 4 days—comparison with historical control group of young subjects. Bl Deutschland No. 140.35, Unpublished report U92-0574/UL-FS 49, March 8, 1992.

57. Woodhouse UW, Wynne HA: Age-related changes in liver size and hepatic blood flow. Clin Pharmacokinet 15:287-294, 1988.

58. Chen Z, Slinker BK: The sinus node inhibitor UL-FS 49 lacks significant inotropic effect. J Cardiovasc Pharmacol 19:264, 1992.

59. Forest MC, Cheval B, Brial A: Comparison of the electrophysiological effects of UL-FS 49 and verapamil in canine cardiac purkinje fibers. J Mol Cell Cardiol 23(Suppl IV):S26, 1991.

60. Kobinger W, Lillie C: Cardiovascular characterization of UL-FS 49 CL, 1,3,4,5-tetrahydro-7,8-dimethoxy-3-[3-[[2-(3,4-dimethoxyphenyl)-ethyl]-methylamino]propyl]-2H-3-benzapin-2-one-hydrochloride, a new "specific bradycardic agent." Eur J Pharmacol 104:9, 1984.

61. Bril A: Antiarrhythmic effects of UL-FS 49 in anesthetized rabbits.[Abstract D-12.] The Pharmacologist 32:116, 1990.

62. Breall JA, Watanabe J, Grossman W: Effect of Zatebradine on contractility, relaxation and coronary blood flow. J Am Coll Cardiol 21:471, 1993.

63. Braun E, Roth B, Ball HA: Effects of the bradycardic agent UL-FS 49 in the anesthetized mini pig [abstract 44P]. Eur J Pharmacol 104:9, 1984.

64. Krumpl G, Winkler M, Schneider W, et al: Comparison of the haemodynamic effects of the selective bradycardic agent UL-FS 49, with those of propranolol during treadmill exercise in dogs. Br J Pharmacol 94:55, 1988.

65. Taggart P, Sutton PMI, Lab MJ, et al: Beat-to-beat response of repolarization to transient aortic occlusion in man. J Mol Cell Cardiol 22:282, 1990.

66. Krumpl G, Schneider W, Raberger G: Can exercise-induced regional contractile dysfunction be prevented by selective bradycardic agents? Arch Pharmacol 334:540, 1986.

67. Vatner S, Baig H, Manders WT, et al: Effects of propranolol on regional myocardial function, electrograms, and blood flow in conscious dogs with myocardial ischemia. J Clin Invest 60:353, 1977.

68. Lillie C, Kobinger W: Investigations into the bradycardic effects of UL-FS 49 (1,3,4,5-tetrahydro-7,8-dimethoxy-3-[3-[[2-(3,4-dimethoxyphenyl)-ethyl]-methylamino]propyl]-2H-3-benzazepin-2-one-hydrochloride) in isolated guinea pig atria. J Cardiovasc Pharmacol 8:791, 1986.

69. Obrien PD, Warltier DC: Improvement of ischemic myocardial blood flow and contractile function by simultaneous administration of Dobutamine and UL-FS 49, a special bradycardic agent. [Abstract 924-56.] J Am Coll Cardiol 19:133A, 1992.

70. Lasker SM, Hillel Z, Benjamin E, Shiang H: The hemodynamic interaction of epinephrine with the specific Bradycardic Agent UL-FS 49 [abstract]. Anesthesiology 73:A593, 1990.

71. van Woerkens LJ, van der Giessen WJ, Verdouw PD: The selective bradycardic effects of zatebradine (UL-FS 49) do not adversely affect left ventricular function in conscious pigs with chronic coronary artery occlusion. Cardiovasc Drugs Ther 6:59, 1992.

72. Trolese-Monghea Y, Barthelemy J, Laborde P, et al: Influence of amrinone and milrinone on cardiac rhythm in anesthetized dogs after experimental myocardial infarct. J Mol Cell Cardiol 22:S60, 1990.

73. Riley DC, Gross GJ, Kampine JP, et al: Specific bradycardic agents, a new therapeutic modality for anesthesiology: Hemodynamic effects of UL-FS 49 and propranolol in conscious and isoflurane-anesthetized dogs. Anesthesiology 67:707, 1987.

74. Tanoue T, Pajaro OE, Biasucci LM, et al: Effects of a bradycardic agent (UL-FS 49) on diastolic function during isoflurane anesthesia in the dog [abstract]. Anesthesiology 71:A492, 1989.

75. Rose P: Efficacy and tolerance of 5 and 10 mg UL-FS 49 CL i.v. single doses in patients with stable coronary heart disease compared to placebo. Dr. Karl Thomae GmbH, Study No. 140.6, Unpublished report MD-8901/UL-FS (U88-0820), November 10, 1988.

76. Rose P: Efficacy and effects of 2 x 2.5 mg and 2 x 7.5 mg UL-FS 49 p.o. for 4 weeks in patients with stable angina compared to placebo. Dr. Karl Thomae GmbH, Study No. 140.7, Unpublished Report MD-8802/UL-FS 49 (U88-0175), February 15, 1988.

77. Sieber de Moura V: Exercise effect and tolerability of 1 x 2.5 and 1 x 5.0 mg UL-FS 49 CL i.v. in patients with coronary heart disease compared to placebo. Dr. Karl Thomae GmbH, No. 140.9, Unpublished report U92-0395/UL-FS 49, February 9, 1991.

78. Baiker W: Efficacy, duration of action and tolerability of 2 x 1.25 mg, 2 x 2.5 mg and 2 x 5 mg UL-FS 49 CL p.o. for 2 weeks in patients with stable angina compared to placebo. Dr. Karl Thomae GmbH, Study No. 140.16, Unpublished report MD-9102/UL-FS 49 (U91-0459).

79. Duong D: Pharmacodynamic, pharmacokinetic and tolerability study of a single i.v. dose of UL-FS 49 CL (rapid infusion of 5 mg in 5 min., followed by maintenance infusion of 5 mg in 45 min.) compared to placebo in healthy volunteers. Bl Deutschland No. 140.55, Unpublished report U92-0555/UL-FS 49, August 27, 1992.

80. Baiker W: Effects on cardiac stimulus conduction system of 5 mg UL-FS 49 CL i.v. with subsequent infusion of 5 mg UL-FS 49 CL over 95 minutes as maintenance dose compared to placebo. Bl Deutschland, No. 140.14, Unpublished report U92-0628/UL-FS 49.

81. Herberg KW: Effects of p.o. administration of 2.5, 7.5 and 15 mg UL-FS 49 CL, each twice daily for 7 days, versus placebo, on the driving ability in healthy volunteers. Dr. Karl Thomae GmbH, Study 140.18, Unpublished report MD-9002/UL-FS 49 (U89-0651), October 2, 1989.

82. Lutzen L: Determination of the LD$_{50}$ of substance UL-FS 49 CL in the rat following oral administration. Dr. Karl Thomae GmbH, Unpublished report U82-0152, April 6, 1982.

83. Serbedija R: Determination of the ALD$_{50}$ of substance UL-FS 49 CL in the dog following oral administration. Dr. Karl Thomae GmbH, Unpublished report U82-0154, May 12, 1982.

84. Lutzen L: Determination of the ALD$_{50}$ of substance UL-FS 49 CL in the rabbit following intravenous administration. Dr. Karl Thomae GmbH, Unpublished Report U82-0153, April 14, 1982.

85. Wiegleb J, Roth W, Eckenfels A, et al: Toxicity study of UL-FS 49 CL with oral administration to beagle dogs over a period of 12 months. Dr. Karl Thomae GmbH, Unpublished report U89-0283, October 27, 1988.

86. Roth W: UL-FS 49 CL determination of plasma levels in a 12-month chronic toxicity study in beagle dogs doses: 1, 5 and 25 mg/kg p.o. Dr. Karl Thomae GmbH, Unpublished report U88-0649, August 30, 1988.

87. Wiegleb J, Eckenfels A, Bauer M, Puschner H: Toxicity study of UL-FS 49 CL following intravenous administration to beagle dogs over a period of 4 weeks. Dr. Karl Thomae GmbH, Unpublished report U88-0417, March 31, 1988.

88. Roth W: Report: UL-FS 49 CL determination of plasma levels in a 4-week subchronic i.v. toxicity study in the dog. Dr. Karl Thomae GmbH, Unpublished report U88-0380, May 4, 1988.

89. BoSmith RE, Briggs I, Sturgess NC: Inhibition of the hyperpolarisation activated cationic current (I_F) by ICI D7288 in guinea-pig isolated sinoatrial node cells. Br J Pharmacol 108:126P, 1993.

90. Marshall PW, Bramley J, Briggs I: The effects of ICI D7288, a Novelsino-atrial node modulating agent, on guinea pig isolated atria. Br J Pharmacol 107:134P, 1992.

91. BoSmith RE, Briggs I, Danks P, et al: Actions of ICI D7288 on sinoatrial node cellular electrophysiology: Whole-cell currents. Br J Pharmacol 107:381P, 1992.

92. Briggs I, Heapy CG: Actions of ICI D7288 on sinoatrial node cellular electrophysiology: Action potentials. Br J Pharmacol 107:382P, 1992.

93. Rouse W, Johnson IR: Haemodynamic comparison of ICI D7288 and alinidine, propranolol, verapamil and zatebradine. Br J Pharmacol 108(Suppl):138P, 1993.

94. Rouse W, Johnson IR: Haemodynamic actions of ICI D7288, a novel sinoatrial node modulator. Br J Pharmacol 107:383P, 1992.

95. Banning MM, Curtis MJ: Ischaemia-induced and reperfusion-induced arrhythmias in the isolated rat heart are suppressed by cimetidine without haemodynamic or electrocardiographic alteration. Br J Pharmacol 110:121P, 1993.

96. Rouse W, Johnson IR: Haemodynamic comparison of ICI D7288 and alinidine, propranolol, verapamil and zatebradine. Br J Pharmacol 108:4193, 1993.

97. Marshall PW, Rouse W, Briggs I, et al: ICI D7288, a novel sinoatrial node modulator. J Cardiovasc Pharmacol 21:902, 1993.

98. Donovan A: ICI D7288: Ascending dose safety and tolerance study in human volunteers. Study No. 0001. Data on file. Boehringer Pharmaceutical Co., 1992.

99. Donovan A: ICI D7288: Comparative bioavailability study in human volunteers. Study No. 0002. Data on file. Boehringer Pharmaceutical Co., 1992.

100. Donovan A: ICI D7288: Isoprenaline challenge study in human volunteers. Study No. 0003. Data on file. Boehringer Pharmaceutical Co., 1992.

101. Donovan A: ICI D7288: Exercise challenge study in human volunteers. Study No. 0004. Data on file. Boehringer Pharmaceutical Co., 1992.

102. Donovan A: ICI D7288: Repeat dose study in human volunteers. Study No. 0005. Data on file. Boehringer Pharmaceutical Co., 1992.

XV.

Antithrombotic Therapy

A. Principles and Practice of Antithrombotic Therapy

CHAPTER 152

Antithrombotic Therapy for the Prevention of Cardiac and Arterial Thromboembolism

Thomas G. DiSalvo, M.D., Douglas H. Israel, M.D., Bernardo Stein, M.D., James H. Chesebro, M.D., and Valentin Fuster, M.D.

This chapter discusses experimental and clinical evidence supporting the role of antithrombotic therapy in preventing the following:

1. Intracardiac thrombosis and systemic embolization
2. Prosthetic heart valve thromboembolism
3. Arterial thrombosis *in situ* with emphasis on coronary artery disease
4. Saphenous vein bypass graft thrombotic disease

The desirable intensity of anticoagulation differs with the magnitude of thromboembolic risk and pathogenesis of thrombosis. Determination of the prothrombin time depends on the source of the thromboplastin reagent: Human brain thromboplastin is more sensitive than rabbit brain thromboplastin. The international normalized ratio (INR) was introduced by the World Health Organization to standardize prothrombin time.[1, 2]

INTRACARDIAC THROMBOSIS AND SYSTEMIC EMBOLIZATION

As first proposed by Virchow, three broad disturbances predispose to thrombosis: (1) endothelial injury, (2) abnormal rheology of blood flow (including stasis, turbulence, and elevated shear rates found at the site of vascular stenoses), and (3) hypercoagulability. Coronary artery endothelial dysfunction due to atherosclerosis and ventricular subendocardial endothelial dysfunction due to myocardial infarction (MI) predispose to thrombosis in the coronary arteries and ventricular chambers, respectively. Depressed contractility or dyssynergia of myocardial segments predisposes to intraventricular mural thrombosis.

Ventricular Thrombi

Acute Myocardial Infarction

Incidence of Thrombus Formation

Left ventricular mural thrombosis is the major cause of systemic embolization following acute MI (Table 152–1). More than 90% of all mural thrombi arise following acute transmural anterior infarctions that involve the ventricular apex. Mural thrombi occur in 20% of all MIs, 40% of all anterior infarctions, and 60% of large anterior MIs involving the apex with creatine phosphokinase levels in excess of 2000 IU/L.[3] Mural thrombi develop in only 5% of inferior infarctions.[3–12] At postmortem examination of fatal MIs, mural thrombi are demonstrable in 40% to 70% of cases not treated with anticoagulants and in 22% to 24% of cases treated with anticoagulants.[13]

Table 152–1. **Prevalences of Mural Thrombus Formation and Systemic Embolism in Patients With Acute Myocardial Infarction and Chronic Forms of Left Ventricular Dysfunction**

Disorder	Mural Thrombi (%)	Stroke and Embolism (Events per 100 Patient-Years)
Acute myocardial infarction		
All	10–20	1–3
Anterior	30–40	2–6
Large apical	60–70	10–20
Inferior	<5	<1
Chronic ventricular aneurysm	50	1
Dilated cardiomyopathy		
Diffuse	30	3–4
Segmental	15	3

From Fuster V, Verstraete M (eds): Thrombosis in Cardiovascular Disorders. Philadelphia: WB Saunders, 1992.

Pathogenesis

Mural thrombi form following MI because of the combined effects of endocardial endothelial damage and stasis. Striking histopathologic alterations are observed in the ventricular endocardial endothelium following transmural MI.[14] Endothelial separation from the basal lamina due to extensive leukocytic infiltration with subsequent endothelial desquamation and exposure of the underlying denuded basal lamina and subendothelium are intense stimuli to thrombosis. Stasis adjacent to akinetic or dyskinetic segments of the left ventricle activates coagulation factors under conditions of low shear rates, as does the transient hypercoagulable state commonly observed after MI.[15] Finally, the nonendothelialized surface of the evolving thrombus is itself intensely thrombogenic, largely because of the activity of enzymatically active fibrin-bound thrombin.[16]

Diagnosis

In pooled series, two-dimensional echocardiography has a sensitivity of 77% to 95% and a specificity of 88% to 94% for detecting intraventricular thrombi.[17-22] Twenty-five percent of thrombi are apparent within the first 24 hours following infarction, 50% within 2 to 3 days, 75% within 7 days, and the remainder within 10 to 14 days.[3] Echocardiographic resolution of thrombi is not uncommon: fully 20% to 30% of thrombi resolve per year following infarction.[4, 5, 20, 23-25] Most thrombi either stabilize or become undetectable by echocardiography following 1 to 3 months of oral anticoagulation.[4, 5, 20] Anticoagulant therapy accelerates the rate of echocardiographic resolution. Resolution is less common with persistent apical dyskinesis or advanced left ventricular dysfunction.[26] Although transesophageal echocardiography (TEE) is more sensitive in the detection of small apical thrombi than transthoracic echocardiography, to date no large series have compared the relative sensitivities of the two techniques.[27, 28] Newer imaging modalities, such as ultrafast computerized tomography (CT) and magnetic resonance tomography, may have sensitivities equivalent to TEE but also have yet to be compared in large studies. Indium-111 labeled platelet techniques are sensitive in the detection of ventricular thrombi, but imaging requires 48 to 72 hours.[3]

Incidence of Embolism

Embolism is twice as common with echocardiographically demonstrable thrombi.[4, 20] However, up to 24% of patients who experience embolism do not have an echocardiographically detectable thrombus.[29] Overall, approximately 10% of all patients with detectable mural thrombi experience systemic embolism; series report ranges from 5% to 26%.[5] In one study of fatal MI, however, postmortem examination revealed systemic embolism in 50%.[30] In the absence of anticoagulant therapy, stroke occurs in 1% to 3% of all patients with MI, in 2% to 6% of patients with anterior MI, and

in 10% to 20% of patients with large anteroapical infarctions.[17] Risk of stroke is highest in the first 3 months following infarction but persists in the presence of significant left ventricular dysfunction, heart failure, or atrial fibrillation. It is not yet proven that echocardiographically detectable left ventricular thrombosis increases mortality independent of residual left ventricular function.[31]

Risk Factors for Embolism

Embolism risk is greatest in the first week following infarction.[31] Risk increases with infarct size, depression of left ventricular function, and coexistent atrial fibrillation. As the extent of thrombus mobility (due to pedunculation) and the extent of thrombus protuberance into the left ventricular cavity by echocardiography rise, the risk of embolism increases.[32, 33] Thrombus adjacent to hyperkinetic ventricular segments may be at higher risk. By itself, thrombus size does not appear to be as significant a predictor of embolism as mobility and protuberance. Up to 40% of emboli occur in the absence of apparent thrombus mobility or protuberance by echocardiography.[29] Abnormal flow patterns within the left ventricle as detected by pulsed Doppler echocardiography may predict thrombus formation: a free vortex ring flow pattern (representing a delay in onset of blood motion at the apical level compared with the mitral valve inflow level) and an apical rotating flow pattern are highly associated with thrombus formation following anteroapical MI.[34]

Clinical Trials of Antithrombotic Therapy

In pooled results of three large trials of heparin and orally administered anticoagulants in MI, cerebral embolism was reduced from 3% to 1%.[35-37] Anticoagulation decreases the incidence of noncerebral arterial embolism in survivors of MI.[5, 19, 22, 35, 38, 39] Immediate anticoagulation after hospital admission effectively reduces the incidence of left ventricular mural thrombus,[35] but warfarin therapy begun after detection of thrombus may not lessen the incidence of systemic emboli.[40] In an echocardiographic series, early (within 48 hours of symptom onset) thrombus formation following MI was an independent predictor of increased in-hospital mortality in a multivariate model (42.5% versus 13%, $p < .008$) despite similar Killip class.[41] Deferring the decision to anticoagulate until echocardiography is performed may cause therapy to be postponed while it is most valuable.

The intensity of anticoagulation is important. Turpie et al. randomized 221 patients following thrombolysis to subcutaneously administered heparin, 12,500 IU or 5000 IU every 12 hours.[42] Thrombi were significantly decreased in the high-dose heparin group (11% versus 32%, $p = .0004$). In the SCATI trial, 200 of the 771 patients randomized to heparin (12,500 IU subcutaneously) or no heparin underwent initial and follow-up echocardiograms to detect left ventricular thrombus.[43] Heparin significantly decreased ventricular thrombus on the predischarge echocardiogram (18% versus 37%, $p < .01$).

A meta-analysis has addressed the role of anticoagulant and thrombolytic therapy in the prevention of mural thrombosis and embolism.[29] In 11 studies, the pooled odds ratio (OR) of embolism was significantly increased for cases of MI with echocardiographically detected mural thrombus over the OR for cases without (OR 5.45, 95% confidence interval 3.02 to 9.83). Anticoagulant therapy significantly decreased embolism (OR 0.14, 95% confidence interval 0.04 to 0.52) and echocardiographically detectable mural thrombus (OR 0.32, 95% confidence interval 0.2 to 0.52). Thrombolytic therapy decreased mural thrombus formation (OR 0.48, 95% confidence interval 0.29 to 0.79), but antiplatelet therapy alone did not (OR 1.43, 95% confidence interval 0.04 to 56.8).

Trials of Thrombolytic Therapy

The only randomized trial to date of thrombolytic agents with and without heparin in the prevention of ventricular mural thrombosis showed no difference between streptokinase alone, streptokinase plus heparin, t-PA alone, or t-PA plus heparin in the prevention of thrombi at hospital discharge.[44] In this small substudy of GISSI-2, use of heparin—although it did not result in fewer thrombi overall—did result in significantly fewer thrombi that were protuberant in shape. This study lacked statistical power because of the small sample size. Studies of thrombolytic therapy administered within 24 hours of symptom onset of MI, the period during which many thrombi form, have yielded conflicting results. In the LATE trial, there was no difference in the incidence of ischemic stroke among groups.[45] In the EMERAS trial, there was significant reduction in ischemic stroke over the 35 day follow-up period.[46] Thrombolytic agents likely decrease intraventricular thrombus formation by ameliorating segmental left ventricular asynergy and improving overall left ventricular function.

The presence of an apical mobile ventricular thrombus following MI is not an indication for thrombolytic therapy in an attempt to lyse the thrombus. In a report of four such patients treated with streptokinase in the dose employed in thrombosed prosthetic valves (375,000 IU bolus followed by 70,000 IU/hr and heparin, 1000 IU/hr), one transient ischemic attack and one death from a large embolic stroke occurred.[47] Lysis of the thrombus stalk at the point of attachment to the ventricular wall was the likely mechanism.

Treatment Recommendations (Table 152–2)

Without waiting for echocardiographic evidence of thrombus, patients with Q-wave anterior infarction or extensive inferior infarction involving the apex should receive immediate intravenous heparin therapy (5000 IU intravenous bolus followed by a 1000-U/hr continuous intravenous infusion) or adjusted high-dose subcutaneously administered heparin (12,500 IU every 12 hours) to maintain the activated

Table 152–2. Antithrombotic Therapy for the Prevention of Ventricular Thrombi

Cardiac Disease	Recommendations
AMI	IV heparin acutely after large anterior AMI or inferior AMI involving the apex
	Warfarin for 3 months (PT 1.5 times control, INR 2.0 to 3.0)
LV aneurysm	IV heparin followed by warfarin for only 3 months after AMI (PT 1.5 times control, INR 2.0 to 3.0)
	Long-term warfarin (INR 2.0 to 3.0) if LV dysfunction is severe or after embolic event
Dilated cardiomyopathy	Long-term warfarin (PT 1.5 times control, INR 2.0 to 3.0)

AMI, acute myocardial infarction; INR, international normalized ratio; LV, left ventricular; PT, prothrombin time.

partial thromboplastin time (aPTT) at 1.5 to 2.0 times control (see Table 152–1). Simultaneously, orally administered anticoagulants should be begun and overlapped for at least 3 days with heparin to allow for depletion of all vitamin K–dependent clotting factors. Oral anticoagulation with intermediate intensity is advised (prothrombin time 1.5 to 2.0 times control, INR 2.5 to 3.5). A lower intensity of anticoagulation (prothrombin time 1.3 to 1.5 times control, INR 2 to 3) may be sufficient.[35] Warfarin may be discontinued after 3 months unless there is cardiac failure, atrial fibrillation, or extensive left ventricular dysfunction, in which case warfarin should be continued indefinitely. Although routine long-term therapy with warfarin is efficacious in the secondary prevention of MI, in lower-risk patients,[48] therapy with aspirin is less costly, simpler, and equally effective. Thrombolysis is not considered standard therapy for left ventricular thrombus complicating MI: one fatality has been reported to date. Rarely, surgery with excision of the thrombus has been performed in patients with large mobile thrombi or recurrent emboli despite adequate anticoagulation.

Left Ventricular Aneurysm

Thrombus within a left ventricular aneurysm is found in 48% to 95% of surgical patients undergoing aneurysmectomy.[39, 49] In autopsy series, thrombus is found within left ventricular aneurysms in 49% of cases.[50] After the first 3 months following infarction and aneurysm formation, however, clinically manifest embolism is infrequent, occurring with an event rate of 0.35 per 100 patient-years. Intraaneurysmal thrombi form during the acute phase of MI and persist, undergoing organization and reendothelialization. Ultimately, the thrombi become laminated and adherent to the underlying aneurysmal sac.[3] Because the thrombus is contained within the noncontractile aneurysmal cul-de-sac and does not usually protrude into the left ventricle, it is protected from contact with the circulation. Given the risk of complications from long-term anticoagulation and the considerably lower risk of embolism in this setting compared with acute MI or dilated cardiomyopathy, long-term anticoagulation is not recommended. Whether the occasional patient with a mobile or protuberant aneurysm-associated thrombus benefits from long-term anticoagulant therapy has not been addressed. Antiplatelet therapy has not been studied in this setting.

Treatment Recommendations (see Table 152–2)

The 1% or 2% per year risk of bleeding complications associated with orally administered anticoagulants outweighs the benefits of anticoagulation in chronic left ventricular aneurysm. Routine anticoagulation is not advised beyond the first 3 months following infarction in the presence of a ventricular aneurysm (see Table 152–1). Patients with chronic left ventricular aneurysms who experience emboli or who have a significantly reduced ejection fraction (less than 35%), clinical congestive heart failure, or atrial fibrillation should undergo anticoagulation.

Dilated Cardiomyopathy

Incidence of Thrombus Formation and Embolic Risk

Intracavitary mural thrombi are found in 30% to 50% of patients with dilated cardiomyopathy (DCM) of any etiology at postmortem examination.[51] Echocardiography detects left ventricular thrombi in up to 36% of cases.[25] Clinical embolism occurs in approximately 10% to 20% of all patients with DCM regardless of etiology (see Table 152–1). In the retrospective Mayo Clinic study, the rate of clinical emboli complicating DCM was moderately high, at 3.5% per year.[52] Embolism occurred in 14% of patients in sinus rhythm and in 33% of patients in atrial fibrillation. Patients receiving anticoagulants in this study had no thromboemboli in 101 patient-years of follow-up. In a small series of serial echocardiography in patients with nonischemic DCM, the presence of a previously detected thrombus, particularly if protuberant, was associated with increased embolism.[53] Magnetic resonance imaging reveals a high incidence of brain parenchymal abnormalities, likely embolic in origin, in neurologically asymptomatic patients with DCM.[54] Pulmonary emboli occur with the same frequency (11%) as systemic emboli do.[55]

Pathogenesis

Abnormal intracavitary blood flow patterns resulting in stasis and abnormalities of hemostasis both contribute to the pathogenesis of intracavitary thrombosis in DCM. By echocardiographic pulsed wave Doppler flow sampling, lower inflow velocities at the ventricular apex, generally lower flow velocities throughout the ventricle, and significantly lower systolic flow velocity at the apex have been observed in patients with DCM and ventricular thrombi compared with patients with DCM and no ventricular thrombi.[56] Elevations of fibrinogen, plasma viscosity, whole blood

viscoelasticity, and red cell aggregation have been reported in DCM in the absence of diuretic-induced hemoconcentration,[57] as have significantly elevated plasma levels of β-thromboglobulin, D-dimers, and thrombin–antithrombin III complexes (indicative of platelet activation, fibrinolytic activity, and thrombin activation, respectively).[58] Ventricular thrombi in DCM tend to be small, multiple, and not necessarily localized to the most dyskinetic regions. Unlike acute MI, ventricular thrombosis may be a diffuse process throughout the ventricular chamber. Importantly, because of chronic alterations in intraventricular blood flow patterns and stasis, thromboembolism poses a continuous risk.

Treatment Recommendations (see Table 152–2)

Anticoagulation in DCM has not been studied in a prospective, randomized way. However, in view of the chronic risk of embolism and the efficacy of anticoagulation in preventing emboli in our study,[52] long-term anticoagulation with warfarin (prothrombin time 1.5 to 2.0 times control, INR 2.0 to 3.0) is recommended regardless of the etiology of cardiomyopathy once the ejection fraction falls below 35% (see Table 152–1). This indication becomes stronger in the presence of atrial fibrillation, decompensated cardiac failure, or prolonged bed rest.

Atrial Thrombi

Although incompletely understood, stasis is important to atrial thrombosis, particularly in the setting of a dilated, fibrillating atrium. Loss of mechanical atrial contraction predisposes to sluggish flow, long local residence time of coagulation proteins, and the formation of red cell rouleaux, platelet clumps, and eventually fibrin-rich thrombi. This process of rouleaux and platelet clump formation can be detected frequently in dilated, fibrillating atria by the appearance of spontaneous atrial contrast or "smoke" by two-dimensional echocardiography, even in the absence of apparent atrial thrombus.

Valvular Heart Disease

Mitral Valve Disease

Incidence

Embolism is more frequent in rheumatic mitral valve disease than in any other type of common heart disease.[59] The greatest risk of thromboembolism occurs in isolated mitral stenosis or combined mitral stenosis and regurgitation. Thrombi occur most commonly in the left atrial appendage. The incidence of embolism in nonanticoagulated patients varies from 1% to 5% per year.[60–68] Over the entire course of rheumatic mitral disease, the incidence of systemic embolism is approximately 27%.[59] Seventy-five percent of emboli involve the cerebral circulation, and emboli may be the presenting symptom of rheumatic mitral disease in up to 12.4% of cases.[69, 70]

Before the advent of anticoagulation, thromboembolism accounted for 16% to 19% of mortality in mitral stenosis.[62, 67] In Wood's experience, emboli occurred 1.5 times more commonly in mitral stenosis than in rheumatic mitral regurgitation.[70] Isolated mitral regurgitation carries a smaller but still substantial risk of systemic thromboembolism. The risk of embolism is greater with increasing severity of valvular regurgitation and in patients with mixed mitral stenosis and regurgitation.[62] Embolism may complicate the clinical course in as many as 14% to 18% of such patients.[61] Overall, in a 10-year follow-up period, 2.9 events occurred per 100 patient-years.[60]

Risk Factors for Embolism

Atrial fibrillation increases the risk of embolism 6 to 18 times in rheumatic mitral disease and is by far the most important risk factor.[59] Other risk factors include history of embolism, older age, and low cardiac index.[59] Left atrial size, mitral calcification, mitral valve area, and clinical functional classification do not correlate well with risk of embolism: embolism may occur with minor degrees of valvular disease, including in asymptomatic patients. Left atrial enlargement does not appear to be an independent risk factor for embolism but does increase the risk of atrial fibrillation. Because most emboli occur shortly after the onset of atrial fibrillation (a third occur within 1 month, and two thirds occur within 1 year), the physician is responsible for anticipating atrial fibrillation and beginning oral anticoagulation before the onset of atrial fibrillation.[61] Emboli recur commonly (30% to 65% of the time), usually within 6 months, and are associated with substantial mortality.[61, 66] Mitral valvuloplasty does not appear to decrease the incidence of subsequent embolism.[59]

Clinical Trials

No randomized, primary prevention trials of orally administered anticoagulants in rheumatic mitral valve disease have been performed (Table 152–3). Retrospective studies document the efficacy of orally administered anticoagulants in preventing recurrence of emboli.[61, 71–73]

Treatment Recommendations (Table 152–4)

Patients with mitral stenosis, mitral regurgitation, or mixed lesions in atrial fibrillation are at high risk for thromboembolism. Long-term anticoagulation with warfarin is advised (prothrombin time to 1.5 to 2 times control, INR 2.5 to 3.5; see Table 152–2). Atrial fibrillation should be anticipated in patients in sinus rhythm who have left atrial dilatation of more than 50 to 55 mm by echocardiography. These patients should undergo prophylactic anticoagulation in an attempt to lower the high risk of embolism immediately after the onset of atrial fibrillation. Patients with previous episodes of embolism or impaired left ventricular systolic function (ejection fraction less than

Table 152–3. Valvular Heart Disease: Indications for Anticoagulation

Medium risk*
1. Atrial fibrillation (chronic or paroxysmal) in mitral regurgitation or after anticoagulation for 1 year in mitral stenosis
2. Sinus rhythm with a very large left atrium (>55 mm by M-mode echocardiography)
3. Presence of heart failure or severe left ventricular dysfunction

High risk†
4. Atrial fibrillation (chronic or paroxysmal) in mitral stenosis during the first year of anticoagulation
5. History of previous systemic embolism

---

*International normalized ratio = 2.0 to 3.0.[17] Prothrombin time to 1.3 to 1.5 times control for usual North American thromboplastins.
†International normalized ratio = 3.0 to 4.5[17] Prothrombin time to 1.5 to 1.8 times control.
Modified from Chesebro JH, Adams PC, Fuster V: Antithrombotic therapy in patients with valvular heart disease and prosthetic heart valves. J Am Coll Cardiol 8:41B, 1986. Reprinted with permission from the American College of Cardiology.

35%) should undergo anticoagulation. The number of patients requiring anticoagulation increases with age. If disease is hemodynamically insignificant, no anticoagulation is required, provided none of the other risk factors for thromboembolism previously discussed are present. Platelet inhibitor therapy may be efficacious in low-risk patients, but evidence is not conclusive to date.[74] Aspirin, 325 mg daily, is recommended in the event of strong contraindications to warfarin. In patients with recurrent embolism despite warfarin, low-dose aspirin (80 to 160 mg/day) may be considered in combination with warfarin. At present, patients prior to percutaneous mitral valvuloplasty are usually treated with warfarin for several weeks prior

Table 152–4. Antithrombotic Therapy in Valvular Heart Disease and Nonvalvular Atrial Fibrillation

Cardiac Disease	Recommendation
Mitral stenosis	Long-term warfarin (PT 1.5 to 2 times control, INR 3 to 4.5) if atrial fibrillation is present
	Consider warfarin for patients in sinus rhythm with large LA (>50 mm by M-mode echocardiogram)
Mitral regurgitation	Long-term warfarin in high-risk patients (atrial fibrillation, LV dysfunction, prior embolic events)
Mitral valve prolapse	Aspirin, 325 mg/day, if neurologic events of unclear etiology occur
	Warfarin in case of obvious embolic event*
Aortic valve disease	No therapy needed in the absence of other risk factors for thromboembolism
Nonvalvular atrial fibrillation	Long-term warfarin (PT 1.2 to 1.5 times control, INR 2 to 3)
	Aspirin, 325 mg/day, in low-risk patients (lone atrial fibrillation)†

INR, international normalized ratio; LA, left atrium; LV, left ventricular; PT, prothrombin time.
*This therapy needs to be submitted to clinical trials.
†A randomized trial of low-dose warfarin, aspirin, and placebo is under way.

to the procedure to decrease their chances of embolism during the procedure.

Mitral Valve Prolapse

Incidence and Mechanism of Thromboembolism

Mitral valve prolapse (MVP) is a common condition, occurring in 6% of women and 4% of men.[59] MVP is uncommonly associated with transient and permanent ischemic events.[75] In an early case-control study, Barnett et al. found that MVP was much more frequent (OR 9.33, $p < .001$) in a group of patients under age 45 with transient ischemia or partial stroke than in an older group of patients.[76] Although MVP has been reported in as many as 40% of young patients with transient ischemia or stroke,[59–61] the overall incidence of stroke is low in the population of young adults with MVP and has been estimated at 1 in 6000/year.[59]

Stroke results from embolism in the setting of MVP because of several mechanisms: (1) fibrinous nonbacterial thrombotic endocarditis of the mitral valve (seen only with significant mitral regurgitation and valvular redundancy), (2) endothelial denudation of the mitral valve with subsequent formation of leaflet fibrin thrombi, and (3) mural thrombosis of the atrium due to mitral regurgitation. Most cerebral emboli are small and result in transient ischemic attacks or small strokes.[77] In the individual patient, it is often difficult to establish a causal relationship between valvular disease and cerebral ischemia. Common causes of cerebral ischemia must be excluded before implicating MVP, especially in elderly patients.[3]

Thromboembolic Risk Factors

Embolic risk due to MVP is clearly related to the severity of prolapse, leaflet redundancy, and degree of mitral regurgitation. A follow-up study of 237 patients (mean 6 years) showed that patients with redundant mitral valve leaflets as identified by echocardiography experienced significantly more complications than those without redundant leaflets.[78] In this study, 10 patients had cerebral emboli, but only 2 experienced cerebral emboli in the absence of other risk factors for embolization (atrial fibrillation, endocarditis, ventricular thrombus). A retrospective echocardiographic series of 465 patients showed that infective endocarditis, moderate-to-severe mitral incompetence, mitral valve replacement, but not stroke (7.5% versus 5.8%, $p = $ NS) were more common in patients with mitral-valve leaflet thickening and redundancy than in those without.[79] This study made no attempt to determine the etiology of stroke. The retrospective nature of this study and possible selection bias limits its generalizability to the population of patients with MVP, especially as regards the risk of embolic stroke.

Treatment Recommendations (see Table 152–4)

Routine prophylactic antithrombotic therapy is unwarranted in patients with MVP, given the low incidence of embolism in this common condition. If other risk factors for embolism are also present in patients with MVP (chronic or paroxysmal atrial fibrillation, left atrial size >55 mm, significant mitral regurgitation, heart failure or severe left ventricular dysfunction, history of previous systemic embolism), appropriate prophylactic antithrombotic therapy is warranted. After a mild or transient embolic event in a patient with MVP, oral anticoagulation for 3 to 6 months is indicated while other possible causes of cerebral ischemia are investigated. If no other cause of cerebral ischemia is found, and if risk factors for future embolism as discussed are absent, patients may be treated with long-term aspirin therapy (80 to 325 mg/day). If risk factors for embolism are present, long-term anticoagulation with warfarin (INR 2 to 3) is indicated. If a questionable neurologic event occurs in a patient with MVP, it is appropriate to use aspirin in a dose of 80 to 325 mg/day. Other causes of cerebral ischemia should be investigated.

Mitral Annular Calcification

The clinical syndrome of mitral annular calcification is associated with mitral stenosis and regurgitation, calcific aortic stenosis, conduction disturbances, arrhythmias, embolic phenomena, and endocarditis.[59] Embolic events occur with and without atrial fibrillation. Emboli may be composed of either fibrin clots or calcium spicules. In the Framingham study, the presence of mitral annular calcification in multivariate analysis was associated with a relative risk of stroke of 2.10 (95% confidence interval 1.24 to 3.57, $p = .006$). This effect was independent of other risk factors for stroke, but whether mitral annular calcification itself contributed causally to risk of stroke or was a marker of increased risk could not be determined from the study.[80] Prior data from the Framingham study also indicated that the presence of mitral annular calcification increased the risk of atrial fibrillation 12-fold.[81] There have been no trials of antithrombotic therapy in patients with mitral annular calcification alone. At present, treatment of these patients should be based on the presence of associated valvular stenosis or regurgitation, atrial fibrillation, or prior embolism.

Aortic Valve Disease

Clinical thromboemboli are much less common in aortic valve disease, being most frequently seen with concomitant atrial fibrillation, mitral valve disease, or infective endocarditis.[82–84] Few long-term data pinpoint the incidence of embolism in disorders of the aortic valve. In a series of 68 patients with moderate to severe aortic incompetence followed for 10 years, emboli complicated the clinical course in 4.4% of patients, with an overall event rate of 0.83% per 100 patient-years.[85] Autopsy studies have documented platelet deposition on abnormal aortic valvular endothelium in aortic stenosis, perhaps accounting for some of the neurologic symptoms seen in these patients.[86] However, many if not most emboli in aortic stenosis are calcific, frequently small and subclinical. Pathologic study has detected calcareous emboli, largely clinically silent, in up to 19% of patients with aortic stenosis.[87] Calcific emboli occur independently of the severity of the lesion; they may be the initial presenting feature of aortic stenosis and may lead to transient or permanent monocular blindness as a result of retinal artery involvement.[88] Detection of cerebral or central retinal artery emboli in patients with aortic stenosis may be obscured by the frequent occurrence of transient neurologic symptoms due to arrhythmias and altered hemodynamics in this disorder. Great care must be taken during cardiac catheterization and cardiac surgery not to dislodge emboli from the calcareous aortic valve.

Treatment Recommendations (see Table 152–4)

There is a low risk of embolism in either aortic stenosis or regurgitation. Despite evidence that some emboli occur because of platelet deposition on abnormal aortic valve endothelium, no study supports a role for platelet inhibitor therapy or anticoagulants in aortic valve disease. There is no effective therapy for the calcific emboli that occur not infrequently in aortic stenosis. Recurrence of calcific emboli may warrant aortic valve replacement. Patients with aortic valve disease and other risk factors for embolism as detailed in previous discussions should undergo anticoagulation.

Nonvalvular Atrial Fibrillation

Incidence

Nonvalvular atrial fibrillation (NVAF) is the most common cardiac disorder predisposing to cardiogenic embolism.[89] The prevalence of NVAF is 0.4% in all adults, 0.5% in adults under the age of 60, and 10% in adults older than the age of 75.[90] The cumulative 22-year incidence of NVAF in the Framingham study was 21.5 cases per 1000 men and 17.1 cases per 1000 women.[91] In the United States, over 1 million adults are thus affected. In the Framingham study, the presence of NVAF doubled overall mortality and cardiovascular mortality.[91] Because the mean age of onset is 64 years, NVAF is a common significant cause of morbidity and mortality in the elderly.[71]

Incidence of Stroke

Of patients with NVAF, 25% to 35% suffer stroke, accounting for 75,000 strokes per year. In patients with NVAF and cerebral ischemia, 50% to 70% of episodes are embolic.[90] NVAF is found in 45% of all patients with cardioembolic stroke. In the Framingham study, the incidence of stroke in patients with NVAF rose from 2.6 per 1000 at ages 25 to 34 to 37.9 at ages 55 to 64 for men, and from 2.2 per 1000 at ages 25 to 34 to 29.9 per 1000 at ages 55 to 64 for women.[91] There is a high incidence of silent cerebral infarcts as documented by CT of the brain in patients with NVAF as well.[92]

Risk Factors for Stroke

In the absence of anticoagulation, the risk of stroke in NVAF is approximately 5% per year.[90, 93] High risk occurs with coexisting rheumatic mitral valvular disease, a mechanical prosthetic valve, and thromboembolism within the previous 2 years (Table 152–5).[3] The presence of other cardiac disease (hypertension, mitral regurgitation, congestive heart failure, ischemic heart disease), older age, recent onset of NVAF, history of previous thromboembolism beyond 2 years also increase the risk of embolism.[90, 95] Paroxysmal NVAF may confer a slight reduction in risk of embolism compared with sustained NVAF, although this reduction is unlikely to be substantial.[90, 96] In the SPAF and BAATAF trials of anticoagulant therapy of NVAF, paroxysmal NVAF conferred the same risk of embolism as did sustained NVAF in the control groups.[97, 98] Thyrotoxicosis also likely increases the baseline risk of embolism due to NVAF, although large studies have not been reported.[94] Of thyrotoxic patients, 10% to 30% develop NVAF.[89]

Low-risk patients with NVAF include those with "lone" atrial fibrillation: patients under the age of 60 who lack any signs, symptoms, or history of cardiovascular disease and who have structurally normal hearts by echocardiography. Patients with lone fibrillation account for 2.7% to 11.4% of all patients with NVAF.[89] Two long-term follow-up studies have investigated the risk of stroke in patients with lone NVAF. In a 30-year follow-up study of 97 patients from the Mayo Clinic, there was no difference in survival or survival free of stroke among patients with isolated, recurrent, or chronic lone NVAF.[99] The cumulative actuarial stroke risk was 1.3%, with a calculated stroke event rate of 0.35% per 100 patient-years. In a smaller 30-year follow-up case-control study from the Framingham study, patients with lone atrial fibril-

Table 152–5. **Risk Factors for Stroke in NVAF**

High risk

   Rheumatic mitral valve disease
   Mechanical prosthetic valve
   Recent prior thromboembolism (within 2 years)
   Congestive heart failure
   Significant left ventricular dysfunction

Medium risk

   Advanced age
   Hypertension
   Mitral regurgitation
   Ischemic heart disease
   Recent-onset NVAF
   Thyrotoxicosis
   Remote prior thromboembolism (>2 years)
   Increased LA size (>50 mm)

Low risk

   "Lone" atrial fibrillation

LA, left atrium; NVAF, nonvalvular atrial fibrillation.

lation experienced a fourfold increase in stroke (age-adjusted percentage, 28% versus 7%, $p < .01$). However, the number of patients with lone atrial fibrillation in this study was small (n = 43), and only 3 were under the age of 60. Thus, lone atrial fibrillation in patients over the age of 60 increases risk of stroke.[100]

Echocardiographic Risk Factors

Some, but not all, of the early echocardiographic studies of NVAF implicated left atrial size as a risk factor for embolism.[101] Left atrial size has been shown to increase with increasing duration of atrial fibrillation.[102] Although the issue of left atrial size and embolic risk in NVAF has not been resolved conclusively, left atrial size likely does contribute to risk.[103] In an echocardiographic substudy of 568 patients in the SPAF trial, both left atrial size by M-mode echocardiography and degree of left ventricular dysfunction by two-dimensional echocardiography were independent predictors of embolism in a multivariate model.[104] In a prospective study of TEE to detect atrial thrombi prior to cardioversion, left atrial dimension was significantly greater in the group with left atrial thrombi than in the group without.[105] The finding of left atrial spontaneous contrast or "smoke" (caused by stasis of atrial blood and red cell rouleaux and platelet clump formation) has been shown to be a marker of previous thromboembolism in patients with NVAF or mitral valve disease.[106] The incidence of spontaneous echo contrast was significantly higher in the group with left atrial thrombi.[107] Left atrial size increases embolic risk due to mechanical prosthetic valves.[106] Thus, left atrial dimension, spontaneous atrial contrast, and diminished left ventricular func-

tion by echocardiography appear to define higher-risk patients with NVAF.

Clinical Trials

Five prospective trials have addressed the role of anticoagulant and antiplatelet therapy in NVAF: the Atrial Fibrillation, Aspirin, Anticoagulation study (AFASAK),[103] the Stroke Prevention in Atrial Fibrillation study (SPAF),[98] the Boston Area Anticoagulation Trial for Atrial Fibrillation (BAATAF),[97] the Canadian Atrial Fibrillation Anticoagulation study (CAFA),[108] and the Stroke Prevention in Nonrheumatic Atrial Fibrillation study (SPINAF).[109] All five studies compared warfarin with placebo (Table 152–6); the AFASAK and SPAF study also included an arm of aspirin alone. All studies were stopped prematurely; interim analysis of AFASAK, SPAF, BAATAF, and SPINAF revealed sufficient evidence of the efficacy of warfarin in the prevention of stroke in NVAF, and CAFA was stopped once the results of the other four studies were published. These trials will be briefly discussed in turn followed by a discussion of their implications.

In the AFASAK trial, 1007 patients were randomized to either high-dose warfarin (target INR 2.8 to 4.2), aspirin 75 mg/day, or placebo. Warfarin therapy was not blinded. Of the eligible subjects, 40% were randomized, a higher percentage than in other studies. Subjects were older (mean age 74) and had a higher incidence of congestive heart failure (52%) than in the other studies. Of the warfarin-assigned subjects, 38% were withdrawn from therapy, but on an intention-to-treat analysis, warfarin still provided a significant benefit. In multivariate analysis, only prior MI predicted stroke. In the AFASAK study, warfarin provided significant protection against stroke,

Table 152–6. **Trials of Antithrombotic Therapy in Atrial Fibrillation**

Trial	AFASAK	SPAF	BAATAF	SPINAF	CAFA
Patients	1007	1330	420	525	383
F/U (years)	1.2	1.3	2.3	1.8	1.3
% CHF	51	19	28	30	20
INR Target	2.8–4.2	2.0–3.5	1.5–2.7	1.4–2.8	2.0–3.0
ASA Dose	75 qd	325 qd	—	—	—
Primary Event Rate, Placebo	6.25%	6.3%/yr	2.98%/yr	4.3%/yr	5.2%
Primary Event Rate, Warfarin	1.49%*	2.3%/yr*	0.41%/yr*	0.9%/yr*	3.5%
Primary Event Rate, ASA	5.97%	3.6%/yr	—	—	—
Major Bleeds, Placebo	0.0%	1.6/yr	0.4%	0.9%	0.5%
Major Bleeds, Warfarin	0.3%	1.5/yr	0.9%	1.5%	1.5%
Major Bleeds, Aspirin	0.3%	1.4/yr	—	—	—
CVA, Placebo	4.7%	7.39%	2.98%/yr	4.3%/yr	4.7%
CVA, Warfarin	1.49%*	3.34%*	0.41%/yr*	0.9%/yr*	3.2%
CVA, Aspirin	4.48%	4.35%	—	—	—
Primary Event†	CVA, TIA, emboli	CVA, non-CNS emboli	Ischemic CVA	CVA	N-L CVA, non-CNS emboli, ICH

*Statistically significant at $p <= 0.05$.

†F/U, follow-up; CHF, congestive heart failure; INR, international normalized ratio; CVA, cerebrovascular accident; TIA, transient ischemic event; CNS, central nervous system; NL, nonlacunar; ICH, intracranial hemorrhage.

but aspirin did not. There were significantly fewer vascular deaths in the warfarin group than in the other two groups. There was no increase in serious bleeding complications in the warfarin group.

In the SPAF trial, 1330 subjects were randomized to warfarin (target INR 1.7 to 4.5), aspirin 75 mg/day, or placebo. Only 10% of eligible subjects were randomized. Warfarin therapy was not blinded. Unlike in the AFASAK trial, subjects were younger (mean age 67) with a significantly lower prevalence of congestive heart failure (19%). Of these subjects, 34% had paroxysmal NVAF; in the control group, there was no difference in stroke incidence in these subjects compared with subjects with sustained NVAF. Of the warfarin-treated subjects, 11% were withdrawn from therapy. In multivariate analysis, risk of stroke was increased by recent (within 3 months) congestive heart failure, history of hypertension, and previous arterial thromboembolism.[95] In the SPAF trial, aspirin was efficacious in subjects under the age of 75 (stroke incidence 2.2% versus 6.2%, risk reduction 65%, $p = .0042$) but not in subjects over age 75 (stroke incidence 7.4% versus 7.4%, $p = $ NS). In addition, aspirin did not confer protection against severe stroke.

In the BAATAF trial, subjects were randomized to low-dose warfarin (target INR 1.5 to 2.7) or placebo. Aspirin use was allowed in the placebo group and was taken by 46% of subjects. Aspirin use in the placebo group did not appear to protect against stroke. In the study overall, 35% of subjects had paroxysmal NVAF; there was no difference in the incidence in stroke between subjects with paroxysmal NVAF and subjects with sustained NVAF. Also, 10% of subjects were withdrawn from warfarin. Mitral annular calcification (30% of patients) increased stroke risk, as did older age and the presence of clinical heart disease. There was no difference in major bleeding events or intracerebral hemorrhages between groups but minor bleeding was increased in the warfarin group. Significantly, total mortality was decreased in the warfarin group (rate ratio 0.38, $p = .005$). The BAATAF trial follow-up of 2.2 years was the longest of the five trials.

In the SPINAF trial, 571 subjects were randomized to low-dose warfarin (target INR 1.2 to 1.5) or placebo. The SPINAF trial was the only trial among the five to employ a double-blind strategy with regard to warfarin therapy. In 228 subjects over the age of 70, warfarin conferred significant benefit (stroke rate 0.9% versus 4.8%, $p = .02$). There were no differences in total mortality between groups. More strokes occurred among subjects with a prior history of stroke. Minor bleeding was significantly increased in the warfarin groups, but major bleeding, including intracranial hemorrhage, was not increased.

The CAFA trial was stopped early after 378 of a planned 630 subjects were enrolled in a double-blind, placebo-controlled trial of warfarin (target INR 2 to 3) versus placebo. Twenty-six percent of these subjects discontinued warfarin. Because of the small sample size enrolled, the trial was unable to show a statistically significant reduction in stroke (3.5% versus 5.2%,

$p = .17$) before it was stopped early upon the publication of AFASAK and SPAF. There was more major bleeding in the warfarin group (2.5% versus 0.5%) and two deaths due to hemorrhage (one fatal intracranial hemorrhage, one ruptured aortic aneurysm). However, there was only one intracranial hemorrhage in the treatment group compared with none in the placebo group. There were no deaths from bleeding in the placebo group.

The key results of these five trials may be summarized as follows (Table 152–7):[89, 90, 93] (1) the risk of stroke from NVAF in nonanticoagulated patients is approximately 5% per year, (2) the risk of stroke in NVAF is decreased to 2% per year (or by 60%) by warfarin, (3) high-dose and low-dose warfarin are equally efficacious in the prevention of stroke in NVAF, (4) aspirin (325 mg/day) is likely efficacious in preventing stroke in patients under the age of 75, especially in the absence of congestive heart failure, (5) neither high-dose nor low-dose warfarin in carefully selected and monitored patients increases the risk of life-threatening bleeding or intracranial hemorrhage, although the yearly risk of bleeding that is severe enough to require hospitalization, transfusion, or surgery is 1% to 2%, (6) the risk of cerebral hemorrhage due to warfarin in these carefully selected and monitored patients was approximately 0.3% per year, no higher than in aspirin-treated or placebo-treated patients, (7) high-dose and low-dose warfarin in carefully selected and monitored patients increases the risk of minor bleeding, (8) approximately 30% of carefully selected and monitored patients will discontinue warfarin over 1 to 2 years of follow-up, (9) for every 1000 patients treated with warfarin for NVAF, warfarin will prevent 20 to 30 ischemic strokes at a cost of 4 to 6 major bleeding episodes per year, and (10) two of the trials observed a decrease in vascular mortality with warfarin, including the trial with the longest follow-up.

Current Role of Aspirin

At present, an unresolved issue in the therapy for NVAF is the efficacy of aspirin compared with warfa-

---

Table 152–7. Conclusions from the Five Recent Randomized Trials of Long-Term Warfarin Therapy in NVAF

1. In absence of anticoagulation, the incidence of stroke is 5% per year in NVAF
2. Warfarin decreases the incidence of stroke in NVAF by 60% to 2% per year
3. Low-dose warfarin (INR 2 to 3) is equivalent to high-dose warfarin (INR 3 to 4.5)
4. Major noncerebral bleeding complications are not increased by warfarin*
5. Risk of intracerebral hemorrhage (0.3% per year) is not increased by warfarin*
6. Risk or minor bleeding is increased by warfarin*
7. Up to 30% of patients are withdrawn or withdraw*

*Among carefully selected and monitored patients in these controlled clinical trials.

rin in the prevention of stroke. The AFASAK trial observed no benefit from aspirin (75 mg/day) in a relatively elderly population with a high prevalence of heart failure. In contrast, the SPAF trial observed benefit from aspirin (325 mg/day) similar to the benefit of warfarin in a younger population with a much lower prevalence of congestive heart failure. Aspirin may be less efficacious than warfarin in the prevention of the relatively fibrin-rich atrial thrombi that form in the left atrium during NVAF under sluggish flow and low shear conditions; this difference in efficacy is likely more pronounced in the setting of congestive heart failure.[110] In the AFASAK study, more stasis-induced and therefore aspirin "resistant" thrombi may have formed than in the SPAF study. The lower dose of aspirin in the AFASAK study or relative lack of efficacy of this low dose in older patients may have contributed to the disparate results of the trials as well.[89] Ongoing trials of warfarin versus aspirin in the prevention of stroke in NVAF will soon resolve this issue.

Safety of Warfarin in NVAF

The safety and practicality of widespread warfarin therapy in NVAF is an important issue. As mentioned, NVAF occurs in 2.5% of those older than age 60 and in 10% of those older than 75. In patients not as carefully screened and monitored during warfarin therapy as those in the five trials discussed earlier, the incidence of bleeding complications from warfarin therapy will probably increase compared with the incidence of complications reported in the trials: It is unlikely that the safety of warfarin therapy in general clinical practice will be similar to that reported from these carefully controlled clinical trials.[93] In routine clinical practice, one third of all prothrombin times drawn to monitor warfarin therapy either exceed or fall short of the therapeutic range.[110] Compliance with long-term warfarin therapy is likely to be less than that observed in these controlled trials, wherein up to 30% of patients either withdrew of were withdrawn from warfarin. Thus, before recommending long-term warfarin therapy for the prevention of stroke in patients with NVAF, the prescribing physician must discuss the risks, benefits, and discomforts of long-term therapy with the patient and address all absolute and relative contraindications to long-term warfarin therapy.

There have been no randomized trials of anticoagulant or antiplatelet agents in the prevention of thromboembolism following an initial thromboembolic event in a patient with NVAF. However, because risk of recurrent thromboembolism is high in these patients according to observational and retrospective studies, long-term anticoagulant therapy is reasonable and recommended.[89] No trials have addressed the role of anticoagulants or antiplatelets agents in the therapy in NVAF in DCM or congenital heart disease. Patients with DCM should be treated with anticoagulants because their risk of stroke is appreciable, as has been discussed. Patients with NVAF and atrial septal defects, ventricular septal defects, corrected transposition of the arteries, or Ebstein's anomaly are at significant risk of thromboembolism according to observational studies and should receive anticoagulants.[89]

Role of Antithrombotic Therapy at the Time of Cardioversion

The role of anticoagulation around the time of cardioversion of NVAF is evolving.[111] In older retrospective observational studies, the incidence of embolism without anticoagulation around the time of electrical cardioversion was observed to be higher than with anticoagulation (5% to 7% versus 0.8% to 1.6%, respectively).[89, 105, 111] There are no large prospective studies of the risk of embolism following chemical conversion of atrial fibrillation, although older, smaller studies suggest a risk of 1.2% to 1.5% in all patients.[112] Embolism may occur hours to days after cardioversion, because the normal mechanical atrial activity and coordinated atrial contraction that dislodge atrial thrombi may not return for up to 2 weeks following restoration of normal atrial electrical activity and electrocardiographic normal sinus rhythm.[111] It is hypothesized, but not proven, that 1 to 2 weeks are required for an atrial thrombus to organize and adhere securely to the atrial appendage or atrial wall, making dislodgement and embolism less likely. Three weeks of anticoagulation prior to attempted cardioversion and 4 weeks of anticoagulation following successful cardioversion have been recommended.[89] Patients with atrial fibrillation of less than 2 days' duration are thought to be at low risk of embolism, and cardioversion is often attempted without prophylactic anticoagulant therapy. This approach has not been evaluated in large prospective clinical studies but appears to be reasonably safe in retrospective studies.

Studies of TEE in patients with atrial fibrillation of greater than 2 days' duration prior to cardioversion have reported a prevalence of atrial thrombi between 13% and 19%.[105] Nearly all thrombi are in the atrial appendage. In a small study, the presence of a left atrial appendage thrombus was a marker of increased embolism, although anticoagulant therapy usually resulted in partial or complete eradication of the thrombus.[113] The finding of spontaneous atrial contrast in the right or left atrium is significantly associated with coexistent atrial thrombus; this finding should prompt a search for thrombus. Though some studies have reported that patients without thrombus seen by TEE may be safely cardioverted (direct-current) with minimal antithrombotic therapy (in some studies, 24 hours of heparin precardioversion and no antithrombotic therapy afterward), other studies have reported embolism following a negative TEE and cardioversion without anticoagulation.[105, 111, 114] Although TEE is superior to transthoracic echocardiography in detecting atrial thrombus, especially in the atrial appendage, TEE may still miss small thrombi of 1 to 2 mm, not provide optimal imaging of the left atrial appendage in all patients, and misinterpret small muscle ridges in the atrial appendage as thrombi.[110] The sensitivity of TEE in the detection of small atrial thrombi has not yet been established. Currently, TEE cannot be recommended routinely prior to attempted cardioversion of atrial fibrillation. TEE may be useful to screen high-risk patients prior to cardioversion (prior embolism, mechanical prosthesis, mitral stenosis).[115]

Treatment Recommendations (see Table 152–4)

All patients lacking contraindication to long-term warfarin therapy with sustained or paroxysmal NVAF (except patients younger than age 60 with lone NVAF) should be treated with low-dose warfarin therapy indefinitely (target INR 2 to 3). Patients at highest risk include those with prior thromboembolism, significant left ventricular dysfunction, or congestive heart failure; in such patients, higher-dose warfarin is indicated (target INR 2.5 to 3.5). Patients at higher-than-baseline risk include the elderly and those with recent-onset fibrillation, thyrotoxicosis, enlarged left atria, and coexistent hypertensive or ischemic heart disease. Patients under the age of 60 with no signs, symptoms, or history of cardiovascular disease and structurally normal hearts by echocardiography have lone atrial fibrillation and do not require long-term anticoagulant therapy. Patients older than the age of 60 with lone atrial fibrillation are at risk of thromboembolism and should be treated with warfarin. Patients who have contraindications to long-term warfarin or who are poor candidates for warfarin should be treated with aspirin (325 mg) once a day indefinitely.

It is also recommended that warfarin (INR 2.0 to 3.0) be administered for 3 weeks prior to elective cardioversion in patients who have had atrial fibrillation for longer than 2 days and that warfarin be continued for 4 weeks following successful cardioversion. Use of aspirin before cardioversion in low-risk patients (i.e., lone atrial fibrillation) may be a reasonable compromise, but no evidence is available to assess its efficacy. Anticoagulation is not necessary for patients without other risk factors for thromboembolism who have been in atrial fibrillation for less than 2 days prior to cardioversion.

Native Valve Endocarditis

In the preantibiotic era, native valve endocarditis (NVE) was complicated by clinically apparent emboli in 70% to 97% of cases.[116] In the antibiotic era, emboli still occur in approximately 30% of cases. Most emboli occur either at presentation or during the first 7 to 10 days of antibiotic therapy.[117] Cerebral emboli occur in 11% to 19% of cases.[118] Platelets likely play a pivotal role in the propagation of vegetations: in the classic studies of the very earliest lesions of experimental NVE, large friable masses of platelets were seen supported by slender fibrin strands.[119] In animals, trials of aspirin,[120] anticoagulants,[121] and fibrinolytic agents[122] have proved disappointing. Anticoagulants and fibrinolytic agents have in experimental models led to increased bacteremia, fever, septicemia, embolism,

and death, perhaps because of disruption of the protective encapsulating fibrin-rich and platelet-rich vegetation that contains the infection and shields highly thrombogenic bacterial cell-wall surfaces from circulating blood.

Early clinical experience in nonrandomized retrospective studies in humans showed no improvement in survival with the addition of heparin or warfarin to antibiotic therapy in NVE.[123] Bleeding complications, especially intracranial hemorrhage and death, were increased. Pooled series revealed similar results, and as a consequence routine anticoagulation with heparin or warfarin in NVE was abandoned. These early trials differed significantly, however, in the range of anticoagulation employed and methods of determining the degree of anticoagulation, particularly compared with current practices. Despite the uncontrolled nature of most of these studies, there have been no trials since the mid-1940s of anticoagulant therapy for NVE given these observations. It appears advisable to discontinue anticoagulation in patients with NVE because the risk of cerebral hemorrhage may outweigh the somewhat lower risk of thromboembolism. The use of aspirin in this setting seems a reasonable but unproven compromise.

PROSTHETIC HEART VALVES AND THROMBOEMBOLISM

Thromboembolism in patients with prosthetic heart valves is decreased but not eradicated with antithrombotic therapy. Orally administered anticoagulants have been the mainstay of therapy in prevention of thromboembolism from cardiac valvular prostheses, but platelet inhibitors have an important adjuvant role. Antithrombotic therapy is based on assessment of pathogenesis and risk in patients with prosthetic heart valves.

Mechanical Prosthetic Valves

Pathogenesis of Thromboembolism

Perioperative tissue injury and stasis, turbulent flow through the newly implanted prosthesis, and the inherent thrombogenicity of the valvular prosthetic materials all predispose to perioperative thrombus formation on mechanical prosthetic heart valves (Table 152–8). Activation of both platelets and factor XII (via contact activation of the extrinsic coagulation cascade pathway) and platelet adhesion to perivalvular structures and prosthetic materials occur intraoperatively. Continued platelet activation and thrombin generation ensue as soon as blood flows through the implanted valve.[124] It is possible to image platelet deposition on the Dacron sewing ring used in all types of valvular prosthesis by indium-111 platelet scintigraphy within 24 hours of surgery.[125, 126] Inhibition of thrombin, the most potent platelet agonist known, is required in addition to inhibition of platelets to prevent thrombosis on prosthetic vascular surfaces.[127] Thrombin inhibition prevents experimental arterial

Table 152–8. **Prosthetic Heart Valves and Systemic Embolism Pathophysiology and Risk Stratification**

Type	Thrombi			Emboli 100 Patient-Years§ No Anticoagulation (Anticoagulation)
	*Injury**	*Flow†*	*Coagulation‡*	
Mitral mechanical	+ +	+ +	+	5 (2.5)
Aortic mechanical	+ +	+	+	4 (2)
Mitral bioprosthesis	+	+	0	2 (1)
Aortic bioprosthesis	+	0	0	1 (0.5)

*Suture-prosthesis (early).
†Atrial fibrillation (left atrium size), design of prothesis (thrombosis-emboli).
‡Adequacy anticoagulation, previous thromboembolism, others.
§Collection methods and analysis (that is, prospective, timing, source).
From Fuster V, Verstraete M (eds): Thrombosis in Cardiovascular Disorders. Philadelphia: WB Saunders, 1992.

thrombus formation in deep arterial injury and limits platelet deposition to a monolayer.

Decreased platelet survival is directly related to the prosthetic valve surface area and correlates with increased thromboembolic risk.[128–130] Decreased platelet survival following prosthetic valve replacement has been documented and signifies ongoing platelet aggregation. Experimentally, platelet inhibitors normalize platelet survival in this setting, providing a rationale for combination therapy with anticoagulants.[128–130] There is also evidence for persistent thrombin activity following prosthetic valve replacement. Fibrinopeptide A, a circulating peptide cleaved from fibrinogen by thrombin in the process of fibrin generation and thus a marker of *in vivo* thrombin activity, remains elevated in patients with mechanical prosthetic valves receiving orally administered warfarin with prothrombin times at recommended INR ranges (3.0 to 4.5).[131] Early thrombus formation may increase the subsequent risk of thromboembolism.[124] Beyond the perioperative period, persistent platelet aggregation and thrombin activity continue to place the patient with a mechanical prosthetic valve at chronic risk of thromboembolism.

Risk Factors for Thromboembolism

The most important risk factor for thromboembolism is the variability and intensity of long-term anticoagulation with warfarin (Table 152–9). In patients with mitral valve prostheses, the thromboembolic event rate in adequately anticoagulated patients is half that of adequately anticoagulated patients.[132–139] Fully half of all thromboembolic complications occur with inadequate anticoagulation, and half of the bleeding complications of warfarin occur with excessive anticoagulation.[133, 138, 139] Fibrinopeptide A levels and the level of anticoagulation are inversely related.[131] The variability of the prothrombin time is likely as important as the intensity.[140]

The location of the mechanical prosthetic valve influences thromboembolic risk (see Table 152–8). Valves in the aortic position are at lowest risk, those in the mitral position at higher risk, and double valves in the mitral and aortic positions at highest risk. Studies of all models of mechanical prosthetic

valves in the aortic position have documented a high risk of embolism in the absence of long-term anticoagulation or therapy with platelet inhibitors alone, despite early reports that the St. Jude model (and similar bileaflet, low-profile models) in the aortic position had a low incidence of thromboembolism in the absence of antithrombotic therapy or with antiplatelet therapy alone.[124] Atrial fibrillation increases the risk of thromboembolism from mechanical or bioprosthetic valves.[140–142] Left atrial size greater than 50 to 55 mm by M-mode echocardiography despite normal sinus rhythm increases risk,[105] as does previous thromboembolism and left ventricular dysfunction. Finally, older valve design (due to less favorable hemodynamic valve profile and construction from more thrombogenic materials) and year of valve replacement operation prior to 1980 (due to referral for valve replacement later in the course of chronic valvular heart disease) also increase risk.[124]

Incidence of Thromboembolism

The risk of thromboembolism is highest during the first postoperative year, likely because of variability in anticoagulation and the presence of nonendothelialized, thrombogenic, exposed perivalvular tissues and prosthetic surfaces.[124] The cumulative risk of thromboembolism increases directly with time after

Table 152–9. **Risk Factors for Prosthetic Valve Thromboembolism**

1. Variability and intensity of anticoagulation
2. Prosthetic valve location (MV + AV > MV > AV)*
3. Atrial fibrillation
4. LA size > 50–55 mm despite sinus rhythm
5. Previous thromboembolism
6. Congestive heart failure
7. Significant left ventricular dysfunction
8. Older valve model/design†
9. Valve replacement before 1980
10. Cumulative time after operation‡

*MV, mitral valve; AV, aortic valve; LA, left atrium.
†Due to increased turbulence of older designs and increased thrombogenicity of materials.
‡Risk of thromboembolism increases cumulatively with time after operation.

Table 152–10. **Approximate Incidence of Thromboembolism by Valve Type and Location (Events per 100 Patient-Years of Follow-up)***

Valve Type	Position	Incidence (%)
Starr-Edwards	Aortic	2
	Mitral	3
St. Jude/Hall-Medtronic	Aortic	1.5
	Mitral	2.5
Björk-Shiley	Aortic	2
	Mitral	2.5
Bioprosthetic†	Aortic	1
	Mitral	2

*Assuming therapeutic warfarin therapy.
†First 3 months following surgery, assuming therapeutic warfarin therapy.

operation: risk persists indefinitely. Accurate absolute rates of thromboembolism are difficult to derive from longitudinal studies of valve replacement because of variations in the definitions of thromboembolism, thromboembolic events, variability of follow-up, lack of standardization in the measurement and reporting of prothrombin times, heterogeneity of patient populations, and modification in valve models. In general, in patients who have undergone anticoagulation, the various valve models are associated with the following approximate risks of thromboembolism expressed as percentages of thromboembolic events per 100 patient-years of follow-up (Table 152–10): Starr-Edwards—2% aortic position, 3% mitral position; St. Jude and Hall-Medtronic—1.5% aortic position, 2.5% mitral position; Björk-Shiley—2% aortic position, 2.5% mitral position; bioprosthetic valves—1% aortic position, 2% mitral position.[124, 143]

From the Mayo Clinic, 302 patients were followed for 10 to 19 years with mitral or aortic Starr-Edwards valves. Of these patients, 34% experienced embolism by 10 years, 42% by 15 years (Fig. 152–1). Embolism involved the cerebral circulation in 85% of cases, 10% of which were fatal and 50% of which left a permanent neurologic deficit. Although no significant difference emerged between event rates with mitral versus aortic prostheses in this study (3.9% versus 3.7% per 100 patient-years, respectively), other studies have found greater thromboembolic risk in mitral Starr-Edwards prostheses. This appears to apply mostly to the older Starr-Edwards 6000 model with a larger

inlet orifice than that found in later models. The incidence of emboli from early Starr-Edwards aortic prostheses (model 1000) does not appear to be significantly different from those of later 1200 and 1260 models.[144] Overall, the incidence of emboli from early Starr-Edwards valves appears greater than that of valves replaced at a later date. This probably reflects both improvements in valve design (less turbulence and thrombogenic materials) and patient-related variables (earlier operation with better ventricular function, less atrial fibrillation).[145]

Starr-Edwards prostheses implanted more recently are associated with only slightly greater thromboembolic risk than other mechanical prostheses are. In three studies, the incidence of thromboembolism with Björk-Shiley valves was only slightly lower than that reported with Starr-Edwards valves.[133, 138, 139] The major difference is the risk of thrombotic valvular dysfunction or stenosis in Björk-Shiley valves leading to heart failure that may be subacute, acute, or occasionally fulminant in onset. Valvular thrombosis *in situ* may occur in up to 5% to 6% of Björk-Shiley mitral prostheses and in 2% to 3% of aortic prostheses; as discussed later, the occurrence of valvular thrombosis depends critically on inadequate anticoagulation. The St. Jude and Hall-Medtronic valves (Fig. 152–2) are low-profile, bileaflet valves designed to maximize hemodynamic performance for a given annulus size.[146] As a result of more favorable hemodynamics, such models appear to have lower rates of thromboembolism. However, anticoagulation is still mandatory. In a large study of 815 St. Jude valves implanted in 785 patients, the overall rate of thromboembolism was 2.6% per patient-year in warfarin-treated patients, 9.2% per patient-year in aspirin-treated patients, and 15.6% per patient-year in patients without any antithrombotic therapy.[147]

Clinical Trials of Antithrombotic Therapy

The recommendation of long-term antithrombotic therapy following prosthetic heart valve replacement is based largely on retrospective, observational data. Such studies are flawed, as has been discussed, by varying definitions of thromboembolism, varying measurements of anticoagulation efficacy, and varying follow-up.[124] It is clear from such studies, however imperfect, that therapy with long-term anticoagulants

Figure 152–1. Percentage of survivors free of thromboembolism plotted against time (years) in patients with isolated Starr-Edwards mitral or aortic prostheses. The number of patients seen at each follow-up interval is given below the horizontal axis. MVR, mitral valve replacement; AVR, aortic valve replacement. (Reproduced with permission from Fuster V, Pumphrey CW, McGoon MD, et al: Systemic thromboembolism in mitral and aortic Starr-Edwards prostheses. Circulation 66[Suppl I]:I-157, 1982. Copyright 1982, American Heart Association, Inc.)

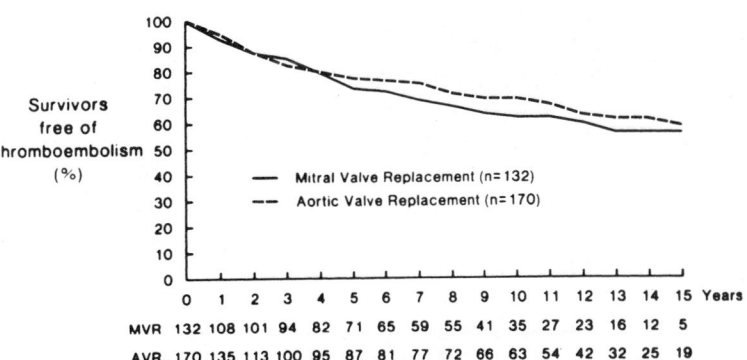

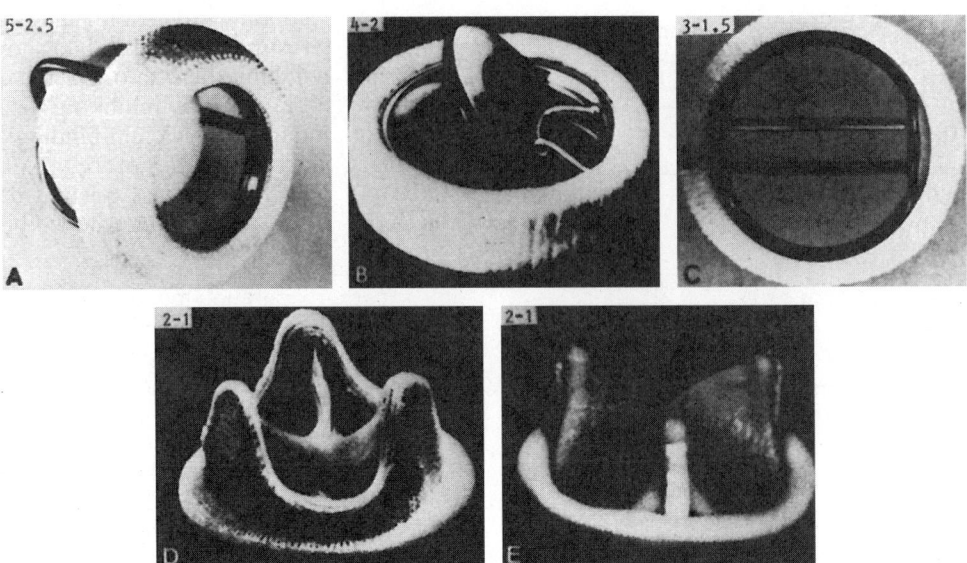

Figure 152–2. Popular types of valve prostheses. *A,* Starr-Edwards prosthesis; *B,* Björk-Shiley tilting disk prosthesis; *C,* bileaflet St. Jude prosthesis in fully open position (there are two lateral major flow orifices and a minor central orifice); *D,* porcine heterograft (frame-mounted glutaraldehyde-preserved, or Hancock model); *E,* bovine pericardial valve (frame-mounted glutaraldehyde-preserved, or Ionescu-Shiley model). For each prosthesis, the incidence of thromboembolism is shown in the upper corner in nonanticoagulated *(left)* and anticoagulated *(right)* patients.

significantly decreases the risk of thromboembolism from mechanical prosthetic heart valves. With regard to warfarin dosage, the following conclusions may be drawn from the available large prospective studies: (1) a target INR of 2.5 to 3.5 appears adequate to prevent thromboembolism in most instances,[148] (2) an INR above 3.5 is associated with excess bleeding but no additional protection against thromboembolism,[149] and (3) an INR below 1.8 confers inadequate protection against thromboembolism.[150] Saour et al. randomized 258 patients with mechanical prosthetic valves of various types to moderate-intensity (target INR 2.65, prothrombin time 1.5) or high-intensity (target INR 9, prothrombin time 2.5) warfarin therapy. After follow-up of approximately 420 patient-years per group, there was no difference in the incidence of

thromboembolism (4.0 versus 3.7 events per 100 patient-years) but significantly decreased bleeding (6.2 versus 12.1 events per 100 patient-years), including major bleeding (0.95 versus 2.1 events per 100 patient-years) in the moderate-intensity warfarin group compared with the high-intensity warfarin group.[148]

Therapy with combined anticoagulant and antiplatelet agents is more efficacious than therapy with anticoagulants alone (Table 152–11). Five trials have shown that the combination of the antiplatelet agent dipyridamole (375 to 400 mg/day) and warfarin is superior to warfarin alone in reducing the incidence of thromboembolism from mechanical prosthetic valves.[124, 150] Use of dipyridamole in combination with warfarin does not increase bleeding. Dipyridamole has been approved by the Food and Drug Adminis-

Table 152–11. Antithrombotic Therapy in Patients with Mechanical Prosthetic Heart Valves

Reference	Method	Follow-Up (yr)	Treatment Group	Dose (mg/day)	Patients	Thromboembolism (%/yr)
Dale et al.	PR, R, B	1	AC + P		38	9
			AC + ASA	1000	39	2
			ASA	1000	77	15
Sullivan et al.	PR, R	1	AC + P		84	14
			AC + D	400	79	1
Kasahara et al.	PR, R	1 to 3 (mean 2.5)	AC		39	21
			AC + D	400	40	5
Groupe PACTE	PR, R	1	AC		154	5
			AC + D	375	136	3
Rajah et al.	PR, R	1 to 2	AC		87	13
			AC + D	300	78	4
Altman et al.	PR, R	2	AC		65	20
			AC + ASA	500	57	5
Turpie et al.	PR, R, B	2	AC + P		184	2.84
			AC + ASA	500	186	1.08

AC, warfarin; ASA, aspirin; D, dipyridamole; PR, prospective; R, randomized.

tration (FDA) for use in patients with mechanical prosthetic valves at high risk of thromboembolism. Aspirin also has additive benefit to warfarin in the prevention of thromboembolism. The combination of aspirin (500 to 1000 mg daily) and warfarin significantly increased the incidence of major hemorrhage requiring transfusion or hospitalization.[133, 151, 152] However, aspirin in lower doses appears safer. Turpie et al., in a double-blind, placebo-controlled trial, randomized 370 patients with mechanical prosthetic valves of various types to warfarin (target INR 3.0 to 4.5) plus aspirin (100 mg/day) or warfarin (target INR 3.0 to 4.5) plus placebo.[153] After an average follow-up of 2.5 years, the combination of warfarin plus aspirin compared with warfarin alone significantly decreased major systemic embolism or death from vascular causes (1.9% versus 8.5%, risk reduction 77%, $p < .001$), total mortality (2.8% versus 7.4%, risk reduction 63%, $p = .01$) while increasing overall bleeding (35% versus 22%, $p = .02$) but not major, life-threatening, or fatal bleeding. There was no difference in the incidence of intracranial hemorrhage. Thus, in this preliminary study, low-dose aspirin appears to be superior to dipyridamole in combination with warfarin, although aspirin increases the incidence of bleeding complications. Further studies are currently underway to establish the optimal doses and safety of aspirin and warfarin in combination in this setting. Ticlopidine has not been studied in the prevention of prosthetic heart valve thromboembolism.

Antiplatelet agents alone are ineffective in reducing thromboembolism from mechanical prosthetic valves. This has been clearly shown for St. Jude valves[146, 147, 154–156] and Björk-Shiley valves.[157]

Bioprosthetic Valves

Incidence of Thromboembolism

Thromboembolism is less frequent from bioprosthetic valves but still occurs, especially in the early postoperative period.[124] Incidence varies with the coexistence of other risk factors for thromboembolism, including the variability and intensity of anticoagulation. Eight percent to 16% of patients with bioprostheses in the aortic position, and 31% to 79% of patients with bioprostheses in the mitral position, are on long-term anticoagulation because of prior embolization, atrial fibrillation, left ventricular systolic failure, or left atrial enlargement.[158] Thus, the incidence of embolism in this population due to valvular thrombosis alone and not these other contributing factors is difficult to establish.

Clinical Trials

There have been no randomized prospective trials of antithrombotic therapy for the prevention of thromboembolism following bioprosthetic valve replacement. The highest risk of thromboembolism occurs within the first 3 months of operation; this risk may be as high as 12% without postoperative, intravenous

administration of heparin followed by warfarin.[159] This risk is markedly reduced by postoperative anticoagulation.[160, 161] In the study of Heras et al., there was no difference in long-term bioprosthetic aortic valve thromboembolism between patients who had and had not undergone anticoagulation but a significant difference in bioprosthetic mitral valve thromboembolism between patients who had and had not undergone anticoagulation (1.2% per year versus 4.3% per year, $p < .05$).[161] Although some studies have reported similar risks of thromboembolism from bioprosthetic and mechanical valves,[158] this conclusion may be biased by the older age and baseline increased thromboembolic risk of patients selected for bioprosthetic valve implantation. In addition to valve location and adequacy of anticoagulation, atrial fibrillation, left ventricular systolic dysfunction, and marked enlargement of the left atrium increase the risk of bioprosthetic valve thromboembolism.[158] There is a lesser incidence of valve thrombosis with bioprosthetic valves than mechanical prosthetic valves.

Platelet inhibitor therapy has not been adequately tested in patients with bioprosthetic heart valves, but one uncontrolled study using postoperative aspirin (500 or 1000 mg) in two different patient groups found a low incidence of thromboembolism (0.3% and 1.3%, respectively), suggesting possible benefit.[162] Although bioprostheses are frequently chosen to avoid the need for long-term oral anticoagulation, it is interesting that some data show that warfarin may inhibit the rate of calcific degeneration of these valves by inhibiting γ-carboxylation of glutamate, a calcium-binding amino acid. One study found significantly less calcium on porcine bioprostheses that were removed because of degeneration of function in patients on warfarin than in untreated patients.[163]

Prosthetic Valve Thrombosis

Prosthetic valve thrombosis has been reported in mechanical and bioprosthetic valves of all types but is fortunately rare, with an annual incidence of 0.1% to 0.5%.[164] Björk-Shiley valves in the mitral position are at highest risk. In general, the Björk-Shiley valve has twice the risk of thrombosis compared with other models.[143] Bioprosthetic valve thrombosis is commonest the first 3 months following surgery and occurs in the setting of suboptimal anticoagulation in 50% to 70% of cases.[124] Valve thrombosis may occur within 3 weeks or less of discontinuation of orally administered warfarin in anticipation of noncardiac surgery.[165]

New congestive heart failure or pulmonary edema, insidious or sudden in onset, in a patient with a mechanical or bioprosthetic heart valve should always prompt consideration of prosthetic dysfunction, including valve thrombosis.[150] New-onset angina may occur in half of such patients; MI is uncommon. A new murmur is present in 90%, and abnormal (absent or decreased) opening or closing clicks are present in 60%. Doppler echocardiography or cinefluoroscopy is useful in establishing the diagnosis. Urgent valve replacement in this setting carries a 2% to 4% mortality rate in low-risk groups and a 25% to 40% mortality rate in high-risk groups (mitral valve thrombosis, New York Heart Association class IV heart failure, emergency surgery, increased age, long surgical cross-clamp time).[164]

Over 100 patients who have been treated with thrombolytic agents for valve thrombosis have been reported to date, although thrombolytic agents have not yet been approved for this purpose.[164] Patients with tricuspid valve thrombosis or patients with aortic or mitral valve thrombosis at prohibitive risk of surgical replacement may be considered for thrombolytic therapy. Streptokinase has been administered in an intravenous loading dose of 250,000 to 500,000 IU over 30 minutes followed by infusion of 100,000 IU/hr for 9 to 96 hours or 150,000 IU/hr for 10 hours. t-PA has also been used in various dosing regimens. Because thrombolytic agents activate thrombin and platelets, simultaneous heparin infusion (aPTT 1.5 to 2.0 times control) should be administered for 5 to 7 days, followed by warfarin (target INR 3.0 to 4.5). In series to date, thrombolytic agents are ineffective in 20% to 40%, systemic emboli occur in 0% to 20%, bleeding occurs in 5% to 10%, and acute mortality occurs in 13% to 18%.[164] There appears to be an increased incidence of embolism following thrombolytic therapy for Björk-Shiley but not St. Jude valves.[165] Series to date are small, and no firm recommendations can be made at present. Therapy should be individualized and based on the relative risks of surgery and thrombolytic agents.

Treatment Recommendations (Table 152–12)[166]

Mechanical Prosthetic Valves

All patients should receive heparin subcutaneously begun 6 hours after surgery to prolong the aPTT to the upper limit of normal. Warfarin should be begun 24 to 48 hours after operation (down the nasogastric tube if necessary) in all patients, with a target INR of 2.5 to 3.5. Once the chest tubes are removed, heparin should be administered intravenously to maintain the aPTT at 1.5 to 2.0 times control until warfarin is within the therapeutic range.

All routine patients should receive warfarin therapy with a target INR of 2.5 to 3.5 indefinitely. High-risk patients (valve implanted before 1980, previous thromboembolism, anticoagulation decreased or stopped because of bleeding, poor patient compliance, high variability in prothrombin times, patient population with an incidence of thromboembolism more than 2.0% per year on warfarin alone) should receive high-dose warfarin alone (target INR 3.0 to 4.5) or medium-dose warfarin (target INR 2.5 to 3.5) in combination with antiplatelet therapy. Dipyridamole (350 to 400 mg/day) is approved by the FDA for use in combination with warfarin and will not increase bleeding. One study to date supports the use of low-dose aspirin (100 mg/day) rather than dipyridamole as combination therapy with medium-dose warfarin in high-risk patients: although mortality was decreased in these carefully selected and monitored patients, bleeding was more common.[153] Ongoing studies may demonstrate the increased efficacy of combined warfarin and low-dose aspirin in all patients with prosthetic heart valves; it is premature to recommend the combination of warfarin and aspirin in all patients. Patients who are not at high risk and who experience bleeding problems with warfarin should be treated with low-dose warfarin (INR 2.0 to 3.0) plus either low-dose aspirin (80 to 100 mg/day) or dipyridamole (375 to 400 mg/day). Patients who cannot tolerate or have absolute contraindication to warfarin should be treated with aspirin (100 to 325 mg/day) plus dipyridamole (375 to 400 mg/day), although this combination has not been evaluated. A patient who has recurrent thromboembolism while on adequate warfarin and antiplatelet therapy should be considered for another valve replacement. In patients with bleeding during anticoagulation when the prothrombin time is not beyond twice control (INR ≤ 4.5), secondary causes of bleeding should be evaluated.

Bioprosthetic Valve Replacement

Warfarin should be administered to all patients within 24 to 48 hours of operation to prolong the prothrombin time to INR 3.0 to 4.5 for 3 months. Patients at

Table 152–12. **Antithrombotic Therapy for Prosthetic Heart Valves—1993**

Value	Grade-Situation	Therapy
Mechanical	Routine	MD warfarin
	Old prosthesis, TE	HD warfarin, or MD warfarin + LD ASA? or + Dip 400 mg/day
	ACRx problems (bleeding)	LD warfarin + Dip 400 mg/day or LD warfarin + LD ASA
	Recurrent embolism	Consider reoperation
Bioprosthetic	AVR routine–NSR	LD warfarin for 3 months (then ASA?)
	MVR routine–NSR	LD warfarin for 3 months (then ASA?)
	AF, LA thrombus, TE	HD warfarin for 3 months then LD warfarin

HD warfarin, high-dose warfarin (INR, 3.0–4.5); MD warfarin, medium-dose warfarin (INR 2.5–3.5); LD warfarin, low-dose warfarin (INR 2.0–3.0); ACRx, anticoagulant therapy; AF, atrial fibrillation; LD ASA, low-dose (80–100 mg/day); AVR, aortic valve replacement; Dip, dipyridamole; LA, left atrium; MVR, mitral valve replacement; NSR, normal sinus rhythm; TE, previous thromboembolism.
From Israel O, Sharma SK, Fuster V: Antithrombotic therapy in prosthetic heart valve replacement. Am Heart J 127:400–411, 1994.

high risk of thromboembolism (previous thromboembolism, left atrial thrombus) should be treated indefinitely. Patients with moderate risk of thromboembolism (left ventricular dysfunction, atrial fibrillation, enlarged left atrium greater than 50 mm by M-mode echocardiography) should receive warfarin for 3 months as described earlier followed by warfarin at a dose to prolong the INR to 2.0 to 3.0 indefinitely after 3 months. For aortic or mitral bioprosthetic valve replacement at low risk of thromboembolism (without any of the risk factors cited), patients may be treated with aspirin (80 mg/day) indefinitely after they have been on warfarin for 3 months (target INR 3.0 to 4.5).

Clinical Problems with Anticoagulants

Noncardiac Surgery

Orally administered anticoagulants may be safely discontinued for 5 to 10 days prior to noncardiac surgery in a patient with a prosthetic heart valve.[167] Dipyridamole or aspirin, if administered concurrently, should be continued, and intravenously administered heparin should be begun to maintain the activated thromboplastin time at 2 times control when the prothrombin time drops below 1.5 times control. Heparin should be continued until 4 to 5 hours preoperatively. Subcutaneously administered heparin (15,000 IU/day in two or three divided doses) should be continued during and immediately after surgery except in brain or intraocular operations. As soon as possible after surgery, subcutaneously administered heparin should then be increased to 12,500 IU twice a day. As soon as is feasible, a continuous intravenous infusion of heparin should be begun to maintain the aPTT at 1.5 to 2 times control. Orally administered warfarin should be begun as soon as possible postoperatively, and heparin should be discontinued once the prothrombin time is within range.

Prosthetic Valve Endocarditis

Patients with prosthetic valve endocarditis incur an approximately 50% risk of thromboembolism in the absence of anticoagulant therapy.[168–170] The pooled results of three nonrandomized studies suggest a sixfold to ninefold reduction of this risk with anticoagulant therapy at the cost of an approximately 14% incidence of intracranial hemorrhage.[168, 169, 171] The presence of mycotic aneurysms predisposes to intracranial hemorrhage during endocarditis. In the absence of evidence of intracranial hemorrhage or large cerebral infarction during endocarditis, full anticoagulation should be continued. Upon hospitalization, patients should be switched from warfarin to intravenously administered heparin in case emergency surgery becomes necessary or bleeding occurs.

Prosthetic Heart Valve and Acute Cerebral Embolism

Not infrequently, a patient with a prosthetic heart valve in need of long-term anticoagulation experiences a cerebral ischemic event consistent with cerebral embolism. The physician in this setting faces the dilemma of whether to continue anticoagulation to prevent recurrent embolism while risking hemorrhagic infarct transformation or to discontinue anticoagulation to prevent hemorrhagic transformation while risking recurrent embolism. Pooled data of 15 studies indicate that the risk of recurrence of embolism in patients with acute aseptic cardiogenic cerebral embolism is 10% to 12% over the next 2 weeks (or approximately 1% per day).[74] Patients with NVAF are at lower risk. In the absence of anticoagulation, approximately 20% of cardiogenic embolic cerebral infarctions undergo hemorrhagic transformation by CT. Of all hemorrhagic transformations, 75% are apparent on CT by 48 hours following embolism and are frequently asymptomatic.[74]

Immediate anticoagulation after acute cardiogenic cerebral embolism results in a two-thirds reduction in the risk of recurrent cerebral embolism.[74] In the presence of immediate anticoagulation, 1% to 24% of cerebral infarctions undergo symptomatic hemorrhagic transformation with deterioration in neurologic status. The differing reported rates of transformation with immediate anticoagulation reflect differences in the intensity of anticoagulation, size of the infarct, blood pressure, and other patient-related variables. Large infarcts incur a greater risk of hemorrhagic transformation for up to 7 days.[172] Hemorrhagic transformation is more frequent in the presence of hypertension and in the elderly.

Thus, although anticoagulants reduce recurrent embolism, they also increase symptomatic hemorrhagic transformation. During the first 2 weeks, the overall risk of recurrent embolism is approximately equal to the overall risk of spontaneous hemorrhagic transformation; however, a key distinction is that the risk of spontaneous hemorrhagic transformation sharply declines after 48 hours, whereas the risk of recurrent embolism is evenly distributed over the first 2 weeks. This temporal distinction in risk is exploited in current recommendations of anticoagulant therapy following a cerebral embolism.[74] Anticoagulation with heparin is recommended after a small- to medium-sized embolic stroke if a CT brain scan performed 48 hours after the event fails to reveal hemorrhage and if severe hypertension (blood pressure greater than or equal to 180/100) is absent. Heparin should be followed by warfarin with a target INR of 2.0 to 3.0 indefinitely. In patients with large cerebral infarcts or with severe hypertension, anticoagulation with heparin should be postponed for 5 to 14 days until repeat CT brain scan then excludes hemorrhagic transformation and blood pressure is controlled. When used in patients with embolic strokes, intravenously administered heparin should be administered without an initial or subsequent bolus. The aPTT should be maintained at 1.5 to 2.0 times control. Patients with NVAF and no other risk factors for embolism whose CT brain scan results at 48 hours are negative may be treated with orally administered warfarin alone; intravenously administered heparin is likely unnecessary given the lower incidence of recurrent embolism in these patients.

Prosthetic Heart Valve and Pregnancy

Warfarin, a known and potent teratogen, causes fetal wastage in up to 80% of all first-trimester pregnancies. In infants who survive to term, there is a distressingly high incidence of congenital anomalies, including nasal hypoplasia, stippling of bones (chondrodysplasia punctata or Conradi's syndrome), mental retardation, optic atrophy, microcephaly, spasticity, and hypotonia.[124] Warfarin crosses the placenta, and late gestational use may lead to hemorrhagic complications in the fetus. Pregnancy should therefore be well-planned and anticipated in women with prosthetic heart valves who require anticoagulant therapy, because warfarin is contraindicated during pregnancy.

Adjusted-dose subcutaneously administered heparin (aPTT at 1.5 times control, adjusted by drawing aPTTs midway between the 8-hour dosing intervals) successfully prevents maternal thromboembolic complications and congenital anomalies in live-born infants.[173] However, of 18 pregnancies, 9 spontaneous abortions were attributed to exposure to warfarin before the recognition of pregnancy. Ideally, warfarin should be switched to subcutaneously administered heparin before or immediately at the time of suspected conception. Adjusted-dose subcutaneously administered heparin should be continued throughout the pregnancy (aPTT 1.5 to 2 times control). Most women will require 10,000 to 20,000 IU administered every 8 to 12 hours as adjusted by aPTTs drawn halfway between doses. Doses of 5000 IU every 12 hours are not sufficient to prevent thromboembolism from prosthetic heart valves.[124] Outpatient subcutaneously administered heparin is continued up to the week before delivery, at which time intravenously administered heparin is begun and continued until labor. During labor, low-dose heparin (5000 IU every 8 hours) is recommended. Following delivery, intravenously administered heparin and warfarin should be resumed. It is safe to resume warfarin therapy during breast feeding, because active warfarin metabolites do not enter breast milk.[174] Platelet inhibitor therapy should be avoided during pregnancy: Aspirin may allow premature closure of the ductus arteriosus, and neither dipyridamole nor sulfinpyrazone is approved. Bioprosthetic heart valves are preferred for women of child-bearing age who wish to bear children, although the risk of bioprosthetic calcification under the age of 35 and short durability of the valve (10 to 15 years) must be kept in mind.

ARTERIAL THROMBOSIS
Pathogenesis

Vascular Injury

Three types of vascular injury important in the pathophysiology of atherosclerosis and the acute coronary syndromes have been proposed.[175] Type I injury consists of alteration in vascular endothelial function without macroscopic morphologic alteration (Table 152–13). Type I injury may result from turbulent coronary flow patterns at branch points or bifurcations in the coronary arterial tree, hypercholesterolemia, exposure to circulating vasoactive amines or immune complexes, infection, tobacco or exposure to other substances injurious to vascular endothelium and leads to the accumulation of lipids and monoctyes.[176] Type II injury is caused by toxic monocyte and macrophage products and results in platelet adhesion to the injured endothelium. Release of monocyte and platelet growth factors (PDGF, EDGF, TGF-β, and somatomedin C in the case of platelets) results in fibrointimal proliferation and formation of a fibrotic capsule that overlies the lipid-filled atherosclerotic lesion. Type III injury results from disruption of this fibrotic capsule. Circulating blood is exposed to the lipid core and extracellular matrix of the atherosclerotic lesion in superficial plaque disruption (superficial type III injury). If disruption extends to the underlying arterial media (deep type III injury), blood is exposed to subendothelial collagen and subendothelial matrix tissue in addition to the lipid core and extracellular matrix of the plaque.

After either superficial or deep type III injury at high arterial shear rates, platelet deposition on these

Table 152–13. **The Three Types of Vascular Injury**

Type	Mechanism	Depth	Consequence(s)
I	Mild endothelial injury (blood flow, hypercholesterolemia, immune complexes, infection, tobacco)	Endothelium	Lipid + monocyte accumulation only in endothelium
II	Plaque fissure PTCA, CABG, cardiac transplantation; release of toxic macrophage or monocyte products	Endothelial denudation, intimal damage; internal elastic lamina intact; media spared	*Acute:* single or double layer of platelet deposition. *Chronic:* myointimal hyperplasia
III	Plaque rupture; PTCA, CABG	Endothelial denudation with exposure of intima, lipid core, ECM, (superficial) or media (deep)	Platelet adhesion, aggregation, thrombin generation; mural or possibly occlusive thrombus formation

CABG, coronary artery bypass graft; ECM, extracellular matrix; PTCA, percutaneous coronary angioplasty.

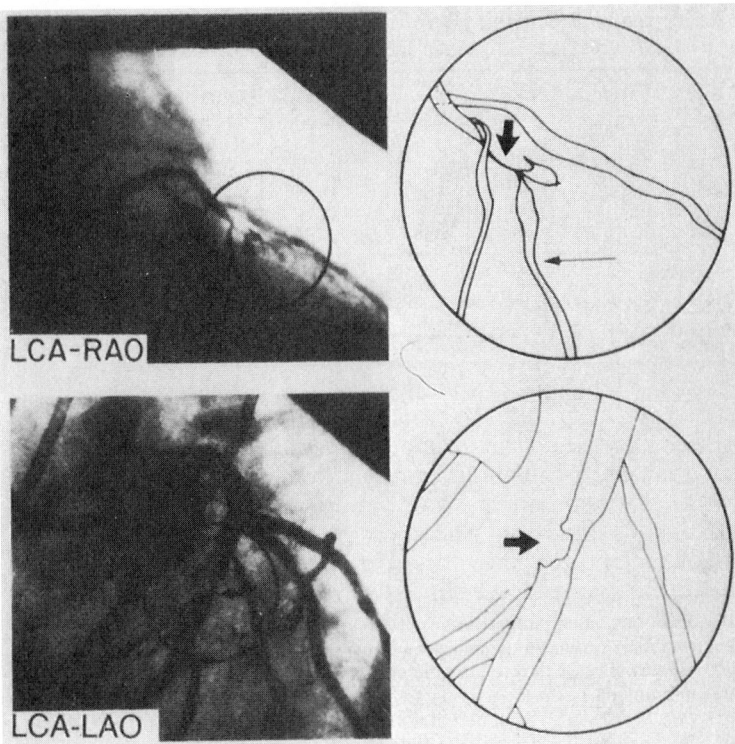

Figure 152–3. Coronary arteriograms and accompanying schematic diagrams of the left anterior descending arteries in two patients with complex eccentric plaques—the end result of plaque rupture and thrombosis. Both patients had unstable angina.

highly thrombogenic surfaces is maximal within 5 to 10 minutes.[177–179] Nonocclusive or occlusive intraluminal thrombosis may occur. The size, extent, and adherence of the thrombus depends on the depth of arterial injury. Superficial type III injury results in the formation of mural thrombus that may be dislodged by the high shear forces of arterial blood flow. Deep type III injury and the exposure of fibrillar collagen in particular results in the formation of a larger, much more tightly adherent thrombus.

Thrombosis and the Progression of Atherosclerosis

This sequence of vascular injury, plaque disruption, and resultant thrombosis is important in the progression of atherosclerosis and provocation of the acute coronary syndromes. Usually, the progression of atherosclerosis in a given lesion is likely rapid.[175] Recurrent minor plaque fissuring (relatively superficial type III injury) results in the formation of nonocclusive mural thrombi that may undergo organization and fibrotic incorporation into the underlying atheroma. Postmortem studies have provided evidence for this process. Of patients with coronary artery disease, 17% have plaques with fissures (often resealed) at postmortem examination; some are associated with thrombi, and previously healed fissures may exhibit incorporated thrombus.[180, 181] In patients dying of unstable angina pectoris or MI, layered thrombi overlying fissured plaques are common.[182] This finding suggests that acute coronary syndromes may be caused by repetitive episodes of mural thrombosis.[175]

Plaque Disruption

The most common cause of atherosclerotic plaque disruption is fissuring or ulceration, although rupture of the coronary vasa vasorum with resultant plaque hemorrhage occasionally occurs.[175, 183] Lipid-rich plaques are prone to disruption more than are lipid-poor plaques. Changes in intraluminal pressure, vascular tone, and shear rates; increased turbulence due to progressive lesion stenosis; and capsule torsion by cardiac contraction all contribute to capsule disruption. The low tensile strength and concentration of mechanical stress forces at the edges of lipid-rich plaques makes disruption more likely at the junction with the arterial wall, where the capsule lacks collagen support. Macrophages within the plaque secrete collagenase and elastase, enzymes that digest the plaque extracellular matrix and may predispose to plaque fissuring and disruption. High macrophage content may predispose to plaque disruption. Platelet deposition increases with increased degree of underlying stenosis following plaque disruption due to the increased arterial shear rates found at significantly stenotic lesions and shear-induced platelet activation.[178]

Thrombosis and the Acute Coronary Syndromes

Thrombosis after plaque disruption in unstable angina and non–Q-wave MI is dynamic and repetitive (Fig. 152–3 and Table 152–14).[175] In unstable angina, transient partial or total thrombotic occlusions (10 to 20 minutes in duration) subsequently undergo spontaneous or pharmacologically enhanced fibrinolysis.

Table 152–14. **Proposed Hypothesis of Pathogenesis of the Acute and Subacute Coronary Syndromes**

Syndrome	Plaque Damage	Thrombus	
		Fixed	Labile
Unstable angina	+	+ *	+ + +
Non–Q-wave myocardial infarction	+ +	+ *	+ +
Q-wave myocardial infarction	+ + +	+ + +†	+

*Vasoconstriction (may contribute to coronary occlusion).
†Collaterals (may decrease extension of infarction).
+ = Mild; + + = moderate; + + + = severe.
From Fuster V, Verstraete M (eds): Thrombosis in Cardiovascular Disorders. Philadelphia: WB Saunders, 1992.

Angioscopic studies in unstable angina usually reveal nonocclusive platelet-rich mural thrombi.[184] Thrombus microemboli are common in the coronary microcirculation of patients who succumb during unstable angina, supporting the concept of intermittent thrombus formation, endogenous lysis, fragmentation, and downstream embolization.[182] In animal models of the acute coronary syndromes, cyclic coronary artery flow variations correspond to intermittent thrombosis and the cyclic release of the vasoactive platelet products thromboxane A_2 and serotonin from platelet-rich mural thrombi. Cyclic flow variations are ameliorated by potent antiplatelet agents.[185] In unstable angina in humans, there is a temporal relationship between chest pain episodes and transcardiac increases in thromboxane A_2 and serotonin.[185] Fibrinopeptide A levels are also increased in unstable angina, indicative of ongoing thrombin activity.[186]

The pathophysiology of non–Q-wave MI is similar to that of unstable angina except that in non–Q-wave MI, coronary occlusion lasts longer; spontaneous or enhanced fibrinolysis occurs not within 10 to 20 minutes as in unstable angina but within 2 hours of the onset of occlusion, resulting in a varying degree of nontransmural myocardial necrosis. Supporting this concept is the observation that three fourths of infarct-related vessels are patent at angiography shortly following non–Q-wave MI.[175]

In Q-wave MI, deeper arterial injury or extensive ulceration of the plaque leads to larger, more adherent thrombus formation and persistent arterial occlusion. Endogenous or exogenous thrombolysis is incomplete. Although angiographic follow-up studies show that arteries with severe stenoses are 3 times more likely to occlude than arteries with less-severe stenoses, MI infrequently results from the occlusion of highly stenotic arteries due to the presence of well-formed collaterals.[175, 187] In up to half of cases of MI, the infarct-related artery may lack a previous significant stenosis (greater than 50%); in up to two thirds of cases, the infarct-related artery may have lacked a hemodynamically significant stenosis (greater than 70%).[188]

Residual Thrombus After Plaque Disruption

Mural thrombus predisposes to residual stenosis (if incorporated into the atherosclerotic lesion) and re-current occlusion.[180, 189, 190] Three mechanisms contribute.[175] First, residual thrombus may encroach on the vascular lumen, increasing the degree of lesion stenosis, in turn increasing shear-induced platelet activation and deposition. Second, the exposed surface of the residual thrombus is itself potently thrombogenic. In animal models of arterial balloon injury, the surface of residual thrombus is 2 to 4 times more thrombogenic than deep arterial injury.[179] Fibrin-bound thrombin exposed on the residual thrombus surface is enzymatically active and inaccessible to heparin because of heparin's size; in this manner, heparin alone may be incapable of preventing thrombus propagation. Selective thrombin inhibitors such as hirudin, which are 10 times smaller than heparin, can inhibit fibrin-bound thrombin and can more completely prevent mural thrombus formation and propagation following deep arterial injury.[127] Third, fibrinolysis itself activates platelets and thrombin.

In animal models, inhibition of both platelets and thrombin is necessary to prevent reocclusion following successful thrombolysis.[191] The presence of systemic risk factors for thrombosis such as a primary hypercoagulable state, high circulating levels of catecholamines, enhanced platelet reactivity due to smoking, hypercholesterolemia, elevated levels of homocysteine of apolipoprotein A, or defective endogenous fibrinolytic mechanisms all enhance the risk of recurrent occlusion.[175] These systemic thrombogenic risk factors may also modify the extent and duration of thrombus deposition following plaque disruption.

Thrombosis and Vasoconstriction

Following type II or III injury, the release of thromboxane A_2 and serotonin from deposited, activated platelets promotes vasoconstriction of the already compromised coronary artery. Vasospasm contributes to intermittent coronary occlusion observed during thrombolysis[192] in addition to the cyclic flow variations in unstable angina.[185] Thrombin promotes vasoconstriction via direct, potent effect on platelet activation, aggregation, and secretion. Normal vascular endothelium constitutively elaborates vasodilatory substances, the most important of which are endothelium-derived relaxant factor (nitric oxide) and prostacyclin. In addition to potent vasodilating properties, both prostacyclin and nitric oxide possess platelet antiaggregatory properties and thus antagonize the proaggregatory effects of thromboxane A_2 and thrombin.[193] In the physiologic basal state, constitutive production of nitric oxide is likely the most important mechanism whereby normal vascular endothelium modulates arterial tone. Nitric oxide also inhibits platelet aggregation, although the physiologic importance of this mechanism in preventing thrombosis has not yet been fully elucidated. Following type I, II, or III injury, vascular endothelium may produce relatively more vasoconstricting substances (such as endothelins) than vasodilating substances (prostacyclin and nitric oxide). Atherosclerotic coronary arteries exhibit increased basal vascular tone and altered, even paradoxical vasoconstrictor responses to normally endothelium-dependent vasodilating substances such as acetylcholine.[194] Exaggerated vasoconstrictive responses of atherosclerotic coronaries may be invoked via the release of vasoconstrictors such as thromboxane A_2 and serotonin from platelets and thrombin-mediated vasoconstriction at the site of plaque disruption and thrombosis. By further reducing the lumen of the injured vessel, thereby increasing arterial shear rates, vasoconstriction predisposes to augmented shear-induced platelet adhesion and aggregation.

Role of Platelets and Thrombin in the Myofibrotic Response to Vascular Injury

Platelets and thrombin are important in the myofibrotic atherosclerotic response following vascular injury. Pigs lacking von Willebrand factor (a protein important for platelet adhesion and aggregation) are resistant to spontaneous atherosclerosis and thrombosis following arterial balloon injury; thrombocytopenic rabbits after arterial balloon injury develop less intimal thickening.[175] Three phases of the myofibrotic response following balloon-arterial injury have been proposed.[195] Phase I, which occurs minutes after injury and lasts for up to 24 hours, consists of platelet deposition on the injured arterial surface and resultant thrombus formation. Phase II, which occurs 4 days to 14 days following injury, consists of smooth muscle hypertrophy, proliferation, and migration from the media into the intima. Platelets induce smooth muscle migration and proliferation via the secretion of PDGF and other growth and chemotactic factors. Phase III, which occurs 14 days to 3 months following injury, consists of progressive intimal thickening due to continued smooth muscle proliferation and extracellular matrix accumulation. Platelets initiate (phase I) and likely play an important role in sustaining (phase II) the three-phase myofibrotic response to vascular injury.

Thrombin is produced during phase I and is incorporated into the thrombus and extracellular matrix by binding to fibrin. Fibrin-bound thrombin remains enzymatically active and continues to activate platelets and coagulation factors. As the thrombus is remodeled or lysed, this "reservoir" of slowly exposed and released fibrin-bound thrombin remains active. This may represent an additional mechanism whereby thrombin-activated platelets stimulate smooth muscle migration during phase II. By itself, thrombin is a potent stimulus of smooth muscle migration and proliferation.[175] Thrombin is the most potent platelet agonist known.

Antithrombotic Therapy in Coronary Artery Disease (Table 152–15)

No available antiplatelet agent completely prevents platelet adhesion to the subendothelium following vascular injury. If the principal cause of progression of coronary artery atherosclerotic lesions is intimal hyperplasia related to chronic and subtle endothelial damage mediated by platelet and monocyte vessel wall interactions,[176] then antithrombotic therapy in its present form may be insignificant in halting such progression. If, however, progression is more related to recurrent plaque rupture,[175] nonocclusive mural thrombosis, and subsequent organization and incorporation of the thrombus into the growing lesion, antiplatelet agents may play an important role.

Chronic Stable Angina Pectoris

Because plaque rupture appears to be a random event in the protracted natural history of coronary artery disease and because platelet-rich thrombosis occurs at the site of plaque disruption, the prophylactic use of platelet inhibitors in patients with stable angina pectoris has a theoretical rationale. A 5-year prospective, randomized, double-blind, placebo-controlled trial of 370 patients has investigated the efficacy of aspirin (975 mg/day) plus dipyridamole (225 mg/day) in the angiographic progression of coronary artery disease.[196] Two angiograms performed mean 4.6 years apart showed that aspirin plus dipyridamole decreased new lesion formation by 12% (23% versus 35%, $p = .04$) but did not prevent preexistent lesion

Table 152–15. **Coronary Artery Disease Antithrombotic Therapy—1994**

Syndrome	Risk	ASA	A/C	A/C + ASA	
				<1 wk	≥1 wk
Unstable angina	High	+	+	+[1]	±*
MI (acute)—no lysis	High	+	±	?[1]	?[2]
MI (acute)—lysis	High	+	±	±[1]	?[2]
MI (acute)—LV-Ant	Medium	−	+	−	−
PTCA	High	+	+	+	−
SVBC	High	+	±	?*	?*
MI (>1 month–3 years)	Medium	±	+		?[2]
Chronic/stable CAD	Medium	+	+		?*
Primary prevention	Low	±*	?		−

*Evolving approach in high risk: need of trials.
[1]GUSTO II (hirudin).
[2]CARS (A/C + ASA low dose and fixed).

Table 152–16. **Aspirin in the Primary Prevention of Myocardial Infarction in the Setting of Chronic Angina Pectoris**

Study	Patients	ASA Dose (mg)	Follow-Up (Months)	MI Reduction	p-Value*
PHS	333	325 qod	60	87%	0.001
SAPAT	2035	75 qd	50	34%	0.003
Chesebro	370	975 qd	60	44%	0.05

ASA, aspirin; MI, myocardial infarction; PHS, Physicians' Health Study.
*For MI reduction.

progression. Patients treated with aspirin plus dipyridamole experienced fewer MIs (5.3% versus 12.1%, $p = .05$); no difference was observed in mortality or cardiac death.

Clinical Studies

Two clinical trials have evaluated aspirin in chronic stable angina pectoris (Table 152–16). In a double-blind, placebo-controlled study of 333 male physicians with chronic stable angina and no prior MI enrolled in the larger Physicians Health Study, use of aspirin (325 mg every other day for 60 months) resulted in a 87% risk reduction of first MI ($p < .001$) in a proportional hazards model.[197] Stroke was significantly increased in the aspirin group (relative risk 5.4, 95% confidence interval 1.3 to 22.1, $p = .02$). Aspirin use did not affect the frequency or severity of stable angina episodes. In the prospective, double-blind, placebo-controlled Swedish Angina Pectoris Aspirin Trial (SAPAT), 2035 patients with stable angina pectoris and no prior MI were randomized to aspirin (75 mg/day) or placebo with a median follow-up of 50 months.[198] The aspirin group experienced a significant 34% reduction ($p = .003$) in the primary combined end point, MI and sudden death. A significant 39% reduction ($p = .006$) in the incidence of first MI alone was observed. A significant 32% reduction ($p = .001$) in vascular events including MI occurred. There was an insignificant 25% reduction in stroke in the aspirin group. Extrapolating from their data, the authors calculated that aspirin therapy over 10,000 patient-years would prevent 118 vascular events at the cost of 10 fatal hemorrhagic episodes.

In the first Antiplatelet Trialists' Collaboration meta-analysis of 25 trials of antiplatelet agents in patients with a history of transient ischemic attack, occlusive stroke, unstable angina, or MI, antiplatelet therapy reduced nonfatal MI by 32% ($p < .0001$), vascular mortality by 15% ($p = .0003$), and nonfatal stroke by 27% ($p < .0001$).[199] In the second Antiplatelet Trialists' Collaboration, antiplatelet agents reduced the combined end point of nonfatal MI, nonfatal stroke, and vascular mortality by one fourth, and the individual end points of nonfatal MI by 34% and vascular death by 17%.[200]

Current Recommendations (Table 152–17)

Based on the three trials cited and the results of the Antiplatelet Trialists' Collaboration meta-analysis, all patients with stable chronic angina pectoris should receive aspirin (160 to 325 mg/day) indefinitely. Patients with clear clinical or laboratory evidence of coronary artery disease who do not experience angina should also receive aspirin (160 to 325 mg/day) indefinitely.

Unstable Angina

Antiplatelet Agents in Unstable Angina

Convincing evidence of the benefit of aspirin in unstable angina derives from several double-blind, randomized, placebo-controlled trials (Table 152–18). In the Veterans Administration Cooperative Study, 1266 men with unstable angina of recent onset were randomized to 325 mg of aspirin daily (as Alka-Seltzer) or placebo.[201] During 12 weeks of follow-up, death and MI in the aspirin group were significantly reduced (5% versus 10%, respectively). Gastrointestinal side effects and bleeding were not increased from this buffered aspirin preparation. In the Canadian Multicenter Trial of unstable angina, 555 men and women were randomized to aspirin (325 mg four times daily), sulfinpyrazone (200 mg four times daily), both aspirin and sulfinpyrazone, or neither.[202] At 18 months of follow-up, death or nonfatal MI was reduced by 51% in the groups receiving aspirin alone or in combination (Fig. 152–4). No benefit was seen with sulfinpyrazone alone, and no additional benefit

Table 152–17. **Antithrombotic Therapy in Coronary Artery Disease**

Coronary Event	Recommendations
Stable angina	Aspirin, 325 mg/day
Unstable angina	*Acute phase:* IV heparin plus low-dose aspirin, 75–100 mg
	Chronic phase: aspirin, 325 mg/day
Non–Q-wave MI	*Acute phase:* IV heparin plus low-dose aspirin
	Chronic phase: aspirin, 325 mg/day
Q-wave MI: absence of thrombolytic therapy	Aspirin, 325 mg/day, in acute and chronic phases. IV heparin in acute phase
Q-wave MI: presence of thrombolytic therapy	Aspirin, 325 mg on admission, then 75–100 mg/day combined with adjunctive heparin* (aPTT 2–3 times control) for 2–7 days Aspirin, 325 mg/day thereafter

aPTT, activated partial thromboplastin time; MI, myocardial infarction.
*Heparin has not yet been shown to be efficacious adjunctive therapy with streptokinase.

Table 152–18. **Antiplatelet Therapy in Unstable Angina**

Study	VA	Canadian	Theroux	Ticlopidine	RISC
Patients	1266	555	479	652	796
Design	R, PC	R, PC	R, PC	R	R, PC
Therapy	ASA 325 qd or placebo	ASA 325 qid, ASA + S, S	ASA 325 qd or IV heparin	Ticlopidine 250 mg bid	ASA 75 mg qd or ASA 75 mg qp + IV heparin
Follow-up	12 weeks, 1 year	18 months, 24 months	6 days	6 months	5 days, 3 months
Primary end point	Death, MI	Death, MI	RAP, death, MI	Death, nonfatal MI	Death, MI
Reduction, primary end point, first F/U	51%*	—	38%†	46%*	57%*
Reduction, primary end point, second F/U	43%*	71%*	—	—	64%*

VA, Veterans Administration; R, randomized; PC, placebo-controlled; MI, myocardial infarction; RAP, refractory angina pectoris; F/U, follow-up; ASA, aspirin.

*Significant at p value $\leq .05$.
†Nearly significant p value $= .066$.

accrued from sulfinpyrazone compared with aspirin alone. At 24 months of follow-up, the aspirin group had a 71% reduction in risk of cardiac death (3% versus 11.7%) compared with the groups not receiving aspirin. Gastrointestinal side effects and hemorrhage were significantly more common in aspirin-treated patients, owing to the higher dose. Two other large trials from the Montreal Heart Institute have also shown that aspirin is efficacious in unstable angina.[203, 204]

Ticlopidine has been shown to be efficacious in unstable angina.[205] In a double-blind, randomized trial of conventional therapy (excluding heparin or aspirin) versus conventional therapy plus ticlopidine (250 mg twice daily) begun within 48 hours of admission and continued through the 6-month follow-up period, intention-to-treat analysis showed that conventional therapy plus ticlopidine resulted in a 46% reduction in the primary combined end point of vascular death and nonfatal MI (7.3% versus 13.6%, $p = .009$). Ticlopidine reduced fatal and nonfatal MI by 53% (5.1% versus 10.9%, $p = .006$) and nonfatal MI alone by 46% (4.8% versus 8.9%, $p = .039$), but not

new Q-wave MI. Adverse effects from ticlopidine included gastrointestinal upset in 5% and skin reaction in 2% of patients. Neutropenia did not occur, unlike in other large trials of the drug in which the incidence of neutropenia was approximately 1%. Ticlopidine's greater expense, high incidence of adverse effects (including neutropenia), and delayed onset of antiplatelet action compared with aspirin all favor the use of aspirin as the first-line antiplatelet agent in unstable angina.[17] Ticlopidine may be considered in aspirin-intolerant or allergic patients; however, its delayed onset of antiplatelet action should be borne in mind. A pilot study of the platelet glycoprotein IIb/IIIa antagonist c7E3 has appeared: this potent antiplatelet antibody does not appear to increase bleeding in heparin- and aspirin-treated patients.[206]

Anticoagulants in Unstable Angina

Four small, uncontrolled trials in the early 1960s concluded that anticoagulants reduced the incidence of MI and death in unstable angina, and anticoagulation therapy became standard practice.[207] More recent tri-

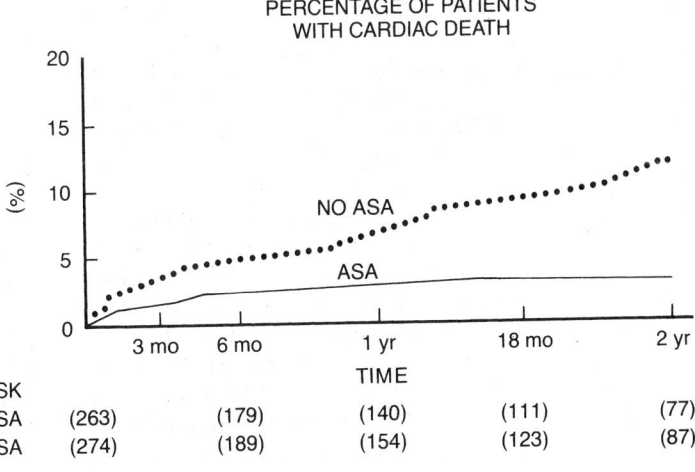

Figure 152–4. Efficacy of aspirin versus no aspirin in reducing fatal myocardial infarction in patients with unstable angina. The Canadian Multicenter Trial. (From Cairns JA, Gent M, Singer J, et al: Aspirin, sulfinpyrazone, or both in unstable angina. N Engl J Med 313:1369, 1985.)

als have clearly established the efficacy of heparin in unstable angina. Telford and Wilson in a double-blind, placebo-controlled trial randomized 214 patients with unstable angina to intravenously administered heparin (5000-IU bolus every 6 hours), atenolol (100 mg/day), both heparin and atenolol, or placebo.[208] Heparin but not atenolol prevented transmural MI ($p = .024$ for heparin), which occurred in 2% of the heparin-alone group, 4% of the heparin-plus-atenolol group, 13% of the atenolol-alone group, and 17% of the placebo group. In a smaller study, Williams et al. treated 102 patients with open-label intravenously administered heparin (10,000 IU every 6 hours for 48 hours) followed by warfarin for 6 months.[209] The combined end point, recurrent unstable angina, MI, or death was reduced from 34% to 12% in the heparin-warfarin group ($p < .05$). In a double-blind study, Neri Serneri et al. randomized 97 patients with refractory unstable angina to an initial protocol of either bolus heparin (6000 IU every 6 hours), continuous-infusion heparin (5000-IU bolus followed by 1000 IU/hr adjusted to an aPTT of 1.5 to 2.0 times control), or aspirin (325 mg/day).[210] Heparin infusion, the most efficacious of these three antithrombotic regimens, was then compared with alteplase, which became available on the market. Heparin infusion significantly reduced the frequency of angina (from 84% to 94%), episodes of silent ischemia (71% to 77%), and overall duration of ischemia (81% to 86%).

Antiplatelet Agents and Anticoagulants in Unstable Angina

In a double-blind, placebo-controlled trial, Theroux et al. randomized 479 patients with unstable angina at a mean of 8 hours after the last episode of chest pain to aspirin (325 mg/day), intravenously administered heparin (5000-IU bolus followed by 1000 IU/hr adjusted to an aPTT of 1.5 to 2.0 times control), aspirin plus heparin, or placebo.[199] By 6 days, refractory angina, MI, and death occurred in 23%, 12%, and 1.7% of the placebo group, respectively. Heparin alone resulted in a significant decrease in refractory angina (8.5% versus 23%, $p = .002$), MI (0.8% versus 12%, $p < .001$), and the combined end point of "any event" (9.3% versus 26.3%, $p < .001$). Aspirin alone did not decrease refractory angina (16.5% versus 23%, $p = .217$), but it did decrease MI (3.3% versus 12%, $p = .012$); aspirin did not reduce the combined end point of any event (16.5% versus 26.3%, $p = .066$). Combined aspirin and heparin reduced refractory angina (10.7% versus 23%, $p = .011$), MI (1.6% versus 12%, $p = .001$), and any event (11.5% versus 26.3%, $p = .003$). The combination of aspirin and heparin had no greater effect than heparin alone but was associated with more bleeding complications (3.3% versus 1.7%). In a follow-up study, Theroux et al. reported that the discontinuation of heparin resulted in reactivation of unstable angina in 13% of patients at a mean of 9.5 hours after discontinuation of heparin.[211] Rate of reactivation was highest in patients treated with heparin alone and was lower in patients treated with

heparin plus aspirin. The authors recommended that aspirin be administered at least several hours before discontinuation of heparin to prevent reactivation of angina.

The randomized, double-blind, placebo-controlled RISC trial evaluated treatment of unstable angina with aspirin (75 mg/day) versus aspirin (75 mg/day) plus 5 days of intravenously administered heparin (5000-IU bolus every 6 hours for the first 24 hours followed by 3750 IU every 6 hours for 4 days) in 796 men with unstable angina.[212] Aspirin reduced the primary event rate of MI or death at 5 days, 1 month, or 3 months by 57% to 69%. Aspirin alone did not significantly reduce death alone at 5 days, 30 days, or 90 days. Heparin alone did not alter overall event rates of MI or death including during the first 5 days. The combination of aspirin plus heparin did significantly reduce the risk of MI or death by 75% in the first 5 days. The authors were careful to point out that in this trial, heparin was begun relatively late compared with the trial of Theroux et al.; the median delay to heparin following admission was 33 hours, and 81% began therapy more than 24 hours after admission. In addition, heparin was administered in bolus form and not by continuous infusion.

Cohen et al. randomized 358 patients with unstable angina or non–Q-wave MI within 48 hours of admission to orally administered aspirin alone (162.5 mg/day) or orally administered aspirin (162.5 mg/day) plus intravenously administered heparin (100-IU/kg bolus followed by continuous infusion) to maintain the aPTT at 1.5 to 2.0 times control followed by warfarin.[213, 214] There was no difference in the combined total number of primary ischemia end points during the 12-week follow-up period. However, a relatively high withdrawal rate (36%) and unbalanced randomization assignment (only 28% of patients were randomized to aspirin alone) limited the statistical conclusions of the study.

In a later, separate double-blind study, Theroux et al. randomized 484 patients with unstable angina to therapy with either aspirin (325 mg twice a day) or intravenously administered heparin (5000-IU bolus followed by continuous infusion adjusted to maintain the aPTT at 1.5 to 2.0 times control).[204] Therapy was begun at a mean of 8 hours following admission and continued for at least 6 days. Patients on aspirin at the time of hospital admission were excluded. The primary study end point was the occurrence of fatal and nonfatal MI. MI occurred in 0.8% of the heparin-treated patients and in 3.7% of the aspirin-treated patients ($p = .035$), an OR of 0.22 and risk difference of 2.9% (95% confidence interval 0.3% to 5.6%). This study was limited to the acute phase of unstable angina, however, and did not present data on patients after 6 days of the study period.

In a second trial, Cohen et al. randomized 214 patients who had not been taking aspirin prior to the study within 9.5 hours of presenting unstable angina to aspirin (162.5 mg/day) or aspirin (162.5 mg/day) plus intravenously administered heparin (aPTT at 2 times control) followed by warfarin (INR 2 to 3) for 12 weeks.[200] At 2 weeks, total ischemic events (recurrent angina, MI) were significantly reduced in the aspirin-plus-anticoagulant group (10.5% versus 27%, p = .004), and at 12 weeks, total ischemic events were nearly significantly reduced (13% versus 25%, p = .06). Thus, the combination of aspirin and anticoagulants appears more efficacious than either agent alone in both the acute and likely chronic phases of unstable angina in patients who had not been taking aspirin previously. Overview of the results of the Montreal Heart Institute, RISC, and ATACS trials showed that combination heparin and aspirin therapy during the acute phase (5 days) significantly decreased the relative risk of MI or death (RR = 0.44, 95% confidence interval 0.21% to 0.93%) compared with therapy with either agent alone.

In summary, both heparin and aspirin are efficacious in the acute phase of unstable angina (see Table 152–15). Aspirin (75 mg/day) appears to be as effective as higher doses. Heparin alone decreases the incidence of MI during the acute phase of unstable angina compared with therapy with aspirin alone, but the combination of aspirin plus heparin is more efficacious than either agent alone. Heparin is most effective when administered as an intravenous bolus followed by continuous infusion to prolong the aPTT at 1.5 to 2.0 times control; intermittent-bolus heparin administration does not appear to be effective. Subcutaneously administered heparin in unstable angina has not yet been evaluated in large trials.

The duration of heparin therapy in the acute phase of unstable angina is empiric at present. As discussed earlier, the largest trials of heparin have continued therapy for 5 to 6 days. Unstable angina may be reactivated when heparin is discontinued; the incidence of reactivation can be decreased by concurrent or overlapping aspirin therapy. In the chronic phase, aspirin has been proven efficacious. Trials of low-dose aspirin in combination with low-dose warfarin in the chronic phase are currently underway.

Thrombolysis in Unstable Angina

Although theoretically attractive, thrombolysis during unstable angina has not proved efficacious to date. Early studies employed small patient populations and often lacked control groups.[207] Change in the angiographic appearance of the culprit lesion has been the primary end point in most of these studies.[215] Two relatively large trials have appeared to date. In the UNASEM trial (Thrombolysis in Patients with Unstable Angina), 126 patients with angina within 12 hours underwent catheterization within 3 hours of hospital admission.[216] Anistreplase (30 IU) or placebo was administered after the first catheterization, and catheterization was repeated within 12 to 28 hours. There was no significant difference in the angiographic appearance of the lesions or lumen diameter following anistreplase therapy compared with placebo. Most other studies have been unable to show consistent improvement in lumen diameter.[215]

In the TIMI-IIIA trial, 306 patients with unstable angina were randomized following initial angiography to a 90-minute front-loaded infusion of t-PA (0.8 mg/kg) or placebo.[217] All patients received conventional antianginal therapy, including full heparinization. Most patients also received aspirin. The primary study end point was change in angiographic appearance of the culprit lesion and lumen diameter at 18 to 48 hours. There was no advantage of t-PA over the placebo regimen (which included full-dose intravenously administered heparin) in angiographic improvement of the culprit lesion (25% versus 19%, p = .25), lumen diameter (p = .27), or mean change in percentage of stenosis (-6.2% versus -4.6%, p = .16). However, t-PA was associated with a statistically significant percentage increase in the secondary end point of substantial angiographic improvement (15% versus 5%, p = .003); this was especially the case in patients with non–Q-wave MI and in patients with angiographically apparent thrombus. Overall, only 15% of patients treated with t-PA experienced substantial angiographic improvement.

Of interest, thrombus was found at initial angiography in only 35% of patients, even when the angiograms were viewed with sevenfold magnification in multiple views. The authors hypothesized that the low incidence of apparent thrombus at angiography in TIMI-IIIA was due to either the low sensitivity of routine angiography for thrombus detection; the presence of predominantly older, multilayered mural thrombus that may be undetectable by angiography; the presence of intermittent, recurrent thrombus; or a lesser prevalence of thrombus in unstable angina than the high prevalence previously reported in angiographic trials. TIMI-IIIA did not report any clinical outcomes; the ongoing TIMI-IIIB trial (which randomized 1271 patients in a 2 × 2 factorial design to t-PA or placebo without baseline arteriography, then to invasive or conservative revascularization schemes) will provide detailed clinical outcomes information. Preliminary results indicate that death or MI occurred in 11.6% of patients randomized to t-PA and in 10.3% of patients randomized to placebo.[215] Total ischemic events were not improved by t-PA.

Given the intermittent, recurrent nature of thrombosis during unstable angina, it is not surprising that thrombolytic therapy has not proved efficacious in clinical end points in the reported small uncontrolled clinical studies or efficacious in reducing culprit lesion morphology of lumen diameter in the larger angiographic trials. The transient antithrombotic effect of thrombolytic agents, basic differences in pathophysiologic mechanisms compared with MI, and thrombolytic agent activation of platelets and coagulation system factors (which predisposes to recurrent thrombosis) all contribute to the apparent lack of efficacy of thrombolytic agents in unstable angina compared with MI.[215]

Selective Thrombin Inhibitors

Given the efficacy of heparin in unstable angina, thrombin apparently has a potent role in the pathophysiology of unstable angina. Pilot trials of hirudin and argatroban have been reported.[218, 219] Both agents appear efficacious, although in these small preliminary reports, patients may still experience refractory angina or MI despite these potent agents. The incidence of bleeding does not appear to be increased. Reactivation of angina has been reported following discontinuation of argatroban infusion.[219] Large studies are underway to evaluate the role of selective thrombin inhibitors in unstable angina.

Current Recommendations (see Table 152–17)

Many patients who develop unstable angina will be taking aspirin chronically at the time of hospital admission: aspirin should be continued in these patients. Such patients should also be treated with intravenously administered heparin (5000-IU bolus followed by continuous infusion to maintain the aPTT at 1.5 to 2.0 times control). The dose of aspirin should be reduced to 75 mg/day during concurrent heparin therapy. Patients who are not taking aspirin at the time of hospital admission should be treated with intravenously administered heparin (5000-IU bolus followed by continuous infusion to maintain the aPTT at 1.5 to 2.0 times control) and low-dose aspirin (75 to 100 mg/day) in combination. Combination therapy is strongly recommended in high-risk patients with unstable angina: those with suspected non–Q-wave MI, postinfarction angina, electrocardiographic changes with angina, recurrent angina despite aspirin or heparin monotherapy, rest angina, or depressed left ventricular function. To date there are no conclusive data that low-dose aspirin combined with heparin increases major or life-threatening bleeding complications, although minor bleeding complications are increased.

The duration of heparin therapy is empiric at present. Controlled trials to date have treated patients with intravenously administered heparin for 5 to 7 days. In low-risk patients who experience no further angina following 72 hours of heparin therapy, heparin may be discontinued. Heparin should never be discontinued in the absence of overlapping aspirin ther-

apy to prevent reactivation of angina: aspirin (75 to 325 mg) should be started several hours before heparin is discontinued. In aspirin-intolerant or allergic patients, ticlopidine should be started 48 hours prior to heparin discontinuation because of ticlopidine's delayed antiplatelet effect. In high-risk patients, heparin should be continued for 5 to 7 days. Recurrent angina, especially angina at rest or in association with electrocardiographic changes should always prompt evaluation of the aPTT to ensure that heparin therapy is within therapeutic range. In the chronic phase, all patients should receive aspirin (75 to 325 mg/day). In the chronic phase, patients intolerant of aspirin may be treated with ticlopidine (250 mg twice a day), and patients intolerant of ticlopidine should be treated with warfarin (target INR of 2 to 3).

SAPHENOUS VEIN BYPASS GRAFT THROMBOTIC DISEASE
Incidence

Atherothrombotic coronary artery saphenous vein graft (SVG) occlusion remains a vexing problem following coronary artery bypass graft surgery.[220–223] SVG occlusion occurs in 10% to 15% of all grafts within 1 month of surgery and in 25% of all grafts by 1 year. From 2 to 5 years after surgery, approximately 2% to 4% of SVGs occlude per year. Fully 50% of SVGs are occluded 10 years following surgery. The left internal mammary artery (LIMA) has a much lower incidence of occlusion, approximately 10% at 7 to 10 years following surgery.[224]

Pathogenesis

SVG occlusion appears to involve four stages.[225] Stage I consists of an early (within 1 month) phase of postoperative thrombotic occlusion (Figs. 152–5 and 152–6). Stage II consists of an intermediate phase of platelet-mediated intimal hyperplasia and superimposed thrombosis. Stage III consists of a late phase of atherothrombotic occlusion (analogous to the accelerated atherosclerosis following angioplasty or cardiac trans-

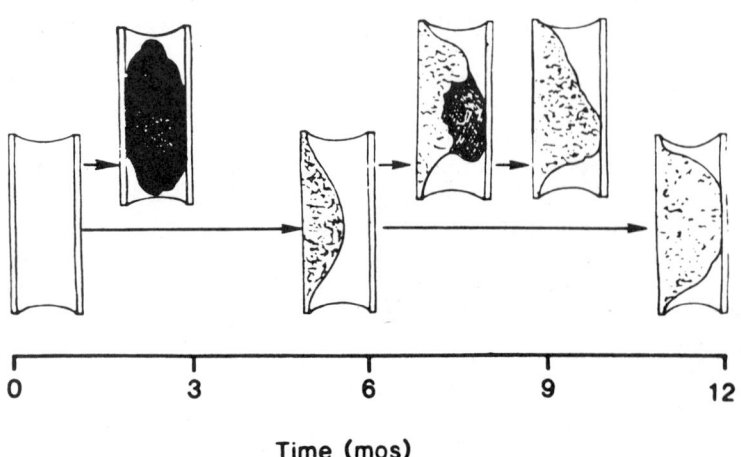

Time (mos)

Figure 152–5. Scheme of the four phases of vein graft disease leading to occlusion within the first postoperative year: (1) early thrombotic occlusion *(high in panel, left),* (2) intermediate phase of intimal hyperplasia *(low in panel, middle),* (3) late phase of occlusion related to intimal hyperplasia *(low in panel, right)* or to complicating thrombosis superimposed on intimal hyperplasia with fibrotic organization of thrombus *(high in panel, right).* The phase of atherosclerotic disease after the first postoperative year is not shown. (From Fuster V, Chesebro JH: Coronary artery bypass grafting: A model for understanding progression of atherosclerotic disease and role of pharmacologic intervention. Adv Prostaglandin Thromboxane Leukotriene Res 13:286, 1985. Reproduced with permission from Raven Press, New York.)

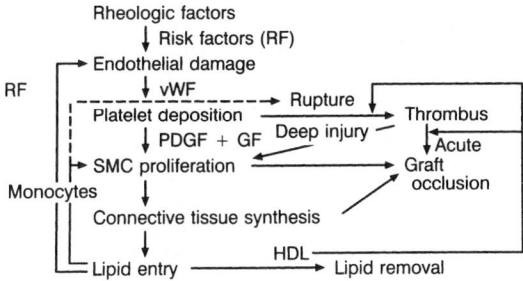

Figure 152–6. Proposed pathogenesis of vein graft occlusion and chronic disease. Acute endothelial damage is due to surgical factors. Late endothelial dysfunction or injury is associated with risk factors. Platelet deposition early is more prominent in regions of deeper injury, especially at the distal anastomotic site where shear forces are higher as the vein joins a smaller coronary artery lumen. Thrombus formation late is related to a ruptured atherosclerotic plaque. Because vein grafts have no branches, thrombus often propagates proximally to fill the whole graft proximal to the site of thrombosis. Accelerated smooth muscle cell (SMC) proliferation occurs early in stage II and appears significantly related to platelet-derived growth factor (PDGF) and probably also other growth factors (GF). Slower and more chronic proliferation may also occur, especially in the presence of abnormal risk factors. Increased connective tissue matrix occurs in the later phases of SMC proliferation. Lipid entry into the vein graft wall marks the beginning of stage III with the formation of a complex lesion that may rupture and lead to spontaneous deep injury and acute thrombosis. High-density lipoprotein cholesterol may remove lipid from the wall and carries an important inhibitor of coagulation, lipoprotein-associated coagulation inhibitor (LACI), which inhibits the interaction between tissue factor and activated factor VII early in the coagulation cascade. Thus, particular attention to maintaining high levels of high-density lipoprotein cholesterol appears important. Elevated low-density lipoprotein and triglycerides may attract monocytes with more foam cell development and increase risk for complex atherosclerotic lesion with plaque rupture. (From Fuster V, Verstraete M [eds]: Thrombosis in Cardiovascular Disorders. Philadelphia: WB Saunders, 1992.)

plantation) occurring near the end of the first year. Stage IV consists of a late phase (beyond 1 year) of progressive atherosclerosis similar to native coronary artery atherosclerosis. Thrombosis is a key mechanism in stages I through III, and antithrombotic therapy plays an important preventive role.

The pathogenesis of SVG occlusion begins with intraoperative trauma to the SVG resulting from vein harvesting, surgical manipulation, temporal delay between vein harvesting and implantation, and vein preservation techniques.[226, 227] Type II vascular injury (endothelial denudation) may occur throughout the length of the harvested SVG; type III vascular injury may occur at sites of anastomosis. Contractile responses of the dissected, free SVG may lead to further endothelial damage due to contraction-generated shear forces operative at the endothelial-media interface.[227] In the past, pressurizing techniques used to prepare the graft prior to implantation led to further graft endothelial damage. Storage of harvested SVGs prior to implantation may also lead to further endothelial injury; physiologic solutions containing electrolytes and albumin result in less endothelial damage than do less physiologic saline solutions.[227] Although the injured or denuded endothelial surfaces of SVGs regenerate within days following surgery, normal en-

dothelial function may not be restored. SVG endothelium may exhibit impaired fibrinolytic activity,[228] and diminished release of the important vasodilating and platelet antiaggregatory substances prostacyclin and nitric oxide.[227, 229] The LIMA is protected from endothelial injury and platelet deposition due to less extensive surgical handling, previous adaptation to arterial shear forces, and preservation of partially intact vasa vasorum.[226]

Lack of conditioning of the SVG to arterial shear forces and further shear-induced endothelial injury upon implantation increases the susceptibility of the SVG to platelet deposition.[226] Platelet deposition on the SVG is immediate and occurs as soon as blood flows through the newly implanted graft: this has been confirmed angioscopically.[230] Platelet deposition is found in approximately 75% of SVGs in both experimental animals and humans who die within 24 hours of coronary artery bypass surgery.[231] SVG platelet deposition is further enhanced by platelet activation that occurs as platelets circulate through the cardiopulmonary bypass pump. Sluggish implanted SVG blood flow may also promote thrombosis. Up to 20% of SVGs show technical faults in distal anastomosis suturing, which may lead to reduced graft flow and increased thrombotic risk.[230] In particular, SVGs with flow of less than 40 ml/min or with a distal anastomosis to a small receiving coronary artery less than 1.5 mm in diameter are at increased risk of occlusion.[226]

If early stage-I thrombotic occlusion does not occur, platelets adherent to the SVG secrete growth factors, chemotactic factors, and mitogens (most importantly PDGF and TGF-β), which attract monocytes and stimulate medial smooth muscle hypertrophy and migration to the intima.[226] Myofibrotic intimal hyperplasia results.[175] Histologically, this myofibrotic process is apparent in SVGs by the first postoperative month.[225, 232] Though the myofibrotic process tends to progress slowly, rapid episodic progression may occur with superimposed thrombosis, and subsequent organization and intimal incorporation or thrombotic occlusion may occur. After the first postoperative year, this process of myofibrotic intimal hyperplasia becomes less important, and subsequent SVG atherothrombotic disease appears indistinguishable from native coronary artery atherosclerosis.[175]

Rationale for Antiplatelet Therapy

Given these clinical and pathophysiologic observations, the rationale for antiplatelet therapy following coronary artery bypass surgery is as follows: (1) to reduce perioperative SVG platelet adhesion and aggregation, (2) reduce acute perioperative thrombotic SVG occlusion and thrombosis, (3) decrease chronic platelet adhesion and aggregation in order to blunt intimal hyperplasia and superimposed thrombosis. In animal models, antiplatelet agents have been shown to reduce acute occlusion and intimal proliferation.[233–236]

Clinical Trials

A meta-analysis of 13 trials of antiplatelet and anticoagulants from 1966 to 1988 in humans showed that early initiation of active treatment was beneficial in preventing SVG occlusion (overall effect size = 0.30, confidence interval 0.21% to 0.38%).[237] In the Mayo Clinic trial, dipyridamole was selected because it possessed the theoretical capability of preventing platelet activation during transit through the cardiopulmonary bypass pump, and because unlike aspirin, dipyridamole experimentally increased platelet survival without increasing perioperative blood loss.[222, 238–240] Nearly 400 patients undergoing coronary artery bypass surgery were randomly assigned to antithrombotic therapy or placebo.[221, 241] Dipyridamole was begun in a dose of 100 mg four times daily 48 hours preoperatively; aspirin, 325 mg, was administered via nasogastric tube within 7 hours postoperatively; combined aspirin and dipyridamole therapy was continued for 1 year after surgery. Early postoperative vein graft angiography performed in 88% of patients a median of 8 days after surgery demonstrated a statistically significant reduction in early graft occlusion in patients treated with platelet inhibitor therapy per distal anastomosis (Fig. 152–7). This finding was constant in more than 50 subsets of patients, including those at high risk for graft occlusion. Bleeding did not differ among treatment groups and placebo groups, and discontinuation of therapy due to side effects (headache or gastrointestinal upset) was required in only 6% of treated patients, compared with 2% of patients receiving placebo. Repeat angiography was performed in 84% of patients about 1 year after surgery (see Fig. 152–7). Of grafts patent up to 1 month postoperatively, the percentage developing late occlusion was decreased from 14% in the group taking placebo to 9% in the treated group.

In the Veterans Administration trial, 772 patients were randomized in a double-blind, placebo-controlled design to one of five groups: (1) aspirin, 325 mg/day, (2) aspirin, 325 mg three times a day, (3) aspirin, 325 mg three times a day plus dipyridamole, 75 mg three times a day, (4) sulfinpyrazone, 267 mg three times a day, or (5) placebo three times a day.[222] Dipyridamole was begun 48 hours prior to surgery. The first dose of aspirin was begun 12 hours before surgery, and aspirin was continued per protocol beginning 6 hours after surgery. On follow-up angiography in 72% of the patients within 60 days of surgery (median 9 days), all aspirin-containing regimens resulted in significantly improved patency compared with placebo ($p < .05$). Aspirin significantly increased chest tube drainage ($p < .02$) and reoperation rate ($p < .01$), but there was no difference between groups in overall or surgical mortality. In the 1-year follow-up study, repeat angiography was performed in 90% of eligible patients.[242] Graft occlusion was significantly decreased by aspirin compared with placebo (15.8% versus 22.6%, $p = .029$). This reduction in occlusion was especially significant for grafts with distal anastomoses less than 2.0 mm in diameter (20.1% versus 32.3%, $p = .008$). In grafts with distal anastomoses greater than 2.0 mm in diameter, there was no difference between aspirin and placebo groups in occlusion rates at 1 year (8.7% versus 9.0%, $p = .918$). In a separate report, the same investigators reported on difference in LIMA patency at 1 year between aspirin and placebo groups.[243]

Five more recent trials have appeared that have helped to clarify the role of combined antiplatelet therapy with aspirin and dipyridamole. Pfisterer et al. randomized 249 patients following bypass surgery to orally administered anticoagulants for 12 months, orally administered anticoagulants for 3 months followed by placebo, low-dose aspirin and dipyridamole for 12 months (dipyridamole, 200 mg twice a day begun 48 hours preoperatively and continued postoperatively; aspirin, 50 mg/day begun the morning of surgery and continued thereafter), or low-dose aspirin

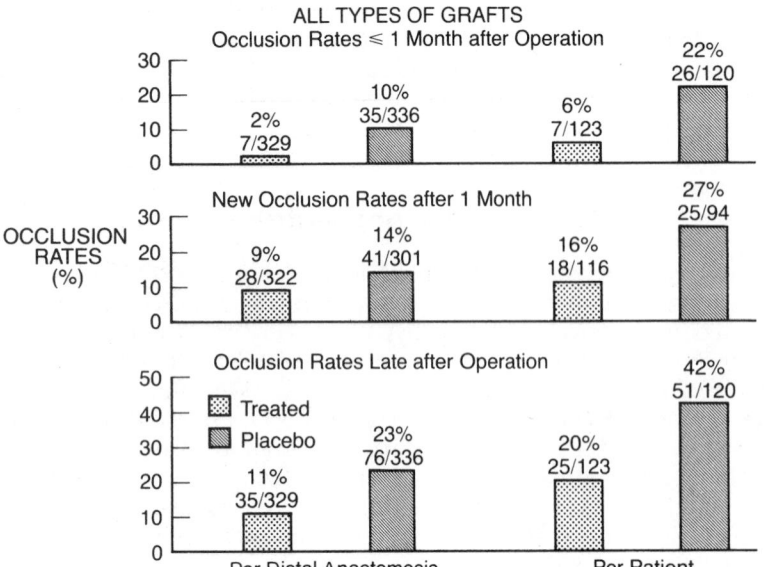

Figure 152–7. Occlusion rates for all types of vein grafts are shown per distal anastomosis and per patient (proportion with at least one occlusion). Occlusions are shown within 1 month, and new occlusions beyond 1 month, from angiography performed at a median of 1 year after operation. Below each percentage is shown the number of distal anastomoses or patients with occlusion per total number of distal anastomoses or patients. (From Chesebro JH, Fuster V, Elveback LR, et al: Effect of dipyridamole and aspirin on late vein graft patency after coronary bypass operations. N Engl J Med 310:209, 1984.)

and dipyridamole as just described for 3 months followed by placebo for 9 months.[244] There were no differences among the groups in the incidence of early graft occlusion at angiography 2 weeks after surgery. New late graft occlusion (between 2 weeks and 1 year) by repeat angiography at 1 year following surgery was significantly reduced by therapy with either anticoagulants or antiplatelet agents. Ekestrom et al. randomized 360 patients in a double-blind, placebo-controlled trial to either dipyridamole (100 mg four times a day for 2 days preoperatively followed by 100 mg four times a day) for 1 year or placebo.[245] Preoperative dipyridamole significantly increased interoperative SVG blood flow. There was a nonsignificant trend toward increased graft patency by repeat angiography 1 year following surgery in the dipyridamole group ($p = .08$).

In the largest reported trial to date, Sanz et al. randomized 1112 consecutive patients in a double-blind, placebo-controlled trial to aspirin (50 mg three times a day), aspirin (50 mg three times a day) plus dipyridamole, or placebo.[246] All patients received dipyridamole (100 mg four times a day) for 48 hours prior to surgery, and assigned treatment was begun 7 hours following surgery. Angiography was performed at mean of 10 days following surgery. Aspirin plus dipyridamole significantly reduced the occlusion rate compared with placebo (12.9% versus 18%, $p = .017$). Aspirin alone resulted in a nearly significant reduction in the rate of occlusion compared with placebo (14% versus 12.9%, $p = .058$). Although mediastinal drainage was slightly higher in the aspirin-plus-dipyridamole group, there was no difference in hospital mortality or reoperation. Gavaghan et al. randomized 237 patients in a double-blind, placebo-controlled trial to either aspirin (324 mg/day) administered first within 1 hour of surgery or placebo.[247] Angiography at 1 week revealed significant reduction in early graft occlusion in the aspirin group compared with placebo (1.6% versus 6.2%, $p = .004$), and angiography at 1 year revealed significant reduction in new late graft occlusion in the aspirin group compared with the placebo group as well (4.3% versus 7.4%, $p = .013$). There was no difference in chest tube drainage or transfusion requirement between groups, but a trend toward increased reoperation in the aspirin group was observed.

In a double-blind, placebo-controlled trial, van der Meer et al. randomized 948 patients to aspirin (50 mg/day) begun the night after surgery (the first dose via the nasogastric tube), dipyridamole and aspirin (as described earlier), or orally administered anticoagulants (acenocoumarol or phenprocoumon) begun on the day before surgery and continued after surgery with a target INR of 2.8 to 4.8.[248] Dipyridamole was administered as an intravenous infusion (5 mg/kg) from 10:00 PM the day prior to surgery until midnight the day following surgery then followed by orally administered dipyridamole (200 mg twice a day in slow-release form) for 1 year. At angiography 1 year following surgery in 86% of enrolled patients, occlusion rate of distal anastomoses was 11% in the aspirin-plus-dipyridamole group versus 15% in the aspirin group (relative risk 0.76, 95% confidence interval 0.54% to 1.05%) and 13% in the orally administered anticoagulant group. There was a significant benefit of aspirin plus dipyridamole in grafts placed into distal vessels with a lumen diameter of 1.5 mm or less (relative risk 0.66, 95% confidence interval 0.49% to 0.90%). Overall clinical events (defined as the combination of MI, thrombosis, major bleeding, or death) occurred in 20.3% of the aspirin-plus-dipyridamole group, in 13.9% of the aspirin group (relative risk 1.46, 95% confidence interval 1.02% to 2.08%), and in 16.9% of the anticoagulant group. The incidence of major bleeding was similar for all three groups.

One trial to date has investigated the role of the antiplatelet agent ticlopidine following bypass surgery. In a double-blind, placebo-controlled trial, 173 patients were randomized to ticlopidine (250 mg twice a day) or placebo.[249] Vein graft angiography was performed at 10 days, 180 days, and 360 days postoperatively. A statistically significant reduction in vein graft occlusion was noted among the patients treated with ticlopidine on day 10 (7.1% versus 13.4%), day 180 (15% versus 24%) and day 360 (15.9% versus 26.1%). Based on this single trial to date, ticlopidine appears to be effective in reducing SVG occlusion.

In the second Antiplatelet Trialists' Collaboration meta-analysis of 20 trials of antiplatelet therapy following coronary artery bypass surgery, antiplatelet agents decreased by 41% the odds of graft occlusion. Antiplatelet therapy was most efficacious when begun before the procedure or within 24 hours after the procedure. There was no difference in efficacy between medium-dose aspirin (75 to 325 mg/day) and higher-dose aspirin, and no added efficacy with dipyridamole in addition to aspirin.[115]

Conclusions from Clinical Trials of Antiplatelet Agents to Date

Antiplatelet therapy reduces the incidence of early (within several weeks) and late (within 1 year) SVG occlusion by 30% to 50%. Low-dose aspirin appears to be as efficacious as higher-dose aspirin. Ticlopidine appears to be effective. Dipyridamole alone is not effective. The efficacy of routine preoperative and intraoperative dipyridamole is uncertain. Antiplatelet therapy is particularly efficacious in grafts at high risk of occlusion, namely those with low-flow (less than 40 ml/min) or with small distal anastomoses (less than 1.5 mm). For antiplatelet therapy to be effective, it must be begun within 48 hours postoperatively. Aspirin begun as early as 1 hour postoperatively results in increased chest tube drainage and a trend toward higher rates of reoperation but not to increased hospital mortality. Aspirin begun preoperatively may result in an increased rate of reoperation for bleeding, although this has not been established yet for low-dose aspirin.

Although there is no conclusive evidence to date that the combination of dipyridamole and aspirin is

Table 152–19. **Antithrombotic Therapy in Coronary Revascularization**

Intervention	Recommendation
SVBG surgery	Aspirin, 325 mg/day, early postoperatively and long-term thereafter; in grafts at high risk* of occlusion, combine low-dose aspirin 75–100 mg/day or low-dose warfarin (INR 2–3)
PTCA (acute occlusion)	Aspirin, 325 mg/day, 24 hours pre-PTCA; 325 mg/day thereafter
	Intravenous heparin 10,000 IU bolus at time of PTCA, then 1000 IU/hr for 4–12 hours in uncomplicated PTCA, 24 hours for complicated PTCA†
PTCA (chronic restenosis)	Current antithrombotic agents are ineffective; aspirin 75–325 mg/day to all for long-term therapy of CAD

PTCA, percutaneous transluminal coronary angioplasty; SVBG, saphenous vein bypass graft.
*Distal anastomosis <1.5 mm or flow <40 mm.
†Multivessel PTCA, suboptimal result, visible thrombus, dissection, intimal flap, preceding unstable angina, acute occlusion.

more efficacious in preventing early and late graft occlusion in all patients than is aspirin alone, in the largest trial to date the combination was more efficacious than aspirin alone. The most recent trial also reported a nearly statistically significant reduction in occlusion with the combination compared with aspirin alone. The combination of aspirin and dipyridamole does appear to significantly lower the incidence of occlusion in grafts with small distal anastomoses (less than 1.5 mm) compared with aspirin alone. The role of aspirin combined with anticoagulants in the prevention of occlusion of these high-risk grafts is theoretically attractive but, to date, of unproven benefit. No currently available therapy prevents late (beyond 1 year) occlusion of SVG, the pathophysiology of which is similar to that of native coronary artery disease.

Current Recommendations (Table 152–19)

Aspirin (160 to 325 mg loading dose 1 hour postoperatively down the nasogastric tube) should be administered followed by daily aspirin (80 to 325 mg) indefinitely thereafter. Patients at high risk of SVG occlusion (SVG blood flow <40 ml/min or distal anastomosis <1.5 mm in diameter) should receive low-dose heparin to maintain the aPTT just above the upper normal value in the recovery room in addition to aspirin as described earlier. The heparin dosage should be increased to prolong the aPTT to 1.5 to 2.0 times control once the chest tubes are removed, and orally administered warfarin should be begun with a target INR of 2.5 to 3.5. When warfarin is given, low-dose aspirin (80 to 100 mg/day) should be used. Patients at high risk of SVG occlusion but who are poor candidates for warfarin should receive aspirin (325 mg/day) and dipyridamole (350 to 400 mg/day) in divided doses. Patients with severe unstable angina awaiting surgery may be treated with low-dose aspirin (80 to 100 mg daily) in addition to intravenously administered heparin up to the time of operation. Patients intolerant of aspirin may be treated with ticlopidine (250 mg twice a day).

Use of the internal mammary artery for coronary artery bypass is encouraged whenever possible. All risk factors for coronary artery disease should be modulated insofar as possible to prevent the late phase of atherosclerotic vein graft disease, as well as to prevent progression of native coronary artery disease.

SUMMARY

Antithrombotic therapy for the prevention of cardiac and arterial thromboembolism is predicated on pathogenesis and thromboembolic risk (Table 152–20). Judicious use of presently available antithrombotic agents significantly decreases morbidity and mortality from

Table 152–20. **Antithrombotic Therapy—1994**

| Pathogenesis | Thromboembolic Risk | | |
	High (>6% per year)	Medium (2–6% per year)	Low (<2% per year)
Arterial system platelets = fibrin	ACS Intervention PI + A/C	Stable CAD Post MI—chronic PI (or A/C)	Primary prevention PI (±)
Cardiac chamber	A-fib[1]—emboli A-fib[1]—M. stenosis	A-fib[1]—valv, nonvalv[2] Ant MI—early Dilated cardiom	A-fib[1, 2]—idiopathic Chronic LV aneurysm
Fibrin	A/C (INR 2.5–3.5)	A/C (INR 2.0–3.0)	No therapy
Prosth valves	Old mech Mech—emboli	Recent mech Bioprostheses—A-fib	Bioprost—NSR
Fibrin > platelets	A/C (INR 3.0–4.5) or (INR 2.5–3.5) + PI[3]?	A/C (Mech—INR 2.5–3.5[4] Bio—INR 2.0–3.0)	No therapy

[1]Cardioversion: 3 weeks before (and so on) v/s TEE and decision made.
[2]ASA if assoc. vasc dis. (AF—marker).
[3]ASA 100 mg/day; Turpie, N Engl J Med 329:524, 1993.
[4]INR 2.0–3.0 + ASA 300 mg/day + Dip; Altman et al, J Thorac Cardiovasc Surg 101:427, 1991.

cardiovascular disease. Novel antithrombotic agents such as selective antithrombins and glycoprotein IIa/IIIb receptor antagonists and combinations of potent antiplatelet agents and anticoagulants may further decrease the burden of cardiovascular disease.

REFERENCES

1. Kirkwood T, Lewis S: Requirements for thromboplastins and plasma used to control oral anticoagulant therapy. WHO Tech Rep Ser 687:81, 1983.
2. Expert Committee on Biological Standardization: Thirty-fourth report. WHO Tech Rep Ser 700:18, 1983.
3. Fuster V, Verstraete M (eds): Thrombosis in Cardiovascular Disorders. Philadephia: WB Saunders, 1992.
4. Keating E, Gross A, Schlamowitz R, et al: Mural thrombi in myocardial infarction: Prospective evaluation by two-dimensional echocardiography. Am J Med 74:989, 1983.
5. Meltzer R, Visser C, Fuster V: Intracardiac thrombi and systemic embolization. Ann Intern Med 104:689, 1986.
6. Mikell F, Asinger R, Elsperger J, et al: Long term prospective evaluation of left ventricular thrombi in acute myocardial infarction [abstract]. Circulation 64(Suppl IV):93, 1981.
7. Visser C, Kan G, Lie K, et al: Left ventricular thrombus following acute myocardial infarction: A prospective serial evalution of 96 patients. Eur Heart J 4:333, 1983.
8. Tramarin R, Pozzoli M, Febo O, et al: Echocardiographic assessment of therapy efficacy in left ventricular thrombosis post myocardial infarction [abstract]. Circulation 68(Suppl III):331, 1983.
9. Tramarin R, Pozzoli M, Vecchio C: Trombosi ventricolare sinistra nell-infarcto miocardio recente: Studio ecocardiographico. G Ital Cardiol 12:397, 1982.
10. Friedman M, Carlson K, Marcus F, et al: Clinical correlations in patients with acute myocardial infarction and left ventricular thrombus detected by two-dimensional echocardiography. Am J Med 72:894, 1982.
11. McEntee C, Van Reet R, Winters W, et al: Incidence and natural history of mural thrombi in acute mycaardial infarction by two-dimensional echocardiography [abstract]. Circulation 64(Suppl IV):93, 1981.
12. Visser C, Kan G, Meltzer R, et al: Long-term follow-up of left ventricular thrombus after myocardial infarction: A two-dimensional echocardiographic study of 96 patients. Chest 86:532, 1984.
13. Hilden T, Iversen K, Raaschou R, et al: Anticoagulants in acute myocardial infarction. Lancet 2:327, 1961.
14. Johnson R, Crissman R, DiDio L: Endocardial alterations in myocardial infarction. Lab Invest 40:183, 1979.
15. Fulton R, Duckett K: Plasma-fibrinogen and thromboembolism after myocardial infarction. Lancet 2:1161, 1976.
16. Fuster V, Dyken M, Vokonas P, et al: Aspirin as a therapeutic agent in cardiovascular disease. Circulation 87:659, 1993.
17. Cairns J, Hirsh J, Lewis H, et al: Antithrombotic agents in coronary artery disease. Chest 102(Suppl 4):456S, 1992.
18. DeMaria A, Bommer W, Neumann A, et al: Left ventricular thrombi identified by cross-sectional echocardiography. Ann Intern Med 90:14, 1979.
19. Ezekowitz M, Wilson D, Smith E, et al: Comparison of indium-111 platelet scintigraphy and two-dimensional echocardiography in the diagnosis of left ventricular thrombi. N Engl J Med 306:1509, 1982.
20. Asinger R, Mikell F, Elsperger J, et al: Incidence of left ventricular thrombosis after acute transmural myocardial infarction: Serial evaluation by two-dimensional echocardiography. N Engl J Med 305:297, 1981.
21. Reeder G, Tajik A, Seward J: Left ventricular mural thrombus: Two-dimensional echocardiographic diagnosis. Mayo Clin Proc 56:82, 1981.
22. Visser C, Kan G, David G, et al: Two-dimensional echocardiography in the diagnosis of left ventricular thrombus: A prospective study of 67 patients with anatomic validation. Chest 83:228, 1983.
23. Funke-Kupper A, Freek W, Verbeugt F, et al: Long term therapy with oral anticoagulants in patients with left ventricular thrombosis after myocardial infarction [abstract]. Circulation 72(Suppl III):458, 1985.
24. Spirito P, Bellotu P, Chiarella R, et al: Prognostic significance and natural history of left ventricular thrombi in patients with acute myocardial infarction: A two-dimensional echocardiographic study. Circulation 72:774, 1985.
25. Stratton J, Resnick A: Increased embolic risk in patients with left ventricular thrombi. Circulation 75:1004, 1987.
26. Funke-Kupper A, Verheugt F, Peels C, et al: Left ventricular thrombus incidence and behavior studied by serial two-dimensional echocardiography in acute anterior myocardial infarction: Left ventricular wall motion, systemic embolism and oral anticoagulation. J Am Coll Cardiol 13:1514, 1989.
27. Black I, Hopkins A, Lee L, et al: Role of transoesophageal echocardiography in evaluation of cardiogenic embolism. Br Heart J 66:302, 1991.
28. Chen C, Koschyk D, Hamm C, et al: Usefulness of transesophageal echocardiography in identifying small left ventricular apical thrombi. J Am Coll Cardiol 21:208, 1993.
29. Vaitkus P, Barnathan E: Embolic potential, prevention and management of mural thrombus complicating anterior mycoardial infarction: A meta-analysis. J Am Coll Cardiol 22:1004, 1993.
30. Hellerstein H, Martin J: Incidence of thromboembolic lesions accompanying myocardial infarction. Am Heart J 32:443, 1946.
31. Lapeyre AI, Steele P, Kazimer F, et al: Systemic embolism in chronic left ventricular aneurysm: Incidence and the role of anticoagulation. J Am Coll Cardiol 6:534, 1985.
32. Johannessen K, Nordrehaug J, von der Lippe G, et al: Risk factor for embolisation in patients with left ventricular thrombi and acute myocardial infarction. Br Heart J 60:104, 1988.
33. Jugdutt B, Sivaram C, Wortman C, et al: Prospective two-dimensional echocardiographic evaluation of left ventricular thrombus and embolism after acute myocardial infarction. J Am Coll Cardiol 13:554, 1989.
34. Delemarre B, Visser C, Bot H, et al: Prediction of apical thrombus formation in acute myocardial infarction based on left ventricular spatial flow pattern. J Am Coll Cardiol 15:355, 1990.
35. Investigators VAC: Anticoagulants in acute myocardial infarction: Results of a cooperative trial. JAMA 225:724, 1973.
36. Drapkin A, Merskey C: Anticoagulant therapy after acute myocardial infarction: Relation of therapeutic benefit to patient's age, sex, and severity of infarction. JAMA 222:541, 1972.
37. Report of the Working Party on Anticoagulant Therapy in Coronary Thrombosis to the Medical Research Council: Assessment of short term anticoagulant administration after cardiac infarction: Report of the Working Party on Anticoagulant Therapy in Coronary Thrombosis to the Medical Research Council. Br Med J 1:335, 1969.
38. Asinger R, Mikell F, Sharma B, et al: Observations on detecting left ventricular thrombus with two dimensional echocardiography: Emphasis on avoidance of false positive diagnosis. Am J Cardiol 47:145, 1981.
39. Reeder G, Lengyel M, Tajik A, et al: Mural thrombus in left ventricular aneurysm: Incidence, role of angiography, and relation between anticoagulation and embolization. Mayo Clin Proc 56:77, 1981.
40. Visser C, Kan G, Meltzer R, et al: Embolic potential of left ventricular thrombi after myocardial infarction: A two-dimensional echocardiographic study of 119 patients. J Am Coll Cardiol 5:1276, 1985.
41. Domenicucci S, Chiarella F, Bellotti P, et al: Early appearance of left ventricular thrombi after anterior myocardial infarction: A marker of higher in-hospital mortality in patients not treated with antithrombotic drugs. Eur Heart J 11:51, 1990.
42. Turpie A, Robinson J, Doyle D, et al: Comparison of high-dose with low-dose subcutaneous heparin to prevent left ventricular thrombosis in patients with acute transmural anterior myocardial infarction. N Engl J Med 320:352, 1989.
43. The SCATI Group: Randomised controlled trial of subcutane-

ous calcium-heparin in acute myocardial infarction. Lancet 2:182, 1989.

44. Vecchio C, Chiarella R, Lupi G, et al: Left ventricular thrombus in acute anterior myocardial infarction after thrombolysis: A GISSI-2 connected study. Circulation 84:512, 1991.

45. The LATE Study Group: Late Assessment of Thrombolytic Efficacy (LATE) study with alteplase 6–24 hours after onset of acute myocardial infarction. Lancet 342:759, 1993.

46. The EMERAS Cooperative Study Group: Randomised trial of late thrombolysis in patients with suspected acute myocardial infarction. Lancet 342:767, 1993.

47. Keren A, Goldberg A, Gottlief S, et al: Natural history of left ventricular thrombi: Their appearance and resolution in the posthospitalization period of acute myocardial infarction. J Am Coll Cardiol 15:790, 1990.

48. Smith P, Arnesen H, Holme I: The effect of warfarin on mortality and reinfarction after myocardial infarction. N Engl J Med 323:147,1990.

49. Cooley D, Hallman G: Surgical treatment of left ventricular aneurysm: Experience with excision of post-infarction lesions in 80 patients. Prog Cardiovasc Dis 11:222, 1968.

50. Cabin H, Roberts W: Left ventricular aneurysm, intra-aneurysmal thrombus and systemic embolus in coronary heart disease. Chest 77:586, 1980.

51. Roberts W, Ferrans V: Pathologic aspects of certain cardiomyopathies. Circ Res 34–35(Suppl II):128, 1974.

52. Fuster V, Gersh B, Giulani E, et al: The natural history of dilated cardiomyopathy. Am J Cardiol 47:525, 1981.

53. Falk R, Foster E, Coats M: Ventricular thrombi and thromboembolism in dilated cardiomyopathy: A prospective follow-up study. Am Heart J 123:136, 1991.

54. Dusleag J, Klein W, Eber B, et al: Frequency of magnetic resonance signal abnormalities of the brain in patients aged <50 years with idiopathic dilated cardiomyopathy. Am J Cardiol 69:1446, 1992.

55. Hamly R: Primary myocardial disease. Medicine 49:55, 1970.

56. Maze S, Kotler M, Parry W: Flow characteristics in the dilated left ventricle with thrombus: Qualitative and quantitative doppler analysis. J Am Coll Cardiol 13:873, 1989.

57. Siostrzonek P, Koppensteiner R, Kreiner G, et al: Abnormal blood rheology in idiopathic dilated cardiomyopathy. Am J Cardiol 69:1497, 1991.

58. Jafri S, Ozawa T, Mammen E, et al: Platelet function, thrombin and fibrinolytic activity in patients with heart failure. Eur Heart J 14:205, 1993.

59. Levine H, Pauker S, Salzman E, et al: Antithrombotic therapy in valvular heart disease. Chest 102(Suppl 4):434S, 1992.

60. Pumphrey C, Fuster V, Chesebro J: Systemic thromboembolism in valvular heart disease and prosthetic heart valves. Modern Concepts in Cardiovascular Disease 51:131, 1982.

61. Szekely P: Systemic embolism and anticoagulant prophylaxis in rheumatic heart disease. Br Med J 1:1209, 1964.

62. Coulshed N, Epstein E, McKendrick C, et al: Systemic embolism in mitral valve disease. Br Heart J 32:26, 1970.

63. Easton J, Sherman D: Management of cerebral embolism of cardiac origin. Stroke 11:433, 1980.

64. Hart R, Miller V: Cerebral infarction in young adults: A practical approach. Stroke 14:110, 1983.

65. Deveral P, Olley P, Smith D, et al: Incidence of systemic embolism before and after mitral valvotomy. Thorax 23:530, 1968.

66. Abernathy W, Willis P: Thromboembolic complications of rheumatic heart disease. Cardiovasc Clin 5:131, 1973.

67. Askey J, Berstein S: The management of rheumatic heart disease in relation to systemic arterial embolism. Prog Cardiovasc Dis 3:220, 1960.

68. Nielson B, Galea E, Hossack K: Thromboembolic complications of mitral valve disease. Aust N Z J Med 8:372, 1978.

69. Selzer A, Cohn K: Natural history of mitral stenosis: A review. Circulation 45:878, 1972.

70. Wood P: Diseases of the Heart and Circulation. Philadephia: JB Lippincott, 1956.

71. Wolf P, Dawber T, Thomas H, et al: Epidemiologic assessment of chronic atrial fibrillation and the risk of stroke. Neurology 28:973, 1978.

72. Wook J, Conn H: Prevention of systemic arterial embolism in chronic rheumatic heart disease by means of protracted anticoagulant therapy. Circulation 10:517, 1954.

73. Adams G, Merrett J, Hutchinson W, et al: Cerebral embolism and mitral stenosis: Survival with and without anticoagulants. J Neurol Neurosurg Psychiatry 37:973, 1974.

74. Sherman D, Dyken M, Fisher M, et al: Cerebral embolism. ACCP-NHLBI National Conference of Antithrombotic Therapy. Chest 89(Suppl 2):82S, 1986.

75. Devereux R, Kramer-Fox R, Kligfield P: Mitral valve prolapse: Causes, clincical manifestations, and management. Ann Intern Med 111:305, 1989.

76. Barnett H, Jonew M, Boughner D, et al: Cerebral ischemic events associated with prolapsing mitral valve. Arch Neurol 33:777, 1976.

77. Jackson A, Boughner D, Barnett H, et al: Mitral valve prolapse and cerebral ischemic events in young patients. Neurology 34:784, 1984.

78. Nishimura R, McGoon M, Shub C, et al: Echocardiographically documented mitral valve prolapse: Long-term follow-up in 237 patients. N Engl J Med 313:1305, 1985.

79. Marks A, Choong C, Sanfilippo A, et al: Identification of high-risk and low-risk subgoups of patients with mitral-valve prolapse. N Engl J Med 320:1031, 1989.

80. Benjamin E, Plehn J, D'Agostino R, et al: Mitral annular calcification and the risk of stroke in an eldery cohort. N Engl J Med 327:374, 1992.

81. Savage D, Garrison R, Castelli W, et al: Prevalence of submitral (annular) calcium and its correlations in a general population-based sample (the Framingham Study). Am J Cardiol 51:1375, 1983.

82. Rotman M, Morris J, Behar V, et al: Aortic valvular disease: Comparison of types and their medical management. Am J Med 51:241, 1971.

83. Kumpe C, Bean W: Aortic stenosis: A study of the clincial and pathologic aspects of 107 proved cases. Medicine 27:139, 1948.

84. Dry T, Willius F: Calcareous disease of the aortic valve: A study of 228 cases. Am Heart J 17:138, 1939.

85. Pumphrey C, Fuster V, Chesebro J: Systemic thromboembolism in valvular heart disease and prosthetic heart valves. Modern Concepts in Cardiovascular Disease 51:131, 1982.

86. Stein P, Sabbah H, Pitha J: Continuing disease process of calcific aortic stenosis: Role of microthrombi and turbulent flow. Am J Cardiol 39:159, 1977.

87. Holley K, Bahn R, McGoon D, et al: Spontaneous calcific embolization associated with calcific stenosis. Circulation 27:197, 1963.

88. Brockmeier L, Adolph R, Gustin B, et al: Calcium emboli to the retinal artery in calcific aortic stenosis. Am Heart J 101:32, 1981.

89. Laupacis A, Albers G, Dunn M, et al: Antithrombotic therapy in atrial fibrillation. Chest 102(Suppl 4):426S, 1992.

90. Nolan J, Bloomfield P: Non-rheumatic atrial fibrillation: Warfarin of aspirin for all? Br Heart J 68:544, 1992.

91. Kannel W, Abbott R, Savage D, et al: Epidemiologic features of chronic atrial fibrillation: The Framingham Study. N Engl J Med 306:1018, 1982.

92. Petersen P, Madsen E, Brun B, et al: Silent cerebral infarction in chronic atrial fibrillation. Stroke 18:1098, 1987.

93. Singer D: Randomized trials of warfarin for atrial fibrillation. N Engl J Med 327:1451, 1992.

94. Petersen P, Hansen J: Stroke in thyrotoxicosis with atrial fibrillation. Stroke 19:15, 1988.

95. The Stroke Prevention in Atrial Fibrillation Investigators: Predictors of thromboembolism in atrial fibrillation: I. Clinical features of patients at risk. Ann Intern Med 116:1, 1992.

96. Petersen P, Godtfredsen J: Embolic complications in paroxysmal atrial fibrillation. Stroke 17:622, 1986.

97. The Boston Area Anticoagulation Trial for Atrial Fibrillation Investigators: The effect of low-dose warfarin on the risk of stroke in patients with nonrheumatic atrial fibrillation. N Engl J Med 323:1505, 1990.

98. The Stroke Prevention in Atrial Fibrillation Investigators: The stroke prevention in atrial fibrillation trial: Final results. Circulation 84:527, 1991.

99. Kopecky S, Bersh B, McGoon M, et al: The natural history of lone atrial fibrillation: A population-based study over three decades. N Engl J Med 317:669, 1987.

100. Brand F, Abbott R, Kannel W, et al: Characteristics and prognosis of lone atrial fibrillation: 30-year follow-up in the Framingham Study. JAMA 254:3449, 1985.

101. Caplan L, D'Cruz I, Hier D, et al: Atrial size, atrial fibrillation, and stroke. Ann Neurol 19:158, 1986.

102. Sanfillipo A, Abascal V, Sheehan M, et al: Atrial enlargement as a consequence of atrial fibrillation: A prospective echocardiographic study. Circulation 82:792, 1990.

103. Petersen P, Godtfredesen J, Boysen G, et al: Placebo-controlled, randomized trial of warfarin and aspirin for prevention of thromboembolic complications in chronic atrial fibrillation: The Copenhagen AFASAK Study. Lancet 1:175.

104. The Stroke Prevention in Atrial Fibrillation Investigators: Predictors of thromboembolism in atrial fibrillation: II. Echocardiographic features of patients at risk. Ann Intern Med 116:6, 1992.

105. Manning W, Silverman D, Gordon S, et al: Cardioversion from atrial fibrillation without prolonged anticoagulation with use of transesophageal echocardiography to exclude the presence of atrial thrombi. N Engl J Med 328:750, 1993.

106. Burchfiel C, Hammermeister K, Krause-Steinrauf H, et al: Left atrial dimension and risk of systemic embolism in patients with a prosthetic heart valve. J Am Coll Cardiol 15:32, 1990.

107. Black I, Hopkins A, Lee L: Left atrial spontaneous echo contrast: A clinical and echocardiographic analysis. J Am Coll Cardiol 18:398, 1991.

108. Connolly S, Laupacis A, Gent M, et al: Canadian Atrial Fibrillation Anticoagulation (CAFA) Study. J Am Coll Cardiol 18:349, 1991.

109. Ezekowitz M, Bridgers S, James K, et al: Warfarin in the prevention of stroke associated with nonrheumatic atrial fibrillation. N Engl J Med 327:1406, 1992.

110. Chesebro J, Fuster V, Halperin J: Atrial fibrillation-risk marker for stroke. N Engl J Med 323:1556, 1990.

111. Daniel W: Should transesophageal echocardiography be used to guide cardioversion? N Engl J Med 328:803, 1992.

112. Goldman M: The management of chronic atrial fibrillation: Indications and method of conversion to normal sinus rhythm. Prog Cardiovasc Dis 2:645, 1960.

113. Grote J, Mugge A, Nikutta P, et al: Follow-up of patients with left atrial appendage thrombi. Circulation 88(Suppl 4):313, 1993.

114. Black I, Fatkin D, Sagar K, et al: Does exclusion of atrial thrombus by transesophageal echocardiography preclude embolism after cardioversion? A multicenter study [abstract]. Circulation 88(Suppl 4):314, 1993.

115. Antiplatelet Trialists' Collaboration: Collaborative overview of randomized trials of antiplatelet therapy—Parts I, II, III. Br Med J 308:81, 159, 235, 1994.

116. Weinstein L, Schlesinger J: Pathoanatomic, pathophisiologic and clinical correlations in endocarditis. N Engl J Med 291:832, 1122, 1974.

117. Kaye D: Infective Endocarditis, 2nd ed. New York: Raven Press, 1992.

118. Salgado A: Central nervous complications of infective endocarditis. Stroke 22:1461, 1991.

119. Durack D: Experimental Bacterial Endocarditis: IV. Structure and evolution of very early lesions. Br J Exp Pathol 56:81, 1974.

120. Levison M, Carrizosa J, Tanphaichitra D, et al: Effect of aspirin on thrombogenesis and on production of experimental aortic valvular Streptococcus viridans endocarditis in rabbits. Blood 49:645, 1977.

121. Thorig L, Thompson J, Eulderink F: Effect of warfarin on the induction and course of experimental Staphylococcus epidermidis endocarditis. Infect Immun 17:504, 1977.

122. Johnson C, Dewar H, Aherne W: Fibrinolytic therapy in subacute bacterial endocarditis: An experimental study. Cardiovasc Res 14:482, 1980.

123. Thill C, Meyer O: Experiences with penicillin and dicumarol in the treatments of subacute bacterial endocarditis. Am J Med Sci 213:300, 1947.

124. Chesebro J, Fuster V: Valvular heart disease and prosthetic heart valves. In Fuster V, Verstraete M (eds): Thrombosis in Cardiovascular Disease. Philadelphia: WB Saunders, 1992.

125. Dewanjee M, Fuster V, Rao S, et al: Noninvasive radiosiotopic technique for detection of platelet deposition on mitral valve prostheses and quantitation of visceral microembolism in dogs. Mayo Clin Proc 58:307, 1983.

126. Dewanjee M, Trastek V, Tago M, et al: Radioisotopic techniques for non-invasive detection of platelet deposition in bovine tissue mitral valve prostheses and in-vitro quantification of visceral microembolism in dogs. Invest Radiol 6:535, 1984.

127. Heras M, Chesebro J, Webster M, et al: Hirudin, heparin, and placebo during deep arterial injury in the pig: The in-vivo role of thrombin in platelet-mediated thrombosis. Circulation 82:1476, 1990.

128. Harker L, Slichter S: Studies of platelet and fibrinogen kinetics in patients with prosthetic heart valves. N Engl J Med 283:1302, 1970.

129. Weily H, Genton E: Altered platelet function in patients with prosthetic mitral valves: Effects of sulfinpyrazone therapy. Circulation 42:967, 1970.

130. Steele P, Rainwater J, Vogel R: Platelet suppressant therapy in patients with prosthetic heart valves: Relationship of clinical effectiveness to alteration of platelet survival time. Circulation 60:910, 1979.

131. Peugo V, Peruzzi P, Baca M, et al: The optimal therapeutic range for oral anticoagulant treatment as suggested by fibrinopeptide A (FpA) levels in patients with heart valve prosthesis. Eur J Clin Invest 19:181, 1989.

132. Barnhorst D, Oxman H, Connolly D, et al: Long-term follow up of isolated replacement of the aortic or mitral valve with the Starr-Edwards prosthesis. Am J Cardiol 35:228, 1975.

133. Chesebro J, Fuster V, Elveback L, et al: Trial of combined warfarin plus dipyridamole or aspirin therapy in prosthetic heart valve replacement: Danger of aspirin compared with dipyridamole. Am J Cardiol 51:1537, 1983.

134. Cleland J, Molloy P: Thromboembolic complications of the cloth covered Starr-Edwards prostheses No. 2300 aortic and No. 6300 mitral. Thorax 28:41, 1973.

135. Friedli B, Aerichide H, Grondin P, et al: Thromboembolic complications of heart valve replacement. Am Heart J 81:702, 1971.

136. Gadboys H, Litwak R, Niemetz J, et al: Role of anticoagulants in preventing embolization from prosthetic heart valves. JAMA 202:134, 1967.

137. Fuster V, Pumphrey C, McGoon M, et al: Systemic thromboembolism in mitral and aortic Starr-Edwards prostheses: A long-term follow-up (10–19 years). Circulation 66(Suppl I):157, 1982.

138. Murphy D, Levine F, Buckley M, et al: A comparative analysis of the Starr-Edwards and Bjork-Shiley prostheses. J Thorac Cardiovasc Surg 86:746, 1983.

139. Perier P, Bessou J, Swanson J, et al: Comparative evaluation of aortic valve replacement with Starr, Bjork, and porcine valve prostheses. Circulation 72(Suppl II):140, 1985.

140. Bjork V, Henze A: Ten years' experience with the Bjork-Shiley tilting disk valve. J Thorac Cardiovasc Surg 78:331, 1979.

141. Dale J, Myhre E: Can acetylsalicylic acid alone prevent arterial thromboembolism? A pilot study in patients with aortic ball valve prosthesis. Acta Med Scand 645(Suppl):73, 1981.

142. Oyer P, Stinson E, Griepp R, et al: Valve replacement with the Starr-Edwards and Hancock prostheses. Ann Surg 186:301, 1977.

143. Grunkemeier G, Rahimtoola S: Artificial heart valves. Annu Rev Med 41:251, 1990.

144. Rubin J, Moore H, Hilison R, et al: A thirteen year experience with aortic valve replacement. Am J Cardiol 40:345, 1977.

145. MacManus Q, Grunkemeier G, Lambert L, et al: Year of operation as a risk factor in the late results of valve replacement. J Thorac Cardiovasc Surg 80:834, 1980.

146. Czer L, Matloff J, Chaux A, et al: The St. Jude valve: Analysis of thromboembolism, warfarin-related hemorrhage, and survival. Am Heart J 114:389, 1987.

147. Myers M, Lawrie G, Crawford E, et al: The St. Jude prosthesis: Analysis of the clinical results in 815 implants and the need for systemic anticoagulation. J Am Coll Cardiol 13:57, 1989.

148. Saour J, Sieck J, Mamo L, et al: Trial of different intensities of anticoagulation in patients with prosthetic heart valves. N Engl J Med 322:428, 1990.

149. Altman R, Rouvier J, Gurfinkel E, et al: Comparison of two levels of anticoagulant therapy in patients with substitute heart valves. J Cardiovasc Surg 101:427, 1991.

150. Stein P, Alpert J, Copeland J, et al: Antithrombotic therapy in patients with mechanical and biological prosthetic heart valves. Chest 102(Suppl 4):445S, 1992.

151. Dale J, Myhre E, Storstein O, et al: Prevention of arterial thromboembolism with acetylsalicylic acid: A controlled clinical study in patients with aortic ball valves. Am Heart J 94:101, 1977.

152. Altman R, Boullon F, Rouvier J, et al: Aspirin and prophylaxis of thromboembolic complications in patients with substitute heart valves. J Thorac Cardiovasc Surg 72:127, 1976.

153. Turpie A, Gent M, Laupacis A, et al: A comparison of aspirin with placebo in patients treated with warfarin after heart-valve replacement. N Engl J Med 329:524, 1993.

154. Ribeiro P, Al Zaibag M, Idris M, et al: Antiplatelet drugs and the incidence of thromboembolic complications of the St. Jude medical aortic prosthesis in patients with rheumatic heart disease. J Thorac Cardiovasc Surg 91:92, 1986.

155. Nair C, Mohiuddin S, Hilleman D, et al: Ten-year results with the St. Jude medical prosthesis. Am J Cardiol 65:217, 1990.

156. Hartz R, LoCiero JI, Kucich V, et al: Comparative study of warfarin versus antiplatelet therapy in patients with a St. Jude medical valve in the aortic position. J Thorac Cardiovasc Surg 1986:684, 1986.

157. Bjork V, Henze A: Management of thomboembolism after aortic valve replacement with the Bjork-Shiley tilting disc valve. Scand J Thorac Cardiovasc Surg 9:183, 1975.

158. Turina J, Hess O, Turina M, et al: Cardiac bioprostheses in the 1990s. Circulation 88:775, 1993.

159. Turpie A, Gunstensen J, Hirsh J, et al: Randomized comparison of two intensities of oral anticoagulant therapy after tissue heart valve replacement. Lancet 1:1242, 1988.

160. Perier P, Deloche A, Chauvaud S, et al: A 10-year comparison of mitral valve replacement with Carpentier-Edwards and Hancock porcine prostheses. Ann Thorac Surg 48:54, 1989.

161. Heras J, Chesebro J, Grill D, et al: Chronic risk of thromboembolism after bioprosthetic valve replacement [abstract]. Eur Heart J 10(Suppl C):260, 1989.

162. Nunez L, Aguado G, Larrea J, et al: Prevention of thromboembolism using aspirin after mitral valve replacement with porcine bioprosthesis. Ann Thorac Surg 37:84, 1984.

163. Stein P, Riddle J, Kemp S, et al: Effect of warfarin on calcification of spontaneously degenerated porcine bioprosthetic valves. J Thorac Cardiovasc Surg 90:119, 1985.

164. McKay C: Prosthetic heart valve thrombosis. Circulation 87:294, 1993.

165. Silber J, Khan S, Matloff J, et al: The St. Jude valve: Thrombolysis as the first line of therapy for cardiac valve thrombosis. Circulation 87:30, 1993.

166. Israel, OH, Sharma SK, Fuster V: Antithrombotic therapy in prosthetic heart valve replacement. Am Heart J 127:400, 1994.

167. Tinker J, Tarhan S: Discontinuing anticoagulant therapy in surgical patients with cardiac valve prostheses: Observations in 180 operations. JAMA 234:738, 1978.

168. Wilson W, Geraci J, Danielson G, et al: Anticoagulant therapy and central nervous system complications in patients with prosthetic valve endocarditis. Circulation 57:1004, 1978.

169. Garvey G, Neu H: Infective endocarditis—an evolving disease: A review of endocarditis at the Columbia-Presbyterian Medical Center 1968–1973. Medicine 57:105, 1978.

170. Block P, DeSanctis R, Weingerg A, et al: Prosthetic valve endocarditis. J Thorac Cardiovasc Surg 60:540, 1970.

171. Karchmer A, Dismukes W, Buckley M, et al: Late prosthetic valve endocarditis: Clinical features influencing therapy. Am J Med 64:199, 1978.

172. Cerebral Embolism Study Group: Immediate anticoagulation of embolic stroke: Brain hemorrhage and management options. Stroke 15:1984.

173. Lee P, Wang R, Chow J, et al: Combined use of warfarin and adjusted subcutaneous heparin during pregnancy with an artificial heart valve. J Am Coll Cardiol 8:221, 1986.

174. Baty J, Breckinridge A, Lewis P, et al: May mothers taking warfarin breast feed their infants? Br J Clin Pharmacol 3:969, 1976.

175. Fuster V, Badimon L, Badimon J, Chesebro J: The pathogenesis of coronary artery disease and the acute coronary syndromes. N Engl J Med 326:242, 310, 1992.

176. Ross R: The pathogenesis of atherosclerosis: A perspective for the 1990s. Nature 362:801, 1993.

177. Lassila R, Badimon J, Vallabhajosula S, et al: Dynamic monitoring of platelet deposition on severely damaged vessel walls in flowing blood: Effects of different stenosis on thrombus growth. Arteriosclerosis 10:306, 1990.

178. Badimon L, Badimon J, Turitto V, et al: Platelet thrombus formation on collagen type I: A model of deep vessel injury; influence of blood rheology, von Willebrand factor, and blood coagulation. Circulation 78:1431, 1988.

179. Badimon L, Badimon J: Mechanism of arterial thrombosis in nonparallel streamlines; platelet thrombi grow at the apex of stenotic severely injured vessel wall: Experimental study in the pig model. J Clin Invest 84:1134, 1989.

180. Davies S, Marchant B, Lyons J, et al: Coronary lesion morphology in acute myocardial infarction: Demonstration of early remodeling after streptokinase treatment. J Am Coll Cardiol 16:1079, 1990.

181. Roberts W, Buja L: The frequency and significance of coronary arterial thrombi and other observations in fatal acute myocardial infarction: A study of 107 necropsy patients. Am J Med 52:425, 1972.

182. Falk E: Unstable angina with fatal outcome: Dynamic coronary thrombosis leading to infarction and/or sudden death: Autposy evidence of recurrent mural thrombosis with peripheral embolization culminating in total vascular occlusion. Circulation 71:699, 1985.

183. Barger A, Beewkes R: Rupture of coronary vasa vasorum as a trigger of actue mycoardial infarction. Am J Cardiol 66:41G, 1990.

184. Mizuno K, Satomura K, Miyamoto A, et al: Angioscopic evaluation of coronary artery thrombi in acute coronary syndromes. N Engl J Med 326:287, 1992.

185. Report of a Meeting of Physicians and Scientists: Thrombus and unstable angina. Lancet 342:1151, 1993.

186. Willerson J, Casscells W: Thrombin inhibitors in unstable angina: Rebound or continuation of angina after argatroban withdrawl. J Am Coll Cardiol 21:1048, 1993.

187. Webster M, Chesebro J, Smith H, et al: Myocardial infarction and coronary artery occlusion: A prospective 5-year angiographic study [abstract]. J Am Coll Cardiol 15(Suppl):218A, 1990.

188. Ambrose J, Tannenbaum M, Alexopolous D, et al: Angiographic progression of coronary artery disease and the development of myocardial infarction. J Am Coll Cardiol 12:56, 1988.

189. Gulba D, Barthels M, Westhoff-Bleck M, et al: Increased thrombin levels during thrombolytic therapy in acute myocardial infarction: Relevance for the success of therapy. Circulation 83:937, 1987.

190. Hackett D, Davies G, Chierchia S, et al: Intermittent coronary occlusion in acute myocardial infarction: Value of combined thrombolytic and vasodilatory therapy. N Engl J Med 317:1055, 1987.

191. Prager N, Torr-Brown S, Sobel B, et al: Maintenance of patency after thrombolysis in stenotic coronary arteries requires combined inhibition of thrombin and platelets. J Am Coll Cardiol 22:296, 1993.

192. Maseri A, L'Abbate A, Baroldi G, et al: Coronary vasospasm as a possible cause of myocardial infarction: A conclusion derived from the study of "preinfarction" angina. N Engl J Med 299:1271, 1978.

193. Vane J, Anggaard E, Botting R: Regulatory functions of the vascular endothelium. N Engl J Med 323:27, 1990.

194. McLenachan J, Williams J, Fish R, et al: Loss of flow-mediated endothelium-dependent dilation occurs early in the development of atherosclerosis. Circulation 84:1273, 1991.

195. Steele P, Chesebro J, Stanson A, et al: Balloon angioplasty: Natural history of the pathophysiologic response to injury in a pig model. Circ Res 57:105, 1985.

196. Chesebro J, Webster M, Smith H, et al: Antiplatelet therapy in coronary disease progression: Reduced infarction and new lesion formation [abstract]. Circulation 80(Suppl II):266, 1989.
197. Ridker P, Manson J, Gaziano M, et al: Low-dose aspirin therapy for chronic stable angina: A randomized, placebo-controlled clinical trial. Ann Intern Med 114:835, 1991.
198. Juul-Moller S, Edvardsson N, Jahnmatz B, et al: Double-blind trial of aspirin in primary prevention of myocardial infarciton in patients with stable chronic angina pectoris. Lancet 340:1421, 1992.
199. Antiplatelet Trialists' Collaboration: Secondary prevention of vascular disease by prolonged antiplatelet treatment. Br Med J 296:320, 1988.
200. Cohen M, Adams PC, Parry G, et al: Combination antithrombotic therapy in unstable rest angina and non-Q-wave infarction in nonprior aspirin users: Primary end points analysis from the ATACS trial. Circulation 89:81, 1994.
201. Lewis H, Davis J, Archibald D, et al: Protective effects of aspirin against acute myocardial infarction and death in men with unstable angina. N Engl J Med 309:396, 1983.
202. Cairns J, Gent M, Singer J, et al: Aspirin, sulfinpyrazone, or both in unstable angina. N Engl J Med 313:1369, 1985.
203. Theroux P, Ouimet H, McCans J, et al: Aspirin, heparin, of both to treat acute unstable angina. N Engl J Med 319:1105, 1988.
204. Theroux P, Waters D, Qiu S, et al: Aspirin versus heparin to prevent myocardial infarction during the acute phase of unstable angina. Circulation 88:2045, 1993.
205. Balsano F, Rizzon P, Violi F, et al: Antiplatelet treatment with ticlopidine in unstable angina: A controlled, multicenter study. Circulation 82:17, 1990.
206. Simoons ML, Jan de Boer MJ, van den Brand MJBM, et al: Randomized trial of a GPIIb/IIIa platelet receptor blocker in refractory unstable angina. Circulation 89:596, 1994.
207. Cairns J, Cohen M: Unstable angina-antithrombotics and thrombolytics. In Fuster V, Verstraete M (eds): Thrombosis in Cardiovascular Disease. Philadelphia: WB Saunders, 1992.
208. Telford A, Wilson C: Trial of heparin versus atenolol in prevention of myocardial infarciton in intermediate coronary syndrome. Lancet 1:1225, 1981.
209. Williams D, Kirby M, McPherson K, et al: Anticoagulant treatment in unstable angina pectoris. Br J Clin Pract 40:114, 1986.
210. Neri Serneri G, Gensini G, Poggesi L, et al: Effect of heparin, aspirin, or alteplase in reduction of myocardial ischaemia in refractory unstable angina pectoris. Lancet 335:615, 1990.
211. Theroux P, Waters D, Lam J, et al: Reactivation of unstable angina after the discontinuation of heparin. N Engl J Med 327:141, 1992.
212. The RISC Group: Risk of myocardial infarction and death during treatment with low dose aspirin and intravenous heparin in men with unstable coronary artery disease. Lancet 336:827, 1990.
213. Cohen M, Xiong J, Parry G, et al: Prospective comparison of unstable angina versus non-Q wave myocardial infarction during antithrombotic therapy. J Am Coll Cardiol 22:1388, 1993.
214. Cohen M, Adams P, Hawkins L, et al: Usefulness of antithrombotic therapy in resting angina pectoris or non-Q wave myocardial infarction in preventing death and myocardial infarction (a pilot study from the antithrombotic therapy in acute coronary syndromes group). Am J Cardiol 66:1287, 1990.
215. Theroux P, Lidon R: Unstable angina: Pathogenesis, diagnosis, and treatment. Curr Prob Cardiol 17:157, 1993.
216. Bar F, Verheugt F, Col J, et al: Thrombolysis in patients with unstable angina improves the angiographic but not the clinical outcome: Results of UNASEM, a multicenter, randomized, placebo-controlled, clinical trial with anistreplase. Circulation 86:131, 1992.
217. The TIMI IIIA Investigators: Early effects of tissue-type plasminogen activator added to conventional therapy on the culprit lesion in patients presenting with ischemic cardiac pain at rest: Results of the Thrombolysis in Myocardial in Ischemia (TIMI IIIA) trial. Circulation 87:38, 1993.
218. Lidon R, Theroux P, Juneau M, et al: Initial experience with a direct antithrombin, hirulog, in unstable angina. Circulation 88:1495, 1993.
219. Gold H, Torres F, Garabedian H, et al: Evidence for a rebound coagulation phenomenon after cessation of a 4-hour infusion of a specific thrombin inhibitor in patients with unstable angina pectoris. J Am Coll Cardiol 21:1039, 1993.
220. Buring J, Hennekens C: Antiplatelet therapy to prevent coronary artery bypass graft occlusion. Circulation 82:1046, 1990.
221. Chesebro J, Clements I, Fuster V, et al: A platelet inhibitor drug trial in coronary artery bypass operations: Benefit of perioperative dipyridamole and aspirin therapy on early postoperative vein graft patency. N Engl J Med 307:73, 1982.
222. Goldman S, Copeland J, Moritz T, et al: Improvement in early saphenous vein graft patency after coronary artery bypass surgery with antiplatelet therapy: Results of a Veterans Administration Cooperative Study. Circulation 77:1324, 1988.
223. Verstraete M, Brown B, Chesebro J, et al: Evaluation of antiplatelet agents in the prevention of aorto-coronary bypass occlusion. Eur Heart J 7:4, 1986.
224. Spencer F: The internal mammary artery: The ideal coronary bypass graft? N Engl J Med 314:50,1986.
225. Ip J, Fuster V, Badimon L, et al: Syndromes of accelerated atherosclerosis: Role of vascular injury and smooth muscle cell proliferation. J Am Coll Cardiol 15:1667, 1990.
226. Chesebro J, Goldman S: Coronary artery bypass surgery: Antithrombotic therapy. In Fuster V, Verstraete M (eds): Thrombosis in Cardiovascular Disorders. Philadelphia: WB Saunders, 1992.
227. Luscher T: Vascular biology of coronary bypass grafts. Coronary Artery Dis 3:157, 1992.
228. Malone J, Gervin A, Kischer C, et al: Venous fibrinolytic activity and histologic features with distension. Surg Forum 29:479, 1978.
229. Angelini G, Breckenridge I, Psaila J, et al: Preparation of human saphenous vein for coronary arery bypass grafting impairs its capacity to produce prostacyclin. Cardiovasc Res 21:28, 1987.
230. Grundfest W, Litvack F, Sherman T, et al: Delineation of peripheral and coronary detail by intraoperative angioscopy. Ann Surg 202:394, 1985.
231. Bulkley B, Hutchins G: Pathology of coronary artery bypass graft surgery. Arch Pathol Lab Med 102:273, 1978.
232. Unni K, Kottke B, Titus J, et al: Pathologic changes in aortocoronary saphenous vein grafts. Am J Cardiol 34:526, 1974.
233. Fuster V, Dewanjee M, Kaye M, et al: Noninvasive radioisotope technique for detection of platelet deposition in coronary artery bypass grafts in dogs and its reduction with platelet inhibitors. Circulation 60:1508, 1979.
234. Dobrin P, Golan J, Fareed J, et al: Pre- vs post-operative pharmacologic inhibition of platelets: Effect on intimal hyperplasia in canine autogenous vein grafts. J Cardiovasc Surg 33:705, 1992.
235. Josa M, Lie J, Bianco R, et al: Reduction of thrombosis in canine coronary artery bypass vein grafts with dipyridamole and aspirin. Am J Cardiol 47:1248, 1981.
236. Metke M, Lie J, Fuster V, et al: Reduction of intimal thickening in canine coronary bypass vein grafts with dipyridamole and aspirin. Am J Cardiol 43:1144, 1979.
237. Henderson W, Goldman S, Copeland J, et al: Antiplatelet or anticoagulant therapy after coronary artery bypass surgery: A meta-analysis of clinical trials. Ann Intern Med 111:743, 1989.
238. Fuster V, Chesebro J: Role of platelets and platelet inhibitors in aortocoronary vein graft disease. Circulation 72:227, 1986.
239. Torosian M, Michaelson E, Morganroth J, et al: Aspirin and coumadin related bleeding after coronary arery bypass surgery. Ann Intern Med 89:325, 1978.
240. Weber M: Trial of anticoagulant vs. preoperative low dose aspirin in aortocoronary bypass operation. Presented at the International Workshop on Antithrombotic Therapy in Coronary Artery Disease. Munich, FRG, January, 1986.
241. Chesebro J, Fuster V, Elveback L, et al: Effect of dipyridamole and aspirin on late vein graft patency after coronary bypass operations. N Engl J Med 310:209, 1984.
242. Goldman S, Copeland J, Moritz T, et al: Saphenous vein graft patency 1 year after coronary artery bypass surgery and effects of antiplatelet therapy: Results of a Veterans Administration Cooperative Study. Circulation 80:1190, 1989.

243. Goldman S, Copeland J, Moritz T, et al: Internal mammary artery and saphenous vein graft patency: Effects of aspirin. Circulation 82(Suppl IV):237, 1990.
244. Pfisterer M, Burkart F, Jockers G, et al: Trial of low-dose aspirin plus dipyridamole versus anticoagulants for prevention of arotocoronary vein graft occlusion. Lancet 1:1, 1989.
245. Ekestrom S, Gunnes S, Brodin U: Effect of dipyridamole on blood flow and patency of aortocoronary vein bypass grafts. Scand J Thorac Cardiovasc Surg 24:191, 1990.
246. Sanz G, Pajaron A, Alegria E, et al: Prevention of early aortocoronary bypass occlusion by low-dose aspirin and dipyridamole. Circulation 82:765, 1990.
247. Gavaghan T, Gebski V, Baron D: Immediate postoperative aspirin improves vein graft patency early and late after coronary artery bypass surgery: A placebo-controlled, randomized study. Circulation 83:1526, 1991.
248. van der Meer J, Hillege H, Kootstra G, et al: Prevention of one-year vein-graft occlusion after aortocoronary bypass surgery: A comparison of low-dose aspirin, low-dose aspirin plus dipyridamole, and oral anticoagulants. Lancet 342:257, 1993.
249. Limet R, David J, Magotteau P, et al: Prevention of aortocoronary bypass graft occlusion. Beneficial effect of ticlopidine on early and late patency rates of venous coronary bypass grafts: A double-blind study. J Thorac Cardiovasc Surg 94:773, 1987.

CHAPTER 153

Thrombolytic Therapy in Acute Myocardial Infarction

David J. Moliterno, M.D., and Eric J. Topol, M.D.

Numerous studies have demonstrated that in most subjects with myocardial infarction the inciting pathophysiologic event is an occlusive coronary arterial thrombus.[1-6] Restoration of antegrade perfusion with thrombolytic agents has been intensely studied over the past decade, and the benefit of this therapy is incontrovertible. Timely thrombolytic intervention limits myocardial necrosis and is associated with a reduction in infarct size[7, 8] and left ventricular dilation[9] and with improved left ventricular function[10-19] and survival.[20-24] These striking benefits along with the ability for rapid implementation have led to widespread acceptance of thrombolytic agents as standard therapy to restore myocardial perfusion in acute myocardial infarction, thus establishing the current "thrombolytic era." The conventional use of thrombolytic agents reduces periinfarction mortality approximately 25% to 30%, and refinement of this interventional therapy aggressively continues. Issues regarding patient selection, dose administration, and adjunctive therapies remain under investigation to find even better therapeutic approaches for patients with acute coronary syndromes. This chapter reviews the use of thrombolytic agents during acute myocardial infarction with particular attention to the results of randomized clinical trials.

THROMBOLYTIC AGENTS

Thrombolysis is mediated by plasmin, a nonspecific serine protease that causes fibrinolysis by degrading fibrinogen and fibrin clot. All thrombolytic agents act directly or indirectly as plasminogen activators converting the proenzyme plasminogen to plasmin. Figure 153–1 schematically depicts the fibrinolytic agents in two general groups as fibrin-specific or nonfibrin-specific activators. Tissue-type plasminogen activator (t-PA) and single-chain urokinase-type plasminogen activator (scu-PA) belong to the former group; streptokinase (SK), anistreplase (APSAC), and urokinase (UK) belong to the latter. For a detailed review of these thrombolytic agents, please see their respective chapters.

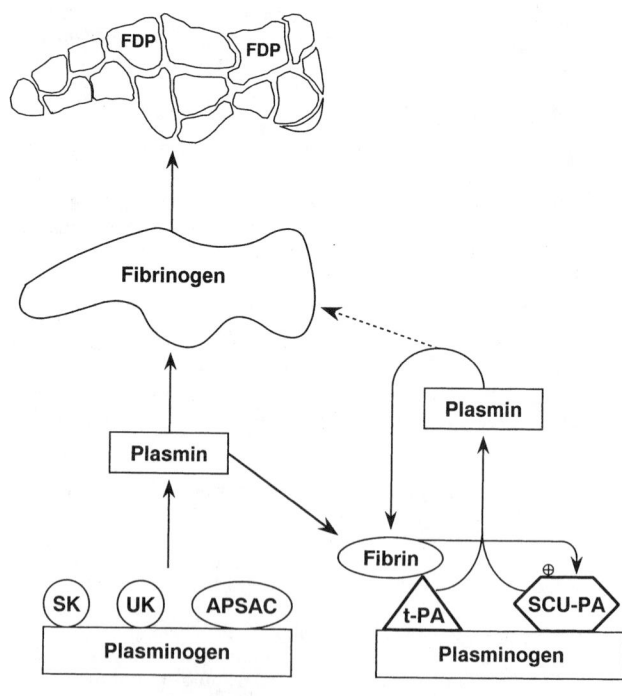

Circulating Blood   **Clot Surface**

Figure 153–1. Schematic representation of the action of fibrinolytic enzymes. Streptokinase (SK), urokinase (UK), and anisoylated plasminogen-streptokinase activator complex (APSAC) work predominantly on circulating plasminogen, whereas tissue-type plasminogen activator (t-PA) and single-chain urokinase-type plasminogen activator (scu-PA) are relatively clot selective. (From Topol EJ: Clinical use of streptokinase and urokinase therapy for acute myocardial infarction. Heart Lung 16:760, 1987.)

Table 153–1. **Infarct Artery Patency at 90 Minutes**

Study/Author	Agent	n	Dose	Patency
ECSG-1[19]	None	65	NA	21% (13/62)
Charbonnier et al.[72]	SK	58	1.5 mU	51% (27/53)
ECSG-2[73]	SK	65	1.0 mU	55% (34/62)
Hogg et al.[74]	SK	63	1.5 mU	53% (31/58)
Lopez-Sendon et al.[75]	SK	25	1.5 mU	60% (15/25)
PRIMI[76]	SK	203	1.5 mU	64% (124/194)
Stack et al.[77]	SK	216	1.5 mU	44% (95/216)
TIMI-1[55]	SK	159	1.5 mU	43% (63/146)
Pooled	**SK**	**789**		**52% (389/754)**
CRAFT[78]	UK	202	3 mU/90 min	53% (105/198)
GAUS[79]	UK	121	3 mU/90 min	66% (77/117)
Mathey et al.[80]	UK	50	2 mU bolus	60% (30/50)
TAMI-5[34]	UK	95	3 mU/90 min	65% (62/95)
Pooled	**UK**	**468**		**60% (274/460)**
Charbonnier et al.[72]	APSAC	58	30 mg	72% (38/54)
Hogg et al.[74]	APSAC	65	30 mg	55% (32/60)
Lopez-Sendon et al.[75]	APSAC	22	30 mg	86% (19/22)
Relik-van Wely et al.[81]	APSAC	156	30 mg	73% (106/145)
TAPS[82]	APSAC	210	30 mg	70% (142/202)
Pooled	**APSAC**	**511**		**70% (337/483)**
CRAFT[78]	t-PA	206	100 mg/3 hr	63% (126/199)
ECSG-1[19]	t-PA	64	0.75 mg/kg/90 min	61% (38/62)
ECSG-2[73]	t-PA	64	0.75 mg/kg/90 min	70% (43/61)
GAUS[79]	t-PA	124	70 mg/90 min	69% (84/121)
Johns et al.[83]	t-PA	68	1 mg/kg/90 min	77% (52/68)
KAMIT[32]	t-PA	107	100 mg/3 hr	64% (65/102)
RAAMI[84]	t-PA	138	100 mg/3 hr	75% (92/122)
Smalling et al.[85]	t-PA	91	1.25 mg/kg/3 hr	70% (61/87)
TAMI-3[86]	t-PA	134	1.5 mg/kg/4 hr	79% (104/131)
TAMI-4[87]	t-PA	50	100 mg/3 hr	52% (26/50)
TAMI-5[34]	t-PA	95	100 mg/3 hr	71% (67/95)
TIMI-1[55]	t-PA	157	80 mg/3 hr	70% (100/143)
TIMI-2A[88]	t-PA	133	100 mg/6 hr	75% (90/131)
Topol et al.[89]	t-PA	75	1.25 mg/kg/3 hr	69% (49/71)
Topol et al.[90]	t-PA	142	1 mg/kg/hr, 100–150	72% (102/142)
Pooled	**t-PA**	**1648**		**70% (1107/1585)**
Gemmill et al.[91]	accl t-PA	33	70 mg/90 min	87% (26/30)
Neuhaus et al.[92]	accl t-PA	80	100 mg/90 min	91% (67/74)
RAAMI[84]	accl t-PA	143	100 mg/90 min	82% (105/128)
TAMI-7[93]	accl t-PA	61	1.25 mg/kg/90 min	84% (51/61)
TAPS[82]	accl t-PA	210	100 mg/90 min	84% (168/199)
Pooled	**accl t-PA**	**527**		**85% (417/492)**
Bonnet et al.[33]	SK + t-PA	34	1.0 mU/0.5 hr + 50 mg/0.5 hr	82% (28/34)
GUSTO-1[71]	SK + t-PA	299	1.0 mU/hr + 1 mg/kg/hr	73% (218/299)
KAMIT[32]	SK + t-PA	109	1.5 mU/hr + 50 mg/hr	79% (81/102)
Pooled	**SK + t-PA**	**442**		**75% (327/435)**

COMBINATION PLASMINOGEN ACTIVATORS

Because the thrombolytic agents have relatively different advantages and disadvantages—fibrin specificity, biologic half-life, cost, side effect profile—it has been proposed that the combination of two or more agents at low dose may be beneficial.[25] Several small studies assessing combination therapies have shown similar[26–31] or slightly improved[32, 33] rates of early infarct artery patency (Table 153–1), and others[32, 34] have demonstrated a low incidence of infarct vessel reocclusion without an increased incidence of bleeding complications.[27, 28, 30–33] In the GUSTO trial,[35] 10,328 patients received recombinant tissue plasminogen activator (rt-PA) (1 mg/kg, up to 90 mg) combined with streptokinase (1 million units). As will be discussed later, the early infarct artery patency rate and 1-month mortality were not improved compared with accelerated t-PA or streptokinase-only regimens.

PATIENT SELECTION

Timely administration of thrombolytic therapy is clearly indicated in the majority of patients presenting with acute myocardial infarction, and the identification of appropriate candidates continues to improve. The reasons for underutilization include a previously more restricted application of therapy because risk-to-benefit ratios were uncertain in some patient subgroups, such as those with advanced age, late entry, severe hypertension, previous cerebrovascular event, or an uncomplicated inferior infarction.

Advanced Age

Until recently, being elderly was considered a relative contraindication to thrombolytic therapy. In addition to being the single most important demographic predictor of mortality, advanced age is associated with a high risk of serious bleeding complications during thrombolytic therapy. Whereas the rate of stroke for patients younger than age 65 years is approximately 0.75%, with no difference between thrombolytic agents, as age increases, the rate of stroke does so as well (streptokinase 1.4% and t-PA 2.1%).[36] Meta-analysis of large patient trials has shown the overall 35-day mortality rate of all postinfarction patients aged 65 to 74 years to be approximately 15%, which is several-fold higher than younger cohorts.[36]

Although it was initially feared that elderly patients receiving thrombolytic therapy would have a prohibitively high incidence of serious bleeding complications, a net benefit of mortality reduction has become apparent. In both the ISIS-3 and GUSTO trials,[30, 35, 37] 14% of patients enrolled were 75 years or older; this contrasts markedly to before 1990, when the same figure in the United States was less than 1%. In these thrombolytic therapy trials, the greatest margin of benefit (absolute risk reduction) for all patient age groups was found in subjects 65 to 74 years of age. Specifically, those receiving therapy had a 5-week mortality of 14.1% compared with the control group mortality of 16.5%. Beyond 75 years of age, mortality is reduced, but pooled results indicate the absolute benefit (number of lives saved per 1000 patients treated) is not statistically significant.[38] The analysis presented is based on more than 5000 patients aged 75 years or older. The reduction of absolute benefit in this cohort is linked, in part, to the increase in bleeding complications or "early hazard" (death within 24 hours of thrombolytic therapy).

In balance, elderly patients merit serious consideration for thrombolytic therapy. Although comorbidity needs to be taken into account, patients should no longer be excluded from treatment solely on the basis of age.

Late Entry

Delayed presentation, i.e., after the traditional 6-hour time window, also had been an exclusion criterion from therapy. In response to early data from streptokinase use,[20] it was believed that thrombolytic therapy benefit was limited to patients presenting shortly after the onset of symptoms. However, the meta-analysis in the Fibrinolytic Therapy Trialists' Collaboration[36] systematically pooled data from 52,892 patients enrolled into eight placebo-controlled trials (not including the LATE trial)[20–24, 39] and showed significant benefit up to 12 hours, but not beyond this time point. In light of data from this large meta-analysis and the LATE trial,[40] there is consensus that the "window of treatment" be extended to 12 hours. Some patients presenting 12 to 24 hours after symptom onset may derive benefit from treatment, particularly if there has been a stuttering pattern of chest pain, continued presence of ischemic pain, a large myocardial infarction, or persistent or pronounced ST-segment elevation. Although no trial has directly addressed whether treatment benefit exists for such patients, it seems prudent to weigh the potential benefits of reperfusion therapy. A synthesis of the major thrombolytic trials, shown in Figure 153–2, displays a two-step decrement in mortality over time rather than a linear relationship. This may represent the multifactorial benefit of a patent infarct artery related to myocardial salvage, geometry, and electrical stability.

Electrocardiographic Criteria

Patients presenting with ST-segment elevation or bundle branch block clearly benefited from thrombolytic therapy. In fact, the entrance criteria for GISSI and GUSTO trials included ST-segment elevation of 2 mm or more in precordial leads or 1 mm or more in limb leads. Mortality data according to electrocardiographic presentation are shown in Figure 153–3.[36] As might be expected, there is no advantage for patients with chest pain and a normal electrocardiogram (ECG) or with minor T-wave changes to receive thrombolytic therapy. These patients have a very low mortality in treated and control groups.[23, 24] Patients with chest pain and focal ST-segment depression generally have unfavorable baseline characteristics, a high mortality, and receive little or no survival benefit

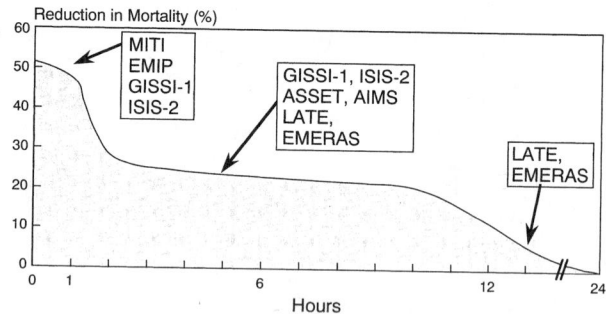

Figure 153–2. Mortality reduction (%) derived from thrombolytic therapy as a function of the elapsed time between symptom onset and initiation of thrombolytic agent. Clinical trials from which these data are extrapolated are noted. A greater than 50% reduction in mortality is noted during the "golden first hour," after which mortality benefit declines to a plateau of approximately 25% reduction until 12 hours after symptom onset. Beyond 12 hours, significant survival benefit has not been demonstrated with thrombolytic administration. AIMS, Anistreplase Intervention Mortality Study;[22] ASSET, Anglo-Scandinavian Study of Early Thrombolysis;[23] EMERAS, Estudio Multicéntrico Estreptoquinasa Repúblicas de America del Sur;[94] EMIP, European Myocardial Infarction Project;[95] GISSI-1, Gruppo Italiano per lo Studio della Sopravvivenza nell'Infarto Miocardico;[20] ISIS-2, Second International Study of Infarct Survival;[21] LATE, Late Assessment of Thrombolytic Efficacy;[40] MITI, Myocardial Infarction Triage and Intervention Trial.[7] (Reproduced with permission from Lincoff AM, Topol EJ: The illusion of reperfusion. Does anyone achieve optimal reperfusion during acute myocardial infarction? Circulation 88:1361, 1993. Copyright 1993, American Heart Association.)

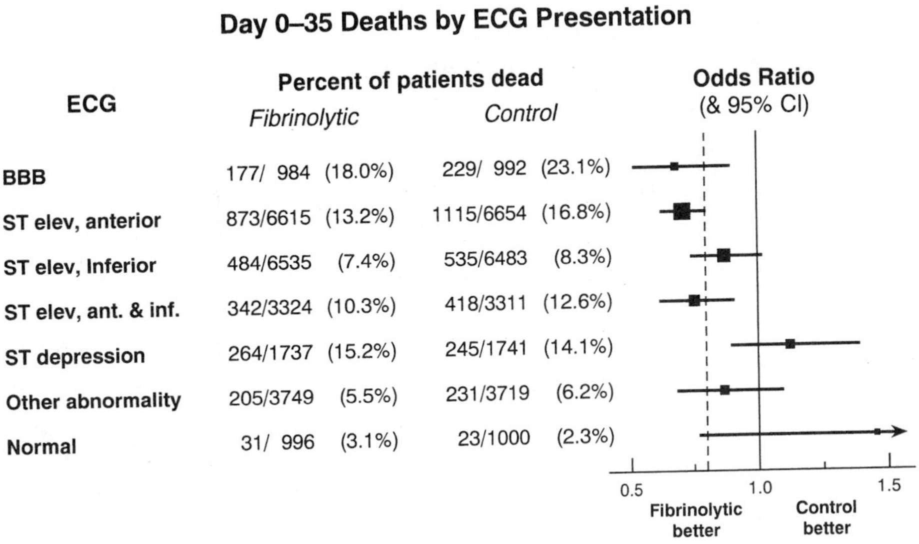

Day 0–35 Deaths by ECG Presentation

ECG	Percent of patients dead Fibrinolytic	Control	Odds Ratio (& 95% CI)
BBB	177/ 984 (18.0%)	229/ 992 (23.1%)	
ST elev, anterior	873/6615 (13.2%)	1115/6654 (16.8%)	
ST elev, Inferior	484/6535 (7.4%)	535/6483 (8.3%)	
ST elev, ant. & inf.	342/3324 (10.3%)	418/3311 (12.6%)	
ST depression	264/1737 (15.2%)	245/1741 (14.1%)	
Other abnormality	205/3749 (5.5%)	231/3719 (6.2%)	
Normal	31/ 996 (3.1%)	23/1000 (2.3%)	

Figure 153–3. Odds ratio and confidence interval of survival for ECG presentation from the collaborative fibrinolytic trials. Only ST elevation and bundle branch block (BBB) were associated with improved survival. (From Fibrinolytic Therapy Trialists' [FTT] Collaborative Group: Indications for fibrinolytic therapy in suspected acute myocardial infarction: Collaborative overview of mortality and major morbidity results from randomized trials of more than 1,000 patients. Lancet 343:311, 1994. © by The Lancet Ltd, 1994.)

from thrombolysis. These patients may benefit from a more aggressive approach, including early diagnostic catheterization and coronary intervention; a large proportion actually have unstable angina and not acute myocardial infarction. Patients with chest pain and prior myocardial infarction, as evident on the admission electrocardiogram, receive benefit from thrombolytic therapy. The pooled analysis of patients with prior infarction indicated a mortality of 516 in 3663 control group patients (14.1%) compared with 81 of 3893 thrombolytic treated patients (12.4%) ($p < .02$).[36]

Admission Blood Pressure

A history of hypertension is not an exclusion for thrombolytic intervention. This is a common presenting demographic feature, and regardless of the prior severity of blood pressure, no trial has convincingly shown an associated excessive risk of thrombolytic therapy. Elevated blood pressure is a risk for intracranial hemorrhage; however, a reduction in cardiac-related deaths and overall mortality has been demonstrated in hypertensive subjects receiving thrombolytic therapy. This information was a meaningful outgrowth of a large meta-analysis[36] that showed that the risk of cerebral hemorrhage increased with systolic arterial pressure of more than 150 mmHg and further increased when pressure exceeded 175 mmHg (Table 153–2). The increased stroke rate associated with a systolic arterial pressure of 175 mmHg or higher may account for the lack of significant mortality reduction observed in some studies (Fig. 153–4).[38] It is not known whether promptly controlling the blood pressure with antihypertensive agents after presentation improves the prognosis for those with severe hypertension. The benefit of thrombolytic therapy in patients with marked elevation of diastolic arterial pressure (≥ 120 mmHg) is uncertain. In these situations, in which an otherwise good candidate for reperfusion therapy has marked arterial hypertension and the clinical setting is feasible, it may

be prudent to recommend primary angioplasty rather than thrombolysis.

Hypotension is a similarly difficult area to discern true benefit from thrombolysis. Low arterial pressure on presentation can stem from cardiogenic shock or hypervagotonia; the former may be associated with large anterior myocardial infarctions, whereas the latter more often accompanies inferior infarctions. Figure 153–4 suggests that patients with systolic blood pressure of less than 100 mmHg on admission benefit from thrombolysis despite a very high mortality rate in both the treatment and control groups.[41] The high mortality (30%) in the control group suggests that patients in cardiogenic shock were included. Contrasting these data, subgroup analyses of the GISSI-1[20] and GISSI-2[42] trials according to Killip class revealed no apparent mortality reduction with streptokinase versus placebo for both Killip class III and IV.[43] Furthermore, in GISSI-2, there was no mortality difference between Killip class IV subjects receiving streptokinase or t-PA and the historical control group mortality from GISSI-1 (Fig. 153–5).

It remains unsettled whether thrombolysis improves prognosis in cardiogenic shock.[43] Prewitt et

Table 153–2. **Direct Comparison of SK vs t-PA: Cerebral Hemorrhage Days 0–35, Subdivided by Systolic Blood Pressure**

Prerandomization Systolic BP (mmHg)	SK		t-PA		Diff/sd (z-score)
<100	3/1529	0.2%	6/1459	0.4%	1.0
100–124	12/6980	0.2%	21/7006	0.3%	1.5
125–149	17/7903	0.2%	32/7884	0.4%	2.1*
150–174	24/6396	0.4%	48/6385	0.8%	2.9*
175+	8/1649	0.3%	27/1653	1.6%	3.2†
ALL	64/24,457	0.3%	134/24,387	0.5%	5.0†

*2p<.05.
†2p<.001.

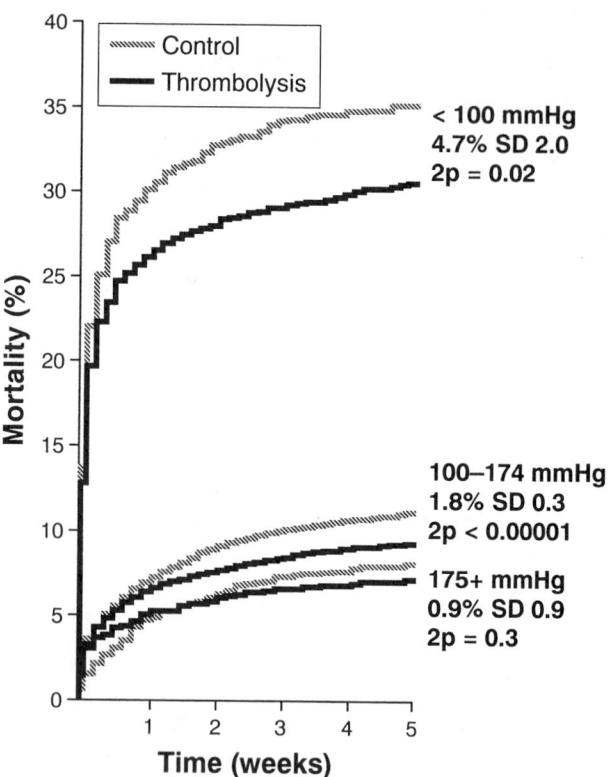

Day 0–35 Deaths
Subdivided by Systolic Blood Pressure

Figure 153–4. Survival curves subdivided by admission systolic arterial pressure. For patients with markedly abnormal systolic blood pressure (<100 mmHg or >175 mmHg), no statistically significant survival benefit from thrombolysis was demonstrable. (From Fibrinolytic Therapy Trialists' [FTT] Collaborative Group: Indications for fibrinolytic therapy in suspected acute myocardial infarction: Collaborative overview of mortality and major morbidity results from randomized trials of more than 1,000 patients. Lancet 343:311, 1994. © by The Lancet Ltd, 1994.)

al.[44] have shown in an experimental model that perfusion is quantitatively linked with thrombolysis. It is plausible that diminished perfusion in the setting of cardiogenic shock could lead to inadequate delivery of thrombolytic agent to the occlusive thrombus and thereby limit efficacy. On the other hand, primary angioplasty for cardiogenic shock has been associated with favorable results[45] and should be considered the procedure of choice in Killip class IV patients suitable for reperfusion therapy. Thrombolysis is indicated if primary angioplasty is not available.

Other Categories

A number of additional diagnoses or demographic factors—cardiopulmonary resuscitation, diabetes, recent stroke—have been touted as contraindications to thrombolytic therapy, but often there are limited or no data supporting the recommendation.[46–52] Patients who have had cardiopulmonary resuscitation remain excellent candidates for thrombolytic therapy, provided there has not been prolonged (>10 minutes)

resuscitation or extensive chest trauma from manual compressions.[53] On the other hand, a recent summary of thrombolytic trials has linked an association with concomitant coumadin therapy at admission with intracerebral hemorrhage[54] following t-PA. Diabetes is not a contraindication to thrombolysis, and patients with known, active diabetic retinopathy have received therapy without untoward sequelae. The only absolute contraindication for thrombolytic therapy is active significant bleeding. Although patients with uncontrolled active bleeding are not appropriate candidates for thrombolytic therapy, many patients may have a history of an "ulcer" or rectal bleeding from hemorrhoids that should not preclude them from therapy. Recent stroke (<6 months), major surgery, and trauma constitute relative contraindications, but there are inadequate data for meaningful recommendations. A past central nervous system event of any kind, including arteriovenous malformation or neoplasm, represents an important relative contraindication. Central venous punctures, particularly of the internal jugular vein, can lead to tracheal compression during thrombolysis, such that patients with noncompressible punctures should be considered for thrombolysis only if there is no alternative. Importantly, if a patient is considered a good candidate for reperfusion but there is a lingering concern over one or more of the relative contraindications, he or she should be considered for direct angioplasty. Patients with prior coronary artery bypass grafting are suitable for thrombolytic therapy, but their response to therapy may be reduced by extensive clot burden in vein grafts. In suitable hospitals, patients with prior bypass grafting should alternatively be considered for primary angioplasty.

CLINICAL END POINT ASSESSMENT

Much of the foundational work for the development of thrombolytic therapy was based on pathophysiologic theory, basic science, and animal model research. Once the administration of exogenous thrombolysis was possible, it became necessary to develop an assessment of clinical end points to compare and contrast different thrombolytic drug regimens. Various meaningful end points—infarct artery patency, reocclusion/reinfarction, cerebrovascular accident, left ventricular function, and mortality—have been assessed in numerous clinical trials (Table 153–3). These end points help evaluate existing therapies, establish new therapies, and guide the development of future agents and regimens.

Infarct Artery Patency

It is well established that myocardial infarction results when patency of an epicardial coronary artery is compromised by an occlusive thrombus. The primary aim of any thrombolytic agent, therefore, is to restore antegrade coronary flow by degrading this thrombus. As previously mentioned, antegrade flow restoration is associated with improved ventricular function and

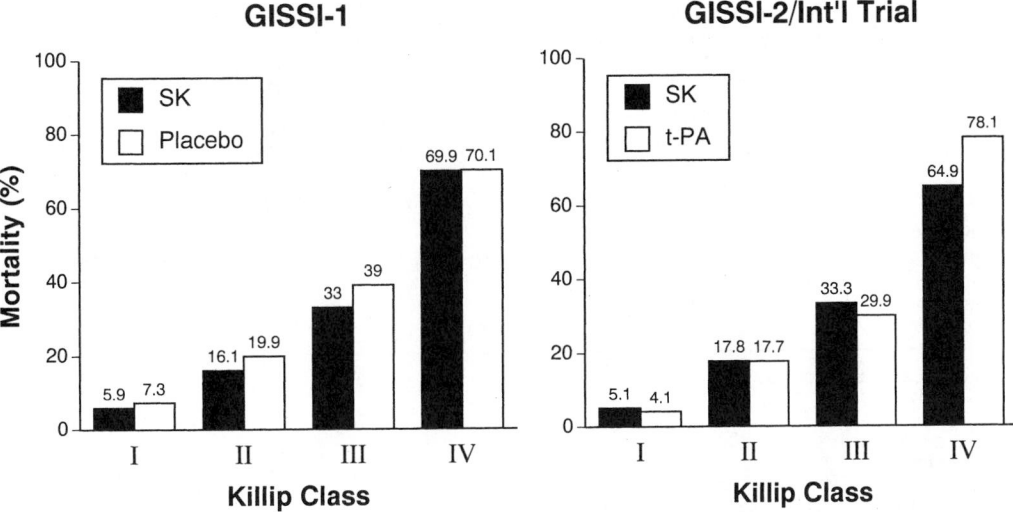

Figure 153–5. No difference in survival for streptokinase versus placebo (GISSI-1) or patients treated with streptokinase versus t-PA (GISSI-2) in cardiogenic shock or Killip classes III, IV. (Data from Bates ER, Topol EJ: Limitations of thrombolytic therapy for acute myocardial infarction complicated by congestive heart failure and cardiogenic shock. J Am Coll Cardiol 18:1077, 1991.)

geometry and improved short- and long-term survival. Information from angiography performed in the early hours of myocardial infarction demonstrated that endogenous thrombolysis occurs in some individuals with a patency rate of 20% to 35% at 24 hours.[5, 9] Unfortunately, endomyocardial myocardial necrosis may begin within minutes of ischemia, and irreparable transmural damage may occur within several hours of ischemia. For these reasons, it seems logical to restore antegrade perfusion promptly and to use arterial patency as an end point assessment of thrombolytic therapy. Table 153–4 displays rates of infarct artery patency in a number of major clinical trials and will be discussed later in this chapter.

Unfortunately, it is difficult to optimally define and standardize "infarct artery patency." A "90-minute" end point of infarct artery patency was arbitrarily picked by trialists in 1984 because this interval was convenient and feasible to assess and was believed to be clinically representative as an index of clot-dissolving capacity.[55–57] Furthermore, the TIMI (Thrombolysis in Myocardial Infarction) investigators defined arterial flow in a four-level grading scale (i.e., TIMI grades 0 to 3). Although TIMI grades 2 and 3 both were considered to represent arterial patency,

they differed in the rate of coronary arterial flow. After years of angiographic reperfusion studies, it has become clear that this arbitrary lumping and relatively late (90-minute rather than 60-minute) assessment of patency were misleading. Additionally, there are problems with intermittent vessel patency and reocclusion. In short, even though early infarct artery patency is a highly desirable goal of thrombolytic intervention, it is a rather complex end point with multiple historical definitions. For these reasons, other end points or clinical outcomes (left ventricular function, reinfarction, survival) have gained more attention in major thrombolytic trials.

Reocclusion and Reinfarction

Like the initial coronary arterial occlusion, reocclusion, unless quickly ameliorated, can produce myocardial ischemia. Among patients with reocclusion, approximately one half clinically experience reinfarction. It is not surprising, therefore, that subjects with reocclusion have an associated mortality approximately twice that of those whose vessel remains patent.[58] It is interesting to note that t-PA, the agent with the highest rate of early infarct artery patency, has the

Table 153–3. **Clinical End Points in Comparative Thrombolytic Trials**

End Point	n	GISSI-2/International		ISIS-3			GUSTO-1		
		SK 10,396	t-PA 10,372	SK 13,607	t-PA 13,569	APSAC 13,599	SK 20,173	t-PA† 10,344	SK + t-PA 10,328
Death (%)		8.5	8.9	10.6	10.3	10.5	7.3	6.3*	7.0
Reinfarction (%)		3.0	2.6	3.5	2.9*	3.6	3.7	4.0	4.0
Any stroke (%)		0.9	1.3*	1.0	1.4*	1.3	1.3	1.6	1.7
Hemmorhagic stroke (%)		0.3	0.4	0.2	0.7*	0.6	0.5	0.7*	0.9
Non-CNS bleeds (%)		0.9	0.6*	4.5	5.2*	5.4	6.0	5.4*	6.1

SK, streptokinase; t-PA, tissue-type plasminogen activator; APSAC, anistreplase.
Statistical comparisons are only listed for SK vs. t-PA; *$p < .05$.
†Accelerated dose tissue-type plasminogen activator.

Table 153–4. **Rate of Patency and Complete Reperfusion Among Treatment Groups**

	SK (SQ)	SK (IV)	t-PA	t-PA + SK
Patency (TIMI 2 or 3)				
At 90 minutes	159/293 (54%)	171/283 (60%)	236/292 (81%)	218/299 (73%)[a, b, c]
At 180 minutes	77/106 (73%)	72/97 (74%)	71/93 (76%)	77/91 (85%)
At 24 hours	64/83 (77%)	74/92 (80%)	89/104 (86%)	87/93 (94%)[d]
At 5–7 days	67/93 (72%)	80/96 (83%)	70/83 (84%)	71/89 (80%)[e]
Complete Reperfusion (TIMI 3)				
At 90 minutes	85/293 (29%)	922/283 (33%)	157/292 (54%)	114/299 (38%)
At 180 minutes	37/106 (35%)	40/97 (41%)	40/93 (43%)	48/91 (53%)[b, f]
At 24 hours	42/83 (51%)	38/92 (41%)	47/104 (45%)	56/93 (60%)
At 5–7 days	47/93 (51%)	55/96 (57%)	48/83 (58%)	49/89 (55%)

SQ, subcutaneous heparin; IV, intravenous heparin.
[a] t-PA vs. t-PA + SK: $p<.04$.
[b] t-PA vs. SK (IV + SQ): $p<.001$.
[c] SK(IV + SQ) vs. t-PA + SK: $p<.001$.
[d] SK(SQ) vs. t-PA + SK: $p<.001$.
[e] t-PA vs. SK(SQ): $p<.04$.
[f] t-PA vs. SK + t-PA: $p<.0001$.

highest reocclusion. Like patency, the definition of reocclusion may be vulnerable, because it is difficult to differentiate primary from recurrent and partial from complete vessel occlusion without serial angiography.

Left Ventricular Function

Left ventricular ejection fraction has been long recognized as an important predictor of survival after infarction[59] because of its parallel association with mortality. Because the functional goal of thrombolysis is to minimize myocardial necrosis, left ventricular systolic function should be an ideal clinical end point. Compared with placebo, all thrombolytic agents improve regional and global ventricular function, with an approximately 5% higher left ventricular ejection fraction in treated groups.[60] This relative improvement in ejection fraction is relatively constant over the days to weeks after myocardial infarction.[61]

Unfortunately, ventricular function, like the previously discussed end points, has fallen short of being an ideal surrogate marker for survival for several reasons. Using data from nine placebo-controlled thrombolytic trials,[10, 11, 13–17, 24, 62] a disparity between ejection fraction and survival becomes apparent (Fig. 153–6).[63] The problems are, first, a significant amount of data is missing (because patients were critically ill or died early) or technically inadequate.[63] Second, there is a lack of correlation between ejection fraction improvement and time to therapy, except for patients treated in the first hour of symptom onset. Third, there is compensatory non–infarct zone hyperkinesis so that global ejection fraction tends to be insensitive to infarct zone dysfunction and little change in ejection fraction occurs over weeks to months. Finally, the accurate assessment of baseline ventricular volumes and function complicates thrombolytic administration.

Why then does left ventricular systolic function parallel survival? Interestingly, left ventricular function is more closely associated with vessel patency than with treatment with thrombolysis per se (Fig.

153–7). Several studies have shown that early infarct artery patency, regardless of thrombolysis, is associated with greater preservation of global left ventricular function.[64–66] From this, it has been suggested that to benefit ventricular function substantially, thrombolysis must be given early in the course of symptoms. Indeed, patients treated early (within 3 hours) demonstrate a greater ejection fraction than those treated

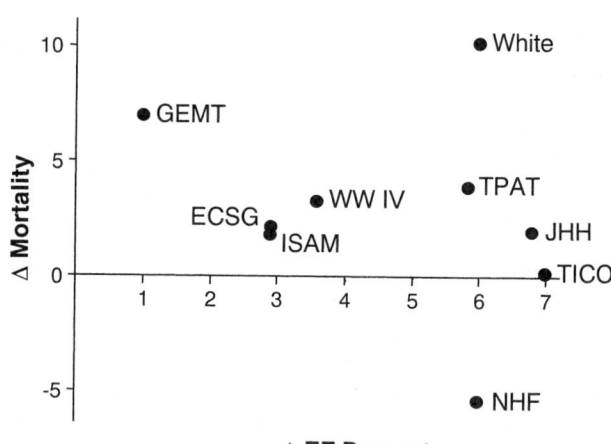

Δ EF Percent

Figure 153–6. Scatterplot showing relation of ejection fraction improvement to mortality reduction in nine placebo-controlled intravenous thrombolytic therapy reperfusion trials. The graph demonstrates lack of clear association (except possibly a paradoxically inverse one). Trials that have demonstrated the greatest ejection fraction improvement (ΔEF) over placebo have tended to exhibit the least mortality reduction. It is important to note that these were trials of left ventricular ejection fraction and were not intended to detect differences of mortality. Trial abbreviations and references are as follows: ECSG, European Cooperative Study Group;[15] GEMT, German Eminase Multicenter Trial;[62] ISAM, Intravenous Streptokinase in Acute Myocardial Infarction;[24] JHH, Johns Hopkins Hospital Trial;[10] NHF, National Heart Foundation Trial;[13] TICO, Thrombolysis in Coronary Occlusion Trial;[17] TPAT, Tissue Plasminogen Activator–Toronto Trial;[11] WWIV, Western Washington Intravenous Streptokinase Trial;[14] and White et al.[16] (Reproduced with permission from Califf RM, Harrelson-Woodlief L, Topol EJ: Left ventricular ejection fraction may not be useful as an endpoint for thrombolytic therapy comparative trials. Circulation 82:1847, 1990. Copyright 1990, American Heart Association.)

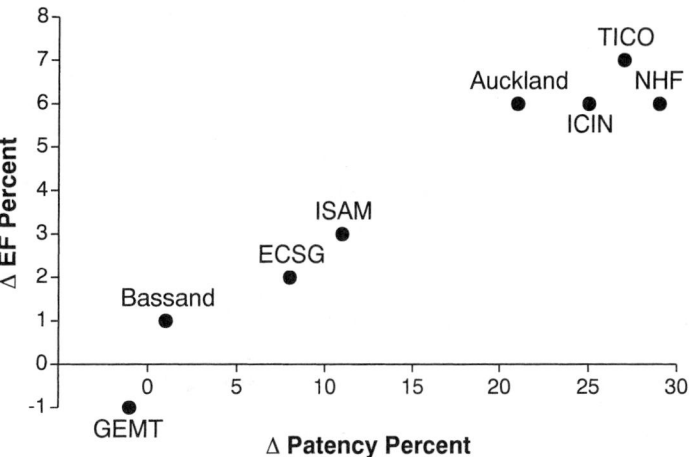

Figure 153–7. Data from various placebo-controlled thrombolytic trials at angiography 10 to 30 days after acute myocardial infarction. Differences in ejection fraction (EF) in favor of thrombolysis coincide with differences between patency rates of the infarct artery in thrombolysis and control groups. Trial abbreviations and references are as follows: GISSI, Gruppo Italiano per lo Studio della Sopravvivenza nell' Infarto Miocardico[20]; ISAM, Intravenous Streptokinase in Acute Myocardial Infarction[24]; ISIS-2, Second International Study of Infarct Survival[21]; AIMS, Anistreplase Intervention Mortality Study[22]; ASSET, Anglo-Scandinavian Study of Early Thrombolysis.[23] (Modified from Schröder R, Neuhaus KL, Linderer T, et al: Impact of late coronary artery reperfusion on left ventricular function one month after acute myocardial infarction [Results of the ISAM study]. Am J Cardiol 64:878, 1989. Adapted with permission from American Journal of Cardiology.)

later. Further interesting insight was provided by The Western Washington Trial,[14] in which intracoronary streptokinase was administered approximately 5 hours after symptomatic myocardial ischemia commenced. Despite similar ventricular function among subject groups, those with complete reperfusion had only a 2.5% mortality compared with 15% in subjects with minimal or no reperfusion. This study and others[67–69] have provided evidence that the importance of the "open artery" is independent of ventricular function. In summary, left ventricular function better estimates early infarct artery patency, whereas vessel patency independently influences long-term survival.

Mortality

Saving lives, or mortality reduction, is the gold standard end point assessment for thrombolytic therapy. It is obviously an objective end point and represents the culmination of many divergent effects that thrombolytic therapy can have—early reperfusion and myocardial salvage, late reperfusion and avoidance of malignant arrhythmias, or fatal intracerebral stroke. When considering the lifesaving potential of thrombolytic agents in large-scale trials, it is important to consider (1) the percentage mortality reduction, (2) the number of lives actually saved, and (3) whether the survival benefit was assessed short term or long term. The survival benefit of thrombolysis appears maximally demonstrable at approximately 1 month after treatment and persists over a year. Finally, it is important to appreciate the outcome measures mortality does not encompass, such as nonfatal stroke and overall quality of life.

Large-scale, randomized thrombolytic trials require an enormous effort and resource consumption but have contributed much to our understanding of myocardial reperfusion therapy with respect to these end points. The "big five" randomized controlled trials[20–24] (i.e., thrombolytic therapy versus placebo or conventional care) are summarized in Figure 153–8. The landmark Gruppo Italiano per lo Studio della Sopravvivenza nell'Infarto Miocardico (GISSI-1)[20] was the first to show that thrombolytic therapy saves

lives—approximately one in five patients treated in the trial of nearly 12,000 patients. The largest placebo-controlled trial, the Second International Study of Infarct Survival (ISIS-2)[21] enrolled 17,187 patients in a 2 × 2 factorial design with streptokinase and aspirin and demonstrated the additive effect of adjunct therapies—in this case, aspirin. Although these five controlled trials with more than 28,000 patients were heterogeneous with respect to entry criteria, thrombolytic agent used, adjunctive therapies, and duration of follow-up, their results were concordant, with an overall 27% risk reduction of death (see Fig. 153–8).

These pivotal placebo-controlled trials set the template for "mega-trials" to assess comparative thrombolytic regimens, including GISSI-2/International, ISIS-3, and GUSTO trials.[35, 37, 42] Each of these trials assessed various clinical events but kept mortality as the primary end point. Although it might have been faster or easier to use surrogate measures such as infarct vessel patency or ejection fraction as primary end points, this was undesirable owing to the inconsistent correlation with these parameters and long-term survival.

MAJOR CLINICAL TRIALS
GISSI-2/International

The Italian investigators in GISSI-2[70] combined forces with investigators from 13 other countries to enroll 20,891 patients with suspected acute myocardial infarction.[42] Entry criteria included admission to the coronary care unit within 6 hours from symptom onset and electrocardiographic ST-segment elevation of 1 mm or more in limb leads or 2 mm or more in precordial leads. Patients were randomly assigned to either t-PA (alteplase, 100 mg over 3 hours, conventional dosing) or streptokinase (1.5 million U over 60 minutes, conventional dosing). The trial was a 2 × 2 factorial design, with adjunct assignment to either subcutaneous heparin (12,500 U beginning 12 hours after thrombolytic therapy and twice daily subsequently) or no heparin. All patients, in the absence of contraindications, were to receive aspirin and β-

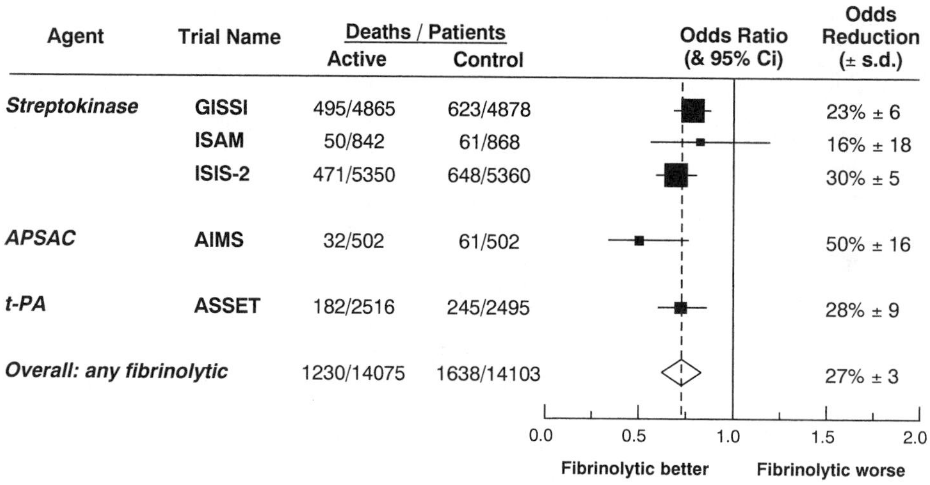

Agent	Trial Name	Deaths / Patients		Odds Ratio (& 95% Ci)	Odds Reduction (± s.d.)
		Active	Control		
Streptokinase	GISSI	495/4865	623/4878		23% ± 6
	ISAM	50/842	61/868		16% ± 18
	ISIS-2	471/5350	648/5360		30% ± 5
APSAC	AIMS	32/502	61/502		50% ± 16
t-PA	ASSET	182/2516	245/2495		28% ± 9
Overall: any fibrinolytic		1230/14075	1638/14103		27% ± 3

0.0 0.5 1.0 1.5 2.0
Fibrinolytic better   Fibrinolytic worse

Figure 153–8. Reductions in the odds of early death among patients treated within 6 hours; overview of currently available data from the five largest randomized controlled trials of thrombolytic versus control. (From Granger CB, Califf RM, Topol EJ: Thrombolytic therapy for acute myocardial infarction. Drugs 44:293, 1992.)

adrenergic blockade as soon as possible. The protocol did not recommend intravenous heparin, and it was rarely used. The results for mortality (see Table 153–3) demonstrate no difference between streptokinase (8.5%) and t-PA (8.9%), with or without subcutaneous heparin.[42, 70] There was a greater incidence of total strokes in the t-PA group (1.3% versus 0.9%), although the ability to discern hemorrhagic versus nonhemorrhagic strokes was incomplete. There was a higher incidence of major bleeds with streptokinase than t-PA (0.9% versus 0.6%). In summary, (1) no difference in major cardiac complications or in-hospital mortality was detected between subjects receiving t-PA or SK, and (2) an increase in overall stroke rate was noted for t-PA compared with SK.

ISIS-3

The Third International Study of Infarct Survival (ISIS-3),[37] similar to the GISSI-2/International trial, was a very large multinational project specifically aimed at comparing different thrombolytic regimens. This study contained a third arm to include the latest addition to the thrombolytic drug list, anistreplase (APSAC). In addition to recruiting the largest number of subjects ever in a thrombolytic trial (n = 41,299), several differences in ISIS-3 made it distinct from previous trials. First, the study was conducted in a double-blinded and fully placebo-controlled fashion in that each subject received all three "agents"; one of which was real, the other two were placebo solutions. Second, the double-strand form of t-PA, duteplase (0.6 mU/kg), was used instead of alteplase. Third, heparin administration was randomized (3×2), given subcutaneously, and initiated 4 rather than 12 hours after starting the thrombolytic infusion. Fourth, patient entry criteria were broad, and in each case the responsible physician deemed the indication for thrombolytic therapy "clear" (randomization to one of the three thrombolytic agents) or "uncertain" (equal randomization between thrombolytic agent and open control). The definitions or criteria for "clear" and "uncertain" indications for therapy were

left solely to the physician responsible for each case. For example, patients could be enrolled into either category with no electrocardiographic changes or with ST-segment depression, with hypertension, advanced age, or after more than 6 hours from symptom onset. This "simplified" enrollment strategy attracted participation from 914 hospitals and perhaps represents a "real life" approach to thrombolysis in myocardial infarction.

The 41,299 subjects initially reported on included those subjects who were to receive thrombolytic therapy whether for "clear" or "uncertain" indications. The mean randomization time was 4 hours. Several "minor" differences were noted among the agents' reported side effects: t-PA was associated with the least reports of allergic complications and hypotension, whereas SK was associated with the fewest noncerebral bleeds compared with the other two thrombolytic drugs. With respect to major clinical events in hospital, t-PA was associated with less reinfarctions but again more total strokes (t-PA 1.4%, SK 1.0%, APSAC 1.3%) as compared with SK. Despite these differences, there was no significant mortality difference among the randomized patients at 35 days (t-PA 10.3%, SK 10.6%, APSAC 10.5%). This finding was the same whether all patients were included or only the GISSI-2 equivalent patients (i.e., those entering within 6 hours from symptom onset with ST-segment elevation). These observations, therefore, reinforce those of the GISSI-2/International study; and combining the data, it can be seen that conventionally dosed t-PA was associated with 5 per 1000 fewer reinfarctions but 4 per 1000 more total strokes as compared with SK. The main results demonstrating equivalence of mortality reduction are summarized in Table 153–3.

GUSTO-1

The global utilization of streptokinase and tissue-type plasminogen activator for occluded vessels (GUSTO) trial[35] was designed to test new, aggressive thrombolytic strategies developed to reduce mortality by establishing early and sustained infarct artery patency. The GUSTO investigators reported their findings in 41,022 subjects randomized into four treatment arms: (1) accelerated, weight-adjusted alteplase t-PA with intravenous heparin; (2) combination t-PA (1 mg/kg in 60 minutes) plus 1 million U of streptokinase, administered simultaneously, with intravenous heparin; (3) streptokinase, 1.5 million U over 60 minutes with intravenous heparin; or (4) streptokinase, 1.5 million U over 60 minutes with high-dose subcutaneous heparin as used in the ISIS-3[37] trial. Subjects enrolled in this study had 20 minutes or more of chest pain, ST-segment elevation of 0.1 mV or more in two or more limb leads, or 0.2 mV or more in two or more contiguous precordial leads, and presented to a participating hospital within 6 hours of symptom onset. The diagnosis of acute myocardial infarction was confirmed in 97% or more of subjects.

The four groups were similar regarding clinical characteristics and baseline variables. The two streptokinase-only treatment groups were similar in major clinical outcomes—mortality and stroke—and can be referred to collectively. Considering the primary end point, mortality, the accelerated t-PA regimen reduced mortality 19% compared with streptokinase-only strategies at 24 hours. At the 30-day end point (Fig. 153–9), accelerated t-PA continued to reduce mortality more than streptokinase (10 additional lives saved per 1000, risk reduction of 14%) and the combination therapy (7 additional lives saved per 1000, risk reduction 10%). These findings are very important in that they represent the first reduction in mortality in a large-scale comparative thrombolytic trial since the addition of aspirin in ISIS-2.[21] The 1% absolute mortality reduction seen with accelerated t-PA (see Table 153–3, Fig. 153–9) should be viewed in light of its comparison to previously established, active thrombolytic regimens as opposed to placebo or control (inactive treatment). The 10 additional lives saved per 1000 represent an improvement of 40% beyond the

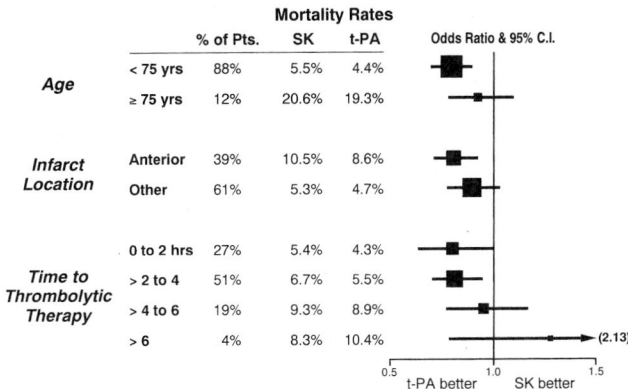

Figure 153–10. Subgroup analysis from GUSTO-1 comparing streptokinase-only strategies with accelerated t-PA. Advanced age and anterior infarction location had among the highest mortality rates, yet were benefited most by the aggressive strategy of accelerated t-PA. (Data from The GUSTO Angiographic Investigators: The comparative effects of tissue plasminogen activator, streptokinase, or both on coronary artery patency, ventricular function, and survival after acute myocardial infarction. N Engl J Med 329:1615, 1993.)

initial gain of thrombolytics over placebo (GISSI-1, ISIS-2, ASSET, ISAM, AIMS).

Considering total strokes, t-PA was associated with an excess of 2 strokes per 1000 treated patients and combination therapy with an excess of 3 per 1000 treated patients when compared with streptokinase strategies. However, when considering the combined end point—mortality or disabling stroke—accelerated t-PA demonstrated a more favorable outcome (12% risk reduction) compared with streptokinase strategies. Interestingly, subgroup analyses of the GUSTO study patients (Fig. 153–10) mirrored findings from previous trials showing that those with advanced age or anterior infarctions have among the highest mortality rates yet are benefited most by aggressive treatment strategies (in this study, accelerated t-PA). A consistent pattern of fewer complications was noted for the accelerated t-PA strategy, particularly regarding allergic reactions, ventricular dysfunction, and life-threatening arrhythmias. No differences were noted among the four strategies for recurrent ischemia or need for coronary revascularization.

Within the GUSTO trial, a 2431-patient substudy was incorporated that randomized subjects to coronary angiography at 90 minutes, 3 hours, 24 hours, or 5 to 7 days, including serial assessment of the early group patients.[71] For the first time within a large-scale mortality trial, the angiographic component allowed for tracking of early and sustained patency with mortality outcomes. Thus, the primary goal of the trial was to test the hypothesis that early and sustained infarct vessel patency is the key determinant of survival after thrombolytic therapy.

The early (90-minute) infarct artery patency rates observed in GUSTO-1 were in complete agreement and strongly confirmed pooled data from the 14 corresponding studies listed in Table 153–1. Specifically, accelerated t-PA was associated with the highest patency rate (81%) compared with SK alone (57%) and

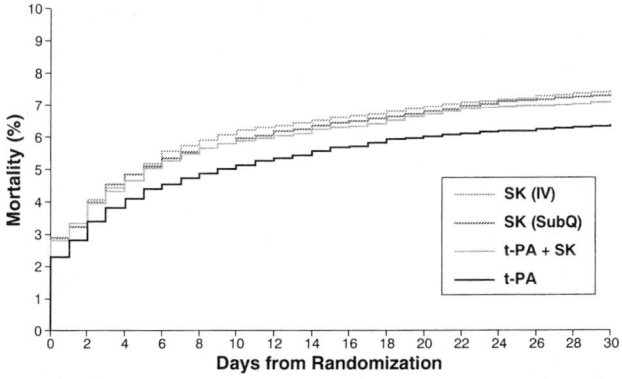

Figure 153–9. Percentage mortality associated with the four GUSTO treatment strategies. Accelerated t-PA was associated with lowest mortality throughout the study period, with an absolute reduction of 1% relative to the other established therapies. (Data from The GUSTO Investigators: An international randomized trial comparing four thrombolytic strategies for acute myocardial infarction. N Engl J Med 329:673, 1993.)

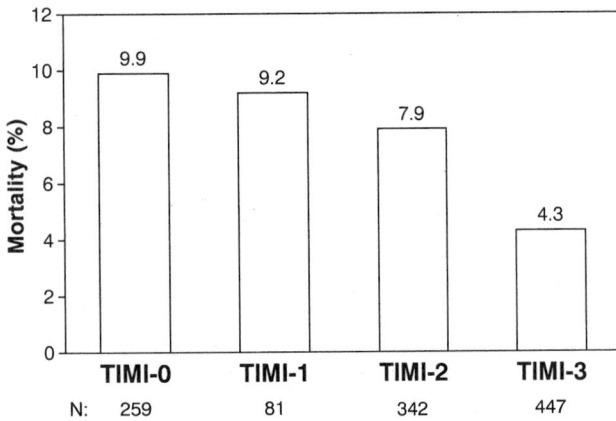

Figure 153–11. Relation of infarct artery patency/perfusion to mortality from the GUSTO angiographic substudy. Closed arteries (TIMI 0 or 1) were associated with higher mortality rates than open arteries (TIMI 2 or 3), and myocardium with partial reperfusion (TIMI 2) had a higher associated mortality rate compared with myocardium with complete reperfusion (TIMI 3). (Data from The GUSTO Angiographic Investigators: The comparative effects of tissue plasminogen activator, streptokinase, or both on coronary artery patency, ventricular function, and survival after acute myocardial infarction. N Engl J Med 329:1615, 1993.)

t-PA + SK (73%). As displayed in Table 153–4, the accelerated t-PA group had both the highest rate of patent vessels (TIMI 2 or 3) and complete reperfusion (TIMI 3) at 90 minutes, although equilibration among the groups occurred over the ensuing hours. Minor benefit in regional and global ventricular function was noted for those receiving accelerated t-PA. Further important insight was yielded from the GUSTO angiographic substudy when the 90-minute TIMI flow grade, independent of treatment assignment, was analyzed to assess its influence on 30-day mortality. Not surprisingly, closed infarct-related arteries (TIMI 0 or 1) had a higher mortality than open arteries (TIMI 2 or 3); however, a further reduction in mortality was demonstrated from TIMI 2 (partial reperfusion) to TIMI 3 (complete reperfusion) (Fig. 153–11). These observations highlight the importance of rapid, complete, and sustained reperfusion of the involved myocardium and reestablish the links among early patency, ventricular function, and survival.

SUMMARY AND FUTURE DIRECTION

Numerous studies have demonstrated that timely thrombolytic intervention restores antegrade coronary artery blood flow, limits myocardial necrosis, and improves short- and long-term survival. These striking benefits have firmly established the current "thrombolytic era." Although differences exist among currently available thrombolytic agents, our sole focus should not be to identify the best agent, but rather to find the best strategy to ensure that the maximum percentage of candidates receives timely therapy and achieves rapid, complete myocardial reperfusion. Although conventional use of thrombolytic agents does reduce periinfarction mortality by approximately 25% to 30%, added benefit from more aggressive regimens,

such as seen in GUSTO-1, show us we must not become complacent toward further clinical investigations of better therapeutic approaches. Indeed, we have entered an era of "enhanced reperfusion." In the future, addition of potent antithrombotic adjunctive therapies (e.g., antiplatelet agents and antithrombins) currently under intense investigation promises to further enhance current strategies. By further systematic improvement in achieving very early, complete, and sustained myocardial reperfusion in the future, we will undoubtedly further improve the prognosis of patients with acute myocardial infarction.

REFERENCES

1. Davies MJ, Woolf N, Robertson WB: Pathology of acute myocardial infarction with particular reference to occlusive coronary thrombi. Br Heart J 38:659, 1976.
2. Silver MD, Baroldi G, Mariani F: The relationship between acute occlusive coronary thrombi and myocardial infarction studied in 100 consecutive patients. Circulation 61:219, 1980.
3. Buja LM, Willerson JT: Clinicopathologic correlates of acute ischemic heart disease syndromes. Am J Cardiol 47:343, 1981.
4. Cowley MJ, Hastillo A, Vetrovec GW, et al: Effects of intracoronary streptokinase in acute myocardial infarction. Am Heart J 102:1149, 1981.
5. DeWood MA, Spores J, Notske R, et al: Prevalence of total coronary occlusion during the early hours of transmural myocardial infarction. N Engl J Med 303:897, 1980.
6. Bertrand ME, Lefebvre JM, Laisne CL, et al: Coronary arteriography in acute transmural myocardial infarction. Am Heart J 97:61, 1979.
7. Weaver WD, Cerqueira M, Hallstrom AP, et al: Prehospital-initiated vs hospital-initiated thrombolytic therapy. The Myocardial Infarction Triage and Intervention Trial. JAMA 270:1211, 1993.
8. Simoons ML, Serryts PW, van den Brand M, et al: Early thrombolysis in acute myocardial infarction: Limitation of infarct size and improved survival. J Am Coll Cardiol 7:717, 1986.
9. Topol EJ, Califf RM, Vandormael M, et al: A randomized trial of late reperfusion therapy for acute myocardial infarction. Circulation 85:2090, 1992.
10. Guerci AD, Gerstenblith G, Brinker JA, et al: A randomized trial of intravenous tissue plasminogen activator for acute myocardial infarction with subsequent randomization to elective coronary angioplasty. N Engl J Med 317:1613, 1987.
11. Armstrong PW, Baigrie RS, Daly PA, et al: Tissue plasminogen activator: Toronto (TPAT) placebo-controlled randomized trial in acute myocardial infarction. J Am Coll Cardiol 13:1469, 1989.
12. Bassand JP, Machecourt J, Cassagnes J, et al: Multicenter trial of intravenous anisoylated plasminogen streptokinase activator complex (APSAC) in acute myocardial infarction: Effects on infarct size and left ventricular function. J Am Coll Cardiol 13:988, 1989.
13. National Heart Foundation of Australia Coronary Thrombolysis Group: Coronary thrombolysis and myocardial salvage by tissue plasminogen activator given up to 4 hours after onset of myocardial infarction. Lancet 1:203, 1988.
14. Kennedy JW, Martin GV, Davis KB, et al: The Western Washington intravenous streptokinase in acute myocardial infarction randomized trial. Circulation 77:345, 1988.
15. Van de Werf F, Arnold AE: Intravenous tissue plasminogen activator and size of infarct, left ventricular function, and survival in acute myocardial infarction (ECSG-4). Br Med J 297:1374, 1988.
16. White HD, Norris RM, Brown MA, et al: Effect of intravenous streptokinase on left ventricular function and early survival after acute myocardial infarction. N Engl J Med 317:850, 1987.
17. O'Rourke M, Baron D, Keogh A, et al: Limitation of myocardial infarction by early infusion of recombinant tissue-type plasminogen activator. Circulation 77:1311, 1988.

18. Bassand JP, Faivre R, Becque O, et al: Effects of early high-dose streptokinase intravenously on left ventricular function in acute myocardial infarction. Am J Cardiol 60:435, 1987.

19. Verstraete M, Brower RW, Collen D, et al: Double-blind randomized trial of intravenous tissue-type plasminogen activator versus placebo in acute myocardial infarction (ECSG-1). Lancet 2:965, 1985.

20. Gruppo Italiano per lo Studio della Sopravvivenza nell'Infarto Miocardico (GISSI): Effectiveness of intravenous thrombolytic treatment in acute myocardial infarction. Lancet 1:397, 1986.

21. ISIS-2 (Second International Study of Infarct Survival) Collaborative Group: Randomized trial of intravenous streptokinase, oral aspirin, both, or neither among 17,187 cases of suspected acute myocardial infarction; ISIS-2. Lancet 2:349, 1988.

22. AIMS Trial Study Group: Effect of intravenous APSAC on mortality after acute myocardial infarction: Preliminary report of a placebo-controlled clinical trial. Lancet 1:842, 1988.

23. Wilcox RG, von der Lippe G, Olsson CG, et al: Trial of tissue plasminogen activator for mortality reduction in acute myocardial infarction. Lancet 2:525, 1988.

24. ISAM Study Group: A prospective trial of intravenous streptokinase in acute myocardial infarction (ISAM). Mortality, morbidity and infarct size at 21 days. N Engl J Med 314:1465, 1986.

25. Collen D, Stassen JM, Stump DC, et al: Synergism of thrombolytic agents in vivo. Circulation 74:838, 1986.

26. Collen D, Stump DC, Van de Werf F: Coronary thrombolysis in patients with acute myocardial infarction by intravenous infusion of synergic thrombolytic agents. Am Heart J 58:1083, 1986.

27. Topol EJ, Califf RM, George BS, et al: Coronary arterial thrombolysis with combined infusion of recombinant tissue-type plasminogen activator and urokinase in patients with acute myocardial infarction (TAMI-2). Circulation 77:1100, 1988.

28. Urokinase and Alteplase in Myocardial Infarction Collaborative Group (URALMI): Combination of urokinase and alteplase in the treatment of myocardial infarction. Coron Artery Dis 2:225, 1991.

29. Kirshenbaum JM, Bahr RD, Flaherty JT, et al: Clot-selective coronary thrombolysis with low-dose synergistic combinations of single-chain urokinase-type plasminogen activator and recombinant tissue-type plasminogen activator. Am J Cardiol 68:1564, 1991.

30. Granger CB, Kalbfleisch J, Califf R, et al: The Global Utilization of Streptokinase and Tissue Plasminogen Activator for Occluded Coronary Arteries (GUSTO) pilot study: Combined streptokinase and t-PA [abstract]. Circulation 84(Suppl II):II-573, 1991.

31. Grines CL, Nissen SE, Booth DC, et al: A new thrombolytic regimen for acute myocardial infarction using combination half dose tissue-type plasminogen activator with full dose streptokinase: A pilot study. J Am Coll Cardiol 14:573, 1989.

32. Grines CL, Nissen SE, Booth DC, et al: A prospective, randomized trial comparing combination half-dose tissue-type plasminogen activator and streptokinase with full-dose tissue-type plasminogen activator. Circulation 84:540, 1991.

33. Bonnet JL, Bory M, D'Houdain F, et al: Association of tissue plasminogen activator and streptokinase in acute myocardial infarction: Preliminary data [abstract]. Circulation 80(Suppl II):II-343, 1989.

34. Califf RM, Topol EJ, Stack RS, et al: Evaluation of combination thrombolytic therapy and timing of cardiac catheterization in acute myocardial infarction: Results of thrombolysis and angioplasty in myocardial infarction—Phase 5 randomized trial. Circulation 83:1543, 1991.

35. The GUSTO Investigators: An international randomized trial comparing four thrombolytic strategies for acute myocardial infarction. N Engl J Med 329:673, 1993.

36. Fibrinolytic Therapy Trialists' (FTT) Collaborative Group: Indications for fibrinolytic therapy in suspected acute myocardial infarction: Collaborative overview of mortality and major morbidity results from all randomized trials of more than 1,000 patients. Lancet 343:311, 1994.

37. ISIS-3 (Third International Study of Infarct Survival) Collaborative Group: ISIS-3. A randomized comparison of streptokinase vs tissue plasminogen activator vs anistreplase and of aspirin plus heparin vs aspirin alone among 41,299 cases of suspected acute myocardial infarction. Lancet 339:753, 1992.

38. Califf RM, Topol EJ, Stump D, et al: Hemorrhagic complications associated with the use of intravenous tissue plasminogen activator in treatment of acute myocardial infarction. Am J Med 85:353, 1988.

39. Rossi P, Bolognese L, on behalf of Urochinasi per via Sistemica nell'Infarto Miocardico (USIM) Collaborate Group: Comparison of intravenous urokinase plus heparin versus heparin alone in acute myocardial infarction. Am J Cardiol 68:585, 1991.

40. Wilcox RG, for the LATE Steering Committee: Late assessment of thrombolytic efficacy with alteplase 6–24 hours after onset of acute myocardial infarction. Lancet 342:759, 1993.

41. Hsia J, Hamilton WP, Kleiman N, et al: A comparison between heparin and low-dose aspirin as adjunctive therapy with tissue plasminogen activator for acute myocardial infarction. N Engl J Med 323:1433, 1990.

42. The International Study Group: In-hospital mortality and clinical course of 20,891 patients with suspected acute myocardial infarction randomized between alteplase and streptokinase with or without heparin. Lancet 336:71, 1990.

43. Bates ER, Topol EJ: Limitations of thrombolytic therapy for acute myocardial infarction complicated by congestive heart failure and cardiogenic shock. J Am Coll Cardiol 18:1077, 1991.

44. Prewitt RM, Downes AMT, Gu S, et al: Effects of hydralazine and increased cardiac output on recombinant tissue plasminogen activator-induced thrombolysis in canine pulmonary embolism. Chest 99:708, 1991.

45. Gacioch GM, Ellis SG, Lee L, et al: Cardiogenic shock complicating acute myocardial infarction: The use of coronary angioplasty and the integration of the new support devices into patient management. J Am Coll Cardiol 19:647, 1992.

46. Muller DW, Topol EJ: Selection of patients with acute myocardial infarction for thrombolytic therapy. Ann Intern Med 113:949, 1990.

47. Cragg DR, Friedman HZ, Bonema JD, et al: Outcome of patients with acute myocardial infarction who are ineligible for thrombolytic therapy. Ann Intern Med 115:173, 1991.

48. Lee TH, Weisberg MC, Brand DA, et al: Candidates for thrombolysis among emergency room patients with acute chest pain. Potential true- and false-positive rates. Ann Intern Med 119:957, 1989.

49. Eisenberg MS, Ho MT, Schaeffer S, et al: A community survey of the potential use of thrombolytic agents for acute myocardial infarction. Ann Emerg Med 18:838, 1989.

50. Murray N, Lyons J, Layton C, et al: What proportion of patients with myocardial infarction are suitable for thrombolysis? Br Heart J 57:144, 1987.

51. Doorey AJ, Michelson EL, Weber FJ, Dreifus LS: Thrombolytic therapy of acute myocardial infarction: Emerging challenges of implementation. J Am Coll Cardiol 10:1357, 1987.

52. Jagger JD, Davies MK, Murray RG, et al: Eligibility for thrombolytic therapy in acute myocardial infarction. Lancet 1:34, 1987.

53. Tenaglia AN, Califf R, Candela RJ, et al: Thrombolytic therapy in patients requiring cardiopulmonary resuscitation. Am J Cardiol 68:1015, 1991.

54. DeJaegere PP, Arnold AA, Balk AH, et al: Intracranial hemorrhage in association with thrombolytic therapy: Incidence and clinical predictive factors. J Am Coll Cardiol 19:289, 1992.

55. Chesebro HJ, Knatterud G, Roberts R, et al: Thrombolysis in Myocardial Infarction (TIMI) Trial, Phase I: A comparison between intravenous tissue plasminogen activator and intravenous streptokinase. Circulation 76:142, 1987.

56. Timmis AD, Griffin B, Crick J, et al: Anisoylated plasminogen streptokinase activator complex in acute myocardial infarction: A placebo-controlled arteriographic coronary recanalization study. J Am Coll Cardiol 10:205, 1987.

57. Collen D, Topol EJ, Tiefenbrunn AJ, et al: Coronary thrombolysis with recombinant human tissue-type plasminogen activator: A prospective, randomized, placebo-controlled trial. Circulation 70:1012, 1984.

58. Ohman EM, Califf RM, Topol EJ, et al: Consequences of reocclusion following successful reperfusion therapy in acute myocardial infarction. Circulation 82:781, 1990.

59. The Multicenter Postinfarction Research Group: Risk stratification and survival after myocardial infarction. N Engl J Med 309:331, 1983.

60. Schröder R, Neuhaus KL, Linderer T, et al: Impact of late coronary artery reperfusion on left ventricular function one month after acute myocardial infarction (Results of the ISAM study). Am J Cardiol 64:878, 1989.

61. Granger CB, Califf RM, Topol EJ: Thrombolytic therapy for acute myocardial infarction. A review. Drugs 44:293, 1992.

62. Kasper W, Meinertz T, Wollschläger H, et al: Coronary thrombolysis during acute myocardial infarction by intravenous BRL 26921, a new anisoylated plasminogen-streptokinase activator complex. Am J Cardiol 58:418, 1986.

63. Califf RM, Harrelson-Woodlief L, Topol EJ: Left ventricular ejection fraction may not be useful as an endpoint for thrombolytic therapy comparative trials. Circulation 82:1847, 1990.

64. Sheehan FH, Braunwald E, Canner P, et al: The effect of intravenous thrombolytic therapy on left ventricular function: A report on tissue-type plasminogen activator and streptokinase from the Thrombolysis in Myocardial Infarction (TIMI phase I) Trial. Circulation 75:817, 1987.

65. Morgan CD, Roberts RS, Haq A, et al: Coronary patency, infarct size and left ventricular function after thrombolytic therapy for acute myocardial infarction: Results from the tissue-plasminogen activator: Toronto (TPAT) Placebo-controlled Trial. J Am Coll Cardiol 17:451, 1991.

66. Harrison JK, Califf RM, Woodlief LH, et al: Systolic left ventricular function after reperfusion therapy for acute myocardial infarction. Analysis of determinants of improvement. The TAMI Study Group. Circulation 87:1531, 1993.

67. Cigarroa RG, Lange RA, Hillis LD: Prognosis after acute myocardial infarction in patients with and without residual anterograde coronary blood flow. Am J Cardiol 64:155, 1989.

68. Lange RA, Cigarroa RG, Hillis LD: Influence of residual antegrade coronary blood flow on survival after myocardial infarction in patients with multivessel coronary artery disease. Coron Artery Dis 1:59, 1990.

69. Trappe HJ, Lichtlen PR, Klein H, et al: Natural history of single vessel disease. Risk of sudden coronary death in relation to coronary anatomy and arrhythmia profile. Eur Heart J 10:514, 1989.

70. Gruppo Italiano per lo Studio della Sopravvivenza nell'Infarto Miocardico: GISSI-2. A factorial randomized trial of alteplase versus streptokinase and heparin versus no heparin among 14,490 patients with acute myocardial infarction. Lancet 336:65, 1990.

71. The GUSTO Angiographic Investigators: The comparative effects of tissue plasminogen activator, streptokinase, or both on coronary artery patency, ventricular function, and survival after acute myocardial infarction. N Engl J Med 329:1615, 1993.

72. Charbonnier B, Cribier A, Monassier JP, et al: Etude eurpeenne multicentrique et randomisee de l'APSAC versus streptokinase dans l'infarctus du myocarde. Arch Mal Coeur 82:1565, 1989.

73. Verstraete M, Bory M, Collen D, et al: Randomized trial of intravenous recombinant tissue-type plasminogen activator versus intravenous streptokinase in acute myocardial infarction (ECSG-2). Lancet 1:842, 1985.

74. Hogg KJ, Gemmill JD, Burns JM, et al: Angiographic patency study of anistreplase versus streptokinase in acute myocardial infarction. Lancet 335:254, 1990.

75. Lopez-Sendon J, Searbra-Gomes R, Macaya C, et al: Intravenous anisoylated plasminogen streptokinase activator complex versus intravenous streptokinase in myocardial infarction. A randomized multicenter study [abstract]. Circulation 78(Suppl II):277, 1988.

76. PRIMI Trial Study Group: Randomized double-blind trial of recombinant prourokinase against streptokinase in acute myocardial infarction. Lancet 1:863, 1989.

77. Stack RS, O'Connor CM, Mark DB, et al: Coronary perfusion during acute myocardial infarction with a combined therapy of coronary angioplasty and high-dose intravenous streptokinase. Circulation 77:151, 1988.

78. Whitlow PL, Bashore TM: Catheterization/Rescue Angioplasty Following Thrombolysis (CRAFT) Study: Acute myocardial infarction treated with recombinant tissue plasminogen activator versus urokinase [abstract]. J Am Coll Cardiol 17(Suppl):276A, 1991.

79. Neuhaus KL, Tebbe U, Gottwik M, et al: Intravenous recombinant tissue plasminogen activator (rt-PA) and urokinase in acute myocardial infarction: Results of the German Activator Urokinase Study (GAUS). J Am Coll Cardiol 12:581, 1988.

80. Mathey DG, Schofer J, Sheehan FH, et al: Intravenous urokinase in acute myocardial infarction. Am J Cardiol 55:878, 1985.

81. Relik-van Wely L, Visser RF, van der Pol J, et al: Angiographically assessed coronary arterial patency and reocclusion in patients with acute myocardial infarction treated with anistreplase: Results of the Anistreplase Reocclusion Multicenter Study (ARMS). Am J Cardiol 68:296, 1991.

82. Neuhaus KL, Von Essen R, Tebbe U, et al: Improved thrombolysis in acute myocardial infarction with front-loaded administration of alteplase: Results of the rt-PA-APSAC Patency Study (TAPS). J Am Coll Cardiol 19:885, 1992.

83. Johns JA, Gold HK, Leinbach RC, et al: Prevention of coronary artery reocclusion and reduction in late coronary artery stenosis after thrombolytic therapy in patients with acute myocardial infarction. Circulation 78:546, 1988.

84. Carney RJ, Murphy GA, Brandt TR, et al: Randomized angiographic trial of recombinant tissue-type plasminogen activator (alteplase) in myocardial infarction. J Am Coll Cardiol 20:17, 1992.

85. Smalling RW, Schumacher R, Morris D, et al: Improved infarct-related arterial patency after high dose, weight-adjusted, rapid infusion of tissue-type plasminogen activator in myocardial infarction: Results of multicenter randomized trial of two dosage regimens. J Am Coll Cardiol 15:915, 1990.

86. Topol EJ, George GS, Kereiakes DJ, et al: A randomized controlled trial of intravenous tissue plasminogen activator and early intravenous heparin in acute myocardial infarction (TAMI-3). Circulation 79:281, 1989.

87. Topol EJ, Ellis SG, Califf RM, et al: Combined tissue-type plasminogen activator and prostacyclin therapy for acute myocardial infarction. J Am Coll Cardiol 14:877, 1989.

88. TIMI Research Group: Immediate vs. delayed catheterization and angioplasty following thrombolytic therapy for acute myocardial infarction. TIMI II A results. JAMA 260:2849, 1988.

89. Topol EJ, Morris DC, Smalling RW, et al: A multicenter, randomized, placebo-controlled trial of a new form of intravenous recombinant tissue-type plasminogen activator (Activase) in acute myocardial infarction. J Am Coll Cardiol 9:1205, 1987.

90. Topol EJ, Bates ER, Walton JA, et al: Community hospital administration of intravenous tissue plasminogen activator in acute myocardial infarction: Improved timing, thrombolytic efficacy and ventricular function. J Am Coll Cardiol 10:1173, 1987.

91. Gemmill JD, Hogg KJ, MacIntyre PD, et al: A pilot study of the efficacy and safety of bolus administration of alteplase in acute myocardial infarction. Br Heart J 66:134, 1991.

92. Neuhaus KL, Feuerer W, Jeep-Tebbe S, et al: Improved thrombolysis with a modified dose regimen of recombinant tissue-type plasminogen activator. J Am Coll Cardiol 14:1566, 1989.

93. Wall TC, Califf RM, George BS, et al: Accelerated plasminogen activator dose regimens for coronary thrombolysis. J Am Coll Cardiol 19:482, 1992.

94. EMERAS (Estudio Multicéntrico Estreptoquinasa Repúblicas de America del Sur) Collaborative Group: Randomized trial of late thrombolysis in patients with suspected myocardial infarction. Lancet 342:767, 1993.

95. The European Myocardial Infarction Project Group: Pre-hospital thrombolytic therapy in patients with suspected acute myocardial infarction. N Engl J Med 329:383, 1993.

B. Platelet Inhibitors

CHAPTER 154

Acetylsalicylic Acid

Carlo Patrono, M.D.

Acetylsalicylic acid (ASA) is a salicylate ester of acetic acid in which the carboxyl group of salicylic acid is retained and substitution is made in the OH group. This compound, synthesized by Hoffman at Bayer AG, was introduced into medicine in 1899 under the name aspirin.

ASA has a wide spectrum of pharmacologic effects that are dependent on a number of variables, including dosage. Thus, while an antiplatelet effect has been demonstrated with doses as low as 0.5 to 1 mg/kg, the analgesic and antipyretic effects require at least 5 to 10 mg/kg, and an antiinflammatory effect can be appreciated only at daily dosages greater than 30 mg/kg and may require 80 to 100 mg/kg.[1] Similarly, relatively rare uses of the drug have been described, such as the treatment of Bartter's syndrome or closure of a patent ductus arteriosus in neonates, with dosages as high as 80 to 100 mg/kg.[1] Except for the latter, all therapeutic uses of ASA were introduced before the fundamental discovery of Vane and his associates of its mechanism of action in 1971.[2] As a consequence, use of ASA as an analgesic, antipyretic, antirheumatic, or antithrombotic drug was largely based on empirical observations and was adjusted by a process of trial and error.

Although it has long been known that platelet function can be inhibited by oral doses of ASA 10 to 50 times lower than those required to obtain other pharmacologic effects,[3] this fact has been regarded more as a scientific curiosity than as a guideline for its use as an antiplatelet agent.

MECHANISM OF ACTION

ASA induces a long-lasting functional defect in platelets, detectable clinically as prolongation of the bleeding time. This appears to be primarily, if not exclusively, related to permanent inactivation by ASA of a key enzyme in platelet arachidonate metabolism. This enzyme is known as prostaglandin (PG) H synthase and is responsible for the generation of PGH_2, the precursor of thromboxane (TX) A_2.[4] In human platelets, TXA_2 provides a mechanism for amplifying the activation signal, by virtue of its being synthesized and released in response to a variety of platelet activators (e.g., collagen, adenosine diphosphate, platelet activating factor, and thrombin) and in turn inducing irreversible aggregation.[5]

ASA selectively acetylates the hydroxyl group of a single serine residue at position 529 (Ser529) within the polypeptide chain of platelet PGH synthase.[6, 7] This enzyme exhibits two distinct catalytic activities, a bis-oxygenase (cyclooxygenase) involved in PGG_2 formation and a hydroperoxidase, allowing a net two-electron reduction of the 15-hydro-peroxyl group of PGG_2 to yield PGH_2.[8] As a consequence of O-acetylation of Ser529 by ASA, the cyclooxygenase activity is permanently lost, while the hydroperoxidase activity is unaffected (Fig. 154–1). Recently, an inducible form of PGH-synthase has been identified.[9] ASA modifies the cyclooxygenase activity of the inducible enzyme, though less efficiently than in the constitutive enzyme.[10] The relevance of acetylation of PGH_2 to the pharmacologic effects of ASA remains to be investigated.

Reduced formation of various eicosanoids (that is, TXA_2 as well as PGE_2 and PGI_2) in different tissues can probably account for the variety of pharmacologic effects of ASA that form the basis for both its therapeutic use and its toxicity.[2] Because inactivation of PGH synthase by ASA is irreversible, *de novo* synthesis of the enzyme is required to restore normal eicosanoid formation. This occurs within hours in nucleated cells but cannot adequately take place in platelets, which derive from fragmentation of the megakaryocyte cytoplasm and can only synthesize small amounts of protein. Thus, the duration of platelet and extra-platelet effects of a single dose of the drug varies considerably, ranging from several days to a few hours, respectively.[11]

Alternative explanations have been considered to explain the protective effect of ASA against vascular thrombotic events.[12–14] Thus, ASA can acetylate other proteins, including the lysine residues of fibrinogen, although at higher concentrations and over longer time periods than required for acetylation of PGH synthase. N-Acetylated fibrinogen facilitates plasminogen activation and is much less effective in supporting platelet aggregation than unmodified fibrinogen.[14] However, both the dose-response relationship and the consequent clinical relevance of these additional effects of the drug remain to be established.

PHARMACOKINETICS

The pharmacokinetics of ASA have been reviewed by Pedersen and FitzGerald.[15] Orally ingested ASA is absorbed rapidly, partly from the stomach but mostly from the upper small intestine. This occurs primarily by passive diffusion of the nondissociated lipid-soluble ASA across gastrointestinal membranes. ASA is also hydrolyzed by gastric and jejunal esterases and is therefore absorbed in part as salicylate. Such a presystemic metabolism contributes to a variable sys-

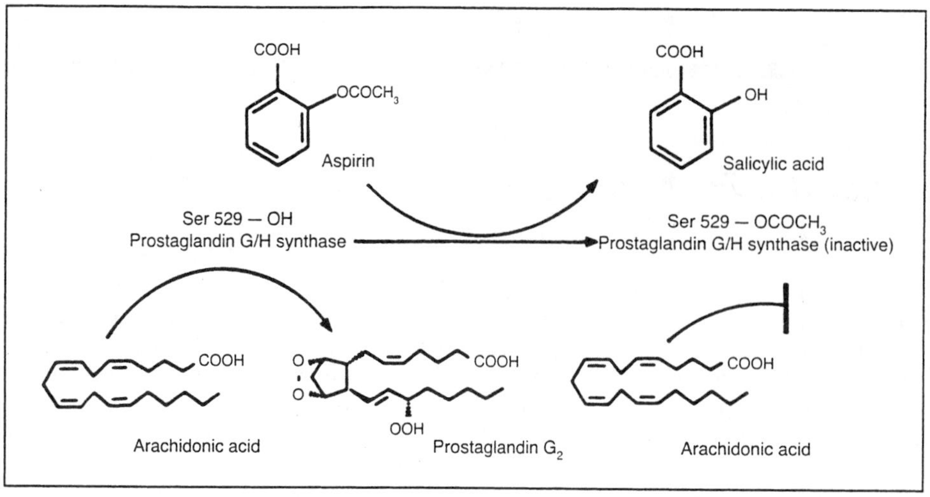

Figure 154–1. Acetylation by aspirin of the hydroxyl group of a serine residue at position 529 (Ser529) in the polypeptide chain of human platelet prostaglandin (PG) G/H-synthase, and the resulting inactivation of cyclooxygenase catalytic activity. Blockade by aspirin of PGG_2 formation will result in suppression of PGH_2 and thromboxane A_2 biosynthesis. (Reprinted by permission from Patrono C: Aspirin as an antiplatelet drug. N Engl J Med 330:1287, 1994. Copyright 1994, Massachusetts Medical Society.)

temic bioavailability as a function of fluid and food ingestion. Systemic bioavailability of regular ASA tablets is on the order of 40% to 50% in a range of doses from 20 to 1300 mg.[16] A considerably lower bioavailability has been reported for enteric-coated tablets and sustained-release microencapsulated preparations.[15] Thus, different pharmaceutical formulations may deliver little or no measurable ASA to the systemic circulation.

The absorbed ester is rapidly hydrolyzed to salicylate in plasma, the liver, the lungs, and erythrocytes. The plasma half-life of ASA is approximately 15 minutes; the half-life for salicylate is dose dependent and ranges between 2 and 12 hours. Hydrolysis of the ester is associated with transfer of the acetyl group to a number of proteins that are covalently acetylated. These include human plasma albumin, hormones, enzymes (e.g., PGH synthases), hemoglobin, and several proteins present in cell membranes.[1, 15]

With the notable exception of PGH synthase, the functional correlate of these acetylation processes is largely unknown. The extent to which proteins other than PGH synthase are acetylated by ASA probably varies with dosage and systemic bioavailability of the intact drug. As discussed earlier, the contribution of these processes to the antithrombotic effect of ASA is entirely speculative.

Salicylate is further metabolized to salicyluric acid (the glycine conjugate), to the ether or phenolic glucuronide, and to the ester or acyl glucuronide. In addition, a small fraction is oxidized to 2,3-dihydroxybenzoic, 2,5-dihydroxybenzoic acid (gentisic acid) and 2,3,5-trihydroxybenzoic acid. With the possible exception of gentisic acid, no pharmacologic effects have been ascribed to these metabolites.

Salicylates are excreted mainly by the kidneys. The pharmacokinetics of ASA has been approximated by an open, two-compartment model with first-order absorption and elimination and metabolism from the central compartment.[17]

PHARMACODYNAMICS

Methods for assessment *ex vivo* or *in vivo* of pharmacologic inhibition of platelet cyclooxygenase activity are now readily available.[18] The vast majority of studies assessing ASA pharmacodynamics in humans have relied on measurements of serum TXB_2 as a reflection of thrombin-induced platelet TXA_2 production during whole blood clotting.[19] This method evaluates the capacity of platelets to synthesize TXB_2 in response to virtually maximal stimulation and by no means reflects the actual production rate of TXB_2 *in vivo*, which is several orders of magnitude lower.[20] When given orally to healthy subjects, ASA inhibits TXA_2 production and TXA_2-dependent platelet function in a dose- and time-dependent fashion.[21, 22] A linear inhibition of platelet cyclooxygenase activity is found after single doses in the range of 10 to 100 mg.[21] Moreover, such a dose-response relationship is similar in healthy subjects and in patients with atherosclerosis[23] when assessed by the same technique of determination of TXB_2 production *ex vivo* in whole blood. No sex-related difference in the platelet effect of ASA has been described. Following oral administration, serum TXB_2 levels are significantly reduced as early as 5 minutes after dosing. Inasmuch as no ASA can be detected in peripheral venous blood at this time, acetylation of cyclooxygenase during the first 5 minutes may occur by exposure of platelets to the drug in the presystemic circulation.[16] Serum TXB_2 concentrations are maximally suppressed at between 30 and 60 minutes after ASA and remain stable thereafter up to 24 hours, reflecting irreversible enzyme inactivation. Evidence has been presented that the recovery of unacetylated platelet PGH synthase and of cyclooxygenase activity after a single dose of ASA (100 mg) does not occur for approximately 48 hours.[19, 24]

The 2-day lag in the return of functioning enzyme to the circulation has been interpreted as evidence that ASA acetylates PGH synthase in the megakaryocyte. At variance with these biochemical findings, platelet aggregation and secretion occur as early as 4 hours after ingestion of ASA (650 mg) in response to a combination of arachidonate with epinephrine, collagen, or ADP.[25] This finding may suggest the early entry into the circulation of platelets originating from megakaryocytes in which PGH synthase has not been completely acetylated. However, the clinical observation that the antithrombotic effect of 300 to 325 mg ASA given every 24 hours is not appreciably different from that of the same dose given b.i.d., t.i.d., or q.i.d. (see later) would contradict the biologic relevance of *in vitro* platelet aggregation studies using pairs of aggregating agents to maximize platelet response.

Because of irreversible enzyme inactivation and lack of *de novo* enzyme synthesis in platelets, acetylation of platelet PGH synthase and consequent inhibition of TXA_2 production by low-dose ASA is cumulative on repeated dosing.[21, 24] As shown in Figure 154–2, a log-linear relationship exists between the oral ASA dose and the percentage of inhibition of platelet TXB_2 production after both single and repeated daily dosing. However, based on steady-state measurements performed during repeated daily dosing, the dose-response curve is shifted to the left when compared with single dosing by a factor of 8 (ID_{50}: 3.2 and 26 mg, respectively) (see Fig. 154–2).[18]

This finding in healthy subjects suggests that the fractional dose of ASA necessary for achieving a given level of acetylation by virtue of cumulative effects approximately equals the fractional daily platelet turnover (i.e., 10% to 15%).[18] Thus, for a given dose of the drug, both the rate at which cumulative acetylation occurs and its maximal extent would depend essentially on the rate of platelet turnover and the dosing interval.

Regarding inhibition of TXA_2-dependent platelet function, daily administration of 50 mg to patients with coronary artery disease is associated with time-dependent biochemical and functional changes that are indistinguishable from those achieved with 324 mg daily.[26] This observation implies not that the clinical effects to be expected from the former are identical to those achieved with the latter (see later) but that the measurable *ex vivo* and *in vivo* platelet effects of a standard dose of ASA can be fully reproduced by a dose of the drug suppressing platelet cyclooxygenase activity by more than 95%. The only difference is related to the different rate at which such maximal effect is achieved, that is, virtually instantaneously versus several days. Such a potential disadvantage of low-dose ASA can be overcome by a loading dose (e.g., 120 mg) followed by a daily maintenance dose (e.g., 30 to 50 mg).[18]

Much of the interest in establishing the lowest fully effective antiplatelet regimen of the drug derived from the appreciation in the late 1970s that eicosanoids synthesized via the same cyclooxygenase pathway in other cell types might participate in the homeostatic maintenance of important bodily functions. Thus, PGI_2, a vasodilator and antiaggregatory eicosanoid produced by the vascular endothelium and smooth muscle cells, by the gastric mucosa, and by kidney glomeruli, was shown to contribute to platelet–vessel wall homeostasis, gastric cytoprotection, and modulation of glomerular hemodynamics.[1, 11, 27]

Chronic inhibition of cyclooxygenase activity in these tissues might be expected to increase thrombogenicity of the vessel wall, to disrupt the integrity of the gastric mucosa, and to impair renal function. While evidence for the first event is difficult to obtain in humans because of the concomitant antiplatelet effect of the drug, the pattern of side effects associated with long-term administration of high doses of ASA is consistent with the other two expectations, that is, gastric and renal toxicity.

The mechanism of action of ASA and the markedly different renewal rate of PGH synthase in platelets (as a function of platelet turnover) *vis-à-vis* other cell types (as a function of *de novo* enzyme synthesis), theoretically allow us to dissociate the desired antiplatelet effect from the unwanted vascular, gastric, and renal effects. In fact, evidence derived from large-scale clinical trials, as reviewed in detail later, indicates that the incidence of side effects is dose related in the range of doses tested so far (i.e., 30 to 1500 mg) with no apparent difference in antithrombotic efficacy.[28]

This clinical observation is consistent with the demonstration that a single daily administration of 300 to 325 mg will inhibit extra-platelet cyclooxygenase activity substantially less (i.e., only for 4 to 6 hours after administration) than a b.i.d., t.i.d., or q.i.d. regimen. This does not appear to be the case for vascular cyclooxygenase activity, which is equally and profoundly suppressed in the dose range of 300 to 1300 mg.[22] In fact, it has been difficult to demonstrate clearcut separation of platelet and vascular effects of ASA, and different investigators have obtained somewhat different results depending on the particular approach used to monitor PGI_2 production *in vivo* or *ex vivo*.[11] Only studies relying on measurement of urinary derivatives of PGI_2 (i.e., 6-keto-$PGF_{1\alpha}$ and 2,3-dinor-6-keto-$PGF_{1\alpha}$) have indicated a substantial sparing (i.e., no statistically significant changes) of vascular PGI_2 production during daily administration of 20 to 40 mg.[21, 22] The mechanism or mechanisms by

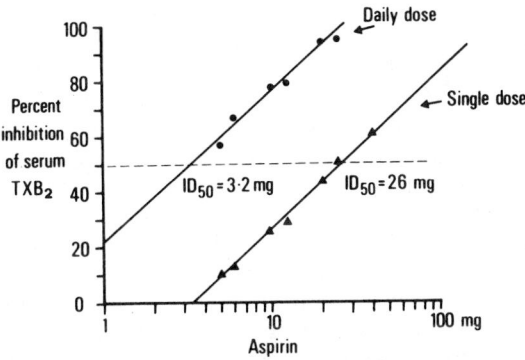

Figure 154–2. Dose dependence of the inhibition of platelet thromboxane B_2 (TXB_2) production by aspirin. Serum TXB_2 was measured before and after single (Δ) or daily ($\cdot$) administration of aspirin (5 to 40 mg) in four healthy subjects. Individual data are expressed as a percentage of inhibition, with each subject serving as his or her own control. Daily dosing values represent measurements obtained at steady-state inhibition. ID_{50}, 50% inhibitory dose. (Reproduced with permission from Patrono C, Ciabattoni G, Patrignani P, et al: Clinical pharmacology of platelet cyclooxygenase inhibition. Circulation 72:1177, 1985. Copyright 1985, American Heart Association, Inc.)

which biochemical selectivity might be related to dose are unclear. Both a differential "sensitivity" of the platelet and endothelial PGH synthase to ASA and presystemic acetylation of the platelet enzyme (as discussed earlier) might contribute to this effect.[11, 15]

ACETYLSALICYLIC ACID AND THE SECONDARY PREVENTION OF VASCULAR OCCLUSIVE DISEASE

The results of randomized clinical trials of ASA and other antiplatelet drugs in the prevention of cardiovascular and cerebrovascular disease have been extensively reviewed recently.[28-30] Besides considering individual studies, of greatest interest for assessing the value of antiplatelet therapy is the recently completed second overview of the Antiplatelet Trialists' Collaboration.[31-33]

The Research Group on Instability in Coronary Artery Disease in Southeast Sweden (RISC) has examined the effects of ASA 75 mg/day given to 796 men with unstable coronary artery disease (unstable angina or non-Q-wave myocardial infarction).[34] The risk of myocardial infarction and death was reduced by ASA compared with placebo treatment. At 5 days and thereafter, the treatment with ASA reduced the event rate by 57% to 69%. However, no apparent effects were detected during the first 2 days of this study in contrast with the marked reduction in the risk of fatal and nonfatal myocardial infarction recorded in the early phase of unstable angina, when patients were given an ASA dose of 325 mg twice a day.[35] Although a different trial design and relatively small numbers might account for the apparent discrepancy between the two studies, one should also consider the fact discussed earlier that when given at doses lower than 2 mg/kg the effect of ASA on platelet PGH synthase is cumulative upon repeated daily dosing and may require several days to fully inhibit TX-dependent platelet function. Thus, in the setting of acute coronary instability, a loading dose of approximately 160 mg is recommended before initiation of a low-dose regimen.[28, 30] In patients with unstable angina, stopping heparin may reactivate acute coronary syndromes, but concomitant treatment with ASA may markedly reduce the incidence and severity of reactivation events.[36]

The medium-term (3 months) and long-term (1 year) effects of ASA on the risk for myocardial infarction and death recorded in the Swedish study with 75 mg/day are at least of the same order of magnitude as the effects described by the Veterans Administration Cooperative Study using 324 mg/day and by the Canadian Multicenter Trial using 1300 mg/day in patients with unstable angina.[34, 37-39] Thus, no apparent dose dependence in antithrombotic efficacy is observed over a 17-fold range of daily doses of the drug, consistently with the dose requirement for inhibition of platelet TX production indicating a ceiling effect at 30 mg/day (see Fig. 154–2). The comparable efficacy of 75 mg/day to that of much

higher doses is also consistent with the observation that low-dose ASA can largely suppress episodes of enhanced TX biosynthesis in patients with unstable angina.[40]

The rather impressive protection afforded by ASA against vascular occlusive events in patients with unstable angina might be related to the importance of TXA_2-dependent platelet activation in amplifying the hemostatic consequences of sudden fissuring of a coronary atherosclerotic plaque. This concept is consistent with the results of ISIS-2, a randomized trial of intravenous streptokinase, oral aspirin, both, or neither among 17,187 patients entering the hospital up to 24 hours after the onset of suspected acute myocardial infarction.[41] One month of enteric-coated ASA (160 mg/day) was associated with a 23% reduction in 5-week vascular mortality and 50% reductions in reinfarction and in stroke. In terms of vascular mortality, ASA was equally effective as streptokinase (odds reduction: 25% $\pm$ 4%), and their separate effects appeared to be additive in patients receiving both (odds reduction: 42% $\pm$ 5%).

Based on the results of subgroup analysis of the RISC study, ASA reduced the risk of myocardial infarction in patients with "silent" as well as "symptomatic" ischemia at a predischarge exercise test, thereby suggesting that a common pathogenetic mechanism contributes to persistent, complete vascular occlusion in both types of patients.[42] There is uncertainty whether ASA affects the incidence or severity of myocardial ischemia after an episode of coronary instability, with some of the studies reporting no statistically significant changes and other describing both short-term and long-term beneficial effects.[28] Such a variable response may reflect the relatively minor role of TXA_2 biosynthesis in the mechanism(s) responsible for spontaneous myocardial ischemia, different trial designs (e.g., clinical versus electrocardiographic end points) or variable degrees of inhibition by ASA of the biosynthesis of vasodilator PGI_2, in the range of 20 to 1300 mg/day doses employed in these studies.[22, 40] Thus, the presence or absence of pain should not dictate the use of ASA in unstable angina: available evidence suggests that ASA reduces the incidence of myocardial infarction and death in patients with this syndrome regardless of any effect on episodes of transient ischemia.

The ability of ASA (300 to 1500 mg daily), alone or in combination with dipyridamole, to reduce the risk of recurrent cardiovascular complications in patients who survived a myocardial infarction has been studied in eight trials involving over 16,000 patients.[31] An overview of these trials suggests that ASA, started weeks to years after the infarction, can reduce the risk of fatal and nonfatal vascular events by one fourth.[31]

At variance with the results obtained in primary prevention studies (see below), ASA is effective in secondary stroke prevention.[43] In 1991, three large European studies of ASA prophylaxis were published.[44-46] Thus, additional information on approximately 7000 patients with transient ischemic attacks or minor stroke is now available. In this type of patient, the risk of serious cardiac events (i.e., fatal and nonfatal myocardial infarction, sudden cardiac death) is about the same as the risk of stroke.[43] Therefore, the composite outcome of stroke, myocardial infarction, and vascular death has been considered for comparative analysis of these studies. Indirect comparisons have not shown any difference in efficacy between 75 mg, 300 mg, and 1200 mg of ASA daily.[44, 45] The few direct comparisons have not shown any statistically significant difference between 300 and 1200 mg daily or between 30 and 283 mg, although a small difference one way or the other may have been missed because of limited sample size.[44, 46]

Skepticism on the efficacy of lower doses has been aired both in recent editorials and in scientific meetings where the subject of stroke prevention by ASA was thoroughly reviewed.[47] This in part reflects emphasis being placed on earlier studies with inadequate sample size. Also it reflects, to some extent, a widely held view among neurologists whereby the mechanism(s) of action and the dose dependence of the antithrombotic effect of ASA would differ in cerebrovascular versus cardiovascular disease.[47] Although no convincing experimental evidence is available to support this contention, there are several valid reasons for favoring low-dose versus high-dose ASA in cerebrovascular disease. These include (1) equal efficacy of lower and higher doses is biologically plausible; (2) the clinical results of the Swedish and Dutch studies are consistent with recent biochemical measurements demonstrating complete suppression of enhanced TXA_2 biosynthesis by low-dose ASA administration (50 mg daily for 7 days) in patients with acute ischemic stroke;[48] (3) the efficacy of ASA at daily doses of 162.5 to 325 mg in preventing stroke has been established in other high-risk categories, such as patients with suspected acute myocardial infarction and patients with nonvalvular atrial fibrillation;[41, 49] and (4) the indirect comparison of different regimens carried out by the second overview of the Antiplatelet Trialists' Collaboration.[31] In this analysis, ASA regimens were by far the most widely tested, accounting for two thirds of the data in more than 70,000 patients. Overall, ASA was associated with a highly significant 25% SD 2% reduction ($2 p < .00001$) in vascular events, with at least as great an effect in trials of 75 to 325 mg daily as in trials of 500 to 1500 mg daily.[31]

In summary, repeated episodes of TXA_2-dependent platelet activation occur in patients with acute ischemic syndromes affecting the coronary or the cerebral circulation. Low-dose ASA (i.e., less than 100 mg daily) can effectively suppress enhanced TXA_2 biosynthesis in these settings.[40, 48] Evidence is now available from at least two unconfounded, randomized, placebo-controlled trials to demonstrate that the long-term administration of ASA 75 mg daily is effective in reducing the risk of vascular death, nonfatal myocardial infarction, or nonfatal stroke among high-risk patients recruited into the trials because of an episode of coronary instability, a transient ischemic attack, or

a minor stroke.[34, 45] The extent of protection afforded by low-dose ASA against these important vascular events is comparable with that previously demonstrated in the same clinical conditions with doses 4 to 20 times higher, and to the average risk reduction suggested by a large overview of all ASA trials in high-risk patients.[31] The absolute risk reductions associated with such secondary prevention are quite substantial ranging from a 1-year benefit of about 15 vascular events avoided per 1000 patients actually treated to a 1-month benefit of approximately 40 per 1000 (Fig. 154–3).[31] No convincing argument exists to use a different dose in patients with cerebrovascular disease than in patients with coronary heart disease. Although even lower doses (e.g., 30 mg daily) might be equally effective, their routine use should await further clinical testing as well as the availability of properly designed pharmaceutical preparations. At present, a single loading dose of 200 to 300 mg is recommended followed by daily administration of 75 to 100 mg, which in most countries represents the smallest size commercially available.

ASA AND THE PRIMARY PREVENTION OF VASCULAR OCCLUSIVE DISEASE

The efficacy of ASA (75 to 650 mg) for the primary prevention of occlusive vascular disease has been studied in four trials of approximately 33,000 subjects with an average annual risk of 0.7% to 3.8% of having an important vascular event if untreated.[50–53] Two studies in more than 27,000 healthy male physicians addressed the possibility that long-term administration of ASA might protect against thrombotic vascular events among low-risk subjects.[50, 51] An overview of these trials suggests that the nonsignificant reduction (10% SD 6%; $2 p = .08$) in major vascular events represents the balance between a definite reduction in nonfatal MI (29% SD 8% decrease; $2 p < .0005$), a possible increase in nonfatal stroke (21% SD 13% increase; NS: due at least in part to an excess of hemorrhagic strokes) and no apparent effect on vascular mortality (2% SD 10% reduction).[31] The net absolute benefit of primary prevention with ASA in such low-risk individuals is of only 4 vascular events per 1000 subjects treated for approximately 5 years (Fig. 154–3).[31]

In the Swedish Angina-Pectoris Aspirin Trial (SAPAT) of 2035 patients with chronic stable angina and without a previous myocardial infarction treated with 75 mg daily or placebo, ASA reduced the occurrence of MI and sudden death by 34% (95% confidence interval, 24% to 49%).[52] The reduction in secondary outcome events (all cardiovascular events, cardiovascular death, all cause mortality, stroke) ranged from 22% to 32%. In this medium-risk population, treatment of 1000 patients with ASA for 4 years may avoid approximately 50 important vascular events, an absolute benefit at least 10-fold greater than that obtained in the low-risk American and British doctors' trials.

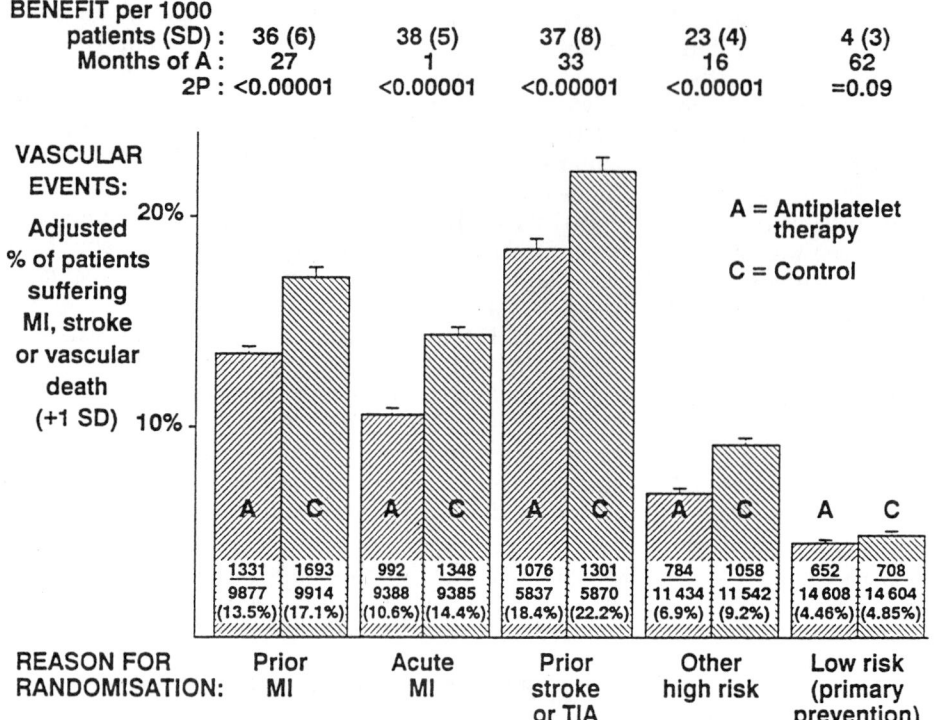

BENEFIT per 1000

patients (SD) :	36 (6)	38 (5)	37 (8)	23 (4)	4 (3)
Months of A :	27	1	33	16	62
2P :	<0.00001	<0.00001	<0.00001	<0.00001	=0.09

VASCULAR EVENTS:

Adjusted % of patients suffering MI, stroke or vascular death (+1 SD)

A = Antiplatelet therapy

C = Control

	1331	1693	992	1348	1076	1301	784	1058	652	708
	9877	9914	9388	9385	5837	5870	11 434	11 542	14 608	14 604
	(13.5%)	(17.1%)	(10.6%)	(14.4%)	(18.4%)	(22.2%)	(6.9%)	(9.2%)	(4.46%)	(4.85%)

REASON FOR RANDOMISATION:	Prior MI	Acute MI	Prior stroke or TIA	Other high risk	Low risk (primary prevention)

Figure 154–3. Absolute effects of antiplatelet therapy (145 trials) on vascular events (myocardial infarction, stroke or vascular death) in four main high-risk categories of patients and in low-risk patients (primary prevention). Adjusted totals have been calculated after converting any unevenly randomized trials to even ones by counting their control groups more than once, for calculation of adjusted percentages and of events prevented per 1000 patients allocated antiplatelet treatment. Months of A: Mean of scheduled antiplatelet duration. (From Antiplatelet Trialists' Collaboration: Collaborative overview of randomised trials of antiplatelet treatment. Part I: Prevention of death, myocardial infarction and stroke by prolonged antiplatelet therapy in various categories of patients. Br Med J 308:81, 1994. By permission of the British Medical Association.)

Patients with insulin-dependent and non–insulin-dependent diabetes mellitus have an increased risk for macrovascular complications, including myocardial infarction and stroke. In a subgroup analysis performed by the Antiplatelet Trialists' Collaboration on approximately 1000 major vascular events in over 4500 diabetic patients, the benefit of antiplatelet therapy was similar to that in the vast majority of nondiabetic patients entered into primary and secondary prevention trials.[31] The results of the Early Treatment Diabetic Retinopathy Study (ETDRS) also demonstrated a beneficial effect of ASA.[53] In this trial of 3711 patients with diabetes (49% with a history of cardiovascular disease) given ASA (650 mg daily) or a placebo and followed for an average of 5 years, ASA treatment was associated with a significant ($p = .01$) 28% reduction in MI, a nonsignificant 16% increase in stroke, and a significant ($p = .05$) 18% reduction in important vascular events. However, for the entire duration of follow-up of 7 years, the differences were smaller.[53]

Additional direct evidence is needed regarding whether the beneficial effects of long-term ASA prophylaxis outweigh the hazards in primary prevention. At least four randomized, placebo-controlled trials of low-dose ASA (40 to 75 mg daily) involving more than 65,000 subjects are currently under way.[28]

MAINTENANCE OF ARTERIAL OR VASCULAR GRAFT PATENCY

The systematic overview of the Antiplatelet Trialists' Collaboration provides unequivocal evidence that antiplatelet therapy greatly reduces, by nearly one half, the odds of arterial or graft occlusion among patients who have undergone a range of vascular operations.[32] Similar-size effects were observed after coronary artery surgery or angioplasty, after peripheral vessel surgery or angioplasty, and after formation of a hemodialysis shunt or fistula. Different ASA regimens were tested in these trials, and some direct comparisons of the effects on occlusion are available, although these are generally too small to be reliable. Thus, although there is a trend toward a slightly larger effect with ASA doses of less than 325 mg per day than with higher doses, this result is not statistically significant.[32] Only three placebo-controlled trials have examined the effects of doses of ASA in the range of 100 to 160 mg daily.[54–56] Their results are compatible with the size of the effect suggested by the overview. Moreover, biochemical measurements performed in patients undergoing elective coronary angioplasty demonstrate equal efficacy of low-dose ASA (75 mg daily for 5 days before the procedure) and doses up to 1300 mg in preventing the transient increase in TXA_2 biosynthesis associated with the procedure.[57] Because continuing ASA therapy long term (i.e., beyond 1 year after the operation) is justified to prevent important vascular events in these high-risk patients, irrespective of any additional effects on vascular patency, there seems to be no good reason to use a different ASA regimen than the one recommended earlier.

SIDE EFFECTS

Persons who regularly take nonsteroidal antiinflammatory drugs have an increased risk of serious gastrointestinal complications, such as bleeding, perforation, or other adverse events resulting in hospitalization or death.[58] The variables that influence the overall incidence of gastrointestinal side effects, including upper gastrointestinal symptoms, during prolonged ASA therapy include the dose and dosing interval, duration of treatment, plain versus enteric-coated formulations, and type of assessment. Therefore, it is not surprising that the results of different studies vary widely. Among trials in which the daily dose of ASA was 900 to 1300 mg (given as 300 or 325 mg t.i.d. or q.i.d.), the incidence of stomach pain, heartburn, and nausea was 40% to 60% higher among the patients who received ASA compared with a placebo (24% to 44% versus 15% to 32%).[28, 29] The increase in incidence of these upper gastrointestinal symptoms in patients with cerebrovascular disease treated with ASA 300 mg daily during an average follow-up of 4 years was smaller (31% versus 26%).[44] In contrast, the frequency of gastrointestinal symptoms in patients with unstable angina treated with one Alka-Seltzer® tablet (containing 324 mg of ASA) or a placebo for 12 weeks was similar.[38] Likewise, the frequency of gastrointestinal symptoms was comparably low (4% to 13% and 3% to 11%) during 12 to 50 months of therapy in patients given 75 mg aspirin or a placebo in three Swedish studies.[37, 45, 52] In the ongoing Thrombosis Prevention Trial, interim safety results for the first 3667 subjects followed up, on average, for 1.1 years demonstrated no excess of gastrointestinal symptoms in those treated with enteric-coated, controlled-release aspirin 75 mg daily as compared with a placebo.[59]

Although a dose-response relationship for upper gastrointestinal symptoms was noted in the United Kingdom Transient Ischemic Attack ASA trial (placebo, 26%; 300 mg, 31%; 1200 mg, 41%), the increased incidence of constipation was not dose dependent (placebo, 2%; 300 mg, 6%; 1200 mg, 7%).[44] This finding is consistent with the similar threefold increase in the incidence of constipation with aspirin 75 mg daily in the Thrombosis Prevention Trial.[59] Thus, both the mechanism(s) and the dose dependence for the two types of adverse effects appear to be different.

Overall, in the antiplatelet trials there was an increase in hemorrhagic strokes from 0.2% to 0.3%. The proportion of strokes attributed to hemorrhagic causes was greater in primary prevention studies than in the trials of high-risk patients.[31] Given the relatively small number of such hemorrhagic events, any comparison among different ASA regimens is rather meaningless. However, a dose-response relationship for extracranial hemorrhagic events has been found in placebo-controlled ASA trials, the comparison of 300 mg and 1200 mg in the United Kingdom trial, and the comparison of 30 and 283 mg in the Dutch trial.[44, 46, 60]

The excess of gastrointestinal hemorrhages associated with the higher doses (1200 mg, 5% versus 300 mg, 3%) may have reflected more profound gastric mucosal damage and thus a higher risk of bleeding from more prevalent erosions.[44] Doses lower than 100

mg daily are also associated with bleeding complications.[45, 59]

Regular use of nonsteroidal antiinflammatory drugs may increase the risk for chronic renal disease in some high-risk groups and impair blood pressure control in patients with essential hypertension.[17, 27, 61, 62] These effects appear to be related to the ability of most inhibitors of PGH synthase to reduce the renal synthesis of vasodilator PGI_2 and PGE_2. ASA is a relatively weak inhibitor of renal PG synthesis and is unlikely to exert any clinically relevant effect at doses of 75 to 100 mg daily.[63] However, in the United Kingdom Transient Ischemic Attack trial, the patients treated with 300 and 1200 mg ASA daily had slightly higher systolic blood pressures than the placebo-treated group.[44] Thus, there seems to be no rationale nor existing information to contraindicate the use of low-dose ASA for patients with mild impairment of renal function or essential hypertension. In contrast, episodes of bronchial asthma can occur in "intolerant" patients even in response to a single 30-mg dose, possibly reflecting the involvement of platelets in this adverse reaction. The antiplatelet drug ticlopidine is now available for use in such ASA-intolerant patients.

In summary, the different pharmacologic effects of ASA on platelets, vessel walls, stomach, and kidneys are characterized by somewhat different dose-response relationships and markedly different duration.[11] Therefore, it is not surprising that the antiplatelet effect of the drug can be separated at least in part from its other actions on the basis of reduced dosage and prolonged dosing interval. The limited results from direct comparisons of different doses of ASA are consistent with the cross-sectional impression that both gastrointestinal toxicity and hemorrhagic complications are dose related. Regular use of the lowest effective dose (i.e., 75 to 100 mg daily) as well as the development of enteric-coated formulations should minimize, although not abolish, the risk of serious adverse events associated with long-term administration of the drug.

Acknowledgment

I wish to thank Alessandra Migliavacca for expert editorial assistance.

REFERENCES

1. Flower RJ, Moncada S, Vane JR: Analgesic-antipyretics and anti-inflammatory agents; drugs employed in the treatment of gout. In Goodman GA, Goodman LS, Rall TW, et al (eds): Goodman and Gilman's The Pharmacological Basis of Therapeutics, 7th ed. New York: Macmillan, 1985, pp 674–715.
2. Vane JR: Inhibition of prostaglandin synthesis as a mechanism of action for aspirin-like drugs. Nature (New Biol) 231:232, 1971.
3. O'Brien JR: Effects of salicylates on human platelets. Lancet 1:779, 1968.
4. Hamberg M, Svensson J, Samuelsson B: Thromboxanes: A new group of biologically active compounds derived from prostaglandin endoperoxides. Proc Natl Acad Sci USA 72:2294, 1975.
5. FitzGerald GA: Mechanisms of platelet activation: Thrombox-

ane A2 as an amplifying signal for other agonists. Am J Cardiol 68:11B, 1991.

6. Roth GJ, Stanford N, Majerus PW: Acetylation of prostaglandin synthetase by aspirin. Proc Natl Acad Sci USA 72:3073, 1975.

7. DeWitt DL, Smith WL: Primary structure of prostaglandin G/H-synthase from sheep vesicular gland determined from complementary DNA sequence. Proc Natl Acad Sci USA 85:1412, 1988.

8. Smith WL, Marnett LJ: Prostaglandin endoperoxide synthase: Structure and catalysis. Biochim Biophys Acta 1083:1, 1991.

9. Smith WL: Prostanoid biosynthesis and mechanisms of action. Am J Physiol 263:F181, 1992.

10. Meade EA, Smith WL, DeWitt DL: Differential inhibition of prostaglandin endoperoxide synthase (cyclooxygenase) isozymes by aspirin and other non-steroidal antiinflammatory drugs. J Biol Chem 268:6610, 1993.

11. Patrono C: Aspirin and human platelets: From clinical trials to acetylation of cyclooxygenase and back. Trends Pharmacol Sci 10:453, 1989.

12. Bjornsson TD, Schneider DE, Berger H Jr: Aspirin acetylates fibrinogen and enhances fibrinolysis. Fibrinolytic effect is independent of changes in plasminogen activator levels. J Pharmacol Exp Ther 250:154, 1989.

13. Ratnatunga CP, Edmondson SF, Rees GM, Kovacs IB: High-dose aspirin inhibits shear-induced platelet reaction involving thrombin generation. Circulation 85:1077, 1992.

14. Ezratty AM, Simon DI, Loscalzo J: Acetylated fibrinogen facilitates plasminogen activation and attenuates platelet aggregation [abstract]. Clin Res 40:201A, 1992.

15. Pedersen AK, FitzGerald GA: The human pharmacology of platelet inhibition: Pharmacokinetics relevant to drug action. Circulation 72:1164, 1985.

16. Pedersen AK, FitzGerald GA: Dose-related kinetics of aspirin: Presystemic acetylation of platelet cyclooxygenase. N Engl J Med 311:1206, 1984.

17. Rowland M, Riegelman S: Pharmacokinetics of acetylsalicylic acid and salicylic acid after intravenous administration in man. J Pharmacol Sci 57:1313, 1968.

18. Patrono C, Ciabattoni G, Patrignani P, et al: Clinical pharmacology of platelet cyclooxygenase inhibition. Circulation 72:1177, 1985.

19. Patrono C, Ciabattoni G, Pinca E, et al: Low-dose aspirin and inhibition of thromboxane B2 production in healthy subjects. Thromb Res 17:317, 1980.

20. Patrono C, Ciabattoni G, Pugliese F, et al: Estimated rate of thromboxane secretion into the circulation of normal humans. J Clin Invest 77:590, 1986.

21. Patrignani P, Filabozzi P, Patrono C: Selective cumulative inhibition of platelet thromboxane production by low-dose aspirin in healthy subjects. J Clin Invest 69:1366, 1982.

22. FitzGerald GA, Oates JA, Hawiger J, et al: Endogenous biosynthesis of prostacyclin and thromboxane and platelet function during chronic administration of aspirin in man. J Clin Invest 71:676, 1983.

23. Weksler BB, Pett SB, Alonso D, et al: Differential inhibition by aspirin of vascular and platelet prostaglandin synthesis in atherosclerotic patients. N Engl J Med 308:800, 1983.

24. Burch JW, Stanford N, Majerus PW: Inhibition of platelet prostaglandin synthetase by oral aspirin. J Clin Invest 61:314, 1978.

25. Di Minno G, Silver MJ, Murphy S: Monitoring the entry of new platelets into the circulation after ingestion of aspirin. Blood 61:1081, 1983.

26. De Caterina R, Giannessi D, Boem A, et al: Equal antiplatelet effects of aspirin 50 or 324 mg/day in patients after acute myocardial infarction. Thromb Haemost 54:528, 1985.

27. Patrono C, Dunn MJ: The clinical significance of inhibition of renal prostaglandin synthesis. Kidney Int 32:1, 1987.

28. Patrono C: Aspirin as an antiplatelet drug. N Engl J Med 330:1287, 1984.

29. Hirsh J, Dalen JE, Fuster V, et al: Aspirin and other platelet-active drugs. The relationship between dose, effectiveness, and side effects. Chest 102(Suppl):327S, 1992.

30. Fuster V, Dyken ML, Vokonas PS, Hennekens C: Aspirin as a therapeutic agent in cardiovascular disease. Circulation 87:659, 1993.

31. Antiplatelet Trialists' Collaboration: Collaborative overview of randomised trials of antiplatelet treatment. Part I: Prevention of death, myocardial infarction and stroke by prolonged antiplatelet therapy in various categories of patients. Br Med J 308:81, 1994.

32. Antiplatelet Trialists' Collaboration: Collaborative overview of randomised trials of antiplatelet treatment. Part II: Maintenance of vascular graft or arterial patency by antiplatelet therapy. Br Med J 308:159, 1994.

33. Antiplatelet Trialists' Collaboration: Collaborative overview of randomised trials of antiplatelet treatment. Part III: Reduction in venous thrombosis and pulmonary embolism by antiplatelet prophylaxis among surgical and medical patients. Br Med J 308:235, 1994.

34. The RISC Group: Risk of myocardial infarction and death during treatment with low dose aspirin and intravenous heparin in men with unstable coronary heart disease. Lancet 336:827, 1990.

35. Théroux P, Ouimet H, McCans J, et al: Aspirin, heparin, or both to treat acute unstable angina. N Engl J Med 319:1105, 1988.

36. Théroux P, Waters D, Lam J, et al: Reactivation of unstable angina after the discontinuation of heparin. N Engl J Med 327:141, 1992.

37. Wallentin LC and the Research Group on Instability in Coronary Artery Disease in Southeast Sweden: Aspirin (75 mg/day) after an episode of unstable coronary artery disease: Long term effects on the risk for myocardial infarction, occurrence of severe angina and the need for revascularization. J Am Coll Cardiol 18:1587, 1991.

38. Lewis HD Jr, Davis JW, Archibald DG, et al: Protective effects of aspirin against acute myocardial infarction and death in men with unstable angina: Results of a Veterans Administration Cooperative Study. N Engl J Med 309:396, 1983.

39. Cairns JA, Gent M, Singer J, et al: Aspirin, sulfinpyrazone, or both in unstable angina. N Engl J Med 313:1369, 1985.

40. Vejar M, Fragasso G, Hackett D, et al: Dissociation of platelet activation and spontaneous myocardial ischemia in unstable angina. Thromb Haemost 63:163, 1990.

41. Second International Study of Infarct Survival Collaborative Group: Randomized trial of intravenous streptokinase, oral aspirin, both or neither among 17,187 cases of suspected acute myocardial infarction: ISIS-2. Lancet 2:349, 1988.

42. Nyman I, Larson H, Wallentin L, et al: Prevention of serious cardiac events by low-dose aspirin in patients with silent myocardial ischemia. Lancet 340:497, 1992.

43. Warlow C: Secondary prevention of stroke. Lancet 339:724, 1992.

44. The United Kingdom Transient Ischaemic Attack (UK-TIA) Aspirin Trial: Final results. J Neurol Neurosurg Psychiatry 54:1044, 1991.

45. The SALT Collaborative Group: Swedish Aspirin Low-dose Trial (SALT) of 75 mg aspirin as secondary prophylaxis after cerebrovascular ischaemic events. Lancet 338:1345, 1991.

46. The Dutch TIA Trial Study Group: A comparison of two doses of aspirin (30 mg vs. 283 mg a day) in patients after a transient ischemic attack or minor ischemic stroke. N Engl J Med 325:1261, 1991.

47. Dyken ML, Barnett HJM, Easton JD, et al: Low-dose aspirin and stroke. "It ain't necessarily so." Stroke 23:1395, 1992.

48. Koudstaal PJ, Ciabattoni G, van Gijn J, et al: Increased thromboxane biosynthesis in patients with acute cerebral ischemia. Stroke 24:219, 1993.

49. Stroke Prevention in Atrial Fibrillation Investigators: Stroke Prevention in Atrial Fibrillation Study. Final results. Circulation 84:527, 1991.

50. Peto R, Gray R, Collins R, et al: Randomised trial of prophylactic daily aspirin in British male doctors. Br Med J 296:313, 1988.

51. The Steering Committee of the Physicians' Health Study Research Group: Final report on the aspirin component of the ongoing Physicians' Health Study. N Engl J Med 321:129, 1989.

52. Juul-Moller S, Edvardsson N, Jahrmatz B, et al: For the Swedish Angina Pectoris Aspirin Trial (SAPAT) Group: Double-blind trial of aspirin in primary prevention of myocardial infarction in patients with stable angina pectoris. Lancet 340:1421, 1992.

53. ETDRS Investigators: Aspirin effects on mortality and morbidity in patients with diabetes mellitus. Early Treatment Diabetic Retinopaty Study Report 14. JAMA 268:1292, 1992.
54. Harter H, Burch J, Majerus PW, et al: Prevention of thrombosis in patients on hemodialysis by low-dose aspirin. N Engl J Med 301:577, 1979.
55. Lorenz RL, von Schacky C, Weber M, et al: Improved aortocoronary bypass patency by low-dose aspirin (100 mg daily). Effects on platelet aggregation and thromboxane formation. Lancet 1:1261, 1984.
56. Sanz G, Parajou A, Alegria E, et al: Prevention of early aorto-coronary bypass occlusion by low-dose aspirin and dipyridamole. Circulation 82:765, 1990.
57. Ciabattoni G, Sharom Ujang M, Sritara P, et al: Aspirin, but not heparin, suppresses the transient increase in thromboxane biosynthesis associated with cardiac catheterization or coronary angioplasty. J Am Coll Cardiol 21:1377, 1993.
58. Gabriel SE, Jaakkimainen L, Bombardier C: Risk for serious gastrointestinal complications related to use of nonsteroidal anti-inflammatory drugs. A meta-analysis. Ann Intern Med 115:787, 1991.
59. Meade TW, Roderick PJ, Brennan PJ, et al: Extra-cranial bleeding and other symptoms due to low dose aspirin and low intensity oral anticoagulation. Thromb Haemost 68:1,1992.
60. Roderick PJ, Wilkes HC, Meade TW: The gastrointestinal toxicity of aspirin: An overview of randomised controlled trials. Br J Clin Pharmacol 35:219, 1993.
61. Oates JA, FitzGerald GA, Branch RA, et al: Clinical implications of prostaglandin and thromboxane A2 formation (second of two parts). N Engl J Med 319:761, 1988.
62. Sandler DP, Burr R, Weinberg CR: Nonsteroidal anti-inflammatory drugs and the risk for chronic renal disease. Ann Intern Med 115:165, 1991.
63. Minuz P, Barrow SE, Cockcroft JR, Ritter JM: Effects of nonsteroidal antiinflammatory drugs on prostacyclin and thromboxane biosynthesis in patients with mild essential hypertension. Br J Clin Pharmacol 30:519, 1990.

CHAPTER 155

Dipyridamole

Thomas G. DiSalvo, M.D., Mark W. I. Webster, M.B., Ch.B., F.R.A.C.P., James H. Chesebro, M.D., and Valentin Fuster, M.D.

Dipyridamole is a pyrimidopyrimidine compound with antithrombotic and vasodilating actions. It has been used in an array of cardiovascular conditions to prevent thromboembolism. Dipyridamole usually is combined with aspirin, a drug that acts independently to inhibit platelet function. There is increasing evidence that the effect of dipyridamole plus aspirin on biologic surfaces is due to the effects of aspirin alone. The most compelling current indication for dipyridamole is in combination with warfarin, to prevent thromboembolism from mechanical prosthetic valve surfaces, because dipyridamole is most effective against thrombus formation on prosthetic material. Because of the widespread use of dipyridamole since the 1970s, it is worthwhile reviewing the large amount of clinical information compiled regarding the efficacy of this drug on mechanical prosthetic, but not biologic, surfaces.

PHARMACODYNAMICS

The exact mechanism of the antithrombotic action of dipyridamole remains obscure (Table 155–1). Early *in vitro* studies showed that dipyridamole inhibits cyclic adenosine monophosphate (cAMP) phosphodiesterase and hence reduces the breakdown of intracellular cAMP.[1-3] Dipyridamole also activates adenylate cyclase indirectly by modulating the activity of prostacyclin and other platelet-inhibiting eicosanoids.[4-7] However, both these effects occur at plasma levels considerably above those achieved with the usual oral dose of dipyridamole and are thus not likely to account for dipyridamole's antithrombotic action *in vivo*.[1]

Dipyridamole's effects on adenosine metabolism likely determine both the antithrombotic and vasodilating actions of dipyridamole. Dipyridamole inhibits the facilitated transport of adenosine into vascular endothelium and erythrocytes.[8, 9] This inhibition of transport is dose-dependent and occurs at therapeutic plasma concentrations of dipyridamole.[9, 10] In addition, dipyridamole inhibits adenosine deaminase, the enzyme responsible for conversion of adenosine into inactive inosine.[11] By inhibiting both the cellular uptake and enzymatic degradation of adenosine, dipyridamole increases adenosine concentrations in human plasma and in the myocardial effluent and myocardial interstitium of laboratory animals.[12, 13]

Based on *ex vivo* studies of whole blood, it has been suggested that dipyridamole's antithrombotic action may stem from increased systemic and local adenosine concentrations. Adenosine binds to platelet mem-

Table 155–1. **Putative Mechanisms of Dipyridamole's Antithrombotic Effect**

A. Decreases platelet aggregability
  1. At therapeutic serum concentrations:
    a. Increased circulating and interstitial adenosine levels
      i. Inhibits intracellular transport
      ii. Inhibits adenosine deaminase
    b. Potentiates nitric oxide platelet inhibition
    c. Stimulates platelet cGMP production
    d. Inhibits platelet aggregation by oxygen-derived free radicals
  2. At supratherapeutic serum concentrations:
    a. Inhibits cAMP phosphodiesterase
    b. Modulates PGI_2 production
B. Decreases platelet adhesion to prosthetic surfaces
C. Increases platelet survival
D. Increases red blood cell deformability

brane adenosine A2 receptors.[14] A2 receptors are coupled to adenyl cyclase via the guanine nucleotide-binding protein Gs.[10] Activation of the A2 receptor by adenosine ultimately results in increased platelet cAMP content and inhibition of platelet aggregation. Adenosine has been shown to inhibit platelet aggregation in several models, including during myocardial ischemia in dogs.[14, 15]

Dipyridamole has also been shown to potentiate platelet inhibition by nitric oxide (NO).[16, 17] NO is both a potent inhibitor of platelet aggregation and an inhibitor of platelet adhesion under flow conditions.[18] NO inhibits platelet activation by stimulating guanylate cyclase and increasing platelet cyclic guanosine monophosphate (cGMP) content.[19] Dipyridamole at therapeutic plasma levels preferentially inhibits cGMP phosphodiesterase rather than cAMP phosphodiesterase. This cGMP phosphodiesterase–inhibiting effect is synergistic with prostacyclin-induced increase in platelet cAMP content, because cGMP suppresses the degradation of cAMP.[16, 17] When NO at subthreshold concentration is combined with varying concentrations of dipyridamole in rabbit and human platelet-rich plasma, dipyridamole causes concentration-dependent platelet inhibition.[16, 17] This inhibition is more pronounced in the presence of prostacyclin.

In isolated animal and human platelet preparations, dipyridamole has no effect on platelet activation or aggregation.[16] In whole blood, dipyridamole has no effect on platelet activation or aggregation unless red blood cell injury is enhanced, and the concentration of free adenine nucleotides is increased.[17] These results are not unexpected if the inhibition of adenosine uptake and catabolism and potentiation of NO effects underlie dipyridamole's antiplatelet effects.

Dipyridamole has also been reported to inhibit platelet aggregation induced by oxygen-derived free radicals, inhibit red cell–induced platelet activation in whole blood ex vivo, and reduce platelet recruitment induced by activated platelets in collagen-stimulated whole blood.[20–22] Several reports suggest that dipyridamole increases erythrocyte deformability.[23, 24]

Despite these disparate ex vivo observations, the effect of dipyridamole on platelet aggregability, activation, and adhesion in vivo is still uncertain. In animal models of arterial stenosis or injury, dipyridamole does not reduce platelet aggregation or mural thrombosis.[25, 26] Studies of platelet aggregability in dipyridamole-treated volunteers are conflicting. One such study found that dipyridamole (200 mg administered daily for 10 days to healthy volunteers) significantly inhibited spontaneous, platelet activation factor, and collagen-induced platelet aggregation.[27] Most studies, however, have not found that orally administered dipyridamole inhibits aggregability or have found only weak effects on aggregation at moderately high doses (300 to 450 mg/day).[28, 29]

In contrast, animal studies have shown that dipyridamole inhibits platelet adhesion to prosthetic surfaces. Platelet adherence to a polytetrafluoroethylene (PTFE) graft in rabbit aorta was significantly reduced by both aspirin and dipyridamole, with a combina-

tion of the two being most effective.[30] In a dog model, low-dose aspirin (1 mg/kg/day) had no effect on graft patency at 1 week in dogs undergoing carotid artery replacement with either PTFE or Dacron end-to-end grafts.[31] Graft patency with both prosthetic materials was improved when a higher dose of aspirin (approximately 15 mg/kg/day) was combined with dipyridamole. Dipyridamole alone significantly reduced thrombus formation and platelet deposition in PTFE grafts in dogs.[32] In the baboon, platelet consumption in a Dacron arteriovenous cannula was significantly reduced by dipyridamole.[33] Aspirin enhanced this effect but was ineffective when given alone. Platelet consumption depended on the dose of dipyridamole, with 10 mg/kg/day being more effective than 2.5 mg/kg/day. At the higher dose, dipyridamole plasma levels were 30 times less than those obtained in humans because of poor drug absorption. Studies of ex vivo platelet adhesion to rabbit subendothelium and rat aorta in human volunteers receiving dipyridamole are conflicting, but the studies involved very small numbers of volunteers.[8]

In human subjects, dipyridamole prolongs the shortened platelet survival times associated with prosthetic heart valves, prosthetic grafts, and following arterial thromboembolism in vivo.[34–36] Reduced platelet survival has been used as an in vivo index of the interaction between platelets and the prosthetic material, between platelets and the arterial wall, or both.[34, 37] Thus, prolongation of shortened survival time with dipyridamole appears to reflect an in vivo antiplatelet effect. However, many of these studies involve small numbers of patients and uncontrolled data. In one study, dipyridamole had no effect on platelet survival when combined with orally administered anticoagulant agents for 3 months in 55 patients after valve replacement, although survival times were not measured before treatments and were not abnormally short in the control group.[37] Dipyridamole has been shown to decrease platelet activation associated with cardiopulmonary bypass in several studies.[38]

In accord with this experimental evidence, dipyridamole likely has a limited effect on biologic surfaces in human subjects. As reviewed later, most clinical trials in myocardial infarction, angina, stroke, angioplasty, and coronary artery bypass surgery have not documented an advantage of the combination of dipyridamole and aspirin over aspirin alone. This observation was confirmed in the second Antiplatelet Trialists' Collaboration meta-analysis.[39]

PHARMACOKINETICS

Following oral administration, absorption of dipyridamole varies highly, with peak plasma concentrations varying by up to 15 times with 50-mg, 75-mg, or 100-mg preparations.[8] Absorption is decreased by food or a gastric pH greater than 4. In plasma, dipyridamole is 91% to 99% bound to albumin and α_1-acid glycoprotein.[40–42] Elimination is primarily by biliary excretion as a glucuronide conjugate.[41] The steady-state elimination half-life is approximately 10 hours with a small amount of enterohepatic circulation.[43]

There is some evidence for a possible pharmacokinetic interaction with aspirin. Coadministration of aspirin and dipyridamole in rabbits increased the plasma levels of both drugs.[44] One short-term study in human subjects found that adding dipyridamole (75 mg) to aspirin (1 g) produced a small but significant increase in peak plasma concentration and in the area under the aspirin plasma concentration-time curve.[45] This finding has not been confirmed by others, and its clinical significance is unclear.[46] No data indicate that such an interaction leads to synergistic antithrombotic effects.[8, 47]

In contrast, the pharmacokinetic interaction with endogenous and exogenous adenosine is of definite clinical importance.[48–50] As has been described, dipyridamole increases endogenous adenosine concentration by inhibiting intracellular adenosine transport and enzymatic degradation. Intravenously administered dipyridamole (0.56 mg/kg bolus, 5 μg/kg/min infusion) significantly increased the AH interval, increased the cycle length at which pacing-induced atrioventricular (AV) nodal Wenckebach's occurred, decreased SVT cycle length, and by itself terminated and prevented reinduction of SVT in one of six patients.[51] In the other five patients, dipyridamole reduced fourfold the dose of exogenous adenosine necessary to terminate SVT (68 ± 15 to 17 ± 6 μg/kg). These effects of dipyridamole on AV nodal conduction were completely reversed by the adenosine antagonist aminophylline. Because exogenous adenosine in usual intravenous bolus dose (6 μg) has been reported to cause profound bradycardia and asystole in patients receiving orally administered dipyridamole, the adenosine dose used to terminate SVT should be reduced to one fourth the usual dose in these patients.[48, 51]

ADVERSE EFFECTS

Nausea and abdominal discomfort are the main adverse effects of dipyridamole.[52, 53] These effects occur in approximately 10% of patients receiving 400 mg/day of dipyridamole but often subside with continued use. Because of dipyridamole's vasodilating effects, headaches occur in up to 10% of patients with this dose and may prompt discontinuance in up to a third of affected patients.

Myocardial ischemia and angina may be precipitated by dipyridamole in those with coronary artery disease because of its inhibition of adenosine uptake and degradation and resultant adenosine-induced coronary "steal."[11] Increased levels of adenosine activate adenosine A_2 receptors on coronary artery endothelium, causing potent coronary artery vasodilation and marked enhancement of regional myocardial flow. This effect is used with thallium (201Tl) imaging as a diagnostic test for coronary artery disease in patients unable to exercise adequately. Dipyridamole and adenosine enhance flow in myocardial regions subtended by atherosclerotic coronary arteries much less than in regions subtended by normal arteries.[54, 55] This results in a significant endocardial-to-epicardial flow gradient and a phenomenon of transmural "coronary steal" with resultant subendocardial ischemia in the absence of change in total coronary blood flow. In up to 25% of patients with coronary artery disease, dipyridamole (300 mg orally or 0.56 mg/kg intravenously) may precipitate myocardial ischemia.[11, 56] Ischemia is rapidly ameliorated by intravenously administered aminophylline (100 mg), a potent nonselective adenosine A1 and A2 receptor antagonist. Provocation of myocardial ischemia by adequately spaced therapeutic orally administered doses of dipyridamole (50 to 100 mg every 6 hours) is uncommon and has not been prominent in large studies. In a study of patients with mechanical prosthetic heart valves, only 1 of 181 patients receiving dipyridamole (400 mg/day) had angina that required coronary artery bypass grafting.[57–59] Though angina was not an end point in the large Persantine-Aspirin Reinfarction Study (PARIS), the persantine plus aspirin group (n = 810) had no detectable increase or change in angina compared with the aspirin (n = 810) or placebo (n = 406) groups while taking dipyridamole (75 mg three times daily for 41 months).[60] In a small randomized, double-blind, crossover trial of dipyridamole (75 mg every 8 hours for 2 weeks), no change occurred in self-reported angina frequency, exercise treadmill performance, or ischemia by ambulatory electrocardiographic monitoring.[61] Of interest, theophylline has been shown to improve exercise capacity and exercise-induced myocardial ischemia in several reports, as has bamifylline, a selective adenosine A1 receptor antagonist.[62] Redistribution of coronary flow toward the hypoperfused subendocardium has been hypothesized as the mechanism.

Dipyridamole is not associated with gastritis or gastroduodenal ulcers and does not increase the risk of bleeding even when combined with anticoagulants.[8]

CLINICAL STUDIES

Dipyridamole is combined with anticoagulants or other antiplatelet agents in current clinical practice. The major indication for dipyridamole is in patients with mechanical prosthetic heart valves who are on anticoagulant therapy but who remain at high risk for arterial thromboembolism. Given that dipyridamole's antiplatelet effects on prosthetic surfaces is superior to that of aspirin, dipyridamole may be considered for use in such instances.

PROSTHETIC HEART VALVES

Patients with prosthetic heart valves have a medium to high long-term risk of thromboembolism.[63] Perioperative tissue injury, stasis, and turbulence of flow, as well as the inherent thrombogenicity of the prosthetic valve surface and Dacron swing ring, all promote thrombosis as soon as blood begins to flow through the newly implanted valve. By 24 hours after valve replacement, indium-111–labeled platelets adhere to the sewing ring.[64] Long-term follow-up studies show a continued risk of thromboembolism. With the Starr-Edwards valve, 34% of patients experience an embolic event within 10 years.[65] In anticoagulated patients with the St. Jude valve, the least thrombogenic model, thromboembolism still occurs at a rate of 2.0% per patient-year and 3.9% per patient-year with valves in the aortic and mitral positions, respectively.[66] Platelet survival is often shortened in patients with prosthetic heart valves and may indicate increased risk of arterial thromboembolism.[34, 35, 66] Because dipyridamole (400 mg/day) has been shown to prolong platelet survival in patients with prosthetic valves, this may be a significant advantage to dipyridamole's use.

Other risk factors for prosthetic valve thromboembolism include the mitral position, double valves, atrial fibrillation, left atrium size greater than 50 mm with sinus rhythm, previous thromboembolism, left ventricular dysfunction, operation prior to 1980 (because of changes in valve design, changes in flow characteristics, and generally earlier valve replacement in the course of chronic valvular heart disease today).[63] However, the single most important risk factor for prosthetic valve thromboembolism is clearly the adequacy of long-term anticoagulation. Both the intensity and variability of the prothrombin times are important. Many studies have documented that long-term oral anticoagulation is often suboptimal. In a series of measurements of 12,000 prothrombin times in patients with prosthetic valves, only 65% were in the therapeutic range (30% too low, 5% too high).[67] At the time of an embolic event, approximately one half of prothrombin times were less than 1.5 times control in one study.[68] Given these observations on the inadequacies of long-term anticoagulation, and dipyridamole's inhibition of platelet adhesion to prosthetic surfaces and prolongation of platelet survival, dipyridamole has been combined with anticoagulant agents to prevent prosthetic valve thromboembolism. Dipyridamole has been approved by the United States Food and Drug Administration for this specific use.

Five trials have shown that dipyridamole added to oral anticoagulation decreases thromboembolism from prosthetic valves compared with oral anticoagulation alone (Table 155–2).[67, 69–72] Only two trials were placebo-controlled, and only one of these was sufficiently large to establish dipyridamole's efficacy with high statistical power.[72] This latter trial randomized 163 patients prospectively to dipyridamole (400 mg/day) or placebo. Warfarin was begun on postoperative day 4 and dipyridamole on postoperative day 10. Warfarin dose was chosen to maintain the prothrombin time twice normal. During 1 year of follow-up, thromboembolism occurred in 14.3% of patients in the placebo group and in 1.3% in the dipyridamole group ($p < .01$). Though this study was initially criticized for failure to report prothrombin times in both groups, a subsequent report of 4000 prothrombin times collected during the study showed no differences in level of anticoagulation between the two groups.[73] However, data analysis was not performed on an "intention-to-treat" basis. The four other studies also showed fewer thromboembolic events with dipyridamole plus anticoagulants.

Studies of aspirin combined with anticoagulants have consistently shown a decrease in thromboembolism compared with anticoagulants alone but a significantly increased risk of gastrointestinal bleeding with aspirin doses of 500 to 1000 mg/day.[27, 67] A randomized, double-blind, placebo-controlled trial of aspirin (100 mg/day) plus warfarin (target international normalized ratio [INR] 3.0 to 4.5) in 370 patients with prosthetic valves showed that the addition of aspirin reduced the risk of systemic embolism by 77% ($p < .001$), reduced the combined end point of major systemic embolism, nonfatal intracranial hemorrhage, or death from hemorrhage or vascular causes by 61% ($p = .005$) or death from any cause by 63% ($p = .01$).[74] Bleeding risk increased by 55% in the aspirin group ($p = .02$); major bleeding risk increased by 27% in the aspirin group ($p = .43$). Most of the bleeding was minor (hematuria, epistaxis, bruising). Three patients in each group had fatal intracerebral hemorrhages, but all five nonfatal intracranial hemorrhages occurred in the aspirin group. The authors concluded that the considerable benefit of combined treatment

Table 155–2. **Dipyridamole Therapy in Patients with Mechanical Prosthetic Heart Valves**

Study (Reference)	Methods	Follow-Up (yr)	Treatment Group	Dose (mg/day)	Patients (No.)	Thromboembolic Events (%/yr)
Sullivan et al.[72]	Prospective, randomized	1	A/C + placebo		84	14
			A/C + D	400	79	1
Kasahara[70]	Prospective, randomized	1 to 3 (mean 30 mo)	A/C		39	21
			A/C + D	400	40	5
Groupe de Recherche PACTE[69]	Prospective, randomized	1	A/C		154	5
			A/C + D	375	136	3
Rajah et al.[71]	Prospective, randomized	1 to 2	A/C		87	13
			A/C + D	300	78	4
Chesebro et al.[67]	Prospective, randomized to groups 2 and 3	0 to 2	A/C		183	1.2
			A/C + D	400	181	0.5
			A/C + ASA*	500	170	1.8

A/C, anticoagulant; ASA, aspirin; D, dipyridamole.
*Excessive bleeding (major events), 6.5%/yr required stopping ASA.

with aspirin (100 mg/day) and warfarin outweighed the increase in bleeding.

Current Recommendations

In patients at acceptably low risk of perioperative bleeding, begin intravenously administered heparin 6 hours after operation (600 to 700 units/hour to maintain the activated partial thromboplastin time [aPTT] at the upper limit of normal) and continue until chest tubes are removed. Then use intravenously administered heparin to prolong the aPTT to 1.5 to 2.0 times the upper limit of control. Start warfarin 24 to 48 hours after the operation and adjust to prolong the prothrombin time to 1.5 to 2.0 times control (target INR, 3.0 to 4.5) and continue indefinitely.

All patients with mechanical prosthetic valves should receive warfarin indefinitely. Patients at high risk for thromboembolism (previous thromboembolism, atrial fibrillation, enlarged left atrium, depressed left ventricular function, surgery before 1980, variable prothrombin times) should receive supplemental antiplatelet therapy. Because one well-done trial supports the concept that low-dose aspirin (100 mg/day) decreases thromboembolism and all-cause mortality, albeit with an increased risk of nonfatal bleeding, and because dipyridamole in combination with Coumadin has not been proven to decrease mortality, combination therapy with aspirin and warfarin may be preferable to dipyridamole and warfarin in high-risk patients.[74] The combination of aspirin and warfarin is superior to the combination of dipyridamole and warfarin in reducing the incidence of myocardial infarction and stroke but may not provide additional protection against thromboembolism from prosthetic surfaces. For patients unwilling to accept an increased risk of bleeding due to aspirin or patients intolerant of aspirin, dipyridamole may be used. Begin dipyridamole (50 mg four times a day) at the same time as warfarin and increase over 2 to 3 days to 350 to 400 mg/day in four divided doses (5 to 6 mg/kg/day). Gastrointestinal upset or headache may be reduced by giving dipyridamole with food. In high-risk patients intolerant of aspirin and dipyridamole, sulfinpyrazone may be used (800 mg/day), although this drug has never been studied in a randomized trial. Ticlopidine to date has not been studied in this setting.

PROSTHETIC ARTERIAL GRAFTS

In a large study of lower extremity reconstructions with PTFE grafts, only 12% of the grafts were patent at 6 years.[75] The high occlusion rate of prosthetic arterial grafts mandates antithrombotic therapy.[76] Early prosthetic graft occlusion may occur because of technical problems at operation or thrombosis. At operation, vessel dissection and trauma, the application of vascular clamps, endarterectomy, and the placement of suture lines all predispose to acute thrombosis. In addition, reconstruction of small arteries (less than 6 mm in diameter) carrying low flow

(less than 200 mg/min) is associated with increased risk of thrombotic occlusion. Late prosthetic graft occlusion is often due to neointimal hyperplasia at suture lines with or without superimposed thrombosis.

Unlike prosthetic grafts in animals, prosthetic arterial grafts in human subjects are not completely covered by vascular endothelium. Studies of indium-111–labeled platelets show continued deposition of labeled platelets on prosthetic vascular grafts in human subjects even years after operation.[77] Antiplatelet therapy with aspirin and dipyridamole reduce platelet deposition and improve the patency of both Dacron and PTFE grafts.[78-81] Studies using good animal models, including primates, provide a sound experimental basis for recommending the combination of dipyridamole and aspirin rather than aspirin alone.[30, 31, 33]

There have been no trials of dipyridamole alone in the prevention of prosthetic arterial graft thrombosis in humans. Five trials have investigated the role of aspirin plus dipyridamole.[80-84] Two studies with low statistical power showed that aspirin and dipyridamole administered preoperatively significantly reduced prosthetic graft occlusion.[80, 84] A large study of aspirin and dipyridamole administered postoperatively showed no difference in occlusion rates.[83] Preoperative dipyridamole administration followed by intraoperative, intravenous dipyridamole administration and then postoperative, oral dipyridamole administration was shown to significantly reduce prosthetic graft occlusion when combined with postoperative, oral aspirin administration.[81] Occlusion rates of saphenous vein bypass grafts were not reduced in a trial of preoperative and postoperative combined aspirin and dipyridamole.[82] In this trial, wound hematomas and the need for transfusion were increased twofold.

Thus, antiplatelet therapy with aspirin and dipyridamole, when begun preoperatively (either as dipyridamole alone or in the combination), has been shown to reduce thrombotic occlusion of prosthetic vascular grafts but not peripheral saphenous vein grafts. Therapy begun postoperatively may have no effect. Dipyridamole has not been studied alone, but because dipyridamole inhibits platelet adhesion to prosthetic surfaces and is synergistic with aspirin in this regard, it is reasonable to recommend combined therapy with aspirin and dipyridamole.[76]

Current Recommendations

Ideally, begin aspirin (325 mg/day) preoperatively. If bleeding is of sufficient concern, instead of aspirin, begin dipyridamole (100 mg four times a day) 1 day preoperatively. Dextran 40 administered intravenously during the operation (500 ml at 100 ml/hour, followed by 500 ml at 75 ml/hour and then 500 ml/day for 3 days) has been shown to decrease occlusion at 1 week.[76] Though many surgeons use intravenously administered heparin intraoperatively, no controlled studies of this practice have been reported. Nonetheless, intraoperative heparin administration likely reduces prosthetic graft thrombosis. As reported in one study, intravenously administered dipyridamole may be of benefit intraoperatively if tolerated. Aspirin (325 mg) plus dipyridamole (75 mg three times a day) should be started down the nasogastric tube 8 hours after surgery and orally thereafter. Patients with complex reconstructions of small vessels with low flow, or those with successful thrombectomy following initial reconstruction, may benefit from long-term warfarin therapy.[76]

AORTOCORONARY SAPHENOUS VEIN BYPASS GRAFTS

Occlusion of saphenous vein bypass grafts occurs in 10% to 15% of grafts in the first month, 16% to 26% within the first year, 2% per year for the next 5 years, and 5% per year for the next 5 years.[85] At 5 to 7 years, 37% of grafts are occluded; at 12 years, 55% are occluded.[86] Grafts at particularly high risk for early thrombotic occlusion have low flow rates (less than 40 ml/min) and a distal anastomosis with a small coronary artery (less than 1.5 mm in diameter).[85] Occlusion within the first month is usually due to thrombosis. Graft endothelial injury during harvesting and deep arterial injury in the receiving coronary artery due to arteriotomy and suturing are all potent stimuli to thrombus formation.[85] Platelet deposition on the denuded endothelial surfaces of the vein graft and distal anastomotic site begins as soon as blood flows through the graft.[87] Mural thrombus is found histologically in three quarters of grafts of animals or patients who die within 24 hours of operation.[88] Because platelet deposition is critical to graft thrombosis and occlusion, it is not surprising that trials of antiplatelet therapy after coronary artery bypass have established a clear role for antiplatelet therapy.[47] Antiplatelet therapy reduces graft occlusion in the first few weeks following operation by 50% to 70% and at 1 year by 30% to 56%.[85] Antiplatelet therapy must be begun preoperatively or at most within 24 to 48 hours postoperatively. Graft occlusion is not reduced when antiplatelet therapy is begun more than 48 hours postoperatively.[85]

Both aspirin and ticlopidine have been clearly shown in large, randomized, double-blind, placebo-controlled trials to reduce occlusion of saphenous vein grafts (SVGs).[85] The role of dipyridamole in addition to aspirin is uncertain. Dipyridamole administered preoperatively reduces platelet activation by the prosthetic materials in the heart-lungs bypass oxygenator, maintains the platelet count, and reduces myocardial platelet deposition and cardiac thromboxane release without increasing the risk of bleeding during operation.[89–92] Dipyridamole also significantly increases vein graft blood flow.[93] Despite these effects of dipyridamole, clinical trials have not shown that dipyridamole plus aspirin aids graft survival compared with aspirin alone except in grafts with low flow and distal anastomoses less than 1.5 mm.[39, 85]

Brown et al.[94] randomized 147 patients in a double-blind, placebo-controlled trial of aspirin (325 mg three times a day) plus dipyridamole (75 mg three times a

day), aspirin (325 mg three times a day), or placebo. This small trial showed a statistically significant reduction in graft occlusion for both treatment groups over placebo but no difference in graft occlusion rates in the treatment groups themselves. A multicenter Veterans Administration study compared aspirin (325 mg/day), aspirin (325 mg three times a day) plus dipyridamole (75 mg three times a day), sulfinpyrazone (267 mg three times a day), and placebo in 555 patients in a randomized, double-blind, placebo-controlled trial.[95] All aspirin groups showed statistically significant higher SVG patency rates by angiography (in 72% of patients randomized) at 60 days (91.9% to 93.5% versus 85.2%, $p < .05$). There was no difference in patency between the aspirin plus dipyridamole group and either aspirin alone group. Dipyridamole was begun 48 hours preoperatively, and aspirin was begun 72 hours preoperatively. Intravenously administered dipyridamole was not given intraoperatively. Perioperative bleeding complications (chest tube drainage, transfusion requirement, and reoperation rate) were significantly greater in the groups receiving aspirin. The 1-year patency results of this trial were published separately.[96] The occlusion rates at 1 year for all grafts were 22.6% for placebo, 13.2% for aspirin at 325 mg four times a day, 16.8% for aspirin at 325 mg three times a day, 17.5% for aspirin at 325 mg plus dipyridamole at 75 mg three times a day, 18.2% for sulfinpyrazone at 267 mg three times a day, and 15.8% overall for all aspirin-containing groups. There was no difference in occlusion rates between the aspirin plus dipyridamole group and the aspirin-alone groups. Aspirin (325 mg once daily) conferred a statistically significant reduction in occlusion compared with placebo ($p = .05$), as did all the aspirin-containing groups pooled together ($p = .029$) Aspirin prevented occlusion in grafts to vessels with diameters of less than 2.0 mm compared with placebo (20.1 versus 32.3%, $p = .008$). For vessels with diameter of greater than 2.0 mm, aspirin conferred no benefit. In addition, for all grafts shown to be patent by earlier study, there was no difference in occlusion rates at 1 year between aspirin groups and placebo (8.7 versus 9.4%, $p = .763$).

The Mayo Clinic placebo-controlled trial was the first to begin therapy before operation.[57] Patients received dipyridamole at 100 mg four times a day for 2 days preoperatively followed by dipyridamole at 75 mg three times a day started 1 hour postoperatively and aspirin at 325 mg three times a day started 7 hours postoperatively and continued for 1 year. There was no increased risk of bleeding with combination therapy. Early (median, 8 days) and late (1 year) angiography was performed in 88% and 84% of subjects, respectively. Angiography showed significantly less graft occlusion in the treatment group than in the placebo group (3% versus 9% at 10 days, 3% versus 10% at 1 month, 11% versus 25% at 1 year, respectively). There was not an aspirin-only group in this study. Ekestrom et al.[93] randomized 360 patients to dipyridamole (100 mg four times a day for 2 days preoperatively, 5 mg/kg/24 hours perioperatively, and 100 mg four times a day orally for 1 year postoperatively) or placebo. Twenty-eight percent of patients receiving dipyridamole were withdrawn, as were 31% receiving placebo. The high rate of withdrawal was due to cardiovascular and cerebrovascular events; these were more common in the placebo group. Dipyridamole increased the intraoperatively measured blood flow in the saphenous vein graft ($p < .01$). Angiography performed 1 year postoperatively showed a statistically insignificant trend toward greater patency in the dipyridamole group (51% versus 47%, $p = .08$). Agnew et al.[97] randomized 101 patients to either aspirin at 100 mg once daily or aspirin at 100 mg once daily plus dipyridamole at 300 mg once daily 36 hours before surgery and continued for 1 year. Thirty-seven patients withdrew, 14 because of drug effects. Angiography at 9 weeks and 1 year showed no significant differences in patency rates (93% and 87%, and 90% and 98%, in the aspirin-alone and aspirin-plus-dipyridamole groups, respectively).

Two large, randomized, double-blind, placebo-controlled trials have suggested possible roles for dipyridamole. Sanz et al.[98] randomized 1112 consecutive patients to aspirin (50 mg three times a day), aspirin (50 mg three times a day) plus dipyridamole (75 mg three times a day), or placebo. All patients received dipyridamole (100 mg four times a day) for 48 hours preoperatively, and assigned treatment began 7 hours after surgery. Angiography was performed in 83% of patients within 28 days of operation (mean 10 days). Occlusion rates compared with placebo were 12.9% versus 18% ($p = .017$) for the aspirin plus dipyridamole group and 14% versus 18% ($p = .058$) for the aspirin-alone group. Although chest tube drainage was significantly higher in the aspirin plus dipyridamole group, the hospital mortality or reoperation rates were not different. Logistic regression analysis showed that diameter of the distal vessel of less than 1.5 mm and angiographic quality of the distal vessel were independent predictors of occlusion controlling for antiplatelet therapy. In distal vessels of less than 1.0 mm, the occlusion rates in the placebo, aspirin, and combined therapy groups were 49%, 36.3%, and 32.7%, respectively.

Van der Meer et al.[99] randomized 948 patients to aspirin (50 mg four times a day) begun at midnight after the operation; dipyridamole (5 mg/kg intravenously) from 10 PM the day before operation until midnight the day after operation, then at 200 mg orally twice a day plus aspirin at 50 mg four times a day; or orally administered acenocoumarol or phenprocoumon anticoagulants begun on the day before operation and continued postoperatively with a target INR of 2.8 to 4.8. Repeat angiography in 78% of the patients at 1 year showed occlusion rates of 11% in the aspirin plus dipyridamole group, 15% in the aspirin group (RR 0.76, CI$_{95}$ 0.54 to 1.05), and 13% in the anticoagulant group (NS). Though occlusion rates tended to be lower in the dipyridamole plus aspirin group, there was a significant benefit of aspirin plus dipyridamole in grafts in vessels with lumen diameter of 1.5 mm or less compared with aspirin alone

(17% versus 11%—RR 0.66, CI$_{95}$ 0.47 to 0.94) but not compared with anticoagulants (13%). There was a statistically significant increase in chest tube drainage ($p = .012$) and a trend toward higher median transfusion requirement ($p = .07$), but no difference in rates of early reoperation or operative mortality between the aspirin plus dipyridamole groups and the other groups. Combined clinical outcome events, defined as myocardial infarction, thrombosis, major bleeding, or death, were higher in the aspirin plus dipyridamole group than in the aspirin-alone group (RR 1.46, CI$_{95}$ 1.02 to 2.08), though the incidence of individual outcome events did not differ. The improvement in patency achieved by aspirin plus dipyridamole was offset, in the authors' view, by an increase in overall clinical rate, prompting their conclusion that dipyridamole does not improve overall clinical outcome following bypass surgery.

In summary, trials of 1-year patency of bypass grafts comparing dipyridamole and aspirin combined with aspirin alone have shown no consistent benefit of combined therapy except in grafts with distal vessels less than 1.5 mm in diameter. In these grafts, combined therapy may help prevent occlusion. However, anticoagulants also appear to prevent occlusion in distal vessels with diameters less than 1.5 mm and are comparable with aspirin plus dipyridamole. Preoperative and interoperative dipyridamole combined with aspirin begun preoperatively or 6 hours after operation appears to increase chest tube drainage and transfusion requirement, but not early reoperation or early mortality.

Beyond 1 month after operation, accelerated atherosclerosis of vein grafts predisposes to occlusion. Following initial endothelial disruption and injury at the time of surgery and damage due to increased shear forces of pulsatile arterial flow, perioperative mural thrombosis may occur.[85] Platelet deposition and secretion of growth and chemotactic factors for smooth muscle cells and leukocytes may promote graft smooth muscle proliferation and extracellular matrix synthesis, which is the main cause of graft occlusion between 1 and 12 months after operation.

Current Recommendations

Preoperative dipyridamole administration is of uncertain value and does not need to be routine. If patients have not been treated with aspirin preoperatively, start aspirin at 160 mg/day down the nasogastric tube 1 hour postoperatively and continue at 80 to 325 mg indefinitely. Low-dose aspirin may be adequate, although this has been addressed in only one large trial to date. Patients at high risk of graft occlusion (flow less than 40 ml/min or coronary artery luminal diameter less than 1.5 mm) should be considered for combination therapy with orally administered anticoagulant agents (begun on postoperative day 1) and low-dose aspirin (80 mg/day). Heparin may be administered at low dose in these high-risk patients to maintain the aPTT at just above normal in the recovery room and until the chest tubes are removed, when heparin dosage may be increased to prolong the aPTT to 1.5 to 2.0 times control until the prothrombin time is within range on warfarin (INR 3.0 to 4.5 times control). For high-risk patients intolerant of warfarin or at high risk of anticoagulant-induced bleeding, aspirin at 325 mg/day plus dipyridamole at 300 to 400 mg/day is reasonable. Although one trial has shown that the antiplatelet agent ticlopidine reduced graft occlusion by day 10, the delayed onset of action of this agent (2 to 4 days) and the lack of data regarding efficacy in high-risk grafts argues against its use in high-risk patients at present.

CORONARY ARTERY DISEASE/ISCHEMIC HEART DISEASE

Dipyridamole's effect of elevating plasma and myocardial adenosine levels has prompted research into the use of dipyridamole in ischemic heart disease and myocardial infarction, because adenosine has been shown to have diverse and beneficial myocardial protective effects.[15] Current understanding of the possible roles of adenosine in ischemic heart disease will be reviewed briefly followed by discussion of the trials to date of dipyridamole in ischemic heart disease.

Adenosine is a ubiquitous endogenous nucleoside produced continuously during myocardial ischemia by cardiomyocytes, primarily via the dephosphorylation of AMP to adenosine by cytosolic 5'-nucleotidase.[15] AMP is in turn derived from adenosine triphosphate (ATP), adenosine diphosphate (ADP), or cAMP. Adenosine is itself removed in three ways: phosphorylation to AMP by adenosine kinase, degradation to inosine by adenosine deaminase, or circulatory washout. Dipyridamole inhibits both the transport of adenosine across cell membranes and adenosine deaminase and thus increases adenosine concentrations in plasma, myocardial interstitium, and likely within cardiomyocytes.[12]

Both endogenous and exogenous adenosine provide myocardial protection during myocardial ischemia by multiple beneficial effects on myocardial metabolism, blood flow, microvascular function, infiltrating neutrophils, neutrophil toxic products, and the degree and extent of endothelial injury.[15] Because of these protective, homeostatic effects, adenosine has been called a "retaliatory" metabolite during ischemia.[100] Adenosine may ameliorate myocardial stunning and hasten functional recovery by decreasing free radical injury, increasing perfusion, and supplying substrate for ATP biosynthesis via the purine salvage pathway.[101] In most, but not all, studies in dogs, adenosine limits regional reperfusion injury, reduces infarct size, and increases myocardial salvage when experimental occlusion of the left anterior descending coronary artery is less than 3 hours old.[102] Adenosine may hasten recovery of ventricular performance following global ischemic injury, use of cardioplegia during cardiopulmonary bypass, or transplantation of stored donor hearts.[15] In animals, adenosine by itself appears to be an important mediator of ischemic preconditioning and limits resultant infarct size.[103, 104]

The cardioprotective effects of adenosine stem from multiple mechanisms. Following the consumption of ATP during ischemia, adenosine replenishes exhausted purine precursor pools and stimulates ATP biosynthesis via the purine salvage pathway.[101] Enhanced ATP formation has been shown in experimental animals with the infusion of adenosine. Adenosine increases total coronary blood flow via stimulation of coronary artery endothelium adenosine A_2 receptors and resultant coronary artery vasodilation.[105] In the presence of normal coronary arteries, subepicardial and subendocardial flow both increase. In the presence of obstructive coronary artery lesions, however, particularly if collateral channels are well developed, transmural "coronary steal" may result with subendocardial ischemia relative to the subepicardium. Adenosine inhibits norepinephrine release and attenuates the effects of released norepinephrine.[101] Adenosine enhances anaerobic glycolysis and diminishes myocardial oxygen demand. By promoting vasodilation in the microcirculation, inhibiting neutrophil chemotaxis, adhesion, and production of toxic superoxide anions, and inhibiting platelet aggregation and release of platelet-derived vasoconstrictors, adenosine mollifies endothelial injury in the microcirculation.[101] In dogs, adenosine attenuates markedly the pathologic ultrastructural changes in reperfused myocardial vascular beds.[102] Adenosine may also promote angiogenesis in rats.[106]

In view of these wide-ranging effects of adenosine, dipyridamole has been shown to limit reperfusion injury in some animal models.[15] However, the existence of myocardial reperfusion injury in humans is controversial and has yet to be clearly shown. In rabbits, dipyridamole has been shown to potentiate the myocardial infarct size–limiting effect of ischemic preconditioning.[107] However, none of these effects has yet been shown in humans.

Available trials of dipyridamole in ischemic heart disease are few except for two large, well-designed trials of dipyridamole alone in combination with aspirin in the secondary prevention of myocardial infarction.[60, 108] No trials of dipyridamole in asymptomatic coronary artery disease have been reported. The use of dipyridamole in stable angina pectoris has been reported in one small, double-blind, randomized, crossover trial of dipyridamole (75 mg three times a day) versus placebo for 2 weeks in 15 men.[61] The usual long-term orally administered antianginal agents were continued. No differences in frequency of self-reported angina, exercise performance, or ischemia as determined by ambulatory electrocardiography were found between groups. Large studies of dipyridamole in the secondary prevention of myocardial infarction and following coronary artery bypass have shown that dipyridamole does not decrease the frequency or severity of angina when combined with aspirin or the usual antianginal medications. No evidence thus supports the use of dipyridamole to decrease angina or improve exercise tolerance in coronary artery disease. This is not surprising, because adenosine and dipyridamole may invoke a phenomenon of coronary artery "steal" in the setting of epicardial coronary artery disease.[11] Theophylline, a nonselective adenosine antagonist, and bamifylline, a selective adenosine A_1 antagonist, have both been shown in small studies to improve exercise duration, time to angina, and time to ST depression in patients with known coronary artery disease, presumably by decreasing transmural "steal" and relative subendocardial ischemia.[62, 109] No studies of dipyridamole in unstable angina have appeared.

An early randomized trial of dipyridamole (100 mg four times a day) versus placebo for 28 days following myocardial infarction in 103 patients, 75% of whom began treatment within 3 days of infarction, showed no benefit of dipyridamole.[108] These patients were not treated with anticoagulant agents or aspirin. In the current era of thrombolytic therapy, a trial of intravenously administered heparin with orally administered aspirin and dipyridamole following t-PA administration for acute myocardial infarction randomized patients to 7 to 10 days of heparin following t-PA or 24 hours of heparin followed by aspirin (300 mg/day) and dipyridamole (300 mg/day).[110] At 7 to 10 days, the infarct-related artery was patent in 80.2% of the aspirin plus dipyridamole group. Although no studies of conjunctive antithrombotic therapy following lytic therapy have randomized patients to aspirin versus aspirin plus dipyridamole, this patency rate of aspirin plus dipyridamole is similar to patency rates reported with aspirin alone following thrombolytic therapy.[111] Because thrombolysis activates platelets (likely via the generation of thrombin), antiplatelet therapy with aspirin is currently recommended as conjunctive therapy following thrombolysis.[111] The role of dipyridamole in combination with aspirin following thrombolysis is not yet settled.

Pilot studies have appeared suggesting that dipyridamole via its effects on adenosine metabolism may improve recovery of ventricular function when given by intravenous infusion during thrombolysis. In one study, 174 patients undergoing thrombolysis within 6 hours of onset of myocardial infarction were randomized following t-PA and heparin to placebo or dipyridamole (400 mg/day intravenously followed by 300 mg/day orally).[112] At 1 month, left ventricular ejection fraction, left ventricular end-diastolic pressure, and regional wall motion in the infarct zone were all significantly improved in those with complete occlusion or residual stenosis greater than 50% of the infarct-related artery in the dipyridamole-treated group. No differences were found in patients with residual stenosis of less than 50%. There was a statistically insignificant trend toward lower mortality and serious arrhythmias but higher bleeding complications in the dipyridamole group, although dipyridamole appeared to be safe during thrombolysis. Further large studies are needed to corroborate this preliminary finding and establish dipyridamole's safety during acute infarction before it can be recommended.

Dipyridamole has been most thoroughly studied in the secondary prevention of myocardial infarction. Two large trials, both from the PARIS research group, have examined the efficacy of aspirin, with or without dipyridamole, in the secondary prevention of myocardial infarction.[60, 108] In PARIS I, 2026 patients were randomized to one of three groups: aspirin (324 mg three times a day) plus dipyridamole (75 mg three times a day, n = 810), aspirin alone (324 mg three times a day, n = 810), or placebo (n = 406). Patients entered the study between 8 weeks and 5 years after a Q-wave or non–Q wave infarction and were followed up for an average of 41 months. Comparing the groups taking aspirin plus dipyridamole or aspirin alone with the group receiving placebo, the total mortality rate was reduced by 16% and 18%, the coronary mortality rate by 24% and 21%, and the rate of nonfatal myocardial infarction combined with fatal coronary disease by 25% and 24%, respectively. None of these reductions were statistically significant, in part because the smaller placebo group reduced the statistical power of the study. Although gastrointestinal side effects were significantly more frequent in both groups receiving aspirin, these effects were not increased in those also taking dipyridamole. Headache was the only side effect more common in the combined treatment group.

PARIS II compared dipyridamole plus aspirin (in a dose similar to that of PARIS I) with placebo in 3128 patients. Patients were randomized earlier, 4 weeks to 4 months following their infarct, and followed up for 2 years. Coronary events were significantly reduced (24%), but coronary mortality and total mortality showed only a small, nonsignificant reduction (6% and 3%, respectively). A group randomized to either aspirin or dipyridamole alone was not included in this study.

Pooled analyses of trials of aspirin with large groups of patients and doses ranging from 300 to 1500 mg/day clearly show that antiplatelet therapy with aspirin reduces cardiovascular end points by 15% to 25%.[39, 113] This reduction is the same order of magnitude seen with combined aspirin and dipyridamole treatment in the two PARIS studies. Further, both active treatment groups in PARIS I showed a similar reduction in cardiac end points.

Current Recommendations

There is no convincing evidence that dipyridamole confers additional therapeutic benefit when combined with aspirin compared with aspirin alone in the therapy of asymptomatic coronary artery disease, chronic stable angina pectoris, unstable angina pectoris, or acute myocardial infarction or in the secondary prevention of myocardial infarction. Future studies are necessary to evaluate the possible role of dipyridamole in infarct size limitation, myocardial salvage, and preservation of ventricular function in the presence of persistently occluded infarct-related arteries as suggested by small animal studies and pilot studies in humans.

PERCUTANEOUS TRANSLUMINAL CORONARY ANGIOPLASTY

Successful acute dilatation of a coronary artery stenosis by percutaneous transluminal coronary angioplasty (PTCA) may result from one of four mechanisms: tearing, fracturing, or cracking of the atherosclerotic plaque; dissection of the intima with extension into the media and production of an intimal flap; redistribution and compression of plaque; or distention and stretching of the disease-free arc of the vessel.[114] In human subjects, angioscopy immediately following angioplasty shows intimal disruption and dissection, clefts in atheromas, and adherent mural thrombus in nearly all dilated arteries.[115] Postmortem studies in animals and humans following angioplasty reveal endothelial denudation, dissection, plaque disruption, and a high incidence of platelet-rich mural thrombus within hours. Mural thrombus results from the exposure of several profoundly thrombogenic substrates, including subendothelial collagen, tissue factor, elastic tissue, and smooth muscle cells, by deep arterial injury and fatty gruel by plaque disruption. The amount of platelet deposition, which largely determines the size of the resultant thrombus, is determined by the depth of arterial injury and arterial shear forces. Mural thrombosis formation is responsible for most of the up to 5% incidence of abrupt occlusion following angioplasty. Preprocedure platelet activation predicts abrupt occlusion.[116]

Given the intense stimuli present for platelet adhesion, activation, and aggregation following deep arterial injury during angioplasty, it is not surprising that in experimental porcine models, preprocedure antiplatelet therapy with aspirin plus dipyridamole alone or preprocedure antiplatelet therapy combined with heparin reduces but does not inhibit platelet adhesion or mural thrombus formation on deeply injured arteries.[25, 117–120] In these models, dipyridamole alone does not reduce platelet deposition of the formation of mural thrombus. The combination of high-dose aspirin (20 mg/kg/day) with dipyridamole (100 mg intravenously during 90 minutes) was no better than low-dose aspirin (1 mg/kg/day) in the prevention of mural thrombosis.[25, 118] Thus, no data in animals support dipyridamole's role in preventing platelet adhesion of mural thrombus formation following angioplasty.

Antiplatelet therapy, however, has been unquestionably shown to decrease the incidence of abrupt occlusion following angioplasty. A retrospective analysis of 300 patients undergoing successful angioplasty found that, compared with patients receiving no antiplatelet therapy, the combination of aspirin and dipyridamole reduced the incidence of thrombus formation and the need for emergency revascularization surgery.[121] Patients receiving either aspirin or dipyridamole alone showed an intermediate benefit, but numbers in both groups were small, and neither drug alone yielded results significantly different from those of either placebo or the combined treatment. The benefit of antiplatelet therapy in reducing acute occlusion

following angioplasty in this retrospective study was confirmed in a randomized, double-blind trial comparing placebo with aspirin (330 mg twice or three times a day) plus dipyridamole (75 mg three times a day) begun 24 hours prior to angioplasty.[122] The periprocedural Q-wave myocardial infarction rate in these 376 patients was significantly reduced in the active treatment group (6.9% versus 1.6%, $p = .0113$), as was the incidence of acute occlusion and the need for early revascularization. In the 249 patients who underwent follow-up angiography at 4 to 7 months, there was no difference in restenosis rates (33.7% versus 38.6%, respectively). A subsequent study showed that aspirin alone achieves comparable reductions in rates of acute occlusion. Lembo et al.[123] randomized 232 patients to either aspirin (325 mg three times a day) or aspirin (325 mg) plus dipyridamole (75 mg three times a day); 87% received at least one dose before PTCA. The results were not analyzed on an intention-to-treat basis. Rates of acute complications comparing the aspirin alone and aspirin plus dipyridamole groups were as follows: Q-wave myocardial infarction, 1.7% versus 4.3% ($p = .24$); emergency coronary artery bypass surgery, 2.6% versus 6.1% ($p = .19$); death, 0% versus 1% ($p = .31$).

No studies have shown a decrease in restenosis at 6 months following angioplasty with aspirin plus dipyridamole or aspirin alone.[47, 124] In a randomized, double-blind, placebo-controlled trial in 207 patients, Chesebro et al.[125] found no difference in restenosis at 6-month follow-up angiography in 85% of patients with aspirin (325 mg/day) plus dipyridamole (100 mg three times a day) begun 1 day prior to angioplasty versus placebo. In a randomized, double-blind, placebo-controlled trial in 236 patients, White et al.[126] found no difference in restenosis at 6-month follow-up angiography in 75% of patients with either aspirin (325 mg twice a day) plus dipyridamole (75 mg three times a day) or ticlopidine (250 mg three times a day) begun 4 to 5 days before angioplasty versus placebo. In a small trial (n = 72) lacking a placebo control group, Okamoto et al.[127] randomized patients to either aspirin (300 mg/day) plus dipyridamole (150 mg/day) or trapidil (600 mg/day), a platelet-derived growth factor inhibitor. Follow-up angiography in all patients showed restenosis (defined as loss of 50% gain following angioplasty) in 41.7% and 19.4% of the aspirin plus dipyridamole and trapidil groups, respectively ($p < .05$). Although the rates of restenosis in the latter trial in the aspirin-dipyridamole group are comparable to those of other trials, the trial suffers from the same limitations as most of the extant clinical trials of pharmacologic agents in preventing restenosis: small sample size, inconstant dosing and duration of preprocedure regimens, varying definitions of angiographic restenosis, and lack of biochemical validation of antiplatelet effects.[124]

Current Recommendations

No convincing data show that dipyridamole decreases either acute occlusion or chronic restenosis following angioplasty. Because antiplatelet therapy clearly decreases the rate of acute occlusion following angioplasty, patients should commence aspirin alone (325 mg/day) on at least the day prior to angioplasty and receive intravenously administered heparin for 16 to 24 hours after angioplasty. Because aspirin has been shown to aid in the secondary prevention of myocardial infarction in high-risk patients, such as those undergoing angioplasty, aspirin should be continued indefinitely in these patients.

CEREBROVASCULAR DISEASE

A number of studies have examined the role of antiplatelet therapy in the secondary prevention of transient ischemic attacks (TIAs) or strokes.[47, 128] The four largest trials of aspirin following TIA or minor stroke showed a 20% to 50% reduction in the incidence of recurrent stroke. Of the more than 10 randomized, placebo-controlled trials reported, only two have failed to show benefit from aspirin. Meta-analysis by the Antiplatelet Trialists' Collaboration showed a 22% reduction in stroke with aspirin following TIA or minor stroke.[39] Although the role for aspirin in acute stroke remains to be established, it is clear that aspirin is efficacious in the secondary prevention of stroke in patients with TIAs or previous minor stroke. Aspirin has not been shown to decrease the incidence of cardiogenic embolic stroke conclusively, and its role in nonvalvular atrial fibrillation is still controversial.[47] Ticlopidine has been shown in several trials to be effective in the secondary prevention of stroke and is superior to aspirin in patients with TIAs.[39, 47] Ticlopidine's greater cost, gastrointestinal side effects, 10% elevation in serum cholesterol levels, and 1% to 2% risk of neutropenia render it second-line therapy for patients intolerant of aspirin.[47]

No study has demonstrated the benefit of dipyridamole alone or the combination of dipyridamole plus aspirin in the secondary prevention of ischemic stroke compared with aspirin alone. The European Stroke Prevention Study (ESPS) randomized 2500 patients with either complete stroke (60%), TIA (33%), or reversible ischemic neurologic deficit (6%) to aspirin (325 mg three times a day) plus dipyridamole (75 mg three times a day) or placebo.[129] At 2-year follow-up, there was a 33% reduction in event rate (stroke and death) and 31% reduction in mortality in the treatment group. Though an aspirin-alone group was not included in the study, the results of the ESPS study are similar to subsequent studies of aspirin alone. Two French studies compared aspirin plus dipyridamole with aspirin alone and with placebo in patients with cerebral ischemic events. The Accidents Ischemiques Cerebraux Lies a l'Atherosclerose study randomized 604 patients, 84% of whom had suffered a completed stroke.[130] At the end of 3 years of follow-up, the rate of fatal and nonfatal cerebral infarcts for both treated groups was 10.5%, significantly lower than the 18% rate of the placebo group. The second French study had a similar design and also showed no reduction in cerebral events in those receiving

dipyridamole over and above that seen with aspirin.[131] The American-Canadian Cooperative Study Group trial randomized 890 patients with carotid-territory TIAs to aspirin (325 mg four times a day) plus dipyridamole (75 mg four times a day) or aspirin (325 mg four times a day) plus placebo.[132] At mean 2-year follow-up, no difference was observed between the two groups in the cumulative relative risk of either fatal or nonfatal stroke (RR = 1.02, CI_{95} 0.77 to 1.35) by life-table analysis. Thus, there is no evidence that dipyridamole combined with aspirin is more effective than aspirin alone in the secondary prevention of stroke. Dipyridamole has not been studied in the primary prevention of stroke or during the acute phase of stroke.

Although preliminary data from the North American Symptomatic Carotid Endarterectomy Trial suggest that high-dose aspirin (1300 mg/day) may prevent ipsilateral stroke following carotid endarterectomy, there are as yet no conclusive data that antiplatelet therapy following recurrent stenosis of the endarterectomized carotid artery is efficacious.[133] Relatively high-dose (650 mg twice a day), but not low-dose (50 to 100 mg four times a day), aspirin has been shown to decrease combined TIA, stroke, retinal hemorrhage, and death from stroke. A small study of 163 patients randomized to aspirin (325 mg three times a day) plus dipyridamole (75 mg three times a day) or placebo failed to show that aspirin plus dipyridamole decreased recurrent stenosis following carotid endarterectomy as detected by duplex ultrasound studies.[134]

Current Recommendations

There is no evidence that dipyridamole alone or in combination with aspirin aids the secondary prevention of stroke or prevention of recurrent restenosis following carotid endarterectomy compared with aspirin alone. Dipyridamole has not been studied in acute stroke.

PERIPHERAL VASCULAR DISEASE

There is as yet no definitive evidence that antithrombotic therapy influences the natural history of peripheral vascular disease, although ticlopidine may relieve symptoms and improve walking distance in patients with intermittent claudication.[76] Meta-analysis shows that antiplatelet therapy with aspirin reduces vascular mortality by 15% ($p < .0003$) and nonfatal stroke and myocardial infarction by 30% ($p < .0001$) in patients with peripheral vascular disease.[39] In a placebo-controlled trial of aspirin plus dipyridamole versus aspirin plus placebo in patients with peripheral vascular disease, serial angiography at 2 years showed reduced disease progression in the aspirin plus dipyridamole group.[135] This trial has been criticized, however, because of worse baseline disease in the aspirin-placebo group. Small studies have shown that indium-111–labeled platelet deposition is reduced by aspirin plus dipyridamole but not by either agent alone.[136, 137] Combined aspirin plus dipyridamole has also been shown to reduce early reocclusion in some, but not all, studies of peripheral arterial reconstructive surgery.[76]

Current Recommendations

There is no definite evidence to show that dipyridamole is efficacious either alone or combined with aspirin in the therapy of peripheral vascular disease, except possibly in patients with underlying arterial reconstructive surgery with prosthetic graft materials, as discussed previously.

SUMMARY

Animal models of thrombosis suggest that dipyridamole is most effective in preventing thrombosis on prosthetic surfaces. Clinical trials support this finding; the most consistent benefit is shown when dipyridamole is combined with warfarin to prevent thromboembolism from prosthetic heart valves. Dipyridamole has been approved by the FDA for this use. Therapy should begin with 50 mg four times a day on the first postoperative day and should increase to 100 mg four times a day (or 5 to 6 mg/kg per day in four divided doses in patients weighing less than 60 kg). The safety and efficacy of low-dose aspirin in combination with warfarin to prevent thromboembolism from mechanical prosthetic valves may supplant the combination of dipyridamole with warfarin in high-risk patients.

Although dipyridamole inhibits platelet interaction with the heart-lung bypass machine during coronary artery bypass graft operations, its routine perioperative use is not recommended. Similarly, although dipyridamole may reduce platelet deposition on peripheral arterial synthetic bypass grafts, it has not yet been clearly shown to prevent prosthetic graft occlusion, except in grafts with low flow and small distal anastomoses.

Headache and nausea from dipyridamole can be ameliorated by administering the drug after meals to slow absorption. The vasodilating effect can be rapidly reversed by intravenously administered aminophylline (100 mg) should the rare side effect of angina occur.

REFERENCES

1. Best L, McGuire M, Jones P, et al: Mode of action of dipyridamole on human platelets. Thromb Res 16:367, 1979.
2. McElroy F, Philp R: Relative potencies of dipyridamole and related agents as inhibitors of cyclic nucleotide phosphodiesterases: Possible explanation of mechanism of inhibition of platelet function. Life Sci 17:1479, 1975.
3. Mills D: The role of cyclic nucleotides in platelets. In Kebabian JW, Nathanson JA (eds): Cyclic Nucleotides: Part II: Physiology and Pharmacology. Berlin: Springer-Verlag, 1982, pp 723–761.
4. Masotti G, Pogessi L, Galanti G, et al: Stimulation of prostacyclin by dipyridamole. Lancet 1:1412, 1979.
5. Mehta J, Mehta P, Pepine C, et al: Platelet function studies in coronary artery disease: Effect of dipyridamole. Am J Cardiol 47:1111, 1981.
6. Moncada S, Korbut R: Dipyridamole and other phosphodiesterase inhibitors act as antithrombotic agents by potentiating endogenous prostacyclin. Lancet 1:1286, 1978.
7. Van de Velde V, Blut H, Weisenberger H, et al: Dipyridamole stimulates prostacyclin production in isolated rat aortic tissue. Arch Int Pharmacodyn Ther 256:327, 1982.
8. Fitzgerald G: Dipyridamole. N Engl J Med 316:1247, 1987.
9. Schrader J, Berne R, Rubio R: Uptake and metabolism of adenosine by human erythrocyte ghosts. Am J Physiol 223:159, 1972.
10. Dawicki D, Agarwal K, Parks R: Role of adenosine uptake and metabolism by blood cells in the antiplatelet actions of dipyridamole, dilazep, and nitrobenzylthioinosine. Biochem Pharmacol 34:3965, 1985.
11. Verani M: Pharmacologic stress myocardial perfusion imaging. Curr Prob Cardiol 18:481, 1993.
12. Wang T, Mentzer R, Van Wylen D: Interstitial adenosine with dipyridamole: Effect on adenosine receptor blockade and adenosine deaminase. Am J Physiol 263:H552, 1992.
13. German D, Kredich N, Bjornsson T: Oral dipyridamole increases plasma adenosine levels in human beings. Clin Pharmacol Ther 45:80, 1989.
14. Kitakaze M, Hori M, Sato H, et al: Endogenous adenosine inhibits platelet aggregation during myocardial ischemia in dogs. Circ Res 69:1402, 1991.
15. Ely S, Berne R: Protective effects of adenosine in myocardial ischemia. Circulation 85:893, 1992.
16. Bult H, Fret H, Jordaens F, et al: Dipyridamole potentiates platelet inhibition by nitric oxide. Thromb Haemos 66:343, 1991.
17. Bult H, Fret H, Jordaens F, et al: Dipyridamole potentiates the anti-aggregating and vasodilator activity of nitric oxide. Eur J Pharmacol 199:1, 1991.
18. Radomski M, Moncada S: Regulation of vascular homeostasis by nitric oxide. Thromb Haemos 70:36, 1993.
19. Graaf J, Banga J, Moncada S, et al: Nitric oxide functions as an inhibitor of platelet adhesion under flow conditions. Circulation 85:2284, 1992.
20. de la Cruz J, Garcia P, Sanchez de la Cuesta F: Dipyridamole inhibits platelet aggregation induced by oxygen-derived free radicals. Thromb Res 66:277, 1992.
21. Saniabadi A, Tomiak R, Lowe R, et al: Dipyridamole inhibits red cell-induced platelet activation. Atherosclerosis 76:149, 1989.
22. Saniabadi A, Fisher T, McLaren M, et al: Effect of dipyridamole alone and in combination with aspirin on whole blood platelet aggregation, PGI2 generation, and red cell deformability ex vivo in humans. Cardiovasc Res 25:177, 1991.
23. Saniabadi A, Fisher T, Lau S, et al: Dipyridamole increases human red blood cell deformability. Eur J Clin Pharmacol 42:651, 1992.
24. Saniabadi A, Fisher T, Rimmer A, et al: A study of dipyridamole on erythrocyte deformability using an improved filtration technique. Clinical Hemorrheology 10:263, 1990.
25. Steele P, Chesebro J, Fuster V: The natural history of arterial balloon angioplasty in pigs and intervention with platelet-inhibitor therapy: Implications for clinical trials [abstract]. Clin Res 32:209A, 1984.
26. Folts J, Rowe G: Dipyridamole alone or with low-dose aspirin does not inhibit thrombus formation in stenosed canine coronary arteries nor does it protect against renewal of thrombus formation by epinephrine. J Vasc Med Biol 4:225, 1989.
27. Stein P, Alpert J, Copeland J, et al: Antithrombotic therapy in patients with mechanical and biological prosthetic heart valves. Chest 102(Suppl 4):445S, 1992.
28. Harker L, Fuster V: Pharmacology of platelet inhibitors. J Am Coll Cardiol 8:21B, 1986.
29. Gregov D, Jenkins A, Duncan E: Dipyridamole: Pharmacokinetics and effects on aspects of platelet function in humans. Br J Clin Pharmacol 34:3965, 1987.
30. Fujitam R, Merdestgaard A, Marcus C, et al: Perioperative suppression of platelet adherence to small-diameter polytetrafluoroethylene grafts. J Surg Res 44:455, 1988.
31. McDaniel M, Huntsman W, Mett T, et al: Effect of a selective thromboxane synthase inhibitor on arterial graft patency and platelet deposition in dogs. Arch Surg 122:887, 1987.

32. Pumphrey C, Fuster V, Dewanjee M, et al: Comparison of the antithrombotic action of calcium antagonist drugs with dipyridamole in dogs. Am J Cardiol 51:591, 1983.

33. Hanson S, Harker L, Bjornsson T: Effect of platelet-modifying drugs on arterial thromboembolism in baboons. Aspirin potentiated the antithrombotic actions of dipyridamole and sulfinpyrazone by mechanism(s) independent of platelet cyclooxygenase inhibition. J Clin Invest 75:1591, 1985.

34. Harker L, Slichter S: Studies of platelet and fibrinogen kinetics in patients with prosthetic heart valves. N Engl J Med 283:534, 1970.

35. Harker L, Slichter S: Studies of platelet and fibrinogen kinetics in patients with prosthetic heart valves. N Engl J Med 283:1302, 1970.

36. Harker L, Slichter S: Platelet and fibrinogen consumption in humans. N Engl J Med 287:999, 1972.

37. Schbath J, Boissel J, Mathy B, et al: Drugs effect on platelet-survival times: Comparison of two pyrimido-pyrimidine derivatives in patients with aortic or mitral replacement. Thromb Haemos 51:45, 1984.

38. Theo K, Christakis G, Weisel R, et al: Dipyridamole preserved platelets and reduced blood loss after cardiopulmonary bypass. J Thorac Cardiovasc Surg 96:322, 1988.

39. Collaboration AT: Collaborative overview of randomized trials of antiplatelet therapy. Br Med J 308:81, 159, 235, 1994.

40. Dresse A, Chevolet C, Delapierre D, et al: Pharmacokinetics of oral dipyridamole (Persantine) and its effect on platelet adenosine uptake in humans. Eur J Clin Pharmacol 23:229, 1982.

41. Beisenhertz G, Koss F, Schule A, et al: Das Schicksal des 2,6-Bis(diathanolamino)-4, 8-dipiperidino-pyrimido (5,4-d)-pyrimidinum menschlichen und tierischen Organismus. Arzneimittelforshung 10:307, 1960.

42. Mahony C, Wolfram K, Cocchetto D, et al: Dipyridamole kinetics. Clin Pharmacol Ther 31:330, 1982.

43. Mahoney C, Cox J, Bjornsson T: Plasma dipyridamole concentrations after two different dosage regimens in patients. J Clin Pharmacol 23:123, 1983.

44. Buchanan M, Rosenfeld J, Gent M, et al: Increased dipyridamole plasma concentrations associated with salicylate administration: Relationship to effects on platelet aggregation in vivo. Thromb Res 15:813, 1979.

45. Nitelius E, Melander A, Wahlin-Boll E: Pharmacokinetic interaction of acetylsalicylic acid and dipyridamole. Br J Clin Pharmacol 19:379, 1985.

46. Rosenfeld J, Buchanan M, Reilly P, et al: Dipyridamole disposition after chronic administration: Effect of aspirin. Thromb Res 4(Suppl):317, 1983.

47. Fuster V, Dyken M, Vokonas P, et al: Aspirin as a therapeutic agent in cardiovascular disease. Circulation 87:659, 1993.

48. Barker M: Clinical use of adenosine for arrhythmias. Coronary Art Disease 3:1127, 1992.

49. Pelleg A: Mechanisms of action and the therapeutic potential of adenosine and its analogues in the treatment of cardiac arrhythmias. Coronary Art Dis 4:109, 1993.

50. Watt A, Bernard M, Webster J, et al: Intravenous adenosine in the treatment of supraventricular tachycardia: A dose-ranging study and interaction with dipyridamole. Br J Clin Pharmacol 21:227, 1986.

51. Lerman B, Wesley R, Belardinelli L: Electrophysiologic effects of dipyridamole on atrioventricular nodal conduction and supraventricular tachycardia: Role of endogenous adenosine. Circulation 80:1536, 1989.

52. Hirsh J, Fuster V, Salzman E: Antiplatelet agents: The relationship among dose, side effects, and antithrombotic effectiveness. Chest 89(Suppl):4S, 1986.

53. Stein B, Fuster V: Pharmacology of platelet inhibitors. In Fuster V, Verstraete M (eds): Thrombosis in Cardiovascular Disorders. Philadelphia: WB Saunders, 1992.

54. Keltz T, Innerfield M, Gitler B, et al: Dipyridamole-induced myocardial ischemia. JAMA 257:1515, 1987.

55. Feldman R, Nichols W, Pepine C, et al: Acute effect of intravenous dipyridamole on regional coronary hemodynamics and metabolism. Circulation 64:333, 1981.

56. Homma S, Callahan R, Ameer B, et al: Usefulness of oral dipyridamole suspension for stress thallium imaging without exercise in the detection of coronary artery disease. Am J Cardiol 57:503, 1986.

57. Chesebro J, Clements I, Fuster V, et al: A platelet inhibitor drug trial in coronary artery bypass operations. Benefit of perioperative dipyridamole and aspirin therapy on early postoperative vein-graft patency. N Engl J Med 307:73, 1982.

58. Chesebro J, Fuster V, Elveback L: Effect of dipyridamole and aspirin on late vein-graft patency after coronary bypass operations. N Engl J Med 310:209, 1984.

59. Chesebro J, Fuster V, Elveback L: Reply to letter to the editor. N Engl J Med 310:1534, 1984.

60. Persantine-Aspirin Reinfarction Study Research Group: Persantine and aspirin in coronary heart disease. Circulation 62:449, 1980.

61. Barbour M, Garber C, Agarwal K: Effect of dipyridamole therapy on myocardial ischemia in patients with stable angina pectoris receiving concurrent anti-ischemic therapy. Am J Cardiol 69:449, 1992.

62. Barbour M, Garber C, Ahlberg A, et al: Effects of intravenous theophylline on exercise-induced myocardial ischemia: II. A concentration-dependent phenomenon. J Am Coll Cardiol 22:1155, 1993.

63. Chesebro J, Fuster V: Valvular heart disease and prosthetic heart valves in thrombosis. In Fuster V, Verstraete M (eds): Cardiovascular Disorders. Philadelphia: WB Saunders, 1992.

64. Dewanjee M, Trastek V, Tago M, et al: Radio-isotopic techniques for noninvasive detection of platelet deposition in bovine tissue mitral-valve prosthesis and in vitro quantification of visceral microembolism in dogs. Invest Radiol 6:535, 1983.

65. Fuster V, Pumphrey C, McGoon M, et al: Systemic thromboembolism in mitral and aortic Starr-Edwards prostheses. A 10-19 year follow-up. Circulation 66(Suppl I):157, 1982.

66. Myers M, Lawrie G, Crawford E, et al: The St. Jude prosthesis: Analysis of the clinical results in 815 implants and the need for systemic anticoagulation. J Am Coll Cardiol 13:57, 1989.

67. Chesebro J, Fuster V, McGoon D, et al: Trial of combined warfarin plus dipyridamole or aspirin therapy in prosthetic heart valve replacement: Danger of aspirin compared with dipyridamole. Am J Cardiol 51:1537, 1983.

68. Bjork V, Henze A: Ten years' experience with the Bjork-Shiley tilting disk valve. J Thorac Cardiovasc Surg 78:331, 1979.

69. Groupe de Recherche PACTE: Prevention des accidents thromboemboliques systemiques chez les proteurs de prothesis valvulaires artificielles; essai cooperatif controle du dipyridamole. Coeur 9:915, 1978.

70. Kasahara T: Clinical effect of dipyridamole ingestion after prosthetic heart valve replacement-especially on the blood coagulation system. J Jpn Assoc Thorac Surg 25:1007, 1977.

71. Rajah J, Sreeharan N, Joseph A, et al: A prospective trial of dipyridamole and warfarin in heart valve patients. Acta Therapeutica 6(Suppl 93):54, 1980.

72. Sullivan J, Harker D, Gorlin R: Pharmacologic control of the thromboembolic complications of cardiac-valve replacement. N Engl J Med 284:1391, 1971.

73. Ranhosky A: Dipyridamole. N Engl J Med 317:1734, 1987.

74. Turpie A, Gent M, Laupacis A, et al: A comparison of aspirin with placebo in patients treated with warfarin after heart-valve replacement. N Engl J Med 329:524, 1993.

75. Veith F, Gupta S, Ascer E, et al: Six-year prospective multicenter randomized comparison of autologous saphenous vein and expanded polytetrafluoroethylene grafts in infra-inguinal arterial reconstructions. J Vasc Surg 3:104, 1986.

76. Clagett G, Graor R, Salzman E: Antithrombotic therapy in peripheral arterial occlusive disease. Chest 102(Suppl 4):516S, 1992.

77. Stratton J, Ritchie J: Reduction of indium-111 platelet deposition on Dacron vascular grafts in humans by aspirin plus dipyridamole. Circulation 73:325, 1986.

78. Rosenthal D, Mittenthal M, Ruben D, et al: The effects of aspirin, dipyridamole, and warfarin in femorodistal reconstruction: Long-term results. Am Surg 53:477, 1987.

79. Pumphrey C, Chesebro J, Dewanjee M, et al: In vivo quantification of platelet deposition on human peripheral arterial bypass grafts using indium-111-labeled platelets. Am J Cardiol 51:796, 1983.

80. Goldman M, Hall H, Dyken J, et al: Does 111-indium platelet-deposition predict patency in prosthetic arterial grafts? Br J Surg 70:635, 1983.

81. Clyne C, Archer T, Atuhaire L, et al: Random control trial of a short course of aspirin and dipyridamole (Persantin) for femorodistal grafts. Br J Surg 74:246, 1987.

82. McCollum K, Alexander C, Kenchington G, et al: Antiplatelet drugs in femoropliteal vein bypasses: A multicenter trial. Surgery 13:150, 1991.

83. Kohler T, Kaufman J, Kocoyanis G, et al: Effect of aspirin and dipyridamole on the patency of lower extremity bypass grafts. Surgery 96:462, 1984.

84. Green R, Roedersheimer R, De Weese J: Effects of aspirin and dipyridamole on expanded polytetrafluoroethylene graft patency. Surgery 92:1016, 1982.

85. Chesebro J, Goldman S: Coronary artery bypass surgery: Antithrombotic therapy. In Fuster V, Verstraete M (eds): Thrombosis in Cardiovascular Disorders. Philadelphia: WB Saunders, 1992.

86. Fuster V, Chesebro J: Role of platelets and platelet inhibitors in aortocoronary artery vein-graft disease. Circulation 2:227, 1986.

87. Fuster V, Dewanjee M, Kaye M, et al: Noninvasive radioisotope technique for detection of platelet deposition in coronary artery bypass grafts in dogs and its reduction with platelet inhibitors. Circulation 60:1508, 1979.

88. Bulkley B, Hutchins G: Pathology of coronary artery bypass graft surgery. Arch Pathol Lab Med 102:273, 1978.

89. Feinberg H, Rosenbaum D, Levitsky S, et al: Platelet deposition after surgically induced myocardial ischemia: An etiologic factor for reperfusion injury. J Thorac Cardiovasc Surg 84:815, 1982.

90. Nuntinsen L, Pihlajaniemi R, Saarela E, et al: The effect of dipyridamole on the thrombocyte count and bleeding tendency in open-heart surgery. J Thorac Cardiovasc Surg 74:295, 1977.

91. Teoh K, Christakis G, Weisel R, et al: Prevention of myocardial platelet deposition and thromboxane release with dipyridamole. Circulation 74(Suppl III):145, 1986.

92. Teoh K, Christakis C, Weisel R, et al: Blood conservation with membrane oxygenators and dipyridamole. Ann Thorac Surg 44:40, 1987.

93. Ekestrom S, Gunnes S, Brodin V: Effect of dipyridamole on blood flow and patency of aortocoronary vein bypass grafts. Scand J Thorac Cardiovasc Surg 24:191, 1990.

94. Brown B, Cukingnan R, De Rouen T, et al: Improved graft patency in patients treated with platelet-inhibiting therapy after coronary artery bypass surgery. Circulation 72:138, 1985.

95. Goldman S, Copeland J, Moritz T, et al: Improvement in early saphenous vein graft patency after coronary artery bypass surgery with antiplatelet therapy: Results of a Veterans Administration Cooperative Study. Circulation 77:1324, 1988.

96. Goldman S, Copeland J, Moritz T, et al: Saphenous vein graft patency 1 year after coronary artery bypass surgery and effects of antiplatelet therapy: Results of a Veterans Administration Cooperative Study. Circulation 80:1190, 1989.

97. Agnew T, French J, Neutze J, et al: The role of dipyridamole in addition to low-dose aspirin in the prevention of occlusion of coronary artery bypass grafts. Aust N Z J Med 22:665, 1992.

98. Sanz G, Pajaron A, Alegria E, et al: Prevention of early aortocoronary bypass occlusion by low-dose aspirin and dipyridamole. Circulation 82:765, 1990.

99. van der Meer J, Hillege H, Kootstra G, et al: Prevention of one-year vein-graft occlusion after aortocoronary bypass surgery: A comparison of low-dose aspirin, low-dose aspirin plus dipyridamole, and oral anticoagulants. Lancet 342:257, 1993.

100. Newby A, Worku Y, Meghji P, et al: Adenosine: A retaliatory metabolite or not? News Physiol Sci 56:67, 1990.

101. Forman M, Velasco C, Vitola J, et al: Salvage of ischemic myocardium after reperfusion with adenosine. Coronary Artery Disease 3:1135, 1992.

102. Babbitt D, Virmani R, Foman M: Intracoronary adenosine administered after reperfusion limits vascular injury after prolonged ischemia in the canine model. Circulation 80:1388, 1989.

103. Mullane K: Myocardial preconditioning: Part of the adenosine revival. Circulation 85:845, 1992.

104. Thornton J, Liu G, Olsson R, et al: Intravenous pretreatment with an alpha-1 selective adenosine analogue protects the heart against infarction. Circulation 85:659, 1992.

105. Belarinelli L, Linden J, Berne R: The cardiac effects of adenosine. Prog Cardiovasc Dis 32:73, 1989.

106. Meininger C, Schelling M, Granger H: Adenosine and hypoxia stimulate proliferation and migration of endothelial cells. Am J Physiol 255:H554, 1988.

107. Miura T, Ogawa T, Iwamoto T, et al: Dipyridamole potentiates the myocardial infarct-size limiting effect of ischemic preconditioning. Circulation 86:979, 1992.

108. Klimt C, Knatterud G, Stamler J, et al: Persantine-aspirin reinfarction study. Part II. Secondary coronary prevention with persantine and aspirin. J Am Coll Cardiol 7:251, 1986.

109. Gaspardone A, Crea R, Iamele M, et al: Bamiphylline improves exercise-induced myocardial ischemia through a novel mechanism of action. Circulation 88:502, 1993.

110. Thompson P, Aylward P, Federman J, et al: A randomized comparison of intravenous heparin with oral aspirin and dipyridamole 24 hours after recombinant tissue-type plasminogen activator for acute myocardial infarction. Circulation 83:1534, 1991.

111. Anderson H, Willerson J: Thrombolysis in acute myocardial infarction. N Engl J Med 329:703, 1993.

112. Rousseau M, van Eyll C, Hayashida W, et al: Intravenous dipyridamole infusion during thrombolysis improves the recovery of left ventricular function [abstract]. Circulation 88:158, 1993.

113. Willard J, Lange R, Hillis L: The use of aspirin in ischemic heart disease. N Engl J Med 327:175, 1992.

114. Ip J, Fuster V, Israel D, et al: The role of platelets, thrombin, and hyperplasia in restenosis following coronary angioplasty. J Am Coll Cardiol 17:77B, 1991.

115. Mizuno K, Mujamoto A, Shibuya T, et al: Changes of angioscopic macromorphology following coronary angioplasty [abstract]. Circulation 78(Suppl II):289, 1988.

116. Tschoepe D, Schultheib H, Kolarov P, et al: Platelet membrane activation markers are predictive for increased risk of acute ischemic events after PTCA. Circulation 88:37, 1993.

117. Lam J, Chesebro J, Steele P, et al: Antithrombotic therapy for deep arterial injury by angioplasty: Efficacy of common platelet inhibition compared with thrombin inhibition in pigs. Circulation 84:814, 1991.

118. Lam J, Chesebro J, Steele P, et al: Is vasospasm related to platelet deposition? Relationship in a porcine preparation of arterial injury in vivo. Circulation 75:243, 1987.

119. Steele P, Chesebro J, Stanson A, et al: Balloon angioplasty: Natural history of the pathophysiologic response to injury in a pig model. Circ Res 57:105, 1985.

120. Wilentz J, Sanborn T, Haudenschild C, et al: Platelet accumulation in experimental angioplasty: Time course and relation to vascular injury. Circulation 75:636, 1987.

121. Barnathan E, Schwartz J, Taylor L, et al: Aspirin and dipyridamole in the prevention of acute coronary thrombosis complicating coronary angioplasty. Circulation 76:125, 1987.

122. Schwartz L, Bourassa M, Lesperance J, et al: Aspirin and dipyridamole in the prevention of acute coronary thrombosis complicating coronary angioplasty. N Engl J Med 318:1714, 1988.

123. Lembo N, Black A, Roubin G, et al: Effect of pretreatment with aspirin versus aspirin plus dipyridamole on frequency and type of acute complications of percutaneous transluminal coronary angioplasty. Am J Cardiol 65:422, 1990.

124. Franklin S, Faxon D: Pharmacologic prevention of restenosis after coronary angioplasty: Review of the randomized clinical trials. Coronary Art Dis 4:232, 1993.

125. Chesebro J, Webster M, Reeder G, et al: Coronary angioplasty: Antiplatelet therapy reduces acute complications but not restenosis [abstract]. Circulation 80(Suppl II):64, 1989.

126. White C, Knudson M, Schmidt K, et al: Neither ticlopidine nor aspirin-dipyridamole prevents restenosis post PTCA: Results from a randomized placebo-controlled multicenter trial. Circulation 76(Suppl IV):213, 1987.

127. Okamoto S, Inden M, Setsuda M, et al: Effects of trapidil (triazolopyrimidine), a platelet-derived growth factor antagonist, in preventing restenosis after percutaneous transluminal coronary angioplasty. Am Heart J 123:1439, 1992.

128. Sherman D, Dyken M, Fisher M, et al: Antithrombotic therapy for cerebrovascular disorders. Chest 102(Suppl 4):529S, 1992.

129. The ESPS Group: The European Stroke Prevention Study: Principal end-points. Lancet 2:1351, 1987.

130. Bousser M, Eschwege E, Haugenau M, et al: "AICLA" controlled trial of aspirin and dipyridamole in the secondary prevention of atherothrombotic cerebral ischemia. Stroke 14:5, 1983.

131. Guiraud-Chaumeil B, Rascol A, David J, et al: Prevention des recidives des accidents vasculaires cerebraux ischmiques par les anti-agregants plaquettaires. Rev Neurol (Paris) 138:367, 1982.

132. American-Canadian Co-Operative Study Group: Persantine aspirin trial in cerebral ischemia. Part II. Endpoint results. Stroke 16:406, 1985.

133. North American Symptomatic Carotid Endarterectomy Trial (NASCET) Investigators: Clinical alert: Benefit of carotid endarterectomy for patients with high-grade stenosis of the internal carotid artery. Stroke 22:816, 1991.

134. Harker S, Bernstein E, Dilley R, et al: Failure of aspirin plus dipyridamole to prevent stenosis after carotid endarterectomy. Ann Intern Med 116:731, 1992.

135. Hess H, Mietaschk A, Deichsel G: Drug-induced inhibition of platelet function delays progression of peripheral occlusive arterial disease. A prospective double-blind arteriographically controlled trial. Lancet 1:415, 1985.

136. Harjola P, Meurala M, Frick M: Prevention of early reocclusion by dipyridamole and ASA in arterial reconstructive surgery. J Cardiovasc Surg 22:141, 1981.

137. Sinzinger H, O'Grady J, Firscha P: Platelet deposition on human atherosclerotic lesions is decreased by low-dose aspirin in combination with dipyridamole. J Intern Med Res 16:39, 1988.

CHAPTER 156

Ticlopidine Hydrochloride

John W. Harbison, M.D.

Ticlopidine hydrochloride (Ticlid), a thienopyridine derivative whose only pharmacologic effect is the inhibition of platelet aggregation, was discovered in the early 1970s by a French pharmaceutical research team during a search for more active and better tolerated antiinflammatory agents.[1]

The subsequent investigation and development of ticlopidine's antiplatelet effect was closely related to evolving knowledge of the etiology and treatment of cerebrovascular disease. It was around this time that the role of platelets in arterial thrombosis emerged. In 1967, Weiss and Aledort noted the impact of aspirin on platelets.[2] Subsequently, a number of retrospective studies suggested that patients treated with aspirin for other indications had a reduced incidence of coronary and cerebral vascular events.[3] This sequence led directly to the development of platelet inhibition as a new treatment strategy in preventing myocardial infarction (MI) and stroke. In the 1970s, a series of large prospective clinical trials were begun to validate this strategy using aspirin, followed in the 1980s with similar trials using ticlopidine. The results of these trials established the efficacy of platelet inhibition by both aspirin and ticlopidine in preventing vascular thrombotic events.

MECHANISM OF ACTION

Ticlopidine is structurally different from other platelet inhibitors and has a unique mechanism of action that has not been fully characterized despite extensive study. It is administered orally and has a time- and dose-dependent onset of platelet inhibition. When ticlopidine is given at the recommended dose, 250 mg twice daily, its peak effect is seen between 8 and 11 days. It is known to broadly inhibit platelet aggrega-

tion mediated by several interdependent pathways, which include induction by adenosine diphosphate (ADP), collagen, thrombin, serotonin, arachidonic acid, epinephrine, and platelet activating factor.[4] This effect is irreversible and lasts for the life of the platelet. Ticlopidine and its stable metabolites appear to be inactive; when added *in vitro* to platelet-rich plasma, they fail to inhibit platelet aggregation. If platelets from untreated patients are added to plasma from patients treated with ticlopidine, platelet aggregation is not inhibited. When resuspended in plasma from either treated or untreated patients, however, platelets from patients treated with ticlopidine will not aggregate with ADP induction. These studies clearly show that the ticlopidine effect is permanently associated with the platelet. Current theory, incorporating the delayed onset of aggregation inhibition already discussed and its apparent restriction to the platelet, suggests that ticlopidine may act on platelets during megakaryocytopoiesis and subsequent platelet production in the bone marrow.[4]

Platelet inhibition by currently recommended ticlopidine dosing (250 mg b.i.d.) is primarily the result of ADP activation, mediated through the platelet membrane GPIIb/IIIa fibrinogen binding receptor, where it prevents the binding of fibrin to platelets at the end of the coagulation cascade. Studies of both the platelet ADP receptor and the GPIIb/IIIa fibrinogen receptor indicate that the ticlopidine effect occurs by inhibition of signal transduction rather than by structural alteration of either receptor.[4]

In summary, ticlopidine is a unique platelet inhibitor that requires oral dosing and has a time- and dose-dependent onset of effect. This effect is likely based on the action of a metabolite of ticlopidine at the level of megakaryocytopoiesis in the bone marrow, where the capacity of the GPIIb/IIIa fibrinogen binding receptor on the platelet membrane for normal signal transduction is affected without structural changes in the receptor, and binding of fibrin to the platelet membrane is prevented. This effect on the so-called final common pathway of platelet activation is irreversible and lasts for the life of the platelet.

PHARMACODYNAMICS

Peak plasma levels following single oral doses in healthy volunteers using radioactive labeling are reached in 1.5 to 2 hours.[5] Inhibition of platelet aggregation can be detected within 2 days, and maximal inhibition is achieved by 8 to 11 days. ADP-induced platelet aggregation, the principal mechanism mediating ticlopidine action, is reduced by a median value of 70% by the recommended total daily dose of 500 mg.

Platelet inhibition by ticlopidine is dose- and time-dependent. Although maximal inhibition is achieved more rapidly with a total daily dose of 750 mg, median inhibition is not increased (70.5%). Doses of 250 mg daily result in only modest reductions of median inhibition of platelet aggregation (64.3%). Median inhibition is substantially reduced with doses of ticlopidine of 125 mg daily (46.3%).[5] Although it is important to understand the dose-dependent effect of ticlopidine on platelet aggregation inhibition, it is also important to recognize that no studies have correlated platelet inhibition with the clinically relevant benefit of ticlopidine, the reduction of vascular thromboembolic events. Bleeding time is prolonged approximately twofold. Both the bleeding time and platelet function return to normal within 10 days to 2 weeks following ticlopidine withdrawal, reflecting the fact that the effect is irreversible and lasts for the life of the platelet.

PHARMACOKINETICS

Ticlopidine is rapidly absorbed orally. Animal studies in several species using radioactive labeling show absorption to be complete. Although similar studies have not been done in humans, indirect data suggest that absorption in humans is complete as well.[5] Administration with food, a critical strategy in avoiding the adverse effects of gastrointestinal intolerance and particularly diarrhea, is estimated to increase plasma levels by 20%. Unfortunately, plasma levels correlate quite poorly with platelet inhibition and, as previously noted inhibition, have not been correlated with clinical effect.[5]

Ticlopidine binds reversibly to plasma proteins, primarily serum albumin and lipoproteins. It also binds irreversibly to plasma proteins. This has been most extensively studied with the metabolite 2-hydroxy ticlopidine. It is not clear whether the phenomena of irreversible binding is related to ticlopidine's mechanism of action or is associated with adverse effects.[5]

Ticlopidine is extensively metabolized by the liver.

Neither ticlopidine nor any of the identified metabolites, however, have been correlated with the therapeutic inhibition of platelet aggregation. Indirect evidence suggests that metabolism in the bone marrow during megakaryocytopoiesis may be the basis for the resultant platelet inhibition.

Studies of the excretion of metabolized ticlopidine using radioactive labels show that 60% of the labeled dose is recovered in the urine; 23% is identified in the feces.[5]

Ticlopidine is well tolerated in patients with mild or moderate impairment of renal function. Its use is not recommended in patients with more advanced renal failure or in patients with hepatic failure.

CLINICAL STUDIES

Ticlopidine's inhibition of platelet aggregation was identified in the 1970s while the platelet's role in arterial thromboembolism was unfolding and the strategy of using agents to inhibit platelet aggregation to prevent vascular thromboembolic events was evolving. Several large prospective clinical trials of antiplatelet agents in coronary artery and cerebrovascular disease were underway, and in 1978 the Canadian cooperative study group showed that aspirin significantly reduced the risk of stroke and death in patients with transient cerebral ischemia.[6] This effect, however, appeared to be gender-dependent, with no apparent benefit for women. No data were available by the early 1980s to conclusively show that aspirin prevented recurrent stroke in patients with completed stroke.

A series of prospective clinical trials was begun in the 1980s to investigate ticlopidine's effect in reducing vascular thromboembolic events in patients with symptomatic cerebrovascular, coronary artery, and peripheral vascular disease.

TRANSIENT ISCHEMIC ATTACKS AND STROKE

Two large, well-conceived prospective clinical trials of ticlopidine in stroke prevention have been published.[7, 8] Their results demonstrate a significant reduction in the incidence of stroke following both transient ischemia and completed ischemic stroke in patients receiving ticlopidine.

The Ticlopidine Aspirin Stroke Study (TASS) was a North American, multicenter, randomized, double-blind comparison of ticlopidine (500 mg daily) with aspirin (1300 mg daily) in reduction of stroke and death in patients presenting with transient ischemic attacks (TIAs), amaurosis fugax (AF), resolving ischemic neurologic deficit (RIND), or minor stroke in the 90 days prior to randomization. Prospective patients were excluded if their qualifying symptoms were due to migraine, hematologic disorders, or cardiogenic emboli; they had a history of peptic ulcer, gastrointestinal bleeding, aspirin intolerance, or hypersensitivity or life-threatening disease; they were of child-bearing potential; they had a continuing need for aspirin or anticoagulation; or they could not give informed consent. Of the 3069 patients included in the study, 1529 were assigned to ticlopidine and 1540 to aspirin. The mean age of the participants was 63, 80% were Caucasian, and 64% were males. Demographic characteristics were well-balanced between the two study groups and accurately reflected the stroke risk profile of patients in other North American stroke studies. Half of qualifying events were TIAs; only 6% of patients had isolated AF. Significantly, 23% presented with minor strokes, 12% presented with a RIND, and 15% had more than one type of qualifying event. Seventy percent of symptoms were in the carotid distribution, 25% in the vertebrobasilar. The vascular distribution was uncertain in 5%. Treatment compliance reflected that 89% of patients took 75% of the medication 90% of the time. At study's end, only between 2% and 3% of patients were lost to follow-up, which lasted from 2 to 6 years. All but 12 patients were subsequently accounted for.

The primary end point, nonfatal stroke or death from any cause, occurred in 306 patients receiving ticlopidine and in 349 receiving aspirin. The most frequent end point was nonfatal stroke, occurring in 156 patients receiving ticlopidine and in 189 receiving aspirin. The severity, type, and distribution of first stroke was similar in both treatment groups; most were carotid atherothrombotic events. Hemorrhagic stroke occurred in only seven patients, three receiving ticlopidine and four receiving aspirin. An intent-to-treat analysis for the primary end point of death from all causes and nonfatal stroke revealed a 12% risk reduction (95% confidence interval, -2% to 26%) at 3 years in favor of ticlopidine ($p = .048$). For the secondary end point of fatal or nonfatal stroke, there was a 21% risk reduction (95% confidence interval, 4% to 30%) in favor of ticlopidine at 3 years ($p = .024$). In the first year, when stroke risk is greatest, there was a statistically significant 42% risk reduction for the primary end point of all-cause death and nonfatal stroke and a 47% risk reduction for the secondary end point of fatal and nonfatal stroke in favor of ticlopidine. An additional important result was that the benefit of ticlopidine was observed in both men and women. TASS was the first clinical trial in which an antiplatelet agent, ticlopidine, was conclusively shown to reduce stroke risk in women.

Since the initial TASS publication, a number of subgroups from the TASS have been analyzed.[9-13] Subgroup analysis must be viewed with caution. It represents *post hoc* analysis and as such may reflect bias. In addition, the numbers of patients and end point events in subgroups are rarely sufficient for statistical significance. On the other hand, subgroup analysis may reveal trends that may be compared with the overall population and allow studies and comparisons of populations that may not otherwise be examined because of the enormous costs of clinical trials. Specific TASS subgroups selected for analysis were women, nonwhite patients, and patients whose qualifying event was a minor completed stroke. The entire TASS population was also analyzed by the vascular distribution of their qualifying symptoms. The results showed that the benefit of ticlopidine when compared with aspirin in stroke prevention was maintained irrespective of gender, ethnic origins, or vascular distribution. In patients with minor stroke, a clear trend in favor of ticlopidine over aspirin was noted. This in conjunction with the results of the Canadian-American Ticlopidine Study (CATS), which will be discussed shortly, suggests that ticlopidine is superior to aspirin in preventing second or recurrent stroke in patients with a completed ischemic stroke.

The CATS was a smaller, multicenter, randomized, double-blind trial of ticlopidine in prevention of recurrent or second stroke. Participating patients had experienced a moderate to major thromboembolic stroke of either atherothrombotic or lacunar origin within the 4 months prior to randomization. Patients were excluded if their stroke was of cardioembolic origin, if they were likely to be demented or bedridden, had severe comorbidity, required long-term anticoagulant or antiplatelet use, or they could not give informed consent. As previously noted, in 1980, there was no conclusive evidence that aspirin prevented recurrent stroke. For this reason, the CATS was placebo-based. Over 3 years, 1072 patients were enrolled. Nineteen were judged to be ineligible and were excluded from analysis. Of the remaining 1053 patients, 528 were randomized to placebo, and 525 received ticlopidine (500 mg total daily dose). The demographic characters of both groups were comparable: 62% were male, the mean age was 65 years, and substantial cardiovascular comorbidity was present. Of the qualifying strokes, 74% were atherothrombotic and 26% were lacunar. Between 70% and 80% were in the carotid distribution, with the remainder of vertebrobasilar origin. In keeping with the character of the qualifying event, 70% of patients required assistance in the acts of daily living. Average follow-up was 2 years, and mean compliance was 90% when on the study drug. Forty percent of the placebo group and 52% of the ticlopidine group stopped the study medication prior to the end of the trial. Efficacy analysis was based on the occurrence of the first event of a vascular composite of recurrent stroke, MI, or vascular death. End points occurring more than 28 days following permanent stopping of the study drug were not included in the analysis. The most frequent first event was recurrent stroke. The placebo group experienced 118 events, an average yearly rate of 15.3%, whereas the ticlopidine group experienced 74 events, an average yearly rate of 10.8%. This resulted in a risk reduction of 30.2% (95% confidence interval 7.5% to 48.3%) in the incidence of stroke, MI, or vascular death associated with the use of ticlopidine ($p = .006$). The risk reduction with ticlopidine for fatal and nonfatal stroke was 33.5% ($p = .008$). Ticlopidine was the first antiplatelet agent to be clearly shown effective in reducing recurrent stroke, and, as in TASS, the benefit was consistent for both men and women.

MYOCARDIAL INFARCTION, UNSTABLE ANGINA, AORTOCORONARY BYPASS, AND ANGIOPLASTY

Ticlopidine has not been definitively studied in clinical trials specific for prevention of MI. Data of limited clinical value regarding cardiovascular end points are available from the TASS and CATS trials. In TASS, which compared ticlopidine (500 mg daily) to aspirin (1300 mg daily) in the prevention of stroke or death in patients with transient or minor completed cerebral ischemia, data are available on reduction of cardiovascular death as a subgroup of the primary end point of all causes of death. Intention-to-treat analysis shows that cardiovascular death accounted for 89 deaths in the group treated with ticlopidine and 78 deaths in the aspirin-treated group. Cardiovascular death was further divided into acute MI (21 ticlopidine versus 14 aspirin), sudden death (44 versus 41), and other (24 versus 23). Although cardiovascular death was the most common overall cause of death, there was no significant difference in its frequency between the two treatment groups.

CATS, a placebo-controlled efficacy trial of ticlopidine in the reduction of second or recurrent stroke in patients with an initial completed moderate or major ischemic stroke, utilized a primary end point consisting of the first occurrence of recurrent stroke, MI, or vascular death. Not surprisingly, the most frequent first event was recurrent stroke. MI occurred first in 13 patients receiving ticlopidine and in 12 patients on placebo. Vascular death occurred first in 8 patients receiving ticlopidine and in 18 patients on placebo. The number of events in both MI and vascular death are so small that they preclude any clinically relevant analysis.

Although neither the TASS nor the CATS study provided adequate data regarding ticlopidine's role in the prevention of MI, a randomized trial in unstable angina is more helpful.[14] In a multicenter Italian trial, 652 patients under age 75 with unstable angina consecutively admitted to a coronary care unit were randomized within 48 hours to either conventional therapy, consisting of calcium antagonists (86.2% of patients) combined with nitrates, β-blockers (72.4%), or both or conventional therapy plus ticlopidine (500 mg total daily dose) and followed for up to 6 months.

Unstable angina was defined as (1) new onset or sudden worsening of effort angina without increased physical activity during the preceding month, (2) new onset of worsening of angina at rest within the preceding month and still present during the week before admission with at least five episodes, at least one of which lasted more than 15 minutes, or (3) angina at rest with at least one episode lasting longer than 15 minutes in the 12 hours prior to admission. Patients had to show electrocardiographic changes consisting of transient ST-segment depression, ischemic T-wave inversion during the anginal attack or in the hours immediately following without enzyme elevation, or

both. The principal end points were fatal or nonfatal MI or vascular death.

Exclusion criteria consisted of acute or recent (within 6 weeks) MI, aortocoronary bypass within 3 months, use of either antiplatelet or anticoagulant agents within the preceding 4 days, age greater than 75, peptic ulcer symptoms or hemorrhagic risk, other cardiac disease (tachyarrhythmia, congestive heart failure, valvular heart disease), severe comorbidity (severe hypertension, hepatic or renal failure, hypotension, respiratory failure, hematologic disorders, or thyrotoxicosis), fever (temperature $\geq 39°C$), known ticlopidine allergy, pregnancy or use of high-dose oral contraceptives, and probable poor compliance.

The two study groups were homogeneous and predominately male (71.8%). Coronary risk factors were common (90.3% of patients had one risk factor, 26.7% had three), and coronary artery disease history was present in 65.3% of patients (angina 48.4%, MI 33.1%).

Outcome events were evaluated in a blinded manner, and data were analyzed using an intent-to-treat technique. The primary end points of vascular death and nonfatal MI were reached in 13.6% of patients treated with conventional therapy and in 7.3% of patients treated with conventional therapy and ticlopidine. This constituted a risk reduction of 46.3% ($p = .009$). Vascular mortality alone was observed in 4.7% of patients receiving conventional therapy and in 2.5% of patients receiving conventional therapy plus ticlopidine. This resulted in a nonsignificant risk reduction of 46.3% ($p = .139$). Nonfatal MI occurred in 8.9% of patients treated conventionally and in 4.8% of patients receiving ticlopidine in addition to conventional therapy for a risk reduction of 46.1% ($p = .039$). Finally, conventional therapy plus ticlopidine resulted in a 53.2% risk reduction in fatal and nonfatal MI ($p = .006$) when compared with conventional therapy alone (fatal and nonfatal MI incidence was 10.9% in conventional therapy and 5.1% with ticlopidine added). These data clearly show that the antiplatelet effect of ticlopidine significantly reduces the early occurrence of fatal and nonfatal MI in patients with unstable angina, a phase of coronary artery disease in which platelet aggregation is recognized as very important. Ticlopidine's ability to reduce vascular mortality was not clearly shown, and the study design leaves unanswered the relative merits of aspirin and ticlopidine in this setting. Further study of both antiplatelet agents is needed to establish their relative merits.

Ticlopidine's capacity to maintain the patency of aortocoronary bypass grafts has been studied both in the laboratory[15] and in the clinical setting.[16–18] The limited data available have been reviewed by Balsano and Violi.[19] Ticlopidine improved Dacron arterial graft patency in a single study in mongrel dogs.[15] Its use in the clinical setting is based on three small trials that provide promising results. Chevigne et al.[16] evaluated ticlopidine (500 mg total daily dose) in a randomized, placebo-controlled, double-blind study of 77 patients undergoing coronary bypass grafting and followed for 3 months for graft patency documented by thallium myocardial scintigraphy and angiography. Intent-to-treat analysis failed to achieve significance (10.1% occlusion rate with ticlopidine versus 20.3% with placebo), whereas on treatment analysis was significant ($p < .02$) (7.1 % occlusion rate with ticlopidine versus 21.8% with placebo). Limet et al.[17] studied 175 patients following coronary bypass surgery given ticlopidine (500 mg total daily dose) at 48 hours in a double-blind placebo control trial that analyzed graft patency at 10, 180, and 360 days. Ticlopidine proved significantly better than placebo at each interval (occlusion rates: 10 days, 7.1% [ticlopidine] versus 13.4% [placebo], $p < .05$; 180 days, 15% versus 24%, $p < .02$; and 360 days, 15% versus 26%, $p < .01$) and reduced intercurrent events (death, MI, stroke, unstable angina, and pulmonary embolism) at 1 year (6.9% in the ticlopidine group and 14% with placebo). In the third trial, Rothlin et al.[18] in 166 patients following coronary bypass surgery compared ticlopidine (500 mg total daily dose) with acenocoumarol with a prothrombin activity of 20% to 25% in a randomized but unblinded study of graft patency documented at 3 months by coronary angiography. Graft occlusion occurred with essentially the same frequency in both the ticlopidine group (43%) and the acenocoumarol group (42%).

Two trials have studied ticlopidine's value in preventing early occlusion and late restenosis following angioplasty.[20, 21] White et al.[20] compared aspirin (325 mg) plus dipyridamole (75 mg three times daily) and ticlopidine (500 mg total daily dose) with placebo in a double-blind study of 333 patients who underwent angioplasty. End points were early occlusion and late restenosis documented by coronary angiography at 6 months. Both aspirin plus dipyridamole and ticlopidine significantly reduced the early complications of abrupt occlusion, thrombosis, and dissection compared with placebo (placebo 14% versus aspirin + dipyridamole 5% or ticlopidine 2%—both $p < .005$); on the other hand, neither antiplatelet agent had greater effect than placebo in reducing late restenosis (placebo 25%, aspirin + dipyridamole 33%, ticlopidine 39%) and did not appear to influence late clinical events (MI and cardiac death). Bertrand et al.[21] compared ticlopidine (500 mg total daily dose) with placebo in a double-blind trial of reduction of acute closure and late restenosis (confirmed by angiography at 6 months) in 266 patients undergoing angioplasty. Ticlopidine significantly reduced acute closure (16.2% in placebo group versus 5.1% in the ticlopidine group, $p < .01$), but as in White's study, had no effect on the reduction of restenosis (40.7% in placebo group versus 49.6% in ticlopidine group). Clearly, antiplatelet agents, including ticlopidine, help to reduce early coronary occlusion following angioplasty but have no role in preventing late restenosis. These results are in keeping with the recognized role of platelet aggregation in early occlusion and a different mechanism resulting in restenosis.

PERIPHERAL ARTERIAL DISEASE

Atherosclerosis is a generalized, systemic disease that affects the entire vascular tree. Current estimates suggest that 2% of middle-aged men and 1% of middle-aged women have peripheral arterial disease as manifested by intermittent claudication, with the incidence in women increasing, possibly because of their increasing habit of smoking, the most prevalent risk factor for peripheral vascular disease.[22] The risk of symptomatic cardiovascular and cerebrovascular disease in these patients is substantial. Studies show a 30% to 50% prevalence of the signs and symptom of coronary artery disease in patients with newly diagnosed peripheral arterial disease,[22, 23] and the Framingham study identified an annual mortality rate of 39/1000 compared to 10/1000 in men free of disease.[23]

Peripheral vascular thromboembolism is thought to involve platelet aggregation in much the same manner as is found in the coronary and cerebrovascular arterial trees. Trials of antiplatelet agents in peripheral arterial disease therefore commonly use stroke and MI as well as peripheral vascular events as part of a composite end point.

Ticlopidine has been studied in a number of small trials in patients with peripheral arterial disease using this composite end point of peripheral vascular events (blood flow impairment resulting in either vascular reconstruction or amputation), MI, and stroke. The number of patients involved, however, has been too small to achieve statistical significance. Boissel et al.,[24] in a metaanalysis of four of these placebo-controlled studies involving 611 patients followed for 6 to 12 months, showed that ticlopidine treatment resulted in a significant reduction of cardiovascular events (ticlopidine 3% versus placebo 9%, $p = .006$).

The effect of ticlopidine treatment in preventing cardiovascular and cerebrovascular morbidity and mortality in patients with peripheral arterial disease confirmed by abnormal arm ankle systolic blood pressure gradients was studied further in the Swedish Ticlopidine Multicentre Study (STIMS).[25] The trial recruited 687 patients under age 70 with intermittent claudication by World Health Organization (WHO) criteria, 266 of whom completed the study (146 of 340 placebo-treated patients and 120 of 346 patients treated with ticlopidine) with a median of 5.6 years follow-up to the composite end point of MI, stroke or TIA, death, or study completion. History of preceding vascular disease and expected vascular risk factors was well-documented.

Using an efficacy analysis and excluding events that occurred more than 15 days after permanent discontinuation of drug, the incidence of MI, stroke, and TIA was 13.8% in patients treated with ticlopidine and 22.4% in patients receiving placebo ($p = .017$). There were 89 deaths in patients receiving placebo and 64 in patients taking ticlopidine. The resulting 29% reduction of mortality in the ticlopidine-treated patients ($p = .015$) was entirely explained by a decline in fatal MI (31 in patients treated with ticlopidine and 54 in patients receiving placebo, a risk reduction of 26% [$p < .01$]).

Although the data regarding the reduction of cardiovascular and cerebrovascular events by ticlopidine in patients with peripheral arterial disease are limited, the trend is favorable. Larger trials recruiting thousands of patients would clearly be valuable in firmly establishing ticlopidine's role in peripheral arterial disease.

DIABETIC RETINOPATHY

A limited number of clinical trials have investigated the benefit of ticlopidine in altering the course of diabetic retinopathy.[26, 27] The Ticlopidine Microangiopathy of Diabetes Trial (TIMAD) was a French, multicenter, randomized, double-blind, placebo-controlled study of the effect of ticlopidine on the progression of nonproliferative diabetic retinopathy. The basis for the investigation was the well-established observation of platelet aggregates in the small vessels of the retina in diabetic retinopathy wherein small vessel occlusion may be a key pathologic mechanism. Prior trials using aspirin had been disappointing.[28] The TIMAD study followed 435 patients for 3 years and evaluated the mean yearly increase in microaneurysms defined by fluorescein angiography. Ticlopidine resulted in a significantly smaller yearly increase in microaneurysms than did placebo (0.48 ± 5.79 in the ticlopidine group versus 1.44 ± 4.67 in the placebo group, $p = .03$). In insulin-treated diabetics, ticlopidine significantly reduced yearly microaneurysm progression (0.23 ± 6.66 in those treated with ticlopidine versus 1.57 ± 5.29 with placebo, $p = .03$). Overall progression of retinopathy was significantly reduced by ticlopidine compared with placebo ($p = .04$). Ticlopidine may be a promising new treatment modality in nonproliferative diabetic retinopathy.

CLINICAL USE

Indications for clinical use of ticlopidine should be derived from an analysis of the results of patient trials, its adverse effects profile, and its cost. Haynes et al.[29] carried out a comprehensive, independent analysis of these data and recommended use of ticlopidine in a range of clinical settings. Their findings suggested that ticlopidine was appropriate when antiplatelet treatment was indicated. These included patients with recent TIAs, completed stroke, and unstable angina. They felt that the data for ticlopidine's use in peripheral vascular disease was less conclusive. Because aspirin is effective and inexpensive, it is likely to remain the most commonly used antiplatelet agent despite the modest superiority of ticlopidine when the two agents are directly compared in clinical trials. There are several settings, however, in which ticlopidine is the appropriate antiplatelet agent for initial use. Ticlopidine should be used in patients requiring antiplatelet therapy who are either allergic to or intolerant of aspirin because of a past history of peptic ulcer disease or gastrointestinal hemorrhage. Ticlopidine should replace aspirin in patients who continue to have vascular symptoms or events while on regular aspirin therapy. The results of the antiplatelet trialists' collaboration not withstanding, ticlopidine seems appropriate in women with TIAs

and in both men and women who have experienced a completed moderate or major ischemic stroke. Finally, useful evidence from subgroup analysis in TASS shows trends supporting the previously noted modest ticlopidine superiority over aspirin in nonwhite patients[11] and patients who have experienced a minor completed stroke.[12] Because of the marked difference of cost between aspirin (≤25 cents a day) and ticlopidine (≤$2.50 to $2.75 a day), it is also reasonable to involve the patient in drug selection.

ADVERSE EFFECTS

Data on the tolerance and safety of ticlopidine are primarily derived from the 4000 patients involved in the TASS and CATS trials over a 5.8-year time frame. Additional data are available from extensive European and Japanese postmarketing surveillance experience.

During the trials, side effects were reported in 60% of the patients receiving ticlopidine (≥2000), 53.2% of the patients receiving aspirin (≥1500), and 34.3% of the patients receiving placebo (≥500). This included any reported side effect, whether or not it was related to the study drug. It seems likely that the high incidence of adverse effects is related at least in part to the advanced age of the study population, the incidence of associated illness, the use of multiple additional drugs, and the long duration of the study. This may also be reflected by the greater than one-third incidence of adverse effects in patients receiving placebo over only a 3-year period in the CATS trial. The comparative adverse effects data in aspirin-treated patients from the TASS study are likely to be understated, because nearly 10% of qualified patients were excluded from participation because of aspirin sensitivity.

The most frequent side effects reported with ticlopidine were diarrhea, occurring in approximately 20% of patients, and a morbilliform, or less frequently, urticarial rash, observed in 11.5% of patients. Other mild adverse effects included nausea 11.4%, dyspepsia 10.5%, gastrointestinal pain 6.9%, vomiting 4.0%, flatulence 2.4%, anorexia 2.2%, pruritus 3.3%, dizziness 3.4%, headache 3.1%, purpura 3.3%, and asthenia 3.6%. In general, gastrointestinal side effects occurred less frequently with ticlopidine than with aspirin. These side effects tended to occur early in ticlopidine use, generally in the first 10 to 20 days, and often remitted with temporary withdrawal or reduction of the dose. Diarrhea was often related to failure of the patient to take the drug at meal time or with an adequate meal. Ticlopidine use was terminated prematurely in 20.9% of patients who felt their symptoms or signs were severe. This was most common with diarrhea (6.3%). In general, with careful attention to adequate food intake with dosing, the judicious use of brief drug withdrawal and or reduced dosing and commitment to drug use on the part of both the patient and physician, the early mild adverse effects of ticlopidine can be weathered. Once past the early adverse experience, the long-term use of ticlopidine is remarkably free of side effects.

The severe adverse effects of ticlopidine consisted primarily of neutropenia and gastrointestinal hemorrhage. Additional rare severe side effects are discussed later. The incidence of severe adverse effects with ticlopidine was similar to that of aspirin in the TASS trial (approximately 1.5%). The profile of events with the two agents, however, was quite different, with neutropenia characteristic of ticlopidine and gastrointestinal hemorrhage characteristic of aspirin. It should again be recalled that 10% of all patients eligible for participation in TASS were excluded because of a history of peptic ulcer disease, gastrointestinal hemorrhage, or simply aspirin sensitivity. Their exclusion seems likely to have resulted in some reduction in the reported gastrotoxicity of aspirin in the TASS study.

Some degree of neutropenia, defined as an absolute neutrophil count (ANC) of less than 1200, occurred in 2.4% of the 2043 patients receiving ticlopidine in the TASS and CATS trials. Mild (ANC of 800 to 1200) and moderate (ANC of 450 to 800) neutropenia did not require drug termination during the trials and often spontaneously remitted. Severe neutropenia, occurring in 17 patients (0.8%), did result in drug termination. All severe neutropenia occurred in the first 3 months of drug use (specifically between day 26 and day 62). Postmarketing data from the Syntex complete blood count (CBC) monitoring program (≧ 10,000 patients) suggests the incidence of severe neutropenia may actually be slightly lower at 0.5%. Experience clearly shows, however, that the incidence of severe neutropenia, though small, is consistent and usually restricted to the first 3 months of therapy. Regular biweekly CBC monitoring has proven effective in identifying neutropenia and must be regarded as mandatory. If the ANC falls below 1200, the frequency of CBC monitoring should be increased to every other day until the ANC returns to a normal range. If the ANC falls below 800, monitoring should be daily until the neutropenia remits. As previously noted, if the ANC falls below 450, the drug should be permanently terminated. Daily monitoring must continue until the neutrophil count is greater than 1200. This usually requires 4 to 21 days, depending on the nadir of neutropenia. More frequent monitoring is required as well if there is an infection or if the most recent ANC has shown rapid decline (≥30%). If either the patient or the physician feels uncomfortable or is unwilling to comply with the increased monitoring required by a declining ANC, the drug should be discontinued. Even in this setting, monitoring must continue until the ANC is solidly normal. Routine monitoring is not ordinarily required beyond 3 months unless the patient is symptomatic. The risk of neutropenia should not deter use of ticlopidine when CBC monitoring is rigorous.

Ticlopidine's sole pharmacologic effect, platelet inhibition, is associated with a twofold increase in bleeding time. It is therefore logical, as with aspirin, to expect a variety of possible hemorrhagic adverse events. Such events were reported in 8.3% of patients receiving ticlopidine, 10% of patients receiving aspirin, and 3% of patients receiving placebo in the TASS and CATS trials. The most frequent events were purpura, epistaxis, hematuria, and petechiae.

The most common severe hemorrhagic event was gastrointestinal bleeding. Upper gastrointestinal bleeding occurred in 1.5% of ticlopidine patients and 3.1% of aspirin patients. It resulted in drug termination in 0.5% of ticlopidine patients and 1.6% of patients treated with aspirin. Peptic ulcer was diagnosed in 0.6% of ticlopidine patients and 2.9% of aspirin patients, leading to drug termination in 0.05% of ticlopidine patients and 1.2% of aspirin patients. Again, prescreening for aspirin sensitivity seems likely to have lessened the incidence of both gastrointestinal hemorrhage and peptic ulcer in the TASS patients assigned aspirin.

A frequent concern in the use of antiplatelet agents in the prevention of ischemic stroke is that the incidence of intracranial hemorrhage may be inadvertently promoted. Careful study of the incidence of intracranial hemorrhage, hemorrhagic infarction, and subarachnoid hemorrhage in the TASS and CATS populations does not indicate any increase with either ticlopidine or aspirin.

Rare serious adverse events that are felt to be caused by ticlopidine are pancytopenia, hemolytic anemia with associated reticulocytosis, allergic pneumonitis that was associated with acute neuropathy, hepatitis, cholestatic jaundice, and thrombotic thrombocytopenia purpura (TTP). For a number of these adverse events, only one or, at most, a few cases have been documented.

Serious adverse events that were noted rarely in the trials and are not clearly caused by ticlopidine include systemic lupus erythematosus, vasculitis, serum sickness arthropathy, myositis, and nephrotic syndrome.

All severe adverse events require withdrawal of ticlopidine. The drug should not be used again. In the single case of TTP in the stroke prevention trials, plasmapheresis was used and proven effective. Additional cases of TTP have been reported during postmarketing experience with ticlopidine. For a more comprehensive discussion of ticlopidine side effects, the reader is directed to Molony.[30]

PRECAUTIONS AND CONTRAINDICATIONS

Ticlopidine is contraindicated in patients known to be hypersensitive. It should be avoided in hematopoietic disorders that manifest neutropenia or thrombocytopenia. It should not be used in patients with active pathologic bleeding such as a bleeding peptic ulcer or intracranial bleeding or in patients with disorders of hemostasis. It is also contraindicated in severe hepatic failure.

Ticlopidine should be used cautiously in patients at increased risk of bleeding for any reason. If elimination of the antiplatelet effect is desired, ticlopidine should be withdrawn 10 to 14 days prior to planned elective surgery. A prolonged bleeding time can be normalized within 2 hours following intravenous injection of 20 mg of methylprednisolone. The effect of ticlopidine on bleeding can be reversed with platelet transfusions.

Although ticlopidine appears to be tolerated in patients with mild renal impairment, it should not be used in patients with significant renal failure.

DRUG INTERFERENCE

Ticlopidine at therapeutic doses results in a 30% increased plasma half-life of antipyrine, a model compound for hepatic metabolism, suggesting that a reduction in clearance of drugs similarly metabolized is likely.[31] This effect has been documented by an observed increase in the elimination half-life of theophylline from 8.6 to 12.2 hours.[32] In a similar vein, drugs that reduce hepatic metabolism are likely to alter ticlopidine metabolism. An example is the 50% reduction of single-dose clearance of ticlopidine that results with long-term use of cimetidine. Administration of ticlopidine after antacids results in a 20% decrease in plasma area under the curve for ticlopidine.[33] The clinical significance of these interactions, however, is unclear.

A drug interaction of considerable clinical interest is the simultaneous use of aspirin and ticlopidine. Limited data show that combined use of aspirin and ticlopidine does not alter the ticlopidine-mediated inhibition of ADP-induced platelet aggregation but does potentiate aspirin's effect on collagen-induced platelet aggregation, and the bleeding time is more prolonged than with either drug independently.[34, 35] The clinical effects of the combined use of aspirin and ticlopidine have not been fully investigated, and this combination cannot be recommended.

DOSAGE

The recommended dose of ticlopidine and the dose used in all clinical trials is 250 mg twice daily with meals. Utilization of the drug with meals is quite important because it enhances absorption, increases plasma levels, and reduces the common side effect of diarrhea. Although a total daily dose of 750 mg achieves maximal platelet inhibition earlier ($\geq$8 days) than the recommended 500-mg daily dose ($\geq$11 days), it does not improve platelet inhibition. A ticlopidine dose of 250 mg daily results in a modest decline in the 60% to 70% maximal platelet inhibition achieved with either 500 or 750 mg daily.

REFERENCES

1. Panak E, Verry M: Overview of ticlopidine development. *In* Hass WK, Easton JD (eds): Ticlopidine, Platelets and Vascular Disease. New York: Springer-Verlag, 1993, pp 13–25.
2. Weiss HJ, Aledort LM: Impaired platelet/connective tissue reaction after aspirin ingestion. Lancet 2:495, 1967.
3. Craven LL: Prevention of coronary and cerebral thrombosis. Miss Valley Med J 78:213, 1956.
4. Harker LA, Bruno JJ: Ticlopidine's mechanism of action on human platelets. *In* Hass WK, Easton JD (eds): Ticlopidine Platelets, and Vascular Disease. New York: Springer-Verlag, 1993, pp 41–59.
5. Teitelbaum P: Pharmacodynamics and pharmacokinetics of Ticlopidine. *In* Hass WK, Easton JD (eds): Ticlopidine, Platelets and Vascular Disease. New York: Springer-Verlag, 1993, pp 27–40.
6. Canadian Cooperative Study Group: A randomized trial of aspirin and sulfinpyrazone in threatened stroke. N Engl J Med 299:53, 1978.
7. Hass WK, Easton JD, Adams HP, et al: A randomized trial comparing ticlopidine hydrochloride with aspirin for the prevention of stroke in high-risk patients. N Engl J Med 321:501, 1989.
8. Gent M, Blakely JA, Easton JD, et al: The Canadian American Ticlopidine study (CATS) in thromboembolic stroke. Lancet 1:1215, 1989.
9. Hershey LA: Stroke prevention in women: Role of aspirin versus ticlopidine. Am J Med 91:288, 1991.
10. Grotta JC, Norris JW, Kamm B: Prevention of stroke with ticlopidine: Who benefits most? Neurology 42:111, 1992.
11. Weisberg LA: The efficacy and safety of ticlopidine and aspirin in non-whites: Analysis of patient subgroup from the Ticlopidine Aspirin Stroke Study. Neurology 43:27, 1993.
12. Harbison JW: Ticlopidine versus aspirin for the prevention of recurrent stroke. Analysis of patients with minor stroke from the Ticlopidine Aspirin Stroke Study. Stroke 23:1723, 1992.
13. Pryse-Phillips W: Ticlopidine aspirin stroke study: Outcome by vascular distribution of the qualifying event. J Stroke Cerebrovasc Dis 3:49, 1993.
14. Balsano F, Rizzon P, Violi F, et al: Antiplatelet treatment with ticlopidine in unstable angina. A controlled multicenter clinical trial. Circulation 82:17, 1990.
15. Walter P, Geronlanos S, Rothlin M, et al: Dierasterelek tronenoposchen oberflichenveran-derungen der gefassunflache gewobener dacrongefassprothensen uach vara breichung von Ticlopidine. Folia Angiol 29:20, 1987.
16. Chevigne M, David JL, Rigo P, et al: Effect of ticlopidine on saphenous vein bypass patency rates: A double-blind study. Ann Thorac Surg 37:371, 1984.
17. Limet R, David JL, Magotteaux P, et al: Prevention of aortocoronary bypass graft occlusion. Beneficial effect of ticlopidine on early and late patency rates of venous coronary bypass grafts: A double blind study. Ann Thorac Surg 94:773, 1987.
18. Rothlin ME, Pflunger N, Speiser K, et al: Platelet inhibitors versus anticoagulants for prevention of aortocoronary bypass graft occlusion. Eur Heart J 6:168, 1985.
19. Balsano F, Violi F: Clinical trials of Ticlopidine in patients with coronary artery disease. *In* Hass WK, Easton JD (eds): Ticlopidine, Platelets and Vascular Disease. New York: Springer-Verlag, 1993, pp 85–98.
20. White CW, Chaitman B, Lasser TA, et al: Antiplatelet agents are effective in reducing the immediate complications of PTCA: Results from ticlopidine multicenter study. Circulation 76 (Suppl IV):1591, 1987.
21. Bertrand ME, Allain H, LaBlanche JM, et al: Results of a randomized trial of Ticlopidine versus placebo for prevention of acute closure and restenosis after coronary angioplasty (PTCA) the TACT study. XII Congress of the European Society of Cardiology Abstract Suppl, 1990, p 2022.
22. Reunanen A, Takkunen H, Aromaa A: Prevalence of intermittent claudication and its effect on mortality. Acta Med Scand 211:249, 1982.
23. Kannel WB, Shurtleff D: The natural history of atherosclerosis obliterans. Cardiovasc Clin 37:3, 1971.
24. Boissel JC, Peyrieux JC, Destors JM: Is it possible to reduce the risk of cardiovascular events in subjects suffering from intermittent claudication of the lower limbs? Thromb Haemost 62:681, 1989.
25. Janzon L, Bergqvist D, Boberg J, et al: Prevention of myocardial

infarction and stroke in patients with intermittent claudication; effects of ticlopidine. Results from STIMS, the Swedish Ticlopidine Multicentre Study. J lntern Med 227:301, 1990.

26. The TIMAD Study Group: Ticlopidine treatment reduces the progression of nonproliferative diabetic retinopathy. Arch Ophthalmol 108:1577, 1990.

27. Belgian Ticlopidine Retinopathy Study Group: Clinical study of ticlopidine in diabetic retinopathy. Ophthalmologica 204:4, 1992.

28. The DAMAD Study Group: Effect of aspirin alone and aspirin plus dipyridamole in early diabetic retinopathy: A multicenter randomized controlled clinical trial. Diabetes 38:491, 1989.

29. Haynes RB, Sandler RS, Larson EB, et al: A critical appraisal of Ticlopidine, a new antiplatelet agent. Effectiveness and clinical indications for prophylaxis of atherosclerotic events. Arch Intern Med 152:1376, 1992.

30. Molony BA: An analysis of the side effects of Ticlopidine. In Hass WK, Easton JD (eds): Ticlopidine, Platelets and Vascular Disease. New York: Springer-Verlag, 1993, pp 117–139.

31. Thebault JJ, Blatrix CE, Blanchard JF, et al: Effect of treatment on liver metabolizing enzymes in man. Br J Clin Pharm 10:311, 1980.

32. Colli A, Buccino G, Cocciolo M, et al: Ticlopidine Theophylline interaction. Clin Pharm Ther 41:358, 1987.

33. Shah J, Fratis A, Ellis D, et al: Effect of food and antacids on absorption of orally administered Ticlopidine Hydrochloride. J Clin Pharm 30:733, 1990.

34. Thebault JJ, Blatrix CE, Blanchard JF, et al: The interactions of Ticlopidine and aspirin in normal subjects. J Int Med Res 5:405, 1977.

35. Uchiyama S, Sone R, Nagayama T, et al: Combination therapy with low-dose aspirin and Ticlopidine in cerebral ischemia. Stroke 20:1643, 1989.

C. Anticoagulants

CHAPTER 157

Heparin

Marc Verstraete, M.D., Ph.D., F.R.C.P., F.A.C.P. (Honorary)

HISTORY

In 1906, J. McLean, a medical student, left San Francisco (recently devastated by an earthquake) to join the physiologist W. Howell at Johns Hopkins in Baltimore. While studying thromboplastin extracts from several tissues, McLean accidentally found that some of these so-called hepatophosphatides had anticoagulant activity.[1] Two years later, the same laboratory described the characteristics of this novel anticoagulant and named it *heparin* because of its abundant occurrence in the liver.[2] This rather crude material could be injected into animals without causing ill effects and prolonged the whole blood clotting time. The substance subsequently was developed as a drug for clinical use by research groups in Toronto and Stockholm, headed by Charles H. Best and Erik Jorpes, respectively.

Considerably later, it was discovered that heparin was effective as an anticoagulant but only in the presence of a plasma component that at that time was called *heparin cofactor*;[3-5] it since has been isolated[6,7] and renamed *antithrombin*.

CHEMISTRY

Heparin consists of a simple chain constructed of repeating disaccharide units, all of which contain glucosamine and uronic acid; the latter may be glucuronic acid or iduronic acid. The iduronic acid residues and possibly the glucuronic acid residues are sulfated to a varying degree (one to three sulfate groups per disaccharide unit), mainly at the C2 position. The glucosamine moieties are ester-sulfated to a variable extent at the C3 and the C6 positions.

The sulfur content is about 10%. Because of its large number of acid groups, heparin is a strong acid. A combination of chemical properties is required for coagulation inhibiting activity: free carboxyl groups, O-sulfate ester groups from hexuronic acid, and sulfamino groups on glucosamine.[8-12]

The biosynthesis of heparin is initiated by attachment of a carbohydrate-protein linkage region to the serine residues of a specific polypeptide chain.[11] How the complex events leading from this core protein to the final product are regulated is not completely clear. Heparin proteoglycan, or macromolecular heparin, thus consists of a core protein of unknown size with variable numbers of mucopolysaccharide chains of molecular weight 30,000 to 100,000.[13]

Heparin exerts the main part of its anticoagulant action via a plasmaprotein called *antithrombin III*. The active center serine of thrombin and other serine coagulation enzymes is inhibited by an arginine reactive center on the antithrombin III molecule; heparin complexes to lysine binding sites on antithrombin III and produces a conformational change at the arginine reactive center, which converts antithrombin III from a slow, progressive inhibitor to a very rapid inhibitor. Preparation of heparin fragments by chemical or enzymatic degradation has led to the isolation of a pentasaccharide sequence required for the binding of heparin to antithrombin III.[14-16] Disruption of a single disulfide bridge in antithrombin III leads to a reduced affinity for heparin and a corresponding loss of inhibitory activity in the presence but not in the absence of heparin.[17] This observation indicates that heparin and thrombin bind at different sites of the antithrombin III molecule.[18] Seven arginine residues thought to be required for heparin binding are located at the amino terminal part of antithrombin III.[19] This labile α-helix is separated widely from the protease binding domain in the carboxyl terminal end.[20]

PHARMACOLOGY
Mode of Action

The principal role of heparin as an anticoagulant is due to its ability to accelerate the formation of a molecular complex between antithrombin III and serine proteases of the coagulation system, thereby blocking the enzymatic activity of coagulation factors. The term *antithrombin III* is a misnomer for several reasons. One reason is that acting in concert with heparin, this protein inhibits not only thrombin but also the activated forms of numerous coagulation factors (IX, X, XI, and XII) as well as of plasmin and kallikrein. However, the inhibition of thrombin and factor Xa is particularly important and is clinically relevant.

The inhibition of thrombin by antithrombin III alone is a slow process. Direct binding of heparin to γ-aminolysyl residues of the antithrombin III molecule is responsible for a 1000-fold acceleration of thrombin–antithrombin III complex formation, whereas interaction between thrombin (active center serine) and heparin–antithrombin III (reactive site arginine) provides an additional 4- to 15-fold further acceleration.[20] However, during this catalytic interaction, the 1:1 stoichiometry of the enzyme-inhibitor reaction is unaffected. After covalent binding of antithrombin III to the active serine center of coagulation enzymes, heparin then dissociates from the ternary complex and can be reutilized. The remaining antithrombin III–thrombin complexes are removed by the endothelial system. Evidence suggests that a three-way complex is required in which heparin, antithrombin III, and thrombin bind to each other for maximal heparin-enhanced inhibition of thrombin by antithrombin. At least 18 saccharides per heparin molecule are required to enable heparin to bind to thrombin and antithrombin III simultaneously and thereby inhibit thrombin.[21–23] The binding of thrombin to heparin is indeed electrostatic and strongly depends on the length of the heparin molecule. In contrast, very small heparin fragments, containing 6 saccharides that nonetheless possess the high-affinity pentasaccharide sequence, can inhibit activated factor X by antithrombin III.

Heparin Fractions with High or Low Affinity for Antithrombin III

In pharmaceutical-grade heparin, most anticoagulant activity is accounted for by a small functional fraction of the molecules, the one third with high affinity to antithrombin III. The remaining molecules have only a limited anticoagulant effect at therapeutic concentrations but may still increase bleeding in experimental animals,[24] inhibit the activation of prothrombin by factor Xa,[25, 26] or potentiate the action of high-affinity, low-molecular-weight fractions.[27] Furthermore, heparin molecules with low affinity for antithrombin III appear to inhibit hyperplasia of vascular smooth muscle,[28] activation of lipoprotein lipase,[29] suppression of aldosterone secretion, and induction of platelet aggregation.[30]

At higher than therapeutic concentrations, heparin and heparin-like mucopolysaccharides and high- or low-affinity heparins have an additional effect by catalyzing the inhibition of thrombin by a second plasma protein, heparin cofactor II.[31] The latter anticoagulant is specific for thrombin.

Low- versus High-Molecular-Weight Heparin

Heparins of low molecular weight are obtained by chemical or enzymatic depolymerization of unfractionated commercial-grade heparin and have a mean molecular weight range between less than 4000 and about 6500 daltons. Low-molecular-weight heparins contain the unique pentasaccharide required for binding to antithrombin III, but in a lower proportion than the commercial-grade heparin does.

Fragments below 16 to 20 monosaccharide units per heparin molecule (molecular weight <5000 daltons), although containing the essential pentasaccharide binding sequence to antithrombin III, are not long enough to bind also to thrombin; they therefore inhibit only factor Xa.[32] Even a synthetic pentasaccharide containing only 5 monosaccharide units (about 1700 daltons) contains the domain that binds to antithrombin III and possesses a high specific activity *in vitro* against factor Xa but little activity against thrombin.[15] Heparin preparations weighing more than 5000 daltons maintain their inhibitory property against factor Xa but gain, with increasing chain length, a progressively stronger inhibitory capacity against thrombin. The unexpected discovery that heparins of low molecular weight essentially lack the ability to prolong clotting time (indicating no thrombin inhibition) but still can potentiate the inhibition of factor Xa raised the hope of a dissociation of the antithrombotic property (anti–factor Xa) from the anticoagulant property (inhibition of thrombin), which then would avoid the hemorrhage-inducing effect of unfractionated heparin. According to this hypothesis, a low-molecular-weight heparin with high anti–factor Xa activity and little effect on the activated partial thromboplastin time (aPTT) would have an antithrombotic effect without causing bleeding. It was shown in animal experiments that anti–factor Xa activity is a prerequisite, but not sufficient in itself, for a thrombosis-preventing effect. Heparin molecules, large enough to retain some thrombin-blocking action, are also necessary; some other factors, possibly a molecular-weight-dependent vascular wall interaction, must also contribute to the antithrombotic effect.[33–36] An advantage of heparins of low molecular weight is that they interact less with platelets, von Willebrand factor, and endothelial cells than does high-molecular-weight heparin.[37] Reduced bleeding therefore may be more related to a decreased effect on platelets than to the reduced antithrombin property of low-molecular-weight heparin.[38, 39]

PHARMACOKINETICS
Unfractionated Heparin

After intravenous injection, heparin undergoes a rapid phase of elimination due to equilibration, followed by a more gradual disappearance.[40] The disappearance of the anticoagulant activity of heparin is compatible with a model based on the combination of a saturable mechanism (most probably rapid uptake by the endothelium and desulfatation by mononuclear phagocytes) and a linear (that is, unsaturable), mechanism (most probably elimination by the kidney).[41, 42] The faster disappearance of the thrombin inhibitor activity (anti–factor IIa activity) than the anti–factor Xa activity on the initial clearance phase also suggests an earlier elimination mechanism of large molecules having a high ratio of anti–factor IIa to anti–factor Xa. Thus, in practice, the dose-response relation of heparin is not linear and increases disproportionally in intensity and duration as the dose increases.[41] After bolus injection of 25 U/kg, the half-life of heparin is approximately 30 minutes, 60 minutes after a bolus dose of 100 U/kg, and 150 minutes after a bolus dose of 400 U/kg.[41]

CLINICAL USE OF HEPARIN
Indications

Postoperative Prevention of Deep Venous Thrombosis

The incidence of proximal deep venous thrombosis (DVT) in the limbs and pelvis is estimated to be 0.4% in patients at low risk (uncomplicated surgery in patients under 40 years of age with no other risk factors for venous thromboembolism), 2% to 8% in moderately high-risk patients (surgery in patients over 40 years lasting at least 30 minutes), and 10% to 20% in high-risk patients (major surgery in patients over 40 years old plus previous DVT, pulmonary embolism, or any orthopedic surgery).[43] The incidence of calf vein thrombosis is 2%, 10% to 40%, 40% to 80%, respectively, in the three groups of thrombotic risk. Leg elevation, early ambulation, and graduated compression stockings can serve as effective prevention in low-risk patients. *Miniheparin prevention* is a term applied to subcutaneous administration of 5000 U of concentrated heparin (20,000 U/ml) every 8 to 12 hours. Numerous well-conducted trials with objective diagnostic end points established the validity of miniheparin in the prevention of DVT and pulmonary embolism in patients at medium thrombotic risk. To this effect, the first dose of heparin usually is given 2 hours before surgery. An injection of standard unfractionated heparin, subcutaneously every 8 hours is associated with a slightly higher but still acceptable rate of bleeding complications compared with a scheme of injections at 12-hour intervals. The superiority with regard to antithrombotic protection of the higher dose in patients at lower thrombotic risk has not been demonstrated unequivocally.

In high-risk patients—including those with hip fracture or those who have undergone elective operations of the hip or knee, open urologic operations, gynecologic malignancy, and major amputation—a dose of 5000 U of heparin given at 8-hour intervals is not sufficient. One can monitor the dose of subcutaneous heparin in order to maintain the aPTT around 50 to 70 seconds, which improves prophylaxis but not at the cost of increased postoperative bleeding. The addition of dihydroergotamine, 0.5 mg, to each 5000 U of unfractionated heparin results in greater antithrombotic protection, also in patients undergoing traumatic or elective orthopedic surgery.[44, 45] Dihydroergotamine increases the sympathetic tone in veins and the venous flow rate in the legs and pelvic region. The greater efficacy of the combination of heparin and dihydroergotamine than of heparin alone could therefore be an accelerated venous return, although there are other explanations for this phenomenon. The use of dihydroergotamine, however, may occasionally result in leg ischemia due to arterial spasm, especially in patients with major trauma, in patients with obstructive arterial disease, and during pregnancy. In those patients, the risk outweighs the potential benefit.

Several clinical trials have established that heparin of low molecular weight given subcutaneously once or twice daily offers better protection against distal and proximal DVT and pulmonary embolism than subcutaneous unfractionated heparin, even in patients at high thrombotic risk.

During Pregnancy

Women needing prolonged oral anticoagulation should be placed on minidoses of heparin in case of desired pregnancy because of the teratogenic effects of warfarin (Coumarin) derivatives that should not be given during the first trimester. Also, from week 36 onward, heparin should be used again for prophylaxis. Heparin does not cross the placenta. The starting dose to be used in pregnant patients with prosthetic heart valves is approximately 10,000 U subcutaneously every 12 hours. The dose is adjusted based on the aPTT obtained at the mid-dose interval (6 hours) and aimed at 1.5 to 2.5 times the control value.

In Bedridden Patients at Risk for Deep Venous Thrombosis

Low-dose heparin prophylaxis is often recommended for elderly patients with severe heart failure as well as for paralyzed patients. Compared with placebo, low-molecular-weight heparins reduce the incidence of positive fibrinogen leg scanning from 21% to 6%.

Treatment of Deep Venous Thrombosis

Heparin is the initial and essential treatment for all recent proximal vein thromboses not treated with thrombolytic agents. The treatment of calf vein thrombosis is controversial, because only 20% of cases extend into proximal venous segments and rarely are associated with major pulmonary embolism, provided that they remain confined to the calf. Proximal extension of calf vein thrombosis can be investigated with noninvasive tests. If this monitoring is unavailable, all venous thromboses, irrespective of their site, should be treated with heparin. A bolus injection of 5000 to 10,000 U of unfractionated heparin is given initially, followed by a constant maintenance infusion of approximately 1300 U/hour; a more optimal dosage is to adapt to body weight (15 to 20 U heparin per kilogram and per hour). Both intermittent and constant intravenous infusion are effective. Heparin of low molecular weight also has been given intravenously, and it seems to be as effective as unfractionated heparin.[46] Further experience will determine whether the latter drug also minimizes the risk of bleeding.

Thirteen randomized and objectively documented clinical trials show that fixed doses of low-molecular-weight heparin, administered by the subcutaneous route, are at least as effective and safe as a continuous intravenous infusion of unfractionated heparin for the initial treatment of established DVT.[47]

To prevent recurrence of venous thrombosis, orally administered anticoagulants (Coumarin) usually are given for 3 to 6 months in those with persisting risk factors. A practical alternative is adjusted-dose prophylaxis with subcutaneous unfractionated heparin.[48a] This preventive measure is associated with a lower risk of bleeding than oral anticoagulation given at doses producing an international normalized ratio of 3.0 to 4.5. Six months of prophylactic oral anticoagulation after a first episode of venous thromboembolism led to a lower recurrence rate (9.5% versus 18.1%) than did treatment lasting for 6 weeks.[48b]

Treatment of Acute Pulmonary Embolism

Pulmonary embolism is a form of arterial obstruction caused by an embolus from a peripheral vein. For treatment purposes, pulmonary embolism may be considered in four different clinical categories:

1. The emboli may be large and immediately fatal
2. The emboli may be large and cause collapse, hypotension, progressive deterioration, or death
3. The emboli may cause collapse followed by partial recovery but residual major hemodynamic problems
4. The emboli may be small and produce no lasting hemodynamic effects

An initial injection of 10,000 to 20,000 U of heparin is followed by 30,000 to 40,000 U per 24 hours as soon as the diagnosis is suspected. The duration of treatment depends on the confirmation of diagnosis and evaluation of hemodynamic evolution. For emboli in category 4, this dose is the treatment of choice, supplemented by investigation of the peripheral veins.[44] Prior to discharge, the patient should be switched to orally administered anticoagulants for 3 to 6 months to prevent further embolism. Of the

relatively small group in category 3, the choice is between surgical embolectomy and thrombolytic therapy. Because the necessary surgical facilities often are unavailable, thrombolytic treatment will be started, especially in patients with underlying cardiac or respiratory disease. The rapidly deteriorating patient (category 2) needs immediate relief from pulmonary artery obstruction; while awaiting surgery, the patient can receive thrombolytic treatment.

The difference in hemodynamic improvement achieved with heparin or thrombolytic drugs clearly favors thrombolytic drugs in massive pulmonary embolism with major hemodynamic problems.

Treatment of Acute Myocardial Infarction

The treatment of choice in the first 6 to 12 hours after acute myocardial infarction (AMI) is intravenous thrombolysis because this treatment was shown to improve the ventricular function and survival. Concomitant intravenously administered heparin and, most often, aspirin have been used to prevent reocclusion after successful coronary recanalization; both drugs are essential if alteplase is used. Whether either or both of these drugs can be replaced by other antithrombotics is still unclear. Left ventricular thrombi are a common complication of transmural anterior infarction associated with severe abnormalities of motion in the apical wall. Thrombi have been identified in 32% to 70% of such patients with two-dimensional echocardiography. Thrombus mobility and protrusion are the two echocardiographic characteristics most helpful in identifying patients with left ventricular thrombi who are at risk of embolism.[50]

High-dose heparin reduces the incidence of thrombus[51] and may alter its morphologic pattern favorably, but high-dose heparin (12,500 U twice daily) prevents the formation of thrombus no better than low-dose (5000 U twice daily) subcutaneously administered heparin.[52] Notwithstanding the inability of heparin to fully prevent formation of left ventricular thrombus, the drug was shown to prevent systemic embolism when given in the first days after AMI and followed by orally administered anticoagulants for 3 to 6 months.[53] Most emboli form in the first 4 months. Several studies indicate that left ventricular thrombi resolve on therapy with anticoagulants.

Unfractionated heparin followed by orally administered anticoagulants has been used in patients with AMI, but there is no convincing evidence that anticoagulation improves the short-term prognosis of the infarction per se. Venous thromboembolism, however, is reduced significantly. Prophylactic low-dose heparin can be recommended in patients with myocardial infarction at high thrombotic risk (advanced age, severity of infarct, duration of immobility, obesity, a history of DVT) to ensure that these patients do not have to cope with pulmonary embolism in addition to myocardial infarction.

Treatment of Unstable Angina

Several large-scale trials using aspirin in patients with unstable angina have shown marked reductions of

AMI and cardiac death, both in the short term and the long term. There is some evidence that the addition of heparin to aspirin improves the short-term outcome.[48]

In Patients with Atrial Fibrillation

Among patients with atrial fibrillation, a small subgroup (2.7%) has lone atrial fibrillation with no recognizable cardiovascular disorder; the incidence of thromboembolism in this group is small (1.3% of patients younger than 60 years had a stroke over a 15-year period on a cumulative actuarial basis), and anticoagulants are of no avail.[54] However, patients with valvular heart disease, especially if the left atrium is enlarged, who have paroxysmal or chronic atrial fibrillation run a considerable risk of systemic embolism (one to four events per 100 patient-years). The protective effect (60% risk reduction) of long-term oral anticoagulation is rather convincing, but there is no need to start with heparin.

Treatment of Acute Occlusion in Limb Arteries

Unfractionated heparin treatment is initiated at a therapeutic dosage to prevent extension of the thrombosis or recurrence of embolism. An arterial embolism in young patients usually is removed under local anesthesia with the Fogarty catheter. The same procedure can be tried without delay in patients with acute occlusions superimposed on atheromatous plaques. If surgical intervention is impractical for technical reasons or because of the poor general condition of the patient, systemic or local thrombolytic treatment with streptokinase, urokinase, or t-PA can be considered.[55]

Treatment of Cerebral Embolism

Nonseptic cerebral embolism of cardiac origin is a common cause of stroke. The risks of early anticoagulant treatment with heparin remain controversial. Spontaneous hemorrhagic transformation, most frequently associated with large embolic infarcts, is estimated at up to 20% in this group, exceeding the 12% risk of early recurrent embolism.[56, 57] In a double-blind controlled trial, 225 patients with parietal stable thrombotic stroke were randomly assigned to receive continuous intravenously administered heparin or placebo for 7 days. Prophylaxis was started within 7 days of acute onset of thrombotic stroke with danaparoid. Prophylaxis was started with a loading dose of 1000 anti–factor Xa units intravenously followed by a fixed dose of 750 anti–factor Xa units subcutaneously twice daily for 14 days.[58, 59] Venous thrombosis documented with venography occurred in 4% of patients treated with the trial medication and in 28% of patients given placebo.

Precautions and Adverse Effects

Bleeding is the most frequent complication of heparin and is a direct extension of its therapeutic action. Spontaneous bleeding is most likely in subjects older than 60 years of age (risk × 3), in the presence of underlying morbidity (×4), in heavy drinkers (×7), in women (×2), and in patients with a blood urea nitrogen value over 50 mg/100 ml (×1.5). There is a consensus that the average incidence of major bleeding is 6.8% among patients given continuous heparin infusions and 14.2% among patients given intermittent intravenous injections of unfractionated heparin. When continuous intravenously administered unfractionated heparin is compared with subcutaneously administered unfractionated heparin, the average bleeding incidence is 5.2% and 4.1%, respectively.[60] Postoperative or posttraumatic bleeding is more common than spontaneous bleeding.[61] Other complications are uncommon, but osteoporosis can occur with full doses continued for 6 months or more. Thrombocytopenia is recognized with increasing frequency as much with unfractionated heparin as with low-molecular-weight heparins.[62, 63]

Contraindications

Anticoagulant drugs, including heparin, should not be used in unreliable outpatients or in patients in whom there is a definite risk of hemorrhage that cannot be avoided by careful adjustment of dosage, particularly when the bleeding could occur in certain tissues (e.g., eyes, brain, central nervous system). Arterial hypertension inadequately responding to antihypertensive treatment is an absolute contraindication. The presence of hemostatic defect obviously contraindicates the initiation of full-dose heparin.

Interference with Other Drugs

Many drugs inhibit platelet aggregation, so much so that prudence is obligatory if they are given concomitantly with heparin. This is particularly true for aspirin and ticlopidine.

Because of the formation of relatively insoluble complexes, heparin should not be mixed in the infusion fluid with most antibiotics and a number of psychotropic drugs.

Use in Patients with Impaired Organ Function

Heparin is partially degraded in the liver and is partially eliminated by the kidneys in unchanged form. Elimination might be prolonged after larger doses in patients with chronic renal failure or severe liver disease,[64] but the clinical importance of any alteration in clearance is not known. However, with intravenous administration, variability in clearance between patients is sufficiently marked to make laboratory control of dosage mandatory.[65]

Dosage and Administration

Heparin is not absorbed when given by mouth and must be given parenterally. Absorption from intramuscular sites is variable. Heparin may be given intravenously by continuous infusion or by intermittent injection. Major bleeding is less frequent with continuous infusion, at least at dosages that effectively prevent thromboembolism.[66] Moreover, continuous infusion reduces the dosage of the drug. Accelerated clearance of heparin in patients with pulmonary embolism makes it more difficult to attain adequate concentrations for any duration with usual intermittent regimens. It is uncertain how intense the anticoagulant effect of heparin must be to prevent thrombosis in humans. In rabbits, venous thrombus extension is prevented by heparin levels between 0.3 and 0.5 U/ml.[67] The relationship of the degree of effect to bleeding complications is also uncertain.[61]

When given by continuous intravenous infusion, standard dosage of unfractionated heparin is a loading dose of 5000 U (sometimes 10,000 U) given as bolus, followed by 15 to 20 U/kg/hour in normal saline or 5% dextrose with an automatic infusion pump. The rate of the infusion is regulated subsequently to keep the aPTT at about twice the baseline level.

Given intermittently, the usual intravenous dose of standard unfractionated heparin is 10,000 U at 6-hour intervals or 15,000 U at 8-hour intervals. Some use 5000 to 10,000 U every 4 hours. Intermittent injection is preferred by some because laboratory monitoring can be ignored. However, in the experience of most investigators, failure to monitor the appropriate coagulation parameters increases the risk of bleeding. Individuals vary widely in the anticoagulant response to a given dose of heparin or in the dose required to produce a particular anticoagulant response.[61] The wide variation in clearance of heparin among individuals and in different types of patients also suggests the desirability of monitoring intravenous heparin therapy so that dosage can be adjusted appropriately.

Concentrated aqueous heparin usually contains between 20,000 and 25,000 U/ml and is given subcutaneously in a skinfold raised from the abdominal wall. The "full" dose of this subcutaneous slow-release heparin administration is 20,000 to 30,000 U per 24 hours, administered in one or two injections. In the low-dose regimen, 5000 U of concentrated heparin is given subcutaneously at 8- or 12-hour intervals for the prophylaxis of DVT. In most cases, it causes only slight, if any, prolongation of clotting times and no clinically significant bleeding, except in a few cases after major orthopedic surgery, when 5000 U is given every 8 hours.

Monitoring of Therapy

The anticoagulant response of all antithrombotic drugs can be measured reasonably well; therefore, therapy can be governed by appropriate laboratory control of the desired anticoagulant effect, but it is not always required. Some monitoring is desirable with continuous infusion of heparin. However, monitoring is not essential for short-term, intravenous administration or with long-term subcutaneous administration. The major therapeutic usefulness of laboratory control is to ensure the presence of at least some anticoagulant effect at all times during treatment. As coagulation must be inhibited continuously to inhibit fibrin deposition or impede extension of the thrombus, the ideal test and intensity of orally administered anticoagulant effect have not been established. Some suggested desirable ranges of clotting tests are given in Table 157–1. A heparin dose adjustment nomogram has been developed for a specific aPTT reagent for which the therapeutic range is 1.9 to 2.7 times control (based on a heparin level of 0.2 to 0.4 U/ml plasma). This nomogram is not applicable to all aPTT systems but can be adapted to other systems by the local laboratory.[68]

SOCIOECONOMIC CONSIDERATIONS

It has been documented that the technical diagnosis of DVT with impedance plethysmography and leg scanning is as cost-effective as is venography. Considering the major cost of hospitalization, outpatient noninvasive diagnosis of DVT should be emphasized. Prevention with low-dose, unfractionated heparin be-

Table 157–1. **Heparin Dose Adjustment Protocol**

Patient's aPTT†	Dosing Instructions*			
	Repeat Bolus Dose	Stop Infusion (minutes)	Change Rate (Dose) of Infusion ml/hr‡ (U/24 hr)§	Timing of Next aPTT
<50	5000 U	0	+3 (+2880)	6 hr
50–59	0	0	+3 (+2880)	6 hr
60–85‡	0	0	0	**Next morning**
86–95	0	0	−2 (−1920)	Next morning
96–120	0	30	−2 (−1920)	6 hr
>120	0	60	−4 (−3840)	6 hr

*Starting dose of 5000 U IV bolus followed by 32,000 U every 24 hr as a continuous infusion. First aPTT performed 6 hours after the bolus injection; dosage was adjusted according to protocol, and the aPTT was repeated as indicated in the right-hand column.

†Normal range for aPTT with Dade Actin FS reagent in 27–35 seconds.

‡Therapeutic range of 60–85 seconds equivalent to a heparin level of 0.2–0.4 U/ml by protamine titration or 0.35–0.7 U/ml as an anti–factor Xa level. The therapeutic range will vary with the responsiveness of the aPTT reagent to heparin.

§Heparin concentration 40 U/ml.

aPTT, activated partial thromboplastin time.

comes considerably less expensive. The practical convenience of a single subcutaneous injection of low-molecular-weight heparin for the prevention and treatment of DVT has to be considered. Its clinical effectiveness, low bleeding incidence, and safety without laboratory monitoring have to be balanced against its price.

REFERENCES

1. McLean J: The thromboplastic action of cephalin. Am J Physiol 41:250, 1916.
2. Howell W, Holt E: Two new factors on blood coagulation: Heparin and pro-antithrombin. Am J Physiol 48:328, 1918.
3. Brinkhous KM, Smith HP, Warner ED, et al: The inhibition of blood clotting: An unidentified substance which acts in conjunction with heparin to prevent the conversion of prothrombin to thrombin. Am J Physiol 125:683, 1939.
4. Waugh DF, Fitzgerald MA: Quantitative aspects of antithrombin and heparin in plasma. Am J Physiol 184:627, 1956.
5. Monkhouse FC, France ES, Seegers WH: Studies on the antithrombin and heparin cofactor activities of a fraction absorbed from plasma by aluminum hydroxide. Circ Res 3:397, 1955.
6. Abildgaard U: Highly purified antithrombin III with heparin cofactor activity prepared by disc gel electrophoresis. Scand J Clin Lab Invest 21:89, 1968.
7. Rosenberg RD, Damus PS: The purification and mechanism of action of human antithrombin-heparin cofactor. J Biol Chem 248:6490, 1973.
8. Jorpes JE, Boström H, Mutt V: The linkage of the aminogroup in heparin. J Biol Chem 183:607, 1950.
9. Cifonelli JA: The relationship of molecular weight and sulfate content and distribution to anticoagulant activity of heparin preparations. Carbohydr Res 37:145, 1974.
10. Danihefsky I: Synthesis and properties of heparin derivatives. Adv Exp Med Biol 52:105, 1975.
11. Lindahl U, Höök M, Backström G, et al: Structure and biosynthesis of heparin-like polysaccharides. Fed Proc 36:19, 1977.
12. Jacobson I, Backström G, Höök M, et al: Biosynthesis of heparin: Assay and properties of the microsomal uronosyl C-5 epimerase. J Biol Chem 254:2975, 1979.
13. Robinson HC, Honer AA, Höök M, et al: A proteoglycan form of heparin and its degradation to single chain molecules. J Biol Chem 253:6687, 1978.
14. Lindahl U, Backström G, Thunberg L: The antithrombin-binding sequence in heparin. J Biol Chem 258:9826, 1983.
15. Choay J, Petitou M, Lormeau JC, et al: Structure activity relationships in heparin: A synthetic pentasaccharide with high affinity for antithrombin III and eliciting high anti factor Xa activity. Biochem Biophys Res Comm 116:492, 1983.
16. Lindhardt RJ, Grant A, Cooney CL, et al: Differential anticoagulant activity of heparin fragment prepared using microbial heparinase. J Biol Chem 257:7310, 1982.
17. Longas MO, Ferguson WS, Finlay TH: A disulfide bond in antithrombin is required for heparin accelerated thrombin inactivation. J Biol Chem 255:3436, 1980.
18. Jorgensen AM, Borders CL, Fish WW: Arginine residues are critical for the heparin cofactor activity of antithrombin III. Biochem J 231:59, 1985.
19. Blackburn MN, Smith RL, Carson J, et al: The heparin binding site of antithrombin III: Identification of a critical tryptophan in the amino acid sequence. J Biol Chem 259:939, 1984.
20. Griffith MJ: Heparin-catalyzed inhibitor/protease reactions: Kinetic evidence for a common mechanism of action of heparin. Proc Natl Acad Sci U S A 80:5460, 1983.
21. Pletcher CH, Nelsestuen GL: Two-substrate reaction model for the heparin-catalyzed bovine antithrombin/protease reaction. J Biol Chem 258:1086, 1983.
22. Hoylaerts M, Owen WG, Collen D: Involvement of heparin chain length in the heparin-catalyzed inhibition of thrombin by antithrombin III. J Biol Chem 259:5670, 1984.
23. Pletcher CH, Cunningham M, Nelsestuen GL: Kinetic analysis
of various fractions and heparin substitutes in the thrombin inhibition reaction. Biochim Biophys Acta 838:106, 1985.
24. Ockelford P, Carter CJ, Cerskus A, et al: Comparison of the in vivo haemorrhagic and antithrombotic effects of a low antithrombin III affinity heparin fraction. Thromb Res 27:679, 1982.
25. Walker FJ, Esmon CT: Interactions between heparin and factor Xa, inhibition of prothrombin activation. Biochim Biophys Acta 585:405, 1979.
26. Ofosu FA, Blajchman MA, Hirsh J: The inhibition by heparin of the intrinsic pathway activation of factor X in the absence of antithrombin III. Thromb Res 20:391, 1980.
27. Barrowcliffe TW, Merton RE, Havercroft SJ, et al: Low affinity heparin potentiates the action of high affinity heparin oligosaccharides. Thromb Res 34:124, 1984.
28. Rosenberg RD, Reilly C, Fritze L: Atherogenic regulation by heparin-like molecules. Ann N Y Acad Sci 454:270, 1985.
29. Bengtsson-Olivecrona G, Olivecrona T: Binding of active and inactive forms of lipoprotein lipase to heparin: Effects of pH. Biochem J 226:409, 1985.
30. Zucker MG: Heparin and platelet function. Fed Proc 36:47, 1977.
31. Tollefsen DM, Blank MK: Detection of a new heparin-dependent inhibitor of thrombin in human plasma. J Clin Invest 68:589, 1981.
32. Oosta GM, Gardner WT, Beeler DL, et al: Multiple functional domains of the heparin molecule. Proc Natl Acad Sci U S A 78:829, 1981.
33. Holmer E, Mattson C, Nilsson S: Anticoagulant and antithrombotic effects of heparin and low molecular weight heparin fragments in rabbits. Thromb Res 25:475, 1982.
34. Ockelford PA, Carter CJ, Mitchell L, et al: Discordance between the anti-Xa activity and the antithrombotic activity of an ultra-low molecular weight heparin fraction. Thromb Res 28:401, 1982.
35. Thomas DP, Merton RE, Barrowcliffe TW, et al: Effects of heparin oligosaccharides with high affinity for antithrombin III in experimental venous thrombosis. Thromb Haemost 47:244, 1982.
36. Ofosu FA, Blajchman MA, Modi GJ, et al: The importance of thrombin inhibition for the expression of the anticoagulant activities of heparin, dermatan sulphate, low molecular weight heparin and pentosan sulphate. Br J Haematol 60:695, 1985.
37. Salzman EW, Rosenberg RD, Smith MH, et al: Effect of heparin and heparin fractions on platelet aggregation. J Clin Invest 65:64, 1980.
38. Cade JF, Buchanan MR, Boneu B, et al: A comparison of the antithrombotic and hemorrhagic effects of low molecular weight heparin fractions: The influence of the method of preparation. Thromb Res 35:613, 1984.
39. Aiach M, Michaud A, Balian JL, et al: A new low molecular weight heparin derivative: In vitro and in vivo studies. Thromb Res 31:611, 1983.
40. Olsson P, Lagergren H, Ek S: The elimination from plasma of intravenous heparin: An experimental study on dogs and humans. Acta Med Scand 173:619, 1963.
41. De Swart CAM, Nymeyer B, Roelofs JMN, et al: Kinetics of intravenously administered heparin in normal humans. Blood 60:1251, 1982.
42. Simon TL, Hyers TIM, Gaston JP, et al: Heparin pharmacokinetics. Increased requirements in pulmonary embolism. Br J Haematol 39:111, 1978.
43. Gallus AS, Salzman EW, Hirsh J: Prevention of venous thromboembolism. In Colman RW, Hirsh J, Marder VJ, et al (eds): Haemostasis and Thrombosis, 2nd ed. Philadelphia: JB Lippincott, 1994, pp 1331–1345.
44. Kakkar VV, Stamatakis JD, Bently PD, et al: Prophylaxis for postoperative deep venous thrombosis: Synergistic effect of heparin and dihydroergotamine. JAMA 241:39, 1979.
45. Kakkar VV, Fox PJ, Murray WJG, et al: Heparin and dihydroergotamine prophylaxis against thromboembolism after hip arthroplasty. J Bone Joint Surg [Br] 67(Suppl 4):838, 1985.
46. Verstraete M: Curative treatment of subcutaneous unfractionated and low molecular weight heparins in established deep vein thrombosis. In Boccolon H (ed): Vascular Medicine. Amsterdam: Elsevier Science Publisher, 1993, pp 49–55.

47. Hirsh J, Siragusa S, Cosmi B, Ginsberg JS: Low molecular weight heparins (LMWH) in the treatment of patients with acute venous thromboembolism. Thromb Haemost 74:360–363, 1995.
48. Cohen M, Adams PC, Parry G, et al: Combination antithrombotic therapy in unstable rest angina and non-Q-wave infarction in nonprior aspirin users. Circulation 89:81–88, 1994.
48a. Hull R, Delmore T, Genton E, et al: Warfarin sodium versus low-dose heparin in the long-term treatment of venous thrombosis. N Engl J Med 301:855, 1980.
48b. Schulman S, Rhedin AS, Lindmarker P, et al: A comparison of six weeks with six months of oral anticoagulant therapy after a first episode of venous thromboembolism. N Engl J Med 332:1661, 1995.
49. Hyers TM, Hull RD, Weg JG: Antithrombotic therapy for venous thromboembolic disease. Chest 102:408S, 1992.
50. Cairns JA, Hirsh J, Lewis HD, et al: Antithrombotic agents in coronary artery disease. Chest 102:457S, 1992.
51. Gueret P, Dubourg O, Ferrier A, et al: Effects of full-dose heparin anticoagulation on the development of left ventricular thrombosis in acute transmural myocardial infarction. J Am Coll Cardiol 8:419, 1986.
52. Davis MJE, Ireland MA: Effect of early anticoagulation on the frequency of left ventricular thrombi after anterior wall acute myocardial infarction. Am J Cardiol 57:1244, 1986.
53. Weinreich DJ, Burke JF, Pauletto FJ: Left ventricular mural thrombi complicating acute myocardial infarction: Long-term follow-up with serial echocardiography. Ann Intern Med 100:789, 1984.
54. Kopecky SL, Gersh BJ, McGoon MD, et al: The natural history of lone atrial fibrillation: A population-based study over three decades. N Engl J Med 317:669, 1987.
55. Verhaeghe R, Bounameaux H: Peripheral arterial occlusion: Thromboembolism and antithrombotic therapy. In Fuster V, Verstraete M (eds): Thrombosis in Cardiovascular Disorders. Philadelphia: WB Saunders, 1992, p 423.
56. Cerebral Embolism Study Group: Immediate anticoagulation of embolic stroke: A randomized trial. Stroke 14:668, 1983.
57. Cerebral Embolism Study Group: Immediate anticoagulation of embolic stroke: Brain haemorrhage and management options. Stroke 15:779, 1984.
58. Duke RJ, Bloch RF, Turpie AGG, et al: Intravenous heparin for the prevention of stroke progression in acute stable stroke: A randomized controlled trial. Ann Intern Med 105:825, 1986.
59. Turpie AGG, Levine MN, Hirsh J, et al: Double-blind randomized trial of Org 10172 low-molecular-weight heparinoid in prevention of deep-vein thrombosis in thrombotic stroke. Lancet 1:523, 1987.
60. Levine MN, Hirsh J, Kelton JG: Heparin-induced bleeding. In Lane DA, Lindahl U (eds): Heparin: Chemical and Biological Properties. Clinical Applications. London: Edward Arnold, 1989, pp 517–532.
61. Basu D, Gallus A, Hirsh J, et al: A prospective study of the value of monitoring heparin treatment with the activated partial thromboplastin time. N Engl J Med 287:324, 1972.
62. Warrentin TE, Kelton JG: Heparin-induced thrombocytopenia. Ann Rev Med 40:31, 1989.
63. Chong BH, Ismail F, Cade J, et al: Heparin-induced thrombocytopenia. Studies with a low molecular weight heparin Org 10172. Blood 73:1592, 1989.
64. Teien AN: Heparin elimination in patients with liver cirrhosis. Thromb Haemost 38:701, 1977.
65. Simon TL, Hyers TM, Gaston JP, et al: Heparin pharmacokinetics: Increased requirements in pulmonary embolism. Br J Haematol 39:111, 1978.
66. Salzman EW, Deykin D, Shapiro RM, et al: Management of heparin therapy: Controlled prospective trial. N Engl J Med 191:1046, 1975.
67. Chiu HM, Hirsh J, Yung WL: Relationship between the anticoagulant and antithrombotic effects of heparin in experimental venous thrombosis. Blood 49:171, 1977.
68. Hirsh J, Dalen JE, Deykin D, Poller L: Heparin: Mechanism of action, pharmacokinetics, dosing considerations, monitoring, efficacy, and safety. Chest 102:337S, 1992.

CHAPTER 158

Logiparin in the Prevention and Treatment of Deep Vein Thrombosis

Russell D. Hull, M.B.B.S., M.Sc., and Graham F. Pineo, M.D.

Logiparin (Novo Nordisk A/S) is a low-molecular-weight heparin that is available for use in several European countries and is currently under review for approval in North America. Logiparin has been used in experimental models of thrombosis in animals and in clinical trials for the prevention and treatment of deep vein thrombosis. This chapter reviews published data regarding the pharmacology and pharmacokinetics of Logiparin as well as reports on the efficacy and safety of Logiparin in the prevention and treatment of deep vein thrombosis.

CHEMISTRY AND PHARMACOLOGY

Logiparin is derived from heparin sodium USP from porcine mucosa by enzymatic depolymerization. The mean molecular weight of Logiparin is 4500 ± 1500.

As with unfractionated heparin, Logiparin has both anti–factor IIa (antithrombin) and anti–factor Xa activity. As is seen with other low-molecular-weight heparins, the anti–factor Xa activity is greater than the anti–factor IIa activity. Thus, when the international standard for low-molecular-weight heparin (National Institute for Biological Standards and Controls) is used, the anti–factor Xa activity is approximately 80 IU/ml, whereas the anti–factor IIa activity and the activated partial thromboplastin time (aPTT) activity are about 50 IU/ml.[1, 2] Toxicity studies have been performed in animals. In acute toxicity studies with Logiparin given intravenously or subcutaneously, major bleeding was directly correlated with dosage, but there were no other toxic effects. Long-term toxicity studies demonstrated no toxicity with daily subcutaneous injections for up to 1 year. Logiparin as measured by anti–factor Xa and anti–factor IIa activity was shown not to cross the placental barrier.[3] When compared with unfractionated heparin, Logiparin was shown to cause the same degree of reduction in mineral bone mass in rats,[4] suggesting that long-term use of Logiparin may cause osteopenia. Liver enzymes are transiently elevated with the use of unfractionated heparin; this has also been observed with the use of Logiparin. Additionally, thrombocytopenia has occurred in 1% to 2% of patients treated with Logiparin,[5, 6] although thrombosis as a complication has not been reported.

The effects of Logiparin can be neutralized by protamine sulphate.[7]

PHARMACODYNAMICS
Bioavailability

Subcutaneous injection of different factor Xa doses of Logiparin showed a dose-related response with regard to factor Xa and factor IIa activity. Peak values occurred at 4 hours after subcutaneous injection, and factor Xa activity and body weight were strongly correlated. Therefore, Logiparin is best administered according to the body weight of the patient.[5, 8] The half-life of Logiparin varies with the dose given and the assay method used.[9] The anti–factor Xa activity persists for more than 12 hours, making once-daily administration of Logiparin possible.

Logiparin is well absorbed after subcutaneous injection. The half-life of absorption following subcutaneous injection is 200 minutes. The bioavailability of a similar low-molecular-weight heparin (Fragmin-Kabi) was reported to be approximately 90% of an equivalent intravenous dose.[10] Repeated daily subcutaneous injections of various doses of Logiparin did not demonstrate any evidence of drug accumulation in normal volunteers.[11] Based on these findings, clinical trials have been designed that use daily subcutaneous injections of Logiparin individualized by body weight.

Animal Studies

The effect of Logiparin on thrombosis and hemostasis has been demonstrated in animals.[12–14] It was shown that inhibition of factor Xa correlated well with antithrombotic activity. Logiparin had less effect than unfractionated heparin in a rat-tail bleeding time model.[13]

CLINICAL TRIALS USING LOGIPARIN
Prophylaxis of Postoperative Deep Venous Thrombosis

Logiparin in two doses (2500 or 3500 factor Xa units administered subcutaneously once daily) was compared with subcutaneously administered heparin (5000 units twice a day) in a double-blind study in patients undergoing general surgery.[15] Venographically proven deep vein thrombosis occurred in 5.6% of patients receiving 2500 factor Xa units, in 2.3% receiving 3500 factor Xa units, and in 3.0% receiving unfractionated heparin.

The incidence of bleeding in these same three groups was 2.1%, 3.0%, and 3.3%, respectively.

Logiparin was compared with placebo[16] or dextran[17, 18] in the prevention of deep vein thrombosis following hip fracture or total hip replacement. Logiparin, 50 factor Xa units per kilogram, was given 2 hours before surgery and then once daily and compared with a placebo in a double-blind trial.[16] Venographically proven deep vein thrombosis occurred in 45 (46%) of 97 patients receiving a placebo and in 30 (31%) of 93 patients on Logiparin ($p = .02$). Major bleeding occurred in one patient on placebo and in no patients on Logiparin.

Mätzch et al. compared Logiparin with dextran in two separate studies.[17, 18] Logiparin, 35 factor Xa units per kilogram, starting 2 hours preoperatively and then given once daily for 7 days, resulted in a deep vein thrombosis rate, as measured by fibrinogen uptake and phlebography, of 27.6% compared with a rate of 38.7% for patients receiving dextran (odds ratio = 0.61). There was no major bleeding in either group. Logiparin, 50 factor Xa units per kilogram, starting 2 hours preoperatively and given once daily for 7 days, resulted in a deep vein thrombosis rate, detected by fibrinogen uptake and phlebography, of 18.3% compared with a rate of 29.3% for patients on dextran ($p = .46$). Major bleeding occurred in 3.3% of patients receiving Logiparin and in 8.3% of patients receiving dextran.

Logiparin, 75 factor Xa units per kilogram, once daily, starting 18 to 24 hours postoperatively, was compared with a less-intense formulation of warfarin, starting the night of surgery and adjusted to maintain an international normalized ratio (INR) of 2 to 3 in patients undergoing total hip or total knee replacement.[6] The trial, maintained in double-blind fashion throughout, as well as all efficacy and safety end points, was adjudicated by an independent committee. Bilateral ascending venography was performed on day 14 or at the time of discharge from the hospital, whichever occurred first, and all venograms were interpreted independently. The pooled results for hip and knee replacement patients are shown in Table 158–1.[6] Patients undergoing total hip and knee replacement were analyzed separately.

PATIENTS UNDERGOING HIP REPLACEMENT

Adequate bilateral venograms were obtained in 337 patients (82.9%) receiving Logiparin and in 343 pa-

Table 158–1. **Incidence of All DVT, Proximal DVT, Major Bleeding, and Wound Hematoma Following Hip and Knee Replacement (Pooled Data)**

	Logiparin ($n = 715$)	Warfarin ($n = 721$)	p
All DVT	185 (31.4%)	231 (37.4%)	0.03
Proximal DVT	36 (6.1%)	47 (7.6%)	NS
Major bleeding	20 (2.8%)	9 (1.2%)	0.04
Wound hematoma	48 (6.7%)	26 (3.6%)	0.01

NS, not significant.

tients (87.1%) receiving warfarin. The overall rate of deep vein thrombosis in patients on Logiparin was 17.3%, and the rate of proximal thrombosis was 4.0%.[6] The overall rate of deep vein thrombosis in patients on warfarin was 19.9%, and the rate for proximal thrombosis was 3.2%. For all deep vein thromboses, the observed difference favoring Logiparin was 2.6% (95% confidence interval, −2.8% to 8.0%). For proximal deep vein thrombosis, the observed difference was 0.7% favoring warfarin (95% confidence interval, −1.9% to 2.3%). Wound hematomas occurred in 23 (5.8%) of patients on Logiparin and in 10 (2.5%) of patients on warfarin ($p = .036$).[6]

PATIENTS UNDERGOING KNEE REPLACEMENT

Adequate bilateral venograms were obtained in 78.5% of patients on Logiparin and 82.7% of patients on warfarin. The overall deep vein thrombosis rate of patients on Logiparin was 116 of 317 (36.6%); the thrombosis rate of those on warfarin was 154 of 324 (47.5%) ($p = .007$, risk reduction = 23%).[6] Proximal deep venous thrombosis occurred in 20 patients (6.5%) given Logiparin and in 34 patients (10.5%) given warfarin ($p = .08$, risk reduction = 38%). Major bleeding occurred in nine patients (2.8%) receiving Logiparin and in three patients (0.9%) receiving warfarin ($p = .134$). The difference equals 1.9% in favor of warfarin (95% confidence interval, −0.2% to 4.0%). Minor bleeding occurred in five patients (1.6%) on Logiparin and in five patients (1.5%) on warfarin. Wound hematomas occurred in 28 patients on Logiparin (8.8%) and in 19 patients on warfarin (5.9%) ($p > .105$).[6]

The frequencies of venous thrombosis and bleeding complications observed in patients undergoing hip replacement who received low-molecular-weight heparin[6] are similar to those reported previously.[19] The frequency of deep vein thrombosis in patients treated with low-molecular-weight heparin is similar to that of patients observed in a large, unblinded trial comparing low-molecular-weight heparin with warfarin sodium.[20] However, the frequency of deep vein thrombosis was higher than the frequency reported in another multicenter trial evaluating knee replacement surgery.[21] Despite this improvement, the rates remain high and support the continued need for case finding with venography. Results of this trial[6] indicate that further studies are required with the use of low-molecular-weight heparin, pneumatic leg compression,[22] or both in order to find the optimal method of prophylaxis.

In the study comparing low-molecular-weight heparin with warfarin sodium, prophylaxis was started postoperatively.[6] It is possible that the observed frequency of venous thrombosis could be decreased by using preoperative prophylaxis with low-molecular-weight heparin without unnecessarily compromising safety.[16–18] (Which type of prophylaxis should be used in patients undergoing total hip replacement patients should be further evaluated in randomized trials.)

This study[6] showed that low-molecular-weight heparin given as a single daily subcutaneous injection was effective when compared with warfarin sodium prophylaxis and avoided the need for monitoring. The reduction in rates of venous thrombosis with low-molecular-weight heparin was offset by the increase in bleeding complications and wound hematomas.

TREATMENT OF DEEP VEIN THROMBOSIS

In a dose-finding study, Logiparin, 75 factor Xa units per kilogram given twice daily or 150 factor Xa units per kilogram given once daily, along with warfarin, was given to patients with deep vein thrombosis for 5 days.[23] Venographic assessment using the Marder score[24] on repeat venograms showed improvement in many patients. It was concluded that a single dose of 150 to 200 factor Xa units per kilogram per day would probably appropriate for the treatment of deep vein thrombosis.

A multicenter, double-blind clinical trial compared a fixed dose of Logiparin, 175 factor Xa units per kilogram administered subcutaneously, with a continuous intravenous infusion of heparin adjusted to maintain an aPTT 1.5 to 2.5 times the mean normal control value.[5] All patients had venographically proven proximal vein thrombosis, and at the time of entry all underwent ventilation/perfusion lung scans and impedance plethysmography. All patients were started on warfarin on day 2, which was continued for 3 months with the dose adjusted to produce an INR of 2 to 3. Venous thromboembolism (recurrence or extension of deep vein thrombosis or pulmonary embolism), major and minor bleeding, thrombocytopenia, and death were the possible outcomes documented objectively.

New episodes of venous thromboembolism occurred in 6 of 213 patients receiving Logiparin (2.8%) and in 15 of 219 patients intravenously receiving heparin (6.9%, $p = .07$, 95% confidence interval for the difference = 0.02% to 8.1%). Major bleeding associated with initial therapy occurred in one patient receiving Logiparin (0.5%) and in 11 patients receiving intravenously administered heparin (5%), constituting a reduction in risk of 95% ($p = .006$). During long-term warfarin therapy, major hemorrhage occurred in five patients who had received Logiparin (2.3%) and in none of those receiving intravenously administered heparin ($p = .028$). The explanation for this is that unfractionated heparin had uncovered sites of bleeding during the initial treatment phase, whereas Logiparin, which is less hemorrhagic, did not cause bleeding during that time. However, long-term warfarin therapy led to bleeding in patients who had received Logiparin.

Ten patients (4.7%) who received Logiparin died, compared with 21 patients (9.6%) who received intravenously administered heparin, constituting a risk reduction of 51% ($p = .049$). The most striking difference was in abrupt death in patients with metastatic carcinoma; most of these deaths occurred within the first 3 weeks. The majority were not associated with thromboembolism or bleeding. The results of this trial were compared with those published by Prandoni et al.[25] When the two studies were combined, there was a statistically significant decrease in cancer deaths in the group receiving low-molecular-weight heparin compared with the group receiving unfractionated heparin.[26] This decrease in mortality rate, particularly in patients with metastatic carcinoma, was unexpected and requires confirmation by additional prospective, randomized trials.

Logiparin was shown to be more effective and safer than unfractionated heparin when both were used for 6 days at the initiation of anticoagulant therapy for proximal venous thrombosis. Long-term use of Logiparin in place of warfarin might have a greater impact on recurrent thromboembolic events, bleeding, and death, particularly in patients with metastatic carcinoma.

Cost-effectiveness analyses are being performed on data from the prophylaxis[6] and the treatment trial[5] involving the use of Logiparin. With a decrease in inhospital expenses related to complications of venous thromboembolism, Logiparin should prove more cost-effective than intravenously administered heparin. The fact that one third of patients with proximal deep vein thrombosis required admission to the hospital simply for initial diagnosis and blinding of the study indicates that most of these patients could be treated in an outpatient setting, resulting in major cost savings. It is therefore predicted that Logiparin will be highly cost-effective in the treatment of venous thrombosis.

CONCLUSION

Logiparin has been shown to be an effective and safe agent in the prevention and treatment of venous thromboembolism. The simplicity and convenience of a once-daily subcutaneous injection of a weight-adjusted dose of Logiparin, without the need for laboratory monitoring, makes this agent very attractive for both prevention and treatment of venous thrombosis. Further studies are needed to demonstrate the usefulness of Logiparin in other settings in which antithrombotic agents are required.

REFERENCES

1. Barrowcliffe TW, Curtis AD, Tomlinson TP, et al: Standardization of low molecular weight heparins: A collaborative study. Thromb Haemost 54:675, 1985.
2. National Institute for Biological Standards and Control Data Sheet: 1st International Standard for Low Molecular Weight Heparin (Established in 1987, Code no. 85/600), London, 1987.
3. Omri A, Delaloye JF, Andersen H, et al: Low molecular weight heparin Novo (LHN-1) does not cross the placenta during the second trimester of pregnancy. Thromb Haemost 61:55, 1989.
4. Mätzsch T, Bergqvist D, Hedner U, et al: Induction of osteoporosis by standard heparin and low molecular weight heparin in rats [abstract]. Thromb Haemost 58:36, 1987.
5. Hull RD, Raskob GE, Pineo GF, et al: Subcutaneous low molecular weight heparin compared with continuous intravenous

6. Hull RD, Raskob GE, Pineo GF, et al: A comparison of subcutaneous low-molecular-weight heparin with warfarin sodium for prophylaxis against deep-vein thrombosis after hip or knee implantation. N Engl J Med 329:1370, 1993.
7. Diness V, Østergaard PB: Neutralization of a low molecular weight heparin (LHN-1) and conventional heparin by protamine sulfate in rats. Thromb Haemost 56:318, 1986.
8. Mätzsch T, Bergqvist D, Hedner U, et al: Effects of an enzymatically depolymerized heparin as compared with conventional heparin in healthy volunteers. Thromb Haemostasis 57:97, 1987.
9. Bouchelouche PN, Østergaard PB, Mortensen SÅ, et al: Comparative pharmacokinetics of a low molecular weight heparin (LHN-1, Novo) and conventional heparin after intravenous injection [abstract]. Thromb Res (Suppl VI):89, 1986.
10. Bratt G, Tornebohm E, Widlund L, et al: Low molecular weight heparin (Kabi 2165; Fragmin): Pharmacokinetics after intravenous and subcutaneous administration in human volunteers. Thromb Res 42:613, 1986.
11. Johnston RV, Orr M, Rumley A, et al: A study of the antithrombotic potential of low molecular weight heparin LHN-1 (Novo) in normal volunteers [abstract]. Thromb Haemost 58:119, 1987.
12. Bergqvist D, Nilsson B, Hedner U, et al: The effect of heparin fragments of different molecular weights on experimental thrombosis and haemostasis. Thromb Res 38:589, 1985.
13. Diness V, Nielsen JL, Pedersen PC, et al: A comparison of the antithrombotic and haemorrhagic effects of a low molecular weight heparin (LHN-1) and conventional heparin. Thromb Haemost 55:410, 1986.
14. Østergaard PB, Nilsson B, Bergqvist D, et al: The effect of low molecular weight heparin on experimental thrombosis and haemostasis—the influence of production method. Thromb Res 45:739, 1987.
15. Liezorovicz A, Picolet H, Peyrieux JC, et al, and the HBPM Research Group: Prevention of perioperative deep vein thrombosis in general surgery: A multicentre double blind study comparing two doses of Logiparin and standard heparin. Br J Surg 78:412, 1991.
16. Lassen MR, Borris LC, Christiansen HM, et al: Prevention of thromboembolism in hip fracture patients. Comparison of low dose heparin and low molecular weight heparin combined with dihydroergotamine. Arch Orthop Trauma Surg 108:10, 1989.
17. Mätzsch T, Bergqvist D, Fredin H, et al: Safety and efficacy of a low molecular weight heparin (Logiparin) versus dextran as prophylaxis against thrombosis after total hip replacement. Acta Chir Scand 543(Suppl):80, 1988.
18. Mätzsch T, Bergqvist D, Fredin H, et al: Comparison of the thromboprophylactic effect of a low molecular weight heparin versus dextran in total hip replacement. Thrombosis and Haemorrhagic Disorders 3:25, 1991.
19. Levine MN, Hirsh J, Gent M, et al: Prevention of deep-vein thrombosis after elective hip surgery. A randomized trial comparing low molecular weight heparin with standard unfractionated heparin. Ann Intern Med 114:545, 1991.
20. Heit J, Kessler C, Mammen E, et al, for the RD Heparin Study Group: Efficacy of RD heparin (a LMWH) and warfarin for prevention of deep vein thrombosis after hip or knee replacement [abstract]. Blood 78(1):187, 1991.
21. Leclerc JR, Geerts WH, Desjardins L, Jobin F, et al: Prevention of deep vein thrombosis after major knee surgery—a randomized, double-blind trial comparing a low-molecular-weight heparin fragment (Enoxaparin) to placebo. Thromb Haemost 67:417, 1992.
22. Hull RD, Delmore TJ, Hirsh J, et al: Effectiveness of intermittent pulsatile elastic stockings for the prevention of calf and thigh vein thrombosis in patients undergoing elective knee surgery. Thromb Res 16:37, 1979.
23. Siegbahn A, Shams Y-H, Boberg J, et al: Subcutaneous treatment of deep vein thrombosis with low molecular weight heparin. A dose finding study with LMWH-Novo. Thromb Res 55:767, 1989.
24. Marder VJ, Soulen RL, Archartakarn V, et al: Quantitative veno-

heparin in the treatment of proximal-vein thrombosis. N Engl J Med 326:975, 1992.

graphic assessment of deep vein thrombosis in the evaluation of streptokinase and heparin therapy. J Lab Clin Med 89:1018, 1977.

25. Prandoni P, Lensing AW, Buller HR, et al: Comparison of subcutaneous low molecular weight heparin with intravenous

standard heparin in proximal deep vein thrombosis. Lancet 339:441, 1992.

26. Green D, Hull RD, Brant R, et al: Lower mortality in cancer patients treated with low molecular weight versus standard heparin. Lancet 339:1476, 1992.

CHAPTER 159

Fraxiparine (Nadroparin Calcium)

Henri Bounameaux, M.D.

HISTORY

Heparin was discovered in 1916 by J. McLean in animal liver extracts. The substance was administered to humans as an anticoagulant drug as early as the 1930s. The standard preparations of heparin are highly heterogeneous, with molecular weights ranging from 5000 or less to more than 30,000, and the biologic activities of the various components of heparin parallel their molecular weight distribution. It was therefore postulated that more homogeneous heparin preparations might be associated with less variable patient response, thereby avoiding the cumbersome *ex vivo* monitoring tests. Low-molecular-weight (LMW) fractions were obtained in the 1970s from crude heparin by a variety of methods. In contrast with heparin, LMW heparins (LMWHs) have a restricted molecular weight distribution with an average of around 5000, and these fractions exhibit a preferential inhibitory effect on activated factor X (FXa) rather than thrombin.[1] The hypothesis that FXa inhibition might confer antithrombotic potency while thrombin inhibition would be responsible for the anticoagulant, hemorrhagic potential led to the development of LMWH preparations with a view toward achieving an improved efficacy-to-safety ratio.[2] Among the preparations that were developed in Europe in the eighties, nadroparin calcium, initially referred to as CY 216, has been marketed as Fraxiparine (Sanofi-Winthrop, Gentilly, France). The differences among the various LMWH brands in molecular size, affinity for antithrombin III, and many other properties make it necessary to examine each of them to establish their specific characteristics.

CHEMISTRY

Nadroparin calcium is prepared from porcine sodium heparin by controlled nitrous acid depolymerization, reduction of terminal groups with sodium borohydride, purification, and exchange of sodium for calcium. Its chemical structure is thus related to that of unfractionated heparin (UFH) (see Chapter 157). Briefly, it consists of linear polysaccharides with alternating iduronic acid or glucuronate units and N-acetylglucosamine units joined by 1–4 linkages. In UFH, the chain lengths can vary from 5 to 100 or more, and the polysaccharidic sequences occur at random. The mean molecular weight of nadroparin calcium is 4500, with 90% of the molecular components being between 2000 and 8000.[3]

PHARMACOLOGY
Mode of Action

Among the numerous polysaccharidic sequences of heparin, there is one sequence with a specific function: the pentasaccharide that causes the heparin to bind with high affinity to antithrombin III.[4] This binding induces a 1000-fold increase in biologic activity of the inhibitor. Material containing the pentasaccharide has been called high-affinity material (HAM). All HAM heparin molecules catalyze the antithrombin III–dependent FXa inactivation but only those HAM molecules that are longer than 17 sugar units (which is called the "critical length") are able of catalyzing thrombin inhibition.[5] Apart from these anticoagulant actions, which result in an inhibition of prothrombin activation, standard heparin also exhibits a high affinity for platelet factor 4 (PF_4), a protein that is released by the α-granules upon platelet activation.

Approximately one fourth of the nadroparin molecules exhibit the pentasaccharide sequence specific for binding to antithrombin III.[3] However, the lack of correlation between the apparent plasma activity of the compound and its antithrombotic action[6] suggests that the antiprotease activity only partially reflects its therapeutic potential. Thus, low-affinity material (LAM) inhibits vascular smooth muscle cell proliferation,[7] lipoprotein lipase activation,[8] and platelet aggregation.[9]

Comparison of Nadroparin and Unfractionated Heparin

Compared with UFH, nadroparin, like other LMWHs, is enriched in material below the critical length (BCLM, after Hemker)[6] of 17 sugar units, which means that its anti-FXa activity is relatively more important than its antithrombin activity. Moreover, because the biologic half-life of BCLM *in vivo* is longer than that of material that is above the critical length (ACLM), the BCLM fraction of LMWH survives longer in the circulation. In addition, released PF_4 neutralizes ACLM but not BCLM very efficiently. All these mechanisms contribute to a prolonged biologic anti-FXa activity of LMWH in plasma compared with UFH. The specific activity of nadroparin in terms of anti-FXa activity is 200 Institut Choay units (ICU)/mg and 50 U/mg in the aPTT assay (anti-FXa/antithrombin ratio, 4.0:1). One anti-FXa IU of nadroparin corresponds approximately to 2.6 anti-FXa ICU.[10]

PHARMACOKINETICS
Absorption

Plasma concentrations of nadroparin calcium are usually measured by indirect *ex vivo* plasma measurement of anti-FXa activity. Using amidolytic assays, single subcutaneous doses of 3750 to 22,500 ICU anti-FXa (corresponding to 1440 to 8650 IU anti-FXa) resulted in dose-related plasma anti-FXa activities of 0.36 to 2.38 ICU/ml (0.14 to 0.92 IU/ml) in healthy subjects.[11] Maximal anti-FXa activity was detected in plasma 3.4 hours after subcutaneous administration with large interindividual variations.[12] Repeated subcutaneous administrations over 5 days did not produce a significant increase in maximal anti-FXa activity.[13] The estimated bioavailability of nadroparin is 98% (compared with 25% for UFH).[14]

Distribution and Elimination

The apparent volume of distribution of nadroparin in healthy subjects ranged between 41 and 71 ml/kg.[12] The drug does not appear to cross the placenta, but this statement is based on the study of seven women who terminated their pregnancy in the third trimester and who were given 17,500 ICU (6730 IU) of nadroparin as a single subcutaneous dose 3 hours before abortion. Fetal blood sampling did not show any anti-FXa activity.[15]

Nadroparin is eliminated by a nonsaturable renal mechanism. Plasma clearance in healthy volunteers occurs at a rate of about 19 ml/min (1.1 L/hr).[12] The half-life of the plasma anti-FXa activity was between 2.2 and 3.6 hours after intravenous administration and approximately 3.5 hours after subcutaneous application.[16] Thus, compared with UFH, the plasma half-life of the anti-FXa activity for nadroparin appears to be prolonged by a factor of two.

CLINICAL USE
Indications

Prevention of Venous Thromboembolism

The improved bioavailability and prolonged half-life of nadroparin compared with UFH means that, like other LMWHs, nadroparin can be given as one single subcutaneous injection instead of two or three in the prophylactic setting. Recently, two meta-analyses compared subcutaneous low doses of LMWH and UFH for prevention of postoperative venous thromboembolism.[17, 18] The main results of these analyses are presented in Table 159–1. Briefly, in patients undergoing general surgery, there was a statistically marginally significant[17] to nonsignificant[18] greater efficacy of LMWH regarding incidence of postoperative deep venous thrombosis (DVT) and pulmonary embolism (PE) compared with UFH. However, both pooled analyses were consistent with a clinically relevant reduction of the postoperative thromboembolic risk following general surgery when LMWHs were used. The risk reduction might be as high as 21% for DVT and 56% for PE compared with UFH. In patients who underwent total hip arthroplasty, both meta-analyses agreed on the superiority of LMWH with respect to the incidence of postoperative DVT (risk reduction 17% to 32%) and PE (risk reduction approximately 50%).

The results of any meta-analysis can be influenced or even flawed by many factors, including publication bias and heterogeneity of the pooled studies. In addition, in the particular case of LMWH, one additional

Table 159–1. **Prophylactic Use of LMWH Following Surgery: Summary of Two Meta-analyses**

Critical Event	Outcomes/Patients		(95% CI) Relative Risk
	LMWH	*UFH*	
General Surgery			
DVT			
Nurmohamed et al.[17]	184/3467	230/3411	0.79 (0.65–0.95)
Leizorovicz et al.[18]	248/5108	267/4575	0.86 (0.72–1.04)
PE			
Nurmohamed et al.[17]	9/2888	20/2843	0.44 (0.21–0.95)
Leizorovicz et al.[18]	12/4841	25/4305	0.62 (0.33–1.15)
Bleedings			
Nurmohamed et al.[17]	52/1977	51/1966	1.01 (0.70–1.48)
Leizorovicz et al.[18]	649/5108	596/4575	1.02 (0.90–1.16)
Orthopedic Surgery			
DVT			
Nurmohamed et al.[17]	93/672	132/622	0.68 (0.54–0.86)
Leizorovicz et al.[18]	224/1369	256/1323	0.83 (0.68–1.02)
PE			
Nurmohamed et al.[17]	10/590	24/582	0.43 (0.22–0.82)
Leizorovicz et al.[18]	17/1239	28/1236	0.53 (0.27–1.03)
Bleedings			
Nurmohamed et al.[17]	6/672	8/622	0.75 (0.26–2.14)
Leizorovicz et al.[18]	145/1236	143/1187	1.09 (0.76–1.58)

LMWH, low-molecular-weight heparin; UFH, unfractionated heparin; 95% CI, 95% confidence interval; DVT, deep venous thrombosis; PE, pulmonary embolism.

concern is the heterogeneity of the drug itself. Thus, a meta-analysis of clinical results conducted with different LMWH compounds might not be appropriate. However, it provides an overview and may be very helpful if the pooled results are not immediately advocated to support the use of one particular brand. Results of studies that used nadroparin compared with UFH, dalteparin, and placebo are displayed in Table 159–2. In all these studies,[19-25] nadroparin was administered as one daily subcutaneous injection of 7500 ICU (3075 IU), or according to a weight-adjusted regimen[21] (41 IU/kg during the first 3 days followed by 62 IU/kg from the fourth to the tenth postoperative day). The diagnostic end points for DVT were either fibrinogen uptake tests confirmed by phlebography[19, 20, 23] or systematic phlebography.[21, 22, 24] Symptoms and signs of PE had to be confirmed by an objective method (ventilation/perfusion lung scan, pulmonary angiography, or autopsy). In the only placebo-controlled study in general surgery patients,[25] the mortality was significantly ($p < .05$) lowered by the nadroparin prophylaxis. In all other comparative trials with UFH or dalteparin, the thromboprophylactic effect of nadroparin was found to be either superior[19, 20] or at least equivalent[21-24] to that of the control prophylaxis. In addition, in the two hip-surgery trials, a statistically significant, selective reduction in proximal DVT was observed.

Preliminary data are also available regarding the use of nadroparin in the prophylaxis of venous thromboembolism in patients undergoing neurosurgery[26] or ophthalmologic surgery[27] as well as in outpatients immobilized in plaster casts.[28] However, these data are insufficient to support the use of the drug in these settings, but the frequency of clinically relevant bleeding complications was very low, encouraging further research in these areas.

Treatment of Venous Thromboembolism

The classic treatment of established DVT consists of the continuous intravenous infusion of UFH at a dosage monitored to prolong the aPTT by a factor of 1.5 to 2.5. Nadroparin calcium (two daily subcutaneous injections at weight-adjusted doses) was compared with this regimen in three randomized trials that assessed either phlebographic[29, 30] or phlebographic and clinical end points[31] (Table 159–3). In these trials, nadroparin was found to be at least as effective and safe as the classic UFH regimen.

In a pooled analysis of the two therapeutic trials with clinically relevant follow-up end points (symptomatic recurrent thromboembolism and major bleedings),[31] including one study using nadroparin,[31] Lensing et al.[34] showed that LMWHs are associated with a statistically significant ($p = .015$) and clinically relevant reduction in the risk of thromboembolic recurrence (odds ratio 0.38, 95% confidence interval: 0.20 to 0.85). On the other hand, the same analysis suggested a highly significant ($p = .003$) and clinically relevant reduction in the risk of major bleeding, which was reduced in these two trials by more than 80% (odds ratio: 0.14, 95% confidence interval: 0.03 to 0.62).[33] A meta-analysis of all 13 trials of LMWHs in the treatment of established DVT concluded that use of LMWH instead of UFH is associated with a significant 44% decrease in the incidence of recurrent thromboembolism ($p = .02$) and 48% reduction in clot progression ($p = .01$). Total mortality and major bleedings were also reduced, albeit not significantly.[34] The main additional advantages of the novel regimens compared with the classic intravenous therapy with UFH are first, the subcutaneous application, which allows a greater mobility of the patient, and second, the absence of laboratory controls of the anticoagulant effect, because the LMWHs were given according to body weight.

Preliminary data regarding the use of nadroparin in patients with established, nonmassive pulmonary embolism[32] are already available from a dose-ranging study, which showed that at day 8, the improvement in the pulmonary vascular obstruction and the frequency of major bleedings were similar in the group of patients given 400 ICU (160 IU)/kg/day (n = 35) in two subcutaneous applications of nadroparin and in the group of patients treated with continuous intra-

Table 159–2. **Prophylactic Use of Nadroparin Following Surgery: Efficacy and Safety Data**

Study	Type of Surgery	Dosage*		DVT		PE		Bleedings	
		N	C	N	C	N	C	N	C
Versus UFH									
Kakkar and Murray[19]	General	1×3075	2×5000	5/200	15/200	0/200	1/200	10/200	7/200
EFS Group[20]	General	1×3075	3×5000	27/968	42/941	2/968	5/941	150/968	144/941
Leyvraz et al.[21]	Hip	weight†	APTT†	22/203	28/206	1/203	4/206	1/203	3/206
GHAT Group[22]	Hip	1×4000	3×5000	45/137	47/136	2/167	6/168	11/167	8/168
Dahan et al.[23]	Oncologic	1×3075	3×5000	0/50	0/50	0/50	0/50	3/50	2/50
Versus LMWH dalteparin									
Bounameaux et al.[24]	General	1×3075	1×2500	15/92	30/93	ND	ND	ND	ND
Versus placebo									
Pezzuoli et al.[25]	General	1×3075	placebo	ND	ND	2/2247	8/2251	173/2247	69/2251

N, nadroparin; C, controls; LMWH, low-molecular-weight heparin; UFH, unfractionated heparin; ND, not determined; DVT, deep venous thrombosis; PE, pulmonary embolism.
*Nadroparin and controls (UFH or dalteparin sodium) dosages expressed in anti-FXa IU.
†Dosage adapted either to weight (nadroparine) or to APTT (UFH).

Table 159–3. **Therapeutic Use of Nadroparin Calcium in Established DVT or PE**

Study	Dosage		Phlebographic Result or Pulmonary Vascular Obstruction	Recurrent VTE		Major Bleedings	
	N	UFH		N	UFH	N	UFH
DVT							
Lopaciuk et al.[29]	2×225 ICU/kg*	APTT‡	N=UFH	0/74	3/72	0/74	1/72
European Multicentre Group[30]	2×225 ICU/kg*	APTT‡	N>UFH	2/85	0/81	2/85	4/81
Prandoni et al.[31]	2×225 ICU/kg*	APTT‡	N>UFH	6/85	12/85	1/85	3/85
PE							
Théry et al.[32]	2×200 ICU/kg†	APTT‡	N=UFH	0/35	0/35	0/33	2/35

N, nadroparin calcium; UFH, unfractionated heparin; DVT, deep venous thrombosis; PE, pulmonary embolism.
*†Corresponding to 87 (*) IU/kg b.i.d. or 77 (†) IU/kg b.i.d.
‡Doses adjusted to maintain the APTT 1.5–2 times control values.

venous UFH (n = 33). These data need to be confirmed in larger trials.

Use in Extracorporeal Circuits

Anticoagulation is required to prevent fibrin deposition and thrombus formation in the extracorporal tubing system and membranes in cases of hemodialysis, hemofiltration, and cardiac bypass surgery. It has been shown that a single predialysis intravenous bolus injection (for an hematocrit of less than 30%) of 200 to 250 ICU/kg (approximately 80 to 100 IU/kg) nadroparin provides an adequate and safe anticoagulation during chronic hemodialysis in adults[36] and in children.[37] Data are scarce regarding its use in cardiac bypass surgery.

Acute Ischemic Stroke

A randomized double-blind, placebo-controlled trial comparing two dosages of fraxiparine with placebo in the treatment of ischemic stroke[37a] showed a significant dose-dependent effect among the three study groups in favor of low-molecular-weight heparin (p = .005) with regard to primary measures of outcome (death or dependency regarding activities of daily living) 6 months after randomization. The authors concluded that, for patients with ischemic stroke treatment within 48 hours of the onset of symptoms, fraxiparine was effective in improving outcomes at 6 months. This study is an important step forward in the management of acute ischemic stroke—a disease for which until now no efficacious treatment has been available.

Other Indications

Some authors have advocated the use of LMWHs in the presence of heparin-associated thrombocytopenia. Because LMWHs can induce heparin-associated thrombocytopenia (see later) and because some episodes of heparin-associated thrombocytopenia have been reported under LMWH after discontinuation of UFH, this practice cannot be recommended.

At the present time, there are no clinical data regarding the use of nadroparin in the treatment of arterial thromboembolic disease (acute myocardial infarction, unstable angina, cerebral embolism, and pe-

ripheral arterial thrombosis). Following percutaneous transluminal coronary angioplasty, one preliminary report shows that nadroparin is well tolerated when administered as one daily subcutaneous injection of 6150 IU during 28 days, but the sample size of the study does not allow any conclusions regarding the efficacy of this treatment to prevent restenosis.[38]

Precautions and Adverse Effects

Following both general and orthopedic surgery, the incidence of major bleeding was almost identical when the meta-analyses of the comparative trials of LMWH and UFH are considered (see Table 159–1). In all thromboprophylactic trials in which nadroparin was used (see Table 159–2), the frequency of bleeding complications was similar in the nadroparin and UFH groups. However, when compared with a placebo,[25] nadroparin prophylaxis was associated with a statistically significant ($p < .01$) 2.5-fold increase of hemorrhages, necessitating the interruption of treatment. In rare cases, minor hematoma or necrosis at the injection site has occurred. When nadroparin was used at higher dosages for treatment of established DVT, the frequency of bleeding complications was lower (see Table 159–3) than that observed with intravenous UFH.

Other complications such as osteoporosis (after administration over months), allergic reactions, and thrombocytopenia are uncommon and probably less common than with UFH. However, some cases of nadroparin-induced thrombocytopenia associated with thromboembolic complications resulting from *in vivo* platelet aggregation have been reported,[39] which renders regular platelet counts (once to twice weekly) mandatory during administration.

Drugs should generally be given with great caution during pregnancy. However, both UFH and LMWHs, which do not cross the placenta, are not expected to cause direct adverse effects to the fetus.[40]

Contraindications

Nadroparin, like other anticoagulant drugs, should not be administered, especially at therapeutic dosages, to patients with active bleeding, in patients at particular risk of bleeding in certain locations (e.g., brain, eyes), and in patients with a known hemostatic

Table 159–4. **Dosage Recommendations for the Various Indications of Nadroparin**

Indication	Administration	Daily Dosage*
Prevention of Venous Thromboembolism		
General surgery	Subcutaneous, once daily	3075 IU starting 2–12 hr before surgery
Medical patients	Subcutaneous, once daily	3075 IU
Orthopedic surgery	Subcutaneous, once daily	40 IU/kg for 3 days starting 12 hr before surgery followed by 60 IU/kg
Treatment of Deep Venous Thrombosis (DVT)		
	Subcutaneous, in two injections	400 IU/kg

*Expressed as anti-FXa international units (1 IU corresponds approximately to 2.6 anti-FXa Institut Choay units, ICU).

defect. Other contraindications include hypersensitivity to heparins, gastric or duodenal ulcer, and proliferative retinitis. However, in all cases, the individual benefit-to-risk ratio should be carefully weighed.

Interactions with Other Drugs

Because of the additional hemorrhagic risk, drugs that inhibit platelet function should be administered concomitantly with nadroparin only with care. This is particularly true for aspirin and ticlopidine. Physicochemical incompatibility (visible flocculation) has been observed when nadroparin was mixed with the combination of sulfamethoxazole and trimethoprim, with streptomycin, or with amiodarone.

Use in Patients with Impaired Liver or Kidney Function

In elderly patients with renal failure (creatinine clearance as low as < 10 ml/min), clearance of nadroparin was reduced and plasma half-life of the anti-FXa activity was prolonged from 2.2 hours in young healthy volunteers to 3 to 4.6 hours. However, there was no correlation between any clearance variable and the degree of impairment of renal function.[41] Despite this absence of correlation, with a mean half-life of 3.6 hours in patients with a creatinine clearance of less than 10 ml/min, these authors advised monitoring plasma anti-FXa activity in patients with renal insufficiency given nadroparin.

Dosage, Administration, and Neutralization

Nadroparin calcium is usually administered by the subcutaneous route in one or two daily injections in the prophylactic and therapeutic setting, respectively. The possibility of treating patients with established proximal DVT with one single daily injection of nadroparin is presently being tested in a multicenter trial. Dosage recommendations are given in Table 159–4. Intravenous administration is also possible, especially for preventing clot formation in extracorporeal circuits. Following surgery, prophylaxis is recommended to continue for at least 7 days. However, it has been recognized that one fourth of all postoperative pulmonary embolisms following general surgery occur during the month after discharge from the hospital,[42] thus suggesting that prophylaxis be continued for a longer period in some patients. In such cases and also in patients who have undergone hip replacement,

administration of low-dose warfarin with a targeted international normalized ratio (INR) of 1.5 to 2.0 might be considered a cost-effective alternative to prolonged administration of LMWH. In the therapeutic setting, oral anticoagulation should be started on the first or second treatment day and nadroparin administered until the INR is within the therapeutic range of 2.0 to 3.0 on 2 consecutive days, which usually occurs after 5 to 7 days. The total duration of anticoagulation after proximal DVT should be approximately 3 months.

In case of overdosage of nadroparin, protamine chlorhydrate partially neutralizes the anticoagulant effect: 1000 IU of nadroparin will be largely neutralized by the slow intravenous injection of 600 antiheparin units of protamine chlorhydrate.

SOCIOECONOMIC CONSIDERATIONS

Systematic prevention of postoperative venous thromboembolism with subcutaneous low-dose UFH is more cost-effective than diagnostic screening and selective treatment of patients with proven DVT.[43] Because LMWHs are at least as safe and probably more effective than UFH in this setting, the convenience of a once-daily regimen for LMWHs in general and nadroparin in particular over regimens requiring two or three daily injections is obvious. In the therapeutic setting, the novel therapeutic scheme offers the possibility of home treatment of established DVT, the safety of which is presently being assessed in a large international trial using nadroparin calcium. If safe, outpatient treatment of DVT will reduce considerably the treatment costs. Even when the drug is administered to hospitalized patients, a comparative analysis of the costs of a continuous intravenous infusion of UFH and a subcutaneous administration of nadroparin revealed no difference, even though the price of nadroparin was 10 times higher than that of UFH. In addition, the LMWH regimen would save 1 hour of costly nursing time per patient per week.[44]

REFERENCES

1. Lane DA, Mac Gregor IR, van Ross M, et al: Molecular weight dependence of the anticoagulant properties of heparin: Intravenous and subcutaneous administration of fractionated heparins to man. Thromb Res 16:651, 1975.
2. Choay J: L'héparine et ses métamorphoses. Nouv Rev Fr Hematol 23:253, 1981.

3. Lormeau JC: Physicochemical and biological characteristics of CY216. *In* Breddin K, Fareed J, Samama M (eds): Fraxiparine, First International Symposium. Stuttgart: Schattauer, 1989, p l3.

4. Choay J, Petitou M, Lormeau JC, et al: Structure activity relationships in heparin: A synthetic pentasaccharide with high affinity for antithrombin III and eliciting high anti-factor Xa activity. Biochem Biophys Res Commun 116:492, 1983.

5. Hemker HC, Beguin S: Mode of action of low-molecular-weight heparins in plasma and its consequences for the clinical laboratory. *In* Bounameaux H (ed): Low-molecular-weight Heparins for Prophylaxis and Treatment of Thromboembolic Disease. New York: Marcel Dekker, 1994, p 21.

6. Ockelford PA, Carter CJ, Mitchell T, et al: Discordance between the anti Xa activity and antithrombotic activity of an ultra low molecular weight heparin fraction. Thromb Res 28:401, 1982.

7. Rosenberg RD, Reilly C, Fritze L: Atherogenic regulation by heparin-like molecules. Ann NY Acad Sci 454:270, 1985.

8. Bengtsson-Olivecrona G, Olivecrona T: Binding of active and inactive forms of lipoprotein lipase to heparin: Effects of pH. Biochem J 226:409, 1985.

9. Zucker MG: Heparin and platelet function. Fed Proc 36:47, 1977.

10. Thomas DP: Biological standards and heparin. Thromb Haemost 62:648, 1989.

11. Freedman MD, Leese P, Prasad R, Hayden D: An evaluation of the biological response to Fraxiparine (a low molecular weight heparin) in the healthy individual. J Clin Pharmacol 30:720, 1990.

12. Rostin M, Montastruc JL, Hoiun G, et al: Pharmacodynamics of CY 216 in healthy volunteers: Inter-individual variations. Fundam Clin Pharmacol 4:17, 1990.

13. Pogliani EM, Bucciarelli P, Bregani R, et al: Effect on haemostasis of repeated subcutaneous administration of CY 216 in volunteers. Thromb Haemost 65:1358, 1991.

14. Harenberg J, Würzner B, Zimmermann R, Schettler G: Bioavailability and antagonization of the low molecular weight heparin CY216 in man. Thromb Res 44:549, 1986.

15. Forestier F, Daffos F, Rainaut M, Toulemonde F: Low molecular weight heparin (CY 216) does not cross the placenta during the third trimester of pregnancy. Thromb Haemost 57:234, 1987.

16. Baradell LB, Buckley MM: Nadroparin calcium: A review of its pharmacology and clinical applications in the prevention and treatment of thromboembolic disorders. Drugs 44:858, 1992.

17. Nurmohamed MT, Rosendaal FR, Büller HR, et al: Low-molecular-weight heparin versus standard heparin in general and orthopedic surgery: A meta-analysis. Lancet 340:152, 1992.

18. Leizorovicz A, Haugh MC, Chapuis FR, et al: Low molecular weight heparin in prevention of perioperative thrombosis. Br Med J 305:13, 1992.

19. Kakkar W, Murray WJG: Efficacy and safety of low molecular weight heparin (CY216) in preventing postoperative venous-thrombo-embolism: A cooperative study. Br J Surg 72:786, 1985.

20. European Fraxiparin Study (EFS) Group: Comparison of a low molecular weight heparin and unfractionated heparin for the prevention of deep vein thrombosis in patients undergoing abdominal surgery. Br J Surg 75:1058, 1988.

21. Leyvraz P, Bachmann F, Hoek J, et al: Prevention of deep vein thrombosis after hip replacement: Randomized comparison between unfractionated heparin and low molecular weight heparin. Br Med J 303:543, 1991.

22. The German Hip Arthroplasty Trial (GHAT) Group: Prevention of deep vein thrombosis with low molecular weight heparin in patients undergoing total hip replacement. Arch Orthop Trauma Surg 111:110, 1992.

23. Dahan M, Levasseur P, Bogaty J, et al: Prevention of postoperative deep vein thrombosis (DVT) in malignant patients by Fraxiparine (a low molecular weight heparin). Thromb Haemost 62:519, 1989.

24. Bounameaux H, Huber O, Khabiri E, et al: Unexpectedly high rate of phlebographic deep venous thrombosis following elective general abdominal surgery among patients given prophylaxis with low-molecular-weight heparin. Arch Surg 128:326, 1993.

25. Pezzuoli G, Neri Serneri GG, Settembrini P, et al: Prévention de l'embolie pulmonaire mortelle en chirurgie générale par le CY 216, héparine de bas poids moléculaire: essai multicentrique, randomisé, en double insu, contrôlé contre placebo (Etude STEP). Int Surg 74:205, 1989.

26. Rem JA, Gratzl O, Faes JM: Feasibility of LMWH CY 216 in neurosurgery on patients undergoing lumbar disc operation. A randomised, prospective, double-blind pilot-study. Thromb Haemost 65:926, 1991.

27. Morin Y, Limon S: Etude de la tolérance en chirurgie opthalmologique du CY 216 employé pour la prévention des thromboses veineuses profondes des membres inférieurs. J Fr Opthalmol 11:747, 1988.

28. Spannagel U, Kujath P: Low molecular weight heparin for the prevention of thromboembolism in outpatients immobilized by plaster cast. Semin Thromb Hemost 19(Suppl 1):131, 1993.

29. Lopaciuk S, Meissener AJ, Filipecki S, et al: Subcutaneous low molecular weight heparin versus subcutaneous unfractionated heparin in the treatment of deep vein thrombosis: A Polish multicenter trial. Thromb Haemost 68:14, 1992.

30. Collaborative European Multicentre Study Group: A randomised trial of subcutaneous low molecular weight heparin (CY 216) compared with intravenous unfractionated heparin in the treatment of deep vein thrombosis. Thromb Haemost 65:251, 1991.

31. Prandoni P, Lensing AW, Büller HR, et al: Comparison of subcutaneous low molecular weight heparin with intravenous standard heparin in proximal deep vein thrombosis. Lancet 339:441, 1992.

32. Théry C, Simonneau G, Meyer G, et al: Randomized trial of subcutaneous low molecular-weight heparin CY 216 (Fraxiparine) compared with intravenous unfractionated heparin in the curative treatment of submassive pulmonary embolism. A dose-ranging study. Circulation 85:1380, 1992.

33. Hull RD, Raskob GE, Pineo GF, et al: Subcutaneous low-molecular-weight heparin compared with continuous intravenous heparin in the treatment of proximal-vein thrombosis. N Engl J Med 326:975, 1992.

34. Lensing AW, Prins M, Koopman MMW, Büller HR: Which heparin for proximal deep-vein thrombosis? Lancet 340:311, 1992.

35. Leizorovicz A, Simonneau G, Decousus H: Comparison of low molecular weight heparin and unfractionated heparin in the treatment of DVT: A meta-analysis. Thromb Haemost 69:647, 1993.

36. Nurmohamed MT, ten Cate J, Stevens P, et al: Long-term efficacy and safety of a low-molecular weight heparin in chronic hemodialysis patients. A comparison with standard heparin. Trans Am Soc Artif Intern Organs 37:M459, 1991.

37. Schlegel N, Macher MA, Hurtaud MF, et al: The use of CY 216 in paediatric haemodialysis. *In* Breddin K, Fareed J, Samama M (eds): First International Fraxiparine Symposium. Stuttgart: Schattauer, 1989, p 177.

37a. Kay R, Wong KS, Ling Y, et al: Low-molecular-weight heparin for the treatment of acute ischemic stroke. N Engl J Med 333:1588, 1995.

38. Amann FW, Neuenschwander Ch, Meyer BJ: Fraxiparin for prevention of restenosis after percutaneous transluminal coronary angioplasty. Semin Thromb Hemost 19(Suppl 1):160, 1993.

39. Lecompte T, Luo SK, Stieltjes N, et al: Thrombocytopenia associated with low-molecular-weight heparin. Lancet 338:1217, 1991.

40. Maternal and Neonatal Haemostasis Working Party of the Haemostasis and Thrombosis Task: Guidelines on the prevention, investigation and management of thrombosis associated with pregnancy. J Clin Pathol 46:489, 1993.

41. Goudable C, Saivin S, Houin G, et al: Pharmacokinetics of a low molecular weight heparin (Fraxiparine) in various stages of chronic renal failure. Nephron 59:543, 1991.

42. Huber O, Bounameaux H, Borst F, Rohner A: Postoperative pulmonary embolism after hospital discharge. An underestimated risk. Arch Surg 127:310, 1992.

43. Colditz GA: Cost-effectiveness. *In* Goldhaber SZ (ed): Prevention of Venous Thromboembolism. New York: Marcel Dekker, 1993, p 541.

44. Lévesque H, Cailleux N, Vasse D, et al: Letter to the Editor. Lancet 341:824, 1993.

CHAPTER 160

Hirudin

Marc Verstraete, M.D., Ph.D., F.R.C.P., F.A.C.P. (Honorary)

HISTORY

Hirudin is produced by the salivary glands of medicinal leeches. Leeches are segmented worms (annelids) that evolved from earthworms. They have a sucker at each end: the one at the head houses the mouth, and the larger one at the tail is employed in crawling. The leech's scientific name, *Hirudo medicinalis*, reflects the animal's medical utility in the once widespread practice of blood-letting, or phlebotomy. The leech fastens itself to the skin and secretes the content of the salivary glands into the sucked blood. Without anticoagulation, the blood flow would cease because of clotting and the leech would be prevented from further sucking.

Nicander of Colophon (200 to 130 BC) may have been the first person to use the leech, followed by Themison of Laodicea (123 to 43 BC), a pupil of Asclepiades.[1] The second-century Greek physician Galen mentioned leeching, and the practice was detailed by the medieval Islamic philosopher Avicenna. By the Middle Ages, the use of leeches had developed into such a common treatment for most maladies that the word "leech" assumed multiple meanings: any medical procedure, poultice, drug, even the physician himself. In fact, in old English, *laece* means physician.[2] The popularity of leeching peaked in the late eighteenth century. Some 30 to 40 million leeches were imported each year into France alone. The demand was so great that leeches were extensively fished to near-extinction in Western Europe. Their use peaked in the 1830s in France with Broussais, the "most sanguinary" physician in history.[3] He applied so many leeches simultaneously to the abdomen of one patient that it looked like a "black glittering coat of mail."[4] During this time, French physicians commonly prescribed the number of leeches to be applied to newly hospitalized patients even before seeing the patient.[5] It was Haycraft,[6] working in Schmiedeberg's pharmacologic laboratory in Strasbourg, who discovered the anticoagulant property in leeches. In the first studies, aqueous extracts of the homogenized heads of leeches were used containing only minute amounts of the active principle. Its protein nature was recognized by Markwardt,[7] who also described the selective thrombin inhibitory property of the polypeptide. The name was coined by Jacoby in 1904.[8]

CHEMISTRY

Natural hirudins represent a family of several variants of structurally related isoproteins that share 85% amino acid sequence homology. Their complete primary and secondary structure has been described.[9–11]

Hirudin is composed of 64 to 66 amino acids with a molecular weight of approximately 7000 (Fig. 160–1).

The N-terminal moiety (residue 1 to 39) of the single-chain polypeptide is stabilized by three disulfide bridges. Number and localization of the S-S bridges are strictly conserved in all variants. Striking similarity is found for the C-terminal portion starting at position 40 in all isoforms.[13] The C-terminal moiety (residue 40 to 65) is highly acidic: the last 9-C terminal residues contain four Glu residues and one Tyr residue. This Tyr residue in the antepenultimate position 63 is sulfated. The N-terminal amino acids Val-Val can be replaced by Ile-Tyr. Although some of the hirudin variants differ in primary amino acid sequence, they share identical biologic activity toward thrombin.[14] The three-dimensional structure of hirudin in solution has been elucidated by nuclear magnetic resonance techniques.[15, 16] Hirudin is composed of three domains: a central core made up of residues 3 to 30, 37 to 46, and 56 to 57 containing β-pleated sheets stabilized by the three disulfide bridges; a protruding "finger" (residues 31 to 36) consisting of the tip of an antiparallel β-sheet; and an exposed loop (residues 47 to 55). The structure of the C-terminal end (residues 57 to 65) is too mobile to be determined by nuclear magnetic resonance.

The antithrombin function of hirudin is lost during reduction of the disulfide bridges, the splitting off of the acidic C-terminal segment, or by proteolytic

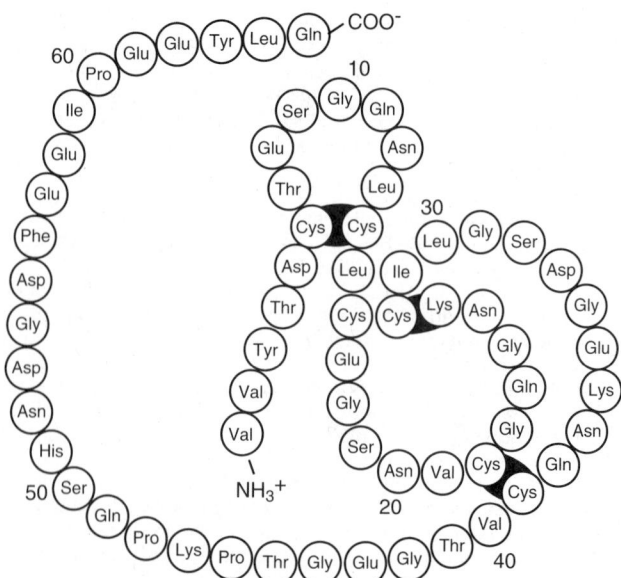

Figure 160–1. Structure of desulfatohirudin. (From Talbot M: Biology of recombinant hirudin [CGP 39393]: A new prospect in the treatment of thrombosis. Semin Thromb Hemost 15:293, 1989.)

1490

degradation. The minimal sequence with maximal anticoagulatory activity was found to contain the 12 residues that correspond to the amino acids in positions 53 to 64 of desulfatohirudin.

With advanced methods of peptide isolation and genetic engineering, cloning and expression of a DNA coding for hirudin has been obtained in *Escherichia coli,* yeast, *Bacillus subtilis,* and other systems.[17-25] The polypeptide can be highly purified from the broth to homogeneity by absorption on macroreticular resins, ion exchange chromatography, and gel filtration.[22]

Recombinant hirudins may exhibit several amino acid variations: All lack the sulfate group of Tyr 63; hence, these hirudins are designated desulfatohirudins (international non-proprietary name: desurin). Desurins are water-soluble and highly stable in lyophilized form or in solution in plasma.[12]

At least 12 commercial sources are reported to provide natural or recombinant hirudin.[14, 26]

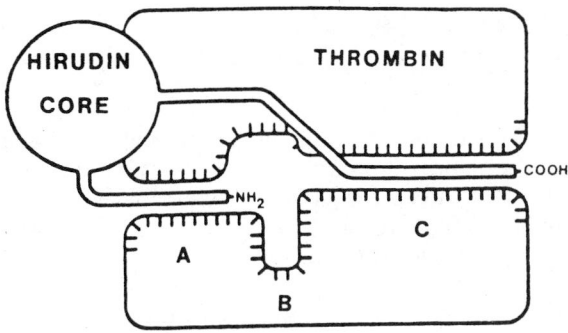

Figure 160–2. Interaction between hirudin and thrombin in the complex. Hirudin binds with its three N-terminal residues to the active site cleft of thrombin (A), but the primary specificity pocket of thrombin (B) is not occupied by hirudin. The carboxyl tail of hirudin (residues 55 to 65) binds along the anion-binding exosite of thrombin (C). (Modified from Grütter MG, Priestle JP, Rahvel J, et al: Crystal structure of the thrombin-hirudin complex: A novel mode of serine protease inhibition. EMBO J 9:2361, 1990, by permission of Oxford University Press.)

PHARMACOLOGY

Hirudin is a potent inhibitor of thrombin. The affinity of hirudin is in fact high enough to cause it to displace thrombin, also from cellular receptors. This neutralizing reaction is even faster than that between human thrombin and its main physiologic substrate, fibrinogen. In the equimolar, noncovalent complex, all biologic functions of thrombin are blocked, including its effects on vascular endothelium, vasoconstriction, and other nonhemostatic cellular events. The dissociation equilibrium constant (K_i) of 20 fM found for the human thrombin/natural hirudin complex indicates that hirudin is the most potent thrombin inhibitor known.[27] Absence of the sulfate group at residue Tyr 63 in recombinant hirudin leads to a tenfold increase of the K_i value. Because the thrombin-hirudin complex formation is essentially irreversible, this difference is highly unlikely to have any pharmacologic significance. A schematic diagram of the hirudin-thrombin complex is shown in Figure 160–2. The carboxyl tail of the hirudin molecule (residues 48 to 65) wraps around thrombin along its putative fibrinogen secondary binding site, whereby hirudin has numerous interactions with the thrombin molecule in this area. The core region of hirudin closes off the active site pocket of thrombin, and the three amino-terminal residues of hirudin are bound in a hydrophobic cleft of thrombin, but the primary specificity pocket itself is not directly involved in the binding. The tripeptide sequence 46 to 48 of hirudin seems to be important in facilitating the hirudin amino terminus/thrombin active site cleft interaction, but not because of its thrombin substrate-like sequence.[14]

Hirudin is specific for α-thrombin, because prothrombin activated with the nonenzymatic protein staphylocoagulase (resulting in an activity of 20% compared with α-thrombin) is not blocked by hirudin.[29] The same holds for snake venoms, such as batroxobin, which catalyze the release of fibrinopeptides of fibrinogen.[30] It is interesting to note that recombinant hirudin blocks endothelial thrombomodulin.[27]

Hirudin exhibits a selectivity of greater than four orders of magnitude for thrombin over all other proteolytic enzymes tested.[31, 32] Recombinant desulfate HV1 type hirudin has no effect on the digestive enzymes trypsin and chymotrypsin (at 12 μM), on the coagulation enzymes factor Xa, kallikrein, or plasmin (at 22 μM), or on any of the elements of the complement pathway.[12]

Hirudin not only prevents fibrinogen conversion to fibrin by immediately blocking any thrombin generated but also inhibits the thrombin-catalyzed activation of factors V, VIII, XIII and thrombin-induced platelet activation.[7, 35] In particular, hirudin is significantly more potent than unfractionated heparin in preventing thrombin activation of factor VIII.[34, 35]

By instantaneous inhibition of the small amount of thrombin generated after activation of the clotting system, the autocatalytic reaction that would otherwise lead to the accelerated generation of further thrombin is prevented. In fact, thrombin generation is remarkably amplified (by 280,000 times)[36] by formation of the prothrombinase complex produced by the binding of factors Va, Xa, and Ca^{2+} to the phospholipid of the platelet membrane. However, hirudin suppresses this feedback effect of thrombin. Unlike heparin, hirudin can displace thrombin bound to platelet thrombus receptors[37] and blocks the action of fibrin-bound thrombin in which the antithrombin III–binding sites are masked.[38, 39]

The activity of hirudin can be measured in antithrombin units (AT-U): 1 AT-U is the amount of hirudin that neutralizes one international unit of thrombin.[40] One microgram of pure hirudin inhibits about 5 μg of human thrombin. Pure hirudin contains approximately 10,000 to 15,000 AT-U/mg protein, depending on the thrombin used for the standardization.

PHARMACOKINETIC STUDIES IN ANIMALS

After intravenous bolus administration of 0.5 to 1 mg/kg of natural hirudin in rats, rabbits, and dogs, values at 10 to 15 minutes for the distribution and at 50 to 65 minutes for the elimination half-lives were obtained.[41] Similar values were found with recombinant desulfatohirudin in rats and dogs.[22, 42–49] The pharmacokinetic data can best be described by an open two-compartment model with first-order kinetics.

In the case of recombinant hirudin infusion in the dog, plateau values were reached within 30 to 60 minutes.[43]

In nephrectomized dogs, approximately 80% of an intravenously administered recombinant hirudin dose was distributed into extravascular compartments within 60 minutes. After this distribution phase, the blood levels of hirudin remained nearly constant for at least 4 hours,[45] showing nearly complete renal excretion of unmodified hirudin.

After intravenous (and subcutaneous) administration of natural hirudin or recombinant desulfated hirudin, the pharmacokinetic data from different studies in dogs[43, 45, 46] are similar. Only the renal excretion is increased by 20% to 25% with recombinant hirudin, presumably because of the absence of sulfation on Tyr 63.[44]

Following intravenous injection, radioactive-labeled recombinant[125] iododesulfatohirudin is uniformly distributed in all organs, but the peak radioactivity in the kidneys reflects an extensive renal excretion.[47, 48] The renal clearance of hirudin approximates the creatinine clearance, which suggests a glomerular filtration. Seventy-five percent of the injected dose of hirudin (intravenous or subcutaneous) is recovered unchanged in the urine 1 hour after administration, and 95% is recovered unchanged after 5 hours.[49] Natural (sulfated) or recombinant (nonsulfated) hirudin preparations, given intravenously to dogs, were isolated from urine and compared with the administered preparation by reversed-phase high-performance liquid chromatography, amino acid sequencing, and composition analysis.[50, 51] The cumulative urinary excretion was rapid and complete for sulfated and nonsulfated hirudin. It was shown that, in humans, 30% to 40% of the administered hirudins are eliminated in active form by glomerular filtration.

Up to 85% of natural hirudin and recombinant desulfated hirudin is adsorbed after subcutaneous administration in rats, rabbits, and dogs.[52] Peak plasma hirudin levels are reached after 1 to 2 hours, and the apparent elimination half-life is between 1.9 and 5.7 hours.[48, 53–55]

There is some absorption of recombinant hirudin after intratracheal instillation in rats with an elimination half-life of about 3.3 hours.[46] Rectal or intraduodenal administration of either natural or recombinant hirudin in dogs did not generate detectable plasma levels of either compound.[46]

Hirudin does not seem to pass through the blood-brain barrier, and there is only slight transfer through the placenta in rabbits.[46]

PHARMACODYNAMIC STUDIES IN HUMANS

Two hours after a single subcutaneous injection of recombinant hirudin (0.1 mg/kg), the activated partial thromboplastin time is prolonged to almost twice the basal value. The intersubject coefficient of variation of the weight-adjusted hirudin dose level remained within 20% of the mean value, even when the drug was readministered 1 month later in these immunocompetent volunteers, suggesting that recombinant hirudin does not elicit neutralizing antibodies. When four dose levels were tested, the mean activated partial thromboplastin time (aPTT) was maximally prolonged to 1.42, 1.70, 1.75, and 2.05 times the mean baseline values for the 0.1-, 0.3-, 0.5-, and 0.75-mg/kg subcutaneous doses of hirudin, respectively (Fig. 160–3).[56] Onset of effect occurred within the first 30 minutes of administration; plasma levels were sustained for 4 to 6 hours after the dose. Although the duration of the effect of aPTT was slightly longer at the higher doses, the mean aPTT had returned to approximately baseline values for all four dose levels tested by 24 hours after single dosing. The prolongation of aPTT was related to plasma hirudin concentration, whether measured by a functional or an immunologic method. Doubling of the aPTT is obtained at about 400 ng of desulfatohirudin per milliliter of plasma (two-step thrombin chromogenic assay method), which corresponds to approximately 60 nmol/L.

When 0.3 or 0.5 mg/kg of hirudin was subcutaneously injected at 8-hour intervals for 3 consecutive days in human volunteers, the mean aPTT prolongation, obtained 3 hours after dosing, was dose-dependent and ranged from 1.67 to 1.88 times baseline values.[56] The aPTT changes are reproducible and parallel with the concentrations of recombinant hirudin. With three times daily subcutaneous administration of recombinant hirudin for 3 days, the mean aPTT and plasma concentrations of recombinant hirudin remained elevated at the end of each dosing interval. Prolongation of aPTT and plasma concentrations of recombinant hirudin suggest no cumulative pharmacodynamic and pharmacokinetic effects. Values returned to baseline 16 hours after the eighth subcutaneous injection, irrespective of the dose level. When the same two dose levels were administered twice daily, the mean aPTT obtained 3 hours after dosing was dose-dependent and ranged from 1.5 to 2.5 times baseline. The aPTT values for the sixth-day administration of two dose levels of recombinant hirudin administered subcutaneously every 12 hours are reproducible and parallel with the changes in the plasma concentration of recombinant desulfatohirudin.

After intravenous bolus injection and infusion of ascending doses of recombinant hirudin for 6 and 72 hours, the aPTT followed a parabolic function with

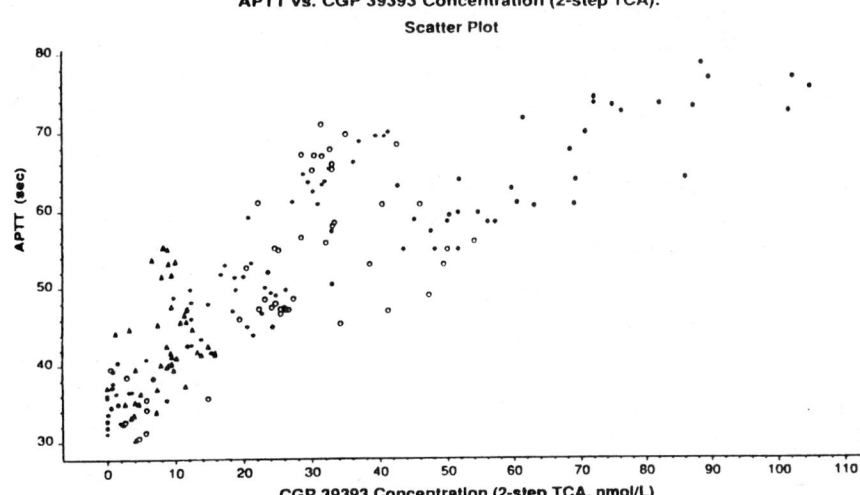

APTT vs. CGP 39393 Concentration (2-step TCA):
Scatter Plot

Figure 160–3. Scatter plots of correlation between activated partial thromboplastin time (aPTT) (*top*) or thrombin time (TT) (*bottom*) and plasma concentration of recombinant desulfatohirudin (CGP 39393). L, liter; TCA, thrombin chromogenic assay. (From Verstraete M, Nurmohead M, Kienast J, et al: Biologic effects of recombinant hirudin [CGP 39393] in human volunteers. J Am Coll Cardiol 22:1080, 1993. Reprinted with permission from the American College of Cardiology.)

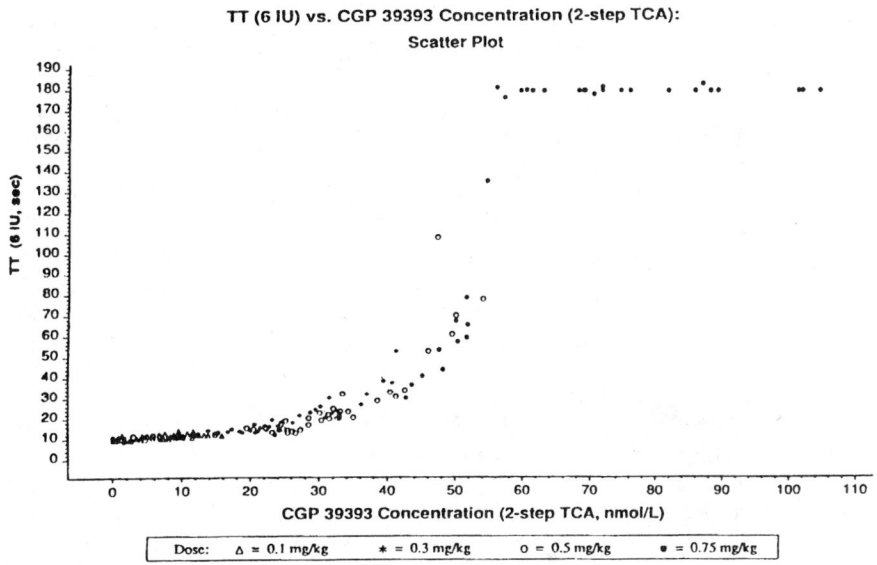

TT (6 IU) vs. CGP 39393 Concentration (2-step TCA):
Scatter Plot

| Dose: | Δ = 0.1 mg/kg | ★ = 0.3 mg/kg | o = 0.5 mg/kg | ● = 0.75 mg/kg |

doubled and quadrupled values at hirudin plasma concentrations of 100 and 1000 nmol/L, respectively.[57] The dose-response curve for prolongation of the aPTT is shallow at plasma levels of hirudin considered to be therapeutic. Whereas thrombin times were very sensitive to low hirudin plasma levels with unmeasurable clotting times at hirudin plasma concentrations greater than 30 nmol/L (bovine thrombin 3 IU/ml) and 60 nmol/L (bovine thrombin 6 IU/ml), the prothrombin time was prolonged by a factor of only 1.3 above baseline at 300 nmol/L. Thus, the aPTT appears to be most suitable for monitoring the anticoagulant effect of hirudin over a broad concentration range.

Although the aPTT is a simple and cheap method that can be automated, this test is hampered by problems of standardization, which make the results considerably dependent on the sensitivity of the reagent and instrument used. This was amply demonstrated in a comparison of 10 reagents used in one laboratory to assay hirudin added *in vitro* to normal plasma.[58]

PHARMACOKINETIC STUDIES IN HUMANS

After subcutaneous injection of six ascending doses of desulfatohirudin in human volunteers (0.1 to 0.75 mg/kg), the plasma clearance was between 1.5 and 1.7 ml/kg/min, and apparent elimination half-life was between 2 and 2.4 hours.[56]

Mean peak concentrations after intravenous bolus injections of 0.1, 0.3, 0.5, and 1.0 mg/kg were 154, 443, 764, and 1691 nmol/L, respectively. Intravenous infusions of 0.1 mg/kg/hr for 6 hours and of 0.2 and 0.3 mg/kg/hr for 6 hours and 72 hours resulted in mean steady-state levels of 78, 227, and 312 nmol/L, respectively.[57] Elimination was multiexponential and dose-independent. Concordant pharmacokinetic parameters were obtained from both intravenous bolus and infusion experiments (overall average total plasma clearance, 2.20 ml/kg/min; mean residence time, 2.12 hours; volume at steady state, 0.27 L/kg). The concentration in plasma after an intravenous infusion of ascending doses (0.1 mg/kg/hr, 0.2 mg/kg/hr, and 0.3 mg/kg/hr desulfatohirudin) during 6 or 72 hours rose steeply and reached 88 ± 14% of the steady-state concentration at 4 hours. This corresponds to three half-lives for a drug following first-order kinetics or a one-compartment model. When the same recombinant desulfatohirudin was used in volunteers with established atherosclerosis, terminal half-life was again 2 to 3 hours.[59] Pharmacokinetic values were similar in studies using another recombinant HV1 desulfatohirudin injected in human volunteers at lower doses (0.01 to 0.1 mg/kg).[49, 60]

IMMUNOLOGIC RESPONSE TO HIRUDIN

Hirudin, being a protein produced by the leech *Hirudo medicinalis*, has the theoretic potential to elicit an immunologic response and/or allergic reaction, including systemic anaphylaxis in humans.

Repeated administration in 263 fully immunocompetent healthy subjects, including those with a history of previous allergy and high levels of total IgE, resulted in type I allergic reactions mediated through IgA or IgE in 0.22% (95% confidence intervals 0.01 to 1.23).[61] In the same study, specific antibodies directed against hirudin appeared in 1 of 263 volunteers. Other human studies show that the risk of allergenicity appears to be low and have detected no signs of sensitization.[46, 52, 56–59] In brief, desulfatohirudin appears to be a very weak immunogen.

NEUTRALIZATION OF HIRUDIN

Hirudin, like all potent anticoagulants currently available, can result in unwanted bleeding. The use of hirudin in clinical situations, particularly postoperatively, is thus tempered by the absence of an effective antidote similar to the availability of vitamin K and protamine sulfate for the reversal of the biologic effects of coumarin drugs and heparin, respectively.

The hemorrhagic effect of recombinant hirudin is markedly reduced in a concentration-dependent manner by addition of increasing concentrations of a prothrombin complex concentrate. When factor-eight-inhibitor-bypassing-actively (FEIBA) as a source of prothrombin complex was administered 5 minutes after hirudin by a 25-U/kg slow infusion, the original bleeding response was reduced by 50%.[62] This suggests that prothrombin complex concentrates may be useful in reversing the hemorrhagic effect of hirudin. Desmopressin (1-deamino-8-D-arginine-vasopressin), a vasopressin analogue, increases coagulation factors (e.g., factor VIII) *in vivo* by a yet undefined mechanism. A 15-minute infusion of 0.3 μg of desmopressin per kilogram can reduce the hirudin effect in humans.

Three monoclonal antibodies (IgG-κ) against hirudin have been obtained and characterized.[63] They were detected toward continuous overlapping epitopes that are likely to be located in the C-terminal region of the protein. One of the monoclonal antibodies interferes with the interaction of hirudin with α-thrombin. Whether monoclonal or polyclonal antibodies against hirudin could be used to neutralize hirudin *in vivo* is still to be carefully evaluated. Other possibilities are acetylated thrombin derivatives and meizothrombin (which are not prothrombic but still bind to hirudin).[64] Also, recombinant factor VIIa will generate new thrombin, which after complex formation can exhaust circulating hirudin. Other possibilities currently being explored are cleaving enzymes and binding to inert peptides or proteins.

CLINICAL USE

Recombinant hirudin has been used in several arterial thrombotic models in animals without concomitant antiplatelet drugs. At doses prolonging the aPTT to two to three times baseline values, hirudin prevented heparin-resistant, platelet-rich thrombus formation at the site of coronary angioplasty in the pig;[65, 66] in baboons, it substantially reduced platelet deposition in chronic venous shunts grafted with endarterectomized segments of aorta.[67, 68] It was shown to speed thrombolysis with recombinant tissue-type plasminogen activator of occlusive platelet-rich thrombi and decrease reocclusion in a pig carotid endarterectomy model,[69] in models of coronary thrombosis,[67, 70, 71] and in other thrombosis models.[72, 73]

In minipigs, recombinant hirudin and aspirin also significantly reduce platelet and fibrin deposition in coronary stents compared with the reduction achieved with combined heparin, dextran, and aspirin.[74]

Initial phase II studies of hirudin in conjunction with thrombolytic therapy have been encouraging. TIMI-5 was a dose-ranging, pilot trial of hirudin versus heparin in conjunction with front-loaded alteplase and aspirin in 246 patients with acute myocardial infarction.[75] Patients received either intravenously administered heparin or hirudin at one of four ascending doses administered as a bolus followed by an intravenous infusion for 5 days (0.05–0.2 mg/kg/hr). Death or recurrent myocardial infarction occurred during hospitalization in 11 of 62 (6.8%) of hirudin-treated patients compared with 14 of 84 (16.7%) of heparin-treated patients (*p* = .02). The primary end point, TIMI grade 3 flow at 90 minutes and at 18 to 36 hours of catheterization, was achieved in 62% of hirudin-treated patients compared with 49% of heparin-treated patients (*p* = .07). Patients in the TIMI-6 trial[76] were treated with streptokinase and aspirin and then randomized to receive either desirudin or heparin. In this pilot trial, desirudin appeared to be as safe as heparin when given with streptokinase and aspirin to patients with acute myocardial infarction. Although this study was not prospectively designed to detect differences in efficacy, a trend toward lower rates of death, reinfarction, cardiogenic shock, and congestive heart failure was observed with the higher doses of desirudin (0.3 mg/kg bolus followed by 0.1 mg/kg/hr infusion; 0.6 mg/kg bolus followed by 0.2 mg/kg/hr infusion) when compared with the lowest dose (0.15 mg/kg bolus followed by 0.05 mg/kg/hr infusion).

The risk of bleeding, particularly from hemorrhagic stroke, associated with high-dose recombinant hirudin and heparin, has become apparent during the course of three large, phase III clinical trials—TIMI-9A,[77] GUSTO IIa,[78] and HIT-III.[79] In the first two, desirudin was administered as a 0.6 mg/kg IV bolus followed by a fixed-dose infusion of 0.2 mg/kg/hr for 96 (TIMI-9A) or 72 to 120 hours (GUSTO IIa). In HIT-III, patients were randomized to a 48- to 72-hour infusion of a different recombinant desirudin (0.4 mg/kg IV bolus, followed by 0.15 mg/kg/hr) or heparin. A front-loaded alteplase protocol was used in all three trials, and all received aspirin; 15% of patients in TIMI-9A received streptokinase. In HIT-III, but not GUSTO IIa and TIMI-9A, the dose of desirudin was adjusted to achieve aPPT values 2 to 3.5 times baseline.

In GUSTO,[80] intracranial bleeding occurred in 0.5% (with streptokinase) and 0.7% (with t-PA) of patients treated with concomitant intravenous (IV) heparin. Intracranial bleeding rates of 0.9% and 1.9% with t-PA (with heparin or desirudin) and the astonishingly high rates of 2.7% and 3.2% with streptokinase (with heparin or desirudin) in GUSTO IIa are up to five times greater than in GUSTO—as are rates of 1.9% and 1.7% in patients given t-PA with heparin or desirudin in TIMI-9A. Because 50% of patients had aPTT values below the target range of 60 to 85 seconds, a weight-adjusted heparin regimen was used in GUSTO IIa and TIMI-9A (patients < 80 kg or ≥ 80 kg received heparin at 1000 or 1300 IU/hr, respectively), and the drug was titrated to achieve a higher aPTT range of 60 to 90 seconds. Compared with GUSTO, this strategy resulted in a 20% increase in the total amount of heparin given.

In HIT-III, the dose of heparin was also adjusted according to body weight: 70 IU/kg followed by 15 IU/kg/hr. Intracranial bleeding rates in this trial were 2.7% in the group receiving recombinant hirudin and 0% in the group receiving heparin. All hemorrhagic strokes in HIT-III occurred within 24 hours of the start of treatment. In TIMI-9A and HIT-III, patients with major bleeding treated with recombinant hirudin tended to have higher median aPTT values 12 hours after the start of treatment than did those without major bleeding.

In view of these results and of the observation that infusion of desirudin at a dose of 0.1 mg/kg/hr appears to be as effective as higher doses, in both unstable angina[76] and myocardial infarction,[75] trials have now restarted (GUSTO IIb and TIMI-9B, in which to date more than 10,000 patients have been enrolled) using lower doses (e.g., 0.1 mg/kg IV bolus of desirudin, followed by 0.1 mg/kg/hr; or 1000 IU/hr heparin, without weight adjustment). In addition, dosage of both drugs will be adjusted to achieve target aPTT values of 55 to 85 seconds (TIMI-9B) and 60 to 85 seconds (GUSTO IIb), since aPTT values above 100 seconds are clearly associated with an increased risk of intracerebral hemorrhage. Down-titra-

tion of desirudin and adjustment to aPTT values only two to three times baseline may take better advantage of the lower anticoagulant/antithrombin ratio of desirudin compared with heparin clearly established in preclinical studies, in which desirudin was more effective than heparin at aPTT ratios several times lower than those achieved with high-dose heparin.

In a double-blind multicenter trial, the effects of desulfatohirudin relative to unfractionated heparin were assessed in 113 patients with stable angina undergoing percutaneous transluminal coronary balloon angioplasty (PTCA).[81] Prior to PTCA, 20 mg of desulfatohirudin was administered as a bolus, followed by continuous infusion at a rate of 0.16 mg/kg/hr, or 10,000 IU heparin was administered as a bolus and continued at a rate of 12 IU/kg/hr for 24 hours. Infusion was adjusted to aPTT levels (85–120 seconds). In comparison with patients treated with heparin, patients who received hirudin had a lower incidence of thrombotic events (10.3% versus 1.4% of acute myocardial infarction and/or emergency coronary artery bypass surgery). The relative risk of postprocedural ischemia, as measured by ST-segment changes on 24-hour Holter ambulatory electrocardiographic monitoring, was significantly reduced in the hirudin cohort. Because hirudin appeared to be safe and effective in this pilot study, a large European multicenter trial in patients with stable angina undergoing PTCA is now in progress.

A double-blind randomized large-scale trial in patients due to undergo PTCA was conducted in Europe:[82] patients with recent onset angina, worsening angina, or angina at rest began treatment before PTCA, with heparin (10,000 IU IV bolus followed by 15 IU/kg/hr for 24 hours) or desirudin. Desirudin was given either as a 40 mg IV bolus followed by IV infusion of 0.2 mg/kg/hr for 24 hours, or as a 40-mg IV bolus, plus IV infusion of 0.2 mg/kg/hr for 24 hours, followed by a 40-mg subcutaneous dose twice daily for 3 consecutive days. Quantitative coronary angiography was performed immediately before and after PTCA and again 6 months later. The incidence of early (< 96 hours) major adverse cardiac events was significantly ($p < .01$) reduced by the regimen of desirudin that incorporated subcutaneous desirudin for 3 days. At 7 months' follow-up, there were no statistically significant differences in event-free survival ($p = .5$) or minimal-lumen diameter among the three groups.[83]

An open ascending dose-finding pilot trial after hip replacement has been completed.[84] Forty-eight patients undergoing an elective total hip replacement received 10, 15, 20, or 40 mg of desulfatohirudin subcutaneously twice a day. The first injection took place preoperatively, and the prophylaxis continued for a mean of 11 days (range, 7 to 12 days). Blood loss and transfusion requirements were recorded preoperatively and postoperatively, and all patients underwent bilateral ascending phlebography. A first and second set of 12 patients, each receiving 10 and 20 mg, respectively, did not present severe bleeding complications or other adverse events that would preclude the fur-

ANTITHROMBOTIC THERAPY

ther administration of hirudin. However, 2 of 3 patients receiving 40 mg had significantly increased blood loss during the first days, leading to the discontinuation of this dose level. The study was then continued with 9 additional patients on 20 mg and 12 new patients on 15 mg twice a day. Median bleeding volume (1050, 1250, or 1240 ml) or transfusion requirements perioperatively were similar in the 10-, 15-, and 20-mg hirudin groups. Measurements of aPTT done 2 hours post injection were prolonged by a mean of 7 to 12 seconds in the three treatment groups. The thromboembolic rate was 42% in the 10-mg, 9% in the 15-mg, and 10% in the 20-mg group. The prophylactic effect of 15 or 20 mg compares very favorably with previous results obtained in the same hospital with either standard or low-molecular-weight heparin. A large, multicenter, double-blind randomized trial has evaluated the efficacy and safety of three doses of hirudin (10 mg, 15 mg, or 20 mg twice a day) versus unfractionated heparin (5000 IU three times a day) in patients undergoing elective hip replacement. Of the 1120 patients recruited, 837 had evaluable phlebograms. The results indicate that hirudin 15 mg and 20 mg twice daily offers safe and effective prophylaxis. Interestingly, the rates of proximal deep vein thrombosis at these two doses are 3.1% and 2.4%, respectively, compared with 19.6% for unfractioned heparin.

A pilot trial on treatment with recombinant hirudin has been published.[86] Ten patients with clinical signs of deep venous thrombosis of less than 14 days were included, and the diagnosis was confirmed by venography. All patients were treated with a bolus injection of 0.07 mg/kg followed by 0.05 mg/kg/hr for 5 days. The score on the repeat venogram (day 5) remained unchanged, and there was no recurrence of thrombosis, death, or major bleedings in this open trial. In another pilot trial, the same recombinant hirudin as in the previous trial was administered subcutaneously at a dose of 0.75 mg/kg twice daily for 5 days to 10 patients with recent deep vein thrombosis[94]; standard heparin and acenocaumarol were subsequently given. Lower limb venography was repeated after 5 days, and showed no changes when compared with the pretreatment phlebogram. A dose-ranging study comparing subcutaneous recombinant hirudin with heparin is required to establish whether one drug gives better results than the other.

Although several large-scale, multicenter clinical trials with hirudin are in progress, published reports on its therapeutic use are limited. In addition to the proper assessment of hirudin's therapeutic and bleeding risks, the optimal dose and duration of hirudin therapy and the possibility of a rebound phenomenon similar to the one described following an infusion of argatroban[88] still have to be carefully investigated.

PRECAUTIONS AND ADVERSE EFFECTS

Tolerability and safety measurements (physical examination, hemodynamic variables, electrocardiogram, routine clinical chemistry, and hematologic values) were not influenced by administration of single or repeated subcutaneous doses,[56] intravenous bolus doses, or infusions[57] of ascending doses of recombinant desulfated hirudin. Apart from its anticoagulant effect, hirudin is pharmacologically inert and well tolerated.

Desulfatohirudin exhibits a moderate influence in the mainly platelet-mediated "primary hemostasis." Hirudin inhibits thrombin-induced platelet aggregation but has no effect on aggregation induced by other agonists.[88] In human volunteers receiving an intravenous bolus dose of 1.0 mg/kg of desulfatohirudin, bleeding time was prolonged by less than two times. The continuous infusion of recombinant hirudin resulting in 200 to 400 nmol/L steady-state plasma concentration had no effect on bleeding time in healthy human volunteers.[57] Also, in a group of patients with established atherosclerosis, a 6-hour intravenous infusion of ascending doses of desulfatohirudin (0.02 to 0.3 mg/kg/hr) was not associated with a significant prolongation of the bleeding time when measured 30 minutes before the end of infusion.[59] Because bleeding time occasionally has been prolonged in some volunteers, more clinical experience is needed before it is possible to judge this issue.[89, 90]

It should be noted that hirudin inhibits the binding of thrombin to endothelial thrombomodulin, which may result in reduced activation of protein C.

REFERENCES

1. Stillé A, Maisch JM: Hirudo. *In* The National Dispensary, 3rd ed. Philadelphia: Henry C. Lea's Son, 1884, pp 766–768.
2. Dirckx J: The language of medicine. Its evolution, structure, and dynamics, 2nd ed. New York: Praeger, 1983, p 28.
3. Castiglioni A, Krumbhaar EB: A History of Medicine, 2nd ed. New York: Alfred A. Knopf, 1958, pp 698–712.
4. King J: Hirudo medicinalis. *In* The American Dispensatory, 8th ed. Cincinnati: Wilstach, Baldwin, 1870, pp 424–426.
5. Singer C, Underwood EA: A Short History of Medicine, 2nd ed. New York: Oxford University Press, 1962, pp 280–287.
6. Haycraft JB: On the action of secretion obtained from the medicinal leech on the coagulation of the blood. Proc R Soc Lond 36:478, 1884.
7. Markwardt F: Untersuchungen über Hirudin. Naturwissenschaften 52:537, 1955.
8. Petersen TE, Roberts HR, et al: Primary structure of hirudin, a thrombin-specific inhibitor. *In* Peeters H (ed): Protides of the Biological Fluids (Proceedings of the 23rd colloquium held in Brugge, 1975). Oxford: Pergamon Press, 1976, pp 145–149.
9. Dodt J: Hirudine, die Thromboinhibitoren des Blutegels "Hirudo medicinalis." Dissertation zur Erlangung der Doktorwurde am Fachbereich Chemie und Pharmazie des Ludwig-Maximilian Universitat München, München, 1984.
10. Dodt J, Müller H-P, Seemüller U, Chang J-Y: The complete amino acid sequence of hirudin, a thrombin specific inhibitor. FEBS Lett 165:180, 1984.
11. Dodt J, Seemüller U, Maschler R, Fritz H: The complete covalent structure of hirudin. Biol Chem Hoppe-Seyler 366:379, 1985.
12. Talbot M: Biology of recombinant hirudin (CGP 39393): A new prospect in the treatment of thrombosis. Semin Thromb Hemost 15(3):293, 1989.
13. Scharf M, Engels J, Tripier D: Primary structures of new "isohirudins." FEBS Lett 225:105, 1989.
14. Bichler J, Fritz H: Hirudin, a new therapeutic tool? Ann Hematol 63:67, 1991.

15. Sukumaran DK, Clare GM, Presus A, et al: Proton nuclear magnetic resonance study of hirudin: Resonance assignment and secondary structure. Biochemistry 26:333, 1987.

16. Clore GM, Sukumaran DK, Nilges M, et al: The conformation of hirudin in solution. A study using nuclear magnetic resonance, distance geometry and restrained molecular dynamics. EMBO J 6:529, 1987.

17. Bergmann C, Dodt J, Köhler S, et al: Chemical synthesis and expression of a gene coding for hirudin, the thrombin-specific inhibitor from the leech *Hirudo medicinalis*. Biol Chem Hoppe-Seyler 367:731, 1986.

18. Dodt J, Machleidt W, Seemüller U, et al: Isolation and characterization of hirudin isoinhibitors and sequence analysis of hirudin PA. Biol Chem Hoppe-Seyler 367:803, 1986.

19. Fortkamp E, Rieger M, Heisterberg-Moutses G, et al: Cloning and expression in *Escherichia coli* of a synthetic DNA for hirudin, the blood coagulation inhibitor in the leech. DNA 5:511, 1986.

20. Harvey RP, Degryse E, Stefani L, et al: Cloning and expression of a cDNA coding for the anticoagulant hirudin from the blood-sucking leech, *Hirudo medicinalis*. Proc Natl Acad Sci U S A 83:1084, 1986.

21. Courtney M, Loison G, Lemoine Y, et al: Production and evaluation of recombinant hirudin. Semin Thromb Hemost 15:288, 1989.

22. Meyhack B, Heim J, Rink H, et al: Desulphatohirudin, a specific thrombin inhibitor: Expression and secretion in yeast [abstract]. Thromb Res 7(Suppl):3, 1987.

23. Roitsch C, Riehl-Bellon N, Carvallo D, et al: Characterization of hirudins isolated from *Hirudo medicinalis* [abstract]. Thromb Res 7(Suppl):32, 1987.

24. Tripier D: Isolation and sequence analysis of new hirudin [abstract]. Thromb Res Suppl 7:31, 1987.

25. Johnson P, Sze P, Winant R, et al: Biochemistry and genetic engineering of hirudin. Semin Thromb Hemost 15:302, 1989.

26. Fareed J, Walenga J M, Hoppenstead D A, Pifarre R: Developmental perspectives for recombinant hirudin as an antithrombotic agent. Biol Clin Hematol 11:1431, 1989.

27. Stone S, Hofsteenge J: The kinetics of the inhibition of thrombin by hirudin. Biochemistry 25:4622, 1986.

28. Grütter MG, Priestle JP, Rahvel J, et al: Crystal structure of the thrombin-hirudin complex: A novel mode of serine protease inhibition. EMBO J 9:2361, 1990.

29. Kawabata S-L, Morita T, Miyata T, et al: Difference in enzymatic properties between "staphylothrombin" and free-thrombin. Ann N Y Acad Sci 485:27, 1986.

30. Walsmann P, Markwardt F: Biochemische und pharmakologische Aspekte des Thrombininhibitors Hirudin. Pharmazie 26:653, 1981.

31. Bagdy D, Barabas E, Graf L, et al: Hirudin. *In* Lorand L (ed): Methods in Enzymology, Vol 45: Proteolytic Enzymes. New York: Academic Press, 1976, pp 669–678.

32. Markwardt F: Hirudin as an inhibitor of thrombin. *In* Perlman GE, Lorand L (eds): Methods in Enzymology, Vol 19. Proteolytic Enzymes. New York: Academic Press, 1970, pp 924–932.

33. Kaiser B, Markwardt F: Antithrombotic and haemorrhagic effects of synthetic and naturally occurring thrombin inhibitors. Thromb Res 43:613, 1986.

34. Gray E, Watton J, Barrowcliffe TW, Thomas DP: Anticoagulant and antithrombotic effects of recombinant hirudin [abstract]. Thromb Haemost 62(Suppl 1):187, 1989.

35. Pieters J, Lindhout T, Hemker HC: In situ–generated thrombin is the only enzyme that effectively activates factor VIII and factor V in thromboplastin-activated plasma. Blood 74:1021, 1989.

36. Mann KG: Prothrombin and thrombin. *In* Colman RW, Hirsh J, Marder VJ, Salzman EW (eds): Hemostasis and Thrombosis: Basic Principles and Clinical Practice. Philadelphia: JB Lippincott, 1993, pp 184–199.

37. Tam SW, Fenton JW, Detwiler TC: Dissociation of thrombin from platelets by hirudin. J Biol Chem 254:8723, 1979.

38. Hogg PJ, Jackson CM: Fibrin monomer protects thrombin from inactivation by heparin-antithrombin III: Implications for heparin efficacy. Proc Natl Acad Sci U S A 86:3619, 1989.

39. Weltz JJ, Hudoba M, Massel D, et al: Clot-bound thrombin is protected from inhibition by heparin-antithrombin III but is susceptible to inactivation by antithrombin III-independent inhibitors. J Clin Invest 86:385, 1990.

40. Markwardt F: Versuche zur pharmakologischen Charakterisierung des Hirudins. Naunyn-Schmiedebergs Arch Pharmacol 234:516, 1958.

41. Markwardt F, Hauptmann J, Nowak G, et al: Pharmacological studies on the antithrombotic action of hirudin in experimental animals. Thromb Haemost 47:226, 1982.

42. Grossenbacher HH, Auden JAL, Bill K, et al: Isolation and characterization of recombinant desulphato-hirudin from yeast, a highly selective thrombin inhibitor [abstract]. Thromb Res 7(Suppl):34, 1987.

43. Markwardt F: Development of hirudin as an antithrombotic agent. Semin Thromb Hemost 15:269, 1989.

44. Markwardt F, Kaiser B, Nowak G: Studies on antithrombotic effects of recombinant hirudin. Thromb Res 54:377, 1989.

45. Nowak G, Markwardt F, Fink E: Pharmacokinetic studies with recombinant hirudin in dogs. Folia Haematol, Leipzig 115:70, 1988.

46. Markwardt F, Fink G, Kaiser B, et al: Pharmacological survey of recombinant hirudin. Pharmazie 43:202, 1988.

47. Richter M, Walsmann P, Cyranka U, Markwardt F: 125I-Markierung von Hirudin. Pharmazie 41:510, 1986.

48. Richter M, Cyranka U, Nowak G, Walsmann P: Pharmacokinetics of 125I-hirudin in rats and dogs. Folia Haematol 115:64, 1988.

49. Markwardt F, Nowak G, Stürzebecher J, Vogel G: Clinico-pharmacological studies with recombinant hirudin. Thromb Res 52:393, 1988.

50. Henschen A, Markwardt F, Walsmann P: Identification by HPLC analysis of the unaltered forms of hirudin and desulfated hirudin after kidney passage [abstract]. Thromb Res 7(Suppl): 37, 1987.

51. Henschen A, Markwardt F, Walsmann P: Evidence for the identity of hirudin isolated after kidney passage with the starting material. Folia Haematol, Leipzig 115:59, 1988.

52. Bichler J, Siebeck M, Fichtl B, Fritz H: Pharmacokinetics, effect on clotting parameters and assessment of the immunoallergic potential of hirudin in man after single subcutaneous and intravenous bolus administration [abstract]. Thromb Haemost 62(Suppl 1):533, 1989.

53. Nowak G, Markwardt F: Pharmacokinetic studies with hirudin [abstract]. Thromb Res 7(Suppl):36, 1987.

54. Markwardt F, Nowak G, Sturzebecher J, et al: Pharmacokinetics and anticoagulant effect of hirudin in man. Thromb Haemost 52:160, 1984.

55. Markwardt F, Nowak G, Stürzebecher U, Walsmann P: Studies on the pharmacokinetics of hirudin. Biomed Biochim Acta 46:237, 1987.

56. Verstraete M, Nurmohead M, Kienast J, et al: Biologic effects of recombinant hirudin (CGP 39393) in human volunteers. J Am Coll Cardiol 22:1080, 1993.

57. Marbet GA, Verstraete M, Kienast J, et al: Clinical pharmacology of intravenously administered recombinant desulfatohirudin (CGP 39393) in healthy volunteers. J Cardiovasc Pharmacol 22:364, 1993.

58. Tripodi A, Chantarangkul V, Arbini AA, et al: Effects of hirudin on activated partial thromboplastin time determined with ten different reagents. Thromb Haemost 70:286, 1993.

59. Zoldhelyi P, Webster MWI, Fuster V, et al: Recombinant hirudin in patients with chronic, stable coronary artery disease. Safety, half-life, and effect on coagulation parameters. Circulation 88:2015, 1993.

60. Meyer BH, Luus HG, Müller FO, et al. The pharmacology of recombinant hirudin, a new anticoagulant. S Afr Med J 78:268, 1990.

61. Close P, Bichler J, Kerry R, et al: Weak allergenicity of recombinant hirudin CGP 39393 in immunocompetent volunteers. Coron Art Dis 5:943, 1994.

62. Walenga JM, Pifarre R, Hoppensteadt DA, Fareed J: Development of recombinant hirudin as a therapeutic anticoagulant and antithrombotic agent: Some objective considerations. Semin Thromb Hemost 15:316, 1989.

63. Spinner S, Stöffler G, Fink E: Quantitative enzyme-linked immunosorbent assay (ELISA) for hirudin. J Immunol Meth 87:79, 1988.

64. Brüggener E, Walsman P, Markwardt F: Neutralization of hirudin anticoagulant activity by DIP-thrombin. Pharmazie 44:648, 1989.

65. Heras M, Chesebro JH, Penny WJ, et al: Effects of thrombin inhibition on the development of acute platelet-thrombus deposition during angioplasty in pigs. Heparin versus recombinant hirudin, a specific thrombin inhibitor. Circulation 79:657, 1989.

66. Heras M, Chesebro JH, Webster MWI, et al: Hirudin, heparin or placebo during deep arterial injury in the pig: The in vivo role of thrombin in platelet-mediated thrombosis. Circulation 82:1476, 1990.

67. Haskel EJ, Prager NA, Sobel BE, Abendschein DR: Relative efficacy of antithrombin compared with antiplatelet agents in accelerating coronary thrombolysis and preventing early reocclusion. Circulation 83:1048, 1991.

68. Haskel EJ, Torr SR, Day KC, et al: Prevention of arterial reocclusion after thrombolysis with recombinant lipoprotein-associated coagulation inhibitor. Circulation 84:821, 1991.

69. Mruk JS, Chesebro JH, Webster MWI, et al: Hirudin markedly enhances thrombolysis with rt-PA [abstract]. Circulation 82(Suppl III):111, 1990.

70. Rudd MA, George D, Johnstone MT, et al: Effect of thrombin inhibition on the dynamics of thrombolysis and on platelet function during thrombolytic therapy. Circ Res 70:829, 1992.

71. Kaiser B, Simon A, Markwardt F: Antithrombotic effects of recombinant hirudin in experimental angioplasty and intravascular thrombolysis. Thromb Haemost 63:44, 1990.

72. Sitko GR, Ramjit DR, Stabilito II, et al: Conjunctive enhancement of enzymatic thrombolysis and prevention of thrombotic reocclusion with the selective factor Xa inhibitor, tick anticoagulant peptide: Comparison to hirudin and heparin in a canine model of acute coronary thrombosis. Circulation 85:805, 1992.

73. Rigel DF, Olson RW, Lappe RW: Comparison of hirudin and heparin as adjuncts to streptokinase thrombolysis in a canine model of coronary thrombosis. Circ Res 72:1091, 1993.

74. Buchwald AB, Sandrock D, Unterberg CA, et al: Platelet and fibrin deposition on coronary stents in minipigs: Effects of hirudin versus heparin. J Am Coll Cardiol 21:249, 1993.

75. Canon CP, McCabe CH, Henry TD, et al: Recombinant desulfatohirudin compared with heparin in conjunction with alteplase and aspirin for acute myocardial infarction. Results of the Thrombolysis in Myocardial Infarction (TIMI) 5 trial. J Am Coll Cardiol 23:993, 1994.

76. Lee LV, for the TIMI-6 investigators: Initial experience with hirudin and streptokinase in acute myocardial infarction: Results of the thrombolysis in myocardial infarction (TIMI) 6 trial. J Am Coll Cardiol 75:7, 1995.

77. Antman E, for the TIMI-9A investigators: Hirudin in myocardial infarction: Safety report from the thrombolysis and thrombin inhibition in myocardial infarction (TIMI-9A) trial. Circulation 90:1624, 1994.

78. GUSTO IIa Investigators (global use of strategies to open occluded coronary arteries): Randomised trial of intravenous heparin versus recombinant hirudin for acute coronary syndromes. Circulation 90:1631, 1994.

79. Neuhaus KL, von Essen R, Tebbe U, et al: Safety observations from the pilot phase of the randomised r-hirudin for improvement of thrombolysis (HIT-III) study. Circulation 90:1638, 1994.

80. The GUSTO Investigators: An international randomised trial comparing four thrombolytic strategies for acute myocardial infarction. N Engl J Med 329:673, 1993.

81. van den Bos AA, Deckers JW, Heyndrickx GR, et al: PTCA with hirudin associated with less acute complications than with heparin. Circulation 86(Suppl I):1, 1992.

82. Serruys PW, Fox KAA, Herrman JPR, et al: HELVETICA Investigators. Recombinant hirudin (CGP 39 393) reduces the incidence of major adverse cardiac events, reported within the first 96 hours post angioplasty in unstable patients (Braunwald classification) pretreated by heparin [abstract]. J Am Coll Cardiol 23:90A, 1995.

83. Serruys PW, Herrman JPR, Simon R, et al, for the HELVETICA Investigators: A comparison of hirudin with heparin in the prevention of restenosis after coronary angioplasty. N Engl J Med 333:757, 1995.

84. Eriksson BI, Kälebo P, Lindbratt S, et al: Direct thrombin inhibition with rec-hirudin CGP 39393 as prophylaxis of thromboembolic complications after total hip replacement. Thromb Haemost 72:227, 1994.

85. Eriksson BI, Ekman S, Kälebo P, et al: Prevention of deep-vein thrombosis after total hip replacement: Direct thrombin inhibitor with recombinant hirudin. CGP 39393. Lancet 347:635, 1996.

86. Parent F, Bridey F, Dreyfus M, et al: Treatment of severe venous thrombo-embolism with intravenous hirudin (HBW023). An open pilot study. Thromb Haemost 70:386, 1993.

87. Schiele F, Vuillemenot A, Kramarz P, et al: A pilot study of subcutaneous recombinant hirudin (HBW 023) in the treatment of deep vein thrombosis. Thromb Haemost 71:558, 1994.

88. Gold HK, Torres FW, Garabedian HD, et al: Evidence for a dose-related rebound coagulation phenomenon following cessation of a 4-hour infusion of a specific thrombin inhibitor in patients with unstable angina pectoris. J Am Coll Cardiol 21:1039, 1993.

89. Markwardt F: Hirudin: The promising antithrombotic. Cardiovasc Drug Rev 10:211, 1992.

90. Marki WE, Wallis RB: The anticoagulant and antithrombotic properties of hirudins. Thromb Haemost 64:344, 1990.

CHAPTER 161

Hirulog*

Christopher P. Cannon, M.D.

HISTORY

Hirulog is a polypeptide that was designed based on structural studies of hirudin, the naturally occurring 65-amino-acid anticoagulant derived from the saliva of the leech *Hirudo medicinalis*.[1] As discussed in the previous chapter, leeches were used for medicinal purposes dating back to approximately 200 BC, although they were of greatest popularity in the late 18th century in France.[2] The anticoagulant activity of the leech was discovered by Haycraft in 1884,[3] and its protein nature was isolated by Markwardt.[4] Studies of the interaction of thrombin and hirudin reported two major sites where hirudin binds to thrombin: the catalytic site and the substrate recognition site (also known as the anion-binding exosite).[5, 6] The carboxyl-terminal region of hirudin was found to be necessary for binding, notably a 12-amino-acid peptide.[7] The amino-terminal region of hirudin was found to interact with the catalytic site of thrombin.[6]

Hirulog brand direct thrombin inhibitor (Biogen, Inc., Cambridge, MA), herein referred to as Hirulog.

Hirulog was designed by Maraganore et al. in 1990 based on these observations.[1] Hirulog, a direct thrombin inhibitor, was produced to contain three domains: the 12-amino-acid carboxyl-terminus derived from hirudin; a 4-amino-acid sequence, D-Phe-Pro-Arg-Pro, which binds to the catalytic site of thrombin; and a linker region with the optimal length to allow binding of both inhibitory sites.[1] Hirulog is produced synthetically, and since 1990, has undergone extensive experimental and clinical evaluation and has shown promise as a potent antithrombotic agent.

CHEMISTRY

Hirulog is a 20-amino-acid polypeptide with three domains, as shown in Figure 161–1: (1) The carboxyl-terminal domain contains 12 amino acids, which correspond to the Tyr-sulfated residues 53 to 64 of hirudin.[7] This 12-amino-acid polypeptide, known as "hirugen,"[7] binds in a competitive manner to the substrate recognition site of thrombin[8] and thereby inhibits thrombin reaction with fibrinogen, but not the catalytic properties of thrombin.[7, 9] (2) The amino-terminal sequence D-Phe-Pro-Arg-Pro interacts with thrombin's active catalytic site. (3) An intervening tetraglycyl "spacer" linking the amino and carboxyl terminal sequences.[1] The linker domain allows the two inhibitory moieties to bind to their cognate sites in thrombin within the intermolecular distance of 18 A. X-ray crystallographic studies have confirmed these binding relationships.[6, 10, 11] The molecular weight of Hirulog is 2180. Hirulog is made by a multiple-step synthetic chemical process and is formulated either as a frozen phosphate-buffered mannitol solution with a pH of 5.5 to 7.5 or, more recently, as a lyophilized powder with sodium hydroxide mannitol at a pH of 5.0 to 6.0.

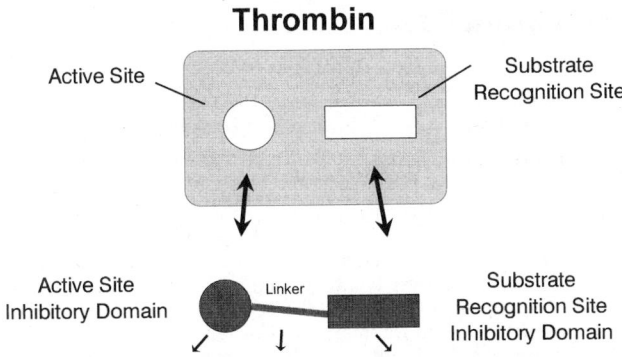

Thrombin

Active Site

Substrate Recognition Site

Active Site Inhibitory Domain

Linker

Substrate Recognition Site Inhibitory Domain

D-Phe-Pro-Arg-Pro - (Gly)4 - Asn-Gly-Asp-Phe-Glu-Glu-Ile-Pro-Glu-Glu-Tyr-Leu

Hirulog

Figure 161–1. The structure of Hirulog and its interaction with thrombin. Hirulog contains three domains: (1) an active site inhibitor domain, which binds to the active catalytic site of thrombin; (2) a substrate recognition site inhibitory domain, which binds to the site where thrombin binds to fibrinogen or the platelet membrane receptor; (3) a linker domain. (Adapted with permission from Cannon CP, Maraganore JM, Loscalzo J, et al: Anticoagulant effects of Hirulog, a novel thrombin inhibitor, in patients with coronary artery disease. Am J Cardiol 71:778, 1993.)

Other hirudin-derived peptides were constructed and tested,[1] although it is the above-described Hirulog (known initially as Hirulog-1) that had the most favorable binding characteristics.[1] Other lengths of the linker domain were tested, as well as use of only the "hirugen" compound,[7] which did not inhibit the active catalytic site of thrombin.

PHARMACOLOGY

Hirulog is a highly potent and specific thrombin inhibitor that binds to thrombin in a 1:1 complex (see Fig. 161–1), inhibiting all known hemostatic and non-hemostatic actions of thrombin.[1, 12] Hirulog inhibits thrombin-mediated formation of fibrin, amplification of coagulation by factor V, activation of platelets, and proliferation of smooth muscle cells.[13, 14] Because Hirulog acts independently of antithrombin III, it remains effective even when plasma antithrombin III is quantitatively or qualitatively deficient.[13] Hirulog can escape neutralization by platelet factors, such as platelet factor 4,[15] and, perhaps most importantly, Hirulog can inhibit both soluble and clot-bound thrombin.[13, 16] Finally, Hirulog provides a constant and predictable degree of anticoagulation.[12, 17, 18]

Interaction with Thrombin

The binding of Hirulog to thrombin occurs in a four-step process: (1) The carboxyl-terminal region of Hirulog binds to the substrate recognition site of thrombin with a dissociation constant of 0.75 μM (Data on file, Biogen, Inc.). (2) An intramolecular conformational change occurs to form a second intermediate conformation with a rate constant of about 300 s^{-1}, which is the rate-limiting step. (3) A very rapid step, formation of a third intermediate conformation, occurs with the amino-terminus of Hirulog binding to the active site. (4) A final intramolecular step is identified with a rate constant of 30 s^{-1}. Active site interactions of Hirulog, described by the final step, increase the stability of the Hirulog-thrombin complex by 400-fold. A value of 4.3×10^8 M^{-1} s^{-1} was determined as the effective second-order rate constant for complex formation (K_{ass}). The effective dissociation rate constant (K_{diss}) can be calculated from the expression $K_{diss} = K_i(K_{ass})$ to be 0.8 s^{-1} (Data on file, Biogen, Inc.). Hirulog can also be cleaved at the Arg_3-Pro_4 bond after interactions with thrombin.[19] However, the rate of thrombin cleavage of Hirulog was 0.01 s^{-1}. Thus, it can be concluded that under the conditions of the assay, the major pathway of dissociation of Hirulog from the complex does not involve the release of cleaved inhibitor.

Kinetic studies showed Hirulog to inhibit thrombin activity (tested with hydrolysis of tripeptidyl *p*-nitroanilide substrates) with a K_i of 2.3 nM, while the carboxyl-terminal hirudin peptide(s), e.g., hirugen, failed to inhibit thrombin cleavage of small substrates.[1] The formation of the Hirulog:thrombin complex was also studied using steady-state and rapid kinetics at 37°C. The inhibition constant (K_i) for Hirulog was found to be 1.9 nM , a value in agreement with that previously determined.[1]

The interaction of Hirulog and thrombin has also been studied with x-ray crystallographic studies.[11, 20] The amino-terminal sequence D-Phe-Pro-Arg was observed to bind to thrombin's active site, with the orientation of the peptide backbone running antiparallel to thrombin residues $Ser2_{14}$-$Gly2_{16}$. The side chain of D-Phe1 lies in the middle of a hydrophobic pocket formed by thrombin residues His_{57}, Tyr_{60A}, Trp_{60D}, Leu_{99}, Ile_{174}, and Trp_{215}. The side chain of Arg_3 was located in the primary specificity pocket of thrombin in an extended conformation. The guanidinium group of Arg_3 formed a doubly hydrogen-bonded ion pair with thrombin residue $Asp1_{89}$. The carboxyl-terminal amino acids of Hirulog observed in the crystallographic structure bind to the substrate recognition site of thrombin in a manner analogous to that observed in the hirudin:thrombin and hirugen:thrombin complexes.[6, 11] Both electrostatic and van der Waals' contacts accommodated the interactions of the Hirulog carboxyl-terminal moiety with thrombin's substrate recognition site. Together, these studies demonstrated that interaction of Hirulog with thrombin is achieved through multiple contacts across the near full diameter of thrombin, which accounts for the high affinity and specificity of the complex.

Specificity for Thrombin

As could be predicted by its structure, Hirulog is very specific for thrombin as compared with other serine proteinases. The specificity of Hirulog was examined by measuring the ability of Hirulog to inhibit the activity of 15 other serine proteinases, including plasmin, tissue-type plasminogen activator, activated protein C, and factor Xa. Results demonstrate that Hirulog concentrations more than 26,000-fold greater than those required for thrombin inhibition are required for inhibition of other serine proteinases (Data on file, Biogen, Inc.). Thus, at Hirulog concentrations employed in clinical studies, Hirulog would remain pharmacologically specific for thrombin.

Inhibition of Clot-Bound Thrombin

Weitz et al.[16] have reported that clot-bound thrombin is resistant to inactivation by heparin while remaining susceptible to inactivation by direct thrombin inhibitors such as hirudin and hirugen. The effects of Hirulog on soluble and clot-bound thrombin were measured using a radioimmunoassay for detecting levels of fibrinopeptide A (FPA), the fragment released from thrombin cleavage of fibrinogen.[13] At a Hirulog concentration of 1.0 μM, both soluble and clot-bound thrombin activity were inhibited by the same degree (Fig. 161–2). In contrast, at a heparin concentration that inhibited the same amount of soluble thrombin, only minimal inhibition of clot-bound thrombin was achieved.[13]

Inhibition of Thrombin-Induced Amplification Reaction

In addition to inhibiting thrombin's action in cleaving fibrinogen, part of the anticoagulant activity of Hirulog can be ascribed to its inhibition of thrombin-induced activation of coagulation factors V and VIII.[14] Thrombin is the physiologic activator of both coagulation factors, resulting in generation of activated factor V (Va) and factor VIII (VIIIa), which participate in the prothrombinase complex (Va/Xa/prothrombin) and tenase complex (VIIIa/IXa/X), respectively. In assays measuring generation of factor Xa from the tenase complex, Hirulog was observed to inhibit intrinsic and extrinsic activation of factor X in a concentration-dependent manner.[14] Thus, by inhibiting thrombin-induced activation of factor VIII, Hirulog was found to inhibit tenase complex activity and thereby decrease the rate of subsequent generation of new thrombin (and thus inhibit this positive feedback loop for thrombin generation).

Antiplatelet Effects

In addition to its anticoagulant effects, the antithrombotic activities of Hirulog may also result from inhibition of thrombin-induced activation of platelets. Thrombin is the most potent physiologic agonist for

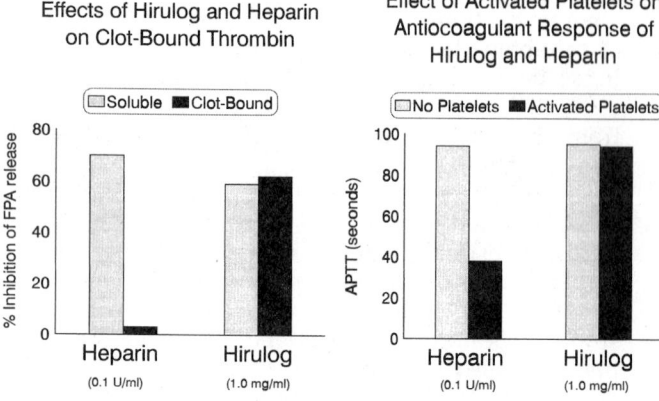

Figure 161–2. The effect of Hirulog on soluble and clot-bound thrombin (*left*), using a radioimmunoassay for detecting levels of fibrinopeptide A (FPA). The ability to inhibit clot-bound and matrix-bound thrombin is preserved, whereas clot-bound thrombin is resistant to neutralization by the heparin–antithrombin III complex. (Data from Maraganore JM, Chao BH, Weitz JI, et al: Comparison of antithrombin activities of heparin and hirulog-1: Basis for improved antithrombotic properties of direct thrombin inhibitors [abstract]. Thromb Haemost 65:829, 1991.) The right panel demonstrates the preservation of Hirulog's anticoagulant activity in the presence of activated platelets, in contrast with the inhibition of anticoagulant activity of heparin. APTT, activated partial thromboplastin time. (Adapted from Maraganore JM: Pre-clinical clinical studies on hirulog: A potent and specific direct thrombin inhibitor. *In* Claeson G, Scully MF, Kakkar VV, Deadman J [eds]: Design of Synthetic Inhibitors of Thrombin. New York: Plenum Press, 1993, pp 227–236.)

platelet activation, stimulating aggregation and release reactions.[21, 22] Thrombin activation of platelets occurs through a specific thrombin receptor.[23, 24] Thrombin binds to the thrombin receptor via its substrate recognition site and then cleaves a sessile bond in the receptor, leaving a 5-amino-acid sequence that itself stimulates the platelet.[23, 24] In in vitro studies, Hirulog was found to inhibit both thrombin-induced platelet aggregation and granule release reactions. The effects of Hirulog were specific for thrombin, with no measurable effect of Hirulog toward collagen- and ADP-induced platelet aggregation responses (Data on file, Biogen, Inc.).

Stability of Anticoagulant Response

The anticoagulant effects of heparin are known to be variable[25, 26] and appear to be related in part to neutralization of heparin by circulating plasma factors and by proteins released by activated platelets.[25, 27–29] The anticoagulant effects of Hirulog were measured in human plasma samples from which platelets were removed and in samples with collagen-activated platelets. As shown in Figure 161–2, heparin had a markedly inhibited anticoagulant response in the presence of activated platelets, whereas the anticoagulant response of Hirulog was unaffected by the presence of activated platelets, indicating the absence of any detectable platelet-derived neutralization activity.[13]

These findings were then examined in a clinical study of patients across the spectrum of ischemic heart disease.[15] Plasma samples were obtained from four groups of subjects: normal volunteers, patients with stable coronary artery disease, patients with unstable angina, and those with acute myocardial infarction. Fixed amounts of Hirulog or heparin were added to each sample at concentrations that would prolong the activated partial thromboplastin time (aPTT) to 400% of baseline in normal plasma. Overall, a lower degree of variability was found in Hirulog-treated samples (standard deviation 12% of the mean) compared with heparin-treated samples (standard deviation 30% of the mean).[15] Furthermore, in patients treated with heparin, the aPTT response was attenuated in patients with unstable angina (290% of baseline) and acute myocardial infarction (230% of baseline) ($p < .001$).[15] In contrast, Hirulog provided a stable anticoagulant response across the full spectrum of ischemic syndromes (377% and 354% of baseline, respectively). Thus, the in vitro and in vivo studies suggest that Hirulog has a predictable and stable anticoagulant response.

PHARMACOKINETICS

The pharmacokinetics of Hirulog were evaluated in a study by Fox et al.[17] When administered intravenously as a bolus, peak plasma concentration was achieved at the earliest time point tested, 2 minutes.[17] There was a dose-dependent increase in the plasma concentration. The total body clearance time was 43 ± 9 minutes, and the half-life was 36 ± 33 minutes.[17] After subcutaneous injection, the maximal plasma levels were lower than those achieved by intravenous injection, but were sustained for a longer period of time.[17] Peak concentration after subcutaneous injection was reached between 1 and 2 hours. The bioavailability of subcutaneously administered Hirulog ranged from 40% to 80%.

The maximal cumulative urinary excretion of Hirulog was approximately 20% after either intravenous or subcutaneous injection, with two thirds of the urinary excretion occurring in the first 2 hours.[17] The remainder of Hirulog elimination appears to be from protein metabolism, with at least two metabolites that are excreted in the urine. In animal studies, rats were given ^{14}C- and ^{3}H-labeled Hirulog. ^{3}H radioactivity disappeared from blood and was detected only in the kidneys and urine. Levels of ^{14}C also decreased initially from blood but remained at a low constant level for at least 24 hours. Concentrations were found in the kidney, spleen, and thymus (Data on file, Biogen, Inc.). Together with the pharmacokinetic data, these findings suggest that both renal and metabolic clearance account for the rapid clearance of Hirulog from the body.[17] Of note, there is only a modest change in Hirulog half-life in patients with renal dysfunction (Data on file, Biogen, Inc.).

PHARMACODYNAMICS
Anticoagulant Effects

As a direct thrombin inhibitor, Hirulog inhibits thrombin's cleavage of fibrinogen to fibrin in the formation of fibrin clot. The anticoagulant activity of Hirulog can be measured with several plasma assays, including activated partial thromboplastin time (aPTT), prothrombin time (PT), thrombin time (TT), and activated clotting time (ACT). All assays demonstrate a dose-dependent increase in the assay time.[12, 17, 30, 31] The TT is too sensitive a test, with all doses having a TT of more than 400 seconds. The aPTT, PT, and ACT are useful measures of Hirulog dose in that a clear dose response is seen. The aPTT ranged from 1.6 times control at a dose of 0.05 mg/kg/hr up to 4 times control at 1.0 mg/kg/hr.[12, 17] Similarly, the ACT ranged from 192 seconds at a dose of 0.2 mg/kg/hr up to 375 seconds at 2.2 mg/kg/hr.[12, 30] Of interest, elevation of the PT is roughly proportional to that of the aPTT, in contrast to heparin, which prolongs the aPTT to a much greater degree than it does the PT.

In correlating Hirulog plasma concentration and anticoagulant response, a curvilinear relationship is observed in the relationship of plasma levels with prolongation of aPTT.[17] At lower doses, the increase in plasma level rises linearly; at higher doses, the increase in aPTT is less. Additional clinical studies in patients with coronary artery disease have also demonstrated a good correlation between Hirulog plasma levels and anticoagulant activity.[12, 30, 31] In one study, Hirulog was administered intravenously to 55 patients and there was found to be a very close correlation between the dose infused and aPTT (r = 0.95) and Hirulog plasma level (r = 0.91).[31] In patients treated with intravenous Hirulog, the half-life of Hirulog's effect on the aPTT was found to be approximately 40 minutes,[12] which matched that of the pharmacokinetic study.[17]

More direct measurement of the anticoagulant effects of Hirulog can be made by evaluating fibrinopeptide A (FPA)—a marker of thrombin activity. At doses of 0.2 mg/kg/hr or higher, Hirulog was found to inhibit FPA generation.[12, 31, 32] As has been shown with heparin[33] and argatroban,[34] fibrinopeptide levels rose after discontinuation of Hirulog, although recurrent ischemia or other clinical events were not observed during the 24- to 48-hour period after discontinuation of Hirulog.[31, 32] Thrombin–antithrombin III complexes were found to be unchanged by Hirulog administration in one study of patients with unstable angina.[35] Similarly, bleeding times have not been found to change significantly with Hirulog.[17]

Antiplatelet and Antithrombotic Effects—Experimental Studies

The effects of Hirulog on acute platelet-dependent thrombosis were determined in experimental studies. In a baboon arteriovenous shunt model, arterial thrombus formation was measured using autologous [111]indium-labeled platelets, and deposition of fibrin was measured by [125]iodine-labeled fibrinogen.[36] Hirulog showed dose-dependent inhibition of platelet deposition and fibrin accumulation. At the higher dose level, the effect of Hirulog corresponded to a 76% inhibition of platelet deposition on the endarterectomized segment.[36] In a similar experiment in which flow conditions were varied to mimic arterial and venous flow, the highest dose of Hirulog showed an essentially complete interruption of thrombus formation for both arterial and venous flow conditions.[37] These studies also demonstrated that fibrin deposition is inhibited at a lower dose of Hirulog than that required for platelet deposition,[36, 37] a finding that has been observed with other anticoagulants.[38, 39]

The effects of Hirulog on tissue-type plasminogen activator (t-PA)–induced fibrinolysis of an experimental thrombus were measured in a rat aorta model.[40] Hirulog was found to both speed the time to reperfusion and decrease reocclusion.[40] A similar finding was observed with the Hirulog component hirugen.[41] The effects of Hirulog on t-PA–induced thrombolysis of experimental coronary artery thrombus were studied in a dog model.[42] Animals received t-PA alone, t-PA and Hirulog, t-PA and ridogrel (a combined thromboxane A_2 receptor and synthetase inhibitor), or t-PA combined with both Hirulog and ridogrel. Reperfusion of the occluded coronary artery occurred in one of seven dogs treated with t-PA alone at an average time of 86 ± 4 minutes, in seven of nine dogs treated with t-PA and Hirulog at an average time of 53 ± 11 minutes, in one of eight dogs treated with t-PA and ridogrel at 85 ± 5 minutes, and in seven of eight dogs treated with t-PA, Hirulog, and ridogrel at 37 ±

10 minutes.[42] Thus, the combination of t-PA and Hirulog showed a significant effect on occurrence of and time to reperfusion as compared with the other study groups. The occurrence of reocclusion was also measured in the dogs with reestablished coronary blood flow. Reocclusion time was delayed by the combination of t-PA with Hirulog but was further delayed by the addition of the antiplatelet agent ridogrel.

Thus, experimental studies show that Hirulog is able to decrease thrombus formation and enhance thrombolysis, thereby laying the groundwork for clinical studies with Hirulog in patients with acute ischemic syndromes.

CLINICAL USE
Unstable Angina

Two pilot trials examined the usefulness of Hirulog in patients with unstable angina.[31, 32] One study treated 55 patients with one of three ascending doses of Hirulog, 0.25, 0.5, and 1.0 mg/kg/hr. Clinical success was defined as the absence of myocardial infarction, recurrent refractory angina, or hemodynamic deterioration. Overall clinical success was achieved in 87.5% of patients.[31] A second study treated 20 patients with a 5-day infusion of Hirulog, at 0.2 mg/kg/hr, with a similar rate of clinical success, with only one patient having recurrent ischemia.[32]

The Thrombin Inhibition in Myocardial Ischemia (TIMI) 7 trial was a multicenter, randomized, double-blind, dose-ranging trial of Hirulog in patients with unstable angina.[18] Patients received a 72-hour intravenous infusion of one of four doses of Hirulog: 0.02, 0.25, 0.5, or 1.0 mg/kg/hr. Comparing the patients who received the lowest dose of Hirulog (n = 160) with patients who collectively received one of the higher doses of Hirulog (n = 250), the incidence of death or myocardial infarction (MI) through hospital discharge was 10.0% in the low-dose group and 3.2% in the aggregate high-dose group ($p < .008$)[18] (Fig. 161–3). At 42 days, death or MI occurred in 12.5% of the low-dose group compared with 5.2% of the higher dose group ($p < .013$). Because all patients received aspirin, this trial demonstrated that the combination of aspirin and an anticoagulant appears to be beneficial, and thus supports the use of combination antithrombotic therapy in unstable angina and non–Q-wave MI.

Angioplasty

Hirulog was also tested during coronary angioplasty in a dose-ranging trial.[30] Two hundred ninety-one patients were enrolled, and 279 received the study drug. Patients received aspirin and were treated with intravenous Hirulog at increasing doses given as a bolus followed by an infusion for 4 hours. The five doses ranged from 0.15 mg/kg bolus and 0.6 mg/kg/hr infusion to 0.55 mg/kg bolus and 2.2 mg/kg/hr infusion. The primary end point, abrupt closure (or death or MI) within 24 hours of the procedure, occurred

Figure 161–3. Effect of higher doses of Hirulog compared with lower doses. In the TIMI 7 trial of unstable angina, patients treated with the higher doses (0.25, 0.5, and 1 mg/kg/hr) had a lower rate of death or myocardial infarction (MI) through hospital discharge than those treated with a lower dose (0.02 mg/kg/hr). In patients undergoing routine percutaneous transluminal coronary angioplasty (PTCA), those at the higher two doses (1.8 and 2.2 mg/kg/hr) also had a lower rate of abrupt closure events (abrupt closure, death, or MI) compared with patients treated with the lower doses (0.6, 1.0, and 1.4 mg/kg/hr). (Data from Fuchs J, Cannon CP, and the TIMI 7 Investigators: Hirulog in the treatment of unstable angina: Results of the TIMI 7 trial. Circulation 92:727, 1995; and Topol EJ, Bonan R, Jewitt D, et al: Use of a direct antithrombin, Hirulog, in place of heparin during coronary angioplasty. Circulation 87:1622, 1994.)

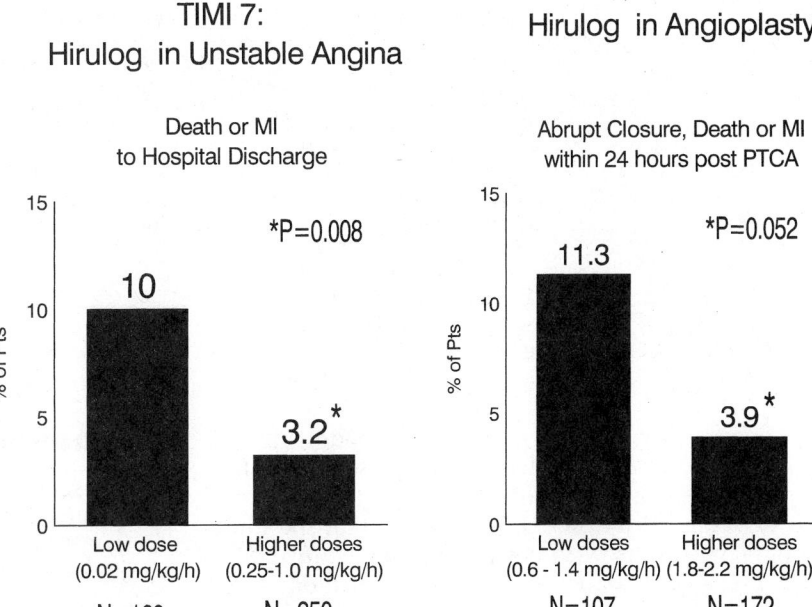

in 11.3% of patients in the three lower dose groups compared with 3.9% in the two higher dose groups ($p = .052$) (see Fig. 161–3). A phase III, double-blind randomized trial was conducted in 4088 patients with unstable and postinfarction angina undergoing angioplasty.[43] In the overall group, Hirulog had a similar rate of death, MI, abrupt closure, or need for urgent repeat revascularization in-hospital, 11.4%, versus 12.3% for heparin ($p = $ NS). However, in the prestratified group of postinfarction patients, Hirulog led to a lower adverse event rate, 9.0% versus 14.5% for heparin ($p = .03$). In addition, Hirulog had a lower rate of major hemorrhage, 3.8% versus 9.8% ($p < .001$). Thus, Hirulog appeared promising in high-risk patients undergoing percutaneous transluminal coronary angioplasty (PTCA).

Acute Myocardial Infarction

A pilot trial of Hirulog as adjunctive treatment to streptokinase for acute myocardial infarction was performed.[44] Forty-five patients were enrolled; 30 pa-tients received Hirulog at 0.5 mg/kg/hr for 12 hours, then 0.1 mg/kg/hr for 5 days, and 15 patients received a heparin infusion (without a bolus) at 1000 U/hr titrated to an aPTT of 2 to 2.5 times control. Patency of the infarct-related artery at 90 minutes after the start of thrombolysis was significantly higher in Hirulog-treated patients: 77% compared with 47% of heparin-treated patients ($p < .05$) (Fig. 161–4).[44] TIMI grade 3 flow[45] was present in 67% of Hirulog-treated patients compared with 40% of heparin-treated patients ($p = .08$).[44] At 120 minutes, similar improvements were present. Clinical events also tended to be lower in Hirulog-treated patients. The incidence of a composite end point (death, recurrent MI, severe congestive heart failure or cardiogenic shock, recurrent ischemia, or stroke) occurred in 7% of the Hirulog group compared with 27% of the heparin group ($p = .06$) (see Fig. 161–4).[44]

When these studies are considered together, Hirulog has shown very promising results in improving clinical outcome in the early pilot trials of unstable angina, acute MI, and angioplasty. Additional studies

Figure 161–4. Effects of Hirulog compared with heparin as adjunctive therapy with streptokinase for acute myocardial infarction. Patients treated with Hirulog had a higher rate of infarct-related artery patency and of TIMI grade 3 flow compared with heparin-treated patients at 90 minutes after thrombolytic-antithrombotic therapy. Clinical events also tended to be lower: the incidence of a composite end point (death, recurrent MI, severe congestive heart failure or cardiogenic shock, recurrent ischemia, or stroke) was 7% for Hirulog-treated patients and 27% for heparin-treated patients. (Data from Lidon R-M, Theroux P, Lesperance J, et al: A pilot, early angiographic patency study using a direct thrombin inhibitor as adjunctive therapy to streptokinase in acute myocardial infarction. Circulation 89:1567, 1994.)

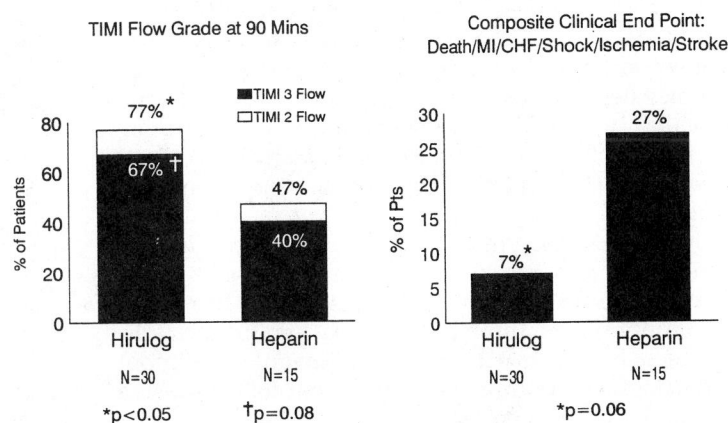

Table 161–1. **Incidence of Hemorrhagic Events in Trials of Hirulog**

Study	Indication	Number of Patients	Major Hemorrhage (%)	Minor Hemorrhage (%)
Cannon et al.[12]	Cardiac catheterization	30	3.3	6.6
Topol et al.[30]	Angioplasty	279	0.3	2.8
Sharma et al.[32]	Unstable angina	20	0	5.0
Lidon et al.[31]	Unstable angina	55	0	5.5
TIMI 7[18]	Unstable angina	410	0.2	—
Lidon et al.[44]	Acute myocardial infarction	30	13.0	67.0
All studies		824	0.8	8.2

—, not reported.
Total for minor hemorrhage based on 414 patients.

are ongoing for the prevention of deep venous thrombosis with subcutaneous Hirulog and comparing Hirulog with heparin as adjunctive therapy to thrombolysis in acute MI (HERO-1). It is hoped that the initial promising results with Hirulog will be confirmed in the larger comparative trials, so that Hirulog would represent an advance in the treatment of these acute ischemic syndromes.

Precautions and Adverse Effects

Studies to date have shown Hirulog to be well tolerated. The principal adverse effect of this anticoagulant, as with any other anticoagulant, is bleeding, although the initial experience has shown a low incidence of major hemorrhage (Table 161–1). Overall, major hemorrhage occurred in 7 of 824 (0.8%) patients treated, with a slightly higher percentage of major hemorrhage, as expected, in patients receiving concomitant thrombolytic therapy.[44] Bleeding was observed most often at an instrumented site (i.e., at the arterial access site for cardiac catheterization).[12, 30, 44] In published reports to date, no patient has suffered an intracranial hemorrhage. Other adverse experiences reported include nausea, vomiting, and headache, but their relationship to the drug is not yet clear.[17, 30] No anaphylactic reactions have been reported with Hirulog.[12, 30–32, 44]

Immunogenic Response

Because Hirulog is a polypeptide derived from the leech protein hirudin, the potential exists for an immunogenic response. However, both animal (Data on file, Biogen, Inc.) and human studies have failed to shown an antigenic response.[12, 17, 30] One subject had an elevated titer of antibodies before treatment with Hirulog, which did not change after administration of Hirulog. One other subject of 84 tested developed a low titer (<1:15) after 9 days of Hirulog administration.[17]

Indeed, Hirulog may be a useful alternative for patients who develop an immune response to heparin.[46] In a select group of patients with a history of heparin-induced thrombocytopenia and thrombosis, Hirulog has been used as an anticoagulant without inducing an immune-mediated thrombocytopenia (Data on file, Biogen Inc.).

Neutralization of Hirulog

At present, there is no antidote for Hirulog. Theoretic antidotes include antibodies to Hirulog or altered (inactive) thrombin derivatives, which are currently under investigation.[47] In clinical use, however, given the relatively short half-life, the effect of Hirulog rapidly disappears after discontinuation of the drug, which may explain the favorable safety profile observed to date.

Acknowledgments

The author would like to thank John Maraganore, Ph.D., at Biogen, Inc., who has made available unpublished data for this review.

REFERENCES

1. Maraganore JM, Bourdon P, Jablonski J, et al: Design and characterization of hirulogs: A novel class of bivalent peptide inhibitors of thrombin. Biochemistry 29:7095, 1990.
2. Adams SL: The medicinal leech: A page from the annelids of internal medicine. Ann Intern Med 109:399, 1988.
3. Haycraft JB: On the action of secretion obtained from the medicinal leech on coagulation of the blood. Proc R Soc Lond 36:478, 1884.
4. Markwardt F: Isolierung uber Hirudin. Naturwissenschaften 42:537, 1955.
5. Fenton JW, Olson TA, Zabinski MP, et al: Anion-binding of human alpha-thrombin and fibrin(ogen) recognition. Biochemistry 27:7106, 1988.
6. Rydel TJ, Ravichandran KG, Tulinsky A, et al: The structure of a complex of recombinant hirudin and human alpha-thrombin. Science 249:277, 1990.
7. Maraganore JM, Chao B, Joseph ML, et al: Anticoagulant activity of synthetic hirudin peptides. J Biol Chem 264:8692, 1989.
8. Naski MC, Fenton JW, Maraganore JM, et al: The COOH-terminal domain of hirudin: An exosite-directed competitive inhibitor of the action of alpha-thrombin on fibrinogen. J Biol Chem 265:13484, 1990.
9. Krstenansky JL, Mao SJT: Antithrombin properties of C-terminus of hirudin using synthetic unsulfated N-alpha-acetyl-hirudin45–65. FEBS Lett 211:10, 1987.
10. Grutter MG, Priestle JP, Rahuel J, et al: Crystal structure of the thrombin-hirudin complex: A novel mode of serine protease inhibition. EMBO J 9:2361, 1990.
11. Skrzypczak-Jankun E, Carperos VE, Ravichandran KG, et al: Structure of the hirugen and hirulog-1 complexes of alpha-thrombin. J Mol Biol 221:1379, 1992.
12. Cannon CP, Maraganore JM, Loscalzo J, et al: Anticoagulant effects of Hirulog, a novel thrombin inhibitor, in patients with coronary artery disease. Am J Cardiol 71:778, 1993.
13. Maraganore JM, Chao BH, Weitz JI, et al: Comparison of antithrombin activities of heparin and hirulog-1: Basis for im-

proved antithrombotic properties of direct thrombin inhibitors [abstract]. Thromb Haemost 65:829, 1991.

14. Ofosu FA, Fenton JW, Maraganore J, et al: Inhibition of the amplification reactions of blood coagulation by site-specific inhibitors of alpha-thrombin. Biochem J 283:893, 1992.

15. Maraganore JM, Bourdon P, Adelman B, et al: Heparin variability and resistance: Comparisons with a direct thrombin inhibitor [abstract]. Circulation 86(Suppl I):I-386, 1992.

16. Weitz JI, Hudoba M, Massel D, et al: Clot-bound thrombin is protected from inhibition by heparin-antithrombin III but is susceptible to inactivation by antithrombin III-independent inhibitors. J Clin Invest 86:385, 1990.

17. Fox I, Dawson A, Loynds P, et al: Anticoagulant activity of Hirulog™, a direct thrombin inhibitor, in humans. Thromb Haemost 69:157, 1993.

18. Fuchs J, Cannon CP, and the TIMI 7 Investigators: Hirulog in the treatment of unstable angina: Results of the thrombin inhibition in myocardial ischemia (TIMI) 7 trial. Circulation 92:727, 1995.

19. Witting JI, Bourdon P, Brezniak DV, et al: Thrombin-specific inhibition by and slow cleavage of hirulog-1. Biochem J 283:737, 1992.

20. Qiu X, Padmanabhan K, Caerperos VE, et al: The structure of the hirulog-3 thrombin complex and the nature of the S′ subsites of substrates and inhibitors. Biochemistry 31:11689, 1993.

21. Harker LA: Pathogenesis of thrombosis. In Williams WJ, Beutler E, Erslev AJ, Lichtman MA (eds): Hematology, Vol 1, 4th ed. New York: McGraw-Hill, 1990, pp 1559–1569.

22. Fuster V, Badimon L, Badimon JJ, et al: The pathophysiology of coronary artery disease and the acute coronary syndromes. N Engl J Med 326:242, 1992.

23. Vu TK, Hung DT, Wheaton I, et al: Molecular cloning of a functional thrombin receptor reveals a novel proteolytic mechanism of receptor activation. Cell 64:1057, 1991.

24. Coughlin SR, Vu TH, Hung DT, et al: Characterization of a functional thrombin receptor: Issues and opportunities. J Clin Invest 89:351, 1992.

25. Hirsh J: Heparin. N Engl J Med 324:1565, 1991.

26. Ogilby JD, Untereker WJ, Corin WJ, et al: Variability of effective anticoagulation for PTCA is dependent upon heparin potency [abstract]. Circulation 84(Suppl II):II-592, 1991.

27. Bock PE, Juscombe M, Marshall SE, et al: The multiple complexes formed by the interaction of platelet factor 4 with heparin. Biochem J 191:769, 1980.

28. Lijnen HR, Hoylaerts M, Collens D: Heparin binding properties of human histidine-rich glycoprotein: Mechanism and role in the neutralization of heparin in plasma. J Biol Chem 258:3803, 1983.

29. Preissner KT, Muller-Berghaus G: Neutralization and binding of heparin by S-protein/vitronectin in the inhibition of factor Xa by antithrombin III. J Biol Chem 262:12247, 1987.

30. Topol EJ, Bonan R, Jewitt D, et al: Use of a direct antithrombin, Hirulog, in place of heparin during coronary angioplasty. Circulation 87:1622, 1993.

31. Lidon R-M, Theroux P, Juneau M, et al: Initial experience with a direct antithrombin, Hirulog, in unstable angina: Anticoagu-

lant, antithrombotic and clinical effects. Circulation 88:1495, 1993.

32. Sharma GVRK, Lapsey D, Vita JA, et al: Usefulness and tolerability of Hirulog, a direct thrombin-inhibitor, in unstable angina pectoris. Am J Cardiol 72:1357, 1993.

33. Granger CB, Miller JM, Bovill EG, et al: Rebound increase in thrombin generation and activity after cessation of intravenous heparin in patients with acute coronary syndromes. Circulation 91:1929, 1995.

34. Gold HK, Torres FW, Garabedian HD, et al: Evidence of a rebound coagulation phenomenon after cessation of a 4-hour infusion of a specific thrombin inhibitor in patients with unstable angina pectoris. J Am Coll Cardiol 21:1039, 1993.

35. Lidon R-M, Theroux P, Ghitescu M: Anticoagulants and antithrombotic effects of Hirulog™ in unstable angina [abstract]. Circulation 88(Part 2):I-201, 1993.

36. Kelly AB, Maraganore JM, Bourdon P, et al: Antithrombotic effects of synthetic peptides targeting various functional domains of thrombin. Proc Natl Acad Sci U S A 89:6040, 1992.

37. Cadroy Y, Maraganore JM, Hanson SR, et al: Selective inhibition by a synthetic hirudin peptide of fibrin-dependent thrombosis in baboons. Proc Natl Acad Sci U S A 88:1177, 1991.

38. Heras M, Chesebro JH, Penny WJ, et al: Effects of thrombin inhibition on the development of acute platelet-thrombus deposition during angioplasty in pigs: Heparin versus recombinant hirudin, a specific thrombin inhibitor. Circulation 79:657, 1989.

39. Heras M, Chesebro JH, Webster MWI, et al: Hirudin, heparin and placebo during deep arterial injury in the pig: The in vivo role of thrombin in platelet-mediated thrombosis. Circulation 82:1476, 1990.

40. Klement P, Borm A, Hirsh J, et al: The effects of thrombin inhibitors on tissue plasminogen activator induced thrombolysis in a rat model. Thromb Haemost 68:64, 1992.

41. Yao SK, McNatt J, Anderson HJ, et al: Thrombin inhibition enhances tissue-type plasminogen activator-induced thrombolysis and delays reocclusion. Am J Physiol 262(2 Pt 2):H374, 1992.

42. Yao S-K, Ober JC, Ferguson JJ, et al: Combination of inhibition of thrombin and blockade of thromboxane A2 synthetase and receptors enhances thrombolysis and delays reocclusion in canine coronary arteries. Circulation 86:1993, 1992.

43. Bittl JA, Strony J, Brinker JA, et al: Hirulog compared with heparin during coronary angioplasty for unstable or post-infarction angina. N Engl J Med (In press).

44. Lidon R-M, Theroux P, Lesperance J, et al: A pilot, early angiographic patency study using a direct thrombin inhibitor as adjunctive therapy to streptokinase in acute myocardial infarction. Circulation 89:1567, 1994.

45. Chesebro JH, Knatterud G, Roberts R, et al: Thrombolysis in Myocardial Infarction (TIMI) Trial, Phase 1: A comparison between intravenous tissue plasminogen activator and intravenous streptokinase. Circulation 76:142, 1987.

46. Warkentin TE: Heparin-induced thrombocytopenia. Annu Rev Med 40:31, 1989.

47. Bruggener E, Walsman P, Markwardt F: Neutralization of hirudin anticoagulant action by DIP-thrombin. Pharmazie 44:648, 1989.

CHAPTER 162

Danaparoid

Alexander G. G. Turpie, M.D., F.R.C.P., F.A.C.P., F.A.C.C., F.R.C.P.C.

Danaparoid (Orgaran; Org 10172) is a low-molecular-weight (LMW) heparinoid with antithrombotic activity similar to that of heparin and related compounds. Danaparoid is a mixture of glycosaminoglycans derived from porcine intestinal mucosa with an average molecular weight of approximately 6000 daltons. Although derived from the same raw material as heparin and LMW heparins, danaparoid differs from these compounds in a number of ways.[1] Danaparoid consists mainly of heparan sulfate (84%), a small quantity of dermatan sulfate (12%), and a minor amount of chondroitin sulfate (4%). Approximately 4.5% to 5% of the heparan sulfate molecules in danaparoid have a high affinity for antithrombin III (AT-III). Danaparoid does not contain any heparin or heparin fragments, which is a unique feature of this anticoagulant when compared with heparin and related compounds. The main chemical difference between danaparoid and heparin is in the composition of the major repeating units of the polysaccharide chains, which in the case of heparan sulfate, the principal component of danaparoid, contains mostly glucuronic acid, whereas the major repeating unit of heparin and LMW heparins is iduronic acid 2-sulphate.[2] In addition, danaparoid contains mostly N-acetyl-glucosamine, whereas heparin and LMW heparins contain mainly glucosamine-N-sulfate, the result being less sulfation and a lower charge density in danaparoid. The main anticoagulant activity of danaparoid is through inhibition of activated coagulation factors by high-affinity heparan sulfate, but the dermatan sulfate component contributes to its antithrombotic activity by inactivating thrombin directly by combining with heparin cofactor II.[3]

Danaparoid has been extensively studied in a wide range of *in vitro* experiments and in experimental models of thrombosis in animals. These studies have shown that danaparoid has important antithrombotic activity with minimal bleeding potential.[1]

EFFECT OF DANAPAROID ON COAGULATION

The main glycosaminoglycan constituents of danaparoid contribute to its pharmacologic activity in a number of ways. The heparan sulfate fraction with high affinity for AT-III selectively inhibits activated factor X (factor Xa). Danaparoid has a more selective inhibitory effect on factor Xa than heparin or the LMW heparins, which results in greater anti-Xa to anti-IIa activity.[1] The low-affinity heparin sulfate fraction has no effect on activated coagulation factors but contributes to the antithrombotic activity of danaparoid by an endothelial cellular mechanism.[4]

EFFECT OF DANAPAROID IN EXPERIMENTAL THROMBOSIS AND HEMOSTASIS IN ANIMAL MODELS

Vogel et al.[5] have compared the antithrombotic effects of danaparoid with those of heparin and LMW heparin in a rat venous stasis model in which thrombus formation was induced by a combination of stasis and hypercoagulability. In this model, danaparoid, heparin, and LMW heparin had similar antithrombotic activity with identical dose-response curves. Similar results were obtained in an arteriovenous shunt model in rats, in which danaparoid and heparin inhibited thrombus formation equally.[6] In contrast, in a model of thrombosis in rabbits, Boneu et al.[7] demonstrated that danaparoid was more effective

than both heparin and LMW heparin in inhibiting extension of an existing thrombus, suggesting that danaparoid may be more effective clinically than heparin and LMW heparin when thrombi may already be present.

Danaparoid has also been compared with both heparin and LMW heparin in a number of bleeding models in experimental animals. Using a rabbit ear bleeding model, Cade et al.[8] demonstrated that danaparoid caused significantly less bleeding than either heparin or LMW heparin at equivalent antithrombotic doses. In a modification of the rabbit ear bleeding model, Meuleman[1] reported that danaparoid, given intravenously at dosages of up to five times those used to obtain effective antithrombotic activity, resulted in only a slight increase in blood loss. In the subdermal bleeding model in rats, Meuleman et al.[6] have confirmed the low bleeding potential of danaparoid compared with that of heparin. These studies showed that in contrast with heparin, danaparoid causes significantly less blood loss than heparin, and the amount of blood loss was relatively low even when high doses of danaparoid were used.

EFFECT OF DANAPAROID ON PLATELETS

Inhibition of platelet function has been shown to cause increased bleeding in a number of studies. The bleeding associated with heparin therapy is partly due to impairment of primary hemostatic platelet plug formation by heparin. The improved risk/benefit ratio of danaparoid is due not only to its selective inhibition of coagulation but also to its minimal effect on physiologic platelet function, a key factor in the maintenance of hemostasis and the reduction of bleeding. Meuleman et al.[6] compared the effects of danaparoid and heparin in terms of *in vivo* platelet adhesion in the rat arteriovenous shunt model and found that at effective antithrombotic doses, heparin inhibited platelet deposition, but danaparoid had only a minimal inhibitory effect.

Pharmacologic studies[9] have confirmed the lack of an inhibitory effect on normal platelet function by danaparoid in healthy volunteers in whom bleeding time was significantly prolonged 10 minutes after an intravenous injection of heparin, but not after danaparoid administration.[1, 9] Studies in human volunteers have also shown that danaparoid is a less potent activator of platelets than heparin is, which causes platelet aggregation by a direct, nonspecific interaction with platelets, which leads to functional changes.[11]

In addition to a direct effect on platelets, heparin causes immune-mediated thrombocytopenia via heparin-induced antibodies against platelets.[10, 11] Although uncommon, heparin-induced thrombocytopenia occasionally results in severe or life-threatening paradoxic thromboembolic complications. Danaparoid has been shown to have low cross-reactivity with the heparin-induced antibody,[12] suggesting that it may be useful in patients who have heparin-associated thrombocytopenia.

TOXICITY OF DANAPAROID

Studies in both rats and dogs have shown that danaparoid has low toxicity.[6] In rats, the LD_{50} after a single subcutaneous injection is approximately 15,200 anti-Xa U/kg, and in dogs, intravenous doses up to 28,000 anti-Xa U/kg are well tolerated without significant adverse effects. The long-term administration of danaparoid to both rats and dogs at doses of 1600 anti-Xa U/kg/day given intravenously for 6 months or subcutaneously for 6 weeks has been shown to be nontoxic.

Administration of danaparoid to pregnant female rabbits does not exacerbate postimplantation fetal loss or produce teratogenicity. Sexually mature female rats treated with danaparoid were unaffected in terms of fertility, gestation, and fetal growth *in utero*. Thus, danaparoid appears to be free of any embryotoxic or teratogenic effects in experimental animals.[6]

PHARMACOKINETICS OF DANAPAROID IN HUMANS

The pharmacokinetics of danaparoid have been studied by monitoring the kinetics of its biologic activities by measurement of plasma anti-Xa activity or thrombin generation inhibition (TGI). Standard coagulation tests, such as activated partial thromboplastin time (aPPT), prothrombin time (PT), and thrombin clotting time (TT), are of little value in the evaluation of the pharmacokinetics of danaparoid, because at therapeutic dosages, danaparoid has no effect or only a minimal effect on these tests.

After subcutaneous injection of danaparoid in humans, plasma anti-Xa activity increases relatively rapidly, with peak plasma anti-Xa levels occurring within approximately 4 to 5 hours and maximum TGI activity returning 2 to 3 hours after injection.[13] The kinetics of danaparoid after intravenous or subcutaneous administration are linear, which contrasts with the non-linear pharmacokinetics of heparin.[14] This property of danaparoid results in more predictable plasma levels in clinical practice.

In humans, the bioavailability of danaparoid after subcutaneous administration is almost 100% in contrast with heparin, which has a bioavailability of only 20% to 30% after subcutaneous injection.[15, 16] In addition, after subcutaneous injection, intraindividual and interindividual variations in heparin concentration are substantial.[17] The total distribution volume of the anti-Xa activity of danaparoid is approximately 9 L.[15] In addition, in contrast with heparin, heparin neutralizing factor does not neutralize danaparoid. These properties of danaparoid suggest that danaparoid may have a clinical advantage over heparin.

Danaparoid is predominantly cleared from the circulation by the kidneys, which accounts for at least 40% to 50% of the total plasma clearance of its anti-Xa activity.[14] The importance of the kidneys in the excretion of the anti-Xa activity has been confirmed in renal failure patients on long-term hemodialysis in whom accumulation of danaparoid has been reported. The elimination half-life of the anti-Xa activity is approximately 25 hours, and the thrombin generation–inhibiting activity is eliminated with a half-life of approximately 7 hours. Although these data suggest that once-daily dosing with danaparoid may be sufficient, clinical experience has shown that twice-daily dosing is optimal for danaparoid.

CLINICAL EVALUATION OF DANAPAROID

The safety and efficacy of danaparoid have been studied for the prophylaxis of deep vein thrombosis (DVT) in a number of large-scale trials in patients at high risk for venous thromboembolism and bleeding, such as patients undergoing orthopedic surgery or cancer surgery or those with nonhemorrhagic stroke.

Thrombosis Prophylaxis in Elective Hip Surgery

Venous thromboembolism is a major complication of patients undergoing orthopedic surgery. In the absence of prophylaxis, patients undergoing hip surgery have a 40% to 60% incidence of calf vein thrombosis, a 20% incidence of proximal vein thrombosis, and a 1% to 5% incidence of fatal pulmonary embolism.[18]

Danaparoid has been evaluated for the prevention of DVT in patients undergoing total hip replacement in two studies, one in which it was compared with placebo and in the other with heparin in combination with dihydroergotamine (DHE). In the placebo-controlled trial reported by Hoek et al.,[19] danaparoid was given subcutaneously in a dose of 750 anti-Xa U twice daily starting preoperatively. The efficacy of danaparoid was assessed by bilateral venography performed at day 10 and interpreted by an independent panel of experts unaware of the treatment groups. In this study, the incidence of DVT was reduced from 56 (57%) of 99 placebo-treated patients to 15 (15%) of 97 patients treated with danaparoid ($p < .001$). The frequency of proximal DVT was 25% and 8.2% in the placebo- and danaparoid-treated groups, respectively ($p < .005$). Major bleeding complications were not seen in either group, but six patients (6.2%) in the danaparoid group developed wound hematomas, although they were minor and none required surgical intervention. In the second study reported by Leyvraz et al.,[20] danaparoid was given in a dose of 750 anti-Xa U twice daily and was compared with heparin-DHE (5000 U heparin + 0.5 mg DHE) given twice daily. In this randomized and assessor-blind trial, subcutaneously given prophylaxis was started 2 hours prior to surgery and continued for up to 10 days. The frequency of DVT was determined by bilateral venography at day 10, which was performed in all patients and interpreted by a panel of experts blinded to treatment. The incidence of DVT was reduced from 44 (32%) of 139 patients in the heparin-DHE group to

Table 162–1. **Randomized Trials of Danaparoid in the Prevention of DVT Following Orthopedic Surgery**

	No.		Total DVT	Proximal DVT
Elective Hip Replacement				
Hoek et al., 1992[19]	97	Danaparoid	15 (15%)	8 (8%)
	99	Placebo	56 (57%)	25 (25%)
		p value	<.0001	<.005
Leyvraz et al., 1992[20]	145	Danaparoid	25 (17%)	7 (4.8%)
	139	Heparin/DHE	44 (32%)	9 (6.5%)
		p value	.007	—
Fracture Hip Surgery				
Gerhart et al., 1991[21]	107	Danaparoid	14 (13%)	5 (4.7%)
	155	Dextran	40 (35%)	10 (8.7%)
		p value	<.001	—
Bergqvist et al., 1991[22]	132	Danaparoid	9 (7%)	3 (2.2%)
	131	Warfarin	28 (21%)	7 (5.3%)
		p value	<.001	—

DVT, deep vein thrombosis; DHE, dihydroergotamine.

25 (17%) of 145 patients in the danaparoid group (p < .05). Major bleeding occurred in one patient in each group, and there was no difference in the incidence of minor bleeding between the groups.

The results of these studies, shown in Table 162–1, indicate that danaparoid is effective and safe in the prevention of DVT in patients undergoing total hip replacement.

Thrombosis Prophylaxis in Fractured Hip Surgery

Venous thromboembolism is a major complication in patients undergoing surgery for fracture of the hip.[18] Danaparoid has been investigated for the prevention of DVT in patients with hip fractures in two studies. In the first study, reported by Bergqvist et al.,[22] danaparoid (750 anti-factor Xa U) given twice daily subcutaneously was compared with dextran in a randomized assessor-blind study. Prophylaxis was started on admission to hospital and was continued for 10 days. In this study, DVT was diagnosed by bilateral venography performed in all patients at the end of the study period or earlier if detected by fibrinogen leg scanning. DVT occurred in 14 (13.1%) of 107 patients receiving danaparoid compared with 40 (34.8%) of 115 patients given dextran (p < .001). Proximal DVT occurred in 4.7% of the patients on danaparoid and in 8.7% of the patients on dextran. Pulmonary embolism occurred in 3.1% and 0% in the dextran and danaparoid groups, respectively. No major bleeds occurred in either group, and there was no difference in perioperative or total blood loss between the two groups. In the second study, carried out by Gerhart et al.,[21] danaparoid was compared with warfarin. In this study, danaparoid was started on admission and given twice daily in doses of 750 anti-Xa U given subcutaneously and continued until the ninth postoperative day. In the danaparoid-treated group, warfarin was started on the seventh postoperative day and continued until discharge on day 14. The combination treatment with danaparoid and warfarin was compared with warfarin given alone, which was started

on admission and given for 14 days or until the patients' discharge from the hospital. The frequency of DVT was assessed by fibrinogen leg scanning and impedance plethysmography and confirmed whenever possible by ultrasonography or ascending venography. The frequency of DVT was reduced from 28 (21%) of 131 patients treated with warfarin alone to 9 (7%) of 132 patients who were treated with danaparoid (p < .001). Eight of the patients in the danaparoid group suffered major bleeding episodes, four of which occurred during the period in which danaparoid alone was given and four of which occurred after warfarin was started, compared with five episodes in the patients in the warfarin-alone group. There was no difference in intraoperative blood loss or transfusion requirements between the two treatment groups.

These studies, the results of which are shown in Table 162–1, indicate that danaparoid is effective in the prevention of DVT in patients undergoing surgery for fracture of the hip.

Abdominothoracic Surgery for Cancer

Patients who undergo surgery for malignant disease are at high risk for venous thromboembolism. Danaparoid given in a dose of 750 anti-Xa U twice daily subcutaneously was shown to be as effective as 5000 U of heparin given three times daily subcutaneously in the prevention of DVT in a prospective, single-blind, randomized study of 121 patients undergoing surgery for gastrointestinal tract cancer reported by Blum et al.[23] In this study, venographically detected DVT occurred in 11% of the danaparoid-treated patients and in 10% of the heparin-treated patients with no significant difference in bleeding complications between the two groups. In a randomized, double-blind, multicenter DVT prevention trial of 490 patients undergoing elective surgery for malignant abdominal or thoracic disease, Gallus et al.[24] reported that the incidence of DVT based on an intent-to-treat analysis was reduced from 14.9% in the patients allocated to treatment with heparin in a dose of 5000 U given twice daily subcutaneously to 10.4% in the

Table 162–2. **Randomized Trials of Danaparoid in the Prevention of DVT in Cancer Surgery**

	No.		Total DVT
Blum et al., 1989[23]	63	Danaparoid	7 (11%)
	58	Heparin	6 (10%)
Gallus et al., 1993[24]	241	Danaparoid	25 (10.4%)
	249	Heparin	37 (14.9%)

DVT, deep vein thrombosis.

patients allocated to danaparoid in a dose of 750 anti-Xa U given twice daily subcutaneously. This trend toward less DVT in the danaparoid-treated patients was not statistically significant ($p > .1$). The results of these studies suggest that danaparoid is at least as effective as standard low-dose heparin in high-risk patients undergoing elective surgery for malignant disease. The results are shown in Table 162–2.

Ischemic Stroke

Venous thromboembolism is a common complication in patients with acute ischemic stroke. Without prophylaxis, DVT occurs in 60% to 70% of patients with dense hemiplegia (usually in the paralyzed limb), and 1% to 2% suffer fatal pulmonary embolism.[25] Several methods to prevent DVT have been proved safe and effective in high-risk medical patients. Two small randomized trials of low-dose heparin prophylaxis in patients with acute ischemic stroke have been reported, both of which show a significant benefit of treatment.[26, 27] However, the studies were too small to provide convincing evidence that low-dose heparin is safe, and heparin is not widely used in stroke patients because of concern about intracranial hemorrhage. Danaparoid has been evaluated for the prevention of DVT in patients with ischemic stroke in two studies.[28, 29] In both of these studies, danaparoid given in doses of 750 anti-Xa U twice daily subcutaneously was compared in double-blind, randomized trials with placebo and, in the second study, with low-dose heparin. In the placebo-controlled study reported by Turpie et al.,[28] patients were monitored by fibrinogen leg scanning and impedance plethysmography; when either test was positive, the occurrence of DVT was confirmed by venography. In this study, the incidence of DVT was reduced from 7 (28%) of 25 patients in the placebo group to 2 (4%) of 50 patients in the danaparoid group ($p < .005$). The corresponding rates

of proximal DVT were 16% and 0%, respectively ($p = .01$). One major and one minor hemorrhage occurred in the danaparoid group and in the placebo-treated patients, respectively. In the second study by Turpie et al.,[29] in which danaparoid was compared with standard heparin, the occurrence of DVT, which was detected by fibrinogen leg scanning and confirmed by ascending venography, was reduced from 13 (31.0%) of 42 patients in the heparin-treated group to 4 (8.9%) of 45 in the danaparoid-treated group ($p < .012$); the corresponding rates of proximal DVT were 11.9% and 4.4% in the heparin- and danaparoid-treated groups, respectively ($p = .255$). There was no significant difference in the frequency of bleeding complications in the two groups. The results of these two studies, shown in Table 162–3, demonstrate that danaparoid is an effective agent for prevention of DVT in patients with acute ischemic stroke without causing increased bleeding. In the direct comparison with heparin, danaparoid was shown to be more effective. Danaparoid is currently being evaluated for the prevention of stroke progression in a large-scale multicenter trial in North America.[30]

HEPARIN-INDUCED THROMBOCYTOPENIA

Heparin-induced thrombocytopenia (HIT) is an uncommon complication that follows the administration of unfractionated heparin.[11, 12, 31] Some patients with HIT experience paradoxic thrombosis, which can give rise to a major morbidity and mortality. HIT is associated with the presence of a platelet-activating antibody, but its mechanism of action is poorly understood.[32] In comparison with heparins and LMW heparins, danaparoid has low cross-reactivity against this antibody in the platelet aggregation test (12% versus approximately 80% for LMW heparins), which suggests that danaparoid may be useful as an antithrombotic agent in HIT patients. This is supported by favorable clinical results as measured by improved thrombocytopenia and effective anticoagulation for prevention of DVT or extension of existing thrombosis in a compassionate-use program involving 161 patients.[33] The low cross-reactivity of danaparoid with the heparin-induced antibody and its safe and effective use in HIT patients is likely because of its unique composition without any heparin component.

Table 162–3. **Randomized Trials of Danaparoid in the Prevention of DVT in Ischemic Stroke**

	No.		Total DVT	Proximal DVT
Turpie et al., 1987[28]	50	Danaparoid	2 (4%)	0 (0%)
	25	Placebo	7 (28%)	4 (16%)
		p value	.005	.01
Turpie et al., 1992[29]	45	Danaparoid	4 (8.9%)	2 (4.4%)
	42	Heparin	13 (31%)	5 (11.9%)
		p value	.014	.255

DVT, deep vein thrombosis.

SUMMARY

Danaparoid is an effective antithrombotic agent for the prevention of DVT in high-risk patients. It has pharmacologic and pharmacokinetic advantages over standard heparin that may result in its having greater therapeutic efficacy and safety than heparin. Danaparoid has an additional advantage over unfractionated heparin and LMW heparins in that it does not cross-react with antibodies to heparin or LMW heparin and thus may be less likely to produce thrombocytopenia. Further studies with danaparoid are under way.

REFERENCES

1. Meuleman DG: Organan (Org 10172): Its pharmacological profile in experimental models. Haemostasis 22:58, 1992.
2. Gordon DL, Linhardt R, Adams HP: Low-molecular-weight heparins and heparinoids and their use in acute or progressing ischaemic stroke. Clin Neuropharmacol 13:522, 1990.
3. Casu B: Structural features of chondroitin sulphates, dermatan sulfate and heparan sulfate. Semin Thromb Haemost 17(Suppl 1):9, 1991.
4. Nurmohamed MT, Fareed J, Hoppensteadt D, et al: Pharmacological and clinical studies with Lomoparan, a low molecular weight glycosaminoglycan. Semin Thromb Hemost 17(Suppl 2):205, 1991.
5. Vogel GMT, Meuleman DG, Bourgendien FGN, et al: Comparison of two experimental thrombosis models in rats: Effects of four glycosaminoglycans. Thromb Res 54:399, 1989.
6. Meuleman DG, van Dinther T, Hobbelen PMJ, et al: Effects of the low molecular weight heparinoid Org 10172 in experimental thrombosis and bleeding models: Comparison with heparin. Thromb Haemorrhagic Disord 2(1):25, 1990.
7. Boneu B, Buchanan MR, Cade JF, et al: Effects of heparin, its low molecular weight fractions and other glycosaminoglycans on thrombus growth in vivo. Thromb Res 40:81, 1985.
8. Cade JF, Buchanan MR, Boneu B, et al: A comparison of the antithrombotic and haemorrhagic effects of low molecular weight heparin fraction: The influence of the method of preparation. Thromb Res 35:613, 1984.
9. Mikhailidis DP, Fonseca VA, Barrados J, et al: Platelet activation following intravenous injection of a conventional heparin: Absence of effect with a low molecular weight heparinoid (Org 10172). Br J Clin Pharmacol 24:415, 1987.
10. Atkinson JLD, Sundt TM, Kazmier FJ, et al: Heparin-induced thrombocytopenia and thrombosis in ischaemic stroke. Mayo Clin Proc 63:353, 1988.
11. Chong BH, Pitney WR, Castaldi PA: Heparin-induced thrombocytopenia—Association of thrombotic complications with a heparin-dependent IgG antibody which induces platelet aggregation, release and thromboxane synthesis. Lancet 2:1246, 1983.
12. Chong BH, Magnani HN: Organan in heparin-induced thrombocytopenia. Haemostasis 22:85, 1992.
13. Donhof M, de Boer A, Magnani HN, et al: Pharmacokinetic considerations on Organan Org 10172 therapy. Haemostasis 22:73, 1992.
14. Bradbrook ID, Magnani HN, Moelker CT, et al: ORG 10172: A low molecular weight heparinoid anticoagulant with a long half-life in man. Br J Clin Pharmacol 23:667, 1987.
15. Stiekema JCJ, Wijnand HP, van Dinther THG, et al: Safety and pharmacokinetics of the low molecular weight heparinoid Org 10172 administered to healthy elderly volunteers. Br J Pharmacol 27:39, 1989.
16. Frei U, Wilks MF, Boehmer S, et al: Gastrointestinal blood loss in haemodialysis patients during use of a low molecular weight heparinoid. Nephrol Dial Transplant 3:435, 1988.
17. Kroon C, de Boer A, Kroon JM, et al: Influence of skin thickness on heparin absorption. Lancet 337:945, 1991.
18. Turpie AGG: Thromboprophylaxis in orthopaedic surgery. Orthopaedics International Edition 1(5):396, 1993.
19. Hoek JA, Nurmohamed MT, Hamelynck KJ, et al: Prevention of deep vein thrombosis following total hip replacement by low molecular weight heparinoid. Thromb Haemost 67:28, 1992.
20. Leyvraz P, Bachmann F, Bohnet J, et al: Thromboembolic prophylaxis in total hip replacement: A comparison between the low molecular weight heparinoid Lomoparan and heparin dihydroergoramine. Br J Surg 79(9):911, 1992.
21. Gerhart TN, Yett HS, Robertson LK, et al: Low-molecular-weight heparinoid compared with warfarin for prophylaxis of deep-vein thrombosis in patients who are operated on for fracture of the hip. J Bone Joint Surg [Am] 73:494, 1991.
22. Bergqvist D, Kettunen K, Fredin H, et al: Thromboprophylaxis in patients with hip fractures: A prospective, randomized, comparative study between ORG 10172 and dextran 70. Surgery 109:617, 1991.
23. Blum A, Desruennes E, Elias A, et al: DVT prophylaxis in surgery for digestive tract cancer comparing the LMW heparinoid ORG 10172 (Lomoparan) with calcium heparin [abstract]. Thromb Haemost 62(1):126, 1989.
24. Gallus A, Cade J, Ockelford P, et al: Organan (Org 10172) or heparin for preventing venous thrombosis after elective surgery for malignant disease? A double-blind, randomised, multicenter comparison. Thromb Haemost 70(4):562, 1993.
25. Warlow C, Ogston D, Douglas AS: Venous thrombosis following strokes. Lancet 1:1305, 1972.
26. McCarthy ST, Robertson D, Turner JJ, et al: Low-dose heparin as a prophylaxis against deep vein thrombosis after acute stroke. Lancet 2:800, 1977.
27. McCarthy ST, Turner J: Low-dose subcutaneous heparin in the prevention of deep vein thrombosis and pulmonary emboli following acute stroke. Age Ageing 15:84, 1986.
28. Turpie AGG, Levine MN, Hirsh J, et al: A double-blind randomized trial of Org 10172 low molecular weight heparinoid in the prevention of deep vein thrombosis in patients with thrombotic stroke. Lancet 1:523, 1987.
29. Turpie AGG, Gent M, Cote R, et al: A low-molecular weight heparinoid compared with unfractionated heparin in the prevention of deep vein thrombosis in patients with acute ischemic stroke. Ann Intern Med 117(5):353, 1992.
30. Adams HP, Woolson R, Biller J, et al: Studies of Org 10172 in patients with acute ischemic stroke. Haemostasis 22:99, 1992.
31. King DE, Kelton JG: Heparin-induced thrombocytopenia. Ann Intern Med 100:535, 1984.
32. Chong BH, Ismail F, Chesterman CN, et al: Heparin-induced thrombocytopenia: Mechanism of interaction of the heparin-dependent antibody with platelets. Br J Haematol 73:235, 1989.
33. Magnani HN: Heparin-induced thrombocytopenia (HIT): An overview of 230 patients treated with Organan (Org 10172). Thromb Haemost 70(4):554, 1993.

CHAPTER 163

Enoxaparin (Lovenox)

Alexander G. G. Turpie, M.D., F.R.C.P., F.A.C.P., F.A.C.C., F.R.C.P.C.

Heparin may be fractionated or depolymerized into a number of components with varying molecular weights. The component of heparin that has a molecular weight of 2000 to 5000 has been designated the low-molecular-weight fraction or fragment. Several low-molecular-weight heparins have been developed and evaluated for clinical use. Each low-molecular-weight heparin is prepared differently and has a different molecular composition and a different average molecular weight. Clinical studies have shown that each low-molecular-weight heparin is efficacious and safe in the management of a number of thromboembolic disorders, but because each of the low-molecular-weight heparins is different, each one has to be evaluated separately in each clinical indication. Enoxaparin is one such low-molecular-weight heparin and is approved for clinical use in North America.[1, 2]

PHARMACOLOGY: ENOXAPARIN/HEPARIN

Enoxaparin is prepared by partial alkaline depolymerization of the benzyl ester of unfractionated porcine heparin. Enoxaparin consists of homogeneous short chains of uniform length that range in molecular weight from 2000 to 8000 with an average weight of 4500.[2] Low-molecular-weight heparins, such as enoxaparin, contain the pentasaccharide sequence required to bind antithrombin III (AT-III), but their binding capacity is lower than that of the standard heparins from which they are derived.[3] As with heparin, the major anticoagulant effect of enoxaparin is production of a conformational change in AT-III that accelerates its inactivation of thrombin and activated coagulation factors X and IX.[1] However, there is a major difference between the anticoagulant effect of heparin and that of low-molecular-weight heparins such as enoxaparin. Of the activated coagulation enzymes, thrombin is the most sensitive to inhibition by heparin, both because AT-III inhibits thrombin more rapidly than activated factor X and because activated factor X is protected from inhibition by the AT-III heparin complex when it is bound to phospholipid in the prothrombinase complex. Heparin potentiates the inactivation of thrombin by serving as a template to which both AT-III and thrombin bind to form a ternary complex. In contrast, the accelerated inactivation of factor X by the AT-III heparin complex does not require ternary complex formation, but is achieved by the binding of heparin to AT-III alone.[1] The inhibitory action of the various heparins on activated factor X and thrombin is inversely proportional to the length of the polysaccharide chains. Low-molecular-weight heparin molecules such as enoxaparin that have fewer than 18 saccharides (molecular weight < 5400) are unable to bind to thrombin and AT-III simultaneously and thus cannot catalyze the inactivation of thrombin by AT-III. However, heparins do not have to bind to AT-III and factor X simultaneously; therefore, the low-molecular-weight heparins can retain their ability to catalyze the inhibition of factor X by AT-III. Enoxaparin has a higher ratio of anti–factor Xa to antithrombin activity (3:1) than unfractionated heparin does (1:1). Thus, at equivalent anti-Xa activity, enoxaparin has an attenuated effect on thrombin as compared with unfractionated heparin.[1]

Brace et al.[4] reported that the antithrombin and anti–factor Xa activities for enoxaparin were 34 U/mg and 118 U/mg, respectively. Enoxaparin is almost completely absorbed after subcutaneous injection, with maximum plasma anti–factor Xa activity occurring 3 to 5 hours after injection. In healthy volunteers, the bioavailability of enoxaparin after subcutaneous administration exceeds 90% and is more than three times greater than that of unfractionated heparin (30%). After subcutaneous injection, the half-life of the anti-Xa activity produced by enoxaparin is about 4.5 hours compared with a dose-dependent half-life of only 1 hour for intravenously administered unfractionated heparin.[4] *Ex vivo*, enoxaparin has minimal effect on the activated partial thromboplastin time (aPTT) and thrombin clotting time. Because of this and because of the predictable pharmacokinetics and stable dose response with enoxaparin, monitoring with coagulation tests is unnecessary.

Heparin and its derivatives inhibit platelet function to varying degrees, depending on their molecular weight.[5] Low-molecular-weight heparins (molecular weight < 5000) have fewer inhibitory effects on platelet aggregation or on binding of fibrinogen to platelets. It has been suggested that the reduced platelet reactivity reported with low-molecular-weight heparins is due to a reduction in their ability to bind with platelets, which results from the smaller molecules having lower affinity for platelet binding sites and from a reduction in the number of binding sites on the molecule. Studies of the platelet-binding capacities of the various heparin fractions have shown that, in general, the amount of heparin bound increased with increasing molecular size. Enoxaparin, like other heparin fragments, especially those with a strong affinity for AT-III, has been shown to have reduced platelet interaction compared with standard heparin, hence its potential to cause less hemorrhage.[6]

In addition to its actions on factor Xa and thrombin, the administration of enoxaparin is associated with increased fibrinolytic activity, possibly by facilitating the release of t-PA from the vascular endothelium. In a study by Vinazzer and Woler,[1] enoxaparin in doses ranging from 30 to 90 mg given subcutaneously resulted in increased fibrinolytic activity measured as a significant decrease in euglobulin lysis time.

The molecular size of heparin and its fragments influences their ability to bind to plasma proteins and endothelial cells. The plasma bioavailability and pharmacokinetics of enoxaparin differ from those of unfractionated heparin, possibly because of their different binding characteristics to plasma proteins and endothelial cells. Because enoxaparin has a low affinity for heparin-binding proteins and endothelial cells, its plasma recovery and clearance depend on the dose administered and plasma concentration achieved. The reduced binding of enoxaparin to endothelial cells may contribute to its greater bioavailability and longer plasma half-life, which at therapeutic doses is approximately two to four times longer than that of unfractionated heparin.[1, 3]

ANTITHROMBOTIC ACTIVITY OF ENOXAPARIN

Cade et al.[7] assessed the antithrombotic effects of enoxaparin in a thrombosis model in New Zealand white rabbits. In this study, enoxaparin markedly reduced thrombus formation at a dose of 10 anti–factor Xa U/kg, and completely inhibited thrombus formation at 20 anti–factor Xa U/kg, a dose that gave circulating anti–factor Xa levels of 0.1 to 0.2 U/ml. The hemorrhagic effects of enoxaparin were also studied by Cade et al.[7] using a microvascular bleeding model in animals. Enoxaparin was found to cause much less bleeding than standard heparin at equivalent antithrombotic doses. In addition, the inhibitory effects of enoxaparin on thrombus formation were obtained with minimal increases in aPTT and thrombin clotting time.

CLINICAL EVALUATION OF ENOXAPARIN

Venous thromboembolism is a common complication in hospitalized patients. In the absence of prophylaxis, patients with general medical illnesses and patients undergoing major general surgery have a 10% to 40% incidence of calf vein thrombosis, a 2% to 8% incidence of proximal vein thrombosis, and a 0.1% to

0.8% incidence of fatal pulmonary embolism. Patients undergoing orthopedic procedures and who do not receive prophylaxis are at very high risk for venous thromboembolism: 40% to 80% develop calf vein thrombosis, 10% to 20% develop proximal vein thrombosis, and 1% to 5% suffer fatal pulmonary embolism. Thus, the morbidity and mortality of thromboembolic disease are major problems in hospitalized patients.[8] Several methods of thrombosis prophylaxis have been evaluated in high-risk patients, including low-dose unfractionated heparin, adjusted-dose unfractionated heparin, oral anticoagulants, antiplatelet drugs, intermittent pneumatic compression devices, and low-molecular-weight heparins. Low-dose heparin prophylaxis is the most widely recommended and utilized form of prophylaxis for moderate- and high-risk patients. A metaanalysis showed that low-dose heparin was effective in reducing the risk of venous thrombosis in general surgical patients, in orthopedic patients, and in patients undergoing urologic procedures, with a risk reduction in each category of approximately 65%.[9] Despite the evidence that low-dose heparin is effective, prophylaxis is not universally used, largely because of a perception that there is a significant increased risk in bleeding complications. In addition, in about 30% to 35% of patients, low-dose heparin is ineffective.

Low-molecular-weight heparins have been evaluated for the prevention of venous thromboembolism in randomized clinical trials in general surgical patients, in orthopedic patients, in spinal cord injured patients, and in medical patients.[10] The data from the general surgical studies demonstrate that low-molecular-weight heparins effectively prevent deep vein thrombosis (DVT), and in doses that yield an antithrombotic effect equal to or greater than that of standard unfractionated heparin, the risk of bleeding complications is similar (Table 163–1). Patients undergoing orthopedic procedures provide a much more rigorous test of the efficacy and safety of low-molecular-weight heparin fragments in the prevention of DVT. Before the introduction of low-molecular-weight heparins, a number of methods of thrombosis prophylaxis were evaluated in patients undergoing orthopedic procedures, but none was ideal.[11] Low-dose subcutaneous heparin is only 50% effective, aspirin has been shown to be of no benefit overall when venography was used to detect venous thrombosis, and dextran, which provides about a 50% risk reduc-

Table 163–1. **Frequency of Deep Vein Thrombosis and Major Bleeding in Randomized Trials Comparing LMWH with Unfractionated Heparin in General Surgery**

| | Patients | | Outcomes | | |
	LMWH	Heparin	LMWH	Heparin	RR (CI$_{95}$)
Deep vein thrombosis	3467	3411	184	230	0.79 (0.65–0.95)
Pulmonary embolism	2888	2843	9	20	0.44 (0.21–0.95)
Major bleeding	1977	1966	52	51	1.01 (0.70–1.48)

LMWH, low-molecular-weight heparin; RR, relative risk.

Table 163–2. Frequency of Deep Vein Thrombosis and Major Bleeding in Randomized Trials Comparing LMWH with Unfractionated Heparin in Orthopedic Surgery

	Patients		Outcomes		
	LMWH	Heparin	LMWH	UFH	RR (CI$_{95}$)
Deep vein thrombosis	672	622	93	132	0.68 (0.54–0.86)
Pulmonary embolism	590	582	10	24	0.43 (0.22–0.82)
Major bleeding	672	622	6	8	0.75 (0.26–2.14)

LMWH, low-molecular-weight heparin; UFH, unfractionated heparin; RR, relative risk.

tion, is not widely used because of the frequency of side effects, including heart failure and allergic reactions. Orally administered anticoagulants, which are widely used but require careful monitoring, result in an approximately 60% risk reduction in venous thrombosis. Several studies have demonstrated the safety and efficacy of low-molecular-weight heparin in patients undergoing elective and emergency orthopedic procedures. In the 1992 meta-analysis of studies involving orthopedic patients,[10] low-molecular-weight heparins were shown to be either as effective as or superior to unfractionated heparin in the prevention of DVT, with some reduction in bleeding (Table 163–2). Thus, there is solid evidence from randomized clinical trials that low-molecular-weight heparins are highly effective in the prevention of DVT in high-risk surgical patients. Although the various low-molecular-weight heparins have differences in terms of specific activity and pharmacokinetics, there is no evidence from studies to date that there are major differences between them with regard to efficacy.

Enoxaparin in the Prevention of DVT in High-Risk Surgery

Enoxaparin has been extensively evaluated in high-risk medical and surgical patients and has been shown to be highly effective in the prevention of DVT.

Most studies that evaluate enoxaparin in the prophylaxis of DVT have been in high-risk orthopedic patients (Table 163–3). Several studies with enoxaparin in the prophylaxis of DVT in patients undergoing hip replacement surgery were conducted in North America. Turpie et al.[12] conducted a double-blind, randomized study to compare enoxaparin given in a subcutaneous dose of 30 mg twice daily with placebo for the prevention of DVT in patients undergoing elective hip replacement surgery. Treatment was begun 12 to 24 hours postoperatively and continued for 14 days. The patients were screened for DVT with ^{125}I-fibrinogen leg scanning and impedance plethysmography. However, the frequency of DVT detected by the screening tests and confirmed by venography was unexpectedly low in the first 24 patients who were randomized, and therefore venography was carried out routinely in the remaining 76 patients at the end of treatment. In this latter group, venous thrombosis occurred in 4 (10.8%) of the 37 enoxaparin-treated patients and in 20 (51.3%) of the 39 placebo-treated patients ($p = .0002$). The corresponding rates of proximal vein thrombosis were 2 (5.4%) and 9 (23.1%) in the enoxaparin- and placebo-treated patients, respectively ($p = .029$). For all patients who were randomized in the trial, venous thrombosis occurred in 6 (12%) of the 50 enoxaparin-treated patients and in 21 (42%) of the 50 placebo-treated patients ($p = .0007$). The corresponding rates of proximal DVT were 2 (4%) and 10 (20%) in the enoxaparin- and placebo-treated patients, respectively ($p = .014$). Bleeding complications occurred in 2 of the 50 pa-

Table 163–3. Randomized Clinical Trials of Enoxaparin in Prevention of DVT in Orthopedic Patients

Author	Surgery	Treatment	Total DVT %	Proximal DVT %	Major Hemorrhage
Turpie et al., 1986[12]	Elective hip	Enoxaparin 30 mg twice daily	12	4	2
		Placebo	42	20	4
Planes et al., 1988[16]	Elective hip	Enoxaparin 40 mg once daily	12.5	7.5	2
		Heparin 5000 U thrice daily	25	18.5	0
Levine et al., 1991[14]	Elective hip	Enoxaparin 30 mg twice daily	17	5	3
		Heparin 7500 U twice daily	19	6.5	6
Danish Study Group, 1991[17]	Elective hip	Enoxaparin 40 mg once daily	6.5	2	—
		Dextran 70	22	5	—
Leclerc et al., 1992[13]	Elective knee	Enoxaparin 30 mg twice daily	17	0	2
		Placebo	58	19	0
Colwell et al., 1994[15]	Elective hip	Enoxaparin 30 mg twice daily	5	2	4
		Enoxaparin 40 mg once daily	15	4	1
		Heparin 5000 U thrice daily	12	5	6

DVT, deep vein thrombosis.

tients in the enoxaparin group (one major, one minor) and in 2 of the 50 patients in the placebo group (two major), and there was no difference in the postoperative hemoglobin fall or red cell transfusion requirements between the two treatment groups.

Leclerc et al.[13] performed a similar study in patients undergoing total knee replacement or tibial osteotomy. In this study, 131 patients were randomized to receive 30 mg of enoxaparin twice daily or placebo begun postoperatively; outcomes were to be assessed by bilateral venography at day 14 or at the time of discharge from the hospital, whichever came first. Venography was performed in 95 of the patients randomized. DVT, detected by venography, occurred in 35 (65%) of 54 patients in the placebo group and in 8 (20%) of 41 patients in the enoxaparin group, a risk reduction of 71% ($p < .0001$). For the entire study group of 131 patients, DVT was diagnosed either by venography or by noninvasive tests in 37 (58%) of 64 patients in the placebo group and in 11 (17%) of 65 patients in the enoxaparin group, a risk reduction of 71% ($p < .001$). Proximal vein thrombosis occurred in 19% of the placebo-treated patients and in none of the enoxaparin-treated patients ($p < .001$). Bleeding complications occurred in 5 (8%) of 65 patients in the placebo group and in 4 (6%) of 66 patients in the enoxaparin group ($p = .71$). There were no differences in the amount of blood loss, hemoglobin fall, or number of units of packed red cells transfused in patients in the two treatment groups.

These two placebo-controlled studies confirmed the safety and efficacy of enoxaparin in the prevention of DVT in high-risk orthopedic patients.

Two North American studies have compared enoxaparin with unfractionated heparin in the treatment of DVT in orthopedic patients. Levine and colleagues[14] compared the efficacy of enoxaparin with a high dose of standard heparin for the prevention of postoperative DVT in a double-blind, randomized study in 665 patients who underwent elective hip surgery. Patients were randomized to either fixed doses of 30 mg of enoxaparin given twice daily or 7500 IU of unfractionated heparin given twice daily subcutaneously. Treatment was begun 12 to 24 hours following surgery and was continued for 14 days. Venography was planned between days 10 and 14 in all patients, or sooner if the patient was ready for hospital discharge or had a positive screening test. For the 521 patients with evaluable venograms, thrombosis was detected in 50 (19.4%) of the 258 patients in the enoxaparin treatment group compared with 61 (23.2%) of the patients in the unfractionated heparin treatment group. Proximal DVT occurred in 14 (5.4%) of the patients who received enoxaparin and in 17 (6.5%) of the patients who received unfractionated heparin. For the entire group of 665 patients, venous thrombosis, diagnosed by venography or detected by a screening test, occurred in 57 (17.1%) of the 333 patients given enoxaparin and in 63 (19%) of the 332 patients given unfractionated heparin. The corresponding rates for proximal thrombosis were 16 (4.8%) and 18 (5.4%), respectively. Thus, there was no difference in the incidence of DVT in the two groups. However, hemorrhagic complications occurred almost twice as often in the unfractionated heparin group. Bleeding occurred in 17 (5.1%) of the enoxaparin-treated patients and in 31 (9.3%) of the unfractionated heparin–treated patients ($p = .035$), and major bleeding episodes occurred in 11 (3.3%) of the enoxaparin-treated patients and in 19 (5.7%) of the unfractionated heparin–treated patients. Thus, this study showed that for equivalent efficacy using high doses of unfractionated heparin, enoxaparin caused significantly less bleeding.

Colwell et al.[15] carried out a randomized, open-label, multicenter study to compare the efficacy of enoxaparin and unfractionated heparin in the prophylaxis of DVT in 604 patients who underwent elective hip replacement surgery. In this study, patients were randomized to one of three treatment groups: enoxaparin, 30 mg twice daily (194 patients); enoxaparin, 40 mg once daily (203 patients); and unfractionated heparin, 5000 IU every 8 hours (207 patients). All three dosage regimens were administered subcutaneously and begun within 24 hours following surgery and were continued for up to 7 days. Patients were screened for DVT with noninvasive tests and underwent bilateral contrast venography at the end of the study or earlier if clinically indicated. For all randomized patients, DVT occurred in 9 (6%) of the patients treated with enoxaparin, 30 mg twice daily; in 30 (15%) of the 230 patients treated with enoxaparin, 40 mg once daily; and in 24 (12%) of the 207 patients treated with unfractionated heparin. The rate of DVT was statistically significantly lower in the group given 30 mg of enoxaparin twice daily compared with the group given 40 mg of enoxaparin once daily ($p = .0002$) and the group given unfractionated heparin ($p = .0278$). Proximal vein DVT developed in 2% of the patients given 30 mg of enoxaparin twice daily, in 4% of the patients given 40 mg of enoxaparin once daily, and in 5% of the patients given unfractionated heparin. Eight (4%) of the patients given 30 mg of enoxaparin twice daily and 3 (1%) of the patients given 40 mg of enoxaparin twice daily had major bleeding episodes, as compared with 13 (6%) of the patients given unfractionated heparin. This study demonstrated that enoxaparin given in a dose of 30 mg twice daily was more effective than a 40-mg once-daily regimen of enoxaparin and a standard fixed dose of unfractionated heparin with no increase in the risk of bleeding.

The prophylaxis studies carried out with enoxaparin in Europe used daily doses of 40 mg once daily and, in contrast with the North American trials, used a preoperative dose. Planes et al.[16] carried out a double-blind, randomized trial in patients undergoing elective hip replacement comparing enoxaparin given subcutaneously in a dose of 40 mg once daily with standard unfractionated heparin administered at a dose of 5000 U every 8 hours. In this study, treatment regimens began 12 hours preoperatively with enoxaparin and 2 hours preoperatively with standard unfractionated heparin, and they were continued for 15 days or until discharge. Venography was performed in all patients. Two hundred thirty-seven patients were included in the study: 113 received unfractionated heparin and 124 received enoxaparin. The incidence of total DVT was reduced from 25% in the heparin group to 12.5% in the enoxaparin group ($p = .03$). The incidence of proximal DVT was reduced from 18.5% in the unfractionated heparin group to 7.5% in the enoxaparin group ($p = .014$). There were two major bleeding episodes and one minor bleed in the enoxaparin group compared with two minor bleeds in the unfractionated heparin group. Patients who received enoxaparin required fewer red blood cell transfusions and had significantly higher hemoglobin levels on postoperative days 3 and 4 than the heparin-treated patients. Thus, prophylaxis with enoxaparin, 40 mg once daily, was found to be safe and more effective than standard, low-dose unfractionated heparin in preventing DVT in patients undergoing elective hip replacement.

The Danish Enoxaparin Study Group[17] compared enoxaparin in a dose of 40.6 mg once daily with dextran 70 in the prevention of DVT in 246 patients undergoing elective hip replacement. DVT diagnosed by ascending venography occurred in 7 (6.5%) of 108 enoxaparin-treated patients and in 24 (21.6%) of 111 dextran-treated patients ($p = .0013$). In this study, postoperative blood loss and the number of patients transfused were higher in the dextran-treated patients.

Thus, the two European studies that tested enoxaparin given once daily, but with a preoperative dose, showed that enoxaparin was more effective than standard treatments in the prevention of DVT in high-risk orthopedic patients.

Samama et al.[18] evaluated enoxaparin for the prevention of DVT in general surgical patients in a multicenter European trial. In this study, which was an open-label comparison with low-dose heparin, both regimens were found to have similar efficacy, with DVT occurring in 13 (3%) of the 448 enoxaparin-treated patients and in 20 (5%) of the 437 heparin-treated patients.

The approved regimen for DVT prophylaxis in orthopedic patients in North America is 30 mg twice daily given subcutaneously and begun postoperatively. Whether this regimen is equivalent to or better than the once-daily regimen with a preoperative dose requires further evaluation in randomized clinical trials.

Treatment of Venous Thromboembolism

Unfractionated heparin has been the mainstay of treatment for venous thromboembolism for the past several decades.[3] The evidence for the use of heparin in the initial treatment of venous thromboembolism comes from two studies. The superiority of heparin over no antithrombotic treatment was shown in the classic study by Barritt and Jordan[19] that demonstrated a better clinical outcome in patients with pulmonary embolism treated with heparin followed by

orally administered anticoagulants compared with those who did not receive antithrombotic treatment. Convincing evidence for the benefits of initial heparin in the treatment of DVT comes from a study by Brandjes et al.[20] that compared orally administered anticoagulants alone with continuous intravenously administered heparin followed by orally administered anticoagulants. In this study, the clinical outcome was significantly better in the patients who received heparin as the initial treatment. Heparin is usually administered by continuous intravenous infusion, but it can also be given by subcutaneous injection, provided the patient receives an initial bolus intravenously.[21] Intermittent intravenous administration of heparin is another option that is probably comparable in efficacy but is associated with more bleeding than with either continuous intravenous infusion or subcutaneous injections.[3] In the treatment of venous thromboembolism, the heparin dose is usually titrated to obtain a desired level of anticoagulation referred to as the therapeutic range, usually an aPTT 1.5 to 2.5 times control. Several studies of heparin therapy in patients with venous and arterial thrombosis have shown that the risk of recurrent thromboembolic events is 4- to 12-fold higher if the anticoagulant response, assessed with a sensitive aPTT, is less than the lower limit of the therapeutic range, usually 1.5 times control.[22] In patients with venous thromboembolism, treatment with intravenously administered heparin is usually started with a bolus of 5000 to 7500 U followed by a continuous infusion of 30,000 to 35,000 U per 24 hours to prolong the aPTT to 1.5 to 2.0 times control. The duration of heparin treatment in patients with venous thromboembolism has conventionally been 10 days in North America but, more recently, shorter 4- to 5-day regimens have been shown to be effective. The duration of heparin therapy has been the subject of two trials, one in patients with submassive venous thromboembolism reported by Gallus et al.[23] and the other in patients with proximal DVT reported by Hull et al.[24] The results of both studies showed that the discontinuation of heparin after 5 days of treatment—provided that orally administered anticoagulation started at the same time or shortly after the start of heparin therapy was in the therapeutic range for more than 24 hours—is effective and safe. For secondary prophylaxis after the initial treatment, oral anticoagulant therapy or, in selected patients, adjusted-dose subcutaneously administered heparin (midinterval aPTT 1.5 to 2.0 times control) is effective.

A number of randomized studies have evaluated low-molecular-weight heparins in the initial management of venous thromboembolism and have shown that these drugs, administered either intravenously with dose adjustments or subcutaneously in fixed doses, are at least as effective and probably more effective than continuous intravenously administered, adjusted-dose unfractionated heparin.[25] Two of the studies assessed major clinical end points during long-term follow-up after treatment with either unfractionated heparin or low-molecular-weight heparin.[26, 27] Both studies reported a lower incidence of recurrent venous thromboembolism and major bleeding complications in patients randomized to fixed-dose, subcutaneously administered low-molecular-weight heparin compared with those randomized to standard unfractionated heparin treatment. In addition, both trials reported a lower incidence of mortality due to causes unrelated to venous thromboembolism in the patients treated with low-molecular-weight heparin. Low-molecular-weight heparins have not been formally evaluated in treatment of patients with pulmonary embolism.

Simonneau and colleagues[28] compared fixed-dose, weight-adjusted enoxaparin with standard intravenously administered unfractionated heparin in the treatment of proximal vein thrombosis in a prospective randomized trial. In this study, 67 patients were randomized to receive enoxaparin and 67 to heparin, and the primary outcome of efficacy was a change in thrombus size on repeat venography. In addition, the rates of recurrent thromboembolism in the two groups were compared. The results of the study showed that there was a significantly greater reduction in thrombus mass in the enoxaparin-treated patients than in the heparin-treated patients on repeat venography after a 7- to 10-day treatment ($p < .002$). In addition, there were significantly fewer recurrent thromboembolic events ($p < .002$) in enoxaparin-treated patients (1 of 67) than in heparin-treated patients (5 of 67). There were no serious bleeding complications in either group. Thus, enoxaparin, like the other low-molecular-weight heparins, appears to be an effective treatment in the initial management of proximal vein thromboembolism. Because it was given in a fixed dose without monitoring, this raises the possibility that enoxaparin may be useful for the outpatient management of patients with proximal vein thrombosis. This hypothesis is currently being tested in a randomized trial.

SUMMARY

The pharmacology and pharmacokinetics of enoxaparin, a low-molecular-weight heparin approved for clinical use in North America for the prevention of DVT in high-risk orthopedic patients, offer a number of advantages over standard unfractionated heparin. The clinical evaluation of enoxaparin in randomized clinical trials indicates that it is at least as effective as, if not more effective than, unfractionated heparin in the prevention and treatment of venous thromboembolism.

REFERENCES

1. Vinazzer H, Woler M: A new low-molecular-weight heparin fragment (PK 10169): In vitro and in vivo studies. Thromb Res 40(2):135, 1985.
2. Buckley MM, Sorkin EM: Enoxaparin: A review of its pharmacology and clinical applications in the prevention and treatment of thromboembolic disorders. Drugs 44(3):465, 1992.
3. Hirsh J: Drug therapy. Heparin. N Engl J Med 324(22):1565, 1991.
4. Brace LD, Fareed J, Tomeo J, et al: Biochemical and pharmaco-
logical studies on the interaction of PK 10169 and its subfractions with human platelets. Haemostasis 16:93, 1986.
5. Salzman EW, Rosenberg RD, Smith MH, et al: Effect of heparin and heparin fractions on platelet aggregation. J Clin Invest 65:64, 1980.
6. Holmer E, Lindahl U, Backstrom G, et al: Anticoagulant activities and effects on platelets of a heparin fragment with high affinity for antithrombin. Thromb Res 18(6):861, 1980.
7. Cade JF, Buchanan MR, Boneu B, et al: A comparison of the antithrombotic and haemorrhagic effects of low-molecular-weight heparin fractions: The influence of the method of preparation. Thromb Res 35(6):613, 1984.
8. Turpie AGG: Thromboprophylaxis in orthopaedic surgery. Orthopaedics International 1(5):396, 1993.
9. Collins R, Scrimgeour A, Yusuf S, et al: Reduction in fatal pulmonary embolism and venous thrombosis by perioperative administration of subcutaneous heparin. Overview of results of randomized trials in general, orthopedic and urologic surgery. N Engl J Med 318:1162, 1988.
10. Nurmohamed MT, Rosendaal FR, Büller HR, et al: Low-molecular-weight heparin versus standard heparin in general and orthopaedic surgery: A meta-analysis. Lancet 340:152, 1992.
11. Mohr DN, Silverstein MD, Murtaugh PA, et al: Prophylactic agents for venous thrombosis in elective hip surgery. Meta-analysis of studies using venographic assessment. Arch Intern Med 153:2221, 1993.
12. Turpie AGG, Levine MN, Hirsh J, et al: A randomized controlled trial of a low-molecular-weight heparin (enoxaparin) to prevent deep vein thrombosis in patients undergoing elective hip surgery. N Engl J Med 315(15):925, 1986.
13. Leclerc JR, Geerts WH, Desjardins L, et al: Prevention of deep vein thrombosis after major knee surgery—a randomized, double-blind trial comparing a low-molecular-weight heparin fragment (enoxaparin) to placebo. Thromb Haemost 67(4):417, 1992.
14. Levine MN, Hirsh J, Gent M, et al: Prevention of deep vein thrombosis after elective hip surgery. A randomized trial comparing low-molecular-weight heparin with standard unfractionated heparin. Ann Intern Med 114:545, 1991.
15. Colwell CW, Spiro TE, Trowbridge AA, et al: Use of enoxaparin, a low-molecular-weight heparin, and unfractionated heparin for the prevention of deep venous thrombosis after elective hip replacement. J Bone Joint Surg [Am] 76(1):3, 1994.
16. Planes A, Vochelle N, Mazas F, et al: Prevention of postoperative venous thrombosis: A randomized trial comparing unfractionated heparin with low-molecular-weight heparin in patients undergoing total hip replacement. Thromb Haemost 60(3):407, 1988.
17. The Danish Enoxaparin Study Group: Low-molecular-weight heparin (enoxaparin) vs dextran 70. The prevention of postoperative deep vein thrombosis after total hip replacement. Arch Intern Med 151:1621, 1991.
18. Samama M, Bernard P, Bonnardot JP, et al: Low-molecular-weight heparin compared with unfractionated heparin in prevention of postoperative thrombosis. Br J Surg 75:128, 1988.
19. Barritt DW, Jordan SC: Anticoagulant drugs in the treatment of pulmonary embolism. A controlled trial. Lancet 1:1309, 1960.
20. Brandjes DPM, Büller HR, Heijboer H, et al: Comparative trial of heparin and oral anticoagulants in the initial treatment of proximal deep-vein thrombosis (DVT) [abstract]. Thromb Haemost 65(6):703, 1991.
21. Hommes DW, Bura A, Mazzolai L, et al: Subcutaneous heparin compared with continuous intravenous heparin administration in the initial treatment of deep vein thrombosis. Ann Intern Med 116:279, 1992.
22. Prins MH, Hirsh J: Heparin as an adjunctive treatment after thrombolytic therapy or acute myocardial infarction. Am J Cardiol 67:3A, 1991.
23. Gallus A, Jackaman J, Tillet J, et al: Safety and efficacy of warfarin started early after submassive venous thrombosis or pulmonary embolism. Lancet 2:1293, 1986.
24. Hull RD, Raskob GE, Rosenblood D, et al: Heparin for 5 days as compared within 10 days in the initial treatment of proximal venous thrombosis. N Engl J Med 322:1260, 1990.
25. Prins MH, Turpie AGG: Diagnosis and treatment of venous thromboembolism. *In* Bloom AL, Forbes CD, Thomas DP, Tud-

denham EG (eds): Haemostasis and Thrombosis. New York: Churchill Livingstone, 1994, pp 1381–1414.
26. Hull RD, Raskob GE, Pineo GF, et al: Subcutaneous low-molecular-weight heparin compared with continuous intravenous heparin in the treatment of proximal vein thrombosis. N Engl J Med 326:975, 1992.
27. Prandoni P, Lensing AWA, Büller HR, et al: Comparison of

subcutaneous low-molecular-weight heparin with intravenous standard in proximal deep vein thrombosis. Lancet 339:441, 1992.
28. Simonneau G, Charbonnier B, Decousus H, et al: Subcutaneous low-molecular-weight heparin compared with continuous intravenous unfractionated heparin in the treatment of proximal deep vein thrombosis. Arch Intern Med 153:1541, 1993.

CHAPTER 164

Warfarin

Edward E. Genton, M.D.

Warfarin has been used clinically for antithrombotic prophylaxis for more than 50 years. During this time, acceptance of the drug by physicians has fluctuated greatly, largely because of the inadequacy of clinical trials until the 1970s. Only recently has conclusive information about the efficacy of oral anticoagulation for primary and secondary prophylaxis in various thrombotic states been presented. This new information has enhanced understanding of the optimal approach of administering the drug and monitoring its use to achieve maximum benefit with minimal adverse effects.

HISTORY

Chemicals with anticoagulant actions were first discovered during the search for the cause of hemorrhaging in cattle found to occur after ingestion of sweet clover that had spoiled. The animals were found to be deficient in prothrombin, and in 1939, Karl Paul Link isolated dicumarol from the sweet clover; some investigators thereafter synthesized the compound, 3-3-methyl *bis* 4 hydroxycoumarin ($C_{19}H_{15}NaO_4$). Within a few years, Link had synthesized a number of related compounds. For the past several decades, one of these compounds, warfarin, has become the most widely used orally administered anticoagulant drug because of its favorable pharmacodynamic properties, including good absorption, predictable effects, and a desirable duration of action.[1]

CHEMISTRY

Warfarin is the generic name for 3 (α-acetonylbenzyl)-4-hydroxycoumarin and has a molecular weight of 330.3.

PHARMACOLOGY

Warfarin and other coumarin anticoagulant derivatives act by inhibiting the hepatic synthesis of the vitamin K–dependent coagulation factors, which include factors VII, IX, X, and II and proteins C and S. The drug is not a direct inhibitor of vitamin K, but acts by interfering with cyclic interconversion of vitamin K in liver microsomes. This inhibits a vitamin K–mediated effect on the synthesis of these coagulation factors. Vitamin K promotes the carboxylation of N-terminal glutamic acid residues in these coagulation factor molecules. The carboxylation increases affinity for calcium ions on that site, and calcium serves as the bridge for binding to phospholipids, which forms a complex and greatly accelerates the enzymatic effect of these activated vitamin K–dependent factors. Noncarboxylated factors, which are formed with a vitamin K deficiency or during anticoagulant therapy, do not bind with calcium and therefore do not complex with phospholipids and, hence, lack coagulant activity. During anticoagulant therapy, the liver synthesizes immunologically detectable proteins that are biologically inactive.[1, 2]

PHARMACOKINETICS

Warfarin administered orally is completely absorbed. Although food consumption does not affect bioavailability, it may delay the rate of absorption. Peak absorption usually occurs within 2 to 4 hours, with more than 90% of the drug bound to plasma albumin. There is some anticoagulant effect within 24 hours, but the peak effect of a dose occurs at approximately 36 hours and, in some circumstances, may be delayed for as long as 72 to 96 hours. The half-life of warfarin is approximately 2½ days.

Metabolism and excretion of warfarin vary considerably among individuals, primarily because of the variability in half-life due to natural differences in metabolism or because of the effect of diseases or drug-induced alterations in the metabolic half-life. The drug is metabolized by hepatic microsomal enzymes to inactive metabolites that are excreted into bile, travel through an enterohepatic circulation, are partially reabsorbed, and eventually are excreted into urine.

Several coagulation tests—including the one-stage prothrombin time, the thrombotest, and the activated partial thromboplastin time—are sensitive to decreased activity of vitamin K–dependent coagulation factors. The prothrombin time detects decreased activity of factors II, VII, and X, but not factor IX; the thrombotest detects decreased activity of all four coagulation factors; and the activated partial thromboplastin time is sensitive to factors II, IX, and X, but not factor VII. The prothrombin time is the most commonly employed test for monitoring warfarin therapy. It involves the addition of a tissue thromboplastin derived from various sources, most often human brain or rabbit brain or lung tissue, to citrated plasma. The sensitivity of these thromboplastins to levels of vitamin K–dependent clotting factors varies considerably, and this variation must be considered to avoid inappropriate changes in warfarin dosage when interpreting prothrombin time results.

The effect of warfarin on the prothrombin time depends on the depression of procoagulant vitamin K–dependent factors II, VII, and X. The rate of reduction of the individual factors depends on their half-life in plasma. This varies from 6 hours for factor VII to approximately 60 hours for factor II. Although the prothrombin time may be prolonged within 24 hours if large doses of warfarin are given because of suppression of factor VII, this would not afford antithrombotic prophylaxis, which requires a decrease in the other factors that would not occur for several days. In addition, protein C, like factor VII, has quite a short half-life, and this naturally occurring antithrombotic protein, if rapidly depressed, may result in a thrombotic tendency before the other coagulation factors become depressed and produce an anticoagulant state.[2]

CLINICAL USE
Indications

Conclusive evidence establishes the effectiveness of warfarin, both for primary and for secondary prophylaxis, to prevent venous or arterial thromboembolism. The drug should not be used during an active thrombotic state to prevent propagation or embolization. In these instances, heparin is more effective because of its direct action to inhibit thrombin, in contrast with warfarin's indirect action to decrease the concentration of vitamin K–dependent clotting factors. Warfarin is used for secondary prophylaxis to prevent recurrence after an initial course of heparin therapy. Before discontinuing heparin, the two drugs should be combined to allow sufficient time for all of the vitamin K factors to decline in the plasma, even though the prothrombin time might have been prolonged earlier from a prompt fall in factor VII level. Note that heparin may prolong the prothrombin time by its antithrombin action in the prothrombin time. To assess the warfarin effects in patients on combined therapy, the prothrombin time should be drawn when heparin effect is minimal and the partial thromboplastin time is in the "therapeutic" range.

Warfarin is clinically indicated for conditions caused by or associated with thrombotic episodes or recurrent thromboembolism. These include venous thromboembolism, cerebrovascular disease, and cardiac disorders, which are described in more detail in the following sections.

Venous Thromboembolism (Deep Vein Thrombosis or Pulmonary Embolism)

Warfarin is very effective for primary prophylaxis in medical or surgical conditions associated with a moderate to high risk for venous thrombosis. The intensity of the prothrombin time prolongations (international normalized ratio [INR] level) correlates with the intensity of the thrombotic provocation. Thus, patients with knee or hip replacement or hip fracture are likely to develop thrombosis and should be maintained at a higher INR level than should patients who have undergone general abdominal surgery or gynecologic procedures.

Warfarin is indicated in patients with established venous thrombosis or pulmonary embolism for secondary prophylaxis of recurrent thrombosis after a 5- to 10-day course of heparin. As noted earlier, heparin should overlap the initiation of warfarin for 3 to 5 days, until all affected coagulation factors have decreased. The duration of warfarin therapy depends on the clinical circumstances, and the drug should be continued until the provocation for the initial thrombotic event is eliminated. In most patients, this occurs within 3 to 4 months, but it can take much longer in some patients. Occasionally, lifetime anticoagulation is indicated.

Cerebrovascular Disease

Warfarin reduces the risk of recurrent transient ischemic attacks, whether the embolus has arisen in the heart or from extracranial arteries. In patients with recurrent ischemic attack, long-term drug therapy may be indicated and is often preceded by a course of heparin therapy. Less certain is the effect of long-term warfarin therapy to prevent recurrent stroke.

Cardiac Disorders

A major indication for warfarin therapy is to prevent systemic emboli in patients with atrial fibrillation. This indication is especially strong in patients with mitral valvular disease of any cause. Patients with atrial fibrillation of an uncertain duration prior to cardioversion benefit from a 3- to 4-week course of warfarin therapy to decrease the likelihood of embolization after sinus rhythm is restored.

Similarly, patients who undergo cardiac valvular replacement benefit from warfarin therapy. After tissue valve placement, the indicated course of anticoagulation is only 2 to 3 months; patients with mechanical heart valves, however—especially valves in the mitral position—remain at high risk for thromboembolism and should receive permanent warfarin treatment.

Other patients with cardiac disease, including those with ventricular aneurysms or cardiomyopathy, may benefit from anticoagulant therapy. Clinical trials have indicated that recurrence of myocardial infarction may be decreased with oral anticoagulant therapy; however, this is not routinely used in the United States.

DOSAGE AND ADMINISTRATION

The dose of warfarin to initiate anticoagulation must be individualized, and the maintenance dose should be determined by serial prothrombin times so that it can be adjusted to the level of anticoagulation appropriate for the patient's disease state. Treatment should begin in most patients, if the baseline prothrombin time is normal, with a dose of 10 mg daily for 2 days. Even smaller initial doses may be appropriate in patients with prolonged prothrombin times at baseline; patients with hepatic dysfunction, congestive heart failure, or debilitation; patients older than 80 years; or patients taking drugs known to increase warfarin action. The daily maintenance dose will usually range between 2 mg and 10 mg, but may require up to 25 mg, as determined by daily prothrombin times, until the desired intensity of anticoagulation (INR) is achieved. Thereafter, the interval between prothrombin times is gradually lengthened according to the stability of the patient's control, but seldom for more than 3 to 4 weeks, because many factors, such as diet, physical activity, and climate, may affect warfarin control.

Much has been done to standardize warfarin therapy: properly designed clinical trials have established both conditions in which the treatment is effective and the levels of anticoagulation required to prevent thrombus. Progress has also been made toward standardizing the reporting of the prothrombin time. As has been discussed, the tissue thromboplastin reagent used in prothrombin time varies considerably in its sensitivity to activate the coagulation sequence, depending on the tissue source of the reagent. To decrease the problems related to this lack of standardization, a system of reporting results based on thromboplastin standards has been developed. A standardized thromboplastin reagent derived from human brain tissue has been established by the World Health Organization and assigned an international sensitivity index (ISI) of one. Commercial thromboplastins are compared with this reagent and assigned an ISI accordingly. Reports of the prothrombin time results obtained with the reagents should be standardized, expressing the result as if it were obtained with the standard thromboplastin. This calculation is called the INR and is calculated from the following formula: INR = observed prothrombin ratio (patient plasma/control plasma) raised to the power of the ISI of the thromboplastin reagent used. For simplicity, the INR may be obtained in the laboratories from a standard nomogram. The use of INR values in controlling dose ensures maximum safety and effectiveness regardless of which thromboplastin is used, thus permitting interpretation of data from various laboratories.

The INR system has been used in reporting trial results in numerous clinical conditions; national organizations in North America and Europe have used these results to make recommendations on the intensity of anticoagulation appropriate for patients in various disease groups[2-4] (Table 164–1).

PRECAUTIONS AND ADVERSE EFFECTS

A major complication of warfarin therapy is hemorrhage, which develops with anticoagulant therapy in approximately 5% to 10% of cases per year; about one-half of cases involve major bleeds, 1% of which are life-threatening. Bleeding correlates with the intensity of the anticoagulant effect, and bleeding complications in patients with prothrombin times in the therapeutic range are frequently related to local lesions, such as gastrointestinal ulcerations or carcinomas. When prothrombin time is prolonged excessively, bleeding may be spontaneous and involve numerous sites, most often the kidney; fatal bleeds, however, most frequently relate to intercerebral or gastrointestinal bleeding.[5]

The management of excessive anticoagulation depends on the prothrombin time and the urgency of the situation. Most patients with a prothrombin time of 30 seconds or less, but longer than desired, can be managed in the absence of bleeding by withholding the dose for the appropriate amount of time. The length of time for a fall in prothrombin time is reasonably predictable by the patient's maintenance dose. Thus, patients requiring a high maintenance dose can be assumed to be rapid metabolizers and to require less time for prothrombin time to be reduced to the therapeutic range, whereas patients on low maintenance doses are slow metabolizers and may require more time for prothrombin times to be corrected. When prothrombin times exceed 30 seconds (INR > 7), it is desirable to promptly decrease the degree of anticoagulation, because such levels have no thera-

Table 164–1. **Therapeutic Range (INR) for Warfarin**

	British Society for Haematology	NIHLB American College of Chest Physicians
Venous thromboembolism		
Primary Prophylaxis		
General surgery	2.0–2.5	2.0–3.0
Hip surgery and fracture	2.0–3.0	2.0–3.0
Secondary Prevention		
DVT and PE	2.0–3.0	2.0–3.0
Recurrent DVT	3.0–4.5	2.0–3.0
Cerebrovascular TIA	2.0–3.0	
Peripheral artery disease	3.0–4.5	2.0–3.0
Cardiac disease		
Atrial fibrillation	2.0–3.0	2.0–3.0
Valvular lesions	2.0–3.0	2.0–3.0
Tissue heart valves	2.0–3.0	2.0–3.0
Prosthetic heart valves	3.0–4.5	3.0–4.5

NIHLB, National Institutes of Health, Lung and Blood; DVT, deep venous thrombosis; PE, pulmonary embolism; TIA, transient ischemic attack.

peutic value and these patients can experience serious adverse consequences. Vitamin K administration effectively reverses warfarin effects. If the patient is to be continued on warfarin, it is important to administer a dose of vitamin K that will reduce the prothrombin time to safe levels but not entirely eliminate the warfarin effect. This can usually be accomplished by the parenteral administration of 1 or 2 mg of vitamin K_1 (AquaMEPHYTON, Konakion). The effect is usually evident within 6 to 8 hours. Occasionally, an additional dose of vitamin K is required because warfarin's duration of action in plasma may cause the prothrombin time to rise again. In urgent situations in which warfarin effects must be reversed promptly, such as serious bleeding, fresh frozen plasma may have to be administered. This plasma provides coagulation factors immediately, and the effect may be measured with serial prothrombin times. Although the dose required to reverse the effect in a particular patient may vary, approximately 15 ml of fresh frozen plasma per kilogram of body weight is usually effective.[1, 3–5]

When invasive procedures are necessary in patients on warfarin therapy, one must decide whether a dose adjustment to prevent bleeding is indicated. Many procedures, including relatively bloodless procedures such as dental work and procedures in which good hemostasis is usual (e.g., cholecystectomy or appendectomy), may be performed without interrupting anticoagulation (INR 2.0 to 2.5) or, at most, by only reducing the INR slightly. More invasive procedures require anticoagulants to be discontinued or the level of anticoagulation to be reduced considerably to an INR level of 2.0 or less. In most patients on anticoagulation therapy for prior venous thromboembolism, cardiomyopathy, or atrial fibrillation, warfarin may be safely interrupted for a few days. In other cases, such as patients with prosthetic heart valves, particularly with mitral valve prosthesis, anticoagulation should not be interrupted. In these cases, the warfarin therapy may be suspended, and after 2 or 3 days when the prothrombin time is decreasing, heparin therapy may be initiated, continued until a few hours before the planned surgery, and resumed at an appropriate time postoperatively. Warfarin may then be resumed and heparin stopped after a few days. In emergency situations, such as after trauma or unanticipated major surgery, it may be necessary to reverse the anticoagulant effects, partially or completely, with plasma, as described in the prior section.

Nonhemorrhagic side effects with warfarin are unusual but include skin necrosis, adrenal hemorrhage, and dermatitis. Skin necrosis may be severe and lead to extensive damage, including gangrenous necrosis. This gangrenous complication is seen within the first 1 or 2 weeks of warfarin therapy and usually involves areas of the body with a lot of subcutaneous fat, such as breasts, thighs, and buttocks. Although the cause of this rare complication is not definite, it might relate to the reduced levels of protein C that, when creating a thrombotic state, may allow thrombosis in the microcirculation and hemorrhaging in the involved tissues. Dermatitis is a macula papular eruption that is usually mild and limited but that may be extensive.

The use of warfarin during pregnancy may result in fetal abnormality. When the drug is given during the first trimester of pregnancy, a syndrome of chondrodysplasia punctata is seen in approximately 10% to 15% of fetuses. The syndrome includes stippling of tarsal bones and vertebral bodies and, often, nasal hypoplasia. Some cases of microcephaly with blindness have been reported when the drug is given during the second or third trimesters of pregnancy. *Post partum*, the drug does not enter breast milk in an active form, and breastfeeding does not endanger the infant.

CONTRAINDICATIONS

Obviously, careful case selection for warfarin administration is important, and numerous medical conditions contraindicate the use of this drug. These include aneurysms (cerebral or dissecting), active bleeding disorder, cerebral vascular hemorrhage (confirmed or suspected), blood dyscrasias associated with hemorrhage or thrombocytopenia, severe uncontrolled hypertension, recent (2–3 weeks) trauma (especially to the central nervous system) or neurosurgery, ulceration or active lesions of the gastrointestinal, respiratory, or urinary tracts, and severe vasculitis. Drugs must be administered with caution in patients with a variety of medical disorders that might increase the patient's response to the anticoagulant and, thereby, increase the risk of bleeding. These include a debility of any cause, dysfunction from primary or secondary hepatic disorders, and conditions associated with vitamin K deficiency.

INTERFERENCE WITH OTHER DRUGS

Warfarin interacts with numerous other drugs, resulting in an increase or decrease of anticoagulant effects. If an interacting drug being taken at the onset of warfarin therapy is continued without interruption, the maintenance dose of warfarin is established by serial protimes, and no problem may result. However, if drugs with interactions are begun or discontinued without frequent sampling of protimes, serious difficulties can result. There are numerous mechanisms of interaction, including (1) inhibition of enzymatic metabolism of warfarin, (2) accelerated metabolism of warfarin by stimulation of hepatic microsome activity, (3) alteration of hepatocyte synthesis or catabolism of a procoagulant protein, (4) increased receptor affinity for warfarin, (5) decreased absorption from the gastrointestinal tract, (6) decreased vitamin K synthesis in the gastrointestinal tract, and (7) displacement of warfarin from plasma protein that increases the amount of drug entering hepatocytes.

Furthermore, the likelihood of bleeding complications may be increased by agents that alter platelet function, produce thrombocytopenia, inhibit coagulation pathways, or cause gastrointestinal tract ulcerations.[2, 3]

Organ dysfunction may result in altered warfarin effects. Most notably, hepatic dysfunction may increase the sensitivity to warfarin effect, as may hyperthyroidism, which by increasing the turnover of coagulation factors increases sensitivity to warfarin.

Because warfarin may also affect the action of numerous other drugs, a possibility that is seldom considered, it is good practice to suspect a possible change in the degree of anticoagulation in all patients on warfarin when any drug is added or removed. Furthermore, more frequent prothrombin times should be obtained to detect such changes.

REFERENCES

1. Ansell JE: Oral anticoagulant therapy—50 years later. Arch Intern Med 153:586, 1993.
2. United States Pharmacopeial: Anticoagulants (systemic). In Drug Information for the Healthcare Professional, Vol I, 14th ed. Rockville, MD: United States Pharmacopeial Convention, 1994, pp 228–239.
3. British Society for Haematology, British Committee for Standards in Haematology, Haemostasis and Thrombosis Task Force: Guidelines on oral anticoagulation. J Clin Pathol 43:177, 1990.
4. Second American College of Chest Physicians and the National Heart, Lung and Blood Institute. National Conference on Antithrombotic Therapy. Chest 89(Suppl):1S, 1986.
5. Levine HJ, Hirsh J, Landefeld VS, et al: Hemorrhagic complications of anticoagulant treatment. Chest 102(Suppl):352S, 1992.

D. Thrombolytic Agents

CHAPTER 165

Streptokinase*

Sol Sherry, M.D., and Victor J. Marder, M.D.

Streptokinase (SK) is a bacterial protein secreted into the culture fluid during the growth phase of β hemolytic streptococci. The SK used for therapeutic thrombolysis is derived from a nonpathogenic, group C (Lancefield) strain of the organism. Originally named streptococcal fibrinolysin and discovered by Tillett and Garner[1] in the early 1930s, its clinical investigation began in the late 1940s[2] and extended through the 1950s.[3-5] Although extensively studied abroad during the next two decades and used clinically by practitioners there, its approval for physician use in the United States for the management of acute deep vein thrombosis (DVT) and of acute pulmonary embolism (PE) took place in 1977. Subsequently, accepted indications have included arterial thrombosis and embolism, clotted external dialysis shunts, and intracoronary and intravenous administration for acute myocardial infarction (MI). Streptokinase was the first thrombolytic agent developed for clinical use, has served as the standard-bearer for thrombolytic therapy, and provides the basis for comparison with other thrombolytic agents.

PHARMACOLOGY
Mechanism of Action

Streptokinase is a single-chain protein containing little carbohydrate and without a disulfide bond; it consists of 415 amino acid residues and has a molecular weight of 45,000 to 50,000.[6, 7] Although SK has considerable homology with serine proteases,[7] it is not an enzyme; consequently, its ability to activate plasminogen is indirect. A two-step reaction is involved in which SK reacts immediately and stoichiometrically on a 1:1 basis with plasminogen or plasmin to form an SK-plasminogen or SK-plasmin complex; an active site is exposed in the plasminogen or plasmin portion of the complex, and it becomes a highly efficient enzyme activator for plasminogen, catalytically converting it rapidly to plasmin. The SK-plasminogen complex also can be degraded to a SK-plasmin complex with the retention of activator activity[8] (Fig. 165–1). In vivo, the activator complex formed by SK has a half-life of approximately 23 minutes.[9]

Plasmin is a nonspecific proteolytic enzyme. When it is formed on a fibrin surface (i.e., through activation of fibrin-bound plasminogen), fibrinolysis is the result; when it is formed in plasma (i.e., through activation of plasma plasminogen), fibrinogenolysis occurs.[10] Although SK can form a complex with the plasminogen bound to fibrin, fibrin provides no specific binding sites for SK. Consequently, when SK is introduced in the circulation, two independent actions take place: activation of fibrin-bound plasminogen and activation of plasma plasminogen.

Effects of Plasma Plasminogen Activation

During therapy, when sufficient SK has been administered to overcome anti-SK antibody (the only inhibitor to the action of SK or its activator complex), prompt and extensive activation of plasma plasminogen takes place. The hyperplasminemic state that results, although transient, produces an anticoagulant state in which levels of fibrinogen and factors V and

*This work was supported in part by grant HL-30616 from the National Heart, Lung and Blood Institute, National Institutes of Health, Bethesda, MD.

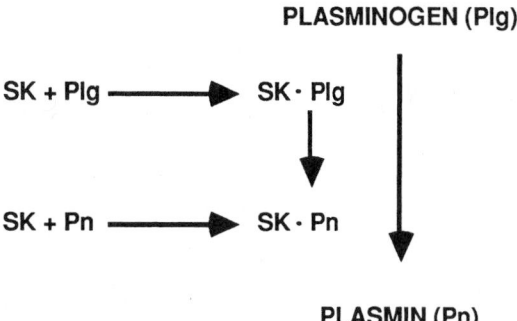

PLASMINOGEN (Plg)

Figure 165–1. Two-step mechanism by which streptokinase activates plasminogen.

VIII fall precipitously, the former often to levels of 100 mg/dl or less. The breakdown products of fibrinogen proteolysis (FDPs) that are formed also impede normal clotting. These effects significantly prolong the activated partial thromboplastin time (aPTT), the thrombin clotting time, and the prothrombin time, assays frequently used in laboratory monitoring during SK therapy because they provide indirect evidence of a clot-dissolving state.

Hemostasis is impaired, primarily because of the degradation of fibrinogen.[9] Usually, no native fibrinogen is in the circulation; the circulating clottable protein is fragment X,[9] a smaller molecule resulting from the initial action of plasmin on fibrinogen (Fig. 165–2).[11] The hemostatic defect not only increases the risk of a bleeding episode, but, should bleeding occur, its severity is likely to be enhanced. Because the hemostatic defect diminishes the likelihood of rethrom-

bosis, it counterbalances the danger of a bleeding episode in terms of the risk:benefit ratio of therapy. The state of anticoagulation produced by the hemostatic defect is a useful attribute during and for some time after thrombolytic therapy because a thrombogenic stimulus or an inadequate flow rate may persist. The presence of an anticoagulated state avoids the necessity for the simultaneous use of heparin, an agent that can add significantly to the bleeding risk.[12–14]

Fibrinogen is an elongated, elliptical molecule and is the major determinant of plasma viscosity, and, at low shear rates, it may increase blood viscosity by bridging red blood cells together into clumps.[15] Thus, the extensive hypofibrinogenemic state is associated with a reduction in blood and plasma viscosity,[16–18] thereby improving flow rates through large and small vessels and reducing afterload.[16] The reduction of blood viscosity may be of benefit to patients with acute MI because an increase in blood viscosity is usually associated with this disorder.[19]

After SK therapy is completed, restoration of the plasma to the normal state depends on synthesis of new fibrinogen and clearing of the FDPs. The half-life of FDPs in the circulation is approximately 6 or 7 hours,[9] with higher molecular weight forms clearing more slowly than more degraded fragments.[20]

The effects of plasminogen activators on plasmin-susceptible proteins in plasma are often referred to as the *lytic state*, that is, the plasma proteolytic state.[21] The lytic state is the end result of free plasmin in the circulation, in turn caused by the action of the plasminogen activator on plasminogen. Whereas the lytic state is quantitated by the concentration of plasma plasminogen, fibrinogen, factors V and VIII,

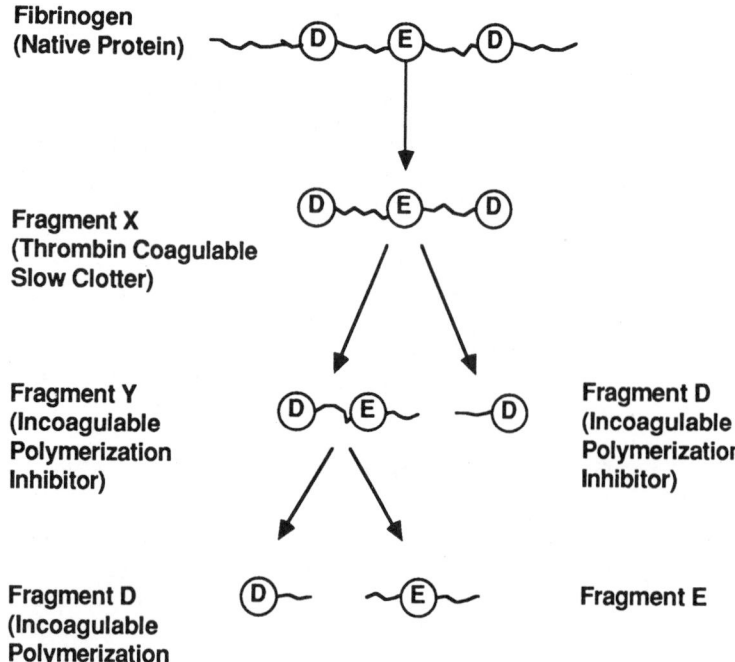

Fibrinogen (Native Protein)

Fragment X (Thrombin Coagulable Slow Clotter)

Fragment Y (Incoagulable Polymerization Inhibitor)

Fragment D (Incoagulable Polymerization Inhibitor)

Fragment D (Incoagulable Polymerization Inhibitor)

Fragment E

Figure 165–2. Schema of degradation of fibrinogen by plasmin, with the sequential formation of fragment X (a slow thrombin coagulable protein), fragments Y and D (inhibitors of the conversion of fibrinogen to fibrin), and the end-products fragments D and E.

and FDPs, plasminogen activator activity in plasma can be measured by the euglobulin lysis time,[22] unheated fibrin plate assay,[23] or release of radioactively labeled fibrin fragments from isotopically labeled clots[24] or from fibrin films.[25] Also, assays of D-dimer,[26] a specific fragment of cross-linked fibrin, or of small peptides cleaved from fibrinogen by plasmin (e.g., $B\beta_{1-42}$) or by thrombin (e.g., fibrinopeptide A), have been applied to the monitoring of therapy[27-30] (Fig. 165-3). Such assays could theoretically reflect processes of increased thrombus formation, thrombolysis, or degradation of circulating fibrinogen or soluble fibrin, but such application has not been proven to be applicable for routine monitoring of thrombolytic therapy.

Factors Influencing the Lysis of Thrombi and Emboli

Although the presence of thrombolytic activity in the circulation is a prerequisite for clot lysis, a poor correlation exists between the level of thrombolytic activity, as determined by direct or indirect methods, and success in clot dissolution;[27-36] this is because several variable factors are critical in determining the success of therapy.

Therapeutic thrombolysis depends on penetration or diffusion of an activator into the clot with activation of fibrin-bound plasminogen. The rate of lysis *in vitro* is a direct function of proximate concentrations of activator and fibrin-bound plasminogen, with the solubilizing process beginning at the surface and progressing inward.[37] *In vivo*, this relationship is influenced greatly by anatomic and biologic factors that are not controllable. These factors include (1) the surface area of clot exposed to activator, (2) the concentration of clot plasminogen, and (3) perhaps most importantly, the age of the thrombus or embolus.

Total occlusions of coronary arteries (grade 0 as defined in the TIMI 1 study),[38] which expose a small surface area to the blood, are not as readily dissolved as when there is penetration of blood into (grade 1) and especially around the clot (grade 2), or when the vessel is only partially occluded (grade 3). Similarly, nonocclusive deep vein thrombi appear to be more readily dissolved by thrombolytic agents such as SK[39] or tissue-type plasminogen activator (t-PA)[40] than are thrombi that totally occlude the vein.

That old thrombi or emboli are more resistant to lysis by SK than fresh clots has been known for a long time.[41] In DVT and PE, this resistance is a matter of days, but resistance to lysis in coronary thrombosis appears to occur within hours.[42-44] The several factors that are operative include (1) rapid chemical cross-linking of the fibrin polymers with their increased resistance to lysis;[45] (2) formation of ultra-large fibrin α chain polymers, as for example induced by the presence of a high concentration of factor XIII or large numbers of platelets;[46] (3) cross-linking of antiplasmin to fibrin by factor XIII;[47] (4) clot retraction, during which serum is squeezed out and fibrin becomes more compacted; and (5) progressive impaction of the thrombus so as to occlude the vessel totally. This progressive resistance to lysis by SK in coronary artery thrombosis is not as evident with t-PA[38] because, in contrast with SK, t-PA binds to fibrin and works longer and more effectively on older or more lysis-resistant fibrin.

Adverse Reactions

As an antigen infused into patients previously exposed to hemolytic streptococcal infections, SK is responsible for a variety of adverse reactions,[48, 49] but the incidence of side effects is not great and they are infrequently severe. Anaphylaxis occurs in less than 0.5% of patients, and angioneurotic edema, periorbital edema, and bronchospasm occur in less than 2%. Rarely, serum sickness, hypersensitivity vasculitis, and renal failure secondary to interstitial nephritis

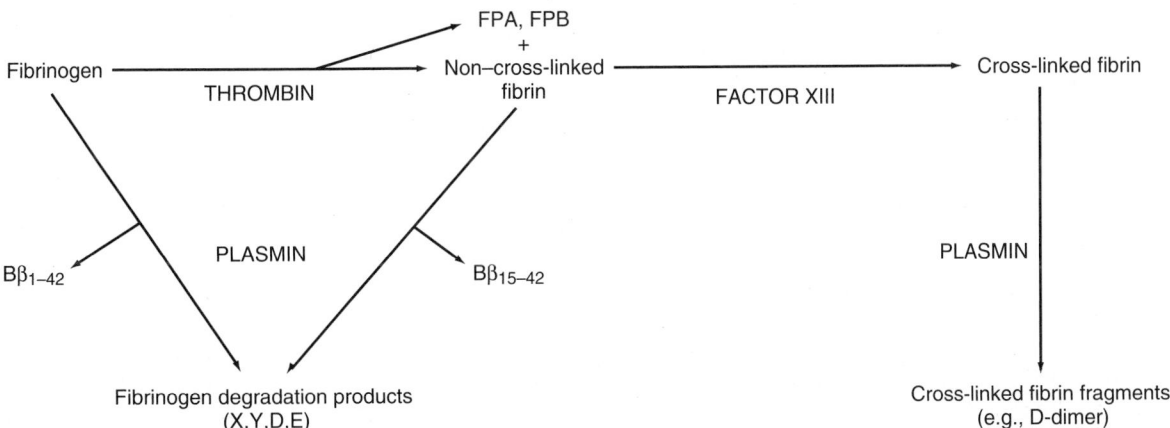

Figure 165–3. Derivation of fibrinopeptides A and B (FPA,FPB) and of fibrinogen and cross-linked fibrin degradation products by action of thrombin, factor XIII, and plasmin on fibrinogen. Degradation products from fibrinogen and non–cross-linked fibrin are identical except for relatively minor differences relative to fibrinopeptide cleavage. In addition to D-dimer, other cross-linked fibrin fragments include high-molecular-weight polymers of cross-linked α chain.

may accompany SK therapy, especially with repeated administration.[50-52] The most common adverse reaction is fever, which is occasionally severe. This delayed hypersensitivity type reaction occurs in 5% to 30% of patients, depending on the duration of treatment (more if continued for days) and whether intravenous hydrocortisone is used for premedication. When fever occurs, it is controlled readily by acetaminophen. Although aspirin and other platelet-active antipyretics were initially not recommended because of a presumed increase in bleeding risk, aspirin is now widely used to prevent rethrombosis after fibrinolytic therapy for acute MI. Other minor reactions, such as urticaria, rash, flushing, itching, musculoskeletal pain, nausea, and headache, also have been described. None of the reactions (mild or severe) has been fatal, and all are managed with antihistamines or steroids.

Probably unrelated to the antigenicity of SK is acute hypotension, which may occur when SK is infused rapidly in high concentration (e.g., more than 750,000 U in 30 minutes).[53] This transient phenomenon may be due to the release of bradykinin after plasmin activation of the kallikrein enzyme system.

Bleeding Complications

As with all thrombolytic agents, bleeding episodes are a complication of SK therapy.[54] It has become increasingly evident that the major cause of bleeding is lysis of hemostatic plugs at sites of previous invasive procedures or internal vascular injury.[55, 56] Thrombolytic therapy can disaggregate platelets[57, 58] and dissolve fibrin in a hemostatic plug at least as readily as the fibrin of a thrombus. Another contributing factor to bleeding episodes is the use of heparin in conjunction with or immediately after thrombolytic therapy.[12-14, 59-65] For example, delayed subcutaneous heparin added to thrombolytic therapy of acute MI is associated with a higher incidence of bleeding, including an increase in intracranial hemorrhage from 0.4% to 0.6%.[66-68] Furthermore, intravenous heparin causes more bleeding than does subcutaneous heparin when administered with aspirin plus a thrombolytic agent (SK, anistreplase, or t-PA).[68, 69] Higher dosages of intravenous heparin (and hirudin) increase the bleeding risk even more, as for example in the GUSTO-IIa[70] and the TIMI-9A[71] trials, which showed intracranial hemorrhage rates with SK and t-PA of approximately 2%, resulting in early termination of the studies and reassessment of anticoagulant dosages. Heparin therapy apparently adds significantly to the bleeding problem after a hemostatic plug is dissolved by the thrombolytic agent, because the hemostatic defect induced by heparin alone is not sufficient to induce this degree of hemorrhagic problem. For example, the incidence of intracranial hemorrhage using heparin (plus aspirin) was 0.3% in GUSTO-IIa, versus 1.8% for heparin plus aspirin used in addition to a thrombolytic agent.[70]

Bleeding, including severe bleeding, is most frequent when invasive procedures such as arterial catheterization are part of the treatment protocol.[63, 64] In contrast, in the absence of invasive procedures, SK therapy (e.g., for PE and DVT) has been associated with an incidence of major bleeding of approximately 9%,[31] slightly higher than the 5% associated with full-dose heparin therapy,[72] and a 1% incidence of cerebral hemorrhage (twice that reported for heparin).[55] The relative risk of bleeding with a thrombolytic agent over heparin in DVT has been calculated from pooled trials as 2.9.[73] The intracoronary administration of SK also has been associated with a similar incidence of severe bleeding (4.8%),[74] primarily due to hemorrhage from the site of catheter insertion in the femoral artery. In the trials with high-dose, brief-duration, intravenous SK for acute MI, when invasive procedures were not performed as part of the protocol, the incidence of severe bleeding in the absence of compulsory anticoagulation has been approximately 0.3% to 0.5%; with compulsory anticoagulation, it has averaged 0.5% to 1%.[66-68, 75-80]

Many bleeding complications can be avoided by patient selection, elimination of invasive procedures, limited duration of therapy, and judicious use of anticoagulation.[55, 56, 81, 82] Known cerebrovascular disease, recent head trauma or cardiopulmonary resuscitation, chest or head surgery within 10 days, or any recently active bleeding lesion presents clearly increased risks of serious hemorrhagic complication; they are generally considered as absolute contraindications to SK therapy. Other less-stringent contraindications are an increased risk of bleeding in patients with recent (10 days or less) less serious surgical procedures, trauma, or impaired constitutional or acquired hemostatic mechanisms.

Rethrombosis

Ten percent to 20% of arteries reperfused with SK are subject to early rethrombosis despite anticoagulant therapy. The most important factors that predispose to rethrombosis are essentially the same as those that led to the initial occlusive event, the presence of a thrombogenic stimulus and altered flow dynamics due to residual thrombus or underlying atherostenotic lesion. A persisting thrombogenic stimulus can result from reexposure of the ruptured atheromatous plaque, which precipitated the original event,[83] or from undissolved thrombus,[84, 85] which possesses surface-bound thrombin activity.[86] The thrombogenic stimulus and flow dynamics are interrelated factors (e.g., in the presence of a fully patent vessel with normal flow, the effects of a thrombogenic stimulus even of moderate proportions may be diluted or washed away). Conversely, a ruptured plaque or a clot that possesses only a mild thrombogenic stimulus but also causes luminal encroachment and altered hemodynamics[87] may lead to dyskinetic and even static zones of flow, thereby predisposing to recurrent formation of thrombus.

Several approaches have been suggested to reduce the incidence of rethrombosis after successful reperfusion of coronary or peripheral arterial occlusions.

They include (1) the thrombolytic approach, which extends the duration of therapy to minimize the amount of residual thrombus;[88] (2) the antithrombotic approach, employing heparin, or more specific anti-thrombins such as hirudin[89] or Hirulog,[90] or antiplate-let agents such as aspirin or newer agents such as the monoclonal antibody against platelet glycoprotein IIb/IIIa;[91] (3) the vasodilator approach, using nitro-glycerin,[92] isosorbide dinitrate,[93] or prostaglandin E1, which also provides prostacyclin-like actions of dila-tation and platelet inhibition;[94] and (4) the mechanical or surgical approach by use of angioplasty[95–101] or bypass graft surgery,[102–107] often in conjunction with antithrombotic agents.

Although the rationale of using mechanical or sur-gical intervention to complete or correct a process of partial or failed thrombolytic reperfusion is self-evi-dent in conceptual simplicity and a seemingly natural back-up procedure, the results have not been gratify-ing for routine application in patients with acute MI. The principal application of this approach would seem to be in cases of clinical deterioration that neces-sitate immediate intervention, for example, to reverse cardiogenic shock. In fact, a more appropriate use of angioplasty appears to be as initial treatment of the acute MI patient, as an alternative—not as a rescue or follow-up measure—to thrombolytic agents.[108–111]

The ideal antithrombotic regimen to follow success-ful reperfusion has not been established.[112] Although a number of new antithrombotic approaches[113–117] have been considered, a combination of aspirin at doses of 160 mg/day or higher plus heparin, delayed until 4 hours after SK infusion,[118] is still the usual recom-mended regimen. Heparin does not improve survival in patients with acute MI treated with SK,[66–68, 119] and because it probably contributes to bleeding and possi-bly rethrombosis,[13] the minimal dosage of heparin that is required still needs to be established by appro-priate clinical trial.

Bleeding complications during surgery performed shortly after thrombolytic infusion are a definite pos-sibility, although relatively uncommon.[74] Although plasminogen activators in the circulation are rapidly cleared,[55] the plasma proteolytic state as manifested by hypofibrinogenemia can last for hours at nadir levels and require 36 to 48 hours for physiologic correction.[120] Thus, reversal of the plasminogen acti-vator effect with antifibrinolytic agents, correction of hypofibrinogenemia with cryoprecipitate,[121] and transfusion of platelets to correct the prolonged bleed-ing time induced by fibrinolysis may well prevent the bleeding complications that have occurred under such circumstances.[103, 122–124]

Laboratory Monitoring

Repetitive assays of blood coagulation and fibrinoly-sis are of little value in SK therapy. Because the infor-mation is predictive of neither a successful outcome[31, 33, 34] nor a complicating bleed, it cannot be used to guide therapy. However, limited monitoring is recom-mended when SK is administered by systemic infu-sion for the management of acute pulmonary embo-lism, DVT, or acute arterial thrombosis and embolism. In these situations, an initial screen that includes the bleeding time, prothrombin time, and aPTT will de-termine the patients' suitability for thrombolytic ther-apy. Clearly, patients with constitutional or acquired hemostatic defects are at higher risk of bleeding dur-ing thrombolytic therapy.[31] For patients who have been on heparin therapy, it is desirable to wait until the aPTT is in the range of two times normal or less before instituting SK therapy. A fibrinogen assay is also recommended as a baseline for comparison with a later determination. Three or 4 hours after the initia-tion of SK therapy, blood is drawn again for determi-nations of aPTT and fibrinogen levels. In the presence of an active thrombolytic state, the aPTT is signifi-cantly prolonged and the fibrinogen significantly re-duced. A fibrinogen assay is the more sensitive test because it is influenced by both hypofibrinogenemia and the clot-inhibiting activity of FDPs. The absence of a significant change in the aPTT or fibrinogen level indicates that the patient is resistant to SK, and it is prudent to discontinue therapy with this particular agent. The infusion can be continued without the need for further assays in the 90% to 95% of patient who respond as anticipated.[56] For the management of deep vein thrombosis or pulmonary embolism, the aPTT is assayed at 2 to 4 hours after termination of the SK infusion and just prior to the institution of heparin therapy. When it is in the range of two times normal or less, heparin administration is started.

When SK is administered locally by direct perfu-sion of an obstructed vessel for coronary thrombolysis or for the dissolution of other arterial thrombi or emboli, there is even less need to monitor the throm-bolytic state. Although lower dosages are used, the local concentration of activator is higher than with systemic administration. Thus, the duration of ther-apy frequently is much shorter or is tailored to the desired therapeutic effect, i.e., the establishment of reperfusion as documented by diagnostic imaging techniques. Because of the presence of the catheter in a coronary artery, heparin is administered concur-rently.

No reason exists for monitoring when SK is admin-istered intravenously in acute MI. The amount given, 1,500,000 U, is sufficient to overcome resistance in almost every patient (except those recently treated with SK), and the duration of therapy (1 hour) is short. Patients with acute MI generally receive 12,500 U of heparin subcutaneously beginning at 4 hours after SK,[68] but a lower dose, more in line with the 5000 U delivered subcutaneously twice a day as pro-phylaxis against deep vein thrombosis, may prove to be safer and as effective.

Dosage, Therapeutic Regimens, and Guidelines

Protocols for patient selection and SK treatment schedules for various indications have been the subject of several articles and book chapters.[55, 72, 125–128]

THERAPEUTIC RESULTS IN ACUTE MYOCARDIAL INFARCTION
Early Studies with Intravenous Streptokinase

Streptokinase was the first plasminogen activator that was successfully applied to the therapy for acute MI. The initial pilot study was reported in 1958, with the drug administered intravenously over a 30-hour period with encouraging results.[129] Subsequently, from 1963 to 1979, there were 19 additional trials with intravenous SK, usually involving a 24-hour period of treatment; the results of all these trials have been reviewed by Yusuf et al.,[130] and eight trials that met more rigid inclusion criteria[131-138] were analyzed by Stampfer et al.[139] Pooling of the results (meta-analysis), a basis for analysis when individual sample sizes are inadequate for mortality studies,[140] suggests a 20% to 22% reduction in the odds of death using the intravenous route of administration. Nevertheless, for a number of reasons,[141] these observations were not considered by some to be a significant therapeutic approach for treating acute MI even as late as 1980.[142]

Intracoronary Administration

Intracoronary administration of preparations containing SK is also not a recent innovation. In 1960, Boucek and Murphy[143] developed a novel method for the use of their preparation for local perfusion, and Chazov et al.[144] in 1976 were the first to use coronary catheterization to instill SK directly into the coronary artery. Nevertheless, it remained for DeWood et al.[145] to establish coronary thrombosis as the responsible culprit in the pathogenesis of most cases of acute transmural MI and for Rentrop et al.[146] to demonstrate that intracoronary administration of SK into the obstructed coronary artery early after the onset of ischemia frequently resulted in rapid reperfusion.

The latter observation soon was confirmed by others[147] who infused 2000 U/min for periods of 60 to 90 minutes. When therapy was initiated within 3 hours of onset of a protracted ischemic event, on average 75% of occluded vessels were reperfused in 30 minutes; serious bleeding complications were low (4.8%) and originated primarily at the catheter insertion site. A significant incidence of reocclusion (18%) was related to underlying residual stenosis,[87, 95, 148] with unlysed thrombus as a prominent deterrent to adequate reflow.[84, 85] However, ventriculography showed a 55% return of function of the initially stunned myocardium, which, in the absence of reperfusion, would have been expected to undergo necrosis and irreversible loss of function.[74] Studies with thallium-201 scintigraphy demonstrated that coronary thrombolysis was associated with improved regional perfusion.[149] However, consistent with the observations by Reimer and Jennings[150] on the progression of irreversible necrosis as a function of time in experimental coronary occlusion in dogs and those of Bergman et al.[151] on positron emission tomography, there is little evidence of myocardial salvage when therapy is begun more than 4 hours after the onset of infarct. Along with timely reperfusion, there is a rapid disappearance of chest pain, early peaking of the MB fraction of creatine phosphokinase, appearance of reperfusion arrhythmias, and rapid reduction of the injury current on the electrocardiogram.[147] Registries of experience with intracoronary SK[152, 153] strongly suggested improved mortality rates and provided the basis for several randomized trials that produced short-term[154, 155] and long-term[155, 156] evidence of a reduction in mortality, especially among patients with anterior infarcts.

High-Dose Intravenous Streptokinase

The technical problems associated with intracoronary thrombolysis, including delay in initiating therapy and limited availability of trained personnel and catheterization laboratories at all times, as well as its high cost, led to the adoption of intravenous use of SK for general use. Dose-ranging studies of intravenous SK have not been exhaustive,[157, 158] but the dose that has been studied most extensively and that has been generally accepted for routine use is 1,500,000 U infused over 1 hour. This SK dose floods the circulation with high levels of activator activity, at the end of which infusion the plasma contains an activity equivalent to 65 U/ml of SK.[9] Recovery from the lytic state begins 4 hours later and is complete within 36 to 48 hours.[33] Antibodies to SK are neutralized during the infusion but begin to reappear on the fifth day and rapidly rise to a peak of 1000 or more U/ml of blood at 2 to 4 weeks before slowly receding to pretreatment levels, usually by 6 to 12 months. Variations of this thrombolytic regimen have utilized, for example, combinations of either full or attenuated dosages of SK with a reduced amount of t-PA.[118, 159] Totally unexploited as a therapeutic option is the potential of genetically engineered mutants of cloned SK.[160, 161] For example, the selection of a fragment lacking the amino terminal 13 amino acid residues would likely be less antigenic than wild-type SK,[162] but to date, there has been no report that has evaluated the efficacy of this or other potentially advantageous forms.[163]

Several factors influence the incidence of restored blood flow (average time, 45 minutes) as mediated by intravenous SK. On the basis of limited data,[74] the incidence of successful reperfusion increases with increasing dosage up to 750,000 U; thereafter the incidence reaches a plateau, although a dose of 3,000,000 U has been claimed to produce the best results in patency (80%).[157] The advantage of administering a large dose, for example 1.5 million units, is not only to ensure a maximum effect but also to maintain thrombolytic activity in the circulation for several hours[9] so as to effect more complete lysis of the thrombus. In addition to the nature of the vascular occlusion (complete or partial), a most important determinant of success is the duration of symptoms before therapy is initiated. Analysis of the data obtained in various studies in which recanalization or patency rates were measured[42, 44, 151] demonstrates a strong correlation when therapy is carried out within 3 hours of ischemic pain, and a reasonable estimate of the frequency of reperfusion is 65%.[55, 164]

Achieving a patent coronary artery is probably the major determinant of successful thrombolytic therapy. For example, a review of the literature showed that achievement of patency after intracoronary SK treatment was clearly associated with a lowered mortality, 2.5% of the 76% of patients (538/712) with patent vessels versus 14% in the 24% of patients with vessels that remained occluded (174/712).[154, 165] Given that the incidence of rapid, "spontaneous" lysis of coronary artery thrombi within 90 minutes is only 15% or less[145] in comparison with rates of 40% to 80% with plasminogen activator therapy, the decided advantages in preserved ventricular function and survival would appear to reflect this more effective rapid reperfusion to the ischemic myocardium. However, in the consideration of the relative efficacy of different plasminogen activators or various regimens of activators, considerable controversy exists as to the relevance of early patency at 90 or 180 minutes. For example, SK use results in a lower incidence of patent vessels than t-PA (60% versus 30%) by angiographic study at 90 minutes after initiation of therapy.[63] Yet, this same study does not demonstrate an advantage for t-PA over SK in ventricular function,[166] suggesting either that treatment (and reperfusion) was too late to achieve a relative benefit in function or that the 90-minute "snapshot" of the vessel is not an absolute indicator of a functional result.[167]

The "open artery" hypothesis as based on the correlation of duration of experimental coronary artery occlusion with ventricular damage[149-151, 168] is a fundamental tenet of the approach to thrombolytic therapy. Therefore, new approaches that may achieve more rapid reperfusion of the occluded coronary artery might achieve better ventricular function and/or survival benefit as well. A recent study compared adjunctive anticoagulant use of intravenous heparin with intravenous Hirulog, a more potent antithrombin agent, and noted a significant increase in the 90-minute patency from 40% to 77%, a result similar to that attained with t-PA.[169] Although there is debate[170, 171] as to whether ventricular function is an important measure of response to thrombolytic treatment, improved function clearly results from the use

of SK as opposed to placebo,[77-80, 155, 172] but only if SK is administered within the first 3 to 4 hours after symptom onset. Improved function appears to be correlated with vessel patency,[173-178] but the relationship is inexact. Thus, the clearly higher 90-minute patency using t-PA compared with SK in the GUSTO-1 angiographic substudy[179] was not translated to better ventricular function at the 90-minute observation point, as reflected by equal values for ejection fraction, end-systolic volume index, wall motion, and number of abnormal chords. Although there is no clear distinction in function between SK- and t-PA–treated patients,[63, 180, 181] a clearly patent vessel (TIMI-2, 1 or 0)[182] induced by treatment with any plasminogen activator results in better ventricular function measurements than is attained with patients whose coronary arteries remain nonpatent.[179]

Mortality Reduction

There have been five randomized trials comparing mortality rates in patients with an acute evolving myocardial infarction assigned either to a placebo control group or to a group receiving 1,500,000 U of streptokinase over a 30- to 60-minute period.[75, 77-79, 183-186] Table 165–1 summarizes the results in those patients who received thrombolytic therapy within 3 hours of symptom onset and who were evaluated for short-term survival at 3 to 4 weeks after treatment. Two of the studies[77, 79] showed a trend that was not statistically significant toward a survival benefit using streptokinase. The 20% advantage (5.2% versus 6.5%) in survival in the ISAM trial[79] was, however, associated with significantly better ventricular function. The Western Washington Trial[77] showed a marked 54% improved survival, but the numbers were insufficient to reach significant values at 14 days after treatment; follow-up at 2 years in patients who had anterior myocardial infarctions did show a significant (20%) advantage in the streptokinase-treated group. A study reported by White et al.[78] was also quite small, but the dramatic difference in mortality (3.7% versus 12.5%) among only 219 patients in the trial reached statistical significance for the 70% survival advantage with streptokinase. By far, the weight of evidence is provided by two much larger studies, the study of the Gruppo Italiano per lo Studio della Streptochinasi

Table 165–1. **Short-term Mortality Reduction Using SK (versus Placebo) Administered in First 3 Hours After Acute Myocardial Infarction**

Study	Year	No.	Mortality (%)		Survival Benefit (%)
			Streptokinase	*Placebo*	
ISAM[79, 186]	1985 and 1987	940	5.2	6.5	20 (NS)
GISSI[75, 185]	1986 and 1987	6094	9.2	12.0	23 (.0005)
White et al[78]	1987	219	3.7	12.5	70 (.012)
Western Washington[77]	1988	194	5.2	11.3	54 (NS)
ISIS-2[183, 184]	1987 and 1988	5108	8.1	12.2	34 (<.0001)

Follow-up at approximately 3–4 weeks after treatment. Overall reduction of approximately 30% in favor of treatment with streptokinase.

nell'Infarto Miocardica (GISSI),[75, 185] which entered more than 6000 patients within 3 hours of symptoms, and the Second International Study of Infarct Survival (ISIS-2),[183, 184] which compared more than 5000 patients treated in this time frame. The GISSI results showed a 23% survival advantage with streptokinase (9.2% versus 12% mortality), which was highly significant ($p = .0005$), and likewise, the ISIS-2 experience showed an increase of 34% in survival (12.2% mortality versus 8.1% with streptokinase, $p < .0001$). The overall experience of the five trials summarized in Table 165–1 is a reduction of 29% for patients treated within 3 hours of symptom onset, as evaluated at approximately 3 to 4 weeks after such therapy.

Delay Before Therapy

Clearly, the earlier that patients are treated with thrombolytic therapy after symptom onset, the better the results. The GISSI study showed that treatment provided during the first hour reduced mortality significantly by 47% as compared with 23% when treatment was delayed for up to 3 hours and only 17%, still a significant reduction ($p = .03$), when treatment was provided at 3 to 6 hours after symptom onset. Similar results were obtained in the ISIS-2 trial, which showed a 35% reduced mortality with treatment in the first 4 hours, as compared with a 17% reduction with treatment provided at 5 to 24 hours. The data on survival versus delay in administration of thrombolytic therapy have been summarized for all of the plasminogen activator studies by the Fibrinolytic Therapy Trials' Collaborative Group,[128] which demonstrated a straight-line relationship between lives saved and delay after symptom onset, from a high value of 35 lives/1000 in the first hour to about 20 for those treated between 7 and 12 hours and a nonstatistically significant trend in favor of thrombolytic treatment (approximately 6 lives/1000) between 12 and 24 hours after symptom onset. Follow-up at 1 or 2 years after treatment[184–186] clearly shows that the survival advantage achieved at about 1 month is maintained long term. Although individual reports suggest that intracoronary SK administration can reduce mortality,[154–156, 187, 188] a retrospective analysis of eight randomized studies of the intracoronary route (versus placebo) by Furberg[189] showed no advantage in mortality (11% versus 12.4%, $p = .64$) at 2 to 54 weeks after the infarction. It is likely that the greater delay required to provide intracoronary therapy accounts for this suboptimal response.

In distinction to the marginal[128] or frank absence of benefit if SK[190] or other thrombolytic agent[191] is administered more than 12 hours after symptom onset, efforts to minimize the time delay before treatment appear to translate into a survival advantage. Thus, administration of plasminogen activator in the ambulance or even at home can cut an average of approximately 1 hour from the usual time delay before treatment, with an overall decrease in mortality of approximately 17%.[192] Although no study has specifically used SK as the thrombolytic agent, the use

of the related plasminogen activator, anisoylated SK-plasmin activator complex (APSAC, anistreplase), has shown the most gratifying results, for example, in the European Myocardial Infarction Project (EMIP)[193] and the Grampian Region Early Anistreplase Trial (GREAT).[194, 195] The EMIP study evaluated 2750 patients treated in the ambulance versus 2719 patients treated 55 minutes later in the hospital and showed a 15% reduction ($p = .08$) in mortality. The GREAT trial was considerably smaller, but treatment at home for 163 patients was administered 130 minutes earlier than for the 148 patients treated in the hospital (median delays, 110 minutes versus 240 minutes). Although the initial survival comparison showed only a trend ($p = .1$) in favor of the earlier-treated group,[194] follow-up at 1 year showed a significantly reduced mortality rate for home therapy (10.4% versus 21.6%, $p = .007$).[195] Although APSAC is especially amenable for rapid intravenous administration,[55, 196] it is reasonable to expect that similar effective initiation and completion of activator treatment in sufficiently large trials of other agents would also prove useful despite the absence of conclusive evidence to date.[197]

Percutaneous Transluminal Coronary Angioplasty (PTCA)

Direct or primary PTCA has been studied in comparison with intracoronary SK[198] or intravenous SK,[199, 200] although the largest experience of PTCA with a thrombolytic agent used intravenous t-PA.[108] The collective experience of these trials,[127, 192] as well as a prospective registry comparison,[201] suggests that the results are equally effective regarding ejection fraction and survival but that reinfarction and the incidence of hemorrhagic strokes are less common with PTCA than with thrombolytic treatment. This approach is limited by availability of an operational facility to handle acute emergencies efficiently and would seem best suited to patients with contraindications to thrombolytic therapy who present especially early after symptom onset. PTCA performed routinely immediately after prior thrombolytic treatment offers no advantage and probably causes more complications (reocclusion, reinfarction, death) than when PTCA is performed only as clinically indicated.[96, 98–101]

Adjunctive Antithrombotic Therapy

Given the distinct biochemical effects of the different plasminogen activators on blood coagulation and fibrinolytic components,[33, 55] the issue of optimal adjunctive antithrombotic therapy must be considered separately for each agent. The most incontrovertible aspect is the requirement for aspirin administration to patients receiving a thrombolytic agent, as documented for SK in the ISIS-2 trial.[183, 184] In this four-arm design of aspirin, SK, both agents, or neither agent in 17,187 patients treated within 24 hours of pain, the 35-day vascular mortality was 10.4% ($p < .0001$) for SK alone, 10.7% ($p < .00001$) for aspirin alone, and 8% ($p < .00001$) for 160 mg aspirin per day for 30 days in addition to standard SK, compared with 13.2% for neither agent. The effect of aspirin alone was constant for patients treated within the first 4 hours and during the 13 to 24–hour interval, about 20% to 25% reduction compared with the placebo group (Table 165–2). In contrast and as cited previously, the results of SK alone were better for patients treated early rather than late, 35% reduced mortality in the first 4 hours versus 21% at 13 to 24 hours' delay. The benefits that accrued from SK or aspirin alone were additive at both the early and late time periods, indicating independent but complementary modes of action (53% reduction in vascular deaths at 0 to 4 hours and 38% at 13 to 24 hours). The additional advantage in survival afforded by aspirin was also associated with a significant reduction in the number of reinfarctions without an increase in the number of intracranial hemorrhages over the number induced by SK alone.

Given the additional benefit of aspirin to clinical results with SK, the overriding issue now would be whether heparin further contributes positively to survival outcome.[202] This issue is succinctly summarized by Ridker et al.,[69] who distinguished the relevance of disparate studies of various plasminogen activators, variable regimens of both aspirin and heparin, and different end points of benefit (e.g., vascular patency versus mortality). Considerable emphasis has been placed on two trials of coronary artery patency after t-PA that compared intravenous heparin adjunctive treatment with placebo.[203, 204] These studies showed significantly higher coronary artery patency rates for patients receiving heparin, 82% versus 52% and 71% versus 44%. However, these patients received either a low (80 mg/day) dosage of aspirin[203] or no aspirin at all,[204] thereby putting into question the contribution of heparin had there been optimal aspirin administration. By contrast, trials of similar design showed no difference in patency at 90 minutes after t-PA initiation with or without intravenous heparin[205] or no difference between heparin or aspirin at 7 days after t-PA,[206] and one study that did allow for full-dose aspirin in addition to heparin showed only a small difference at 3.3 days (83% versus 75%).[207]

Similar trials using APSAC (DUCCS-1)[208] or SK (OSIRIS)[209] compared patency results with or without IV heparin in patients who received therapeutic dosages of aspirin. The DUCCS-1 results were most impressive in that combined clinical outcome, left ventricular function and coronary artery patency (80%

versus 73%, p = .26), were no different with or without heparin, but intravenous heparin caused significantly more bleeding (32% versus 17%, p = .006). The preliminary OSIRIS data showed a transiently higher patency rate (by noninvasive technology) at 90 minutes (77% versus 60%, p < .05), but this difference was not apparent at 120 minutes (82% versus 72%; p, NS [not significant]) or at 24 hours (86% versus 87%; p, NS).

The more important clinical evaluations of heparin administration in addition to adequate aspirin in patients receiving a thrombolytic agent come from the megatrials of GISSI-2/International Study Group,[66, 67] ISIS-3,[68] and GUSTO.[119] The first two of these studies compared no heparin with delayed subcutaneous heparin delivered either at 12 hours[66, 67] or at 4 hours[68] after thrombolytic initiation. The results are in essential agreement, namely that 35-day mortality is not decreased (10.0% versus 10.2%; p, NS), but the incidence of major bleeding (requiring transfusion) and of intracranial hemorrhage was increased (0.5% versus 0.4%). To answer the question whether the subcutaneous heparin administration in these trials was administered too little and too late, the GUSTO study directly compared subcutaneous heparin (12,500 U b.i.d.) delayed until 4 hours after initiation of therapy with immediate intravenous heparin (5000-U bolus, then 1000 U/hr for patients less than 80 kg body weight or 1200 U/hr for those more than 80 kg body weight) in patients receiving SK and adequate aspirin.[68] This comparison of approximately 20,000 patients showed no significant difference in 30-day mortality (7.2% for subcutaneous heparin versus 7.4% for intravenous heparin) or hemorrhagic stroke (0.53% versus 0.59%), clearly indicating that the use of intravenous heparin does not provide a clinical advantage over the more conservative subcutaneous heparin regimen. In fact, the trend in clinical result was generally in favor of the subcutaneous heparin group, despite the fact that a significant number of patients assigned to receive only subcutaneous heparin were given intravenous heparin, especially in the United States.

Of great importance are the subsequent trials of GUSTO-IIa[70] and TIMI-9A,[71] which used a slightly higher dosage of intravenous heparin for patients treated with thrombolytic therapy (SK or t-PA) and aspirin. These studies were suspended because of an unacceptably high incidence of intracranial hemorrhage of 2.7% and 1.6% in patients receiving SK (as well as in patients who received t-PA), and the studies were restarted at intravenous heparin dosages as originally used in GUSTO-I.[119] Acceptable safety has apparently been reestablished, but a full understanding of the high intracranial hemorrhage rate in GUSTO-IIa and TIMI-9A is not evident, because the published original dosages and guidelines for anticoagulant management for these studies were not very different from those of GUSTO-I.

It would seem evident from the available data that intravenous heparin at any dosage is not needed for SK plus aspirin regimens, because mortality is not

Table 165–2. **Effect of Delay After Symptom Onset on Response to SK and Aspirin***

	Reduction in Vascular Mortality (35 Days) (%)		
Delay (hrs)	Aspirin	SK	Aspirin + SK
0–4	25	35	53
5–24	21	17	33
Overall	33	25	42

*All the results, as reported in the ISIS-2 trial,[184] were highly statistically significant.

improved, the intracranial hemorrhage rate is increased, and the margin of safety for an excessive intracranial rate is narrow. In fact, there is little evidence for any benefit of even delayed subcutaneous use (at 12,500 U b.i.d.) in such patients, and perhaps only a venous prophylactic dose of 5000 U b.i.d. would be safer with regard to the occurrence of intracranial hemorrhage.

Newer Approaches

The potential for more rapid and lasting vascular reperfusion has generated an active search[113] for more effective antithrombotic approaches to supplant the currently used agents, namely, aspirin as the antiplatelet agent and heparin as the antithrombin inhibitor. Many approaches are under current assessment but the greatest interest is generated toward agents that interfere with fibrinogen binding to the platelet IIb/IIIa receptor as a means of limiting platelet aggregation, most notably using the monoclonal antibody 7E3[210] and the hirudin/Hirulog family of specific inhibitors of thrombin.[116, 211] The hirudin-type agents have been tested for safety and efficacy relative to heparin in a variety of vascular thrombotic disturbances, including unstable angina, post-PTCA reocclusion, and for adjunctive treatment along with plasminogen activators. The synthetic inhibitor Hirulog has been compared with heparin as adjunct to SK for patients with acute MI, and the effect on 90-minute and 120-minute coronary artery patency has been striking.[169] As compared with heparin, Hirulog produced greater TIMI grade 2 + 3 patency at 90 minutes (77% versus 47%, $p = .05$) and at 120 minutes (87% versus 47%, $p < .01$). Among the values at 120 minutes, Hirulog induced a 77% TIMI-3 result, compared with only 40% using heparin. These data are equivalent to those obtained with front-loaded t-PA plus heparin[179] or hirudin,[89] the latter results being TIMI 2 + 3 flow rates of 82%, including 65% for TIMI-3.

In the TIMI-6 study,[212] SK plus hirudin at dosages of 0.1 and 0.2 mg/kg/hr was associated with fewer adverse clinical outcomes (death, reinfarction, congestive heart failure, shock) than was obtained with SK plus heparin. A higher dosage of hirudin (e.g., 0.6 mg/kg bolus followed by 0.2 mg/kg/hr) was chosen for large clinical trials comparing hirudin with heparin (using either SK or t-PA), although the TIMI-5 trial showed no patency advantage and a suggestive higher rate of bleeding, compared with lower dosages.[89] As noted previously for the heparin-treated patients, excessive intracranial hemorrhage rates occurred as well for patients receiving hirudin plus t-PA or SK, 1.7% to 1.8% in the TIMI-9A trial[71] and 1.7% and 3.2%, respectively, in the GUSTO-IIa trial.[70] Thus, although there is reasonable anticipation of improved outcome using hirudin or Hirulog rather than heparin, the dosage schedules have first to be optimized to lessen the incidence of hemorrhagic complications. At a lower dosage of hirudin or heparin, intracranial hemorrhage appears to be within an ac-

ceptable range.[70, 71] Using such conservative dose schedules, the main predictors of an increased rate of intracranial hemorrhage appear to be a relatively advanced age of older than 65 years, asthenia (which tends to exaggerate the effect of blood concentration of t-PA more so than SK), hypertension, and exposure to t-PA rather than SK.[213]

The possibility of accelerated thrombolysis is especially interesting for agents that cause a more profound lytic state (low fibrinogen, low plasminogen) such as occurs with SK, urokinase (UK), or APSAC.[55] If the lower 90-minute reperfusion rates using SK rather than t-PA in patients with acute MI[63, 179] are partly explained by the strikingly lower plasminogen concentration, which hypothetically decelerates the thrombolytic action of SK, then repletion of the plasma plasminogen concentration might allow for sustained and progressive clot lysis[214–217] and improved clinical outcome. Such improved response to fibrinolytic therapy would ensue regardless of the specific plasminogen activator or antithrombotic agent used. Clinical trials that test the concept of plasminogen supplementation to maximize thrombolytic potential have been reported for deep vein thrombosis,[218] pulmonary embolism,[219] peripheral arterial occlusion,[220, 221] and acute MI.[222] The results of some studies have been positive, but none has yet met appropriate standards for a valid comparison of treatment without plasminogen, and appropriate randomized and prospective trials are needed to fully evaluate this potential therapeutic modality.

COMPARISON OF PLASMINOGEN ACTIVATORS (Table 165–3)
Acute Deep Vein Thrombosis (DVT)

The rationale for use of thrombolytic therapy in acute DVT of the lower extremities is to prevent the development of dependent venous hypertension, a common occurrence when patients are treated with anticoagulants alone. Although anticoagulants prevent extension and embolization, they do not mediate

Table 165–3. **Comparison of Different Plasminogen Activators**

Indication	Results
DVT	Most extensive information using SK, which includes extensive lysis in >50%. Probably equivalent results using t-PA and other plasminogen activators.
PE	No difference in results of trials comparing SK with UK, or UK with t-PA, strongly suggesting that all three agents produce equivalent results.
PAO	No direct comparison of SK with other plasminogen activators. Noncomparative studies show higher reperfusion and lower bleeding rates with t-PA and UK.
MI	Entirely equivalent mortality results in two of three megatrials and marginal survival advantage for t-PA over SK in one third. Consistently higher intracranial hemorrhage rate with t-PA than with SK.

rapid resolution of the underlying thrombus. Consequently, venous valvular function is impaired permanently, and this defect leads to pooling of blood, dependent edema, and, in more severe cases, a post-phlebitic insufficiency syndrome.[223] Approximately 60% to 70% of patients with symptomatic proximal vein thrombosis who are treated with heparin followed by oral anticoagulants develop the post-thrombotic syndrome at 5 years.[224] This is not surprising, because although heparin prevents recurrent venous thromboembolism, it does not produce substantial lysis of most proximal vein thrombi. Thus, in studies comparing thrombus size on venography before and after heparin treatment in patients with symptomatic proximal vein thrombosis, complete lysis occurred in less than 10% and partial lysis in only 20% to 25% of cases; in contrast, thrombolytic therapy produces complete or substantial thrombolysis at venography in up to 70% of patients.[225-238]

Most studies comparing thrombolytic with heparin therapy include patients whose symptoms occurred within 7 days of treatment. The long time interval between onset of symptoms and initiation of treatment is an important limitation, because it is likely that prevention of permanent damage to venous valves requires prompt dissolution of the thrombus and because a fresh thrombus is more responsive to lysis. SK was used in all of the studies, except two that used t-PA.[230, 231] A statistically significant reduction of thrombus size in favor of thrombolytic therapy was demonstrated, with moderate or significant thrombolysis achieved 2.9 times more often among these patients than among patients treated with heparin (62.2% versus 21.5%; 95% confidence interval, 1.9 to 4.5 times).[239, 240]

There have not been direct comparative trials of one plasminogen activator versus another, but the results obtained using t-PA versus heparin[230, 231] suggest that rapid lysis of DVT can be attained significantly more often and to a greater degree than with heparin, roughly equivalent to the results with SK. Pilot studies of t-PA,[241, 242] urokinase,[243] and prourokinase[244] support but do not prove the general conclusion that plasminogen activators in general all are capable of effective lysis of DVT.

Prevention of the post-thrombotic syndrome by thrombolytic therapy has been investigated in only two studies that assessed the outcome measures blindly.[229, 231] Elliot et al. investigated 41 patients at a mean follow-up period of 19 months.[229] Two of 21 (10%) of the heparin-treated patients available for follow-up were asymptomatic; the remaining 19 (90%) had evidence of post-thrombotic syndrome (severe manifestations in 5 and moderate manifestations in 14). Of the 20 SK-treated patients available for follow-up, 12 (60%) had no evidence of the post-thrombotic syndrome; of the other eight (40%, $p < .0001$), two had severe and six had moderate clinical evidence of the post-thrombotic syndrome. Turpie et al. performed long-term follow-up at 2 to 3 years in 19 heparin-treated patients and 27 patients treated with t-PA.[231] Patients who complained of persistent pain

and swelling of the legs and who had evidence of reflux on Doppler ultrasonography were considered to have the post-thrombotic syndrome. Three (25%) of the 12 patients in whom more than 50% lysis was achieved had symptoms of the post-thrombotic syndrome, compared with 19 (56%) of the 34 patients in whom less than 50% or no lysis was achieved. Other studies have been generally supportive of this conclusion,[234, 237, 245-247] although opinions are not universally in agreement.[248]

Thus, there is clear evidence that both SK and t-PA are more effective than heparin in producing thrombolysis of acute DVT. However, two considerations may interfere with prevention of venous valvular damage. First, older DVT is more resistant to lysis, so the best results are obtained when treatment is begun within 7 days and especially within the first 1 or 2 days after onset of symptoms. Second, the integrity of the vein wall should be reestablished (i.e., all or almost all of the thrombus should be dissolved) if venous valvular damage is to be prevented. In the presence of an extensive clot of indeterminable age, lysis of 90% or more usually requires several days of therapy. Thrombolytic therapy is contraindicated when there is a risk of serious bleeding.

Current recommendations for treatment of DVT are to administer SK at 250,000 U IV as a loading dose followed by a sustaining infusion of 100,000 U/hr for a period of up to 3 days, depending on adequate restoration of blood flow. Urokinase has been administered as a loading dose of 2200 U/lb, followed by the same dose each hour for the duration of therapy. The dosage of t-PA is yet to be fully established.[241, 242, 249] After thrombolytic therapy, anticoagulation is used to prevent reocclusion and to allow maximal vascular reconstruction.

Acute Pulmonary Embolism (PE)

The rationale for the use of SK in patients with acute PE is to reduce acute morbidity, reperfuse the pulmonary vascular bed, and prevent late consequences such as persistent perfusion defects, reduced pulmonary capillary blood volume, and chronic pulmonary hypertension.[250, 251] Thrombolytic therapy is more effective than heparin in achieving rapid lysis of acute PE. However, the clinical benefits of thrombolytic therapy have been difficult to demonstrate unequivocally because the randomized studies reported to date lack the statistical power to demonstrate clinically important differences. The effectiveness of thrombolytic therapy has been evaluated in randomized trials comparing the effects of different thrombolytic agents with heparin on early lysis of PE and on morbidity and mortality; studies have also compared the relative efficacy and safety of the different thrombolytic agents and regimens.

Trials Comparing Thrombolytic Therapy with Heparin

Six methodologically rigorous randomized trials have compared thrombolytic therapy with heparin for the treatment of acute PE.[31, 252–257] The first and largest of the studies was the Urokinase Pulmonary Embolism Trial (UPET).[31, 253] Patients who received a 12-hour infusion of UK showed greater resolution of PE at repeat angiography 24 hours later than did the group who received heparin alone. In addition, UK produced significantly greater improvement in hemodynamics and greater resolution of the perfusion lung scan at 24 hours after therapy. However, by 5 days, the degree of resolution of perfusion scans was equivalent for the UK and heparin groups. There was no difference in mortality (6% versus 7% at 2 weeks) or short-term morbidity in the two treatment groups. Mortality was high in the subgroup of patients who presented with massive PE and shock, four of nine UK patients (44%) versus one of five heparin patients (20%) died in the 2-week observation period.

Two studies compared 72-hour infusions of SK with heparin control.[252, 254] Patients treated with SK had significantly greater improvement of angiographic abnormalities and pulmonary artery pressure than did patients who received heparin. Similar results were obtained for patients treated with t-PA versus heparin.[255–257] In addition, one such trial demonstrated improvement of right ventricular wall motion at 24 hours in 39% of patients treated with t-PA versus 17% of heparin-treated patients, with worsening in 2% and 17%, respectively.[257] Although these studies have not demonstrated any clear-cut difference in recurrence of PE, one trial[257] detected five such recurrences (two fatal and three nonfatal) with heparin therapy as opposed to none in the treated group.

Only one randomized trial assessed long-term effects of thrombolytic therapy.[258, 259] Diffusion lung capacity and lung capillary volumes were studied at 2 weeks, 1 year, and 7 years after entry into comparative studies of thrombolytic efficacy.[31, 62] A consistent finding was that thrombolytic therapy induced significantly higher diffusion lung capacity and lung capillary volumes, as well as lower pulmonary artery pressure and pulmonary vascular resistance, than did heparin, although the clinical significance of these findings is uncertain.

Trials Comparing Various Thrombolytic Regimens

Four randomized studies have compared different thrombolytic regimens for the treatment of PE.[62, 260–263] The largest study was the multicenter USPET trial of 167 patients that compared 24 hours of SK with 12 or 24 hours of UK, each treatment of which was followed by heparin. There was no difference in thrombolytic efficacy, bleeding, or mortality among the three regimens, and each produced significant improvement in pulmonary angiographic and lung scan resolution as well as in reduction of pulmonary artery pressure, compared with a historic heparin arm.[31] A similar trial (UKEP) compared two dose schedules of UK over 24 or 12 hours, finding no difference in resolution of angiographic abnormalities or reduction of pulmonary artery pressure. Similarly, no difference

has been demonstrated for administration of a thrombolytic agent (t-PA) directly into the occluded pulmonary artery, as compared with systemic intravenous administration.[261] SK has also been administered directly into the pulmonary artery in a feasibility study.[264] In addition to the equivalence of UK and SK,[62] UK has been found equivalent to t-PA as well. Initial trials compared t-PA infusion for 2 hours with 24 hours of UK,[262] with significantly greater resolution of angiographic abnormalities and pulmonary artery pressures with the shorter infusion of t-PA, although the 24-hour lung scan studies were equivalent. Comparison of t-PA and UK in which both agents were administered in large dosages for 2 hours showed totally equivalent results by angiographic improvement, perfusion scan changes, and safety.

Thus, thrombolytic therapy leads to more rapid resolution of both radiographic (pulmonary angiography and perfusion lung scan) and hemodynamic abnormalities caused by acute PE than does heparin alone.[252–255] These benefits are short-lived: by 5 to 7 days, the degree of resolution of perfusion defects in patients who received thrombolytic therapy is similar to that achieved in patients treated with heparin alone.[253, 256] Patients who present in shock might be expected to benefit most from the effects of early resolution of PE. Despite the lack of clear evidence from randomized trials that thrombolytic therapy improves clinical outcome, especially to decrease mortality, the consistent finding of more rapid resolution supports its use in critically ill, hemodynamically compromised patients with acute PE. The available plasminogen activators (SK, UK, t-PA) that have been studied have approximately equal efficacy, but further research is needed to clarify the precise role for thrombolytic therapy in the management of these patients, especially regarding subgroups that are most likely to benefit.

Peripheral Arterial Occlusion (PAO)

Fibrinolytic therapy is a viable, even preferred, alternative to surgical intervention in the initial treatment of acute PAO. Occlusions of peripheral arteries are more likely to respond dramatically to fibrinolytic therapy if treatment is instituted within hours of the onset of symptoms[265–267] and if the disease is due to embolic material rather than in situ thrombosis.[72, 268–273] Amery et al.[267] used high-dose SK by systemic administration to achieve a 77% clearing of vessels in acute occlusion of less than 12 hours, but patency was achieved in only 20% of patients with chronic in situ thrombostenotic lesions.

Regional Infusion

The regional approach to treatment appears to recanalize occluded vessels more efficiently than the systemic approach.[215, 269, 274–278] This approach has several theoretical advantages, including (1) delivery of the agent to the intended site, (2) higher local concentrations achieved with lower dosages (e.g., 5000 to 10,000

U of SK per hour), (3) ability to tailor duration of therapy to the desired therapeutic objective using serial angiography, and (4) maximal therapy using guide wires, progressive advancement of catheter, and follow-up angioplasty. Dotter et al.[279] first applied this approach and obtained gratifying reperfusion results, albeit with a significant incidence of bleeding complication. Although the issue of increased efficacy of regional versus systemic therapy has never been addressed in a randomized and controlled trial, virtually all of the recent clinical studies of thrombolytic treatment for PAO have used the regional approach, sometimes with angioplasty or bypass surgery to ensure long-term patency.[274–277, 280–284] In earlier studies, graft occlusions appeared to be less amenable to thrombolysis than were thrombosed native arteries, perhaps best exemplified in the study of Sicard et al.,[280] who showed approximately 50% the success rate with graft thrombi as with native vessel thrombi. In studies since 1985, success rates have been similar, perhaps because the graft occlusions are now treated earlier and more aggressively than heretofore.[278, 285, 286] Some investigators have suggested that UK instead of SK produces better results in terms of avoiding bleeding,[285–287] the majority of which occurs at arteriotomy sites for angiography and catheterization.

Thrombolytic Therapy Versus Surgery as Initial Therapy

Fibrinolytic therapy after unsuccessful surgical repair carries the added risk of bleeding from the surgical wound or through the graft itself.[288] However, the perioperative period is a relative but not absolute contraindication. For example, Quinones-Baldrich et al.[289] reported on 23 patients with residual distal thrombus who received intraoperative regional SK or UK, of whom 76% demonstrated angiographic and clinical improvement without major bleeding complications. Comerota et al.[290] similarly used intraoperative therapy in 38 patients with residual tibial thrombus, achieving lysis in 28 patients, clinical benefit in 18, and a major bleeding complication in only one patient.

The recent report by Ouriel et al.[291] suggests that initial treatment of PAO should use a thrombolytic approach rather than surgical repair. In this trial, 114 patients with life-threatening ischemia of less than 7 days' duration were randomly assigned to intra-arterial, catheter-directed thrombolytic therapy (with UK) or to operative intervention. Thrombolytic therapy dissolved the occluding thrombus in 40 (70%) patients, decreased the need for operative intervention by 36% over a 12-month period, and provided the opportunity to perform a subsequent limited procedure to correct a focal stenotic lesion. Although the cumulative limb salvage rate was similar in the two treatment groups (82% at 12 months), the cumulative survival rate was significantly improved in patients randomized to thrombolysis (84% versus 58% at 12 months, $p = .01$). The mortality differences seem to be primarily attributable to an increased frequency of

in-house hospital cardiopulmonary complications in the operative treatment group (49% versus 16%, $p = .001$). Thrombolytic therapy resulted in hemorrhagic complications in approximately 20% of patients, half of which were major, including a case of lethal intracranial hemorrhage. These data support the use of intraarterial thrombolytic therapy as the initial intervention in patients with PAO, followed by aggressive management of lesions unmasked by thrombolysis.

Comparison of Agents

Table 165–4 shows the relative rates of reperfusion and major bleeding complication associated with SK, UK, and t-PA, based on combined data from noncomparative clinical trials reported between 1983 and 1990. Both UK and t-PA were associated with apparently higher reperfusion rates (80% and 85% versus 64%) and a lower incidence of major bleeding complication (7% and 4% versus 26%) compared with SK. However, these results must be viewed as presumptive at best, because no study compared SK directly with UK or t-PA in a prospective and randomized manner. Further, the SK studies predominated the period prior to 1985, and t-PA was applied only since that time.[292] One comparative trial showed no difference between UK and t-PA,[293] but as yet there has been no comparison of UK or t-PA with SK.

Acute Myocardial Infarction (MI)

As noted earlier, SK decreases the short-term (5 weeks) and long-term (6 to 12 months) mortality in patients with acute MI, in comparison with placebo.[75, 183–186] Similar results accrue with APSAC and with t-PA, as shown in the AIMS[294, 295] and ASSET[296, 297] trials, respectively. However, any statement regarding relative benefit in survival and risk in bleeding, especially intracranial hemorrhage, would depend on direct comparisons of agents, given the variation in clinical results in patients of different age, delay before treatment, site of MI, and other risk factors that influence outcome.[298] Such comparisons have been made in three major trials, namely the ISG/GISSI-2,[66, 67] ISIS-3,[68] and GUSTO.[119] Each of these studies used mortality as the major clinical end point, and generally they were similar in patient characteristics, although there were specific differences in therapeutic approach. As summarized in Table 165–5, just over 100,000 patients were randomized in the three studies, two of which compared SK with t-PA and one of which (ISIS-3) included a group treated with APSAC as well. The

Table 165–4. **Outcomes Using SK, UK, or t-PA in PAO (1983–1990)[292]***

	SK (%)	UK (%)	t-PA (%)
Reperfusion	64	80	85
Bleeding	26	7	4

*None of the studies summarized in this analysis directly compared results obtained with SK versus UK or SK versus t-PA.

Table 165–5. **Thrombolytic Megatrials of Acute MI**

	ISG-GISSI-2 (66, 67)	ISIS-3 (68)	GUSTO (119)	
	(1990)	(1992)	(1993)	
Clinical presentation				
Total no. of patients	20,891	41,299	41,021	
Age				
>70 years	23%	26%		
<75 years			12%	
Delay until therapy				
Limit (hours)	6	24	6	
Median (hours)	?	4	2.8	
Infarct location				
Anterior	31%	35%	39%	
Inferior	34%	34%		
Treatment regimens				
Aspirin (mg/d)	300–325	162	160–325	
Heparin*			SK	t-PA
Initial dose at	12 hours	4 hours	12 hours	Immediate
Route	SQ	SQ	SQ	IV
Dosage (b.i.d.)	12,500	12,500	12,500	5000 bolus, 1000/hr
t-PA				
Type	Alteplase	Duteplase	Alteplase	
Dosage	100 mg/3 hours	100 mg/4 hours	100 mg/1.5 hours	
Overall results (all patients)				
Mortality				
In-hospital	8.8%	7.7%		
5 weeks	9.4%	10.4%	7.0%	
Strokes (all)	1.1%	1.2%	1.45%	

*One half of the patients in ISG/GISSI-2 and in ISIS-3 received SQ heparin. The groups illustrated in GUSTO represent two of the four treatments, the others being SK with immediate IV heparin and combined t-PA and SK treatment with IV heparin.

GUSTO trial had four treatment groups, only two of which are included here for comparison, namely, those using SK with subcutaneous heparin as described in ISIS-3 and an "accelerated" regimen of t-PA over 90 minutes[299, 300] instead of the previously utilized 3 to 4 hours. The t-PA–treated patients in GUSTO also received immediate intravenous heparin instead of delayed subcutaneous heparin as used in the ISIS-3 and ISG/GISSI-2 studies. The latter trials further randomized patients to receive subcutaneous heparin or no heparin, but because the results were essentially the same for SK, t-PA, and APSAC with and without the subcutaneous heparin, these subgroups are considered together in this analysis. The clinical presentations in the three trials were quite similar with regard to location of infarct (anterior versus inferior) and age of the patient population, but patients were treated on average sooner in GUSTO

Table 165–6. **Comparison of SK, t-PA, and APSAC in Megatrials of Acute MI**

	SK (%)	t-PA (%)	APSAC (%)
ISG/GISSI-2 (66, 67)			
Mortality (in-hospital)	8.5	8.9	
Intracranial hemorrhage	0.5	0.8	
ISIS-3 (68)			
Mortality (35 days)	10.6	10.3	10.5
Intracranial hemorrhage	0.24	0.66	0.55
GUSTO (119)			
Mortality (30 days)	7.2	6.3	
Intracranial hemorrhage	0.49	0.72	

than in ISIS-3. The overall 5-week mortality was approximately the same in the ISG/GISSI-2 and ISIS-3 trials (9.4% versus 10.4%) but apparently much lower in GUSTO (7%), perhaps reflecting the shorter delay until treatment and other more favorable prognostic patient attributes. The overall stroke rates were similar, between 1.1% and 1.45%.

The direct comparisons of SK and t-PA in ISG/GISSI-2 and in ISIS-3 show entirely equivalent results in 35-day mortality, 8.5% versus 8.9% and 10.0% versus 10.3%, the latter also being equivalent to the result with APSAC (10.5%) (Table 165–6). The incidence of intracranial hemorrhage was consistently higher with t-PA than with SK, 0.8% versus 0.5% in ISG/GISSI-2 and 0.66% versus 0.24% in ISIS-3. In the GUSTO study, the 30-day mortality was slightly lower with t-PA than with SK (6.3% versus 7.2%), a difference that did reach statistical significance. On the other hand, the rate of intracranial hemorrhage was again higher with t-PA than with SK (0.72% versus 0.49%). In a third arm of the GUSTO study, patients receiving SK with immediate intravenous heparin had a slightly (but not statistically significant) higher overall mortality as well as a higher rate of intracranial hemorrhage, clearly indicating that the use of intravenous heparin rather than delayed subcutaneous heparin with streptokinase presented a greater risk to the patient. Streptokinase-treated patients tended to have a higher incidence of cardiovascular problems, including hypotension and arrhythmias, but t-PA–treated patients in the GUSTO study were subjected to coronary artery bypass graft procedures more often (8/1000 treated).

The benefit:risk ratio for using the t-PA regimen versus the SK regimen translates to 10 fewer nonstroke deaths using t-PA but four extra lethal or permanent deficit strokes with t-PA in comparison with SK. The small difference in the number of patients alive and without neurologic deficit at 5 weeks (924/1000 for t-PA versus 930/1000 for SK, $p = .09$) suggests that the data do not present a clear-cut choice of one agent over the other.

REFERENCES

1. Tillett WS, Garner RL: The fibrinolytic activity of hemolytic streptococci. J Exp Med 58:485, 1933.
2. Tillett WS, Sherry S: The effect in patients of streptococcal fibrinolysin (streptokinase) and streptococcal desoxyribonuclease on fibrinous, purulent and sanguineous pleural exudations. J Clin Invest 28:173, 1949.
3. Johnson AJ, Tillett WS: Lysis in rabbits of intravascular blood clots by the streptococcal fibrinolytic system (streptokinase). J Exp Med 95:449, 1952.
4. Fletcher AP, Alkjaersig N, Sherry S: The maintenance of a sustained thrombolytic state in man. I. Induction and effects. J Clin Invest 38:1096, 1959.
5. Fletcher AP, Sherry S, Alkjaersig N, et al: The maintenance of a sustained thrombolytic state in man. II. Clinical observations on patients with myocardial infarction and other thromboembolic disorders. J Clin Invest 38:1111, 1959.
6. Castellino FJ, Sodetz JM, Brockway NJ, et al: Streptokinase. Methods Enzymol 45:244, 1976.
7. Jackson KW, Tang J: Complete amino acid sequence of streptokinase and its homology with serine proteases. Biochemistry 21:6220, 1982.
8. Tang J, Jackson KW: The streptokinase-plasminogen interaction: A model for binding activation of serine-protease zymogens. In Bradshaw RA, Hill RL, Tang J, et al (eds): Proteins in Biology and Medicine. New York: Academic Press, 1982, pp 363–377.
9. Mentzer RL, Budzynski AZ, Sherry S: High-dose, brief-duration intravenous infusion of streptokinase in acute myocardial infarction: Description of effects in the circulation. Am J Cardiol 57:1220, 1986.
10. Alkjaersig N, Fletcher AP, Sherry S: The mechanism of clot dissolution by plasmin. J Clin Invest 38:1086, 1959.
11. Marder VJ, Shulman NR, Carroll WR: High molecular weight derivatives of human fibrinogen produced by plasmin. I. Physicochemical and immunological characterization. J Biol Chem 244:2111, 1969.
12. Schulman S, Lockner D, Granqvist D, et al: A comparative randomized trial of low dose versus high dose streptokinase in deep vein thrombosis of the thigh. Thromb Haemost 51:261, 1984.
13. Timmis GC, Mannem EF, Ramos RG, et al: Hemorrhage vs rethrombosis after thrombolysis for acute myocardial infarction. Arch Intern Med 146:667, 1986.
14. Hirsh J: The use of anticoagulation in patients treated with streptokinase. In Martin M, Schoop W, Hirsh J (eds): New Concepts in Streptokinase Dosimetry. Bern: Hans Huber, 1978, pp 135–140.
15. Merrill EW: Rheology of blood. Physiol Rev 49:863, 1969.
16. Verstraete M, Van de Loo J, Jesdinsky HJ: Streptokinase in acute myocardial infarction. Acta Med Scand Suppl 648:5, 1981.
17. Jan K-M, Reinhart W, Chien S, et al: Altered rheological properties of blood following administration of tissue plasminogen activator and streptokinase in patients with acute myocardial infarction [abstract]. Circulation 72(Suppl II):II-47, 1985.
18. Arntz R, Hertz J, Schafer H, et al: Hemorrheology in acute myocardial infarction: Effects of high dose intravenous streptokinase [abstract]. Circulation 72(Suppl II):II-417, 1985.
19. Jan K-M, Chien S, Bigger JT Jr: Observations on blood viscosity changes after acute myocardial infarction. Circulation 51:1079, 1975.
20. Fletcher AP, Alkjaersig N, Sherry S: Pathogenesis of the coagulation defect developing during pathological plasma proteolytic ("fibrinolytic") states. I. The significance of fibrinogen proteolysis and circulating fibrinogen breakdown products. J Clin Invest 41:896, 1962.
21. Sherry S, Fletcher AP, Alkjaersig N: Fibrinolysis and fibrinolytic activity in man. Physiol Rev 39:343, 1959.
22. Sherry S, Lindemeyer RI, Fletcher AP, et al: Studies on enhanced fibrinolytic activity in man. J Clin Invest 38:810, 1959.
23. Astrup T, Mullertz S: The fibrin plate method for estimating fibrinolytic activity. Arch Biochem 40:346, 1952.
24. Sawyer WE, Fletcher AP, Alkjaersig N, et al: Studies on the thrombolytic activity of human plasma. J Clin Invest 39:426, 1960.
25. Moroz L, Gilmore NJ: A rapid and sensitive 125 I-fibrin solid phase fibrinolytic assay for plasmin. Blood 46:543, 1975.
26. Rylatt DB, Black AS, Cottis LE, et al: An immunoassay for human D dimer using monoclonal antibodies. Thromb Res 31:767, 1983.
27. Jaffe AS, Eisenberg PR, Wilner GD: In vivo assessment of thrombosis and fibrinolysis during acute myocardial infarction. Prog Hematol 15:71, 1987.
28. Owen J, Friedman KD, Grossman BA, et al: Quantitation of fragment X formation during thrombolytic therapy with streptokinase and tissue plasminogen activator. J Clin Invest 79:1642, 1987.
29. Brenner B, Francis CW, Totterman S, et al: Quantitation of venous clot lysis with the D-dimer immunoassay during fibrinolytic therapy requires correction for soluble fibrin degradation. Circulation 81:1818, 1990.
30. Francis CW, Marder VJ: Physiologic regulation and pathologic disorders of fibrinolysis. In Colman RW, Marder VJ, Salzman EW, Hirsh J (eds): Hemostasis and Thrombosis: Basic Principles and Clinical Practice, 3rd ed. Philadelphia: JB Lippincott, 1994, pp 1076–1103.
31. The Urokinase Pulmonary Embolism Trial: A national cooperative study. Circulation 47(Suppl II):II-1, 1973.
32. Rothbard RL, Fitzpatrick PG, Francis CW, et al: Relationship of lytic state to successful reperfusion with standard and low dose intracoronary streptokinase. Circulation 71:562, 1985.
33. Marder VJ: Relevance of changes in blood fibrinolytic and coagulation parameters during thrombolytic therapy. Am J Med 83(2A):15, 1987.
34. Rao AK, Pratt C, Berke A, et al: Thrombolysis in Myocardial Infarction (TIMI) Trial. Phase 1: Hemorrhagic manifestations and changes in plasma fibrinogen and the fibrinolytic system in patients treated with recombinant tissue plasminogen activator and streptokinase. J Am Coll Cardiol 11:1, 1988.
35. Hirsch DR, Goldhaber SZ: Laboratory parameters to monitor safety and efficacy during thrombolytic therapy. Chest 99:113S, 1991.
36. Brenner B, Francis CW, Fitzpatrick PG, et al: Relation of plasma D-dimer concentrations to coronary artery reperfusion before and after thrombolytic treatment in patients with acute myocardial infarction. Am J Cardiol 63:1179, 1989.
37. Francis CW, Markham RE Jr, Marder VJ: Demonstration of in situ fibrin degradation in pathologic thrombi. Blood 63:1216, 1984.
38. Chesebro JH, Knatterud G, Roberts R, et al: Thrombolysis in Myocardial Infarction (TIMI) Trial, Phase I: A comparison between intravenous tissue plasminogen activator and intravenous streptokinase: Clinical findings through hospital discharge. Circulation 76:142, 1987.
39. Théry C, Bauchart JJ, Lesenne M, et al: Predictive factors of effectiveness of streptokinase in deep venous thrombosis. Am J Cardiol 69:117, 1992.
40. Meyerovitz MF, Polak JF, Goldhaber SZ: Short-term response to thrombolytic therapy in deep venous thrombosis: Predictive value of venographic appearance. Radiology 184:345, 1992.
41. Hess H: Zur Streptokinase Therapie akuter Verschlusse von Gliedmassengefassen. In Hiemeyer V (ed): Therapeutische und Experimentelle Fibrinolyse. Stuttgart: F.K. Schattauer Verlag, 1969, pp 275–277.

42. Schroder R, Biamino G, Enz-Dudiger L, et al: Intravenous short-term infusion of streptokinase in acute myocardial infarction. Circulation 63:536, 1983.

43. Sherry S: Recombinant tissue plasminogen activator (rt-PA): Is it the thrombolytic agent of choice for an evolving acute myocardial infarction? Am J Cardiol 59:984, 1987.

44. Anderson JL, Rothbard RL, Hackworthy RA, et al: Randomized reperfusion comparison of intravenous thrombolytic therapy with anisoylated plasminogen streptokinase activator complex (APSAC) and intracoronary therapy with streptokinase in acute myocardial infarction. J Am Coll Cardiol 11:1153, 1988.

45. Gormsen J, Fletcher AP, Alkjaersig N, et al: The enzymatic lysis of plasma clots: The influence of fibrin stabilization on lysis rates. Arch Biochem Biophys 120:654, 1967.

46. Francis CW, Marder VJ: Increased resistance to plasmic degradation of fibrin with highly cross-linked α-polymer chains formed at high factor XIII concentrations. Blood 71:1361, 1988.

47. Reed GL, Matsueda GR, Haber E: Platelet factor XIII increases the fibrinolytic resistance of platelet-rich clots by accelerating the cross linking of alpha 1-antiplasmin to fibrin. Thromb Haemost 68:315, 1992.

48. Marbet G, Eichlisberger H, Duckert F, et al: Side effects of thrombolytic therapy with porcine plasmin and low dose streptokinase. Thromb Haemost 48:196, 1982.

49. Thayer CF: Results of postmarketing surveillance program on streptokinase. Curr Ther Res 30:129, 1981.

50. Totty WG, Romano T, Benian GM, et al: Serum sickness following streptokinase therapy. AJR 138:143, 1982.

51. Manoharan A, Ramsay D, Davis S, et al: Hypersensitivity vasculitis associated with streptokinase. Aust N Z J Med 16:815, 1986.

52. Pick RA, Joswig BC, Cheung AK, et al: Acute renal failure following repeated streptokinase therapy for pulmonary embolism. West J Med 138:878, 1983.

53. Lew AS, Laramee P, Cercek B, et al: The hypotensive effect of intravenous streptokinase in patients with acute myocardial infarction. Circulation 72:1321, 1985.

54. Sherry S: What are the reasons for bleeding in thrombolysis? In Kakkar VV, Kennedy JW, Mettinger KL (eds): Coronary Thrombolysis: Current Answers to Critical Questions. London: Current Medical Literature, 1988, pp 127–131.

55. Marder VJ, Sherry S: Thrombolytic therapy: Current status. N Engl J Med 318:1512, 1988.

56. Marder VJ: The use of thrombolytic agents: Choice of patient, drug administration, laboratory monitoring. Ann Intern Med 90:802, 1979.

57. Vaughan DE, Loscalzo J: Disaggregation of platelets: A comparison of tissue plasminogen activator, streptokinase and urokinase [abstract]. Circulation 74(Suppl II):II-95, 1986.

58. Silverstein RL, Leung LL, Harpel PC, Nachman RL: Platelet thrombospondin forms a trimolecular complex with plasminogen and histidine rich glycoprotein. J Clin Invest 75:2065, 1985.

59. Ganz W, Geft I, Shah PK, et al: Intravenous streptokinase in evolving acute myocardial infarction. Am J Cardiol 53:1209, 1984.

60. Sherry S: Intravenous streptokinase in acute myocardial infarction [letter]. N Engl J Med 315:1356, 1986.

61. Hillis D, Borer J, Braunwald E, et al: High-dose intravenous streptokinase for acute myocardial infarction: Preliminary results of a multicenter trial. J Am Coll Cardiol 6:957, 1985.

62. Urokinase-Streptokinase Embolism Trial: Phase 2 results: A cooperative study. JAMA 229:1606, 1974.

63. The TIMI Study Group: The Thrombolysis in Myocardial Infarction (TIMI) Trial. Phase I findings. N Engl J Med 312:932, 1985.

64. European Cooperative Study Group for Recombinant Tissue-Type Plasminogen Activator: Randomized trial of intravenous recombinant tissue-type plasminogen activator versus intravenous streptokinase in acute myocardial infarction. Lancet 1:842, 1985.

65. Sherry S, Bell WR, Duckert FH, et al: Thrombolytic therapy in thrombosis: A National Institutes of Health Consensus Development Conference. Ann Intern Med 93:141, 1980.

66. Gruppo Italiano per lo Studio della Sopravvivenza nell'Infarto

Miocardico (GISSI): GISSI-2: A factorial randomized trial of alteplase versus streptokinase and heparin versus no heparin among 12,490 patients with acute myocardial infarction. Lancet 336:65, 1990.

67. The International Study Group: In-hospital mortality and clinical course of 20,891 patients with suspected acute myocardial infarction randomized between alteplase and streptokinase with or without heparin. Lancet 336:71, 1990.

68. ISIS-3 (Third International Study of Infarct Survival) Collaborative Group: ISIS-3: A randomized comparison of streptokinase vs tissue plasminogen activator vs anistreplase and of aspirin plus heparin vs aspirin alone among 41,299 cases of suspected acute myocardial infarction. Lancet 339:753, 1992.

69. Ridker PM, Hebert PR, Fuster V, et al: Are both aspirin and heparin justified as adjuncts to thrombolytic therapy for acute myocardial infarction? Lancet 341:1574, 1993.

70. The Global Use of Strategies to Open Occluded Coronary Arteries (GUSTO) IIa Investigators: Randomized trial of intravenous heparin versus recombinant hirudin for acute coronary syndromes. Circulation 90:1631, 1994.

71. Antman EM for the TIMI 9A Investigators: Hirudin in acute myocardial infarction. Safety report from the Thrombolysis and Thrombin Inhibition in Myocardial Infarction (TIMI) 9A Trial. Circulation 90:1624, 1994.

72. Marder VJ, Bell WR: Fibrinolytic therapy. In Colman RW, Hirsh J, Marder VJ, et al (eds): Hemostasis and Thrombosis: Basic Principles in Clinical Practice. Philadelphia: JB Lippincott, 1987, pp 1393–1437.

73. Goldhaber SZ, Burning JE, Lipnick RJ, et al: Pooled analyses of randomized trials of streptokinase and heparin in phlebographically documented acute deep venous thrombosis. Am J Med 76:393, 1984.

74. Spann JF, Sherry S: Coronary thrombolysis for evolving myocardial infarction. Drugs 28:465, 1984.

75. Gruppo Italiano per lo Studio della Streptochinasi nell'Infarto Miocardica (GISSI): Effectiveness of intravenous thrombolytic treatment in acute myocardial infarction. Lancet 1:397, 1986.

76. Collins R, Conway M, Alexopoulos D, et al: Randomized factorial trial of high-dose intravenous streptokinase, of oral aspirin and of intravenous heparin in acute myocardial infarction. Eur Heart J 8:634, 1987.

77. Kennedy JW, Martin GV, Davis KB, et al: The Western Washington Intravenous Streptokinase in Acute Myocardial Infarction Randomized Trial. Circulation 77:345, 1988.

78. White HD, Norris RM, Brown MA, et al: Effect of intravenous streptokinase on left ventricular function and early survival after acute myocardial infarction. N Engl J Med 317:850, 1987.

79. The I.S.A.M. Study Group: A prospective trial of intravenous streptokinase in acute myocardial infarction (I.S.A.M.). Mortality, morbidity and infarct size at 21 days. N Engl J Med 314:1465, 1985.

80. Schreiber TL, Miller DH, Silvasi DA, et al: Randomized double-blind trial of intravenous streptokinase for acute myocardial infarction. Am J Cardiol 58:47, 1986.

81. Bell WR, Meek AG: Guidelines for the use of thrombolytic agents. N Engl J Med 306:1268, 1982.

82. Sharma GVBRK, Cella G, Parise AF, Sasahara AA: Thrombolytic therapy. N Engl J Med 306:1268, 1982.

83. Constantinides P: Plaque fissures in human coronary thrombosis. J Atheroscler Res 6:1, 1966.

84. Gash A, Spann JF, Sherry S, et al: Factors influencing reocclusion after coronary thrombolysis for acute myocardial infarction. Am J Cardiol 57:175, 1986.

85. Brown BG, Gallery CA, Badger RS, et al: Incomplete lysis of thrombus in the moderate underlying atherosclerotic lesion during intracoronary infusion of streptokinase for acute myocardial infarction: Quantitative angiographic observations. Circulation 73:653, 1986.

86. Francis CW, Markham RE Jr, Barlow GH, et al: Thrombin activity of fibrin thrombi and soluble plasmic derivatives. J Lab Clin Med 102:220, 1983.

87. Harrison DG, Ferguson DW, Collins SM, et al: Rethrombosis after reperfusion with streptokinase: Importance of geometry of residual lesions. Circulation 69:991, 1984.

88. Gold HK, Leinbach RC, Garabedian HD, et al: Acute coronary

reocclusion after thrombolysis with recombinant human tissue-type plasminogen activator: Prevention by a maintenance infusion. Circulation 73:347, 1986.

89. Cannon CP, McCabe CH, Henry TR, et al: A pilot trial of recombinant desulfatohirudin compared with heparin in conjunction with tissue-type plasminogen activator and aspirin for acute myocardial infarction: Results of the Thrombosis in Myocardial Infarction (TIMI) 5 trial. J Am Coll Cardiol 23:993, 1994.

90. Lidon RM, Theroux P, Juneau M, et al: Initial experience with a direct antithrombin, Hirulog, in unstable angina: Anticoagulant, antithrombotic and clinical effects. Circulation 88:1495, 1993.

91. Topol RJ, Califf RM, Weisman HF, et al, on behalf of the EPIC Investigators: Randomized trial of coronary intervention with antibody against platelet IIb/IIIa integrin for reduction of clinical restenosis: Results at 6 months. Lancet 343:881, 1994.

92. Rentrop KP, Feit F, Lanke H, et al: Effects of intracoronary streptokinase and intracoronary nitroglycerin infusion on coronary angiographic patterns and mortality in patients with acute myocardial infarction. N Engl J Med 311:1457, 1984.

93. Hackett D, Davies G, Chiercha S, et al: Intermittent coronary occlusion in acute myocardial infarction: Value of combined thrombolytic and vasodilator therapy. N Engl J Med 317:1055, 1987.

94. Sharma B, Wyeth RP, Lane GE, et al: Combined intracoronary prostaglandin E1 and streptokinase in acute myocardial infarction [abstract]. J Am Coll Cardiol 7(Suppl A):208A, 1986.

95. Serruys PW, Wigns W, van den Brand M, et al: Is transluminal coronary angioplasty mandatory after successful thrombolysis? Quantitative coronary angiographic study. Br Heart J 50:257, 1983.

96. Topol EJ, Califf RM, George BS, et al: A randomized trial of immediate versus delayed elective angioplasty after intravenous tissue plasminogen activator in acute myocardial infarction. N Engl J Med 317:581, 1987.

97. Erbel R, Tiberius P, Karl-Jurgen H, et al: Percutaneous transluminal coronary angioplasty after thrombolytic therapy: A prospective controlled randomized trial. J Am Coll Cardiol 8:485, 1986.

98. The TIMI Research Group: Intermediate vs delayed catheterization and angioplasty following thrombolytic therapy for acute myocardial infarction. JAMA 260:2849, 1988.

99. The TIMI Study Group: Comparison of invasive and conservative strategies after treatment with intravenous tissue plasminogen activator in acute myocardial infarction: Results of the Thrombolysis in Myocardial Infarction (TIMI) phase II trial. N Engl J Med 320:618, 1989.

100. Simoons ML, Arnold AE, Betriu A, et al: Thrombolysis with tissue plasminogen activator in acute myocardial infarction: No additional benefit from immediate PTCA. Lancet 1:197, 1988.

101. Arnold AE, Simoons ML, Van de Werf F, et al: Recombinant tissue-type plasminogen activator and immediate angioplasty in acute myocardial infarction: One year follow-up. Circulation 86:111, 1992.

102. Sutton JM, Taylor GJ, Mikell FL, et al: Thrombolytic therapy followed by early revascularization for acute myocardial infarction. Am J Cardiol 57:1227, 1986.

103. Anderson JL, Battistessa SA, Clayton PD, et al: Coronary bypass surgery early after thrombolytic therapy for acute myocardial infarction. Ann Thorac Surg 41:176, 1986.

104. Wellons HA Jr, Schneider JA, Mikell FL, et al: Early operative intervention after thrombolytic therapy for acute myocardial infarction. J Vasc Surg 2:186, 1985.

105. Mathey DG, Rodewald G, Rentrop P, et al: Intracoronary streptokinase thrombolytic recanalization and subsequent surgical bypass of remaining atherosclerotic stenosis in acute myocardial infarction: Complimentary combined approach affecting reduced infarct size, preventing reinfarction and improving left ventricular function. Am Heart J 102:1194, 1981.

106. Kereiakes DJ, Califf RM, George BS, et al: Coronary bypass surgery improves global and regional left ventricular function following thrombolytic therapy for acute myocardial infarction. Am Heart J 122:390, 1991.

107. Moosvi AR, Khaja F, Villanueva L, et al: Early revascularization improves survival in cardiogenic shock complicating acute myocardial infarction. J Am Coll Cardiol 19:907, 1992.

108. Grines CL, Browne KF, Marco J, et al: A comparison of immediate angioplasty with thrombolytic therapy for acute myocardial infarction. N Engl J Med 328:673, 1993.

109. Zilstra F, de Boer MJ, Hoorntje JC, et al: A comparison of immediate coronary angioplasty with intravenous streptokinase in acute myocardial infarction. N Engl J Med 328:680, 1993.

110. Gibbons RJ, Holmes DR, Reeder GS, et al: Immediate angioplasty compared with the administration of a thrombolytic agent followed by conservative treatment for myocardial infarction. N Engl J Med 328:685, 1993.

111. de Boer MJ, Hoorntje JC, Ottervanger JP, et al: Immediate angioplasty versus intravenous streptokinase in acute myocardial infarction: Left ventricular ejection fraction, hospital mortality and reinfarction. J Am Coll Cardiol 23:1004, 1994.

112. Sherry S: Following coronary thrombolysis. In Wessler S, Becker CG, Nemerson Y (eds): The New Dimensions of Warfarin Prophylaxis. New York: Plenum Publishing, 1987, pp 255–263.

113. Popma JJ, Topol EJ: Adjuncts to thrombolysis for myocardial reperfusion. Ann Intern Med 115:34, 1991.

114. Coller BS: Platelets and thrombolytic therapy. N Engl J Med 322:33, 1990.

115. Willerson JT, Golino P, McNatt J, et al: Role of new antiplatelet agents as adjunctive therapies in thrombolysis. Am J Cardiol 67:12A, 1991.

116. Lefkovits J, Topol EJ: Direct thrombin inhibitors in cardiovascular medicine. Circulation 90:1522, 1994.

117. Bang NU: Leeches, snakes, ticks, and vampire bats and today's cardiovascular drug development. Circulation 84:436, 1991.

118. Marder VJ, Hirsh J, Bell WR: Rationale and practical basis of thrombolytic therapy. In Colman RW, Marder VJ, Salzman EW, Hirsh J (eds): Hemostasis and Thrombosis: Basic Principles and Clinical Practice, 3rd ed. Philadelphia: JB Lippincott, 1994, pp 1514–1542.

119. The GUSTO Investigators: An international randomized trial comparing four thrombolytic strategies for acute myocardial infarction. N Engl J Med 329:673, 1993.

120. Marder VJ: Comparison of thrombolytic agents: Selected hematologic, vascular and clinical events. Am J Cardiol 64:2A, 1989.

121. Rubin R, Sherry S: Drug interactions involving fibrinolytic therapy. In Petrie JC (ed): Gastrointestinal, Hematological and Infectious Disease Therapy. Amsterdam: Elsevier, 1985, pp 67–84.

122. Skinner JR, Phillips SJ, Zeff RH, et al: Immediate coronary bypass following failed streptokinase infusion in evolving myocardial infarction. J Thorac Cardiovasc Surg 87:567, 1984.

123. Kay P, Ahmad A, Floten S, et al: Emergency coronary artery bypass surgery after intracoronary thrombolysis for evolving myocardial infarction. Br Heart J 53:260, 1985.

124. Mantia AM, Lolley DM, Stullken EH Jr, et al: Coronary artery bypass grafting within 24 hours after intracoronary streptokinase thrombolysis. J Cardiothorac Anesth 1:392, 1987.

125. Verstraete M, Tygat G, Amery A, et al: Thrombolytic therapy with streptokinase using a standard dosage. Thromb Diath Haemorrh 21(Suppl):493, 1966.

126. Spann JF, Sherry S, Rubin RN: Techniques of achieving pulmonary, peripheral and coronary thrombolysis. In Hurst JW, Logue RB, Rackley CE, et al (eds): The Heart. New York: McGraw-Hill, 1985, pp 1916–1922.

127. International Society and Federation of Cardiology and World Health Organization Task Force on Myocardial Reperfusion: Reperfusion in acute myocardial infarction. Circulation 90:2091, 1994.

128. Fibrinolytic Therapy Trialists' (FTT) Collaborative Group: Indications for fibrinolytic therapy in suspected acute myocardial infarction: Collaborative overview of early mortality and major morbidity results from all randomized trials of more than 1000 patients. Lancet 343:311, 1994.

129. Fletcher AP, Alkjaersig N, Smyniotis FE, et al: The treatment of patients suffering from early myocardial infarction with

massive and prolonged streptokinase therapy. Trans Assoc Am Physicians 71:287, 1958.

130. Yusuf S, Collins R, Peto R, et al: Intravenous and intracoronary fibrinolytic therapy in acute myocardial infarction: Overview of results on mortality, reinfarction and side-effects from 33 randomized controlled trials. Eur Heart J 6:556, 1985.

131. Dewar HA, Stephenson P, Horler AR, et al: Fibrinolytic therapy of coronary thrombosis: Controlled trial of 75 cases. Br Med J 1:915, 1963.

132. Amery A, Roeber G, Bermeulen HJ, et al: Single-blind randomized multicentre trial comparing heparin and streptokinase treatment in recent myocardial infarction. Acta Med Scand Suppl 505:5, 1969.

133. Heikenheimo R, Ahrenberg P, Honkapohja H, et al: Fibrinolytic treatment in acute myocardial infarction. Acta Med Scand 189:7, 1971.

134. Dioguardi N, Mannucci PM, Lotto A, et al: Controlled trial of streptokinase and heparin in acute myocardial infarction. Lancet 2:891, 1971.

135. Bett JHN, Biggs JC, Castaldi PA, et al: Australian multicentre trial of streptokinase in acute myocardial infarction. Lancet 1:57, 1973.

136. Aber CP, Bass NM, Berry CL, et al: Streptokinase in acute myocardial infarction: A controlled multicentre study in the United Kingdom. Br Med J 2:1100, 1976.

137. European Co-operative Study Group for Streptokinase Treatment in Acute Myocardial Infarction: Streptokinase in acute myocardial infarction. N Engl J Med 301:797, 1979.

138. Breddin K, Ehrly AM, Fechler L, et al: Die Kurzzeitfibrinolyse beim akuten Myokardinfarkt. Dtsch Med Wochenschr 98:861, 1973.

139. Stampfer MJ, Goldhaber SZ, Yusuf S, et al: Effect of intravenous streptokinase on acute myocardial infarction: Pooled results from randomized trials. N Engl J Med 307:1180, 1982.

140. L'Abbe KA, Detsky AS, O'Rourke K: Meta-analysis in clinical research. Ann Intern Med 107:224, 1987.

141. Sherry S, Gustafson E: The current and future use of thrombolytic therapy. Ann Rev Pharmacol Toxicol 25:413, 1985.

142. Braunwald E: Treatment of the patient after myocardial infarction. The last decade and the next. N Engl J Med 302:290, 1980.

143. Boucek RJ, Murphy WP Jr: Segmental perfusion of the coronary arteries with fibrinolysin in man following a myocardial infarction. Am J Cardiol 6:525, 1960.

144. Chazov EL, Mateeva LS, Mazaeo AV, et al: Intracoronary administration of fibrinolysin in acute myocardial infarction. Ter Arkh 48:8, 1976.

145. DeWood MA, Spores J, Natske R, et al: Prevalence of total coronary occlusion during the early hours of transmural myocardial infarction. N Engl J Med 303:897, 1980.

146. Rentrop P, Blanke H, Karsch FR, et al: Acute myocardial infarction: Intracoronary application of nitroglycerin and streptokinase. Clin Cardiol 2:354, 1979.

147. Mason DT (ed): Symposium on Intracoronary Thrombolysis in Acute Myocardial Infarction. Am Heart J 102:1123, 1981.

148. Gold HK, Cowley MJ, Palacios IF, et al: Combined intracoronary streptokinase infusion and coronary angioplasty during acute myocardial infarction. Am J Cardiol 53:122C, 1984.

149. Markis JE, Malagold M, Parker A, et al: Myocardial salvage after intracoronary thrombolysis with streptokinase in acute myocardial infarction. N Engl J Med 305:777, 1981.

150. Reimer KA, Jennings RB: The wavefront phenomenon of myocardial ischemic death: Transmural progression of necroses within the framework of ischemic bed size (myocardium at risk) and collateral flow. Lab Invest 40:633, 1979.

151. Bergman SR, Lercha RA, Fox FAA, et al: Temporal dependence of beneficial effects of coronary thrombolysis characterized by position tomography. Am J Med 73:573, 1982.

152. Kennedy JW, Gensini GG, Timmis GC, et al: Acute myocardial infarction treated with intracoronary streptokinase: A report of the Society for Cardiac Angiography. Am J Cardiol 55:871, 1985.

153. Weinstein J: Treatment of myocardial infarction with intracoronary streptokinase: Efficiency and safety data from 209 United States cases in the Hoechst-Roussel registry. Am Heart J 104:894, 1982.

154. Kennedy JW, Ritchie JL, Davis JB, et al: Western Washington randomized trial of intracoronary streptokinase in acute myocardial infarction. N Engl J Med 309:1477, 1983.

155. Simoons ML, Serruys PW, Van den Brand M, et al: Early thrombolysis in acute myocardial infarction: Limitations of infarct size and improved survival. J Am Coll Cardiol 7:717, 1986.

156. Kennedy JW, Ritchie JL, Davis JB, et al: The Western Washington randomized trial of intracoronary streptokinase in acute myocardial infarction: A 12-month follow-up report. N Engl J Med 312:1073, 1985.

157. Six AJ, Louwerenburg HW, Braams R, et al: A double-blind randomized multicenter dose-ranging trial of intravenous streptokinase in acute myocardial infarction. Am J Cardiol 65:119, 1990.

158. Col JJ, Col-De Beys CM, Renkin JP, et al: Pharmacokinetics, thrombolytic efficacy and hemorrhagic risk of different streptokinase regimens in heparin-treated acute myocardial infarction. Am J Cardiol 63:1185, 1989.

159. Grines CL, Nissen SE, Booth DC, et al: A prospective, randomized trial comparing combination half-dose tissue-type plasminogen activator and streptokinase with full-dose tissue-type plasminogen activator. Circulation 84:540, 1991.

160. Malke H, Ferretti JJ: Streptokinase: Cloning, expression, and excretion by Escherichia coli. Proc Natl Acad Sci USA 81:3557, 1984.

161. Malke H, Lorenz D, Ferretti JJ: Streptokinase: Expression of altered forms. In Ferretti JJ, Curtiss R III (eds): Streptococcal Genetics. Washington, DC: American Society for Microbiology, pp 143–149.

162. Reed GL, Kussie P, Parhami-Seren B: A functional analysis of the antigenicity of streptokinase using monoclonal antibody mapping and recombinant streptokinase fragments. J Immunol 150:4407, 1993.

163. Marder VJ: Recombinant streptokinase: Opportunity for an improved agent [letter to the editor]. Blood Coagul Fibrinolysis 4:1039, 1993.

164. Sherry S: Appraisal of various thrombolytic agents in the treatment of acute myocardial infarction. In Sherry S, Solomon HA (eds): Thrombolytic Therapy in Cardiovascular Diseases: Current Practices and Future Directions. Am J Med 83(Suppl 2A):31, 1987.

165. Marder VJ, Francis CW: Thrombolytic therapy for acute transmural myocardial infarction. Intracoronary versus intravenous. Am J Med 77:921, 1984.

166. Sheehan FH, Braunwald E, Canner P, et al: The effect of intravenous thrombolytic therapy on left ventricular function: A report on tissue-type plasminogen activator and streptokinase from the Thrombolysis in Myocardial Infarction (TIMI Phase I) Trial. Circulation 75:817, 1987.

167. Sherry S, Marder VJ: Streptokinase and recombinant tissue plasminogen activator (rt-PA) are equally effective in treating acute myocardial infarction. Ann Intern Med 114:417, 1991.

168. Blumgart HL, Gilligan R, Schlesinger MJ: Experimental studies on the effect of temporary occlusion of coronary arteries. II. The production of myocardial infarction. Am Heart J 22:374, 1941.

169. Lidón R-M, Théroux P, Lespérance J, et al: A pilot, early angiographic patency study using a direct thrombin inhibitor as adjunctive therapy to streptokinase in acute myocardial infarction. Circulation 89:1567, 1994.

170. Norris RM, White HD: Therapeutic trials in coronary thrombosis should measure left ventricular function as an endpoint of treatment. Lancet 1:104, 1988.

171. Califf RM, Harrelson WL, Topol EJ: Left ventricular ejection fraction may not be useful as an end point of thrombolytic therapy in comparative trials. Circulation 82:1847, 1990.

172. Bassand JP, Faivre R, Becque O, et al: Intravenous streptokinase versus heparin in recent acute myocardial infarction. Haemostasis 16(Suppl 3):130, 1986.

173. Neuhaus KL, Tebbe U, Sauer G, et al: Hochdosierte intravenose Kurzinfusion von Streptokinase beim akuten Myokardinfarkt. In Trubestein G, Etzel F (eds): Fibrinolytische Therapie. Stuttgart: FK Shattauer Verlag, 1983, pp 425–430.

174. Spann JF, Sherry S, Carabello BA, et al: Coronary thrombolysis

by intravenous streptokinase in acute myocardial infarction: Acute and follow-up studies. Am J Cardiol 53:655, 1984.

175. Schwarz F, Hofmann H, Schuler G, et al: Thrombolysis in acute myocardial infarction: Effect of intravenous followed by intracoronary streptokinase application on estimates of infarct size. Am J Cardiol 53:1505, 1984.

176. Tebbe V, Sauer G, Kreuzer H, et al: Effects of nonsurgical reperfusion on regional left ventricular function in patients with acute myocardial infarction. In Sigwart V, Heutzen PL (eds): Ventricular Wall Motion. Stuttgart: G Thieme Verlag, 1984, pp 210–217.

177. Valentine RP, Pitts DE, Brooks-Brunn JA, et al: Intravenous versus intracoronary streptokinase in acute myocardial infarction. Am J Cardiol 55:309, 1985.

178. Granger CB, Califf RM, Topol EJ: Thrombolytic therapy for acute myocardial infarction: A review. Drugs 44:293, 1992.

179. The GUSTO Angiographic Investigators: The effects of tissue plasminogen activator, streptokinase, or both on coronary artery patency, ventricular function, and survival after acute myocardial infarction. N Engl J Med 329:1615, 1993.

180. Magnani B: Plasminogen Activator Italian Multicenter Study (PAIMS): Comparison of intravenous recombinant single-chain human tissue-type plasminogen activator (rt-PA) with intravenous streptokinase in acute myocardial infarction. J Am Coll Cardiol 13:19, 1989.

181. White HD, Rivers JT, Maslowski AH, et al: Effect of intravenous streptokinase as compared with that of tissue plasminogen activator on left ventricular function after first myocardial infarction. N Engl J Med 320:817, 1989.

182. Karagounis L, Sorensen SG, Menlove RL, et al: Does thrombolysis in myocardial infarction (TIMI) perfusion grade 2 represent a mostly patent artery or a mostly occluded artery? Enzymatic and electrocardiographic evidence from the TEAM-2 study. J Am Coll Cardiol 19:1, 1992.

183. ISIS Steering Committee: Intravenous streptokinase given within 0–4 hours of onset of myocardial infarction reduced mortality in ISIS-2. Lancet 1:502, 1987.

184. ISIS-2 (The Second International Study of Infarct Survival). Randomized trial of intravenous streptokinase, oral aspirin, both, or neither among 17,187 cases of suspected acute myocardial infarction: ISIS-2 (Second International Study of Infarct Survival) Collaborative Group. Lancet 2:349, 1988.

185. Gruppo Italiano per lo Studio della Streptochinasi nell'Infarto Miocardico (GISSI). Long-term effects of intravenous thrombolysis in acute myocardial infarction: Final report of the GISSI study. Lancet 2:871, 1987.

186. Schroder R, Neuhaus K-L, Leizorovicz A, et al: A prospective placebo-controlled double-blind multicenter trial of intravenous streptokinase in acute myocardial infarction (ISAM): Long-term mortality and morbidity. J Am Coll Cardiol 9:197, 1987.

187. Anderson JL, Marshall HW, Bray BE, et al: A randomized trial of intracoronary streptokinase in the treatment of acute myocardial infarction. N Engl J Med 308:1312, 1983.

188. Khaja F, Walton JA Jr, Brymer JF, et al: Intracoronary fibrinolytic therapy in acute myocardial infarction: Report on a prospective randomized trial. N Engl J Med 308:1305, 1983.

189. Furberg CD: Clinical value of intracoronary streptokinase. Am J Cardiol 53:626, 1984.

190. EMERAS (Estudio Multicéntrico Estreptoquinasa Republicas de America del Sur) Collaborative Group: Randomized trial of late thrombolysis in patients with suspected acute myocardial infarction. Lancet 342:767, 1993.

191. LATE Study Group: Late assessment of thrombolytic efficacy (LATE) study with alteplase 6–24 hours after onset of acute myocardial infarction. Lancet 342:759, 1993.

192. Le Feuvre C, Yusuf S, Flather M, Farkouh M: Maximizing benefits of therapies in acute myocardial infarction. Am J Cardiol 72:145G, 1993.

193. The European Myocardial Infarction Project Group: Prehospital thrombolytic therapy in patients with suspected acute myocardial infarction. N Engl J Med 329:383, 1993.

194. GREAT Group: Feasibility, safety, and efficacy of domiciliary thrombolysis by general practitioners. Grampian Region Early Anistreplase Trial. Br J Med 305:548, 1992.

195. Rawles J, on behalf of the GREAT Group: Halving of mortality at 1 year by domiciliary thrombolysis in the Grampian Region Early Anistreplase Trial (GREAT). J Am Coll Cardiol 23:1, 1994.

196. Smith RAG, Dupe RJ, English PD, Green J: Fibrinolysis with acyl-enzymes: A new approach to thrombolytic therapy. Nature 290:505, 1981.

197. Weaver WD, Eisenberg MS, Martin JS, et al: Myocardial Infarction Triage and Intervention Project—Phase I: Patient characteristics and feasibility of pre-hospital initiation of thrombolytic therapy. J Am Coll Cardiol 15:925, 1990.

198. O'Neill WO, Timmis GC, Bourdillon AD, et al: A prospective randomized clinical trial of intracoronary streptokinase versus coronary angioplasty for acute myocardial infarction. N Engl J Med 314:812, 1986.

199. Zijlstra F, de Boer MJ, Hoorntje JC, et al: Comparison of immediate coronary angioplasty with intravenous streptokinase in acute myocardial infarction. N Engl J Med 328:680, 1993.

200. Ribeiro EE, Silva LA, Carngiro R, et al: Randomized trial of direct coronary angioplasty versus intravenous streptokinase in acute myocardial infarction. J Am Coll Cardiol 22:376, 1993.

201. Rogers WJ, Dean LS, Moore PB, et al, for the Alabama Registry of Myocardial Ischemia Investigators: Comparison of primary angioplasty versus thrombolytic therapy for acute myocardial infarction. Am J Cardiol 74:111, 1994.

202. Topol EJ, Califf RM: Intravenous heparin, thrombolytics, and medical marketing. Personal communication, 1990.

203. Hsia J, Hamilton WP, Kleinman N, et al, for the Heparin-Aspirin Reperfusion Trial (HART) investigators: A comparison between heparin and low-dose aspirin as adjunctive therapy with tissue plasminogen activator for acute myocardial infarction. N Engl J Med 323:1433, 1990.

204. Bleich SD, Nichols TC, Schumacher RR, et al: The effect of heparin on coronary arterial patency after thrombolysis with tissue plasminogen activator in acute myocardial infarction. Am J Cardiol 66:1412, 1990.

205. Topol EJ, George BS, Kereiakes DJ, et al (TAMI Study Group): A randomized controlled trial of intravenous tissue plasminogen activator and early intravenous heparin in acute myocardial infarction. Circulation 79:281, 1989.

206. Thompson PL, Aylward PE, Federman J, et al: A randomized comparison of intravenous heparin with oral aspirin and dipyridamole 24 hours after recombinant tissue-type plasminogen activator for acute myocardial infarction. Circulation 83:1534, 1991.

207. de Bono DP, Simoons ML, Tijssen J, et al: Effect of early intravenous heparin on coronary patency, infarct size, and bleeding complications after alteplase thrombolysis: Results of a randomized double blind European Cooperative Study Group trial. Br Heart J 67:122, 1992.

208. O'Connor CM, Meese R, Carney R, et al, for the DUCCS Study Group: A randomized trial of intravenous heparin in conjunction with anistreplase (anisoylated plasminogen streptokinase activator complex) in acute myocardial infarction: The Duke University Clinical Cardiology Study (DUCCS) 1. J Am Coll Cardiol 23:11, 1994.

209. Col J, Decoster O, Hanique G, et al: Infusion of heparin conjunct to streptokinase accelerates reperfusion of acute myocardial infarction: Results of a double-blind randomized study (OSIRIS) [abstract]. Circulation 86:I-259, 1992.

210. Coller BS, Folts JD, Scudder LE, Smith SR: Antithrombotic effect of a monoclonal antibody to the platelet glycoprotein IIb/IIIa receptor in an experimental animal model. Blood 68:783, 1986.

211. Maraganore JM, Bourdon P, Jablonski J, et al: Design and characterization of hirulog: A novel class of bivalent peptide inhibitors of thrombin. Biochemistry 29:7095, 1990.

212. Lee LV, McCabe CH, Antman EM, et al, for the TIMI 6 Investigators: Initial experience with hirudin and streptokinase in acute myocardial infarction: Results of the TIMI 6 trial [abstract]. J Am Coll Cardiol (special issue):344A, 1994.

213. Simoons ML, Maggioni AP, Knatterud G, et al: Individual risk assessment for intracranial haemorrhage during thrombolytic therapy. Lancet 342:1523, 1993.

214. Ljungberg J, Hedner U: Potentiated thrombolysis in a Chandler system using rt-PA and lys-plasminogen. Thromb Res 53:569, 1989.
215. Badylak SF, Voytik SL, Henkin J, et al: The beneficial effect of lys-plasminogen upon the thrombolytic efficacy of urokinase in a dog model of peripheral arterial thrombosis. Haemostasis 21:278, 1991.
216. Önundarson PT, Francis CW, Marder VJ: Depletion of plasminogen in vitro or during thrombolytic therapy limits fibrinolytic potential. J Lab Clin Med 120:120, 1992.
217. Torr SR, Nachowiak DA, Fujii S, Sobel BE: "Plasminogen steal" and clot lysis. J Am Coll Cardiol 19:1085, 1992.
218. Kakker VV, Sagar S, Lewis M: Treatment of deep-vein thrombosis with intermittent streptokinase and plasminogen infusion. Lancet 2:674, 1975.
219. Ellis DA, Neville E, Hall RJC: Subacute massive pulmonary embolism treated with plasminogen and streptokinase. Thorax 38:903, 1983.
220. Giraud CL, Joffre F, Tasrini J, et al: Indications et résultats de l'association urokinase-lys plasminogen dans la pathologie ischémique aigue des membres inferieurs. J Mal Vasc (Paris) 10:321, 1985.
221. Tilsner V: Klinische Erfahrungen bei der Anwendung von Lys-Plasminogen zur Behandlung von arteriellen Gefäβverschlüssen (Clinical experience with lys-plasminogen in the treatment of arterial occlusions). Ellipse 22:301, 1990.
222. deProst D, Guerot C, Laffay N, et al: Intra-coronary thrombolysis with streptokinase or lys-plasminogen/urokinase in acute myocardial infarction: Effects on recanalization and blood fibrinolysis. Thromb Haemost 50:792, 1983.
223. Immelman EJ, Jeffery PC: The post-phlebitic syndrome. Pathophysiology, prevention and management. Clin Chest Med 5:537, 1984.
224. Lensing AWA, Hirsh J: Natural history of minimal calf DVT. Rationale and results of thrombolytic therapy. In Bernstein (ed): Vascular Diagnosis, 4th ed. St. Louis: Mosby–Year Book, 1990, pp 779–781.
225. Porter J, Seaman AJ, Common HC, et al: Comparison of heparin and streptokinase in the treatment of venous thrombosis. Am Surg 41:511, 1975.
226. Robertson BR, Nillson IM, Nylander G: Thrombolytic effect of streptokinase as evaluated by phlebography of deep venous thrombi of the leg. Acta Chir Scand 136:173, 1970.
227. Kakkar VV, Franc C, Howe CT, et al: Treatment of deep vein thrombosis: A trial of heparin, streptokinase and arvin. Br Med J 1:806, 1969.
228. Tsapogas MJ, Peabody RA, Wu KT, et al: Controlled study of thrombolytic therapy in deep vein thrombosis. Surgery 74:973, 1973.
229. Elliot MS, Immelman EJ, Benatar JSR, et al: A comparative randomized trial of heparin versus streptokinase in the treatment of acute proximal venous thrombosis: An interim report of a prospective trial. Br J Surg 66:838, 1979.
230. Goldhaber SZ, Meyerovitz MF, Green D, et al: Randomized controlled trial of tissue plasminogen activator in proximal DVT. Am J Med 88:235, 1990.
231. Turpie AGG, Levine MN, Hirsh J, et al: Tissue plasminogen activator vs heparin in DVT. Results of a randomized trial. Chest 97:172S, 1990.
232. Browse NL, Thomas ML, Pim HP: Streptokinase and deep vein thrombosis. Br Med J 3:707, 1968.
233. Tibbutt DA, Williams EW, Walker MW, et al: Controlled trial of ancrod and streptokinase in the treatment of deep vein thrombosis of lower limb. Br J Haematol 27:407, 1974.
234. Rssch J, Dotter CT, Seaman AJ, et al: Healing of deep venous thrombosis: Venographic findings in a randomized study comparing streptokinase and heparin. Am J Roentgenol 127:553, 1976.
235. Marder VJ, Soulen RL, Atichartakarn V, et al: Quantitative venographic assessment of deep vein thrombosis in the evaluation of streptokinase and heparin therapy. J Lab Clin Med 89:1018, 1977.
236. Arnesen H, Heilo A, Jakobsen E, et al: A prospective study of streptokinase and heparin in the treatment of deep vein thrombosis. Acta Med Scand 203:457, 1978.
237. Watz R, Savidge GF: Rapid thrombolysis and preservation of valvular venous function in high deep vein thrombosis. Acta Med Scand 205:293, 1979.
238. Duckert F, Müller G, Nyman D, et al: Treatment of deep vein thrombosis with streptokinase. Br Med J 1:479, 1975.
239. Hirsh J, Marder VJ, Salzman EW, Hull R: Treatment of venous thromboembolism. In Colman RW, Hirsh J, Marder VJ, Salzman EW (eds): Hemostasis and Thrombosis. Basic Principles and Clinical Practice, 3rd ed. Philadelphia: JB Lippincott, 1994, pp 1346–1366.
240. Francis CW, Marder VJ: Fibrinolytic therapy for venous thrombosis. Prog Cardiovasc Dis 34:193, 1991.
241. Bounameaux H, Banga JD, Bluhmki E, et al: Double-blind, randomized comparison of systemic continuous infusion of 0.25 versus 0.50 mg/kg/24 h of alteplase over 3 to 7 days for treatment of deep venous thrombosis in heparinized patients: Results of the European Thrombolysis with rt-PA in Venous Thrombosis (ETTT) Trial. Thromb Haemost 67:306, 1992.
242. Marder VJ, Brenner B, Totterman S, et al: Comparison of dosage schedules of rt-PA in the treatment of proximal deep vein thrombosis. J Lab Clin Med 119:485, 1992.
243. D'Angelo A, Mannucci PM: Outcome of treatment of deep-vein thrombosis with urokinase: Relationship to dosage, duration of therapy, age of the thrombus and laboratory changes. Thromb Haemost 51:236, 1984.
244. Moia M, Mannucci PM, Pini M, Prandoni P: A pilot study of pro-urokinase in the treatment of deep vein thrombosis. Thromb Haemost 72:430, 1994.
245. Kakkar VV, Howe CT, Laws JW, et al: Late results of treatment of deep vein thrombosis. Br Med J 1:810, 1981.
246. Bieger R, Boekhout-Mussert RJ, Hohmann F, et al: Is streptokinase useful in the treatment of deep venous thrombosis? Acta Med Scand 199:81, 1976.
247. Arnesen H, Hoiseth A, Ly B: Streptokinase or heparin in the treatment of deep vein thrombosis. Acta Med Scand 211:65, 1982.
248. Sidorov J: Streptokinase vs heparin for deep venous thrombosis. Can lytic therapy be justified? Arch Intern Med 149:1841, 1989.
249. Verhaeghe R, Besse P, Bounameaux H, Marbet GA: Multicenter pilot study of the efficacy and safety of systemic rt-PA administration in the treatment of deep vein thrombosis of the lower extremities and/or pelvis. Thromb Res 55:5, 1989.
250. Dalen JE, Alpert JS: Natural history of pulmonary embolism. In Sasahara AA, Sonnenblick EH, Lesch M (eds): Pulmonary Emboli. New York: Grune and Stratton, 1975, pp 77–88.
251. deSoyza NDB, Murphy ML: Persistent post-embolic pulmonary hypertension. Chest 62:665, 1972.
252. Tibbutt DA, Davies JA, Anderson JA, et al: Comparison by controlled clinical trial of streptokinase and heparin in treatment of life-threatening pulmonary embolism. Br Med J 1:343, 1974.
253. Urokinase Pulmonary Embolism Trial: Phase 1 results. JAMA 214:2163, 1970.
254. Ly B, Arnesen H, Eie H, Hol R: A controlled clinical trial of streptokinase and heparin in the treatment of major pulmonary embolism. Acta Med Scand 203:465, 1978.
255. Tissue plasminogen activator for the treatment of acute pulmonary embolism: a collaborative study by the PIOPED investigators. Chest 97:528, 1990.
256. Levine M, Hirsh J, Weitz J, et al: A randomized trial of a single bolus dosage regimen of recombinant tissue plasminogen activator in patients with acute pulmonary embolism. Chest 98:1473, 1990.
257. Goldhaber SZ, Haire WD, Feldstein ML, et al: Alteplase versus heparin in acute pulmonary embolism: Randomized trial assessing right-ventricular function and pulmonary perfusion. Lancet 341:507, 1993.
258. Sharma GVRK, Burleson VA, Sasahara AA: Effect of thrombolytic therapy on pulmonary-capillary blood volume in patients with pulmonary embolism. N Engl J Med 303:842, 1980.
259. Sharma GVRK, Folland ED, McIntyre KM, Sasahara AA: Long-term hemodynamic benefit of thrombolytic therapy in pulmonary embolic disease. J Am Coll Cardiol 15:65A, 1990.
260. The UKEP Study Research Group: The UKEP study—

Multicentre clinical trial on two local regimens of urokinase in massive pulmonary embolism. Eur Heart J 8:2, 1987.

261. Verstraete M, Miller GAH, Bounameaux H, et al: Intravenous and intrapulmonary recombinant tissue-type plasminogen activator in the treatment of acute massive pulmonary embolism. Circulation 77:353, 1988.

262. Goldhaber SZ, Kessler CM, Heit JA, et al: Randomized controlled trial of recombinant tissue plasminogen activator versus urokinase in the treatment of acute pulmonary embolism. Lancet 2:293, 1988.

263. Goldhaber SZ, Kessler CM, Heit JA, et al: Recombinant tissue-type plasminogen activator versus a novel dosing regimen of urokinase in acute pulmonary embolism. A randomized controlled multicenter trial. J Am Coll Cardiol 20:24, 1992.

264. Demeter SL, Fuenning C: Intra-pulmonary artery streptokinase. Angiology 34:70, 1983.

265. Schmutzler R, Koller F: Thrombolytic therapy. In Poller L (ed): Recent Advances in Blood Coagulation. London: J&A Churchill, 1969.

266. Cotton LT, Flute PT, Tsapogas MJC: Popliteal artery thrombosis treated with streptokinase. Lancet 2:1081, 1962.

267. Amery A, Deloof W, Vermylen J, Verstraete M: Outcome of recent thromboembolic occlusions of limb arteries treated with streptokinase. Br Med J 4:639, 1970.

268. Marder VJ, Francis CW: An assessment of regional versus systemic thrombolytic treatment of peripheral and coronary artery thrombosis. Prog Hemost Thromb 7:325, 1984.

269. Verstraete M: Biochemical and clinical aspects of thrombolysis. Semin Hematol 15:35, 1978.

270. Poliwoda H, Alexander K, Buhl V, et al: Treatment of chronic arterial occlusions with streptokinase. N Engl J Med 280:689, 1969.

271. Samama M, Cormier JM, Abastado M, et al: La thrombolyse par la streptokinase, 2me partie: A propos de 66 observations. Coagulation 2:221, 1969.

272. Chesterman CN, Briggs JC: Thrombolytic therapy with streptokinase. Med J Aust 57:839, 1970.

273. Martin M: Thrombolytic therapy in arterial thromboembolism. Prog Cardiovasc Dis 21:351, 1979.

274. Hess H, Ingrisch H, Mietaschk A, Rath H: Local low-dose thrombolytic therapy of peripheral arterial occlusions. N Engl J Med 307:1627, 1982.

275. Katzen BT, van Breda A: Low-dose streptokinase in the treatment of arterial occlusions. AJR 136:1171, 1981.

276. Dardik H, Sussman BC, Kahn M, et al: Lysis of arterial clot by intravenous or intra-arterial administration of streptokinase. Surg Gynecol Obstet 158:137, 1984.

277. Hargrove WC III, Barker CF, Berkowitz HD, et al: Treatment of acute peripheral arterial and graft thromboses with low-dose streptokinase. Surgery 92:981, 1982.

278. Pernes JM, Augusto deA, Vitoux JF, et al: Local thrombolysis in peripheral arteries and bypass grafts. J Vasc Surg 6:372, 1987.

279. Dotter CT, Rosch J, Seaman AJ: Selective clot lysis with low-dose streptokinase. Radiology 111:31, 1974.

280. Sicard GA, Schier JJ, Totty WG, et al: Thrombolytic therapy for acute arterial occlusion. J Vasc Surg 2:65, 1985.

281. Pernes JM, Brenot P, Raynaud A, et al: Results of in situ arterial thrombolysis by the combination of urokinase and lysyl plasminogen in acute arterial occlusive diseases of the lower limb. J Radiol 66:385, 1985.

282. Boyles PW, Meyer WH, Graff J, et al: Comparative effectiveness of intravenous and intra-arterial fibrinolysin therapy. Am J Cardiol 6:439, 1960.

283. Hallatt JW Jr, Yrizarry JM, Greenwood LH: Regional low-dosage thrombolytic therapy for peripheral arterial occlusions. Surg Gynecol Obstet 156:148, 1983.

284. Chesterman CN, Nash T, Biggs JC: Small-vessel thrombosis following vascular injury: Successful treatment with a low-dose intra-arterial infusion of streptokinase. Br J Surg 58:582, 1971.

285. Gardiner GA Jr, Koltun W, Kandarpa K, et al: Thrombolysis of occluded femoropopliteal grafts. AJR 147:621, 1986.

286. Belkin M, Belkin B, Bucknam CA, et al: Intra-arterial fibrinolytic therapy—efficacy of streptokinase vs. urokinase. Arch Surg 121:769, 1986.

287. McNamara TO, Fischer JR: Thrombolysis of peripheral arterial and graft occlusions: Improved results using high-dose urokinase. AJR 144:769, 1985.

288. Rabe FE, Becker GJ, Richmond BD, et al: Contrast extravasation through Dacron grafts: A sequela of low-dose streptokinase therapy. Am J Radiol 138:917, 1982.

289. Quinones-Baldrich WJ, Baker JD, Busuttil RW, et al: Intraoperative infusion of lytic drugs for thrombotic complications of revascularization. J Vasc Surg 10:408, 1989.

290. Comerota AJ, White JV, Grosh JD: Intraoperative intra-arterial thrombotic therapy for salvage of limbs in patients with distal arterial thrombosis. Surg Gynecol Obstet 169:283, 1989.

291. Ouriel K, Shortell CK, DeWeese JA, et al: A comparison of thrombolytic therapy with operative revascularization in the initial treatment of acute peripheral arterial ischemia. J Vasc Surg 19:1021, 1994.

292. Strandness DE Jr, Salzman EW, Shortell CK, Marder VJ: Management of peripheral arterial disease. In Colman RW, Hirsh J, Marder VJ, Salzman EW (eds): Hemostasis and Thrombosis: Basic Principles and Clinical Practice, 3rd ed. Philadelphia: JB Lippincott, 1994, p 1396.

293. The STILE Investigators: Results of a prospective randomized trial evaluating surgery versus thrombolysis for ischemia of the lower extremity. Ann Surg 220:251, 1994.

294. AIMS Trial Study Group: Effect of intravenous APSAC on mortality after acute myocardial infarction: Preliminary report of a placebo-controlled clinical trial. Lancet 1:545, 1988.

295. AIMS Trial Study Group: Long-term effects of intravenous anistreplase in acute myocardial infarction: Final report of the AIMS study. Lancet 335:427, 1990.

296. Wilcox RG, von der Lippe G, Olsson CG, et al, for the ASSET (Angelo-Scandinavian Study of Early Thrombolysis) Study Group: Trial of tissue plasminogen activator for mortality reduction in acute myocardial infarction: Anglo-Scandinavian Study of Early Thrombolysis (ASSET). Lancet 2:525, 1988.

297. Wilcox RG, von der Lippe, Olsson CG, et al, for the Anglo-Scandinavian Study of Early Thrombolysis: Effects of alteplase in acute myocardial infarction: 6-month results from the ASSET study: Anglo-Scandinavian Study of Early Thrombolysis. Lancet 335:1175, 1990.

298. Pietrolungo JF, Topol EJ: Thrombolytic therapy for acute myocardial infarction. In Comerota AJ (ed): Thrombolytic Therapy for Peripheral Vascular Disease. Philadelphia: JB Lippincott, 1995, p 349.

299. Neuhaus KL, Feuerer W, Jeep TS, et al: Improved thrombolysis with a modified dose regimen of recombinant tissue-type plasminogen activator. J Am Coll Cardiol 14:1566, 1989.

300. Wall TC, Califf RM, George BS, et al: Accelerated plasminogen activator dose regimens for coronary thrombolysis: the TAMI-7 study group. J Am Coll Cardiol 19: 482, 1992.

CHAPTER 166

Urokinase

Robert B. Rutherford, M.D., and Anthony J. Comerota, M.D.

Thrombolyic therapy can now be applied using a variety of agents, the best known of which are urokinase (UK), streptokinase (SK), and tissue-type plasminogen activator (t-PA). This chapter reviews the clinical applications of UK, not only *vis a vis* other thrombolytic agents but in the broader context of comparing thrombolytic therapy with thrombectomy or anticoagulant therapy alone. The pharmacology, dosage, and techniques of the administration of UK are also discussed, but the focus is on the indications, contraindications, success, and complication rates of lytic therapy in the form of urokinase infusion. Thrombolytic therapy for coronary artery thrombosis or thrombotic stroke is not considered here.

GENERAL COMMENTS CONCERNING LYTIC THERAPY AND UROKINASE

As pointed out by Astrup in 1958, in the blood circulating through vessels, there is a "dynamic equilibrium" between the coagulation and fibrinolytic systems, which attempts to maintain a safe position between the extremes of thrombosis and hemorrhage. In the fibrolytic system, plasminogen is activated to plasmin, which in turn breaks down fibrin, under an intricate system of checks and balances provided by a number of inhibitors and activators whose individual nature and mechanism of interaction are important but beyond the scope of this chapter. Suffice it to say that UK (and SK for that matter) are exogenous plasminogen activators that produce fibrinolysis by activating the body's natural fibrinolytic system.

UK was originally purified and concentrated from urine, hence its name. Eventually it was produced from renal cell cultures, an expensive process that at times has caused difficulties in keeping up with the increasing demands for this drug. Fortunately, recombinant DNA techniques have been developed and ultimately should ease the problems of increasing demand and high cost. UK's action is tempered by the same inhibitors and antiactivators that control spontaneous fibrinolysis (Fig. 166–1). The plasmin produced has a nonspecific proteolytic effect, digesting not only fibrin and fibrinogen but also prothrombin and factors V and VIII, particularly after α_2-antiplasmin levels are reduced. Even tissue-type plasminogen activator, which might seem to be a more natural approach to activating the fibrinolytic system, can, in excess, seriously disturb this intrinsic system of checks and balances. Thus, any of the current lytic agents represents the proverbial "two-edged

sword" in that, by dissolving clot, it can also produce hemorrhage.

Fortunately, the risk of serious hemorrhage has been mitigated by the natural protection offered by these same inhibitors and by the coagulation system itself, and there appears to be an initial "golden period" during which they are able to prevent serious hemorrhage. For this reason, it is an understood goal of modern lytic therapy to effectively lyse the offending pathologic thrombus *before* these protective mechanisms are overcome by lytic excesses. This time constraint placed significant limitations on *systemic* lytic therapy (SLT), but this problem has now largely been solved by the localized delivery of lytic agents via percutaneously introduced and angiographically positioned catheters. This localized delivery of the lytic agent, so-called catheter-directed lytic therapy (CDLT), not only is more rapidly effective but produces significantly fewer systemic effects. This, in turn, has allowed even higher doses of lytic agents to be introduced, speeding up the process and allowing it to be completed well within this "golden period." This approach has been called "high-dose UK," in contrast with previous "low-dose" protocols. It also

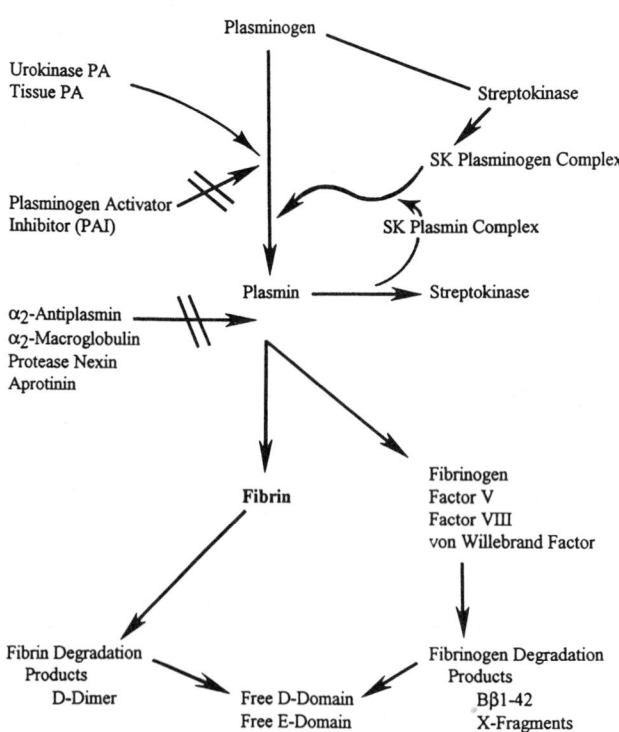

Figure 166–1. Simplified scheme of the fibrinolytic system. (From Quiñones-Baldrich WJ: Principles of thrombolytic therapy. *In* Rutherford RB [ed]: Vascular Surgery, 4th ed. Philadelphia: WB Saunders, 1995, p 335.)

represents a significant advantage of UK over SK, in that the latter must first combine with plasminogen to form an activator complex that, in turn, activates plasminogen. This gives a dose-response curve in which the lytic effect rises and falls with increasing dose. As a result, the lytic effect of SK is not as predictable and controllable, and it cannot be deliberately and reliably used in a high-dose regimen like UK. The longer durations of lytic therapy characteristically reported with SK may be in part related to this characteristic and explain its significantly higher rate of bleeding complications. But even t-PA, with the theoretical advantages offered by its greater affinity for thrombus-bound fibrin and fibrinogen as opposed to circulating fibrinogen, does not appear to have reduced the frequency of bleeding complications associated with lytic therapy.[1, 2] Finally, although SK is notorious for producing allergic reactions, other lytic agents are not free of this, and mild allergic responses to UK have been reported.

Comparative data on UK, SK, and t-PA are presented throughout this chapter, but to go beyond these general observations in their comparison would risk appearing proprietary. The reader should understand that the optimal dose and the mode of delivery have not been systematically determined for any of these agents and that many, if not most, comparisons between them are flawed. All can be effective if used carefully and can produce hemorrhagic complications if not. Nevertheless, at this time in the United States, UK has clearly become the lytic drug of choice for peripheral vascular applications, whereas t-PA remains popular with cardiologists for the management of acute coronary occlusions. UK's higher cost compared with SK appears to be offset by its shorter duration of infusion and fewer serious bleeding complications, the latter adding to cost by requiring additional treatments and prolonging hospital stay. Thus, in spite of high cost, the ability of short-duration, high-dose UK therapy to increase efficacy and reduce complications has been irresistible to clinicians.

CHEMISTRY

Although it is generally accepted that urokinase is a double-chain polypeptide with a molecular weight of 54,000 to 57,000, in its early history several investigators observed that urokinase could exist in several molecular weights.[3, 4] Molecular weights of about 22,000, 33,000, and 54,000 were confirmed, depending on the assay and purification technique used.

The complete primary amino acid sequence of urokinase has been characterized clearly.[5, 6] Three active site residues are His 204, Asp 255, and Ser 256. Plasmin and kallikrein cleave prourokinase (single-chain urokinase plasminogen activator [scuPA]) at position 156, which then produces urokinase in its two-chain form.[7] The two chains are held together by a disulfide bond that is important for the fibrinolytic activity of urokinase.

PHARMACOLOGY

Human plasminogen is produced by the liver as a single-chain glycoprotein with a molecular weight of approximately 90,000 and a plasma concentration of 20 mg/dl.[8, 9] The native plasminogen molecule has an amino acid terminal glutamic acid, GLU-plasminogen. GLU-plasminogen is degraded in the plasma by removal of an 8-kD peptide-forming molecule with amino acid terminal lysine, valine, and methionine, which is commonly designated Lys-plasminogen.[10] Lys-plasminogen has a much higher affinity for fibrin both in purified systems and in plasma.[11, 12]

Urokinase converts the inactive forms of plasminogen to plasmin, with greater affinity for the fibrin-bound Lys-plasminogen. The conversion is due to the cleavage of a single Arg 560–Val 561 bond.[13] This results in a two-chain plasmin molecule composed of an A-chain (heavy chain) from the amino-terminal end of the plasminogen and a B-chain (light chain) from the carboxyl-terminal end of the plasminogen.[14] The A-chain appears to be important in binding, and the B-chain contains the active catalytic site.

Activation of fibrin-bound plasminogen allows fibrinolysis to occur in a relatively inhibitor-free environment, because there are no competing substrates for fibrin-bound plasmin. During therapy with urokinase, circulating plasminogen is activated to form free plasmin, which then degrades fibrin, fibrinogen, and factors V and VIII and affects platelet function. Although the action of plasmin is limited by inhibitors such as α_2-antiplasmin and α_2-macroglobulin, it can stimulate considerable fibrinogen proteolysis, subsequent hypofibrinogenemia, altered platelet function, and the anticoagulant effect of the fibrin and fibrinogen breakdown products.

PHARMACOKINETICS

In early studies using *in vitro* incubation systems, it was shown that, although the total amount of plasmin generated was independent of the urokinase concentration, the rate of the reaction depended on its concentration.[15] Furthermore, it was observed that enzymatic conversion by urokinase proceeded essentially according to first-order kinetics. However, as clinical experience was gained, there appeared to be little correlation between serum levels of urokinase and the rate and extent of thrombolysis, which probably are due in part to circulating urokinase inhibitors.[16] Effective thrombolysis seems to depend on a variety of local factors, such as those listed below:

1. Accessibility of urokinase to the plasminogen-containing thrombus
2. Amount of plasminogen within the clot
3. Concentration of urokinase surrounding the thrombus
4. Age of the clot (fresh clots dissolve more easily than older ones)

Wun et al.[17] showed that urokinase is present in plasma in a circulating concentration of at least 5 to

10 μg/L, which is sufficient to generate substantial levels of plasmin, particularly if activation is localized to specific sites.

Urokinase is cleared rapidly by the liver, with approximately 3% to 5% cleared by the kidneys.[18] It has a half-life of about 16 minutes, which might be prolonged in patients with hepatic dysfunction.

Although UK induces clotting defects that persist after discontinuation of the drug infusion, evidence suggests that coagulation parameters do not deteriorate as much with UK as with SK and normalize more rapidly with UK than with SK.

EFFECTS ON PATHOPHYSIOLOGY AND CLINICAL USE
Deep Venous Thrombosis of the Lower Extremities

In managing deep venous thrombosis (DVT) of the lower extremities, there are three basic therapeutic options: thrombectomy, thrombolysis, or anticoagulant therapy alone. The choice should be considered in relation to the three major therapeutic goals: (1) reducing the risk of pulmonary embolism; (2) reducing acute morbidity; and (3) mitigating late postphlebitic sequelae. Of these, anticoagulant therapy is by far the most commonly used, and each of the other two therapies is superimposed on a background of anticoagulant therapy, so it serves as the control, if not the gold standard, in this setting.

The primary role of anticoagulant therapy in preventing pulmonary embolism is not challenged. It is in relation to the other two therapeutic goals that it falls short. It does little for acute morbidity other than preventing progression by clot propagation. Nevertheless, concomitant elevation of the extremities plus heparinization suffices to control acute morbidity in the majority of the cases. However, this does not suffice in some cases of phlegmasia cerulea dolens, because the extensiveness of the iliofemoral venous thrombosis blocks most of the tributaries that serve as collateral pathways. In these severe cases, prompt clot removal would quickly decrease pain and swelling, shorten hospital stay, and prevent progression to a compartment compression syndrome and even venous gangrene.

Anticoagulant therapy alone also does little in reducing late postthrombotic sequelae, e.g., pain and swelling with activity, stasis dermatitis, and venous ulceration. It simply limits clot propagation while collaterals develop and/or spontaneous recanalization of thrombosed segments occurs, through the action of naturally occurring plasmin. Potentially, prompt clot removal not only relieves obstruction and preserves functioning valves in the involved *proximal* segment, but prevents secondary *distal* valve incompetence that develops because of dilation in the chronically congested venous segments below the proximal obstruction.

The key question is how successful is either thrombectomy or thrombolysis in relieving acute morbidity or preventing postthrombotic sequelae relative to anticoagulant therapy alone and compared with each other (Table 166–1). Only prompt and atraumatic removal of thrombus is likely to restore venous patency and preserve the function of the delicate venous valves. Practically, this can be achieved only by *early* intervention in cases with less extensive proximal venous thrombosis, i.e., phlegmasia alba dolens of recent onset. Also, for practical reasons, intervention cannot be justified for the reason of preventing long-term postphlebitic sequelae in either elderly patients or those with serious chronic intercurrent disease. Thus, thrombectomy or thrombolysis essentially vie for the same patients at two ends of the DVT disease spectrum: younger healthy, active patients with relatively recent onset of phlegmasia alba dolens (i.e., early, limited iliofemoral venous thrombosis) and, at the other extreme, patients with massive iliofemoral venous thrombosis and phlegmasia cerulea dolens that has progressed to the point of unrelenting pain, compartment compression syndrome, or imminent venous gangrene.

Unfortunately, thrombectomy and thrombolysis have not been compared with each other in prospective randomized trials in either of these two settings. Thrombectomy has been shown to be more efficacious than anticoagulant therapy, in both regards, in a Scandinavian prospective randomized trial in which symptomatic, venographic, and functional assessments were done at 6 months[19] and again at 5 years.[20] Lytic therapy, in the form of systemic SK therapy, has also been shown to be statistically significantly better

Table 166–1. **Potential Advantages and Disadvantages of Thrombectomy and Thrombolysis**

Thrombectomy	Thrombolysis
Faster clot removal; difficulty clearing small branches/tributaries	Less traumatic to patient, to endothelium; more complete clot removal
Requires anesthesia; significant blood loss	Little or no sedation, analgesia; risk of remote hemorrhage from systemic thrombolysis
Surgical wound morbidity	Puncture site complications
Operating room costs, longer hospitalization	Requires intensive care monitoring, but shorter hospital stay
Appropriate management of underlying lesion(s) not readily apparent (requires completion arteriography/angioscopy)	Clears and images distal tree, allowing planned attack on underlying lesion
Precludes all but "one-shot" intraoperative thrombolytic therapy for 10–14 days	Does not preclude quick change to surgical intervention
Effectiveness more limited by duration (age) of clot (3–5 days)	May lyse clot readily up to 2 weeks or beyond

than anticoagulant therapy alone in a number of trials. In many of these, venous patency was the only major end point, and, as reported by Comerota[21] in summarizing the results of 13 such trials (Table 166–2), significant or complete lysis was proved (venographically) to occur in 45%, with partial lysis in another 18%, whereas only 4% of heparinized patients had complete lysis, 14% had partial lysis, and 82% had no lysis or were worse. The importance of achieving complete lysis was shown in a study by Jeffrey et al.[22] in which complete lysis was achieved in 55% of SK-treated patients versus 5% for heparinized patients. In a 5- to 10-year follow-up of these patients, those with complete lysis had only a 9% incidence of reflux at the critical popliteal level, compared with 77% for those with incomplete lysis. Three other major trials of systemic SK versus heparin therapy for acute lower extremity DVT have been reported with long-term follow-up. Two of the trials, a Scandinavian trial reported by Amesen et al.[23] and a South African trial reported by Elliot et al.,[24] observed very significant advantages to the use of SK therapy using the clinical criteria of edema, stasis pigmentation, and ulceration. However, in another trial, Kakkar and Lawrence,[25] using foot volumetry as the primary index of venous reflux, could not show a significant difference between heparin- and SK-treated patients at 2 years.

In spite of the convincing evidence from these many trials of the superiority of systemic lytic therapy (particularly UK) over heparin anticoagulation, this approach has not gained popularity and wide usage for the treatment of DVT, probably because of concern over possible bleeding complications, the lack of complete lysis in many cases, and widespread apathy regarding late postphlebitic sequelae, which lack the immediate and dramatic impact of acute pulmonary embolism. However, attitudes appear to be changing now with the advent of catheter-directed high-dose UK therapy. Based on the successful technology developed for intraarterial infusions of UK in treating arterial thromboembolism, direct venous access to the thrombosed iliofemoral venous segment was ultimately attempted by several routes: from above via the internal jugular vein; from the opposite extremity via the iliofemoral segment; and from below via the popliteal or lesser saphenous veins. Even direct puncture of the femoral veins guided by duplex scan or angiography with road mapping has been success-

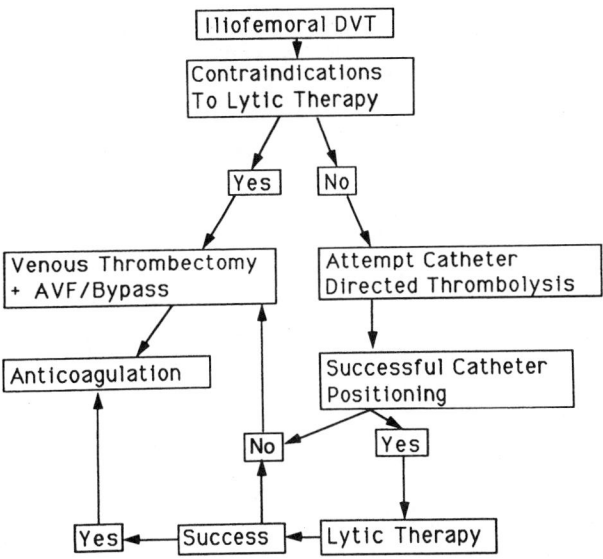

Figure 166–2. Algorithm for treating iliofemoral venous thrombosis. (From Comerota AJ: Venous thromboembolism. *In* Rutherford RB [ed]: Vascular Surgery, 4th ed. Philadelphia: WB Saunders, 1995, p 1809.)

fully accomplished. Using such access, either singly or in combination, an initial personal communication from M. D. Dake has now burgeoned into a small published series (e.g., 15 to 30 cases) with very high initial success rates for achieving patency.[26] Unfortunately, this catheter-directed approach is so recent in application that sufficiently large series with objective long-term follow-up have not yet been reported. Nevertheless, the high rate of prompt restoration of patency can be expected to translate into better long-term functional outcome and allow thrombolytic therapy to vie with thrombectomy for the two groups of patients previously outlined.

In choosing between these two treatment methods, assuming that the patient has been selected for intervention for the two major indications presented earlier, the choice of therapy is usually determined by relative contraindications to one or the other method of clot removal. A selective approach, based on contraindications to thrombolytic therapy and success in achieving catheter access and producing satisfactory thrombolysis, is outlined in algorithmic form in Figure 166–2. In this scheme, if thrombolytic therapy is not contraindicated (Table 166–3), catheter access would be attempted, and, if this could be achieved, lytic therapy would be done. If catheter access was not achieved, or if lytic therapy did not show satisfactory dissolution of clot, based on serial angiographic control, then thrombectomy would be carried out. Although this approach seems rational, based on current evidence, clinical trials with long-term functional follow-up will obviously be needed to confirm this recommendation.

Deep Venous Thrombosis of the Upper Extremeties

As with the lower extremity, intervention can be currently justified only for *proximal* vein thrombosis.

Table 166–2. Phlebographic Outcome of Anticoagulation Versus Thrombolytic Therapy for Acute DVT: Results of Pooled Data from 13 Reports

Treatment	Number of Patients	None/Worse	Partial	Significant/Complete
Heparin	254	82%	14%	4%
Lytic therapy	337	37%	18%	45%

From Comerota AJ: Venous thromboembolism. *In* Rutherford RB (ed): Vascular Surgery, 4th ed. Philadelphia: WB Saunders, 1995, p 1800.

Table 166–3. **Contraindications to Systemic Lytic Therapy**

Absolute
  Active internal bleeding
  Recent (<2 mo) cerebrovascular accident
  Intracranial pathology

Relative: Major
  Recent (<10 days) major surgery, obstetric delivery, or organ biopsy
  Thrombus of left side of the heart
  Active peptic ulcer or gastrointestinal pathology
  Recent major trauma
  Uncontrolled hypertension

Relative: Minor
  Minor surgery or trauma
  Recent cardiopulmonary resuscitation
  Atrial fibrillation with mitral valve disease
  Bacterial endocarditis
  Hemostatic defects, i.e., renal or liver disease
  Diabetic hemorrhagic retinopathy
  Pregnancy

Contraindications to Streptokinase
  Known allergy
  Recent streptococcal infection
  Previous therapy within 6 months

Data from NIH Consensus Development Conference: Thrombolytic therapy in treatment. Ann Intern Med 93:141, 1980.

Furthermore, subclavian/axillary vein thrombosis (SAVT) should be separated into primary ("spontaneous") or secondary (catheter-induced) thrombosis for treatment purposes. In spontaneous or effort/position-induced SAVT, obstructive symptoms (pain and swelling with activity) are the more important considerations; distal reflux with stasis dermatitis and ulceration are almost never seen in the upper extremity. In primary SAVT, similar to ileofemoral venous thrombosis (IFVT), only active, healthy patients with recent onset symptoms are usually considered candidates for intervention and thrombus removal; phlegmasia cerulea dolens with the threat of gangrene is almost unheard of in the upper extremity. However, with SAVT, the initial choice of catheter-directed thrombolysis over thrombectomy is better supported by clinical experience. Catheter access is easier to achieve in the upper extremity (via the antecubital and/or basilic veins), the thrombotic mass is smaller, and there are at least a few sizeable experiences with long-term follow-up on which to base this preference. After a number of encouraging but limited reports appeared in the literature (typically 3 to 5 initially successful cases without long-term follow-up), Kunkel and Machleder[27] reported the first large experience, with 25 patients with primary SAVT, treated with lytic therapy. The use of SK was only partially successful, but all the UK-treated patients were successfully lysed. In an evolving protocol, patients with successful lysis were stabilized with anticoagulant therapy and studied with positional venography. Extrinsic compression and/or residual defects, indicating an underlying thoracic outlet compression, were seen in close to 75% of the patients. Asymptomatic thoracic outlet compression was demonstrated in many of the patients on the contralateral side as well. This approach of initial thrombolysis with subsequent surgical relief of thoracic outlet compression where demonstrable has now reached more than 50 cases and, when presented by Machleder,[28] close to 80% of patients were successfully carried through the complete protocol and the majority (approximately 70%) underwent successful rehabilitation and returned to their former professional or sports-related activities.

Primarily because of this gratifying experience, thrombectomy has now generally been abandoned for thrombolysis using high-dose UK as initial treatment, unless there are specific contraindications to lytic therapy. To avoid an extended period of time away from work and two hospitalizations, a number of surgeons have shortened the interval between lysis and thoracic outlet decompression. J. E. Molina reported in a personal communication that his group has proceeded with surgical correction of underlying lesions promptly after thrombolysis. Their experience is particularly interesting in that it demonstrates that the longer the delay between onset of treatment and thrombolysis, the greater the likelihood of an organic stricture requiring angioplasty or reconstruction rather than simple thoracic outlet decompression.

Secondary SAVT, related to indwelling venous access procedures, has become increasingly common in this day and age when long-term antibiotic and cancer chemotherapy, hemodialysis access, transvenous pacemakers, and the like are commonplace therapies. Because the majority of these patients are chronically ill, do not use their upper extremities regularly in their daily activities, and may have limited longevity, aggressive intervention is not often warranted. Surgical thrombectomy rarely succeeds in achieving lasting patency in this setting where associated trauma and inflammation play a major role in thrombosis. However, in a small but significant number of these patients, preserving venous access may be critical to continued treatment with life-sustaining measures. In this circumstance, UK infusions have produced sufficiently gratifying results to justify their continued selective use, and here, two reported experiences are worthy of comment. Fraschini et al.[29] reported on 30 patients undergoing cancer chemotherapy who experienced 35 episodes of central venous catheter–related axillosubclavian vein thrombosis. After a loading dose of 500 IU/kg of UK over 10 minutes, the same dose was infused hourly, being increased up to 2000 IU/kg/hr in those who did not respond to the lower dose. The catheters had been in place for an average duration of 1 month, and treatment was started with significant delays after symptoms developed. UK was administered for 3 days, and then the response was assessed venographically. In spite of this, 25 of the 30 patients had complete lysis, one had partial lysis, and only four patients showed no response. Sixteen of the 30 patients were able to retain the same intravenous catheter for use. In a similar subsequent experience reported by Haire et al.,[30] 30 patients with venographically proven thrombosis were treated with 40,000 U of UK per hour for 12 hours through the occluded catheter. Sixteen had complete lysis, 14 had partial lysis, and 28 of 30 were able to retain use of the indwelling catheter. There were no significant bleeding complications. These experiences would suggest that where continued venous access is critical, it can safely be restored with UK infusions in a majority of patients.

Pulmonary Embolism

Pulmonary embolism would seem to be an obvious application of thrombolytic therapy, and it was one of the first. But even after a number of well-conducted prospective clinical trials, and a consensus statement by the National Institutes of Health that thrombolytic therapy is underutilized in this setting,[31] this approach has not gained the expected popularity. There are two potential goals of thrombolytic therapy for pulmonary embolism. One is to prevent *immediate* death, and the other to reduce the likelihood of *late* hemodynamic sequelae, primarily pulmonary hypertension. The other major clinical consideration, of course, is the prevention of recurrent pulmonary embolism, but this is generally adequately handled by anticoagulant therapy alone, initially with vena cava filters being placed for recurrence under adequate anticoagulant therapy or for prophylaxis when anticoagulant therapy is contraindicated. However, it should be pointed out that thrombolytic therapy, when applied to deep venous thrombosis, potentially offers a dual benefit in also preventing pulmonary embolism (by removing the venous thrombus).

Current data suggest that thrombolysis is used in less than 10% of patients with pulmonary embolism, even though the Thrombolysis in Pulmonary Embolism (TIPE) trial[32] indicated that close to 50% of patients should be eligible for thrombolytic therapy. The probable reasons for this underutilization are fear of bleeding complications, problems in diagnosis, and inexperience with the method. The general impression derived from the original trials with thrombolytic therapy versus heparin alone for pulmonary embolism was that the former produced faster clot dissolution but that the ultimate degree of clearing of the pulmonary tree was not significantly different. This early conclusion seems to have influenced clinicians to apply lytic therapy only for massive or submassive pulmonary embolism. However, there is some evidence that patients treated with lytic therapy have lower pulmonary pressures and vascular resistance than those treated with heparin and Coumadin alone. The UK pulmonary embolism trial (UPET)[33] and the UK-SK pulmonary embolism trial (USPET)[34] provided some perspective on this issue. In the UPET trial, UK showed more improvement as demonstrated by lung scans and angiograms and in pulmonary hemodynamics than heparin. However, by 7 days and beyond (up to 6 months), there were no significant differences in these same parameters. Bleeding complications occurred in 45% of UK-treated and 27% of heparinized patients. In the USPET trial, there were mean differences in pulmonary hemodynamics favoring lytic therapy, but these were not statistically significant.

In regard to long-term outcome, however, Sharma et al.[35] observed 40 UPET patients and found that pulmonary capillary blood volume and pulmonary diffusing capacity were better for UK-treated than for heparin-treated patients at 2 weeks and at 1 year. In another long-term study by Sharma et al.,[36] 23 patients randomized to UK or heparin underwent right-sided heart catheterization an average of 7 years after their pulmonary embolus. Twice as many heparin- as UK-treated patients fell into the New York Heart Association classes III or IV, and many heparin-treated patients had persistently elevated resting pulmonary artery wedge pressures and higher pulmonary vascular resistances, whereas they were, on average, normal in the UK-treated group. More recently, Molina et al.[37] have designed a catheter-directed protocol using UK infused at the rate of 2000 IU/kg/hr after a bolus injection. Eleven of 13 patients showed greater than 90% clearance at 12 hours, and more than 98% showed clearance at 24 hours. All patients had significant lysis. Most interventionalists now "lace" the clot with bolus injections of UK during pulmonary angiography, then pull back the catheter and continue with a systemic intravenous infusion thereafter. On the basis of these and other reports, thrombolysis is now recommended for the following patients with proven pulmonary embolism: (1) those who are hemodynamically unstable; (2) those with marked pulmonary hypertension and/or right-sided heart failure; (3) those with significant recurrent pulmonary embolism; and, many now add, (4) those with more than two-segment or lobar embolization. These recommendations presume that the pulmonary emboli are of recent onset, although the temporal definition of this has now been stretched up to 14 days.[38]

Arterial Thromboembolism

It is clear that UK (and other thrombolytic agents) can frequently lyse clots in peripheral arteries. What remain to be answered are (1) how competitive is this approach with other therapeutic options in terms of success and complication rates, durability, and cost effectiveness; and (2) when does the degree and duration of ischemia preclude clot removal by lytic therapy and favor surgical thromboembolectomy? Additionally, (3) does the nature of the arterial occlusion (i.e., thrombus versus embolus) and (4) does the duration of occlusion affect this choice of therapy? In answering these questions, it should be pointed out at the outset that only direct, intraarterial infusion of lytic agents (i.e., current "state of the art," catheter-directed lytic therapy) are considered and discussed here. Systemic lytic therapy is no longer being applied in this setting.

As with venous thromboembolism, there are basically three different therapeutic options to be considered in the management of arterial thromboembolism, namely, thrombectomy, thrombolysis, and anticoagulant therapy, with the last being used only to prevent clot propagation and recurrence, not to restore patency. The degree or severity of ischemia plays the major role in the choice between the two forms of clot removal. For practical purposes, in cases of acute extremity thromboembolism, the degree of ischemia can best be divided into three categories, viable, threatened, and irreversible.[39] The distinguishing features of these three categories are outlined in Table 166–4. If these definitions are carefully applied, their practical implication is that thrombolytic therapy can and should be used only in the least ischemic group. In this "viable" group, it is presumed that, if there is no further deteriorization (i.e., clot propagation is prevented by heparinization), there should be no tissue loss or irreversible nerve damage, and clot removal is indicated for a better functional outcome. In contrast, a "threatened" extremity would be expected to progress to such an undesirable outcome, and thus ultimately major or minor amputation, without prompt, successful revascularization. In the final "irreversible" category, the ischemia is too profound and advanced for the limb to be salvaged by *any* therapeutic intervention, and major amputation is inevitable in surviving patients, regardless of treatment, and, in fact, revascularization could lead to rhabdomyolysis, renal shutdown, and even pulmonary embolism. Thus, although heparinization would be applied in all categories to prevent progression, recurrence, and/or secondary *venous* thromboembolism, prompt surgical revascularization would be mandated only in the intermediate or "threatened" category in which there is not time for lytic therapy and thrombectomy and thrombolysis would compete only in the potentially viable group. Thus, if this threatening degree of ischemia is evidenced by persistent ischemic rest pain, detectable sensory or motor deficit, and/or the absence of detectable Doppler arterial signals in the pedal arteries, prompt surgical revascularization would be indicated; otherwise, lytic therapy could be tried.

These decisions are clear-cut in principle, but separation into the appropriate category is not always as clear-cut clinically, even in the hands of experts. For decision making, the separation between "viable" and "threatened" is the critical one, and this is obfuscated by the presence in some patients of numbness without detectable sensory deficit. Now that thrombolytic therapy has been speeded up with the use of high-dose UK, this decision has become even more critical, because complete lysis may be achieved in 4 to 6 hours and partial lysis with symptomatic improvement in even less time. Therefore, most now include such patients in the potentially viable category. Thus, it is recommended that, in addition to those with clearly viable limbs, those with initial numbness or with a subjective sensation of numbness in whom careful examination shows no detectable sensory deficit (using light touch, two-point discrimination and proprioception testing) be included in those who can undergo formal angiography with UK therapy, *providing they are closely monitored for changing status.*

In patients in whom the degree of ischemia allows time for lytic therapy, it offers a number of advantages over thrombectomy as the *initial* treatment. Both thrombectomy and thrombolysis can restore flow through the involved segment and then provide angiographic imaging of the distal arterial tree, but thrombectomy begins as a blind procedure and, only if completely successful, does it allow visualization of the underlying lesions and appropriate therapy to be directed against them. Thrombolytic therapy, on the other hand, being guided by serial angiography, usually gives better visualization of the underlying lesions and the distal runoff vessels and allows the most appropriate therapy, be it an endovascular procedure or a vascular surgical reconstruction to be carried out under optimal conditions with advance planning. It also allows discrete and localized lesions responsible for the acute thrombosis, i.e., those favorable to percutaneous transluminal angioplasty (PTA), to be treated at the same session, without unnecessary surgery having been performed.

The advantages of this approach are primarily seen with arterial thromboses. There are theoretical objections to treating peripheral arterial emboli with thrombolytic therapy: (1) although the embolus may be recent, the original clot itself may be relatively old and not amenable to lysis; (2) emboli may be quickly and simply removed surgically by balloon catheter embolectomy without need for balloon dilation or bypass of an underlying lesion; and (3) excessive lytic therapy might produce a systemic lytic effect that, in turn, would raise the risk of recurrent embolism. There is some logic to these objections. Beyond that, McNamara and Fischer[40] have shown that thrombo-

Table 166–4. **Clinical Categories of Acute Limb Ischemia**

Category	Description	Capillary Return	Muscle Weakness	Sensory Loss	Doppler Signals	
					Arterial	*Audible*
Viable	Not immediately threatened	Intact	None	None	Audible (AP >30 mmHg)	Audible
Threatened	Salvageable if promptly treated	Intact, slow	Mild, partial	Mild, incomplete	Inaudible	Audible
Irreversible	Major tissue loss, amputation regardless of treatment	Absent (marbling)	Profound, paralysis (rigor)	Profound, anesthetic	Inaudible	Inaudible

lytic therapy is not as successful for emboli as for thrombi. Although in their experience, the majority of emboli did lyse, the emboli required twice the dose and twice the duration of infusion and thus could be expected to produce a higher complication rate. However, the risk of causing recurrent embolism has not been realized often enough in clinical reports to convince most authorities that they are not chance occurrences, because recurrent embolism can occur even with anticoagulant therapy. Nevertheless, if an arterial embolus rather than a thrombus is known to have occurred, surgical embolectomy is normally preferred, except in patients who are prohibitive anesthetic risks.

It is fortuitous, in terms of decision making, that emboli, lodging as they do on an "unprepared" arterial tree, without adequate collateral development, usually cause severe enough ischemia to require prompt surgical revascularization. In contrast, a severely stenotic arterial segment stimulates collateral development, so that when this segment finally thromboses, the resulting ischemia is relatively less and usually allows time for formal angiographic study and lytic therapy. Thus, in clinical practice, these two groups, emboli and thrombi, usually are diverted toward surgical embolectomy and thrombolytic therapy, respectively, by the severity of the associated ischemia. With this in mind, the categorical approach shown in the algorithm in Figure 166–3 can be used to guide therapy.

Arterial Graft Occlusion

Bypass grafts have a significant 5-year failure rate, varying from 10% to 70%, depending on their location, the type of graft, and the severity of disease in the distal "runoff" vessels, among other factors. The failure rate is clearly worse for distal than proximal bypasses and for prosthetic rather than autogenous vein grafts. In clinical presentation, thrombosis of a bypass graft is more akin to acute arterial thrombosis of, rather than embolism to, a native artery and, as discussed previously, involves the same choice of treatment options, governed primarily by the severity of ischemia. Thrombolysis holds the same advantages over thrombectomy in this setting, namely less morbidity, less endothelial trauma, and more complete removal of thrombus in the distal arterial tree with better angiographic visualization. Again, speed is the main feature favoring thrombectomy, and, because with graft occlusion, the patient usually returns to the preoperative level of ischemia (e.g., claudication or chronic critical ischemia rather than acute limb-threatening ischemia), thrombolytic therapy is an appropriate choice. The main exception here would be late graft occlusions where there had been significant progression of disease in the adjacent arterial segments; but even then, there is usually time for formal arteriography and lytic therapy. However, a most important advantage of lytic therapy here is the lack of endothelial trauma. Thrombectomy of vein grafts can have devastating delayed effects (recurrent stricture), and thrombectomy often disturbs and disrupts the mature pseudointimal lining of a prosthetic graft. For these reasons, lytic therapy is preferred to thrombectomy, if the associated ischemia is not threatening. Because of the stated similarities between thrombosis of grafts and native arteries, the two are usually grouped together in reported experiences of thrombolytic therapy for peripheral arterial occlusions.

RESULTS
Acute Peripheral Arterial or Graft Occlusion

The initial success rate of lytic therapy is relatively similar between thrombosed native arteries and bypass grafts and, over the last decade, has gradually improved from approximately 60% to 75% to close to 80% to 90%. This can be attributed to improving technology and possibly the shift from SK to UK, and particularly to high-dose UK. Tables 166–5[40–48] and 166–6[49–53] show these trends. It will be seen that UK

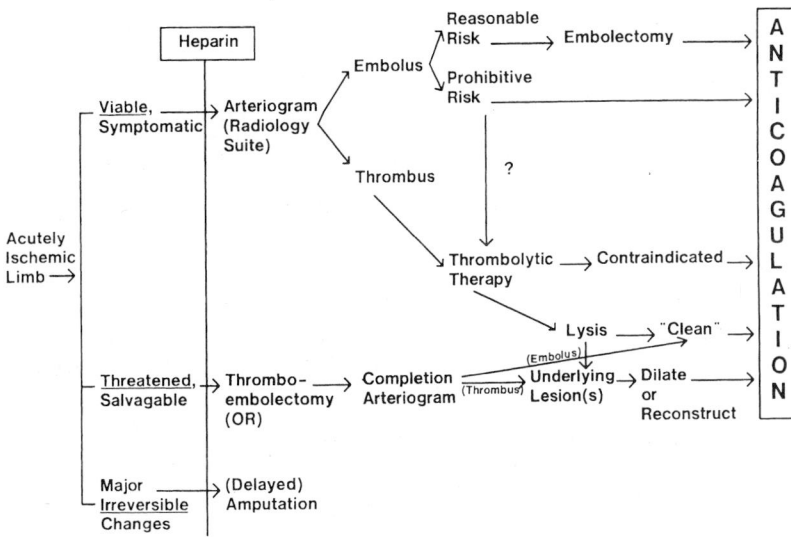

Figure 166–3. Algorithm showing selective arrangement of the acutely ischemic limbs based on severity of ischemia, diagnostic findings, and the underlying lesion shown by thrombectomy or thrombolysis. (From Gardiner GA, Sullivan KL: Catheter directed thrombolysis for the failed lower extremity bypass graft. Semin Vasc Surg 5:99, 1992.)

Table 166–5. **Results of Thrombolytic Therapy for Arterial Occlusion**

Author/Year	Number of Patients		Success (%)		Significant Complications (%)	
	SK	UK	SK	UK	SK	UK
Berni et al., 1983[41]	16	—	75	—	25	—
Kakkasseril et al., 1985[42]	35	—	43	—	37	—
Seeger et al., 1987[43]	25	—	47	—	25	—
Belkin et al., 1986[44]	25	12	50	100	48	0
Van Breda et al., 1987[45]	24	24	63	80	33	8
Traughber et al., 1987[46]	10	20	80	90	50	10
Sicard et al., 1988[47]	33	35	42	74	42	14
McNamara and Fischer, 1985[40]	—	85	—	81	—	4
Price et al., 1988[48]	2	15	50	88	—	5

also appears better than SK in terms of lower complication (bleeding) rates, but this could be in part attributable to the generally longer infusion periods associated with SK therapy. However, in an experience reported by Gardiner et al.,[54] SK had a 48% success rate, a mean infusion time of 48 hours, and a 41% complication rate, whereas UK had an 84% success rate, a 22-hour mean infusion time, and a 19% complication rate. This report also showed that although the success rate was better for bypasses that had been implanted for more than 12 months (71% versus 44% for grafts implanted fewer than 12 months), there was no difference in initial success of lytic therapy for durations of occlusion up to 28 days, beyond which there was a significant drop. Gardiner and Sullivan[55] reported a higher success rate (83% versus 71%) and a lower complication rate (9% versus 23%) for high-dose versus low-dose UK.

Although the initial results of catheter-directed lytic therapy (CDLT) for grafts are as good, if not better, than for native arteries,[51] the long-term patency of reopened grafts is not as good.[56, 57] The long-term patency of thrombosed native vessels treated with thrombolytic therapy is good as long as an underlying lesion is found that is favorable to surgical revision or PTA. Overall long-term patency of 50% or more have been commonly reported, but in this subgroup with discrete underlying stenoses, it is much higher.[58] In contrast, the overall long-term patency for similarly treated thrombosed grafts is low, close to 20% in some

series.[56, 57] This is not significantly different from the results reported earlier for thrombectomy and should not be considered an indictment of the method of clot removal. Rather, it reflects the fact that a thrombosed graft has failed for a reason, and unless that reason is correctable and is corrected in a durable manner, it will fail again. Gardiner and Sullivan and colleagues[55, 59] have shown much better patency for thrombolysed grafts when the underlying lesion was corrected. Thus, although the same principle holds true for both thrombosed grafts and native vessels, the latter are more likely to have localized arteriosclerotic plaques as the underlying cause. The thrombosed artery also has an endothelial lining and, for most of its length, normal compliance. In contrast, prosthetic grafts characteristically do not endothelialize, and they, and even vein grafts, become poorly compliant with the passage of time after implantation. Finally, they are more likely to have obstructive lesions, which by nature do not respond well to balloon dilation (e.g., neointimal hyperplasia or a fibrous stricture).

Subacute and Chronic Arterial Occlusions

Although most of the previous comments and the supporting data refer to acute arterial occlusion, it has become apparent that some arterial thromboses may respond to catheter-directed UK infusions after a considerable delay in treatment. It was once thought

Table 166–6. **Thrombolysis in Lower Extremity Ischemia: Recent Results**

Author/Year	Agent/Dose	N*	Lytic Success (%)	Significant Complications (%)
Sullivan et al., 1989[49]	UK—low dose	35	71	22.9
	UK—high dose	23	83	8.7
Meyerovitz et al., 1990[50]	rt–PA	16	50†	31
	UK	16	38†	12.5
Cragg et al., 1991[51]	UK—high dose	17	58	
	artery graft	18	83	NG
	UK—low dose	17	71	
	artery graft	20	80	NG
Valji et al., 1991[52]	UK—artery	23	100	4 (overall)
	UK—graft	25	96	
LeBlang et al., 1992[53]	UK—low dose	132	95	7

*Infusions.
†At 24 hours.
NG, not given.

that arterial thrombi more than 2 weeks of age did not respond well to lytic agents (and delay does correlate with failure to respond to lytic treatment); however, many late thromboses do respond weeks and even months after thrombosis, so much so that it is now common thinking among interventional radiologists that if a guidewire will "pass" (i.e. traverse the occlusion), lysis is likely using high-dose UK. Motarjeme[60] and others have preferentially applied this to chronic occlusions with some success. This is probably because many chronic occlusions consist mainly of thrombosis superimposed on a discrete stenosis (termed a thrombus-dominant occlusive lesion), and these usually respond to UK and balloon angioplasty. In contrast, if the plaque is extensive and the stenosis long and irregular (a plaque-dominant occlusive lesion), one would not expect a good response to this approach. In reports of success of this approach, most of the latter lesions have probably been excluded, because balloon dilation was not applied after lysis. Although initial patency rates after successful intervention for chronic occlusive lesions have been encouraging, it remains to be seen how durable these late interventions really are. Comerota et al.[61] have carried this approach one step further, by applying a closed system infusion of UK using tourniquet control to patients in limb salvage situations in whom angiography shows no open runoff vessels, but in whom the final occlusive event is thought to have involved these same vessels. Their achievement of 50% initial limb salvage in this otherwise hopeless group of patients is a further testimony to the potential effectiveness of UK in lysing subacute and chronic arterial thrombi.

Thrombosed Arteriovenous Fistulas and Shunts

The various forms of hemodialysis access, and their revisions, are now among the most common surgical procedures performed in major hospitals in the United States. Although arteriovenous (AV) fistulas generally last longer than AV shunts using polytetrafluoroethylene (PTFE) grafts, the latter's other practical advantages have led to their greater utilization. One-year primary patency rates for PTFE AV shunts now approach 60% to 70%. Secondary patencies are significantly higher, thanks to thrombectomy or thrombolysis. With the advent of newer catheters for delivering thrombolytic agents (e.g., pulse spray catheters[52, 62]), the use of cross-catheter techniques[63] and high-dose UK, and the ability to visualize and treat by balloon angioplasty most of the underlying lesions causing thrombosis (usually neointimal hyperplasia involving the venous outflow segment), thrombolysis has become the preferred initial management of AV shunt thrombosis. It is also preferred for fistulas, where blind balloon thrombectomy could damage the endothelium of the venous outflow tract. Thrombectomy also suffers in comparison, primarily because of the inability to readily visualize and deal with the underlying lesions, the need for and cost of operating time, and the limitations placed by the fresh surgical wound on immediate use of the AV shunt for hemodialysis. Like other failed arterial grafts, the durability of thrombolysis (or thrombectomy, for that matter) depends on the ability to detect and successfully treat the underlying cause of thrombosis.

SUMMARY

Catheter-directed UK infusions can now successfully remove thrombus and restore patency in a high percentage of cases of venous, arterial, and graft thromboses and do so less traumatically and with lower morbidity than thrombectomy and, by clearing the involved segment and distal vascular bed, allow the underlying causative lesions to be visualized and their appropriate management carefully planned and deliberately carried out. It is also apparent that the long-term success of this approach depends on the ability to determine and correct the causes of thrombosis in the first place. Finally, urokinase, particularly when used in a high-dose protocol, gives faster, safer, and more complete lysis of thrombosed native vessels and grafts than other lytic regimens.

REFERENCES

1. Graor RA, Risius B, Lucas FV, et al: Thrombolysis with recombinant human tissue type plasminogen activator in patients with peripheral artery and bypass occlusions. Circulation 74(Suppl 1):15, 1986.
2. De Jaegere PP, Arnold M, Balk AH, et al: Intracranial hemorrhage in association with thrombolytic therapy: Incidence and clinical predictive factors. J Am Coll Cardiol 19:289, 1992.
3. White WF, Barlow GH, Mozen MM: The isolation and characterization of plasminogen activators (urokinase) from human urine. Biochemistry 5:2160, 1966.
4. Duckert F: Urokinase. In Markwadt F (ed): Fibrinolytics and Antifibrinolytics. New York: Springer-Verlag, 1978, pp 209–307.
5. Gunzler WA, Steffens GJ, Otting F, et al: The primary structure of high molecular mass urokinase from human urine: The complete amino-acid sequence of the A chain. Hoppe Seylers Z Physiol Chem 363:1155, 1982.
6. Steffens GJ, Gunzler WA, Otting F, et al: The complete amino-acid sequence of low molecular mass urokinase from human urine. Hoppe Seylers Z Physiol Chem 363:1043, 1982.
7. Ichinose A, Frijikawa K, Suyanma T: The activation of pro-urokinase by plasma Kalikrein and its inactivation by thrombin. J Biol Chem 261:3486, 1986.
8. Collen D: On the regulation and control of fibrinolysis. Thromb Haemost 43:77, 1980.
9. Bohmfalk JR, Fuller GM: Plasminogen is synthesized by primary cultures of rat hepatocytes. Science 209:408, 1980.
10. Wallen P, Wiman B: Characterization of human plasminogen. II. Separation and partial characterization of different forms of human plasminogen. Biochem Biophys Acta 257:122, 1972.
11. Pennica D, Holmes WE, Kohr WJ, et al: Cloning and expression of human tissue-type plasminogen activator CDNA in E. coli. Nature 301:214, 1983.
12. Ryken DC, Collen D: Purification and characterization of the plasminogen activator secreted by human melanoma cells in culture. J Biol Chem 256:7035, 1981.
13. Robbins KC, Summaria L, Hsieh B, et al: The peptide chains of human plasmin: Mechanism of activation of human plasminogen to plasmin. J Biol Chem 242:2333, 1967.
14. Groshop WR, Summaria L, Robbins KC: Studies on the active center of human plasmin: Partial amino acid sequence of peptide containing the active center serine residue. J Biol Chem 244:3590, 1969.

15. Celander DR, Guest MM: The biochemistry and physiology of urokinase. Am J Cardiol 6:409, 1960.

16. Podor TJ, Schleef RR, Loskutoff DJ: A competitive radioimmunoassay (RIA) for a fast acting inhibitor to plasminogen activator. Thromb Haemost 54(Suppl 1):218, 1985.

17. Wun TC, Scheluning WD, Reich E: Isolation and characterization of urokinase from human plasma. J. Biol Chem 257(6):3276, 1982.

18. Sherry S, Gustafson E: The current and future use of thrombolytic therapy. Annu Rev Pharmacol Toxicol 25:413, 1985.

19. Plate G, Einarsson E, Ohlin P, et al: Thrombectomy with temporary arteriovenous fistula in acute iliofemoral venous thrombosis. J Vasc Surg 1:867, 1984.

20. Plate G, Akesson H, Einarsson E, et al: Long term results of venous thrombectomy combined with a temporary arteriovenous fistula. Eur J Vasc Surg 4:483, 1994.

21. Comerota AJ: Venous thromboembolism. *In* Rutherford RB (ed): Vascular Surgery, 4th ed. Philadelphia: WB Saunders, 1995, pp 1785–1814.

22. Jeffrey P, Immelman E, Amoore J: Treatment of deep vein thrombosis with heparin or streptokinase: Long term venous function assessment [abstract no. S20.3]. London, Proceedings of the Second International Vascular Symposium, 1986.

23. Amesen H, Hoiseth A, Ly B: Streptokinase or heparin in the treatment of deep vein thrombosis: Follow up results of a prospective study. Acta Med Scand 211:65, 1982.

24. Elliot MS, Immelman EJ, Jeffery P, et al: A comparative randomized trial of heparin versus streptokinase in the treatment of acute proximal venous thrombosis: An interim report of a prospective trial. Br J Surg 66:838, 1979.

25. Kakkar W, Lawrence D: Hemodynamic and clinical assessment after therapy for acute deep vein thrombosis: A prospective study. Am J Surg 150:28, 1985.

26. Semba CP, Dake MD, Enstrom RJ, et al: Iliofemoral venous thrombosis: Treatment with regional thrombolysis [abstract]. J Vasc Intervent Radiol 4:54, 1993.

27. Kunkel JM, Machleder HL: Treatment of Paget-Schroetter syndrome: A staged multidisciplinary approach. Arch Surg 124:1153, 1989.

28. Machleder HL: Evaluation of a new treatment for Paget-Schroetter syndrome: Spontaneous thrombosis of the axillary-subclavian vein. J Vasc Surg 17:305, 1993.

29. Fraschini G, Jadeja J, Lawson M, et al: Local infusion of urokinase for the lysis of thrombosis associated with permanent central venous catheters in cancer patients. J Clin Oncol 5:672, 1987.

30. Haire WD, Lieberman RP, Lund GB, et al: Obstructed central venous catheters: Restoring function with a 12 hour infusion of low dose urokinase. Cancer 66:2279, 1990.

31. Ton DE, Wagner HN Jr: Recovery of pulmonary arterial blood flow in patients with pulmonary embolism: Thrombolytic therapy in thrombosis. A National Institutes of Health Consensus Development Conference. Ann Intern Med 93:141, 1967.

32. Terrin M, Goldhaber SZ, Thompson B, and the TIPE Investigators: Selection of patients with acute pulmonary embolism for thrombolytic therapy: Thrombolysis in pulmonary embolism (TIPE) patient study. Chest 95(Suppl):279S, 1989.

33. Urokinase pulmonary embolism trial phase 1 results: A cooperative study. JAMA 214:2163, 1970.

34. Urokinase-streptokinase embolism trial phase 2 results: A cooperative study. JAMA 229:1606, 1974.

35. Sharma GVRK, Burleson VA, Sasahara A: Effect of thrombolytic therapy on pulmonary capillary blood volume in patients with pulmonary embolism. N Engl J Med 303:842, 1980.

36. Sharma GVRK, Folland ED, McIntyre KM, Sasahara M: Long-term hemodynamic benefit of thrombolytic therapy in pulmonary embolic disease. J Am Coll Cardiol 15:65a, 1990.

37. Molina JE, Hunter DW, Yedlicka JW, Cerra FB: Thrombolytic therapy for postoperative pulmonary embolism. Am J Surg 163:375, 1992.

38. Goldhaber SZ: Evolving concepts in thrombolytic therapy for pulmonary embolism. Chest 101(4 Suppl):183S, 1992.

39. Rutherford RB, Flanigan DP, Gupta SK, et al: Suggested standards for reports dealing with lower extremity ischemia. J Vasc Surg 4:80, 1986.

40. McNamara TO, Fischer JR: Thrombolysis of peripheral arterial and graft occlusions: Improved results using high dose urokinase. AJR 144:769, 1985.

41. Berni GA, Bandyk DF, Zierler RE, et al: Streptokinase treatment of acute arterial occlusion. Ann Surg 198:185, 1983.

42. Kakkasseril JS, Cranley JJ, Anbaugh JJ, et al: Efficacy of low-dose streptokinase in acute arterial occlusion and graft thrombosis. Arch Surg 120:427, 1985.

43. Seeger JM, Flynn TC, Quintessenza JA: Intraarterial streptokinase in the treatment of acute arterial thrombosis. Surg Gynecol Obstet 164:303, 1987.

44. Belkin M, Belkin B, Bucknam CA, et al: Intraarterial fibrinolytic therapy. Efficacy of streptokinase vs urokinase. Arch Surg 121:769, 1986.

45. van Breda A, Katzen BT, Deutsch AF: Urokinase vs streptokinase in local thrombolysis. Radiology 165:109, 1987.

46. Traughber PD, Cook PS, Micklos TJ, Miller FJ: Intraarterial fibrinolytic therapy for popliteal and tibial artery obstruction: Comparison of streptokinase and urokinase. AJR 149:453, 1987.

47. Sicard GA, Schier JJ, Totty WG, et al: Thrombolytic therapy for acute arterial occlusion. J Vasc Surg 2:65, 1985. (Updated with unpublished data.)

48. Price C, Jacocks MA, Tytle T: Thrombolytic therapy in acute arterial thrombosis. Am J Surg 156:488, 1988.

49. Sullivan KL, Gardiner GA Jr, Shapiro MJ, et al: Acceleration of thrombolysis with a high-dose transthrombus bolus technique. Radiology 173:805, 1989.

50. Meyerovitz MF, Goldhaber SZ, Reagan K, et al: Recombinant tissue-type plasminogen activator versus urokinase in peripheral arterial and graft occlusions: A randomized trial. Radiology 175:75, 1990.

51. Cragg AH, Smith TP, Corson JD, et al: Two urokinase dose regimens in native arterial and graft occlusions: Initial results of a prospective randomized trial. Radiology 178:681, 1991.

52. Valji K, Roberts AC, Davis GB, Bookstein JJ: Pulsed-spray thrombolysis of arterial and bypass graft occlusions. Am J Radiol 156:617, 1991.

53. LeBlang SD, Becker GJ, Benenati JF, et al: Low-dose urokinase regimen for the treatment of lower extremity arterial and graft occlusions: Experience in 132 patients. J Vasc Intervent Radiol 3:475, 1992.

54. Gardiner GA, Harrington DP, Koltun W, et al: Salvage of occluded arterial bypass grafts by means of thrombolysis. J Vasc Surg 9:426, 1989.

55. Gardiner GA, Sullivan KL: Catheter directed thrombolysis for the failed lower extremity bypass graft. Semin Vasc Surg 5:99, 1992.

56. Rutherford RB, Rosales C: Options in the management of graft thrombosis. Acta Chir Scand 529(Suppl):101, 1985.

57. Durham JD, Gellar SC, Abbott WM, et al: Regional infusion of urokinase into occluded lower extremity bypass grafts: Long term clinical results. Radiology 172:83, 1989.

58. McNamara TO, Bomberger RA: Factors affecting initial and 6 month patency rates after intraarterial thrombolysis with high dose urokinase. Am J Surg 152:709, 1986.

59. Sullivan KL, Gardiner GA Jr, Kandarpa K, et al: Efficacy of thrombolysis in infrainguinal bypass grafts. Circulation 83(Suppl 1):99, 1991.

60. Motarjeme A: Thrombolytic therapy in arterial occlusion and graft thrombosis. Semin Vasc Surg 2:155, 1989.

61. Comerota AJ, White JV, Grosh JD: Intraoperative, intraarterial thrombolytic therapy for salvage of limbs in patients with distal arterial thrombosis. Surg Gynecol Obstet 169:283, 1989. (Updated with unpublished data.)

62. Bookstein JJ, Fellmeth B, Roberts A, et al: Pulsed spray pharmacomechanical thrombolysis: Preliminary clinical results. AJR 152:1097, 1989.

63. Kumpe DA, Cohen MAH: Treatment of failing and failed hemodialysis access sites: Comparison of surgical treatment with thrombolysis/angioplasty. Semin Vasc Surg 5:118, 1992.

Anisoylated Plasminogen-Streptokinase Activator Complex (APSAC)

Jeffrey L. Anderson, M.D., and Robert M. Califf, M.D.

HISTORY

Realization that thrombolytic agents such as streptokinase may play an important therapeutic role in acute cardiovascular diseases directed attention in the late 1970s to the development of more efficient, effective, and safer drugs. Chemists at Beecham Laboratories (London) speculated that temporary masking of the catalytic center of the plasminogen-streptokinase activator complex might confer functional advantages over streptokinase. The active site was acylated with a number of groups, from which the anisoylated compound was selected.[1] The focus on development of anisoylated plasminogen-streptokinase activator complex (APSAC)—generic name anistreplase—has been for treatment of acute myocardial infarction (AMI). Therapeutic evaluation of APSAC in other conditions involving pathologic intravascular thrombosis has begun and may be anticipated.

STRUCTURE AND CHEMISTRY

Structure

The *p*-anisoylated derivative of human lys-plasminogen-streptokinase complex,[1, 2] APSAC is prepared by acylation of the serine residue that resides in the center of the active site on plasminogen in the 1:1 plasminogen-streptokinase complex (Fig. 167–1). APSAC has a molecular weight of 131,000.

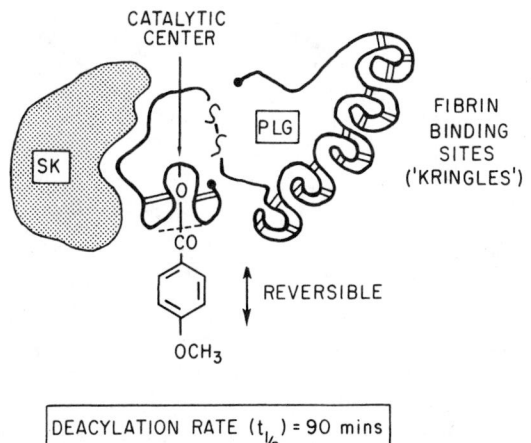

Figure 167–1. Structure of APSAC. SK, streptokinase; PLG, plasminogen. (Modified from Ferres H: Preclinical pharmacological evaluation of anisoylated plasminogen streptokinase activator complex. Drugs 33[Suppl 3]:39, 1987.)

Chemistry

APSAC is prepared by the reaction of streptokinase and human lys-plasminogen in the presence of an excess of the acylating agent *p*-amidinophenyl *p'*-anisate HCl (APAN).[1-3] Acylation is specific at the active site of plasminogen with little, if any, nondiscriminant acylation of other parts of the activator molecule.

APSAC is enzymatically inactive in the protected acyl-form and is stable in lyophilized form for at least 1 year at 5°C. When APSAC is placed in solution, deacylation occurs by simple ester hydrolysis, following pseudo-first-order kinetics in a temperature-dependent fashion. Products of this deacylation reaction are *p*-anisic acid and free activator complex in equimolar amounts. The free complex is a potent activator of plasminogen, promoting the formation of the active fibrinolytic enzyme plasmin.

The biologic potency of APSAC is expressed in units of fibrinolytic activity. The size of 1 U was selected to correspond to about 1 mg of drug. For clinical trials, APSAC is formulated in vials containing 30 U of lyophilized compound in a mixture of human albumin plus stabilizing and solubilizing agents. Vials of APSAC must be stored at 5°C until use. APSAC is reconstituted at room temperature with physiologic saline or sterile water at the time of clinical application. The reconstituted solution should be used within 30 minutes and must not be added to solutions of other infused medications.

PHARMACOLOGY
Rationale

Intravenous administration of streptokinase as a thrombolytic agent has certain disadvantages.[1, 3] On injection, streptokinase rapidly forms a complex with plasminogen in a 1:1 molar ratio. The activator complex is then subject to rapid degradation by plasma antiactivators. Simultaneously, vigorous but nonspecific systemic fibrinogenolysis and plasminemia occur. Bleeding risk increases and activity, which might otherwise be directed toward pathologic clot, is wasted in the circulation.

To improve the kinetic properties of the plasminogen-streptokinase complex, Smith et al.[1] undertook temporary chemical protection of the active site with acyl-blocking groups. Potential advantages of APSAC, based on biochemical considerations and preclinical studies, include (1) controlled and prolonged plasma clearance, (2) greater lytic potency and semiselectivity for clot, (3) superior clot retention, and (4) ability to be administered by simple, rapid injection without adverse effects.[1-3]

In the acyl form, the rates of nonspecific systemic neutralization of activator complex by plasmin inhibitors and antiactivators and degradation by autodigestion are attenuated substantially, resulting in greater persistence of fibrinolytic activity. However, the fibrin-binding sites on plasminogen are not affected by acylation and are active immediately on injection, allowing circulating APSAC to bind rapidly to fibrin clot. This property confers semiselective clot fibrinolytic activity on APSAC at lower doses (<10 mg). Given APSAC's controlled activation, semiselective binding to clot, and continued, long duration of fibrinolytic activity, greater reductions in intravascular thrombus mass (and reocclusion rates) were predicted.

Fibrin (Clot) Binding

The fibrin-binding capacity of APSAC has been compared by two methods with that of tissue-type plasminogen activator (t-PA), known to have strong fibrin affinity, and urokinase, known to have little specific affinity for fibrin.[3, 4] One method compared concentration of t-PA in human plasma and serum after the plasma was clotted by thrombin. Another assessed the relative uptakes of t-PA into human clots preformed *in vitro*. In both systems, APSAC and t-PA exhibited similarly high degrees of fibrin binding, whereas urokinase demonstrated little or no fibrin affinity. Similar experiments have shown APSAC to be at least as highly bound to forming clot as streptokinase-plasmin is.

Stability in Plasma and Molecular Integrity

Fibrinogenolysis takes place in human plasma by activation of plasminogen by streptokinase-plasmin. Sodium dodecyl sulfate (SDS)–polyacylamide gel electrophoresis, used to examine this autodigestion process, showed that acylation of streptokinase-plasminogen renders the active complex less susceptible to fast proteolytic degradation.[3, 5]

Further experiments were performed *in vitro* to determine the extent to which the streptokinase moiety in APSAC could dissociate from the complex, prematurely activating nonacylated plasminogen in the bloodstream. Tritium-labeling experiments showed that such exchange does not occur over at least 1 hour at 37°C.[6] This result demonstrates the molecular integrity of APSAC and indicates that generation of fibrinolytic activity is controlled by the rate of deacylation from APSAC's catalytic center.

Fibrin Semiselectivity

The structure of APSAC suggests the possibility of semiselectivity by binding of APSAC to clot followed by activation at the site of clot by deacylation.[1] This increased bioavailability of APSAC at the site of clot may help explain its greater thrombolytic efficacy in

animal models and humans.[3] Although little systemic activation is observed with small doses of APSAC (≤7.5 mg), at clinical doses (30 mg = 30 U), deacylation is substantial both for APSAC attached to thrombus and for excess, unbound (circulating) APSAC. After administration of 30 U of APSAC, systemic plasminemia and degradation of circulating coagulation factors (fibrinogen, α_2-antiplasmin) result and are comparable in extent with those of equivalent doses of streptokinase (1,000,000 to 1,500,000 U).[7-9]

Thrombolytic Efficacy and Platelet Effects

Preclinical experiments have shown that APSAC has greater lytic potency than streptokinase, which may be attributed to greater bioavailability at the site of thrombus because of APSAC's longer-lasting activity in the bloodstream and its superior properties of fibrin binding and clot retention.[2, 3] In a guinea pig *in vivo* pulmonary embolism model, the dose-response curve for APSAC was shifted substantially to the left of that for streptokinase-plasmin for equivalent bolus doses of both agents (Fig. 167–2).[3]

A comparison of thrombus retention and sustained activity of various plasminogen activators was evaluated in an *in vitro* experiment by immersion of preformed human thrombi for 1 minute in plasma containing equivalent concentrations of urokinase, streptokinase, and APSAC, followed by observation of clot lysis for over 5 hours.[10] Eventual thrombolysis was greater than 60% for APSAC but less than 10% of clot mass for urokinase and streptokinase, suggesting that APSAC had superior clot penetration and retention and continued thrombolytic activity.

APSAC, t-PA, or streptokinase was incubated in human plasma with 300,000 platelets/mm[3] for up to 90 minutes in clinically relevant concentrations.[11]

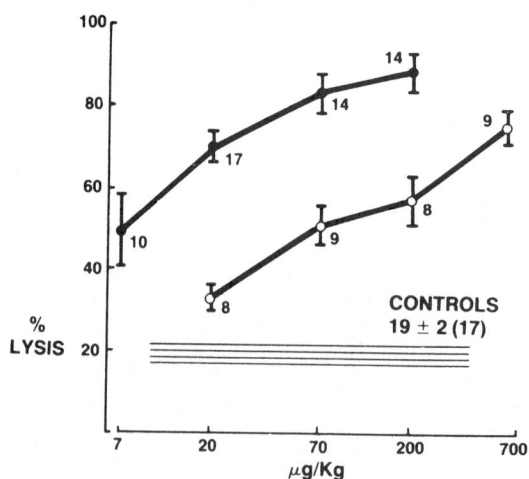

Figure 167–2. Comparison of thrombolytic efficacy on pulmonary embolism of intravenous injections of APSAC (*solid circles*) and streptokinase-plasmin (*open circles*) in guinea pigs at 4 hours. Values are mean ± SE. Numbers of animals receiving each dose are given. (From Ferres H: Preclinical pharmacological evaluation of anisoylated plasminogen streptokinase activator complex. Drugs 33[Suppl 3]:44, 1987.)

APSAC markedly inhibited platelet aggregation in response to both adenosine diphosphate (ADP) and collagen; inhibition was achieved earlier than with streptokinase. t-PA was less inhibitory, and effects were achieved only with extended incubation.

Effects of Acylation on Plasma Clearance Rates in Animal Models

Plasma clearance rates of APSAC, measured by a calibrated fibrin plate assay of total potential fibrinolytic activity (activity resulting from both acylated and nonacylated forms), have been measured *in vivo* in animal species and humans (Table 167–1). In guinea pigs, acylation increases the half-life of plasma clearance markedly, from 1.5 to 92 minutes.[3, 13] In dogs, clearance half-life is 60 minutes.[3] In rabbits, the 2.5-minute clearance half-life is increased 19-fold to 47 minutes.[3, 13] These substantial gains in bioavailability of active enzyme by acylation in animals are proportionately more dramatic than those seen in humans but are directionally similar.

Effect of Acylation on Systemic Plasmin Flux and Hemodynamic Effects

Intravenous administration of a potent plasminogen activator may cause excessive lowering of blood pressure by the rapid generation of plasmin, which generates kallikrein from prekallikrein, resulting in the formation of bradykinin, a potent vasodilator. In dogs, the ability of APSAC to delay the onset and slow the rate of plasmin generation has been implicated in explaining the substantially reduced hypotensive effect of APSAC compared with streptokinase-plasmin.[3, 14]

Summary of Preclinical Pharmacology

The important pharmacologic features of APSAC, demonstrated by preclinical investigations, include the following: (1) Acylation of the active site does not interfere with the high fibrin-binding capacity of APSAC. (2) Systemic activation of the fibrinolytic system is attenuated at low doses but only modestly attenuated at high doses (although the rate of activation is slowed) compared with streptokinase. (3) Acylation provides partial protection against autodigestion of APSAC in human plasma. (4) The streptokinase component of APSAC does not exchange with excess plasminogen in human plasma, indicating the integrity of the APSAC molecule. (5) Acylation has a marked effect on the rate at which plasminogen activator activity is cleared from the bloodstream, substantially improving bioavailability. (6) A proportionate increase in thrombolytic efficacy is seen in animal species in which the activator clearance is slowed and bioavailability improved. (7) Acylation attenuates the adverse hemodynamic consequences of potent plasminogen activator administration.

PHARMACOKINETICS

Although APSAC contains streptokinase, it exhibits a different pharmacokinetic profile, with a substantially longer plasma clearance half-life of fibrinolytic activity. The half-life of fibrinolytic activity is similar to that for deacylation, suggesting that deacylation is the limiting step in clearance.[3] It is also consistent with less neutralization by plasma inhibitors (which cannot interact with the acylated activator), slower proteolytic autodegradation, and slower clearance by the liver of the acylated form than of streptokinase. Table 167–1 compares plasma clearance of total potential fibrinolytic activity in a system of calibrated human fibrin plates in humans and animals.

Initial studies of APSAC measured the deacylation rate in a glycerol-containing buffer and determined the half-life to be about 40 minutes.[1] More recently, a radiochemical method for determining deacylation rate has allowed measurement of this rate in non–glycerol-containing buffer, plasma, whole blood, and plasma clots.[12] In these studies, the deacylation half-life at 37°C was determined to be 105 minutes in both human plasma and whole blood and about 120 minutes in clotted human plasma. The deacylation half-life was almost 150 minutes in phosphate-buffered albumin. The effect of acylation on the stability of APSAC compared with streptokinase and streptokinase-plasmin, as measured by total fibrinolytic activity in human plasma, is shown in Figure 167–3.[5] The half-life of fibrinolytic activity in these experiments was more than 120 minutes for APSAC, compared with 15 to 20 minutes for streptokinase.

These values obtained *in vitro* are similar to clearance half-lives (clearance of total potential fibrinolytic activity) found in patients with AMI (i.e., 90 to 105 minutes for APSAC[13, 15] and 18 to 23 minutes for streptokinase[16, 17]). Thus, clearance of these activators from the circulation appears to be determined largely by processes that can be examined *in vitro*.

Table 167–1. **Comparative Plasma Clearance Half-Lives for APSAC and Streptokinase-Plasmin in Various Species**

	Half-Life* (min)			
Agent	Guinea Pig	Rabbit	Dog	Human
Streptokinase-plasmin	2	3	—	15
APSAC	92	47	60	90

*Plasma clearance of total potential fibrinolytic activity (in acylated plus free enzyme). Measured by euglobulin precipitates on calibrated human fibrin plates during 24 hours at 37°C.

From Ferres H, Hibbs M, Smith RAG: Deacylation studies in vitro on anisoylated plasminogen streptokinase activator complex. Drugs 33(Suppl 3):80, 1987.

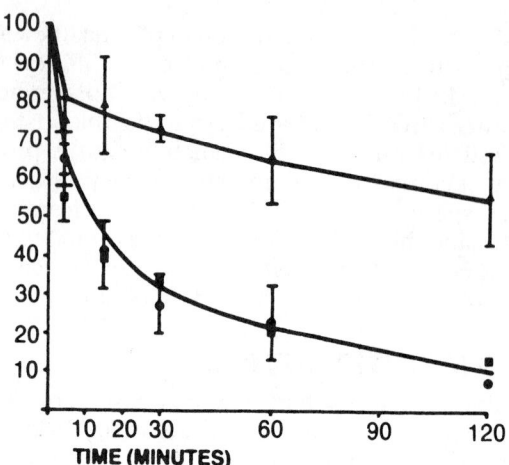

Figure 167–3. Stability of APSAC (8×10^8 M, *triangles*) compared with streptokinase (8×10^8 M, *squares*) and streptokinase-plasmin (8×10^8 M, *circles*) in human plasma *in vitro* (mean ± SE). (From Ferres H: Preclinical pharmacological evaluation of anisoylated plasminogen streptokinase activator complex. Drugs 33[Suppl 3]:42, 1987.)

In a comparative trial involving 24 AMI patients, both terminal half-life (1.2 versus 0.6 hours) and mean residence times (1.6 versus 0.8 hours) were twice as great with APSAC as with streptokinase, using a functional bioassay.[18]

As anticipated from its clearance half-life, APSAC generates plasma fibrinolytic activity for about 6 hours. However, substantially longer periods are required (1 or 2 days) to regenerate plasma clotting factors.[7–9, 19] In a dose of 30 U, APSAC was shown to reduce plasma fibrinogen levels (measured as thrombin-clottable protein) to 32% of pretreatment values at 90 minutes with recovery to 79% of baseline value by 24 hours in one large study.[20] Similarly, plasminogen and α_2-antiplasmin levels fell to 22% and 18% of initial values, respectively, at 90 minutes after APSAC administration, with recovery to 45% and 65%, respectively, by 24 hours.[20] Systemic lytic effects may be important to clinical outcome. In one study,[21] a systemic nonlytic state was associated with reperfusion failure in APSAC-treated AMI patients.

Despite previous concerns, there appears to be only a poor correlation between reductions in circulating fibrinogen after streptokinase and APSAC administration and clinical bleeding events.[9, 22, 23] Effects of these agents on physiologic clots rather than new clot formation may be more important in the usual situation.[22] Moreover, persistent effects on plasma and fibrin-clot formation and viscosity[24] may help to reduce the risk of coronary reocclusion and improve circulation to ischemic myocardium.

The effects of renal, hepatic, and other metabolic diseases on plasma pharmacokinetics of APSAC have not been determined. Because APSAC is given as a single dose and because initial degradation is primarily by enzymatic degradation in plasma, it is likely that hepatic and renal dysfunction probably exert indirect but few substantial direct effects on pharmacokinetics.

EFFECTS ON PATHOPHYSIOLOGY
Effects on Hemodynamics

Green et al.[14] showed that rapid intravenous injections of streptokinase but not APSAC lead to unacceptable hypotension in dogs. Equivalent doses of streptokinase-plasmin (comparable with a 2,000,000-U dose of streptokinase in humans) and APSAC (50 U) were given by intravenous bolus injection. Profound hypotension followed streptokinase administration within 3 minutes, characterized by 50% reductions in mean blood pressure. APSAC injections did not affect blood pressure. Streptokinase injections were associated with abrupt generation of large quantities of plasmin, which causes activation of the kininogen system with production of the vasodilator bradykinin, whereas generation of plasmin after APSAC was more gradual.

In human studies, Lew et al.[25] administered streptokinase in a dose of 750,000 U over 30 minutes and measured blood pressure changes in a consecutive series of 98 patients with AMI. The maximum blood pressure fall occurred at 15 minutes and consisted of a mean decline of 35 mmHg in systolic and 19 mmHg in diastolic blood pressure (24-mmHg mean fall). After a 2- to 4-minute rapid injection of 30 U of APSAC (equivalent to 1,100,000 U of streptokinase), mean blood pressure declined by a median of 10 mmHg (mean, 14 mmHg) in 240 patients with AMI in a multicenter United States trial.[20] Clinical hypotension after administration of APSAC was reported in this trial in 20% of patients but was typically transient (resolving within 15 minutes) and without lasting consequences. A direct comparison of blood pressure effects of the two drugs, both administered intravenously but over differing but clinically recommended periods (i.e., about 3 minutes versus 60 minutes), showed a similar profile except for a small (4- to 5-mmHg), transient, early (at 5 to 10 minutes) differential fall in blood pressure after the much more rapidly administered APSAC.[26]

Effects on Ventricular Function

APSAC is not known to have any direct negative (or positive) inotropic effects on ventricular function. However, important indirect effects on function may result from reperfusion. It is well established that timely reperfusion by a number of thrombolytic agents, when accomplished within 2 to 4 hours of the onset of symptoms, leads to improved ventricular function.[27–33] Improvement in function is less likely when reperfusion is delayed beyond 4 to 6 hours. Studies with APSAC also have noted a beneficial effect on left ventricular function.[34, 35] Been et al.[34] studied left ventricular function by radionuclide ventriculography in 91 patients given APSAC or placebo within 4 hours of the onset of AMI. Left ventricular function was measured at 10 days and at 6 months, and benefit correlated with timing of treatment and site of infarction. Bassand et al.[35] measured the effects of therapy on left ventricular function in 231 patients randomized to APSAC or heparin at 3.1 ± 1.0 hours after the onset of symptoms of a first AMI. Left ventricular ejection fraction, determined by contrast angiography on day 4 in 209 patients, was significantly greater after APSAC (53% ± 13%) than after heparin (47% ± 12%) (p = .002). At 3 weeks, the difference (determined by radionuclide ventriculography) remained significant for the anterior infarct group. Ejection fraction and infarct size were inversely related. Infarct size, determined by thallium-201 computed tomography, was reduced by 31% overall (p < .01), 33% for the anterior and 16% for the inferior infarct groups.

Effects on Electrophysiology

APSAC has no direct myocardial electrophysiologic effects. Indirect effects might be expected as a consequence of reperfusion (e.g., reperfusion arrhythmias) and ventricular myocardial salvage.

Effects on Coronary Blood Flow

The major effects of APSAC relate to changes in coronary blood flow as a result of thrombolysis and are discussed in detail in the clinical study section. In several studies, coronary perfusion formed the primary outcome variable. In doses causing systemic fibrinogenolysis, APSAC also reduces blood viscosity,[24] similar to the demonstrated effects of streptokinase. Sherry[36] and others have postulated that this reduced viscosity improves microcirculatory flow in ischemic myocardium. Microcirculatory effects remain to be well documented and quantified in careful clinical trials.

Effects on Peripheral Vascular Resistance and Blood Pressure

By generating plasmin and bradykinin, APSAC acts as a vasodilator, reducing vascular resistance and blood pressure, a potentially beneficial effect. The hypotensive effects of APSAC are discussed in the hemodynamic and clinical trial sections. Generally, hypotensive effects are transient, usually resolving within 10 to 15 minutes.

Other Pathophysiologic Effects

APSAC causes no consistent endocrine or metabolic effects and does not affect renal function directly. Indirect effects on renal function may occur as a result of changes in cardiac function and effects on peripheral vascular resistance. Effects on blood chemistry are discussed later. Rarely, cholesterol emboli have been noted with or without APSAC (or any other thrombolytic agent).

CLINICAL TRIALS AND USE
Clinical Experience and Drug Indications

APSAC was approved for thrombolytic therapy of AMI in Belgium and Germany in 1986, in the United Kingdom in 1989, and in the United States in 1990. Although thrombolytic therapy for AMI is the only currently approved indication, future applications could include the treatment of other pathologic vascular thrombotic syndromes such as pulmonary embolism[37] and peripheral venous and arterial thrombosis.[38] Efficacy and safety results with APSAC are summarized in the following sections.[39, 40]

Initial Clinical Perfusion Trials and Dose-Ranging Information

Kasper et al.[41] demonstrated the ability of APSAC to cause thrombolysis when administered by the intracoronary route; they observed reperfusion in 15 of 22 patients (68%) at a mean of 42 ± 37 minutes after intracoronary administration of the drug. However, the unique features of APSAC favor its development for intravenous use, as was suggested by several early trials in patients with AMI.[15, 39–47] Initial experience used a range of intravenous doses (5 to 30 U) and suggested dose-response behavior. In these trials, coronary patency rates of about 30% to 40% were observed with 5 to 10 U, 40% to 50% with 15 U, 60% with 20 to 25 U, and up to 80% with 30 U. Larger doses (≥10 U) caused substantial systemic fibrinogenolysis but lower reocclusion rates. In a U.S. dose-ranging trial, Marder et al.[19] administered doses of 5, 15, and 30 U of APSAC to 29 AMI patients with documented coronary occlusion. Reperfusion occurred in 21% of patients (3 of 14 patients) given 5 U, 43% (3 of 7 patients) given 15 U, and 60% (9 of 15 patients) given 30 U. In an angiographically controlled clinical trial versus placebo, APSAC (30 U) achieved reperfusion in 9 of 16 patients (56%), compared with 1 of 11 (9%) with placebo (p < .05).[48] On the basis of these and other data, a dose of 30 U of APSAC has generally been used in subsequent trials.

Controlled Reperfusion Comparisons of APSAC versus Intracoronary Administration of Streptokinase

Until November 1987, intracoronary administration of streptokinase was the approved standard thrombolytic regimen in the United States for comparisons with new regimens.

A multicenter, randomized United States trial compared the reperfusion potential of intravenously administered APSAC and intracoronary streptokinase administration in AMI patients who could be studied angiographically within 6 hours of the onset of symptoms.[20] After coronary occlusion (TIMI flow grade 0 or 1) had been confirmed by coronary angiography, patients were randomized to receive either APSAC, 30 U by intravenous injection over 2 to 4 minutes, or streptokinase, 20,000-U bolus followed by 2000 U/min for 60 minutes via the intracoronary route. Treatment was given at a mean of 3.4 hours (range 0.4 to 6) after onset of AMI. Both groups also received heparin for at least 24 hours. Reperfusion was evaluated angiographically over 90 minutes, and success was defined as advancement of grade 0 or 1 flow to grade 2 or 3 flow. Rates of reperfusion for the two regimens were 51% (59 of 115 patients) at 90 minutes after intravenous APSAC administration and 60% (67 of 111 patients) after 60 minutes of intracoronary streptokinase administration (p = NS). Reperfusion occurred at 43 ± 23 minutes after intravenous and 31 ± 17 minutes after intracoronary therapy. Success of intravenous therapy depended on time to treatment: intravenous APSAC therapy yielded rates of reperfusion identical to those of intracoronary therapy when given within 4 hours of symptom onset (60% for each regimen) but lower rates of reperfusion when administered later (33% versus 61%, p < .03) (Fig. 167–4). Reperfusion success for both therapies was substantially greater when even minimal initial flow was present (78% reperfusion rates for grade 1 and 48% for grade 0 flow). Additional interventions were given frequently when indicated (intracoronary guidewire or angioplasty procedures or bypass surgery in 97 of 240 patients) and were well tolerated, and reocclusion and mortality rates during the in-hospital course were low.

A Dutch trial comparing APSAC with intracoronary streptokinase administration used a higher infusion rate of intracoronary streptokinase (250,000 U over 1 hour) and achieved a shorter mean time to treatment (2.4 hours).[49, 50] Among 85 randomly assigned patients, reperfusion success was achieved in 64% of evaluable patients treated with APSAC and 68% treated with streptokinase (p = NS). Both groups subsequently received heparin. Among patients not receiving early mechanical intervention, reocclusion

at 24 hours was observed in only one APSAC-treated patient and in three streptokinase-treated patients. Bleeding and other adverse events were comparable in both groups.

The reperfusion potential of intravenously administered APSAC is thus 60% to 65% when given within 4 hours of symptom onset to patients with AMI and coronary occlusion, approximately comparable with that of intracoronary streptokinase administration.

Comparisons of Intravenously Administered APSAC and Intravenously Administered Streptokinase

The 90-minute reperfusion potential of intravenously administered APSAC and of intravenously administered streptokinase in patients with AMI and coronary occlusion can be compared indirectly by comparing results from the U.S. APSAC multicenter study and the TIMI study.[20, 51] The overall reperfusion rate with APSAC was higher than with streptokinase (51% versus 31%), as was reperfusion after early therapy (≤4 hours of symptoms, 60% versus 44%) and later therapy (4 to 6 hours of symptoms, 33% versus 24%) (see Fig. 167–4).

A European patency study directly compared intravenously administered APSAC and intravenously administered streptokinase: 116 patients with AMI were randomly assigned within 6 hours of the onset of symptoms to receive either APSAC, 30 U given over 5 minutes, or streptokinase, 1,500,000 U infused over 1 hour.[52] Patency, defined as coronary flow grade 2 or 3, was determined angiographically in 107 patients at an average of 98 minutes after initiation of treatment. APSAC achieved a patency rate of 70% (38 of 54 patients) and streptokinase achieved a rate of 51% (27 of 53 patients, p < .05). Both agents caused comparable falls in circulating fibrinogen levels, and clinical outcomes were similar. These results are similar to the comparison between standard-dose, intravenously administered t-PA and streptokinase in an earlier European patency trial (respective patency rates of 70% and 55%).[53]

A large double-blind patency trial of intravenously administered APSAC and intravenously administered streptokinase was performed in the United States in 370 patients younger than 76 years who were entered within 4 hours of onset of symptoms and randomized to APSAC (30 U over 2 to 5 minutes) or streptokinase (1.5 million U over 1 hour).[26] Coronary patency was determined angiographically at a median of 2.1 hours later. Overall patency rates (TIMI grades 2 and 3) were high after both APSAC (72%) and streptokinase (73%), although patent arteries showed "complete" (grade 3) perfusion more often after APSAC (83% versus 72%, p = .03). Reocclusion within 1 day, defined angiographically, was low (APSAC, 1 of 96 patients; streptokinase, 2 of 94 patients). In-hospital mortality (5.9% versus 7.1%), stroke (0.5% versus 1.6%), and other adverse event rates did not differ significantly.

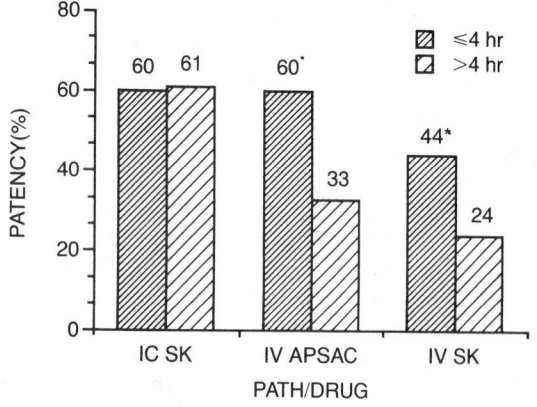

Figure 167– 4. Comparisons of reperfusion rates of streptokinase (SK) administered via the intracoronary route (IC SK), intravenously administered APSAC (IV APSAC), and intravenously administered streptokinase (IV SK) for AMI patients treated early (≤4 hours) and late (>4 hours) after onset of symptoms. *, p < .05 versus ≤4 hours. (Data for IC SK and IV APSAC from Anderson JL, Rothbard RL, Hackworthy RA, et al: Multicenter reperfusion trial of intravenous anisoylated plasminogen streptokinase activator complex [APSAC] in acute myocardial infarction: Controlled comparison with intracoronary streptokinase. J Am Coll Cardiol 11[6]:53, 1988; data for IV SK from Chesebro JH, Knatterud G, Roberts R, et al: Thrombolysis in myocardial infarction [TIMI] trial, phase I: A comparison between intravenous tissue plasminogen activator and intravenous streptokinase. Circulation 76:142, 1987.)

Reocclusion and Reinfarction
Potential after APSAC

Reocclusion may be an important morbid event, often leading to reinfarction and loss of clinical benefit. However, little information is available, because assessment requires a second angiographic study. The Anistreplase Reperfusion and Reocclusion Multicenter Study (ARMS) was designed to specifically study reocclusion in 156 AMI patients successfully treated with APSAC within 4 hours of symptom onset.[54] Initial (90-minute) patency was 73%; 96% of initially patent arteries (102 of 106) remained patent at the 24-hour angiogram, and only four (4%) had reoccluded. Information on reocclusion within 1 to 3 days has been summarized for 289 patients treated in several other clinical studies; angiographic reocclusion was documented in only nine (3.1%).[55] These rates are lower than those reported for conventional-dose t-PA and similar to or lower than rates for streptokinase.

Clinical reinfarction during hospitalization after APSAC has been summarized from a relatively large patient database (n = 1058).[55] Early hospital reinfarction (within 1 to 3 days) was noted in 3.7% of patients, and reinfarction occurring at any time during hospitalization was noted in 8.5%. In the ISIS-3 experience,[56] reinfarction after APSAC was reported in 3.5% of patients, identical to the rate for streptokinase.

Overall Patency Profile after
APSAC and Other Thrombolytics

Granger et al. performed an overview of patency studies of thrombolytic regimens to assess overall patency profiles.[57] Patency (TIMI 2/3) after APSAC administration averaged 61% at 60 minutes (n = 260), 70% at 90 minutes (n = 511), 74% at 2 to 3 hours (n = 232), 80% at 1 day (n = 854), and 85% at 3 to 21 days (n = 344) (Fig. 167–5). Patency was greater than that following nonthrombolytic therapy at all time

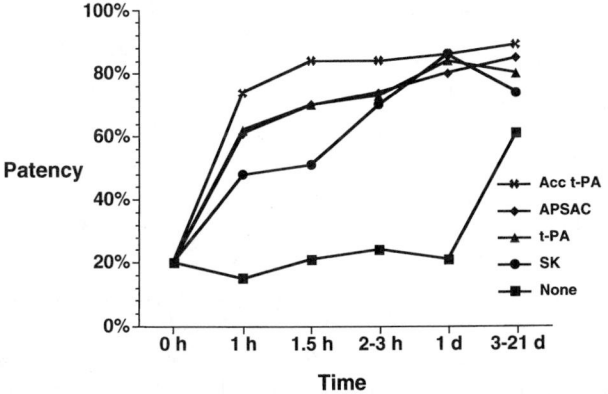

Figure 167–5. Patency profiles of thrombolytic drugs at various times after treatment. APSAC and t-PA track together. Streptokinase (SK) initially tracks behind and accelerated (Acc) t-PA ahead. All tend to merge by 1 day. (Modified from Granger CB, Califf RM, Topol EJ: Thrombolytic therapy for acute myocardial infarction: A review. Drugs 44:293, 1992.)

points, greater than patency after streptokinase administration at 60 and 90 minutes, virtually identical to patency after standard regimens of rt-PA at all time points, but less than that of accelerated-dose alteplase at 60 and 90 minutes. In an independent patency overview, early (90 to 240 minutes) and late patency (≥1 day) after APSAC administration averaged 72.1% (n = 767) and 84.5% (n = 1042), respectively.[58] The early patency rate was favorable compared with that of streptokinase, and the late patency rate was favorable compared with that of standard-dose rt-PA.[58]

Functional and Patency Comparisons of
APSAC and Tissue-Type Plasminogen Activator

To determine the relative clinical efficacy and safety of t-PA[59] and APSAC, a direct, randomized comparison trial (TEAM-3) was undertaken.[60]

A total of 325 patients with AMI, 75 years or younger and in whom symptom duration was 4 hours or less and the ST segment was elevated, were enrolled and randomized to blindly receive standard doses of APSAC (30 U for 2 to 5 minutes) or rt-PA (100 mg over 3 hours), each with aspirin and intravenously administered heparin. Time to treatment averaged 2.7 hours. The specific comparisons of interest were (1) left ventricular ejection fraction, (2) clinical morbidity and need for mechanical intervention, and (3) coronary patency. Rest ejection fraction, the primary end point, measured at discharge and at 1 month, favored rt-PA by small differences (2 to 4 percentage points, $p < .05$ to .01) that were due to differences in infarct zone function and end-systolic volumes. However, convalescent ejection fractions were excellent in both groups (mean, >50%), and exercise responses were comparable. Clinical outcomes were also comparable and favorable, as assessed by the clinical morbidity index, and the 1-day coronary artery patency rate (TIMI grades 2/3) was similarly high in both groups (APSAC 89%, rt-PA 86%). Bleeding episodes and transfusion requirements were somewhat greater after the APSAC plus heparin than the rt-PA plus heparin regimen, suggesting that intravenously administered heparin given shortly after APSAC administration should probably be avoided (see later). One possible explanation for the difference in global ejection fraction between agents is that thrombolysis may proceed more rapidly after treatment with fibrin-selective than after treatment with non–fibrin-selective agents, a difference that may influence myocardial salvage in the early hours (i.e., <2 to 3 hours) after coronary occlusion.

In another, smaller randomized trial comparing the functional outcome after APSAC and rt-PA administration in 183 French patients, ejection fractions averaged 50% after APSAC and 52% after rt-PA at the 5-day angiographic study (p = NS) and 48% and 47%, respectively, at the radionuclide study conducted at 18 ± 5 days (p = NS).[61] As in the TEAM-3 study, clinical outcomes were similar in the two groups.[61]

The rT-PA–APSAC Patency Study (TAPS) compared the kinetics of reperfusion with a front-loaded regimen of rt-PA (100 mg over 90 minutes) and with APSAC (30 U over 5 minutes) in 421 patients with AMI who were treated at a mean of 2.6 hours after symptom onset.[62] Patency was achieved faster after rt-PA than after APSAC administration as demonstrated by coronary angiography at 60 minutes (TIMI grade 2/3 73% versus 60%, $p < .01$) and at 90 minutes (84% versus 70%, $p < .001$), whereas later patency rates (at 1 to 2 days) favored APSAC (rt-PA 85%, APSAC 93%, $p < .03$), as did the reocclusion rate within 1 to 2 days (rt-PA 10.3%, APSAC 2.5%, $p < .01$). Bleeding and morbidity and mortality rates were greater after APSAC administration, but comparisons were confounded by the aggressive use of intravenously administered heparin with APSAC and the greater use of interventions in the APSAC group at the 90-minute angiogram.

Combination therapy using fibrin-selective and non–fibrin-selective agents has been proposed for clinical testing. The TIMI-4 trial compared three regimens for AMI in 367 patients: front-loaded rt-PA, APSAC, or both (each in slightly reduced dosage), each given with intravenously administered and aspirin.[63] A composite end point was used and was defined as the sum of death, intracranial hemorrhage, severe heart failure or shock, ejection fraction below 40%, reinfarction, major spontaneous hemorrhage, TIMI flow below 2 at 90 minutes or 1 day, reocclusion (confirmed by radionuclide [MIBI] testing), or anaphylaxis during the hospital stay. The combination regimen achieved the worst score (54% reaching one of the unsatisfactory outcome end points versus 41% for rt-PA, $p < .06$), with trends to greater hemorrhagic events and greater in-hospital mortality without improved patency.[63] The rt-PA alone regimen showed the best composite outcome, including the highest patency rate at 90 minutes (84%). The addition of intravenously administered heparin to the APSAC regimen, now believed to be unnecessary when aspirin is given (see later), may have added to morbidity in the APSAC arm.

Effects of APSAC Therapy on Mortality after AMI Compared with Placebo and Other Thrombolytics

Although early trials with APSAC were too small to assess mortality effects, pooling the controlled trials in a meta-analysis yielded strong suggestive evidence for a mortality benefit of APSAC therapy.[39] In these trials, 708 patients received nonthrombolytic therapy (standard therapy, placebo, or heparin), and 1386 received APSAC (more than 85% received 30 U). The early mortality rate (in hospital or within 1 month) was 6.1% after APSAC and 12.3% after standard therapy ($p < .001$).

A randomized mortality trial (APSAC Intervention Mortality Study, or AIMS) followed and confirmed the potential for APSAC to reduce mortality.[64, 65] In this multicenter trial coordinated in the United Kingdom, patients presenting within 6 hours of AMI were randomly assigned to 30 U of APSAC or placebo together with heparin and subsequent warfarin (Coumarin) and other standard therapy (e.g., β-blockade); patients were then followed for mortality outcome (at 1 month and at 1 year). AIMS was stopped early by the safety monitoring board after 1258 patients had been entered because of substantial mortality differences in favor of thrombolytic therapy (Fig. 167–6). After 30 days, mortality after APSAC was 6.4% compared with 12.1% after placebo ($p = .0006$), an actuarial odds reduction in mortality of 51% (95% confidence interval, 26% to 67%). One-year mortality rates showed a similar contrast: 11.1% for APSAC versus 17.8% for placebo, an odds reduction of 43% ($p = .0007$). Reductions in mortality were large, both in patients treated relatively late (4 to 6 hours after symptom onset) and in those treated earlier (<4 hours after symptom onset), and these reductions occurred in both patients who were over age 65 years and younger patients (Table 167–2). APSAC also provided safe therapy. The overall incidence of stroke was 8 in the APSAC group and 4 in the placebo group (absolute difference −0.5%). The absolute differential rates of anaphylaxis, hemorrhage, and transfusion were 0.6%, 9.7%, and 0%, respectively.

The ISIS-3 trial was a randomized, blinded comparison of streptokinase (1.5 million U over 1 hour) versus t-PA (duteplase, 0.60 million U/kg over 4 hours) versus APSAC (30 U over 3 minutes) among 41,299 patients with suspected AMI presenting within 24 hours of symptom onset. Median time to randomization was 4 hours.[56] Mortality rates were comparable among the three thrombolytic regimens at the 5-week end point (streptokinase 10.6%, t-PA 10.3%, APSAC 10.5%) and at 6 months (14.0%, 14.1%, 13.7%, respectively). The risk of cerebral hemorrhage with APSAC (0.55%) was intermediate between that of streptokinase (0.24%) and t-PA (0.66%). APSAC was associated with a slightly but significantly greater risk of allergy than streptokinase was; t-PA had the fewest reports of allergy, and streptokinase had the fewest reports of noncerebral hemorrhage. Transfusions were compara-

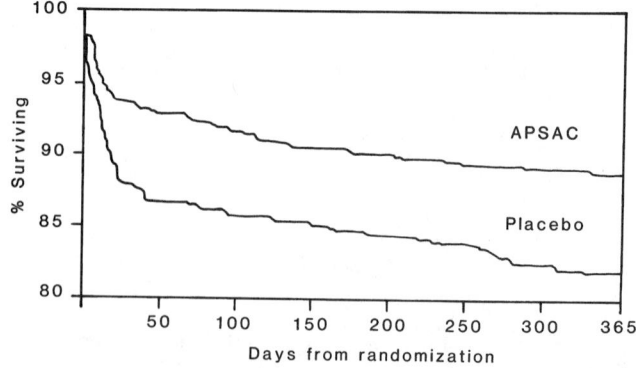

Figure 167–6. One-year survival curves of acute myocardial infarction patients randomly assigned to treatment with anistreplase (APSAC) or placebo in the AIMS trial. The curves are significantly different ($p = .0007$). (From AIMS Trial Study Group: Long-term effects of intravenous anistreplase in acute myocardial infarction: Final report of the AIMS study. Lancet 335:427, 1990. © by The Lancet Ltd., 1990.)

Table 167–2. **Survival Effects after AMI for Patients Given APSAC or Placebo: The AIMS Trial**

Criterion	Therapy	Patients	30-Day Mortality (%)	Change* (%)	Estimated 1-Year Mortality (%)	Change* (%)
All Patients	APSAC	624	6.4	−47	11.1	−38
	Placebo	634	12.1		17.8	
Time to Therapy (hr)						
0–4	APSAC	414	5.1	−46	8.9	−43
	Placebo	410	9.5		15.6	
4–6	APSAC	196	8.2	−44	14.3	−27
	Placebo	204	14.7		19.6	
Age (yr)						
<60	APSAC	372	4.0	−34	7.5	−32
	Placebo	379	6.1		11.1	
≤60	APSAC	252	9.9	−54	16.3	−42
	Placebo	254	21.3		28.0	

AIMS, APSAC in Myocardial Infarction Study; AMI, acute myocardial infarction; APSAC, anisoylated plasminogen-streptokinase activator complex.
*At end of observation period risk reduction.
Data from AIMS Trial Study Group: Effect of intravenous APSAC on mortality after acute myocardial infarction: Preliminary report of a placebo-controlled clinical trial. Lancet 1:545, 1988; and AIMS Trial Study Group: Long-term effects of intravenous anistreplase in acute myocardial infarction: Final report of the AIMS study. Lancet 335:427, 1990.

ble among agents, however. ISIS-3 showed that when the three agents were given at a similar (and relatively late) time from symptom onset, their mortality outcomes were not significantly different. However, the design of ISIS-3 did not allow evaluation of the primary advantage of APSAC over the other thrombolytic agents, namely, the greater ease and time-efficiency of its administration (versus streptokinase and t-PA), as well as its greater thrombolytic efficiency (versus streptokinase) when given early after symptom onset.

Emergency Department and Prehospital Use of APSAC

One of the most promising approaches to improving the efficacy of thrombolytic therapy is the earlier treatment of patients with AMI, with a goal of therapy within the first 60 to 90 minutes after symptom onset. APSAC is particularly well suited to the acute care setting, given its ease of administration. The Virginia Thrombolytic Therapy Study Group found that urban hospital location, teaching hospital status, a high case volume of AMI patients, stocking and starting of drug in the emergency department, and decision to treat by an emergency physician were factors correlating with reduced hospital delay to therapy.[66] In addition, the use of a simple, single-injection thrombolytic regimen with APSAC resulted in shorter drug processing time (9 ± 4 versus 23 ± 16 minutes) and total hospital time to therapy (33 ± 16 versus 66 ± 43 minutes) than with a more complex infusion regimen of rt-PA therapy. APSAC has also been evaluated in the prehospital setting and has resulted in a further improvement in mortality benefit (see later).

Intuitively, prehospital initiation of thrombolytic therapy is the most promising approach to reducing overall time to therapy and hence, optimizing outcome, but this approach is complicated by strategic challenges and safety concerns. APSAC's simple, sin-gle-injection regimen is well suited to use in the prehospital setting and was tested in the 163-center European Myocardial Infarction Project (EMIP).[67] The objective of EMIP was to demonstrate whether additional mortality benefit at 30 days could be achieved by the earlier administration of thrombolytic agent before admission rather than in the hospital. The size of EMIP was reduced from the proposed sample size of 10,000 patients because of funding problems, but the results are nonetheless of interest. A total of 5469 patients who were attended in the field by emergency medical personnel within 6 hours of the onset of symptoms were randomly assigned to receive double-blind therapy with either APSAC before admission followed by placebo in the hospital (prehospital group) or placebo in the field followed by APSAC in the hospital (hospital group). The prehospital group received thrombolytic therapy a median of 55 minutes earlier than the hospital group did. (The median overall symptom-to-treatment time was 130 minutes in the prehospital and 190 minutes in the in-hospital group.) ST elevation was present in 87.2% of patients on presentation, and AMI was subsequently confirmed in 87.8%. At 30 days, death from cardiac causes was reduced by 16% by prehospital therapy (8.3% versus 9.8%, $p < .05$), and overall mortality was reduced by 13% (9.7% versus 11.1%, $p = .08$). The overall incidence of adverse events, except for symptomatic hypotension, was similar for both groups, although certain events occurred more frequently before hospitalization in the prehospital group (i.e., ventricular fibrillation, bradycardia, hypotension, and shock). Reduction in cardiac mortality was related to the length of time between the prehospital and the in-hospital injections: risk was reduced significantly in the prehospital group for those in whom the interval between injections was longer than 90 minutes (relative risk 0.55, $p = .04$).

In a smaller, randomized British prehospital study (GREAT),[68] APSAC could be administered by general practitioners in patients' homes an average of 101 minutes after onset of symptoms compared with 240 minutes when given in the hospital. The 3-month mortality rate was less in patients given thrombolytic therapy at home (13 of 163, 8.0%) than in the hospital (23 of 148, 15.5%) (risk reduction 49%, $p = .04$).

Adverse Effects, Precautions, and Contraindications

The adverse potential of APSAC is generally similar to or slightly greater than that of standard doses of streptokinase. These adverse effects are most commonly hemorrhagic and allergic. Selected adverse event rates in the placebo-controlled AIMS trial are shown in Table 167–3. The hemodynamic effects of APSAC have been discussed.

Bleeding

As expected, bleeding after APSAC has been reported more commonly in studies requiring invasive procedures (coronary angiography). In a comparative trial of APSAC and intracoronary streptokinase,[20] bleeding events were reported after APSAC in 33% of patients, but 58% of bleeding events occurred at the catheter insertion site. Hematocrit fell by more than 10 percentage points within 24 hours of treatment in 19% of patients receiving APSAC and similarly in 15% of patients given low doses of streptokinase administered via the intracoronary route. Transfusions unrelated to coronary bypass surgery were required in 21 (17%) of APSAC-treated patients. In worldwide experience with 5275 patients, 14.6% of patients receiving APSAC (30 U) were reported to experience hemorrhagic events, but these were severe in only 1.6%.[39, 40] Most of these events occurred at the site of arterial puncture; gastrointestinal bleeding, hemoptysis, and hematemesis were reported infrequently (generally at a rate of <1%). Event rates were higher in studies requiring angiography (22% versus 13%).

Of concern with all thrombolytic agents is the risk of cerebrovascular accidents. Potentially hemorrhagic cerebrovascular accidents were reported in 30 (0.57%) of 5275 patients.[39, 40] This incidence is approximately comparable (i.e., 0.5% ± 0.3%) with that reported for intravenously administered streptokinase[27, 69, 70] and t-PA.[59]

The size of ISIS-3 (41,299 patients) allows an excellent opportunity to assess and compare relatively uncommon adverse events of therapy among various thrombolytic regimens, including APSAC.[56] APSAC led to slightly more hemorrhagic events than did streptokinase, as might be expected because of APSAC's greater fibrinolytic efficiency. Noncerebral bleeds were reported in 5.4% of patients after APSAC, in 5.2% after t-PA, but in 4.5% after streptokinase; a similar and smaller percentage required transfusion after each regimen, however (1.0%, 0.8%, and 0.9%, respectively). The risk of cerebral hemorrhage was also somewhat greater after APSAC than streptokinase (0.55% versus 0.24%) but tended to be less than the risk after t-PA (0.66%).

In an overview of clinical trials, respective rates of total and hemorrhagic stroke were 0.91% and 0.38% for APSAC, 0.69% and 0.17% for streptokinase, and 1.27% and 0.50% for t-PA (alteplase).[58]

Potential Allergic Events

Because APSAC contains streptokinase, a known antigen, occasional allergy or hypersensitivity might be expected. Of 1152 patients treated with 30 U of APSAC, 61 (5%) developed a possible allergic reaction.[39] Serious allergic reactions, such as anaphylaxis and bronchoconstriction, occurred rarely (11 of 5275 patients, 0.2% incidence) and responded to symptomatic treatment.[39, 64] Purpuric skin rashes are another uncommon reported adverse manifestation of therapy (1% incidence).[39, 64] More commonly, fever, flushing, or chills have been observed (5% to 10% of patients).[20]

In the ISIS-3 experience,[56] allergic reactions were reported in 5.1% of patients after APSAC compared with 3.6% after streptokinase and 0.8% after t-PA. Most of these reactions were minor, with only 0.5%, 0.3%, and 0.1%, respectively, of patients developing severe or persistent symptoms. Hypotension was reported in a similar percentage of patients after APSAC (12.5%) and streptokinase (11.8%) and less commonly after t-PA (7.1%); about half of these epi-

Table 167–3. Other Clinical Events after AMI in Patients given APSAC or Placebo: The AIMS Trial[65]

Event (n)	APSAC (n = 624)	Placebo (n = 634)	Absolute % Change (%A minus %P)
Cardiogenic shock	16	29	−2.0 ($p = .07$)
Cardiac rupture	5	13	−1.2 ($p = .09$)
Cardiac failure	131	154	−3.3 ($p = .2$)
Ventricular fibrillation	41	46	−0.7 ($p = .7$)
Pericarditis	43	98	−8.6 ($p < .001$)
Reinfarction (in-hospital)	38	30	1.4 ($p = .3$)
Hemorrhage (any)	86	26	9.7 ($p < .001$)
Transfusion	5	5	0.0 ($p = 1.0$)
Anaphylaxis	4	0	0.6 ($p = .06$)
Other allergy	11	17	−0.9 ($p = .3$)
Stroke	8	4	0.7 ($p = .4$)
Stroke or TIA	13	5	1.0 ($p = .06$)

AMI, acute myocardial infarction; TIA, transient ischemic attack.

sodes required treatment. Thus, potentially allergic or hypotensive reactions can occur with APSAC but are rarely severe, and they occur at a rate similar to or slightly greater than that of streptokinase.

Despite the small risk of allergy, routine (prophylactic) administration of corticosteroids is generally not indicated because of the uncertain effect on myocardial infarct healing and because APSAC generally is well tolerated without such therapy.

Other Adverse Events

Other, occasionally reported adverse experiences of uncertain cause include dyspnea, headache, flushing, and chest pain. They may relate to symptoms of myocardial infarction and to the vasodilating effects of APSAC and other therapy.

Arrhythmias have often been reported after APSAC but are common during the course of AMI, particularly in association with reperfusion, and have been reported in about 15% of both actively treated and placebo-receiving groups. Symptomatic hypotension was reported in the pharmaceutical database among 8% of APSAC-treated patients and 5% of placebo-treated patients during the course of therapy.[39] Effects of APSAC therapy on parameters of blood coagulation result from its therapeutic effects and have been reviewed earlier (see section on pharmacokinetics).[7–9, 19, 20]

After treatment with APSAC, the mean decline in hemoglobin concentration has averaged 10% during the first 24 hours, with a maximum decline of 15.6% (after 3 days) and a return toward normal within 1 week. In these patients, the fall may result from frequent blood testing and hemodilution as well as from hemorrhage.

Other effects of APSAC on blood test results have been unremarkable, but liver function has risen transiently after active and control treatments, making it difficult to separate drug effects from changes associated with AMI. No instances of transmission of infectious agents by plasminogen-containing APSAC have been reported.

Contraindications

Absolute and relative contraindications to APSAC are similar to those for streptokinase (Table 167–4). Absolute contraindications include active internal bleeding, known allergy to APSAC or streptokinase, and a history (particularly recent) of intracranial pathology. Other (relative) contraindications are also summarized in Table 167–4.

Interference with Other Drugs

No known pharmacologic interaction with APSAC and other commonly used cardiovascular drugs has been described. Pharmacodynamic interactions may occur with other drugs causing vasodilation and hypotension during early AMI and agents such as heparin and aspirin, which predispose to hemorrhage.

Table 167–4. **Contraindications to Thrombolytic Therapy**

Absolute Contraindications
Active internal bleeding
History of cerebrovascular accident or disease (especially recent); neurologic procedure or surgery within 2 mo

Relative Contraindications
Known hemostatic deficiencies and coagulation defects, including those associated with advanced hepatic or renal disease
Recent major surgery (especially <10 days)
Recent gastrointestinal bleeding or active ulcer disease (<6 mo)
Cardiopulmonary resuscitation, especially if traumatic (e.g., rib fractures); traumatic intubation
Recent organ biopsy, puncture of noncompressible blood vessel, thoracentesis, paracentesis, lumbar puncture
Pregnancy, early postpartum period
Uncontrolled hypertension (BP ≥190/115 mmHg)
Other conditions associated with known bleeding risks (e.g., advanced age [≥75 yr], full-dose anticoagulant therapy, diabetic hemorrhagic retinopathy)
Known allergy to streptokinase, recent streptokinase therapy (<12 mo), recent streptococcal infection (<12 mo)

BP, blood pressure.

Adjunctive Heparin and Aspirin Therapy with APSAC

The relative risk/benefit ratio of using heparin as adjunctive therapy with non–fibrin-selective thrombolytic therapies such as APSAC has been controversial, especially when combined with aspirin. APSAC not only provides long-lasting fibrinolytic activity (half-life 90 to 120 minutes) but also generates large amounts of fibrin degradation products associated with long-lasting antithrombotic effects. Most early studies of APSAC used heparin without aspirin, beginning about 6 hours after APSAC. After ISIS-2,[70] which demonstrated an additive mortality benefit of aspirin with streptokinase, studies of APSAC added aspirin to thrombolytic therapy and generally continued to use heparin. In APSAC comparisons with rt-PA, heparin, believed to be necessary for rt-PA, was also used earlier and more aggressively with APSAC. However, in these latter studies, rates of hemorrhage increased without improved clinical outcomes. Specifically in ISIS-3,[56] mortality was identical after APSAC plus aspirin and after APSAC plus aspirin and subcutaneously administered heparin (10.5%, all patients; 9.9%, <6 hours in patients with ST elevation), but cerebral hemorrhage was greater in those randomized to subcutaneously administered heparin (0.71% versus 0.40%). In a nonrandomized ISIS-3 comparison, patients who received heparin intravenously with APSAC (n = 1612) had increased rates of cerebral hemorrhage (0.9%) and transfused bleeds (2.7%) than did patients receiving only subcutaneously administered heparin (n = 6304) (0.5%, 0.9%, respectively) and those receiving no heparin (n = 5683) (0.5%, 0.7%, respectively). (The 5-week mortality rate was 10.0% in those receiving intravenously administered heparin, 8.3% in the subcutaneously administered heparin group, and 13.1% in the group not receiving heparin, but interpretation is complicated by the lack of randomization.)

O'Connor et al. performed a randomized trial of intravenously administered heparin versus no heparin in conjunction with APSAC and aspirin in 250 AMI patients.[71] Rates of post-AMI nonhemorrhagic complications (death, stroke, reinfarction, heart failure, or recurrent ischemia) were similar in both groups (40% versus 38%); bleeding complications were twice as common in the heparin group (33%) than in the group not receiving heparin (16%) and often occurred 2 days or more after APSAC. Life-threatening bleeds occurred in 4.7% of heparin and in 0.8% of patients not receiving heparin. Thus, withholding heparin after APSAC given with aspirin resulted in half the bleeding rate without leading to an increase in nonhemorrhagic adverse clinical outcomes. These results, taken together with the ISIS-3 and other observational data, suggest that intravenously administered heparin should not be routinely used after APSAC and aspirin therapy. In patients at higher risk, subcutaneous heparin therapy appears to be safer than intravenously administered heparin (ISIS-3), but survival outcome has not been shown to improve.

A follow-up study by O'Connor et al. randomized 162 patients presenting within 12 hours of the onset of symptoms to front-loaded t-PA with weight-adjusted heparin or APSAC without heparin. The study included a factorial design with 325 mg versus 81 mg of aspirin. The study was terminated early by the Safety and Data Monitoring Committee after results of the GUSTO-1 trial were known in conjunction with the findings that the composite end point favored t-PA (25.4% versus 31.3% for APSAC) and that more patients in the APSAC-treated group had bleeding complications. Overall, the rate of bleeding was 15% in the accelerated t-PA group using weight-adjusted heparin dosing compared with 21% in the APSAC group. Of APSAC-treated patients, 5% had life-threatening bleeding compared with none of the t-PA–treated patients. Aspirin appeared to have no effect on these differences. None of these differences is statistically significant, although in conjunction with the TEAM-3 study[60] and the TIMI-4 study,[65] they raise the question of whether front-loaded t-PA leads to less systemic bleeding than does APSAC with or without heparin. These findings do not provide insight into intracranial hemorrhage rates, which can only be estimated from larger studies.

Angioplasty and Surgery after APSAC

Angioplasty has been performed frequently after APSAC therapy without unusual difficulty or reported excessive bleeding. Bypass surgery has also been well tolerated; as expected, early surgery increases the frequency of transfusion (from 12% to 21%) to a degree similar to that after streptokinase.[55]

An additional question is whether coronary angioplasty is routinely indicated in patients with significant residual stenosis after thrombolysis. This was

investigated in the Should We Intervene Following Thrombolysis? (SWIFT) study.[72] SWIFT entered 933 and randomized 833 patients to either a conservative or an invasive approach taken 1 to 2 days after therapy. In the intervention group, angioplasty was undertaken in 134 patients with an initial success rate of 88%, and bypass surgery was undertaken in 42 patients for a 47% intervention rate in the invasive group. Hospital stay was longer by a day in the intervention group ($p < .001$). Three-month mortality rates were low but favored the conservative care group (3.2% versus 4.8%). By 12 months, mortality rates were 5.0% versus 5.8% and reinfarction rates were 12.9% versus 15.1%, respectively ($p = $ NS). Thus, SWIFT suggested that the conservative approach may be best for most patients, with the invasive approach being reserved for those with specific clinical indications. (Similar results have been found for t-PA.)

APSAC in Unstable Angina and Other Thromboembolic Conditions

Unstable angina may be a precursor to AMI and may involve coronary thrombosis. Whether thrombolytics are useful in this setting has been studied. To study the use of APSAC in unstable angina, 159 patients were enrolled in a double-blind, placebo-controlled multicenter trial.[73] Angiography was performed at baseline and at 12 to 28 hours. APSAC caused a decrease in the diameter of stenosis between angiograms compared with placebo (11% versus 3% change, $p < .01$), a difference explained by reopening of occluded vessels. However, an overall benefit in clinical outcome could not be demonstrated, and bleeding complications were more frequent in patients who received thrombolytic therapy (21 versus 7 patients, $p = .001$). Thus, based on this and other trials (with t-PA), thrombolytic therapy cannot be recommended routinely for patients with unstable angina.

APSAC has not been formally tested for other thromboembolic conditions, but case reports indicate its potential utility in massive pulmonary embolism and peripheral arterial and venous thrombosis or thromboembolism.[37, 38]

Dosage, Indications, Administration, Reuse, and Cost

APSAC is marketed as a vial of lyophilized powder (see section on chemistry) containing 30 U (approximately 30 mg) of APSAC.

APSAC is indicated for use in the management of AMI in adults, lysis of thrombi obstructing coronary arteries, reduction of infarct size, improvement of ventricular function after AMI, and reduction of mortality associated with AMI.

APSAC is reconstituted with 5 ml of sterile water or saline and injected within 30 minutes of reconstitution. APSAC should be administered by slow intravenous injection in increments over 2 to 5 minutes with constant monitoring of blood pressure and electrocardiographic changes. APSAC generally reaches its maximum hypotensive effect within 5 to 15 minutes. The optimal concomitant therapeutic regimen continues to be studied, but most patients receiving APSAC receive aspirin.[70] Intravenous heparin therapy, used routinely in the past, may increase risk more than benefit. Concurrent therapy with other drugs commonly used in patients with AMI (i.e., lidocaine, nitroglycerin, β-blocker) has been generally given as needed without difficulty.

APSAC, like streptokinase, is antigenic; potentially neutralizing antibodies develop within 4 to 5 days after administration and persist for over 1 to 4 years.[74, 75] Thus, reuse is not recommended after 4 days, perhaps indefinitely (at least, within 1 to 4 years). On the other hand, pretherapy measurement of antistreptococcal antibodies in those without prior receipt of drug does not appear to be necessary as a screening test; no difference in outcome by level of preformed antibody titer has been found.[76]

The cost of APSAC is approximately $1500 per dose, compared with about $300 for streptokinase and $2300 for alteplase.

In summary, APSAC provides the advantage of the greatest ease of administration among thrombolytics: a single, simple injection without the requirement for intravenously administered heparin when given with aspirin. This convenience and simplicity of administration may be particularly valuable in emergency ward and prehospital use. APSAC is also a more efficient and long-lasting thrombolytic than streptokinase, but it is more expensive.

REFERENCES

1. Smith RAG, Dupe RJ, English PD, et al: Fibrinolysis with acyl-enzymes: A new approach to thrombolytic therapy. Nature 290:505, 1981.
2. Anderson JL, Boissel J-P, Chamberlain DA (eds): Symposium on anisoylated plasminogen streptokinase activator complex (APSAC). Drugs 33(Suppl 3):1, 1987.
3. Ferres H: Preclinical pharmacological evaluation of anisoylated plasminogen streptokinase activator complex. Drugs 33(Suppl 3):33, 1987.
4. Fears R, Ferres H, Standring R: Evidence for the progressive uptake of anisoylated plasminogen streptokinase activator complex by clots in human plasma in vitro. Drugs 33(Suppl 3):51, 1987.
5. Fears R, Ferres H, Standring R: The protective effect of acylation on the stability of anisoylated plasminogen streptokinase activator complex in human plasma. Drugs 33(Suppl 3):57, 1987.
6. Smith RAG: Non-exchange of streptokinase from anisoylated plasminogen streptokinase activator complex and other acylated streptokinase-plasminogen complexes. Drugs 33(Suppl 3):75, 1987.
7. Monassier JP (on behalf of the IRS II Study Group), Hanssen M: Haematological effects of anisoylated plasminogen streptokinase activator complex and streptokinase in patients with acute myocardial infarction: Interim report of the IRS II study. Drugs 33(Suppl 3):247, 1987.
8. Samama M, Conard J, Verdy E, et al: Biological study of intravenous anisoylated plasminogen streptokinase activator complex in acute myocardial infarction. Drugs 33(Suppl 3):268, 1987.
9. Marder VJ, Kinsalle PA, Brown MJ: Fibrinogen concentration and coronary artery reperfusion after intravenous anisoylated plasminogen streptokinase activator complex or intracoronary streptokinase therapy. Drugs 33(Suppl 3):237, 1987.
10. Fears R, Green J, Smith RAG, et al: Induction of a sustained fibrinolytic response by BRL 26921 in vitro. Thromb Res 38:251, 1985.
11. Fears R, Ferres H, Greenwood HC: Comparison of the effects of streptokinase, t-PA and APSAC on human platelet aggregation in vitro in the absence and presence of aspirin. Thromb Res 15:259, 1990.
12. Ferres H, Hibbs M, Smith RAG: Deacylation studies in vitro on anisoylated plasminogen streptokinase activator complex. Drugs 33(Suppl 3):80, 1987.
13. Nunn B, Esmail A, Fears R, et al: Pharmacokinetic properties of anisoylated plasminogen streptokinase activator complex and other thrombolytic agents in animals and in humans. Drugs 33(Suppl 3):88, 1987.
14. Green J, Dupe RJ, Smith RAG, et al: Comparison of the hypotensive effects of streptokinase-(human) plasminutesactivator complex and BRL 26921 (p-anisoylated streptokinase-plasminogen activator complex) in the dog after high dose bolus administration. Thromb Res 36:29, 1984.
15. Doenecke P, Schwerdt H, Hellstern P, et al: Bolus injection of anisoylated plasminogen-streptokinase activator complex (BRL 26921): A new approach to intravenous thrombolytic treatment of acute myocardial infarction. Klin Wochenschr 64:682, 1986.
16. Martin M: Streptokinase in Chronic Arterial Disease. Boca Raton, FL: CRC Press, 1982.
17. Mentzer RL, Budzynski AZ, Sherry S: High-dose, brief-duration intravenous infusion of streptokinase in acute myocardial infarction: Description of effects in circulation. Am J Cardiol 57:1220, 1986.
18. Gemmill JD, Hogg KJ, Burns JM, et al: A comparison of the pharmacokinetic properties of streptokinase and anistreplase in acute myocardial infarction. Br J Clin Pharmacol 31:143, 1991.
19. Marder VJ, Rothbard RL, Fitzpatrick PG, et al: Rapid lysis of coronary artery thrombi with anisoylated plasminogen-streptokinase activator complex: Treatment by bolus intravenous injection. Ann Intern Med 104:304, 1986.
20. Anderson JL, Rothbard RL, Hackworthy RA, et al: Multicenter reperfusion trial of intravenous anisoylated plasminogen streptokinase activator complex (APSAC) in acute myocardial infarction: Controlled comparison with intracoronary streptokinase. J Am Coll Cardiol 11(6):53, 1988.
21. Brügemann J, van der Meer J, Takens BH, Hillege H, Lie KI. A systemic non-lytic state and local thrombolytic failure of anistreplase in acute myocardial infarction. Br Heart J 64:355, 1990.
22. Marder VJ, Francis CW: Physiological balance of haemostasis and bleeding. Drugs 33(Suppl 3):13, 1987.
23. Rao AK, Pratt C, Berke A, et al: Thrombolysis in myocardial infarction (TIMI) trial, phase I: Hemorrhagic manifestations and changes in plasma fibrinogen and the fibrinolytic system in patients treated with recombinant tissue plasminogen activator and streptokinase. J Am Coll Cardiol 11:1, 1988.
24. Hoffman JJ, Bonnier JJ, Melman PG, Bartholomeus I: Blood viscosity during thrombolytic therapy with anistreplase in acute myocardial infarction. Am J Cardiol 71:14, 1993.
25. Lew AS, Laramee P, Cercek B, et al: The hypotensive effect of intravenous streptokinase in patients with acute myocardial infarction. Circulation 72:1321, 1985.
26. Anderson JL, Sorensen SG, Moreno FL, et al, and the TEAM-2 Study Investigators: Multicenter patency trial of intravenous anistreplase with streptokinase in acute myocardial infarction. Circulation 83:126, 1991.
27. ISAM Study Group: A prospective trial of intravenous streptokinase in acute myocardial infarction (ISAM): Mortality, morbidity, and infarct size at 21 days. N Engl J Med 14:1465, 1986.
28. White HD, Norris RM, Brown MA, et al: Effect of intravenous streptokinase on left ventricular function and early survival after acute myocardial infarction. N Engl J Med 317:850, 1987.
29. Guerci AD, Gerstenblith G, Brinker JA, et al: A randomized trial of intravenous tissue plasminogen activator for acute myocardial infarction with subsequent randomization to elective coronary angioplasty. N Engl J Med 317:1613, 1987.
30. O'Rourke M, Norris R (for the TICO Group): Improved LV

ejection fraction at 21 days following coronary occlusion treated by early intravenous rt-PA infusion [abstract]. J Am Coll Cardiol 11(Suppl A):105A, 1988.

31. Mathey DG, Schofer J, Sheehan FH, et al: Intravenous urokinase in acute myocardial infarction. Am J Cardiol 55:878, 1985.

32. Spann JF, Sherry S: Coronary thrombolysis for evolving myocardial infarction. Drugs 28:465, 1984.

33. Anderson JL: Principles of thrombolytic therapy: Intracoronary administration. In Anderson JL (ed): Acute Myocardial Infarction, New Management Strategies. Rockville, MD: Aspen, 1987, pp 157–184.

34. Been M, Muir AL, De Bono DP: Left ventricular function after anisoylated plasminogen streptokinase activator complex. Drugs 33(Suppl 3):191, 1987.

35. Bassand J-P, Machecourt J, Cassagnes J, et al: Multicenter trial of intravenous anisoylated plasminogen streptokinase activator complex (APSAC) in acute myocardial infarction: Effects on infarct size and left ventricular function. J Am Coll Cardiol 13:988, 1989.

36. Sherry S: Recombinant tissue plasminogen activator (rt-PA): Is it the thrombolytic agent of choice for an evolving acute myocardial infarction? Am J Cardiol 59:984, 1987.

37. Schalij MJ, van de Meeberg PC, Marsman JW, Maingay D: Pulmonary embolism treated with a single dose of anisoylated lys-plasminogen streptokinase activator complex and systemic heparinization: A report of two cases. Neth J Med 40:69, 1992.

38. Pires LA, Jay G: Upper-extremity deep-vein thrombosis: Thrombolytic therapy with anistreplase. Ann Emerg Med 22:748, 1993.

39. Johnson ES, Cregeen RJ: An interim report of the efficacy and safety of anisoylated plasminogen streptokinase activator complex (APSAC). Drugs 33(Suppl 3):298, 1987.

40. Cregeen R: Report to the US FDA Advisory Committee, Bureau of Biologics. Anistreplase Review Meeting, Bethesda, MD, October 31, 1989.

41. Kasper W, Erbel R, Meinertz T, et al: Intracoronary thrombolysis with an acylated streptokinase plasminogen activator (BRL 26921) in patients with acute myocardial infarction. J Am Coll Cardiol 4:357, 1984.

42. Been M, De Bono DP, Boulton FE, et al: Clinical effects of intravenous APSAC: Anisoylated plasminogen-streptokinase activator complex (BRL 26921) in acute myocardial infarction. Int J Cardiol 11:53, 1986.

43. Hillis WS, Hornung RS: The use of BRL 26921 (APSAC) as fibrinolytic therapy in acute myocardial infarction. Eur Heart J 6:909, 1985.

44. Been M, De Bono DP, Muir AL, et al: Coronary thrombolysis with intravenous anisoylated plasminogen-streptokinase complex BRL 26921. Br Heart J 53:253, 1985.

45. Ikram S, Lewis S, Buckwall C, et al: Treatment of acute myocardial infarction with anisoylated plasminogen streptokinase activator complex. Br Med J 293:786, 1986.

46. Kasper W, Meinertz T, Wollschlager H, et al: Coronary thrombolysis during acute myocardial infarction by intravenous BRL 26921, a new anisoylated plasminogen-streptokinase activator complex. Am J Cardiol 58:418, 1986.

47. Jackson D: Summary of early clinical experience with anisoylated plasminogen streptokinase activator complex in the treatment of acute myocardial infarction. Drugs 33(Suppl 3):104, 1987.

48. Timmis AD, Griffin B, Crick JCP, et al: Anisoylated plasminogen-streptokinase activator complex in acute myocardial infarction: A placebo-controlled arteriographic coronary recanalization study. J Am Coll Cardiol 10:205, 1987.

49. Bonnier JJRM (report of the Dutch Multicentre Invasive Reperfusion Study Group): Comparison of intravenous anisoylated plasminogen streptokinase activator complex with intracoronary streptokinase in acute myocardial infarction. Drugs 33(Suppl 3):151, 1987.

50. Bonnier JJRM, Visser RF, Klomps HC, et al: Intravenous APSAC versus intracoronary streptokinase in acute myocardial infarction. Am J Cardiol 62:25, 1988.

51. Chesebro JH, Knatterud G, Roberts R, et al: Thrombolysis in myocardial infarction (TIMI) trial, phase I: A comparison between intravenous tissue plasminogen activator and intravenous streptokinase. Circulation 76:142, 1987.

52. Pacouret G, Charbonnier B, Curien ND, et al: Invasive reperfusion study. II: Multicentre European randomized trial of anistreplase vs streptokinase in acute myocardial infarction. Eur Heart J 12:179, 1991.

53. Verstraete M, Bernard R, Bory M, et al: Randomized trial of intravenous recombinant tissue-type plasminogen activator versus intravenous streptokinase in acute myocardial infarction. Lancet 1:842, 1985.

54. Relik-van Wely L, Visser RF, van der Pol JM, et al: Angiographically assessed coronary arterial patency and reocclusion in patients with acute myocardial infarction treated with anistreplase: Results of the anistreplase reocclusion multicenter study (ARMS). Am J Cardiol 68:296, 1991.

55. Anderson JL: Review of anistreplase (APSAC) for AMI. In Andersen JL (ed): Modern Management of AMI in the Community Hospital. New York: Marcel Dekker, 1991, p 162.

56. ISIS-3 Collaborative Group: ISIS-3: A randomised comparison of streptokinase vs tissue plasminogen activator vs anistreplase and of aspirin plus heparin vs aspirin alone among 41,299 cases of suspected acute myocardial infarction. Lancet 339:753, 1992.

57. Granger CB, Califf RM, Topol EJ: Thrombolytic therapy for acute myocardial infarction: A review. Drugs 44:293, 1992.

58. Baxter-Jones CS, White HD, Anderson JL: An overview of the patency and stroke rates following thrombolysis with streptokinase, alteplase, and anistreplase used to treat an acute myocardial infarction. J Interven Cardiol 6:15, 1993.

59. Braunwald E, Knatterud GL, Passamani ER, et al: Announcement of protocol change in thrombolysis in myocardial infarction trial [letter]. J Am Coll Cardiol 9:467, 1987.

60. Andersen JL, Becker LC, Sorensen SG, et al, and the TEAM-3 Investigators: Anistreplase versus alteplase in acute myocardial infarction: Comparative effects on left ventricular function, morbidity and 1-day coronary artery patency. J Am Coll Cardiol 20:753, 1992.

61. Bassand JP, Cassagnes J, Machecourt J, et al: Comparative effects of APSAC and rt-PA on infarct size and left ventricular function in acute myocardial infarction: A multicenter randomized study. Circulation 84:1107, 1991.

62. Neuhaus K-L, von Essen R, Tebbe U, et al. Improved thrombolysis in acute myocardial infarction with front-loaded administration of alteplase: Results of the rt-PA–APSAC Patency Study (TAPS). J Am Coll Cardiol 19:885, 1992.

63. Cannon CP, McCabe CH, Diver DJ, et al, and the TIMI 4 Investigators: Comparison of front-loaded recombinant tissue-type plasminogen activator, anistreplase, and combination thrombolytic therapy for acute myocardial infarction: Results of the thrombolysis in myocardial infarction (TIMI) 4 Trial. J Am Coll Cardiol 24:1602, 1994.

64. AIMS Trial Study Group: Effect of intravenous APSAC on mortality after acute myocardial infarction: Preliminary report of a placebo-controlled clinical trial. Lancet 1:545, 1988.

65. AIMS Trial Study Group: Long-term effects of intravenous anistreplase in acute myocardial infarction: Final report of the AIMS study. Lancet 335:427, 1990.

66. Gonzalez ER, Jones LA, Ornato JP, et al: Hospital delays and problems with thrombolytic administration in patients receiving thrombolytic therapy: A multicenter prospective assessment. Virginia Thrombolytic Study Group. Ann Emerg Med 21:1215, 1992.

67. The European Myocardial Infarction Project Group (EMIP): Prehospital thrombolytic therapy in patients with suspected acute myocardial infarction. N Engl J Med 329:383, 1993.

68. GREAT Group: Feasibility, safety, and efficacy of domiciliary thrombolysis by general practitioners: Grampian region early anistreplase trial. Br Med J 305:548, 1992.

69. Italian Group for the Study of Streptokinase in Myocardial Infarction (GISSI): Effectiveness of intravenous thrombolytic treatment in acute myocardial infarction. Lancet 1:397, 1986.

70. ISIS-2 Collaborative Group: Randomized trial of intravenous streptokinase, oral aspirin, both, or neither among 17,187 cases of suspected acute myocardial infarction: ISIS-2. Lancet 2:349, 1988.

71. O'Connor CM, Meese R, Carney R, et al, for the DUCCS 1 Investigators: A randomized trial of intravenous heparin in conjunction with the anistreplase in acute myocardial in-

farction: The Duke University Clinical Cardiology Study (DUCCS 1). J Am Coll Cardiol 23:11, 1994.

72. SWIFT Trial Study Group: SWIFT trial of delayed elective intervention vs conservative treatment after thrombolysis with anistreplase in acute myocardial infarction. Br Med J 302:555, 1991.

73. Bär FW, Verheugt FW, Col J, et al: Thrombolysis in patients with unstable angina improves the angiographic but not the clinical outcome: Results of UNASEM, a multicenter, randomized, placebo-controlled, clinical trial with anistreplase. Circulation 86:131, 1992.

74. Fears R, Ferres H, Glasgow E, et al: Monitoring of streptokinase resistance titre in acute myocardial infarction patients up to 30

months after giving streptokinase or anistreplase and related studies to measure specific antistreptokinase IgG. Br Heart J 68:167, 1992.

75. Lee HS, Cross S, Davidson R, et al: Raised levels of antistreptokinase antibody and neutralization titres from 4 days to 54 months after administration of streptokinase or anistreplase. Eur Heart J 14:84, 1993.

76. Fears R, Hearn J, Standring R, et al: Lack of influence of pretreatment antistreptokinase antibody on efficacy in a multicenter patency comparison of intravenous streptokinase and anistreplase in acute myocardial infarction. Am Heart J 124:305, 1992.

CHAPTER 168

Tissue-Type Plasminogen Activator

Alan J. Tiefenbrunn, M.D., F.A.C.C.

Tissue-type plasminogen activator (t-PA) is the primary if not sole physiologic activator of plasminogen. This protein is elaborated by vascular endothelium and also can be found in diverse tissues including uterus, prostate, lung, ovary, muscle, spleen, and liver.[1] t-PA was identified first in 1947[2] but was not isolated for another two decades. In the early 1980s, Rijken and Collen and their coworkers[3, 4] succeeded in isolating and purifying t-PA from a melanoma cell tissue culture in quantities not only sufficient for characterization of the protein but also adequate for pharmacologic study. Studies in rabbits with jugular

Table 168–1. **Components of the Fibrinolytic System**

Components	Description
Plasminogen	A proenzyme of plasmin
Plasmin	The active enzyme that hydrolyzes fibrin (or fibrinogen)
Tissue and vascular activators of plasminogen	Enzymes in tissues that convert plasminogen to plasmin
Blood plasminogen activator	Plasminogen activator present in blood, probably identical to vascular plasminogen activator
Streptokinase	A streptococcal protein that forms complexes with circulating plasminogen, thereby forming an activator in human plasma
Urokinase	A plasminogen activator isolated from urine that hydrolyzes plasminogen
Hageman's factor, high-molecular-weight kininogen, prekallikrein	Plasma proteins involved in intrinsic activation of plasminogen
α_2-Antiplasmin	The fast-reacting plasmin inhibitor in human plasma
α_2-Macroglobulin	The slow-reacting plasmin adsorbent in human plasma
Plasminogen activator inhibitors	Inhibitors of t-PA and urokinase, present in plasma

Compiled from references 11 and 12.

vein thrombosis demonstrated a dose-dependent thrombolytic effect after infusion of t-PA.[5] Lysis of femoral vein thrombosis in dogs was demonstrated with the melanoma-derived t-PA.[6] In animal studies, t-PA was found to have a higher specific thrombolytic effect than urokinase. In addition, it was found to elicit clot lysis without systemic fibrinogenolysis.

The first pharmacologic administration of t-PA to human subjects was for the treatment of iliofemoral thrombosis.[7] Treatment was successful despite the fact that the thrombus was 6 weeks old and the dose of t-PA administered was relatively small (7.5 mg over 24 hours). Subsequently, the ability to lyse intracoronary thrombosis was demonstrated in dogs,[8] which led to a pilot study of t-PA in humans with evolving myocardial infarction. Again, only relatively small doses (10 to 12 mg over 30 to 60 minutes) were employed because of the laborious procedures required to produce large quantities of t-PA. Nevertheless, six of seven patients treated with intracoronary or intravenous t-PA exhibited angiographic criteria of coronary clot lysis without significant concomitant fibrinogenolysis.[9] The successful cloning of the t-PA gene facilitated production of large quantities of recombinant t-PA and made large-scale production and application of this novel pharmacologic agent feasible.[10]

BIOCHEMISTRY
Fibrinolytic System

Both physiologic and pharmacologic fibrinolysis involves plasminogen and its activation to form plasmin. The major components of the fibrinolytic system are listed in Table 168–1;[11, 12] and the potential means of activating plasminogen and the subsequent fate of plasmin are diagrammed in Figure 168–1.[13]

Wild-type human t-PA generally occurs as a single-chain molecule, with a molecular weight of approximately 64,000. The molecule can be cleaved proteolytically to yield a two-subunit form. Both forms activate

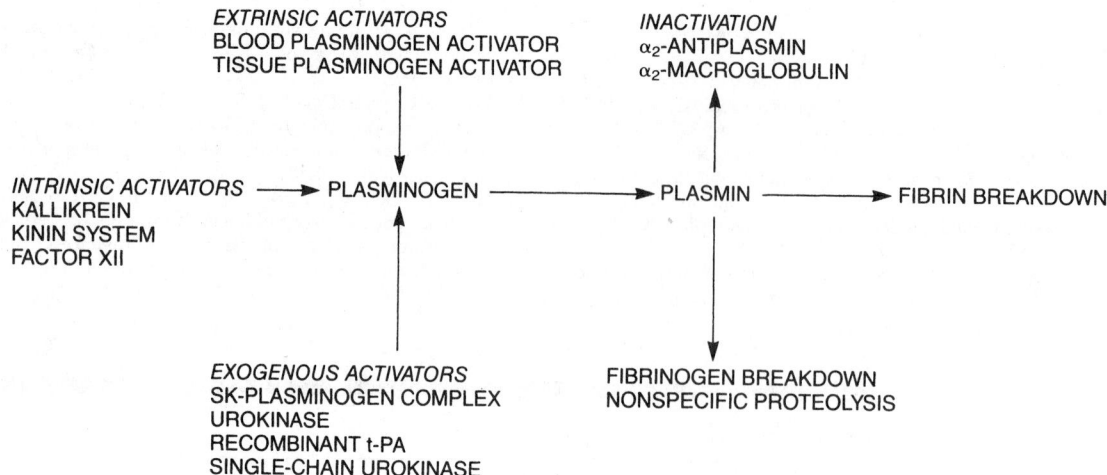

Figure 168–1. Activation of plasminogen and the fate of plasmin. (From Tiefenbrunn AJ, Robison AK, Sobel BE: Clinical pharmacology of coronary thrombolysis. Cardiol Clin 5[1]:126, 1987.)

plasminogen equally, with no significant difference of affinity or catalytic efficacy.[14] The single-chain form is less reactive with low-molecular-weight substrates and inhibitors and appears to be converted to the double-chain form on the fibrin surface of clots.[12]

Plasminogen is a glycoprotein with a molecular weight of approximately 88,000. It circulates in plasma in a concentration of approximately 2 μM.[15] Activation involves peptide bond cleavage and formation of two-chain molecules that spontaneously convert to an active proteolytic enzyme, plasmin. Detectable levels of plasmin are never present in the circulation under physiologic circumstances because the molecule is inactivated rapidly by α2-antiplasmin or bound by α2-macroglobulin.

The high affinity of t-PA for fibrin and fibrin-bound plasminogen relative to circulating plasminogen results in local production of plasmin and local fibrinolytic activity.[16] t-PA is subject to inhibition by a specific, rapid-acting inhibitor, plasminogen activator inhibitor (PAI).[17, 18] In addition, t-PA is cleared relatively rapidly from the circulation by the liver and persists in the circulation for only a few minutes.[19, 20] Thus, with physiologic fibrinolysis, plasminemia and rampant nonspecific proteolysis are avoided by multiple mechanisms:

1. Presence of an inactive circulating plasmin precursor, plasminogen, which has a high affinity for fibrin.

2. Preferential binding of plasminogen activator to fibrin-bound plasminogen.

3. Inhibition of plasminogen activator in the circulation by PAI.

4. Relatively rapid clearance of plasminogen activator that is not fibrin bound (plasma half-life of a few minutes).

5. Rapid inactivation of plasmin elaborated into the circulation (plasma half-life of less than 0.1 second).

Clot Selectivity

The preference of t-PA for fibrin-bound plasminogen depends on the reaction kinetics of the interaction of t-PA with fibrin-bound, as opposed to free, plasminogen. As indicated in Figure 168–2,[21] the Michaelis constant associated with the reaction of t-PA with fibrin-bound plasminogen is much lower than that for circulating plasminogen,[21, 22] indicating that this reaction is favored whenever limited amounts of the respective moieties are available. A corollary to this observation is the fact that the reaction in plasma will proceed when an excess of t-PA is provided. Thus, the fibrin specificity of t-PA is a relative and dose-dependent, rather than an absolute, phenomenon. If massive amounts of t-PA are administered, significant activation of plasminogen occurs in the circulation.

When plasminogen combines with fibrin, lysine-binding sites of the plasminogen molecule become occupied. These sites remain occupied when plasminogen is converted to plasmin by the action of t-PA. The lysine-binding sites mediate the interaction of plasmin with α2-antiplasmin, and, when they are unavailable for additional binding, inactivation of the molecule by α2-antiplasmin is greatly inhibited.[16]

Study of patients receiving t-PA for treatment of acute myocardial infarction (AMI) demonstrates prolonged elaboration of cross-linked fibrin degradation products (XL-FDPs), a marker of fibrin (as opposed to fibrinogen) breakdown.[23] This process is shown graphically in Figure 168–3. Concentrations of XL-FDPs in plasma several hours after administration of t-PA are higher and more persistent than corresponding values in patients treated with streptokinase. Occupation of lysine-binding sites probably contributes to the observation that t-PA–induced fibrinolytic activity persists much longer than would be predicted by its plasma half-life.

In addition, the Michaelis constant (Km) for plasmin activation decreases approximately tenfold after onset of fibrin degradation.[24, 25] This positive feedback is thought to result from exposure of strong plasminogen-binding sites during fibrin degradation and results in a further increase in the rate of plasmin formation. Thus, the ternary complex of t-PA, fibrin, and fibrin-bound plasminogen results in potent local fibrinolytic effects.

In plasma

$$t\text{-}PA + \text{plasminogen} \underset{k_{-1}}{\overset{k_1}{\rightleftharpoons}} [t\text{-}PA \cdot \text{plasminogen}] \overset{k_2}{\rightarrow} t\text{-}PA + \text{plasmin}$$

$$\frac{k_{-1}}{k_1} = K_M{}^a = 65 \ \mu M$$

In fibrin

$$t\text{-}PA + [\text{plasminogen} \cdot \text{fibrin}] \underset{k_{-3}}{\overset{k_3}{\rightleftharpoons}} [t\text{-}PA \cdot \text{plasminogen} \cdot \text{fibrin}] \overset{k_4}{\rightarrow} [t\text{-}PA \cdot \text{plasmin} \cdot \text{fibrin}]$$

$$\frac{k_{-3}}{k_3} = K_M = 0.14 \ \mu M$$

Figure 168–2. Reactions involved in the activation of plasminogen by t-PA in the circulation and on fibrin clots. [a], Michaelis constant. Brackets surrounding two or more constituents joined by a dot symbolize a complex. The symbols k_x and k_{-x} refer to forward and reverse rate constants, respectively. (Reprinted from Tiefenbrunn AJ, Sobel BE: Pharmacodynamics of activation of plasminogen with t-PA. *In* Sobel BE, Collen D, Grossbard EB [eds]: Tissue Plasminogen Activator in Thrombolytic Therapy. New York: Marcel Dekker, 1987, pp 25–39, by courtesy of Marcel Dekker, Inc.)

Interaction with Heparin

Initial studies of both streptokinase and t-PA for treatment of AMI were performed in the cardiac catheterization suite, where intravenous heparin was administered before initiation of the lytic agent. Heparin does not have intrinsic fibrinolytic activity. However, heparin may potentiate the thrombolytic effect of t-PA by decreasing incorporation of new fibrin in the dynamic process of fibrin formation and degradation within thrombus.[26] The third Thrombolysis and Angioplasty in Myocardial Infarction (TAMI-3) trial did not demonstrate higher angiographic patency rates at 90 minutes in patients who received intravenous heparin in combination with t-PA compared with those who received t-PA alone.[27] However, this study did not exclude the possibility of accelerated thrombolysis in the presence of heparin, because angiography earlier than 90 minutes was not performed.

Antithrombin therapy is very important, however, after thrombolysis with t-PA. After the use of any thrombolytic agent, reocclusion is a potential problem because the milieu of exposed collagen and platelet products at a site of disrupted atheroma is highly thrombogenic. Reocclusion is related to both local and systemic factors, including the concentration of the lytic agent,[28] an increase in plasminogen activator inhibitor level,[17, 18] decreased prostacyclin (PGI$_2$)-mediated inhibition of platelet aggregation,[29] and plasmin-mediated thrombin activation.[30, 31] t-PA has a very short circulating half-life, and therefore reocclusion needs to be prevented either by prolonged infusions[32] or by inhibition of thrombosis through combined antiplatelet therapy with aspirin and antithrombin therapy using heparin.

A series of trials have now confirmed the importance of intravenous heparin after therapy with t-PA, documenting significantly higher angiographic patency rates in patients receiving conjunctive heparin therapy.[33–35] The importance of effective heparinization has been emphasized by analyzing patency rates in patients receiving heparin but with and with-

Figure 168–3. Levels of cross-linked fibrin degradation products (XL-FDP) after treatment with streptokinase or t-PA in patients with AMI. The numbers in the bars indicate the number of patient samples in each time period. Sample intervals indicate the time after initiation of infusion of activator. (From Eisenberg PR, Sherman LA, Tiefenbrunn AJ, et al: Sustained fibrinolysis after administration of t-PA despite its short half-life in the circulation. Thromb Haemost 57:35, 1987.)

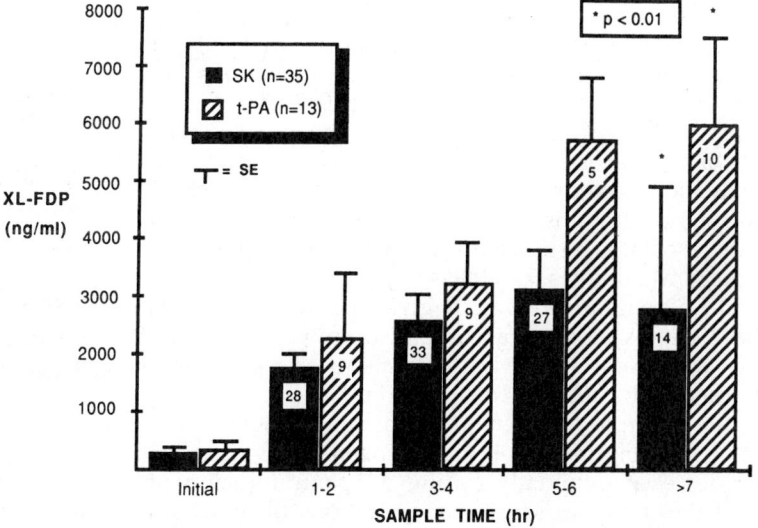

out therapeutic levels. In the Heparin or Aspirin Re-occlusion Trial (HART), patients treated with intravenous t-PA followed by intravenous heparin resulting in a consistently therapeutic partial thromboplastin time (PTT) had a 5% chance of having an occluded vessel at angiography 18 hours after treatment. Patients receiving t-PA and intravenous heparin, but without a therapeutic PTT, had a 50% chance of having an occluded vessel.[33]

PHARMACODYNAMICS
Interactions of Tissue-Type Plasminogen Activator

Because t-PA is a naturally occurring human protein with a specific function, its pharmacologic actions are specific and limited even when administered in large doses. It is nonallergenic and has no known hemodynamic, neuromuscular, or gastrointestinal effects. Only the effects of t-PA on fibrin clot and the consequences of plasminogen activation in the circulation are clinically significant.

Plasminogen activation in the circulation and the subsequent fate of plasmin become important when large pharmacologic doses of t-PA are administered. Circulating inhibitors of t-PA are present in small amounts and are overwhelmed rapidly.[18] α_2-Antiplasmin, an efficient inhibitor of plasmin, is present in blood in a molar concentration about half that of plasminogen and therefore may be depleted when elaboration of plasmin continues.[36] α_2-Macroglobulin, which adsorbs or engulfs plasmin molecules, reacts relatively slowly and is not of major importance during physiologic plasminogen activation. However, with consumption of α_2-antiplasmin, α_2-macroglobulin provides continued protection against plasminemia.[12, 36]

Dose-Dependent Effects

A computer simulation has been developed to characterize the impact of specific doses and durations of infusion of t-PA on the components of the hemostatic and fibrinolytic systems.[36] The computer program developed for simulation uses reiterative solutions for the interactive differential chemical equations involved, calculating estimated concentrations of each chemical moiety at each selected time point. Given all of the pertinent reactions involving plasminogen activation and subsequent plasmin interactions, starting concentrations of the constituent proteins, and rate constants estimated from *in vitro* studies, the program estimates the effects of a given concentration of t-PA maintained over a given period. Its results have been validated by comparison of predicted values with data obtained in patients receiving selected regimens of t-PA.

An example of the results that can be obtained is shown in Figure 168–4. Plasminogen levels are seen to decrease minimally during a 1-hour infusion of t-PA, resulting in serum concentrations of less than

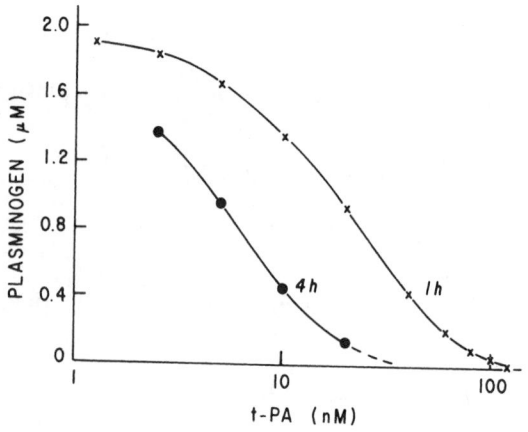

Figure 168–4. Simulated concentrations of plasminogen in plasma (plotted on the ordinate) as a function of prevailing concentrations of t-PA throughout infusions for 1 or 4 hours. The t-PA values on the abscissa are plotted on a logarithmic scale. The simulation indicates marked diminution of plasma plasminogen at the end of a 4-hour infusion even when plasma concentrations of t-PA do not exceed 10 nM. Anticipated diminution of plasminogen is modest at the end of a 1-hour infusion with a plasma concentration of this magnitude. However, even a brief infusion of 1 hour is anticipated to lead to marked depletion of plasma plasminogen when the prevailing concentration of t-PA approaches 100 nM. (Reproduced with permission from Tiefenbrunn AJ, Graor RA, Robison SK, et al: Pharmacodynamics of tissue-type plasminogen activator characterized by computer-assisted simulation. Circulation 73:1291, 1986. Copyright 1986, American Heart Association.)

10 nM. However, with larger concentrations of t-PA, a relatively rapid diminution of anticipated plasminogen levels occurs. As expected, maintenance of a given concentration of t-PA for the longer interval of 4 hours can result in significant depletion of plasminogen even with relatively low prevailing plasma t-PA concentrations.

The predictions and clinical observations obtained to support them emphasize the relative selectivity of t-PA for fibrin-bound plasminogen and document the loss of clot selectivity with excessive pharmacologic administration of t-PA. In addition to producing undesirable plasminemia, large doses of t-PA may result in consumption of plasminogen to the extent that plasminogen activation on the fibrin clot is impaired by lack of substrate. *In vitro* studies have demonstrated depression of thrombolysis with suprapharmacologic levels of t-PA, accompanied by depletion of clot-associated plasminogen ("plasminogen steal" phenomenon). The rate of thrombolysis and the clot-associated plasminogen level return to baseline values after plasminogen supplementation.[37]

PHARMACOKINETICS
Measurement of Tissue-Type Plasminogen Activator

Studies of pharmacokinetics require reliable assays for t-PA. Epitopes of t-PA protein may be quantified with either immunoradiometric assays[38] or enzyme-linked immunosorbent assays.[39] Such assays are specific for t-PA. They measure the amount of protein, independent of its enzymatic activity.[1]

The functional activity of t-PA can be determined with fibrin plate assays or with amidolytic assays with results quantified with reference to comparison with standard curves.[1] Such assays define effects of the plasmin generated. Thus, they are not specific for t-PA, as opposed to other generators of plasmin. Immunologic and functional assays for t-PA activity yield comparable results in patients given pharmacologic doses of t-PA.[19, 20] Thus, there do not appear to be active metabolites that are undetected by immunologic assay nor immunologically reactive fragments devoid of functional activity under these circumstances. However, apparent functional activity may be decreased by inhibitors or α_2-antiplasmin in samples. Recombinant t-PA ^{125}I has been used for assessing distribution volume and the fate of t-PA.[20]

Distribution and Clearance

Early Studies

Estimates of pharmacokinetics of the melanoma cell t-PA first used in humans[7] indicated an initial half-life of 2.4 minutes with a t-PA clearance of 847 ml/min.[40] The first pharmacologic study of recombinant t-PA in patients employed a monoexponential, single-compartment model as a first approximation of clearance and yielded estimates of a plasma half-life of 8.3 minutes based on functional activity and protein antigen.[19] Results demonstrated a linear relationship between dose (expressed as micrograms per kilograms per minute) and plateau plasma levels, corroborated later by others.[41-43] Considerable individual variation was noted. Subsequent studies have shown that continuous intravenous infusion of t-PA without an initial bolus elicits 90% of the plateau plasma level within 30 minutes, confirming the importance of the short initial (α-phase) half-life.[19, 41]

One- and Two-Chain Tissue-Type Plasminogen Activator

As noted previously, t-PA occurs in either a one- or two-chain form, each having similar or identical catalytic effects on plasminogen activation.[14] The early recombinant t-PA produced by Genentech (lot G11021) consisted of predominantly (approximately 95%) two-chain t-PA. When the production process was altered to produce larger quantities of t-PA, the product obtained (lot G11035) comprised approximately 80% single-chain t-PA. Although there is no difference in plasminogen activation or fibrin specificity of the two forms of t-PA, the predominantly single-chain t-PA has a significantly shorter half-life in humans (4.3 minutes, α-phase; 36.5 minutes, β-phase) compared with values for the predominantly double-chain preparation (5.2 minutes, α-phase; 46.2 minutes, β-phase).[44] Accordingly, continuous intravenous infusion of the predominantly single-chain form (G11035) results in an approximately one-third lower

plasma concentration than that seen with corresponding infusions of the predominantly double-chain form (G11021). Thus, a higher dose of the single-chain form of t-PA is required to elicit the same plasma level. This difference has led to some confusion in comparing early studies of t-PA that used G11021 (predominantly double-chain)—the Genentech pilot study,[45] the initial European cooperative studies of t-PA versus placebo[46] and versus streptokinase,[47] the Thrombolysis in Myocardial Infarction Phase I (TIMI I) study,[48] and studies performed in 1985 or later, including the TIMI open-label studies and TIMI II, which employed G11035 t-PA (predominantly single-chain).

Multicompartment Models

Frequent blood sampling over prolonged intervals has clarified our understanding of the kinetics of t-PA in humans. Verstraete et al.[43] used a two-compartment model to estimate clearance and half-life over a range of doses of G11021 t-PA. t-PA clearance estimates ranged from 420 ml/min to 800 ml/min. α-Phase half-life was 5.2 minutes, and β-phase half-life was 55 minutes.

A two-compartment model was used in another study of G11021 t-PA in patients with myocardial infarction.[42] The α-phase half-life was found to be 5.3 minutes and the β-phase half-life to be 46 minutes. An apparent volume of distribution of 7.3 L was observed, considerably larger than plasma volume.

The pharmacokinetics of G11021 t-PA were compared with those of G11035 t-PA by the same investigators.[44] G11021 (predominantly double-chain) t-PA had a longer half-life. Whether this difference in clearance is related directly to the number of chains or other factors, such as glycosylation, remains unclear.[20] Clearance was 732 ml/min for the G11035 t-PA and 555 ml/min for the G11021 t-PA. However, a combination of compartment-dependent and compartment-independent models suggests that a t-PA clearance of 550 ml/min appears reasonable as an estimate of clearance of available (predominantly single-chain) t-PA for prediction of steady-state plasma concentrations.[20]

Metabolism

Several studies in rabbits[49, 50] and mice[51] have documented that removal of t-PA from plasma and its subsequent breakdown occur primarily in the liver. Within 20 minutes, approximately half of t-PA labeled with ^{125}I given to rabbits is taken up by the liver.[49] Decreases in fibrinolytic activity parallel disappearance of ^{125}I-labeled t-PA, indicating that few if any functional metabolites are released by the liver. There is no change in clearance of t-PA with blockade of the reticuloendothelial system or bilateral nephrectomy.[51] However, no appreciable clearance of ^{125}I-labeled t-PA is observed after hepatectomy.[49] Large doses of unlabeled t-PA administered concomitantly with ^{125}I-labeled t-PA do not affect clearance, suggesting that hepatic binding and catabolism are not saturated by usual pharmacologic doses.[51] There appears to be no difference in metabolism of melanoma cell t-PA or recombinant DNA-produced t-PA.[52]

CLINICAL APPLICATIONS
Acute Myocardial Infarction

Tissue-type plasminogen activator became available for clinical trials during a period of great enthusiasm for opening occluded coronary arteries during evolving myocardial infarction. The goal of such therapy includes not only reperfusing the infarct-related artery, but opening this vessel as quickly as possible and preserving patency once it is achieved. Because t-PA in this application appeared to offer significant theoretic advantages over available thrombolytic agents, initial studies were comparative.

The first Thrombolysis in Myocardial Infarction (TIMI-I) trial, sponsored by the National Institutes of Health, is a recanalization study comparing angiographic patency rates after administration of intravenous t-PA or streptokinase.[48] This and other controlled studies documented that coronary artery patency is restored within 90 minutes in approximately 75% of patients with AMI treated with intravenous t-PA.[45–48, 53] This patency rate is comparable with that seen with intracoronary streptokinase and significantly higher than the 45% to 55% patency rate usually associated with intravenous streptokinase.[53] In addition, thrombolysis is observed earlier during infusion of intravenous t-PA than during treatment with intravenous streptokinase.[48] As opposed to streptokinase, older clots (> 4 hours) appear to be just as susceptible to lysis by t-PA as fresh thrombi.[48] Subsequent studies have demonstrated a "catch-up" phenomenon: patients treated with intravenous streptokinase demonstrate increased patency rates over time such that angiographic patency rates at 24 hours are comparable to those seen in patients receiving t-PA.[54]

Controlled studies of streptokinase in AMI, including the GISSI-I trial,[55, 56] the ISIS-2 trial,[57] and the Western Washington trial,[58] have consistently demonstrated mortality benefits in patients receiving thrombolytic therapy. Mortality benefit is associated with successful reperfusion[58, 59] and is sustained for at least one year.[56] Similarly, controlled studies of t-PA in AMI have documented improved left ventricular function[60–63] and improved survival.[64, 65]

It is intuitive and evident from animal studies that maximal clinical benefit is associated with prompt reperfusion.[66–69] Indeed, both the GISSI-I and ISIS-2 trials demonstrated a marked decrement in the observed mortality benefit with increasing time from onset of symptoms until treatment could be instituted.[55, 57] In GISSI-I, mortality was reduced by approximately 47% among patients receiving treatment within 1 hour of the onset of symptoms compared with a mortality reduction of only 17% in those patients treated between 3 and 6 hours after onset of symptoms. While maximum benefit is clearly associated with early treatment, the Late Assessment of

Thrombolytic Efficacy trial (LATE), presented at the European Society of Cardiology Meeting in September 1992, demonstrated a 27% reduction in mortality (8.7% versus 11.9%) in patients treated with t-PA 6 to 12 hours after symptom onset compared with patients receiving only intravenous heparin and aspirin.

Because intravenous t-PA works more rapidly than intravenous streptokinase, improved clinical outcome with this agent might be expected. A review of noncomparative trials using either t-PA or a nonspecific lytic agent such as streptokinase did suggest overall lower mortality rates for those patients receiving t-PA.[70] Three large, multicenter trials have now been performed to evaluate the relative mortality impact of different thrombolytic regimens. The GISSI-2/rt-PA/ streptokinase International Mortality Trial[71, 72] compared streptokinase with alteplase (the recombinant t-PA that is discussed in this chapter). The ISIS-3 trial[73] compared streptokinase with anisoylated plasminogen streptokinase activator complex (APSAC) and duteplase, a double-chain form of recombinant t-PA. These trials failed to demonstrate any mortality benefit for the fibrin-specific agents. However, patients enrolled in these studies did not receive effective antithrombin therapy with intravenous heparin; they received either no heparin or a subcutaneous regimen, probably leading to excessively high reocclusion rates in patients receiving the fibrin-specific agents.

A third large trial, the Global Utilization of Streptokinase or t-PA for Occluded Coronary Arteries study (GUSTO) was presented at the American Federation of Clinical Research meeting in April 1993 and subsequently published in September 1993.[73a] In this study, more than 41,000 patients were randomized to receive t-PA, streptokinase, or a combination of both agents. Half of the streptokinase-treated patients were treated with subcutaneous heparin. All of the other patients received an aggressive intravenous heparin regimen for at least 48 hours. All patients received oral aspirin. This trial did demonstrate a highly significant reduction in mortality among patients treated with t-PA compared with those receiving streptokinase or combination therapy. Mortality was reduced by 19%, from 2.8% to 2.3%, at 24 hours in patients receiving t-PA compared with those receiving streptokinase ($p <$ .05). A 14% reduction in mortality, from 7.3% with streptokinase to 6.3% with t-PA, was observed at 30 days ($p <$ .001). Mortality at 30 days in patients receiving combination therapy was 7.0%, which is also significantly higher than the mortality observed with t-PA alone ($p <$ .05). Results were consistent in all subgroup analyses, including age, sex, time to treatment, infarct location, and Killip class at presentation. The angiographic substudy of the GUSTO trial correlated significantly higher 90-minute angiographic patency rates in patients receiving t-PA with the lower mortality rate observed.

Pulmonary Embolism

Pulmonary embolism has been treated successfully with infusions of t-PA, with both angiographic and hemodynamic improvement.[74–76] Studies large enough to demonstrate an impact on mortality or development of chronic pulmonary hypertension have not been performed. However, t-PA may be especially valuable in treating massive pulmonary embolism with associated right ventricular hemodynamic compromise.[75, 76] In comparative trials, patients treated with t-PA have demonstrated more rapid angiographic and hemodynamic improvement than patients treated with urokinase.[77, 78] Pulmonary embolism, like myocardial infarction, is an indication for t-PA that has been approved by the Food and Drug Administration (FDA).

Acute Ischemic Stroke

In a study from the National Institute of Neurological Disorders and Stroke, the effects of t-PA on ischemic stroke were assessed in a randomized double-blind trial.[78a] Despite an increased incidence of symptomatic intracerebral hemorrhage, treatment with intravenous t-PA within 3 hours of the onset of ischemic stroke improved clinical outcome at 3 months. As compared with patients given placebo, patients treated with t-PA were more than 30% more likely to have minimal or no disability. Symptomatic intracerebral hemorrhage occurred in 6.4% of patients given t-PA versus 0.6% of patients with placebo. Mortality at 3 months was 17% in the t-PA group versus 21% in the placebo group. Although the potential risks associated with thrombolysis should be borne in mind, this study is an important step toward the treatment of acute ischemic stroke, a disease for which until now no efficacious therapy has been available.

Other Indications

Other indications for t-PA that are under investigation include peripheral arterial occlusive disease, deep venous thrombosis, unstable angina, embolic stroke, and adjunctive therapy during coronary artery angioplasty.[79–85]

ADVERSE EFFECTS AND PRECAUTIONS
Hemorrhage

The major potentially serious complication of therapy with t-PA is bleeding. Although t-PA is clot selective in a dose-dependent fashion, it is not selective for pathologic, as opposed to protective, thrombi. Spontaneous bleeding is unusual; blood loss not related to vascular trauma occurred in 2% of patients treated with a total dose of 80 mg t-PA in the TIMI-I trial.[48] However, bleeding from surgical wounds, vascular access sites, peptic ulcer sites, or nascent leaky vascular aneurysms can be anticipated. The most worrisome complication is intracranial bleeding. This occurred in 11 of 582 patients in the TIMI-II study given a total dose of 150 mg single-chain t-PA.[86] However, the incidence of intracranial bleeding in the TIMI-II

trial was only 0.5% among 2952 patients receiving 100 mg t-PA, an incidence similar to that seen with conventionally treated myocardial infarction.[86] Patients older than the age of 75 years were excluded from the TIMI-II trial. The incidence of intracranial bleeding in the GUSTO trial was 0.5% among more than 8500 patients younger than the age of 75 years receiving 100 mg t-PA in a front-loaded regimen. Advanced age or long-standing and uncontrolled systemic hypertension increase the risk of intracranial bleeding.[87]

Avoidance of bleeding complications is critically dependent on proper patient selection and a thorough understanding of the mechanisms of action of thrombolytic agents.[88] Laboratory monitoring of fibrinogen levels, protamine-corrected thrombin time, and other indices of hemostasis during thrombolytic therapy may be important in titrating heparin and deciding when invasive procedures can be undertaken safely,[89, 90] but it is of limited value during the early, high-dose treatment for AMI. Fibrinogenolysis occurs in improperly collected samples,[36] and laboratory results usually cannot be obtained promptly enough to guide initial treatment effectively.

Treatment of Bleeding Complications

Detailed recommendations for managing patients with bleeding complications are available.[88, 91] Superficial bleeding is best managed by direct compression. Serious bleeding or anticipated urgent surgery may require discontinuation of t-PA, heparin, and aspirin, with associated risk of rethrombosis. Because of the short circulating half-life of t-PA, near normal hemostasis returns relatively quickly in many patients. The effect of heparin may be rapidly reversed by administration of protamine sulfate. In patients who exhibit a marked fall of fibrinogen with associated hemorrhage after administration of t-PA, treatment with cryoprecipitate or fresh frozen plasma may be required to replace clotting factors. Cryoprecipitate replaces fibrinogen and factor VIII and has the theoretic advantage over fresh frozen plasma of not supplying additional plasminogen that may then be converted to plasmin. Depending on the severity of hemorrhage and hemodynamic status, transfusion may be required. ε-aminocaproic acid blocks binding of plasminogen to fibrin,[92] but systemic administration is of limited value after an infusion of t-PA has been discontinued and may be associated with precipitation of thrombosis.

Contraindications
Absolute Contraindications

In several clinical situations (Table 168–2), administration of t-PA or any thrombolytic agent is strongly contraindicated and can be justified only under unusual circumstances.[90] These absolute contraindications to thrombolytic therapy fit into two major categories: pathologic conditions of the central nervous

Table 168–2. **Contraindications to Thrombolytic Therapy**

Absolute Contraindications	Relative Contraindications
Potential Central Nervous System Bleeding	Systemic hypertension
Known intracranial pathology (e.g., neoplasm, aneurysm, arteriovenous malformation)	Recent surgery (including organ biopsy or puncture of noncompressible vessels)
History of intracranial bleeding (e.g., subdural hematoma)	History of gastrointestinal or gastrourinary bleeding
Recent intracranial surgery	Trauma
Recent surgery near spinal cord	Pregnancy
Recent severe head or back trauma	Postpartum state
Severe systemic hypertension (>180/110)	Active menstruation
	Acute pericarditis
Potential Massive Hemorrhage	Cerebrovascular disease
Active internal bleeding	Hemorrhagic retinopathy
Immediate postoperative period	Septic thrombophlebitis
Severe thrombocytopenia	Bacterial endocarditis
Hepatic failure	Hepatic dysfunction
Documented bleeding diathesis	Chronic steroid therapy (or other reason to suspect vascular fragility)
	History of skin grafting
	Minor hemostatic defects

system, where even a small amount of bleeding may be devastating, and active or anticipated bleeding that would be difficult to control and could lead to major hemorrhage. These situations include severe systemic hypertension (arterial blood pressure greater than 180/110 mmHg) or intracranial pathologic conditions that may predispose a patient to bleeding, such as neoplasm, arteriovenous malformation, or aneurysm. A history of intracranial bleeding or recent (within 2 months) intracranial or back surgery (e.g., disc repair) or trauma are contraindications as well. Active internal bleeding or a documented diathesis for significant bleeding are additional contraindications to thrombolytic agents.

Relative Contraindications

In many patients at relatively increased risk for thrombolytic therapy, the potential benefits must be weighed carefully against inherent risk (see Table 168–2). Systemic hypertension, especially if it is severe, uncontrolled, or long standing, constitutes a relative contraindication, as does recent (within 10 days) major surgery or significant trauma. Although no studies are available, women who are pregnant, postpartum, or menstruating may be at increased risk of bleeding. Other relative contraindications include acute pericarditis, minor hemostatic defects, history of cerebrovascular disease, hemorrhagic retinopathy, septic thrombophlebitis, bacterial endocarditis, hepatic dysfunction, and any other condition in which bleeding is a potential hazard or would be particularly difficult to manage because of its location. Although older individuals are more likely to have specific contraindications, advanced age is no longer considered an intrinsic contraindication to thrombolytic therapy.[68, 93]

DOSAGE AND ADMINISTRATION
General Considerations

Although functional t-PA activity persists in thrombi, its short plasma half-life dictates administration by continuous intravenous infusion. Plasma level generally is proportionate to infusion rate. Desired dose depends on the therapeutic goals. Because plateau levels are reached relatively quickly, an initial bolus of t-PA is indicated only when rapid onset of peak plasma levels is advantageous, as in the treatment of evolving myocardial infarction.

Although blood level is proportional to dose, there is wide variation in individual response.[44] Weight-adjusted dosing is recommended for smaller patients (<65 kg) to avoid overdosage and excess risk of bleeding complications.

The dose does not have to be altered because of age or renal dysfunction. However, hepatic dysfunction may result not only in prolongation of the half-life of t-PA but also may decrease clearance of FDPs and increase the time for restoration of circulating fibrinogen and plasminogen. These factors, combined with disordered hemostasis related to clotting factor deficiencies, lead to significantly increased risk in patients with severe liver dysfunction.

Acute Myocardial Infarction

The initial FDA-approved regimen for intravenous t-PA in the treatment of AMI is 60 mg/hr (of which 6 to 10 mg is given as a bolus over 1 to 2 minutes) followed by 20 mg/hr for 2 hours, for a total dose of 100 mg. A total dose of 1.25 mg/kg administered over 3 hours is recommended for patients weighing less than 65 kg. Higher doses evaluated in the TIMI series of trials demonstrated more rapid lysis but no increase in angiographic patency rates at 90 minutes.[94, 95] An unacceptably high rate of intracranial bleeding (1.30%) was associated with a 150-mg dose that was not weight adjusted.[86]

More recent studies have demonstrated improved patency rates of 74% at 60 minutes and approximately 80% to 90% at 90 minutes with accelerated or "front-loaded" t-PA regimens in which the standard 100-mg dose is administered over 90 minutes with approximately two thirds of the dose given over the first 30 minutes.[96-99] This type of regimen, adjusted for patient weight, was employed in the GUSTO trial, specifically, a 15-mg bolus followed by 50 mg over 30 minutes and the remaining 35 mg over the next hour in a typical 80-kg patient. The intracranial bleeding rate with this regimen in the GUSTO trial was 0.7% overall and 0.5% for patients younger than 75 years, comparable with that observed with longer drug infusions in earlier studies. Largely on the basis of the GUSTO trial results, this accelerated t-PA regimen was approved by the FDA in April 1995. As discussed above, conjunctive intravenous heparin is essential following thrombolytic therapy with t-PA and was associated with a low angiographic reocclusion rate (approximately 6%) in the GUSTO trial when continued for at least 48 hours.

Repeat infusions of t-PA have been employed for clinically manifest re-infarction with complete resolution of ischemic symptoms in 44 of 52 patients (85%). A full dose of t-PA (100 or 120 mg over 3 hours) was initiated less than 1 hour after completion of the first thrombolytic infusion in 35 of these patients.[100]

Pulmonary Embolism

The recommended dose of t-PA for treatment of pulmonary embolism is an intravenous infusion of 100 mg over 2 hours. Direct intrapulmonary infusion of t-PA appears to offer no advantage over peripheral intravenous administration.[101]

COST

Tissue-type plasminogen activator is a protein synthesized by recombinant DNA technology and expressed in a mammalian cell line. Although t-PA is more expensive than other available agents, its superiority in treating patients with acute myocardial infarction or pulmonary embolism has now been documented. Thrombolytic therapy is only one step in a rapidly evolving, aggressive, and expensive approach to the management of myocardial infarction, which now often includes early cardiac catheterization and percutaneous transluminal coronary angioplasty (PTCA) or bypass surgery. Preliminary data suggest that a significant fraction of patients with AMI benefit from this approach. Deciding prospectively which patients are most likely to benefit is difficult even when only medical factors are considered. Thus, physicians will be required to exercise judgment based on their knowledge, the clinical situation, compassion, and full consideration of relevant medical and societal issues.

REFERENCES

1. Robison AK, Collen D: Activation of the fibrinolytic system. Cardiol Clin 5:13, 1987.
2. Astrup T, Permin PM: Fibrinolysis in animal organism. Nature 159:681, 1947.
3. Rijken DC, Collen D: Purification and characterization of the plasminogen activator secreted by human melanoma cells in culture. J Biol Chem 256:7035, 1981.
4. Collen D, Rijken DC, Van Damme J, et al: Purification of human tissue-type plasminogen activator in centigram quantities from human melanoma cell culture fluid and its conditioning for use in vivo. Thromb Haemost 48:294, 1982.
5. Collen D, Stassen JM, Verstraete M: Thrombolysis with human extrinsic (tissue-type) plasminogen activator in rabbits with experimental jugular vein thrombosis. J Clin Invest 71:368, 1983.
6. Korninger C, Matsuo O, Suy R, et al: Thrombolysis with human extrinsic (tissue-type) plasminogen activator in dogs with femoral vein thrombosis. J Clin Invest 69:573, 1982.
7. Weimar W, Stibbe J, Van Seyen AJ, et al: Specific lysis of an iliofemoral thrombus by administration of extrinsic (tissue-type) plasminogen activator. Lancet 2:1018, 1981.
8. Bergmann SR, Fox KAA, Ter-Pogossian MM, et al: Clot-selective coronary thrombolysis with tissue-type plasminogen activator. Science 220:1181, 1983.
9. VandeWerf F, Ludbrook PA, Bergmann SR, et al: Coronary thrombolysis with tissue-type plasminogen activator in patients with evolving myocardial infarction. N Engl J Med 310:609, 1984.
10. Pennica D, Holmes WE, Kohr WJ, et al: Cloning and expression of human tissue-type plasminogen activator cDNA in E. coli. Nature 301:214, 1983.
11. Tiefenbrunn AJ, Sobel BE: Factors contributing to the emergence of coronary thrombolysis. Cardiol Clin 5:49, 1987.
12. Collen D: Biological properties of plasminogen activators. In Sobel BE, Collen D, Grossbard EB (eds): Tissue Plasminogen Activator in Thrombolytic Therapy. New York: Marcel Dekker, 1987, pp 3–24.
13. Tiefenbrunn AJ, Robison AK, Sobel BE: Clinical pharmacology of coronary thrombolysis. Cardiol Clin 5:125, 1987.
14. Rijken DC, Hoylaerts M, Collen D: Fibrinolytic properties of one-chain and two-chain human extrinsic (tissue-type) plasminogen activator. J Biol Chem 257:2920, 1982.
15. Kline DL, Reddy KNN (eds): Fibrinolysis. Boca Raton, FL: CRC Press, 1980.
16. Collen D: On the regulation and control of fibrinolysis. Thromb Haemost 43:77, 1980.
17. Lucore CL, Fujii S, Sobel BE: Dependence of fibrinolytic activity on the concentration of free rather than total tissue-type plasminogen activator in plasma after pharmacologic administration. Circulation 79:1204, 1989.
18. Lucore CL, Sobel BE: Interactions of tissue-type plasminogen activator with plasma inhibitors and their pharmacologic implications. Circulation 77:660, 1988.
19. Tiefenbrunn AJ, Robison AK, Kurnik PB, et al: Clinical pharmacology in patients with evolving myocardial infarction of tissue-type plasminogen activator produced by recombinant DNA technology. Circulation 71:110, 1985.
20. Baughman RA: Pharmacokinetics of tissue plasminogen activator. In Sobel BE, Collen D, Grossbard EB (eds): Tissue Plasminogen Activator in Thrombolytic Therapy. New York: Marcel Dekker, 1987, pp 41–53.
21. Tiefenbrunn AJ, Sobel BE: Pharmacodynamics of activation of plasminogen with t-PA. In Sobel BE, Collen D, Grossbard EB (eds): Tissue Plasminogen Activator in Thrombolytic Therapy. New York: Marcel Dekker, 1987, pp 25–39.
22. Hoylaerts M, Rijken DC, Lijnen HR, et al: Kinetics of the activation of plasminogen by human tissue plasminogen activator: Role of fibrin. J Biol Chem 257:2912, 1982.
23. Eisenberg PR, Sherman LA, Tiefenbrunn AJ, et al: Sustained fibrinolysis after administration of t-PA despite its short half-life in the circulation. Thromb Haemost 57:35, 1987.
24. Suenson E, Lutzen O, Thorsen S: Initial plasmin-degradation of fibrin as the basis of a positive feedback mechanism in fibrinolysis. Eur J Biochem 140:513, 1984.
25. Ranby M, Bergsdorf N, Norrman B, et al: Tissue plasminogen activator kinetics. In Davidson JF, Bachmann F, Bouvier CA, et al (eds): Progress in Fibrinolysis, Vol 6. Edinburgh: Churchill Livingstone, 1983, pp 182–184.
26. Cercek B, Lew AS, Hod H, et al: Enhancement of thrombolysis with tissue-type plasminogen activator by pretreatment with heparin. Circulation 74:583, 1986.
27. Topol EJ, George BS, Kereiakes DJ, et al, and the TAMI Study

Group: A randomized controlled trial of intravenous tissue plasminogen activator and early intravenous heparin in acute myocardial infarction. Circulation 79:281, 1989.

28. Gold HK, Leinbach RC, Garabedian HD: Acute coronary reocclusion after thrombolysis with recombinant human tissue-type plasminogen activator: Prevention by a maintenance infusion. Circulation 73:347, 1986.

29. Shebuski RJ, Ohlstein EH: Attenuation of platelet responsiveness to prostacyclin (PGI$_2$) after tissue-type plasminogen activator (tPA). Circulation 76(Suppl IV):IV338, 1987.

30. Eisenberg PR, Miletich J: Induction of marked thrombin activity by pharmacologic concentrations of plasminogen activators in nonanticoagulated whole blood. Thromb Res 55:635, 1989.

31. Sobel BE, Hirsh J: Principles and practice of coronary thrombolysis and conjunctive treatment. Am J Cardiol 68:382, 1991.

32. Verstraete M, Arnold A, Brower RW, et al: Acute coronary thrombolysis with recombinant human tissue-type plasminogen activator: Initial patency and influence of maintained infusion on reocclusion rate. Am J Cardiol 60:231, 1987.

33. Hsia J, Hamilton WP, Kleiman N, et al, for the Heparin-Aspirin Reperfusion Trial (HART) Investigators: A comparison between heparin and low-dose aspirin as adjunctive therapy with tissue plasminogen activator for acute myocardial infarction. N Engl J Med 323:1433, 1990.

34. Bleich SD, Nichols TC, Schumacher RR, et al: Effect of heparin on coronary arterial patency after thrombolysis with tissue plasminogen activator in acute myocardial infarction. Am J Cardiol 66:1412, 1990.

35. deBono DP, Simoons ML, Tijssen J, et al, for the European Cooperative Study Group: Effect of early intravenous heparin on coronary patency, infarct size and bleeding complications after alteplase thrombolysis: Results of a randomized double blind European Cooperative Study Group trial. Br Heart J 67:122, 1992.

36. Tiefenbrunn AJ, Graor RA, Robison AK, et al: Pharmacodynamics of tissue-type plasminogen activator characterized by computer-assisted simulation. Circulation 73:1291, 1986.

37. Torr SR, Nachowiak DA, Fujii S, Sobel BE: "Plasminogen Steal" and clot lysis. J Am Coll Cardiol 19:1085, 1992.

38. Rijken DC, Juhan-Vague I, DeCock F, et al: Measurement of human tissue-type plasminogen activator by a two-site immunoradiometric assay. J Lab Clin Med 101:274, 1983.

39. Holvoet P, Cleemput H, Collen D: Assay of human tissue-type plasminogen activator (t-PA) with an enzyme-linked immunosorbent assay (ELISA) based on three murine monoclonal antibodies to t-PA. Thromb Haemost 54:684, 1985.

40. Matsuo O: Turnover of tissue plasminogen activator in man. Thromb Haemost 48:242, 1982.

41. Topol EJ, Bell WR, Weisfeldt ML: Coronary thrombolysis with recombinant tissue-type plasminogen activator. Ann Intern Med 103:837, 1985.

42. Garabedian HD, Gold HK, Leinbach RC, et al: Dose-dependent thrombolysis, pharmacokinetics and hemostatic effects of recombinant human tissue-type plasminogen activator for coronary thrombolysis. Am J Cardiol 58:673, 1986.

43. Verstraete M, Bounameaux H, deCock F, et al: Pharmacokinetics and systemic fibrinolytic effects of recombinant human tissue-type plasminogen activator (rt-PA) in humans. J Pharmacol Exp Ther 235:506, 1985.

44. Garabedian HD, Gold HK, Leinbach RC, et al: Comparative properties of two clinical preparations of recombinant human tissue-type plasminogen activator in patients with acute myocardial infarction. J Am Coll Cardiol 9:599, 1987.

45. Collen D, Topol EJ, Tiefenbrunn AJ, et al: Coronary thrombolysis with recombinant human tissue-type plasminogen activator: A prospective, randomized, placebo-controlled trial. Circulation 70:1012, 1984.

46. Verstraete M, Bleifeld W, Brower RW, et al: Double-blind randomised trial of intravenous tissue-type plasminogen activator versus placebo in acute myocardial infarction. Lancet 2:965, 1985.

47. Verstraete M, Bernard R, Bory M, et al: Randomised trial of intravenous recombinant tissue-type plasminogen activator versus intravenous streptokinase in acute myocardial infarction. Lancet 1:842, 1985.

48. Chesebro JH, Knatterud G, Roberts R, et al: Thrombolysis in myocardial infarction (TIMI) trial, phase I: A comparison between intravenous tissue plasminogen activator and intravenous streptokinase. Circulation 76:142, 1987.

49. Korninger C, Stassen JM, Collen D: Turnover of human extrinsic (tissue-type) plasminogen activator in rabbits. Thromb Haemost 46:658, 1981.

50. Nilsson S, Einarsson M, Ekvarn S, et al: Turnover of tissue plasminogen activator in normal and hepatectomized rabbits. Thromb Res 39:511, 1985.

51. Fuchs HE, Berger H, Pizzo SV: Catabolism of human tissue plasminogen activator in mice. Blood 65:539, 1985.

52. Bounameaux H, Verstraete M, Collen D: Comparative pharmacokinetics of human tissue-type plasminogen activator (tPA) obtained from cell culture (Bowes melanoma) or by recombinant DNA technology. Thromb Haemost 54:61, 1985.

53. Tiefenbrunn AJ, Sobel BE: Invited Review: The impact of coronary thrombolysis on myocardial infarction. Fibrinolysis 3:1, 1989.

54. Sherry S, Marder VJ: Streptokinase and recombinant tissue plasminogen activator (rt-PA) are equally effective in treating acute myocardial infarction. Ann Intern Med 114:417, 1991.

55. Gruppo Italiano per lo Studio della Streptochinasi nell'Infarto Miocardico (GISSI): Effectiveness of intravenous thrombolytic treatment in acute myocardial infarction. Lancet 1:397, 1986.

56. Gruppo Italiano per lo Studio della Streptochinasi nell'Infarto Miocardico (GISSI): Long-term effects of intravenous thrombolysis in acute myocardial infarction: Final report of the GISSI study. Lancet 2:871, 1987.

57. ISIS-2 (Second International Study of Infarct Survival) Collaborative Group: Randomized trial of intravenous streptokinase, oral aspirin, both, or neither among 17,187 cases of suspected acute myocardial infarction: ISIS-2. Lancet 2:349, 1988.

58. Kennedy JW, Ritchie JD, Davis KB, et al: The Western Washington randomized trial of intracoronary streptokinase in acute myocardial infarction: A 12-month follow-up report. N Engl J Med 312:1073, 1985.

59. Ohman EM, Califf RM, Topol EJ, et al, and the TAMI Study Group: Consequences of reocclusion after successful reperfusion therapy in acute myocardial infarction. Circulation 82:781, 1990.

60. Sheehan FH, Braunwald E, Canner P, et al: The effect of intravenous thrombolytic therapy on left ventricular function: A report on tissue-type plasminogen activator and streptokinase from the Thrombolysis in Myocardial Infarction (TIMI phase I) trial. Circulation 75:817, 1987.

61. National Heart Foundation of Australia Coronary Thrombolysis Group: Coronary thrombolysis and myocardial salvage by tissue plasminogen activator given up to 4 hours after onset of myocardial infarction. Lancet 1:203, 1988.

62. O'Rourke M, Baron D, Keogh A: Limitation of myocardial infarction by early infusion of recombinant tissue-type plasminogen activator. Circulation 77:1311, 1988.

63. Guerci AD, Gerstenblith G, Brinker JA, et al: A randomized trial of intravenous tissue plasminogen activator for acute myocardial infarction with subsequent randomization to elective coronary angioplasty. N Engl J Med 317:1613, 1987.

64. Wilcox RG, Olsson CG, Skene AM, et al: Trial of tissue plasminogen activator for mortality reduction in acute myocardial infarction. Lancet 2:525, 1988.

65. Van de Werf F, Arnold AE: Intravenous tissue plasminogen activator and size of infarct, left ventricular function, and survival in acute myocardial infarction. Br Med J 297:1374, 1988.

66. Reimer KA, Lowe JE, Rasmussen M, Jennings RB: The wave front phenomenon of ischemic cell death: I. Myocardial infarct size versus duration of coronary occlusion in dogs. Circulation 56:786, 1977.

67. Bergmann SR, Lerch RA, Fox KAAS, et al: Temporal dependence of beneficial effects of coronary thrombolysis characterized by positron tomography. Am J Med 73:573, 1932.

68. Tiefenbrunn AJ: Clinical benefits of thrombolytic therapy in acute myocardial infarction. Am J Cardiol 69:3A, 1992.

69. Tiefenbrunn AJ, Sobel BE: Timing of coronary recanalization: Paradigms, paradoxes, and pertinence. Circulation 85:2311, 1992.

70. Tiefenbrunn AJ, Sobel BE: Invited review: Thrombolysis and myocardial infarction. Fibrinolysis 5:1, 1991.

71. Gruppo Italiano per lo Studio della Sopravvivenza nell'Infarto Miocardico: GISSI2: A factorial randomized trial of alteplase versus streptokinase and heparin versus no heparin among 12,490 patients with acute myocardial infarction. Lancet 336:65, 1990.

72. The International Study Group: In-hospital mortality and clinical course of 20,891 patients with suspected acute myocardial infarction randomized between alteplase and streptokinase with or without heparin. Lancet 336:71, 1990.

73. ISIS-3 (Third International Study of Infarct Survival) Collaborative Group: ISIS-3: A randomized comparison of streptokinase vs tissue plasminogen activator vs anistreplase and of aspirin plus heparin vs aspirin alone among 41,299 cases of suspected acute myocardial infarction. Lancet 339:753, 1992.

73a. The GUSTO Investigators: An international randomized trial comparing four thrombolytic strategies for acute myocardial infarction. N Engl J Med 329:673, 1993.

74. Goldhaber SZ, Vaughan DE, Markis JE: Acute pulmonary embolism treated with tissue plasminogen activator. Lancet 2:886, 1986.

75. Bounameaux H, Vermylen J, Collen D: Thrombolytic treatment with recombinant tissue-type plasminogen activator in a patient with massive pulmonary embolism. Ann Intern Med 103:64, 1985.

76. Come PC, Markis JE: Reversal of right ventricular dysfunction in patients after intravenous tissue plasminogen activator for acute pulmonary embolism. J Am Coll Cardiol 9:40A, 1987.

77. Goldhaber SZ, Kessler CM, Heit J, et al: A randomized controlled trial of recombinant tissue plasminogen activator versus urokinase in the treatment of acute pulmonary embolism. Lancet 2:293, 1988.

78. Meyer G, Sors H, Charbonnier B, et al: Effects of intravenous urokinase versus alteplase on total pulmonary resistance in acute massive pulmonary embolism: A European multicenter double-blind trial. J Am Coll Cardiol 19:239, 1992.

78a. The National Institute of Neurological Disorders and Stroke, rt-PA Stroke Study Group: Tissue plasminogen activator for acute ischemic stroke. N Engl J Med 333:1581, 1995.

79. Graor RA, Risius B: Thrombolysis with recombinant human tissue-type plasminogen activator in patients with peripheral artery and bypass graft thrombosis. In Sobel BE, Collen D, Grossbard EB (eds): Tissue Plasminogen Activator in Thrombolytic Therapy. New York: Marcel Dekker, 1987, pp 171–204.

80. Turpie AGG, Jay RM, Carter CJ, et al: A randomized trial of recombinant tissue plasminogen activator for the treatment of proximal deep vein thrombosis. Circulation 72(Suppl III):III193, 1985.

81. Gold HK, Johns JA, Leinbach RC, et al: A randomized, blinded, placebo-controlled trial of recombinant human tissue-type plasminogen activator in patients with unstable angina pectoris. Circulation 75:1192, 1987.

82. Scrutinio D, Biasco MG, Rizzon P: Thrombolysis in unstable angina: Results of clinical studies. Am J Cardiol 68:99B, 1991.

83. Brott TG, Haley EC Jr, Levy DE, et al: Urgent therapy for stroke: Part I, pilot study of tissue plasminogen activator administered within 90 minutes. Stroke 23:632, 1992.

84. Haley EC Jr, Levy DE, Brott TG, et al: Urgent therapy for stroke: Part II, pilot study of tissue plasminogen activator administered within 91–180 minutes from onset. Stroke 23:641, 1992.

85. Tiefenbrunn AJ: Intracoronary thrombolysis. Chest 101:1484, 1992.

86. The TIMI Study Group: Comparison in invasive and conservative strategies after treatment with intravenous tissue plasminogen activator in acute myocardial infarction. Results of the Thrombolysis in Myocardial Infarction (TIMI) phase II trial: N Engl J Med 320:618, 1989.

87. Sloan M, Gore J: Ischemic stroke and intracranial hemorrhage following thrombolytic therapy for acute myocardial infarction: A risk-benefit analysis. Am J Cardiol 69:21A, 1192.

88. Califf RM, Fortin DF, Tenaglia AN, Sane DC: Clinical risks of thrombolytic therapy. Am J Cardiol 69:12A, 1992.

89. Shafer KE, Santoro SA, Sobel BE, et al: Monitoring activity of fibrinolytic agents: A therapeutic challenge. Am J Med 76:879, 1984.

90. Eisenberg PR, Jaffe AS: Coronary thrombolysis: Practical considerations. Cardiol Clin 5:129, 1987.

91. Sane DC, Califf RM, Topol EJ, et al: Bleeding during thrombolytic therapy for acute myocardial infarction: Mechanism and management. Ann Intern Med 111:1010, 1989.

92. Griffin JD, Ellman L: Epsilon-aminocaproic acid (EACA). Semin Thromb Hemost 5:27, 1978.

93. Grines CL, DeMaria AN: Optimal utilization of thrombolytic therapy for acute myocardial infarction: Concepts and controversies. J Am Coll Cardiol 16:223, 1990.

94. Passamani ER: Thrombolysis in myocardial infarction: The NHLBI Experience. In Sobel BE, Collen D, Grossbard EB (eds): Tissue Plasminogen Activator in Thrombolytic Therapy. New York: Marcel Dekker, 1987, pp 75–86.

95. Mueller HS, Rao AK, Forman SA, et al: Thrombolysis in myocardial infarction (TIMI): Comparative studies of coronary reperfusion and systemic fibrinogenolysis with two forms of recombinant tissue-type plasminogen activator. J Am Coll Cardiol 10:479, 1987.

96. Neuhaus KL, Feuerer W, Jeep-Tebbe S, et al: Improved thrombolysis with a modified dose regimen of recombinant tissue-type plasminogen activator. J Am Coll Cardiol 14:1566, 1989.

97. Carney RJ, Murphy GA, Brandt TR, et al, for the RAAMI Study Investigators: Randomized angiographic trial of recombinant tissue-type plasminogen activator (alteplase) in myocardial infarction. J Am Coll Cardiol 20:17, 1992.

98. Wall TC, Califf RM, George BS, et al, for the TAMI-7 Study Group: Accelerated plasminogen activator dose regimens for coronary thrombolysis. J Am Coll Cardiol 19:482, 1992.

99. Neuhaus KL, Von Essen R, Tebbe U, et al: Improved thrombolysis in acute myocardial infarction with front-loaded administration of alteplase: Results of the rt-PA-APSAC Patency Study (TAPS). J Am Coll Cardiol 19:885, 1992.

100. Barbash GI, Hod H, Roth A, et al: Repeat infusions of recombinant tissue-type plasminogen activator in patients with acute myocardial infarction and early recurrent myocardial ischemia. J Am Coll Cardiol 16:779, 1990.

101. Verstraete M, Miller AH, Bounameaux H: Intravenous and intrapulmonary recombinant tissue-type plasminogen activator in the treatment of acute massive pulmonary embolism. Circulation 77:353, 1988.

CHAPTER 169

Single-Chain Urokinase-Type Plasminogen Activator (Prourokinase)

H. Roger Lijnen, Ph.D., David C. Stump, M.D., and Désiré Collen, M.D., Ph.D.

HISTORY

In the early 1950s, it was recognized that urine contains a fibrinolytically active component designated urokinase,[1] which, after its purification, was characterized as a two-chain molecule.[2, 3] Urokinase (UK) was found to be a potent activator of plasminogen, which, when given to patients, could cause a fibrinolytically active state in blood, leading to therapeutic thrombolysis.[4] However, two major limitations hampered its widespread use: (1) like streptokinase, UK activates plasminogen without fibrin specificity and thus causes systemic fibrinolysis characterized by fibrinogen degradation, hemostatic breakdown, and increased risk of bleeding, and (2) the concentration of UK in urine and conditioned kidney cell culture media is low, its isolation is tedious, and thus the cost of a therapeutic dose is high. Because of these drawbacks, UK has never enjoyed a significant clinical role compared with streptokinase.

In 1973, Bernik[5] reported that the conditioned media of some cultured human cells contained a previously unrecognized latent UK-like activity. In 1977, Nolan et al.[6] identified an inactive form of a plasminogen activator in human embryonic kidney cell cultures with the following properties: (1) it reacted with anti-urokinase antibodies; (2) unlike urokinase, it did not bind to benzamidine-Sepharose; and (3) it could be activated, without change in molecular weight, by trypsin. Based on these observations, the authors concluded that they had identified a proenzyme form of urokinase. In the early 1980s, a single-chain form of urokinase was isolated from both urine[7] and conditioned human cell culture media[8, 9] by adsorption to and elution from immobilized fibrin. This chromatographic behavior led to the speculation that this single-chain UK had a specific affinity for fibrin and thereby might constitute a more fibrin-specific plasminogen activator than UK itself.

Single-chain UK was also purified from human plasma[10] and conditioned human cell culture media[11, 12] and was biochemically characterized as a proenzyme form of the active two-chain enzyme, hence the adoption of the designation prourokinase. More recently, development of improved purification methods for prourokinase (pro-UK) from human urine[13, 14] and human cell culture systems,[15–19] and its molecular cloning and expression,[20] have facilitated further characterization of its biochemical and biologic properties and its investigation as a relatively fibrin-specific thrombolytic agent in humans.[21] However, its mechanism of action has now been shown to be distinct from that of tissue-type plasminogen activator (t-PA)[22]

and not to be dependent on specific binding to fibrin.[22, 23] The specific binding of single-chain UK to fibrin, which was initially observed during its purification from urine, was later shown to be pH-dependent, with an optimum at pH 6.5.[24] In addition, a strong and specific interaction with fibrin has been reported in the presence of Zn^{2+}.[25]

The designation urokinase-type plasminogen activator (u-PA) was adopted by the International Committee on Thrombosis and Haemostasis to distinguish urokinase-like plasminogen activators from tissue-type plasminogen activators (t-PA). The single-chain form of u-PA is designated scu-PA or prourokinase, whereas the two-chain form is designated tcu-PA or urokinase (UK).[26]

BIOCHEMISTRY

The amino acid sequence of scu-PA determined by both peptide[27, 28] and cDNA[20, 29] sequencing is represented in Figure 169–1. It comprises 411 amino acids in a single polypeptide chain and contains the serine protease active site triad His, Asp, and Ser at positions 204, 255, and 356, respectively (indicated by asterisks in Fig. 169–1). The molecule contains an NH_2-terminal growth factor domain and a triple disulfide bonded kringle structure homologous to the five kringles found in plasminogen and the two kringles in t-PA. Conversion of scu-PA to tcu-PA occurs after proteolytic cleavage at position Lys158-Ile159.[27] Proteases that cleave the Lys158-Ile159 peptide bond in scu-PA include plasmin,[27] kallikrein,[30] trypsin,[30] cathepsin B,[31] human T cell–associated serine proteinase-1,[32] and thermolysin.[33] A fully active tcu-PA derivative is obtained after additional proteolysis by plasmin at position Lys135-Lys136.[28] In addition, a low molecular weight form of scu-PA (scu-PA-32k) can be obtained by selective cleavage at position Glu143-Leu144;[19] this cleavage can be obtained with the matrix metalloproteinase Pump-1.[34] In contrast, scu-PA is converted to an inactive two-chain molecule by thrombin after proteolytic cleavage at position Arg156-Phe157.[30] This inactive derivative can be reactivated by extensive treatment with plasmin, resulting in removal of the dipeptide Phe157-Lys158.[35] Inactivation of scu-PA by thrombin is strongly enhanced in the presence of thrombomodulin,[36] and this effect is dependent on the O-linked glucosaminoglycan of thrombomodulin.[37] This cofactor effect of thrombomodulin on the inactivation of scu-PA by thrombin has been confirmed in a perfused rabbit heart model.[38]

The cDNA sequence of u-PA contains an open read-

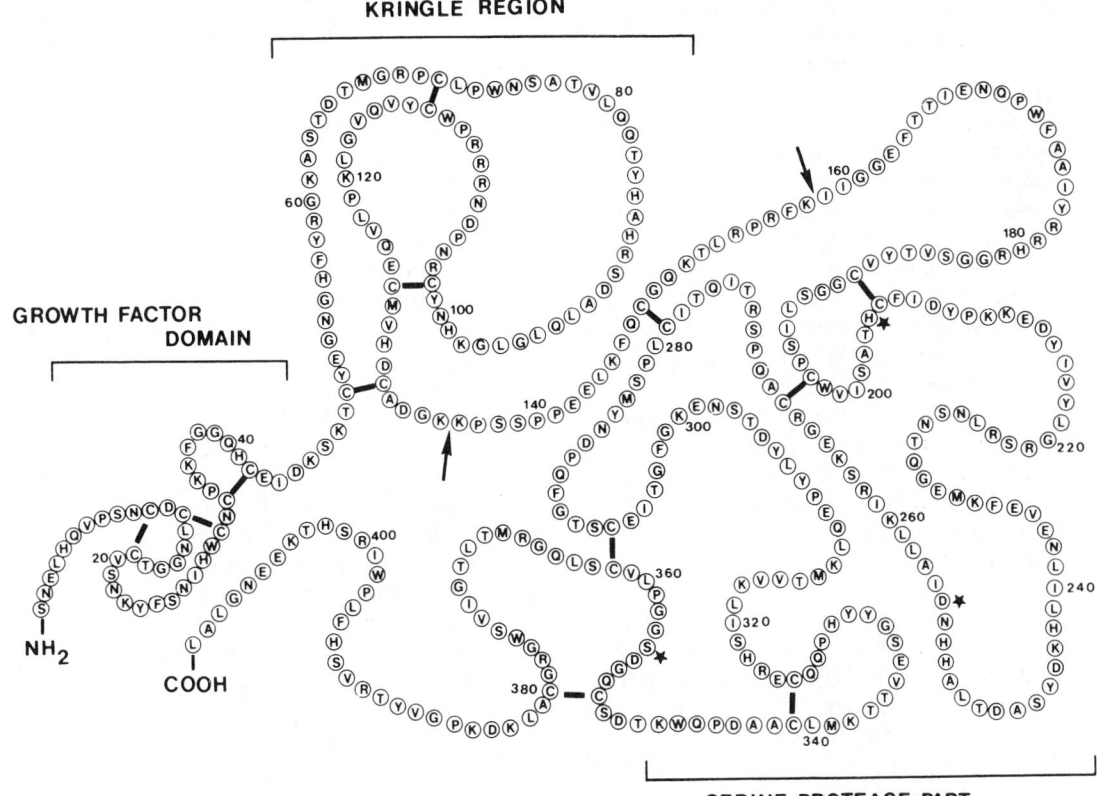

Figure 169–1. Schematic representation of the primary structure of single-chain urokinase-type plasminogen activator (scu-PA). Proteolytic cleavage sites are denoted by arrows for conversion to two-chain (158–159) and low-molecular-weight (135–136) urokinase forms. Asterisks denote the active-site amino acid residues. (Adapted from data in Holmes WE, Pennica D, Blaber M, et al: Cloning and expression of the gene for pro-urokinase in Escherichia coli. Biotechnology 3:923, 1985; and Günzler WA, Steffens GJ, Otting F, et al: The primary structure of high molecular mass urokinase from human urine. The complete amino acid sequence of the A chain. Hoppe-Seyler's Z Physiol Chem 363:133, 1982.)

ing frame that starts with ATG at nucleotide positions 77 to 79 and extends for 1293 nucleotides until a TGA stop codon is reached at positions 1370 to 1372.[20] The open reading frame is preceded by at least 76 nucleotides of 5'-untranslated mRNA, and the cDNA extends for another 932 nucleotides beyond the stop codon. The human u-PA gene is 6.4 kb long and located on chromosome 10.[39] It contains 11 exons, and the intron-exon organization of the gene closely resembles that of the t-PA gene.[40] However, exons III, VIII, and IX of t-PA are totally missing and exon IV partially missing in the u-PA gene; this accounts for the absence of a finger domain and a second kringle in u-PA. Exon II of the u-PA gene codes for a signal peptide consisting of 20 amino acids; exons III and IV code for the growth factor domain and exons V and VI for the kringle region. The 5' region of exon VII, which codes for the peptide connecting the light and the heavy chain, is 39 bp longer than the corresponding exon X of the t-PA gene. The 3' region of exon VII and exons VIII to XI code for the heavy chain.

All the molecular forms of u-PA (except the thrombin inactivated species) cause plasminogen-dependent lysis on fibrin films with specific activities of 50,000 to 100,000 international units (IU) per milligram as calibrated against the International Reference Preparation of Urokinase (66/46). In contrast, scu-PA displays very low activity toward low-molecular-weight chromogenic substrates (<1000 IU/mg), whereas by conversion to tcu-PA full amidolytic activity is generated. However, scu-PA appears to have some intrinsic plasminogen-activating potential, which represents 0.5% or less of the catalytic efficiency of tcu-PA.[41, 42] This intrinsic activity has been confirmed in studies using noncleavable mutants of scu-PA obtained by substitution of Lys158 with nonbasic amino acids.[43, 44] Other investigators, however, have claimed that scu-PA has no measurable intrinsic amidolytic or plasminogen activator activities.[45] Recently, the occurrence of a transitional state of scu-PA with a higher catalytic efficiency against native plasminogen than tcu-PA has been postulated.[46] Furthermore, it has been reported that fibrin fragment E-2 selectively promotes the activation of plasminogen by scu-PA[47] mainly by enhancing the catalytic rate constant of the activation.[48]

PHARMACOLOGY

Clot-specific activation of the fibrinolytic system requires that the plasminogen-activating potential of a plasminogen activator is fibrin dependent. Indeed, under physiologic conditions, free plasmin in circulating blood is rapidly neutralized by the presence of its main natural inhibitor, α_2-antiplasmin. However, at the fibrin surface, this inhibition occurs only slowly because of masking by fibrin of the lysine-binding sites of plasmin, which mediate the rapid interaction between plasmin and α_2-antiplasmin.[49, 50] Thus, efficient, fibrin-specific plasminogen activation will occur only at or in the vicinity of the fibrin surface.

tcu-PA has no fibrin specificity and activates fibrin-bound and circulating plasminogen relatively indiscriminately. Extensive plasminogen activation and depletion of α_2-antiplasmin may occur after patients with thromboembolic disease are treated with tcu-PA, leading to degradation of several plasma proteins including fibrinogen, factor V, and factor VIII.

In contrast with tcu-PA, scu-PA has a significant fibrin specificity. Several hypotheses for the mechanism of plasminogen activation and fibrin specificity of clot lysis with scu-PA in a plasma milieu have been proposed. One hypothesis claims that scu-PA has some intrinsic plasminogen activating potential ($\leq 0.5\%$ that of tcu-PA) that is counteracted by a competitive inhibitory mechanism in plasma, which is reversed by fibrin.[22] Alternatively, scu-PA was claimed to be inactive toward circulating native plasminogen (Glu-plasminogen) but active toward conformationally altered plasminogen (Lys-plasminogen) bound to partially digested fibrin.[51, 52] Third, scu-PA has been proposed to be a genuine proenzyme with negligible activity toward plasminogen,[11, 12, 45] and fibrinolysis with scu-PA would thus entirely depend on generation of tcu-PA.

The mechanism of plasminogen activation and fibrin specificity of scu-PA in in vitro plasma systems was recently reinvestigated by direct comparison of the relative catalytic efficiency and fibrinolytic potency of scu-PA, tcu-PA, and a plasmin-resistant mutant of scu-PA (scu-PA K158E). Using plasmin-mediated fibrin clot lysis as an endpoint, scu-PA had a 2000-fold higher fibrinolytic potency than scu-PA K158E, but only a 2.5-fold lower potency than tcu-PA. This suggests that conversion of scu-PA to tcu-PA during clot lysis constitutes a primary positive

feedback system.[42] Binding of plasminogen to fibrin or predigestion of fibrin by plasmin was found to result in relatively minor additional acceleration of fibrinolysis. Using an ELISA specific for two-chain forms of u-PA, it was shown that clot lysis with scu-PA in human plasma does not require extensive systemic conversion of scu-PA to tcu-PA. Systemic fibrinogen breakdown, however, occurs only secondarily to extensive systemic conversion of scu-PA to tcu-PA, resulting in a marked plasminogen activation and α_2-antiplasmin consumption.[53] Taken together, these data[42, 53] suggest that the clot selectivity of scu-PA may be mediated by preferential conversion of scu-PA to tcu-PA at the fibrin surface. Other authors have recently confirmed that local activation of scu-PA on the fibrin surface induces far more lysis and less nonspecific effects than systemic conversion to tcu-PA and that local activation is well correlated with the fibrinolytic activity of scu-PA.[54]

This mechanism of plasminogen activation and fibrin dissolution with scu-PA in a plasma milieu in vitro may, however, not be identical to its physiologic mechanism of action. It has indeed been reported that plasmin-resistant mutants of scu-PA have only a three- to fivefold lower in vivo thrombolytic potency than wild-type scu-PA,[55] suggesting that with respect to in vivo thrombolysis, conversion of scu-PA to tcu-PA may play a less important role.

Interaction of scu-PA with different cell types may also modulate its activity. Binding of scu-PA to platelets,[56, 57] monocytes,[58] and endothelial cells[59] has been reported. scu-PA is expressed in the apical endothelial cell membrane.[60]

PHARMACOKINETICS

The pharmacokinetics of natural (from urinary or cell culture origin) and recombinant scu-PA have been studied in several animal models (Table 169–1). The disappearance of u-PA is adequately represented by a two-compartment mammillary model composed of a central (intravascular) and a peripheral (interstitial) compartment, with clearance occurring from the central compartment. The turnover in blood of all uroki-

Table 169–1. **Pharmacokinetic Properties of scu-PA**

Species	scu-PA	Number	Administration	Postinjection Half-Life (min)		Clearance Site	Reference
				Early	Late		
Rabbit	Natural	2	IV bolus	5	360	—	Gurewich et al.[41]
Dog	Natural	1	IV bolus	5	360	—	Gurewich et al.[41]
Rabbit	Recombinant	3	IV bolus	3–6	—	Liver	Collen et al.[61]
Squirrel monkey	Recombinant	3	IV bolus	3.5	—	Liver	Collen et al.[61]
Rabbit	Natural	6	IV bolus	3	18	Liver (primary) Kidney (secondarily)	Stump et al.[62]
Rabbit	Natural (scu-PA-32k)	3	IV bolus	3	18	Liver (primary) Kidney (secondarily)	Stump et al.[62]
Squirrel monkey	Natural	3	IV bolus	3	20	Liver	Stump et al.[62]
Dog	Natural	6	30-min IV infusion	7	—	—	Collen et al.[63]
Baboon	Recombinant	6	60-min IV infusion	5	—	—	Flameng et al.[64]
Rabbit	Natural	3	4-hr IV infusion	6	—	—	Stump et al.[62]
Human	Natural	4	60-min IV infusion	4	—	—	Van de Werf et al.[21]
Human	Recombinant	17	60-min IV infusion	8	48	—	Van de Werf et al.[65]

Table 169–2. **Thrombolytic Properties of scu-PA in Animal Models of Thrombosis**

Animal Model	scu-PA Type	Number	Administration	Results	Fibrinogen	Reference
Dogs with saphenous vein thrombosis	Natural	6	3000 IU/kg IV	100% lysis in 1.5 hr	—	Sumi et al.[8]
Rabbits with IV fibrin clots	Natural	8	100,000–200,000 IU/hr over 5 hr	12%–53% lysis	Normal	Gurewich et al.[41]
Dogs with IV fibrin clots	Natural	3	75,000 IU/hr over 6 hr	90% lysis	Normal	Gurewich et al.[41]
Rabbits with jugular vein thrombosis	Recombinant	9	30,000–120,000 IU/kg IV over 4 hr	14%–60% lysis	Normal	Collen et al.[69]
	Natural	5	480,000 IU/kg IV over 4 hr	34% lysis	80% of baseline	Matsuo et al.[67]
	Natural	13	8700–35,000 IU/kg IV over 4 hr	13%–34% lysis	Normal	Stump et al.[68]
	Natural (scu-PA-32k)	9	9000–36,000 IU/kg IV over 4 hr	15%–40% lysis	Normal	Stump et al.[68]
Dogs with coronary artery thrombosis	Natural	6	20 μg/kg/min IV over 30 min	Reperfusion 23 ± 2 min	Normal	Collen et al.[63]
		2	10 μg/kg/min IV over 30 min	No reperfusion	—	Collen et al.[63]
	Recombinant	4	20 μg/kg/min IV over 30 min	Reperfusion at 14 ± 3 min	Normal	Van de Werf et al.[70]
		4	8 μg/kg/min IV over 30 min	Reperfusion in 3 at 18 ± 3 min	Normal	Van de Werf et al.[70]
		7	4 μg/kg/min IV over 30 min	Reperfusion in 2 at 25 and 27 min	Normal	Van de Werf et al.[70]
		4	2 μg/kg/min IV over 30 min	No reperfusion	—	Van de Werf et al.[70]
Baboons with coronary artery thrombosis	Recombinant	6	20 μg/kg/min IV over 60 min	Reperfusion 21 ± 4 min	Normal	Flameng et al.[64]

IU, international units; IV, intravenous.

nase species occurs with an initial half-life of approximately 3 to 7 minutes.[41, 61–64] Because similar turnover rates were observed for ^{125}I-labeled tracer, enzymatic activity, and antigen, this short half-life seems to be an inherent property of the urokinase molecule. The main mechanism of removal of urokinase from the blood appears to occur by hepatic clearance of the molecule. Experimental hepatectomy indeed markedly prolonged the initial half-life of scu-PA (from 3 minutes to 20–30 minutes).[61] scu-PA is taken up in the liver via a recognition site on parenchymal cells and is subsequently degraded in the lysosomes.[66]

The rapid clearance of u-PA apparently is not mediated via carbohydrate receptors, because very similar turnover characteristics were observed for both the scu-PA and tcu-PA forms of unglycosylated recombinant molecules and of glycosylated natural molecules. It does not occur via reaction with plasma protease inhibitors and subsequent rapid clearance of the complexes, because active site blocked tcu-PA and scu-PA, which do not react with plasma protease inhibitors, have the same half-life as the active tcu-PA forms.[61] In addition, the similar half-life observed for natural scu-PA-32k indicates that clearance of scu-PA is not mediated via the NH$_2$-terminal kringle-containing portion of the molecule.[62]

Following intravenous infusion of natural or recombinant scu-PA in patients with acute myocardial infarction, a biphasic disappearance rate was observed with initial half-lives in plasma (post-infusion) of 4 minutes or 8 minutes, respectively.[21, 65] This short half-life suggests that the maintenance of a therapeutic level of the agent in plasma may require its continuous infusion.

THROMBOLYTIC PROPERTIES
Animal Models

The thrombolytic properties of scu-PA have now been studied in several animal models of thrombosis, with the results shown in Table 169–2. Significant thrombolysis could be achieved in rabbits with a ^{125}I-labeled jugular vein thrombus with a 4-hour intravenous infusion of 480,000 IU/kg[67] or in a dose-dependent manner with 7500 to 36,000 IU/kg of natural scu-PA.[68] Thrombolysis occurred in the absence of α$_2$-antiplasmin consumption or fibrinogen degradation, which is suggestive of a considerable degree of clot selectivity. Very similar profiles of efficacy and specificity were observed with recombinant scu-PA[69] and with the low molecular weight scu-PA-32k.[68]

Both natural and recombinant scu-PA have also been studied in animal models of coronary artery thrombosis. Natural scu-PA given intravenously to dogs with a 1-hour-old copper coil–induced left anterior descending coronary artery thrombosis caused reperfusion in all of six animals after 23 ± 2 minutes when infused at 20 μg/kg/min and was not associated with systemic fibrinolytic activation.[63] In this model, recombinant scu-PA induced reperfusion in all of four animals after 14 ± 3 minutes at 20 μg/kg/min, in three of four animals after 18 ± 3 minutes at 8 μg/kg/min, but in only two of seven animals after 25 and 27 minutes at 4 μg/kg/min.[70] Recombinant scu-PA also caused no significant fibrinogen degradation, even at the highest dose. Very similar results were obtained with recombinant scu-PA in open-chest baboons with a 45-minute-old thrombus in the left anterior descending coronary artery.[64] Intravenous infusion of 20 μg/kg/min caused reperfusion in all of six animals after 21 ± 4 minutes in the absence of systemic fibrinolytic breakdown. Thus, in these mammalian animal models, multiple molecular forms of scu-PA displayed dose-related thrombolytic efficacy with a high degree of fibrin specificity.

Several approaches to enhance the thrombolytic potency of scu-PA were investigated in animal models. Thus, it was shown that administration of heparin enhances clot lysis induced by scu-PA in rabbits with jugular vein thrombosis[71] or with femoral artery thrombosis[72] and in dogs with femoral artery thrombosis.[73] Taprostene, a stable prostacyclin analogue, was also found to enhance the thrombolytic efficacy of scu-PA in a rabbit pulmonary embolism model.[74] Systemic administration of Lys-plasminogen in dogs with arterial thrombosis resulted in enhanced thrombolytic efficiency of a single IV bolus injection of scu-PA.[75] Interestingly, thrombin-inactivated scu-PA, which is totally inactive in plasma *in vitro*, has a significant thrombolytic activity *in vivo* in rabbits with jugular vein thrombosis.[76, 77]

The investigation of scu-PA has led to the recognition that the molecular interactions that regulate its biologic activity are different from those of t-PA and tcu-PA. The question was therefore raised whether combinations of these plasminogen activators might act synergistically with scu-PA.[22] Although initial investigation in a ^{125}I-plasma clot model *in vitro* showed no demonstrable synergism for fibrinolysis between scu-PA and t-PA or scu-PA and tcu-PA,[22, 78] contrasting results were obtained *in vivo*. In a rabbit jugular vein thrombosis model, significant synergism between scu-PA and t-PA was observed, because infusion of the agents in combination yielded significantly higher thrombolytic efficacy than was expected on the basis of the additive effects of these agents when used alone.[79] However, the effects of scu-PA and tcu-PA in combination were only additive.[79]

Human Studies

The encouraging results of animal studies with scu-PA formed the basis for its preliminary investigation in patients with early acute myocardial infarction (AMI), with the results shown in Table 169–3. The first six patients with AMI and angiographically confirmed coronary artery occlusion were treated within 5 hours of onset of symptoms.[21] Intravenous infusion of natural scu-PA from human cell cultures at a dose of 40 mg over 60 minutes resulted in reperfusion of the infarct-related vessel in four of six patients. A fifth patient was reperfused following additional intracoronary infusion of 20 mg over 30 minutes. No degrada-

tion of plasma fibrinogen was observed in five of the patients, but the remaining individual experienced a drop to 25% of baseline. In addition, three of the five patients with normal fibrinogen displayed some evidence of systemic fibrinolytic activation as evident from significant consumption of α_2-antiplasmin, causing a decrease to 40% of the baseline value.

The first 17 patients treated with intravenous recombinant scu-PA from *Escherichia coli* achieved somewhat less encouraging results.[66] Eight patients received 40 mg over 1 hour, causing reperfusion in six, but with persistent delayed opacification of the coronary artery during angiography in four and residual intraluminal thrombus in three. Plasma fibrinogen levels fell only slightly to a mean of 80% of the baseline value, but in one patient the levels fell to below 50%. Nine patients were treated with 70 mg over 1 hour, with reperfusion occurring in seven after 46 ± 17 minutes, but again, residual thrombus was observed in two. At the higher dose, more pronounced fibrinogen degradation occurred, to a mean of 45% of the baseline value, but including severe degradation to below 25% in four patients. Additional follow-up studies with both natural[80, 81] and recombinant[82] scu-PA have largely confirmed the results of these first pilot studies. With a total of 107 patients reported in these studies, who were treated with intravenous scu-PA at doses from 40 to 80 mg over 60 to 90 minutes, the cumulative reperfusion rate was 62% in association with modest overall fibrinolytic activation and fibrinogen degradation. Fibrinolytic activation can, however, be very extensive in some patients.

In a more extensive study (PRIMI trial), 401 patients with AMI of less than 4 hours duration were randomized to receive intravenous treatment with either 80 mg recombinant scu-PA (saruplase) or 1.5×10^6 IU streptokinase administered over 60 minutes.[83] Angiographic patency rates were higher at 60 minutes in saruplase-treated patients (72% versus 48%; $p < .001$), but did not differ significantly at 90 minutes (71% versus 64%; $p = .15$). Fibrinogen levels dropped markedly in both groups, but the decrease was delayed and less pronounced with saruplase.[84] Thus, it would appear that scu-PA will be at best similar to

Table 169–3. **Thrombolytic Properties of scu-PA in Humans**

Clinical Setting	scu-PA Type	Number	Administration (IV over 60 Minutes)	Results	Fibrinogen (% Baseline)	Side Effects	Reference
Acute myocardial infarction; <5 hr duration	Natural	6	40 mg	Reperfusion in 4	Normal in 5	None	Van de Werf et al.[21]
		(2)	(+ 20 mg IC)	(Reperfusion in 1)	25% in 1	None	Van de Werf et al.[21]
Acute myocardial infarction; <6 hr duration	Recombinant	8	40 mg	Reperfusion in 6 (delayed opacification in 4 and residual thrombus in 3)	89% (50% in 1)	None	Van de Werf et al.[65]
		9	70 mg	Reperfusion in 7 in 46 ± 17 min (residual thrombus in 2)	45% (<50% in 5 and <25% in 4)	None	Van de Werf et al.[65]
		12	40 mg	Reperfusion in 6 in 58 ± 17 min	Normal	None	Diefenbach et al.[82]
		12	80 mg	Reperfusion in 9 in 44 ± 30 min	<100 mg/dl in 2	None	Diefenbach et al.[82]
	Natural	8	30 mg	Reperfusion in 2 in 30 and 45 min	—	None	Welzel and Wolf[80]
		21	50 mg	Reperfusion in 11 in 42 ± 15 min	60%–90% of baseline	None	Welzel and Wolf[80]
		20	68 mg	Reperfusion in 14 in 60 min	60%–90% of baseline	None	Welzel and Wolf[80]
		19	62.5 mg (over 90 min)	Reperfusion in 9 in 61 ± 19 min	$94\% \pm 7\%$ of baseline	None	Loscalzo[81]

IC, intracoronary.

t-PA in terms of both its thrombolytic efficacy and its relative fibrin specificity.

Preliminary investigation of combinations of thrombolytic agents in human subjects has been encouraging. In three patients with acute myocardial infarction, intravenous infusion over 60 minutes of 3 mg of scu-PA and 10 mg of t-PA, doses which represent only 5% to 15% of the therapeutic dose of each used singly, resulted in coronary artery reperfusion after 40 ± 14 minutes.[85] In addition, no systemic consumption of α_2-antiplasmin or degradation of fibrinogen was observed. These initial results have been confirmed using combinations of 10 mg of scu-PA and 10 mg of t-PA in nine patients with AMI, producing stable coronary artery reperfusion in seven.[86] Two subsequent studies have confirmed that combination therapy may allow substantial reduction in the total dose of thrombolytic agent while still achieving effective and fibrin-specific coronary thrombolysis. Bode et al. studied the effects of simultaneous infusions of 12 mg rt-PA over 30 minutes and 48 mg scu-PA over 40 minutes in 38 patients with AMI. Patency, assessed angiographically, was achieved in 19 of 31 patients (61%) at 60 minutes and in 27 of 33 patients (82%) at 90 minutes. At 120 minutes, fibrinogen levels were 91% ± 17% of the preinfusion level, whereas plasminogen and α_2-antiplasmin levels had decreased to 65% ± 13% and 32% ± 21%, respectively. Kirshenbaum et al.[88] investigated the effect of simultaneous infusion of low-dose rt-PA (10 mg as a bolus followed by 10 mg infused over 60 minutes) and scu-PA (4 mg as a bolus followed by 12 mg infused over 60 minutes) on coronary arterial thrombolysis in 23 patients treated within 6 hours of symptoms of AMI. Infarct artery patency at 90 minutes was achieved in 16 patients (70%), with a decrease in fibrinogen levels from 370 ± 210 to 320 ± 190 mg/dl, and residual plasminogen and α_2-antiplasmin levels of 69% ± 24% and 77% ± 24%, respectively.

Despite the lack of demonstrable synergism between scu-PA and tcu-PA in vitro or in rabbits in vivo, this combination has shown promise in small clinical pilot studies. Indeed, the addition of a 200,000-unit bolus injection of tcu-PA before 50 mg of scu-PA given intravenously over 1 hour caused reperfusion after 22 ± 14 minutes in 10 of 13 patients with coronary occlusion.[80] Subsequent small clinical trials in patients with AMI have confirmed a synergistic interaction between low-dose tcu-PA and scu-PA.[89–92] These promising initial results have formed the basis for a multicenter dose-finding trial for thrombolysis with urokinase preactivated scu-PA in patients with AMI.[93] This study revealed, however, that the reopening of the occluded coronary arteries with the combination therapy was achieved relatively slowly, and it was concluded that urokinase-preactivated scu-PA does not seem to offer significant advantages.[93]

NEWER DEVELOPMENTS

Several approaches to improve the thrombolytic profile of recombinant scu-PA (rscu-PA) by site-specific mutagenesis of selected amino acids or by deletion mutagenesis of domain structures have been evaluated. So far, however, mutants or variants with improved thrombolytic potency have not been reported (for references, see Lijnen and Collen[94]). Alternative strategies include the construction of recombinant chimeric plasminogen activators or of complexes between rscu-PA and monoclonal antibodies.

Recombinant Chimeric Plasminogen Activators

Recombinant chimeric plasminogen activators have been constructed primarily using different regions of t-PA and scu-PA, although alternative combinations have also been evaluated to some extent (for references, see Lijnen and Collen[94]). The rationale for the construction of recombinant chimeric molecules between t-PA and scu-PA is based on two observations. First, the structures in t-PA responsible for its fibrin affinity are apparently localized in the A-chain. Second, the fibrin specificity of scu-PA is not dependent on the NH_2-terminal 143 amino acids but is preserved when the Lys158-Ile159 peptide bond is intact. Chimeric proteins consisting of parts of the A-chain of t-PA (amino acids Ser1 through Arg275) and containing scu-PA-32k (amino acids Leu144 through Leu411) might thus combine the mechanisms of fibrin selectivity of both molecules. Chimeric molecules of t-PA and u-PA were produced by splicing of cDNA fragments encoding the A-chain of t-PA with cDNA fragments encoding scu-PA-32k. The functional properties (specific activity and catalytic efficiency for plasminogen activation) of these recombinant t-PA/u-PA chimeric plasminogen activators were similar to those of u-PA (tcu-PA or scu-PA), but their affinity for fibrin was lower than that of rt-PA (for references, see Lijnen and Collen[94]).

In vivo evaluation of chimeric plasminogen activators has been performed in animal models of thrombosis.[95–97] One of these variants ($K_1K_2P_u$) was found to have a markedly enhanced thrombolytic potency toward venous and arterial thrombi.[97] $K_1K_2P_u$ consists of kringles 1 and 2 of rt-PA (amino acids Ser1-Gln3 and Asp87-Phe274) and of the serine proteinase part of rscu-PA (amino acids Ser138-Leu411). The delayed plasma clearance of $K_1K_2P_u$ with relatively preserved specific thrombolytic activity suggested that a significant reduction of the total amount of material required for thrombolytic therapy and its administration by bolus injection may be possible.

A small feasibility study of coronary thrombolysis with $K_1K_2P_u$ has been performed in patients with acute myocardial infarction with thrombotic coronary artery occlusion.[98] An intravenous bolus injection of 10 mg $K_1K_2P_u$ was given over 5 minutes in two patients, and in four patients a second 10-mg bolus injection of $K_1K_2P_u$ was given 15 minutes after the first one. Arteriography of the occluded coronary artery was repeated at 10-minute intervals and the study was terminated after the 30-minute angiogram. At 30 minutes all patients were also given 320 mg aspirin, and a continuous intravenous infusion of heparin (1000 units/hr) was started. Clot lysis within 30 minutes was not achieved after intravenous injection of a single bolus of 10 mg $K_1K_2P_u$ in two patients, but was obtained in two of the four patients given two 10-mg boluses of $K_1K_2P_u$. The patients without recanalization at 30 minutes were immediately given 100 mg recombinant t-PA (rt-PA) over 90 minutes. At 24 hours, all patients had patent infarct-related coronary arteries, with residual stenoses of 40% to 90%. Administration of $K_1K_2P_u$ did not induce an overt systemic lytic state in any of the patients as shown by unchanged levels of fibrinogen and α_2-antiplasmin. In the patients given a single bolus injection of $K_1K_2P_u$, $K_1K_2P_u$-related antigen increased to 2 to 3 μg/ml and disappeared from plasma with an initial half-life of approximately 9 minutes and a terminal half-life of 70 minutes, corresponding to a plasma clearance of approximately 50 ml/min. After the second bolus injection in four patients, the plasma level increased to approximately 4 to 5 μg/ml and $K_1K_2P_u$ disappeared from plasma at a rate similar to that observed after the first bolus.

Although the small number of patients studied precludes valid estimation of the frequency of coronary recanalization with $K_1K_2P_u$ and of the adequacy of the dose used, this pilot experience suggests that two bolus injections of 10 mg $K_1K_2P_u$ may produce fibrin-specific coronary thrombolysis.

Complexes Between Monoclonal Antibodies and scu-PA

The fibrin specificity of scu-PA may be improved by targeting of the agent to a fibrin clot by conjugation with monoclonal antibodies that are fibrin-specific and do not cross-react with fibrinogen. Monoclonal antibodies that have been used for this purpose include antibodies against the B-chain of fibrin and against cross-linked fibrin fragment D-dimer.[99, 100]

Chemical conjugates of scu-PA with a murine monoclonal antibody directed against human cross-linked fibrin fragment D-dimer (MA-15C5) had a three- to sixfold enhanced thrombolytic potency in venous thrombosis models in rabbits[77] and baboons.[101] From these studies, it was concluded that the increased thrombolytic potency of scu-PA/MA-15C5 was the result of, on the one hand, a reduction of the thrombolytic potency resulting from chemical coupling of scu-PA to the antibody molecule, and, on the other hand, an enhancement of the thrombolytic potency resulting from fibrin-targeting by the specific idiotype. A recombinant chimeric plasminogen activator, rscu-PA-32k/MA-15C5Hu, which consists of humanized MA-15C5 (MA-15C5Hu) and rscu-PA-32k, had an 11-fold higher thrombolytic potency than rscu-PA in rabbits with jugular vein thrombosis.[102, 103] Alternatively, a single-chain chimeric plasminogen activator consisting of a synthetic single-chain variable region (Fv) fragment of MA-15C5 and scu-PA-33k (Ala132 through Leu411 of scu-PA), was found to have a 10-fold increased specific thrombolytic activity

and a sixfold increased thrombolytic potency compared with scu-PA in a hamster pulmonary embolism model.[104] These smaller fragments may be preferred moieties for the construction of recombinant chimeric scu-PA/antibody proteins for fibrin-targeted thrombolytic therapy.

Antibody targeting with fibrin-specific monoclonal antibodies thus appears to have the potential to increase the concentration of plasminogen activator in the vicinity of a thrombus, thereby leading to enhanced clot lysis. The use of such agents may allow a significant reduction of the total dose of plasminogen activator required for thrombolytic therapy, with, it is hoped, reduced systemic side effects. It was indeed shown that the thrombolytic potency of rscu-PA/anti-fibrin conjugates was determined by their clearance and by the rate and extent of initial binding to the emboli as well as by changes in binding during clot lysis. Thus, clot targeting reduces the dose required to obtain maximal clot lysis, but the minimal lag phase and the maximal rate of lysis appear to be independent of the nature of the plasminogen activator or of targeting. These observations suggest that there may be intrinsic limitations to the maximal achievable speed of thrombolysis.[105]

An alternative approach may consist in the use of bispecific monoclonal antibodies. Thus, rscu-PA/MA-FU1-74, an immunoconjugate of rscu-PA with a bispecific monoclonal antibody directed against u-PA and against the β-chain of human fibrin, was found to have a fivefold higher thrombolytic potency than unconjugated rscu-PA in baboons with femoral vein thrombosis. This is the result of both fibrin targeting by the specific idiotype of the antibody and of a slower plasma clearance.[106] It remains to be shown whether any of these approaches may be clinically useful.

CONCLUSIONS

The biochemical and biologic characterization of single-chain urokinase-type plasminogen activator (scu-PA, prourokinase) has revealed that it is a more fibrin-specific plasminogen activator than the more widely investigated tcu-PA (urokinase). Its mechanism of action is quite distinct from that of t-PA, and its clinical potential appears to be, at best, comparable with that of t-PA.

REFERENCES

1. Williams JRB: The fibrinolytic activity of urine. Br J Exp Pathol 32:530, 1951.
2. Plough J, Kjeldgaard KO: Urokinase: An activator of plasminogen from human urine. I. Isolation and properties. Biochim Biophys Acta 24:278, 1964.
3. White WF, Barlow GH, Mozen MM: The isolation and characterization of plasminogen activators (urokinase) from human urine. Biochemistry 5:2160, 1966.
4. Fletcher AP, Alkjaersig N, Sherry S, et al: The development of urokinase as a thrombolytic agent. Maintenance of a sustained thrombolytic state in man by its intravenous infusion. J Lab Clin Med 65:713, 1965.

5. Bernik MB: Increased plasminogen activator (urokinase) in tissue culture after fibrin deposition. J Clin Invest 42:823, 1973.

6. Nolan C, Hall L, Barlow G, et al: Plasminogen activator from human embryonic kidney cell cultures. Evidence for a proactivator. Biochim Biophys Acta 496:384, 1977.

7. Husain S, Gurewich V, Lipinski B: Purification and partial characterization of a single-chain high-molecular-weight form of urokinase from human urine. Arch Biochem Biophys 220:31, 1983.

8. Sumi H, Maruyama M, Matsuo O, et al: Higher fibrin-binding and thrombolytic properties of single polypeptide chain, high molecular weight urokinase. Thromb Haemost 47:297, 1982.

9. Kohno T, Hopper P, Lillquist JS, et al: Kidney plasminogen activator: A precursor form of human urokinase with high fibrin affinity. Biotechnology 2:628, 1984.

10. Wun TC, Schleuning WD, Reich E: Isolation and characterization of urokinase from human plasma. J Biol Chem 257:3276, 1982.

11. Nielsen LS, Hansen JG, Skriver L, et al: Purification of zymogen to plasminogen activator from human glioblastoma cells by affinity chromatography with monoclonal antibody. Biochemistry 21:6410, 1982.

12. Wun TC, Ossowski L, Reich E: A proenzyme form of human urokinase. J Biol Chem 257:7262, 1982.

13. Stump DC, Thienpont M, Collen D: Urokinase-related proteins in human urine. Isolation and characterization of single chain urokinase (prourokinase) and urokinase-inhibitor complex. J Biol Chem 261:1267, 1986.

14. Wojta J, Kirchheimer JC, Turcu L, et al: Monoclonal antibodies against human high molecular weight urinary urokinase: Application for affinity purification of urinary prourokinase. Thromb Haemost 55:347, 1986.

15. Eaton DL, Scott RW, Baker JB: Purification of human fibroblast urokinase proenzyme and analysis of its regulation by proteases and protease nexin. J Biol Chem 259:6241, 1984.

16. Kasai S, Arimura H, Nishida M, et al: Proteolytic cleavage of single-chain pro-urokinase induces conformational change which follows activation of the zymogen and reduction of its high affinity for fibrin. J Biol Chem 260:12377, 1985.

17. Stump DC, Lijnen HR, Collen D: Purification and characterization of single chain urokinase-type plasminogen activator (scu-PA) from human cell cultures. J Biol Chem 261:1274, 1986.

18. Wijngaards G, Rijken DC, van Wezel AL, et al: Characterization and fibrin-binding properties of different molecular forms of pro-urokinase from a monkey kidney cell culture. Thromb Res 42:749, 1986.

19. Stump DC, Lijnen H, Collen D: Purification and characterization of a novel low molecular weight form of single chain urokinase-type plasminogen activator. J Biol Chem 261:17120, 1986.

20. Holmes WE, Pennica D, Blaber M, et al: Cloning and expression of the gene for pro-urokinase in *Escherichia coli.* Biotechnology 3:923, 1985.

21. Van de Werf F, Nobuhara M, Collen D: Coronary thrombolysis with human single chain urokinase-type plasminogen activator (scu-PA) in patients with acute myocardial infarction. Ann Intern Med 104:345, 1986.

22. Lijnen HR, Zamarron C, Blaber M, et al: Activation of plasminogen by pro-urokinase. I. Mechanism. J Biol Chem 261:1253, 1986.

23. Gurewich V, Pannell R: Inactivation of single-chain urokinase (pro-urokinase) by thrombin and thrombin-like enzymes: Relevance of the findings to the interpretation of fibrin-binding experiments. Blood 69:769, 1987.

24. Pannell R, Angles-Cano E, Gurewich V: The pH dependence of the binding of pro-urokinase to fibrin/celite. Thromb Haemost 64:556, 1990.

25. Husain SS: Fibrin affinity of urokinase-type plasminogen activator. Evidence that Zn^{2+} mediates strong and specific interaction of single-chain urokinase with fibrin. J Biol Chem 268:8574, 1993.

26. Report of the Subcommittee on Fibrinolysis of the International Society of Thrombosis and Haemostasis, San Diego. Thromb Haemost 54:893, 1985.

27. Günzler WA, Steffens GJ, Otting F, et al: The primary structure of high molecular mass urokinase from human urine. The complete amino acid sequence of the A chain. Hoppe-Seyler's Z Physiol Chem 363:1155, 1982.

28. Günzler WA, Steffens GJ, Otting F, et al: Structural relationship between human high and low molecular mass urokinase. Hoppe-Seyler's Z Physiol Chem 363:133, 1982.

29. Verde P, Stoppelli MP, Galeffi P, et al: Identification and primary sequence of an unspliced human urokinase poly-(a)$^+$RNA. Proc Natl Acad Sci USA 81:4727, 1984.

30. Ichinose A, Fujikawa K, Suyama T: The activation of pro-urokinase by plasma kallikrein and its inactivation by thrombin. J Biol Chem 261:3486, 1986.

31. Kobayashi H, Schmitt M, Goretzki L, et al: Cathepsin B efficiently activates the soluble and the tumor cell receptor-bound form of the proenzyme urokinase-type plasminogen activator (Pro-uPA). J Biol Chem 266:5147, 1991.

32. Brunner G, Vettel U, Jobstmann S, et al: A T-cell-related proteinase expressed by T-lymphoma cells activates their endogenous pro-urokinase. Blood 79:2099, 1992.

33. Marcotte PA, Henkin J: Characterization of the activation of pro-urokinase by thermolysin. Biochim Biophys Acta 1160:105, 1993.

34. Marcotte PA, Kozan IM, Dorwin SA, et al: The matrix metalloproteinase Pump-1 catalyzes formation of low molecular weight (pro)urokinase in cultures of normal human kidney cells. J Biol Chem 267:13803, 1992.

35. Lijnen HR, Van Hoef B, Collen D: Activation with plasmin of two-chain urokinase-type plasminogen activator derived from single-chain urokinase-type plasminogen activator by treatment with thrombin. Eur J Biochem 169:359, 1987.

36. de Munk GA, Groeneveld E, Rijken DC: Acceleration of the thrombin inactivation of single chain urokinase-type plasminogen activator (pro-urokinase) by thrombomodulin. J Clin Invest 88:1680, 1991.

37. de Munk GA, Parkinson JF, Groeneveld E, et al: Role of the glycosaminoglycan component of thrombomodulin in its acceleration of the inactivation of single-chain urokinase-type plasminogen activator by thrombin. Biochem J 290:655, 1993.

38. Molinari A, Giorgetti C, Lansen J: Thrombomodulin is a cofactor for thrombin degradation of recombinant single-chain urokinase plasminogen activator "in vitro" and in a perfused rabbit heart model. Thromb Haemost 67:226, 1992.

39. Rajput B, Degen SF, Reich E, et al: Chromosomal locations of human tissue plasminogen activator and urokinase genes. Science 230:672, 1985.

40. Riccio A, Grimaldi G, Verde P, et al: The human urokinase-plasminogen activator gene and its promoter. Nucleic Acids Res 13:2759, 1985.

41. Gurewich V, Pannell R, Louie S, et al: Effective and fibrin-specific clot lysis by a zymogen precursor form of urokinase (pro-urokinase). A study in vitro and in two animal species. J Clin Invest 73:1731, 1984.

42. Lijnen HR, Van Hoef B, De Cock F, et al: The mechanism of plasminogen activation and fibrin dissolution by single-chain urokinase-type plasminogen activator in a plasma milieu in vitro. Blood 73:1864, 1989.

43. Nelles L, Lijnen HR, Collen D, et al: Characterization of recombinant human single chain urokinase-type plasminogen activator mutants produced by site-specific mutagenesis of Lys 158. J Biol Chem 262:5682, 1987.

44. Lijnen HR, Van Hoef B, Nelles L, et al: Plasminogen activation with single-chain urokinase-type plasminogen activator (scu-PA). Studies with active site mutagenized plasminogen (Ser740 -> Ala) and plasmin resistant scu-PA (Lys158 -> Glu). J Biol Chem 265:5232, 1990.

45. Husain SS: Single-chain urokinase-type plasminogen activator does not possess measurable intrinsic amidolytic or plasminogen activator activities. Biochemistry 30:5797, 1991.

46. Liu JN, Pannell R, Gurewich V: A transitional state of pro-urokinase that has a higher catalytic efficiency against Glu-plasminogen than urokinase. J Biol Chem 267:15289, 1992.

47. Liu JN, Gurewich V: A comparative study of the promotion of tissue plasminogen activator and pro-urokinase-induced plasminogen activation by fragments D and E-2 of fibrin. J Clin Invest 88:2012, 1991.

48. Liu JN, Gurewich V: Fragment E-2 from fibrin substantially enhances pro-urokinase-induced Glu-plasminogen activation. A kinetic study using the plasmin-resistant mutant pro-urokinase Ala-158-rpro-UK. Biochemistry 31:6311, 1992.

49. Wiman B, Collen D: Molecular mechanism of physiological fibrinolysis. Nature 272:549, 1978.

50. Collen D: On the regulation and control of fibrinolysis. Thromb Haemost 43:77, 1980.

51. Pannell R, Gurewich V: Pro-urokinase: A study of its stability in plasma and of a mechanism for its selective fibrinolytic effect. Blood 67:1215, 1986.

52. Gurewich V: The sequential, complementary and synergistic activation of fibrin-bound plasminogen by tissue plasminogen activator and pro-urokinase. Fibrinolysis 3:59, 1989.

53. Declerck PJ, Lijnen HR, Verstreken M, et al: A monoclonal antibody specific for two-chain urokinase-type plasminogen activator. Application to the study of the mechanism of clot lysis with single-chain urokinase-type plasminogen activator in plasma. Blood 75:1794, 1990.

54. Giorgetti C, Molinari A, Bonomini L, et al: The role of urokinase generation during clot lysis by pro-urokinase in a plasma milieu. Fibrinolysis 7:183, 1993.

55. Collen D, Mao J, Stassen JM, et al: Thrombolytic properties of Lys-158 mutants of recombinant single chain urokinase-type plasminogen activator (scu-PA) in rabbits with jugular vein thrombosis. J Vasc Med Biol 1:46, 1989.

56. Vaughan D, Van Houtte E, Collen D: Urokinase binds to platelets through a specific saturable and low affinity mechanism. Fibrinolysis 4:141, 1990.

57. Gurewich V, Johnstone M, Loza JP, et al: Pro-urokinase and prekallikrein are both associated with platelets. Implications for the intrinsic pathway of fibrinolysis and for therapeutic thrombolysis. FEBS Lett 318:317, 1993.

58. Manchanda N, Schwartz BS: Single chain urokinase. Augmentation of enzymatic activity upon binding to monocytes. J Biol Chem 266:14580, 1991.

59. Barnathan ES, Kuo A, Rosenfeld L, et al: Interaction of single-chain urokinase-type plasminogen activator with human endothelial cells. J Biol Chem 265:2865, 1990.

60. Lee SW, Kahn ML, Dichek DA: Expression of an anchored urokinase in the apical endothelial cell membrane. J Biol Chem 267:13020, 1992.

61. Collen D, De Cock F, Lijnen HR: Biological and thrombolytic properties of proenzyme and active forms of human urokinase. II. Turnover of natural and recombinant urokinase in rabbits and squirrel monkeys. Thromb Haemost 52:24, 1984.

62. Stump DC, Kieckens L, De Cock F, et al: Pharmacokinetics of single chain forms of urokinase-type plasminogen activator. J Pharmacol Exp Ther 242:245, 1987.

63. Collen D, Stump DC, Van de Werf F, et al: Coronary thrombolysis in dogs with intravenously administered human pro-urokinase. Circulation 72:384, 1985.

64. Flameng W, Vanhaecke J, Stump DC, et al: Coronary thrombolysis by intravenous infusion of recombinant single chain urokinase-type plasminogen activator or recombinant urokinase in baboons. J Am Coll Cardiol 8:118, 1986.

65. Van de Werf F, Vanhaecke J, De Geest H, et al: Coronary thrombolysis with recombinant single-chain urokinase-type plasminogen activator (rscu-PA) in patients with acute myocardial infarction. Circulation 74:1066, 1986.

66. Kuiper J, Rijken DC, de Munk GAW, et al: In vivo and in vitro interaction of high and low molecular weight single-chain urokinase-type plasminogen activator with rat liver cells. J Biol Chem 267:1589, 1992.

67. Matsuo O, Bando H, Okada K, et al: Thrombolytic effect of single-chain pro-urokinase in a rabbit jugular vein thrombosis model. Thromb Res 42:187, 1986.

68. Stump DC, Stassen JM, Demarsin E, et al: Comparative thrombolytic properties of single chain forms of urokinase-type plasminogen activator. Blood 69:592, 1987.

69. Collen D, Stassen JM, Blaber M, et al: Biological and thrombolytic properties of proenzyme and active forms of human urokinase. III. Thrombolytic properties of natural and recombinant urokinase in rabbits with experimental jugular vein thrombosis. Thromb Haemost 54:27, 1984.

70. Van de Werf F, Jang IK, Collen D: Thrombolysis with recombinant human single chain urokinase-type plasminogen activator (rscu-PA). Dose-response in dogs with coronary artery thrombosis. J Cardiovasc Pharmacol 9:91, 1987.

71. Stassen JM, Juhan-Vague I, Alessi MC, et al: Potentiation by heparin fragments of thrombolysis induced with human tissue-type plasminogen activator or human single-chain urokinase-type plasminogen activator. Thromb Haemost 58:947, 1987.

72. Schneider J: Heparin and the thrombin inhibitor argatroban enhance fibrinolysis by infused or bolus-injected saruplase (r-scu-PA) in rabbit femoral artery thrombosis. Thromb Res 64:677, 1991.

73. Burke SE, Lubbers NL, Nelson RA, et al: Recombinant pro-urokinase requires heparin for optimal clot lysis and restoration of blood flow in a canine femoral artery thrombosis model. Thromb Haemost 69:375, 1993.

74. Schneider J: Taprostene, a stable prostacyclin analogue, enhances the thrombolytic efficacy of saruplase (recombinant single-chain urokinase-type plasminogen activator) in rabbits with pulmonary embolized thrombi. Prostaglandins 41:595, 1991.

75. Badylak SF, Voytik SL, Henkin J, et al: Enhancement of the thrombolytic efficacy of prourokinase by Lys-plasminogen in a dog model of arterial thrombosis. Thromb Res 62:115, 1991.

76. Abercrombie DM, Buchinski B, Salvato KA, et al: Fibrin specific thrombolysis by two-chain urokinase-type plasminogen activator cleaved after arginine 156 by thrombin. Thromb Haemost 64:426, 1990.

77. Collen D, Dewerchin M, Stassen JM, et al: Thrombolytic and pharmacokinetic properties of conjugates of urokinase-type plasminogen activator with a monoclonal antibody specific for crosslinked fibrin. Fibrinolysis 3:197, 1989.

78. Collen D, De Cock F, Demarsin E, et al: Absence of synergism between tissue-type plasminogen activator (t-PA) and single chain urokinase-type plasminogen activator (scu-PA) on clot lysis in a plasma milieu in vitro. Thromb Haemost 56:35, 1986.

79. Collen D, Stassen JM, Stump DC, et al: Synergism of thrombolytic agents in vivo. Circulation 74:838, 1986.

80. Welzel D, Wolf H: Clinical research on single-chain urokinase-type plasminogen activator (scu-PA) in Germany. Results in patients with acute myocardial infarction (AMI) [abstract 160]. Thromb Haemost 58:47, 1987.

81. Loscalzo J: The efficacy and relative fibrin selectivity of pro-urokinase in patients with acute myocardial infarction [abstract 774]. Thromb Haemost 58:209, 1987.

82. Diefenbach C, Erbel R, Meyer J, et al: Dose-finding study of thrombolysis in acute myocardial infarction by single-chain prourokinase [abstract 770]. Thromb Haemost 58:208, 1987.

83. PRIMI Trial Study Group: Randomised double-blind trial of recombinant pro-urokinase against streptokinase in acute myocardial infarction. Lancet 1:863, 1989.

84. Ostermann H, Schmitz-Huebner U, Windeler J, et al: Rate of fibrinogen breakdown related to coronary patency and bleeding complications in patients with thrombolysis in acute myocardial infarction. Results from the PRIMI trial. Eur Heart J 13:1225, 1992.

85. Collen D, Stump DC, Van de Werf F: Coronary thrombolysis in patients with acute myocardial infarction by intravenous infusion of synergic thrombolytic agents. Am Heart J 112:1083, 1986.

86. Collen D, Van de Werf F: Coronary arterial thrombolysis with low dose synergistic combinations of recombinant tissue-type plasminogen activator (rt-PA) and recombinant single chain urokinase-type plasminogen activator (scu-PA) for acute myocardial infarction. Am J Cardiol 60:431, 1987.

87. Bode C, Schuler G, Nordt T, et al: Intravenous thrombolytic therapy with a combination of single-chain urokinase-type plasminogen activator and recombinant tissue-type plasminogen activator in acute myocardial infarction. Circulation 81:907, 1990.

88. Kirshenbaum JM, Bahr RD, Flaherty JT, et al: Clot-selective coronary thrombolysis with low-dose synergistic combinations of single-chain urokinase-type plasminogen activator and recombinant tissue-type plasminogen activator. Am J Cardiol 68:1564, 1991.

89. Gulba DCL, Fischer K, Barthels M, et al: Low dose urokinase preactivated natural prourokinase for thrombolysis in acute myocardial infarction. Am J Cardiol 63:1025, 1989.

90. Bode C, Schoenermark S, Schuler G, et al: Efficacy of intravenous prourokinase and a combination of prourokinase and urokinase in acute myocardial infarction. Am J Cardiol 61:971, 1988.

91. Kasper W, Hohnloser SH, Engler H, et al: Coronary reperfusion studies with pro-urokinase in acute myocardial infarction: Evidence for synergism of low dose urokinase. J Am Coll Cardiol 16:733, 1990.

92. Pindur G, Koehler M, Sen S, et al: Fibrinolytic effects of pro-urokinase combined with low-dose urokinase compared to high-dose urokinase in patients with acute myocardial infarction. Thromb Res 67:191, 1992.

93. Gulba DC, Bode C, Sen S, et al: Multicenter dose-finding trial for thrombolysis with urokinase preactivated pro-urokinase (TCL 598) in acute myocardial infarction. Cathet Cardiovasc Diagn 26:177, 1992.

94. Lijnen HR, Collen D: Strategies for the improvement of thrombolytic agents. Thromb Haemost 66:88, 1991.

95. Agnelli G, Pascucci C, Colucci M, et al: Thrombolytic activity of two chimeric recombinant plasminogen activators (FK2tu-PA and K2tu-PA) in rabbits. Thromb Haemost 68:331, 1992.

96. Robinson JH, Browne MJ, Carey JE, et al: A recombinant, chimeric enzyme with a novel mechanism of action leading to greater potency and selectivity than tissue-type plasminogen activator. Circulation 86:548, 1992.

97. Collen D, Lu HR, Lijnen HR, et al: Thrombolytic and pharmacokinetic properties of chimeric tissue-type and urokinase-type plasminogen activators. Circulation 84:1216, 1991.

98. Van de Werf F, Lijnen HR, Collen D: Coronary thrombolysis with $K_1K_2P_u$, a chimeric tissue-type and urokinase-type plasminogen activator. A feasibility study in six patients with acute myocardial infarction. Coron Art Dis 4:929, 1993.

99. Bode C, Runge MS, Schönermark S, et al: Conjugation to antifibrin Fab' enhances fibrinolytic potency of single-chain urokinase plasminogen activator. Circulation 81:1974, 1990.

100. Dewerchin M, Collen D: Enhancement of the thrombolytic potency of plasminogen activators by conjugation with clot-specific monoclonal antibodies. Bioconjugate Chemistry 2:293, 1991.

101. Collen D, Dewerchin M, Rapold HJ, et al: Thrombolytic and pharmacokinetic properties of a conjugate of recombinant single chain urokinase-type plasminogen activator with a monoclonal antibody specific for cross-linked fibrin in a baboon venous thrombosis model. Circulation 82:1744, 1990.

102. Dewerchin M, Van Damme AM, Holvoet P, et al: Thrombolytic and pharmacokinetic properties of a recombinant chimeric plasminogen activator consisting of a fibrin fragment D-dimer specific humanized monoclonal antibody and a truncated single-chain urokinase. Thromb Haemost 68:170, 1992.

103. Van Damme AM, Dewerchin M, Lijnen HR, et al: Characterization of a recombinant chimeric plasminogen activator composed of a fibrin fragment D-dimer specific humanized monoclonal antibody and a truncated single-chain urokinase. Eur J Biochem 205:139, 1992.

104. Holvoet P, Laroche Y, Stassen JM, et al: Pharmacokinetic and thrombolytic properties of chimeric plasminogen activators consisting of a single-chain Fv fragment of a fibrin-specific antibody fused to single-chain urokinase. Blood 81:696, 1993.

105. Holvoet P, Dewerchin M, Stassen JM, et al: Thrombolytic profiles of clot-targeted plasminogen activators: Parameters determining potency and initial and maximal rates. Circulation 87:1007, 1993.

106. Imura Y, Stassen JM, Kurokawa T, et al: Thrombolytic and pharmacokinetic properties of an immunoconjugate of single chain urokinase-type plasminogen activator (u-PA) and a bispecific monoclonal antibody against fibrin and against u-PA in baboons. Blood 79:2322, 1992.

CHAPTER 170

Saruplase

Frits W. Bär, M.D., and Frank Vermeer, M.D.

Since the early 1980s, thrombolytic therapy has become a cornerstone in the treatment of acute myocardial infarction; artery patency can be restored in most patients by thrombolytic agents, which reduces mortality and morbidity.[1-4] However, in a clinically significant proportion of patients (15% to 45%), this therapy will not result in normalization of coronary flow.[5-9] Several reasons account for why thrombolysis is not always successful. In some patients, local concentrations of the thrombolytic agent may be inadequate. In other patients, instead of a thrombus, an occluding dissection of the intimal wall is present. Furthermore, arterial thrombosis involves activation of platelets and the coagulation system with formation of fibrin.[10] Treatment of thrombotic vascular occlusions with plasminogen activators is not targeted at the platelet component of an established thrombus. The success of thrombolytic therapy may be impaired by many other factors, including platelet activation and aggregation on the surface of the residual thrombus, on which thrombin activity is reexposed.[11] At least some thrombolytic agents may even directly promote platelet aggregation at an early phase, which could further detract from their efficacy.[12-15] The choice of the thrombolytic agent seems to be important to confront some of the complications mentioned above, not only because some agents promote platelet aggregation, but also because there are suggestions that several thrombolytic agents have different profiles in terms of speed of reperfusion and chance of reocclusion.[7, 16-19] Further, one study[7] also suggests differences in bleeding complications, and another[4] shows different stroke frequencies. The above-mentioned findings indicate that it is worthwhile to study new thrombolytic agents with a view toward improving efficacy and decreasing side effects.

TYPES OF THROMBOLYTIC AGENTS
Currently Available Drugs

Currently, four thrombolytic medications are on the market in Europe and the United States: streptokinase, urokinase, anistreplase, and alteplase, each with its individual advantages and disadvantages.

Saruplase

Saruplase is the name for recombinant unglycosylated full-length human form of single-chain urokinase-type plasminogen activator (scu-PA). Saruplase has the same amino acid sequence as native scu-PA but, in contrast, lacks a carbohydrate side chain because of its production by means of recombinant bacteria. Effective and clot-specific lysis has been observed both *in vitro* and *in vivo*. The biochemistry of saruplase is well elucidated (Fig. 170–1). Preclinical results have been described elsewhere.[20–22]

Clinical Experiences with Saruplase

Clinical studies have been performed in the indications of acute myocardial infarction and pulmonary embolism. In this chapter, only the trials in patients with acute myocardial infarction are discussed.

Dose-Finding Studies

Two studies[23, 24] were performed to determine a suitable dose regimen for the use of saruplase in the treatment of acute myocardial infarction. Both were reperfusion studies, and recruited patients were suffering from their first myocardial infarction. Before treatment was begun, a coronary angiography had to show the culprit coronary artery to be totally obstructed. The patients were to be treated within 6 hours of the onset of symptoms with saruplase. Efficacy was judged as the number of patients with an open culprit artery after 60 or 90 minutes.

In the first study of saruplase in humans,[23] 17 patients were treated with either 40 mg of saruplase (10-mg intravenous bolus plus 30-mg intravenous infusion over 60 minutes, n = 8) or 70 mg of saruplase (10-mg intravenous bolus plus 60-mg intravenous infusion over 60 minutes, n = 9). By the end of the infusion, in the 40-mg group, three of eight patients had complete reperfusion, three had partial reperfusion, and two had no reperfusion. In the 70-mg group, six of nine patients had complete reperfusion, one had partial reperfusion, and two had no reperfusion. As could be expected, the hemostatic system was more disturbed in patients treated with the 70-mg dose.

In the second study,[24] 24 patients were treated with either 40 mg of saruplase (10-mg intravenous bolus plus 30-mg intravenous infusion over 60 minutes, n = 12) or 80 mg of saruplase (20-mg intravenous bolus plus 60-mg intravenous infusion over 60 minutes, n = 12). By the end of the infusion period (60 minutes), reperfusion had occurred in 3 of 12 patients in the 40-mg group compared with 7 of 12 patients in the 80-mg group. Thirty minutes later (at 90 minutes), reperfusion was observed in 4 of 12 patients in the 40-mg group and in 10 of 12 patients in the 80-mg group. The greatest changes in plasminogen, α_2-antiplasmin, fibrinogen, and fibrinogen degradation products were observed in both groups at 2 hours after saruplase was started. At all times, the changes were more pronounced in the 80-mg group. It was concluded that an 80-mg dose of saruplase is superior to 40 mg in achieving reperfusion, though the larger dose leads to a more profound systemic lytic state.

Thereafter, all saruplase trials used 80 mg of saruplase (20-mg intravenous bolus and 60 mg given as a 1-hour infusion).

Interaction Studies

Two interaction studies[25, 26] have been performed, one looking at the effect of a heparin bolus given before

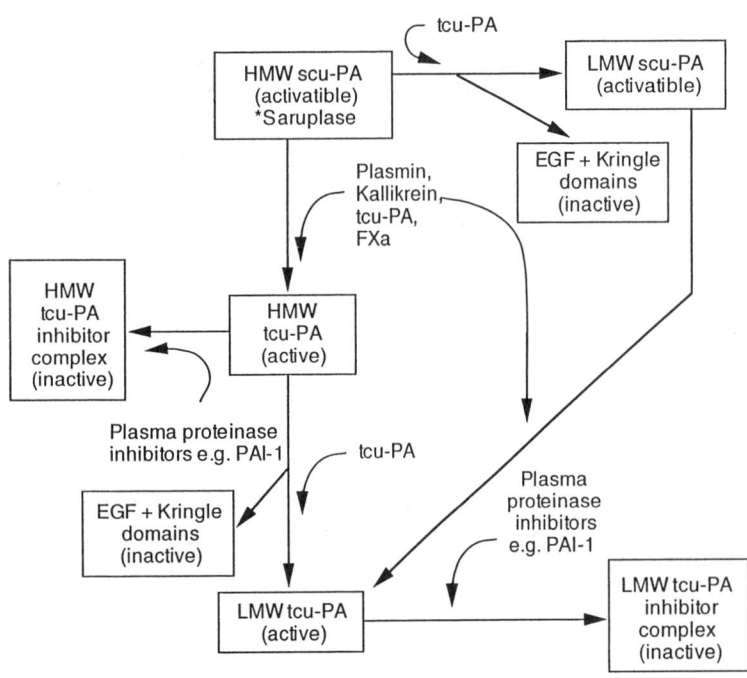

Figure 170 –1. Derivatives of saruplase potentially generated *in vivo*. EGF, epidermal growth factor; HMW, high-molecular-weight; LMW, low-molecular-weight.

starting saruplase and one investigation of the effect of the concomitant administration of a prostacyclin analogue (taprostene).

Heparin and Saruplase (LIMITS Study)

A number of experiments in animal models had shown that conjunctive heparin probably could improve the efficacy of saruplase; early in the development of saruplase, it was decided to test this hypothesis in patients. Therefore, a study[25] was conducted in which consenting patients were randomized to receive a single bolus of either heparin (5000 IU intravenously, n = 56) or placebo (n = 62) immediately before starting thrombolytic therapy with saruplase (80 mg). Starting 30 minutes after completion of the saruplase infusion, all patients received a 5-day, uninterrupted infusion of heparin titrated against the activated partial thromboplastin time (aPTT).

Between the 6th and 12th hours after starting thrombolytic therapy, the patients received a second bolus of heparin (5000 IU intravenously) and underwent coronary angiography. Patency rates were 78.6% in the group given heparin before saruplase and 56.5% in the control group. Some evidence of earlier recanalization in the heparin group was corroborated by an earlier time to peak concentration (8 hours versus 10.05 hours) of the mean plasma creatine kinase (CK-MB) activity in these patients.

The in-hospital mortality rate was 5.4% in the pre-lysis heparin group and 14.5% in the control group. Bleeding occurred in 14.3% and 8.1% of patients, respectively. Most bleeding events occurred during the saruplase infusion phase and at puncture sites. No cerebrovascular event or allergic reaction was reported. There was no significant difference between the two groups in the changes in plasma levels of the hemostatic parameters (fibrinogen and fibrin- and fibrinogen-degradation products). Thrombin–antithrombin III levels were lower ($p = .003$) in the heparin group, suggesting lower thrombin generation.

Thus, the risk-to-benefit ratio of saruplase therapy appeared to be improved with pretreatment heparin. Consequently, it was strongly recommended that therapy with saruplase be preceded by an intravenous bolus of 5000 IU of heparin.

Taprostene and Saruplase (START Study)

Taprostene is a prostacyclin analogue that inhibits platelet aggregation.[27-30] After successful thrombolysis, the exposed ruptured plaque promotes platelet aggregation. Therefore, it was thought that the use of an inhibitor of platelet aggregation might be a useful adjuvant to thrombolytic therapy in patients suffering from acute myocardial infarction. This hypothesis was tested in the START study.[26] Within 4 hours of the onset of symptoms, patients were randomly allocated either to saruplase (80 mg) plus placebo or to saruplase (80 mg) plus taprostene treatment. Doses of taprostene were as follows: 6.25 ng/kg/min (S + T1), 12.5 ng/kg/min (S + T2), or 25.0 ng/kg/min (S +

T3) intravenous infusion for 48 hours followed by 24 hours of tapering. All patients received heparin and saruplase (80 mg). Acetylsalicylic acid (aspirin), which at the time of the study was not proven to be beneficial, was not permitted until discharge. The culprit coronary artery was assessed angiographically at 90 minutes and at 32 to 48 hours after start of saruplase.

The patency rates (TIMI grade 2 or 3 perfusion) were 75% (S + P); 75% (S + T1); 67% (S + T2); and 82% (S + T3) ($p = .71$). Angioplasty (percutaneous transluminal coronary angioplasty—PTCA) was needed in 12 of 20 patients with TIMI grade 0 or 1 perfusion and in one patient with TIMI grade 2 perfusion. The infarct-related artery remained occluded in 3 of these 13 patients; hence, final patency rates at the end of the first catheterization were 95% (S + P), 92% (S + T1), 75% (S + T2), and 86% (S + T3) ($p = .26$). At the second angiogram (at 32 to 48 hours), patency decreased in S + P to 79% but remained unchanged in S + T1 at 92% or improved to 82% in S + T2 and to 94% in S + T3. Therefore, taprostene cotherapy did not enhance lysis per se, but patency after lysis followed by PTCA may be prolonged. Among the seven deaths in hospital (8.8%), four were from cardiogenic shock, and one each followed severe thrombotic stroke, heart failure, and severe arrhythmia/pneumonia. Stroke, bleeding, and hypotension rates were not discernibly different among the small treatment groups. The safety of saruplase therapy seemed unaffected by taprostene cotherapy, but only large differences could have been detected in this small study.

Placebo-Controlled Studies

Placebo-controlled studies with saruplase have not been performed, because earlier studies with other thrombolytic agents already demonstrated that thrombolytic therapy is superior to placebo.

Comparative Studies

Saruplase has been compared with several other thrombolytic agents. Five comparative efficacy studies have assessed patency. Two were versus streptokinase[7] (COMPASS—not yet published), one was versus urokinase,[31, 32] and two studies were versus alteplase.[33, 34]

Streptokinase Versus Saruplase (PRIMI Study)

In a randomized trial,[7] 401 patients with a first acute myocardial infarction were treated within 4 hours after onset of symptoms with saruplase (80 mg, n = 198) or streptokinase (1.5 million IU infusion in 60 minutes, n = 203). Angiograms of the culprit artery were taken at 60 minutes, 90 minutes, and 24 to 36 hours. Patency rates at 60 minutes were 71.8% for saruplase patients and 48.0% for streptokinase patients ($p < .001$); at 90 minutes, these rates were 71.2% and 63.9% ($p = .15$). Between 90 minutes and 24 to 36 hours, reocclusion rates dropped from 5.0% to 4.4% (Fig. 170–2).

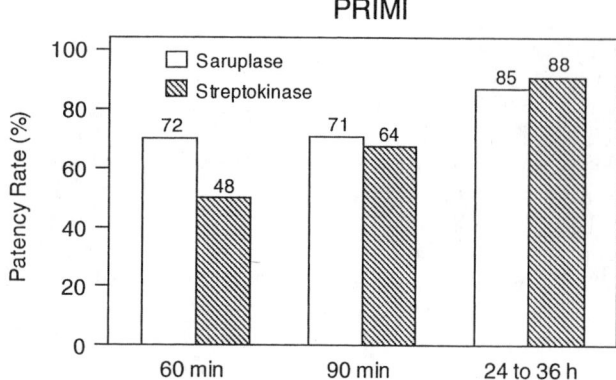

Figure 170–2. Patency data of 198 patients treated with saruplase and 203 patients treated with streptokinase from the PRIMI trial. Patency rates are given at 60 minutes, at 90 minutes, and at 24 to 36 hours after the start of the thrombolytic agent. At 60 minutes, the difference in patency significantly ($p < .001$) favors saruplase.

Table 170–1. Adverse Event Data of PRIMI Study Comparing Saruplase (20-mg Intravenous Bolus, 60 mg as 1-Hour Infusion) with Streptokinase (1.5 million U over 1-Hour) in Patients with Acute Myocardial Infarction

Adverse Events	Saruplase n = 198	Streptokinase n = 203
Reocclusion	5.0%	4.8%
Mortality:		
Hospital	3.5%	4.9%
1 year	6.3%	5.6%
Bleeding:		
Total	14.1%	24.6%
Severe	4.0%	11.3%
Stroke:		
Ischemic	0.5%	0.5%
Hemorrhagic	1.0%	0.5%

In streptokinase patients, lower fibrinogen, plasminogen, and α_2-antiplasmin as well as higher fibrin-(ogen) degradation product levels (all p values $< .001$) were observed (Fig. 170–3).

Bleeding complications were less common in saruplase patients than in the streptokinase patients (14.1% versus 24.6%, $p < .01$). Major bleeding was observed in 4.0% of the saruplase patients and in 11.3% of the streptokinase patients ($p < .01$). Three patients had intracranial bleeding (saruplase, two patients; streptokinase, one patient). Other safety data were comparable (Table 170–1). Hospital mortality rates were low in both treatment groups (saruplase, 3.5%; streptokinase, 4.9%). At discharge, both treatment groups were comparable in terms of functional state. The total 1-year mortality rate was 6.3% in saruplase patients compared with 5.6% in streptokinase patients.

A further study (Comparative Trial of Saruplase versus Streptokinase [COMPASS]) was performed comparing saruplase and streptokinase in more than 3000 patients with mortality at 30 days; this end-point study has recently been completed.

Urokinase Versus Saruplase (SUTAMI Study)

Although urokinase has long been available for use as a thrombolytic medication, it is not often used in myocardial infarction. It was decided that a comparative study[31, 32] between urokinase and saruplase should be performed because saruplase could be directly compared with its metabolite, bearing in mind that the metabolite of saruplase is not glycosylated, whereas the marketed urokinase is.

In this study, patients suffering from an acute myocardial infarction within 6 hours of onset were randomly treated with saruplase (80 mg, n = 272) or urokinase (1.5 million IU intravenous bolus plus 1.5 million U in 60 minutes, n = 271). Heparin was started 3 hours after the thrombolytic therapy infusions were completed. Angiography was performed at 24 to 72 hours. The patency rates at that time were 75.4% and 74.2%, respectively ($p = .77$). There was a slightly higher ejection fraction at the angiography performed at 24 to 72 hours in the saruplase treatment group (55.2%) compared with the urokinase treatment group (53.4%) ($p = .09$). Estimated infarct size as judged from the cumulative lactate dehydrogenase release was the same for both treatment groups.

Both treatments caused a similar disturbance of the hemostatic system. The median fibrinogen concentration fell from 3.00 g/L to 0.35 g/L in the saruplase treatment group and from 3.20 g/L to 0.44 g/L in the urokinase treatment group. The median fibrinogen degradation product concentrations rose from 0.43 mg/L to 160 mg/L for saruplase-treated patients and from 0.45 mg/L to 89 mg/L for urokinase-treated patients.

Bleeding complications were reported in 10.7% of the patients and were the same in both groups (Table 170–2). The incidence of stroke was higher in the saruplase-treated patients (seven patients vs. two patients). There were three hemorrhagic strokes (1.1%) in the saruplase group and none in the urokinase group ($p = .25$). There were four ischemic cerebral events (1.5%) in the saruplase group and two in the urokinase group (0.7%) ($p = .69$). In contrast, the hospital mortality rate was higher in the urokinase treatment group. The mortality rate was 4.4% in the

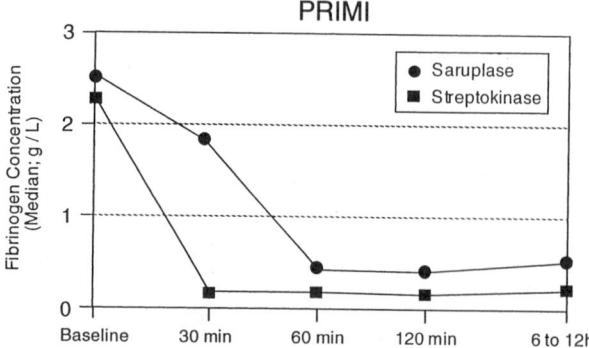

Figure 170–3. Fibrinogen concentrations versus time of the 198 patients treated with saruplase and the 203 patients treated with streptokinase in the PRIMI trial. Decrease of fibrinogen in the saruplase group is less pronounced than in the streptokinase group. After start of medication, differences are highly significant ($p < .0001$) at all given time points.

Table 170–2. **Adverse Event Data of Study Comparing Saruplase (20-mg Intravenous Bolus, 60 mg as 1-Hour Infusion) with Urokinase (1.5 million U as Intravenous Bolus plus 1.5 million U in 60 Minutes) in Patients with Acute Myocardial Infarction**

Adverse Events	Saruplase n = 272	Urokinase n = 271
Reinfarction	6.9%	4.7%
Mortality:		
Hospital	4.4%	8.1%
1 year	7.5%	11.7%
Bleeding:		
Total	10.7%	10.7%
Severe	3.3%	2.6%
Stroke:		
Ischemic	1.5%	0.7%
Hemorrhagic	1.1%	0.0%

saruplase group and 8.1% in the urokinase group (p = .08). There were 2.9% deaths due to a cardiovascular cause in the saruplase group and 7.7% in the urokinase group (p = .01). During the 1 year of subsequent follow-up, this mortality difference persisted. The rates at 1 year were 7.5% for the saruplase-treated group and 11.7% for the urokinase-treated group. In the 1 year follow-up phase, the reinfarction rates and classification of functional status (New York Heart Association [NYHA] and Canadian Cardiovascular Society [CCS]) did not differ between the two treatment groups.

In conclusion, in this study wherein there was no pretreatment with heparin, the efficacy and safety profiles of saruplase and urokinase were very similar in many respects.

Alteplase Versus Saruplase

Two studies have compared saruplase and alteplase.[33] The first was a pilot study examining the effect of the thrombolytic medication on the hemostatic system. Angiography at 24 to 72 hours indicated a higher patency rate in the saruplase-treated patients, which could have been due to a higher reocclusion rate in the alteplase-treated patients. Therefore, a confirmatory study was performed to compare the rates of reocclusion between an angiography at 90 minutes and a control angiography at 24 to 40 hours.

Alteplase Versus Saruplase Pilot Study (SAT study). In the SAT study,[33] 52 patients with acute myocardial infarction were treated within 4 hours after onset of symptoms with either saruplase (80 mg, n = 24) or alteplase (10 mg intravenous bolus followed by an infusion of 50 mg over 60 minutes and then 40 mg over 120 minutes, n = 28). Heparin treatment (5000 IU intravenous bolus followed by infusion at the initial dose of 1000 IU/hr) was started 30 minutes after the end of thrombolytic treatment. Antiplatelet drugs were not allowed during the first 5 days.

The primary aim of this study was to evaluate and to compare the changes induced in the levels of fibrinogen, fibrin(ogen) degradation products, plasminogen, α_2-antiplasmin, and D-dimer. Fibrinogen,

plasminogen, and α_2-antiplasmin levels were consistently and significantly higher and fibrin(ogen) degradation product levels were consistently and significantly lower in the alteplase group than in the saruplase group at the end of the infusion of the thrombolytic medication as well as at 1 hour and 12 to 18 hours thereafter (Fig. 170–4). For D-dimer, no significant intergroup difference was observed. In the saruplase group, 86% of patients had a fibrinogen level of 1 g/L or less on at least one assessment, as opposed to 26% of patients in the alteplase group (p < .001). Nadir levels of fibrinogen were observed at the end of the infusion (66% of baseline) in the alteplase group and at 2 hours after the infusion (22% of baseline) in the saruplase group.

In the saruplase group, 5 of 24 patients experienced at least one bleeding complication compared with 8 of 28 patients in the alteplase group. Multiple bleeding complications occurred in 4% of the patients from the saruplase group versus 14% of the patients from the alteplase group. Major bleeding was reported in 4 patients from the alteplase group and in no patients of the saruplase group. One patient in the alteplase group suffered a hemorrhagic stroke.

Thus, although saruplase induced significantly more systemic activation of the fibrinolytic system, bleeding complications were more frequent in the alteplase group.

Evaluation of coronary patency at 24 to 72 hours was a secondary aim of this study. The patency rates were 88% in the saruplase group and 61% in the alteplase group (p = .06).

Alteplase Versus Saruplase Confirmatory Study (SESAM Study). Following the pilot study, a second angiography study was performed on a larger group of patients with acute myocardial infarction within 6 hours of onset.[34] They were treated with saruplase (80 mg, n = 236) or alteplase (100 mg/3 hr, n = 237) using dose regimens similar to those of the pilot study. In contrast with the pilot study, a heparin bolus (5000 IU) was given intravenously before the start of the thrombolytic medication, and heparin infusion was continued thereafter. Also, aspirin was already started before study medication.

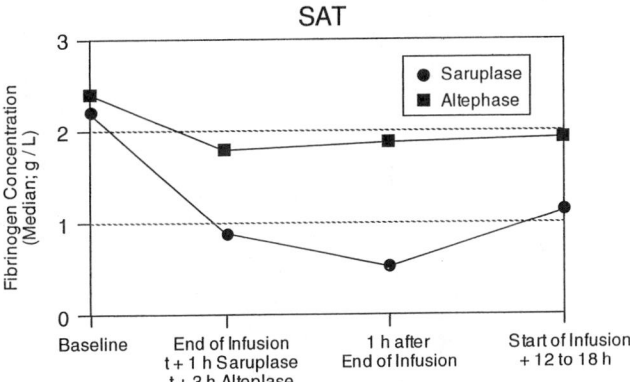

Figure 170–4. Fibrinogen concentrations versus time of the 24 patients treated with saruplase and the 28 patients treated with alteplase of the SAT study. Decrease of fibrinogen level in the saruplase group is significantly lower than in the alteplase group at the end of the infusion period up to 12 to 18 hours.

Angiographic data showed that at 45 minutes, 74.6% of the saruplase-treated and 68.9% of the alteplase-treated patients had an open vessel ($p = .22$); at 60 minutes, these figures were 79.9% and 75.3%, respectively ($p = .26$). Patients with a TIMI grade 3 flow at 60 minutes did not have to undergo angiography at 90 minutes. Therefore, for purposes of determining patency rate at 90 minutes, these patients were included as patients with an open vessel; the rates were 82.2% for saruplase-treated patients versus 81.5% for alteplase-treated patients (Fig. 170–5). The reocclusion rate of patent infarct-related arteries between the first catheterization and a control angiography at 24 to 40 hours was 1.2% for saruplase and 2.4% for alteplase. Adverse event rates for the two study medications were similar (Table 170–3).

In conclusion, patency can be achieved rapidly with saruplase. Patency rates obtained with saruplase and alteplase in this study are as good as those obtained using front-loaded alteplase regimens.[39] The reocclusion rates with both saruplase and alteplase therapy within 24 to 40 hours are low when adequate conjunctive medication is given. Conjunctive medication does not give rise to an appreciable increased bleeding or stroke risk.

Open-Label Safety Studies (PASS Study)

An open-label study in 1698 patients assessed the applicability and safety of saruplase in the routine treatment of patients with acute myocardial infarction.[36] Patients were included within 6 hours after onset of symptoms. Concomitant medication, including nitroglycerin, aspirin, and heparin, was given according to local routine.

The hospital mortality rate was 5.4% (Table 170–4). Total and major bleeding complications occurred in 4.9% and 1.2% of patients, respectively. Cerebrovascular events occurred in 0.9% of patients. In 0.5% of patients, a hemorrhagic stroke occurred, and in 0.4% an ischemic stroke occurred, including two ischemic events classified as transient ischemic attack. Allergic reactions were reported in 0.6% of the patients, probably caused by concomitant medication.

The incidence of definite reinfarction after saruplase infusion was 2.9% during hospital stay. Coronary angiography was performed within 72 hours in 347 of 1698 patients (20.4%) and revealed a patency rate of 70.0%.

Another open-label study (COMPASS) involving over 3000 patients has ended. Results of this trial will be available in the near future.

CONCLUSIONS

Saruplase has shown to be a fast acting, effective, and safe drug when given to patients with acute myocardial infarction. Its efficacy and safety profile is at least as good as those of any available thrombolytic agent. At present, saruplase therapy is administered in a dose of 80 mg (20-mg bolus + 60-mg intravenous infusion over 60 minutes). Whether different saruplase regimes are as effective is unclear. The results of a pilot study using different bolus doses will be available soon (Bolus Administration of Saruplase in Europe [BASE] pilot study).

Table 170–3. Adverse Event Data of SESAM Study Comparing Saruplase (20-mg Intravenous Bolus, 60 mg as 1-Hour Infusion) with Alteplase (10 mg as Intravenous Bolus, Infusion of 50 mg in 60 Minutes and 40 mg in 120 Minutes) in Patients with Acute Myocardial Infarction

Adverse Events	Saruplase n = 236	Alteplase n = 237
Reinfarction	4.2%	4.2%
Mortality:		
Hospital	4.7%	3.8%
Bleeding:		
Total	42.8%	39.7%
Severe	9.3%	8.4%
Stroke:		
Ischemic	0.8%	1.3%
Hemorrhagic	0.8%	0.8%

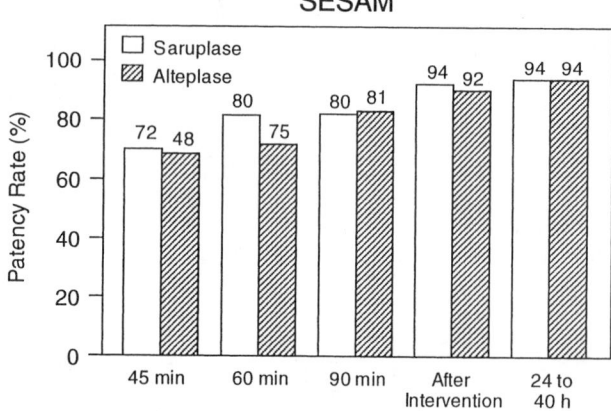

SESAM

Saruplase / Alteplase

	45 min	60 min	90 min	After Intervention	24 to 40 h
Saruplase	72	80	80	94	94
Alteplase	48	75	81	92	94

Figure 170–5. Patency data of 236 patients treated with saruplase and 237 patients treated with alteplase of the SESAM trial. Patency rates are given at 45 minutes, at 60 minutes, at 90 minutes before any intracoronary intervention, at the last view of the first catheterization (including additional percutaneous transluminal coronary angioplasty if performed), and at 24 to 40 hours. Note that the patency rates at the different time points are not significantly different.

Table 170–4. Adverse Event Data of Open PASS Study of Saruplase (20 mg as Intravenous Bolus, 60 mg as 1-Hour Infusion) in 1698 Patients with Acute Myocardial Infarction

Adverse Events	n	%
Hospital mortality	92	5.4
Total bleedings	84	4.9
Major bleedings	20	1.2
Cerebrovascular accident:	15	0.9
Hemorrhagic	8	0.5
Ischemic	7	0.4
Reinfarction	50	2.9

Saruplase seems to be most effective when combined with heparin. Therefore, a 5000-IU intravenous bolus of heparin given prior to saruplase administration is recommended. Continuation of heparin is advised as an infusion up to 48 hours, titrated according to the aPTT. No comparative trial of saruplase with and without aspirin has been performed, and no recommendation can be made. Experience with other thrombolytic agents suggests that concomitant use is advisable.

Acknowledgments

Mrs. Margriet Muytjens typed this manuscript without complaints. Mr. Gwyn Hopkins provided us with the most recent information.

REFERENCES

1. Vermeer F, Simoons M, Bär FW, et al: Which patients benefit most from early thrombolytic therapy with intracoronary streptokinase? Circulation 74:1379, 1986.
2. Dalen JE, Gore JM, Braunwald E, et al: Six and twelve month follow-up of the phase I thrombolysis in myocardial infarction (TIMI) trial. Am J Cardiol 62:179, 1988.
3. Gruppo italiano per lo studio della streptochinase: nell' infarto miocardio (GISSI): Effectiveness of intravenous thrombolytic treatment in acute myocardial infarction. Lancet 1:397, 1986.
4. ISIS 2 (second International Study of Infarct Survival) Collaborative Group: Randomized trial of intravenous streptokinase, oral aspirin, both, or neither among 17,187 cases of suspected acute myocardial infarction: ISIS-2. Lancet 2:349, 1988.
5. The TIMI Study Group: The thrombolysis in myocardial infarction (TIMI) trial. N Engl J Med 312:932, 1985.
6. Van de Werf F, Arnold AER: Intravenous tissue plasminogen activator and size of infarct, left ventricular function, and survival in acute myocardial infarction. Br Med J 297:1374, 1988.
7. PRIMI Trial Study Group: Randomized double-blind trial of recombinant pro-urokinase against streptokinase in acute myocardial infarction. Lancet 1:863, 1989.
8. Mathey DG, Schofer J, Sheehan FH, et al: Intravenous urokinase in acute myocardial infarction. Am J Cardiol 55:878, 1985.
9. Marder VJ, Rothbarth RL, Fitzpatrick PG, Francis CW: Rapid lysis of coronary artery thrombi with anisoylated plasminogen streptokinase activator complex: Treatment by bolus intravenous injection. Ann Intern Med 104:304, 1986.
10. Matthias FR: Blood Coagulation Disorders. Hemorrhagic Diatheses and Thromboembolic Disease. Berlin: Springer, 1987, p 30.
11. Badimon L, Lassila R, Badimon J, et al: Residual thrombus is more thrombogenic than severely damaged vessel wall [abstract]. Circulation 78(Suppl 2):119, 1988.
12. Ohlstein EH, Storer B, Fujita T, Shebuski RJ: Tissue type plasminogen activator and streptokinase induce platelet hyperaggregability in rabbit. Thromb Res 46:575, 1987.
13. Rudd MA, George D, Amarante P, et al: Temporal effects of thrombolytic agents on platelet function in vivo and their modulation by prostaglandins. Circ Res 67(5):1175, 1990.
14. Kerins DM, Roy L, FitzGerald GA, Fitzgerald DJ: Platelet activation and depressed prostacyclin (PGI$_2$ biosynthesis following reperfusion with tissue-type plasminogen activator (t-PA) in man [abstract]. Circulation 78:508, 1988.
15. Fitzgerald DJ, Catella F, Roy L, FitzGerald GA: Marked platelet activation in vivo after intravenous streptokinase in patients with acute myocardial infarction. Circulation 77:142, 1988.
16. Relik-van Wely L, Visser RF, Van der Pol J, et al: Angiographically assessed coronary arterial patency and reocclusion in patients with acute myocardial infarction treated with anistreplase: Results of the anistreplase reocclusion multicentre study (ARMS). Am J Cardiol 68:296, 1991.

17. Bonnier HJRM, Visser RF, Klomps HC, et al: Comparison of intravenous anisoylated plasminogen streptokinase activator complex and intracoronary streptokinase in acute myocardial infarction. Am J Cardiol 62:2530, 1988.
18. Chesebro JH, Knatterud G, Roberts R, et al: Thrombolysis in myocardial infarction (TIMI) trial, phase I. A comparison between intravenous tissue plasminogen activator and intravenous streptokinase. Circulation 76:142, 1987.
19. Simoons ML, Arnold AER, Betrin A, et al: Thrombolysis with tissue plasminogen activator in acute myocardial infarction: No additional benefit from immediate percutaneous coronary angiography. Lancet 2:197, 1988.
20. Collen D, Stump DC, van de Werf F, et al: Coronary thrombolysis in dogs with intravenously administered human pro-urokinase (pro-UK). Circulation 72:384, 1985.
21. Van de Werf F, Jang IK, Collen D, et al: Thrombolysis with recombinant human single-chain urokinase-type plasminogen activator (rscu-PA): dose-response in dogs with coronary artery thrombosis. J Cardiovasc Pharmacol 9:91, 1987.
22. Flameng W, Vanhaecke J, Stump DC, et al: Coronary thrombolysis by intravenous infusion of recombinant single chain urokinase-type plasminogen activator or recombinant urokinase in baboons: Effect on regional blood flow, infarct size and hemostasis. J Am Coll Cardiol 8:118, 1986.
23. Van der Werf F, Vanhaecke J, De Geest H, et al: Coronary thrombolysis with recombinant single chain urokinase-type plasminogen activator in patients with acute myocardial infarction. Circulation 74:1066, 1986.
24. Diefenbach C, Erbel R, Pop T, et al: Recombinant single-chain urokinase-type plasminogen activator during acute myocardial infarction. Am J Cardiol 61:966, 1988.
25. Tebbe U, Massberg I, Windeler J, Barth H: Fur die LIMITS-studien-gruppe: Einfluss von Heparin auf die Thrombolytische Wirksamkeit von Saruplase beim Akutem Myocardinfarkt. Z Kardiol 80(Suppl 3):32, 1991.
26. Bär FW, Meyer J, Michels R, et al: The effect of taprostene in patients with acute myocardial infarction treated with thrombolytics: Results of the START study. Eur Heart J 14:1118, 1993.
27. Barth H, Lintz W, Michel G, et al: Inhibition of platelet aggregation by intravenous administration of the biochemically stable prostacyclin analogue CG4203 in man. Naunyn Schmiedebergs Arch Pharmacol (Suppl 324), 1983.
28. Groves R, Schneider J, Flohe L: Cooperative action of the prostacyclin analogue taprostene and the fibrinolytic pro-urokinase (r-scu-PA) in experimental artery thrombosis. *In* Schror K, Sisszinger M (eds): Prostaglandins in Clinical Research: Cardiovascular System. New York: AR Liss, 1989, p 603.
29. Flohe L, Bohlke H, Frankus E, et al: Designing prostacyclin analogues. Drug Res 33:1240, 1983.
30. Kaliman J, Fitscha P, Barth H, Sinzinger H: Clinical and platelet effects of CG 4203, a stable PGI$_2$ analogue. Abstracts 6th International Conference on Prostaglandins and Related Compounds, Florence (Italy), June 3–6 1986, p 443.
31. Hoffmann JJML, Vijgen M, Nieuwenhuizen A: Comparison of the specificity of four fibrinogen assays during thrombolytic therapy. Fibrinolysis 4:121, 1990.
32. Michels R, Hoffmann H, Windler J, et al: A double-blind multicentre comparison of the efficacy and safety of saruplase in the treatment of acute myocardial infarction. Report of the SUTAMI study group. Submitted for publication.
33. The Belgian Saruplase Alteplase Trial Group: Effects of alteplase and saruplase on hemostatic variables: A single-blind, randomized trial in patients with acute myocardial infarction. Coronary Artery Dis 2:349, 1991.
34. The SESAM investigators: Early patency and reocclusion in acute myocardial infarction. A comparison between the thrombolytic agents saruplase and alteplase. Results of the SESAM trial. J Am Coll Cardiol 954:405a, 1994.
35. The GUSTO Angiographic Investigators: The effects of tissue plasminogen activator, streptokinase, or both on coronary artery patency, ventricular function, and survival after acute myocardial infarction. N Engl J Med 329:1615, 1993.
36. Vermeer F, Bär FW, Windeler J, Schenkel W: Saruplase, a new fibrin specific thrombolytic agent. Final results of the PASS study (1698 patients) [abstract]. Circulation 88:292, 1993.

XVI.

Cellular Antiischemic Agents

CHAPTER 171

Trimetazidine: Experimental Aspects

Joël de Leiris, Ph.D., and Lionel H. Opie, M.D., D.Phil., F.R.C.P.

Trimetazidine is a representative of a new group of pharmaceutical compounds with a myocardial antiischemic effect,[1] achieved independently of any changes in the oxygen demand-supply equation. The proposal is that it has a metabolic protective effect. This chapter first reviews animal experimental data favoring trimetazidine's use, then reviews the pharmacokinetics of this agent in humans and evidence for its clinical use.

EXPERIMENTAL BACKGROUND
Acidosis and Depression of Energy Metabolism

The classic effect of the poor washout of metabolites caused by ischemia is the accumulation of protons. The latter are derived not from glycolysis itself but from the adenosine triphosphate (ATP) turnover associated with the production of lactate and from a variety of proton-producing metabolic cycles.[2]

The effects of trimetazidine on ischemic acidosis have been studied in isolated Langendorff-perfused rat hearts submitted to normothermic low-flow global ischemia (with a residual coronary flow of 0.2 ml/min^{-1} during ischemia) by the noninvasive technique of phosphorus-31 nuclear magnetic resonance (^{31}P-NMR) spectroscopy.[3]

Under ischemic conditions, acidosis developed rapidly in controls, and the pH fell from 7.08 under normoxic conditions to 6.05 ± 0.25 after 24 minutes of ischemia. When trimetazidine was added to the perfusate at a concentration of 6.10^{-7} mol/L^{-1}, ischemia-induced intracellular acidosis developed more slowly and the pH appeared to significantly improve at the end of the ischemic period (pHi = 6.35 ± 0.25; $p < .05$ vs. control hearts). Furthermore, the cellular content in phosphorylated compounds (ATP and creatine phosphate [CP]) recovered faster in the trimetazidine-perfused group following reperfusion (Fig. 171–1). Similar results were obtained in rat or chick embryo myocardial cell cultures subjected to transient hypoxia. Trimetazidine also protects mitochondrial function during reperfusion of ischemic hypertrophied rat myocardium without directly interfering

with the electron transfer process at the level of respiratory chain.[4] In every case, the antiischemic effect was obtained in the presence of doses of trimetazidine that did not modify the cardiac hemodynamic characteristics and that were within the range of therapeutic levels observed in treated patients with cardiovascular disorders (1.5×10^{-7} mol/L^{-1}). The exact mechanism by which trimetazidine improves cardiac energetics and protects the mitochondrial activity has not yet been fully elucidated.

Trimetazidine does not directly affect the sarcolemmal calcium channel or the various membrane systems involved in the maintenance of ionic homeostasis of the normal heart.[5] However, use of trimetazidine to prevent the myocardial acidosis that

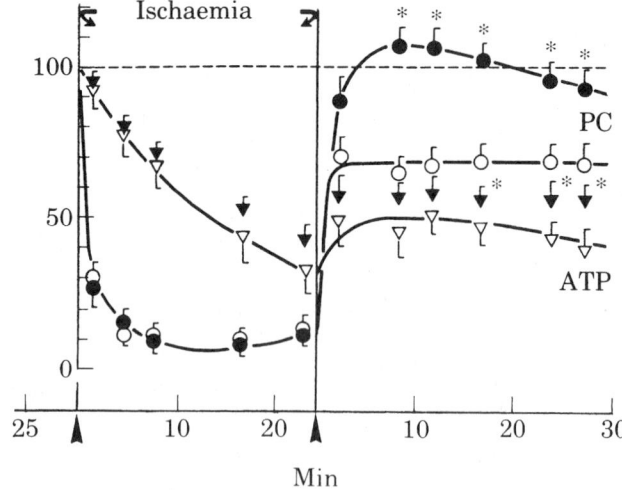

Figure 171–1. Changes in myocardial concentrations of phosphorylated compounds during ischemia and reperfusion: effects of 6.10^{-7} M trimetazidine on phosphocreatine (PC) and adenosine triphosphate (ATP) concentrations are expressed as percentages of the preischemic values. Hearts were subjected to global partial ischemia (residual flow rate 0.2 ml/min^{-1}) for 24 minutes at 37°C. Values shown on the graph constitute means plus or minus standard error of the mean. The symbol * indicates a significant difference ($p < .05$) between values determined for control hearts (*open symbols*, n = 11) and values determined for trimetazidine-perfused hearts (*shaded symbols*, n = 9). (From Lavanchy N, Martin J, Rossi A: Anti-ischemic effects of trimetazidine: ^{31}PNMR spectroscopy in the isolated rat heart. Arch Int Pharmacodyn Ther 286:97, 1987.)

occurs in hypoxic myocardial cells is accompanied by a reduction in the sodium influx usually observed under pathophysiologic conditions.[5] This suggests that by lessening the availability of internal protons, trimetazidine decreases the exchange of extracellular sodium for protons so that intracellular sodium rises less rapidly, followed by a lower rate of sodium-calcium exchange. Thus, trimetazidine may indirectly limit the calcium overload in ischemic myocardium, at least temporarily.

Calcium Overload

The mild negative inotropic and chronotropic effects of trimetazidine have only been described at high doses of trimetazidine. Indeed, at doses between 3 and 10 mg/kg^{-1} administered intravenously in open-chest dogs, there is little alteration in heart rate and coronary flow, whereas dP/dt$_{max}$ decreases in a dose-dependent manner.[6] Although some authors have attributed these findings to an antagonistic effect on calcium channels,[7] it now seems well established that trimetazidine does not exert any such effect.[5] It may nevertheless indirectly limit calcium overload during ischemia via the mechanisms suggested earlier.

Trimetazidine improved the viability of myocardial cells isolated from the adult rat ventricular myocardium subjected to hypoxia in the presence of a raised extracellular calcium concentration.[8] In the absence of trimetazidine in the incubation medium, hypoxic stress in the presence of calcium actually led to a reduction of almost 60% in the number of viable myocardial cells, whereas the addition of trimetazidine (10^{-7} mol/L^{-1}) was accompanied by a significant rise in the number of viable cells associated with a better maintenance of the cellular ATP level. The addition of adenosine diphosphate (ADP) to the incubation medium of a normoxic culture of mitochondria isolated from adult rat hearts induced physiologic synthesis of ATP, but when calcium was added to the incubation medium, ATP synthesis was inhibited variably. The addition of trimetazidine, however, limited this inhibition and restored ADP phosphorylation in a dose-dependent manner.[8] This study of mitochondrial function suggested that trimetazidine might directly act on the calcium-dependent processes responsible for oxidative regulation at the mitochondrial level.[8]

Boucher et al.[9] have studied the effect of trimetazidine (either added to the perfusion fluid or given as pretreatment to the animals) on the development of ischemic contracture in experimental low-flow ischemia (residual flow = 0.2 ml/min^{-1}) of isolated Langendorff-perfused rat hearts. Ischemic contracture was measured by a water-filled intraventricular balloon. Trimetazidine pretreatment alone (3 mg/kg^{-1} by mouth twice a day for 5 days) did not exert any measurable cardioprotective effect. However, addition to the perfusate of trimetazidine (10^{-6} mol/L^{-1}) reduced ischemic contracture in both pretreated and control groups (Fig. 171–2) and improved postischemic recovery of developed pressure. In addition,

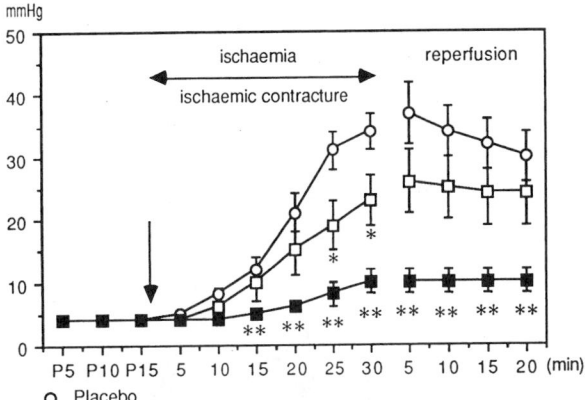

Figure 171–2. Effects of the addition of trimetazidine (TMZ) (10^{-6} mol/L^{-1}) to the perfusate of isolated Langendorff-perfused rat hearts on diastolic pressure measured during 15 minutes of normoxic perfusion (P), 30 minutes of low-flow ischemia (residual flow: 0.2 ml/min), and 20 minutes of reperfusion. Note lessened ischemic contracture (trimetazidine 10^{-6} mol/L^{-1}) and almost complete abolition of both the ischemic and the reperfusion rise of diastolic pressure when pretreatment (3 mg/kg^{-1}/day^{-1} by mouth for 5 days) was combined with trimetazidine (10^{-6} mol/L^{-1}). (From Boucher FR, Hearse DJ, Opie LH: Effects of trimetazidine on ischemic contracture in isolated perfused rat hearts. J Cardiovasc Pharmacol 24:45, 1994.)

glucose utilization remained unchanged in the different groups, indicating that the mechanism of the anti-ischemic action of trimetazidine (10^{-6} M) does not depend on glycolytic flux rate.

In a model of short-duration regional ischemia induced *ex vivo* by temporary left coronary artery ligation in the isolated Langendorff-perfused rat heart, the preventive administration of trimetazidine (10 mg/kg^{-1} by mouth 48, 24, and 6 hours before perfusion) reduced myocardial calcium accumulation as measured in cardiac tissue samples by atomic absorption spectroscopy during the reperfusion period (calcium content in the left ventricle: 10.9 ± 0.8 mmol/kg^{-1} dry weight in the placebo group vs. 7.7 ± 0.3 mmol/kg^{-1} dry weight in the trimetazidine-treated group) (Rochette et al., unpublished data) (Fig. 171–3). The mechanism involved might be a protective effect of trimetazidine on mitochondrial activity, as hypothesized by others,[4, 8] and/or an antiradical effect.

Oxygen-Reactive Intermediates

Maupoil et al.[10] have used electron spin resonance (ESR) spectroscopy to directly measure free-radical generation in isolated Langendorff-perfused rat hearts subjected to a 10-minute period of normothermic low-flow global ischemia (residual coronary flow = 10% of initial value in normoxia—i.e., 1.2 ml/min^{-1}) followed by 20 seconds of reflow. ESR spectra were directly obtained from frozen cardiac tissue samples at different temperatures (−173°C, −83°C, and −33°C). The addition of trimetazidine (10^{-5} mol/L^{-1}) to the perfusate did not significantly decrease the total

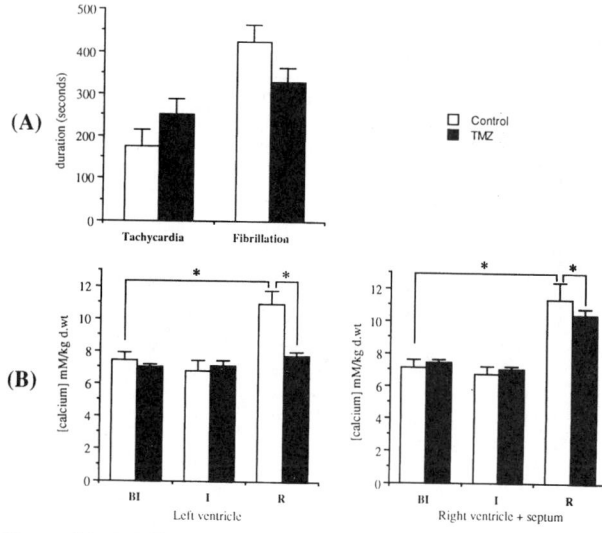

Figure 171–3. Effects of a trimetazidine pretreatment (intraperitoneal administration of 10 mg/kg⁻¹ at 48, 24, and 6 hours prior to excision of the heart) on calcium content in the left ventricle (*left panel*) and in the rest of the heart (right ventricle plus interventricular septum—*right panel*) in isolated Langendorff-perfused rat hearts submitted to regional ischemia (10 minutes) and reperfusion (10 minutes). Open bars, controls; black bars, trimetazidine; BI, before ischemia; I, end of 10 minutes of ischemia; R, during 10 minutes of reperfusion; *, $p < .05$ (means ± SEM). (From Rochette et al., unpublished data.)

amount of oxygen-derived free radicals, although the mean value fell.

Charlon et al.[11] demonstrated that daily intraperitoneal administration of trimetazidine at a dose of 2.5 mg/kg⁻¹ for 5 days interacted (directly or through one of its metabolites) with certain oxygen-derived free radicals produced at the early stage of reperfusion (30 seconds) in isolated Langendorff-perfused rat hearts previously subjected to 10 minutes of normothermic global ischemia. This interaction, demonstrated by ESR spectroscopy in the presence of the spin trap PBN (N-tert-butyl-alphaphenylnitrone, 56 mM), was accompanied by a significant reduction in tissue accumulation of malondialdehyde (MDA), an index of lipid peroxidation, whereas the activity of the enzymes involved in the antiradical defense system was not altered in response to treatment.[11] In a pig model of reperfusion injury, however, trimetazidine did not appear to modify free-radical production or stunning.[12]

An original model allowing evaluation of the antiradical activity of various drugs was applied in humans by Maridonneau-Parini and Harpey.[13] Red blood cells from healthy volunteers were incubated in the presence of phenazine methosulfate (an intracellular oxygen free-radical generating system) and diethyldithiocarbamate (a superoxide dismutase inhibitor). Intracellular loss of potassium and membrane malondialdehyde content, used to quantify radical attack on the incubated erythrocytes, appeared to be significantly reduced when the subjects had received trimetazidine as pretreatment (40 to 60 mg/day, by mouth, for 7 days). However, this effect was not observed when trimetazidine was simply added

in vitro to isolated erythrocytes from untreated volunteers. It is therefore possible that the antiradical activity of trimetazidine is mediated by one of its metabolites or that it needs a longer duration of *in vitro* incubation to exhibit a significant effect.

Finally, in a model of cardiac hypertrophy induced in rats by subcutaneous injection of monocrotaline (105 mg/kg⁻¹), an alkaloid with high cardiac toxicity, Guarnieri and Muscari[4] showed that long-term administration of trimetazidine significantly reduced the mitochondrial formation of superoxide anions and the accumulation of malondialdehyde and lipofuscin after a 40-minute normoxic *ex vivo* perfusion of the heart (Fig. 171–4), as well as after 20 minutes of ischemia followed by 20 minutes of reperfusion (Fig. 171–5).[4]

Inflammatory Process

Characteristic features of an inflammatory response, including cellular edema formation, have been described in ischemic myocardial tissue for many years.[14]

This cellular infiltration occurs in two phases: an early phase of infiltration by neutrophils (24 to 48 hours) followed by a phase of infiltration by mononuclear cells. This inflammatory response may aggravate the ischemic lesions and extend necrosis in cases of permanent ischemia. It has also been demonstrated, in various experimental models of coronary ligations, that procedures such as neutrophil depletion and/or the administration of substances that inhibit leukocyte infiltration are accompanied by a reduction in the size of the myocardial infarct.[15] Williams et al.[16] have

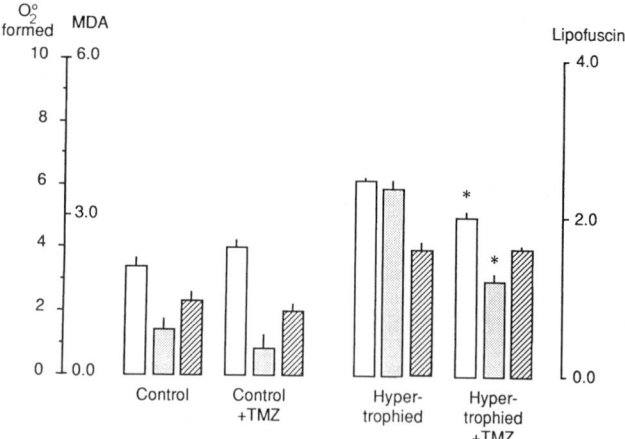

Figure 171– 4. Effect of the addition of trimetazidine (1 mmol/L) to the perfusate of isolated rat hearts on superoxide anions O₂° mitochondrial generation and lipoperoxidative damage after 40 minutes of aerobic perfusion. Data are expressed as mean ± SEM (n = 6). *, $p < .05$, significance of difference between the untreated versus the corresponding trimetazidine-treated group.

$\square$ = O₂° formed (nmol O₂°·min⁻¹·mg prot⁻¹);

= MDA (nmol·mg prot⁻¹); = lipofuscin (relative fluorescence U·g pror⁻¹)

(From Guarnieri C, Muscari C: Effect of trimetazidine on mitochondrial function and oxidative damage during reperfusion of ischemic hypertrophied myocardium. Pharmacology 46:324, 1993.)

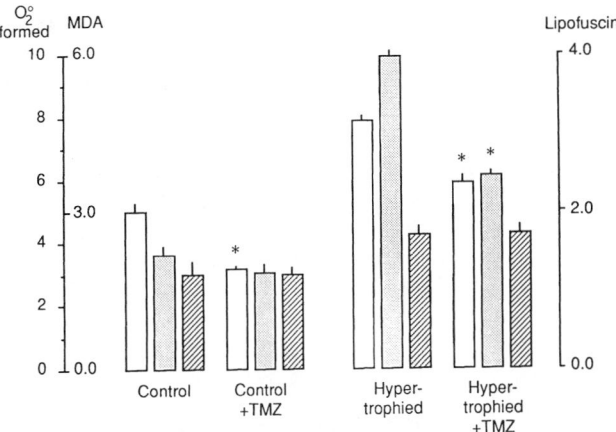

Figure 171–5. Effect of the addition of trimetazidine (1 μmol/L) to the perfusate of isolated rat hearts on $O_2^°$ mitochondrial generation and lipoperoxidative damage after 20 minutes of ischemia followed by 20 minutes of reperfusion. Data are expressed as mean ± SEM (n = 6). *, $p < .05$, significance of difference between the untreated versus the corresponding trimetazidine-treated group.

= $O_2^°$ formed (nmol $O_2^° \cdot min^{-1} mg\ prot^{-1}$);

= MDA (nmol·mg $prot^{-1}$);

= lipofuscin (relative fluorescence U·g $prot^{-1}$).

(From Guarnieri C, Muscari C: Effect of trimetazidine on mitochondrial function and oxidative damage during reperfusion of ischemic hypertrophied myocardium. Pharmacology 46:324, 1993.)

developed a model of temporary coronary artery occlusion (30 minutes) and reperfusion (3 hours) in the rabbit that enabled them to estimate leukocyte infiltration by using ^{111}In-labeled neutrophils. They observed a significant effect of trimetazidine, administered intravenously at a dose of 2.5 mg/kg[-1], 10 minutes prior to coronary ligation. These conditions led to a reduction in the accumulation of ^{111}In neutrophils into the zone at risk, an effect that might contribute to limitation of the final extent of necrosis.[17]

Effect on Platelets

In a relatively high concentration, trimetazidine attenuates the influx of calcium into platelets induced by exposure to thrombin.[18]

Summary of Experimental Data

There are several possible mechanisms of action by which trimetazidine promotes preservation of membrane structures and cellular function, thereby allowing the postischemic myocardial cell more rapidly to reconstitute its energetic pool during reperfusion. The mechanisms are limitation of intracellular acidosis, correction of disturbances of transmembrane ion exchanges leading to calcium overload, prevention of an excessive production of free radicals, inhibition of the inflammatory reaction, and an effect on platelets.

PHARMACOKINETICS AND PHARMACOLOGIC PROPERTIES

Most of the information stems from a review article written by Goupit[19] and from in-house studies in

which the plasma concentration was determined by high-performance liquid chromatography and fluorescence detection.[20]

Absorption

Following oral administration of 40 mg of trimetazidine, the blood level rapidly increases to reach a peak between 2 and 3 hours and then gradually decreases with a terminal half-life of about 6 hours. The bioavailability of orally administered trimetazidine is approximately 90%.

Metabolism

The major route of elimination is urinary, with about 60% of the administered dose being eliminated in the unchanged form. The rest is metabolized. Little is known of the properties of the metabolites, which are, however, only present in weak concentrations.

Plasma Protein Binding

Approximately 16% is bound to plasma proteins, chiefly albumin.

Plasma Levels

In one study, plasma levels measured at the end of the treatment period ranged between 70 and 200 ng/ml. Two of ten subjects did not respond to treatment despite high plasma levels, whereas in the other anginal patients, the plasma level correlated with the increase in work.[21]

Volume of Distribution

The large volume of distribution of trimetazidine is supported by the recovery in animal experiments of radioactive trimetazidine from a large variety of internal organs.

DOSE

The standard dose used in humans has been 20 mg three times daily.

SIDE EFFECTS

Although almost no serious side effects have been reported, 6 of 71 patients in the multicenter European study[22] stopped their medication for a variety of reasons, compared with 12 of 78 patients in the propranolol group.[23] Unexpectedly, the patients in the trimetazidine group had a greater incidence of sedation or drowsiness than those in the propranolol group, although the difference did not reach statistical significance. In the relatively small series of Dalla-Volta et al.,[24] trimetazidine had fewer side effects than did nifedipine in capsule form.

CONCURRENT DISEASE

There are few or no studies concerning the use of trimetazidine in patients with renal or hepatic disease or in elderly patients.

DRUG INTERACTIONS

Trimetazidine has no significant effects on the kinetics of two commonly used drugs, namely theophylline and digoxin.[25] Also, trimetazidine does not alter the rate of metabolism of antipyrine, which is used as an index of a possible effect of trimetazidine as an inducer or inhibitor of drug hydroxylation reactions. The low plasma protein binding of trimetazidine suggests that it is not likely to interact with other highly bound drugs such as warfarin.

ANGINA PECTORIS

The current conventional approach to the treatment of angina pectoris is to use drugs that either vasodilate (nitrates and calcium antagonists) or alter the rate-pressure product (β-blockers). Increasingly, mechanical revascularization, either by angioplasty or by surgery, is undertaken in suitable patients. It is attractive to have a further line of approach that involves drugs, such as trimetazidine and ranolazine,[26] that do not alter hemodynamic parameters. Trimetazidine has been studied in five trials involving 280 patients (Table 171–1).[21, 22, 24, 27, 28]

TRIMETAZIDINE AS MONOTHERAPY

The first and basic issue is whether trimetazidine works as monotherapy. When given over 4 weeks, trimetazidine reduces the incidence of angina and improves exercise tolerance.[29]

Trimetazidine monotherapy has also been compared with nifedipine or propranolol in double-blind control studies. For example, the changes in exercise capacity in patients with angina were similar in patients treated with trimetazidine and patients treated with nifedipine; washout of both agents gave similar results.[24]

In a relatively large European study involving 149 patients,[23] trimetazidine (20 mg, three times daily) was compared with propranolol (40 mg, three times daily) in patients with stable angina pectoris and documented coronary artery disease. Dose titration was possible after 2 weeks. The number of anginal attacks was reduced equally by both drugs, and exercise duration was increased equally, as was the time to 1-mm ST depression. In contrast with propranolol, trimetazidine did not alter the rate-pressure product, whereas propranolol reduced both heart rate and blood pressure.

TRIMETAZIDINE AS PART OF COMBINATION THERAPY

In patients already treated by nifedipine or β-blockade, the addition of trimetazidine (20 mg, three times daily) reduces anginal attacks and improves exercise capacity.[29]

SAFETY

In several trials, trimetazidine has been tested as an antianginal agent, both as monotherapy and combined with existing antianginal hemodynamic-based therapy, without evident adverse effects. No long-term outcome trials on trimetazidine nor any carefully monitored reports on long-term safety are yet available, however. Nonetheless, it appears that trimetazidine is a safe drug with apparently few side effects or adverse consequences.[23]

PERCUTANEOUS TRANSLUMINAL CORONARY ANGIOPLASTY

In a study involving 20 patients undergoing percutaneous transluminal coronary angioplasty (PTCA), there were two repetitive balloon inflations between which the patients received either trimetazidine (6 mg via the intracoronary route) or placebo. Trimetazidine decreased the start and the extent of maximum ST-segment shift during the second dilation.[30]

CARDIAC SURGERY

In a small group of cardiac surgical patients undergoing coronary bypass, 19 patients were put into a dou-

Table 171–1. **Comparative Effects of Trimetazidine (TMZ) and Other Antianginal Agents in Chronic Stable Effort Angina**

Author	Trial Design	Patients (n)	Drug Test Period	TMZ Daily Dose	Comparative Drug	End Point	Result
Sellier et al.[27]	Pl, DB, CO	10	Acute	60 mg single oral dose	Placebo	Ex	TMZ > Pl
Sellier[21]	Pl, R	32	4 weeks	60 mg	Placebo	Clin, Ex	TMZ > Pl
Passeron[28]	Pl, R	54	2 weeks	60 mg	Placebo	Clin, Ex	TMZ > Pl
Dalla Volta et al.[24]	DB, CO, Pl run-in and washout	35	6 weeks	60 mg	Nifedipine, 40 mg	Clin, Ex	TMZ > N
Sellier et al.[22]	DB, R, Pl run-in	149	12 weeks	67 mg (mean)	Propranolol, 132 mg (mean)	Clin, Ex	TMZ = Pl

CO, cross-over; DB, double-blind; Pl, placebo; R, randomized; Clin, clinical; Ex, exercise test.

ble-blind, placebo-controlled study. Ten received trimetazidine (20 mg per tablet three times daily) before cardiac surgery, as well as trimetazidine (110^{-6} M) in the cardioplegic solution. The trimetazidine group had a better stroke work index before surgery than did the placebo group; however, there were no differences in stroke work between the groups during surgery.[31]

EUROPEAN MYOCARDIAL INFARCTION PROJECT—FREE RADICAL STUDY EMIP-FR PILOT STUDY GROUP

In a pilot study involving 136 patients undergoing thrombolytic therapy and randomized either to 40 mg of trimetazidine as an intravenous bolus followed by an infusion at 60 mg/day for 2 days or to placebo, there were no major differences in major or minor adverse events. The conclusion was that the agent was safe and the study acceptable. Therefore, a large-scale European study[32] is underway.

There are reservations to the term free radical in the title of the study because there is no certain evidence that trimetazidine in low concentrations has any effect on free-radical formation in the heart. In fact, in one study in which generation of oxygen-derived free radicals was measured in the heart,[10] trimetazidine (10^{-5} M) only modestly inhibited free-radical production, without reaching statistical significance, whereas another study's results were negative.[12] This observation does not detract from the general concept that in other tissues, trimetazidine may inhibit free-radical formation.[1] For example, oral pretreatment with trimetazidine can protect red blood cells against oxidative stress.[21] A possible alternative mechanism of action is inhibition of neutrophil infiltration in the damaged myocardium.[16]

OTHER POSSIBLE INDICATIONS FOR TRIMETAZIDINE

In a relatively small study involving 20 patients with severe ischemic cardiomyopathy, 9 were randomized to trimetazidine and 11 to placebo. They were studied over 6 months in a double-blind manner.[33] All patients were receiving long-acting nitrates. In the trimetazidine group, symptoms improved and ejection fraction increased.[33] It would be of interest to study more patients for a longer period.

SUMMARY

Trimetazidine has been studied in a variety of situations in which protection against ischemia was tested. It is best studied, however, in chronic stable effort angina. The overall evidence gathered on 280 patients in five trials suggests that trimetazidine is a useful antianginal agent as an additive or alternative to conventional agents, such as β-blockers or calcium antagonists. It acts independently of hemodynamic

changes, presumably in a metabolic manner, and it seems to have relatively few adverse effects. Long-term outcome studies in anginal patients are still awaited. A large European trial will determine whether trimetazidine given at the time of thrombolytic reperfusion can improve the outcome.

Acknowledgments

We thank Professor L. Rochette of Dijon, France, for kindly providing unpublished data (see Fig. 171–3).

REFERENCES

1. Harpey C, Clauser P, Labrid C, et al: Trimetazidine, a cellular anti-ischemic agent. Cardiovasc Drug Rev 6:292, 1988.
2. Dennis SC, Gevers W, Opie LH: Protons in ischemia: where do they come from; where do they go to? J Mol Cell Cardiol 23:1077, 1991.
3. Lavanchy N, Martin J, Rossi A: Anti-ischemic effects of trimetazidine: ^{31}PNMR spectroscopy in the isolated rat heart. Arch Int Pharmacodyn Ther 286:97, 1987.
4. Guarnieri C, Muscari C: Effect of trimetazidine on mitochondrial function and oxidative damage during reperfusion of ischemic hypertrophied myocardium. Pharmacology 46:324, 1993.
5. Renaud JF: Internal pH, Na^+ and Ca^{2+} regulation by trimetazidine during cardiac cell acidosis. Cardiovasc Drugs Ther 1:677, 1988.
6. Takenaka F, Sakanashi M, Watanabe A: Effects of trimetazadine in the coronary circulation and myocardial metabolism in the dog. Pharmacometrics 11:429, 1976.
7. Kiyosue T, Nakamura S, Arita M: Effects of trimetazidine on action potentials and membrane currents of guinea-pig ventricular myocytes. J Mol Cell Cardiol 18:1301, 1986.
8. Cruz C, Zaoui A, Ayoub S: Altération des myocytes isolés des ventricules de rat adulte: protection par la trimétazidine. Le Concours Médical 36:3470, 1987.
9. Boucher FR, Hearse DJ, Opie LH: Effects of trimetazidine on ischemic contracture in isolated perfused rat hearts. J Cardiovasc Pharmacol 24:45, 1994.
10. Maupoil V, Rochette L, Tabard A, et al: Evolution of free radical formation during low-flow ischemia and reperfusion in isolated rat heart. Cardiovasc Drugs Ther 4:791, 1990.
11. Charlon V, Boucher F, Clauser P, et al: Effect of a 5 day trimetazidine pretreatment in a model of ischemic and reperfused isolated rat heart. Adv Exp Med Biol 264:377, 1990.
12. Koning MMG, Krams R, Xiao CS, et al: Intracoronary trimetazidine does not improve recovery of regional function in a porcine model of repeated ischemia. Cardiovasc Drugs Ther 7:801, 1993.
13. Maridonneau-Parini I, Harpey C: Effect of trimetazidine on membrane damage induced by oxygen free radicals in human red cells. Br J Clin Pharmacol 20:148, 1985.
14. Mallory GK, White PD, Salcedo-Salgar J: The speed of healing of myocardial infarction: A study of the pathologic anatomy in seventy-two cases. Am Heart J 18:647, 1939.
15. Romson JL, Hook BG, Kunkel SL, et al: Reduction of the extent of ischemic myocardial injury by neutrophil depletion in the dog. Circulation 67:1016, 1983.
16. Williams FM, Tanda K, Kus M, Williams TJ: Trimetazidine inhibits neutrophil accumulation after myocardial ischemia and reperfusion in rabbits. J Cardiovasc Pharmacol 22:828, 1993.
17. Belcher P, Drake-Holland AJ, Hynd JW, Noble MIM: Trimetazidine reduces myocardial infarct size, relative to area at risk, after temporary coronary artery occlusion in the rabbit. Br J Pharmacol 107:265, 1992.
18. Astarie-Dequeker C, Joulin Y, Devynck MA: Inhibitory effect of trimetazidine on thrombin-induced aggregation and calcium entry into human platelets. Cardiovasc Pharmacol 23:401, 1994.
19. Goupit P: Pharmacocinétique de la trimetazidine. Le Concours Médical 109(Suppl 36):3447, 1987.

20. Courte S, Bromet N: Trace determination of trimetazidine in plasma by high-performance liquid chromatography using fluorescence detection. J Chromatogr 224:162, 1981.
21. Sellier P: Effets de la trimetazidine sur les parametres ergometique dans l'angor d'effort: Etude multicentrique controlee a double insu contre placebo. Arch Mal Coeur et Vaiss 9:1371, 1986.
22. Sellier P, Detry JM, Pennaforte S: Comparative antianginal effects of trimetazidine and propranolol: The Trimetazidine European Multicentre Study [abstract]. Eur Heart J 14(Suppl):298, 1993.
23. Detry JM, Sellier P, Pennaforte S, et al: Trimetazidine: A new concept in the treatment of angina: Comparison with propranolol in patients with stable angina. Br J Clin Pharmacol 37:279, 1994.
24. Dalla-Volta S, Maraglino G, Della-Valentina P, et al: Comparison of trimetazidine with nifedipine in effort angina: A double-blind, crossover study. Cardiovasc Drugs Ther 4:853, 1988.
25. Edeki TI, Johnston A, Campbell DB, et al: An examination of the possible pharmacokinetic interaction of trimetazidine with theophylline, dioxin and antipyrine. Proceedings of the British Pharmacological Society, July 6–8, 1988, p 657.
26. Rousseau MF, Visser FG, Bax JJ, et al: Is modulation of myocardial metabolism as effective as beta-blockade in exercise-induced angina? J Am Coll Cardiol 23:484A, 1994.
27. Sellier P, Andouin P, Payen B, et al: Acute effects of trimetazidine evaluated by exercise testing. Eur J Clin Pharmacol 33:105, 1987.
28. Passeron J: Efficacite de la trimetazidine dans l'angor d'effort stable de l'insuffisant coronarien chronique. Presse Med 35:1775, 1986.
29. Detry JM: Clinical features of an anti-anginal drug in angina pectoris. Eur Heart J 14(Suppl G):18, 1993.
30. Kober G, Pennaforte S, Buck T, et al: Myocardial cytoprotection during percutaneous transluminal coronary angioplasty. Eur Heart J 14(Suppl G):12, 1993.
31. Fabiani JN, Farah B, Vuilleminot T, et al: Chromosomal aberrations and neutrophil activation induced by reperfusion in the ischemic human heart. Eur Heart J 14(Suppl G):12, 1993.
32. EMIP-FR Pilot Study Group: Free radicals, reperfusion and myocardial infarction therapy: European Myocardial Infarction Project—Free radicals pilot-study. Eur Heart J 14(Suppl G):48, 1993.
33. Brottier L, Barat JL, Combe C, et al: Therapeutic value of a cardioprotective agent in patients with severe ischemic cardiomyopathy. Eur Heart J 11:207, 1990.

CHAPTER 172

Ranolazine

Franz C. Aepfelbacher, M.D., Carl J. Pepine, M.D., and Franz H. Messerli, M.D.

Accepted pharmacologic management of ischemic heart disease with nitrates, calcium antagonists, and β-blockers has focused on improving the balance between myocardial oxygen supply and demand. However, in many patients, these drugs, alone or in combination, do not sufficiently protect against acute or chronic events associated with this disease. Therefore, alternative strategies to protect the myocardium from ischemia are widely investigated. A very promising alternative approach is the improvement of cardiac efficiency through manipulation of myocardial energy metabolism. The two main sources of energy in the myocardium are free fatty acids and glucose. Whereas heart muscle will use mostly free fatty acids as an energy source, it has been shown that cardiac efficiency is greater when glucose is utilized, particularly when coronary flow is impaired.[1] Several reasons might account for this effect: (1) the ratio between adenosine triphosphate (ATP) production and oxygen consumption is higher for glucose than for free fatty acids; however, this only partly explains the observed increase in efficiency; (2) ATP production by anaerobic glycolysis is enhanced with glucose-utilization; and (3) free fatty acids have been shown to uncouple oxidative phosphorylation, thereby causing oxygen that is not used for the generation of ATP to be consumed. All three of these mechanisms allow the heart to use oxygen more sparingly while maintaining ATP generation at the same level.

A variety of different agents have demonstrated that in patients with ischemic heart disease, modulation of myocardial energy metabolism results in greater cardiac efficiency[2-6] (Table 172–1); however, most of these agents are not suitable for long-term treatment. Ranolazine, a new drug with a similar mechanism of action, was developed by Syntex Pharmaceuticals and is undergoing clinical trials as an antiischemic agent. So far, the results are very promising and indicate that this drug could herald a novel class of antianginal agents.

CHEMISTRY

Ranolazine [(±)-N-(2,6dimethyl-phenyl)-4[2-hydroxy-3-(2-methoxyphenoxy)-propyl]-1-piperazine acetamide dihydrochloride] is chemically derived from pipera-

Table 172–1. **Metabolic Modulating Agents That Improve Cardiac Efficiency in Ischemic Heart Disease**

Agent	Mechanism of Action
Glucose-insulin-potassium	Increased glucose uptake and metabolism, reduction of arterial free fatty acids
Dichloroacetate	Activation of pyruvate dehydrogenase (PDH), leading to increased glucose utilization
L-Carnitine	Fatty acid carrier in mitochondria, regulation of adenosine triphosphate (ATP) production, stimulation of PDH
Ribose	Acceleration of ATP production
4-Bromochrotonic acid	Inhibition of fatty acid utilization

zine and has a molecular weight of 500.48. It is a white crystalline powder, 100% soluble in water, and is stable to light and temperature.

PHARMACOLOGY

Brown et al. have investigated the pharmacologic profile of ranolazine in animal models.[7] From these data, it appears that ranolazine has negligible affinity (pKi <5) for α_1-, β_1-, and β_2-adrenoceptors and a series of other receptors (D_1, M_1, M_2, $5HT_1$, A_1, A_2) and weak affinity for α_2-, D_2-, and $5HT_2$-receptors. Calcium antagonist effects were weak compared with those of nicardipine and thus seem unlikely to contribute to the mechanism of action; passive membrane permeabilities to Na^+ and K^+ were also unaffected. The antiischemic properties of ranolazine are therefore thought to be due to its activation of pyruvate dehydrogenase (PDH), a key enzyme complex in respiratory fuel selection.[8] Under ordinary conditions, only about 30% of this enzyme complex is in an active (dephosphorylated) form. Activation of PDH improves the efficiency of oxygen utilization by switching myocardial energy substrate utilization away from fatty acids toward glucose, thereby producing more ATP per mole of oxygen.[9] This hypothesis is supported by the findings that ranolazine decreases free fatty acid uptake[10] and increased glucose oxidation[11] during pacing-induced ischemia. Other possible mechanisms of action of ranolazine include retarding the inhibition of anaerobic glycolysis, resulting in a delay of the consequences of ischemia, and preventing the paradoxic increase in mitochondrial oxygen uptake during the early phase of ischemia through inhibition of NADH dehydrogenase.[12]

PHARMACOKINETICS

The pharmacokinetics of ranolazine have been determined in both patients with ischemic heart disease and healthy male volunteers (Data on file, Syntex Pharmaceuticals, Palo Alto, CA). Following single intravenous administration, elimination was biexponential, with a rapid distribution phase and a longer elimination phase. Mean terminal elimination half-life and systemic clearance of ranolazine ranged from 1.40 to 2.17 hours and 5.18 to 9.85 ml/min/kg in volunteers and from 1.35 to 4.15 hours and 5.60 to 10.4 ml/min/kg in patients, respectively. After oral administration of 10 to 120 mg, ranolazine is rapidly absorbed with a bioavailability of approximately 30% to 55%, and peak plasma levels are achieved within 1 hour of dosing. Single oral doses of up to 2000 mg have been well tolerated in volunteers.

Following multiple oral doses, there was no evidence of accumulation of ranolazine over a 28-day period, and pharmacokinetics were similar to those following single oral administration (Data on file, Syntex Pharmaceuticals).

When ranolazine was administered during a high-fat meal, peak levels were slightly lower and trough levels were at least twofold higher, but there were no significant differences in either the extent of drug availability or the elimination half-life (Data on file, Syntex Pharmaceuticals).

EFFECTS ON PATHOPHYSIOLOGY

Although the exact mechanism of action has yet to be defined, several animal studies demonstrated a beneficial effect of ranolazine in the reduction of metabolic and electrophysiologic consequences of myocardial ischemia and in renal transplantation.

Metabolic Effects

In an animal model using male baboons, ranolazine clearly inhibited the peripheral appearance of clinically used enzymatic markers of myocardial damage (creatine kinase, lactate dehydrogenase) after ligation of the left anterior descending coronary artery for 30 minutes, indicating a protective effect on the myocardium during ischemia.[13] Furthermore, in a study using isolated guinea pig hearts, ranolazine preserved tissue ATP during ischemia,[8] which was associated with an increase in active pyruvate dehydrogenase.

The impact of ranolazine on modulation of α_1-adrenoceptors has been investigated in rat left ventricle.[14] Ranolazine prevented upregulation of α_1-adrenoreceptors during ischemia, probably because of inhibition of synthesis of acyl carnitines, lipid mediators said to cause ischemic damage.

Electrophysiologic Effects

A study using anesthetized dogs compared the effects of ranolazine on myocardial conduction with those of the standard antianginal compounds nicardipine, nifedipine, and verapamil.[15] Ranolazine had no significant effects on intraatrial, intraventricular, and atrioventricular (AV) conduction parameters and did not affect reestablishment of sinus rhythm after atrial pacing, whereas all calcium antagonists significantly prolonged AV conduction and reestablishment of sinus rhythm.

Other studies demonstrated a significant decrease in ischemia-induced ST-segment elevations[16] and a reduction of reperfusion-induced cardiac fibrillation and cardiac failure[17] when ranolazine was given prior to the ischemic event.

Effect on Hemodynamics

The available data demonstrate that ranolazine, at the concentrations used, is essentially free of action on heart rate, arterial pressure, and myocardial contractility,[11, 13, 16, 17] supporting the hypothesis that the principal action of ranolazine is exerted through a modulation of myocardial metabolism.

Effect on Renal Preservation

The effect of ranolazine during preservation and reperfusion of kidneys after 24 hours of cold storage was investigated in a porcine model of renal autotransplantation.[18] When ranolazine was administered prior to organ retrieval and then added to the storage solution, post-transplant function improved overall as reflected by a significantly higher glomerular filtration rate, a more rapid return to normal tubular function and effective renal plasma flow, and improved function of the loop of Henle.

CLINICAL USE

Ranolazine is currently undergoing phase III clinical trials as an antianginal compound, and some published studies have investigated its efficacy, safety, and tolerability in humans. In a double-blind, crossover, randomized, placebo-controlled study, the antianginal properties of ranolazine were assessed in 106 patients with chronic stable angina pectoris treated with a β-blocker or diltiazem.[12] When given as a single oral dose of 240 mg, ranolazine significantly improved exercise duration, time to angina, and time to 1-mm ST-segment depression compared with placebo. There was a positive relationship between plasma level and efficacy of the drug: below plasma levels of 500 ng/ml, time to angina was improved in only 40% of patients; however, this percentage rose to 67% for plasma levels above 500 ng/ml.

Plasma ranolazine concentrations were significantly higher in patients taking diltiazem than in patients taking β-blockers. Although the mechanism responsible for this difference is unknown, a plausible explanation is that diltiazem and ranolazine share a common metabolic pathway that may become saturated when both drugs are used together. No serious side effects were reported in this study, but 21% of patients reported symptoms such as mild headache, dizziness, or fatigue after a single dose of 240 mg of ranolazine, compared with 8% after placebo. No clinically significant differences were found in laboratory evaluations.

Another double-blind, crossover study compared the effects of ranolazine and atenolol on exercise duration, time to angina, and ST-segment depression in 158 patients with angina pectoris. Whereas both drugs significantly improved the times to angina and ST-segment depression, ranolazine also increased exercise duration and the maximal pressure rate product (Fig. 172–1). This would indicate that clinical improvement in exercise-induced ischemia with ranolazine was greater than with atenolol.[19]

A large multicenter study including over 300 patients with chronic stable angina is under way in the United States. The results will be available soon.

DOSAGE AND ADMINISTRATION

Ranolazine can be given both orally and intravenously. A slow-release formulation has been developed and is being used in the U.S. multicenter trial.

Single oral doses of 10, 60, and 120 mg had no effect on exercise duration in patients with angina pectoris; a significant improvement was observed after administration of 240 mg,[12] and 400 mg three

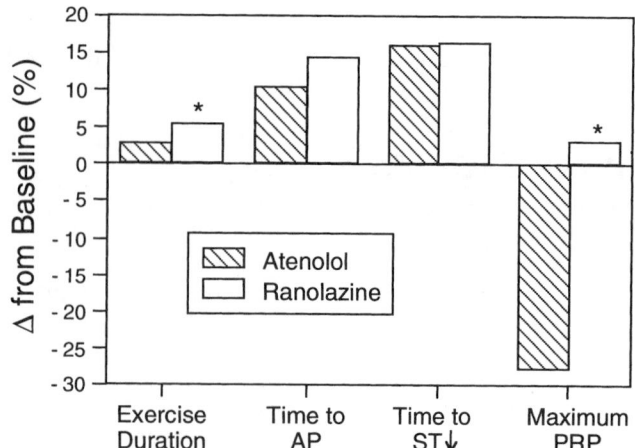

Figure 172–1. Antiischemic properties of atenolol and ranolazine in patients with exercise-induced angina. Time to AP, time to angina; time to ST, time to ST-segment depression (≤0.1 mV); maximum PRP, maximal pressure rate product; *, $p \leq .05$ versus atenolol.

times daily proved to be even more effective.[19] Single doses of up to 2000 mg were well-tolerated; however, further studies are needed to determine the maximal effective dose and potential adverse effects associated with long-term treatment.

SUMMARY

Ranolazine differs from other antianginal agents (e.g., β-blockers, calcium antagonists) in that it does not affect systemic hemodynamics. It seems to act principally via a modulation of myocardial metabolism, shifting substrate utilization toward carbohydrates rather than fatty acids. This allows the heart to use oxygen more efficiently. Although the results of a large, ongoing multicenter clinical trial have to be awaited, the available data indicate that ranolazine is efficacious and safe and that it could become a novel addition to the arsenal of antianginal agents.

REFERENCES

1. Burckhoff D, Weiss RG, Schulman SP, et al: Influence of metabolic substrate on rat heart rate function and metabolism at different coronary flows. Am J Physiol 30:H741, 1991.
2. Stanley AW, Moraski RE, Russell RO, et al: Effects of glucose-insulin-potassium on myocardial substrate availability and utilization in stable coronary artery disease. Am J Cardiol 36:929, 1975.
3. Wargovich TJ, Macdonald RG, Hill JA, et al: Myocardial metabolic and hemodynamic effects of dichloroacetate in coronary artery disease. Am J Cardiol 61:65, 1988.
4. Pepine CJ: The therapeutic potential of carnitine in cardiovascular disorders. Clin Ther 13:2, 1991.
5. Pliml W, von Arnim T, Staeblein A, et al: Effects of ribose on exercise-induced ischaemia in stable coronary artery disease. Lancet 340:507, 1992.
6. Hutter JF, Schweickhardt C, Piper HM, et al: Inhibition of fatty acid oxydation and decrease of oxygen consumption of working rat heart by 4-bromochrotonic acid. J Mol Cell Cardiol 16:105, 1984.
7. Brown CM, Clarke B, Dye A, et al: Pharmacological profile of ranolazine, a metabolic modulator active in ischaemia. Br J Pharmacol 93:247P, 1988.

8. Clarke B, Spedding M, Patmore L, et al: Protective effects of ranolazine in guinea-pig hearts during low-flow ischaemia and their association with increases in active pyruvate dehydrogenase. Br J Pharmacol 109:748, 1993.

9. Allely MC, Alps BJ, Kilpatrick AT: The effects of the novel anti-anginal compound RS 43285 on [lactic acid], [K+] and pH in a canine model of transient myocardial ischemia. Biochem Soc Trans 15:1057, 1987.

10. Pouleur H, Hue L, Harlow BJ, et al: Metabolic pathways modulation: A new approach to treat myocardial ischemia? Circulation 80(Suppl 2):52, 1989.

11. Collins-Nakai RL, Barr R, Humen D, et al: Ranolazine stimulates glucose oxidation in isolated working rat hearts [abstract]. Can J Cardiol 9:104E, 1993.

12. Cocco G, Rousseau MF, Bouvy T, et al: Effects of a new metabolic modulator, ranolazine, on exercise tolerance in angina pectoris patients treated with beta-blocker or diltiazem. J Cardiovasc Pharmacol 20(1):131, 1992.

13. Allely MC, Alps BJ: Prevention of myocardial enzyme release by ranolazine in a primate model of ischemia with reperfusion. Br J Pharmacol 99:5, 1991.

14. Allely MC, Brown CM, Kenny BA, et al: Modulation of alpha 1 adrenoceptors in rat left ventricle by ischaemia and acyl carnitines: Protection by ranolazine. J Cardiovasc Pharmacol 21(6):869, 1993.

15. Allely MC, Alps BJ: The effects of the novel anti-anginal compound RS43285 on myocardial conduction in the anaesthetized dog. Br J Pharmacol 93:375, 1988.

16. Allely MC, Alps BJ: The effects of the novel anti-anginal agent ranolazine in a canine model of transient myocardial ischaemia. Br J Pharmacol 93:246P, 1988.

17. Ferrandon P, Pascal J-C, Armstrong JM: Protective effects of the novel anti-ischaemic agent ranolazine (RS-43285) in perfused rat hearts. Br J Pharmacol 93:247P, 1988.

18. Lodge JPA, Lam FT, Perry SL, et al: Ranolazine—A new drug with beneficial effects on renal preservation. Transplantation 50:755, 1990.

19. Rousseau MF, Visser FG, Bax JJ, et al: Is modulation of myocardial metabolism as effective as beta-blockade in exercise-induced angina? [abstract]. J Am Coll Cardiol 23:268A, 1994.

XVII.

Other Drugs for the Treatment of Cardiovascular Disorders

Editors: Giuseppe Mancia and Lennart Hansson

CHAPTER 173

Pentoxifylline

John A. Spittell, Jr., M.D., M.A.C.P., F.A.C.C.

HISTORY

Interest in the factors influencing blood viscosity, which is inversely related to arterial blood flow, has led investigators to study rheologic and biochemical aspects of persons with occlusive peripheral arterial disease and intermittent claudication.[1] Because of the findings of decreased deformability and filterability of erythrocytes (increasing blood viscosity) in persons with atherosclerotic disease and intermittent claudication and the hypothesis that increased blood viscosity adversely affects microcirculation and tissue perfusion, some investigators have focused on the rheology of the microcirculation and agents that may influence it. Pentoxifylline is one agent so studied.[2] An extensive review of the properties and early therapeutic trials of pentoxifylline has been published.[3]

CHEMISTRY

Pentoxifylline, a methylxanthine and an analogue of theobromine, is a water- and alcohol-soluble crystalline powder. It was synthesized in 1964 and was introduced as a therapeutic agent in 1972.[4]

PHARMACOLOGY

Pentoxifylline has been characterized as a hemorrheologically active compound that promotes blood flow and improves tissue perfusion principally as a result of its effect on the microcirculation.[5] Its clinical pharmacology and pharmacokinetics have been reviewed.[6]

PHARMACOKINETICS

Pentoxifylline is rapidly absorbed after oral administration. Peak plasma concentration is reached in less than 1 half-hour and then declines rapidly because of a plasma half-life of 0.39 to 0.84 hour.[7] Absorption

after oral intake appears to be complete, and when the drug is administered with food, absorption, though delayed, still appears to be complete. When pentoxifylline is administered as a sustained-release tablet (the commercially available form), the peak plasma concentration of the drug is reached in about 3 hours. After extensive metabolism with enterohepatic recycling, the metabolites of pentoxifylline are rapidly excreted in the urine; thus, renal clearance of pentoxifylline is decreased in patients with renal insufficiency.[3]

EFFECTS ON PATHOPHYSIOLOGY

The mechanisms by which pentoxifylline is thought to improve perfusion in the microcirculation include its effects on blood viscosity, erythrocyte deformability, platelet aggregation, and plasma fibrinogen concentration.[8, 9] More recently, additional mechanisms involving leukocyte filterability and function have been proposed as the basis of the therapeutic effects of pentoxifylline.[10-14] In addition to possible influence on the complex interactions of blood cells and the endothelium, there is some experimental evidence that long-term treatment with pentoxifylline enhances relaxation of canine femoral arteries by an endothelium-dependent mechanism that requires the metabolism of arachidonic acid.[15]

In addition to the hematocrit and plasma viscosity, erythrocyte deformability affects blood viscosity and its flow in capillaries. Significantly increased blood viscosity and impaired erythrocyte deformability have been found in patients with occlusive peripheral arterial disease;[1] the latter effect, related to impaired elasticity of the erythrocyte cell membrane, is believed to result from depletion of intracellular adenosine triphosphate (ATP) and calcium ion accumulation. Other factors that are reported to impair red blood cell deformability are abnormal plasma osmolarity and an acid pH.[16] Pentoxifylline is reported to increase red blood cell deformability in patients with occlusive peripheral arterial disease by several investigators,[17, 18] although others disagree.[19] Pentoxifylline is also reported to increase red blood cell deformability in patients with cerebrovascular disease.[20]

A decrease in platelet adhesion and aggregation reportedly occurs in experimental animals[21] and in patients with peripheral[22] and cerebral vascular disease[20] treated with pentoxifylline. The antiplatelet effect of pentoxifylline appears to be an indirect one that results from the stimulation of prostacyclin formation in blood vessel walls and reduction of synthesis of thromboxane by pentoxifylline. Of note in this regard is the fact that pentoxifylline does not prolong the bleeding time.[22]

Increased fibrinogen levels found in patients with intermittent claudication have been reported to be decreased by pentoxifylline as a result of either increased fibrinolysis[22] or decreased production of fibrinogen, perhaps as a result of the inhibiting effect of pentoxifylline on tumor necrosis factor (TNF),[10] which is a potent inducer of fibrinogen synthesis.[24] Similar reduction of fibrinogen levels has been reported in patients with cerebrovascular disease treated with pentoxifylline.[20]

Pentoxifylline is reported to increase tissue partial oxygen pressure in ischemic limb muscles,[25] but there are no other clinically significant hemodynamic effects of orally administered pentoxifylline.[26]

Blood glucose, serum insulin, and free fatty acid levels are reported to be unchanged in persons receiving pentoxifylline,[3, 27] and the drug has no effect on the endogenous secretion of catecholamines in healthy persons.[28] *In vitro* and *in vivo* studies demonstrating the ability of pentoxifylline to inhibit cytokines and their effects on platelets, endothelium smooth muscle cells, and collagen suggest that the drug, acting as an "anticytokine," may have a therapeutic role in hyperplastic arterial diseases—atherosclerosis and restenosis—as well as in inflammation.[29]

CLINICAL USE

Pentoxifylline has been approved by the United States Food and Drug Administration for the symptomatic treatment of intermittent claudication. The recommended dose is 400 mg three times per day, preferably taken with meals. Although walking distance is improved in some patients as early as 2 weeks after the start of therapy, continued improvement may be noted for up to 12 weeks after initiation of treatment. Multiple studies have reported improvement in about 50% to 60% of patients with occlusive peripheral arterial disease,[29-34] but others have reported no change in claudication or walking distance.[18, 19] This discrepancy in results may be explained by a study that identified a "target population" in whom improved initial and maximal walking distances is likely with the use of pentoxifylline; this target population was characterized as persons having their claudication for

more than 1 year and a supine ankle systolic pressure 80% or less than the supine brachial systolic pressure.[35]

Some studies of the effect of pentoxifylline in special circumstances are of interest. Most persons with atherosclerotic occlusive arterial disease are smokers; one study reported that smoking tends to reduce plasma concentrations of pentoxifylline and its metabolite.[36] Such an effect, if confirmed, could explain failure of the drug if the patient continues to smoke while taking it. When pentoxifylline was evaluated in combination with an exercise program, it was reported to be clinically effective in claudicants.[37] Concerning the long-term use of pentoxifylline, it has been reported that 54% of patients who had been receiving the drug for more than 1 year could be successfully weaned off the drug by gradual reduction of the dose over a 3-month period.[38] A double-blind, placebo-controlled trial of pentoxifylline combined with other antianginal therapy in patients with stable angina pectoris showed no improvement in exercise tolerance.[39] In a randomized trial in persons with prior myocardial infarction and silent ischemia with exercise, pentoxifylline was reported to diminish exercise-induced electrocardiographic changes; however,[40] in both of these studies, the drug was well-tolerated.

The most common side effects noted with pentoxifylline in the recommended dose are indigestion and nausea, which can often be lessened by taking the drug during a meal or reducing the dose. Less-common side effects are dizziness and headache. There is a report of an acute psychotic reaction associated with the intravenous infusion of 60 mg of pentoxifylline in 5% dextrose; the same report states that high parenteral doses of pentoxifylline may enhance the hypoglycemic activity of insulin in diabetic patients.[41] If side effects continue despite lowered dosage, pentoxifylline should be discontinued.

Blood counts should be monitored in patients treated with pentoxifylline, because aplastic anemia has been reported with its use in two patients.[42] When pentoxifylline is prescribed for patients who are receiving anticoagulants orally, frequent monitoring of the prothrombin time is recommended; however, interaction with warfarin has not been observed in animals[43] or humans.[44] A study with rats has shown inhibition of pentoxifylline clearance by cimetidine,[45] but the clinical significance of this interaction needs clarification. When patients receive antihypertensive therapy, frequent monitoring of the blood pressure is recommended to detect any added effect of pentoxifylline. No interaction of pentoxifylline with other commonly used cardiovascular drugs or antidiabetic agents has been noted. The concomitant use of pentoxifylline in patients receiving theophylline does not interfere with assays of serum theophylline concentration.[46]

Pentoxifylline should not be used in persons who have shown intolerance to methylxanthines such as caffeine, theophylline, and theobromine.

Pentoxifylline is approved in the United States *only*

for the symptomatic treatment of intermittent claudication due to occlusive peripheral arterial disease. However, with its proposed beneficial effect on the microcirculation and tissue perfusion, it is not surprising that the agent has been tried in other vascular conditions. The limited trials of pentoxifylline in stable angina pectoris[39] and in silent myocardial ischemia[41] have already been noted. In a trial of pentoxifylline in 12 men with impotence due to mild to moderate penile vascular insufficiency, penile brachial indices were regularly increased, and 9 men were able to reestablish coital function; there were no complications of therapy.[47] Improvement in or healing of trophic leg ulcer,[49] livedo vasculitis,[49] and leg ulcer due to beta-thalassemia[51] has been reported. Studies on the use of pentoxifylline in the management of venous stasis ulcer have been extended; the earlier report of benefit[51] has been confirmed in a double-blind, randomized, prospective, placebo-controlled parallel group study that showed that pentoxifylline used in combination with compression bandaging significantly improved the healing of venous stasis ulcers.[52] The improved healing is believed to be related to the effect of pentoxifylline on leukocytes, which have been shown to accumulate in the microcirculation in the dependent legs of persons with venous hypertension.[52] Symptomatic improvement has been reported in patients with primary Raynaud syndrome,[54] patients with diabetic neuropathy,[55] and one patient with mesenteric insufficiency.[56] Studies in patients with cerebrovascular disease have reported increased regional cerebral blood flow[57] with the use of pentoxifylline. In a double-blind, randomized, placebo-controlled study of 80 patients with vascular dementia, the pentoxifylline group experienced significant improvement in both short- and long-term memory compared with the placebo group.[58] The incidence of transient ischemic attacks was reduced in patients who were receiving pentoxyifylline.[20, 59]

Continuous intravenous infusion of pentoxifylline (1200 mg/day for 15 days) has been reported to be safe and effective in relieving pain at rest as well as in increasing walking distance in 22 patients with severe occlusive arterial disease.[60] Interestingly, intravenously administered pentoxifylline enhanced the antiplatelet (antiaggregatory) effect of prostacyclin.[61]

SOCIOECONOMIC CONSIDERATIONS

Pentoxifylline may offer an alternative to restoration of pulsatile flow by arterial surgery or transluminal angioplasty for persons with intermittent claudication due to occlusive peripheral arterial disease. However, its availability should not lessen the emphasis on important conservative measures for all persons with occlusive peripheral arterial disease (i.e., interdiction of tobacco, protection of the affected limb from trauma, fastidious foot care, and a regular walking program).

The cost of pentoxifylline is in the range of $30 or more per month; its benefit must therefore be evaluated in light of its cost to the patient, because maintenance of symptomatic improvement may require continued use of the drug.

In this context, Stergachis et al. assessed the medical outcomes and costs associated with the treatment of patients with occlusive peripheral arterial disease and reported that pentoxifylline may reduce the risk of vascular surgery for patients with occlusive peripheral arterial disease.[62]

REFERENCES

1. Dormandy JA, Hoare E, Colley J, et al: Clinical, haemodynamic, rheological and biochemical findings in 126 patients with intermittent claudication. Br Med J 4:576, 1973.
2. Marcel GA: Hemorrheological agents. *In* Spittell JA (ed): Pharmacological Approach to the Treatment of Limb Ischemia. Philadelphia: College of Physicians, 1983, pp 125–140.
3. Ward A, Clissold SP: Pentoxifylline: A review of its pharmacodynamic and pharmacokinetic properties, and its therapeutic efficacy. Drugs 34:50, 1987.
4. Theis H, Lebrach F, Muller R: A 5-year review of clinico-experimental and therapeutic experience with pentoxifylline. Pharmatherapeutica 2(Suppl 1):150, 1978.
5. Muller R: Hemorrheology and peripheral vascular diseases: A new therapeutic approach. J Med 12:209, 1981.
6. Dettelbach HR, Aviado DM: Clinical pharmacology of pentoxifylline with special reference to its hemorrheologic effect for the treatment of intermittent claudication. J Clin Pharmacol 25:8, 1985.
7. Smith RV, Waller ES, Doluisio JT, et al: Pharmacokinetics of orally administered pentoxifylline in humans. J Pharm Sci 75:47, 1986.
8. Spittell JA: Pentoxifylline and intermittent claudication. Ann Intern Med 102:126, 1985.
9. Barnes AJ, Locke P, Scudder PR, et al: Is hyperviscosity a treatable component of diabetic microcirculatory disease? Lancet 2:789, 1977.
10. Soria J, Giovannangeli I, Jolchine E, Chassoux G: Pentoxifylline, fibrinogen, and leukocytes. Blood Coagul Fibrinolysis 1:485, 1990.
11. Cummings DM, Ballas SK, Ellison MJ: Lack of effect of pentoxifylline on red blood cell deformability. J Clin Pharmacol 32:1050, 1992.
12. Novick WJ: Pentoxifylline and leukocyte function. Critical Care Report 2:236, 1991.
13. Nash GB, Loosemore T, Thomas PRS, Dormandy JA: Effects of acute Trental infusion on white blood cell rheology in patients with critical leg ischemia. Clin Hemorheology 11:309, 1991.
14. Ciuffetti G, Mercuri M, Lombardini R, et al: Use of pentoxifylline as an inhibitor of free radical generation in peripheral vascular disease. Clin Pharmacol 41:511, 1991.
15. Kim CH, Miller VM, Sandberg SM, Edwards BS: Chronic pentoxifylline administration results in endothelium dependent, cyclooxygenase dependent vasodilatation [abstract]. J Am Coll Cardiol 21:313A, 1993.
16. Marcel GA: Red cell deformability: Physiological, clinical and pharmacological aspects. J Med 10:409, 1979.
17. Angelkort B, Maurin N, Boateng K: Influence of pentoxifylline on erythrocyte deformability in peripheral occlusive arterial disease. Curr Med Res Opin 6:255, 1979.
18. Donaldson DR, Hall TJ, Kester RC, et al: Does oxypentifylline (Trental) have a place in the treatment of intermittent claudication? Curr Med Res Opin 9:35, 1984.
19. Gallus AS, Gleadow F, Dupont P, et al: Intermittent claudication: A double-blind crossover trial of pentoxifylline. Aust N Z J Med 15:402, 1985.
20. Ott E, Fazekas F, Valetitsch E, et al: The rationale of rheological pharmacological strategy. Clin Hemorrheol 6:35, 1986.
21. Zinzadse KI, Gulishwili LN, Tavchedlidse TD, et al: The effect of pentoxifylline on the flow properties of blood in experimental atherosclerosis in rabbits. Pharmatherapeutica 2:118, 1978.

22. Angelkort B, Kresivetter H: Influence of risk factors and coagulation phenomena on the fluidity of blood in chronic arterial occlusive disease. Scand J Clin Lab Invest 156(Suppl):185, 1981.

23. Matzky R, Darius H, Schror K: The release of prostacyclin (PG12) by pentoxifylline from human vascular tissue. Arzneimittelforschung 32:1315, 1982.

24. Gresser I, Demlers FD, Tran-Quangs N, et al: Tumor necrosis factor induces acute phase proteins in rates. J Biol Regul Homeost Agents 1:173, 1987.

25. Ehrly AM, Saeger-Lorenz K: Influence of pentoxifylline on muscle tissue oxygen tension (pO2) of patients with intermittent claudication before and after pedal ergometer exercise. Angiology 38:93, 1987.

26. Nordhus O, Ekestrom S, Liljequist EI: Effects of pentoxifylline on central hemodynamics in patients with congestive heart failure. Scand J Thorac Cardiovasc Surg 20:217, 1986.

27. Heidrich H, Schirop T: Blood glucose and serum insulin levels following acute and chronic pentoxifylline administration. Acta Diabetol 17:15, 1980.

28. Nudemberg F, Chamberlain J, Haja P, et al: Influence of intravenously administered pentoxifylline on endogenous secretion of catecholamines. IRCS Med Sci (Hematology) 10:466, 1982.

29. Libby P, Clinton SK: Cytokines as mediators of vascular pathology. Nauv Rev Fr Hematol 34(Suppl):S47, 1992.

30. Porter JM, Cutter BS, Lee BY, et al: Pentoxifylline efficacy in the treatment of intermittent claudication: Multicenter controlled double-blind trial with objective assessment of chronic occlusive arterial disease patients. Am Heart J 113:864, 1982.

31. Lee BY, Berkowitz P, Savitsky JP, et al: Pentoxifylline treatment of moderate to severe chronic occlusive arterial disease. Clin Cardiol 8:161, 1985.

32. Reich T, Gillings D: Effects of pentoxifylline on severe claudication. Angiology 38:651, 1987.

33. Johnson WC, Sentissi JM, Baldwin D, et al: Treatment of claudication with pentoxifylline: Are benefits related to improvement in viscosity? J Vasc Surg 6:211, 1987.

34. Schwartz RW, Logan NM, Johnson PJ, et al: Pentoxifylline increases extremity blood flow in diabetic atherosclerotic patients. Arch Surg 124:434, 1989.

35. Lindgarde F, Jelnes R, Bjorkman H, et al: Conservative drug treatment in patients with moderately severe chronic occlusive peripheral arterial disease. Circulation 80:1549, 1989.

36. Mauro VF, Mauro LS, Hageman JH: Comparison of pentoxifylline pharmacokinetics between smokers and nonsmokers. J Clin Pharmacol 32:1054, 1992.

37. Ernst E, Kollar L, Resch KL: Does pentoxifylline prolong the walking distance in exercised claudicants? A placebo-controlled double-blind trial. Angiology 43:121, 1992.

38. Johnson WC, Hamilton J, Baldwin D, Walker N: Pentoxifylline treatment of chronic claudication: Are patients dependent on therapy? J Vasc Surg 16:484, 1992.

39. Strauss WE, Parisi AF: Safety and efficacy of pentoxifylline in stable angina pectoris. Am J Cardiol 71:342, 1993.

40. Marin JA, Menegazzo A, Coude M: Effect of oral pentoxifylline in exercised-induced silent myocardial ischemia. Curr Ther Res 52:839, 1992.

41. Jani AP, Diwan SK, Gupta OP, Jajoo VN: Acute psychotic reaction to pentoxifylline. J Assoc Physicians India 40:479, 1992.

42. Mass RD, Venook AP, Linker CA: Pentoxifylline and aplastic anemia. Ann Intern Med 107:427, 1987.

43. Luke DR, O'Donnell MP, Keane WF, et al: Lack of pharmacodynamic interaction between pentoxifylline and warfarin in the rat. Res Commun Chem Pathol Pharmacol 54:65, 1986.

44. Ingerslev J, Mowitzen C, Stenbjerg S: Pentoxifylline does not interfere with stable coumarin anticoagulant therapy: A clinical study. Pharmatherapeutica 4:595, 1986.

45. Luke DR, Rocci ML, Hoholick C: Inhibition of pentoxifylline clearance by cimetidine. J Pharm Sci 75:155, 1986.

46. Cummings DM, Rocci ML, Green P, et al: Interference potential of pentoxifylline and its major metabolite with theophylline assays. Am J Pharm 42:2717, 1985.

47. Korenman SG, Viosca SP: Treatment of vasculogenic sexual dysfunction with pentoxifylline. J Am Geriatr Soc 41:363, 1993.

48. Steruitzky R, Seige K: Clinical investigation of the effects of pentoxifylline in patients with severe peripheral occlusive vascular disease. Curr Med Res Opin 9:602, 1985.

49. Bard JW: Trental termed drug of choice for treatment of livedo vasculitis. Skin Allergy News 18:17, 1987.

50. Tercedor J, Herranz MT, Rodenas JM, et al: Pentoxifylline treatment for Betathalassemia intermedia leg ulcer. Int J Dermatol 31:747, 1992.

51. Burton CS: Pentoxifylline helps prevent leg ulcers in venous insufficiency. Int Med News 20:13, 1987.

52. Colgan M, Dormandy JA, Jones PW, et al: Oxypentifylline treatment of venous ulcers of the leg. Br Med J 300:972, 1990.

53. Thomas PRS, Nash GB, Dormandy JA: White cell accumulation in dependent legs of patients with venous hypertension: A possible mechanism for trophic changes in the skin. Br Med J 296:1693, 1988.

54. Neirotti M, Longo F, Macchione C, et al: Functional vascular disorders: Treatment with pentoxifylline. Angiology 38:575, 1987.

55. Cohen KL, Harris S: Pentoxifylline and diabetic neuropathy. Ann Intern Med 107:600, 1987.

56. Maurelis PG, Doumanian H: Pentoxifylline for mesenteric ischemia. Am J Gastroenterol 82:175, 1987.

57. Hartman A: Comparative randomized study of cerebral blood flow after long-term administration of pentoxifylline and codergocrine mesylate in patients with chronic cerebrovascular disease. Curr Med Res Opin 9:475, 1985.

58. Blume J, Ruhlmann KV, de la Haye R, Rettig K: Treatment of chronic cerebrovascular disease in elderly patients with pentoxifylline. J Med 23:417, 1992.

59. Herskovitz E, Famulari A, Tamoroff L, et al: Preventive treatment of cerebral transient ischemia: Comparative randomized trial of pentoxifylline vs. conventional anti-aggregants. Eur Neurol 24:73, 1985.

60. Angelides NS: Continuous infusion treatment with pentoxifylline in patients with severe peripheral vascular occlusive disease. Angiology 37:555, 1986.

61. Maurique RV, Maurique V: Platelet resistance to prostacyclin: Enhancement of the antiaggregatory effect of prostacyclin by pentoxifylline. Angiology 38:101, 1987.

62. Stergachis A, Steingold S, Luce BR, et al: Medical care and cost outcomes after pentoxifylline treatment of peripheral arterial disease. Arch Intern Med 152:1220, 1992.

CHAPTER 174

Fish Oils

Carl J. Lavie, M.D., F.A.C.C., F.A.C.P., F.A.C.C.P.,
and Richard V. Milani, M.D., F.A.C.C.

Substantial data indicate that serum lipids, including elevated levels of low-density lipoprotein cholesterol (LDL-C) and triglyceride-rich lipoproteins and low levels of high-density lipoprotein cholesterol (HDL-C), are strongly related to the pathogenesis and progression of coronary artery disease (CAD).[1-3] Platelets also play a pivotal role in the pathogenesis of atherosclerosis and acute atherosclerotic events, both by involvement in the early pathophysiologic steps in the atherosclerosis process and in its complications.[4, 5] Numerous other risk factors for atherosclerosis, including arterial pressure, also need to be addressed for optimal primary and secondary prevention of atherosclerosis in general and particularly in CAD.[6]

Epidemiologic and interventional studies have provided evidence that fish and fish oils containing high quantities of omega-3 fatty acids may improve platelet function and other aspects of the cardiovascular profile.[7, 8] Substantial epidemiologic data indicate higher CAD morbidity and mortality associated with high fat consumption (particularly from saturated fat and cholesterol), whereas societies that consume a very high percentage of fat from marine sources have strikingly low CAD morbidity and mortality in comparison with societies consuming other forms of fat.

CLASSES OF FATTY ACIDS

In general, fatty acids can be classified according to the degree of saturation and unsaturation site in the molecule of carbon-carbon double bonds. It is well-known that polyunsaturated fatty acids have fewer adverse affects on serum lipids than the saturated fatty acids. Interest has grown in the different types of polyunsaturated fatty acids compared with saturated

fatty acids (Table 174–1).[7] The prototype of the omega-9 fatty acid, oleic acid, has been shown to be neutral and possibly beneficial on plasma lipids. Humans are unable to synthesize fatty acids with double bonds more distal from the carboxyl end of the fatty acids than the ninth carbon atom. This is why linoleic acid, which is the parent compound of the omega-6 fatty acids, is an essential fatty acid from which arachidonic acid (AA), which is the precursor of prostaglandins and leukotrienes (Fig. 174–1), is formed.[9] Likewise, α-linolenic acid is the parent compound of the omega-3 fatty acids and is now emerging as an essential fatty acid and the precursor of eicosapentaenoic acid (EPA) and docosahexaenoic acid (DHA). In humans, EPA and DHA are both synthesized from α-linolenic acid and/or are ingested from marine sources or dietary supplements. The biologic and clinical effects of these fatty acids, EPA and DHA, is the subject of this chapter.

EPIDEMIOLOGIC STUDIES

Much of the enthusiasm regarding omega-3 fatty acids is derived from epidemiologic studies demonstrating an inverse relationship between consumption of fish and death from CAD.[7, 8, 10, 11] As early as 1944, Sinclair pointed out the rarity of CAD and other evidence of atherosclerosis in Greenland Eskimos, despite a diet high in fat and cholesterol.[12] However, the Greenland Eskimos consumed a diet very high in fatty fish, including whale, seal, and walrus. Sinclair observed that the Eskimos tended to bruise and bleed easily, and Bang and Dyerberg subsequently demonstrated that the Eskimos had reduced platelet counts (50,000 to 80,000 mm³ lower) and decreased platelet aggregation, resulting in prolonged bleeding times.[13]

Table 174–1. **Major Classes of Fatty Acids**

Family*	Fatty Acids	Formula†	Source
I Omega-9	Oleic acid	C16:1	Olive oil, other vegetable oils, animal fats
II Omega-6	Linoleic acid	C18:2	Vegetable oils
	Arachidonic acid	C20:4	Poultry, meats
III Omega-3	α-Linolenic acid	C18:3	Marine and land plants‡
	EPA	C20:5	Marine oils and fish
	DHA	C22:6	Marine oils and fish
IV Saturated fats	Palmitic acid	C16:0	Animal and vegetable fats
	Stearic acid	C18:0	Butter, lard, palm oil, palm kernel oil, coconut oil

*The omega number refers to the position of the first double bond from the methyl end of the molecule.
†The notation shows the total number of carbon atoms and total number of double bonds.
‡A particularly good source is rape-seed, commercially available as canola oil.
EPA, eicosapentaenoic acid; DHA, docosahexaenoic acid.
Adapted from Lavie CJ, Squires RW, Gau GT: Preventive cardiology: What is the role of fish and fish oils in primary and secondary prevention? J Cardiopulm Rehab 7:527, 1987.

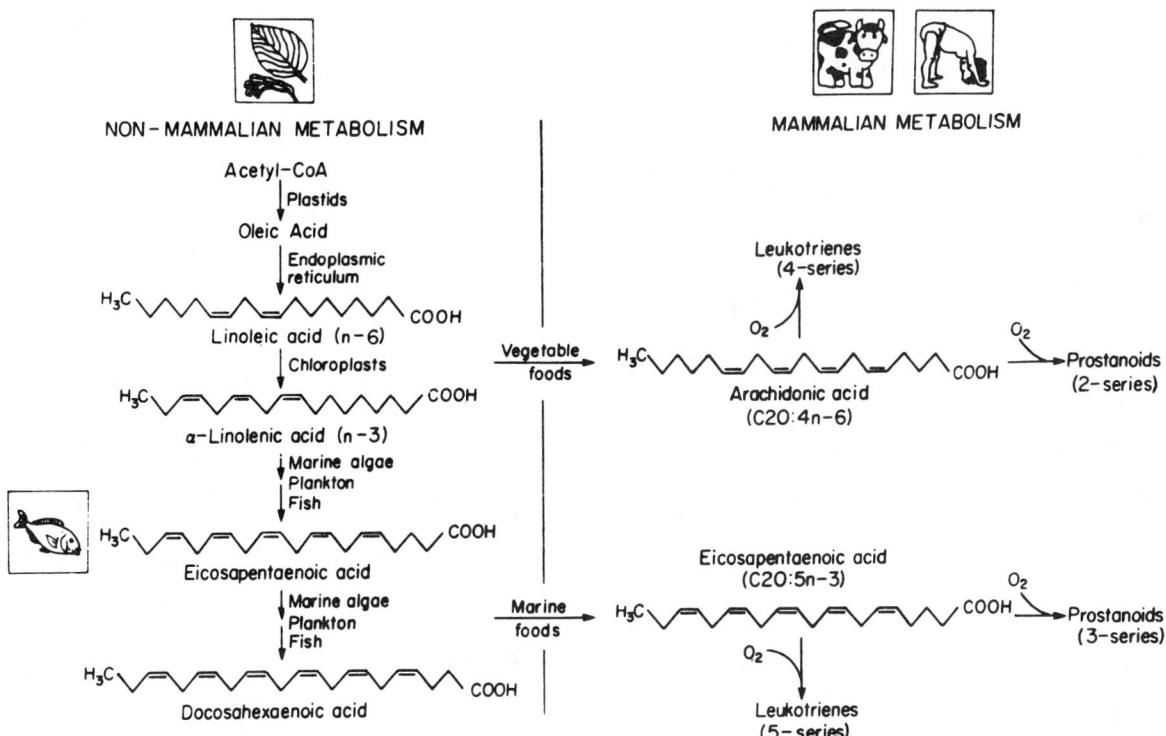

Figure 174–1. The origins and metabolism of omega-6 and omega-3 polyunsaturated fatty acids in nonmammals and mammals and the biosynthesis of eicosanoids, prostanoids, and leukotrienes from the omega-6 and omega-3 precursors, arachidonic acid, and eicosapentaenoic acid, respectively. The prostanoids and leukotrienes produced from these parent 20-carbon fatty acids are of different series. (From Leaf A, Weber PC: Omega-3 fatty acids and cardiovascular disease. *In* Braunwald E [ed]: Heart Disease: A Textbook of Cardiovascular Medicine, 4th ed, Supplement Update 3. Philadelphia: WB Saunders, 1992, p 52.)

In addition, the Eskimos, who eat approximately 500 g of fish a day (compared with only 10 to 20 g/day in westernized society), had considerably higher contents of omega-3 fatty acids and lower levels of AA in plasma, platelets, and red blood cell membranes than did a group of Danish controls. Interestingly, associated with their reduced rate of CAD, the Greenland Eskimos also had more favorable lipid profiles and lower levels of arterial pressure.

The Japanese eat approximately 100 g/day of fish, which is considerably more than do most people from westernized society but considerably less than do the Greenland Eskimos. Despite a high prevalence of hypertension and tobacco abuse, the Japanese have a low risk of atherosclerosis and CAD. Even within Japan, groups that eat more fish have higher levels of omega-3 and lower levels of AA in the plasma and in platelets and red blood cell membranes; likewise, they have a lower prevalence of hypertension, other cardiovascular disease, and all-cause mortality than groups consuming less fish.[7, 8, 11]

In westernized society, there is also evidence that increased consumption of fish is associated with decreased CAD mortality. In the Zutphen study from the Netherlands, the 20-year mortality rate was 50% lower among those who ate 30 g of fish per day (approximately two fish meals per week) than among those who did not eat fish.[14] The difference was evident regardless of the fish eaten (fatty or lean) and was independent of age, cholesterol level, and blood pressure level. Interestingly, the ingestion of this fairly small quantity of fish would not be expected to have any appreciable effect on plasma lipids (with the possible exception of slightly reducing triglyceride levels) or to alter platelet function. Therefore, the reason for the decrease in CAD mortality associated with fish consumption in this study and in a subsequent Western Electric Company study remains uncertain.[15] Data from two other population studies, however, failed to demonstrate a significant association between cardiovascular mortality and consumption of fish;[16, 17] however, in these two populations, most persons eat fish two or more times per week and have a lower overall incidence of CAD than do populations that consume less fish.

CLINICAL EFFECTS
Platelets

As mentioned earlier, Dyerburg and colleagues initiated the idea that the changes in the metabolism of eicosanoids induced by omega-3 fatty acids may have important antiplatelet effects.[18] EPA and DHA compete with AA in several sites, including competition for the enzyme cyclooxygenase (Fig. 174–2).[8] In general, EPA is converted by platelets into thromboxane A_3 (TXA_3). Unlike TXA_2, which is produced by platelets from AA and is a potent vasoconstrictor and stimulator in platelet aggregation, TXA_3 is essentially

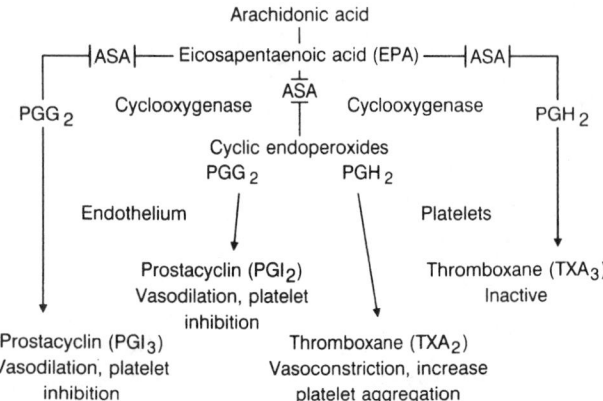

Figure 174–2. The effects of fish oils containing eicosapentaenoic acid (EPA) on prostaglandin biosynthesis and platelet function. (From Lavie CJ, Squires RW, Gau GT: Preventive cardiology: What is the value of antiplatelet agents and fish oils? Southern Medical Journal 81:1146, 1988.)

inactive. The endothelium converts EPA to prostacyclin I_3 (PGI$_3$), which, like PGI$_2$ produced in endothelial cells from AA, is a potent vasodilator and inhibitor of platelet aggregation. There is also some evidence that EPA directly inhibits the enzyme thromboxane synthetase and thus decreases TXA$_2$ production. Therefore, the net effect of a diet high in omega-3 fatty acids and lower in omega-6 fatty acids is the high concentration of physiologically active PGI$_2$ and PGI$_3$ in endothelium and a low concentration of TXA$_2$ and physiologically inactive TXA$_3$ in platelets, resulting in a state of vasodilation and platelet inhibition. Additionally, circulating neutrophils as well as monocytes/macrophages are involved in leukotriene metabolism.[9] Arachidonic acid also yields the 4-series of leukotrienes, of which LTB$_4$ is strongly chemotactic, whereas EPA yields the 5-series of leukotrienes, and LTB$_5$ is weakly chemotactic. Through these actions, fish oils manifest antiinflammatory effects that may be important in thrombosis and atherosclerosis.

Platelets and thrombosis play major roles in the complications of CAD.[4, 5, 8] Although platelets play a major role in the pathogenesis of atherosclerosis, thrombus formation on an atherosclerotic plaque clearly is the pathophysiologic mechanism present in acute coronary syndromes, including unstable angina, acute myocardial infarction, and sudden cardiac ischemic death. Although this mechanism likely explains the reduced rate of CAD in Greenland Eskimos and in Japan, the clinical effects must be compared with other proven antiplatelet therapy. For example, low doses of aspirin (80 to 325 mg/day), which irreversibly acetylates the enzyme cyclooxygenase, probably have as potent, or even more potent, effects on platelets than large doses of omega-3 fatty acids.

Lipids

Nearly 20 years ago, Dyerburg and Bang demonstrated that LDL-C was lower and HDL-C was higher in the Greenland Eskimos than in Danish controls.[18]

Since then, numerous studies have assessed the effects of omega-3 fatty acids on plasma lipids.[7–11, 19–24] The major consistent effect observed with fish oils has been significant reductions in very low-density lipoproteins (VLDLs) and triglycerides due to inhibition of hepatic triglyceride synthesis. Because VLDLs are a precursor of LDLs, a reduction in LDL-C occurs in some patients with hypertriglyceridemia, but this has not been a universally consistent finding in individuals with hypercholesterolemia without hypertriglyceridemia. The effects of omega-3 fatty acids have varied, reducing total cholesterol and raising HDL-C in some but not all studies. In individuals ingesting fish oils, there is also a blunted rise in total cholesterol and LDL-C following a cholesterol-rich meal.[9] In addition, feeding fish oil has resulted in the formation of smaller low-density lipoprotein particles with less cholesterol content that may be less atherogenic, without necessarily reducing total cholesterol and LDL-C levels.[25]

Arterial Pressure

Several studies indicate that omega-3 fatty acids cause a modest reduction in levels of arterial pressure in both normotensive subjects and mildly hypertensive patients.[26–28] Studies have demonstrated some reduction in the vasospastic response to circulating catecholamines and possibly to angiotensin.[7] Several reports demonstrate that omega-3 fatty acids exert significant antihypertensive effects in patients with cyclosporine-induced hypertension.[29] We recently reported the hemodynamic profile for cardiac transplant recipients with cyclosporine-induced hypertension,[30] as well as the effects of omega-3 fatty acids in these patients.[29] Compared with placebo, omega-3 fatty acids led to significant reductions in arterial pressure and systemic vascular resistance (by approximately 20% to 25%) in cardiac transplant recipients with cyclosporine-induced hypertension. Therapy with fish oils was also associated with a mild reduction in left ventricular mass (not significant statistically) and mild improvements in some parameters of diastolic left ventricular filling.

Restenosis Following Percutaneous Transluminal Coronary Angioplasty

Several randomized trials suggested that omega-3 fatty acids reduced the rate of restenosis following percutaneous transluminal coronary angioplasty (PTCA), although other trials failed to demonstrate a significant protective effect.[31] This raised the debate regarding the need for high doses of fish oils, as well as pretreatment days to weeks prior to PTCA. Nevertheless, a metaanalysis suggested an approximately 15% to 30% reduction in the rate of restenosis following PTCA in patients treated with various protocols using fish oils, leading to a large National Institutes of Health–sponsored randomized trial to further elucidate the benefits of this therapy. However, preliminary data from this large, randomized, prospec-

Table 174–2. **Potential Inhibition of Human Atherosclerosis by Fish Oils**

Inhibits platelets
Increases vasodilatation
Produces beneficial lipid effects
Lowers arterial pressure
Modifies leukotriene production to reduce inflammatory
  components of atherosclerosis
Increases fibrinolytic activity
Reduces vascular response to catecholamines
Decreases blood viscosity
Increases red blood cell deformability
Reduces formation of interleukin-1 and tumor necrosis factor

Table 174–3. **Evidence of Fish Oils to Prevent Atherosclerosis in Animal Models**

Inhibits intimal hyperplasia
Increases endothelial-dependent vasorelaxation
Reduces infarct size
Prevents fatal arrhythmias following coronary occlusion

tive study failed to confirm any benefit of fish oils following PTCA.[32] Therefore, as with numerous other therapeutic modalities tested to reduce restenosis following PTCA, fish oils do not appear to confer any substantial benefit and should not be routinely recommended to patients following PTCA.

Atherosclerosis

Numerous properties, some of which are discussed above, suggest a potential role of omega-3 fatty acids for inhibiting atherosclerosis in humans (Table 174–2). Besides potential mechanisms to inhibit atherosclerosis per se, it is known that plaque rupture and thrombus formation on the atherosclerotic plaque is the final pathogenic event involved in acute coronary syndromes (as discussed earlier). One interesting mechanism by which fish oils may inhibit this process is by reducing triglyceride levels, which, therefore, may lead to a reduction in the level of plasminogen activator, thereby increasing circulating fibrinolytic activity.[9] Fish oils have many properties in the blood similar to those induced by long-term exercise, leading not only to increased fibrinolytic activity but also to reduced whole-blood viscosity and increased red blood cell deformability, all of which improve tissue perfusion at a cellular level.[7-9, 33]

Evidence from animal studies for an action of omega-3 fatty acids to reduce atherosclerosis also is convincing (Table 174–3).[9, 34, 35] Therefore, these agents could have significant antiatherosclerotic effects in humans. Unfortunately, preliminary data from an an-

giographic trial in humans failed to demonstrate any effects on angiographically diagnosed CAD.[36] Although fish oils still might inhibit human atherosclerosis if more sophisticated studies were employed (e.g., intravascular ultrasound and/or angioscopy), there is currently no support for the routine use of omega-3 fatty acids to prevent or reduce atherosclerosis.

Other Potential Cardiovascular Effects

Fish oils also have known immunologic effects, including producing significant reductions in levels in tumor necrosis factor (TNF). Data have demonstrated high levels of TNF in the cardiac cachexia of end-stage congestive heart failure (CHF).[37] In a small, placebo-controlled, randomized study of patients with severe CHF, we demonstrated 50% to 70% reductions in TNF and interleukin-1 following administration of fish oils, whereas both of these factors increased following placebo therapy.[38] Although larger studies over longer periods are clearly needed, we believe our preliminary data suggest a potential role for fish oils for the cardiac cachexia of severe CHF.

Ingestion of EPA and DHA has also been shown to prevent ventricular fibrillation during both coronary artery occlusion and reperfusion in conscious dogs. Similarly, acute infusions of 10% emulsion of fish oil concentrate have been shown to prevent ventricular fibrillation in animals known to be susceptible to sudden cardiac death. The mechanism is likely due to blunting of cytosolic calcium levels, which rise after induction of ischemia. Omega-3 fatty acids therefore have important effects on the calcium channel that prevent ischemia-induced dysrhythmias in animals.

Table 174–4. **Daily Doses of Fish Oils Needed to Affect Platelets and Lipids***

Blood Component Affected	EPA (g)	Cod Liver Oil† (ml)	Promega‡ (Tablets)	Max EPA§ (Tablets)
Triglycerides	0.7–1.1	3.0–5.0	2.0–3.0	4.0–6.0
HDL cholesterol	1.5–2.0	7.0–10.0	4.0–6.0	8.0–12.0
Cholesterol	2.0–3.0	10.0–15.0	6.0–8.0	12.0–16.0
Platelets	3.0–4.0	15.0–20.0	8.0–12.0	16.0–24.0

*Fish oil capsules containing up to 50% omega-3 fatty acids and having small amounts of cholesterol, vitamin A, and vitamin D are now also marketed.
†Three grams of EPA in each tablespoon.
‡Each 1-g tablet contains about 350 mg of EPA.
§Each 1-g tablet contains about 180 mg of EPA.
EPA, eicosapentaenoic acid; DHA, docosahexaenoic acid; HDL, high-density lipoprotein.
Adapted from Lavie CJ, Squires RW, Gau GT: Preventive cardiology: What is the role of fish and fish oils in primary and secondary prevention? J Cardiopulm Rehab 7:530, 1987.

Table 174–5. **Cholesterol and Calories in Fish and Dietary Supplements Supplying 1 g Eicosapentaenoic Acid (EPA) and Docosahexanoic Acid (DHA)***

Fish or Supplement	Fat† (g)	EPA + DHA† (g)	Cholesterol† (mg)	Calories‡ (number)	Amount to Supply About 1 g EPA + DHA (g)	Cholesterol (mg)	Calories (number)
Salmon							
(steamed)	6.6	1.0	74	199	100	74	199
Trout	3.4	0.5	57	131	200	114	262
Crab (broiled)	1.3	0.4	78	127	250	195	317
Cod							
(steamed)	0.7	0.2	37	82	500	185	410
(fried)	—	—	—	204	—	—	1020
Flounder							
(steamed)	1.0	0.2	46	53	500	230	265
(fried)	—	—	—	214	—	—	1070
Shrimp							
(broiled)	1.3	0.2	128	114	500	640	570
Lobster							
(broiled)	0.9	0.2	95	119	500	475	595
Cod-liver oil	100	22	500	930	5 (about 4 ml)	25	46
Max EPA	100	30	450	930	3 (3–4 capsules)	14	30

*Fish oil capsules containing up to 50% omega-3 fatty acids and having small amounts of cholesterol, vitamin A, and vitamin D are now also marketed.
†Values are per 100-g portion (Data from Reed SA).
Adapted from Lavie CJ, Squires RW, Gau GT: Preventive cardiology: What is the role of fish and fish oils in primary and secondary prevention? J Cardiopulm Rehab 7:530, 1987.

DOSES OF OMEGA-3 FATTY ACIDS

If one decides to prescribe omega-3 fatty acids for a variety of theoretical effects, no good data are available on the exact dose necessary to provide beneficial effects. In addition, the dose needed would vary considerably depending on several other factors, including the exact effect desired, the amount of omega-6 fatty acids in the diet, and the duration of treatment. For example, Greenland Eskimos ingest approximately 5 to 10 g/day of omega-3 fatty acids for a lifetime, and most clinical studies use high doses (e.g., 2 to 10 g/day). We have combined data from numerous studies in order to give an idea of the amount of EPA (or the dose of fish, fish oil, capsules, or cod-liver oil) needed to inhibit platelets or have favorable effects on the blood lipid profile (Tables 174–4 and 174–5).[7, 39] Although this type of analysis is difficult, because much depends on the dose, source, and population being studied, these data emphasize that fairly high doses (e.g., above 20 ml of cod-liver oil or 5 to 10 fish oil tablets) are needed daily to produce potential beneficial effects.

ADVERSE EFFECTS

The potential adverse affects of ingesting fish oils should also be emphasized (Table 174–6). Although all of these adverse effects are only relative, the proven beneficial effects in humans are also only minimal. This paucity in proven benefits must be strongly considered in light of the potential toxicity and high cost of this therapy.

CONCLUSIONS

Although some epidemiologic studies and small intervention trials with omega-3 fatty acids appear promising, the effects on platelets appear less promising than those induced by low doses of aspirin, the lipid effects are less impressive than those produced by other nonprescription agents (e.g., psyllium and nicotinic acid), and large-scale trials to date have not demonstrated protection against human atherosclerosis. Although it seems reasonable to eat more fish (as long as it is not fried using atherogenic fat), the use of supplemental fish oils is expensive and potentially dangerous and should be considered experimental. Controlled trials are still needed to assess both the efficacy and safety of supplemental fish oils before these substances are routinely recommended by physicians or other allied health professionals to patients for either primary or secondary prevention of cardiovascular diseases.

Table 174–6. **Potential Adverse Effects of Fish Oils**

Bleeding
Immune suppression
Increased cerebral vascular incidents
Weight gain
Paradoxical increase in levels of low-density lipoprotein cholesterol
Glucose intolerance in patients with baseline insulin resistance and hypertriglyceridemia
Vitamin A and D toxicity
Increased autooxidation and lipid peroxidation (possibly increasing requirements for antioxidants)
Increased carcinogenesis
Mercury, chlorinated hydrocarbons (e.g., pesticides) may be concentrated in natural, unprepared fish oils
Foul fish smell

REFERENCES

1. Lavie CJ, Gau GT, Squires RW, et al: Management of lipids in primary and secondary prevention of cardiovascular diseases. Mayo Clin Proc 63:605, 1988.

2. Lavie CJ, O'Keefe JH, Blond L, et al: High-density lipoprotein cholesterol: Recommendations for routine testing and treatment. Postgrad Med J 87:36, 1990.

3. Lavie CJ: Lipid and lipoprotein fractions and coronary artery disease [editorial]. Mayo Clin Proc 68:618, 1993.

4. Lavie CJ, Genton E: Hemostasis, thrombosis, and antiplatelet therapy: Implications for prevention of cardiovascular diseases. Cardiovasc Rev Rep 12(2):24, 1991.

5. Lavie CJ, Schmieder R, Genton E: Antiplatelet therapy for cardiovascular diseases. Cardiovasc Rev Rep 8:64, 1987.

6. Lavie CJ, Messerli FH: Hypertension and target organ disease. In Messerli FH (ed): The ABC's of Antihypertensive Therapy. New York: Authors' Publishing House, Raven Press, 1994, p 175.

7. Lavie CJ, Squires RW, Gau GT: Preventive cardiology: What is the role of fish and fish oils in primary and secondary prevention? J Cardiopulmonary Rehabil 7:526, 1987.

8. Lavie CJ, Squires RW, Gau GT: Preventive cardiology: What is the value of antiplatelet agents and fish oils? South Med J 81:1145, 1988.

9. Leaf A, Weber PC: Omega-3 fatty acids and cardiovascular disease. In Braunwald E (ed): Heart Disease: A Textbook of Cardiovascular Medicine, 4th ed, Supplement Update 3. Philadelphia: WB Saunders, 1992, p 49.

10. Lavie CJ, Squires RW, Gau GT: Preventive cardiology: What is the role of risk factor modification, exercise, fish, and aspirin therapy? Postgrad Med J 81:52, 1987.

11. Leaf A, Weber PC: Cardiovascular effects of n-3 fatty acids. N Engl J Med 318:549, 1988.

12. Lavie CJ, Milani RV: National cholesterol education program's recommendations, and implications of "missing" high-density lipoprotein cholesterol in cardiac rehabilitation programs. Am J Cardiol 68:1087, 1991.

13. Bang HO, Dyerberg J: Plasma lipids and lipoproteins in greenlandic west coast eskimos. Acta Med Scand 192:85, 1972.

14. Kromhout D, Bosschieter EB, Coulander CDL: The inverse relation between fish consumption and 20-year mortality from coronary heart disease. N Engl J Med 312:1205, 1985.

15. Skekelle RB, Paul O, Shyrock AM, et al: Fish consumption and mortality from coronary heart disease [letter]. N Engl J Med 313:820, 1985.

16. Volset SE, Heuch I, Bjelk E: Fish consumption and mortality from coronary heart disease [letter]. N Engl J Med 313:820, 1985.

17. Curb JD, Reed DM: Fish consumption and mortality from coronary heart disease [letter]. N Engl J Med 313:821, 1985.

18. Dyerberg J, Bang HO, Hjørne N: Fatty acid composition of the plasma lipids in Greenland Eskimos. Am J Clin Nutr 28:958, 1975.

19. Schectman G, Kaul S, Cherayil GD, et al: Can the hypotriglyceridemic effect of fish oil concentrate be sustained? Ann Intern Med 110:346, 1989.

20. Huff MW, Telford DE: Dietary fish oil increases conversion of very low density lipoprotein apoprotein B to low density lipoprotein. Arteriosclerosis 9(1):58, 1989.

21. Schectman G, Kaul S, Kissebah AH: Heterogeneity of low density lipoprotein responses to fish-oil supplementation in hypertriglyceridemic subjects. Arteriosclerosis 9:345, 1989.

22. Davidson MH, Burns JH, Subbaiah PV, et al: Marine oil capsule therapy for the treatment of hyperlipidemia. Arch Intern Med 151:1732, 1991.

23. Harris WS, Dujovne CA, Zucker M, et al: Effects of a low saturated fat, low cholesterol fish oil supplement in hypertriglyceridemic patients. Ann Intern Med 109:465, 1988.

24. Wilt TJ, Lofgren RP, Nichol KL, et al: Fish oil supplementation does not lower plasma cholesterol in men with hypercholesterolemia. Ann Intern Med 111:900, 1989.

25. Mehta J, Lawson D, Saldeen T: Reduction in plasminogen activator inhibitort-1 (PAI-1) with omega-3 polyunsaturated fatty acid (PUFA) intake. Am Heart J 116:1201, 1988.

26. Radack K, Deck C, Huster G: The effects of low doses of n-3 fatty acid supplementation on blood pressure in hypertensive subjects. Arch Intern Med 151:1173, 1991.

27. Knapp HR, Fitzgerald G: The antihypertensive effects of fish oil: A controlled study of polyunsaturated fatty acid supplements in essential hypertension. N Engl J Med 320:1037, 1989.

28. Bfnaa KH, Bjerve KS, Straume B, et al: Effect of eicosapentaenoic and docosahexaenoic acids on blood pressure in hypertension: A population-based intervention trial from the Tromsf Study. N Engl J Med 322:795, 1990.

29. Ventura H, Milani T, Lavie C, et al: Cyclosporine-induced hypertension: Efficacy of Omega-3 fatty acids in patients after cardiac transplantation. Circulation 88:281, 1993.

30. Ventura HO, Lavie CJ, Messerli FH, et al: Cardiovascular adaptation to cyclosporine-induced hypertension. J Hum Hypertens 8:233, 1994.

31. Gapinski JP, VanRuiswyk JV, Heudebert GR, et al: Preventing restenosis with fish oil following coronary angioplasty. Arch Intern Med 153:1595, 1993.

32. Jacobs AK, Weiner BH, Raizner A, et al: The impact of fish oil on restenosis following coronary angioplasty: the fish oil restenosis trial (FORT) [abstract]. J Am Coll Cardiol 23:59A, 1994.

33. Lavie CJ, Milani RV, Squires RW, et al: Exercise and the heart: Good, benign or evil? Postgrad Med J 91:130, 1992.

34. Endres S, Kelly VE, Dinarello CA: Effects of dietary Omega-3 fatty acids on the in vitro production of human interleukin-1 [abstract]. J Leukoc Biol 42:617, 1987.

35. Prickett JD, Robinson DR, Steinberg AD: Dietary enrichment with the polyunsaturated fatty acid eiosapentaenoic acid prevents proteinuria and prolongs survival in NZB × NZW F₁ mice. J Clin Invest 68:556, 1981.

36. Sacks FM, Stone PH, Gibson CM, et al: Lack of anti-atherosclerotic effect of fish oil in patients with coronary disease: A controlled quantitative coronary angiographic trial [abstract]. J Am Coll Cardiol 23:264A, 1994.

37. Levine B, Kalman J, Mayer L, et al: Elevated circulating levels of tumor necrosis factor in severe chronic heart failure. N Engl J Med 323:236, 1990.

38. Milani RV, Endres S, Ventura HO, et al: Suppression of tumor necrosis factor synthesis by n-3 fatty acids in end-stage congestive heart failure [abstract]. J Am Coll Cardiol 23:453A, 1994.

39. Reed SA: More on fish oil [letter]. N Engl J Med 316:625, 1987.

CHAPTER 175

Magnesium EDTA Chelation

Martin Rubin, Ph.D.

The complex pathophysiologic cascade of the development of atherosclerosis, with its major stages of lipid oxidation initiating vascular wall damage, ensuing coagulation, and underlying cell death with calcification, poses a therapeutic challenge. That these individual processes exist simultaneously at varied sites limits the applicability of therapeutic agents targeted to one or another component of the disease progression. In this respect, EDTA chelation therapy has an implicit advantage in that it can favorably influence all facets of the disease development. Thus, it can also provide an alternative to the combination of drugs administered to attain a multiplicity of therapeutic effects.

The term "chelation" stems from the Greek *chele*, meaning "a claw." It represents the linkage of a polyvalent metal and an organic molecule in a ring chelate structure. Such compounds, exemplified in biologic systems by the chelation of iron in the heme portion of hemoglobin, are characteristic of the binding of polyvalent cations *in vivo*. The chelating compound ethylenediaminetetraacetic acid, EDTA, was invented in Germany in the mid-1930s. It was developed as a substitute for citric acid to maintain the solubility of Ca^{2+} and Mg^{2+} in the alkaline solutions used in the textile and photographic industries.

A continued, sustained expansion in industrial, agricultural, and pharmaceutical applications of EDTA chelation followed the 1952 publication of *The Chemistry of Metal Chelate Compounds*.[1] By 1989, EDTA production reached an international annual level of 40 tons.[2]

CHEMISTRY

At pH 7.4, Na_2EDTA in solution has its dibasic structure. In the presence of metal ions such as Mg^{2+}, the characteristic chelate ring forms rapidly (Fig. 175–1). The log value binding constants of polyvalent cations range from 8.7 for Mg^{2+}, 10.6 for Ca^{2+}, 16.5 for Zn^{2+}, 18.0 for Pb^{2+}, and 18.8 for Cu^{2+} to 25.0 for Fe^{3+}. Thus, for example, the EDTA chelation of Ca^{2+} is about 100 times greater than that for Mg^{2+} and $10^{14.4}$ times greater for iron than for calcium. In mixtures of polyvalent metal ions, the extent of their individual EDTA chelation depends not only on their relative binding constants but also on their concentrations.

EDTA metal binding in biologic systems will be influenced by its concentration, metabolism, and excretion, as well as the presence of other metal binding ligands, including amino acids, peptides, and proteins. All these factors can vary individually during the progression of pathologic processes.

METABOLISM, PHARMACOLOGY, AND TOXICITY

The initial clinical utilization of the intravenous infusion of Na_2EDTA for therapy of atherosclerotic disease has been superseded since the 1960s by its magnesium chelate, $Na_2MgEDTA$. Although both compounds have the same spectrum of polyvalent metal binding *in vivo*, the infusion of the Mg chelate is significantly less painful. By the simultaneous release of Mg^{2+} and plasma calcium chelation with hypocalcemia, the usual pharmacologic consequences of intravenous Mg^{2+} administration are enhanced. These include hypotension and cutaneous vasodilation.[3]

The symptoms and extent of Na_2EDTA hypocalcemia are a function of its dose and rapidity of administration. Acutely toxic levels in animals result in hypocalcemic tetany and death. Repletion from the body calcium stores is rapid.[4-9] Studies in animals and observations in patients have documented renal tubular damage following large doses of Na_2EDTA.[10-13] The administration of 9.5 g in 60 minutes to patients with multiple myeloma and malignant myeloma resulted in death from renal failure in 4 days.[14] Repetitive daily doses of 5 g/day to a patient with carcinomatosis and another with vitamin D intoxication resulted in death with severe damage to the proximal convoluted tubules characterized by some epithelial loss with dilated and vacuolated cells.[15]

Since the 1960s, intravenous infusion of $Na_2MgEDTA$ to thousands of patients has essentially eliminated acute toxic responses. This has been attained by limiting the dose to a maximum of 3.0 g for patients weighing 70 kg or more with infusion periods of 1.5 to 3 hours. Two such treatments per week for 15 consecutive weeks are followed by a rest period of 4 to 6 weeks. Courses of therapy may then be repeated.

It is of interest that the hypocalcemic response to EDTA administration stimulates the hormonal output of the parathyroid gland.[16] Studies have established that "parathyroid hormone" is a mixture of polypeptides of closely related structure.[17] One of these isomers has the unique property of increasing collateral blood flow.[18] This pharmacologic response comple-

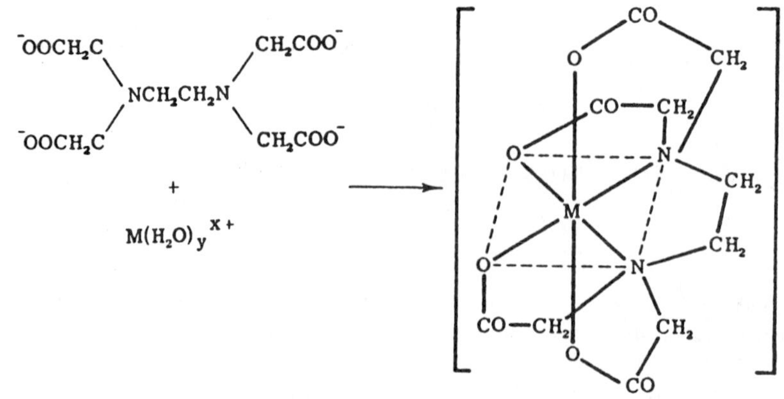

Figure 175–1. EDTA metal chelation reaction.

ments the cutaneous vasodilation associated with intravenous Mg^{2+} released by MgEDTA administration.[19]

ATHEROSCLEROSIS AND VASCULAR CALCIFICATION THERAPY

Antioxidant

Since the 1950s, EDTA has been added to foods and drugs as an inhibitor of their oxidation. *In vivo*, the formation of reactive free radicals by oxidative withdrawal of an electron from a saturated molecule is a common and essential step in the normal pathways of cell physiology. Because such free radicals are very reactive and potentially injurious, their metabolic occurrence and possible generation by low-molecular-weight iron complexes are usually controlled and restricted by a variety of endogenous systems. This capability is enhanced by the presence of ascorbic acid in aqueous compartments and vitamin E and carotene in lipid environments. When the protective mechanisms are inadequate in cells, tissues, and body fluids, the uncontrolled generation of free radicals leads to oxidized lipoproteins, their uptake by macrophages, the formation of foam cells, generation of fatty streaks, and calcification.

Although studies have delineated the complexity of atherogenesis, its initiation clearly is in the uncontrolled formation of oxidatively modified lipid-laden, low-density lipoprotein (LDL) and lipoprotein (a). This may occur in plasma or in the subendothelial space. The oxidized LDL is taken up by macrophages, which form the foam cells characteristic of the fatty streak. An extensive continuing literature documents that the oxidation of LDL depends on the presence and concentration of ferric or cupric ions in plasma and is completely inhibited by their EDTA chelation.[20-32] *In vivo*, this is followed by urinary excretion of the metal chelates. It is of interest to note that in the 1950s the intravenous administration of 3 to 4 g of $Na_2CaEDTA$ to patients with primary hemochromatosis and transfusional siderosis increased the urinary iron output by 8 to 10 times over controls. Infusion of Na_2EDTA and $Na_2MgEDTA$ yielded analogous results.[33-37]

Anticoagulant

The industrial applicability of EDTA for calcium chelation was extended to blood collection in Germany in 1942.[38] This was independently confirmed in 1951 and rapidly attained worldwide acceptance for this purpose.[39-45] When EDTA is added to whole blood as an anticoagulant, its optimal molecular ratio to blood calcium is approximately 1.1:1. *In vivo*, however, its applicability for the therapeutic inhibitory control of the multiplicity of calcium-dependent stages of the coagulation cascade is more complex. Since the mid-1980s, there has been a major expansion in the detailed knowledge of the multiplicity of factors involved in the normal and pathologic processes of the coagulation cascade. Current studies suggest that the most significant of these involve the calcium-dependent function of the platelet glycoprotein GPIIb/IIIa. While anchored within the platelet, its molecular structure extends its two calcium-binding arms beyond the cell membrane into the plasma. These provide for calcium chelation at its micromolar level and at less-specific binding sites for Ca^{2+} in the usual plasma millimolar concentration. The two extension arms of the GPIIb/IIIa glycoproteins can enter into calcium chelation with plasma proteins or with fibrinogen in pathogenic platelet clots.[46, 47] These platelet linkages are modified and disrupted at reduced yet physiologic Ca^{2+} concentrations by the presence of EDTA. This results in the dissociation of the GPIIb/IIIa into its individual GPIIb and GPIIIa monomers, which can subsequently form irreversibly aggregates.[48]

Decalcification Capability

Although calcium antagonists can inhibit the continued cellular uptake and disposition of calcium, surgical intervention has been required for its removal from calcified vascular areas. Two major calcium sources, however, provide for its plasma repletion during the hypocalcemia and urinary chelated calcium excretion characteristic of the 90-g total $Na_2MgEDTA$ infusion in a biweekly, 15-week course of therapy. Isotopic ^{45}Ca studies have established that one of these is the skeletal system and the other consists of "soft tissue" calcium. Studies in the early clinical literature of EDTA chelation provided what appeared to be significant evidence of the dissolution of tissue calcification following the hypocalcemia and therapeutic response to repetitive intravenous administration of Na_2EDTA.[49-64] Because of the current availability of radiographic ultrafast computed tomography (CT) cardiac scanning, it is possible to obtain unambiguous records of the decrement in cardiac calcification resulting from long-term repetitive infusion of $Na_2MgEDTA$ (Figs. 175–2 and 175–3). The patient was treated with a total of 48 3.0-g intravenous infusions of $Na_2MgEDTA$. It is of interest that there was a simultaneous major improvement in the patient's clinical status. Analogous results were observed in the treatment of a second patient at a different geographic location. Thirty infusions of 3.0 g of $Na_2MgEDTA$ were administered during a period of 7 months. The patient had a history of myocardial infarction and a five-vessel bypass operation 14 years prior to the present course of $Na_2MgEDTA$ chelation therapy. Ultrafast CT obtained through the coronary arteries for evaluation of calcification revealed "216 lesions for a total calcium score of 15872." The radiologic impression was "extensive multivessel coronary artery disease. This corresponds to a 91% specificity and a 74% positive predicted value based on the patient's age." The CT scan at the completion of 30 $Na_2MgEDTA$ infusions in 7 months of therapy was as follows: "There are 118 lesions and a total calcium score of 7970." The radiologic impression was "exten-

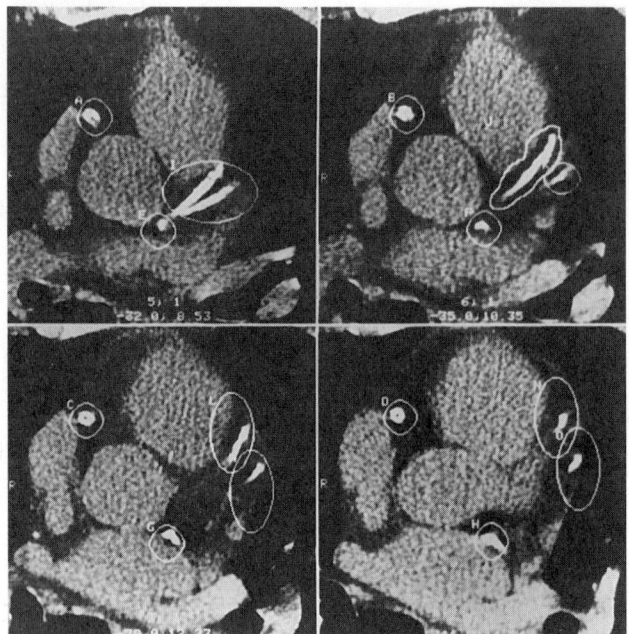

Figure 175–2. Pretreatment ultrafast CT cardiac calcification scan.

sive multivessel coronary artery disease. There has been a significant reduction in the number of lesions and in the total calcium score from the prior examination."[65]

SUMMARY

The multicomponent complexity of the pathophysiologic atherosclerotic cascade, occurring in a given individual in different stages at multiple sites, challenges the potential therapeutic efficacy of highly targeted drugs.

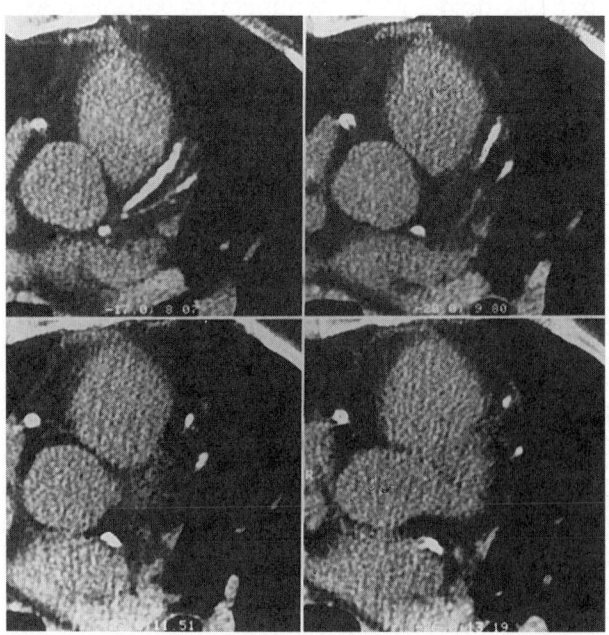

Figure 175–3. Posttreatment Na$_2$MgEDTA ultrafast CT cardiac calcification scan.

In contrast, repetitive intravenous infusion of Na$_2$MgEDTA promotes the restoration of the plasma and tissue balance and metabolism of essential minerals such as calcium, iron, and magnesium. This, in turn, permits the functional improvement of damaged vascular areas. A current example of this therapeutic capability is cardiac decalcification attained by the repetitive intravenous infusion of Na$_2$MgEDTA.

REFERENCES

1. Martell AE, Calvin M: Chemistry of the Metal Chelate Compounds. New York: Prentice Hall, 1952.
2. Hart JR: Ethylenediaminetetraacetic acid and related chelating agents. Ullmann's Encyclopedia of Industrial Chemistry, Vol A 10, New York: VCH Publishers, 1987, p 95.
3. Popovici A, Geshickter CF, Rubin M: The treatment of essential hypertension by magnesium chelate solution. Bull Georgetown Univ Med Ctr 5:108, 1951.
4. Popovici A, Geshickter CF, Reinovsky A, Rubin M: Experimental control of serum calcium levels in vivo. Proc Soc Exp Biol Med 74:415, 1950.
5. Rubin M: Chelating agents in the study of calcium metabolism. Fifth Conference on Metabolic Interrelations, Josiah Macy Jr. Foundation, New York, 1954, p 355.
6. Spencer H, Vankinscott V, Levin I, Lazlo D: Removal of calcium in man by ethylenediaminetetraacetic acid: A metabolic study. J Clin Invest 31:1023, 1952.
7. Sodder A, Toribara T: Changes in serum and spinal fluid calcium effected by dosodium ethylenediaminetetraacetate. J Lab Clin Med 58:542, 1961.
8. Spencer H, Greenberg J, Berger E, et al: Studies on the effect of ethylenediaminetetraacetic acid in hypercalcemia. J Lab Clin Med 47:29, 1956.
9. Spencer H, Vankinscott V, Levin I, Lazlo D: Removal of calcium in man by ethylenediaminetetraacetic acid (EDTA). J Clin Invest 31:1023, 1952.
10. Foreman H, Finnegan C, Lushbough CC: Nephrotoxic hazard from uncontrolled edathamel calcium-disodium therapy. JAMA 160:1042, 1956.
11. Foreman H: Toxic side effects of ethylenediaminetetraacetic acid. J Chronic Dis 16:319, 1963.
12. Meltzer L, Kitchell J, Palmon F: The long term use, side effects and toxicity of disodium ethylenediaminetetraacetic acid (EDTA). Am J Med Sci 242:11, 1961.
13. Schwartz S, Hayer JR, Johnson CV, Doolan PD: The nephrotoxicity of ethylenediaminetetraacetic acid. Biochem Pharmacol 15:377, 1966.
14. Holland JF, Danielson E, Sahagian-Edwards A: Use of ethylenediaminetetraacetic acid in hypercalcemic patients. Proc Soc Exp Biol Med 84:359, 1953.
15. Dudley MD, Ritchie AC, Schilling A, Baker WH: Pathologic changes associated with the use of sodium ethylenediaminetetraacetate in the treatment of hypocalcemia. N Engl J Med 252:332, 1955.
16. Kaiser W, Ponsold W: Concerning the possibility of relative parathyroid hormone insufficiency through the infusion of ethylenediaminetetraacetate (EDTA). Klin Wochr 37:1183, 1959.
17. Burtis WJ: Parathyroid hormone-related protein: Structure, function and measurement. Clin Chem 38:2171, 1992.
18. Pang PKT, Yang MCM, Keutmann HT, Kenny AD: Structure activity relationship of parathyroid hormone: Separation of hypotensive and hypercalcemic properties. Endocrinology 112:284, 1983.
19. Winkler AW, Smith PK, Hoff HE: Intravenous magnesium sulfate in the treatment of nephritic convulsions in adults. J Clin Invest 21:207, 1943.
20. Schwartz CJ, Valente AJ, Sprague EA: A modern view of atherogenesis. Am J Cardiol 71:9B, 1993.
21. Morel DW, Hessler JR, Chisolm GM: Low density lipoprotein cytotoxicity induced by free radical peroxidation of lipid. J Lipid Res 24:1070, 1983.

22. Morel DW, DiCorleto PE, Chisolm GM: Endothelial and smooth muscle cells alter low density lipoprotein in vitro by free radical oxidation. Arteriosclerosis 4:357, 1984.

23. Steinbrecher UP, Parathasarathy S, Leake DS, et al: Modification of low density lipoprotein by endothelial cells involves lipid peroxidation and degradation of low density phospholipids. Proc Natl Acad Sci U S A 83:3883, 1984.

24. Steinberg D, Parathasarathy S, Carew TE, et al: Beyond cholesterol modifications of low-density lipoprotein. N Engl J Med 320:917, 1989.

25. Palinski W, Yla-Herthula S, Rosenfeld ME, et al: Antisera and monoconal antibodies specific for epitopes generated during oxidative modification of low density lipoprotein. Arteriosclerosis 10:325, 1990.

26. Thomas CE, Jackson RL: Lipid hydroperoxide involvement in copper-dependent and independent oxidation of low density lipoproteins. J Pharm Exp Ther 256:1182, 1991.

27. Steinbrecher UP, Zhang H, Lougheed M: Role of oxidatively modified LDL in atherosclerosis. Free Radic Biol Med 9:155, 1990.

28. Parathasarathy S, Steinbrecher UP, Barnett J, et al: Essential role of phospholipase A2 activity in endothelial cell-induced modificaiton of low density lipoprotein. Proc Natl Acad Sci U S A 82:3000, 1985.

29. Aust S, Morehouse LA, Thomas CE: Role of metals in oxygen radical reactions. J Free Radic Biol Med 1:3, 1985.

30. Heinecke J: Free radical modification of low-density lipoprotein: Mechanisms and biological consequences. J Free Radic Biol Med 3:65, 1987.

31. Morel DW, Hessler JR, Chisolm GM: Low density lipoprotein cytotoxicity by free radical peroxidation of lipid. J Lipid Res 24:1070, 1983.

32. Olwin JH, Koppel JL: Reduction of elevated plasma lipid levels in atherosclerosis following EDTA chelation therapy. Proc Soc Exp Biol Med 128:1137, 1968.

33. Wishinsky H, Weinberg T, Prevost EM, et al: Ethylenediaminetetraacetic acid in the mobilization and removal of iron in a case of hemochromatosis. J Lab Clin Med 42:550, 1953.

34. Figuera WG, Adams WS, Bassett SH, et al: Effect of disodium calcium versenate in iron excretion in man. Am J Med 17:101, 1954.

35. Figuera WG, Adams WS, Davis FW, Bassett SH: A study of the effect of disodium calcium versenate (CaEDTA) on iron excretion in man. J Lab Clin Med 46:534, 1955.

36. Kleckner MS, Kark RM, Baker LA, et al: Clinical features, pathology and therapy of hemochromatosis. JAMA 157:1471, 1955.

37. McMahon FG: A comparison of the effect of Fe^{+++} specific, versenol, and calcium disodium versenate on urinary iron excretion in a patient with hemochromatosis. J Lab Clin Med 48:589, 1956.

38. Dyckerhoff H, Marx R, Ludwig B: On the mode of action and use of an organic substance that arrests coagulation. Z Ges Exptl Med 110:412, 1942.

39. Klapheke MA, Rubin M: Sodium ethylenediaminetetraacetate as an anticoagulant for routine laboratory procedures. Bull Georgetown Univ Med Ctr 5:33, 1951.

40. Proescher F: Anticoagulant properties of ethylenediaminetetraacetic acid. Proc Soc Exp Biol Med 76:619, 1951.

41. Dillard GHL, Brecher G, Cronkhite EP: Separation, concentration and transfusion of platelets. Proc Soc Exp Biol Med 78:796, 1951.

42. Grant RA, Zucker MB: EDTA induced increase in platelet surface charge associated with loss of aggregability: Assessment by partition in aequeous two-phase polymer systems and electrophoretic mobility. Blood 52:515, 1978.

43. Zucker MB, Grant RA: Nonreversible loss of platelet agreeability induced by calcium deprivation. Blood 52:505, 1987.

44. Stein B: Platelet inhibitor agents in cardiovascular disease: An update. J Am Coll Cardiol 14:813, 1989.

45. Becker RC, Gore JM: Adjuvant antiplatelet strategies in coronary thrombosis. Circulation 83:1115, 1991.

46. Phillips D, Charo IF, Parise LV, Fitzgerald LA: The platelet membrane glycoprotein IIb-IIIa complex. Blood 71:831, 1988.

47. Steiner B, Consot D, Trzeciak A, et al: Ca2+-dependent binding of a synthetic arg-gly-asp (RGD) peptide to a single site on the purified platelet glycoprotein IIb-IIIa complex. J Biol Chem 264:13102, 1989.

48. Fitzgerald LA, Phillips DR: Calcium regulation of the platelet membrane glycoprotein IIb-IIIa complex. J Biol Chem 260:11366, 1985.

49. Klein R, Harris SB: Treatment of scleroderma, sclerodactylia and calcinosis by chelation (EDTA). Am J Med Sci 19:798, 1955.

50. Clarke NE, Clarke CN, Mosher RE: The in vivo dissolution of metastatic calcium: An approach to atherosclerosis. Am J Med Sci 229:142, 1955.

51. Clarke NE, Clarke CN, Mosher RE: Treatment of angina pectoris with disodium ethylene diamine tetraacetic acid. Am J Med Sci 232:654, 1956.

52. Clarke NE: Atherosclerosis, occlusive vascular disease and EDTA. Am J Cardiol 6:233, 1960.

53. Clarke NE: Treatment of occlusive vascular disease with disodium ethylene diamine tetraacetic acid (EDTA). Am J Med Sci 6:732, 1960.

54. Boyle AJ, Clarke NE, Mosher RE, McCann DS: Chelation therapy in circulatory and sclerosing diseases. Fed Proc 20(Suppl 10):243, 1961.

55. Wilder JW, DeJode JR, Ahlstein SW, Howard JM: Mobilization of atherosclerotic plaque calcium with EDTA utilizing the isolation perfusion principle. Surgery 52:793, 1962.

56. Aronov DM: First experience with the treatment of atherosclerosis patients with calcinosis of the arteries with trilon BC disodium salt of EDTA. Klin Med (Mosk) 41:19, 1963.

57. Lamar CP: Chelation therapy of occlusive arteriosclerosis in diabetic patients. Angiology 15:379, 1964.

58. Lamar CP: Chelation endarterectomy for occlusive atherosclerosis. J Am Geriatr Soc 14:272, 1966.

59. Wartman A, Lampe TL, McCann DS, Boyle AJ: Plaque reversal with MgEDTA in experimental atherosclerosis: elastin and collagen metabolism. J Atherscl Res 7:331, 1967.

60. Brucknerova O, Tulacek J, Krojzl O: Chelates in the treatment of obliterating arteriopathies. Unitr Lek 9:841, 1968.

61. Nikitina EK, Abramova MA: Treatment of atherosclerosis with trilon-B (EDTA). Kardiologics 12:137, 1972.

62. Brucknerova O, Tulacek J: Chelates in the treatment of occlusive atherosclerosis. Initr Lek 18:729, 1972.

63. Wissler RW, Vesselinovitch D: Regression of atherosclerosis in experimental animals and man. Modern Concepts of Cardiovascular Disease 46:27, 1977.

64. Brucknerova O, Malinovska V: First clinical experience with combined treatment with chelation III and glucagon in ischemic disease of the lower extremities. Cas Lek Cesk 119(29–30):814, 1980.

65. Rubin M, Scarchilli AJ, Rozema T, Casdorph R: Cardiac decalcification by $Na_2MgEDTA$. Am Chem Soc Med Chem Aug 23, 1994.

CHAPTER 176

Perfluorochemicals, Specifically Fluosol

John M. Elliott, M.B., Ch.B., Ph.D., F.R.A.C.P., Andrew I. MacIsaac, M.B., B.S., F.R.A.C.P., and Patrick L. Whitlow, M.D., F.A.C.C.

Early in the search for blood substitutes, fluorocarbons, or perfluorochemicals, were demonstrated to have excellent oxygen-carrying capacity. Fluorocarbons are hydrophobic, nonpolar molecules that must be emulsified before suspension into water-based solutions. Much of the initial development of fluorocarbons was preoccupied with optimizing such emulsions. However, the fluorocarbons possess several other useful characteristics. They are acellular, sterile, and chemically inert, and they are excreted unchanged from the lungs. The emulsions have a low viscosity, the emulsified particles are small enough to pass through capillaries, and some are radiopaque whether imaged by conventional radiography, ultrasonography, or magnetic resonance imaging.

The oxygen carried by fluorocarbons is simply dissolved within the emulsified particles rather than chemically bound and is readily available to diffuse across any concentration gradient. The availability of this oxygen for diffusion was graphically demonstrated by early reports that a mouse could breathe and survive if submerged in fluid containing oxygenated fluorocarbons[1] and that rats could survive after all their blood had been replaced by fluid containing emulsified perfluorotributyline.[2]

Subsequently, an emulsion containing three parts of perfluorotributyline ($C_9F_{21}N$) and seven parts of perfluorodecalin ($C_{10}F_{18}$) was developed and administered to normal volunteers[3] and to anemic patients[4] without important adverse effects. This emulsion was produced commercially as Fluosol (Alpha Therapeutic Corp., Los Angeles, CA) and was extensively investigated in animal and clinical studies. Following reports that Fluosol reduced symptoms and signs of ischemia during coronary artery occlusion in animals[5-7] and balloon angioplasty in humans,[8-14] Fluosol became the first fluorocarbon approved by the Food and Drug Administration (FDA) for support of balloon angioplasty.

The fluorocarbons have considerable potential in many aspects of clinical medicine.[15, 16] It is therefore appropriate to review the experience with Fluosol in detail and discuss the potential of other fluorocarbons under investigation.

CHEMISTRY

Fluosol contains two fluorocarbons, perfluorodecalin and perfluorotributylamine (or perfluorotripropylamine), coated with egg yolk phospholipid and a detergent Pluronic F-68 (poloxamer 188) in a 20% emulsion by weight. The formulas and relevant characteristics of these and other well-studied fluorocarbons are presented in Figure 176–1.

Fluosol is supplied as four separate components that must be mixed before administration: the emulsion, two separate electrolyte solutions, and oxygenating equipment. The emulsion is packaged in a plastic bag and frozen for long-term storage because of the instability of perfluorodecalin at room temperature. Prior to use, the emulsion is thawed by immersing the bag in warm water. Then the two separate electrolyte solutions are added. This solution is then equilibrated to 37°C and oxygenated just prior to use with a small cylinder containing 95% oxygen and 5% carbon dioxide. The method of preparation is rather labor-intensive and takes 10 to 20 minutes to complete.

The final composition of Fluosol when prepared for intracoronary administration is presented in Table 176–1. The mean diameter of the emulsified particles is 270 nm; the osmolality of the solution is 410 mOsm/L, and the pH is 7.3. The stability of Fluosol depends on the stage of preparation of the final mixture. Fluosol must be administered within 7 days of thawing the emulsion (provided that it is then refrigerated), within 24 hours of mixing with the electrolyte solutions, and within 8 hours of oxygenation.

PHARMACOLOGY

The oxygen contained in oxygenated Fluosol is dissolved within the emulsified particles. The amount of oxygen dissolved in each milliliter of Fluosol therefore depends on the partial pressure of oxygen (P_{O_2}) at which the Fluosol is oxygenated and the concentration of the emulsified particles. If oxygenated at a P_{O_2} of 100 mmHg, Fluosol will contain one twentieth and release one tenth of the oxygen as the same volume of blood with a hematocrit of 45 and oxygenated at

Table 176–1. **Composition of Fluosol Emulsion**

Component	Concentration (g/100 ml)
Perfluorodecalin	14.0
Perfluorotripropylamine	6.0
Poloxamer 188	2.72
Glycerin USP	0.80
Sodium chloride USP	0.60
Egg yolk phospholipids	0.40
Sodium bicarbonate USP	0.21
Dextrose USP, anhydrous	0.18
Magnesium chloride 6H_2O USP	0.043
Calcium chloride 2H_2O USP	0.036
Potassium chloride USP	0.034
Potassium oleate	0.032

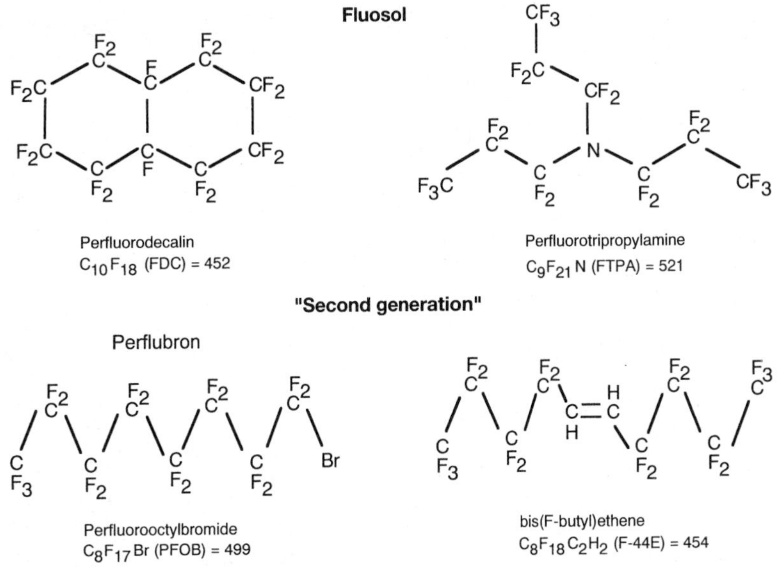

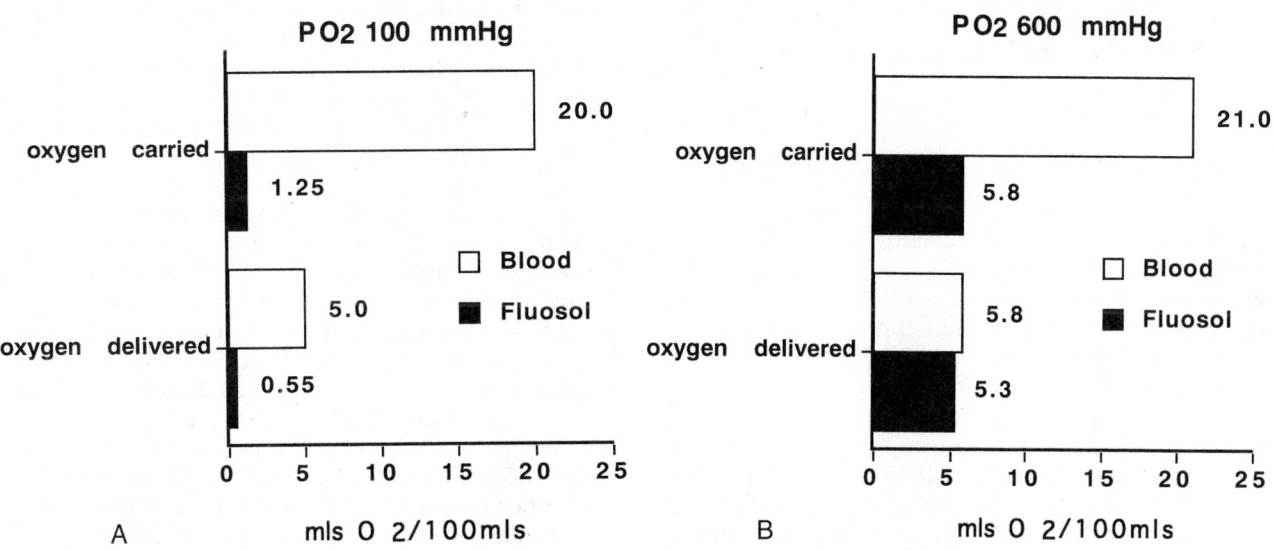

Figure 176–1. Formulas and characteristics of selected fluorocarbons. Fluosol contains an emulsion of three parts of perfluorotributyline and seven parts of perfluorodecalin. (Adapted from Riess JG: Fluorocarbon-based in vivo oxygen transport and delivery systems. Vox Sang 61:225, 1991. Used with permission of S. Karger AG, Basel).

the same partial pressure. However, if the Fluosol is oxygenated at a P_{O_2} of 600 mmHg prior to delivery, it will carry one quarter the volume of oxygen but release the same amount of oxygen as blood (Fig. 176–2). Oxygenated Fluosol will release more oxygen than blood with lower hematocrits.[17]

The viscosity of Fluosol is substantially lower than that of whole blood and is relatively independent of flow rate and shear rate (Fig. 176–3). Also, the particle size of the Fluosol emulsion is only 2% of that of an erythrocyte. These two properties enable rapid infusion through a small lumen (as exists within an angioplasty balloon) and maximize flow through a partially occluded microcirculation. Potentially, the small emulsion particles may carry and deliver oxygen to tissues that cannot be reached by erythrocytes.

PHARMACOKINETICS

Ninety-eight percent of the fluorocarbons contained in Fluosol are excreted unchanged from the lungs.

Most are excreted directly from the blood, but small amounts are taken up by the reticuloendothelial tissues of the liver, spleen, and bone marrow and later released and excreted. The half-life in the circulation is dose-dependent and on the order of 4 to 8 hours in human subjects.[17]

Fluorocarbon concentrations in the liver and spleen peak at 96 hours after administration; the tissue half-life of perfluorotributyline is 65 days, almost 10 times that of perfluorodecalin. Because repeated dosing will result in further accumulation, it is recommended that Fluosol not be readministered within 6 months. The Pluronic F-68 (poloxamer 188) used to emulsify the fluorocarbons is not metabolized and is cleared by the kidney. At least half the dose is cleared within 30 minutes.[17]

Fluosol may prolong the action of lipid-soluble anesthetics, and augment the hepatotoxic effects of carbon tetrachloride. There is little potential for drug interactions with the short infusions and low total

Figure 176–2. Volumes of oxygen carried and delivered by 100 ml of blood (at hematocrit 45) compared with Fluosol (20%) oxygenated at 100 mmHg (*A*) and at 600 mmHg (*B*).

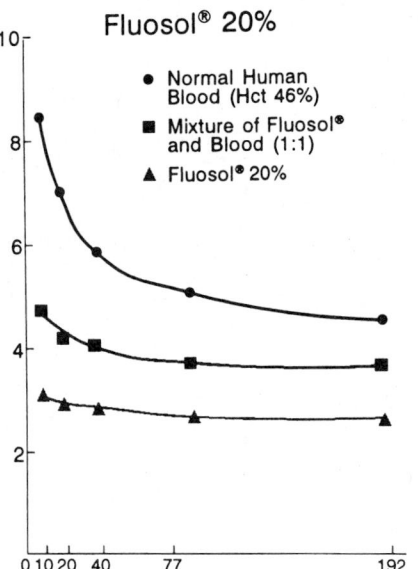

Figure 176–3. Comparison of the viscosity of whole blood (hematocrit 46%), Fluosol (20%), and a 1:1 blood:Fluosol mixture at 37°C in relation to changes in shear rate. (From Cleman MW, LaSala JM: Pharmacologically protected percutaneous transluminal coronary angioplasty. *In* Topol EJ [ed]: Textbook of Interventional Cardiology. Philadelphia: WB Saunders, 1992, p 512. Courtesy of Alpha Therapeutics, Los Angeles.)

dose (<5 ml/kg) used during balloon angioplasty. However, if Fluosol is infused for longer periods with larger cumulative doses, the unbound concentrations of warfarin and prednisolone and other highly protein-bound drugs may increase. Fluosol has no effect on carcinogenesis and no demonstrated effect on fertility or teratogenesis in animal studies. However, administration in pregnant women is not recommended. Fluosol has been found in breast milk. Although it is not absorbed orally, administration to breastfeeding women is not recommended. Contraindications include known allergy to any components such as egg proteins. Between 1% and 2% of patients have reacted to a test dose of 0.5 ml of Fluosol (product information, Alpha Therapeutics).

ANIMAL AND CLINICAL STUDIES

Fluosol was approved by the FDA in 1989 for the prevention of myocardial ischemia during percutaneous coronary angioplasty. This is achieved by infusion of oxygenated Fluosol directly into the distal coronary vascular bed via the internal lumen of the inflated angioplasty balloon. Prior to this approval, a number of animal studies had demonstrated beneficial effects in preserving ventricular function during and reducing infarct size after transient occlusion of coronary arteries. Further studies have demonstrated the mechanisms of this benefit. Subsequent randomized multicenter clinical studies confirmed benefit during balloon angioplasty[13] but not after thrombolysis for acute myocardial infarction.[18]

Myocardial Ischemia During Coronary Occlusion

Early reports correlated histologic evidence of reduction in ischemic damage with elevations in intramyocardial gas tensions during infusion of oxygenated fluorocarbons.[19, 20] Roberts et al.[5] confirmed that oxygenated Fluosol reduced ultrastructural myocardial changes indicative of ischemia after balloon occlusion of the left anterior descending (LAD) coronary artery in open chest dogs. Subsequent studies reported beneficial effects on left ventricular function in closed chest canine preparations. Tokioka et al.[7] reported that regional hypokinesis during 2-minute occlusions of the LAD coronary artery was partly prevented by oxygenated Fluosol but not by unoxygenated Fluosol. Positive dP/dt and negative dP/dt were also well preserved. Robalino et al.[6] compared the effects of active distal coronary artery perfusion with oxygenated Fluosol (30 ml/min) with passive blood perfusion using a perfusion balloon and a control group with no distal coronary perfusion during 30-minute balloon occlusion of the LAD coronary artery. Infusion of Fluosol was begun 10 minutes after the artery was occluded. The regional wall motion score, assessed by two-dimensional echocardiography, was better preserved in both the Fluosol-treated group and the passive perfusion group compared with controls ($p < .001$) (Table 176–2). There was no apparent difference in the tendency to arrhythmias. Left ventricular end-diastolic pressure was increased in the Fluosol group ($p < .01$), probably because of the volume of Fluosol infused (600 ml over 20 minutes in 20-kg dogs).

An early clinical study compared the effects of distal coronary artery infusion of oxygenated Fluosol with oxygenated Ringer's lactate solutions in 34 patients using a single-blind, randomized, crossover design.[8] The results were analyzed in 29 patients. During Fluosol perfusion, the mean time to onset of angina was delayed by 8 seconds ($p < .05$), the mean duration of angina was reduced by 7 seconds ($p < .05$), the onset of ST-segment changes was delayed, and the rise in ST segments was reduced by 38%. As a result, longer balloon inflations were possible during infusion of Fluosol. Small but significant increases in wedge pressures were also noted.

In a similar study,[9] regional wall motion assessed by 2D echocardiography and electrocardiographic ST changes were documented during balloon angioplasty of proximal LAD coronary artery stenoses. Regional wall motion was better preserved during infusion of oxygenated Fluosol. Other single-center studies reported similar findings.[10, 11] Young et al. reported that perfusion of oxygenated Fluosol in 12 patients was accompanied by decreased lactate release into the great cardiac vein compared with nonoxygenated Fluosol. Lactate release still occurred, suggesting that other factors may be important in preserving left ventricular function during Fluosol infusion.

Bell et al.[12] carefully assessed the effect of Fluosol on indices of diastolic function during 60-second bal-

Table 176–2. **Cardiovascular Effects of Fluosol**

Observed Effect	Mechanism	Clinical Implication
During-transient occlusion ↓ Angina Preservation of regional wall motion and left ventricular function	↑ O₂ delivery ↓ Viscosity	Useful adjunct to PTCA in high-risk patients
↑ Pulmonary artery wedge pressure	↑ Fluid load	Cautious use in patient with severely impaired left ventricular function
Following prolonged occlusion ↓ Myocardial Infarction Size	↓ Neutrophil adhesion Preservation of endothelial function ↑ O₂ delivery (?) ↓ Viscosity	Not useful as an adjunct to thrombolysis overall, though may be effective in high-risk subgroup Role as an adjunct to PTCA in acute myocardial infarction uncertain

PTCA, percutaneous transluminal coronary angioplasty.

loon inflations in 10 patients using a single-blind, randomized, crossover design. Although patients reported less severe pain, there was no significant difference in ventricular relaxation during oxygenated Fluosol (P_{O_2} >600 mmHg) compared with no perfusion.

Cowley et al.[14] have assessed the efficacy of Fluosol as adjunctive therapy during balloon angioplasty of 38 patients with unstable angina or high-risk lesions. The target lesion was in the LAD coronary artery in half of the patients. Mean ejection fraction (two-dimensional echocardiography) was greater than 50%. Cardiac output, left ventricular ejection fraction, and regional wall motion were better maintained during infusion of Fluosol into the distal coronary compared with no infusion (Fig. 176–4).

A large multicenter trial was reported in 1990 in which 245 patients undergoing balloon angioplasty were randomized to either distal coronary artery perfusion with oxygenated Fluosol (P_{O_2} >600 mmHg) or no perfusion.[13] During all procedures, the infusion pump was loaded with Fluosol and connected to the lumen of the catheter. Neither the patient nor the physician knew whether the infusion was turned on. Effects on chest pain and ST-segment changes were analyzed in 205 patients. Regional wall motion and global left ventricular function were assessed in 24 patients by two-dimensional echocardiography and analyzed at a central laboratory using both the radial shortening and centerline methods. Important exclusions included the presence of distal collateral vessels, severe lesions in the same artery distal to the treated segment, recent myocardial infarction, and heart failure.

The groups were well-matched, with a mean baseline ejection fraction of 58%. The target lesion was in the LAD coronary artery in 57% of the control group and in 50% of the Fluosol group. Severe angina during balloon inflation was reported by 21% of the patients who received Fluosol, compared with 34% of controls ($p < .05$), regional wall motion was better preserved (-61 ± 335 U versus -561 ± 224 U, $p < .0001$), and left ventricular ejection fraction was better maintained (54% to 51% versus 58% to 37%, $p < .001$) (Fig. 176–5). There was no significant difference in ST-segment shifts. Relevant to this, Schaer et al.[21] had demonstrated that infusion of Fluosol or Ringer's lactate into the LAD artery of dogs with closed chests produced ST-segment elevation without any changes in regional wall motion (assessed by ventriculography). The mechanism of the ST-segment elevation induced by Fluosol in the absence of ischemic abnormality of wall motion is not known.

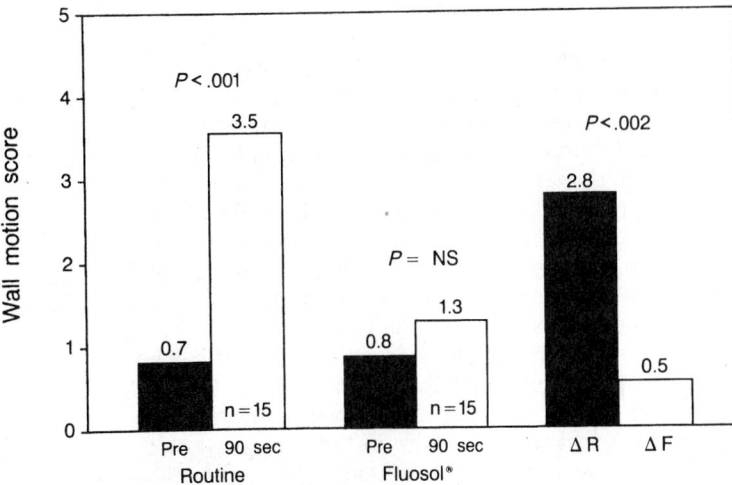

Figure 176–4. Regional left ventricular dysfunction scores at baseline and after 90 seconds of coronary artery occlusion during routine balloon angioplasty (left-hand bars) and during balloon angioplasty with distal perfusion of oxygenated Fluosol (middle bars). The right-hand bars represent the change in dysfunction score in each group. (Reproduced with permission from Cowley MJ, Snow FR, DiSciascio G, et al: Perfluorochemical perfusion during coronary angioplasty in unstable and high-risk patients. Circulation 81:4, 1990. Copyright 1990, American Heart Association.)

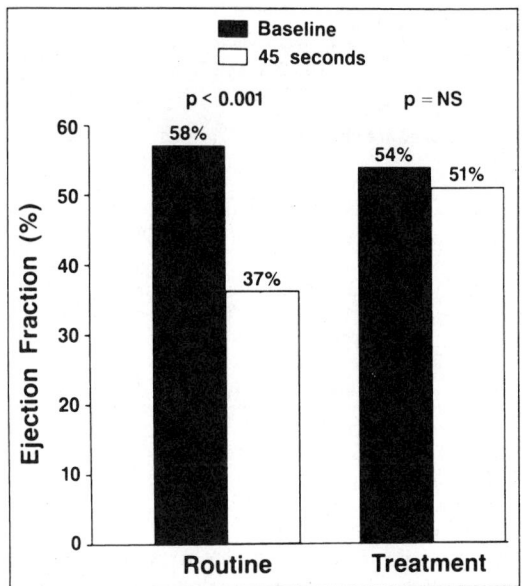

Figure 176–5. Global left ventricular ejection fraction in patients treated with intracoronary oxygenated Fluosol during balloon angioplasty (treatment) compared with controls. (Reprinted from Kent KM, Cleman MW, Cowley MJ, et al: Reduction of myocardial ischemia during percutaneous transluminal coronary angioplasty with oxygenated Fluosol. Am J Cardiol 66:279–284, 1990.)

Ongoing trials include (1) a multicenter, open-label, parallel trial in which patients with an ejection fraction of less than 30% or blood pressure of less than 90 mmHg are randomized to routine balloon angioplasty or to balloon angioplasty with perfusion of the distal coronary bed with oxygenated Fluosol and (2) a study in which patients with high-risk, complex lesions are randomized to balloon angioplasty with or without intracoronary infusion of Fluosol at 40 ml/min. These trials will help to determine whether Fluosol is more or less useful in "high-risk" patients than in "low-risk" patients such as those entered in the study by Kent and others.[13]

Effects of Fluosol on Myocardial Infarction Size

A number of animal studies reported by Forman et al.,[22–24] Virmani et al.,[25, 26] and others[19, 20] have assessed the effect of Fluosol given via the intravenous or intracoronary routes during or after temporary coronary artery occlusion on the size of subsequent myocardial infarction. These studies have consistently demonstrated that infarct size is reduced in animals that have received oxygenated Fluosol. Reduction in infarct size was reported at 24 hours and at 1 week after coronary artery occlusion in dogs[22, 23] and in the rabbit.[25] Benefit was demonstrated in the rabbit at intravenous doses greater than 15 ml/kg started while the coronary artery was still occluded.[26] The same group has explored the mechanism of this reduction in infarct size. Histologic examination of the reperfused vascular bed 24 hours after coronary occlusion confirmed a decrease in neutrophil infiltration

in the dogs that had received Fluosol intravenously.[27] In a second study, a 40% lesser dose of Fluosol significantly reduced infarct size when compared with an equal volume of oxygenated Ringer's lactate in dogs.[28] Serial microsphere injections suggested a significantly higher blood flow in the inner two thirds of the myocardium in the ischemic zone after 3 hours of reperfusion. Reduced microvascular injury and reduced neutrophil plugging (Fig. 176–6) were also reported.[29]

Administration of Fluosol results in decreased adherence of neutrophils to endothelial cells. This property is probably specific to the fluorocarbon content of Fluosol in that other components, such as the Pluronic F-68, glycerol, and egg yolk phospholipids, had no effect in one study;[30] however, the Pluronic F-68 might have been responsible.[31] Activation and deposition of complement on the surface of the Fluosol particles with a consequent fall in circulating complement levels have been described.[32]

The reduction in infarct size in these animal studies has been encouraging and suggests that Fluosol may be useful as adjunctive therapy in reperfusion with thrombolytics or by mechanical means. Whether the mechanism is due to reduction in "reperfusion injury,"[31] to reduction in ischemic injury (by improved oxygen delivery to periinfarct regions, improved collateral circulation, improved reflow due to low viscosity) independent of effects on neutrophil

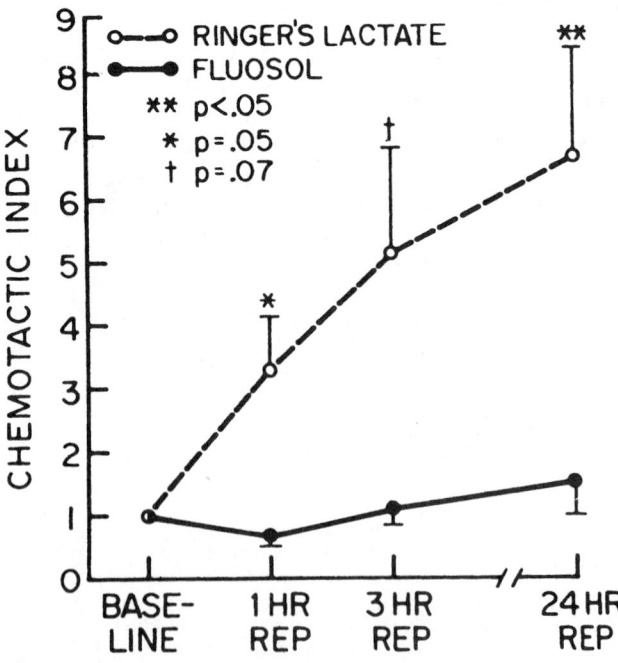

Figure 176–6. Comparison of the effect of intravenously administered Fluosol and Ringer's lactate infusions on neutrophil chemotaxis to zymosan *ex vivo.* Heparinized blood samples were taken before and after 90 minutes of coronary occlusion in anesthetized dogs. HR, hour. (From Forman MB, Pitarys CJ, Vildibill HD, et al: Pharmacologic perturbation of neutrophils by Fluosol results in a sustained reduction in infarct size in the canine model of reperfusion. J Am Coll Cardiol 19:205, 1992. Reprinted with permission from the American College of Cardiology.)

function, or to preservation of endothelial cell function is still not certain.

Forman et al.[24] reported a pilot study in 12 patients undergoing urgent balloon angioplasty for acute myocardial infarction in whom the LAD coronary artery was occluded on initial angiography. These patients were randomized to balloon angioplasty alone or to angioplasty followed by infusion of oxygenated Fluosol at 40 ml/min for 30 minutes. Oxygen treatment in the angioplasty alone group was not specified. Twelve days after intervention, regional ventricular function was significantly better in the Fluosol group.

However, this benefit was not confirmed in the Ninth Thrombolysis in Acute Infarction Trial,[18, 33] in which 430 patients were randomized to tissue-type plasminogen activator (t-PA) plus Fluosol and oxygen or to t-PA without Fluosol and oxygen. Fluosol and oxygen (100% by nonrebreathing mask) were administered for 12 hours. There was no significant difference in mortality, reinfarction, heart failure, or recurrent ischemia in the hospital or in left ventricular ejection fraction on ventriculography (Table 176–3).

OTHER FLUOROCARBONS

Fluosol can be regarded as a first-generation fluorocarbon. Attempts to improve stability and oxygen-carrying capacity have involved the testing of many second-generation agents emulsified with different detergents or surfactants.[16] The structure of several of these agents is presented in Figure 176–1.

Perfluorooctylbromide (Perflubron) and *bis*(F-butyl)-ethene have a linear structure that is associated with better oxygen-carrying capacity. Indeed, Perflubron can carry three to four times as much oxygen as Fluosol and can deliver more oxygen than whole blood. Perflubron was initially selected for further investigation because it is radiopaque when imaged by conventional radiography, ultrasonography, computerized tomography, or magnetic resonance techniques. It is also rapidly excreted. Perflubron can be prepared in concentrated emulsions (up to 90% by weight) that have a low viscosity and are stable at room temperature for 1 year.[34] Perflubron is rapidly excreted following intravenous administration. *Bis*(F-butyl)ethene is also both easily produced and rapidly excreted.

Pluronic F-68 has been associated with transient hypotension. Other nuisance symptoms such as facial flushing, back pain, and chills may be prevented by cyclooxygenase inhibition. Newer fluorocarbons have been emulsified with lecithins, which do not activate complement and are stable and autoclavable. Other advances in the development of fluorocarbons have been well-summarized by Riess.[34]

OTHER CLINICAL APPLICATIONS

Fluorocarbons as Contrast Agents

Evidence of the potential of fluorocarbons as radiographic contrast agents was first reported over 20 years ago (Table 176–4).[35] Fluorocarbon emulsions enhance perfused tissues when imaged by ultrasonography, enhancing contrast between normal tissues and tumors, and improve the detection of perfusion defects in the liver, spleen, and kidneys.[36] Enhancement may depend more on the emulsifier used than on the fluorocarbon.[37]

Perflubron increases the signal-to-noise ratio for Doppler signal processing of blood flow in vessels and enhances perfused tissues during its capillary phase. It is also highly reflective when stationary in tissue.[38]

Resuscitation

The initial stimulus for the development of fluorocarbons was the hope that acellular fluids could be injected in acute blood loss to alleviate hypoxia and hypovolemic shock. Fluosol has been used in the severely anemic patient, but dosing limitations have reduced its efficacy.[39] Fluosol has not been approved by the FDA for use in hypovolemic shock.

Cardioplegia

Studies in dogs[40] and piglets[41] have demonstrated beneficial effects of Fluosol when it is infused into

Table 176–3. **End Points of the TAMI-9 Study**

End Point	Control (n = 219)	Fluosol (n = 211)
Death	3.7%	5.6%
Reinfarction	4.2%	2.4%
Congestive heart failure	31%	45%
Recurrent ischemia	11%	6%
Infarct size*	$16.3 \pm 1.1\%$	$15.1 \pm 1.0\%$
Left ventricular ejection fraction†	$52.1 \pm 1.1\%$	$51.3 \pm 0.9\%$

*Expressed as a percentage of the left ventricle (control, n = 155; fluosol, n = 149).

†Control, n = 157; fluosol, n = 140.

Adapted from Werns SW. Free radical scavengers and leukocyte inhibitors. *In* Topol EJ (ed): Textbook of Interventional Cardiology. Philadelphia: WB Saunders, 1993, p 137.

Table 176–4. **Clinical Applications of Fluosol and Other Fluorocarbons**

Cardiovascular
  Coronary angioplasty
  Reperfusion
  Cardioplegia
Blood substitute
  Hypovolemic shock
  Blood dyscrasias
Organ and tissue preservation
  Donor tissues for transplantation
  Microcirculatory disturbances
Contrast agent for tissue imaging
  Ultrasonography
  Radiology
  Computed tomography
  Magnetic resonance imaging
Ventilatory failure
  Preterm neonates

transplanted hearts just prior to resuming whole-blood perfusion. Ventricular function, adenosine triphosphate levels, mitochondrial function, and ultrastructural architecture are improved when compared with control organs reperfused with whole blood. Perfusion with Fluosol also reduced the efflux of the MB (predominant isoenzyme in myocardium) fraction of creatine kinase from the transplanted hearts (Fig. 176–7).

Blood Diseases

Oxygenated fluorocarbons and Pluronic F-68 both reduce the incidence of sickling and reduce the adherence of red cells to endothelial cells when cultured with hypoxic red cells from patients with sickle cell anemia.[42]

Immature Lungs

Fluorocarbon emulsions can act as wetting agents when administered directly into the airways and may improve lung compliance in premature babies with deficient alveolar surfactant.[43]

FUTURE DIRECTIONS AND SUMMARY

Animal and clinical studies have demonstrated that Fluosol and other fluorocarbons can transport and deliver clinically meaningful quantities of oxygen.

Furthermore, fluorocarbon emulsions have a low viscosity and are radiopaque. Fluosol has proved useful in reducing myocardial ischemia during balloon angioplasty of the coronary arteries. There is also experimental evidence that Fluosol reduces the extent of myocardial infarction following prolonged coronary artery occlusion. However, a large clinical study failed to demonstrate any benefit for Fluosol when used as an adjunct to thrombolysis.

New fluorocarbon emulsions that may overcome some of the limitations of Fluosol continue to be developed. More concentrated emulsions such as Perflubron have an oxygen-carrying capacity equivalent to blood and an oxygen delivery capacity that exceeds that of blood. Newer emulsions are stable at room temperature and promise to be more convenient to use in routine and emergency situations. Further development of surfactants will be specific to the intended use of the emulsion.

Potential clinical applications of fluorocarbons encompass many branches of medicine, including their use as nontoxic contrast agents in diagnostic radiology. The concept that the emergency physician could reach for one emulsion that could both resuscitate and assist in diagnostic imaging of a patient in shock is exciting. Despite this promise, however, widespread clinical utilization of Fluosol and other fluorocarbons is yet to be established.

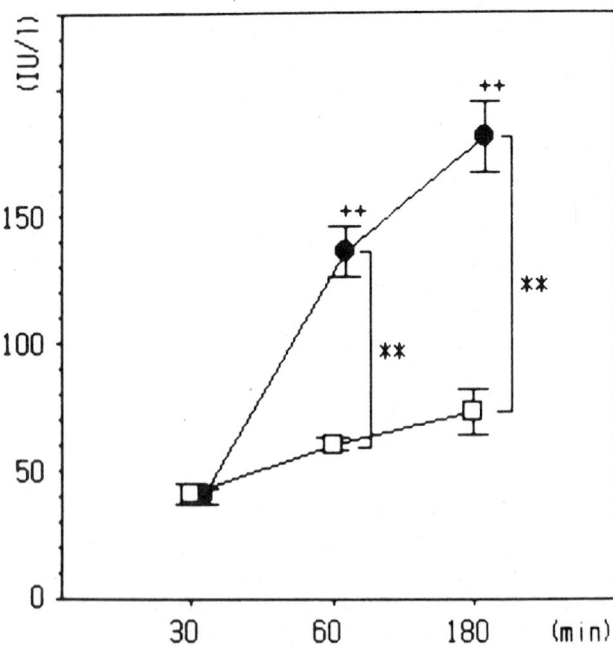

Figure 176–7. Efflux of creatine kinase MB fraction from orthotopically transplanted dog hearts during the first 180 minutes after whole blood reperfusion with (open squares, n = 7) or without (solid circles, n = 8) pretreatment with 200 ml of Fluosol. (From Ueda K, Genda T, Hirata I, et al: Beneficial effect of fluorocarbon reperfusion on postoperative cardiac dysfunction of transplanted heart. J Heart Lung Transplant 11:646, 1992.)

REFERENCES

1. Clark LC, Gollan F: Survival of mammals breathing organic liquids equilibrated with oxygen at atmospheric pressure. Science 152:1755, 1966.
2. Geyer RP: Fluorocarbon-polyol artificial blood substitutes. N Engl J Med 289:1077, 1973.
3. Ohyanagi H, Toshima K, Sekita M, et al: Clinical studies of perfluorochemical whole blood substitutes: Safety of Fluosol-DA(20%) in normal human volunteers. Clin Ther 2:306, 1979.
4. Tremper KK, Freidman AE, Levine EM, et al: The preoperative treatment of severely anemic patients with perflurochemical oxygen transport fluid, Fluosol-DA. N Engl J Med 307:277, 1982.
5. Roberts CS, Anderson HV, Carboni AA, et al: Usefulness of intracoronary infusion of fluorocarbon distal to prolonged coronary occlusion by angioplasty balloon in dogs. Am J Cardiol 57:1202, 1986.
6. Robalino BD, Marwick T, Lafont A, et al: Protection against ischemia during prolonged balloon inflation by distal coronary perfusion with use of an autoperfusion catheter or Fluosol. J Am Coll Cardiol 20:1378, 1992.
7. Tokioka H, Miyazaki A, Fung P, et al: Effects of intracoronary infusion of arterial blood or Fluosol-DA 20% on regional myocardial metabolism and function during brief coronary artery occlusions. Circulation 75:473, 1987.
8. Anderson HV, Leimgruber PP, Roubin GS, et al: Distal coronary artery perfusion during percutaneous transluminal coronary angioplasty. Am Heart J 110:720, 1985.
9. Clemans M, Jaffee CC, Wohlgelernter D: Prevention of ischemia during percutaneous transluminal coronary angioplasty by transcatheter infusion of oxygenated Fluosol-DA 20%. Circulation 74:555, 1986.
10. Jaffe CC, Wohlgelernter D, Cabin H, et al: Preservation of left ventricular ejection fraction during percutaneous transluminal coronary angioplasty by distal transcatheter coronary perfusion of oxygenated Fluosol DA 20%. Am Heart J 115:1156, 1988.
11. Young LH, Jaffe CC, Revkin JH, et al: Metabolic and functional

effects of perfluorocarbon distal perfusion during coronary angioplasty. Am J Cardiol 65:986, 1990.

12. Bell MR, Nishimura RA, Holmes DJ, et al: Does intracoronary infusion of Fluosol-DA 20% prevent left ventricular diastolic dysfunction during coronary balloon angioplasty? J Am Coll Cardiol 16:959, 1990.

13. Kent KM, Cleman MW, Cowley MJ, et al: Reduction of myocardial ischemia during percutaneous transluminal coronary angioplasty with oxygenated Fluosol. Am J Cardiol 66:279, 1990.

14. Cowley MJ, Snow FR, DiSciascio G, et al: Perfluorochemical perfusion during coronary angioplasty in unstable and high-risk patients. Circulation 81:4, 1990.

15. Lowe KC: Synthetic oxygen transport fluids based on perfluorochemicals: Applications in medicine and biology. Vox Sang 60:129, 1991.

16. Riess JG: Fluorocarbon-based in vivo oxygen transport and delivery systems. Vox Sang 61:225, 1991.

17. Garrelts JC: Fluosol: An oxygen-delivery fluid for use in percutaneous transluminal coronary angioplasty. Drug Intell Clin Pharm 24:1105, 1990.

18. Wall TC, Califf RM, Blankenship J, et al: Intravenous Fluosol in the treatment of acute myocardial infarction. Results of the Thrombolysis and Angioplasty in Myocardial Infarction 9 Trial. TAMI 9 Research Group. Circulation 90:114, 1994.

19. Glogar DH, Klonar RA, Muller J, et al: Fluorocarbons reduce myocardial ischemic damage after coronary occlusion. Science 211:1439, 1981.

20. Rude RE, Glogar D, Khuri SF: Effects of intravenous fluorocarbons during and without oxygen enhancement on acute myocardial ischemic injury assessed by measurement of intramyocardial gas tensions. Am Heart J 195:60, 1982.

21. Schaer GL, Krucoff MW, Green C, Visner MS: Dissociation of ST segment elevation and regional wall motion with open-artery, intracoronary Fluosol. Am Heart J 118:679, 1989.

22. Forman MB, Puett DW, Wilson BH, et al: Beneficial longterm effects of intracoronary perfluorochemical on infarct size and ventricular function in a canine reperfusion model. J Am Coll Cardiol 95:1082, 1987.

23. Forman MB, Bingham S, Kopelman HA, et al: Reduction of infarct size with intracoronary perfluorochemical in a canine preparation of reperfusion. Circulation 71:1060, 1985.

24. Forman MB, Perry JM, Wilson BH, et al: Demonstration of myocardial reperfusion injury in humans: Results of a pilot study utilizing acute coronary angioplasty with perfluorochemical in anterior myocardial infarction. J Am Coll Cardiol 18:911, 1991.

25. Virmani R, Osmialowski AF, Kolodgie FD, et al: The effect of perfluorochemical fluosol-DA (20%) on myocardial infarct healing in the rabbit. Am J Cardiovasc Pathol 3:69, 1990.

26. Rice HE, Virmani R, Hart CL, et al: Dose-dependent reduction of myocardial infarct size with the perfluorochemical Fluosol-DA. Am Heart J 120:1039, 1990.

27. Bajaj AK, Cobb MA, Virmani R, et al: Limitation of myocardial reperfusion injury by intravenous perfluorochemicals. Role of neutrophil activation. Circulation 79:645, 1989.

28. Forman MB, Pitarys CJ, Vildibill HD, et al: Pharmacologic perturbation of neutrophils by Fluosol results in a sustained reduction in infarct size in the canine model of reperfusion. J Am Coll Cardiol 19:205, 1992.

29. Kolodgie FD, Virmani R, Farb A: Limitation of no reflow injury by blood-free reperfusion with oxygenated perfluorochemical (Fluosol-DA 20%). J Am Coll Cardiol 18:215, 1991.

30. Babbitt DG, Forman MB, Jones R, et al: Prevention of neutrophil-mediated injury to endothelial cells by perfluorochemical. Am J Pathol 136:451, 1990.

31. Forman MB, Ingram DA, Murray JJ: Role of perfluorochemical emulsions in the treatment of myocardial reperfusion injury. Am Heart J 124:1347, 1992.

32. Hong F, Shastri KA, Logue GL, et al: Complement activation by artificial blood substitute Fluosol: In vitro and in vivo studies. Transfusion 31:642, 1991.

33. Werns SW: Free radical scavengers and leukocyte inhibitors. In Topol EJ (ed): Textbook of Interventional Cardiology. Philadelphia: WB Saunders, 1993, p 137.

34. Riess JG: Fluorocarbon-based oxygen carriers: New orientations. Artif Organs 15:408, 1991.

35. Long DM, Liu M, Szanto PS, et al: Efficacy and toxicity studies with radiopaque perfluorocarbon. Radiology 105:323, 1972.

36. Coley BD, Mattrey RF, Roberts A, et al: Potential role of PFOB enhanced sonography of the kidney. II: Detection of partial infarction. Kidney Int 39:740, 1991.

37. Satterfield R, Tarter VM, Schumacher DJ, et al: Comparison of different perfluorocarbons as ultrasound contrast agents. Invest Radiol 28:325, 1993.

38. Andre MP, Steinbach G, Mattrey RF: Enhancement of the echogenicity of flowing blood by the contrast agent Perflubron. Invest Radiol 28:502, 1993.

39. Gould SA, Rosen AL, Sehgal LR, et al: Fluosol-DA as a red cell substitute in acute anemia. N Engl J Med 314:1653, 1986.

40. Ueda K, Genda T, Hirata I, et al: Beneficial effect of fluorocarbon reperfusion on postoperative cardiac dysfunction of transplanted heart. J Heart Lung Transplant 11:646, 1992.

41. Martin SM, Laks H, Drinkwater DC, et al: Perfluorochemical reperfusion yields improved myocardial recovery after global ischemia. Ann Thorac Surg 55:954, 1993.

42. Smith CM, Hebbel RP, Tukey DP, et al: Pluronic F-68 reduces the endothelial adherence and improves the rheology of liganded sickle erythrocytes. Blood 69:1631, 1987.

43. Greenspan JS, Wolfson MR, Rubenstein SD, et al: Liquid ventilation of human preterm neonates. J Pediatr 117:106, 1990.

CHAPTER 177

c7E3 Fab (abciximab)

Benedict R. Lucchesi, M.D., Ph.D.

OVERVIEW

c7E3 Fab (abciximab—ReoPro) is one of the first available receptor-specific antiplatelet agents. Produced by monoclonal antibody technology, c7E3 Fab binds to the glycoprotein IIb/IIIa (GPIIb/IIIa) receptor on the surface of platelets, blocking platelet aggregation and *in vivo* thrombus formation. Clinical trials of c7E3 Fab have shown that it reduces the incidence of vessel occlusion after percutaneous transluminal coronary angioplasty (PTCA). Currently, c7E3 Fab is indicated

for prevention of cardiac ischemic complications (death, myocardial infarction [MI], or need for urgent reintervention) during or after PTCA or directional coronary atherectomy in patients at high risk for acute coronary artery thrombosis.

HISTORY AND RATIONALE FOR DRUG DEVELOPMENT

Since its first use in coronary disease in the late 1970s, PTCA has gained widespread acceptance as a nonsurgical method of coronary revascularization.[1–3] As interventional cardiologists have gained experience with the procedure and as the catheter technology has improved, the use of PTCA in patient groups at high risk for complications has increased.[3] Vessel occlusion is the major complication of PTCA; it may occur acutely (abrupt closure) or after a delay of 1 to 6 months (restenosis).[2–4] Reported in approximately 2% to 10% of cases, acute vessel closure usually occurs in the catheterization laboratory or within the first 24 hours following the procedure.[3, 5–12] Associated with significant and sustained reduction in flow through the treated vessel, acute closure is considered the primary contributor to angioplasty-related morbidity and mortality.[1–3]

Vessel closure also limits the efficacy of PTCA in the long term, and a restenosis rate of approximately 30% to 40% has been reported consistently since the introduction of the procedure.[13–17] Restenosis (>50% narrowing of the lumen diameter at the site of PTCA) typically occurs within 1 to 3 months of PTCA; in 95% of patients who experience restenosis, the event occurs within 6 months after coronary angioplasty.[1]

A number of pharmacologic agents, most commonly antiplatelet and antithrombotic drugs, have been administered with PTCA in an effort to reduce the occlusion rate.[1, 6] Currently, the standard PTCA regimen includes adjunctive therapy with low-dose aspirin for reduced risk of platelet aggregation and heparin for its antithrombotic properties.[1] Because platelet-rich thrombi are often found in patients with occlusion, improved antiplatelet agents are being actively sought.[6]

"Antiplatelet" is a relatively broad term; antiplatelet agents may inhibit either platelet adhesion or platelet aggregation through a variety of metabolic pathways.[18] Although it is a relatively weak antiplatelet agent, aspirin has been shown to reduce the incidence of restenosis by inhibiting platelet aggregation and subsequent thrombus formation.[1] As the sole antiplatelet strategy, however, aspirin is insufficient to stop the platelet response to vascular injury.[5, 19, 20] This is probably due to its mechanism of action: aspirin inhibits thromboxane A_2 synthesis, thereby blocking one of the pathways to platelet aggregation, but it does not affect the several other metabolic pathways that contribute to this vital step in hemostasis.[20]

Today, PTCA is being used in increasing numbers of patients with risk factors for cardiovascular thrombosis, such as multivessel or diffuse disease, unstable angina, and complex lesions.[3, 7–9] Clearly, the rates of both short- and long-term occlusive complications will only increase as more high-risk patients undergo the procedure. Because platelet aggregation is thought to constitute one of the primary mechanisms underlying vessel occlusion, a number of antiplatelet agents with increased potency—such as c7E3 Fab—are under investigation in an attempt to reduce the incidence of peri- and post-procedural occlusion.[1, 19]

GPIIb/IIIa Receptor

Since the late 1970s, a number of lines of research have pointed to the importance of the GPIIb/IIIa receptor as the final common pathway to platelet aggregation.[18] Advances in the understanding of platelet physiology have provided the basis for the rational design of newer agents, such as c7E3 Fab, that block this important receptor, neutralizing thrombin and reducing the incidence of thrombotic complications.[18]

In the late 1970s, studies of Glanzmann's thrombasthenia provided the first indication that GPIIb/IIIa was the specific platelet receptor responsible for mediating platelet aggregation.[21] Platelets from patients with this disorder, a congenital defect resulting in a lack of functional GPIIb/IIIa receptors, are incapable of either fibrinogen binding or platelet aggregation.[21, 22] This evidence, combined with later investigations in normal platelets showing that the binding of adhesive proteins is enhanced after platelet activation, led to the conclusion that a conformational change after platelet activation is required for aggregation.[21, 23–26] Research also showed that platelet aggregation depends on the function of the GPIIb/IIIa receptor, which binds fibrinogen and/or von Willebrand factor, allowing subsequent platelet-platelet binding and aggregate formation.[18, 21, 23]

The first cell surface adhesion receptor, or integrin, to be identified, GPIIb/IIIa is one of the most abundant cell surface proteins and is found only on platelets and cells of megakaryocytic potential.[23, 25–27] Electron microscopy has shown that GPIIb/IIIa is a heterodimer consisting of a globular head with two tails that descend into the cell membrane.[23]

Because adhesive proteins are present in the normal circulation at levels that are sufficient for platelet aggregation, a number of complex mechanisms regulate the activation of the GPIIb/IIIa receptor.[28] These involve not only agonists such as thrombin, adenosine diphosphate (ADP), and serotonin but also transducing mechanisms that depend on arachidonic acid, protein C, and perhaps other agents.[28] This explains why GPIIb/IIIa is one of a limited number of integrin receptors that become capable of binding to their natural ligands only after activation.[23, 24] On platelets that have not been activated, GPIIb/IIIa receptors are randomly dispersed and capable only of binding fibrinogen at a low level.[23] Platelet activation allows GPIIb/IIIa to form patches on the platelet surface that have an increased affinity for fibrinogen and can bind with other adhesive proteins, including fibronectin, von Willebrand factor, and vitronectin.[29] Because linking of platelets does not occur until sufficient adhesive proteins bind to GPIIb/IIIa, this step appears necessary for platelet aggregation.[21, 30] The final common pathway for platelet aggregation involves the cross-linking by fibrinogen of the GPIIb/IIIa receptors and adjacent platelets,[25, 26, 31] a process that is not inhibited completely by aspirin and/or antithrombins.[32–34] Platelet adherence and deposition after arterial wall injury are time-limited phenomena.[35, 36] A superficially denuded vascular surface becomes nonreactive to platelets when platelet deposition is inhibited for 8 hours, whereas deeper vascular lesions may increase platelet deposition 10-fold in normal arteries and 20- to 30-fold in atherosclerotic vessels.[23, 37, 38]

c7E3 Fab is one of the first GPIIb/IIIa antagonists developed for clinical use. Immunoprecipitation and immunoaffinity purification studies have shown that it is a competitive inhibitor of fibrinogen and von Willebrand binding.[29] When bound to platelets, c7E3 Fab blocks the binding of the adhesive proteins, inhibiting platelet aggregation at the final common pathway.[29]

Development of c7E3 Fab

Monoclonal antibodies have emerged as an important new class of agents because of their high specificity for the targeted protein.[39] Investigation of various monoclonal antibodies has contributed significantly to the understanding of physiology at the molecular level, which in turn has led to the application of monoclonal antibodies in a wide variety of diagnostic and therapeutic areas.[39] One of the first monoclonal antibodies to be widely used in clinical cardiology, c7E3 Fab is a unique antiplatelet agent that has shown promise in reducing ischemic complications after PTCA.[5, 19, 31, 40]

The development of c7E3 Fab began in the early 1980s, when Coller et al.[31] responded to the mounting evidence that the binding of fibrinogen to platelets was critical for platelet aggregation by searching for a murine monoclonal antibody capable of inhibiting platelet aggregation. A number of clones that targeted GPIIb/IIIa were identified by this group; the murine 7E3 cell line was chosen for further study because the antibody it produces was cross-reactive with platelets from nonhuman species, facilitating the study of the role of GPIIb/IIIa in thrombosis.[31] Initial investigation showed that the 7E3 antibody had activity against human, primate, and canine platelets as well as the ability to bind to GPIIb/IIIa receptors on both resting and activated platelets.[31, 40] In 1986, a live culture of the cell line 7E3 was received at Centocor, Inc., for use as the master cell bank that would eventually lead to the production of c7E3 Fab.[40]

The native murine 7E3 antibody molecule is a member of the immunoglobulin G (IgG) class. Because the surface of the platelets is host to a vast number of GPIIb/IIIa receptors, and because the binding of large numbers of IgG molecules to the cell surface can potentially cause platelet destruction, the original 7E3 molecule was not considered for in vivo applications. Two fragments, the F(ab')$_2$ and Fab fragments of 7E3, were employed for early animal and human testing.[40] Preparations of the fragments were each equally effective in binding to platelets and inhibiting platelet aggregation after injection in monkeys.[40] Although there were no striking differences in the safety or pharmacodynamic profiles for murine 7E3 F(ab')$_2$ and murine 7E3 Fab in animals or human subjects, preliminary results suggested that the Fab fragment was less immunogenic.[40] To maximize compatibility with the human immune system, a cell line producing a chimeric antibody that combined a mu-

rine antibody binding sequence with a human constant nonbinding antibody sequence was genetically engineered. The chimeric antibody retains the heavy- and light-chain variable regions that confer its specificity for the GPIIb/IIIa receptor. The constant domains were replaced by human IgG$_1$ heavy-chain and light-chain regions, respectively. The modification in the antibody reduces the amount of foreign protein that is administered to a patient, diminishing the potential for an immune response to the antibody-based therapy.[40, 41] Chimeric 7E3 (c7E3) possessed equivalent antiplatelet activity compared with the original murine antibody, and it too has been developed as a Fab fragment (c7E3 Fab), associated with extremely low levels of human antimouse antibodies (HAMA) and human antichimeric antibodies (HACA),[31] known as c7E3 Fab.[40]

PHARMACOLOGY AND PHARMACOKINETICS

A number of in vitro and in vivo studies have been conducted to establish the physiologic activity of 7E3 and its fragments, including aggregation responses, platelet function, plasma clearance, and receptor blockade.[28, 29, 31, 40, 42-72] These studies have shown that c7E3 Fab (abciximab) exhibits a number of features that facilitate its use as a therapeutic antiplatelet agent. First, c7E3 Fab binds to resting platelets and does not require prior activation of the platelet to bind GPIIb/IIIa receptors.[31, 40] In addition, administration of c7E3 Fab does not lead to an increased rate of platelet clearance or interfere with other receptor-mediated pathways or other important platelet functions.[40] Furthermore, the interaction of c7E3 Fab with platelets is readily quantified, and the blockade of GPIIb/IIIa receptors can be correlated directly to the inhibition of platelet aggregation.[47] Finally, c7E3 Fab is a poor immunogen and leads to a low incidence of induced human immune responses.[40]

Mechanism of Action

c7E3 Fab binds to the intact heterodimer structure of GPIIb/IIIa, preventing binding of the natural macromolecular ligands.[40] Platelet binding occurs within minutes and produces transient yet total inhibition of platelet aggregation.[40]

As briefly mentioned earlier, platelet adhesion can be mediated by other glycoprotein surface receptors, such as GPIa/IIb, in addition to GPIIb/IIIa. An early study by Mickelson et al.[66] showed that c7E3 Fab–induced inhibition of the GPIIb/IIIa receptor does not entirely prevent platelet adhesion. These authors and others speculated that competitive inhibition of platelet-fibrinogen-platelet binding was the primary means by which c7E3 Fab decreased aggregation.[51, 66] Another study showed that c7E3 Fab–bound platelets retain a limited ability to adhere to the subendothelial surfaces via binding to von Willebrand factor.[43] Thus, although c7E3 Fab blocks the accumulation of multiple layers of platelets, the initial layer of platelet deposition occurs, and the risk for hemorrhage is reduced.[43]

Aggregation Responses

The results of *in vitro* platelet aggregation assays showed that c7E3 Fab inhibited GPIIb/IIIa-dependent platelet aggregation in a dose-dependent fashion.[40] As shown in Figure 177–1, both the rate and the final extent of platelet aggregation are correlated with the dosage.[40] Subsequent *in vivo* studies of platelet aggregation in response to ADP in animal models confirmed this correlation and showed that the response was also directly related to the number of bound c7E3 Fab molecules per platelet.[43]

In vitro, c7E3 Fab had no other effect on known platelet functions.[40] Investigation revealed that saturation binding of GPIIb/IIIa receptors with c7E3 Fab did not provoke either degranulation or shape change, indicating that the agent does not stimulate platelet activation. Furthermore, c7E3 Fab binding did not impede degranulation during exposure to platelet agonists.[40]

Antiplatelet Activity and Impact on Platelet Function

Testing in dogs and nonhuman primates showed that c7E3 Fab was an effective antiplatelet agent *in vivo* and that the number of circulating platelets remained stable during administration of the agent.[43, 48, 51, 58, 65] Flow cytometry was used to assess platelet function and monitor the distribution of c7E3 Fab on the platelets of monkeys for extended periods after treatment.[40] After administration, c7E3 Fab was detectable for a 10-day period, during which all circulating platelets possessed some bound c7E3 Fab. Only when the levels fell below the threshold of detection were platelets without bound c7E3 Fab observed.[40]

According to the data from these investigations, the

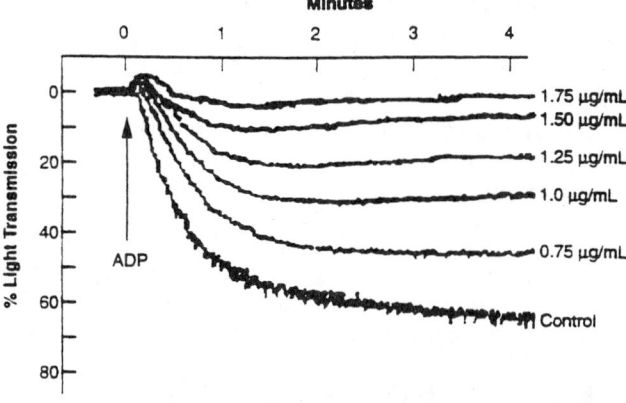

Figure 177–1. Inhibition of platelet aggregation at different concentrations of abciximab. Individual *in vitro* tests each used a separate aliquot of single-donor, platelet-rich plasma preincubated with saline diluent or different concentrations of abciximab. Curves represent the change in light transmission that occurred over approximately 4 minutes after addition of adenosine diphosphate (10 μmol/L). (Courtesy of Centocor, Inc., data on file, 1994.)

continual redistribution of c7E3 Fab on platelets slowly decreases the level of receptor blockade.[40] It is thought that the progressive decline in bound c7E3 Fab molecules per platelet is attributable to the addition of new platelets to the circulation and drug clearance.[28] Because of the diminishing levels and because c7E3 Fab binding is reversible, platelet function is restored within several hours of treatment.

Plasma Clearance

c7E3 Fab is quickly cleared from the plasma after bolus injection because of rapid platelet binding.[31] Clearance may also be due to the small size of the molecule, which may allow rapid glomerular filtration.[40] In humans, the initial half-life after a c7E3 Fab bolus is less than 10 minutes, whereas the second phase half-life is about 30 minutes.[40]

Platelet-bound c7E3 Fab can be detected for as long as 3 weeks, although at steadily diminishing levels. Within a few hours, recovery of unoccupied platelet receptors allows the return of platelet function.[60] Therefore, a low-dose continuous infusion after bolus injection has been used to sustain the therapeutic effect of c7E3 Fab, which requires high levels of receptor blockade. Bolus injection combined with a 72-hour continuous infusion has been shown to produce relatively constant free plasma concentrations.[54] After cessation of infusion, the level of c7E3 Fab decreases rapidly for 6 hours and then continues to decline at a slower rate.[40, 54] The time to recovery of platelet function is not related to the duration of infusion but rather is similar to that observed after a bolus dose.[40]

Receptor Blockade

Iodine-125 radiolabeling showed that each molecule of c7E3 Fab binds to a single GPIIb/IIIa receptor and that there is a direct correlation between the numbers of bound molecules and occupied receptors.[31, 40] An average blockade of about 82% was attained within 2 minutes after injection.[31, 40] The radiolabeling studies also showed the reversibility of binding and the progressive diminution of bound molecules per platelet. By 24 hours after bolus injection, the level of receptor blockade had decreased by approximately 50%.[31, 40] Continuous infusion extended high-level receptor blockade, but unoccupied receptors were detectable immediately after the infusion ceased.[40]

A sizable fraction of injected antibody binds to platelets and thus does not leave the vascular compartment. In dogs, approximately 20% of the injected antibody becomes bound to platelets at a dose of 0.81 mg/kg, the dose of antibody required to nearly saturate receptor sites.[31, 43] The dose required to nearly saturate GPIIb/IIIa receptor sites in primates and human subjects is only 0.20 to 0.25 mg/kg; at these doses, nearly 60% of the injected antibody is bound to platelets.[47, 55, 60]

The attachment of a large fraction of injected 7E3 F(ab′)₂ antibody onto circulating platelets and the distribution of unattached antibody into extravascular tissues result in a rapid decline in free 7E3 F(ab')$_2$ plasma concentrations. This allows rapid reversal of the 7E3 effect within minutes after 7E3 injection by the infusion of normal platelets, because the plasma concentration of 7E3 is too low to inhibit the new platelets.

Bates et al.[51] demonstrated that a single injection of murine 7E3 F(ab')$_2$ that could prevent platelet aggregation could also preclude thrombus formation in response to deep arterial wall injury. Furthermore, despite the return of platelet activity within the next 3 hours, as determined by *ex vivo* platelet aggregation, the platelets did not interact with the injured vessel wall. Temporary platelet inhibition prevents the acute response of the platelet to vessel wall injury and subsequent thrombus formation, allowing time for the injured vessel wall to become nonreactive; this process is referred to as "passivation." It remains to be determined whether the observation of passivation after inhibition of the platelet GPIIb/IIIa receptor is applicable to clinical situations such as angioplasty or thrombolytic therapy.

IN VIVO STUDIES
Effect on Thrombus Formation

An animal model designed to simulate the vascular abnormalities in patients with unstable angina and transient ischemic attacks was initially used to assess the antithrombotic potential of 7E3.[31, 44, 39] The model was characterized by cyclic flow reductions supposedly due to the formation of loosely bound platelet aggregates at the site of vessel wall injury. Thus, platelet thrombi form and embolize to give rise to the repetitive cyclic alterations in blood flow. Doses of 7E3 that did not completely inhibit *ex vivo* platelet aggregation were able to abolish *in vivo* platelet thrombus formation in this model.

Interactions between platelets and injured vascular endothelium contribute to thrombotic occlusion. In an experimental model of coronary artery thrombosis, 7E3 F(ab')$_2$ was given to dogs with direct current-induced intimal injury and critical stenosis of the left circumflex coronary artery.[73] In this model, injury to the vessel wall results in the spontaneous formation of an occlusive platelet-dependent arterial thrombus. Oscillations in coronary blood flow preceded occlusive thrombosis in control animals but did not occur with 7E3 F(ab')$_2$ treatment. The resulting thrombus mass recovered from the coronary artery 30 minutes after occlusion was significantly smaller in the antibody-treated group. After treatment, the *ex vivo* aggregation of platelets from the 7E3 F(ab')$_2$–treated animals was inhibited, whereas platelets from the control animals continued to aggregate *ex vivo* throughout the period of the experimental protocol. When platelets were labeled with indium-111, the thrombus and vascular endothelium in the antibody-treated dogs showed less accumulation of radioactivity than did those in the control group. 7E3 F(ab')$_2$ did not affect hemodynamic values or the circulating platelet count during the experimental protocol. In conclusion, this study showed that antibody to the platelet GPIIb/IIIa receptor prevented thrombotic coronary artery occlusion, inhibited *ex vivo* platelet aggregation, minimized platelet deposition on injured vascular endothelium and within formed thrombi, and stabilized coronary blood flow in the presence of arterial intimal injury.

In Combination with Thrombolytics

The significance of inhibiting the platelet GPIIb/IIIa receptor was demonstrated in a canine model of heparin and tissue plasminogen activator (t-PA)-induced reperfusion of severely stenosed and thrombosed coronary arteries.[59, 70–72] Additional studies were done in a long-term canine model to determine whether 7E3 F(ab')$_2$ could prevent coronary artery rethrombosis after successful thrombolysis with recombinant t-PA (rt-PA).[32] A vessel wall of the circumflex coronary artery was injured by a current applied to its intimal surface. The resulting occlusive thrombus was aged for 30 minutes, and rt-PA was administered. Animals were allocated to receive either placebo or a single dose of 7E3 as the sole adjunctive agent. *Ex vivo* platelet function and coronary artery blood flow velocity were recorded on each of 5 consecutive days. Reocclusion and mortality were reduced significantly in animals treated with 7E3 compared with the placebo-treated group. Significant inhibition of *ex vivo* platelet aggregation persisted for 48 hours after a single injection of 7E3. Thus, 7E3 F(ab')$_2$ was effective as the sole adjunctive agent with rt-PA in the prevention of rethrombosis. This study is unique in that it examined the efficacy of GPIIb/IIIa inhibition in an experimental model for an extended time, demonstrating the duration of antiplatelet therapy.

A preliminary study in human subjects indicated that the use of murine 7E3 F(ab')$_2$ resulted in antibody formation against the murine immunoglobulin.[60] This led to the development of the chimeric antibody c7E3 Fab (c7E3 Fab) discussed previously. The antithrombotic efficacy of 7E3 Fab was studied in a nonhuman primate model of arterial thrombosis.[33] The primary end point in the study was occlusive thrombus formation resulting from continuous anodal current injury to the intimal surface of the carotid arteries in cynomolgus monkeys. c7E3 Fab inhibition of the GPIIb/IIIa receptor was reported to be safe and effective for the prevention of primary thrombus formation, whereas treatment with aspirin, heparin, or a combination of the two agents failed to protect against occlusive thrombus formation in the nonhuman primate.

Toxicology

Both short- and long-term toxicology studies in nonhuman primates showed that c7E3 Fab lacked significant toxicity when administered in single doses, as multiple doses for as long as 3 days, or as continuous infusion for up to 4 days.[55, 56]

Neuropharmacology and Cardiovascular Effects

The activity of c7E3 Fab is highly targeted to platelets; no adverse effects have been shown on any neurologic or cardiovascular parameters tested, including seizure activity, barbiturate-induced sleeping time or duration, responses to a variety of autonomic nervous system agonists, heart rate, blood pressure, and electrocardiographic activity.[40]

CLINICAL EXPERIENCE

Clinical trials have shown that the antiplatelet activity of c7E3 Fab is indeed sufficient to significantly reduce the incidence of vessel occlusion after PTCA.[5, 19] The agent is currently indicated for prevention of acute cardiac ischemic complications (death, MI, or need for urgent reintervention) during or after PTCA or directional coronary atherectomy in patients at high risk for acute coronary artery thrombosis. Patient groups considered to be at high risk include those with acute MI, unstable angina, or other identifiable clinical factors and angiographically defined coronary anatomic characteristics that have been associated with an increased incidence of acute coronary artery thrombosis during and after PTCA.

The dosing, safety, and efficacy of c7E3 Fab in the prevention of ischemic complications following PTCA have been evaluated in several clinical trials. These studies have enrolled a variety of subjects, including normal volunteers, patients with stable or unstable angina, patients undergoing elective and emergency PTCA, and patients with acute MI.[5, 19, 40, 42, 54, 60, 64, 67, 69]

Clinical Trials

Dosing

The phase I dosing studies of c7E3 Fab showed that the agent was well-tolerated and helped to establish the optimal dosing regimen.[42, 64, 68, 69, 71, 75, 76] In a dose-ranging study, Wagner et al.[67] reported that nearly complete platelet inhibition is achieved at c7E3 Fab doses of 0.25 mg/kg and higher. Subsequent phase I and II studies demonstrated that the inhibitory action of c7E3 Fab could be prolonged via continuous infusions for up to 3 days.[54] In addition, the studies suggested that optimal results in high-risk patients might be attained with a bolus dose followed by a 12-hour infusion of c7E3 Fab.[42] These studies confirmed preclinical data suggesting that the potent antiplatelet effect would be readily reversible by transfusion of platelets.[42, 69] By reducing the level of bound c7E3 Fab per platelet and allowing binding of the natural ligands, platelet infusion reestablishes the normal hemostatic mechanisms. Therefore, infusion allows patients to safely undergo immediate emergency coronary artery bypass surgery (CABG) when necessary.

c7E3 Fab produced a dose-dependent blockade of GPIIb/IIIa receptors in other phase I studies.[60, 64] Gold et al.[60] showed that a single dose of c7E3 Fab of 0.2 mg/kg could induce profound platelet inhibition in patients with unstable angina without producing unacceptable adverse effects. Notably, these investigators were also able to correlate the extent of platelet inhibition with a reduction in unstable angina symptoms. Angina was absent during the 12 hours following c7E3 Fab injection and returned only when bleeding times normalized.[60]

Bleeding Times

Before clinical testing, a standard-template bleeding-time test was used to assess bleeding times in animals treated with c7E3 Fab plus anticoagulant and thrombolytic agents.[59, 61, 70, 71] These studies showed that c7E3 Fab produced a dose-dependent increase in bleeding time.[40, 44] Baseline bleeding times of 1 to 3 minutes were prolonged to an average of 28 minutes after a c7E3 Fab dose of 0.25 mg/kg.[40, 59, 61, 70] The bleeding time was often extended to 30 minutes or longer when pharmacologic doses were achieved (at levels adequate to almost completely inhibit platelet aggregation).[40, 59, 61, 70, 71]

As expected from the preclinical data, therapeutically effective doses of c7E3 Fab (sufficient to block 80% or more of the platelet GPIIb/IIIa receptors) prolonged the bleeding time to more than 30 minutes in human subjects.[42, 54] Normalization of bleeding time (return to ≤10 minutes) occurred within 16 to 20 hours post treatment, whereas normalization of *ex vivo* platelet aggregation in response to ADP (return to at least 80% of baseline) occurred by 50 hours.[42] Other studies showed that an increase in bleeding time did not predict hemorrhagic events.[53] In a group of patients who received intravenously administered c7E3 Fab (bolus-plus-infusion regimen) while enrolled in the TAMI-8 acute MI and high-risk PTCA trials, bleeding times were not found to correlate with bleeding events in either the presence or the absence of thrombolysis.[53]

Efficacy

Phase II studies evaluated the efficacy of c7E3 Fab in two high-risk categories: unstable angina and acute MI.[42, 64, 68, 69] Separately, these studies of both the murine and the chimeric 7E3 antibodies showed that the agents had potent antiaggregatory action.[42, 64, 68, 69] In addition, they showed that c7E3 Fab could be administered safely with heparin and aspirin and supported the concept that effective blockade of the GPIIb/IIIa receptor could reduce the complications of PTCA.[42, 64, 68] Because an early study by Ellis et al.[42] showed that the murine antibody was associated with a risk for development of HAMA, later studies were conducted with c7E3 Fab, the chimeric version of the 7E3 antibody.[64, 68]

To assess the overall impact of c7E3 Fab in phase II trials, the combined patient population was analyzed using a composite end point that included all causes of mortality, MI, and urgent invasive coronary intervention.[40] According to this analysis, c7E3 Fab therapy had a positive effect in reducing the incidence of the composite end-point events.[40] Death, MI, or urgent invasive coronary intervention was reported in 9 of 49 patients (18.4%) in the control groups, compared with 8 of 137 patients (5.8%) in c7E3 Fab–treated patients (p = .017).[40]

Whereas these studies evaluated the overall safety and efficacy of c7E3 Fab, Anderson et al.[50] specifically examined the effect of c7E3 Fab on post-PTCA cyclic variations in coronary blood flow. These variations often precede thrombotic occlusion and have been attributed to repetitive accumulation and subsequent dislodging of platelet aggregates at the site of endothelial injury. Coronary blood flow was monitored for 30 minutes after angioplasty in 27 patients; those who experienced cyclic flow received c7E3 Fab, and flow monitoring continued for another 30 minutes.[50] Notably, c7E3 Fab abolished cyclic variations and stabilized flow in four of five patients within 1 minute.[50]

Phase III: The EPIC Trial

In 1991, the EPIC (Evaluation of 7E3 for the Prevention of Ischemic Complications) trial was initiated. This multicenter, randomized, double-blind, placebo-controlled trial was designed to evaluate the efficacy of c7E3 Fab in high-risk patients undergoing coronary balloon angioplasty or directional coronary atherectomy.[5, 19] In this large study (n = 2099), c7E3 Fab therapy was associated with a significant reduction in post-PTCA occlusive complications in both the short and the long term.[5, 19] Although c7E3 Fab therapy was generally well-tolerated, it was correlated with an increased risk of bleeding, primarily at the local vascular access site.[5, 19] Risk/benefit analysis for c7E3 Fab showed that immediate and long-term benefits to the high-risk patients enrolled in the trial far outweighed the transient risk of bleeding.

Study Design

The study was double-blinded and included three treatment arms of bolus plus 12-hour continuous infusion: c7E3 Fab bolus plus placebo infusion, c7E3 Fab bolus plus c7E3 Fab infusion, and placebo bolus plus placebo infusion.[5] The approach to PTCA was standard and included an adjunctive regimen of high-dose intravenously administered heparin and orally administered aspirin.[5] Platelet counts were measured at 30 minutes and at 2, 12, and 24 hours after the start of study medications and then daily until hospital discharge to monitor the risk for thrombocytopenia.[5]

The baseline demographic variables were comparable among groups, and all enrolled patients were at increased risk for acute complications of angioplasty because of high proportions of diabetes, recent MIs, advanced age, or female sex. Most patients had one- or two-vessel disease and good left ventricular function.[5]

Acute postprocedural follow-up lasted 30 days to determine the incidence of primary composite end points defined as the first occurrence of any one of the following events: death from any cause, MI, or need for urgent coronary reintervention (PTCA, CABG, intracoronary stent placement, or intraaortic balloon pump placement).

Follow-up was completed for all but 10 patients (0.5%). The intent-to-treat method of statistical analysis was used, and all enrolled patients were included in the safety and efficacy analyses. However, 61 patients (2.9%) did not receive the assigned study treatment, 41 patients (2.0%) did not undergo PTCA, and 45 patients (2.1%) did not meet study entry criteria, primarily because of disease of the left main coronary artery.[5]

Reduction in Primary End Points

The c7E3 Fab bolus-plus-infusion regimen was associated with a significant reduction (34.8% reduction; p = .008 versus placebo) in the incidence of primary end points. The rate of primary end points was also reduced in the c7E3 Fab bolus-plus-placebo infusion group, but the difference was not statistically significant (p = .43 versus placebo). The beneficial effect of bolus-plus-infusion c7E3 Fab was observed in all patient types, including older patients, women, those with stable coronary disease, and those with acute unstable coronary syndromes.[5]

The primary end-point rates are broken down by component in Table 177–1. The greatest impact of bolus-plus-infusion c7E3 Fab therapy could be seen in the reduction in MI (39.4%, p = .013) and need for urgent intervention (49.1%, p = .003). The c7E3 Fab bolus-plus-placebo infusion regimen, which produced

Table 177–1. **EPIC Trial Primary End-Point Events by Component**

Response	Total (n = 2099)	Placebo (n = 696)	Bolus (n = 695)	Bolus + Infusion (n = 708)	Dose p value
Death	33 (1.6%)	12 (1.7%)	9 (1.3%)	12 (1.7%)	0.964
% Reduction vs. placebo			24.8%	1.6%	
			p = .511	p = .963	
Myocardial infarction	140 (6.7%)	60 (8.6%)	43 (6.2%)	37 (5.2%)	0.013
% Reduction vs. placebo			28.2%	39.4%	
			p = .091	p = .014	
Urgent intervention	126 (6.0%)	54 (7.8%)	44 (6.4%)	28 (4.0%)	0.003
% Reduction vs. placebo			17.2%	1%	
			p = .300	p = .003	

only short-term blockade, was associated with an insignificant trend in the same direction.[5]

Reduction in Nonfatal Ischemic Events

Because one of the most notable effects of c7E3 Fab related to a reduction in MI, a separate analysis was performed to quantify the type and severity of MIs by treatment group. The EPIC investigators required at least a threefold increase in myocardial creatine kinase activity to classify an event as an MI because the significance of isolated enzyme elevations is controversial and may not assist in determining overall patient prognosis.[5] As shown in Table 177–2, c7E3 Fab reduced the incidence of both Q-wave infarctions and infarctions associated with large enzyme elevations; furthermore, a dose-response effect was observed. All types of MI, including those associated with moderate enzyme elevations, large enzyme elevations, and Q-wave development, were affected similarly by c7E3 Fab therapy. This finding, in combination with the reduction in the need for emergency coronary revascularization procedures, was one of the most significant results of the study in clinical terms.[5]

Analysis of the need for urgent repeat angioplasty showed that the timing of nonfatal ischemic events was different in the three treatment groups (Fig. 177–2). Administered as bolus alone, c7E3 Fab delayed the onset of ischemic complications by approximately 4 to 6 hours. This finding corresponds well with the platelet aggregation data from pharmacologic studies.[59, 69] As discussed previously, approximately 50% of platelet function is recovered within this period.[47] Sustained inhibition was correlated with both a delay in time to a primary end point and the significant reduction in events. As shown in Figure 177–2, ischemic events did not occur in this group until after approximately 11 hours and then quickly reached a plateau. These data suggest that complete and sustained inhibition of platelet aggregation is necessary for a therapeutic effect. After approximately 12 hours, the clinical event rate no longer depends on recovery of platelet function.[5, 19, 40]

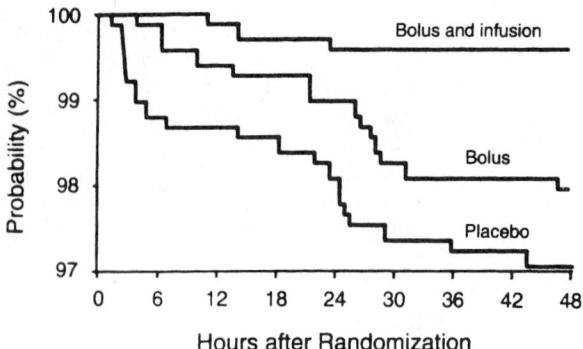

Figure 177–2. Kaplan-Meier plot demonstrating length of time to urgent repeat percutaneous revascularization procedures following percutaneous transluminal coronary angioplasty. Notice that although events began to occur shortly after the index procedure in the placebo group, there was a slight lag of 6 to 12 hours for patients who received abciximab bolus alone and a markedly longer lag before urgent repeat procedures were needed in patients who received abciximab bolus plus infusion. (Reprinted by permission from EPIC Investigators: Use of a monoclonal antibody directed against the platelet glycoprotein IIb/IIIa receptor in high-risk coronary angioplasty. N Engl J Med 330:959, 1994. Copyright 1994, Massachusetts Medical Society.)

Efficacy: Restenosis

To evaluate the effect of c7E3 Fab on the rate of clinical restenosis (defined by an ischemic event or the need for repeat revascularization), the double-blind follow-up was extended to 6 months.[19] At 6 months, the primary end point was a composite of death, nonfatal MI, and the need for a repeat revascularization (PTCA, CABG, or both); stenting or the use of an intraaortic balloon pump was not included as an outcome after the 30-day follow-up period.[19]

As with the findings in the acute phase of the study, events were significantly reduced in patients who received the c7E3 Fab bolus-plus-infusion regimen (23%, $p = .001$) compared with the other treatment arms (Fig. 177–3). Although most acute events occurred within 48 hours, regardless of the treatment group, long-term follow-up revealed that a substantial portion of events occurred after the initial 30 days.

Table 177–2. **Effect of Abciximab on Myocardial Infarction**

Response	Total (n = 2099)	Placebo (n = 696)	Bolus (n = 695)	Bolus + Infusion (n = 708)	Dose p value
Q wave	293 (1.4%)	16 (2.3%)	7 (1.0%)	6 (0.8%)	0.020
% Reduction vs. placebo			56.3%	63.1%	
			$p = .090$	$p = .032$	
Large non–Q wave*	68 (3.2%)	28 (4.0%)	19 (2.7%)	21 (3.0%)	0.265
% Reduction vs. placebo			32.0%	26.3%	
			$p = .235$	$p = .310$	
Small non–Q wave	43 (2.0%)	16 (2.3%)	17 (2.4%)	10 (1.4%)	0.239
% Reduction vs. placebo			−6.4%	38.6%	
			$p = .862$	$p = .240$	
All myocardial infarctions†	140 (6.7%)	60 (8.6%)	43 (6.2%)	37 (5.2%)	0.011
% Reduction vs. placebo			28.2%	39.4%	
			$p = .101$	$p = .015$	

*Enzymes ≥5 × upper limit of normal.
†p Values do not match those in Table 177–1 because log-rank statistics were used in Table 177–1 and x^2 statistics were used in this table.

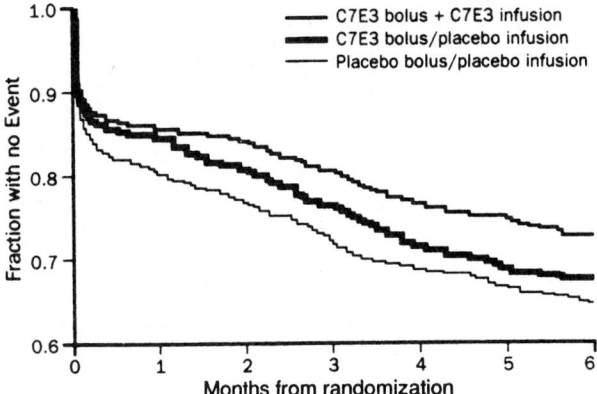

Figure 177–3. Kaplan-Meier plot of all events (death, myocardial infarction, coronary revascularization) during 6-month follow-up. (Adapted from Topol EJ, Califf RM, Weisman HF, et al: Randomised trial of coronary intervention with antibody against platelet IIb/IIIa integrin for reduction of clinical restenosis: Results at six months. Lancet 343:883, 1994. © by The Lancet Ltd., 1994.)

This observation and the stability in the restenosis rates following PTCA underline the need for an intervention that can reduce both short- and long-term complications.[19]

A subanalysis of the need for subsequent target vessel revascularization showed a 26% reduction in patients who received the c7E3 Fab bolus-plus-infusion regimen compared with patients in the other two arms (Fig. 177–4). A separate analysis of patient types showed that the composite events were significantly reduced in patients with acute coronary syndromes at baseline as well as in those with stable angina but high-risk angiographic morphology. However, the repeat revascularization rate was significantly reduced only in patients with stable angina.[19]

Adverse Events

The benefit of c7E3 Fab therapy was accompanied by an increase in the number of major bleeding events.[5]

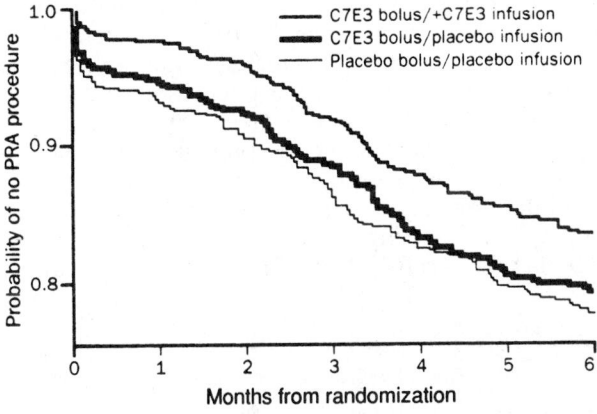

Figure 177–4. Need for subsequent revascularization of target vessel by either coronary angioplasty or coronary artery bypass surgery. Repeat revascularization was significantly ($p = .007$) reduced in the abciximab bolus-plus-infusion group. (Adapted from Topol EJ, Califf RM, Weisman HF, et al: Randomised trial of coronary intervention with antibody against platelet IIb/IIIa integrin for reduction of clinical restenosis: Results at six months. Lancet 343:883, 1994. © by The Lancet Ltd., 1994.)

However, bleeding was generally transient, manageable, and confined to the local vascular access site.

The occurrence of stroke and other major bleeding events was used to evaluate bleeding complications, classified using criteria developed by the Thrombolysis in Myocardial Infarction (TIMI) study group. Major bleeding events were defined as intracranial hemorrhage or a decrease in hemoglobin of more than 5 g/dl, and minor bleeding events were defined as spontaneous gross hematuria or hematemesis, observed blood loss with a decrease in hemoglobin of more than 3 g/dl, or, in the absence of blood loss, a decrease in hemoglobin of more than 4 g/dl. Table 177–3 presents the bleeding complications observed in the EPIC trial.[5]

Although substantial blood loss was documented, bleeding occurred primarily at the femoral puncture site. There was no significant difference in nadir hematocrits or the rate of life-threatening complications among the patient groups, and the need for surgical intervention was not increased in c7E3 Fab–treated patients.[5] Adverse events other than bleeding and associated consequences were infrequent (Table 177–4).[5]

Clinical Guidelines for c7E3 Fab Therapy

As the experience with c7E3 Fab therapy increases, a number of simple guidelines that can be incorporated into the routine practice of PTCA have evolved to maximize clinical outcome and minimize the risk for adverse effects.

Patient Selection

Many patients at high risk for ischemic complications after PTCA, including those with unstable angina, evolving MI, and clinical or angiographic characteristics indicating high risk, are good candidates for c7E3 Fab therapy. c7E3 Fab is contraindicated in patients with active internal bleeding; a history of cerebrovascular accident within 2 years, major surgery, or gastrointestinal/genitourinary bleeding within 6 weeks;

Table 177–3. **Bleeding Complications in the EPIC Trial**

	Placebo (n = 696)	Bolus (n = 695)	Bolus + Infusion (n = 708)
Major bleeding	46 (8%)*	76 (11%)	99 (14%)*
Site of major bleeding			
Groin	20	49	58
Need for surgical repair	7 (1.0%)	16 (2.3%)	6 (0.8%)
Retroperitoneal	3	3	12
Coronary artery†	23	21	26
Intracranial	2	1	3
Hematemesis	0	5	11
Transfusions			
Red cells	49 (7%)	92 (13%)	109 (15%)
Platelets	18 (3%)	29 (4%)	39 (6%)

*$p = .001$ placebo vs. bolus + infusion group.
†Bleeding during coronary artery bypass graft surgery.

Table 177–4. **Overall Adverse Events Related to Abciximab Therapy**

	Total (n = 2038)	Placebo (n = 681)	Bolus (n = 679)	Bolus + Infusion (n = 678)
Hypotension	119 (5.8%)	21 (3.1%)	46 (6.8%)	52 (7.7%)
Nausea	84 (4.1%)	23 (3.4%)	21 (3.1%)	40 (5.9%)
Vomiting	63 (3.1%)	18 (2.6%)	18 (2.7%)	27 (4.0%)
Thrombocytopenia	27 (1.3%)	3 (0.4%)	8 (1.2%)	16 (2.4%)
Hematoma	27 (1.3%)	7 (1.0%)	11 (1.6%)	9 (1.3%)
Bradycardia	25 (1.2%)	3 (0.4%)	12 (1.8%)	10 (1.5%)
Fever	23 (1.1%)	6 (0.9%)	7 (1.0%)	10 (1.5%)
Vascular disorder	21 (1.0%)	4 (0.6%)	12 (1.8%)	5 (0.7%)

intracranial or intraspinal surgery or trauma; intracranial neoplasm; arteriovenous malformation or aneurysm; known bleeding disorders or severe uncontrolled hypertension; a history of vasculitis or administration of oral anticoagulants within 7 days; or thrombocytopenia. Caution should be employed when c7E3 Fab is used with other drugs affecting hemostasis.[74]

Anticoagulation

Bleeding in patients treated with c7E3 Fab has been correlated with three factors: age greater than 65 years, female sex, and the extent of heparin anticoagulation. Thus, it seemed prudent to examine the effect of heparin dosing in patients who received c7E3 Fab therapy. Patients enrolled in the EPIC study received intravenously administered heparin in an initial bolus of 10,000 to 12,000 U plus incremental bolus doses of up to 3000 U at 15-minute intervals to maintain an activated clotting time (ACT) of between 300 and 350 seconds.[5] This dosage was given regardless of the patient's weight. Analysis of the correlation between weight and bleeding showed that lighter patients who received c7E3 Fab experienced more bleeding episodes. In fact, in patients who weighed less than 76.8 kg, the rate of bleeding was 21% in c7E3 Fab–treated patients, compared with 7% of placebo-treated patients. In the heaviest patients (weight >89.9 kg), however, the incidence of bleeding was comparable between groups (9% in c7E3 Fab–treated patients versus 6% in the placebo group).[5]

Because the results of the EPIC trial suggested that weight was inversely related to the number of bleeding episodes, it is likely that future regimens including c7E3 Fab would employ adjusted dosages of antithrombotic drugs.[5] During PTCA, the ACT should be regularly monitored and the dosage of heparin should be adjusted to achieve an ACT of 300 to 350 seconds during the procedure.[5]

Procedural Modifications: Guidelines for Vascular Sheath Management

A number of modifications to the practice of PTCA may be used to minimize the risk of bleeding complications. To establish vascular access, a technique that punctures only the anterior wall reduces the number of puncture wounds, thereby decreasing the potential for bleeding complications. If bleeding from the access site is unstoppable with mild pressure, a sheath of the next largest size should be tried. A venous sheath should be used only when clinically indicated, as in the case of patients who require a temporary pacemaker or administration of pressors or fluids to maintain blood pressure. In the EPIC trial, most bleeding episodes occurred secondary to CABG or at the vascular access site in the groin. Prompt removal of the vascular sheath may diminish the risk for bleeding by reducing the risk for wound-site injury.[75]

Ongoing Clinical Investigations

Two additional large-scale studies are currently underway. These are phase II and phase III trials designed to evaluate the clinical outcome of angioplasty in patients treated with c7E3 Fab plus either standard weight-adjusted heparin or low-dose weight-adjusted heparin. The results of the EPIC trial make it seem likely that weight adjustment and/or reduction of the heparin dose will increase the safety profile of c7E3 Fab while maintaining clinical efficacy after PTCA.

Drug Interactions

c7E3 Fab has been studied in combination with medications commonly used in the treatment of angina, MI, and hypertension to evaluate the risk for possible interactions. No adverse drug interactions have been observed when c7E3 Fab was given to patients receiving warfarin, β-adrenergic receptor blockers, calcium antagonists, angiotensin-converting enzyme inhibitors, intravenously and orally administered nitrates, and aspirin. Bleeding times were increased in some patients who received both c7E3 Fab and heparin.[40]

Use of Thrombolytics, Anticoagulants, and Other Antiplatelet Agents

c7E3 Fab should be used with caution in patients receiving other agents that affect hemostasis, such as heparin, orally administered anticoagulants, thrombolytics, and antiplatelet agents other than aspirin. Early data indicate that c7E3 Fab may be beneficial in certain subsets of patients receiving thrombolytic agents; the results of these studies are reviewed later.

If symptoms do not resolve after c7E3 Fab therapy, the procedure of choice is repeat PTCA to salvage the situation. If this is not successful, and if the angiogram suggests thrombosis, administering adjunctive thrombolytic therapy via the intracoronary route could be considered. However, a systemic lytic state should be avoided.[74]

Dosage and Administration

c7E3 Fab is intended as an adjunct to standard heparin and aspirin therapy. When given as a single dose, the antiaggregatory effect of c7E3 Fab lasts for up to 12 hours.[29] The results of the EPIC trial indicated that the single-dose regimen alone was not accompanied by a significant reduction in ischemic events.[5, 18] However, use of an intravenous 0.25 mg/kg bolus followed by a 10 µg/min continuous intravenous infusion for 12 hours was shown to be effective; this is the currently recommended regimen for c7E3 Fab dosing.[5]

SOCIOECONOMIC CONSIDERATIONS

Cost containment is a major consideration today when evaluating new therapeutic options. To understand the impact of a new therapy that is designed to prevent complications, it follows that it is important to understand the economic consequences of the complications themselves. Two recent studies evaluating the cost impact of abrupt closure and restenosis are reviewed in the following sections to provide a framework for discussing the economic substudy conducted during the EPIC trial of c7E3 Fab.[75, 76]

Costs of Abrupt Closure

Bendan et al.[75] conducted a prospective study of 545 patients to evaluate the costs associated with abrupt closure after balloon angioplasty and directional atherectomy. Not surprisingly, abrupt closure was associated with higher costs compared to no post-PTCA complications ($24,042 and $11,017, respectively), and the average length of hospital stay was significantly longer in patients with abrupt closure (9 and 5 days, respectively). In those who experienced abrupt closure, increased costs were attributed to emergency coronary bypass surgery (31%) and MI (41%).[75]

Costs of Restenosis

To determine the impact of restenosis, Hillegass et al.[77] evaluated the need for bypass surgery, repeat PTCA, and more intensive medical therapy within 1 year of PTCA. They found that the break-even cost of a new therapy was directly correlated with the degree to which therapy reduced the risk for restenosis. According to their calculations, an intervention that reduced the relative risk of restenosis by 20% would reduce the overall costs of the procedure if it were priced at less than $1300 per patient treated. They speculated that "highly effective" new interventions would reduce overall costs, even at a cost of $3000 to $6000 per patient treated.[76]

EQOL Evaluation of Economic Benefits of c7E3 Fab

Potential economic benefit of c7E3 Fab bolus-plus-infusion therapy was demonstrated in clinical trials by a decreased incidence of ischemic events after PTCA in high-risk patients[5] and the reduced occurrence of MI and need for revascularization procedures (32% reduction in MI, $p = .018$ versus placebo; 22.8% reduction in PTCA or CABG, $p = .004$ versus placebo).[5] An economic subanalysis of the EPIC trial, called EQOL, included an evaluation of direct costs and resource consumption in both the acute and long-term phases of the study.[40]

Overall, EQOL showed that the mean total baseline hospital costs in c7E3 Fab–treated patients were similar to those in the placebo group ($11,198 and $11,259, respectively).[41] In the c7E3 Fab group, the savings due to fewer acute complications were offset by costs associated with bleeding episodes. However, improved periprocedural management (see earlier section, Clinical Guidelines for c7E3 Fab Therapy) to prevent or minimize bleeding should result in an additional reduction in the overall costs associated with c7E3 Fab therapy, leading to an immediate cost reduction.[40]

The evaluation of long-term costs from restenosis included evaluation of follow-up hospitalizations. Hospitalization, primarily attributable to cardiac revascularization, was reported in 26% of the c7E3 Fab group versus 32% of placebo-treated patients. The difference in average hospital costs was significant: $2909 for c7E3 Fab–treated patients and $3665 ($p <.01$) for controls.[40]

Although these preliminary data suggest that c7E3 Fab therapy will be cost-effective, additional information is required to evaluate the costs associated with its use in clinical practice.[40]

INVESTIGATIONAL USES OF c7E3 FAB

In addition to its use as adjunctive therapy for PTCA, c7E3 Fab has also undergone preliminary investigation in patients with refractory unstable angina and as combination therapy with thrombolytic agents.[60, 62, 64–66, 68, 70–72] Early studies showed that c7E3 Fab had an inhibitory effect on *in vivo* platelet thrombus formation and relieved angina in patients with unstable angina.[29, 60] Subsequently, Simoons et al.[68] demonstrated that c7E3 Fab facilitated PTCA and helped to reduce MI in a group of 60 patients with refractory unstable angina. Equally promising results have been attained in studies evaluating the combination of c7E3 Fab with thrombolytic agents.[62, 64, 65, 70–72] In both animals and humans, c7E3 Fab reduced or prevented reocclusion after thrombolysis.[62, 64, 65, 70–72] The studies in human subjects indicate that inhibition of platelet aggregation after thrombolysis warrants further investigation.[62, 64, 65, 70–72]

CONCLUSIONS

Clinical data demonstrate the beneficial effect of sustained blockade of the GPIIb/IIIa receptor in high-risk patients undergoing PTCA.[5, 19] After vessel dilatation, the c7E3 Fab bolus-plus-infusion regimen preserves coronary flow by preventing acute thrombotic closure, ultimately reducing the need for repeat procedures as well as the incidence of MI and death.[5, 19]

The binding of c7E3 Fab to GPIIb/IIIa receptors is both dose- and time-dependent; its antiaggregatory effects diminish over time and soon revert to baseline.[5, 42] It is not surprising, therefore, that the administration of a single bolus dose did not produce a significant reduction in ischemic complications.[5, 19] However, a bolus of 0.25 mg/kg plus a 10-μg/min infusion for 12 hours significantly improves clinical outcomes and reduces the need for repeat revascularization procedures.[5]

Although c7E3 Fab therapy is generally well tolerated, an increase in bleeding events within the first 36 hours constituted the major adverse consequence.[5] However, the bleeding was transient and manageable, usually occurred at the vascular access site, and was not associated with long-term consequences.[5, 19] Adherence to the clinical guidelines discussed in this chapter should minimize the risk of bleeding.

Acute ischemic complications account for most of the morbidity and mortality associated with PTCA. Inasmuch as c7E3 Fab therapy significantly reduces the incidence of these complications, it seems likely that the overall risk/benefit ratio of c7E3 Fab therapy will be highly favorable.

REFERENCES

1. Landau C, Lange RA, Hillis DL: Percutaneous transluminal coronary angioplasty. N Engl J Med 330:981, 1994.
2. Scott NA, Weintraub WS, Carlin SF, et al: Recent changes in the management and outcome of acute closure after percutaneous transluminal coronary angioplasty. Am J Cardiol 71:1159, 1993.
3. de Feyter P, van den Brand M, Jaarman GJ, et al: Acute coronary occlusion during and after percutaneous transluminal coronary angioplasty: Frequency, prediction, clinical course, management, and follow-up. Circulation 83:927, 1991.
4. Califf RM, Ohman M, Fried DJ, et al: Restenosis: The clinical issues. In Topol EJ (ed): Textbook of Interventional Cardiology. Philadelphia: WB Saunders, 1990, pp 363–394.
5. EPIC Investigators: Use of a monoclonal antibody directed against the platelet glycoprotein IIb/IIIa receptor in high-risk coronary angioplasty. N Engl J Med 330:956, 1994.
6. Satler LF, Leon MB, Kent KM, et al: Strategies for acute occlusion after coronary angioplasty. J Am Coll Cardiol 19:936, 1992.
7. Lincoff AM, Popma JJ, Ellis SG, et al: Abrupt vessel closure complicating coronary angioplasty: Clinical angiographic and therapeutic profile. J Am Coll Cardiol 19:926, 1992.
8. Gaul G, Hollman J, Simpfendorfer C, et al: Acute occlusion in multiple lesion coronary angioplasty: Frequency and management. J Am Coll Cardiol 13:283, 1989.
9. Ellis SG, Roubin GS, King SB III, et al: Angiographic and clinical predictors of acute closure after native vessel coronary angioplasty. Circulation 77:372, 1988.
10. Detre KM, Holmes DR Jr, Holubkov R, et al: Incidence and consequences of periprocedural occlusion: The 1985–1986 National Heart, Lung, and Blood Institute Percutaneous Transluminal Coronary Angioplasty Registry. Circulation 82:739, 1990.
11. Kahn JK, Rutherford BD, McConahay DR, et al: Outcome following emergency coronary artery bypass grafting for failed elective balloon coronary angioplasty in patients with prior coronary bypass. Am J Cardiol 66:285, 1990.
12. Holmes DR Jr, Holubkov R, Vlietstra RE, et al: Comparison of complications during percutaneous transluminal coronary angioplasty from 1977 to 1981 and from 1985 to 1986: The National Heart, Lung, and Blood Institute Percutaneous Transluminal Coronary Angioplasty Registry. J Am Coll Cardiol 12:1149, 1988.
13. Leimgruber PP, Roubin GS, Hollman J, et al: Restenosis after successful coronary angioplasty in patients with single vessel disease. Circulation 73:710, 1986.
14. Levine S, Ewels CJ, Rosing DR, et al: Coronary angioplasty: Clinical and angiographic follow-up. Am J Cardiol 55:673, 1985.
15. Holmes DR, Vlietstra RE, Smith HC, et al: Restenosis after percutaneous transluminal coronary angioplasty (PTCA): A report from the PTCA Registry of the National Heart, Lung, and Blood Institute. Am J Cardiol 53:77c, 1984.
16. Mabin TA, Holmes DR, Smith HC, et al: Follow-up clinical results in patients undergoing percutaneous transluminal coronary angioplasty. Circulation 71:754, 1985.
17. Nobuyoshi M, Kimura T, Ohishi H, et al: Restenosis after percutaneous transluminal coronary angioplasty: Pathologic observations in 20 patients. J Am Coll Cardiol 17:433, 1991.
18. Coller BS: Antiplatelet agents in the prevention and therapy of thrombosis. Annu Rev Med 43:171, 1992.
19. Topol EJ, Califf RM, Weisman HF, et al: Randomised trial of coronary intervention with antibody against platelet IIb/IIIa integrin for reduction of clinical restenosis: results at six months. Lancet 343:881, 1994.
20. Barnathan ES, Schwartz JS, Taylor L, et al: Aspirin and dipyridamole in the prevention of acute coronary thrombosis complicating coronary angioplasty. Circulation 76:125, 1987.
21. Nichols AJ, Ruffolo RR Jr, Huffman WF, et al: Development of GPIIb/IIIa antagonists as antithrombotic drugs. Trends Pharmacol Sci 13:413, 1992.
22. Mustard JF, Kinlough-Rathbone RL, Packham MA, et al: Comparison of fibrinogen association with normal and thrombasthenic platelets on exposure to ADP or chymotrypsin. Blood 54:987, 1979.
23. Phillips DR, Charo IF, Scarborough RM: GPIIb-IIIa: the responsive integrin. Cell 65:359, 1991.
24. Niiya K, Hodson E, Baer R, et al: Increased surface expression of the membrane glycoprotein IIb/IIIa complex induced by platelet activation: Relationship to the binding of fibrinogen and platelet aggregation. Blood 70:475, 1987.
25. Kieffer N, Phillips DR: Platelet membrane glycoproteins: functions in cellular interactions. Annu Rev Cell Biol 6:329, 1990.
26. Plow EF, Ginsberg MH: Cellular adhesion: GPIIb/IIIa as a prototypic adhesion receptor. In Coller BS (ed): Progress in Hemostasis and Thrombosis. Philadelphia: WB Saunders, 1989, pp 117–156.
27. Smyth SS, Joneckis CC, Parise LV: Regulation of vascular integrins. Blood 81:2827, 1993.
28. Coller BS: Inhibitors of the platelet glycoprotein IIb/IIIa receptor as conjunctive therapy for coronary artery thrombolysis. Coronary Artery Dis 3:1016, 1992.
29. Ellis SG, Bates ER, Schaible T, et al: Prospects for the use of antagonists to the platelet glycoprotein IIb/IIIa receptor to prevent postangioplasty restenosis and thrombosis. J Am Coll Cardiol 17:89b, 1991.
30. Jang I-K, Fuster V, Gold HK: Antiplatelets. Coronary Artery Dis 3:1092, 1992.
31. Coller BS, Scudder LE, Beer J, et al: Monoclonal antibodies to platelet glycoprotein IIb/IIIa as antithrombotic agents. Ann N Y Acad Sci 614:193, 1991.
32. Rote WE, Mu D-X, Bates ER, et al: Prevention of rethrombosis after coronary thrombolysis in a chronic canine model. I: Adjunctive therapy with monoclonal antibody 7E3 F(ab')$_2$ fragment. J Cardiovasc Pharmacol 23:194, 1994.

33. Rote WE, Nedelman MS, Mu D-X, et al: Chimeric 7E3 prevents carotid artery thrombosis in cynomolgus monkeys. Stroke 25:1223, 1994.

34. Rote WE, Mu D-X, Bates ER, et al: Prevention of rethrombosis after coronary thrombolysis in a chronic canine model. II: Adjunctive therapy with r-hirudin. J Cardiovasc Pharmacol 23:203, 1994.

35. Baumgartner HR: The role of blood flow in platelet adhesion, fibrin deposition and formation of mural thrombi. Microvacs Res 5:167, 1973.

36. Groves HM, Kinlough-Rathbone RL, Richardson M, et al: Platelet interaction with damaged rabbit aorta. Lab Invest 40:194, 1979.

37. Groves HM, Kinlough-Rathbone RL, Mustard JF: Development of nonthrombogenicity of injured rabbit aortas despite inhibition of platelet adherence. Arteriosclerosis 6:189, 1986.

38. Steele PM, Chesebro JH, Stanson AW, et al: Balloon angioplasty: Natural history of the pathophysiological response to injury in a pig model. Circ Res 57:105, 1985.

39. Azrin MA: The use of antibodies in clinical cardiology. Am Heart J 124:753, 1992.

40. Centocor Corporation, data on file, 1994.

41. Jordan RE, Knight DM, Wagner C, et al: A dramatic reduction in the immunogenicity of the anti-GPIIb/IIIa monoclonal antibody, 7E3 Fab, by humanization of the murine constant domains. Circulation 86(Suppl 1):411a, 1992.

42. Ellis SG, Tcheng JE, Navetta FI, et al: Safety and antiplatelet effect of murine monoclonal antibody 7E3 Fab directed against platelet glycoprotein IIb/IIIa in patients undergoing elective coronary angioplasty. Coron Artery Dis 4:167, 1993.

43. Coller BS, Scudder LE: Inhibition of dog platelet function by in vivo infusion of F(ab')$_2$ fragments of a monoclonal antibody to the platelet glycoprotein IIb/IIIa receptor. Blood 66:1456, 1985.

44. Coller BS, Folts JD, Smith SR, et al: Abolition of in vivo platelet thrombus formation in primates with monoclonal antibodies to the platelet GPIIb/IIIa receptor: correlation with bleeding time, platelet aggregation, and blockade of GPIIb/IIIa receptors. Circulation 80:1766, 1989.

45. Coller BS, Peerscke EI, Scudder LE, et al: A murine monoclonal antibody that completely blocks the binding of fibrinogen to platelets produces a thrombasthenic-like state in normal platelets and binds to glycoproteins IIb and/or IIIa. J Clin Invest 72:325, 1983.

46. Coller BS, Folts JD, Scudder LE, et al: Antithrombotic effect of a monoclonal antibody to the platelet glycoprotein IIb/IIIa receptor in an experimental animal model. Blood 68:783, 1986.

47. Coller BS, Scudder LE, Berger HJ, et al: Inhibition of human platelet function in vivo with a monoclonal antibody: With observations on the newly dead as experimental subjects. Ann Intern Med 109:635, 1988.

48. Rote W, Nedelman MA, Mu D-X, et al: Efficacy of chimeric Fab fragment 7E3 versus aspirin and heparin for the prevention of carotid thrombosis in a non-human primate [abstract]. J Am Coll Cardiol 21:109a, 1993.

49. Anderson HV, Revana M, Rosales O, et al: Intravenous administration of monoclonal antibody to the platelet GPIIb/IIIa receptor to treat abrupt closure during coronary angioplasty. Am J Cardiol 69:1373, 1992.

50. Anderson HV, Kirkeeide RL, Krishnaswami A, et al: Cyclic flow variations after coronary angioplasty in humans: Clinical and angiographic characteristics and elimination with 7E3 monoclonal antiplatelet antibody. J Am Coll Cardiol 23:1031, 1994.

51. Bates ER, Walsh DG, Mu D-X, et al: Sustained inhibition of the vessel wall-platelet interaction after deep coronary artery injury by temporary inhibition of the platelet glycoprotein IIb/IIIa receptor. Coronary Artery Dis 3:67, 1992.

52. Bates ER, McGillem MJ, Mickelson JK, et al: A monoclonal antibody against the platelet glycoprotein IIb/IIIa receptor complex prevents platelet aggregation and thrombosis in a canine model of coronary angioplasty. Circulation 84:2463, 1991.

53. Bernardi MM, Califf RM, Kleiman N, et al: Prolonged bleeding times do not predict hemorrhagic events in patients receiving the 7E3 glycoprotein IIb/IIIa platelet antibody [abstract]. Circulation 86(Suppl 1):260, 1992.

54. Bhattacharya S, Weisman HF, Morris KG, et al: Chimeric (humanised) monoclonal antiplatelet antibody 7E3 produces prolonged dose-dependent inhibition of platelet function [abstract]. Clin Res 39:196, 1991.

55. Cavagnaro J, Serabian MA, Shealy DJ, et al: Pharmacokinetic analysis of murine monoclonal antibody 7E3 F(Ab')$_2$ in monkeys [abstract]. Blood 70(Suppl 1):349A, 1987.

56. Cavagnaro J, Serabian MA, Coller BS, et al: Long-term toxicologic evaluation of anti-platelet monoclonal antibody 7E3 F(Ab')$_2$ in monkeys [abstract]. Blood 70(Suppl 1):337A, 1987.

57. Coller BS: A new murine monoclonal antibody reports on activation-dependent change in the conformation and/or microenvironment of the platelet glycoprotein IIb/IIIa complex. J Clin Invest 76:101, 1985.

58. Coller BS, Peerschke EI, Seligsohn U, et al: Studies on the binding of an autoimmune and two murine monoclonal antibodies to the platelet glycoprotein IIb/IIIa complex receptor [abstract]. J Lab Clin Med 107:384, 1986.

59. Gold HK, Coller BS, Yasuda T, et al: Rapid and sustained coronary artery recanalization with combined bolus injection of recombinant tissue-type plasminogen activator and monoclonal antiplatelet GPIIb/IIIa antibody in a canine preparation. Circulation 77:670, 1988.

60. Gold HK, Gimple LW, Yasuda T, et al: Pharmacodynamic study of F(ab')$_2$ fragments of murine monoclonal antibody 7E3 directed against human platelet glycoprotein IIb/IIIa in patients with unstable angina pectoris. J Clin Invest 86:651, 1990.

61. Gold HK, Coller B, Yasuda T, et al: A monoclonal antibody to the platelet receptor GPIIb/IIIa (7E3) accelerates thrombolysis with recombinant tissue-type plasminogen activator (rt-PA) and prevents coronary reocclusion [abstract]. Circulation 77(Suppl 4):377, 1988.

62. Iuliucci JD, Treacy G, Cornell S, et al: Potent anti-thrombotic activity and safety of antiplatelet monoclonal antibody 7E3 Fab combined with thrombolytic and anticoagulant drugs [abstract]. Circulation 82(Suppl 3):602, 1990.

63. Jordan R, Wagner C, McAleer MF, et al: Evaluation of the potency and immunogenicity of 7E3 F(ab')$_2$ and Fab fragments in monkeys [abstract]. Circulation 82(Suppl 3):661, 1990.

64. Kleiman NS, Ohman EM, Calif RM, et al: Profound inhibition of platelet aggregation with monoclonal antibody 7E3 Fab after thrombolytic therapy. Results of the thrombolysis and angioplasty in myocardial infarction (TAMI) 8 pilot study. J Am Coll Cardiol 22:381, 1993.

65. Kohmura C, Gold HK, Yasuda T, et al: A novel chimeric human/murine GPIIb/IIIa antiplatelet antibody enhances thrombolysis in the baboon [abstract]. J Am Coll Cardiol 21:85a, 1993.

66. Mickelson JK, Simpson PJ, Cronin M, et al: Antiplatelet antibody [7E3 F(ab')$_2$] prevents rethrombosis after recombinant tissue-type plasminogen activator-induced coronary artery thrombolysis in a canine model. Circulation 81:617, 1990.

67. Wagner CL, Weisman HF, Gray JW, et al: Molecular pharmacology of chimeric 7E3 monoclonal Fab fragment binding to platelet GPIIb/IIIa receptors. Arteriosler Thromb 11:1594a, 1991.

68. Simoons ML, Jan de Boer M, van den Brand MJBM, et al: Randomized trial of a GPIIb/IIIa platelet receptor blocker in refractory unstable angina. Circulation 89:596, 1994.

69. Tcheng JE, Kleiman NS, Miller MJ, et al: Chimeric antiplatelet GPIIb/IIIa receptor antibody (C-7E3) in elective PTCA: Safety and platelet function inhibition [abstract]. Circulation 84:590, 1991.

70. Yasuda T, Gold HK, Fallon J, et al: Monoclonal antibody against the platelet GP IIb/IIIa receptor prevents coronary artery reocclusion following reperfusion with recombinant tissue-type plasminogen activator in dogs. J Clin Invest 81:1284, 1988.

71. Yasuda T, Gold HK, Yaoita H, et al: Comparative effects of aspirin, a synthetic thrombin inhibitor and a monoclonal antiplatelet glycoprotein IIb/IIIa antibody on coronary artery reperfusion, reocclusion, and bleeding with recombinant tissue-type plasminogen activator in a canine preparation. J Am Coll Cardiol 16:714, 1990.

72. Yasuda T, Gold HK, Leinbach RC, et al: Lysis of plasminogen activator-resistant platelet-rich coronary artery thrombus with combined bolus injection of recombinant tissue-type plasminogen activator and antiplatelet GPIIb/IIIa antibody. J Am Coll Cardiol 16:1728, 1990.

73. Mickelson JK, Simpson PJ, Lucchesi BR: Antiplatelet monoclonal F(ab')2 antibody directed against the platelet GPIIb/IIIa receptor complex prevents coronary artery thrombosis in the canine heart. J Mol Cell Cardiol 21:393, 1989.
74. Abciximab. Manufacturer's prescribing information.
75. Bendan LG, Holmes DR, Davidson-Ray L, et al: Economic impact of abrupt closure following percutaneous intervention: The CAVEAT experience [abstract]. J Am Coll Cardiol 23:434a, 1994.
76. Hillegass WB, Peterson ED, Jollis JG: What cost of therapies to reduce restenosis is justified? Circulation 88:1, 1993.

CHAPTER 178

Nicorandil

Henry Purcell, M.B., Deven J. Patel, M.B.B.S., M.R.C.P., David Mulcahy, M.D., and Kim Fox, M.D.

The relief of chest discomfort remains one of the primary objectives in the management of patients with angina pectoris. β-Blockers, calcium antagonists, and nitrates are indicated and widely used for this purpose, but these agents all have limitations and are therefore not a complete answer to the problem.[1] There is a need to augment and perhaps even replace these conventional antianginal agents, and a number of alternative compounds are currently under clinical investigation. Among these are drugs that modulate potassium (K^+) channel activity in cell membranes, in particular the potassium channel opener nicorandil.

Potassium channels are ubiquitous and diverse. Of these, the adenosine triphosphate (ATP)–sensitive channels have been the focus of much recent attention. Activation of these channels is inhibited by physiologic levels of intracellular ATP, and they open only when ATP levels fall below a critical concentration. Thus, activation of these channels in the heart may provide endogenous cardioprotection under conditions in which cardiac metabolism is compromised, as would occur during myocardial ischemia.[2] Exogenous agents, such as drugs, also modulate K^+-ATP channel activity; sulphonylureas (e.g., glibenclamide) block these channels and reduce K^+ ion loss, and therefore have potential antiarrhythmic properties. Glibenclamide has been shown to significantly reduce ventricular ectopy and nonsustained ventricular tachycardia, whereas K^+ channel openers, such as nicorandil, and older drugs like diazoxide and minoxidil, which enhance K^+ ion loss, could aggravate ischemic injury.[3] Animal studies that we reviewed suggest the opposite, however, that nicorandil reduces myocardial stunning and infarct size. By enhancing K^+ efflux during myocardial repolarization, shortening the action potential and effective refractory period, K^+ channel openers may be proarrhythmic.[4] Although this potential for profibrillatory activity has been demonstrated in animal models,[5] this has not been observed in humans.[6] Conversely, K^+ channel openers may be regarded as reinforcing the intrinsic propensity of the cardiomyocyte to overcome ischemic stress, in that they enhance the endogenous low ATP activation of K^+ channels and thus afford a degree of cardioprotection, possibly through ischemic preconditioning.[7]

A variety of K^+ activators have been characterized,[8] but most clinical experience in the treatment of angina pectoris has been acquired with nicorandil,[9] which was originally developed in Japan, where it has been in clinical use for several years. More recently, this agent has been studied in the United States and Europe, where it will soon be available.

PHARMACOLOGY

Nicorandil is a nicotinamide nitrate ester. The nitrate moiety in its chemical structure may in part contribute to the antiischemic action, but it is different from conventional nitrates and appears to have a dual mechanism of action, functioning as a hybrid between a nitrate and a K^+ channel activator.[10] Nicorandil induces vascular smooth muscle relaxation by increasing intracellular cyclic guanosine monophosphate (cGMP) levels. Potassium channel opening hyperpolarizes vascular cell membranes, causing calcium (Ca^{2+}) ion channels to close and a consequent reduction in intracellular Ca^{2+} concentration (i.e., indirect calcium antagonism) that results in further smooth muscle relaxation and vasodilation.[11] These effects of vascular smooth muscle relaxation have been demonstrated at therapeutic doses of nicorandil. The effects of nicorandil on myocardial tissue depend on the presence of ischemia. In nonischemic myocardium, nicorandil at therapeutic doses has no negative inotropic effect,[11] but at much higher concentrations, these ATP-sensitive K^+ channels can be activated, leading to negative inotropy. In ischemic myocardial cells, shortening of the action potential is the main effect owing to K^+ efflux aggravated by reduced extracellular washout.

PHARMACOKINETICS

Pharmacokinetics of nicorandil have been determined from studies in human volunteers and patients.[12, 13] The drug is rapidly absorbed from the gut, with peak plasma concentrations occurring after 30 to 60 minutes, and it is not significantly affected by food. Plasma concentration reaches steady state after 4 days of regular dosing. Maximal concentration and area under the curve of the plasma concentration time curve are linearly related in a dose range of 5 to 40 mg. Nicorandil does not undergo significant hepatic first-pass metabolism. Absolute bioavailability after oral administration is between 75% and 80%. The drug is weakly bound to plasma protein, with more than 75% remaining unbound in the systemic circulation. The apparent volume of distribution is approximately 1.4 L/kg body weight, with distribution occurring within 20 minutes after intravenous dosing. Nicorandil is almost entirely metabolized in the liver, and it is excreted mainly as metabolites in urine, with only approximately 1% of the initial dose being excreted unchanged. Elimination is biphasic, consisting of a rapid phase with an elimination half-life of 1 hour involving some 96% of the dose and 85% to 90% of its metabolites. This is followed by a slower phase, giving an overall half-life of 12 hours. This latter phase may be due to the slow release of nicorandil from vascular endothelium. No significant drug interactions are known to occur.

EFFECTS ON PATHOPHYSIOLOGY
Effects on Hemodynamics

The hemodynamic performance of nicorandil has been reviewed by Suryapranata.[14] Unlike conventional nitrates, nicorandil reduces both preload and afterload in a dose-dependent fashion. It increases coronary blood flow and is not negatively inotropic. These effects occur without significant increases in heart rate. In patients with ischemic heart disease, nicorandil dilates both stenotic and nonstenotic coronary arteries. Wolf et al.[15] have studied the effects of a 12-hour infusion of nicorandil in 21 healthy volunteers, using a placebo-controlled, crossover design. Compared with placebo, nicorandil caused a blood pressure fall in the standing position and a nonsignificant increase in heart rate; cardiac output increased slightly at lower doses. These hemodynamic changes correlated poorly with plasma nicorandil concentrations. Total doses, shown in an earlier study to be well tolerated after bolus injections, were poorly tolerated when extended over 12 hours, with headaches reflecting the duration of nicorandil exposure with no evidence of a tolerance phenomenon. Belz et al.[16] have shown that a single sublingual dose of nicorandil (60 mg) produced an equivalent preload reduction compared with isosorbide dinitrate (ISDN) (20 mg SL), but greater afterload reduction. Peak effect of nicorandil was at 60 minutes and was sustained after 4 hours, by which time the hemodynamic effects in the ISDN group had almost completely disappeared. A further study[17] showed that nicorandil (15, 30, 60 mg SL) increased heart rate and produced dose-dependent reductions in peripheral resistance, whereas ISDN (5 mg) produced less intense effects.

Kobayashi et al.[18] compared the hemodynamic effects of nicorandil 2 mg IV, nitroglycerin (GTN) 0.3 mg SL, nifedipine 10 mg SL, and propranolol 0.1 mg/kg IV in 41 patients with ischemic heart disease. Nicorandil decreased arterial pressure, cardiac output (CO), and pulmonary artery pressure without changing heart rate. Resting coronary sinus flow (CSF) was increased by nicorandil and nifedipine, with nicorandil showing the highest CSF/CO ratio and a greater reduction in coronary resistance. Nicorandil did not, however, alter CSF during rapid atrial pacing. Myocardial norepinephrine release was increased by nitroglycerin and nifedipine, but not by nicorandil and propranolol. Nicorandil also produced a reduction in preload and afterload, and, in contrast with nitroglycerin and nifedipine, it did not cause a reflex increase in heart rate or myocardial sympathetic activation.

Coltart and Signy[19] have confirmed the reduction in preload using nicorandil 40 mg SL and PO, in a study of 15 patients undergoing cardiac catheterization for investigation of chest pain. Afterload was also reduced, and total peripheral resistance was maximally lowered at 30 minutes.

Nicorandil has also been studied in patients with chronic congestive heart failure. Cohen Solal et al.[20] investigated the magnitude and time course of the acute hemodynamic effects of a single oral dose of nicorandil, 40 to 80 mg, in 11 patients with severe heart failure (New York Heart Association [NYHA] class III or IV).[20] Maximum hemodynamic changes were seen 30 minutes after dosing and persisted for 3 hours. Pulmonary wedge pressure, mean arterial pressure, and diastolic blood pressure all were significantly reduced by nicorandil, with a nonsignificant decrease in systolic blood pressure. Nicorandil also caused a 55% increase in cardiac index by 30 minutes, entirely as a result of an increase in stroke volume, because heart rate did not change significantly. The calculated systemic vascular resistance index decreased by 36%. Higher doses of nicorandil than those used in patients with myocardial ischemia were required to achieve these effects, and nicorandil 40 mg had only a weak action. These higher doses were well tolerated by patients in the supine position, but the authors urge caution when using such doses in ambulant patients, for fear of inducing hypotension. Other workers have also shown a dose-related, but short lived, improvement in cardiac function in heart failure patients treated with nicorandil.[21] Further investigation of nicorandil in this indication is warranted, as the drug does appear to have a useful role in unloading the failing heart. Issues relating to tolerance of nicorandil are addressed later.

Effects on Ventricular Function

Silke et al.[22] have studied the effects of nicorandil on left ventricular hemodynamics at rest and during exercise-induced angina pectoris. Nicorandil 20 mg was compared with placebo in a double-blind study of 20 patients with coronary artery disease. At rest, nicorandil reduced systolic and diastolic systemic arterial blood pressure without changing heart rate, cardiac output, or stroke volume indices. Pulmonary artery wedge pressure was also reduced without change in cardiac contractility. On exercise, nicorandil reduced mean arterial pressure and left ventricular filling pressure without altering cardiac stroke volume indices or heart rate. The effects of sublingual nicorandil 5 mg were investigated in pacing-induced ischemia in 11 patients with coronary artery disease.[23] The drug favorably modified both the symptomatic and hemodynamic responses to transient ischemia.

These effects were mainly due to a reduction of preload and to an improvement of regional function of the ischemic myocardium.

Effects on Electrophysiology

The electrophysiologic effects of K[+] opener drugs have been described earlier. There is limited information on the electrophysiologic effects of nicorandil in humans; however, some clinical studies have been conducted using Holter monitoring.[13] Chikamatsu et al.[24] have investigated the electrophysiologic effects of nicorandil 4 mg IV in eight patients with sinoatrial disease, five with atrioventricular block, and seven with paroxysmal supraventricular tachycardia. The drug did not change sinoatrial conduction time. The duration of both the sinus node cycle and the sinus node recovery time was shortened. Because nicorandil did not exhibit negative chronotropic effects, these authors conclude that it can be used safely in these conditions. In general, clinical studies[25] suggest that nicorandil used at therapeutic doses does not adversely affect cardiac conduction and that it is not proarrhythmic. This is confirmed by Japanese long-term experience with the drug.[26] Further large-scale studies of nicorandil in high-risk groups, such as patients with unstable angina, are currently under way in Europe.

Effects on Coronary Blood Flow

Nicorandil increases coronary blood flow and decreases coronary vascular resistance, with little effect on myocardial oxygen demand.[27] Furthermore, nicorandil at antiischemic doses induces a significant increase in the coronary artery diameter of nonstenotic, as well as stenotic, coronary segments, indicating that it also has a significant vasodilatory effect on epicardial as well as resistance vessels.[28] Ten patients undergoing coronary angioplasty were randomized into two groups. In the first group, nicorandil 6 μg/kg was administered intracoronary (IC) followed by ISDN 2 mg IC. In the second group, the order of treatment was reversed, with ISDN given first followed by nicorandil, so as to examine the additive effects of the two agents. Quantitative coronary angiography was performed at baseline and after each drug administration. In nonstenotic coronary segments, the mean coronary diameter increased significantly after either nicorandil (+12%) or ISDN (+17%). In stenotic segments, however, nicorandil produced a 20% increase in arterial diameter compared with only an 8% increase with ISDN. Furthermore, there was a significant additional 13% increase in diameter of the stenotic segment when nicorandil was administered after ISDN; no such additional effect was seen when the ISDN was given after nicorandil. The vasodilatory action of nicorandil is associated with lower increases in cGMP than conventional nitrates,[29] which suggests that it has additional vasorelaxant properties independent of cGMP production that may be explained by its K[+] channel opening.[10]

Berwing et al.,[30] using myocardial contrast echocardiography, have recently shown in 10 patients with coronary artery disease that nicorandil 20 mg PO significantly improved regional perfusion and wall motion abnormalities.[30]

Effects on Arteries and Veins

Nicorandil is a potent vasodilator of the coronary and peripheral vascular beds.[31] It dilates large coronary vessels and venous capacitance vessels, creating what is widely described as a balanced hemodynamic profile. In contrast with conventional nitrates, nicorandil causes sustained increases in coronary blood flow and decreases in systemic vascular resistance, as a result of dilatation of coronary and systemic resistance vessels.[14] Data from animal experiments show that a significant increase in coronary blood flow occurs only at relatively high active concentrations, and therefore a coronary steal phenomenon is probably not expected at the usual clinical doses.[32] Because of its effects in reducing preload and afterload, it influences two of the main determinants of oxygen demand without impairing myocardial contractility and thus, by reducing cardiac workload, has a potentially useful role in a number of cardiovascular conditions.

Other Effects

Clinical experience with nicorandil suggests that, during long-term treatment, it does not induce edema (unlike other K[+] openers such as pinacidil), cause weight gain, or adversely affect blood lipid or glucose levels.[33] Effects on specific organ systems are reviewed in the section on drug safety.

Although reflex stimulation of the sympathetic-adrenergic system can restrict the use of many vasodilators, there is no indication that this occurs with nicorandil.[34] Similarly, no activation of the renin-angiotensin-aldosterone system could be detected with nicorandil at doses of 10 to 30 mg.[35]

Clinical studies with nicorandil have shown no relevant pharmacokinetic modifications in patients with hepatic[36] or renal failure,[37] and therefore special dose adjustments are unnecessary in these conditions.

CLINICAL USE

Nicorandil is intended for use in the treatment of patients with ischemic heart disease. The following section reviews some representative studies that have been conducted in a wide range of heart disease patients.

Stable Angina Pectoris

The antianginal effectiveness of nicorandil has been assessed in open studies as well as in comparative studies against placebo or other antianginal agents. Early open studies have shown that nicorandil in doses of 5 mg three or four times daily is effective in patients with exercise-induced and rest angina.[38] In these studies, anginal attacks were significantly reduced in 37.5% to 100% (mean, 76%) of patients 2 to 8 weeks after treatment. Some of these open studies, however, were conducted with small numbers of patients and are further limited by the fact that patients were sometimes receiving other antianginal medication.

Camm and Maltz[39] evaluated the efficacy and safety of single doses of nicorandil, 20, 40, and 60 mg, and placebo in eight patients with exertional angina, in a double blind, randomized crossover study. Significant dose-dependent effects on blood pressure were observed at 2 and 6 hours after treadmill exercise testing, both at rest and at peak exercise. Resting diastolic blood pressure (DBP) decreased -7, -14, and -21 mmHg from baseline, with the three increasing doses at 2 hours after administration. The only significant increase in heart rate, $+13$ beats/min, occurred with the 60-mg dose. Significant improvement in exercise capacity, compared with placebo, was maintained at 6 hours after administration, although there was no consistent effect on double product with nicorandil. The incidence of side effects, mainly headache, appeared to be dose-related, and the 20-mg single dose was considered to be the most effective in terms of antianginal activity and tolerability. Dose-ranging studies have been reported[25] in which nicorandil doses of 10 and 20 mg twice daily have improved exercise capacity at peak and trough (12 hours), and therefore these doses have been used in most major controlled trials.

Meany et al.[40] conducted a randomized double-blind parallel group study over 4 weeks, comparing nicorandil 5 or 10 mg twice daily, increasing to 10 or 20 mg twice daily after 1 week, and placebo, in 46 patients with chronic stable angina. The principal effect of nicorandil was an improvement in exercise capacity after initial and prolonged dosing. Single doses of nicorandil 5 and 10 mg significantly increased time to onset of angina and exercise duration compared with placebo. After 2 weeks of treatment, time to onset of angina was significantly increased with the 10- and 20-mg doses of the drug. Exercise duration, time to 1-mm ST depression, and total exercise work increased in the nicorandil groups, although not significantly. There was no significant change in hemodynamic parameters at rest, peak exercise, or recovery.

Thadani et al.[41] recently reported results of a placebo-controlled study of nicorandil monotherapy in 83 patients with relatively mild exercise-induced angina. After 1 week of single-blind placebo therapy, patients were randomized to 2 weeks of double-blind treatment of either nicorandil 10 mg twice daily or placebo. Frequency of angina was similar in both groups, and there was no significant improvement in total exercise duration or time to ischemia.

Comparative Studies
with Other Antianginal Agents

Doring[42] has reported results from two double-blind randomized studies in 129 patients, comparing the antianginal and antiischemic efficacy of nicorandil with isosorbide-5-mononitrate (IS-5-MN) and ISDN. The first study was a crossover design with 4 weeks on each randomized treatment comparing 20 mg IS-5-MN and 20 mg nicorandil twice daily. Both agents were equally effective, with prolongation of exercise tolerance and reduced anginal attack rates. Twenty-five patients reported headache in the nicorandil group as compared with 21 with IS-5-MN. The majority of nicorandil-treated patients rated their headaches as mild, with only three patients requiring analgesics, compared with seven with IS-5-MN.

In the second study, comparing nicorandil and ISDN, both agents were administered in two parallel groups of patients at a dose of 10 mg three times daily for 2 weeks and then 20 mg three times daily for 4 weeks. In this study also, both drugs improved exercise capacity and reduced ST-segment depression equally well, with higher doses of both agents showing greater efficacy. A similar statistical analysis as that undertaken for the first study on the incidence of headache was not possible, but the author concludes that the overall pattern of adverse events, predominantly headaches, was similar. No tolerance to nitrate or nicorandil was observed in either study.

Other comparative studies have been conducted between nicorandil and β-blockers, including propranolol,[43] metoprolol,[44] and atenolol.[45] Raftery et al.[45] reported a randomized, double-blind, parallel study of nicorandil and atenolol in 37 patients with exercise-induced angina. At the end of a single-blind placebo period, patients were randomized and received either atenolol 50 mg once daily or nicorandil 10 mg twice daily for 3 weeks. On the third week, the dosage was increased, to nicorandil 20 mg twice daily or atenolol 100 mg once daily, for the final 3-week phase. Treadmill exercise testing was performed immediately before and 2 hours after dosing at the end of the placebo period and at the end of weeks 3 and 6 of active treatment. Increase in total exercise duration was seen with both drugs, and although the antianginal activity of both agents was similar, their effects on the double product were clearly different. Atenolol induced a decrease in peak rate pressure product, but this was almost unchanged with nicorandil, reflecting the different mechanism of action of the β-blocker and K^+ channel activator. One patient with severe three-vessel disease died suddenly after 3 days' treatment with nicorandil 10 mg twice daily. The most frequent adverse effect reported was headache, which led to discontinuation of treatment in one patient on atenolol and five on nicorandil. There was no attenuation of antiischemic activity with either drug, and effectiveness was sustained over a 6-week treatment period. The authors consider that nicorandil may be suitable for patients for whom β-blockade is contraindicated, and that the combination of the two drugs remains to be explored.

Commonly used calcium antagonists have also been compared with nicorandil in exertional angina. Ulvenstam et al.,[46] in an 8-week study, randomized 58 patients who were receiving ISDN to nicorandil 10 mg twice daily for 4 weeks, increasing to 20 mg twice daily or a fixed dose of nifedipine 20 mg twice daily. Nifedipine and nicorandil 10 mg twice daily showed equal efficacy in increasing total exercise duration, time to angina, and time to 1-mm ST depression; but nicorandil 20 mg twice daily produced a greater improvement in exercise performance, although this failed to reach statistical significance because of the small numbers of patients in the study. A more marked effect on resting hemodynamics was seen with nifedipine, which also produced more vasodilator side effects. Thirteen patients experienced headache in the nicorandil group, which had four withdrawals, compared with nine and three, respectively, with nifedipine. The frequency of headache was greatest during the prestudy treatment phase with ISDN.

Guermonprez et al.[47] compared the efficacy and safety of nicorandil 20 mg twice daily and diltiazem 60 mg three times daily, in a double-blind, randomized, parallel group study in 123 patients with exertional angina. The duration of the study was 3 months, and exercise testing was performed on placebo (day 0) and at the end of the study (day 90). Both agents were found to reduce the frequency of anginal attacks and consumption of nitroglycerin tablets. Maximum exercise capacity, the amount of work performed before reaching the ischemic threshold, and work to onset of angina significantly increased for both groups on day 90. The rate pressure product was unchanged or slightly decreased at the ischemic threshold. No significant differences between the two agents were evident for any of these parameters. Approximately the same number of patients experienced at least one adverse event (nicorandil, 31%; diltiazem, 30.2%), and withdrawal rates were similar. At the end of the 3-month period, some 45% of nicorandil patients and 43% of those taking diltiazem continued treatment under double-blind conditions for 1 year, which in the view of these authors was an indirect reflection of the investigators' judgment of the risk-to-benefit ratio of this therapy.

In summary, nicorandil, administered at doses of between 10 and 20 mg twice daily to patients with stable exertional angina, appears to be safe and to have comparable efficacy to the three major groups of established antianginal drugs. Tachyphylaxis has not been observed in clinical trials. Adverse events commonly occur in up to one third of patients taking nicorandil, the principal problem being headache, which is severe enough to warrant withdrawal from studies in only approximately 10% of cases.[48] It is reassuring that there are no abnormal electrocardiographic or biochemical findings. As with all small studies, there are limitations in assessing differences among antianginal agents.[49] Clearly, larger studies are required to establish the antiischemic efficacy of nicorandil as monotherapy in patients with chronic stable angina, as well as its effects on episodes of transient ambulatory myocardial ischemia in daily life. Furthermore, in view of its unique properties, its role in combination therapy needs to be addressed.

Coronary Spasm and Unstable Angina

Nicorandil may have a role to play in the management of coronary vasospasm and unstable angina. Aizawa et al.[50] assessed the effects of nicorandil 4 mg IV in 10 patients who had spontaneous and ergonovine-induced coronary spasm. Prompt and complete relief of spasm was achieved in all cases. The drug had minimal chronotropic effects but reduced mean aortic pressure and end-diastolic pressure by 6% and 18%, respectively, and produced a 7% decrease in coronary vascular resistance. Lablanche et al.[51] compared single oral doses of nicorandil 30 mg, nifedipine 10 mg, or placebo during coronary angiography in 13 patients with vasospastic angina. Both agents were shown to prevent ergometrine-induced coronary spasm. Fukami et al., in a preliminary report,[52] evaluated the effects of nicorandil IV between 1 mg/hr and a maximum of 6 mg/hr in 33 consecutive patients with unstable angina who also received calcium antagonists and/or β-blockers and who were refractory to nitrates. Complete abolition of pain occurred in 19 patients, and there was "considerable reduction" of pain in three; however, the details of the duration of infusion or concomitant antianginal therapy are not disclosed in this abstract. From these and other reports from Japanese workers, it appears that nicorandil exhibits "spasmolytic activity." The safety and efficacy of nicorandil in unstable angina are currently being assessed in a large multicenter trial in the United Kingdom.

Coronary Angioplasty

Nicorandil may also have a role in coronary angioplasty. Saito et al.[53] assessed the efficacy and safety of nitroglycerin, verapamil, and nicorandil on the intracoronary ECG and hemodynamic variables during coronary angioplasty in 40 patients with proximal coronary stenoses. After two 30-second balloon inflations, patients received one of these agents or 30 ml saline intracoronary. Five minutes after injection a third inflation was performed. Nicorandil, unlike verapamil and nitroglycerin, did not significantly change systemic hemodynamics, and no adverse effects were noted. Although both nicorandil and verapamil reduced the extent of myocardial ischemia during brief occlusion, nicorandil was deemed to be safer and more efficacious than verapamil. The incidence of negative U waves was significantly reduced by verapamil (30%) and nicorandil (20%) compared with saline (60%) and nitroglycerin (50%). Kitazume et al.[54] reported in an abstract the combined effects of aspirin, ticlopidine, and nicorandil in prevention of restenosis after coronary angioplasty. Analysis of follow-up angiograms after a mean of 28 weeks revealed that the combination of all three agents significantly reduced restenosis rates, which were 16% as compared with aspirin alone (38%) or aspirin in combination with ticlopidine (27%).

Heart Failure and Tolerance

In view of the effect of nicorandil in reducing preload and afterload and its dose-related improvement in hemodynamic performance,[20, 21] it may be a potentially useful agent in the treatment of cardiac failure. In a study by Galie et al.,[55] of nine patients with heart failure, single oral doses of nicorandil, 40 or 60 mg, decreased pulmonary capillary wedge pressure (PCWP) without increasing heart rate. Tsutamoto et al.[56] investigated hemodynamics after administration of nitroglycerin and nicorandil in 25 patients with heart failure, to determine whether tolerance developed during continuous intravenous infusions of both drugs. Doses were titrated to achieve a reduction in PCWP of 20% or more within 1 hour, and infusion was maintained at a constant rate for 24 hours. In the nitrate group, PCWP was not significantly different from baseline by 12 hours; but in the nicorandil group, it was significantly lower than baseline up to 24 hours, indicating that tolerance to nitroglycerin developed within 12 hours, whereas nicorandil continues to remain effective for 24 hours. These same workers have investigated the lack of development of tolerance with nicorandil[57] in a study of 15 patients with chronic heart failure. They measured both hemodynamics and blood levels of cGMP during nitroglycerin and nicorandil infusions. In the nitroglycerin group, cGMP levels returned to baseline at 12 hours and PCWP increased, indicating tolerance. Although cGMP levels had returned to baseline after 24 hours in the nicorandil group, PCWP continued to decrease for 24 hours. These findings suggest that the effects of nitroglycerin are dependent on its activation of cGMP, whereas nicorandil, in view of its K^+ channel opening, is hemodynamically active when cGMP formation is no longer stimulated. There appears to be little evidence of cross-tolerance between nicorandil and conventional nitrates,[13] and a review of the clinical data suggests that tolerance development seems to be of no practical importance for long-term therapy with nicorandil.[34]

Other Potential Indications

Nicorandil may possess a number of interesting "cardioprotective" properties. Auchampach et al.[58] have shown in the anesthetized dog that nicorandil attenuates myocardial stunning as a direct effect of K^+-ATP channel activation in ischemic myocardium. Gross et al.,[59] in several dog models of reversible ischemic injury, have shown that nicorandil administration enhances recovery of regional systolic shortening, a measure of contractile function, during reperfusion after a single episode of 10 to 15 minutes of coronary artery occlusion. In further experiments on myocardial infarction, these workers have shown that infarct size was significantly smaller in dogs pretreated with nicorandil, compared with control animals or those pretreated with nifedipine.

Under experimental conditions, nicorandil inhibits neutrophil infiltration into damaged cardiac tissue.[60]

During reperfusion injury, neutrophil infiltration can lead to production of superoxide radicals. Nicorandil has been shown to produce a concentration-dependent inhibition of superoxide anion production in human neutrophils.[59] Nicorandil also shares with other nitrates the ability to inhibit agonist-induced platelet aggregation.[61]

These and other observations suggest that nicorandil may have important ancillary properties of benefit to the patient with coronary artery disease. At present, however, these actions of nicorandil remain unproven in the clinical setting.

Precautions and Adverse Effects

Nicorandil is contraindicated in patients who have shown purported hypersensitivity or idiosyncrasy to it. It is also contraindicated in cardiogenic shock, hypotension, and left ventricular failure with low filling pressures.

An extensive European development program has provided a large database of clinical experience with nicorandil.[33] Safety has been assessed in 1680 subjects, with 458 patient-years of exposure to nicorandil. From an analysis of 1152 patients, a 36.4% incidence of headache has been recorded. A long-term study with 255 patients has shown an 8.5% drop-out rate related to headache.[33] The majority of headaches were experienced during the first week or two of therapy and gradually diminished with continued treatment. Progressive up-titration of nicorandil from a dose of 5 mg twice daily can reduce the rate of withdrawal of study patients by two thirds. Other side effects, including dizziness, hypotension, palpitation, and gastrointestinal disturbances, have been reported in less than 3% of subjects. The European experience of adverse events with nicorandil concurs with that of Japan, although the overall incidence of adverse events is lower in European studies.

Edema and weight gain do not significantly change during nicorandil therapy, and blood parameters, including glucose, cholesterol, and triglyceride levels, are not significantly affected.[33]

Nicorandil has been administered to patients with a range of other cardiovascular drugs without any significant interactions being identified. This may be because nicorandil is weakly bound to plasma proteins, and therefore displacement of nicorandil from plasma protein by other drugs does not significantly alter its plasma concentration. Similarly, nicorandil does not induce or inhibit drug-metabolizing enzymes that might subsequently change metabolism.

Elderly Patients

Approximately one third of patients enrolled in the nicorandil clinical trial program were 65 years or older, and age-specific side effects were not identified. Results of a large multicenter Study of Nicorandil in Angina Pectoris in the Elderly (SNAPE), comparing 10 mg nicorandil twice daily with ISMN 20 mg twice daily, in chronic stable angina patients older than 65 years have not as yet been reported. Although a higher incidence of hepatic and renal impairment in elderly patients has been noted, these patients have not been specifically recruited into clinical trials, and pharmaco-kinetic studies have not shown relevant modifications in patients with hepatic or renal failure.[36, 37]

DISCUSSION

Our understanding of K^+-ATP–sensitive channel openers is at an early and exciting stage. Nicorandil is a novel agent of this class. While we assume that its action is in part similar to that of a calcium antago-nist,[11] nicorandil clearly also acts in part as a nitrodila-tor. It has been argued that unlike a "pure" K^+ chan-nel opener, such as cromakalim, nicorandil exerts its action entirely as a nitrate.[62] As we have shown, how-ever, it does not appear to function solely as a nitrate, and we must therefore keep an open mind regarding its precise mode of action.[63]

Nicorandil is currently undergoing assessment for the management of ischemic heart disease. Evidence to date suggests that the drug is safe, that it is not proarrhythmic, and that it has an acceptable side ef-fect profile. The principal side effect, headache, can be minimized by dose titration. Although comparative studies of monotherapy in angina pectoris show that nicorandil has similar efficacy to other antianginal agents, further larger studies are required to identify more subtle and smaller differences between agents. Studies of combination therapy for angina pectoris with nicorandil have not been performed as yet to any great extent. Nicorandil possesses antiplatelet ac-tivity and other potentially useful properties for man-agement of myocardial ischemia.[64] Although nicoran-dil acts in part as a nitrate, tolerance has not been observed in the short term. Further studies will estab-lish its efficacy in longer-term therapy. It should be useful in a variety of patient groups, including the elderly and those with poor left ventricular func-tion,[65-67] and particularly beneficial in patients who cannot tolerate β-blockers. We believe that further investigation of this interesting new agent is merited in order to establish its role in cardiovascular therapy.

REFERENCES

1. Campbell RWF: The deficiencies of current medical therapy for the management of angina pectoris. Postgrad Med J 67:S37, 1991.
2. Wilde AAM, Janse MJ: Electrophysiological effects of ATP sen-sitive potassium channel modulation: Implications for arrhyth-mogenesis. Cardiovasc Res 28:16, 1994.
3. Tosaki A, Faha AH: Adenosine triphosphate-sensitive potas-sium channel blocking agent ameliorates, but the opening agent aggravates, ischemia/reperfusion injury. J Am Coll Cardiol 23:487, 1994.
4. Siegl P: Blockers of ATP sensitive potassium current are of potential benefit in ischaemic heart disease. Cardiovasc Res 28:31, 1994.
5. Chi L, Black SC, Kuo PI, et al: Actions of pinacidil at a reduced potassium concentration: A direct cardiac effect involving the ATP-dependent potassium channel. J Cardiovasc Pharmacol 21:179, 1993.

6. Gross GJ, Auchampach JA: Role of ATP dependent potassium channels in myocardial ischaemia. Cardiovasc Res 26:1011, 1992.
7. Cavero I, Premmereur J: ATP sensitive potassium channel openers are of potential benefit in ischaemic heart disease. Cardiovasc Res 28:31, 1994.
8. Hamilton TC, Weston AH: Cromakalim, nicorandil and pinaci-dil: Novel drugs which open potassium channels in smooth muscle. Gen Pharmacol 20:1, 1989.
9. Purcell H, Fox K: Potassium channel activators in the manage-ment of ischaemic heart disease: A focus on nicorandil. Br J Clin Pract 47:150, 1993.
10. Taira N: Nicorandil as a hybrid between nitrates and potassium channel activators. Am J Cardiol 63:18J, 1989.
11. Escande D, Henry P: Potassium channels as pharmacological targets in cardiovascular medicine. Eur Heart J 14(Suppl B):2, 1993.
12. Frydman AM, Chapelle P, Diekmann H, et al: Pharmacokinetics of nicorandil. Am J Cardiol 63:25J, 1989.
13. Frampton J, Buckley MM, Fitton A: Nicorandil: A review of its pharmacology and therapeutic efficacy in angina pectoris. Drugs 4:625, 1992.
14. Suryapranata H: The cardiovascular profile of nicorandil. Rev Contemp Pharmacother 4:207, 1993.
15. Wolf DL, Hearron AE, Metzler CM, et al: The pharmacokinetics and haemodynamic effects of continuous nicorandil infusion in healthy volunteers. Eur J Clin Pharmacol 45:437, 1993.
16. Belz GG, Matthews JH, Beck A, et al: Hemodynamic effects of nicorandil, isosorbide dinitrate, and dihydralazine in healthy volunteers. J Cardiovasc Pharmacol 7:1107, 1985.
17. Belz GG, Matthews JH, Heinrich J, et al: Controlled comparison of the pharmacodynamic effects of nicorandil (SG-75) and iso-sorbide dinitrate in man. Eur J Clin Pharmacol 26:681, 1984.
18. Kobayashi K, Hakuta T, Yoshimura H, et al: Effects of nicoran-dil on coronary hemodynamics in ischemic heart disease: Com-parison with nitroglycerine, nifedipine, and propranolol. J Cardiovasc Pharmacol 10(Suppl 8):S109, 1987.
19. Coltart DJ, Signy M: Acute hemodynamic effects of single-dose nicorandil in coronary artery disease. Am J Cardiol 63:34J, 1989.
20. Cohen Solal A, Jaeger P, Bouthier J, et al: Hemodynamic action of nicorandil in chronic congestive heart failure. Am J Cardiol 63:44J, 1989.
21. Tice FD, Binkley PF, Cody RJ, et al: Hemodynamic effects of nicorandil in congestive heart failure. Am J Cardiol 65:1361, 1990.
22. Silke B, Verma SP, Ali MS, et al: Effects of nicorandil on left ventricular hemodynamics and volume at rest and during exer-cise-induced angina pectoris. Am J Cardiol 63:49J, 1989.
23. Kambara H, Nakamura Y, Tamaki S, et al: Beneficial effects of nicorandil on cardiovascular hemodynamics and left ventricu-lar function. J Cardiovasc Pharmacol 10(Suppl 8):S104, 1987.
24. Chikamatsu H, Hishida H, Matsuyama H, et al: Electrophysio-logic effects of nicorandil, an antianginal drug in man. Acta Pharmacol Toxicol 59(Suppl V):179, 1986.
25. Krumenacker M, Roland E: Clinical profile of nicorandil: An overview of its hemodynamic properties and therapeutic effi-cacy. J Cardiovasc Pharmacol 20(Suppl 3):S93, 1992.
26. Purcell H, Mulcahy D, Fox K: The clinical profile of nicorandil. Rev Contemp Pharmacother 4:215, 1993.
27. Suryapranata H: Coronary haemodynamics and vasodilatory profile of a potassium channel opener in patients with coronary artery disease. Eur Heart J 14(Suppl B):16, 1993.
28. Suryapranata H, MacLeod D: Nicorandil and cardiovascular performance in patients with coronary artery disease. J Cardio-vasc Pharmacol 20(Suppl 3):S45, 1992.
29. Holzmann S: Cyclic GMP as possible mediator of coronary arterial relaxation by nicorandil (SG 75). J Cardiovasc Pharma-col 5:364, 1983.
30. Berwing K, Strasser R, Schlepper M, et al: The effect of nicoran-dil (potassium channel opener) on regional perfusion, wall motion abnormality, and coronary stenoses in patients with coronary artery disease [abstract]. Circulation 88(Part 2):348, 1993.
31. Treese N, Erbel R, Meyer J: Acute effects of nicorandil in coronary artery disease. J Cardiovasc Pharmacol 20(Suppl 3):S52, 1992.

32. Hashimoto K, Kinoshita, Ohbayashi Y: Coronary effects of nicorandil in comparison with nitroglycerin in chronic conscious dogs. Cardiovasc Drugs Ther 5:131, 1991.

33. Roland E: Safety profile of an anti-anginal agent with potassium channel opening activity: An overview. Eur Heart J 14(Suppl B):48, 1993.

34. Neuss H: The safety profile of nicorandil. Rev Contemp Pharmacother 4:221, 1993.

35. Leonetti G, Fruscio M, Gradnik R, et al: Nicorandil, a new vasodilator drug, in patients with essential hypertension. J Hypertens 7(Suppl):292, 1989.

36. Jungbluth GL, Della-Coletta AA, Blum RA, et al: Comparative pharmacokinetics and bioavailability of nicorandil in subjects with stabilized cirrhosis and matched healthy volunteers. Clin Pharmacol Ther 49(2):181, 1991.

37. Molinaro M, Villa G, Regazzi MB, et al: Pharmacokinetics of nicorandil in patients with normal and impaired renal function. Eur J Clin Pharmacol 42:203, 1992.

38. Kinoshita M, Saki K: Pharmacology and therapeutic effects of nicorandil. Cardiovasc Drugs Ther 4:1075, 1990.

39. Camm AJ, Maltz MB: A controlled single-dose study of the efficacy, dose response and duration of action of nicorandil in angina pectoris. Am J Cardiol 63:61J, 1989.

40. Meany TB, Richardson P, Camm AJ, et al: Exercise capacity after single and twice-daily doses of nicorandil in chronic stable angina pectoris. Am J Cardiol 63:66J, 1989.

41. Thadani U, Strauss W, Glasser SP, et al: Evaluation of antianginal and anti-ischemic efficacy of nicorandil; results of a multicenter study [abstract]. J Am Coll Cardiol 1A:267A, 1994.

42. Doring D: Antianginal and anti-ischemic efficacy of nicorandil in comparison with isosorbide-5 mononitrate and isosorbide dinitrate: Results from two multicenter, double-blind, randomized studies with stable coronary heart disease patients. J Cardiovasc Pharmacol 20(Suppl 3):S74, 1992.

43. Meeter K, Kelder JC, Tijssen JGP, et al: Efficacy of nicorandil versus propranolol in mild stable angina of effort: A long-term, double-blind, randomized study. J Cardiovasc Pharmacol 20(Suppl 3):S59, 1992.

44. Di Somma S, Liquori V, Verdecchia P, et al: A double-blind comparison of nicorandil and metoprolol in patients with effort stable angina [abstract]. Eur Heart J 11(Suppl):80, 1990.

45. Raftery EB, Lahiri A, Hughes LO, et al: A double-blind comparison of a beta-blocker and a potassium channel opener in exercise induced angina. Eur Heart J 14(Suppl B):35, 1993.

46. Ulvenstam G, Diderholm E, Frithz G, et al: Antianginal and anti-ischemic efficacy of nicorandil compared with nifedipine in patients with angina pectoris and coronary heart disease: A double-blind, randomized, multicenter study. J Cardiovasc Pharmacol 20:S67, 1992.

47. Guermonprez JL, Blin P, Peterlongo F: A double-blind comparison of the long-term efficacy of a potassium channel activator and a calcium antagonist in stable angina pectoris. Eur Heart J 14(Suppl B):30, 1993.

48. Why HJF, Richardson PJ: A potassium channel opener as monotherapy in chronic stable angina pectoris: Comparison with placebo. Eur Heart J 14(Suppl B):25, 1993.

49. Ford I: Angina clinical trial methodology. Postgrad Med J 67(Suppl 3):S2, 1991.

50. Aizawa T, Ogasawara K, Nakamura A, et al: Effect of nicorandil on coronary spasm. Am J Cardiol 63:75J, 1989.

51. Lablanche J-M, Bauters C, Leroy F, et al: Prevention of coronary spasm by nicorandil: Comparison with nifedipine. J Cardiovasc Pharmacol 20:S82, 1992.

52. Fukami K, Haze K, Sumiyoshi T, et al: Beneficial effects of intravenous nicorandil in refractory unstable angina. Eur Heart J 9(Suppl):64, 1988.

53. Saito S, Tamura Y, Moriuchi M, et al: Comparative efficacy and safety of nitroglycerin, verapamil and nicorandil during coronary angioplasty [abstract]. J Am Coll Cardiol 17:377A, 1991.

54. Kitazume H, Kuko I, Iwama T, et al: Combined use of aspirin, ticlopidine and nicorandil prevented restenosis after coronary angioplasty [abstract]. Circulation 78(Suppl 11):633, 1988.

55. Galie N, Varani E, Maiello L: Usefulness of nicorandil in congestive heart failure. Am J Cardiol 65:343, 1990.

56. Tsutamoto T, Kinoshita M, Nakae I, et al: Absence of hemodynamic tolerance to nicorandil in patients with severe congestive heart failure. Am Heart J 127:866, 1994.

57. Tsutamoto T, Kinoshita M, Hisanaga T, et al: Comparison of hemodynamic effects and plasma cyclic guanosine monophosphate of nicorandil and nitroglycerin in patients with congestive heart failure. Am J Cardiol 75:1162, 1995.

58. Auchampach JA, Cavero I, Gross GJ: Nicorandil attenuates myocardial dysfunction associated with transient ischemia by opening ATP-dependent potassium channels. J Cardiovasc Pharmacol 20:765, 1992.

59. Gross GJ, Auchampach JA, Maruyama M, et al: Cardioprotective effects of nicorandil. J Cardiovasc Pharmacol 20(Suppl 3):S22, 1992.

60. Galie N, Guarnieri C, Ussia GP, et al: Limitation of myocardial infarct size by nicorandil after sustained ischemia in pigs. J Cardiovasc Pharmacol 26:477, 1995.

61. Jaraki O, Strauss WE, Francis S, et al: Antiplatelet effects of a novel antianginal agent, nicorandil. J Cardiovasc Pharmacol 23:24, 1994.

62. Satoh K, Mori T, Yamada N, et al: Nicorandil as a nitrate, and cromakalim as a potassium channel opener, dilate isolated porcine large coronary arteries in an agonist-nonselective manner. Cardiovasc Drugs Ther 7:691, 1993.

63. Knight C, Purcell H, Fox K: Potassium channel openers; clinical applications in ischaemic heart disease: Overview of clinical efficacy of nicorandil. Cardiovasc Drugs Ther 9:229, 1995.

64. Ogino K, Osaki S, Noguchi N, et al: Nicorandil suppressed myocardial purine metabolism during exercise in patients with angina pectoris. Eur J Clin Pharmacol 48:189, 1995.

65. Fox KM: Anti-anginal actions and tolerability of nicorandil. Presentation during IFECC lll International Forum for the Evaluation of Cardiovascular Care. Monte Carlo, 1994.

66. Schlepper M, Thormann J, Berwing K, et al: Effects of nicorandil on regional perfusion and left ventricular function. Cardiovasc Drugs Ther 9(Suppl 2):203, 1995.

67. Koike A, Hiroe M, Yajima T, et al: Effects of nicorandil on kinetics of oxygen uptake at the onset of exercise in patients with coronary artery disease. Am J Cardiol 76:449, 1995.

CHAPTER 179

Molsidomine

Werner Rudolph, M.D., and Donald Hall, M.D.

Molsidomine (N-ethoxycarbonyl-3-morpholino sydnonimine) is a vasodilator with an action similar to that of the organic nitrates. It is a prodrug, converted in the liver to SIN-1 (3-morpholino sydnonimine), which undergoes spontaneous ring opening to SIN-1A (N-morpholino-N-N-nitroso-aminoacetonitrile), the active drug, resulting in the release of nitric oxide, its active principal. After oral administration, absorption is nearly complete. The onset of action can be detected within 10 to 15 minutes; maximal plasma concentrations are reached after approximately 60 minutes. Molsidomine is extensively metabolized, and 90% of its metabolites are excreted by the kidneys. Molsidomine has been in clinical use for several years in Europe and Japan. Estimates of its usage from 1987 to 1992 in Germany alone amount to approximately 1 million patient-years.

MECHANISM OF ACTION

The antiischemic effect of molsidomine is attributable to its vasodilating properties. According to current concepts, this is the result of direct stimulation by SIN-lA and/or its degradation product nitric oxide of guanylate cyclase with increased generation of cyclic guanosine monophosphate (cGMP) from guanylyl triphosphate (GTP), which leads to relaxation of smooth muscle. There is predominant dilation of venous capacitance vessels, with a decrease in venous return to the heart. Owing to the predominant vasodilation of venous capacitance vessels, there is a reduction of myocardial wall tension as reflected by a decrease in ventricular filling pressures and volumes and, consequently, a decrease in myocardial oxygen requirements. In the coronary arterial system, molsidomine affects dilation of stenotic regions in epicardial vessels that are still capable of dilation as well as in collateral vessels. Thus, in hypoperfused, poststenotic regions, there is an increased oxygen supply as a result of a reduction in the extravascular component of the coronary artery resistance resulting from the diminished myocardial wall tension as well as from direct dilation of collateral vessels and, when possible, dilation of stenotic coronary lesions. Myocardial contractility and heart rate, further determinants of myocardial oxygen requirements, remain essentially unchanged. Increases in the ejection fraction and regional ventricular wall motion are attributable to improved loading conditions as well as enhanced perfusion of poststenotic myocardial regions.[1, 2] Accordingly, the antiischemic effect can be anticipated regardless of whether the primary mechanism of ischemia is an increased myocardial oxygen requirement or a reduction in myocardial oxygen supply resulting from increased coronary arterial tone. Additionally, these mechanisms render themselves well suited for use in the presence of impaired ventricular function and heart failure. Moreover, in vitro studies have shown that the substance is a potent activator of soluble thrombocyte guanylate cyclase, thereby leading to inhibition of platelet aggregation.[3, 4]

CLINICAL USE
Ischemic Heart Disease

Exertional Angina Pectoris

In the appropriate dosage, molsidomine is clearly an effective antiischemic and antianginal agent. Several dosing regimens have been tested in controlled studies using randomized, double-blind, crossover protocols.[5-7] Early studies showed that on administration of 2 mg of the non-sustained-release form of molsidomine three times daily, there were only slight but significant decreases in the rate of anginal attacks and nitrate consumption of 17% and 18%, respectively. ST-segment depression was reduced by 45% and 9% at 1 and 3 hours, but subsequent testing at 5 and 8 hours showed no significant changes. Because these effects were evanescent and only of a modest magnitude, higher doses were considered necessary. On increasing the dosage to 3 mg three times daily, however, the effects were not more marked. Only through doubling the frequency of administration, that is to 2 mg six times daily, was there a more pronounced reduction in the rate of anginal attacks and nitrate consumption of 38% and 36%, respectively. While on this regimen, testing at 1 hour after administration of a 4-mg dose showed a 57% reduction in the amount of ST-segment depression.

The sustained-release formulation has been shown to yield the most beneficial effects. Administration of 8 mg molsidomine in sustained-release form three times daily resulted in a highly significant 93% reduction in the rate of anginal attacks and an 83% decrease in the use of sublingual nitroglycerin capsules. One hour after administration, ST-segment depression was reduced 74% to 83%. At 2 hours, the reduction of 67% is comparable to that observed after administration of 120 mg isosorbide dinitrate in sustained-release form.[8] At 5 hours, the reduction of 44% to 51% was still significant. Eight hours after the molsidomine dose, the reduction in ST-segment depression was diminished and ranged between 10% and 30%. During long-term treatment, at 1 and 5 hours after the 8-mg sustained-release dose, there were comparably significant reductions in ST-segment depression[9] (Fig. 179–1). Thus, in contrast with continuous treatment with nitrates during which tolerance invariably develops, the effects of molsidomine remain essentially intact.

Established Tolerance to the Antiischemic Effects of Nitrates

Even during the established state of nitrate tolerance, the effects of molsidomine are maintained. In patients in whom nitrate tolerance was induced through transdermal patches employing a release rate of 20 mg/24 hr, the marked reduction in ST-segment depression of 71% at 2.5 hours after application declined clearly to 25% and 14% at 10 and 24 hours.[10] At 2.5 hours after a second patch application, in association with increasing plasma concentrations, the reduction in ST-segment depression amounted to only 20% and is clearly indicative of tolerance. At 1.5 hours after an 8-mg dose of molsidomine in sustained-release form with no concomitant nitrate treatment, there was a 56% reduction in ST-segment depression; in the state of established nitrate tolerance, ST-segment depression was reduced by 76% (Fig. 179–2). Consequently, it can even be assumed that the residual effect of nitroglycerin and the effect of molsidomine are additive.

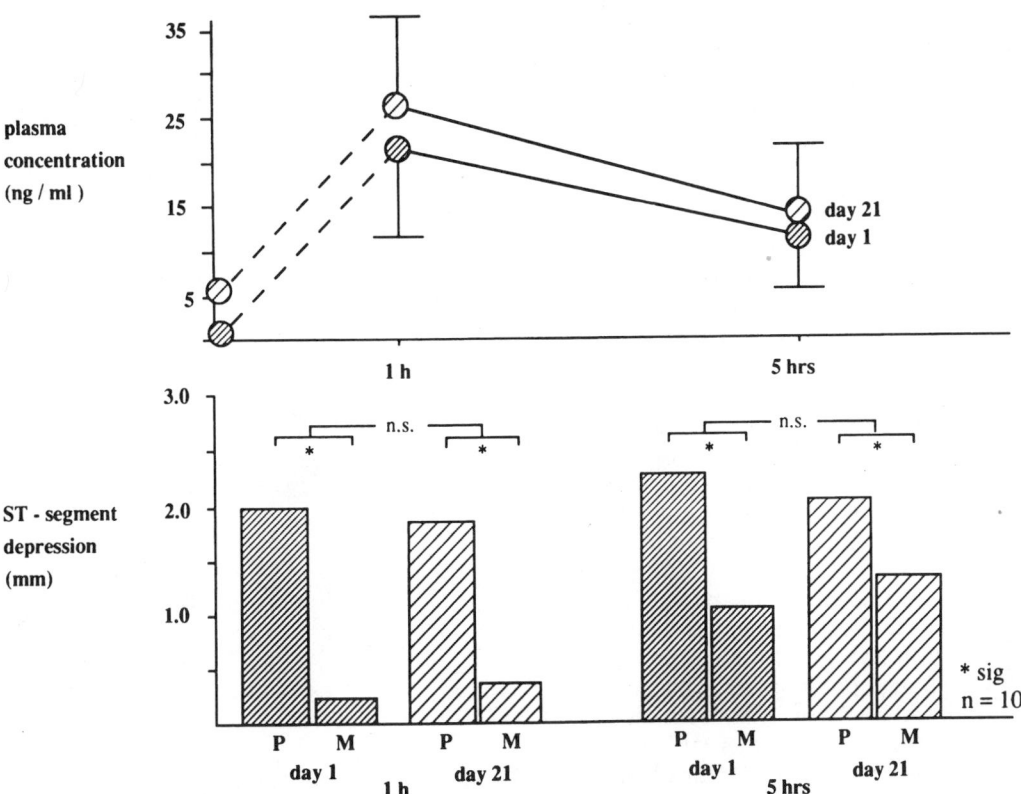

Figure 179–1. Plasma concentrations and ST-segment depression at comparable workloads at 1 and 5 hours after oral administration of 8 mg molsidomine (M) in sustained-release form as compared with placebo (P) after initial administration and during long-term treatment with 8 mg three times daily. (*, *p* < .05) (From Rudolph W, Dirschinger W: Clinical comparison of nitrates and sydnonimines. Eur Heart J 12[Suppl E]:33, 1991.)

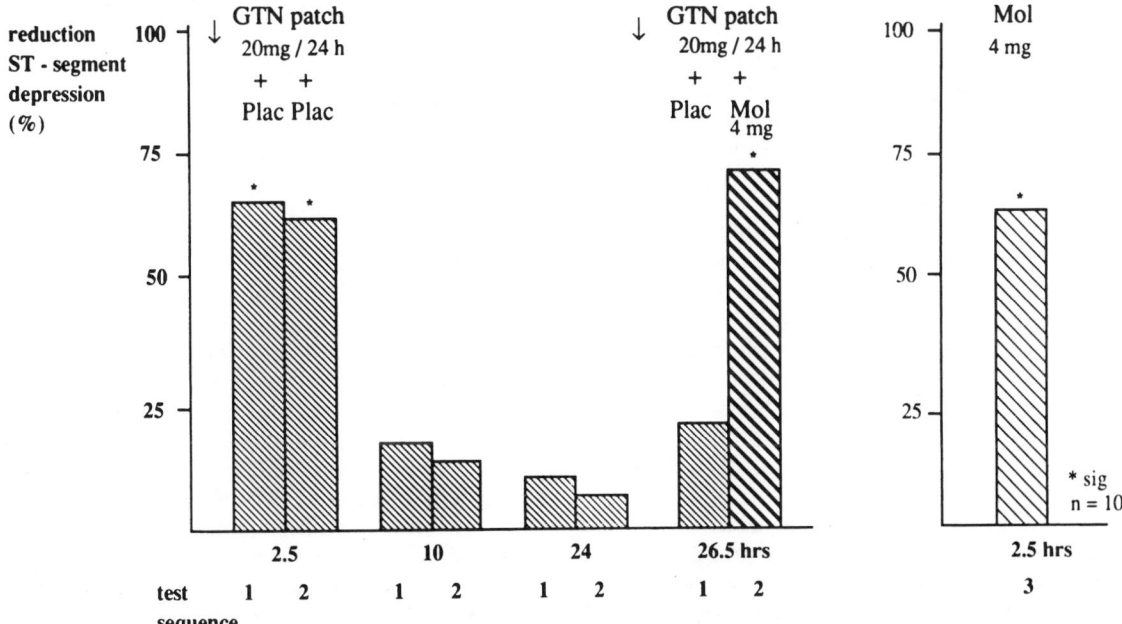

Figure 179–2. Reduction in exercise-induced ST-segment depression after initial and second application of a nitroglycerin (GTN) patch with a delivery rate of 20 mg/24 hr together with placebo (Plac), or second patch application together with 4 mg molsidomine (Mol), as well as reduction in ST-segment depression after administration of 4 mg molsidomine alone. (*, *p* < .05) (Reproduced with permission from Rudolph W, Dirschinger W: Clinical comparison of nitrates and sydnonimines. Eur Heart J 12[Suppl E]:33, 1991.)

Clinical Relevance of Nitric Oxide Release Mechanism

The fact that the antiischemic effects of molsidomine are preserved in the state of established nitroglycerin tolerance confirms the clinical relevance of the differences between the mechanism of nitric oxide (NO) release. Both organic nitrates and SIN-1, through NO-mediated stimulation of guanylyl cyclase, effect increased conversion of GTP to cGMP, resulting in relaxation of vascular smooth muscle. The reason molsidomine is not associated with tolerance development appears to be that at the molecular level only molsidomine leads directly to NO delivery, whereas organic nitrates are dependent on enzyme-catalyzed reduction processes. This difference is important because the tolerance phenomena that develop during continuous administration of organic nitrates appear attributable to depletion of sulfhydryl groups as electron donors or to other mechanisms such as inactivation of key enzymes of biotransformation (e.g., cytochrome P-450).[11] However, *in vitro* studies with excessively high drug concentrations indicate that another site in the nitrate bioconversion cascade, most likely at the level of NO generation, may also be responsible for tolerance phenomena. This may also account for the observation of attenuated action to high-dose molsidomine in experimental studies, as well as on very rare occasions in humans.[12, 13] However, in the beginning of the treatment, mechanisms of physiologic counterregulation have also to be taken into account.

Heart Failure

Hemodynamic Profile

Most studies dealing with the effects of molsidomine in heart failure have been concerned only with hemodynamics or ventricular function, and most were uncontrolled. From early studies of its mechanism of action in coronary artery disease, however, its basic usefulness could be predicted. The results of a double-blind, randomized, placebo-controlled study characterize its general hemodynamic profile[14] (Fig. 179–3). On use of 4 mg in non-sustained-release form every 6 hours as well as a single oral dose of 16 mg in sustained-release form, there were significant decreases in mean pulmonary artery pressure of 5% to 15% up to 12 hours after administration. The mean right atrial pressure showed initial decreases at 1 and 2 hours after the 4-mg dose of 36% and 34%, respectively, whereas those of the 16-mg dose in sustained-release form amounted to 22% and 24%; at 6 and 12 hours, decreases ranged from 13% to 22%. Over the same time period, the two dosing regimens led to reductions in total pulmonary resistance ranging from 4% to 18%. There were no meaningful changes in cardiac output, arterial blood pressure, and heart rate. Overall, the 16-mg dose of molsidomine in sustained-release form showed most favorable effects.

Additionally, it has been shown that the acute he-

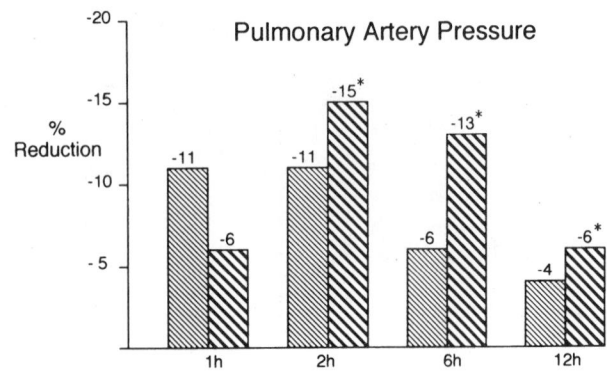

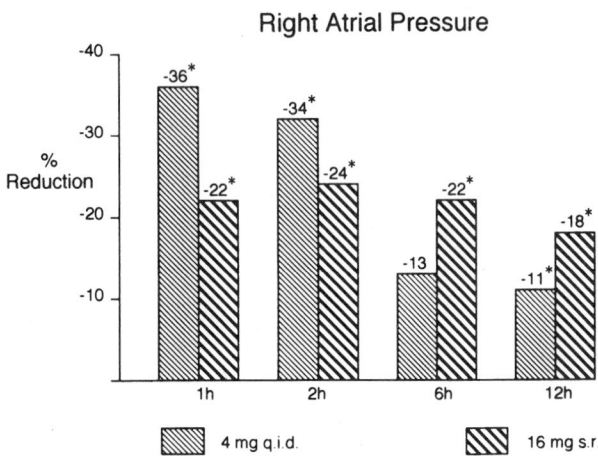

Figure 179–3. Percentage reduction in mean pulmonary artery pressure and mean right atrial pressure at 1, 2, 6, and 12 hours (h) after molsidomine, 4 mg four times daily and 16 mg in sustained-release form once daily, as compared with placebo. (*, $p < .05$)

modynamic effects are maintained without attenuation for periods of 7 and 21 days, such that on use of molsidomine for treatment of heart failure, as in coronary artery disease, there is no evidence of tolerance development.

No data are available from controlled studies dealing with symptoms, exercise tolerance, or mortality in patients with heart failure.

Counterregulatory Mechanisms

During long-term therapy at clinically employed dosages, there is no evidence of counterregulatory mechanisms to attenuate the action. Counterregulatory activity can be observed, however, on use of very high intravenous doses. In a controlled study, after administration of 12 mg over 30 minutes followed by an infusion of 6 mg/hr for 24 hours, plasma concentrations increased up to 300 ng/ml, whereas the usual maximal concentrations achieved with an 8-mg dose in sustained-release form range between 20 and 25 ng/ml. This led initially to a decrease in diastolic pulmonary artery pressure of approximately 30%, which leveled off after 8 to 24 hours at approximately 25%. This attenuation of action of molsidomine must be regarded as indicative of counterregulatory activity. It is associated with a decrease in hematocrit and increases in plasma volume and body weight. There were also significant increases in plasma renin concentration, plasma renin activity, and aldosterone concentrations with no significant changes in the concentrations of epinephrine, norepinephrine, vasopressin, cGMP, or atrial natriuretic peptide (ANP). Accordingly, it can be assumed that undesired counterregulatory activity would be anticipated only when excessively high doses of molsidomine are given that render plasma concentrations a factor of 10 to 15 times higher than during the usual oral administration.

Therapeutic Uses

Indications and Recommended Dosage

In coronary artery disease, molsidomine is an efficacious drug that elicits antiischemic and antianginal effects comparable to those of long-acting nitrates (e.g., isosorbide dinitrate) with the advantage, as pointed out, that its continuous use is not associated with tolerance development. At the time of maximal effect, between 1 and 2 hours after administration, an approximately 80% to 90% reduction in ST-segment depression can be anticipated; at 5 hours, the extent of reduction is approximately 50%. Because of the dissipation of action between the 5th and 8th hours on use of the formulation currently marketed, around-the-clock antiischemic treatment can best be achieved with 8 mg molsidomine in sustained-release form every 6 hours. In this regard, molsidomine is well suited for adjunctive use in the acute setting of treatment of unstable angina pectoris. Because the majority of patients, however, do not require uninterrupted antiischemic protection, the usual period of physical activities during which anginal complaints may be precipitated can readily be covered with three 8-mg doses, one in the morning, one at midday, and one in the late afternoon. Molsidomine can appropriately be regarded as an alternative or adjunct to nitrate interval treatment, in particular to bridge the therapeutic gap prerequisite to effective nitrate use.

In heart failure, a 16-mg dose in sustained-release form can be used beneficially to provide continuous reduction of filling pressures with administration on a twice-daily basis.

Precautions and Contraindications

Molsidomine should not be administered in the presence of acute circulatory compromise (shock, vascular collapse, inadequate filling pressure) or severe hypotension (systolic blood pressure less than 100 mmHg). In acute myocardial infarction, molsidomine should be given only under strict supervision of the physician, and circulatory parameters should be monitored continuously. Molsidomine should not be given during the first trimester of pregnancy and should not be given to any person with known hypersensitivity to its constituent drug. Because molsidomine is primarily metabolized in the liver, patients with hepatic

insufficiency should be monitored because of possible underdosing of its active metabolite. Caution is advised for persons operating motorized vehicles or machines.

Side Effects

Molsidomine has a low incidence of adverse reactions. Based on drug surveillance studies encompassing several thousand patients, the most frequently reported side effect was headache (2.9%). Other adverse reactions, all reported with an incidence of less than 0.1%, include flush, dizziness, hypotension, and palpitations. Gastrointestinal complaints can encompass nausea and loss of appetite. In rare instances, allergic skin reactions have been reported.

Drug Interactions

Patients receiving antihypertensive drugs, β-adrenergic blockers, calcium antagonists, or phenothiazines and molsidomine concomitantly should be observed for possible additive hypotensive effects. Aspirin at a dosage of up to 1 g does not appear to interfere with the hemodynamic effect of molsidomine.

REFERENCES

1. Fleck E, Dirschinger J, Rudolph W: Hemodynamic effects of molsidomine in coronary artery disease. Herz 4:285, 1979.
2. Bassenge E: Pharmacologic basis of treatment with molsidomine. Herz 7:296, 1982.
3. Rosen R, Bernards W, Jumpertz K, et al: Interaction between thrombocytes and the coronary system in the presence of SIN 1 and nitroglycerin after endothelial damage. Z Kardiol 80(Suppl 5):23, 1991.
4. Groves PH, Lewis MJ, Cheadle HA, Penny WJ: SIN-1 reduces platelet adhesion and platelet thrombus formation in a porcine model of balloon angioplasty. Circulation 87:590, 1993.
5. Mannes A, Goebel G, Kafka W, Rudolph W: Treatment of angina pectoris with molsidomine. Herz 3:172, 1978.
6. Blasini R, Brugmann U, Mannes A, Rudolph W: Long-term treatment of angina pectoris with molsidomine. Herz 7:307, 1982.
7. Rudolph W, Dirschinger J: Effectiveness of molsidomine in the long-term treatment of exertional angina pectoris and chronic congestive heart failure. Am Heart J 109:670, 1985.
8. Rudolph W, Dirschinger J: Clinical comparison of nitrates and sydnonimines. Eur Heart J 12(Suppl E):33, 1991.
9. Beyerle A, Reiniger G, Rudolph W: Molsidomine, a nitrate-like substance with marked anti-ischemic and antianginal efficacy and no tolerance development during long-term treatment. J Am Coll Cardiol 7:178A, 1986.
10. Beyerle A, Lehmann G, Reiniger G, Rudolph W: No loss of action with the nitrate-like substance molsidomine during established nitrate tolerance. J Vascular Med Biol 4:260, 1993.
11. Schroder H: Cytochrome P-450 mediates bioactivation of organic nitrates. J Pharmacol Exp Ther 262:298, 1992.
12. Henry P, Horowitz J, Louis W: Nitroglycerin-induced tolerance affects multiple sites in the organic nitrate bioconversion cascade. J Pharmacol Exp Ther 248:762, 1989.
13. Wagner F, Gohlke C, Jaehnchen E, Roskamm J: Comparison of anti-ischemic effects of molsidomine and ISDN during acute and subchronic therapy. Eur Heart J 10:792, 1989.
14. Lehmann G, Reiniger G, Beyerle A, et al: Hemodynamic effects of two dosing regimens of molsidomine in patients with heart failure. Z Kardiol 82(Suppl 3):55, 1993.

CHAPTER 180

Ketanserin

Roland E. Schmieder, M.D., and A. E. Doyle, M.D.

HISTORY

It has been known for many years that serum or defibrinated blood contains a vasoconstrictor agent. Two independent lines of research led to the identification of this substance as 5-hydroxytryptamine (5HT). Rapport et al.[1-3] succeeded in isolating and identifying this material, which they named *serotonin*, from beef blood. The structure was subsequently confirmed by the synthesis of 5HT by Hamlin and Fischer in 1951.[4]

Working independently, Erspamer and his collaborators studied the nature of the chromaffin material present in epithelial cells of mammalian gastrointestinal mucosa,[5] and, in 1952, enteramine was also identified as 5HT.[6] Subsequent studies identified platelets as well as the enterochromaffin cells as a rich store of 5HT.

Ketanserin was demonstrated to bind to 5HT2-receptors[7] and to be a selective antagonist to the action of 5HT at these receptor sites. At higher concentrations, ketanserin also binds to α_1-adrenoreceptors and may therefore inhibit α_1-mediated contractions of vascular smooth muscle.

CHEMISTRY

Ketanserin is 3-[2-[4-(4-fluorobenzoyl)-1-piperidinyl] ethyl]-2,4[1H,3H]-quinazolinedione.

PHARMACOLOGY
Receptor Binding Sites

Evidence suggests heterogeneity of receptors that bind 5HT. Peroutka and Snyder[8] defined two types of receptors in brain based on radioligand binding. The 5HT1-receptor was preferentially labeled by 5HT, whereas the antagonist spiperone had a higher affinity for the 5HT2-receptor. Cohen et al.[9] provided evidence that the contraction of vascular smooth muscle induced by serotonin was mediated by 5HT2-receptors and that this contraction could be inhibited by the serotonin antagonist spiperone.

Early radioligand binding studies using ketanserin demonstrated high selectivity of ketanserin for the 5HT2-receptor and almost no affinity for the 5HT1-receptor.[7] In the same study, ketanserin showed a moderate binding affinity for the α_1-adrenoreceptor and the histamine-1 receptor, but none for α_2-adrenoreceptors.

Effects on Smooth Muscle

Early studies confirmed the pharmacologic specificity of ketanserin for the 5HT2-receptor by demonstrating

that ketanserin did not inhibit contractions induced by 5HT in the rat fundus or guinea pig ileum, which are mediated via other 5HT-receptors.[10] The same workers reported that ketanserin was an effective antagonist of the constrictor effects of serotonin on isolated vascular smooth muscle.

Subsequently, Van Nueten et al.[11] studied the inhibiting effect of ketanserin on contractile responses to serotonin and to aggregating platelets in vascular smooth muscle from various sites in different species. Ketanserin caused a dose-dependent inhibition of contractile responses to 5HT and to aggregating platelets in rat caudal artery and canine basilar, carotid, and coronary arteries and in gastrosplenic and saphenous veins. Ketanserin also inhibited the amplification by serotonin of vasoconstriction caused by other agents, such as norepinephrine or angiotensin II. At rather larger doses, ketanserin also caused a dose-dependent inhibition of the contractile responses of the rat caudal artery to norepinephrine. It has been shown that the constrictor responses to serotonin are exaggerated in blood vessels from aging animals.[12] Van Nueten et al.[11] noted a dose-dependent fall in blood pressure in spontaneously hypertensive rats, which they thought could be attributed either to the effects on 5HT- or α-adrenoreceptor–induced contraction or to a combination of the two.

The mechanism of the fall in blood pressure in spontaneously hypertensive rats was also studied by Fozard[13] and by Kalkman et al.[14] Fozard found that intravenous ketanserin induced an immediate fall in blood pressure and heart rate that was dose dependent. The fall in heart rate could be abolished by section of the vasosympathetic trunk, which did not affect the hypotensive response. In rats, at doses that caused the fall in blood pressure, ketanserin caused inhibition of the pressor responses to stimulation of the spinal cord and to phenylephrine, but the responses to norepinephrine and to angiotensin were less affected. Blood pressure responses to 5HT were inhibited at much lower doses of ketanserin. Using a 5HT antagonist, Fozard found no depressor effect nor any inhibition of the pressor response to phenylephrine or spinal stimulation; he concluded that the antihypertensive effect of ketanserin was probably due mainly to α_1-adrenoreceptor blockade.

Kalkman et al.[14] also concluded that the major mechanism of the antihypertensive action in spontaneously hypertensive rats was likely to be due to α_1-adrenoreceptor blockade because, at effective doses, ketanserin blocked the pressor action of the selective α_1-agonist methoxamine.

On the other hand, Pettersson et al.[15] studied hypertensive rats given ketanserin orally for 6 weeks. At the end of this time, blood pressure had fallen by 16%, but pressor responses to phenylephrine were unaffected, even though the pressor response to 5HT was almost abolished. These authors concluded that the chronic antihypertensive effect was not caused by α_1-blockade.

Central Nervous System Effects

Some evidence suggests an inhibiting action of ketanserin on sympathetic vascular tone due to an effect within the central nervous system. Phillips et al.[16] found that the intravenous administration of ketanserin induced a sustained fall in both blood pressure and heart rate in anesthetized dogs. There was no inhibition of responses to intraarterial norepinephrine or to preganglionic stimulation of the sectioned cervical sympathetic nerve, thus excluding an effect on α-adrenoreceptors or ganglion block. However, systemic pressor effects of intravenous nicotine and of common carotid artery occlusion, both of which induce a pressor response via central stimulation of the sympathetic nervous system, were inhibited.

Ramage[17] gave a 30-minute infusion of ketanserin to anesthetized cats and noted a fall in blood pressure and heart rate with decreased peripheral resistance and reduced preganglionic sympathetic nerve activity, consistent in part with reduced central sympathetic outflow.

McCall and Schuette[18] also found evidence for a reduction in central sympathetic nervous discharge with a fall in blood pressure and heart rate. This effect could be prevented by pretreatment with reserpine, which causes depletion of central catecholamines, but not by pretreatment with the serotonin synthesis inhibitor parachlorophenylalanine. The authors concluded that ketanserin acted by reducing central sympathetic outflow, probably by an action on central α_1-receptors.

These data support the possibility of a central inhibition of sympathetic outflow as a component in the antihypertensive action of ketanserin, in addition to its peripheral action. The relative magnitude of the two effects remains uncertain.

PHARMACOKINETICS

Absorption after oral administration is substantially complete.[19] However, bioavailability is between 16% and 60%,[20] owing to extensive hepatic metabolism. After a single oral dose, the terminal half-life is approximately 9 hours, but at steady-state conditions after prolonged administration of a single daily dose of 40 mg, the terminal half-life reaches approximately 24 hours. The major metabolites are 6-hydroxy ketanserin and ketanserol; the latter appears to be oxidized back to ketanserin, which extends the terminal half-life. The rate of elimination is determined by hepatic blood flow, hepatic clearance, and protein binding. The half-life is prolonged in patients with hepatic disease or renal failure; in the latter, retention of ketanserol with subsequent reoxidation to ketanserin prolongs the half-life. No pharmacokinetic interactions between ketanserin and β-blocking drugs, digoxin, or cimetidine have been found.

PATHOPHYSIOLOGIC EFFECTS
Hemodynamics

Acute Administration

The administration of ketanserin, 10 mg IV, to hypertensive patients to induce a hemodynamic pattern consistent with dilation of both resistance and capacitance vessels was reported by Wenting et al.[21] Mean arterial pressure fell by 22% in 30 patients, cardiac output rose, and calculated total peripheral resistance fell. Stroke volume fell as a result of the associated increase in heart rate. Plasma norepinephrine level rose sharply.

Right atrial pressure, pulmonary arterial pressure, and pulmonary capillary wedge pressure also fell. Pulmonary vascular resistance was not altered. Forearm blood flow and digital skin temperature increased markedly after ketanserin administration. Rectal temperature and skin temperature of the forehead remained constant.

Glomerular filtration rate remained constant, and renal blood flow rose slightly despite the decrease in blood pressure.

Prior treatment with prazosin greatly reduced the hypotensive effect of ketanserin, and the pressor response to bolus injections of phenylephrine was reduced after administration of ketanserin. Intravenous administration of ketanserin to four patients with autonomic insufficiency caused a fall of arterial pressure, whereas 20 mg of phentolamine had no effect.

Chronic Administration

The hemodynamic data after chronic oral administration of ketanserin are less clear-cut than the data after acute intravenous administration, and, in some cases, they are conflicting. Omvik and Lund-Johansen[22] studied 13 patients with mild or moderate hypertension treated for 9 months with ketanserin. Heart rate and cardiac output were moderately decreased with no change in stroke volume or total peripheral resistance. Fagard et al.[23] found a fall in heart rate with a significant increase in stroke volume and a fall in total peripheral resistance. de Leeuw and Birkenhager[24] also found a fall in heart rate, but they noted no change in cardiac output or renal vascular resistance.

The number of patients in whom chronic hemodynamic studies have been performed probably is too small to allow definitive conclusions. Most authors agree that blood pressure falls with a small fall in heart rate. The fall in heart rate would be consistent with a centrally mediated reduction in sympathetic outflow.

Effects on Ventricular Function and Structure

Ketanserin has been found to prolong the action potential of ventricular muscle in rabbits and to depress conduction.[25] This effect is consistent with a weak class III antiarrhythmic action. In both volunteers and patients, the QT_c interval was reported to lengthen in a dose-dependent manner. An average increase of QT_c interval of 12 msec was found with administration of ketanserin, 40 mg twice daily, whereas no significant increase was seen with 20 mg twice daily. In a few patients, arrhythmias associated with a prolonged QT interval have been reported. All patients had other possible contributing factors to the development of the arrhythmias.[26]

Effects on Coronary Arteries

Studies in animals have shown that serotonin constricts coronary arteries if the endothelium is damaged, but dilates coronary segments if the endothelium is intact. In humans, serotonin has a vasodilatory effect on normal coronary arteries, but again when the endothelium is damaged, as in coronary artery disease, serotonin exerts a vasoconstrictive effect.[27] The reduction of coronary blood flow by approximately 60% after serotonin administration was blunted by ketanserin.[27] Subsequent studies revealed that ketanserin inhibited coronary vasoconstriction in proximal, but not distal, arteriosclerotic arteries.[28] This action of ketanserin may prevent myocardial ischemia owing to the vasoconstrictive action of serotonin released after intracoronary activation of platelets. Of interest, vasoconstriction of coronary arteries was abolished only in the presence of ketanserin and thromboxane receptor antagonists.[29] The clinical implication of these findings remains to be determined.

Effects on Arteries and Veins

Ketanserin is a vasodilator drug causing relaxation of vascular smooth muscle in both arteries and veins. As already stated, ketanserin appears to have affinity for both the 5HT2-receptor and the α_1-adrenoreceptor. From the use of the drug in patients with Raynaud's phenomenon and with intermittent claudication and their subsequent improvement, evidence suggests that dilation of vascular beds can occur even when vascular disease is advanced.[30-32] This may be a direct effect on vascular 5HT2-receptors, or it may be mediated by the antagonism of ketanserin against 5HT released from platelets adhering to diseased blood vessels. It has been proposed[32-34] that platelets adhering to atherosclerotic plaques may release serotonin, which not only may induce local effects but also may cause constriction in vascular beds, including collateral vessels distal to the site of adhesion. Such a mechanism might explain the apparently beneficial effects of ketanserin that have been reported in some studies in patients with peripheral vascular disease.

Effects on Thrombocytes

Endogenous 5-hydroxytryptamine, released from the platelet-dense granules, has been shown to potentiate adenosine 5-diphosphate (ADT)–induced aggregation in human platelet-rich plasma.[35] Conversely, ketanserin inhibited potentiation by 5-hydroxytryptamine in the absence and presence of aspirin. Although aspirin caused substantial inhibition of aggregation by ADP, further inhibition occurred when ketanserin was also present.[35] These findings may help to explain the beneficial outcome in studies examining coronary and peripheral arteriosclerosis.

Effects on Fluid Volume State and Electrolytes

No consistent changes result from ketanserin treatment in either body weight or plasma volume. Effects on electrolytes are not significant.

Endocrine and Metabolic Effects

After acute administration, small increases occur in both plasma renin and plasma norepinephrine.

Prolonged oral administration has no consistent effect on plasma renin, aldosterone, or catecholamine levels. Ketanserin has no effect on the levels of pituitary hormones or thyroid function and does not affect glucose levels.

Either lipid levels are unchanged or total cholesterol and triglyceride levels are decreased, and the low-density lipoprotein/high-density lipoprotein (LDL/HDL) ratio is decreased.[26, 31, 36] One mechanism by which plasma LDL level is reduced by ketanserin is the direct induction of upregulation of LDL receptors.[36]

Effects on Renal Function

Given acutely, ketanserin increases renal blood flow without altering glomerular filtration rate.

Long-term effects on renal function are insignificant.

Effects on the Central Nervous System

Serotoninergic neurons are present in several areas of the central nervous system, and 5HT2-receptors were originally characterized in brain tissue. Large doses of ketanserin induce somnolence and electroencephalographic alterations, which suggest that the drug reaches the brain. Serotoninergic neurons are located in the brain stem and are concerned with the regulation of blood pressure,[37] and pharmacologic evidence suggests that a central action may mediate the antihypertensive effect of ketanserin. However, this suggestion is countered by the fact that ketanserin induces no fall in circulating norepinephrine such as occurs after administration of clonidine.[26]

Aside from somnolence, dizziness, and dry mouth, major central nervous system symptoms have not been reported.

Effects on Platelets and Red Blood Cells

Ketanserin inhibits *ex vivo* platelet aggregation and the release reaction induced by serotonin. It also reduces the platelet aggregation that occurs when intraplatelet products including serotonin are released after stimulation with such agents as collagen, epinephrine, and adenosine diphosphate. However, the primary aggregation induced by nonserotoninergic agents (e.g., epinephrine, adenosine diphosphate) is not affected by ketanserin treatment.[38] Bleeding time is slightly prolonged but remains within normal limits.[32] Treatment with ketanserin improves red blood cell deformability.[33]

CLINICAL USES
Indications

Hypertension

The antihypertensive action of ketanserin has been studied extensively in a large number of controlled trials against placebo and in comparison with other antihypertensive agents. The data have been summarized by Breckenridge,[39] using data made available by the Janssen International data base, and more recently by Vanhoutte et al.[26] In both placebo-controlled, crossover studies and parallel studies in patients with mild to moderate hypertension, ketanserin lowered both systolic and diastolic blood pressure significantly more than did placebo.[40] The average decrease in blood pressure with ketanserin was approximately 15/12.5 mmHg. The magnitude of the decrease in blood pressure was in part dependent on the initial level of blood pressure, with larger decreases occurring with higher initial blood pressures. Woittiez et al.[40] reported smaller decreases in blood pressure. Using 40 mg of ketanserin twice daily in 18 patients, Schalekamp et al.[41] found significantly lower blood pressures over the whole 24-hour period in the ketanserin-treated group than in the group receiving placebo.

It has been suggested that the magnitude of the fall in blood pressure becomes larger with continued administration. Breckenridge[39] reported that the decreases in diastolic pressure were larger after 3 months than after 2 weeks of administration. Similar results were obtained by Mauersberger.[42]

It has been claimed that the decrease in blood pressure is greater in patients older than 60 years than in younger patients independent of the starting blood pressure.[39, 43–46]

The efficacy of ketanserin has been compared with that of metoprolol and hydrochlorothiazide,[45] pindolol,[47] propranolol,[48] atenolol,[49] and prazosin[50] in patients with mild to moderate hypertension. In all studies, ketanserin proved to be as effective as the reference drug (Fig. 180–1). The usual dose of ketanserin is 40 mg twice daily.

Ketanserin has been used successfully in combination with β-blocking drugs[39] and thiazides.

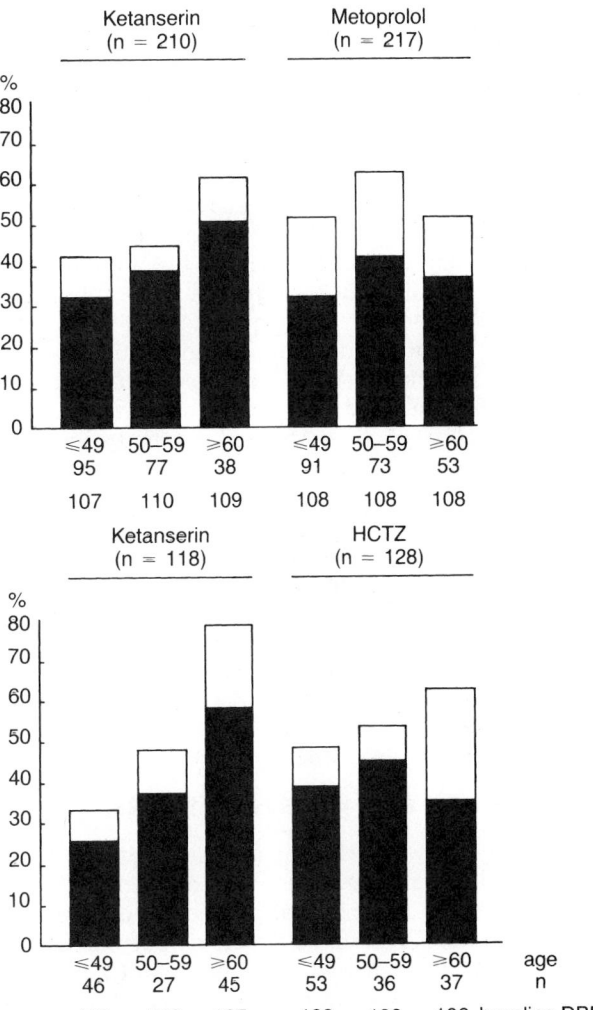

Figure 180–1. Response rate in hypertensive patients as a function of age for ketanserin, metoprolol, and hydrochlorothiazide (HCTZ). The bars give the total response rates, subdivided to show normalization ■ and partial response □. DBP, diastolic blood pressure. (From Rosendorff C, Murray GD [for the International Study Group]: Ketanserin versus metoprolol and hydrochlorothiazide in essential hypertension: Only ketanserin's hypotensive effect is age-related. J Hypertens 4[Suppl 1]:S109, 1986.)

To summarize, ketanserin is an antihypertensive drug that seems to be as effective as thiazide diuretics or β-blocking drugs. Its antihypertensive action is progressive for several weeks, and evidence suggests that it is more effective in elderly patients than in younger patients.

Vascular Disease

A number of reports suggest that ketanserin can reduce symptoms in patients with intermittent claudication.[51] Although not all studies have confirmed improvement, in a pooled analysis of 13 placebo-controlled studies in claudicants, 25% of patients treated with ketanserin doubled their walking distance, compared with 13% of placebo-treated patients.[52] Although these results are not confirmed, they are of considerable potential importance.

Heistad et al.[53] have shown that vasoconstrictor responses to serotonin are markedly potentiated in atherosclerotic monkeys. The normal vasodilator response to 5HT was reversed, with constriction of major arteries and a diversion of blood flow from distal to proximal vessels. Methysergide and ketanserin antagonized these changes. These findings, and the possible beneficial effect of ketanserin, raise the possibility that ketanserin might, by antagonizing 5HT-induced constriction, induce a favorable effect on vascular disease in humans. The possibility that ketanserin might reduce the incidence of vascular events was explored in a large placebo-controlled study in 3899 patients with intermittent claudication (PACK trial),[54] as preliminary evidence had suggested such an effect.[53] The trial neither confirmed nor refuted the original hypothesis. Although overall there was no difference in mortality, an adverse interaction occurred between potassium-wasting diuretics and ketanserin. Subgroup analyses[54] indicated that when patients taking potassium-wasting diuretics and antiarrhythmics were excluded, fewer patients had a morbid cardiovascular event with ketanserin than with placebo, and multiple events were fewer with ketanserin.

Precautions and Adverse Effects

Ketanserin has weak class II antiarrhythmic activity in some animal preparations.[25] Dose-dependent prolongation of the QT_c interval has been noted in humans. In the PACK trial, increased risk of ventricular tachycardia and increased mortality, mainly because of sudden death, were observed when ketanserin was combined with potassium-wasting diuretics, probably owing to QT-interval prolongation by ketanserin in the presence of diuretic-induced hypokalemia. No adverse interaction was observed when ketanserin was combined with potassium-sparing diuretics.[54]

Renal or Hepatic Insufficiency

The terminal half-life of ketanserin is prolonged in patients with renal or hepatic failure. In such patients, the dose should be smaller than in patients without these disabilities.

Central Nervous System Effects

Ketanserin induces somnolence, occasional dizziness, fatigue, and loss of concentration in some patients, mainly during the initial days of treatment. At doses of 40 mg twice daily these symptoms are unusual, but they increase in frequency and severity with larger doses. No major neurologic adverse effects have been reported.

Contraindications

Although no teratogenic effects have been noted, administration in early pregnancy should be avoided.

Interference with Other Drugs

As mentioned earlier, at a dose of 40 mg twice daily, ketanserin had a negative interaction with potassium-wasting diuretics in the PACK trial. No such interaction occurred when a potassium-sparing diuretic was included in the treatment regimen.

Place in the Antihypertensive Spectrum

Ketanserin is an effective antihypertensive drug suitable for monotherapy, as a step I drug, or for combination with β-blocking drugs. It has no major first-dose effect[55] and rarely causes hypotensive reactions. As in the case of most other antihypertensive drugs, patients with higher initial blood pressures have larger decreases in blood pressure. The antihypertensive effect appears to increase with continued administration over a period of several weeks. Ketanserin has been claimed to be particularly effective in patients aged 60 years or older. There are no orthostatic effects, reflex tachycardia does not occur, and side effects at the recommended maximum dose of 40 mg twice daily are infrequent. Responses to the drug vary from one individual to the next, and no factors other than initial blood pressure and age to predict a favorable response or likely ineffectiveness have been identified.

Unconfirmed preliminary data suggest that ketanserin may reduce the frequency of cardiac, cerebral, and peripheral complications of atherosclerosis, possibly via an action on 5HT2-receptors, because there is experimental evidence for increased sensitivity to 5HT in patients with atherosclerosis. If these findings are confirmed, ketanserin would have a unique place in the treatment of hypertension, because most existing drugs appear not to reduce morbidity or mortality from vascular disease in patients with hypertension. Consistent with this action, ketanserin does not raise serum cholesterol or reduce HDL cholesterol.

Initiation of antihypertensive drug treatment with ketanserin should be considered in patients with mild to moderate hypertension, particularly those older than 60 years or with clinical evidence of atherosclerosis.

DOSAGE

Initial dose of ketanserin is 20 mg daily by mouth, increasing after a few weeks to a maximum of 40 mg twice daily, if needed. Larger doses induce little additional fall in blood pressure but may increase side effects. Administration every 12 hours appears to control blood pressure over a 24-hour period.

SOCIOECONOMIC CONSIDERATIONS

Few data are available on compliance. However, side effects are not common and the dosage schedule is simple, which are factors likely to favor compliance.

Ketanserin has only recently been made available in a few countries. Details regarding cost of the drug are not widely available.

REFERENCES

1. Rapport MM, Green AA, Page IH: Partial purification of the vasoconstrictor in beef serum. J Biol Chem 174:735, 1948.
2. Rapport MM, Green AA, Page IH: Serum vasoconstrictor (Serotonin) III: Chemical inactivation. J Biol Chem 176:1243, 1948.
3. Rapport MM: Serum vasoconstrictor (Serotonin) V: The presence of creatinine in the complex: A proposed structure of the vasoconstrictor principle. J Biol Chem 180:961, 1949.
4. Hamlin KE, Fischer EE: The synthesis of 5-hydroxytryptamine. J Am Chem Soc 73:5007, 1951.
5. Erspamer V: Pharmakologische Studien uber Enteramin. Naunyn Schmiedebergs Arch Exp Pathol Pharmacol 196:346, 1940.
6. Erspamer V, Asero B: Identification of enteramine, the specific hormone of the enterochromaffin cell system as 5-hydroxytryptamine. Nature 169:800, 1952.
7. Leysen JE, Awouters F, Kennis L, et al: Receptor binding profile of R41468, a novel antagonist at 5HT2 receptors. Life Sci 28:1015, 1981.
8. Peroutka SJ, Snyder SH: Multiple serotonin receptors: Differential binding of [³H]5-hydroxytryptamine, [³H] lysergic acid, diethylamide and [³H] spiroperidol. Mol Pharmacol 16:687, 1979.
9. Cohen ML, Fuller RW, Wiley KS: Evidence for 5HT2 receptors mediating contraction in vascular smooth muscle. J Pharmacol Exp Ther 218:421, 1981.
10. Van Nueten JM, Vanhoutte PM: Selectivity of calcium antagonism and serotonin antagonism with respect to venous and arterial tissues. Angiology 32:476, 1981.
11. Van Nueten JM, Janssen PAJ, Van Beek J, et al: Vascular effects of ketanserin (R41468), a novel antagonist of 5HT2 receptors. J Pharmacol Exp Ther 218:217, 1981.
12. De Mey C, Vanhoutte PM: Effect of age and spontaneous hypertension on the tachyphylaxis to 5-hydroxytryptamine and angiotensin II in the isolated rat kidney. Hypertension 3:718, 1981.
13. Fozard JR: Mechanism of the hypotensive effect of ketanserin. J Cardiovasc Pharmacol 4:829, 1982.
14. Kalkman HO, Timmermans PBMWH, Van Zwieten PA: Characterization of the antihypertensive properties of ketanserin (R41468) in rats. J Pharmacol Exp Ther 222:227, 1982.
15. Pettersson A, Persson B, Henning M, et al: Antihypertensive effects of chronic 5-hydroxytryptamine (5HT2) receptor blockade with ketanserin in the spontaneously hypertensive rat. Naunyn Schmiedebergs Arch Pharmacol 327:43, 1984.
16. Phillips CA, Mylecharane EJ, Markus JK, et al: Hypotensive actions of ketanserin in dogs: Involvement of a centrally mediated inhibition of sympathetic vascular tone. Eur J Pharmacol 111:319, 1985.
17. Ramage AG: Effects of ketanserin and methysergide on the cardiovascular system of the cat. Br J Pharmacol 80:608P, 1983.
18. McCall RB, Schuette MR: Evidence for an alpha-1 receptor mediated central sympathoinhibitory action of ketanserin. J Pharmacol Exp Ther 228:704, 1984.
19. Riemann IW, Okonkwo RO, Kloz U: Pharmacokinetics of ketanserin in man. Eur J Clin Pharmacol 25:73, 1983.
20. Hedner T, Pettersson A, Persson B: Blood pressure reduction and pharmacokinetics of ketanserin in hypertensive patients. J Hypertens 4(Suppl 1):S91, 1986.
21. Wenting GT, Woittiez AJJ, Man in't Veld AJ, et al: 5-HT, alpha-adrenoceptors and blood pressure: Effects of ketanserin in essential hypertension and autonomic insufficiency. Hypertension 6:100, 1984.
22. Omvik P, Lund-Johansen P: Long term effects on central haemodynamics and body fluid volumes of ketanserin in essential hypertension: Studies at rest and during dynamic exercise. J Hypertens 1:405, 1983.
23. Fagard R, Fiocchi R, Lijner P, et al: Haemodynamic response to chronic ketanserin treatment in essential hypertension. J Cardiovasc Pharmacol 7(Suppl 7):S128, 1985.
24. de Leeuw PW, Birkenhager WH: Chronic effects of serotonin inhibition in hypertensive patients: Hemodynamic and humoral findings. J Cardiovasc Pharmacol 7(Suppl 7):S137, 1985.
25. Saman S, Thaudroyen F, Opie LH: Serotonin and the heart: Effects of ketanserin on myocardial function, heart rate and arrhythmias. J Cardiovasc Pharmacol 7(Suppl 7):S70, 1985.
26. Vanhoutte PM, Amery A, Birkenhager W, et al: Serotonergic mechanisms in hypertension: Focus on the effects of ketanserin. Hypertension 11:111, 1988.
27. Golino P, Piscione F, Willerson JT, et al: Divergent effects of seotonin on coronary-artery dimensions and blood flow in patients with coronary atherosclerosis and control patients. N Engl J Med 324:641, 1991.
28. McFadden EP, Bauters C, Lablanche JM, et al: Effect of ketanserin on proximal and distal coronary constrictor responses to intracoronary infusion of serotonin in patients with stable angina, patients with variant angina, and control patients. Circulation 86:187, 1992.
29. Yang ZH, Stulz P, von Segesser L, et al: Different interactions of platelets with arterial and venous coronary bypass vessels. Lancet 337:939, 1991.
30. Bounameaux HM, Holditch T, Hellemans H, et al: Placebo controlled, double-blind, two centre trial of ketanserin in intermittent claudication. Lancet 2:1265, 1985.
31. Amery A, Fagard R, Fiocchi R, et al: Ketanserin: A new hypotensive drug? J Cardiovasc Pharmacol 7(Suppl 7):S176, 1985.
32. Longstaff J, Gush R, Williams EH, et al: Effects of ketanserin on peripheral blood flow, hemorrheology, and platelet function in patients with Reynaud's phenomenon. J Cardiovasc Pharmacol 7(Suppl 7):S99, 1985.
33. Bogar L, Matrai A, Walker RT, et al: Haemorrheological effects of a 5-HT2-receptor antagonist (ketanserin). Clin Haemorrheology 5:115, 1985.
34. Vanhoutte PM, Luscher TF: Serotonin and the blood vessel wall. J Hypertens 4(Suppl 1):S29, 1986.
35. Vanags, DM, Rodgers SE, Duncan EM, et al: Potentiation of ADP-induced aggregation in human platelet rich plasma by 5-hydroxytryptamine and adrenaline. Br J Pharmacol 106:917, 1992.
36. Suzukawa M, Nakamura H: Effect of ketanserin tartrate on HMG CoA reductase and LDL receptor activity in cultured human skin fibroblasts. Eur J Clin Pharmacol 39:217, 1990.
37. Howe PRC, Kuhn DM, Minson JB, et al: Evidence for a bulbospinal serotonergic pressor pathway in the rat brain. Brain Res 270:29, 1983.
38. De Clerck F, Xhonneux B: Continuous inhibition of platelet S2-serotonergic receptors during chronic administration of ketanserin in humans. J Cardiovasc Pharmacol 7(Suppl 7):S23, 1985.
39. Breckenridge A: Ketanserin: A new antihypertensive agent. J Hypertens 4(Suppl 1):S13, 1986.
40. Woittiez AJJ, Wenting GJ, Van den Meiracker AH, et al: Chronic effect of ketanserin in mild to moderate hypertension. Hypertension 8:167, 1986.
41. Schalekamp MADH, Woittiez AJJ, Wenting GJ, et al: Ketanserin: Hemodynamic effects and mechanism of action. J Hypertens 4(Suppl 1):S7, 1986.
42. Mauersberger H: Long term safety and efficiency of ketanserin in essential hypertension: Ketanserin versus or in combination with metoprolol. J Hypertens 4(Suppl 1):S73, 1986.
43. De CrCe J, Hoing M, De Ryck M, et al: The acute antihypertensive effect of ketanserin increases with age. J Cardiovasc Pharmacol 7(Suppl 7):S126, 1985.
44. Hedner T, Persson B, Berglund G: A comparative and long term evaluation of ketanserin in the treatment of essential hypertension. J Cardiovasc Pharmacol 7(Suppl 7):S148, 1985.
45. Rosendorff C, Murray GD (for the International Study Group): Ketanserin versus metoprolol and hydrochlorothiazide in essential hypertension: Only ketanserin's hypotensive effect is age-related. J Hypertens 4(Suppl 1):S109, 1986.
46. Cameron HA, Walker PC, Ramsay LE: Ketanserin in essential hypertension: Use as monotherapy and in combination with a diuretic or β-adrenoceptor antagonist. Br J Clin Pharmacol 24:705, 1987.
47. Gordin A, Saraste K, Turanlahti N, et al: Comparison of ketan-

serin and pindolol in hypertension. J Hypertens 4(Suppl 1):S61, 1986.

48. Dona G, Ribeiro A, Tammaro AE: Ketanserin in the treatment of mild hypertension in elderly patients: Preliminary results of a controlled double-blind trial. J Hypertens 4(Suppl 1):S89, 1986.

49. Kirch W, Ohnhaus EE: Double-blind comparison of ketanserin with atenolol: Antihypertensive activity and effect in platelet function. J Hypertens 4(Suppl 1):S67, 1986.

50. Rosenthal J, Koehle W, Gruebel B, et al: Moderate essential hypertension control: A double blind crossover study between a serotonin antagonist and a post-synaptic alpha-blocker. J Hypertens 4(Suppl 1):S85, 1986.

51. Clement DL, Duprez D: Effect of ketanserin in the treatment of patients with intermittent claudication: Results from 13 pla-

cebo-controlled parallel group studies. J Cardiovasc Pharmacol 10(Suppl 3):S89, 1987.

52. Thulesius O, Lundvall J, Kroese A, et al: Ketanserin in intermittent claudication: Effect on walking distance, blood pressure and cardiovascular complications. J Cardiovasc Pharmacol 9:728, 1987.

53. Heistad DD, Armstrong ML, Marcus ML, et al: Augmented responses to vasoconstrictor stimuli in hypercholesterolaemic and atherosclerotic monkeys. Circ Res 54:711, 1984.

54. The PACK Trial Group: Prevention of atherosclerotic complications with ketanserin. Br Med J 298:424, 1989.

55. Marwood JF, Stokes GS: Studies on the mechanism of the hypotensive effect of ketanserin. Clin Exp Pharmacol Physiol 11:125, 1984.

CHAPTER 181

Thyroid Hormone (T_4 and T_3)

John D. Klemperer, M.D., Kaie Ojamaa, Ph.D., and Irwin Klein, M.D.

HISTORY

Thyroid hormone has profound effects on almost all organ systems. Cardiovascular manifestations of thyroid disease have been recognized for more than a century,[1] and a wide range of effects on the heart and peripheral circulation have been described.[2-4] The approach to applied pharmacology of thyroid hormone has been unique in that most of our knowledge has arisen from analysis of disease states. The thyroid gland is the source of the two major hormones, tetraiodothyronine (levothyroxine, T_4) and triiodothyronine (liothyronine, T_3), of which T_3 is the biologically active compound. Because oral T_4 preparations are the treatment of choice for replacement therapy in chronic hypothryoidism, extensive clinical experience with this compound has been gained. The response of the heart and systemic circulation to chronic therapy is well documented. In contrast, the clinical spectrum of T_3 therapy has been expanding, with emphasis directed at its acute action on cardiovascular physiology. Accumulating experimental and clinical evidence suggest that T_3 may act as both a novel inotropic agent and vasodilator. The current status of the drug's applicability is evolving, but T_3 may prove to be a useful agent in the armamentarium of endocrinologists, cardiologists, cardiac surgeons, and anesthesiologists alike.

CHEMISTRY

The synthesis of the thyroid hormones occurs within the thyroid gland on thyroglobulin and involves the iodination of thyroglobulin-bound tyrosine residues with subsequent couplings of monoiodotyrosine and diiodotyrosine moities to yield both T_4 and T_3.[5] The molecular formula of T_3 is $C_{15}H_{12}I_3NO_4$. In normal subjects, 85% of T_3 available to body tissues is derived from peripheral conversion of T_4 via the 5'-monodeiodinase enzyme present primarily in the kidney and liver. The remaining available T_3 is directly produced and secreted by the thyroid gland. The biologically inactive metabolite, reverse T_3 (rT_3), is derived from T_4 by a second enzyme, 5-monodeiodinase.[5] Structurally, triiodothyronine is distinct from known cardioactive agents with the exception of the bipyridine compound milrinone, with which it shares some structural homolog.[6] T_3 is available as a sodium liothyronine preparation for oral and parenteral use, marketed under the brand names Cytomel and Triostat, respectively.

PHARMACOLOGY AND MECHANISM OF ACTION

Triiodothyronine assumes a central role in the regulation of basal metabolism and tissue oxygen consumption.[7] In addition, significant effects on the cardiovascular system are mediated by T_3. The cardiovascular actions of T_3 can be attributed to (1) direct effects on the heart, (2) effects on the peripheral circulatory system, and (3) interaction with the sympathoadrenal axis.

T_3 has well-characterized nuclear and potential extranuclear actions, and the separation of hemodynamic effects into chronic and acute categories parallels this distinction. It is important to recognize that differences between the short- and long-term effects of T_3 have significant therapeutic implications. Long-term hyperthyroidism is characterized by a hyperdynamic cardiovascular state associated with identifiable changes in myocardial gene expression, including a shift in the predominance of myosin isoforms in animals,[8-10] and an increase in sarcoplasmic reticulum (SR) Ca-ATPase levels.[11, 12] However, the T_3-induced shift in myosin isoenzymes has not been found in the ventricles of all large animal models and has not been demonstrated in human hearts. It has also been difficult to separate the alterations in gene expression induced by T_3 acting directly on the myocyte from an indirect response mediated by changes in cardiac work. Klein et al.[8, 13, 14] have addressed this question using a heterotopic transplant model to distinguish the direct effects of T_3 on cardiac myocyte growth and gene expression and the indirect effects mediated by alterations in peripheral hemodynamics and cardiac loading conditions.

Many of the biologic effects of T_3 can be attributed to genomic changes mediated by specific nuclear T_3 receptors. However, attention has been recently directed toward the acute, non-nuclear-mediated effects of T_3 on the heart and peripheral circulation.[15] Accumulating experimental evidence supports a direct role for T_3 action at the subcellular level independent of the cell nucleus. Acute effects such as stimulation of sarcolemmal[6, 16, 17] and SR Ca-ATPase activity,[18, 19] sugar transport,[20] and alteration in sodium channel activity[21] have been identified in several in vitro systems. Evidence also exists that T_3 may act directly on vascular smooth muscle and function as a vasodilator.[22, 23] As will be discussed, the extranuclear actions of T_3 assume potential therapeutic relevance in certain clinical situations.

Some of the long-term manifestations of chronic hyperthyroidism are similar to a hyperadrenergic state, and an interaction with catecholamines has been proposed to be a potential mechanism of the action of the thyroid hormones. In experimental models, thyroid hormone treatment was associated with increased β-adrenergic receptor density, expression of the stimulatory subunit of the guanosine triphosphate (GTP)–binding protein (G_i), and β-adrenergic agonist sensitivity.[24, 25] However, studies in human subjects have produced conflicting results concerning β-adrenergic receptor responsiveness. Liggett et al.[26] found no alteration in catecholamine sensitivity in human subjects made hyperthyroid, whereas Martin et al.[27] reported increased left ventricular shortening velocity to β-adrenergic stimulation in hyperthyroid patients. This important issue remains to be resolved.

PHARMACOKINETICS

Circulating T_4 and T_3 are primarily bound to blood proteins, with only 0.02% and 0.2%, respectively, representing the free fraction. The greater biologic potency of T_3 compared with T_4 is attributed in part to its 10-fold higher binding affinity for the nuclear receptors. The half-life of T_3 may be significantly decreased in certain disease states.[28] When T_3 is given orally, it is 95% absorbed within 4 hours.[29] However, absorption may be impaired in severe hypothyroidism. Intravenous administration of T_3 may be indicated when rapid onset of effects are desirable or normal T_4 metabolism is impaired. Both T_4 and T_3 undergo hepatic conjugation before elimination.[5]

CLINICAL CONDITIONS OF LOW SERUM T₃ LEVELS

Hypothyroidism, characterized by low serum T_4 and T_3 levels and elevated thyroid-stimulating hormone (TSH) levels, is a common endocrine disorder that affects approximately 8% of the adult female population and a lower percentage of the adult male population. The classic symptoms include fatigue, cold intolerance, weight gain, and deepened voice.[30] Characteristic hemodynamic changes also become evident with long-standing hypothyroidism, including low cardiac index, decreased intravascular volume, increased systemic vascular resistance (SVR), and, in a subset of patients, hypertension.[2, 30] In the extreme case, myxedema coma may result in hemodynamic collapse and cardiogenic shock. Treatment of myxedema coma employs either T_4 or T_3 administered parenterally at doses from 100 to 300 μg/day for the former and 75 to 200 μg/day for the latter.[31]

A variety of disease states (Table 181–1) may produce the "euthyroid sick syndrome," a condition resulting from impaired conversion of T_4 to T_3 with subsequent low serum T_3 levels, low to normal T_4 levels, normal TSH levels, and characteristically elevated reverse T_3 (rT_3) levels.[32] Interest has focused recently on the use of T_3 supplementation to improve hemodynamic performance in specific patient populations with the low T_3 syndrome.[29] As will be discussed, administration of T_3 in the settings of cardiopulmonary bypass, cardiac transplantation, and congestive heart failure have shown the most promise to date.

PHYSIOLOGIC EFFECTS
Effects on Hemodynamics

Triiodothyronine-mediated changes in hemodynamics occur via the pathways described in previous sections. The extent and nature of the effects on cardiovascular hemodynamics are determined by whether there is chronic versus acute exposure to T_3. Hyperthyroidism is characterized by a hyperdynamic circulation that results from both direct genetic changes within the myocardium and changes in peripheral vascular tone.[2, 3, 23] These effects on the heart and peripheral circulation cannot be easily distinguished, as cardiac output and systemic vascular resistance are interdependent.[23] In an early study by Graettinger et al.,[33] the high cardiac index and low systemic vascular resistance of hyperthyroidism and the opposite findings in hypothyroidism were detailed. One of the first responses in hypothyroid patients to T_3 administration was a decrease in systemic vascular resistance,[23, 34] which may reflexively alter cardiac output. Theilen

Table 181–1. **Conditions Resulting in the Euthyroid Sick Syndrome**

Amiodarone therapy	Hypothermia
Burns	Myocardial infarction
Cardiopulmonary bypass	Prolonged stay in intensive care unit
Cirrhosis	Sepsis
Chronic renal failure	Starvation/protein-calorie
Congestive heart failure	malnutrition
Diabetic ketoacidosis	Trauma
	Widespread malignancy

and Wilson[35] found that the elevated cardiac output of hyperthyroidism could be diminished by abolishing the changes in SVR with the administration of phenylephrine. In a more recent study, acute administration of T_3 to normal animals produced a significant decrease in peripheral vascular resistance and an increase in stroke volume and cardiac output.[36]

Ventricular Function and Structure

Contractility

Prolonged treatment with thyroid hormone (whether T_4 or T_3) increased the maximal developed tension and rate of developed tension in isolated cat papillary muscles[37] and in the isolated working rat heart.[38] Studies in hyperthyroid human subjects have also described enhanced left ventricular systolic and diastolic function.[39] Because changes in ventricular loading conditions were not controlled, it is not possible to attribute all of the enhanced performance to a direct cardiac effect. Still, in addition to the known effects of thyroid hormone on SVR, much of this improved contractility can arise from increases in SR Ca^{2+}-ATPase activity.[40]

The acute effects of T_3 administration display several unique features. In animal models, acute T_3 treatment had no effect on the intrinsic contractility of the normal heart.[46] However, an inotropic effect became evident within minutes after the postischemic-reperfused heart was treated with T_3. This acute augmentation of postischemic left ventricular function has been shown in models of warm[41, 42] and hypothermic ischemia.[43]

Energetics

The linear relationship between left ventricular pressure-volume area and myocardial oxygen consumption (PVA-MVO_2 relationship) provides a sophisticated method for analyzing the efficiency of myocardial oxygen utilization in response to changes in work. For the chronic hyperthyroid heart, conflicting, although perhaps species-dependent, data have been presented. Isolated rabbit hearts demonstrated a decreased conversion efficiency,[44] whereas isolated canine hearts showed no change compared with the euthyroid state.[45] The authors of this chapter completed a study in 1994 in which the effects of acute T_3 treatment on the efficiency of myocardial oxygen utilization were analyzed using an *ex vivo* canine heart model of hypothermic global ischemia.[43] Acute T_3 treatment had significant inotropic action without associated oxygen-wasting effects, as seen for instance with traditional β-adrenergic agonists.[43]

Structure

Experimental hyperthyroidism results in cardiac hypertrophy. The excess thyroid hormone leads to a consistent increase in left ventricular weight.[46–48] This effect, however, is attenuated both by β-adrenergic

blockade[47] and under conditions in which the hemodynamic loading of hyperthyroidism is prevented, suggesting that the hypertrophic response is at least partially mediated by the imposed increase in cardiac work.[8, 48]

Diastolic Function

Left ventricular diastolic function is influenced by thyroid hormone status.[3, 4, 39, 49] Hypothyroidism and myxedema are associated with diastolic abnormalities, including prolonged ventricular relaxation time,[50] which is reversible with replacement therapy.[51] In comparison, hyperthyroid patients demonstrate an enhanced diastolic relaxation rate as assessed by two-dimensional echocardiographic Doppler ultrasound.[39] Acute effects of T_3 on ventricular diastolic function have been examined in animal models with divergent results. In a model employing normothermic ischemia-reperfusion injury, improvement in contractility after T_3 treatment was associated with restoration of diastolic function.[52]

Effects on Coronary Flow

Limited data exist regarding the direct effects of triiodothyronine on the coronary vasculature. Acute administration of T_3 decreased coronary vascular resistance, which resulted in increased coronary flow through a range of diastolic loading conditions in the postischemic reperfused canine heart.[43] In an isolated rat heart model, however, T_3 did not alter coronary flow.[53] Methodologic differences between the two studies may account for this discrepancy. Clinical data pertaining to the effects of T_3 on coronary blood flow are not available.

Effects on Arteries and Veins

As discussed previously, hyperthyroidism is associated with decreased peripheral vascular resistance.[2, 23] Accumulating evidence supports the concept that T_3 may function acutely as a novel vasodilator with direct effects on vascular smooth muscle cells. Recent studies using both vascular smooth muscle strips[22] and cell cultures[23] have demonstrated a rapid relaxation in response to T_3. The characterization of the vasodilatory effects of T_3 (on both peripheral and coronary vessels) is far from complete, but it represents an important area of investigation and potential therapeutic benefit.

Effects on Fluid Volume

Studies in both animals[53, 54] and human subjects[55] have documented an increased blood volume in hyperthyroidism and the opposite with hypothyroidism. In extreme cases, this can lead to edema formation. Much of this change can be accounted for by alteration in the renin-angiotensin-aldosterone system, the activity of which correlates directly with serum levels of thyroid hormone.[34] In hyperthyroidism, the expanded plasma volume results from increased renal sodium absorption, and appears to reflect a chronic effect of T_4 and T_3. The alterations in blood volume are responsive to appropriate therapy of thyroid disease states.

CLINICAL USE
Approved Indications

Although oral triiodothyronine (Cytomel) is approved for replacement or supplemental therapy of hypothyroidism,[29] there are almost no situations in which its use is preferred to that of T_4. Oral levothyroxine (Synthroid, Levothroid) is the standard and most appropriate therapy for the long-term treatment of hypothyroidism.[56] Intravenous T_3 (Triostat) is approved for the treatment of myxedema coma[57] and, similar to intravenous T_4, can successfully reverse the associated cardiovascular and other organ system complications.[58]

Experimental Use

Apart from the acute treatment of severe hypothyroidism, the potential benefits of parenteral T_3 therapy are being evaluated in a variety of clinical settings.[29] The rationale for use in these conditions arises from documentation of the associated euthyroid sick state along with a substantial body of relevant experimental literature. Several areas of active investigation are discussed here.

Cardiopulmonary Bypass

Cardiopulmonary bypass (CPB) results in a euthyroid sick state with a 50% to 75% decrease in free and total serum T_3 that persists for up to 24 hours postoperatively.[59, 60] The mechanism by which T_3 levels decrease has not been fully characterized but is associated with hypothermia, hemodilution, and a generalized inflammatory response possibly resulting in (1) decreased peripheral conversion of T_4 to T_3, (2) altered volume of distribution, and (3) a shortened half-life. The rationale for T_3 supplementation is based on experimental and limited clinical data that suggest that T_3 may have acute hemodynamic benefits in the immediate post-bypass period. In animal models of experimental CPB, T_3 treatment has resulted in improvement in postischemic cardiac function and ability to successfully terminate bypass. In a porcine model,[61] 100% of the animals treated with 6 μg of T_3 at reperfusion after 3 hours of cardioplegic arrest could be effectively removed from bypass, while four of six untreated animals did not survive. A study of T_3 administration to nonhuman primates also demonstrated an increased cardiac index, a decreased SVR, and maintenance of myocardial ATP levels after prolonged cardiopulmonary bypass.[62]

The results of two small clinical trials have been published. Novitzky et al.[63] administered T_3 (4 to 10 μg IV) to 12 patients experiencing difficulty being removed from bypass or in whom low cardiac output was unresponsive to inotropic or intraaortic balloon pump (IABP) support. Striking improvement was reported within hours of T_3 treatment, with discontinuation of IABP in all five patients. A placebo-controlled study, conducted by the same investigators,[64] was performed in 33 patients undergoing coronary artery bypass graft (CABG) surgery. Intravenous T_3 (0.1 to 0.2 μg/kg), given after aortic cross-clamp removal and repeated at intervals during the initial 24 hours postoperatively, restored physiologic serum T_3 levels and reduced the need for inotropic support in patients with preoperative ejection fractions less than 30%. T_3 treatment enhanced the cardiac output and lowered the SVR in patients with ejection fractions of more than 40%. Ongoing larger scale clinical trials should further define the circumstances in which pharmacologic T_3 supplementation may be of benefit in the cardiac surgery patient.

Cardiac Transplantation

The administration of T_3 to brain-dead organ donors was among the first clinical applications of T_3 therapy in which the drug was targeted specifically at improving hemodynamic performance. Low free and total T_3 levels occur shortly after brain death in both experimental animals[65] and human subjects.[66-68] Experimental evidence suggests that T_3 replacement improves the hemodynamic stability of the donor and the function of cardiac allografts.[69] Furthermore, several transplant centers have reported the benefits of hormonal supplementation in their potential organ donors. In one study,[70] prolonged survival after brain death was reported in subjects who were dosed with T_3 (1 to 1.5 μg/kg). Intravenous T_3 (0.2 μg/hr) administered with cortisol and insulin in brain-dead donors reduced the need for inotropic agents, corrected metabolic derangements, and improved cardiovascular hemodynamics that significantly improved the acceptability rate of the donor hearts for transplantation.[66, 71] Although these and other studies[72] have suggested a benefit in administering T_3 to organ donors, findings of other investigators[73] have not supported this view.

Congestive Heart Failure

Although hypothyroidism is infrequently the sole cause of heart failure, the euthyroid sick syndrome has been described in patient populations with advanced heart failure.[74] A low T_3/rT_3 ratio was identified as an independent poor prognostic indicator in this patient population.[74, 75] Whether the low T_3 levels definitely contribute to the deterioration of cardiac function in this subset of patients or are merely a marker of disease severity has not been determined. The therapeutic potential of intravenous T_3 supplementation in congestive heart failure is currently being addressed.[73]

ADVERSE EFFECTS AND PRECAUTIONS

Intravenous and oral T_3 therapy are well tolerated. To date no adverse effects of acute intravenous T_3 administration have been reported. Intravenous T_3 administration to normal volunteers in doses of 10 to 50 μg over 3 to 6 hours was not associated with any adverse effects or significant changes in measured hemodynamic parameters (Freed MI, unpublished observations). This dose is similar to that given for daily physiologic replacement and is extremely well tolerated at the same time that TSH levels are acutely suppressed (Freed MI, unpublished observations). The range of pathologic cardiovascular responses[2-4] (i.e., atrial fibrillation, other tachyarrhythmias, aggravation of angina pectoris, or even heart failure) associated with chronic clinical hyperthyroidism may prompt concern regarding the use of T_3 in patients undergoing heart surgery or with congestive failure. However, it is important to recognize that acute T_3 repletion in the setting of low serum T_3 levels is fundamentally different from the situation presented by the natural disease state. Indeed, data in coronary bypass surgery patients showed that the T_3-treated groups experienced fewer arrhythmias, both ventricular and supraventricular, than placebo-matched controls.[64] In this trial, patients treated with bolus doses of 0.2 μg/kg experienced no significant adverse reactions. Although not the treatment of choice, adverse reactions associated with T_3 during treatment of chronic hypothyroidism are rare and generally signal therapeutic overdosage with associated symptoms of hyperthyroidism.[57]

Precautions for the use of T_3 as a cardioactive agent are similar to those for other substances undergoing investigation. Although the drug has been well tolerated in the various clinical trials to date, appropriate cardiac monitoring should be conducted during administration. In the setting of cardiopulmonary bypass or cardiac transplantation, such monitoring is routinely employed.

CONTRAINDICATIONS

True allergic or idiosyncratic reactions to T_3 have not been reported with the oral or parenteral forms of delivery. T_3 is generally contraindicated in patients with adrenal cortical insufficiency before glucocorticoid replacement.[31, 56]

DRUG INTERACTIONS

There is evidence, as stated previously, to suggest that T_3 may sensitize patients to the effects of catecholamines. This should be kept in mind when coadministering T_3 and exogenous catecholamines.[56] Again, the eported clinical trials[63, 64] did not document problematic interactions between acute T_3 administration and routine β-adrenergic agonist therapy. The antiarrhythmic agent amiodarone inhibits the peripheral conversion of T_4 to T_3 and may produce change in serum T_3 and rT_3 similar to that seen with the euthy-

roid sick syndrome.[76] Thyroid hormones may increase the catabolism of vitamin K–dependent clotting factors,[57] and adjustments in long-term anticoagulant therapy may be necessary during the initial phase of thyroid replacement therapy.

DOSAGE AND ADMINISTRATION

T_3 is not the treatment of choice for long-term oral replacement in patients with hypothyroidism. When used in selected circumstances, oral T_3 is initiated at 25 μg/day given in divided doses progressing to a total maintenance dose of 25 to 75 μg/day. In older patients or patients suspected of having coronary artery disease, the recommended starting dose is 5 μg daily with a more gradual increase to maintenance dosing. The parenteral formula of T_3 can be used for the treatment of myxedema coma/precoma. An intravenous T_3 regimen of 50 μg/day is effective in reversing metabolic and myocardial function abnormalities.[77] Intravenous T_3 has been given to cardiac surgery patients in bolus doses of 0.1 to 0.2 μg/kg after removal of the aortic cross-clamp and at regular intervals for the initial 24-hour postoperative period. Current trials are under way in cardiac surgery patients, using doses up to 0.8 μg/kg bolus followed by a continuous infusion.

SOCIOECONOMIC CONSIDERATIONS

Long-term replacement therapy with oral T_3 compares favorably with T_4-based regimens with respect to cost. However, the need for multiple daily doses owing to the short half-life and the variability of clinical response makes the drug less desirable. The cost effectiveness of T_3 supplementation in cardiac surgery patients has not been addressed. Although T_3 therapy is likely to be more expensive on a dose-related basis than standard inotropic support, this must be evaluated in light of potential reductions in the need for and duration of traditional vasoactive agent support, ventilator dependence, and intensive care unit monitoring. These issues can be addressed only through prospective clinical trials.

REFERENCES

1. Graves RJ: Clinical lectures. Lond Med Surg J 7(Pt 2):516, 1835.
2. Klein I: Thyroid hormone and the cardiovascular system. Am J Med 88:631, 1990.
3. Dillmann W: Biochemical basis of thyroid action in the heart. Am J Med 88:626, 1990.
4. Polikar R, Burger AG, Scherrer U, et al: The thyroid and the heart. Circulation 87:1435, 1993.
5. Haynes RC Jr: Thyroid and antithyroid drugs. In Gilman AG, Rall TW, Nies AS, et al (eds): Goodman and Gilman's The Pharmacological Basis of Therapeutics, 8th ed. New York: Pergamon Press, 1990, pp 1361–1374.
6. Mylotte KM, Cody V, Davis PJ, et al: Milrinone and thyroid hormone stimulate myocardial membrane Ca^{2+} activity and share structural homologies. Proc Natl Acad Sci U S A 82:7974, 1985.

7. Oppenheimer JH, Schwartz HL, Mariash CN, et al: Advances in our understanding of thyroid hormone action at the cellular level. Endocr Rev 8:288, 1987.

8. Klein I, Hong C: Effects of thyroid hormone on the cardiac size and myosin content of the heterotopically transplanted rat heart. J Clin Invest 77:1694, 1986.

9. Martin AF, Pagani ED, Solaro RJ: Thyroxine-induced redistribution of isoenzymes of rabbit ventricular myosin. Circ Res 50:117, 1982.

10. Hoh JFY, McGrath PA, Hale PT: Electrophoretic analysis of multiple forms of cardiac myosin: Effect of lipopolysectomy and thyroxine replacement. J Moll Cell Cardiol 10:1053, 1978.

11. Rohrer D, Dillmann WH: Thyroid hormone markedly increases the mRNA coding for sarcoplasmic reticulum Ca²⁺-ATPase in the rat heart. J Biol Chem 263:941, 1988.

12. Arai M, Otsu K, MacLennan DH, et al: Effect of thyroid hormone on the expression of mRNA encoding sarcoplasmic reticulum proteins. Circ Res 69:266, 1991.

13. Klein I, Hong C, Schreiber SS: Isovolumic loading prevents atrophy of the heterotopically transplanted rat heart. Circ Res 69:1421, 1991.

14. Ojamaa K, Petrie JF, Balkman C, et al: Posttranscriptional modification of myosin heavy-chain gene expression in the hypertrophied rat myocardium. Proc Natl Acad Sci U S A 91:3468, 1994.

15. Davis PJ, Davis FB: Acute cellular actions of thyroid hormone and myocardial function. Ann Thorac Surg 56:S16, 1993.

16. Rudinger A, Mylotte KM, Davis PJ, et al: Rabbit myocardial membrane Ca²⁺ activity: Stimulation in vitro by thyroid hormone. Arch Biochem Biophys 229:379, 1984.

17. Kim D, Smith TW: Effects of thyroid hormone on calcium handling in cultured chick ventricular cells. J Physiol (Lond) 364:131, 1985.

18. Suko J: The calcium pump of sarcoplasmic reticulum. Functional alterations at different levels of thyroid state in rabbits. J Physiol 228:563, 1973.

19. Warnick PR, Davis FB, Cody V, et al: Stimulation in vitro of rabbit skeletal muscle sarcoplasmic reticulum Ca²⁺-ATPase activity by thyroid hormone and bipyridines [abstract 356]. Proceedings of the 70th Annual Meeting of the Endocrine Society, New Orleans, LA, 1988.

20. Segal J: Action of the thyroid hormone at the level of the plasma membrane. Endocr Res 15:619, 1989.

21. Harris DR, Green WL, Craelius W: Acute thyroid hormone promotes slow inactivation of sodium current in neonatal cardiac myocytes. Biochim Biophys Acta 1045:175, 1991.

22. Ishikawa T, Chijiwa T, Hagiwara M, et al: Thyroid hormones directly interact with vascular smooth muscle strips. Mol Pharmacol 35:760, 1985.

23. Ojamaa K, Balkman C, Klein I: Acute effects of triiodothyronine on arterial smooth muscle cells. Ann Thorac Surg 56:S61, 1993.

24. Williams LT, Lefkowitz RJ, Watanabe AM: Thyroid hormone regulation of beta-adrenergic receptor number. J Biol Chem 252:2787, 1977.

25. Bilezkian JP, Loeb JN: The influence of hyperthyroidism and hypothyroidism on the beta-adrenergic responsiveness of the turkey erythrocyte. J Clin Invest 63:184, 1979.

26. Liggett SB, Shah SD, Cryer PE: Increased fat and skeletal muscle β-adrenergic receptors but unaltered metabolic and hemodynamic sensitivity to epinephrine in vivo in experimental human thyrotoxicosis. J Clin Invest 83:803, 1989.

27. Martin WH, Spina RJ, Korte E: Effect of hyperthyroidism of short duration on cardiac sensitivity to β-adrenergic stimulation. J Am Coll Cardiol 15:94, 1990.

28. Sypniewski E: Comparative pharmacology of the thyroid hormones. Ann Thorac Surg 56:S2, 1993.

29. Klein I, Ojamaa O, Powell S: Potential clinical applications for parenteral thyroid hormone therapy. Hosp Form 28:848, 1993.

30. Klein I, Levey GS: Unusual manifestations of hypothyroidism. Ann Intern Med 144:123, 1984.

31. Klein I, Levey GS: Treatment of thyroid storm and myxedema coma. Topics in Emergency Medicine 5:33, 1984.

32. Wartofsky L, Burman KD: Alterations in thyroid function in patients with systemic illness: The "euthyroid sick syndrome." Endocr Rev 3:164, 1982.

33. Graettinger JS, Muenster JJ, Selverstone LA, et al: A correlation of clinical and hemodynamic studies in patients with hyperthyroidism and without congestive heart failure. J Clin Invest 38:1316, 1959.

34. Klein I: Thyroid hormone and blood pressure regulation. In Laragh JH, Brenner BM (eds): Hypertension: Pathophysiology, Diagnosis and Treatment. New York: Raven Press, 1989, p 166.

35. Theilen EO, Wilson WR: Hemodynamic effects of peripheral vasoconstriction in normal and thyrotoxic subjects. J Appl Physiol 22:207, 1967.

36. Kapitola J, Vilimovska D: Inhibition of the early circulatory effects of triiodothyronine in rats by propranolol. Physiol Bohemoslov 30:347, 1981.

37. Buccino RA, Spann JF, Pool PE, et al: Influence of the thyroid state on the intrinsic contractile properties and energy stores of the myocardium. J Clin Invest 46:1669, 1967.

38. Marriott ML, McNeill JH: Effect of thyroid hormone treatment on responses of the isolated working rat heart. Can J Physiol Pharmacol 61:1382, 1983.

39. Mintz G, Pizzarello R, Klein I: Enhanced left ventricular diastolic function in hyperthyroidism: Noninvasive assessment and response to treatment. J Clin Endocrinol Metab 73:146, 1991.

40. Klein I, Ojamaa K: Thyroid hormone and the cardiovascular system: From theory to practice [editorial; comment]. J Clin Endocrinol Metab 78:1026, 1994.

41. Dyke CM, Yeh T Jr, Lehman JD, et al: Triiodothyronine-enhanced left ventricular function after ischemic injury. Ann Thorac Surg 52:14, 1991.

42. Holland FW, Brown PS Jr, Clark RE: Acute severe postischemic myocardial depression reversed by triiodothyronine. Ann Thorac Surg 54:301, 1992.

43. Klemperer JD, Zelano J, Helm RE, et al: Triiodothyronine improves left ventricular function without oxygen wasting effects following global hypothermic ischemia. J Thorac Cardiovasc Surg 109:457, 1995.

44. Goto Y, Slinker BK, LeWinter MM: Decreased contractile efficiency and increased non-mechanical energy cost in hyperthyroid rabbit heart: Relation between O₂ consumption and systolic pressure-volume area or force-time integral. Circ Res 66:999, 1990.

45. Suga H, Tanaka N, Ohgoshi Y, et al: Hyperthyroid dog left ventricle has the same oxygen consumption versus pressure-volume area (PVA) relation as euthyroid dog. Heart Vessels 6:71, 1991.

46. Sanford CF, Griffen EE, Wildenthal K: Synthesis and degradation of myocardial protein during the development and regression of thyroxine-induced cardiac hypertrophy in rats. Circ Res 43:688, 1978.

47. Klein I: Thyroxine-induced cardiac hypertrophy: Time course of development and inhibition by propranolol. Endocrinology 123:203, 1988.

48. Ojamaa K, Samarel AM, Kupfer JM, et al: Thyroid hormone effects on cardiac gene expression independent of cardiac growth and protein synthesis. Am J Physiol 263:E534, 1992.

49. Friedman MJ, Okada RD, Ewy GA, et al: Left ventricular systolic and diastolic function in hyperthyroidism. Am Heart J 104:1303, 1982.

50. Wieshammer S, Keck FS, Waitzinger J, et al: Acute hypothyroidism slows the rate of left ventricular diastolic relaxation. Can J Physiol Pharmacol 67:1007, 1989.

51. Vora J, O'Malley BP, Petersen S, et al: Reversible abnormalities of myocardial relaxation in hypothyroidism. J Clin Endocrinol Metab 61:269, 1985.

52. Kadletz M, Mullen PG, Ding M, et al: Effect of triiodothyronine on postischemic myocardial function in the isolated heart. Ann Thorac Surg 57:657, 1994.

53. Gay R, Lee RW, Appleton C, et al: Control of cardiac function and venous return in thyrotoxic calves. Am J Physiol 252:H467, 1987.

54. Goldman S, Olajos M, Morkin E: Control of cardiac output in thyrotoxic calves: Evaluation of changes in the systemic circulation. J Clin Invest 73:358, 1984.

55. Gibson JG, Harris AW: Clinical studies of the blood volume. V: Hyperthyroidism and myxedema. J Clin Invest 18:59, 1939.

56. Levey GS, Klein I: Disorders of the thyroid. In Stein's Text of Medicine, 4th ed. St. Louis: Mosby, 1994, pp 1323–1349.

57. Triostat prescribing information. Philadelphia: Smith Kline Beecham Pharmaceuticals, January 1992.
58. MacKerrow SD, Osborn LA, Levy H, et al: Myxedema-associated cardiogenic shock treated with intravenous triiodothyronine. Ann Intern Med 177:1014, 1992.
59. Holland FW, Brown PS, Weintraub BD, Clark RE: Cardiopulmonary bypass and thyroid function: A "euthyroid sick syndrome." Ann Thorac Surg 52:46, 1991.
60. Robuschi G, Medici D, Fesani F, et al: Cardiopulmonary bypass: "A low T4 and T3 syndrome" with blunted thyrotropin (TSH) response to thyrotropic-releasing hormone (TRH). Horm Res 23:151, 1986.
61. Novitzky D, Human PA, Cooper DKC, et al: Inotropic effect of triiodothyronine following myocardial ischemia and cardiopulmonary bypass: An experimental study in pigs. Ann Thorac Surg 45:50, 1988.
62. Novitzky D, Huma PA, Cooper DKC: Effect of triiodothyronine (T3) on myocardial high energy phosphates and lactate after ischemia and cardiopulmonary bypass: An experimental study in baboons. J Thorac Cardiovasc Surg 96:600, 1988.
63. Novitzky D, Cooper DKC, Swanepoel A: Inotropic effect of triiodothyronine (T3) in low cardiac output following cardioplegic arrest and cardiopulmonary bypass: Initial experience in patients undergoing open heart surgery. Eur J Cardiothorac Surg 3:140, 1989.
64. Novitzky D, Cooper DKC, Barton CI, et al: Triiodothyronine as an inotropic agent after open heart surgery. J Thorac Cardiovasc Surg 98:972, 1989.
65. Novitzky D, Wilcomb WN, Cooper DKC, et al: Electrocardiographic, hemodynamic, and endocrine changes occurring during experimental brain death in Chacma a baboon. J Heart Transplant 4:63, 1984.
66. Novitzky D: Triiodothyronine replacement, the euthyroid sick syndrome, and organ transplantation. Transplant Proc 23:2460, 1991.
67. Sazonetsa IE, Kozlov IA, Moisuc YG, et al: Hormonal response to brain death. Transplant Proc 23:2467, 1991.
68. Gifford RRM, Weaver AS, Burg JE, et al: Thyroid hormone levels in heart and kidney cadaver donors. J Heart Transplant 5:249, 1986.
69. Novitzky D, Wicomb WN, Cooper DKC, et al: Improved cardiac function following hormonal therapy in brain-dead pigs: Relevance to organ donation. Cryobiology 24:1, 1987.
70. Taniguchi S, Kitamura S, Kawachi K, et al: Effects of hormonal supplements on the maintenance of cardiac function in potential donor patients after cerebral death. Eur J Cardiothorac Surg 6:96, 1992.
71. Novitzky D, Cooper DKC, Chaffin JS, et al: Improved cardiac allograft function following triiodothyronine therapy to both donor and recipient. Transplantation 49:311, 1990.
72. Garcia-Fages LC, Antolin M, Cabrer C, et al: Effects of substitutive triiodothyronine therapy on intracellular nucleotide levels in donor organs. Transplant Proc 23:2495, 1991.
73. Cohen S, Coarin JP, Jacquens Y, et al: Effects of triiodothyronine on hemodynamic status and myocardial function in brain dead donors. Anesthesiology 75:A1018, 1991.
74. Hamilton MA, Stevenson LW, Luu M, et al: Altered thyroid hormone metabolism in advanced heart failure. J Am Coll Cardiol 16:91, 1990.
75. Hamilton M: Prevalence and clinical implications of abnormal thyroid hormone metabolism in advanced heart failure. Ann Thorac Surg 56:S48, 1993.
76. Amico JA, Richardson V, Alpert B, et al: Clinical and chemical assessment of thyroid function during therapy with amiodarone. Ann Intern Med 144:487, 1984.
77. Ladenson PW, Goldenheim PD, Ridgeway EC: Rapid pituitary and peripheral tissue responses to intravenous L-triiodothyronine in hypothyroidism. J Clin Endocrin Metab 56:1252, 1983.

Index

Note: Page numbers in *italics* refer to illustrations; page numbers followed by t refer to tables.

abciximab. See *c7E3 Fab.*
Absorption of drugs. See also specific drugs.
  age-related changes in, 225
Accelerated idioventricular rhythm, 202
  with acute myocardial infarction, 132
ACE inhibitor(s). See *Angiotensin-converting enzyme (ACE) inhibitor(s)*; specific drugs.
Acebutolol, 183t, 496–499
  adverse effects of, 498–499
  chemical properties of, *475*, 496
  cost of, 548t
  drug interactions with, 348t
  during pregnancy and lactation, 498
  effects of, 467t, 472t, 497, *497*
    serum lipid, 499
  exercise's interaction with, 256
  for hypertension, 497–498
  intrinsic sympathomimetic activity of, 98, 497
  pharmacodynamics of, 467t, 472t
  pharmacokinetics of, 496, *496*, 553t
  pharmacology of, 496–497
  receptor selectivity of, 337t, 496–497, *558*
Acetazolamide, history of, 396, *396*
  in chronic renal failure, 363
  quinidine interaction with, 1365t
Acetylator phenotype, procainamide metabolism and, 1343
  procainamide-induced lupus and, 1345
Acetylcholine, arterial relaxation in response to, endothelium and, 832–833, *832, 833*
  for primary pulmonary hypertension, 85
N-Acetylprocainamide (NAPA), 1342
  accumulation of, in organ dysfunction, 239, 1346
Acetysalicylic acid. See *Aspirin (ASA).*
α_1-Acid glycoprotein (α_{1A}Gp), disopyramide binding to, 1283
Acid-base management. See also *Metabolic acidosis; Metabolic alkalosis.*
  in cardiopulmonary resuscitation, 218–219
Actin, in myocardial contraction, 1147
Action potential(s), duration of, afterdepolarizations and, 59
  slow response, 60
Activated partial thromboplastin time (aPTT), hirudin's effects on, 1492–1493, *1493*
  Hirulog's effects on, 1501–1502
  in monitoring streptokinase therapy, 1525
Adalat. See *Nifedipine.*
Adenoma, adrenal, amiloride for, 449
  spironolactone for, 455
Adenosine, 1239–1246
  adverse effects of, 1245
  antiarrhythmic effects of, mechanisms of, 1240, *1241*
  clinical effects of, 1240–1245, *1242–1244*
  dipyridamole interaction with, 1453
  during pregnancy, 274t, 275

Adenosine *(Continued)*
  endogenous, cardiac effects of, 217
    cardioprotective effects of, in ischemic heart disease, 1458
    dipyridamole interaction with, 1451–1452, 1453
    formation, metabolism, and function of, 1240
  for AV nodal reentrant tachycardia, 187
  for paroxysmal atrial tachycardia with myocardial infarction, 131
  for paroxysmal supraventricular tachycardia, 1242
  for primary pulmonary hypertension, 88
  for supraventricular tachycardias, 195
  for Wolff-Parkinson-White syndrome, 189
  in wide-complex tachycardia diagnosis, 203, *1244*, 1245–1246, *1245*
  inotropic effects of, mechanisms of, 44, 45t
Adenosine triphosphate (ATP), in regulation of nitric oxide formation and/or release, 837
Adenosine-blocking drug(s), in cardiopulmonary resuscitation, 217
ADH. See *Vasopressin.*
Adrenal adenoma, amiloride for, 449
  spironolactone for, 455
Adrenal hyperplasia, amiloride for, 449
  spironolactone for, 455
Adrenaline. See *Epinephrine (adrenaline).*
α-Adrenergic agonist(s). See also specific drugs.
  selectivity of, 336t
α_1-Adrenergic agonist(s). See also specific drugs.
  for heart failure, 344
  for postural hypotension, 99
α_2-Adrenergic agonist(s), 341–342. See also specific drugs.
β-Adrenergic agonist(s), 343–344
  for heart failure, 343, 1148
  in elderly persons, 230
  inotropic action of, attenuation of response to, in heart failure, 1147–1148
  mechanisms of, 44, 45t, 1147
  selectivity of, 337t
α-Adrenergic blocker(s), 661–687. See also specific drugs.
  calcium antagonist interactions with, 348t
  dopamine with, hypotension due to, 1164
  for hypertension, as initial therapy, 68, 69t, 71t
  for primary pulmonary hypertension, 86
  noncompetitive, 608
  postural hypotension due to, 96
  selectivity of, 336t
α_1-Adrenergic blocker(s), 342–343, *342*, 608–612. See also specific drugs.
  adverse effects of, 611–612
  clinical use of, 609–611

α_1-Adrenergic blocker(s) *(Continued)*
  during pregnancy, 271
  effects of, hemodynamic, 609
    metabolic, 611
  for hypertension, 609–611
    advantages of, 612
  in organ dysfunction, 242
  mode of action of, 609
  pharmacokinetics of, 610
  withdrawal of, 612
α_2-Adrenergic blocker(s), 343. See also specific drugs.
$\alpha\beta$-Adrenergic blocker(s), 568–598. See also specific drugs.
β-Adrenergic blocker(s), 465–598. See also specific drugs.
  ACE inhibitor with, for hypertension, 702
  adverse effects of, 479, 479t
  after myocardial infarction, 141, 292–294, *293, 294*, 301–302, 478, *478*
  ancillary properties of, 337, 337t, 344, 542
  antiarrhythmic effects of, 469, 469t, 470t
  antiatherogenic effect of, 481
  antihypertensive effects of, mechanisms of, 465–466, 466t, 477
  cardioselective, 344, 522–566
    decrease in serum potassium due to, 547
  central nervous system symptoms due to, 487, 534, 547
  chemical properties of, *475*, 475
  circadian pattern of cardiac disease and, 312–313, *312*
  classification of, 558t
  contraindications to, 480, 541
  cost of, 481, 548t
  delayed vasodilating effect of, 476
  drug interactions with, 348t, 352, 480
    with amiloride, 450
    with amiodarone, 1253
    with antiarrhythmic drugs, 347–349
    with bepridil, 1057
    with calcium antagonists, 347, 348t, 352, 555, 893, 893t
    with digoxin, 1142
    with disopyramide, 347–349, 349t, 351
    with dopamine, 1164
    with flecainide, 347–349, 348t, 349t
    with isradipine, 1017
    with lidocaine, 348t, 349t, 351, 352
    with mexiletine, 1326
    with moricizine, 1332
    with nifedipine, 348t, 973, 975
    with nitroglycerin, 871–872
    with NSAIDs, 348t, 350, 480
    with quinidine, 349t, 1365t
    with triamterene, 440
    with verapamil, 348t, 352, 480, 922
  during lactation, 276
  during pregnancy, 271–272, 271t, 274t, 480
  effects of, 467t, 472t, 476–479, *478*
  exercise's interaction with, 252–253, 253t, 255–256

β-Adrenergic blocker(s) *(Continued)*
for angina, 252t, 466–469, *468*
amlodipine with, 1036
calcium antagonists with, 32–34, 32t, 37, 468, 893, 893t
diltiazem with, 943
guidelines for, 36
in combined therapy, 31–34, *32*, 32t, 468
in triple therapy, 35–36
mechanism of action of, 27t, 30–31, 30t
unstable, 34–35
for cardiac disorders, 465–472
for congestive heart failure, 11
for hypertension, 474–481
ACE inhibitor with, 702
as initial therapy, 68, 69t, 71t, 480
clinical use of, 480–481
clonidine with, 625
dosage and administration of, 481
felodipine with, 1042
indapamide with, 428
nicardipine with, 989
nitrendipine with, 1002
socioeconomic considerations with, 481
with myocardial infarction, 129
for hypertrophic cardiomyopathy, nifedipine with, 976
for multifocal atrial tachycardia, 191
for myocardial infarction, 6, 133, 140–141
for atrial fibrillation with, 131
for hypertension with, 129
mechanism of action of, 7
for myocardial ischemia, nifedipine with, 972, 975
for postural hypotension, 98
for stress-related coronary artery disease prevention, 264
for stress-related sudden death prevention, 264
heart rate–reducing effect of, 1387
hemodynamic response to stress and, 265, 266
in black persons, 283–284, 284t
in cardiopulmonary resuscitation, 215
in combined therapy, for angina, 31–34, *32*, 32t, 468
using fixed combinations, 331–332
with amlodipine, 1036
with calcium antagonists, 32–34, 32t, 37, 332, 468, 893, 893t
with clonidine, 625, 626
with diuretics, 331–332
with felodipine, 1042
with guanabenz, 630, 631
with indapamide, 428
with mexiletine, 1327
with nifedipine, 972, 975
with nitrates, 31–32, *32*, 32t, 468
in elderly persons, 226–227, 231
in organ dysfunction, 241–242, 480
indications for, 465t, 466t, 480, 544–546
intrinsic sympathomimetic activity of, 337t, 344, 476, 542
membrane-stabilizing activity of, 469, 542
noncardioselective, 483–520
pharmacodynamics of, 467t, 472t
pharmacokinetics of, 476, 542–543, 553t
pharmacology of, 475–476, 476t, 540–542
precautions with, 480
principles and practice of therapy with, 465–481
selectivity of, 337t, 344, 541–542, 541t
solubility of, 542, 542t

β-Adrenergic blocker(s) *(Continued)*
thermoregulation and, 256–257
ultrashort-acting, 507–514
with coronary angioplasty, 308
withdrawal of, 531, 548
Adrenergic nerve varicosity, presynaptic receptors of, 335, *336*, 1190, *1190*
Adrenergic neuroeffector junction, 540
Adrenergic synapse, *336*
Adrenoreceptor(s), 335–338, 540–541, 541t
blockade of. See *Adrenergic blocker(s);* specific drugs.
classification of, 335, 540–541, 541t
in central nervous system, 338
postsynaptic, function of, 337–338
presynaptic, function of, 337
vascular, function and distribution of, 337–338, *338*
α-Adrenoreceptor(s), 602, 643
agonists and antagonists of, 335–336, 336t
central, 602–603
diltiazem interaction with, 934
postsynaptic, 335, *336*
types of, 541, 541t, 662
α₁-Adrenoreceptor(s), 643
agonists and antagonists of, 335–336, 336t
in central nervous system, 338
postsynaptic, 337–338, *338*
upregulation of, in myocardial ischemia, 341
α₂-Adrenoreceptor(s), 643
agonists and antagonists of, 335–336, 336t
in central nervous system, 338
postsynaptic, 337–338, *338*
presynaptic, 335, *336*, 337
β-Adrenoreceptor(s), agonists and antagonists of, 336–337, 337t
amiodarone's effects on, 1248
downregulation of, in heart failure, 341, 1147–1148
in response to amrinone, 1169
organ distribution of, 475t
postsynaptic, 336–337
presynaptic, 337
propafenone's effects on, 1350, 1352
sotalol's effects on, 1369
types of, 540–541, 541t
upregulation of, in response to propranolol, 484
β₁-Adrenoreceptor(s), agonists and antagonists of, 336–337, 337t
downregulation of, in congestive heart failure, 341
in heart, 338
β₂-Adrenoreceptor(s), agonists and antagonists of, 336–337, 337t
diminished sensitivity of, in old age, 341
postsynaptic, 338
presynaptic, 337
Adult respiratory distress syndrome (ARDS), 126–127, 126t
AF-DX116 (muscarinic antagonist), 340, 345
African American(s). See *Black person(s).*
Afterdepolarization(s), arrhythmia due to, 58–60, *59*
after myocardial infarction, diltiazem for, 942
causes of, 59
delayed, 59
arrhythmia due to, 14, 59
early, 60
as mechanism of arrhythmia, 14

Afterdepolarization(s) *(Continued)*
drugs causing, 59–60
Afterload, changes in, effects on pressure-volume loop, 45, *45*
reduction of, effects of, 869
vasodilators' effects on, mechanisms of, 43
"Afterload mismatch," prevention of, with β-blocker/calcium antagonist therapy in angina, 34, 37
Agmatine, 653–654
insulin secretion and, 657
Agranulocytosis, due to procainamide, 1345
AICD. See *Cardioverter-defibrillator, implantable.*
Alcohol. See *Ethanol.*
Aldactazide (hydrochlorothiazide/spironolactone), for hypertension, dose and side effects of, 374t
Aldactone. See *Spironolactone.*
Aldomet. See *Methyldopa.*
Aldosterone, ACE inhibitors' effects on, 692
ibopamine's effects on, 1201
renal potassium handling and, 445, *445*
Aldosterone receptor(s), 454
Aldosteronism, ACE inhibitors in evaluation of, 698
amiloride for, 449
during pregnancy, 270–271
ramipril use in, 769
spironolactone for, 455
Alinidine, 1387, 1388
Alkaline solution(s), dopamine interaction with, 211
epinephrine interaction with, 209–210
Alkalosis. See *Metabolic alkalosis.*
Allergy. See also *Hypersensitivity reaction(s).*
to contrast agent, premedication for, with coronary angioplasty, 309
to sulfite, dobutamine and, 1158
Allopurinol, warfarin interaction with, 350t, 353
Alpha blocker(s). See *α-Adrenergic blocker(s).*
Alprenolol, chemical properties of, *475*
in cardioprotection after acute myocardial infarction, *293*
pharmacokinetics of, 553t
receptor selectivity of, 337t
Alteplase. See *Tissue-type plasminogen activator (alteplase).*
Ambulatory monitoring, exercise testing vs., in antiischemic therapy evaluation, 37
in antiarrhythmic therapy evaluation, 1218
Amiloride, 443–451
advantages of, 450–451
adverse effects of, 374t, 449–450
chemical properties of, 444, *444*
contraindications to, 450
dosage and administration of, 374t, 451
drug interactions with, 446, 450
with digoxin, 351
during pregnancy and lactation, 450
effects of, 446–448, 448t
hydrochlorothiazide with, 374t, 448t, 451
in organ dysfunction, 247, 450
indications for, 448–449
mechanism of action of, 362, 444–445, *444*, *445*
pharmacokinetics of, 445–446
socioeceonomic considerations with, 451
ε-Aminocaproic acid, for bleeding due to tissue-type plasminogen activator, 1573

Aminoglycoside(s), ototoxicity of, loop
  diuretic interaction with, 361, 365
  procainamide interaction with, 1346
Aminophylline, in cardiopulmonary
  resuscitation, 217
Amiodarone, 1247–1258
  adverse effects of, 183t, 1256–1257
  arrhythmia aggravation by, 1235t, 1257
  chemical properties of, 1247, *1248*
  contraindications to, 1257–1258
  cost of, 1367t
  dosage for, 183t, 1252t
  drug interactions with, 204, 349t, 1252–
    1253
    with digoxin, 1142, 1252
    with diltiazem, 933, 1253
    with diuretics, 352
    with flecainide, 349t, 1253, 1315
    with nadroparin, 1488
    with phenytoin, 204, 1253, 1340
    with procainamide, 1253, 1346
    with quinidine, 204, 349t, 1253, 1365t
    with warfarin, 307, 350t, 353, 1252–
      1253
  during lactation, 1256
  during pregnancy, 274t, 275, 1256
  effects of, 1248–1251, *1249–1251*, 1382t
  for angina, diltiazem with, 943
    mechanism of action of, 1248
  for arrhythmias, after myocardial in-
    farction, 64, 132, 295–296, 1254–1255
    flecainide vs., 1309
    in congestive heart failure, 55, 1255
    mechanism of action of, 15, 1249–1251,
      1249–1251
  for atrial fibrillation, 194, 1253–1254
  for atrial flutter, 192, 1253–1254
  for ventricular tachyarrhythmias, 203,
    1255–1256
    mexiletine with, 1328
    propafenone with, 1356–1357
  in cardiopulmonary resuscitation, 216
  in children, 1256
  in combined therapy, with mexiletine,
    1328
    with propafenone, 1355, 1356–1357
  in elderly persons, 231
  in organ dysfunction, 236, 241, 1258
  indications for, 1253–1256
  intravenous, dosage for, 183t
    for atrial fibrillation, 1254
    indications for, 1253
  oral, dosage for, 183t, 1252t
    indications for, 1252t, 1253
  pharmacokinetics of, 1251–1252, 1252t
  response to outpatient dobutamine infu-
    sion and, 1155
  thyroid hormone interaction with, 1660
Amlodipine, 1024–1038
  advantages of, 1038
  adverse effects of, 1036–1037, 1037t
  cost of, 949t
  dosage and administration of, 1037–1038
  effects of, 909t, 1024–1029
    in animal studies, 1026–1029, *1027*
    in clinical studies, 1028, 1029
    in *in vitro* and mechanistic studies,
      1024–1026, *1025*
    renal, 1028–1029
  exercise's interaction with, 253
  for angina, guidelines for, 37
    in combined therapy, 1036
    therapeutic trials of, 1034–1036, *1035*
  for heart failure, 1036
  for hypertension, in combined therapy,
    1028, 1034

Amlodipine (Continued)
  therapeutic trials of, 1030–1034, *1031,
    1032*
  in elderly persons, 227–228, 1030, 1032
    dosage for, 1038
  in organ dysfunction, 246, 1030, 1038
  pharmacokinetics of, 1029–1030, 1030t
  therapeutic trials of, 1030–1036
Amlodipine/benazepril, 332–333, *333*, 1034
Amphetamine, for postural hypotension,
  99
Ampicillin, β-blocker interaction with, 480
Amrinone, 1167–1175
  adverse effects of, 1173
  chemical properties of, 1167
  clinical use of, 1172–1174
  comparison of, to other drugs, 1173–1174
  contraindications to, 1173
  disopyramide interaction with, 1173
  dobutamine vs., 1154, 1173–1174
  dobutamine with, for acute heart failure,
    1149, 1149t
    for chronic heart failure, 1154
    for dilated cardiomyopathy, 1173
    hemodynamic effects of, 50t
  dosage and administration of, 1174
  effects of, 1169–1172
    biochemical, 1172
    electrophysiologic, 1171
    hemodynamic, 49, 49t, 1149t, 1188t
    immunomodulating, 1188t
    in combined therapy, 50t
    metabolic, 1172
    noncoronary vasomotor, 1171
    on congestive heart failure, 1169–1170
    on coronary blood flow, 1170
  for heart failure, 12, 54, 1148, 1172
    in combined therapy, 50t, 1149, 1149t,
      1154, 1173
    with acute myocardial infarction, 136–
      137
  for left ventricular failure, 52
  for pulmonary edema, 50, 125
  for pulmonary hypertension, 87
  in cardiopulmonary resuscitation, 211–
    212
  in neonates, 1173
  in organ dysfunction, 1168, 1173
  indications for, 1172–1173
  mechanism of action of, 125, 1167–1168
  pharmacokinetics of, 1168–1169
  tolerance to, 1169
Amyl nitrite, 866, 867, 878
  adverse effects of, 878
  chemical properties of, 876–877
  effects of, 877–878
  methemoglobinemia produced by, for cy-
    anide toxicity, 869
  pharmacokinetics of, 877
Anemia, aplastic, due to pentoxifylline,
    1605
  hemolytic, due to methyldopa, 619
    due to procainamide, 1345
  hypoplastic, due to procainamide, 1345
  sickle cell, fluorocarbons' effects on red
    cells in, 1624
Anesthesia, arrhythmias associated with,
    phenytoin for, 1339
  cardiac problems with. See *Surgery.*
  hypotensive. See *Hypotensive anesthesia.*
Anesthetic(s), halogenated, diltiazem
    interaction with, 948
  dopamine interaction with, 1164
  inhalation, β-blocker interaction with,
    480
    verapamil interaction with, 922

Aneurysm, ventricular, ventricular
    thrombus with, 171, 171t, 1395t,
    1397–1398, 1397t
Angina pectoris. See also *Myocardial
    ischemia.*
  acebutolol for, 498
  amlodipine for, 1028
    therapeutic trials of, 1034–1036, *1035*
  antithrombotic therapy in, 174–175, 175t,
    1415–1416, 1416t
  aspirin for, 174–175, 175t, 1415–1417,
    1416t, 1447
  atenolol for, 544, 548
  bepridil for, 892, 1055–1057, 1056t
  β-blockers for, 252t, 466–469, *468*
    guidelines for, 36
    in combined therapy, 31–34, *32*, 32t,
      468, 893, 893t, 943, 1036
    in triple therapy, 35–36
    mechanisms of action of, 27t, 30–31,
      30t
  betaxolol for, 554
  bisoprolol for, 560–561, *560, 561*
  calcium antagonists for, 891–893
    guidelines for, 36
    in combined therapy, 32–34, 32t
    in triple therapy, 35–36
    mechanisms of action of, 891, 892t
  carvedilol's effects in, 593–594, 593t, *594,
    598*
  combined therapy for, 27–37
    evaluation of, 37
    experience with, 31–36, *32*, 32t
    goals of, 29
    guidelines and principles of, 36–37
    with three drugs, 35–36
  diltiazem for, 892, 942–944, 949
    guidelines for, 37
    in combined therapy, 32t, 33, 943
  dipyridamole for, 1458–1459
  emerging concepts in therapy for, 8–10
  felodipine for, 1043
  gallopamil for, 928
  in black persons, 280
  isosorbide mononitrate for, 883, *883*
    in controlled-release form, 886, 886t,
      887, 888
  isradipine for, 1020–1021
  metoprolol for, 530–531, *531*
  mibefradil's effects in, 1012, 1014
  molsidomine for, 1646–1648, *1647*
  nadolol for, 502–503
  nicardipine for, 984–988, *985–987*, 987t,
    988t
    adverse effects of, 987, 988
  nicorandil for, 1640–1642
  nifedipine for, 37, 974–975
    in combined therapy, 32–33, 32t
    in triple therapy, 35
  nisoldipine for, 1007
  nitrendipine for, 1003
  nitroglycerin for, 871–872
  pharmacologic management of, 252t
  pindolol for, 518, 520
  propranolol for, 487–488
    in combined therapy, 31–34, *32*, *34–35*
    in triple therapy, 35
  ranolazine for, 1602, *1602*
  rationale for therapy for, 9
  refractory hypertension with, 151
  sympathetic activity and, 466–467
  timolol for, 495
  trimetazidine for, 1598, 1598t
  unstable, antithrombotic therapy in, 108–
    109, 109t, 114, 175, 175t, 1415t–1417t,
    1416–1420, *1417*

Angina pectoris (Continued)
APSAC for, 1564
aspirin for, 108, 109, 109t, 114, 175, 175t, 1415t–1417t, 1416–1420, 1417, 1446
bepridil use in, 1057
β-blockers for, 34–35, 468–469
c7E3 Fab for, 1635
calcium antagonists for, 892
clinical presentation of, 9
combined therapy for, 34–35
diltiazem for, 943
esmolol for, 510–511
guidelines for therapy for, 36
heparin for, 108, 109, 109t, 175, 175t, 1416t, 1418–1419, 1420, 1476–1477
Hirulog for, 108, 1502, 1503
nicorandil for, 1642
nifedipine for, 974
nitroglycerin for, 872
pathophysiology of, 28
propranolol for, 34–35, 488
thrombolytic therapy for, 108, 1419
thrombosis after plaque disruption in, 1413–1414, 1414t
ticlopidine for, 1417, 1420, 1468
verapamil for, 920
variant, amlodipine for, 1036
β-blockers for, 468–469, 544
calcium antagonists for, 892
diltiazem for, 943, 949
felodipine for, 1043
metoprolol for, 531
nicardipine for, 988
nicorandil for, 1642
nifedipine for, 892, 974
nitrendipine for, 1003
propranolol for, 488
verapamil for, 892, 920
guidelines for, 37
in combined therapy, 32t, 33
zatebradine for, 1389
Angioedema, due to captopril, 736
due to ramipril, 768
due to trandolapril, 786
Angioplasty. See Coronary angioplasty; Percutaneous transluminal coronary angioplasty (PTCA).
Angioscope, 304
Angiotensin I, 690, 727
discovery of, 726
Angiotensin II, actions of, in kidney, 695
as neuropeptide, 795
discovery of, 726
in congestive heart failure, 711–712
in hypertension, 691–692
nitric oxide interaction with, 838
norepinephrine interaction with, 694
Angiotensin II analogue(s), 690–691, 691. See also Saralasin.
Angiotensin II receptor(s), types of, 819–820, 820t
Angiotensin II receptor inhibitor(s), 817–824. See also Losartan.
Angiotensin-converting enzyme (ACE), ACE inhibitor binding to, in tissue, comparative potencies of, 796–797, 797
captopril binding to, 727, 727
discovery of, 726
induction of, by ACE inhibitor therapy, 692
lisinopril binding to, 750, 751
trandolapril binding to, 785
Angiotensin-converting enzyme (ACE) inhibitor(s), 690–816. See also specific drugs.

Angiotensin-converting enzyme (ACE) inhibitor(s) (Continued)
adverse effects of, 701–702, 701
after myocardial infarction, 139, 296–297, 300–301, 300
effects of, 718–719, 719
in combined therapy, 719–720
approved uses for, 788
bradykinin accumulation and, 693–694
calcium antagonists with, for hypertension, 702, 732
in fixed combinations, 332–333
chemical classes of, 794
differences in ACE binding by, 801, 802
clinical applications of, 697–700
comparative tissue and plasma ACE binding potency of, 796–797, 797
cough due to, 285, 701, 747
diuretics with, decline in renal function with, 364
for hypertension, 72, 701, 702
hemodynamic effects of, 50
in black persons, 284, 285
in congestive heart failure, 387
in diabetic nephropathy, 363
in fixed combinations, 332
dosage and administration of, 700–701
drug interactions with, 352–353
with aspirin, 350, 353
with diuretics, 350
with NSAIDs, 350
with triamterene, 440
during lactation, 277
during pregnancy, 272, 698–699
effects of, 691–697
hemodynamic, 47, 48, 695–696, 695, 696
in tissue, 795–796, 796
metabolic, 696–697, 697
on pressor and depressor systems, 692–695
on renal function, 47–48, 697–698
on renin-angiotensin system, 691–692, 692
exercise training–like effect of, 258
exercise's interaction with, 257–258
for angina, 36
for congestive heart failure, 12, 53–54, 700, 711–716
as treatment, 712–715, 714, 715
in prevention, 715, 717–720
for coronary artery disease, 700
for hypertension, 697–700, 698
as initial therapy, 68, 69t, 71t, 702
calcium antagonists with, 702, 732
diuretics with, 72, 701, 702
in combined therapy, 702
nitrendipine with, 1002
for hypertensive emergencies, 154t, 155t, 158, 699
for peripheral vascular disease, 700
for pulmonary hypertension, 86
future directions for, 737–738, 791–792
hemodynamic response to stress and, 266
in black persons, 284–285, 285t
in chronic obstructive lung disease, 700
in congestive heart failure, very-low-dose, 387
in diabetes mellitus, 700
in elderly persons, 228–229
in fixed combinations, with calcium antagonists, 332–333
in renal insufficiency, 722–725, 722t, 724, 724t, 725

Angiotensin-converting enzyme (ACE) inhibitor(s) (Continued)
indapamide with, 428–429
mechanism of action of, 691–692, 692
pharmacokinetics of, 722–723, 723t
in renal insufficiency, 723–725, 724, 724t, 725
phosphodiesterase inhibitors with, hemodynamic effects of, 50t
principles and practice of therapy with, 690–725
prostaglandin metabolism and, 693
spironolactone with, 456
sympathetic activity and, 693–694
thrombolysis with, after myocardial infarction, 719–720
Angiotensinogen, 726, 727
Anisotropic conduction, 60
reentry and, 14, 61
Anisoylated plasminogen streptokinase activator complex. See Anistreplase (APSAC).
Anistreplase (APSAC), 1553–1565
adverse effects of, 1562–1563, 1562t
aspirin or heparin with, 1563–1564
chemical properties of, 1553, 1553
clinical trials of, 1557–1562, 1558–1560, 1561t
contraindications to, 1563, 1563t
cost of, 1565
dosage and administration of, 1564–1565
drug interactions with, 1563
effects of, 1556–1557
emergency department and prehospital use of, 1561–1562
for myocardial infarction, comparative trials of, 1431t, 1438, 1438, 1533–1535, 1534t, 1557–1561, 1558, 1559
timing of, 1528
in elderly persons, 231
indications for, 1557, 1564
neutralizing antibodies to, 1565
patency profile of, 1559, 1559
pharmacokinetics of, 1555–1556, 1555t, 1556
pharmacology of, 1553–1555, 1554
reocclusion and reinfarction potential after, 1559
survival effects of, 1560–1561, 1560, 1561t
ANP. See Atrial natriuretic peptide (ANP).
Antacids, drug interactions with, with fosinopril, 808
with mexiletine, 1326
with pravastatin, 1125
with quinidine, 1363, 1365t
with ticlopidine, 1472
α-Antiadrenergic drug(s), 601–687. See also specific drugs.
centrally-acting, 616–659
during lactation, 276
during pregnancy, 271
exercise's interaction with, 254–255
for hypertension, 69t, 70, 608
hemodynamic effects of, 601–602
in elderly persons, 227
peripherally-acting. See α-Adrenergic blocker(s); specific drugs.
principles and practice of therapy with, 601–612
Antianginal drug(s). See Antiischemic therapy; specific drugs.
Antiarrhythmic device(s), 1216–1217, 1217, 1222, 1222–1223. See also Cardioverter-defibrillator; Pacemaker.
Antiarrhythmic drug(s), 183t, 1207–1391. See also specific drugs and classes of drugs.

Antiarrhythmic drug(s) *(Continued)*
adverse effects of, 1222–1224, *1224*
after myocardial infarction, 295–296
aggravation of arrhythmia by. See *Arrhythmia(s), drug-induced aggravation of.*
atrial flutter and, 192
classification of, 1220–1221, 1220t, 1333
clinical considerations with use of, 1220–1226
combined therapy with, 1225
cost of, 1367t
drug interactions with, 349t, 352, 1222
with bepridil, 1058
with β-blockers, 480
with digoxin, 349t, 352, 1141–1142
with verapamil, 922
during lactation, 277
during pregnancy, 273–275, 274t
exercise's interaction with, 258–259
in elderly persons, 230–231
long-term therapy with, 1225–1226
metabolism of, 1221–1222
monitoring blood levels of, 1221
new and investigational, 1224–1225
patient surveillance during therapy with, 1219–1220, 1221
principles and practice of therapy with, 1207–1238
selection of, 1217–1220, *1219, 1220*
basis for, 58–64
electrophysiologic vs. electrocardiographic monitoring for, 1375–1376, *1375*
Antibiotic(s). See also specific drugs.
digoxin interaction with, 1138, 1142
Anticholinergic drug(s), 345
drug interactions with, with disopyramide, 349t
with mexiletine, 1326
with procainamide, 1346
Anticholinergic effects, due to disopyramide, 1285
Anticoagulant(s), 101t, 1473–1592. See also *Antithrombotic therapy;* specific drugs.
after embolic stroke, 168, 168t, 1411–1412
after myocardial infarction, 292, *292,* 299–300, *300*
for ventricular thrombus prevention, 171, 171t, 1396–1397
after saphenous vein bypass graft, 1457–1458
drug interactions with, with ciprofibrate, 1096
with fenofibrate, 1090
with gemfibrozil, 1101
with HMG-CoA reductase inhibitors, 1112
with quinidine, 1365t
with thyroid hormone, 1660
for deep venous thrombosis, limitations of, 1544
thrombolytic therapy vs., 1545, 1545t
in atrial fibrillation, 195
in dilated cardiomyopathy, 171, 171t
in mitral valve disease, 172, 172t, 1399–1400, 1399t
in pulmonary hypertension, 83
in unstable angina, 1417–1418
in valvular heart disease, indications for, 1399t
oral, in thromboembolism prevention, 163
pentoxifylline use with, 1605
platelet inhibitors with, experience and recommendations for, 106–113

Anticoagulant(s) *(Continued)*
in vaso-occlusive disease, 101–102
with coronary angioplasty, 306–307
with left ventricular aneurysm, 171, 171t
with prosthetic heart valves, 173–174, 174t
clinical problems with, 1411–1412
Anticonvulsant(s). See also specific drugs.
felodipine interaction with, 1044
Antidepressant(s), tricyclic. See *Tricyclic antidepressant(s).*
Antidiuretic hormone. See *Vasopressin.*
Antifungal agent(s). See also specific drugs.
digoxin interaction with, 1142
Antihypertensive therapy, 66–74. See also *Hypertension;* specific drugs and classes of drugs.
adverse effects of, 67, 67t
available drugs for, 67, 67t, 996t
combination tablets for, 73, 330–333, 331t, *333,* 333t
comparative trials of, 67
cost of, 70–71, 287, 430t, 949t
demographic characteristics affecting response to, 70, 71t
dose adjustment for, in organ dysfunction, 241
drug selection for, 67–73, 379–380, 380t, 626t
during lactation, 276–277
during pregnancy, 270–273, 273t
effects of, 17, *17*
emerging concepts in, 16–18
exercise's interaction with, 254–258
for hypertensive emergencies, 153–158, 154t–156t
future of, 18
hemodynamic response to stress and, 265–266
history of, 17
ideal drug for, characteristics of, 373–375, 375t, 618
in black persons. See under *Black person(s).*
individualized approach to, 68–70, 71t
Joint National Committee recommendations for, 68, *68,* 68t
objectives of, 461
parenteral, desirable drug properties for, 996–997, 996t
drugs available for, 996t
poor response to, 73–74, 73t
reactive sodium retention in, 70, 71
reduction or termination of, 74
rebound hypertension after, 152
stepped-care approach to, 17–18
fixed combinations as initial therapy in, 330–333, 331t, *333,* 333t
initial drug selection in, 379–380, 380t
substitution vs., 70
two drugs as initial therapy in, 72–73
Antiischemic therapy. See also *Angina pectoris; Myocardial ischemia;* specific drugs.
cellular agents for, 1594–1602
cost of, 949t
evaluation of, 37
exercise's interaction with, 251–254, 252t
experience with, 31–36, *32,* 32t
guidelines and principles of, 36–37
intentions of, 29
mechanisms of action in, 27t, 29–31, 30t
with coronary angioplasty, 307–308
Antinuclear antibodies, with betaxolol, 555
with labetalol, 576

Antinuclear antibodies *(Continued)*
with procainamide, 1345–1346
Antioxidant(s), for hyperlipidemia, 24
in cardiovascular disease prevention, 324–329
naturally occurring, 326, *326*
nutritional, 326–328, *326, 327,* 327t
α_2-Antiplasmin, in fibrinolytic system, 1567t, *1568,* 1570
Antiplatelet agent(s). See *Platelet inhibitor(s);* specific drugs.
Antipyrine, spironolactone interaction with, 458
Antitachycardia device(s), 1216–1217, *1217,* 1222, *1222–1223.* See also *Cardioverter-defibrillator; Pacemaker.*
Antithrombin(s), selective, 102. See also specific drugs.
Antithrombin III, 1473, 1474
Antithrombotic therapy, 1395–1592. See also *Thrombolytic therapy;* specific drugs and classes of drugs.
after coronary angioplasty, 111
after coronary artery bypass surgery, 1422–1424, 1424t
after myocardial infarction, 171, 171t, 1396–1397, 1397t, 1416t
experience and recommendations for, 110–111, 113–114
combined, 101–116
experience and recommendations for, 106–115, 114t, 115t
future directions in, 115–116, 115t
with anticoagulant and platelet inhibitor, 101–102, 106–113
with platelet inhibitors, 102–106, 113–115
drug interactions in, 350t, 353
for thromboembolism prevention, 1395–1425, 1424t
in acute myocardial infarction, 1416t
experience and recommendations for, 109–110, 109t
in atrial fibrillation, experience and recommendations for, 107–108
in cerebral ischemia, 113, 168, 168t
in coronary artery disease, 174–176, 175t, 1415–1420, 1415t, 1416t
experience and recommendations for, 108
in dilated cardiomyopathy, 171, 171t
in left ventricular aneurysm, 171, 171t
in mitral valve prolapse, 172, 172t, 1399t, 1400
in nonvalvular atrial fibrillation, 172t, 173, 1399t, 1402–1405
clinical trials of, 1402–1403, 1402t, 1403t
in peripheral vascular disease, experience and recommendations for, 112–113, 114–115
in unstable angina, experience and recommendations for, 108–109, 109t, 114
in valvular heart disease, 172, 172t, 1399t
principles and practice of, 1395–1440
with coronary artery bypass surgery, 1456–1458
experience and recommendations for, 111–112, 114
with prosthetic arterial grafts, 1455–1456
with prosthetic heart valves, 173–174, 174t, 1405–1412, 1453–1455, 1454t
bioprosthetic, 1409, 1410–1411, 1410t
clinical problems with, 1411–1412
experience and recommendations for, 106–107, 106t, 107t

1668 INDEX

Antithrombotic therapy (Continued)
  mechanical, 1407–1409, 1408t, 1410, 1410t
  with thrombolytic therapy, 1528–1530, 1529t
Anxiety, nadolol for, 503
  propranolol for, 489
Aortic aneurysm, dissecting, β-blockers for, 471, 546
  hypertensive emergency with, 150–151
Aortic dissection, β-blockers for, 471
  nitroprusside for, 862–863
  propranolol for, 489
Aortic impedance, 43
Aortic isthmus stenosis, urapidil use in, 678
Aortic regurgitation, nitroprusside for, 862
  thromboembolism risk in, 1400, 1401
Aortic stenosis, bretylium use in, 1270
  combined therapy for acute pulmonary edema with, 50–51
  dobutamine use in, 1158
  milrinone use in, 1183
  nitrate use in, 870
  thromboembolism in, 1399t, 1400–1401
Aplastic anemia, due to pentoxifylline, 1605
Apoprotein(s), bile acid sequestrants' effects on, 1070
  fibrates' effects on, 1076
  lipid-regulating therapy guidelines and, 76
Apresoline. See Hydralazine.
Aprindine, amiodarone interaction with, 1253
APSAC. See Anistreplase (APSAC).
aPTT. See Activated partial thromboplastin time (aPTT).
AQ-A39 (specific bradycardic agent), 1387
Arachidonic acid, 1608, 1608t, 1609
ARDS (adult respiratory distress syndrome), 126–127, 126t
Arfonad (trimethaphan), for hypertensive emergencies, 154t, 155t, 158
Argatroban, 102
  for unstable angina, 108, 1420
L-Arginine, nitric oxide formation from, 833–835, 834
Arginine vasopressin. See Vasopressin.
Arlix. See Piretanide.
Arrhythmia(s). See also specific arrhythmias.
  after myocardial infarction, sudden death and, 295
  atenolol for, 545
  β-blockers for, 469, 469t, 470t
  betaxolol for, 554
  calcium antagonists for, 893–894, 893t
  catheter ablation of. See Catheter ablation.
  diltiazem for, 945–946
    advantages and disadvantages of, 949
    mechanism of action of, 942
  dobutamine use with, 1158
  dofetilide's effects on, in preclinical studies, 1297–1298, 1298
  drug-induced aggravation of, 201, 1229–1238
    causes of, 15, 1237–1238
    definition of, 1229–1233, 1230, 1230t, 1231
    due to amiodarone, 1235t, 1257
    due to disopyramide, 1235t, 1286
    due to dobutamine, 1158
    due to dofetilide, 1298, 1301
    due to dopamine, 1163
    due to flecainide, 1235, 1235t, 1237, 1312–1314, 1313t

Arrhythmia(s) (Continued)
  due to mexiletine, 1235t, 1329
  due to milrinone, 1182
  due to moricizine, 1336
  due to procainamide, 1234, 1235t, 1344–1345
  due to propafenone, 1233, 1235, 1235t, 1354–1355
  due to sotalol, 1376–1377
  incidence of, 1234–1236, 1235t
  risk factors for, 1236–1237, 1236t, 1237
  types of, 1229t
  due to diuretic-induced electrolyte abnormalities, 386–387, 447
  due to magnesium deficiency, 364
  emerging concepts in therapy for, 13–16
  exercise and, 258–259
  ibopamine and, 1199, 1203
  in black persons, 280
  in children, amiodarone for, 1256
    bretylium safety in, 1270
    propafenone for, 1353, 1357
  in congestive heart failure, 55
  in digitalis toxicity, 1143
    management of, 1144
  in pulmonary edema, 121
  labetalol's effects on, 571–572
  mechanisms of, 14, 58–61
  metoprolol for, 531–532
  nadolol for, 503
  nonpharmacologic treatment of, 16, 1216–1217, 1217, 1222, 1222–1223. See also Cardioverter-defibrillator; Pacemaker.
  pharmacologic treatment of. See Antiarrhythmic drug(s); specific drugs and classes of drugs.
  pindolol for, 518–519
    dosage and administration of, 520
  propranolol for, 488
  stress as risk factor for, 262–263
  thiazides and, 414–415
  with acute myocardial infarction, 130–132, 130t, 527
Arterial compliance, 828
Arterial graft(s). See also Coronary artery bypass surgery; Saphenous vein graft(s); Vascular graft(s).
  prosthetic, antithrombotic therapy with, 1455–1456
  thrombolytic therapy for occlusion of, 1549–1551, 1550t
Arterial hypertrophy, in hypertension, 830
Arterial lesion(s). See also Vascular injury.
  in atherosclerosis, 1412–1413, 1412t. See also Atherosclerotic plaque(s).
  in hypertension, dietary potassium and, 461–462
Arterial pressure, mean, reduction of, to limit infarct size, 718
Arterial stenosis, vasodilatation in, 830–831, 831
Arterial thromboembolism, heparin for, 1477
  therapeutic options for, 1547–1548
  thrombolytic therapy for, 1547–1549, 1548t, 1549
    after delay, 1550–1551
    drawbacks of, 1548–1549
    results with, 1549–1551, 1550t
Arterial thrombosis, 174–176, 175t, 1412–1420
  pathogenesis of, 1412–1415, 1412t, 1413, 1414t
  recurrent, after streptokinase therapy, 1524–1525

Arterial thrombosis (Continued)
  thrombolytic therapy for, comparative trials of, 1530t, 1532–1533, 1533t
Arteriolar dilator(s), 853–857. See also Vasodilator(s); specific drugs.
  hemodynamic effects of, 11, 43, 46, 47, 853–854
Arteriolitis, fibrinoid necrosing, in accelerated and malignant hypertension, 149
Arteriovenous fistula(s), thrombosed, thrombolytic therapy for, 1551
Arteriovenous shunt(s), thrombosed, thrombolytic therapy for, 1551
  urapidil use in presence of, 678
ASA (acetylsalicylic acid). See Aspirin (ASA).
Ascites, furosemide for, 392, 456
  spironolactone for, 456
Ascorbic acid (vitamin C), in atherosclerosis prevention, 326, 327–328, 327t
Aspirin (ASA), 1443–1449
  adverse effects of, 1448–1449
    dose and, 1445
  after coronary artery bypass surgery, 112, 176, 176t, 1422, 1423, 1424, 1424t
    dipyridamole with, 1422–1424, 1456–1457, 1458
  after myocardial infarction, 110–111, 113–114, 291–292, 298–299, 298, 299, 1446, 1448
    dipyridamole with, 1459
  as antiplatelet agent, effects of, 102–103
    limitations of, 1626
  circadian pattern of cardiac disease and, 312
  dipyridamole with, after coronary artery bypass surgery, 1422–1424, 1456–1457, 1458
    after myocardial infarction, 1459
    in cerebrovascular disease, 1461
    in peripheral vascular disease, 1461–1462
    in stable angina, 1415–1416
    with coronary angioplasty, 177, 1460
    with prosthetic arterial graft, 1455, 1456
    with thrombolytic therapy, 1459
  drug interactions with, 350t, 353
    with ACE inhibitors, 350, 353
    with dipyridamole, 1453
    with enalapril, 745
    with nadroparin, 1488
    with probenecid, 350t, 351, 353
    with spironolactone, 458
    with sulfinpyrazone, 350t, 351, 353
    with ticlopidine, 1472
  during pregnancy, 1412
  for vascular occlusive disease, in primary prevention, 1447–1448, 1448
    in secondary prevention, 1446–1447, 1448
  heparin with, for acute myocardial infarction, 1416t
    for unstable angina, 1416t, 1418–1419, 1420
  in acute myocardial infarction, 109, 109t, 110, 175, 175t, 1416t
  in atrial fibrillation, 107–108
  in cerebrovascular disease, 113, 168, 168t, 1446–1447, 1448, 1461
  in chronic coronary artery disease, 37, 108, 1447, 1448
  in mitral valve disease, 1399

Aspirin (ASA) (Continued)
 in mitral valve prolapse, 172, 172t, 1399t, 1400
 in nonvalvular atrial fibrillation, 172t, 173, 1399t, 1402t, 1403–1404, 1405
 in organ dysfunction, 236, 247
 in peripheral vascular disease, 113, 114–115
  dipyridamole with, 1461–1462
 in stable angina, 174, 175t, 1416, 1416t, 1447
  dipyridamole with, 1415–1416
 in thromboembolism prevention, 163
 in unstable angina, 108, 109, 109t, 114, 175, 175t, 1416–1417, 1416t, 1417, 1417t, 1420, 1446
  anticoagulants with, 1415t, 1416t, 1418–1419, 1420
 low-dose slow-release preparations of, 299
 mechanism of action of, 1443
 pharmacodynamics of, 1444–1446, 1445
  in uremia, 236
 pharmacokinetics of, 1443–1444
 thrombolytic therapy with, 298
 with coronary angioplasty, 111, 176t, 177, 305, 308t, 309, 309t, 1460, 1461
 with coronary artery bypass surgery, 114
 with prosthetic heart valves, 173–174, 174t
  bioprosthetic, 1409, 1410t, 1411
  in combined therapy, 106–107, 106t, 107t
  warfarin with, 1408t, 1409, 1410, 1410t, 1454–1455
 with thrombolytic therapy, 5, 1525, 1528–1530, 1529t, 1563–1564
  dipyridamole with, 1459
 with vascular graft, 1448
  dipyridamole with, 1455, 1456
Asthma. See also Bronchospasm; Chronic obstructive pulmonary disease (COPD).
 ACE inhibitor use in, 700
 aspirin use in, 1449
 β-blocker use in, 480, 541, 542
 bisoprolol use in, 565
 esmolol use in, 512, 513
 labetalol use in, 573
 propafenone use in, 1354
 propranolol use in, 490
Asystole, due to verapamil, 922
 with acute myocardial infarction, 131
Atenolol, 540–548
 adverse effects of, 479, 546–547
 after myocardial infarction, 301, 470
 central nervous system symptoms due to, 544, 547
 chemical properties of, 475, 540
 contraindications to, 547
 cost of, 430t, 548, 548t, 949t
 dosage and administration of, 548
 drug interactions with, 547
  with disopyramide, 1285
  with quinidine, 1365t
 during lactation, 276, 276t
 during pregnancy, 272, 545
 effects of, 467t, 472t, 543–544
 exercise's interaction with, 253, 255
 for angina, 544, 548
  nicorandil vs., 1641
 for hypertension, 545, 548
  mechanisms of action of, 544–545
 in black persons, 284t
 in organ dysfunction, 241, 547–548
 indications for, 544–546
 pharmacokinetics of, 542–543, 553t

Atenolol (Continued)
 pharmacology of, 467t, 472t, 540–542
 precautions with, 546–547
 receptor selectivity of, 337t
 socioeconomic considerations with, 548
 type A behavior and, 264
Atherectomy catheter(s), 304
Atherogenic lipoprotein phenotype, 1087
Atherosclerosis. See also Atherosclerotic plaque(s); Coronary artery disease.
 antioxidants in prevention of, 324–329
 β-blockers in prevention of, 481
 calcium antagonists in prevention of, 901–906
  animal studies of, 903–906, 904, 905
  clinical studies of, 906, 911t
 diltiazem's effects on, 937–938
 doxazosin's effects on, 683–684
 endogenous nitric oxide in, 843–845
 experimental, calcium antagonists in, 903–906, 904, 905
  effects of drugs on, 902–903
 fish oils' effects on, 1611, 1611t
 isradipine's effects on, 1017, 1019–1020
 lacidipine's effects on, 1050
 lovastatin's effects on, 1110
 magnesium EDTA chelation for, 1615–1616, 1616
 metoprolol's effects on, 533–534
 pathogenesis of, 902
  mechanisms of cholesterol deposition in, 532–533
  vascular injury in, 1412, 1412t
 pravastatin's effects on, 1126
 probucol's effects on, 1102
 progression of, thrombosis in, 1413
 simvastatin's effects on, 1116
 trandolapril's effects on, 786
 vasoconstriction in, 1414–1415
 vasodilatation in, 830–831, 831
Atherosclerotic plaque(s). See also Atherosclerosis.
 calcium antagonists' effect on, 31
 development of, 28, 28, 902
 disruption of, 1413, 1413
  acute coronary syndromes and, 1413–1414, 1414t
  in initiation of coronary thrombosis, 9, 28, 28
  residual thrombus after, 1414
 lipid-regulating therapy's effects on, 24
ATP (adenosine triphosphate), in regulation of nitric oxide formation and/or release, 837
Atrial fibrillation, 193–194, 194, 1208–1209, 1208
 adenosine's effects on, 1241
 amiodarone for, 1253–1254
 antithrombotic therapy with, 107–108, 172t, 1477
  warfarin for, 1518
 β-blockers for, 470t
 calcium antagonists for, 893
 differential diagnosis of, 185t
 digoxin for, 194, 196, 1139–1140
 diltiazem for, 131, 893, 946, 1209
  mechanism of action of, 942
 disopyramide for, 1288–1290, 1289
 dofetilide for, 1300
 drug treatment for, 63, 193–194, 195–196
 due to adenosine, 1245
 esmolol for, 509–510
 flecainide's effects in, 1310–1311
 in acute myocardial infarction, 131
 in valvular heart disease, embolism and, 172, 1399

Atrial fibrillation (Continued)
 metoprolol for, 532
 milrinone use in, 1183
 moricizine for, 1336
 nonvalvular, antithrombotic therapy in, 172t, 173, 1399t, 1402–1405, 1402t, 1403t
  embolism in, 172–173, 1401–1405, 1401t
 prevention of, 14–15
 propafenone for, 1357–1358
 quinidine for, 15, 1362, 1364, 1366–1367
 sotalol for, 1372–1373, 1383
 d-sotalol for, 1383
 verapamil for, 920
Atrial flutter, 192–193, 1209–1210, 1209
 adenosine's effects on, 1241
 amiodarone for, 1253–1254
 atypical, 192
 β-blockers for, 470t
 calcium antagonists for, 894
 differential diagnosis of, 185t
 disopyramide for, 1289–1290
 dofetilide for, 1300
 drug selection for, 62–63
 due to antiarrhythmic drugs, 1233, 1233
 esmolol for, 509–510
 flecainide's effects in, 1310
 in acute myocardial infarction, 131
 metoprolol for, 532
 prevention of, 14–15
 procainamide for, 1344
 propafenone for, 1357–1358
 quinidine for, 1362, 1364
 sotalol for, 1372–1373
 d-sotalol for, 1383
 verapamil for, 920
Atrial natriuretic peptide (ANP), ACE inhibitors' effects on, 693
 in acute renal failure, in animal models, 359
 in chronic renal failure, 362
 in response to congestive heart failure, 44
 response to, in nephrotic syndrome, 363
Atrial septal defect, pulmonary hypertension with, 90
Atrial tachycardia(s), 184, 1210, 1210. See also specific arrhythmias.
 automatic, adenosine's effects on, 1242
 β-blockers for, 470t
 chaotic, 191–192, 191
  drug treatment of, 196
 drug selection for, 62
 ectopic, differential diagnosis of, 185t
  moricizine for, 1336
 fetal, drug treatment for, 275
 flecainide's effects in, 1310
 metoprolol for, 532
 nadolol for, 503
 paroxysmal, in acute myocardial infarction, 131
  with AV block, 190–191
 procainamide for, 1344
 with long RP interval, 1212, 1214, 1215
Atrial thrombosis, 171–173, 172t, 1398
 echocardiographic detection of, 1402, 1404–1405
Atrioventricular (AV) block, β-blocker use in, 546
 due to antiarrhythmic drugs, 1232, 1233
 due to disopyramide, 1286
 due to pindolol, 519
 due to procainamide, 1224, 1224
 due to propafenone, 1354
 due to verapamil, 921–922

Atrioventricular (AV) block *(Continued)*
  with acute myocardial infarction, 130–131
Atrioventricular (AV) junction, defined, 196
Atrioventricular junctional arrhythmia(s), 196–197, *197.* See also specific arrhythmias.
Atrioventricular junctional tachycardia(s), 196
  differential diagnosis of, 185t
  ectopic, adenosine's effects on, 1243
  management of, 197
  nonpreexcited, adenosine's effects on, 1242, *1243*
    verapamil for, 1242
  preexcited, adenosine's effects on, 1242–1243
Atrioventricular nodal reentrant tachycardia (AVNRT), *184,* 185–187, *186,* 1210–1211, *1211*
  adenosine's effects on, 1242
  AV reentrant tachycardia vs., 187, 1210–1212, *1211, 1212*
  differential diagnosis of, 185t
  disopyramide for, 1288
  dofetilide for, 1300–1301
  flecainide's effects on, 1310, 1311–1312
  propafenone for, 1357
  sotalol for, 1373
  treatment of, 61–62, 1212, *1213*
  with long RP interval, 1212–1215, *1214*
Atrioventricular (AV) node, digitalis' effects on, 1137
  drug interactions involving, 347
  in supraventricular tachycardia, 14
Atrioventricular reentrant tachycardia (AVRT), 1211–1212, *1211, 1212*
  adenosine's effects on, 1242, *1243*
  AV nodal reentrant tachycardia vs., 187, 1210–1212, *1211, 1212*
  differential diagnosis of, 185t
  disopyramide for, 1288–1289
  dofetilide for, 1300–1301
  flecainide's effects on, 1310, 1311
  in Wolff-Parkinson-White syndrome, 187–188, *188*
    management of, 189
  propafenone for, 1357
  treatment of, 189, 195, 1212, *1213*
  with "concealed bypass tract," 188–189, *189*
  with long RP interval, 1212, *1214*
Atrioventricular reentry, atypical, drug selection for, 62
Atromid. See *Clofibrate.*
Atropine, 345
  for bradycardia with acute myocardial infarction, 130
  for digitalis toxicity, 1144
  in cardiopulmonary resuscitation, 216–217
    endotracheal administration of, 207, 216–217
  mexiletine interaction with, 1320
Automatic implantable cardioverter-defibrillator. See *Cardioverter-defibrillator, implantable.*
Automaticity, abnormal, arrhythmia due to, 58
  digitalis' effects on, 1137
  triggered, 58–60, *59*
    after myocardial infarction, diltiazem for, 942
Autonomic neuropathy, postural hypotension due to, 96

Autonomic neuropathy *(Continued)*
  β-blockers for, 98
    caffeine in management of, 99
    octreotide for, 100
Autoregulation, of regional blood flow, 827
  "structural," in hypertension, 830
AVNRT. See *Atrioventricular nodal reentrant tachycardia (AVNRT).*
AVP. See *Vasopressin.*
AVRT. See *Atrioventricular reentrant tachycardia (AVRT).*
Azapropazone, dose adjustment for, in organ dysfunction, 248
Azepexole, receptors stimulated by, 336t, 342
Azotemia. See also *Renal failure; Renal insufficiency.*
  diuretic-induced, in congestive heart failure, 384
  due to amiloride, 449
  with treatment of hypertensive emergencies, 149

Bacitracin, procainamide interaction with, 1346
Balloon angioplasty. See also *Coronary angioplasty.*
  after myocardial infarction, 140
  percutaneous. See *Percutaneous transluminal coronary angioplasty (PTCA).*
Balloon catheter extraction, for lower extremity embolectomy, 169
Balloon counterpulsation. See *Intraaortic balloon counterpulsation.*
Balloon valvuloplasty, for pulmonary hypertension in mitral stenosis, 90
Bamifylline, exercise-induced myocardial ischemia and, 1453, 1459
Barbiturate(s), drug interactions with, 350
  with antiarrhythmic drugs, 352
  with aspirin, 350t
  with disopyramide, 1285
  with guanabenz, 631
  with quinidine, 1365t
  with warfarin, 307
Bartter's syndrome, amiloride for, 449
  triamterene for, 439
Bed rest, deconditioning due to, dobutamine and, 1156
Benazepril, 788–792
  adverse effects of, 792, 792t
  amlodipine in fixed combination with, 332–333, *333,* 1034
  chemical properties of, 788, *789*
  clinical applications of, 791–792
  cost of, 430t
  drug interaction studies with, 792, 792t
  during lactation, 790
  effects of, 790–791
  for hypertension, 790, 791–792, *792*
    mechanism of action of, in animal models, 788, 789t
  in organ dysfunction, 245, 789–790, *790*
  pharmacokinetics of, 789–790, *789, 790*
  pharmacology of, 788
Benazeprilat, amlodipine with, for hypertension, 1028
  chemical properties of, 788, *789*
  pharmacokinetics of, 723t, 789–790, *789, 790*
  pharmacology of, 788
Bendrofluazide, adverse lipid effects of, 377
Bendroflumethiazide, for hypertension, dose and side effects of, 374t

Bendroflumethiazide *(Continued)*
  racial differences in response to, 281
Benzarone, *1248*
Benzazepine, antihypertensive activity of, 343
Benziodarone, 1247, *1248*
Benzodiazepine(s), guanabenz interaction with, 631
  postural hypotension due to, 96
Benzthiazide, for hypertension, dose and side effects of, 374t
N-Benzylimidazole(s), 818
Bepridil, 1053–1058
  adverse effects of, 1057–1058
  arrhythmia aggravation by, 1057–1058, 1234, 1235t
  β-blockers with, 1057
  chemical properties of, 1053, *1053*
  clinical applications of, 1056–1057, 1056t
  contraindications to, 1057–1058
  cost of, 1058
  diuretic use with, 1057
  dosage and administration of, 1057, 1057t
  drug interactions with, 1058
  effects of, 892t, 1054–1056, 1054t, *1055*
  for angina, 892, 1055–1057, 1056t
  for ventricular arrhythmias, 894
  in elderly persons, 1058
  in organ dysfunction, 246, 1058
  pharmacokinetics of, 1054
  pharmacology of, 1053–1054, 1053t
  precautions with, 1057–1058
Beta blocker(s). See β*-Adrenergic blocker(s).*
Beta-carotene, in atherosclerosis prevention, *326,* 327t, 328
Betapace. See *Sotalol.*
Betaxolol, 550–556
  advantages of, 555
  adverse effects of, 555, 555t
  chemical properties of, 550
  contraindications to, 554
  cost of, 548t
  drug interactions with, 555
  during pregnancy, 272, 555
  effects of, 467t, 472t, 551–552
  in organ dysfunction, 554–555
  indications for, 553–554, 555t
  pharmacodynamics of, 467t, 472t, 550–551
  pharmacokinetics of, 552–553, 553t
  precautions with, 554–555
  receptor selectivity of, 550–551
Bethanidine, arrhythmia aggravation by, 1235t
Bezafibrate, chemical properties of, *1084*
  pharmacology of, 1077
B-HT 920 (α₂-agonist), 336t
B-HT 933 (α₂-agonist), 336t, 342
Bile acid metabolism, bile acid sequestrants' effects on, 1068–1069
Bile acid sequestrant(s), 1067–1073. See also specific drugs.
  adverse effects of, 77–78, 1071–1073, 1072t
  chemical properties of, 1067, *1068*
  clinical trials of, 1073
  contraindications to, 1070, 1072
  dosage and administration of, 1070–1071
  drug interactions with, 78, 1072
    with digitalis, 1142
    with lovastatin, 1112
  for hyperlipidemia, 21, 77–78
    mechanism of action of, 80t
  formulations of, 1070
  in children, 1072

Bile acid sequestrant(s) *(Continued)*
  in combined therapy, with fibrate, 1090
    with fluvastatin, 1134
    with lovastatin, 1112, 1113
    with nicotinic acid, 1064–1065
    with pravastatin, 1123, 1124
    with simvastatin, 1117, 1117t
    with statin, 80, 80t
  indications for, 1070, 1071t
  pharmacology of, 1067–1068
  serum lipid effects of, 1068–1070
Biphenyl carboxylic acid(s), 818
bis(F-butyl)-ethene, 1623
Bisoprolol, 557–566
  advantages of, 565–566
  adverse effects of, 564
  central nervous system symptoms due to, 564
  chemical properties of, 557
  clinical applications of, 560–564
  dosage and administration of, 566
  during pregnancy and lactation, 560
  effects of, electrophysiologic, 467t, 563
    hemodynamic, 467t, 559
    noncardiac, 472t, 565, 566
  exercise's interaction with, 253t
  hydrochlorothiazide with, for hypertension, 563
    in fixed combination, 73, 332
  in chronic obstructive lung disease, 564–565
  in diabetes mellitus, 565
  in hyperthyroidism, 565
  in organ dysfunction, 560
  pharmacodynamics of, 467t, 472t, 557–559, *558*
  pharmacokinetics of, 559–560, *560*
  receptor selectivity of, 337t, 557–559, *558*
  withdrawal of, 564
Bisoprolol/hydrochlorothiazide, 73, 332
Björk-Shiley prosthesis, thromboembolism risk with, 1407, 1407t, *1408*, 1409, 1410
Black person(s), cardiovascular disease in, epidemiology of, 280
  cardiovascular therapy in, 280–287
    socioeconomic considerations in, 286–287
  hypertension in, 280–287
    benefits of therapy of, 286, 287t
    captopril for, 284, 285t, 732
    drug therapy for, 281–286
    labetalol for, 284t, 574
    nitrendipine for, 286t, 1002
    pathophysiology of, 280–281
Bleeding. See *Hemorrhage.*
Bleeding time, c7E3 Fab effect on, 1630
Blocadren. See *Timolol.*
Blood flow, regional. See also *Cerebral blood flow; Coronary blood flow; Renal blood flow.*
  control of, 827
Blood pressure. See also *Hypertension; Hypotension.*
  during pregnancy, 269, 270
  mean arterial, reduction of, to limit infarct size, 718
  neural control of, 94–95, *94*, 601, 602, 616
  response of, to standing, 94–95. See also *Postural hypotension.*
Bone marrow depression, due to procainamide, 1345
Boots, intermittent pneumatic compression, in thromboembolism prevention, 1163
Bopindolol, duration of action of, 481
Bowditch effect, 1386

Bradyarrhythmia, antiarrhythmic drug–induced, 1233
Bradyasystole, 216–217
Bradycardia, due to adenosine, 1240
  due to nadolol, 503, 504
  ventricular arrhythmia due to, 1216, *1216*
  with acute myocardial infarction, 130–131
Bradycardic agent(s), 1386–1391. See also *Zatebradine.*
  clinical uses of, 1391
Bradykinin, accumulation of, with captopril therapy, 727
  ACE inhibitors' effects on, 693–694
  in regulation of nitric oxide formation, 836
  potentiation of, by ramipril, 756, 757
    cardoprotective effect and, 762–763, *762*
Braking phenomenon, with loop diuretics, 390, *390*
  with thiazides, 384, 414
Breast cancer, estrogen replacement therapy and, 322
Breast milk. See *Lactation.*
Bretylium, 183t, 1264–1271
  adverse effects of, 1270–1271
  chemical properties of, 1264
  clinical use of, 1269–1271
  cost of, 1271
  dosage and administration of, 1271
  drug interactions with, 1271
    with dopamine, 211
  during pregnancy and lactation, 1270
  effects of, 1266–1269, *1268*, 1268t
  for ventricular tachycardia, 203, 1269–1270
    with myocardial infarction, 132
  in cardiopulmonary resuscitation, 213–214
  in children, 1270
  in organ dysfunction, 1270, 1271
  indications for, 1269–1270
  pharmacokinetics of, 1265–1266, *1265*, *1266*, 1266t
  pharmacology of, 1265
  precautions with, 1270
Bretylol. See *Bretylium.*
Brevibloc. See *Esmolol.*
4-Bromochrotonic acid, effects of, on myocardial energy metabolism, 1600t
Bromocriptine, postural hypotension due to, 96
  receptor selectivity of, 339
Bronchospasm. See also *Asthma.*
  β-blockers and, 541, 542, 546
  due to adenosine, 1245
  due to propafenone, 1354
  esmolol and, 512–513
  labetalol and, 573
  pindolol and, 519
Bucindolol, 467t, 472t
Bullous dermatitis, due to furosemide, 365
Bumetanide, 396–401
  adverse effects of, 401
  chemical properties of, 397
  clinical use of, 399–401
  dosage and administration of, 401
  effects of, 398–399
  for hypertension, 399
    dose and side effects of, 374t
  for pulmonary edema, 124
  history of, 396–397, *396*
  in organ dysfunction, 246, 400–401
  NSAID interaction with, 398

Bumetanide *(Continued)*
  ototoxicity of, 361
  pharmacokinetics of, 397
  pharmacology of, 397–398, *406*
  site and mechanism of action of, 398
Bumex. See *Bumetanide.*
Bupivacaine, diltiazem interaction with, 948
Burn(s), hypertensive emergency with, 152

c7E3 Fab, 1625–1636
  adverse effects of, 1633, 1633t, 1634t
  clinical experience with, 1630–1635, 1631t–1634t, *1632*, *1633*
  contraindications to, 1633–1634
  development of, 1626–1627
  dosage and administration of, 1635
  drug interactions with, 1634
  guidelines for use of, 1633–1634
  in vivo studies of, 1629–1630
  investigational uses of, 1635–1636
  mechanism of action of, 1627–1628
  pharmacokinetics of, 1628
  pharmacology of, 1627–1629, *1628*
  rationale for, 1625–1626
  reversal of, 1630
  safety of, 1629–1630
  socioeconomic considerations with, 1635
Caffeine, for postural hypotension, 97, 99
Calan. See *Verapamil.*
Calcific embolus(i), in aortic valve disease, 1401
Calcification, vascular, in atherosclerosis, 1615
  magnesium EDTA chelation for, 1615–1616, *1616*
Calcium, excretion of, bumetanide's effect on, 399
  thiazides' effects on, 414
  in cardiopulmonary resuscitation, 217, 218
  in myocardial contraction, 1147
  in nitric oxide–induced vascular relaxation, 840
  in pathogenesis of atherosclerosis, 902
  in regulation of nitric oxide formation and/or release, 834, 836
  intracellular, amrinone's effects on, 1167–1168
    digitalis' effects on, 1136, *1137*
    intracellular accumulation of, in ischemic myocardial damage, 973
    in reperfusion injury, 6
    trimetazidine's effects on, 1595, *1595*, *1596*
  metabolism of, in hypertensive black persons, 281
  mitochondrial transport of, gallopamil's effects on, 926
  renal reabsorption of, furosemide's effects on, 389
Calcium antagonist(s), 891–1058. See also specific drugs.
  adverse effects of, 922t
  after myocardial infarction, 294–295, 302, 910
  classification of, 915
  clinical applications of, 891–898, 891t
  dihydropyridine. See *Dihydropyridine(s);* specific drugs.
  dopamine with, hypotension due to, 1164
  drug interactions with, 348t, 352

Calcium antagonist(s) *(Continued)*
  with amiodarone, 1253
  with atenolol, 547
  with β-blockers, 347, 348t, 352, 555,
    893, 893t
  with digoxin, 348t, 1142
  with mexiletine, 1326
  with propranolol, 491
  during lactation, 276–277
  during pregnancy, 272
  effects of, electrophysiologic, 909
    hemodynamic, 30t, 31, 48, 908–912,
      909t, 1387
    renal, 48, 911–912
  exercise's interaction with, 252t, 253–254
  factors limiting efficacy of, 1009, *1009*
  for acute myocardial infarction, 6–7, 31,
    895
    guidelines for, 36–37
  for angina, 891–893
    β-blockers with, 32–34, 32t, 37, 468,
      893, 893t
    guidelines for, 36
    in combined therapy, 32–34, 32t, 892–
      893, 893t
    in triple therapy, 35–36
    mechanisms of action of, 27t, 30t, 31,
      891, 892t
    nitrates with, 32t, 33
  for arrhythmias, 893–894, 893t
  for atherosclerosis prevention, 228, 901–
    906
    animal studies of, 31, 903–906, *904,
      905*
    clinical studies of, 31, 906, 911t
  for cerebral arterial spasm, 897
  for congestive heart failure, 896–897, 909
    due to diastolic dysfunction, 55–56
  for dementia, 897
  for hypertension, 894–895
    ACE inhibitors with, 332–333, 702, 732
    as initial therapy, 68, 69t, 71t
    cardiac effects of, 908–912, 909t
    in fixed combinations, 332–333
  for hypertensive emergencies, 156, 895
  for hypertrophic cardiomyopathy, 895–
    896
  for prevention of reperfusion injury, 6–7,
    31
  for pulmonary hypertension, in chronic
    lung disease, 89
    in collagen vascular diseases, 90
    primary, 86–87, 897
  for "silent" myocardial ischemia, 895
  for stroke, 897
  hemodynamic response to stress and,
    266
  hypertensive heart disease and, 911
  in black persons, 285–286, 286t
  in cardiopulmonary resuscitation, 219
  in elderly persons, 227–228
  in organ dysfunction, 245–246
  pharmacokinetics of, 31
  principles and practice of therapy with,
    891–912
  use dependency of, 934
  with coronary angioplasty, 307–308, 308t,
    309, 309t
Calcium channel(s), bepridil's effects on,
    1053–1054
  diltiazem's effects on, 933–934
  gallopamil's effects on, 926
  indapamide binding to, 421
  isradipine's effects on, 1016
  L- and T-type voltage-operated, blocking
    of, by mibefradil, 1010

Calcium channel(s) *(Continued)*
  characteristics of, 1010t
  verapamil's effects on, 916–917
  vesnarinone's effects on, 1186
Calcium channel agonist(s), inotropic
    effects of, mechanisms of, 44, 45t
Calcium channel blocker(s). See *Calcium
    antagonist(s)*; specific drugs.
Calcium chloride, in cardiopulmonary
    resuscitation, 217, 218
Calcium entry blocker(s). See *Calcium
    antagonist(s)*; specific drugs.
Calcium gluceptate, in cardiopulmonary
    resuscitation, 217
Calcium gluconate, in cardiopulmonary
    resuscitation, 217
Calcium paradox, 936
Calculus(i), renal, thiazides for, 417–418
  triamterene and, 439
Calmodulin, bepridil's effects on, 1054
cAMP. See *Cyclic adenosine monophosphate
    (cAMP)*.
Cancer. See *Malignancy(ies)*.
Canrenone, 454, *455*
  mechanism of action of, 362
Capoten. See *Captopril*.
Captopril, 726–738
  adverse effects of, 701, 735–736, 735t
  after myocardial infarction, 296, 300, 735
    effects of, 718, 719, *719*
    ventricular remodeling and, 715
  chemical properties of, 726–727, *727*
  clinical applications of, 731–735
  cost of, 949t
  discovery of, 17
  diuretic with, for hypertension, 732
    precautions with, 735, 737
  dosage and administration of, 700, 736–
    737
  drug interactions with, with amiloride,
    450
    with β-blockers, 348t
    with furosemide, 351
    with indomethacin, 693
    with probenecid, 351
    with procainamide, 349t
  during lactation, 276t, 277
  during pregnancy, 272, 698
  exercise's interaction with, 257
  for congestive heart failure, 12, 53, 387,
    734–735
    furosemide with, 393
    in combined therapy, 54
    pharmacokinetics of, 729
  for hypertension, 731–734, *733*
    advantages of, 737
    amlodipine with, 1034
    as initial therapy, 731
    drawbacks of, 794
    in combined therapy, 732
    in elderly persons, 732–733
    quality of life with, 734, *734*
  for hypertensive emergencies, 154t, 155t,
    699
  for peripheral vascular disease, 700
  for primary pulmonary hypertension, 86
  hemodynamic effects of, 47t, 729–730
  hydralazine with, for chronic heart fail-
    ure, 54
    hemodynamic effects of, 47t
  in black persons, 284, 285t, 732
  in children, 734
  in diabetes mellitus, 700, 733, *733*
  in elderly persons, 732–733
  in organ dysfunction, 244, 701, 722t, 729,
    737

Captopril *(Continued)*
  pharmacokinetics of, 723t, 728–729
  pharmacology of, 727–728, *727, 728*
  prazosin with, for chronic heart failure,
    54
    hemodynamic effects of, 47t
  prostaglandin metabolism and, 693, 727–
    728, *728*
Carbamazepine, drug interactions with,
    with calcium antagonists, 348t
    with diltiazem, 933
    with phenytoin, 1340
    with verapamil, 922
Carbidopa/L-dopa, postural hypotension
    and, 96–97
Carbohydrate metabolism. See also
    Diabetes mellitus; Insulin resistance.
  acebutolol's effects on, 498
  α₁-blockers' effects on, 611
  diltiazem's effects on, 939
  diuretics' effects on, 365, 377–378, 416–
    417
  doxazosin's effects on, 684–685
  labetalol's effects on, 572
  nadolol's effects on, 504
  pindolol's effects on, 518, 519
  propranolol's effects on, 486–487, 490
  terazosin's effects on, 668
Carbon monoxide, vascular effects of, 837
Carbonic anhydrase inhibitor(s). See also
    Acetazolamide.
  history of, 396
Carcinoma. See also *Malignancy(ies)*.
  estrogen replacement therapy and, 322
  prostatic, estrogens for, cardiovascular
    events and, 321
Cardene. See *Nicardipine*.
Cardiac catheterization, in acute
    pulmonary edema management,
    indications for, 122
  mitral stenosis detection during, dobu-
    tamine for, 1157
Cardiac glycoside(s). See also *Digitalis;
    Digitoxin; Digoxin*.
  history of, 1136
Cardiac insufficiency. See *Congestive heart
    failure*.
Cardiac output, neurohumoral response to
    drop in, 1140
Cardiac transplantation, amrinone for
    patients awaiting, 1172–1173
  diltiazem's effects after, 940
  dobutamine after, 1156
  triiodothyronine for donor in, 1659
Cardiogenic shock, thrombolytic therapy
    in presence of, 1433–1434, *1435*
  with acute myocardial infarction, 137
Cardiomyopathy(ies), dilated. See *Dilated
    cardiomyopathy*.
  hypertrophic. See *Hypertrophic cardiomy-
    opathy*.
  restrictive, amrinone use in, 1173
Cardioplegia, fluorocarbons in, 1623–1624,
    1624
Cardiopulmonary bypass, diltiazem with,
    937
  triiodothyronine with, 1659
Cardiopulmonary resuscitation (CPR),
    206–219
  acid-base management in, 218–219
  active compression and decompression,
    212
  adjunctive techniques in, 212
  bradyasystole management in, 216–217
  cerebral protection during and after, 219
  pharmacokinetics and pharmacodynam-
    ics in, 206–208

Cardiopulmonary resuscitation (CPR) (Continued)
  pulseless electrical activity management in, 217–218
  refractory or recurrent ventricular fibrillation management in, 212–216
  vasopressors in, 208–210, 209t
Cardiovascular system, age-related changes in, 225
Cardioversion, for atrial fibrillation, 194
  for nonvalvular atrial fibrillation, antithrombotic therapy at time of, 1404–1405
  for paroxysmal atrial tachycardia with myocardial infarction, 131
  for ventricular tachycardia, 202
Cardioverter-defibrillator, implantable, 16, 64, 204, 204
  flecainide use with, 1315
  tiered, 1222, 1222–1223
Cardizem. See Diltiazem.
Cardura. See Doxazosin.
Carmoxirole, 1189–1193
  adverse effects of, 1193
  chemical properties of, 1190
  clinical use of, 1193
  effects of, 1192–1193, 1192, 1193
  pharmacokinetics of, 1191, 1191t
  pharmacology of, 1190–1191, 1191t
L-Carnitine, effects of, on myocardial energy metabolism, 1600t
β-Carotene, in atherosclerosis prevention, 326, 327t, 328
Carteolol, cost of, 548t
  dose adjustment for, in organ dysfunction, 241–242
  effects of, 467t, 472t
  pharmacodynamics of, 467t, 472t
Carvedilol, 583–598
  chemical properties of, 583, 588
  clinical applications of, 598
  clinical studies of, 589–598
    in congestive heart failure, 595–598, 596, 596t, 597
    in exercise-induced angina, 593–594, 593t, 594
    in hypertension, 590–592, 591, 591t, 592t
    in normal volunteers, 589–590, 589, 590
    side effect profile in, 594–595, 595
  effects of, 467t, 472t, 585–586
  hypotensive effect of, in animal models, 584–585, 585, 586
    in clinical studies, 589–592, 589–591, 591t, 593t
  mechanism of, 584–585, 585, 586
  pharmacodynamics of, 467t, 472t, 583–584, 584, 584t
  pharmacokinetics of, 587–589, 587, 588, 588t, 589t
Catalase, 326, 326
Catapres. See Clonidine.
Cataracts, fluvastatin and, 1129, 1133
  lovastatin and, 1111–1112, 1124
  pravastatin and, 1124
  simvastatin and, 1117, 1124
Catecholamine(s). See also specific substances.
  afterdepolarizations due to, 59
  drug interactions with, arrhythmia aggravation and, 1238
    with adenosine, 1240
    with bretylium, 1271
    with triiodothyronine, 1660
  in response to congestive heart failure, 11

Catecholamine(s) (Continued)
  tachycardias dependent on, drug selection for, 63–64
Catecholamine assay(s), labetalol interference with, 572
Catheter(s), atherectomy, 304
  central venous. See Central venous line.
Catheter ablation, 16
  for atrial fibrillation, 1208, 1209, 1209
  for atrial flutter, 1210
  for AV node reentry tachycardia, 1212
  for AV reciprocating tachycardia, 189, 1212, 1213
  for refractory ventricular arrhythmia, 64
  for supraventricular tachycardias, 196
Catheter extraction, for lower extremity embolus, 169
CEB (calcium entry blocker). See Calcium antagonist(s); specific drugs.
Cellular antiischemic agent(s), 1594–1602
Central nervous system, ACE inhibitor's effects on, 767–768
  adrenoreceptors in, 338
  degenerative diseases of, postural hypotension in, 96
Central venous line, drug administration through, during cardiopulmonary resuscitation, 206–207
  thrombosis associated with, urokinase for, 1546–1547
Cerebral arterial spasm, calcium antagonists for, 897
Cerebral blood flow, ACE inhibitors' effects on, 696
  autoregulation of, 827
  felodipine's effects on, 1042
  fosinopril's effects on, 807
  isradipine's effects on, 1017
  nicardipine's effects on, 982, 990
Cerebral embolism, 167–168, 168t. See also Stroke.
  acute, in prosthetic heart valve patient, 1411–1412
  anticoagulation and, 1411–1412
  heparin for, 1477
Cerebral ischemia. See also Stroke; Transient ischemic attack(s) (TIA).
  antithrombotic therapy in, 113
Cerebrovascular accident(s). See Stroke.
Cerebrovascular disease, dipyridamole for, 1461
  nicardipine for, 990–991
  pentoxifylline for, 1606
  warfarin for, 1518
CETP (cholesteryl ester transfer protein), 1088–1089
cGMP (cyclic guanosine monophosphate), in nitric oxide–induced vascular relaxation, 833, 834, 835, 837, 840
CGS 13080 (thromboxane synthetase inhibitor), for primary pulmonary hypertension, 88
CGS 14824A. See Benazepril.
Chest pain, recurrent, with acute myocardial infarction, 139–140
Chest thump, for ventricular tachycardia, 202, 203
  in cardiopulmonary resuscitation, 217
Child(ren). See also Neonate(s).
  arrhythmias in, amiodarone for, 1256
    bretylium safety in, 1270
    propafenone for, 1353, 1357
    verapamil for, 893
  dobutamine use in, 1152–1153
  hypercholesterolemia in, bile acid sequestrants for, 1072

Child(ren) (Continued)
  simvastatin for, 1118
  hypertension in, captopril for, 734
    enalapril for, 744–745
    minoxidil for, 855
Chloride transport, in thick ascending limb of loop of Henle, 398
Chlorothiazide, chemical properties of, 413
  for hypertension, dose and side effects of, 374t
Chlorpromazine, β-blocker interaction with, 480
  dopamine interaction with, 1164
  postural hypotension due to, 96
Chlorthalidone, 412–418
  adverse lipid effects of, 377
  chemical properties of, 413
  combination tablets containing, 418t
  during lactation, 276t
  for hypertension, dose and side effects of, 374t
  history of, 412
  in black persons, 282–283
  in organ dysfunction, 247
  serum potassium and, 415, 415
Cholecystokinin, release of, due to cholestyramine, 1072
Cholesterol. See also High-density lipoprotein cholesterol (HDL-C); Hypercholesterolemia; Lipid metabolism; Low-density lipoprotein cholesterol (LDL-C).
  deposition of, in arterial tissue, mechanisms of, 532–533
  metabolism of, bile acid sequestrants' effects on, 1068–1069
    clofibrate's effects on, 1076
  serum levels of, diuretics' effects on, 375–377, 376t, 417
    goals for lipid-regulating therapy, 20
    total mortality and, 22
  synthesis of, 1107, 1109
  fenofibrate's effects on, 1088
Cholesteryl ester transfer protein (CETP), 1088–1089
Cholestyramine, 1067–1073
  adverse effects of, 1071–1073, 1072t
  chemical properties of, 1067, 1068
  clinical trials of, 1073
  dosage and administration of, 1070–1071
  drug interactions with, 1072
    with digoxin, 351, 352
    with pravastatin, 1125
    with warfarin, 350t, 351, 353
  fluvastatin with, dosage and administration of, 1134
  for hyperlipidemia, 1132, 1132t
  safety of, 1133
  for hyperlipidemia, as initial drug, 77–78
    fluvastatin with, 1132, 1132t
    pravastatin with, 1124, 1125
    simvastatin with, 1117
  formulations of, 1070
  in elderly persons, 231–232
  indications for, 1070, 1071t
  pharmacology of, 1067–1068
  serum lipid effects of, 1068–1070
Cholinergic drug(s), quinidine interaction with, 1365t
Cholinergic receptor(s), in cardiovascular system, 340
Chondrodysplasia punctata, due to intrauterine warfarin exposure, 1520
Chondroitin sulfate A, in experimental atherosclerosis, 903

Chronic obstructive pulmonary disease
(COPD). See also *Asthma.*
ACE inhibitor use in, 700
β-blocker use in, 534
bisoprolol use in, 564–565
digoxin use in, 1141
esmolol use in, 512–513
pulmonary hypertension in, treatment
of, 88–89
Cibenzoline, arrhythmia aggravation by,
1235t
Cigarettes, drug interactions with, with
calcium antagonists, 348t
with diltiazem, 352, 933
with mexiletine, 1320
with nifedipine, 352
with pentoxifylline, 1605
with propranolol, 491
Cilazapril, 810–812
Cilazaprilat, 810
pharmacokinetics of, 723t, 810–811
Cimetidine, drug interactions with, 350
with amiloride, 446
with antiarrhythmic drugs, 352
with β-blockers, 348t, 480
with calcium antagonists, 348t
with diltiazem, 352, 933
with felodipine, 1044
with flecainide, 1315
with fluvastatin, 1134
with lidocaine, 349t
with metoprolol, 352
with mexiletine, 1320, 1326
with moricizine, 1332
with nifedipine, 352, 973
with pentoxifylline, 1605
with phenytoin, 1340
with pindolol, 519
with pravastatin, 1125
with procainamide, 349t, 351, 1346
with propafenone, 1354
with propranolol, 352, 491
with quinidine, 1365t
with ticlopidine, 1472
with verapamil, 916, 922
with warfarin, 307, 350t, 353
for contrast allergy, with coronary angioplasty, 309
Cinchonism, due to quinidine, 1364
Ciprofibrate, 1092–1097
advantages of, 1096, 1097
adverse effects of, 1095–1096, 1096t
carcinogenicity of, 1093
chemical properties of, *1084,* 1092, *1092*
clinical use of, 1094–1095, *1094,* 1095t
contraindications to, 1096
dosage and administration of, 1096–1097
drug interactions with, 1096
in organ dysfunction, 1096
indications for, 1094–1095
pharmacokinetics of, 1093–1094, 1094t
pharmacology of, 1077, 1092–1093, *1093*
Circadian pattern of cardiac disease,
311–315
drug therapy guided by, 314–315
drug therapy's effects on, 312–313, *312*
epidemiologic findings of, 311, *312*
triggering events and, 314
Cirrhosis, bumetanide in, 401
spironolactone in, 456
torsemide in, pharmacokinetics and
pharmacodynamics of, 406t, 408–
410, *409*
triamterene in, 439
Claudication, acebutolol in presence of,
498

Claudication *(Continued)*
ketanserin for, 1653–1654
pentoxifylline for, 1605–1606
Clofibrate, 1075–1080
adverse effects of, 1078–1079
carcinogenicity of, 1077, 1079
chemical properties of, 1075–1076, *1075,*
1084, 1098
contraindications to, 1079
dosage and administration of, 1080
drug interactions with, 1079
during lactation, 1079
during pregnancy, 1079
in combined therapy, 1076–1077
in elderly persons, 232
in organ dysfunction, 1078, 1079
indications for, 1078
patient selection for, 1079–1080
pharmacokinetics of, 1078
pharmacology of, 1076–1078
precautions with, 1078–1079
serum lipid effects of, 1076
socioeconomic considerations with, 1080
Clofibrate analogue(s). See also specific
drugs.
pharmacology of, 1077
Clofibric acid, 1075–1076, *1075*
Clonidine, 605–608, 622–627
adverse effects of, 607, 625–626
chemical properties of, *628*
clinical applications of, 625
cost of, 649
drug interactions with, with atenolol,
547
with β-blockers, 480
during lactation, 276, 276t
during pregnancy, 271
effects of, 623–624
hemodynamic, 606, 607, 623–624
on renin-aldosterone axis, 606, 624
exercise's interaction with, 255
for hypertension, 607, 625, 627
for hypertensive emergencies, 154t, 155t,
157, 625
for postural hypotension, 98–99
hemodynamic response to stress and,
266
in elderly persons, 227
in organ dysfunction, 242, 622, 623
mechanism of action of, 605, 622–623
pharmacokinetics of, 622
receptors stimulated by, 336t, 342
sites of action of, 603
transdermal, 255, 624–625
adverse effects of, 625–626
dosage and administration of, 627
in combined therapy, 625
pharmacokinetics of, 622
Clonidine withdrawal syndrome, 608, 626
labetalol for, 575
Clonidine-displacing substance, 653–654
Clopidogrel, 105
Coagulopathy, due to nicotinic acid, 1065
Cocaine, cardiotoxicity due to, esmolol for,
512
hypertension and, 280
vasoconstriction due to, 350
Codeine, quinidine interaction with, 1365t
Coenzyme Q10 (CoQ10), HMG-CoA
reductase inhibitors' effects on, 1125
inotropic effects of, mechanisms of, 44,
45t
Cognitive appraisal, in stress response, 262
Colcemide, in experimental atherosclerosis,
903
Colestid. See *Colestipol.*

Colestipol, 1067–1073
adverse effects of, 1071–1073
chemical properties of, 1067, *1068*
clinical trials of, 1073
drug interactions with, 1072
with pravastatin, 1125
for hyperlipidemia, as initial drug, 77–78
dosage and administration of, 1070–
1071
fibrate with, 1090
fluvastatin with, 1134
formulations of, 1070
indications for, 1070, 1071t
pharmacology of, 1067–1068
serum lipid effects of, 1068–1070
Collagen vascular disease(s), pulmonary
hypertension in, treatment of, 89–90
Coma, myxedema, 1657, 1660
Combination therapy. See also specific
disorders and drugs.
for angina, 27–37
evaluation of, 37
experience with, 31–36, *32,* 32t
goals of, 29
guidelines and principles of, 36–37
with three drugs, 35–36
for congestive heart failure, 43–56
clinical applications of, 50–56
expected systemic hemodynamic effects of, 50t
rationale for, 45–46, *46*
for hyperlipidemia, 21–22, 79–81, 79t, 80t
Compactin. See *Mevastatin.*
Compensatory pause, with premature
ventricular systole, 198
Compliance, arterial, 828
venous, 828
Compression boots, intermittent
pneumatic, in thromboembolism
prevention, 163
Compression stockings, graduated, in
thromboembolism prevention, 163
Conduction, anisotropic, 60
reentry and, 14, 61
drug interactions affecting, 347
slowed, in reentrant arrhythmia, 60, *60*
Congenital heart disease, nitroprusside for,
863
nonvalvular atrial fibrillation in, anticoagulants with, 1404
pulmonary hypertension in, treatment
of, 90–91
surgery for, phenytoin for arrhythmias
after, 1339–1340
thromboembolism in, 169–170
Congestive heart failure, ACE inhibitors
for, 12, 53–54, 700, 711–716
as treatment, 712–715, *714, 715*
in prevention, 715, 717–720
very-low-dose, 387
acute, hypertensive emergency with, 151
inotropic therapy for, 1148–1149, 1149t
vasodilators for, 11
after myocardial infarction, 134–137
ACE inhibitors for prevention of, 715,
717–720
captopril for prevention of, 735
cardioprotective effect of β-blockade
in, 294, *294*
pathogenesis of, 715, 717
α₁-agonists in treatment of, 344
α₁-blockers for, 611
amiodarone for, 55, 1255
amlodipine for, 1036
amrinone for, 12, 52, 54, 1148, 1172
after myocardial infarction, 136–137

Congestive heart failure (Continued)
  dobutamine with, 50t, 1149, 1149t, 1154
  dopamine with, 50t
  effects of, 1169–1170
  atenolol use in, 546
  benazepril for, 791
  benefits of exercise in, 258
  β-agonists for, 343, 1148
  β-blocker use in, 294, 294, 546
  β-receptor downregulation in, 341, 1147–1148
  bisoprolol for, 563–564
  bumetanide in, 399–400
  calcium antagonists for, 55–56, 896–897, 909
  captopril for, 12, 53, 387, 734–735
    effects of, 730
    in combined therapy, 54, 393
    pharmacokinetics of, 729
  carvedilol for, 595–598, 596, 596t, 597
  choice of therapeutic modality for, 43–47
  chronic, combined therapy for, 53–56, 55t
    dobutamine for, 1153–1155
    sudden death in, 55
  cilazapril for, 811
  combined therapy for, 43–56
    clinical applications of, 50–56
    expected systemic hemodynamic effects of, 50t
    rationale for, 45–46, 46
  decompensated, cytokines in pathogenesis of, 1186
  defined, 711
  digoxin for, 53, 136, 1140
    predictors of response to, 386
  diltiazem for, 946–947
  disopyramide use in, 1284
  diuretics for, 383–387
    ACE inhibitors with, 387
    adverse effects of, 53
    complications of, 386–387
    mechanisms of action of, 383–386
    rationale for, 46–47
  L-dopa for, 345, 1164–1165
  dopamine for, 136, 1163
    in combined therapy, 48, 50t, 1149, 1149t, 1163
  dopaminergic agonists for, 1164
  doxazosin for, 685–686
  due to bepridil, 1058
  due to disopyramide, 1281, 1286
  due to mexiletine, 1329
  due to minoxidil, 855
  due to moricizine, 1334, 1336
  due to propafenone, 1354
  due to sotalol, 1370
  during pregnancy, 270
  emerging concepts in therapy for, 10–13
  enalapril for, 12, 54, 387, 745–747, 745t
    dosage for, 745–746, 748
    survival with, 712–714, 714, 715
  experimental, mibefradil's effects in, 1013
  felodipine for, 1043
  fish oils' effects on, 1611
  flecainide use in, 1315
  functional effects of pulmonary congestion in, 385–386
  furosemide for, 392–393
    after myocardial infarction, 134
    extrarenal actions of, 385
    in combined therapy, 387, 393, 413
    resistance to, 384
  future needs for, 12–13

Congestive heart failure (Continued)
  hepatic drug elimination in, 235–236
  hydralazine for, 53
    captopril with, 54
    nitrates with, 53, 873, 879
  ibopamine for, 54, 1165
    clinical efficacy of, 1201–1203, 1201t, 1202t
  in black persons, 280
  indapamide for, 429
  inotropic therapy for, 44–45, 45t, 1148
    indications for, 1146–1147
    new agents for, 12
    oral agents for, 1149–1150
  isosorbide dinitrate for, 873
    hydralazine with, 53, 873, 879
  isosorbide mononitrate for, in controlled-release form, 887–888, 889
  isradipine for, 1020
  left ventricular, acute, combined therapy for, 51–53
    dobutamine for, 1155–1156
  lisinopril for, 752
  losartan for, 823, 823t
  metolazone for, furosemide with, 413
  mibefradil for, 1014
  milrinone for, 12, 1148, 1182, 1183
    adverse effects of, 230
    after myocardial infarction, 136–137
    long-term therapy with, 1149–1150
  molsidomine for, 1648–1649, 1648
  nadolol and, 503, 504
  neurohumoral activation in, 11
  nicardipine for, 990
  nicorandil for, 1643
    effects of, 1639
  nitrates for, 873
    hydralazine with, 53, 873, 879
  nitroglycerin for, 872–873
    with myocardial infarction, 135–136
  nitroprusside for, 861–862
    in combined therapy, 1149, 1149t, 1155
    with myocardial infarction, 135–136
  pathophysiology of, 10–11, 43
  perindopril for, 782
  pindolol use in, 519
  preload reduction in, effects of, 869
  propafenone use in, 1351–1352
  propranolol in, 489, 490
  quinapril for, 799
  ramipril for, 759, 768
    after myocardial infarction, 715
    renal effects of, 766–767
  renin-angiotensin system in, 11, 44, 711–712
    tissue, 712, 796
  severe refractory, mortality rate with, 54
  spironolactone in, 456
  terazosin for, 670
  thiazides' effects in, 414
  torsemide in, 404–405
    pharmacokinetics and pharmacodynamics of, 406t, 409, 410
  trandolapril for, 786
  triamterene for, 438
  triiodothyronine for, 1659
  urapidil for, 678
  vasodilator therapy for, 11–12, 43–44, 44t, 830
    survival with, 712, 713–714, 713, 715
  verapamil use in, 918
Constipation. See also Gastrointestinal symptoms.
  due to bile acid sequestrants, 1071–1072
Continuous positive airway pressure (CPAP), for acute pulmonary edema, 123

Contraceptive(s), oral, phenytoin interaction with, 1340
Contractility, changes in, effects on pressure-volume loop, 45, 46
Contrast agent(s), fluorocarbons as, 1623
  premedication for allergy to, with coronary angioplasty, 309
Coombs' test, positive, due to methyldopa, 619
COPD. See Chronic obstructive pulmonary disease (COPD).
Coping, in stress response, 262
CoQ10. See Coenzyme Q10 (CoQ10).
Cordarone. See Amiodarone.
Corneal microdeposits, due to amiodarone, 1257
Coronary angioplasty, after APSAC therapy, 1564
  as rescue measure for failed thrombolysis, 1525
  aspirin for graft patency maintenance after, 1448
  balloon, after myocardial infarction, 140
  for acute myocardial infarction, 4
  indications for, 6
  percutaneous transluminal. See Percutaneous transluminal coronary angioplasty (PTCA).
  ticlopidine for prevention of occlusion after, 1469
Coronary artery bypass surgery. See also Saphenous vein graft(s).
  after APSAC therapy, 1564
  antiplatelet therapy after, 1421–1424
    clinical trials of, 1422–1424
    rationale for, 1421
  antithrombotic therapy after, 111–112, 114, 1424t
  diltiazem with, 944
  graft occlusion rates after, 1422
  graft patency maintenance after, aspirin for, 1448
    ticlopidine for, 1468–1469
  graft thrombosis after, 112
  hypertension after, esmolol for, 511–512
  immediate, for acute myocardial infarction, 4
  low output syndrome after, amrinone for, 1172
  supraventricular tachyarrhythmias after, sotalol for, 1373
  triiodothyronine with, 1659
  trimetazidine with, 1598–1599
Coronary artery disease. See also Atherosclerosis.
  ACE inhibitors for, 700
  after menopause, 316. See also Estrogen replacement therapy.
  antithrombotic therapy in, 174–176, 175t, 1415–1420, 1415t, 1416t
    experience and recommendations for, 108
  diltiazem for, 942–944
    advantages and disadvantages of, 948
  dipyridamole for, 1458–1459
  dobutamine for left ventricular failure in, 1155–1156
  due to minoxidil, 856
  fish oils and, epidemiologic studies of, 1608–1609
  in black persons, 280
  labetalol for, 575
  metoprolol for, for primary prevention, 523–527, 524, 526
    for secondary prevention, 527–531, 528–530

Coronary artery disease (Continued)
  molsidomine for, 1646–1648, 1647
  nicorandil's effects in, 1639–1640
  pathophysiology of, 27–29, 28
  prevention of stress-induced effects in, 264
  sex-specific differences in, 316
  simvastatin for, mortality benefit from, 1116
  stress as risk factor for, 263
  ticlopidine for, 1468–1469
  ventricular tachycardia in, adenosine's effects on, 1244–1245
  drug selection for, 64
Coronary artery embolus(i), 169
Coronary artery spasm. See also Angina pectoris, variant.
  ergonovine-induced, nitroprusside for, 863
  in pathogenesis of acute myocardial infarction, 9
  verapamil for, 898
Coronary artery stenosis(es), concentric, 28
  dynamic, 28–29
  eccentric, 28, 28
Coronary artery thrombosis, 3
  factors influencing lysis of, 1523
  initiation of, 9, 28, 28, 313–314
Coronary blood flow, autoregulation of, 827
  calcium antagonists' effects on, in hypertension, 908–909
  heart rate and, 1386
Coronary embolus(i), 169
Coronary steal syndrome, due to adenosine, 1458, 1459
  due to arteriolar dilation, 869
  due to dipyridamole, 1453
  due to nitroprusside, 860
Corticosteroid(s). See also specific drugs.
  amiloride interaction with, 450
Corynanthine, receptor selectivity of, 336t
Cough, due to ACE inhibitors, 285, 701, 747
  due to benazepril, 792
  due to captopril, 736
  due to fosinopril, 807
  due to ramipril, 768
  due to trandolapril, 786
  losartan and, 823
Coumarin. See also Warfarin.
  clofibrate interaction with, 1079
Countershock, for ventricular tachycardia with myocardial infarction, 132
CPAP (continuous positive airway pressure), for acute pulmonary edema, 123
CPR. See Cardiopulmonary resuscitation (CPR).
Cryoprecipitate, for bleeding due to tissue-type plasminogen activator, 1573
Crystalloid(s), with coronary angioplasty, 309
CS–514. See Pravastatin.
CVA (cerebrovascular accident). See Stroke.
CY 216. See Nadroparin.
Cyanide toxicity, amyl or sodium nitrite in treatment of, 869
  due to nitroprusside, 859
  management of, 864
Cyclic adenosine monophosphate (cAMP), amrinone's effects on, 1167–1168
  in myocardial contraction, 1178
  milrinone's effects on, 1178, 1178
  platelet, antiplatelet drugs increasing, 104–105

Cyclic guanosine monophosphate (cGMP), in nitric oxide–induced vascular relaxation, 833, 834, 835, 837, 840
Cyclooxygenase, 103
Cyclooxygenase inhibitor(s), antiplatelet therapy with, 103
Cyclopropane, dopamine interaction with, 1164
Cyclosporine, drug interactions with, 350
  with digoxin, 1142
  with diltiazem, 352, 940, 948
  with lovastatin, 1111, 1113
  with nicardipine, 350, 996
  with propafenone, 1354
  with simvastatin, 1118
  with verapamil, 922
Cystic fibrosis, amiloride in, 449
Cytochrome P-450 reductase, nitric oxide synthase and, 837
Cytokines, stimulation of nitric oxide production by, in leukocytes, 839
  in vascular smooth muscle cells, 840
  vesnarinone's effects on, 1186
Cytomel. See Triiodothyronine (T₃).
Cytostatic agent(s), calcium antagonist interactions with, 348t

Dacarel. See Nicardipine.
Danaparoid, 1505–1510
  chemical properties of, 1505–1506
  clinical evaluation of, 1507–1509, 1508t, 1509t
  during pregnancy, 1507
  in organ dysfunction, 1507
  pharmacokinetics of, 1507
  pharmacology of, 1506–1507
  toxicity of, 1507
DCA. See Dichloroacetate (DCA).
Debrisoquin, genetic difference in metabolism of, 1352
  quinidine interaction with, 1354
Deconditioning, due to bed rest, dobutamine and, 1156
Deep venous thrombosis (DVT), factors influencing lysis of, 1523
  prevention of, 160–163, 161t, 162t, 165–166
    danaparoid for, 1507–1509, 1508t, 1509t
    enoxaparin for, 1513–1515, 1513t
    heparin for, 1475, 1476
    hirudin for, 1495–1496
    Logiparin for, 1481–1482, 1481t
    low-molecular-weight heparin for, 1512–1513, 1512t, 1513t
    nadroparin for, 1485–1486, 1485t, 1486t
  treatment of, 163–164, 166, 166t
    heparin for, 1475–1476, 1515–1516
    hirudin for, 1496
    Logiparin for, 1482–1483
    nadroparin for, 1486–1487, 1487t
    options for, 1544–1545, 1544t
    outpatient, 1488
    thrombolytic therapy for, comparative trials of, 1530–1531, 1530t
    urokinase for, 1544–1547, 1544t–1546t, 1545
DEFIANT II study, 1007
Defibrillation threshold, dofetilide's effects on, 1301
Demadex. See Torsemide.
Dementia, calcium antagonists for, 897
Depression, propranolol and, 490
N-Depropylpropafenone, 1352

Dermatitis, bullous, due to furosemide, 365
Desethylamiodarone, 1252
Desipramine, propafenone interaction with, 1354
Desmopressin, for hirudin neutralization, 1494
Desulfatohirudin, 1490, 1491. See also Hirudin.
Desurin, 1490, 1491. See also Hirudin.
Dextran, antiplatelet effect of, 105
  for prosthetic arterial graft occlusion prevention, 1455
  for thromboembolism prevention, 163
  with coronary angioplasty, 306, 309, 309t
DHA. See Docosahexaenoic acid (DHA).
Diabetes insipidus, lithium-induced, amiloride for, 449
Diabetes mellitus, aspirin for vascular occlusive disease prevention in, 1448
  β-blocker use in, 541–542, 546–547
  bisoprolol use in, 565
  cilazapril use in, 811
  diltiazem's effects on renal function in, 939
  diuretic use in, 226
  due to nicotinic acid, 1064
  enalapril use in, 744
  hyperlipidemia in, 22–23
    pravastatin for, 1125
    simvastatin for, 1117
  hypertension in, ACE inhibitors for, 700
    acebutolol for, 498
    captopril for, 700, 733, 733
    diuretic therapy for, 377–378
    enalapril for, 744
    indapamide for, 424t, 429
    isradipine for, 1018
    thiazides for, 417
  lipid-lowering therapy in, 1099–1100, 1100, 1100t
  nadolol use in, 504
  nifedipine use in, 975
  pentoxifylline use in, 1605
  pindolol use in, 519
  postural hypotension due to neuropathy in, octreotide for, 100
Diabetic nephropathy, captopril for, 733, 733
  ramipril use in, 767
  verapamil's effects in, 919, 919
Diabetic retinopathy, ticlopidine for, 1470
Diacetolol, 496, 496
Dialysis, digoxin and, 1141
  thrombosis of access device for, thrombolytic therapy for, 1551
Dialysis disequilibrium syndrome, osmotic diuretic for, 363–364
Diarrhea. See also Gastrointestinal symptoms.
  due to bile acid sequestrants, 1072
  due to quinidine, 1364
    treatment's effects on drug absorption, 1363
Diastolic dysfunction, nifedipine for, 976
Diazepam, with coronary angioplasty, 309
Diazoxide, for hypertension, disadvantages of, 996
  severe, during pregnancy, 273, 273t
  for hypertensive emergencies, 154t, 155t, 156–157
  for primary pulmonary hypertension, 86
Dibenzyline (phenoxybenzamine), for hypertensive emergencies, 154t, 155t, 158
Dibutyryl cAMP, hemodynamic effects of, 48
  inotropic effects of, mechanisms of, 44, 45t

Dibutyryl cAMP (Continued)
Dichloroacetate (DCA), effects of, on myocardial energy metabolism, 1600t
in cardiopulmonary resuscitation, 219
Dichloroisoprenaline, chemical properties of, 475
Dicumarol, phenytoin interaction with, 1340
Diet, antioxidants in, 326–328, 326, 327, 327t
  fiber in. See Fiber, dietary.
  lipid-lowering therapy using, 19
  potassium in, cardiovascular health and, 461–464
  salt increase in, for postural hypotension, 97
  sodium restriction in, as adjunct to diuretic therapy, 390–391
Diflunisal, dose adjustment for, in organ dysfunction, 247–248
Digibind, for digitalis toxicity, 1143t, 1144, 1144t
Digitalis, 1136–1144. See also Digitoxin; Digoxin.
  chemical properties of, 1136
  dosing regimens for, 1138, 1138t
  drug interactions with, with betaxolol, 555
    with calcium, 217
    with felodipine, 1043–1044
    with indapamide, 429
    with triamterene, 438
  during lactation, 277
  during pregnancy, 274
  exercise's interaction with, 258
  for chronic heart failure, 53
  in elderly persons, 229–230
  intoxication with. See Digitalis toxicity.
  mechanism of action of, 44, 45t, 1136–1137, 1137
  quinidine syncope and, 1229, 1234, 1364
Digitalis toxicity, 1142–1144
  bretylium use in, 1270, 1271
  clinical manifestations of, 1143
  during pregnancy, 274
  factors predisposing to, 1142t
  in elderly persons, 1142–1143
  management of, 1143–1144, 1143t, 1144t
  mechanism of triggered activity in, 59
  paroxysmal atrial tachycardia with AV block in, 190–191
  phenytoin for, 1144, 1339
  ventricular tachyarrhythmias due to, 203
  verapamil use in, 347, 352
Digitoxin. See also Digitalis.
  bile acid sequestrant interaction with, 1142
  dosing regimens for, 1138t
  during pregnancy, 274
  pharmacokinetics of, 1139
  quinidine interaction with, 1364
Digoxin, 183t. See also Digitalis.
  after myocardial infarction, 1140–1141
  antiarrhythmic drugs having little or no pharmacokinetic interaction with, 349t
  clinical applications of, 1139–1140
  cost of, 1140
  dosing regimens for, 1138, 1138t
  drug interactions with, 195, 230, 349t, 351, 352, 1141–1142, 1142t
    with amiodarone, 1142, 1252
    with antiarrhythmic drugs, 352, 1141–1142
    with bepridil, 1058
    with calcium antagonists, 348t, 1142

Digoxin (Continued)
  with diltiazem, 230, 352, 933, 1142
  with esmolol, 513
  with flecainide, 195, 230, 349t, 1315
  with nadolol, 504
  with nicardipine, 980
  with nifedipine, 352, 973
  with nitrendipine, 352, 1000
  with pindolol, 520
  with prazosin, 351
  with propafenone, 349t, 351, 352, 1353
  with propranolol, 491
  with quinidine, 258, 349t, 1141–1142, 1364, 1365t
  with simvastatin, 1118
  with spironolactone, 351, 458
  with verapamil, 352, 922, 1142
  during lactation, 276t, 277, 1141
  during pregnancy, 274, 274t, 1141
  exercise's interaction with, 258
  for atrial fibrillation, 194, 196, 1139–1140
    esmolol with, 510
    quinidine with, 1362, 1364
    with acute myocardial infarction, 131
  for heart failure, 53, 1140
    predictors of response to, 386
    with acute myocardial infarction, 136
  for pulmonary hypertension, 83
  for supraventricular tachycardias, 195, 196
  gelatin capsule formulation of, 1137, 1138t
  hemodynamic effects of, 48–49, 1188t
  in elderly persons, 229–230
  in organ dysfunction, 236–237, 1141
  in Wolff-Parkinson-White syndrome, 187–188, 189
  measuring serum levels of, 237, 1138–1139
    after digoxin-specific antibody therapy, 1144
  pharmacokinetics of, 1137–1139, 1137
  precautions with, 1140–1141
Digoxin-like immunoreactive factor(s), interference in drug assays by, 237
Digoxin-specific antibodies, for digitalis toxicity, 1143t, 1144, 1144t
Dihydrodigoxin, digoxin metabolism to, 1138
Dihydroergotamine, for postural hypotension, 99–100
  heparin with, for postoperative deep vein thrombosis prevention, 1475
Dihydropyridine(s). See also Calcium antagonist(s); specific drugs.
  β-blockers in fixed combinations with, 332
  drug interactions with, 352
  during lactation, 277
  for angina, guidelines for, 37
  for congestive heart failure, 896
  in black persons, 285–286
  in elderly persons, 227–228
  in experimental atherosclerosis, 903
  pharmacokinetics of, 1030t
Dilacor. See Diltiazem.
Dilated cardiomyopathy, β-blockers for, 471, 546
  β-receptor downregulation in, 341
  bisoprolol for, 564
  diltiazem for, 946–947
  metoprolol for, 532, 546
  propranolol for, 489
  ventricular tachycardia associated with, adenosine's effects on, 1245
  ventricular thrombosis in, 171, 171t, 1395t, 1397t, 1398

Diltiazem, 183t, 931–950
  advantages and disadvantages of, 948–949
  adverse effects of, 286, 922t, 947
  after myocardial infarction, 295, 302, 943–944
  chemical properties of, 931, 931
  clinical applications of, 942–947
  contraindications to, 948
  cost of, 949–950, 949t, 1058
  dosage and administration of, 949
  drug interactions with, 348t, 352, 933, 948
    with amiodarone, 933, 1253
    with β-blockers, 348t, 480
    with cyclosporine, 350, 352, 940, 948
    with digoxin, 230, 352, 933, 1142
    with flecainide, 349t
    with propranolol, 491, 933
    with quinidine, 349t
    with ranolazine, 1602
  during lactation, 276–277, 276t, 948
  during pregnancy, 948
  effects of, cardioprotective, 910, 936–937, 943–944
    cardiovascular, 30t, 31, 909t, 934–938
    cellular, 933–934
    diuretic, 938, 942
    electrophysiologic, 935–936
    endocrine and metabolic, 939
    hemodynamic, 892t, 934–935
    renal, 48, 938–939
  exercise's interaction with, 252t, 253
  for accessory pathway tachycardia, 894
  for angina, 892, 942–944
    dosage and administration of, 949
    guidelines for, 37
    in combined therapy, 32t, 33, 943
    mechanism of action of, 940–941
    nicorandil vs., 1642
  for arrhythmias, 945–946
    advantages and disadvantages of, 949
    mechanism of action of, 942
  for atherosclerosis prevention, animal studies of, 903, 906, 937–938
    clinical studies of, 906, 911t
  for atrial fibrillation, 893, 946, 1209
    mechanism of action of, 942
    with acute myocardial infarction, 131
  for atrial flutter, 894
  for hypertension, 944–945
    advantages and disadvantages of, 945, 948–949
    dosage and administration of, 949
    mechanism of action of, 941–942
  for paroxysmal supraventricular tachycardia, 893–894, 945–946
    dosage and administration of, 949
  for pulmonary hypertension, 87
    effects of, 939–940
  for "silent" myocardial ischemia, 895, 943
  for supraventricular tachycardias, 195
    mechanism of action of, 942
  in black persons, 285, 286t
  in elderly persons, 228, 231
  in organ dysfunction, 246, 933, 948
  left ventricular mass reduction by, 911t
  overdosage with, 947
  pharmacokinetics of, 931–933, 932, 932t
  precautions with, 948
  receptor sites for, 933–934
  socioeconomic considerations with, 949–950, 949t
  use dependency of, 934
  withdrawal of, 947

Diltiazem (Continued)
in angina, 892
Dimethyl-arginine, asymmetric, 835
Diphenhydramine hydrochloride, with coronary angioplasty, 309
Diphosphonate(s), in experimental atherosclerosis, 903
Dipropyldopamine, receptors stimulated by, 345
Dipyridamole, 1451–1462
adverse effects of, 1453
after coronary angioplasty, 111, 177
after coronary artery bypass surgery, 112, 176, 176t, 1422–1424, 1456–1457, 1458
after myocardial infarction, 113–114, 1459
after thrombolytic therapy, 1459
aspirin interaction with, 1453
clinical uses of, 1453–1462
for angina, 1415–1416
for cerebrovascular disease, 113, 1461
for coronary artery disease, 1458–1459
for peripheral vascular disease, 113, 114–115, 1461–1462
for prosthetic arterial graft occlusion prevention, 1455, 1456
for thromboembolism prevention, 163
with prosthetic heart valves, 106, 106t, 107, 173, 174, 174t, 1408–1409, 1408t, 1410, 1410t, 1453–1455, 1454t
in combined antithrombotic therapy, 113
mechanism of action of, 1451–1452, 1451t
pharmacokinetics of, 1452–1453
with coronary angioplasty, 305–306, 309t, 1460–1461
with coronary artery bypass surgery, 114
Disintegrin(s), antiplatelet effect of, 105–106
Disopyramide, 183t, 1273–1291
adverse effects of, 1285–1286
arrhythmia aggravation by, 1235t, 1286
chemical properties of, 1273, 1274
clinical efficacy of, 1286–1291
contraindications to, 1281
cost of, 1367t
diagnostic use of, in syncope, 1290
drug interactions with, 349t, 351, 1285
with amrinone, 1173
with β-blockers, 347–349, 349t, 351
with calcium antagonists, 348t
with diuretics, 352
with nadolol, 504
with propranolol, 491
with quinidine, 349t, 1285
with verapamil, 349t, 351, 922
during lactation, 276t, 277, 1283, 1286
during pregnancy, 274, 274t, 1283, 1286
effects of, 1274–1281
electrophysiologic, 1274–1280, 1275–1278, 1279t
hemodynamic, 1280–1281, 1281
for ventricular arrhythmias, 1287–1288, 1287
mexiletine vs., 1325, 1325t
mexiletine with, 1328
quinidine vs., 1287–1288, 1287, 1365, 1365t
for ventricular ectopy, 1286–1287
flecainide vs., 1286–1287, 1309
propafenone vs., 1355
heart failure due to, 1281, 1286
in elderly persons, 230
in organ dysfunction, 237, 1284–1285, 1284t

Disopyramide (Continued)
intramuscular, 1282
intravenous, 1282
overdose of, 1286
pharmacokinetics of, 1281–1284, 1282
in organ dysfunction, 1284–1285, 1284t
receptors affected by, 351
rectal administration of, 1282
Distribution of drugs. See also specific drugs.
age-related changes in, 225
Diucardin (hydroflumethiazide), for hypertension, dose and side effects of, 374t
Diulo. See Metolazone.
Diuretic(s), 357–464. See also specific drugs and classes of drugs.
ACE inhibitors with, for congestive heart failure, 387
for hypertension, 701, 702
hemodynamic effects of, 50
in black persons, 284, 285
in fixed combinations, 332
bepridil use with, 1057
braking phenomenon with, 384, 390, 390, 414
captopril with, for hypertension, 732
precautions with, 735, 737
classification of, by site of action, 385
combined regimens of, in chronic renal failure, 362–363
dietary sodium restriction with, 390–391
drug interactions with, with ACE inhibitors, 350
with amiodarone, 349t, 352
with antiarrhythmic drugs, 352
with digoxin, 1142
with mexiletine, 1327
with NSAIDs, 350
with probenecid, 351
with procainamide, 1346
with quinidine, 349t, 352
with rilmenidine, 640
with sotalol, 349t, 352
during lactation, 276
during pregnancy, 270–271
electrolyte abnormalities due to, 386–387
exercise's interaction with, 254
fixed combinations containing, 73, 331–332
for acute left ventricular failure, 52
for acute myocardial infarction, 129
for congestive heart failure, 383–387
ACE inhibitors with, 387
adverse effects of, 53, 386–387
mechanisms of action of, 383–386
rationale for, 46–47
for hypertension, 371–380
ACE inhibitors with, 701, 702
as initial drug, 68, 69t, 71t, 373–375, 375t, 379–380, 380t
as second drug, 71–72
captopril with, 732, 735, 737
clinical trials of, 373–375, 375t
enalapril with, 744
mechanism of action of, 371–373, 372
nitrendipine with, 1002
prazosin with, 664
preparations and dosages of, 373, 374t
quality of life issues with, 379
ramipril with, 769–770, 770t, 771
safety of, 375–379
for hypertensive emergencies, 154t, 155t, 158
for pulmonary hypertension, 83
glucose intolerance due to, 365, 377–378

Diuretic(s) (Continued)
hemodynamic effects of, 49–50
hemodynamic response to stress and, 265, 266
high-ceiling, 388. See also Loop diuretic(s); specific drugs.
hyperuricemia due to, 377
hypokalemia due to, 378, 378t, 415–416, 415
glucose intolerance and, 365, 438
in chronic renal failure, 364
in congestive heart failure, 386–387
ventricular arrhythmias and, 414–415, 447
in black persons, 281–283, 282t, 283t
ACE inhibitors with, 284, 285
in elderly persons, 226
in renal failure, 357–365
complications of, 364–365
indications for, 363–364
pharmacology of, 360–363
indications for, 417t
lipid effects of, 375–377, 376t
loop. See Loop diuretic(s); specific drugs.
low-ceiling, 413, 413
mercurial, 389
mortality due to, in patients with abnormal ECG, 282, 282t
nitrates with, hemodynamic effects of, 50
osmotic. See also Mannitol.
in chronic renal failure, 360
postural hypotension due to, 96
potassium-sparing. See Potassium-sparing diuretic(s); specific drugs.
potassium-wasting. See also specific drugs and classes of drugs.
digitalis toxicity with, 352
ketanserin interaction with, 1654
principles and practice of therapy with, 357–387
resistance to. See Diuretic resistance.
thiazide. See Thiazide diuretic(s); specific drugs.
Diuretic resistance, factors affecting, 391, 391t
in congestive heart failure, 384
malabsorption in, 392–393
in hypoalbuminemia, 400
Diuril. See Chlorothiazide.
Dobutamine, 1151–1158
adverse effects of, 1158
amrinone vs., 1154, 1173–1174
bed rest–induced deconditioning and, 1156
chemical properties of, 1151
clinical uses of, 1153–1157
comparison of, to other drugs, 1154–1155
contraindications to, 1158
diagnostic applications of, 1156–1157
dosage and administration of, 1158
drug interactions with, 1158
during pregnancy, 1158
effects of, 48, 49t, 1149t, 1152–1153, 1188t
in combined therapy, 50t
for cardiogenic shock, 137
for dilated cardiomyopathy, amrinone with, 1173
for heart failure, acute, 1149, 1149t
chronic, 54, 1153–1155
dopamine with, 48, 1163
intermittent therapy with, 12
outpatient infusion of, 1155
with myocardial infarction, 136
for hypotension with right ventricular infarction, 138

Dobutamine *(Continued)*
  for left ventricular dysfunction after
      myocardial infarction, vasodilator
      with, 1156
  for left ventricular failure, 52, 53, 1155–
      1156
  for low-output state, after cardiac sur-
      gery, 1156
    with right ventricular infarction, 51
  for pulmonary edema, 50, 125
  in cardiopulmonary resuscitation, 211
  in children, 1152–1153
  in elderly persons, 1153
  in organ dysfunction, 1158
  milrinone vs., 1179–1180
  pharmacokinetics of, 1152
  pharmacology of, 1148, 1151–1152
  phosphodiesterase inhibitors with, for
      acute heart failure, 1149, 1149t
    hypotension due to, 49
  precautions with, 1157–1158
  receptor activity of, 337t, 343–344, 1151–
      1152
Dobutrex. See *Dobutamine.*
Docosahexaenoic acid (DHA), 1608, 1608t,
      1609. See also *Fish oil(s); Omega-3 fatty
      acid(s).*
  antiplatelet therapy with, 103–104
  for prevention of ventricular fibrillation,
      1611
  sources of, 1612t
Dofetilide, 1296–1302
  adverse effects of, 1301
  chemical properties of, 1296
  clinical studies of, 1298–1301, *1299–1301*
  mechanism of action of, 1296
  pharmacokinetics of, 1298, *1299, 1300*
  pharmacology of, in clinical studies,
      1298–1301, *1301*
    in preclinical studies, 1296–1298, *1296,
      1298*
  proarrhythmic effect of, 1298, 1301
Domperidone, 339
L-Dopa, 1164–1165
  carbidopa with, postural hypotension
      and, 96–97
  for heart failure, 54, 345, 1164–1165
  hemodynamic effects of, 49
  postural hypotension due to, 96–97
  vasodilators with, hemodynamic effects
      of, 50t
Dopamine, 1162–1165
  amrinone vs., 1174
  chemical properties of, 1162, *1195*
  dobutamine vs., 1154
  dosage and administration of, 1163
  drug interactions with, 1163–1164
    in cardiopulmonary resuscitation, 211
  for cardiogenic shock, 137, 1163
  for heart failure, 1163
    acute, 1149, 1149t
    with acute myocardial infarction, 136
  for left ventricular failure, 52
  for low-output state, after cardiac sur-
      gery, nitroprusside with, 862
    with right ventricular infarction, 51,
      52t
  for pulmonary edema, 125
  for pulmonary hypertension in congeni-
      tal heart disease, 91
  for renal failure, 360, 1163
    atrial natriuretic peptide with, 359
    in animal models, 358
    with heart failure, dobutamine with,
      48
  hemodynamic effects of, 48, 49t, 1149t

Dopamine *(Continued)*
    in combined therapy, 50t
  hypertension and, 1165
  in cardiopulmonary resuscitation, 210–
      211
  pharmacology of, 1148, 1162–1163, *1162*
  receptors stimulated by, 339, 345, 1162–
      1163, *1162*
Dopamine receptor(s), 338–339, 339t, 1162,
      1162, 1189, *1190*, 1190t, 1194–1195
Dopaminergic agonist(s), 339t, 345
  for heart failure, 1164
Dopexamine, 345, 1164
Doxazosin, 681–687
  adverse effects of, 611, 612, 686
  chemical properties of, 681, *681*
  clinical applications of, 685–686
  cost of, 949t
  dosage and administration of, 610–611
  effects of, 682–685
    hemodynamic, 609, 682–683
    serum lipid, 611, 684
  for hypertension, 610, 685
    advantages of, 686–687
    in elderly persons, 227
    in organ dysfunction, 242
  mechanism of action of, 609, 681, 682
  pharmacokinetics of, 681–682, *682*
  receptor selectivity of, 336t, 342–343,
      681, 682
Dressler's syndrome, 130
Drug(s). See also specific drugs and classes
      of drugs.
  dosage changes for, in organ dysfunc-
      tion, 234–235, 234t, 235t, 236
  interactions of, 347–353
    cholinergic, 351
    during cardiopulmonary resuscitation,
      208
    involving gastrointestinal tract, 351
    involving heart, 347–350
    involving kidneys, 351
    involving liver, 350–351
    involving peripheral circulation, 350
    involving plasma protein binding, 351
    of antiarrhythmic drugs, 349t
    of β-blockers, 348t
    of calcium antagonists, 348t
  monitoring concentrations of, limitations
      of, 234
  pharmacokinetics and pharmacodynam-
      ics of, age-related changes in, 225–
      226
    during cardiopulmonary resuscitation,
      206–208
    in organ dysfunction, 235–236
  postural hypotension due to, 96–97
DuP 753. See *Losartan.*
DVT. See *Deep venous thrombosis (DVT).*
Dyazide. See *Triamterene/hydrochlorothiazide.*
Dynacirc. See *Isradipine.*
Dynamite, 866
Dyrenium. See *Triamterene.*
Dysbetalipoproteinemia, bile acid
      sequestrants' effects in, 1069
  clofibrate for, 1078
  nicotinic acid's effects on, 1063
Dysgeusia, due to captopril, 736
Dyslipidemia. See *Hyperlipidemia(s).*
Dyspepsia, due to fluvastatin, 1133

E-3174 (losartan metabolite), 819, 821
Echocardiography, dobutamine with, for
      coronary artery disease detection, 1157

Echocardiography *(Continued)*
  in atrial thrombus detection, 1402, 1404–
      1405
  in ventricular thrombus detection, after
      myocardial infarction, 1396
Eclampsia, 150
  labetalol for, 576
  urapidil for, 678
Edecrin. See *Ethacrynic acid.*
Edema, due to felodipine, 1043
  due to lacidipine, 1051
  due to minoxidil, 855
  due to nitrendipine, 1003
  furosemide for, dosage and administra-
      tion of, 395
  in arteriolar wall, in hypertension, 371
  in chronic renal failure, diuretic therapy
      for, 363
  in liver failure, amiloride for, 449
  pulmonary. See *Pulmonary edema.*
  refractory, in congestive heart failure,
      383–384, 385
  thiazides for, 414
  torsemide for, 404–405
EDRF (endothelium-derived relaxing
      factor), 833, *834*. See also *Nitric oxide
      (NO).*
  identity of, 868
EDTA chelation, 1613–1616
  applications of, 1615–1616, *1616*
  chemistry of, 1614, *1614*
  pharmacology of, 1614–1615
Efaroxan, 652
EHDP (ethane-1-hydroxy-1,1-
      diphosphonate), in experimental
      atherosclerosis, 903
Eicosapentaenoic acid (EPA), 1608, 1608t,
      1609. See also *Fish oil(s); Omega-3 fatty
      acid(s).*
  antiplatelet therapy with, 103–104
  for prevention of ventricular fibrillation,
      1611
  platelet effects of, 1609–1610, *1610*
  sources of, 1612t
Eisenmenger's reaction, treatment of
      pulmonary hypertension in, 90, 91
Elderly person(s), ACE inhibitor therapy
      in, 228–229
  amlodipine use in, 227–228, 1030
  antiadrenergic therapy in, 227
  antiarrhythmic therapy in, 230–231
  bepridil use in, 1058
  β-blocker therapy in, 226–227, 231
  calcium antagonist therapy in, 227–228
  cardiovascular drug therapy in, 225–232
  digitalis therapy in, 229–230
  digitalis toxicity in, 1142–1143
  diuretic therapy in, 226
  dobutamine use in, 1153
  enalapril use in, 228–229, 743
  endogenous hemodynamic and neurohu-
      moral response to vasodilatation in,
      829
  felodipine use in, 227–228, 1041
  hypertension in, amlodipine for, 1032,
      1038
    captopril for, 732–733
    felodipine for, 1042
    isolated systolic, 73–74, 228–229
    labetalol for, 574
    lacidipine for, 1049, *1049*
    metoprolol for, 525
    nifedipine for, 975–976
    trandolapril for, 785
  ibopamine use in, 1196
  inotropic therapy in, 229–230

Elderly person(s) (Continued)
lacidipine use in, 1048
lipid-lowering therapy in, 231–232
lovastatin use in, 1108–1109
nicorandil use in, 1643–1644
nitrate therapy in, 230
pharmacokinetics in, 225–226
pravastatin use in, 1125
sotalol use in, 231, 1371
thrombolytic therapy in, 231, 1432
zatebradine use in, 1388
Electroconvulsive therapy, esmolol for
tachycardia and hypertension with,
512
Electrophysiologic testing, drug-induced
arrhythmia aggravation criteria on,
1229, 1231
in arrhythmia evaluation, 61, 199–200,
200
after acute myocardial infarction, 296
with antiarrhythmic therapy, 1218–1219,
1219, 1220
Elimination of drugs. See also specific
drugs.
age-related changes in, 225
hepatic, 235–236
renal, 235
Embolectomy, for lower extremity
embolus, 168–169
pulmonary, 165
Embolism. See also Thromboembolism.
calcific, in aortic valve disease, 1401
cerebral. See Cerebral embolism.
coronary, 169
lower extremity, 168–169
mesenteric, 169
pulmonary. See Pulmonary embolism (PE).
EMD45609. See Carmoxirole.
Emergencies, cardiovascular. See also
Cardiopulmonary resuscitation (CPR);
specific conditions.
drug treatment of, 119–219
Enalapril, 742–748
adverse effects of, 701–702, 747–748, 747t
after myocardial infarction, 296
effects of, 718–719, 719
approved uses of, 742–743
clinical applications of, 744–747
cost of, 949t
dosage and administration of, 700–701
drug interactions with, with amiloride,
450
with aspirin, 745
during lactation, 276t, 277
during pregnancy, 698, 743, 744
effects of, 47t, 743–744
exercise's interaction with, 257
for congestive heart failure, 12, 54, 387,
745–747, 745t
dosage for, 745–746, 748
survival with, 712–714, 714, 715
for hypertension, 744–745
amlodipine with, 1034
indapamide with, 428–429
for hypertensive emergencies, 155t
for pulmonary hypertension, in congenital heart disease, 91
in black persons, 284, 285t
in children, 744–745
in elderly persons, 228–229, 743
in organ dysfunction, 244, 701, 722t, 725,
743
mechanism of action of, 743
pharmacokinetics of, 743
socioeconomic considerations with, 748
Enalaprilat, for hypertension,
disadvantages of, 996

Enalaprilat (Continued)
for hypertensive emergencies, 154t
hemodynamic effects of, 1149t
pharmacokinetics of, 723t, 743
Encainide, arrhythmia aggravation by,
1235, 1235t, 1236–1237
for ventricular ectopy, flecainide vs.,
1309
moricizine vs., 1334–1335
propafenone vs., 1355
in elderly persons, 231
in organ dysfunction, 240
Encephalopathy, hypertensive, 149–150
felodipine for, 1043
Endocardial catheter ablation. See Catheter
ablation.
Endocarditis, native valve,
thromboembolism with, 1405
prosthetic valve, anticoagulant therapy
in, 1411
Endometrial carcinoma, estrogen
replacement therapy and, 322
Endothelin, production of, nitrates' effects
on, 846
nitric oxide's effects on, 837–838, 838
regulation of, 838
Endothelium, acetylcholine-induced
arterial relaxation and, 832–833, 832,
833
alterations in, in atherosclerosis, 844–845
in hyperlipidemia, 843–844
in hypertension, 842–843, 844
defective, nitrate action in presence of,
846
function of, estrogens' effects on, 321–
322
lovastatin's effects on, 1110
mibefradil's effects on, 1012
ramipril's effects on, 765–766
injury to, in pathogenesis of atherosclerosis, 902, 1412–1413, 1412t
vasoconstriction after, 1414–1415
normal, antithrombotic activity of, 1414
probucol's protective effects for, 1103–
1104, 1104
Endothelium-derived relaxing factor
(EDRF), 833, 834. See also Nitric oxide
(NO).
identity of, 868
Endotracheal drug administration, in
cardiopulmonary resuscitation,
207–208
Enduron (methyclothiazide), for
hypertension, dose and side effects of,
374t
Energy metabolism, during myocardial
ischemia, 1600, 1600t
ranolazine's effects on, 1601
trimetazidine's effects on, 1594–1595,
1594
Enflurane, diltiazem interaction with, 948
Enoxaparin, 1511–1516
chemical properties of, 1511
clinical evaluation of, 1512–1516, 1513t
pharmacokinetics of, 1512
pharmacology of, 1511–1512
Enoximone, adverse effects of, in severe
heart failure, 230
for chronic heart failure, 54
for left ventricular failure, 52
for pulmonary edema, 50
hemodynamic effects of, 49, 49t
EPA. See Eicosapentaenoic acid (EPA).
Epinephrine (adrenaline), auto-oxidation
of, with alkaline drugs, 209–210
for ventricular tachycardia with myocardial infarction, 132

Epinephrine (adrenaline) (Continued)
hemodynamic effects of, 49t
ibopamine's effects on, 1200–1201, 1200t
in cardiopulmonary resuscitation, 208–
210, 209t
endotracheal administration of, 207
for cerebral protection, 219
receptors stimulated by, 336t, 337, 337t,
341–342, 343
therapeutic uses of, 342
Epinine, 1195, 1195
hemodynamic effects of, 1198, 1198
pharmacokinetics of, 1196
Epoprostenol, for hypertension during
pregnancy, 273
Eptastatin. See Pravastatin.
Ergonovine, coronary artery spasm due to,
nitroprusside for, 863
Ergot alkaloid(s), dopamine interaction
with, 1164
for postural hypotension, 99–100
Ergotamine, β-blocker interaction with,
480
for postural hypotension, 100
Ergotism, nitroprusside for, 863
Erythrityl tetranitrate, adverse effects of,
878
chemical properties of, 876, 877
effects of, 877–878
oral, 879
pharmacokinetics of, 877
sublingual, 878
Erythrocyte(s), fluorocarbons' effects on, in
sickle cell anemia, 1624
impaired deformability of, in occlusive
peripheral arterial disease, 1604–
1605
Erythromycin, drug interactions with, with
digoxin, 351, 1142
with disopyramide, 1285
with lovastatin, 1111
Esidrix. See Hydrochlorothiazide.
Esmolol, 183t, 507–514
adverse effects of, 512–513
chemical properties of, 507, 507
clinical applications of, 509–512
dosage and administration of, 513–514
drug interactions with, 513
during pregnancy, 274t, 275, 514
effects of, 467t, 472t, 508–509
for acute myocardial infarction, 133
for atrial fibrillation, 193, 509–510
with acute myocardial infarction, 131
for hypertension, disadvantages of, 996
perioperative, 511–512
for myocardial ischemia, 510–511
for supraventricular tachycardias, 195,
509–510
in organ dysfunction, 508
pharmacodynamics of, 467t, 472t, 508–
509
pharmacokinetics of, 507–508
pharmacology of, 508t
withdrawal of, 513–514
Esophageal varices, nadolol for, 503
Estrogen(s). See also Estrogen replacement
therapy.
endothelial nitric oxide release and, 839
for prostatic carcinoma, cardiovascular
events and, 321
Estrogen replacement therapy, after
surgical menopause, 320
age and, 320
angiographic studies of, 317–318
community-based studies of, 317
extracardiovascular risks and benefits of,
322

Estrogen replacement therapy *(Continued)*
  for hyperlipidemia, 22, 79
  hospital-based studies of, 316–317
  in low-risk women, 320
  lipid effects of, 317, 318, 320–321
  prospective studies of, 318–319
  survival in coronary artery disease and,
    319–320
ET. See *Erythrityl tetranitrate.*
Ethacrynic acid, advantages of, 373
  for hypertension, dose and side effects
    of, 374t
  history of, 396
  in chronic renal failure, indications for
    use of, 361
Ethane-1-hydroxy-1,1-diphosphonate
    (EHDP), in experimental
    atherosclerosis, 903
Ethanol, drug interactions with, with
    calcium antagonists, 348t
  with guanabenz, 631
  with isosorbide mononitrate, 884
  with warfarin, 307
  intoxication with, due to intravenous ni-
    troglycerin, 870
  postural hypotension and, 97
Ethmozine. See *Moricizine.*
Ethylenediaminetetraacetic acid, chelation
    therapy with. See *EDTA chelation.*
Etmozin. See *Moricizine.*
Euthyroid sick syndrome, 1657, 1657t
  due to cardiopulmonary bypass, 1659
  in heart failure, 1659
Eutonyl (pargyline hydrochloride),
    dopamine interaction with, 211
"Excitable gap," in reentry, 61
Exercise, antianginal agents' interaction
    with, 251–254, 252t
  antihypertensive drugs' interaction with,
    254–258
  arrhythmias and, 258–259
  cardiovascular drug therapy interacting
    with, 250–259
  for dyslipidemia, 19
  hemodynamics of hypertension during,
    254
  in heart failure patient, 258
  normal response to, 251
  timing of, circadian pattern of cardiac
    disease and, 314–315
Exercise fatigue, due to β-blockers, 256
  due to propranolol, 490
Exercise testing, after coronary
    angioplasty, 308–309
  dobutamine stress testing vs., 1156–1157
  Holter monitoring vs., in antiischemic
    therapy evaluation, 37
  in detection of drug-induced arrhythmia
    aggravation, 1236
  with antiarrhythmic therapy, 1218
Exercise tolerance, in chronic congestive
    heart failure, α-adrenergic blockers'
    effects on, 48
Exna (benzthiazide), for hypertension,
    dose and side effects of, 374t
Extracellular fluid volume. See also
    Hypovolemia; Plasma volume.
  excessively rapid reduction in, due to di-
    uretic therapy in chronic renal fail-
    ure, 364
Extracorporeal circuits, anticoagulation in,
    nadroparin for, 1487
Extrasystole(s), ventricular. See *Ventricular
    premature complexes.*

Factor Xa, danaparoid's effect on, 1506

Factor Xa *(Continued)*
  enoxaparin's effect on, 1511
  heparin's effect on, 1474
  Logiparin's effect on, 1480
  nadroparin's effect on, 1485
Fascicular tachycardia, adenosine's effects
    on, 1243
Fatigue, due to β-blockers, 256
  due to propranolol, 490
Fatty acid(s), classes of, 1608, 1608t
  clofibrate's effects on metabolism of,
    1077–1078
  "fraudulent," fibrates as, 1092–1093,
    1093
  omega-3. See *Omega-3 fatty acid(s).*
Fatty streaks, 28, 28
  in pathogenesis of atherosclerosis, 902
Felodipine, 1040–1044
  adverse effects of, 1043
  chemical properties of, 1040
  clinical applications of, 1042–1043
  contraindications to, 1044
  diuretic effect of, 1040, 1041–1042
  dosage and administration of, 1044
  drug interactions with, 1043–1044
  during pregnancy, 1044
  effects of, 909t, 1041–1042
  in elderly persons, 227–228, 1041, 1042
  in organ dysfunction, 246, 1042–1043
  left ventricular mass reduction by, 911t
  pharmacokinetics of, 1030t, 1040–1041
  pharmacology of, 1040
  vascular selectivity of, 1040, 1041
Fenofibrate, 78, 1083–1090
  adverse effects of, 1089–1090, 1089t
  carcinogenicity of, 1089
  chemical properties of, 1083, 1084
  clinical efficacy of, 1085, 1085t
  drug interactions with, 1090
  in combined therapy, 1090
  in organ dysfunction, 1084, 1090
  pharmacokinetics of, 1084–1085, 1084,
    1085t
  pharmacology of, 1077
  serum lipid effects of, 1085–1089, 1086
Fenoldopam, 339, 345
  for heart failure, 1164
  receptors stimulated by, 337t
Fenoterol, receptors stimulated by, 337t
Fentanyl, diltiazem interaction with, 948
  nicardipine interaction with, 996
Fetal hydantoin syndrome, 274
Fetal tachycardia, amiodarone for, 1256
  digoxin for, 1141
  quinidine for, 275
  verapamil for, 275
Fiber, dietary, digitalis interaction with,
    1142
  with bile acid sequestrants, 1071–1072
  with nicotinic acid, 1065
Fibric acid derivative(s). See also specific
    drugs.
  adverse effects of, 78
  carcinogenic action of, 1077
  chemical properties of, 1084
  for hyperlipidemia, 23, 78–79
    bile acid sequestrant with, 1090
    lovastatin with, 1112
    mechanism of action of, 80t
    nicotinic acid with, 81, 1064
    statin with, 81, 1079, 1090
  in combined therapy, 1090
    skeletal muscle disorders due to, 1079,
      1100, 1112
  lipid effects of, 80t, 1076
Fibrinogen, 1522
  aspirin's effect on, 1443

Fibrinogen *(Continued)*
  ciprofibrate's effects on, 1094
  degradation of, by plasmin, 1521–1522,
    1523
  pentoxifylline's effects on, 1605
  simvastatin's effects on, 1116
Fibrinogen assay, in monitoring
    streptokinase therapy, 1525
Fibrinogen degradation products,
    anticoagulant effects of, 1521–1522
  half-life of, 1522
Fibrinoid necrotizing arteriolitis, in
    accelerated and malignant
    hypertension, 149
Fibrinolytic system, 1542, 1567t, 1568, 1568
Fibrinolytic therapy. See *Thrombolytic
    therapy;* specific drugs.
Fibrin-specific monoclonal antibodies,
    single-chain urokinase-type
    plasminogen activator complexes
    with, 1583–1584
Filter, inferior vena cava, in pulmonary
    embolism prevention, 163
First-dose phenomenon, with α₁-blockers,
    611
  with prazosin, 664
  with terazosin, 671
Fish oil(s), 1608–1612
  adverse effects of, 1612, 1612t
  clinical effects of, 1609–1611, 1610, 1611t
  coronary artery disease and, epidemio-
    logic studies of, 1608–1609
  dose of, 1611t, 1612, 1612t
  pravastatin with, for hyperlipidemia,
    1124
"Fist pacing," for ventricular tachycardia,
    202, 203
  in cardiopulmonary resuscitation, 217
Flavonoids, felodipine interaction with,
    1044
Flecainide, 183t, 1304–1316
  adverse effects of, 1312–1314, 1313t
  arrhythmia aggravation by, 1235, 1235t,
    1237, 1312–1314, 1313t
  chemical properties of, 1304
  clinical use of, 1314–1316
  cost of, 1367t
  dosage and administration of, 1315t,
    1316
  drug interactions with, 349t, 1315
    with amiodarone, 349t, 1253, 1315
    with β-blockers, 347–349, 348t, 349t
    with digoxin, 195, 230, 349t, 1315
  during lactation, 276t, 277
  effects of, 1306–1312
    antiarrhythmic, 1307–1312
    electrocardiographic, 1307
    electrophysiologic, 1306–1307, 1307t
    hemodynamic, 1312
    on left ventricular function, 1312
  for atrial flutter, 192, 1310
  for ventricular ectopy, 1308, 1309
    moricizine vs., 1309, 1334–1335
    propafenone vs., 1355
    quinidine vs., 1309, 1365t, 1366
  for ventricular tachyarrhythmia, 203,
    1307–1309
  in elderly persons, 231
  in organ dysfunction, 240, 1305, 1315
  indications for, 1314–1315
  pharmacokinetics of, 1304–1306, 1306
  plasma concentrations of, 1315–1316
  precautions with, 1315
  use dependency of, 1306, 1309
    proarrhythmic effect and, 1314
Florinef (fludrocortisone), for postural
    hypotension, 97

Flosequinan, for congestive heart failure, 12

Fludex. See *Indapamide.*

Fludrocortisone, for postural hypotension, 97

Fluid retention. See also *Edema.*
due to minoxidil, 855, *856*

Fluid therapy, in cardiopulmonary resuscitation, 207, 212

Fluorocarbon(s), 1618–1624. See also *Fluosol.*
adverse effects of, 1623
clinical applications of, 1623–1624, 1623t
second-generation, *1619,* 1623

Fluosol, 1618–1624
adverse effects of, 1623
animal and clinical studies of, 1620–1623
cardiovascular effects of, 1620–1621, *1621,* 1621t, *1622*
chemical properties of, 1618, 1618t, *1619*
clinical applications of, 1623–1624, 1623t
drug interactions with, 1619–1620
during pregnancy and lactation, 1620
pharmacokinetics of, 1619–1620
pharmacology of, 1618–1619, *1619, 1620*

Flushing, due to nicotinic acid, 1065

Fluvastatin, 1128–1134
adverse effects of, 1132–1133
animal studies of, 1129–1130
cataracts and, 1129, 1133
chemical properties of, 1128
cost of, 1134
dosage and administration of, 1134
drug interactions with, 1133–1134
for hyperlipidemia, 1130–1132, *1131,* 1131t, *1132*
animal studies of, 1128
as initial drug, 76–77
in combined therapy, 1132, 1132t
in organ dysfunction, 1129, 1134
indications for, 1130
LDL cholesterol reduction with, 77t
pharmacokinetics of, 1128–1129, *1129*
tissue selectivity of, 1129, *1130*

Foam cell(s), in pathogenesis of atherosclerosis, 324–325, *325,* 902

Fogarty balloon catheter extraction, for lower extremity embolus, 169

Foramen ovale, patent, paradoxical embolism and, 169, 170

Forrester classification, of acute myocardial infarction patients, 133, 134t

Forskolin, mechanism of action of, 44, 45t, *1178*

Fosinopril, 801–808
adverse effects of, 807
chemical properties of, 801–802, *802*
clinical applications of, 807–808
contraindications to, 807–808
dosage and administration of, 808
during lactation, 808
during pregnancy, 807–808
effects of, 803–807, 806t, 807t
exercise's interaction with, 257
for hypertension, clinical use of, 807
efficacy of, 804–805, *804,* 805t, *806*
in organ dysfunction, 245, 722t, 725, 803, *804,* 808
pharmacokinetics of, 802–803, *803, 804*
socioeconomic considerations with, 808
tissue ACE inhibition by, 802

Fosinoprilat, chemical properties of, 802, *802*
pharmacokinetics of, 723t, 802–803, *803, 804*
in renal insufficiency, 723–724, *724,* 724t, 803, *804*

Fraxiparine. See *Nadroparin.*

Free radicals, 324
in pathogenesis of atherosclerosis, 1615
indapamide's effects on, 421–422
trimetazidine's effects on, 1595–1596, *1596, 1597,* 1599

Fresh frozen plasma, for bleeding due to tissue-type plasminogen activator, 1573
for warfarin reversal, 1520

Furosemide, 388–395
adverse effects of, 374t, 394, 394t
in hypertensive emergency management, 153
bullous dermatitis due to, 365
clinical use of, 392–393
determinants of response to, 390–392, 391t
dosage and administration of, 395
dose adjustment for, in organ dysfunction, 246–247
drug interactions with, with captopril, 351
with metolazone, 418
effects of, acute, 389–390
chronic, 390, *390*
hemodynamic, 49, 361–362
vascular, 389–390
for ascites, 392
spironolactone with, 456
for congestive heart failure, 392–393
ACE inhibitor with, 387
extrarenal actions of, 385
metolazone with, 413
with acute myocardial infarction, 134
for edema, dosage and administration of, 395
for hypertension, dosage and administration of, 374t, 395
with reduced renal function, 393
for hypertensive emergencies, 154t
adverse effects of, 153
for hyponatremia, 393
for hyporeninemic hypoaldosteronism, 363, 393
for nephrotic syndrome, 393
for pulmonary edema, 50, 124
for renal failure, acute, 359–360
chronic, 361
in animal models, 358
prophylactic use of, 393
history of, 396, *396*
in black persons, 282, 283t
indications for, 392, 392t
ototoxicity of, 361, 365
pharmacokinetics of, 390
aging's effects on, 391–392
in renal insufficiency, 400
pharmacology of, 389, *406*
precautions with, 392
resistance to, 391
in congestive heart failure, 384
ventricular function deterioration due to, 50
with coronary angioplasty, 309

Fusion beat(s), with premature ventricular systole, 198

GADPH (glyceraldehyde-3-phosphate-dehydrogenase), nitric oxide's effects on, 837, 845

Galactorrhea, due to methyldopa, 604, 619

Gallbladder disease, due to ciprofibrate, 1095

Gallbladder disease (*Continued*)
due to clofibrate, 1079
due to fenofibrate, 1089
due to gemfibrozil, 1101
fluvastatin and, 1133
in animal studies, 1130

Gallopamil, 926–929
effects of, 909t, 927–928
in elderly persons, 228

Gangrene, due to dopamine, 1163

Gangrenous necrosis, due to warfarin, 1520

Gastrointestinal symptoms. See also *Nausea.*
due to amiodarone, 1257
due to amrinone, 1173
due to aspirin, 1448–1449
due to bile acid sequestrants, 1071–1072
due to disopyramide, 1285
due to ibopamine, 1203
due to mexiletine, 1329
due to phenytoin, 1340
due to procainamide, 1345
due to quinidine, 1364
treatment's effects on drug absorption, 1363
due to ticlopidine, 1470

Gastrointestinal tract, diltiazem's effects on, 940
drug interactions involving, 351
malignancies of, enalapril and, 747

Gemfibrozil, 1098–1101
adverse effects of, 1100–1101
chemical properties of, *1084,* 1098, *1098*
clinical trials of, 1099–1100, *1099, 1100,* 1100t
contraindications to, 1101
for hyperlipidemia, as initial drug, 78–79
nicotinic acid with, 1064
pravastatin with, 1100, 1123
in combined therapy, 1100
myopathy due to, 1100, 1111
indications for, 1101
lipid effects of, 1076
mechanism of action of, 1098–1099
pharmacokinetics of, 1098

Gene therapy, for hyperlipidemia, 24–25

Gentamicin, diltiazem interaction with, 933

Gingival hyperplasia, due to amlodipine, 1037
due to phenytoin, 1340

Glomerulonephritis, acute, hypertensive emergency with, 151

Glucagon, inotropic effects of, mechanisms of, 45t

Glucose, in fluid therapy during cardiopulmonary resuscitation, 207

Glucose intolerance. See also *Carbohydrate metabolism; Diabetes mellitus; Insulin resistance.*
diuretic-induced, 365, 377–378
triamterene and, 438, 440

Glutathione peroxidase, 326, *326*

Glutathione S-transferase, in nitroglycerin metabolism, 868

Glyceraldehyde-3-phosphate-dehydrogenase (GADPH), nitric oxide's effects on, 837, 845

Glyceryl trinitrate. See *Nitroglycerin.*

Glycine xylide, accumulation of, in renal insufficiency, 238

Glycoprotein IIb/IIIa receptor, 1626–1627
monoclonal antibodies to. See also *c7E3 Fab.*
antiplatelet effect of, 105

Glycoside(s), cardiac. See also *Digitalis; Digitoxin; Digoxin.*

Glycoside(s) (Continued)
history of, 1136
Glycoside receptor(s), in heart, 340
Gout. See also Hyperuricemia.
diuretic therapy and, 226, 377
due to intravenous nitroglycerin, 870
α_{1A}Gp (α_1-acid glycoprotein),
disopyramide binding to, 1283
GP IIb/IIIa receptor. See Glycoprotein IIb/
IIIa receptor.
G_1-protein, milrinone's effects on, 1178
Graduated compression stockings, in
thromboembolism prevention, 163
Grapefruit juice, felodipine interaction
with, 1044
GTN (glyceryl trinitrate). See Nitroglycerin.
Guanabenz, 628–632
adverse effects of, 608, 630
chemical properties of, 628, 628
clinical applications of, 630
contraindications to, 630–631
cost of, 631–632, 649
drug interactions with, 631
during pregnancy, 630
effects of, 629–630
hemodynamic, 606, 607, 629
exercise's interaction with, 255
for hypertension, 607, 630, 631
as initial therapy, 69t
in elderly persons, 227
in organ dysfunction, 243, 631
mechanism of action of, 605, 628–629
pharmacokinetics of, 629
withdrawal of, 608, 630
Guanethidine, for hypertensive
emergencies, 154t, 155t, 158
in experimental atherosclerosis, 902
Guanfacine, 642–650
adverse effects of, 607–608, 648
chemical properties of, 643
clinical applications of, 648–649
clinical studies of, 644–648, 646t, 647t
drug interactions with, 649
effects of, 606, 644
exercise's interaction with, 255
for hypertension, 607, 649
in organ dysfunction, 242–243
mechanism of action of, 605, 643
pharmacokinetics of, 643–644
receptor selectivity of, 336t, 342, 643
socioeconomic considerations with, 649
withdrawal of, 608, 648
Guanylyl cyclase, activation of, by nitric
oxide, 833, 834, 835
Guncotton, 866

Hageman's factor, in fibrinolytic system,
1567t
Hall-Medtronic prosthesis, thromboembolism risk with, 1407, 1407t
Halofenate, propranolol interaction with,
491
Halogenated anesthetic(s), diltiazem
interaction with, 948
dopamine interaction with, 1164
Haloperidol, dopamine interaction with,
1164
Halothane, calcium antagonist interactions
with, 348t
diltiazem interaction with, 948
HDL-C. See High-density lipoprotein
cholesterol (HDL-C).
Head injury, hypertensive emergency with,
150

Headache. See also Migraine.
due to isosorbide mononitrate, 883
in controlled-release form, 888
due to nicorandil, 1643
due to nitroglycerin, 869
Heart, drug interactions involving, 347–350
Heart block. See also Atrioventricular (AV)
block.
diltiazem and, 947
with acute myocardial infarction, 130–
131
Heart disease, congenital. See Congenital
heart disease.
hypertensive, 910–911
ischemic. See Atherosclerosis; Coronary
artery disease.
Heart failure. See Congestive heart failure.
Heart rate, 1386
pharmacologic reduction in, 1386–1387
Heart sound(s), third, response to digoxin
and, in congestive heart failure, 386
Heart transplantation. See Cardiac
transplantation.
Heat, postural hypotension and, 97
Hemodialysis access, thrombosed,
thrombolytic therapy for, 1551
Hemolytic anemia, due to methyldopa,
619
due to procainamide, 1345
Hemopericardium, with acute myocardial
infarction, 129–130
Hemorrhage, due to APSAC, 1562
due to c7E3 Fab, 1633, 1633t
due to heparin, 1477
due to hirudin, 1495
due to Hirulog, 1504, 1504t
due to nadroparin, 1486t, 1487
due to streptokinase, 1524
due to ticlopidine, 1471
due to tissue-type plasminogen activator, 1573
due to warfarin, 1519–1520
intracranial. See Intracranial hemorrhage;
Stroke.
Heparin, 1473–1479
adjusted-dose subcutaneous, for pregnant prosthetic heart valve patient,
1412
in thromboembolism prevention, 162
adverse effects of, 1477
after coronary artery bypass surgery,
112, 1424, 1424t, 1457–1458
after embolic stroke, 168, 168t
after myocardial infarction, 171t, 299–
300, 300, 1396–1397, 1397t
antithrombin effect of, 105
chemical properties of, 1473
clinical use of, 1475–1478
contraindications to, 1477
dosage and administration of, 1477–1478
drug interactions with, 1477
with c7E3 Fab, 1634
during pregnancy, 1412, 1475
fixed low-dose subcutaneous, in thromboembolism prevention, 161–162
for cerebral embolism, 1411
for deep venous thrombosis, 163–164,
166, 166t
for embolism prevention, 161–163, 165
after myocardial infarction, 171t
in acute myocardial infarction, 162t,
175, 175t
in unstable angina, 175, 175t
secondary, 169
with prosthetic heart valves, 1412,
1455

Heparin (Continued)
for lower extremity embolus, 168
for myocardial infarction, 109–110, 109t,
129
aspirin with, 1416t
saruplase with, 1589, 1593
for peripheral vascular disease, 113
for pulmonary embolism, 164, 166, 166t
for unstable angina, 108, 109, 109t, 1416t,
1418, 1420, 1476–1477
aspirin with, 1416t, 1418–1419, 1420
for venous thromboembolism treatment,
1515–1516
for ventricular thrombus prevention,
after myocardial infarction, 1396–
1397, 1397t
in organ dysfunction, 1477
indications for, 1475–1477
low-molecular-weight, 102, 1474. See
also Logiparin; Nadroparin.
for thromboembolism prevention,
162–163, 1512–1513, 1512t, 1513t
for thromboembolism treatment, 1515–
1516
mode of action of, 1474
monitoring therapy with, 1478, 1478t
pharmacokinetics of, 1475
pharmacology of, 1474
platelet effects of, 102
resistance to, due to intravenous nitroglycerin, 870
socioeconomic considerations with,
1478–1479
thrombocytopenia due to, 1477
danaparoid use in, 1509
unfractionated, 101–102
nadroparin calcium vs., 1484
warfarin with, overlapping therapy
with, 1518
with coronary angioplasty, 111, 176t, 177,
306–307, 308t, 309, 309t
with noncardiac surgery in prosthetic
heart valve patient, 1411
with thrombolytic therapy, 5, 1525,
1529–1530
bleeding due to, 1524
for prosthetic valve thrombosis, 1410
in acute myocardial infarction, 109t,
110, 111t, 175–176, 175t
with APSAC, 1563–1564
with tissue-type plasminogen activator, 110, 111t, 299–300, 300, 1569–
1570
Hepatic blood flow, vasodilators' effects
on, 48
Hepatic dysfunction. See also Liver failure.
dose adjustments in, 234, 235t, 236. See
also specific drugs.
drugs not requiring dosage change in,
235t
Hepatomegaly, due to clofibrate, 1078
due to fenofibrate, 1089
Hepatotoxicity, due to fluvastatin, in
animal studies, 1129
due to lovastatin, 1111
due to nicotinic acid, 1065
High-density lipoprotein cholesterol (HDL-
C), bile acid sequestrants' effects on,
1070
estrogen replacement therapy and, 317,
318, 320–321
fenofibrate's effects on, 1088–1089
gemfibrozil's effects on, 1098
lipid-regulating therapy guidelines using, 75–76, 76t
low levels of, 22–23

High-density lipoprotein cholesterol (HDL-C) *(Continued)*
 "isolated," nicotinic acid's effects on, 1062–1063
 probucol's effects on, 1104–1105
High-molecular-weight kininogen, in fibrinolytic system, 1567t
Hirsutism, spironolactone for, 456–457
Hirudin, 102, 1490–1496
 antithrombin effect of, 105, 1491, *1491*
 chemical properties of, 1490–1491, *1490*
 clinical use of, 1494–1496
 for unstable angina, 108, 1420, 1495
 immunologic response to, 1494
 neutralization of, 1494
 pharmacodynamics of, 1492–1493, *1493*
 pharmacokinetics of, 1493–1494
  in animals, 1492
 safety of, 1496
 with coronary angioplasty, 111, 1495
 with thrombolytic therapy, 1494–1495, 1530
Hirulog, 102, 1498–1504
 adverse effects of, 1504, 1504t
 chemical properties of, 1499, *1499*
 clinical use of, 1502–1504, *1503*
 for unstable angina, 108, 1502, *1503*
 immunogenic response to, 1504
 neutralization of, 1504
 pharmacodynamics of, 1501–1502
 pharmacokinetics of, 1501
 pharmacology of, 1499–1501, *1499, 1500*
 with coronary angioplasty, 111, 1502–1503
 with thrombolytic therapy, 1530
His bundle tachycardia, adenosine's effects on, 1243
His-Purkinje system, disopyramide for evaluation of, in syncope, 1290
HMG-CoA (3-hydroxy-3-methylglutaryl coenzyme A), *1108, 1115*
HMG-CoA reductase inhibitor(s). See also specific drugs.
 adverse effects of, 77
 bile acid sequestrant with, 80, 80t
 cataracts and, 1124
 drug interactions with, with anticoagulants, 1112
  with ciprofibrate, 1096
 fibrates with, 81, 1090
  myopathy due to, 81, 1079
 for hyperlipidemia, 21, 76–77, 77t
  comparative efficacy of, 1118t
  mechanism of action of, 80t
 in organ dysfunction, 248
 nicotinic acid with, 80–81, 1065
 relative inhibitory activity of, 1108, 1109t
Holiday heart, 193
Holter monitoring. See *Ambulatory monitoring.*
Homeopathy, 866
Hormone replacement therapy. See also *Estrogen replacement therapy.*
 endometrial carcinoma and, 322
 serum lipids and, 320, 321
Hostility, β-blockers' effects on, 264
 coronary artery disease and, 263
5-HT. See *Serotonin (5-HT).*
Hydralazine, β-blocker interaction with, 348t, 480
 captopril with, for chronic heart failure, 54
  hemodynamic effects of, 47t
 dose adjustment for, in organ dysfunction, 243–244

Hydralazine *(Continued)*
 during lactation, 276t
 during pregnancy, 273, 273t
 exercise's interaction with, 48, 257
 fluid retention due to, 50
 for hypertensive emergencies, 154t, 155t, 157
 for left ventricular failure due to ventricular septal rupture, 53
 for pulmonary hypertension, in chronic lung disease, 89
  in congenital heart disease, 91
  primary, 86
 hemodynamic effects of, 47, 47t, 48
 isosorbide dinitrate with, for congestive heart failure, 53, 873, 879
 nitrates with, for congestive heart failure, 53, 873, 879
  hemodynamic effects of, 47t
 renal function and, 47
Hydrochlorothiazide. See also *Thiazide diuretic(s).*
 adverse effects of, 418
 chemical properties of, *413*
 combination tablets containing, 73, 332, 418t. See also specific combinations.
  with potassium-sparing diuretics, 331
 cost of, 430t, 548t, 949t
 drug interactions with, with guanabenz, 631
  with rilmenidine, 640
 during lactation, 276t
 for hypertension, amlodipine with, 1034
  benazepril with, 790, 791, *792*
  bisoprolol with, 73, 332, 563
  captopril with, 284, 732
  diltiazem with, 945
  dose and side effects of, 374t
  lisinopril with, 752
  moexipril with, 815, 815t
  ramipril with, 770, 770t, 771
  in black persons, 281–283, 282t, 283t
   ACE inhibitor with, 284, 732
  in organ dysfunction, 247
  serum potassium and, 415, *415*
  time-course of urinary sodium excretion in response to, *414*
  triamterene with. See *Triamterene/hydrochlorothiazide.*
Hydrochlorothiazide/amiloride, 374t, 448t, 451
Hydrochlorothiazide/spironolactone, for hypertension, dose and side effects of, 374t
Hydrochlorothiazide/triamterene. See *Triamterene/hydrochlorothiazide.*
HydroDIURIL. See *Hydrochlorothiazide.*
Hydroflumethiazide, for hypertension, dose and side effects of, 374t
Hydromox (quinethazone), for hypertension, dose and side effects of, 374t
3-Hydroxy-3-methylglutaryl coenzyme A (HMG-CoA), *1108, 1115*
3-Hydroxy-3-methylglutaryl coenzyme A reductase inhibitor(s). See *HMG-CoA reductase inhibitor(s); specific drugs.*
5-Hydroxypropafenone, 1352
4-Hydroxypropranolol, 484
5-Hydroxytryptamine. See *Serotonin (5-HT).*
Hygroton. See *Chlorthalidone.*
Hyperaldosteronism. See *Aldosteronism.*
Hypercalcemia, bumetanide for emergency treatment of, 399
 with thiazides, 416

Hyperchloremic metabolic acidosis, due to spironolactone, 457
Hypercholesterolemia. See also *Cholesterol; Hyperlipidemia(s); Lipid metabolism.*
 ciprofibrate for, 1094, *1094*, 1095t
 familial, gene therapy for, 24
  xanthoma regression in, due to probucol, 1102
 HMG-CoA reductase inhibitors for, comparative efficacy of, 1118t
 in children, bile acid sequestrants for, 1072
 simvastatin for, 1118
 lovastatin for, 1110–1111
 pravastatin for, 1121–1124, *1122*
 simvastatin for, 1116–1117, 1117t
Hyperglycemia. See also *Carbohydrate metabolism; Diabetes mellitus; Insulin resistance.*
 diuretic-induced, 365, 377–378
  triamterene and, 438, 440
 outcome of cardiopulmonary resuscitation and, 207
Hyperinsulinemia, lipid abnormalities and, 684, 685
Hyperkalemia, due to amiloride, 449–450
 due to digitalis toxicity, 1143
 due to potassium-sparing diuretics, in chronic renal failure, 364
 due to spironolactone, 457
 due to triamterene, 439
Hyperlipidemia(s). See also *Dysbetalipoproteinemia; Hypercholesterolemia; Hypertriglyceridemia; Lipid metabolism.*
 ciprofibrate for, 1094–1095, *1094*, 1095t
 due to diuretics, 365
 endogenous nitric oxide in, 844
 fluvastatin for, 1130–1132, *1131*, 1131t, *1132*
  in combined therapy, 1132, 1132t
 gemfibrozil for, clinical trials of, 1099–1100, *1099, 1100*, 1100t
 lovastatin for, 1110–1111
  in combined therapy, 1112
 nicotinic acid's effects in, 1062–1063
 pravastatin for, 1121–1124, *1122*, 1122t
 simvastatin for, 1116–1117, 1117t
 treatment of. See *Lipid-regulating therapy; specific drugs and classes of drugs.*
Hypersensitivity reaction(s). See also *Allergy.*
 due to methyldopa, 619
 to APSAC, 1562–1563
 to streptokinase, 1523–1524
Hypertension. See also *Antihypertensive therapy; specific drugs and classes of drugs.*
 accelerated, 149
 ACE inhibitors for, 697–700, *698*
  as initial drug, 68, 69t, 71t, 702
  calcium antagonists with, 332–333, 702, 732
  diuretics with, 72, *701*, 702
  in combined therapy, 702
 acebutolol for, 497–498
 after renal transplantation, captopril for, 734
 α-adrenoreceptor hyperreactivity in, 341
 α₁-blockers for, 609–611
  advantages of, 612
  as initial therapy, 68, 69t, 71t
 amiloride for, 374t, 448–449, 450–451
 amlodipine for, in combined therapy, 1028, 1034
  therapeutic trials of, 1030–1034, *1031, 1032*

Hypertension (*Continued*)
  angiotensin II's role in, 691–692
  arterial hypertrophy in, 830
  atenolol for, 544–545, 548
  benazepril for, 790, 791–792, *792*
    mechanism of action of, in animal
      models, 788, 789t
  β-blockers for, 474–481
    ACE inhibitor with, 702
    as initial therapy, 68, 69t, 71t, 480
    clinical use of, 480–481
    clonidine with, 625
    indapamide with, 428
    mechanism of action of, 465–466, 466t,
      477
    nicardipine with, 989
    nitrendipine with, 1002
  betaxolol for, 553–554
  bisoprolol for, 561–563, *562*
  calcium antagonists for, 894–895
    ACE inhibitors with, 332–333, 702, 732
    as initial therapy, 68, 69t, 71t
    cardiac effects of, 908–912, 909t
    in fixed combinations, 332–333
  captopril for, 731–734, *733*
    advantages of, 737
    amlodipine with, 1034
    as initial therapy, 731
    drawbacks of, 794
    in combined therapy, 732
    in elderly persons, 732–733
    quality of life with, 734, *734*
  carmoxirole for, 1192, *1192*, 1193, *1193*
  carvedilol for, 598
    clinical studies of, 590–592, *591*, 591t,
      592t
  centrally-acting antiadrenergic drugs for,
    608
  chronic, shift in vascular autoregulation
    in, 148, *148*
  cilazapril for, 811
  clonidine for, 607, 625, 627
  diazoxide for, disadvantages of, 996
    during pregnancy, 273, 273t
  diltiazem for, 944–945
    advantages and disadvantages of, 945,
      948–949
    dosage and administration of, 949
    mechanism of action of, 941–942
  diuretics for, 371–380
    ACE inhibitors with, 72, *701*, 702
    as initial drug, 68, 69t, 71t, 373–375,
      375t, 379–380, 380t
    as second drug, 71–72
    captopril with, 732, 735, 737
    clinical trials of, 373–375, 375t
    enalapril with, 744
    mechanism of action of, 371–373, *372*
    nitrendipine with, 1002
    prazosin with, 664
    preparations and dosages of, 373, 374t
    quality of life issues with, 379
    ramipril with, 771
    safety of, 375–379
  dopamine and, 1165
  doxazosin for, 610, 685
    advantages of, 686–687
  during pregnancy. See *Preeclampsia; Pregnancy*.
  emergency treatment of. See *Hypertensive
    emergencies*.
  enalapril for, 744–745
    amlodipine with, 1034
    indapamide with, 428–429
  enalaprilat for, disadvantages of, 996
  endogenous nitric oxide and, 842–843,
    844

Hypertension (*Continued*)
  endothelial alterations in, 842–843, *844*
  esmolol for, disadvantages of, 996
    perioperative, 511–512
  essential, natural history of, 16–17, *17*
  felodipine for, 1042–1043
  fish oils' effects on, 1610
  fosinopril for, clinical use of, 807
    efficacy of, 804–805, *804*, 805t, *806*
  furosemide for, dosage and administration of, 374t, 395
    with reduced renal function, 393
  guanabenz for, 607, 630, 631
    as initial therapy, 69t
  guanfacine for, 607, 648–649
  hemodynamics of, during exercise, 254
  in African Americans. See under *Black
    person(s)*.
  in children, captopril for, 734
    enalapril for, 744–745
    minoxidil for, 855
  in chronic renal failure, diuretic therapy
    for, 363
  in diabetes mellitus, ACE inhibitors for,
    700
    acebutolol for, 498
    captopril for, 733, *733*
    diuretic therapy for, 377–378
    enalapril for, 744
    indapamide for, 424t, 429
    isradipine for, 1018
    thiazides for, 417
  in elderly persons. See under *Elderly person(s)*.
  in renal parenchymal disease, captopril
    for, 733
  indapamide for, 374t, 430–431
    effects of, 422, 423t, *427*, 428
    in diabetes mellitus, 424t, 429
    isolated systolic, 73–74
    crossover drug trial in, 228–229
  isradipine for, 1017–1020, *1018*
  ketanserin for, 1653, *1653*
    advantages of, 1654
    mechanisms of action of, 1650–1651
  labetalol for, 573–575, 575t
    disadvantages of, 996
    in black persons, 284t, 574
    in elderly persons, 574
    mechanisms of action of, 570–571, 570t
  lacidipine for, 1048–1049, *1048*, *1049*
  lisinopril for, 751–752, *752*
  losartan for, clinical trials of, 821–823,
    821t, 822t
  malignant, 149
  methyldopa for, 604, 605
    as initial therapy, 69t
    during pregnancy, 271, 604
  metoprolol for, 523–527, *524*
    effects of very-long-term treatment
      with, 525–527, *526*
    in elderly, 525
  mibefradil for, 1014
    in animal models, 1011–1012, *1011*,
      1012
  minoxidil for, 854–855
  moexipril for, 814–815
  moxonidine for, 607, 657–659
  nadolol for, 502, 504–505
  nicardipine for, 988–990, *989*
    intravenous, *995*, 997–998, *997*, *998*
  nifedipine for, 975–976
    benazepril with, 791
  nisoldipine for, 1007
  nitrendipine for, 1001–1003, *1002*
    in black persons, 286t, 1002

Hypertension (*Continued*)
  nitroprusside for, disadvantages of, 996
  pathophysiology of, in black persons,
    280–281
  perindopril for, 782
  perioperative, esmolol for, 511–512
    intravenous nicardipine for, 998–999
    labetalol for, 576
    severe, 151
    urapidil for, 678
  pindolol for, 518
    dosage and administration of, 520
  prazosin for, 664–665
  propranolol for, 488–489, 491–492
    clonidine with, 625
    minoxidil with, 855
  pulmonary. See *Pulmonary hypertension*.
  quinapril for, 797–799
  ramipril for, 759, 760, 761t, 768, 770t
    advantages of, 770–771
    in combined therapy, 769–770, 770t,
      771
  rebound, after cessation of antihypertensive therapy, 152
  renovascular, ACE inhibitor use in, 697–
    698, *698*
    captopril for, 734
    severe, 152
  resistant, 73–74, 73t
  rilmenidine for, 607, 640, 641
  spironolactone for, 374t, 454–455
  stress and, 264–267
  target-organ disease in, 18
  terazosin for, 610, 667–670, 671
  thiazides for, 373, 374t, 414
    lisinopril with, 751–752
    triamterene with, 438
  thrombolytic therapy in presence of,
    1433, 1433t, *1434*
  tissue-type plasminogen activator use in,
    1573–1574
  torsemide for, 374t, 402–404
  trandolapril for, 785–786
  triamterene for, 374t, 438
  urapidil for, 610, 675–678, 677t
  vasodilatation in, 830
  verapamil for, 921
    amlodipine with, 1034
  with acute myocardial infarction, 129
Hypertensive emergencies, 148–158
  ACE inhibitors for, 154t, 155t, 158, 699
  calcium antagonists for, 156, 895
  classification of, 148–149
  clonidine for, 154t, 155t, 157, 625
  conditions associated with, 149–153, 149t
  defined, 148–149
  isradipine for, 1019
  labetalol for, 154t, 155t, 157, 574–575,
    575t
  management of, 153–158, 154t–156t
  minoxidil for, 154t, 155t, 157, 855
  nicardipine for, 895
  nifedipine use in, 154t, 155t, 156, 976
  nitroprusside for, 154t, 155–156, 155t,
    860–861
  urapidil for, 677–678
Hypertensive encephalopathy, 149–150
  felodipine for, 1043
Hypertensive heart disease, 910–911
Hypertensive urgencies, defined, 149
Hyperthyroidism. See also *Thyrotoxic crisis;
    Thyrotoxicosis*.
  bisoprolol use in, 565
  cardiovascular effects of, 1657–1659
  catecholamine sensitivity in, 1657
  change in myocardial gene expression
    in, 1656–1657

Hyperthyroidism (Continued)
  digoxin use in, 1141
  due to amiodarone, 1257
Hypertrichosis, due to minoxidil, 856–857
Hypertriglyceridemia, 22–23. See also
    Hyperlipidemia(s); Lipid metabolism;
    Triglycerides.
  ciprofibrate for, 1094
  clofibrate for, 1078
  combined therapy for, 81
  nicotinic acid's effects on, 1062
  therapy aimed at, 23
    guidelines for, 76, 76t
Hypertrophic cardiomyopathy, β-blockers
    for, 470–471, 545–546
  calcium antagonists for, 895–896
  combined therapy for, 55–56, 55t
  diltiazem for, 946
  hypertensive, treatment of, 286
  isosorbide mononitrate use in, 883
  milrinone use in, 1183
  nifedipine for, 976
  nitrate use in, 870
  obstructive, amrinone use in, 1173
    disopyramide for, 1291, *1291*
    dobutamine use in, 1158
  propranolol for, 489
  pulmonary venous congestion in, com-
      bined therapy for, 51
  verapamil for, 895–896, 921
    adverse effects of, 896
Hyperuricemia. See also *Gout.*
  due to diuretics, 377
    in chronic renal failure, 365
  due to triamterene, 437, 439–440
Hypoalbuminemia, furosemide resistance
    in, 391, 393
  loop diuretic pharmacokinetics in, 400
Hypoaldosteronism, hyporeninemic. See
    Hyporeninemic hypoaldosteronism.
Hypocalcemia, due to EDTA chelation,
    1614–1615
  due to furosemide, 394
Hypoglycemia, due to disopyramide,
    1285–1286
Hypoglycemic agent(s), oral, β-blocker
    interaction with, 480
  ciprofibrate interaction with, 1096
  fenofibrate interaction with, 1090
  pindolol interaction with, 520
Hypokalemia, diuretic-induced, 378, 378t,
    415–416, *415*
  glucose intolerance and, 365, 438
  in chronic renal failure, 364
  in congestive heart failure, 386–387
  ventricular arrhythmias and, 414–415,
    447
  due to digitalis toxicity, 1143
  due to dobutamine, 1158
  paroxysmal atrial tachycardia with AV
    block in, 190–191
  treatment of, in cardiopulmonary resusci-
    tation, 215
  ventricular arrhythmia due to, 1216
Hypokalemic periodic paralysis,
    triamterene for, 439
Hypomagnesemia, due to diuretic therapy
    in chronic renal failure, 364
  treatment of, in cardiopulmonary resusci-
    tation, 215
Hyponatremia, due to amiloride, 449
  due to diuretic therapy, in chronic renal
    failure, 364–365
  due to furosemide, 394
  due to thiazides, 416
  furosemide for, 393

Hypoplastic anemia, due to procainamide,
    1345
Hyporeninemic hypoaldosteronism,
    diuretic therapy for, 363
  furosemide for, 393
  potassium-sparing diuretic use in, 373
Hypotension, amrinone use in, 1173
  dopamine for, 1163
  due to ACE inhibition, 701, *701*
  due to ACE inhibitor/diuretic therapy,
    701, 702
  due to amrinone, 1170, 1173
  due to APSAC, 1556, 1562–1563
  due to bretylium, 214, 1270
  due to captopril, 735
  due to esmolol, 512
  due to milrinone, 1183
  due to phenytoin, 1340
  due to quinidine, 1364
  due to ramipril, 769
  due to streptokinase, 1524
  due to trandolapril, 786
  due to verapamil, 922
  induced. See *Hypotensive anesthesia.*
  postural. See *Postural hypotension.*
  thrombolytic therapy in presence of,
    1433, 1433t, *1434*
  with acute myocardial infarction, man-
    agement of, 133–134
  with right ventricular infarction, manage-
    ment of, 138
Hypotensive anesthesia, esmolol for, 512
  labetalol for, 576
  nitroprusside for, 863
Hypothalamus theory, 265
Hypothyroidism, 1657
  amiodarone-induced, 1257
    in renal insufficiency, 236, 241
  diastolic function in, 1658
  digoxin use in, 1141
Hypovolemia. See also *Extracellular fluid*
    volume; Plasma volume.
  postural hypotension due to, 95–96
    initial nonpharmacologic therapies for,
      97
  pulseless electrical activity due to, 218
Hypoxemia, systemic, vasodilators' effects
    on, in pulmonary hypertension, 85
Hypoxia, adenosine production in
    response to, 1240

Ibopamine, 345, 1194–1203
  adverse effects of, 1203
  chemical properties of, 1195, *1195*
  effects of, 1196–1201
    hemodynamic, 49t, 1196–1199, 1197t,
      1198
    on electrophysiology, 1199
    on neurohumoral system, 1199–1201,
      1200t
    on renal function, 1199
  for heart failure, 54, 1165
    clinical efficacy of, 1201–1203, 1201t,
      1202t
  in elderly persons, 1196
  in organ dysfunction, 1196, 1199
  mechanism of action of, 1195–1196
  pharmacokinetics of, 1196
  pharmacology of, in animal studies, 1195
  vasodilators with, hemodynamic effects
    of, 50t
Ibuprofen. See also *Nonsteroidal anti-*
    inflammatory drug(s) (NSAID).
  for postural hypotension, 97

Ibuprofen (Continued)
  in antiplatelet therapy, 104
ICD. See *Cardioverter-defibrillator,*
    implantable.
ICI 118,551 (β-blocker), receptor selectivity
    of, 337t
Idazoxan, receptor selectivity of, 336t
Idioventricular rhythm, accelerated, 202
  with myocardial infarction, 132
IL-1 (interleukin-1), secretion of, by
    macrophages, probucol's effects on,
    1104
IL-6 (interleukin-6), vesnarinone's effects
    on, 1186
Iloprost, tissue-type plasminogen activator
    interaction with, 104
Imdur. See *Isosorbide mononitrate, controlled-*
    release (Imdur).
Imidazoline receptor(s), 338, 602, 605–606,
    652–654, *652, 653*
  central, 636
  peripheral, 636
  renal, 652, 656
  rilmenidine's affinity for, 606, 634
Imipramine, for ventricular ectopy,
    flecainide vs., 1309
    moricizine vs., 1334–1335
  for ventricular tachyarrhythmias, 1326t
Immune hemolytic anemia, due to
    methyldopa, 619
  due to procainamide, 1345
Implantable cardioverter-defibrillator. See
    under *Cardioverter-defibrillator.*
Impotence, due to propranolol, 490
  pentoxifylline for, 1606
Inandione anticoagulant(s), gemfibrozil
    interaction with, 1101
Indacrinone, in hyperuricemia, 365
Indapamide, 420–431
  chemical properties of, 420, *421*
  cost of, 430, 430t
  drug interactions with, 429–430
  effects of, 421–428, 423t, 424t
    diuretic, 422
    metabolic, 423t, 424–427, 424t, *425, 426*
    renal, 427–428
  for hypertension, 374t
    effects of, 422, 423t, 427, 428
    in combined therapy, 428–429
    in diabetic patients, 424t, 429
    in stepped therapy, 430–431
  in elderly persons, 429
  in renal failure, 361, 429
  indications and dose for, 429
  pharmacokinetics of, 421
  pharmacology of, 421
Indecainide, arrhythmia aggravation by,
    1235t
Inderal. See *Propranolol.*
Indoline(s), 420. See also *Indapamide.*
Indomethacin, drug interactions with, with
    β-blockers, 348t
    with captopril, 693
    with triamterene, 440
  for postural hypotension, 97
Indoramin, for hypertension, 610
Infant(s). See *Child(ren); Neonate(s).*
Infarct artery patency, as end point for
    thrombolytic therapy, 1431t,
    1434–1435, 1436t, 1437, *1437*
Inferior vena cava filter, in pulmonary
    embolism prevention, 163
Inflammation, in myocardial ischemia,
    trimetazidine's effects on, 1596–1597
Inhalation anesthetic(s), β-blocker
    interaction with, 480

Inhalation anesthetic(s) *(Continued)*
  verapamil interaction with, 922
Inocor. See *Amrinone.*
Inosine, inotropic effects of, mechanisms
    of, 44, 45t
Inotropic agent(s), 1136–1203. See also
    specific drugs.
  classification of, 1149, 1149t
  for heart failure, 44–45
    acute, 1148–1149, 1149t
    vasodilators with, 45–46, 46t, 50t
    with acute myocardial infarction, 136–
      137
  goals of therapy with, 1147
  hemodynamic effects of, 48–49, 49t, 50t,
    1188t
  immunomodulating effects of, 1188t
  in elderly persons, 229–230
  mechanisms of action of, 44–45, 45t,
    1147–1148
  new, 12
  oral, 1149–1150
  patient selection for, 1146–1147
  principles and practice of therapy with,
    1146–1150
INR (international normalized ratio), for
    prothrombin time reporting, 1395,
    1519
Insulin, β-blocker interaction with, 480
  for hyperglycemia, in cardiopulmonary
    resuscitation, 207
  pindolol interaction with, 520
Insulin resistance. See also *Carbohydrate
    metabolism; Diabetes mellitus.*
  diuretic-induced, 365, 377–378
    triamterene and, 438, 440
  in hypertension, captopril's effects on,
    737–738
    ramipril's effects on, 766
Interatrial reentrant tachycardia, 185t, 190
Interleukin-1 (IL-1), secretion of, by
    macrophages, probucol's effects on,
    1104
Interleukin-6 (IL-6), vesnarinone's effects
    on, 1186
Intermittent pneumatic compression boots,
    in thromboembolism prevention, 163
International normalized ratio (INR), for
    prothrombin time reporting, 1395,
    1519
Interstitial nephritis, due to diuretics, 365
Interventricular septum, rupture of. See
    Ventricular septal rupture.
Intraaortic balloon counterpulsation, for
    cardiogenic shock, 137
  for left ventricular failure due to ventric-
    ular septal rupture, 53
Intraatrial reentrant tachycardia, 185t, 190
  adenosine's effects on, 1241, *1242*
Intracranial hemorrhage. See also *Stroke.*
  due to tissue-type plasminogen activa-
    tor, 5, 1573
  with thrombolytic therapy, 5
Intracranial mass, hypertensive emergency
    with, 150
Intrinsic sympathomimetic activity (ISA),
    of β-blockers, 337t, 344, 476, 542
IS–5-MN. See *Isosorbide mononitrate.*
ISA (intrinsic sympathomimetic activity),
    of β-blockers, 337t, 344, 476, 542
Ischemia, cerebral. See also *Stroke;
    Transient ischemic attack(s) (TIA).*
  antithrombotic therapy in, 113
  limb, algorithm for management of, *1549*
    classification of, 1548, 1548t
  myocardial. See *Angina pectoris; Myocar-
    dial infarction; Myocardial ischemia.*

Ischemic heart disease. See *Atherosclerosis;
    Coronary artery disease.*
ISDN. See *Isosorbide dinitrate.*
Ismelin. See *Guanethidine.*
ISMO. See *Isosorbide mononitrate.*
Isoamyl nitrite, chemical properties of, 876
Isocarboxazid, dopamine interaction with,
    211
Isoflurane, calcium antagonist interactions
    with, 348t
Isoniazid, phenytoin interaction with, 1340
Isoprenaline, 343
  chemical properties of, *517*
  receptor selectivity of, 337t
Isoproterenol, for congestive heart failure,
    amrinone vs., 1174
    dobutamine vs., 1154
  for primary pulmonary hypertension, 85
  hemodynamic effects of, 49t, 1149t
  in cardiopulmonary resuscitation, 212
  mechanism of action of, *1178*
Isoptin. See *Verapamil.*
Isosorbide dinitrate, adverse effects of, 878
  chemical properties of, 876, 877
  chewable, 878
  for angina, in triple therapy, 35
    nicorandil vs., 1641
  for congestive heart failure, 873
    hydralazine with, 53, 873, 879
  oral, 879
    drawbacks of, 888
  pharmacokinetics of, 877
  pharmacology of, 877–878
  sublingual, 878
  tolerance to, 880
Isosorbide mononitrate, 881–884
  adverse effects of, 878, 883
  chemical properties of, 876, 877, 881
  clinical applications of, 883
  contraindications to, 883–884
  controlled-release (Imdur), 885–889
    advantages of, 889
    adverse effects of, 888, 888t
    after myocardial infarction, 301
    clinical applications of, 886–889
    drug interactions with, 888
    pharmacokinetics of, 885, *886*, 886t
    cost of, 884
  dosage and administration of, 884
  drug interactions with, 884
  during pregnancy, 882, 884
  effects of, 882
  for angina, nicorandil vs., 1641
  for myocardial infarction, 872, 879
  in organ dysfunction, 248, 884
  oral, 878
    drawbacks of, 888
  overdosage with, 883
  pharmacokinetics of, 877, 881–882
  pharmacology of, 877–878, 881
  tolerance to, 880, 881
Isradipine, 1016–1021
  adverse effects of, 1020
  chemical properties of, 1016
  clinical applications of, 1017–1021
  cost of, 949t
  diuretic effect of, 1018
  drug interactions with, 1017
  effects of, 909t, 1016–1017, *1018*
  exercise's interaction with, 253
  for atherosclerosis prevention, clinical
    studies of, 911t
    effects of, 1017, 1019–1020
  for hypertension, 1017–1020, *1018*
  for hypertensive emergencies, 1019
  in black persons, 286t

Isradipine *(Continued)*
  in elderly persons, 227–228
  in organ dysfunction, 246
  left ventricular mass reduction by, 911t
  pharmacokinetics of, 1016
  slow-release formulation of, 1018

Junctional tachycardia. See *Atrioventricular
    junctional tachycardia(s).*

Kallikrein-kinin system, ACE inhibitors'
    interaction with, 693–694
Kaolin-pectin, quinidine interaction with,
    1365t
Ketamine, diltiazem interaction with, 948
Ketanserin, 1650–1655
  adverse effects of, 1654
  chemical properties of, 1650
  clinical uses of, 1653–1654, *1653*
  contraindications to, 1654
  dosage and administration of, 1654
  during pregnancy, 1654
  effects of, 1651–1653
    on platelets, 105, 1652
  for hypertension, 1653, *1653*
    advantages of, 1654
    mechanisms of action of, 345, 1650–
      1651
  in organ dysfunction, 246, 1651, 1654
  pharmacokinetics of, 1651
  pharmacology of, 1650–1651
  socioeconomic considerations with,
    1654–1655
Ketoconazole, quinidine interaction with,
    1365t
Khellin, 1247, *1248*
Kidney(s). See also *Renal* entries.
  drug elimination by, mechanisms of, 235
Killip classification, of acute myocardial
    infarction patients, 133, 133t
Kininogen, high-molecular-weight, in
    fibrinolytic system, 1567t

Labetalol, 568–578
  adverse effects of, 576
  chemical properties of, 569
  clinical applications of, 573–576, 577
  contraindications to, 576
  cost of, 548t, 577–578
  dosage and administration of, 576–577
  drug interactions with, 348t
  during lactation, 571
  during pregnancy, 271, 273, 273t, 571,
    575–576
  effects of, 467t, 571–573
    antiarrhythmic, 571–572
    antihypertensive, 570–571, 570t
    hemodynamic, 569–570, 570t
    noncardiac, 472t, 572–573
  for hypertension, disadvantages of, 996
    during pregnancy, 271, 273, 273t, 575–
      576
  in black persons, 284t, 574
  in elderly persons, 574
  for hypertensive emergencies, 154t, 155t,
    157, 574–575, 575t
  in elderly persons, 226–227, 574
  in organ dysfunction, 571
  pharmacodynamics of, 467t, 472t, 571
  pharmacokinetics of, 553t, 571

Labetalol (Continued)
  pharmacology of, 569–571, 569t
  postural hypotension due to, 96
  receptor selectivity of, 336t, 569
  socioeconomic considerations with, 577–578
  withdrawal of, 575
Lacidipine, 1047–1051
  adverse effects of, 1051, 1051t
  animal studies of, 1047–1048
  cardiovascular effects of, 1049–1051, 1050
  for hypertension, efficacy of, 1048–1049, 1048, 1049
  in elderly persons, 1048, 1049, 1049
  in organ dysfunction, 1048
  pharmacokinetics of, 1048
  vascular selectivity of, 1047–1048
Lactation, acebutolol use during, 498
  amiloride use during, 450
  amiodarone use during, 1256
  benazepril use during, 790
  bisoprolol use during, 560
  bretylium use during, 1270
  cardiac drug therapy during, 275–277, 276t
  clofibrate use during, 1079
  digoxin use during, 276t, 277, 1141
  diltiazem use during, 276–277, 276t, 948
  disopyramide use during, 276t, 277, 1283, 1286
  Fluosol use during, 1620
  fosinopril use during, 808
  labetalol use during, 571
  lovastatin use during, 1112
  moxonidine use during, 654
  nadolol use during, 276, 276t, 504
  ramipril use during, 758, 769
  rilmenidine use during, 640
  simvastatin use during, 1118
  urapidil use during, 678
  warfarin use during, 1412, 1520
Lanthanum, in experimental atherosclerosis, 903
Lasix. See Furosemide.
LCAT. See Lecithin-cholesterol acyltransferase (LCAT).
LDL. See Low-density lipoprotein (LDL).
Leading circle model of reentry, 61
Lecithin-cholesterol acyltransferase (LCAT), 1088–1089
  bile acid sequestrants' effects on, 1070
  fenofibrate's effects on, 1089
Leeches, 1490
Left ventricular aneurysm, ventricular thrombus with, 171, 171t, 1395t, 1397–1398, 1397t
Left ventricular failure. See also Congestive heart failure.
  acute, combined therapy for, 51–53
  dobutamine for, 1155–1156
Left ventricular function. See also Myocardial function.
  as end point for thrombolytic therapy, 1436–1437, 1436, 1437
Left ventricular hypertrophy, ACE inhibitors' effects on, 699–700
  acebutolol for, 498
  adverse effects of diuretics in, 226
  after myocardial infarction, compensatory function of, 715, 717
    tissue renin-angiotensin system in, 712, 715
  atenolol's effects on, 543
  β-blockers for, 471–472
    effects of, 477–478

Left ventricular hypertrophy (Continued)
  calcium antagonists' effects on, 910, 911t
  captopril's effects on, 731–732
  clonidine's effects on, 623
  doxazosin's effects on, 683
  enalapril's effects on, 744
  felodipine's effects on, 1041
  guanfacine's effects on, 644
  indapamide's effects in, 422
  isradipine's effects on, 1019
  lacidipine's effects on, 1050, 1050
  methyldopa's effects on, 618–619
  metoprolol's effects on, 525–526, 526
  moxonidine's effects on, 656
  nitrendipine's effects on, 1002
  perindopril's effects on, 778–779, 779t
  prazosin's effects on, 662
  ramipril's effects on, 763–764
  rilmenidine's effects on, 638
  terazosin's effects on, 670
  trandolapril's effects on, 786
  urapidil's effects on, 674, 675t
Left ventricular tachycardia, idiopathic, drug selection for, 63
Left-to-right shunt, with ventricular septal rupture, determinants of, 53
Lergotrile mesylate, 339
Leukocyte(s), nitric oxide production by, 839
Leukopenia, due to bepridil, 1058
  due to ibopamine, 1203
  due to procainamide, 1345
Levine, Samuel, on quinidine therapy, 1226
Levodopa. See L-Dopa.
Levothyroxine. See Thyroxine (T4).
Libenzapril, elimination kinetics of, 723t
Liddle's syndrome, triamterene for, 439
Lidocaine, 183t
  arrhythmia aggravation by, 1235t
  drug interactions with, 349t
    with β-blockers, 348t, 349t, 351, 352
    with propranolol, 491
  during lactation, 277
  during pregnancy, 274, 274t
  for digitalis toxicity, 1144
  for ventricular tachycardia, 203
    with acute myocardial infarction, 132
  in cardiopulmonary resuscitation, 212–213
    endotracheal administration of, 208
  in elderly persons, 231
  in organ dysfunction, 238
  prophylactic, in acute myocardial infarction, 213
Limb blood flow, vasodilators' effects on, 48
Limb ischemia, algorithm for management of, 1549
  classification of, 1548, 1548t
Linoleic acid, 1608, 1608t, 1609
α-Linolenic acid, 1608, 1608t, 1609
Liothyronine. See Triiodothyronine (T3).
Lipid metabolism. See also Hyperlipidemia(s); Lipid-regulating therapy; specific lipids.
  abnormalities of, hyperinsulinemia and, 684, 685
  ACE inhibitors' effects on, 696
  acebutolol's effects on, 499
  α1-blockers' effects on, 611
  atenolol's effects on, 547
  β-blockers' effects on, 479
  betaxolol's effects on, 552
  bile acid sequestrants' effects on, 1068–1070
  bisoprolol's effects on, 565, 566

Lipid metabolism (Continued)
  centrally-acting antiadrenergic drugs' effects on, 607
  ciprofibrate's effects on, 1093
  clofibrate's effects on, 1076
  clonidine's effects on, 624
  diltiazem's effects on, 939
  diuretics' effects on, 375–377, 376t
  doxazosin's effects on, 684
  fenofibrate's effects on, 1085–1089, 1086
  fish oils' effects on, 1610
    dose required for, 1611t
  fluvastatin's effects on, 1131t
  gemfibrozil's effects on, 1098–1099
  guanabenz's effects on, 630
  indapamide's effects on, 424–426, 425, 426
  isradipine's effects on, 1019
  lovastatin's effects on, 1110
  metoprolol's effects on, 532–533
  nadolol's effects on, 502
  nicotinic acid's effects on, 1061–1062
  pravastatin's effects on, 1126
  prazosin's effects on, 663–664
  probucol's effects on, 1104–1105
  simvastatin's effects on, 1115
  terazosin's effects on, 667–668, 670
  urapidil's effects on, 675
Lipid peroxidation, dietary potassium and, 462–463
Lipidil. See Fenofibrate.
Lipid-regulating therapy, 75–81, 1061–1134. See also specific drugs and classes of drugs.
  aimed at LDL cholesterol, 20–22
    guidelines for, 75, 75t, 76t, 1062
    total mortality and, 22
  aimed at triglycerides, 22–23
    guidelines for, 76, 76t
  clinical events vs. lesion regression with, 23–24
  considerations in, 25t
  dietary, 19
  drug classes used for, 19
    mechanisms of action of, 80t
  emerging concepts in, 19–25
  future directions in, 24–25
  goals for, 20
  in elderly persons, 231–232
  initial drug choice for, 76–79, 76t
  initiation of, 19–20
  patient selection for, 75–76, 75t
  stepwise approach to, 19, 19t
  tactics for enhancing adherence to, 20t
  with drug combinations, 21–22, 79–81, 79t, 80t
Lipoprotein(s). See Lipid metabolism; specific lipoproteins, e.g., Low-density lipoprotein (LDL).
Lipoprotein lipase, fenofibrate's effects on, 1085–1086, 1086
Lipoprotein(a) (Lp(a)) , estrogen replacement therapy and, 320–321
  lipid-regulating therapy guidelines and, 76
  nicotinic acid's effects on, 21, 1062, 1063
Lisinopril, 750–753
  after myocardial infarction, 296
  chemical properties of, 750, 751, 789
  effects of, 47t, 751
  in black persons, 284
  in organ dysfunction, 244–245, 722t, 750
  pharmacokinetics of, 723t, 750, 751
Lithium, drug interactions with, with calcium antagonists, 348t
    with indapamide, 429–430

Lithium *(Continued)*
  with spironolactone, 458
  with thiazides, 418
  with verapamil, 922
 nephrogenic diabetes insipidus due to, amiloride for, 449
Liver, amiodarone's effects on, 1257
 ciprofibrate's effects on function of, 1095
 drug elimination by, mechanisms of, 235–236
 drug interactions involving, 350–351
Liver enzyme elevations, due to amrinone, 1173
  due to ciprofibrate, 1095
  due to fluvastatin, 1133
  due to labetalol, 576
  due to lovastatin, 1111
  due to moricizine, 1336
  due to nicotinic acid, 1065
  due to pravastatin, 1124, 1125
  due to simvastatin, 1117
  due to statins, 77
Liver failure. See *Hepatic dysfunction.*
 amiloride for edema in, 449
Loading dose, adjustment in, in organ dysfunction, 236
Local anesthetic effect, of β-blockers, 469, 542
  of propranolol, 484
Logiparin, 1480–1483, 1481t
Long QT syndrome, β-blockers in, 471
 torsades de pointes in, 200, 201–202, *201*
Long RP tachycardia, 1212–1215, *1214*
Lonitem. See *Minoxidil.*
Loop diuretic(s), 388–411, 388t. See also *Diuretic(s); specific drugs.*
  for hypertension, 373, 374t
  for pulmonary edema, 124
  for renal failure, potassium-sparing diuretic with, 363
   thiazide with, 362–363
  in elderly persons, 226
  in renal failure, acute, 359–360
   chronic, 361–362
   in animal models, 358
  mechanism of action of, 388–389
  NSAID interaction with, 391
  ototoxicity of, 361, 365
  pharmacokinetics of, aging's effects on, 391–392
   in hypoalbuminemia, 400
  pharmacology of, 389
  response to, chronic, 390, *390*
   determinants of, 390–392, 391t
   urinary excretion rate vs. response curves for, *406*
Lopid. See *Gemfibrozil.*
Lopressor. See *Metoprolol.*
Lorcainide, arrhythmia aggravation by, 1235t
Losartan, 817–824
  active metabolite of, 819
  adverse effects of, 823
  clinical efficacy of, 821–823, 821t, 822t
  effects of, antihypertensive, 820–821, *820*
   hemodynamic, 823–824, 823t, *824*
   metabolic, 823
  history of, 817–818, *818*
  pharmacology of, 818–819, *819*
Losartan/hydrochlorothiazide, 332
Lotensin. See *Benazepril.*
Lotrel (amlodipine/benazepril), 332–333, *333*, 1034
Lovastatin, 1107–1113
  adverse effects of, 1111–1112
  cataracts and, 1111–1112, 1124

Lovastatin *(Continued)*
  chemical properties of, 1107, *1108, 1115*
  contraindications to, 1112
  dosage and administration of, 1112–1113
  drug interactions with, 1112
  during lactation, 1112
  during pregnancy, 1112
  effects of, 1110
  for hyperlipidemia, 1110–1111
   as initial drug, 76–77
   clofibrate with, 1076–1077
   comparative efficacy of, 1118t
   in combined therapy, 1112, 1113
  in elderly persons, 1108–1109
  in organ dysfunction, 248, 1112
  indications for, 1110–1111
  LDL cholesterol reduction with, 77t
  myopathy due to, 1111
   with clofibrate, 1079
   with fibrate, 1112
   with gemfibrozil, 1100, 1111
   with nicotinic acid, 1065, 1111, 1112
  pharmacokinetics of, 1108–1109
  pharmacology of, 1107–1108, 1109t
  sleep disturbances due to, 1124
  socioeconomic considerations with, 1113
Lovenox. See *Enoxaparin.*
Low-density lipoprotein (LDL). See also *Lipid metabolism; Low-density lipoprotein cholesterol (LDL-C).*
  arterial uptake of, 324–325, *325*, 532
  β-blockers' effects on, 533
  fenofibrate's effects on, 1086–1087, *1086*
  heterogeneity of, 23, 1086–1087
  oxidative modification of, EDTA chelation's effects on, 1615
   endothelial effects of, 325–326, 843–844
   in pathogenesis of atherosclerosis, 325–326, *325*, 1615
   probucol's effects on, 1102–1103, 1105
  receptors for. See *Low-density lipoprotein receptor(s).*
  structure of, probucol's effects on, 1104
Low-density lipoprotein cholesterol (LDL-C). See also *Cholesterol; Lipid metabolism; Low-density lipoprotein (LDL).*
  bile acid sequestrants' effects on, 1069
  drug therapy emphasizing, 20–22
   guidelines for, 75, 75t, 76t, 1062
  gemfibrozil's effects on, 1099
  hepatic uptake of, 324
  nicotinic acid's effects on, 1062
Low-density lipoprotein receptor(s), arterial LDL uptake and, 324–325
  lovastatin's effect on, 1107–1108
  response to bile acid sequestrants and, 1069
  simvastatin's effects on, 1114–1115
Lozol. See *Indapamide.*
Lp(a). See *Lipoprotein(a) (Lp(a)).*
Lung transplantation, diltiazem's effects after, 940
Lupus-like syndrome, due to procainamide, 1345–1346
Lytic state, 1522
Lytic therapy. See *Thrombolytic therapy.*

α_2-Macroglobulin, in fibrinolytic system, 1567t, *1568*, 1570
Macrophage(s), interleukin–1 secretion by, probucol's effects on, 1104
  low-density lipoprotein–activated, in disruption of atherosclerotic plaque, 9

Magnesium, adverse effects of, 215
  after myocardial infarction, 6, 142, 301
  deficiency of. See *Hypomagnesemia; Magnesium deficiency.*
  excretion of, bumetanide's effect on, 399
   triamterene's effects on, 436–437
  for digitalis toxicity, 1144
  for sudden death prevention, 264
  hemodynamic response to stress and, 266–267
  renal reabsorption of, furosemide's effects on, 389
Magnesium deficiency. See also *Hypomagnesemia.*
  cardiovascular toxicity of, 364
  diuretic-induced, 386
   in chronic renal failure, 364
  due to furosemide, 394
  due to thiazides, 416
Magnesium EDTA chelation, for atherosclerosis, 1615–1616, *1616*
  pharmacology of, 1614–1615
Magnesium sulfate, for preeclampsia, 273
  for torsades de pointes, 201
  in cardiopulmonary resuscitation, 215
Mahaim tachycardia(s), adenosine's effects on, 1243
  drug selection for, 62
Malignancy(ies), due to ciprofibrate, 1093
  due to clofibrate, 1077, 1079
  due to fenofibrate, 1089
  estrogen replacement therapy and, 322
  gastrointestinal tract, enalapril and, 747
  prostatic, estrogens for, cardiovascular events and, 321
Malignant hypertension, 149
Mannitol, in acute renal failure, 359
  in animal models, 357–358
  in chronic renal failure, 360
  with coronary angioplasty, 309
MAO inhibitor. See *Monoamine oxidase (MAO) inhibitor(s).*
Marplan (isocarboxazid), dopamine interaction with, 211
Maxzide. See *Triamterene/hydrochlorothiazide.*
Mean arterial pressure, reduction of, to limit infarct size, 718
Mechanical ventilation, for acute pulmonary edema, indications for, 123
  for adult respiratory distress syndrome, 127
Mefenamic acid, dose adjustment for, in organ dysfunction, 248
Membrane-stabilizing activity, of β-blockers, 469, 542
  of propranolol, 484
Menopause, coronary heart disease after, 316. See also *Estrogen replacement therapy.*
  surgical, estrogen replacement therapy after, 320
Mercurial diuretic(s), 389
Mesenteric embolus(i), 169
Metabolic acidosis, complicating diuretic therapy, in chronic renal failure, 365
  due to amiloride, 446
  hyperchloremic, due to spironolactone, 457
  in myocardial ischemia, trimetazidine's effects on, 1594–1595, *1594*
Metabolic alkalosis, due to furosemide, 394
  hypokalemic, with thiazides, 416
Metabolism of drugs. See also specific drugs.
  age-related changes in, 225

Meta-O-dealkylated flecainide, 1305, *1306*

Methemoglobinemia, due to nitroglycerin, 869

Methoxamine, hemodynamic effects of, 48
  in cardiopulmonary resuscitation, 209
  receptor selectivity of, 336t

Methyclothiazide, for hypertension, dose and side effects of, 374t

Methyldopa, 603–605, 616–619
  adverse effects of, 604, 619
  cost of, 649
  during lactation, 276, 276t
  during pregnancy, 271, 604
  effects of, 603–604, 617–619
  exercise's interaction with, 254–255
  for hypertension, 604, 605
    as initial therapy, 69t
    during pregnancy, 271, 604
  for hypertensive emergencies, 154t, 155t, 157–158
  in elderly persons, 227, 604
  in organ dysfunction, 242, 617
  mechanisms of action of, 603, 616–617
  pharmacokinetics of, 617
  withdrawal of, 604, 619

α-Methylnorepinephrine (methylnoradrenaline), 617
  receptors stimulated by, 342

Methylphenidate, for postural hypotension, 99

Metocloparamide, dopamine interaction with, 1164
  mexiletine interaction with, 1320

Metolazone, 412–418
  chemical properties of, 412, *413*
  for hypertension, dose and side effects of, 374t
  for nephrolithiasis, 417–418
  furosemide interaction with, 418
  furosemide with, in congestive heart failure, 413
  history of, 412
  in chronic renal failure, 361, 417
  mechanism of action of, 412

Metoprolol, 183t, 522–536
  adverse effects of, 479, 528, 534
  after myocardial infarction, 293, 294, 301, 470, 529–530, *529, 530*
  chemical properties of, *475, 507*
  cost of, 530, 548t, 949t
  drug interactions with, 348t
    with cimetidine, 352
    with propafenone, 1354
    with quinidine, 1365t
    with verapamil, 350, 352
  during lactation, 276, 276t
  during pregnancy, 272
  effects of, antiarrhythmic, 531–532
    antiatherogenic, 533–534
    cardiac, 467t
    noncardiac, 472t
    serum lipid, 532–533
  exercise's interaction with, 255–256
  for acute myocardial infarction, 133, 141, 527–529, *528*
  for atrial fibrillation with acute myocardial infarction, 131
  for dilated cardiomyopathy, 532
  for hypertension, 523–527, *524*
    effects of very-long-term treatment with, 525–527, *526*
    in elderly, 525
  in organ dysfunction, 534
  once-daily controlled-release system for, 535–536, *535*
  pharmacodynamics of, 467t, 472t, 522–523

Metoprolol (*Continued*)
  pharmacokinetics of, 522–523, 553t
  receptor selectivity of, 337t, 523, *558*
  socioeconomic considerations with, 530, 534–535
  withdrawal of, 531

Mevastatin, 1114, 1120
  chemical properties of, *1115*
  inhibitory activity of, relative to lovastatin, 1109t

Mevinolin. See *Lovastatin.*

Mexiletine, 183t, 1319–1329, 1320t
  adverse effects of, 1328–1329, 1328t
  arrhythmia aggravation by, 1235t, 1329
  clinical experience with, 1321–1329
    after myocardial infarction, 1324–1325, 1324t
    with invasive evaluation, 1323–1324, 1323t
    with noninvasive evaluation, 1321–1323, 1322t
  comparison of, with other antiarrhythmic agents, 1325–1326, 1325t, *1326,* 1326t
  cost of, 1367t
  drug interactions with, 349t, 1320, 1326–1328, 1327t
  during lactation, 276t, 277
  effects of, electrophysiologic, 1319
    hemodynamic, 1320–1321, *1322*
  for atrial fibrillation, disopyramide with, 1289
  for ventricular ectopy, 1321–1323, 1322t
    disopyramide with, 1286
    propafenone vs., 1355
    quinidine vs., 1325, 1325t, 1365t, 1366
    quinidine with, 1327–1328
  for ventricular tachyarrhythmias, 203, 1322–1324, 1322t
    in combined therapy, 1328
    propafenone with, 1328, 1357
    quinidine with, 1367
  in combined therapy, 1327–1328
  in elderly persons, 231
  in organ dysfunction, 238, 1320
  pharmacokinetics of, 1319–1320, 1320t

Mexitil. See *Mexiletine.*

Mibefradil, 1009–1014
  chemical properties of, 1009
  clinical applications of, 1014
  effects of, in animal studies, 1011–1013, *1011, 1012*
    in clinical studies, 1013–1014
  pharmacokinetics of, 1013
  pharmacology of, 1009–1011, *1009, 1011*

Microalbuminuria, in diabetes, indapamide's effect on, 429

Midamor. See *Amiloride.*

Midodrine, for postural hypotension, 99

Migraine, calcium antagonists for, 897
  diltiazem's effects on, 940
  propranolol for, 489

Milrinone, 1177–1184
  adverse effects of, 125, 230, 1182–1183, 1183t
  clinical use of, 1182–1183
  contraindications to, 1183
  dosage and administration of, 243, 1183
  effects of, 1178–1182
    hemodynamic, 49, 49t, 125, 1149t, 1178–1180, *1179, 1180,* 1188t
    immunomodulating, 1188t
    on electrophysiology, 1181–1182, 1181t
    on myocardial oxygen consumption, 1182
    on renal function, 1182

Milrinone (*Continued*)
  on vasculature, 1182
  on ventricular function, 1180–1181
  for acute left ventricular failure, 52
  for heart failure, 12, 1182, 1183
    acute, dobutamine with, 1149t
    adverse effects of, 230, 1148
    amrinone vs., 1174
    chronic, 53, 54
    dobutamine vs., 1179–1180
    long-term therapy with, 1149–1150
    with acute myocardial infarction, 136–137
  for pulmonary edema, 50, 125
  in organ dysfunction, 243, 1183
  indications for, 1182
  pharmacokinetics of, 1178
  pharmacology of, 125, 1177–1178, *1178*
  precautions with, 1182–1183

Mineralocorticoid(s), for postural hypotension, 97

Miniheparin prevention, for postoperative deep venous vein thrombosis, 1475

Minipress. See *Prazosin.*

Minoxidil, 853–857
  adverse effects of, 855–857
  effects of, 47t, 853–854, *854,* 855t
  exercise tolerance and, 48
  fluid retention due to, 50, 855, *856*
  for hypertension, 854–855
  for hypertensive emergencies, 154t, 155t, 157, 855
  in children, 855
  in organ dysfunction, 244
  pharmacokinetics of, 853

Mitral annular calcification, thromboembolism in, 1400

Mitral regurgitation, left ventricular failure due to, combined therapy for, 52
  nitroprusside for, 862
  thromboembolism in, 171–172, 172t, 1398–1400, 1399t

Mitral stenosis, acute pulmonary edema with, combined therapy for, 50–51
  detection of, during cardiac catheterization, dobutamine for, 1157
  pulmonary hypertension in, treatment of, 90
  thromboembolism in, 171–172, 172t, 1398–1400, 1399t

Mitral valve prolapse, β-blockers for, 471
  propranolol for, 489
  thromboembolism in, 172, 172t, 1399t, 1400

Mitral valve surgery, for pulmonary hypertension in mitral stenosis, 90

Mitral valvuloplasty, balloon, for pulmonary hypertension in mitral stenosis, 90
  percutaneous, warfarin prior to, 1399–1400

Moduretic (hydrochlorothiazide/amiloride), 374t, 451

Moexipril, 813–816
  adverse effects of, 815, 815t
  chemical properties of, 813
  contraindications to, 816
  dosage and administration of, 815–816
  for hypertension, 814–815
  in organ dysfunction, 814, 816
  pharmacokinetics of, 814
  withdrawal of, 815

Moexiprilat, 813–814

Molsidomine, 1645–1649
  adverse effects of, 1649
  chemical properties of, 1645

Molsidomine (*Continued*)
clinical use of, 1646–1649, *1647, 1648*
contraindications to, 1649
dosage and administration of, 1649
drug interactions with, 1649
during pregnancy, 1649
in organ dysfunction, 1649
indications for, 1649
mechanism of action of, 1646
pharmacokinetics of, 1645
Monoamine oxidase (MAO) inhibitor(s),
dopamine interaction with, 211, 1164
tyramine interaction with, hypertensive
emergency due to, 152
tyramine with, for postural hypotension,
99
vasoconstriction due to, 350
Monoclonal antibodies, against GP IIb/IIIa
receptor complex. See also *c7E3 Fab.*
antiplatelet effect of, 105
fibrin-specific, single-chain urokinase-
type plasminogen activator complexes with, 1584
Monoket. See *Isosorbide mononitrate.*
Moricizine, 183t, 1331–1337
adverse effects of, 1336–1337, 1337t
arrhythmia aggravation by, 1234, 1235t,
1336
chemical properties of, 1332
clinical efficacy of, 1334–1336, 1334t,
1335, 1335t
cost of, 1367t
drug interactions with, 1332
effects of, 1332–1334, 1333t
for ventricular arrhythmias, 203, 1335–
1336
for ventricular ectopy, 1334–1335, 1334t,
1335t
flecainide vs., 1309, 1334–1335
propafenone vs., 1355
heart failure due to, 1334, 1336
in organ dysfunction, 240
pharmacokinetics of, 1332
Morphine, esmolol interaction with, 513
for myocardial infarction, 128
for pulmonary edema, 50, 123–124
mexiletine interaction with, 1320
Moxonidine, 651–659
adverse effects of, 608, 658–659, *658, 659*
chemical properties of, 652
clinical studies of, 657–659
during lactation, 654
effects of, 654–657, *654, 655*, 655t
hemodynamic, 606, 654–655, *654, 655*,
655t
for hypertension, 607
advantages of, 659
clinical studies of, 657–659
in organ dysfunction, 658
mechanisms of action of, 652
pharmacokinetics of, 654, 654t
receptor selectivity of, 605, 652
withdrawal of, 659
Muscarinic receptor(s), drug interactions
involving, 351
in cardiovascular system, 340
Muscle disorder(s). See *Myopathy.*
Muzolamine, in acute renal failure, in
animal models, 358
metabolism of, 361
Myasthenia gravis, procainamide use in,
1346
quinidine interaction with treatment of,
351
Mykrox. See *Metolazone.*
Myocardial function. See also *Left
ventricular function.*

Myocardial function (*Continued*)
drug interactions involving, 347–349
Myocardial infarction, ACE inhibitors
after, 229, 296–297
effects of, 718–719, *719*
in combined therapy, 719–720
acute, 128–142
acute pulmonary edema with, combined therapy for, 51
antithrombotic therapy for, 109–110,
109t, 175–176, 175t, 1416t
complications of, 129–140, 130t
congestive heart failure with, combined therapy for, 51, 52t
conventional management of, 128–129
diltiazem for, 943
disopyramide pharmacokinetics during, 1284
emerging concepts in therapy for, 3–7
Forrester classification in, 133, 134t
guidelines for therapy for, 36–37
hemodynamic monitoring in, 133–134,
134t
heparin for, 1476
historical background of, 3
isosorbide mononitrate for, in controlled-release form, 872, 879,
886–887, 888–889
Killip classification in, 133, 133t
lidocaine use in, 213
limitation of size of, 140–142, 717–718
metoprolol for, 527–529, *528*
milrinone for, 1182
modern management of, 5–6
molsidomine use in, 1649
nifedipine use in, 973–974
nitrates for, 872
nitroglycerin for, 872
nitroprusside use in, 11, 861
recurrent chest pain with, 139–140
research in progress on, 6–7
sequence of events in, 3–4
after coronary angioplasty, c7E3 Fab's effects on, 1632, 1632t
Fluosol's effect on, 1622–1623
amiodarone after, 1254–1255
antiarrhythmic therapy after, 295–296
anticoagulant therapy after, 292, *292*
antiplatelet therapy after, 291–292
antithrombotic therapy after, 110–111,
113–114
APSAC for, clinical trials of, 1557–1562,
1558–1560, 1561t
aspirin after, 1446, *1448*, 1459
bepridil use after, 1058
β-blockers after, 292–294, *293, 294*, 478,
478
effects of, 469–470, 470t
calcium antagonists after, 294–295, 895,
910
cardioprotection after, 291–297
circadian pattern of. See *Circadian pattern
of cardiac disease.*
congestive heart failure after, 134–137
ACE inhibitors for prevention of, 715,
717–720
captopril for prevention of, 735
pathogenesis of, 715, 717
digoxin use after, 1140–1141
diltiazem after, 228, 295, 302, 943–944
dipyridamole after, 1459
disopyramide after, 1288
left ventricular dysfunction after, dobutamine for, 1155–1156
metoprolol after, 529–530, *529, 530*
mexiletine after, 1324–1325, 1324t

Myocardial infarction (*Continued*)
nadolol after, 503
nisoldipine after, 1007
non–Q-wave, antithrombotic therapy for,
109t, 1416t
recurrent chest pain with, 140
thrombosis after plaque disruption in,
1414, 1414t
premature ventricular systoles after, 197
propranolol after, 488
ramipril after, 762–763, *763*, 768
refractory hypertension with, 151
right atrial, 138
right ventricular, 137–138
combined therapy for heart failure
with, 51, 52t
saruplase for, clinical studies of, 1587–
1592
sotalol after, 1374
d-sotalol after, 1384
streptokinase for, 1526–1530, 1527t, 1529t
Hirulog with, 1503, *1503*
intracoronary administration of, 1526
intravenous administration of, 1526–
1527
mortality reduction with, 1527–1528,
1527t
timing of, 1528, 1529t
theory of onset of, 313–314
thromboembolism prevention in, 161, 162t
thrombolytic therapy for, 1430–1440
comparative trials of, 1530t, 1533–
1535, 1534t
hirudin with, 1494–1495
thrombosis after plaque disruption in,
1414, 1414t
tissue-type plasminogen activator for,
1572
dosage and administration of, 1574–
1575
heparin with, 110, 111t, 299–300, *300*,
1569–1570
metoprolol with, 528–529
single-chain urokinase-type plasminogen activator with, 1582
treatment strategies after, 298–302
triggering of, 313, 315
circadian pattern and, 314
ventricular thrombosis after, 170–171,
171t, 1395–1397, 1395t
antithrombotic therapy for, 1396–1397,
1397t
treatment recommendations for, 1397,
1397t
verapamil after, 228, 920, *920*
Myocardial ischemia. See also *Angina
pectoris; Myocardial infarction.*
α_1-receptor upregulation in, 341
amlodipine for, 1026–1027
arrhythmias induced by, diltiazem for,
mechanism of action of, 942
drug selection for, 64
causes of, 10t
diltiazem for, 936–937
dosage and administration of, 949
mechanism of action of, 940–941, 942
drug-induced arrhythmia aggravation
and, 1237, *1237*
due to dipyridamole, 1453
enalapril's effects on, 746
esmolol for, 510–511
gallopamil for, 926–927
heart rate and, 1386
mibefradil's effects in, in animal studies,
1012–1013
nicardipine's effects in, 984–985, *985–987*

Myocardial ischemia (Continued)
  nifedipine for, 973–975
  nitroprusside for, 861
    problems with, 860
  pathogenesis of, 8–9, 27–29, 28
  ranolazine's effects in, 1601, 1602
  "silent," 27, 29
    atenolol for, 544
    β-blockers for prevention of, 470
    calcium antagonists for, 895
    diltiazem for, 895, 943
  transient. See also Circadian pattern of car-
      diac disease.
    timing and triggers of, 311
  trimetazidine's effects on, 1594–1597,
      1594–1597
Myocardial lesion(s), hemorrhagic and
    necrotic, due to minoxidil, 856
Myocardial oxygen consumption, β-
    blockers' effects on, 467, 468
  determinants of, 467
  heart rate and, 1386
  milrinone's effects on, 1182
Myocardial rupture, with acute myocardial
    infarction, 138–139
Myocyte resting potential, 58
Myoglobinuria, mannitol in, in animal
    models, 358
Myopathy, due to clofibrate, 1079
  due to lovastatin, 1111
    with clofibrate, 1079
    with gemfibrozil, 1100, 1111
    with nicotinic acid, 1065, 1111, 1112
  due to nicotinic acid, 1065
  due to pravastatin, 1124, 1125
  due to simvastatin, 1117
  due to statin therapy, 77
    with nicotinic acid, 1065
  fluvastatin and, 1133, 1134
Myosin, in myocardial contraction, 1147
Myxedema coma, 1657, 1660

Naclex (benzthiazide), for hypertension,
    dose and side effects of, 374t
Nadolol, 500–505
  adverse effects of, 503
  chemical properties of, 475, 501
  clinical use of, 502–505
  contraindications to, 503–504
  cost of, 505, 548t
  dosage and administration of, 505
  drug interactions of, 504
  during lactation, 276, 276t, 504
  effects of, 467t, 472t, 501–502
  in black persons, 283, 284t
  in organ dysfunction, 241, 504
  indications for, 502–503
  pharmacodynamics of, 467t, 472t
  pharmacokinetics of, 501, 553t
  pharmacology of, 501
  psychiatric uses of, 503
  socioeconomic considerations with, 505
Nadroparin, 1484–1488
  adverse effects of, 1487
  chemical properties of, 1484
  clinical use of, 1485–1488, 1485t–1488t
  contraindications to, 1487–1488
  dosage and administration of, 1488,
      1488t
  drug interactions with, 1488
  during pregnancy, 1485, 1487
  for acute ischemic stroke, 1487
  in organ dysfunction, 1488
  indications for, 1485–1487
  mode of action of, 1484

Nadroparin (Continued)
  overdose of, 1488
  pharmacokinetics of, 1485
  pharmacology of, 1484
  socioeconomic considerations with, 1488
  unfractionated heparin vs., 1484
NAPA (N-acetylprocainamide), 1342
  accumulation of, in organ dysfunction,
      239, 1346
Naproxen, dose adjustment for, in organ
    dysfunction, 248
Narcotic(s). See also Morphine; Opiate(s).
  mexiletine interaction with, 1326
Nardil (phenelzine sulfate), dopamine
    interaction with, 211
Natrilix. See Indapamide.
Naturetin. See Bendroflumethiazide.
Nausea. See also Gastrointestinal symptoms.
  due to bretylium, 1270
  due to carmoxirole, 1193
  due to nicotinic acid, 1065
Necrosing arteriolitis, fibrinoid, in
    accelerated and malignant
    hypertension, 149
Necrosis, due to dopamine, 1163
  due to warfarin, 1520
Neointima formation, in pathogenesis of
    atherosclerosis, 902
  mibefradil's effects on, 1013
  nitric oxide's effects on, 841–842
Neonate(s), amrinone use in, 1173
  nitroprusside use in, 863
  premature, fluorocarbons as pulmonary
      wetting agents in, 1624
Neo-Synephrine. See Phenylephrine.
Nephrolithiasis, thiazides for, 417–418
  triamterene and, 439
Nephrotic syndrome, bumetanide in, 400
  diuretic therapy in, 363
  furosemide in, 393
  hyperlipidemia in, pravastatin for, 1125
  spironolactone in, 456
  triamterene in, 438
Nerdipina. See Nicardipine.
Neurohumoral activation, in response to
    congestive heart failure, 11
Neurologic complaints, due to
    amiodarone, 1257
  due to mexiletine, 1329
  due to phenytoin, 1340
  due to procainamide, 1346
Neuromuscular blocking agent(s),
    quinidine interaction with, 1365t
  verapamil interaction with, 922
Neurotransmitter(s), of sympathetic
    nervous system, 602
Neutropenia, due to ACE inhibitors, 285
  due to captopril, 736
  due to ticlopidine, 1471
  due to vesnarinone, 1187
Neutrophil chemotaxis, after balloon
    angioplasty, Fluosol's effect on, 1622,
    1622
Niacin. See Nicotinic acid.
Nicardipine, 979–991
  adverse effects of, in angina pectoris,
      987, 988
    in hypertension, 989
  approved uses for, 979
  chemical properties of, 980
  clinical applications of, 986–991
  dosage and administration of, 991
  drug interactions with, with
      cyclosporine, 350, 996
    with digoxin, 980
  effects of, hemodynamic, 892t, 909t, 982,
      983, 984

Nicardipine (Continued)
  in animal studies, 981–982
  in clinical studies, 982–985, 983–987
  in in vitro studies, 981
  for angina, 986–988, 987t, 988t
    effects of, 984–985, 985–987
  for atherosclerosis prevention, 31
    animal studies of, 903, 906
    clinical studies of, 906, 911t
  for hypertension, 988–990, 989
  for hypertensive emergencies, 895
  in black persons, 286t
  in elderly persons, 227
  in organ dysfunction, 980–981, 991
  intravenous, 995–999
    adverse effects of, 999
    clinical applications of, 996–997
    contraindications to, 996
    dosage and administration of, 997–
        999, 997
    drug interactions with, 996
    effects of, 995–996, 995
    for moderate hypertension, 995, 997,
        997
    for severe hypertension, 997–998, 997,
        998
    in organ dysfunction, 996
    pharmacokinetics of, 995
    precautions with, 996
  pharmacokinetics of, 980–981, 980, 1030t
  with coronary angioplasty, 308
Nicodel. See Nicardipine.
Nicorandil, 1638–1644
  adverse effects of, 1642, 1643
  cardioprotective properties of, 1643
  clinical use of, 1640–1644
  comparative studies of, 1641–1642
  contraindications to, 1643
  effects of, 1639–1640
  in elderly persons, 1643–1644
  in organ dysfunction, 1640
  pharmacokinetics of, 1638–1639
  pharmacology of, 1638
Nicotinamide, 1061. See also Nicotinic acid.
Nicotinic acid, 1061–1066, 1066t
  adverse effects of, 78, 1064t, 1065
  dosage and administration of, 1064
  for hyperlipidemia, 21, 23, 78, 1062–1063
    bile acid sequestrants with, 1064–1065
    fibric acid derivative with, 81
    fluvastatin with, 1132, 1133–1134
    gemfibrozil with, 1064
    in combined therapy, 1064–1065
    lovastatin with, 1112
    mechanism of action of, 80t
    statin with, 80–81, 1065
  in elderly persons, 232
  major studies with, 1063–1064
  mechanism of action of, 1061–1062
  myopathy due to, 1065
    in combined therapy, 1065, 1111, 1112
  pharmacokinetics of, 1061
  sustained-release, 78, 1064
    adverse effects of, 1065
Nicotinuric acid, 1061
Nifedipine, 972–977
  adverse effects of, 286t, 922t, 972–973
    in acute myocardial infarction, 129
    in pulmonary hypertension, 976
    mechanisms of, 975
  after myocardial infarction, 294
  approved uses for, 977
  chemical properties of, 972, 1000
  clinical applications of, 973–977
  cost of, 949t
  drug interactions with, 348t, 352, 973

Nifedipine *(Continued)*
  with β-blockers, 348t, 973, 975
  with diltiazem, 933
  with prazosin, 350, 352
  with propranolol, 351, 352
  with quinidine, 349t, 1364
  during lactation, 276t, 277
  during pregnancy, 272, 973
  effects of, 972
    hemodynamic, 30t, 31, 892t, 909t, 972
    renal, 48, 972
  exercise's interaction with, 252t, 253, 254
  for angina, 974–975
    at rest, 892, 974
    guidelines for, 37
    in combined therapy, 32–33, 32t
    in triple therapy, 35
    nicorandil vs., 1642
  for atherosclerosis prevention, 31
    animal studies of, 903, 905–906
    clinical studies of, 906, 911t
  for congestive heart failure, 896
    hemodynamic effects in, 47
  for hypertension, 975–976
    benazepril with, 791
  for hypertensive emergencies, 154t, 155t,
      156, 976
  for hypertrophic cardiomyopathy, 976
  for migraine, 897
  for myocardial ischemia, 973–975
    β-blockers with, 972, 975
    "silent," 895
  for pulmonary hypertension, 86–87, 976
    in chronic lung disease, 89
  in black persons, 285–286
  in diabetes mellitus, 975
  in elderly persons, 227, 975–976
  in organ dysfunction, 246
  left ventricular mass reduction by, 911t
  pharmacokinetics of, 31, 972, 1030t
  sublingual administration of, 227
  sustained-delivery formulation of, 972
    for stable angina, 892
  with coronary angioplasty, 308
  withdrawal of, 975
    in angina, 892
Nimodipine, for cerebral arterial spasm, 897
  for migraine, 897
  pharmacokinetics of, 1030t
Nipride. See *Nitroprusside.*
Nisoldipine, 1005–1008
  adverse effects of, 1008
  chemical properties of, 1005
  effects of, 1006–1007
    renal, 48
  in elderly persons, 227
  indications for, 1007
  pharmacokinetics of, 1005–1006
  pharmacology of, 1005
  post-myocardial infarction, 1007
Nitrate(s), 832–847. See also specific drugs.
  after myocardial infarction, 301
  contraindications to, 870
  drug interactions with, with calcium an-
      tagonists, 348t
    with diltiazem, 948
  effects of, 27t, 29–30, 30t
    hemodynamic, 47, 47t, 48
    in diseased vessels, 846
    vascular, heterogeneity of, 846
    with diuretics, 50
  exercise's interaction with, 251–252, 252t
  for acute left ventricular failure, 52
  for angina, β-blockers with, 31–32, 32,
      32t, 468
    calcium antagonists with, 32t, 33, 893,
      893t

Nitrate(s) *(Continued)*
    guidelines for, 36
    in combined therapy, 31–32, 32, 32t, 34
    in triple therapy, 35–36
  for heart failure, 873
    hydralazine with, 53, 873, 879
  for myocardial infarction, 872
    guidelines for, 36
  for pulmonary edema, 50
  in elderly persons, 230
  long-acting, 876–880. See also specific
      drugs.
    adverse effects of, 878
    available preparations of, 878–879
    chemical properties of, 876–877
    clinical applications of, 879
    effects of, 877–878
    indications for, 878, 879
    pharmacokinetics of, 877
    regimen selection for, 889
    tolerance to, 879–880
  nitric oxide generated by, endogenous ni-
      tric oxide and, 845–846, 845
  pharmacodynamics of, 867–868
  pharmacokinetics of, 30
  rebound on withdrawal of, 870
  resistance to, 870
  short-acting, indications for, 878
  tolerance to, 846–847, 873–874
    molsidomine in presence of, 1646–
      1648, 1647
  with coronary angioplasty, 307, 308t,
      309, 309t
Nitrendipine, 999–1003
  adverse effects of, 1003
  chemical properties of, 1000
  clinical applications of, 1001–1003
  digoxin interaction with, 352, 1000
  during lactation, 276t, 277
  during pregnancy, 272
  effects of, 909t, 1000–1001, 1000, 1001
  for angina, 1003
  for hypertension, 1001–1003, 1002
    in black persons, 286t, 1002
  in elderly persons, 227
  in organ dysfunction, 1000
  left ventricular mass reduction by, 911t
  mechanisms of action of, 1001
  pharmacokinetics of, 999–1000, 1030t
  vascular selectivity of, 1000–1001
Nitric oxide (NO), antiproliferative effects
    of, 841–842, 841
  as endothelium-derived relaxing factor,
      833
  basal activity of, 835, 836
  endogenous, in ischemia, 845
    therapeutic nitrates and, 845–846, 845
  endothelial effects of, 837–838, 838
  endothelial release of, factors influenc-
      ing, 835–837
    heterogeneity in, 838–839
    in hyperlipidemia, 844
    sex hormones and, 839
  for pulmonary hypertension, 88
  formation of, 833–835, 834
    in hypertension, 842–843, 843
    negative feedback mechanisms regulat-
      ing, 837
  humoral effects of, 838
  hypertension and, 842–843, 843
  in atherosclerosis, 28, 844–845
  in clinical arena, 842–845
  in hyperlipidemia, 844
  nonendothelial cells releasing, 839–840
  platelet inhibition by, 835, 840–841, 841
    dipyridamole's effects on, 1452

Nitric oxide (NO) *(Continued)*
    platelet-derived, 840
  release of, by molsidomine, 1645, 1648
  renin-angiotensin system and, 838
  vascular effects of, 29–30, 840
Nitric oxide synthase, 833–835, 834
  oxidative cofactors of, 837
  superoxide generation and, 837, 845
Nitro-Bid. See *Nitroglycerin.*
Nitroglycerin, 865–874
  adverse effects of, 869–870
  available preparations of, 870–871
  β-blocker interaction with, 871–872
  buccal, 867, 870
  chemical properties of, 866–867
  clinical applications of, 871–873
  contraindications to, 870
  during pregnancy, for severe hyperten-
      sion, 273, 273t
  effects of, 29–30, 860t, 868–869
    in combined therapy, 50t
    in diseased vessels, 846
    regional, 47, 48
    systemic, 47t
    vascular, heterogeneity of, 846, 868–
      869
  exercise's interaction with, 251–252, 252t
  for acute left ventricular failure, 52
  for angina, 871–872
  for congestive heart failure, 872–873
    with acute myocardial infarction, 135–
      136
  for hypertensive emergencies, 154t, 155t,
      156
  for intravenous use, 867, 871
    adverse effects of, 870
  for low-output state with right ventricu-
      lar infarction, 52t
  for myocardial infarction, 129, 872
    guidelines for, 36
    to inhibit ventricular remodeling, 139
    to limit infarct size, 141–142
  for pulmonary edema, 50, 123
  for pulmonary hypertension, 86
    after mitral valve replacement, 90
  history of, 865–866
  in organ dysfunction, 248
  mechanism of action of, 868
  nitroprusside vs., 860t, 861
  oral, 871
  pharmacodynamics of, 867–868
  pharmacokinetics of, 867
  rebound on withdrawal of, 870, 873, 874
  resistance to, 870
  sublingual, 870
  tolerance to, 873–874
  transdermal, 867, 871
    adverse effects of, 869
    drawbacks of, 889
  translingual, 870
  transmucosal, 867, 870
  with coronary angioplasty, 307, 309
Nitroglycerin ointment, 871
  adverse effects of, 869
Nitrol. See *Nitroglycerin.*
Nitropress. See *Nitroprusside.*
Nitroprusside, 858–864
  adverse effects of, 863–864, 864t
  amrinone vs., 1174
  chemical properties of, 859
  clinical applications of, 860–863
  contraindications to, 863t
  cyanide toxicity due to, 859
    management of, 864
  dobutamine vs., 1154–1155
  dobutamine with, for acute heart failure,
      1149, 1149t

Nitroprusside (Continued)
  for chronic heart failure, 1155
  hemodynamic effects of, 50t
  dopamine with, for acute heart failure, 1149, 1149t
    for postcardiotomy low-output states, 862
    in cardiopulmonary resuscitation, 210
  dosage and administration of, 859–860
  during pregnancy, 861
    for severe hypertension, 273, 273t
  effects of, 860, 860t, 1149t
    in combined therapy, 50t
    systemic, 47t
  for aortic dissection, 862–863
  for congenital heart disease, 863
  for heart failure, acute, 11, 861–862, 1149, 1149t
    chronic, dobutamine with, 1155
    with acute myocardial infarction, 135–136, 862
  for hypertension, disadvantages of, 996
    during pregnancy, 273, 273t
  for hypertensive emergencies, 154t, 155–156, 155t, 860–861
  for hypotensive anesthesia, 863
  for left ventricular failure, 52
  for low-output state, after cardiotomy, dopamine with, 862
    with right ventricular infarction, 52t
  for myocardial infarction, 129, 861
  for myocardial ischemia, 861
    problems with, 860
  for pulmonary edema, 50, 124
  for pulmonary hypertension, 86, 863
    in congenital heart disease, 91
  in organ dysfunction, 243
  mechanism of action of, 859
  metabolic degradation of, 859
  nitroglycerin vs., 860t, 861
  renal function and, 47
  thiocyanate toxicity due to, 156, 863
  withdrawal of, 864
NO. See Nitric oxide (NO).
Noise, blood pressure and, 265
Nonsteroidal anti-inflammatory drug(s) (NSAID). See also specific drugs.
  diuretic resistance and, in congestive heart failure, 384
  dose adjustment for, in organ dysfunction, 247–248
  drug interactions with, with antihypertensive drugs, 350
    with β-blockers, 348t, 350, 480
    with bumetanide, 398
    with diuretics, 350
    with indapamide, 430
    with loop diuretics, 362, 391
    with propranolol, 491
  in antiplatelet therapy, 104
Nonvalvular atrial fibrillation, antithrombotic therapy in, 172t, 173, 1399t, 1402–1405, 1402t, 1403t
  embolism in, 172–173, 1401–1405, 1401t
Norepinephrine (noradrenaline), angiotensin II interaction with, 694
  digitalis' effect on, 1140
  for cardiogenic shock, 137
  for congestive heart failure, with acute myocardial infarction, 136
  hemodynamic effects of, 48, 49t, 1149t
    with nitroprusside, 50t
  ibopamine's effects on, 1200, 1200t
  in blood pressure regulation, 616
  in blood pressure response to standing, 94–95, 94

Norepinephrine (noradrenaline) (Continued)
  infusion pump for, for postural hypotension, 99
  moxonidine's effects on, 656
  receptors stimulated by, 336t, 337, 337t, 341–342, 343
  therapeutic uses of, 342
Normodyne. See Labetalol.
Norpace. See Disopyramide.
Norvasc. See Amlodipine.
Norverapamil, 916
NSAID. See Nonsteroidal anti-inflammatory drug(s) (NSAID); specific drugs.
Nucleus tractus solitarii, 651, 652
  methyldopa action at, 617
Nystagmus, due to phenytoin, 1340–1341

Obesity, hypertension and, in black women, 282
Octreotide, for postural hypotension, 100
Oleic acid, 1608, 1608t, 1609
Omega-3 fatty acid(s), 1608, 1608t, 1609. See also Fish oil(s).
  antiplatelet therapy with, 103–104
  dose of, 1611t, 1612, 1612t
Omega-6 fatty acid(s), 1608, 1608t, 1609
Omeprazole, fluvastatin interaction with, 1134
OPC-8212. See Vesnarinone.
OPC-18,790 (vesnarinone analogue), 1148
Opiate(s). See also Morphine; Narcotic(s).
  for acute pulmonary edema, 50
Orciprenaline, 343
  receptor selectivity of, 337t
Oretic. See Hydrochlorothiazide.
Org 10172. See Danaparoid.
Organ failure, cardiovascular drug therapy in, 234–248
  dose adjustments in, 234, 234t, 235t. See also specific drugs.
  drugs not requiring dosage change in, 235t
Orgaran. See Danaparoid.
Orthostatic hypotension. See Postural hypotension.
Osmotic diuretic(s). See also Mannitol.
  in chronic renal failure, 360
Osteoporosis, due to heparin, 1477
  estrogen replacement therapy and, 322
Ototoxicity, of loop diuretics, 361, 365
Ouabain, diltiazem interaction with, 933
Oxidative modification hypothesis, 324–326, 325, 1615
Oxprenolol, after acute myocardial infarction, 293
  chemical properties of, 475
  during lactation, 276, 276t
  effects of, 467t, 472t
  exercise's interaction with, 253t
  for stress-induced arrhythmias, 264
  pharmacodynamics of, 467t, 472t
  pharmacokinetics of, 553t
  receptor selectivity of, 337t
Oxygen therapy, for adult respiratory distress syndrome, 126, 127
  for myocardial infarction, 128–129
  for pulmonary edema, 122–123
  for pulmonary hypertension, in chronic lung disease, 88–89
    primary, 87
Oxygen-derived free radicals. See Free radicals.

Pacemaker, antitachycardia, cardioverter-defibrillator with, 16, 204, 204

Pacemaker (Continued)
  flecainide use with, 1315
Pacing, "fist," for ventricular tachycardia, 202, 203
  in cardiopulmonary resuscitation, 217
  for atrial flutter, 192
  for AV nodal reentrant tachycardia, 187
  for AV reciprocating tachycardia, 189
  for bradycardia with myocardial infarction, 130–131
  for ventricular tachycardia, 203
  in cardiopulmonary resuscitation, 217
Papillary muscle rupture, with acute myocardial infarction, 139
Paracentesis, for ascites, diuresis vs., 392
Paradoxical embolism, 169–170, 170t
Parathyroid hormone, diltiazem's effects on, 939
Pargyline hydrochloride, dopamine interaction with, 211
Parkinsonism, postural hypotension in, 96–97
  α₁-adrenergic agonists for, 99
Parnate (tranylcypromine sulfate), dopamine interaction with, 211
Paroxysmal atrial tachycardia, in acute myocardial infarction, 131
  with AV block, 190–191
Paroxysmal sinus node reentrant tachycardia, 1207
Paroxysmal supraventricular tachycardia, 184–185
  adenosine's effects on, 1242, 1243
  amiodarone for, 1253
  calcium antagonists for, 893–894
  diltiazem for, 893–894, 945–946
    dosage and administration of, 949
  propranolol for, 488
  sotalol for, 1371–1372
  verapamil for, 893–894, 920, 1242
Passivation, after vascular injury, 1629
Patent foramen ovale, paradoxical embolism and, 169, 170
PD 123177 (angiotensin receptor antagonist), 820
PE. See Pulmonary embolism (PE).
PEEP (positive end-expiratory pressure), for adult respiratory distress syndrome, 127
Penbutolol, 467t, 472t
  cost of, 548t
  exercise's interaction with, 253t
  receptor selectivity of, 558
Pentaerythritol tetranitrate, actions of, 877–878
  adverse effects of, 878
  chemical properties of, 876, 877
  oral, 879
  pharmacokinetics of, 877
Pentazocine, adverse effects of, in acute myocardial infarction, 128
Pentoxifylline, 1604–1606
Peptic ulcer disease, due to nicotinic acid, 1065
Percutaneous transluminal coronary angioplasty (PTCA), antithrombotic therapy with, 305–307
  experience and recommendations for, 111
  c7E3 Fab with, 1630–1635, 1631t–1634t, 1632, 1633
  devices for, 303, 304
  diltiazem with, 944
  dipyridamole with, 1460–1461
  Fluosol with, 1620–1623, 1621, 1621t, 1622

Percutaneous transluminal coronary angioplasty (PTCA) (Continued)
hirudin with, 1495
Hirulog with, 1502–1503, 1503
morphologic effects of, 303, 304
nicorandil with, 1642
pharmacologic management with, 303–
309
goals of, 303
recommendations for, 308t, 309, 309t
risk factor modification after, 308–309
stent placement with, 305
drug therapy with, 309t
trimetazidine with, 1598
vessel occlusion after, 305, 1626
acute thrombotic, 176–177, 176t
costs of, 1635
fish oils' effects on, 1610–1611
prevention of, 308
Perdipine. See Nicardipine.
Perflubron, 1623
Perfluorochemical(s). See Fluorocarbon(s);
Fluosol.
Performance anxiety, propranolol for, 489
Pergolide mesylate, 339
Pericardial effusion, due to minoxidil, 856
Pericardial tamponade, pulseless electrical
activity due to, 218
Pericarditis, with acute myocardial
infarction, 129–130
Perindopril, 775–782
adverse effects of, 781
chemical properties of, 775–776, 776
clinical use of, 781–782
dosage and administration of, 781–782
effects of, 778–781, 779–781, 779t
pharmacokinetics of, 777–778, 778t
pharmacology of, 776–777
Perindoprilat, chemical properties of, 776,
776
pharmacokinetics of, 723t, 777–778, 778t
pharmacology of, 776–777
Perioperative hypertension. See under
Hypertension.
Perioperative tachycardia, esmolol for, 511
Peripheral circulation, drug interactions
involving, 350
Peripheral vascular disease, ACE
inhibitors for, 700
antithrombotic therapy in, 112–113, 114–
115
β-blocker use in, 546
dipyridamole for, 1461–1462
ketanserin for, 1653–1654
nifedipine for, 976–977
pentoxifylline for, 1605–1606
ticlopidine for, 1469–1470
Peripheral vascular reconstructive surgery,
antithrombotic therapy after, 112–113
Peroxisome proliferation, hepatic, due to
ciprofibrate, 1093, 1095
due to clofibrate, 1077–1078
due to fenofibrate, 1089
Peroxisome proliferator-activated receptor
(PPAR), 1077, 1089
fibrate interaction with, 1092, 1093, 1093
Persantine. See Dipyridamole.
PET. See Pentaerythritol tetranitrate.
PG. See Prostaglandin(s); specific
prostaglandins.
Pharmacodynamics. See also specific drugs
and classes of drugs.
during cardiopulmonary resuscitation,
206–208
in organ dysfunction, 236
Pharmacokinetics. See also specific drugs
and classes of drugs.

Pharmacokinetics (Continued)
age-related changes in, 225–226
during cardiopulmonary resuscitation,
206–208
in organ dysfunction, 235–236
Phenelzine sulfate, dopamine interaction
with, 211
Phenindione, in thromboembolism
prevention, 163
Phenobarbital, drug interactions with, with
calcium antagonists, 348t
with mexiletine, 1327
with propranolol, 491
Phenothiazine(s), drug interactions with,
with amiodarone, 349t
with isosorbide mononitrate, 884
with sotalol, 349t
Phenoxybenzamine, for hypertensive
emergencies, 154t, 155t, 158
Phenoxyethylamine(s), 583
Phentolamine, for hypertensive
emergencies, 154t, 155t, 158
for left ventricular failure due to ventricular septal rupture, 53
receptor selectivity of, 336t
Phenylbutazone, fenofibrate interaction
with, 1090
Phenylephrine, for postural hypotension,
99
hemodynamic effects of, 48
in cardiopulmonary resuscitation, 209
Phenylpropanolamine, for postural
hypotension, 99
Phenytoin, 183t, 1338–1341
adverse effects of, 1340
clinical use of, for cardiac arrhythmias,
1339–1340
dosage and administration of, 1340–1341
drug interactions with, 350, 1340
with amiodarone, 204, 1253, 1340
with antiarrhythmic drugs, 352
with aspirin, 350t
with calcium antagonists, 348t
with clofibrate, 1079
with disopyramide, 349t, 1285
with dopamine, 211
with mexiletine, 349t, 1320, 1327
with nifedipine, 973
with propranolol, 491
with quinidine, 1365t
during pregnancy, 274, 274t
for digitalis toxicity, 1144, 1339
in organ dysfunction, 238–239
pharmacokinetics of, 1338–1339
socioeconomic considerations with, 1341
Pheochromocytoma, ACE inhibitor use in,
698
β-blocker use in, 546
dopamine use in, 1163
hypertensive emergency with, 152
labetalol for, 575
propranolol use in, 488
Phlebitis, due to intravenous phenytoin,
1339
Phosphodiesterase inhibitor(s). See also
Amrinone; Milrinone.
adverse effects of, in severe heart failure, 230
fluid retention due to, 50
for acute left ventricular failure, 52
for heart failure, 12, 54, 1148
dobutamine with, 49
for pulmonary edema, 50, 125
hemodynamic effects of, 49, 49t
with ACE inhibitors, 50t
inotropic effects of, mechanisms of, 44,
45t, 1147

Phosphodiesterase inhibitor(s) (Continued)
pharmacology of, 1148
Photodermatitis, due to
hydrochlorothiazide, 418
Photosensitivity, due to amiodarone, 1257
Pimobendan, for heart failure, 1148
hemodynamic effects of, 49t
mechanism of action of, 44, 45t, 1148
Pindolol, 516–520
adverse reactions to, 519, 520t
after myocardial infarction, 293
chemical properties of, 475, 516, 517
contraindications to, 519
cost of, 548t
dosage and administration of, 520
drug interactions with, 519–520
with isradipine, 1017
during lactation, 276
during pregnancy, 519
effects of, cardiac, 467t, 517
noncardiac, 472t, 517–518
exercise's interaction with, 253t
for postural hypotension, 98
in black persons, 284t
in organ dysfunction, 520
indications for, 518–519
pharmacodynamics of, 467t, 472t
pharmacokinetics of, 516–517, 553t
pharmacology of, 516
precautions with, 519
receptor selectivity of, 337t
withdrawal of, 519
Pirbuterol, hemodynamic effects of, 49t
receptor selectivity of, 337t
Pirenzepine, 340
Piretanide, in acute renal failure, in animal
models, 358
ototoxicity of, 361
ramipril with, for hypertension, 770t,
771
urinary excretion rate vs. response
curves for, 406
Pirmenol, for ventricular
tachyarrhythmias, 1326t
Plaque. See Atherosclerotic plaque(s).
Plasma, fresh frozen, for bleeding due to
tissue-type plasminogen activator,
1573
for warfarin reversal, 1520
Plasma renin activity (PRA),
antihypertensive therapy choice and,
70
β-blockers' effects on, 465–466
ibopamine's effects on, 1201
in hypertension, in black persons, 280–
281
labetalol's effects on, 572
nisoldipine's effects on, 1007
Plasma volume. See also Extracellular fluid
volume; Hypovolemia.
diuretics' effects on, 371, 372, 372
in hypertension, in black persons, 280
Plasmin, 1521, 1567t, 1568
Plasminogen, 1567t, 1568
activation of, 1568, 1568
by streptokinase, 1521–1523, 1522
by urokinase, 1543
chemical properties of, 1543, 1568
depletion of, with large doses of tissue-
type plasminogen activator, 1570
fibrin-bound, single-chain urokinase-
type plasminogen activator's preference for, 1579–1580
tissue-type plasminogen activator's
preference for, 1568, 1569
supplemental, as adjunct to thrombolytic
therapy, 1530

Plasminogen activator(s). See also specific drugs.
comparative trials of, 1530–1535, 1530t, 1533t, 1534t
recombinant chimeric, 1583–1584
Plasminogen activator activity, measurement of, in plasma, 1522–1523
Plasminogen activator inhibitor, 1568
Plasminogen steal phenomenon, with large doses of tissue-type plasminogen activator, 1570
Platelet(s), APSAC's effects on, 1554–1555
aspirin's effect on, 1444–1446, 1445
mechanism of, 1443, 1444
c7E3 Fab's effects on, 1627–1628, 1628
captopril's effects on, 727–728
clofibrate's effects on, 1078
danaparoid's effects on, 1506–1507
diltiazem's effects on, 938
dipyridamole's effects on, 1451–1452, 1451t
doxazosin's effects on, 683
enalapril's effects on, 744
enoxaparin's effect on, 1511
fish oils' effects on, 1609–1610, 1610
dose required for, 1611t
GPIIb/IIIa receptor in aggregation of, 1626–1627
heparin's effects on, 102
Hirulog's effects on, 1500–1501
in atherosclerosis, 902
in myofibrotic response to vascular injury, 1415
in prosthetic valve thromboembolism, 1405–1406
in saphenous vein graft thrombosis, 1421
isradipine's effects on, 1019
ketanserin's effects on, 1652, 1653
lacidipine's effects on, 1050
nitric oxide release stimulated by, 840
nitric oxide's effects on, 833, 835, 840–841, 841
nitroprusside's effects on, 860
pentoxifylline's effects on, 1605
ticlopidine's effects on, 105
elimination of, 1471–1472
mechanism of, 1465–1466
verapamil's effects on, 917
Platelet infusion, for c7E3 Fab reversal, 1630
Platelet inhibitor(s), 103t, 1443–1472. See also Antithrombotic therapy; specific drugs.
after myocardial infarction, 291–292
anticoagulants with, experience and recommendations for, 106–113
in vaso-occlusive disease, 101–102
combined therapy with, experience and recommendations for, 113–115
in vaso-occlusive disease, 102–106
theoretical considerations in, 113
for peripheral vascular disease, 1461–1462
for thromboembolism prevention, 163
for unstable angina, 1416–1417
rationale for use of, 9
with coronary angioplasty, 305–306, 1460–1461
with saphenous vein graft, 1421–1424, 1456–1458
Pluronic F–68, adverse effects of, 1623
in Fluosol, 1618, 1622
Pneumatic compression boots, in thromboembolism prevention, 163
Pneumonitis, amiodarone-induced, 1256–1257

Pneumothorax, pulseless electrical activity due to, 218
Poiseuille law, 826–827, 827
Polythiazide, for hypertension, dose and side effects of, 374t
Portacaval shunt, metoprolol use with, 534
propranolol bioavailability in presence of, 485
Positive end-expiratory pressure (PEEP), for adult respiratory distress syndrome, 127
Postmyocardial infarction syndrome, 130
Postoperative hypertension. See Hypertension, perioperative.
Post-thrombotic syndrome, prevention of, by thrombolytic therapy, 1531
Postural dizziness, due to nitroglycerin, 869
Postural hypotension, 94–100
causes of, 95–97, 95t
drug therapy for, 97–100
drug-induced, 96–97
due to ACE inhibitors, 694–695
due to α_1-blockers, 609, 611
due to bretylium, 1270
due to carvedilol, 594–595
due to isradipine, 1020
initial nonpharmacologic therapies for, 97
neurogenic, 96
Potassium. See also Hyperkalemia; Hypokalemia.
ACE inhibitors' effects on, 696–697, 697
amiloride's effect on, 444–445, 444, 445
bepridil and, 1057
β-blockers' effects on, 547
bumetanide's effect on, 399
dietary, cardiovascular health and, 461–464
digitalis' effects on, 1136–1137, 1137
for digitalis toxicity, 1144
furosemide's effects on, 389, 394
indapamide's effects on, 422–423, 423t, 424t
renal handling of, 398, 444–445, 444, 445
situations calling for monitoring of, 440t
tissue deficits of, due to diuretic therapy, 386
trandolapril's effects on, 786
triamterene's effects on, 436–437
verapamil's effects on, 916
Potassium canrenoate, mechanism of action of, 362
Potassium channel opener(s), 1638. See also Nicorandil.
Potassium chloride, for prevention of diuretic-induced hypokalemia, limitations of, 378
in cardiopulmonary resuscitation, 215
Potassium supplement(s), 461–464
with diuretic therapy, in black persons, 283
limitations of, 378
Potassium-sparing diuretic(s), 435–464. See also Diuretic(s); specific drugs.
dose and side effects of, 373, 374t
drug interactions with, with ACE inhibitors, 353
with digoxin, 351
with ramipril, 769
in chronic renal failure, 362, 364
loop diuretics with, 363
magnesium-sparing effects of, 386
thiazides with, for hypertension, dose and side effects of, 374t
in fixed combinations, 331

Potassium-sparing diuretic(s) (Continued)
indications for, 378, 378t
Potassium-wasting diuretic(s). See also Diuretic(s); specific drugs.
digitalis toxicity with, 352
ketanserin interaction with, 1654
PPAR (peroxisome proliferator-activated receptor), 1077, 1089
fibrate interaction with, 1092, 1093, 1093
PRA. See Plasma renin activity (PRA).
Practolol, adverse effects of, 479
after myocardial infarction, 293
receptor selectivity of, 337t
Pravastatin, 1120–1126
adverse effects of, 1124–1125
animal studies of, 1120–1121, 1120, 1121
cataracts and, 1124
chemical properties of, 1120
dosage and administration of, 1125
drug interactions with, 1125
for hyperlipidemia, 1121–1124, 1122, 1122t
as initial drug, 76–77
bile acid sequestrant with, 1123, 1124, 1125
comparative efficacy of, 1118t
gemfibrozil with, 1100, 1123
in combined therapy, 1123–1124
in elderly persons, 1125
in organ dysfunction, 248, 1125
indications for, 1121
inhibitory activity of, relative to lovastatin, 1108, 1109t
LDL cholesterol reduction with, 77t
pharmacokinetics of, 1121
tissue selectivity of, 1120–1121, 1121
Prazosin, 661–665
adverse effects of, 611–612, 664
chemical properties of, 661, 666, 681
clinical applications of, 664
cost of, 949t
dosage and administration of, 610
drug interactions with, 352
with β-blockers, 480
with digoxin, 351
with nifedipine, 350, 352
with verapamil, 350, 352
during pregnancy, 271
effects of, 662–664
hemodynamic, 47, 47t, 48, 609, 662–663
serum lipid, 611, 663–664
exercise tolerance and, 48
exercise's interaction with, 257
for heart failure, 611
captopril with, 54
for hypertension, 609–610, 664
advantages of, 665
dosage and administration of, 664
in combined therapy, 664–665
in elderly persons, 227
in organ dysfunction, 242, 662
mechanism of action of, 609, 662
pharmacokinetics of, 662
postural hypotension due to, 96
pulmonary vascular response to, 86
receptor selectivity of, 336t, 342, 662
Precordial thump, for ventricular tachycardia, 202, 203
in cardiopulmonary resuscitation, 217
Prednisolone, Fluosol interaction with, 1620
Prednisone, with coronary angioplasty, 309
Preeclampsia. See also Eclampsia.
diuretic use and, 270
labetalol for, 576

Preeclampsia (Continued)
   nitroprusside for, 861
   treatment of, 273, 273t
   urapidil for, 678
Pregnancy, acebutolol use in, 498
   amiloride use in, 450
   amiodarone use in, 274t, 275, 1256
   antiarrhythmic therapy in, 273–275, 274t
   antihypertensive therapy in, 270–273, 273t
   aspirin use in, 1412
   atenolol use in, 272, 545
   β-blocker use in, 271–272, 271t, 274t, 480
   betaxolol use in, 272, 555
   bisoprolol use in, 560
   blood pressure in, 269, 270
   bretylium use in, 1270
   captopril use in, 272, 698
   cardiac disease in, 270
   cardiovascular therapy in, 269–275
   clofibrate use in, 1079
   congestive heart failure in, 270
   danaparoid use in, 1507
   digoxin use in, 274, 274t, 1141
   diltiazem use in, 948
   disopyramide use in, 274, 274t, 1283, 1286
   dobutamine use in, 1158
   enalapril use in, 698, 743, 744
   esmolol use in, 274t, 275, 514
   felodipine use in, 1044
   Fluosol use in, 1620
   fosinopril use in, 807–808
   guanabenz use in, 630
   hemodynamic effects of, 269–270, 269t
   heparin use in, 1412, 1475
   hypertension in. See also Eclampsia; Pre-
      eclampsia.
      ACE inhibitor use in, 272, 698–699
      adverse effects of β-blockers in, 271t
      isradipine for, 1019
      labetalol for, 271, 273, 273t, 575–576
      methyldopa for, 271, 604
      nitroprusside for, 273, 273t, 861
      nonpharmacologic treatment of, 270
      severe, treatment of, 273, 273t
   in prosthetic heart valve patient, antico-
      agulation in, 1412
   isosorbide mononitrate use in, 882, 884
   ketanserin use in, 1654
   labetalol use in, 271, 571
   lovastatin use in, 1112
   molsidomine use in, 1649
   nadroparin use in, 1485, 1487
   nifedipine use in, 272, 973
   nitroprusside use in, 273, 273t, 861
   pindolol use in, 519
   procainamide use in, 274, 274t, 1346
   propranolol use in, 272, 489
   ramipril use in, 758, 769
   rilmenidine use in, 640
   simvastatin use in, 1118
   trandolapril use in, 786
   triamterene use in, 440
   urapidil use in, 678
   warfarin use in, 1412, 1520
Prekallikrein, in fibrinolytic system, 1567t
Preload reduction, effects of, 868–869
Premature infant(s), fluorocarbons as
   pulmonary wetting agents in, 1624
Premature ventricular contractions. See
   Ventricular ectopy; Ventricular premature
   complexes.
Prenalterol, for chronic heart failure, 54
   for postural hypotension, 98
   hemodynamic effects of, 48, 49t

Prenalterol (Continued)
   receptors stimulated by, 337t, 344
Pressure-volume loop, effects of afterload
      changes on, 45, 45
   effects of contractility changes on, 45, 46
Prinzmetal's angina. See Angina pectoris,
   variant.
Probenecid, drug interactions with, 350t,
   351, 353
Probucol, 22, 79, 1102–1105
   clofibrate interaction with, 1077
Procainamide, 183t, 1341–1348
   advantages of, 1346–1347
   adverse effects of, 1344–1346
   arrhythmia aggravation by, 1234, 1235t,
      1344–1345
   AV block due to, 1224, 1224
   chemical properties of, 1342
   clinical use of, 1343–1344
   contraindications to, 1346
   cost of, 1367t
   dosage and administration of, 1348
   drug interactions with, 349t, 1346
      with amiloride, 446
      with amiodarone, 204, 1253, 1346
      with β-blockers, 348t
      with cimetidine, 351
      with flecainide, 349t
      with verapamil, 922
   during pregnancy, 274, 274t, 1346
   effects of, 1343
   exercise's interaction with, 259
   for atrial fibrillation, 194
   for ventricular arrhythmias, 203, 1326t,
      1343–1344
      mexiletine vs., 1325, 1325t
      propafenone with, 1356
      quinidine with, 1367
      with acute myocardial infarction, 132
   in cardiopulmonary resuscitation, 214–
      215
   in elderly persons, 230
   in organ dysfunction, 239, 1342, 1346
   indications for, 1343–1344
   metabolism of, 1221, 1342
   pharmacokinetics of, 1342–1343, 1343t
   pharmacology of, 1342
   precautions with, 1344–1346
   socioeconomic considerations with, 1348
   therapeutic blood level of, 1343
Procardia. See Nifedipine.
Progestin(s), in hormone replacement
      therapy, endometrial carcinoma and,
      322
   serum lipids and, 320, 321
Programmed electrical stimulation. See
      also Electrophysiologic testing; Pacing.
   in automatic rhythms, 58
   in reentrant arrhythmia, 61
   in triggered rhythms, 59, 60
Pronethalol, 475, 483–484
Propafenone, 183t, 1349–1358
   adverse effects of, 1354–1355
   arrhythmia aggravation by, 1233, 1235,
      1235t, 1354–1355
   chemical properties of, 1349
   clinical efficacy of, 1355–1358
   cost of, 1367t
   dosage and administration of, 1353
   drug interactions with, 349t, 1353–1354
      with digoxin, 349t, 351, 352, 1353
   effects of, electrophysiologic, 1350–1351
      hemodynamic, 1351–1352
   for atrial flutter, 192
   for ventricular arrhythmias, 203, 1326t,
      1355–1357

Propafenone (Continued)
   in combined therapy, 1356–1357
   mexiletine with, 1328, 1357
   quinidine vs., 1355, 1366
   quinidine with, 1356, 1367
   genetic differences in metabolism of,
      1352, 1353
   in children, 1353, 1357
   in elderly persons, 231
   in organ dysfunction, 241, 1353
   overdose of, 1355
   pharmacokinetics of, 1352–1353
   pharmacology of, 1350
Propranolol, 183t, 483–492
   adverse effects of, 490
   after myocardial infarction, 293–294, 293,
      294, 470, 488
   bioavailability of, after oral dosing, 485
   chemical properties of, 475, 484, 507, 517
   clinical use of, 487–492
   contraindications to, 490–491
   cost of, 548t, 949t
   dosage and administration of, 492
   drug interactions with, 348t, 491
      with cimetidine, 352
      with diltiazem, 491, 933
      with isradipine, 1017
      with lovastatin, 1112
      with propafenone, 1354
      with quinidine, 1365t
   during lactation, 276, 276t
   during pregnancy, 272, 489
   effects of, 485–487
      antiarrhythmic, 488
      cardiac, 467t, 485–486
      central nervous system, 487, 490
      hemodynamic, 476, 477, 485
      noncardiac, 472t
   exercise's interaction with, 253, 253t,
      255–256
   for angina, 487–488
      diltiazem with, 943
      in combined therapy, 31–34, 32, 34–35
      in triple therapy, 35
      unstable, 34–35, 488
   for atrial fibrillation, 194, 488
      with acute myocardial infarction, 131
   for hypertension, 488–489, 491–492
      clonidine with, 625
      mechanism of action of, 488–489
      minoxidil with, 855
      with moricizine, 1332
      with nifedipine, 351, 352
   for hypertensive emergencies, 154t, 155t,
      157
   for hypertrophic cardiomyopathy, 471,
      489
      nifedipine with, 976
   for myocardial infarction, 133
   for postural hypotension, 98
   for supraventricular tachycardias, 195,
      488
   for ventricular arrhythmias, 203, 488
      propafenone vs., 1355
   history of, 483–484
   in black persons, 283, 284, 284t
   in experimental atherosclerosis, 902
   in organ dysfunction, 242, 491
   indications for, 487–489
   membrane-stabilizing activity of, 484
   pharmacodynamics of, 467t, 472t
      carvedilol vs., 584t
   pharmacokinetics of, 484–485, 553t
   pharmacology of, 484
      esmolol vs., 508t
   psychiatric uses of, 489

Propranolol (Continued)
  receptor selectivity of, 337t, *558*
  thermoregulation and, 256–257
  vasoconstriction due to, 486
  with coronary angioplasty, 308
D-Propranolol, 467t, 472t
Propylbutyl dopamine, 345, 1164
Prostacyclin (PGI₂), antiplatelet therapy
  with, 104–105
  for pulmonary hypertension, after mitral
    valve replacement, 90
    primary, 87–88
  metoprolol's effects on synthesis of, 534
Prostaglandin(s), ACE inhibitors' effects
  on, 693
  captopril's effects on, 693, 727–728, *728*
  for pulmonary hypertension, 87–88
  indapamide's effects on, 421
  vasodilator, in response to congestive
    heart failure, 44
Prostaglandin E (PGE), triamterene's
  effects on, 437
Prostaglandin E₁ (PGE₁), antiplatelet
  therapy with, 104
Prostaglandin E₂ (PGE₂), amiloride's effect
  on, 450
Prostaglandin H synthase, aspirin's effect
  on, 1443, *1444*
Prostaglandin H₂ receptor antagonist(s),
  antiplatelet therapy with, 104
Prostaglandin I₂. See *Prostacyclin (PGI₂).*
Prostaglandin inhibitor(s). See also
  Nonsteroidal anti-inflammatory drug(s)
  (NSAID); specific drugs.
  for postural hypotension, 97–98
Prostatic carcinoma, estrogens for,
  cardiovascular events and, 321
Prostatic hypertrophy, benign, α₁-blockers
  for, 611
  doxazosin for, 686
  prazosin for, 664
  terazosin for, 670–671
Prosthetic arterial graft(s), antithrombotic
  therapy with, 1455–1456
  thrombolytic therapy for occlusion of,
    1549–1551, 1550t
Prosthetic heart valve(s), antithrombotic
  therapy for, clinical problems
    with, 1411–1412
  experience and recommendations for,
    106–107, 106t, 107t
  with bioprosthesis, 1409, 1410–1411,
    1410t
  with mechanical valve, 1407–1409,
    1408t, 1410, 1410t
  pregnancy in presence of, anticoagula-
    tion during, 1412
  thromboembolism with, 173–174, 174t,
    1405–1412
    dipyridamole for prevention of, 1453–
      1455, 1454t
    incidence of, 1406–1407, *1407*, 1407t,
      1408, 1409
    pathogenesis of, 1405–1406, 1406t
    risk factors for, 173, 173t, 174, 1406,
      1406t, 1454
    warfarin for prevention of, 1518
    with bioprosthesis, *1408*, 1409
    with mechanical valve, 1405–1409,
      1407t, *1408*, 1408t
Prosthetic materials, dipyridamole's effects
  on platelet adhesion to, 1452
Prosthetic valve endocarditis,
  anticoagulant therapy in, 1411
Prosthetic valve thrombosis, 1409–1410
Protamine chlorhydrate, for nadroparin
  overdose, 1488

Prothrombin complex concentrate(s), for
  hirudin neutralization, 1494
Prothrombin time, for monitoring warfarin
  therapy, 1518
  standardization of, 1395, 1519
Protriptyline, for bretylium-induced
  hypotension, 1270
Prourokinase. See *Single-chain urokinase-*
  type plasminogen activator.
Provitamin A, in atherosclerosis
  prevention, *326*, 327t, 328
Pseudoaneurysm, with acute myocardial
  infarction, 139
Psychotic reaction, due to pentoxifylline,
  1605
PTCA. See *Percutaneous transluminal*
  coronary angioplasty (PTCA).
Pteridine(s), 435
Pulmonary edema, acute, 119–127
  combined therapy for, 50–51
  cardiogenic, 119–125
    clinical aspects of, 120–122
    noncardiogenic vs., 121
    pathophysiology of, 119–120, *120*, 120t
    pharmacologic therapy for, 123–125
    respiratory care in, 122–123
    steps in therapy of, 122
  noncardiac, 126–127, 126t
Pulmonary embolectomy, 165
Pulmonary embolism (PE), factors
  influencing lysis of, 1523
  prevention of, 160–163, 161t, 162t, 165–
    166
    nadroparin for, 1485–1486, 1485t, 1486t
  thrombolytic therapy for, 1547
    comparative trials of, 1530t, 1531–1532
    tissue-type plasminogen activator in,
      164, 165, 166, 166t, 1532, 1572–
      1573, 1575
  treatment of, 164–165, 166, 166t
    dobutamine for, 1156
    heparin for, 1476
    nadroparin for, 1487, 1487t
Pulmonary hypertension, amrinone for,
  1172–1173
  bretylium use in, 1270
  combined therapy for, 82–91
  diltiazem's effects in, 939–940
  due to minoxidil, 856
  in chronic lung disease, 88–89
  in collagen vascular diseases, 89–90
  in congenital heart disease, 90–91
  in mitral stenosis, 90
  mibefradil for, 1013
  nifedipine for, 976
  nitroprusside for, 863
  primary, calcium antagonists for, 897
    vasodilators for, 85–88
Pulmonary vascular resistance, in
  assessment of vasodilator effects,
  84–85, *84*
Pulseless electrical activity, treatment of,
  217–218
Pyridostigmine, drug interactions with,
  351
  with disopyramide, 349t, 351
  for anticholinergic effects of disopyr-
    amide, 1285
Pyridoxine, L-dopa with, for heart failure,
  1165

QT interval, prolongation of. See also *Long*
  QT syndrome.
  by probucol, 1105

QT interval (Continued)
  drug interactions causing, 349–350
  procainamide use in, 1346
  risk for arrhythmia aggravation and,
    1236
Quadriplegia, hypertensive crisis in, 153
  postural hypotension in, 96
Questran. See *Cholestyramine.*
Quinapril, 794–800
  adverse effects of, 799–800
  for congestive heart failure, 799
  for hypertension, 797–799
  in organ dysfunction, 245, 795
  pharmacokinetics of, 794–795
  plasma and tissue ACE binding potency
    of, 796–797, *797*
  tissue ACE inhibition by, 795–796, *796*
Quinaprilat, 794
  plasma and tissue ACE binding potency
    of, 796–797, *797*
Quinethazone, for hypertension, dose and
  side effects of, 374t
Quinidine, 183t, 1362–1367
  adverse effects of, 1364
  arrhythmia aggravation by, 1229, *1230*,
    1234–1235, 1235t, 1364
  clinical use of, 1364
  comparative trials of, 1365–1367, 1365t
  contraindications to, 1364–1365
  cost of, 1367t
  dosage and administration of, 1363
  drug interactions with, 349t, 351, 1364,
    1365t
    with amiodarone, 204, 349t, 1253,
      1365t
    with bretylium, 1271
    with calcium antagonists, 348t
    with debrisoquin, 1354
    with digoxin, 258, 349t, 1141–1142,
      1364, 1365t
    with disopyramide, 349t, 1285
    with diuretics, 349t, 352
    with procainamide, 1346
    with propafenone, 1354
    with verapamil, 349t, 350, 352, 922,
      1364, 1365t
    with warfarin, 349t, 350, 350t, 353
  during lactation, 276t, 277
  during pregnancy, 275
  exercise's interaction with, 258, 259
  for atrial fibrillation, 15, 1362, 1364
    sotalol vs., 1365t, 1372–1373
  for ventricular arrhythmias, 1326t, 1364
    moricizine vs., 1334, 1335t, 1336
    propafenone with, 1356, 1367
  for ventricular ectopy, flecainide vs.,
    1309, 1365t, 1366
    mexiletine vs., 1325, 1325t, 1365t, 1366
    mexiletine with, 1327–1328
    propafenone vs., 1355
  in combined therapy, 1367
  in elderly persons, 230
  in organ dysfunction, 239–240, 1363,
    1365
  monitoring therapy with, 1363
  pharmacokinetics of, 1363
  pharmacology of, 1362–1363, 1362t
  use of, 1226
Quinidine syncope, 1229, *1230*, 1234–1235,
  1364
Quinidine-like effect, of β-blockers, 469,
  542
  of propranolol, 484
Quinine, digoxin interaction with, 351

Radiofrequency catheter ablation. See
  Catheter ablation.

Ramipril, 755–771
  adverse effects of, 768–769, 769t
  after myocardial infarction, 300–301, 300, 715
  bradykinin potentiation by, 756–757
    cardioprotective effect and, 762–763, 762
  chemical properties of, 755, 755
  clinical applications of, 768
  contraindications to, 769
  dosage and administration of, 771
  drug interactions with, 769–770
  during lactation, 758, 769
  during pregnancy, 758, 769
  effects of, 758–768
    on arteries and veins, 764–766, 765
    on central nervous system, 767–768
    on coronary blood flow, 764
    on hemodynamics, 758–760, 759
    on metabolism, 766
    on renal function, 766–767, 770
    on ventricular function and structure, 760–764, 762, 763
  for congestive heart failure, 759, 768
    after myocardial infarction, 715
  for hypertension, 759, 760, 761t, 768, 770t
    advantages of, 770–771
    in combined therapy, 769–770, 770t, 771
  in organ dysfunction, 758, 769
    dose adjustment for, 245, 722t, 771
  pharmacokinetics of, 757–758, 757t
  pharmacology of, 755–757
  socioeconomic considerations with, 771
Ramiprilat, chemical properties of, 755, 755
  in organ dysfunction, 758
  pharmacokinetics of, 757–758, 757t
  pharmacology of, 755–757
Ranitidine, drug interactions with, with calcium antagonists, 348t
    with fluvastatin, 1134
    with nifedipine, 973
    with triamterene, 440
Ranolazine, 1600–1602, 1602
Rash, due to captopril, 735–736
Rauwolscine, receptor selectivity of, 336t
Raynaud's phenomenon, diltiazem's effects on, 940
  due to β-blockers, 546
  nicardipine for, 991
  nifedipine for, 976–977
Reactive oxygen species. See Free radicals.
Rebound hypertension, 152
Rebound phenomena, with β-blocker withdrawal, 531
  with nitroglycerin withdrawal, 870, 873, 874
Recanalization, after coronary thrombosis. See also Coronary angioplasty; Coronary artery bypass surgery; Thrombolytic therapy.
  beneficial effects of, 4
Receptor(s), 334–346
  adrenergic. See Adrenoreceptor(s).
  cholinergic, in cardiovascular system, 340
  dopaminergic, 338–339, 339t, 1162, 1162, 1189, 1190, 1190t, 1194–1195
  experimental methods for study of, 334–335
  glycoside, in heart, 340
  imidazoline. See Imidazoline receptor(s).
  low-density lipoprotein. See Low-density lipoprotein receptor(s).
  muscarinic, drug interactions involving, 351

Receptor(s) (Continued)
  in cardiovascular system, 340
  serotonergic, 1650
    in cardiovascular system, 339–340
  transfer of signals triggered by, 335
  types of, 335–340
  up- and downregulation of, 340–341
Reentrant arrhythmia(s), 14, 60–61, 60. See also specific arrhythmias.
Regitine. See Phentolamine.
Rejection, after cardiac transplantation, dobutamine for, 1156
Renal artery stenosis, ACE inhibitor use in, 697–698, 698
  captopril use in, 730, 734, 736
  enalapril use in, 744
  ramipril use in, 767, 769
Renal blood flow, age-related changes in, 225
  autoregulation of, 827
  diltiazem's effects on, 938
  dopamine to increase, 1163
  in black persons, 280
Renal calculus(i), thiazides for, 417–418
  triamterene and, 439
Renal disease, ACE inhibitor use in, 699
  aspirin and, 1449
  in hypertension, calcium antagonists' effects on, 911–912
  parenchymal, captopril use in, 733
Renal failure. See also Renal insufficiency.
  ACE inhibitor use in, 699
  acute, animal models of, 357–359
    diuretics in, 357–360
    furosemide in prophylaxis of, 393
  captopril pharmacokinetics in, 729
  chronic, diuretics in, 360–365
    hypertensive emergency with, 151–152
  digoxin use in, 236–237, 1141
  diuretics in, 357–365
  dose adjustments in, 234, 234t, 236. See also specific drugs.
  drug metabolites accumulating in, 234–235, 235t
  drugs not requiring dosage change in, 235t
Renal function, age-related changes in, 225
  drug interactions involving, 351
  in heart failure, vasodilators' effects on, 47–48
  metoprolol's effects on, 526–527
  ramipril's effects on, 766–767
Renal insufficiency. See also Renal failure.
  ACE inhibitor elimination patterns in, 723–725, 724, 724t, 725
  ACE inhibitor use in, 722–725
    dose adjustment for, 722t
  bumetanide in, 400–401
  captopril for hypertension in, 732
  disopyramide use in, 1284, 1284t
  due to ACE inhibitors, 158
  due to captopril, 736
  due to enalapril, 747–748
  hyperlipidemia in, simvastatin for, 1117
  loop diuretic pharmacokinetics in, 400
  ramipril use in, 767
  thiazides' efficacy in, 417
  torsemide in, pharmacokinetics and pharmacodynamics of, 406t, 407–408, 408, 410
Renal transplantation, captopril use after, 734
  diltiazem's effects after, 940
  hypertension after, 152
  ranolazine's effects on renal preservation for, 1601–1602

Renal tubular acidosis, type IV. See Hyporeninemic hypoaldosteronism.
Renese (polythiazide), for hypertension, dose and side effects of, 374t
Renin, 727
  ACE inhibitors' effects on, 692
  centrally-acting antiadrenergic drugs' effects on, 606
  discovery of, 726
  in blood pressure response to standing, 95
  measurement of, in renal artery stenosis, 698
  nitric oxide's effects on production of, 838
  plasma. See Plasma renin activity (PRA).
  tumor production of, ACE inhibitor use with, 698
Renin hypothesis, 817
Renin inhibitor(s), 818
Renin-angiotensin-aldosterone system, 727, 727
  ACE inhibitors' effects on, 691–692, 692
  activation of, in response to congestive heart failure, 11, 44
  approaches to inhibition of, 690–691, 691
  brain, 795
  circulating, action of, during cardiovascular decompensation, 795
  clonidine's effects on, 624
  in congestive heart failure, 711–712
  minoxidil's effects on, 854
  nitric oxide and, 838
  ramipril's effects on, 766
  tissue, 795
    ACE inhibitors' effects on, 728, 795–796, 796
    in congestive heart failure, 712, 796
    in ventricular remodeling after myocardial infarction, 712, 715
Renovascular hypertension. See under Hypertension.
Reocclusion, after angioplasty. See under Coronary angioplasty; Percutaneous transluminal coronary angioplasty (PTCA).
  after thrombolysis, as end point for therapy, 1435–1436
  factors in, 1569
Reperfusion injury, mechanisms of, 6
  nicorandil's effects on, 1643
  nitric oxide in, 837, 845
  prevention of, 6–7
    diltiazem for, 936, 937
    gallopamil for, 927
    ramipril for, 760, 762
Reserpine, atenolol interaction with, 547
  betaxolol interaction with, 555
  for hypertension, as initial therapy, 68
  for hypertensive emergencies, 154t, 155t, 157–158
  in experimental atherosclerosis, 902
Resin(s). See Bile acid sequestrant(s); specific drugs.
Respiratory failure, dobutamine for, 1156
Resting potential, of myocardial cells, 58
Restrictive cardiomyopathy, amrinone use in, 1173
Resuscitation. See also Cardiopulmonary resuscitation (CPR).
  fluorocarbons in, 1623
Reversed rate dependency, 1369–1370
Rheumatic heart disease, congestive heart failure due to, during pregnancy, 270
  thromboembolism in, 171–172, 1398–1399

Ribose, effects of, on myocardial energy metabolism, 1600t
Ridogrel, antiplatelet therapy with, 104
Rifampicin, drug interactions with, 350
  with antiarrhythmic drugs, 352
  with mexiletine, 1320
Rifampin, drug interactions with, 350
  with aspirin, 350t
  with calcium antagonists, 348t
  with disopyramide, 1285
  with mexiletine, 1327
  with propafenone, 1354
  with propranolol, 491
  with quinidine, 1365t
  with verapamil, 922
Right atrial infarction, 138
Right ventricular infarction, 137–138
  congestive heart failure with, combined therapy for, 51, 52t
Right ventricular outflow tract tachycardia, adenosine's effects on, 1243–1244, 1244
Rilmenidine, 633–641
  adverse effects of, 608, 639–640, 639, 640
  binding of, to imidazoline receptor, 606, 634
  chemical properties of, 633
  clinical applications of, 640
  contraindications to, 640
  drug interactions with, 640
  during pregnancy and lactation, 640
  effects of, 637–640, 638
    central, 635–636, 635
    hemodynamic, 606, 607, 637, 638
    in animals, 634–635, 634, 635
    peripheral, 636
  for hypertension, 607, 640
    advantages of, 641
    dosage and administration of, 641
  in organ dysfunction, 637, 640
  mechanism of action of, 636
  pharmacokinetics of, 636–637, 637t
  precautions with, 640
  receptor selectivity of, 633–634
  withdrawal of, 638
Rimiterol, receptor selectivity of, 337t
Risk factor modification, after coronary angioplasty, 308–309
Ritodrine, receptor selectivity of, 337t
RMS-415. See Pravastatin.
Ro 40-5967. See Mibefradil.
Rotating tourniquet, for pulmonary edema, 50
RP interval, long, tachycardia with, 1212–1215, 1214
Rythmodan. See Disopyramide.
Rythmol. See Propafenone.

S-9490. See Perindopril.
S-9780. See Perindoprilat.
St. Jude prosthesis, thromboembolism risk with, 1407, 1407t, 1408, 1454
Salbutamol, hemodynamic effects of, 49t
  receptors stimulated by, 337t, 344
Salicylate, metabolism of, 1444
Salt, dietary, for postural hypotension, 97
Saluron (hydroflumethiazide), for hypertension, dose and side effects of, 374t
Saphenous vein graft(s). See also Coronary artery bypass surgery.
  antithrombotic therapy with, 1456–1458
  thrombotic disease of, 112, 1420–1424
    acute, 176, 176t
    antiplatelet therapy for, 1421–1424

Saphenous vein graft(s) (Continued)
    antithrombotic therapy for, 1422–1424, 1424t
    incidence of, 1420
    pathogenesis of, 1420–1421, 1420, 1421
Saralasin, 817
  exercise's interaction with, 257
  sodium depletion with, 691, 691
Saruplase, 1588–1593
  chemical properties of, 1588
  comparative studies of, 1589–1592, 1589–1592, 1590t, 1591t, 1592t
  for myocardial infarction, heparin with, 1589, 1593
    taprostene with, 1589
  metabolism of, 1588
  safety of, 1592, 1592t
Scavenger receptor, LDL cholesterol uptake by, 325
Sch 23390 (dopaminergic receptor antagonist), 339
Scleroderma renal crisis, captopril for, 734
scu-PA. See Single-chain urokinase-type plasminogen activator.
Seasonal variation in cardiac disease, 314
Sedative(s), adverse effects of, in hypertensive emergency management, 153–155
  mexiletine interaction with, 1326
Seizure, postural hypotension vs., 95
Selenium, in atherosclerosis prevention, 327t, 328
Septic shock, dobutamine for, 1156
Sequential nephron blockade, in refractory edema in congestive heart failure, 384–385
Serotonin (5-HT), distribution of, 339
  effects of, on coronary arteries, 1652
  platelet function and, 105
Serotonin receptor(s), 1650
  in cardiovascular system, 339–340
Serotonin receptor blocker(s), 345
Serpasil. See Reserpine.
Sex hormone(s), endothelial nitric oxide release and, 839
Shear stress, endothelial nitric oxide release and, 837
Shock, bretylium use in, 1270
  cardiogenic, thrombolytic therapy in presence of, 1433–1434, 1435
    with acute myocardial infarction, 137
  dobutamine for, 1156
  dopamine for, 1163
Shy-Drager syndrome, postural hypotension in, 96–97
  α_1-adrenergic agonists for, 99
  β-blockers for, 98
  fludrocortisone for, 97
Sick sinus syndrome, adenosine and, 1240
  calcium antagonist use in, precautions with, 894
  disopyramide's effects in, 1278–1279
  pindolol for, 519
  propranolol use in, adverse effects of, 490
Sickle cell anemia, fluorocarbons' effects on red cells in, 1624
Simvastatin, 1114–1119
  adverse effects of, 1117
  cataracts and, 1117, 1124
  chemical properties of, 1114, 1115
  contraindications to, 1118
  dosage and administration of, 1118, 1118t
  drug interactions with, 1118
  during pregnancy and lactation, 1118

Simvastatin (Continued)
  effects of, 1115–1116
  for coronary artery disease, mortality benefit from, 1116
  for hyperlipidemia, 1116–1117, 1117t
    as initial drug, 76–77
    comparative efficacy of, 1118t
    in combined therapy, 1117, 1117t
    in renal insufficiency, 1117
    total mortality with, 22
  in children, 1118
  in elderly persons, 231
  in organ dysfunction, 248, 1118
  indications for, 1116
  inhibitory activity of, relative to lovastatin, 1108, 1109t
  LDL cholesterol reduction with, 77, 77t
  pharmacokinetics of, 1115, 1116
  pharmacology of, 1114–1115
  socioeconomic considerations with, 1118–1119
Sinemet (carbidopa/L-dopa), postural hypotension and, 96–97
Single-chain urokinase-type plasminogen activator, 1578–1584. See also Saruplase.
  biochemical properties of, 1578–1579, 1579
  fibrin specificity of, 1579–1580
  newer developments in, 1583–1584
  pharmacokinetics of, 1580–1581, 1580t
  pharmacology of, 1579–1580
  thrombolytic properties of, 1581–1583, 1581t, 1582t
  tissue-type plasminogen activator with, 1582
Sinorphan, in chronic renal failure, 362
Sinus bradycardia, due to adenosine, 1240
  with acute myocardial infarction, 130
Sinus node, depression of automaticity of, by antiarrhythmic drugs, 1232, 1233
  drug interactions involving, 347
Sinus node inhibitor(s), 1386–1391. See also Zatebradine.
  clinical uses of, 1391
Sinus node reentrant tachycardia, 190
  adenosine's effects on, 1241–1242
  differential diagnosis of, 185t
  paroxysmal, 1207
Sinus tachycardia, 182–184, 1207–1208, 1207t
  β-blockers for, 470t, 545
  due to adenosine, 1240–1241
  noncompensatory, 194
  nonparoxysmal inappropriate, 1207–1208
  propranolol for, 488
  with acute myocardial infarction, 131
SK. See Streptokinase.
Skeletal muscle blood flow, vasodilators' effects on, 48
Skeletal muscle disorder(s). See Myopathy.
SK&F 83566 (dopaminergic receptor antagonist), 339
SK&F 86466 (α_2-antagonist), antihypertensive activity of, 343
Skin necrosis, due to warfarin, 1520
Sleep disturbance, due to lovastatin, 1124
Slowed conduction, in reentrant arrhythmia, 60, 60
Smoking. See Cigarettes.
Smooth muscle, vascular. See Vascular smooth muscle.
SOD (superoxide dismutase), 326, 326
Sodium, dietary restriction of, as adjunct to diuretic therapy, 390–391
  renal potassium handling and, 444–445, 444, 445

Sodium (*Continued*)
  renal reabsorption of, in congestive
    heart failure, 383, 384–385
  retention of, due to minoxidil, 855
    reactive, in antihypertensive therapy,
      70, 71
  transport of, in thick ascending limb of
    loop of Henle, 398
Sodium balance, negative, diuretics for
    induction of, in chronic renal failure,
    363
Sodium bicarbonate, drug interactions
    with, with calcium, 217
  with dopamine, 211
  with epinephrine, 209–210
  with mexiletine, 1326, 1327
  with quinidine, 1365t
  in cardiopulmonary resuscitation, 218–
    219
Sodium EDTA chelation, toxicity of, 1614
Sodium nitrite, methemoglobinemia
    produced by, for cyanide toxicity, 869
Sodium nitroprusside. See *Nitroprusside.*
Sodium/potassium ATPase, digitalis'
    effects on, 1136–1137, *1137*
  in cardiac cells, as glycoside receptor,
    340
Somatostatin, for postural hypotension,
    100
Sotalol, 183t, 1224, 1369–1377
  adverse effects of, 1376–1377
  after myocardial infarction, *293, 295*
  chemical properties of, *475*
  clinical use of, 1371–1376
  contraindications to, 1376
  cost of, 548t, 1367t
  dosage and administration of, 1377
  drug interactions with, 349t, 1371
    with diuretics, 349t, 352
    with thiazides, 349–350
  during lactation, 276t, 277
  effects of, antiarrhythmic, 469, 1371,
    1382t
    cardiac, 467t
    noncardiac, 472t
  for atrial fibrillation, 1372–1373, 1383
    quinidine vs., 1365t, 1372–1373
  for atrial flutter, 192
  for ventricular tachyarrhythmias, 203,
    1326t
    chronic, in ischemic heart disease, 64
    quinidine vs., 1366
  heart failure due to, 1370
  in elderly persons, 231, 1371
  in organ dysfunction, 1371
  pharmacodynamics of, 467t, 472t
  pharmacokinetics of, 553t, 1370–1371,
    1371t
  pharmacology of, 1369–1370
  receptor selectivity of, 337t
d-Sotalol, 1224, 1380–1384
  effects of, antiarrhythmic, 1382–1384
    electrophysiologic, 1380–1381, *1380,
      1381,* 1382t
    inotropic and hemodynamic, 1381–
      1382
  pharmacokinetics of, 1382
Spinal cord, high transection of, postural
    hypotension due to, 96
Spirapril, isradipine interaction with, 1017
Spironolactone, 454–458
  ACE inhibitor with, 456
  actions of, 457
  adverse effects of, 457–458
  clinical uses of, 454–458
  digoxin interaction with, 351, 458
  dose adjustment for, in organ dysfunc-
    tion, 247

Spironolactone (*Continued*)
  for hypertension, 454–455
    dose and side effects of, 374t
  for primary hyperaldosteronism, during
    pregnancy, 270–271
  hydrochlorothiazide with, for hyperten-
    sion, dose and side effects of, 374t
  mechanism of action of, 362, 454
  pharmacokinetics of, 454, *455*
SQ 31,000. See *Pravastatin.*
ST 567 (alinidine), 1387, 1388
Starr-Edwards prosthesis,
    thromboembolism risk with, 1407,
    1407, 1407t, *1408,* 1454
Statin(s). See *HMG-CoA reductase
    inhibitor(s); specific drugs.*
Steroid hormone(s), pravastatin's effects
    on, 1124–1125
Stockings, graduated compression, in
    thromboembolism prevention, 163
Streptokinase, 1521–1535
  adverse effects of, 1523–1524
  antithrombotic therapy with, 1528–1530,
    1529t
  chemical properties of, 1521
  clinical trials using, 1431t, 1436t, 1437–
    1440, *1438, 1439*
  contraindications to, 1524
  for coronary embolus, 169
  for deep venous thrombosis, 1531, 1544–
    1545
  for myocardial infarction, *298,* 1526–
    1530, 1527t, 1529t
    comparative trials of, 1533–1535, 1534t
    heparin with, 110
    mortality reduction with, 1527–1528,
      1527t
    saruplase vs., 1589–1590, *1589, 1590,
      1590*
    timing of, 1528, 1529t
  for peripheral arterial occlusion, 1532–
    1533, 1533t
    results with, 1549–1550, 1550t
  for prosthetic valve thrombosis, 1410
  for pulmonary embolism, 164, 165, 166,
    166t, 1531, 1532
  in elderly persons, 231
  in fibrinolytic system, 1567t, *1568*
  intracoronary, APSAC vs., 1557–1558,
    1558
    for myocardial infarction, 1526
  intravenous, APSAC vs., 1558
    effectiveness of, 4
    for myocardial infarction, 1526–1527
  mechanism of action of, 1521, *1522*
  monitoring therapy with, 1525
  mortality rates with, 1559
  patency profile of, *1559*
  pharmacology of, 1521–1523, *1522, 1523*
  rethrombosis after, 1524–1525
  with coronary angioplasty, 307
Streptomycin, nadroparin interaction with,
    1488
Stress, as risk factor for cardiac diseases,
    262–263
  cardiovascular therapy and, 262–267
  drug therapy for cardiac effects of, 263–
    264
  hypertension and, 264–267
Stress response, 262, 264
Stress testing. See also *Exercise testing.*
  dobutamine for, 1156–1157
Stroke, after myocardial infarction, 170–171
  risk of, 1396
  embolic, 167–168, 168t
    hemorrhagic transformation of, 167,
      168, 168t
    heparin for, 1477

Stroke (*Continued*)
  in mitral valve prolapse, 1400
  hemorrhagic, due to APSAC, 1562
    due to aspirin, 1449
    thrombolytic therapy and, 5
  hypertension with, 150
  in nonvalvular atrial fibrillation, 172–
    173, 1401–1404, 1401t–1403t
  ischemic, danaparoid for thromboembo-
    lism prevention in, 1477, 1509, 1509t
    nadroparin for, 1487
    nicardipine's protective effect in, 982
    nimodipine for, 897
    tissue-type plasminogen activator for,
      1573
  prevention of, aspirin for, 1446–1447,
    1448
    dipyridamole for, 1461
    ticlopidine for, 1466–1467
Subarachnoid hemorrhage, cerebral arterial
    spasm with, calcium antagonists for,
    897
Subclavian/axillary vein thrombosis,
    urokinase for, 1546
Succinylcholine, esmolol interaction with,
    513
  procainamide interaction with, 1346
Sudden death, circadian pattern of. See
    Circadian pattern of cardiac disease.
  due to diuretic-induced electrolyte abnor-
    malities, 386–387
  due to ketanserin, 1654
  due to outpatient dobutamine infusion,
    1155
  in chronic heart failure, 55
  prevention of, 263–264
    amiodarone for, 1254–1255
    β-blockers for, mechanism of action
      of, 524–525
    disopyramide for, 1288
  stress as risk factor for, 262–263
  ventricular arrhythmias and, 197–198, 295
Sulfamethoxazole/trimethoprim,
    nadroparin interaction with, 1488
Sulfanilamide, antihypertensive effects of,
    discovery of, 17
Sulfinpyrazone, antiplatelet effect of, 105
  drug interactions with, 350t
    with aspirin, 350t, 351, 353
    with calcium antagonists, 348t
    with thiazides, 351
    with warfarin, 350t, 351, 353
  for thromboembolism prevention, with
    prosthetic heart valves, 1455
Sulfite allergy, dobutamine and, 1158
Sulfonamide(s), phenytoin interaction
    with, 1340
Sulfonylurea(s). See *Hypoglycemic agent(s),
    oral.*
Sulmazole, inotropic effects of,
    mechanisms of, 44, 45t
Sulotroban, antiplatelet therapy with, 104
Superoxide anion(s), endogenous
    formation of, 324, *325*
  nitric oxide synthase and, 837, 845
Superoxide dismutase (SOD), 326, *326*
Support garments, in postural hypotension
    management, 97
Supraventricular arrhythmia(s). See also
    *Supraventricular tachycardia(s); specific
    arrhythmias.*
  AV node–dependent, 1207t, 1210–1215
  AV node–independent, 1207t, 1208–1210
  drug-induced aggravation of, 1233–1234,
    1233, 1233t

Supraventricular arrhythmia(s) (Continued)
 flecainide for, 1314–1315
  effects of, 1309–1312
 moricizine for, 1336
 principles and practice of therapy for, 14–15, 1207–1215
 procainamide for, 1344
 propafenone for, 1357–1358
 d-sotalol for, 1383
 verapamil for, 920
Supraventricular tachycardia(s), 182–197, 184t
 after coronary artery bypass surgery, sotalol for, 1373
 amrinone use in, 1173
 clinical classification of, 1207, 1207t
 clinical features of, 182
 differential diagnosis of, 182–184, 184, 185t
 diltiazem for, 195
  mechanism of action of, 942
 drug selection for, 61–63
 drug treatment of, 194–196
 electrocardiographic features of, 182–184
 esmolol for, 509–510
  dosage and administration of, 513–514
 fetal, digoxin for, 1141
  verapamil for, 275
 nadolol for, 503
 paroxysmal. See Paroxysmal supraventricular tachycardia.
 quinidine for, 1364
 sotalol for, 1371–1373
 with acute myocardial infarction, 131
Surgery. See also Coronary artery bypass surgery.
 arrhythmia ablation by, 16
 cardiac, dobutamine for low cardiac output states after, 1156
 cardiothoracic, prophylactic digoxin use with, 1141
 cardiovascular instability with, esmolol for, 511–512
  metoprolol for, 531
 for congenital heart disease, phenytoin for arrhythmias after, 1339–1340
 hypertension with, esmolol for, 511–512
  intravenous nicardipine for, 998–999
  labetalol for, 576
  urapidil for, 678
 in presence of ventricular dysfunction, milrinone for, 1182
 in presence of warfarin therapy, 1520
 noncardiac, in prosthetic heart valve patient, 1411
 peripheral vascular reconstructive, antithrombotic therapy after, 112–113
 soon after thrombolytic therapy, prevention of bleeding in, 1525
Sympathetic inhibitor(s), for hypertensive emergencies, 154t, 155t, 157–158
Sympathetic nervous system, ACE inhibitors' interaction with, 694–695
 activation of, in response to congestive heart failure, 11, 44
 in blood pressure regulation, 601, 602, 616
 in blood pressure response to standing, 94–95, 94
 in progression of heart failure, 1140
 inadequate response of, postural hypotension due to, 96
 ketanserin's effects on, 1651
 peripheral, receptor types in, 335–339. See also Adrenoreceptor(s).
 transmitter substances of, 602

Symptom monitoring, with antiarrhythmic therapy, 1218
Syncope, disopyramide for His-Purkinje system evaluation in, 1290
 neurocardiogenic, esmolol for predicting β-blocker efficacy in, 512
 quinidine, 1229, 1230, 1234–1235, 1364
 vasovagal, disopyramide for, 1290–1291
Syndrome X, dyslipidemia associated with, 23
Synvinolin. See Simvastatin.

T₃. See Triiodothyronine (T₃).
T₄. See Thyroxine (T₄).
Tachyarrhythmia(s). See also Atrial tachycardia(s); Supraventricular tachycardia(s); Ventricular tachycardia(s); specific arrhythmias.
 acute, 182–204
Tachycardia(s). See also Atrial tachycardia(s); Supraventricular tachycardia(s); Ventricular tachycardia(s); specific arrhythmias.
 acceleration of, due to adenosine, 1245
 fetal, amiodarone for, 1256
 perioperative, esmolol for, 511
 wide-complex, adenosine in diagnosis of, 203, 1244, 1245–1246, 1245
Tambocor. See Flecainide.
Taprostene, saruplase with, for myocardial infarction, 1589
Tenex. See Guanfacine.
Tenormin. See Atenolol.
Teprotide, 691, 726
Terazosin, 665–671
 adverse effects of, 611–612, 671
 chemical properties of, 665–666, 666
 clinical applications of, 667–671
 dosage and administration of, 610
 for benign prostatic hypertrophy, 611, 670–671
 for hypertension, 610, 667–670
 hemodynamic effects of, 609
 in organ dysfunction, 242, 667
 mechanism of action of, 609, 666, 667
 pharmacokinetics of, 666–667, 667
 receptor selectivity of, 336t, 342–343, 666
 withdrawal of, 669
Terbutaline, receptors stimulated by, 337t, 344
Testosterone, endothelial nitric oxide release and, 839
Tetracycline, digoxin interaction with, 351, 1142
Tetraiodothyronine. See Thyroxine (T₄).
Tetralogy of Fallot, β-blockers in, 471
Thalitone. See Chlorthalidone.
Thallium scintigraphy, dobutamine for, 1157
THAM, in cardiopulmonary resuscitation, 219
Theophylline, drug interactions with, with β-blockers, 480
 with calcium antagonists, 348t
 with moricizine, 1332
 with phenytoin, 1340
 with propafenone, 1354
 with ticlopidine, 1472
 with verapamil, 350
 exercise-induced myocardial ischemia and, 1453, 1459
Therapeutic ratio, 235
Thermoregulation, β-blockade's effects on, 256–257

Thiazide diuretic(s), 412–431, 413t. See also Diuretic(s); specific drugs.
 chemical properties of, 412–413, 413
 clinical use of, 417–418, 417t
 dose equivalencies for, 282
 drug interactions with, 418
  with aspirin, 350t, 353
  with probenecid, 351
  with sotalol, 349–350
  with sulfinpyrazone, 351
 during lactation, 276
 during pregnancy, 270
 effects of, 414–417, 415
  on carbohydrate metabolism, 365, 377, 416–417
  on lipid metabolism, 365, 417, 424–426, 426
 exercise's interaction with, 254
 for hypertension, 414
  dose and side effects of, 373, 374t
  lisinopril with, 751–752
  triamterene with, 438
 for nephrolithiasis, 417–418
 history of, 396, 412
 hyponatremia due to, 365, 416
 in acute renal failure, in animal models, 358
 in black persons, 282–283
 in chronic renal failure, 360–361
  loop diuretic with, 362–363
 in elderly persons, 226
 mechanism of action of, 412
 pharmacology and pharmacokinetics of, 413–414, 413, 414
 potassium-sparing diuretics with, for hypertension, dose and side effects of, 374t
  in fixed combinations, 331
  indications for, 378, 378t
 sudden death due to, magnesium depletion and, 264
Thick ascending limb of loop of Henle, transport system in, 398
Thiocyanate toxicity, with nitroprusside therapy, 156, 863
7-α-Thiomethylspironolactone, 454, 455
Thiophene(s), in experimental atherosclerosis, 903
Thorazine. See Chlorpromazine.
Thrombectomy, for arterial graft occlusion, drawbacks of, 1549
 for arterial thromboembolism, limitations of, 1548
 for deep venous thrombosis, 1544, 1544t, 1545
Thrombin, heparin's effects on, mode of action of, 1474
 hirudin's effects on, 1491, 1491
 Hirulog's effects on, 1499–1501, 1499, 1500
 in myofibrotic response to vascular injury, 1415
 in pathogenesis of prosthetic valve thromboembolism, 1405–1406
 in platelet activation, 105
 vascular effects of, 840–841, 841
Thrombin inhibitor(s), selective, for unstable angina, 1419–1420
Thrombocyte(s). See Platelet(s).
Thrombocytopenia, amrinone use in, 1173
 due to amrinone, 1173
 due to heparin, 1477
  danaparoid use in, 1509
 due to milrinone, 1183
 due to nadroparin, 1487
 due to procainamide, 1345

Thromboembolism. See also *Deep venous thrombosis (DVT).*
acute, 160–177
antithrombotic therapy for prevention of, 1395–1425
arterial. See *Arterial thromboembolism.*
cerebral. See *Cerebral embolism.*
coronary artery, 169
lower extremity, 168–169
mesenteric, 169
paradoxical, 169–170, 170t
pulmonary. See *Pulmonary embolism (PE).*
systemic, 166–170
  sequelae of, 166
  sources of, 166, 167t, 170–177
venous. See *Venous thromboembolism.*
with prosthetic heart valves. See under *Prosthetic heart valve(s).*
with ventricular thrombus after myocardial infarction, 1396
Thrombolytic therapy. See also specific drugs.
adjunctive treatment with, 6, 109t, 110
  expected improvements in, 7
c7E3 Fab with, 1635–1636
  in vivo studies of, 1629
catheter-directed, 1542
classification of agents used in, 1430, *1430*
clinical end point assessment in, 1434–1437, 1435t, *1436–1438*, 1436t
clinical trials of, 1431t, 1437–1440, *1439*, *1440*
combined therapy in, 1431, 1431t
comparative trials of, 1530–1535, 1530t, 1533t, 1534t
conjunctive interventions with, 5
  expected improvements in, 7
contraindications to, 6, 1434, 1546t, 1573–1574, 1574t
dipyridamole with, 1459
dipyridamole/aspirin after, 1459
door-to-needle time for, 6, 1432, *1432*
  strategies for reducing, 7
factors influencing, 1523, 1543
Fluosol with, 1623, 1623t
for arterial thromboembolism, 1547–1549, 1548t, *1549*
for coronary embolus, 169
for deep venous thrombosis, 1544–1545, 1544t, *1545*, 1545t
  comparative trials of, 1530–1531, 1530t
for embolism prevention, after myocardial infarction, 171
for lower extremity embolus, 169
for myocardial infarction, 298, *298*, 1430–1440
  ACE inhibitors with, 719–720
  adjunctive therapy with, 109t, 110
  antithrombotic therapy with, 175–176, 175t
  beneficial effects of, 4
  comparative trials of, 1530t, 1533–1535, 1534t
  indicators of failure of, 6
  metoprolol with, 528–529
  recurrent chest pain with, 140
  to limit infarct size, 140
for peripheral arterial occlusion, 1549–1551, 1550t
  comparative trials of, 1530t, 1532–1533, 1533t
for prosthetic valve thrombosis, 1410
for pulmonary embolism, 164–165, 166, 166t, 1547
  comparative trials of, 1530t, 1531–1532

Thrombolytic therapy (*Continued*)
for stroke, 167
for thrombosed hemodialysis access, 1551
for unstable angina, 108, 1419
for ventricular thrombus prevention, after myocardial infarction, 1397
hirudin with, 1494–1495
Hirulog's effects on, 1502
in elderly persons, 231, 1432
intracoronary administration of, 4
intravenous administration of, effectiveness of, 4
mechanisms of action of, *1430*
patency profiles of agents used in, 1559, *1559*
patient selection for, 1431–1434, *1432–1435*
problems with, 1542–1543
reocclusion after, as therapeutic end point, 1435–1436
  factors in, 1569
safety of, 5
survival benefit of, 1437, *1438*
with coronary angioplasty, *305, 307*
Thrombosis, arterial. See *Arterial thrombosis.*
atrial, 171–173, 172t, 1398
  echocardiographic detection of, 1402, 1404–1405
coronary, 3
  factors influencing lysis of, 1523
  initiation of, 9, 28, *28*, 313–314
disturbances predisposing to, 1395
intracardiac, in valvular heart disease, 1398–1401, *1399t*
of hemodialysis access, thrombolytic therapy for, 1551
prosthetic valve, 1409–1410
saphenous vein graft, 112, 1420–1424. See also under *Saphenous vein graft(s).*
venous. See *Deep venous thrombosis (DVT).*
ventricular. See *Ventricular thrombus(i).*
Thrombotic thrombocytopenic purpura, due to ticlopidine, 1471
Thromboxane A_2 receptor antagonist(s), antiplatelet therapy with, 104
Thromboxane B_2, aspirin's effect on, 1444, *1445*
Thromboxane synthetase inhibitor(s), antiplatelet therapy with, 104
  for pulmonary hypertension, after mitral valve replacement, 90
  primary, 88
Thyroid gland, fluvastatin's effects on, in animal studies, 1129–1130
Thyroid hormone(s), 1656–1660. See also *Thyroxine (T_4); Triiodothyronine (T_3).*
adverse effects of, 1660
biochemical properties of, 1656
clinical use of, 1659
contraindications to, 1660
dosage and administration of, 1660
drug interactions with, 1660
effects of, 1657–1659
pharmacokinetics of, 1657
pharmacology of, 1656–1657
precautions with, 1660
socioeconomic considerations with, 1660
Thyrotoxic crisis, bisoprolol for, 565
  esmolol for, 512
Thyrotoxicosis, nonvalvular atrial fibrillation in, 1401
  propranolol for, 489

Thyroxine (T_4), 1656
approved uses for, 1659
effects of, 1658–1659
pharmacokinetics of, 1657
propranolol's effects on metabolism of, 487
TIA. See *Transient ischemic attack(s) (TIA).*
Ticlid. See *Ticlopidine.*
Ticlopidine, 1465–1472
adverse effects of, 1470–1471
after coronary artery bypass surgery, 1423, 1424, 1458
antiplatelet effect of, 105, 1465–1466
  elimination of, 1471–1472
clinical studies of, 1466–1470
contraindications to, 1471
dosage and administration of, 1472
drug interactions with, 1472
  with nadroparin, 1488
for cerebrovascular disease, 168, 168t, 1461, 1466–1467
for coronary artery disease, 1468–1469
for diabetic retinopathy, 1470
for peripheral arterial disease, 1469–1470
for unstable angina, 1417, 1420, 1468
in organ dysfunction, 248, 1466
indications for, 1470
mechanism of action of, 1465–1466
pharmacodynamics of, 1466
pharmacokinetics of, 1466
precautions with, 1471–1472
with coronary angioplasty, 111, 177, 306
Ticrynafen, 365
Tigramin, antiplatelet effect of, 105
Tilt testing, for neurocardiogenic syncope, esmolol in, 512
  in assessment of drug efficacy, limitations of, 1291
Timolol, 494–495
after myocardial infarction, 293–294, *293*, 470, 495
chemical properties of, 475
clinical use of, 495
cost of, 548t
during lactation, 276, 276t
effects of, 467t, 472t, 494–495
for acute myocardial infarction, 141
pharmacokinetics of, 494, 553t
pharmacology of, 467t, 472t, 494
quinidine interaction with, 1365t
receptor selectivity of, 337t
Tissue-type plasminogen activator (alteplase), 1567–1575
adverse effects of, 1573
biochemical properties of, 1567–1568
c7E3 Fab after, *in vivo* studies of, 1629
clinical applications of, 1572–1573
clinical trials using, 1431t, 1436t, 1437–1440, *1438, 1439*
clot selectivity of, *1430*, 1568, *1569*
contraindications to, 1573–1574, 1574t
cost of, 1575
dosage and administration of, 1574–1575
drug interactions with, with doxazosin, 683
  with Hirulog, 1502
  with iloprost, 104
effectiveness of, 4–5
for deep venous thrombosis, 1531
for ischemic stroke, 1573
for myocardial infarction, 1572
  APSAC vs., 1559–1560
  comparative trials of, 1533–1535, 1534t, 1591–1592, *1591, 1592*, 1592t
  dosage and administration of, 1574–1575
  Fluosol with, 1623, 1623t

Tissue-type plasminogen activator (alteplase) (Continued)
Tissue-type plasminogen activator (alteplase) (Continued)
  heparin with, 110, 111t, 299–300, 300, 1569–1570
  metoprolol with, 528–529
  single-chain urokinase-type plasminogen activator with, 1582
  for peripheral arterial occlusion, 1533, 1533t
  for pulmonary embolism, 164, 165, 166, 166t, 1532, 1572–1573
  dosage and administration of, 1575
  for unstable angina, 108, 1419
  in elderly persons, 231, 1432
  in organ dysfunction, 1574
  intracranial bleeding with, 5, 1573
  large doses of, plasminogen depletion with, 1570
  measurement of, 1570–1571
  mortality rates with, 1559
  patency profile of, 1559
  pharmacodynamics of, 1570, 1570
  pharmacokinetics of, 1570–1572
  single-chain vs. double-chain, 1571
  with coronary angioplasty, 307
TNF. See Tumor necrosis factor (TNF).
Tobacco. See Cigarettes.
Tocainide, 183t
  arrhythmia aggravation by, 1235t
  cost of, 1367t
  dose adjustment for, in organ dysfunction, 238
  drug interactions with, 349t
  for ventricular arrhythmia, 203
    mexiletine vs., 1325, 1325t, 1326
    propafenone vs., 1355
    quinidine vs., 1365–1366, 1365t
  in elderly persons, 231
α-Tocopherol (vitamin E), in atherosclerosis prevention, 326, 327, 327, 327t
Tolazoline, for pulmonary hypertension, in congenital heart disease, 91
  primary, 85
  receptor selectivity of, 336t
Tolbutamide, clofibrate interaction with, 1079
Tonocard. See Tocainide.
Torasemide. See Torsemide.
Torsades de pointes, 200–202, 201
  bretylium for, 1269–1270
  drug interactions causing, 349–350
  drug-induced, 1235
    due to bepridil, 1056, 1057–1058
    due to disopyramide, 1286
    due to dofetilide, 1301
    due to procainamide, 1344
    due to propafenone, 1355
    due to quinidine, 1229, 1235
    due to sotalol, 1376–1377
  in bradycardia/tachycardia syndrome, 1216
  in quinidine syncope, 1364
  phenytoin for, 1340
  treatment of, in cardiopulmonary resuscitation, 216
Torsemide, 402–411
  chemical properties of, 403
  dose adjustment for, in organ dysfunction, 246
  for edematous disorders, 404–405
  for hypertension, 402–404
    dose and side effects of, 374t
  hemodynamic effects of, 405

Torsemide (Continued)
  metabolism of, 361
  pharmacokinetics and pharmacodynamics of, in cirrhosis, 406t, 408–410, 409
    in congestive heart failure, 406t, 409, 410
    in elderly persons, 406–407, 406t, 408
    in healthy persons, 405–406, 406, 406t, 407
    in renal insufficiency, 406t, 407–408, 408, 410
  pharmacology of, 404
  urinary excretion rate vs. response curves for, 406
Tourniquet, rotating, for pulmonary edema, 50
Toxic shock, dobutamine for, 1156
t-PA. See Tissue-type plasminogen activator (alteplase).
Trandate injection. See Labetalol.
Trandolapril, 784–787
Trandolaprilat, 784
Transaminase elevation. See Liver enzyme elevations.
Transient ischemic attack(s) (TIA), antithrombotic therapy after, 168, 168t
  dipyridamole for, 1461
  ticlopidine for, 1466–1467
Transluminal coronary angioplasty, percutaneous. See Percutaneous transluminal coronary angioplasty (PTCA).
Transplantation, cardiac. See Cardiac transplantation.
  lung, diltiazem's effects after, 940
  renal. See Renal transplantation.
Tranylcypromine sulfate, dopamine interaction with, 211
Treadmill testing. See Exercise testing.
Tremor, familial essential, propranolol for, 489
Triamterene, 435–441
  adverse effects of, 439–440, 439t
  contraindications to, 440
  drug interactions with, 440
    with digitalis, 438
    with digoxin, 351
  during pregnancy, 440
  effects of, 436–438
  for hypertension, 438
    dose and side effects of, 374t
  formulations of, 441t
  hydrochlorothiazide with. See Triamterene/hydrochlorothiazide.
  in organ dysfunction, 247, 436
  indications for, 438–439
  mechanism of action of, 362
  pharmacokinetics of, 435–436
  pharmacology of, 435
Triamterene/hydrochlorothiazide, cost of, 430t
  dose and side effects of, 374t
  formulations of, 441t
  variation in bioavailability of, 436
Tricyclic antidepressant(s), drug interactions with, with amiodarone, 349t
  with bepridil, 1058
  with guanfacine, 649
  with isosorbide mononitrate, 884
  with quinidine, 1365t
  with rilmenidine, 640
  with sotalol, 349t
Triggered rhythm(s), 58–60, 59
  after myocadial infarction, diltiazem for, 942

Triggering events for cardiac disease, 313, 315
  circadian pattern of disease and, 314
Triglycerides. See also Hypertriglyceridemia; Lipid metabolism.
  bile acid sequestrants' effects on, 1069, 1070
  bisoprolol's effects on, 565, 566
  clofibrate's effects on, 1076
  diuretics' effects on, 375–377, 376t
  fenofibrate's effects on, 1085–1086, 1086
  fish oils' effects on, 1610, 1611
    dose required for, 1611t
  gemfibrozil's effects on, 1099
Triiodothyronine (T_3), adverse effects of, 1660
  approved uses for, 1659
  biochemical properties of, 1656
  contraindications to, 1660
  dosage and administration of, 1660
  drug interactions with, 1660
  effects of, 1657–1659
    acute, 1657
    long-term, 1656–1657
  experimental uses for, 1659
  low serum levels of. See also Hypothyroidism.
    clinical conditions of, 1657, 1657t
  pharmacokinetics of, 1657
  pharmacology of, 1656–1657
  precautions with, 1660
  socioeconomic considerations with, 1660
Trimazosin, exercise tolerance and, 48
  hemodynamic effects of, 47t
  in elderly persons, 227
  receptor selectivity of, 336t
Trimetazidine, 1594–1599
  adverse effects of, 1597
  dose of, 1597
  for angina, 1598, 1598t
  mechanisms of action of, 1594–1597, 1594–1597
  pharmacokinetics of, 1597
Trimethaphan, for hypertensive emergencies, 154t, 155t, 158
Trimethoprim/sulfamethoxazole, nadroparin interaction with, 1488
Triostat. See Triiodothyronine (T_3).
Tromethamine, in cardiopulmonary resuscitation, 219
Tropomyosin, in myocardial contraction, 1147
Tumor necrosis factor (TNF), fish oils' effects on, 1611
  vesnarinone's effects on, 1186
TXA. See Thromboxane entries.
Type A behavior, β-blockers' effects on, 264
  coronary artery disease and, 263
Tyramine, for postural hypotension, 99
  monoamine oxidase inhibitor interaction with, hypertensive emergency due to, 152

UK. See Urokinase.
UK-14,304 (α$_2$-agonist), 336t
UK-68,798. See Dofetilide.
Ulcer(s), gastrointestinal, due to nicotinic acid, 1065
  venous stasis, pentoxifylline for, 1606
UL-FS 49. See Zatebradine.
Unidirectional block, in reentry, 60–61, 60
Urapidil, 673–678
  adverse effects of, 611, 612, 678

Urapidil (Continued)
  clinical applications of, 675–678, 677t
  contraindications to, 678
  dosage and administration of, 611
  during pregnancy and lactation, 678
  effects of, 609, 674–675, 675t
    on serum lipids, 611
  for hypertension, 610, 675–678, 677t
  for hypertensive emergencies, 677–678
  in organ dysfunction, 674
  mechanism of action of, 609, 673
  pharmacokinetics of, 673–674
  receptor selectivity of, 343, 673
Urate excretion. See also Gout;
    Hyperuricemia.
  drug interactions affecting, 351
  losartan's effects on, 823
Urine concentration, bumetanide's effects
    on, 399
Urine dilution, bumetanide's effects on,
    398–399
Urodilatin, in acute renal failure, in animal
    models, 359
Urokinase, 1542–1551
  advantages of, 1543
  catheter-directed therapy with, for deep
      venous thrombosis, 1545, 1545
  chemical properties of, 1543
  clinical use of, 1544–1549
  for deep venous thrombosis, 1531, 1544–
      1547, 1544t–1546t, 1545
  for myocardial infarction, saruplase vs.,
      1590–1591, 1590t
  for peripheral arterial occlusion, 1533,
      1533t
    results with, 1549–1551, 1550t
  for pulmonary embolism, 164, 165, 166,
      166t, 1532, 1547
  for subclavian/axillary vein thrombosis,
      1546–1547
  in fibrinolytic system, 1567t, 1568
  intracoronary, for coronary embolus, 169
  pharmacokinetics of, 1543–1544
  pharmacology of, 1543
  with coronary angioplasty, 307
Urokinase-type plasminogen activator. See
    Single-chain urokinase-type plasminogen
    activator.
Use dependency, of antiarrhythmic drugs,
    aggravation of arrhythmia due to,
    1232, 1233, 1314
  of calcium antagonists, 934

Valvular heart disease. See also specific
    disorders.
  anticoagulation in, indications for, 1399t
  antithrombotic therapy in, 1399t
    experience and recommendations for,
        106–107, 106t, 107t
  intracardiac thrombosis in, 1398–1401,
      1399t
Valvuloplasty, balloon, for pulmonary
    hypertension in mitral stenosis, 90
  percutaneous mitral, warfarin prior to,
      1399–1400
Vascular calcification, in atherosclerosis,
    1615
  magnesium EDTA chelation for, 1615–
      1616, 1616
Vascular graft(s). See also Arterial graft(s);
    Coronary artery bypass surgery;
    Saphenous vein graft(s).
  aspirin for maintenance of patency of,
      1448

Vascular injury, due to percutaneous
    transluminal coronary angioplasty,
    1460
  during coronary artery bypass surgery,
      1421
  in pathogenesis of atherosclerosis, 1412–
      1413, 1412t
  myofibrotic response to, platelets and
      thrombin in, 1415
  passivation after, 1629
  vasoconstriction after, 1414–1415
Vascular resistance, calculation of, 826
    problems with, 826–827
  pulmonary, in assessment of vasodilator
      effects, 84–85, 84
Vascular smooth muscle, ketanserin's
    effects on, 1650–1651, 1652
  nitric oxide production by, 840
  nitric oxide's antiproliferative effects on,
      841, 841
  verapamil's effects on, 917
Vascular wall, ramipril's effects on,
    764–766, 765
Vasculitis, disseminated, hypertensive
    crisis due to, 153
Vasoconstriction, α_1- vs. α_2-mediated,
    337–338
  thrombosis and, 1414–1415
Vasodilation, 826–847
  due to diuretics, mechanisms of, 371–372
  due to nitroglycerin, dose-related vaso-
      selectivity of, 868–869
  endogenous hemodynamic and neurohu-
      moral response to, 828–829
    aging's effect on, 829
  endothelium-dependent, 832–833, 832,
      833
  in atherosclerosis, 830–831, 831
  in congestive heart failure, 830
  in hypertension, 830
  in large arteries, 827–828
  in small arteries, problems in assessment
      of, 826–827
  in veins, problems in assessment of, 828
  peripheral, in preservation of left ventric-
      ular performance, 33–34
  postural hypotension in, 96
  principles and practice of, 826–831
Vasodilator(s), 826–889. See also specific
    drugs.
  arteriolar, 853–857
    hemodynamic effects of, 11, 43, 46,
        853–854
  arteriolar and venous, 858–889
  dopamine with, for heart failure, 1163
    hypotension due to, 1163–1164
  during pregnancy, 273
  exercise's interaction with, 257
  for congestive heart failure, 11–12, 44t
    dopamine with, 1163
    inotropic drugs with, 45–46, 46t
    rationale for, 43–44
    survival with, 712, 713–714, 713, 715
    with acute myocardial infarction, 134–
        136
  for hypertension, clonidine with, 625
  for hypertensive emergencies, 154t, 155–
      157, 155t
  for left ventricular dysfunction after
      myocardial infarction, dobutamine
      with, 1156
  for left ventricular failure, acute, 52
    due to ventricular septal rupture, 53
  for preservation of left ventricular func-
      tion, after myocardial infarction,
      300–302

Vasodilator(s) (Continued)
  for pulmonary hypertension, 83–88
    in chronic lung disease, 89
    in collagen vascular diseases, 89–90
    in congenital heart disease, 91
    monitoring effects of, 84–85, 84
    primary, 85–88
  hemodynamic classification of, 829
  hemodynamic effects of, in combined
      therapy, 50t
    regional, 47–48
    systemic, 47, 47t
  indirect, as initial therapy for hyperten-
      sion, 68, 69t
  reflex mechanisms triggered by, adrener-
      gic blockers' effects on, 342
Vasonase. See Nicardipine.
Vaso-occlusive disease, aspirin in, in
    primary prevention, 1447–1448, 1448
  in secondary prevention, 1446–1447,
      1448
  combined therapy in, 101–116
    experience and recommendations for,
        106–115
Vasopressin, ACE inhibitors' effects on,
    692–693
  captopril's effects on, 728
  increased levels of, in response to heart
      failure, 11, 44
Vasopressor(s), in cardiopulmonary
    resuscitation, 208–212
Vasotec. See Enalapril.
Vasovagal syncope, disopyramide for,
    1290–1291
Venodilator(s). See also Vasodilator(s);
    specific drugs.
  effects of, 11, 12, 43, 46, 47
Venous compliance, 828
"Venous paradox," in closed-chest
    compression, 218
Venous stasis ulcer, pentoxifylline for, 1606
Venous thromboembolism, prevention of,
    low-molecular-weight heparin for,
    1512–1513, 1512t, 1513t
  nadroparin for, 1485–1486, 1485t, 1486t
  warfarin for, 1518
  risk of, 1512
  treatment of, enoxaparin for, 1516
    nadroparin for, 1486–1487, 1487t
Venous thrombosis. See Deep venous
    thrombosis (DVT).
Ventilation, mechanical. See Mechanical
    ventilation.
Ventricular aneurysm, ventricular
    thrombus with, 171, 171t, 1395t,
    1397–1398, 1397t
Ventricular arrhythmia(s). See also specific
    arrhythmias.
  antiarrhythmic therapy for, 15
    patient selection for, 1215–1216
    principles and practice of, 1215–1226
  calcium antagonists for, 894
  disopyramide's effects on, in animal
      studies, 1277–1278
  drug selection for, 63–64
  due to digitalis toxicity, 1143
    management of, 1144
  due to milrinone, 1181
  flecainide for, 1314
    effects of, 1307–1309
  metoprolol for, 532
    after myocardial infarction, 530
  mexiletine for, clinical experience with,
      1321–1324, 1322t, 1323t
  moricizine for, 1335–1336
  nadolol for, 503

Ventricular arrhythmia(s) *(Continued)*
  phenytoin for, 1339–1340
  probucol's effects on, 1105
  procainamide for, 1343–1344
  propranolol for, 488
  sotalol for, 1373–1376
  d-sotalol for, 1383–1384
  with acute myocardial infarction, 131–132
Ventricular ectopy. See also *Ventricular premature complexes.*
  adverse effects of diuretics in, 226
  moricizine for, 1334, 1334t, *1335*
  propafenone for, 1355
  quinidine for, 1364
Ventricular extrasystoles. See *Ventricular ectopy; Ventricular premature complexes.*
Ventricular fibrillation, 202–204, *204*
  amiodarone for, 1255–1256
  β-blockers for, 470t, 545
  bretylium for, 1269
  dofetilide's effects on, in preclinical studies, 1298, *1298*
  fish oils for prevention of, 1611
  propafenone for, 1355–1357
  refractory or recurrent, treatment of, 212–216
  sotalol for, 1374–1376, *1375*
  d-sotalol for, 1383–1384
  with acute myocardial infarction, 131–132
Ventricular flutter, 202–204
  ventricular tachycardia vs., 198–199
Ventricular premature complexes, 197–198, 200. See also *Ventricular ectopy.*
  β-blockers for, 470t, 545
  disopyramide for, 1286–1287
  drug selection for, 63
  due to digitalis toxicity, 1143
  moricizine for, 1334
  nadolol for, 503
  sotalol's effects on, 1374
Ventricular remodeling, after myocardial infarction, 138–139, 715, 717
  ACE inhibitors' effects on, 715
Ventricular septal rupture, left ventricular failure due to, combined therapy for, 53
  with acute myocardial infarction, 139
Ventricular tachycardia(s), 197–204
  amiodarone for, 1255–1256
  β-blockers for, 470t
  bidirectional, 199
  bretylium for, 1269–1270
  clinical features of, 197–198
  disopyramide for, 1286–1288, *1287*
  dofetilide for, 1300
  drug selection for, 63
  due to ketanserin, 1654
  electrocardiographic features of, 198
  esmolol for, 510
  flecainide's effects in, 1308–1309
  idiopathic, drug selection for, 63
  in dilated cardiomyopathy, adenosine's effects on, 1245
  in ischemic heart disease, adenosine's effects on, 1244–1245
  chronic, drug selection for, 64
  nonsustained, 198, 200. See also *Ventricular ectopy; Ventricular premature complexes.*
  polymorphic, 200–202, *201*
  propafenone for, 1355–1357
  quinidine for, 1364
  reentrant, phenytoin for, 1340
  sotalol for, 1374–1376, *1375*
  d-sotalol for, 1383–1384
  sustained, 198–200, *200*

Ventricular tachycardia(s) *(Continued)*
  clinical features of, 198
  electrocardiographic features of, 198–200, *200*
  with structurally normal heart, adenosine's effects on, 1243–1244
Ventricular thrombus(i), 170–171, 171t, 1395–1398, 1395t
  after myocardial infarction, 1395–1397, 1395t
    treatment recommendations for, 1397, 1397t
  heparin for prevention of, 1476
Ventrolateral medulla, 651–652, *652*
Verapamil, 183t, 915–923
  adverse effects of, 286, 922, 922t
    in digitalis poisoning, 347, 352
    in hypertrophic cardiomyopathy, 896
  after myocardial infarction, 294–295, 302
  arrhythmia aggravation by, 1235t
  chemical properties of, 915
  chronobiologic release of, 916
  clinical applications of, 919–921, 919t
  contraindications to, 922
  cost of, 430t, 949t
  dosage and administration of, 923
  drug interactions with, 348t, 352, 922–923
    with β-blockers, 348t, 352, 480, 922
    with cimetidine, 916
    with digoxin, 352, 922–923, 1142
    with disopyramide, 349t, 351, 922
    with flecainide, 349t
    with lidocaine, 349t
    with metoprolol, 350, 352
    with nadolol, 504
    with prazosin, 350, 352
    with propranolol, 491
    with quinidine, 349t, 350, 352, 922, 1364, 1365t
    with theophylline, 350
  during lactation, 276t, 277
  during pregnancy, 274t, 275
  effects of, 917–919
    cardioprotective, 910
    cardiovascular, 30t, 31, 909t
    electrophysiologic, 909, 917, 918
    hemodynamic, 892t, 917–918, 918t
  exercise's interaction with, 252t, 253, 254
  for accessory pathway tachycardia, 894
  for angina, 892
    guidelines for, 37
    in combined therapy, 32t, 33
  for atherosclerosis prevention, animal studies of, 903–905, *904, 905*
    clinical studies of, 906, 911t
    mechanism of action of, 906
  for atrial fibrillation, 893, 1209
  for atrial flutter, 894
  for congestive heart failure, problems with, 918
  for coronary artery disease, 921–922
  for coronary artery spasm, 898
  for hypertension, 921
    amlodipine with, 1034
  for hypertrophic cardiomyopathy, 895–896, 920–921
    adverse effects of, 896
  for migraine, 897
  for multifocal atrial tachycardia, 191
  for paroxysmal supraventricular tachycardia, 893–894, 920
    adenosine vs., 1242
  for "silent" myocardial ischemia, 895
  for supraventricular tachycardias, 195, 196

Verapamil *(Continued)*
  for Wolff-Parkinson-White syndrome, 187–188, 189
  in black persons, 285, 286t
  in elderly persons, 228, 231
  in organ dysfunction, 246, 916
  left ventricular mass reduction by, 911t
  pharmacokinetics of, 31, 915–916, 916t
  pharmacology of, 915–916
  ventricular fibrillation due to, 203
  withdrawal of, in angina, 892
Verelan. See *Verapamil.*
Very-low-density lipoprotein (VLDL). See also *Lipid metabolism.*
  bile acid sequestrants' effects on, 1069
  fenofibrate's effects on, 1085–1086, *1086*
  fish oils' effects on, 1610
  gemfibrozil's effects on, 1099
  nicotinic acid's effects on, 1061–1062
  simvastatin's effects on, 1114–1115
Vesnarinone, 1148, 1185–1188
  adverse effects of, 1187
  chemical properties of, 1185
  clinical trials of, 1187–1188, 1188t
  for heart failure, 12, 54–55
    long-term therapy with, 1150
  hemodynamic effects of, 44–45, 45t, 49t
  in elderly persons, 230
  pharmacokinetics of, 1186–1187, 1187t
  pharmacology of, 1185–1186, 1188t
Vest, to increase intrathoracic pressure in cardiopulmonary resuscitation, 212
Visual disturbances, due to zatebradine, 1390
Vitamin(s). See also specific vitamins.
  bile acid sequestrants' effects on absorption of, 1072–1073
Vitamin C, in atherosclerosis prevention, *326,* 327–328, 327t
Vitamin E, in atherosclerosis prevention, *326,* 327, *327,* 327t
Vitamin K, for warfarin reversal, 1520
  warfarin interaction with, 1517
VLDL. See *Very-low-density lipoprotein (VLDL).*
Volume loading, in cardiopulmonary resuscitation, 212

Warfarin, 102, 1517–1521
  adverse effects of, 1519–1520
  after coronary artery bypass surgery, 112, 176t, 1424, 1424t, 1458
  after embolic stroke, 168, 168t
  after myocardial infarction, 110–111, 171, 171t, 292, *292,* 1397, 1397t
  chemical properties of, 1517
  clinical use of, 1518–1519
  contraindications to, 1520
  dosage and administration of, 1519, 1519t
  drug interactions with, 307, 350t, 353, 1520–1521
    with amiodarone, 307, 350t, 353, 1252–1253
    with β-blockers, 480
    with cholestyramine, 350t, 351, 353
    with Fluosol, 1620
    with gemfibrozil, 1101
    with propafenone, 1353–1354
    with quinidine, 349t, 350, 350t, 353
    with simvastatin, 1118
    with spironolactone, 458
    with sulfinpyrazone, 350t, 351, 353
  during pregnancy and lactation, 1412, 1520

Warfarin (Continued)
  for cerebral embolism, 1411
  for deep venous thrombosis, 164, 166,
    166t
      Logiparin vs., for prevention, 1481t,
        1482
  for prosthetic valve thrombosis, thrombo-
    lytic therapy with, 1410
  for pulmonary embolism, 166, 166t
  for unstable angina, 1420
  heparin with, overlapping therapy with,
    1518
  in atrial fibrillation, 107
  in cyanotic congenital heart disease, 170
  in dilated cardiomyopathy, 171, 171t,
    1397t, 1398
  in mitral valve disease, 172, 172t, 1399–
    1400, 1399t
  in mitral valve prolapse, 172, 172t, 1399t,
    1400
  in nonvalvular atrial fibrillation, 172t,
    173, 1399t, 1405
      clinical trials of, 1402–1403, 1402t,
        1403t
      safety of, 1404
  in organ dysfunction, 1521
  in peripheral vascular disease, 113
  in thromboembolism prevention, 163
  indications for, 1518
  pharmacokinetics of, 1517–1518
  pharmacology of, 1517
  precautions with, 1519–1520
  reversal of effects of, 1520
  with coronary angioplasty, 307, 308t,
    309t
  with prosthetic heart valves, 173–174,
    174t, 1455
      aspirin with, 1408t, 1409, 1410, 1410t,
        1454–1455

Warfarin (Continued)
      dipyridamole with, 1454, 1455
      in combined therapy, 106–107, 106t,
        107t
      with bioprosthesis, 1409, 1410–1411,
        1410t
      with mechanical valve, 1408–1409,
        1408t, 1410, 1410t
Weight loss, for dyslipidemia, 19
Weight-reduction program(s), potassium
    excretion with, in patient on diuretic
    therapy, 254
Wernicke's encephalopathy, due to
    intravenous nitroglycerin, 870
Wide-complex tachycardia, adenosine in
    diagnosis of, 203, 1244, 1245–1246,
    1245
WIN40680. See Amrinone.
Wolff-Parkinson-White syndrome, 187–189,
    188
  adenosine's effects on tachycardia in,
    1242–1243
  amiodarone for, 1253
  calcium antagonists for, 894
  differential diagnosis of, 185t
  disopyramide for, 1288–1289, 1289
  drug selection for, 62
  electrocardiographic characteristics of,
    188
  flecainide's effects in, 1311
  procainamide for, 1344
  propafenone for, 1357
  quinidine for, 1364
  sotalol for, 1373
  tachycardia management in, 189
Women, cardiovascular disease in,
    estrogen replacement therapy and,
    316–322. See also Estrogen replacement
    therapy.

WPW. See Wolff-Parkinson-White syndrome.
Wytensin. See Guanabenz.

Xamoterol, for postural hypotension, 98
  receptor selectivity of, 337t
Xanthoma(s), regression of, due to
    probucol, 1102

Yohimbine, for hypertension, limitations
    of, 343
  for postural hypotension, 98–99
  receptor selectivity of, 336t

Zaroxolyn. See Metolazone.
Zatebradine, 1387–1390
  adverse effects of, 1390
  animal studies of, 1388–1389
  chemical properties of, 1387
  clinical studies of, 1389–1390
  clinical uses of, 1391
  pharmacodynamics of, 1387–1388
  pharmacokinetics of, 1388
  toxicity of, 1390
ZD7288. See Zeneca.
Zebeta. See Bisoprolol.
Zeneca, 1387, 1390–1391
Ziac (bisoprolol/hydrochlorothiazide), 73,
  332
Zinc depletion, with thiazides, 416
Zinc ion, in angiotensin-converting
  enzyme function, 801
Zocor. See Simvastatin.
Zofenoprilat, elimination kinetics of, 723t